OPTUM360°®

ICD-10-CM Professional for Hospitals

The complete official code set

Codes valid from October 1, 2019
through September 30, 2020

2020

THE NEW WEBSITE HAS
LAUNCHED
VISIT OPTUM360

Publisher's Notice

The *ICD-10-CM Professional for Hospitals: The Complete Official Code Set* is designed to be an accurate and authoritative source regarding coding and every reasonable effort has been made to ensure accuracy and completeness of the content. However, Optum360 makes no guarantee, warranty, or representation that this publication is accurate, complete or without errors. It is understood that Optum360 is not rendering any legal or other professional services or advice in this publication and that Optum360 bears no liability for any results or consequences that may arise from the use of this book.

Acknowledgments

Marianne Randall, CPC, *Product Manager*
Karen Schmidt, BSN, *Technical Director*
Anita Schmidt, BS, RHIA, AHIMA-approved ICD-10-CM/PCS
    Trainer, *Clinical Technical Editor*
Karen Krawzik, RHIT, CCS, AHIMA-approved ICD-10-CM/PCS
    Trainer, *Clinical Technical Editor*
Peggy Willard, CCS, AHIMA-approved ICD-10-CM/PCS
    Trainer, *Clinical Technical Editor*
Leanne Patterson, CPC, *Clinical Technical Editor*
LaJuana Green, RHIA, CCS, *Clinical Technical Editor*
Stacy Perry, *Manager, Desktop Publishing*
Lisa Singley, *Project Manager*
Tracy Betzler, *Senior Desktop Publishing Specialist*
Hope M. Dunn, *Senior Desktop Publishing Specialist*
Katie Russell, *Desktop Publishing Specialist*
Kate Holden, *Editor*

Our Commitment to Accuracy

Optum360 is committed to producing accurate and reliable materials.

To report corrections, please visit www.optum360coding.com/accuracy or email accuracy@optum.com. You can also reach customer service by calling 1.800.464.3649, option 1.

Anita Schmidt, BS, RHIA, AHIMA-approved ICD-10-CM/PCS Trainer

Ms. Schmidt has expertise in ICD-10-CM/PCS, DRG, and CPT with more than 15 years' experience in coding in multiple settings, including inpatient, observation, and same-day surgery. Her experience includes analysis of medical record documentation, assignment of ICD-10-CM and PCS codes, and DRG validation. She has conducted training for ICD-10-CM/PCS and electronic health record. She has also collaborated with clinical documentation specialists to identify documentation needs and potential areas for physician education. Most recently she has been developing content for resource and educational products related to ICD-10-CM, ICD-10-PCS, DRG, and CPT. Ms. Schmidt is an AHIMA-approved ICD-10-CM/PCS trainer and is an active member of the American Health Information Management Association (AHIMA) and the Minnesota Health Information Management Association.

Peggy Willard, CCS, AHIMA-approved ICD-10-CM/PCS Trainer

Ms. Willard has 18 years of experience in the healthcare field. Her expertise is in ICD-10-CM and ICD-10-PCS, including in-depth analysis of medical record documentation, ICD-10-CM/PCS code and DRG assignment, as well as clinical documentation improvement (CDI). In recent years Ms. Willard has been responsible for the creation and development of several products for Optum360 Coding Solutions that are designed to assist with appropriate application of the ICD-10-CM and ICD-10-PCS coding systems. She has several years of prior experience in Level I adult and pediatric trauma hospital and inpatient rehabilitation facility (IRF) coding, specializing in ICD-9-CM diagnosis and procedural coding, with emphasis in conducting coding audits, and conducting coding training for coding staff and clinical documentation specialists. Ms. Willard is an AHIMA-approved ICD-10 CM/PCS trainer and is an active member of the American Health Information Management Association (AHIMA) and the Minnesota Health Information Management Association (MHIMA).

2020 ICD-10-CM Official Guidelines for Coding and Reporting

Optum360 is pleased to provide you with this 2020 ICD-10-CM code book that INCLUDES the 2020 Official Guidelines for Coding and Reporting.

Contents

Preface iii
    ICD-10-CM Official Preface iii
    Characteristics of ICD-10-CM iii

How to Use ICD-10-CM Professional for Hospitals 2020 iv
    Introduction iv
    What's New for 2020 iv
    Conversion Table iv
    10 Steps to Correct Coding iv
    Official ICD-10-CM Guidelines for Coding and Reporting iv
    Indexes iv
        Index to Diseases and Injuries iv
        Neoplasm Table iv
        Table of Drugs and Chemicals v
        External Causes Index v
        Index Notations v
    Tabular List of Diseases vi
        Code and Code Descriptions vi
        Tabular Notations vi
        Official Notations vi
        Optum360 Notations vii
        Icons vii
        Color Bars ix
        Footnotes ix
    Chapter-Level Notations ix
    Illustrations x

What's New for 2020 xi
    Official Updates xi
    Proprietary Updates xv

Conversion Table of ICD-10-CM Codes xvi

10 Steps to Correct Coding xviii

**ICD-10-CM Official Guidelines for Coding
and Reporting** .... Coding Guidelines-1

ICD-10-CM Index to Diseases and Injuries 1

ICD-10-CM Neoplasm Table 330

ICD-10-CM Table of Drugs and Chemicals 349

ICD-10-CM Index to External Causes 398

ICD-10-CM Tabular List of Diseases and Injuries 433
    Chapter 1.   Certain Infectious and Parasitic Diseases
        (A00-B99) 433
    Chapter 2.   Neoplasms (C00-D49) 461
    Chapter 3.   Diseases of the Blood and Blood-forming
        Organs and Certain Disorders Involving the
        Immune Mechanism (D50-D89) 503
    Chapter 4.   Endocrine, Nutritional and Metabolic Diseases
        (E00-E89) 515
    Chapter 5.   Mental, Behavioral, and Neurodevelopmental
        Disorders (F01-F99) 541

    Chapter 6.   Diseases of the Nervous System (G00-G99) 569
    Chapter 7.   Diseases of the Eye and Adnexa (H00-H59) 593
    Chapter 8.   Diseases of the Ear and Mastoid Process
        (H60-H95) 631
    Chapter 9.   Diseases of the Circulatory System (I00-I99) 643
    Chapter 10.   Diseases of the Respiratory System (J00-J99) 691
    Chapter 11.   Diseases of the Digestive System (K00-K95) 709
    Chapter 12.   Diseases of the Skin and Subcutaneous Tissue
        (L00-L99) 735
    Chapter 13.   Diseases of the Musculoskeletal System and
        Connective Tissue (M00-M99) 759
    Chapter 14.   Diseases of the Genitourinary System (N00-N99) ..853
    Chapter 15.   Pregnancy, Childbirth and the Puerperium
        (O00-O9A) 873
    Chapter 16.   Certain Conditions Originating in the Perinatal
        Period (P00-P96) 917
    Chapter 17.   Congenital Malformations, Deformations and
        Chromosomal Abnormalities (Q00-Q99) 931
    Chapter 18.   Symptoms, Signs and Abnormal Clinical and
        Laboratory Findings Not Elsewhere
        Classified (R00-R99) 953
    Chapter 19.   Injury, Poisoning and Certain Other Consequences
        of External Causes (S00-T88) 975
    Chapter 20.   External Causes of Morbidity (V00-Y99)................ 1211
    Chapter 21.   Factors Influencing Health Status and Contact
        With Health Services (Z00-Z99) 1273

Illustrations Illustrations-1
    Chapter 3.   Diseases of the Blood and Blood-forming Organs and
        Certain Disorders Involving the Immune
        Mechanism (D50-D89) Illustrations-1
        Red Blood Cells Illustrations-1
        White Blood Cell Illustrations-1
        Platelet Illustrations-2
        Coagulation Illustrations-2
        Spleen Anatomical Location and
          External Structures Illustrations-3
        Spleen Interior Structures Illustrations-3
    Chapter 4.   Endocrine, Nutritional and Metabolic
        Diseases (E00-E89) Illustrations-4
        Endocrine System Illustrations-4
        Thyroid Illustrations-5
        Thyroid and Parathyroid Glands Illustrations-5
        Pancreas Illustrations-6
        Anatomy of the Adrenal Gland Illustrations-6
        Structure of an Ovary Illustrations-7
        Testis and Associated Structures Illustrations-7
        Thymus Illustrations-8
    Chapter 6.   Diseases of the Nervous System
        (G00-G99) Illustrations-9
        Brain Illustrations-9
        Cranial Nerves Illustrations-9
        Peripheral Nervous System Illustrations-10
        Spinal Cord and Spinal Nerves Illustrations-11
        Nerve Cell Illustrations-12
    Chapter 7.   Diseases of the Eye and Adnexa
        (H00-H59) Illustrations-13
        Eye Illustrations-13

Posterior Pole of Globe/Flow of Aqueous Humor	Illustrations–13
Lacrimal System	Illustrations–14
Eye Musculature	Illustrations–14
Eyelid Structures	Illustrations–14
Chapter 8. Diseases of the Ear and Mastoid Process (H60–H95)	Illustrations–15
Ear Anatomy	Illustrations–15
Chapter 9. Diseases of the Circulatory System (I00–I99)	Illustrations–16
Anatomy of the Heart	Illustrations–16
Heart Cross Section	Illustrations–16
Heart Valves	Illustrations–17
Heart Conduction System	Illustrations–17
Coronary Arteries	Illustrations–18
Arteries	Illustrations–19
Veins	Illustrations–20
Internal Carotid and Vertebral Arteries and Branches	Illustrations–21
External Carotid Artery and Branches	Illustrations–21
Branches of Abdominal Aorta	Illustrations–22
Portal Venous Circulation	Illustrations–22
Lymphatic System	Illustrations–23
Axillary Lymph Nodes	Illustrations–24
Lymphatic System of Head and Neck	Illustrations–24
Lymphatic Capillaries	Illustrations–25
Lymphatic Drainage	Illustrations–25
Chapter 10. Diseases of the Respiratory System (J00–J99)	Illustrations–26
Respiratory System	Illustrations–26
Upper Respiratory System	Illustrations–27
Lower Respiratory System	Illustrations–27
Paranasal Sinuses	Illustrations–27
Lung Segments	Illustrations–28
Alveoli	Illustrations–28
Chapter 11. Diseases of the Digestive System (K00–K95)	Illustrations–29
Digestive System	Illustrations–29
Omentum and Mesentery	Illustrations–30
Peritoneum and Retroperitoneum	Illustrations–30
Chapter 12. Diseases of the Skin and Subcutaneous Tissue (L00–L99)	Illustrations–31
Nail Anatomy	Illustrations–31
Skin and Subcutaneous Tissue	Illustrations–31
Chapter 13. Diseases of the Musculoskeletal System and Connective Tissue (M00–M99)	Illustrations–32
Bones and Joints	Illustrations–32
Shoulder Anterior View	Illustrations–33
Shoulder Posterior View	Illustrations–33
Elbow Anterior View	Illustrations–33
Elbow Posterior View	Illustrations–33
Hand	Illustrations–33
Hip Anterior View	Illustrations–34
Hip Posterior View	Illustrations–34
Knee Anterior View	Illustrations–34
Knee Posterior View	Illustrations–34
Foot	Illustrations–34
Muscles	Illustrations–35
Chapter 14. Diseases of the Genitourinary System (N00–N99)	Illustrations–36
Urinary System	Illustrations–36
Male Genitourinary System	Illustrations–37
Female Internal Genitalia	Illustrations–37
Female Genitourinary Tract Lateral View	Illustrations–37
Chapter 15. Pregnancy, Childbirth and the Puerperium (O00–O9A)	Illustrations–38
Term Pregnancy – Single Gestation	Illustrations–38
Twin Gestation–Dichorionic–Diamniotic (DI-DI)	Illustrations–38
Twin Gestation–Monochorionic–Diamniotic (MO-DI)	Illustrations–39
Twin Gestation–Monochorionic–Monoamniotic (MO-MO)	Illustrations–39
Chapter 19. Injury, Poisoning and Certain Other Consequences of External Causes (S00-T88)	Illustrations–40
Types of Fractures	Illustrations–40
Salter-Harris Fracture Types	Illustrations–40

Preface

ICD-10-CM Official Preface

This FY 2020 update of the International Statistical Classification of Diseases and Related Health Problems, 10th revision, Clinical Modification (ICD-10-CM) is being published by the United States government in recognition of its responsibility to promulgate this classification throughout the United States for morbidity coding. The International Statistical Classification of Diseases and Related Health Problems, 10th Revision (ICD-10), published by the World Health Organization (WHO), is the foundation of ICD-10-CM. ICD-10 continues to be the classification used in cause-of-death coding in the United States. The ICD-10-CM is comparable with the ICD-10. The WHO Collaborating Center for the Family of International Classifications in North America, housed at the Centers for Disease Control and Prevention's National Center for Health Statistics (NCHS), has responsibility for the implementation of ICD and other WHO-FIC classifications and serves as a liaison with the WHO, fulfilling international obligations for comparable classifications and the national health data needs of the United States. The historical background of ICD and ICD-10 can be found in the Introduction to the International Classification of Diseases and Related Health Problems (ICD-10), 2010, World Health Organization, Geneva, Switzerland.

ICD-10-CM is the United States' clinical modification of the World Health Organization's ICD-10. The term "clinical" is used to emphasize the modification's intent: to serve as a useful tool in the area of classification of morbidity data for indexing of health records, medical care review, and ambulatory and other health care programs, as well as for basic health statistics. To describe the clinical picture of the patient the codes must be more precise than those needed only for statistical groupings and trend analysis.

Characteristics of ICD-10-CM

ICD-10-CM far exceeds its predecessors in the number of concepts and codes provided. The disease classification has been expanded to include health-related conditions and to provide greater specificity at the sixth and seventh character level. The sixth and seventh characters are not optional and are intended for use in recording the information documented in the clinical record.

ICD-10-CM extensions, interpretations, modifications, addenda, or errata other than those approved by the Centers for Disease Control and Prevention are not to be considered official and should not be utilized. Continuous maintenance of the ICD-10-CM is the responsibility of the aforementioned agencies. However, because the ICD-10-CM represents the best in contemporary thinking of clinicians, nosologists, epidemiologists, and statisticians from both public and private sectors, when future modifications are considered, advice will be sought from all stakeholders.

All official authorized addenda since the last complete update (October 1, 2019) have been included in this revision. For more detailed information please see the complete official authorized addenda to ICD-10-CM, including the "ICD-10-CM Official Guidelines for Coding and Reporting," and a description of the ICD-10-CM updating and maintenance process.

How to Use ICD-10-CM Professional for Hospitals 2020

Introduction

ICD-10-CM Professional for Hospitals: The Complete Official Code Set is your definitive coding resource, combining the work of the National Center for Health Statistics (NCHS), Centers for Medicare and Medicaid Services (CMS), American Hospital Association (AHA), and Optum360 experts to provide the information you need for coding accuracy.

The International Classification of Diseases, 10th Revision, Clinical Modification (ICD-10-CM), is an adaptation of ICD-10, copyrighted by the World Health Organization (WHO). The development and maintenance of this clinical modification (CM) is the responsibility of the NCHS as authorized by WHO. Any new concepts added to ICD-10-CM are based on an established update process through the collaboration of WHO's Update and Revision Committee and the ICD-10-CM Coordination and Maintenance Committee.

In addition to the ICD-10-CM classification, other official government source information has been included in this manual. Depending on the source, updates to information may be annual or quarterly. This manual provides the most current information that was available at the time of publication. For updates to the source documents that may have occurred after this manual was published, please refer to the following:

- **National Center for Health Statistics (NCHS), International Classification of Diseases, Tenth Revision, Clinical Modification (ICD-10-CM)**

    https://www.cdc.gov/nchs/icd/icd10cm.htm

    https://www.cms.gov/Medicare/Coding/ICD10/2020-ICD-10-CM.html

- **Centers for Medicare and Medicaid Services (CMS) Inpatient Prospective Payment System Proposed Rule, FY2020**

    https://www.cms.gov/Medicare/Medicare-Fee-for-Service-Payment/AcuteInpatientPPS/IPPS-Regulations-and-Notices.html

- **Centers for Medicare and Medicaid Services (CMS) Inpatient Prospective Payment Final Rule Data Files, FY2019 - Definition of Medicare Code Edits, version 36 and ICD-10 MS-DRG Definitions Manual, version 36R1**

    https://www.cms.gov/Medicare/Medicare-Fee-for-Service-Payment/AcuteInpatientPPS/MS-DRG-Classifications-and-Software.html

- **Centers for Medicare & Medicaid Services (CMS) Risk Adjustment Model, version 24**

    https://www.cms.gov/Medicare/Health-Plans/MedicareAdvtgSpecRateStats/Risk-Adjustors.html

- **Centers for Medicare & Medicaid Services (CMS) Long-term Care Hospital Prospective Payment System Final Rule and Data Files**

    https://www.cms.gov/Medicare/Medicare-Fee-for-Service-Payment/LongTermCareHospitalPPS/LTCHPPS-Regulations-and-Notices-Items/LTCH-PPS-CMS-1694-F.html

- **American Hospital Association (AHA) Coding Clinics**

    https://www.codingclinicadvisor.com/

The official NCHS ICD-10-CM classification includes three main sections: the guidelines, the indexes, and the tabular list, all of which make up the bulk of this coding manual. To complement the classification, Optum360's coding experts have incorporated Medicare-related coding edits and proprietary features, such as supplementary notations, coding tools, and appendixes, into a comprehensive and easy-to-use reference. This publication is organized as follows:

What's New for 2020

This section provides a high-level overview of the changes made to the ICD-10-CM official code set for fiscal 2020, identifying codes that have been added and deleted from the classification, codes that had validity changes as a result of these additions and deletions, as well as codes that had revisions to their descriptions. All changes are based on the 2020 official addendum, posted June 20, 2019, by the National Center for Health Statistics (NCHS), the agency charged with maintaining and updating ICD-10-CM. NCHS is part of the Centers for Disease Control and Prevention (CDC).

Conversion Table

The conversion table was developed by National Center for Healthcare Statistics (NCHS) to help facilitate data retrieval as new codes are added to the ICD-10-CM classification. This table provides a crosswalk from each FY 2020 new code to the equivalent code(s) assigned prior to October 1, 2019, for that particular diagnosis or condition. For the full conversion table, including code crosswalks before October 1, 2019, refer to the 2020 Conversion Table zip file at https://www.cms.gov/Medicare/Coding/ICD10/2020-ICD-10-CM.html.

10 Steps to Correct Coding

This step-by-step tutorial walks the coder through the process of finding the correct code — from locating the code in the official indexes to verifying the code in the tabular section — while following applicable conventions, guidelines, and instructional notes. Specific examples are provided with detailed explanations of each coding step along with advice for proper sequencing.

Official ICD-10-CM Guidelines for Coding and Reporting

This section provides the full official conventions and guidelines regulating the appropriate assignment and reporting of ICD-10-CM codes. These conventions and guidelines are published by the U.S. Department of Health and Human Services (DHHS) and approved by the cooperating parties (American Health Information Management Association [AHIMA], National Center for Health Statistics [NCHS], Centers for Disease Control and Prevention [CDC], and the American Hospital Association [AHA]).

Indexes

Index to Diseases and Injuries

The Index to Diseases and Injuries is arranged in alphabetic order by terms specific to a disease, condition, illness, injury, eponym, or abbreviation as well as terms that describe circumstances other than a disease or injury that may require attention from a health care professional.

Neoplasm Table

The Neoplasm Table is arranged in alphabetic order by anatomical site. Codes are then listed in individual columns based upon the histological behavior (malignant, in situ, benign, uncertain, or unspecified) of the neoplasm.

Table of Drugs and Chemicals

The Table of Drugs and Chemicals is arranged in alphabetic order by the specific drug or chemical name. Codes are listed in individual columns based upon the associated intent (poisoning, adverse effect, or underdosing).

External Causes Index

The External Causes Index is arranged in alphabetic order by main terms that describe the cause, the intent, the place of occurrence, the activity, and the status of the patient at the time the injury occurred or health condition arose.

Index Notations

With

The word "with" or "in" should be interpreted to mean "associated with" or "due to." The classification presumes a causal relationship between the two conditions linked by these terms in the index. These conditions should be coded as related even in the absence of provider documentation explicitly linking them unless the documentation clearly states the conditions are unrelated or when another guideline specifically requires a documented linkage between two conditions (e.g., the sepsis guideline for "acute organ dysfunction that is not clearly associated with the sepsis"). For conditions not specifically linked by these relational terms in the classification or when a guideline requires explicit documentation of a linkage between two conditions, provider documentation must link the conditions to code them as related.

The word "with" in the index is sequenced immediately following the main term, not in alphabetical order.

> **Dermatopolymyositis** M33.9Ø
> with
> myopathy M33.92
> respiratory involvement M33.91
> specified organ involvement NEC M33.99
> in neoplastic disease — *see also* Neoplasm D49.9 *[M36.Ø]*

See

When the instruction "see" follows a term in the index, it indicates that another term must be referenced to locate the correct code.

> **Hematoperitoneum** — *see* Hemoperitoneum

See Also

The instructional note "see also" simply provides alternative terms the coder may reference that may be useful in determining the correct code but are not necessary to follow if the main term supplies the appropriate code.

> **Hematinuria** — *see also* Hemaglobinuria
> malarial B5Ø.8

Default Codes

In the index, the default code is the code listed next to the main term and represents the condition most commonly associated with that main term. This code may be assigned when documentation does not support reporting a more specific code. Alternatively, it may provide an unspecified code for the condition.

> **Headache** R51
> allergic NEC G44.89
> associated with sexual activity G44.82
> chronic daily R51

Parentheses

Parentheses in the indexes enclose nonessential modifiers, supplementary words that may be present or absent in the statement of a disease without affecting the code.

> **Pseudomeningocele** (cerebral) (infective) (post-traumatic) G96.19
> postprocedural (spinal) G97.82

Brackets

ICD-10-CM has a coding convention addressing code assignment for manifestations that occur as a result of an underlying condition. This convention requires the underlying condition to be sequenced first, followed by the code or codes for the associated manifestation. In the index, italicized codes in brackets identify manifestation codes.

> **Polyneuropathy** (peripheral) G62.9
> alcoholic G62.1
> amyloid (Portuguese) E85.1 *[G63]*
> transthyretin-related (ATTR) familial E85.1 *[G63]*

Shaded Guides

Exclusive vertical shaded guides in the Index to Diseases and Injuries and External Causes Index help the user easily follow the indent levels for the subentries under a main term. Sequencing rules may apply depending on the level of indent for separate subentries.

> **Hemicrania**
> congenital malformation QØØ.Ø
> continua G44.51
> meaning migraine — *see also* Migraine G43.9Ø9
> paroxysmal G44.Ø39
> chronic G44.Ø49
> intractable G44.Ø41
> not intractable G44.Ø49
> episodic G44.Ø39
> intractable G44.Ø31
> not intractable G44.Ø39
> intractable G44.Ø31
> not intractable G44.Ø39

Following References

The Index to Diseases and Injuries includes following references to assist in locating out-of-sequence codes in the tabular list. Out-of-sequence codes contain an alphabetic character (letter) in the third- or 4th-character position. These codes are placed according to the classification rules — according to condition — not according to alphabetic or numeric sequencing rules.

> **Carcinoma** (malignant) — *see also* Neoplasm, by site, malignant
> neuroendocrine — *see also* Tumor, neuroendocrine
> high grade, any site C7A.1 (*following* C75)
> poorly differentiated, any site C7A.1 (*following* C75)

Additional Character Required

The Index to Diseases and Injuries, Neoplasm Table, and External Causes Index provide an icon after certain codes to signify to the user that additional characters are required to make the code valid. The tabular list should be consulted for appropriate character selection.

> **Fall, falling** (accidental) W19 ☑
> building W2Ø.1 ☑

Tabular List of Diseases

ICD-10-CM codes and descriptions are arranged numerically within the tabular list of diseases with 19 separate chapters providing codes associated with a particular body system or nature of injury or disease. There is also a chapter providing codes for external causes of an injury or health conditions and finally a chapter for codes that address encounters with healthcare facilities for circumstances other than a disease or injury.

Code and Code Descriptions

ICD-10-CM is an alphanumeric classification system that contains categories, subcategories, and valid codes. The first character is always a letter with any additional characters represented by either a letter or number. A three-character category without further subclassification is equivalent to a valid three-character code. Valid codes may be three, four, five, six, or seven characters in length, with each level of subdivision after a three-character category representing a subcategory. The final level of subdivision is a valid code.

Boldface

Boldface type is used for all codes and descriptions in the tabular list.

Italics

Italicized type is used to identify manifestation codes, those codes that should not be reported as first-listed diagnoses.

Deleted Text

~~Strikethrough~~ on a code and code description indicates a deletion from the classification for the current year.

Key Word

Green font is used throughout the Tabular List of Diseases to differentiate the key words that appear in similar code descriptions in a given category or subcategory. The key word convention is used only in those categories in which there are multiple codes with very similar descriptions with only a few words that differentiate them.

For example, refer to the list of codes below from category H55:

> ☑4ᵗʰ **H55 Nystagmus and other** irregular eye movements
>   ☑5ᵗʰ **H55.0 Nystagmus**
>   **H55.00 Unspecified nystagmus**
>   **H55.01** Congenital **nystagmus**
>   **H55.02** Latent **nystagmus**
>   **H55.03** Visual deprivation **nystagmus**
>   **H55.04** Dissociated **nystagmus**
>   **H55.09 Other forms of nystagmus**

The portion of the code description that appears in green font in the tabular list helps the coder quickly identify the key terms and the correct code. This convention is especially useful when the codes describe laterality, such as the following codes from subcategory H40.22:

> ☑6ᵗʰ **H40.22** Chronic **angle-closure glaucoma**
>   Chronic primary angle-closure glaucoma
>   ☑7ᵗʰ **H40.221 Chronic angle-closure glaucoma,** right **eye**
>   ☑7ᵗʰ **H40.222 Chronic angle-closure glaucoma,** left **eye**
>   ☑7ᵗʰ **H40.223 Chronic angle-closure glaucoma,** bilateral
>   ☑7ᵗʰ **H40.229 Chronic angle-closure glaucoma, unspecified eye**

Tabular Notations

Official parenthetical notes as well as Optum360's supplementary notations are provided at the chapter, code block, category, subcategory, and individual code level to help the user assign proper codes. The information in the notation can apply to one or more codes depending on where the citation is placed.

Official Notations

Includes Notes

The word INCLUDES appears immediately under certain categories to further define, clarify, or give examples of the content of a code category.

Inclusion Terms

Lists of inclusion terms are included under certain codes. These terms indicate some of the conditions for which that code number may be used. Inclusion terms may be synonyms with the code title, or, in the case of "other specified" codes, the terms may also provide a list of various conditions included within a classification code. The inclusion terms are not exhaustive. The index may provide additional terms that may also be assigned to a given code.

Excludes Notes

ICD-10-CM has two types of excludes notes. Each note has a different definition for use. However, they are similar in that they both indicate that codes excluded from each other are independent of each other.

Excludes 1

An EXCLUDES 1 note is a "pure" excludes. It means "NOT CODED HERE!" An Excludes 1 note indicates mutually exclusive codes: two conditions that cannot be reported together. An Excludes1 note indicates that the code excluded should never be used at the same time as the code above the Excludes1 note. An Excludes1 is used when two conditions cannot occur together, such as a congenital form versus an acquired form of the same condition.

An exception to the Excludes 1 definition is when the two conditions are unrelated to each other. If it is not clear whether the two conditions involving an Excludes 1 note are related or not, query the provider. For example, code F45.8 Other somatoform disorders, has an Excludes 1 note for "sleep related teeth grinding (G47.63)" because "teeth grinding" is an inclusion term under F45.8. Only one of these two codes should be assigned for teeth grinding. However, psychogenic dysmenorrhea is also an inclusion term under F45.8, and a patient could have both this condition and sleep-related teeth grinding. In this case, the two conditions are clearly unrelated to each other, so it would be appropriate to report F45.8 and G47.63 together.

Excludes 2

An EXCLUDES 2 note means "NOT INCLUDED HERE." An Excludes 2 note indicates that although the excluded condition is not part of the condition it is excluded from, a patient may have both conditions at the same time. Therefore, when an Excludes 2 note appears under a code, it may be acceptable to use both the code and the excluded code together if supported by the medical documentation.

Note

The term "NOTE" appears as an icon and precedes the instructional information. These notes function as alerts to highlight coding instructions within the text.

Code First/Use additional code

These instructional notes provide sequencing instruction. They may appear independently of each other or to designate certain etiology/manifestation paired codes. These instructions signal the coder that an additional code should be reported to provide a more complete picture of that diagnosis.

In etiology/manifestation coding, ICD-10-CM requires the underlying condition to be sequenced first, followed by the manifestation. In these situations, codes with "In diseases classified elsewhere" in the code description are never permitted as a first-listed or principal diagnosis code and must be sequenced following the underlying condition code.

Code Also

A "code also" note alerts the coder that more than one code may be required to fully describe the condition. The sequencing depends on the circumstances of the encounter. Factors that may determine sequencing include severity and reason for the encounter.

Revised Text

The revised text ▶◀ "bow ties" alert the user to changes in official notations for the current year. Revised text may include the following:

- A change in a current parenthetical description

- A change in the code(s) associated with a current parenthetical note

- A change in how a current parenthetical note is classified (e.g., an Excludes 1 note that changed to an Excludes 2 note)

- Addition of a new parenthetical note(s) to a code

Deleted Text

~~Strikethrough~~ on official notations indicate a deletion from the classification for the current year.

Optum360 Notations

AHA Coding Clinic Citations

Coding Clinics are official American Hospital Associated (AHA) publications that provide coding advice specific to ICD-10-CM and ICD-10-PCS.

These citations identify the year, quarter, and page number of one or more Coding Clinic publications that may have coding advice relevant to a particular code or group of codes. With the most current citation listed first, these notations are preceded by the symbol **AHA:** and appear in purple type.

> **I15.1** **Hypertension secondary to** other renal disorders
> **AHA:** 2016, 3Q, 22

Definitions

Definitions explain a specific term, condition, or disease process in layman's terms. These notations are preceded by the symbol **DEF:** and appear in purple type.

> ✓5ᵗʰ **M51.4 Schmorl's nodes**
> **DEF:** Irregular bone defect in the margin of the vertebral body that causes herniation into the end plate of the vertebral body.

Coding Tips

The tips in the tabular list offer coding advice that is not readily available within the ICD-10-CM classification. It may relate official coding guidelines, indexing nuances, or advice from AHA's Coding Clinic for ICD-10-CM/PCS. These notations are preceded by the symbol **TIP:** and appear in brown type.

> **P15.8 Other specified birth injuries**
> **TIP:** Use for any injury of newborn from scalpel.

CC Excludes Notations

The assignment of an MS-DRG or MS-LTC-DRG often depends on the presence or absence of a secondary diagnosis code that is designated as an MCC or CC. However, in some instances the MCC or CC designation for that secondary diagnosis code is negated due to its relationship with the principal diagnosis.

To save space in this coding manual and provide a more comprehensive reference for the user, the CC Exclusion notations have been restructured. Instead of the individual codes being listed in the reference, which can in many cases be extensive, only the principal diagnosis collection (PDX collection) number is provided. A PDX collection contains a specific list of ICD-10-CM codes and their official descriptions that when used as

principal diagnosis would render the MCC/CC designation ineffective. Each PDX collection is provided in an easily searchable data file which can be accessed at the following:

https://www.optum360coding.com/ProductUpdates/
Title: "2020 ICD-10-CM for Hospitals CC Excludes Data File"
Password: OptumCCExcl20

Similar to the parenthetical notes, the CC Exclusion notations are provided at the category, subcategory, and/or code level. If a CC Exclusion notation is found at the category or subcategory level, all the CC and/or MCC codes in that category or subcategory share the same PDX collection listed in that notation. For example:

> ✓5ᵗʰ **G43.6** Persistent **migraine** aura with cerebral infarction
> Code also the type of cerebral infarction (I63.-)
> **CC Excl: For CC codes in subcategory G43.6, unless otherwise noted:** PDX collection 584

Often a CC exclusion reference is specific to laterality for CC/MCC codes in a category or subcategory. Where possible, a CC exclusion reference is placed at the category or subcategory level with the PDX collection identified for the right, left, or unspecified side. For example:

> ✓4ᵗʰ **S58** Traumatic amputation **of elbow and forearm**
> An amputation not identified as partial or complete should be coded to complete.
> *EXCLUDES 1* traumatic amputation of wrist and hand (S68.-)
> The appropriate 7th character is to be added to each code from category S58.
> A initial encounter
> D subsequent encounter
> S sequela
> **CC Excl: For CC codes in category S58:**
> **Right side:** PDX collection 1266
> **Left side:** PDX collection 1267
> **Unspecified side:** PDX collection 1268

Where possible a "see" reference may also be used, referring the user to a previously designated CC excludes notation. For example:

> ✓5ᵗʰ **S72.0** Fracture of head and neck **of femur**
> *EXCLUDES 2* physeal fracture of upper end of femur (S79.0-)
> **AHA:** 2016, 3Q, 16
> **CC Excl: For CC/MCC codes in subcategory S72.0:**
> **Right side:** See code S72.001
> **Left side:** See code S72.002
> **Unspecified side:** See code S72.009

Note: CC Excludes notations in chapters 13 and 19 apply to 7th character A, unless otherwise noted.

Certain codes may also have no principal diagnosis codes to which they would be excluded from functioning as a CC or MCC. These are identified as follows:

> **I16.1** **Hypertensive** emergency   CC
> **CC Excl:** No Excl

Icons

Note: The following icons are placed to the left of the code.

● **New Code**
Codes that have been added to the classification system for the current year.

▲ **Revised Code Title**
Codes that have had a change to their description or validity change for the current year. For additional information on codes with validity changes, see the "What's New" section.

☑ **Additional Characters Required**

✓4ᵗʰ This symbol indicates that the code requires a 4th character.

✓5ᵗʰ This symbol indicates that the code requires a 5th character.

✓6ᵗʰ This symbol indicates that the code requires a 6th character.

✓7ᵗʰ This symbol indicates that the code requires a 7th character.

> **✓5ᵗʰ H60.3 Other infective otitis externa**
> > **✓6ᵗʰ H60.31 Diffuse** otitis externa
> > > H60.311 Diffuse otitis externa, right ear
> > > H60.312 Diffuse otitis externa, left ear
> > > H60.313 Diffuse otitis externa, bilateral
> > > H60.319 Diffuse otitis externa, unspecified ear

✓x7ᵗʰ Placeholder Alert

This symbol indicates that the code requires a 7th character following the placeholder "X". Codes with fewer than six characters that require a 7th character must contain placeholder "X" to fill in the empty character(s).

> **✓x7ᵗʰ T16.1 Foreign body in right ear**

Optum360 has provided a searchable data file that includes each edit listed below and all ICD-10-CM codes associated with that edit. These comprehensive lists are based on FY 2020 IPPS final rule official files, effective October 1, 2019:

- Age
- Sex
- Hospital-acquired condition (HAC)
- CC
- MCC
- HIV
- Manifestation code
- Unacceptable diagnosis
- Questionable diagnosis

This data file can be accessed at the following:

https://www.optum360coding.com/ProductUpdates/
Title: "2020 ICD-10-CM for Hospital IPPS Data File"
Password: OptumIPPS20

Note: The following icons are placed to the right of the code description.

Age Edits

Codes intended for a specific age group based on CMS MCE designations, v36.

N Newborn Age: 0

These diagnoses are intended for newborns and neonates and the patient's age must be 0 years.

> **N47.0 Adherent prepuce, newborn**   N♂

P Pediatric Age: 0-17

These diagnoses are intended for children and the patient's age must be between 0 and 17 years.

> **L21.1 Seborrheic infantile dermatitis**   P

M Maternity Age: 9-64

These diagnoses are intended for childbearing patients between the age of 9 and 64 years.

> **O02.9 Abnormal product of conception, unspecified**   M♀

A Adult Age: 15-124

These diagnoses are intended for patients between the age of 15 and 124 years.

> **R54 Age-related physical debility**   A
> > Frailty
> > Old age
> > Senescence
> > Senile asthenia
> > Senile debility
> > **EXCLUDES 1** age-related cognitive decline (R41.81)
> >   sarcopenia (M62.84)
> >   senile psychosis (F03)
> >   senility NOS (R41.81)

Sex Edits

Codes intended for a specific sex based on CMS MCE designations, v36.

♂ Male diagnosis only

> **Q98.0 Klinefelter syndrome karyotype 47, XXY**   ♂

♀ Female diagnosis only

> **N35.12 Postinfective urethral stricture, not elsewhere classified, female**   ♀

H1-H14 Hospital Acquired Condition (HAC)

These codes identify conditions that are high cost or high volume or both, are either a complication or comorbidity (CC) or major complication or comorbidity (MCC) that as a secondary diagnosis results in assignment of a case to a higher-paying MS-DRG. These conditions are reasonably preventable through the application of evidence-based guidelines. If the condition is not present on admission (meaning it developed during the hospital admission), the case will not group to the higher-paying MS-DRG based solely upon the reporting of the HAC code. Many of these HACs are conditional, and are based on reporting the specific diagnosis code(s) in combination with certain procedure codes, notated in footnotes.

Note: Hospital-acquired conditions do not impact MS-LTC-DRG assignment.

> **N15.1 Renal and perinephric abscess**   MCC H6
> > **CC Excl:** PDX collection 919

CC CC Condition

This symbol designates a complication or comorbidity diagnosis that may affect DRG assignment. A complication or comorbidity diagnosis, CC condition, is defined as a significant acute disease, a significant acute manifestation of a chronic disease, an advanced or end-stage chronic disease, or a chronic disease associated with systemic physiological decompensation and debility that have consistently greater impact on hospital resources.

> **G90.59 Complex regional pain syndrome I of other specified site**   CC

MCC MCC Condition

This symbol designates a major complication or comorbidity diagnosis that may affect DRG assignment. An MCC condition meets the same criteria as a CC condition but is associated with a higher acuity level and hospital resource consumption is expected to be higher than that for a CC condition. There are fewer conditions that meet the criteria as an MCC than those for a CC condition.

> **✓7ᵗʰ S35.238 Other injury of inferior mesenteric artery**   MCC

HIV **HIV-related Condition**
This symbol indicates that the condition is considered a major HIV-related diagnosis. When the condition is coded in combination with a diagnosis of human immunodeficiency virus (HIV), code B20, the case will move from MS-DRG/MS-LTC-DRG 977 to MS-DRGs/MS-LTC-DRGs 974-976.

| G96.9 | Disorder of central nervous system, unspecified | **HIV** |

HCC **CMS-HCC Condition**
Identify conditions that are considered a CMS-HCC (hierarchical condition category) diagnosis.

The HCC codes represented in this manual have been updated to reflect the 2020 Initial ICD-10-CM Mappings for CMS-HCC Model v24. Midyear final mappings were not available at the time this publication went to print; refer to the following CMS website for final mappings: https://www.cms.gov/Medicare/Health-Plans/MedicareAdvtgSpecRateStats/Risk-Adjustors.html.

| Y62.2 | Failure of sterile precautions during kidney dialysis and other perfusion | **HCC** |

SW **Severe Wound Diagnosis**
This symbol indicates that the condition is considered a severe wound diagnosis. Depending on the facility from which the patient is discharged, these conditions may not require that the payment rate for that admission be adjusted.

| L89.014 | Pressure ulcer of right elbow, stage 4 | **CC** **HCC** **SW** |

Color Bars

Manifestation Code
Codes defined as manifestation codes appear in italic type, with a blue color bar over the code description. A manifestation cannot be reported as a first-listed code; it is sequenced as a secondary diagnosis with the underlying disease code listed first.

| G32.89 | *Other specified degenerative disorders of nervous system in diseases classified elsewhere*
Degenerative encephalopathy in diseases classified elsewhere |

Unacceptable Principal Diagnoses
Unacceptable principal diagnoses will appear with a purple color bar over the code description. These codes do not describe a current illness or injury, but a circumstance which influences a patient's health status. They are considered an unacceptable principal diagnosis for *inpatient* admission.

| **✓7th** T48.5X5 | Adverse effect of other anti-common-cold drugs |

Questionable Admission Diagnoses
Questionable admission diagnoses will appear with a yellow color bar over the code description. These codes, although not unacceptable as a PDx, may be considered a "questionable admission" when used as PDx in an acute care hospital.

| E66.09 | Other obesity due to excess calories |

Wrong Procedure Performed Edit
An orange color bar over the code title indicates the Wrong Procedure Performed edit. This edit was created to identify cases in which wrong surgeries occurred. Any claim with a code from Y65.51-Y65.53 will be denied and returned to the provider. A surgical or other invasive procedure is considered to be a wrong procedure if one of the following is true:

- The procedure was performed on the wrong site.
- The procedure was performed on the wrong patient.
- The incorrect procedure was performed on a patient.

| Y65.51 | Performance of wrong procedure (operation) on correct patient
Wrong device implanted into correct surgical site
EXCLUDES 1 *performance of correct procedure (operation) on wrong side or body part (Y65.53)* |

Unspecified Diagnosis
Codes that appear with a gray color bar over the alphanumeric code identify unspecified diagnoses. These codes should be used in limited circumstances, when neither the diagnostic statement nor the documentation provides enough information to assign a more specific diagnosis code. The abbreviation NOS, "not otherwise specified," in the tabular list may be interpreted as "unspecified."

| G03.9 | Meningitis, unspecified
Arachnoiditis (spinal) NOS |

Footnotes
Certain codes in the tabular section have a numerical superscript located to the upper left of the code. This numerical superscript corresponds to a specific footnote description.

For example:

| [1] R57.1 | Hypovolemic shock | |

For convenience, the footnote descriptions are provided on the front cover.

The following list also provides the footnote descriptions of all numerical superscripts found in the Tabular List of Diseases:

1 These codes are considered major complication/comorbidity (MCC) conditions only if the patient is discharged alive.

2 This condition is considered an MCC only when reported as an initial encounter for an open fracture (7th character B or C specific to category).

3 This condition is considered a CC only when reported as an initial encounter for a fracture (7th character A, B, or C specific to category) or a subsequent encounter for nonunion or malunion fracture (7th character K, M, N, P, Q, or R specific to category).

4 This condition is considered a CC only when reported as a subsequent encounter for a nonunion or malunion fracture (7th character K, M, N, P, Q, or R specific to category).

5 This condition is considered a CC only when reported as an initial encounter or subsequent encounter (7th character A or D).

6 This condition is considered an HCC when reported as initial encounter (7th character A, B, or C specific to category).

7 This condition is considered an HCC when reported as initial encounter (7th character A or B specific to category) or as a sequela.

8 This condition is considered an HCC when reported as a sequela.

Chapter-Level Notations

Chapter-Specific Guidelines with Coding Examples
Each chapter begins with the Official Guidelines for Coding and Reporting specific to that chapter, where provided. Coding examples specific to outpatient care settings have been provided to illustrate the coding and/or sequencing guidance in these guidelines.

Muscle and Tendon Table
ICD-10-CM categorizes certain muscles and tendons in the upper and lower extremities by their action (e.g., extension or flexion) as well as their anatomical location. The Muscle/Tendon table is provided at the beginning of chapter 13 and chapter 19 to help users when code selection depends on the action of the muscle and/or tendon.

Note: This table is not all-inclusive, and proper code assignment should be based on the provider's documentation.

Illustrations

This section includes illustrations of normal anatomy with ICD-10-CM-specific terminology.

Official Updates

The official ICD-10-CM addendum was posted to the Centers for Medicare and Medicaid Services (CMS) website on June 20, 2019, identifying the changes to the ICD-10-CM code set for fiscal 2020, effective October 1, 2019, to September 30, 2020. These changes were made by the agency charged with maintaining and updating the ICD-10-CM code set, the National Center for Health Statistics (NCHS), a section of the Centers for Disease Control and Prevention (CDC). A summary of the changes is provided below:

15 Codes with a Change in Validity

Note: Validity changes are the result of codes being added to or deleted from the classification. Codes that change from valid to invalid allow the creation of a new subcategory to which new codes can be assigned that provide greater detail about the condition. Codes that change from invalid to valid are the result of codes being deleted from a subcategory in the classification, when the detail provided in those codes is no longer required.

Valid to Invalid

D81.3	I48.1	I48.2	Q66.0	Q66.1
Q66.21	Q66.22	Q66.3	Q66.4	Q66.7
Q66.9	Q79.6	Q87.1	R82.8	

Invalid to Valid
H81.4

7 Codes Deleted from the Classification

H81.41	Vertigo of central origin, right ear
H81.42	Vertigo of central origin, left ear
H81.43	Vertigo of central origin, bilateral
H81.49	Vertigo of central origin, unspecified ear
T67.0XXA	Heatstroke and sunstroke, initial encounter
T67.0XXD	Heatstroke and sunstroke, subsequent encounter
T67.0XXS	Heatstroke and sunstroke, sequela

273 New Codes Added to the Classification

D75.A	Glucose-6-phosphate dehydrogenase (G6PD) deficiency without anemia
D81.30	Adenosine deaminase deficiency, unspecified
D81.31	Severe combined immunodeficiency due to adenosine deaminase deficiency
D81.32	Adenosine deaminase 2 deficiency
D81.39	Other adenosine deaminase deficiency
I26.93	Single subsegmental pulmonary embolism without acute cor pulmonale
I26.94	Multiple subsegmental pulmonary emboli without acute cor pulmonale
I48.11	Longstanding persistent atrial fibrillation
I48.19	Other persistent atrial fibrillation
I48.20	Chronic atrial fibrillation, unspecified
I48.21	Permanent atrial fibrillation
I80.241	Phlebitis and thrombophlebitis of right peroneal vein
I80.242	Phlebitis and thrombophlebitis of left peroneal vein
I80.243	Phlebitis and thrombophlebitis of peroneal vein, bilateral
I80.249	Phlebitis and thrombophlebitis of unspecified peroneal vein
I80.251	Phlebitis and thrombophlebitis of right calf muscular vein
I80.252	Phlebitis and thrombophlebitis of left calf muscular vein
I80.253	Phlebitis and thrombophlebitis of calf muscular vein, bilateral
I80.259	Phlebitis and thrombophlebitis of unspecified calf muscular vein
I82.451	Acute embolism and thrombosis of right peroneal vein
I82.452	Acute embolism and thrombosis of left peroneal vein
I82.453	Acute embolism and thrombosis of peroneal vein, bilateral
I82.459	Acute embolism and thrombosis of unspecified peroneal vein
I82.461	Acute embolism and thrombosis of right calf muscular vein
I82.462	Acute embolism and thrombosis of left calf muscular vein
I82.463	Acute embolism and thrombosis of calf muscular vein, bilateral
I82.469	Acute embolism and thrombosis of unspecified calf muscular vein
I82.551	Chronic embolism and thrombosis of right peroneal vein
I82.552	Chronic embolism and thrombosis of left peroneal vein
I82.553	Chronic embolism and thrombosis of peroneal vein, bilateral
I82.559	Chronic embolism and thrombosis of unspecified peroneal vein
I82.561	Chronic embolism and thrombosis of right calf muscular vein
I82.562	Chronic embolism and thrombosis of left calf muscular vein
I82.563	Chronic embolism and thrombosis of calf muscular vein, bilateral
I82.569	Chronic embolism and thrombosis of unspecified calf muscular vein
L89.006	Pressure-induced deep tissue damage of unspecified elbow
L89.016	Pressure-induced deep tissue damage of right elbow
L89.026	Pressure-induced deep tissue damage of left elbow
L89.106	Pressure-induced deep tissue damage of unspecified part of back
L89.116	Pressure-induced deep tissue damage of right upper back
L89.126	Pressure-induced deep tissue damage of left upper back
L89.136	Pressure-induced deep tissue damage of right lower back
L89.146	Pressure-induced deep tissue damage of left lower back
L89.156	Pressure-induced deep tissue damage of sacral region
L89.206	Pressure-induced deep tissue damage of unspecified hip
L89.216	Pressure-induced deep tissue damage of right hip
L89.226	Pressure-induced deep tissue damage of left hip
L89.306	Pressure-induced deep tissue damage of unspecified buttock
L89.316	Pressure-induced deep tissue damage of right buttock
L89.326	Pressure-induced deep tissue damage of left buttock
L89.46	Pressure-induced deep tissue damage of contiguous site of back, buttock and hip
L89.506	Pressure-induced deep tissue damage of unspecified ankle
L89.516	Pressure-induced deep tissue damage of right ankle
L89.526	Pressure-induced deep tissue damage of left ankle

L89.606	Pressure-induced deep tissue damage of unspecified heel
L89.616	Pressure-induced deep tissue damage of right heel
L89.626	Pressure-induced deep tissue damage of left heel
L89.816	Pressure-induced deep tissue damage of head
L89.896	Pressure-induced deep tissue damage of other site
L89.96	Pressure-induced deep tissue damage of unspecified site
N63.15	Unspecified lump in the right breast, overlapping quadrants
N63.25	Unspecified lump in the left breast, overlapping quadrants
N99.85	Post endometrial ablation syndrome
Q66.00	Congenital talipes equinovarus, unspecified foot
Q66.01	Congenital talipes equinovarus, right foot
Q66.02	Congenital talipes equinovarus, left foot
Q66.10	Congenital talipes calcaneovarus, unspecified foot
Q66.11	Congenital talipes calcaneovarus, right foot
Q66.12	Congenital talipes calcaneovarus, left foot
Q66.211	Congenital metatarsus primus varus, right foot
Q66.212	Congenital metatarsus primus varus, left foot
Q66.219	Congenital metatarsus primus varus, unspecified foot
Q66.221	Congenital metatarsus adductus, right foot
Q66.222	Congenital metatarsus adductus, left foot
Q66.229	Congenital metatarsus adductus, unspecified foot
Q66.30	Other congenital varus deformities of feet, unspecified foot
Q66.31	Other congenital varus deformities of feet, right foot
Q66.32	Other congenital varus deformities of feet, left foot
Q66.40	Congenital talipes calcaneovalgus, unspecified foot
Q66.41	Congenital talipes calcaneovalgus, right foot
Q66.42	Congenital talipes calcaneovalgus, left foot
Q66.70	Congenital pes cavus, unspecified foot
Q66.71	Congenital pes cavus, right foot
Q66.72	Congenital pes cavus, left foot
Q66.90	Congenital deformity of feet, unspecified, unspecified foot
Q66.91	Congenital deformity of feet, unspecified, right foot
Q66.92	Congenital deformity of feet, unspecified, left foot
Q79.60	Ehlers-Danlos syndrome, unspecified
Q79.61	Classical Ehlers-Danlos syndrome
Q79.62	Hypermobile Ehlers-Danlos syndrome
Q79.63	Vascular Ehlers-Danlos syndrome
Q79.69	Other Ehlers-Danlos syndromes
Q87.11	Prader-Willi syndrome
Q87.19	Other congenital malformation syndromes predominantly associated with short stature
R11.15	Cyclical vomiting syndrome unrelated to migraine
R82.81	Pyuria
R82.89	Other abnormal findings on cytological and histological examination of urine
S02.121A	Fracture of orbital roof, right side, initial encounter for closed fracture
S02.121B	Fracture of orbital roof, right side, initial encounter for open fracture
S02.121D	Fracture of orbital roof, right side, subsequent encounter for fracture with routine healing
S02.121G	Fracture of orbital roof, right side, subsequent encounter for fracture with delayed healing
S02.121K	Fracture of orbital roof, right side, subsequent encounter for fracture with nonunion
S02.121S	Fracture of orbital roof, right side, sequela
S02.122A	Fracture of orbital roof, left side, initial encounter for closed fracture
S02.122B	Fracture of orbital roof, left side, initial encounter for open fracture
S02.122D	Fracture of orbital roof, left side, subsequent encounter for fracture with routine healing
S02.122G	Fracture of orbital roof, left side, subsequent encounter for fracture with delayed healing
S02.122K	Fracture of orbital roof, left side, subsequent encounter for fracture with nonunion
S02.122S	Fracture of orbital roof, left side, sequela
S02.129A	Fracture of orbital roof, unspecified side, initial encounter for closed fracture
S02.129B	Fracture of orbital roof, unspecified side, initial encounter for open fracture
S02.129D	Fracture of orbital roof, unspecified side, subsequent encounter for fracture with routine healing
S02.129G	Fracture of orbital roof, unspecified side, subsequent encounter for fracture with delayed healing
S02.129K	Fracture of orbital roof, unspecified side, subsequent encounter for fracture with nonunion
S02.129S	Fracture of orbital roof, unspecified side, sequela
S02.831A	Fracture of medial orbital wall, right side, initial encounter for closed fracture
S02.831B	Fracture of medial orbital wall, right side, initial encounter for open fracture
S02.831D	Fracture of medial orbital wall, right side, subsequent encounter for fracture with routine healing
S02.831G	Fracture of medial orbital wall, right side, subsequent encounter for fracture with delayed healing
S02.831K	Fracture of medial orbital wall, right side, subsequent encounter for fracture with nonunion
S02.831S	Fracture of medial orbital wall, right side, sequela
S02.832A	Fracture of medial orbital wall, left side, initial encounter for closed fracture
S02.832B	Fracture of medial orbital wall, left side, initial encounter for open fracture
S02.832D	Fracture of medial orbital wall, left side, subsequent encounter for fracture with routine healing
S02.832G	Fracture of medial orbital wall, left side, subsequent encounter for fracture with delayed healing
S02.832K	Fracture of medial orbital wall, left side, subsequent encounter for fracture with nonunion
S02.832S	Fracture of medial orbital wall, left side, sequela
S02.839A	Fracture of medial orbital wall, unspecified side, initial encounter for closed fracture
S02.839B	Fracture of medial orbital wall, unspecified side, initial encounter for open fracture
S02.839D	Fracture of medial orbital wall, unspecified side, subsequent encounter for fracture with routine healing
S02.839G	Fracture of medial orbital wall, unspecified side, subsequent encounter for fracture with delayed healing
S02.839K	Fracture of medial orbital wall, unspecified side, subsequent encounter for fracture with nonunion
S02.839S	Fracture of medial orbital wall, unspecified side, sequela

S02.841A	Fracture of lateral orbital wall, right side, initial encounter for closed fracture
S02.841B	Fracture of lateral orbital wall, right side, initial encounter for open fracture
S02.841D	Fracture of lateral orbital wall, right side, subsequent encounter for fracture with routine healing
S02.841G	Fracture of lateral orbital wall, right side, subsequent encounter for fracture with delayed healing
S02.841K	Fracture of lateral orbital wall, right side, subsequent encounter for fracture with nonunion
S02.841S	Fracture of lateral orbital wall, right side, sequela
S02.842A	Fracture of lateral orbital wall, left side, initial encounter for closed fracture
S02.842B	Fracture of lateral orbital wall, left side, initial encounter for open fracture
S02.842D	Fracture of lateral orbital wall, left side, subsequent encounter for fracture with routine healing
S02.842G	Fracture of lateral orbital wall, left side, subsequent encounter for fracture with delayed healing
S02.842K	Fracture of lateral orbital wall, left side, subsequent encounter for fracture with nonunion
S02.842S	Fracture of lateral orbital wall, left side, sequela
S02.849A	Fracture of lateral orbital wall, unspecified side, initial encounter for closed fracture
S02.849B	Fracture of lateral orbital wall, unspecified side, initial encounter for open fracture
S02.849D	Fracture of lateral orbital wall, unspecified side, subsequent encounter for fracture with routine healing
S02.849G	Fracture of lateral orbital wall, unspecified side, subsequent encounter for fracture with delayed healing
S02.849K	Fracture of lateral orbital wall, unspecified side, subsequent encounter for fracture with nonunion
S02.849S	Fracture of lateral orbital wall, unspecified side, sequela
S02.85XA	Fracture of orbit, unspecified, initial encounter for closed fracture
S02.85XB	Fracture of orbit, unspecified, initial encounter for open fracture
S02.85XD	Fracture of orbit, unspecified, subsequent encounter for fracture with routine healing
S02.85XG	Fracture of orbit, unspecified, subsequent encounter for fracture with delayed healing
S02.85XK	Fracture of orbit, unspecified, subsequent encounter for fracture with nonunion
S02.85XS	Fracture of orbit, unspecified, sequela
T50.911A	Poisoning by multiple unspecified drugs, medicaments and biological substances, accidental (unintentional), initial encounter
T50.911D	Poisoning by multiple unspecified drugs, medicaments and biological substances, accidental (unintentional), subsequent encounter
T50.911S	Poisoning by multiple unspecified drugs, medicaments and biological substances, accidental (unintentional), sequela
T50.912A	Poisoning by multiple unspecified drugs, medicaments and biological substances, intentional self-harm, initial encounter
T50.912D	Poisoning by multiple unspecified drugs, medicaments and biological substances, intentional self-harm, subsequent encounter
T50.912S	Poisoning by multiple unspecified drugs, medicaments and biological substances, intentional self-harm, sequela
T50.913A	Poisoning by multiple unspecified drugs, medicaments and biological substances, assault, initial encounter
T50.913D	Poisoning by multiple unspecified drugs, medicaments and biological substances, assault, subsequent encounter
T50.913S	Poisoning by multiple unspecified drugs, medicaments and biological substances, assault, sequela
T50.914A	Poisoning by multiple unspecified drugs, medicaments and biological substances, undetermined, initial encounter
T50.914D	Poisoning by multiple unspecified drugs, medicaments and biological substances, undetermined, subsequent encounter
T50.914S	Poisoning by multiple unspecified drugs, medicaments and biological substances, undetermined, sequela
T50.915A	Adverse effect of multiple unspecified drugs, medicaments and biological substances, initial encounter
T50.915D	Adverse effect of multiple unspecified drugs, medicaments and biological substances, subsequent encounter
T50.915S	Adverse effect of multiple unspecified drugs, medicaments and biological substances, sequela
T50.916A	Underdosing of multiple unspecified drugs, medicaments and biological substances, initial encounter
T50.916D	Underdosing of multiple unspecified drugs, medicaments and biological substances, subsequent encounter
T50.916S	Underdosing of multiple unspecified drugs, medicaments and biological substances, sequela
T67.01XA	Heatstroke and sunstroke, initial encounter
T67.01XD	Heatstroke and sunstroke, subsequent encounter
T67.01XS	Heatstroke and sunstroke, sequela
T67.02XA	Exertional heatstroke, initial encounter
T67.02XD	Exertional heatstroke, subsequent encounter
T67.02XS	Exertional heatstroke, sequela
T67.09XA	Other heatstroke and sunstroke, initial encounter
T67.09XD	Other heatstroke and sunstroke, subsequent encounter
T67.09XS	Other heatstroke and sunstroke, sequela
Y35.009A	Legal intervention involving unspecified firearm discharge, unspecified person injured, initial encounter
Y35.009D	Legal intervention involving unspecified firearm discharge, unspecified person injured, subsequent encounter
Y35.009S	Legal intervention involving unspecified firearm discharge, unspecified person injured, sequela
Y35.019A	Legal intervention involving injury by machine gun, unspecified person injured, initial encounter
Y35.019D	Legal intervention involving injury by machine gun, unspecified person injured, subsequent encounter
Y35.019S	Legal intervention involving injury by machine gun, unspecified person injured, sequela
Y35.029A	Legal intervention involving injury by handgun, unspecified person injured, initial encounter
Y35.029D	Legal intervention involving injury by handgun, unspecified person injured, subsequent encounter
Y35.029S	Legal intervention involving injury by handgun, unspecified person injured, sequela
Y35.039A	Legal intervention involving injury by rifle pellet, unspecified person injured, initial encounter
Y35.039D	Legal intervention involving injury by rifle pellet, unspecified person injured, subsequent encounter

What's New for 2020

Y35.039S	Legal intervention involving injury by rifle pellet, unspecified person injured, sequela
Y35.049A	Legal intervention involving injury by rubber bullet, unspecified person injured, initial encounter
Y35.049D	Legal intervention involving injury by rubber bullet, unspecified person injured, subsequent encounter
Y35.049S	Legal intervention involving injury by rubber bullet, unspecified person injured, sequela
Y35.099A	Legal intervention involving other firearm discharge, unspecified person injured, initial encounter
Y35.099D	Legal intervention involving other firearm discharge, unspecified person injured, subsequent encounter
Y35.099S	Legal intervention involving other firearm discharge, unspecified person injured, sequela
Y35.109A	Legal intervention involving unspecified explosives, unspecified person injured, initial encounter
Y35.109D	Legal intervention involving unspecified explosives, unspecified person injured, subsequent encounter
Y35.109S	Legal intervention involving unspecified explosives, unspecified person injured, sequela
Y35.119A	Legal intervention involving injury by dynamite, unspecified person injured, initial encounter
Y35.119D	Legal intervention involving injury by dynamite, unspecified person injured, subsequent encounter
Y35.119S	Legal intervention involving injury by dynamite, unspecified person injured, sequela
Y35.129A	Legal intervention involving injury by explosive shell, unspecified person injured, initial encounter
Y35.129D	Legal intervention involving injury by explosive shell, unspecified person injured, subsequent encounter
Y35.129S	Legal intervention involving injury by explosive shell, unspecified person injured, sequela
Y35.199A	Legal intervention involving other explosives, unspecified person injured, initial encounter
Y35.199D	Legal intervention involving other explosives, unspecified person injured, subsequent encounter
Y35.199S	Legal intervention involving other explosives, unspecified person injured, sequela
Y35.209A	Legal intervention involving unspecified gas, unspecified person injured, initial encounter
Y35.209D	Legal intervention involving unspecified gas, unspecified person injured, subsequent encounter
Y35.209S	Legal intervention involving unspecified gas, unspecified person injured, sequela
Y35.219A	Legal intervention involving injury by tear gas, unspecified person injured, initial encounter
Y35.219D	Legal intervention involving injury by tear gas, unspecified person injured, subsequent encounter
Y35.219S	Legal intervention involving injury by tear gas, unspecified person injured, sequela
Y35.299A	Legal intervention involving other gas, unspecified person injured, initial encounter
Y35.299D	Legal intervention involving other gas, unspecified person injured, subsequent encounter
Y35.299S	Legal intervention involving other gas, unspecified person injured, sequela
Y35.309A	Legal intervention involving unspecified blunt objects, unspecified person injured, initial encounter
Y35.309D	Legal intervention involving unspecified blunt objects, unspecified person injured, subsequent encounter
Y35.309S	Legal intervention involving unspecified blunt objects, unspecified person injured, sequela
Y35.319A	Legal intervention involving baton, unspecified person injured, initial encounter
Y35.319D	Legal intervention involving baton, unspecified person injured, subsequent encounter
Y35.319S	Legal intervention involving baton, unspecified person injured, sequela
Y35.399A	Legal intervention involving other blunt objects, unspecified person injured, initial encounter
Y35.399D	Legal intervention involving other blunt objects, unspecified person injured, subsequent encounter
Y35.399S	Legal intervention involving other blunt objects, unspecified person injured, sequela
Y35.409A	Legal intervention involving unspecified sharp objects, unspecified person injured, initial encounter
Y35.409D	Legal intervention involving unspecified sharp objects, unspecified person injured, subsequent encounter
Y35.409S	Legal intervention involving unspecified sharp objects, unspecified person injured, sequela
Y35.419A	Legal intervention involving bayonet, unspecified person injured, initial encounter
Y35.419D	Legal intervention involving bayonet, unspecified person injured, subsequent encounter
Y35.419S	Legal intervention involving bayonet, unspecified person injured, sequela
Y35.499A	Legal intervention involving other sharp objects, unspecified person injured, initial encounter
Y35.499D	Legal intervention involving other sharp objects, unspecified person injured, subsequent encounter
Y35.499S	Legal intervention involving other sharp objects, unspecified person injured, sequela
Y35.819A	Legal intervention involving manhandling, unspecified person injured, initial encounter
Y35.819D	Legal intervention involving manhandling, unspecified person injured, subsequent encounter
Y35.819S	Legal intervention involving manhandling, unspecified person injured, sequela
Y35.831A	Legal intervention involving a conducted energy device, law enforcement official injured, initial encounter
Y35.831D	Legal intervention involving a conducted energy device, law enforcement official injured, subsequent encounter
Y35.831S	Legal intervention involving a conducted energy device, law enforcement official injured, sequela
Y35.832A	Legal intervention involving a conducted energy device, bystander injured, initial encounter
Y35.832D	Legal intervention involving a conducted energy device, bystander injured, subsequent encounter
Y35.832S	Legal intervention involving a conducted energy device, bystander injured, sequela
Y35.833A	Legal intervention involving a conducted energy device, suspect injured, initial encounter
Y35.833D	Legal intervention involving a conducted energy device, suspect injured, subsequent encounter
Y35.833S	Legal intervention involving a conducted energy device, suspect injured, sequela

Y35.839A	Legal intervention involving a conducted energy device, unspecified person injured, initial encounter
Y35.839D	Legal intervention involving a conducted energy device, unspecified person injured, subsequent encounter
Y35.839S	Legal intervention involving a conducted energy device, unspecified person injured, sequela
Y35.99XA	Legal intervention, means unspecified, unspecified person injured, initial encounter
Y35.99XD	Legal intervention, means unspecified, unspecified person injured, subsequent encounter
Y35.99XS	Legal intervention, means unspecified, unspecified person injured, sequela
Z01.020	Encounter for examination of eyes and vision following failed vision screening without abnormal findings
Z01.021	Encounter for examination of eyes and vision following failed vision screening with abnormal findings
Z11.7	Encounter for testing for latent tuberculosis infection
Z22.7	Latent tuberculosis
Z71.84	Encounter for health counseling related to travel
Z86.002	Personal history of in-situ neoplasm of other and unspecified genital organs
Z86.003	Personal history of in-situ neoplasm of oral cavity, esophagus and stomach
Z86.004	Personal history of in-situ neoplasm of other and unspecified digestive organs
Z86.005	Personal history of in-situ neoplasm of middle ear and respiratory system
Z86.006	Personal history of melanoma in-situ
Z86.007	Personal history of in-situ neoplasm of skin
Z86.15	Personal history of latent tuberculosis infection
Z96.82	Presence of neurostimulator

30 Code Descriptions Revised

Note: Each code is listed with its revised description only. Please refer to the full FY 2020 official addenda code files at https://www.cms.gov/Medicare/Coding/ICD10/2020-ICD-10-CM.html for the specific changes made to the codes listed.

B96.21	Shiga toxin-producing Escherichia coli [E. coli] [STEC] O157 as the cause of diseases classified elsewhere
B96.22	Other specified Shiga toxin-producing Escherichia coli [E. coli] [STEC] as the cause of diseases classified elsewhere
B96.23	Unspecified Shiga toxin-producing Escherichia coli [E. coli] [STEC] as the cause of diseases classified elsewhere
G43.A0	Cyclical vomiting, in migraine, not intractable
G43.A1	Cyclical vomiting, in migraine, intractable
I70.238	Atherosclerosis of native arteries of right leg with ulceration of other part of lower leg
I70.248	Atherosclerosis of native arteries of left leg with ulceration of other part of lower leg
J44.0	Chronic obstructive pulmonary disease with (acute) lower respiratory infection
M50.120	Mid-cervical disc disorder, unspecified level
M66.88	Spontaneous rupture of other tendons, other sites

M67.839	Other specified disorders of synovium and tendon, unspecified wrist
M77.50	Other enthesopathy of unspecified foot and ankle
M77.51	Other enthesopathy of right foot and ankle
M77.52	Other enthesopathy of left foot and ankle
N35.814	Other anterior urethral stricture, male
R82.993	Hyperuricosuria
T40.906A	Underdosing of unspecified psychodysleptics [hallucinogens], initial encounter
T40.906D	Underdosing of unspecified psychodysleptics [hallucinogens], subsequent encounter
T40.906S	Underdosing of unspecified psychodysleptics [hallucinogens], sequela
T40.996A	Underdosing of other psychodysleptics [hallucinogens], initial encounter
T40.996D	Underdosing of other psychodysleptics [hallucinogens], subsequent encounter
T40.996S	Underdosing of other psychodysleptics [hallucinogens], sequela
T44.1X6A	Underdosing of other parasympathomimetics [cholinergics], initial encounter
T44.1X6D	Underdosing of other parasympathomimetics [cholinergics], subsequent encounter
T44.1X6S	Underdosing of other parasympathomimetics [cholinergics], sequela
V43.13XA	Car passenger injured in collision with pick-up truck in nontraffic accident, initial encounter
V43.13XD	Car passenger injured in collision with pick-up truck in nontraffic accident, subsequent encounter
V43.13XS	Car passenger injured in collision with pick-up truck in nontraffic accident, sequela
Z45.42	Encounter for adjustment and management of neurostimulator
Z68.43	Body mass index (BMI) 50.0-59.9, adult

Proprietary Updates

The following proprietary features have also been added:

- 40+ new definitions that describe, in lay terms, a specific condition or disease process

- 40+ new coding tips that provide coding advice beyond the code classification

- Updated *AHA Coding Clinic* references through second quarter 2019

Conversion Table of ICD-10-CM Codes

Code Assignment Beginning 10/1/2019	Previous Code(s) Assignment
D75.A	D55.0
D81.30	D81.3
D81.31	D81.3
D81.32	D81.3
D81.39	D81.3
H81.4	H81.41–H81.43; H81.49
I26.93	I26.99
I26.94	I26.99
I48.11	I48.1
I48.19	I48.1
I48.20	I48.2
I48.21	I48.2
I80.241	I80.291
I80.242	I80.292
I80.243	I80.293
I80.249	I80.299
I80.251	I80.291
I80.252	I80.292
I80.253	I80.293
I80.259	I80.299
I82.451	I80.491
I82.452	I80.492
I82.453	I80.493
I82.459	I80.499
I82.461	I80.491
I82.462	I80.492
I82.463	I80.493
I82.469	I80.499
I82.551	I80.591
I82.552	I80.592
I82.553	I80.593
I82.559	I80.599
I82.561	I80.591
I82.562	I80.592
I82.563	I80.593
I82.569	I80.599
L89.006	L89.000
L89.016	L89.010
L89.026	L89.020
L89.106	L89.100
L89.116	L89.110
L89.126	L89.120
L89.136	L89.130
L89.146	L89.140
L89.156	L89.150
L89.206	L89.200
L89.216	L89.210

Code Assignment Beginning 10/1/2019	Previous Code(s) Assignment
L89.226	L89.220
L89.306	L89.300
L89.316	L89.310
L89.326	L89.320
L89.46	L89.45
L89.506	L89.500
L89.516	L89.510
L89.526	L89.520
L89.606	L89.600
L89.616	L89.610
L89.626	L89.620
L89.816	L89.810
L89.896	L89.890
L89.96	L89.95
N63.15	N63.11–N63.14
N63.25	N63.21–N63.24
N99.85	N99.89
Q66.00	Q66.0
Q66.01	Q66.0
Q66.02	Q66.0
Q66.10	Q66.1
Q66.11	Q66.1
Q66.12	Q66.1
Q66.211	Q66.21
Q66.212	Q66.21
Q66.219	Q66.21
Q66.221	Q66.22
Q66.222	Q66.22
Q66.229	Q66.22
Q66.30	Q66.3
Q66.31	Q66.3
Q66.32	Q66.3
Q66.40	Q66.4
Q66.41	Q66.4
Q66.42	Q66.4
Q66.70	Q66.7
Q66.71	Q66.7
Q66.72	Q66.7
Q66.90	Q66.9
Q66.91	Q66.9
Q66.92	Q66.9
Q79.60	Q79.6
Q79.61	Q79.6
Q79.62	Q79.6
Q79.63	Q79.6
Q79.69	Q79.6
Q87.11	Q87.1
Q87.19	Q87.1

Code Assignment Beginning 10/1/2019	Previous Code(s) Assignment
R11.15	K31.89 and a code from R11-
R82.81	R82.8
R82.89	R82.8
S02.121A	S02.19A*
S02.121B	S02.19B*
S02.121D	S02.19D*
S02.121G	S02.19G*
S02.121K	S02.19K*
S02.121S	S02.19S*
S02.122A	S02.19A*
S02.122B	S02.19B*
S02.122D	S02.19D*
S02.122G	S02.19G*
S02.122K	S02.19K*
S02.122S	S02.19S*
S02.129A	S02.19A*
S02.129B	S02.19B*
S02.129D	S02.19D*
S02.129G	S02.19G*
S02.129K	S02.19K*
S02.129S	S02.19S*
S02.831A	S02.81XA
S02.831B	S02.81XB
S02.831D	S02.81XD
S02.831G	S02.81XG
S02.831K	S02.81XK
S02.831S	S02.81XS
S02.832A	S02.82XA
S02.832B	S02.82XB
S02.832D	S02.82XD
S02.832G	S02.82XG
S02.832K	S02.82XK
S02.832S	S02.82XS
S02.839A	S02.80XA
S02.839B	S02.80XB
S02.839D	S02.80XD
S02.839G	S02.80XG
S02.839K	S02.80XK
S02.839S	S02.80XS
S02.841A	S02.81XA
S02.841B	S02.81XB
S02.841D	S02.81XD
S02.841G	S02.81XG
S02.841K	S02.81XK
S02.841S	S02.81XS
S02.842A	S02.82XA
S02.842B	S02.82XB
S02.842D	S02.82XD

Code Assignment Beginning 10/1/2019	Previous Code(s) Assignment	Code Assignment Beginning 10/1/2019	Previous Code(s) Assignment	Code Assignment Beginning 10/1/2019	Previous Code(s) Assignment
S02.842G	S02.82XG	Y35.019A	None	Y35.409A	None
S02.842K	S02.82XK	Y35.019D	None	Y35.409D	None
S02.842S	S02.82XS	Y35.019S	None	Y35.409S	None
S02.849A	S02.80XA	Y35.029A	None	Y35.419A	None
S02.849B	S02.80XB	Y35.029D	None	Y35.419D	None
S02.849D	S02.80XD	Y35.029S	None	Y35.419S	None
S02.849G	S02.80XG	Y35.039A	None	Y35.499A	None
S02.849K	S02.80XK	Y35.039D	None	Y35.499D	None
S02.849S	S02.80XS	Y35.039S	None	Y35.499S	None
S02.85XA	S02.80XA	Y35.049A	None	Y35.819A	None
S02.85XB	S02.80XB	Y35.049D	None	Y35.819D	None
S02.85XD	S02.80XD	Y35.049S	None	Y35.819S	None
S02.85XG	S02.80XG	Y35.099A	None	Y35.831A	Y35.891A
S02.85XK	S02.80XK	Y35.099D	None	Y35.831D	Y35.891D
S02.85XS	S02.80XS	Y35.099S	None	Y35.831S	Y35.891S
T50.911A	T50.991A	Y35.109A	None	Y35.832A	Y35.892A
T50.911D	T50.991D	Y35.109D	None	Y35.832D	Y35.892D
T50.911S	T50.991S	Y35.109S	None	Y35.832S	Y35.892S
T50.912A	T50.992A	Y35.119A	None	Y35.833A	Y35.893A
T50.912D	T50.992D	Y35.119D	None	Y35.833D	Y35.893D
T50.912S	T50.992S	Y35.119S	None	Y35.833S	Y35.893S
T50.913A	T50.993A	Y35.129A	None	Y35.839A	None
T50.913D	T50.993D	Y35.129D	None	Y35.839D	None
T50.913S	T50.993S	Y35.129S	None	Y35.839S	None
T50.914A	T50.994A	Y35.199A	None	Y35.99XA	None
T50.914D	T50.994D	Y35.199D	None	Y35.99XD	None
T50.914S	T50.994S	Y35.199S	None	Y35.99XS	None
T50.915A	T50.995A	Y35.209A	None	Z01.020	Z01.00
T50.915D	T50.995D	Y35.209D	None	Z01.021	Z01.01
T50.915S	T50.995S	Y35.209S	None	Z11.7	Z11.1
T50.916A	T50.996A	Y35.219A	None	Z22.7	R76.11
T50.916D	T50.996D	Y35.219D	None	Z71.84	Z71.89
T50.916S	T50.996S	Y35.219S	None	Z86.002	Z86.008
T67.01XA	T67.0XXA	Y35.299A	None	Z86.003	Z86.008
T67.01XD	T67.0XXD	Y35.299D	None	Z86.004	Z86.008
T67.01XS	T67.0XXS	Y35.299S	None	Z86.005	Z86.008
T67.02XA	T67.0XXA	Y35.309A	None	Z86.006	Z86.008
T67.02XD	T67.0XXD	Y35.309D	None	Z86.007	Z86.008
T67.02XS	T67.0XXS	Y35.309S	None	Z86.15	R76.11
T67.09XA	T67.0XXA	Y35.319A	None	Z96.82	Z96.89
T67.09XD	T67.0XXD	Y35.319D	None		
T67.09XS	T67.0XXS	Y35.319S	None		
Y35.009A	None	Y35.399A	None		
Y35.009D	None	Y35.399D	None		
Y35.009S	None	Y35.399S	None		

* These codes are listed exactly as found in the official conversion table from the CDC.

10 Steps to Correct Coding

Follow the 10 steps below to correctly code encounters for health care services.

Step 1: Identify the reason for the visit or encounter (i.e., a sign, symptom, diagnosis and/or condition).

The medical record documentation should accurately reflect the patient's condition, using terminology that includes specific diagnoses and symptoms or clearly states the reasons for the encounter.

Choosing the main term that best describes the reason chiefly responsible for the service provided is the most important step in coding. If symptoms are present and documented but a definitive diagnosis has not yet been determined, code the symptoms. *For outpatient cases, do not code conditions that are referred to as "rule out," "suspected," "probable," or "questionable."* Diagnoses often are not established at the time of the initial encounter/visit and may require two or more visits to be established. Code only what is documented in the available outpatient records and only to the highest degree of certainty known at the time of the patient's visit. For inpatient medical records, uncertain diagnoses may be reported if documented at the time of discharge.

Step 2: After selecting the reason for the encounter, consult the alphabetic index.

The most critical rule is to begin code selection in the alphabetic index. Never turn first to the tabular list. The index provides cross-references, essential and nonessential modifiers, and other instructional notations that may not be found in the tabular list.

Step 3: Locate the main term entry.

The alphabetic index lists conditions, which may be expressed as nouns or eponyms, with critical use of adjectives. Some conditions known by several names have multiple main entries. Reasons for encounters may be located under general terms such as admission, encounter, and examination. Other general terms such as history, status (post), or presence (of) can be used to locate other factors influencing health.

Step 4: Scan subterm entries.

Scan the subterm entries, as appropriate, being sure to review continued lines and additional subterms that may appear in the next column or on the next page. Shaded vertical guidelines in the index indicate the indentation level for each subterm in relation to the main terms.

Step 5: Pay close attention to index instructions.

- Parentheses ( ) enclose nonessential modifiers, terms that are supplementary words or explanatory information that may or may not appear in the diagnostic statement and do not affect code selection.

- Brackets [ ] enclose manifestation codes that can be used only as secondary codes to the underlying condition code immediately preceding it. If used, manifestation codes must be reported with the appropriate etiology codes.

- Default codes are listed next to the main term and represent the condition most commonly associated with the main term or the unspecified code for the main term.

- "*See*" cross-references, identified by italicized type and "code by" cross-references indicate that another term *must be referenced* to locate the correct code.

- "*See also*" cross-references, identified by italicized type, provide alternative terms that may be useful to look up but *are not mandatory.*

- "Omit code" cross-references identify instances when a code is not applicable depending on the condition being coded.

- "With" subterms are listed out of alphabetic order and identify a presumed causal relationship between the two conditions they link.

- "Due to" subterms identify a relationship between the two conditions they link.

- "NEC," abbreviation for "not elsewhere classified," follows some main terms or subterms and indicates that there is no specific code for the condition even though the medical documentation may be very specific.

- "NOS," abbreviation for "not otherwise specified," follows some main terms or subterms and is the equivalent of unspecified; NOS signifies that the information in the medical record is insufficient for assigning a more specific code.

- *Following* references help coders locate alphanumeric codes that are out of sequence in the tabular section.

- Check-additional-character symbols flag codes that require additional characters to make the code valid; the characters available to complete the code should be verified in the tabular section.

Step 6: Choose a potential code and locate it in the tabular list.

To prevent coding errors, always use both the alphabetic index (to identify a code) and the tabular list (to verify a code), as the index does not include the important instructional notes found in the tabular list. An added benefit of using the tabular list, which groups like things together, is that while looking at one code in the list, a coder might see a more specific one that would have been missed had the coder relied solely on the alphabetic index. Additionally, many of the codes require a fourth, fifth, sixth, or seventh character to be valid, and many of these characters can be found only in the tabular list.

Step 7: Read all instructional material in the tabular section.

The coder must follow any Includes, Excludes 1 and Excludes 2 notes, and other instructional notes, such as "Code first" and "Use additional code," listed in the tabular list for the chapter, category, subcategory, and subclassification levels of code selection that direct the coder to use a different or additional code. Any codes in the tabular range A00.0- through T88.9- may be used to identify the diagnostic reason for the encounter. The tabular list encompasses many codes describing disease and injury classifications (e.g., infectious and parasitic diseases, neoplasms, symptoms, nervous and circulatory system etc.).

Codes that describe symptoms and signs, as opposed to definitive diagnoses, should be reported when an established diagnosis has not been made (confirmed) by the physician. Chapter 18 of the ICD-10-CM code book, "Symptoms, Signs, and Abnormal Clinical and Laboratory Findings, Not Elsewhere Classified" (codes R00.--R99), contains many, but not all, codes for symptoms.

ICD-10-CM classifies encounters with health care providers for circumstances other than a disease or injury in chapter 21, "Factors Influencing Health Status and Contact with Health Services" (codes Z00–Z99). Circumstances other than a disease or injury often are recorded as chiefly responsible for the encounter.

A code is invalid if it does not include the full number of characters (greatest level of specificity) required. Codes in ICD-10-CM can contain from three to seven alphanumeric characters. A three-character code is to be used only if the category is not further subdivided into four-, five-, six-, or seven-character codes. Placeholder character X is used as part of an alphanumeric code to allow for future expansion and as a placeholder for empty characters in a code that requires a seventh character but has no fourth, fifth, or sixth character. Note that certain categories require seventh characters that apply to all codes in that category. Always check the category level for applicable seventh characters for that category.

Step 8: Consult the official ICD-10-CM conventions and guidelines.

The *ICD-10-CM Official Guidelines for Coding and Reporting* govern the use of certain codes. These guidelines provide both general and chapter-specific coding guidance.

Step 9: Confirm and assign the code.

Having reviewed all relevant information concerning the possible code choices, assign the code that most completely describes the condition.

Repeat steps 1 through 9 for all additional documented conditions that meet the following criteria:

- They exist at the time of the visit *AND*

- They require or affect patient care, treatment, or management

Step 10: Sequence codes correctly.

Sequencing is the order in which the codes are listed on the claim. List first the ICD-10-CM code for the diagnosis, condition, problem, or other reason for the encounter/visit that is shown in the medical record to be chiefly responsible for the services provided. List additional codes that describe any coexisting conditions. Follow the official coding guidelines (see the guidelines, section II, "Selection of Principal Diagnosis"; section III, "Reporting Additional Diagnoses"; and section IV, "Diagnostic Coding and Reporting Guidelines for Outpatient Services") on proper sequencing of codes.

Coding Examples

Diagnosis: Anorexia

Step 1: The reason for the encounter was the condition, anorexia.

Step 2: Consult the alphabetic index.

Step 3: Locate the main term "Anorexia."

Step 4: Two possible subterms are available, "hysterical" and "nervosa." Neither is documented in this instance, however, so they cannot be used in code selection.

Step 5: The code listed next to the main term is called the default code selection. Because the two subentries (essential modifiers) do not apply in this instance, the default code (R63.0) should be used.

Step 6: Turn to code R63.0 in the tabular list and read all instructional notes.

Step 7: The Excludes 1 note at code R63.0 indicates that anorexia nervosa and loss of appetite determined to be of nonorganic origin should be reported with a code from chapter 5. The diagnostic statement does not describe the condition as anorexia nervosa, however, and does not indicate that the anorexia is of a nonorganic origin. There is no further division of the category past the fourth-character subcategory. Therefore, code R63.0 is at the highest level of specificity.

Step 8: Review of official guideline I.C.18 indicates that a symptom code is appropriate when a more definitive diagnosis is not documented.

Step 9: The default code, R63.0 Anorexia, is the correct code selection.

Repeat steps 1 through 9 for any concomitant diagnoses.

Step 10: Since anorexia is listed as the chief reason for the health care encounter, the first-listed, or principal, diagnosis is R63.0. Note that this is a chapter 18 symptom code but can be assigned for both inpatient and outpatient records since the provider did not establish a more definitive diagnosis, according to sections II.A and IV.D.

Diagnosis: Acute bronchitis

Step 1: The reason for the encounter was the condition, acute bronchitis.

Step 2: Consult the alphabetic index.

Step 3: Locate the main term "Bronchitis."

Step 4: There is a subterm for "acute or subacute." Additional subterms are not included in the diagnostic statement.

Step 5: Review the instructional notes. Nonessential modifiers (with bronchospasm or obstruction) are terms that do not affect code assignment. Since no other subterms indented under "acute" apply here, the code listed next to this subentry—in this case J20.9—should be chosen.

Step 6: Turn to code J20.9 in the tabular list and read all instructional notes.

Step 7: The Includes note under category J20 lists alternative terms for acute bronchitis. Note that the list is not exhaustive but is only a representative selection of diagnoses that are included in the subcategory. The Excludes 1 note refers to category J40 for bronchitis and tracheobronchitis NOS. There are several conditions in the Excludes 2 notes that, if applicable, can be coded in addition to this code.

Note that the codes included in J20 represent acute bronchitis due to various infectious organisms that could be selected if identified in the documentation. In this case, the organism was not identified and there is no further division of the category past the fourth character subcategory. Therefore, code J20.9 is at the highest level of specificity.

Step 8: Review of official guideline I.C.10 provides no additional information affecting the code selected.

Step 9: Assign code J20.9 Acute bronchitis, unspecified.

Repeat steps 1 through 9 for any concomitant diagnoses.

Step 10: In the absence of additional diagnoses that may affect sequencing, code J20.9 should be sequenced as the first-listed, or principal, diagnosis.

Diagnosis: Cerebellar ataxia in myxedema

Step 1: The reason for the encounter was the condition, cerebellar ataxia.

Step 2: Consult the alphabetic index.

Step 3: Locate the main term "Ataxia."

Step 4: Available subterms include "cerebellar (hereditary)," with additional indented subterms for "in" and "myxedema," all essential modifiers that are included in the diagnostic statement. Two codes are provided, E03.9 and G13.2, the latter of which is in brackets.

Step 5: Note the nonessential modifier (in parentheses) after the subterm cerebellar includes the term "hereditary." Because it is in parentheses, this term is not required in the diagnostic statement for this subentry to apply. The brackets around G13.2 identify this code as a manifestation of the condition described by code E03.9 and indicate that the two must be reported together and sequencing rules apply.

Step 6: Locate codes E03.9 and G13.2 in the tabular list, and read all instructional notes.

Step 7: For code E03.9, there are no instructional notes in the tabular list at the category E03 or code level that indicate that this condition should be coded elsewhere in the classification or that additional codes are required. Without further information from the diagnostic statement, myxedema, not otherwise specified (NOS), is appropriately reported with code E03.9 Hypothyroidism, unspecified, according to the inclusion term at this code.

Code G13.2 in the tabular list has an instructional note to "Code first underlying disease," which includes conditions found in category E03.-. Based on this note, codes E03.9 and G13.2 are to be coded together, with G13.2 listed only as a secondary diagnosis. This correlates with what the alphabetic index indicated. As there is no further division of codes in category G13 beyond the fourth character, G13.2 is at the highest level of specificity.

Step 8: Although there are some general conventions, such as how to interpret brackets in the alphabetic index, no chapter-specific guidelines apply to this coding scenario.

Step 9: Assign codes E03.9 Hypothyroidism, unspecified, and G13.2 Systemic atrophy primarily affecting the central nervous system in myxedema.

Repeat steps 1 through 9 for any concomitant diagnoses.

Step 10: Based on the alphabetic index and tabular instructional notations, code E03.9 should be sequenced as the first-listed, or principal, diagnosis followed by G13.2 as a secondary diagnosis.

Diagnosis: Decubitus ulcer of right elbow with skin loss and necrosis of subcutaneous tissue

Step 1: The reason for the encounter was the condition, decubitus ulcer.

Step 2: Consult the alphabetic index.

Step 3: Locate the main term "Ulcer."

Step 4: For the subterm "decubitus," there is no code provided or additional subterms indented, but a cross-reference is listed.

Step 5: The italicized cross-reference instructs the coder to "*see* Ulcer, pressure, by site."

Repeat steps 3 through 5 for the cross-reference.

Step 3: Locate the main term "Ulcer."

Step 4: Review the subentries for the subterm "pressure." The next level of indent lists either the site of the ulcer or the specific stage of the ulcer (stage 1–4, unstageable, and unspecified stages). The diagnostic statement provides the site, right elbow, and the extent of tissue damage (skin loss and necrosis of subcutaneous tissue) but does not specifically state that the ulcer is stage 1, stage 2, etc. Nonessential modifiers (in parentheses) at each stage include a description of the typical extent of damage at each stage. For example, stage 1 describes "pre-ulcer skin changes limited to persistent focal edema." Based on the documentation in the record, the coder can correlate the documentation to the nonessential modifiers and choose the specific stage from the index. The coder can also go directly to the body site, choosing the stage of the ulcer after reviewing the code options and instructional notations in the tabular list.

The diagnostic statement indicates that the extent of the damage to the elbow includes skin loss and necrosis of subcutaneous tissue, coinciding with the nonessential modifier next to the subentry "stage 3." The body site of elbow (L89.0-) is listed as another level of indent with other body sites.

Step 5: Note that code L89.0 is followed by a dash and an additional-character-required icon, which indicate that more characters are needed to complete the code. From here, the tabular listing for L89.0- can be consulted.

Step 6: Locate code L89.0- in the tabular list and read all instructional notes.

Step 7: The tabular listing at category L89 has an Includes note for "decubitus ulcer," which confirms that category L89 is the appropriate category to represent what is documented in the diagnostic statement.

Several Excludes 2 notes are also listed at the category level. Excludes 2 notes represent conditions that can occur concomitantly with the decubitus ulcer and can be coded in addition to code L89, if supported by the documentation.

The subcategory codes under L89.0 indicate that the fifth character describes laterality. Locate the right elbow at subcategory L89.01. See that an additional sixth character to specify the stage of the ulcer is now needed to complete the code. The stage can be determined either by the specific documentation of the stage (e.g., stage 1, stage 2) or, in this case, a description that matches one of the inclusion terms that follow

each stage code. For example, the diagnostic description in this case of "skin loss and necrosis of the subcutaneous tissue" matches the inclusion term under L89.013 Pressure ulcer of right elbow, stage 3. No additional characters are required because code L89.013 is at its highest level of specificity.

Step 8: The official guidelines contain quite a bit of information relating to pressure ulcers in chapter-specific guideline I.C.12 as well as information in general guideline I.B.14. These and any other pertinent guidelines should be reviewed to ensure appropriate code assignment.

Step 9: Assign code L89.013 Pressure ulcer of right elbow, stage 3.

Repeat steps 1 through 9 for any concomitant diagnoses.

Step 10: Since the decubitus ulcer is listed as the chief reason for the health care encounter, the first-listed, or principal, diagnosis is L89.013. However, according to the code first instructional note at the L89 category level, gangrene (I96) would be sequenced before the pressure ulcer if it were documented.

Diagnosis: Emergency department visit for bimalleolar fracture of the right ankle due to trauma

Step 1: The reason for the encounter was the condition, bimalleolar fracture.

Step 2: Consult the alphabetic index.

Step 3: Locate the main term "Fracture." Note that many main terms represent fractures: "Fracture, burst," "Fracture, chronic," "Fracture, insufficiency," "Fracture, nontraumatic NEC," "Fracture, pathological," and "Fracture, traumatic." Since the diagnostic statement specifically states that this fracture was the result of trauma, the main term "Fracture, traumatic" should be used.

Step 4: Subterms that should be referenced are "ankle" and "bimalleolar (displaced)," which lists code S82.84-.

Step 5: A nonessential modifier (in parentheses) next to the term bimalleolar for "displaced" indicates that S82.84- is the default category unless the fracture is specifically identified as "nondisplaced."

Note that code S82.84- is followed by a dash and an additional-character icon, both of which indicate that more characters are required. From here, the tabular list can be consulted.

Step 6: Locate code S82.84- in the tabular list and read all instructional notes.

Step: 7 The instructional notes at category S82 indicate that fractures not specified as displaced or nondisplaced default to displaced and that fractures not designated as open or closed default to closed. Additional instructional notes can be found at the category level but none pertain to the current scenario.

Read through the subcategory codes under S82.84, and note that the sixth character specifies displaced or nondisplaced and laterality. Based on the index nonessential modifier (displaced) and the code note at category S82, code selection should identify a displaced fracture of the right side. A displaced bimalleolar fracture of the right lower leg is coded to S82.841.

To complete the code, a seventh character must be assigned to identify the type of encounter (initial, subsequent, or sequela) and whether the fracture is open or closed. Most of the codes in category S82 require a seventh character represented in the list at the category level. However, it is important to note that some subcategories have their own specific set of seventh characters. In this instance, subcategory S82.84- does not have a unique set of seventh characters and the list provided at the category level should be used. Without documentation of the fracture being open, the tabular notation indicates that the default is closed. Character A, representing "initial encounter for closed fracture," listed in the box at the category level is the most appropriate option.

Step 8: Assign code S82.841A Displaced bimalleolar fracture of right lower leg, initial encounter for closed fracture.

Repeat steps 1 through 9 for any concomitant diagnoses.

Step 9: Review chapter-specific guideline I.C.19. and any other official conventions or guidelines to ensure appropriate code assignment.

Step 10: Additional codes can be applied to relate the specific cause of the injury, the place of occurrence, the activity of the patient at the time of the injury, and the patient's status, when this information is available in the record. However, coding this information is voluntary and reporting requirements depend on state mandates and/or facility-specific reporting requirements. If assigned, the external cause codes should be reported as secondary diagnoses only with the injury (fracture) sequenced first. Most codes in chapter 20, "External Causes of Morbidity," require a seventh character to identify the type of encounter. The seventh character assigned to an external cause code should match the seventh character of the code assigned for the associated injury or condition for the encounter.

2020 ICD-10-CM Official Guidelines for Coding and Reporting

Narrative changes appear in **bold** text

Items underlined have been moved within the guidelines since the FY 2019 version

Italics are used to indicate revisions to heading changes

The Centers for Medicare and Medicaid Services (CMS) and the National Center for Health Statistics (NCHS), two departments within the U.S. Federal Government's Department of Health and Human Services (DHHS) provide the following guidelines for coding and reporting using the International Classification of Diseases, 10th Revision, Clinical Modification (ICD-10-CM). These guidelines should be used as a companion document to the official version of the ICD-10-CM as published on the NCHS website. The ICD-10-CM is a morbidity classification published by the United States for classifying diagnoses and reason for visits in all health care settings. The ICD-10-CM is based on the ICD-10, the statistical classification of disease published by the World Health Organization (WHO).

These guidelines have been approved by the four organizations that make up the Cooperating Parties for the ICD-10-CM: the American Hospital Association (AHA), the American Health Information Management Association (AHIMA), CMS, and NCHS.

These guidelines are a set of rules that have been developed to accompany and complement the official conventions and instructions provided within the ICD-10-CM itself. The instructions and conventions of the classification take precedence over guidelines. These guidelines are based on the coding and sequencing instructions in the Tabular List and Alphabetic Index of ICD-10-CM, but provide additional instruction. Adherence to these guidelines when assigning ICD-10-CM diagnosis codes is required under the Health Insurance Portability and Accountability Act (HIPAA). The diagnosis codes (Tabular List and Alphabetic Index) have been adopted under HIPAA for all healthcare settings. A joint effort between the healthcare provider and the coder is essential to achieve complete and accurate documentation, code assignment, and reporting of diagnoses and procedures. These guidelines have been developed to assist both the healthcare provider and the coder in identifying those diagnoses that are to be reported. The importance of consistent, complete documentation in the medical record cannot be overemphasized. Without such documentation accurate coding cannot be achieved. The entire record should be reviewed to determine the specific reason for the encounter and the conditions treated.

The term encounter is used for all settings, including hospital admissions. In the context of these guidelines, the term provider is used throughout the guidelines to mean physician or any qualified health care practitioner who is legally accountable for establishing the patient's diagnosis. Only this set of guidelines, approved by the Cooperating Parties, is official.

The guidelines are organized into sections. Section I includes the structure and conventions of the classification and general guidelines that apply to the entire classification, and chapter-specific guidelines that correspond to the chapters as they are arranged in the classification. Section II includes guidelines for selection of principal diagnosis for non-outpatient settings. Section III includes guidelines for reporting additional diagnoses in non-outpatient settings. Section IV is for outpatient coding and reporting. It is necessary to review all sections of the guidelines to fully understand all of the rules and instructions needed to code properly.

Section I. Conventions, general coding guidelines and chapter specific guidelines 3

A. Conventions for the ICD-10-CM 3
1. The Alphabetic Index and Tabular List 3
2. Format and Structure: 3
3. Use of codes for reporting purposes 3
4. Placeholder character 3
5. 7th Characters 3
6. Abbreviations 3
   a. Alphabetic Index abbreviations 3
   b. Tabular List abbreviations 3
7. Punctuation 3
8. Use of "and". 3
9. Other and Unspecified codes 3
   a. "Other" codes 3
   b. "Unspecified" codes 3
10. Includes Notes 3
11. Inclusion terms 3
12. Excludes Notes 3
   a. Excludes1 3
   b. Excludes2 4
13. Etiology/manifestation convention ("code first", "use additional code" and "in diseases classified elsewhere" notes) 4
14. "And" 4
15. "With" 4
16. "See" and "See Also" 4
17. "Code also" note 4
18. Default codes 4
19. Code assignment and Clinical Criteria 4

B. General Coding Guidelines 4
1. Locating a code in the ICD-10-CM 4
2. Level of Detail in Coding 4
3. Code or codes from A00.0 through T88.9, Z00-Z99.8 4
4. Signs and symptoms 4
5. Conditions that are an integral part of a disease process 4
6. Conditions that are not an integral part of a disease process ... 4
7. Multiple coding for a single condition 5
8. Acute and Chronic Conditions 5
9. Combination Code 5
10. Sequela (Late Effects) 5
11. Impending or Threatened Condition 5
12. Reporting Same Diagnosis Code more than Once 5
13. Laterality 5
14. Documentation *by Clinicians Other than the Patient's Provider* ... 5
15. Syndromes 5
16. Documentation of Complications of Care 5
17. Borderline Diagnosis 6
18. Use of Sign/Symptom/Unspecified Codes 6
19. Coding for Healthcare Encounters in Hurricane Aftermath ... 6
   a. Use of External Cause of Morbidity Codes 6
   b. Sequencing of External Causes of Morbidity Codes 6
   c. Other External Causes of Morbidity Code Issues 6
   d. Use of Z codes 6

C. Chapter-Specific Coding Guidelines 6

In addition to general coding guidelines, there are guidelines for specific diagnoses and/or conditions in the classification. Unless otherwise indicated, these guidelines apply to all health care settings. Please refer to Section II for guidelines on the selection of principal diagnosis 6
1. Chapter 1: Certain Infectious and Parasitic Diseases (A00-B99) ... 6
   a. Human Immunodeficiency Virus (HIV) Infections 6
   b. Infectious agents as the cause of diseases classified to other chapters 7
   c. Infections resistant to antibiotics 7
   d. Sepsis, Severe Sepsis, and Septic Shock 7
   e. Methicillin Resistant Staphylococcus aureus (MRSA) Conditions 8
   f. Zika virus infections 8
2. Chapter 2: Neoplasms (C00-D49) 8
   General guidelines 8
   a. Treatment directed at the malignancy 9
   b. Treatment of secondary site 9
   c. Coding and sequencing of complications 9
   d. Primary malignancy previously excised 9
   e. Admissions/Encounters involving chemotherapy, immunotherapy and radiation therapy 9
   f. Admission/encounter to determine extent of malignancy ... 9
   g. Symptoms, signs, and abnormal findings listed in Chapter 18 associated with neoplasms 9
   h. Admission/encounter for pain control/management 9
   i. Malignancy in two or more noncontiguous sites 10
   j. Disseminated malignant neoplasm, unspecified 10
   k. Malignant neoplasm without specification of site 10
   l. Sequencing of neoplasm codes 10
   m. Current malignancy versus personal history of malignancy ... 10
   n. Leukemia, Multiple Myeloma, and Malignant Plasma Cell Neoplasms in remission versus personal history 10
   o. Aftercare following surgery for neoplasm 10
   p. Follow-up care for completed treatment of a malignancy ... 10
   q. Prophylactic organ removal for prevention of malignancy ... 10
   r. Malignant neoplasm associated with transplanted organ ... 10
3. Chapter 3: Disease of the blood and blood-forming organs and certain disorders involving the immune mechanism (D50-D89) 10
4. Chapter 4: Endocrine, Nutritional, and Metabolic Diseases (E00-E89) 10
   a. Diabetes mellitus 10
5. Chapter 5: Mental, Behavioral and Neurodevelopmental disorders (F01–F99) 11
   a. Pain disorders related to psychological factors 11

b. Mental and behavioral disorders due to psychoactive
substance use 11
c. Factitious Disorder 11
6. Chapter 6: Diseases of the Nervous System (G00-G99) 11
a. Dominant/nondominant side 11
b. Pain - Category G89 11
7. Chapter 7: Diseases of the Eye and Adnexa (H00-H59) 12
a. Glaucoma 12
b. Blindness 13
8. Chapter 8: Diseases of the Ear and Mastoid Process (H60-H95) 13
9. Chapter 9: Diseases of the Circulatory System (I00-I99) 13
a. Hypertension 13
The classification presumes a causal relationship between
hypertension and heart involvement and between hypertension
and kidney involvement, as the two conditions are linked by the
term "with" in the Alphabetic Index. These conditions should be
coded as related even in the absence of provider documentation
explicitly linking them, unless the documentation clearly states
the conditions are unrelated 13
For hypertension and conditions not specifically linked by
relational terms such as "with," "associated with" or "due to"
in the classification, provider documentation must link the
conditions in order to code them as related 13
b. Atherosclerotic Coronary Artery Disease and Angina 13
c. Intraoperative and Postprocedural Cerebrovascular Accident ...13
d. Sequelae of Cerebrovascular Disease 14
e. Acute myocardial infarction (AMI) 14
10. Chapter 10: Diseases of the Respiratory System (J00-J99) 14
a. Chronic Obstructive Pulmonary Disease [COPD] and Asthma 14
b. Acute Respiratory Failure 14
c. Influenza due to certain identified influenza viruses 14
d. Ventilator associated Pneumonia 15
11. Chapter 11: Diseases of the Digestive System (K00-K95) 15
12. Chapter 12: Diseases of the Skin and Subcutaneous Tissue
(L00-L99) 15
a. Pressure ulcer stage codes 15
b. Non-Pressure Chronic Ulcers 15
13. Chapter 13: Diseases of the Musculoskeletal System and
Connective Tissue (M00-M99) 15
a. Site and laterality 15
b. Acute traumatic versus chronic or recurrent musculoskeletal
conditions 15
c. Coding of Pathologic Fractures 16
d. Osteoporosis 16
14. Chapter 14: Diseases of Genitourinary System (N00-N99) 16
a. Chronic kidney disease 16
15. Chapter 15: Pregnancy, Childbirth, and the Puerperium
(O00-O9A) 16
a. General Rules for Obstetric Cases 16
b. Selection of OB Principal or First-listed Diagnosis 16
c. Pre-existing conditions versus conditions due to the
pregnancy 17
d. Pre-existing hypertension in pregnancy 17
e. Fetal Conditions Affecting the Management of the Mother 17
f. HIV Infection in Pregnancy, Childbirth and the Puerperium 17
g. Diabetes mellitus in pregnancy 17
h. Long term use of insulin and oral hypoglycemics 17
i. Gestational (pregnancy induced) diabetes 17
j. Sepsis and septic shock complicating abortion, pregnancy,
childbirth and the puerperium 17
k. Puerperal sepsis 17
l. Alcohol, tobacco *and drug* use during pregnancy, childbirth
and the puerperium 17
m. Poisoning, toxic effects, adverse effects and underdosing in a
pregnant patient 18
n. Normal Delivery, Code O80 18
o. The Peripartum and Postpartum Periods 18
p. Code O94, Sequelae of complication of pregnancy,
childbirth, and the puerperium 18
q. Termination of Pregnancy and Spontaneous abortions 18
r. Abuse in a pregnant patient 18
16. Chapter 16: Certain Conditions Originating in the Perinatal
Period (P00-P96) 18
a. General Perinatal Rules 18
b. Observation and Evaluation of Newborns for Suspected
Conditions not Found 19
c. Coding Additional Perinatal Diagnoses 19

d. Prematurity and Fetal Growth Retardation 19
e. Low birth weight and immaturity status 19
f. Bacterial Sepsis of Newborn 19
g. Stillbirth 19
17. Chapter 17: Congenital malformations, deformations, and
chromosomal abnormalities (Q00-Q99) 19
18. Chapter 18: Symptoms, signs, and abnormal clinical and
laboratory findings, not elsewhere classified (R00-R99) 19
a. Use of symptom codes 19
b. Use of a symptom code with a definitive diagnosis code 19
c. Combination codes that include symptoms 19
d. Repeated falls 19
e. Coma scale 20
f. Functional quadriplegia 20
g. SIRS due to Non-Infectious Process 20
h. Death NOS 20
i. NIHSS Stroke Scale 20
19. Chapter 19: Injury, poisoning, and certain other consequences of
external causes (S00-T88) 20
a. Application of 7th Characters in Chapter 19 20
b. Coding of Injuries 20
c. Coding of Traumatic Fractures 20
d. Coding of Burns and Corrosions 21
e. Adverse Effects, Poisoning, Underdosing and Toxic Effects 21
f. Adult and child abuse, neglect and other maltreatment 22
g. Complications of care 22
20. Chapter 20: External Causes of Morbidity (V00-Y99) 22
a. General External Cause Coding Guidelines 23
b. Place of Occurrence Guideline 23
c. Activity Code 23
d. Place of Occurrence, Activity, and Status Codes Used with
other External Cause Code 23
e. If the Reporting Format Limits the Number of External
Cause Codes 23
f. Multiple External Cause Coding Guidelines 23
g. Child and Adult Abuse Guideline 23
h. Unknown or Undetermined Intent Guideline 23
i. Sequelae (Late Effects) of External Cause Guidelines 23
j. Terrorism Guidelines 24
k. External cause status 24
21. Chapter 21: Factors influencing health status and contact with
health services (Z00-Z99) 24
a. Use of Z codes in any healthcare setting 24
b. Z Codes indicate a reason for an encounter 24
c. Categories of Z Codes 24

Section II. Selection of Principal Diagnosis 28
A. Codes for symptoms, signs, and ill-defined conditions 28
B. Two or more interrelated conditions, each potentially meeting
the definition for principal diagnosis 28
C. Two or more diagnoses that equally meet the definition for
principal diagnosis 28
D. Two or more comparative or contrasting conditions 29
E. A symptom(s) followed by contrasting/comparative diagnoses 29
F. Original treatment plan not carried out 29
G. Complications of surgery and other medical care ...29
H. Uncertain Diagnosis 29
I. Admission from Observation Unit 29
1. Admission Following Medical Observation 29
2. Admission Following Post-Operative Observation 29
J. Admission from Outpatient Surgery 29
K. Admissions/Encounters for Rehabilitation 29

Section III. Reporting Additional Diagnoses 29
A. Previous conditions 29
B. Abnormal findings 29
C. Uncertain Diagnosis 29

**Section IV. Diagnostic Coding and Reporting Guidelines for
Outpatient Services 30**
A. Selection of first-listed condition 30
1. Outpatient Surgery 30
2. Observation Stay 30
B. Codes from A00.0 through T88.9, Z00-Z99 30
C. Accurate reporting of ICD-10-CM diagnosis codes 30
D. Codes that describe symptoms and signs 30
E. Encounters for circumstances other than a disease or injury 30
F. Level of Detail in Coding 30

1. ICD-10-CM codes with 3, 4, 5, 6 or 7 characters 30
2. Use of full number of characters required for a code 30
G. ICD-10-CM code for the diagnosis, condition, problem, or other reason for encounter/visit 30
H. Uncertain diagnosis 30
I. Chronic diseases 30
J. Code all documented conditions that coexist 30
K. Patients receiving diagnostic services only 30
L. Patients receiving therapeutic services only 30
M. Patients receiving preoperative evaluations only 31
N. Ambulatory surgery 31
O. Routine outpatient prenatal visits 31
P. Encounters for general medical examinations with abnormal findings 31
Q. Encounters for routine health screenings 31

Appendix I. Present on Admission Reporting Guidelines 31

Section I. Conventions, general coding guidelines and chapter specific guidelines

The conventions, general guidelines and chapter-specific guidelines are applicable to all health care settings unless otherwise indicated. The conventions and instructions of the classification take precedence over guidelines.

A. Conventions for the ICD-10-CM

The conventions for the ICD-10-CM are the general rules for use of the classification independent of the guidelines. These conventions are incorporated within the Alphabetic Index and Tabular List of the ICD-10-CM as instructional notes.

1. The Alphabetic Index and Tabular List

The ICD-10-CM is divided into the Alphabetic Index, an alphabetical list of terms and their corresponding code, and the Tabular List, a structured list of codes divided into chapters based on body system or condition. The Alphabetic Index consists of the following parts: the Index of Diseases and Injury, the Index of External Causes of Injury, the Table of Neoplasms and the Table of Drugs and Chemicals.

See Section I.C2. General guidelines
See Section I.C.19. Adverse effects, poisoning, underdosing and toxic effects

2. Format and Structure:

The ICD-10-CM Tabular List contains categories, subcategories and codes. Characters for categories, subcategories and codes may be either a letter or a number. All categories are 3 characters. A three-character category that has no further subdivision is equivalent to a code. Subcategories are either 4 or 5 characters. Codes may be 3, 4, 5, 6 or 7 characters. That is, each level of subdivision after a category is a subcategory. The final level of subdivision is a code. Codes that have applicable 7th characters are still referred to as codes, not subcategories. A code that has an applicable 7th character is considered invalid without the 7th character.

The ICD-10-CM uses an indented format for ease in reference.

3. Use of codes for reporting purposes

For reporting purposes only codes are permissible, not categories or subcategories, and any applicable 7th character is required.

4. Placeholder character

The ICD-10-CM utilizes a placeholder character "X". The "X" is used as a placeholder at certain codes to allow for future expansion. An example of this is at the poisoning, adverse effect and underdosing codes, categories T36-T50.

Where a placeholder exists, the X must be used in order for the code to be considered a valid code.

5. 7th Characters

Certain ICD-10-CM categories have applicable 7th characters. The applicable 7th character is required for all codes within the category, or as the notes in the Tabular List instruct. The 7th character must always be the 7th character in the data field. If a code that requires a 7th character is not 6 characters, a placeholder X must be used to fill in the empty characters.

6. Abbreviations

a. Alphabetic Index abbreviations

NEC "Not elsewhere classifiable"

This abbreviation in the Alphabetic Index represents "other specified." When a specific code is not available for a condition, the Alphabetic Index directs the coder to the "other specified" code in the Tabular List.

NOS "Not otherwise specified"

This abbreviation is the equivalent of unspecified.

b. Tabular List abbreviations

NEC "Not elsewhere classifiable"

This abbreviation in the Tabular List represents "other specified". When a specific code is not available for a condition, the Tabular List includes an NEC entry under a code to identify the code as the "other specified" code.

NOS "Not otherwise specified"

This abbreviation is the equivalent of unspecified.

7. Punctuation

[ ] Brackets are used in the Tabular List to enclose synonyms, alternative wording or explanatory phrases. Brackets are used in the Alphabetic Index to identify manifestation codes.

( ) Parentheses are used in both the Alphabetic Index and Tabular List to enclose supplementary words that may be present or absent in the statement of a disease or procedure without affecting the code number to which it is assigned. The terms within the parentheses are referred to as nonessential modifiers. The nonessential modifiers in the Alphabetic Index to Diseases apply to subterms following a main term except when a nonessential modifier and a subentry are mutually exclusive, the subentry takes precedence. For example, in the ICD-10-CM Alphabetic Index under the main term Enteritis, "acute" is a nonessential modifier and "chronic" is a subentry. In this case, the nonessential modifier "acute" does not apply to the subentry "chronic".

: Colons are used in the Tabular List after an incomplete term which needs one or more of the modifiers following the colon to make it assignable to a given category.

8. Use of "and"

See Section I.A.14. Use of the term "And"

9. Other and Unspecified codes

a. "Other" codes

Codes titled "other" or "other specified" are for use when the information in the medical record provides detail for which a specific code does not exist. Alphabetic Index entries with NEC in the line designate "other" codes in the Tabular List. These Alphabetic Index entries represent specific disease entities for which no specific code exists so the term is included within an "other" code.

b. "Unspecified" codes

Codes titled "unspecified" are for use when the information in the medical record is insufficient to assign a more specific code. For those categories for which an unspecified code is not provided, the "other specified" code may represent both other and unspecified.

See Section I.B.18 Use of Signs/Symptom/Unspecified Codes

10. Includes Notes

This note appears immediately under a three character code title to further define, or give examples of, the content of the category.

11. Inclusion terms

List of terms is included under some codes. These terms are the conditions for which that code is to be used. The terms may be synonyms of the code title, or, in the case of "other specified" codes, the terms are a list of the various conditions assigned to that code. The inclusion terms are not necessarily exhaustive. Additional terms found only in the Alphabetic Index may also be assigned to a code.

12. Excludes Notes

The ICD-10-CM has two types of excludes notes. Each type of note has a different definition for use but they are all similar in that they indicate that codes excluded from each other are independent of each other.

a. Excludes1

A type 1 Excludes note is a pure excludes note. It means "NOT CODED HERE!" An Excludes1 note indicates that the code excluded should never be used at the same time as the code above the Excludes1 note. An Excludes1 is used when two conditions cannot occur together, such as a congenital form versus an acquired form of the same condition.

An exception to the Excludes1 definition is the circumstance when the two conditions are unrelated to each other. If it is not clear whether the two conditions involving an Excludes1 note are related or not, query the provider. For example, code F45.8, Other somatoform disorders, has an Excludes1 note for "sleep related teeth grinding (G47.63)," because "teeth grinding" is an inclusion term under F45.8. Only one of these two codes should be assigned for teeth grinding. However psychogenic dysmenorrhea is also an inclusion term under F45.8, and a patient could have both this condition and sleep related teeth grinding. In this case, the two conditions are clearly unrelated to each other, and so it would be appropriate to report F45.8 and G47.63 together.

b. Excludes2

A type 2 Excludes note represents "Not included here." An excludes2 note indicates that the condition excluded is not part of the condition represented by the code, but a patient may have both conditions at the same time. When an Excludes2 note appears under a code, it is acceptable to use both the code and the excluded code together, when appropriate.

13. Etiology/manifestation convention ("code first", "use additional code" and "in diseases classified elsewhere" notes)

Certain conditions have both an underlying etiology and multiple body system manifestations due to the underlying etiology. For such conditions, the ICD-10-CM has a coding convention that requires the underlying condition be sequenced first, if applicable, followed by the manifestation. Wherever such a combination exists, there is a "use additional code" note at the etiology code, and a "code first" note at the manifestation code. These instructional notes indicate the proper sequencing order of the codes, etiology followed by manifestation.

In most cases the manifestation codes will have in the code title, "in diseases classified elsewhere." Codes with this title are a component of the etiology/ manifestation convention. The code title indicates that it is a manifestation code. "In diseases classified elsewhere" codes are never permitted to be used as first-listed or principal diagnosis codes. They must be used in conjunction with an underlying condition code and they must be listed following the underlying condition. See category F02, Dementia in other diseases classified elsewhere, for an example of this convention.

There are manifestation codes that do not have "in diseases classified elsewhere" in the title. For such codes, there is a "use additional code" note at the etiology code and a "code first" note at the manifestation code, and the rules for sequencing apply.

In addition to the notes in the Tabular List, these conditions also have a specific Alphabetic Index entry structure. In the Alphabetic Index both conditions are listed together with the etiology code first followed by the manifestation codes in brackets. The code in brackets is always to be sequenced second.

An example of the etiology/manifestation convention is dementia in Parkinson's disease. In the Alphabetic Index, code G20 is listed first, followed by code F02.80 or F02.81 in brackets. Code G20 represents the underlying etiology, Parkinson's disease, and must be sequenced first, whereas code F02.80 and F02.81 represent the manifestation of dementia in diseases classified elsewhere, with or without behavioral disturbance.

"Code first" and "Use additional code" notes are also used as sequencing rules in the classification for certain codes that are not part of an etiology/ manifestation combination.

See Section I.B.7. Multiple coding for a single condition.

14. "And"

The word "and" should be interpreted to mean either "and" or "or" when it appears in a title.

For example, cases of "tuberculosis of bones", "tuberculosis of joints" and "tuberculosis of bones and joints" are classified to subcategory A18.0, Tuberculosis of bones and joints.

15. "With"

The word "with" or "in" should be interpreted to mean "associated with" or "due to" when it appears in a code title, the Alphabetic Index (either under a main term or subterm), or an instructional note in the Tabular List. The classification presumes a causal relationship between the two conditions linked by these terms in the Alphabetic Index or Tabular List. These conditions should be coded as related even in the absence of provider documentation explicitly linking them, unless the documentation clearly states the conditions are unrelated or when another guideline exists that specifically requires a documented linkage between two conditions (e.g., sepsis guideline for "acute organ dysfunction that is not clearly associated with the sepsis").

For conditions not specifically linked by these relational terms in the classification or when a guideline requires that a linkage between two conditions be explicitly documented, provider documentation must link the conditions in order to code them as related.

The word "with" in the Alphabetic Index is sequenced immediately following the main term **or subterm**, not in alphabetical order.

16. "See" and "See Also"

The "see" instruction following a main term in the Alphabetic Index indicates that another term should be referenced. It is necessary to go to the main term referenced with the "see" note to locate the correct code.

A "see also" instruction following a main term in the Alphabetic Index instructs that there is another main term that may also be referenced that may provide additional Alphabetic Index entries that may be useful. It is not necessary to follow the "see also" note when the original main term provides the necessary code.

17. "Code also" note

A "code also" note instructs that two codes may be required to fully describe a condition, but this note does not provide sequencing direction. The sequencing depends on the circumstances of the encounter.

18. Default codes

A code listed next to a main term in the ICD-10-CM Alphabetic Index is referred to as a default code. The default code represents that condition that is most commonly associated with the main term, or is the unspecified code for the condition. If a condition is documented in a medical record (for example, appendicitis) without any additional information, such as acute or chronic, the default code should be assigned.

19. Code assignment and Clinical Criteria

The assignment of a diagnosis code is based on the provider's diagnostic statement that the condition exists. The provider's statement that the patient has a particular condition is sufficient. Code assignment is not based on clinical criteria used by the provider to establish the diagnosis.

B. General Coding Guidelines

1. Locating a code in the ICD-10-CM

To select a code in the classification that corresponds to a diagnosis or reason for visit documented in a medical record, first locate the term in the Alphabetic Index, and then verify the code in the Tabular List. Read and be guided by instructional notations that appear in both the Alphabetic Index and the Tabular List.

It is essential to use both the Alphabetic Index and Tabular List when locating and assigning a code. The Alphabetic Index does not always provide the full code. Selection of the full code, including laterality and any applicable 7th character can only be done in the Tabular List. A dash (-) at the end of an Alphabetic Index entry indicates that additional characters are required. Even if a dash is not included at the Alphabetic Index entry, it is necessary to refer to the Tabular List to verify that no 7th character is required.

2. Level of Detail in Coding

Diagnosis codes are to be used and reported at their highest number of characters available.

ICD-10-CM diagnosis codes are composed of codes with 3, 4, 5, 6 or 7 characters. Codes with three characters are included in ICD-10-CM as the heading of a category of codes that may be further subdivided by the use of fourth and/or fifth characters and/or sixth characters, which provide greater detail.

A three-character code is to be used only if it is not further subdivided. A code is invalid if it has not been coded to the full number of characters required for that code, including the 7th character, if applicable.

3. Code or codes from A00.0 through T88.9, Z00-Z99.8

The appropriate code or codes from A00.0 through T88.9, Z00-Z99.8 must be used to identify diagnoses, symptoms, conditions, problems, complaints or other reason(s) for the encounter/visit.

4. Signs and symptoms

Codes that describe symptoms and signs, as opposed to diagnoses, are acceptable for reporting purposes when a related definitive diagnosis has not been established (confirmed) by the provider. Chapter 18 of ICD-10-CM, Symptoms, Signs, and Abnormal Clinical and Laboratory Findings, Not Elsewhere Classified (codes R00.0 - R99) contains many, but not all, codes for symptoms.

See Section I.B.18 Use of Signs/Symptom/Unspecified Codes

5. Conditions that are an integral part of a disease process

Signs and symptoms that are associated routinely with a disease process should not be assigned as additional codes, unless otherwise instructed by the classification.

6. Conditions that are not an integral part of a disease process

Additional signs and symptoms that may not be associated routinely with a disease process should be coded when present.

7. Multiple coding for a single condition

In addition to the etiology/manifestation convention that requires two codes to fully describe a single condition that affects multiple body systems, there are other single conditions that also require more than one code. "Use additional code" notes are found in the Tabular List at codes that are not part of an etiology/manifestation pair where a secondary code is useful to fully describe a condition. The sequencing rule is the same as the etiology/manifestation pair, "use additional code" indicates that a secondary code should be added, if known.

For example, for bacterial infections that are not included in chapter 1, a secondary code from category B95, Streptococcus, Staphylococcus, and Enterococcus, as the cause of diseases classified elsewhere, or B96, Other bacterial agents as the cause of diseases classified elsewhere, may be required to identify the bacterial organism causing the infection. A "use additional code" note will normally be found at the infectious disease code, indicating a need for the organism code to be added as a secondary code.

"Code first" notes are also under certain codes that are not specifically manifestation codes but may be due to an underlying cause. When there is a "code first" note and an underlying condition is present, the underlying condition should be sequenced first, if known.

"Code, if applicable, any causal condition first" notes indicate that this code may be assigned as a principal diagnosis when the causal condition is unknown or not applicable. If a causal condition is known, then the code for that condition should be sequenced as the principal or first-listed diagnosis.

Multiple codes may be needed for sequela, complication codes and obstetric codes to more fully describe a condition. See the specific guidelines for these conditions for further instruction.

8. Acute and Chronic Conditions

If the same condition is described as both acute (subacute) and chronic, and separate subentries exist in the Alphabetic Index at the same indentation level, code both and sequence the acute (subacute) code first.

9. Combination Code

A combination code is a single code used to classify:

> Two diagnoses, or
>
> A diagnosis with an associated secondary process (manifestation)
>
> A diagnosis with an associated complication

Combination codes are identified by referring to subterm entries in the Alphabetic Index and by reading the inclusion and exclusion notes in the Tabular List.

Assign only the combination code when that code fully identifies the diagnostic conditions involved or when the Alphabetic Index so directs. Multiple coding should not be used when the classification provides a combination code that clearly identifies all of the elements documented in the diagnosis. When the combination code lacks necessary specificity in describing the manifestation or complication, an additional code should be used as a secondary code.

10. Sequela (Late Effects)

A sequela is the residual effect (condition produced) after the acute phase of an illness or injury has terminated. There is no time limit on when a sequela code can be used. The residual may be apparent early, such as in cerebral infarction, or it may occur months or years later, such as that due to a previous injury. Examples of sequela include: scar formation resulting from a burn, deviated septum due to a nasal fracture, and infertility due to tubal occlusion from old tuberculosis. Coding of sequela generally requires two codes sequenced in the following order: the condition or nature of the sequela is sequenced first. The sequela code is sequenced second.

An exception to the above guidelines are those instances where the code for the sequela is followed by a manifestation code identified in the Tabular List and title, or the sequela code has been expanded (at the fourth, fifth or sixth character levels) to include the manifestation(s). The code for the acute phase of an illness or injury that led to the sequela is never used with a code for the late effect.

See Section I.C.9. Sequelae of cerebrovascular disease

See Section I.C.15. Sequelae of complication of pregnancy, childbirth and the puerperium

See Section I.C.19. Application of 7th characters for Chapter 19

11. Impending or Threatened Condition

Code any condition described at the time of discharge as "impending" or "threatened" as follows:

> If it did occur, code as confirmed diagnosis.

If it did not occur, reference the Alphabetic Index to determine if the condition has a subentry term for "impending" or "threatened" and also reference main term entries for "Impending" and for "Threatened."

> If the subterms are listed, assign the given code.

> If the subterms are not listed, code the existing underlying condition(s) and not the condition described as impending or threatened.

12. Reporting Same Diagnosis Code More than Once

Each unique ICD-10-CM diagnosis code may be reported only once for an encounter. This applies to bilateral conditions when there are no distinct codes identifying laterality or two different conditions classified to the same ICD-10-CM diagnosis code.

13. Laterality

Some ICD-10-CM codes indicate laterality, specifying whether the condition occurs on the left, right or is bilateral. If no bilateral code is provided and the condition is bilateral, assign separate codes for both the left and right side. If the side is not identified in the medical record, assign the code for the unspecified side.

When a patient has a bilateral condition and each side is treated during separate encounters, assign the "bilateral" code (as the condition still exists on both sides), including for the encounter to treat the first side. For the second encounter for treatment after one side has previously been treated and the condition no longer exists on that side, assign the appropriate unilateral code for the side where the condition still exists (e.g., cataract surgery performed on each eye in separate encounters). The bilateral code would not be assigned for the subsequent encounter, as the patient no longer has the condition in the previously-treated site. If the treatment on the first side did not completely resolve the condition, then the bilateral code would still be appropriate.

14. Documentation *by Clinicians Other than the Patient's Provider*

Code assignment is based on the documentation by patient's provider (i.e., physician or other qualified healthcare practitioner legally accountable for establishing the patient's diagnosis). There are a few exceptions, such as codes for the Body Mass Index (BMI), depth of non-pressure chronic ulcers, pressure ulcer stage, coma scale, and NIH stroke scale (NIHSS) codes, code assignment may be based on medical record documentation from clinicians who are not the patient's provider (i.e., physician or other qualified healthcare practitioner legally accountable for establishing the patient's diagnosis), since this information is typically documented by other clinicians involved in the care of the patient (e.g., a dietitian often documents the BMI, a nurse often documents the pressure ulcer stages, and an emergency medical technician often documents the coma scale). However, the associated diagnosis (such as overweight, obesity, acute stroke, or pressure ulcer) must be documented by the patient's provider. If there is conflicting medical record documentation, either from the same clinician or different clinicians, the patient's attending provider should be queried for clarification.

For social determinants of health, such as information found in categories Z55-Z65, Persons with potential health hazards related to socioeconomic and psychosocial circumstances, code assignment may be based on medical record documentation from clinicians involved in the care of the patient who are not the patient's provider since this information represents social information, rather than medical diagnoses.

The BMI, coma scale, NIHSS codes and categories Z55-Z65 should only be reported as secondary diagnoses.

15. Syndromes

Follow the Alphabetic Index guidance when coding syndromes. In the absence of Alphabetic Index guidance, assign codes for the documented manifestations of the syndrome. Additional codes for manifestations that are not an integral part of the disease process may also be assigned when the condition does not have a unique code.

16. Documentation of Complications of Care

Code assignment is based on the provider's documentation of the relationship between the condition and the care or procedure, unless otherwise instructed by the classification. The guideline extends to any complications of care, regardless of the chapter the code is located in. It is important to note that not all conditions that occur during or following medical care or surgery are classified as complications. There must be a cause-and-effect relationship between the care provided and the condition, and an indication in the documentation that it is a complication. Query the provider for clarification, if the complication is not clearly documented.

17. **Borderline Diagnosis**

If the provider documents a "borderline" diagnosis at the time of discharge, the diagnosis is coded as confirmed, unless the classification provides a specific entry (e.g., borderline diabetes). If a borderline condition has a specific index entry in ICD-10-CM, it should be coded as such. Since borderline conditions are not uncertain diagnoses, no distinction is made between the care setting (inpatient versus outpatient). Whenever the documentation is unclear regarding a borderline condition, coders are encouraged to query for clarification.

18. **Use of Sign/Symptom/Unspecified Codes**

Sign/symptom and "unspecified" codes have acceptable, even necessary, uses. While specific diagnosis codes should be reported when they are supported by the available medical record documentation and clinical knowledge of the patient's health condition, there are instances when signs/symptoms or unspecified codes are the best choices for accurately reflecting the healthcare encounter. Each healthcare encounter should be coded to the level of certainty known for that encounter.

If a definitive diagnosis has not been established by the end of the encounter, it is appropriate to report codes for sign(s) and/or symptom(s) in lieu of a definitive diagnosis. When sufficient clinical information isn't known or available about a particular health condition to assign a more specific code, it is acceptable to report the appropriate "unspecified" code (e.g., a diagnosis of pneumonia has been determined, but not the specific type). Unspecified codes should be reported when they are the codes that most accurately reflect what is known about the patient's condition at the time of that particular encounter. It would be inappropriate to select a specific code that is not supported by the medical record documentation or conduct medically unnecessary diagnostic testing in order to determine a more specific code.

19. **Coding for Healthcare Encounters in Hurricane Aftermath**

a. **Use of External Cause of Morbidity Codes**

An external cause of morbidity code should be assigned to identify the cause of the injury(ies) incurred as a result of the hurricane. The use of external cause of morbidity codes is supplemental to the application of ICD-10-CM codes. External cause of morbidity codes are never to be recorded as a principal diagnosis (first-listed in non-inpatient settings). The appropriate injury code should be sequenced before any external cause codes. The external cause of morbidity codes capture how the injury or health condition happened (cause), the intent (unintentional or accidental; or intentional, such as suicide or assault), the place where the event occurred, the activity of the patient at the time of the event, and the person's status (e.g., civilian, military). They should not be assigned for encounters to treat hurricane victims' medical conditions when no injury, adverse effect or poisoning is involved. External cause of morbidity codes should be assigned for each encounter for care and treatment of the injury. External cause of morbidity codes may be assigned in all health care settings. For the purpose of capturing complete and accurate ICD-10-CM data in the aftermath of the hurricane, a healthcare setting should be considered as any location where medical care is provided by licensed healthcare professionals.

b. **Sequencing of External Causes of Morbidity Codes**

Codes for cataclysmic events, such as a hurricane, take priority over all other external cause codes except child and adult abuse and terrorism and should be sequenced before other external cause of injury codes. Assign as many external cause of morbidity codes as necessary to fully explain each cause. For example, if an injury occurs as a result of a building collapse during the hurricane, external cause codes for both the hurricane and the building collapse should be assigned, with the external causes code for hurricane being sequenced as the first external cause code. For injuries incurred as a direct result of the hurricane, assign the appropriate code(s) for the injuries, followed by the code X37.0-, Hurricane (with the appropriate 7th character), and any other applicable external cause of injury codes. Code X37.0- also should be assigned when an injury is incurred as a result of flooding caused by a levee breaking related to the hurricane. Code X38.-, Flood (with the appropriate 7th character), should be assigned when an injury is from flooding resulting directly from the storm. Code X36.0.-, Collapse of dam or man-made structure, should not be assigned when the cause of the collapse is due to the hurricane. Use of code X36.0- is limited to collapses of man-made structures due to earth surface movements, not due to storm surges directly from a hurricane.

c. **Other External Causes of Morbidity Code Issues**

For injuries that are not a direct result of the hurricane, such as an evacuee that has incurred an injury as a result of a motor vehicle accident, assign the appropriate external cause of morbidity code(s) to

describe the cause of the injury, but do not assign code X37.0-, Hurricane. If it is not clear whether the injury was a direct result of the hurricane, assume the injury is due to the hurricane and assign code X37.0-, Hurricane, as well as any other applicable external cause of morbidity codes. In addition to code X37.0-, Hurricane, other possible applicable external cause of morbidity codes include:

　　W54.0-, Bitten by dog

　　X30-, Exposure to excessive natural heat

　　X31-, Exposure to excessive natural cold

　　X38-, Flood

d. **Use of Z codes**

Z codes (other reasons for healthcare encounters) may be assigned as appropriate to further explain the reasons for presenting for healthcare services, including transfers between healthcare facilities. The ICD-10-CM Official Guidelines for Coding and Reporting identify which codes may be assigned as principal or first-listed diagnosis only, secondary diagnosis only, or principal/first-listed or secondary (depending on the circumstances). Possible applicable Z codes include:

　　Z59.0,　Homelessness

　　Z59.1,　Inadequate housing

　　Z59.5,　Extreme poverty

　　Z75.1,　Person awaiting admission to adequate facility elsewhere

　　Z75.3,　Unavailability and inaccessibility of health-care facilities

　　Z75.4,　Unavailability and inaccessibility of other helping agencies

　　Z76.2,　Encounter for health supervision and care of other healthy infant and child

　　Z99.12, Encounter for respirator [ventilator] dependence during power failure

The external cause of morbidity codes and the Z codes listed above are not an all-inclusive list. Other codes may be applicable to the encounter based upon the documentation. Assign as many codes as necessary to fully explain each healthcare encounter. Since patient history information may be very limited, use any available documentation to assign the appropriate external cause of morbidity and Z codes.

C. Chapter-Specific Coding Guidelines

In addition to general coding guidelines, there are guidelines for specific diagnoses and/or conditions in the classification. Unless otherwise indicated, these guidelines apply to all health care settings. Please refer to Section II for guidelines on the selection of principal diagnosis.

1. **Chapter 1: Certain Infectious and Parasitic Diseases (A00-B99)**

a. **Human Immunodeficiency Virus (HIV) Infections**

1) **Code only confirmed cases**

Code only confirmed cases of HIV infection/illness. This is an exception to the hospital inpatient guideline Section II, H.

In this context, "confirmation" does not require documentation of positive serology or culture for HIV; the provider's diagnostic statement that the patient is HIV positive, or has an HIV-related illness is sufficient.

2) **Selection and sequencing of HIV codes**

(a) **Patient admitted for HIV-related condition**

If a patient is admitted for an HIV-related condition, the principal diagnosis should be B20, Human immunodeficiency virus [HIV] disease followed by additional diagnosis codes for all reported HIV-related conditions.

(b) **Patient with HIV disease admitted for unrelated condition**

If a patient with HIV disease is admitted for an unrelated condition (such as a traumatic injury), the code for the unrelated condition (e.g., the nature of injury code) should be the principal diagnosis. Other diagnoses would be B20 followed by additional diagnosis codes for all reported HIV-related conditions.

(c) **Whether the patient is newly diagnosed**

Whether the patient is newly diagnosed or has had previous admissions/encounters for HIV conditions is irrelevant to the sequencing decision.

(d) **Asymptomatic human immunodeficiency virus**
Z21, Asymptomatic human immunodeficiency virus [HIV] infection status, is to be applied when the patient without any documentation of symptoms is listed as being "HIV positive," "known HIV," "HIV test positive," or similar terminology. Do not use this code if the term "AIDS" is used or if the patient is treated for any HIV-related illness or is described as having any condition(s) resulting from his/her HIV positive status; use B20 in these cases.

(e) **Patients with inconclusive HIV serology**
Patients with inconclusive HIV serology, but no definitive diagnosis or manifestations of the illness, may be assigned code R75, Inconclusive laboratory evidence of human immunodeficiency virus [HIV].

(f) **Previously diagnosed HIV-related illness**
Patients with any known prior diagnosis of an HIV-related illness should be coded to B20. Once a patient has developed an HIV-related illness, the patient should always be assigned code B20 on every subsequent admission/encounter. Patients previously diagnosed with any HIV illness (B20) should never be assigned to R75 or Z21, Asymptomatic human immunodeficiency virus [HIV] infection status.

(g) **HIV Infection in Pregnancy, Childbirth and the Puerperium**
During pregnancy, childbirth or the puerperium, a patient admitted (or presenting for a health care encounter) because of an HIV-related illness should receive a principal diagnosis code of O98.7-, Human immunodeficiency [HIV] disease complicating pregnancy, childbirth and the puerperium, followed by B20 and the code(s) for the HIV-related illness(es). Codes from Chapter 15 always take sequencing priority.

Patients with asymptomatic HIV infection status admitted (or presenting for a health care encounter) during pregnancy, childbirth, or the puerperium should receive codes of O98.7- and Z21.

(h) **Encounters for testing for HIV**
If a patient is being seen to determine his/her HIV status, use code Z11.4, Encounter for screening for human immunodeficiency virus [HIV]. Use additional codes for any associated high risk behavior.

If a patient with signs or symptoms is being seen for HIV testing, code the signs and symptoms. An additional counseling code Z71.7, Human immunodeficiency virus [HIV] counseling, may be used if counseling is provided during the encounter for the test.

When a patient returns to be informed of his/her HIV test results and the test result is negative, use code Z71.7, Human immunodeficiency virus [HIV] counseling.

If the results are positive, see previous guidelines and assign codes as appropriate.

b. **Infectious agents as the cause of diseases classified to other chapters**
Certain infections are classified in chapters other than Chapter 1 and no organism is identified as part of the infection code. In these instances, it is necessary to use an additional code from Chapter 1 to identify the organism. A code from category B95, Streptococcus, Staphylococcus, and Enterococcus as the cause of diseases classified to other chapters, B96, Other bacterial agents as the cause of diseases classified to other chapters, or B97, Viral agents as the cause of diseases classified to other chapters, is to be used as an additional code to identify the organism. An instructional note will be found at the infection code advising that an additional organism code is required.

c. **Infections resistant to antibiotics**
Many bacterial infections are resistant to current antibiotics. It is necessary to identify all infections documented as antibiotic resistant. Assign a code from category Z16, Resistance to antimicrobial drugs, following the infection code only if the infection code does not identify drug resistance.

d. **Sepsis, Severe Sepsis, and Septic Shock**
1) **Coding of Sepsis and Severe Sepsis**
(a) **Sepsis**
For a diagnosis of sepsis, assign the appropriate code for the underlying systemic infection. If the type of infection or causal organism is not further specified, assign code A41.9, Sepsis, unspecified organism.

A code from subcategory R65.2, Severe sepsis, should not be assigned unless severe sepsis or an associated acute organ dysfunction is documented.

(i) **Negative or inconclusive blood cultures and sepsis**
Negative or inconclusive blood cultures do not preclude a diagnosis of sepsis in patients with clinical evidence of the condition; however, the provider should be queried.

(ii) **Urosepsis**
The term urosepsis is a nonspecific term. It is not to be considered synonymous with sepsis. It has no default code in the Alphabetic Index. Should a provider use this term, he/she must be queried for clarification.

(iii) **Sepsis with organ dysfunction**
If a patient has sepsis and associated acute organ dysfunction or multiple organ dysfunction (MOD), follow the instructions for coding severe sepsis.

(iv) **Acute organ dysfunction that is not clearly associated with the sepsis**
If a patient has sepsis and an acute organ dysfunction, but the medical record documentation indicates that the acute organ dysfunction is related to a medical condition other than the sepsis, do not assign a code from subcategory R65.2, Severe sepsis. An acute organ dysfunction must be associated with the sepsis in order to assign the severe sepsis code. If the documentation is not clear as to whether an acute organ dysfunction is related to the sepsis or another medical condition, query the provider.

(b) **Severe sepsis**
The coding of severe sepsis requires a minimum of 2 codes: first a code for the underlying systemic infection, followed by a code from subcategory R65.2, Severe sepsis. If the causal organism is not documented, assign code A41.9, Sepsis, unspecified organism, for the infection. Additional code(s) for the associated acute organ dysfunction are also required.

Due to the complex nature of severe sepsis, some cases may require querying the provider prior to assignment of the codes.

2) **Septic shock**
(a) **Septic shock generally refers to circulatory failure associated with severe sepsis, and therefore, it represents a type of acute organ dysfunction.**
For cases of septic shock, the code for the systemic infection should be sequenced first, followed by code R65.21, Severe sepsis with septic shock or code T81.12, Postprocedural septic shock. Any additional codes for the other acute organ dysfunctions should also be assigned. As noted in the sequencing instructions in the Tabular List, the code for septic shock cannot be assigned as a principal diagnosis.

3) **Sequencing of severe sepsis**
If severe sepsis is present on admission, and meets the definition of principal diagnosis, the underlying systemic infection should be assigned as principal diagnosis followed by the appropriate code from subcategory R65.2 as required by the sequencing rules in the Tabular List. A code from subcategory R65.2 can never be assigned as a principal diagnosis.

When severe sepsis develops during an encounter (it was not present on admission), the underlying systemic infection and the appropriate code from subcategory R65.2 should be assigned as secondary diagnoses.

Severe sepsis may be present on admission, but the diagnosis may not be confirmed until sometime after admission. If the documentation is not clear whether severe sepsis was present on admission, the provider should be queried.

4) **Sepsis *or* severe sepsis with a localized infection**
If the reason for admission is sepsis or severe sepsis and a localized infection, such as pneumonia or cellulitis, a code(s) for the underlying systemic infection should be assigned first and the

code for the localized infection should be assigned as a secondary diagnosis. If the patient has severe sepsis, a code from subcategory R65.2 should also be assigned as a secondary diagnosis. If the patient is admitted with a localized infection, such as pneumonia, and sepsis/severe sepsis doesn't develop until after admission, the localized infection should be assigned first, followed by the appropriate sepsis/severe sepsis codes.

5) Sepsis due to a postprocedural infection

(a) Documentation of causal relationship

As with all postprocedural complications, code assignment is based on the provider's documentation of the relationship between the infection and the procedure.

(b) Sepsis due to a postprocedural infection

For infections following a procedure, a code from T81.40, to T81.43 Infection following a procedure, or a code from O86.00 to O86.03, Infection of obstetric surgical wound, that identifies the site of the infection should be coded first, if known. Assign an additional code for sepsis following a procedure (T81.44) or sepsis following an obstetrical procedure (O86.04). Use an additional code to identify the infectious agent. If the patient has severe sepsis, the appropriate code from subcategory R65.2 should also be assigned with the additional code(s) for any acute organ dysfunction.

For infections following infusion, transfusion, therapeutic injection, or immunization, a code from subcategory T80.2, Infections following infusion, transfusion, and therapeutic injection, or code T88.0-, Infection following immunization, should be coded first, followed by the code for the specific infection. If the patient has severe sepsis, the appropriate code from subcategory R65.2 should also be assigned, with the additional codes(s) for any acute organ dysfunction.

(c) Postprocedural infection and postprocedural septic shock

If a postprocedural infection has resulted in postprocedural septic shock, assign the codes indicated above for sepsis due to a postprocedural infection, followed by code T81.12-, Postprocedural septic shock. Do not assign code R65.21, Severe sepsis with septic shock. Additional code(s) should be assigned for any acute organ dysfunction.

6) Sepsis and severe sepsis associated with a noninfectious process (condition)

In some cases a noninfectious process (condition), such as trauma, may lead to an infection which can result in sepsis or severe sepsis. If sepsis or severe sepsis is documented as associated with a noninfectious condition, such as a burn or serious injury, and this condition meets the definition for principal diagnosis, the code for the noninfectious condition should be sequenced first, followed by the code for the resulting infection. If severe sepsis is present, a code from subcategory R65.2 should also be assigned with any associated organ dysfunction(s) codes. It is not necessary to assign a code from subcategory R65.1, Systemic inflammatory response syndrome (SIRS) of non-infectious origin, for these cases.

If the infection meets the definition of principal diagnosis, it should be sequenced before the non-infectious condition. When both the associated non-infectious condition and the infection meet the definition of principal diagnosis, either may be assigned as principal diagnosis.

Only one code from category R65, Symptoms and signs specifically associated with systemic inflammation and infection, should be assigned. Therefore, when a non-infectious condition leads to an infection resulting in severe sepsis, assign the appropriate code from subcategory R65.2, Severe sepsis. Do not additionally assign a code from subcategory R65.1, Systemic inflammatory response syndrome (SIRS) of non-infectious origin.

See Section I.C.18. SIRS due to non-infectious process

7) Sepsis and septic shock complicating abortion, pregnancy, childbirth, and the puerperium

See Section I.C.15. Sepsis and septic shock complicating abortion, pregnancy, childbirth and the puerperium

8) Newborn sepsis

See Section I.C.16. f. Bacterial sepsis of Newborn

e. Methicillin Resistant Staphylococcus aureus (MRSA) Conditions

1) Selection and sequencing of MRSA codes

(a) Combination codes for MRSA infection

When a patient is diagnosed with an infection that is due to methicillin resistant *Staphylococcus aureus* (MRSA), and that infection has a combination code that includes the causal organism (e.g., sepsis, pneumonia) assign the appropriate combination code for the condition (e.g., code A41.02, Sepsis due to Methicillin resistant Staphylococcus aureus or code J15.212, Pneumonia due to Methicillin resistant Staphylococcus aureus). Do not assign code B95.62, Methicillin resistant Staphylococcus aureus infection as the cause of diseases classified elsewhere, as an additional code, because the combination code includes the type of infection and the MRSA organism. Do not assign a code from subcategory Z16.11, Resistance to penicillins, as an additional diagnosis.

See Section C.1. for instructions on coding and sequencing of sepsis and severe sepsis.

(b) Other codes for MRSA infection

When there is documentation of a current infection (e.g., wound infection, stitch abscess, urinary tract infection) due to MRSA, and that infection does not have a combination code that includes the causal organism, assign the appropriate code to identify the condition along with code B95.62, Methicillin resistant Staphylococcus aureus infection as the cause of diseases classified elsewhere for the MRSA infection. Do not assign a code from subcategory Z16.11, Resistance to penicillins.

(c) Methicillin susceptible Staphylococcus aureus (MSSA) and MRSA colonization

The condition or state of being colonized or carrying MSSA or MRSA is called colonization or carriage, while an individual person is described as being colonized or being a carrier. Colonization means that MSSA or MSRA is present on or in the body without necessarily causing illness. A positive MRSA colonization test might be documented by the provider as "MRSA screen positive" or "MRSA nasal swab positive".

Assign code Z22.322, Carrier or suspected carrier of Methicillin resistant Staphylococcus aureus, for patients documented as having MRSA colonization. Assign code Z22.321, Carrier or suspected carrier of Methicillin susceptible Staphylococcus aureus, for patients documented as having MSSA colonization. Colonization is not necessarily indicative of a disease process or as the cause of a specific condition the patient may have unless documented as such by the provider.

(d) MRSA colonization and infection

If a patient is documented as having both MRSA colonization and infection during a hospital admission, code Z22.322, Carrier or suspected carrier of Methicillin resistant Staphylococcus aureus, and a code for the MRSA infection may both be assigned.

f. Zika virus infections

1) Code only confirmed cases

Code only a confirmed diagnosis of Zika virus (A92.5, Zika virus disease) as documented by the provider. This is an exception to the hospital inpatient guideline Section II, H. In this context, "confirmation" does not require documentation of the type of test performed; the **provider's** diagnostic statement that the condition is confirmed is sufficient. This code should be assigned regardless of the stated mode of transmission.

If the provider documents "suspected", "possible" or "probable" Zika, do not assign code A92.5. Assign a code(s) explaining the reason for encounter (such as fever, rash, or joint pain) or Z20.821, Contact with and (suspected) exposure to Zika virus.

2. Chapter 2: Neoplasms (C00-D49)
General guidelines

Chapter 2 of the ICD-10-CM contains the codes for most benign and all malignant neoplasms. Certain benign neoplasms, such as prostatic adenomas, may be found in the specific body system chapters. To properly code a neoplasm it is necessary to determine from the record if the neoplasm is benign, in-situ, malignant, or of uncertain histologic behavior. If malignant, any secondary (metastatic) sites should also be determined.

Primary malignant neoplasms overlapping site boundaries

A primary malignant neoplasm that overlaps two or more contiguous (next to each other) sites should be classified to the subcategory/code .8 ('overlapping lesion'), unless the combination is specifically indexed elsewhere. For multiple neoplasms of the same site that are not contiguous such as tumors in different quadrants of the same breast, codes for each site should be assigned.

Malignant neoplasm of ectopic tissue

Malignant neoplasms of ectopic tissue are to be coded to the site of origin mentioned, e.g., ectopic pancreatic malignant neoplasms involving the stomach are coded to malignant neoplasm of pancreas, unspecified (C25.9).

The neoplasm table in the Alphabetic Index should be referenced first. However, if the histological term is documented, that term should be referenced first, rather than going immediately to the Neoplasm Table, in order to determine which column in the Neoplasm Table is appropriate. For example, if the documentation indicates "adenoma," refer to the term in the Alphabetic Index to review the entries under this term and the instructional note to "see also neoplasm, by site, benign." The table provides the proper code based on the type of neoplasm and the site. It is important to select the proper column in the table that corresponds to the type of neoplasm. The Tabular List should then be referenced to verify that the correct code has been selected from the table and that a more specific site code does not exist.

See Section I.C.21. Factors influencing health status and contact with health services, Status, for information regarding Z15.0, codes for genetic susceptibility to cancer.

a. Treatment directed at the malignancy
If the treatment is directed at the malignancy, designate the malignancy as the principal diagnosis.

The only exception to this guideline is if a patient admission/encounter is solely for the administration of chemotherapy, immunotherapy or external beam radiation therapy, assign the appropriate Z51.-- code as the first-listed or principal diagnosis, and the diagnosis or problem for which the service is being performed as a secondary diagnosis.

b. Treatment of secondary site
When a patient is admitted because of a primary neoplasm with metastasis and treatment is directed toward the secondary site only, the secondary neoplasm is designated as the principal diagnosis even though the primary malignancy is still present.

c. Coding and sequencing of complications
Coding and sequencing of complications associated with the malignancies or with the therapy thereof are subject to the following guidelines:

1) Anemia associated with malignancy
When admission/encounter is for management of an anemia associated with the malignancy, and the treatment is only for anemia, the appropriate code for the malignancy is sequenced as the principal or first-listed diagnosis followed by the appropriate code for the anemia (such as code D63.0, Anemia in neoplastic disease).

2) Anemia associated with chemotherapy, immunotherapy and radiation therapy
When the admission/encounter is for management of an anemia associated with an adverse effect of the administration of chemotherapy or immunotherapy and the only treatment is for the anemia, the anemia code is sequenced first followed by the appropriate codes for the neoplasm and the adverse effect (T45.1X5-, Adverse effect of antineoplastic and immunosuppressive drugs).

When the admission/encounter is for management of an anemia associated with an adverse effect of radiotherapy, the anemia code should be sequenced first, followed by the appropriate neoplasm code and code Y84.2, Radiological procedure and radiotherapy as the cause of abnormal reaction of the patient, or of later complication, without mention of misadventure at the time of the procedure.

3) Management of dehydration due to the malignancy
When the admission/encounter is for management of dehydration due to the malignancy and only the dehydration is being treated (intravenous rehydration), the dehydration is sequenced first, followed by the code(s) for the malignancy.

4) Treatment of a complication resulting from a surgical procedure
When the admission/encounter is for treatment of a complication resulting from a surgical procedure, designate the complication as the principal or first-listed diagnosis if treatment is directed at resolving the complication.

d. Primary malignancy previously excised
When a primary malignancy has been previously excised or eradicated from its site and there is no further treatment directed to that site and there is no evidence of any existing primary malignancy at that site, a code from category Z85, Personal history of malignant neoplasm, should be used to indicate the former site of the malignancy. Any mention of extension, invasion, or metastasis to another site is coded as a secondary malignant neoplasm to that site. The secondary site may be the principal or first-listed **diagnosis** with the Z85 code used as a secondary code.

e. Admissions/Encounters involving chemotherapy, immunotherapy and radiation therapy
1) Episode of care involves surgical removal of neoplasm
When an episode of care involves the surgical removal of a neoplasm, primary or secondary site, followed by adjunct chemotherapy or radiation treatment during the same episode of care, the code for the neoplasm should be assigned as principal or first-listed diagnosis.

2) Patient admission/encounter solely for administration of chemotherapy, immunotherapy and radiation therapy
If a patient admission/encounter is solely for the administration of chemotherapy, immunotherapy or external beam radiation therapy assign code Z51.0, Encounter for antineoplastic radiation therapy, or Z51.11, Encounter for antineoplastic chemotherapy, or Z51.12, Encounter for antineoplastic immunotherapy as the first-listed or principal diagnosis. If a patient receives more than one of these therapies during the same admission more than one of these codes may be assigned, in any sequence.

The malignancy for which the therapy is being administered should be assigned as a secondary diagnosis.

If a patient admission/encounter is for the insertion or implantation of radioactive elements (e.g., brachytherapy) the appropriate code for the malignancy is sequenced as the principal or first-listed diagnosis. Code Z51.0 should not be assigned.

3) Patient admitted for radiation therapy, chemotherapy or immunotherapy and develops complications
When a patient is admitted for the purpose of external beam radiotherapy, immunotherapy or chemotherapy and develops complications such as uncontrolled nausea and vomiting or dehydration, the principal or first-listed diagnosis is Z51.0, Encounter for antineoplastic radiation therapy, or Z51.11, Encounter for antineoplastic chemotherapy, or Z51.12, Encounter for antineoplastic immunotherapy followed by any codes for the complications.

When a patient is admitted for the purpose of insertion or implantation of radioactive elements (e.g., brachytherapy)and develops complications such as uncontrolled nausea and vomiting or dehydration, the principal or first-listed diagnosis is the appropriate code for the malignancy followed by any codes for the complications.

f. Admission/encounter to determine extent of malignancy
When the reason for admission/encounter is to determine the extent of the malignancy, or for a procedure such as paracentesis or thoracentesis, the primary malignancy or appropriate metastatic site is designated as the principal or first-listed diagnosis, even though chemotherapy or radiotherapy is administered.

g. Symptoms, signs, and abnormal findings listed in Chapter 18 associated with neoplasms
Symptoms, signs, and ill-defined conditions listed in Chapter 18 characteristic of, or associated with, an existing primary or secondary site malignancy cannot be used to replace the malignancy as principal or first-listed diagnosis, regardless of the number of admissions or encounters for treatment and care of the neoplasm.

See section I.C.21. Factors influencing health status and contact with health services, Encounter for prophylactic organ removal.

h. Admission/encounter for pain control/management
See Section I.C.6. for information on coding admission/encounter for pain control/management.

i. **Malignancy in two or more noncontiguous sites**
A patient may have more than one malignant tumor in the same organ. These tumors may represent different primaries or metastatic disease, depending on the site. Should the documentation be unclear, the provider should be queried as to the status of each tumor so that the correct codes can be assigned.

j. **Disseminated malignant neoplasm, unspecified**
Code C80.0, Disseminated malignant neoplasm, unspecified, is for use only in those cases where the patient has advanced metastatic disease and no known primary or secondary sites are specified. It should not be used in place of assigning codes for the primary site and all known secondary sites.

k. **Malignant neoplasm without specification of site**
Code C80.1, Malignant (primary) neoplasm, unspecified, equates to Cancer, unspecified. This code should only be used when no determination can be made as to the primary site of a malignancy. This code should rarely be used in the inpatient setting.

l. **Sequencing of neoplasm codes**
1) **Encounter for treatment of primary malignancy**
If the reason for the encounter is for treatment of a primary malignancy, assign the malignancy as the principal/first-listed diagnosis. The primary site is to be sequenced first, followed by any metastatic sites.

2) **Encounter for treatment of secondary malignancy**
When an encounter is for a primary malignancy with metastasis and treatment is directed toward the metastatic (secondary) site(s) only, the metastatic site(s) is designated as the principal/first-listed diagnosis. The primary malignancy is coded as an additional code.

3) **Malignant neoplasm in a pregnant patient**
When a pregnant woman has a malignant neoplasm, a code from subcategory O9A.1-, Malignant neoplasm complicating pregnancy, childbirth, and the puerperium, should be sequenced first, followed by the appropriate code from Chapter 2 to indicate the type of neoplasm.

4) **Encounter for complication associated with a neoplasm**
When an encounter is for management of a complication associated with a neoplasm, such as dehydration, and the treatment is only for the complication, the complication is coded first, followed by the appropriate code(s) for the neoplasm.

The exception to this guideline is anemia. When the admission/encounter is for management of an anemia associated with the malignancy, and the treatment is only for anemia, the appropriate code for the malignancy is sequenced as the principal or first-listed diagnosis followed by code D63.0, Anemia in neoplastic disease.

5) **Complication from surgical procedure for treatment of a neoplasm**
When an encounter is for treatment of a complication resulting from a surgical procedure performed for the treatment of the neoplasm, designate the complication as the principal/first-listed diagnosis. See **the** guideline regarding the coding of a current malignancy versus personal history to determine if the code for the neoplasm should also be assigned.

6) **Pathologic fracture due to a neoplasm**
When an encounter is for a pathological fracture due to a neoplasm, and the focus of treatment is the fracture, a code from subcategory M84.5, Pathological fracture in neoplastic disease, should be sequenced first, followed by the code for the neoplasm.

If the focus of treatment is the neoplasm with an associated pathological fracture, the neoplasm code should be sequenced first, followed by a code from M84.5 for the pathological fracture.

m. **Current malignancy versus personal history of malignancy**
When a primary malignancy has been excised but further treatment, such as an additional surgery for the malignancy, radiation therapy or chemotherapy is directed to that site, the primary malignancy code should be used until treatment is completed.

When a primary malignancy has been previously excised or eradicated from its site, there is no further treatment (of the malignancy) directed to that site, and there is no evidence of any existing primary malignancy at that site, a code from category Z85, Personal history of malignant neoplasm, should be used to indicate the former site of the malignancy.

Subcategories Z85.0 – Z85.7 should only be assigned for the former site of a primary malignancy, not the site of a secondary malignancy. Codes from subcategory Z85.8-, may be assigned for the former site(s) of either a primary or secondary malignancy included in this subcategory.
See Section I.C.21. Factors influencing health status and contact with health services, History (of)

n. **Leukemia, Multiple Myeloma, and Malignant Plasma Cell Neoplasms in remission versus personal history**
The categories for leukemia, and category C90, Multiple myeloma and malignant plasma cell neoplasms, have codes indicating whether or not the leukemia has achieved remission. There are also codes Z85.6, Personal history of leukemia, and Z85.79, Personal history of other malignant neoplasms of lymphoid, hematopoietic and related tissues. If the documentation is unclear as to whether the leukemia has achieved remission, the provider should be queried.
See Section I.C.21. Factors influencing health status and contact with health services, History (of)

o. **Aftercare following surgery for neoplasm**
See Section I.C.21. Factors influencing health status and contact with health services, Aftercare

p. **Follow-up care for completed treatment of a malignancy**
See Section I.C.21. Factors influencing health status and contact with health services, Follow-up

q. **Prophylactic organ removal for prevention of malignancy**
See Section I.C. 21, Factors influencing health status and contact with health services, Prophylactic organ removal

r. **Malignant neoplasm associated with transplanted organ**
A malignant neoplasm of a transplanted organ should be coded as a transplant complication. Assign first the appropriate code from category T86.-, Complications of transplanted organs and tissue, followed by code C80.2, Malignant neoplasm associated with transplanted organ. Use an additional code for the specific malignancy.

3. **Chapter 3: Disease of the blood and blood-forming organs and certain disorders involving the immune mechanism (D50-D89)**
Reserved for future guideline expansion

4. **Chapter 4: Endocrine, Nutritional, and Metabolic Diseases (E00-E89)**
a. **Diabetes mellitus**
The diabetes mellitus codes are combination codes that include the type of diabetes mellitus, the body system affected, and the complications affecting that body system. As many codes within a particular category as are necessary to describe all of the complications of the disease may be used. They should be sequenced based on the reason for a particular encounter. Assign as many codes from categories E08 – E13 as needed to identify all of the associated conditions that the patient has.

1) **Type of diabetes**
The age of a patient is not the sole determining factor, though most type 1 diabetics develop the condition before reaching puberty. For this reason type 1 diabetes mellitus is also referred to as juvenile diabetes.

2) **Type of diabetes mellitus not documented**
If the type of diabetes mellitus is not documented in the medical record the default is E11.-, Type 2 diabetes mellitus.

3) **Diabetes mellitus and the use of insulin and oral hypoglycemics**
If the documentation in a medical record does not indicate the type of diabetes but does indicate that the patient uses insulin, code E11.-, Type 2 diabetes mellitus, should be assigned. An additional code should be assigned from category Z79 to identify the long-term (current) use of insulin or oral hypoglycemic drugs. If the patient is treated with both oral medications and insulin, only the code for long-term (current) use of insulin should be assigned. Code Z79.4 should not be assigned if insulin is given temporarily to bring a type 2 patient's blood sugar under control during an encounter.

4) **Diabetes mellitus in pregnancy and gestational diabetes**
See Section I.C.15. Diabetes mellitus in pregnancy.
See Section I.C.15. Gestational (pregnancy induced) diabetes

5) Complications due to insulin pump malfunction

(a) Underdose of insulin due to insulin pump failure

An underdose of insulin due to an insulin pump failure should be assigned to a code from subcategory T85.6, Mechanical complication of other specified internal and external prosthetic devices, implants and grafts, that specifies the type of pump malfunction, as the principal or first-listed code, followed by code T38.3X6-, Underdosing of insulin and oral hypoglycemic [antidiabetic] drugs. Additional codes for the type of diabetes mellitus and any associated complications due to the underdosing should also be assigned.

(b) Overdose of insulin due to insulin pump failure

The principal or first-listed code for an encounter due to an insulin pump malfunction resulting in an overdose of insulin, should also be T85.6-, Mechanical complication of other specified internal and external prosthetic devices, implants and grafts, followed by code T38.3X1-, Poisoning by insulin and oral hypoglycemic [antidiabetic] drugs, accidental (unintentional).

6) Secondary diabetes mellitus

Codes under categories E08, Diabetes mellitus due to underlying condition, E09, Drug or chemical induced diabetes mellitus, and E13, Other specified diabetes mellitus, identify complications/manifestations associated with secondary diabetes mellitus. Secondary diabetes is always caused by another condition or event (e.g., cystic fibrosis, malignant neoplasm of pancreas, pancreatectomy, adverse effect of drug, or poisoning).

(a) Secondary diabetes mellitus and the use of insulin or oral hypoglycemic drugs

For patients with secondary diabetes mellitus who routinely use insulin or oral hypoglycemic drugs, an additional code from category Z79 should be assigned to identify the long-term (current) use of insulin or oral hypoglycemic drugs. If the patient is treated with both oral medications and insulin, only the code for long-term (current) use of insulin should be assigned. Code Z79.4 should not be assigned if insulin is given temporarily to bring a secondary diabetic patient's blood sugar under control during an encounter.

(b) Assigning and sequencing secondary diabetes codes and its causes

The sequencing of the secondary diabetes codes in relationship to codes for the cause of the diabetes is based on the Tabular List instructions for categories E08, E09 and E13.

(i) Secondary diabetes mellitus due to pancreatectomy

For postpancreatectomy diabetes mellitus (lack of insulin due to the surgical removal of all or part of the pancreas), assign code E89.1, Postprocedural hypoinsulinemia. Assign a code from category E13 and a code from subcategory Z90.41, Acquired absence of pancreas, as additional codes.

(ii) Secondary diabetes due to drugs

Secondary diabetes may be caused by an adverse effect of correctly administered medications, poisoning or sequela of poisoning.

See section I.C.19.e for coding of adverse effects and poisoning, and section I.C.20 for external cause code reporting.

5. Chapter 5: Mental, Behavioral and Neurodevelopmental disorders (F01–F99)

a. Pain disorders related to psychological factors

Assign code F45.41, for pain that is exclusively related to psychological disorders. As indicated by the Excludes 1 note under category G89, a code from category G89 should not be assigned with code F45.41.

Code F45.42, Pain disorders with related psychological factors, should be used with a code from category G89, Pain, not elsewhere classified, if there is documentation of a psychological component for a patient with acute or chronic pain.

See Section I.C.6. Pain

b. Mental and behavioral disorders due to psychoactive substance use

1) In Remission

Selection of codes for "in remission" for categories F10-F19, Mental and behavioral disorders due to psychoactive substance use (categories F10-F19 with -.11, -.21) requires the provider's clinical judgment. The appropriate codes for "in remission" are assigned only on the basis of provider documentation (as defined in the Official Guidelines for Coding and Reporting), unless otherwise instructed by the classification.

Mild substance use disorders in early or sustained remission are classified to the appropriate codes for substance abuse in remission, and moderate or severe substance use disorders in early or sustained remission are classified to the appropriate codes for substance dependence in remission.

2) Psychoactive Substance Use, Abuse and Dependence

When the provider documentation refers to use, abuse and dependence of the same substance (e.g. alcohol, opioid, cannabis, etc.), only one code should be assigned to identify the pattern of use based on the following hierarchy:

- If both use and abuse are documented, assign only the code for abuse
- If both abuse and dependence are documented, assign only the code for dependence
- If use, abuse and dependence are all documented, assign only the code for dependence
- If both use and dependence are documented, assign only the code for dependence.

3) Psychoactive Substance Use, Unspecified

As with all other unspecified diagnoses, the codes for unspecified psychoactive substance use (F10.9-, F11.9-, F12.9-, F13.9-, F14.9-, F15.9-, F16.9-, F18.9-, F19.9-) should only be assigned based on provider documentation and when they meet the definition of a reportable diagnosis (see Section III, Reporting Additional Diagnoses). These codes are to be used only when the psychoactive substance use is associated with a physical, mental or behavioral disorder, and such a relationship is documented by the provider.

c. Factitious Disorder

Factitious disorder imposed on self or Munchausen's syndrome is a disorder in which a person falsely reports or causes his or her own physical or psychological signs or symptoms. For patients with documented factitious disorder on self or Munchausen's syndrome, assign the appropriate code from subcategory F68.1-, Factitious disorder imposed on self.

Munchausen's syndrome by proxy (MSBP) is a disorder in which a caregiver (perpetrator) falsely reports or causes an illness or injury in another person (victim) under his or her care, such as a child, an elderly adult, or a person who has a disability. The condition is also referred to as "factitious disorder imposed on another" or "factitious disorder by proxy." The perpetrator, not the victim, receives this diagnosis. Assign code F68.A, Factitious disorder imposed on another, to the perpetrator's record. For the victim of a patient suffering from MSBP, assign the appropriate code from categories T74, Adult and child abuse, neglect and other maltreatment, confirmed, or T76, Adult and child abuse, neglect and other maltreatment, suspected.

See Section I.C.19.f. Adult and child abuse, neglect and other maltreatment

6. Chapter 6: Diseases of the Nervous System (G00-G99)

a. Dominant/nondominant side

Codes from category G81, Hemiplegia and hemiparesis, and subcategories G83.1, Monoplegia of lower limb, G83.2, Monoplegia of upper limb, and G83.3, Monoplegia, unspecified, identify whether the dominant or nondominant side is affected. Should the affected side be documented, but not specified as dominant or nondominant, and the classification system does not indicate a default, code selection is as follows:

- For ambidextrous patients, the default should be dominant.
- If the left side is affected, the default is non-dominant.
- If the right side is affected, the default is dominant.

b. Pain - Category G89

1) General coding information

Codes in category G89, Pain, not elsewhere classified, may be used in conjunction with codes from other categories and chapters to provide more detail about acute or chronic pain and neoplasm-related pain, unless otherwise indicated below.

If the pain is not specified as acute or chronic, post-thoracotomy, postprocedural, or neoplasm-related, do not assign codes from category G89.

A code from category G89 should not be assigned if the underlying (definitive) diagnosis is known, unless the reason for the encounter is pain control/ management and not management of the underlying condition.

When an admission or encounter is for a procedure aimed at treating the underlying condition (e.g., spinal fusion, kyphoplasty), a code for the underlying condition (e.g., vertebral fracture, spinal stenosis) should be assigned as the principal diagnosis. No code from category G89 should be assigned.

(a) Category G89 Codes as Principal or First-Listed Diagnosis

Category G89 codes are acceptable as principal diagnosis or the first-listed code:

- When pain control or pain management is the reason for the admission/encounter (e.g., a patient with displaced intervertebral disc, nerve impingement and severe back pain presents for injection of steroid into the spinal canal). The underlying cause of the pain should be reported as an additional diagnosis, if known.

- When a patient is admitted for the insertion of a neurostimulator for pain control, assign the appropriate pain code as the principal or first-listed diagnosis. When an admission or encounter is for a procedure aimed at treating the underlying condition and a neurostimulator is inserted for pain control during the same admission/encounter, a code for the underlying condition should be assigned as the principal diagnosis and the appropriate pain code should be assigned as a secondary diagnosis.

(b) Use of Category G89 Codes in Conjunction with Site Specific Pain Codes

(i) Assigning Category G89 and Site-Specific Pain Codes

Codes from category G89 may be used in conjunction with codes that identify the site of pain (including codes from chapter 18) if the category G89 code provides additional information. For example, if the code describes the site of the pain, but does not fully describe whether the pain is acute or chronic, then both codes should be assigned.

(ii) Sequencing of Category G89 Codes with Site-Specific Pain Codes

The sequencing of category G89 codes with site-specific pain codes (including chapter 18 codes), is dependent on the circumstances of the encounter/admission as follows:

- If the encounter is for pain control or pain management, assign the code from category G89 followed by the code identifying the specific site of pain (e.g., encounter for pain management for acute neck pain from trauma is assigned code G89.11, Acute pain due to trauma, followed by code M54.2, Cervicalgia, to identify the site of pain).

- If the encounter is for any other reason except pain control or pain management, and a related definitive diagnosis has not been established (confirmed) by the provider, assign the code for the specific site of pain first, followed by the appropriate code from category G89.

2) Pain due to devices, implants and grafts
See Section I.C.19. Pain due to medical devices

3) Postoperative Pain
The provider's documentation should be used to guide the coding of postoperative pain, as well as *Section III. Reporting Additional Diagnoses and Section IV. Diagnostic Coding and Reporting in the Outpatient Setting.*

The default for post-thoracotomy and other postoperative pain not specified as acute or chronic is the code for the acute form.

Routine or expected postoperative pain immediately after surgery should not be coded.

(a) Postoperative pain not associated with specific postoperative complication
Postoperative pain not associated with a specific postoperative complication is assigned to the appropriate postoperative pain code in category G89.

(b) Postoperative pain associated with specific postoperative complication
Postoperative pain associated with a specific postoperative complication (such as painful wire sutures) is assigned to the appropriate code(s) found in Chapter 19, Injury, poisoning, and certain other consequences of external causes. If appropriate, use additional code(s) from category G89 to identify acute or chronic pain (G89.18 or G89.28).

4) Chronic pain
Chronic pain is classified to subcategory G89.2. There is no time frame defining when pain becomes chronic pain. The provider's documentation should be used to guide use of these codes.

5) Neoplasm Related Pain
Code G89.3 is assigned to pain documented as being related, associated or due to cancer, primary or secondary malignancy, or tumor. This code is assigned regardless of whether the pain is acute or chronic.

This code may be assigned as the principal or first-listed code when the stated reason for the admission/encounter is documented as pain control/pain management. The underlying neoplasm should be reported as an additional diagnosis.

When the reason for the admission/encounter is management of the neoplasm and the pain associated with the neoplasm is also documented, code G89.3 may be assigned as an additional diagnosis. It is not necessary to assign an additional code for the site of the pain.

See Section I.C.2 for instructions on the sequencing of neoplasms for all other stated reasons for the admission/encounter (except for pain control/pain management).

6) Chronic pain syndrome
Central pain syndrome (G89.0) and chronic pain syndrome (G89.4) are different than the term "chronic pain," and therefore codes should only be used when the provider has specifically documented this condition.

See Section I.C.5. Pain disorders related to psychological factors

7. Chapter 7: Diseases of the Eye and Adnexa (H00-H59)

a. Glaucoma

1) Assigning Glaucoma Codes
Assign as many codes from category H40, Glaucoma, as needed to identify the type of glaucoma, the affected eye, and the glaucoma stage.

2) Bilateral glaucoma with same type and stage
When a patient has bilateral glaucoma and both eyes are documented as being the same type and stage, and there is a code for bilateral glaucoma, report only the code for the type of glaucoma, bilateral, with the seventh character for the stage.

When a patient has bilateral glaucoma and both eyes are documented as being the same type and stage, and the classification does not provide a code for bilateral glaucoma (i.e. subcategories H40.10 and H40.20) report only one code for the type of glaucoma with the appropriate seventh character for the stage.

3) Bilateral glaucoma stage with different types or stages
When a patient has bilateral glaucoma and each eye is documented as having a different type or stage, and the classification distinguishes laterality, assign the appropriate code for each eye rather than the code for bilateral glaucoma.

When a patient has bilateral glaucoma and each eye is documented as having a different type, and the classification does not distinguish laterality (i.e. subcategories H40.10 and H40.20), assign one code for each type of glaucoma with the appropriate seventh character for the stage.

When a patient has bilateral glaucoma and each eye is documented as having the same type, but different stage, and the classification does not distinguish laterality (i.e. subcategories H40.10 and H40.20), assign a code for the type of glaucoma for each eye with the seventh character for the specific glaucoma stage documented for each eye.

4) Patient admitted with glaucoma and stage evolves during the admission

If a patient is admitted with glaucoma and the stage progresses during the admission, assign the code for highest stage documented.

5) Indeterminate stage glaucoma

Assignment of the seventh character "4" for "indeterminate stage" should be based on the clinical documentation. The seventh character "4" is used for glaucomas whose stage cannot be clinically determined. This seventh character should not be confused with the seventh character "0", unspecified, which should be assigned when there is no documentation regarding the stage of the glaucoma.

b. Blindness

If "blindness" or "low vision" of both eyes is documented but the visual impairment category is not documented, assign code H54.3, Unqualified visual loss, both eyes. If "blindness" or "low vision" in one eye is documented but the visual impairment category is not documented, assign a code from H54.6-, Unqualified visual loss, one eye. If "blindness" or "visual loss" is documented without any information about whether one or both eyes are affected, assign code H54.7, Unspecified visual loss.

8. Chapter 8: Diseases of the Ear and Mastoid Process (H60-H95)

Reserved for future guideline expansion

9. Chapter 9: Diseases of the Circulatory System (I00-I99)

a. Hypertension

The classification presumes a causal relationship between hypertension and heart involvement and between hypertension and kidney involvement, as the two conditions are linked by the term "with" in the Alphabetic Index. These conditions should be coded as related even in the absence of provider documentation explicitly linking them, unless the documentation clearly states the conditions are unrelated.

For hypertension and conditions not specifically linked by relational terms such as "with," "associated with" or "due to" in the classification, provider documentation must link the conditions in order to code them as related.

1) Hypertension with Heart Disease

Hypertension with heart conditions classified to I50.- or I51.4-I51.7, I51.89, I51.9, are assigned to a code from category I11, Hypertensive heart disease. Use additional code(s) from category I50, Heart failure, to identify the type(s) of heart failure in those patients with heart failure.

The same heart conditions (I50.-, I51.4-I51.7, I51.89, I51.9) with hypertension are coded separately if the provider has documented they are unrelated to the hypertension. Sequence according to the circumstances of the admission/encounter.

2) Hypertensive Chronic Kidney Disease

Assign codes from category I12, Hypertensive chronic kidney disease, when both hypertension and a condition classifiable to category N18, Chronic kidney disease (CKD), are present. CKD should not be coded as hypertensive if the provider indicates the CKD is not related to the hypertension.

The appropriate code from category N18 should be used as a secondary code with a code from category I12 to identify the stage of chronic kidney disease.

See Section I.C.14. Chronic kidney disease.

If a patient has hypertensive chronic kidney disease and acute renal failure, an additional code for the acute renal failure is required.

3) Hypertensive Heart and Chronic Kidney Disease

Assign codes from combination category I13, Hypertensive heart and chronic kidney disease, when there is hypertension with both heart and kidney involvement. If heart failure is present, assign an additional code from category I50 to identify the type of heart failure.

The appropriate code from category N18, Chronic kidney disease, should be used as a secondary code with a code from category I13 to identify the stage of chronic kidney disease.

See Section I.C.14. Chronic kidney disease.

The codes in category I13, Hypertensive heart and chronic kidney disease, are combination codes that include hypertension, heart

disease and chronic kidney disease. The Includes note at I13 specifies that the conditions included at I11 and I12 are included together in I13. If a patient has hypertension, heart disease and chronic kidney disease, then a code from I13 should be used, not individual codes for hypertension, heart disease and chronic kidney disease, or codes from I11 or I12.

For patients with both acute renal failure and chronic kidney disease, an additional code for acute renal failure is required.

4) Hypertensive Cerebrovascular Disease

For hypertensive cerebrovascular disease, first assign the appropriate code from categories I60-I69, followed by the appropriate hypertension code.

5) Hypertensive Retinopathy

Subcategory H35.0, Background retinopathy and retinal vascular changes, should be used with a code from category I10- I15, Hypertensive disease to include the systemic hypertension. The sequencing is based on the reason for the encounter.

6) Hypertension, Secondary

Secondary hypertension is due to an underlying condition. Two codes are required: one to identify the underlying etiology and one from category I15 to identify the hypertension. Sequencing of codes is determined by the reason for admission/encounter.

7) Hypertension, Transient

Assign code R03.0, Elevated blood pressure reading without diagnosis of hypertension, unless patient has an established diagnosis of hypertension. Assign code O13.-, Gestational [pregnancy-induced] hypertension without significant proteinuria, or O14.-, Pre-eclampsia, for transient hypertension of pregnancy.

8) Hypertension, Controlled

This diagnostic statement usually refers to an existing state of hypertension under control by therapy. Assign the appropriate code from categories I10-I15, Hypertensive diseases.

9) Hypertension, Uncontrolled

Uncontrolled hypertension may refer to untreated hypertension or hypertension not responding to current therapeutic regimen. In either case, assign the appropriate code from categories I10-I15, Hypertensive diseases.

10) Hypertensive Crisis

Assign a code from category I16, Hypertensive crisis, for documented hypertensive urgency, hypertensive emergency or unspecified hypertensive crisis. Code also any identified hypertensive disease (I10-I15). The sequencing is based on the reason for the encounter.

11) Pulmonary Hypertension

Pulmonary hypertension is classified to category I27, Other pulmonary heart diseases. For secondary pulmonary hypertension (I27.1, I27.2-), code also any associated conditions or adverse effects of drugs or toxins. The sequencing is based on the reason for the encounter, except for adverse effects of drugs (See Section I.C.19.e.).

b. Atherosclerotic Coronary Artery Disease and Angina

ICD-10-CM has combination codes for atherosclerotic heart disease with angina pectoris. The subcategories for these codes are I25.11, Atherosclerotic heart disease of native coronary artery with angina pectoris and I25.7, Atherosclerosis of coronary artery bypass graft(s) and coronary artery of transplanted heart with angina pectoris.

When using one of these combination codes it is not necessary to use an additional code for angina pectoris. A causal relationship can be assumed in a patient with both atherosclerosis and angina pectoris, unless the documentation indicates the angina is due to something other than the atherosclerosis.

If a patient with coronary artery disease is admitted due to an acute myocardial infarction (AMI), the AMI should be sequenced before the coronary artery disease.

See Section I.C.9. Acute myocardial infarction (AMI)

c. Intraoperative and Postprocedural Cerebrovascular Accident

Medical record documentation should clearly specify the cause-and-effect relationship between the medical intervention and the cerebrovascular accident in order to assign a code for intraoperative or postprocedural cerebrovascular accident.

Proper code assignment depends on whether it was an infarction or hemorrhage and whether it occurred intraoperatively or postoperatively. If it was a cerebral hemorrhage, code assignment depends on the type of procedure performed.

d. Sequelae of Cerebrovascular Disease

1) Category I69, Sequelae of Cerebrovascular disease
Category I69 is used to indicate conditions classifiable to categories I60-I67 as the causes of sequela (neurologic deficits), themselves classified elsewhere. These "late effects" include neurologic deficits that persist after initial onset of conditions classifiable to categories I60-I67. The neurologic deficits caused by cerebrovascular disease may be present from the onset or may arise at any time after the onset of the condition classifiable to categories I60-I67.

Codes from category I69, Sequelae of cerebrovascular disease, that specify hemiplegia, hemiparesis and monoplegia identify whether the dominant or nondominant side is affected. Should the affected side be documented, but not specified as dominant or nondominant, and the classification system does not indicate a default, code selection is as follows:

- For ambidextrous patients, the default should be dominant.
- If the left side is affected, the default is non-dominant.
- If the right side is affected, the default is dominant.

2) Codes from category I69 with codes from I60-I67
Codes from category I69 may be assigned on a health care record with codes from I60-I67, if the patient has a current cerebrovascular disease and deficits from an old cerebrovascular disease.

3) Codes from category I69 and Personal history of transient ischemic attack (TIA) and cerebral infarction (Z86.73)
Codes from category I69 should not be assigned if the patient does not have neurologic deficits.

See Section I.C.21. 4. History (of) for use of personal history codes

e. Acute myocardial infarction (AMI)

1) Type 1 ST elevation myocardial infarction (STEMI) and non-ST elevation myocardial infarction (NSTEMI)
The ICD-10-CM codes for type 1 acute myocardial infarction (AMI) identify the site, such as anterolateral wall or true posterior wall. Subcategories I21.0-I21.2 and code I21.3 are used for type 1 ST elevation myocardial infarction (STEMI). Code I21.4, Non-ST elevation (NSTEMI) myocardial infarction, is used for type 1 non ST elevation myocardial infarction (NSTEMI) and nontransmural MIs.

If a type 1 NSTEMI evolves to STEMI, assign the STEMI code. If a type 1 STEMI converts to NSTEMI due to thrombolytic therapy, it is still coded as STEMI.

For encounters occurring while the myocardial infarction is equal to, or less than, four weeks old, including transfers to another acute setting or a postacute setting, and the myocardial infarction meets the definition for "other diagnoses" (see Section III, Reporting Additional Diagnoses), codes from category I21 may continue to be reported. For encounters after the 4 week time frame and the patient is still receiving care related to the myocardial infarction, the appropriate aftercare code should be assigned, rather than a code from category I21. For old or healed myocardial infarctions not requiring further care, code I25.2, Old myocardial infarction, may be assigned.

2) Acute myocardial infarction, unspecified
Code I21.9, Acute myocardial infarction, unspecified, is the default for unspecified acute myocardial infarction or unspecified type. If only type 1 STEMI or transmural MI without the site is documented, assign code I21.3, ST elevation (STEMI) myocardial infarction of unspecified site.

3) AMI documented as nontransmural or subendocardial but site provided
If an AMI is documented as nontransmural or subendocardial, but the site is provided, it is still coded as a subendocardial AMI.

See Section I.C.21.3 for information on coding status post administration of tPA in a different facility within the last 24 hours.

4) Subsequent acute myocardial infarction
A code from category I22, Subsequent ST elevation (STEMI) and non-ST elevation (NSTEMI) myocardial infarction, is to be used when a patient who has suffered a type 1 or unspecified AMI has a new AMI within the 4 week time frame of the initial AMI. A code from category I22 must be used in conjunction with a code from

category I21. The sequencing of the I22 and I21 codes depends on the circumstances of the encounter.

Do not assign code I22 for subsequent myocardial infarctions other than type 1 or unspecified. For subsequent type 2 AMI assign only code I21.A1. For subsequent type 4 or type 5 AMI, assign only code I21.A9.

If a subsequent myocardial infarction of one type occurs within 4 weeks of a myocardial infarction of a different type, assign the appropriate codes from category I21 to identify each type. Do not assign a code from I22. Codes from category I22 should only be assigned if both the initial and subsequent myocardial infarctions are type 1 or unspecified.

5) Other Types of Myocardial Infarction
The ICD-10-CM provides codes for different types of myocardial infarction. Type 1 myocardial infarctions are assigned to codes I21.0-I21.4.

Type 2 myocardial infarction (myocardial infarction due to demand ischemia or secondary to ischemic **im**balance), is assigned to code I21.A1, Myocardial infarction type 2 with the underlying cause **coded first**. Do not assign code I24.8, Other forms of acute ischemic heart disease, for the demand ischemia. **If** a type 2 AMI is described as NSTEMI or STEMI, only assign code I21.A1. Codes I21.01-I21.4 should only be assigned for type 1 AMIs.

Acute myocardial infarctions type 3, 4a, 4b, 4c and 5 are assigned to code I21.A9, Other myocardial infarction type.

The "Code also" and "Code first" notes should be followed related to complications, and for coding of postprocedural myocardial infarctions during or following cardiac surgery.

10. Chapter 10: Diseases of the Respiratory System (J00-J99)

a. Chronic Obstructive Pulmonary Disease [COPD] and Asthma

1) Acute exacerbation of chronic obstructive bronchitis and asthma
The codes in categories J44 and J45 distinguish between uncomplicated cases and those in acute exacerbation. An acute exacerbation is a worsening or a decompensation of a chronic condition. An acute exacerbation is not equivalent to an infection superimposed on a chronic condition, though an exacerbation may be triggered by an infection.

b. Acute Respiratory Failure

1) Acute respiratory failure as principal diagnosis
A code from subcategory J96.0, Acute respiratory failure, or subcategory J96.2, Acute and chronic respiratory failure, may be assigned as a principal diagnosis when it is the condition established after study to be chiefly responsible for occasioning the admission to the hospital, and the selection is supported by the Alphabetic Index and Tabular List. However, chapter-specific coding guidelines (such as obstetrics, poisoning, HIV, newborn) that provide sequencing direction take precedence.

2) Acute respiratory failure as secondary diagnosis
Respiratory failure may be listed as a secondary diagnosis if it occurs after admission, or if it is present on admission, but does not meet the definition of principal diagnosis.

3) Sequencing of acute respiratory failure and another acute condition
When a patient is admitted with respiratory failure and another acute condition, (e.g., myocardial infarction, cerebrovascular accident, aspiration pneumonia), the principal diagnosis will not be the same in every situation. This applies whether the other acute condition is a respiratory or nonrespiratory condition. Selection of the principal diagnosis will be dependent on the circumstances of admission. If both the respiratory failure and the other acute condition are equally responsible for occasioning the admission to the hospital, and there are no chapter-specific sequencing rules, the guideline regarding two or more diagnoses that equally meet the definition for principal diagnosis *(Section II, C.)* may be applied in these situations.

If the documentation is not clear as to whether acute respiratory failure and another condition are equally responsible for occasioning the admission, query the provider for clarification.

c. Influenza due to certain identified influenza viruses
Code only confirmed cases of influenza due to certain identified influenza viruses (category J09), and due to other identified influenza virus (category J10). This is an exception to the hospital inpatient guideline Section II, H. (Uncertain Diagnosis).

In this context, "confirmation" does not require documentation of positive laboratory testing specific for avian or other novel influenza A or other identified influenza virus. However, coding should be based on the provider's diagnostic statement that the patient has avian influenza, or other novel influenza A, for category J09, or has another particular identified strain of influenza, such as H1N1 or H3N2, but not identified as novel or variant, for category J10.

If the provider records "suspected" or "possible" or "probable" avian influenza, or novel influenza, or other identified influenza, then the appropriate influenza code from category J11, Influenza due to unidentified influenza virus, should be assigned. A code from category J09, Influenza due to certain identified influenza viruses, should not be assigned nor should a code from category J10, Influenza due to other identified influenza virus.

d. Ventilator associated Pneumonia

1) Documentation of Ventilator associated Pneumonia

As with all procedural or postprocedural complications, code assignment is based on the provider's documentation of the relationship between the condition and the procedure.

Code J95.851, Ventilator associated pneumonia, should be assigned only when the provider has documented ventilator associated pneumonia (VAP). An additional code to identify the organism (e.g., Pseudomonas aeruginosa, code B96.5) should also be assigned. Do not assign an additional code from categories J12-J18 to identify the type of pneumonia.

Code J95.851 should not be assigned for cases where the patient has pneumonia and is on a mechanical ventilator and the provider has not specifically stated that the pneumonia is ventilator-associated pneumonia. If the documentation is unclear as to whether the patient has a pneumonia that is a complication attributable to the mechanical ventilator, query the provider.

2) Ventilator associated Pneumonia Develops after Admission

A patient may be admitted with one type of pneumonia (e.g., code J13, Pneumonia due to Streptococcus pneumonia) and subsequently develop VAP. In this instance, the principal diagnosis would be the appropriate code from categories J12-J18 for the pneumonia diagnosed at the time of admission. Code J95.851, Ventilator associated pneumonia, would be assigned as an additional diagnosis when the provider has also documented the presence of ventilator associated pneumonia.

11. Chapter 11: Diseases of the Digestive System (K00-K95)
Reserved for future guideline expansion

12. Chapter 12: Diseases of the Skin and Subcutaneous Tissue (L00-L99)

a. Pressure ulcer stage codes

1) Pressure ulcer stages

Codes in category L89, Pressure ulcer, identify the site and stage of the pressure ulcer.

The ICD-10-CM classifies pressure ulcer stages based on severity, which is designated by stages 1-4, **deep tissue pressure injury,** unspecified stage and unstageable.

Assign as many codes from category L89 as needed to identify all the pressure ulcers the patient has, if applicable.

See Section I.B.14 for pressure ulcer stage documentation by clinicians other than patient's provider

2) Unstageable pressure ulcers

Assignment of the code for unstageable pressure ulcer (L89.--0) should be based on the clinical documentation. These codes are used for pressure ulcers whose stage cannot be clinically determined (e.g., the ulcer is covered by eschar or has been treated with a skin or muscle graft). This code should not be confused with the codes for unspecified stage (L89.--9). When there is no documentation regarding the stage of the pressure ulcer, assign the appropriate code for unspecified stage (L89.--9).

3) Documented pressure ulcer stage

Assignment of the pressure ulcer stage code should be guided by clinical documentation of the stage or documentation of the terms found in the Alphabetic Index. For clinical terms describing the stage that are not found in the Alphabetic Index, and there is no documentation of the stage, the provider should be queried.

4) Patients admitted with pressure ulcers documented as healed

No code is assigned if the documentation states that the pressure ulcer is completely healed **at the time of admission.**

5) Pressure ulcers documented as healing

Pressure ulcers described as healing should be assigned the appropriate pressure ulcer stage code based on the documentation in the medical record. If the documentation does not provide information about the stage of the healing pressure ulcer, assign the appropriate code for unspecified stage.

If the documentation is unclear as to whether the patient has a current (new) pressure ulcer or if the patient is being treated for a healing pressure ulcer, query the provider.

For ulcers that were present on admission but healed at the time of discharge, assign the code for the site and stage of the pressure ulcer at the time of admission.

6) Patient admitted with pressure ulcer evolving into another stage during the admission

If a patient is admitted to an inpatient hospital with a pressure ulcer at one stage and it progresses to a higher stage, two separate codes should be assigned: one code for the site and stage of the ulcer on admission and a second code for the same ulcer site and the highest stage reported during the stay.

7) Pressure-induced deep tissue damage

For pressure-induced deep tissue damage or deep tissue pressure injury, assign only the appropriate code for pressure-induced deep tissue damage (L89.--6).

b. Non-Pressure Chronic Ulcers

1) Patients admitted with non-pressure ulcers documented as healed

No code is assigned if the documentation states that the non-pressure ulcer is completely healed **at the time of admission.**

2) Non-pressure ulcers documented as healing

Non-pressure ulcers described as healing should be assigned the appropriate non-pressure ulcer code based on the documentation in the medical record. If the documentation does not provide information about the severity of the healing non-pressure ulcer, assign the appropriate code for unspecified severity.

If the documentation is unclear as to whether the patient has a current (new) non-pressure ulcer or if the patient is being treated for a healing non-pressure ulcer, query the provider.

For ulcers that were present on admission but healed at the time of discharge, assign the code for the site and severity of the non-pressure ulcer at the time of admission.

3) Patient admitted with non-pressure ulcer that progresses to another severity level during the admission

If a patient is admitted to an inpatient hospital with a non-pressure ulcer at one severity level and it progresses to a higher severity level, two separate codes should be assigned: one code for the site and severity level of the ulcer on admission and a second code for the same ulcer site and the highest severity level reported during the stay.

See Section I.B.14 for pressure ulcer stage documentation by clinicians other than patient's provider

13. Chapter 13: Diseases of the Musculoskeletal System and Connective Tissue (M00-M99)

a. Site and laterality

Most of the codes within Chapter 13 have site and laterality designations. The site represents the bone, joint or the muscle involved. For some conditions where more than one bone, joint or muscle is usually involved, such as osteoarthritis, there is a "multiple sites" code available. For categories where no multiple site code is provided and more than one bone, joint or muscle is involved, multiple codes should be used to indicate the different sites involved.

1) Bone versus joint

For certain conditions, the bone may be affected at the upper or lower end, (e.g., avascular necrosis of bone, M87, Osteoporosis, M80, M81). Though the portion of the bone affected may be at the joint, the site designation will be the bone, not the joint.

b. Acute traumatic versus chronic or recurrent musculoskeletal conditions

Many musculoskeletal conditions are a result of previous injury or trauma to a site, or are recurrent conditions. Bone, joint or muscle conditions that are the result of a healed injury are usually found in chapter 13. Recurrent bone, joint or muscle conditions are also usually found in chapter 13. Any current, acute injury should be coded to the appropriate injury code from chapter 19. Chronic or recurrent conditions should generally be coded with a code from chapter 13. If it is difficult to determine from the documentation in the record which code is best to describe a condition, query the provider.

c. Coding of Pathologic Fractures

7th character A is for use as long as the patient is receiving active treatment for the fracture. While the patient may be seen by a new or different provider over the course of treatment for a pathological fracture, assignment of the 7th character is based on whether the patient is undergoing active treatment and not whether the provider is seeing the patient for the first time.

7th character D is to be used for encounters after the patient has completed active treatment for the fracture and is receiving routine care for the fracture during the healing or recovery phase. The other 7th characters, listed under each subcategory in the Tabular List, are to be used for subsequent encounters for treatment of problems associated with the healing, such as malunions, nonunions, and sequelae.

Care for complications of surgical treatment for fracture repairs during the healing or recovery phase should be coded with the appropriate complication codes.

See Section I.C.19. Coding of traumatic fractures.

d. Osteoporosis

Osteoporosis is a systemic condition, meaning that all bones of the musculoskeletal system are affected. Therefore, site is not a component of the codes under category M81, Osteoporosis without current pathological fracture. The site codes under category M80, Osteoporosis with current pathological fracture, identify the site of the fracture, not the osteoporosis.

1) Osteoporosis without pathological fracture

Category M81, Osteoporosis without current pathological fracture, is for use for patients with osteoporosis who do not currently have a pathologic fracture due to the osteoporosis, even if they have had a fracture in the past. For patients with a history of osteoporosis fractures, status code Z87.310, Personal history of (healed) osteoporosis fracture, should follow the code from M81.

2) Osteoporosis with current pathological fracture

Category M80, Osteoporosis with current pathological fracture, is for patients who have a current pathologic fracture at the time of an encounter. The codes under M80 identify the site of the fracture. A code from category M80, not a traumatic fracture code, should be used for any patient with known osteoporosis who suffers a fracture, even if the patient had a minor fall or trauma, if that fall or trauma would not usually break a normal, healthy bone.

14. Chapter 14: Diseases of Genitourinary System (N00-N99)

a. Chronic kidney disease

1) Stages of chronic kidney disease (CKD)

The ICD-10-CM classifies CKD based on severity. The severity of CKD is designated by stages 1-5. Stage 2, code N18.2, equates to mild CKD; stage 3, code N18.3, equates to moderate CKD; and stage 4, code N18.4, equates to severe CKD. Code N18.6, End stage renal disease (ESRD), is assigned when the provider has documented end-stage-renal disease (ESRD).

If both a stage of CKD and ESRD are documented, assign code N18.6 only.

2) Chronic kidney disease and kidney transplant status

Patients who have undergone kidney transplant may still have some form of chronic kidney disease (CKD) because the kidney transplant may not fully restore kidney function. Therefore, the presence of CKD alone does not constitute a transplant complication. Assign the appropriate N18 code for the patient's stage of CKD and code Z94.0, Kidney transplant status. If a transplant complication such as failure or rejection or other transplant complication is documented, see section I.C.19.g for information on coding complications of a kidney transplant. If the documentation is unclear as to whether the patient has a complication of the transplant, query the provider.

3) Chronic kidney disease with other conditions

Patients with CKD may also suffer from other serious conditions, most commonly diabetes mellitus and hypertension. The sequencing of the CKD code in relationship to codes for other contributing conditions is based on the conventions in the Tabular List.

See I.C.9. Hypertensive chronic kidney disease.

See I.C.19. Chronic kidney disease and kidney transplant complications.

15. Chapter 15: Pregnancy, Childbirth, and the Puerperium (O00-O9A)

a. General Rules for Obstetric Cases

1) Codes from chapter 15 and sequencing priority

Obstetric cases require codes from chapter 15, codes in the range O00-O9A, Pregnancy, Childbirth, and the Puerperium. Chapter 15 codes have sequencing priority over codes from other chapters. Additional codes from other chapters may be used in conjunction with chapter 15 codes to further specify conditions. Should the provider document that the pregnancy is incidental to the encounter, then code Z33.1, Pregnant state, incidental, should be used in place of any chapter 15 codes. It is the provider's responsibility to state that the condition being treated is not affecting the pregnancy.

2) Chapter 15 codes used only on the maternal record

Chapter 15 codes are to be used only on the maternal record, never on the record of the newborn.

3) Final character for trimester

The majority of codes in Chapter 15 have a final character indicating the trimester of pregnancy. The timeframes for the trimesters are indicated at the beginning of the chapter. If trimester is not a component of a code, it is because the condition always occurs in a specific trimester, or the concept of trimester of pregnancy is not applicable. Certain codes have characters for only certain trimesters because the condition does not occur in all trimesters, but it may occur in more than just one.

Assignment of the final character for trimester should be based on the provider's documentation of the trimester (or number of weeks) for the current admission/encounter. This applies to the assignment of trimester for pre-existing conditions as well as those that develop during or are due to the pregnancy. The provider's documentation of the number of weeks may be used to assign the appropriate code identifying the trimester.

Whenever delivery occurs during the current admission, and there is an "in childbirth" option for the obstetric complication being coded, the "in childbirth" code should be assigned.

4) Selection of trimester for inpatient admissions that encompass more than one trimester

In instances when a patient is admitted to a hospital for complications of pregnancy during one trimester and remains in the hospital into a subsequent trimester, the trimester character for the antepartum complication code should be assigned on the basis of the trimester when the complication developed, not the trimester of the discharge. If the condition developed prior to the current admission/encounter or represents a pre-existing condition, the trimester character for the trimester at the time of the admission/encounter should be assigned.

5) Unspecified trimester

Each category that includes codes for trimester has a code for "unspecified trimester." The "unspecified trimester" code should rarely be used, such as when the documentation in the record is insufficient to determine the trimester and it is not possible to obtain clarification.

6) 7th character for Fetus Identification

Where applicable, a 7th character is to be assigned for certain categories (O31, O32, O33.3 - O33.6, O35, O36, O40, O41, O60.1, O60.2, O64, and O69) to identify the fetus for which the complication code applies.

Assign 7th character "0":

- For single gestations
- When the documentation in the record is insufficient to determine the fetus affected and it is not possible to obtain clarification.
- When it is not possible to clinically determine which fetus is affected.

b. Selection of OB Principal or First-listed Diagnosis

1) Routine outpatient prenatal visits

For routine outpatient prenatal visits when no complications are present, a code from category Z34, Encounter for supervision of normal pregnancy, should be used as the first-listed diagnosis. These codes should not be used in conjunction with chapter 15 codes.

2) **Supervision of High-Risk Pregnancy**
Codes from category O09, Supervision of high-risk pregnancy, are intended for use only during the prenatal period. For complications during the labor or delivery episode as a result of a high-risk pregnancy, assign the applicable complication codes from Chapter 15. If there are no complications during the labor or delivery episode, assign code O80, Encounter for full-term uncomplicated delivery.

For routine prenatal outpatient visits for patients with high-risk pregnancies, a code from category O09, Supervision of high-risk pregnancy, should be used as the first-listed diagnosis. Secondary chapter 15 codes may be used in conjunction with these codes if appropriate.

3) **Episodes when no delivery occurs**
In episodes when no delivery occurs, the principal diagnosis should correspond to the principal complication of the pregnancy which necessitated the encounter. Should more than one complication exist, all of which are treated or monitored, any of the complication codes may be sequenced first.

4) **When a delivery occurs**
When an obstetric patient is admitted and delivers during that admission, the condition that prompted the admission should be sequenced as the principal diagnosis. If multiple conditions prompted the admission, sequence the one most related to the delivery as the principal diagnosis. A code for any complication of the delivery should be assigned as an additional diagnosis. In cases of cesarean delivery, if the patient was admitted with a condition that resulted in the performance of a cesarean procedure, that condition should be selected as the principal diagnosis. If the reason for the admission was unrelated to the condition resulting in the cesarean delivery, the condition related to the reason for the admission should be selected as the principal diagnosis.

5) **Outcome of delivery**
A code from category Z37, Outcome of delivery, should be included on every maternal record when a delivery has occurred. These codes are not to be used on subsequent records or on the newborn record.

c. **Pre-existing conditions versus conditions due to the pregnancy**
Certain categories in Chapter 15 distinguish between conditions of the mother that existed prior to pregnancy (pre-existing) and those that are a direct result of pregnancy. When assigning codes from Chapter 15, it is important to assess if a condition was pre-existing prior to pregnancy or developed during or due to the pregnancy in order to assign the correct code.

Categories that do not distinguish between pre-existing and pregnancy-related conditions may be used for either. It is acceptable to use codes specifically for the puerperium with codes complicating pregnancy and childbirth if a condition arises postpartum during the delivery encounter.

d. **Pre-existing hypertension in pregnancy**
Category O10, Pre-existing hypertension complicating pregnancy, childbirth and the puerperium, includes codes for hypertensive heart and hypertensive chronic kidney disease. When assigning one of the O10 codes that includes hypertensive heart disease or hypertensive chronic kidney disease, it is necessary to add a secondary code from the appropriate hypertension category to specify the type of heart failure or chronic kidney disease.

See Section I.C.9. Hypertension.

e. **Fetal Conditions Affecting the Management of the Mother**
1) **Codes from categories O35 and O36**
Codes from categories O35, Maternal care for known or suspected fetal abnormality and damage, and O36, Maternal care for other fetal problems, are assigned only when the fetal condition is actually responsible for modifying the management of the mother, i.e., by requiring diagnostic studies, additional observation, special care, or termination of pregnancy. The fact that the fetal condition exists does not justify assigning a code from this series to the mother's record.

2) **In utero surgery**
In cases when surgery is performed on the fetus, a diagnosis code from category O35, Maternal care for known or suspected fetal abnormality and damage, should be assigned identifying the fetal condition. Assign the appropriate procedure code for the procedure performed.

No code from Chapter 16, the perinatal codes, should be used on the mother's record to identify fetal conditions. Surgery performed in utero on a fetus is still to be coded as an obstetric encounter.

f. **HIV Infection in Pregnancy, Childbirth and the Puerperium**
During pregnancy, childbirth or the puerperium, a patient admitted because of an HIV-related illness should receive a principal diagnosis from subcategory O98.7-, Human immunodeficiency [HIV] disease complicating pregnancy, childbirth and the puerperium, followed by the code(s) for the HIV-related illness(es).

Patients with asymptomatic HIV infection status admitted during pregnancy, childbirth, or the puerperium should receive codes of O98.7- and Z21, Asymptomatic human immunodeficiency virus [HIV] infection status.

g. **Diabetes mellitus in pregnancy**
Diabetes mellitus is a significant complicating factor in pregnancy. Pregnant women who are diabetic should be assigned a code from category O24, Diabetes mellitus in pregnancy, childbirth, and the puerperium, first, followed by the appropriate diabetes code(s) (E08-E13) from Chapter 4.

h. **Long term use of insulin and oral hypoglycemics**
See section I.C.4.a.3 for information on the long term use of insulin and oral hypoglycemic.

i. **Gestational (pregnancy induced) diabetes**
Gestational (pregnancy induced) diabetes can occur during the second and third trimester of pregnancy in women who were not diabetic prior to pregnancy. Gestational diabetes can cause complications in the pregnancy similar to those of pre-existing diabetes mellitus. It also puts the woman at greater risk of developing diabetes after the pregnancy. Codes for gestational diabetes are in subcategory O24.4, Gestational diabetes mellitus. No other code from category O24, Diabetes mellitus in pregnancy, childbirth, and the puerperium, should be used with a code from O24.4.

The codes under subcategory O24.4 include diet controlled, insulin controlled, and controlled by oral hypoglycemic drugs. If a patient with gestational diabetes is treated with both diet and insulin, only the code for insulin-controlled is required. If a patient with gestational diabetes is treated with both diet and oral hypoglycemic medications, only the code for "controlled by oral hypoglycemic drugs" is required. Code Z79.4, Long-term (current) use of insulin or code Z79.84, Long-term (current) use of oral hypoglycemic drugs, should not be assigned with codes from subcategory O24.4.

An abnormal glucose tolerance in pregnancy is assigned a code from subcategory O99.81, Abnormal glucose complicating pregnancy, childbirth, and the puerperium.

j. **Sepsis and septic shock complicating abortion, pregnancy, childbirth and the puerperium**
When assigning a chapter 15 code for sepsis complicating abortion, pregnancy, childbirth, and the puerperium, a code for the specific type of infection should be assigned as an additional diagnosis. If severe sepsis is present, a code from subcategory R65.2, Severe sepsis, and code(s) for associated organ dysfunction(s) should also be assigned as additional diagnoses.

k. **Puerperal sepsis**
Code O85, Puerperal sepsis, should be assigned with a secondary code to identify the causal organism (e.g., for a bacterial infection, assign a code from category B95-B96, Bacterial infections in conditions classified elsewhere). A code from category A40, Streptococcal sepsis, or A41, Other sepsis, should not be used for puerperal sepsis. If applicable, use additional codes to identify severe sepsis (R65.2-) and any associated acute organ dysfunction.

l. **Alcohol, tobacco and drug use during pregnancy, childbirth and the puerperium**
1) **Alcohol use during pregnancy, childbirth and the puerperium**
Codes under subcategory O99.31, Alcohol use complicating pregnancy, childbirth, and the puerperium, should be assigned for any pregnancy case when a mother uses alcohol during the pregnancy or postpartum. A secondary code from category F10, Alcohol related disorders, should also be assigned to identify manifestations of the alcohol use.

2) **Tobacco use during pregnancy, childbirth and the puerperium**
Codes under subcategory O99.33, Smoking (tobacco) complicating pregnancy, childbirth, and the puerperium, should

be assigned for any pregnancy case when a mother uses any type of tobacco product during the pregnancy or postpartum. A secondary code from category F17, Nicotine dependence, should also be assigned to identify the type of nicotine dependence.

3) Drug use during pregnancy, childbirth and the puerperium
Codes under subcategory O99.32, Drug use complicating pregnancy, childbirth, and the puerperium, should be assigned for any pregnancy case when a mother uses drugs during the pregnancy or postpartum. This can involve illegal drugs, or inappropriate use or abuse of prescription drugs. Secondary code(s) from categories F11-F16 and F18-F19 should also be assigned to identify manifestations of the drug use.

m. Poisoning, toxic effects, adverse effects and underdosing in a pregnant patient
A code from subcategory O9A.2, Injury, poisoning and certain other consequences of external causes complicating pregnancy, childbirth, and the puerperium, should be sequenced first, followed by the appropriate injury, poisoning, toxic effect, adverse effect or underdosing code, and then the additional code(s) that specifies the condition caused by the poisoning, toxic effect, adverse effect or underdosing.
See Section I.C.19. Adverse effects, poisoning, underdosing and toxic effects.

n. Normal Delivery, Code O80
1) Encounter for full term uncomplicated delivery
Code O80 should be assigned when a woman is admitted for a full-term normal delivery and delivers a single, healthy infant without any complications antepartum, during the delivery, or postpartum during the delivery episode. Code O80 is always a principal diagnosis. It is not to be used if any other code from chapter 15 is needed to describe a current complication of the antenatal, delivery, or **postnatal** period. Additional codes from other chapters may be used with code O80 if they are not related to or are in any way complicating the pregnancy.

2) Uncomplicated delivery with resolved antepartum complication
Code O80 may be used if the patient had a complication at some point during the pregnancy, but the complication is not present at the time of the admission for delivery.

3) Outcome of delivery for O80
Z37.0, Single live birth, is the only outcome of delivery code appropriate for use with O80.

o. The Peripartum and Postpartum Periods
1) Peripartum and Postpartum periods
The postpartum period begins immediately after delivery and continues for six weeks following delivery. The peripartum period is defined as the last month of pregnancy to five months postpartum.

2) Peripartum and postpartum complication
A postpartum complication is any complication occurring within the six-week period.

3) Pregnancy-related complications after 6 week period
Chapter 15 codes may also be used to describe pregnancy-related complications after the peripartum or postpartum period if the provider documents that a condition is pregnancy related.

4) Admission for routine postpartum care following delivery outside hospital
When the mother delivers outside the hospital prior to admission and is admitted for routine postpartum care and no complications are noted, code Z39.0, Encounter for care and examination of mother immediately after delivery, should be assigned as the principal diagnosis.

5) Pregnancy associated cardiomyopathy
Pregnancy associated cardiomyopathy, code O90.3, is unique in that it may be diagnosed in the third trimester of pregnancy but may continue to progress months after delivery. For this reason, it is referred to as peripartum cardiomyopathy. Code O90.3 is only for use when the cardiomyopathy develops as a result of pregnancy in a woman who did not have pre-existing heart disease.

p. Code O94, Sequelae of complication of pregnancy, childbirth, and the puerperium
1) Code O94
Code O94, Sequelae of complication of pregnancy, childbirth, and the puerperium, is for use in those cases when an initial

complication of a pregnancy develops a sequelae requiring care or treatment at a future date.

2) After the initial postpartum period
This code may be used at any time after the initial postpartum period.

3) Sequencing of Code O94
This code, like all sequela codes, is to be sequenced following the code describing the sequelae of the complication.

q. Termination of Pregnancy and Spontaneous abortions
1) Abortion with Liveborn Fetus
When an attempted termination of pregnancy results in a liveborn fetus, assign code Z33.2, Encounter for elective termination of pregnancy and a code from category Z37, Outcome of Delivery.

2) Retained Products of Conception following an abortion
Subsequent encounters for retained products of conception following a spontaneous abortion or elective termination of pregnancy, without complications are assigned O03.4, Incomplete spontaneous abortion without complication, or code O07.4, Failed attempted termination of pregnancy without complication. This advice is appropriate even when the patient was discharged previously with a discharge diagnosis of complete abortion. If the patient has a specific complication associated with the spontaneous abortion or elective termination of pregnancy in addition to retained products of conception, assign the appropriate complication **code (e.g., O03.-, O04.-, O07.-)** instead of code O03.4 or O07.4

3) Complications leading to abortion
Codes from Chapter 15 may be used as additional codes to identify any documented complications of the pregnancy in conjunction with codes in categories in O04, O07 and O08.

r. Abuse in a pregnant patient
For suspected or confirmed cases of abuse of a pregnant patient, a code(s) from subcategories O9A.3, Physical abuse complicating pregnancy, childbirth, and the puerperium, O9A.4, Sexual abuse complicating pregnancy, childbirth, and the puerperium, and O9A.5, Psychological abuse complicating pregnancy, childbirth, and the puerperium, should be sequenced first, followed by the appropriate codes (if applicable) to identify any associated current injury due to physical abuse, sexual abuse, and the perpetrator of abuse.
See Section I.C.19. Adult and child abuse, neglect and other maltreatment.

16. Chapter 16: Certain Conditions Originating in the Perinatal Period (P00-P96)
For coding and reporting purposes the perinatal period is defined as before birth through the 28th day following birth. The following guidelines are provided for reporting purposes.

a. General Perinatal Rules
1) Use of Chapter 16 Codes
Codes in this chapter are <u>never</u> for use on the maternal record. Codes from Chapter 15, the obstetric chapter, are never permitted on the newborn record. Chapter 16 codes may be used throughout the life of the patient if the condition is still present.

2) Principal Diagnosis for Birth Record
When coding the birth episode in a newborn record, assign a code from category Z38, Liveborn infants according to place of birth and type of delivery, as the principal diagnosis. A code from category Z38 is assigned only once, to a newborn at the time of birth. If a newborn is transferred to another institution, a code from category Z38 should not be used at the receiving hospital.

A code from category Z38 is used only on the newborn record, not on the mother's record.

3) Use of Codes from other Chapters with Codes from Chapter 16
Codes from other chapters may be used with codes from chapter 16 if the codes from the other chapters provide more specific detail. Codes for signs and symptoms may be assigned when a definitive diagnosis has not been established. If the reason for the encounter is a perinatal condition, the code from chapter 16 should be sequenced first.

4) Use of Chapter 16 Codes after the Perinatal Period
Should a condition originate in the perinatal period, and continue throughout the life of the patient, the perinatal code should continue to be used regardless of the patient's age.

5) Birth process or community acquired conditions
If a newborn has a condition that may be either due to the birth process or community acquired and the documentation does not indicate which it is, the default is due to the birth process and the code from Chapter 16 should be used. If the condition is community-acquired, a code from Chapter 16 should not be assigned.

6) Code all clinically significant conditions
All clinically significant conditions noted on routine newborn examination should be coded. A condition is clinically significant if it requires:

- clinical evaluation; or
- therapeutic treatment; or
- diagnostic procedures; or
- extended length of hospital stay; or
- increased nursing care and/or monitoring; or
- has implications for future health care needs

Note: The perinatal guidelines listed above are the same as the general coding guidelines for "additional diagnoses," except for the final point regarding implications for future health care needs. Codes should be assigned for conditions that have been specified by the provider as having implications for future health care needs.

b. Observation and Evaluation of Newborns for Suspected Conditions not Found

1) Use of Z05 codes
Assign a code from category Z05, Observation and evaluation of newborns and infants for suspected conditions ruled out, to identify those instances when a healthy newborn is evaluated for a suspected condition that is determined after study not to be present. Do not use a code from category Z05 when the patient has identified signs or symptoms of a suspected problem; in such cases code the sign or symptom.

2) Z05 on other than the birth record
A code from category Z05 may also be assigned as a principal or first-listed code for readmissions or encounters when the code from category Z38 code no longer applies. Codes from category Z05 are for use only for healthy newborns and infants for which no condition after study is found to be present.

3) Z05 on a birth record
A code from category Z05 is to be used as a secondary code after the code from category Z38, Liveborn infants according to place of birth and type of delivery.

c. Coding Additional Perinatal Diagnoses

1) Assigning codes for conditions that require treatment
Assign codes for conditions that require treatment or further investigation, prolong the length of stay, or require resource utilization.

2) Codes for conditions specified as having implications for future health care needs
Assign codes for conditions that have been specified by the provider as having implications for future health care needs.
Note: This guideline should not be used for adult patients.

d. Prematurity and Fetal Growth Retardation
Providers utilize different criteria in determining prematurity. A code for prematurity should not be assigned unless it is documented. Assignment of codes in categories P05, Disorders of newborn related to slow fetal growth and fetal malnutrition, and P07, Disorders of newborn related to short gestation and low birth weight, not elsewhere classified, should be based on the recorded birth weight and estimated gestational age.

When both birth weight and gestational age are available, two codes from category P07 should be assigned, with the code for birth weight sequenced before the code for gestational age.

e. Low birth weight and immaturity status
Codes from category P07, Disorders of newborn related to short gestation and low birth weight, not elsewhere classified, are for use for a child or adult who was premature or had a low birth weight as a newborn and this is affecting the patient's current health status.
See Section I.C.21. Factors influencing health status and contact with health services, Status.

f. Bacterial Sepsis of Newborn
Category P36, Bacterial sepsis of newborn, includes congenital sepsis. If a perinate is documented as having sepsis without documentation

of congenital or community acquired, the default is congenital and a code from category P36 should be assigned. If the P36 code includes the causal organism, an additional code from category B95, Streptococcus, Staphylococcus, and Enterococcus as the cause of diseases classified elsewhere, or B96, Other bacterial agents as the cause of diseases classified elsewhere, should not be assigned. If the P36 code does not include the causal organism, assign an additional code from category B96. If applicable, use additional codes to identify severe sepsis (R65.2-) and any associated acute organ dysfunction.

g. Stillbirth
Code P95, Stillbirth, is only for use in institutions that maintain separate records for stillbirths. No other code should be used with P95. Code P95 should not be used on the mother's record.

17. Chapter 17: Congenital malformations, deformations, and chromosomal abnormalities (Q00-Q99)
Assign an appropriate code(s) from categories Q00-Q99, Congenital malformations, deformations, and chromosomal abnormalities when a malformation/deformation or chromosomal abnormality is documented. A malformation/deformation/or chromosomal abnormality may be the principal/first-listed diagnosis on a record or a secondary diagnosis.

When a malformation/deformation or chromosomal abnormality does not have a unique code assignment, assign additional code(s) for any manifestations that may be present.

When the code assignment specifically identifies the malformation/deformation or chromosomal abnormality, manifestations that are an inherent component of the anomaly should not be coded separately. Additional codes should be assigned for manifestations that are not an inherent component.

Codes from Chapter 17 may be used throughout the life of the patient. If a congenital malformation or deformity has been corrected, a personal history code should be used to identify the history of the malformation or deformity. Although present at birth, **a** malformation/deformation/or chromosomal abnormality may not be identified until later in life. Whenever the condition is diagnosed by the **provider**, it is appropriate to assign a code from codes Q00-Q99. For the birth admission, the appropriate code from category Z38, Liveborn infants, according to place of birth and type of delivery, should be sequenced as the principal diagnosis, followed by any congenital anomaly codes, Q00- Q99.

18. Chapter 18: Symptoms, signs, and abnormal clinical and laboratory findings, not elsewhere classified (R00-R99)
Chapter 18 includes symptoms, signs, abnormal results of clinical or other investigative procedures, and ill-defined conditions regarding which no diagnosis classifiable elsewhere is recorded. Signs and symptoms that point to a specific diagnosis have been assigned to a category in other chapters of the classification.

a. Use of symptom codes
Codes that describe symptoms and signs are acceptable for reporting purposes when a related definitive diagnosis has not been established (confirmed) by the provider.

b. Use of a symptom code with a definitive diagnosis code
Codes for signs and symptoms may be reported in addition to a related definitive diagnosis when the sign or symptom is not routinely associated with that diagnosis, such as the various signs and symptoms associated with complex syndromes. The definitive diagnosis code should be sequenced before the symptom code.

Signs or symptoms that are associated routinely with a disease process should not be assigned as additional codes, unless otherwise instructed by the classification.

c. Combination codes that include symptoms
ICD-10-CM contains a number of combination codes that identify both the definitive diagnosis and common symptoms of that diagnosis.

When using one of these combination codes, an additional code should not be assigned for the symptom.

d. Repeated falls
Code R29.6, Repeated falls, is for use for encounters when a patient has recently fallen and the reason for the fall is being investigated.

Code Z91.81, History of falling, is for use when a patient has fallen in the past and is at risk for future falls. When appropriate, both codes R29.6 and Z91.81 may be assigned together.

e. Coma scale
The coma scale codes (R40.2-) can be used in conjunction with traumatic brain injury codes, acute cerebrovascular disease or sequelae of cerebrovascular disease codes. These codes are primarily for use by trauma registries, but they may be used in any setting

where this information is collected. The coma scale may also be used to assess the status of the central nervous system for other non-trauma conditions, such as monitoring patients in the intensive care unit regardless of medical condition. The coma scale codes should be sequenced after the diagnosis code(s).

These codes, one from each subcategory, are needed to complete the scale. The 7th character indicates when the scale was recorded. The 7th character should match for all three codes.

At a minimum, report the initial score documented on presentation at your facility. This may be a score from the emergency medicine technician (EMT) or in the emergency department. If desired, a facility may choose to capture multiple coma scale scores.

Assign code R40.24, Glasgow coma scale, total score, when only the total score is documented in the medical record and not the individual score(s).

Do not report codes for individual or total Glasgow coma scale scores for a patient with a medically induced coma or a sedated patient.

See Section I.B.14 for coma scale documentation by clinicians other than patient's provider

f.   **Functional quadriplegia**
   GUIDELINE HAS BEEN DELETED EFFECTIVE OCTOBER 1, 2017

g.   **SIRS due to Non-Infectious Process**
   The systemic inflammatory response syndrome (SIRS) can develop as a result of certain non-infectious disease processes, such as trauma, malignant neoplasm, or pancreatitis. When SIRS is documented with a noninfectious condition, and no subsequent infection is documented, the code for the underlying condition, such as an injury, should be assigned, followed by code R65.10, Systemic inflammatory response syndrome (SIRS) of non-infectious origin without acute organ dysfunction, or code R65.11, Systemic inflammatory response syndrome (SIRS) of non-infectious origin with acute organ dysfunction. If an associated acute organ dysfunction is documented, the appropriate code(s) for the specific type of organ dysfunction(s) should be assigned in addition to code R65.11. If acute organ dysfunction is documented, but it cannot be determined if the acute organ dysfunction is associated with SIRS or due to another condition (e.g., directly due to the trauma), the provider should be queried.

h.   **Death NOS**
   Code R99, Ill-defined and unknown cause of mortality, is only for use in the very limited circumstance when a patient who has already died is brought into an emergency department or other healthcare facility and is pronounced dead upon arrival. It does not represent the discharge disposition of death.

i.   **NIHSS Stroke Scale**
   The NIH stroke scale (NIHSS) codes (R29.7- -) can be used in conjunction with acute stroke codes (I63) to identify the patient's neurological status and the severity of the stroke. The stroke scale codes should be sequenced after the acute stroke diagnosis code(s).

   At a minimum, report the initial score documented. If desired, a facility may choose to capture multiple stroke scale scores.

   See Section I.B.14 for NIHSS stroke scale documentation by clinicians other than patient's provider

19. **Chapter 19: Injury, poisoning, and certain other consequences of external causes (S00-T88)**

a.   **Application of 7th Characters in Chapter 19**
   Most categories in chapter 19 have a 7th character requirement for each applicable code. Most categories in this chapter have three 7th character values (with the exception of fractures): A, initial encounter, D, subsequent encounter and S, sequela. Categories for traumatic fractures have additional 7th character values. While the patient may be seen by a new or different provider over the course of treatment for an injury, assignment of the 7th character is based on whether the patient is undergoing active treatment and not whether the provider is seeing the patient for the first time.

   For complication codes, active treatment refers to treatment for the condition described by the code, even though it may be related to an earlier precipitating problem. For example, code T84.50XA, Infection and inflammatory reaction due to unspecified internal joint prosthesis, initial encounter, is used when active treatment is provided for the infection, even though the condition relates to the prosthetic device, implant or graft that was placed at a previous encounter.

   7th character "A", initial encounter is used for each encounter where the patient is receiving active treatment for the condition.

7th character "D" subsequent encounter is used for encounters after the patient has completed active treatment of the condition and is receiving routine care for the condition during the healing or recovery phase.

The aftercare Z codes should not be used for aftercare for conditions such as injuries or poisonings, where 7th characters are provided to identify subsequent care. For example, for aftercare of an injury, assign the acute injury code with the 7th character "D" (subsequent encounter).

7th character "S", sequela, is for use for complications or conditions that arise as a direct result of a condition, such as scar formation after a burn. The scars are sequelae of the burn. When using 7th character "S", it is necessary to use both the injury code that precipitated the sequela and the code for the sequela itself. The "S" is added only to the injury code, not the sequela code. The 7th character "S" identifies the injury responsible for the sequela. The specific type of sequela (e.g. scar) is sequenced first, followed by the injury code.

See Section I.B.10 Sequelae, (Late Effects)

b.   **Coding of Injuries**
   When coding injuries, assign separate codes for each injury unless a combination code is provided, in which case the combination code is assigned. Codes from category T07, Unspecified multiple injuries should not be assigned in the inpatient setting unless information for a more specific code is not available. Traumatic injury codes (S00-T14.9) are not to be used for normal, healing surgical wounds or to identify complications of surgical wounds.

   The code for the most serious injury, as determined by the provider and the focus of treatment, is sequenced first.

1)   **Superficial injuries**
   Superficial injuries such as abrasions or contusions are not coded when associated with more severe injuries of the same site.

2)   **Primary injury with damage to nerves/blood vessels**
   When a primary injury results in minor damage to peripheral nerves or blood vessels, the primary injury is sequenced first with additional code(s) for injuries to nerves and spinal cord (such as category S04), and/or injury to blood vessels (such as category S15). When the primary injury is to the blood vessels or nerves, that injury should be sequenced first.

3)   **Iatrogenic injuries**
   Injury codes from Chapter 19 should not be assigned for injuries that occur during, or as a result of, a medical intervention. Assign the appropriate complication code(s).

c.   **Coding of Traumatic Fractures**
   The principles of multiple coding of injuries should be followed in coding fractures. Fractures of specified sites are coded individually by site in accordance with both the provisions within categories S02, S12, S22, S32, S42, S49, S52, S59, S62, S72, S79, S82, S89, S92 and the level of detail furnished by medical record content.

   A fracture not indicated as open or closed should be coded to closed. A fracture not indicated whether displaced or not displaced should be coded to displaced.

   More specific guidelines are as follows:

1)   **Initial vs. subsequent encounter for fractures**
   Traumatic fractures are coded using the appropriate 7th character for initial encounter (A, B, C) for each encounter where the patient is receiving active treatment for the fracture. The appropriate 7th character for initial encounter should also be assigned for a patient who delayed seeking treatment for the fracture or nonunion.

   Fractures are coded using the appropriate 7th character for subsequent care for encounters after the patient has completed active treatment of the fracture and is receiving routine care for the fracture during the healing or recovery phase.

   Care for complications of surgical treatment for fracture repairs during the healing or recovery phase should be coded with the appropriate complication codes.

   Care of complications of fractures, such as malunion and nonunion, should be reported with the appropriate 7th character for subsequent care with nonunion (K, M, N,) or subsequent care with malunion (P, Q, R).

   Malunion/nonunion: The appropriate 7th character for initial encounter should also be assigned for a patient who delayed seeking treatment for the fracture or nonunion.

The open fracture designations in the assignment of the 7th character for fractures of the forearm, femur and lower leg, including ankle are based on the Gustilo open fracture classification. When the Gustilo classification type is not specified for an open fracture, the 7th character for open fracture type I or II should be assigned (B, E, H, M, Q).

A code from category M80, not a traumatic fracture code, should be used for any patient with known osteoporosis who suffers a fracture, even if the patient had a minor fall or trauma, if that fall or trauma would not usually break a normal, healthy bone.

See Section I.C.13. Osteoporosis.

The aftercare Z codes should not be used for aftercare for traumatic fractures. For aftercare of a traumatic fracture, assign the acute fracture code with the appropriate 7th character.

2) Multiple fractures sequencing
Multiple fractures are sequenced in accordance with the severity of the fracture.

3) Physeal fractures
For physeal fractures, assign only the code identifying the type of physeal fracture. Do not assign a separate code to identify the specific bone that is fractured.

d. Coding of Burns and Corrosions
The ICD-10-CM makes a distinction between burns and corrosions. The burn codes are for thermal burns, except sunburns, that come from a heat source, such as a fire or hot appliance. The burn codes are also for burns resulting from electricity and radiation. Corrosions are burns due to chemicals. The guidelines are the same for burns and corrosions.

Current burns (T20-T25) are classified by depth, extent and by agent (X code). Burns are classified by depth as first degree (erythema), second degree (blistering), and third degree (full-thickness involvement). Burns of the eye and internal organs (T26-T28) are classified by site, but not by degree.

1) Sequencing of burn and related condition codes
Sequence first the code that reflects the highest degree of burn when more than one burn is present.

a. When the reason for the admission or encounter is for treatment of external multiple burns, sequence first the code that reflects the burn of the highest degree.

b. When a patient has both internal and external burns, the circumstances of admission govern the selection of the principal diagnosis or first-listed diagnosis.

c. When a patient is admitted for burn injuries and other related conditions such as smoke inhalation and/or respiratory failure, the circumstances of admission govern the selection of the principal or first-listed diagnosis.

2) Burns of the same anatomic site
Classify burns of the same anatomic site and on the same side but of different degrees to the subcategory identifying the highest degree recorded in the diagnosis (e.g., for second and third degree burns of right thigh, assign only code T24.311-).

3) Non-healing burns
Non-healing burns are coded as acute burns.
Necrosis of burned skin should be coded as a non-healed burn.

4) Infected *burn*
For any documented infected burn site, use an additional code for the infection.

5) Assign separate codes for each burn site
When coding burns, assign separate codes for each burn site. Category T30, Burn and corrosion, body region unspecified is extremely vague and should rarely be used.

Codes for burns of "multiple sites" should only be assigned when the medical record documentation does not specify the individual sites.

6) Burns and corrosions classified according to extent of body surface involved
Assign codes from category T31, Burns classified according to extent of body surface involved, or T32, Corrosions classified according to extent of body surface involved, when the site of the burn is not specified or when there is a need for additional data. It is advisable to use category T31 as additional coding when needed to provide data for evaluating burn mortality, such as that needed by burn units. It is also advisable to use category T31 as an additional code for reporting purposes when there is mention

of a third-degree burn involving 20 percent or more of the body surface.

Categories T31 and T32 are based on the classic "rule of nines" in estimating body surface involved: head and neck are assigned nine percent, each arm nine percent, each leg 18 percent, the anterior trunk 18 percent, posterior trunk 18 percent, and genitalia one percent. Providers may change these percentage assignments where necessary to accommodate infants and children who have proportionately larger heads than adults, and patients who have large buttocks, thighs, or abdomen that involve burns.

7) Encounters for treatment of sequela of burns
Encounters for the treatment of the late effects of burns or corrosions (i.e., scars or joint contractures) should be coded with a burn or corrosion code with the 7th character "S" for sequela.

8) Sequelae with a late effect code and current burn
When appropriate, both a code for a current burn or corrosion with 7th character "A" or "D" and a burn or corrosion code with 7th character "S" may be assigned on the same record (when both a current burn and sequelae of an old burn exist). Burns and corrosions do not heal at the same rate and a current healing wound may still exist with sequela of a healed burn or corrosion.

See Section I.B.10 Sequela (Late Effects)

9) Use of an external cause code with burns and corrosions
An external cause code should be used with burns and corrosions to identify the source and intent of the burn, as well as the place where it occurred.

e. Adverse Effects, Poisoning, Underdosing and Toxic Effects
Codes in categories T36-T65 are combination codes that include the substance that was taken as well as the intent. No additional external cause code is required for poisonings, toxic effects, adverse effects and underdosing codes.

1) Do not code directly from the Table of Drugs
Do not code directly funderdosinrom the Table of Drugs and Chemicals. Always refer back to the Tabular List.

2) Use as many codes as necessary to describe
Use as many codes as necessary to describe completely all drugs, medicinal or biological substances.

3) If the same code would describe the causative agent
If the same code would describe the causative agent for more than one adverse reaction, poisoning, toxic effect or underdosing, assign the code only once.

4) If two or more drugs, medicinal or biological substances
If two or more drugs, medicinal or biological substances are **taken**, code each individually unless a combination code is listed in the Table of Drugs and Chemicals.

If multiple unspecified drugs, medicinal or biological substances were taken, assign the appropriate code from subcategory T50.91, Poisoning by, adverse effect of and underdosing of multiple unspecified drugs, medicaments and biological substances.

5) The occurrence of drug toxicity is classified in ICD-10-CM as follows:

(a) Adverse Effect
When coding an adverse effect of a drug that has been correctly prescribed and properly administered, assign the appropriate code for the nature of the adverse effect followed by the appropriate code for the adverse effect of the drug (T36-T50). The code for the drug should have a 5th or 6th character "5" (for example T36.0X5-) Examples of the nature of an adverse effect are tachycardia, delirium, gastrointestinal hemorrhaging, vomiting, hypokalemia, hepatitis, renal failure, or respiratory failure.

(b) Poisoning
When coding a poisoning or reaction to the improper use of a medication (e.g., overdose, wrong substance given or taken in error, wrong route of administration), first assign the appropriate code from categories T36-T50. The poisoning codes have an associated intent as their 5th or 6th character (accidental, intentional self-harm, assault and undetermined. If the intent of the poisoning is unknown or unspecified, code the intent as accidental intent. The undetermined

intent is only for use if the documentation in the record specifies that the intent cannot be determined. Use additional code(s) for all manifestations of poisonings.

If there is also a diagnosis of abuse or dependence of the substance, the abuse or dependence is assigned as an additional code.

Examples of poisoning include:

(i)   Error was made in drug prescription
Errors made in drug prescription or in the administration of the drug by provider, nurse, patient, or other person.

(ii) Overdose of a drug intentionally taken
If an overdose of a drug was intentionally taken or administered and resulted in drug toxicity, it would be coded as a poisoning.

(iii) Nonprescribed drug taken with correctly prescribed and properly administered drug
If a nonprescribed drug or medicinal agent was taken in combination with a correctly prescribed and properly administered drug, any drug toxicity or other reaction resulting from the interaction of the two drugs would be classified as a poisoning.

(iv) Interaction of drug(s) and alcohol
When a reaction results from the interaction of a drug(s) and alcohol, this would be classified as poisoning.

See Section I.C.4. if poisoning is the result of insulin pump malfunctions.

(c) Underdosing
Underdosing refers to taking less of a medication than is prescribed by a provider or a manufacturer's instruction. Discontinuing the use of a prescribed medication on the patient's own initiative (not directed by the patient's provider) is also classified as an underdosing. For underdosing, assign the code from categories T36-T50 (fifth or sixth character "6").

Codes for underdosing should never be assigned as principal or first-listed codes. If a patient has a relapse or exacerbation of the medical condition for which the drug is prescribed because of the reduction in dose, then the medical condition itself should be coded.

Noncompliance (Z91.12-, Z91.13- and Z91.14-) or complication of care (Y63.6-Y63.9) codes are to be used with an underdosing code to indicate intent, if known.

(d) Toxic Effects
When a harmful substance is ingested or comes in contact with a person, this is classified as a toxic effect. The toxic effect codes are in categories T51-T65.

Toxic effect codes have an associated intent: accidental, intentional self-harm, assault and undetermined.

f. Adult and child abuse, neglect and other maltreatment
Sequence first the appropriate code from categories T74, Adult and child abuse, neglect and other maltreatment, confirmed) or T76, Adult and child abuse, neglect and other maltreatment, suspected) for abuse, neglect and other maltreatment, followed by any accompanying mental health or injury code(s).

If the documentation in the medical record states abuse or neglect it is coded as confirmed (T74.-). It is coded as suspected if it is documented as suspected (T76.-).

For cases of confirmed abuse or neglect an external cause code from the assault section (X92-Y09) should be added to identify the cause of any physical injuries. A perpetrator code (Y07) should be added when the perpetrator of the abuse is known. For suspected cases of abuse or neglect, do not report external cause or perpetrator code.

If a suspected case of abuse, neglect or mistreatment is ruled out during an encounter code Z04.71, Encounter for examination and observation following alleged physical adult abuse, ruled out, or code Z04.72, Encounter for examination and observation following alleged child physical abuse, ruled out, should be used, not a code from T76.

If a suspected case of alleged rape or sexual abuse is ruled out during an encounter code Z04.41, Encounter for examination and observation following alleged adult rape or code Z04.42, Encounter for examination and observation following alleged child rape, should be used, not a code from T76.

If a suspected case of forced sexual exploitation or forced labor exploitation is ruled out during an encounter, code Z04.81, Encounter for examination and observation of victim following forced sexual exploitation, or code Z04.82, Encounter for examination and observation of victim following forced labor exploitation, should be used, not a code from T76.

See Section I.C.15. Abuse in a pregnant patient.

g. Complications of care
1) General guidelines for complications of care
(a) Documentation of complications of care
See Section I.B.16. for information on documentation of complications of care.

2) Pain due to medical devices
Pain associated with devices, implants or grafts left in a surgical site (for example painful hip prosthesis) is assigned to the appropriate code(s) found in Chapter 19, Injury, poisoning, and certain other consequences of external causes. Specific codes for pain due to medical devices are found in the T code section of the ICD-10-CM. Use additional code(s) from category G89 to identify acute or chronic pain due to presence of the device, implant or graft (G89.18 or G89.28).

3) Transplant complications
(a) Transplant complications other than kidney
Codes under category T86, Complications of transplanted organs and tissues, are for use for both complications and rejection of transplanted organs. A transplant complication code is only assigned if the complication affects the function of the transplanted organ. Two codes are required to fully describe a transplant complication: the appropriate code from category T86 and a secondary code that identifies the complication.

Pre-existing conditions or conditions that develop after the transplant are not coded as complications unless they affect the function of the transplanted organs.

See I.C.21. for transplant organ removal status

See I.C.2. for malignant neoplasm associated with transplanted organ.

(b) Kidney transplant complications
Patients who have undergone kidney transplant may still have some form of chronic kidney disease (CKD) because the kidney transplant may not fully restore kidney function. Code T86.1- should be assigned for documented complications of a kidney transplant, such as transplant failure or rejection or other transplant complication. Code T86.1- should not be assigned for post kidney transplant patients who have chronic kidney (CKD) unless a transplant complication such as transplant failure or rejection is documented. If the documentation is unclear as to whether the patient has a complication of the transplant, query the provider.

Conditions that affect the function of the transplanted kidney, other than CKD, should be assigned a code from subcategory T86.1, Complications of transplanted organ, Kidney, and a secondary code that identifies the complication.

For patients with CKD following a kidney transplant, but who do not have a complication such as failure or rejection, *see section I.C.14. Chronic kidney disease and kidney transplant status.*

4) Complication codes that include the external cause
As with certain other T codes, some of the complications of care codes have the external cause included in the code. The code includes the nature of the complication as well as the type of procedure that caused the complication. No external cause code indicating the type of procedure is necessary for these codes.

5) Complications of care codes within the body system chapters
Intraoperative and postprocedural complication codes are found within the body system chapters with codes specific to the organs and structures of that body system. These codes should be sequenced first, followed by a code(s) for the specific complication, if applicable.

Complication codes from the body system chapters should be assigned for intraoperative and postprocedural complications (e.g., the appropriate complication code from chapter 9 would be assigned for a vascular intraoperative or postprocedural complication) unless the complication is specifically indexed to a T code in chapter 19.

20. Chapter 20: External Causes of Morbidity (V00-Y99)

The external causes of morbidity codes should never be sequenced as the first-listed or principal diagnosis.

External cause codes are intended to provide data for injury research and evaluation of injury prevention strategies. These codes capture how the injury or health condition happened (cause), the intent (unintentional or accidental; or intentional, such as suicide or assault), the place where the event occurred the activity of the patient at the time of the event, and the person's status (e.g., civilian, military).

There is no national requirement for mandatory ICD-10-CM external cause code reporting. Unless a provider is subject to a state-based external cause code reporting mandate or these codes are required by a particular payer, reporting of ICD-10-CM codes in Chapter 20, External Causes of Morbidity, is not required. In the absence of a mandatory reporting requirement, providers are encouraged to voluntarily report external cause codes, as they provide valuable data for injury research and evaluation of injury prevention strategies.

a. General External Cause Coding Guidelines

1) Used with any code in the range of A00.0-T88.9 Z00-Z99

An external cause code may be used with any code in the range of A00.0-T88.9, Z00-Z99, classification that represents a health condition due to an external cause. Though they are most applicable to injuries, they are also valid for use with such things as infections or diseases due to an external source, and other health conditions, such as a heart attack that occurs during strenuous physical activity.

2) External cause code used for length of treatment

Assign the external cause code, with the appropriate 7th character (initial encounter, subsequent encounter or sequela) for each encounter for which the injury or condition is being treated.

Most categories in chapter 20 have a 7th character requirement for each applicable code. Most categories in this chapter have three 7th character values: A, initial encounter, D, subsequent encounter and S, sequela. While the patient may be seen by a new or different provider over the course of treatment for an injury or condition, assignment of the 7th character for external cause should match the 7th character of the code assigned for the associated injury or condition for the encounter.

3) Use the full range of external cause codes

Use the full range of external cause codes to completely describe the cause, the intent, the place of occurrence, and if applicable, the activity of the patient at the time of the event, and the patient's status, for all injuries, and other health conditions due to an external cause.

4) Assign as many external cause codes as necessary

Assign as many external cause codes as necessary to fully explain each cause. If only one external code can be recorded, assign the code most related to the principal diagnosis.

5) The selection of the appropriate external cause code

The selection of the appropriate external cause code is guided by the Alphabetic Index of External Causes and by Inclusion and Exclusion notes in the Tabular List.

6) External cause code can never be a principal diagnosis

An external cause code can never be a principal (first-listed) diagnosis.

7) Combination external cause codes

Certain of the external cause codes are combination codes that identify sequential events that result in an injury, such as a fall which results in striking against an object. The injury may be due to either event or both. The combination external cause code used should correspond to the sequence of events regardless of which caused the most serious injury.

8) No external cause code needed in certain circumstances

No external cause code from Chapter 20 is needed if the external cause and intent are included in a code from another chapter (e.g. T36.0X1- Poisoning by penicillins, accidental (unintentional)).

b. Place of Occurrence Guideline

Codes from category Y92, Place of occurrence of the external cause, are secondary codes for use after other external cause codes to identify the location of the patient at the time of injury or other condition.

Generally, a place of occurrence code is assigned only once, at the initial encounter for treatment. However, in the rare instance that a new injury occurs during hospitalization, an additional place of occurrence code may be assigned. No 7th characters are used for Y92.

Do not use place of occurrence code Y92.9 if the place is not stated or is not applicable.

c. Activity Code

Assign a code from category Y93, Activity code, to describe the activity of the patient at the time the injury or other health condition occurred.

An activity code is used only once, at the initial encounter for treatment. Only one code from Y93 should be recorded on a medical record.

The activity codes are not applicable to poisonings, adverse effects, misadventures or sequela.

Do not assign Y93.9, Unspecified activity, if the activity is not stated.

A code from category Y93 is appropriate for use with external cause and intent codes if identifying the activity provides additional information about the event.

d. Place of Occurrence, Activity, and Status Codes Used with other External Cause Code

When applicable, place of occurrence, activity, and external cause status codes are sequenced after the main external cause code(s). Regardless of the number of external cause codes assigned, generally there should be only one place of occurrence code, one activity code, and one external cause status code assigned to an encounter. However, in the rare instance that a new injury occurs during hospitalization, an additional place of occurrence code may be assigned.

e. If the Reporting Format Limits the Number of External Cause Codes

If the reporting format limits the number of external cause codes that can be used in reporting clinical data, report the code for the cause/intent most related to the principal diagnosis. If the format permits capture of additional external cause codes, the cause/intent, including medical misadventures, of the additional events should be reported rather than the codes for place, activity, or external status.

f. Multiple External Cause Coding Guidelines

More than one external cause code is required to fully describe the external cause of an illness or injury. The assignment of external cause codes should be sequenced in the following priority:

If two or more events cause separate injuries, an external cause code should be assigned for each cause. The first-listed external cause code will be selected in the following order:

External codes for child and adult abuse take priority over all other external cause codes.

See Section I.C.19., Child and Adult abuse guidelines.

External cause codes for terrorism events take priority over all other external cause codes except child and adult abuse.

External cause codes for cataclysmic events take priority over all other external cause codes except child and adult abuse and terrorism.

External cause codes for transport accidents take priority over all other external cause codes except cataclysmic events, child and adult abuse and terrorism.

Activity and external cause status codes are assigned following all causal (intent) external cause codes.

The first-listed external cause code should correspond to the cause of the most serious diagnosis due to an assault, accident, or self-harm, following the order of hierarchy listed above.

g. Child and Adult Abuse Guideline

Adult and child abuse, neglect and maltreatment are classified as assault. Any of the assault codes may be used to indicate the external cause of any injury resulting from the confirmed abuse.

For confirmed cases of abuse, neglect and maltreatment, when the perpetrator is known, a code from Y07, Perpetrator of maltreatment and neglect, should accompany any other assault codes.

See Section I.C.19. Adult and child abuse, neglect and other maltreatment

h. Unknown or Undetermined Intent Guideline

If the intent (accident, self-harm, assault) of the cause of an injury or other condition is unknown or unspecified, code the intent as accidental intent. All transport accident categories assume accidental intent.

1) Use of undetermined intent
External cause codes for events of undetermined intent are only for use if the documentation in the record specifies that the intent cannot be determined.

i. Sequelae (Late Effects) of External Cause Guidelines
1) Sequelae external cause codes
Sequela are reported using the external cause code with the 7th character "S" for sequela. These codes should be used with any report of a late effect or sequela resulting from a previous injury.
See Section I.B.10 Sequela (Late Effects)

2) Sequela external cause code with a related current injury
A sequela external cause code should never be used with a related current nature of injury code.

3) Use of sequela external cause codes for subsequent visits
Use a late effect external cause code for subsequent visits when a late effect of the initial injury is being treated. Do not use a late effect external cause code for subsequent visits for follow-up care (e.g., to assess healing, to receive rehabilitative therapy) of the injury when no late effect of the injury has been documented.

j. Terrorism Guidelines
1) Cause of injury identified by the Federal Government (FBI) as terrorism
When the cause of an injury is identified by the Federal Government (FBI) as terrorism, the first-listed external cause code should be a code from category Y38, Terrorism. The definition of terrorism employed by the FBI is found at the inclusion note at the beginning of category Y38. Use additional code for place of occurrence (Y92.-). More than one Y38 code may be assigned if the injury is the result of more than one mechanism of terrorism.

2) Cause of an injury is suspected to be the result of terrorism
When the cause of an injury is suspected to be the result of terrorism a code from category Y38 should not be assigned. Suspected cases should be classified as assault.

3) Code Y38.9, Terrorism, secondary effects
Assign code Y38.9, Terrorism, secondary effects, for conditions occurring subsequent to the terrorist event. This code should not be assigned for conditions that are due to the initial terrorist act.

It is acceptable to assign code Y38.9 with another code from Y38 if there is an injury due to the initial terrorist event and an injury that is a subsequent result of the terrorist event.

k. External Cause Status
A code from category Y99, External cause status, should be assigned whenever any other external cause code is assigned for an encounter, including an Activity code, except for the events noted below. Assign a code from category Y99, External cause status, to indicate the work status of the person at the time the event occurred. The status code indicates whether the event occurred during military activity, whether a non-military person was at work, whether an individual including a student or volunteer was involved in a non-work activity at the time of the causal event.

A code from Y99, External cause status, should be assigned, when applicable, with other external cause codes, such as transport accidents and falls. The external cause status codes are not applicable to poisonings, adverse effects, misadventures or late effects.

Do not assign a code from category Y99 if no other external cause codes (cause, activity) are applicable for the encounter.

An external cause status code is used only once, at the initial encounter for treatment. Only one code from Y99 should be recorded on a medical record.

Do not assign code Y99.9, Unspecified external cause status, if the status is not stated.

21. Chapter 21: Factors influencing health status and contact with health services (Z00-Z99)
Note: The chapter specific guidelines provide additional information about the use of Z codes for specified encounters.

a. Use of Z Codes in Any Healthcare Setting
Z codes are for use in any healthcare setting. Z codes may be used as either a first-listed (principal diagnosis code in the inpatient setting) or secondary code, depending on the circumstances of the encounter. Certain Z codes may only be used as first-listed or principal diagnosis.

b. Z Codes Indicate a Reason for an Encounter
Z codes are not procedure codes. A corresponding procedure code must accompany a Z code to describe any procedure performed.

c. Categories of Z Codes
1) Contact/Exposure
Category Z20 indicates contact with, and suspected exposure to, communicable diseases. These codes are for patients who do not show any sign or symptom of a disease but are suspected to have been exposed to it by close personal contact with an infected individual or are in an area where a disease is epidemic.

Category Z77, Other contact with and (suspected) exposures hazardous to health, indicates contact with and suspected exposures hazardous to health.

Contact/exposure codes may be used as a first-listed code to explain an encounter for testing, or, more commonly, as a secondary code to identify a potential risk.

2) Inoculations and vaccinations
Code Z23 is for encounters for inoculations and vaccinations. It indicates that a patient is being seen to receive a prophylactic inoculation against a disease. Procedure codes are required to identify the actual administration of the injection and the type(s) of immunizations given. Code Z23 may be used as a secondary code if the inoculation is given as a routine part of preventive health care, such as a well-baby visit.

3) Status
Status codes indicate that a patient is either a carrier of a disease or has the sequelae or residual of a past disease or condition. This includes such things as the presence of prosthetic or mechanical devices resulting from past treatment. A status code is informative, because the status may affect the course of treatment and its outcome. A status code is distinct from a history code. The history code indicates that the patient no longer has the condition.

A status code should not be used with a diagnosis code from one of the body system chapters, if the diagnosis code includes the information provided by the status code. For example, code Z94.1, Heart transplant status, should not be used with a code from subcategory T86.2, Complications of heart transplant. The status code does not provide additional information. The complication code indicates that the patient is a heart transplant patient.

For encounters for weaning from a mechanical ventilator, assign a code from subcategory J96.1, Chronic respiratory failure, followed by code Z99.11, Dependence on respirator [ventilator] status.

The status Z codes/categories are:

Z14   Genetic carrier

Genetic carrier status indicates that a person carries a gene, associated with a particular disease, which may be passed to offspring who may develop that disease. The person does not have the disease and is not at risk of developing the disease.

Z15   Genetic susceptibility to disease

Genetic susceptibility indicates that a person has a gene that increases the risk of that person developing the disease.

Codes from category Z15 should not be used as principal or first-listed codes. If the patient has the condition to which he/she is susceptible, and that condition is the reason for the encounter, the code for the current condition should be sequenced first. If the patient is being seen for follow-up after completed treatment for this condition, and the condition no longer exists, a follow-up code should be sequenced first, followed by the appropriate personal history and genetic susceptibility codes. If the purpose of the encounter is genetic counseling associated with procreative management, code Z31.5, Encounter for genetic counseling, should be assigned as the first-listed code, followed by a code from category Z15. Additional codes should be assigned for any applicable family or personal history.

Z16   Resistance to antimicrobial drugs

This code indicates that a patient has a condition that is resistant to antimicrobial drug treatment. Sequence the infection code first.

Z17   Estrogen receptor status

Z18   Retained foreign body fragments

Z19   Hormone sensitivity malignancy status

Z21   Asymptomatic HIV infection status

This code indicates that a patient has tested positive for HIV but has manifested no signs or symptoms of the disease.

Z22   Carrier of infectious disease

Carrier status indicates that a person harbors the specific organisms of a disease without manifest symptoms and is capable of transmitting the infection.

Z28.3   Underimmunization status

Z33.1   Pregnant state, incidental

This code is a secondary code only for use when the pregnancy is in no way complicating the reason for visit. Otherwise, a code from the obstetric chapter is required.

Z66   Do not resuscitate

This code may be used when it is documented by the provider that a patient is on do not resuscitate status at any time during the stay.

Z67   Blood type

Z68   Body mass index (BMI)

BMI codes should only be assigned when **there is an associated, reportable diagnosis (such as obesity).** Do not assign BMI codes during pregnancy.

See Section I.B.14 for BMI documentation by clinicians other than the patient's provider.

Z74.01   Bed confinement status

Z76.82   Awaiting organ transplant status

Z78   Other specified health status

Code Z78.1, Physical restraint status, may be used when it is documented by the provider that a patient has been put in restraints during the current encounter. Please note that this code should not be reported when it is documented by the provider that a patient is temporarily restrained during a procedure.

Z79   Long-term (current) drug therapy

Codes from this category indicate a patient's continuous use of a prescribed drug (including such things as aspirin therapy) for the long-term treatment of a condition or for prophylactic use. It is not for use for patients who have addictions to drugs. This subcategory is not for use of medications for detoxification or maintenance programs to prevent withdrawal symptoms in patients with drug dependence (e.g., methadone maintenance for opiate dependence). Assign the appropriate code for the drug dependence instead.

Assign a code from Z79 if the patient is receiving a medication for an extended period as a prophylactic measure (such as for the prevention of deep vein thrombosis) or as treatment of a chronic condition (such as arthritis) or a disease requiring a lengthy course of treatment (such as cancer). Do not assign a code from category Z79 for medication being administered for a brief period of time to treat an acute illness or injury (such as a course of antibiotics to treat acute bronchitis).

Z88   Allergy status to drugs, medicaments and biological substances

Except: Z88.9, Allergy status to unspecified drugs, medicaments and biological substances status

Z89   Acquired absence of limb

Z90   Acquired absence of organs, not elsewhere classified

Z91.0-   Allergy status, other than to drugs and biological substances

Z92.82   Status post administration of tPA (rtPA) in a different facility within the last 24 hours prior to admission to a current facility

Assign code Z92.82, Status post administration of tPA (rtPA) in a different facility within the last 24 hours prior to admission to current facility, as a secondary diagnosis when a patient is received by transfer into a facility and documentation indicates they were administered tissue

plasminogen activator (tPA) within the last 24 hours prior to admission to the current facility.

This guideline applies even if the patient is still receiving the tPA at the time they are received into the current facility.

The appropriate code for the condition for which the tPA was administered (such as cerebrovascular disease or myocardial infarction) should be assigned first.

Code Z92.82 is only applicable to the receiving facility record and not to the transferring facility record.

Z93   Artificial opening status

Z94   Transplanted organ and tissue status

Z95   Presence of cardiac and vascular implants and grafts

Z96   Presence of other functional implants

Z97   Presence of other devices

Z98   Other postprocedural states

Assign code Z98.85, Transplanted organ removal status, to indicate that a transplanted organ has been previously removed. This code should not be assigned for the encounter in which the transplanted organ is removed. The complication necessitating removal of the transplant organ should be assigned for that encounter.

See section I.C19. for information on the coding of organ transplant complications.

Z99   Dependence on enabling machines and devices, not elsewhere classified

Note: Categories Z89-Z90 and Z93-Z99 are for use only if there are no complications or malfunctions of the organ or tissue replaced, the amputation site or the equipment on which the patient is dependent.

4)   **History (of)**

There are two types of history Z codes, personal and family. Personal history codes explain a patient's past medical condition that no longer exists and is not receiving any treatment, but that has the potential for recurrence, and therefore may require continued monitoring.

Family history codes are for use when a patient has a family member(s) who has had a particular disease that causes the patient to be at higher risk of also contracting the disease.

Personal history codes may be used in conjunction with follow-up codes and family history codes may be used in conjunction with screening codes to explain the need for a test or procedure. History codes are also acceptable on any medical record regardless of the reason for visit. A history of an illness, even if no longer present, is important information that may alter the type of treatment ordered.

The history Z code categories are:

Z80   Family history of primary malignant neoplasm

Z81   Family history of mental and behavioral disorders

Z82   Family history of certain disabilities and chronic diseases (leading to disablement)

Z83   Family history of other specific disorders

Z84   Family history of other conditions

Z85   Personal history of malignant neoplasm

Z86   Personal history of certain other diseases

Z87   Personal history of other diseases and conditions

Z91.4-   Personal history of psychological trauma, not elsewhere classified

Z91.5   Personal history of self-harm

Z91.81   History of falling

Z91.82   Personal history of military deployment

Z92   Personal history of medical treatment

Except: Z92.0, Personal history of contraception

Except: Z92.82, Status post administration of tPA (rtPA) in a different facility within the last 24 hours prior to admission to a current facility

5)   **Screening**

Screening is the testing for disease or disease precursors in seemingly well individuals so that early detection and treatment can be provided for those who test positive for the disease (e.g., screening mammogram).

The testing of a person to rule out or confirm a suspected diagnosis because the patient has some sign or symptom is a diagnostic examination, not a screening. In these cases, the sign or symptom is used to explain the reason for the test.

A screening code may be a first-listed code if the reason for the visit is specifically the screening exam. It may also be used as an additional code if the screening is done during an office visit for other health problems. A screening code is not necessary if the screening is inherent to a routine examination, such as a pap smear done during a routine pelvic examination.

Should a condition be discovered during the screening then the code for the condition may be assigned as an additional diagnosis.

The Z code indicates that a screening exam is planned. A procedure code is required to confirm that the screening was performed.

The screening Z codes/categories:

Z11   Encounter for screening for infectious and parasitic diseases
Z12   Encounter for screening for malignant neoplasms
Z13   Encounter for screening for other diseases and disorders
       Except: Z13.9, Encounter for screening, unspecified
Z36   Encounter for antenatal screening for mother

6) **Observation**

There are three observation Z code categories. They are for use in very limited circumstances when a person is being observed for a suspected condition that is ruled out. The observation codes are not for use if an injury or illness or any signs or symptoms related to the suspected condition are present. In such cases the diagnosis/symptom code is used with the corresponding external cause code.

The observation codes are to be used as principal diagnosis only. The only exception to this is when the principal diagnosis is required to be a code from category Z38, Liveborn infants according to place of birth and type of delivery. Then a code from category Z05, Encounter for observation and evaluation of newborn for suspected diseases and conditions ruled out, is sequenced after the Z38 code. Additional codes may be used in addition to the observation code, but only if they are unrelated to the suspected condition being observed.

Codes from subcategory Z03.7, Encounter for suspected maternal and fetal conditions ruled out, may either be used as a first-listed or as an additional code assignment depending on the case. They are for use in very limited circumstances on a maternal record when an encounter is for a suspected maternal or fetal condition that is ruled out during that encounter (for example, a maternal or fetal condition may be suspected due to an abnormal test result). These codes should not be used when the condition is confirmed. In those cases, the confirmed condition should be coded. In addition, these codes are not for use if an illness or any signs or symptoms related to the suspected condition or problem are present. In such cases the diagnosis/symptom code is used.

Additional codes may be used in addition to the code from subcategory Z03.7, but only if they are unrelated to the suspected condition being evaluated.

Codes from subcategory Z03.7 may not be used for encounters for antenatal screening of mother. *See Section I.C.21. Screening.*

For encounters for suspected fetal condition that are inconclusive following testing and evaluation, assign the appropriate code from category O35, O36, O40 or O41.

The observation Z code categories:

Z03   Encounter for medical observation for suspected diseases and conditions ruled out
Z04   Encounter for examination and observation for other reasons
       Except: Z04.9, Encounter for examination and observation for unspecified reason
Z05   Encounter for observation and evaluation of newborn for suspected diseases and conditions ruled out

7) **Aftercare**

Aftercare visit codes cover situations when the initial treatment of a disease has been performed and the patient requires continued care during the healing or recovery phase, or for the long-term consequences of the disease. The aftercare Z code should not be used if treatment is directed at a current, acute disease. The diagnosis code is to be used in these cases. Exceptions to this rule are codes Z51.0, Encounter for antineoplastic radiation therapy, and codes from subcategory Z51.1, Encounter for antineoplastic chemotherapy and immunotherapy. These codes are to be first-listed, followed by the diagnosis code when a patient's encounter is solely to receive radiation therapy, chemotherapy, or immunotherapy for the treatment of a neoplasm. If the reason for the encounter is more than one type of antineoplastic therapy, code Z51.0 and a code from subcategory Z51.1 may be assigned together, in which case one of these codes would be reported as a secondary diagnosis.

The aftercare Z codes should also not be used for aftercare for injuries. For aftercare of an injury, assign the acute injury code with the appropriate 7th character (for subsequent encounter).

The aftercare codes are generally first-listed to explain the specific reason for the encounter. An aftercare code may be used as an additional code when some type of aftercare is provided in addition to the reason for admission and no diagnosis code is applicable. An example of this would be the closure of a colostomy during an encounter for treatment of another condition.

Aftercare codes should be used in conjunction with other aftercare codes or diagnosis codes to provide better detail on the specifics of an aftercare encounter visit, unless otherwise directed by the classification. The sequencing of multiple aftercare codes depends on the circumstances of the encounter.

Certain aftercare Z code categories need a secondary diagnosis code to describe the resolving condition or sequelae. For others, the condition is included in the code title.

Additional Z code aftercare category terms include fitting and adjustment, and attention to artificial openings.

Status Z codes may be used with aftercare Z codes to indicate the nature of the aftercare. For example, code Z95.1, Presence of aortocoronary bypass graft, may be used with code Z48.812, Encounter for surgical aftercare following surgery on the circulatory system, to indicate the surgery for which the aftercare is being performed. A status code should not be used when the aftercare code indicates the type of status, such as using Z43.0, Encounter for attention to tracheostomy, with Z93.0, Tracheostomy status.

The aftercare Z category/codes:

Z42   Encounter for plastic and reconstructive surgery following medical procedure or healed injury
Z43   Encounter for attention to artificial openings
Z44   Encounter for fitting and adjustment of external prosthetic device
Z45   Encounter for adjustment and management of implanted device
Z46   Encounter for fitting and adjustment of other devices
Z47   Orthopedic aftercare
Z48   Encounter for other postprocedural aftercare
Z49   Encounter for care involving renal dialysis
Z51   Encounter for other aftercare and medical care

8) **Follow-up**

The follow-up codes are used to explain continuing surveillance following completed treatment of a disease, condition, or injury. They imply that the condition has been fully treated and no longer exists. They should not be confused with aftercare codes, or injury codes with a 7th character for subsequent encounter, that explain ongoing care of a healing condition or its sequelae. Follow-up codes may be used in conjunction with history codes to provide the full picture of the healed condition and its treatment. The follow-up code is sequenced first, followed by the history code.

A follow-up code may be used to explain multiple visits. Should a condition be found to have recurred on the follow-up visit, then the diagnosis code for the condition should be assigned in place of the follow-up code.

The follow-up Z code categories:

Z08   Encounter for follow-up examination after completed treatment for malignant neoplasm

Z09   Encounter for follow-up examination after completed treatment for conditions other than malignant neoplasm

Z39   Encounter for maternal postpartum care and examination

9) Donor

Codes in category Z52, Donors of organs and tissues, are used for living individuals who are donating blood or other body tissue. These codes are only for individuals donating for others, not for self-donations. They are not used to identify cadaveric donations.

10) Counseling

Counseling Z codes are used when a patient or family member receives assistance in the aftermath of an illness or injury, or when support is required in coping with family or social problems.

The counseling Z codes/categories:

Z30.0-   Encounter for general counseling and advice on contraception

Z31.5   Encounter for procreative genetic counseling

Z31.6-   Encounter for general counseling and advice on procreation

Z32.2   Encounter for childbirth instruction

Z32.3   Encounter for childcare instruction

Z69   Encounter for mental health services for victim and perpetrator of abuse

Z70   Counseling related to sexual attitude, behavior and orientation

Z71   Persons encountering health services for other counseling and medical advice, not elsewhere classified

Note: Code Z71.84, Encounter for health counseling related to travel, is to be used for health risk and safety counseling for future travel purposes.

Z76.81   Expectant mother prebirth pediatrician visit

11) Encounters for Obstetrical and Reproductive Services

See Section I.C.15. Pregnancy, Childbirth, and the Puerperium, for further instruction on the use of these codes.

Z codes for pregnancy are for use in those circumstances when none of the problems or complications included in the codes from the Obstetrics chapter exist (a routine prenatal visit or postpartum care). Codes in category Z34, Encounter for supervision of normal pregnancy, are always first-listed and are not to be used with any other code from the OB chapter.

Codes in category Z3A, Weeks of gestation, may be assigned to provide additional information about the pregnancy. Category Z3A codes should not be assigned for pregnancies with abortive outcomes (categories O00-O08), elective termination of pregnancy (code Z33.2), nor for postpartum conditions, as category Z3A is not applicable to these conditions. The date of the admission should be used to determine weeks of gestation for inpatient admissions that encompass more than one gestational week.

The outcome of delivery, category Z37, should be included on all maternal delivery records. It is always a secondary code. Codes in category Z37 should not be used on the newborn record.

Z codes for family planning (contraceptive) or procreative management and counseling should be included on an obstetric record either during the pregnancy or the postpartum stage, if applicable.

Z codes/categories for obstetrical and reproductive services:

Z30   Encounter for contraceptive management

Z31   Encounter for procreative management

Z32.2   Encounter for childbirth instruction

Z32.3   Encounter for childcare instruction

Z33   Pregnant state

Z34   Encounter for supervision of normal pregnancy

Z36   Encounter for antenatal screening of mother

Z3A   Weeks of gestation

Z37   Outcome of delivery

Z39   Encounter for maternal postpartum care and examination

Z76.81   Expectant mother prebirth pediatrician visit

12) Newborns and Infants

See Section I.C.16. Newborn (Perinatal) Guidelines, for further instruction on the use of these codes.

Newborn Z codes/categories:

Z76.1   Encounter for health supervision and care of foundling

Z00.1-   Encounter for routine child health examination

Z38   Liveborn infants according to place of birth and type of delivery

13) Routine and Administrative Examinations

The Z codes allow for the description of encounters for routine examinations, such as, a general check-up, or, examinations for administrative purposes, such as, a pre-employment physical. The codes are not to be used if the examination is for diagnosis of a suspected condition or for treatment purposes. In such cases the diagnosis code is used. During a routine exam, should a diagnosis or condition be discovered, it should be coded as an additional code. Pre-existing and chronic conditions and history codes may also be included as additional codes as long as the examination is for administrative purposes and not focused on any particular condition.

Some of the codes for routine health examinations distinguish between "with" and "without" abnormal findings. Code assignment depends on the information that is known at the time the encounter is being coded. For example, if no abnormal findings were found during the examination, but the encounter is being coded before test results are back, it is acceptable to assign the code for "without abnormal findings." When assigning a code for "with abnormal findings," additional code(s) should be assigned to identify the specific abnormal finding(s).

Pre-operative examination and pre-procedural laboratory examination Z codes are for use only in those situations when a patient is being cleared for a procedure or surgery and no treatment is given.

The Z codes/categories for routine and administrative examinations:

Z00   Encounter for general examination without complaint, suspected or reported diagnosis

Z01   Encounter for other special examination without complaint, suspected or reported diagnosis

Z02   Encounter for administrative examination

      Except: Z02.9, Encounter for administrative examinations, unspecified

Z32.0-   Encounter for pregnancy test

14) Miscellaneous Z *Codes*

The miscellaneous Z codes capture a number of other health care encounters that do not fall into one of the other categories. Certain of these codes identify the reason for the encounter; others are for use as additional codes that provide useful information on circumstances that may affect a patient's care and treatment.

Prophylactic Organ Removal

For encounters specifically for prophylactic removal of an organ (such as prophylactic removal of breasts due to a genetic susceptibility to cancer or a family history of cancer), the principal or first-listed code should be a code from category Z40, Encounter for prophylactic surgery, followed by the appropriate codes to identify the associated risk factor (such as genetic susceptibility or family history).

If the patient has a malignancy of one site and is having prophylactic removal at another site to prevent either a new primary malignancy or metastatic disease, a code for the malignancy should also be assigned in addition to a code from subcategory Z40.0, Encounter for prophylactic surgery for risk factors related to malignant neoplasms. A Z40.0 code should not be assigned if the patient is having organ removal for treatment of a malignancy, such as the removal of the testes for the treatment of prostate cancer.

Miscellaneous Z codes/categories:

Z28   Immunization not carried out

       Except: Z28.3, Underimmunization status

Z29   Encounter for other prophylactic measures

Z40   Encounter for prophylactic surgery

Z41   Encounter for procedures for purposes other than remedying health state

       Except: Z41.9, Encounter for procedure for purposes other than remedying health state, unspecified

Z53   Persons encountering health services for specific procedures and treatment, not carried out

Z55   Problems related to education and literacy

Z56   Problems related to employment and unemployment

Z57   Occupational exposure to risk factors

Z58   Problems related to physical environment

Z59   Problems related to housing and economic circumstances

Z60   Problems related to social environment

Z62   Problems related to upbringing

Z63   Other problems related to primary support group, including family circumstances

Z64   Problems related to certain psychosocial circumstances

Z65   Problems related to other psychosocial circumstances

Z72   Problems related to lifestyle

       Note: These codes should be assigned only when the documentation specifies that the patient has an associated problem

Z73   Problems related to life management difficulty

Z74   Problems related to care provider dependency

       Except: Z74.01, Bed confinement status

Z75   Problems related to medical facilities and other health care

Z76.0   Encounter for issue of repeat prescription

Z76.3   Healthy person accompanying sick person

Z76.4   Other boarder to healthcare facility

Z76.5   Malingerer [conscious simulation]

Z91.1-   Patient's noncompliance with medical treatment and regimen

Z91.83   Wandering in diseases classified elsewhere

Z91.84-   Oral health risk factors

Z91.89   Other specified personal risk factors, not elsewhere classified

See Section I.B.14 for Z55-Z65 Persons with potential health hazards related to socioeconomic and psychosocial circumstances, documentation by clinicians other than the patient's provider.

15) **Nonspecific Z Codes**

Certain Z codes are so non-specific, or potentially redundant with other codes in the classification, that there can be little justification for their use in the inpatient setting. Their use in the outpatient setting should be limited to those instances when there is no further documentation to permit more precise coding. Otherwise, any sign or symptom or any other reason for visit that is captured in another code should be used.

Nonspecific Z codes/categories:

Z02.9   Encounter for administrative examinations, unspecified

Z04.9   Encounter for examination and observation for unspecified reason

Z13.9   Encounter for screening, unspecified

Z41.9   Encounter for procedure for purposes other than remedying health state, unspecified

Z52.9   Donor of unspecified organ or tissue

Z86.59   Personal history of other mental and behavioral disorders

Z88.9   Allergy status to unspecified drugs, medicaments and biological substances status

Z92.0   Personal history of contraception

16) **Z Codes That May Only be Principal/First-Listed Diagnosis**

The following Z codes/categories may only be reported as the principal/first-listed diagnosis, except when there are multiple encounters on the same day and the medical records for the encounters are combined:

Z00   Encounter for general examination without complaint, suspected or reported diagnosis

       Except: Z00.6

Z01   Encounter for other special examination without complaint, suspected or reported diagnosis

Z02   Encounter for administrative examination

Z03   Encounter for medical observation for suspected diseases and conditions ruled out

Z04   Encounter for examination and observation for other reasons

Z33.2   Encounter for elective termination of pregnancy

Z31.81   Encounter for male factor infertility in female patient

Z31.83   Encounter for assisted reproductive fertility procedure cycle

Z31.84   Encounter for fertility preservation procedure

Z34   Encounter for supervision of normal pregnancy

Z39   Encounter for maternal postpartum care and examination

Z38   Liveborn infants according to place of birth and type of delivery

Z40   Encounter for prophylactic surgery

Z42   Encounter for plastic and reconstructive surgery following medical procedure or healed injury

Z51.0   Encounter for antineoplastic radiation therapy

Z51.1-   Encounter for antineoplastic chemotherapy and immunotherapy

Z52   Donors of organs and tissues

       Except: Z52.9, Donor of unspecified organ or tissue

Z76.1   Encounter for health supervision and care of foundling

Z76.2   Encounter for health supervision and care of other healthy infant and child

Z99.12   Encounter for respirator [ventilator] dependence during power failure

Section II. Selection of Principal Diagnosis

The circumstances of inpatient admission always govern the selection of principal diagnosis. The principal diagnosis is defined in the Uniform Hospital Discharge Data Set (UHDDS) as "that condition established after study to be chiefly responsible for occasioning the admission of the patient to the hospital for care."

The UHDDS definitions are used by hospitals to report inpatient data elements in a standardized manner. These data elements and their definitions can be found in the July 31, 1985, Federal Register (Vol. 50, No, 147), pp. 31038-40.

Since that time the application of the UHDDS definitions has been expanded to include all non-outpatient settings (acute care, short term, long term care and psychiatric hospitals; home health agencies; rehab facilities; nursing homes, etc). The UHDDS definitions also apply to hospice services (all levels of care).

In determining principal diagnosis, coding conventions in the ICD-10-CM, the Tabular List and Alphabetic Index take precedence over these official coding guidelines.

(See Section I.A., Conventions for the ICD-10-CM)

The importance of consistent, complete documentation in the medical record cannot be overemphasized. Without such documentation the application of all coding guidelines is a difficult, if not impossible, task.

A. **Codes for symptoms, signs, and ill-defined conditions**

Codes for symptoms, signs, and ill-defined conditions from Chapter 18 are not to be used as principal diagnosis when a related definitive diagnosis has been established.

B. **Two or more interrelated conditions, each potentially meeting the definition for principal diagnosis.**

When there are two or more interrelated conditions (such as diseases in the same ICD-10-CM chapter or manifestations characteristically associated with a certain disease) potentially meeting the definition of principal diagnosis, either condition may be sequenced first, unless the circumstances of the admission, the therapy provided, the Tabular List, or the Alphabetic Index indicate otherwise.

C. Two or more diagnoses that equally meet the definition for principal diagnosis

In the unusual instance when two or more diagnoses equally meet the criteria for principal diagnosis as determined by the circumstances of admission, diagnostic workup and/or therapy provided, and the Alphabetic Index, Tabular List, or another coding guidelines does not provide sequencing direction, any one of the diagnoses may be sequenced first.

D. Two or more comparative or contrasting conditions

In those rare instances when two or more contrasting or comparative diagnoses are documented as "either/or" (or similar terminology), they are coded as if the diagnoses were confirmed and the diagnoses are sequenced according to the circumstances of the admission. If no further determination can be made as to which diagnosis should be principal, either diagnosis may be sequenced first.

E. A symptom(s) followed by contrasting/comparative diagnoses

GUIDELINE HAS BEEN DELETED EFFECTIVE OCTOBER 1, 2014

F. Original treatment plan not carried out

Sequence as the principal diagnosis the condition, which after study occasioned the admission to the hospital, even though treatment may not have been carried out due to unforeseen circumstances.

G. Complications of surgery and other medical care

When the admission is for treatment of a complication resulting from surgery or other medical care, the complication code is sequenced as the principal diagnosis. If the complication is classified to the T80-T88 series and the code lacks the necessary specificity in describing the complication, an additional code for the specific complication should be assigned.

H. Uncertain Diagnosis

If the diagnosis documented at the time of discharge is qualified as "probable," "suspected," "likely," "questionable," "possible," or "still to be ruled out," **"compatible with," "consistent with,"** or other similar terms indicating uncertainty, code the condition as if it existed or was established. The bases for these guidelines are the diagnostic workup, arrangements for further workup or observation, and initial therapeutic approach that correspond most closely with the established diagnosis.

Note: This guideline is applicable only to inpatient admissions to short-term, acute, long-term care and psychiatric hospitals.

I. Admission from Observation Unit

1. Admission Following Medical Observation

When a patient is admitted to an observation unit for a medical condition, which either worsens or does not improve, and is subsequently admitted as an inpatient of the same hospital for this same medical condition, the principal diagnosis would be the medical condition which led to the hospital admission.

2. Admission Following Post-Operative Observation

When a patient is admitted to an observation unit to monitor a condition (or complication) that develops following outpatient surgery, and then is subsequently admitted as an inpatient of the same hospital, hospitals should apply the Uniform Hospital Discharge Data Set (UHDDS) definition of principal diagnosis as "that condition established after study to be chiefly responsible for occasioning the admission of the patient to the hospital for care."

J. Admission from Outpatient Surgery

When a patient receives surgery in the hospital's outpatient surgery department and is subsequently admitted for continuing inpatient care at the same hospital, the following guidelines should be followed in selecting the principal diagnosis for the inpatient admission:

- If the reason for the inpatient admission is a complication, assign the complication as the principal diagnosis.
- If no complication, or other condition, is documented as the reason for the inpatient admission, assign the reason for the outpatient surgery as the principal diagnosis.
- If the reason for the inpatient admission is another condition unrelated to the surgery, assign the unrelated condition as the principal diagnosis.

K. Admissions/Encounters for Rehabilitation

When the purpose for the admission/encounter is rehabilitation, sequence first the code for the condition for which the service is being performed. For example, for an admission/encounter for rehabilitation for right-sided dominant hemiplegia following a cerebrovascular infarction, report code I69.351, Hemiplegia and hemiparesis following cerebral infarction affecting right dominant side, as the first-listed or principal diagnosis.

If the condition for which the rehabilitation service is being provided is no longer present, report the appropriate aftercare code as the first-listed or principal diagnosis, unless the rehabilitation service is being provided following an injury. For rehabilitation services following active treatment of an injury, assign the injury code with the appropriate seventh character for subsequent encounter as the first-listed or principal diagnosis. For example, if a patient with severe degenerative osteoarthritis of the hip, underwent hip replacement and the current encounter/admission is for rehabilitation, report code Z47.1, Aftercare following joint replacement surgery, as the first-listed or principal diagnosis. If the patient requires rehabilitation post hip replacement for right intertrochanteric femur fracture, report code S72.141D, Displaced intertrochanteric fracture of right femur, subsequent encounter for closed fracture with routine healing, as the first-listed or principal diagnosis.

See Section I.C.21.c.7, Factors influencing health states and contact with health services, Aftercare.

See Section I.C.19.a for additional information about the use of 7th characters for injury codes.

Section III. Reporting Additional Diagnoses

GENERAL RULES FOR OTHER (ADDITIONAL) DIAGNOSES

For reporting purposes the definition for "other diagnoses" is interpreted as additional conditions that affect patient care in terms of requiring:

clinical evaluation; or
therapeutic treatment; or
diagnostic procedures; or
extended length of hospital stay; or
increased nursing care and/or monitoring.

The UHDDS item #11-b defines Other Diagnoses as "all conditions that coexist at the time of admission, that develop subsequently, or that affect the treatment received and/or the length of stay. Diagnoses that relate to an earlier episode which have no bearing on the current hospital stay are to be excluded." UHDDS definitions apply to inpatients in acute care, short-term, long term care and psychiatric hospital setting. The UHDDS definitions are used by acute care short-term hospitals to report inpatient data elements in a standardized manner. These data elements and their definitions can be found in the July 31, 1985, Federal Register (Vol. 50, No, 147), pp. 31038-40.

Since that time the application of the UHDDS definitions has been expanded to include all non-outpatient settings (acute care, short term, long term care and psychiatric hospitals; home health agencies; rehab facilities; nursing homes, etc). The UHDDS definitions also apply to hospice services (all levels of care).

The following guidelines are to be applied in designating "other diagnoses" when neither the Alphabetic Index nor the Tabular List in ICD-10-CM provide direction. The listing of the diagnoses in the patient record is the responsibility of the attending provider.

A. Previous conditions

If the provider has included a diagnosis in the final diagnostic statement, such as the discharge summary or the face sheet, it should ordinarily be coded. Some providers include in the diagnostic statement resolved conditions or diagnoses and status-post procedures from previous admission that have no bearing on the current stay. Such conditions are not to be reported and are coded only if required by hospital policy.

However, history codes (categories Z80-Z87) may be used as secondary codes if the historical condition or family history has an impact on current care or influences treatment.

B. Abnormal findings

Abnormal findings (laboratory, x-ray, pathologic, and other diagnostic results) are not coded and reported unless the provider indicates their clinical significance. If the findings are outside the normal range and the attending provider has ordered other tests to evaluate the condition or prescribed treatment, it is appropriate to ask the provider whether the abnormal finding should be added.

Please note: This differs from the coding practices in the outpatient setting for coding encounters for diagnostic tests that have been interpreted by a provider.

C. Uncertain Diagnosis

If the diagnosis documented at the time of discharge is qualified as "probable," "suspected," "likely," "questionable," "possible," or "still to be ruled out," **"compatible with," "consistent with,"** or other similar terms indicating uncertainty, code the condition as if it existed or was established. The bases for these guidelines are the diagnostic workup, arrangements for further workup or observation, and initial therapeutic approach that correspond most closely with the established diagnosis.

Note: This guideline is applicable only to inpatient admissions to short-term, acute, long-term care and psychiatric hospitals.

Section IV. Diagnostic Coding and Reporting Guidelines for Outpatient Services

These coding guidelines for outpatient diagnoses have been approved for use by hospitals/ providers in coding and reporting hospital-based outpatient services and provider-based office visits. Guidelines in Section I, Conventions, general coding guidelines and chapter-specific guidelines, should also be applied for outpatient services and office visits.

Information about the use of certain abbreviations, punctuation, symbols, and other conventions used in the ICD-10-CM Tabular List (code numbers and titles), can be found in Section IA of these guidelines, under "Conventions Used in the Tabular List." Section I.B. contains general guidelines that apply to the entire classification. Section I.C. contains chapter-specific guidelines that correspond to the chapters as they are arranged in the classification. Information about the correct sequence to use in finding a code is also described in Section I.

The terms encounter and visit are often used interchangeably in describing outpatient service contacts and, therefore, appear together in these guidelines without distinguishing one from the other.

Though the conventions and general guidelines apply to all settings, coding guidelines for outpatient and provider reporting of diagnoses will vary in a number of instances from those for inpatient diagnoses, recognizing that:

The Uniform Hospital Discharge Data Set (UHDDS) definition of principal diagnosis does not apply to hospital-based outpatient services and provider-based office visits.

Coding guidelines for inconclusive diagnoses (probable, suspected, rule out, etc.) were developed for inpatient reporting and do not apply to outpatients.

A. Selection of first-listed condition

In the outpatient setting, the term first-listed diagnosis is used in lieu of principal diagnosis.

In determining the first-listed diagnosis the coding conventions of ICD-10-CM, as well as the general and disease specific guidelines take precedence over the outpatient guidelines.

Diagnoses often are not established at the time of the initial encounter/visit. It may take two or more visits before the diagnosis is confirmed.

The most critical rule involves beginning the search for the correct code assignment through the Alphabetic Index. Never begin searching initially in the Tabular List as this will lead to coding errors.

1. Outpatient Surgery

When a patient presents for outpatient surgery (same day surgery), code the reason for the surgery as the first-listed diagnosis (reason for the encounter), even if the surgery is not performed due to a contraindication.

2. Observation Stay

When a patient is admitted for observation for a medical condition, assign a code for the medical condition as the first-listed diagnosis.

When a patient presents for outpatient surgery and develops complications requiring admission to observation, code the reason for the surgery as the first reported diagnosis (reason for the encounter), followed by codes for the complications as secondary diagnoses.

B. Codes from A00.0 through T88.9, Z00-Z99

The appropriate code(s) from A00.0 through T88.9, Z00-Z99 must be used to identify diagnoses, symptoms, conditions, problems, complaints, or other reason(s) for the encounter/visit.

C. Accurate reporting of ICD-10-CM diagnosis codes

For accurate reporting of ICD-10-CM diagnosis codes, the documentation should describe the patient's condition, using terminology which includes specific diagnoses as well as symptoms, problems, or reasons for the encounter. There are ICD-10-CM codes to describe all of these.

D. Codes that describe symptoms and signs

Codes that describe symptoms and signs, as opposed to diagnoses, are acceptable for reporting purposes when a diagnosis has not been established (confirmed) by the provider. Chapter 18 of ICD-10-CM, Symptoms, Signs, and Abnormal Clinical and Laboratory Findings Not Elsewhere Classified (codes R00-R99) contain many, but not all codes for symptoms.

E. Encounters for circumstances other than a disease or injury

ICD-10-CM provides codes to deal with encounters for circumstances other than a disease or injury. The Factors Influencing Health Status and Contact with Health Services codes (Z00-Z99) are provided to deal with occasions when circumstances other than a disease or injury are recorded as diagnosis or problems.

See Section I.C.21. Factors influencing health status and contact with health services.

F. Level of Detail in Coding

1. ICD-10-CM codes with 3, 4, 5, 6 or 7 characters

ICD-10-CM is composed of codes with 3, 4, 5, 6 or 7 characters. Codes with three characters are included in ICD-10-CM as the heading of a category of codes that may be further subdivided by the use of fourth, fifth, sixth or seventh characters to provide greater specificity.

2. Use of full number of characters required for a code

A three-character code is to be used only if it is not further subdivided. A code is invalid if it has not been coded to the full number of characters required for that code, including the 7th character, if applicable.

G. ICD-10-CM code for the diagnosis, condition, problem, or other reason for encounter/visit

List first the ICD-10-CM code for the diagnosis, condition, problem, or other reason for encounter/visit shown in the medical record to be chiefly responsible for the services provided. List additional codes that describe any coexisting conditions. In some cases the first-listed diagnosis may be a symptom when a diagnosis has not been established (confirmed) by the **provider**.

H. Uncertain diagnosis

Do not code diagnoses documented as "probable", "suspected," "questionable," "rule out," **"compatible with," "consistent with,"** or "working diagnosis" or other similar terms indicating uncertainty. Rather, code the condition(s) to the highest degree of certainty for that encounter/visit, such as symptoms, signs, abnormal test results, or other reason for the visit.

Please note: This differs from the coding practices used by short-term, acute care, long-term care and psychiatric hospitals.

I. Chronic diseases

Chronic diseases treated on an ongoing basis may be coded and reported as many times as the patient receives treatment and care for the condition(s)

J. Code all documented conditions that coexist

Code all documented conditions that coexist at the time of the encounter/visit, and require or affect patient care treatment or management. Do not code conditions that were previously treated and no longer exist. However, history codes (categories Z80-Z87) may be used as secondary codes if the historical condition or family history has an impact on current care or influences treatment.

K. Patients receiving diagnostic services only

For patients receiving diagnostic services only during an encounter/visit, sequence first the diagnosis, condition, problem, or other reason for encounter/visit shown in the medical record to be chiefly responsible for the outpatient services provided during the encounter/visit. Codes for other diagnoses (e.g., chronic conditions) may be sequenced as additional diagnoses.

For encounters for routine laboratory/radiology testing in the absence of any signs, symptoms, or associated diagnosis, assign Z01.89, Encounter for other specified special examinations. If routine testing is performed during the same encounter as a test to evaluate a sign, symptom, or diagnosis, it is appropriate to assign both the Z code and the code describing the reason for the non-routine test.

For outpatient encounters for diagnostic tests that have been interpreted by a physician, and the final report is available at the time of coding, code any confirmed or definitive diagnosis(es) documented in the interpretation. Do not code related signs and symptoms as additional diagnoses.

Please note: This differs from the coding practice in the hospital inpatient setting regarding abnormal findings on test results.

L. Patients receiving therapeutic services only

For patients receiving therapeutic services only during an encounter/visit, sequence first the diagnosis, condition, problem, or other reason for encounter/visit shown in the medical record to be chiefly responsible for the outpatient services provided during the encounter/visit. Codes for other diagnoses (e.g., chronic conditions) may be sequenced as additional diagnoses.

The only exception to this rule is that when the primary reason for the admission/encounter is chemotherapy or radiation therapy, the appropriate Z code for the service is listed first, and the diagnosis or problem for which the service is being performed listed second.

M. Patients receiving preoperative evaluations only

For patients receiving preoperative evaluations only, sequence first a code from subcategory Z01.81, Encounter for pre-procedural examinations, to describe the pre-op consultations. Assign a code for the condition to describe the reason for the surgery as an additional diagnosis. Code also any findings related to the pre-op evaluation.

N. Ambulatory surgery

For ambulatory surgery, code the diagnosis for which the surgery was performed. If the postoperative diagnosis is known to be different from the preoperative diagnosis at the time the diagnosis is confirmed, select the postoperative diagnosis for coding, since it is the most definitive.

O. Routine outpatient prenatal visits

See Section I.C.15. Routine outpatient prenatal visits.

P. Encounters for general medical examinations with abnormal findings

The subcategories for encounters for general medical examinations, Z00.0- and encounter for routine child health examination, Z00.12-, provide codes for with and without abnormal findings. Should a general medical examination result in an abnormal finding, the code for general medical examination with abnormal finding should be assigned as the first-listed diagnosis. An examination with abnormal findings refers to a condition/diagnosis that is newly identified or a change in severity of a chronic condition (such as uncontrolled hypertension, or an acute exacerbation of chronic obstructive pulmonary disease) during a routine physical examination. A secondary code for the abnormal finding should also be coded.

Q. Encounters for routine health screenings

See Section I.C.21. Factors influencing health status and contact with health services, Screening

Appendix I. Present on Admission Reporting Guidelines

Introduction

These guidelines are to be used as a supplement to the *ICD-10-CM Official Guidelines for Coding and Reporting* to facilitate the assignment of the Present on Admission (POA) indicator for each diagnosis and external cause of injury code reported on claim forms (UB-04 and 837 Institutional).

These guidelines are not intended to replace any guidelines in the main body of the *ICD-10-CM Official Guidelines for Coding and Reporting*. The POA guidelines are not intended to provide guidance on when a condition should be coded, but rather, how to apply the POA indicator to the final set of diagnosis codes that have been assigned in accordance with Sections I, II, and III of the official coding guidelines. Subsequent to the assignment of the ICD-10-CM codes, the POA indicator should then be assigned to those conditions that have been coded.

As stated in the Introduction to the *ICD-10-CM Official Guidelines for Coding and Reporting*, a joint effort between the healthcare provider and the coder is essential to achieve complete and accurate documentation, code assignment, and reporting of diagnoses and procedures. The importance of consistent, complete documentation in the medical record cannot be overemphasized. Medical record documentation from any provider involved in the care and treatment of the patient may be used to support the determination of whether a condition was present on admission or not. In the context of the official coding guidelines, the term "provider" means a physician or any qualified healthcare practitioner who is legally accountable for establishing the patient's diagnosis.

These guidelines are not a substitute for the provider's clinical judgment as to the determination of whether a condition was/was not present on admission. The provider should be queried regarding issues related to the linking of signs/symptoms, timing of test results, and the timing of findings.

Please see the CDC website for the detailed list of ICD-10-CM codes that do not require the use of a POA indicator (https://www.cdc.gov/nchs/icd/icd10cm.htm). The codes and categories on this exempt list are for circumstances regarding the healthcare encounter or factors influencing health status that do not represent a current disease or injury or that describe conditions that are always present on admission.

General Reporting Requirements

All claims involving inpatient admissions to general acute care hospitals or other facilities that are subject to a law or regulation mandating collection of present on admission information.

Present on admission is defined as present at the time the order for inpatient admission occurs -- conditions that develop during an outpatient encounter, including emergency department, observation, or outpatient surgery, are considered as present on admission.

POA indicator is assigned to principal and secondary diagnoses (as defined in Section II of the Official Guidelines for Coding and Reporting) and the external cause of injury codes.

Issues related to inconsistent, missing, conflicting or unclear documentation must still be resolved by the provider.

If a condition would not be coded and reported based on UHDDS definitions and current official coding guidelines, then the POA indicator would not be reported.

Reporting Options

    Y - Yes

    N - No

    U - Unknown

    W – Clinically undetermined

    Unreported/Not used – (Exempt from POA reporting)

Reporting Definitions

    Y = present at the time of inpatient admission

    N = not present at the time of inpatient admission

    U = documentation is insufficient to determine if condition is present on admission

    W = provider is unable to clinically determine whether condition was present on admission or not

Timeframe for POA Identification and Documentation

There is no required timeframe as to when a provider (per the definition of "provider" used in these guidelines) must identify or document a condition to be present on admission. In some clinical situations, it may not be possible for a provider to make a definitive diagnosis (or a condition may not be recognized or reported by the patient) for a period of time after admission. In some cases it may be several days before the provider arrives at a definitive diagnosis. This does not mean that the condition was not present on admission. Determination of whether the condition was present on admission or not will be based on the applicable POA guideline as identified in this document, or on the provider's best clinical judgment.

If at the time of code assignment the documentation is unclear as to whether a condition was present on admission or not, it is appropriate to query the provider for clarification.

Assigning the POA Indicator

Condition is on the "Exempt from Reporting" list

    Leave the "present on admission" field blank if the condition is on the list of ICD-10-CM codes for which this field is not applicable. This is the only circumstance in which the field may be left blank.

POA Explicitly Documented

    Assign Y for any condition the provider explicitly documents as being present on admission.

    Assign N for any condition the provider explicitly documents as not present at the time of admission.

Conditions diagnosed prior to inpatient admission

    Assign "Y" for conditions that were diagnosed prior to admission (example: hypertension, diabetes mellitus, asthma)

Conditions diagnosed during the admission but clearly present before admission

    Assign "Y" for conditions diagnosed during the admission that were clearly present but not diagnosed until after admission occurred.

    Diagnoses subsequently confirmed after admission are considered present on admission if at the time of admission they are documented as suspected, possible, rule out, differential diagnosis, or constitute an underlying cause of a symptom that is present at the time of admission.

Condition develops during outpatient encounter prior to inpatient admission

    Assign Y for any condition that develops during an outpatient encounter prior to a written order for inpatient admission.

Documentation does not indicate whether condition was present on admission

    Assign "U" when the medical record documentation is unclear as to whether the condition was present on admission. "U" should not be routinely assigned and used only in very limited circumstances. Coders are encouraged to query the providers when the documentation is unclear.

Documentation states that it cannot be determined whether the condition was or was not present on admission

Assign "W" when the medical record documentation indicates that it cannot be clinically determined whether or not the condition was present on admission.

Chronic condition with acute exacerbation during the admission

If a single code identifies both the chronic condition and the acute exacerbation, see POA guidelines pertaining to codes that contain multiple clinical concepts.

If a single code only identifies the chronic condition and not the acute exacerbation (e.g., acute exacerbation of chronic leukemia), assign "Y."

Conditions documented as possible, probable, suspected, or rule out at the time of discharge

If the final diagnosis contains a possible, probable, suspected, or rule out diagnosis, and this diagnosis was based on signs, symptoms or clinical findings suspected at the time of inpatient admission, assign "Y."

If the final diagnosis contains a possible, probable, suspected, or rule out diagnosis, and this diagnosis was based on signs, symptoms or clinical findings that were not present on admission, assign "N".

Conditions documented as impending or threatened at the time of discharge

If the final diagnosis contains an impending or threatened diagnosis, and this diagnosis is based on symptoms or clinical findings that were present on admission, assign "Y".

If the final diagnosis contains an impending or threatened diagnosis, and this diagnosis is based on symptoms or clinical findings that were not present on admission, assign "N".

Acute and Chronic Conditions

Assign "Y" for acute conditions that are present at time of admission and N for acute conditions that are not present at time of admission.

Assign "Y" for chronic conditions, even though the condition may not be diagnosed until after admission.

If a single code identifies both an acute and chronic condition, see the POA guidelines for codes that contain multiple clinical concepts.

Codes That Contain Multiple Clinical Concepts

Assign "N" if at least one of the clinical concepts included in the code was not present on admission (e.g., COPD with acute exacerbation and the exacerbation was not present on admission; gastric ulcer that does not start bleeding until after admission; asthma patient develops status asthmaticus after admission).

Assign "Y" if all of the clinical concepts included in the code were present on admission (e.g., duodenal ulcer that perforates prior to admission).

For infection codes that include the causal organism, assign "Y" if the infection (or signs of the infection) were present on admission, even though the culture results may not be known until after admission (e.g., patient is admitted with pneumonia and the provider documents Pseudomonas as the causal organism a few days later).

Same Diagnosis Code for Two or More Conditions

When the same ICD-10-CM diagnosis code applies to two or more conditions during the same encounter (e.g. two separate conditions classified to the same ICD-10-CM diagnosis code):

Assign "Y" if all conditions represented by the single ICD-10-CM code were present on admission (e.g. bilateral unspecified age-related cataracts).

Assign "N" if any of the conditions represented by the single ICD-10-CM code was not present on admission (e.g. traumatic secondary and recurrent hemorrhage and seroma is assigned to a single code T79.2, but only one of the conditions was present on admission).

Obstetrical conditions

Whether or not the patient delivers during the current hospitalization does not affect assignment of the POA indicator. The determining factor for POA assignment is whether the pregnancy complication or obstetrical condition described by the code was present at the time of admission or not.

If the pregnancy complication or obstetrical condition was present on admission (e.g., patient admitted in preterm labor), assign "Y".

If the pregnancy complication or obstetrical condition was not present on admission (e.g., 2nd degree laceration during delivery, postpartum hemorrhage that occurred during current hospitalization, fetal distress develops after admission), assign "N".

If the obstetrical code includes more than one diagnosis and any of the diagnoses identified by the code were not present on admission assign "N". (e.g., Category O11, Pre-existing hypertension with pre-eclampsia)

Perinatal conditions

Newborns are not considered to be admitted until after birth. Therefore, any condition present at birth or that developed in utero is considered present at admission and should be assigned "Y". This includes conditions that occur during delivery (e.g., injury during delivery, meconium aspiration, exposure to streptococcus B in the vaginal canal).

Congenital conditions and anomalies

Assign "Y" for congenital conditions and anomalies except for categories Q00-Q99, Congenital anomalies, which are on the exempt list. Congenital conditions are always considered present on admission.

External cause of injury codes

Assign "Y" for any external cause code representing an external cause of morbidity that occurred prior to inpatient admission (e.g., patient fell out of bed at home, patient fell out of bed in emergency room prior to admission)

Assign "N" for any external cause code representing an external cause of morbidity that occurred during inpatient hospitalization (e.g., patient fell out of hospital bed during hospital stay, patient experienced an adverse reaction to a medication administered after inpatient admission).

A

Aarskog's syndrome Q87.19
Abandonment — *see* Maltreatment
Abasia (-astasia) (hysterical) F44.4
Abderhalden-Kaufmann-Lignac syndrome (cystinosis) E72.04
Abdomen, abdominal — *see also* condition
  muscle deficiency syndrome Q79.4
  angina K55.1
  acute R10.0
Abdominalgia — *see* Pain, abdominal
Abduction contracture, hip or other joint — *see* Contraction, joint
Aberrant (congenital) — *see also* Malposition, congenital
  hepatic duct Q44.5
  endocrine gland NEC Q89.2
  breast Q83.8
  artery (peripheral) Q27.8
    basilar NEC Q28.1
    cerebral Q28.3
    coronary Q24.5
    digestive system Q27.8
    eye Q15.8
    lower limb Q27.8
    precerebral Q28.1
    pulmonary Q25.79
    renal Q27.2
    retina Q14.1
    specified site NEC Q27.8
    subclavian Q27.8
    upper limb Q27.8
    vertebral Q28.1
  adrenal gland Q89.1
  pancreas Q45.3
  parathyroid gland Q89.2
  pituitary gland Q89.2
  sebaceous glands, mucous membrane, mouth, congenital Q38.6
  spleen Q89.09
  subclavian artery Q27.8
  thymus (gland) Q89.2
  thyroid gland Q89.2
  vein (peripheral) NEC Q27.8
    cerebral Q28.3
    digestive system Q27.8
    lower limb Q27.8
    precerebral Q28.1
    specified site NEC Q27.8
    upper limb Q27.8
Aberration
  distantial — *see* Disturbance, visual
  mental F99
Abetalipoproteinemia E78.6
Abiotrophy R68.89
Ablatio, ablation
  retinae — *see* Detachment, retina
Ablepharia, ablepharon Q10.3
Abnormal, abnormality, abnormalities — *see also* Anomaly
  acid-base balance (mixed) E87.4
  albumin R77.0
  alphafetoprotein R77.2
  alveolar ridge K08.9
  anatomical relationship Q89.9
  apertures, congenital, diaphragm Q79.1
  auditory perception H93.29- ☑
    diplacusis — *see* Diplacusis
    hyperacusis — *see* Hyperacusis
    recruitment — *see* Recruitment, auditory
    threshold shift — *see* Shift, auditory threshold
  autosomes Q99.9
    fragile site Q95.5
  basal metabolic rate R94.8
  biosynthesis, testicular androgen E29.1
  bleeding time R79.1
  blood level (of)
    cobalt R79.0
    copper R79.0
    iron R79.0
    lithium R78.89
    magnesium R79.0

Abnormal, abnormality, abnormalities — *continued*
  blood level — *continued*
    mineral NEC R79.0
    zinc R79.0
  blood pressure
    elevated R03.0
    low reading (nonspecific) R03.1
  blood sugar R73.09
  blood-gas level R79.81
  bowel sounds R19.15
    absent R19.11
    hyperactive R19.12
  brain scan R94.02
  breathing R06.9
  caloric test R94.138
  cerebrospinal fluid R83.9
    cytology R83.6
    drug level R83.2
    enzyme level R83.0
    hormones R83.1
    immunology R83.4
    microbiology R83.5
    nonmedicinal level R83.3
    specified type NEC R83.8
  chemistry, blood R79.9
    C-reactive protein R79.82
    drugs — *see* Findings, abnormal, in blood
    gas level R79.81
    minerals R79.0
    pancytopenia D61.818
    PTT R79.1
    specified NEC R79.89
    toxins — *see* Findings, abnormal, in blood
  chest sounds (friction) (rales) R09.89
  chromosome, chromosomal Q99.9
    with more than three X chromosomes, female Q97.1
    analysis result R89.8
      bronchial washings R84.8
      cerebrospinal fluid R83.8
      cervix uteri NEC R87.89
      nasal secretions R84.8
      nipple discharge R89.8
      peritoneal fluid R85.89
      pleural fluid R84.8
      prostatic secretions R86.8
      saliva R85.89
      seminal fluid R86.8
      sputum R84.8
      synovial fluid R89.8
      throat scrapings R84.8
      vagina R87.89
      vulva R87.89
      wound secretions R89.8
    dicentric replacement Q93.2
    ring replacement Q93.2
    sex Q99.8
      female phenotype Q97.9
        specified NEC Q97.8
      male phenotype Q98.9
        specified NEC Q98.8
      structural male Q98.6
    specified NEC Q99.8
  clinical findings NEC R68.89
  coagulation D68.9
    newborn, transient P61.6
    profile R79.1
    time R79.1
  communication — *see* Fistula
  conjunctiva, vascular H11.41- ☑
  coronary artery Q24.5
  cortisol-binding globulin E27.8
  course, eustachian tube Q17.8
  creatinine clearance R94.4
  cytology
    anus R85.619
      atypical squamous cells cannot exclude high grade squamous intraepithelial lesion (ASC-H) R85.611
      atypical squamous cells of undetermined significance (ASC-US) R85.610
      cytologic evidence of malignancy R85.614

Abnormal, abnormality, abnormalities — *continued*
  cytology — *continued*
    anus — *continued*
      high grade squamous intraepithelial lesion (HGSIL) R85.613
      human papillomavirus (HPV) DNA test
        high risk positive R85.81
        low risk positive R85.82
      inadequate smear R85.615
      low grade squamous intraepithelial lesion (LGSIL) R85.612
      satisfactory anal smear but lacking transformation zone R85.616
      specified NEC R85.618
      unsatisfactory smear R85.615
    female genital organs — *see* Abnormal, Papanicolaou (smear)
  dark adaptation curve H53.61
  dentofacial NEC — *see* Anomaly, dentofacial
  development, developmental Q89.9
    central nervous system Q07.9
  diagnostic imaging
    abdomen, abdominal region NEC R93.5
    biliary tract R93.2
    bladder R93.41
    breast R92.8
    central nervous system NEC R90.89
    cerebrovascular NEC R90.89
    coronary circulation R93.1
    digestive tract NEC R93.3
    gastrointestinal (tract) R93.3
    genitourinary organs R93.89
    head R93.0
    heart R93.1
    intrathoracic organ NEC R93.89
    kidney R93.42- ☑
    limbs R93.6
    liver R93.2
    lung (field) R91.8
    musculoskeletal system NEC R93.7
    renal pelvis R93.41
    retroperitoneum R93.5
    site specified NEC R93.89
    skin and subcutaneous tissue R93.89
    skull R93.0
    testis R93.81- ☑
    ureter R93.41
    urinary organs specified NEC R93.49
  direction, teeth, fully erupted M26.30
  ear ossicles, acquired NEC H74.39- ☑
    ankylosis — *see* Ankylosis, ear ossicles
    discontinuity — *see* Discontinuity, ossicles, ear
    partial loss — *see* Loss, ossicles, ear (partial)
  Ebstein Q22.5
  echocardiogram R93.1
  echoencephalogram R90.81
  echogram — *see* Abnormal, diagnostic imaging
  electrocardiogram [ECG] [EKG] R94.31
  electroencephalogram [EEG] R94.01
  electrolyte — *see* Imbalance, electrolyte
  electromyogram [EMG] R94.131
  electro-oculogram [EOG] R94.110
  electrophysiological intracardiac studies R94.39
  electroretinogram [ERG] R94.111
  erythrocytes
    congenital, with perinatal jaundice D58.9
  feces (color) (contents) (mucus) R19.5
  finding — *see* Findings, abnormal, without diagnosis
  fluid
    amniotic — *see* Abnormal, specimen, specified
    cerebrospinal — *see* Abnormal, cerebrospinal fluid
    peritoneal — *see* Abnormal, specimen, digestive organs
    pleural — *see* Abnormal, specimen, respiratory organs
    synovial — *see* Abnormal, specimen, specified
    thorax (bronchial washings) (pleural fluid) — *see* Abnormal, specimen, respiratory organs
    vaginal — *see* Abnormal, specimen, female genital organs
  form
    teeth K00.2

▽ Subterms under main terms may continue to next column or page   ☑ Additional Character Required — Refer to the Tabular List for Character Selection   1

Aarskog's syndrome — Abnormal, abnormality, abnormalities

Abnormal, abnormality, abnormalities —
continued
form — *continued*
    uterus — *see* Anomaly, uterus
function studies
    auditory R94.120
    bladder R94.8
    brain R94.09
    cardiovascular R94.30
    ear R94.128
    endocrine NEC R94.7
    eye NEC R94.118
    kidney R94.4
    liver R94.5
    nervous system
        central NEC R94.09
        peripheral NEC R94.138
    pancreas R94.8
    placenta R94.8
    pulmonary R94.2
    special senses NEC R94.128
    spleen R94.8
    thyroid R94.6
    vestibular R94.121
gait — *see* Gait
    hysterical F44.4
gastrin secretion E16.4
globulin R77.1
    cortisol-binding E27.8
    thyroid-binding E07.89
glomerular, minor — *see also* N00-N07 with fourth
        character .0 N05.0
glucagon secretion E16.3
glucose tolerance (test) (non-fasting) R73.09
gravitational (G) forces or states (effect of) T75.81 ☑
hair (color) (shaft) L67.9
    specified NEC L67.8
hard tissue formation in pulp (dental) K04.3
head movement R25.0
heart
    rate R00.9
        specified NEC R00.8
    shadow R93.1
    sounds NEC R01.2
hemoglobin (disease) — *see also* Disease, hemoglobin
        D58.2
    trait — *see* Trait, hemoglobin, abnormal
histology NEC R89.7
immunological findings R89.4
    in serum R76.9
        specified NEC R76.8
increase in appetite R63.2
involuntary movement — *see* Abnormal, movement,
        involuntary
jaw closure M26.51
karyotype R89.8
kidney function test R94.4
knee jerk R29.2
leukocyte (cell) (differential) NEC D72.9
liver function test R94.5
loss of
    height R29.890
    weight R63.4
mammogram NEC R92.8
    calcification (calculus) R92.1
    microcalcification R92.0
Mantoux test R76.11
movement (disorder) — *see also* Disorder, movement
    head R25.0
    involuntary R25.9
        fasciculation R25.3
        of head R25.0
        spasm R25.2
        specified type NEC R25.8
        tremor R25.1
myoglobin (Aberdeen) (Annapolis) R89.7
neonatal screening P09
oculomotor study R94.113
palmar creases Q82.8
Papanicolaou (smear)
    anus R85.619
        atypical squamous cells cannot exclude high
            grade squamous intraepithelial lesion
            (ASC-H) R85.611
        atypical squamous cells of undetermined signif-
            icance (ASC-US) R85.610
        cytologic evidence of malignancy R85.614

Abnormal, abnormality, abnormalities —
continued
Papanicolaou — *continued*
    anus — *continued*
        high grade squamous intraepithelial lesion
            (HGSIL) R85.613
        human papillomavirus (HPV) DNA test
            high risk positive R85.81
            low risk postive R85.82
        inadequate smear R85.615
        low grade squamous intraepithelial lesion (LGSIL)
            R85.612
        satisfactory anal smear but lacking transforma-
            tion zone R85.616
        specified NEC R85.618
        unsatisfactory smear R85.615
    bronchial washings R84.6
    cerebrospinal fluid R83.6
    cervix R87.619
        atypical squamous cells cannot exclude high
            grade squamous intraepithelial lesion
            (ASC-H) R87.611
        atypical squamous cells of undetermined signif-
            icance (ASC-US) R87.610
        cytologic evidence of malignancy R87.614
        high grade squamous intraepithelial lesion
            (HGSIL) R87.613
        inadequate smear R87.615
        low grade squamous intraepithelial lesion (LGSIL)
            R87.612
        non-atypical endometrial cells R87.618
        satisfactory cervical smear but lacking transfor-
            mation zone R87.616
        specified NEC R87.618
        thin preparaton R87.619
        unsatisfactory smear R87.615
    nasal secretions R84.6
    nipple discharge R89.6
    peritoneal fluid R85.69
    pleural fluid R84.6
    prostatic secretions R86.6
    saliva R85.69
    seminal fluid R86.6
    sites NEC R89.6
    sputum R84.6
    synovial fluid R89.6
    throat scrapings R84.6
    vagina R87.629
        atypical squamous cells cannot exclude high
            grade squamous intraepithelial lesion
            (ASC-H) R87.621
        atypical squamous cells of undetermined signif-
            icance (ASC-US) R87.620
        cytologic evidence of malignancy R87.624
        high grade squamous intraepithelial lesion
            (HGSIL) R87.623
        inadequate smear R87.625
        low grade squamous intraepithelial lesion (LGSIL)
            R87.622
        specified NEC R87.628
        thin preparation R87.629
        unsatisfactory smear R87.625
    vulva R87.69
    wound secretions R89.6
partial thromboplastin time (PTT) R79.1
pelvis (bony) — *see* Deformity, pelvis
percussion, chest (tympany) R09.89
periods (grossly) — *see* Menstruation
phonocardiogram R94.39
plantar reflex R29.2
plasma
    protein R77.9
        specified NEC R77.8
    viscosity R70.1
pleural (folds) Q34.0
posture R29.3
product of conception O02.9
    specified type NEC O02.89
prothrombin time (PT) R79.1
pulmonary
    artery, congenital Q25.79
    function, newborn P28.89
    test results R94.2
pulsations in neck R00.2
pupillary H21.56- ☑
    function (reaction) (reflex) — *see* Anomaly, pupil,
        function
radiological examination — *see* Abnormal, diagnostic
    imaging

Abnormal, abnormality, abnormalities —
continued
red blood cell(s) (morphology) (volume) R71.8
reflex — *see* Reflex
renal function test R94.4
response to nerve stimulation R94.130
retinal correspondence H53.31
retinal function study R94.111
rhythm, heart — *see also* Arrhythmia
saliva — *see* Abnormal, specimen, digestive organs
scan
    kidney R94.4
    liver R93.2
    thyroid R94.6
secretion
    gastrin E16.4
    glucagon E16.3
semen, seminal fluid — *see* Abnormal, specimen, male
    genital organs
serum level (of)
    acid phosphatase R74.8
    alkaline phosphatase R74.8
    amylase R74.8
    enzymes R74.9
        specified NEC R74.8
    lipase R74.8
    triacylglycerol lipase R74.8
shape
    gravid uterus — *see* Anomaly, uterus
sinus venosus Q21.1
size, tooth, teeth K00.2
spacing, tooth, teeth, fully erupted M26.30
specimen
    digestive organs (peritoneal fluid) (saliva) R85.9
        cytology R85.69
        drug level R85.2
        enzyme level R85.0
        histology R85.7
        hormones R85.1
        immunology R85.4
        microbiology R85.5
        nonmedicinal level R85.3
        specified type NEC R85.89
    female genital organs (secretions) (smears) R87.9
        cytology R87.69
            cervix R87.619
                human papillomavirus (HPV) DNA test
                    high risk positive R87.810
                    low risk positive R87.820
                inadequate (unsatisfactory) smear
                    R87.615
                non-atypical endometrial cells R87.618
                specified NEC R87.618
            vagina R87.629
                human papillomavirus (HPV) DNA test
                    high risk positive R87.811
                    low risk positive R87.821
                inadequate (unsatisfactory) smear
                    R87.625
            vulva R87.69
        drug level R87.2
        enzyme level R87.0
        histological R87.7
        hormones R87.1
        immunology R87.4
        microbiology R87.5
        nonmedicinal level R87.3
        specified type NEC R87.89
    male genital organs (prostatic secretions) (semen)
        R86.9
        cytology R86.6
        drug level R86.2
        enzyme level R86.0
        histological R86.7
        hormones R86.1
        immunology R86.4
        microbiology R86.5
        nonmedicinal level R86.3
        specified type NEC R86.8
    nipple discharge — *see* Abnormal, specimen, spec-
        ified
    respiratory organs (bronchial washings) (nasal secre-
        tions) (pleural fluid) (sputum) R84.9
        cytology R84.6
        drug level R84.2
        enzyme level R84.0
        histology R84.7
        hormones R84.1
        immunology R84.4

Abnormal, abnormality, abnormalities — *continued*
  specimen — *continued*
    respiratory organs — *continued*
      microbiology R84.5
      nonmedicinal level R84.3
      specified type NEC R84.8
    specified organ, system and tissue NOS R89.9
      cytology R89.6
      drug level R89.2
      enzyme level R89.0
      histology R89.7
      hormones R89.1
      immunology R89.4
      microbiology R89.5
      nonmedicinal level R89.3
      specified type NEC R89.8
    synovial fluid — *see* Abnormal, specimen, specified
    thorax (bronchial washings) (pleural fluids) — *see* Abnormal, specimen, respiratory organs
    vagina (secretion) (smear) R87.629
    vulva (secretion) (smear) R87.69
    wound secretion — *see* Abnormal, specimen, specified
    spermatozoa — *see* Abnormal, specimen, male genital organs
  sputum (amount) (color) (odor) R09.3
  stool (color) (contents) (mucus) R19.5
    bloody K92.1
    guaiac positive R19.5
  synchondrosis Q78.8
  thermography — *see also* Abnormal, diagnostic imaging R93.89
  thyroid-binding globulin E07.89
  tooth, teeth (form) (size) K00.2
  toxicology (findings) R78.9
  transport protein E88.09
  tumor marker NEC R97.8
  ultrasound results — *see* Abnormal, diagnostic imaging
  umbilical cord complicating delivery O69.9 ☑
  urination NEC R39.198
  urine (constituents) R82.90
    bile R82.2
    cytological examination R82.89
    drugs R82.5
    fat R82.0
    glucose R81
    heavy metals R82.6
    hemoglobin R82.3
    histological examination R82.89
    ketones R82.4
    microbiological examination (culture) R82.79
    myoglobin R82.1
    positive culture R82.79
    protein — *see* Proteinuria
    specified substance NEC R82.998
      chromoabnormality NEC R82.91
    substances nonmedical R82.6
  uterine hemorrhage — *see* Hemorrhage, uterus
  vectorcardiogram R94.39
  visually evoked potential (VEP) R94.112
  white blood cells D72.9
    specified NEC D72.89
  X-ray examination — *see* Abnormal, diagnostic imaging
Abnormity (any organ or part) — *see* Anomaly
Abocclusion M26.29
  hemolytic disease (newborn) P55.1
  incompatibility reaction ABO — *see* Complication(s), transfusion, incompatibility reaction, ABO
Abolition, language R48.8
Aborter, habitual or recurrent — *see* Loss (of), pregnancy, recurrent
Abortion (complete) (spontaneous) O03.9
  with
    retained products of conception — *see* Abortion, incomplete
  attempted (elective) (failed) O07.4
    complicated by O07.30
      afibrinogenemia O07.1
      cardiac arrest O07.36
      chemical damage of pelvic organ(s) O07.34
      circulatory collapse O07.31
      cystitis O07.38
      defibrination syndrome O07.1
      electrolyte imbalance O07.33
      embolism (air) (amniotic fluid) (blood clot) (fat) (pulmonary) (septic) (soap) O07.2
      endometritis O07.0

Abortion — *continued*
  attempted — *continued*
    complicated by — *continued*
      genital tract and pelvic infection O07.0
      hemolysis O07.1
      hemorrhage (delayed) (excessive) O07.1
      infection
        genital tract or pelvic O07.0
        urinary tract tract O07.38
      intravascular coagulation O007.1
      laceration of pelvic organ(s) O07.34
      metabolic disorder O07.33
      oliguria O07.32
      oophoritis O07.0
      parametritis O07.0
      pelvic peritonitis O07.0
      perforation of pelvic organ(s) O07.34
      renal failure or shutdown O07.32
      salpingitis or salpingo-oophoritis O07.0
      sepsis O07.37
      shock O07.31
      specified condition NEC O07.39
      tubular necrosis (renal) O07.32
      uremia O07.32
      urinary tract infection O07.38
      venous complication NEC O07.35
        embolism (air) (amniotic fluid) (blood clot) (fat) (pulmonary) (septic) (soap) O07.2
  complicated (by) (following) O03.80
    afibrinogenemia O03.6
    cardiac arrest O03.86
    chemical damage of pelvic organ(s) O03.84
    circulatory collapse O03.81
    cystitis O03.88
    defibrination syndrome O03.6
    electrolyte imbalance O03.83
    embolism (air) (amniotic fluid) (blood clot) (fat) (pulmonary) (septic) (soap) O03.7
    endometritis O03.5
    genital tract and pelvic infection O03.5
    hemolysis O03.6
    hemorrhage (delayed) (excessive) O03.6
    infection
      genital tract or pelvic O03.5
      urinary tract O03.88
    intravascular coagulation O03.6
    laceration of pelvic organ(s) O03.84
    metabolic disorder O03.83
    oliguria O03.82
    oophoritis O03.5
    parametritis O03.5
    pelvic peritonitis O03.5
    perforation of pelvic organ(s) O03.84
    renal failure or shutdown O03.82
    salpingitis or salpingo-oophoritis O03.5
    sepsis O03.87
    shock O03.81
    specified condition NEC O03.89
    tubular necrosis (renal) O03.82
    uremia O03.82
    urinary tract infection O03.88
    venous complication NEC O03.85
      embolism (air) (amniotic fluid) (blood clot) (fat) (pulmonary) (septic) (soap) O03.7
  failed — *see* Abortion, attempted
  habitual or recurrent N96
    with current abortion — *see* categories O03-O04
    without current pregnancy N96
    care in current pregnancy O26.2- ☑
  incomplete (spontaneous) O03.4
    complicated (by) (following) O03.30
      afibrinogenemia O03.1
      cardiac arrest O03.36
      chemical damage of pelvic organ(s) O03.34
      circulatory collapse O03.31
      cystitis O03.38
      defibrination syndrome O03.1
      electrolyte imbalance O03.33
      embolism (air) (amniotic fluid) (blood clot) (fat) (pulmonary) (septic) (soap) O03.2
      endometritis O03.0
      genital tract and pelvic infection O03.0
      hemolysis O03.1
      hemorrhage (delayed) (excessive) O03.1
      infection
        genital tract or pelvic O03.0
        urinary tract O03.38
      intravascular coagulation O03.1
      laceration of pelvic organ(s) O03.34

Abortion — *continued*
  incomplete — *continued*
    complicated — *continued*
      metabolic disorder O03.33
      oliguria O03.32
      oophoritis O03.0
      parametritis O03.0
      pelvic peritonitis O03.0
      perforation of pelvic organ(s) O03.34
      renal failure or shutdown O03.32
      salpingitis or salpingo-oophoritis O03.0
      sepsis O03.37
      shock O03.31
      specified condition NEC O03.39
      tubular necrosis (renal) O03.32
      uremia O03.32
      urinary infection O03.38
      venous complication NEC O03.35
        embolism (air) (amniotic fluid) (blood clot) (fat) (pulmonary) (septic) (soap) O03.2
  induced (encounter for) Z33.2
    complicated by O04.80
      afibrinogenemia O04.6
      cardiac arrest O04.86
      chemical damage of pelvic organ(s) O04.84
      circulatory collapse O04.81
      cystitis O04.88
      defibrination syndrome O04.6
      electrolyte imbalance O04.83
      embolism (air) (amniotic fluid) (blood clot) (fat) (pulmonary) (septic) (soap) O04.7
      endometritis O04.5
      genital tract and pelvic infection O04.5
      hemolysis O04.6
      hemorrhage (delayed) (excessive) O04.6
      infection
        genital tract or pelvic O04.5
        urinary tract O04.88
      intravascular coagulation O04.6
      laceration of pelvic organ(s) O04.84
      metabolic disorder O04.83
      oliguria O04.82
      oophoritis O04.5
      parametritis O04.5
      pelvic peritonitis O04.5
      perforation of pelvic organ(s) O04.84
      renal failure or shutdown O04.82
      salpingitis or salpingo-oophoritis O04.5
      sepsis O04.87
      shock O04.81
      specified condition NEC O04.89
      tubular necrosis (renal) O04.82
      uremia O04.82
      urinary tract infection O04.88
      venous complication NEC O04.85
        embolism (air) (amniotic fluid) (blood clot) (fat) (pulmonary) (septic) (soap) O04.7
  missed O02.1
  spontaneous — *see* Abortion (complete) (spontaneous)
    threatened O20.0
  threatened (spontaneous) O20.0
  tubal O00.10-
    with intrauterine pregnancy O00.11- ☑
Abortus fever A23.1
Aboulomania F60.7
Abrami's disease D59.8
Abramov-Fiedler myocarditis (acute isolated myocarditis) I40.1
Abrasion T14.8 ☑
  abdomen, abdominal (wall) S30.811 ☑
  alveolar process S00.512 ☑
  ankle S90.51- ☑
  antecubital space — *see* Abrasion, elbow
  anus S30.817 ☑
  arm (upper) S40.81- ☑
  auditory canal — *see* Abrasion, ear
  auricle — *see* Abrasion, ear
  axilla — *see* Abrasion, arm
  back, lower S30.810 ☑
  breast S20.11- ☑
  brow S00.81 ☑
  buttock S30.810 ☑
  calf — *see* Abrasion, leg
  canthus — *see* Abrasion, eyelid
  cheek S00.81 ☑
    internal S00.512 ☑
  chest wall — *see* Abrasion, thorax
  chin S00.81 ☑

⛛ Subterms under main terms may continue to next column or page   ☑ Additional Character Required — Refer to the Tabular List for Character Selection   3

Abnormal, abnormality, abnormalities — Abrasion

Abrasion — *continued*
- clitoris S30.814 ☑
- cornea S05.0- ☑
- costal region — *see* Abrasion, thorax
- dental K03.1
- digit(s)
  - foot — *see* Abrasion, toe
  - hand — *see* Abrasion, finger
- ear S00.41- ☑
- elbow S50.31- ☑
- epididymis S30.813 ☑
- epigastric region S30.811 ☑
- epiglottis S10.11 ☑
- esophagus (thoracic) S27.818 ☑
  - cervical S10.11 ☑
- eyebrow — *see* Abrasion, eyelid
- eyelid S00.21- ☑
- face S00.81 ☑
- finger(s) S60.41- ☑
  - index S60.41- ☑
  - little S60.41- ☑
  - middle S60.41- ☑
  - ring S60.41- ☑
- flank S30.811 ☑
- foot (except toe(s) alone) S90.81- ☑
  - toe — *see* Abrasion, toe
- forearm S50.81- ☑
  - elbow only — *see* Abrasion, elbow
- forehead S00.81 ☑
- genital organs, external
  - female S30.816 ☑
  - male S30.815 ☑
- groin S30.811 ☑
- gum S00.512 ☑
- hand S60.51- ☑
- head S00.91 ☑
  - ear — *see* Abrasion, ear
  - eyelid — *see* Abrasion, eyelid
  - lip S00.511 ☑
  - nose S00.31 ☑
  - oral cavity S00.512 ☑
  - scalp S00.01 ☑
  - specified site NEC S00.81 ☑
- heel — *see* Abrasion, foot
- hip S70.21- ☑
- inguinal region S30.811 ☑
- interscapular region S20.419 ☑
- jaw S00.81 ☑
- knee S80.21- ☑
- labium (majus) (minus) S30.814 ☑
- larynx S10.11 ☑
- leg (lower) S80.81- ☑
  - knee — *see* Abrasion, knee
  - upper — *see* Abrasion, thigh
- lip S00.511 ☑
- lower back S30.810 ☑
- lumbar region S30.810 ☑
- malar region S00.81 ☑
- mammary — *see* Abrasion, breast
- mastoid region S00.81 ☑
- mouth S00.512 ☑
- nail
  - finger — *see* Abrasion, finger
  - toe — *see* Abrasion, toe
- nape S10.81 ☑
- nasal S00.31 ☑
- neck S10.91 ☑
  - specified site NEC S10.81 ☑
  - throat S10.11 ☑
- nose S00.31 ☑
- occipital region S00.01 ☑
- oral cavity S00.512 ☑
- orbital region — *see* Abrasion, eyelid
- palate S00.512 ☑
- palm — *see* Abrasion, hand
- parietal region S00.01 ☑
- pelvis S30.810 ☑
- penis S30.812 ☑
- perineum
  - female S30.814 ☑
  - male S30.810 ☑
- periocular area — *see* Abrasion, eyelid
- phalanges
  - finger — *see* Abrasion, finger
  - toe — *see* Abrasion, toe
- pharynx S10.11 ☑

Abrasion — *continued*
- pinna — *see* Abrasion, ear
- popliteal space — *see* Abrasion, knee
- prepuce S30.812 ☑
- pubic region S30.810 ☑
- pudendum
  - female S30.816 ☑
  - male S30.815 ☑
- sacral region S30.810 ☑
- scalp S00.01 ☑
- scapular region — *see* Abrasion, shoulder
- scrotum S30.813 ☑
- shin — *see* Abrasion, leg
- shoulder S40.21- ☑
- skin NEC T14.8 ☑
- sternal region S20.319 ☑
- submaxillary region S00.81 ☑
- submental region S00.81 ☑
- subungual
  - finger(s) — *see* Abrasion, finger
  - toe(s) — *see* Abrasion, toe
- supraclavicular fossa S10.81 ☑
- supraorbital S00.81 ☑
- temple S00.81 ☑
- temporal region S00.81 ☑
- testis S30.813 ☑
- thigh S70.31- ☑
- thorax, thoracic (wall) S20.91 ☑
  - back S20.41- ☑
  - front S20.31- ☑
- throat S10.11 ☑
- thumb S60.31- ☑
- toe(s) (lesser) S90.416 ☑
  - great S90.41- ☑
- tongue S00.512 ☑
- tooth, teeth (dentifrice) (habitual) (hard tissues) (occupational) (ritual) (traditional) K03.1
- trachea S10.11 ☑
- tunica vaginalis S30.813 ☑
- tympanum, tympanic membrane — *see* Abrasion, ear
- uvula S00.512 ☑
- vagina S30.814 ☑
- vocal cords S10.11 ☑
- vulva S30.814 ☑
- wrist S60.81- ☑

Abrism — *see* Poisoning, food, noxious, plant

Abruptio placentae O45.9- ☑
- with
  - afibrinogenemia O45.01- ☑
  - coagulation defect O45.00- ☑
    - specified NEC O45.09- ☑
  - disseminated intravascular coagulation O45.02- ☑
  - hypofibrinogenemia O45.01- ☑
- specified NEC O45.8- ☑

Abruption, placenta — *see* Abruptio placentae

Abscess (connective tissue) (embolic) (fistulous) (infective) (metastatic) (multiple) (pernicious) (pyogenic) (septic) L02.91
- with
  - diverticular disease (intestine) K57.80
    - with bleeding K57.81
    - large intestine K57.20
      - with
        - bleeding K57.21
        - small intestine K57.40
          - with bleeding K57.41
    - small intestine K57.00
      - with
        - bleeding K57.01
        - large intestine K57.40
          - with bleeding K57.41
  - lymphangitis — *code by* site under Abscess
- abdomen, abdominal
  - cavity K65.1
  - wall L02.211
- abdominopelvic K65.1
- accessory sinus — *see* Sinusitis
- adrenal (capsule) (gland) E27.8
- alveolar K04.7
  - with sinus K04.6
- amebic A06.4
  - brain (and liver or lung abscess) A06.6
  - genitourinary tract A06.82
  - liver (without mention of brain or lung abscess) A06.4
  - lung (and liver) (without mention of brain abscess) A06.5

Abscess — *continued*
- amebic — *continued*
  - specified site NEC A06.89
  - spleen A06.89
- anerobic A48.0
- ankle — *see* Abscess, lower limb
- anorectal K61.2
- antecubital space — *see* Abscess, upper limb
- antrum (chronic) (Highmore) — *see* Sinusitis, maxillary
- anus K61.0
- apical (tooth) K04.7
  - with sinus (alveolar) K04.6
- appendix K35.33
- areola (acute) (chronic) (nonpuerperal) N61.1
  - puerperal, postpartum or gestational — *see* Infection, nipple
- arm (any part) — *see* Abscess, upper limb
- artery (wall) I77.89
- atheromatous I77.2
- auricle, ear — *see* Abscess, ear, external
- axilla (region) L02.41- ☑
  - lymph gland or node L04.2
- back (any part, except buttock) L02.212
- Bartholin's gland N75.1
  - with
    - abortion — *see* Abortion, by type complicated by, sepsis
    - ectopic or molar pregnancy O08.0
    - following ectopic or molar pregnancy O08.0
- Bezold's — *see* Mastoiditis, acute
- bilharziasis B65.1
- bladder (wall) — *see* Cystitis, specified type NEC
- bone (subperiosteal) — *see also* Osteomyelitis, specified type NEC
  - accessory sinus (chronic) — *see* Sinusitis
  - chronic or old — *see* Osteomyelitis, chronic
  - jaw (lower) (upper) M27.2
  - mastoid — *see* Mastoiditis, acute, subperiosteal
  - petrous — *see* Petrositis
  - spinal (tuberculous) A18.01
    - nontuberculous — *see* Osteomyelitis, vertebra
- bowel K63.0
- brain (any part) (cystic) (otogenic) G06.0
  - amebic (with abscess of any other site) A06.6
  - gonococcal A54.82
  - pheomycotic (chromomycotic) B43.1
  - tuberculous A17.81
- breast (acute) (chronic) (nonpuerperal) N61.1
  - newborn P39.0
  - puerperal, postpartum, gestational — *see* Mastitis, obstetric, purulent
- broad ligament N73.2
  - acute N73.0
  - chronic N73.1
- Brodie's (localized) (chronic) M86.8X- ☑
- bronchi J98.09
- buccal cavity K12.2
- bulbourethral gland N34.0
- bursa M71.00
  - ankle M71.07- ☑
  - elbow M71.02- ☑
  - foot M71.07- ☑
  - hand M71.04- ☑
  - hip M71.05- ☑
  - knee M71.06- ☑
  - multiple sites M71.09
  - pharyngeal J39.1
  - shoulder M71.01- ☑
  - specified site NEC M71.08
  - wrist M71.03- ☑
- buttock L02.31
- canthus — *see* Blepharoconjunctivitis
- cartilage — *see* Disorder, cartilage, specified type NEC
- cecum K35.33
- cerebellum, cerebellar G06.0
  - sequelae G09
- cerebral (embolic) G06.0
  - sequelae G09
- cervical (meaning neck) L02.11
  - lymph gland or node L04.0
- cervix (stump) (uteri) — *see* Cervicitis
- cheek (external) L02.01
  - inner K12.2
- chest J86.9
  - with fistula J86.0
  - wall L02.213
- chin L02.01
- choroid — *see* Inflammation, chorioretinal

Abscess — *continued*
circumtonsillar J36
cold (lung) (tuberculous) — *see also* Tuberculosis, abscess, lung
articular — *see* Tuberculosis, joint
colon (wall) K63.0
colostomy K94.02
conjunctiva — *see* Conjunctivitis, acute
cornea H16.31- ☑
corpus
cavernosum N48.21
luteum — *see* Oophoritis
Cowper's gland N34.0
cranium G06.0
cul-de-sac (Douglas') (posterior) — *see* Peritonitis, pelvic, female
cutaneous — *see* Abscess, by site
dental K04.7
with sinus (alveolar) K04.6
dentoalveolar K04.7
with sinus K04.6
diaphragm, diaphragmatic K65.1
Douglas' cul-de-sac or pouch — *see* Peritonitis, pelvic, female
Dubois A50.59
ear (middle) — *see also* Otitis, media, suppurative
acute — *see* Otitis, media, suppurative, acute
external H60.0- ☑
entamebic — *see* Abscess, amebic
enterostomy K94.12
epididymis N45.4
epidural G06.2
brain G06.0
spinal cord G06.1
epiglottis J38.7
epiploon, epiploic K65.1
erysipelatous — *see* Erysipelas
esophagus K20.8
ethmoid (bone) (chronic) (sinus) J32.2
external auditory canal — *see* Abscess, ear, external
extradural G06.2
brain G06.0
sequelae G09
spinal cord G06.1
extraperitoneal K68.19
eye — *see* Endophthalmitis, purulent
eyelid H00.03- ☑
face (any part, except ear, eye and nose) L02.01
fallopian tube — *see* Salpingitis
fascia M72.8
fauces J39.1
fecal K63.0
femoral (region) — *see* Abscess, lower limb
filaria, filarial — *see* Infestation, filarial
finger (any) — *see also* Abscess, hand
nail — *see* Cellulitis, finger
foot L02.61- ☑
forehead L02.01
frontal sinus (chronic) J32.1
gallbladder K81.0
genital organ or tract
female (external) N76.4
male N49.9
multiple sites N49.8
specified NEC N49.8
gestational mammary O91.11- ☑
gestational subareolar O91.11- ☑
gingival — *see* Periodontitis, localized
gland, glandular (lymph) (acute) — *see* Lymphadenitis, acute
gluteal (region) L02.31
gonorrheal — *see* Gonococcus
groin L02.214
gum — *see* Periodontitis, localized
hand L02.51- ☑
head NEC L02.811
face (any part, except ear, eye and nose) L02.01
heart — *see* Carditis
heel — *see* Abscess, foot
helminthic — *see* Infestation, helminth
hepatic (cholangitic) (hematogenic) (lymphogenic) (pylephlebitic) K75.0
amebic A06.4
hip (region) — *see* Abscess, lower limb
horseshoe K61.31
ileocecal K35.33
ileostomy (bud) K94.12
iliac (region) L02.214

Abscess — *continued*
iliac — *continued*
fossa K35.33
infraclavicular (fossa) — *see* Abscess, upper limb
inguinal (region) L02.214
lymph gland or node L04.1
intersphincteric K61.4
intestine, intestinal NEC K63.0
rectal K61.1
intra-abdominal — *see also* Abscess, peritoneum K65.1
following procedure T81.43 ☑
obstetrical O86.03
postprocedural T81.49 ☑
retroperitoneal K68.11
intracranial G06.0
intramammary — *see* Abscess, breast
intramuscular, following procedure T81.42 ☑
obstetrical O86.02
intraorbital — *see* Abscess, orbit
intraperitoneal K65.1
intrasphincteric (anus) K61.4
intraspinal G06.1
intratonsillar J36
ischiorectal (fossa) (specified NEC) K61.39
jaw (bone) (lower) (upper) M27.2
joint — *see* Arthritis, pyogenic or pyemic
spine (tuberculous) A18.01
nontuberculous — *see* Spondylopathy, infective
kidney N15.1
with calculus N20.0
with hydronephrosis N13.6
puerperal (postpartum) O86.21
knee — *see also* Abscess, lower limb
joint M00.9
labium (majus) (minus) N76.4
lacrimal
caruncle — *see* Inflammation, lacrimal, passages, acute
gland — *see* Dacryoadenitis
passages (duct) (sac) — *see* Inflammation, lacrimal, passages, acute
lacunar N34.0
larynx J38.7
lateral (alveolar) K04.7
with sinus K04.6
leg (any part) — *see* Abscess, lower limb
lens H27.8
lingual K14.0
tonsil J36
lip K13.0
Littre's gland N34.0
liver (cholangitic) (hematogenic) (lymphogenic) (pylephlebitic) (pyogenic) K75.0
amebic (due to Entamoeba histolytica) (dysenteric) (tropical) A06.4
with
brain abscess (and liver or lung abscess) A06.6
lung abscess A06.5
loin (region) L02.211
lower limb L02.41- ☑
lumbar (tuberculous) A18.01
nontuberculous L02.212
lung (miliary) (putrid) J85.2
with pneumonia J85.1
due to specified organism (see Pneumonia, in (due to))
amebic (with liver abscess) A06.5
with
brain abscess A06.6
pneumonia A06.5
lymph, lymphatic, gland or node (acute) — *see also* Lymphadenitis, acute
mesentery I88.0
malar M27.2
mammary gland — *see* Abscess, breast
marginal, anus K61.0
mastoid — *see* Mastoiditis, acute
maxilla, maxillary M27.2
molar (tooth) K04.7
with sinus K04.6
premolar K04.7
sinus (chronic) J32.0
mediastinum J85.3
meibomian gland — *see* Hordeolum
meninges G06.2
mesentery, mesenteric K65.1
mesosalpinx — *see* Salpingitis
mons pubis L02.215

Abscess — *continued*
mouth (floor) K12.2
muscle — *see* Myositis, infective
myocardium I40.0
nabothian (follicle) — *see* Cervicitis
nasal J32.9
nasopharyngeal J39.1
navel L02.216
newborn P38.9
with mild hemorrhage P38.1
without hemorrhage P38.9
neck (region) L02.11
lymph gland or node L04.0
nephritic — *see* Abscess, kidney
nipple N61.1
associated with
lactation — *see* Pregnancy, complicated by
pregnancy — *see* Pregnancy, complicated by
nose (external) (fossa) (septum) J34.0
sinus (chronic) — *see* Sinusitis
omentum K65.1
operative wound T81.49 ☑
orbit, orbital — *see* Cellulitis, orbit
otogenic G06.0
ovary, ovarian (corpus luteum) — *see* Oophoritis
oviduct — *see* Oophoritis
palate (soft) K12.2
hard M27.2
palmar (space) — *see* Abscess, hand
pancreas (duct) — *see* Pancreatitis, acute
parafrenal N48.21
parametric, parametrium N73.2
acute N73.0
chronic N73.1
paranephric N15.1
parapancreatic — *see* Pancreatitis, acute
parapharyngeal J39.0
pararectal K61.1
parasinus — *see* Sinusitis
parauterine — *see also* Disease, pelvis, inflammatory N73.2
paravaginal — *see* Vaginitis
parietal region (scalp) L02.811
parodontal — *see* Periodontitis, aggressive, localized
parotid (duct) (gland) K11.3
region K12.2
pectoral (region) L02.213
pelvis, pelvic
female — *see* Disease, pelvis, inflammatory
male, peritoneal K65.1
penis N48.21
gonococcal (accessory gland) (periurethral) A54.1
perianal K61.0
periapical K04.7
with sinus (alveolar) K04.6
periappendicular K35.33
pericardial I30.1
pericecal K35.33
pericemental — *see* Periodontitis, aggressive, localized
pericholecystic — *see* Cholecystitis, acute
pericoronal — *see* Periodontitis, aggressive, localized
peridental — *see* Periodontitis, aggressive, localized
perimetric — *see also* Disease, pelvis, inflammatory N73.2
perinephric, perinephritic — *see* Abscess, kidney
perineum, perineal (superficial) L02.215
urethra N34.0
periodontal (parietal) — *see* Periodontitis, aggressive, localized
apical K04.7
periosteum, periosteal — *see also* Osteomyelitis, specified type NEC
with osteomyelitis — *see also* Osteomyelitis, specified type NEC
acute — *see* Osteomyelitis, acute
chronic — *see* Osteomyelitis, chronic
peripharyngeal J39.0
peripleuritic J86.9
with fistula J86.0
periprostatic N41.2
perirectal K61.1
perirenal (tissue) — *see* Abscess, kidney
perisinuous (nose) — *see* Sinusitis
peritoneum, peritoneal (perforated) (ruptured) K65.1
with appendicitis — *see also* Appendicitis K35.33
pelvic
female — *see* Peritonitis, pelvic, female
male K65.1

Abscess — *continued*
  peritoneum, peritoneal — *continued*
    postoperative T81.49 ☑
    puerperal, postpartum, childbirth O85
    tuberculous A18.31
  peritonsillar J36
  perityphlic K35.33
  periureteral N28.89
  periurethral N34.0
    gonococcal (accessory gland) (periurethral) A54.1
  periuterine — *see also* Disease, pelvis, inflammatory N73.2
  perivesical — *see* Cystitis, specified type NEC
  petrous bone — *see* Petrositis
  phagedenic NOS L02.91
    chancroid A57
  pharynx, pharyngeal (lateral) J39.1
  pilonidal L05.01
  pituitary (gland) E23.6
  pleura J86.9
    with fistula J86.0
  popliteal — *see* Abscess, lower limb
  postcecal K35.33
  postlaryngeal J38.7
  postnasal J34.0
  postoperative (any site) — *see also* Infection, postoperative wound T81.49 ☑
    retroperitoneal K68.11
  postpharyngeal J39.0
  posttonsillar J36
  post-typhoid A01.09
  pouch of Douglas — *see* Peritonitis, pelvic, female
  premammary — *see* Abscess, breast
  prepatellar — *see* Abscess, lower limb
  prostate N41.2
    gonococcal (acute) (chronic) A54.22
  psoas muscle K68.12
  puerperal — *code by* site under Puerperal, abscess
  pulmonary — *see* Abscess, lung
  pulp, pulpal (dental) K04.01
    irreversible K04.02
    reversible K04.01
  rectovaginal septum K63.0
  rectovesical — *see* Cystitis, specified type NEC
  rectum K61.1
  renal — *see* Abscess, kidney
  retina — *see* Inflammation, chorioretinal
  retrobulbar — *see* Abscess, orbit
  retrocecal K65.1
  retrolaryngeal J38.7
  retromammary — *see* Abscess, breast
  retroperitoneal NEC K68.19
    postprocedural K68.11
  retropharyngeal J39.0
  retrouterine — *see* Peritonitis, pelvic, female
  retrovesical — *see* Cystitis, specified type NEC
  root, tooth K04.7
    with sinus (alveolar) K04.6
  round ligament — *see also* Disease, pelvis, inflammatory N73.2
  rupture (spontaneous) NOS L02.91
  sacrum (tuberculous) A18.01
    nontuberculous M46.28
  salivary (duct) (gland) K11.3
  scalp (any part) L02.811
  scapular — *see* Osteomyelitis, specified type NEC
  sclera — *see* Scleritis
  scrofulous (tuberculous) A18.2
  scrotum N49.2
  seminal vesicle N49.0
  septal, dental K04.7
    with sinus (alveolar) K04.6
  serous — *see* Periostitis
  shoulder (region) — *see* Abscess, upper limb
  sigmoid K63.0
  sinus (accessory) (chronic) (nasal) — *see also* Sinusitis
    intracranial venous (any) G06.0
  Skene's duct or gland N34.0
  skin — *see* Abscess, by site
  specified site NEC L02.818
  spermatic cord N49.1
  sphenoidal (sinus) (chronic) J32.3
  spinal cord (any part) (staphylococcal) G06.1
    tuberculous A17.81
  spine (column) (tuberculous) A18.01
    epidural G06.1
    nontuberculous — *see* Osteomyelitis, vertebra
  spleen D73.3

Abscess — *continued*
  spleen — *continued*
    amebic A06.89
  stitch T81.41 ☑
    following an obstetrical procedure O86.01
  subarachnoid G06.2
    brain G06.0
    spinal cord G06.1
  subareolar — *see* Abscess, breast
  subcecal K35.33
  subcutaneous — *see also* Abscess, by site
    following procedure T81.41 ☑
      obstetrical O86.01
    pheomycotic (chromomycotic) B43.2
  subdiaphragmatic K65.1
  subdural G06.2
    brain G06.0
      sequelae G09
    spinal cord G06.1
  sub-fascial, following an obstetrical procedure O86.02
  subgaleal L02.811
  subhepatic K65.1
  sublingual K12.2
    gland K11.3
  submammary — *see* Abscess, breast
  submandibular (region) (space) (triangle) K12.2
    gland K11.3
  submaxillary (region) L02.01
    gland K11.3
  submental L02.01
    gland K11.3
  subperiosteal — *see* Osteomyelitis, specified type NEC
  subphrenic K65.1
    following an obstetrical procedure O86.03
    postoperative T81.43 ☑
  suburethral N34.0
  sudoriparous L75.8
  supraclavicular (fossa) — *see* Abscess, upper limb
  supralevator K61.5
  suprapelvic, acute N73.0
  suprarenal (capsule) (gland) E27.8
  sweat gland L74.8
  tear duct — *see* Inflammation, lacrimal, passages, acute
  temple L02.01
  temporal region L02.01
  temporosphenoidal G06.0
  tendon (sheath) M65.00
    ankle M65.07- ☑
    foot M65.07- ☑
    forearm M65.03- ☑
    hand M65.04- ☑
    lower leg M65.06- ☑
    pelvic region M65.05- ☑
    shoulder region M65.01- ☑
    specified site NEC M65.08
    thigh M65.05- ☑
    upper arm M65.02- ☑
  testis N45.4
  thigh — *see* Abscess, lower limb
  thorax J86.9
    with fistula J86.0
  throat J39.1
  thumb — *see also* Abscess, hand
    nail — *see* Cellulitis, finger
  thymus (gland) E32.1
  thyroid (gland) E06.0
  toe (any) — *see also* Abscess, foot
    nail — *see* Cellulitis, toe
  tongue (staphylococcal) K14.0
  tonsil(s) (lingual) J36
  tonsillopharyngeal J36
  tooth, teeth (root) K04.7
    with sinus (alveolar) K04.6
    supporting structures NEC — *see* Periodontitis, aggressive, localized
  trachea J39.8
  trunk L02.219
    abdominal wall L02.211
    back L02.212
    chest wall L02.213
    groin L02.214
    perineum L02.215
    umbilicus L02.216
  tubal — *see* Salpingitis
  tuberculous — *see* Tuberculosis, abscess
  tubo-ovarian — *see* Salpingo-oophoritis
  tunica vaginalis N49.1
  umbilicus L02.216

Abscess — *continued*
  upper
    limb L02.41- ☑
    respiratory J39.8
  urethral (gland) N34.0
  urinary N34.0
  uterus, uterine (wall) — *see also* Endometritis
    ligament — *see also* Disease, pelvis, inflammatory N73.2
    neck — *see* Cervicitis
  uvula K12.2
  vagina (wall) — *see* Vaginitis
  vaginorectal — *see* Vaginitis
  vas deferens N49.1
  vermiform appendix K35.33
  vertebra (column) (tuberculous) A18.01
    nontuberculous — *see* Osteomyelitis, vertebra
  vesical — *see* Cystitis, specified type NEC
  vesico-uterine pouch — *see* Peritonitis, pelvic, female
  vitreous (humor) — *see* Endophthalmitis, purulent
  vocal cord J38.3
  von Bezold's — *see* Mastoiditis, acute
  vulva N76.4
  vulvovaginal gland N75.1
  web space — *see* Abscess, hand
  wound T81.49 ☑
  wrist — *see* Abscess, upper limb
Absence (of) (organ or part) (complete or partial)
  adrenal (gland) (congenital) Q89.1
    acquired E89.6
  albumin in blood E88.09
  alimentary tract (congenital) Q45.8
    upper Q40.8
  alveolar process (acquired) — *see* Anomaly, alveolar
  ankle (acquired) Z89.44- ☑
  anus (congenital) Q42.3
    with fistula Q42.2
  aorta (congenital) Q25.41
  appendix, congenital Q42.8
  arm (acquired) Z89.20- ☑
    above elbow Z89.22- ☑
      congenital (with hand present) — *see* Agenesis, arm, with hand present
      and hand — *see* Agenesis, forearm, and hand
    below elbow Z89.21- ☑
      congenital (with hand present) — *see* Agenesis, arm, with hand present
      and hand — *see* Agenesis, forearm, and hand
    congenital — *see* Defect, reduction, upper limb
    shoulder (following explantation of shoulder joint prosthesis) (joint) (with or without presence of antibiotic-impregnated cement spacer) Z89.23- ☑
      congenital (with hand present) — *see* Agenesis, arm, with hand present
  artery (congenital) (peripheral) Q27.8
    brain Q28.3
    coronary Q24.5
    pulmonary Q25.79
    specified NEC Q27.8
    umbilical Q27.0
  atrial septum (congenital) Q21.1
  auditory canal (congenital) (external) Q16.1
  auricle (ear), congenital Q16.0
  bile, biliary duct, congenital Q44.5
  bladder (acquired) Z90.6
    congenital Q64.5
  bowel sounds R19.11
  brain Q00.0
    part of Q04.3
  breast(s) (and nipple(s)) (acquired) Z90.1- ☑
    congenital Q83.8
  broad ligament Q50.6
  bronchus (congenital) Q32.4
  canaliculus lacrimalis, congenital Q10.4
  cerebellum (vermis) Q04.3
  cervix (acquired) (with uterus) Z90.710
    with remaining uterus Z90.712
    congenital Q51.5
  chin, congenital Q18.8
  cilia (congenital) Q10.3
    acquired — *see* Madarosis
  clitoris (congenital) Q52.6
  coccyx, congenital Q76.49
  cold sense R20.8
  congenital
    lumen — *see* Atresia
    organ or site NEC — *see* Agenesis

☑ **Additional Character Required** — Refer to the Tabular List for Character Selection   ⚐ Subterms under main terms may continue to next column or page

Absence — continued
  congenital — continued
    septum — see Imperfect, closure
  corpus callosum Q04.0
  cricoid cartilage, congenital Q31.8
  diaphragm (with hernia), congenital Q79.1
  digestive organ(s) or tract, congenital Q45.8
    acquired NEC Z90.49
    upper Q40.8
  ductus arteriosus Q28.8
  duodenum (acquired) Z90.49
    congenital Q41.0
  ear, congenital Q16.9
    acquired H93.8- ☑
    auricle Q16.0
    external Q16.0
    inner Q16.5
    lobe, lobule Q17.8
    middle, except ossicles Q16.4
      ossicles Q16.3
    ossicles Q16.3
  ejaculatory duct (congenital) Q55.4
  endocrine gland (congenital) NEC Q89.2
    acquired E89.89
  epididymis (congenital) Q55.4
    acquired Z90.79
  epiglottis, congenital Q31.8
  esophagus (congenital) Q39.8
    acquired (partial) Z90.49
  eustachian tube (congenital) Q16.2
  extremity (acquired) Z89.9
    congenital Q73.0
    knee (following explantation of knee joint prosthe-sis) (joint) (with or without presence of antibi-otic-impregnated cement spacer) Z89.52- ☑
    lower (above knee) Z89.619
      below knee Z89.51- ☑
    upper — see Absence, arm
  eye (acquired) Z90.01
    congenital Q11.1
    muscle (congenital) Q10.3
  eyeball (acquired) Z90.01
    congenital Q11.1
  eyelid (fold) (congenital) Q10.3
    acquired Z90.01
  face, specified part NEC Q18.8
  fallopian tube(s) (acquired) Z90.79
    congenital Q50.6
  family member (causing problem in home) NEC — see also Disruption, family Z63.32
  femur, congenital — see Defect, reduction, lower limb, longitudinal, femur
  fibrinogen (congenital) D68.2
    acquired D65
  finger(s) (acquired) Z89.02- ☑
    congenital — see Agenesis, hand
  foot (acquired) Z89.43- ☑
    congenital — see Agenesis, foot
  forearm (acquired) — see Absence, arm, below elbow
  gallbladder (acquired) Z90.49
    congenital Q44.0
  gamma globulin in blood D80.1
    hereditary D80.0
  genital organs
    acquired (female) (male) Z90.79
    female, congenital Q52.8
      external Q52.71
      internal NEC Q52.8
    male, congenital Q55.8
  genitourinary organs, congenital NEC
    female Q52.8
    male Q55.8
  globe (acquired) Z90.01
    congenital Q11.1
  glottis, congenital Q31.8
  hand and wrist (acquired) Z89.11- ☑
    congenital — see Agenesis, hand
  head, part (acquired) NEC Z90.09
  heat sense R20.8
  hip (following explantation of hip joint prosthesis) (joint) (with or without presence of antibiotic-impregnated cement spacer) Z89.62- ☑
  hymen (congenital) Q52.4
  ileum (acquired) Z90.49
    congenital Q41.2
  immunoglobulin, isolated NEC D80.3
    IgA D80.2
    IgG D80.3
    IgM D80.4

Absence — continued
  incus (acquired) — see Loss, ossicles, ear
    congenital Q16.3
  inner ear, congenital Q16.5
  intestine (acquired) (small) Z90.49
    congenital Q41.9
      specified NEC Q41.8
    large Z90.49
      congenital Q42.9
        specified NEC Q42.8
  iris, congenital Q13.1
  jejunum (acquired) Z90.49
    congenital Q41.1
  joint
    acquired
      hip (following explantation of hip joint prosthe-sis) (with or without presence of antibiotic-impregnated cement spacer) Z89.62- ☑
      knee (following explantation of knee joint pros-thesis) (with or without presence of antibi-otic-impregnated cement spacer) Z89.52- ☑
      shoulder (following explantation of shoulder joint prosthesis) (with or without presence of antibiotic-impregnated cement spacer) Z89.23- ☑
    congenital NEC Q74.8
  kidney(s) (acquired) Z90.5
    congenital Q60.2
      bilateral Q60.1
      unilateral Q60.0
  knee (following explantation of knee joint prosthesis) (joint) (with or without presence of antibiotic-impregnated cement spacer) Z89.52- ☑
  labyrinth, membranous Q16.5
  larynx (congenital) Q31.8
    acquired Z90.02
  leg (acquired) (above knee) Z89.61- ☑
    below knee (acquired) Z89.51- ☑
    congenital — see Defect, reduction, lower limb
  lens (acquired) — see also Aphakia
    congenital Q12.3
    post cataract extraction Z98.4- ☑
  limb (acquired) — see Absence, extremity
  lip Q38.6
  liver (congenital) Q44.7
  lung (fissure) (lobe) (bilateral) (unilateral) (congenital) Q33.3
    acquired (any part) Z90.2
  menstruation — see Amenorrhea
  muscle (congenital) (pectoral) Q79.8
    ocular Q10.3
  neck, part Q18.8
  neutrophil — see Agranulocytosis
  nipple(s) (with breast(s)) (acquired) Z90.1- ☑
    congenital Q83.2
  nose (congenital) Q30.1
    acquired Z90.09
  organ
    of Corti, congenital Q16.5
    or site, congenital NEC Q89.8
      acquired NEC Z90.89
  osseous meatus (ear) Q16.4
  ovary (acquired)
    bilateral Z90.722
    congenital
      bilateral Q50.02
      unilateral Q50.01
    unilateral Z90.721
  oviduct (acquired)
    bilateral Z90.722
    congenital Q50.6
    unilateral Z90.721
  pancreas (congenital) Q45.0
    acquired Z90.410
      complete Z90.410
      partial Z90.411
      total Z90.410
  parathyroid gland (acquired) E89.2
    congenital Q89.2
  patella, congenital Q74.1
  penis (congenital) Q55.5
    acquired Z90.79
  pericardium (congenital) Q24.8
  pituitary gland (congenital) Q89.2
    acquired E89.3
  prostate (acquired) Z90.79
    congenital Q55.4

Absence — continued
  pulmonary valve Q22.0
  punctum lacrimale (congenital) Q10.4
  radius, congenital — see Defect, reduction, upper limb, longitudinal, radius
  rectum (congenital) Q42.1
    with fistula Q42.0
    acquired Z90.49
  respiratory organ NOS Q34.9
  rib (acquired) Z90.89
    congenital Q76.6
  sacrum, congenital Q76.49
  salivary gland(s), congenital Q38.4
  scrotum, congenital Q55.29
  seminal vesicles (congenital) Q55.4
    acquired Z90.79
  septum
    atrial (congenital) Q21.1
    between aorta and pulmonary artery Q21.4
    ventricular (congenital) Q20.4
  sex chromosome
    female phenotype Q97.8
    male phenotype Q98.8
  skull bone (congenital) Q75.8
    with
      anencephaly Q00.0
      encephalocele — see Encephalocele
      hydrocephalus Q03.9
        with spina bifida — see Spina bifida, by site, with hydrocephalus
      microcephaly Q02
  spermatic cord, congenital Q55.4
  spine, congenital Q76.49
  spleen (congenital) Q89.01
    acquired Z90.81
  sternum, congenital Q76.7
  stomach (acquired) (partial) Z90.3
    congenital Q40.2
  superior vena cava, congenital Q26.8
  teeth, tooth (congenital) K00.0
    acquired (complete) K08.109
      class I K08.101
      class II K08.102
      class III K08.103
      class IV K08.104
      due to
        caries K08.139
          class I K08.131
          class II K08.132
          class III K08.133
          class IV K08.134
        periodontal disease K08.129
          class I K08.121
          class II K08.122
          class III K08.123
          class IV K08.124
        specified NEC K08.199
          class I K08.191
          class II K08.192
          class III K08.193
          class IV K08.194
        trauma K08.119
          class I K08.111
          class II K08.112
          class III K08.113
          class IV K08.114
    partial K08.409
      class I K08.401
      class II K08.402
      class III K08.403
      class IV K08.404
      due to
        caries K08.439
          class I K08.431
          class II K08.432
          class III K08.433
          class IV K08.434
        periodontal disease K08.429
          class I K08.421
          class II K08.422
          class III K08.423
          class IV K08.424
        specified NEC K08.499
          class I K08.491
          class II K08.492
          class III K08.493
          class IV K08.494
        trauma K08.419
          class I K08.411

▽ Subterms under main terms may continue to next column or page   ☑ Additional Character Required — Refer to the Tabular List for Character Selection   7

Absence — Absence

Absence — *continued*
  teeth, tooth — *continued*
    acquired — *continued*
      partial — *continued*
        due to — *continued*
          trauma — *continued*
            class II K08.412
            class III K08.413
            class IV K08.414
  tendon (congenital) Q79.8
  testis (congenital) Q55.0
    acquired Z90.79
  thumb (acquired) Z89.01- ☑
    congenital — *see* Agenesis, hand
  thymus gland Q89.2
  thyroid (gland) (acquired) E89.0
    cartilage, congenital Q31.8
    congenital E03.1
  toe(s) (acquired) Z89.42- ☑
    with foot — *see* Absence, foot and ankle
    congenital — *see* Agenesis, foot
    great Z89.41- ☑
  tongue, congenital Q38.3
  trachea (cartilage), congenital Q32.1
  transverse aortic arch, congenital Q25.49
  tricuspid valve Q22.4
  umbilical artery, congenital Q27.0
  upper arm and forearm with hand present, congenital — *see* Agenesis, arm, with hand present
  ureter (congenital) Q62.4
    acquired Z90.6
  urethra, congenital Q64.5
  uterus (acquired) Z90.710
    with cervix Z90.710
    with remaining cervical stump Z90.711
    congenital Q51.0
  uvula, congenital Q38.5
  vagina, congenital Q52.0
  vas deferens (congenital) Q55.4
    acquired Z90.79
  vein (peripheral) congenital NEC Q27.8
    cerebral Q28.3
    digestive system Q27.8
    great Q26.8
    lower limb Q27.8
    portal Q26.5
    precerebral Q28.1
    specified site NEC Q27.8
    upper limb Q27.8
  vena cava (inferior) (superior), congenital Q26.8
  ventricular septum Q20.4
  vertebra, congenital Q76.49
  vulva, congenital Q52.71
  wrist (acquired) Z89.12- ☑

Absorbent system disease I87.8
Absorption
  carbohydrate, disturbance K90.49
  chemical — *see* Table of Drugs and Chemicals
    through placenta (newborn) P04.9
      environmental substance P04.6
      nutritional substance P04.5
      obstetric anesthetic or analgesic drug P04.0
  drug NEC — *see* Table of Drugs and Chemicals
    addictive
      through placenta (newborn) — *see also* Newborn, affected by, maternal, use of P04.40
        cocaine P04.41
        hallucinogens P04.42
        specified drug NEC P04.49
    medicinal
      through placenta (newborn) P04.19
    through placenta (newborn) P04.19
      obstetric anesthetic or analgesic drug P04.0
  fat, disturbance K90.49
    pancreatic K90.3
  noxious substance — *see* Table of Drugs and Chemicals
  protein, disturbance K90.49
  starch, disturbance K90.49
  toxic substance — *see* Table of Drugs and Chemicals
  uremic — *see* Uremia
Abstinence symptoms, syndrome
  alcohol F10.239
    with delirium F10.231
  cocaine F14.23
  neonatal P96.1
  nicotine — *see* Dependence, drug, nicotine, with, withdrawal
  opioid F11.93

Abstinence symptoms, syndrome — *continued*
  opioid — *continued*
    with dependence F11.23
  psychoactive NEC F19.939
    with
      delirium F19.931
      dependence F19.239
        with
          delirium F19.231
          perceptual disturbance F19.232
        uncomplicated F19.230
      perceptual disturbance F19.932
    uncomplicated F19.930
  sedative F13.939
    with
      delirium F13.931
      dependence F13.239
        with
          delirium F13.231
          perceptual disturbance F13.232
        uncomplicated F13.230
      perceptual disturbance F13.932
    uncomplicated F13.930
  stimulant NEC F15.93
    with dependence F15.23
Abulia R68.89
Abulomania F60.7
Abuse
  adult — *see* Maltreatment, adult
    as reason for
      couple seeking advice (including offender) Z63.0
  alcohol (non-dependent) F10.10
    with
      anxiety disorder F10.180
      intoxication F10.129
        with delirium F10.121
        uncomplicated F10.120
      mood disorder F10.14
      other specified disorder F10.188
      psychosis F10.159
        delusions F10.150
        hallucinations F10.151
      sexual dysfunction F10.181
      sleep disorder F10.182
      unspecified disorder F10.19
    counseling and surveillance Z71.41
    in remission (early) (sustained) F10.11
  amphetamine (or related substance) — *see also* Abuse, drug, stimulant NEC
    stimulant NEC F15.10
      with
        anxiety disorder F15.180
        intoxication F15.129
          with
            delirium F15.121
            perceptual disturbance F15.122
  analgesics (non-prescribed) (over the counter) F55.8
  antacids F55.0
  antidepressants — *see* Abuse, drug, psychoactive NEC
  anxiolytic — *see* Abuse, drug, sedative
  barbiturates — *see* Abuse, drug, sedative
  caffeine — *see* Abuse, drug, stimulant NEC
  cannabis, cannabinoids — *see* Abuse, drug, cannabis
  child — *see* Maltreatment, child
  cocaine — *see* Abuse, drug, cocaine
  drug NEC (non-dependent) F19.10
    with sleep disorder F19.182
    amphetamine type — *see* Abuse, drug, stimulant NEC
    analgesics (non-prescribed) (over the counter) F55.8
    antacids F55.0
    antidepressants — *see* Abuse, drug, psychoactive NEC
    anxiolytics — *see* Abuse, drug, sedative
    barbiturates — *see* Abuse, drug, sedative
    caffeine — *see* Abuse, drug, stimulant NEC
    cannabis F12.10
      with
        anxiety disorder F12.180
        intoxication F12.129
          with
            delirium F12.121
            perceptual disturbance F12.122
          uncomplicated F12.120
        other specified disorder F12.188
        psychosis F12.159
          delusions F12.150
          hallucinations F12.151

Abuse — *continued*
  drug — *continued*
    cannabis — *continued*
      with — *continued*
        unspecified disorder F12.19
      in remission (early) (sustained) F12.11
    cocaine F14.10
      with
        anxiety disorder F14.180
        intoxication F14.129
          with
            delirium F14.121
            perceptual disturbance F14.122
          uncomplicated F14.120
        mood disorder F14.14
        other specified disorder F14.188
        psychosis F14.159
          delusions F14.150
          hallucinations F14.151
        sexual dysfunction F14.181
        sleep disorder F14.182
        unspecified disorder F14.19
      in remission (early) (sustained) F14.11
    counseling and surveillance Z71.51
    hallucinogen F16.10
      with
        anxiety disorder F16.180
        flashbacks F16.183
        intoxication F16.129
          with
            delirium F16.121
            perceptual disturbance F16.122
          uncomplicated F16.120
        mood disorder F16.14
        other specified disorder F16.188
        perception disorder, persisting F16.183
        psychosis F16.159
          delusions F16.150
          hallucinations F16.151
        unspecified disorder F16.19
      in remission (early) (sustained) F16.11
    hashish — *see* Abuse, drug, cannabis
    herbal or folk remedies F55.1
    hormones F55.3
    hypnotics — *see* Abuse, drug, sedative
    in remission (early) (sustained) F19.11
    inhalant F18.10
      with
        anxiety disorder F18.180
        dementia, persisting F18.17
        intoxication F18.129
          with delirium F18.121
          uncomplicated F18.120
        mood disorder F18.14
        other specified disorder F18.188
        psychosis F18.159
          delusions F18.150
          hallucinations F18.151
        unspecified disorder F18.19
      in remission (early) (sustained) F18.11
    laxatives F55.2
    LSD — *see* Abuse, drug, hallucinogen
    marihuana — *see* Abuse, drug, cannabis
    morphine type (opioids) — *see* Abuse, drug, opioid
    opioid F11.10
      with
        intoxication F11.129
          with
            delirium F11.121
            perceptual disturbance F11.122
          uncomplicated F11.120
        mood disorder F11.14
        other specified disorder F11.188
        psychosis F11.159
          delusions F11.150
          hallucinations F11.151
        sexual dysfunction F11.181
        sleep disorder F11.182
        unspecified disorder F11.19
      in remission (early) (sustained) F11.11
    PCP (phencyclidine) (or related substance) — *see* Abuse, drug, hallucinogen
    psychoactive NEC F19.10
      with
        amnestic disorder F19.16
        anxiety disorder F19.180
        dementia F19.17
        intoxication F19.129

☑ **Additional Character Required** — **Refer to the Tabular List for Character Selection**   ᵛᵇˢ **Subterms under main terms may continue to next column or page**

Abuse — *continued*
  drug — *continued*
    psychoactive — *continued*
      with — *continued*
        intoxication — *continued*
          with
            delirium F19.121
            perceptual disturbance F19.122
          uncomplicated F19.120
        mood disorder F19.14
        other specified disorder F19.188
        psychosis F19.159
          delusions F19.150
          hallucinations F19.151
        sexual dysfunction F19.181
        sleep disorder F19.182
        unspecified disorder F19.19
      sedative, hypnotic or anxiolytic F13.10
        with
          anxiety disorder F13.180
          intoxication F13.129
            with delirium F13.121
            uncomplicated F13.120
          mood disorder F13.14
          other specified disorder F13.188
          psychosis F13.159
            delusions F13.150
            hallucinations F13.151
          sexual dysfunction F13.181
          sleep disorder F13.182
          unspecified disorder F13.19
      in remission (early) (sustained) F13.11
    solvent — *see* Abuse, drug, inhalant
    steroids F55.3
    stimulant NEC F15.10
      with
        anxiety disorder F15.180
        intoxication F15.129
          with
            delirium F15.121
            perceptual disturbance F15.122
          uncomplicated F15.120
        mood disorder F15.14
        other specified disorder F15.188
        psychosis F15.159
          delusions F15.150
          hallucinations F15.151
         sexual dysfunction F15.181
        sleep disorder F15.182
        unspecified disorder F15.19
      in remission (early) (sustained) F15.11
    tranquilizers — *see* Abuse, drug, sedative
    vitamins F55.4
  hallucinogens — *see* Abuse, drug, hallucinogen
  hashish — *see* Abuse, drug, cannabis
  herbal or folk remedies F55.1
  hormones F55.3
  hypnotic — *see* Abuse, drug, sedative
  inhalant — *see* Abuse, drug, inhalant
  laxatives F55.2
  LSD — *see* Abuse, drug, hallucinogen
  marihuana — *see* Abuse, drug, cannabis
  morphine type (opioids) — *see* Abuse, drug, opioid
  non-psychoactive substance NEC F55.8
    antacids F55.0
    folk remedies F55.1
    herbal remedies F55.1
    hormones F55.3
    laxatives F55.2
    steroids F55.3
    vitamins F55.4
  opioids — *see* Abuse, drug, opioid
  PCP (phencyclidine) (or related substance) — *see* Abuse, drug, hallucinogen
  physical (adult) (child) — *see* Maltreatment
  psychoactive substance — *see* Abuse, drug, psychoactive NEC
  psychological (adult) (child) — *see* Maltreatment
  sedative — *see* Abuse, drug, sedative
  sexual — *see* Maltreatment
  solvent — *see* Abuse, drug, inhalant
  steroids F55.3
  vitamins F55.4
Acalculia R48.8
  developmental F81.2
Acanthamebiasis (with) B60.10
  conjunctiva B60.12
  keratoconjunctivitis B60.13

Acanthamebiasis — *continued*
  meningoencephalitis B60.11
  other specified B60.19
Acanthocephaliasis B83.8
Acanthocheilonemiasis B74.4
Acanthocytosis E78.6
Acantholysis L11.9
Acanthosis (acquired) (nigricans) L83
  benign Q82.8
  congenital Q82.8
  seborrheic L82.1
    inflamed L82.0
  tongue K14.3
Acapnia E87.3
Acarbia E87.2
Acardia, acardius Q89.8
Acardiacus amorphus Q89.8
Acardiotrophia I51.4
Acariasis B88.0
  scabies B86
Acarodermatitis (urticarioides) B88.0
Acarophobia F40.218
Acatalasemia, acatalasia E80.3
Acathisia (drug induced) G25.71
Accelerated atrioventricular conduction I45.6
Accentuation of personality traits (type A) Z73.1
Accessory (congenital)
  adrenal gland Q89.1
  anus Q43.4
  appendix Q43.4
  atrioventricular conduction I45.6
  auditory ossicles Q16.3
  auricle (ear) Q17.0
  biliary duct or passage Q44.5
  bladder Q64.79
  blood vessels NEC Q27.9
    coronary Q24.5
  bone NEC Q79.8
  breast tissue, axilla Q83.1
  carpal bones Q74.0
  cecum Q43.4
  chromosome(s) NEC (nonsex) Q92.9
    with complex rearrangements NEC Q92.5
      seen only at prometaphase Q92.8
    13 — *see* Trisomy, 13
    18 — *see* Trisomy, 18
    21 — *see* Trisomy, 21
    partial Q92.9
    sex
      female phenotype Q97.8
  coronary artery Q24.5
  cusp(s), heart valve NEC Q24.8
    pulmonary Q22.3
  cystic duct Q44.5
  digit(s) Q69.9
  ear (auricle) (lobe) Q17.0
  endocrine gland NEC Q89.2
  eye muscle Q10.3
  eyelid Q10.3
  face bone(s) Q75.8
  fallopian tube (fimbria) (ostium) Q50.6
  finger(s) Q69.0
  foreskin N47.8
  frontonasal process Q75.8
  gallbladder Q44.1
  genital organ(s)
    female Q52.8
      external Q52.79
      internal NEC Q52.8
    male Q55.8
  genitourinary organs NEC Q89.8
    female Q52.8
    male Q55.8
  hallux Q69.2
  heart Q24.8
    valve NEC Q24.8
      pulmonary Q22.3
  hepatic ducts Q44.5
  hymen Q52.4
  intestine (large) (small) Q43.4
  kidney Q63.0
  lacrimal canal Q10.6
  leaflet, heart valve NEC Q24.8
  ligament, broad Q50.6
  liver Q44.7
    duct Q44.5
  lobule (ear) Q17.0
  lung (lobe) Q33.1

Accessory — *continued*
  muscle Q79.8
  navicular of carpus Q74.0
  nervous system, part NEC Q07.8
  nipple Q83.3
  nose Q30.8
  organ or site not listed — *see* Anomaly, by site
  ovary Q50.31
  oviduct Q50.6
  pancreas Q45.3
  parathyroid gland Q89.2
  parotid gland (and duct) Q38.4
  pituitary gland Q89.2
  preauricular appendage Q17.0
  prepuce N47.8
  renal arteries (multiple) Q27.2
  rib Q76.6
    cervical Q76.5
  roots (teeth) K00.2
  salivary gland Q38.4
  sesamoid bones Q74.8
    foot Q74.2
    hand Q74.0
  skin tags Q82.8
  spleen Q89.09
  sternum Q76.7
  submaxillary gland Q38.4
  tarsal bones Q74.2
  teeth, tooth K00.1
  tendon Q79.8
  thumb Q69.1
  thymus gland Q89.2
  thyroid gland Q89.2
  toes Q69.2
  tongue Q38.3
  tooth, teeth K00.1
  tragus Q17.0
  ureter Q62.5
  urethra Q64.79
  urinary organ or tract NEC Q64.8
  uterus Q51.28
  vagina Q52.10
  valve, heart NEC Q24.8
    pulmonary Q22.3
  vertebra Q76.49
  vocal cords Q31.8
  vulva Q52.79
Accident
  birth — *see* Birth, injury
  cardiac — *see* Infarct, myocardium
  cerebral I63.9
  cerebrovascular (embolic) (ischemic) (thrombotic) I63.9
    aborted I63.9
    hemorrhagic — *see* Hemorrhage, intracranial, intracerebral
    old (without sequelae) Z86.73
      with sequelae (of) — *see* Sequelae, infarction, cerebral
  coronary — *see* Infarct, myocardium
  craniovascular I63.9
  vascular, brain I63.9
Accidental — *see* condition
Accommodation (disorder) — *see also* condition
  hysterical paralysis of F44.89
  insufficiency of H52.4
  paresis — *see* Paresis, of accommodation
  spasm — *see* Spasm, of accommodation
Accouchement — *see* Delivery
Accreta placenta O43.21- ☑
Accretio cordis (nonrheumatic) I31.0
Accretions, tooth, teeth K03.6
Acculturation difficulty Z60.3
Accumulation secretion, prostate N42.89
Acephalia, acephalism, acephalus, acephaly Q00.0
Acephalobrachia monster Q89.8
Acephalochirus monster Q89.8
Acephalogaster Q89.8
Acephalostomus monster Q89.8
Acephalothorax Q89.8
Acerophobia F40.298
Acetonemia R79.89
  in Type 1 diabetes E10.10
    with coma E10.11
Acetonuria R82.4
Achalasia (cardia) (esophagus) K22.0
  congenital Q39.5
  pylorus Q40.0
  sphincteral NEC K59.8

Ache(s) — *see* Pain
Acheilia Q38.6
Achillobursitis — *see* Tendinitis, Achilles
Achillodynia — *see* Tendinitis, Achilles
Achlorhydria, achlorhydric (neurogenic) K31.83
  anemia D50.8
  diarrhea K31.83
  psychogenic F45.8
  secondary to vagotomy K91.1
Achluophobia F40.228
Acholia K82.8
Acholuric jaundice (familial) (splenomegalic) — *see also*
    Spherocytosis
  acquired D59.8
Achondrogenesis Q77.0
Achondroplasia (osteosclerosis congenita) Q77.4
Achroma, cutis L80
Achromat (ism), achromatopsia (acquired) (congenital)
    H53.51
Achromia, congenital — *see* Albinism
Achromia parasitica B36.0
Achylia gastrica K31.89
  psychogenic F45.8
Acid
  burn — *see* Corrosion
  deficiency
    amide nicotinic E52
    ascorbic E54
    folic E53.8
    nicotinic E52
    pantothenic E53.8
  intoxication E87.2
  peptic disease K30
  phosphatase deficiency E83.39
  stomach K30
    psychogenic F45.8
Acidemia E87.2
  argininosuccinic E72.22
  isovaleric E71.110
  metabolic (newborn) P19.9
    first noted before onset of labor P19.0
    first noted during labor P19.1
    noted at birth P19.2
  methylmalonic E71.120
  pipecolic E72.3
  propionic E71.121
Acidity, gastric (high) K30
  psychogenic F45.8
Acidocytopenia — *see* Agranulocytosis
Acidocytosis D72.1
Acidopenia — *see* Agranulocytosis
Acidosis (lactic) (respiratory) E87.2
  in Type 1 diabetes E10.10
    with coma E10.11
  kidney, tubular N25.89
  lactic E87.2
  metabolic NEC E87.2
    with respiratory acidosis E87.4
    hyperchloremic, of newborn P74.421
    late, of newborn P74.0
  mixed metabolic and respiratory, newborn P84
  newborn P84
  renal (hyperchloremic) (tubular) N25.89
  respiratory E87.2
    complicated by
      metabolic
        acidosis E87.4
        alkalosis E87.4
Aciduria
  4-hydroxybutyric E72.81
  argininosuccinic E72.22
  gamma-hydroxybutyric E72.81
  glutaric (type I) E72.3
    type II E71.313
    type III E71.5- ☑
  orotic (congenital) (hereditary) (pyrimidine deficiency)
      E79.8
    anemia D53.0
Acladiosis (skin) B36.0
Aclasis, diaphyseal Q78.6
Acleistocardia Q21.1
Aclusion — *see* Anomaly, dentofacial, malocclusion
Acne L70.9
  artificialis L70.8
  atrophica L70.8
  cachecticorum (Hebra) L70.8
  conglobata L70.1
  cystic L70.0

Acne — *continued*
  decalvans L66.2
  excoriée (des jeunes filles) L70.5
  frontalis L70.2
  indurata L70.0
  infantile L70.4
  keloid L73.0
  lupoid L70.2
  necrotic, necrotica (miliaris) L70.2
  neonatal L70.4
  nodular L70.0
  occupational L70.8
  picker's L70.5
  pustular L70.0
  rodens L70.2
  rosacea L71.9
  specified NEC L70.8
  tropica L70.3
  varioliformis L70.2
  vulgaris L70.0
Acnitis (primary) A18.4
Acosta's disease T70.29 ☑
Acoustic — *see* condition
Acousticophobia F40.298
Acquired — *see also* condition
  immunodeficiency syndrome (AIDS) B20
Acrania Q00.0
Acroangiodermatitis I78.9
Acroasphyxia, chronic I73.89
Acrobystitis N47.7
Acrocephalopolysyndactyly Q87.0
Acrocephalosyndactyly Q87.0
Acrocephaly Q75.0
Acrochondrohyperplasia — *see* Syndrome, Marfan's
Acrocyanosis I73.89
  newborn P28.2
    meaning transient blue hands and feet — *omit code*
Acrodermatitis L30.8
  atrophicans (chronica) L90.4
  continua (Hallopeau) L40.2
  enteropathica (hereditary) E83.2
  Hallopeau's L40.2
  infantile papular L44.4
  perstans L40.2
  pustulosa continua L40.2
  recalcitrant pustular L40.2
Acrodynia — *see* Poisoning, mercury
Acromegaly, acromegalia E22.0
Acromelalgia I73.81
Acromicria, acromikria Q79.8
Acronyx L60.0
Acroparesthesia (simple) (vasomotor) I73.89
Acropathy, thyroid — *see* Thyrotoxicosis
Acrophobia F40.241
Acroposthitis N47.7
Acroscleriasis, acroscleroderma, acrosclerosis — *see*
    Sclerosis, systemic
Acrosphacelus I96
Acrospiroma, eccrine — *see* Neoplasm, skin, benign
Acrostealgia — *see* Osteochondropathy
Acrotrophodynia — *see* Immersion
ACTH ectopic syndrome E24.3
Actinic — *see* condition
Actinobacillosis, actinobacillus A28.8
  mallei A24.0
  muris A25.1
Actinomyces israelii (infection) — *see* Actinomycosis
Actinomycetoma (foot) B47.1
Actinomycosis, actinomycotic A42.9
  with pneumonia A42.0
  abdominal A42.1
  cervicofacial A42.2
  cutaneous A42.89
  gastrointestinal A42.1
  pulmonary A42.0
  sepsis A42.7
  specified site NEC A42.89
Actinoneuritis G62.82
Action, heart
  disorder I49.9
  irregular I49.9
    psychogenic F45.8
Activated protein C resistance D68.51
Activation
  mast cell (disorder) (syndrome) D89.40
    idiopathic D89.42

Activation — *continued*
  mast cell — *continued*
    monoclonal D89.41
    secondary D89.43
    specified type NEC D89.49
Active — *see* condition
Acute — *see also* condition
  abdomen R10.0
  gallbladder — *see* Cholecystitis, acute
Acyanotic heart disease (congenital) Q24.9
Acystia Q64.5
Adair-Dighton syndrome (brittle bones and blue sclera, deafness) Q78.0
Adamantinoblastoma — *see* Ameloblastoma
Adamantinoma — *see also* Cyst, calcifying odontogenic
  long bones C40.90
    lower limb C40.2- ☑
    upper limb C40.0- ☑
  malignant C41.1
    jaw (bone) (lower) C41.1
      upper C41.0
  tibial C40.2- ☑
Adamantoblastoma — *see* Ameloblastoma
Adams-Stokes (-Morgagni) disease or syndrome I45.9
Adaption reaction — *see* Disorder, adjustment
Addiction — *see also* Dependence F19.20
  alcohol, alcoholic (ethyl) (methyl) (wood) (without remission) F10.20
    with remission F10.21
  drug — *see* Dependence, drug
  ethyl alcohol (without remission) F10.20
    with remission F10.21
  heroin — *see* Dependence, drug, opioid
  methyl alcohol (without remission) F10.20
    with remission F10.21
  methylated spirit (without remission) F10.20
    with remission F10.21
  morphine (-like substances) — *see* Dependence, drug, opioid
  nicotine — *see* Dependence, drug, nicotine
  opium and opioids — *see* Dependence, drug, opioid
  tobacco — *see* Dependence, drug, nicotine
Addison-Biermer anemia (pernicious) D51.0
Addisonian crisis E27.2
Addison's
  anemia (pernicious) D51.0
  disease (bronze) or syndrome E27.1
    tuberculous A18.7
  keloid L94.0
Addison-Schilder complex E71.528
Additional — *see also* Accessory
  chromosome(s) Q99.8
    21 — *see* Trisomy, 21
    sex — *see* Abnormal, chromosome, sex
Adduction contracture, hip or other joint — *see*
    Contraction, joint
Adenitis — *see also* Lymphadenitis
  acute, unspecified site L04.9
  axillary I88.9
    acute L04.2
    chronic or subacute I88.1
  Bartholin's gland N75.8
  bulbourethral gland — *see* Urethritis
  cervical I88.9
    acute L04.0
    chronic or subacute I88.1
  chancroid (Hemophilus ducreyi) A57
  chronic, unspecified site I88.1
  Cowper's gland — *see* Urethritis
  due to Pasteurella multocida (P. septica) A28.0
  epidemic, acute B27.09
  gangrenous L04.9
  gonorrheal NEC A54.89
  groin I88.9
    acute L04.1
    chronic or subacute I88.1
  infectious (acute) (epidemic) B27.09
  inguinal I88.9
    acute L04.1
    chronic or subacute I88.1
  lymph gland or node, except mesenteric I88.9
    acute — *see* Lymphadenitis, acute
    chronic or subacute I88.1
  mesenteric (acute) (chronic) (nonspecific) (subacute) I88.0
  parotid gland (suppurative) — *see* Sialoadenitis
  salivary gland (any) (suppurative) — *see* Sialoadenitis
  scrofulous (tuberculous) A18.2

☑ Additional Character Required — Refer to the Tabular List for Character Selection   ▼ Subterms under main terms may continue to next column or page

Adenitis — continued
  Skene's duct or gland — see Urethritis
  strumous, tuberculous A18.2
  subacute, unspecified site I88.1
  sublingual gland (suppurative) — see Sialoadenitis
  submandibular gland (suppurative) — see Sialoadenitis
  submaxillary gland (suppurative) — see Sialoadenitis
  tuberculous — see Tuberculosis, lymph gland
  urethral gland — see Urethritis
  Wharton's duct (suppurative) — see Sialoadenitis
Adenoacanthoma — see Neoplasm, malignant, by site
Adenoameloblastoma — see Cyst, calcifying odontogenic
Adenocarcinoid (tumor) — see Neoplasm, malignant, by site
Adenocarcinoma — see also Neoplasm, malignant, by site
  acidophil
    specified site — see Neoplasm, malignant, by site
    unspecified site C75.1
  adrenal cortical C74.0- ☑
  alveolar — see Neoplasm, lung, malignant
  apocrine
    breast — see Neoplasm, breast, malignant
    in situ
      breast D05.8- ☑
      specified site NEC — see Neoplasm, skin, in situ
      unspecified site D04.9
    specified site NEC — see Neoplasm, skin, malignant
    unspecified site C44.99
  basal cell
    specified site — see Neoplasm, skin, malignant
    unspecified site C08.9
  basophil
    specified site — see Neoplasm, malignant, by site
    unspecified site C75.1
  bile duct type C22.1
    liver C22.1
    specified site NEC — see Neoplasm, malignant, by site
    unspecified site C22.1
  bronchiolar — see Neoplasm, lung, malignant
  bronchioloalveolar — see Neoplasm, lung, malignant
  ceruminous C44.29- ☑
  cervix, in situ — see also Carcinoma, cervix uteri, in situ D06.9
  chromophobe
    specified site — see Neoplasm, malignant, by site
    unspecified site C75.1
  diffuse type
    specified site — see Neoplasm, malignant, by site
    unspecified site C16.9
  duct
    infiltrating
      with Paget's disease — see Neoplasm, breast, malignant
      specified site — see Neoplasm, malignant, by site
      unspecified site (female) C50.91- ☑
        male C50.92- ☑
    specified site — see Neoplasm, malignant, by site
    unspecified site
      female C56.9
      male C61
  eosinophil
    specified site — see Neoplasm, malignant, by site
    unspecified site C75.1
  follicular
    with papillary C73
    moderately differentiated C73
    specified site — see Neoplasm, malignant, by site
    trabecular C73
    unspecified site C73
    well differentiated C73
  Hurthle cell C73
  in
    adenomatous
      polyposis coli C18.9
  infiltrating duct
    with Paget's disease — see Neoplasm, breast, malignant
    specified site — see Neoplasm, by site, malignant
    unspecified site (female) C50.91- ☑
      male C50.92- ☑
  inflammatory
    specified site — see Neoplasm, by site, malignant
    unspecified site (female) C50.91- ☑

Adenocarcinoma — continued
  inflammatory — continued
    unspecified site — continued
      male C50.92- ☑
  intestinal type
    specified site — see Neoplasm, by site, malignant
    unspecified site C16.9
  intracystic papillary
  intraductal
    breast D05.1- ☑
    noninfiltrating
      breast D05.1- ☑
      papillary
        with invasion
          specified site — see Neoplasm, by site, malignant
          unspecified site (female) C50.91- ☑
            male C50.92- ☑
        breast D05.1- ☑
        specified site NEC — see Neoplasm, in situ, by site
        unspecified site D05.1- ☑
      specified site NEC — see Neoplasm, in situ, by site
      unspecified site D05.1- ☑
    papillary
      with invasion
        specified site — see Neoplasm, malignant, by site
        unspecified site (female) C50.91- ☑
          male C50.92- ☑
      breast D05.1- ☑
      specified site — see Neoplasm, in situ, by site
      unspecified site D05.1- ☑
    specified site NEC — see Neoplasm, in situ, by site
    unspecified site D05.1- ☑
  islet cell
    with exocrine, mixed
      specified site — see Neoplasm, malignant, by site
      unspecified site C25.9
    pancreas C25.4
    specified site NEC — see Neoplasm, malignant, by site
    unspecified site C25.4
  lobular
    in situ
      breast D05.0- ☑
      specified site NEC — see Neoplasm, in situ, by site
      unspecified site D05.0- ☑
    specified site — see Neoplasm, malignant, by site
    unspecified site (female) C50.91- ☑
      male C50.92- ☑
  mucoid — see also Neoplasm, malignant, by site
    cell
      specified site — see Neoplasm, malignant, by site
      unspecified site C75.1
  nonencapsulated sclerosing C73
  papillary
    with follicular C73
    follicular variant C73
    intraductal (noninfiltrating)
      with invasion
        specified site — see Neoplasm, malignant, by site
        unspecified site (female) C50.91- ☑
          male C50.92- ☑
      breast D05.1- ☑
      specified site NEC — see Neoplasm, in situ, by site
      unspecified site D05.1- ☑
    serous
      specified site — see Neoplasm, malignant, by site
      unspecified site C56.9
  papillocystic
    specified site — see Neoplasm, malignant, by site
    unspecified site C56.9
  pseudomucinous
    specified site — see Neoplasm, malignant, by site
    unspecified site C56.9
  renal cell C64- ☑
  sebaceous — see Neoplasm, skin, malignant
  serous — see also Neoplasm, malignant, by site

Adenocarcinoma — continued
  serous — see also Neoplasm, malignant, by site — continued
    papillary
      specified site — see Neoplasm, malignant, by site
      unspecified site C56.9
  sweat gland — see Neoplasm, skin, malignant
  water-clear cell C75.0
Adenocarcinoma-in-situ — see also Neoplasm, in situ, by site
  breast D05.9- ☑
Adenofibroma
  clear cell — see Neoplasm, benign, by site
  endometrioid D27.9
    borderline malignancy D39.10
    malignant C56- ☑
  mucinous
    specified site — see Neoplasm, benign, by site
    unspecified site D27.9
  papillary
    specified site — see Neoplasm, benign, by site
    unspecified site D27.9
  prostate — see Enlargement, enlarged, prostate
  serous
    specified site — see Neoplasm, benign, by site
    unspecified site D27.9
  specified site — see Neoplasm, benign, by site
  unspecified site D27.9
Adenofibrosis
  breast — see Fibroadenosis, breast
  endometrioid N80.0
Adenoiditis (chronic) J35.02
  with tonsillitis J35.03
  acute J03.90
    recurrent J03.91
    specified organism NEC J03.80
      recurrent J03.81
    staphylococcal J03.80
      recurrent J03.81
    streptococcal J03.00
      recurrent J03.01
Adenoids — see condition
Adenolipoma — see Neoplasm, benign, by site
Adenolipomatosis, Launois-Bensaude E88.89
Adenolymphoma
  specified site — see Neoplasm, benign, by site
  unspecified site D11.9
Adenoma — see also Neoplasm, benign, by site
  acidophil
    specified site — see Neoplasm, benign, by site
    unspecified site D35.2
  acidophil-basophil, mixed
    specified site — see Neoplasm, benign, by site
    unspecified site D35.2
  adrenal (cortical) D35.00
    clear cell D35.00
    compact cell D35.00
    glomerulosa cell D35.00
    heavily pigmented variant D35.00
    mixed cell D35.00
  alpha-cell
    pancreas D13.7
    specified site NEC — see Neoplasm, benign, by site
    unspecified site D13.7
  alveolar D14.30
  apocrine
    breast D24- ☑
    specified site NEC — see Neoplasm, skin, benign, by site
    unspecified site D23.9
  basal cell D11.9
  basophil
    specified site — see Neoplasm, benign, by site
    unspecified site D35.2
  basophil-acidophil, mixed
    specified site — see Neoplasm, benign, by site
    unspecified site D35.2
  beta-cell
    pancreas D13.7
    specified site NEC — see Neoplasm, benign, by site
    unspecified site D13.7
  bile duct D13.4
    common D13.5
    extrahepatic D13.5
    intrahepatic D13.4
    specified site NEC — see Neoplasm, benign, by site
    unspecified site D13.4

Adenoma — continued
  black D35.00
  bronchial D38.1
    cylindroid type — see Neoplasm, lung, malignant
  ceruminous D23.2- ☑
  chief cell D35.1
  chromophobe
    specified site — see Neoplasm, benign, by site
    unspecified site D35.2
  colloid
    specified site — see Neoplasm, benign, by site
    unspecified site D34
  duct
  eccrine, papillary — see Neoplasm, skin, benign
  endocrine, multiple
    single specified site — see Neoplasm, uncertain
      behavior, by site
    two or more specified sites D44- ☑
    unspecified site D44.9
  endometrioid — see also Neoplasm, benign
    borderline malignancy — see Neoplasm, uncertain
      behavior, by site
  eosinophil
    specified site — see Neoplasm, benign, by site
    unspecified site D35.2
  fetal
    specified site — see Neoplasm, benign, by site
    unspecified site D34
  follicular
    specified site — see Neoplasm, benign, by site
    unspecified site D34
  hepatocellular D13.4
  Hurthle cell D34
  islet cell
    pancreas D13.7
    specified site NEC — see Neoplasm, benign, by site
    unspecified site D13.7
  liver cell D13.4
  macrofollicular
    specified site — see Neoplasm, benign, by site
    unspecified site D34
  malignant, malignum — see Neoplasm, malignant, by
    site
  microcystic
    pancreas D13.6
    specified site NEC — see Neoplasm, benign, by site
    unspecified site D13.6
  microfollicular
    specified site — see Neoplasm, benign, by site
    unspecified site D34
  mucoid cell
    specified site — see Neoplasm, benign, by site
    unspecified site D35.2
  multiple endocrine
    single specified site — see Neoplasm, uncertain
      behavior, by site
    two or more specified sites D44- ☑
    unspecified site D44.9
  nipple D24- ☑
  papillary — see also Neoplasm, benign, by site
    eccrine — see Neoplasm, skin, benign, by site
  Pick's tubular
    specified site — see Neoplasm, benign, by site
    unspecified site
      female D27.9
      male D29.20
  pleomorphic
    carcinoma in — see Neoplasm, salivary gland, ma-
      lignant
      specified site — see Neoplasm, malignant, by
        site
      unspecified site C08.9
  polypoid — see also Neoplasm, benign
    adenocarcinoma in — see Neoplasm, malignant, by
      site
    adenocarcinoma in situ — see Neoplasm, in situ, by
      site
  prostate — see Neoplasm, benign, prostate
  rete cell D29.20
  sebaceous — see Neoplasm, skin, benign
  Sertoli cell
    specified site — see Neoplasm, benign, by site
    unspecified site
      female D27.9
      male D29.20
  skin appendage — see Neoplasm, skin, benign
  sudoriferous gland — see Neoplasm, skin, benign
  sweat gland — see Neoplasm, skin, benign

Adenoma — continued
  testicular
    specified site — see Neoplasm, benign, by site
    unspecified site
      female D27.9
      male D29.20
  tubular — see also Neoplasm, benign, by site
    adenocarcinoma in — see Neoplasm, malignant, by
      site
    adenocarcinoma in situ — see Neoplasm, in situ, by
      site
    Pick's
      specified site — see Neoplasm, benign, by site
      unspecified site
        female D27.9
        male D29.20
  tubulovillous — see also Neoplasm, benign, by site
    adenocarcinoma in — see Neoplasm, malignant, by
      site
    adenocarcinoma in situ — see Neoplasm, in situ, by
      site
  villous — see Neoplasm, uncertain behavior, by site
    adenocarcinoma in — see Neoplasm, malignant, by
      site
    adenocarcinoma in situ — see Neoplasm, in situ, by
      site
  water-clear cell D35.1
Adenomatosis
  endocrine (multiple) E31.20
    single specified site — see Neoplasm, uncertain
      behavior, by site
  erosive of nipple D24- ☑
  pluriendocrine — see Adenomatosis, endocrine
  pulmonary D38.1
    malignant — see Neoplasm, lung, malignant
  specified site — see Neoplasm, benign, by site
  unspecified site D12.6
Adenomatous
  goiter (nontoxic) E04.9
    with hyperthyroidism — see Hyperthyroidism, with,
      goiter, nodular
    toxic — see Hyperthyroidism, with, goiter, nodular
Adenomyoma — see also Neoplasm, benign, by site
  prostate — see Enlarged, prostate
Adenomyometritis N80.0
Adenomyosis N80.0
Adenopathy (lymph gland) R59.9
  generalized R59.1
  inguinal R59.0
  localized R59.0
  mediastinal R59.0
  mesentery R59.0
  syphilitic (secondary) A51.49
  tracheobronchial R59.0
    tuberculous A15.4
      primary (progressive) A15.7
  tuberculous — see also Tuberculosis, lymph gland
    tracheobronchial A15.4
      primary (progressive) A15.7
Adenosalpingitis — see Salpingitis
Adenosarcoma — see Neoplasm, malignant, by site
Adenosclerosis I88.8
Adenosis (sclerosing) breast — see Fibroadenosis, breast
Adenovirus, as cause of disease classified elsewhere
  B97.0
Adentia (complete) (partial) — see Absence, teeth
Adherent — see also Adhesions
  labia (minora) N90.89
  pericardium (nonrheumatic) I31.0
    rheumatic I09.2
  placenta (with hemorrhage) O72.0
    without hemorrhage O73.0
  prepuce, newborn N47.0
  scar (skin) L90.5
  tendon in scar L90.5
Adhesions, adhesive (postinfective) K66.0
  with intestinal obstruction K56.50
    complete K56.52
    incomplete K56.51
    partial K56.51
  abdominal (wall) — see Adhesions, peritoneum
  appendix K38.8
  bile duct (common) (hepatic) K83.8
  bladder (sphincter) N32.89
  bowel — see Adhesions, peritoneum
  cardiac I31.0
    rheumatic I09.2
  cecum — see Adhesions, peritoneum

Adhesions, adhesive — continued
  cervicovaginal N88.1
    congenital Q52.8
    postpartal O90.89
      old N88.1
  cervix N88.1
  ciliary body NEC — see Adhesions, iris
  clitoris N90.89
  colon — see Adhesions, peritoneum
  common duct K83.8
  congenital — see also Anomaly, by site
    fingers — see Syndactylism, complex, fingers
    omental, anomalous Q43.3
    peritoneal Q43.3
    tongue (to gum or roof of mouth) Q38.3
  conjunctiva (acquired) H11.21- ☑
    congenital Q15.8
  cystic duct K82.8
  diaphragm — see Adhesions, peritoneum
  due to foreign body — see Foreign body
  duodenum — see Adhesions, peritoneum
  ear
    middle H74.1- ☑
  epididymis N50.89
  epidural — see Adhesions, meninges
  epiglottis J38.7
  eyelid H02.59
  female pelvis N73.6
  gallbladder K82.8
  globe H44.89
  heart I31.0
    rheumatic I09.2
  ileocecal (coil) — see Adhesions, peritoneum
  ileum — see Adhesions, peritoneum
  intestine — see also Adhesions, peritoneum
    with obstruction K56.50
      complete K56.52
      incomplete K56.51
      partial K56.51
  intra-abdominal — see Adhesions, peritoneum
  iris H21.50- ☑
    anterior H21.51- ☑
    goniosynechiae H21.52- ☑
    posterior H21.54- ☑
    to corneal graft T85.898 ☑
  joint — see Ankylosis
    knee M23.8X ☑
    temporomandibular M26.61- ☑
  labium (majus) (minus), congenital Q52.5
  liver — see Adhesions, peritoneum
  lung J98.4
  mediastinum J98.59
  meninges (cerebral) (spinal) G96.12
    congenital Q07.8
    tuberculous (cerebral) (spinal) A17.0
  mesenteric — see Adhesions, peritoneum
  nasal (septum) (to turbinates) J34.89
  ocular muscle — see Strabismus, mechanical
  omentum — see Adhesions, peritoneum
  ovary N73.6
    congenital (to cecum, kidney or omentum) Q50.39
  paraovarian N73.6
  pelvic (peritoneal)
    female N73.6
      postprocedural N99.4
    male — see Adhesions, peritoneum
    postpartal (old) N73.6
    tuberculous A18.17
  penis to scrotum (congenital) Q55.8
  periappendiceal — see also Adhesions, peritoneum
  pericardium (nonrheumatic) I31.0
    focal I31.8
    rheumatic I09.2
    tuberculous A18.84
  pericholecystic K82.8
  perigastric — see Adhesions, peritoneum
  periovarian N73.6
  periprostatic N42.89
  perirectal — see Adhesions, peritoneum
  perirenal N28.89
  peritoneum, peritoneal (postinfective) K66.0
    with obstruction (intestinal) K56.50
      complete K56.52
      incomplete K56.51
      partial K56.51
    congenital Q43.3
    pelvic, female N73.6
      postprocedural N99.4

Adhesions, adhesive — *continued*
  peritoneum, peritoneal — *continued*
    postpartal, pelvic N73.6
    postprocedural K66.0
    to uterus N73.6
  peritubal N73.6
  periureteral N28.89
  periuterine N73.6
  perivesical N32.89
  perivesicular (seminal vesicle) N50.89
  pleura, pleuritic J94.8
    tuberculous NEC A15.6
  pleuropericardial J94.8
  postoperative (gastrointestinal tract) K66.0
    with obstruction — *see also* Obstruction, intestine, postoperative K91.30
    due to foreign body accidentally left in wound — *see* Foreign body, accidentally left during a procedure
    pelvic peritoneal N99.4
    urethra — *see* Stricture, urethra, postprocedural
    vagina N99.2
  postpartal, old (vulva or perineum) N90.89
  preputial, prepuce N47.5
  pulmonary J98.4
  pylorus — *see* Adhesions, peritoneum
  sciatic nerve — *see* Lesion, nerve, sciatic
  seminal vesicle N50.89
  shoulder (joint) — *see* Capsulitis, adhesive
  sigmoid flexure — *see* Adhesions, peritoneum
  spermatic cord (acquired) N50.89
    congenital Q55.4
  spinal canal G96.12
  stomach — *see* Adhesions, peritoneum
  subscapular — *see* Capsulitis, adhesive
  temporomandibular M26.61- ☑
  tendinitis (*see also* Tenosynovitis, specified type NEC)
    shoulder — *see* Capsulitis, adhesive
  testis N44.8
  tongue, congenital (to gum or roof of mouth) Q38.3
    acquired K14.8
  trachea J39.8
  tubo-ovarian N73.6
  tunica vaginalis N44.8
  uterus N73.6
    internal N85.6
    to abdominal wall N73.6
  vagina (chronic) N89.5
    postoperative N99.2
  vitreomacular H43.82- ☑
  vitreous H43.89
  vulva N90.89
Adiaspiromycosis B48.8
Adie (-Holmes) pupil or syndrome — *see* Anomaly, pupil, function, tonic pupil
Adiponecrosis neonatorum P83.88
Adiposis — *see also* Obesity
  cerebralis E23.6
  dolorosa E88.2
Adiposity — *see also* Obesity
  heart — *see* Degeneration, myocardial
  localized E65
Adiposogenital dystrophy E23.6
Adjustment
  disorder — *see* Disorder, adjustment
  implanted device — *see* Encounter (for), adjustment (of)
  prosthesis, external — *see* Fitting
  reaction — *see* Disorder, adjustment
Administration of tPA (rtPA) in a different facility within the last 24 hours prior to admission to current facility Z92.82
Admission (for) — *see also* Encounter (for)
  adjustment (of)
    artificial
      arm Z44.00- ☑
        complete Z44.01- ☑
        partial Z44.02- ☑
      eye Z44.2 ☑
      leg Z44.10- ☑
        complete Z44.11- ☑
        partial Z44.12- ☑
    brain neuropacemaker Z46.2
      implanted Z45.42
    breast
      implant Z45.81 ☑
      prosthesis (external) Z44.3 ☑

Admission — *continued*
  adjustment — *continued*
    colostomy belt Z46.89
    contact lenses Z46.0
    cystostomy device Z46.6
    dental prosthesis Z46.3
    device NEC
      abdominal Z46.89
      implanted Z45.89
        cardiac Z45.09
          defibrillator (with synchronous cardiac pacemaker) Z45.02
          pacemaker (cardiac resynchronization therapy (CRT-P)) Z45.018
            pulse generator Z45.010
          resynchronization therapy defibrillator (CRT-D) Z45.02
        hearing device Z45.328
          bone conduction Z45.320
          cochlear Z45.321
        infusion pump Z45.1
        nervous system Z45.49
          CSF drainage Z45.41
          hearing device — *see* Admission, adjustment, device, implanted, hearing device
          neuropacemaker Z45.42
          visual substitution Z45.31
        specified NEC Z45.89
        vascular access Z45.2
        visual substitution Z45.31
    nervous system Z46.2
      implanted — *see* Admission, adjustment, device, implanted, nervous system
    orthodontic Z46.4
    prosthetic Z44.9
      arm — *see* Admission, adjustment, artificial, arm
      breast Z44.3 ☑
      dental Z46.3
      eye Z44.2 ☑
      leg — *see* Admission, adjustment, artificial, leg
      specified type NEC Z44.8
    substitution
      auditory Z46.2
        implanted — *see* Admission, adjustment, device, implanted, hearing device
      nervous system Z46.2
        implanted — *see* Admission, adjustment, device, implanted, nervous system
      visual Z46.2
        implanted Z45.31
    urinary Z46.6
  hearing aid Z46.1
    implanted — *see* Admission, adjustment, device, implanted, hearing device
  ileostomy device Z46.89
  intestinal appliance or device NEC Z46.89
  neuropacemaker (brain) (peripheral nerve) (spinal cord) Z46.2
    implanted Z45.42
  orthodontic device Z46.4
  orthopedic (brace) (cast) (device) (shoes) Z46.89
  pacemaker (cardiac resynchronization therapy (CRT-P))
    cardiac Z45.018
      pulse generator Z45.010
    nervous system Z46.2
      implanted Z45.42
  portacath (port-a-cath) Z45.2
  prosthesis Z44.9
    arm — *see* Admission, adjustment, artificial, arm
    breast Z44.3 ☑
    dental Z46.3
    eye Z44.2 ☑
    leg — *see* Admission, adjustment, artificial, leg
    specified NEC Z44.8
  spectacles Z46.0
  aftercare — *see also* Aftercare Z51.89
    postpartum
      immediately after delivery Z39.0
      routine follow-up Z39.2
    radiation therapy (antineoplastic) Z51.0
  attention to artificial opening (of) Z43.9
    artificial vagina Z43.7
    colostomy Z43.3
    cystostomy Z43.5

Admission — *continued*
  attention to artificial opening — *continued*
    enterostomy Z43.4
    gastrostomy Z43.1
    ileostomy Z43.2
    jejunostomy Z43.4
    nephrostomy Z43.6
    specified site NEC Z43.8
      intestinal tract Z43.4
      urinary tract Z43.6
    tracheostomy Z43.0
    ureterostomy Z43.6
    urethrostomy Z43.6
  breast augmentation or reduction Z41.1
  breast reconstruction following mastectomy Z42.1
  change of
    dressing (nonsurgical) Z48.00
    neuropacemaker device (brain) (peripheral nerve) (spinal cord) Z46.2
      implanted Z45.42
    surgical dressing Z48.01
  circumcision, ritual or routine (in absence of diagnosis) Z41.2
  clinical research investigation (control) (normal comparison) (participant) Z00.6
  contraceptive management Z30.9
  cosmetic surgery NEC Z41.1
  counseling — *see also* Counseling
    dietary Z71.3
    gestational carrier Z31.7
    HIV Z71.7
    human immunodeficiency virus Z71.7
    nonattending third party Z71.0
    procreative management NEC Z31.69
  delivery, full-term, uncomplicated O80
    cesarean, without indication O82
  desensitization to allergens Z51.6
  dietary surveillance and counseling Z71.3
  ear piercing Z41.3
  examination at health care facility (adult) — *see also* Examination Z00.00
    with abnormal findings Z00.01
    clinical research investigation (control) (normal comparison) (participant) Z00.6
    dental Z01.20
      with abnormal findings Z01.21
    donor (potential) Z00.5
    ear Z01.10
      with abnormal findings NEC Z01.118
    eye Z01.00
      with abnormal findings Z01.01
      following failed vision screening Z01.020
        with abnormal findings Z01.021
    general, specified reason NEC Z00.8
    hearing Z01.10
      with abnormal findings NEC Z01.118
      infant or child (over 28 days old) Z00.129
        with abnormal findings Z00.121
    postpartum checkup Z39.2
    psychiatric (general) Z00.8
      requested by authority Z04.6
    vision Z01.00
      with abnormal findings Z01.01
      following failed vision screening Z01.020
        with abnormal findings Z01.021
      infant or child (over 28 days old) Z00.129
        with abnormal findings Z00.121
  fitting (of)
    artificial
      arm — *see* Admission, adjustment, artificial, arm
      eye Z44.2 ☑
      leg — *see* Admission, adjustment, artificial, leg
    brain neuropacemaker Z46.2
      implanted Z45.42
    breast prosthesis (external) Z44.3 ☑
    colostomy belt Z46.89
    contact lenses Z46.0
    cystostomy device Z46.6
    dental prosthesis Z46.3
    dentures Z46.3
    device NEC
      abdominal Z46.89
      nervous system Z46.2
        implanted — *see* Admission, adjustment, device, implanted, nervous system
      orthodontic Z46.4
      prosthetic Z44.9
        breast Z44.3 ☑

▽ Subterms under main terms may continue to next column or page   ☑ Additional Character Required — Refer to the Tabular List for Character Selection   13

Adhesions, adhesive — Admission

Admission — *continued*
  fitting — *continued*
    device — *continued*
      prosthetic — *continued*
        dental Z46.3
        eye Z44.2 ☑
      substitution
        auditory Z46.2
          implanted — *see* Admission, adjustment,
            device, implanted, hearing device
        nervous system Z46.2
          implanted — *see* Admission, adjustment,
            device, implanted, nervous system
        visual Z46.2
          implanted Z45.31
  hearing aid Z46.1
  ileostomy device Z46.89
  intestinal appliance or device NEC Z46.89
  neuropacemaker (brain) (peripheral nerve) (spinal
    cord) Z46.2
    implanted Z45.42
  orthodontic device Z46.4
  orthopedic device (brace) (cast) (shoes) Z46.89
  prosthesis Z44.9
    arm — *see* Admission, adjustment, artificial, arm
    breast Z44.3 ☑
    dental Z46.3
    eye Z44.2 ☑
    leg — *see* Admission, adjustment, artificial, leg
    specified type NEC Z44.8
  spectacles Z46.0
  follow-up examination Z09
  intrauterine device management Z30.431
    initial prescription Z30.014
  mental health evaluation Z00.8
    requested by authority Z04.6
  observation — *see* Observation
  Papanicolaou smear, cervix Z12.4
    for suspected malignant neoplasm Z12.4
  plastic and reconstructive surgery following medical
    procedure or healed injury NEC Z42.8
  plastic surgery, cosmetic NEC Z41.1
  postpartum observation
    immediately after delivery Z39.0
    routine follow-up Z39.2
  poststerilization (for restoration) Z31.0
    aftercare Z31.42
  procreative management Z31.9
  prophylactic (measure) — *see also* Encounter, prophy-
    lactic measures
    organ removal Z40.00
      breast Z40.01
      fallopian tube(s) Z40.03
        with ovary(s) Z40.02
      ovary(s) Z40.02
      specified organ NEC Z40.09
      testes Z40.09
    vaccination Z23
  psychiatric examination (general) Z00.8
    requested by authority Z04.6
  radiation therapy (antineoplastic) Z51.0
  reconstructive surgery following medical procedure or
    healed injury NEC Z42.8
  removal of
    cystostomy catheter Z43.5
    drains Z48.03
    dressing (nonsurgical) Z48.00
    implantable subdermal contraceptive Z30.46
    intrauterine contraceptive device Z30.432
    neuropacemaker (brain) (peripheral nerve) (spinal
      cord) Z46.2
      implanted Z45.42
    staples Z48.02
    surgical dressing Z48.01
    sutures Z48.02
    ureteral stent Z46.6
  respirator [ventilator] use during power failure Z99.12
  restoration of organ continuity (poststerilization) Z31.0
    aftercare Z31.42
  sensitivity test — *see also* Test, skin
    allergy NEC Z01.82
    Mantoux Z11.1
  tuboplasty following previous sterilization Z31.0
    aftercare Z31.42
  vasoplasty following previous sterilization Z31.0
    aftercare Z31.42
  vision examination Z01.00
    with abnormal findings Z01.01

Admission — *continued*
  vision examination — *continued*
    following failed vision screening Z01.020
      with abnormal findings Z01.021
    infant or child (over 28 days old) Z00.129
      with abnormal findings Z00.121
    waiting period for admission to other facility Z75.1
Adnexitis (suppurative) — *see* Salpingo-oophoritis
Adolescent X-linked adrenoleukodystrophy E71.521
Adrenal (gland) — *see* condition
Adrenalism, tuberculous A18.7
Adrenalitis, adrenitis E27.8
  autoimmune E27.1
  meningococcal, hemorrhagic A39.1
Adrenarche, premature E27.0
Adrenocortical syndrome — *see* Cushing's, syndrome
Adrenogenital syndrome E25.9
  acquired E25.8
  congenital E25.0
  salt loss E25.0
Adrenogenitalism, congenital E25.0
Adrenoleukodystrophy E71.529
  neonatal E71.511
  X-linked E71.529
    Addison only phenotype E71.528
    Addison-Schilder E71.528
    adolescent E71.521
    adrenomyeloneuropathy E71.522
    childhood cerebral E71.520
    other specified E71.528
Adrenomyeloneuropathy E71.522
Adventitious bursa — *see* Bursopathy, specified type
  NEC
Adverse effect — *see* Table of Drugs and Chemicals,
  categories T36-T50, with 6th character 5
Advice — *see* Counseling
Adynamia (episodica) (hereditary) (periodic) G72.3
Aeration lung imperfect, newborn — *see* Atelectasis
Aerobullosis T70.3 ☑
Aerocele — *see* Embolism, air
Aerodermectasia
  subcutaneous (traumatic) T79.7 ☑
Aerodontalgia T70.29 ☑
Aeroembolism T70.3 ☑
Aerogenes capsulatus infection A48.0
Aero-otitis media T70.0 ☑
Aerophagy, aerophagia (psychogenic) F45.8
Aerophobia F40.228
Aerosinusitis T70.1 ☑
Aerotitis T70.0 ☑
Affection — *see* Disease
Afibrinogenemia — *see also* Defect, coagulation D68.8
  acquired D65
  congenital D68.2
  following ectopic or molar pregnancy O08.1
  in abortion — *see* Abortion, by type, complicated by,
    afibrinogenemia
  puerperal O72.3
African
  sleeping sickness B56.9
  tick fever A68.1
  trypanosomiasis B56.9
    gambian B56.0
    rhodesian B56.1
Aftercare — *see also* Care Z51.89
  following surgery (for) (on)
    amputation Z47.81
    attention to
      drains Z48.03
      dressings (nonsurgical) Z48.00
        surgical Z48.01
      sutures Z48.02
    circulatory system Z48.812
    delayed (planned) wound closure Z48.1
    digestive system Z48.815
    explantation of joint prosthesis (staged procedure)
      hip Z47.32
      knee Z47.33
      shoulder Z47.31
    genitourinary system Z48.816
    joint replacement Z47.1
    neoplasm Z48.3
    nervous system Z48.811
    oral cavity Z48.814
    organ transplant
      bone marrow Z48.290
      heart Z48.21
      heart-lung Z48.280

Aftercare — *continued*
  following surgery — *continued*
    organ transplant — *continued*
      kidney Z48.22
      liver Z48.23
      lung Z48.24
      multiple organs NEC Z48.288
      specified NEC Z48.298
    orthopedic NEC Z47.89
    planned wound closure Z48.1
    removal of internal fixation device Z47.2
    respiratory system Z48.813
    scoliosis Z47.82
    sense organs Z48.810
    skin and subcutaneous tissue Z48.817
    specified body system
      circulatory Z48.812
      digestive Z48.815
      genitourinary Z48.816
      nervous Z48.811
      oral cavity Z48.814
      respiratory Z48.813
      sense organs Z48.810
      skin and subcutaneous tissue Z48.817
      teeth Z48.814
    specified NEC Z48.89
    spinal Z47.89
    teeth Z48.814
  fracture — *code to* fracture with seventh character D
  involving
    removal of
      drains Z48.03
      dressings (nonsurgical) Z48.00
      staples Z48.02
      surgical dressings Z48.01
      sutures Z48.02
  neuropacemaker (brain) (peripheral nerve) (spinal cord)
    Z46.2
    implanted Z45.42
  orthopedic NEC Z47.89
  postprocedural — *see* Aftercare, following surgery
After-cataract — *see* Cataract, secondary
Agalactia (primary) O92.3
  elective, secondary or therapeutic O92.5
Agammaglobulinemia (acquired) (secondary) (nonfamilial) D80.1
  with
    immunoglobulin-bearing B-lymphocytes D80.1
    lymphopenia D81.9
  autosomal recessive (Swiss type) D80.0
  Bruton's X-linked D80.0
  common variable (CVAgamma) D80.1
  congenital sex-linked D80.0
  hereditary D80.0
  lymphopenic D81.9
  Swiss type (autosomal recessive) D80.0
  X-linked (with growth hormone deficiency) (Bruton)
    D80.0
Aganglionosis (bowel) (colon) Q43.1
Age (old) — *see* Senility
Agenesis
  adrenal (gland) Q89.1
  alimentary tract (complete) (partial) NEC Q45.8
    upper Q40.8
  anus, anal (canal) Q42.3
    with fistula Q42.2
  aorta Q25.41
  appendix Q42.8
  arm (complete) Q71.0- ☑
    with hand present Q71.1- ☑
  artery (peripheral) Q27.9
    brain Q28.3
    coronary Q24.5
    pulmonary Q25.79
    specified NEC Q27.8
    umbilical Q27.0
  auditory (canal) (external) Q16.1
  auricle (ear) Q16.0
  bile duct or passage Q44.5
  bladder Q64.5
  bone Q79.9
  brain Q00.0
    part of Q04.3
  breast (with nipple present) Q83.8
    with absent nipple Q83.0
  bronchus Q32.4
  canaliculus lacrimalis Q10.4
  carpus — *see* Agenesis, hand

14

☑ **Additional Character Required** — Refer to the Tabular List for Character Selection   Ⓦ **Subterms under main terms may continue to next column or page**

Agenesis — *continued*
- cartilage Q79.9
- cecum Q42.8
- cerebellum Q04.3
- cervix Q51.5
- chin Q18.8
- cilia Q10.3
- circulatory system, part NOS Q28.9
- clavicle Q74.0
- clitoris Q52.6
- coccyx Q76.49
- colon Q42.9
  - specified NEC Q42.8
- corpus callosum Q04.0
- cricoid cartilage Q31.8
- diaphragm (with hernia) Q79.1
- digestive organ(s) or tract (complete) (partial) NEC Q45.8
  - upper Q40.8
- ductus arteriosus Q28.8
- duodenum Q41.0
- ear Q16.9
  - auricle Q16.0
  - lobe Q17.8
- ejaculatory duct Q55.4
- endocrine (gland) NEC Q89.2
- epiglottis Q31.8
- esophagus Q39.8
- eustachian tube Q16.2
- eye Q11.1
  - adnexa Q15.8
- eyelid (fold) Q10.3
- face
  - bones NEC Q75.8
  - specified part NEC Q18.8
- fallopian tube Q50.6
- femur — *see* Defect, reduction, lower limb, longitudinal, femur
- fibula — *see* Defect, reduction, lower limb, longitudinal, fibula
- finger (complete) (partial) — *see* Agenesis, hand
- foot (and toes) (complete) (partial) Q72.3- ☑
- forearm (with hand present) — *see* Agenesis, arm, with hand present
  - and hand Q71.2- ☑
- gallbladder Q44.0
- gastric Q40.2
- genitalia, genital (organ(s))
  - female Q52.8
    - external Q52.71
    - internal NEC Q52.8
  - male Q55.8
- glottis Q31.8
- hair Q84.0
- hand (and fingers) (complete) (partial) Q71.3- ☑
- heart Q24.8
  - valve NEC Q24.8
    - pulmonary Q22.0
- hepatic Q44.7
- humerus — *see* Defect, reduction, upper limb
- hymen Q52.4
- ileum Q41.2
- incus Q16.3
- intestine (small) Q41.9
  - large Q42.9
    - specified NEC Q42.8
- iris (dilator fibers) Q13.1
- jaw M26.09
- jejunum Q41.1
- kidney(s) (partial) Q60.2
  - bilateral Q60.1
  - unilateral Q60.0
- labium (majus) (minus) Q52.71
- labyrinth, membranous Q16.5
- lacrimal apparatus Q10.4
- larynx Q31.8
- leg (complete) Q72.0- ☑
  - with foot present Q72.1- ☑
  - lower leg (with foot present) — *see* Agenesis, leg, with foot present
    - and foot Q72.2- ☑
- lens Q12.3
- limb (complete) Q73.0
  - lower — *see* Agenesis, leg
  - upper — *see* Agenesis, arm
- lip Q38.0
- liver Q44.7
- lung (fissure) (lobe) (bilateral) (unilateral) Q33.3

Agenesis — *continued*
- mandible, maxilla M26.09
- metacarpus — *see* Agenesis, hand
- metatarsus — *see* Agenesis, foot
- muscle Q79.8
  - eyelid Q10.3
  - ocular Q15.8
- musculoskeletal system NEC Q79.8
- nail(s) Q84.3
- neck, part Q18.8
- nerve Q07.8
- nervous system, part NEC Q07.8
- nipple Q83.2
- nose Q30.1
- nuclear Q07.8
- organ
  - of Corti Q16.5
  - or site not listed — *see* Anomaly, by site
- osseous meatus (ear) Q16.1
- ovary
  - bilateral Q50.02
  - unilateral Q50.01
- oviduct Q50.6
- pancreas Q45.0
- parathyroid (gland) Q89.2
- parotid gland(s) Q38.4
- patella Q74.1
- pelvic girdle (complete) (partial) Q74.2
- penis Q55.5
- pericardium Q24.8
- pituitary (gland) Q89.2
- prostate Q55.4
- punctum lacrimale Q10.4
- radioulnar — *see* Defect, reduction, upper limb
- radius — *see* Defect, reduction, upper limb, longitudinal, radius
- rectum Q42.1
  - with fistula Q42.0
- renal Q60.2
  - bilateral Q60.1
  - unilateral Q60.0
- respiratory organ NEC Q34.8
- rib Q76.6
- roof of orbit Q75.8
- round ligament Q52.8
- sacrum Q76.49
- salivary gland Q38.4
- scapula Q74.0
- scrotum Q55.29
- seminal vesicles Q55.4
- septum
  - atrial Q21.1
  - between aorta and pulmonary artery Q21.4
  - ventricular Q20.4
- shoulder girdle (complete) (partial) Q74.0
- skull (bone) Q75.8
  - with
    - anencephaly Q00.0
    - encephalocele — *see* Encephalocele
    - hydrocephalus Q03.9
      - with spina bifida — *see* Spina bifida, by site, with hydrocephalus
    - microcephaly Q02
- spermatic cord Q55.4
- spinal cord Q06.0
- spine Q76.49
- spleen Q89.01
- sternum Q76.7
- stomach Q40.2
- submaxillary gland(s) (congenital) Q38.4
- tarsus — *see* Agenesis, foot
- tendon Q79.8
- testicle Q55.0
- thymus (gland) Q89.2
- thyroid (gland) E03.1
  - cartilage Q31.8
- tibia — *see* Defect, reduction, lower limb, longitudinal, tibia
- tibiofibular — *see* Defect, reduction, lower limb, specified type NEC
- toe (and foot) (complete) (partial) — *see* Agenesis, foot
- tongue Q38.3
- trachea (cartilage) Q32.1
- ulna — *see* Defect, reduction, upper limb, longitudinal, ulna
- upper limb — *see* Agenesis, arm
- ureter Q62.4
- urethra Q64.5

Agenesis — *continued*
- urinary tract NEC Q64.8
- uterus Q51.0
- uvula Q38.5
- vagina Q52.0
- vas deferens Q55.4
- vein(s) (peripheral) Q27.9
  - brain Q28.3
  - great NEC Q26.8
  - portal Q26.5
- vena cava (inferior) (superior) Q26.8
- vermis of cerebellum Q04.3
- vertebra Q76.49
- vulva Q52.71
Ageusia R43.2
Agitated — *see* condition
Agitation R45.1
Aglossia (congenital) Q38.3
Aglossia-adactylia syndrome Q87.0
Aglycogenosis E74.00
Agnosia (body image) (other senses) (tactile) R48.1
- developmental F88
- verbal R48.1
  - auditory R48.1
    - developmental F80.2
- visual (object) R48.3
Agoraphobia F40.00
- with panic disorder F40.01
- without panic disorder F40.02
Agrammatism R48.8
Agranulocytopenia — *see* Agranulocytosis
Agranulocytosis (chronic) (cyclical) (genetic) (infantile) (periodic) (pernicious) — *see also* Neutropenia D70.9
- congenital D70.0
- cytoreductive cancer chemotherapy sequela D70.1
- drug-induced D70.2
  - due to cytoreductive cancer chemotherapy D70.1
- due to infection D70.3
- secondary D70.4
  - drug-induced D70.2
    - due to cytoreductive cancer chemotherapy D70.1
Agraphia (absolute) R48.8
- with alexia R48.0
- developmental F81.81
Ague (dumb) — *see* Malaria
Agyria Q04.3
Ahumada-del Castillo syndrome E23.0
Aichomophobia F40.298
AIDS (related complex) B20
Ailment heart — *see* Disease, heart
Ailurophobia F40.218
AIN — *see* Neoplasia, intraepithelial, anal
Ainhum (disease) L94.6
AIPHI (acute idiopathic pulmonary hemorrhage in infants (over 28 days old)) R04.81
Air
- anterior mediastinum J98.2
- compressed, disease T70.3 ☑
- conditioner lung or pneumonitis J67.7
- embolism (artery) (cerebral) (any site) T79.0 ☑
  - with ectopic or molar pregnancy O08.2
  - due to implanted device NEC — *see* Complications, by site and type, specified NEC
  - following
    - abortion — *see* Abortion by type, complicated by, embolism
    - ectopic or molar pregnancy O08.2
  - infusion, therapeutic injection or transfusion T80.0 ☑
  - in pregnancy, childbirth or puerperium — *see* Embolism, obstetric
  - traumatic T79.0 ☑
- hunger, psychogenic F45.8
- rarefied, effects of — *see* Effect, adverse, high altitude
- sickness T75.3 ☑
Airplane sickness T75.3 ☑
Akathisia (drug-induced) (treatment-induced) G25.71
- neuroleptic induced (acute) G25.71
- tardive G25.71
Akinesia R29.898
Akinetic mutism R41.89
Akureyri's disease G93.3
Alactasia, congenital E73.0
Alagille's syndrome Q44.7
Alastrim B03

▽ Subterms under main terms may continue to next column or page   ☑ Additional Character Required — Refer to the Tabular List for Character Selection   **15**

Agenesis — Alastrim

Albers-Schönberg syndrome Q78.2
Albert's syndrome — *see* Tendinitis, Achilles
Albinism, albino E70.30
  with hematologic abnormality E70.339
    Chédiak-Higashi syndrome E70.330
    Hermansky-Pudlak syndrome E70.331
    other specified E70.338
  I E70.320
  II E70.321
  ocular E70.319
    autosomal recessive E70.311
    other specified E70.318
    X-linked E70.310
  oculocutaneous E70.329
    other specified E70.328
    tyrosinase (ty) negative E70.320
    tyrosinase (ty) positive E70.321
  other specified E70.39
Albinismus E70.30
Albright (-McCune)(-Sternberg) syndrome Q78.1
Albuminous — *see* condition
Albuminuria, albuminuric (acute) (chronic) (subacute)
    — *see also* Proteinuria R80.9
  complicating pregnancy — *see* Proteinuria, gestational
  with
    gestational hypertension — *see* Pre-eclampsia
    pre-existing hypertension — *see* Hypertension,
      complicating pregnancy, pre-existing,
      with, pre-eclampsia
  gestational — *see* Proteinuria, gestational
  with
    gestational hypertension — *see* Pre-eclampsia
    pre-existing hypertension — *see* Hypertension,
      complicating pregnancy, pre-existing,
      with, pre-eclampsia
  orthostatic R80.2
  postural R80.2
  pre-eclamptic — *see* Pre-eclampsia
  scarlatinal A38.8
Albuminurophobia F40.298
Alcaptonuria E70.29
Alcohol, alcoholic, alcohol-induced
  addiction (without remission) F10.20
    with remission F10.21
  amnestic disorder, persisting F10.96
    with dependence F10.26
  anxiety disorder F10.980
  bipolar and related disorder F10.94
  brain syndrome, chronic F10.97
    with dependence F10.27
  cardiopathy I42.6
  counseling and surveillance Z71.41
    family member Z71.42
  delirium (acute) (tremens) (withdrawal) F10.231
    with intoxication F10.921
      in
        abuse F10.121
        dependence F10.221
  dementia F10.97
    with dependence F10.27
  depressive disorder F10.94
  deterioration F10.97
    with dependence F10.27
  hallucinosis (acute) F10.951
    in
      abuse F10.151
      dependence F10.251
  insanity F10.959
  intoxication (acute) (without dependence) F10.129
    with
      delirium F10.121
      dependence F10.229
        with delirium F10.221
        uncomplicated F10.220
      uncomplicated F10.120
  jealousy F10.988
  Korsakoff's, Korsakov's, Korsakow's F10.26
  liver K70.9
    acute — *see* Disease, liver, alcoholic, hepatitis
  major neurocognitive disorder, amnestic-confabulatory
    type F10.96
  major neurocognitive disorder, nonamnestic-confabu-
    latory type F10.97
  mania (acute) (chronic) F10.959
  mild neurocognitive disorder F10.988
  paranoia, paranoid (type) psychosis F10.950
  pellagra E52

Alcohol, alcoholic, alcohol-induced — *continued*
  poisoning, accidental (acute) NEC — *see* Table of Drugs
    and Chemicals, alcohol, poisoning
  psychosis — *see* Psychosis, alcoholic
  psychotic disorder F10.959
  sexual dysfunction F10.981
  sleep disorder F10.982
  withdrawal (without convulsions) F10.239
    with delirium F10.231
Alcoholism (chronic) (without remission) F10.20
  with
    psychosis — *see* Psychosis, alcoholic
    remission F10.21
  Korsakov's F10.96
    with dependence F10.26
Alder (-Reilly) **anomaly or syndrome** (leukocyte granu-
    lation) D72.0
Aldosteronism E26.9
  familial (type I) E26.02
  glucocorticoid-remediable E26.02
  primary (due to (bilateral) adrenal hyperplasia) E26.09
  primary NEC E26.09
  secondary E26.1
  specified NEC E26.89
Aldosteronoma D44.10
Aldrich (-Wiskott) **syndrome** (eczema-thrombocytope-
    nia) D82.0
Alektorophobia F40.218
Aleppo boil B55.1
Aleukemic — *see* condition
Aleukia
  congenital D70.0
  hemorrhagica D61.9
    congenital D61.09
  splenica D73.1
Alexia R48.0
  developmental F81.0
  secondary to organic lesion R48.0
Algoneurodystrophy M89.00
  ankle M89.07- ☑
  foot M89.07- ☑
  forearm M89.03- ☑
  hand M89.04- ☑
  lower leg M89.06- ☑
  multiple sites M89.0- ☑
  shoulder M89.01- ☑
  specified site NEC M89.08
  thigh M89.05- ☑
  upper arm M89.02- ☑
Algophobia F40.298
Alienation, mental — *see* Psychosis
Alkalemia E87.3
Alkalosis E87.3
  metabolic E87.3
    with respiratory acidosis E87.4
    of newborn P74.41
  respiratory E87.3
Alkaptonuria E70.29
Allen-Masters syndrome N83.8
Allergy, allergic (reaction) (to) T78.40 ☑
  air-borne substance NEC (rhinitis) J30.89
  alveolitis (extrinsic) J67.9
    due to
      Aspergillus clavatus J67.4
      Cryptostroma corticale J67.6
      organisms (fungal, thermophilic actinomycete)
        growing in ventilation (air conditioning)
        systems J67.7
    specified type NEC J67.8
  anaphylactic reaction or shock T78.2 ☑
  angioneurotic edema T78.3 ☑
  animal (dander) (epidermal) (hair) (rhinitis) J30.81
  bee sting (anaphylactic shock) — *see* Toxicity, venom,
    arthropod, bee
  biological — *see* Allergy, drug
  colitis — *see also* Colitis, allergic K52.29
  dander (animal) (rhinitis) J30.81
  dandruff (rhinitis) J30.81
  dental restorative material (existing) K08.55
  dermatitis — *see* Dermatitis, contact, allergic
  diathesis — *see* History, allergy
  drug, medicament & biological (any) (external) (inter-
    nal) T78.40 ☑
    correct substance properly administered — *see* Ta-
      ble of Drugs and Chemicals, by drug, adverse
      effect

Allergy, allergic — *continued*
  drug, medicament & biological — *continued*
    wrong substance given or taken NEC (by accident)
      — *see* Table of Drugs and Chemicals, by drug,
      poisoning
  due to pollen J30.1
  dust (house) (stock) (rhinitis) J30.89
    with asthma — *see* Asthma, allergic extrinsic
  eczema — *see* Dermatitis, contact, allergic
  epidermal (animal) (rhinitis) J30.81
  feathers (rhinitis) J30.89
  food (any) (ingested) NEC T78.1 ☑
    anaphylactic shock — *see* Shock, anaphylactic, due
      to food
    dermatitis — *see* Dermatitis, due to, food
    dietary counseling and surveillance Z71.3
    in contact with skin L23.6
    rhinitis J30.5
    status (without reaction) Z91.018
      eggs Z91.012
      milk products Z91.011
      peanuts Z91.010
      seafood Z91.013
      specified NEC Z91.018
  gastrointestinal — *see also* specific type of allergic re-
    action
    meaning colitis — *see also* Colitis, allergic K52.29
    meaning gastroenteritis — *see also* Gastroenteritis,
      allergic K52.29
    meaning other adverse food reaction not elsewhere
      classified T78.1 ☑
  grain J30.1
  grass (hay fever) (pollen) J30.1
    asthma — *see* Asthma, allergic extrinsic
  hair (animal) (rhinitis) J30.81
  history (of) — *see* History, allergy
  horse serum — *see* Allergy, serum
  inhalant (rhinitis) J30.89
    pollen J30.1
  kapok (rhinitis) J30.89
  medicine — *see* Allergy, drug
  milk protein — *see also* Allergy, food Z91.011
    anaphylactic reaction T78.07 ☑
    dermatitis L27.2
    enterocolitis syndrome K52.21
    enteropathy K52.22
    gastroenteritis K52.29
    gastroesophageal reflux — *see also* Reaction, ad-
      verse, food K21.9
      with esophagitis K21.0
    proctocolitis K52.82
  nasal, seasonal due to pollen J30.1
  pneumonia J82
  pollen (any) (hay fever) J30.1
    asthma — *see* Asthma, allergic extrinsic
  primrose J30.1
  primula J30.1
  proctocolitis K52.82
  purpura D69.0
  ragweed (hay fever) (pollen) J30.1
    asthma — *see* Asthma, allergic extrinsic
  rose (pollen) J30.1
  seasonal NEC J30.2
  Senecio jacobae (pollen) J30.1
  serum — *see also* Reaction, serum T80.69 ☑
    anaphylactic shock T80.59 ☑
  shock (anaphylactic) T78.2 ☑
    due to
      administration of blood and blood products
        T80.51 ☑
      adverse effect of correct medicinal substance
        properly administered T88.6 ☑
      immunization T80.52 ☑
      serum NEC T80.59 ☑
      vaccination T80.52 ☑
  specific NEC T78.49 ☑
  tree (any) (hay fever) (pollen) J30.1
    asthma — *see* Asthma, allergic extrinsic
  upper respiratory J30.9
  urticaria L50.0
  vaccine — *see* Allergy, serum
  wheat — *see* Allergy, food
Allescheriasis B48.2
Alligator skin disease Q80.9
Allocheiria, allochiria R20.8
Almeida's disease — *see* Paracoccidioidomycosis
Alopecia (hereditaria) (seborrheica) L65.9

Alopecia — *continued*
  androgenic L64.9
    drug-induced L64.0
    specified NEC L64.8
  areata L63.9
    ophiasis L63.2
    specified NEC L63.8
    totalis L63.0
    universalis L63.1
  cicatricial L66.9
    specified NEC L66.8
  circumscripta L63.9
  congenital, congenitalis Q84.0
  due to cytotoxic drugs NEC L65.8
  mucinosa L65.2
  postinfective NEC L65.8
  postpartum L65.0
  premature L64.8
  specific (syphilitic) A51.32
  specified NEC L65.8
  syphilitic (secondary) A51.32
  totalis (capitis) L63.0
  universalis (entire body) L63.1
  X-ray L58.1
Alpers' disease G31.81
Alpine sickness T70.29 ☑
Alport syndrome Q87.81
ALTE (apparent life threatening event) **in newborn and infant** R68.13
Alteration (of), **Altered**
  awareness
    transient R40.4
    unintended under general anesthesia, during procedure T88.53 ☑
  mental status R41.82
  pattern of family relationships affecting child Z62.898
  sensation
    following
      cerebrovascular disease I69.998
        cerebral infarction I69.398
        intracerebral hemorrhage I69.198
        nontraumatic intracranial hemorrhage NEC I69.298
        specified disease NEC I69.898
        subarachnoid hemorrhage I69.098
Alternating — *see* condition
Altitude, high (effects) — *see* Effect, adverse, high altitude
Aluminosis (of lung) J63.0
Alveolitis
  allergic (extrinsic) — *see* Pneumonitis, hypersensitivity
  due to
    Aspergillus clavatus J67.4
    Cryptostroma corticale J67.6
  fibrosing (cryptogenic) (idiopathic) J84.112
  jaw M27.3
  sicca dolorosa M27.3
Alveolus, alveolar — *see* condition
Alymphocytosis D72.810
  thymic (with immunodeficiency) D82.1
Alymphoplasia, thymic D82.1
Alzheimer's disease or sclerosis — *see* Disease, Alzheimer's
Amastia (with nipple present) Q83.8
  with absent nipple Q83.0
Amathophobia F40.228
Amaurosis (acquired) (congenital) — *see also* Blindness
  fugax G45.3
  hysterical F44.6
  Leber's congenital H35.50
  uremic — *see* Uremia
Amaurotic idiocy (infantile) (juvenile) (late) E75.4
Amaxophobia F40.248
Ambiguous genitalia Q56.4
Amblyopia (congenital) (ex anopsia) (partial) (suppression) H53.00- ☑
  anisometropic — *see* Amblyopia, refractive
  deprivation H53.01- ☑
  hysterical F44.6
  nocturnal — *see also* Blindness, night
    vitamin A deficiency E50.5
  refractive H53.02- ☑
  strabismic H53.03- ☑
  suspect H53.04- ☑
  tobacco H53.8
  toxic NEC H53.8
  uremic — *see* Uremia
Ameba, amebic (histolytica) — *see also* Amebiasis

Ameba, amebic — *continued*
  abscess (liver) A06.4
Amebiasis A06.9
  with abscess — *see* Abscess, amebic
  acute A06.0
  chronic (intestine) A06.1
    with abscess — *see* Abscess, amebic
  cutaneous A06.7
  cutis A06.7
  cystitis A06.81
  genitourinary tract NEC A06.82
  hepatic — *see* Abscess, liver, amebic
  intestine A06.0
  nondysenteric colitis A06.2
  skin A06.7
  specified site NEC A06.89
Ameboma (of intestine) A06.3
Amelia Q73.0
  lower limb — *see* Agenesis, leg
  upper limb — *see* Agenesis, arm
Ameloblastoma — *see also* Cyst, calcifying odontogenic
  long bones C40.9- ☑
    lower limb C40.2- ☑
    upper limb C40.0- ☑
  malignant C41.1
    jaw (bone) (lower) C41.1
      upper C41.0
  tibial C40.2- ☑
Amelogenesis imperfecta K00.5
  nonhereditaria (segmentalis) K00.4
Amenorrhea N91.2
  hyperhormonal E28.8
  primary N91.0
  secondary N91.1
Amentia — *see* Disability, intellectual
  Meynert's (nonalcoholic) F04
American
  leishmaniasis B55.2
  mountain tick fever A93.2
Ametropia — *see* Disorder, refraction
AMH (asymptomatic microscopic hematuria) R31.21
Amianthosis J61
Amimia R48.8
Amino-acid disorder E72.9
  anemia D53.0
Aminoacidopathy E72.9
Aminoaciduria E72.9
Amnesia R41.3
  anterograde R41.1
  auditory R48.8
  dissociative F44.0
    with dissociative fugue F44.1
  hysterical F44.0
  postictal in epilepsy — *see* Epilepsy
  psychogenic F44.0
  retrograde R41.2
  transient global G45.4
Amnes(t)ic syndrome (post-traumatic) F04
  induced by
    alcohol F10.96
      with dependence F10.26
    psychoactive NEC F19.96
      with
        abuse F19.16
        dependence F19.26
    sedative F13.96
      with dependence F13.26
Amnion, amniotic — *see* condition
Amnionitis — *see* Pregnancy, complicated by
Amok F68.8
Amoral traits F60.89
Amphetamine (or other stimulant) **-induced**
  anxiety disorder F15.980
  bipolar and related disorder F15.94
  delirium F15.921
  depressive disorder F15.94
  obsessive-compulsive and related disorder F15.988
  psychotic disorder F15.959
  sexual dysfunction F15.981
  sleep disorder F15.982
  stimulant withdrawal F15.23
Ampulla
  lower esophagus K22.8
  phrenic K22.8
Amputation — *see also* Absence, by site, acquired
  neuroma (postoperative) (traumatic) — *see* Complications, amputation stump, neuroma

Amputation — *continued*
  stump (surgical)
    abnormal, painful, or with complication (late) — *see* Complications, amputation stump
    healed or old NOS Z89.9
  traumatic (complete) (partial)
    arm (upper) (complete) S48.91- ☑
      at
        elbow S58.01- ☑
          partial S58.02- ☑
        shoulder joint (complete) S48.01- ☑
          partial S48.02- ☑
      between
        elbow and wrist (complete) S58.11- ☑
          partial S58.12- ☑
        shoulder and elbow (complete) S48.11- ☑
          partial S48.12- ☑
      partial S48.92- ☑
    breast (complete) S28.21- ☑
      partial S28.22- ☑
    clitoris (complete) S38.211 ☑
      partial S38.212 ☑
    ear (complete) S08.11- ☑
      partial S08.12- ☑
    finger (complete) (metacarpophalangeal) S68.11- ☑
      index S68.11- ☑
      little S68.11- ☑
      middle S68.11- ☑
      partial S68.12- ☑
        index S68.12- ☑
        little S68.12- ☑
        middle S68.12- ☑
        ring S68.12- ☑
      ring S68.11- ☑
      thumb — *see* Amputation, traumatic, thumb
      transphalangeal (complete) S68.61- ☑
        index S68.61- ☑
        little S68.61- ☑
        middle S68.61- ☑
        partial S68.62- ☑
          index S68.62- ☑
          little S68.62- ☑
          middle S68.62- ☑
          ring S68.62- ☑
        ring S68.61- ☑
    foot (complete) S98.91- ☑
      at ankle level S98.01- ☑
        partial S98.02- ☑
      midfoot S98.31- ☑
        partial S98.32- ☑
      partial S98.92- ☑
    forearm (complete) S58.91- ☑
      at elbow level (complete) S58.01- ☑
        partial S58.02- ☑
      between elbow and wrist (complete) S58.11- ☑
        partial S58.12- ☑
      partial S58.92- ☑
    genital organ(s) (external)
      female (complete) S38.211 ☑
        partial S38.212 ☑
      male
        penis (complete) S38.221 ☑
          partial S38.222 ☑
        scrotum (complete) S38.231 ☑
          partial S38.232 ☑
        testes (complete) S38.231 ☑
          partial S38.232 ☑
    hand (complete) (wrist level) S68.41- ☑
      finger(s) alone — *see* Amputation, traumatic, finger
      partial S68.42- ☑
      thumb alone — *see* Amputation, traumatic, thumb
      transmetacarpal (complete) S68.71- ☑
        partial S68.72- ☑
    head
      ear — *see* Amputation, traumatic, ear
      nose (partial) S08.812 ☑
        complete S08.811 ☑
      part S08.89 ☑
        scalp S08.0 ☑
    hip (and thigh) (complete) S78.91- ☑
      at hip joint (complete) S78.01- ☑
        partial S78.02- ☑
      between hip and knee (complete) S78.11- ☑
        partial S78.12- ☑

⬙ Subterms under main terms may continue to next column or page   ☑ Additional Character Required — Refer to the Tabular List for Character Selection   17

Alopecia — Amputation

Amputation — *continued*
  traumatic — *continued*
    hip — *continued*
      partial S78.92- ☑
    labium (majus) (minus) (complete) S38.21- ☑
      partial S38.21- ☑
    leg (lower) S88.91- ☑
      at knee level S88.01- ☑
        partial S88.02- ☑
      between knee and ankle S88.11- ☑
        partial S88.12- ☑
      partial S88.92- ☑
    nose (partial) S08.812 ☑
      complete S08.811 ☑
    penis (complete) S38.221 ☑
      partial S38.222 ☑
    scrotum (complete) S38.231 ☑
      partial S38.232 ☑
    shoulder — *see* Amputation, traumatic, arm
      at shoulder joint — *see* Amputation, traumatic,
        arm, at shoulder joint
    testes (complete) S38.231 ☑
      partial S38.232 ☑
    thigh — *see* Amputation, traumatic, hip
    thorax, part of S28.1 ☑
      breast — *see* Amputation, traumatic, breast
    thumb (complete) (metacarpophalangeal)
      S68.01- ☑
      partial S68.02- ☑
      transphalangeal (complete) S68.51- ☑
        partial S68.52- ☑
    toe (lesser) S98.13- ☑
      great S98.11- ☑
        partial S98.12- ☑
      more than one S98.21- ☑
        partial S98.22- ☑
      partial S98.14- ☑
    vulva (complete) S38.211 ☑
      partial S38.212 ☑
Amputee (bilateral) (old) Z89.9
Amsterdam dwarfism Q87.19
Amusia R48.8
  developmental F80.89
Amyelencephalus, amyelencephaly Q00.0
Amyelia Q06.0
Amygdalitis — *see* Tonsillitis
Amygdalolith J35.8
Amyloid heart (disease) E85.4 [I43]
Amyloidosis (generalized) (primary) E85.9
  with lung involvement E85.4 [J99]
  familial E85.2
  genetic E85.2
  heart E85.4 [I43]
  hemodialysis-associated E85.3
  light chain (AL) E85.81
  liver E85.4 [K77]
  localized E85.4
  neuropathic heredofamilial E85.1
  non-neuropathic heredofamilial E85.0
  organ limited E85.4
  Portuguese E85.1
  pulmonary E85.4 [J99]
  secondary systemic E85.3
  senile systemic (SSA) E85.82
  skin (lichen) (macular) E85.4 [L99]
  specified NEC E85.89
  subglottic E85.4 [J99]
  wild-type transthyretin-related (ATTR) E85.82
Amylopectinosis (brancher enzyme deficiency) E74.03
Amylophagia — *see* Pica
Amyoplasia congenita Q79.8
Amyotonia M62.89
  congenita G70.2
Amyotrophia, amyotrophy, amyotrophic G71.8
  congenita Q79.8
  diabetic — *see* Diabetes, amyotrophy
  lateral sclerosis G12.21
  neuralgic G54.5
  spinal progressive G12.25
Anacidity, gastric K31.83
  psychogenic F45.8
Anaerosis of newborn P28.89
Analbuminemia E88.09
Analgesia — *see* Anesthesia
Analphalipoproteinemia E78.6
Anaphylactic
  purpura D69.0

Anaphylactic — *continued*
  shock or reaction — *see* Shock, anaphylactic
Anaphylactoid shock or reaction — *see* Shock, anaphylactic
Anaphylactoid syndrome of pregnancy O88.01- ☑
Anaphylaxis — *see* Shock, anaphylactic
Anaplasia cervix — *see also* Dysplasia, cervix N87.9
Anaplasmosis, human A77.49
Anarthria R47.1
Anasarca R60.1
  cardiac — *see* Failure, heart, congestive
  lung J18.2
  newborn P83.2
  nutritional E43
  pulmonary J18.2
  renal N04.9
Anastomosis
  aneurysmal — *see* Aneurysm
  arteriovenous ruptured brain I60.8
    intracerebral I61.8
    intraparenchymal I61.8
    intraventricular I61.5
    subarachnoid I60.8
  intestinal K63.89
    complicated NEC K91.89
      involving urinary tract N99.89
  retinal and choroidal vessels (congenital) Q14.8
Anatomical narrow angle H40.03- ☑
Ancylostoma, ancylostomiasis (braziliense) (caninum)
  (ceylanicum) (duodenale) B76.0
  Necator americanus B76.1
Andersen's disease (glycogen storage) E74.09
Anderson-Fabry disease E75.21
Andes disease T70.29 ☑
Andrews' disease (bacterid) L08.89
Androblastoma
  benign
    specified site — *see* Neoplasm, benign, by site
    unspecified site
      female D27.9
      male D29.20
  malignant
    specified site — *see* Neoplasm, malignant, by site
    unspecified site
      female C56.9
      male C62.90
  specified site — *see* Neoplasm, uncertain behavior, by
    site
  tubular
    with lipid storage
      specified site — *see* Neoplasm, benign, by site
      unspecified site
        female D27.9
        male D29.20
    specified site — *see* Neoplasm, benign, by site
    unspecified site
      female D27.9
      male D29.20
  unspecified site
    female D39.10
    male D40.10
Androgen insensitivity syndrome — *see also* Syndrome, androgen insensitivity E34.50
Androgen resistance syndrome — *see also* Syndrome,
  androgen insensitivity E34.50
Android pelvis Q74.2
  with disproportion (fetopelvic) O33.3 ☑
    causing obstructed labor O65.3
Androphobia F40.290
Anectasis, pulmonary (newborn) — *see* Atelectasis
Anemia (essential) (general) (hemoglobin deficiency)
  (infantile) (primary) (profound) D64.9
  with (due to) (in)
    disorder of
      anaerobic glycolysis D55.2
      pentose phosphate pathway D55.1
    koilonychia D50.9
  achlorhydric D50.8
  achrestic D53.1
  Addison (-Biermer) (pernicious) D51.0
  agranulocytic — *see* Agranulocytosis
  amino-acid-deficiency D53.0
  aplastic D61.9
    congenital D61.09
    drug-induced D61.1
    due to
      drugs D61.1
      external agents NEC D61.2

Anemia — *continued*
  aplastic — *continued*
    due to — *continued*
      infection D61.2
      radiation D61.2
    idiopathic D61.3
    red cell (pure) D60.9
      chronic D60.0
      congenital D61.01
      specified type NEC D60.8
      transient D60.1
    specified type NEC D61.89
    toxic D61.2
  aregenerative
    congenital D61.09
  asiderotic D50.9
  atypical (primary) D64.9
  Baghdad spring D55.0
  Balantidium coli A07.0
  Biermer's (pernicious) D51.0
  blood loss (chronic) D50.0
    acute D62
  bothriocephalus B70.0 [D63.8]
  brickmaker's B76.9 [D63.8]
  cerebral I67.89
  childhood D58.9
  chlorotic D50.8
  chronic
    blood loss D50.0
    hemolytic D58.9
      idiopathic D59.9
    simple D53.9
  chronica congenita aregenerativa D61.09
  combined system disease NEC D51.0 [G32.0]
    due to dietary vitamin B12 deficiency D51.3 [G32.0]
  complicating pregnancy, childbirth or puerperium —
    see Pregnancy, complicated by (management
    affected by), anemia
  congenital P61.4
    aplastic D61.09
    due to isoimmunization NOS P55.9
    dyserythropoietic, dyshematopoietic D64.4
    following fetal blood loss P61.3
    Heinz body D58.2
    hereditary hemolytic NOS D58.9
    pernicious D51.0
    spherocytic D58.0
  Cooley's (erythroblastic) D56.1
  cytogenic D51.0
  deficiency D53.9
    2, 3 diphosphoglycurate mutase D55.2
    2, 3 PG D55.2
    6 phosphogluconate dehydrogenase D55.1
    6-PGD D55.1
    amino-acid D53.0
    combined B12 and folate D53.1
    enzyme D55.9
      drug-induced (hemolytic) D59.2
      glucose-6-phosphate dehydrogenase (G6PD)
        D55.0
      glycolytic D55.2
      nucleotide metabolism D55.3
      related to hexose monophosphate (HMP) shunt
        pathway NEC D55.1
      specified type NEC D55.8
    erythrocytic glutathione D55.1
    folate D52.9
      dietary D52.0
      drug-induced D52.1
    folic acid D52.9
      dietary D52.0
      drug-induced D52.1
    G SH D55.1
    G6PD D55.0
    GGS-R D55.1
    glucose-6-phosphate dehydrogenase D55.0
    glutathione reductase D55.1
    glyceraldehyde phosphate dehydrogenase D55.2
    hexokinase D55.2
    iron D50.9
      secondary to blood loss (chronic) D50.0
    nutritional D53.9
      with
        poor iron absorption D50.8
        specified deficiency NEC D53.8
    phosphofructo-aldolase D55.2
    phosphoglycerate kinase D55.2
    PK D55.2
    protein D53.0

Anemia — *continued*
  deficiency — *continued*
    pyruvate kinase D55.2
    transcobalamin II D51.2
    triose-phosphate isomerase D55.2
    vitamin B12 NOS D51.9
      dietary D51.3
      due to
        intrinsic factor deficiency D51.0
        selective vitamin B12 malabsorption with
          proteinuria D51.1
      pernicious D51.0
      specified type NEC D51.8
  Diamond-Blackfan (congenital hypoplastic) D61.01
  dibothriocephalus B70.0 *[D63.8]*
  dimorphic D53.1
  diphasic D53.1
  Diphyllobothrium (Dibothriocephalus) B70.0 *[D63.8]*
  due to (in) (with)
    antineoplastic chemotherapy D64.81
    blood loss (chronic) D50.0
      acute D62
    chemotherapy, antineoplastic D64.81
    chronic disease classified elsewhere NEC D63.8
    chronic kidney disease D63.1
    deficiency
      amino-acid D53.0
      copper D53.8
      folate (folic acid) D52.9
        dietary D52.0
        drug-induced D52.1
      molybdenum D53.8
      protein D53.0
      zinc D53.8
    dietary vitamin B12 deficiency D51.3
    disorder of
      glutathione metabolism D55.1
      nucleotide metabolism D55.3
    drug — *see* Anemia, by type — *see also* Table of
      Drugs and Chemicals
    end stage renal disease D63.1
    enzyme disorder D55.9
    fetal blood loss P61.3
    fish tapeworm (D.latum) infestation B70.0 *[D63.8]*
    hemorrhage (chronic) D50.0
      acute D62
    impaired absorption D50.9
    loss of blood (chronic) D50.0
      acute D62
    myxedema E03.9 *[D63.8]*
    Necator americanus B76.1 *[D63.8]*
    prematurity P61.2
    selective vitamin B12 malabsorption with protein-
      uria D51.1
    transcobalamin II deficiency D51.2
  Dyke-Young type (secondary) (symptomatic) D59.1
  dyserythropoietic (congenital) D64.4
  dyshematopoietic (congenital) D64.4
  Egyptian B76.9 *[D63.8]*
  elliptocytosis — *see* Elliptocytosis
  enzyme-deficiency, drug-induced D59.2
  epidemic — *see also* Ancylostomiasis B76.9 *[D63.8]*
  erythroblastic
    familial D56.1
    newborn — *see also* Disease, hemolytic P55.9
    of childhood D56.1
  erythrocytic glutathione deficiency D55.1
  erythropoietin-resistant anemia (EPO resistant anemia)
    D63.1
  Faber's (achlorhydric anemia) D50.9
  factitious (self-induced blood letting) D50.0
  familial erythroblastic D56.1
  Fanconi's (congenital pancytopenia) D61.09
  favism D55.0
  fish tapeworm (D. latum) infestation B70.0 *[D63.8]*
  folate (folic acid) deficiency D52.9
  glucose-6-phosphate dehydrogenase (G6PD) deficiency
    D55.0
  glutathione-reductase deficiency D55.1
  goat's milk D52.0
  granulocytic — *see* Agranulocytosis
  Heinz body, congenital D58.2
  hemolytic D58.9
    acquired D59.9
      with hemoglobinuria NEC D59.6
      autoimmune NEC D59.1
      infectious D59.4
      specified type NEC D59.8

Anemia — *continued*
  hemolytic — *continued*
    acquired — *continued*
      toxic D59.4
    acute D59.9
      due to enzyme deficiency specified type NEC
        D55.8
      Lederer's D59.1
    autoimmune D59.1
      drug-induced D59.0
    chronic D58.9
      idiopathic D59.9
    cold type (secondary) (symptomatic) D59.1
    congenital (spherocytic) — *see* Spherocytosis
    due to
      cardiac conditions D59.4
      drugs (nonautoimmune) D59.2
        autoimmune D59.0
      enzyme disorder D55.9
        drug-induced D59.2
      presence of shunt or other internal prosthetic
        device D59.4
    familial D58.9
    hereditary D58.9
      due to enzyme disorder D55.9
        specified type NEC D55.8
      specified type NEC D58.8
    idiopathic (chronic) D59.9
    mechanical D59.4
    microangiopathic D59.4
    nonautoimmune D59.4
      drug-induced D59.2
    nonspherocytic
      congenital or hereditary NEC D55.8
        glucose-6-phosphate dehydrogenase deficien-
          cy D55.0
        pyruvate kinase deficiency D55.2
        type
          I D55.1
          II D55.2
      type
        I D55.1
        II D55.2
    secondary D59.4
      autoimmune D59.1
    specified (hereditary) type NEC D58.8
    Stransky-Regala type — *see also* Hemoglobinopathy
      D58.8
    symptomatic D59.4
      autoimmune D59.1
    toxic D59.4
    warm type (secondary) (symptomatic) D59.1
  hemorrhagic (chronic) D50.0
    acute D62
  Herrick's D57.1
  hexokinase deficiency D55.2
  hookworm B76.9 *[D63.8]*
  hypochromic (idiopathic) (microcytic) (normoblastic)
    D50.9
    due to blood loss (chronic) D50.0
      acute D62
    familial sex-linked D64.0
    pyridoxine-responsive D64.3
    sideroblastic, sex-linked D64.0
  hypoplasia, red blood cells D61.9
    congenital or familial D61.01
  hypoplastic (idiopathic) D61.9
    congenital or familial (of childhood) D61.01
  hypoproliferative (refractive) D61.9
  idiopathic D64.9
    aplastic D61.3
    hemolytic, chronic D59.9
  in (due to) (with)
    chronic kidney disease D63.1
    end stage renal disease D63.1
    failure, kidney (renal) D63.1
    neoplastic disease — *see also* Neoplasm D63.0
  intertropical — *see also* Ancylostomiasis D63.8
  iron deficiency D50.9
    secondary to blood loss (chronic) D50.0
      acute D62
    specified type NEC D50.8
  Joseph-Diamond-Blackfan (congenital hypoplastic)
    D61.01
  Lederer's (hemolytic) D59.1
  leukoerythroblastic D61.82
  macrocytic D53.9
    nutritional D52.0
    tropical D52.8

Anemia — *continued*
  malarial — *see also* Malaria B54 *[D63.8]*
  malignant (progressive) D51.0
  malnutrition D53.9
  marsh — *see also* Malaria B54 *[D63.8]*
  Mediterranean (with other hemoglobinopathy) D56.9
  megaloblastic D53.1
    combined B12 and folate deficiency D53.1
    hereditary D51.1
    nutritional D52.0
    orotic aciduria D53.0
    refractory D53.1
    specified type NEC D53.1
  megalocytic D53.1
  microcytic (hypochromic) D50.9
    due to blood loss (chronic) D50.0
      acute D62
    familial D56.8
  microdrepanocytosis D57.40
  microelliptopoikilocytic (Rietti-Greppi- Micheli) D56.9
  miner's B76.9 *[D63.8]*
  myelodysplastic D46.9
  myelofibrosis D75.81
  myelogenous D64.89
  myelopathic D64.89
  myelophthisic D61.82
  myeloproliferative D47.Z9 (*following* D47.4)
  newborn P61.4
    due to
      ABO (antibodies, isoimmunization, maternal/fetal
        incompatibility) P55.1
      Rh (antibodies, isoimmunization, maternal/fetal
        incompatibility) P55.0
    following fetal blood loss P61.3
    posthemorrhagic (fetal) P61.3
  nonspherocytic hemolytic — *see* Anemia, hemolytic,
    nonspherocytic
  normocytic (infectional) D64.9
    due to blood loss (chronic) D50.0
      acute D62
    myelophthisic D61.82
  nutritional (deficiency) D53.9
    with
      poor iron absorption D50.8
      specified deficiency NEC D53.8
    megaloblastic D52.0
  of prematurity P61.2
  orotaciduric (congenital) (hereditary) D53.0
  osteosclerotic D64.89
  ovalocytosis (hereditary) — *see* Elliptocytosis
  paludal — *see also* Malaria B54 *[D63.8]*
  pernicious (congenital) (malignant) (progressive) D51.0
  pleochromic D64.89
    of sprue D52.8
  posthemorrhagic (chronic) D50.0
    acute D62
    newborn P61.3
  postoperative (postprocedural)
    due to (acute) blood loss D62
      chronic blood loss D50.0
    specified NEC D64.9
  postpartum O90.81
  pressure D64.89
  progressive D64.9
    malignant D51.0
    pernicious D51.0
  protein-deficiency D53.0
  pseudoleukemica infantum D64.89
  pure red cell D60.9
    congenital D61.01
  pyridoxine-responsive D64.3
  pyruvate kinase deficiency D55.2
  refractory D46.4
    with
      excess of blasts D46.20
        1 (RAEB 1) D46.21
        2 (RAEB 2) D46.22
        in transformation (RAEB T) — *see* Leukemia,
          acute myeloblastic
      hemochromatosis D46.1
      sideroblasts (ring) (RARS) D46.1
    megaloblastic D53.1
    sideroblastic D46.1
    sideropenic D50.9
    without ring sideroblasts, so stated D46.0
    without sideroblasts without excess of blasts D46.0
  Rietti-Greppi-Micheli D56.9
  scorbutic D53.2

⊽ **Subterms under main terms may continue to next column or page**   ☑ **Additional Character Required — Refer to the Tabular List for Character Selection**   19

Anemia — *continued*
  secondary to
    blood loss (chronic) D50.0
      acute D62
    hemorrhage (chronic) D50.0
      acute D62
  semiplastic D61.89
  sickle-cell — *see* Disease, sickle-cell
  sideroblastic D64.3
    hereditary D64.0
    hypochromic, sex-linked D64.0
    pyridoxine-responsive NEC D64.3
    refractory D46.1
    secondary (due to)
      disease D64.1
      drugs and toxins D64.2
    specified type NEC D64.3
  sideropenic (refractory) D50.9
    due to blood loss (chronic) D50.0
      acute D62
  simple chronic D53.9
  specified type NEC D64.89
  spherocytic (hereditary) — *see* Spherocytosis
  splenic D64.89
  splenomegalic D64.89
  stomatocytosis D58.8
  syphilitic (acquired) (late) A52.79 *[D63.8]*
  target cell D64.89
  thalassemia D56.9
  thrombocytopenic — *see* Thrombocytopenia
  toxic D61.2
  tropical B76.9 *[D63.8]*
    macrocytic D52.8
  tuberculous A18.89 *[D63.8]*
  vegan D51.3
  vitamin
    B12 deficiency (dietary) pernicious D51.0
    B6-responsive D64.3
  von Jaksch's D64.89
  Witts' (achlorhydric anemia) D50.8
Anemophobia F40.228
Anencephalus, anencephaly Q00.0
Anergasia — *see* Psychosis, organic
Anesthesia, anesthetic R20.0
  complication or reaction NEC — *see also* Complications,
    anesthesia T88.59 ☑
    due to
      correct substance properly administered — *see*
        Table of Drugs and Chemicals, by drug,
        adverse effect
      overdose or wrong substance given — *see* Table
        of Drugs and Chemicals, by drug, poison-
        ing
    unintended awareness under general anesthesia
      during procedure T88.53 ☑
      personal history of Z92.84
  cornea H18.81- ☑
  dissociative F44.6
  functional (hysterical) F44.6
  hyperesthetic, thalamic G89.0
  hysterical F44.6
  local skin lesion R20.0
  sexual (psychogenic) F52.1
  shock (due to) T88.2 ☑
  skin R20.0
  testicular N50.9
Anetoderma (maculosum) (of) L90.8
  Jadassohn-Pellizzari L90.2
  Schweniger-Buzzi L90.1
Aneurin deficiency E51.9
Aneurysm (anastomotic) (artery) (cirsoid) (diffuse) (false)
    (fusiform) (multiple) (saccular) I72.9
  abdominal (aorta) I71.4
    ruptured I71.3
    syphilitic A52.01
  aorta, aortic (nonsyphilitic) I71.9
    abdominal I71.4
      ruptured I71.3
    arch I71.2
      ruptured I71.1
    arteriosclerotic I71.9
      ruptured I71.8
    ascending I71.2
      ruptured I71.1
    congenital Q25.43
    descending I71.9
      abdominal I71.4
        ruptured I71.3

Aneurysm — *continued*
  aorta, aortic — *continued*
    descending — *continued*
      ruptured I71.8
      thoracic I71.2
        ruptured I71.1
    root Q25.43
    ruptured I71.8
    sinus, congenital Q25.43
    syphilitic A52.01
    thoracic I71.2
      ruptured I71.1
    thoracoabdominal I71.6
      ruptured I71.5
    thorax, thoracic (arch) I71.2
      ruptured I71.1
    transverse I71.2
      ruptured I71.1
    valve (heart) — *see also* Endocarditis, aortic I35.8
  arteriosclerotic I72.9
    cerebral I67.1
      ruptured — *see* Hemorrhage, intracranial, sub-
        arachnoid
  arteriovenous (congenital) — *see also* Malformation,
    arteriovenous
    acquired I77.0
      brain I67.1
        ruptured — *see* Aneurysm, arteriovenous,
          brain, ruptured
      coronary I25.41
      pulmonary I28.0
    brain Q28.2
      ruptured I60.8
        intracerebral I61.8
        intraparenchymal I61.8
        intraventricular I61.5
        subarachnoid I60.8
    peripheral — *see* Malformation, arteriovenous, pe-
      ripheral
    precerebral vessels Q28.0
    specified site NEC — *see also* Malformation, arteri-
      ovenous
      acquired I77.0
  basal — *see* Aneurysm, brain
  basilar (trunk) I72.5
  berry (congenital) (nonruptured) I67.1
    ruptured I60.7
  brain I67.1
    arteriosclerotic I67.1
      ruptured — *see* Hemorrhage, intracranial, sub-
        arachnoid
    arteriovenous (congenital) (nonruptured) Q28.2
      acquired I67.1
        ruptured — *see* Aneurysm, arteriovenous,
          brain, ruptured I60.8
      ruptured — *see* Aneurysm, arteriovenous, brain,
        ruptured I60.8
    berry (congenital) (nonruptured) I67.1
      ruptured — *see* Hemorrhage, intracranial,
        subarachnoid I60.7
    congenital Q28.3
      ruptured I60.7
    meninges I67.1
      ruptured I60.8
    miliary (congenital) (nonruptured) I67.1
      ruptured — *see also* Hemorrhage, intracranial,
        subarachnoid I60.7
    mycotic I33.0
      ruptured — *see* Aneurysm, arteriovenous, brain,
        ruptured I60.8
    syphilitic (hemorrhage) A52.05
  cardiac (false) — *see also* Aneurysm, heart I25.3
  carotid artery (common) (external) I72.0
    internal (intracranial) I67.1
      extracranial portion I72.0
      ruptured into brain I60.0- ☑
    syphilitic A52.09
      intracranial A52.05
  cavernous sinus I67.1
    arteriovenous (congenital) (nonruptured) Q28.3
      ruptured I60.8
  celiac I72.8
  central nervous system, syphilitic A52.05
  cerebral — *see* Aneurysm, brain
  chest — *see* Aneurysm, thorax
  circle of Willis I67.1
    congenital Q28.3
      ruptured I60.6

Aneurysm — *continued*
  circle of Willis — *continued*
    ruptured I60.6
  common iliac artery I72.3
  congenital (peripheral) Q27.8
    aorta (root) (sinus) Q25.43
    brain Q28.3
      ruptured I60.7
    coronary Q24.5
    digestive system Q27.8
    lower limb Q27.8
    pulmonary Q25.79
    retina Q14.1
    specified site NEC Q27.8
    upper limb Q27.8
  conjunctiva — *see* Abnormality, conjunctiva, vascular
  conus arteriosus — *see* Aneurysm, heart
  coronary (arteriosclerotic) (artery) I25.41
    arteriovenous, congenital Q24.5
    congenital Q24.5
    ruptured — *see* Infarct, myocardium
    syphilitic A52.06
    vein I25.89
  cylindroid (aorta) I71:9
    ruptured I71.8
    syphilitic A52.01
  ductus arteriosus Q25.0
  endocardial, infective (any valve) I33.0
  femoral (artery) (ruptured) I72.4
  gastroduodenal I72.8
  gastroepiploic I72.8
  heart (wall) (chronic or with a stated duration of over
    4 weeks) I25.3
    valve — *see* Endocarditis
  hepatic I72.8
  iliac (common) (artery) (ruptured) I72.3
  infective I72.9
    endocardial (any valve) I33.0
  innominate (nonsyphilitic) I72.8
    syphilitic A52.09
  interauricular septum — *see* Aneurysm, heart
  interventricular septum — *see* Aneurysm, heart
  intrathoracic (nonsyphilitic) I71.2
    ruptured I71.1
    syphilitic A52.01
  lower limb I72.4
  lung (pulmonary artery) I28.1
  mediastinal (nonsyphilitic) I72.8
    syphilitic A52.09
  miliary (congenital) I67.1
    ruptured — *see* Hemorrhage, intracerebral, sub-
      arachnoid, intracranial
  mitral (heart) (valve) I34.8
  mural — *see* Aneurysm, heart
  mycotic I72.9
    endocardial (any valve) I33.0
    ruptured, brain — *see* Hemorrhage, intracerebral,
      subarachnoid
  myocardium — *see* Aneurysm, heart
  neck I72.0
  pancreaticoduodenal I72.8
  patent ductus arteriosus Q25.0
  peripheral NEC I72.8
    congenital Q27.8
      digestive system Q27.8
      lower limb Q27.8
      specified site NEC Q27.8
      upper limb Q27.8
  popliteal (artery) (ruptured) I72.4
  precerebral
    congenital (nonruptured) Q28.1
    specified site, NEC I72.5
  pulmonary I28.1
    arteriovenous Q25.72
      acquired I28.0
    syphilitic A52.09
    valve (heart) — *see* Endocarditis, pulmonary
  racemose (peripheral) I72.9
    congenital — *see* Aneurysm, congenital
  radial I72.1
  Rasmussen NEC A15.0
  renal (artery) I72.2
  retina — *see also* Disorder, retina, microaneurysms
    congenital Q14.1
    diabetic — *see* E08-E13 with .3-
  sinus of Valsalva Q25.49
  specified NEC I72.8
  spinal (cord) I72.8

☑ **Additional Character Required — Refer to the Tabular List for Character Selection**   ▧ **Subterms under main terms may continue to next column or page**

Aneurysm — *continued*
  spinal — *continued*
    syphilitic (hemorrhage) A52.09
  splenic I72.8
  subclavian (artery) (ruptured) I72.8
    syphilitic A52.09
  superior mesenteric I72.8
  syphilitic (aorta) A52.01
    central nervous system A52.05
    congenital (late) A50.54 *[I79.0]*
    spine, spinal A52.09
  thoracoabdominal (aorta) I71.6
    ruptured I71.5
    syphilitic A52.01
  thorax, thoracic (aorta) (arch) (nonsyphilitic) I71.2
    ruptured I71.1
    syphilitic A52.01
  traumatic (complication) (early), specified site — *see* Injury, blood vessel
  tricuspid (heart) (valve) I07.8
  ulnar I72.1
  upper limb (ruptured) I72.1
  valve, valvular — *see* Endocarditis
  venous — *see also* Varix I86.8
    congenital Q27.8
      digestive system Q27.8
      lower limb Q27.8
      specified site NEC Q27.8
      upper limb Q27.8
  ventricle — *see* Aneurysm, heart
  vertebral artery I72.6
  visceral NEC I72.8
Angelman syndrome Q93.51
Anger R45.4
Angiectasis, angiectopia I99.8
Angiitis I77.6
  allergic granulomatous M30.1
  hypersensitivity M31.0
  necrotizing M31.9
    specified NEC M31.8
  nervous system, granulomatous I67.7
Angina (attack) (cardiac) (chest) (heart) (pectoris) (syndrome) (vasomotor) I20.9
  with
    atherosclerotic heart disease — *see* Arteriosclerosis, coronary (artery),
    documented spasm I20.1
  abdominal K55.1
  accelerated — *see* Angina, unstable
  agranulocytic — *see* Agranulocytosis
  angiospastic — *see* Angina, with documented spasm
  aphthous B08.5
  crescendo — *see* Angina, unstable
  croupous J05.0
  cruris I73.9
  de novo effort — *see* Angina, unstable
  diphtheritic, membranous A36.0
  equivalent I20.8
  exudative, chronic J37.0
  following acute myocardial infarction I23.7
  gangrenous diphtheritic A36.0
  intestinal K55.1
  Ludovici K12.2
  Ludwig's K12.2
  malignant diphtheritic A36.0
  membranous J05.0
    diphtheritic A36.0
    Vincent's A69.1
  mesenteric K55.1
  monocytic — *see* Mononucleosis, infectious
  of effort — *see* Angina, specified NEC
  phlegmonous J36
    diphtheritic A36.0
  post-infarctional I23.7
  pre-infarctional — *see* Angina, unstable
  Prinzmetal — *see* Angina, with documented spasm
  progressive — *see* Angina, unstable
  pseudomembranous A69.1
  pultaceous, diphtheritic A36.0
  spasm-induced — *see* Angina, with documented spasm
  specified NEC I20.8
  stable I20.8
  stenocardia — *see* Angina, specified NEC
  stridulous, diphtheritic A36.2
  tonsil J36
  trachealis J05.0
  unstable I20.0
  variant — *see* Angina, with documented spasm

Angina — *continued*
  Vincent's A69.1
  worsening effort — *see* Angina, unstable
Angioblastoma — *see* Neoplasm, connective tissue, uncertain behavior
Angiocholecystitis — *see* Cholecystitis, acute
Angiocholitis — *see also* Cholecystitis, acute K83.09
Angiodysgenesis spinalis G95.19
Angiodysplasia (cecum) (colon) K55.20
  with bleeding K55.21
  duodenum (and stomach) K31.819
    with bleeding K31.811
  stomach (and duodenum) K31.819
    with bleeding K31.811
Angioedema (allergic) (any site) (with urticaria) T78.3 ☑
  hereditary D84.1
Angioendothelioma — *see* Neoplasm, uncertain behavior, by site
  benign D18.00
    intra-abdominal D18.03
    intracranial D18.02
    skin D18.01
    specified site NEC D18.09
  bone — *see* Neoplasm, bone, malignant
  Ewing's — *see* Neoplasm, bone, malignant
Angioendotheliomatosis C85.8- ☑
Angiofibroma — *see also* Neoplasm, benign, by site
  juvenile
    specified site — *see* Neoplasm, benign, by site
    unspecified site D10.6
Angiohemophilia (A) (B) D68.0
Angioid streaks (choroid) (macula) (retina) H35.33
Angiokeratoma — *see* Neoplasm, skin, benign
  corporis diffusum E75.21
Angioleiomyoma — *see* Neoplasm, connective tissue, benign
Angiolipoma — *see also* Lipoma
  infiltrating — *see* Lipoma
Angioma — *see also* Hemangioma, by site
  capillary I78.1
  hemorrhagicum hereditaria I78.0
  intra-abdominal D18.03
  intracranial D18.02
  malignant — *see* Neoplasm, connective tissue, malignant
  plexiform D18.00
    intra-abdominal D18.03
    intracranial D18.02
    skin D18.01
    specified site NEC D18.09
  senile I78.1
  serpiginosum L81.7
  skin D18.01
  specified site NEC D18.09
  spider I78.1
  stellate I78.1
  venous Q28.3
Angiomatosis Q82.8
  bacillary A79.89
  encephalotrigeminal Q85.8
  hemorrhagic familial I78.0
  hereditary familial I78.0
  liver K76.4
Angiomyolipoma — *see* Lipoma
Angiomyoliposarcoma — *see* Neoplasm, connective tissue, malignant
Angiomyoma — *see* Neoplasm, connective tissue, benign
Angiomyosarcoma — *see* Neoplasm, connective tissue, malignant
Angiomyxoma — *see* Neoplasm, connective tissue, uncertain behavior
Angioneurosis F45.8
Angioneurotic edema (allergic) (any site) (with urticaria) T78.3 ☑
  hereditary D84.1
Angiopathia, angiopathy I99.9
  cerebral I67.9
    amyloid E85.4 *[I68.0]*
  diabetic (peripheral) — *see* Diabetes, angiopathy
  peripheral I73.9
    diabetic — *see* Diabetes, angiopathy
    specified type NEC I73.89
  retinae syphilitica A52.05
  retinalis (juvenilis)
    diabetic — *see* Diabetes, retinopathy
    proliferative — *see* Retinopathy, proliferative
Angiosarcoma — *see also* Neoplasm, connective tissue, malignant

Angiosarcoma — *continued*
  liver C22.3
Angiosclerosis — *see* Arteriosclerosis
Angiospasm (peripheral) (traumatic) (vessel) I73.9
  brachial plexus G54.0
  cerebral G45.9
  cervical plexus G54.2
  nerve
    arm — *see* Mononeuropathy, upper limb
      axillary G54.0
      median — *see* Lesion, nerve, median
      ulnar — *see* Lesion, nerve, ulnar
    axillary G54.0
    leg — *see* Mononeuropathy, lower limb
    median — *see* Lesion, nerve, median
    plantar — *see* Lesion, nerve, plantar
    ulnar — *see* Lesion, nerve, ulnar
Angiospastic disease or edema I73.9
Angiostrongyliasis
  due to
    Parastrongylus
      cantonensis B83.2
      costaricensis B81.3
  intestinal B81.3
Anguillulosis — *see* Strongyloidiasis
Angulation
  cecum — *see* Obstruction, intestine
  coccyx (acquired) — *see also* subcategory M43.8 ☑
    congenital NEC Q76.49
  femur (acquired) — *see also* Deformity, limb, specified type NEC, thigh
    congenital Q74.2
  intestine (large) (small) — *see* Obstruction, intestine
  sacrum (acquired) — *see also* subcategory M43.8 ☑
    congenital NEC Q76.49
  sigmoid (flexure) — *see* Obstruction, intestine
  spine — *see* Dorsopathy, deforming, specified NEC
  tibia (acquired) — *see also* Deformity, limb, specified type NEC, lower leg
    congenital Q74.2
  ureter N13.5
    with infection N13.6
  wrist (acquired) — *see also* Deformity, limb, specified type NEC, forearm
    congenital Q74.0
Angulus infectiosus (lips) K13.0
Anhedonia R45.84
  sexual F52.0
Anhidrosis L74.4
Anhydration E86.0
Anhydremia E86.0
Anidrosis L74.4
Aniridia (congenital) Q13.1
Anisakiasis (infection) (infestation) B81.0
Anisakis larvae infestation B81.0
Aniseikonia H52.32
Anisocoria (pupil) H57.02
  congenital Q13.2
Anisocytosis R71.8
Anisometropia (congenital) H52.31
Ankle — *see* condition
Ankyloblepharon (eyelid) (acquired) — *see also* Blepharophimosis
  filiforme (adnatum) (congenital) Q10.3
  total Q10.3
Ankyloglossia Q38.1
Ankylosis (fibrous) (osseous) (joint) M24.60
  ankle M24.67- ☑
  arthrodesis status Z98.1
  cricoarytenoid (cartilage) (joint) (larynx) J38.7
  dental K03.5
  ear ossicles H74.31- ☑
  elbow M24.62- ☑
  foot M24.67- ☑
  hand M24.64- ☑
  hip M24.65- ☑
  incostapedial joint (infectional) — *see* Ankylosis, ear ossicles
  jaw (temporomandibular) M26.61- ☑
  knee M24.66- ☑
  lumbosacral (joint) M43.27
  postoperative (status) Z98.1
  produced by surgical fusion, status Z98.1
  sacro-iliac (joint) M43.28
  shoulder M24.61- ☑
  spine (joint) — *see also* Fusion, spine
    spondylitic — *see* Spondylitis, ankylosing

Ankylosis — continued
  surgical Z98.1
  temporomandibular M26.61- ☑
  tooth, teeth (hard tissues) K03.5
  wrist M24.63- ☑
Ankylostoma — see Ancylostoma
Ankylostomiasis — see Ancylostomiasis
Ankylurethria — see Stricture, urethra
Annular — see also condition
  detachment, cervix N88.8
  organ or site, congenital NEC — see Distortion
  pancreas (congenital) Q45.1
Anodontia (complete) (partial) (vera) K00.0
  acquired K08.10 ☑
Anomaly, anomalous (congenital) (unspecified type)
  Q89.9
  abdominal wall NEC Q79.59
  acoustic nerve Q07.8
  adrenal (gland) Q89.1
  Alder (-Reilly) (leukocyte granulation) D72.0
  alimentary tract Q45.9
    upper Q40.9
  alveolar M26.70
    hyperplasia M26.79
      mandibular M26.72
      maxillary M26.71
    hypoplasia M26.79
      mandibular M26.74
      maxillary M26.73
    ridge (process) M26.79
    specified NEC M26.79
  ankle (joint) Q74.2
  anus Q43.9
  aorta (arch) NEC Q25.40
    coarctation (preductal) (postductal) Q25.1
  aortic cusp or valve Q23.9
  appendix Q43.8
  apple peel syndrome Q41.1
  aqueduct of Sylvius Q03.0
    with spina bifida — see Spina bifida, with hydro-
      cephalus
  arm Q74.0
  arteriovenous NEC
    coronary Q24.5
    gastrointestinal Q27.33
      acquired — see Angiodysplasia
  artery (peripheral) Q27.9
    basilar NEC Q28.1
    cerebral Q28.3
    coronary Q24.5
    digestive system Q27.8
    eye Q15.8
    great Q25.9
      specified NEC Q25.8
    lower limb Q27.8
    peripheral Q27.9
      specified NEC Q27.8
    pulmonary NEC Q25.79
    renal Q27.2
    retina Q14.1
    specified site NEC Q27.8
    subclavian Q27.8
      origin Q25.48
    umbilical Q27.0
    upper limb Q27.8
    vertebral NEC Q28.1
  aryteno-epiglottic folds Q31.8
  atrial
    bands or folds Q20.8
    septa Q21.1
  atrioventricular
    excitation I45.6
    septum Q21.0
  auditory canal Q17.8
  auricle
    ear Q17.8
      causing impairment of hearing Q16.9
    heart Q20.8
  Axenfeld's Q15.0
  back Q89.9
  band
    atrial Q20.8
    heart Q24.8
    ventricular Q24.8
  Bartholin's duct Q38.4
  biliary duct or passage Q44.5
  bladder Q64.70
    absence Q64.5

Anomaly, anomalous — continued
  bladder — continued
    diverticulum Q64.6
    exstrophy Q64.10
      cloacal Q64.12
      extroversion Q64.19
      specified type NEC Q64.19
      supravesical fissure Q64.11
    neck obstruction Q64.31
    specified type NEC Q64.79
  bone Q79.9
    arm Q74.0
    face Q75.9
    leg Q74.2
    pelvic girdle Q74.2
    shoulder girdle Q74.0
    skull Q75.9
      with
        anencephaly Q00.0
        encephalocele — see Encephalocele
        hydrocephalus Q03.9
          with spina bifida — see Spina bifida, by
            site, with hydrocephalus
        microcephaly Q02
  brain (multiple) Q04.9
    vessel Q28.3
  breast Q83.9
  broad ligament Q50.6
  bronchus Q32.4
  bulbus cordis Q21.9
  bursa Q79.9
  canal of Nuck Q52.4
  canthus Q10.3
  capillary Q27.9
  cardiac Q24.9
    chambers Q20.9
      specified NEC Q20.8
    septal closure Q21.9
      specified NEC Q21.8
    valve NEC Q24.8
      pulmonary Q22.3
  cardiovascular system Q28.8
  carpus Q74.0
  caruncle, lacrimal Q10.6
  cascade stomach Q40.2
  cauda equina Q06.3
  cecum Q43.9
  cerebral Q04.9
    vessels Q28.3
  cervix Q51.9
  Chédiak-Higashi (-Steinbrinck) (congenital gigantism
    of peroxidase granules) E70.330
  cheek Q18.9
  chest wall Q67.8
    bones Q76.9
  chin Q18.9
  chordae tendineae Q24.8
  choroid Q14.3
    plexus Q07.8
  chromosomes, chromosomal Q99.9
    D (1) — see condition, chromosome 13
    E (3) — see condition, chromosome 18
    G — see condition, chromosome 21
    sex
      female phenotype Q97.8
      gonadal dysgenesis (pure) Q99.1
      Klinefelter's Q98.4
      male phenotype Q98.9
      Turner's Q96.9
    specified NEC Q99.8
  cilia Q10.3
  circulatory system Q28.9
  clavicle Q74.0
  clitoris Q52.6
  coccyx Q76.49
  colon Q43.9
  common duct Q44.5
  communication
    coronary artery Q24.5
    left ventricle with right atrium Q21.0
  concha (ear) Q17.3
  connection
    portal vein Q26.5
    pulmonary venous Q26.4
      partial Q26.3
      total Q26.2
    renal artery with kidney Q27.2
  cornea (shape) Q13.4
  coronary artery or vein Q24.5

Anomaly, anomalous — continued
  cranium — see Anomaly, skull
  cricoid cartilage Q31.8
  cystic duct Q44.5
  dental
    alveolar — see Anomaly, alveolar
    arch relationship M26.20
      specified NEC M26.29
  dentofacial M26.9
    alveolar — see Anomaly, alveolar
    dental arch relationship M26.20
      specified NEC M26.29
    functional M26.50
      specified NEC M26.59
    jaw size M26.00
      macrogenia M26.05
      mandibular
        hyperplasia M26.03
        hypoplasia M26.04
      maxillary
        hyperplasia M26.01
        hypoplasia M26.02
      microgenia M26.06
      specified type NEC M26.09
    jaw-cranial base relationship M26.10
      asymmetry M26.12
        maxillary M26.11
      specified type NEC M26.19
    malocclusion M26.4
      dental arch relationship NEC M26.29
      jaw size — see Anomaly, dentofacial, jaw size
      jaw-cranial base relationship — see Anomaly,
        dentofacial, jaw-cranial base relationship
    specified type NEC M26.89
    temporomandibular joint M26.60- ☑
      adhesions M26.61- ☑
      ankylosis M26.61- ☑
      arthralgia M26.62- ☑
      articular disc M26.63- ☑
      specified type NEC M26.69
    tooth position, fully erupted M26.30
      specified NEC M26.39
  dermatoglyphic Q82.8
  diaphragm (apertures) NEC Q79.1
  digestive organ(s) or tract Q45.9
    lower Q43.9
    upper Q40.9
  distance, interarch (excessive) (inadequate) M26.25
  distribution, coronary artery Q24.5
  ductus
    arteriosus Q25.0
    botalli Q25.0
  duodenum Q43.9
  dura (brain) Q04.9
    spinal cord Q06.9
  ear (external) Q17.9
    causing impairment of hearing Q16.9
    inner Q16.5
    middle (causing impairment of hearing) Q16.4
    ossicles Q16.3
  Ebstein's (heart) (tricuspid valve) Q22.5
  ectodermal Q82.9
  Eisenmenger's (ventricular septal defect) Q21.8
  ejaculatory duct Q55.4
  elbow Q74.0
  endocrine gland NEC Q89.2
  epididymis Q55.4
  epiglottis Q31.8
  esophagus Q39.9
  eustachian tube Q17.8
  eye Q15.9
    anterior segment Q13.9
      specified NEC Q13.89
    posterior segment Q14.9
      specified NEC Q14.8
    ptosis (eyelid) Q10.0
    specified NEC Q15.8
  eyebrow Q18.8
  eyelid Q10.3
    ptosis Q10.0
  face Q18.9
    bone(s) Q75.9
  fallopian tube Q50.6
  fascia Q79.9
  femur NEC Q74.2
  fibula NEC Q74.2
  finger Q74.0
  fixation, intestine Q43.3

☑ Additional Character Required — Refer to the Tabular List for Character Selection ▼ Subterms under main terms may continue to next column or page

Anomaly, anomalous — *continued*

flexion (joint) NOS Q74.9
  hip or thigh Q65.89
foot NEC Q74.2
  varus (congenital) Q66.3- ☑
foramen
  Botalli Q21.1
  ovale Q21.1
forearm Q74.0
forehead Q75.8
form, teeth K00.2
fovea centralis Q14.1
frontal bone — *see* Anomaly, skull
gallbladder (position) (shape) (size) Q44.1
Gartner's duct Q52.4
gastrointestinal tract Q45.9
genitalia, genital organ(s) or system
  female Q52.9
    external Q52.70
    internal NOS Q52.9
  male Q55.9
    hydrocele P83.5
    specified NEC Q55.8
genitourinary NEC
  female Q52.9
  male Q55.9
Gerbode Q21.0
glottis Q31.8
granulation or granulocyte, genetic (constitutional)
    (leukocyte) D72.0
gum Q38.6
gyri Q07.9
hair Q84.2
hand Q74.0
hard tissue formation in pulp K04.3
head — *see* Anomaly, skull
heart Q24.9
  auricle Q20.8
  bands or folds Q24.8
  fibroelastosis cordis I42.4
  obstructive NEC Q22.6
  patent ductus arteriosus (Botalli) Q25.0
  septum Q21.9
    auricular Q21.1
    interatrial Q21.1
    interventricular Q21.0
      with pulmonary stenosis or atresia, dextraposition of aorta and hypertrophy of right ventricle Q21.3
    specified NEC Q21.8
    ventricular Q21.0
      with pulmonary stenosis or atresia, dextraposition of aorta and hypertrophy of right ventricle Q21.3
  tetralogy of Fallot Q21.3
  valve NEC Q24.8
    aortic
      bicuspid valve Q23.1
      insufficiency Q23.1
      stenosis Q23.0
        subaortic Q24.4
    mitral
      insufficiency Q23.3
      stenosis Q23.2
    pulmonary Q22.3
      atresia Q22.0
      insufficiency Q22.2
      stenosis Q22.1
        infundibular Q24.3
        subvalvular Q24.3
    tricuspid
      atresia Q22.4
      stenosis Q22.4
  ventricle Q20.8
heel NEC Q74.2
Hegglin's D72.0
hemianencephaly Q00.0
hemicephaly Q00.0
hemicrania Q00.0
hepatic duct Q44.5
hip NEC Q74.2
hourglass stomach Q40.2
humerus Q74.0
hydatid of Morgagni
  female Q50.5
  male (epididymal) Q55.4
    testicular Q55.29
hymen Q52.4
hypersegmentation of neutrophils, hereditary D72.0

Anomaly, anomalous — *continued*

hypophyseal Q89.2
ileocecal (coil) (valve) Q43.9
ileum Q43.9
ilium NEC Q74.2
integument Q84.9
  specified NEC Q84.8
interarch distance (excessive) (inadequate) M26.25
intervertebral cartilage or disc Q76.49
intestine (large) (small) Q43.9
  with anomalous adhesions, fixation or malrotation Q43.3
iris Q13.2
ischium NEC Q74.2
jaw — *see* Anomaly, dentofacial
  alveolar — *see* Anomaly, alveolar
jaw-cranial base relationship — *see* Anomaly, dentofacial, jaw-cranial base relationship
jejunum Q43.8
joint Q74.9
  specified NEC Q74.8
Jordan's D72.0
kidney(s) (calyx) (pelvis) Q63.9
  artery Q27.2
  specified NEC Q63.8
Klippel-Feil (brevicollis) Q76.1
knee Q74.1
labium (majus) (minus) Q52.70
labyrinth, membranous Q16.5
lacrimal apparatus or duct Q10.6
larynx, laryngeal (muscle) Q31.9
  web (bed) Q31.0
lens Q12.9
leukocytes, genetic D72.0
  granulation (constitutional) D72.0
lid (fold) Q10.3
ligament Q79.9
  broad Q50.6
  round Q52.8
limb Q74.9
  lower NEC Q74.2
    reduction deformity — *see* Defect, reduction, lower limb
  upper Q74.0
lip Q38.0
liver Q44.7
  duct Q44.5
lower limb NEC Q74.2
lumbosacral (joint) (region) Q76.49
  kyphosis — *see* Kyphosis, congenital
  lordosis — *see* Lordosis, congenital
lung (fissure) (lobe) Q33.9
mandible — *see* Anomaly, dentofacial
maxilla — *see* Anomaly, dentofacial
May (-Hegglin) D72.0
meatus urinarius NEC Q64.79
meningeal bands or folds Q07.9
  constriction of Q07.8
  spinal Q06.9
meninges Q07.9
  cerebral Q04.8
  spinal Q06.9
meningocele Q05.9
mesentery Q45.9
metacarpus Q74.0
metatarsus NEC Q74.2
middle ear Q16.4
  ossicles Q16.3
mitral (leaflets) (valve) Q23.9
  insufficiency Q23.3
  specified NEC Q23.8
  stenosis Q23.2
mouth Q38.6
Müllerian — *see also* Anomaly, by site
  uterus NEC Q51.818
multiple NEC Q89.7
muscle Q79.9
  eyelid Q10.3
musculoskeletal system, except limbs Q79.9
myocardium Q24.8
nail Q84.6
narrowness, eyelid Q10.3
nasal sinus (wall) Q30.8
neck (any part) Q18.9
nerve Q07.9
  acoustic Q07.8
  optic Q07.8
nervous system (central) Q07.9

Anomaly, anomalous — *continued*

nipple Q83.9
nose, nasal (bones) (cartilage) (septum) (sinus) Q30.9
  specified NEC Q30.8
ocular muscle Q15.8
omphalomesenteric duct Q43.0
opening, pulmonary veins Q26.4
optic
  disc Q14.2
  nerve Q07.8
opticociliary vessels Q13.2
orbit (eye) Q10.7
organ Q89.9
  of Corti Q16.5
origin
  artery
    innominate Q25.8
    pulmonary Q25.79
    renal Q27.2
    subclavian Q25.48
osseous meatus (ear) Q16.1
ovary Q50.39
oviduct Q50.6
palate (hard) (soft) NEC Q38.5
pancreas or pancreatic duct Q45.3
papillary muscles Q24.8
parathyroid gland Q89.2
paraurethral ducts Q64.79
parotid (gland) Q38.4
patella Q74.1
Pelger-Huët (hereditary hyposegmentation) D72.0
pelvic girdle NEC Q74.2
pelvis (bony) NEC Q74.2
  rachitic E64.3
penis (glans) Q55.69
pericardium Q24.8
peripheral vascular system Q27.9
Peter's Q13.4
pharynx Q38.8
pigmentation L81.9
  congenital Q82.8
pituitary (gland) Q89.2
pleural (folds) Q34.0
portal vein Q26.5
  connection Q26.5
position, tooth, teeth, fully erupted M26.30
  specified NEC M26.39
precerebral vessel Q28.1
prepuce Q55.69
prostate Q55.4
pulmonary Q33.9
  artery NEC Q25.79
  valve Q22.3
    atresia Q22.0
    insufficiency Q22.2
    specified type NEC Q22.3
    stenosis Q22.1
      infundibular Q24.3
      subvalvular Q24.3
  venous connection Q26.4
    partial Q26.3
    total Q26.2
pupil Q13.2
  function H57.00
    anisocoria H57.02
    Argyll Robertson pupil H57.01
    miosis H57.03
    mydriasis H57.04
    specified type NEC H57.09
    tonic pupil H57.05- ☑
pylorus Q40.3
radius Q74.0
rectum Q43.9
reduction (extremity) (limb)
  femur (longitudinal) — *see* Defect, reduction, lower limb, longitudinal, femur
  fibula (longitudinal) — *see* Defect, reduction, lower limb, longitudinal, fibula
  lower limb — *see* Defect, reduction, lower limb
  radius (longitudinal) — *see* Defect, reduction, upper limb, longitudinal, radius
  tibia (longitudinal) — *see* Defect, reduction, lower limb, longitudinal, tibia
  ulna (longitudinal) — *see* Defect, reduction, upper limb, longitudinal, ulna
  upper limb — *see* Defect, reduction, upper limb
refraction — *see* Disorder, refraction
renal Q63.9

Anomaly, anomalous — *continued*
  renal — *continued*
    artery Q27.2
    pelvis Q63.9
      specified NEC Q63.8
  respiratory system Q34.9
    specified NEC Q34.8
  retina Q14.1
  rib Q76.6
    cervical Q76.5
  Rieger's Q13.81
  rotation — *see* Malrotation
    hip or thigh Q65.89
  round ligament Q52.8
  sacroiliac (joint) NEC Q74.2
  sacrum NEC Q76.49
    kyphosis — *see* Kyphosis, congenital
    lordosis — *see* Lordosis, congenital
  saddle nose, syphilitic A50.57
  salivary duct or gland Q38.4
  scapula Q74.0
  scrotum — *see* Malformation, testis and scrotum
  sebaceous gland Q82.9
  seminal vesicles Q55.4
  sense organs NEC Q07.8
  sex chromosomes NEC — *see also* Anomaly, chromosomes
    female phenotype Q97.8
    male phenotype Q98.9
  shoulder (girdle) (joint) Q74.0
  sigmoid (flexure) Q43.9
  simian crease Q82.8
  sinus of Valsalva Q25.49
  skeleton generalized Q78.9
  skin (appendage) Q82.9
  skull Q75.9
    with
      anencephaly Q00.0
      encephalocele — *see* Encephalocele
      hydrocephalus Q03.9
        with spina bifida — *see* Spina bifida, by site, with hydrocephalus
      microcephaly Q02
  specified organ or site NEC Q89.8
  spermatic cord Q55.4
  spine, spinal NEC Q76.49
    column NEC Q76.49
      kyphosis — *see* Kyphosis, congenital
      lordosis — *see* Lordosis, congenital
    cord Q06.9
    nerve root Q07.8
  spleen Q89.09
    agenesis Q89.01
  stenonian duct Q38.4
  sternum NEC Q76.7
  stomach Q40.3
  submaxillary gland Q38.4
  tarsus NEC Q74.2
  tendon Q79.9
  testis — *see* Malformation, testis and scrotum
  thigh NEC Q74.2
  thorax (wall) Q67.8
    bony Q76.9
  throat Q38.8
  thumb Q74.0
  thymus gland Q89.2
  thyroid (gland) Q89.2
    cartilage Q31.8
  tibia NEC Q74.2
    saber A50.56
  toe Q74.2
  tongue Q38.3
  tooth, teeth K00.9
    eruption K00.6
    position, fully erupted M26.30
    spacing, fully erupted M26.30
  trachea (cartilage) Q32.1
  tragus Q17.9
  tricuspid (leaflet) (valve) Q22.9
    atresia or stenosis Q22.4
    Ebstein's Q22.5
  Uhl's (hypoplasia of myocardium, right ventricle) Q24.8
  ulna Q74.0
  umbilical artery Q27.0
  union
    cricoid cartilage and thyroid cartilage Q31.8
    thyroid cartilage and hyoid bone Q31.8
    trachea with larynx Q31.8

Anomaly, anomalous — *continued*
  upper limb Q74.0
  urachus Q64.4
  ureter Q62.8
    obstructive NEC Q62.39
      cecoureterocele Q62.32
      orthotopic ureterocele Q62.31
  urethra Q64.70
    absence Q64.5
    double Q64.74
    fistula to rectum Q64.73
    obstructive Q64.39
      stricture Q64.32
    prolapse Q64.71
    specified type NEC Q64.79
  urinary tract Q64.9
  uterus Q51.9
    with only one functioning horn Q51.4
  uvula Q38.5
  vagina Q52.4
  valleculae Q31.8
  valve (heart) NEC Q24.8
    coronary sinus Q24.5
    inferior vena cava Q24.8
    pulmonary Q22.3
    sinus coronario Q24.5
    venae cavae inferioris Q24.8
  vas deferens Q55.4
  vascular Q27.9
    brain Q28.3
    ring Q25.45
  vein(s) (peripheral) Q27.9
    brain Q28.3
    cerebral Q28.3
    coronary Q24.5
    developmental Q28.3
    great Q26.9
      specified NEC Q26.8
  vena cava (inferior) (superior) Q26.9
  venous — *see* Anomaly, vein(s)
  venous return Q26.8
  ventricular
    bands or folds Q24.8
    septa Q21.0
  vertebra Q76.49
    kyphosis — *see* Kyphosis, congenital
    lordosis — *see* Lordosis, congenital
  vesicourethral orifice Q64.79
  vessel(s) Q27.9
    optic papilla Q14.2
    precerebral Q28.1
  vitelline duct Q43.0
  vitreous body or humor Q14.0
  vulva Q52.70
  wrist (joint) Q74.0
Anomia R48.8
Anonychia (congenital) Q84.3
  acquired L60.8
Anophthalmos, anophthalmus (congenital) (globe) Q11.1
  acquired Z90.01
Anopia, anopsia H53.46- ☑
  quadrant H53.46- ☑
Anorchia, anorchism, anorchidism Q55.0
Anorexia R63.0
  hysterical F44.89
  nervosa F50.00
    atypical F50.9
    binge-eating type F50.2
      with purging F50.02
    restricting type F50.01
Anorgasmy, psychogenic (female) F52.31
  male F52.32
Anosmia R43.0
  hysterical F44.6
  postinfectional J39.8
Anosognosia R41.89
Anosteoplasia Q78.9
Anovulatory cycle N97.0
Anoxemia R09.02
  newborn P84
Anoxia (pathological) R09.02
  altitude T70.29 ☑
  cerebral G93.1
    complicating
      anesthesia (general) (local) or other sedation T88.59 ☑
        in labor and delivery O74.3

Anoxia — *continued*
  cerebral — *continued*
    complicating — *continued*
      anesthesia or other sedation — *continued*
        in pregnancy O29.21- ☑
        postpartum, puerperal O89.2
      delivery (cesarean) (instrumental) O75.4
    during a procedure G97.81
    newborn P84
    resulting from a procedure G97.82
    due to
      drowning T75.1 ☑
      high altitude T70.29 ☑
    heart — *see* Insufficiency, coronary
    intrauterine P84
    myocardial — *see* Insufficiency, coronary
    newborn P84
    spinal cord G95.11
    systemic (by suffocation) (low content in atmosphere) — *see* Asphyxia, traumatic
Anteflexion — *see* Anteversion
Antenatal
  care (normal pregnancy) Z34.90
  screening (encounter for) of mother — *see also* Encounter, antenatal screening Z36.9
Antepartum — *see* condition
Anterior — *see* condition
Antero-occlusion M26.220
Anteversion
  cervix — *see* Anteversion, uterus
  femur (neck), congenital Q65.89
  uterus, uterine (cervix) (postinfectional) (postpartal, old) N85.4
    congenital Q51.818
    in pregnancy or childbirth — *see* Pregnancy, complicated by
Anthophobia F40.228
Anthracosilicosis J60
Anthracosis (lung) (occupational) J60
  lingua K14.3
Anthrax A22.9
  with pneumonia A22.1
  cerebral A22.8
  colitis A22.2
  cutaneous A22.0
  gastrointestinal A22.2
  inhalation A22.1
  intestinal A22.2
  meningitis A22.8
  pulmonary A22.1
  respiratory A22.1
  sepsis A22.7
  specified manifestation NEC A22.8
Anthropoid pelvis Q74.2
  with disproportion (fetopelvic) O33.0
Anthropophobia F40.10
  generalized F40.11
Antibodies, maternal (blood group) — *see* Isoimmunization, affecting management of pregnancy
  anti-D — *see* Isoimmunization, affecting management of pregnancy, Rh
  newborn P55.0
Antibody
  anticardiolipin R76.0
    with
      hemorrhagic disorder D68.312
      hypercoagulable state D68.61
  antiphosphatidylglycerol R76.0
    with
      hemorrhagic disorder D68.312
      hypercoagulable state D68.61
  antiphosphatidylinositol R76.0
    with
      hemorrhagic disorder D68.312
      hypercoagulable state D68.61
  antiphosphatidylserine R76.0
    with
      hemorrhagic disorder D68.312
      hypercoagulable state D68.61
  antiphospholipid R76.0
    with
      hemorrhagic disorder D68.312
      hypercoagulable state D68.61
Anticardiolipin syndrome D68.61
Anticoagulant, circulating (intrinsic) — *see also* Disorder, hemorrhagic D68.318
  drug-induced (extrinsic) — *see also* Disorder, hemorrhagic D68.32

Anticoagulant, circulating — *continued*
iatrogenic D68.32
Antidiuretic hormone syndrome E22.2
Antimonial cholera — *see* Poisoning, antimony
Antiphospholipid
antibody
with hemorrhagic disorder D68.312
syndrome D68.61
Antisocial personality F60.2
Antithrombinemia — *see* Circulating anticoagulants
Antithromboplastinemia D68.318
Antithromboplastinogenemia D68.318
Antitoxin complication or reaction — *see* Complications, vaccination
Antlophobia F40.228
Antritis J32.0
maxilla J32.0
acute J01.00
recurrent J01.01
stomach K29.60
with bleeding K29.61
Antrum, antral — *see* condition
Anuria R34
calculous (impacted) (recurrent) — *see also* Calculus, urinary N20.9
following
abortion — *see* Abortion by type complicated by, renal failure
ectopic or molar pregnancy O08.4
newborn P96.0
postprocedural N99.0
postrenal N13.8
traumatic (following crushing) T79.5 ☑
Anus, anal — *see* condition
Anusitis K62.89
Anxiety F41.9
depression F41.8
episodic paroxysmal F41.0
generalized F41.1
hysteria F41.8
neurosis F41.1
panic type F41.0
reaction F41.1
separation, abnormal (of childhood) F93.0
specified NEC F41.8
state F41.1
Aorta, aortic — *see* condition
Aortectasia — *see* Ectasia, aorta
with aneurysm — *see* Aneurysm, aorta
Aortitis (nonsyphilitic) (calcific) I77.6
arteriosclerotic I70.0
Doehle-Heller A52.02
luetic A52.02
rheumatic — *see* Endocarditis, acute, rheumatic
specific (syphilitic) A52.02
syphilitic A52.02
congenital A50.54 *[I79.1]*
Apathetic thyroid storm — *see* Thyrotoxicosis
Apathy R45.3
Apeirophobia F40.228
Apepsia K30
psychogenic F45.8
Aperistalsis, esophagus K22.0
Apertognathia M26.29
Apert's syndrome Q87.0
Aphagia R13.0
psychogenic F50.9
Aphakia (acquired) (postoperative) H27.0- ☑
congenital Q12.3
Aphasia (amnestic) (global) (nominal) (semantic) (syntactic) R47.01
acquired, with epilepsy (Landau-Kleffner syndrome) — *see* Epilepsy, specified NEC
auditory (developmental) F80.2
developmental (receptive type) F80.2
expressive type F80.1
Wernicke's F80.2
following
cerebrovascular disease I69.920
cerebral infarction I69.320
intracerebral hemorrhage I69.120
nontraumatic intracranial hemorrhage NEC I69.220
specified disease NEC I69.820
subarachnoid hemorrhage I69.020
primary progressive G31.01 *[F02.80]*
with behavioral disturbance G31.01 *[F02.81]*
progressive isolated G31.01 *[F02.80]*

Aphasia — *continued*
progressive isolated — *continued*
with behavioral disturbance G31.01 *[F02.81]*
sensory F80.2
syphilis, tertiary A52.19
Wernicke's (developmental) F80.2
Aphonia (organic) R49.1
hysterical F44.4
psychogenic F44.4
Aphthae, aphthous — *see also* condition
Bednar's K12.0
cachectic K14.0
epizootic B08.8
fever B08.8
oral (recurrent) K12.0
stomatitis (major) (minor) K12.0
thrush B37.0
ulcer (oral) (recurrent) K12.0
genital organ(s) NEC
female N76.6
male N50.89
larynx J38.7
Apical — *see* condition
Apiphobia F40.218
Aplasia — *see also* Agenesis
abdominal muscle syndrome Q79.4
alveolar process (acquired) — *see* Anomaly, alveolar
congenital Q38.6
aorta (congenital) Q25.41
axialis extracorticalis (congenita) E75.29
bone marrow (myeloid) D61.9
congenital D61.01
brain Q00.0
part of Q04.3
bronchus Q32.4
cementum K00.4
cerebellum Q04.3
cervix (congenital) Q51.5
congenital pure red cell D61.01
corpus callosum Q04.0
cutis congenita Q84.8
erythrocyte congenital D61.01
extracortical axial E75.29
eye Q11.1
fovea centralis (congenital) Q14.1
gallbladder, congenital Q44.0
iris Q13.1
labyrinth, membranous Q16.5
limb (congenital) Q73.8
lower — *see* Defect, reduction, lower limb
upper — *see* Agenesis, arm
lung, congenital (bilateral) (unilateral) Q33.3
pancreas Q45.0
parathyroid-thymic D82.1
Pelizaeus-Merzbacher E75.29
penis Q55.5
prostate Q55.4
red cell (with thymoma) D60.9
acquired D60.9
due to drugs D60.9
adult D60.9
chronic D60.0
congenital D61.01
constitutional D61.01
due to drugs D60.9
hereditary D61.01
of infants D61.01
primary D61.01
pure D61.01
due to drugs D60.9
specified type NEC D60.8
transient D60.1
round ligament Q52.8
skin Q84.8
spermatic cord Q55.4
spleen Q89.01
testicle Q55.0
thymic, with immunodeficiency D82.1
thyroid (congenital) (with myxedema) E03.1
uterus Q51.0
ventral horn cell Q06.1
Apnea, apneic (of) (spells) R06.81
newborn NEC P28.4
obstructive P28.4
sleep (central) (obstructive) (primary) P28.3
prematurity P28.4
sleep G47.30
central (primary) G47.31

Apnea, apneic — *continued*
sleep — *continued*
central — *continued*
idiopathic G47.31
in conditions classified elsewhere G47.37
obstructive (adult) (pediatric) G47.33
hypopnea G47.33
primary central G47.31
specified NEC G47.39
Apneumatosis, newborn P28.0
Apocrine metaplasia (breast) — *see* Dysplasia, mammary, specified type NEC
Apophysitis (bone) — *see also* Osteochondropathy
calcaneus M92.8
juvenile M92.9
Apoplectiform convulsions (cerebral ischemia) I67.82
Apoplexia, apoplexy, apoplectic
adrenal A39.1
heart (auricle) (ventricle) — *see* Infarct, myocardium
heat T67.01 ☑
hemorrhagic (stroke) — *see* Hemorrhage, intracranial
meninges, hemorrhagic — *see* Hemorrhage, intracranial, subarachnoid
uremic N18.9 *[I68.8]*
Appearance
bizarre R46.1
specified NEC R46.89
very low level of personal hygiene R46.0
Appendage
epididymal (organ of Morgagni) Q55.4
intestine (epiploic) Q43.8
preauricular Q17.0
testicular (organ of Morgagni) Q55.29
Appendicitis (pneumococcal) (retrocecal) K37
with
gangrene K35.891
perforation NOS K35.32
peritoneal abscess K35.33
peritonitis NEC K35.33
generalized (with perforation or rupture) K35.20
with abscess K35.21
localized K35.30
with
gangrene K35.31
perforation K35.32
and abscess K35.33
rupture (with localized peritonitis) K35.32
acute (catarrhal) (fulminating) (gangrenous) (obstructive) (retrocecal) (suppurative) K35.80
with
gangrene K35.891
peritoneal abscess K35.33
peritonitis NEC K35.33
generalized (with perforation or rupture) K35.20
with abscess K35.21
localized K35.30
with
gangrene K35.31
perforation K35.32
and abscess K35.33
specified NEC K35.890
with gangrene K35.891
amebic A06.89
chronic (recurrent) K36
exacerbation — *see* Appendicitis, acute
gangrenous — *see* Appendicitis, acute
healed (obliterative) K36
interval K36
neurogenic K36
obstructive K36
recurrent K36
relapsing K36
ruptured NOS (with localized peritonitis) K35.32
subacute (adhesive) K36
subsiding K36
suppurative — *see* Appendicitis, acute
tuberculous A18.32
Appendicopathia oxyurica B80
Appendix, appendicular — *see also* condition
epididymis Q55.4
Morgagni
female Q50.5
male (epididymal) Q55.4
testicular Q55.29
testis Q55.29
Appetite
depraved — *see* Pica

Appetite — *continued*
  excessive R63.2
  lack or loss — *see also* Anorexia R63.0
    nonorganic origin F50.89
    psychogenic F50.89
  perverted (hysterical) — *see* Pica
Apple peel syndrome Q41.1
Apprehension state F41.1
Apprehensiveness, abnormal F41.9
Approximal wear K03.0
Apraxia (classic) (ideational) (ideokinetic) (ideomotor) (motor) (verbal) R48.2
  following
    cerebrovascular disease I69.990
      cerebral infarction I69.390
      intracerebral hemorrhage I69.190
      nontraumatic intracranial hemorrhage NEC I69.290
      specified disease NEC I69.890
      subarachnoid hemorrhage I69.090
  oculomotor, congenital H51.8
Aptyalism K11.7
Apudoma — *see* Neoplasm, uncertain behavior, by site
Aqueous misdirection H40.83- ☑
Arabicum elephantiasis — *see* Infestation, filarial
Arachnitis — *see* Meningitis
Arachnodactyly — *see* Syndrome, Marfan's
Arachnoiditis (acute) (adhesive) (basal) (brain) (cerebrospinal) — *see* Meningitis
Arachnophobia F40.210
Arboencephalitis, Australian A83.4
Arborization block (heart) I45.5
ARC (AIDS-related complex) B20
Arch
  aortic Q25.49
  bovine Q25.49
Arches — *see* condition
Arcuate uterus Q51.810
Arcuatus uterus Q51.810
Arcus (cornea) senilis — *see* Degeneration, cornea, senile
Arc-welder's lung J63.4
Areflexia R29.2
Areola — *see* condition
Argentaffinoma — *see also* Neoplasm, uncertain behavior, by site
  malignant — *see* Neoplasm, malignant, by site
  syndrome E34.0
Argininemia E72.21
Arginosuccinic aciduria E72.22
Argyll Robertson phenomenon, pupil or syndrome (syphilitic) A52.19
  atypical H57.09
  nonsyphilitic H57.09
Argyria, argyriasis
  conjunctival H11.13- ☑
  from drug or medicament — *see* Table of Drugs and Chemicals, by substance
Argyrosis, conjunctival H11.13- ☑
Arhinencephaly Q04.1
Ariboflavinosis E53.0
Arm — *see* condition
Arnold-Chiari disease, obstruction or syndrome (type II) Q07.00
  with
    hydrocephalus Q07.02
      with spina bifida Q07.03
    spina bifida Q07.01
      with hydrocephalus Q07.03
  type III — *see* Encephalocele
  type IV Q04.8
Aromatic amino-acid metabolism disorder E70.9
  specified NEC E70.8
Arousals, confusional G47.51
Arrest, arrested
  cardiac I46.9
    complicating
      abortion — *see* Abortion, by type, complicated by, cardiac arrest
      anesthesia (general) (local) or other sedation — *see* Table of Drugs and Chemicals, by drug
      in labor and delivery O74.2
      in pregnancy O29.11- ☑
        postpartum, puerperal O89.1
      delivery (cesarean) (instrumental) O75.4
    due to
      cardiac condition I46.2
      specified condition NEC I46.8

Arrest, arrested — *continued*
  cardiac — *continued*
    intraoperative I97.71- ☑
    newborn P29.81
    personal history, successfully resuscitated Z86.74
    postprocedural I97.12- ☑
      obstetric procedure O75.4
  cardiorespiratory — *see* Arrest, cardiac
  circulatory — *see* Arrest, cardiac
  deep transverse O64.0 ☑
  development or growth
    bone — *see* Disorder, bone, development or growth
    child R62.50
    tracheal rings Q32.1
  epiphyseal
    complete
      femur M89.15- ☑
      humerus M89.12- ☑
      tibia M89.16- ☑
      ulna M89.13- ☑
      forearm M89.13- ☑
        specified NEC M89.13- ☑
      ulna — *see* Arrest, epiphyseal, by type, ulna
      lower leg M89.16- ☑
        specified NEC M89.168
      tibia — *see* Arrest, epiphyseal, by type, tibia
    partial
      femur M89.15- ☑
      humerus M89.12- ☑
      tibia M89.16- ☑
      ulna M89.13- ☑
    specified NEC M89.18
  granulopoiesis — *see* Agranulocytosis
  growth plate — *see* Arrest, epiphyseal
  heart — *see* Arrest, cardiac
  legal, anxiety concerning Z65.3
  physeal — *see* Arrest, epiphyseal
  respiratory R09.2
    newborn P28.81
  sinus I45.5
  spermatogenesis (complete) — *see* Azoospermia
    incomplete — *see* Oligospermia
  transverse (deep) O64.0 ☑
Arrhenoblastoma
  benign
    specified site — *see* Neoplasm, benign, by site
    unspecified site
      female D27.9
      male D29.20
  malignant
    specified site — *see* Neoplasm, malignant, by site
    unspecified site
      female C56.9
      male C62.90
  specified site — *see* Neoplasm, uncertain behavior, by site
  unspecified site
    female D39.10
    male D40.10
Arrhythmia (auricle) (cardiac) (juvenile) (nodal) (reflex) (sinus) (supraventricular) (transitory) (ventricle) I49.9
  block I45.9
  extrasystolic I49.49
  newborn
    bradycardia P29.12
    occurring before birth P03.819
      before onset of labor P03.810
      during labor P03.811
    tachycardia P29.11
  psychogenic F45.8
  specified NEC I49.8
  vagal R55
  ventricular re-entry I47.0
Arrillaga-Ayerza syndrome (pulmonary sclerosis with pulmonary hypertension) I27.0
Arsenical pigmentation L81.8
  from drug or medicament — *see* Table of Drugs and Chemicals
Arsenism — *see* Poisoning, arsenic
Arterial — *see* condition
Arteriofibrosis — *see* Arteriosclerosis
Arteriolar sclerosis — *see* Arteriosclerosis
Arteriolith — *see* Arteriosclerosis
Arteriolitis I77.6
  necrotizing, kidney I77.5
  renal — *see* Hypertension, kidney
Arteriolosclerosis — *see* Arteriosclerosis

Arterionephrosclerosis — *see* Hypertension, kidney
Arteriopathy I77.9
  cerebral autosomal dominant, with subcortical infarcts and leukoencephalopathy (CADASIL) I67.850
Arteriosclerosis, arteriosclerotic (diffuse) (obliterans) (of) (senile) (with calcification) I70.90
  aorta I70.0
  arteries of extremities — *see* Arteriosclerosis, extremities
  brain I67.2
  bypass graft
    coronary — *see* Arteriosclerosis, coronary, bypass graft
    extremities — *see* Arteriosclerosis, extremities, bypass graft
  cardiac — *see* Disease, heart, ischemic, atherosclerotic
  cardiopathy — *see* Disease, heart, ischemic, atherosclerotic
  cardiorenal — *see* Hypertension, cardiorenal
  cardiovascular — *see* Disease, heart, ischemic, atherosclerotic
  carotid — *see also* Occlusion, artery, carotid I65.2- ☑
  central nervous system I67.2
  cerebral I67.2
  cerebrovascular I67.2
  coronary (artery)
    due to
      calcified coronary lesion (severely) I25.84
      lipid rich plaque I25.83
    bypass graft I25.810
      with
        angina pectoris I25.709
          with documented spasm I25.701
          specified type NEC I25.708
          unstable I25.700
        ischemic chest pain I25.709
      autologous artery I25.810
        with
          angina pectoris I25.729
            with documented spasm I25.721
            specified type I25.728
            unstable I25.720
          ischemic chest pain I25.729
      autologous vein I25.810
        with
          angina pectoris I25.719
            with documented spasm I25.711
            specified type I25.718
            unstable I25.710
          ischemic chest pain I25.719
      nonautologous biological I25.810
        with
          angina pectoris I25.739
            with documented spasm I25.731
            specified type I25.738
            unstable I25.730
          ischemic chest pain I25.739
      specified type NEC I25.810
        with
          angina pectoris I25.799
            with documented spasm I25.791
            specified type I25.798
            unstable I25.790
          ischemic chest pain I25.799
    native vessel
      with
        angina pectoris I25.119
          with documented spasm I25.111
          specified type NEC I25.118
          unstable I25.110
        ischemic chest pain I25.119
    transplanted heart I25.811
      bypass graft I25.812
        with
          angina pectoris I25.769
            with documented spasm I25.761
            specified type I25.768
            unstable I25.760
          ischemic chest pain I25.769
      native coronary artery I25.811
        with
          angina pectoris I25.759
            with documented spasm I25.751
            specified type I25.758
            unstable I25.750
          ischemic chest pain I25.759
  extremities (native arteries) I70.209
    bypass graft I70.309

Arteriosclerosis, arteriosclerotic — *continued*
- extremities — *continued*
  - bypass graft — *continued*
    - autologous vein graft I70.409
      - leg I70.409
        - with
          - gangrene (and intermittent claudication, rest pain and ulcer) I70.469
          - intermittent claudication I70.419
          - rest pain (and intermittent claudication) I70.429
        - bilateral I70.403
          - with
            - gangrene (and intermittent claudication, rest pain and ulcer) I70.463
            - intermittent claudication I70.463
            - rest pain (and intermittent claudication) I70.423
          - specified type NEC I70.493
        - left I70.402
          - with
            - gangrene (and intermittent claudication, rest pain and ulcer) I70.462
            - intermittent claudication I70.412
            - rest pain (and intermittent claudication) I70.422
            - ulceration (and intermittent claudication and rest pain) I70.449
              - ankle I70.443
              - calf I70.442
              - foot site NEC I70.445
              - heel I70.444
              - lower leg NEC I70.448
              - midfoot I70.444
              - thigh I70.441
            - specified type NEC I70.492
        - right I70.401
          - with
            - gangrene (and intermittent claudication, rest pain and ulcer) I70.461
            - intermittent claudication I70.411
            - rest pain (and intermittent claudication) I70.421
            - ulceration (and intermittent claudication and rest pain) I70.439
              - ankle I70.433
              - calf I70.432
              - foot site NEC I70.435
              - heel I70.434
              - lower leg NEC I70.438
              - midfoot I70.434
              - thigh I70.431
            - specified type NEC I70.491
          - specified type NEC I70.499
        - specified NEC I70.408
          - with
            - gangrene (and intermittent claudication, rest pain and ulcer) I70.468
            - intermittent claudication I70.418
            - rest pain (and intermittent claudication) I70.428
            - ulceration (and intermittent claudication and rest pain) I70.45
          - specified type NEC I70.498
      - leg I70.309
        - with
          - gangrene (and intermittent claudication, rest pain and ulcer) I70.369
          - intermittent claudication I70.319
          - rest pain (and intermittent claudication) I70.329
        - bilateral I70.303
          - with
            - gangrene (and intermittent claudication, rest pain and ulcer) I70.363
            - intermittent claudication I70.313
            - rest pain (and intermittent claudication) I70.323
          - specified type NEC I70.393
        - left I70.302
          - with
            - gangrene (and intermittent claudication, rest pain and ulcer) I70.362
            - intermittent claudication I70.312
            - rest pain (and intermittent claudication) I70.322

Arteriosclerosis, arteriosclerotic — *continued*
- extremities — *continued*
  - bypass graft — *continued*
    - leg — *continued*
      - left — *continued*
        - with — *continued*
          - ulceration (and intermittent claudication and rest pain) I70.349
            - ankle I70.343
            - calf I70.342
            - foot site NEC I70.345
            - heel I70.344
            - lower leg NEC I70.348
            - midfoot I70.344
            - thigh I70.341
          - specified type NEC I70.392
      - right I70.301
        - with
          - gangrene (and intermittent claudication, rest pain and ulcer) I70.361
          - intermittent claudication I70.311
          - rest pain (and intermittent claudication) I70.321
          - ulceration (and intermittent claudication and rest pain) I70.339
            - ankle I70.333
            - calf I70.332
            - foot site NEC I70.335
            - heel I70.334
            - lower leg NEC I70.338
            - midfoot I70.334
            - thigh I70.331
          - specified type NEC I70.391
        - specified type NEC I70.399
    - nonautologous biological graft I70.509
      - leg I70.509
        - with
          - gangrene (and intermittent claudication, rest pain and ulcer) I70.569
          - intermittent claudication I70.519
          - rest pain (and intermittent claudication) I70.529
        - bilateral I70.503
          - with
            - gangrene (and intermittent claudication, rest pain and ulcer) I70.563
            - intermittent claudication I70.513
            - rest pain (and intermittent claudication) I70.523
          - specified type NEC I70.593
        - left I70.502
          - with
            - gangrene (and intermittent claudication, rest pain and ulcer) I70.562
            - intermittent claudication I70.512
            - rest pain (and intermittent claudication) I70.522
            - ulceration (and intermittent claudication and rest pain) I70.549
              - ankle I70.543
              - calf I70.542
              - foot site NEC I70.545
              - heel I70.544
              - lower leg NEC I70.548
              - midfoot I70.544
              - thigh I70.541
            - specified type NEC I70.592
        - right I70.501
          - with
            - gangrene (and intermittent claudication, rest pain and ulcer) I70.561
            - intermittent claudication I70.511
            - rest pain (and intermittent claudication) I70.521
            - ulceration (and intermittent claudication and rest pain) I70.539
              - ankle I70.533
              - calf I70.532
              - foot site NEC I70.535
              - heel I70.534
              - lower leg NEC I70.538
              - midfoot I70.534
              - thigh I70.531
            - specified type NEC I70.591
          - specified type NEC I70.599
        - specified NEC I70.508

Arteriosclerosis, arteriosclerotic — *continued*
- extremities — *continued*
  - bypass graft — *continued*
    - nonautologous biological graft — *continued*
      - specified — *continued*
        - with
          - gangrene (and intermittent claudication, rest pain and ulcer) I70.568
          - intermittent claudication I70.518
          - rest pain (and intermittent claudication) I70.528
          - ulceration (and intermittent claudication and rest pain) I70.55
        - specified type NEC I70.598
    - nonbiological graft I70.609
      - leg I70.609
        - with
          - gangrene (and intermittent claudication, rest pain and ulcer) I70.669
          - intermittent claudication I70.619
          - rest pain (and intermittent claudication) I70.629
        - bilateral I70.603
          - with
            - gangrene (and intermittent claudication, rest pain and ulcer) I70.663
            - intermittent claudication I70.613
            - rest pain (and intermittent claudication) I70.623
          - specified type NEC I70.693
        - left I70.602
          - with
            - gangrene (and intermittent claudication, rest pain and ulcer) I70.662
            - intermittent claudication I70.612
            - rest pain (and intermittent claudication) I70.622
            - ulceration (and intermittent claudication and rest pain) I70.649
              - ankle I70.643
              - calf I70.642
              - foot site NEC I70.645
              - heel I70.644
              - lower leg NEC I70.648
              - midfoot I70.644
              - thigh I70.641
            - specified type NEC I70.692
        - right I70.601
          - with
            - gangrene (and intermittent claudication, rest pain and ulcer) I70.661
            - intermittent claudication I70.611
            - rest pain (and intermittent claudication) I70.621
            - ulceration (and intermittent claudication and rest pain) I70.639
              - ankle I70.633
              - calf I70.632
              - foot site NEC I70.635
              - heel I70.634
              - lower leg NEC I70.638
              - midfoot I70.634
              - thigh I70.631
            - specified type NEC I70.691
          - specified type NEC I70.699
        - specified NEC I70.608
          - with
            - gangrene (and intermittent claudication, rest pain and ulcer) I70.668
            - intermittent claudication I70.618
            - rest pain (and intermittent claudication) I70.628
            - ulceration (and intermittent claudication and rest pain) I70.65
          - specified type NEC I70.698
    - specified graft NEC I70.709
      - leg I70.709
        - with
          - gangrene (and intermittent claudication, rest pain and ulcer) I70.769
          - intermittent claudication I70.719
          - rest pain (and intermittent claudication) I70.729
        - bilateral I70.703

Arteriosclerosis, arteriosclerotic — *continued*
  extremities — *continued*
    bypass graft — *continued*
      specified graft — *continued*
        leg — *continued*
          bilateral — *continued*
            with
              gangrene (and intermittent claudication, rest pain and ulcer) I70.763
              intermittent claudication I70.713
              rest pain (and intermittent claudication) I70.723
            specified type NEC I70.793
          left I70.702
            with
              gangrene (and intermittent claudication, rest pain and ulcer) I70.762
              intermittent claudication I70.712
              rest pain (and intermittent claudication) I70.722
              ulceration (and intermittent claudication and rest pain) I70.749
                ankle I70.743
                calf I70.742
                foot site NEC I70.745
                heel I70.744
                lower leg NEC I70.748
                midfoot I70.744
                thigh I70.741
            specified type NEC I70.792
          right I70.701
            with
              gangrene (and intermittent claudication, rest pain and ulcer) I70.761
              intermittent claudication I70.711
              rest pain (and intermittent claudication) I70.721
              ulceration (and intermittent claudication and rest pain) I70.739
                ankle I70.733
                calf I70.732
                foot site NEC I70.735
                heel I70.734
                lower leg NEC I70.738
                midfoot I70.734
                thigh I70.731
            specified type NEC I70.791
        specified type NEC I70.799
      specified NEC I70.708
        with
          gangrene (and intermittent claudication, rest pain and ulcer) I70.768
          intermittent claudication I70.718
          rest pain (and intermittent claudication) I70.728
          ulceration (and intermittent claudication and rest pain) I70.75
        specified type NEC I70.798
    specified NEC I70.308
      with
        gangrene (and intermittent claudication, rest pain and ulcer) I70.368
        intermittent claudication I70.318
        rest pain (and intermittent claudication) I70.328
        ulceration (and intermittent claudication and rest pain) I70.35
      specifiec type NEC I70.398
    leg I70.209
      with
        gangrene (and intermittent claudication, rest pain and ulcer) I70.269
        intermittent claudication I70.219
        rest pain (and intermittent claudication) I70.229
      bilateral I70.203
        with
          gangrene (and intermittent claudication, rest pain and ulcer) I70.263
          intermittent claudication I70.213
          rest pain (and intermittent claudication) I70.223
        specified type NEC I70.293
      left I70.202

Arteriosclerosis, arteriosclerotic — *continued*
  extremities — *continued*
    leg — *continued*
      left — *continued*
        with
          gangrene (and intermittent claudication, rest pain and ulcer) I70.262
          intermittent claudication I70.212
          rest pain (and intermittent claudication) I70.222
          ulceration (and intermittent claudication and rest pain) I70.249
            ankle I70.243
            calf I70.242
            foot site NEC I70.245
            heel I70.244
            lower leg NEC I70.248
            midfoot I70.244
            thigh I70.241
        specified type NEC I70.292
      right I70.201
        with
          gangrene (and intermittent claudication, rest pain and ulcer) I70.261
          intermittent claudication I70.211
          rest pain (and intermittent claudication) I70.221
          ulceration (and intermittent claudication and rest pain) I70.239
            ankle I70.233
            calf I70.232
            foot site NEC I70.235
            heel I70.234
            lower leg NEC I70.238
            midfoot I70.234
            thigh I70.231
        specified type NEC I70.291
      specified type NEC I70.299
    specified site NEC I70.208
      with
        gangrene (and intermittent claudication, rest pain and ulcer) I70.268
        intermittent claudication I70.218
        rest pain (and intermittent claudication) I70.228
        ulceration (and intermittent claudication and rest pain) I70.25
        specified type NEC I70.298
  generalized I70.91
  heart (disease) — *see* Arteriosclerosis, coronary (artery), kidney — *see* Hypertension, kidney
  medial — *see* Arteriosclerosis, extremities
  mesenteric (artery) K55.1
  Mönckeberg's — *see* Arteriosclerosis, extremities
  myocarditis I51.4
  peripheral (of extremities) — *see* Arteriosclerosis, extremities
  pulmonary (idiopathic) I27.0
  renal (arterioles) — *see also* Hypertension, kidney
    artery I70.1
  retina (vascular) I70.8 [H35.0-] ☑
  specified artery NEC I70.8
  spinal (cord) G95.19
  vertebral (artery) I67.2
Arteriospasm I73.9
Arteriovenous — *see* condition
Arteritis I77.6
  allergic M31.0
  aorta (nonsyphilitic) I77.6
    syphilitic A52.02
  aortic arch M31.4
  brachiocephalic M31.4
  brain I67.7
    syphilitic A52.04
  cerebral I67.7
    in systemic lupus erythematosus M32.19
    listerial A32.89
    syphilitic A52.04
    tuberculous A18.89
  coronary (artery) I25.89
    rheumatic I01.8
      chronic I09.89
    syphilitic A52.06
  cranial (left) (right), giant cell M31.6
  deformans — *see* Arteriosclerosis
  giant cell NEC M31.6
    with polymyalgia rheumatica M31.5
  necrosing or necrotizing M31.9

Arteritis — *continued*
  necrosing or necrotizing — *continued*
    specified NEC M31.8
  nodosa M30.0
  obliterans — *see* Arteriosclerosis
  pulmonary I28.8
  rheumatic — *see* Fever, rheumatic
  senile — *see* Arteriosclerosis
  suppurative I77.2
  syphilitic (general) A52.09
    brain A52.04
    coronary A52.06
    spinal A52.09
  temporal, giant cell M31.6
  young female aortic arch syndrome M31.4
Artery, arterial — *see also* condition
  abscess I77.89
  single umbilical Q27.0
Arthralgia (allergic) — *see also* Pain, joint
  in caisson disease T70.3 ☑
  temporomandibular M26.62- ☑
Arthritis, arthritic (acute) (chronic) (nonpyogenic) (subacute) M19.90
  allergic — *see* Arthritis, specified form NEC
  ankylosing (crippling) (spine) — *see also* Spondylitis, ankylosing
    sites other than spine — *see* Arthritis, specified form NEC
  atrophic — *see* Osteoarthritis
    spine — *see* Spondylitis, ankylosing
  back — *see* Spondylopathy, inflammatory
  blennorrhagic (gonococcal) A54.42
  Charcot's — *see* Arthropathy, neuropathic
    diabetic — *see* Diabetes, arthropathy, neuropathic
    syringomyelic G95.0
  chylous (filarial) — *see also* category M01 B74.9
  climacteric (any site) NEC — *see* Arthritis, specified form NEC
  crystal (-induced) — *see* Arthritis, in, crystals
  deformans — *see* Osteoarthritis
  degenerative — *see* Osteoarthritis
  due to or associated with
    acromegaly E22.0
    brucellosis — *see* Brucellosis
    caisson disease T70.3 ☑
    diabetes — *see* Diabetes, arthropathy
    dracontiasis — *see also* category M01 B72
    enteritis NEC
      regional — *see* Enteritis, regional
    erysipelas — *see also* category M01 A46
    erythema
      epidemic A25.1
      nodosum L52
    filariasis NOS B74.9
    glanders A24.0
    helminthiasis — *see also* category M01 B83.9
    hemophilia D66 [M36.2]
    Henoch- (Schönlein) purpura D69.0 [M36.4]
    human parvovirus — *see also* category M01 B97.6
    infectious disease NEC M01 ☑
    leprosy (see also category M01) — *see also* Leprosy A30.9
    Lyme disease A69.23
    mycobacteria — *see also* category M01 A31.8
    parasitic disease NEC — *see also* category M01 B89
    paratyphoid fever (see also category M01) — *see also* Fever, paratyphoid A01.4
    rat bite fever — *see also* category M01 A25.1
    regional enteritis — *see* Enteritis, regional
    respiratory disorder NOS J98.9
    serum sickness — *see also* Reaction, serum T80.69 ☑
    syringomyelia G95.0
    typhoid fever A01.04
  epidemic erythema A25.1
  febrile — *see* Fever, rheumatic
  gonococcal A54.42
  gouty (acute) — *see* Gout
  in (due to)
    acromegaly — *see also* subcategory M14.8- E22.0
    amyloidosis — *see also* subcategory M14.8- E85.4
    bacterial disease — *see also* subcategory M01 A49.9
    Behçet's syndrome M35.2
    caisson disease — *see also* subcategory M14.8- T70.3 ☑
    coliform bacilli (Escherichia coli) — *see* Arthritis, in, pyogenic organism NEC

28

☑ **Additional Character Required** — Refer to the Tabular List for Character Selection   ▽ **Subterms under main terms may continue to next column or page**

Arthritis, arthritic — *continued*
  in — *continued*
    crystals M11.9
      dicalcium phosphate — *see* Arthritis, in, crystals, specified type NEC
      hydroxyapatite M11.0- ☑
      pyrophosphate — *see* Arthritis, in, crystals, specified type NEC
      specified type NEC M11.80
        ankle M11.87- ☑
        elbow M11.82- ☑
        foot joint M11.87- ☑
        hand joint M11.84- ☑
        hip M11.85- ☑
        knee M11.86- ☑
        multiple sites M11.8- ☑
        shoulder M11.81- ☑
        vertebrae M11.88
        wrist M11.83- ☑
    dermatoarthritis, lipoid E78.81
    dracontiasis (dracunculiasis) — *see also* category M01 B72
    endocrine disorder NEC — *see also* subcategory M14.8- E34.9
    enteritis, infectious NEC — *see also* category M01 A09
      specified organism NEC — *see also* category M01 A08.8
    erythema
      multiforme — *see also* subcategory M14.8- L51.9
      nodosum — *see also* subcategory M14.8- L52
    gout — *see* Gout
    helminthiasis NEC — *see also* category M01 B83.9
    hemochromatosis — *see also* subcategory M14.8- E83.118
    hemoglobinopathy NEC D58.2 *[M36.3]*
    hemophilia NEC D66 *[M36.2]*
    Hemophilus influenzae M00.8- ☑ *[B96.3]*
    Henoch (-Schönlein) purpura D69.0 *[M36.4]*
    hyperparathyroidism NEC — *see also* subcategory M14.8- E21.3
    hypersensitivity reaction NEC T78.49 ☑ *[M36.4]*
    hypogammaglobulinemia — *see also* subcategory M14.8- D80.1
    hypothyroidism NEC — *see also* subcategory M14.8- E03.9
    infection — *see* Arthritis, pyogenic or pyemic
      spine — *see* Spondylopathy, infective
    infectious disease NEC M01
    leprosy — *see also* category M01 A30.9
    leukemia NEC C95.9- ☑ *[M36.1]*
    lipoid dermatoarthritis E78.81
    Lyme disease A69.23
    Mediterranean fever, familial — *see also* subcategory M14.8- M04.1
    Meningococcus A39.83
    metabolic disorder NEC — *see also* subcategory M14.8- E88.9
    multiple myelomatosis C90.0- ☑ *[M36.1]*
    mumps B26.85
    mycosis NEC — *see also* category M01 B49
    myelomatosis (multiple) C90.0- ☑ *[M36.1]*
    neurological disorder NEC G98.0
    ochronosis — *see also* subcategory M14.8- E70.29
    O'nyong-nyong — *see also* category M01 A92.1
    parasitic disease NEC — *see also* category M01 B89
    paratyphoid fever — *see also* category M01 A01.4
    Pseudomonas — *see* Arthritis, pyogenic, bacterial NEC
    psoriasis L40.50
    pyogenic organism NEC — *see* Arthritis, pyogenic, bacterial NEC
    Reiter's disease — *see* Reiter's disease
    respiratory disorder NEC — *see also* subcategory M14.8- J98.9
    reticulosis, malignant — *see also* subcategory M14.8- C86.0
    rubella B06.82
    Salmonella (arizonae) (cholerae-suis) (enteritidis) (typhimurium) A02.23
    sarcoidosis D86.86
    specified bacteria NEC — *see* Arthritis, pyogenic, bacterial NEC
    sporotrichosis B42.82
    syringomyelia G95.0
    thalassemia NEC D56.9 *[M36.3]*
    tuberculosis — *see* Tuberculosis, arthritis

Arthritis, arthritic — *continued*
  in — *continued*
    typhoid fever A01.04
    urethritis, Reiter's — *see* Reiter's disease
    viral disease NEC — *see also* category M01 B34.9
  infectious or infective — *see also* Arthritis, pyogenic or pyemic
    spine — *see* Spondylopathy, infective
  juvenile M08.90
    with systemic onset — *see* Still's disease
    ankle M08.97- ☑
    elbow M08.92- ☑
    foot joint M08.97- ☑
    hand joint M08.94- ☑
    hip M08.95- ☑
    knee M08.96- ☑
    multiple sites M08.99
    pauciarticular M08.40
      ankle M08.47- ☑
      elbow M08.42- ☑
      foot joint M08.47- ☑
      hand joint M08.44- ☑
      hip M08.45- ☑
      knee M08.46- ☑
      shoulder M08.41- ☑
      vertebrae M08.48
      wrist M08.43- ☑
    psoriatic L40.54
    rheumatoid — *see* Arthritis, rheumatoid, juvenile
    shoulder M08.91- ☑
    specified type NEC M08.80
      ankle M08.87- ☑
      elbow M08.82- ☑
      foot joint M08.87- ☑
      hand joint M08.84- ☑
      hip M08.85- ☑
      knee M08.86- ☑
      multiple site M08.89
      shoulder M08.81- ☑
      specified joint NEC M08.88
      vertebrae M08.88
      wrist M08.83- ☑
    wrist M08.93- ☑
  meaning osteoarthritis — *see* Osteoarthritis
  meningococcal A39.83
  menopausal (any site) NEC — *see* Arthritis, specified form NEC
  mutilans (psoriatic) L40.52
  mycotic NEC — *see also* category M01 B49
  neuropathic (Charcot) — *see* Arthropathy, neuropathic
    diabetic — *see* Diabetes, arthropathy, neuropathic
    nonsyphilitic NEC G98.0
    syringomyelic G95.0
  ochronotic — *see also* subcategory M14.8- E70.29
  palindromic (any site) — *see* Rheumatism, palindromic
  pneumococcal M00.10
    ankle M00.17- ☑
    elbow M00.12- ☑
    foot joint — *see* Arthritis, pneumococcal, ankle
    hand joint M00.14- ☑
    hip M00.15- ☑
    knee M00.16- ☑
    multiple site M00.19
    shoulder M00.11- ☑
    vertebra M00.18
    wrist M00.13- ☑
  postdysenteric — *see* Arthropathy, postdysenteric
  postmeningococcal A39.84
  postrheumatic, chronic — *see* Arthropathy, postrheumatic, chronic
  primary progressive — *see also* Arthritis, specified form NEC
    spine — *see* Spondylitis, ankylosing
  psoriatic L40.50
  purulent (any site except spine) — *see* Arthritis, pyogenic or pyemic
    spine — *see* Spondylopathy, infective
  pyogenic or pyemic (any site except spine) M00.9
    bacterial NEC M00.80
      ankle M00.87- ☑
      elbow M00.82- ☑
      foot joint — *see* Arthritis, pyogenic, bacterial NEC, ankle
      hand joint M00.84- ☑
      hip M00.85- ☑
      knee M00.86- ☑
      multiple site M00.89

Arthritis, arthritic — *continued*
  pyogenic or pyemic — *continued*
    bacterial — *continued*
      shoulder M00.81- ☑
      vertebra M00.88
      wrist M00.83- ☑
    pneumococcal — *see* Arthritis, pneumococcal
    spine — *see* Spondylopathy, infective
    staphylococcal — *see* Arthritis, staphylococcal
    streptococcal — *see* Arthritis, streptococcal NEC
      pneumococcal — *see* Arthritis, pneumococcal
  reactive — *see* Reiter's disease
  rheumatic — *see also* Arthritis, rheumatoid
    acute or subacute — *see* Fever, rheumatic
  rheumatoid M06.9
    with
      carditis — *see* Rheumatoid, carditis
      endocarditis — *see* Rheumatoid, carditis
      heart involvement NEC — *see* Rheumatoid, carditis
      lung involvement — *see* Rheumatoid, lung
      myocarditis — *see* Rheumatoid, carditis
      myopathy — *see* Rheumatoid, myopathy
      pericarditis — *see* Rheumatoid, carditis
      polyneuropathy — *see* Rheumatoid, polyneuropathy
      rheumatoid factor — *see* Arthritis, rheumatoid, seropositive
      splenoadenomegaly and leukopenia — *see* Felty's syndrome
      vasculitis — *see* Rheumatoid, vasculitis
      visceral involvement NEC — *see* Rheumatoid, arthritis, with involvement of organs NEC
    juvenile (with or without rheumatoid factor) M08.00
      ankle M08.07- ☑
      elbow M08.02- ☑
      foot joint M08.07- ☑
      hand joint M08.04- ☑
      hip M08.05- ☑
      knee M08.06- ☑
      multiple site M08.09
      shoulder M08.01- ☑
      vertebra M08.08
      wrist M08.03- ☑
    seronegative M06.00
      ankle M06.07- ☑
      elbow M06.02- ☑
      foot joint M06.07- ☑
      hand joint M06.04- ☑
      hip M06.05- ☑
      knee M06.06- ☑
      multiple site M06.09
      shoulder M06.01- ☑
      vertebra M06.08
      wrist M06.03- ☑
    seropositive M05.9
      specified NEC M05.80
        ankle M05.87- ☑
        elbow M05.82- ☑
        foot joint M05.87- ☑
        hand joint M05.84- ☑
        hip M05.85- ☑
        knee M05.86- ☑
        multiple sites M05.89
        shoulder M05.81- ☑
        vertebra — *see* Spondylitis, ankylosing
        wrist M05.83- ☑
      without organ involvement M05.70
        ankle M05.77- ☑
        elbow M05.72- ☑
        foot joint M05.77- ☑
        hand joint M05.74- ☑
        hip M05.75- ☑
        knee M05.76- ☑
        multiple sites M05.79
        shoulder M05.71- ☑
        vertebra — *see* Spondylitis, ankylosing
        wrist M05.73- ☑
    specified type NEC M06.80
      ankle M06.87- ☑
      elbow M06.82- ☑
      foot joint M06.87- ☑
      hand joint M06.84- ☑
      hip M06.85- ☑
      knee M06.86- ☑
      multiple site M06.89

Arthritis, arthritic — *continued*
rheumatoid — *continued*
specified type — *continued*
shoulder M06.81- ✓
vertebra M06.88
wrist M06.83- ✓
spine — *see* Spondylitis, ankylosing
rubella B06.82
scorbutic — *see also* subcategory M14.8- E54
senile or senescent — *see* Osteoarthritis
septic (any site except spine) — *see* Arthritis, pyogenic
or pyemic
spine — *see* Spondylopathy, infective
serum (nontherapeutic) (therapeutic) — *see*
Arthropathy, postimmunization
specified form NEC M13.80
ankle M13.87- ✓
elbow M13.82- ✓
foot joint M13.87- ✓
hand joint M13.84- ✓
hip M13.85- ✓
knee M13.86- ✓
multiple site M13.89
shoulder M13.81- ✓
specified joint NEC M13.88
wrist M13.83- ✓
spine — *see also* Spondylopathy, inflammatory
infectious or infective NEC — *see* Spondylopathy,
infective
Marie-Strümpell — *see* Spondylitis, ankylosing
pyogenic — *see* Spondylopathy, infective
rheumatoid — *see* Spondylitis, ankylosing
traumatic (old) — *see* Spondylopathy, traumatic
tuberculous A18.01
staphylococcal M00.00
ankle M00.07- ✓
elbow M00.02- ✓
foot joint — *see* Arthritis, staphylococcal, ankle
hand joint M00.04- ✓
hip M00.05- ✓
knee M00.06- ✓
multiple site M00.09
shoulder M00.01- ✓
vertebra M00.08
wrist M00.03- ✓
streptococcal NEC M00.20
ankle M00.27- ✓
elbow M00.22- ✓
foot joint — *see* Arthritis, streptococcal, ankle
hand joint M00.24- ✓
hip M00.25- ✓
knee M00.26- ✓
multiple site M00.29
shoulder M00.21- ✓
vertebra M00.28
wrist M00.23- ✓
suppurative — *see* Arthritis, pyogenic or pyemic
syphilitic (late) A52.16
congenital A50.55 [M12.80]
syphilitica deformans (Charcot) A52.16
temporomandibular M26.69
toxic of menopause (any site) — *see* Arthritis, specified
form NEC
transient — *see* Arthropathy, specified form NEC
traumatic (chronic) — *see* Arthropathy, traumatic
tuberculous A18.02
spine A18.01
uratic — *see* Gout
urethritica (Reiter's) — *see* Reiter's disease
vertebral — *see* Spondylopathy, inflammatory
villous (any site) — *see* Arthropathy, specified form
NEC
Arthrocele — *see* Effusion, joint
Arthrodesis status Z98.1
Arthrodynia — *see also* Pain, joint
Arthrodysplasia Q74.9
Arthrofibrosis, joint — *see* Ankylosis
Arthrogryposis (congenital) Q68.8
multiplex congenita Q74.3
Arthrokatadysis M24.7
Arthropathy — *see also* Arthritis M12.9
Charcot's — *see* Arthropathy, neuropathic
diabetic — *see* Diabetes, arthropathy, neuropathic
syringomyelic G95.0
cricoarytenoid J38.7
crystal (-induced) — *see* Arthritis, in, crystals
diabetic NEC — *see* Diabetes, arthropathy

Arthropathy — *continued*
distal interphalangeal, psoriatic L40.51
enteropathic M07.60
ankle M07.67- ✓
elbow M07.62- ✓
foot joint M07.67- ✓
hand joint M07.64- ✓
hip M07.65- ✓
knee M07.66- ✓
multiple site M07.69
shoulder M07.61- ✓
vertebra M07.68
wrist M07.63- ✓
following intestinal bypass M02.00
ankle M02.07- ✓
elbow M02.02- ✓
foot joint M02.07- ✓
hand joint M02.04- ✓
hip M02.05- ✓
knee M02.06- ✓
multiple site M02.09
shoulder M02.01- ✓
vertebra M02.08
wrist M02.03- ✓
gouty — *see also* Gout
in (due to)
Lesch-Nyhan syndrome E79.1 [M14.8-] ✓
sickle-cell disorders D57- ✓ [M14.8-] ✓
hemophilic NEC D66 [M36.2]
in (due to)
hyperparathyroidism NEC E21.3 [M14.8-] ✓
metabolic disease NOS E88.9 [M14.8-] ✓
in (due to)
acromegaly E22.0 [M14.8-] ✓
amyloidosis E85.4 [M14.8-] ✓
blood disorder NOS D75.9 [M36.3]
diabetes — *see* Diabetes, arthropathy
endocrine disease NOS E34.9 [M14.8-] ✓
erythema
multiforme L51.9 [M14.8-] ✓
nodosum L52 [M14.8-] ✓
hemochromatosis E83.118 [M14.8-] ✓
hemoglobinopathy NEC D58.2 [M36.3]
hemophilia NEC D66 [M36.2]
Henoch-Schönlein purpura D69.0 [M36.4]
hyperthyroidism E05.90 [M14.8-] ✓
hypothyroidism E03.9 [M14.8-] ✓
infective endocarditis I33.0 [M12.80]
leukemia NEC C95.9- ✓ [M36.1]
malignant histiocytosis C96.A [M36.1]
metabolic disease NOS E88.9 [M14.8-] ✓
multiple myeloma C90.0- ✓ [M36.1]
neoplastic disease NOS (*see also* Neoplasm)
D49.9 [M36.1]
nutritional deficiency — *see also* subcategory
M14.8- E63.9
psoriasis NOS L40.50
sarcoidosis D86.86
syphilis (late) A52.77
congenital A50.55 [M12.80]
thyrotoxicosis — *see also* subcategory M14.8-
E05.90
ulcerative colitis K51.90 [M07.60]
viral hepatitis (postinfectious) NEC B19.9 [M12.80]
Whipple's disease — *see also* subcategory M14.8-
K90.81
Jaccoud — *see* Arthropathy, postrheumatic, chronic
juvenile — *see* Arthritis, juvenile
psoriatic L40.54
mutilans (psoriatic) L40.52
neuropathic (Charcot) M14.60
ankle M14.67- ✓
diabetic — *see* Diabetes, arthropathy, neuropathic
elbow M14.62- ✓
foot joint M14.67- ✓
hand joint M14.64- ✓
hip M14.65- ✓
knee M14.66- ✓
multiple site M14.69
nonsyphilitic NEC G98.0
shoulder M14.61- ✓
syringomyelic G95.0
vertebra M14.68
wrist M14.63- ✓
osteopulmonary — *see* Osteoarthropathy, hypertrophic, specified NEC

Arthropathy — *continued*
postdysenteric M02.10
ankle M02.17- ✓
elbow M02.12- ✓
foot joint M02.17- ✓
hand joint M02.14- ✓
hip M02.15- ✓
knee M02.16- ✓
multiple site M02.19
shoulder M02.11- ✓
vertebra M02.18
wrist M02.13- ✓
postimmunization M02.20
ankle M02.27- ✓
elbow M02.22- ✓
foot joint M02.27- ✓
hand joint M02.24- ✓
hip M02.25- ✓
knee M02.26- ✓
multiple site M02.29
shoulder M02.21- ✓
vertebra M02.28
wrist M02.23- ✓
postinfectious NEC B99 ✓ [M12.80]
in (due to)
enteritis due to Yersinia enterocolitica
A04.6 [M12.80]
syphilis A52.77
viral hepatitis NEC B19.9 [M12.80]
postrheumatic, chronic (Jaccoud) M12.00
ankle M12.07- ✓
elbow M12.02- ✓
foot joint M12.07- ✓
hand joint M12.04- ✓
hip M12.05- ✓
knee M12.06- ✓
multiple site M12.09
shoulder M12.01- ✓
specified joint NEC M12.08
vertebrae M12.08
wrist M12.03- ✓
psoriatic NEC L40.59
interphalangeal, distal L40.51
reactive M02.9
in (due to)
infective endocarditis I33.0 [M02.9]
specified type NEC M02.80
ankle M02.87- ✓
elbow M02.82- ✓
foot joint M02.87- ✓
hand joint M02.84- ✓
hip M02.85- ✓
knee M02.86- ✓
multiple site M02.89
shoulder M02.81- ✓
vertebra M02.88
wrist M02.83- ✓
specified form NEC M12.80
ankle M12.87- ✓
elbow M12.82- ✓
foot joint M12.87- ✓
hand joint M12.84- ✓
hip M12.85- ✓
knee M12.86- ✓
multiple site M12.89
shoulder M12.81- ✓
specified joint NEC M12.88
vertebrae M12.88
wrist M12.83- ✓
syringomyelic G95.0
tabes dorsalis A52.16
tabetic A52.16
transient — *see* Arthropathy, specified form NEC
traumatic M12.50
ankle M12.57- ✓
elbow M12.52- ✓
foot joint M12.57- ✓
hand joint M12.54- ✓
hip M12.55- ✓
knee M12.56- ✓
multiple site M12.59
shoulder M12.51- ✓
specified joint NEC M12.58
vertebrae M12.58
wrist M12.53- ✓
Arthropyosis — *see* Arthritis, pyogenic or pyemic

✓ Additional Character Required — Refer to the Tabular List for Character Selection   Subterms under main terms may continue to next column or page

Arthrosis (deformans) (degenerative) (localized) — *see also* Osteoarthritis M19.90
  spine — *see* Spondylosis
Arthus' phenomenon or reaction T78.41 ☑
  due to
    drug — *see* Table of Drugs and Chemicals, by drug
Articular — *see* condition
Articulation, reverse (teeth) M26.24
Artificial
  insemination complication — *see* Complications, artificial, fertilization
  opening status (functioning) (without complication) Z93.9
    anus (colostomy) Z93.3
    colostomy Z93.3
    cystostomy Z93.50
      appendico-vesicostomy Z93.52
      cutaneous Z93.51
      specified NEC Z93.59
    enterostomy Z93.4
    gastrostomy Z93.1
    ileostomy Z93.2
    intestinal tract NEC Z93.4
    jejunostomy Z93.4
    nephrostomy Z93.6
    specified site NEC Z93.8
    tracheostomy Z93.0
    ureterostomy Z93.6
    urethrostomy Z93.6
    urinary tract NEC Z93.6
    vagina Z93.8
  vagina status Z93.8
Arytenoid — *see* condition
Asbestosis (occupational) J61
Ascariasis B77.9
  with
    complications NEC B77.89
    intestinal complications B77.0
    pneumonia, pneumonitis B77.81
Ascaridosis, ascariasis — *see* Ascariasis
Ascaris (infection) (infestation) (lumbricoides) — *see* Ascariasis
Ascending — *see* condition
ASC-H (atypical squamous cells cannot exclude high grade squamous intraepithelial lesion on cytologic smear)
  anus R85.611
  cervix R87.611
  vagina R87.621
Aschoff's bodies — *see* Myocarditis, rheumatic
Ascites (abdominal) R18.8
  cardiac — *see also* Failure, heart, right I50.810
  chylous (nonfilarial) I89.8
    filarial — *see* Infestation, filarial
  due to
    cirrhosis, alcoholic K70.31
    hepatitis
      alcoholic K70.11
      chronic active K71.51
    S. japonicum B65.2
  heart — *see also* Failure, heart, right I50.810
  malignant R18.0
  pseudochylous R18.8
  syphilitic A52.74
  tuberculous A18.31
ASC-US (atypical squamous cells of undetermined significance on cytologic smear)
  anus R85.610
  cervix R87.610
  vagina R87.620
Aseptic — *see* condition
Asherman's syndrome N85.6
Asialia K11.7
Asiatic cholera — *see* Cholera
Asimultagnosia (simultanagnosia) R48.3
Askin's tumor — *see* Neoplasm, connective tissue, malignant
Asocial personality F60.2
Asomatognosia R41.4
Aspartylglucosaminuria E77.1
Asperger's disease or syndrome F84.5
Aspergilloma — *see* Aspergillosis
Aspergillosis (with pneumonia) B44.9
  bronchopulmonary, allergic B44.81
  disseminated B44.7
  generalized B44.7
  pulmonary NEC B44.1
    allergic B44.81
    invasive B44.0

Aspergillosis — *continued*
  specified NEC B44.89
  tonsillar B44.2
Aspergillus (flavus) (fumigatus) (infection) (terreus) — *see* Aspergillosis
Aspermatogenesis — *see* Azoospermia
Aspermia (testis) — *see* Azoospermia
Asphyxia, asphyxiation (by) R09.01
  antenatal P84
  birth P84
  bunny bag — *see* Asphyxia, due to, mechanical threat to breathing, trapped in bed clothes
  crushing S28.0 ☑
  drowning T75.1 ☑
  gas, fumes, or vapor — *see* Table of Drugs and Chemicals
  inhalation — *see* Inhalation
  intrauterine P84
  local I73.00
    with gangrene I73.01
  mucus — *see also* Foreign body, respiratory tract, causing asphyxia
  newborn P84
  pathological R09.01
  postnatal P84
    mechanical — *see* Asphyxia, due to, mechanical threat to breathing
  prenatal P84
  reticularis R23.1
  strangulation — *see* Asphyxia, due to, mechanical threat to breathing
  submersion T75.1 ☑
  traumatic T71.9 ☑
    due to
      crushed chest S28.0 ☑
      foreign body (in) — *see* Foreign body, respiratory tract, causing asphyxia
      low oxygen content of ambient air T71.20 ☑
        due to
          being trapped in
            low oxygen environment T71.29 ☑
            in car trunk T71.221 ☑
              circumstances undetermined T71.224 ☑
              done with intent to harm by another person T71.223 ☑
                self T71.222 ☑
            in refrigerator T71.231 ☑
              circumstances undetermined T71.234 ☑
              done with intent to harm by another person T71.233 ☑
                self T71.232 ☑
      cave-in T71.21 ☑
      mechanical threat to breathing (accidental) T71.191 ☑
        circumstances undetermined T71.194 ☑
        done with intent to harm by
          another person T71.193 ☑
          self T71.192 ☑
        hanging T71.161 ☑
          circumstances undetermined T71.164 ☑
          done with intent to harm by
            another person T71.163 ☑
            self T71.162 ☑
        plastic bag T71.121 ☑
          circumstances undetermined T71.124 ☑
          done with intent to harm by
            another person T71.123 ☑
            self T71.122 ☑
        smothering
          in furniture T71.151 ☑
            circumstances undetermined T71.154 ☑
            done with intent to harm by
              another person T71.153 ☑
              self T71.152 ☑
          under
            another person's body T71.141 ☑
              circumstances undetermined T71.144 ☑
              done with intent to harm T71.143 ☑
            pillow T71.111 ☑
              circumstances undetermined T71.114 ☑
              done with intent to harm by another person T71.113 ☑

Asphyxia, asphyxiation — *continued*
  traumatic — *continued*
    due to — *continued*
      mechanical threat to breathing — *continued*
        smothering — *continued*
          under — *continued*
            pillow — *continued*
              done with intent to harm by — *continued*
                self T71.112 ☑
          trapped in bed clothes T71.131 ☑
            circumstances undetermined T71.134 ☑
            done with intent to harm by
              another person T71.133 ☑
              self T71.132 ☑
    vomiting, vomitus — *see* Foreign body, respiratory tract, causing asphyxia
Aspiration
  amniotic (clear) fluid (newborn) P24.10
    with
      pneumonia (pneumonitis) P24.11
      respiratory symptoms P24.11
  blood
    newborn (without respiratory symptoms) P24.20
      with
        pneumonia (pneumonitis) P24.21
        respiratory symptoms P24.21
      specified age NEC — *see* Foreign body, respiratory tract
  bronchitis J69.0
  food or foreign body (with asphyxiation) — *see* Asphyxia, food
  liquor (amnii) (newborn) P24.10
    with
      pneumonia (pneumonitis) P24.11
      respiratory symptoms P24.11
  meconium (newborn) (without respiratory symptoms) P24.00
    with
      pneumonitis (pneumonitis) P24.01
      respiratory symptoms P24.01
  milk (newborn) (without respiratory symptoms) P24.30
    with
      pneumonia (pneumonitis) P24.31
      respiratory symptoms P24.31
    specified age NEC — *see* Foreign body, respiratory tract
  mucus — *see also* Foreign body, by site, causing asphyxia
    newborn P24.10
      with
        pneumonia (pneumonitis) P24.11
        respiratory symptoms P24.11
  neonatal P24.9
    specific NEC (without respiratory symptoms) P24.80
      with
        pneumonia (pneumonitis) P24.81
        respiratory symptoms P24.81
  newborn P24.9
    specific NEC (without respiratory symptoms) P24.80
      with
        pneumonia (pneumonitis) P24.81
        respiratory symptoms P24.81
  pneumonia J69.0
  pneumonitis J69.0
  syndrome of newborn — *see* Aspiration, by substance, with pneumonia
  vernix caseosa (newborn) P24.80
    with
      pneumonia (pneumonitis) P24.81
      respiratory symptoms P24.81
  vomitus — *see also* Foreign body, respiratory tract
    newborn (without respiratory symptoms) P24.30
      with
        pneumonia (pneumonitis) P24.31
        respiratory symptoms P24.31
Asplenia (congenital) Q89.01
  postsurgical Z90.81
Assam fever B55.0
Assault, sexual — *see* Maltreatment
Assmann's focus NEC A15.0
Astasia (-abasia) (hysterical) F44.4
Asteatosis cutis L85.3
Astereognosia, astereognosis R48.1
Asterixis R27.8
  in liver disease K71.3
Asteroid hyalitis — *see* Deposit, crystalline
Asthenia, asthenic R53.1

▽ Subterms under main terms may continue to next column or page   ☑ Additional Character Required — Refer to the Tabular List for Character Selection   31

Arthrosis — Asthenia, asthenic

Asthenia, asthenic — *continued*
  cardiac — *see also* Failure, heart I50.9
    psychogenic F45.8
  cardiovascular — *see also* Failure, heart I50.9
    psychogenic F45.8
  heart — *see also* Failure, heart I50.9
    psychogenic F45.8
  hysterical F44.4
  myocardial — *see also* Failure, heart I50.9
    psychogenic F45.8
  nervous F48.8
  neurocirculatory F45.8
  neurotic F48.8
  psychogenic F48.8
  psychoneurotic F48.8
  psychophysiologic F48.8
  reaction (psychophysiologic) F48.8
  senile R54
Asthenopia — *see also* Discomfort, visual
  hysterical F44.6
  psychogenic F44.6
Asthenospermia — *see* Abnormal, specimen, male
  genital organs
Asthma, asthmatic (bronchial) (catarrh) (spasmodic)
  J45.909
  with
    chronic obstructive bronchitis J44.9
      with
        acute lower respiratory infection J44.0
        exacerbation (acute) J44.1
    chronic obstructive pulmonary disease J44.9
      with
        acute lower respiratory infection J44.0
        exacerbation (acute) J44.1
    exacerbation (acute) J45.901
    hay fever — *see* Asthma, allergic extrinsic
    rhinitis, allergic — *see* Asthma, allergic extrinsic
    status asthmaticus J45.902
  allergic extrinsic J45.909
    with
      exacerbation (acute) J45.901
      status asthmaticus J45.902
  atopic — *see* Asthma, allergic extrinsic
  cardiac — *see* Failure, ventricular, left
  cardiobronchial I50.1
  childhood J45.909
    with
      exacerbation (acute) J45.901
      status asthmaticus J45.902
  chronic obstructive J44.9
    with
      acute lower respiratory infection J44.0
      exacerbation (acute) J44.1
  collier's J60
  cough variant J45.991
  detergent J69.8
  due to
    detergent J69.8
    inhalation of fumes J68.3
  eosinophilic J82
  extrinsic, allergic — *see* Asthma, allergic extrinsic
  grinder's J62.8
  hay — *see* Asthma, allergic extrinsic
  heart I50.1
  idiosyncratic — *see* Asthma, nonallergic
  intermittent (mild) J45.20
    with
      exacerbation (acute) J45.21
      status asthmaticus J45.22
  intrinsic, nonallergic — *see* Asthma, nonallergic
  Kopp's E32.8
  late-onset J45.909
    with
      exacerbation (acute) J45.901
      status asthmaticus J45.902
  mild intermittent J45.20
    with
      exacerbation (acute) J45.21
      status asthmaticus J45.22
  mild persistent J45.30
    with
      exacerbation (acute) J45.31
      status asthmaticus J45.32
  Millar's (laryngismus stridulus) J38.5
  miner's J60
  mixed J45.909
    with
      exacerbation (acute) J45.901

Asthma, asthmatic — *continued*
  mixed — *continued*
    with — *continued*
      status asthmaticus J45.902
  moderate persistent J45.40
    with
      exacerbation (acute) J45.41
      status asthmaticus J45.42
  nervous — *see* Asthma, nonallergic
  nonallergic (intrinsic) J45.909
    with
      exacerbation (acute) J45.901
      status asthmaticus J45.902
  persistent
    mild J45.30
      with
        exacerbation (acute) J45.31
        status asthmaticus J45.32
    moderate J45.40
      with
        exacerbation (acute) J45.41
        status asthmaticus J45.42
    severe J45.50
      with
        exacerbation (acute) J45.51
        status asthmaticus J45.52
  platinum J45.998
  pneumoconiotic NEC J64
  potter's J62.8
  predominantly allergic J45.909
  psychogenic F54
  pulmonary eosinophilic J82
  red cedar J67.8
  Rostan's I50.1
  sandblaster's J62.8
  sequoiosis J67.8
  severe persistent J45.50
    with
      exacerbation (acute) J45.51
      status asthmaticus J45.52
  specified NEC J45.998
  stonemason's J62.8
  thymic E32.8
  tuberculous — *see* Tuberculosis, pulmonary
  Wichmann's (laryngismus stridulus) J38.5
  wood J67.8
Astigmatism (compound) (congenital) H52.20- ☑
  irregular H52.21- ☑
  regular H52.22- ☑
Astraphobia F40.220
Astroblastoma
  specified site — *see* Neoplasm, malignant, by site
  unspecified site C71.9
Astrocytoma (cystic)
  anaplastic
    specified site — *see* Neoplasm, malignant, by site
    unspecified site C71.9
  fibrillary
    specified site — *see* Neoplasm, malignant, by site
    unspecified site C71.9
  fibrous
    specified site — *see* Neoplasm, malignant, by site
    unspecified site C71.9
  gemistocytic
    specified site — *see* Neoplasm, malignant, by site
    unspecified site C71.9
  juvenile
    specified site — *see* Neoplasm, malignant, by site
    unspecified site C71.9
  pilocytic
    specified site — *see* Neoplasm, malignant, by site
    unspecified site C71.9
  piloid
    specified site — *see* Neoplasm, malignant, by site
    unspecified site C71.9
  protoplasmic
    specified site — *see* Neoplasm, malignant, by site
    unspecified site C71.9
  specified site NEC — *see* Neoplasm, malignant, by site
  subependymal D43.2
    giant cell
      specified site — *see* Neoplasm, uncertain behavior, by site
      unspecified site D43.2
  specified site — *see* Neoplasm, uncertain behavior, by site
  unspecified site D43.2
  unspecified site C71.9

Astroglioma
  specified site — *see* Neoplasm, malignant, by site
  unspecified site C71.9
Asymbolia R48.8
Asymmetry — *see also* Distortion
  between native and reconstructed breast N65.1
  face Q67.0
  jaw (lower) — *see* Anomaly, dentofacial, jaw-cranial
    base relationship, asymmetry
Asynergia, asynergy R27.8
  ventricular I51.89
Asystole (heart) — *see* Arrest, cardiac
At risk
  for
    dental caries Z91.849
      high Z91.843
      low Z91.841
      moderate Z91.842
    falling Z91.81
Ataxia, ataxy, ataxic R27.0
  acute R27.8
  brain (hereditary) G11.9
  cerebellar (hereditary) G11.9
    with defective DNA repair G11.3
    alcoholic G31.2
    early-onset G11.1
      in
        alcoholism G31.2
        myxedema E03.9 *[G13.2]*
        neoplastic disease — *see also* Neoplasm
          D49.9 *[G32.81]*
        specified disease NEC G32.81
    late-onset (Marie's) G11.2
  cerebral (hereditary) G11.9
  congenital nonprogressive G11.0
  family, familial — *see* Ataxia, hereditary
  following
    cerebrovascular disease I69.993
      cerebral infarction I69.393
      intracerebral hemorrhage I69.193
      nontraumatic intracranial hemorrhage NEC
        I69.293
      specified disease NEC I69.893
      subarachnoid hemorrhage I69.093
  Friedreich's (heredofamilial) (cerebellar) (spinal) G11.1
  gait R26.0
    hysterical F44.4
  general R27.8
  gluten M35.9 *[G32.81]*
    with celiac disease K90.0 *[G32.81]*
  hereditary G11.9
    with neuropathy G60.2
    cerebellar — *see* Ataxia, cerebellar
    spastic G11.4
    specified NEC G11.8
    spinal (Friedreich's) G11.1
  heredofamilial — *see* Ataxia, hereditary
  Hunt's G11.1
  hysterical F44.4
  locomotor (progressive) (syphilitic) (partial) (spastic)
    A52.11
    diabetic — *see* Diabetes, ataxia
  Marie's (cerebellar) (heredofamilial) (late- onset) G11.2
  nonorganic origin F44.4
  nonprogressive, congenital G11.0
  psychogenic F44.4
  Roussy-Lévy G60.0
  Sanger-Brown's (hereditary) G11.2
  spastic hereditary G11.4
  spinal
    hereditary (Friedreich's) G11.1
    progressive (syphilitic) A52.11
  spinocerebellar, X-linked recessive G11.1
  telangiectasia (Louis-Bar) G11.3
Ataxia-telangiectasia (Louis-Bar) G11.3
Atelectasis (massive) (partial) (pressure) (pulmonary)
  J98.11
  newborn P28.10
    due to resorption P28.11
    partial P28.19
    primary P28.0
    secondary P28.19
  primary (newborn) P28.0
  tuberculous — *see* Tuberculosis, pulmonary
Atelocardia Q24.9
Atelomyelia Q06.1

Atheroembolism
- of
  - extremities
    - lower I75.02- ☑
    - upper I75.01- ☑
  - kidney I75.81
  - specified NEC I75.89

Atheroma, atheromatous — see also Arteriosclerosis I70.90
- aorta, aortic I70.0
  - valve — see also Endocarditis, aortic I35.8
- aorto-iliac I70.0
- artery — see Arteriosclerosis
- basilar (artery) I67.2
- carotid (artery) (common) (internal) I67.2
- cerebral (arteries) I67.2
- coronary (artery) I25.10
  - with angina pectoris — see Arteriosclerosis, coronary (artery),
- degeneration — see Arteriosclerosis
- heart, cardiac — see Disease, heart, ischemic, atherosclerotic
- mitral (valve) I34.8
- myocardium, myocardial — see Disease, heart, ischemic, atherosclerotic
- pulmonary valve (heart) — see also Endocarditis, pulmonary I37.8
- tricuspid (heart) (valve) I36.8
- valve, valvular — see Endocarditis
- vertebral (artery) I67.2

Atheromatosis — see Arteriosclerosis

Atherosclerosis — see also Arteriosclerosis
- coronary
  - artery I25.10
    - with angina pectoris — see Arteriosclerosis, coronary (artery),
    - due to
      - calcified coronary lesion (severely) I25.84
      - lipid rich plaque I25.83
  - transplanted heart I25.811
    - bypass graft I25.812
      - with angina pectoris — see Arteriosclerosis, coronary (artery),
    - native coronary artery I25.811
      - with angina pectoris — see Arteriosclerosis, coronary (artery),

Athetosis (acquired) R25.8
- bilateral (congenital) G80.3
- congenital (bilateral) (double) G80.3
- double (congenital) G80.3
- unilateral R25.8

Athlete's
- foot B35.3
- heart I51.7

Athrepsia E41

Athyrea (acquired) — see also Hypothyroidism
- congenital E03.1

Atonia, atony, atonic
- bladder (sphincter) (neurogenic) N31.2
- capillary I78.8
- cecum K59.8
  - psychogenic F45.8
- colon — see Atony, intestine
- congenital P94.2
- esophagus K22.8
- intestine K59.8
  - psychogenic F45.8
- stomach K31.89
  - neurotic or psychogenic F45.8
- uterus (during labor) O62.2
  - with hemorrhage (postpartum) O72.1
  - postpartum (with hemorrhage) O72.1
    - without hemorrhage O75.89

Atopy — see History, allergy

Atransferrinemia, congenital E88.09

Atresia, atretic
- alimentary organ or tract NEC Q45.8
  - upper Q40.8
- ani, anus, anal (canal) Q42.3
  - with fistula Q42.2
- aorta (ring) Q25.29
- aortic (orifice) (valve) Q23.0
  - arch Q25.21
    - congenital with hypoplasia of ascending aorta and defective development of left ventricle (with mitral stenosis) Q23.4
  - in hypoplastic left heart syndrome Q23.4
- aqueduct of Sylvius Q03.0

Atresia, atretic — continued
- aqueduct of Sylvius — continued
  - with spina bifida — see Spina bifida, with hydrocephalus
- artery NEC Q27.8
  - cerebral Q28.3
  - coronary Q24.5
  - digestive system Q27.8
  - eye Q15.8
  - lower limb Q27.8
  - pulmonary Q25.5
  - specified site NEC Q27.8
  - umbilical Q27.0
  - upper limb Q27.8
- auditory canal (external) Q16.1
- bile duct (common) (congenital) (hepatic) Q44.2
  - acquired — see Obstruction, bile duct
- bladder (neck) Q64.39
  - obstruction Q64.31
- bronchus Q32.4
- cecum Q42.8
- cervix (acquired) N88.2
  - congenital Q51.828
  - in pregnancy or childbirth — see Anomaly, cervix, in pregnancy or childbirth
    - causing obstructed labor O65.5
- choana Q30.0
- colon Q42.9
  - specified NEC Q42.8
- common duct Q44.2
- cricoid cartilage Q31.8
- cystic duct Q44.2
  - acquired K82.8
    - with obstruction K82.0
- digestive organs NEC Q45.8
- duodenum Q41.0
- ear canal Q16.1
- ejaculatory duct Q55.4
- epiglottis Q31.8
- esophagus Q39.0
  - with tracheoesophageal fistula Q39.1
- eustachian tube Q17.8
- fallopian tube (congenital) Q50.6
  - acquired N97.1
- follicular cyst N83.0- ☑
- foramen of
  - Luschka Q03.1
    - with spina bifida — see Spina bifida, with hydrocephalus
  - Magendie Q03.1
    - with spina bifida — see Spina bifida, with hydrocephalus
- gallbladder Q44.1
- genital organ
  - external
    - female Q52.79
    - male Q55.8
  - internal
    - female Q52.8
    - male Q55.8
- glottis Q31.8
- gullet Q39.0
  - with tracheoesophageal fistula Q39.1
- heart valve NEC Q24.8
  - pulmonary Q22.0
  - tricuspid Q22.4
- hymen Q52.3
  - acquired (postinfective) N89.6
- ileum Q41.2
- intestine (small) Q41.9
  - large Q42.9
    - specified NEC Q42.8
- iris, filtration angle Q15.0
- jejunum Q41.1
- lacrimal apparatus Q10.4
- larynx Q31.8
- meatus urinarius Q64.33
- mitral valve Q23.2
  - in hypoplastic left heart syndrome Q23.4
- nares (anterior) (posterior) Q30.0
- nasopharynx Q34.8
- nose, nostril Q30.0
  - acquired J34.89
- organ or site NEC Q89.8
- osseous meatus (ear) Q16.1
- oviduct (congenital) Q50.6
  - acquired N97.1
- parotid duct Q38.4
  - acquired K11.8

Atresia, atretic — continued
- pulmonary (artery) Q25.5
  - valve Q22.0
- pulmonic Q22.0
- pupil Q13.2
- rectum Q42.1
  - with fistula Q42.0
- salivary duct Q38.4
  - acquired K11.8
- sublingual duct Q38.4
  - acquired K11.8
- submandibular duct Q38.4
  - acquired K11.8
- submaxillary duct Q38.4
  - acquired K11.8
- thyroid cartilage Q31.8
- trachea Q32.1
- tricuspid valve Q22.4
- ureter Q62.10
  - pelvic junction Q62.11
  - vesical orifice Q62.12
- ureteropelvic junction Q62.11
- ureterovesical orifice Q62.12
- urethra (valvular) Q64.39
  - stricture Q64.32
- urinary tract NEC Q64.8
- uterus Q51.818
  - acquired N85.8
- vagina (congenital) Q52.4
  - acquired (postinfectional) (senile) N89.5
- vas deferens Q55.3
- vascular NEC Q27.8
  - cerebral Q28.3
  - digestive system Q27.8
  - lower limb Q27.8
  - specified site NEC Q27.8
  - upper limb Q27.8
- vein NEC Q27.8
  - digestive system Q27.8
  - great Q26.8
  - lower limb Q27.8
  - portal Q26.5
  - pulmonary Q26.4
    - partial Q26.3
    - total Q26.2
  - specified site NEC Q27.8
  - upper limb Q27.8
- vena cava (inferior) (superior) Q26.8
- vesicourethral orifice Q64.31
- vulva Q52.79
  - acquired N90.5

Atrichia, atrichosis — see Alopecia

Atrophia — see also Atrophy
- cutis senilis L90.8
  - due to radiation L57.8
- gyrata of choroid and retina H31.23
- senilis R54
  - dermatological L90.8
    - due to radiation (nonionizing) (solar) L57.8
- unguium L60.3
  - congenita Q84.6

Atrophie blanche (en plaque) (de Milian) L95.0

Atrophoderma, atrophodermia (of) L90.9
- diffusum (idiopathic) L90.4
- maculatum L90.8
  - et striatum L90.8
    - due to syphilis A52.79
  - syphilitic A51.39
- neuriticum L90.8
- Pasini and Pierini L90.3
- pigmentosum Q82.1
- reticulatum symmetricum faciei L66.4
- senile L90.8
  - due to radiation (nonionizing) (solar) L57.8
- vermiculata (cheeks) L66.4

Atrophy, atrophic (of)
- adrenal (capsule) (gland) E27.49
  - primary (autoimmune) E27.1
- alveolar process or ridge (edentulous) K08.20
- anal sphincter (disuse) N81.84
- appendix K38.8
- arteriosclerotic — see Arteriosclerosis
- bile duct (common) (hepatic) K83.8
- bladder N32.89
  - neurogenic N31.8
- blanche (en plaque) (of Milian) L95.0
- bone (senile) NEC — see also Disorder, bone, specified type NEC

Atrophy, atrophic — *continued*
- bone — *see also* Disorder, bone, specified type — *continued*
  - due to
    - tabes dorsalis (neurogenic) A52.11
- brain (cortex) (progressive) G31.9
  - frontotemporal circumscribed G31.01 [F02.80]
    - with behavioral disturbance G31.01 [F02.81]
  - senile NEC G31.1
- breast N64.2
  - obstetric — *see* Disorder, breast, specified type NEC
- buccal cavity K13.79
- cardiac — *see* Degeneration, myocardial
- cartilage (infectional) (joint) — *see* Disorder, cartilage, specified NEC
- cerebellar — *see* Atrophy, brain
- cerebral — *see* Atrophy, brain
- cervix (mucosa) (senile) (uteri) N88.8
  - menopausal N95.8
- Charcot-Marie-Tooth G60.0
- choroid (central) (macular) (myopic) (retina) H31.10- ☑
  - diffuse secondary H31.12- ☑
  - gyrate H31.23
  - senile H31.11- ☑
- ciliary body — *see* Atrophy, iris
- conjunctiva (senile) H11.89
- corpus cavernosum N48.89
- cortical — *see* Atrophy, brain
- cystic duct K82.8
- Déjérine-Thomas G23.8
- disuse NEC — *see* Atrophy, muscle
- Duchenne-Aran G12.21
- ear H93.8- ☑
- edentulous alveolar ridge K08.20
- endometrium (senile) N85.8
  - cervix N88.8
- enteric K63.89
- epididymis N50.89
- eyeball — *see* Disorder, globe, degenerated condition, atrophy
- eyelid (senile) — *see* Disorder, eyelid, degenerative
- facial (skin) L90.9
- fallopian tube (senile) N83.32- ☑
  - with ovary N83.33- ☑
- fascioscapulohumeral (Landouzy- Déjérine) G71.02
- fatty, thymus (gland) E32.8
- gallbladder K82.8
- gastric K29.40
  - with bleeding K29.41
- gastrointestinal K63.89
- glandular I89.8
- globe H44.52- ☑
- gum — *see* Recession, gingival
- hair L67.8
- heart (brown) — *see* Degeneration, myocardial
- hemifacial Q67.4
  - Romberg G51.8
- infantile E41
  - paralysis, acute — *see* Poliomyelitis, paralytic
- intestine K63.89
- iris (essential) (progressive) H21.26- ☑
  - specified NEC H21.29
- kidney (senile) (terminal) — *see also* Sclerosis, renal N26.1
  - congenital or infantile Q60.5
    - bilateral Q60.4
    - unilateral Q60.3
  - hydronephrotic — *see* Hydronephrosis
- lacrimal gland (primary) H04.14- ☑
  - secondary H04.15- ☑
- Landouzy-Déjérine G71.02
- laryngitis, infective J37.0
- larynx J38.7
- Leber's optic (hereditary) H47.22
- lip K13.0
- liver (yellow) K72.90
  - with coma K72.91
  - acute, subacute K72.00
    - with coma K72.01
  - chronic K72.10
    - with coma K72.11
- lung (senile) J98.4
- macular (dermatological) L90.8
  - syphilitic, skin A51.39
    - striated A52.79
- mandible (edentulous) K08.20
  - minimal K08.21
  - moderate K08.22

Atrophy, atrophic — *continued*
- mandible — *continued*
  - severe K08.23
- maxilla K08.20
  - minimal K08.24
  - moderate K08.25
  - severe K08.26
- muscle, muscular (diffuse) (general) (idiopathic) (primary) M62.50
  - ankle M62.57- ☑
  - Duchenne-Aran G12.21
  - foot M62.57- ☑
  - forearm M62.53- ☑
  - hand M62.54- ☑
  - infantile spinal G12.0
  - lower leg M62.56- ☑
  - multiple sites M62.59
  - myelopathic — *see* Atrophy, muscle, spinal
  - myotonic G71.11
  - neuritic G58.9
  - neuropathic (peroneal) (progressive) G60.0
  - pelvic (disuse) N81.84
  - peroneal G60.0
  - progressive (bulbar) G12.21
    - adult G12.1
    - infantile (spinal) G12.0
    - spinal G12.25
      - adult G12.1
      - infantile G12.0
  - pseudohypertrophic G71.02
  - shoulder region M62.51- ☑
  - specified site NEC M62.58
  - spinal G12.9
    - adult form G12.1
    - Aran-Duchenne G12.21
    - childhood form, type II G12.1
    - distal G12.1
    - hereditary NEC G12.1
    - infantile, type I (Werdnig-Hoffmann) G12.0
    - juvenile form, type III (Kugelberg- Welander) G12.1
    - progressive G12.25
    - scapuloperoneal form G12.1
    - specified NEC G12.8
  - syphilitic A52.78
  - thigh M62.55- ☑
  - upper arm M62.52- ☑
- myocardium — *see* Degeneration, myocardial
- myometrium (senile) N85.8
  - cervix N88.8
- myopathic NEC — *see* Atrophy, muscle
- myotonia G71.11
- nail L60.3
- nasopharynx J31.1
- nerve — *see also* Disorder, nerve
  - abducens — *see* Strabismus, paralytic, sixth nerve
  - accessory G52.8
  - acoustic or auditory H93.3 ☑
  - cranial G52.9
    - eighth (auditory) H93.3 ☑
    - eleventh (accessory) G52.8
    - fifth (trigeminal) G50.8
    - first (olfactory) G52.0
    - fourth (trochlear) — *see* Strabismus, paralytic, fourth nerve
    - second (optic) H47.20
    - sixth (abducens) — *see* Strabismus, paralytic, sixth nerve
    - tenth (pneumogastric) (vagus) G52.2
    - third (oculomotor) — *see* Strabismus, paralytic, third nerve
    - twelfth (hypoglossal) G52.3
  - hypoglossal G52.3
  - oculomotor — *see* Strabismus, paralytic, third nerve
  - olfactory G52.0
  - optic (papillomacular bundle)
    - syphilitic (late) A52.15
      - congenital A50.44
  - pneumogastric G52.2
  - trigeminal G50.8
  - trochlear — *see* Strabismus, paralytic, fourth nerve
  - vagus (pneumogastric) G52.2
- neurogenic, bone, tabetic A52.11
- nutritional E41
- old age R54
- olivopontocerebellar G23.8
- optic (nerve) H47.20
  - glaucomatous H47.23- ☑

Atrophy, atrophic — *continued*
- optic — *continued*
  - hereditary H47.22
    - primary H47.21- ☑
    - specified type NEC H47.29- ☑
  - syphilitic (late) A52.15
    - congenital A50.44
- orbit H05.31- ☑
- ovary (senile) N83.31- ☑
  - with fallopian tube N83.33- ☑
- oviduct (senile) — *see* Atrophy, fallopian tube
- palsy, diffuse (progressive) G12.22
- pancreas (duct) (senile) K86.89
- parotid gland K11.0
- pelvic muscle N81.84
- penis N48.89
- pharynx J39.2
- pluriglandular E31.8
  - autoimmune E31.0
- polyarthritis M15.9
- prostate N42.89
- pseudohypertrophic (muscle) G71.02
- renal — *see also* Sclerosis, renal N26.1
- retina, retinal (postinfectional) H35.89
- rhinitis J31.0
- salivary gland K11.0
- scar L90.5
- sclerosis, lobar (of brain) G31.09 [F02.80]
  - with behavioral disturbance G31.09 [F02.81]
- scrotum N50.89
- seminal vesicle N50.89
- senile R54
  - due to radiation (nonionizing) (solar) L57.8
- skin (patches) (spots) L90.9
  - degenerative (senile) L90.8
  - due to radiation (nonionizing) (solar) L57.8
  - senile L90.8
- spermatic cord N50.89
- spinal (acute) (cord) G95.89
  - muscular — *see* Atrophy, muscle, spinal
  - paralysis G12.20
    - acute — *see* Poliomyelitis, paralytic
    - meaning progressive muscular atrophy G12.25
- spine (column) — *see* Spondylopathy, specified NEC
- spleen (senile) D73.0
- stomach K29.40
  - with bleeding K29.41
- striate (skin) L90.6
  - syphilitic A52.79
- subcutaneous L90.9
- sublingual gland K11.0
- submandibular gland K11.0
- submaxillary gland K11.0
- Sudeck's — *see* Algoneurodystrophy
- suprarenal (capsule) (gland) E27.49
  - primary E27.1
- systemic affecting central nervous system in
  - myxedema E03.9 [G13.2]
  - neoplastic disease — *see also* Neoplasm D49.9 [G13.1]
  - specified disease NEC G13.8
- tarso-orbital fascia, congenital Q10.3
- testis N50.0
- thenar, partial — *see* Syndrome, carpal tunnel
- thymus (fatty) E32.8
- thyroid (gland) (acquired) E03.4
  - with cretinism E03.1
  - congenital (with myxedema) E03.1
- tongue (senile) K14.8
  - papillae K14.4
- trachea J39.8
- tunica vaginalis N50.89
- turbinate J34.89
- tympanic membrane (nonflaccid) H73.82- ☑
  - flaccid H73.81- ☑
- upper respiratory tract J39.8
- uterus, uterine (senile) N85.8
  - cervix N88.8
  - due to radiation (intended effect) N85.8
    - adverse effect or misadventure N99.89
- vagina (senile) N95.2
- vas deferens N50.89
- vascular I99.8
- vertebra (senile) — *see* Spondylopathy, specified NEC
- vulva (senile) N90.5
- Werdnig-Hoffmann G12.0
- yellow — *see* Failure, hepatic

☑ **Additional Character Required** — Refer to the Tabular List for Character Selection   ▽ **Subterms under main terms may continue to next column or page**

Attack, attacks
- with alteration of consciousness (with automatisms) — *see* Epilepsy, localization-related, symptomatic, with complex partial seizures
- Adams-Stokes I45.9
- akinetic — *see* Epilepsy, generalized, specified NEC
- angina — *see* Angina
- atonic — *see* Epilepsy, generalized, specified NEC
- benign shuddering G25.83
- cataleptic — *see* Catalepsy
- coronary — *see* Infarct, myocardium
- cyanotic, newborn P28.2
- drop NEC R55
- epileptic — *see* Epilepsy
- heart — *see* infarct, myocardium
- hysterical F44.9
- jacksonian — *see* Epilepsy, localization-related, symptomatic, with simple partial seizures
- myocardium, myocardial — *see* Infarct, myocardium
- myoclonic — *see* Epilepsy, generalized, specified NEC
- panic F41.0
- psychomotor — *see* Epilepsy, localization-related, symptomatic, with complex partial seizures
- salaam — *see* Epilepsy, spasms
- schizophreniform, brief F23
- shuddering, benign G25.83
- Stokes-Adams I45.9
- syncope R55
- transient ischemic (TIA) G45.9
  - specified NEC G45.8
- unconsciousness R55
  - hysterical F44.89
- vasomotor R55
- vasovagal (paroxysmal) (idiopathic) R55
- without alteration of consciousness — *see* Epilepsy, localization-related, symptomatic, with simple partial seizures

Attention (to)
- artificial
  - opening (of) Z43.9
    - digestive tract NEC Z43.4
      - colon Z43.3
      - ilium Z43.2
      - stomach Z43.1
    - specified NEC Z43.8
    - trachea Z43.0
    - urinary tract NEC Z43.6
      - cystostomy Z43.5
      - nephrostomy Z43.6
      - ureterostomy Z43.6
      - urethrostomy Z43.6
    - vagina Z43.7
- colostomy Z43.3
- cystostomy Z43.5
- deficit disorder or syndrome F98.8
  - with hyperactivity — *see* Disorder, attention-deficit hyperactivity
- gastrostomy Z43.1
- ileostomy Z43.2
- jejunostomy Z43.4
- nephrostomy Z43.6
- surgical dressings Z48.01
- sutures Z48.02
- tracheostomy Z43.0
- ureterostomy Z43.6
- urethrostomy Z43.6

Attrition
- gum — *see* Recession, gingival
- tooth, teeth (excessive) (hard tissues) K03.0

Atypical, atypism — *see also* condition
- cells (on cytolgocial smear) (endocervical) (endometrial) (glandular)
  - cervix R87.619
  - vagina R87.629
- cervical N87.9
- endometrium N85.9
  - hyperplasia N85.00
- parenting situation Z62.9

Auditory — *see* condition

Aujeszky's disease B33.8

Aurantiasis, cutis E67.1

Auricle, auricular — *see also* condition
- cervical Q18.2

Auriculotemporal syndrome G50.8

Austin Flint murmur (aortic insufficiency) I35.1

Australian
- Q fever A78
- X disease A83.4

Autism, autistic (childhood) (infantile) F84.0
- atypical F84.9
- spectrum disorder F84.0

Autodigestion R68.89

Autoerythrocyte sensitization (syndrome) D69.2

Autographism L50.3

Autoimmune
- disease (systemic) M35.9
- inhibitors to clotting factors D68.311
- lymphoproliferative syndrome [ALPS] D89.82
- thyroiditis E06.3

Autointoxication R68.89

Automatism G93.89
- with temporal sclerosis G93.81
- epileptic — *see* Epilepsy, localization-related, symptomatic, with complex partial seizures
- paroxysmal, idiopathic — *see* Epilepsy, localization-related, symptomatic, with complex partial seizures

Autonomic, autonomous
- bladder (neurogenic) N31.2
- hysteria seizure F44.5

Autosensitivity, erythrocyte D69.2

Autosensitization, cutaneous L30.2

Autosome — *see* condition by chromosome involved

Autotopagnosia R48.1

Autotoxemia R68.89

Autumn — *see* condition

Avellis' syndrome G46.8

Aversion
- oral R63.3
  - newborn P92.- ☑
  - nonorganic origin F98.2 ☑
- sexual F52.1

Aviator's
- disease or sickness — *see* Effect, adverse, high altitude
- ear T70.0 ☑

Avitaminosis (multiple) — *see also* Deficiency, vitamin E56.9
- B E53.9
  - with
    - beriberi E51.11
    - pellagra E52
- B2 E53.0
- B6 E53.1
- B12 E53.8
- D E55.9
  - with rickets E55.0
- G E53.0
- K E56.1
- nicotinic acid E52

AVNRT (atrioventricular nodal re-entrant tachycardia) I47.1

AVRT (atrioventricular nodal re-entrant tachycardia) I47.1

Avulsion (traumatic)
- blood vessel — *see* Injury, blood vessel
- bone — *see* Fracture, by site
- cartilage — *see also* Dislocation, by site
  - symphyseal (inner), complicating delivery O71.6
- external site other than limb — *see* Wound, open, by site
- eye S05.7- ☑
- head (intracranial)
  - external site NEC S08.89 ☑
  - scalp S08.0 ☑
- internal organ or site — *see* Injury, by site
- joint — *see also* Dislocation, by site
  - capsule — *see* Sprain, by site
- kidney S37.06- ☑
- ligament — *see* Sprain, by site
- limb — *see also* Amputation, traumatic, by site
  - skin and subcutaneous tissue — *see* Wound, open, by site
- muscle — *see* Injury, muscle
- nerve (root) — *see* Injury, nerve
- scalp S08.0 ☑
- skin and subcutaneous tissue — *see* Wound, open, by site
- spleen S36.032 ☑
- symphyseal cartilage (inner), complicating delivery O71.6
- tendon — *see* Injury, muscle
- tooth S03.2 ☑

Awareness of heart beat R00.2

Axenfeld's
- anomaly or syndrome Q15.0
- degeneration (calcareous) Q13.4

Axilla, axillary — *see also* condition
- breast Q83.1

Axonotmesis — *see* Injury, nerve

Ayerza's disease or syndrome (pulmonary artery sclerosis with pulmonary hypertension) I27.0

Azoospermia (organic) N46.01
- due to
  - drug therapy N46.021
  - efferent duct obstruction N46.023
  - infection N46.022
  - radiation N46.024
  - specified cause NEC N46.029
  - systemic disease N46.025

Azotemia R79.89
- meaning uremia N19

Aztec ear Q17.3

Azygos
- continuation inferior vena cava Q26.8
- lobe (lung) Q33.1

B

Baastrup's disease — *see* Kissing spine

Babesiosis B60.0

Babington's disease (familial hemorrhagic telangiectasia) I78.0

Babinski's syndrome A52.79

Baby
- crying constantly R68.11
- floppy (syndrome) P94.2

Bacillary — *see* condition

Bacilluria R82.71

Bacillus — *see also* Infection, bacillus
- abortus infection A23.1
- anthracis infection A22.9
- coli infection — *see also* Escherichia coli B96.20
- Flexner's A03.1
- mallei infection A24.0
- Shiga's A03.0
- suipestifer infection — *see* Infection, salmonella

Back — *see* condition

Backache (postural) M54.9
- sacroiliac M53.3
- specified NEC M54.89

Backflow — *see* Reflux

Backward reading (dyslexia) F81.0

Bacteremia R78.81
- with sepsis — *see* Sepsis

Bactericholia — *see* Cholecystitis, acute

Bacterid, bacteride (pustular) L40.3

Bacterium, bacteria, bacterial
- agent NEC, as cause of disease classified elsewhere B96.89
- in blood — *see* Bacteremia
- in urine — *see* Bacteriuria

Bacteriuria, bacteruria R82.71
- asymptomatic R82.71

Bacteroides
- fragilis, as cause of disease classified elsewhere B96.6

Bad
- heart — *see* Disease, heart
- trip
  - due to drug abuse — *see* Abuse, drug, hallucinogen
  - due to drug dependence — *see* Dependence, drug, hallucinogen

Baelz's disease (cheilitis glandularis apostematosa) K13.0

Baerensprung's disease (eczema marginatum) B35.6

Bagasse disease or pneumonitis J67.1

Bagassosis J67.1

Baker's cyst — *see* Cyst, Baker's

Bakwin-Krida syndrome (metaphyseal dysplasia) Q78.5

Balancing side interference M26.56

Balanitis (circinata) (erosiva) (gangrenosa) (phagedenic) (vulgaris) N48.1
- amebic A06.82
- candidal B37.42
- due to Haemophilus ducreyi A57
- gonococcal (acute) (chronic) A54.23
- xerotica obliterans N48.0

Balanoposthitis N47.6
- gonococcal (acute) (chronic) A54.23
- ulcerative (specific) A63.8

Balanorrhagia — *see* Balanitis

Balantidiasis, balantidiosis A07.0

Bald tongue K14.4

Baldness — *see also* Alopecia
- male-pattern — *see* Alopecia, androgenic

Balkan grippe A78
Balloon disease — see Effect, adverse, high altitude
Balo's disease (concentric sclerosis) G37.5
Bamberger-Marie disease — see Osteoarthropathy, hypertrophic, specified type NEC
Bancroft's filariasis B74.0
Band(s)
  adhesive — see Adhesions, peritoneum
  anomalous or congenital — see also Anomaly, by site
    heart (atrial) (ventricular) Q24.8
      intestine Q43.3
      omentum Q43.3
  cervix N88.1
  constricting, congenital Q79.8
  gallbladder (congenital) Q44.1
  intestinal (adhesive) — see Adhesions, peritoneum
  obstructive
    intestine K56.50
      complete K56.52
      incomplete K56.51
      partial K56.51
    peritoneum K56.50
      complete K56.52
      incomplete K56.51
      partial K56.51
  periappendiceal, congenital Q43.3
  peritoneal (adhesive) — see Adhesions, peritoneum
  uterus N73.6
    internal N85.6
    vagina N89.5
Bandemia D72.825
Bandl's ring (contraction), complicating delivery O62.4
Bangkok hemorrhagic fever A91
Bang's disease (brucella abortus) A23.1
Bankruptcy, anxiety concerning Z59.8
Bannister's disease T78.3 ☑
  hereditary D84.1
Banti's disease or syndrome (with cirrhosis) (with portal hypertension) K76.6
Bar, median, prostate — see Enlargement, enlarged, prostate
Barcoo disease or rot — see Ulcer, skin
Barlow's disease E54
Barodontalgia T70.29 ☑
Baron Münchausen syndrome — see Disorder, factitious
Barosinusitis T70.1 ☑
Barotitis T70.0 ☑
Barotrauma T70.29 ☑
  odontalgia T70.29 ☑
  otitic T70.0 ☑
  sinus T70.1 ☑
Barraquer (-Simons) **disease or syndrome** (progressive lipodystrophy) E88.1
Barré-Guillain disease or syndrome G61.0
Barrel chest M95.4
Barré-Liéou syndrome (posterior cervical sympathetic) M53.0
Barrett's
  disease — see Barrett's, esophagus
  esophagus K22.70
    with dysplasia K22.719
      high grade K22.711
      low grade K22.710
    without dysplasia K22.70
  syndrome — see Barrett's, esophagus
  ulcer K22.10
    with bleeding K22.11
    without bleeding K22.10
Bársony (-Polgár) (-Teschendorf) **syndrome** (corkscrew esophagus) K22.4
Barth syndrome E78.71
Bartholinitis (suppurating) N75.8
  gonococcal (acute) (chronic) (with abscess) A54.1
Bartonellosis A44.9
  cutaneous A44.1
  mucocutaneous A44.1
  specified NEC A44.8
  systemic A44.0
Barton's fracture S52.56- ☑
Bartter's syndrome E26.81
Basal — see condition
Basan's (hidrotic) ectodermal dysplasia Q82.4
Baseball finger — see Dislocation, finger
Basedow's disease (exophthalmic goiter) — see Hyperthyroidism, with, goiter
Basic — see condition

Basilar — see condition
Bason's (hidrotic) ectodermal dysplasia Q82.4
Basopenia — see Agranulocytosis
Basophilia D72.824
Basophilism (cortico-adrenal) (Cushing's) (pituitary) E24.0
Bassen-Kornzweig disease or syndrome E78.6
Bat ear Q17.5
Bateman's
  disease B08.1
  purpura (senile) D69.2
Bathing cramp T75.1 ☑
Bathophobia F40.248
Batten (-Mayou) **disease** E75.4
  retina E75.4 [H36]
Batten-Steinert syndrome G71.11
Battered — see Maltreatment
Battey Mycobacterium infection A31.0
Battle exhaustion F43.0
Battledore placenta O43.19- ☑
Baumgarten-Cruveilhier cirrhosis, disease or syndrome K74.69
Bauxite fibrosis (of lung) J63.1
Bayle's disease (general paresis) A52.17
Bazin's disease (primary) (tuberculous) A18.4
Beach ear — see Swimmer's, ear
Beaded hair (congenital) Q84.1
Béal conjunctivitis or syndrome B30.2
Beard's disease (neurasthenia) F48.8
Beat(s)
  atrial, premature I49.1
  ectopic I49.49
  elbow — see Bursitis, elbow
  escaped, heart I49.49
  hand — see Bursitis, hand
  knee — see Bursitis, knee
  premature I49.40
    atrial I49.1
    auricular I49.1
    supraventricular I49.1
Beau's
  disease or syndrome — see Degeneration, myocardial
  lines (transverse furrows on fingernails) L60.4
Bechterev's syndrome — see Spondylitis, ankylosing
Becker's
  cardiomyopathy I42.8
  disease
    idiopathic mural endomyocardial disease I42.3
    myotonia congenita, recessive form G71.12
  dystrophy G71.01
  pigmented hairy nevus D22.5
Beck's syndrome (anterior spinal artery occlusion) I65.8
Beckwith-Wiedemann syndrome Q87.3
Bed confinement status Z74.01
Bed sore — see Ulcer, pressure, by site
Bedbug bite(s) — see Bite(s), by site, superficial, insect
Bedclothes, asphyxiation or suffocation by — see Asphyxia, traumatic, due to, mechanical, trapped
Bednar's
  aphthae K12.0
  tumor — see Neoplasm, malignant, by site
Bedridden Z74.01
Bedsore — see Ulcer, pressure, by site
Bedwetting — see Enuresis
Bee sting (with allergic or anaphylactic shock) — see Toxicity, venom, arthropod, bee
Beer drinker's heart (disease) I42.6
Begbie's disease (exophthalmic goiter) — see Hyperthyroidism, with, goiter
Behavior
  antisocial
    adult Z72.811
    child or adolescent Z72.810
  disorder, disturbance — see Disorder, conduct
  disruptive — see Disorder, conduct
  drug seeking Z76.5
  inexplicable R46.2
  marked evasiveness R46.5
  obsessive-compulsive R46.81
  overactivity R46.3
  poor responsiveness R46.4
  self-damaging (life-style) Z72.89
  sleep-incompatible Z72.821
  slowness R46.4
  specified NEC R46.89
  strange (and inexplicable) R46.2
  suspiciousness R46.5
  type A pattern Z73.1

Behavior — continued
  undue concern or preoccupation with stressful events R46.6
  verbosity and circumstantial detail obscuring reason for contact R46.7
Behçet's disease or syndrome M35.2
Behr's disease — see Degeneration, macula
Beigel's disease or morbus (white piedra) B36.2
Bejel A65
Bekhterev's syndrome — see Spondylitis, ankylosing
Belching — see Eructation
Bell's
  mania F30.8
  palsy, paralysis G51.0
    infant or newborn P11.3
  spasm G51.3- ☑
Bence Jones albuminuria or proteinuria NEC R80.3
Bends T70.3 ☑
Benedikt's paralysis or syndrome G46.3
Benign — see also condition
  prostatic hyperplasia — see Hyperplasia, prostate
Bennett's fracture (displaced) S62.21- ☑
Benson's disease — see Deposit, crystalline
Bent
  back (hysterical) F44.4
  nose M95.0
    congenital Q67.4
Bereavement (uncomplicated) Z63.4
Bergeron's disease (hysterical chorea) F44.4
Berger's disease — see Nephropathy, IgA
Beriberi (dry) E51.11
  heart (disease) E51.12
  polyneuropathy E51.11
  wet E51.12
    involving circulatory system E51.11
Berlin's disease or edema (traumatic) S05.8X- ☑
Berlock (berloque) **dermatitis** L56.2
Bernard-Horner syndrome G90.2
Bernard-Soulier disease or thrombopathia D69.1
Bernhardt (-Roth) **disease** — see Mononeuropathy, lower limb, meralgia paresthetica
Bernheim's syndrome — see Failure, heart, right
Bertielliasis B71.8
Berylliosis (lung) J63.2
Besnier-Boeck (-Schaumann) **disease** — see Sarcoidosis
Besnier's
  lupus pernio D86.3
  prurigo L20.0
Bestiality F65.89
Best's disease H35.50
Betalipoproteinemia, broad or floating E78.2
Beta-mercaptolactate-cysteine disulfiduria E72.09
Betting and gambling Z72.6
  pathological (compulsive) F63.0
Bezoar T18.9 ☑
  intestine T18.3 ☑
  stomach T18.2 ☑
Bezold's abscess — see Mastoiditis, acute
Bianchi's syndrome R48.8
Bicornate or bicornis uterus Q51.3
  in pregnancy or childbirth O34.00
    causing obstructed labor O65.5
Bicuspid aortic valve Q23.1
Biedl-Bardet syndrome Q87.89
Bielschowsky (-Jansky) **disease** E75.4
Biermer's (pernicious) anemia or disease D51.0
Biett's disease L93.0
Bifid (congenital)
  apex, heart Q24.8
  clitoris Q52.6
  kidney Q63.8
  nose Q30.2
  patella Q74.1
  scrotum Q55.29
  toe NEC Q74.2
  tongue Q38.3
  ureter Q62.8
  uterus Q51.3
  uvula Q35.7
Biforis uterus (suprasimplex) Q51.3
Bifurcation (congenital)
  gallbladder Q44.1
  kidney pelvis Q63.8
  renal pelvis Q63.8
  rib Q76.6
  tongue, congenital Q38.3
  trachea Q32.1

☑ **Additional Character Required** — Refer to the Tabular List for Character Selection
☷ **Subterms under main terms may continue to next column or page**

Bifurcation — *continued*
  ureter Q62.8
  urethra Q64.74
  vertebra Q76.49
Big spleen syndrome D73.1
Bigeminal pulse R00.8
Bilateral — *see* condition
Bile
  duct — *see* condition
  pigments in urine R82.2
Bilharziasis — *see also* Schistosomiasis
  chyluria B65.0
  cutaneous B65.3
  galacturia B65.0
  hematochyluria B65.0
  intestinal B65.1
  lipemia B65.9
  lipuria B65.0
  oriental B65.2
  piarhemia B65.9
  pulmonary NOS B65.9 *[J99]*
    pneumonia B65.9 *[J17]*
  tropical hematuria B65.0
  vesical B65.0
Biliary — *see* condition
Bilirubin metabolism disorder E80.7
  specified NEC E80.6
Bilirubinemia, familial nonhemolytic E80.4
Bilirubinuria R82.2
Biliuria R82.2
Bilocular stomach K31.2
Binswanger's disease I67.3
Biparta, bipartite
  carpal scaphoid Q74.0
  patella Q74.1
  vagina Q52.10
Bird
  face Q75.8
  fancier's disease or lung J67.2
Birth
  complications in mother — *see* Delivery, complicated
  compression during NOS P15.9
  defect — *see* Anomaly
  immature (less than 37 completed weeks) — *see* Preterm, newborn
    extremely (less than 28 completed weeks) — *see* Immaturity, extreme
  inattention, at or after — *see* Maltreatment, child, neglect
  injury NOS P15.9
    basal ganglia P11.1
    brachial plexus NEC P14.3
    brain (compression) (pressure) P11.2
    central nervous system NOS P11.9
    cerebellum P11.1
    cerebral hemorrhage P10.1
    external genitalia P15.5
    eye P15.3
    face P15.4
    fracture
      bone P13.9
        specified NEC P13.8
      clavicle P13.4
      femur P13.2
      humerus P13.3
      long bone, except femur P13.3
      radius and ulna P13.3
      skull P13.0
      spine P11.5
      tibia and fibula P13.3
    intracranial P11.2
      laceration or hemorrhage P10.9
        specified NEC P10.8
    intraventricular hemorrhage P10.2
    laceration
      brain P10.1
      by scalpel P15.8
      peripheral nerve P14.9
    liver P15.0
    meninges
      brain P11.1
      spinal cord P11.5
    nerve
      brachial plexus P14.3
      cranial NEC (except facial) P11.4
      facial P11.3
      peripheral P14.9
      phrenic (paralysis) P14.2

Birth — *continued*
  injury — *continued*
    paralysis
      facial nerve P11.3
      spinal P11.5
    penis P15.5
    rupture
      spinal cord P11.5
    scalp P12.9
    scalpel wound P15.8
    scrotum P15.5
    skull NEC P13.1
      fracture P13.0
    specified type NEC P15.8
    spinal cord P11.5
    spine P11.5
    spleen P15.1
    sternomastoid (hematoma) P15.2
    subarachnoid hemorrhage P10.3
    subcutaneous fat necrosis P15.6
    subdural hemorrhage P10.0
    tentorial tear P10.4
    testes P15.5
    vulva P15.5
  lack of care, at or after — *see* Maltreatment, child, neglect
  neglect, at or after — *see* Maltreatment, child, neglect
  palsy or paralysis, newborn, NOS (birth injury) P14.9
  premature (infant) — *see* Preterm, newborn
  shock, newborn P96.89
  trauma — *see* Birth, injury
  weight
    low (2499 grams or less) — *see* Low, birthweight
      extremely (999 grams or less) — *see* Low, birthweight, extreme
    4000 grams to 4499 grams P08.1
    4500 grams or more P08.0
Birthmark Q82.5
Birt-Hogg-Dube syndrome Q87.89
Bisalbuminemia E88.09
Biskra's button B55.1
Bite(s) (animal) (human)
  abdomen, abdominal
    wall S31.159 ☑
      with penetration into peritoneal cavity S31.659 ☑
      epigastric region S31.152 ☑
        with penetration into peritoneal cavity S31.652 ☑
      left
        lower quadrant S31.154 ☑
          with penetration into peritoneal cavity S31.654 ☑
        upper quadrant S31.151 ☑
          with penetration into peritoneal cavity S31.651 ☑
      periumbilic region S31.155 ☑
        with penetration into peritoneal cavity S31.655 ☑
      right
        lower quadrant S31.153 ☑
          with penetration into peritoneal cavity S31.653 ☑
        upper quadrant S31.150 ☑
          with penetration into peritoneal cavity S31.650 ☑
      superficial NEC S30.871 ☑
        insect S30.861 ☑
  alveolar (process) — *see* Bite, oral cavity
  amphibian (venomous) — *see* Venom, bite, amphibian
  animal — *see also* Bite, by site
    venomous — *see* Venom
  ankle S91.05- ☑
    superficial NEC S90.57- ☑
      insect S90.56- ☑
  antecubital space — *see* Bite, elbow
  anus S31.835 ☑
    superficial NEC S30.877 ☑
      insect S30.867 ☑
  arm (upper) S41.15- ☑
    lower — *see* Bite, forearm
    superficial NEC S40.87- ☑
      insect S40.86- ☑
  arthropod NEC — *see* Venom, bite, arthropod
  auditory canal (external) (meatus) — *see* Bite, ear
  auricle, ear — *see* Bite, ear
  axilla — *see* Bite, arm

Bite(s) — *continued*
  back — *see also* Bite, thorax, back
    lower S31.050 ☑
      with penetration into retroperitoneal space S31.051 ☑
    superficial NEC S30.870 ☑
      insect S30.860 ☑
  bedbug — *see* Bite(s), by site, superficial, insect
  breast S21.05- ☑
    superficial NEC S20.17- ☑
      insect S20.16- ☑
  brow — *see* Bite, head, specified site NEC
  buttock S31.805 ☑
    left S31.825 ☑
    right S31.815 ☑
    superficial NEC S30.870 ☑
      insect S30.860 ☑
  calf — *see* Bite, leg
  canaliculus lacrimalis — *see* Bite, eyelid
  canthus, eye — *see* Bite, eyelid
  centipede — *see* Toxicity, venom, arthropod, centipede
  cheek (external) S01.45- ☑
    internal — *see* Bite, oral cavity
    superficial NEC S00.87 ☑
      insect S00.86 ☑
  chest wall — *see* Bite, thorax
  chigger B88.0
  chin — *see* Bite, head, specified site NEC
  clitoris — *see* Bite, vulva
  costal region — *see* Bite, thorax
  digit(s)
    hand — *see* Bite, finger
    toe — *see* Bite, toe
  ear (canal) (external) S01.35- ☑
    superficial NEC S00.47- ☑
      insect S00.46- ☑
  elbow S51.05- ☑
    superficial NEC S50.37- ☑
      insect S50.36- ☑
  epididymis — *see* Bite, testis
  epigastric region — *see* Bite, abdomen
  epiglottis — *see* Bite, neck, specified site NEC
  esophagus, cervical S11.25 ☑
    superficial NEC S10.17 ☑
      insect S10.16 ☑
  eyebrow — *see* Bite, eyelid
  eyelid S01.15- ☑
    superficial NEC S00.27- ☑
      insect S00.26- ☑
  face NEC — *see* Bite, head, specified site NEC
  finger(s) S61.259 ☑
    with
      damage to nail S61.359 ☑
    index S61.258 ☑
      with
        damage to nail S61.358 ☑
      left S61.251 ☑
        with
          damage to nail S61.351 ☑
      right S61.250 ☑
        with
          damage to nail S61.350 ☑
      superficial NEC S60.478 ☑
        insect S60.46- ☑
    little S61.25- ☑
      with
        damage to nail S61.35- ☑
      superficial NEC S60.47- ☑
        insect S60.46- ☑
    middle S61.25- ☑
      with
        damage to nail S61.35- ☑
      superficial NEC S60.47- ☑
        insect S60.46- ☑
    ring S61.25- ☑
      with
        damage to nail S61.35- ☑
      superficial NEC S60.47- ☑
        insect S60.46- ☑
    superficial NEC S60.479 ☑
      insect S60.469 ☑
    thumb — *see* Bite, thumb
  flank — *see* Bite, abdomen, wall
  flea — *see* Bite, by site, superficial, insect
  foot (except toe(s) alone) S91.35- ☑
    superficial NEC S90.87- ☑

⬆ Subterms under main terms may continue to next column or page   ☑ Additional Character Required — Refer to the Tabular List for Character Selection   **37**

Bifurcation — Bite

Bite(s) — *continued*
   foot(s alone) — *continued*
      superficial — *continued*
         insect S90.86- ☑
      toe — *see* Bite, toe
   forearm S51.85- ☑
      elbow only — *see* Bite, elbow
      superficial NEC S50.87- ☑
         insect S50.86- ☑
   forehead — *see* Bite, head, specified site NEC
   genital organs, external
      female S31.552 ☑
         superficial NEC S30.876 ☑
            insect S30.866 ☑
         vagina and vulva — *see* Bite, vulva
      male S31.551 ☑
         penis — *see* Bite, penis
         scrotum — *see* Bite, scrotum
         superficial NEC S30.875 ☑
            insect S30.865 ☑
         testes — *see* Bite, testis
   groin — *see* Bite, abdomen, wall
   gum — *see* Bite, oral cavity
   hand S61.45- ☑
      finger — *see* Bite, finger
      superficial NEC S60.57- ☑
         insect S60.56- ☑
      thumb — *see* Bite, thumb
   head S01.95 ☑
      cheek — *see* Bite, cheek
      ear — *see* Bite, ear
      eyelid — *see* Bite, eyelid
      lip — *see* Bite, lip
      nose — *see* Bite, nose
      oral cavity — *see* Bite, oral cavity
      scalp — *see* Bite, scalp
      specified site NEC S01.85 ☑
         superficial NEC S00.87 ☑
            insect S00.86 ☑
         superficial NEC S00.97 ☑
            insect S00.96 ☑
      temporomandibular area — *see* Bite, cheek
   heel — *see* Bite, foot
   hip S71.05- ☑
      superficial NEC S70.27- ☑
         insect S70.26- ☑
   hymen S31.45 ☑
   hypochondrium — *see* Bite, abdomen, wall
   hypogastric region — *see* Bite, abdomen, wall
   inguinal region — *see* Bite, abdomen, wall
   insect — *see* Bite, by site, superficial, insect
   instep — *see* Bite, foot
   interscapular region — *see* Bite, thorax, back
   jaw — *see* Bite, head, specified site NEC
   knee S81.05- ☑
      superficial NEC S80.27- ☑
         insect S80.26- ☑
   labium (majus) (minus) — *see* Bite, vulva
   lacrimal duct — *see* Bite, eyelid
   larynx S11.015 ☑
      superficial NEC S10.17 ☑
         insect S10.16 ☑
   leg (lower) S81.85- ☑
      ankle — *see* Bite, ankle
      foot — *see* Bite, foot
      knee — *see* Bite, knee
      superficial NEC S80.87- ☑
         insect S80.86- ☑
      toe — *see* Bite, toe
      upper — *see* Bite, thigh
   lip S01.551 ☑
      superficial NEC S00.571 ☑
         insect S00.561 ☑
   lizard (venomous) — *see* Venom, bite, reptile
   loin — *see* Bite, abdomen, wall
   lower back — *see* Bite, back, lower
   lumbar region — *see* Bite, back, lower
   malar region — *see* Bite, head, specified site NEC
   mammary — *see* Bite, breast
   marine animals (venomous) — *see* Toxicity, venom, marine animal
   mastoid region — *see* Bite, head, specified site NEC
   mouth — *see* Bite, oral cavity
   nail
      finger — *see* Bite, finger
      toe — *see* Bite, toe

Bite(s) — *continued*
   nape — *see* Bite, neck, specified site NEC
   nasal (septum) (sinus) — *see* Bite, nose
   nasopharynx — *see* Bite, head, specified site NEC
   neck S11.95 ☑
      involving
         cervical esophagus — *see* Bite, esophagus, cervical
         larynx — *see* Bite, larynx
         pharynx — *see* Bite, pharynx
         thyroid gland S11.15 ☑
         trachea — *see* Bite, trachea
      specified site NEC S11.85 ☑
         superficial NEC S10.87 ☑
            insect S10.86 ☑
      superficial NEC S10.97 ☑
         insect S10.96 ☑
      throat S11.85 ☑
         superficial NEC S10.17 ☑
            insect S10.16 ☑
   nose (septum) (sinus) S01.25 ☑
      superficial NEC S00.37 ☑
         insect S00.36 ☑
   occipital region — *see* Bite, scalp
   oral cavity S01.552 ☑
      superficial NEC S00.572 ☑
         insect S00.562 ☑
   orbital region — *see* Bite, eyelid
   palate — *see* Bite, oral cavity
   palm — *see* Bite, hand
   parietal region — *see* Bite, scalp
   pelvis S31.050 ☑
      with penetration into retroperitoneal space S31.051 ☑
      superficial NEC S30.870 ☑
         insect S30.860 ☑
   penis S31.25 ☑
      superficial NEC S30.872 ☑
         insect S30.862 ☑
   perineum
      female — *see* Bite, vulva
      male — *see* Bite, pelvis
   periocular area (with or without lacrimal passages) — *see* Bite, eyelid
   phalanges
      finger — *see* Bite, finger
      toe — *see* Bite, toe
   pharynx S11.25 ☑
      superficial NEC S10.17 ☑
         insect S10.16 ☑
   pinna — *see* Bite, ear
   poisonous — *see* Venom
   popliteal space — *see* Bite, knee
   prepuce — *see* Bite, penis
   pubic region — *see* Bite, abdomen, wall
   rectovaginal septum — *see* Bite, vulva
   red bug B88.0
   reptile NEC — *see also* Venom, bite, reptile
      nonvenomous — *see* Bite, by site
      snake — *see* Venom, bite, snake
   sacral region — *see* Bite, back, lower
   sacroiliac region — *see* Bite, back, lower
   salivary gland — *see* Bite, oral cavity
   scalp S01.05 ☑
      superficial NEC S00.07 ☑
         insect S00.06 ☑
   scapular region — *see* Bite, shoulder
   scrotum S31.35 ☑
      superficial NEC S30.873 ☑
         insect S30.863 ☑
   sea-snake (venomous) — *see* Toxicity, venom, snake, sea snake
   shin — *see* Bite, leg
   shoulder S41.05- ☑
      superficial NEC S40.27- ☑
         insect S40.26- ☑
   snake — *see also* Venom, bite, snake
      nonvenomous — *see* Bite, by site
   spermatic cord — *see* Bite, testis
   spider (venomous) — *see* Toxicity, venom, spider
      nonvenomous — *see* Bite, by site, superficial, insect
   sternal region — *see* Bite, thorax, front
   submaxillary region — *see* Bite, head, specified site NEC
   submental region — *see* Bite, head, specified site NEC

Bite(s) — *continued*
   subungual
      finger(s) — *see* Bite, finger
      toe — *see* Bite, toe
   superficial — *see* Bite, by site, superficial
   supraclavicular fossa S11.85 ☑
   supraorbital — *see* Bite, head, specified site NEC
   temple, temporal region — *see* Bite, head, specified site NEC
   temporomandibular area — *see* Bite, cheek
   testis S31.35 ☑
      superficial NEC S30.873 ☑
         insect S30.863 ☑
   thigh S71.15- ☑
      superficial NEC S70.37- ☑
         insect S70.36- ☑
   thorax, thoracic (wall) S21.95 ☑
      back S21.25- ☑
         with penetration into thoracic cavity S21.45- ☑
      breast — *see* Bite, breast
      front S21.15- ☑
         with penetration into thoracic cavity S21.35- ☑
      superficial NEC S20.97 ☑
         back S20.47- ☑
         front S20.37- ☑
         insect S20.96 ☑
            back S20.46- ☑
            front S20.36- ☑
   throat — *see* Bite, neck, throat
   thumb S61.05- ☑
      with
         damage to nail S61.15- ☑
      superficial NEC S60.37- ☑
         insect S60.36- ☑
   thyroid S11.15 ☑
      superficial NEC S10.87 ☑
         insect S10.86 ☑
   toe(s) S91.15- ☑
      with
         damage to nail S91.25- ☑
      great S91.15- ☑
         with
            damage to nail S91.25- ☑
      lesser S91.15- ☑
         with
            damage to nail S91.25- ☑
      superficial NEC S90.47- ☑
         great S90.47- ☑
         insect S90.46- ☑
            great S90.46- ☑
   tongue S01.552 ☑
   trachea S11.025 ☑
      superficial NEC S10.17 ☑
         insect S10.16 ☑
   tunica vaginalis — *see* Bite, testis
   tympanum, tympanic membrane — *see* Bite, ear
   umbilical region S31.155 ☑
   uvula — *see* Bite, oral cavity
   vagina — *see* Bite, vulva
   venomous — *see* Venom
   vocal cords S11.035 ☑
      superficial NEC S10.17 ☑
         insect S10.16 ☑
   vulva S31.45 ☑
      superficial NEC S30.874 ☑
         insect S30.864 ☑
   wrist S61.55- ☑
      superficial NEC S60.87- ☑
         insect S60.86- ☑
Biting, cheek or lip K13.1
Biventricular failure (heart) I50.82
Björck (-Thorson) **syndrome** (malignant carcinoid) E34.0
Black
   death A20.9
   eye S00.1- ☑
   hairy tongue K14.3
   heel (foot) S90.3- ☑
   lung (disease) J60
   palm (hand) S60.22- ☑
Blackfan-Diamond anemia or syndrome (congenital hypoplastic anemia) D61.01
Blackhead L70.0
Blackout R55
Bladder — *see* condition
Blast (air) (hydraulic) (immersion) (underwater)
   blindness S05.8X- ☑

Blast — *continued*
  injury
    abdomen or thorax — *see* Injury, by site
    ear (acoustic nerve trauma) — *see* Injury, nerve,
      acoustic, specified type NEC
    syndrome NEC T70.8 ☑
Blastoma — *see* Neoplasm, malignant, by site
  pulmonary — *see* Neoplasm, lung, malignant
Blastomycosis, blastomycotic B40.9
  Brazilian — *see* Paracoccidioidomycosis
  cutaneous B40.3
  disseminated B40.7
  European — *see* Cryptococcosis
  generalized B40.7
  keloidal B48.0
  North American B40.9
  primary pulmonary B40.0
  pulmonary B40.2
    acute B40.0
    chronic B40.1
  skin B40.3
  South American — *see* Paracoccidioidomycosis
  specified NEC B40.89
Bleb(s) R23.8
  emphysematous (lung) (solitary) J43.9
  endophthalmitis H59.43
  filtering (vitreous), after glaucoma surgery Z98.83
  inflamed (infected), postprocedural H59.40
    stage 1 H59.41
    stage 2 H59.42
    stage 3 H59.43
  lung (ruptured) J43.9
    congenital — *see* Atelectasis
    newborn P25.8
  subpleural (emphysematous) J43.9
Blebitis, postprocedural H59.40
  stage 1 H59.41
  stage 2 H59.42
  stage 3 H59.43
Bleeder (familial) (hereditary) — *see* Hemophilia
Bleeding — *see also* Hemorrhage
  anal K62.5
  anovulatory N97.0
  atonic, following delivery O72.1
  capillary I78.8
    puerperal O72.2
  contact (postcoital) N93.0
  due to uterine subinvolution N85.3
  ear — *see* Otorrhagia
  excessive, associated with menopausal onset N92.4
  familial — *see* Defect, coagulation
  following intercourse N93.0
  gastrointestinal K92.2
  hemorrhoids — *see* Hemorrhoids
  intermenstrual (regular) N92.3
    irregular N92.1
  intraoperative — *see* Complication, intraoperative,
    hemorrhage
  irregular N92.6
  menopausal N92.4
  newborn, intraventricular — *see* Newborn, affected
    by, hemorrhage, intraventricular
  nipple N64.59
  nose R04.0
  ovulation N92.3
  perimenopausal N92.4
  postclimacteric N95.0
  postcoital N93.0
  postmenopausal N95.0
  postoperative — *see* Complication, postprocedural,
    hemorrhage
  preclimacteric N92.4
  pre-pubertal vaginal N93.1
  puberty (excessive, with onset of menstrual periods)
    N92.2
  rectum, rectal K62.5
    newborn P54.2
  tendencies — *see* Defect, coagulation
  throat R04.1
  tooth socket (post-extraction) K91.840
  umbilical stump P51.9
  uterus, uterine NEC N93.9
    climacteric N92.4
    dysfunctional or functional N93.8
    menopausal N92.4
    preclimacteric or premenopausal N92.4
    unrelated to menstrual cycle N93.9
  vagina, vaginal (abnormal) N93.9

Bleeding — *continued*
  vagina, vaginal — *continued*
    dysfunctional or functional N93.8
    newborn P54.6
    pre-pubertal N93.1
  vicarious N94.89
Blennorrhagia, blennorrhagic — *see* Gonorrhea
Blennorrhea (acute) (chronic) — *see also* Gonorrhea
  inclusion (neonatal) (newborn) P39.1
  lower genitourinary tract (gonococcal) A54.00
  neonatorum (gonococcal ophthalmia) A54.31
Blepharelosis — *see* Entropion
Blepharitis (angularis) (ciliaris) (eyelid) (marginal)
  (nonulcerative) H01.009
  herpes zoster B02.39
  left H01.006
    lower H01.005
    upper H01.004
    upper and lower H01.00B
  right H01.003
    lower H01.002
    upper H01.001
    upper and lower H01.00A
  squamous H01.029
    left H01.026
      lower H01.025
      upper H01.024
      upper and lower H01.02B
    right H01.023
      lower H01.022
      upper H01.021
      upper and lower H01.02A
  ulcerative H01.019
    left H01.016
      lower H01.015
      upper H01.014
      upper and lower H01.01B
    right H01.013
      lower H01.012
      upper H01.011
      upper and lower H01.01A
Blepharochalasis H02.30
  congenital Q10.0
  left H02.36
    lower H02.35
    upper H02.34
  right H02.33
    lower H02.32
    upper H02.31
Blepharoclonus H02.59
Blepharoconjunctivitis H10.50- ☑
  angular H10.52- ☑
  contact H10.53- ☑
  ligneous H10.51- ☑
Blepharophimosis (eyelid) H02.529
  congenital Q10.3
  left H02.526
    lower H02.525
    upper H02.524
  right H02.523
    lower H02.522
    upper H02.521
Blepharoptosis H02.40- ☑
  congenital Q10.0
  mechanical H02.41- ☑
  myogenic H02.42- ☑
  neurogenic H02.43- ☑
  paralytic H02.43- ☑
Blepharopyorrhea, gonococcal A54.39
Blepharospasm G24.5
  drug induced G24.01
Blighted ovum O02.0
Blind — *see also* Blindness
  bronchus (congenital) Q32.4
  loop syndrome K90.2
    congenital Q43.8
  sac, fallopian tube (congenital) Q50.6
  spot, enlarged — *see* Defect, visual field, localized,
    scotoma, blind spot area
  tract or tube, congenital NEC — *see* Atresia, by site
Blindness (acquired) (congenital) (both eyes) H54.0X- ☑
  blast S05.8X- ☑
  color — *see* Deficiency, color vision
  concussion S05.8X- ☑
  cortical H47.619
    left brain H47.612
    right brain H47.611
  day H53.11

Blindness — *continued*
  due to injury (current episode) S05.9- ☑
    sequelae — *code to* injury with seventh character
      S
  eclipse (total) — *see* Retinopathy, solar
  emotional (hysterical) F44.6
  face H53.16
  hysterical F44.6
  legal (both eyes) (USA definition) H54.8
  mind R48.8
  night H53.60
    abnormal dark adaptation curve H53.61
    acquired H53.62
    congenital H53.63
    specified type NEC H53.69
    vitamin A deficiency E50.5
  one eye (other eye normal) H54.40
    left (normal vision on right) H54.42- ☑
      low vision on right H54.12- ☑
      low vision, other eye H54.10
    right (normal vision on left) H54.41- ☑
      low vision on left H54.11- ☑
  psychic R48.8
  river B73.01
  snow — *see* Photokeratitis
  sun, solar — *see* Retinopathy, solar
  transient — *see* Disturbance, vision, subjective, loss,
    transient
  traumatic (current episode) S05.9- ☑
  word (developmental) F81.0
    acquired R48.0
    secondary to organic lesion R48.0
Blister (nonthermal)
  abdominal wall S30.821 ☑
  alveolar process S00.522 ☑
  ankle S90.52- ☑
  antecubital space — *see* Blister, elbow
  anus S30.827 ☑
  arm (upper) S40.82- ☑
  auditory canal — *see* Blister, ear
  auricle — *see* Blister, ear
  axilla — *see* Blister, arm
  back, lower S30.820 ☑
  beetle dermatitis L24.89
  breast S20.12- ☑
  brow S00.82 ☑
  calf — *see* Blister, leg
  canthus — *see* Blister, eyelid
  cheek S00.82 ☑
    internal S00.522 ☑
  chest wall — *see* Blister, thorax
  chin S00.82 ☑
  costal region — *see* Blister, thorax
  digit(s)
    foot — *see* Blister, toe
    hand — *see* Blister, finger
  due to burn — *see* Burn, by site, second degree
  ear S00.42- ☑
  elbow S50.32- ☑
  epiglottis S10.12 ☑
  esophagus, cervical S10.12 ☑
  eyebrow — *see* Blister, eyelid
  eyelid S00.22- ☑
  face S00.82 ☑
  fever B00.1
  finger(s) S60.429 ☑
    index S60.42- ☑
    little S60.42- ☑
    middle S60.42- ☑
    ring S60.42- ☑
  foot (except toe(s) alone) S90.82- ☑
    toe — *see* Blister, toe
  forearm S50.82- ☑
    elbow only — *see* Blister, elbow
  forehead S00.82 ☑
  fracture — *omit code*
  genital organ
    female S30.826 ☑
    male S30.825 ☑
  gum S00.522 ☑
  hand S60.52- ☑
  head S00.92 ☑
    ear — *see* Blister, ear
    eyelid — *see* Blister, eyelid
  lip S00.521 ☑
  nose S00.32 ☑

Index

Blister — Body, bodies

Blister — *continued*
  head — *continued*
    oral cavity S00.522 ✓
    scalp S00.02 ✓
    specified site NEC S00.82 ✓
  heel — *see* Blister, foot
  hip S70.22- ✓
  interscapular region S20.429 ✓
  jaw S00.82 ✓
  knee S80.22- ✓
  larynx S10.12 ✓
  leg (lower) S80.82- ✓
    knee — *see* Blister, knee
    upper — *see* Blister, thigh
  lip S00.521 ✓
  malar region S00.82 ✓
  mammary — *see* Blister, breast
  mastoid region S00.82 ✓
  mouth S00.522 ✓
  multiple, skin, nontraumatic R23.8
  nail
    finger — *see* Blister, finger
    toe — *see* Blister, toe
  nasal S00.32 ✓
  neck S10.92 ✓
    specified site NEC S10.82 ✓
    throat S10.12 ✓
  nose S00.32 ✓
  occipital region S00.02 ✓
  oral cavity S00.522 ✓
  orbital region — *see* Blister, eyelid
  palate S00.522 ✓
  palm — *see* Blister, hand
  parietal region S00.02 ✓
  pelvis S30.820 ✓
  penis S30.822 ✓
  periocular area — *see* Blister, eyelid
  phalanges
    finger — *see* Blister, finger
    toe — *see* Blister, toe
  pharynx S10.12 ✓
  pinna — *see* Blister, ear
  popliteal space — *see* Blister, knee
  scalp S00.02 ✓
  scapular region — *see* Blister, shoulder
  scrotum S30.823 ✓
  shin — *see* Blister, leg
  shoulder S40.22- ✓
  sternal region S20.329 ✓
  submaxillary region S00.82 ✓
  submental region S00.82 ✓
  subungual
    finger(s) — *see* Blister, finger
    toe(s) — *see* Blister, toe
  supraclavicular fossa S10.82 ✓
  supraorbital S00.82 ✓
  temple S00.82 ✓
  temporal region S00.82 ✓
  testis S30.823 ✓
  thermal — *see* Burn, second degree, by site
  thigh S70.32- ✓
  thorax, thoracic (wall) S20.92 ✓
    back S20.42- ✓
    front S20.32- ✓
  throat S10.12 ✓
  thumb S60.32- ✓
  toe(s) S90.42- ✓
    great S90.42- ✓
  tongue S00.522 ✓
  trachea S10.12 ✓
  tympanum, tympanic membrane — *see* Blister, ear
  upper arm — *see* Blister, arm (upper)
  uvula S00.522 ✓
  vagina S30.824 ✓
  vocal cords S10.12 ✓
  vulva S30.824 ✓
  wrist S60.82- ✓
Bloating R14.0
Bloch-Sulzberger disease or syndrome Q82.3
Block, blocked
  alveolocapillary J84.10
  arborization (heart) I45.5
  arrhythmic I45.9
  atrioventricular (incomplete) (partial) I44.30
    with atrioventricular dissociation I44.2
      complete I44.2

Block, blocked — *continued*
  atrioventricular — *continued*
    complete — *continued*
      congenital Q24.6
    congenital Q24.6
    first degree I44.0
    second degree (types I and II) I44.1
    specified NEC I44.39
    third degree I44.2
    types I and II I44.1
  auriculoventricular — *see* Block, atrioventricular
  bifascicular (cardiac) I45.2
  bundle-branch (complete) (false) (incomplete) I45.4
    bilateral I45.2
    left I44.7
      with right bundle branch block I45.2
      hemiblock I44.60
        anterior I44.4
        posterior I44.5
      incomplete I44.7
        with right bundle branch block I45.2
    right I45.10
      with
        left bundle branch block I45.2
        left fascicular block I45.2
      specified NEC I45.19
    Wilson's type I45.19
  cardiac I45.9
  conduction I45.9
    complete I44.2
  fascicular (left) I44.60
    anterior I44.4
    posterior I44.5
    right I45.0
    specified NEC I44.69
  foramen Magendie (acquired) G91.1
    congenital Q03.1
      with spina bifida — *see* Spina bifida, by site, with hydrocephalus
  heart I45.9
    bundle branch I45.4
      bilateral I45.2
    complete (atrioventricular) I44.2
    congenital Q24.6
    first degree (atrioventricular) I44.0
    second degree (atrioventricular) I44.1
    specified type NEC I45.5
    third degree (atrioventricular) I44.2
  hepatic vein I82.0
  intraventricular (nonspecific) I45.4
    bundle branch
      bilateral I45.2
  kidney N28.9
    postcystoscopic or postprocedural N99.0
  Mobitz (types I and II) I44.1
  myocardial — *see* Block, heart
  nodal I45.5
  organ or site, congenital NEC — *see* Atresia, by site
  portal (vein) I81
  second degree (types I and II) I44.1
  sinoatrial I45.5
  sinoauricular I45.5
  third degree I44.2
  trifascicular I45.3
  tubal N97.1
  vein NOS I82.90
  Wenckebach (types I and II) I44.1
Blockage — *see* Obstruction
Blocq's disease F44.4
Blood
  constituents, abnormal R78.9
  disease D75.9
  donor — *see* Donor, blood
  dyscrasia D75.9
    with
      abortion — *see* Abortion, by type, complicated by, hemorrhage
      ectopic pregnancy O08.1
      molar pregnancy O08.1
    following ectopic or molar pregnancy O08.1
    newborn P61.9
    puerperal, postpartum O72.3
  flukes NEC — *see* Schistosomiasis
  in
    feces K92.1
      occult R19.5
    urine — *see* Hematuria
  mole O02.0

Blood — *continued*
  occult in feces R19.5
  pressure
    decreased, due to shock following injury T79.4 ✓
    examination only Z01.30
    fluctuating I99.8
    high — *see* Hypertension
      borderline R03.0
      incidental reading, without diagnosis of hypertension R03.0
    low — *see also* Hypotension
      incidental reading, without diagnosis of hypotension R03.1
  spitting — *see* Hemoptysis
  staining cornea — *see* Pigmentation, cornea, stromal
  transfusion
    reaction or complication — *see* Complications, transfusion
  type
    A (Rh positive) Z67.10
      Rh negative Z67.11
    AB (Rh positive) Z67.30
      Rh negative Z67.31
    B (Rh positive) Z67.20
      Rh negative Z67.21
    O (Rh positive) Z67.40
      Rh negative Z67.41
    Rh (positive) Z67.90
      negative Z67.91
  vessel rupture — *see* Hemorrhage
  vomiting — *see* Hematemesis
Blood-forming organs, disease D75.9
Bloodgood's disease — *see* Mastopathy, cystic
Bloom (-Machacek)(-Torre) **syndrome** Q82.8
Blount's disease or osteochondrosis — *see* Osteochondrosis, juvenile, tibia
Blue
  baby Q24.9
  diaper syndrome E72.09
  dome cyst (breast) — *see* Cyst, breast
  dot cataract Q12.0
  nevus D22.9
  sclera Q13.5
    with fragility of bone and deafness Q78.0
  toe syndrome I75.02- ✓
Blueness — *see* Cyanosis
Blues, postpartal O90.6
  baby O90.6
Blurring, visual H53.8
Blushing (abnormal) (excessive) R23.2
BMI — *see* Body, mass index
Boarder, hospital NEC Z76.4
  accompanying sick person Z76.3
  healthy infant or child Z76.2
  foundling Z76.1
Bockhart's impetigo L01.02
Bodechtel-Guttman disease (subacute sclerosing panencephalitis) A81.1
Boder-Sedgwick syndrome (ataxia-telangiectasia) G11.3
Body, bodies
  Aschoff's — *see* Myocarditis, rheumatic
  asteroid, vitreous — *see* Deposit, crystalline
  cytoid (retina) — *see* Occlusion, artery, retina
  drusen (degenerative) (macula) (retinal) — *see also* Degeneration, macula, drusen
    optic disc — *see* Drusen, optic disc
  foreign — *see* Foreign body
  loose
    joint, except knee — *see* Loose, body, joint
      knee M23.4- ✓
    sheath, tendon — *see* Disorder, tendon, specified type NEC
  mass index (BMI)
    adult
      19.9 or less Z68.1
      20.0-20.9 Z68.20
      21.0-21.9 Z68.21
      22.0-22.9 Z68.22
      23.0-23.9 Z68.23
      24.0-24.9 Z68.24
      25.0-25.9 Z68.25
      26.0-26.9 Z68.26
      27.0-27.9 Z68.27
      28.0-28.9 Z68.28
      29.0-29.9 Z68.29
      30.0-30.9 Z68.30
      31.0-31.9 Z68.31
      32.0-32.9 Z68.32

Body, bodies — *continued*
  mass index — *continued*
    adult — *continued*
      33.0-33.9 Z68.33
      34.0-34.9 Z68.34
      35.0-35.9 Z68.35
      36.0-36.9 Z68.36
      37.0-37.9 Z68.37
      38.0-38.9 Z68.38
      39.0-39.9 Z68.39
      40.0-44.9 Z68.41
      45.0-49.9 Z68.42
      50.0-59.9 Z68.43
      60.0-69.9 Z68.44
      70 and over Z68.45
    pediatric
      5th percentile to less than 85th percentile for age Z68.52
      85th percentile to less than 95th percentile for age Z68.53
      greater than or equal to ninety-fifth percentile for age Z68.54
      less than fifth percentile for age Z68.51
  Mooser's A75.2
  rice — *see also* Loose, body, joint
    knee M23.4- ☑
  rocking F98.4
Boeck's
  disease or sarcoid — *See* Sarcoidosis
  lupoid (miliary) D86.3
Boerhaave's syndrome (spontaneous esophageal rupture) K22.3
Boggy
  cervix N88.8
  uterus N85.8
Boil — *see also* Furuncle, by site
  Aleppo B55.1
  Baghdad B55.1
  Delhi B55.1
  lacrimal
    gland — *see* Dacryoadenitis
    passages (duct) (sac) — *see* Inflammation, lacrimal, passages, acute
  Natal B55.1
  orbit, orbital — *see* Abscess, orbit
  tropical B55.1
Bold hives — *see* Urticaria
Bombé, iris — *see* Membrane, pupillary
Bone — *see* condition
Bonnevie-Ullrich syndrome — *see also* Turner's syndrome Q87.19
Bonnier's syndrome H81.8 ☑
Bonvale dam fever T73.3 ☑
Bony block of joint — *see* Ankylosis
BOOP (bronchiolitis obliterans organized pneumonia) J84.89
Borderline
  diabetes mellitus R73.03
  hypertension R03.0
  osteopenia M85.8- ☑
  pelvis, with obstruction during labor O65.1
  personality F60.3
Borna disease A83.9
Bornholm disease B33.0
Boston exanthem A88.0
Botalli, ductus (patent) (persistent) Q25.0
Bothriocephalus latus infestation B70.0
Botulism (foodborne intoxication) A05.1
  infant A48.51
  non-foodborne A48.52
  wound A48.52
Bouba — *see* Yaws
Bouchard's nodes (with arthropathy) M15.2
Bouffée délirante F23
Bouillaud's disease or syndrome (rheumatic heart disease) I01.9
Bourneville's disease Q85.1
Boutonniere deformity (finger) — *see* Deformity, finger, boutonniere
Bouveret (-Hoffmann) **syndrome** (paroxysmal tachycardia) I47.9
Bovine heart — *see* Hypertrophy, cardiac
Bowel — *see* condition
Bowen's
  dermatosis (precancerous) — *see* Neoplasm, skin, in situ
  disease — *see* Neoplasm, skin, in situ

Bowen's — *continued*
  epithelioma — *see* Neoplasm, skin, in situ
  type
    epidermoid carcinoma-in-situ — *see* Neoplasm, skin, in situ
    intraepidermal squamous cell carcinoma — *see* Neoplasm, skin, in situ
Bowing
  femur — *see also* Deformity, limb, specified type NEC, thigh
    congenital Q68.3
  fibula — *see also* Deformity, limb, specified type NEC, lower leg
    congenital Q68.4
  forearm — *see* Deformity, limb, specified type NEC, forearm
  leg(s), long bones, congenital Q68.5
  radius — *see* Deformity, limb, specified type NEC, forearm
  tibia — *see also* Deformity, limb, specified type NEC, lower leg
    congenital Q68.4
Bowleg(s) (acquired) M21.16- ☑
  congenital Q68.5
  rachitic E64.3
Boyd's dysentery A03.2
Brachial — *see* condition
Brachycardia R00.1
Brachycephaly Q75.0
Bradley's disease A08.19
Bradyarrhythmia, cardiac I49.8
Bradycardia (sinoatrial) (sinus) (vagal) R00.1
  neonatal P29.12
  reflex G90.09
  tachycardia syndrome I49.5
Bradykinesia R25.8
Bradypnea R06.89
Bradytachycardia I49.5
Brailsford's disease or osteochondrosis — *see* Osteochondrosis, juvenile, radius
Brain — *see also* condition
  death G93.82
  syndrome — *see* Syndrome, brain
Branched-chain amino-acid disorder E71.2
Branchial — *see* condition
  cartilage, congenital Q18.2
Branchiogenic remnant (in neck) Q18.0
Brandt's syndrome (acrodermatitis enteropathica) E83.2
Brash (water) R12
Bravais-jacksonian epilepsy — *see* Epilepsy, localization-related, symptomatic, with simple partial seizures
Braxton Hicks contractions — *see* False, labor
Brazilian leishmaniasis B55.2
BRBPR K62.5
Break, retina (without detachment) H33.30- ☑
  with retinal detachment — *see* Detachment, retina
  horseshoe tear H33.31- ☑
  multiple H33.33- ☑
  round hole H33.32- ☑
Breakdown
  device, graft or implant — *see also* Complications, by site and type, mechanical T85.618 ☑
    arterial graft NEC — *see* Complication, cardiovascular device, mechanical, vascular
    breast (implant) T85.41 ☑
    catheter NEC T85.618 ☑
      cystostomy T83.010 ☑
      dialysis (renal) T82.41 ☑
        intraperitoneal T85.611 ☑
      Hopkins T83.018 ☑
      ileostomy T83.018 ☑
      infusion NEC T82.514 ☑
        cranial T85.610- ☑
        epidural T85.610 ☑
        intrathecal T85.610 ☑
        spinal T85.610 ☑
        subarachnoid T85.610 ☑
        subdural T85.610 ☑
      nephrostomy T83.012 ☑
      urethral indwelling T83.011 ☑
      urinary NEC T83.018 ☑
      urostomy T83.018 ☑
    electronic (electrode) (pulse generator) (stimulator)
      bone T84.310 ☑
      cardiac T82.119 ☑
        electrode T82.110 ☑

Breakdown — *continued*
  device, graft or implant — *see also* Complications, by site and type, mechanical — *continued*
    electronic — *continued*
      cardiac — *continued*
        pulse generator T82.111 ☑
        specified type NEC T82.118 ☑
      nervous system — *see* Complication, prosthetic device, mechanical, electronic nervous system stimulator
      urinary — *see* Complication, genitourinary, device, urinary, mechanical
    fixation, internal (orthopedic) NEC — *see* Complication, fixation device, mechanical
    gastrointestinal — *see* Complications, prosthetic device, mechanical, gastrointestinal device
    genital NEC T83.418 ☑
      intrauterine contraceptive device T83.31 ☑
      penile prosthesis (cylinder) (implanted) (pump) (resevoir) T83.410 ☑
      testicular prosthesis T83.411 ☑
    heart NEC — *see* Complication, cardiovascular device, mechanical
    intrathecal infusion pump T85.615 ☑
    joint prosthesis — *see* Complications..., joint prosthesis, internal, mechanical, by site
    nervous system, specified device NEC T85.615 ☑
    ocular NEC — *see* Complications, prosthetic device, mechanical, ocular device
    orthopedic NEC — *see* Complication, orthopedic, device, mechanical
    specified NEC T85.618 ☑
    subcutaneous device pocket
      nervous system prosthetic device, implant, or graft T85.890 ☑
      other internal prosthetic device, implant, or graft T85.898 ☑
    sutures, permanent T85.612 ☑
      used in bone repair — *see* Complications, fixation device, internal (orthopedic), mechanical
    urinary NEC T83.118 ☑
      graft T83.21 ☑
      sphincter, implanted T83.111 ☑
      stent (ileal conduit) (nephroureteral) T83.113 ☑
        ureteral indwelling T83.112 ☑
    vascular NEC — *see* Complication, cardiovascular device, mechanical
    ventricular intracranial shunt T85.01 ☑
  nervous F48.8
  perineum O90.1
  respirator J95.850
    specified NEC J95.859
  ventilator J95.850
    specified NEC J95.859
Breast — *see also* condition
  buds E30.1
    in newborn P96.89
  dense R92.2
  nodule — *see also* Lump, breast N63.0
Breath
  foul R19.6
  holder, child R06.89
  holding spell R06.89
  shortness R06.02
Breathing
  labored — *see* Hyperventilation
  mouth R06.5
    causing malocclusion M26.5 ☑
  periodic R06.3
    high altitude G47.32
Breathlessness R06.81
Breda's disease — *see* Yaws
Breech presentation (mother) O32.1 ☑
  causing obstructed labor O64.1 ☑
  footling O32.8 ☑
    causing obstructed labor O64.8 ☑
  incomplete O32.8 ☑
    causing obstructed labor O64.8 ☑
Breisky's disease N90.4
Brennemann's syndrome I88.0
Brenner
  tumor (benign) D27.9
    borderline malignancy D39.1- ☑
    malignant C56 ☑
    proliferating D39.1- ☑
Bretonneau's disease or angina A36.0
Breus' mole O02.0

☑ Subterms under main terms may continue to next column or page   ☑ Additional Character Required — Refer to the Tabular List for Character Selection   41

Body, bodies — Breus' mole

Brevicollis Q76.49
Brickmakers' anemia B76.9 [D63.8]
Bridge, myocardial Q24.5
Bright red blood per rectum (BRBPR) K62.5
Bright's disease — see also Nephritis
arteriosclerotic — see Hypertension, kidney
Brill (-Zinsser) **disease** (recrudescent typhus) A75.1
Brill-Symmers' disease C82.90
Brion-Kayser disease — see Fever, parathyroid
Briquet's disorder or syndrome F45.0
Brissaud's
infantilism or dwarfism E23.0
motor-verbal tic F95.2
Brittle
bones disease Q78.0
nails L60.3
congenital Q84.6
Broad — see also condition
beta disease E78.2
ligament laceration syndrome N83.8
Broad- or floating-betalipoproteinemia E78.2
Brock's syndrome (atelectasis due to enlarged lymph nodes) J98.19
Brocq-Duhring disease (dermatitis herpetiformis) L13.0
Brodie's abscess or disease M86.8X- ☑
Broken
arches — see also Deformity, limb, flat foot
arm (meaning upper limb) — see Fracture, arm
back — see Fracture, vertebra
bone — see Fracture
implant or internal device — see Complications, by site and type, mechanical
leg (meaning lower limb) — see Fracture, leg
nose S02.2 ☑
tooth, teeth — see Fracture, tooth
Bromhidrosis, bromidrosis L75.0
Bromidism, bromism G92
due to
correct substance properly administered — see Table of Drugs and Chemicals, by drug, adverse effect
overdose or wrong substance given or taken — see Table of Drugs and Chemicals, by drug, poisoning
chronic (dependence) F13.20
Bromidrosiphobia F40.298
Bronchi, bronchial — see condition
Bronchiectasis (cylindrical) (diffuse) (fusiform) (localized) (saccular) J47.9
with
acute
bronchitis J47.0
lower respiratory infection J47.0
exacerbation (acute) J47.1
congenital Q33.4
tuberculous NEC — see Tuberculosis, pulmonary
Bronchiolectasis — see Bronchiectasis
Bronchiolitis (acute) (infective) (subacute) J21.9
with
bronchospasm or obstruction J21.9
influenza, flu or grippe — see Influenza, with, respiratory manifestations NEC
chemical (chronic) J68.4
acute J68.0
chronic (fibrosing) (obliterative) J44.9
due to
external agent — see Bronchitis, acute, due to
human metapneumovirus J21.1
respiratory syncytial virus (RSV) J21.0
specified organism NEC J21.8
fibrosa obliterans J44.9
influenzal — see Influenza, with, respiratory manifestations NEC
obliterans J42
with organizing pneumonia (BOOP) J84.89
obliterative (chronic) (subacute) J44.9
due to fumes or vapors J68.4
due to chemicals, gases, fumes or vapors (inhalation) J68.4
respiratory, interstitial lung disease J84.115
Bronchitis (diffuse) (fibrinous) (hypostatic) (infective) (membranous) J40
with
influenza, flu or grippe — see Influenza, with, respiratory manifestations NEC
obstruction (airway) (lung) J44.9
tracheitis (15 years of age and above) J40

Bronchitis — continued
with — continued
tracheitis — continued
acute or subacute J20.9
chronic J42
under 15 years of age J20.9
acute or subacute (with bronchospasm or obstruction) J20.9
with
bronchiectasis J47.0
chronic obstructive pulmonary disease J44.0
chemical (due to gases, fumes or vapors) J68.0
due to
fumes or vapors J68.0
Haemophilus influenzae J20.1
Mycoplasma pneumoniae J20.0
radiation J70.0
specified organism NEC J20.8
Streptococcus J20.2
virus
coxsackie J20.3
echovirus J20.7
parainfluenzae J20.4
respiratory syncytial (RSV) J20.5
rhinovirus J20.6
viral NEC J20.8
allergic (acute) J45.909
with
exacerbation (acute) J45.901
status asthmaticus J45.902
arachidic T17.528 ☑
aspiration (due to fumes or vapors) J68.0
asthmatic J45.9 ☑
chronic J44.9
with
acute lower respiratory infection J44.0
exacerbation (acute) J44.1
capillary — see Pneumonia, broncho
caseous (tuberculous) A15.5
Castellani's A69.8
catarrhal (15 years of age and above) J40
acute — see Bronchitis, acute
chronic J41.0
under 15 years of age J20.9
chemical (acute) (subacute) J68.0
chronic J68.4
due to fumes or vapors J68.0
chronic J68.4
chronic J42
with
airways obstruction J44.9
tracheitis (chronic) J42
asthmatic (obstructive) J44.9
catarrhal J41.0
chemical (due to fumes or vapors) J68.4
due to
chemicals, gases, fumes or vapors (inhalation) J68.4
radiation J70.1
tobacco smoking J41.0
emphysematous J44.9
mucopurulent J41.1
non-obstructive J41.0
obliterans J44.9
obstructive J44.9
purulent J41.1
simple J41.0
croupous — see Bronchitis, acute
due to gases, fumes or vapors (chemical) J68.0
emphysematous (obstructive) J44.9
exudative — see Bronchitis, acute
fetid J41.1
grippal — see Influenza, with, respiratory manifestations NEC
in those under 15 years age — see Bronchitis, acute
chronic — see Bronchitis, chronic
influenzal — see Influenza, with, respiratory manifestations NEC
mixed simple and mucopurulent J41.8
moulder's J62.8
mucopurulent (chronic) (recurrent) J41.1
acute or subacute J20.9
simple (mixed) J41.8
obliterans J44.9
obstructive (chronic) (diffuse) J44.9
pituitous J41.1
pneumococcal, acute or subacute J20.2

Bronchitis — continued
pseudomembranous, acute or subacute — see Bronchitis, acute
purulent (chronic) (recurrent) J41.1
acute or subacute — see Bronchitis, acute
putrid J41.1
senile (chronic) J42
simple and mucopurulent (mixed) J41.8
smokers' J41.0
spirochetal NEC A69.8
subacute — see Bronchitis, acute
suppurative (chronic) J41.1
acute or subacute — see Bronchitis, acute
tuberculous A15.5
under 15 years of age — see Bronchitis, acute
chronic — see Bronchitis, chronic
viral NEC, acute or subacute — see also Bronchitis, acute J20.8
Bronchoalveolitis J18.0
Bronchoaspergillosis B44.1
Bronchocele meaning goiter E04.0
Broncholithiasis J98.09
tuberculous NEC A15.5
Bronchomalacia J98.09
congenital Q32.2
Bronchomycosis NOS B49 [J99]
candidal B37.1
Bronchopleuropneumonia — see Pneumonia, broncho
Bronchopneumonia — see Pneumonia, broncho
Bronchopneumonitis — see Pneumonia, broncho
Bronchopulmonary — see condition
Bronchopulmonitis — see Pneumonia, broncho
Bronchorrhagia (see Hemoptysis)
Bronchorrhea J98.09
acute J20.9
chronic (infective) (purulent) J42
Bronchospasm (acute) J98.01
with
bronchiolitis, acute J21.9
bronchitis, acute (conditions in J20) — see Bronchitis, acute
due to external agent — see condition, respiratory, acute, due to
exercise induced J45.990
Bronchospirochetosis A69.8
Castellani A69.8
Bronchostenosis J98.09
Bronchus — see condition
Brontophobia F40.220
Bronze baby syndrome P83.88
Brooke's tumor — see Neoplasm, skin, benign
Brown enamel of teeth (hereditary) K00.5
Brown's sheath syndrome H50.61- ☑
Brown-Séquard disease, paralysis or syndrome G83.81
Bruce sepsis A23.0
Brucellosis (infection) A23.9
abortus A23.1
canis A23.3
dermatitis A23.9
melitensis A23.0
mixed A23.8
sepsis A23.9
melitensis A23.0
specified NEC A23.8
suis A23.2
Bruck-de Lange disease Q87.19
Bruck's disease — see Deformity, limb
BRUE (brief resolved unexplained event) R68.13
Brugsch's syndrome Q82.8
Bruise (skin surface intact) — see also Contusion
with
open wound — see Wound, open
internal organ — see Injury, by site
newborn P54.5
scalp, due to birth injury, newborn P12.3
umbilical cord O69.5 ☑
Bruit (arterial) R09.89
cardiac R01.1
Brush burn — see Abrasion, by site
Bruton's X-linked agammaglobulinemia D80.0
Bruxism
psychogenic F45.8
sleep related G47.63
Bubbly lung syndrome P27.0
Bubo I88.8
blennorrhagic (gonococcal) A54.89

☑ **Additional Character Required** — Refer to the Tabular List for Character Selection   ▽ **Subterms under main terms may continue to next column or page**

Bubo — *continued*
  chancroidal A57
  climatic A55
  due to Haemophilus ducreyi A57
  gonococcal A54.89
  indolent (nonspecific) I88.8
  inguinal (nonspecific) I88.8
    chancroidal A57
    climatic A55
    due to H. ducreyi A57
    infective I88.8
  scrofulous (tuberculous) A18.2
  soft chancre A57
  suppurating — *see* Lymphadenitis, acute
  syphilitic (primary) A51.0
    congenital A50.07
  tropical A55
  virulent (chancroidal) A57
Bubonic plague A20.0
Bubonocele — *see* Hernia, inguinal
Buccal — *see* condition
Buchanan's disease or osteochondrosis M91.0
Buchem's syndrome (hyperostosis corticalis) M85.2
Bucket-handle fracture or tear (semilunar cartilage)
    — *see* Tear, meniscus
Budd-Chiari syndrome (hepatic vein thrombosis) I82.0
Budgerigar fancier's disease or lung J67.2
Buds
  breast E30.1
    in newborn P96.89
Buerger's disease (thromboangiitis obliterans) I73.1
Bulbar — *see* condition
Bulbus cordis (left ventricle) (persistent) Q21.8
Bulimia (nervosa) F50.2
  atypical F50.9
  normal weight F50.9
Bulky
  stools R19.5
  uterus N85.2
Bulla (e) R23.8
  lung (emphysematous) (solitary) J43.9
    newborn P25.8
Bullet wound — *see also* Wound, open
  fracture — *code as* Fracture, by site
  internal organ — *see* Injury, by site
Bundle
  branch block (complete) (false) (incomplete) — *see*
    Block, bundle-branch
  of His — *see* condition
Bunion M21.61- ☑
  tailor's M21.62- ☑
Bunionette M21.62- ☑
Buphthalmia, buphthalmos (congenital) Q15.0
Burdwan fever B55.0
Bürger-Grütz disease or syndrome E78.3
Buried
  penis (congenital) Q55.64
    acquired N48.83
  roots K08.3
Burke's syndrome K86.89
Burkitt
  cell leukemia C91.0- ☑
  lymphoma (malignant) C83.7- ☑
    small noncleaved, diffuse C83.7- ☑
    spleen C83.77
    undifferentiated C83.7- ☑
  tumor C83.7- ☑
  type
    acute lymphoblastic leukemia C91.0- ☑
    undifferentiated C83.7- ☑
Burn (electricity) (flame) (hot gas, liquid or hot object)
    (radiation) (steam) (thermal) T30.0
  abdomen, abdominal (muscle) (wall) T21.02 ☑
    first degree T21.12 ☑
    second degree T21.22 ☑
    third degree T21.32 ☑
  above elbow T22.039 ☑
    first degree T22.139 ☑
    left T22.032 ☑
      first degree T22.132 ☑
      second degree T22.232 ☑
      third degree T22.332 ☑
    right T22.031 ☑
      first degree T22.131 ☑
      second degree T22.231 ☑
      third degree T22.331 ☑
    second degree T22.239 ☑

Burn — *continued*
  above elbow — *continued*
    third degree T22.339 ☑
  acid (caustic) (external) (internal) — *see* Corrosion, by
    site
  alimentary tract NEC T28.2 ☑
    esophagus T28.1 ☑
    mouth T28.0 ☑
    pharynx T28.0 ☑
  alkaline (caustic) (external) (internal) — *see* Corrosion,
    by site
  ankle T25.019 ☑
    first degree T25.119 ☑
    left T25.012 ☑
      first degree T25.112 ☑
      second degree T25.212 ☑
      third degree T25.312 ☑
    multiple with foot — *see* Burn, lower, limb, multiple,
      ankle and foot
    right T25.011 ☑
      first degree T25.111 ☑
      second degree T25.211 ☑
      third degree T25.311 ☑
    second degree T25.219 ☑
    third degree T25.319 ☑
  anus — *see* Burn, buttock
  arm (lower) (upper) — *see* Burn, upper, limb
  axilla T22.049 ☑
    first degree T22.149 ☑
    left T22.042 ☑
      first degree T22.142 ☑
      second degree T22.242 ☑
      third degree T22.342 ☑
    right T22.041 ☑
      first degree T22.141 ☑
      second degree T22.241 ☑
      third degree T22.341 ☑
    second degree T22.249 ☑
    third degree T22.349 ☑
  back (lower) T21.04 ☑
    first degree T21.14 ☑
    second degree T21.24 ☑
    third degree T21.34 ☑
    upper T21.03 ☑
      first degree T21.13 ☑
      second degree T21.23 ☑
      third degree T21.33 ☑
  blisters — *code as* Burn, second degree, by site
  breast(s) — *see* Burn, chest wall
  buttock(s) T21.05 ☑
    first degree T21.15 ☑
    second degree T21.25 ☑
    third degree T21.35 ☑
  calf T24.039 ☑
    first degree T24.139 ☑
    left T24.032 ☑
      first degree T24.132 ☑
      second degree T24.232 ☑
      third degree T24.332 ☑
    right T24.031 ☑
      first degree T24.131 ☑
      second degree T24.231 ☑
      third degree T24.331 ☑
    second degree T24.239 ☑
    third degree T24.339 ☑
  canthus (eye) — *see* Burn, eyelid
  caustic acid or alkaline — *see* Corrosion, by site
  cervix T28.3 ☑
  cheek T20.06 ☑
    first degree T20.16 ☑
    second degree T20.26 ☑
    third degree T20.36 ☑
  chemical (acids) (alkalines) (caustics) (external) (inter-
    nal) — *see* Corrosion, by site
  chest wall T21.01 ☑
    first degree T21.11 ☑
    second degree T21.21 ☑
    third degree T21.31 ☑
  chin T20.03 ☑
    first degree T20.13 ☑
    second degree T20.23 ☑
    third degree T20.33 ☑
  colon T28.2 ☑
  conjunctiva (and cornea) — *see* Burn, cornea
  cornea (and conjunctiva) T26.1- ☑
    chemical — *see* Corrosion, cornea

Burn — *continued*
  corrosion (external) (internal) — *see* Corrosion, by site
  deep necrosis of underlying tissue — *code as* Burn,
    third degree, by site
  dorsum of hand T23.069 ☑
    first degree T23.169 ☑
    left T23.062 ☑
      first degree T23.162 ☑
      second degree T23.262 ☑
      third degree T23.362 ☑
    right T23.061 ☑
      first degree T23.161 ☑
      second degree T23.261 ☑
      third degree T23.361 ☑
    second degree T23.269 ☑
    third degree T23.369 ☑
  due to ingested chemical agent — *see* Corrosion, by
    site
  ear (auricle) (external) (canal) T20.01 ☑
    first degree T20.11 ☑
    second degree T20.21 ☑
    third degree T20.31 ☑
  elbow T22.029 ☑
    first degree T22.129 ☑
    left T22.022 ☑
      first degree T22.122 ☑
      second degree T22.222 ☑
      third degree T22.322 ☑
    right T22.021 ☑
      first degree T22.121 ☑
      second degree T22.221 ☑
      third degree T22.321 ☑
    second degree T22.229 ☑
    third degree T22.329 ☑
  epidermal loss — *code as* Burn, second degree, by site
  erythema, erythematous — *code as* Burn, first degree,
    by site
  esophagus T28.1 ☑
  extent (percentage of body surface)
    less than 10 percent T31.0
    10-19 percent T31.10
      with 0-9 percent third degree burns T31.10
      with 10-19 percent third degree burns T31.11
    20-29 percent T31.20
      with 0-9 percent third degree burns T31.20
      with 10-19 percent third degree burns T31.21
      with 20-29 percent third degree burns T31.22
    30-39 percent T31.30
      with 0-9 percent third degree burns T31.30
      with 10-19 percent third degree burns T31.31
      with 20-29 percent third degree burns T31.32
      with 30-39 percent third degree burns T31.33
    40-49 percent T31.40
      with 0-9 percent third degree burns T31.40
      with 10-19 percent third degree burns T31.41
      with 20-29 percent third degree burns T31.42
      with 30-39 percent third degree burns T31.43
      with 40-49 percent third degree burns T31.44
    50-59 percent T31.50
      with 0-9 percent third degree burns T31.50
      with 10-19 percent third degree burns T31.51
      with 20-29 percent third degree burns T31.52
      with 30-39 percent third degree burns T31.53
      with 40-49 percent third degree burns T31.54
      with 50-59 percent third degree burns T31.55
    60-69 percent T31.60
      with 0-9 percent third degree burns T31.60
      with 10-19 percent third degree burns T31.61
      with 20-29 percent third degree burns T31.62
      with 30-39 percent third degree burns T31.63
      with 40-49 percent third degree burns T31.64
      with 50-59 percent third degree burns T31.65
      with 60-69 percent third degree burns T31.66
    70-79 percent T31.70
      with 0-9 percent third degree burns T31.70
      with 10-19 percent third degree burns T31.71
      with 20-29 percent third degree burns T31.72
      with 30-39 percent third degree burns T31.73
      with 40-49 percent third degree burns T31.74
      with 50-59 percent third degree burns T31.75
      with 60-69 percent third degree burns T31.76
      with 70-79 percent third degree burns T31.77
    80-89 percent T31.80
      with 0-9 percent third degree burns T31.80
      with 10-19 percent third degree burns T31.81
      with 20-29 percent third degree burns T31.82
      with 30-39 percent third degree burns T31.83

☷ Subterms under main terms may continue to next column or page   ☑ Additional Character Required — Refer to the Tabular List for Character Selection   **43**

Bubo — Burn

Burn — *continued*

extent — *continued*
  80-89 percent — *continued*
    with 40-49 percent third degree burns T31.84
    with 50-59 percent third degree burns T31.85
    with 60-69 percent third degree burns T31.86
    with 70-79 percent third degree burns T31.87
    with 80-89 percent third degree burns T31.88
  90 percent or more T31.90
    with 0-9 percent third degree burns T31.90
    with 10-19 percent third degree burns T31.91
    with 20-29 percent third degree burns T31.92
    with 30-39 percent third degree burns T31.93
    with 40-49 percent third degree burns T31.94
    with 50-59 percent third degree burns T31.95
    with 60-69 percent third degree burns T31.96
    with 70-79 percent third degree burns T31.97
    with 80-89 percent third degree burns T31.98
    with 90 percent or more third degree burns T31.99
extremity — *see* Burn, limb
eye(s) and adnexa T26.4- ☑
  with resulting rupture and destruction of eyeball T26.2- ☑
  conjunctival sac — *see* Burn, cornea
  cornea — *see* Burn, cornea
  lid — *see* Burn, eyelid
  periocular area — *see* Burn, eyelid
  specified site NEC T26.3- ☑
eyeball — *see* Burn, eye
eyelid(s) T26.0- ☑
  chemical — *see* Corrosion, eyelid
face — *see* Burn, head
finger T23.029 ☑
  first degree T23.129 ☑
  left T23.022 ☑
    first degree T23.122 ☑
    second degree T23.222 ☑
    third degree T23.322 ☑
  multiple sites (without thumb) T23.039 ☑
    with thumb T23.049 ☑
      first degree T23.149 ☑
      left T23.042 ☑
        first degree T23.142 ☑
        second degree T23.242 ☑
        third degree T23.342 ☑
      right T23.041 ☑
        first degree T23.141 ☑
        second degree T23.241 ☑
        third degree T23.341 ☑
      second degree T23.249 ☑
      third degree T23.349 ☑
    first degree T23.139 ☑
    left T23.032 ☑
      first degree T23.132 ☑
      second degree T23.232 ☑
      third degree T23.332 ☑
    right T23.031 ☑
      first degree T23.131 ☑
      second degree T23.231 ☑
      third degree T23.331 ☑
    second degree T23.239 ☑
    third degree T23.339 ☑
  right T23.021 ☑
    first degree T23.121 ☑
    second degree T23.221 ☑
    third degree T23.321 ☑
  second degree T23.229 ☑
  third degree T23.329 ☑
flank — *see* Burn, abdominal wall
foot T25.029 ☑
  first degree T25.129 ☑
  left T25.022 ☑
    first degree T25.122 ☑
    second degree T25.222 ☑
    third degree T25.322 ☑
  multiple with ankle — *see* Burn, lower, limb, multiple, ankle and foot
  right T25.021 ☑
    first degree T25.121 ☑
    second degree T25.221 ☑
    third degree T25.321 ☑
  second degree T25.229 ☑
  third degree T25.329 ☑
forearm T22.019 ☑
  first degree T22.119 ☑

Burn — *continued*

forearm — *continued*
  left T22.012 ☑
    first degree T22.112 ☑
    second degree T22.212 ☑
    third degree T22.312 ☑
  right T22.011 ☑
    first degree T22.111 ☑
    second degree T22.211 ☑
    third degree T22.311 ☑
  second degree T22.219 ☑
  third degree T22.319 ☑
forehead T20.06 ☑
  first degree T20.16 ☑
  second degree T20.26 ☑
  third degree T20.36 ☑
fourth degree — *code as* Burn, third degree, by site
friction — *see* Burn, by site
from swallowing caustic or corrosive substance NEC — *see* Corrosion, by site
full thickness skin loss — *code as* Burn, third degree, by site
gastrointestinal tract NEC T28.2 ☑
  from swallowing caustic or corrosive substance T28.7 ☑
genital organs
  external
    female T21.07 ☑
      first degree T21.17 ☑
      second degree T21.27 ☑
      third degree T21.37 ☑
    male T21.06 ☑
      first degree T21.16 ☑
      second degree T21.26 ☑
      third degree T21.36 ☑
  internal T28.3 ☑
    from caustic or corrosive substance T28.8 ☑
groin — *see* Burn, abdominal wall
hand(s) T23.009 ☑
  back — *see* Burn, dorsum of hand
  finger — *see* Burn, finger
  first degree T23.109 ☑
  left T23.002 ☑
    first degree T23.102 ☑
    second degree T23.202 ☑
    third degree T23.302 ☑
  multiple sites with wrist T23.099 ☑
    first degree T23.199 ☑
    left T23.092 ☑
      first degree T23.192 ☑
      second degree T23.292 ☑
      third degree T23.392 ☑
    right T23.091 ☑
      first degree T23.191 ☑
      second degree T23.291 ☑
      third degree T23.391 ☑
    second degree T23.299 ☑
    third degree T23.399 ☑
  palm — *see* Burn, palm
  right T23.001 ☑
    first degree T23.101 ☑
    second degree T23.201 ☑
    third degree T23.301 ☑
  second degree T23.209 ☑
  third degree T23.309 ☑
  thumb — *see* Burn, thumb
head (and face) (and neck) T20.00 ☑
  cheek — *see* Burn, cheek
  chin — *see* Burn, chin
  ear — *see* Burn, ear
  eye(s) only — *see* Burn, eye
  first degree T20.10 ☑
  forehead — *see* Burn, forehead
  lip — *see* Burn, lip
  multiple sites T20.09 ☑
    first degree T20.19 ☑
    second degree T20.29 ☑
    third degree T20.39 ☑
  neck — *see* Burn, neck
  nose — *see* Burn, nose
  scalp — *see* Burn, scalp
  second degree T20.20 ☑
  third degree T20.30 ☑
hip(s) — *see* Burn, thigh
inhalation — *see* Burn, respiratory tract

Burn — *continued*

inhalation — *see* Burn, respiratory tract — *continued*
  caustic or corrosive substance (fumes) — *see* Corrosion, respiratory tract
internal organ(s) T28.40 ☑
  alimentary tract T28.2
    esophagus T28.1 ☑
  eardrum T28.41 ☑
  esophagus T28.1 ☑
  from caustic or corrosive substance (swallowing) NEC — *see* Corrosion, by site
  genitourinary T28.3 ☑
  mouth T28.0 ☑
  pharynx T28.0 ☑
  respiratory tract — *see* Burn, respiratory tract
  specified organ NEC T28.49 ☑
interscapular region — *see* Burn, back, upper
intestine (large) (small) T28.2 ☑
knee T24.029 ☑
  first degree T24.129 ☑
  left T24.022 ☑
    first degree T24.122 ☑
    second degree T24.222 ☑
    third degree T24.322 ☑
  right T24.021 ☑
    first degree T24.121 ☑
    second degree T24.221 ☑
    third degree T24.321 ☑
  second degree T24.229 ☑
  third degree T24.329 ☑
labium (majus) (minus) — *see* Burn, genital organs, external, female
lacrimal apparatus, duct, gland or sac — *see* Burn, eye, specified site NEC
larynx T27.0 ☑
  with lung T27.1 ☑
leg(s) (lower) (upper) — *see* Burn, lower, limb
lightning — *see* Burn, by site
limb(s)
  lower (except ankle or foot alone) — *see* Burn, lower, limb
  upper — *see* Burn, upper limb
lip(s) T20.02 ☑
  first degree T20.12 ☑
  second degree T20.22 ☑
  third degree T20.32 ☑
lower
  back — *see* Burn, back
  limb T24.009 ☑
    ankle — *see* Burn, ankle
    calf — *see* Burn, calf
    first degree T24.109 ☑
    foot — *see* Burn, foot
    hip — *see* Burn, thigh
    knee — *see* Burn, knee
    left T24.002 ☑
      first degree T24.102 ☑
      second degree T24.202 ☑
      third degree T24.302 ☑
    multiple sites, except ankle and foot T24.099 ☑
      ankle and foot T25.099 ☑
        first degree T25.199 ☑
        left T25.092 ☑
          first degree T25.192 ☑
          second degree T25.292 ☑
          third degree T25.392 ☑
        right T25.091 ☑
          first degree T25.191 ☑
          second degree T25.291 ☑
          third degree T25.391 ☑
        second degree T25.299 ☑
        third degree T25.399 ☑
      first degree T24.199 ☑
      left T24.092 ☑
        first degree T24.192 ☑
        second degree T24.292 ☑
        third degree T24.392 ☑
      right T24.091 ☑
        first degree T24.191 ☑
        second degree T24.291 ☑
        third degree T24.391 ☑
      second degree T24.299 ☑
      third degree T24.399 ☑
    right T24.001 ☑
      first degree T24.101 ☑

Burn — *continued*
  lower — *continued*
    limb — *continued*
      right — *continued*
        second degree T24.201 ☑
        third degree T24.301 ☑
      second degree T24.209 ☑
      thigh — *see* Burn, thigh
      third degree T24.309 ☑
      toe — *see* Burn, toe
  lung (with larynx and trachea) T27.1
  mouth T28.0 ☑
  neck T20.07 ☑
    first degree T20.17 ☑
    second degree T20.27 ☑
    third degree T20.37 ☑
  nose (septum) T20.04 ☑
    first degree T20.14 ☑
    second degree T20.24 ☑
    third degree T20.34 ☑
  ocular adnexa — *see* Burn, eye
  orbit region — *see* Burn, eyelid
  palm T23.059 ☑
    first degree T23.159 ☑
    left T23.052 ☑
      first degree T23.152 ☑
      second degree T23.252 ☑
      third degree T23.352 ☑
    right T23.051 ☑
      first degree T23.151 ☑
      second degree T23.251 ☑
      third degree T23.351 ☑
    second degree T23.259 ☑
    third degree T23.359 ☑
  partial thickness — *code as* Burn, degree, by site
  pelvis — *see* Burn, trunk
  penis — *see* Burn, genital organs, external, male
  perineum
    female — *see* Burn, genital organs, external, female
    male — *see* Burn, genital organs, external, male
  periocular area — *see* Burn, eyelid
  pharynx T28.0 ☑
  rectum T28.2 ☑
  respiratory tract T27.3 ☑
    larynx — *see* Burn, larynx
    specified part NEC T27.2 ☑
    trachea — *see* Burn, trachea
  sac, lacrimal — *see* Burn, eye, specified site NEC
  scalp T20.05 ☑
    first degree T20.15 ☑
    second degree T20.25 ☑
    third degree T20.35 ☑
  scapular region T22.069 ☑
    first degree T22.169 ☑
    left T22.062 ☑
      first degree T22.162 ☑
      second degree T22.262 ☑
      third degree T22.362 ☑
    right T22.061 ☑
      first degree T22.161 ☑
      second degree T22.261 ☑
      third degree T22.361 ☑
    second degree T22.269 ☑
    third degree T22.369 ☑
  sclera — *see* Burn, eye, specified site NEC
  scrotum — *see* Burn, genital organs, external, male
  shoulder T22.059 ☑
    first degree T22.159 ☑
    left T22.052 ☑
      first degree T22.152 ☑
      second degree T22.252 ☑
      third degree T22.352 ☑
    right T22.051 ☑
      first degree T22.151 ☑
      second degree T22.251 ☑
      third degree T22.351 ☑
    second degree T22.259 ☑
    third degree T22.359 ☑
  stomach T28.2 ☑
  temple — *see* Burn, head
  testis — *see* Burn, genital organs, external, male
  thigh T24.019 ☑
    first degree T24.119 ☑
    left T24.012 ☑
      first degree T24.112 ☑
      second degree T24.212 ☑

Burn — *continued*
  thigh — *continued*
    left — *continued*
      third degree T24.312 ☑
    right T24.011 ☑
      first degree T24.111 ☑
      second degree T24.211 ☑
      third degree T24.311 ☑
    second degree T24.219 ☑
    third degree T24.319 ☑
  thorax (external) — *see* Burn, trunk
  throat (meaning pharynx) T28.0 ☑
  thumb(s) T23.019 ☑
    first degree T23.119 ☑
    left T23.012 ☑
      first degree T23.112 ☑
      second degree T23.212 ☑
      third degree T23.312 ☑
    multiple sites with fingers T23.049 ☑
      first degree T23.149 ☑
      left T23.042 ☑
        first degree T23.142 ☑
        second degree T23.242 ☑
        third degree T23.342 ☑
      right T23.041 ☑
        first degree T23.141 ☑
        second degree T23.241 ☑
        third degree T23.341 ☑
      second degree T23.249 ☑
      third degree T23.349 ☑
    right T23.011 ☑
      first degree T23.111 ☑
      second degree T23.211 ☑
      third degree T23.311 ☑
    second degree T23.219 ☑
    third degree T23.319 ☑
  toe T25.039 ☑
    first degree T25.139 ☑
    left T25.032 ☑
      first degree T25.132 ☑
      second degree T25.232 ☑
      third degree T25.332 ☑
    right T25.031 ☑
      first degree T25.131 ☑
      second degree T25.231 ☑
      third degree T25.331 ☑
    second degree T25.239 ☑
    third degree T25.339 ☑
  tongue T28.0 ☑
  tonsil(s) T28.0 ☑
  trachea T27.0 ☑
    with lung T27.1 ☑
  trunk T21.00 ☑
    abdominal wall — *see* Burn, abdominal wall
    anus — *see* Burn, buttock
    axilla — *see* Burn, upper limb
    back — *see* Burn, back
    breast — *see* Burn, chest wall
    buttock — *see* Burn, buttock
    chest wall — *see* Burn, chest wall
    first degree T21.10 ☑
    flank — *see* Burn, abdominal wall
    genital
      female — *see* Burn, genital organs, external, female
      male — *see* Burn, genital organs, external, male
    groin — *see* Burn, abdominal wall
    interscapular region — *see* Burn, back, upper
    labia — *see* Burn, genital organs, external, female
    lower back — *see* Burn, back
    penis — *see* Burn, genital organs, external, male
    perineum
      female — *see* Burn, genital organs, external, female
      male — *see* Burn, genital organs, external, male
    scapula region — *see* Burn, scapular region
    scrotum — *see* Burn, genital organs, external, male
    second degree T21.20 ☑
    specified site NEC T21.09 ☑
      first degree T21.19 ☑
      second degree T21.29 ☑
      third degree T21.39 ☑
    testes — *see* Burn, genital organs, external, male
    third degree T21.30 ☑
    upper back — *see* Burn, back, upper
    vulva — *see* Burn, genital organs, external, female

Burn — *continued*
  unspecified site with extent of body surface involved
    specified
      less than 10 percent T31.0
      10-19 percent (0-9 percent third degree) T31.10
        with 10-19 percent third degree T31.11
      20-29 percent (0-9 percent third degree) T31.20
        with
          10-19 percent third degree T31.21
          20-29 percent third degree T31.22
      30-39 percent (0-9 percent third degree) T31.30
        with
          10-19 percent third degree T31.31
          20-29 percent third degree T31.32
          30-39 percent third degree T31.33
      40-49 percent (0-9 percent third degree) T31.40
        with
          10-19 percent third degree T31.41
          20-29 percent third degree T31.42
          30-39 percent third degree T31.43
          40-49 percent third degree T31.44
      50-59 percent (0-9 percent third degree) T31.50
        with
          10-19 percent third degree T31.51
          20-29 percent third degree T31.52
          30-39 percent third degree T31.53
          40-49 percent third degree T31.54
          50-59 percent third degree T31.55
      60-69 percent (0-9 percent third degree) T31.60
        with
          10-19 percent third degree T31.61
          20-29 percent third degree T31.62
          30-39 percent third degree T31.63
          40-49 percent third degree T31.64
          50-59 percent third degree T31.65
          60-69 percent third degree T31.66
      70-79 percent (0-9 percent third degree) T31.70
        with
          10-19 percent third degree T31.71
          20-29 percent third degree T31.72
          30-39 percent third degree T31.73
          40-49 percent third degree T31.74
          50-59 percent third degree T31.75
          60-69 percent third degree T31.76
          70-79 percent third degree T31.77
      80-89 percent (0-9 percent third degree) T31.80
        with
          10-19 percent third degree T31.81
          20-29 percent third degree T31.82
          30-39 percent third degree T31.83
          40-49 percent third degree T31.84
          50-59 percent third degree T31.85
          60-69 percent third degree T31.86
          70-79 percent third degree T31.87
          80-89 percent third degree T31.88
      90 percent or more (0-9 percent third degree) T31.90
        with
          10-19 percent third degree T31.91
          20-29 percent third degree T31.92
          30-39 percent third degree T31.93
          40-49 percent third degree T31.94
          50-59 percent third degree T31.95
          60-69 percent third degree T31.96
          70-79 percent third degree T31.97
          80-89 percent third degree T31.98
          90-99 percent third degree T31.99
  upper limb T22.00 ☑
    above elbow — *see* Burn, above elbow
    axilla — *see* Burn, axilla
    elbow — *see* Burn, elbow
    first degree T22.10 ☑
    forearm — *see* Burn, forearm
    hand — *see* Burn, hand
    interscapular region — *see* Burn, back, upper
    multiple sites T22.099 ☑
      first degree T22.199 ☑
      left T22.092 ☑
        first degree T22.192 ☑
        second degree T22.292 ☑
        third degree T22.392 ☑
      right T22.091 ☑
        first degree T22.191 ☑
        second degree T22.291 ☑
        third degree T22.391 ☑
      second degree T22.299 ☑
      third degree T22.399 ☑
    scapular region — *see* Burn, scapular region
    second degree T22.20 ☑

Burn — continued

upper limb — continued

shoulder — see Burn, shoulder

third degree T22.30 ☑

wrist — see Burn, wrist

uterus T28.3 ☑

vagina T28.3 ☑

vulva — see Burn, genital organs, external, female

wrist T23.079 ☑

first degree T23.179 ☑

left T23.072 ☑

first degree T23.172 ☑

second degree T23.272 ☑

third degree T23.372 ☑

multiple sites with hand T23.099 ☑

first degree T23.199 ☑

left T23.092 ☑

first degree T23.192 ☑

second degree T23.292 ☑

third degree T23.392 ☑

right T23.091 ☑

first degree T23.191 ☑

second degree T23.291 ☑

third degree T23.391 ☑

second degree T23.299 ☑

third degree T23.399 ☑

right T23.071 ☑

first degree T23.171 ☑

second degree T23.271 ☑

third degree T23.371 ☑

second degree T23.279 ☑

third degree T23.379 ☑

Burnett's syndrome E83.52

Burning

feet syndrome E53.9

sensation R20.8

tongue K14.6

Burn-out (state) Z73.0

Burns' disease or osteochondrosis — see Osteochondrosis, juvenile, ulna

Bursa — see condition

Bursitis M71.9

Achilles — see Tendinitis, Achilles

adhesive — see Bursitis, specified NEC

ankle — see Enthesopathy, lower limb, ankle, specified type NEC

calcaneal — see Enthesopathy, foot, specified type NEC

collateral ligament, tibial — see Bursitis, tibial collateral

due to use, overuse, pressure — see also Disorder, soft tissue, due to use, specified type NEC

specified NEC — see Disorder, soft tissue, due to use, specified NEC

Duplay's M75.0 ☑

elbow NEC M70.3- ☑

olecranon M70.2- ☑

finger — see Disorder, soft tissue, due to use, specified type NEC, hand

foot — see Enthesopathy, foot, specified type NEC

gonococcal A54.49

gouty — see Gout

hand M70.1- ☑

hip NEC M70.7- ☑

trochanteric M70.6- ☑

infective NEC M71.10

abscess — see Abscess, bursa

ankle M71.17- ☑

elbow M71.12- ☑

foot M71.17- ☑

hand M71.14- ☑

hip M71.15- ☑

knee M71.16- ☑

multiple sites M71.19

shoulder M71.11- ☑

specified site NEC M71.18

wrist M71.13- ☑

ischial — see Bursitis, hip

knee NEC M70.5- ☑

prepatellar M70.4- ☑

occupational NEC — see also Disorder, soft tissue, due to, use

olecranon — see Bursitis, elbow, olecranon

pharyngeal J39.1

popliteal — see Bursitis, knee

prepatellar M70.4- ☑

radiohumeral M77.8

rheumatoid M06.20

Bursitis — continued

rheumatoid — continued

ankle M06.27- ☑

elbow M06.22- ☑

foot joint M06.27- ☑

hand joint M06.24- ☑

hip M06.25- ☑

knee M06.26- ☑

multiple site M06.29

shoulder M06.21- ☑

vertebra M06.28

wrist M06.23- ☑

scapulohumeral — see Bursitis, shoulder

semimembranous muscle (knee) — see Bursitis, knee

shoulder M75.5- ☑

adhesive — see Capsulitis, adhesive

specified NEC M71.50

ankle M71.57- ☑

due to use, overuse or pressure — see Disorder, soft tissue, due to, use

elbow M71.52- ☑

foot M71.57- ☑

hand M71.54- ☑

hip M71.55- ☑

knee M71.56- ☑

shoulder — see Bursitis, shoulder

specified site NEC M71.58

tibial collateral M76.4- ☑

wrist M71.53- ☑

subacromial — see Bursitis, shoulder

subcoracoid — see Bursitis, shoulder

subdeltoid — see Bursitis, shoulder

syphilitic A52.78

Thornwaldt, Tornwaldt J39.2

tibial collateral M76.4- ☑

toe — see Enthesopathy, foot, specified type NEC

trochanteric (area) — see Bursitis, hip, trochanteric

wrist — see Bursitis, hand

Bursopathy M71.9

specified type NEC M71.80

ankle M71.87- ☑

elbow M71.82- ☑

foot M71.87- ☑

hand M71.84- ☑

hip M71.85- ☑

knee M71.86- ☑

multiple sites M71.89

shoulder M71.81- ☑

specified site NEC M71.88

wrist M71.83- ☑

Burst stitches or sutures (complication of surgery) T81.31 ☑

external operation wound T81.31 ☑

internal operation wound T81.32 ☑

Buruli ulcer A31.1

Bury's disease L95.1

Buschke's

disease B45.3

scleredema — see Sclerosis, systemic

Busse-Buschke disease B45.3

Buttock — see condition

Button

Biskra B55.1

Delhi B55.1

oriental B55.1

Buttonhole deformity (finger) — see Deformity, finger, boutonniere

Bwamba fever A92.8

Byssinosis J66.0

Bywaters' syndrome T79.5 ☑

C

Cachexia R64

cancerous R64

cardiac — see Disease, heart

dehydration E86.0

due to malnutrition R64

exophthalmic — see Hyperthyroidism

heart — see Disease, heart

hypophyseal E23.0

hypopituitary E23.0

lead — see Poisoning, lead

malignant R64

marsh — see Malaria

nervous F48.8

Cachexia — continued

old age R54

paludal — see Malaria

pituitary E23.0

renal N28.9

saturnine — see Poisoning, lead

senile R54

Simmonds' E23.0

splenica D73.0

strumipriva E03.4

tuberculous NEC — see Tuberculosis

CADASIL (cerebral autosomal dominant arteriopathy with subcortical infarcts and leukoencephalopathy) I67.850

Café, au lait spots L81.3

Caffeine-induced

anxiety disorder F15.980

sleep disorder F15.982

Caffey's syndrome Q78.8

Caisson disease T70.3 ☑

Cake kidney Q63.1

Caked breast (puerperal, postpartum) O92.79

Calabar swelling B74.3

Calcaneal spur — see Spur, bone, calcaneal

Calcaneo-apophysitis M92.8

Calcareous — see condition

Calcicosis J62.8

Calciferol (vitamin D) deficiency E55.9

with rickets E55.0

Calcification

adrenal (capsule) (gland) E27.49

tuberculous E35 [B90.8]

aorta I70.0

artery (annular) — see Arteriosclerosis

auricle (ear) — see Disorder, pinna, specified type NEC

basal ganglia G23.8

bladder N32.89

due to Schistosoma hematobium B65.0

brain (cortex) — see Calcification, cerebral

bronchus J98.09

bursa M71.40

ankle M71.47- ☑

elbow M71.42- ☑

foot M71.47- ☑

hand M71.44- ☑

hip M71.45- ☑

knee M71.46- ☑

multiple sites M71.49

shoulder M75.3- ☑

specified site NEC M71.48

wrist M71.43- ☑

cardiac — see Degeneration, myocardial

cerebral (cortex) G93.89

artery I67.2

cervix (uteri) N88.8

choroid plexus G93.89

conjunctiva — see Concretion, conjunctiva

corpora cavernosa (penis) N48.89

cortex (brain) — see Calcification, cerebral

dental pulp (nodular) K04.2

dentinal papilla K00.4

fallopian tube N83.8

falx cerebri G96.19

gallbladder K82.8

general E83.59

heart — see also Degeneration, myocardial

valve — see Endocarditis

idiopathic infantile arterial (IIAC) Q28.8

intervertebral cartilage or disc (postinfective) — see Disorder, disc, specified NEC

intracranial — see Calcification, cerebral

joint — see Disorder, joint, specified type NEC

kidney N28.89

tuberculous N29 [B90.1]

larynx (senile) J38.7

lens — see Cataract, specified NEC

lung (active) (postinfectional) J98.4

tuberculous B90.9

lymph gland or node (postinfectional) I89.8

tuberculous — see also Tuberculosis, lymph gland B90.8

mammographic R92.1

massive (paraplegic) — see Myositis, ossificans, in, quadriplegia

medial — see Arteriosclerosis, extremities

meninges (cerebral) (spinal) G96.19

metastatic E83.59

Calcification — *continued*
 Mönckeberg's — *see* Arteriosclerosis, extremities
 muscle M61.9
  due to burns — *see* Myositis, ossificans, in, burns
  paralytic — *see* Myositis, ossificans, in, quadriplegia
  specified type NEC M61.40
   ankle M61.47- ☑
   foot M61.47- ☑
   forearm M61.43- ☑
   hand M61.44- ☑
   lower leg M61.46- ☑
   multiple sites M61.49
   pelvic region M61.45- ☑
   shoulder region M61.41- ☑
   specified site NEC M61.48
   thigh M61.45- ☑
   upper arm M61.42- ☑
 myocardium, myocardial — *see* Degeneration, myocardial
 ovary N83.8
 pancreas K86.89
 penis N48.89
 periarticular — *see* Disorder, joint, specified type NEC
 pericardium — *see also* Pericarditis I31.1
 pineal gland E34.8
 pleura J94.8
  postinfectional J94.8
  tuberculous NEC B90.9
 pulpal (dental) (nodular) K04.2
 sclera H15.89
 spleen D73.89
 subcutaneous L94.2
 suprarenal (capsule) (gland) E27.49
 tendon (sheath) — *see also* Tenosynovitis, specified type NEC
  with bursitis, synovitis or tenosynovitis — *see* Tendinitis, calcific
 trachea J39.8
 ureter N28.89
 uterus N85.8
 vitreous — *see* Deposit, crystalline
Calcified — *see* Calcification
Calcinosis (interstitial) (tumoral) (universalis) E83.59
 with Raynaud's phenomenon, esophageal dysfunction, sclerodactyly, telangiectasia (CREST syndrome) M34.1
 circumscripta (skin) L94.2
 cutis L94.2
Calciphylaxis — *see also* Calcification, by site E83.59
Calcium
 deposits — *see* Calcification, by site
 metabolism disorder E83.50
 salts or soaps in vitreous — *see* Deposit, crystalline
Calciuria R82.994
Calculi — *see* Calculus
Calculosis, intrahepatic — *see* Calculus, bile duct
Calculus, calculi, calculous
 ampulla of Vater — *see* Calculus, bile duct
 anuria (impacted) (recurrent) — *see also* Calculus, urinary N20.9
 appendix K38.1
 bile duct (common) (hepatic) K80.50
  with
   calculus of gallbladder — *see* Calculus, gallbladder and bile duct
   cholangitis K80.30
    with
     cholecystitis — *see* Calculus, bile duct, with cholecystitis
     obstruction K80.31
    acute K80.32
     with
      chronic cholangitis K80.36
       with obstruction K80.37
      obstruction K80.33
    chronic K80.34
     with
      acute cholangitis K80.36
       with obstruction K80.37
      obstruction K80.35
   cholecystitis (with cholangitis) K80.40
    with obstruction K80.41
    acute K80.42
     with
      chronic cholecystitis K80.46
       with obstruction K80.47
      obstruction K80.43
     chronic K80.44

Calculus, calculi, calculous — *continued*
 bile duct — *continued*
  with — *continued*
   cholecystitis — *continued*
    chronic — *continued*
     with
      acute cholecystitis K80.46
       with obstruction K80.47
      obstruction K80.45
  biliary — *see also* Calculus, gallbladder
   specified NEC K80.80
    with obstruction K80.81
  bilirubin, multiple — *see* Calculus, gallbladder
  bladder (encysted) (impacted) (urinary) (diverticulum) N21.0
  bronchus J98.09
  calyx (kidney) (renal) — *see* Calculus, kidney
  cholesterol (pure) (solitary) — *see* Calculus, gallbladder
  common duct (bile) — *see* Calculus, bile duct
  conjunctiva — *see* Concretion, conjunctiva
  cystic N21.0
   duct — *see* Calculus, gallbladder
  dental (subgingival) (supragingival) K03.6
  diverticulum
   bladder N21.0
   kidney N20.0
  epididymis N50.89
  gallbladder K80.20
   with
    bile duct calculus — *see* Calculus, gallbladder and bile duct
    cholecystitis K80.10
     with obstruction K80.11
     acute K80.00
      with
       chronic cholecystitis K80.12
        with obstruction K80.13
       obstruction K80.01
     chronic K80.10
      with
       acute cholecystitis K80.12
        with obstruction K80.13
       obstruction K80.11
    specified NEC K80.18
     with obstruction K80.19
    obstruction K80.21
  gallbladder and bile duct K80.70
   with
    cholecystitis K80.60
     with obstruction K80.61
     acute K80.62
      with
       chronic cholecystitis K80.66
        with obstruction K80.67
       obstruction K80.63
     chronic K80.64
      with
       acute cholecystitis K80.66
        with obstruction K80.67
       obstruction K80.65
    obstruction K80.71
  hepatic (duct) — *see* Calculus, bile duct
  ileal conduit N21.8
  intestinal (impaction) (obstruction) K56.49
  kidney (impacted) (multiple) (pelvis) (recurrent) (staghorn) N20.0
   with calculus, ureter N20.2
   congenital Q63.8
  lacrimal passages — *see* Dacryolith
  liver (impacted) — *see* Calculus, bile duct
  lung J98.4
  mammographic R92.1
  nephritic (impacted) (recurrent) — *see* Calculus, kidney
  nose J34.89
  pancreas (duct) K86.89
  parotid duct or gland K11.5
  pelvis, encysted — *see* Calculus, kidney
  prostate N42.0
  pulmonary J98.4
  pyelitis (impacted) (recurrent) N20.0
   with hydronephrosis N13.6
  pyelonephritis (impacted) (recurrent) — *see* category N20 ☑
   with hydronephrosis N13.6
  renal (impacted) (recurrent) — *see* Calculus, kidney
  salivary (duct) (gland) K11.5
  seminal vesicle N50.89
  staghorn — *see* Calculus, kidney

Calculus, calculi, calculous — *continued*
 Stensen's duct K11.5
 stomach K31.89
 sublingual duct or gland K11.5
  congenital Q38.4
 submandibular duct, gland or region K11.5
 submaxillary duct, gland or region K11.5
 suburethral N21.8
 tonsil J35.8
 tooth, teeth (subgingival) (supragingival) K03.6
 tunica vaginalis N50.89
 ureter (impacted) (recurrent) N20.1
  with calculus, kidney N20.2
   with hydronephrosis N13.2
    with infection N13.6
 urethra (impacted) N21.1
 urinary (duct) (impacted) (passage) (tract) N20.9
  with hydronephrosis N13.2
   with infection N13.6
  in (due to)
   lower N21.9
    specified NEC N21.8
 vagina N89.8
 vesical (impacted) N21.0
 Wharton's duct K11.5
 xanthine E79.8 *[N22]*
Calicectasis N28.89
Caliectasis N28.89
California
 disease B38.9
 encephalitis A83.5
Caligo cornea — *see* Opacity, cornea, central
Callositas, callosity (infected) L84
Callus (infected) L84
 bone — *see* Osteophyte
 excessive, following fracture — *code as* Sequelae of fracture
CALME (childhood asymmetric labium majus enlargement) N90.61
Calorie deficiency or malnutrition — *see also* Malnutrition E46
Calvé-Perthes disease — *see* Legg-Calvé-Perthes disease
Calvé's disease — *see* Osteochondrosis, juvenile, spine
Calvities — *see* Alopecia, androgenic
Cameroon fever — *see* Malaria
Camptocormia (hysterical) F44.4
Camurati-Engelmann syndrome Q78.3
Canal — *see also* condition
 atrioventricular common Q21.2
Canaliculitis (lacrimal) (acute) (subacute) H04.33- ☑
 Actinomyces A42.89
 chronic H04.42- ☑
Canavan's disease E75.29
Canceled procedure (surgical) Z53.9
 because of
  contraindication Z53.09
   smoking Z53.01
  left against medical advice (AMA) Z53.29
  patient's decision Z53.20
   for reasons of belief or group pressure Z53.1
   specified reason NEC Z53.29
  specified reason NEC Z53.8
Cancer — *see also* Neoplasm, by site, malignant
 bile duct type liver C22.1
 blood — *see* Leukemia
 breast — *see also* Neoplasm, breast, malignant C50.91- ☑
 hepatocellular C22.0
 lung — *see also* Neoplasm, lung, malignant C34.90
 ovarian — *see also* Neoplasm ovary, malignant C56.9
 unspecified site (primary) C80.1
Cancer (o)phobia F45.29
Cancerous — *see* Neoplasm, malignant, by site
Cancrum oris A69.0
Candidiasis, candidal B37.9
 balanitis B37.42
 bronchitis B37.1
 cheilitis B37.83
 congenital P37.5
 cystitis B37.41
 disseminated B37.7
 endocarditis B37.6
 enteritis B37.82
 esophagitis B37.81
 intertrigo B37.2
 lung B37.1
 meningitis B37.5

Candidiasis, candidal — continued
- mouth B37.0
- nails B37.2
- neonatal P37.5
- onychia B37.2
- oral B37.0
- osteomyelitis B37.89
- otitis externa B37.84
- paronychia B37.2
- perionyxis B37.2
- pneumonia B37.1
- proctitis B37.82
- pulmonary B37.1
- pyelonephritis B37.49
- sepsis B37.7
- skin B37.2
- specified site NEC B37.89
- stomatitis B37.0
- systemic B37.7
- urethritis B37.41
- urogenital site NEC B37.49
- vagina B37.3
- vulva B37.3
- vulvovaginitis B37.3

Candidid L30.2
Candidosis — see Candidiasis
Candiru infection or infestation B88.8
Canities (premature) L67.1
- congenital Q84.2
Canker (mouth) (sore) K12.0
- rash A38.9
Cannabinosis J66.2
Cannabis induced
- anxiety disorder F12.980
- psychotic disorder F12.959
- sleep disorder F12.988
Canton fever A75.9
Cantrell's syndrome Q87.89
Capillariasis (intestinal) B81.1
- hepatic B83.8
Capillary — see condition
Caplan's syndrome — see Rheumatoid, lung
Capsule — see condition
Capsulitis (joint) — see also Enthesopathy
- adhesive (shoulder) M75.0- ☑
- hepatic K65.8
- labyrinthine — see Otosclerosis, specified NEC
- thyroid E06.9
Caput
- crepitus Q75.8
- medusae I86.8
- succedaneum P12.81
Car sickness T75.3 ☑
Carapata (disease) A68.0
Carate — see Pinta
Carbon lung J60
Carbuncle L02.93
- abdominal wall L02.231
- anus K61.0
- auditory canal, external — see Abscess, ear, external
- auricle ear — see Abscess, ear, external
- axilla L02.43- ☑
- back (any part) L02.232
- breast N61.1
- buttock L02.33
- cheek (external) L02.03
- chest wall L02.233
- chin L02.03
- corpus cavernosum N48.21
- ear (any part) (external) (middle) — see Abscess, ear, external
- external auditory canal — see Abscess, ear, external
- eyelid — see Abscess, eyelid
- face NEC L02.03
- femoral (region) — see Carbuncle, lower limb
- finger — see Carbuncle, hand
- flank L02.231
- foot L02.63- ☑
- forehead L02.03
- genital — see Abscess, genital
- gluteal (region) L02.33
- groin L02.234
- hand L02.53- ☑
- head NEC L02.831
- heel — see Carbuncle, foot
- hip — see Carbuncle, lower limb
- kidney — see Abscess, kidney

Carbuncle — continued
- knee — see Carbuncle, lower limb
- labium (majus) (minus) N76.4
- lacrimal
  - gland — see Dacryoadenitis
  - passages (duct) (sac) — see Inflammation, lacrimal, passages, acute
- leg — see Carbuncle, lower limb
- lower limb L02.43- ☑
- malignant A22.0
- navel L02.236
- neck L02.13
- nose (external) (septum) J34.0
- orbit, orbital — see Abscess, orbit
- palmar (space) — see Carbuncle, hand
- partes posteriores L02.33
- pectoral region L02.233
- penis N48.21
- perineum L02.235
- pinna — see Abscess, ear, external
- popliteal — see Carbuncle, lower limb
- scalp L02.831
- seminal vesicle N49.0
- shoulder — see Carbuncle, upper limb
- specified site NEC L02.838
- temple (region) L02.03
- thumb — see Carbuncle, hand
- toe — see Carbuncle, foot
- trunk L02.239
  - abdominal wall L02.231
  - back L02.232
  - chest wall L02.233
  - groin L02.234
  - perineum L02.235
  - umbilicus L02.236
- umbilicus L02.236
- upper limb L02.43- ☑
- urethra N34.0
- vulva N76.4

Carbunculus — see Carbuncle
Carcinoid (tumor) — see Tumor, carcinoid
Carcinoidosis E34.0
Carcinoma (malignant) — see also Neoplasm, by site, malignant
- acidophil
  - specified site — see Neoplasm, malignant, by site
  - unspecified site C75.1
- acidophil-basophil, mixed
  - specified site — see Neoplasm, malignant, by site
  - unspecified site C75.1
- adnexal (skin) — see Neoplasm, skin, malignant
- adrenal cortical C74.0- ☑
- alveolar — see Neoplasm, lung, malignant
  - cell — see Neoplasm, lung, malignant
- ameloblastic C41.1
  - upper jaw (bone) C41.0
- apocrine
  - breast — see Neoplasm, breast, malignant
  - specified site NEC — see Neoplasm, skin, malignant
  - unspecified site C44.99
- basal cell (pigmented) (see also Neoplasm, skin, malignant) C44.91
  - fibro-epithelial — see Neoplasm, skin, malignant
  - morphea — see Neoplasm, skin, malignant
  - multicentric — see Neoplasm, skin, malignant
- basaloid
- basal-squamous cell, mixed — see Neoplasm, skin, malignant
- basophil
  - specified site — see Neoplasm, malignant, by site
  - unspecified site C75.1
- basophil-acidophil, mixed
  - specified site — see Neoplasm, malignant, by site
  - unspecified site C75.1
- basosquamous — see Neoplasm, skin, malignant
- bile duct
  - with hepatocellular, mixed C22.0
    - liver C22.1
  - specified site NEC — see Neoplasm, malignant, by site
  - unspecified site C22.1
- branchial or branchiogenic C10.4
- bronchial or bronchogenic — see Neoplasm, lung, malignant
- bronchiolar — see Neoplasm, lung, malignant
- bronchioloalveolar — see Neoplasm, lung, malignant

Carcinoma — continued
- C cell
  - specified site — see Neoplasm, malignant, by site
  - unspecified site C73
- ceruminous C44.29- ☑
- cervix uteri
  - in situ D06.9
    - endocervix D06.0
    - exocervix D06.1
    - specified site NEC D06.7
- chorionic
  - specified site — see Neoplasm, malignant, by site
  - unspecified site
    - female C58
    - male C62.90
- chromophobe
  - specified site — see Neoplasm, malignant, by site
  - unspecified site C75.1
- cloacogenic
  - specified site — see Neoplasm, malignant, by site
  - unspecified site C21.2
- diffuse type
  - specified site — see Neoplasm, malignant, by site
  - unspecified site C16.9
- duct (cell)
  - with Paget's disease — see Neoplasm, breast, malignant
  - infiltrating
    - with lobular carcinoma (in situ)
      - specified site — see Neoplasm, malignant, by site
      - unspecified site (female) C50.91- ☑
        - male C50.92- ☑
    - specified site — see Neoplasm, malignant, by site
    - unspecified site (female) C50.91- ☑
      - male C50.92- ☑
- ductal
  - with lobular
    - specified site — see Neoplasm, malignant, by site
    - unspecified site (female) C50.91- ☑
      - male C50.92- ☑
- ductular, infiltrating
  - specified site — see Neoplasm, malignant, by site
  - unspecified site (female) C50.91- ☑
    - male C50.92- ☑
- embryonal
  - liver C22.7
- endometrioid
  - specified site — see Neoplasm, malignant, by site
  - unspecified site
    - female C56.9
    - male C61
- eosinophil
  - specified site — see Neoplasm, malignant, by site
  - unspecified site C75.1
- epidermoid — see also Neoplasm, skin, malignant
  - in situ, Bowen's type — see Neoplasm, skin, in situ
- fibroepithelial, basal cell — see Neoplasm, skin, malignant
- follicular
  - with papillary (mixed) C73
  - moderately differentiated C73
  - pure follicle C73
  - specified site — see Neoplasm, malignant, by site
  - trabecular C73
  - unspecified site C73
  - well differentiated C73
- generalized, with unspecified primary site C80.0
- glycogen-rich — see Neoplasm, breast, malignant
- granulosa cell C56- ☑
- hepatic cell C22.0
- hepatocellular C22.0
  - with bile duct, mixed C22.0
  - fibrolamellar C22.0
- hepatocholangiolitic C22.0
- Hurthle cell C73
- in
  - adenomatous
    - polyposis coli C18.9
  - pleomorphic adenoma — see Neoplasm, salivary glands, malignant
  - situ — see Carcinoma-in-situ

☑ **Additional Character Required** — Refer to the Tabular List for Character Selection   ▽ **Subterms under main terms may continue to next column or page**

Index

Carcinoma — *continued*
  infiltrating
    duct
      with lobular
        specified site — *see* Neoplasm, malignant, by
          site
        unspecified site (female) C50.91- ☑
          male C50.92- ☑
      with Paget's disease — *see* Neoplasm, breast,
        malignant
      specified site — *see* Neoplasm, malignant
      unspecified site (female) C50.91- ☑
        male C50.92- ☑
    ductular
      specified site — *see* Neoplasm, malignant
      unspecified site (female) C50.91- ☑
        male C50.92- ☑
    lobular
      specified site — *see* Neoplasm, malignant
      unspecified site (female) C50.91- ☑
        male C50.92- ☑
  inflammatory
    specified site — *see* Neoplasm, malignant
    unspecified site (female) C50.91- ☑
      male C50.92- ☑
  intestinal type
    specified site — *see* Neoplasm, malignant, by site
    unspecified site C16.9
  intracystic
    noninfiltrating — *see* Neoplasm, in situ, by site
  intraductal (noninfiltrating)
    with Paget's disease — *see* Neoplasm, breast, ma-
      lignant
    breast D05.1- ☑
    papillary
      with invasion
        specified site — *see* Neoplasm, malignant, by
          site
        unspecified site (female) C50.91- ☑
          male C50.92- ☑
      breast D05.1- ☑
      specified site NEC — *see* Neoplasm, in situ, by
        site
      unspecified site (female) D05.1- ☑
    specified site NEC — *see* Neoplasm, in situ, by site
    unspecified site (female) D05.1- ☑
  intraepidermal — *see* Neoplasm, in situ
    squamous cell, Bowen's type — *see* Neoplasm, skin,
      in situ
  intraepithelial — *see* Neoplasm, in situ, by site
    squamous cell — *see* Neoplasm, in situ, by site
  intraosseous C41.1
    upper jaw (bone) C41.0
  islet cell
    with exocrine, mixed
      specified site — *see* Neoplasm, malignant, by
        site
      unspecified site C25.9
    pancreas C25.4
    specified site NEC — *see* Neoplasm, malignant, by
      site
    unspecified site C25.4
  juvenile, breast — *see* Neoplasm, breast, malignant
  large cell
    small cell
      specified site — *see* Neoplasm, malignant, by
        site
      unspecified site C34.90
  Leydig cell (testis)
    specified site — *see* Neoplasm, malignant, by site
    unspecified site
      female C56.9
      male C62.90
  lipid-rich (female) C50.91- ☑
    male C50.92- ☑
  liver cell C22.0
  liver NEC C22.7
  lobular (infiltrating)
    with intraductal
      specified site — *see* Neoplasm, malignant, by
        site
      unspecified site (female) C50.91- ☑
        male C50.92- ☑
    noninfiltrating
      breast D05.0- ☑
      specified site NEC — *see* Neoplasm, in situ, by
        site

Carcinoma — *continued*
  lobular — *continued*
    noninfiltrating — *continued*
      unspecified site D05.0- ☑
    specified site — *see* Neoplasm, malignant, by site
    unspecified site (female) C50.91- ☑
      male C50.92- ☑
  medullary
    with
      amyloid stroma
        specified site — *see* Neoplasm, malignant, by
          site
        unspecified site C73
      lymphoid stroma
        specified site — *see* Neoplasm, malignant, by
          site
        unspecified site (female) C50.91- ☑
          male C50.92- ☑
  Merkel cell C4A.9 *(following* C43)
    anal margin C4A.51 *(following* C43)
    anal skin C4A.51 *(following* C43)
    canthus C4A.1- ☑ *(following* C43)
    ear and external auricular canal C4A.2- ☑ *(following*
      C43)
    external auricular canal C4A.2- ☑ *(following* C43)
    eyelid, including canthus C4A.1- ☑ *(following* C43)
    face C4A.30 *(following* C43)
      specified NEC C4A.39 *(following* C43)
    hip C4A.7- ☑ *(following* C43)
    lip C4A.0 *(following* C43)
    lower limb, including hip C4A.7- ☑ *(following* C43)
    neck C4A.4 *(following* C43)
    nodal presentation C7B.1 *(following* C75)
    nose C4A.31 *(following* C43)
    overlapping sites C4A.8 *(following* C43)
    perianal skin C4A.51 *(following* C43)
    scalp C4A.4 *(following* C43)
    secondary C7B.1 *(following* C75)
    shoulder C4A.6- ☑ *(following* C43)
    skin of breast C4A.52 *(following* C43)
    trunk NEC C4A.59 *(following* C43)
    upper limb, including shoulder C4A.6- ☑ *(following*
      C43)
    visceral metastatic C7B.1 *(following* C75)
  metastatic — *see* Neoplasm, secondary, by site
  metatypical — *see* Neoplasm, skin, malignant
  morphea, basal cell — *see* Neoplasm, skin, malignant
  mucoid
    cell
      specified site — *see* Neoplasm, malignant, by
        site
      unspecified site C75.1
  neuroendocrine — *see also* Tumor, neuroendocrine
    high grade, any site C7A.1 *(following* C75)
    poorly differentiated, any site C7A.1 *(following* C75)
  nonencapsulated sclerosing C73
  noninfiltrating
    intracystic — *see* Neoplasm, in situ, by site
    intraductal
      breast D05.1- ☑
      papillary
        breast D05.1- ☑
        specified site NEC — *see* Neoplasm, in situ,
          by site
        unspecified site D05.1- ☑
      specified site — *see* Neoplasm, in situ, by site
      unspecified site D05.1- ☑
    lobular
      breast D05.0- ☑
      specified site NEC — *see* Neoplasm, in situ, by
        site
      unspecified site (female) D05.0- ☑
  oat cell
    specified site — *see* Neoplasm, malignant, by site
    unspecified site C34.90
  odontogenic C41.1
    upper jaw (bone) C41.0
  papillary
    with follicular (mixed) C73
    follicular variant C73
    intraductal (noninfiltrating)
      with invasion
        specified site — *see* Neoplasm, malignant, by
          site
        unspecified site (female) C50.91- ☑
          male C50.92- ☑
      breast D05.1- ☑

Carcinoma — *continued*
  papillary — *continued*
    intraductal — *continued*
      specified site NEC — *see* Neoplasm, in situ, by
        site
      unspecified site D05.1- ☑
    serous
      specified site — *see* Neoplasm, malignant, by
        site
      surface
        specified site — *see* Neoplasm, malignant, by
          site
        unspecified site C56.9
      unspecified site C56.9
  papillocystic
    specified site — *see* Neoplasm, malignant, by site
    unspecified site C56.9
  parafollicular cell
    specified site — *see* Neoplasm, malignant, by site
    unspecified site C73
  pilomatrix — *see* Neoplasm, skin, malignant
  pseudomucinous
    specified site — *see* Neoplasm, malignant, by site
    unspecified site C56.9
  renal cell C64- ☑
  Schmincke — *see* Neoplasm, nasopharynx, malignant
  Schneiderian
    specified site — *see* Neoplasm, malignant, by site
    unspecified site C30.0
  sebaceous — *see* Neoplasm, skin, malignant
  secondary — *see also* Neoplasm, secondary, by site
    Merkel cell C7B.1 *(following* C75)
  secretory, breast — *see* Neoplasm, breast, malignant
  serous
    papillary
      specified site — *see* Neoplasm, malignant, by
        site
      unspecified site C56.9
    surface, papillary
      specified site — *see* Neoplasm, malignant, by
        site
      unspecified site C56.9
  Sertoli cell
    specified site — *see* Neoplasm, malignant, by site
    unspecified site C62.90
      female C56.9
      male C62.90
  skin appendage — *see* Neoplasm, skin, malignant
  small cell
    fusiform cell
      specified site — *see* Neoplasm, malignant, by
        site
      unspecified site C34.90
    intermediate cell
      specified site — *see* Neoplasm, malignant, by
        site
      unspecified site C34.90
    large cell
      specified site — *see* Neoplasm, malignant, by
        site
      unspecified site C34.90
  solid
    with amyloid stroma
      specified site — *see* Neoplasm, malignant, by
        site
      unspecified site C73
    microinvasive
      specified site — *see* Neoplasm, malignant, by
        site
      unspecified site C53.9
  sweat gland — *see* Neoplasm, skin, malignant
  theca cell C56.- ☑
  thymic C37
  unspecified site (primary) C80.1
  water-clear cell C75.0
Carcinoma-in-situ — *see also* Neoplasm, in situ, by site
  breast NOS D05.9- ☑
    specified type NEC D05.8- ☑
  epidermoid — *see also* Neoplasm, in situ, by site
    with questionable stromal invasion
      cervix D06.9
      specified site NEC — *see* Neoplasm, in situ, by
        site
      unspecified site D06.9
    Bowen's type — *see* Neoplasm, skin, in situ
  intraductal
    breast D05.1- ☑
    specified site NEC — *see* Neoplasm, in situ, by site

Carcinoma — Carcinoma-in-situ

Carcinoma-in-situ — continued
  intraductal — continued
    unspecified site D05.1- ☑
  lobular
   · with
      infiltrating duct
        breast (female) C50.91- ☑
          male C50.92- ☑
        specified site NEC — see Neoplasm, malignant
        unspecified site (female) C50.91- ☑
          male C50.92- ☑
      intraductal
        breast D05.8- ☑
        specified site NEC — see Neoplasm, in situ, by site
        unspecified site (female) D05.8- ☑
    breast D05.0- ☑
    specified site NEC — see Neoplasm, in situ, by site
    unspecified site D05.0- ☑
  squamous cell — see also Neoplasm, in situ, by site
    with questionable stromal invasion
      cervix D06.9
      specified site NEC — see Neoplasm, in situ, by site
      unspecified site D06.9
Carcinomaphobia F45.29
Carcinomatosis C80.0
  peritonei C78.6
  unspecified site (primary) (secondary) C80.0
Carcinosarcoma — see Neoplasm, malignant, by site
  embryonal — see Neoplasm, malignant, by site
Cardia, cardial — see condition
Cardiac — see also condition
  death, sudden — see Arrest, cardiac
  pacemaker
    in situ Z95.0
    management or adjustment Z45.018
  tamponade I31.4
Cardialgia — see Pain, precordial
Cardiectasis — see Hypertrophy, cardiac
Cardiochalasia K21.9
Cardiomalacia I51.5
Cardiomegalia glycogenica diffusa E74.02 [I43]
Cardiomegaly — see also Hypertrophy, cardiac
  congenital Q24.8
  glycogen E74.02 [I43]
  idiopathic I51.7
Cardiomyoliposis I51.5
Cardiomyopathy (familial) (idiopathic) I42.9
  alcoholic I42.6
  amyloid E85.4 [I43]
    transthyretin-related (ATTR) familial E85.4 [I43]
  arteriosclerotic — see Disease, heart, ischemic, atherosclerotic
  beriberi E51.12
  cobalt-beer I42.6
  congenital I42.4
  congestive I42.0
  constrictive NOS I42.5
  dilated I42.0
  due to
    alcohol I42.6
    beriberi E51.12
    cardiac glycogenosis E74.02 [I43]
    drugs I42.7
    external agents NEC I42.7
    Friedreich's ataxia G11.1
    myotonia atrophica G71.11 [I43]
    progressive muscular dystrophy G71.09 [I43]
  glycogen storage E74.02 [I43]
  hypertensive — see Hypertension, heart
  hypertrophic (nonobstructive) I42.2
    obstructive I42.1
      congenital Q24.8
  in
    Chagas' disease (chronic) B57.2
      acute B57.0
    sarcoidosis D86.85
  ischemic I25.5
  metabolic E88.9 [I43]
    thyrotoxic E05.90 [I43]
      with thyroid storm E05.91 [I43]
  newborn I42.8
    congenital I42.4
  non-ischemic — see also by cause I42.8
  nutritional E63.9 [I43]
    beriberi E51.12

Cardiomyopathy — continued
  obscure of Africa I42.8
  peripartum O90.3
  postpartum O90.3
  restrictive NEC I42.5
  rheumatic I09.0
  secondary I42.9
  specified NEC I42.8
  stress induced I51.81
  takotsubo I51.81
  thyrotoxic E05.90 [I43]
    with thyroid storm E05.91 [I43]
  toxic NEC I42.7
  transthyretin-related (ATTR) familial amyloid E85.4
  tuberculous A18.84
  viral B33.24
Cardionephritis — see Hypertension, cardiorenal
Cardionephropathy — see Hypertension, cardiorenal
Cardionephrosis — see Hypertension, cardiorenal
Cardiopathia nigra I27.0
Cardiopathy — see also Disease, heart I51.9
  idiopathic I42.9
  mucopolysaccharidosis E76.3 [I52]
Cardiopericarditis — see Pericarditis
Cardiophobia F45.29
Cardiorenal — see condition
Cardiorrhexis — see Infarct, myocardium
Cardiosclerosis — see Disease, heart, ischemic, atherosclerotic
Cardiosis — see Disease, heart
Cardiospasm (esophagus) (reflex) (stomach) K22.0
  congenital Q39.5
    with megaesophagus Q39.5
Cardiostenosis — see Disease, heart
Cardiosymphysis I31.0
Cardiovascular — see condition
Carditis (acute) (bacterial) (chronic) (subacute) I51.89
  meningococcal A39.50
  rheumatic — see Disease, heart, rheumatic
  rheumatoid — see Rheumatoid, carditis
  viral B33.20
Care (of) (for) (following)
  child (routine) Z76.2
  family member (handicapped) (sick)
    creating problem for family Z63.6
    provided away from home for holiday relief Z75.5
    unavailable, due to
      absence (person rendering care) (sufferer) Z74.2
      inability (any reason) of person rendering care Z74.2
  foundling Z76.1
  holiday relief Z75.5
  improper — see Maltreatment
  lack of (at or after birth) (infant) — see Maltreatment, child, neglect
  lactating mother Z39.1
  palliative Z51.5
  postpartum
    immediately after delivery Z39.0
    routine follow-up Z39.2
  respite Z75.5
  unavailable, due to
    absence of person rendering care Z74.2
    inability (any reason) of person rendering care Z74.2
  well-baby Z76.2
Caries
  bone NEC A18.03
  dental (dentino enamel junction) (early childhood) (of dentine) (pre-eruptive) (recurrent) (to the pulp) K02.9
    arrested (coronal) (root) K02.3
    chewing surface
      limited to enamel K02.51
      penetrating into dentin K02.52
      penetrating into pulp K02.53
    coronal surface
      chewing surface
        limited to enamel K02.51
        penetrating into dentin K02.52
        penetrating into pulp K02.53
      pit and fissure surface
        limited to enamel K02.51
        penetrating into dentin K02.52
        penetrating into pulp K02.53
      smooth surface
        limited to enamel K02.61
        penetrating into dentin K02.62
        penetrating into pulp K02.63

Caries — continued
  dental — continued
    pit and fissure surface
      limited to enamel K02.51
      penetrating into dentin K02.52
      penetrating into pulp K02.53
    primary, cervical origin K02.52
    root K02.7
    smooth surface
      limited to enamel K02.61
      penetrating into dentin K02.62
      penetrating into pulp K02.63
  external meatus — see Disorder, ear, external, specified type NEC
  hip (tuberculous) A18.02
  initial (tooth)
    chewing surface K02.51
    pit and fissure surface K02.51
    smooth surface K02.61
  knee (tuberculous) A18.02
  labyrinth H83.8 ☑
  limb NEC (tuberculous) A18.03
  mastoid process (chronic) — see Mastoiditis, chronic
    tuberculous A18.03
  middle ear H74.8 ☑
  nose (tuberculous) A18.03
  orbit (tuberculous) A18.03
  ossicles, ear — see Abnormal, ear ossicles
  petrous bone — see Petrositis
  root (dental) (tooth) K02.7
  sacrum (tuberculous) A18.01
  spine, spinal (column) (tuberculous) A18.01
  syphilitic A52.77
    congenital (early) A50.02 [M90.80]
  tooth, teeth — see Caries, dental
  tuberculous A18.03
  vertebra (column) (tuberculous) A18.01
Carious teeth — see Caries, dental
Carneous mole O02.0
Carnitine insufficiency E71.40
Carotenemia (dietary) E67.1
Carotenosis (cutis) (skin) E67.1
Carotid body or sinus syndrome G90.01
Carotidynia G90.01
Carpal tunnel syndrome — see Syndrome, carpal tunnel
Carpenter's syndrome Q87.0
Carpopedal spasm — see Tetany
Carr-Barr-Plunkett syndrome Q97.1
Carrier (suspected) of
  amebiasis Z22.1
  bacterial disease NEC Z22.39
    diphtheria Z22.2
    intestinal infectious NEC Z22.1
      typhoid Z22.0
    meningococcal Z22.31
    sexually transmitted Z22.4
    specified NEC Z22.39
    staphylococcal (Methicillin susceptible) Z22.321
      Methicillin resistant Z22.322
    streptococcal Z22.338
      group B Z22.330
        complicating pregnancy or delivery O99.82- ☑
    typhoid Z22.0
  cholera Z22.1
  diphtheria Z22.2
  gastrointestinal pathogens NEC Z22.1
  genetic Z14.8
    cystic fibrosis Z14.1
    hemophilia A (asymptomatic) Z14.01
      symptomatic Z14.02
  gestational, pregnant Z33.1
  gonorrhea Z22.4
  HAA (hepatitis Australian-antigen) B18.8
  HB (c)(s)-AG B18.1
  hepatitis (viral) B18.9
    Australia-antigen (HAA) B18.8
    B surface antigen (HBsAg) B18.1
      with acute delta- (super)infection B17.0
    C B18.2
    specified NEC B18.8
  human T-cell lymphotropic virus type-1 (HTLV-1) infection Z22.6
  infectious organism Z22.9
    specified NEC Z22.8
  meningococci Z22.31
  Salmonella typhosa Z22.0
  serum hepatitis — see Carrier, hepatitis

Carrier of — *continued*
staphylococci (Methicillin susceptible) Z22.321
Methicillin resistant Z22.322
streptococci Z22.338
group B Z22.330
complicating pregnancy or delivery O99.82- ☑
syphilis Z22.4
typhoid Z22.0
venereal disease NEC Z22.4
Carrion's disease A44.0
Carter's relapsing fever (Asiatic) A68.1
Cartilage — *see* condition
Caruncle (inflamed)
conjunctiva (acute) — *see* Conjunctivitis, acute
labium (majus) (minus) N90.89
lacrimal — *see* Inflammation, lacrimal, passages
myrtiform N89.8
urethral (benign) N36.2
Cascade stomach K31.2
Caseation lymphatic gland (tuberculous) A18.2
Cassidy (-Scholte) syndrome (malignant carcinoid) E34.0
Castellani's disease A69.8
Castration, traumatic, male S38.231 ☑
Casts in urine R82.998
Cat
cry syndrome Q93.4
ear Q17.3
eye syndrome Q92.8
Catabolism, senile R54
Catalepsy (hysterical) F44.2
schizophrenic F20.2
Cataplexy (idiopathic) — *see* Narcolepsy
Cataract (cortical) (immature) (incipient) H26.9
with
neovascularization — *see* Cataract, complicated
age-related — *see* Cataract, senile
anterior
and posterior axial embryonal Q12.0
pyramidal Q12.0
associated with
galactosemia E74.21 *[H28]*
myotonic disorders G71.19 *[H28]*
blue Q12.0
central Q12.0
cerulean Q12.0
complicated H26.20
with
neovascularization H26.21- ☑
ocular disorder H26.22- ☑
glaucomatous flecks H26.23- ☑
congenital Q12.0
coraliform Q12.0
coronary Q12.0
crystalline Q12.0
diabetic — *see* Diabetes, cataract
drug-induced H26.3- ☑
due to
ocular disorder — *see* Cataract, complicated
radiation H26.8
electric H26.8
extraction status Z98.4- ☑
glass-blower's H26.8
heat ray H26.8
heterochromic — *see* Cataract, complicated
hypermature — *see* Cataract, senile, morgagnian type
in (due to)
chronic iridocyclitis — *see* Cataract, complicated
diabetes — *see* Diabetes, cataract
endocrine disease E34.9 *[H28]*
eye disease — *see* Cataract, complicated
hypoparathyroidism E20.9 *[H28]*
malnutrition-dehydration E46 *[H28]*
metabolic disease E88.9 *[H28]*
myotonic disorders G71.19 *[H28]*
nutritional disease E63.9 *[H28]*
infantile — *see* Cataract, presenile
irradiational — *see* Cataract, specified NEC
juvenile — *see* Cataract, presenile
malnutrition-dehydration E46 *[H28]*
morgagnian — *see* Cataract, senile, morgagnian type
myotonic G71.19 *[H28]*
myxedema E03.9 *[H28]*
nuclear
embryonal Q12.0
sclerosis — *see* Cataract, senile, nuclear
presenile H26.00- ☑
combined forms H26.06- ☑

Cataract — *continued*
presenile — *continued*
cortical H26.01- ☑
lamellar — *see* Cataract, presenile, cortical
nuclear H26.03- ☑
specified NEC H26.09
subcapsular polar (anterior) H26.04- ☑
posterior H26.05- ☑
zonular — *see* Cataract, presenile, cortical
secondary H26.40
Soemmering's ring H26.41- ☑
specified NEC H26.49- ☑
to eye disease — *see* Cataract, complicated
senile H25.9
brunescens — *see* Cataract, senile, nuclear
combined forms H25.81- ☑
coronary — *see* Cataract, senile, incipient
cortical H25.01- ☑
hypermature — *see* Cataract, senile, morgagnian type
incipient (mature) (total) H25.09- ☑
cortical — *see* Cataract, senile, cortical
subcapsular — *see* Cataract, senile, subcapsular
morgagnian type (hypermature) H25.2- ☑
nuclear (sclerosis) H25.1- ☑
polar subcapsular (anterior) (posterior) — *see* Cataract, senile, incipient
punctate — *see* Cataract, senile, incipient
specified NEC H25.89
subcapsular polar (anterior) H25.03- ☑
posterior H25.04- ☑
snowflake — *see* Diabetes, cataract
specified NEC H26.8
toxic — *see* Cataract, drug-induced
traumatic H26.10- ☑
localized H26.11- ☑
partially resolved H26.12- ☑
total H26.13- ☑
zonular (perinuclear) Q12.0
Cataracta — *see also* Cataract
brunescens — *see* Cataract, senile, nuclear
centralis pulverulenta Q12.0
cerulea Q12.0
complicata — *see* Cataract, complicated
congenita Q12.0
coralliformis Q12.0
coronaria Q12.0
diabetic — *see* Diabetes, cataract
membranacea
accreta — *see* Cataract, secondary
congenita Q12.0
nigra — *see* Cataract, senile, nuclear
sunflower — *see* Cataract, complicated
Catarrh, catarrhal (acute) (febrile) (infectious) (inflammation) — *see also* condition J00
bronchial — *see* Bronchitis
chest — *see* Bronchitis
chronic J31.0
due to congenital syphilis A50.03
enteric — *see* Enteritis
eustachian H68.009
fauces — *see* Pharyngitis
gastrointestinal — *see* Enteritis
gingivitis K05.00
nonplaque induced K05.01
plaque induced K05.00
hay — *see* Fever, hay
intestinal — *see* Enteritis
larynx, chronic J37.0
liver B15.9
with hepatic coma B15.0
lung — *see* Bronchitis
middle ear, chronic — *see* Otitis, media, nonsuppurative, chronic, serous
mouth K12.1
nasal (chronic) — *see* Rhinitis
nasobronchial J31.1
nasopharyngeal (chronic) J31.1
acute J00
pulmonary — *see* Bronchitis
spring (eye) (vernal) — *see* Conjunctivitis, acute, atopic
summer (hay) — *see* Fever, hay
throat J31.2
tubotympanal — *see also* Otitis, media, nonsuppurative
chronic — *see* Otitis, media, nonsuppurative, chronic, serous
Catatonia (schizophrenic) F20.2

Catatonic
disorder due to known physiologic condition F06.1
schizophrenia F20.2
stupor R40.1
Cat-scratch — *see also* Abrasion
disease or fever A28.1
Cauda equina — *see* condition
Cauliflower ear M95.1- ☑
Causalgia (upper limb) G56.4- ☑
lower limb G57.7- ☑
Cause
external, general effects T75.89 ☑
Caustic burn — *see* Corrosion, by site
Cavare's disease (familial periodic paralysis) G72.3
Cavernitis (penis) N48.29
Cavernositis N48.29
Cavernous — *see* condition
Cavitation of lung — *see also* Tuberculosis, pulmonary
nontuberculous J98.4
Cavities, dental — *see* Caries, dental
Cavity
lung — *see* Cavitation of lung
optic papilla Q14.2
pulmonary — *see* Cavitation of lung
Cavovarus foot, congenital Q66.1- ☑
Cavus foot (congenital) Q66.7- ☑
acquired — *see* Deformity, limb, foot, specified NEC
Cazenave's disease L10.2
Cecitis K52.9
with perforation, peritonitis, or rupture K65.8
Cecoureterocele Q62.32
Cecum — *see* condition
Celiac
artery compression syndrome I77.4
disease (with steatorrhea) K90.0
infantilism K90.0
Cell(s), cellular — *see also* condition
in urine R82.998
Cellulitis (diffuse) (phlegmonous) (septic) (suppurative) L03.90
abdominal wall L03.311
anaerobic A48.0
ankle — *see* Cellulitis, lower limb
anus K61.0
arm — *see* Cellulitis, upper limb
auricle (ear) — *see* Cellulitis, ear
axilla L03.11- ☑
back (any part) L03.312
breast (acute) (nonpuerperal) (subacute) N61.0
nipple N61.0
broad ligament
acute N73.0
buttock L03.317
cervical (meaning neck) L03.221
cervix (uteri) — *see* Cervicitis
cheek (external) L03.211
internal K12.2
chest wall L03.313
chronic L03.90
clostridial A48.0
corpus cavernosum N48.22
digit
finger — *see* Cellulitis, finger
toe — *see* Cellulitis, toe
Douglas' cul-de-sac or pouch
acute N73.0
drainage site (following operation) T81.49 ☑
ear (external) H60.1- ☑
eosinophilic (granulomatous) L98.3
erysipelatous — *see* Erysipelas
external auditory canal — *see* Cellulitis, ear
eyelid — *see* Abscess, eyelid
face NEC L03.211
finger (intrathecal) (periosteal) (subcutaneous) (subcuticular) L03.01- ☑
foot — *see* Cellulitis, lower limb
gangrenous — *see* Gangrene
genital organ NEC
female (external) N76.4
male N49.9
multiple sites N49.8
specified NEC N49.8
gluteal (region) L03.317

Cellulitis — *continued*
gonococcal A54.89
groin L03.314
hand — *see* Cellulitis, upper limb
head NEC L03.811
face (any part, except ear, eye and nose) L03.211
heel — *see* Cellulitis, lower limb
hip — *see* Cellulitis, lower limb
jaw (region) L03.211
knee — *see* Cellulitis, lower limb
labium (majus) (minus) — *see* Vulvitis
lacrimal passages — *see* Inflammation, lacrimal, passages
larynx J38.7
leg — *see* Cellulitis, lower limb
lip K13.0
lower limb L03.11- ☑
toe — *see* Cellulitis, toe
mouth (floor) K12.2
multiple sites, so stated L03.90
nasopharynx J39.1
navel L03.316
newborn P38.9
with mild hemorrhage P38.1
without hemorrhage P38.9
neck (region) L03.221
nipple (acute) (nonpuerperal) (subacute) N61.0
nose (septum) (external) J34.0
orbit, orbital H05.01- ☑
palate (soft) K12.2
pectoral (region) L03.313
pelvis, pelvic (chronic)
female — *see also* Disease, pelvis, inflammatory N73.2
acute N73.0
following ectopic or molar pregnancy O08.0
male K65.0
penis N48.22
perineal, perineum L03.315
periorbital L03.213
perirectal K61.1
peritonsillar J36
periurethral N34.0
periuterine — *see also* Disease, pelvis, inflammatory N73.2
acute N73.0
pharynx J39.1
preseptal L03.213
rectum K61.1
retroperitoneal K68.9
round ligament
acute N73.0
scalp (any part) L03.811
scrotum N49.2
seminal vesicle N49.0
shoulder — *see* Cellulitis, upper limb
specified site NEC L03.818
submandibular (region) (space) (triangle) K12.2
gland K11.3
submaxillary (region) K12.2
gland K11.3
thigh — *see* Cellulitis, lower limb
thumb (intrathecal) (periosteal) (subcutaneous) (subcuticular) — *see* Cellulitis, finger
toe (intrathecal) (periosteal) (subcutaneous) (subcuticular) L03.03- ☑
tonsil J36
trunk L03.319
abdominal wall L03.311
back (any part) L03.312
buttock L03.317
chest wall L03.313
groin L03.314
perineal, perineum L03.315
umbilicus L03.316
tuberculous (primary) A18.4
umbilicus L03.316
upper limb L03.11- ☑
axilla — *see* Cellulitis, axilla
finger — *see* Cellulitis, finger
thumb — *see* Cellulitis, finger
vaccinal T88.0 ☑
vocal cord J38.3
vulva — *see* Vulvitis
wrist — *see* Cellulitis, upper limb
Cementoblastoma, benign — *see* Cyst, calcifying odontogenic
Cementoma — *see* Cyst, calcifying odontogenic

Cementoperiostitis — *see* Periodontitis
Cementosis K03.4
Central auditory processing disorder H93.25
Central pain syndrome G89.0
Cephalematocele, cephal (o)hematocele
newborn P52.8
birth injury P10.8
traumatic — *see* Hematoma, brain
Cephalematoma, cephalhematoma (calcified)
newborn (birth injury) P12.0
traumatic — *see* Hematoma, brain
Cephalgia, cephalalgia — *see also* Headache
histamine G44.009
intractable G44.001
not intractable G44.009
trigeminal autonomic (TAC) NEC G44.099
intractable G44.091
not intractable G44.099
Cephalic — *see* condition
Cephalitis — *see* Encephalitis
Cephalocele — *see* Encephalocele
Cephalomenia N94.89
Cephalopelvic — *see* condition
Cerclage (with cervical incompetence) in pregnancy — *see* Incompetence, cervix, in pregnancy
Cerebellitis — *see* Encephalitis
Cerebellum, cerebellar — *see* condition
Cerebral — *see* condition
Cerebritis — *see* Encephalitis
Cerebro-hepato-renal syndrome Q87.89
Cerebromalacia — *see* Softening, brain
sequelae of cerebrovascular disease I69.398
Cerebroside lipidosis E75.22
Cerebrospasticity (congenital) G80.1
Cerebrospinal — *see* condition
Cerebrum — *see* condition
Ceroid-lipofuscinosis, neuronal E75.4
Cerumen (accumulation) (impacted) H61.2- ☑
Cervical — *see also* condition
auricle Q18.2
dysplasia in pregnancy — *see* Abnormal, cervix, in pregnancy or childbirth
erosion in pregnancy — *see* Abnormal, cervix, in pregnancy or childbirth
fibrosis in pregnancy — *see* Abnormal, cervix, in pregnancy or childbirth
fusion syndrome Q76.1
rib Q76.5
shortening (complicating pregnancy) O26.87- ☑
Cervicalgia M54.2
Cervicitis (acute) (chronic) (nonvenereal) (senile (atrophic)) (subacute) (with ulceration) N72
with
abortion — *see* Abortion, by type complicated by genital tract and pelvic infection
ectopic pregnancy O08.0
molar pregnancy O08.0
chlamydial A56.09
gonococcal A54.03
herpesviral A60.03
puerperal (postpartum) O86.11
syphilitic A52.76
trichomonal A59.09
tuberculous A18.16
Cervicocolpitis (emphysematosa) — *see also* Cervicitis N72
Cervix — *see* condition
Cesarean delivery, previous, affecting management of pregnancy O34.219
classical (vertical) scar O34.212
low transverse scar O34.211
Céstan (-Chenais) paralysis or syndrome G46.3
Céstan-Raymond syndrome I65.8
Cestode infestation B71.9
specified type NEC B71.8
Cestodiasis B71.9
Chabert's disease A22.9
Chacaleh E53.8
Chafing L30.4
Chagas' (-Mazza) disease (chronic) B57.2
with
cardiovascular involvement NEC B57.2
digestive system involvement B57.30
megacolon B57.32
megaesophagus B57.31
other specified B57.39
megacolon B57.32

Chagas'disease — *continued*
with — *continued*
megaesophagus B57.31
myocarditis B57.2
nervous system involvement B57.40
meningitis B57.41
meningoencephalitis B57.42
other specified B57.49
specified organ involvement NEC B57.5
acute (with) B57.1
cardiovascular NEC B57.0
myocarditis B57.0
Chagres fever B50.9
Chairridden Z74.09
Chalasia (cardiac sphincter) K21.9
Chalazion H00.19
left H00.16
lower H00.15
upper H00.14
right H00.13
lower H00.12
upper H00.11
Chalcosis — *see also* Disorder, globe, degenerative, chalcosis
cornea — *see* Deposit, cornea
crystalline lens — *see* Cataract, complicated
retina H35.89
Chalicosis (pulmonum) J62.8
Chancre (any genital site) (hard) (hunterian) (mixed) (primary) (seronegative) (seropositive) (syphilitic) A51.0
congenital A50.07
conjunctiva NEC A51.2
Ducrey's A57
extragenital A51.2
eyelid A51.2
lip A51.2
nipple A51.2
Nisbet's A57
of
carate A67.0
pinta A67.0
yaws A66.0
palate, soft A51.2
phagedenic A57
simple A57
soft A57
bubo A57
palate A51.2
urethra A51.0
yaws A66.0
Chancroid (anus) (genital) (penis) (perineum) (rectum) (urethra) (vulva) A57
Chandler's disease (osteochondritis dissecans, hip) — *see* Osteochondritis, dissecans, hip
Change(s) (in) (of) — *see also* Removal
arteriosclerotic — *see* Arteriosclerosis
bone — *see also* Disorder, bone
diabetic — *see* Diabetes, bone change
bowel habit R19.4
cardiorenal (vascular) — *see* Hypertension, cardiorenal
cardiovascular — *see* Disease, cardiovascular
circulatory I99.9
cognitive (mild) (organic) R41.89
color, tooth, teeth
during formation K00.8
posteruptive K03.7
contraceptive device Z30.433
corneal membrane H18.30
Bowman's membrane fold or rupture H18.31- ☑
Descemet's membrane
fold H18.32- ☑
rupture H18.33- ☑
coronary — *see* Disease, heart, ischemic
degenerative, spine or vertebra — *see* Spondylosis
dental pulp, regressive K04.2
dressing (nonsurgical) Z48.00
surgical Z48.01
heart — *see* Disease, heart
hip joint — *see* Derangement, joint, hip
hyperplastic larynx J38.7
hypertrophic
nasal sinus J34.89
turbinate, nasal J34.3
upper respiratory tract J39.8
indwelling catheter Z46.6
inflammatory — *see also* Inflammation
sacroiliac M46.1

Change(s) — *continued*
  job, anxiety concerning Z56.1
  joint — *see* Derangement, joint
  life — *see* Menopause
  mental status R41.82
  minimal (glomerular) — *see also* N00-N07 with fourth
    character .0 N05.0
  myocardium, myocardial — *see* Degeneration, myocar-
    dial
  of life — *see* Menopause
  pacemaker Z45.018
    pulse generator Z45.010
  personality (enduring) F68.8
    due to (secondary to)
      general medical condition F07.0
      secondary (nonspecific) F60.89
  regressive, dental pulp K04.2
  renal — *see* Disease, renal
  retina H35.9
    myopic — *see also* Myopia, degenerative H44.2- ☑
  sacroiliac joint M53.3
  senile — *see also* condition R54
  sensory R20.8
  skin R23.9
    acute, due to ultraviolet radiation L56.9
      specified NEC L56.8
    chronic, due to nonionizing radiation L57.9
      specified NEC L57.8
    cyanosis R23.0
    flushing R23.2
    pallor R23.1
    petechiae R23.3
    specified change NEC R23.8
    swelling — *see* Mass, localized
    texture R23.4
  trophic
    arm — *see* Mononeuropathy, upper limb
    leg — *see* Mononeuropathy, lower limb
  vascular I99.9
  vasomotor I73.9
  voice R49.9
    psychogenic F44.4
    specified NEC R49.8
Changing sleep-work schedule, affecting sleep
  G47.26
Changuinola fever A93.1
Chapping skin T69.8 ☑
Charcot-Marie-Tooth disease, paralysis or syndrome
  G60.0
Charcot's
  arthropathy — *see* Arthropathy, neuropathic
  cirrhosis K74.3
  disease (tabetic arthropathy) A52.16
  joint (disease) (tabetic) A52.16
    diabetic — *see* Diabetes, with, arthropathy
  syringomyelic G95.0
  syndrome (intermittent claudication) I73.9
CHARGE association Q89.8
Charley-horse (quadriceps) M62.831
  traumatic (quadriceps) S76.11- ☑
Charlouis' disease — *see* Yaws
Cheadle's disease E54
Checking (of)
  cardiac pacemaker (battery) (electrode(s)) Z45.018
    pulse generator Z45.010
  implantable subdermal contraceptive Z30.46
  intrauterine contraceptive device Z30.431
  wound Z48.0- ☑
    due to injury — code to Injury, by site, using appro-
      priate seventh character for subsequent en-
      counter
Check-up — *see* Examination
Chédiak-Higashi (-Steinbrinck) **syndrome** (congenital
  gigantism of peroxidase granules) E70.330
Cheek — *see* condition
Cheese itch B88.0
Cheese-washer's lung J67.8
Cheese-worker's lung J67.8
Cheilitis (acute) (angular) (catarrhal) (chronic) (exfoliative)
  (gangrenous) (glandular) (infectional) (suppurative)
  (ulcerative) (vesicular) K13.0
  actinic (due to sun) L56.8
    other than from sun L59.8
  candidal B37.83
Cheilodynia K13.0
Cheiloschisis — *see* Cleft, lip
Cheilosis (angular) K13.0
  with pellagra E52

Cheilosis — *continued*
  due to
    vitamin B2 (riboflavin) deficiency E53.0
Cheiromegaly M79.89
Cheiropompholyx L30.1
Cheloid — *see* Keloid
Chemical burn — *see* Corrosion, by site
Chemodectoma — *see* Paraganglioma, nonchromaffin
Chemosis, conjunctiva — *see* Edema, conjunctiva
Chemotherapy (session) (for)
  cancer Z51.11
  neoplasm Z51.11
Cherubism M27.8
Chest — *see* condition
Cheyne-Stokes breathing (respiration) R06.3
Chiari's
  disease or syndrome (hepatic vein thrombosis) I82.0
  malformation
    type I G93.5
    type II — *see* Spina bifida
    net Q24.8
Chicago disease B40.9
Chickenpox — *see* Varicella
Chiclero ulcer or sore B55.1
Chigger (infestation) B88.0
Chignon (disease) B36.8
  newborn (from vacuum extraction) (birth injury) P12.1
Chilaiditi's syndrome (subphrenic displacement, colon)
  Q43.3
Chilblain(s) (lupus) T69.1 ☑
Child
  custody dispute Z65.3
Childbirth — *see* Delivery
Childhood
  cerebral X-linked adrenoleukodystrophy E71.520
  period of rapid growth Z00.2
Chill(s) R68.83
  with fever R50.9
  congestive in malarial regions B54
  without fever R68.83
Chilomastigiasis A07.8
Chimera 46,XX/46,XY Q99.0
Chin — *see* condition
Chinese dysentery A03.9
Chionophobia F40.228
Chitral fever A93.1
Chlamydia, chlamydial A74.9
  cervicitis A56.09
  conjunctivitis A74.0
  cystitis A56.01
  endometritis A56.11
  epididymitis A56.19
  female
    pelvic inflammatory disease A56.11
    pelviperitonitis A56.11
  orchitis A56.19
  peritonitis A74.81
  pharyngitis A56.4
  proctitis A56.3
  psittaci (infection) A70
  salpingitis A56.11
  sexually-transmitted infection NEC A56.8
  specified NEC A74.89
  urethritis A56.01
  vulvovaginitis A56.02
Chlamydiosis — *see* Chlamydia
Chloasma (skin) (idiopathic) (symptomatic) L81.1
  eyelid H02.719
    hyperthyroid E05.90 [H02.719]
      with thyroid storm E05.91 [H02.719]
    left H02.716
      lower H02.715
      upper H02.714
    right H02.713
      lower H02.712
      upper H02.711
Chloroma C92.3- ☑
Chlorosis D50.9
  Egyptian B76.9 [D63.8]
  miner's B76.9 [D63.8]
Chlorotic anemia D50.8
Chocolate cyst (ovary) N80.1
Choked
  disc or disk — *see* Papilledema
  on food, phlegm, or vomitus NOS — *see* Foreign body,
    by site
  while vomiting NOS — *see* Foreign body, by site

Chokes (resulting from bends) T70.3 ☑
Choking sensation R09.89
Cholangiectasis K83.8
Cholangiocarcinoma
  with hepatocellular carcinoma, combined C22.0
  liver C22.1
  specified site NEC — *see* Neoplasm, malignant, by site
  unspecified site C22.1
Cholangiohepatitis K83.8
  due to fluke infestation B66.1
Cholangiohepatoma C22.0
Cholangiolitis (acute) (chronic) (extrahepatic) (gangrenous) (intrahepatic) K83.09
  paratyphoidal — *see* Fever, paratyphoid
  typhoidal A01.09
Cholangioma D13.4
  malignant — *see* Cholangiocarcinoma
Cholangitis (ascending) (recurrent) (secondary) (stenosing) (suppurative) K83.09
  with calculus, bile duct — *see* Calculus, bile duct, with
    cholangitis
  chronic nonsuppurative destructive K74.3
  primary K83.09
    sclerosing K83.01
  sclerosing K83.09
Cholecystectasia K82.8
Cholecystitis K81.9
  with
    calculus, stones in
      bile duct (common) (hepatic) — *see* Calculus,
        bile duct, with cholecystitis
      cystic duct — *see* Calculus, gallbladder, with
        cholecystitis
      gallbladder — *see* Calculus, gallbladder, with
        cholecystitis
      choledocholithiasis — *see* Calculus, bile duct, with
        cholecystitis
      cholelithiasis — *see* Calculus, gallbladder, with
        cholecystitis
    gangrene of gallbladder K82.A1
    perforation of gallbladder K82.A2
  acute (emphysematous) (gangrenous) (suppurative)
    K81.0
    with
      calculus, stones in
        cystic duct — *see* Calculus, gallbladder, with
          cholecystitis, acute
        gallbladder — *see* Calculus, gallbladder, with
          cholecystitis, acute
        choledocholithiasis — *see* Calculus, bile duct,
          with cholecystitis, acute
        cholelithiasis — *see* Calculus, gallbladder, with
          cholecystitis, acute
      chronic cholecystitis K81.2
        with gallbladder calculus K80.12
          with obstruction K80.13
  chronic K81.1
    with acute cholecystitis K81.2
      with gallbladder calculus K80.12
        with obstruction K80.13
  emphysematous (acute) — *see* Cholecystitis, acute
  gangrenous — *see* Cholecystitis, acute
  paratyphoidal, current A01.4
  suppurative — *see* Cholecystitis, acute
  typhoidal A01.09
Cholecystolithiasis — *see* Calculus, gallbladder
Choledochitis (suppurative) K83.09
Choledocholith — *see* Calculus, bile duct
Choledocholithiasis (common duct) (hepatic duct) —
  see Calculus, bile duct
  cystic — *see* Calculus, gallbladder
  typhoidal A01.09
Cholelithiasis (cystic duct) (gallbladder) (impacted)
  (multiple) — *see* Calculus, gallbladder
  bile duct (common) (hepatic) — *see* Calculus, bile duct
  hepatic duct — *see* Calculus, bile duct
  specified NEC K80.80
    with obstruction K80.81
Cholemia — *see also* Jaundice
  familial (simple) (congenital) E80.4
  Gilbert's E80.4
Choleperitoneum, choleperitonitis K65.3
Cholera (Asiatic) (epidemic) (malignant) A00.9
  antimonial — *see* Poisoning, antimony
  classical A00.0
  due to Vibrio cholerae 01 A00.9
    biovar cholerae A00.0

Cholera — *continued*
  due to Vibrio cholerae Ø1 — *continued*
    biovar eltor AØØ.1
    el tor AØØ.1
  el tor AØØ.1
Cholerine — *see* Cholera
Cholestasis NEC K83.1
  with hepatocyte injury K71.Ø
  due to total parenteral nutrition (TPN) K76.89
  pure K71.Ø
Cholesteatoma (ear) (middle) (with reaction) H71.9- ✓
  attic H71.Ø- ✓
  external ear (canal) H6Ø.4- ✓
  mastoid H71.2- ✓
  postmastoidectomy cavity (recurrent) — *see* Complications, postmastoidectomy, recurrent cholesteatoma
  recurrent (postmastoidectomy) — *see* Complications, postmastoidectomy, recurrent cholesteatoma
  tympanum H71.1- ✓
Cholesteatosis, diffuse H71.3- ✓
Cholesteremia E78.ØØ
Cholesterin in vitreous — *see* Deposit, crystalline
Cholesterol
  deposit
    retina H35.89
    vitreous — *see* Deposit, crystalline
  elevated (high) E78.ØØ
    with elevated (high) triglycerides E78.2
    screening for Z13.22Ø
  imbibition of gallbladder K82.4
Cholesterolemia (essential) (pure) E78.ØØ
  familial E78.Ø1
  hereditary E78.Ø1
Cholesterolosis, cholesterosis (gallbladder) K82.4
  cerebrotendinous E75.5
Cholocolic fistula K82.3
Choluria R82.2
Chondritis M94.8X9
  auricular H61.Ø3- ✓
  costal (Tietze's) M94.Ø
  external ear H61.Ø3- ✓
  patella, posttraumatic — *see* Chondromalacia, patella
  pinna H61.Ø3- ✓
  purulent M94.8X- ✓
  tuberculous NEC A18.Ø2
    intervertebral A18.Ø1
Chondroblastoma — *see also* Neoplasm, bone, benign
  malignant — *see* Neoplasm, bone, malignant
Chondrocalcinosis M11.2Ø
  ankle M11.27- ✓
  elbow M11.22- ✓
  familial M11.1Ø
    ankle M11.17- ✓
    elbow M11.12- ✓
    foot joint M11.17- ✓
    hand joint M11.14- ✓
    hip M11.15- ✓
    knee M11.16- ✓
    multiple site M11.19
    shoulder M11.11- ✓
    vertebrae M11.18
    wrist M11.13- ✓
  foot joint M11.27- ✓
  hand joint M11.24- ✓
  hip M11.25- ✓
  knee M11.26- ✓
  multiple site M11.29
  shoulder M11.21- ✓
  specified type NEC M11.2Ø
    ankle M11.27- ✓
    elbow M11.22- ✓
    foot joint M11.27- ✓
    hand joint M11.24- ✓
    hip M11.25- ✓
    knee M11.26- ✓
    multiple site M11.29
    shoulder M11.21- ✓
    vertebrae M11.28
    wrist M11.23- ✓
  vertebrae M11.28
  wrist M11.23- ✓
Chondrodermatitis nodularis helicis or anthelicis — *see* Perichondritis, ear
Chondrodysplasia Q78.9
  with hemangioma Q78.4
  calcificans congenita Q77.3

Chondrodysplasia — *continued*
  fetalis Q77.4
  metaphyseal (Jansen's) (McKusick's) (Schmid's) Q78.8
  punctata Q77.3
Chondrodystrophy, chondrodystrophia (familial) (fetalis) (hypoplastic) Q78.9
  calcificans congenita Q77.3
  myotonic (congenital) G71.13
  punctata Q77.3
Chondroectodermal dysplasia Q77.6
Chondrogenesis imperfecta Q77.4
Chondrolysis M94.35- ✓
Chondroma — *see also* Neoplasm, cartilage, benign
  juxtacortical — *see* Neoplasm, bone, benign
  periosteal — *see* Neoplasm, bone, benign
Chondromalacia (systemic) M94.2Ø
  acromioclavicular joint M94.21- ✓
  ankle M94.27- ✓
  elbow M94.22- ✓
  foot joint M94.27- ✓
  glenohumeral joint M94.21- ✓
  hand joint M94.24- ✓
  hip M94.25- ✓
  knee M94.26- ✓
    patella M22.4- ✓
  multiple sites M94.29
  patella M22.4- ✓
  rib M94.28
  sacroiliac joint M94.259
  shoulder M94.21- ✓
  sternoclavicular joint M94.21- ✓
  vertebral joint M94.28
  wrist M94.23- ✓
Chondromatosis — *see also* Neoplasm, cartilage, uncertain behavior
  internal Q78.4
Chondromyxosarcoma — *see* Neoplasm, cartilage, malignant
Chondro-osteodysplasia (Morquio-Brailsford type) E76.219
Chondro-osteodystrophy E76.29
Chondro-osteoma — *see* Neoplasm, bone, benign
Chondropathia tuberosa M94.Ø
Chondrosarcoma — *see also* Neoplasm, cartilage, malignant
  juxtacortical — *see* Neoplasm, bone, malignant
  mesenchymal — *see* Neoplasm, connective tissue, malignant
  myxoid — *see* Neoplasm, cartilage, malignant
Chordee (nonvenereal) N48.89
  congenital Q54.4
  gonococcal A54.Ø9
Chorditis (fibrinous) (nodosa) (tuberosa) J38.2
Chordoma — *see* Neoplasm, vertebral (column), malignant
Chorea (chronic) (gravis) (posthemiplegic) (senile) (spasmodic) G25.5
  with
    heart involvement IØ2.Ø
      active or acute (conditions in IØ1-) IØ2.Ø
        rheumatic IØ2.9
          with valvular disorder IØ2.Ø
      rheumatic heart disease (chronic) (inactive)(quiescent) — *code to* rheumatic heart condition involved
  drug-induced G25.4
  habit F95.8
  hereditary G1Ø
  Huntington's G1Ø
  hysterical F44.4
  minor IØ2.9
    with heart involvement IØ2.Ø
  progressive G25.5
    hereditary G1Ø
  rheumatic (chronic) IØ2.9
    with heart involvement IØ2.Ø
  Sydenham's IØ2.9
    with heart involvement — *see* Chorea, with rheumatic heart disease
  nonrheumatic G25.5
Choreoathetosis (paroxysmal) G25.5
Chorioadenoma (destruens) D39.2
Chorioamnionitis O41.12- ✓
Chorioangioma D26.7
Choriocarcinoma — *see* Neoplasm, malignant, by site
  combined with
    embryonal carcinoma — *see* Neoplasm, malignant, by site

Choriocarcinoma — *continued*
  combined with — *continued*
    other germ cell elements — *see* Neoplasm, malignant, by site
    teratoma — *see* Neoplasm, malignant, by site
  specified site — *see* Neoplasm, malignant, by site
  unspecified site
    female C58
    male C62.9Ø
Chorioencephalitis (acute) (lymphocytic) (serous) A87.2
Chorioepithelioma — *see* Choriocarcinoma
Choriomeningitis (acute) (lymphocytic) (serous) A87.2
Chorionepithelioma — *see* Choriocarcinoma
Chorioretinitis — *see also* Inflammation, chorioretinal
  disseminated — *see also* Inflammation, chorioretinal, disseminated
    in neurosyphilis A52.19
  Egyptian B76.9 *[D63.8]*
  focal — *see also* Inflammation, chorioretinal, focal
  histoplasmic B39.9 *[H32]*
  in (due to)
    histoplasmosis B39.9 *[H32]*
    syphilis (secondary) A51.43
      late A52.71
    toxoplasmosis (acquired) B58.Ø1
      congenital (active) P37.1 *[H32]*
    tuberculosis A18.53
  juxtapapillary, juxtapapillaris — *see* Inflammation, chorioretinal, focal, juxtapapillary
  leprous A3Ø.9 *[H32]*
  miner's B76.9 *[D63.8]*
  progressive myopia (degeneration) — *see also* Myopia, degenerative H44.2- ✓
  syphilitic (secondary) A51.43
    congenital (early) A5Ø.Ø1 *[H32]*
      late A5Ø.32
    late A52.71
  tuberculous A18.53
Chorioretinopathy, central serous H35.71- ✓
Choroid — *see* condition
Choroideremia H31.21
Choroiditis — *see* Chorioretinitis
Choroidopathy — *see* Disorder, choroid
Choroidoretinitis — *see* Chorioretinitis
Choroidoretinopathy, central serous — *see* Chorioretinopathy, central serous
Christian-Weber disease M35.6
Christmas disease D67
Chromaffinoma — *see also* Neoplasm, benign, by site
  malignant — *see* Neoplasm, malignant, by site
Chromatopsia — *see* Deficiency, color vision
Chromhidrosis, chromidrosis L75.1
Chromoblastomycosis — *see* Chromomycosis
Chromoconversion R82.91
Chromomycosis B43.9
  brain abscess B43.1
  cerebral B43.1
  cutaneous B43.Ø
  skin B43.Ø
  specified NEC B43.8
  subcutaneous abscess or cyst B43.2
Chromophytosis B36.Ø
Chromosome — *see* Anomaly, by chromosome involved
  D (1) — *see* Anomaly, chromosome 13
  E (3) — *see* Anomaly, chromosome 18
  G — *see* Anomaly, chromosome 21
Chromotrichomycosis B36.8
Chronic — *see* condition
  fracture — *see* Fracture, pathological
Churg-Strauss syndrome M3Ø.1
Chyle cyst, mesentery I89.8
Chylocele (nonfilarial) I89.8
  filarial — *see also* Infestation, filarial B74.9 *[N51]*
  tunica vaginalis N5Ø.89
    filarial — *see also* Infestation, filarial B74.9 *[N51]*
Chylomicronemia (fasting) (with hyperprebetalipoproteinemia) E78.3
Chylopericardium I31.3
  acute I3Ø.9
Chylothorax (nonfilarial) I89.8
  filarial — *see also* Infestation, filarial B74.9 *[J91.8]*
Chylous — *see* condition
Chyluria (nonfilarial) R82.Ø
  due to
    bilharziasis B65.Ø
    Brugia (malayi) B74.1
      timori B74.2

Chyluria — *continued*
  due to — *continued*
    schistosomiasis (bilharziasis) B65.0
    Wuchereria (bancrofti) B74.0
  filarial — *see* Infestation, filarial
Cicatricial (deformity) — *see* Cicatrix
Cicatrix (adherent) (contracted) (painful) (vicious) — *see also* Scar L90.5
  adenoid (and tonsil) J35.8
  alveolar process M26.79
  anus K62.89
  auricle — *see* Disorder, pinna, specified type NEC
  bile duct (common) (hepatic) K83.8
  bladder N32.89
  bone — *see* Disorder, bone, specified type NEC
  brain G93.89
  cervix (postoperative) (postpartal) N88.1
  common duct K83.8
  cornea H17.9
    tuberculous A18.59
  duodenum (bulb), obstructive K31.5
  esophagus K22.2
  eyelid — *see* Disorder, eyelid function
  hypopharynx J39.2
  lacrimal passages — *see* Obstruction, lacrimal
  larynx J38.7
  lung J98.4
  middle ear H74.8 ☑
  mouth K13.79
  muscle M62.89
    with contracture — *see* Contraction, muscle NEC
  nasopharynx J39.2
  palate (soft) K13.79
  penis N48.89
  pharynx J39.2
  prostate N42.89
  rectum K62.89
  retina — *see* Scar, chorioretinal
  semilunar cartilage — *see* Derangement, meniscus
  seminal vesicle N50.89
  skin L90.5
    infected L08.89
    postinfective L90.5
    tuberculous B90.8
  specified site NEC L90.5
  throat J39.2
  tongue K14.8
  tonsil (and adenoid) J35.8
  trachea J39.8
  tuberculous NEC B90.9
  urethra N36.8
  uterus N85.8
  vagina N89.8
    postoperative N99.2
  vocal cord J38.3
  wrist, constricting (annular) L90.5
CIDP (chronic inflammatory demyelinating polyneuropathy) G61.81
CIN — *see* Neoplasia, intraepithelial, cervix
CINCA (chronic infantile neurological, cutaneous and articular syndrome) M04.2
Cinchonism — *see* Deafness, ototoxic
  correct substance properly administered — *see* Table of Drugs and Chemicals, by drug, adverse effect
  overdose or wrong substance given or taken — *see* Table of Drugs and Chemicals, by drug, poisoning
Circle of Willis — *see* condition
Circular — *see* condition
Circulating anticoagulants — *see also* Disorder, hemorrhagic D68.318
  due to drugs — *see also* Disorder, hemorrhagic D68.32
  following childbirth O72.3
Circulation
  collateral, any site I99.8
  defective (lower extremity) I99.9
    congenital Q28.9
  embryonic Q28.9
  failure (peripheral) R57.9
    newborn P29.89
  fetal, persistent P29.38
  heart, incomplete Q28.9
Circulatory system — *see* condition
Circulus senilis (cornea) — *see* Degeneration, cornea, senile
Circumcision (in absence of medical indication) (ritual) (routine) Z41.2
Circumscribed — *see* condition
Circumvallate placenta O43.11- ☑

Cirrhosis, cirrhotic (hepatic) (liver) K74.60
  alcoholic K70.30
    with ascites K70.31
  atrophic — *see* Cirrhosis, liver
  Baumgarten-Cruveilhier K74.69
  biliary (cholangiolitic) (cholangitic) (hypertrophic) (obstructive) (pericholangiolitic) K74.5
    due to
      Clonorchiasis B66.1
      flukes B66.3
    primary K74.3
    secondary K74.4
  cardiac (of liver) K76.1
  Charcot's K74.3
  cholangiolitic, cholangitic, cholostatic (primary) K74.3
  congestive K76.1
  Cruveilhier-Baumgarten K74.69
  cryptogenic (liver) K74.69
  due to
    hepatolenticular degeneration E83.01
    Wilson's disease E83.01
    xanthomatosis E78.2
  fatty K76.0
    alcoholic K70.0
  Hanot's (hypertrophic) K74.3
  hepatic — *see* Cirrhosis, liver
  hypertrophic K74.3
  Indian childhood K74.69
  kidney — *see* Sclerosis, renal
  Laennec's K70.30
    with ascites K70.31
    alcoholic K70.30
      with ascites K70.31
    nonalcoholic K74.69
  liver K74.60
    alcoholic K70.30
      with ascites K70.31
      fatty K70.0
    congenital P78.81
    syphilitic A52.74
  lung (chronic) J84.10
  macronodular K74.69
    alcoholic K70.30
      with ascites K70.31
  micronodular K74.69
    alcoholic K70.30
      with ascites K70.31
  mixed type K74.69
  monolobular K74.3
  nephritis — *see* Sclerosis, renal
  nutritional K74.69
    alcoholic K70.30
      with ascites K70.31
  obstructive — *see* Cirrhosis, biliary
  ovarian N83.8
  pancreas (duct) K86.89
  pigmentary E83.110
  portal K74.69
    alcoholic K70.30
      with ascites K70.31
  postnecrotic K74.69
    alcoholic K70.30
      with ascites K70.31
  pulmonary J84.10
  renal — *see* Sclerosis, renal
  spleen D73.2
  stasis K76.1
  Todd's K74.3
  unilobar K74.3
  xanthomatous (biliary) K74.5
    due to xanthomatosis (familial) (metabolic) (primary) E78.2
Cistern, subarachnoid R93.0
Citrullinemia E72.23
Citrullinuria E72.23
Civatte's disease or poikiloderma L57.3
Clam digger's itch B65.3
Clammy skin R23.1
Clap — *see* Gonorrhea
Clarke-Hadfield syndrome (pancreatic infantilism) K86.89
Clark's paralysis G80.9
Clastothrix L67.8
Claude Bernard-Horner syndrome G90.2
  traumatic — *see* Injury, nerve, cervical sympathetic
Claude's disease or syndrome G46.3
Claudicatio venosa intermittens I87.8
Claudication (intermittent) I73.9

Claudication — *continued*
  cerebral (artery) G45.9
  spinal cord (arteriosclerotic) G95.19
    syphilitic A52.09
  venous (axillary) I87.8
Claustrophobia F40.240
Clavus (infected) L84
Clawfoot (congenital) Q66.89
  acquired — *see* Deformity, limb, clawfoot
Clawhand (acquired) — *see also* Deformity, limb, clawhand
  congenital Q68.1
Clawtoe (congenital) Q66.89
  acquired — *see* Deformity, toe, specified NEC
Clay eating — *see* Pica
Cleansing of artificial opening — *see* Attention to, artificial, opening
Cleft (congenital) — *see also* Imperfect, closure
  alveolar process M26.79
  branchial (persistent) Q18.2
    cyst Q18.0
      fistula Q18.0
      sinus Q18.0
  cricoid cartilage, posterior Q31.8
  cyst Q18.0
    fistula Q18.0
    sinus Q18.0
  foot Q72.7 ☑
  hand Q71.6 ☑
  lip (unilateral) Q36.9
    with cleft palate Q37.9
      hard Q37.1
        with soft Q37.5
      soft Q37.3
        with hard Q37.5
    bilateral Q36.0
      with cleft palate Q37.8
        hard Q37.0
          with soft Q37.4
        soft Q37.2
          with hard Q37.4
    median Q36.1
  nose Q30.2
  palate Q35.9
    with cleft lip (unilateral) Q37.9
      bilateral Q37.8
    hard Q35.1
      with
        cleft lip (unilateral) Q37.1
          bilateral Q37.0
        soft Q35.5
          with cleft lip (unilateral) Q37.5
            bilateral Q37.4
    medial Q35.5
    soft Q35.3
      with
        cleft lip (unilateral) Q37.3
          bilateral Q37.2
        hard Q35.5
          with cleft lip (unilateral) Q37.5
            bilateral Q37.4
  penis Q55.69
  scrotum Q55.29
  thyroid cartilage Q31.8
  uvula Q35.7
Cleidocranial dysostosis Q74.0
Cleptomania F63.2
Clicking hip (newborn) R29.4
Climacteric (female) — *see also* Menopause
  arthritis (any site) NEC — *see* Arthritis, specified form NEC
  depression (single episode) F32.89
    recurrent episode F33.8
  male (symptoms) (syndrome) NEC N50.89
  melancholia (single episode) F32.89
    recurrent episode F33.8
  paranoid state F22
  polyarthritis NEC — *see* Arthritis, specified form NEC
  symptoms (female) N95.1
Clinical research investigation (clinical trial) (control subject) (normal comparison) (participant) Z00.6
Clitoris — *see* condition
Cloaca (persistent) Q43.7
Clonorchiasis, clonorchis infection (liver) B66.1
Clonus R25.8
Closed bite M26.29
Clostridium (C.) **perfringens, as cause of disease classified elsewhere** B96.7

Closure
- congenital, nose Q30.0
- cranial sutures, premature Q75.0
- defective or imperfect NEC — *see* Imperfect, closure
- fistula, delayed — *see* Fistula
- foramen ovale, imperfect Q21.1
- hymen N89.6
- interauricular septum, defective Q21.1
- interventricular septum, defective Q21.0
- lacrimal duct — *see also* Stenosis, lacrimal, duct
  - congenital Q10.5
- nose (congenital) Q30.0
  - acquired M95.0
- of artificial opening — *see* Attention to, artificial, opening
- vagina N89.5
- valve — *see* Endocarditis
- vulva N90.5

Clot (blood) — *see also* Embolism
- artery (obstruction) (occlusion) — *see* Embolism
- bladder N32.89
- brain (intradural or extradural) — *see* Occlusion, artery, cerebral
- circulation I74.9
- heart — *see also* Infarct, myocardium
  - not resulting in infarction I51.3
- vein — *see* Thrombosis

Clouded state R40.1
- epileptic — *see* Epilepsy, specified NEC
- paroxysmal — *see* Epilepsy, specified NEC

Cloudy antrum, antra J32.0
Clouston's (hidrotic) **ectodermal dysplasia** Q82.4
Clubbed nail pachydermoperiostosis M89.40 [L62]
Clubbing of finger(s) (nails) R68.3

Clubfinger R68.3
- congenital Q68.1

Clubfoot (congenital) Q66.89
- acquired — *see* Deformity, limb, clubfoot
- equinovarus Q66.0- ☑
- paralytic — *see* Deformity, limb, clubfoot

Clubhand (congenital) (radial) Q71.4- ☑
- acquired — *see* Deformity, limb, clubhand

Clubnail R68.3
- congenital Q84.6

Clump, kidney Q63.1
Clumsiness, clumsy child syndrome F82
Cluttering F80.81
Clutton's joints A50.51 [M12.80]

Coagulation, intravascular (diffuse) (disseminated) — *see also* Defibrination syndrome
- complicating abortion — *see* Abortion, by type, complicated by, intravascular coagulation
- following ectopic or molar pregnancy O08.1

Coagulopathy — *see also* Defect, coagulation
- consumption D65
- intravascular D65
  - newborn P60

Coalition
- calcaneo-scaphoid Q66.89
- tarsal Q66.89

Coalminer's
- elbow — *see* Bursitis, elbow, olecranon
- lung or pneumoconiosis J60

Coalworker's lung or pneumoconiosis J60

Coarctation
- aorta (preductal) (postductal) Q25.1
- pulmonary artery Q25.71

Coated tongue K14.3
Coats' disease (exudative retinopathy) — *see* Retinopathy, exudative

Cocaine-induced
- anxiety disorder F14.980
- bipolar and related disorder F14.94
- depressive disorder F14.94
- obsessive-compulsive and related disorder F14.988
- psychotic disorder F14.959
- sexual dysfunction F14.981
- sleep disorder F14.982

Cocainism — *see* Disorder, cocaine use

Coccidioidomycosis B38.9
- cutaneous B38.3
- disseminated B38.7
- generalized B38.7
- meninges B38.4
- prostate B38.81
- pulmonary B38.2
  - acute B38.0

Coccidioidomycosis — *continued*
- pulmonary — *continued*
  - chronic B38.1
- skin B38.3
- specified NEC B38.89

Coccidioidosis — *see* Coccidioidomycosis
Coccidiosis (intestinal) A07.3
Coccydynia, coccygodynia M53.3
Coccyx — *see* condition
Cochin-China diarrhea K90.1
Cockayne's syndrome Q87.19
Cocked up toe — *see* Deformity, toe, specified NEC
Cock's peculiar tumor L72.3
Codman's tumor — *see* Neoplasm, bone, benign
Coenurosis B71.8
Coffee-worker's lung J67.8
Cogan's syndrome H16.32- ☑
- oculomotor apraxia H51.8

Coitus, painful (female) N94.10
- male N53.12
- psychogenic F52.6

Cold J00
- with influenza, flu, or grippe — *see* Influenza, with, respiratory manifestations NEC
- agglutinin disease or hemoglobinuria (chronic) D59.1
- bronchial — *see* Bronchitis
- chest — *see* Bronchitis
- common (head) J00
- effects of T69.9 ☑
  - specified effect NEC T69.8 ☑
- excessive, effects of T69.9 ☑
  - specified effect NEC T69.8 ☑
- exhaustion from T69.8 ☑
- exposure to T69.9 ☑
  - specified effect NEC T69.8 ☑
- head J00
- injury syndrome (newborn) P80.0
- on lung — *see* Bronchitis
- rose J30.1
- sensitivity, auto-immune D59.1
- symptoms J00
- virus J00

Coldsore B00.1

Colibacillosis A49.8
- as the cause of other disease — *see also* Escherichia coli B96.20
- generalized A41.50

Colic (bilious) (infantile) (intestinal) (recurrent) (spasmodic) R10.83
- abdomen R10.83
  - psychogenic F45.8
- appendix, appendicular K38.8
- bile duct — *see* Calculus, bile duct
- biliary — *see* Calculus, bile duct
- common duct — *see* Calculus, bile duct
- cystic duct — *see* Calculus, gallbladder
- Devonshire NEC — *see* Poisoning, lead
- gallbladder — *see* Calculus, gallbladder
- gallstone — *see* Calculus, gallbladder
  - gallbladder or cystic duct — *see* Calculus, gallbladder
- hepatic (duct) — *see* Calculus, bile duct
- hysterical F45.8
- kidney N23
- lead NEC — *see* Poisoning, lead
- mucous K58.9
  - with diarrhea K58.0
  - psychogenic F54
- nephritic N23
- painter's NEC — *see* Poisoning, lead
- pancreas K86.89
- psychogenic F45.8
- renal N23
- saturnine NEC — *see* Poisoning, lead
- ureter N23
- urethral N36.8
  - due to calculus N21.1
- uterus NEC N94.89
  - menstrual — *see* Dysmenorrhea
- worm NOS B83.9

Colicystitis — *see* Cystitis
Colitis (acute) (catarrhal) (chronic) (noninfective) (hemorrhagic) — *see also* Enteritis K52.9
- allergic K52.29
  - with
    - food protein-induced enterocolitis syndrome K52.21

Colitis — *continued*
- allergic — *continued*
  - with — *continued*
    - proctocolitis K52.82
- amebic (acute) — *see also* Amebiasis A06.0
  - nondysenteric A06.2
- anthrax A22.2
- bacillary — *see* Infection, Shigella
- balantidial A07.0
- Clostridium difficile
  - not specified as recurrent A04.72
  - recurrent A04.71
- coccidial A07.3
- collagenous K52.831
- cystica superficialis K52.89
- dietary counseling and surveillance (for) Z71.3
- dietetic — *see also* Colitis, allergic K52.29
- drug-induced K52.1
- due to radiation K52.0
- eosinophilic K52.82
- food hypersensitivity — *see also* Colitis, allergic K52.29
- giardial A07.1
- granulomatous — *see* Enteritis, regional, large intestine
- indeterminate, so stated K52.3
- infectious — *see* Enteritis, infectious
- ischemic K55.9
  - acute (subacute) — *see also* Ischemia, intestine, acute K55.039
  - chronic K55.1
  - due to mesenteric artery insufficiency K55.1
  - fulminant (acute) — *see also* Ischemia, intestine, acute K55.039
- left sided K51.50
  - with
    - abscess K51.514
    - complication K51.519
      - specified NEC K51.518
    - fistula K51.513
    - obstruction K51.512
    - rectal bleeding K51.511
- lymphocytic K52.832
- membranous
  - psychogenic F54
- microscopic K52.839
  - specified NEC K52.838
- mucous — *see* Syndrome, irritable, bowel
  - psychogenic F54
- noninfective K52.9
  - specified NEC K52.89
- polyposa — *see* Polyp, colon, inflammatory
- protozoal A07.9
- pseudomembranous
  - not specified as recurrent A04.72
  - recurrent A04.71
- pseudomucinous — *see* Syndrome, irritable, bowel
- regional — *see* Enteritis, regional, large intestine
  - infectious A09
- segmental — *see* Enteritis, regional, large intestine
- septic — *see* Enteritis, infectious
- spastic K58.9
  - with diarrhea K58.0
  - psychogenic F54
- staphylococcal A04.8
  - foodborne A05.0
- subacute ischemic — *see also* Ischemia, intestine, acute K55.039
- thromboulcerative — *see also* Ischemia, intestine, acute K55.039
- toxic NEC K52.1
  - due to Clostridium difficile
    - not specified as recurrent A04.72
    - recurrent A04.71
- transmural — *see* Enteritis, regional, large intestine
- trichomonal A07.8
- tuberculous (ulcerative) A18.32
- ulcerative (chronic) K51.90
  - with
    - complication K51.919
      - abscess K51.914
      - fistula K51.913
      - obstruction K51.912
      - rectal bleeding K51.911
      - specified complication NEC K51.918
  - enterocolitis — *see* Enterocolitis, ulcerative
  - ileocolitis — *see* Ileocolitis, ulcerative
  - mucosal proctocolitis — *see* Proctocolitis, mucosal
  - proctitis — *see* Proctitis, ulcerative
  - pseudopolyposis — *see* Polyp, colon, inflammatory

☑ Additional Character Required — Refer to the Tabular List for Character Selection   ▽ Subterms under main terms may continue to next column or page

Colitis — *continued*
  ulcerative — *continued*
    psychogenic F54
    rectosigmoiditis — *see* Rectosigmoiditis, ulcerative
    specified type NEC K51.80
      with
        complication K51.819
          abscess K51.814
          fistula K51.813
          obstruction K51.812
          rectal bleeding K51.811
          specified complication NEC K51.818
Collagenosis, collagen disease (nonvascular) (vascular)
    M35.9
  cardiovascular I42.8
  reactive perforating L87.1
  specified NEC M35.8
Collapse R55
  adrenal E27.2
  cardiorespiratory R57.0
  cardiovascular R57.0
    newborn P29.89
  circulatory (peripheral) R57.9
    during or after labor and delivery O75.1
    following ectopic or molar pregnancy O08.3
    newborn P29.89
  during or
    after labor and delivery O75.1
    resulting from a procedure, not elsewhere classified
        T81.10 ☑
  external ear canal — *see* Stenosis, external ear canal
  general R55
  heart — *see* Disease, heart
  heat T67.1 ☑
  hysterical F44.89
  labyrinth, membranous (congenital) Q16.5
  lung (massive) — *see also* Atelectasis J98.19
    pressure due to anesthesia (general) (local) or other
        sedation T88.2 ☑
      during labor and delivery O74.1
      in pregnancy O29.02- ☑
      postpartum, puerperal O89.09
  myocardial — *see* Disease, heart
  nervous F48.8
  neurocirculatory F45.8
  nose M95.0
  postoperative T81.10 ☑
  pulmonary — *see also* Atelectasis J98.19
    newborn — *see* Atelectasis
  trachea J39.8
  tracheobronchial J98.09
  valvular — *see* Endocarditis
  vascular (peripheral) R57.9
    during or after labor and delivery O75.1
    following ectopic or molar pregnancy O08.3
    newborn P29.89
  vertebra M48.50- ☑
    cervical region M48.52- ☑
    cervicothoracic region M48.53- ☑
    in (due to)
      metastasis — *see* Collapse, vertebra, in, specified
          disease NEC
      osteoporosis — *see also* Osteoporosis M80.88 ☑
        cervical region M80.88 ☑
        cervicothoracic region M80.88 ☑
        lumbar region M80.88 ☑
        lumbosacral region M80.88 ☑
        multiple sites M80.88 ☑
        occipito-atlanto-axial region M80.88 ☑
        sacrococcygeal region M80.88 ☑
        thoracic region M80.88 ☑
        thoracolumbar region M80.88 ☑
      specified disease NEC M48.50- ☑
        cervical region M48.52- ☑
        cervicothoracic region M48.53- ☑
        lumbar region M48.56- ☑
        lumbosacral region M48.57- ☑
        occipito-atlanto-axial region M48.51- ☑
        sacrococcygeal region M48.58- ☑
        thoracic region M48.54- ☑
        thoracolumbar region M48.55- ☑
    lumbar region M48.56- ☑
    lumbosacral region M48.57- ☑
    occipito-atlanto-axial region M48.51- ☑
    sacrococcygeal region M48.58- ☑
    thoracic region M48.54- ☑
    thoracolumbar region M48.55- ☑

Collateral — *see also* condition
  circulation (venous) I87.8
  dilation, veins I87.8
Colles' fracture S52.53- ☑
Collet (-Sicard) syndrome G52.7
Collier's asthma or lung J60
Collodion baby Q80.2
Colloid nodule (of thyroid) (cystic) E04.1
Coloboma (iris) Q13.0
  eyelid Q10.3
  fundus Q14.8
  lens Q12.2
  optic disc (congenital) Q14.2
    acquired H47.31- ☑
Coloenteritis — *see* Enteritis
Colon — *see* condition
Colonization
  MRSA (Methicillin resistant Staphylococcus aureus)
      Z22.322
  MSSA (Methicillin susceptible Staphylococcus aureus)
      Z22.321
  status — *see* Carrier (suspected) of
Coloptosis K63.4
Color blindness — *see* Deficiency, color vision
Colostomy
  attention to Z43.3
  fitting or adjustment Z46.89
  malfunctioning K94.03
  status Z93.3
Colpitis (acute) — *see* Vaginitis
Colpocele N81.5
Colpocystitis — *see* Vaginitis
Colpospasm N94.2
Column, spinal, vertebral — *see* condition .
Coma R40.20
  with
    motor response (none) R40.231 ☑
      abnormal extensor posturing to pain or noxious
          stimuli (< 2 years of age) R40.232 ☑
      abnormal flexure posturing to pain or noxious
          stimuli (0-5 years of age) R40.233 ☑
      extensor posturing to pain or noxious stimuli (2-
          5 years of age) R40.232 ☑
      flexion/decorticate posturing (< 2 years of age)
          R40.233 ☑
      localizes pain (2-5 years of age) R40.235 ☑
      normal or spontaneous movement (< 2 years of
          age) R40.236 ☑
      obeys commands (2-5 years of age) R40.236 ☑
      score of
        1 R40.231 ☑
        2 R40.232 ☑
        3 R40.233 ☑
        4 R40.234 ☑
        5 R40.235 ☑
        6 R40.236 ☑
      withdraws from pain or noxious stimuli (0-5 years
          of age) R40.234 ☑
      withdraws to touch (< 2 years of age) R40.235 ☑
    opening of eyes (never) R40.211 ☑
      in response to
        pain R40.212 ☑
        sound R40.213 ☑
      score of
        1 R40.211 ☑
        2 R40.212 ☑
        3 R40.213 ☑
        4 R40.214 ☑
      spontaneous R40.214 ☑
    verbal response (none) R40.221 ☑
      confused conversation R40.224 ☑
      cooing or babbling or crying appropriately (<2
          years of age) R40.225 ☑
      inappropriate crying or screaming (< 2 years of
          age) R40.223 ☑
      inappropriate words (2-5 years of age)
          R40.224 ☑
      incomprehensible sounds (2-5 years of age)
          R40.222 ☑
      incomprehensible words R40.222 ☑
      irritable cries (< 2 years of age) R40.224 ☑
      moans/grunts to pain; restless (< 2 years old)
          R40.222 ☑
      oriented R40.225 ☑
      score of
        1 R40.221 ☑
        2 R40.222 ☑

Coma — *continued*
  with — *continued*
    verbal response — *continued*
      score of — *continued*
        3 R40.223 ☑
        4 R40.224 ☑
        5 R40.225 ☑
      screaming (2-5 years of age) R40.223 ☑
      uses appropriate words (2-5 years of age)
          R40.225 ☑
  eclamptic — *see* Eclampsia
  epileptic — *see* Epilepsy
  Glasgow, scale score — *see* Glasgow coma scale
  hepatic — *see* Failure, hepatic, by type, with coma
  hyperglycemic (diabetic) — *see* Diabetes, by type, with
      hyperosmolarity, with coma
  hyperosmolar (diabetic) — *see* Diabetes, by type, with
      hyperosmolarity, with coma
  hypoglycemic (diabetic) — *see* Diabetes, by type, with
      hypoglycemia, with coma
    nondiabetic E15
  in diabetes — *see* Diabetes, coma
  insulin-induced — *see* Coma, hypoglycemic
  ketoacidotic (diabetic) — *see* Diabetes, by type, with
      ketoacidosis, with coma
  myxedematous E03.5
  newborn P91.5
  persistent vegetative state R40.3
  specified NEC, without documented Glasgow coma
      scale score, or with partial Glasgow coma scale
      score reported R40.244 ☑
Comatose — *see* Coma
Combat fatigue F43.0
Combined — *see* condition
Comedo, comedones (giant) L70.0
Comedocarcinoma — *see also* Neoplasm, breast, malig-
    nant
  noninfiltrating
    breast D05.8- ☑
    specified site — *see* Neoplasm, in situ, by site
    unspecified site D05.8- ☑
Comedomastitis — *see* Ectasia, mammary duct
Comminuted fracture — *code as* Fracture, closed
Common
  arterial trunk Q20.0
  atrioventricular canal Q21.2
  atrium Q21.1
  cold (head) J00
  truncus (arteriosus) Q20.0
  variable immunodeficiency — *see* Immunodeficiency,
      common variable
  ventricle Q20.4
Commotio, commotion (current)
  brain — *see* Injury, intracranial, concussion
  cerebri — *see* Injury, intracranial, concussion
  retinae S05.8X- ☑
  spinal cord — *see* Injury, spinal cord, by region
  spinalis — *see* Injury, spinal cord, by region
Communication
  between
    base of aorta and pulmonary artery Q21.4
    left ventricle and right atrium Q20.5
    pericardial sac and pleural sac Q34.8
    pulmonary artery and pulmonary vein, congenital
        Q25.72
  congenital between uterus and digestive or urinary
      tract Q51.7
Compartment syndrome (deep) (posterior) (traumatic)
    T79.A0 ☑ (*following* T79.7)
  abdomen T79.A3 ☑ (*following* T79.7)
  lower extremity (hip, buttock, thigh, leg, foot, toes)
      T79.A2 ☑ (*following* T79.7)
  nontraumatic
    abdomen M79.A3 (*following* M79.7)
    lower extremity (hip, buttock, thigh, leg, foot, toes)
        M79.A2- ☑ (*following* M79.7)
    specified site NEC M79.A9 (*following* M79.7)
    upper extremity (shoulder, arm, forearm, wrist,
        hand, fingers) M79.A1- ☑ (*following* M79.7)
  specified site NEC T79.A9 ☑ (*following* T79.7)
  upper extremity (shoulder, arm, forearm, wrist, hand,
      fingers) T79.A1- ☑ (*following* T79.7)
Compensation
  failure — *see* Disease, heart
  neurosis, psychoneurosis — *see* Disorder, factitious
Complaint — *see also* Disease
  bowel, functional K59.9

⏷ Subterms under main terms may continue to next column or page   ☑ Additional Character Required — Refer to the Tabular List for Character Selection   57

Colitis — Complaint

Complaint — *continued*
  bowel, functional — *continued*
    psychogenic F45.8
    intestine, functional K59.9
      psychogenic F45.8
  kidney — *see* Disease, renal
  miners' J6Ø
Complete — *see* condition
Complex
  Addison-Schilder E71.528
  cardiorenal — *see* Hypertension, cardiorenal
  Costen's M26.69
  disseminated mycobacterium avium- intracellulare (DMAC) A31.2
  Eisenmenger's (ventricular septal defect) I27.83
  hypersexual F52.8
  jumped process, spine — *see* Dislocation, vertebra
  primary, tuberculous A15.7
  Schilder-Addison E71.528
  subluxation (vertebral) M99.19
    abdomen M99.19
    acromioclavicular M99.17
    cervical region M99.11
    cervicothoracic M99.11
    costochondral M99.18
    costovertebral M99.18
    head region M99.1Ø
    hip M99.15
    lower extremity M99.16
    lumbar region M99.13
    lumbosacral M99.13
    occipitocervical M99.1Ø
    pelvic region M99.15
    pubic M99.15
    rib cage M99.18
    sacral region M99.14
    sacrococcygeal M99.14
    sacroiliac M99.14
    specified NEC M99.19
    sternochondral M99.18
    sternoclavicular M99.17
    thoracic region M99.12
    thoracolumbar M99.12
    upper extremity M99.17
  Taussig-Bing (transposition, aorta and overriding pulmonary artery) Q2Ø.1
Complication(s) (from) (of)
  accidental puncture or laceration during a procedure (of) — *see* Complications, intraoperative (intraprocedural), puncture or laceration
  amputation stump (surgical) (late) NEC T87.9
    dehiscence T87.81
    infection or inflammation T87.4Ø
      lower limb T87.4- ☑
      upper limb T87.4- ☑
    necrosis T87.5Ø
      lower limb T87.5- ☑
      upper limb T87.5- ☑
    neuroma T87.3Ø
      lower limb T87.3- ☑
      upper limb T87.3- ☑
    specified type NEC T87.89
  anastomosis (and bypass) — *see also* Complications, prosthetic device or implant
    intestinal (internal) NEC K91.89
      involving urinary tract N99.89
    urinary tract (involving intestinal tract) N99.89
    vascular — *see* Complications, cardiovascular device or implant
  anesthesia, anesthetic — *see also* Anesthesia, complication T88.59
    brain, postpartum, puerperal O89.2
    cardiac
      in
        labor and delivery O74.2
        pregnancy O29.19- ☑
      postpartum, puerperal O89.1
    central nervous system
      in
        labor and delivery O74.3
        pregnancy O29.29- ☑
      postpartum, puerperal O89.2
    difficult or failed intubation T88.4 ☑
      in pregnancy O29.6- ☑
    failed sedation (conscious) (moderate) during procedure T88.52 ☑
    general, unintended awareness during procedure T88.53 ☑

Complication(s) — *continued*
  anesthesia, anesthetic — *see also* Anesthesia, complication — *continued*
    hyperthermia, malignant T88.3 ☑
    hypothermia T88.51 ☑
    intubation failure T88.4 ☑
    malignant hyperthermia T88.3 ☑
    pulmonary
      in
        labor and delivery O74.1
        pregnancy NEC O29.Ø9- ☑
      postpartum, puerperal O89.Ø9
    shock T88.2 ☑
    spinal and epidural
      in
        labor and delivery NEC O74.6
          headache O74.5
        pregnancy NEC O29.5X- ☑
      postpartum, puerperal NEC O89.5
        headache O89.4
    unintended awareness under general anesthesia during procedure T88.53 ☑
  anti-reflux device — *see* Complications, esophageal anti-reflux device
  aortic (bifurcation) graft — *see* Complications, graft, vascular
  aortocoronary (bypass) graft — *see* Complications, coronary artery (bypass) graft
  aortofemoral (bypass) graft — *see* Complications, extremity artery (bypass) graft
  arteriovenous
    fistula, surgically created T82.9 ☑
      embolism T82.818 ☑
      fibrosis T82.828 ☑
      hemorrhage T82.838 ☑
      infection or inflammation T82.7 ☑
      mechanical
        breakdown T82.51Ø ☑
        displacement T82.52Ø ☑
        leakage T82.53Ø ☑
        malposition T82.52Ø ☑
        obstruction T82.59Ø ☑
        perforation T82.59Ø ☑
        protrusion T82.59Ø ☑
      pain T82.848 ☑
      specified type NEC T82.898 ☑
      stenosis T82.858 ☑
      thrombosis T82.868 ☑
    shunt, surgically created T82.9 ☑
      embolism T82.818 ☑
      fibrosis T82.828 ☑
      hemorrhage T82.838 ☑
      infection or inflammation T82.7 ☑
      mechanical
        breakdown T82.511 ☑
        displacement T82.521 ☑
        leakage T82.531 ☑
        malposition T82.521 ☑
        obstruction T82.591 ☑
        perforation T82.591 ☑
        protrusion T82.591 ☑
      pain T82.848 ☑
      specified type NEC T82.898 ☑
      stenosis T82.858 ☑
      thrombosis T82.868 ☑
  arthroplasty — *see* Complications, joint prosthesis
  artificial
    fertilization or insemination N98.9
      attempted introduction (of)
        embryo in embryo transfer N98.3
        ovum following in vitro fertilization N98.2
      hyperstimulation of ovaries N98.1
      infection N98.Ø
      specified NEC N98.8
    heart T82.9
      embolism T82.817 ☑
      fibrosis T82.827 ☑
      hemorrhage T82.837 ☑
      infection or inflammation T82.7 ☑
      mechanical
        breakdown T82.512 ☑
        displacement T82.522 ☑
        leakage T82.532 ☑
        malposition T82.522 ☑
        obstruction T82.592 ☑
        perforation T82.592 ☑

Complication(s) — *continued*
  artificial — *continued*
    heart — *continued*
      mechanical — *continued*
        protrusion T82.592 ☑
      pain T82.847 ☑
      specified type NEC T82.897 ☑
      stenosis T82.857 ☑
      thrombosis T82.867 ☑
    opening
      cecostomy — *see* Complications, colostomy
      colostomy — *see* Complications, colostomy
      cystostomy — *see* Complications, cystostomy
      enterostomy — *see* Complications, enterostomy
      gastrostomy — *see* Complications, gastrostomy
      ileostomy — *see* Complications, enterostomy
      jejunostomy — *see* Complications, enterostomy
      nephrostomy — *see* Complications, stoma, urinary tract
      tracheostomy — *see* Complications, tracheostomy
      ureterostomy — *see* Complications, stoma, urinary tract
      urethrostomy — *see* Complications, stoma, urinary tract
  balloon implant or device
    gastrointestinal T85.9 ☑
      embolism T85.818 ☑
      fibrosis T85.828 ☑
      hemorrhage T85.838 ☑
      infection and inflammation T85.79 ☑
      pain T85.848 ☑
      specified type NEC T85.898 ☑
      stenosis T85.858 ☑
      thrombosis T85.868 ☑
    vascular (counterpulsation) T82.9 ☑
      embolism T82.818 ☑
      fibrosis T82.828 ☑
      hemorrhage T82.838 ☑
      infection or inflammation T82.7 ☑
      mechanical
        breakdown T82.513 ☑
        displacement T82.523 ☑
        leakage T82.533 ☑
        malposition T82.523 ☑
        obstruction T82.593 ☑
        perforation T82.593 ☑
        protrusion T82.593 ☑
      pain T82.848 ☑
      specified type NEC T82.898 ☑
      stenosis T82.858 ☑
      thrombosis T82.868 ☑
  bariatric procedure
    gastric band procedure K95.Ø9
      infection K95.Ø1
    specified procedure NEC K95.89
      infection K95.81
  bile duct implant (prosthetic) T85.9 ☑
    embolism T85.818 ☑
    fibrosis T85.828 ☑
    hemorrhage T85.838 ☑
    infection and inflammation T85.79 ☑
    mechanical
      breakdown T85.51Ø ☑
      displacement T85.52Ø ☑
      malfunction T85.51Ø ☑
      malposition T85.52Ø ☑
      obstruction T85.59Ø ☑
      perforation T85.59Ø ☑
      protrusion T85.59Ø ☑
      specified NEC T85.59Ø ☑
    pain T85.848 ☑
    specified type NEC T85.898 ☑
    stenosis T85.858 ☑
    thrombosis T85.868 ☑
  bladder device (auxiliary) — *see* Complications, genitourinary, device or implant, urinary system
  bleeding (postoperative) — *see* Complication, postoperative, hemorrhage
    intraoperative — *see* Complication, intraoperative, hemorrhage
  blood vessel graft — *see* Complications, graft, vascular
  bone
    device NEC T84.9 ☑
      embolism T84.81 ☑
      fibrosis T84.82 ☑

Complication(s) — continued
- bone — continued
  - device — continued
    - hemorrhage T84.83 ☑
    - infection or inflammation T84.7 ☑
    - mechanical
      - breakdown T84.318 ☑
      - displacement T84.328 ☑
      - malposition T84.328 ☑
      - obstruction T84.398 ☑
      - perforation T84.398 ☑
      - protrusion T84.398 ☑
    - pain T84.84 ☑
    - specified type NEC T84.89 ☑
    - stenosis T84.85 ☑
    - thrombosis T84.86 ☑
  - graft — see Complications, graft, bone
  - growth stimulator (electrode) — see Complications, electronic stimulator device, bone
  - marrow transplant — see Complications, transplant, bone, marrow
- brain neurostimulator (electrode) — see Complications, electronic stimulator device, brain
- breast implant (prosthetic) T85.9 ☑
  - capsular contracture T85.44 ☑
  - embolism T85.818 ☑
  - fibrosis T85.828 ☑
  - hemorrhage T85.838 ☑
  - infection and inflammation T85.79 ☑
  - mechanical
    - breakdown T85.41 ☑
    - displacement T85.42 ☑
    - leakage T85.43 ☑
    - malposition T85.42 ☑
    - obstruction T85.49 ☑
    - perforation T85.49 ☑
    - protrusion T85.49 ☑
    - specified NEC T85.49 ☑
  - pain T85.848 ☑
  - specified type NEC T85.898 ☑
  - stenosis T85.858 ☑
  - thrombosis T85.868 ☑
- bypass — see also Complications, prosthetic device or implant
  - aortocoronary — see Complications, coronary artery (bypass) graft
  - arterial — see also Complications, graft, vascular
    - extremity — see Complications, extremity artery (bypass) graft
- cardiac — see also Disease, heart
  - device, implant or graft T82.9 ☑
    - embolism T82.817 ☑
    - fibrosis T82.827 ☑
    - hemorrhage T82.837 ☑
    - infection or inflammation T82.7 ☑
      - valve prosthesis T82.6 ☑
    - mechanical
      - breakdown T82.519 ☑
        - specified device NEC T82.518 ☑
      - displacement T82.529 ☑
        - specified device NEC T82.528 ☑
      - leakage T82.539 ☑
        - specified device NEC T82.538 ☑
      - malposition T82.529 ☑
        - specified device NEC T82.528 ☑
      - obstruction T82.599 ☑
        - specified device NEC T82.598 ☑
      - perforation T82.599 ☑
        - specified device NEC T82.598 ☑
      - protrusion T82.599 ☑
        - specified device NEC T82.598 ☑
    - pain T82.847 ☑
    - specified type NEC T82.897 ☑
    - stenosis T82.857 ☑
    - thrombosis T82.867 ☑
- cardiovascular device, graft or implant T82.9 ☑
  - aortic graft — see Complications, graft, vascular
  - arteriovenous
    - fistula, artificial — see Complication, arteriovenous, fistula, surgically created
    - shunt — see Complication, arteriovenous, shunt, surgically created
  - artificial heart — see Complication, artificial, heart
  - balloon (counterpulsation) device — see Complication, balloon implant, vascular

Complication(s) — continued
- cardiovascular device, graft or implant — continued
  - carotid artery graft — see Complications, graft, vascular
  - coronary bypass graft — see Complication, coronary artery (bypass) graft
  - dialysis catheter (vascular) — see Complication, catheter, dialysis
  - electronic T82.9 ☑
    - electrode T82.9 ☑
      - embolism T82.817 ☑
      - fibrosis T82.827 ☑
      - hemorrhage T82.837 ☑
      - infection T82.7 ☑
      - mechanical
        - breakdown T82.110 ☑
        - displacement T82.120 ☑
        - leakage T82.190 ☑
        - obstruction T82.190 ☑
        - perforation T82.190 ☑
        - protrusion T82.190 ☑
        - specified type NEC T82.190 ☑
      - pain T82.847 ☑
      - specified NEC T82.897 ☑
      - stenosis T82.857 ☑
      - thrombosis T82.867 ☑
    - embolism T82.817 ☑
    - fibrosis T82.827 ☑
    - hemorrhage T82.837 ☑
    - infection T82.7 ☑
    - mechanical
      - breakdown T82.119 ☑
      - displacement T82.129 ☑
      - leakage T82.199 ☑
      - obstruction T82.199 ☑
      - perforation T82.199 ☑
      - protrusion T82.199 ☑
      - specified type NEC T82.199 ☑
    - pain T82.847 ☑
    - pulse generator T82.9 ☑
      - embolism T82.817 ☑
      - fibrosis T82.827 ☑
      - hemorrhage T82.837 ☑
      - infection T82.7 ☑
      - mechanical
        - breakdown T82.111 ☑
        - displacement T82.121 ☑
        - leakage T82.191 ☑
        - obstruction T82.191 ☑
        - perforation T82.191 ☑
        - protrusion T82.191 ☑
        - specified type NEC T82.191 ☑
      - pain T82.847 ☑
      - specified NEC T82.897 ☑
      - stenosis T82.857 ☑
      - thrombosis T82.867 ☑
    - specified condition NEC T82.897 ☑
    - specified device NEC T82.9 ☑
      - embolism T82.817 ☑
      - fibrosis T82.827 ☑
      - hemorrhage T82.837 ☑
      - infection T82.7 ☑
      - mechanical
        - breakdown T82.118 ☑
        - displacement T82.128 ☑
        - leakage T82.198 ☑
        - obstruction T82.198 ☑
        - perforation T82.198 ☑
        - protrusion T82.198 ☑
        - specified type NEC T82.198 ☑
      - pain T82.847 ☑
      - specified NEC T82.897 ☑
      - stenosis T82.857 ☑
      - thrombosis T82.867 ☑
    - stenosis T82.857 ☑
    - thrombosis T82.867 ☑
  - extremity artery graft — see Complication, extremity artery (bypass) graft
  - femoral artery graft — see Complication, extremity artery (bypass) graft
  - heart
    - transplant — see Complication, transplant, heart
    - valve — see Complication, prosthetic device, heart valve
      - graft — see Complication, heart, valve, graft

Complication(s) — continued
- cardiovascular device, graft or implant — continued
  - heart-lung transplant — see Complication, transplant, heart, with lung
  - infection or inflammation T82.7 ☑
  - umbrella device — see Complication, umbrella device, vascular
  - vascular graft (or anastomosis) — see Complication, graft, vascular
  - carotid artery (bypass) graft — see Complications, graft, vascular
  - catheter (device) NEC — see also Complications, prosthetic device or implant
    - cranial infusion
      - infection and inflammation T85.735 ☑
      - mechanical
        - breakdown T85.610 ☑
        - displacement T85.620 ☑
        - leakage T85.630 ☑
        - malfunction T85.690 ☑
        - malposition T85.620 ☑
        - obstruction T85.690 ☑
        - perforation T85.690 ☑
        - protrusion T85.690 ☑
        - specified NEC T85.690 ☑
    - cystostomy T83.9 ☑
      - embolism T83.81 ☑
      - fibrosis T83.82 ☑
      - hemorrhage T83.83 ☑
      - infection and inflammation T83.510 ☑
      - mechanical
        - breakdown T83.010 ☑
        - displacement T83.020 ☑
        - leakage T83.030 ☑
        - malposition T83.020 ☑
        - obstruction T83.090 ☑
        - perforation T83.090 ☑
        - protrusion T83.090 ☑
        - specified NEC T83.090 ☑
      - pain T83.84 ☑
      - specified type NEC T83.89 ☑
      - stenosis T83.85 ☑
      - thrombosis T83.86 ☑
    - dialysis (vascular) T82.9 ☑
      - embolism T82.818 ☑
      - fibrosis T82.828 ☑
      - hemorrhage T82.838 ☑
      - infection and inflammation T82.7 ☑
      - intraperitoneal — see Complications, catheter, intraperitoneal
      - mechanical
        - breakdown T82.41 ☑
        - displacement T82.42 ☑
        - leakage T82.43 ☑
        - malposition T82.42 ☑
        - obstruction T82.49 ☑
        - perforation T82.49 ☑
        - protrusion T82.49 ☑
      - pain T82.848 ☑
      - specified type NEC T82.898 ☑
      - stenosis T82.858 ☑
      - thrombosis T82.868 ☑
    - epidural infusion T85.9 ☑
      - embolism T85.810 ☑
      - fibrosis T85.820 ☑
      - hemorrhage T85.830 ☑
      - infection and inflammation T85.735 ☑
      - mechanical
        - breakdown T85.610 ☑
        - displacement T85.620 ☑
        - leakage T85.630 ☑
        - malfunction T85.610 ☑
        - malposition T85.620 ☑
        - obstruction T85.690 ☑
        - perforation T85.690 ☑
        - protrusion T85.690 ☑
        - specified NEC T85.690 ☑
      - pain T85.840 ☑
      - specified type NEC T85.890 ☑
      - stenosis T85.850 ☑
      - thrombosis T85.860 ☑
    - intraperitoneal dialysis T85.9 ☑
      - embolism T85.818 ☑
      - fibrosis T85.828 ☑
      - hemorrhage T85.838 ☑
      - infection and inflammation T85.71 ☑

Complication(s) — *continued*
catheter — *see also* Complications, prosthetic device
or implant — *continued*
intraperitoneal dialysis — *continued*
mechanical
breakdown T85.611 ☑
displacement T85.621 ☑
leakage T85.631 ☑
malfunction T85.611 ☑
malposition T85.621 ☑
obstruction T85.691 ☑
perforation T85.691 ☑
protrusion T85.691 ☑
specified NEC T85.691 ☑
pain T85.848 ☑
specified type NEC T85.898 ☑
stenosis T85.858 ☑
thrombosis T85.868 ☑
intrathecal infusion
infection and inflammation T85.735 ☑
mechanical
breakdown T85.610 ☑
displacement T85.620 ☑
leakage T85.630 ☑
malfunction T85.690 ☑
malposition T85.620 ☑
obstruction T85.690 ☑
perforation T85.690 ☑
protrusion T85.690 ☑
specified NEC T85.690 ☑
intravenous infusion T82.9 ☑
embolism T82.818 ☑
fibrosis T82.828 ☑
hemorrhage T82.838 ☑
infection or inflammation T82.7 ☑
mechanical
breakdown T82.514 ☑
displacement T82.524 ☑
leakage T82.534 ☑
malposition T82.524 ☑
obstruction T82.594 ☑
perforation T82.594 ☑
protrusion T82.594 ☑
pain T82.848 ☑
specified type NEC T82.898 ☑
stenosis T82.858 ☑
thrombosis T82.868 ☑
spinal infusion
infection and inflammation T85.735 ☑
mechanical
breakdown T85.610 ☑
displacement T85.620 ☑
leakage T85.630 ☑
malfunction T85.690 ☑
malposition T85.620 ☑
obstruction T85.690 ☑
perforation T85.690 ☑
protrusion T85.690 ☑
specified NEC T85.690 ☑
subarachnoid infusion
infection and inflammation T85.735 ☑
mechanical
breakdown T85.610 ☑
displacement T85.620 ☑
leakage T85.630 ☑
malfunction T85.690 ☑
malposition T85.620 ☑
obstruction T85.690 ☑
perforation T85.690 ☑
protrusion T85.690 ☑
specified NEC T85.690 ☑
subdural infusion T85.9 ☑
embolism T85.810 ☑
fibrosis T85.820 ☑
hemorrhage T85.830 ☑
infection and inflammation T85.735 ☑
mechanical
breakdown T85.610 ☑
displacement T85.620 ☑
leakage T85.630 ☑
malfunction T85.610 ☑
malposition T85.620 ☑
obstruction T85.690 ☑
perforation T85.690 ☑
protrusion T85.690 ☑
specified NEC T85.690 ☑

Complication(s) — *continued*
catheter — *see also* Complications, prosthetic device
or implant — *continued*
subdural infusion — *continued*
pain T85.840 ☑
specified type NEC T85.890 ☑
stenosis T85.850 ☑
thrombosis T85.860 ☑
urethral T83.9 ☑
displacement T83.028 ☑
embolism T83.81 ☑
fibrosis T83.82 ☑
hemorrhage T83.83 ☑
indwelling
breakdown T83.011 ☑
displacement T83.021 ☑
infection and inflammation T83.511 ☑
leakage T83.031 ☑
specified complication NEC T83.091 ☑
infection and inflammation T83.511 ☑
leakage T83.038 ☑
malposition T83.028 ☑
mechanical
breakdown T83.011 ☑
obstruction (mechanical) T83.091 ☑
pain T83.84 ☑
perforation T83.091 ☑
protrusion T83.091 ☑
specified type NEC T83.091 ☑
stenosis T83.85 ☑
thrombosis T83.86 ☑
urinary NEC
breakdown T83.018 ☑
displacement T83.028 ☑
infection and inflammation T83.518 ☑
leakage T83.038 ☑
specified complication NEC T83.098 ☑
cecostomy (stoma) — *see* Complications, colostomy
cesarean delivery wound NEC O90.89
disruption O90.0
hematoma O90.2
infection (following delivery) O86.00
chemotherapy (antineoplastic) NEC T88.7 ☑
chin implant (prosthetic) — *see* Complication, prosthetic device or implant, specified NEC
circulatory system I99.8
intraoperative I97.88
postprocedural I97.89
following cardiac surgery — *see also* Infarct,
myocardium, associated with revascularization procedure I97.19- ☑
postcardiotomy syndrome I97.0
hypertension I97.3
lymphedema after mastectomy I97.2
postcardiotomy syndrome I97.0
specified NEC I97.89
colostomy (stoma) K94.00
hemorrhage K94.01
infection K94.02
malfunction K94.03
mechanical K94.03
specified complication NEC K94.09
contraceptive device, intrauterine — *see* Complications,
intrauterine, contraceptive device
cord (umbilical) — *see* Complications, umbilical cord
corneal graft — *see* Complications, graft, cornea
coronary artery (bypass) graft T82.9 ☑
atherosclerosis — *see* Arteriosclerosis, coronary
(artery),
embolism T82.818 ☑
fibrosis T82.828 ☑
hemorrhage T82.838 ☑
infection and inflammation T82.7 ☑
mechanical
breakdown T82.211 ☑
displacement T82.212 ☑
leakage T82.213 ☑
malposition T82.212 ☑
obstruction T82.218 ☑
perforation T82.218 ☑
protrusion T82.218 ☑
specified NEC T82.218 ☑
pain T82.848 ☑
specified type NEC T82.898 ☑
stenosis T82.858 ☑
thrombosis T82.868 ☑

Complication(s) — *continued*
counterpulsation device (balloon), intra- aortic — *see*
Complications, balloon implant, vascular
cystostomy (stoma) N99.518
catheter — *see* Complications, catheter, cystostomy
hemorrhage N99.510
infection N99.511
malfunction N99.512
specified type NEC N99.518
delivery — *see also* Complications, obstetric O75.9
procedure (instrumental) (manual) (surgical) O75.4
specified NEC O75.89
dialysis (peritoneal) (renal) — *see also* Complications,
infusion
catheter (vascular) — *see* Complication, catheter,
dialysis
peritoneal, intraperitoneal — *see* Complications,
catheter, intraperitoneal
dorsal column (spinal) neurostimulator — *see* Complications, electronic stimulator device, spinal cord
drug NEC T88.7 ☑
ear procedure — *see also* Disorder, ear
intraoperative H95.88
hematoma — *see* Complications, intraoperative,
hemorrhage (hematoma) (of), ear
hemorrhage — *see* Complications, intraoperative, hemorrhage (hematoma) (of), ear
laceration — *see* Complications, intraoperative,
puncture or laceration..., ear
specified NEC H95.88
postoperative H95.89
external ear canal stenosis H95.81- ☑
hematoma — *see* Complications, postprocedural,
hematoma (of), ear
hemorrhage — *see* Complications, postprocedural, hemorrhage (of), ear
postmastoidectomy — *see* Complications, postmastoidectomy
seroma — *see* Complications, postprocedural,
seroma (of), mastoid process
specified NEC H95.89
ectopic pregnancy O08.9
damage to pelvic organs O08.6
embolism O08.2
genital infection O08.0
hemorrhage (delayed) (excessive) O08.1
metabolic disorder O08.5
renal failure O08.4
shock O08.3
specified type NEC O08.0
venous complication NEC O08.7
electronic stimulator device
bladder (urinary) — *see* Complications, electronic
stimulator device, urinary
bone T84.9 ☑
breakdown T84.310 ☑
displacement T84.320 ☑
embolism T84.81 ☑
fibrosis T84.82 ☑
hemorrhage T84.83 ☑
infection or inflammation T84.7 ☑
malfunction T84.310 ☑
malposition T84.320 ☑
mechanical NEC T84.390 ☑
obstruction T84.390 ☑
pain T84.84 ☑
perforation T84.390 ☑
protrusion T84.390 ☑
specified type NEC T84.89 ☑
stenosis T84.85 ☑
thrombosis T84.86 ☑
brain T85.9 ☑
embolism T85.810 ☑
fibrosis T85.820 ☑
hemorrhage T85.830 ☑
infection and inflammation T85.731 ☑
mechanical
breakdown T85.110 ☑
displacement T85.120 ☑
leakage T85.190 ☑
malposition T85.120 ☑
obstruction T85.190 ☑
perforation T85.190 ☑
protrusion T85.190 ☑
specified NEC T85.190 ☑
pain T85.840 ☑
specified type NEC T85.890 ☑

Complication(s) — *continued*
 electronic stimulator device — *continued*
  brain — *continued*
   stenosis T85.850 ☑
   thrombosis T85.860 ☑
  cardiac (defibrillator) (pacemaker) — *see* Complications, cardiovascular device or implant, electronic
  generator (brain) (gastric) (peripheral) (sacral) (spinal)
   breakdown T85.113 ☑
   displacement T85.123 ☑
   leakage T85.193 ☑
   malposition T85.123 ☑
   obstruction T85.193 ☑
   perforation T85.193 ☑
   protrusion T85.193 ☑
   specified type NEC T85.193 ☑
  muscle T84.9 ☑
   breakdown T84.418 ☑
   displacement T84.428 ☑
   embolism T84.81 ☑
   fibrosis T84.82 ☑
   hemorrhage T84.83 ☑
   infection or inflammation T84.7 ☑
   mechanical NEC T84.498 ☑
   pain T84.84 ☑
   specified type NEC T84.89 ☑
   stenosis T84.85 ☑
   thrombosis T84.86 ☑
  nervous system T85.9 ☑
   brain — *see* Complications, electronic stimulator device, brain
   cranial nerve — *see* Complications, electronic stimulator device, peripheral nerve
   embolism T85.810 ☑
   fibrosis T85.820 ☑
   gastric nerve — *see* Complications, electronic stimulator device, peripheral nerve
   hemorrhage T85.830 ☑
   infection and inflammation T85.738 ☑
   mechanical
    breakdown T85.118 ☑
    displacement T85.128 ☑
    leakage T85.199 ☑
    malposition T85.128 ☑
    obstruction T85.199 ☑
    perforation T85.199 ☑
    protrusion T85.199 ☑
    specified NEC T85.199 ☑
   pain T85.840 ☑
   peripheral nerve — *see* Complications, electronic stimulator device, peripheral nerve
   sacral nerve — *see* Complications, electronic stimulator device, peripheral nerve
   specified type NEC T85.890 ☑
   spinal cord — *see* Complications, electronic stimulator device, spinal cord
   stenosis T85.850 ☑
   thrombosis T85.860 ☑
   vagal nerve — *see* Complications, electronic stimulator device, peripheral nerve
  peripheral nerve T85.9 ☑
   embolism T85.810 ☑
   fibrosis T85.820 ☑
   hemorrhage T85.830 ☑
   infection and inflammation T85.732 ☑
   mechanical
    breakdown T85.111 ☑
    displacement T85.121 ☑
    leakage T85.191 ☑
    malposition T85.121 ☑
    obstruction T85.191 ☑
    perforation T85.191 ☑
    protrusion T85.191 ☑
    specified NEC T85.191 ☑
   pain T85.840 ☑
   specified type NEC T85.890 ☑
   stenosis T85.850 ☑
   thrombosis T85.860 ☑
  spinal cord T85.9 ☑
   embolism T85.810 ☑
   fibrosis T85.820 ☑
   hemorrhage T85.830 ☑
   infection and inflammation T85.733 ☑

Complication(s) — *continued*
 electronic stimulator device — *continued*
  spinal cord — *continued*
   mechanical
    breakdown T85.112 ☑
    displacement T85.122 ☑
    leakage T85.192 ☑
    malposition T85.122 ☑
    obstruction T85.192 ☑
    perforation T85.192 ☑
    protrusion T85.192 ☑
    specified NEC T85.192 ☑
   pain T85.840 ☑
   specified type NEC T85.890 ☑
   stenosis T85.850 ☑
   thrombosis T85.860 ☑
  urinary T83.9
   embolism T83.81
   fibrosis T83.82
   hemorrhage T83.83
   infection and inflammation T83.598 ☑
   mechanical
    breakdown T83.110 ☑
    displacement T83.120 ☑
    malposition T83.120 ☑
    perforation T83.190 ☑
    protrusion T83.190 ☑
    specified NEC T83.190 ☑
   pain T83.84
   specified type NEC T83.89
   stenosis T83.85
   thrombosis T83.86
 electroshock therapy T88.9 ☑
  specified NEC T88.8 ☑
 endocrine E34.9
  postprocedural
   adrenal hypofunction E89.6
   hypoinsulinemia E89.1
   hypoparathyroidism E89.2
   hypopituitarism E89.3
   hypothyroidism E89.0
   ovarian failure E89.40
    asymptomatic E89.40
    symptomatic E89.41
   specified NEC E89.89
   testicular hypofunction E89.5
 endodontic treatment NEC M27.59
 enterostomy (stoma) K94.10
  hemorrhage K94.11
  infection K94.12
  malfunction K94.13
  mechanical K94.13
  specified complication NEC K94.19
 episiotomy, disruption O90.1
 esophageal anti-reflux device T85.9 ☑
  embolism T85.818 ☑
  fibrosis T85.828 ☑
  hemorrhage T85.838 ☑
  infection and inflammation T85.79 ☑
  mechanical
   breakdown T85.511 ☑
   displacement T85.521 ☑
   malfunction T85.511 ☑
   malposition T85.521 ☑
   obstruction T85.591 ☑
   perforation T85.591 ☑
   protrusion T85.591 ☑
   specified NEC T85.591 ☑
  pain T85.848 ☑
  specified type NEC T85.898 ☑
  stenosis T85.858 ☑
  thrombosis T85.868 ☑
 esophagostomy K94.30
  hemorrhage K94.31
  infection K94.32
  malfunction K94.33
  mechanical K94.33
  specified complication NEC K94.39
 extracorporeal circulation T80.90 ☑
 extremity artery (bypass) graft T82.9 ☑
  arteriosclerosis — *see* Arteriosclerosis, extremities, bypass graft
  embolism T82.818 ☑
  fibrosis T82.828 ☑
  hemorrhage T82.838 ☑
  infection and inflammation T82.7 ☑

Complication(s) — *continued*
 extremity artery graft — *continued*
  mechanical
   breakdown T82.318 ☑
    femoral artery T82.312 ☑
   displacement T82.328 ☑
    femoral artery T82.322 ☑
   leakage T82.338 ☑
    femoral artery T82.332 ☑
   malposition T82.328 ☑
    femoral artery T82.322 ☑
   obstruction T82.398 ☑
    femoral artery T82.392 ☑
   perforation T82.398 ☑
    femoral artery T82.392 ☑
   protrusion T82.398 ☑
    femoral artery T82.392 ☑
  pain T82.848 ☑
  specified type NEC T82.898 ☑
  stenosis T82.858 ☑
  thrombosis T82.868 ☑
 eye H57.9
  corneal graft — *see* Complications, graft, cornea
  implant (prosthetic) T85.9 ☑
   embolism T85.818 ☑
   fibrosis T85.828 ☑
   hemorrhage T85.838 ☑
   infection and inflammation T85.79 ☑
   mechanical
    breakdown T85.318 ☑
    displacement T85.328 ☑
    leakage T85.398 ☑
    malposition T85.328 ☑
    obstruction T85.398 ☑
    perforation T85.398 ☑
    protrusion T85.398 ☑
    specified NEC T85.398 ☑
   pain T85.848 ☑
   specified type NEC T85.898 ☑
   stenosis T85.858 ☑
   thrombosis T85.868 ☑
  intraocular lens — *see* Complications, intraocular lens
  orbital prosthesis — *see* Complications, orbital prosthesis
 female genital N94.9
  device, implant or graft NEC — *see* Complications, genitourinary, device or implant, genital tract
 femoral artery (bypass) graft — *see* Complication, extremity artery (bypass) graft
 fixation device, internal (orthopedic) T84.9 ☑
  infection and inflammation T84.60 ☑
   arm T84.61-
    humerus T84.61- ☑
    radius T84.61- ☑
    ulna T84.61- ☑
   leg T84.629 ☑
    femur T84.62- ☑
    fibula T84.62- ☑
    tibia T84.62- ☑
   specified site NEC T84.89 ☑
   spine T84.63 ☑
  mechanical
   breakdown
    limb T84.119 ☑
     carpal T84.210 ☑
     femur T84.11- ☑
     fibula T84.11- ☑
     humerus T84.11- ☑
     metacarpal T84.210 ☑
     metatarsal T84.213 ☑
     phalanx
      foot T84.213 ☑
      hand T84.210 ☑
     radius T84.11- ☑
     tarsal T84.213 ☑
     tibia T84.11- ☑
     ulna T84.11- ☑
    specified bone NEC T84.218 ☑
    spine T84.216 ☑
   displacement
    limb T84.129 ☑
     carpal T84.220 ☑
     femur T84.12- ☑
     fibula T84.12- ☑
     humerus T84.12- ☑

Index

Complication — Complication

Complication(s) — *continued*
- fixation device, internal — *continued*
  - mechanical — *continued*
    - displacement — *continued*
      - limb — *continued*
        - metacarpal T84.220 ✓
        - metatarsal T84.223 ✓
        - phalanx
          - foot T84.223 ✓
          - hand T84.220 ✓
        - radius T84.12- ✓
        - tarsal T84.223 ✓
        - tibia T84.12- ✓
        - ulna T84.12- ✓
      - specified bone NEC T84.228 ✓
      - spine T84.226 ✓
    - malposition — *see* Complications, fixation device, internal, mechanical, displacement
    - obstruction — *see* Complications, fixation device, internal, mechanical, specified type NEC
    - perforation — *see* Complications, fixation device, internal, mechanical, specified type NEC
    - protrusion — *see* Complications, fixation device, internal, mechanical, specified type NEC
    - specified type NEC
      - limb T84.199 ✓
        - carpal T84.290 ✓
        - femur T84.19- ✓
        - fibula T84.19- ✓
        - humerus T84.19- ✓
        - metacarpal T84.290 ✓
        - metatarsal T84.293 ✓
        - phalanx
          - foot T84.293 ✓
          - hand T84.290 ✓
        - radius T84.19- ✓
        - tarsal T84.293 ✓
        - tibia T84.19- ✓
        - ulna T84.19- ✓
      - specified bone NEC T84.298 ✓
      - vertebra T84.296 ✓
    - specified type NEC T84.89 ✓
    - embolism T84.81 ✓
    - fibrosis T84.82 ✓
    - hemorrhage T84.83 ✓
    - pain T84.84 ✓
    - specified complication NEC T84.89 ✓
    - stenosis T84.85 ✓
    - thrombosis T84.86 ✓
- following
  - acute myocardial infarction NEC I23.8
    - aneurysm (false) (of cardiac wall) (of heart wall) (ruptured) I23.3
    - angina I23.7
    - atrial
      - septal defect I23.1
      - thrombosis I23.6
    - cardiac wall rupture I23.3
    - chordae tendinae rupture I23.4
    - defect
      - septal
        - atrial (heart) I23.1
        - ventricular (heart) I23.2
    - hemopericardium I23.0
    - papillary muscle rupture I23.5
    - rupture
      - cardiac wall I23.3
        - with hemopericardium I23.0
      - chordae tendineae I23.4
      - papillary muscle I23.5
    - specified NEC I23.8
    - thrombosis
      - atrium I23.6
      - auricular appendage I23.6
      - ventricle (heart) I23.6
    - ventricular
      - septal defect I23.2
      - thrombosis I23.6
  - ectopic or molar pregnancy O08.9
    - cardiac arrest O08.81
    - sepsis O08.82
    - specified type NEC O08.89
    - urinary tract infection O08.83
  - termination of pregnancy — *see* Abortion
- gastrointestinal K92.9
  - bile duct prosthesis — *see* Complications, bile duct implant

Complication(s) — *continued*
- gastrointestinal — *continued*
  - esophageal anti-reflux device — *see* Complications, esophageal anti-reflux device
  - postoperative
    - colostomy — *see* Complications, colostomy
    - dumping syndrome K91.1
    - enterostomy — *see* Complications, enterostomy
    - gastrostomy — *see* Complications, gastrostomy
    - malabsorption NEC K91.2
    - obstruction — *see also* Obstruction, intestine, postoperative K91.30
    - postcholecystectomy syndrome K91.5
    - specified NEC K91.89
    - vomiting after GI surgery K91.0
  - prosthetic device or implant
    - bile duct prosthesis — *see* Complications, bile duct implant
    - esophageal anti-reflux device — *see* Complications, esophageal anti-reflux device
    - specified type NEC
      - embolism T85.818 ✓
      - fibrosis T85.828 ✓
      - hemorrhage T85.838 ✓
      - mechanical
        - breakdown T85.518 ✓
        - displacement T85.528 ✓
        - malfunction T85.518 ✓
        - malposition T85.528 ✓
        - obstruction T85.598 ✓
        - perforation T85.598 ✓
        - protrusion T85.598 ✓
        - specified NEC T85.598 ✓
      - pain T85.848 ✓
      - specified complication NEC T85.898 ✓
      - stenosis T85.858 ✓
      - thrombosis T85.868 ✓
- gastrostomy (stoma) K94.20
  - hemorrhage K94.21
  - infection K94.22
  - malfunction K94.23
  - mechanical K94.23
  - specified complication NEC K94.29
- genitourinary
  - device or implant T83.9 ✓
    - genital tract T83.9 ✓
      - infection or inflammation T83.69 ✓
      - intrauterine contraceptive device — *see* Complications, intrauterine, contraceptive device
      - mechanical — *see* Complications, by device, mechanical
      - mesh — *see* Complications, prosthetic device or implant, mesh
      - penile prosthesis — *see* Complications, prosthetic device, penile
      - specified type NEC T83.89 ✓
        - embolism T83.81 ✓
        - fibrosis T83.82 ✓
        - hemorrhage T83.83 ✓
        - pain T83.84 ✓
        - specified complication NEC T83.89 ✓
        - stenosis T83.85 ✓
        - thrombosis T83.86 ✓
      - vaginal mesh — *see* Complications, prosthetic device or implant, mesh
    - urinary system T83.9 ✓
      - cystostomy catheter — *see* Complication, catheter, cystostomy
      - electronic stimulator — *see* Complications, electronic stimulator device, urinary
      - indwelling urethral catheter — *see* Complications, catheter, urethral, indwelling
      - infection or inflammation T83.598 ✓
        - indwelling urethral catheter T83.511 ✓
      - kidney transplant — *see* Complication, transplant, kidney
      - organ graft — *see* Complication, graft, urinary organ
      - specified type NEC T83.89 ✓
        - embolism T83.81 ✓
        - fibrosis T83.82 ✓
        - hemorrhage T83.83 ✓
        - mechanical T83.198 ✓
          - breakdown T83.118 ✓
          - displacement T83.128 ✓
          - malfunction T83.118 ✓

Complication(s) — *continued*
- genitourinary — *continued*
  - device or implant — *continued*
    - urinary system — *continued*
      - specified type — *continued*
        - mechanical — *continued*
          - malposition T83.128 ✓
          - obstruction T83.198 ✓
          - perforation T83.198 ✓
          - protrusion T83.198 ✓
          - specified NEC T83.198 ✓
        - sphincter implant — *see* Complications, implant, urinary sphincter
        - sphincter, implanted T83.191 ✓
        - stent (ileal conduit) (nephroureteral) T83.193 ✓
        - pain T83.84 ✓
        - specified complication NEC T83.89 ✓
        - stenosis T83.85 ✓
        - thrombosis T83.86 ✓
        - ureteral indwelling T83.192 ✓
  - postprocedural
    - pelvic peritoneal adhesions N99.4
    - renal failure N99.0
    - specified NEC N99.89
    - stoma — *see* Complications, stoma, urinary tract
    - urethral stricture — *see* Stricture, urethra, postprocedural
    - vaginal
      - adhesions N99.2
      - vault prolapse N99.3
- graft (bypass) (patch) — *see also* Complications, prosthetic device or implant
  - aorta — *see* Complications, graft, vascular
  - arterial — *see* Complication, graft, vascular
  - bone T86.839
    - failure T86.831
    - infection T86.832
    - mechanical T84.318 ✓
      - breakdown T84.318 ✓
      - displacement T84.328 ✓
      - protrusion T84.398 ✓
      - specified type NEC T84.398 ✓
    - rejection T86.830
    - specified type NEC T86.838
  - carotid artery — *see* Complications, graft, vascular
  - cornea T86.849
    - failure T86.841
    - infection T86.842
    - mechanical T85.398 ✓
      - breakdown T85.318 ✓
      - displacement T85.328 ✓
      - protrusion T85.398 ✓
      - specified type NEC T85.398 ✓
    - rejection T86.840
    - retroprosthetic membrane T85.398 ✓
    - specified type NEC T86.848
  - femoral artery (bypass) — *see* Complication, extremity artery (bypass) graft
  - genital organ or tract — *see* Complications, genitourinary, device or implant, genital tract
  - muscle T84.9 ✓
    - breakdown T84.410 ✓
    - displacement T84.420 ✓
    - embolism T84.81 ✓
    - fibrosis T84.82 ✓
    - hemorrhage T84.83 ✓
    - infection and inflammation T84.7 ✓
    - mechanical NEC T84.490 ✓
    - pain T84.84 ✓
    - specified type NEC T84.89 ✓
    - stenosis T84.85 ✓
    - thrombosis T84.86 ✓
  - nerve — *see* Complication, prosthetic device or implant, specified NEC
  - skin — *see* Complications, prosthetic device or implant, skin graft
  - tendon T84.9 ✓
    - breakdown T84.410 ✓
    - displacement T84.420 ✓
    - embolism T84.81 ✓
    - fibrosis T84.82 ✓
    - hemorrhage T84.83 ✓
    - infection and inflammation T84.7 ✓
    - mechanical NEC T84.490 ✓
    - pain T84.84 ✓
    - specified type NEC T84.89 ✓

Complication(s) — *continued*
graft — *see also* Complications, prosthetic device or implant — *continued*
  tendon — *continued*
    stenosis T84.85 ☑
    thrombosis T84.86 ☑
  urinary organ T83.9 ☑
    embolism T83.81 ☑
    fibrosis T83.82 ☑
    hemorrhage T83.83 ☑
    infection and inflammation T83.598 ☑
      indwelling urethral catheter T83.511 ☑
    mechanical
      breakdown T83.21 ☑
      displacement T83.22 ☑
      erosion T83.24 ☑
      exposure T83.25 ☑
      leakage T83.23 ☑
      malposition T83.22 ☑
      obstruction T83.29 ☑
      perforation T83.29 ☑
      protrusion T83.29 ☑
      specified NEC T83.29 ☑
    pain T83.84 ☑
    specified type NEC T83.89 ☑
    stenosis T83.85 ☑
    thrombosis T83.86 ☑
  vascular T82.9 ☑
    embolism T82.818 ☑
    femoral artery — *see* Complication, extremity artery (bypass) graft
    fibrosis T82.828 ☑
    hemorrhage T82.838 ☑
    mechanical
      breakdown T82.319 ☑
        aorta (bifurcation) T82.310 ☑
        carotid artery T82.311 ☑
        specified vessel NEC T82.318 ☑
      displacement T82.329 ☑
        aorta (bifurcation) T82.320 ☑
        carotid artery T82.321 ☑
        specified vessel NEC T82.328 ☑
      leakage T82.339 ☑
        aorta (bifurcation) T82.330 ☑
        carotid artery T82.331 ☑
        specified vessel NEC T82.338 ☑
      malposition T82.329 ☑
        aorta (bifurcation) T82.320 ☑
        carotid artery T82.321 ☑
        specified vessel NEC T82.328 ☑
      obstruction T82.399 ☑
        aorta (bifurcation) T82.390 ☑
        carotid artery T82.391 ☑
        specified vessel NEC T82.398 ☑
      perforation T82.399 ☑
        aorta (bifurcation) T82.390 ☑
        carotid artery T82.391 ☑
        specified vessel NEC T82.398 ☑
      protrusion T82.399 ☑
        aorta (bifurcation) T82.390 ☑
        carotid artery T82.391 ☑
        specified vessel NEC T82.398 ☑
    pain T82.848 ☑
    specified complication NEC T82.898 ☑
    stenosis T82.858 ☑
    thrombosis T82.868 ☑
heart I51.9
  assist device
    infection and inflammation T82.7 ☑
  following acute myocardial infarction — *see* Complications, following, acute myocardial infarction
  postoperative — *see* Complications, circulatory system
  transplant — *see* Complication, transplant, heart and lung(s) — *see* Complications, transplant, heart, with lung
  valve
    graft (biological) T82.9 ☑
      embolism T82.817 ☑
      fibrosis T82.827 ☑
      hemorrhage T82.837 ☑
      infection and inflammation T82.7 ☑
      mechanical T82.228 ☑
        breakdown T82.221 ☑
        displacement T82.222 ☑

Complication(s) — *continued*
heart — *continued*
  valve — *continued*
    graft — *continued*
      mechanical — *continued*
        leakage T82.223 ☑
        malposition T82.222 ☑
        obstruction T82.228 ☑
        perforation T82.228 ☑
        protrusion T82.228 ☑
      pain T82.847 ☑
      specified type NEC T82.897 ☑
      stenosis T82.857 ☑
      thrombosis T82.867 ☑
    prosthesis T82.9 ☑
      embolism T82.817 ☑
      fibrosis T82.827 ☑
      hemorrhage T82.837 ☑
      infection or inflammation T82.6 ☑
      mechanical T82.09 ☑
        breakdown T82.01 ☑
        displacement T82.02 ☑
        leakage T82.03 ☑
        malposition T82.02 ☑
        obstruction T82.09 ☑
        perforation T82.09 ☑
        protrusion T82.09 ☑
      pain T82.847 ☑
      specified type NEC T82.897 ☑
        mechanical T82.09 ☑
      stenosis T82.857 ☑
      thrombosis T82.867 ☑
hematoma
  intraoperative — *see* Complication, intraoperative, hemorrhage
  postprocedural — *see* Complication, postprocedural, hematoma
hemodialysis — *see* Complications, dialysis
hemorrhage
  intraoperative — *see* Complication, intraoperative, hemorrhage
  postprocedural — *see* Complication, postprocedural, hemorrhage
ileostomy (stoma) — *see* Complications, enterostomy
immunization (procedure) — *see* Complications, vaccination
implant — *see also* Complications, by site and type
  urinary sphincter T83.9 ☑
    embolism T83.81 ☑
    fibrosis T83.82 ☑
    hemorrhage T83.83 ☑
    infection and inflammation T83.591 ☑
    mechanical
      breakdown T83.111 ☑
      displacement T83.121 ☑
      leakage T83.191 ☑
      malposition T83.121 ☑
      obstruction T83.191 ☑
      perforation T83.191 ☑
      protrusion T83.191 ☑
      specified NEC T83.191 ☑
    pain T83.84 ☑
    specified type NEC T83.89 ☑
    stenosis T83.85 ☑
    thrombosis T83.86 ☑
infusion (procedure) T80.90 ☑
  air embolism T80.0 ☑
  blood — *see* Complications, transfusion
  catheter — *see* Complications, catheter
  infection T80.29 ☑
  pump — *see* Complications, cardiovascular, device or implant
  sepsis T80.29 ☑
  serum reaction — *see also* Reaction, serum T80.69 ☑
    anaphylactic shock — *see also* Shock, anaphylactic T80.59 ☑
  specified type NEC T80.89 ☑
inhalation therapy NEC T81.81 ☑
injection (procedure) T80.90 ☑
  drug reaction — *see* Reaction, drug
  infection T80.29 ☑
  sepsis T80.29 ☑
  serum (prophylactic) (therapeutic) — *see* Complications, vaccination
  specified type NEC T80.89 ☑

Complication(s) — *continued*
injection — *continued*
  vaccine (any) — *see* Complications, vaccination
inoculation (any) — *see* Complications, vaccination
insulin pump
  infection and inflammation T85.72 ☑
  mechanical
    breakdown T85.614 ☑
    displacement T85.624 ☑
    leakage T85.633 ☑
    malposition T85.624 ☑
    obstruction T85.694 ☑
    perforation T85.694 ☑
    protrusion T85.694 ☑
    specified NEC T85.694 ☑
intestinal pouch NEC K91.858
intraocular lens (prosthetic) T85.9 ☑
  embolism T85.818 ☑
  fibrosis T85.828 ☑
  hemorrhage T85.838 ☑
  infection and inflammation T85.79 ☑
  mechanical
    breakdown T85.21 ☑
    displacement T85.22 ☑
    malposition T85.22 ☑
    obstruction T85.29 ☑
    perforation T85.29 ☑
    protrusion T85.29 ☑
    specified NEC T85.29 ☑
  pain T85.848 ☑
  specified type NEC T85.898 ☑
  stenosis T85.858 ☑
  thrombosis T85.868 ☑
intraoperative (intraprocedural)
  cardiac arrest — *see also* Infarct, myocardium, associated with revascularization procedure
    during cardiac surgery I97.710
    during other surgery I97.711
  cardiac functional disturbance NEC — *see also* Infarct, myocardium, associated with revascularization procedure
    during cardiac surgery I97.790
    during other surgery I97.791
  hemorrhage (hematoma) (of)
    circulatory system organ or structure
      during cardiac bypass I97.411
      during cardiac catheterization I97.410
      during other circulatory system procedure I97.418
      during other procedure I97.42
    digestive system organ
      during procedure on digestive system K91.61
      during procedure on other organ K91.62
    ear
      during procedure on ear and mastoid process H95.21
      during procedure on other organ H95.22
    endocrine system organ or structure
      during procedure on endocrine system organ or structure E36.01
      during procedure on other organ E36.02
    eye and adnexa
      during ophthalmic procedure H59.11- ☑
      during other procedure H59.12- ☑
    genitourinary organ or structure
      during procedure on genitourinary organ or structure N99.61
      during procedure on other organ N99.62
    mastoid process
      during procedure on ear and mastoid process H95.21
      during procedure on other organ H95.22
    musculoskeletal structure
      during musculoskeletal surgery M96.810
      during non-orthopedic surgery M96.811
      during orthopedic surgery M96.810
    nervous system
      during a nervous system procedure G97.31
      during other procedure G97.32
    respiratory system
      during other procedure J95.62
      during procedure on respiratory system organ or structure J95.61
    skin and subcutaneous tissue
      during a dermatologic procedure L76.01
      during a procedure on other organ L76.02
    spleen
      during a procedure on other organ D78.02

Complication(s) — *continued*
  intraoperative — *continued*
    hemorrhage — *continued*
      spleen — *continued*
        during a procedure on the spleen D78.01
      puncture or laceration (accidental) (unintentional) (of)
        brain
          during a nervous system procedure G97.48
          during other procedure G97.49
        circulatory system organ or structure
          during circulatory system procedure I97.51
          during other procedure I97.52
        digestive system
          during procedure on digestive system K91.71
          during procedure on other organ K91.72
        ear
          during procedure on ear and mastoid process H95.31
          during procedure on other organ H95.32
        endocrine system organ or structure
          during procedure on endocrine system organ or structure E36.11
          during procedure on other organ E36.12
        eye and adnexa
          during ophthalmic procedure H59.21-
          during other procedure H59.22-
        genitourinary organ or structure
          during procedure on genitourinary organ or structure N99.71
          during procedure on other organ N99.72
        mastoid process
          during procedure on ear and mastoid process H95.31
          during procedure on other organ H95.32
        musculoskeletal structure
          during musculoskeletal surgery M96.820
          during non-orthopedic surgery M96.821
          during orthopedic surgery M96.820
        nervous system
          during a nervous system procedure G97.48
          during other procedure G97.49
        respiratory system
          during other procedure J95.72
          during procedure on respiratory system organ or structure J95.71
        skin and subcutaneous tissue
          during a dermatologic procedure L76.11
          during a procedure on other organ L76.12
        spleen
          during a procedure on other organ D78.12
          during a procedure on the spleen D78.11
      specified NEC
        circulatory system I97.88
        digestive system K91.81
        ear H95.88
        endocrine system E36.8
        eye and adnexa H59.88
        genitourinary system N99.81
        mastoid process H95.88
        musculoskeletal structure M96.89
        nervous system G97.81
        respiratory system J95.88
        skin and subcutaneous tissue L76.81
        spleen D78.81
    intraperitoneal catheter (dialysis) (infusion) — *see* Complications, catheter, intraperitoneal
    intrathecal infusion pump
      infection and inflammation T85.738
      mechanical
        breakdown T85.615
        displacement T85.625
        leakage T85.635
        malfunction T85.695
        malposition T85.625
        obstruction T85.695
        perforation T85.695
        protrusion T85.695
        specified NEC T85.695
    intrauterine
      contraceptive device
        embolism T83.81
        fibrosis T83.82
        hemorrhage T83.83
        infection and inflammation T83.69
        mechanical
          breakdown T83.31
          displacement T83.32

Complication(s) — *continued*
  intrauterine — *continued*
    contraceptive device — *continued*
      mechanical — *continued*
        malposition T83.32
        obstruction T83.39
        perforation T83.39
        protrusion T83.39
        specified NEC T83.39
      pain T83.84
      specified type NEC T83.89
      stenosis T83.85
      thrombosis T83.86
    procedure (fetal), to newborn P96.5
  jejunostomy (stoma) — *see* Complications, enterostomy
  joint prosthesis, internal T84.9
    breakage (fracture) T84.01-
    dislocation T84.02-
    fracture T84.01-
    infection or inflammation T84.50
      hip T84.5-
      knee T84.5-
      specified joint NEC T84.59
    instability T84.02-
    malposition — *see* Complications, joint prosthesis, mechanical, displacement
    mechanical
      breakage, broken T84.01-
      dislocation T84.02-
      fracture T84.01-
      instability T84.02-
      leakage — *see* Complications, joint prosthesis, mechanical, specified NEC
      loosening T84.039
        hip T84.03-
        knee T84.03-
        specified joint NEC T84.038
      obstruction — *see* Complications, joint prosthesis, mechanical, specified NEC
      perforation — *see* Complications, joint prosthesis, mechanical, specified NEC
        osteolysis T84.059
          hip T84.05-
          knee T84.05-
          other specified joint T84.058
        periprosthetic T84.059
      protrusion — *see* Complications, joint prosthesis, mechanical, specified NEC
      specified complication NEC T84.099
        hip T84.09-
        knee T84.09-
        other specified joint T84.098
      subluxation T84.02-
      wear of articular bearing surface T84.069
        hip T84.06-
        knee T84.06-
        other specified joint T84.068
    specified joint NEC T84.89
      embolism T84.81
      fibrosis T84.82
      hemorrhage T84.83
      pain T84.84
      specified complication NEC T84.89
      stenosis T84.85
      thrombosis T84.86
      subluxation T84.02-
  kidney transplant — *see* Complications, transplant, kidney
  labor O75.9
    specified NEC O75.89
  liver transplant (immune or nonimmune) — *see* Complications, transplant, liver
  lumbar puncture G97.1
    cerebrospinal fluid leak G97.0
    headache or reaction G97.1
  lung transplant — *see* Complications, transplant, lung
    and heart — *see* Complications, transplant, lung, with heart
  male genital N50.9
    device, implant or graft — *see* Complications, genitourinary, device or implant, genital tract
    postprocedural or postoperative — *see* Complications, genitourinary, postprocedural
    specified NEC N99.89

Complication(s) — *continued*
  mastoid (process) procedure
    intraoperative H95.88
      hematoma — *see* Complications, intraoperative, hemorrhage (hematoma) (of), mastoid process
      hemorrhage — *see* Complications, intraoperative, hemorrhage (hematoma) (of), mastoid process
      laceration — *see* Complications, intraoperative, puncture or laceration, mastoid process
      specified NEC H95.88
    postmastoidectomy — *see* Complications, postmastoidectomy
    postoperative H95.89
      external ear canal stenosis H95.81
      hematoma — *see* Complications, postprocedural, hematoma (of), mastoid process
      hemorrhage — *see* Complications, postprocedural, hemorrhage (of), mastoid process
      postmastoidectomy — *see* Complications, postmastoidectomy
      seroma — *see* Complications, postprocedural, seroma (of), mastoid process
      specified NEC H95.89
  mastoidectomy cavity — *see* Complications, postmastoidectomy
  mechanical — *see* Complications, by site and type, mechanical
  medical procedures — *see also* Complication(s), intraoperative T88.9
  metabolic E88.9
    postoperative E89.89
      specified NEC E89.89
  molar pregnancy NOS O08.9
    damage to pelvic organs O08.6
    embolism O08.2
    genital infection O08.0
    hemorrhage (delayed) (excessive) O08.1
    metabolic disorder O08.5
    renal failure O08.4
    shock O08.3
    specified type NEC O08.0
    venous complication NEC O08.7
  musculoskeletal system — *see also* Complication, intraoperative (intraprocedural), by site
    device, implant or graft NEC — *see* Complications, orthopedic, device or implant
    internal fixation (nail) (plate) (rod) — *see* Complications, fixation device, internal
    joint prosthesis — *see* Complications, joint prosthesis
    post radiation M96.89
      kyphosis M96.2
      scoliosis M96.5
      specified complication NEC M96.89
    postoperative (postprocedural) M96.89
      with osteoporosis — *see* Osteoporosis
      fracture following insertion of device — *see* Fracture, following insertion of orthopedic implant, joint prosthesis or bone plate
      joint instability after prosthesis removal M96.89
      lordosis M96.4
      postlaminectomy syndrome NEC M96.1
        kyphosis M96.3
      pseudarthrosis M96.0
      specified complication NEC M96.89
  nephrostomy (stoma) — *see* Complications, stoma, urinary tract, external NEC
  nervous system G98.8
    central G96.9
    device, implant or graft — *see also* Complication, prosthetic device or implant, specified NEC
      electronic stimulator (electrode(s)) — *see* Complications, electronic stimulator device
      specified NEC
        infection and inflammation T85.738
        mechanical T85.695
          breakdown T85.615
          displacement T85.625
          leakage T85.635
          malfunction T85.695
          malposition T85.625
          obstruction T85.695
          perforation T85.695
          protrusion T85.695
          specified NEC T85.695

☑ Additional Character Required — Refer to the Tabular List for Character Selection   ▽ Subterms under main terms may continue to next column or page

Complication(s) — *continued*
- nervous system — *continued*
  - device, implant or graft — *see also* Complication, prosthetic device or implant, specified — *continued*
    - ventricular shunt — *see* Complications, ventricular shunt
    - electronic stimulator (electrode(s)) — *see* Complications, electronic stimulator device
  - postprocedural G97.82
    - intracranial hypotension G97.2
    - specified NEC G97.82
    - spinal fluid leak G97.0
- newborn, due to intrauterine (fetal) procedure P96.5
- nonabsorbable (permanent) sutures — *see* Complication, sutures, permanent
- obstetric O75.9
  - procedure (instrumental) (manual) (surgical) specified NEC O75.4
  - specified NEC O75.89
  - surgical wound NEC O90.89
    - hematoma O90.2
    - infection O86.00
- ocular lens implant — *see* Complications, intraocular lens
- ophthalmologic
  - postprocedural bleb — *see* Blebitis
- orbital prosthesis T85.9 ☑
  - embolism T85.818 ☑
  - fibrosis T85.828 ☑
  - hemorrhage T85.838 ☑
  - infection and inflammation T85.79 ☑
  - mechanical
    - breakdown T85.31- ☑
    - displacement T85.32- ☑
    - malposition T85.32- ☑
    - obstruction T85.39- ☑
    - perforation T85.39- ☑
    - protrusion T85.39- ☑
    - specified NEC T85.39- ☑
  - pain T85.848 ☑
  - specified type NEC T85.898 ☑
  - stenosis T85.858 ☑
  - thrombosis T85.868 ☑
- organ or tissue transplant (partial) (total) — *see* Complications, transplant
- orthopedic — *see also* Disorder, soft tissue
  - device or implant T84.9 ☑
    - bone
      - device or implant — *see* Complication, bone, device NEC
      - graft — *see* Complication, graft, bone
    - breakdown T84.418 ☑
    - displacement T84.428 ☑
    - electronic bone stimulator — *see* Complications, electronic stimulator device, bone
    - embolism T84.81 ☑
    - fibrosis T84.82 ☑
    - fixation device — *see* Complication, fixation device, internal
    - hemorrhage T84.83 ☑
    - infection or inflammation T84.7 ☑
    - joint prosthesis — *see* Complication, joint prosthesis, internal
    - malfunction T84.418 ☑
    - malposition T84.428 ☑
    - mechanical NEC T84.498 ☑
    - muscle graft — *see* Complications, graft, muscle
    - obstruction T84.498 ☑
    - pain T84.84 ☑
    - perforation T84.498 ☑
    - protrusion T84.498 ☑
    - specified complication NEC T84.89 ☑
    - stenosis T84.85 ☑
    - tendon graft — *see* Complications, graft, tendon
    - thrombosis T84.86 ☑
  - fracture (following insertion of device) — *see* Fracture, following insertion of orthopedic implant, joint prosthesis or bone plate
  - postprocedural M96.89
    - fracture — *see* Fracture, following insertion of orthopedic implant, joint prosthesis or bone plate
    - postlaminectomy syndrome NEC M96.1
      - kyphosis M96.3
      - lordosis M96.4

Complication(s) — *continued*
- orthopedic — *see also* Disorder, soft tissue — *continued*
  - postprocedural — *continued*
    - postradiation
      - kyphosis M96.2
      - scoliosis M96.5
    - pseudarthrosis post-fusion M96.0
    - specified type NEC M96.89
- pacemaker (cardiac) — *see* Complications, cardiovascular device or implant, electronic
- pancreas transplant — *see* Complications, transplant, pancreas
- penile prosthesis (implant) — *see* Complications, prosthetic device, penile
- perfusion NEC T80.90 ☑
- perineal repair (obstetrical) NEC O90.89
  - disruption O90.1
  - hematoma O90.2
  - infection (following delivery) O86.09
- phototherapy T88.9 ☑
  - specified NEC T88.8 ☑
- postmastoidectomy NEC H95.19- ☑
  - cyst, mucosal H95.13- ☑
  - granulation H95.12- ☑
  - inflammation, chronic H95.11- ☑
  - recurrent cholesteatoma H95.0- ☑
- postoperative — *see* Complications, postprocedural
  - circulatory — *see* Complications, circulatory system
  - ear — *see* Complications, ear
  - endocrine — *see* Complications, endocrine
  - eye — *see* Complications, eye
  - lumbar puncture G97.1
    - cerebrospinal fluid leak G97.0
  - nervous system (central) (peripheral) — *see* Complications, nervous system
  - respiratory system — *see* Complications, respiratory system
- postprocedural — *see also* Complications, surgical procedure
  - cardiac arrest — *see also* Infarct, myocardium, associated with revascularization procedure
    - following cardiac surgery I97.120
    - following other surgery I97.121
  - cardiac functional disturbance NEC — *see also* Infarct, myocardium, associated with revascularization procedure
    - following cardiac surgery I97.190
    - following other surgery I97.191
  - cardiac insufficiency
    - following cardiac surgery I97.110
    - following other surgery I97.111
  - chorioretinal scars following retinal surgery H59.81- ☑
  - following cataract surgery
    - cataract (lens) fragments H59.02- ☑
    - cystoid macular edema H59.03- ☑
    - specified NEC H59.09- ☑
    - vitreous (touch) syndrome H59.01- ☑
  - heart failure
    - following cardiac surgery I97.130
    - following other surgery I97.131
  - hematoma (of)
    - circulatory system organ or structure
      - following cardiac bypass I97.631
      - following cardiac catheterization I97.630
      - following other circulatory system procedure I97.638
      - following other procedure I97.621
    - digestive system
      - following procedure on digestive system K91.870
      - following procedure on other organ K91.871
    - ear
      - following other procedure H95.52
      - following procedure on ear and mastoid process H95.51
    - endocrine
      - following endocrine system procedure E89.820
      - following other procedure E89.821
    - eye and adnexa
      - following ophthalmic procedure H59.33- ☑
      - following other procedure H59.34- ☑
    - genitourinary organ or structure
      - following procedure on genitourinary organ or structure N99.840
      - following procedure on other organ N99.841

Complication(s) — *continued*
- postprocedural — *see also* Complications, surgical procedure — *continued*
  - hematoma — *continued*
    - mastoid process
      - following other procedure H95.52
      - following procedure on ear and mastoid process H95.51
    - musculoskeletal structure
      - following musculoskeletal surgery M96.840
      - following non-orthopedic surgery M96.841
      - following orthopedic surgery M96.840
    - nervous system
      - following nervous system procedure G97.61
      - following other procedure G97.62
    - respiratory system
      - following other procedure J95.861
      - following procedure on respiratory system organ or structure J95.860
    - skin and subcutaneous tissue
      - following dermatologic procedure L76.31
      - following procedure on other organ L76.32
    - spleen
      - following procedure on other organ D78.32
      - following procedure on the spleen D78.31
  - hemorrhage (of)
    - circulatory system organ or structure
      - following cardiac bypass I97.611
      - following cardiac catheterization I97.610
      - following other circulatory system procedure I97.618
      - following other procedure I97.620
    - digestive system
      - following procedure on digestive system K91.840
      - following procedure on other organ K91.841
    - ear
      - following other procedure H95.42
      - following procedure on ear and mastoid process H95.41
    - endocrine system
      - following endocrine system procedure E89.810
      - following other procedure E89.811
    - eye and adnexa
      - following ophthalmic procedure H59.31- ☑
      - following other procedure H59.32- ☑
    - genitourinary organ or structure
      - following procedure on genitourinary organ or structure N99.820
      - following procedure on other organ N99.821
    - mastoid process
      - following other procedure H95.42
      - following procedure on ear and mastoid process H95.41
    - musculoskeletal structure
      - following musculoskeletal surgery M96.830
      - following non-orthopedic surgery M96.831
      - following orthopedic surgery M96.830
    - nervous system
      - following nervous system procedure G97.51
      - following other procedure G97.52
    - respiratory system
      - following a respiratory system procedure J95.830
      - following other procedure J95.831
    - skin and subcutaneous tissue
      - following a procedure on other organ L76.22
      - following dermatologic procedure L76.21
    - spleen
      - following procedure on other organ D78.22
      - following procedure on the spleen D78.21
  - seroma (of)
    - circulatory system organ or structure
      - following cardiac bypass I97.641
      - following cardiac catheterization I97.640
      - following other circulatory system procedure I97.648
      - following other procedure I97.622
    - digestive system
      - following procedure on digestive system K91.872
      - following procedure on other organ K91.873
    - ear
      - following other procedure H95.54
      - following procedure on ear and mastoid process H95.53

Index

Complication — Complication

Complication(s) — *continued*
  postprocedural — *see also* Complications, surgical
      procedure — *continued*
    seroma — *continued*
      endocrine system
        following endocrine system procedure
            E89.822
        following other procedure E89.823
      eye and adnexa
        following ophthalmic procedure H59.35- ☑
        following other procedure H59.36- ☑
      genitourinary organ or structure
        following procedure on genitourinary organ
            or structure N99.842
        following procedure on other organ N99.843
      mastoid process
        following other procedure H95.54
        following procedure on ear and mastoid pro-
            cess H95.53
      musculoskeletal structure
        following musculoskeletal surgery M96.842
        following non-orthopedic surgery M96.843
        following orthopedic surgery M96.842
      nervous system
        following nervous system procedure G97.63
        following other procedure G97.64
      respiratory system
        following other procedure J95.863
        following procedure on respiratory system
            organ or structure J95.862
      skin and subcutaneous tissue
        following dermatologic procedure L76.33
        following procedure on other organ L76.34
      spleen
        following procedure on other organ D78.34
        following procedure on the spleen D78.33
    specified NEC
      circulatory system I97.89
      digestive K91.89
      ear H95.89
      endocrine E89.89
      eye and adnexa H59.89
      genitourinary N99.89
      mastoid process H95.89
      metabolic E89.89
      musculoskeletal structure M96.89
      nervous system G97.82
      respiratory system J95.89
      skin and subcutaneous tissue L76.82
      spleen D78.89
  pregnancy NEC — *see* Pregnancy, complicated by
  prosthetic device or implant T85.9 ☑
    bile duct — *see* Complications, bile duct implant
    breast — *see* Complications, breast implant
    bulking agent
      ureteral
        erosion T83.714 ☑
        exposure T83.724 ☑
      urethral
        erosion T83.713 ☑
        exposure T83.723 ☑
    cardiac and vascular NEC — *see* Complications,
        cardiovascular device or implant
    corneal transplant — *see* Complications, graft,
        cornea
    electronic nervous system stimulator — *see* Compli-
        cations, electronic stimulator device
    epidural infusion catheter — *see* Complications,
        catheter, epidural
    esophageal anti-reflux device — *see* Complications,
        esophageal anti-reflux device
    genital organ or tract — *see* Complications, geni-
        tourinary, device or implant, genital tract
      specified NEC T83.79- ☑
    heart valve — *see* Complications, heart, valve,
        prosthesis
    infection or inflammation T85.79 ☑
      intestine transplant T86.892
      liver transplant T86.43
      lung transplant T86.812
      pancreas transplant T86.892
      skin graft T86.822
    intraocular lens — *see* Complications, intraocular
        lens
    intraperitoneal (dialysis) catheter — *see* Complica-
        tions, catheter, intraperitoneal
    joint — *see* Complications, joint prosthesis, internal
    mechanical NEC T85.698 ☑

Complication(s) — *continued*
  prosthetic device or implant — *continued*
    mechanical — *continued*
      dialysis catheter (vascular) — *see also* Complica-
          tion, catheter, dialysis, mechanical
        peritoneal — *see* Complication, catheter, in-
            traperitoneal, mechanical
      gastrointestinal device T85.598 ☑
      ocular device T85.398 ☑
      subdural (infusion) catheter T85.690 ☑
      suture, permanent T85.692 ☑
        that for bone repair — *see* Complications,
            fixation device, internal (orthopedic),
            mechanical
      ventricular shunt
        breakdown T85.01 ☑
        displacement T85.02 ☑
        leakage T85.03 ☑
        malposition T85.02 ☑
        obstruction T85.09 ☑
        perforation T85.09 ☑
        protrusion T85.09 ☑
        specified NEC T85.09 ☑
    mesh
      erosion (to surrounding organ or tissue)
          T83.718 ☑
        urethral (into pelvic floor muscles) T83.712 ☑
        vaginal (into pelvic floor muscles) T83.711 ☑
      exposure (into surrounding organ or tissue)
          T83.728 ☑
        urethral (through urethral wall) T83.722 ☑
        vaginal (into vagina) (through vaginal wall)
            T83.721 ☑
    orbital — *see* Complications, orbital prosthesis
    penile T83.9 ☑
      embolism T83.81 ☑
      fibrosis T83.82 ☑
      hemorrhage T83.83 ☑
      infection and inflammation T83.61 ☑
      mechanical
        breakdown T83.410 ☑
        displacement T83.420 ☑
        leakage T83.490 ☑
        malposition T83.420 ☑
        obstruction T83.490 ☑
        perforation T83.490 ☑
        protrusion T83.490 ☑
        specified NEC T83.490 ☑
      pain T83.84 ☑
      specified type NEC T83.89 ☑
      stenosis T83.85 ☑
      thrombosis T83.86 ☑
    prosthetic materials NEC
      erosion (to surrounding organ or tissue)
          T83.718 ☑
      exposure (into surrounding organ or tissue)
          T83.728 ☑
    skin graft T86.829
      artificial skin or decellularized allodermis
        embolism T85.818 ☑
        fibrosis T85.828 ☑
        hemorrhage T85.838 ☑
        infection and inflammation T85.79 ☑
        mechanical
          breakdown T85.613 ☑
          displacement T85.623 ☑
          malfunction T85.613 ☑
          malposition T85.623 ☑
          obstruction T85.693 ☑
          perforation T85.693 ☑
          protrusion T85.693 ☑
          specified NEC T85.693 ☑
        pain T85.848 ☑
        specified type NEC T85.898 ☑
        stenosis T85.858 ☑
        thrombosis T85.868 ☑
      failure T86.821
      infection T86.822
      rejection T86.820
      specified NEC T86.828
    sling
      urethral (female) (male)
        erosion T83.712 ☑
        exposure T83.722 ☑
    specified NEC T85.9 ☑
      embolism T85.818 ☑

Complication(s) — *continued*
  prosthetic device or implant — *continued*
    specified
      fibrosis T85.828 ☑
      hemorrhage T85.838 ☑
      infection and inflammation T85.79 ☑
      mechanical
        breakdown T85.618 ☑
        displacement T85.628 ☑
        leakage T85.638 ☑
        malfunction T85.618 ☑
        malposition T85.628 ☑
        obstruction T85.698 ☑
        perforation T85.698 ☑
        protrusion T85.698 ☑
        specified NEC T85.698 ☑
      pain T85.848 ☑
      specified type NEC T85.898 ☑
      stenosis T85.858 ☑
      thrombosis T85.868 ☑
    subdural infusion catheter — *see* Complications,
        catheter, subdural
    sutures — *see* Complications, sutures
    urinary organ or tract NEC — *see* Complications,
        genitourinary, device or implant, urinary sys-
        tem
    vascular — *see* Complications, cardiovascular device
        or implant
    ventricular shunt — *see* Complications, ventricular
        shunt (device)
  puerperium — *see* Puerperal
  puncture, spinal G97.1
    cerebrospinal fluid leak G97.0
    headache or reaction G97.1
  pyelogram N99.89
  radiation
    kyphosis M96.2
    scoliosis M96.5
  reattached
    extremity (infection) (rejection)
      lower T87.1X- ☑
      upper T87.0X- ☑
    specified body part NEC T87.2
  reconstructed breast
    asymmetry between native and reconstructed
        breast N65.1
    deformity N65.0
    disproportion between native and reconstructed
        breast N65.1
    excess tissue N65.0
    misshappen N65.0
  reimplant NEC — *see also* Complications, prosthetic
      device or implant
    limb (infection) (rejection) — *see* Complications,
        reattached, extremity
    organ (partial) (total) — *see* Complications, trans-
        plant
    prosthetic device NEC — *see* Complications, pros-
        thetic device
  renal N28.9
    allograft — *see* Complications, transplant, kidney
    dialysis — *see* Complications, dialysis
  respirator
    mechanical J95.850
    specified NEC J95.859
  respiratory system J98.9
    device, implant or graft — *see* Complication, pros-
        thetic device or implant, specified NEC
    lung transplant — *see* Complications, prosthetic
        device or implant, lung transplant
    postoperative J95.89
      air leak J95.812
      Mendelson's syndrome (chemical pneumonitis)
          J95.4
      pneumothorax J95.811
      pulmonary insufficiency (acute) (after nontho-
          racic surgery) J95.2
        chronic J95.3
        following thoracic surgery J95.1
      respiratory failure (acute) J95.821
        acute and chronic J95.822
      specified NEC J95.89
      subglottic stenosis J95.5
      tracheostomy complication — *see* Complica-
          tions, tracheostomy
    therapy T81.89 ☑
  sedation during labor and delivery O74.9

Complication(s) — *continued*
- sedation during labor and delivery — *continued*
  - cardiac O74.2
  - central nervous system O74.3
  - pulmonary NEC O74.1
- shunt — *see also* Complications, prosthetic device or implant
  - arteriovenous — *see* Complications, arteriovenous, shunt
  - ventricular (communicating) — *see* Complications, ventricular shunt
- skin
  - graft T86.829
    - failure T86.821
    - infection T86.822
    - rejection T86.820
    - specified type NEC T86.828
- spinal
  - anesthesia — *see* Complications, anesthesia, spinal
  - catheter (epidural) (subdural) — *see* Complications, spinal, catheter
  - puncture or tap G97.1
    - cerebrospinal fluid leak G97.0
    - headache or reaction G97.1
- stent
  - bile duct — *see* Complications, bile duct prosthesis
  - ureteral indwelling
    - breakdown T83.112 ✓
    - displacement T83.122 ✓
    - leakage T83.192 ✓
    - malposition T83.122 ✓
    - obstruction T83.192 ✓
    - perforation T83.192 ✓
    - protrusion T83.192 ✓
    - specified NEC T83.192 ✓
  - urinary NEC (ileal conduit) (nephroureteral) T83.193 ✓
    - embolism T83.81 ✓
    - fibrosis T83.82 ✓
    - hemorrhage T83.83 ✓
    - infection and inflammation T83.593 ✓
    - mechanical
      - breakdown T83.113 ✓
      - displacement T83.123 ✓
      - leakage T83.193 ✓
      - malposition T83.123 ✓
      - obstruction T83.193 ✓
      - perforation T83.193 ✓
      - protrusion T83.193 ✓
      - specified NEC T83.193 ✓
    - pain T83.84 ✓
    - specified type NEC T83.89 ✓
    - stenosis T83.85 ✓
    - thrombosis T83.86 ✓
  - vascular
    - end stent stenosis — *see* Restenosis, stent
    - in stent stenosis — *see* Restenosis, stent
- stoma
  - digestive tract
    - colostomy — *see* Complications, colostomy
    - enterostomy — *see* Complications, enterostomy
    - esophagostomy — *see* Complications, esophagostomy
    - gastrostomy — *see* Complications, gastrostomy
  - urinary tract N99.528
    - continent N99.538
      - hemorrhage N99.530
      - herniation N99.533
      - infection N99.531
      - malfunction N99.532
      - specified type NEC N99.538
      - stenosis N99.534
    - cystostomy — *see* Complications, cystostomy
    - external NOS N99.528
    - hemorrhage N99.520
    - herniation N99.523
    - incontinent N99.528
      - hemorrhage N99.520
      - herniation N99.523
      - infection N99.521
      - malfunction N99.522
      - specified type NEC N99.528
      - stenosis N99.524
    - infection N99.521
    - malfunction N99.522
    - specified type NEC N99.528
    - stenosis N99.524

Complication(s) — *continued*
- stomach banding — *see* Complication(s), bariatric procedure
- stomach stapling — *see* Complication(s), bariatric procedure
- surgical material, nonabsorbable — *see* Complication, suture, permanent
- surgical procedure (on) T81.9 ✓
  - amputation stump (late) — *see* Complications, amputation stump
  - cardiac — *see* Complications, circulatory system
  - cholesteatoma, recurrent — *see* Complications, postmastoidectomy, recurrent cholesteatoma
  - circulatory (early) — *see* Complications, circulatory system
  - digestive system — *see* Complications, gastrointestinal
  - dumping syndrome (postgastrectomy) K91.1
  - ear — *see* Complications, ear
  - elephantiasis or lymphedema I97.89
    - postmastectomy I97.2
  - emphysema (surgical) T81.82 ✓
  - endocrine — *see* Complications, endocrine
  - eye — *see* Complications, eye
  - fistula (persistent postoperative) T81.83 ✓
  - foreign body inadvertently left in wound (sponge) (suture) (swab) — *see* Foreign body, accidentally left during a procedure
  - gastrointestinal — *see* Complications, gastrointestinal
  - genitourinary NEC N99.89
  - hematoma
    - intraoperative — *see* Complication, intraoperative, hemorrhage
    - postprocedural — *see* Complication, postprocedural, hematoma
  - hemorrhage
    - intraoperative — *see* Complication, intraoperative, hemorrhage
    - postprocedural — *see* Complication, postprocedural, hemorrhage
  - hepatic failure K91.82
  - hyperglycemia (postpancreatectomy) E89.1
  - hypoinsulinemia (postpancreatectomy) E89.1
  - hypoparathyroidism (postparathyroidectomy) E89.2
  - hypopituitarism (posthypophysectomy) E89.3
  - hypothyroidism (post-thyroidectomy) E89.0
  - intestinal obstruction — *see also* Obstruction, intestine, postoperative K91.30
  - intracranial hypotension following ventricular shunting (ventriculostomy) G97.2
  - lymphedema I97.89
    - postmastectomy I97.2
  - malabsorption (postsurgical) NEC K91.2
    - osteoporosis — *see* Osteoporosis, postsurgical malabsorption
  - mastoidectomy cavity NEC — *see* Complications, postmastoidectomy
  - metabolic E89.89
    - specified NEC E89.89
  - musculoskeletal — *see* Complications, musculoskeletal system
  - nervous system (central) (peripheral) — *see* Complications, nervous system
  - ovarian failure E89.40
    - asymptomatic E89.40
    - symptomatic E89.41
  - peripheral vascular — *see* Complications, surgical procedure, vascular
  - postcardiotomy syndrome I97.0
  - postcholecystectomy syndrome K91.5
  - postcommissurotomy syndrome I97.0
  - postgastrectomy dumping syndrome K91.1
  - postlaminectomy syndrome NEC M96.1
    - kyphosis M96.3
  - postmastectomy lymphedema syndrome I97.2
  - postmastoidectomy cholesteatoma — *see* Complications, postmastoidectomy, recurrent cholesteatoma
  - postvagotomy syndrome K91.1
  - postvalvulotomy syndrome I97.0
  - pulmonary insufficiency (acute) J95.2
    - chronic J95.3
    - following thoracic surgery J95.1
  - reattached body part — *see* Complications, reattached
  - respiratory — *see* Complications, respiratory system
  - shock (hypovolemic) T81.19 ✓

Complication(s) — *continued*
- surgical procedure — *continued*
  - spleen (postoperative) D78.89
    - intraoperative D78.81
  - stitch abscess T81.41 ✓
  - subglottic stenosis (postsurgical) J95.5
  - testicular hypofunction E89.5
  - transplant — *see* Complications, organ or tissue transplant
  - urinary NEC N99.89
  - vaginal vault prolapse (posthysterectomy) N99.3
  - vascular (peripheral)
    - artery T81.719 ✓
      - mesenteric T81.710 ✓
      - renal T81.711 ✓
      - specified NEC T81.718 ✓
    - vein T81.72 ✓
  - wound infection T81.49 ✓
- suture, permanent (wire) NEC T85.9 ✓
  - with repair of bone — *see* Complications, fixation device, internal
  - embolism T85.818 ✓
  - fibrosis T85.828 ✓
  - hemorrhage T85.838 ✓
  - infection and inflammation T85.79 ✓
  - mechanical
    - breakdown T85.612 ✓
    - displacement T85.622 ✓
    - malfunction T85.612 ✓
    - malposition T85.622 ✓
    - obstruction T85.692 ✓
    - perforation T85.692 ✓
    - protrusion T85.692 ✓
    - specified NEC T85.692 ✓
  - pain T85.848 ✓
  - specified type NEC T85.898 ✓
  - stenosis T85.858 ✓
  - thrombosis T85.868 ✓
- tracheostomy J95.00
  - granuloma J95.09
  - hemorrhage J95.01
  - infection J95.02
  - malfunction J95.03
  - mechanical J95.03
  - obstruction J95.03
  - specified type NEC J95.09
  - tracheo-esophageal fistula J95.04
- transfusion (blood) (lymphocytes) (plasma) T80.92 ✓
  - air embolism T80.0 ✓
  - circulatory overload E87.71
  - febrile nonhemolytic transfusion reaction R50.84
  - hemochromatosis E83.111
  - hemolysis T80.89 ✓
  - hemolytic reaction (antigen unspecified) T80.919 ✓
  - incompatibility reaction (antigen unspecified) T80.919 ✓
    - ABO T80.30 ✓
      - delayed serologic (DSTR) T80.39 ✓
      - hemolytic transfusion reaction (HTR) (unspecified time after transfusion) T80.319 ✓
        - acute (AHTR) (less than 24 hours after transfusion) T80.310 ✓
        - delayed (DHTR) (24 hours or more after transfusion) T80.311 ✓
      - specified NEC T80.39 ✓
    - acute (antigen unspecified) T80.910 ✓
    - delayed (antigen unspecified) T80.911 ✓
    - delayed serologic (DSTR) T80.89 ✓
    - non-ABO (minor antigens (Duffy) (K) (Kell) (Kidd) (Lewis) (M) (N) (P) (S)) T80.A0 ✓ (*following* T80.4)
      - delayed serologic (DSTR) T80.A9 ✓ (*following* T80.4)
      - hemolytic transfusion reaction (HTR) (unspecified time after transfusion) T80.A19 ✓ (*following* T80.4)
        - acute (AHTR) (less than 24 hours after transfusion) T80.A10 ✓ (*following* T80.4)
        - delayed (DHTR) (24 hours or more after transfusion) T80.A11 ✓ (*following* T80.4)
      - specified NEC T80.A9 ✓ (*following* T80.4)
    - Rh (antigens (C) (c) (D) (E) (e)) (factor) T80.40 ✓
      - delayed serologic (DSTR) T80.49 ✓
      - hemolytic transfusion reaction (HTR) (unspecified time after transfusion) T80.419 ✓

Complication(s) — *continued*
transfusion — *continued*
  incompatibility reaction — *continued*
    Rh — *continued*
      hemolytic transfusion reaction — *continued*
        acute (AHTR) (less than 24 hours after transfusion) T80.410 ☑
        delayed (DHTR) (24 hours or more after transfusion) T80.411 ☑
        specified NEC T80.49 ☑
  infection T80.29 ☑
    acute T80.22- ☑
  reaction NEC T80.89 ☑
  sepsis T80.29 ☑
  shock T80.89 ☑
transplant T86.90
  bone T86.839
    failure T86.831
    infection T86.832
    rejection T86.830
    specified type NEC T86.838
  bone marrow T86.00
    failure T86.02
    infection T86.03
    rejection T86.01
    specified type NEC T86.09
  cornea T86.849
    failure T86.841
    infection T86.842
    rejection T86.840
    specified type NEC T86.848
  failure T86.92
  heart T86.20
    with lung T86.30
    cardiac allograft vasculopathy T86.290
      failure T86.32
      infection T86.33
      rejection T86.31
      specified type NEC T86.39
    failure T86.22
    infection T86.23
    rejection T86.21
    specified type NEC T86.298
  infection T86.93
  intestine T86.859
    failure T86.851
    infection T86.852
    rejection T86.850
    specified type NEC T86.858
  kidney T86.10
    failure T86.12
    infection T86.13
    rejection T86.11
    specified type NEC T86.19
  liver T86.40
    failure T86.42
    infection T86.43
    rejection T86.41
    specified type NEC T86.49
  lung T86.819
    with heart T86.30
      failure T86.32
      infection T86.33
      rejection T86.31
      specified type NEC T86.39
    failure T86.811
    infection T86.812
    rejection T86.810
    specified type NEC T86.818
  malignant neoplasm C80.2
  pancreas T86.899
    failure T86.891
    infection T86.892
    rejection T86.890
    specified type NEC T86.898
  peripheral blood stem cells T86.5
  post-transplant lymphoproliferative disorder (PTLD) D47.Z1 (*following* D47.4)
  rejection T86.91
  skin T86.829
    failure T86.821
    infection T86.822
    rejection T86.820
    specified type NEC T86.828
  specified
    tissue T86.899
      failure T86.891

Complication(s) — *continued*
transplant — *continued*
  specified — *continued*
    tissue — *continued*
      infection Li86.892
      rejection T86.890
      specified type NEC T86.898
    type NEC T86.99
  stem cell (from peripheral blood) (from umbilical cord) T86.5
  umbilical cord stem cells T86.5
trauma (early) T79.9 ☑
  specified NEC T79.8 ☑
ultrasound therapy NEC T88.9 ☑
umbilical cord NEC
  complicating delivery O69.9 ☑
    specified NEC O69.89 ☑
umbrella device, vascular T82.9 ☑
  embolism T82.818 ☑
  fibrosis T82.828 ☑
  hemorrhage T82.838 ☑
  infection or inflammation T82.7 ☑
  mechanical
    breakdown T82.515 ☑
    displacement T82.525 ☑
    leakage T82.535 ☑
    malposition T82.525 ☑
    obstruction T82.595 ☑
    perforation T82.595 ☑
    protrusion T82.595 ☑
  pain T82.848 ☑
  specified type NEC T82.898 ☑
  stenosis T82.858 ☑
  thrombosis T82.868 ☑
urethral catheter — *see* Complications, catheter, urethral, indwelling
vaccination T88.1 ☑
  anaphylaxis NEC T80.52 ☑
  arthropathy — *see* Arthropathy, postimmunization
  cellulitis T88.0 ☑
  encephalitis or encephalomyelitis G04.02
  infection (general) (local) NEC T88.0 ☑
  meningitis G03.8
  myelitis G04.02
  protein sickness T80.62 ☑
  rash T88.1 ☑
  reaction (allergic) T88.1 ☑
    serum T80.62 ☑
  sepsis T88.0 ☑
  serum intoxication, sickness, rash, or other serum reaction NEC T80.62 ☑
    anaphylactic shock T80.52 ☑
  shock (allergic) (anaphylactic) T80.52 ☑
  vaccinia (generalized) (localized) T88.1 ☑
vas deferens device or implant — *see* Complications, genitourinary, device or implant, genital tract
vascular I99.9
  device or implant T82.9 ☑
    embolism T82.818 ☑
    fibrosis T82.828 ☑
    hemorrhage T82.838 ☑
    infection or inflammation T82.7 ☑
    mechanical
      breakdown T82.519 ☑
        specified device NEC T82.518 ☑
      displacement T82.529 ☑
        specified device NEC T82.528 ☑
      leakage T82.539 ☑
        specified device NEC T82.538 ☑
      malposition T82.529 ☑
        specified device NEC T82.528 ☑
      obstruction T82.599 ☑
        specified device NEC T82.598 ☑
      perforation T82.599 ☑
        specified device NEC T82.598 ☑
      protrusion T82.599 ☑
        specified device NEC T82.598 ☑
    pain T82.848 ☑
    specified type NEC T82.898 ☑
    stenosis T82.858 ☑
    thrombosis T82.868 ☑
  dialysis catheter — *see* Complication, catheter, dialysis
  following infusion, therapeutic injection or transfusion T80.1 ☑
  graft T82.9 ☑

Complication(s) — *continued*
vascular — *continued*
  graft — *continued*
    embolism T82.818 ☑
    fibrosis T82.828 ☑
    hemorrhage T82.838 ☑
    mechanical
      breakdown T82.319 ☑
        aorta (bifurcation) T82.310 ☑
        carotid artery T82.311 ☑
        specified vessel NEC T82.318 ☑
      displacement T82.329 ☑
        aorta (bifurcation) T82.320 ☑
        carotid artery T82.321 ☑
        specified vessel NEC T82.328 ☑
      leakage T82.339 ☑
        aorta (bifurcation) T82.330 ☑
        carotid artery T82.331 ☑
        specified vessel NEC T82.338 ☑
      malposition T82.329 ☑
        aorta (bifurcation) T82.320 ☑
        carotid artery T82.321 ☑
        specified vessel NEC T82.328 ☑
      obstruction T82.399 ☑
        aorta (bifurcation) T82.390 ☑
        carotid artery T82.391 ☑
        specified vessel NEC T82.398 ☑
      perforation T82.399 ☑
        aorta (bifurcation) T82.390 ☑
        carotid artery T82.391 ☑
        specified vessel NEC T82.398 ☑
      protrusion T82.399 ☑
        aorta (bifurcation) T82.390 ☑
        carotid artery T82.391 ☑
        specified vessel NEC T82.398 ☑
    pain T82.848 ☑
    specified complication NEC T82.898 ☑
    stenosis T82.858 ☑
    thrombosis T82.868 ☑
  postoperative — *see* Complications, postoperative, circulatory
vena cava device (filter) (sieve) (umbrella) — *see* Complications, umbrella device, vascular
ventilation therapy NEC T81.81 ☑
ventilator
  mechanical J95.850
    specified NEC J95.859
ventricular (communicating) shunt (device) T85.9 ☑
  embolism T85.810 ☑
  fibrosis T85.820 ☑
  hemorrhage T85.830 ☑
  infection and inflammation T85.730 ☑
  mechanical
    breakdown T85.01 ☑
    displacement T85.02 ☑
    leakage T85.03 ☑
    malposition T85.02 ☑
    obstruction T85.09 ☑
    perforation T85.09 ☑
    protrusion T85.09 ☑
    specified NEC T85.09 ☑
  pain T85.840 ☑
  specified type NEC T85.890 ☑
  stenosis T85.850 ☑
  thrombosis T85.860 ☑
wire suture, permanent (implanted) — *see* Complications, suture, permanent

Compressed air disease T70.3 ☑
Compression
  with injury — *code by* Nature of injury
  artery I77.1
    celiac, syndrome I77.4
  brachial plexus G54.0
  brain (stem) G93.5
    due to
      contusion (diffuse) — *see* Injury, intracranial, diffuse
      focal — *see* Injury, intracranial, focal
      injury NEC — *see* Injury, intracranial, diffuse
      traumatic — *see* Injury, intracranial, diffuse
  bronchus J98.09
  cauda equina G83.4
  celiac (artery) (axis) I77.4
  cerebral — *see* Compression, brain
  cervical plexus G54.2

Compression — *continued*
- cord
  - spinal — *see* Compression, spinal
  - umbilical — *see* Compression, umbilical cord
- cranial nerve G52.9
  - eighth H93.3 ☑
  - eleventh G52.8
  - fifth G50.8
  - first G52.0
  - fourth — *see* Strabismus, paralytic, fourth nerve
  - ninth G52.1
  - second — *see* Disorder, nerve, optic
  - seventh G51.8
  - sixth — *see* Strabismus, paralytic, sixth nerve
  - tenth G52.2
  - third — *see* Strabismus, paralytic, third nerve
  - twelfth G52.3
- diver's squeeze T70.3 ☑
- during birth (newborn) P15.9
- esophagus K22.2
- eustachian tube — *see* Obstruction, eustachian tube, cartilaginous
- facies Q67.1
- fracture
  - nontraumatic NOS — *see* Collapse, vertebra
  - pathological — *see* Fracture, pathological
  - traumatic — *see* Fracture, traumatic
- heart — *see* Disease, heart
- intestine — *see* Obstruction, intestine
- laryngeal nerve, recurrent G52.2
  - with paralysis of vocal cords and larynx J38.00
    - bilateral J38.02
    - unilateral J38.01
- lumbosacral plexus G54.1
- lung J98.4
- lymphatic vessel I89.0
- medulla — *see* Compression, brain
- nerve — *see also* Disorder, nerve G58.9
  - arm NEC — *see* Mononeuropathy, upper limb
  - axillary G54.0
  - cranial — *see* Compression, cranial nerve
  - leg NEC — *see* Mononeuropathy, lower limb
  - median (in carpal tunnel) — *see* Syndrome, carpal tunnel
  - optic — *see* Disorder, nerve, optic
  - plantar — *see* Lesion, nerve, plantar
  - posterior tibial (in tarsal tunnel) — *see* Syndrome, tarsal tunnel
  - root or plexus NOS (in) G54.9
    - intervertebral disc disorder NEC — *see* Disorder, disc, with, radiculopathy
      - with myelopathy — *see* Disorder, disc, with, myelopathy
    - neoplastic disease — *see also* Neoplasm D49.9 [G55]
    - spondylosis — *see* Spondylosis, with radiculopathy
  - sciatic (acute) — *see* Lesion, nerve, sciatic
  - sympathetic G90.8
  - traumatic — *see* Injury, nerve
  - ulnar — *see* Lesion, nerve, ulnar
  - upper extremity NEC — *see* Mononeuropathy, upper limb
- spinal (cord) G95.20
  - by displacement of intervertebral disc NEC — *see also* Disorder, disc, with, myelopathy
  - nerve root NOS G54.9
    - due to displacement of intervertebral disc NEC — *see* Disorder, disc, with, radiculopathy
      - with myelopathy — *see* Disorder, disc, with, myelopathy
  - specified NEC G95.29
  - spondylogenic (cervical) (lumbar, lumbosacral) (thoracic) — *see* Spondylosis, with myelopathy NEC
    - anterior — *see* Syndrome, anterior, spinal artery, compression
  - traumatic — *see* Injury, spinal cord, by region
- subcostal nerve (syndrome) — *see* Mononeuropathy, upper limb, specified NEC
- sympathetic nerve NEC G90.8
- syndrome T79.5 ☑
- trachea J39.8
- ulnar nerve (by scar tissue) — *see* Lesion, nerve, ulnar
- umbilical cord
  - complicating delivery O69.2 ☑
    - cord around neck O69.1 ☑

Compression — *continued*
- umbilical cord — *continued*
  - complicating delivery — *continued*
    - prolapse O69.0 ☑
    - specified NEC O69.2 ☑
  - ureter N13.5
  - vein I87.1
  - vena cava (inferior) (superior) I87.1
Compulsion, compulsive
- gambling F63.0
- neurosis F42.8
- personality F60.5
- states F42.8
- swearing F42.8
  - in Gilles de la Tourette's syndrome F95.2
- tics and spasms F95.9
Concato's disease (pericardial polyserositis) A19.9
- nontubercular I31.1
- pleural — *see* Pleurisy, with effusion
Concavity chest wall M95.4
Concealed penis Q55.64
Concern (normal) **about sick person in family** Z63.6
Concrescence (teeth) K00.2
Concretio cordis I31.1
- rheumatic I09.2
Concretion — *see also* Calculus
- appendicular K38.1
- canaliculus — *see* Dacryolith
- clitoris N90.89
- conjunctiva H11.12- ☑
- eyelid — *see* Disorder, eyelid, specified type NEC
- lacrimal passages — *see* Dacryolith
- prepuce (male) N47.8
- salivary gland (any) K11.5
- seminal vesicle N50.89
- tonsil J35.8
Concussion (brain) (cerebral) (current) S06.0X9 ☑
- with
  - loss of consciousness of 30 minutes or less S06.0X1 ☑
  - loss of consciousness of unspecified duration S06.0X9 ☑
- blast (air) (hydraulic) (immersion) (underwater)
  - abdomen or thorax — *see* Injury, blast, by site
  - ear with acoustic nerve injury — *see* Injury, nerve, acoustic, specified type NEC
- cauda equina S34.3 ☑
- conus medullaris S34.02 ☑
- ocular S05.8X- ☑
- spinal (cord)
  - cervical S14.0 ☑
  - lumbar S34.01 ☑
  - sacral S34.02 ☑
  - thoracic S24.0 ☑
- syndrome F07.81
- without loss of consciousness S06.0X0 ☑
Condition — *see* Disease
Conditions arising in the perinatal period — *see* Newborn, affected by
Conduct disorder — *see* Disorder, conduct
Condyloma A63.0
- acuminatum A63.0
- gonorrheal A54.09
- latum A51.31
- syphilitic A51.31
  - congenital A50.07
- venereal, syphilitic A51.31
Conflagration — *see also* Burn
- asphyxia (by inhalation of gases, fumes or vapors) — *see also* Table of Drugs and Chemicals T59.9- ☑
Conflict (with) — *see also* Discord
- family Z73.9
- marital Z63.0
  - involving divorce or estrangement Z63.5
- parent-child Z62.820
  - parent-adopted child Z62.821
  - parent-biological child Z62.820
  - parent-foster child Z62.822
- social role NEC Z73.5
Confluent — *see* condition
Confusion, confused R41.0
- epileptic F05
- mental state (psychogenic) F44.89
- psychogenic F44.89
- reactive (from emotional stress, psychological trauma) F44.89
Confusional arousals G47.51

Congelation T69.9 ☑
Congenital — *see also* condition
- aortic septum Q25.49
- intrinsic factor deficiency D51.0
- malformation — *see* Anomaly
Congestion, congestive
- bladder N32.89
- bowel K63.89
- brain G93.89
- breast N64.59
- bronchial J98.09
- catarrhal J31.0
- chest R09.89
- chill, malarial — *see* Malaria
- circulatory NEC I99.8
- duodenum K31.89
- eye — *see* Hyperemia, conjunctiva
- facial, due to birth injury P15.4
- general R68.89
- glottis J37.0
- heart — *see* Failure, heart, congestive
- hepatic K76.1
- hypostatic (lung) — *see* Edema, lung
- intestine K63.89
- kidney N28.89
- labyrinth H83.8 ☑
- larynx J37.0
- liver K76.1
- lung R09.89
  - active or acute — *see* Pneumonia
- malaria, malarial — *see* Malaria
- nasal R09.81
- nose R09.81
- orbit, orbital — *see also* Exophthalmos
  - inflammatory (chronic) — *see* Inflammation, orbit
- ovary N83.8
- pancreas K86.89
- pelvic, female N94.89
- pleural J94.8
- prostate (active) N42.1
- pulmonary — *see* Congestion, lung
- renal N28.89
- retina H35.81
- seminal vesicle N50.1
- spinal cord G95.19
- spleen (chronic) D73.2
- stomach K31.89
- trachea — *see* Tracheitis
- urethra N36.8
- uterus N85.8
  - with subinvolution N85.3
- venous (passive) I87.8
- viscera R68.89
Congestive — *see* Congestion
Conical
- cervix (hypertrophic elongation) N88.4
- cornea — *see* Keratoconus
- teeth K00.2
Conjoined twins Q89.4
Conjugal maladjustment Z63.0
- involving divorce or estrangement Z63.5
Conjunctiva — *see* condition
Conjunctivitis (staphylococcal) (streptococcal) NOS H10.9
- Acanthamoeba B60.12
- acute H10.3- ☑
  - atopic H10.1- ☑
  - chemical — *see also* Corrosion, cornea H10.21- ☑
  - mucopurulent H10.02- ☑
    - follicular H10.01- ☑
  - pseudomembranous H10.22- ☑
  - serous except viral H10.23- ☑
    - viral — *see* Conjunctivitis, viral
  - toxic H10.21- ☑
- adenoviral (acute) (follicular) B30.1
- allergic (acute) — *see* Conjunctivitis, acute, atopic
  - chronic H10.45
  - vernal H10.44
- anaphylactic — *see* Conjunctivitis, acute, atopic
- Apollo B30.3
- atopic (acute) — *see* Conjunctivitis, acute, atopic
- Béal's B30.2
- blennorrhagic (gonococcal) (neonatorum) A54.31
- chemical (acute) — *see also* Corrosion, cornea H10.21- ☑
- chlamydial A74.0
  - due to trachoma A71.1
  - neonatal P39.1

Conjunctivitis — *continued*
- chronic (nodosa) (petrificans) (phlyctenular) H10.40- ☑
  - allergic H10.45
    - vernal H10.44
  - follicular H10.43- ☑
  - giant papillary H10.41- ☑
  - simple H10.42- ☑
  - vernal H10.44
- coxsackievirus 24 B30.3
- diphtheritic A36.86
- due to
  - dust — *see* Conjunctivitis, acute, atopic
  - filariasis B74.9
  - mucocutaneous leishmaniasis B55.2
- enterovirus type 70 (hemorrhagic) B30.3
- epidemic (viral) B30.9
  - hemorrhagic B30.3
- gonococcal (neonatorum) A54.31
- granular (trachomatous) A71.1
  - sequelae (late effect) B94.0
- hemorrhagic (acute) (epidemic) B30.3
- herpes zoster B02.31
- in (due to)
  - Acanthamoeba B60.12
  - adenovirus (acute) (follicular) B30.1
  - Chlamydia A74.0
  - coxsackievirus 24 B30.3
  - diphtheria A36.86
  - enterovirus type 70 (hemorrhagic) B30.3
  - filariasis B74.9
  - gonococci A54.31
  - herpes (simplex) virus B00.53
    - zoster B02.31
  - infectious disease NEC B99 ☑
  - meningococci A39.89
  - mucocutaneous leishmaniasis B55.2
  - rosacea H10.82- ☑
  - syphilis (late) A52.71
  - zoster B02.31
- inclusion A74.0
- infantile P39.1
  - gonococcal A54.31
- Koch-Weeks' — *see* Conjunctivitis, acute, mucopurulent
- light — *see* Conjunctivitis, acute, atopic
- ligneous — *see* Blepharoconjunctivitis, ligneous
- meningococcal A39.89
- mucopurulent — *see* Conjunctivitis, acute, mucopurulent
- neonatal P39.1
  - gonococcal A54.31
- Newcastle B30.8
- of Béal B30.2
- parasitic
  - filariasis B74.9
  - mucocutaneous leishmaniasis B55.2
- Parinaud's H10.89
- petrificans H10.89
- rosacea H10.82- ☑
- specified NEC H10.89
- swimming-pool B30.1
- trachomatous A71.1
  - acute A71.0
  - sequelae (late effect) B94.0
- traumatic NEC H10.89
- tuberculous A18.59
- tularemic A21.1
- tularensis A21.1
- viral B30.9
  - due to
    - adenovirus B30.1
    - enterovirus B30.3
  - specified NEC B30.8

Conjunctivochalasis H11.82- ☑
Connective tissue — *see* condition
Conn's syndrome E26.01
Conradi (-Hunermann) **disease** Q77.3
Consanguinity Z84.3
- counseling Z71.89
Conscious simulation (of illness) Z76.5
Consecutive — *see* condition
Consolidation lung (base) — *see* Pneumonia, lobar
Constipation (atonic) (neurogenic) (simple) (spastic) K59.00
- chronic K59.09
  - idiopathic K59.04
- drug-induced K59.03
- functional K59.04
- outlet dysfunction K59.02

Constipation — *continued*
- psychogenic F45.8
- slow transit K59.01
- specified NEC K59.09
Constitutional — *see also* condition
- substandard F60.7
Constitutionally substandard F60.7
Constriction — *see also* Stricture
- auditory canal — *see* Stenosis, external ear canal
- bronchial J98.09
- duodenum K31.5
- esophagus K22.2
- external
  - abdomen, abdominal (wall) S30.841 ☑
  - alveolar process S00.542 ☑
  - ankle S90.54- ☑
  - antecubital space — *see* Constriction, external, forearm
  - arm (upper) S40.84- ☑
  - auricle — *see* Constriction, external, ear
  - axilla — *see* Constriction, external, arm
  - back, lower S30.840 ☑
  - breast S20.14- ☑
  - brow S00.84 ☑
  - buttock S30.840 ☑
  - calf — *see* Constriction, external, leg
  - canthus — *see* Constriction, external, eyelid
  - cheek S00.84 ☑
    - internal S00.542 ☑
  - chest wall — *see* Constriction, external, thorax
  - chin S00.84 ☑
  - clitoris S30.844 ☑
  - costal region — *see* Constriction, external, thorax
  - digit(s)
    - foot — *see* Constriction, external, toe
    - hand — *see* Constriction, external, finger
  - ear S00.44- ☑
  - elbow S50.34- ☑
  - epididymis S30.843 ☑
  - epigastric region S30.841 ☑
  - esophagus, cervical S10.14 ☑
  - eyebrow — *see* Constriction, external, eyelid
  - eyelid S00.24- ☑
  - face S00.84 ☑
  - finger(s) S60.44- ☑
    - index S60.44- ☑
    - little S60.44- ☑
    - middle S60.44- ☑
    - ring S60.44- ☑
  - flank S30.841 ☑
  - foot (except toe(s) alone) S90.84- ☑
    - toe — *see* Constriction, external, toe
  - forearm S50.84- ☑
    - elbow only — *see* Constriction, external, elbow
  - forehead S00.84 ☑
  - genital organs, external
    - female S30.846 ☑
    - male S30.845 ☑
  - groin S30.841 ☑
  - gum S00.542 ☑
  - hand S60.54- ☑
  - head S00.94 ☑
    - ear — *see* Constriction, external, ear
    - eyelid — *see* Constriction, external, eyelid
    - lip S00.541 ☑
    - nose S00.34 ☑
    - oral cavity S00.542 ☑
    - scalp S00.04 ☑
    - specified site NEC S00.84 ☑
  - heel — *see* Constriction, external, foot
  - hip S70.24- ☑
  - inguinal region S30.841 ☑
  - interscapular region S20.449 ☑
  - jaw S00.84 ☑
  - knee S80.24- ☑
  - labium (majus) (minus) S30.844 ☑
  - larynx S10.14 ☑
  - leg (lower) S80.84- ☑
    - knee — *see* Constriction, external, knee
    - upper — *see* Constriction, external, thigh
  - lip S00.541 ☑
  - lower back S30.840 ☑
  - lumbar region S30.840 ☑
  - malar region S00.84 ☑
  - mammary — *see* Constriction, external, breast
  - mastoid region S00.84 ☑

Constriction — *continued*
- external — *continued*
  - mouth S00.542 ☑
  - nail
    - finger — *see* Constriction, external, finger
    - toe — *see* Constriction, external, toe
  - nasal S00.34 ☑
  - neck S10.94 ☑
    - specified site NEC S10.84 ☑
    - throat S10.14 ☑
  - nose S00.34 ☑
  - occipital region S00.04 ☑
  - oral cavity S00.542 ☑
  - orbital region — *see* Constriction, external, eyelid
  - palate S00.542 ☑
  - palm — *see* Constriction, external, hand
  - parietal region S00.04 ☑
  - pelvis S30.840 ☑
  - penis S30.842 ☑
  - perineum
    - female S30.844 ☑
    - male S30.840 ☑
  - periocular area — *see* Constriction, external, eyelid
  - phalanges
    - finger — *see* Constriction, external, finger
    - toe — *see* Constriction, external, toe
  - pharynx S10.14 ☑
  - pinna — *see* Constriction, external, ear
  - popliteal space — *see* Constriction, external, knee
  - prepuce S30.842 ☑
  - pubic region S30.840 ☑
  - pudendum
    - female S30.846 ☑
    - male S30.845 ☑
  - sacral region S30.840 ☑
  - scalp S00.04 ☑
  - scapular region — *see* Constriction, external, shoulder
  - scrotum S30.843 ☑
  - shin — *see* Constriction, external, leg
  - shoulder S40.24- ☑
  - sternal region S20.349 ☑
  - submaxillary region S00.84 ☑
  - submental region S00.84 ☑
  - subungual
    - finger(s) — *see* Constriction, external, finger
    - toe(s) — *see* Constriction, external, toe
  - supraclavicular fossa S10.84 ☑
  - supraorbital S00.84 ☑
  - temple S00.84 ☑
  - temporal region S00.84 ☑
  - testis S30.843 ☑
  - thigh S70.34- ☑
  - thorax, thoracic (wall) S20.94 ☑
    - back S20.44- ☑
    - front S20.34- ☑
  - throat S10.14 ☑
  - thumb S60.34- ☑
  - toe(s) (lesser) S90.44- ☑
    - great S90.44- ☑
  - tongue S00.542 ☑
  - trachea S10.14 ☑
  - tunica vaginalis S30.843 ☑
  - uvula S00.542 ☑
  - vagina S30.844 ☑
  - vulva S30.844 ☑
  - wrist S60.84- ☑
- gallbladder — *see* Obstruction, gallbladder
- intestine — *see* Obstruction, intestine
- larynx J38.6
  - congenital Q31.8
    - specified NEC Q31.8
    - subglottic Q31.1
- organ or site, congenital NEC — *see* Atresia, by site
- prepuce (acquired) (congenital) N47.1
- pylorus (adult hypertrophic) K31.1
  - congenital or infantile Q40.0
  - newborn Q40.0
- ring dystocia (uterus) O62.4
- spastic — *see also* Spasm
  - ureter N13.5
- ureter N13.5
  - with infection N13.6
- urethra — *see* Stricture, urethra
- visual field (peripheral) (functional) — *see* Defect, visual field

Constrictive — *see* condition
Consultation
  medical — *see* Counseling, medical
  religious Z71.81
  specified reason NEC Z71.89
  spiritual Z71.81
  without complaint or sickness Z71.9
    feared complaint unfounded Z71.1
    specified reason NEC Z71.89
Consumption — *see* Tuberculosis
Contact (with) — *see also* Exposure (to)
  acariasis Z20.7
  AIDS virus Z20.6
  air pollution Z77.110
  algae and algae toxins Z77.121
  algae bloom Z77.121
  anthrax Z20.810
  aromatic amines Z77.020
  aromatic (hazardous) compounds NEC Z77.028
  aromatic dyes NOS Z77.028
  arsenic Z77.010
  asbestos Z77.090
  bacterial disease NEC Z20.818
  benzene Z77.021
  blue-green algae bloom Z77.121
  body fluids (potentially hazardous) Z77.21
  brown tide Z77.121
  chemicals (chiefly nonmedicinal) (hazardous) NEC
    Z77.098
  cholera Z20.09
  chromium compounds Z77.018
  communicable disease Z20.9
    bacterial NEC Z20.818
    specified NEC Z20.89
    viral NEC Z20.828
    Zika virus Z20.821
  cyanobacteria bloom Z77.121
  dyes Z77.098
  Escherichia coli (E. coli) Z20.01
  fiberglass — *see* Table of Drugs and Chemicals, fiber-
    glass
  German measles Z20.4
  gonorrhea Z20.2
  hazardous metals NEC Z77.018
  hazardous substances NEC Z77.29
  hazards in the physical environment NEC Z77.128
  hazards to health NEC Z77.9
  HIV Z20.6
  HTLV-III/LAV Z20.6
  human immunodeficiency virus (HIV) Z20.6
  infection Z20.9
    specified NEC Z20.89
  infestation (parasitic) NEC Z20.7
  intestinal infectious disease NEC Z20.09
    Escherichia coli (E. coli) Z20.01
  lead Z77.011
  meningococcus Z20.811
  mold (toxic) Z77.120
  nickel dust Z77.018
  noise Z77.122
  parasitic disease Z20.7
  pediculosis Z20.7
  pfiesteria piscicida Z77.121
  poliomyelitis Z20.89
  pollution
    air Z77.110
    environmental NEC Z77.118
    soil Z77.112
    water Z77.111
  polycyclic aromatic hydrocarbons Z77.028
  rabies Z20.3
  radiation, naturally occurring NEC Z77.123
  radon Z77.123
  red tide (Florida) Z77.121
  rubella Z20.4
  sexually-transmitted disease Z20.2
  smallpox (laboratory) Z20.89
  syphilis Z20.2
  tuberculosis Z20.1
  uranium Z77.012
  varicella Z20.820
  venereal disease Z20.2
  viral disease NEC Z20.828
  viral hepatitis Z20.5
  water pollution Z77.111
  Zika virus Z20.821
Contamination, food — *see* Intoxication, foodborne

Contraception, contraceptive
  advice Z30.09
  counseling Z30.09
  device (intrauterine) (in situ) Z97.5
    causing menorrhagia T83.83 ☑
    checking Z30.431
    complications — *see* Complications, intrauterine,
      contraceptive device
    in place Z97.5
    initial prescription Z30.014
    reinsertion Z30.433
    removal Z30.432
    replacement Z30.433
  emergency (postcoital) Z30.012
  initial prescription Z30.019
    barrier Z30.018
    diaphragm Z30.018
    injectable Z30.013
    intrauterine device Z30.014
    pills Z30.011
    postcoital (emergency) Z30.012
    specified type NEC Z30.018
    subdermal implantable Z30.017
    transdermal patch hormonal Z30.016
    vaginal ring hormonal Z30.015
  maintenance Z30.40
    barrier Z30.49
    diaphragm Z30.49
    examination Z30.8
    injectable Z30.42
    intrauterine device Z30.431
    pills Z30.41
    specified type NEC Z30.49
    subdermal implantable Z30.46
    transdermal patch hormonal Z30.45
    vaginal ring hormonal Z30.44
  management Z30.9
    specified NEC Z30.8
  postcoital (emergency) Z30.012
  prescription Z30.019
    repeat Z30.40
  sterilization Z30.2
  surveillance (drug) — *see* Contraception, maintenance
Contraction(s), contracture, contracted
  Achilles tendon — *see also* Short, tendon, Achilles
    congenital Q66.89
  amputation stump (surgical) (flexion) (late) (next
    proximal joint) T87.89
  anus K59.8
  bile duct (common) (hepatic) K83.8
  bladder N32.89
    neck or sphincter N32.0
  bowel, cecum, colon or intestine, any part — *see* Ob-
    struction, intestine
  Braxton Hicks — *see* False, labor
  breast implant, capsular T85.44 ☑
  bronchial J98.09
  burn (old) — *see* Cicatrix
  cervix — *see* Stricture, cervix
  cicatricial — *see* Cicatrix
  conjunctiva, trachomatous, active A71.1
    sequelae (late effect) B94.0
  Dupuytren's M72.0
  eyelid — *see* Disorder, eyelid function
  fascia (lata) (postural) M72.8
    Dupuytren's M72.0
    palmar M72.0
    plantar M72.2
  finger NEC — *see also* Deformity, finger
    congenital Q68.1
    joint — *see* Contraction, joint, hand
  flaccid — *see* Contraction, paralytic
  gallbladder K82.0
  heart valve — *see* Endocarditis
  hip — *see* Contraction, joint, hip
  hourglass
    bladder N32.89
      congenital Q64.79
    gallbladder K82.0
      congenital Q44.1
    stomach K31.89
      congenital Q40.2
      psychogenic F45.8
    uterus (complicating delivery) O62.4
  hysterical F44.4
  internal os — *see* Stricture, cervix
  joint (abduction) (acquired) (adduction) (flexion) (rota-
    tion) M24.50

Contraction(s), contracture, contracted —
  continued
  joint — *continued*
    ankle M24.57- ☑
    congenital NEC Q68.8
      hip Q65.89
    elbow M24.52- ☑
    foot joint M24.57- ☑
    hand joint M24.54- ☑
    hip M24.55- ☑
      congenital Q65.89
    hysterical F44.4
    knee M24.56- ☑
    shoulder M24.51- ☑
    wrist M24.53- ☑
  kidney (granular) (secondary) N26.9
    congenital Q63.8
    hydronephritic — *see* Hydronephrosis
      Page N26.2
    pyelonephritic — *see* Pyelitis, chronic
    tuberculous A18.11
  ligament — *see also* Disorder, ligament
    congenital Q79.8
  muscle (postinfective) (postural) NEC M62.40
    with contracture of joint — *see* Contraction, joint
    ankle M62.47- ☑
    congenital Q79.8
      sternocleidomastoid Q68.0
    extraocular — *see* Strabismus
    eye (extrinsic) — *see* Strabismus
    foot M62.47- ☑
    forearm M62.43- ☑
    hand M62.44- ☑
    hysterical F44.4
    ischemic (Volkmann's) T79.6 ☑
    lower leg M62.46- ☑
    multiple sites M62.49
    pelvic region M62.45- ☑
    posttraumatic — *see* Strabismus, paralytic
    psychogenic F45.8
      conversion reaction F44.4
    shoulder region M62.41- ☑
    specified site NEC M62.48
    thigh M62.45- ☑
    upper arm M62.42- ☑
  neck — *see* Torticollis
  ocular muscle — *see* Strabismus
  organ or site, congenital NEC — *see* Atresia, by site
  outlet (pelvis) — *see* Contraction, pelvis
  palmar fascia M72.0
  paralytic
    joint — *see* Contraction, joint
    muscle — *see also* Contraction, muscle NEC
      ocular — *see* Strabismus, paralytic
  pelvis (acquired) (general) M95.5
    with disproportion (fetopelvic) O33.1
      causing obstructed labor O65.1
    inlet O33.2
    mid-cavity O33.3 ☑
    outlet O33.3 ☑
  plantar fascia M72.2
  premature
    atrium I49.1
    auriculoventricular I49.49
    heart I49.49
    junctional I49.2
    supraventricular I49.1
    ventricular I49.3
  prostate N42.89
  pylorus NEC — *see also* Pylorospasm
    psychogenic F45.8
  rectum, rectal (sphincter) K59.8
  ring (Bandl's) (complicating delivery) O62.4
  scar — *see* Cicatrix
  spine — *see* Dorsopathy, deforming
  sternocleidomastoid (muscle), congenital Q68.0
  stomach K31.89
    hourglass K31.89
      congenital Q40.2
      psychogenic F45.8
    psychogenic F45.8
  tendon (sheath) M62.40
    with contracture of joint — *see* Contraction, joint
    Achilles — *see* Short, tendon, Achilles
    ankle M62.47- ☑
      Achilles — *see* Short, tendon, Achilles
    foot M62.47- ☑

Index

Contraction(s), contracture, contracted — Contusion

Contraction(s), contracture, contracted — *continued*
- tendon — *continued*
  - forearm M62.43- ☑
  - hand M62.44- ☑
  - lower leg M62.46- ☑
  - multiple sites M62.49
  - neck M62.48
  - pelvic region M62.45- ☑
  - shoulder region M62.41- ☑
  - specified site NEC M62.48
  - thigh M62.45- ☑
  - thorax M62.48
  - trunk M62.48
  - upper arm M62.42- ☑
- toe — *see* Deformity, toe, specified NEC
- ureterovesical orifice (postinfectional) N13.5
  - with infection N13.6
- urethra — *see also* Stricture, urethra
  - orifice N32.0
- uterus N85.8
  - abnormal NEC O62.9
  - clonic (complicating delivery) O62.4
  - dyscoordinate (complicating delivery) O62.4
  - hourglass (complicating delivery) O62.4
  - hypertonic O62.4
  - hypotonic NEC O62.2
  - inadequate
    - primary O62.0
    - secondary O62.1
  - incoordinate (complicating delivery) O62.4
  - poor O62.2
  - tetanic (complicating delivery) O62.4
- vagina (outlet) N89.5
- vesical N32.89
  - neck or urethral orifice N32.0
- visual field — *see* Defect, visual field, generalized
- Volkmann's (ischemic) T79.6 ☑

Contusion (skin surface intact) T14.8 ☑
- abdomen, abdominal (muscle) (wall) S30.1 ☑
- adnexa, eye NEC S05.8X- ☑
- adrenal gland S37.812 ☑
- alveolar process S00.532 ☑
- ankle S90.0- ☑
- antecubital space — *see* Contusion, forearm
- anus S30.3 ☑
- arm (upper) S40.02- ☑
  - lower (with elbow) — *see* Contusion, forearm
- auditory canal — *see* Contusion, ear
- auricle — *see* Contusion, ear
- axilla — *see* Contusion, arm, upper
- back — *see also* Contusion, thorax, back
  - lower S30.0 ☑
- bile duct S36.13 ☑
- bladder S37.22 ☑
- bone NEC T14.8 ☑
- brain (diffuse) — *see* Injury, intracranial, diffuse
  - focal — *see* Injury, intracranial, focal
- brainstem S06.38- ☑
- breast S20.0- ☑
- broad ligament S37.892 ☑
- brow S00.83 ☑
- buttock S30.0 ☑
- canthus, eye S00.1- ☑
- cauda equina S34.3
- cerebellar, traumatic S06.37- ☑
- cerebral S06.33- ☑
  - left side S06.32- ☑
  - right side S06.31- ☑
- cheek S00.83 ☑
  - internal S00.532 ☑
- chest (wall) — *see* Contusion, thorax
- chin S00.83 ☑
- clitoris S30.23 ☑
- colon — *see* Injury, intestine, large, contusion
- common bile duct S36.13 ☑
- conjunctiva S05.1- ☑
  - with foreign body (in conjunctival sac) — *see* Foreign body, conjunctival sac
- conus medullaris (spine) S34.139 ☑
- cornea — *see* Contusion, eyeball
  - with foreign body — *see* Foreign body, cornea
- corpus cavernosum S30.21 ☑
- cortex (brain) (cerebral) — *see* Injury, intracranial, diffuse
  - focal — *see* Injury, intracranial, focal
- costal region — *see* Contusion, thorax

Contusion — *continued*
- cystic duct S36.13 ☑
- diaphragm S27.802 ☑
- duodenum S36.420 ☑
- ear S00.43- ☑
- elbow S50.0- ☑
  - with forearm — *see* Contusion, forearm
- epididymis S30.22 ☑
- epigastric region S30.1 ☑
- epiglottis S10.0 ☑
- esophagus (thoracic) S27.812 ☑
  - cervical S10.0 ☑
- eyeball S05.1- ☑
- eyebrow S00.1- ☑
- eyelid (and periocular area) S00.1- ☑
- face NEC S00.83 ☑
- fallopian tube S37.529 ☑
  - bilateral S37.522 ☑
  - unilateral S37.521 ☑
- femoral triangle S30.1 ☑
- finger(s) S60.00 ☑
  - with damage to nail (matrix) S60.10 ☑
  - index S60.02- ☑
    - with damage to nail S60.12- ☑
  - little S60.05- ☑
    - with damage to nail S60.15- ☑
  - middle S60.03- ☑
    - with damage to nail S60.13- ☑
  - ring S60.04- ☑
    - with damage to nail S60.14- ☑
  - thumb — *see* Contusion, thumb
- flank S30.1 ☑
- foot (except toe(s) alone) S90.3- ☑
  - toe — *see* Contusion, toe
- forearm S50.1- ☑
  - elbow only — *see* Contusion, elbow
- forehead S00.83 ☑
- gallbladder S36.122 ☑
- genital organs, external
  - female S30.202 ☑
  - male S30.201 ☑
- globe (eye) — *see* Contusion, eyeball
- groin S30.1 ☑
- gum S00.532 ☑
- hand S60.22- ☑
  - finger(s) — *see* Contusion, finger
  - wrist — *see* Contusion, wrist
- head S00.93 ☑
  - ear — *see* Contusion, ear
  - eyelid — *see* Contusion, eyelid
  - lip S00.531 ☑
  - nose S00.33 ☑
  - oral cavity S00.532 ☑
  - scalp S00.03 ☑
  - specified part NEC S00.83 ☑
- heart — *see also* Injury, heart S26.91 ☑
- heel — *see* Contusion, foot
- hepatic duct S36.13 ☑
- hip S70.0- ☑
- ileum S36.428 ☑
- iliac region S30.1 ☑
- inguinal region S30.1 ☑
- interscapular region S20.229 ☑
- intra-abdominal organ S36.92 ☑
  - colon — *see* Injury, intestine, large, contusion
  - liver S36.112 ☑
  - pancreas — *see* Contusion, pancreas
  - rectum S36.62 ☑
  - small intestine — *see* Injury, intestine, small, contusion
  - specified organ NEC S36.892 ☑
  - spleen — *see* Contusion, spleen
  - stomach S36.32 ☑
- iris (eye) — *see* Contusion, eyeball
- jaw S00.83 ☑
- jejunum S36.428 ☑
- kidney S37.01- ☑
  - major (greater than 2 cm) S37.02- ☑
  - minor (less than 2 cm) S37.01- ☑
- knee S80.0- ☑
- labium (majus) (minus) S30.23 ☑
- lacrimal apparatus, gland or sac S05.8X- ☑
- larynx S10.0 ☑
- leg (lower) S80.1- ☑
  - knee — *see* Contusion, knee
- lens — *see* Contusion, eyeball

Contusion — *continued*
- lip S00.531 ☑
- liver S36.112 ☑
- lower back S30.0 ☑
- lumbar region S30.0 ☑
- lung S27.329 ☑
  - bilateral S27.322 ☑
  - unilateral S27.321 ☑
- malar region S00.83 ☑
- mastoid region S00.83 ☑
- membrane, brain — *see* Injury, intracranial, diffuse
  - focal — *see* Injury, intracranial, focal
- mesentery S36.892 ☑
- mesosalpinx S37.892 ☑
- mouth S00.532 ☑
- muscle — *see* Contusion, by site
- nail
  - finger — *see* Contusion, finger, with damage to nail
  - toe — *see* Contusion, toe, with damage to nail
- nasal S00.33 ☑
- neck S10.93 ☑
  - specified site NEC S10.83 ☑
  - throat S10.0 ☑
- nerve — *see* Injury, nerve
- newborn P54.5
- nose S00.33 ☑
- occipital
  - lobe (brain) — *see* Injury, intracranial, diffuse
    - focal — *see* Injury, intracranial, focal
  - region (scalp) S00.03 ☑
- orbit (region) (tissues) S05.1- ☑
- ovary S37.429 ☑
  - bilateral S37.422 ☑
  - unilateral S37.421 ☑
- palate S00.532 ☑
- pancreas S36.229 ☑
  - body S36.221 ☑
  - head S36.220 ☑
  - tail S36.222 ☑
- parietal
  - lobe (brain) — *see* Injury, intracranial, diffuse
    - focal — *see* Injury, intracranial, focal
  - region (scalp) S00.03 ☑
- pelvic organ S37.92 ☑
  - adrenal gland S37.812 ☑
  - bladder S37.22 ☑
  - fallopian tube — *see* Contusion, fallopian tube
  - kidney — *see* Contusion, kidney
  - ovary — *see* Contusion, ovary
  - prostate S37.822 ☑
  - specified organ NEC S37.892 ☑
  - ureter S37.12 ☑
  - urethra S37.32 ☑
  - uterus S37.62 ☑
- pelvis S30.0 ☑
- penis S30.21 ☑
- perineum
  - female S30.23 ☑
  - male S30.0 ☑
- periocular area S00.1- ☑
- peritoneum S36.81 ☑
- periurethral tissue — *see* Contusion, urethra
- pharynx S10.0 ☑
- pinna — *see* Contusion, ear
- popliteal space — *see* Contusion, knee
- prepuce S30.21 ☑
- prostate S37.822 ☑
- pubic region S30.1 ☑
- pudendum
  - female S30.202 ☑
  - male S30.201 ☑
- quadriceps femoris — *see* Contusion, thigh
- rectum S36.62 ☑
- retroperitoneum S36.892 ☑
- round ligament S37.892 ☑
- sacral region S30.0 ☑
- scalp S00.03 ☑
  - due to birth injury P12.3
- scapular region — *see* Contusion, shoulder
- sclera — *see* Contusion, eyeball
- scrotum S30.22 ☑
- seminal vesicle S37.892 ☑
- shoulder S40.01- ☑
- skin NEC T14.8 ☑
- small intestine — *see* Injury, intestine, small, contusion
- spermatic cord S30.22 ☑

☑ **Additional Character Required — Refer to the Tabular List for Character Selection**   ᴺᴱᶜ **Subterms under main terms may continue to next column or page**

Contusion — *continued*
  spinal cord — *see* Injury, spinal cord, by region
    cauda equina S34.3 ☑
    conus medullaris S34.139 ☑
  spleen S36.029 ☑
    major S36.021 ☑
    minor S36.020 ☑
  sternal region S20.219 ☑
  stomach S36.32 ☑
  subconjunctival S05.1- ☑
  subcutaneous NEC T14.8 ☑
  submaxillary region S00.83 ☑
  submental region S00.83 ☑
  subperiosteal NEC T14.8 ☑
  subungual
    finger — *see* Contusion, finger, with damage to nail
    toe — *see* Contusion, toe, with damage to nail
  supraclavicular fossa S10.83 ☑
  supraorbital S00.83 ☑
  suprarenal gland S37.812 ☑
  temple (region) S00.83 ☑
  temporal
    lobe (brain) — *see* Injury, intracranial, diffuse
      focal — *see* Injury, intracranial, focal
    region S00.83 ☑
  testis S30.22 ☑
  thigh S70.1- ☑
  thorax (wall) S20.20 ☑
    back S20.22- ☑
    front S20.21- ☑
  throat S10.0 ☑
  thumb S60.01- ☑
    with damage to nail S60.11- ☑
  toe(s) (lesser) S90.12- ☑
    with damage to nail S90.22- ☑
    great S90.11- ☑
      with damage to nail S90.21- ☑
  tongue S00.532 ☑
  trachea (cervical) S10.0 ☑
    thoracic S27.52 ☑
  tunica vaginalis S30.22 ☑
  tympanum, tympanic membrane — *see* Contusion, ear
  ureter S37.12 ☑
  urethra S37.32 ☑
  urinary organ NEC S37.892 ☑
  uterus S37.62 ☑
  uvula S00.532 ☑
  vagina S30.23 ☑
  vas deferens S37.892 ☑
  vesical S37.22 ☑
  vocal cord(s) S10.0 ☑
  vulva S30.23 ☑
  wrist S60.21- ☑
Conus (congenital) (any type) Q14.8
  cornea — *see* Keratoconus
  medullaris syndrome G95.81
Conversion hysteria, neurosis or reaction F44.9
Converter, tuberculosis (test reaction) R76.11
Conviction (legal), **anxiety concerning** Z65.0
  with imprisonment Z65.1
Convulsions (idiopathic) — *see also* Seizure(s) R56.9
  apoplectiform (cerebral ischemia) I67.82
  dissociative F44.5
  epileptic — *see* Epilepsy
  epileptiform, epileptoid — *see* Seizure, epileptiform
  ether (anesthetic) — *see* Table of Drugs and Chemicals, by drug
  febrile R56.00
    with status epilepticus G40.901
    complex R56.01
      with status epilepticus G40.901
    simple R56.00
  hysterical F44.5
  infantile P90
    epilepsy — *see* Epilepsy
  jacksonian — *see* Epilepsy, localization-related, symptomatic, with simple partial seizures
  myoclonic G25.3
  newborn P90
  obstetrical (nephritic) (uremic) — *see* Eclampsia
  paretic A52.17
  post traumatic R56.1
  psychomotor — *see* Epilepsy, localization-related, symptomatic, with complex partial seizures
  recurrent R56.9

Convulsions — *continued*
  reflex R25.8
  scarlatinal A38.8
  tetanus, tetanic — *see* Tetanus
  thymic E32.8
Convulsive — *see also* Convulsions
Cooley's anemia D56.1
Coolie itch B76.9
Cooper's
  disease — *see* Mastopathy, cystic
  hernia — *see* Hernia, abdomen, specified site NEC
Copra itch B88.0
Coprophagy F50.89
Coprophobia F40.298
Coproporphyria, hereditary E80.29
Cor
  biloculare Q20.8
  bovis, bovinum — *see* Hypertrophy, cardiac
  pulmonale (chronic) I27.81
    acute I26.09
  triatriatum, triatrium Q24.2
  triloculare Q20.8
    biatrium Q20.4
    biventriculare Q21.1
Corbus' disease (gangrenous balanitis) N48.1
Cord — *see also* condition
  around neck
    complicating delivery O69.81 ☑
      with compression O69.1 ☑
  bladder G95.89
    tabetic A52.19
Cordis ectopia Q24.8
Corditis (spermatic) N49.1
Corectopia Q13.2
Cori's disease (glycogen storage) E74.03
Corkhandler's disease or lung J67.3
Corkscrew esophagus K22.4
Corkworker's disease or lung J67.3
Corn (infected) L84
Cornea — *see also* condition
  donor Z52.5
  plana Q13.4
Cornelia de Lange syndrome Q87.19
Cornu cutaneum L85.8
Cornual gestation or pregnancy O00.80
  with intrauterine pregnancy O00.81
Coronary (artery) — *see* condition
Coronavirus, as cause of disease classified elsewhere B97.29
  SARS-associated B97.21
Corpora — *see also* condition
  amylacea, prostate N42.89
  cavernosa — *see* condition
Corpulence — *see* Obesity
Corpus — *see* condition
Corrected transposition Q20.5
Corrosion (injury) (acid) (caustic) (chemical) (lime) (external) (internal) T30.4
  abdomen, abdominal (muscle) (wall) T21.42 ☑
    first degree T21.52 ☑
    second degree T21.62 ☑
    third degree T21.72 ☑
  above elbow T22.439 ☑
    first degree T22.539 ☑
    left T22.432 ☑
      first degree T22.532 ☑
      second degree T22.632 ☑
      third degree T22.732 ☑
    right T22.431 ☑
      first degree T22.531 ☑
      second degree T22.631 ☑
      third degree T22.731 ☑
    second degree T22.639 ☑
    third degree T22.739 ☑
  alimentary tract NEC T28.7 ☑
  ankle T25.419 ☑
    first degree T25.519 ☑
    left T25.412 ☑
      first degree T25.512 ☑
      second degree T25.612 ☑
      third degree T25.712 ☑
    multiple with foot — *see* Corrosion, lower, limb, multiple, ankle and foot
    right T25.411 ☑
      first degree T25.511 ☑
      second degree T25.611 ☑

Corrosion — *continued*
  ankle — *continued*
    right — *continued*
      third degree T25.711 ☑
    second degree T25.619 ☑
    third degree T25.719 ☑
  anus — *see* Corrosion, buttock
  arm(s) (meaning upper limb(s)) — *see* Corrosion, upper limb
  axilla T22.449 ☑
    first degree T22.549 ☑
    left T22.442 ☑
      first degree T22.542 ☑
      second degree T22.642 ☑
      third degree T22.742 ☑
    right T22.441 ☑
      first degree T22.541 ☑
      second degree T22.641 ☑
      third degree T22.741 ☑
    second degree T22.649 ☑
    third degree T22.749 ☑
  back (lower) T21.44 ☑
    first degree T21.54 ☑
    second degree T21.64 ☑
    third degree T21.74 ☑
    upper T21.43 ☑
      first degree T21.53 ☑
      second degree T21.63 ☑
      third degree T21.73 ☑
  blisters — *code as* Corrosion, second degree, by site
  breast(s) — *see* Corrosion, chest wall
  buttock(s) T21.45 ☑
    first degree T21.55 ☑
    second degree T21.65 ☑
    third degree T21.75 ☑
  calf T24.439 ☑
    first degree T24.539 ☑
    left T24.432 ☑
      first degree T24.532 ☑
      second degree T24.632 ☑
      third degree T24.732 ☑
    right T24.431 ☑
      first degree T24.531 ☑
      second degree T24.631 ☑
      third degree T24.731 ☑
    second degree T24.639 ☑
    third degree T24.739 ☑
  canthus (eye) — *see* Corrosion, eyelid
  cervix T28.8 ☑
  cheek T20.46 ☑
    first degree T20.56 ☑
    second degree T20.66 ☑
    third degree T20.76 ☑
  chest wall T21.41 ☑
    first degree T21.51 ☑
    second degree T21.61 ☑
    third degree T21.71 ☑
  chin T20.43 ☑
    first degree T20.53 ☑
    second degree T20.63 ☑
    third degree T20.73 ☑
  colon T28.7 ☑
  conjunctiva (and cornea) — *see* Corrosion, cornea
  cornea (and conjunctiva) T26.6- ☑
  deep necrosis of underlying tissue — *code as* Corrosion, third degree, by site
  dorsum of hand T23.469 ☑
    first degree T23.569 ☑
    left T23.462 ☑
      first degree T23.562 ☑
      second degree T23.662 ☑
      third degree T23.762 ☑
    right T23.461 ☑
      first degree T23.561 ☑
      second degree T23.661 ☑
      third degree T23.761 ☑
    second degree T23.669 ☑
    third degree T23.769 ☑
  ear (auricle) (external) (canal) T20.41 ☑
    drum T28.91 ☑
    first degree T20.51 ☑
    second degree T20.61 ☑
    third degree T20.71 ☑
  elbow T22.429 ☑
    first degree T22.529 ☑
    left T22.422 ☑

Corrosion — *continued*
  elbow — *continued*
    left — *continued*
      first degree T22.522 ☑
      second degree T22.622 ☑
      third degree T22.722 ☑
    right T22.421 ☑
      first degree T22.521 ☑
      second degree T22.621 ☑
      third degree T22.721 ☑
    second degree T22.629 ☑
    third degree T22.729 ☑
  entire body — *see* Corrosion, multiple body regions
  epidermal loss — *code as* Corrosion, second degree, by site
  epiglottis T27.4 ☑
  erythema, erythematous — *code as* Corrosion, first degree, by site
  esophagus T28.6 ☑
  extent (percentage of body surface)
    less than 10 percent T32.0
    10-19 percent (0-9 percent third degree) T32.10
      with 10-19 percent third degree T32.11
    20-29 percent (0-9 percent third degree) T32.20
      with
        10-19 percent third degree T32.21
        20-29 percent third degree T32.22
    30-39 percent (0-9 percent third degree) T32.30
      with
        10-19 percent third degree T32.31
        20-29 percent third degree T32.32
        30-39 percent third degree T32.33
    40-49 percent (0-9 percent third degree) T32.40
      with
        10-19 percent third degree T32.41
        20-29 percent third degree T32.42
        30-39 percent third degree T32.43
        40-49 percent third degree T32.44
    50-59 percent (0-9 percent third degree) T32.50
      with
        10-19 percent third degree T32.51
        20-29 percent third degree T32.52
        30-39 percent third degree T32.53
        40-49 percent third degree T32.54
        50-59 percent third degree T32.55
    60-69 percent (0-9 percent third degree) T32.60
      with
        10-19 percent third degree T32.61
        20-29 percent third degree T32.62
        30-39 percent third degree T32.63
        40-49 percent third degree T32.64
        50-59 percent third degree T32.65
        60-69 percent third degree T32.66
    70-79 percent (0-9 percent third degree) T32.70
      with
        10-19 percent third degree T32.71
        20-29 percent third degree T32.72
        30-39 percent third degree T32.73
        40-49 percent third degree T32.74
        50-59 percent third degree T32.75
        60-69 percent third degree T32.76
        70-79 percent third degree T32.77
    80-89 percent (0-9 percent third degree) T32.80
      with
        10-19 percent third degree T32.81
        20-29 percent third degree T32.82
        30-39 percent third degree T32.83
        40-49 percent third degree T32.84
        50-59 percent third degree T32.85
        60-69 percent third degree T32.86
        70-79 percent third degree T32.87
        80-89 percent third degree T32.88
    90 percent or more (0-9 percent third degree) T32.90
      with
        10-19 percent third degree T32.91
        20-29 percent third degree T32.92
        30-39 percent third degree T32.93
        40-49 percent third degree T32.94
        50-59 percent third degree T32.95
        60-69 percent third degree T32.96
        70-79 percent third degree T32.97
        80-89 percent third degree T32.98
        90-99 percent third degree T32.99
  extremity — *see* Corrosion, limb
  eye(s) and adnexa T26.9-
    with resulting rupture and destruction of eyeball T26.7-
    conjunctival sac — *see* Corrosion, cornea

Corrosion — *continued*
  eye(s) and adnexa — *continued*
    cornea — *see* Corrosion, cornea
    lid — *see* Corrosion, eyelid
    periocular area — *see* Corrosion eyelid
    specified site NEC T26.8-
  eyeball — *see* Corrosion, eye
  eyelid(s) T26.5-
  face — *see* Corrosion, head
  finger T23.429 ☑
    first degree T23.529 ☑
    left T23.422 ☑
      first degree T23.522 ☑
      second degree T23.622 ☑
      third degree T23.722 ☑
    multiple sites (without thumb) T23.439 ☑
      with thumb T23.449 ☑
        first degree T23.549 ☑
        left T23.442 ☑
          first degree T23.542 ☑
          second degree T23.642 ☑
          third degree T23.742 ☑
        right T23.441 ☑
          first degree T23.541 ☑
          second degree T23.641 ☑
          third degree T23.741 ☑
        second degree T23.649 ☑
        third degree T23.749 ☑
      first degree T23.539 ☑
      left T23.432 ☑
        first degree T23.532 ☑
        second degree T23.632 ☑
        third degree T23.732 ☑
      right T23.431 ☑
        first degree T23.531 ☑
        second degree T23.631 ☑
        third degree T23.731 ☑
      second degree T23.639 ☑
      third degree T23.739 ☑
    right T23.421 ☑
      first degree T23.521 ☑
      second degree T23.621 ☑
      third degree T23.721 ☑
    second degree T23.629 ☑
    third degree T23.729 ☑
  flank — *see* Corrosion, abdomen
  foot T25.429 ☑
    first degree T25.529 ☑
    left T25.422 ☑
      first degree T25.522 ☑
      second degree T25.622 ☑
      third degree T25.722 ☑
    multiple with ankle — *see* Corrosion, lower, limb, multiple, ankle and foot
    right T25.421 ☑
      first degree T25.521 ☑
      second degree T25.621 ☑
      third degree T25.721 ☑
    second degree T25.629 ☑
    third degree T25.729 ☑
  forearm T22.419 ☑
    first degree T22.519 ☑
    left T22.412 ☑
      first degree T22.512 ☑
      second degree T22.612 ☑
      third degree T22.712 ☑
    right T22.411 ☑
      first degree T22.511 ☑
      second degree T22.611 ☑
      third degree T22.711 ☑
    second degree T22.619 ☑
    third degree T22.719 ☑
  forehead T20.46 ☑
    first degree T20.56 ☑
    second degree T20.66 ☑
    third degree T20.76 ☑
  fourth degree — *code as* Corrosion, third degree, by site
  full thickness skin loss — *code as* Corrosion, third degree, by site
  gastrointestinal tract NEC T28.7 ☑
  genital organs
    external
      female T21.47 ☑
        first degree T21.57 ☑
        second degree T21.67 ☑

Corrosion — *continued*
  genital organs — *continued*
    external — *continued*
      female — *continued*
        third degree T21.77 ☑
      male T21.46 ☑
        first degree T21.56 ☑
        second degree T21.66 ☑
        third degree T21.76 ☑
    internal T28.8 ☑
  groin — *see* Corrosion, abdominal wall
  hand(s) T23.409 ☑
    back — *see* Corrosion, dorsum of hand
    finger — *see* Corrosion, finger
    first degree T23.509 ☑
    left T23.402 ☑
      first degree T23.502 ☑
      second degree T23.602 ☑
      third degree T23.702 ☑
    multiple sites with wrist T23.499 ☑
      first degree T23.599 ☑
      left T23.492 ☑
        first degree T23.592 ☑
        second degree T23.692 ☑
        third degree T23.792 ☑
      right T23.491 ☑
        first degree T23.591 ☑
        second degree T23.691 ☑
        third degree T23.791 ☑
      second degree T23.699 ☑
      third degree T23.799 ☑
    palm — *see* Corrosion, palm
    right T23.401 ☑
      first degree T23.501 ☑
      second degree T23.601 ☑
      third degree T23.701 ☑
    second degree T23.609 ☑
    third degree T23.709 ☑
    thumb — *see* Corrosion, thumb
  head (and face) (and neck) T20.40 ☑
    cheek — *see* Corrosion, cheek
    chin — *see* Corrosion, chin
    ear — *see* Corrosion, ear
    eye(s) only — *see* Corrosion, eye
    first degree T20.50 ☑
    forehead — *see* Corrosion, forehead
    lip — *see* Corrosion, lip
    multiple sites T20.49 ☑
      first degree T20.59 ☑
      second degree T20.69 ☑
      third degree T20.79 ☑
    neck — *see* Corrosion, neck
    nose — *see* Corrosion, nose
    scalp — *see* Corrosion, scalp
    second degree T20.60 ☑
    third degree T20.70 ☑
  hip(s) — *see* Corrosion, lower, limb
  inhalation — *see* Corrosion, respiratory tract
  internal organ(s) — *see also* Corrosion, by site T28.90 ☑
    alimentary tract T28.7 ☑
      esophagus T28.6 ☑
    esophagus T28.6 ☑
    genitourinary T28.8 ☑
    mouth T28.5 ☑
    pharynx T28.5 ☑
    specified organ NEC T28.99 ☑
  interscapular region — *see* Corrosion, back, upper
  intestine (large) (small) T28.7 ☑
  knee T24.429 ☑
    first degree T24.529 ☑
    left T24.422 ☑
      first degree T24.522 ☑
      second degree T24.622 ☑
      third degree T24.722 ☑
    right T24.421 ☑
      first degree T24.521 ☑
      second degree T24.621 ☑
      third degree T24.721 ☑
    second degree T24.629 ☑
    third degree T24.729 ☑
  labium (majus) (minus) — *see* Corrosion, genital organs, external, female
  lacrimal apparatus, duct, gland or sac — *see* Corrosion, eye, specified site NEC
  larynx T27.4 ☑

☑ Additional Character Required — Refer to the Tabular List for Character Selection   Subterms under main terms may continue to next column or page

Corrosion — *continued*
  larynx — *continued*
    with lung T27.5 ☑
  leg(s) (meaning lower limb(s)) — *see* Corrosion, lower
      limb
  limb(s)
    lower — *see* Corrosion, lower, limb
    upper — *see* Corrosion, upper limb
  lip(s) T20.42 ☑
    first degree T20.52 ☑
    second degree T20.62 ☑
    third degree T20.72 ☑
  lower
    back — *see* Corrosion, back
    limb T24.409 ☑
      ankle — *see* Corrosion, ankle
      calf — *see* Corrosion, calf
      first degree T24.509 ☑
      foot — *see* Corrosion, foot
      knee — *see* Corrosion, knee
      left T24.402 ☑
        first degree T24.502 ☑
        second degree T24.602 ☑
        third degree T24.702 ☑
      multiple sites, except ankle and foot T24.499 ☑
        ankle and foot T25.499 ☑
          first degree T25.599 ☑
          left T25.492 ☑
            first degree T25.592 ☑
            second degree T25.692 ☑
            third degree T25.792 ☑
          right T25.491 ☑
            first degree T25.591 ☑
            second degree T25.691 ☑
            third degree T25.791 ☑
          second degree T25.699 ☑
          third degree T25.799 ☑
        first degree T24.599 ☑
        left T24.492 ☑
          first degree T24.592 ☑
          second degree T24.692 ☑
          third degree T24.792 ☑
        right T24.491 ☑
          first degree T24.591 ☑
          second degree T24.691 ☑
          third degree T24.791 ☑
        second degree T24.699 ☑
        third degree T24.799 ☑
      right T24.401 ☑
        first degree T24.501 ☑
        second degree T24.601 ☑
        third degree T24.701 ☑
      second degree T24.609 ☑
      thigh — *see* Corrosion, thigh
      third degree T24.709 ☑
  lung (with larynx and trachea) T27.5 ☑
  mouth T28.5 ☑
  neck T20.47 ☑
    first degree T20.57 ☑
    second degree T20.67 ☑
    third degree T20.77 ☑
  nose (septum) T20.44 ☑
    first degree T20.54 ☑
    second degree T20.64 ☑
    third degree T20.74 ☑
  ocular adnexa — *see* Corrosion, eye
  orbit region — *see* Corrosion, eyelid
  palm T23.459 ☑
    first degree T23.559 ☑
    left T23.452 ☑
      first degree T23.552 ☑
      second degree T23.652 ☑
      third degree T23.752 ☑
    right T23.451 ☑
      first degree T23.551 ☑
      second degree T23.651 ☑
      third degree T23.751 ☑
    second degree T23.659 ☑
    third degree T23.759 ☑
  partial thickness — *code as* Corrosion, unspecified degree, by site
  pelvis — *see* Corrosion, trunk
  penis — *see* Corrosion, genital organs, external, male
  perineum
    female — *see* Corrosion, genital organs, external,
        female

Corrosion — *continued*
  perineum — *continued*
    male — *see* Corrosion, genital organs, external, male
  periocular area — *see* Corrosion, eyelid
  pharynx T28.5 ☑
  rectum T28.7 ☑
  respiratory tract T27.7 ☑
    larynx — *see* Corrosion, larynx
    specified part NEC T27.6 ☑
    trachea — *see* Corrosion, larynx
  sac, lacrimal — *see* Corrosion, eye, specified site NEC
  scalp T20.45 ☑
    first degree T20.55 ☑
    second degree T20.65 ☑
    third degree T20.75 ☑
  scapular region T22.469 ☑
    first degree T22.569 ☑
    left T22.462 ☑
      first degree T22.562 ☑
      second degree T22.662 ☑
      third degree T22.762 ☑
    right T22.461 ☑
      first degree T22.561 ☑
      second degree T22.661 ☑
      third degree T22.761 ☑
    second degree T22.669 ☑
    third degree T22.769 ☑
  sclera — *see* Corrosion, eye, specified site NEC
  scrotum — *see* Corrosion, genital organs, external,
      male
  shoulder T22.459 ☑
    first degree T22.559 ☑
    left T22.452 ☑
      first degree T22.552 ☑
      second degree T22.652 ☑
      third degree T22.752 ☑
    right T22.451 ☑
      first degree T22.551 ☑
      second degree T22.651 ☑
      third degree T22.751 ☑
    second degree T22.659 ☑
    third degree T22.759 ☑
  stomach T28.7 ☑
  temple — *see* Corrosion, head
  testis — *see* Corrosion, genital organs, external, male
  thigh T24.419 ☑
    first degree T24.519 ☑
    left T24.412 ☑
      first degree T24.512 ☑
      second degree T24.612 ☑
      third degree T24.712 ☑
    right T24.411 ☑
      first degree T24.511 ☑
      second degree T24.611 ☑
      third degree T24.711 ☑
    second degree T24.619 ☑
    third degree T24.719 ☑
  thorax (external) — *see* Corrosion, trunk
  throat (meaning pharynx) T28.5 ☑
  thumb(s) T23.419 ☑
    first degree T23.519 ☑
    left T23.412 ☑
      first degree T23.512 ☑
      second degree T23.612 ☑
      third degree T23.712 ☑
    multiple sites with fingers T23.449 ☑
      first degree T23.549 ☑
      left T23.442 ☑
        first degree T23.542 ☑
        second degree T23.642 ☑
        third degree T23.742 ☑
      right T23.441 ☑
        first degree T23.541 ☑
        second degree T23.641 ☑
        third degree T23.741 ☑
      second degree T23.649 ☑
      third degree T23.749 ☑
    right T23.411 ☑
      first degree T23.511 ☑
      second degree T23.611 ☑
      third degree T23.711 ☑
    second degree T23.619 ☑
    third degree T23.719 ☑
  toe T25.439 ☑
    first degree T25.539 ☑
    left T25.432 ☑

Corrosion — *continued*
  toe — *continued*
    left — *continued*
      first degree T25.532 ☑
      second degree T25.632 ☑
      third degree T25.732 ☑
    right T25.431 ☑
      first degree T25.531 ☑
      second degree T25.631 ☑
      third degree T25.731 ☑
    second degree T25.639 ☑
    third degree T25.739 ☑
  tongue T28.5 ☑
  tonsil(s) T28.5 ☑
  total body — *see* Corrosion, multiple body regions
  trachea T27.4 ☑
    with lung T27.5 ☑
  trunk T21.40 ☑
    abdominal wall — *see* Corrosion, abdominal wall
    anus — *see* Corrosion, buttock
    axilla — *see* Corrosion, upper limb
    back — *see* Corrosion, back
    breast — *see* Corrosion, chest wall
    buttock — *see* Corrosion, buttock
    chest wall — *see* Corrosion, chest wall
    first degree T21.50 ☑
    flank — *see* Corrosion, abdominal wall
    genital
      female — *see* Corrosion, genital organs, external,
          female
      male — *see* Corrosion, genital organs, external,
          male
    groin — *see* Corrosion, abdominal wall
    interscapular region — *see* Corrosion, back, upper
    labia — *see* Corrosion, genital organs, external, fe-
        male
    lower back — *see* Corrosion, back
    penis — *see* Corrosion, genital organs, external,
        male
    perineum
      female — *see* Corrosion, genital organs, external,
          female
      male — *see* Corrosion, genital organs, external,
          male
    scapular region — *see* Corrosion, upper limb
    scrotum — *see* Corrosion, genital organs, external,
        male
    second degree T21.60 ☑
    shoulder — *see* Corrosion, upper limb
    specified site NEC T21.49 ☑
      first degree T21.59 ☑
      second degree T21.69 ☑
      third degree T21.79 ☑
    testes — *see* Corrosion, genital organs, external,
        male
    third degree T21.70 ☑
    upper back — *see* Corrosion, back, upper
    vagina T28.8 ☑
    vulva — *see* Corrosion, genital organs, external, fe-
        male
  unspecified site with extent of body surface involved
      specified
    less than 10 percent T32.0
    10-19 percent (0-9 percent third degree) T32.10
      with 10-19 percent third degree T32.11
    20-29 percent (0-9 percent third degree) T32.20
      with
        10-19 percent third degree T32.21
        20-29 percent third degree T32.22
    30-39 percent (0-9 percent third degree) T32.30
      with
        10-19 percent third degree T32.31
        20-29 percent third degree T32.32
        30-39 percent third degree T32.33
    40-49 percent (0-9 percent third degree) T32.40
      with
        10-19 percent third degree T32.41
        20-29 percent third degree T32.42
        30-39 percent third degree T32.43
        40-49 percent third degree T32.44
    50-59 percent (0-9 percent third degree) T32.50
      with
        10-19 percent third degree T32.51
        20-29 percent third degree T32.52
        30-39 percent third degree T32.53
        40-49 percent third degree T32.54
        50-59 percent third degree T32.55

Corrosion — *continued*
  unspecified site with extent of body surface involved specified — *continued*
    60-69 percent (Ø-9 percent third degree) T32.6Ø
      with
        10-19 percent third degree T32.61
        20-29 percent third degree T32.62
        30-39 percent third degree T32.63
        40-49 percent third degree T32.64
        50-59 percent third degree T32.65
        60-69 percent third degree T32.66
    70-79 percent (Ø-9 percent third degree) T32.7Ø
      with
        10-19 percent third degree T32.71
        20-29 percent third degree T32.72
        30-39 percent third degree T32.73
        40-49 percent third degree T32.74
        50-59 percent third degree T32.75
        60-69 percent third degree T32.76
        70-79 percent third degree T32.77
    80-89 percent (Ø-9 percent third degree) T32.8Ø
      with
        10-19 percent third degree T32.81
        20-29 percent third degree T32.82
        30-39 percent third degree T32.83
        40-49 percent third degree T32.84
        50-59 percent third degree T32.85
        60-69 percent third degree T32.86
        70-79 percent third degree T32.87
        80-89 percent third degree T32.88
    9Ø percent or more (Ø-9 percent third degree) T32.9Ø
      with
        10-19 percent third degree T32.91
        20-29 percent third degree T32.92
        30-39 percent third degree T32.93
        40-49 percent third degree T32.94
        50-59 percent third degree T32.95
        60-69 percent third degree T32.96
        70-79 percent third degree T32.97
        80-89 percent third degree T32.98
        90-99 percent third degree T32.99
  upper limb (axilla) (scapular region) T22.4Ø ☑
    above elbow — *see* Corrosion, above elbow
    axilla — *see* Corrosion, axilla
    elbow — *see* Corrosion, elbow
    first degree T22.5Ø ☑
    forearm — *see* Corrosion, forearm
    hand — *see* Corrosion, hand
    interscapular region — *see* Corrosion, back, upper
    multiple sites T22.499 ☑
      first degree T22.599 ☑
      left T22.492 ☑
        first degree T22.592 ☑
        second degree T22.692 ☑
        third degree T22.792 ☑
      right T22.491 ☑
        first degree T22.591 ☑
        second degree T22.691 ☑
        third degree T22.791 ☑
      second degree T22.699 ☑
      third degree T22.799 ☑
    scapular region — *see* Corrosion, scapular region
    second degree T22.6Ø ☑
    shoulder — *see* Corrosion, shoulder
    third degree T22.7Ø ☑
    wrist — *see* Corrosion, hand
  uterus T28.8 ☑
  vagina T28.8 ☑
  vulva — *see* Corrosion, genital organs, external, female
  wrist T23.479 ☑
    first degree T23.579 ☑
    left T23.472 ☑
      first degree T23.572 ☑
      second degree T23.672 ☑
      third degree T23.772 ☑
    multiple sites with hand T23.499 ☑
      first degree T23.599 ☑
      left T23.492 ☑
        first degree T23.592 ☑
        second degree T23.692 ☑
        third degree T23.792 ☑
      right T23.491 ☑
        first degree T23.591 ☑
        second degree T23.691 ☑
        third degree T23.791 ☑
      second degree T23.699 ☑
      third degree T23.799 ☑

Corrosion — *continued*
  wrist — *continued*
    right T23.471 ☑
      first degree T23.571 ☑
      second degree T23.671 ☑
      third degree T23.771 ☑
    second degree T23.679 ☑
    third degree T23.779 ☑
Corrosive burn — *see* Corrosion
Corsican fever — *see* Malaria
Cortical — *see* condition
Cortico-adrenal — *see* condition
Coryza (acute) JØØ
  with grippe or influenza — *see* Influenza, with, respiratory manifestations NEC
  syphilitic
    congenital (chronic) A5Ø.Ø5
Costen's syndrome or complex M26.69
Costiveness — *see* Constipation
Costochondritis M94.Ø
Cot death R99
Cotard's syndrome F22
Cotia virus BØ8.8
Cotton wool spots (retinal) H35.81
Cotungo's disease — *see* Sciatica
Cough (affected) (chronic) (epidemic) (nervous) RØ5
  with hemorrhage — *see* Hemoptysis
  bronchial RØ5
    with grippe or influenza — *see* Influenza, with, respiratory manifestations NEC
  functional F45.8
  hysterical F45.8
  laryngeal, spasmodic RØ5
  psychogenic F45.8
  smokers' J41.Ø
  tea taster's B49
Counseling (for) Z71.9
  abuse NEC
    perpetrator Z69.82
    victim Z69.81
  alcohol abuser Z71.41
    family Z71.42
  child abuse
    nonparental
      perpetrator Z69.Ø21
      victim Z69.Ø2Ø
    parental
      perpetrator Z69.Ø11
      victim Z69.Ø1Ø
  consanguinity Z71.89
  contraceptive Z3Ø.Ø9
  dietary Z71.3
  drug abuser Z71.51
    family member Z71.52
  exercise Z71.82
  family Z71.89
  fertility preservation (prior to cancer therapy) (prior to removal of gonads) Z31.62
  for non-attending third party Z71.Ø
    related to sexual behavior or orientation Z7Ø.2
  genetic
    nonprocreative Z71.83
    procreative NEC Z31.5
  gestational carrier Z31.7
  health (advice) (education) (instruction) — *see* Counseling, medical
    risk for travel (international) Z71.84
  human immunodeficiency virus (HIV) Z71.7
  impotence Z7Ø.1
  insulin pump use Z46.81
  medical (for) Z71.9
    boarding school resident Z59.3
    consanguinity Z71.89
    feared complaint and no disease found Z71.1
    human immunodeficiency virus (HIV) Z71.7
    institutional resident Z59.3
    on behalf of another Z71.Ø
      related to sexual behavior or orientation Z7Ø.2
    person living alone Z6Ø.2
    specified reason NEC Z71.89
  natural family planning
    procreative Z31.61
    to avoid pregnancy Z3Ø.Ø2
  perpetrator (of)
    abuse NEC Z69.82
    child abuse
      non-parental Z69.Ø21
      parental Z69.Ø11

Counseling — *continued*
  perpetrator — *continued*
    rape NEC Z69.82
    spousal abuse Z69.12
  procreative NEC Z31.69
    fertility preservation (prior to cancer therapy) (prior to removal of gonads) Z31.62
    using natural family planning Z31.61
  promiscuity Z7Ø.1
  rape victim Z69.81
  religious Z71.81
  safety for travel (international) Z71.84
  sex, sexual (related to) Z7Ø.9
    attitude(s) Z7Ø.Ø
    behavior or orientation Z7Ø.1
    combined concerns Z7Ø.3
    non-responsiveness Z7Ø.1
    on behalf of third party Z7Ø.2
    specified reason NEC Z7Ø.8
  specified reason NEC Z71.89
  spiritual Z71.81
  spousal abuse (perpetrator) Z69.12
    victim Z69.11
  substance abuse Z71.89
    alcohol Z71.41
    drug Z71.51
    tobacco Z71.6
  tobacco use Z71.6
  travel (international) Z71.84
  use (of)
    insulin pump Z46.81
  victim (of)
    abuse Z69.81
    child abuse
      by parent Z69.Ø1Ø
      non-parental Z69.Ø2Ø
    rape NEC Z69.81
Coupled rhythm RØØ.8
Couvelaire syndrome or uterus (complicating delivery) O45.8X- ☑
Cowperitis — *see* Urethritis
Cowper's gland — *see* condition
Cowpox BØ8.Ø1Ø
  due to vaccination T88.1 ☑
Coxa
  magna M91.4- ☑
  plana M91.2- ☑
  valga (acquired) — *see also* Deformity, limb, specified type NEC, thigh
    congenital Q65.81
    sequelae (late effect) of rickets E64.3
  vara (acquired) — *see also* Deformity, limb, specified type NEC, thigh
    congenital Q65.82
    sequelae (late effect) of rickets E64.3
Coxalgia, coxalgic (nontuberculous) — *see also* Pain, joint, hip
  tuberculous A18.Ø2
Coxitis — *see* Monoarthritis, hip
Coxsackie (virus) (infection) B34.1
  as cause of disease classified elsewhere B97.11
  carditis B33.2Ø
  central nervous system NEC A88.8
  endocarditis B33.21
  enteritis AØ8.39
  meningitis (aseptic) A87.Ø
  myocarditis B33.22
  pericarditis B33.23
  pharyngitis BØ8.5
  pleurodynia B33.Ø
  specific disease NEC B33.8
Crabs, meaning pubic lice B85.3
Crack baby PØ4.41
Cracked nipple N64.Ø
  associated with
    lactation O92.13
    pregnancy O92.11- ☑
    puerperium O92.12
Cracked tooth KØ3.81
Cradle cap L21.Ø
Craft neurosis F48.8
Cramp(s) R25.2
  abdominal — *see* Pain, abdominal
  bathing T75.1 ☑
  colic R1Ø.83
    psychogenic F45.8
  due to immersion T75.1 ☑
  fireman T67.2 ☑

Cramp(s) — *continued*
  heat T67.2 ☑
  immersion T75.1 ☑
  intestinal — *see* Pain, abdominal
    psychogenic F45.8
  leg, sleep related G47.62
  limb (lower) (upper) NEC R25.2
    sleep related G47.62
  linotypist's F48.8
    organic G25.89
  muscle (limb) (general) R25.2
    due to immersion T75.1 ☑
    psychogenic F45.8
  occupational (hand) F48.8
    organic G25.89
  salt-depletion E87.1
  sleep related, leg G47.62
  stoker's T67.2 ☑
  swimmer's T75.1 ☑
  telegrapher's F48.8
    organic G25.89
  typist's F48.8
    organic G25.89
  uterus N94.89
    menstrual — *see* Dysmenorrhea
  writer's F48.8
    organic G25.89
Cranial — *see* condition
Craniocleidodysostosis Q74.0
Craniofenestria (skull) Q75.8
Craniolacunia (skull) Q75.8
Craniopagus Q89.4
Craniopathy, metabolic M85.2
Craniopharyngeal — *see* condition
Craniopharyngioma D44.4
Craniorachischisis (totalis) Q00.1
Cranioschisis Q75.8
Craniostenosis Q75.0
Craniosynostosis Q75.0
Craniotabes (cause unknown) M83.8
  neonatal P96.3
  rachitic E64.3
  syphilitic A50.56
Cranium — *see* condition
Craw-craw — *see* Onchocerciasis
Creaking joint — *see* Derangement, joint, specified type
  NEC
Creeping
  eruption B76.9
  palsy or paralysis G12.22
Crenated tongue K14.8
Creotoxism A05.9
Crepitus
  caput Q75.8
  joint — *see* Derangement, joint, specified type NEC
Crescent or conus choroid, congenital Q14.3
CREST syndrome M34.1
Cretin, cretinism (congenital) (endemic) (nongoitrous)
  (sporadic) E00.9
  pelvis
    with disproportion (fetopelvic) O33.0
      causing obstructed labor O65.0
  type
    hypothyroid E00.1
    mixed E00.2
    myxedematous E00.1
    neurological E00.0
Creutzfeldt-Jakob disease or syndrome (with dementia) A81.00
  familial A81.09
  iatrogenic A81.09
  specified NEC A81.09
  sporadic A81.09
  variant (vCJD) A81.01
Crib death R99
Cribriform hymen Q52.3
Cri-du-chat syndrome Q93.4
Crigler-Najjar disease or syndrome E80.5
Crime, victim of Z65.4
Crimean hemorrhagic fever A98.0
Criminalism F60.2
Crisis
  abdomen R10.0
  acute reaction F43.0
  addisonian E27.2
  adrenal (cortical) E27.2
  celiac K90.0

Crisis — *continued*
  Dietl's N13.8
  emotional — *see also* Disorder, adjustment
    acute reaction to stress F43.0
    specific to childhood and adolescence F93.8
  glaucomatocyclitic — *see* Glaucoma, secondary, inflam-
    mation
  heart — *see* Failure, heart
  nitritoid I95.2
    correct substance properly administered — *see* Ta-
      ble of Drugs and Chemicals, by drug, adverse
      effect
    overdose or wrong substance given or taken — *see*
      Table of Drugs and Chemicals, by drug, poi-
      soning
  oculogyric H51.8
    psychogenic F45.8
  Pel's (tabetic) A52.11
  psychosexual identity F64.2
  renal N28.0
  sickle-cell D57.00
    with
      acute chest syndrome D57.01
      splenic sequestration D57.02
  state (acute reaction) F43.0
  tabetic A52.11
  thyroid — *see* Thyrotoxicosis with thyroid storm
  thyrotoxic — *see* Thyrotoxicosis with thyroid storm
Crocq's disease (acrocyanosis) I73.89
Crohn's disease — *see* Enteritis, regional
Crooked septum, nasal J34.2
Cross syndrome E70.328
Crossbite (anterior) (posterior) M26.24
Cross-eye — *see* Strabismus, convergent concomitant
Croup, croupous (catarrhal) (infectious) (inflammatory)
  (nondiphtheritic) J05.0
  bronchial J20.9
  diphtheritic A36.2
  false J38.5
  spasmodic J38.5
    diphtheritic A36.2
  stridulous J38.5
    diphtheritic A36.2
Crouzon's disease Q75.1
Crowding, tooth, teeth, fully erupted M26.31
CRST syndrome M34.1
Cruchet's disease A85.8
Cruelty in children — *see also* Disorder, conduct
Crural ulcer — *see* Ulcer, lower limb
Crush, crushed, crushing T14.8 ☑
  abdomen S38.1 ☑
  ankle S97.0- ☑
  arm (upper) (and shoulder) S47.- ☑
  axilla — *see* Crush, arm
  back, lower S38.1 ☑
  buttock S38.1 ☑
  cheek S07.0 ☑
  chest S28.0 ☑
  cranium S07.1 ☑
  ear S07.0 ☑
  elbow S57.0- ☑
  extremity
    lower
      ankle — *see* Crush, ankle
      below knee — *see* Crush, leg
      foot — *see* Crush, foot
      hip — *see* Crush, hip
      knee — *see* Crush, knee
      thigh — *see* Crush, thigh
      toe — *see* Crush, toe
    upper
      below elbow S67.9- ☑
      elbow — *see* Crush, elbow
      finger — *see* Crush, finger
      forearm — *see* Crush, forearm
      hand — *see* Crush, hand
      thumb — *see* Crush, thumb
      upper arm — *see* Crush, arm
      wrist — *see* Crush, wrist
  face S07.0 ☑
  finger(s) S67.1- ☑
    with hand (and wrist) — *see* Crush, hand, specified
      site NEC
    index S67.19- ☑
    little S67.19- ☑
    middle S67.19- ☑
    ring S67.19- ☑

Crush, crushed, crushing — *continued*
  finger(s) — *continued*
    thumb — *see* Crush, thumb
  foot S97.8- ☑
    toe — *see* Crush, toe
  forearm S57.8- ☑
  genitalia, external
    female S38.002 ☑
      vagina S38.03 ☑
      vulva S38.03 ☑
    male S38.001 ☑
      penis S38.01 ☑
      scrotum S38.02 ☑
      testis S38.02 ☑
  hand (except fingers alone) S67.2- ☑
    with wrist S67.4- ☑
  head S07.9 ☑
    specified NEC S07.8 ☑
  heel — *see* Crush, foot
  hip S77.0- ☑
    with thigh S77.2- ☑
  internal organ (abdomen, chest, or pelvis) NEC T14.8 ☑
  knee S87.0- ☑
  labium (majus) (minus) S38.03 ☑
  larynx S17.0 ☑
  leg (lower) S87.8- ☑
    knee — *see* Crush, knee
  lip S07.0 ☑
  lower
    back S38.1 ☑
    leg — *see* Crush, leg
  neck S17.9 ☑
  nerve — *see* Injury, nerve
  nose S07.0 ☑
  pelvis S38.1 ☑
  penis S38.01 ☑
  scalp S07.8 ☑
  scapular region — *see* Crush, arm
  scrotum S38.02 ☑
  severe, unspecified site T14.8 ☑
  shoulder (and upper arm) — *see* Crush, arm
  skull S07.1 ☑
  syndrome (complication of trauma) T79.5 ☑
  testis S38.02 ☑
  thigh S77.1- ☑
    with hip S77.2- ☑
  throat S17.8 ☑
  thumb S67.0- ☑
    with hand (and wrist) — *see* Crush, hand, specified
      site NEC
  toe(s) S97.10- ☑
    great S97.11- ☑
    lesser S97.12- ☑
  trachea S17.0 ☑
  vagina S38.03 ☑
  vulva S38.03 ☑
  wrist S67.3- ☑
    with hand S67.4- ☑
Crusta lactea L21.0
Crusts R23.4
Crutch paralysis — *see* Injury, brachial plexus
Cruveilhier-Baumgarten cirrhosis, disease or syn-
  drome K74.69
Cruveilhier's atrophy or disease G12.8
Crying (constant) (continuous) (excessive)
  child, adolescent, or adult R45.83
  infant (baby) (newborn) R68.11
Cryofibrinogenemia D89.2
Cryoglobulinemia (essential) (idiopathic) (mixed) (primary) (purpura) (secondary) (vasculitis) D89.1
  with lung involvement D89.1 *[J99]*
Cryptitis (anal) (rectal) K62.89
Cryptococcosis, cryptococcus (infection) (neoformans)
  B45.9
  bone B45.3
  cerebral B45.1
  cutaneous B45.2
  disseminated B45.7
  generalized B45.7
  meningitis B45.1
  meningocerebralis B45.1
  osseous B45.3
  pulmonary B45.0
  skin B45.2
  specified NEC B45.8
Cryptopapillitis (anus) K62.89

Cryptophthalmos Q11.2
  syndrome Q87.0
Cryptorchid, cryptorchism, cryptorchidism Q53.9
  bilateral Q53.20
    abdominal Q53.211
    perineal Q53.22
  unilateral Q53.10
    abdominal Q53.111
    perineal Q53.12
Cryptosporidiosis A07.2
  hepatobiliary B88.8
  respiratory B88.8
Cryptostromosis J67.6
Crystalluria R82.998
Cubitus
  congenital Q68.8
  valgus (acquired) M21.0- ☑
    congenital Q68.8
    sequelae (late effect) of rickets E64.3
  varus (acquired) M21.1- ☑
    congenital Q68.8
    sequelae (late effect) of rickets E64.3
Cultural deprivation or shock Z60.3
Curling esophagus K22.4
Curling's ulcer — see Ulcer, peptic, acute
Curschmann (-Batten) (-Steinert) **disease or syndrome**
  G71.11
Curse, Ondine's — see Apnea, sleep
Curvature
  organ or site, congenital NEC — see Distortion
  penis (lateral) Q55.61
  Pott's (spinal) A18.01
  radius, idiopathic, progressive (congenital) Q74.0
  spine (acquired) (angular) (idiopathic) (incorrect)
    (postural) — see Dorsopathy, deforming
    congenital Q67.5
    due to or associated with
      Charcot-Marie-Tooth disease — see also subcat-
        egory M49.8 G60.0
      osteitis
        deformans M88.88
        fibrosa cystica — see also subcategory M49.8
          E21.0
      tuberculosis (Pott's curvature) A18.01
    sequelae (late effect) of rickets E64.3
    tuberculous A18.01
Cushingoid due to steroid therapy E24.2
  correct substance properly administered — see Table
    of Drugs and Chemicals, by drug, adverse effect
  overdose or wrong substance given or taken — see
    Table of Drugs and Chemicals, by drug, poisoning
Cushing's
  syndrome or disease E24.9
    drug-induced E24.2
    iatrogenic E24.2
    pituitary-dependent E24.0
    specified NEC E24.8
  ulcer — see Ulcer, peptic, acute
Cusp, Carabelli — omit code
Cut (external) — see also Laceration
  muscle — see Injury, muscle
Cutaneous — see also condition
  hemorrhage R23.3
  larva migrans B76.9
Cutis — see also condition
  hyperelastica Q82.8
    acquired L57.4
  laxa (hyperelastica) — see Dermatolysis
  marmorata R23.8
  osteosis L94.2
  pendula — see Dermatolysis
  rhomboidalis nuchae L57.2
  verticis gyrata Q82.8
    acquired L91.8
Cyanosis R23.0
  due to
    patent foramen botalli Q21.1
    persistent foramen ovale Q21.1
  enterogenous D74.8
  paroxysmal digital — see Raynaud's disease
    with gangrene I73.01
  retina, retinal H35.89
Cyanotic heart disease I24.9
  congenital Q24.9
Cycle
  anovulatory N97.0
  menstrual, irregular N92.6
Cyclencephaly Q04.9

Cyclical vomiting, in migraine — see also Vomiting,
  cyclical G43.A0 (following G43.7)
  psychogenic F50.89
Cyclitis — see also Iridocyclitis H20.9
  chronic — see Iridocyclitis, chronic
  Fuchs' heterochromic H20.81- ☑
  granulomatous — see Iridocyclitis, chronic
  lens-induced — see Iridocyclitis, lens-induced
  posterior H30.2- ☑
Cycloid personality F34.0
Cyclophoria H50.54
Cyclopia, cyclops Q87.0
Cyclopism Q87.0
Cyclosporiasis A07.4
Cyclothymia F34.0
Cyclothymic personality F34.0
Cyclotropia H50.41- ☑
Cylindroma — see also Neoplasm, malignant, by site
  eccrine dermal — see Neoplasm, skin, benign
  skin — see Neoplasm, skin, benign
Cylindruria R82.998
Cynanche
  diphtheritic A36.2
  tonsillaris J36
Cynophobia F40.218
Cynorexia R63.2
Cyphosis — see Kyphosis
Cyprus fever — see Brucellosis
Cyst (colloid) (mucous) (simple) (retention)
  adenoid (infected) J35.8
  adrenal gland E27.8
    congenital Q89.1
  air, lung J98.4
  allantoic Q64.4
  alveolar process (jaw bone) M27.40
  amnion, amniotic O41.8X- ☑
  aneurysmal M27.49
  anterior
    chamber (eye) — see Cyst, iris
    nasopalatine K09.1
  antrum J34.1
  anus K62.89
  apical (tooth) (periodontal) K04.8
  appendix K38.8
  arachnoid, brain (acquired) G93.0
    congenital Q04.6
  arytenoid J38.7
  Baker's M71.2- ☑
    ruptured M66.0
    tuberculous A18.02
  Bartholin's gland N75.0
  bile duct (common) (hepatic) K83.5
  bladder (multiple) (trigone) N32.89
  blue dome (breast) — see Cyst, breast
  bone (local) NEC M85.60
    aneurysmal M85.50
      ankle M85.57- ☑
      foot M85.57- ☑
      forearm M85.53- ☑
      hand M85.54- ☑
      jaw M27.49
      lower leg M85.56- ☑
      multiple site M85.59
      neck M85.58
      rib M85.58
      shoulder M85.51- ☑
      skull M85.58
      specified site NEC M85.58
      thigh M85.55- ☑
      toe M85.57- ☑
      upper arm M85.52- ☑
      vertebra M85.58
    solitary M85.40
      ankle M85.47- ☑
      fibula M85.46- ☑
      foot M85.47- ☑
      hand M85.44- ☑
      humerus M85.42- ☑
      jaw M27.49
      neck M85.48
      pelvis M85.45- ☑
      radius M85.43- ☑
      rib M85.48
      shoulder M85.41- ☑
      skull M85.48
      specified site NEC M85.48
      tibia M85.46- ☑

Cyst — continued
  bone — continued
    solitary — continued
      toe M85.47- ☑
      ulna M85.43- ☑
      vertebra M85.48
    specified type NEC M85.60
      ankle M85.67- ☑
      foot M85.67- ☑
      forearm M85.63- ☑
      hand M85.64- ☑
      jaw M27.40
        developmental (nonodontogenic) K09.1
          odontogenic K09.0
        latent M27.0
      lower leg M85.66- ☑
      multiple site M85.69
      neck M85.68
      rib M85.68
      shoulder M85.61- ☑
      skull M85.68
      specified site NEC M85.68
      thigh M85.65- ☑
      toe M85.67- ☑
      upper arm M85.62- ☑
      vertebra M85.68
  brain (acquired) G93.0
    congenital Q04.6
    hydatid B67.99 [G94]
    third ventricle (colloid), congenital Q04.6
  branchial (cleft) Q18.0
  branchiogenic Q18.0
  breast (benign) (blue dome) (pedunculated) (solitary)
    N60.0- ☑
    involution — see Dysplasia, mammary, specified
      type NEC
    sebaceous — see Dysplasia, mammary, specified
      type NEC
  broad ligament (benign) N83.8
  bronchogenic (mediastinal) (sequestration) J98.4
    congenital Q33.0
  buccal K09.8
  bulbourethral gland N36.8
  bursa, bursal NEC M71.30
    with rupture — see Rupture, synovium
    ankle M71.37- ☑
    elbow M71.32- ☑
    foot M71.37- ☑
    hand M71.34- ☑
    hip M71.35- ☑
    multiple sites M71.39
    pharyngeal J39.2
    popliteal space — see Cyst, Baker's
    shoulder M71.31- ☑
    specified site NEC M71.38
    wrist M71.33- ☑
  calcifying odontogenic D16.5
    upper jaw (bone) (maxilla) D16.4
  canal of Nuck (female) N94.89
    congenital Q52.4
  canthus — see Cyst, conjunctiva
  carcinomatous — see Neoplasm, malignant, by site
  cauda equina G95.89
  cavum septi pellucidi — see Cyst, brain
  celomic (pericardium) Q24.8
  cerebellopontine (angle) — see Cyst, brain
  cerebellum — see Cyst, brain
  cerebral — see Cyst, brain
  cervical lateral Q18.0
  cervix NEC N88.8
    embryonic Q51.6
    nabothian N88.8
  chiasmal optic NEC — see Disorder, optic, chiasm
  chocolate (ovary) N80.1
  choledochus, congenital Q44.4
  chorion O41.8X- ☑
  choroid plexus G93.0
    congenital Q04.6
  ciliary body — see Cyst, iris
  clitoris N90.7
  colon K63.89
  common (bile) duct K83.5
  congenital NEC Q89.8
    adrenal gland Q89.1
    epiglottis Q31.8
    esophagus Q39.8
    fallopian tube Q50.4
    kidney Q61.00

☑ **Additional Character Required** — Refer to the Tabular List for Character Selection   ▽ **Subterms under main terms may continue to next column or page**

Cyst — *continued*
- congenital — *continued*
  - kidney — *continued*
    - more than one (multiple) Q61.02
      - specified as polycystic Q61.3
        - adult type Q61.2
        - infantile type NEC Q61.19
          - collecting duct dilation Q61.11
    - solitary Q61.01
  - larynx Q31.8
  - liver Q44.6
  - lung Q33.0
  - mediastinum Q34.1
  - ovary Q50.1
  - oviduct Q50.4
  - periurethral (tissue) Q64.79
  - prepuce Q55.69
  - salivary gland (any) Q38.4
  - sublingual Q38.6
  - submaxillary gland Q38.6
  - thymus (gland) Q89.2
  - tongue Q38.3
  - ureterovesical orifice Q62.8
  - vulva Q52.79
- conjunctiva H11.44- ☑
- cornea H18.89- ☑
- corpora quadrigemina G93.0
- corpus
  - albicans N83.29- ☑
  - luteum (hemorrhagic) (ruptured) N83.1- ☑
- Cowper's gland (benign) (infected) N36.8
- cranial meninges G93.0
- craniobuccal pouch E23.6
- craniopharyngeal pouch E23.6
- cystic duct K82.8
- Cysticercus — *see* Cysticercosis
- Dandy-Walker Q03.1
  - with spina bifida — *see* Spina bifida
- dental (root) K04.8
  - developmental K09.0
  - eruption K09.0
  - primordial K09.0
- dentigerous (mandible) (maxilla) K09.0
- dermoid — *see* Neoplasm, benign, by site
  - with malignant transformation C56.- ☑
  - implantation
    - external area or site (skin) NEC L72.0
    - iris — *see* Cyst, iris, implantation
    - vagina N89.8
    - vulva N90.7
  - mouth K09.8
  - oral soft tissue K09.8
  - sacrococcygeal — *see* Cyst, pilonidal
- developmental K09.1
  - odontogenic K09.0
  - oral region (nonodontogenic) K09.1
  - ovary, ovarian Q50.1
- dura (cerebral) G93.0
  - spinal G96.19
- ear (external) Q18.1
- echinococcal — *see* Echinococcus
- embryonic
  - cervix uteri Q51.6
  - fallopian tube Q50.4
  - vagina Q52.4
- endometrium, endometrial (uterus) N85.8
  - ectopic — *see* Endometriosis
- enterogenous Q43.8
- epidermal, epidermoid (inclusion) (*see also* Cyst, skin) L72.0
  - mouth K09.8
  - oral soft tissue K09.8
- epididymis N50.3
- epiglottis J38.7
- epiphysis cerebri E34.8
- epithelial (inclusion) L72.0
- epoophoron Q50.5
- eruption K09.0
- esophagus K22.8
- ethmoid sinus J34.1
- external female genital organs NEC N90.7
- eyelid (sebaceous) H02.829
  - infected — *see* Hordeolum
  - left H02.826
    - lower H02.825
    - upper H02.824
  - right H02.823
    - lower H02.822

Cyst — *continued*
- eyelid — *continued*
  - right — *continued*
    - upper H02.821
- eye NEC H57.89
  - congenital Q15.8
- fallopian tube N83.8
  - congenital Q50.4
- fimbrial (twisted) Q50.4
- fissural (oral region) K09.1
- follicle (graafian) (hemorrhagic) N83.0- ☑
  - nabothian N88.8
- follicular (atretic) (hemorrhagic) (ovarian) N83.0- ☑
  - dentigerous K09.0
  - odontogenic K09.0
  - skin L72.9
    - specified NEC L72.8
- frontal sinus J34.1
- gallbladder K82.8
- ganglion — *see* Ganglion
- Gartner's duct Q52.4
- gingiva K09.0
- gland of Moll — *see* Cyst, eyelid
- globulomaxillary K09.1
- graafian follicle (hemorrhagic) N83.0- ☑
- granulosal lutein (hemorrhagic) N83.1- ☑
- hemangiomatous D18.00
  - intra-abdominal D18.03
  - intracranial D18.02
  - skin D18.01
  - specified site NEC D18.09
- hemorrhagic M27.49
- hydatid — *see also* Echinococcus B67.90
  - brain B67.99 [G94]
  - liver — *see also* Cyst, liver, hydatid B67.8
  - lung NEC B67.99 [J99]
  - Morgagni
    - female Q50.5
    - male (epididymal) Q55.4
      - testicular Q55.29
  - specified site NEC B67.99
- hymen N89.8
  - embryonic Q52.4
- hypopharynx J39.2
- hypophysis, hypophyseal (duct) (recurrent) E23.6
  - cerebri E23.6
- implantation (dermoid)
  - external area or site (skin) NEC L72.0
  - iris — *see* Cyst, iris, implantation
  - vagina N89.8
  - vulva N90.7
- incisive canal K09.1
- inclusion (epidermal) (epithelial) (epidermoid) (squamous) L72.0
  - not of skin — *code under* Cyst, by site
- intestine (large) (small) K63.89
- intracranial — *see* Cyst, brain
- intraligamentous — *see also* Disorder, ligament
  - knee — *see* Derangement, knee
- intrasellar E23.6
- iris H21.309
  - exudative H21.31- ☑
  - idiopathic H21.30- ☑
  - implantation H21.32- ☑
  - parasitic H21.33- ☑
  - pars plana (primary) H21.34- ☑
    - exudative H21.35- ☑
- jaw (bone) M27.40
  - aneurysmal M27.49
  - developmental (odontogenic) K09.0
  - fissural K09.1
  - hemorrhagic M27.49
  - traumatic M27.49
- joint NEC — *see* Disorder, joint, specified type NEC
- kidney (acquired) N28.1
  - calyceal — *see* Hydronephrosis
  - congenital Q61.00
  - more than one (multiple) Q61.02
    - specified as polycystic Q61.3
      - adult type (autosomal dominant) Q61.2
      - infantile type (autosomal recessive) NEC Q61.19
        - collecting duct dilation Q61.11
  - pyelogenic — *see* Hydronephrosis
  - simple N28.1
  - solitary (single) Q61.01
    - acquired N28.1
- labium (majus) (minus) N90.7

Cyst — *continued*
- labium — *continued*
  - sebaceous N90.7
- lacrimal — *see also* Disorder, lacrimal system, specified NEC
  - gland H04.13- ☑
  - passages or sac — *see* Disorder, lacrimal system, specified NEC
- larynx J38.7
- lateral periodontal K09.0
- lens H27.8
  - congenital Q12.8
- lip (gland) K13.0
- liver (idiopathic) (simple) K76.89
  - congenital Q44.6
  - hydatid B67.8
    - granulosus B67.0
    - multilocularis B67.5
- lung J98.4
  - congenital Q33.0
  - giant bullous J43.9
- lutein N83.1- ☑
- lymphangiomatous D18.1
- lymphoepithelial, oral soft tissue K09.8
- macula — *see* Degeneration, macula, hole
- malignant — *see* Neoplasm, malignant, by site
- mammary gland — *see* Cyst, breast
- mandible M27.40
  - dentigerous K09.0
  - radicular K04.8
- maxilla M27.40
  - dentigerous K09.0
  - radicular K04.8
- medial, face and neck Q18.8
- median
  - anterior maxillary K09.1
  - palatal K09.1
- mediastinum, congenital Q34.1
- meibomian (gland) — *see* Chalazion
  - infected — *see* Hordeolum
- membrane, brain G93.0
- meninges (cerebral) G93.0
  - spinal G96.19
- meniscus, knee — *see* Derangement, knee, meniscus, cystic
- mesentery, mesenteric K66.8
  - chyle I89.8
- mesonephric duct
  - female Q50.5
  - male Q55.4
- milk N64.89
- Morgagni (hydatid)
  - female Q50.5
  - male (epididymal) Q55.4
    - testicular Q55.29
- mouth K09.8
- Müllerian duct Q50.4
  - appendix testis Q55.29
  - cervix Q51.6
  - fallopian tube Q50.4
  - female Q50.4
  - male Q55.29
  - prostatic utricle Q55.4
  - vagina (embryonal) Q52.4
- multilocular (ovary) D39.10
  - benign — *see* Neoplasm, benign, by site
- myometrium N85.8
- nabothian (follicle) (ruptured) N88.8
- nasoalveolar K09.1
- nasolabial K09.1
- nasopalatine (anterior) (duct) K09.1
- nasopharynx J39.2
- neoplastic — *see* Neoplasm, uncertain behavior, by site
  - benign — *see* Neoplasm, benign, by site
- nervous system NEC G96.8
- neuroenteric (congenital) Q06.8
- nipple — *see* Cyst, breast
- nose (turbinates) J34.1
  - sinus J34.1
- odontogenic, developmental K09.0
- omentum (lesser) K66.8
  - congenital Q45.8
- ora serrata — *see* Cyst, retina, ora serrata
- oral
  - region K09.9
    - developmental (nonodontogenic) K09.1
    - specified NEC K09.8

▽ Subterms under main terms may continue to next column or page   ☑ Additional Character Required — Refer to the Tabular List for Character Selection   79

Cyst — Cyst

Cyst — *continued*
oral — *continued*
soft tissue K09.9
specified NEC K09.8
orbit H05.81- ☑
ovary, ovarian (twisted) N83.20- ☑
adherent N83.20- ☑
chocolate N80.1
corpus
albicans N83.29- ☑
luteum (hemorrhagic) N83.1- ☑
dermoid D27.9
developmental Q50.1
due to failure of involution NEC N83.20- ☑
endometrial N80.1
follicular (graafian) (hemorrhagic) N83.0- ☑
hemorrhagic N83.20- ☑
in pregnancy or childbirth O34.8- ☑
with obstructed labor O65.5
multilocular D39.10
pseudomucinous D27.9
retention N83.29- ☑
serous N83.20- ☑
specified NEC N83.29- ☑
theca lutein (hemorrhagic) N83.1- ☑
tuberculous A18.18
oviduct N83.8
palate (median) (fissural) K09.1
palatine papilla (jaw) K09.1
pancreas, pancreatic (hemorrhagic) (true) K86.2
congenital Q45.2
false K86.3
paralabral
hip M24.85- ☑
shoulder S43.43- ☑
paramesonephric duct Q50.4
female Q50.4
male Q55.29
paranephric N28.1
paraphysis, cerebri, congenital Q04.6
parasitic B89
parathyroid (gland) E21.4
paratubal N83.8
paraurethral duct N36.8
paroophoron Q50.5
parotid gland K11.6
parovarian Q50.5
pelvis, female N94.89
in pregnancy or childbirth O34.8- ☑
causing obstructed labor O65.5
penis (sebaceous) N48.89
periapical K04.8
pericardial (congenital) Q24.8
acquired (secondary) I31.8
pericoronal K09.0
periodontal K04.8
lateral K09.0
peripelvic (lymphatic) N28.1
peritoneum K66.8
chylous I89.8
periventricular, acquired, newborn P91.1
pharynx (wall) J39.2
pilar L72.11
pilonidal (infected) (rectum) L05.91
with abscess L05.01
malignant C44.59- ☑
pituitary (duct) (gland) E23.6
placenta O43.19- ☑
pleura J94.8
popliteal — *see* Cyst, Baker's
porencephalic Q04.6
acquired G93.0
postanal (infected) — *see* Cyst, pilonidal
postmastoidectomy cavity (mucosal) — *see* Complications, postmastoidectomy, cyst
preauricular Q18.1
prepuce N47.4
congenital Q55.69
primordial (jaw) K09.0
prostate N42.83
pseudomucinous (ovary) D27.9
pupillary, miotic H21.27- ☑
radicular (residual) K04.8
radiculodental K04.8
ranular K11.8
Rathke's pouch E23.6
rectum (epithelium) (mucous) K62.89
renal — *see* Cyst, kidney

Cyst — *continued*
residual (radicular) K04.8
retention (ovary) N83.29- ☑
salivary gland K11.6
retina H33.19- ☑
ora serrata H33.11- ☑
parasitic H33.12- ☑
retroperitoneal K68.9
sacrococcygeal (dermoid) — *see* Cyst, pilonidal
salivary gland or duct (mucous extravasation or retention) K11.6
Sampson's N80.1
sclera H15.89
scrotum L72.9
sebaceous L72.3
sebaceous (duct) (gland) L72.3
breast — *see* Dysplasia, mammary, specified type NEC
eyelid — *see* Cyst, eyelid
genital organ NEC
female N94.89
male N50.89
scrotum L72.3
semilunar cartilage (knee) (multiple) — *see* Derangement, knee, meniscus, cystic
seminal vesicle N50.89
serous (ovary) N83.20- ☑
sinus (accessory) (nasal) J34.1
Skene's gland N36.8
skin L72.9
breast — *see* Dysplasia, mammary, specified type NEC
epidermal, epidermoid L72.0
epithelial L72.0
eyelid — *see* Cyst, eyelid
genital organ NEC
female N90.7
male N50.89
inclusion L72.0
scrotum L72.9
sebaceous L72.3
sweat gland or duct L74.8
solitary
bone — *see* Cyst, bone, solitary
jaw M27.40
kidney N28.1
spermatic cord N50.89
sphenoid sinus J34.1
spinal meninges G96.19
spleen NEC D73.4
congenital Q89.09
hydatid — *see also* Echinococcus B67.99 *[D77]*
Stafne's M27.0
subarachnoid intrasellar R93.0
subcutaneous, pheomycotic (chromomycotic) B43.2
subdural (cerebral) G93.0
spinal cord G96.19
sublingual gland K11.6
submandibular gland K11.6
submaxillary gland K11.6
suburethral N36.8
suprarenal gland E27.8
suprasellar — *see* Cyst, brain
sweat gland or duct L74.8
synovial — *see also* Cyst, bursa
ruptured — *see* Rupture, synovium
tarsal — *see* Chalazion
tendon (sheath) — *see* Disorder, tendon, specified type NEC
testis N44.2
tunica albuginea N44.1
theca lutein (ovary) N83.1- ☑
Thornwaldt's J39.2
thymus (gland) E32.8
thyroglossal duct (infected) (persistent) Q89.2
thyroid (gland) E04.1
thyrolingual duct (infected) (persistent) Q89.2
tongue K14.8
tonsil J35.8
tooth — *see* Cyst, dental
Tornwaldt's J39.2
trichilemmal (proliferating) L72.12
trichodermal L72.12
tubal (fallopian) N83.8
inflammatory — *see* Salpingitis, chronic
tubo-ovarian N83.8
inflammatory N70.13

Cyst — *continued*
tunica
albuginea testis N44.1
vaginalis N50.89
turbinate (nose) J34.1
Tyson's gland N48.89
urachus, congenital Q64.4
ureter N28.89
ureterovesical orifice N28.89
urethra, urethral (gland) N36.8
uterine ligament N83.8
uterus (body) (corpus) (recurrent) N85.8
embryonic Q51.818
cervix Q51.6
vagina, vaginal (implantation) (inclusion) (squamous cell) (wall) N89.8
embryonic Q52.4
vallecula, vallecular (epiglottis) J38.7
vesical (orifice) N32.89
vitreous body H43.89
vulva (implantation) (inclusion) N90.7
congenital Q52.79
sebaceous gland N90.7
vulvovaginal gland N90.7
wolffian
female Q50.5
male Q55.4
Cystadenocarcinoma — *see* Neoplasm, malignant, by site
bile duct C22.1
endometrioid — *see* Neoplasm, malignant, by site
specified site — *see* Neoplasm, malignant, by site
unspecified site
female C56.9
male C61
mucinous
papillary
specified site — *see* Neoplasm, malignant, by site
unspecified site C56.9
specified site — *see* Neoplasm, malignant, by site
unspecified site C56.9
papillary
mucinous
specified site — *see* Neoplasm, malignant, by site
unspecified site C56.9
pseudomucinous
specified site — *see* Neoplasm, malignant, by site
unspecified site C56.9
serous
specified site — *see* Neoplasm, malignant, by site
unspecified site C56.9
specified site — *see* Neoplasm, malignant, by site
unspecified site C56.9
pseudomucinous
papillary
specified site — *see* Neoplasm, malignant, by site
unspecified site C56.9
specified site — *see* Neoplasm, malignant, by site
unspecified site C56.9
serous
papillary
specified site — *see* Neoplasm, malignant, by site
unspecified site C56.9
specified site — *see* Neoplasm, malignant, by site
unspecified site C56.9
Cystadenofibroma
clear cell — *see* Neoplasm, benign, by site
endometrioid D27.9
borderline malignancy D39.1- ☑
malignant C56.- ☑
mucinous
specified site — *see* Neoplasm, benign, by site
unspecified site D27.9
serous
specified site — *see* Neoplasm, benign, by site
unspecified site D27.9
specified site — *see* Neoplasm, benign, by site
unspecified site D27.9
Cystadenoma — *see also* Neoplasm, benign, by site
bile duct D13.4
endometrioid — *see* Neoplasm, benign, by site

Cystadenoma — *continued*
  endometrioid — *see* Neoplasm, benign, by site —
      continued
    borderline malignancy — *see* Neoplasm, uncertain
        behavior, by site
  malignant — *see* Neoplasm, malignant, by site
  mucinous
    borderline malignancy
      ovary C56.- ☑
      specified site NEC — *see* Neoplasm, uncertain
          behavior, by site
      unspecified site C56.9
    papillary
      borderline malignancy
        ovary C56.- ☑
        specified site NEC — *see* Neoplasm, uncertain
            behavior, by site
        unspecified site C56.9
      specified site — *see* Neoplasm, benign, by site
      unspecified site C27.9
    specified site — *see* Neoplasm, benign, by site
    unspecified site D27.9
  papillary
    borderline malignancy
      ovary C56.- ☑
      specified site NEC — *see* Neoplasm, uncertain
          behavior, by site
      unspecified site C56.9
    lymphomatosum
      specified site — *see* Neoplasm, benign, by site
      unspecified site D11.9
    mucinous
      borderline malignancy
        ovary C56.- ☑
        specified site NEC — *see* Neoplasm, uncertain
            behavior, by site
        unspecified site C56.9
      specified site — *see* Neoplasm, benign, by site
      unspecified site D27.9
    pseudomucinous
      borderline malignancy
        ovary C56.- ☑
        specified site NEC — *see* Neoplasm, uncertain
            behavior, by site
        unspecified site C56.9
      specified site — *see* Neoplasm, benign, by site
      unspecified site D27.9
    serous
      borderline malignancy
        ovary C56.- ☑
        specified site NEC — *see* Neoplasm, uncertain
            behavior, by site
        unspecified site C56.9
      specified site — *see* Neoplasm, benign, by site
      unspecified site D27.9
    specified site — *see* Neoplasm, benign, by site
    unspecified site D27.9
  pseudomucinous
    borderline malignancy
      ovary C56.- ☑
      specified site NEC — *see* Neoplasm, uncertain
          behavior, by site
      unspecified site C56.9
    papillary
      borderline malignancy
        ovary C56.- ☑
        specified site NEC — *see* Neoplasm, uncertain
            behavior, by site
        unspecified site C56.9
      specified site — *see* Neoplasm, benign, by site
      unspecified site D27.9
    specified site — *see* Neoplasm, benign, by site
    unspecified site D27.9
  serous
    borderline malignancy
      ovary C56.- ☑
      specified site NEC — *see* Neoplasm, uncertain
          behavior, by site
      unspecified site C56.9

Cystadenoma — *continued*
  serous — *continued*
    papillary
      borderline malignancy
        ovary C56.- ☑
        specified site NEC — *see* Neoplasm, uncertain
            behavior, by site
        unspecified site C56.9
      specified site — *see* Neoplasm, benign, by site
      unspecified site D27.9
    specified site — *see* Neoplasm, benign, by site
    unspecified site D27.9
Cystathionine synthase deficiency E72.11
Cystathioninemia E72.19
Cystathioninuria E72.19
Cystic — *see also* condition
  breast (chronic) — *see* Mastopathy, cystic
  corpora lutea (hemorrhagic) N83.1- ☑
  duct — *see* condition
  eyeball (congenital) Q11.0
  fibrosis — *see* Fibrosis, cystic
  kidney (congenital) Q61.9
    adult type Q61.2
    infantile type NEC Q61.19
      collecting duct dilatation Q61.11
    medullary Q61.5
  liver, congenital Q44.6
  lung disease J98.4
    congenital Q33.0
  mastitis, chronic — *see* Mastopathy, cystic
  medullary, kidney Q61.5
  meniscus — *see* Derangement, knee, meniscus, cystic
  ovary N83.20- ☑
Cysticercosis, cysticerciasis B69.9
  with
    epileptiform fits B69.0
    myositis B69.81
  brain B69.0
  central nervous system B69.0
  cerebral B69.0
  ocular B69.1
  specified NEC B69.89
Cysticercus cellulose infestation — *see* Cysticercosis
Cystinosis (malignant) E72.04
Cystinuria E72.01
Cystitis (exudative) (hemorrhagic) (septic) (suppurative)
    N30.90
  with
    fibrosis — *see* Cystitis, chronic, interstitial
    hematuria N30.91
    leukoplakia — *see* Cystitis, chronic, interstitial
    malakoplakia — *see* Cystitis, chronic, interstitial
    metaplasia — *see* Cystitis, chronic, interstitial
    prostatitis N41.3
  acute N30.00
    with hematuria N30.01
    of trigone N30.30
      with hematuria N30.31
  allergic — *see* Cystitis, specified type NEC
  amebic A06.81
  bilharzial B65.9 *[N33]*
  blennorrhagic (gonococcal) A54.01
  bullous — *see* Cystitis, specified type NEC
  calculous N21.0
  chlamydial A56.01
  chronic N30.20
    with hematuria N30.21
    interstitial N30.10
      with hematuria N30.11
    of trigone N30.30
      with hematuria N30.31
    specified NEC N30.20
      with hematuria N30.21
  cystic (a) — *see* Cystitis, specified type NEC
  diphtheritic A36.85
  echinococcal
    granulosus B67.39
    multilocularis B67.69
  emphysematous — *see* Cystitis, specified type NEC
  encysted — *see* Cystitis, specified type NEC

Cystitis — *continued*
  eosinophilic — *see* Cystitis, specified type NEC
  follicular — *see* Cystitis, of trigone
  gangrenous — *see* Cystitis, specified type NEC
  glandularis — *see* Cystitis, specified type NEC
  gonococcal A54.01
  incrusted — *see* Cystitis, specified type NEC
  interstitial (chronic) — *see* Cystitis, chronic, interstitial
  irradiation N30.40
    with hematuria N30.41
  irritation — *see* Cystitis, specified type NEC
  malignant — *see* Cystitis, specified type NEC
  of trigone N30.30
    with hematuria N30.31
  panmural — *see* Cystitis, chronic, interstitial
  polyposa — *see* Cystitis, specified type NEC
  prostatic N41.3
  puerperal (postpartum) O86.22
  radiation — *see* Cystitis, irradiation
  specified type NEC N30.80
    with hematuria N30.81
  subacute — *see* Cystitis, chronic
  submucous — *see* Cystitis, chronic, interstitial
  syphilitic (late) A52.76
  trichomonal A59.03
  tuberculous A18.12
  ulcerative — *see* Cystitis, chronic, interstitial
Cystocele (-urethrocele)
  female N81.10
    with prolapse of uterus — *see* Prolapse, uterus
    lateral N81.12
    midline N81.11
    paravaginal N81.12
  in pregnancy or childbirth O34.8- ☑
    causing obstructed labor O65.5
  male N32.89
Cystolithiasis N21.0
Cystoma — *see also* Neoplasm, benign, by site
  endometrial, ovary N80.1
  mucinous
    specified site — *see* Neoplasm, benign, by site
    unspecified site D27.9
  serous
    specified site — *see* Neoplasm, benign, by site
    unspecified site D27.9
  simple (ovary) N83.29- ☑
Cystoplegia N31.2
Cystoptosis N32.89
Cystopyelitis — *see* Pyelonephritis
Cystorrhagia N32.89
Cystosarcoma phyllodes D48.6- ☑
  benign D24- ☑
  malignant — *see* Neoplasm, breast, malignant
Cystostomy
  attention to Z43.5
  complication — *see* Complications, cystostomy
  status Z93.50
    appendico-vesicostomy Z93.52
    cutaneous Z93.51
    specified NEC Z93.59
Cystourethritis — *see* Urethritis
Cystourethrocele — *see also* Cystocele
  female N81.10
    with uterine prolapse — *see* Prolapse, uterus
    lateral N81.12
    midline N81.11
    paravaginal N81.12
  male N32.89
Cytomegalic inclusion disease
  congenital P35.1
Cytomegalovirus infection B25.9
Cytomycosis (reticuloendothelial) B39.4
Cytopenia D75.9
  refractory
    with multilineage dysplasia D46.A (*following* D46.2)
      and ring sideroblasts (RCMD RS) D46.B (*following*
          D46.2)
Czerny's disease (periodic hydrarthrosis of the knee) —
    see Effusion, joint, knee

Cystadenoma — Czerny's disease

D

Da Costa's syndrome F45.8
Daae (-Finsen) **disease** (epidemic pleurodynia) B33.0
Dabney's grip B33.0
Dacryoadenitis, dacryadenitis H04.00- ☑
  acute H04.01- ☑
  chronic H04.02- ☑
Dacryocystitis H04.30- ☑
  acute H04.32- ☑
  chronic H04.41- ☑
  neonatal P39.1
  phlegmonous H04.31- ☑
  syphilitic A52.71
    congenital (early) A50.01
  trachomatous, active A71.1
    sequelae (late effect) B94.0
Dacryocystoblenorrhea — *see* Inflammation, lacrimal, passages, chronic
Dacryocystocele — *see* Disorder, lacrimal system, changes
Dacryolith, dacryolithiasis H04.51- ☑
Dacryoma — *see* Disorder, lacrimal system, changes
Dacryopericystitis — *see* Dacryocystitis
Dacryops H04.11- ☑
Dacryostenosis — *see also* Stenosis, lacrimal
  congenital Q10.5
Dactylitis
  bone — *see* Osteomyelitis
  sickle-cell D57.00
    Hb C D57.219
    Hb SS D57.00
    specified NEC D57.819
  skin L08.9
  syphilitic A52.77
  tuberculous A18.03
Dactylolysis spontanea (ainhum) L94.6
Dactylosymphysis Q70.9
  fingers — *see* Syndactylism, complex, fingers
  toes — *see* Syndactylism, complex, toes
Damage
  arteriosclerotic — *see* Arteriosclerosis
  brain (nontraumatic) G93.9
    anoxic, hypoxic G93.1
      resulting from a procedure G97.82
    child NEC G80.9
    due to birth injury P11.2
  cardiorenal (vascular) — *see* Hypertension, cardiorenal
  cerebral NEC — *see* Damage, brain
  coccyx, complicating delivery O71.6
  coronary — *see* Disease, heart, ischemic
  deep tissue, pressure-induced — *see also* L89 with final character .6
  eye, birth injury P15.3
  liver (nontraumatic) K76.9
    alcoholic K70.9
    due to drugs — *see* Disease, liver, toxic
    toxic — *see* Disease, liver, toxic
  medication T88.7 ☑
  pelvic
    joint or ligament, during delivery O71.6
    organ NEC
      during delivery O71.5
      following ectopic or molar pregnancy O08.6
  renal — *see* Disease, renal
  subendocardium, subendocardial — *see* Degeneration, myocardial
  vascular I99.9
Dana-Putnam syndrome (subacute combined sclerosis with pernicious anemia) — *see* Degeneration, combined
Danbolt (-Cross) **syndrome** (acrodermatitis enteropathica) E83.2
Dandruff L21.0
Dandy-Walker syndrome Q03.1
  with spina bifida — *see* Spina bifida
Danlos' syndrome — *see also* Syndrome, Ehlers-Danlos Q79.60
Darier (-White) **disease** (congenital) Q82.8
  meaning erythema annulare centrifugum L53.1
Darier-Roussy sarcoid D86.3
Darling's disease or histoplasmosis B39.4
Darwin's tubercle Q17.8
Dawson's (inclusion body) **encephalitis** A81.1
De Beurmann (-Gougerot) **disease** B42.1
De la Tourette's syndrome F95.2

De Lange's syndrome Q87.19
De Morgan's spots (senile angiomas) I78.1
De Quervain's
  disease (tendon sheath) M65.4
  syndrome E34.51
  thyroiditis (subacute granulomatous thyroiditis) E06.1
De Toni-Fanconi (-Debré) **syndrome** E72.09
  with cystinosis E72.04
Dead
  fetus, retained (mother) O36.4 ☑
    early pregnancy O02.1
  labyrinth H83.2 ☑
  ovum, retained O02.0
Deaf nonspeaking NEC H91.3
Deafmutism (acquired) (congenital) NEC H91.3
  hysterical F44.6
  syphilitic, congenital — *see also* subcategory H94.8 A50.09
Deafness (acquired) (complete) (hereditary) (partial) H91.9-
  with blue sclera and fragility of bone Q78.0
  auditory fatigue — *see* Deafness, specified type NEC
  aviation T70.0 ☑
    nerve injury — *see* Injury, nerve, acoustic, specified type NEC
  boilermaker's H83.3 ☑
  central — *see* Deafness, sensorineural
  conductive H90.2
    and sensorineural
      mixed H90.8
        bilateral H90.6
    bilateral H90.0
    unilateral H90.1- ☑
      with restricted hearing on the contralateral side H90.A- ☑
  congenital H90.5
    with blue sclera and fragility of bone Q78.0
  due to toxic agents — *see* Deafness, ototoxic
  emotional (hysterical) F44.6
  functional (hysterical) F44.6
  high frequency H91.9- ☑
  hysterical F44.6
  low frequency H91.9- ☑
  mental R48.8
  mixed conductive and sensorineural H90.8
    bilateral H90.6
    unilateral H90.7- ☑
  nerve — *see* Deafness, sensorineural
  neural — *see* Deafness, sensorineural
  noise-induced — *see also* subcategory H83.3 ☑
    nerve injury — *see* Injury, nerve, acoustic, specified type NEC
  nonspeaking H91.3
  ototoxic H91.0 ☑
  perceptive — *see* Deafness, sensorineural
  psychogenic (hysterical) F44.6
  sensorineural H90.5
    and conductive
      bilateral H90.6
      mixed H90.8
        bilateral H90.6
    bilateral H90.3
    unilateral H90.4- ☑
      with restricted hearing on the contralateral side H90.A- ☑
  sensory — *see* Deafness, sensorineural
  specified type NEC H91.8 ☑
  sudden (idiopathic) H91.2- ☑
  syphilitic A52.15
  transient ischemic H93.01- ☑
  traumatic — *see* Injury, nerve, acoustic, specified type NEC
  word (developmental) H93.25
Death (cause unknown) (of) (unexplained) (unspecified cause) R99
  brain G93.82
  cardiac (sudden) (with successful resuscitation) — *code to* underlying disease
    family history of Z82.41
    personal history of Z86.74
  family member (assumed) Z63.4
Debility (chronic) (general) (nervous) R53.81
  congenital or neonatal NOS P96.9
  nervous R53.81
  old age R54
  senile R54
Débove's disease (splenomegaly) R16.1

Decalcification
  bone — *see* Osteoporosis
  teeth K03.89
Decapsulation, kidney N28.89
Decay
  dental — *see* Caries, dental
  senile R54
  tooth, teeth — *see* Caries, dental
Deciduitis (acute)
  following ectopic or molar pregnancy O08.0
Decline (general) — *see* Debility
  cognitive, age-associated R41.81
Decompensation
  cardiac (acute) (chronic) — *see* Disease, heart
  cardiovascular — *see* Disease, cardiovascular
  heart — *see* Disease, heart
  hepatic — *see* Failure, hepatic
  myocardial (acute) (chronic) — *see* Disease, heart
  respiratory J98.8
Decompression sickness T70.3 ☑
Decrease (d)
  absolute neutrophile count — *see* Neutropenia
  blood
    platelets — *see* Thrombocytopenia
    pressure R03.1
      due to shock following
        injury T79.4 ☑
        operation T81.19 ☑
  estrogen E28.39
    postablative E89.40
      asymptomatic E89.40
      symptomatic E89.41
  fragility of erythrocytes D58.8
  function
    lipase (pancreatic) K90.3
    ovary in hypopituitarism E23.0
    parenchyma of pancreas K86.89
    pituitary (gland) (anterior) (lobe) E23.0
      posterior (lobe) E23.0
  functional activity R68.89
  glucose R73.09
  hematocrit R71.0
  hemoglobin R71.0
  leukocytes D72.819
    specified NEC D72.818
  libido R68.82
  lymphocytes D72.810
  platelets D69.6
  respiration, due to shock following injury T79.4 ☑
  sexual desire R68.82
  tear secretion NEC — *see* Syndrome, dry eye
  tolerance
    fat K90.49
    glucose R73.09
    pancreatic K90.3
    salt and water E87.8
  vision NEC H54.7
  white blood cell count D72.819
    specified NEC D72.818
Decubitus (ulcer) — *see* Ulcer, pressure, by site
  cervix N86
Deepening acetabulum — *see* Derangement, joint, specified type NEC, hip
Defect, defective Q89.9
  3-beta-hydroxysteroid dehydrogenase E25.0
  11-hydroxylase E25.0
  21-hydroxylase E25.0
  abdominal wall, congenital Q79.59
  antibody immunodeficiency D80.9
  aorticopulmonary septum Q21.4
  atrial septal (ostium secundum type) Q21.1
    following acute myocardial infarction (current complication) I23.1
    ostium primum type Q21.2
  atrioventricular
    canal Q21.2
    septum Q21.2
  auricular septal Q21.1
  bilirubin excretion NEC E80.6
  biosynthesis, androgen (testicular) E29.1
  bulbar septum Q21.0
  catalase E80.3
  cell membrane receptor complex (CR3) D71
  circulation I99.9
    congenital Q28.9
    newborn Q28.9
  coagulation (factor) — *see also* Deficiency, factor D68.9

☑ **Additional Character Required** — Refer to the Tabular List for Character Selection   ▽ **Subterms under main terms may continue to next column or page**

Defect, defective — *continued*
- coagulation — *see also* Deficiency, factor — *continued*
  - with
    - ectopic pregnancy O08.1
    - molar pregnancy O08.1
  - acquired D68.4
  - antepartum with hemorrhage — *see* Hemorrhage, antepartum, with coagulation defect
  - due to
    - liver disease D68.4
    - vitamin K deficiency D68.4
  - hereditary NEC D68.2
  - intrapartum O67.0
  - newborn, transient P61.6
  - postpartum O99.13
    - with hemorrhage O72.3
  - specified type NEC D68.8
- complement system D84.1
- conduction (heart) I45.9
  - bone — *see* Deafness, conductive
- congenital, organ or site not listed — *see* Anomaly, by site
- coronary sinus Q21.1
- cushion, endocardial Q21.2
- degradation, glycoprotein E77.1
- dental bridge, crown, fillings — *see* Defect, dental restoration
- dental restoration K08.50
  - specified NEC K08.59
- dentin (hereditary) K00.5
- Descemet's membrane, congenital Q13.89
- developmental — *see also* Anomaly
  - cauda equina Q06.3
- diaphragm
  - with elevation, eventration or hernia — *see* Hernia, diaphragm
  - congenital Q79.1
    - with hernia Q79.0
    - gross (with hernia) Q79.0
- ectodermal, congenital Q82.9
- Eisenmenger's Q21.8
- enzyme
  - catalase E80.3
  - peroxidase E80.3
- esophagus, congenital Q39.9
- extensor retinaculum M62.89
- fibrin polymerization D68.2
- filling
  - bladder R93.41
  - kidney R93.42- ☑
  - renal pelvis R93.41
  - stomach R93.3
  - ureter R93.41
  - urinary organs, specified NEC R93.49
- GABA (gamma aminobutyric acid) metabolic E72.81
- Gerbode Q21.0
- glycoprotein degradation E77.1
- Hageman (factor) D68.2
- hearing — *see* Deafness
- high grade F70
- interatrial septal Q21.1
- interauricular septal Q21.1
- interventricular septal Q21.0
  - with dextroposition of aorta, pulmonary stenosis and hypertrophy of right ventricle Q21.3
  - in tetralogy of Fallot Q21.3
- learning (specific) — *see* Disorder, learning
- lymphocyte function antigen-1 (LFA-1) D84.0
- lysosomal enzyme, post-translational modification E77.0
- major osseous M89.70
  - ankle M89.77- ☑
  - carpus M89.74- ☑
  - clavicle M89.71- ☑
  - femur M89.75- ☑
  - fibula M89.76- ☑
  - fingers M89.74- ☑
  - foot M89.77- ☑
  - forearm M89.73- ☑
  - hand M89.74- ☑
  - humerus M89.72- ☑
  - lower leg M89.76- ☑
  - metacarpus M89.74- ☑
  - metatarsus M89.77- ☑
  - multiple sites M89.79
  - pelvic region M89.75- ☑
  - pelvis M89.75- ☑

Defect, defective — *continued*
- major osseous — *continued*
  - radius M89.73- ☑
  - scapula M89.71- ☑
  - shoulder region M89.71- ☑
  - specified NEC M89.78
  - tarsus M89.77- ☑
  - thigh M89.75- ☑
  - tibia M89.76- ☑
  - toes M89.77- ☑
  - ulna M89.73- ☑
- mental — *see* Disability, intellectual
- modification, lysosomal enzymes, post-translational E77.0
- obstructive, congenital
  - renal pelvis Q62.39
  - ureter Q62.39
    - atresia — *see* Atresia, ureter
    - cecoureterocele Q62.32
    - megaureter Q62.2
    - orthotopic ureterocele Q62.31
- osseous, major M89.70
  - ankle M89.77- ☑
  - carpus M89.74- ☑
  - clavicle M89.71- ☑
  - femur M89.75- ☑
  - fibula M89.76- ☑
  - fingers M89.74- ☑
  - foot M89.77- ☑
  - forearm M89.73- ☑
  - hand M89.74- ☑
  - humerus M89.72- ☑
  - lower leg M89.76- ☑
  - metacarpus M89.74- ☑
  - metatarsus M89.77- ☑
  - multiple sites M89.9
  - pelvic region M89.75- ☑
  - pelvis M89.75- ☑
  - radius M89.73- ☑
  - scapula M89.71- ☑
  - shoulder region M89.71- ☑
  - specified NEC M89.78
  - tarsus M89.77- ☑
  - thigh M89.75- ☑
  - tibia M89.76- ☑
  - toes M89.77- ☑
  - ulna M89.73- ☑
- osteochondral NEC — *see also* Deformity M95.8
- ostium
  - primum Q21.2
  - secundum Q21.1
- peroxidase E80.3
- placental blood supply — *see* Insufficiency, placental
- platelets, qualitative D69.1
  - constitutional D68.0
- postural NEC, spine — *see* Dorsopathy, deforming
- reduction
  - limb Q73.8
    - lower Q72.9- ☑
      - absence — *see* Agenesis, leg
      - foot — *see* Agenesis, foot
      - longitudinal
        - femur Q72.4- ☑
        - fibula Q72.6- ☑
        - tibia Q72.5- ☑
      - specified type NEC Q72.89- ☑
      - split foot Q72.7- ☑
    - specified type NEC Q73.8
    - upper Q71.9- ☑
      - absence — *see* Agenesis, arm
        - forearm — *see* Agenesis, forearm
        - hand — *see* Agenesis, hand
      - lobster-claw hand Q71.6- ☑
      - longitudinal
        - radius Q71.4- ☑
        - ulna Q71.5- ☑
      - specified type NEC Q71.89- ☑
- renal pelvis Q63.8
  - obstructive Q62.39
- respiratory system, congenital Q34.9
- restoration, dental K08.50
  - specified NEC K08.59
- retinal nerve bundle fibers H35.89
- septal (heart) NOS Q21.9
  - acquired (atrial) (auricular) (ventricular) (old) I51.0
  - atrial Q21.1

Defect, defective — *continued*
- septal — *continued*
  - atrial — *continued*
    - concurrent with acute myocardial infarction — *see* Infarct, myocardium
    - following acute myocardial infarction (current complication) I23.1
    - ventricular — *see also* Defect, ventricular septal Q21.0
  - sinus venosus Q21.1
- speech R47.9
  - developmental F80.9
  - specified NEC R47.89
- Taussig-Bing (aortic transposition and overriding pulmonary artery) Q20.1
- teeth, wedge K03.1
- vascular (local) I99.9
  - congenital Q27.9
- ventricular septal Q21.0
  - concurrent with acute myocardial infarction — *see* Infarct, myocardium
  - following acute myocardial infarction (current complication) I23.2
  - in tetralogy of Fallot Q21.3
- vision NEC H54.7
- visual field H53.40
  - bilateral
    - heteronymous H53.47
    - homonymous H53.46- ☑
  - generalized contraction H53.48- ☑
  - localized
    - arcuate H53.43- ☑
    - scotoma (central area) H53.41- ☑
      - blind spot area H53.42- ☑
    - sector H53.43- ☑
    - specified type NEC H53.45- ☑
- voice R49.9
  - specified NEC R49.8
- wedge, tooth, teeth (abrasion) K03.1

Deferentitis N49.1
- gonorrheal (acute) (chronic) A54.23

Defibrination (syndrome) D65
- antepartum — *see* Hemorrhage, antepartum, with coagulation defect, disseminated intravascular coagulation
- following ectopic or molar pregnancy O08.1
- intrapartum O67.0
- newborn P60
- postpartum O72.3

Deficiency, deficient
- 3-beta hydroxysteroid dehydrogenase E25.0
- 5-alpha reductase (with male pseudohermaphroditism) E29.1
- 11-hydroxylase E25.0
- 21-hydroxylase E25.0
- abdominal muscle syndrome Q79.4
- AC globulin (congenital) (hereditary) D68.2
  - acquired D68.4
- accelerator globulin (Ac G) (blood) D68.2
- acid phosphatase E83.39
- activating factor (blood) D68.2
- ADA2 (adenosine deaminase 2) D81.32
- adenosine deaminase (ADA) D81.30
  - with severe combined immunodeficiency (SCID) D81.31
  - partial (type 1) D81.39
  - specified NEC D81.39
  - type 1 (without SCID) (without severe combined immunodeficiency) D81.39
  - type 2 D81.32
- aldolase (hereditary) E74.19
- alpha-1-antitrypsin E88.01
- amino-acids E72.9
- anemia — *see* Anemia
- aneurin E51.9
- antibody with
  - hyperimmunoglobulinemia D80.6
  - near-normal immunoglobins D80.6
- antidiuretic hormone E23.2
- anti-hemophilic
  - factor (A) D66
    - B D67
    - C D68.1
  - globulin (AHG) NEC D66
- antithrombin (antithrombin III) D68.59
- ascorbic acid E54
- attention (disorder) (syndrome) F98.8

Deficiency, deficient — *continued*
  attention — *continued*
    with hyperactivity — *see* Disorder, attention-deficit
      hyperactivity
  autoprothrombin
    C D68.2
    I D68.2
    II D67
  beta-glucuronidase E76.29
  biotin E53.8
  biotin-dependent carboxylase D81.819
  biotinidase D81.810
  brancher enzyme (amylopectinosis) E74.03
  C1 esterase inhibitor (C1-INH) D84.1
  calciferol E55.9
    with
      adult osteomalacia M83.8
      rickets — *see* Rickets
  calcium (dietary) E58
  calorie, severe E43
    with marasmus E41
      and kwashiorkor E42
  cardiac — *see* Insufficiency, myocardial
  carnitine E71.40
    due to
      hemodialysis E71.43
      inborn errors of metabolism E71.42
      Valproic acid therapy E71.43
    iatrogenic E71.43
    muscle palmityltransferase E71.314
    primary E71.41
    secondary E71.448
  carotene E50.9
  central nervous system G96.8
  ceruloplasmin (Wilson) E83.01
  choline E53.8
  Christmas factor D67
  chromium E61.4
  clotting (blood) — *see also* Deficiency, coagulation
    factor D68.9
  clotting factor NEC (hereditary) — *see also* Deficiency,
    factor D68.2
  coagulation NOS D68.9
    with
      ectopic pregnancy O08.1
      molar pregnancy O08.1
    acquired (any) D68.4
    antepartum hemorrhage — *see* Hemorrhage, an-
      tepartum, with coagulation defect
    clotting factor NEC — *see also* Deficiency, factor
      D68.2
    due to
      hyperprothrombinemia D68.4
      liver disease D68.4
      vitamin K deficiency D68.4
    newborn, transient P61.6
    postpartum O72.3
    specified NEC D68.8
  cognitive F09
  color vision H53.50
    achromatopsia H53.51
    acquired H53.52
    deuteranomaly H53.53
    protanomaly H53.54
    specified type NEC H53.59
    tritanomaly H53.55
  combined glucocorticoid and mineralocorticoid E27.49
  contact factor D68.2
  copper (nutritional) E61.0
  corticoadrenal E27.40
    primary E27.1
  craniofacial axis Q75.0
  cyanocobalamin E53.8
  debrancher enzyme (limit dextrinosis) E74.03
  dehydrogenase
    long chain/very long chain acyl CoA E71.310
    medium chain acyl CoA E71.311
    short chain acyl CoA E71.312
  diet E63.9
  dihydropyrimidine dehydrogenase (DPD) E88.89
  disaccharidase E73.9
  edema — *see* Malnutrition, severe
  endocrine E34.9
  energy-supply — *see* Malnutrition
  enzymes, circulating NEC E88.09
  ergosterol E55.9
    with
      adult osteomalacia M83.8

Deficiency, deficient — *continued*
  ergosterol — *continued*
    with — *continued*
      rickets — *see* Rickets
  essential fatty acid (EFA) E63.0
  factor — *see also* Deficiency, coagulation
    Hageman D68.2
    I (congenital) (hereditary) D68.2
    II (congenital) (hereditary) D68.2
    IX (congenital) (functional) (hereditary) (with func-
      tional defect) D67
    multiple (congenital) D68.8
      acquired D68.4
    V (congenital) (hereditary) D68.2
    VII (congenital) (hereditary) D68.2
    VIII (congenital) (functional) (hereditary) (with
      functional defect) D66
      with vascular defect D68.0
    X (congenital) (hereditary) D68.2
    XI (congenital) (hereditary) D68.1
    XII (congenital) (hereditary) D68.2
    XIII (congenital) (hereditary) D68.2
  femoral, proximal focal (congenital) — *see* Defect, re-
    duction, lower limb, longitudinal, femur
  fibrinase D68.2
  fibrinogen (congenital) (hereditary) D68.2
    acquired D65
  fibrin-stabilizing factor (congenital) (hereditary) D68.2
    acquired D68.4
  folate E53.8
  folic acid E53.8
  foreskin N47.3
  fructokinase E74.11
  fructose 1,6-diphosphatase E74.19
  fructose-1-phosphate aldolase E74.19
  GABA (gamma aminobutyric acid) transaminase E72.81
  GABA-T (gamma aminobutyric acid transaminase)
    E72.81
  galactokinase E74.29
  galactose-1-phosphate uridyl transferase E74.29
  gammaglobulin in blood D80.1
    hereditary D80.0
  glass factor D68.2
  glucocorticoid E27.49
    mineralocorticoid E27.49
  glucose-6-phosphatase E74.01
  glucose-6-phosphate dehydrogenase
    anemia D55.0
    without anemia D75.A
  glucuronyl transferase E80.5
  glycogen synthetase E74.09
  gonadotropin (isolated) E23.0
  growth hormone (idiopathic) (isolated) E23.0
  Hageman factor D68.2
  hemoglobin D64.9
  hepatophosphorylase E74.09
  homogentisate 1,2-dioxygenase E70.29
  hormone
    anterior pituitary (partial) NEC E23.0
      growth E23.0
    growth (isolated) E23.0
    pituitary E23.0
    testicular E29.1
  hypoxanthine- (guanine)-phosphoribosyltransferase
    (HG- PRT) (total H-PRT) E79.1
  immunity D84.9
    cell-mediated D84.8
      with thrombocytopenia and eczema D82.0
    combined D81.9
    humoral D80.9
    IgA (secretory) D80.2
    IgG D80.3
    IgM D80.4
  immuno — *see* Immunodeficiency
  immunoglobulin, selective
    A (IgA) D80.2
    G (IgG) (subclasses) D80.3
    M (IgM) D80.4
  inositol (B complex) E53.8
  intrinsic
    factor (congenital) D51.0
    sphincter N36.42
      with urethral hypermobility N36.43
  iodine E61.8
    congenital syndrome — *see* Syndrome, iodine-defi-
      ciency, congenital
  iron E61.1
    anemia D50.9
  kalium E87.6

Deficiency, deficient — *continued*
  kappa-light chain D80.8
  labile factor (congenital) (hereditary) D68.2
    acquired D68.4
  lacrimal fluid (acquired) — *see also* Syndrome, dry eye
    congenital Q10.6
  lactase
    congenital E73.0
    secondary E73.1
  Laki-Lorand factor D68.2
  lecithin cholesterol acyltransferase E78.6
  lipocaic K86.89
  lipoprotein (familial) (high density) E78.6
  liver phosphorylase E74.09
  lysosomal alpha-1, 4 glucosidase E74.02
  magnesium E61.2
  major histocompatibility complex
    class I D81.6
    class II D81.7
  manganese E61.3
  menadione (vitamin K) E56.1
    newborn P53
  mental (familial) (hereditary) — *see* Disability, intellec-
    tual
  methylenetetrahydrofolate reductase (MTHFR) E72.12
  mevalonate kinase M04.1
  mineralocorticoid E27.49
    with glucocorticoid E27.49
  mineral NEC E61.8
  molybdenum (nutritional) E61.5
  moral F60.2
  multiple nutrient elements E61.7
  multiple sulfatase (MSD) E75.26
  muscle
    carnitine (palmityltransferase) E71.314
    phosphofructokinase E74.09
  myoadenylate deaminase E79.2
  myocardial — *see* Insufficiency, myocardial
  myophosphorylase E74.04
  NADH diaphorase or reductase (congenital) D74.0
  NADH-methemoglobin reductase (congenital) D74.0
  natrium E87.1
  niacin (amide) (-tryptophan) E52
  nicotinamide E52
  nicotinic acid E52
  number of teeth — *see* Anodontia
  nutrient element E61.9
    multiple E61.7
    specified NEC E61.8
  nutrition, nutritional E63.9
    sequelae — *see* Sequelae, nutritional deficiency
    specified NEC E63.8
  of interleukin 1 receptor antagonist [DIRA] M04.8
  ornithine transcarbamylase E72.4
  ovarian E28.39
  oxygen — *see* Anoxia
  pantothenic acid E53.8
  parathyroid (gland) E20.9
  perineum (female) N81.89
  phenylalanine hydroxylase E70.1
  phosphoenolpyruvate carboxykinase E74.4
  phosphofructokinase E74.19
  phosphomannomutase E74.8
  phosphomannose isomerase E74.8
  phosphomannosyl mutase E74.8
  phosphorylase kinase, liver E74.09
  pituitary hormone (isolated) E23.0
  plasma thromboplastin
    antecedent (PTA) D68.1
    component (PTC) D67
  plasminogen (type 1) (type 2) E88.02
  platelet NEC D69.1
    constitutional D68.0
  polyglandular E31.8
    autoimmune E31.0
  potassium (K) E87.6
  prepuce N47.3
  proaccelerin (congenital) (hereditary) D68.2
    acquired D68.4
  proconvertin factor (congenital) (hereditary) D68.2
    acquired D68.4
  protein — *see also* Malnutrition E46
    anemia D53.0
    C D68.59
    S D68.59
  prothrombin (congenital) (hereditary) D68.2
    acquired D68.4
  Prower factor D68.2

☑ **Additional Character Required** — Refer to the Tabular List for Character Selection
▽ **Subterms under main terms may continue to next column or page**

Deficiency, deficient — *continued*
 pseudocholinesterase E88.09
 PTA (plasma thromboplastin antecedent) D68.1
 PTC (plasma thromboplastin component) D67
 purine nucleoside phosphorylase (PNP) D81.5
 pyracin (alpha) (beta) E53.1
 pyridoxal E53.1
 pyridoxamine E53.1
 pyridoxine (derivatives) E53.1
 pyruvate
  carboxylase E74.4
  dehydrogenase E74.4
 riboflavin (vitamin B2) E53.0
 salt E87.1
 secretion
  ovary E28.39
  salivary gland (any) K11.7
  urine R34
 selenium (dietary) E59
 serum antitrypsin, familial E88.01
 short stature homeobox gene (SHOX)
  with
   dyschondrosteosis Q78.8
   short stature (idiopathic) E34.3
   Turner's syndrome Q96.9
 sodium (Na) E87.1
 SPCA (factor VII) D68.2
 sphincter, intrinsic N36.42
  with urethral hypermobility N36.43
 stable factor (congenital) (hereditary) D68.2
  acquired D68.4
 Stuart-Prower (factor X) D68.2
 succinic semialdehyde dehydrogenase E72.81
 sucrase E74.39
 sulfatase E75.26
 sulfite oxidase E72.19
 thiamin, thiaminic (chloride) E51.9
  beriberi (dry) E51.11
   wet E51.12
 thrombokinase D68.2
  newborn P53
 thyroid (gland) — *see* Hypothyroidism
 tocopherol E56.0
 tooth bud K00.0
 transcobalamine II (anemia) D51.2
 vanadium E61.6
 vascular I99.9
 vasopressin E23.2
 vertical ridge K06.8
 viosterol — *see* Deficiency, calciferol
 vitamin (multiple) NOS E56.9
  A E50.9
   with
    Bitot's spot (corneal) E50.1
    follicular keratosis E50.8
    keratomalacia E50.4
    manifestations NEC E50.8
    night blindness E50.5
    scar of cornea, xerophthalmic E50.6
    xeroderma E50.8
    xerophthalmia E50.7
    xerosis
     conjunctival E50.0
      and Bitot's spot E50.1
     cornea E50.2
      and ulceration E50.3
   sequelae E64.1
  B (complex) NOS E53.9
   with
    beriberi (dry) E51.11
     wet E51.12
    pellagra E52
  B1 NOS E51.9
   beriberi (dry) E51.11
    with circulatory system manifestations E51.11
    wet E51.12
  B12 E53.8
  B2 (riboflavin) E53.0
  B6 E53.1
  C E54
   sequelae E64.2
  D E55.9
   with
    adult osteomalacia M83.8
    rickets — *see* Rickets
   25-hydroxylase E83.32
  E E56.0
  folic acid E53.8
  G E53.0

Deficiency, deficient — *continued*
 vitamin — *continued*
  group B E53.9
   specified NEC E53.8
  H (biotin) E53.8
  K E56.1
   of newborn P53
  nicotinic E52
  P E56.8
  PP (pellagra-preventing) E52
  specified NEC E56.8
  thiamin E51.9
   beriberi — *see* Beriberi
 zinc, dietary E60
Deficit — *see also* Deficiency
 attention and concentration R41.840
  disorder — *see* Attention, deficit
  following
   cerebral infarction I69.310
   cerebrovascular disease I69.910
    specified disease NEC I69.810
   nontraumatic
    intracerebral hemorrhage I69.110
    specified intracranial hemorrhage NEC I69.210
    subarachnoid hemorrhage I69.010
 cognitive
  communication R41.841
  emotional
   following
    cerebral infarction I69.315
    cerebrovascular disease I69.915
     specified disease NEC I69.815
    nontraumatic
     intracerebral hemorrhage I69.115
     specified intracranial hemorrhage NEC I69.215
     subarachnoid hemorrhage I69.015
  following
   cerebral infarction I69.319
   cerebrovascular disease I69.919
    specified disease NEC I69.819
   nontraumatic
    intracerebral hemorrhage I69.119
    specified intracranial hemorrhage NEC I69.219
    subarachnoid hemorrhage I69.019
  social
   following
    cerebral infarction I69.315
    cerebrovascular disease I69.915
     specified disease NEC I69.815
    nontraumatic
     intracerebral hemorrhage I69.115
     specified intracranial hemorrhage NEC I69.215
     subarachnoid hemorrhage I69.015
 cognitive NEC R41.89
  following
   cerebral infarction I69.318
   cerebrovascular disease I69.918
    specified disease NEC I69.818
   nontraumatic
    intracerebral hemorrhage I69.118
    specified intracranial hemorrhage NEC I69.218
    subarachnoid hemorrhage I69.018
 concentration R41.840
 executive function R41.844
  following
   cerebral infarction I69.314
   cerebrovascular disease I69.914
    specified disease NEC I69.814
   nontraumatic
    intracerebral hemorrhage I69.114
    specified intracranial hemorrhage NEC I69.214
    subarachnoid hemorrhage I69.014
 frontal lobe R41.844
  following
   cerebral infarction I69.314
   cerebrovascular disease I69.914
    specified disease NEC I69.814
   nontraumatic
    intracerebral hemorrhage I69.114
    specified intracranial hemorrhage NEC I69.214
    subarachnoid hemorrhage I69.014
 memory
  following
   cerebral infarction I69.311
   cerebrovascular disease I69.911
    specified disease NEC I69.811

Deficit — *continued*
 memory — *continued*
  following — *continued*
   nontraumatic
    intracerebral hemorrhage I69.111
    specified intracranial hemorrhage NEC I69.211
    subarachnoid hemorrhage I69.011
 neurologic NEC R29.818
  ischemic
   reversible (RIND) I63.9
    prolonged (PRIND) I63.9
 oxygen R09.02
 prolonged reversible ischemic neurologic (PRIND) I63.9
 psychomotor R41.843
  following
   cerebral infarction I69.313
   cerebrovascular disease I69.913
    specified disease NEC I69.813
   nontraumatic
    intracerebral hemorrhage I69.113
    specified intracranial hemorrhage NEC I69.213
    subarachnoid hemorrhage I69.013
 visuospatial R41.842
  following
   cerebral infarction I69.312
   cerebrovascular disease I69.912
    specified disease NEC I69.812
   nontraumatic
    intracerebral hemorrhage I69.112
    specified intracranial hemorrhage NEC I69.212
    subarachnoid hemorrhage I69.012
Deflection
 radius — *see* Deformity, limb, specified type NEC, forearm
 septum (acquired) (nasal) (nose) J34.2
 spine — *see* Curvature, spine
 turbinate (nose) J34.2
Defluvium
 capillorum — *see* Alopecia
 ciliorum — *see* Madarosis
 unguium L60.8
Deformity Q89.9
 abdomen, congenital Q89.9
 abdominal wall
  acquired M95.8
  congenital Q79.59
 acquired (unspecified site) M95.9
 adrenal gland Q89.1
 alimentary tract, congenital Q45.9
  upper Q40.9
 ankle (joint) (acquired) — *see also* Deformity, limb, lower leg
  abduction — *see* Contraction, joint, ankle
  congenital Q68.8
  contraction — *see* Contraction, joint, ankle
  specified type NEC — *see* Deformity, limb, foot, specified NEC
 anus (acquired) K62.89
  congenital Q43.9
 aorta (arch) (congenital) Q25.40
  acquired I77.89
 aortic
  arch, acquired I77.89
  cusp or valve (congenital) Q23.8
   acquired — *see also* Endocarditis, aortic I35.8
 arm (acquired) (upper) — *see also* Deformity, limb, upper arm
  congenital Q68.8
  forearm — *see* Deformity, limb, forearm
 artery (congenital) (peripheral) NOS Q27.9
  acquired I77.89
  coronary (acquired) I25.9
   congenital Q24.5
  umbilical Q27.0
 atrial septal Q21.1
 auditory canal (external) (congenital) — *see also* Malformation, ear, external
  acquired — *see* Disorder, ear, external, specified type NEC
 auricle
  ear (congenital) — *see also* Malformation, ear, external
  acquired — *see* Disorder, pinna, deformity
 back — *see* Dorsopathy, deforming
 bile duct (common) (congenital) (hepatic) Q44.5
  acquired K83.8
 biliary duct or passage (congenital) Q44.5
  acquired K83.8

Deformity — *continued*
- bladder (neck) (trigone) (sphincter) (acquired) N32.89
  - congenital Q64.79
- bone (acquired) NOS M95.9
  - congenital Q79.9
  - turbinate M95.0
- brain (congenital) Q04.9
  - acquired G93.89
  - reduction Q04.3
- breast (acquired) N64.89
  - congenital Q83.9
  - reconstructed N65.0
- bronchus (congenital) Q32.4
  - acquired NEC J98.09
- bursa, congenital Q79.9
- canaliculi (lacrimalis) (acquired) — *see also* Disorder, lacrimal system, changes
  - congenital Q10.6
- canthus, acquired — *see* Disorder, eyelid, specified type NEC
- capillary (acquired) I78.8
- cardiovascular system, congenital Q28.9
- caruncle, lacrimal (acquired) — *see also* Disorder, lacrimal system, changes
  - congenital Q10.6
- cascade, stomach K31.2
- cecum (congenital) Q43.9
  - acquired K63.89
- cerebral, acquired G93.89
  - congenital Q04.9
- cervix (uterus) (acquired) NEC N88.8
  - congenital Q51.9
- cheek (acquired) M95.2
  - congenital Q18.9
- chest (acquired) (wall) M95.4
  - congenital Q67.8
  - sequelae (late effect) of rickets E64.3
- chin (acquired) M95.2
  - congenital Q18.9
- choroid (congenital) Q14.3
  - acquired H31.8
  - plexus Q07.8
    - acquired G96.19
- cicatricial — *see* Cicatrix
- cilia, acquired — *see* Disorder, eyelid, specified type NEC
- clavicle (acquired) M95.8
  - congenital Q68.8
- clitoris (congenital) Q52.6
  - acquired N90.89
- clubfoot — *see* Clubfoot
- coccyx (acquired) — *see* subcategory M43.8 ☑
- colon (congenital) Q43.9
  - acquired K63.89
- concha (ear), congenital — *see also* Malformation, ear, external
  - acquired — *see* Disorder, pinna, deformity
- cornea (acquired) H18.70
  - congenital Q13.4
  - descemetocele — *see* Descemetocele
  - ectasia — *see* Ectasia, cornea
  - specified NEC H18.79- ☑
  - staphyloma — *see* Staphyloma, cornea
- coronary artery (acquired) I25.9
  - congenital Q24.5
- cranium (acquired) — *see* Deformity, skull
- cricoid cartilage (congenital) Q31.8
  - acquired J38.7
- cystic duct (congenital) Q44.5
  - acquired K82.8
- Dandy-Walker Q03.1
  - with spina bifida — *see* Spina bifida
- diaphragm (congenital) Q79.1
  - acquired J98.6
- digestive organ NOS Q45.9
- ductus arteriosus Q25.0
- duodenal bulb K31.89
- duodenum (congenital) Q43.9
  - acquired K31.89
- dura — *see* Deformity, meninges
- ear (acquired) — *see also* Disorder, pinna, deformity
  - congenital (external) Q17.9
    - internal Q16.5
    - middle Q16.4
      - ossicles Q16.3
    - ossicles Q16.3
- ectodermal (congenital) NEC Q84.9
- ejaculatory duct (congenital) Q55.4

Deformity — *continued*
- ejaculatory duct — *continued*
  - acquired N50.0
- elbow (joint) (acquired) — *see also* Deformity, limb, upper arm
  - congenital Q68.8
  - contraction — *see* Contraction, joint, elbow
- endocrine gland NEC Q89.2
- epididymis (congenital) Q55.4
  - acquired N50.89
- epiglottis (congenital) Q31.8
  - acquired J38.7
- esophagus (congenital) Q39.9
  - acquired K22.8
- eustachian tube (congenital) NEC Q17.8
- eye, congenital Q15.9
- eyebrow (congenital) Q18.8
- eyelid (acquired) — *see also* Disorder, eyelid, specified type NEC
  - congenital Q10.3
- face (acquired) M95.2
  - congenital Q18.9
- fallopian tube, acquired N83.8
- femur (acquired) — *see* Deformity, limb, specified type NEC, thigh
- fetal
  - with fetopelvic disproportion O33.7 ☑
  - causing obstructed labor O66.3
- finger (acquired) M20.00- ☑
  - boutonniere M20.02- ☑
  - congenital Q68.1
  - flexion contracture — *see* Contraction, joint, hand
  - mallet finger M20.01- ☑
  - specified NEC M20.09- ☑
  - swan-neck M20.03- ☑
- flexion (joint) (acquired) — *see also* Deformity, limb, flexion M21.20
  - congenital NOS Q74.9
    - hip Q65.89
- foot (acquired) — *see also* Deformity, limb, lower leg
  - cavovarus (congenital) Q66.1- ☑
  - congenital NOS Q66.9- ☑
    - specified type NEC Q66.89
  - specified type NEC — *see* Deformity, limb, foot, specified NEC
  - valgus (congenital) Q66.6
    - acquired — *see* Deformity, valgus, ankle
  - varus (congenital) NEC Q66.3- ☑
    - acquired — *see* Deformity, varus, ankle
- forearm (acquired) — *see also* Deformity, limb, forearm
  - congenital Q68.8
- forehead (acquired) M95.2
  - congenital Q75.8
- frontal bone (acquired) M95.2
  - congenital Q75.8
- gallbladder (congenital) Q44.1
  - acquired K82.8
- gastrointestinal tract (congenital) NOS Q45.9
  - acquired K63.89
- genitalia, genital organ(s) or system NEC
  - female (congenital) Q52.9
    - acquired N94.89
    - external Q52.70
  - male (congenital) Q55.9
    - acquired N50.89
- globe (eye) (congenital) Q15.8
  - acquired H44.89
- gum, acquired NEC K06.8
- hand (acquired) — *see* Deformity, limb, hand
  - congenital Q68.1
- head (acquired) M95.2
  - congenital Q75.8
- heart (congenital) Q24.9
  - septum Q21.9
    - auricular Q21.1
    - ventricular Q21.0
  - valve (congenital) NEC Q24.8
    - acquired — *see* Endocarditis
- heel (acquired) — *see* Deformity, foot
- hepatic duct (congenital) Q44.5
  - acquired K83.8
- hip (joint) (acquired) (*see also* Deformity, limb, thigh)
  - congenital Q65.9
  - due to (previous) juvenile osteochondrosis — *see* Coxa, plana
  - flexion — *see* Contraction, joint, hip
- hourglass — *see* Contraction, hourglass
- humerus (acquired) M21.82- ☑

Deformity — *continued*
- humerus — *continued*
  - congenital Q74.0
- hypophyseal (congenital) Q89.2
- ileocecal (coil) (valve) (acquired) K63.89
  - congenital Q43.9
- ileum (congenital) Q43.9
  - acquired K63.89
- ilium (acquired) M95.5
  - congenital Q74.2
- integument (congenital) Q84.9
- intervertebral cartilage or disc (acquired) — *see* Disorder, disc, specified NEC
- intestine (large) (small) (congenital) NOS Q43.9
  - acquired K63.89
- intrinsic minus or plus (hand) — *see* Deformity, limb, specified type NEC, forearm
- iris (acquired) H21.89
  - congenital Q13.2
- ischium (acquired) M95.5
  - congenital Q74.2
- jaw (acquired) (congenital) M26.9
- joint (acquired) NEC M21.90
  - congenital Q68.8
  - elbow M21.92- ☑
  - hand M21.94- ☑
  - hip M21.95- ☑
  - knee M21.96- ☑
  - shoulder M21.92- ☑
  - wrist M21.93- ☑
- kidney(s) (calyx) (pelvis) (congenital) Q63.9
  - acquired N28.89
  - artery (congenital) Q27.2
    - acquired I77.89
- Klippel-Feil (brevicollis) Q76.1
- knee (acquired) NEC — *see also* Deformity, limb, lower leg
  - congenital Q68.2
- labium (majus) (minus) (congenital) Q52.79
  - acquired N90.89
- lacrimal passages or duct (congenital) NEC Q10.6
  - acquired — *see* Disorder, lacrimal system, changes
- larynx (muscle) (congenital) Q31.8
  - acquired J38.7
  - web (glottic) Q31.0
- leg (upper) (acquired) NEC — *see also* Deformity, limb, thigh
  - congenital Q68.8
  - lower leg — *see* Deformity, limb, lower leg
- lens (acquired) H27.8
  - congenital Q12.9
- lid (fold) (acquired) — *see also* Disorder, eyelid, specified type NEC
  - congenital Q10.3
- ligament (acquired) — *see* Disorder, ligament
  - congenital Q79.9
- limb (acquired) M21.90
  - clawfoot M21.53- ☑
  - clawhand M21.51- ☑
  - clubfoot M21.54- ☑
  - clubhand M21.52- ☑
  - congenital, except reduction deformity Q74.9
  - flat foot M21.4- ☑
  - flexion M21.20
    - ankle M21.27- ☑
    - elbow M21.22- ☑
    - finger M21.24- ☑
    - hip M21.25- ☑
    - knee M21.26- ☑
    - shoulder M21.21- ☑
    - toe M21.27- ☑
    - wrist M21.23- ☑
  - foot
    - claw — *see* Deformity, limb, clawfoot
    - club — *see* Deformity, limb, clubfoot
    - drop M21.37- ☑
    - flat — *see* Deformity, limb, flat foot
    - specified NEC M21.6X- ☑
  - forearm M21.93- ☑
  - hand M21.94- ☑
  - lower leg M21.96- ☑
  - specified type NEC M21.80
    - forearm M21.83- ☑
    - lower leg M21.86- ☑
    - thigh M21.85- ☑
    - upper arm M21.82- ☑
  - thigh M21.95- ☑

Deformity — *continued*
- limb — *continued*
  - unequal length M21.70
    - short site is
      - femur M21.75- ☑
      - fibula M21.76- ☑
      - humerus M21.72- ☑
      - radius M21.73- ☑
      - tibia M21.76- ☑
      - ulna M21.73- ☑
    - upper arm M21.92- ☑
  - valgus — *see* Deformity, valgus
  - varus — *see* Deformity, varus
  - wrist drop M21.33- ☑
- lip (acquired) NEC K13.0
  - congenital Q38.0
- liver (congenital) Q44.7
  - acquired K76.89
- lumbosacral (congenital) (joint) (region) Q76.49
  - acquired — *see* subcategory M43.8 ☑
  - kyphosis — *see* Kyphosis, congenital
  - lordosis — *see* Lordosis, congenital
- lung (congenital) Q33.9
  - acquired J98.4
- lymphatic system, congenital Q89.9
- Madelung's (radius) Q74.0
- mandible (acquired) (congenital) M26.9
- maxilla (acquired) (congenital) M26.9
- meninges or membrane (congenital) Q07.9
  - cerebral Q04.8
    - acquired G96.19
  - spinal cord (congenital) G96.19
    - acquired G96.19
- metacarpus (acquired) — *see* Deformity, limb, forearm
  - congenital Q74.0
- metatarsus (acquired) — *see* Deformity, foot
  - congenital Q66.9- ☑
- middle ear (congenital) Q16.4
  - ossicles Q16.3
- mitral (leaflets) (valve) I05.8
  - parachute Q23.2
  - stenosis, congenital Q23.2
- mouth (acquired) K13.79
  - congenital Q38.6
- multiple, congenital NEC Q89.7
- muscle (acquired) M62.89
  - congenital Q79.9
    - sternocleidomastoid Q68.0
- musculoskeletal system (acquired) M95.9
  - congenital Q79.9
  - specified NEC M95.8
- nail (acquired) L60.8
  - congenital Q84.6
- nasal — *see* Deformity, nose
- neck (acquired) M95.3
  - congenital Q18.9
    - sternocleidomastoid Q68.0
- nervous system (congenital) Q07.9
- nipple (congenital) Q83.9
  - acquired N64.89
- nose (acquired) (cartilage) M95.0
  - bone (turbinate) M95.0
  - congenital Q30.9
    - bent or squashed Q67.4
  - saddle M95.0
    - syphilitic A50.57
  - septum (acquired) J34.2
    - congenital Q30.8
  - sinus (wall) (congenital) Q30.8
    - acquired M95.0
  - syphilitic (congenital) A50.57
    - late A52.73
- ocular muscle (congenital) Q10.3
  - acquired — *see* Strabismus, mechanical
- opticociliary vessels (congenital) Q13.2
- orbit (eye) (acquired) H05.30
  - atrophy — *see* Atrophy, orbit
  - congenital Q10.7
  - due to
    - bone disease NEC H05.32- ☑
    - trauma or surgery H05.33- ☑
  - enlargement — *see* Enlargement, orbit
  - exostosis — *see* Exostosis, orbit
- organ of Corti (congenital) Q16.5
- ovary (congenital) Q50.39
  - acquired N83.8
- oviduct, acquired N83.8
- palate (congenital) Q38.5

Deformity — *continued*
- palate — *continued*
  - acquired M27.8
  - cleft (congenital) — *see* Cleft, palate
- pancreas (congenital) Q45.3
  - acquired K86.89
- parathyroid (gland) Q89.2
- parotid (gland) (congenital) Q38.4
  - acquired K11.8
- patella (acquired) — *see* Disorder, patella, specified NEC
- pelvis, pelvic (acquired) (bony) M95.5
  - with disproportion (fetopelvic) O33.0
    - causing obstructed labor O65.0
  - congenital Q74.2
  - rachitic sequelae (late effect) E64.3
- penis (glans) (congenital) Q55.69
  - acquired N48.89
- pericardium (congenital) Q24.8
  - acquired — *see* Pericarditis
- pharynx (congenital) Q38.8
  - acquired J39.2
- pinna, acquired — *see also* Disorder, pinna, deformity
  - congenital Q17.9
- pituitary (congenital) Q89.2
- posture — *see* Dorsopathy, deforming
- prepuce (congenital) Q55.69
  - acquired N47.8
- prostate (congenital) Q55.4
  - acquired N42.89
- pupil (congenital) Q13.2
  - acquired — *see* Abnormality, pupillary
- pylorus (congenital) Q40.3
  - acquired K31.89
- rachitic (acquired), old or healed E64.3
- radius (acquired) — *see also* Deformity, limb, forearm
  - congenital Q68.8
- rectum (congenital) Q43.9
  - acquired K62.89
- reduction (extremity) (limb), congenital — *see also* condition and site Q73.8
  - brain Q04.3
  - lower — *see* Defect, reduction, lower limb
  - upper — *see* Defect, reduction, upper limb
- renal — *see* Deformity, kidney
- respiratory system (congenital) Q34.9
- rib (acquired) M95.4
  - congenital Q76.6
  - cervical Q76.5
- rotation (joint) (acquired) — *see* Deformity, limb, specified site NEC
  - congenital Q74.9
  - hip — *see* Deformity, limb, specified type NEC, thigh
    - congenital Q65.89
- sacroiliac joint (congenital) — *see* subcategory Q74.2
  - acquired — *see* subcategory M43.8 ☑
- sacrum (acquired) — *see* subcategory M43.8 ☑
- saddle
  - back — *see* Lordosis
  - nose M95.0
    - syphilitic A50.57
- salivary gland or duct (congenital) Q38.4
  - acquired K11.8
- scapula (acquired) M95.8
  - congenital Q68.8
- scrotum (congenital) — *see also* Malformation, testis and scrotum
  - acquired N50.89
- seminal vesicles (congenital) Q55.4
  - acquired N50.89
- septum, nasal (acquired) J34.2
- shoulder (joint) (acquired) — *see* Deformity, limb, upper arm
  - congenital Q74.0
  - contraction — *see* Contraction, joint, shoulder
- sigmoid (flexure) (congenital) Q43.9
  - acquired K63.89
- skin (congenital) Q82.9
- skull (acquired) M95.2
  - congenital Q75.8
    - with
      - anencephaly Q00.0
      - encephalocele — *see* Encephalocele
      - hydrocephalus Q03.9
        - with spina bifida — *see* Spina bifida, by site, with hydrocephalus
      - microcephaly Q02

Deformity — *continued*
- soft parts, organs or tissues (of pelvis)
  - in pregnancy or childbirth NEC O34.8- ☑
    - causing obstructed labor O65.5
- spermatic cord (congenital) Q55.4
  - acquired N50.89
  - torsion — *see* Torsion, spermatic cord
- spinal — *see* Dorsopathy, deforming
  - column (acquired) — *see* Dorsopathy, deforming
  - congenital Q67.5
  - cord (congenital) Q06.9
    - acquired G95.89
  - nerve root (congenital) Q07.9
- spine (acquired) — *see also* Dorsopathy, deforming
  - congenital Q67.5
  - rachitic E64.3
  - specified NEC — *see* Dorsopathy, deforming, specified NEC
- spleen
  - acquired D73.89
  - congenital Q89.09
- Sprengel's (congenital) Q74.0
- sternocleidomastoid (muscle), congenital Q68.0
- sternum (acquired) M95.4
  - congenital NEC Q76.7
- stomach (congenital) Q40.3
  - acquired K31.89
- submandibular gland (congenital) Q38.4
- submaxillary gland (congenital) Q38.4
  - acquired K11.8
- talipes — *see* Talipes
- testis (congenital) — *see also* Malformation, testis and scrotum
  - acquired N44.8
  - torsion — *see* Torsion, testis
- thigh (acquired) — *see also* Deformity, limb, thigh
  - congenital NEC Q68.8
- thorax (acquired) (wall) M95.4
  - congenital Q67.8
  - sequelae of rickets E64.3
- thumb (acquired) — *see also* Deformity, finger
  - congenital NEC Q68.1
- thymus (tissue) (congenital) Q89.2
- thyroid (gland) (congenital) Q89.2
  - cartilage Q31.8
    - acquired J38.7
- tibia (acquired) — *see also* Deformity, limb, specified type NEC, lower leg
  - congenital NEC Q68.8
  - saber (syphilitic) A50.56
- toe (acquired) M20.6- ☑
  - congenital Q66.9- ☑
  - hallux rigidus M20.2- ☑
  - hallux valgus M20.1- ☑
  - hallux varus M20.3- ☑
  - hammer toe M20.4- ☑
  - specified NEC M20.5X- ☑
- tongue (congenital) Q38.3
  - acquired K14.8
- tooth, teeth K00.2
- trachea (rings) (congenital) Q32.1
  - acquired J39.8
- transverse aortic arch (congenital) Q25.49
- tricuspid (leaflets) (valve) I07.8
  - atresia or stenosis Q22.4
  - Ebstein's Q22.5
- trunk (acquired) M95.8
  - congenital Q89.9
- ulna (acquired) — *see also* Deformity, limb, forearm
  - congenital NEC Q68.8
- urachus, congenital Q64.4
- ureter (opening) (congenital) Q62.8
  - acquired N28.89
- urethra (congenital) Q64.79
  - acquired N36.8
- urinary tract (congenital) Q64.9
  - urachus Q64.4
- uterus (congenital) Q51.9
  - acquired N85.8
- uvula (congenital) Q38.5
- vagina (acquired) N89.8
  - congenital Q52.4
- valgus NEC M21.00
  - ankle M21.07- ☑
  - elbow M21.02- ☑
  - hip M21.05- ☑
  - knee M21.06- ☑
- valve, valvular (congenital) (heart) Q24.8

Deformity — continued
valve, valvular — continued
acquired — see Endocarditis
varus NEC M21.10
ankle M21.17- ☑
elbow M21.12- ☑
hip M21.15 ☑
knee M21.16- ☑
tibia — see Osteochondrosis, juvenile, tibia
vas deferens (congenital) Q55.4
acquired N50.89
vein (congenital) Q27.9
great Q26.9
vertebra — see Dorsopathy, deforming
vertical talus (congenital) Q66.80
left foot Q66.82
right foot Q66.81
vesicourethral orifice (acquired) N32.89
congenital NEC Q64.79
vessels of optic papilla (congenital) Q14.2
visual field (contraction) — see Defect, visual field
vitreous body, acquired H43.89
vulva (congenital) Q52.79
acquired N90.89
wrist (joint) (acquired) — see also Deformity, limb, forearm
congenital Q68.8
contraction — see Contraction, joint, wrist

Degeneration, degenerative
adrenal (capsule) (fatty) (gland) (hyaline) (infectional) E27.8
amyloid — see also Amyloidosis E85.9
anterior cornua, spinal cord G12.29
anterior labral S43.49- ☑
aorta, aortic I70.0
fatty I77.89
aortic valve (heart) — see Endocarditis, aortic
arteriovascular — see Arteriosclerosis
artery, arterial (atheromatous) (calcareous) — see also Arteriosclerosis
cerebral, amyloid E85.4 [I68.0]
medial — see Arteriosclerosis, extremities
articular cartilage NEC — see Derangement, joint, articular cartilage, by site
atheromatous — see Arteriosclerosis
basal nuclei or ganglia G23.9
specified NEC G23.8
bone NEC — see Disorder, bone, specified type NEC
brachial plexus G54.0
brain (cortical) (progressive) G31.9
alcoholic G31.2
arteriosclerotic I67.2
childhood G31.9
specified NEC G31.89
cystic G31.89
congenital Q04.6
in
alcoholism G31.2
beriberi E51.2
cerebrovascular disease I67.9
congenital hydrocephalus Q03.9
with spina bifida — see also Spina bifida
Fabry-Anderson disease E75.21
Gaucher's disease E75.22
Hunter's syndrome E76.1
lipidosis
cerebral E75.4
generalized E75.6
mucopolysaccharidosis — see Mucopolysaccharidosis
myxedema E03.9 [G32.89]
neoplastic disease — see also Neoplasm D49.6 [G32.89]
Niemann-Pick disease E75.249 [G32.89]
sphingolipidosis E75.3 [G32.89]
vitamin B12 deficiency E53.8 [G32.89]
senile NEC G31.1
breast N64.89
Bruch's membrane — see Degeneration, choroid
capillaries (fatty) I78.8
amyloid E85.89 [I79.8]
cardiac — see also Degeneration, myocardial
valve, valvular — see Endocarditis
cardiorenal — see Hypertension, cardiorenal
cardiovascular — see also Disease, cardiovascular
renal — see Hypertension, cardiorenal
cerebellar NOS G31.9
alcoholic G31.2

Degeneration, degenerative — continued
cerebellar — continued
primary (hereditary) (sporadic) G11.9
cerebral — see Degeneration, brain
cerebrovascular I67.9
due to hypertension I67.4
cervical plexus G54.2
cervix N88.8
due to radiation (intended effect) N88.8
adverse effect or misadventure N99.89
chamber angle H21.21- ☑
changes, spine or vertebra — see Spondylosis
chorioretinal — see also Degeneration, choroid
hereditary H31.20
choroid (colloid) (drusen) H31.10- ☑
atrophy — see Atrophy, choroidal
hereditary — see Dystrophy, choroidal, hereditary
ciliary body H21.22- ☑
cochlear — see subcategory H83.8 ☑
combined (spinal cord) (subacute) E53.8 [G32.0]
with anemia (pernicious) D51.0 [G32.0]
due to dietary vitamin B12 deficiency D51.3 [G32.0]
in (due to)
vitamin B12 deficiency E53.8 [G32.0]
anemia D51.9 [G32.0]
conjunctiva H11.10
concretions — see Concretion, conjunctiva
deposits — see Deposit, conjunctiva
pigmentations — see Pigmentation, conjunctiva
pinguecula — see Pinguecula
xerosis — see Xerosis, conjunctiva
cornea H18.40
calcerous H18.43
band keratopathy H18.42- ☑
familial, hereditary — see Dystrophy, cornea
hyaline (of old scars) H18.49
keratomalacia — see Keratomalacia
nodular H18.45- ☑
peripheral H18.46- ☑
senile H18.41- ☑
specified type NEC H18.49
cortical (cerebellar) (parenchymatous) G31.89
alcoholic G31.2
diffuse, due to arteriopathy I67.2
corticobasal G31.85
cutis L98.8
amyloid E85.4 [L99]
dental pulp K04.2
disc disease — see Degeneration, intervertebral disc NEC
dorsolateral (spinal cord) — see Degeneration, combined
extrapyramidal G25.9
eye, macular — see also Degeneration, macula
congenital or hereditary — see Dystrophy, retina
facet joints — see Spondylosis
fatty
liver NEC K76.0
alcoholic K70.0
grey matter (brain) (Alpers') G31.81
heart — see also Degeneration, myocardial
amyloid E85.4 [I43]
atheromatous — see Disease, heart, ischemic, atherosclerotic
ischemic — see Disease, heart, ischemic
hepatolenticular (Wilson's) E83.01
hepatorenal K76.7
hyaline (diffuse) (generalized)
localized — see Degeneration, by site
infrapatellar fat pad M79.4
intervertebral disc NOS
with
myelopathy — see Disorder, disc, with, myelopathy
radiculitis or radiculopathy — see Disorder, disc, with, radiculopathy
cervical, cervicothoracic — see Disorder, disc, cervical, degeneration
with
myelopathy — see Disorder, disc, cervical, with myelopathy
neuritis, radiculitis or radiculopathy — see Disorder, disc, cervical, with neuritis
lumbar region M51.36
with
myelopathy M51.06

Degeneration, degenerative — continued
intervertebral disc — continued
lumbar region — continued
with — continued
neuritis, radiculitis, radiculopathy or sciatica M51.16
lumbosacral region M51.37
with
neuritis, radiculitis, radiculopathy or sciatica M51.17
sacrococcygeal region M53.3
thoracic region M51.34
with
myelopathy M51.04
neuritis, radiculitis, radiculopathy M51.14
thoracolumbar region M51.35
with
myelopathy M51.05
neuritis, radiculitis, radiculopathy M51.15
intestine, amyloid E85.4
iris (pigmentary) H21.23- ☑
ischemic — see Ischemia
joint disease — see Osteoarthritis
kidney N28.89
amyloid E85.4 [N29]
cystic, congenital Q61.9
fatty N28.89
polycystic Q61.3
adult type (autosomal dominant) Q61.2
infantile type (autosomal recessive) NEC Q61.19
collecting duct dilatation Q61.11
Kuhnt-Junius — see also Degeneration, macula H35.32- ☑
lens — see Cataract
lenticular (familial) (progressive) (Wilson's) (with cirrhosis of liver) E83.01
liver (diffuse) NEC K76.89
amyloid E85.4 [K77]
cystic K76.89
congenital Q44.6
fatty NEC K76.0
alcoholic K70.0
hypertrophic K76.89
parenchymatous, acute or subacute K72.00
with coma K72.01
pigmentary K76.89
toxic (acute) K71.9
lung J98.4
lymph gland I89.8
hyaline I89.8
macula, macular (acquired) (age-related) (senile) H35.30
angioid streaks H35.33
atrophic age-related H35.31- ☑
congenital or hereditary — see Dystrophy, retina
cystoid H35.35- ☑
drusen H35.36- ☑
dry age-related H35.31- ☑
exudative H35.32- ☑
hole H35.34- ☑
nonexudative H35.31- ☑
puckering H35.37- ☑
toxic H35.38- ☑
wet age-related H35.32- ☑
membranous labyrinth, congenital (causing impairment of hearing) Q16.5
meniscus — see Derangement, meniscus
mitral — see Insufficiency, mitral
Mönckeberg's — see Arteriosclerosis, extremities
motor centers, senile G31.1
multi-system G90.3
mural — see Degeneration, myocardial
muscle (fatty) (fibrous) (hyaline) (progressive) M62.89
heart — see Degeneration, myocardial
myelin, central nervous system G37.9
myocardial, myocardium (fatty) (hyaline) (senile) I51.5
with rheumatic fever (conditions in I00) I09.0
active, acute or subacute I01.2
with chorea I02.0
inactive or quiescent (with chorea) I09.0
hypertensive — see Hypertension, heart
rheumatic — see Degeneration, myocardial, with rheumatic fever
syphilitic A52.06
nasal sinus (mucosa) J32.9
frontal J32.1
maxillary J32.0
nerve — see Disorder, nerve

Degeneration, degenerative — *continued*
  nervous system G31.9
    alcoholic G31.2
    amyloid E85.4 *[G99.8]*
    autonomic G90.9
    fatty G31.89
    specified NEC G31.89
  nipple N64.89
  olivopontocerebellar (hereditary) (familial) G23.8
  osseous labyrinth — *see* subcategory H83.8 ☑
  ovary N83.8
    cystic N83.20- ☑
    microcystic N83.20- ☑
  pallidal pigmentary (progressive) G23.0
  pancreas K86.89
    tuberculous A18.83
  penis N48.89
  pigmentary (diffuse) (general)
    localized — *see* Degeneration, by site
    pallidal (progressive) G23.0
  pineal gland E34.8
  pituitary (gland) E23.6
  popliteal fat pad M79.4
  posterolateral (spinal cord) — *see* Degeneration, combined
  pulmonary valve (heart) I37.8
  pulp (tooth) K04.2
  pupillary margin H21.24- ☑
  renal — *see* Degeneration, kidney
  retina H35.9
    hereditary (cerebroretinal) (congenital) (juvenile) (macula) (peripheral) (pigmentary) — *see* Dystrophy, retina
    Kuhnt-Junius — *see also* Degeneration, macula H35.32- ☑
    macula (cystic) (exudative) (hole) (nonexudative) (pseudohole) (senile) (toxic) — *see* Degeneration, macula
    peripheral H35.40
      lattice H35.41- ☑
      microcystoid H35.42- ☑
      paving stone H35.43- ☑
      secondary
        pigmentary H35.45- ☑
        vitreoretinal H35.46- ☑
      senile reticular H35.44- ☑
    pigmentary (primary) — *see also* Dystrophy, retina
      secondary — *see* Degeneration, retina, peripheral, secondary
    posterior pole — *see* Degeneration, macula
  saccule, congenital (causing impairment of hearing) Q16.5
  senile R54
    brain G31.1
    cardiac, heart or myocardium — *see* Degeneration, myocardial
    motor centers G31.1
    vascular — *see* Arteriosclerosis
  sinus (cystic) — *see also* Sinusitis
    polypoid J33.1
  skin L98.8
    amyloid E85.4 *[L99]*
    colloid L98.8
  spinal (cord) G31.89
    amyloid E85.4 *[G32.89]*
    combined (subacute) — *see* Degeneration, combined
    dorsolateral — *see* Degeneration, combined
    familial NEC G31.89
    fatty G31.89
    funicular — *see* Degeneration, combined
    posterolateral — *see* Degeneration, combined
    subacute combined — *see* Degeneration, combined
    tuberculous A17.81
  spleen D73.0
    amyloid E85.4 *[D77]*
  stomach K31.89
  striatonigral G23.2
  suprarenal (capsule) (gland) E27.8
  synovial membrane (pulpy) — *see* Disorder, synovium, specified type NEC
  tapetoretinal — *see* Dystrophy, retina
  thymus (gland) E32.8
    fatty E32.8
  thyroid (gland) E07.89
  tricuspid (heart) (valve) I07.9
  tuberculous NEC — *see* Tuberculosis
  turbinate J34.89

Degeneration, degenerative — *continued*
  uterus (cystic) N85.8
  vascular (senile) — *see* Arteriosclerosis
    hypertensive — *see* Hypertension
  vitreoretinal, secondary — *see* Degeneration, retina, peripheral, secondary, vitreoretinal
  vitreous (body) H43.81- ☑
  Wallerian — *see* Disorder, nerve
  Wilson's hepatolenticular E83.01
Deglutition
  paralysis R13.0
    hysterical F44.4
  pneumonia J69.0
Degos' disease I77.89
Dehiscence (of)
  amputation stump T87.81
  cesarean wound O90.0
  closure of
    cornea T81.31 ☑
    craniotomy T81.32 ☑
    fascia (muscular) (superficial) T81.32 ☑
    internal organ or tissue T81.32 ☑
    laceration (external) (internal) T81.33 ☑
    ligament T81.32 ☑
    mucosa T81.31 ☑
    muscle or muscle flap T81.32 ☑
    ribs or rib cage T81.32 ☑
    skin and subcutaneous tissue (full-thickness) (superficial) T81.31 ☑
    skull T81.32 ☑
    sternum (sternotomy) T81.32 ☑
    tendon T81.32 ☑
    traumatic laceration (external) (internal) T81.33 ☑
  episiotomy O90.1
  operation wound NEC T81.31 ☑
    external operation wound (superficial) T81.31 ☑
    internal operation wound (deep) T81.32 ☑
  perineal wound (postpartum) O90.1
  traumatic injury wound repair T81.33 ☑
  wound T81.30 ☑
    traumatic repair T81.33 ☑
Dehydration E86.0
  newborn P74.1
Déjérine-Roussy syndrome G89.0
Déjérine-Sottas disease or neuropathy (hypertrophic) G60.0
Déjérine-Thomas atrophy G23.8
Delay, delayed
  any plane in pelvis
    complicating delivery O66.9
  birth or delivery NOS O63.9
  closure, ductus arteriosus (Botalli) P29.38
  coagulation — *see* Defect, coagulation
  conduction (cardiac) (ventricular) I45.9
  delivery, second twin, triplet, etc O63.2
  development R62.50
    global F88
    intellectual (specific) F81.9
    language F80.9
      due to hearing loss F80.4
    learning F81.9
    pervasive F84.9
    physiological R62.50
      specified stage NEC R62.0
    reading F81.0
    sexual E30.0
    speech F80.9
      due to hearing loss F80.4
    spelling F81.81
  ejaculation F52.32
  gastric emptying K30
  menarche E30.0
  menstruation (cause unknown) N91.0
  milestone R62.0
  passage of meconium (newborn) P76.0
  primary respiration P28.9
  puberty (constitutional) E30.0
  separation of umbilical cord P96.82
  sexual maturation, female E30.0
  sleep phase syndrome G47.21
  union, fracture — *see* Fracture, by site
  vaccination Z28.9
Deletion(s)
  autosome Q93.9
    identified by fluorescence in situ hybridization (FISH) Q93.89
    identified by in situ hybridization (ISH) Q93.89

Deletion(s) — *continued*
  chromosome
    with complex rearrangements NEC Q93.7
    part of NEC Q93.59
    seen only at prometaphase Q93.89
    short arm
      22q11.2 Q93.81
      4 Q93.3
      5p Q93.4
    specified NEC Q93.89
    long arm chromosome 18 or 21 Q93.89
      with complex rearrangements NEC Q93.7
  microdeletions NEC Q93.88
Delhi boil or button B55.1
Delinquency (juvenile) (neurotic) F91.8
  group Z72.810
Delinquent immunization status Z28.3
Delirium, delirious (acute or subacute) (not alcohol- or drug-induced) (with dementia) R41.0
  alcoholic (acute) (tremens) (withdrawal) F10.921
    with intoxication F10.921
      in
        abuse F10.121
        dependence F10.221
  due to (secondary to)
    alcohol
      intoxication F10.921
        in
          abuse F10.121
          dependence F10.221
      withdrawal F10.231
    amphetamine intoxication F15.921
      in
        abuse F15.121
        dependence F15.221
    anxiolytic
      intoxication F13.921
        in
          abuse F13.121
          dependence F13.221
      withdrawal F13.231
    cannabis intoxication (acute) F12.921
      in
        abuse F12.121
        dependence F12.221
    cocaine intoxication (acute) F14.921
      in
        abuse F14.121
        dependence F14.221
    general medical condition F05
    hallucinogen intoxication F16.921
      in
        abuse F16.121
        dependence F16.221
    hypnotic
      intoxication F13.921
        in
          abuse F13.121
          dependence F13.221
      withdrawal F13.231
    inhalant intoxication (acute) F18.921
      in
        abuse F18.121
        dependence F18.221
    multiple etiologies F05
    opioid intoxication (acute) F11.921
      in
        abuse F11.121
        dependence F11.221
    other (or unknown) substance F19.921
    phencyclidine intoxication (acute) F16.921
      in
        abuse F16.121
        dependence F16.221
    psychoactive substance NEC intoxication (acute) F19.921
      in
        abuse F19.121
        dependence F19.221
    sedative
      intoxication F13.921
        in
          abuse F13.121
          dependence F13.221
      withdrawal F13.231
    unknown etiology R41.0
  exhaustion F43.0
  hysterical F44.89
  postprocedural (postoperative) F05

Delirium, delirious — *continued*
  puerperal F05
  thyroid — *see* Thyrotoxicosis with thyroid storm
  traumatic — *see* Injury, intracranial
  tremens (alcohol-induced) F10.231
    sedative-induced F13.231
Delivery (childbirth) (labor)
  arrested active phase O62.1
  cesarean (for)
    abnormal
      pelvis (bony) (deformity) (major) NEC with dispro-
        portion (fetopelvic) O33.0
        with obstructed labor O65.0
      presentation or position O32.9 ☑
    abruptio placentae — *see also* Abruptio placentae
      O45.9- ☑
    acromion presentation O32.2 ☑
    atony, uterus O62.2
    breech presentation O32.1 ☑
      incomplete O32.8 ☑
    brow presentation O32.3 ☑
    cephalopelvic disproportion O33.9
    cerclage O34.3- ☑
    chin presentation O32.3 ☑
    cicatrix of cervix O34.4- ☑
    contracted pelvis (general)
      inlet O33.2
      outlet O33.3 ☑
    cord presentation or prolapse O69.0 ☑
    cystocele O34.8- ☑
    deformity (acquired) (congenital)
      pelvic organs or tissues NEC O34.8- ☑
      pelvis (bony) NEC O33.0
    disproportion NOS O33.9
    eclampsia — *see* Eclampsia
    face presentation O32.3 ☑
    failed
      forceps O66.5
      induction of labor O61.9
        instrumental O61.1
        mechanical O61.1
        medical O61.0
        specified NEC O61.8
        surgical O61.1
      trial of labor NOS O66.40
        following previous cesarean delivery O66.41
      vacuum extraction O66.5
      ventouse O66.5
    fetal-maternal hemorrhage O43.01- ☑
    hemorrhage (intrapartum) O67.9
      with coagulation defect O67.0
      specified cause NEC O67.8
    high head at term O32.4 ☑
    hydrocephalic fetus O33.6 ☑
    incarceration of uterus O34.51- ☑
    incoordinate uterine action O62.4
    increased size, fetus O33.5 ☑
    inertia, uterus O62.2
      primary O62.0
      secondary O62.1
    lateroversion, uterus O34.59- ☑
    mal lie O32.9 ☑
    malposition
      fetus O32.9 ☑
      pelvic organs or tissues NEC O34.8- ☑
      uterus NEC O34.59- ☑
    malpresentation NOS O32.9 ☑
    oblique presentation O32.2 ☑
    occurring after 37 completed weeks of gestation
      but before 39 completed weeks gestation due
      to (spontaneous) onset of labor O75.82
    oversize fetus O33.5 ☑
    pelvic tumor NEC O34.8- ☑
    placenta previa O44.0- ☑
      complete O44.0- ☑
      with hemorrhage O44.1- ☑
    placental insufficiency O36.51- ☑
    planned, occurring after 37 completed weeks of
      gestation but before 39 completed weeks
      gestation due to (spontaneous) onset of labor
      O75.82
    polyp, cervix O34.4- ☑
      causing obstructed labor O65.5
    poor dilatation, cervix O62.0
    pre-eclampsia O14.94
      mild O14.04
      moderate O14.04

Delivery — *continued*
  cesarean — *continued*
    pre-eclampsia — *continued*
      severe O14.14
        with hemolysis, elevated liver enzymes and
          low platelet count (HELLP) O14.24
    previous
      cesarean delivery O34.219
        classical (vertical) scar O34.212
        low transverse scar O34.211
      surgery (to)
        cervix O34.4- ☑
        gynecological NEC O34.8- ☑
        rectum O34.7- ☑
        uterus O34.29
        vagina O34.6- ☑
    prolapse
      arm or hand O32.2 ☑
      uterus O34.52- ☑
    prolonged labor NOS O63.9
    rectocele O34.8- ☑
    retroversion
      uterus O34.53- ☑
    rigid
      cervix O34.4- ☑
      pelvic floor O34.8- ☑
      perineum O34.7- ☑
      vagina O34.6- ☑
      vulva O34.7- ☑
    sacculation, pregnant uterus O34.59- ☑
    scar(s)
      cervix O34.4- ☑
      cesarean delivery O34.219
        classical (vertical) O34.212
        low transverse O34.211
      transmural uterine O34.29
      uterus O34.29
    Shirodkar suture in situ O34.3- ☑
    shoulder presentation O32.2 ☑
    stenosis or stricture, cervix O34.4- ☑
    streptococcus group B (GBS) carrier state O99.824
    transmural uterine scar O34.29
    transverse presentation or lie O32.2 ☑
    tumor, pelvic organs or tissues NEC O34.8- ☑
      cervix O34.4- ☑
    umbilical cord presentation or prolapse O69.0 ☑
    without indication O82
  completely normal case O80
  complicated O75.9
    by
      abnormal, abnormality (of)
        forces of labor O62.9
          specified type NEC O62.8
        glucose O99.814
        uterine contractions NOS O62.9
      abruptio placentae — *see also* Abruptio placen-
        tae O45.9- ☑
      abuse
        physical O9A.32 (*following* O99)
        psychological O9A.52 (*following* O99)
        sexual O9A.42 (*following* O99)
      adherent placenta O72.0
        without hemorrhage O73.0
      alcohol use O99.314
      anemia (pre-existing) O99.02
      anesthetic death O74.8
      annular detachment of cervix O71.3
      atony, uterus O62.2
      attempted vacuum extraction and forceps O66.5
      Bandl's ring O62.4
      bariatric surgery status O99.844
      biliary tract disorder O26.62
      bleeding — *see* Delivery, complicated by, hem-
        orrhage
      blood disorder NEC O99.12
      cervical dystocia (hypotonic) O62.2
        primary O62.0
        secondary O62.1
      circulatory system disorder O99.42
      compression of cord (umbilical) NEC O69.2 ☑
      condition NEC O99.89
      contraction, contracted ring O62.4
      cord (umbilical)
        around neck
          with compression O69.1 ☑
          without compression O69.81 ☑
        bruising O69.5 ☑
        complication O69.9 ☑

Delivery — *continued*
  complicated — *continued*
    by — *continued*
      cord — *continued*
        complication — *continued*
          specified NEC O69.89 ☑
        compression NEC O69.2 ☑
        entanglement O69.2 ☑
          without compression O69.82 ☑
        hematoma O69.5 ☑
        presentation O69.0 ☑
        prolapse O69.0 ☑
        short O69.3 ☑
        thrombosis (vessels) O69.5 ☑
        vascular lesion O69.5 ☑
      Couvelaire uterus O45.8X- ☑
      damage to (injury to) NEC
        perineum O71.82
        periurethral tissue O71.82
        vulva O71.82
      delay following rupture of membranes (sponta-
        neous) — *see* Pregnancy, complicated by,
        premature rupture of membranes
      depressed fetal heart tones O76
      diabetes O24.92
        gestational O24.429
          diet controlled O24.420
          insulin controlled O24.424
          oral drug controlled (antidiabetic) (hypo-
            glycemic) O24.425
        pre-existing O24.32
          specified NEC O24.82
          type 1 O24.02
          type 2 O24.12
      diastasis recti (abdominis) O71.89
      dilatation
        bladder O66.8
        cervix incomplete, poor or slow O62.0
      disease NEC O99.89
      disruptio uteri — *see* Delivery, complicated by,
        rupture, uterus
      drug use O99.324
      dysfunction, uterus NOS O62.9
        hypertonic O62.4
        hypotonic O62.2
          primary O62.0
          secondary O62.1
        incoordinate O62.4
      eclampsia O15.1
      embolism (pulmonary) — *see* Embolism, obstet-
        ric
      endocrine, nutritional or metabolic disease NEC
        O99.284
      failed
        attempted vaginal birth after previous cesare-
          an delivery O66.41
        induction of labor O61.9
          instrumental O61.1
          mechanical O61.1
          medical O61.0
          specified NEC O61.8
          surgical O61.1
        trial of labor O66.40
      female genital mutilation O65.5
      fetal
        abnormal acid-base balance O68
        acidemia O68
        acidosis O68
        alkalosis O68
        death, early O02.1
        deformity O66.3
        heart rate or rhythm (abnormal) (non-reassur-
          ing) O76
        hypoxia O77.8
        stress O77.9
          due to drug administration O77.1
          electrocardiographic evidence of O77.8
          specified NEC O77.8
          ultrasound evidence of O77.8
      fever during labor O75.2
      gastric banding status O99.844
      gastric bypass status O99.844
      gastrointestinal disease NEC O99.62
      gestational
        diabetes O24.429
          diet controlled O24.420
          insulin (and diet) controlled O24.424

Delivery — continued
  complicated — continued
    by — continued
      gestational — continued
        diabetes — continued
          oral drug controlled (antidiabetic) (hypo-glycemic) O24.425
        edema O12.04
          with proteinuria O12.24
        proteinuria O12.14
      gonorrhea O98.22
      hematoma O71.7
        ischial spine O71.7
        pelvic O71.7
        vagina O71.7
        vulva or perineum O71.7
      hemorrhage (uterine) O67.9
        associated with
          afibrinogenemia O67.0
          coagulation defect O67.0
          hyperfibrinolysis O67.0
          hypofibrinogenemia O67.0
        due to
          low implantation of placenta O44.5- ☑
          low-lying placenta O44.5- ☑
          placenta previa O44.1- ☑
            marginal O44.3- ☑
            partial O44.3- ☑
          premature separation of placenta (normal-ly implanted) — see also Abruptio placentae O45.9- ☑
          retained placenta O72.0
          uterine leiomyoma O67.8
        placenta NEC O67.8
        postpartum NEC (atonic) (immediate) O72.1
          with retained or trapped placenta O72.0
          delayed O72.2
          secondary O72.2
          third stage O72.0
      hourglass contraction, uterus O62.4
      hypertension, hypertensive (pre-existing) — see Hypertension, complicated by, childbirth (labor)
      hypotension O26.5- ☑
      incomplete dilatation (cervix) O62.0
      incoordinate uterus contractions O62.4
      inertia, uterus O62.2
        during latent phase of labor O62.0
        primary O62.0
        secondary O62.1
      infection (maternal) O98.92
        carrier state NEC O99.834
        gonorrhea O98.22
        human immunodeficiency virus (HIV) O98.72
        sexually transmitted NEC O98.32
        specified NEC O98.82
        syphilis O98.12
        tuberculosis O98.02
        viral hepatitis O98.42
        viral NEC O98.52
      injury (to mother) — see also Delivery, complicat-ed, by, damage to O71.9
        nonobstetric O9A.22 (following O99)
          caused by abuse — see Delivery, compli-cated by, abuse
      intrauterine fetal death, early O02.1
      inversion, uterus O71.2
      laceration (perineal) O70.9
        anus (sphincter) O70.4
          with third degree laceration — see also Delivery, complicated, by, lacera-tion, perineum, third degree O70.20
            with mucosa O70.3
          without third degree laceration O70.2 ☑
        bladder (urinary) O71.5
        bowel O71.5
        cervix (uteri) O71.3
        fourchette O70.0
        hymen O70.0
        labia O70.0
        pelvic
          floor O70.1
          organ NEC O71.5
        perineum, perineal O70.9
          first degree O70.0
          fourth degree O70.3
          muscles O70.1

Delivery — continued
  complicated — continued
    by — continued
      laceration — continued
        perineum, perineal — continued
          second degree O70.1
          skin O70.0
          slight O70.0
          third degree O70.20
            with
              both external anal sphincter (EAS) and internal anal sphincter (IAS) torn (IIIc) O70.23
              less than 50% of external anal sphincter (EAS) thickness torn (IIIa) O70.21
              more than 50% external anal sphincter (EAS) thickness torn (IIIb) O70.22
            IIIa O70.21
            IIIb O70.22
            IIIc O70.23
        peritoneum (pelvic) O71.5
        rectovaginal (septum) (without perineal lacer-ation) O71.4
          with perineum — see also Delivery, complicated, by, laceration, per-ineum, third degree O70.20
            with anal or rectal mucosa O70.3
        specified NEC O71.89
        sphincter ani — see Delivery, complicated, by, laceration, anus (sphincter)
        urethra O71.5
        uterus O71.81
          before labor O71.81
        vagina, vaginal (deep) (high) (without per-ineal laceration) O71.4
          with perineum O70.0
          muscles, with perineum O70.1
        vulva O70.0
      liver disorder O26.62
      malignancy O9A.12 (following O99)
      malnutrition O25.2
      malposition, malpresentation
        uterus or cervix O65.5
        placenta O44.0- ☑
          with hemorrhage O44.1- ☑
        without obstruction — see also Delivery, complicated by, obstruction O32.9 ☑
          breech O32.1 ☑
          compound O32.6 ☑
          face (brow) (chin) O32.3 ☑
          footling O32.8 ☑
          high head O32.4 ☑
          oblique O32.2 ☑
          specified NEC O32.8 ☑
          transverse O32.2 ☑
          unstable lie O32.0 ☑
      meconium in amniotic fluid O77.0
      mental disorder NEC O99.344
      metrorrhexis — see Delivery, complicated by, rupture, uterus
      nervous system disorder O99.354
      obesity (pre-existing) O99.214
      obesity surgery status O99.844
      obstetric trauma O71.9
        specified NEC O71.89
      obstructed labor
        due to
          breech (complete) (frank) presentation O64.1 ☑
            incomplete O64.8 ☑
          brow presentation O64.3 ☑
          buttock presentation O64.1 ☑
          chin presentation O64.2 ☑
          compound presentation O64.5 ☑
          contracted pelvis O65.1
          deep transverse arrest O64.0 ☑
          deformed pelvis O65.0
          dystocia (fetal) O66.9
            due to
              conjoined twins O66.3
              fetal
                abnormality NEC O66.3
                ascites O66.3
                hydrops O66.3
                meningomyelocele O66.3
                sacral teratoma O66.3

Delivery — continued
  complicated — continued
    by — continued
      obstructed labor — continued
        due to — continued
          dystocia — continued
            due to — continued
              fetal — continued
                tumor O66.3
                hydrocephalic fetus O66.3
                shoulder O66.0
          face presentation O64.2 ☑
          fetopelvic disproportion O65.4
          footling presentation O64.8 ☑
          impacted shoulders O66.0
          incomplete rotation of fetal head O64.0 ☑
          large fetus O66.2
          locked twins O66.1
          malposition O64.9 ☑
            specified NEC O64.8 ☑
          malpresentation O64.9 ☑
            specified NEC O64.8 ☑
          multiple fetuses NEC O66.6
          pelvic
            abnormality (maternal) O65.9
              organ O65.5
              specified NEC O65.8
            contraction
              inlet O65.2
              mid-cavity O65.3
              outlet O65.3
          persistent (position)
            occipitoiliac O64.0 ☑
            occipitoposterior O64.0 ☑
            occipitosacral O64.0 ☑
            occipitotransverse O64.0 ☑
          prolapsed arm O64.4 ☑
          shoulder presentation O64.4 ☑
        specified NEC O66.8
      pathological retraction ring, uterus O62.4
      penetration, pregnant uterus by instrument O71.1
      perforation — see Delivery, complicated by, lac-eration
      placenta, placental
        ablatio — see also Abruptio placentae O45.9- ☑
        abnormality O43.9- ☑
          specified NEC O43.89- ☑
        abruptio — see also Abruptio placentae O45.9- ☑
        accreta O43.21- ☑
        adherent (with hemorrhage) O72.0
          without hemorrhage O73.0
        detachment (premature) — see also Abruptio placentae O45.9- ☑
        disorder O43.9- ☑
          specified NEC O43.89- ☑
        hemorrhage NEC O67.8
        increta O43.22- ☑
        low (implantation) (lying) O44.4- ☑
          with hemorrhage O44.5- ☑
        malformation O43.10- ☑
        malposition O44.0- ☑
          without hemorrhage O44.1- ☑
        percreta O43.23- ☑
        previa (central) (complete) (lateral) (total) O44.0- ☑
          with hemorrhage O44.1- ☑
          marginal O44.2- ☑
            with hemorrhage O44.3- ☑
          partial O44.2- ☑
            with hemorrhage O44.3- ☑
        retained (with hemorrhage) O72.0
          without hemorrhage O73.0
        separation (premature) O45.9- ☑
          specified NEC O45.8X- ☑
        vicious insertion O44.1- ☑
      precipitate labor O62.3
      premature rupture, membranes — see also Pregnancy, complicated by, premature rupture of membranes O42.90
      prolapse
        arm or hand O32.2 ☑
        cord (umbilical) O69.0 ☑
        foot or leg O32.8 ☑

Delivery — *continued*
  complicated — *continued*
    by — *continued*
      prolapse — *continued*
        uterus O34.52- ☑
      prolonged labor O63.9
        first stage O63.0
        second stage O63.1
      protozoal disease (maternal) O98.62
      respiratory disease NEC O99.52
      retained membranes or portions of placenta O72.2
        without hemorrhage O73.1
      retarded birth O63.9
      retention of secundines (with hemorrhage) O72.0
        without hemorrhage O73.0
        partial O72.2
          without hemorrhage O73.1
      rupture
        bladder (urinary) O71.5
        cervix O71.3
        pelvic organ NEC O71.5
        urethra O71.5
        uterus (during or after labor) O71.1
          before labor O71.0- ☑
      separation, pubic bone (symphysis pubis) O71.6
      shock O75.1
      shoulder presentation O64.4 ☑
      skin disorder NEC O99.72
      spasm, cervix O62.4
      stenosis or stricture, cervix O65.5
      streptococcus group B (GBS) carrier state O99.824
      subluxation of symphysis (pubis) O26.72
      syphilis (maternal) O98.12
      tear — *see* Delivery, complicated by, laceration
      tetanic uterus O62.4
      trauma (obstetrical) — *see also* Delivery, complicated, by, damage to O71.9
        non-obstetric O9A.22 (*following* O99)
        periurethral O71.82
        specified NEC O71.89
      tuberculosis (maternal) O98.02
      tumor, pelvic organs or tissues NEC O65.5
      umbilical cord around neck
        with compression O69.1 ☑
        without compression O69.81 ☑
      uterine inertia O62.2
        during latent phase of labor O62.0
        primary O62.0
        secondary O62.1
      vasa previa O69.4 ☑
      velamentous insertion of cord O43.12- ☑
    specified complication NEC O75.89
  delayed NOS O63.9
    following rupture of membranes
      artificial O75.5
    second twin, triplet, etc. O63.2
  forceps, low following failed vacuum extraction O66.5
  missed (at or near term) O36.4 ☑
  normal O80
  obstructed — *see* Delivery, complicated by, obstructed labor
  precipitate O62.3
  preterm — *see also* Pregnancy, complicated by, preterm labor O60.10 ☑
  spontaneous O80
  term pregnancy NOS O80
  uncomplicated O80
  vaginal, following previous cesarean delivery O34.219
    classical (vertical) scar O34.212
    low transverse scar O34.211
Delusions (paranoid) — *see* Disorder, delusional
Dementia (degenerative (primary)) (old age) (persisting) F03.90
  with
    aggressive behavior F03.91
    behavioral disturbance F03.91
    combative behavior F03.91
    Lewy bodies G31.83 *[F02.80]*
      with behavioral disturbance G31.83 *[F02.81]*
    Parkinsonism G31.83 *[F02.80]*
      with behavioral disturbance G31.83 *[F02.81]*
    Parkinson's disease G20 *[F02.80]*
      with behavioral disturbance G20 *[F02.81]*
    violent behavior F03.91
  alcoholic F10.97
    with dependence F10.27
  Alzheimer's type — *see* Disease, Alzheimer's

Dementia — *continued*
  arteriosclerotic — *see* Dementia, vascular
  atypical, Alzheimer's type — *see* Disease, Alzheimer's, specified NEC
  congenital — *see* Disability, intellectual
  frontal (lobe) G31.09 *[F02.80]*
    with behavioral disturbance G31.09 *[F02.81]*
  frontotemporal G31.09 *[F02.80]*
    with behavioral disturbance G31.09 *[F02.81]*
    specified NEC G31.09 *[F02.80]*
      with behavioral disturbance G31.09 *[F02.81]*
  Huntington's disease or chorea G10
    with dementia G10 *[F02.80]*
  in (due to)
    with behavioral disturbance G31.83 *[F02.81]*
    alcohol F10.97
      with dependence F10.27
    Alzheimer's disease — *see* Disease, Alzheimer's
    arteriosclerotic brain disease — *see* Dementia, vascular
    cerebral lipidoses E75.- *[F02.80]*
      with behavioral disturbance E75.- ☑ *[F02.81]*
    Creutzfeldt-Jakob disease — *see also* Creutzfeldt-Jakob disease or syndrome (with dementia) A81.00
    epilepsy G40.- ☑ *[F02.80]*
      with behavioral disturbance G40.- ☑ *[F02.81]*
    hepatolenticular degeneration E83.01 *[F02.80]*
      with behavioral disturbance E83.01 *[F02.81]*
    human immunodeficiency virus (HIV) disease B20 *[F02.80]*
      with behavioral disturbance B20 *[F02.81]*
    Huntington's disease or chorea G10 *[F02.80]*
      with behavioral disturbance G10 *[F02.81]*
    hypercalcemia E83.52 *[F02.80]*
      with behavioral disturbance E83.52 *[F02.81]*
    hypothyroidism, acquired E03.9 *[F02.80]*
      with behavioral disturbance E03.9 *[F02.81]*
      due to iodine deficiency E01.8 *[F02.80]*
        with behavioral disturbance E01.8 *[F02.81]*
    inhalants F18.97
      with dependence F18.27
    multiple
      etiologies F03 ☑
      sclerosis G35 *[F02.80]*
        with behavioral disturbance G35 *[F02.81]*
    neurosyphilis A52.17 *[F02.80]*
      with behavioral disturbance A52.17 *[F02.81]*
      juvenile A50.49 *[F02.80]*
        with behavioral disturbance A50.49 *[F02.81]*
    niacin deficiency E52 *[F02.80]*
      with behavioral disturbance E52 *[F02.81]*
    paralysis agitans G20 *[F02.80]*
      with behavioral disturbance G20 *[F02.81]*
    Parkinson's disease G20 *[F02.80]*
    pellagra E52 *[F02.80]*
      with behavioral disturbance E52 *[F02.81]*
    Pick's G31.01 *[F02.80]*
      with behavioral disturbance G31.01 *[F02.81]*
    polyarteritis nodosa M30.0 *[F02.80]*
      with behavioral disturbance M30.0 *[F02.81]*
    psychoactive drug F19.97
      with dependence F19.27
      inhalants F18.97
        with dependence F18.27
      sedatives, hypnotics or anxiolytics F13.97
        with dependence F13.27
    sedatives, hypnotics or anxiolytics F13.97
      with dependence F13.27
    systemic lupus erythematosus M32.- ☑ *[F02.80]*
      with behavioral disturbance M32.- ☑ *[F02.81]*
    trypanosomiasis
      African B56.9 *[F02.80]*
        with behavioral disturbance B56.9 *[F02.81]*
    unknown etiology F03 ☑
    vitamin B12 deficiency E53.8 *[F02.80]*
      with behavioral disturbance E53.8 *[F02.81]*
    volatile solvents F18.97
      with dependence F18.27
  infantile, infantilis F84.3
  Lewy body G31.83 *[F02.80]*
    with behavioral disturbance G31.83 *[F02.81]*
  multi-infarct — *see* Dementia, vascular
  paralytica, paralytic (syphilitic) A52.17 *[F02.80]*
    with behavioral disturbance A52.17 *[F02.81]*
    juvenilis A50.45
  paretic A52.17

Dementia — *continued*
  praecox — *see* Schizophrenia
  presenile F03 ☑
    Alzheimer's type — *see* Disease, Alzheimer's, early onset
  primary degenerative F03 ☑
  progressive, syphilitic A52.17
  senile F03 ☑
    with acute confusional state F05
    Alzheimer's type — *see* Disease, Alzheimer's, late onset
    depressed or paranoid type F03 ☑
  vascular (acute onset) (mixed) (multi-infarct) (subcortical) F01.50
    with behavioral disturbance F01.51
Demineralization, bone — *see* Osteoporosis
Demodex folliculorum (infestation) B88.0
Demophobia F40.248
Demoralization R45.3
Demyelination, demyelinization
  central nervous system G37.9
    specified NEC G37.8
  corpus callosum (central) G37.1
  disseminated, acute G36.9
    specified NEC G36.8
  global G35
  in optic neuritis G36.0
Dengue (classical) (fever) A90
  hemorrhagic A91
  sandfly A93.1
Dennie-Marfan syphilitic syndrome A50.45
Dens evaginatus, in dente or invaginatus K00.2
Dense breasts R92.2
Density
  increased, bone (disseminated) (generalized) (spotted) — *see* Disorder, bone, density and structure, specified type NEC
  lung (nodular) J98.4
Dental — *see also* condition
  examination Z01.20
    with abnormal findings Z01.21
  restoration
    aesthetically inadequate or displeasing K08.56
    defective K08.50
      specified NEC K08.59
    failure of marginal integrity K08.51
    failure of periodontal anatomical integrity K08.54
Dentia praecox K00.6
Denticles (pulp) K04.2
Dentigerous cyst K09.0
Dentin
  irregular (in pulp) K04.3
  opalescent K00.5
  secondary (in pulp) K04.3
  sensitive K03.89
Dentinogenesis imperfecta K00.5
Dentinoma — *see* Cyst, calcifying odontogenic
Dentition (syndrome) K00.7
  delayed K00.6
  difficult K00.7
  precocious K00.6
  premature K00.6
  retarded K00.6
Dependence (on) (syndrome) F19.20
  with remission F19.21
  alcohol (ethyl) (methyl) (without remission) F10.20
    with
      amnestic disorder, persisting F10.26
      anxiety disorder F10.280
      dementia, persisting F10.27
      intoxication F10.229
        with delirium F10.221
        uncomplicated F10.220
      mood disorder F10.24
      psychotic disorder F10.259
        with
          delusions F10.250
          hallucinations F10.251
      remission F10.21
      sexual dysfunction F10.281
      sleep disorder F10.282
      specified disorder NEC F10.288
      withdrawal F10.239
        with
          delirium F10.231
          perceptual disturbance F10.232
        uncomplicated F10.230
    counseling and surveillance Z71.41

Dependence — *continued*
  amobarbital — *see* Dependence, drug, sedative
  amphetamine(s) (type) — *see* Dependence, drug,
    stimulant NEC
  amytal (sodium) — *see* Dependence, drug, sedative
  analgesic NEC F55.8
  anesthetic (agent) (gas) (general) (local) NEC — *see*
    Dependence, drug, psychoactive NEC
  anxiolytic NEC — *see* Dependence, drug, sedative
  barbital(s) — *see* Dependence, drug, sedative
  barbiturate(s) (compounds) (drugs classifiable to T42)
    — *see* Dependence, drug, sedative
  benzedrine — *see* Dependence, drug, stimulant NEC
  bhang — *see* Dependence, drug, cannabis
  bromide(s) NEC — *see* Dependence, drug, sedative
  caffeine — *see* Dependence, drug, stimulant NEC
  cannabis (sativa) (indica) (resin) (derivatives) (type) —
    see Dependence, drug, cannabis
  chloral (betaine) (hydrate) — *see* Dependence, drug,
    sedative
  chlordiazepoxide — *see* Dependence, drug, sedative
  coca (leaf) (derivatives) — *see* Dependence, drug, co-
    caine
  cocaine — *see* Dependence, drug, cocaine
  codeine — *see* Dependence, drug, opioid
  combinations of drugs F19.20
  dagga — *see* Dependence, drug, cannabis
  demerol — *see* Dependence, drug, opioid
  dexamphetamine — *see* Dependence, drug, stimulant
    NEC
  dexedrine — *see* Dependence, drug, stimulant NEC
  dextromethorphan — *see* Dependence, drug, opioid
  dextromoramide — *see* Dependence, drug, opioid
  dextro-nor-pseudo-ephedrine — *see* Dependence,
    drug, stimulant NEC
  dextrorphan — *see* Dependence, drug, opioid
  diazepam — *see* Dependence, drug, sedative
  dilaudid — *see* Dependence, drug, opioid
  D-lysergic acid diethylamide — *see* Dependence, drug,
    hallucinogen
  drug NEC F19.20
    with sleep disorder F19.282
    cannabis F12.20
      with
        anxiety disorder F12.280
        intoxication F12.229
          with
            delirium F12.221
            perceptual disturbance F12.222
          uncomplicated F12.220
        other specified disorder F12.288
        psychosis F12.259
          delusions F12.250
          hallucinations F12.251
        unspecified disorder F12.29
        withdrawal F12.23
      in remission F12.21
    cocaine F14.20
      with
        anxiety disorder F14.280
        intoxication F14.229
          with
            delirium F14.221
            perceptual disturbance F14.222
          uncomplicated F14.220
        mood disorder F14.24
        other specified disorder F14.288
        psychosis F14.259
          delusions F14.250
          hallucinations F14.251
        sexual dysfunction F14.281
        sleep disorder F14.282
        unspecified disorder F14.29
        withdrawal F14.23
      in remission F14.21
      withdrawal symptoms in newborn P96.1
    counseling and surveillance Z71.51
    hallucinogen F16.20
      with
        anxiety disorder F16.280
        flashbacks F16.283
        intoxication F16.229
          with delirium F16.221
          uncomplicated F16.220
        mood disorder F16.24
        other specified disorder F16.288
        perception disorder, persisting F16.283
        psychosis F16.259

Dependence — *continued*
  drug — *continued*
    hallucinogen — *continued*
      with — *continued*
        psychosis — *continued*
          delusions F16.250
          hallucinations F16.251
          unspecified disorder F16.29
      in remission F16.21
    in remission F19.21
    inhalant F18.20
      with
        anxiety disorder F18.280
        dementia, persisting F18.27
        intoxication F18.229
          with delirium F18.221
          uncomplicated F18.220
        mood disorder F18.24
        other specified disorder F18.288
        psychosis F18.259
          delusions F18.250
          hallucinations F18.251
        unspecified disorder F18.29
      in remission F18.21
    nicotine F17.200
      with disorder F17.209
        in remission F17.201
        specified disorder NEC F17.208
        withdrawal F17.203
      chewing tobacco F17.220
        with disorder F17.229
          in remission F17.221
          specified disorder NEC F17.228
          withdrawal F17.223
      cigarettes F17.210
        with disorder F17.219
          in remission F17.211
          specified disorder NEC F17.218
          withdrawal F17.213
      specified product NEC F17.290
        with disorder F17.299
          remission F17.291
          specified disorder NEC F17.298
          withdrawal F17.293
    opioid F11.20
      with
        intoxication F11.229
          with
            delirium F11.221
            perceptual disturbance F11.222
          uncomplicated F11.220
        mood disorder F11.24
        other specified disorder F11.288
        psychosis F11.259
          delusions F11.250
          hallucinations F11.251
        sexual dysfunction F11.281
        sleep disorder F11.282
        unspecified disorder F11.29
        withdrawal F11.23
      in remission F11.21
    psychoactive NEC F19.20
      with
        amnestic disorder F19.26
        anxiety disorder F19.280
        dementia F19.27
        intoxication F19.229
          with
            delirium F19.221
            perceptual disturbance F19.222
          uncomplicated F19.220
        mood disorder F19.24
        other specified disorder F19.288
        psychosis F19.259
          delusions F19.250
          hallucinations F19.251
        sexual dysfunction F19.281
        sleep disorder F19.282
        unspecified disorder F19.29
        withdrawal F19.239
          with
            delirium F19.231
            perceptual disturbance F19.232
          uncomplicated F19.230
    sedative, hypnotic or anxiolytic F13.20
      with
        amnestic disorder F13.26
        anxiety disorder F13.280
        dementia, persisting F13.27

Dependence — *continued*
  drug — *continued*
    sedative, hypnotic or anxiolytic — *continued*
      with — *continued*
        intoxication F13.229
          with delirium F13.221
          uncomplicated F13.220
        mood disorder F13.24
        other specified disorder F13.288
        psychosis F13.259
          delusions F13.250
          hallucinations F13.251
        sexual dysfunction F13.281
        sleep disorder F13.282
        unspecified disorder F13.29
        withdrawal F13.239
          with
            delirium F13.231
            perceptual disturbance F13.232
          uncomplicated F13.230
      in remission F13.21
    stimulant NEC F15.20
      with
        anxiety disorder F15.280
        intoxication F15.229
          with
            delirium F15.221
            perceptual disturbance F15.222
          uncomplicated F15.220
        mood disorder F15.24
        other specified disorder F15.288
        psychosis F15.259
          delusions F15.250
          hallucinations F15.251
        sexual dysfunction F15.281
        sleep disorder F15.282
        unspecified disorder F15.29
        withdrawal F15.23
      in remission F15.21
  ethyl
    alcohol (without remission) F10.20
      with remission F10.21
    bromide — *see* Dependence, drug, sedative
    carbamate F19.20
    chloride F19.20
    morphine — *see* Dependence, drug, opioid
  ganja — *see* Dependence, drug, cannabis
  glue (airplane) (sniffing) — *see* Dependence, drug, in-
    halant
  glutethimide — *see* Dependence, drug, sedative
  hallucinogenics — *see* Dependence, drug, hallucinogen
  hashish — *see* Dependence, drug, cannabis
  hemp — *see* Dependence, drug, cannabis
  heroin (salt) (any) — *see* Dependence, drug, opioid
  hypnotic NEC — *see* Dependence, drug, sedative
  Indian hemp — *see* Dependence, drug, cannabis
  inhalants — *see* Dependence, drug, inhalant
  khat — *see* Dependence, drug, stimulant NEC
  laudanum — *see* Dependence, drug, opioid
  LSD (-25) (derivatives) — *see* Dependence, drug, hallu-
    cinogen
  luminal — *see* Dependence, drug, sedative
  lysergic acid — *see* Dependence, drug, hallucinogen
  maconha — *see* Dependence, drug, cannabis
  marihuana — *see* Dependence, drug, cannabis
  meprobamate — *see* Dependence, drug, sedative
  mescaline — *see* Dependence, drug, hallucinogen
  methadone — *see* Dependence, drug, opioid
  methamphetamine(s) — *see* Dependence, drug, stim-
    ulant NEC
  methaqualone — *see* Dependence, drug, sedative
  methyl
    alcohol (without remission) F10.20
      with remission F10.21
    bromide — *see* Dependence, drug, sedative
    morphine — *see* Dependence, drug, opioid
    phenidate — *see* Dependence, drug, stimulant NEC
    sulfonal — *see* Dependence, drug, sedative
  morphine (sulfate) (sulfite) (type) — *see* Dependence,
    drug, opioid
  narcotic (drug) NEC — *see* Dependence, drug, opioid
  nembutal — *see* Dependence, drug, sedative
  neraval — *see* Dependence, drug, sedative
  neravan — *see* Dependence, drug, sedative
  neurobarb — *see* Dependence, drug, sedative
  nicotine — *see* Dependence, drug, nicotine
  nitrous oxide F19.20

Dependence — continued
  nonbarbiturate sedatives and tranquilizers with similar
    effect — see Dependence, drug, sedative
  on
    artificial heart (fully implantable) (mechanical)
      Z95.812
    aspirator Z99.0
    care provider (because of) Z74.9
      impaired mobility Z74.09
      need for
        assistance with personal care Z74.1
        continuous supervision Z74.3
      no other household member able to render care
        Z74.2
      specified reason NEC Z74.8
    machine Z99.89
      enabling NEC Z99.89
      specified type NEC Z99.89
    renal dialysis (hemodialysis) (peritoneal) Z99.2
    respirator Z99.11
    ventilator Z99.11
    wheelchair Z99.3
  opiate — see Dependence, drug, opioid
  opioids — see Dependence, drug, opioid
  opium (alkaloids) (derivatives) (tincture) — see Dependence, drug, opioid
  oxygen (long-term) (supplemental) Z99.81
  paraldehyde — see Dependence, drug, sedative
  paregoric — see Dependence, drug, opioid
  PCP (phencyclidine) (or related substance) — see Dependence, drug, hallucinogen
  pentobarbital — see Dependence, drug, sedative
  pentobarbitone (sodium) — see Dependence, drug, sedative
  pentothal — see Dependence, drug, sedative
  peyote — see Dependence, drug, hallucinogen
  phencyclidine (PCP) (or related substance) — see Dependence, drug, hallucinogen
  phenmetrazine — see Dependence, drug, stimulant NEC
  phenobarbital — see Dependence, drug, sedative
  polysubstance F19.20
  psilocibin, psilocin, psilocyn, psilocyline — see Dependence, drug, hallucinogen
  psychostimulant NEC — see Dependence, drug, stimulant NEC
  secobarbital — see Dependence, drug, sedative
  seconal — see Dependence, drug, sedative
  sedative NEC — see Dependence, drug, sedative
  specified drug NEC — see Dependence, drug
  stimulant NEC — see Dependence, drug, stimulant NEC
  substance NEC — see Dependence, drug
  supplemental oxygen Z99.81
  tobacco — see Dependence, drug, nicotine
    counseling and surveillance Z71.6
  tranquilizer NEC — see Dependence, drug, sedative
  vitamin B6 E53.1
  volatile solvents — see Dependence, drug, inhalant
Dependency
  care-provider Z74.9
  passive F60.7
  reactions (persistent) F60.7
Depersonalization (in neurotic state) (neurotic) (syndrome) F48.1
Depletion
  extracellular fluid E86.9
  plasma E86.1
  potassium E87.6
    nephropathy N25.89
  salt or sodium E87.1
    causing heat exhaustion or prostration T67.4 ☑
    nephropathy N28.9
  volume NOS E86.9
Deployment (current) (military) status Z56.82
  in theater or in support of military war, peacekeeping
    and humanitarian operations Z56.82
  personal history of Z91.82
    military war, peacekeeping and humanitarian deployment (current or past conflict) Z91.82
  returned from Z91.82
Depolarization, premature I49.40
  atrial I49.1
  junctional I49.2
  specified NEC I49.49
  ventricular I49.3
Deposit
  bone in Boeck's sarcoid D86.89
  calcareous, calcium — see Calcification

Deposit — continued
  cholesterol
    retina H35.89
    vitreous (body) (humor) — see Deposit, crystalline
  conjunctiva H11.11- ☑
  cornea H18.00- ☑
    argentous H18.02- ☑
    due to metabolic disorder H18.03- ☑
    Kayser-Fleischer ring H18.04- ☑
    pigmentation — see Pigmentation, cornea
  crystalline, vitreous (body) (humor) H43.2- ☑
  hemosiderin in old scars of cornea — see Pigmentation, cornea, stromal
  metallic in lens — see Cataract, specified NEC
  skin R23.8
  tooth, teeth (betel) (black) (green) (materia alba) (orange) (tobacco) K03.6
  urate, kidney — see Calculus, kidney
Depraved appetite — see Pica
Depressed
  HDL cholesterol E78.6
Depression (acute) (mental) F32.9
  agitated (single episode) F32.2
  anaclitic — see Disorder, adjustment
  anxiety F41.8
    persistent F34.1
  arches — see also Deformity, limb, flat foot
  atypical (single episode) F32.89
    recurrent episode F33.8
  basal metabolic rate R94.8
  bone marrow D75.89
  central nervous system R09.2
  cerebral R29.818
    newborn P91.4
  cerebrovascular I67.9
  chest wall M95.4
  climacteric (single episode) F32.89
    recurrent episode F33.8
  endogenous (without psychotic symptoms) F33.2
    with psychotic symptoms F33.3
  functional activity R68.89
  hysterical F44.89
  involutional (single episode) F32.89
    recurrent episode F33.8
  major F32.9
    with psychotic symptoms F32.3
    recurrent — see Disorder, depressive, recurrent
  manic-depressive — see Disorder, depressive, recurrent
  masked (single episode) F32.89
  medullary G93.89
  menopausal (single episode) F32.89
    recurrent episode F33.8
  metatarsus — see Depression, arches
  monopolar F33.9
  nervous F34.1
  neurotic F34.1
  nose M95.0
  postnatal (NOS) F53.0
  postpartum (NOS) F53.0
  post-psychotic of schizophrenia F32.89
  post-schizophrenic F32.89
  psychogenic (reactive) (single episode) F32.9
  psychoneurotic F34.1
  psychotic (single episode) F32.3
    recurrent F33.3
  reactive (psychogenic) (single episode) F32.9
    psychotic (single episode) F32.3
  recurrent — see Disorder, depressive, recurrent
  respiratory center G93.89
  seasonal — see Disorder, depressive, recurrent
  senile F03 ☑
  severe, single episode F32.2
  situational F43.21
  skull Q67.4
  specified NEC (single episode) F32.89
  sternum M95.4
  visual field — see Defect, visual field
  vital (recurrent) (without psychotic symptoms) F33.2
    with psychotic symptoms F33.3
    single episode F32.2
Deprivation
  cultural Z60.3
  effects NOS T73.9 ☑
    specified NEC T73.8 ☑
  emotional NEC Z65.8
    affecting infant or child — see Maltreatment, child, psychological
  food T73.0 ☑

Deprivation — continued
  protein — see Malnutrition
  sleep Z72.820
  social Z60.4
    affecting infant or child — see Maltreatment, child, psychological
  specified NEC T73.8 ☑
  vitamins — see Deficiency, vitamin
  water T73.1 ☑
Derangement
  ankle (internal) — see Derangement, joint, ankle
  cartilage (articular) NEC — see Derangement, joint, articular cartilage, by site
    recurrent — see Dislocation, recurrent
  cruciate ligament, anterior, current injury — see Sprain, knee, cruciate, anterior
  elbow (internal) — see Derangement, joint, elbow
  hip (joint) (internal) (old) — see Derangement, joint, hip
  joint (internal) M24.9
    ankylosis — see Ankylosis
    articular cartilage M24.10
      ankle M24.17- ☑
      elbow M24.12- ☑
      foot M24.17- ☑
      hand M24.14- ☑
      hip M24.15- ☑
      knee NEC M23.9- ☑
      loose body — see Loose, body
      shoulder M24.11- ☑
      wrist M24.13- ☑
    contracture — see Contraction, joint
    current injury — see also Dislocation
      knee, meniscus or cartilage — see Tear, meniscus
    dislocation
      pathological — see Dislocation, pathological
      recurrent — see Dislocation, recurrent
    knee — see Derangement, knee
    ligament — see Disorder, ligament
    loose body — see Loose, body
    recurrent — see Dislocation, recurrent
    specified type NEC M24.80
      ankle M24.87- ☑
      elbow M24.82- ☑
      foot joint M24.87- ☑
      hand joint M24.84- ☑
      hip M24.85- ☑
      shoulder M24.81- ☑
      wrist M24.83- ☑
    temporomandibular M26.69
  knee (recurrent) M23.9- ☑
    ligament disruption, spontaneous M23.60- ☑
      anterior cruciate M23.61- ☑
      capsular M23.67- ☑
      instability, chronic M23.5- ☑
      lateral collateral M23.64- ☑
      medial collateral M23.63- ☑
      posterior cruciate M23.62- ☑
    loose body M23.4- ☑
    meniscus M23.30- ☑
      cystic M23.00- ☑
        lateral M23.002
          anterior horn M23.04- ☑
          posterior horn M23.05- ☑
          specified NEC M23.06- ☑
        medial M23.005
          anterior horn M23.01- ☑
          posterior horn M23.02- ☑
          specified NEC M23.03- ☑
      degenerate — see Derangement, knee, meniscus, specified NEC
      detached — see Derangement, knee, meniscus, specified NEC
      due to old tear or injury M23.20- ☑
        lateral M23.20- ☑
          anterior horn M23.24- ☑
          posterior horn M23.25- ☑
          specified NEC M23.26- ☑
        medial M23.20- ☑
          anterior horn M23.21- ☑
          posterior horn M23.22- ☑
          specified NEC M23.23- ☑
      retained — see Derangement, knee, meniscus, specified NEC
      specified NEC M23.30- ☑
        lateral M23.30- ☑

Derangement — *continued*
  knee — *continued*
    meniscus — *continued*
      specified — *continued*
        lateral — *continued*
          anterior horn M23.34- ☑
          posterior horn M23.35- ☑
          specified NEC M23.36- ☑
        medial M23.30- ☑
          anterior horn M23.31- ☑
          posterior horn M23.32- ☑
          specified NEC M23.33- ☑
        old M23.8X- ☑
        specified NEC — *see subcategory* M23.8 ☑
  low back NEC — *see* Dorsopathy, specified NEC
  meniscus — *see* Derangement, knee, meniscus
  mental — *see* Psychosis
  patella, specified NEC — *see* Disorder, patella, derangement NEC
  semilunar cartilage (knee) — *see* Derangement, knee, meniscus, specified NEC
  shoulder (internal) — *see* Derangement, joint, shoulder
Dercum's disease E88.2
Derealization (neurotic) F48.1
Dermal — *see* condition
Dermaphytid — *see* Dermatophytosis
Dermatitis (eczematous) L30.9
  ab igne L59.0
  acarine B88.0
  actinic (due to sun) L57.8
    other than from sun L59.8
  allergic — *see* Dermatitis, contact, allergic
  ambustionis, due to burn or scald — *see* Burn
  amebic A06.7
  ammonia L22
  arsenical (ingested) L27.8
  artefacta L98.1
    psychogenic F54
  atopic L20.9
    psychogenic F54
    specified NEC L20.89
  autoimmune progesterone L30.8
  berlock, berloque L56.2
  blastomycotic B40.3
  blister beetle L24.89
  bullous, bullosa L13.9
    mucosynechial, atrophic L12.1
    seasonal L30.8
    specified NEC L13.8
  calorica L59.0
    due to burn or scald — *see* Burn
  caterpillar L24.89
  cercarial B65.3
  combustionis L59.0
    due to burn or scald — *see* Burn
  congelationis T69.1 ☑
  contact (occupational) L25.9
    allergic L23.9
      due to
        adhesives L23.1
        cement L23.5
        chemical products NEC L23.5
        chromium L23.0
        cosmetics L23.2
        dander (cat) (dog) L23.81
        drugs in contact with skin L23.3
        dyes L23.4
        food in contact with skin L23.6
        hair (cat) (dog) L23.81
        insecticide L23.5
        metals L23.0
        nickel L23.0
        plants, non-food L23.7
        plastic L23.5
        rubber L23.5
        specified agent NEC L23.89
    due to
      cement L25.3
      chemical products NEC L25.3
      cosmetics L25.0
      dander (cat) (dog) L23.81
      drugs in contact with skin L25.1
      dyes L25.2
      food in contact with skin L25.4
      hair (cat) (dog) L23.81
      plants, non-food L25.5
      specified agent NEC L25.8
    irritant L24.9

Dermatitis — *continued*
  contact — *continued*
    irritant — *continued*
      due to
        cement L24.5
        chemical products NEC L24.5
        cosmetics L24.3
        detergents L24.0
        drugs in contact with skin L24.4
        food in contact with skin L24.6
        oils and greases L24.1
        plants, non-food L24.7
        solvents L24.2
        specified agent NEC L24.89
  contusiformis L52
  diabetic — *see* E08-E13 with .620
  diaper L22
  diphtheritica A36.3
  dry skin L85.3
  due to
    acetone (contact) (irritant) L24.2
    acids (contact) (irritant) L24.5
    adhesive(s) (allergic) (contact) (plaster) L23.1
      irritant L24.5
    alcohol (irritant) (skin contact) (substances in category T51) L24.2
      taken internally L27.8
    alkalis (contact) (irritant) L24.5
    arsenic (ingested) L27.8
    carbon disulfide (contact) (irritant) L24.2
    caustics (contact) (irritant) L24.5
    cement (contact) L25.3
    cereal (ingested) L27.2
    chemical(s) NEC L25.3
      taken internally L27.8
    chlorocompounds L24.2
    chromium (contact) (irritant) L24.81
    coffee (ingested) L27.2
    cold weather L30.8
    cosmetics (contact) L25.0
      allergic L23.2
      irritant L24.3
    cyclohexanes L24.2
    dander (cat) (dog) L23.81
    Demodex species B88.0
    Dermanyssus gallinae B88.0
    detergents (contact) (irritant) L24.0
    dichromate L24.81
    drugs and medicaments (generalized) (internal use) L27.0
      external — *see* Dermatitis, due to, drugs, in contact with skin
      in contact with skin L25.1
        allergic L23.3
        irritant L24.4
      localized skin eruption L27.1
      specified substance — *see* Table of Drugs and Chemicals
    dyes (contact) L25.2
      allergic L23.4
      irritant L24.89
    epidermophytosis — *see* Dermatophytosis
    esters L24.2
    external irritant NEC L24.9
    fish (ingested) L27.2
    flour (ingested) L27.2
    food (ingested) L27.2
      in contact with skin L25.4
    fruit (ingested) L27.2
    furs (allergic) (contact) L23.81
    glues — *see* Dermatitis, due to, adhesives
    glycols L24.2
    greases NEC (contact) (irritant) L24.1
    hair (cat) (dog) L23.81
    hot
      objects and materials — *see* Burn
      weather or places L59.0
    hydrocarbons L24.2
    infrared rays L59.8
    ingestion, ingested substance L27.9
      chemical NEC L27.8
      drugs and medicaments — *see* Dermatitis, due to, drugs
      food L27.2
      specified NEC L27.8
    insecticide in contact with skin L24.5
    internal agent L27.9

Dermatitis — *continued*
  due to — *continued*
    internal agent — *continued*
      drugs and medicaments (generalized) — *see* Dermatitis, due to, drugs
      food L27.2
    irradiation — *see* Dermatitis, due to, radioactive substance
    ketones L24.2
    lacquer tree (allergic) (contact) L23.7
    light (sun) NEC L57.8
      acute L56.8
      other L59.8
    Liponyssoides sanguineus B88.0
    low temperature L30.8
    meat (ingested) L27.2
    metals, metal salts (contact) (irritant) L24.81
    milk (ingested) L27.2
    nickel (contact) (irritant) L24.81
    nylon (contact) (irritant) L24.5
    oils NEC (contact) (irritant) L24.1
    paint solvent (contact) (irritant) L24.2
    petroleum products (contact) (irritant) (substances in T52.0) L24.2
    plants NEC (contact) L25.5
      allergic L23.7
      irritant L24.7
    plasters (adhesive) (any) (allergic) (contact) L23.1
      irritant L24.5
    plastic (contact) L25.3
    preservatives (contact) — *see* Dermatitis, due to, chemical, in contact with skin
    primrose (allergic) (contact) L23.7
    primula (allergic) (contact) L23.7
    radiation L59.8
      nonionizing (chronic exposure) L57.8
      sun NEC L57.8
        acute L56.8
    radioactive substance L58.9
      acute L58.0
      chronic L58.1
    radium L58.9
      acute L58.0
      chronic L58.1
    ragweed (allergic) (contact) L23.7
    Rhus (allergic) (contact) (diversiloba) (radicans) (toxicodendron) (venenata) (verniciflua) L23.7
    rubber (contact) L24.5
    Senecio jacobaea (allergic) (contact) L23.7
    solvents (contact) (irritant) (substances in category T52) L24.2
    specified agent NEC (contact) L25.8
      allergic L23.89
      irritant L24.89
    sunshine NEC L57.8
      acute L56.8
    tetrachlorethylene (contact) (irritant) L24.2
    toluene (contact) (irritant) L24.2
    turpentine (contact) L24.2
    ultraviolet rays (sun NEC) (chronic exposure) L57.8
      acute L56.8
    vaccine or vaccination L27.0
      specified substance — *see* Table of Drugs and Chemicals
    varicose veins — *see* Varix, leg, with, inflammation
    X-rays L58.9
      acute L58.0
      chronic L58.1
  dyshydrotic L30.1
  dysmenorrheica N94.6
  escharotica — *see* Burn
  exfoliative, exfoliativa (generalized) L26
    neonatorum L00
  eyelid — *see also* Dermatosis, eyelid
    allergic H01.119
      left H01.116
        lower H01.115
        upper H01.114
      right H01.113
        lower H01.112
        upper H01.111
    contact — *see* Dermatitis, eyelid, allergic
    due to
      Demodex species B88.0
      herpes (zoster) B02.39
        simplex B00.59
    eczematous H01.139
      left H01.136

▽ Subterms under main terms may continue to next column or page   ☑ Additional Character Required — Refer to the Tabular List for Character Selection   **95**

Derangement — Dermatitis

Dermatitis — continued
  eyelid — see also Dermatosis, eyelid — continued
    eczematous — continued
      left — continued
        lower H01.135
        upper H01.134
      right H01.133
        lower H01.132
        upper H01.131
  facta, factitia, factitial L98.1
    psychogenic F54
  flexural NEC L20.82
  friction L30.4
  fungus B36.9
    specified type NEC B36.8
  gangrenosa, gangrenous infantum L08.0
  harvest mite B88.0
  heat L59.0
  herpesviral, vesicular (ear) (lip) B00.1
  herpetiformis (bullous) (erythematous) (pustular)
      (vesicular) L13.0
    juvenile L12.2
    senile L12.0
  hiemalis L30.8
  hypostatic, hypostatica — see Varix, leg, with, inflam-
      mation
  infectious eczematoid L30.3
  infective L30.3
  irritant — see Dermatitis, contact, irritant
  Jacquet's (diaper dermatitis) L22
  Leptus B88.0
  lichenified NEC L28.0
  medicamentosa (generalized) (internal use) — see
      Dermatitis, due to drugs
  mite B88.0
  multiformis L13.0
    juvenile L12.2
  napkin L22
  neurotica L13.0
  nummular L30.0
  papillaris capillitii L73.0
  pellagrous E52
  perioral L71.0
  photocontact L56.2
  polymorpha dolorosa L13.0
  pruriginosa L13.0
  pruritic NEC L30.8
  psychogenic F54
  purulent L08.0
  pustular
    contagious B08.02
    subcorneal L13.1
  pyococcal L08.0
  pyogenica L08.0
  repens L40.2
  Ritter's (exfoliativa) L00
  Schamberg's L81.7
  schistosome B65.3
  seasonal bullous L30.8
  seborrheic L21.9
    infantile L21.1
    specified NEC L21.8
  sensitization NOS L23.9
  septic L08.0
  solare L57.8
  specified NEC L30.8
  stasis I87.2
    with
      varicose ulcer — see Varix, leg, with ulcer, with
          inflammation
      varicose veins — see Varix, leg, with, inflamma-
          tion
      due to postthrombotic syndrome — see Syndrome,
          postthrombotic
  suppurative L08.0
  traumatic NEC L30.4
  trophoneurotica L13.0
  ultraviolet (sun) (chronic exposure) L57.8
    acute L56.8
  varicose — see Varix, leg, with, inflammation
  vegetans L10.1
  verrucosa B43.0
  vesicular, herpesviral B00.1
Dermatoarthritis, lipoid E78.81
Dermatochalasis, eyelid H02.839
  left H02.836
    lower H02.835
    upper H02.834

Dermatochalasis, eyelid — continued
  right H02.833
    lower H02.832
    upper H02.831
Dermatofibroma (lenticulare) — see Neoplasm, skin,
    benign
  protuberans — see Neoplasm, skin, uncertain behavior
Dermatofibrosarcoma (pigmented) (protuberans) —
    see Neoplasm, skin, malignant
Dermatographia L50.3
Dermatolysis (exfoliativa) (congenital) Q82.8
  acquired L57.4
  eyelids — see Blepharochalasis
  palpebrarum — see Blepharochalasis
  senile L57.4
Dermatomegaly NEC Q82.8
Dermatomucosomyositis M33.10
  with
    myopathy M33.12
    respiratory involvement M33.11
    specified organ involvement NEC M33.19
Dermatomycosis B36.9
  furfuracea B36.0
  specified type NEC B36.8
Dermatomyositis (acute) (chronic) — see also Der-
    matopolymyositis
  adult — see also Dermatomyositis, specified NEC
      M33.10
  in (due to) neoplastic disease — see also Neoplasm
      D49.9 [M36.0]
  juvenile M33.00
    with
      myopathy M33.02
      respiratory involvement M33.01
      specified organ involvement NEC M33.09
    without myopathy M33.03
  specified NEC M33.10
    with
      myopathy M33.12
      respiratory involvement M33.11
      specified organ involvement NEC M33.19
    without myopathy M33.13
Dermatoneuritis of children — see Poisoning, mercury
Dermatophilosis A48.8
Dermatophytid L30.2
Dermatophytide — see Dermatophytosis
Dermatophytosis (epidermophyton) (infection) (Mi-
    crosporum) (tinea) (Trichophyton) B35.9
  beard B35.0
  body B35.4
  capitis B35.0
  corporis B35.4
  deep-seated B35.8
  disseminated B35.8
  foot B35.3
  granulomatous B35.8
  groin B35.6
  hand B35.2
  nail B35.1
  perianal (area) B35.6
  scalp B35.0
  specified NEC B35.8
Dermatopolymyositis M33.90
  with
    myopathy M33.92
    respiratory involvement M33.91
    specified organ involvement NEC M33.99
  in neoplastic disease — see also Neoplasm
      D49.9 [M36.0]
  juvenile M33.00
    with
      myopathy M33.02
      respiratory involvement M33.01
      specified organ involvement NEC M33.09
  specified NEC M33.10
    myopathy M33.12
    respiratory involvement M33.11
    specified organ involvement NEC M33.19
  without myopathy M33.93
Dermatopolyneuritis — see Poisoning, mercury
Dermatorrhexis — see also Syndrome, Ehlers-Danlos
    Q79.60
  acquired L57.4
Dermatosclerosis — see also Scleroderma
  localized L94.0
Dermatosis L98.9
  Andrews' L08.89
  Bowen's — see Neoplasm, skin, in situ

Dermatosis — continued
  bullous L13.9
    specified NEC L13.8
  exfoliativa L26
  eyelid (noninfectious)
    dermatitis — see Dermatitis, eyelid
    discoid lupus erythematosus — see Lupus, erythe-
        matosus, eyelid
    xeroderma — see Xeroderma, acquired, eyelid
  factitial L98.1
  febrile neutrophilic L98.2
  gonococcal A54.89
  herpetiformis L13.0
    juvenile L12.2
  linear IgA L13.8
  menstrual NEC L98.8
  neutrophilic, febrile L98.2
  occupational — see Dermatitis, contact
  papulosa nigra L82.1
  pigmentary L81.9
    progressive L81.7
    Schamberg's L81.7
  psychogenic F54
  purpuric, pigmented L81.7
  pustular, subcorneal L13.1
  transient acantholytic L11.1
Dermographia, dermographism L50.3
Dermoid (cyst) — see also Neoplasm, benign, by site
  with malignant transformation C56- ☑
  due to radiation (nonionizing) L57.8
Dermopathy
  infiltrative with thyrotoxicosis — see Thyrotoxicosis
  nephrogenic fibrosing L90.8
Dermophytosis — see Dermatophytosis
Descemetocele H18.73- ☑
Descemet's membrane — see condition
Descending — see condition
Descensus uteri — see Prolapse, uterus
Desert
  rheumatism B38.0
  sore — see Ulcer, skin
Desertion (newborn) — see Maltreatment
Desmoid (extra-abdominal) (tumor) — see Neoplasm,
    connective tissue, uncertain behavior
  abdominal D48.1
Despondency F32.9
Desquamation, skin R23.4
Destruction, destructive — see also Damage
  articular facet — see also Derangement, joint, specified
      type NEC
    knee M23.8X- ☑
    vertebra — see Spondylosis
  bone — see also Disorder, bone, specified type NEC
    syphilitic A52.77
  joint — see also Derangement, joint, specified type
      NEC
    sacroiliac M53.3
  rectal sphincter K62.89
  septum (nasal) J34.89
  tuberculous NEC — see Tuberculosis
  tympanum, tympanic membrane (nontraumatic) —
      see Disorder, tympanic membrane, specified NEC
  vertebral disc — see Degeneration, intervertebral disc
Destructiveness — see also Disorder, conduct
  adjustment reaction — see Disorder, adjustment
Desultory labor O62.2
Detachment
  cartilage — see Sprain
  cervix, annular N88.8
    complicating delivery O71.3
  choroid (old) (postinfectional) (simple) (spontaneous)
      H31.40- ☑
    hemorrhagic H31.41- ☑
    serous H31.42- ☑
  ligament — see Sprain
  meniscus (knee) — see also Derangement, knee,
      meniscus, specified NEC
    current injury — see Tear, meniscus
    due to old tear or injury — see Derangement, knee,
        meniscus, due to old tear
  retina (without retinal break) (serous) H33.2- ☑
    with retinal:
      break H33.00- ☑
        giant H33.03- ☑
        multiple H33.02- ☑
        single H33.01- ☑
      dialysis H33.04- ☑

☑ **Additional Character Required** — Refer to the Tabular List for Character Selection   ▽ Subterms under main terms may continue to next column or page

Detachment — *continued*
  retina — *continued*
    pigment epithelium — *see* Degeneration, retina, separation of layers, pigment epithelium detachment
    rhegmatogenous — *see* Detachment, retina, with retinal, break
    specified NEC H33.8
    total H33.05- ☑
    traction H33.4- ☑
  vitreous (body) H43.81 ☑
Detergent asthma J69.8
Deterioration
  epileptic F06.8
  general physical R53.81
  heart, cardiac — *see* Degeneration, myocardial
  mental — *see* Psychosis
  myocardial, myocardium — *see* Degeneration, myocardial
  senile (simple) R54
Deuteranomaly (anomalous trichromat) H53.53
Deuteranopia (complete) (incomplete) H53.53
Development
  abnormal, bone Q79.9
  arrested R62.50
    bone — *see* Arrest, development or growth, bone
    child R62.50
    due to malnutrition E45
  defective, congenital — *see also* Anomaly, by site
    cauda equina Q06.3
    left ventricle Q24.8
      in hypoplastic left heart syndrome Q23.4
    valve Q24.8
      pulmonary Q22.3
  delayed — *see also* Delay, development R62.50
    arithmetical skills F81.2
    language (skills) (expressive) F80.1
    learning skill F81.9
    mixed skills F88
    motor coordination F82
    reading F81.0
    specified learning skill NEC F81.89
    speech F80.9
    spelling F81.81
    written expression F81.81
  imperfect, congenital — *see also* Anomaly, by site
    heart Q24.9
    lungs Q33.6
  incomplete
    bronchial tree Q32.4
    organ or site not listed — *see* Hypoplasia, by site
    respiratory system Q34.9
  sexual, precocious NEC E30.1
  tardy, mental — *see also* Disability, intellectual F79
Developmental — *see* condition
  testing, infant or child — *see* Examination, child
Devergie's disease (pityriasis rubra pilaris) L44.0
Deviation (in)
  conjugate palsy (eye) (spastic) H51.0
  esophagus (acquired) K22.8
  eye, skew H51.8
  midline (jaw) (teeth) (dental arch) M26.29
    specified site NEC — *see* Malposition
  nasal septum J34.2
    congenital Q67.4
  opening and closing of the mandible M26.53
  organ or site, congenital NEC — *see* Malposition, congenital
  septum (nasal) (acquired) J34.2
    congenital Q67.4
  sexual F65.9
    bestiality F65.89
    erotomania F52.8
    exhibitionism F65.2
    fetishism, fetishistic F65.0
      transvestism F65.1
    frotteurism F65.81
    masochism F65.51
    multiple F65.89
    necrophilia F65.89
    nymphomania F52.8
    pederosis F65.4
    pedophilia F65.4
    sadism, sadomasochism F65.52
    satyriasis F52.8
    specified type NEC F65.89
    transvestism F64.1
    voyeurism F65.3

Deviation — *continued*
  teeth, midline M26.29
  trachea J39.8
  ureter, congenital Q62.61
Device
  cerebral ventricle (communicating) in situ Z98.2
  contraceptive — *see* Contraceptive, device
  drainage, cerebrospinal fluid, in situ Z98.2
Devic's disease G36.0
Devil's
  grip B33.0
  pinches (purpura simplex) D69.2
Devitalized tooth K04.99
Devonshire colic — *see* Poisoning, lead
Dextraposition, aorta Q20.3
  in tetralogy of Fallot Q21.3
Dextrinosis, limit (debrancher enzyme deficiency) E74.03
Dextrocardia (true) Q24.0
  with
    complete transposition of viscera Q89.3
    situs inversus Q89.3
Dextrotransposition, aorta Q20.3
d-glycericacidemia E72.59
Dhat syndrome F48.8
Dhobi itch B35.6
Di George's syndrome D82.1
Di Guglielmo's disease C94.0- ☑
Diabetes, diabetic (mellitus) (sugar) E11.9
  with
    amyotrophy E11.44
    arthropathy NEC E11.618
    autonomic (poly)neuropathy E11.43
    cataract E11.36
    Charcot's joints E11.610
    chronic kidney disease E11.22
    circulatory complication NEC E11.59
    complication E11.8
      specified NEC E11.69
    dermatitis E11.620
    foot ulcer E11.621
    gangrene E11.52
    gastroparalysis E11.43
    gastroparesis E11.43
    glomerulonephrosis, intracapillary E11.21
    glomerulosclerosis, intercapillary E11.21
    hyperglycemia E11.65
    hyperosmolarity E11.00
      with coma E11.01
    hypoglycemia E11.649
      with coma E11.641
    ketoacidosis E11.10
      with coma E11.11
    kidney complications NEC E11.29
    Kimmelstiel-Wilson disease E11.21
    loss of protective sensation (LOPS) — *see* Diabetes, by type, with neuropathy
    mononeuropathy E11.41
    myasthenia E11.44
    necrobiosis lipoidica E11.620
    nephropathy E11.21
    neuralgia E11.42
    neurologic complication NEC E11.49
    neuropathic arthropathy E11.610
    neuropathy E11.40
    ophthalmic complication NEC E11.39
    oral complication NEC E11.638
    osteomyelitis E11.69
    periodontal disease E11.630
    peripheral angiopathy E11.51
      with gangrene E11.52
    polyneuropathy E11.42
    renal complication NEC E11.29
    renal tubular degeneration E11.29
    retinopathy E11.319
      with macular edema E11.311
        resolved following treatment E11.37- ☑
      nonproliferative E11.329
        with macular edema E11.321 ☑
        mild E11.329 ☑
          with macular edema E11.321 ☑
        moderate E11.339 ☑
          with macular edema E11.331 ☑
        severe E11.349 ☑
          with macular edema E11.341 ☑
      proliferative E11.359 ☑

Diabetes, diabetic — *continued*
  with — *continued*
    retinopathy — *continued*
      proliferative — *continued*
        with
          combined traction retinal detachment and rhegmatogenous retinal detachment E11.354 ☑
          macular edema E11.351 ☑
          stable proliferative diabetic retinopathy E11.355 ☑
          traction retinal detachment involving the macula E11.352 ☑
          traction retinal detachment not involving the macula E11.353 ☑
        resolved following treatment E09.37 ☑
    skin complication NEC E11.628
    skin ulcer NEC E11.622
  brittle — *see* Diabetes, type 1
  bronzed E83.110
  complicating pregnancy — *see* Pregnancy, complicated by, diabetes
  dietary counseling and surveillance Z71.3
  due to
    autoimmune process — *see* Diabetes, type 1
    immune mediated pancreatic islet beta-cell destruction — *see* Diabetes, type 1
  due to drug or chemical E09.9
    with
      amyotrophy E09.44
      arthropathy NEC E09.618
      autonomic (poly)neuropathy E09.43
      cataract E09.36
      Charcot's joints E09.610
      chronic kidney disease E09.22
      circulatory complication NEC E09.59
      complication E09.8
        specified NEC E09.69
      dermatitis E09.620
      foot ulcer E09.621
      gangrene E09.52
      gastroparalysis E09.43
      gastroparesis E09.43
      glomerulonephrosis, intracapillary E09.21
      glomerulosclerosis, intercapillary E09.21
      hyperglycemia E09.65
      hyperosmolarity E09.00
        with coma E09.01
      hypoglycemia E09.649
        with coma E09.641
      ketoacidosis E09.10
        with coma E09.11
      kidney complications NEC E09.29
      Kimmelstiel-Wilson disease E09.21
      mononeuropathy E09.41
      myasthenia E09.44
      necrobiosis lipoidica E09.620
      nephropathy E09.21
      neuralgia E09.42
      neurologic complication NEC E09.49
      neuropathic arthropathy E09.610
      neuropathy E09.40
      ophthalmic complication NEC E09.39
      oral complication NEC E09.638
      periodontal disease E09.630
      peripheral angiopathy E09.51
        with gangrene E09.52
      polyneuropathy E09.42
      renal complication NEC E09.29
      renal tubular degeneration E09.29
      retinopathy E09.319
        with macular edema E09.311
        resolved following treatment E09.37 ☑
        nonproliferative E09.329 ☑
          with macular edema E09.321 ☑
          mild E09.329 ☑
            with macular edema E09.321 ☑
          moderate E09.339 ☑
            with macular edema E09.331 ☑
          severe E09.349 ☑
            with macular edema E09.341 ☑
        proliferative E09.359 ☑
          with
            combined traction retinal detachment and rhegmatogenous retinal detachment E09.354 ☑
            macular edema E09.351 ☑

▽ Subterms under main terms may continue to next column or page   ☑ Additional Character Required — Refer to the Tabular List for Character Selection   97

Detachment — Diabetes, diabetic

Diabetes, diabetic — *continued*
  due to drug or chemical — *continued*
    with — *continued*
      retinopathy — *continued*
        proliferative — *continued*
          with — *continued*
            stable proliferative diabetic retinopathy E09.355 ☑
            traction retinal detachment involving the macula E09.352 ☑
            traction retinal detachment not involving the macula E09.353 ☑
      skin complication NEC E09.628
      skin ulcer NEC E09.622
  due to underlying condition E08.9
    with
      amyotrophy E08.44
      arthropathy NEC E08.618
      autonomic (poly)neuropathy E08.43
      cataract E08.36
      Charcot's joints E08.610
      chronic kidney disease E08.22
      circulatory complication NEC E08.59
      complication E08.8
        specified NEC E08.69
      dermatitis E08.620
      foot ulcer E08.621
      gangrene E08.52
      gastroparalysis E08.43
      gastroparesis E08.43
      glomerulonephrosis, intracapillary E08.21
      glomerulosclerosis, intercapillary E08.21
      hyperglycemia E08.65
      hyperosmolarity E08.00
        with coma E08.01
      hypoglycemia E08.649
        with coma E08.641
      ketoacidosis E08.10
        with coma E08.11
      kidney complications NEC E08.29
      Kimmelsteil-Wilson disease E08.21
      mononeuropathy E08.41
      myasthenia E08.44
      necrobiosis lipoidica E08.620
      nephropathy E08.21
      neuralgia E08.42
      neurologic complication NEC E08.49
      neuropathic arthropathy E08.610
      neuropathy E08.40
      ophthalmic complication NEC E08.39
      oral complication NEC E08.638
      periodontal disease E08.630
      peripheral angiopathy E08.51
        with gangrene E08.52
      polyneuropathy E08.42
      renal complication NEC E08.29
      renal tubular degeneration E08.29
      retinopathy E08.319
        with macular edema E08.311
        resolved following treatment E08.37 ☑
        nonproliferative E08.329 ☑
          with macular edema E08.321 ☑
          mild E08.329 ☑
            with macular edema E08.321 ☑
          moderate E08.339 ☑
            with macular edema E08.331 ☑
          severe E08.349 ☑
            with macular edema E08.341 ☑
        proliferative E08.359 ☑
          with
            combined traction retinal detachment and rhegmatogenous retinal detachment E08.354 ☑
            macular edema E08.351 ☑
            stable proliferative diabetic retinopathy E08.355 ☑
            traction retinal detachment involving the macula E08.352 ☑
            traction retinal detachment not involving the macula E08.353 ☑
      skin complication NEC E08.628
      skin ulcer NEC E08.622
  gestational (in pregnancy) O24.419
    affecting newborn P70.0
    diet controlled O24.410
    in childbirth O24.429
      diet controlled O24.420
      insulin (and diet) controlled O24.424

Diabetes, diabetic — *continued*
  gestational — *continued*
    in childbirth — *continued*
      oral drug controlled (antidiabetic) (hypoglycemic) O24.425
      insulin (and diet) controlled O24.414
      oral drug controlled (antidiabetic) (hypoglycemic) O24.415
      puerperal O24.439
        diet controlled O24.430
        insulin (and diet) controlled O24.434
        oral drug controlled (antidiabetic) (hypoglycemic) O24.435
  hepatogenous E13.9
  idiopathic — *see* Diabetes, type 1
  inadequately controlled — *code to* Diabetes, by type, with hyperglycemia
  insipidus E23.2
    nephrogenic N25.1
    pituitary E23.2
    vasopressin resistant N25.1
  insulin dependent — *code to* type of diabetes
  juvenile-onset — *see* Diabetes, type 1
  ketosis-prone — *see* Diabetes, type 1
  latent R73.03
  neonatal (transient) P70.2
  non-insulin dependent — *code to* type of diabetes
  out of control — *code to* Diabetes, by type, with hyperglycemia
  phosphate E83.39
  poorly controlled — *code to* Diabetes, by type, with hyperglycemia
  postpancreatectomy — *see* Diabetes, specified type NEC
  postprocedural — *see* Diabetes, specified type NEC
  secondary diabetes mellitus NEC — *see* Diabetes, specified type NEC
  specified type NEC E13.9
    with
      amyotrophy E13.44
      arthropathy NEC E13.618
      autonomic (poly)neuropathy E13.43
      cataract E13.36
      Charcot's joints E13.610
      chronic kidney disease E13.22
      circulatory complication NEC E13.59
      complication E13.8
        specified NEC E13.69
      dermatitis E13.620
      foot ulcer E13.621
      gangrene E13.52
      gastroparalysis E13.43
      gastroparesis E13.43
      glomerulonephrosis, intracapillary E13.21
      glomerulosclerosis, intercapillary E13.21
      hyperglycemia E13.65
      hyperosmolarity E13.00
        with coma E13.01
      hypoglycemia E13.649
        with coma E13.641
      ketoacidosis E13.10
        with coma E13.11
      kidney complications NEC E13.29
      Kimmelsteil-Wilson disease E13.21
      mononeuropathy E13.41
      myasthenia E13.44
      necrobiosis lipoidica E13.620
      nephropathy E13.21
      neuralgia E13.42
      neurologic complication NEC E13.49
      neuropathic arthropathy E13.610
      neuropathy E13.40
      ophthalmic complication NEC E13.39
      oral complication NEC E13.638
      periodontal disease E13.630
      peripheral angiopathy E13.51
        with gangrene E13.52
      polyneuropathy E13.42
      renal complication NEC E13.29
      renal tubular degeneration E13.29
      retinopathy E13.319
        with macular edema E13.311
        resolved following treatment E13.37 ☑
        nonproliferative E13.329 ☑
          with macular edema E13.321 ☑
          mild E13.329 ☑
            with macular edema E13.321 ☑
          moderate E13.339 ☑

Diabetes, diabetic — *continued*
  specified type — *continued*
    with — *continued*
      retinopathy — *continued*
        nonproliferative — *continued*
          moderate — *continued*
            with macular edema E13.331 ☑
          severe E13.349 ☑
            with macular edema E13.341 ☑
        proliferative E13.359 ☑
          with
            combined traction retinal detachment and rhegmatogenous retinal detachment E13.354 ☑
            macular edema E13.351 ☑
            stable proliferative diabetic retinopathy E13.355 ☑
            traction retinal detachment involving the macula E13.352 ☑
            traction retinal detachment not involving the macula E13.353 ☑
      skin complication NEC E13.628
      skin ulcer NEC E13.622
  steroid-induced — *see* Diabetes, due to, drug or chemical
  type 1 E10.9
    with
      amyotrophy E10.44
      arthropathy NEC E10.618
      autonomic (poly)neuropathy E10.43
      cataract E10.36
      Charcot's joints E10.610
      chronic kidney disease E10.22
      circulatory complication NEC E10.59
      complication E10.8
        specified NEC E10.69
      dermatitis E10.620
      foot ulcer E10.621
      gangrene E10.52
      gastroparalysis E10.43
      gastroparesis E10.43
      glomerulonephrosis, intracapillary E10.21
      glomerulosclerosis, intercapillary E10.21
      hyperglycemia E10.65
      hypoglycemia E10.649
        with coma E10.641
      ketoacidosis E10.10
        with coma E10.11
      kidney complications NEC E10.29
      Kimmelsteil-Wilson disease E10.21
      mononeuropathy E10.41
      myasthenia E10.44
      necrobiosis lipoidica E10.620
      nephropathy E10.21
      neuralgia E10.42
      neurologic complication NEC E10.49
      neuropathic arthropathy E10.610
      neuropathy E10.40
      ophthalmic complication NEC E10.39
      oral complication NEC E10.638
      osteomyelitis E10.69
      periodontal disease E10.630
      peripheral angiopathy E10.51
        with gangrene E10.52
      polyneuropathy E10.42
      renal complication NEC E10.29
      renal tubular degeneration E10.29
      retinopathy E10.319
        with macular edema E10.311
        resolved following treatment E10.37 ☑
        nonproliferative E10.329 ☑
          with macular edema E10.321 ☑
          mild E10.329 ☑
            with macular edema E10.321 ☑
          moderate E10.339 ☑
            with macular edema E10.331 ☑
          severe E10.349 ☑
            with macular edema E10.341 ☑
        proliferative E10.359 ☑
          with
            combined traction retinal detachment and rhegmatogenous retinal detachment E10.354 ☑
            macular edema E10.351 ☑
            stable proliferative diabetic retinopathy E10.355 ☑
            traction retinal detachment involving the macula E10.352 ☑

☑ **Additional Character Required** — **Refer to the Tabular List for Character Selection**   ▽ **Subterms under main terms may continue to next column or page**

Diabetes, diabetic — *continued*
  type 1 — *continued*
    with — *continued*
      retinopathy — *continued*
        proliferative — *continued*
          with — *continued*
            traction retinal detachment not involv-
              ing the macula E10.353 ☑
      skin complication NEC E10.628
      skin ulcer NEC E10.622
  type 2 E11.9
    with
      amyotrophy E11.44
      arthropathy NEC E11.618
      autonomic (poly)neuropathy E11.43
      cataract E11.36
      Charcot's joints E11.610
      chronic kidney disease E11.22
      circulatory complication NEC E11.59
      complication E11.8
        specified NEC E11.69
      dermatitis E11.620
      foot ulcer E11.621
      gangrene E11.52
      gastroparalysis E11.43
      gastroparesis E11.43
      glomerulonephrosis, intracapillary E11.21
      glomerulosclerosis, intercapillary E11.21
      hyperglycemia E11.65
      hyperosmolarity E11.00
        with coma E11.01
      hypoglycemia E11.649
        with coma E11.641
      ketoacidosis E11.10
        with coma E11.11
      kidney complications NEC E11.29
      Kimmelstiel-Wilson disease E11.21
      mononeuropathy E11.41
      myasthenia E11.44
      necrobiosis lipoidica E11.620
      nephropathy E11.21
      neuralgia E11.42
      neurologic complication NEC E11.49
      neuropathic arthropathy E11.610
      neuropathy E11.40
      ophthalmic complication NEC E11.39
      oral complication NEC E11.638
      osteomyelitis E11.69
      periodontal disease E11.630
      peripheral angiopathy E11.51
        with gangrene E11.52
      polyneuropathy E11.42
      renal complication NEC E11.29
      renal tubular degeneration E11.29
      retinopathy E11.319
        with macular edema E11.311
        resolved following treatment E11.37 ☑
        nonproliferative E11.329 ☑
          with macular edema E11.321 ☑
          mild E11.329 ☑
            with macular edema E11.321 ☑
          moderate E11.339 ☑
            with macular edema E11.331 ☑
          severe E11.349 ☑
            with macular edema E11.341 ☑
        proliferative E11.359 ☑
          with
            combined traction retinal detachment
              and rhegmatogenous retinal
              detachment E11.354 ☑
            macular edema E11.351 ☑
            stable proliferative diabetic retinopa-
              thy E11.355 ☑
            traction retinal detachment involving
              the macula E11.352 ☑
            traction retinal detachment not involv-
              ing the macula E11.353 ☑
      skin complication NEC E11.628
      skin ulcer NEC E11.622
  uncontrolled
    meaning
      hyperglycemia — *see* Diabetes, by type, with,
        hyperglycemia
      hypoglycemia — *see* Diabetes, by type, with,
        hypoglycemia
Diacyclothrombopathia D69.1
Diagnosis deferred R69

Dialysis (intermittent) (treatment)
  noncompliance (with) Z91.15
  renal (hemodialysis) (peritoneal), status Z99.2
  retina, retinal — *see* Detachment, retina, with retinal,
    dialysis
Diamond-Blackfan anemia (congenital hypoplastic)
  D61.01
Diamond-Gardener syndrome (autoerythrocyte sensi-
  tization) D69.2
Diaper rash L22
Diaphoresis (excessive) R61
Diaphragm — *see* condition
Diaphragmalgia R07.1
Diaphragmatitis, diaphragmitis J98.6
Diaphysial aclasis Q78.6
Diaphysitis — *see* Osteomyelitis, specified type NEC
Diarrhea, diarrheal (disease) (infantile) (inflammatory)
  R19.7
  achlorhydric K31.83
  allergic K52.29
    due to
      colitis — *see* Colitis, allergic
      enteritis — *see* Enteritis, allergic
  amebic — *see also* Amebiasis A06.0
    with abscess — *see* Abscess, amebic
    acute A06.0
    chronic A06.1
    nondysenteric A06.2
  bacillary — *see* Dysentery, bacillary
  balantidial A07.0
  cachectic NEC K52.89
  Chilomastix A07.8
  choleriformis A00.1
  chronic (noninfectious) K52.9
  coccidial A07.3
  Cochin-China K90.1
    strongyloidiasis B78.0
  Dientamoeba A07.8
  dietetic — *see also* Diarrhea, allergic K52.29
  drug-induced K52.1
  due to
    bacteria A04.9
      specified NEC A04.8
    Campylobacter A04.5
    Capillaria philippinensis B81.1
    Clostridium difficile
      not specified as recurrent A04.72
      recurrent A04.71
    Clostridium perfringens (C) (F) A04.8
    Cryptosporidium A07.2
    drugs K52.1
    Escherichia coli A04.4
      enteroaggregative A04.4
      enterohemorrhagic A04.3
      enteroinvasive A04.2
      enteropathogenic A04.0
      enterotoxigenic A04.1
      specified NEC A04.4
    food hypersensitivity — *see also* Diarrhea, allergic
      K52.29
    Necator americanus B76.1
    S. japonicum B65.2
    specified organism NEC A08.8
      bacterial A04.8
      viral A08.39
    Staphylococcus A04.8
    Trichuris trichiuria B79
    virus — *see* Enteritis, viral
    Yersinia enterocolitica A04.6
  dysenteric A09
  endemic A09
  epidemic A09
  flagellate A07.9
  Flexner's (ulcerative) A03.1
  functional K59.1
    following gastrointestinal surgery K91.89
    psychogenic F45.8
  Giardia lamblia A07.1
  giardial A07.1
  hill K90.1
  infectious A09
  malarial — *see* Malaria
  mite B88.0
  mycotic NEC B49
  neonatal (noninfectious) P78.3
  nervous F45.8
  neurogenic K59.1
  noninfectious K52.9

Diarrhea, diarrheal — *continued*
  postgastrectomy K91.1
  postvagotomy K91.1
  protozoal A07.9
    specified NEC A07.8
  psychogenic F45.8
  specified
    bacterium NEC A04.8
    virus NEC A08.39
  strongyloidiasis B78.0
  toxic K52.1
  trichomonal A07.8
  tropical K90.1
  tuberculous A18.32
  viral — *see* Enteritis, viral
Diastasis
  cranial bones M84.88
    congenital NEC Q75.8
  joint (traumatic) — *see* Dislocation
  muscle M62.00
    ankle M62.07- ☑
    congenital Q79.8
    foot M62.07- ☑
    forearm M62.03- ☑
    hand M62.04- ☑
    lower leg M62.06- ☑
    pelvic region M62.05- ☑
    shoulder region M62.01- ☑
    specified site NEC M62.08
    thigh M62.05- ☑
    upper arm M62.02- ☑
  recti (abdomen)
    complicating delivery O71.89
    congenital Q79.59
Diastema, tooth, teeth, fully erupted M26.32
Diastematomyelia Q06.2
Diataxia, cerebral G80.4
Diathesis
  allergic — *see* History, allergy
  bleeding (familial) D69.9
  cystine (familial) E72.00
  gouty — *see* Gout
  hemorrhagic (familial) D69.9
    newborn NEC P53
  spasmophilic R29.0
Diaz's disease or osteochondrosis (juvenile) (talus) —
  see Osteochondrosis, juvenile, tarsus
Dibothriocephalus, dibothriocephaliasis (latus) (infection) (infestation) B70.0
  larval B70.1
Dicephalus, dicephaly Q89.4
Dichotomy, teeth K00.2
Dichromat, dichromatopsia (congenital) — *see* Deficiency, color vision
Dichuchwa A65
Dicroceliasis B66.2
Didelphia, didelphys — *see* Double uterus
Didymytis N45.1
  with orchitis N45.3
Dietary
  inadequacy or deficiency E63.9
  surveillance and counseling Z71.3
Dietl's crisis N13.8
Dieulafoy lesion (hemorrhagic)
  duodenum K31.82
  esophagus K22.8
  intestine (colon) K63.81
  stomach K31.82
Difficult, difficulty (in)
  acculturation Z60.3
  feeding R63.3
    newborn P92.9
      breast P92.5
      specified NEC P92.8
    nonorganic (infant or child) F98.29
  intubation, in anesthesia T88.4 ☑
  mechanical, gastroduodenal stoma K91.89
    causing obstruction — *see also* Obstruction, intes-
      tine, postoperative K91.30
  micturition
    need to immediately re-void R39.191
    position dependent R39.192
    specified NEC R39.198
  reading (developmental) F81.0
    secondary to emotional disorders F93.9
  spelling (specific) F81.81
    with reading disorder F81.89
    due to inadequate teaching Z55.8

Difficult, difficulty — *continued*
- swallowing — *see* Dysphagia
- walking R26.2
- work
  - conditions NEC Z56.5
  - schedule Z56.3

Diffuse — *see* condition
Digestive — *see* condition
Dihydropyrimidine dehydrogenase disease (DPD) E88.89
Diktyoma — *see* Neoplasm, malignant, by site
Dilaceration, tooth K00.4
Dilatation
- anus K59.8
  - venule — *see* Hemorrhoids
- aorta (focal) (general) — *see* Ectasia, aorta
  - with aneuysm — *see* Aneurysm, aorta
  - congenital Q25.44
- artery — *see* Aneurysm
- bladder (sphincter) N32.89
  - congenital Q64.79
- blood vessel I99.8
- bronchial J47.9
  - with
    - exacerbation (acute) J47.1
    - lower respiratory infection J47.0
- calyx (due to obstruction) — *see* Hydronephrosis
- capillaries I78.8
- cardiac (acute) (chronic) — *see also* Hypertrophy, cardiac
  - congenital Q24.8
    - valve NEC Q24.8
      - pulmonary Q22.3
    - valve — *see* Endocarditis
- cavum septi pellucidi Q06.8
- cervix (uteri) — *see also* Incompetency, cervix
  - incomplete, poor, slow complicating delivery O62.0
- colon K59.39
  - congenital Q43.1
  - psychogenic F45.8
  - toxic K59.31
- common duct (acquired) K83.8
  - congenital Q44.5
- cystic duct (acquired) K82.8
  - congenital Q44.5
- duct, mammary — *see* Ectasia, mammary duct
- duodenum K59.8
- esophagus K22.8
  - congenital Q39.5
  - due to achalasia K22.0
- eustachian tube, congenital Q17.8
- gallbladder K82.8
- gastric — *see* Dilatation, stomach
- heart (acute) (chronic) — *see also* Hypertrophy, cardiac
  - congenital Q24.8
  - valve — *see* Endocarditis
- ileum K59.8
  - psychogenic F45.8
- jejunum K59.8
  - psychogenic F45.8
- kidney (calyx) (collecting structures) (cystic) (parenchyma) (pelvis) (idiopathic) N28.89
- lacrimal passages or duct — *see* Disorder, lacrimal system, changes
- lymphatic vessel I89.0
- mammary duct — *see* Ectasia, mammary duct
- Meckel's diverticulum (congenital) Q43.0
  - malignant — *see* Table of Neoplasms, small intestine, malignant
- myocardium (acute) (chronic) — *see* Hypertrophy, cardiac
- organ or site, congenital NEC — *see* Distortion
- pancreatic duct K86.89
- pericardium — *see* Pericarditis
- pharynx J39.2
- prostate N42.89
- pulmonary
  - artery (idiopathic) I28.8
  - valve, congenital Q22.3
- pupil H57.04
- rectum K59.39
- saccule, congenital Q16.5
- salivary gland (duct) K11.8
- sphincter ani K62.89
- stomach K31.89
  - acute K31.0
  - psychogenic F45.8
- submaxillary duct K11.8

Dilatation — *continued*
- trachea, congenital Q32.1
- ureter (idiopathic) N28.82
  - congenital Q62.2
  - due to obstruction N13.4
- urethra (acquired) N36.8
- vasomotor I73.9
- vein I86.8
- ventricular, ventricle (acute) (chronic) — *see also* Hypertrophy, cardiac
  - cerebral, congenital Q04.8
- venule NEC I86.8
- vesical orifice N32.89

Dilated, dilation — *see* Dilatation
Diminished, diminution
- hearing (acuity) — *see* Deafness
- sense or sensation (cold) (heat) (tactile) (vibratory) R20.8
- vision NEC H54.7
- vital capacity R94.2

Diminuta taenia B71.0
Dimitri-Sturge-Weber disease Q85.8
Dimple
- congenital sacral Q82.6
- parasacral Q82.6
- pilonidal or postanal — *see* Cyst, pilonidal

Dioctophyme renalis (infection) (infestation) B83.8
Dipetalonemiasis B74.4
Diphallus Q55.69
Diphtheria, diphtheritic (gangrenous) (hemorrhagic) A36.9
- carrier (suspected) Z22.2
- cutaneous A36.3
- faucial A36.0
- infection of wound A36.3
- laryngeal A36.2
- myocarditis A36.81
- nasal, anterior A36.89
- nasopharyngeal A36.1
- neurological complication A36.89
- pharyngeal A36.0
- specified site NEC A36.89
- tonsillar A36.0

Diphyllobothriasis (intestine) B70.0
- larval B70.1

Diplacusis H93.22- ☑
Diplegia (upper limbs) G83.0
- congenital (cerebral) G80.8
- facial G51.0
- lower limbs G82.20
- spastic G80.1

Diplococcus, diplococcal — *see* condition
Diplopia H53.2
Dipsomania F10.20
- with
  - psychosis — *see* Psychosis, alcoholic
  - remission F10.21

Dipylidiasis B71.1
DIRA (deficiency of interleukin 1 receptor antagonist) M04.8
Direction, teeth, abnormal, fully erupted M26.30
Dirofilariasis B74.8
Dirt-eating child F98.3
Disability, disabilities
- heart — *see* Disease, heart
- intellectual F79
  - with
    - autistic features F84.9
  - mild (I.Q. 50-69) F70
  - moderate (I.Q. 35-49) F71
  - profound (I.Q. under 20) F73
  - severe (I.Q. 20-34) F72
  - specified level NEC F78
- knowledge acquisition F81.9
- learning F81.9
- limiting activities Z73.6
- spelling, specific F81.81

Disappearance of family member Z63.4
Disarticulation — *see* Amputation
- meaning traumatic amputation — *see* Amputation, traumatic

Discharge (from)
- abnormal finding in — *see* Abnormal, specimen
- breast (female) (male) N64.52
- diencephalic autonomic idiopathic — *see* Epilepsy, specified NEC
- ear — *see also* Otorrhea
  - blood — *see* Otorrhagia

Discharge — *continued*
- excessive urine R35.8
- nipple N64.52
- penile R36.9
- postnasal R09.82
- prison, anxiety concerning Z65.2
- urethral R36.9
  - without blood R36.0
  - hematospermia R36.1
- vaginal N89.8

Discitis, diskitis M46.40
- cervical region M46.42
- cervicothoracic region M46.43
- lumbar region M46.46
- lumbosacral region M46.47
- multiple sites M46.49
- occipito-atlanto-axial region M46.41
- pyogenic — *see* Infection, intervertebral disc, pyogenic
- sacrococcygeal region M46.48
- thoracic region M46.44
- thoracolumbar region M46.45

Discoid
- meniscus (congenital) Q68.6
- semilunar cartilage (congenital) — *see* Derangement, knee, meniscus, specified NEC

Discoloration
- nails L60.8
- teeth (posteruptive) K03.7
  - during formation K00.8

Discomfort
- chest R07.89
- visual H53.14- ☑

Discontinuity, ossicles, ear H74.2- ☑
Discord (with)
- boss Z56.4
- classmates Z55.4
- counselor Z64.4
- employer Z56.4
- family Z63.8
- fellow employees Z56.4
- in-laws Z63.1
- landlord Z59.2
- lodgers Z59.2
- neighbors Z59.2
- probation officer Z64.4
- social worker Z64.4
- teachers Z55.4
- workmates Z56.4

Discordant connection
- atrioventricular (congenital) Q20.5
- ventriculoarterial Q20.3

Discrepancy
- centric occlusion maximum intercuspation M26.55
- leg length (acquired) — *see* Deformity, limb, unequal length
  - congenital — *see* Defect, reduction, lower limb
- uterine size date O26.84- ☑

Discrimination
- ethnic Z60.5
- political Z60.5
- racial Z60.5
- religious Z60.5
- sex Z60.5

Disease, diseased — *see also* Syndrome
- absorbent system I87.8
- acid-peptic K30
- Acosta's T70.29 ☑
- Adams-Stokes (-Morgagni) (syncope with heart block) I45.9
- Addison's anemia (pernicious) D51.0
- adenoids (and tonsils) J35.9
- adrenal (capsule) (cortex) (gland) (medullary) E27.9
  - hyperfunction E27.0
  - specified NEC E27.8
- ainhum L94.6
- airway
  - obstructive, chronic J44.9
    - due to
      - cotton dust J66.0
      - specific organic dusts NEC J66.8
  - reactive — *see* Asthma
- akamushi (scrub typhus) A75.3
- Albers-Schönberg (marble bones) Q78.2
- Albert's — *see* Tendinitis, Achilles
- alimentary canal K63.9
- alligator-skin Q80.9
  - acquired L85.0
- alpha heavy chain C88.3

Disease, diseased — *continued*
- alpine T70.29 ☑
- altitude T70.20 ☑
- alveolar ridge
  - edentulous K06.9
    - specified NEC K06.8
- alveoli, teeth K08.9
- Alzheimer's G30.9 *[F02.80]*
  - with behavioral disturbance G30.9 *[F02.81]*
  - early onset G30.0 *[F02.80]*
    - with behavioral disturbance G30.0 *[F02.81]*
  - late onset G30.1 *[F02.80]*
    - with behavioral disturbance G30.1 *[F02.81]*
  - specified NEC G30.8 *[F02.80]*
    - with behavioral disturbance G30.8 *[F02.81]*
- amyloid — *see* Amyloidosis
- Andersen's (glycogenosis IV) E74.09
- Andes T70.29 ☑
- Andrews' (bacterid) L08.89
- angiospastic I73.9
  - cerebral G45.9
  - vein I87.8
- anterior
  - chamber H21.9
  - horn cell G12.29
- antiglomerular basement membrane (anti- GBM) anti-body M31.0
  - tubulo-interstitial nephritis N12
- antral — *see* Sinusitis, maxillary
- anus K62.9
  - specified NEC K62.89
- aorta (nonsyphilitic) I77.9
  - syphilitic NEC A52.02
- aortic (heart) (valve) I35.9
  - rheumatic I06.9
- Apollo B30.3
- aponeuroses — *see* Enthesopathy
- appendix K38.9
  - specified NEC K38.8
- aqueous (chamber) H21.9
- Arnold-Chiari — *see* Arnold-Chiari disease
- arterial I77.9
  - occlusive — *see* Occlusion, by site
    - due to stricture or stenosis I77.1
  - peripheral I73.9
- arteriocardiorenal — *see* Hypertension, cardiorenal
- arteriolar (generalized) (obliterative) I77.9
- arteriorenal — *see* Hypertension, kidney
- arteriosclerotic — *see also* Arteriosclerosis
  - cardiovascular — *see* Disease, heart, ischemic, atherosclerotic
  - coronary (artery) — *see* Disease, heart, ischemic, atherosclerotic
  - heart — *see* Disease, heart, ischemic, atherosclerotic
- artery I77.9
  - cerebral I67.9
  - coronary I25.10
    - with angina pectoris — *see* Arteriosclerosis, coronary (artery)
  - peripheral I73.9
- arthropod-borne NOS (viral) A94
  - specified type NEC A93.8
- atticoantral, chronic H66.20
  - left H66.22
    - with right H66.23
  - right H66.21
    - with left H66.23
- auditory canal — *see* Disorder, ear, external
- auricle, ear NEC — *see* Disorder, pinna
- Australian X A83.4
- autoimmune (systemic) NOS M35.9
  - hemolytic (cold type) (warm type) D59.1
    - drug-induced D59.0
  - thyroid E06.3
- autoinflammatory M04.9
  - NOD2-associated M04.8
  - specified type NEC M04.8
- aviator's — *see* Effect, adverse, high altitude
- Ayerza's (pulmonary artery sclerosis with pulmonary hypertension) I27.0
- Babington's (familial hemorrhagic telangiectasia) I78.0
- bacterial A49.9
  - specified NEC A48.8
  - zoonotic A28.9
    - specified type NEC A28.8
- Baelz's (cheilitis glandularis apostematosa) K13.0
- bagasse J67.1
- balloon — *see* Effect, adverse, high altitude

Disease, diseased — *continued*
- Bang's (brucella abortus) A23.1
- Bannister's T78.3 ☑
- barometer makers' — *see* Poisoning, mercury
- Barraquer (-Simons') (progressive lipodystrophy) E88.1
- Barrett's — *see* Barrett's, esophagus
- Bartholin's gland N75.9
- basal ganglia G25.9
  - degenerative G23.9
    - specified NEC G23.8
  - specified NEC G25.89
- Basedow's (exophthalmic goiter) — *see* Hyperthyroidism, with, goiter (diffuse)
- Bateman's B08.1
- Batten-Steinert G71.11
- Battey A31.0
- Beard's (neurasthenia) F48.8
- Becker
  - idiopathic mural endomyocardial I42.3
  - myotonia congenita G71.12
- Begbie's (exophthalmic goiter) — *see* Hyperthyroidism, with, goiter (diffuse)
- behavioral, organic F07.9
- Beigel's (white piedra) B36.2
- Benson's — *see* Deposit, crystalline
- Bernard-Soulier (thrombopathy) D69.1
- Bernhardt (-Roth) — *see* Mononeuropathy, lower limb, meralgia paresthetica
- Biermer's (pernicious anemia) D51.0
- bile duct (common) (hepatic) K83.9
  - with calculus, stones — *see* Calculus, bile duct
  - specified NEC K83.8
- biliary (tract) K83.9
  - specified NEC K83.8
- Billroth's — *see* Spina bifida
- bird fancier's J67.2
- black lung J60
- bladder N32.9
  - in (due to)
    - schistosomiasis (bilharziasis) B65.0 *[N33]*
  - specified NEC N32.89
- bleeder's D66
- blood D75.9
  - forming organs D75.9
  - vessel I99.9
- Bloodgood's — *see* Mastopathy, cystic
- Bodechtel-Guttmann (subacute sclerosing panen-cephalitis) A81.1
- bone — *see also* Disorder, bone
  - aluminum M83.4
  - fibrocystic NEC
    - jaw M27.49
- bone-marrow D75.9
- Borna A83.9
- Bornholm (epidemic pleurodynia) B33.0
- Bouchard's (myopathic dilatation of the stomach) K31.0
- Bouillaud's (rheumatic heart disease) I01.9
- Bourneville (-Brissaud) (tuberous sclerosis) Q85.1
- Bouveret (-Hoffmann) (paroxysmal tachycardia) I47.9
- bowel K63.9
  - functional K59.9
    - psychogenic F45.8
- brain G93.9
  - arterial, artery I67.9
  - arteriosclerotic I67.2
  - congenital Q04.9
  - degenerative — *see* Degeneration, brain
  - inflammatory — *see* Encephalitis
  - organic G93.9
    - arteriosclerotic I67.2
  - parasitic NEC B71.9 *[G94]*
  - senile NEC G31.1
  - specified NEC G93.89
- breast — *see also* Disorder, breast N64.9
  - cystic (chronic) — *see* Mastopathy, cystic
  - fibrocystic — *see* Mastopathy, cystic
  - Paget's
    - female, unspecified side C50.91- ☑
    - male, unspecified side C50.92- ☑
  - specified NEC N64.89
- Breda's — *see* Yaws
- Bretonneau's (diphtheritic malignant angina) A36.0
- Bright's — *see* Nephritis
  - arteriosclerotic — *see* Hypertension, kidney
- Brill's (recrudescent typhus) A75.1
- Brill-Zinsser (recrudescent typhus) A75.1
- Brion-Kayser — *see* Fever, paratyphoid

Disease, diseased — *continued*
- broad
  - beta E78.2
  - ligament (noninflammatory) N83.9
    - inflammatory — *see* Disease, pelvis, inflammatory
    - specified NEC N83.8
- Brocq-Duhring (dermatitis herpetiformis) L13.0
- Brocq's
  - meaning
    - dermatitis herpetiformis L13.0
    - prurigo L28.2
- bronchopulmonary J98.4
- bronchus NEC J98.09
- bronze Addison's E27.1
  - tuberculous A18.7
- budgerigar fancier's J67.2
- Buerger's (thromboangiitis obliterans) I73.1
- bullous L13.9
  - chronic of childhood L12.2
  - specified NEC L13.8
- Bürger-Grütz (essential familial hyperlipemia) E78.3
- bursa — *see* Bursopathy
- caisson T70.3 ☑
- California — *see* Coccidioidomycosis
- capillaries I78.9
  - specified NEC I78.8
- Carapata A68.0
- cardiac — *see* Disease, heart
- cardiopulmonary, chronic I27.9
- cardiorenal (hepatic) (hypertensive) (vascular) — *see* Hypertension, cardiorenal
- cardiovascular (atherosclerotic) I25.10
  - with angina pectoris — *see* Arteriosclerosis, coronary (artery),
  - congenital Q28.9
  - hypertensive — *see* Hypertension, heart
  - newborn P29.9
    - specified NEC P29.89
  - renal (hypertensive) — *see* Hypertension, cardiorenal
  - syphilitic (asymptomatic) A52.00
- cartilage — *see* Disorder, cartilage
- Castellani's A69.8
- Castleman (unicentric) (multicentric) D47.Z2
  - HHV-8-associated — *see also* Herpesvirus, human, 8 D47.Z2
- cat-scratch A28.1
- Cavare's (familial periodic paralysis) G72.3
- cecum K63.9
- celiac (adult) (infantile) (with steatorrhea) K90.0
- cellular tissue L98.9
- central core G71.2
- cerebellar, cerebellum — *see* Disease, brain
- cerebral — *see also* Disease, brain
  - degenerative — *see* Degeneration, brain
- cerebrospinal G96.9
- cerebrovascular I67.9
  - acute I67.89
    - embolic I63.4- ☑
    - thrombotic I63.3- ☑
  - arteriosclerotic I67.2
  - hereditary NEC I67.858
  - specified NEC I67.89
- cervix (uteri) (noninflammatory) N88.9
  - inflammatory — *see* Cervicitis
  - specified NEC N88.8
- Chabert's A22.9
- Chandler's (osteochondritis dissecans, hip) — *see* Osteochondritis, dissecans, hip
- Charlouis — *see* Yaws
- Chédiak-Steinbrinck (-Higashi) (congenital gigantism of peroxidase granules) E70.330
- chest J98.9
- Chiari's (hepatic vein thrombosis) I82.0
- Chicago B40.9
- Chignon B36.8
- chigo, chigoe B88.1
- childhood granulomatous D71
- Chinese liver fluke B66.1
- chlamydial A74.9
  - specified NEC A74.89
- cholecystic K82.9
- choroid H31.9
  - specified NEC H31.8
- Christmas D67
- chronic bullous of childhood L12.2
- chylomicron retention E78.3

Disease, diseased — *continued*
- ciliary body H21.9
  - specified NEC H21.89
- circulatory (system) NEC I99.8
  - newborn P29.9
  - syphilitic A52.00
    - congenital A50.54
- coagulation factor deficiency (congenital) — *see* Defect, coagulation
- coccidioidal — *see* Coccidioidomycosis
- cold
  - agglutinin or hemoglobinuria D59.1
    - paroxysmal D59.6
  - hemagglutinin (chronic) D59.1
- collagen NOS (nonvascular) (vascular) M35.9
  - specified NEC M35.8
- colon K63.9
  - functional K59.9
    - congenital Q43.2
  - ischemic — *see also* Ischemia, intestine, acute K55.039
- colonic inflammatory bowel, unclassified (IBDU) K52.3
- combined system — *see* Degeneration, combined
- compressed air T70.3 ☑
- Concato's (pericardial polyserositis) A19.9
  - nontubercular I31.1
  - pleural — *see* Pleurisy, with effusion
- conjunctiva H11.9
  - chlamydial A74.0
  - specified NEC H11.89
  - viral B30.9
    - specified NEC B30.8
- connective tissue, systemic (diffuse) M35.9
  - in (due to)
    - hypogammaglobulinemia D80.1 *[M36.8]*
    - ochronosis E70.29 *[M36.8]*
  - specified NEC M35.8
- Conor and Bruch's (boutonneuse fever) A77.1
- Cooper's — *see* Mastopathy, cystic
- Cori's (glycogenosis III) E74.03
- corkhandler's or corkworker's J67.3
- cornea H18.9
  - specified NEC H18.89- ☑
- coronary (artery) — *see* Disease, heart, ischemic, atherosclerotic
  - congenital Q24.5
  - ostial, syphilitic (aortic) (mitral) (pulmonary) A52.03
- corpus cavernosum N48.9
  - specified NEC N48.89
- Cotugno's — *see* Sciatica
- coxsackie (virus) NEC B34.1
- cranial nerve NOS G52.9
- Creutzfeldt-Jakob — *see* Creutzfeldt-Jakob disease or syndrome
- Crocq's (acrocyanosis) I73.89
- Crohn's — *see* Enteritis, regional
- Curschmann G71.11
- cystic
  - breast (chronic) — *see* Mastopathy, cystic
  - kidney, congenital Q61.9
  - liver, congenital Q44.6
  - lung J98.4
    - congenital Q33.0
- cytomegalic inclusion (generalized) B25.9
  - with pneumonia B25.0
  - congenital P35.1
- cytomegaloviral B25.9
  - specified NEC B25.8
- Czerny's (periodic hydrarthrosis of the knee) — *see* Effusion, joint, knee
- Daae (-Finsen) (epidemic pleurodynia) B33.0
- Darling's — *see* Histoplasmosis capsulati
- de Quervain's (tendon sheath) M65.4
  - thyroid (subacute granulomatous thyroiditis) E06.1
- deer fly — *see* Tularemia
- Degos' I77.89
- demyelinating, demyelinizating (nervous system) G37.9
  - multiple sclerosis G35
  - specified NEC G37.8
- dense deposit — *see also* N00-N07 with fourth character .6 N05.6
- deposition, hydroxyapatite — *see* Disease, hydroxyapatite deposition
- Devergie's (pityriasis rubra pilaris) L44.0
- Devic's G36.0
- diaphorase deficiency D74.0
- diaphragm J98.6

Disease, diseased — *continued*
- diarrheal, infectious NEC A09
- digestive system K92.9
  - specified NEC K92.89
- disc, degenerative — *see* Degeneration, intervertebral disc
- discogenic — *see also* Displacement, intervertebral disc NEC
  - with myelopathy — *see* Disorder, disc, with, myelopathy
- diverticular — *see* Diverticula
- Dubois (thymus) A50.59 *[E35]*
- Duchenne-Griesinger G71.01
- ductless glands E34.9
- Duchenne's
  - muscular dystrophy G71.01
  - pseudohypertrophy, muscles G71.01
- Duhring's (dermatitis herpetiformis) L13.0
- duodenum K31.9
  - specified NEC K31.89
- Dupré's (meningism) R29.1
- Dupuytren's (muscle contracture) M72.0
- Durand-Nicholas-Favre (climatic bubo) A55
- Duroziez's (congenital mitral stenosis) Q23.2
- ear — *see* Disorder, ear
- Eberth's — *see* Fever, typhoid
- Ebola (virus) A98.4
- Ebstein's heart Q22.5
- Echinococcus — *see* Echinococcus
- echovirus NEC B34.1
- Eddowes' (brittle bones and blue sclera) Q78.0
- edentulous (alveolar) ridge K06.9
  - specified NEC K06.8
- Edsall's T67.2 ☑
- Eichstedt's (pityriasis versicolor) B36.0
- Eisenmenger's (irreversible) I27.83
- Ellis-van Creveld (chondroectodermal dysplasia) Q77.6
- end stage renal (ESRD) N18.6
  - due to hypertension I12.0
- endocrine glands or system NEC E34.9
- endomyocardial (eosinophilic) I42.3
- English (rickets) E55.0
- enteroviral, enterovirus NEC B34.1
  - central nervous system NEC A88.8
- epidemic B99.9
  - specified NEC B99.8
- epididymis N50.9
- Erb (-Landouzy) G71.02
- Erdheim-Chester (ECD) E88.89
- esophagus K22.9
  - functional K22.4
  - psychogenic F45.8
  - specified NEC K22.8
- Eulenburg's (congenital paramyotonia) G71.19
- eustachian tube — *see* Disorder, eustachian tube
- external
  - auditory canal — *see* Disorder, ear, external
  - ear — *see* Disorder, ear, external
- extrapyramidal G25.9
  - specified NEC G25.89
- eye H57.9
  - anterior chamber H21.9
  - inflammatory NEC H57.89
  - muscle (external) — *see* Strabismus
  - specified NEC H57.89
  - syphilitic — *see* Oculopathy, syphilitic
- eyeball H44.9
  - specified NEC H44.89
- eyelid — *see* Disorder, eyelid
  - specified NEC — *see* Disorder, eyelid, specified type NEC
- eyeworm of Africa B74.3
- facial nerve (seventh) G51.9
  - newborn (birth injury) P11.3
- Fahr (of brain) G23.8
- Fahr Volhard (of kidney) I12.- ☑
- fallopian tube (noninflammatory) N83.9
  - inflammatory — *see* Salpingo-oophoritis
  - specified NEC N83.8
- familial periodic paralysis G72.3
- Fanconi's (congenital pancytopenia) D61.09
- fascia NEC — *see also* Disorder, muscle
  - inflammatory — *see* Myositis
  - specified NEC M62.89
- Fauchard's (periodontitis) — *see* Periodontitis
- Favre-Durand-Nicolas (climatic bubo) A55
- Fede's K14.0
- Feer's — *see* Poisoning, mercury

Disease, diseased — *continued*
- female pelvic inflammatory — *see also* Disease, pelvis, inflammatory N73.9
  - syphilitic (secondary) A51.42
  - tuberculous A18.17
- Fernels' (aortic aneurysm) I71.9
- fibrocaseous of lung — *see* Tuberculosis, pulmonary
- fibrocystic — *see* Fibrocystic disease
- Fiedler's (leptospiral jaundice) A27.0
- fifth B08.3
- file-cutter's — *see* Poisoning, lead
- fish-skin Q80.9
  - acquired L85.0
- Flajani (-Basedow) (exophthalmic goiter) — *see* Hyperthyroidism, with, goiter (diffuse)
- flax-dresser's J66.1
- fluke — *see* Infestation, fluke
- foot and mouth B08.8
- foot process N04.9
- Forbes' (glycogenosis III) E74.03
- Fordyce-Fox (apocrine miliaria) L75.2
- Fordyce's (ectopic sebaceous glands) (mouth) Q38.6
- Forestier's (rhizomelic pseudopolyarthritis) M35.3
  - meaning ankylosing hyperostosis — *see* Hyperostosis, ankylosing
- Fothergill's
  - neuralgia — *see* Neuralgia, trigeminal
  - scarlatina anginosa A38.9
- Fournier (gangrene) N49.3
  - female N76.89
- fourth B08.8
- Fox (-Fordyce) (apocrine miliaria) L75.2
- Francis' — *see* Tularemia
- Franklin C88.2
- Frei's (climatic bubo) A55
- Friedreich's
  - combined systemic or ataxia G11.1
  - myoclonia G25.3
- frontal sinus — *see* Sinusitis, frontal
- fungus NEC B49
- Gaisböck's (polycythemia hypertonica) D75.1
- gallbladder K82.9
  - calculus — *see* Calculus, gallbladder
  - cholecystitis — *see* Cholecystitis
  - cholesterolosis K82.4
  - fistula — *see* Fistula, gallbladder
  - hydrops K82.1
  - obstruction — *see* Obstruction, gallbladder
  - perforation K82.2
  - specified NEC K82.8
- gamma heavy chain C88.2
- Gamna's (siderotic splenomegaly) D73.2
- Gamstorp's (adynamia episodica hereditaria) G72.3
- Gandy-Nanta (siderotic splenomegaly) D73.2
- ganister J62.8
- gastric — *see* Disease, stomach
- gastroesophageal reflux (GERD) K21.9
  - with esophagitis K21.0
- gastrointestinal (tract) K92.9
  - amyloid E85.4
  - functional K59.9
    - psychogenic F45.8
  - specified NEC K92.89
- Gee (-Herter) (-Heubner) (-Thaysen) (nontropical sprue) K90.0
- genital organs
  - female N94.9
  - male N50.9
- Gerhardt's (erythromelalgia) I73.81
- Gibert's (pityriasis rosea) L42
- Gierke's (glycogenosis I) E74.01
- Gilles de la Tourette's (motor-verbal tic) F95.2
- gingiva K06.9
  - plaque induced K05.00
  - specified NEC K06.8
- gland (lymph) I89.9
- Glanzmann's (hereditary hemorrhagic thrombasthenia) D69.1
- glass-blower's (cataract) — *see* Cataract, specified NEC
- salivary gland hypertrophy K11.1
- Glisson's — *see* Rickets
- globe H44.9
  - specified NEC H44.89
- glomerular — *see also* Glomerulonephritis
  - with edema — *see* Nephrosis
  - acute — *see* Nephritis, acute
  - chronic — *see* Nephritis, chronic
  - minimal change N05.0

Disease, diseased — *continued*

glomerular — *see also* Glomerulonephritis — *continued*
    rapidly progressive NØ1.9
glycogen storage E74.ØØ
    Andersen's E74.Ø9
    Cori's E74.Ø3
    Forbes' E74.Ø3
    generalized E74.ØØ
    glucose-6-phosphatase deficiency E74.Ø1
    heart E74.Ø2 *[143]*
    hepatorenal E74.Ø9
    Hers' E74.Ø9
    liver and kidney E74.Ø9
    McArdle's E74.Ø4
    muscle phosphofructokinase E74.Ø9
    myocardium E74.Ø2 *[143]*
    Pompe's E74.Ø2
    Tauri's E74.Ø9
    type Ø E74.Ø9
    type I E74.Ø1
    type II E74.Ø2
    type III E74.Ø3
    type IV E74.Ø9
    type V E74.Ø4
    type VI-XI E74.Ø9
    Von Gierke's E74.Ø1
Goldstein's (familial hemorrhagic telangiectasia) I78.Ø
gonococcal NOS A54.9
graft-versus-host (GVH) D89.813
    acute D89.81Ø
    acute on chronic D89.812
    chronic D89.811
grainhandler's J67.8
granulomatous (childhood) (chronic) D71
Graves' (exophthalmic goiter) — *see* Hyperthyroidism, with, goiter (diffuse)
Griesinger's — *see* Ancylostomiasis
Grisel's M43.6
Gruby's (tinea tonsurans) B35.Ø
Guillain-Barré G61.Ø
Guinon's (motor-verbal tic) F95.2
gum KØ6.9
gynecological N94.9
H (Hartnup's) E72.Ø2
Haff — *see* Poisoning, mercury
Hageman (congenital factor XII deficiency) D68.2
hair (color) (shaft) L67.9
    follicles L73.9
        specified NEC L73.8
Hamman's (spontaneous mediastinal emphysema) J98.2
hand, foot and mouth BØ8.4
Hansen's — *see* Leprosy
Hantavirus, with pulmonary manifestations B33.4
    with renal manifestations A98.5
Harada's H3Ø.81- ☑
Hartnup (pellagra-cerebellar ataxia-renal aminoaciduria) E72.Ø2
Hart's (pellagra-cerebellar ataxia-renal aminoaciduria) E72.Ø2
Hashimoto's (struma lymphomatosa) EØ6.3
Hb — *see* Disease, hemoglobin
heart (organic) I51.9
    with
        pulmonary edema (acute) — *see also* Failure, ventricular, left I5Ø.1
        rheumatic fever (conditions in IØØ)
            active IØ1.9
                with chorea IØ2.Ø
                specified NEC IØ1.8
           inactive or quiescent (with chorea) IØ9.9
              specified NEC IØ9.89
    amyloid E85.4 *[143]*
    aortic (valve) I35.9
    arteriosclerotic or sclerotic (senile) — *see* Disease, heart, ischemic, atherosclerotic
    artery, arterial — *see* Disease, heart, ischemic, atherosclerotic
    beer drinkers' I42.6
    beriberi (wet) E51.12
    black I27.Ø
    congenital Q24.9
        cyanotic Q24.9
        specified NEC Q24.8
    coronary — *see* Disease, heart, ischemic
    cryptogenic I51.9
    fibroid — *see* Myocarditis

Disease, diseased — *continued*

heart — *continued*
    functional I51.89
        psychogenic F45.8
    glycogen storage E74.Ø2 *[143]*
    gonococcal A54.83
    hypertensive — *see* Hypertension, heart
    hyperthyroid — *see also* Hyperthyroidism EØ5.9Ø *[143]*
        with thyroid storm EØ5.91 *[143]*
    ischemic (chronic or with a stated duration of over 4 weeks) I25.9
        atherosclerotic (of) I25.1Ø
            with angina pectoris — *see* Arteriosclerosis, coronary (artery)
            coronary artery bypass graft — *see* Arteriosclerosis, coronary (artery),
        cardiomyopathy I25.5
        diagnosed on ECG or other special investigation, but currently presenting no symptoms I25.6
        silent I25.6
        specified form NEC I25.89
    kyphoscoliotic I27.1
    meningococcal A39.5Ø
        endocarditis A39.51
        myocarditis A39.52
        pericarditis A39.53
    mitral IØ5.9
        specified NEC IØ5.8
    muscular — *see* Degeneration, myocardial
    psychogenic (functional) F45.8
    pulmonary (chronic) I27.9
        in schistosomiasis B65.9 *[152]*
        specified NEC I27.89
    rheumatic (chronic) (inactive) (old) (quiescent) (with chorea) IØ9.9
        active or acute IØ1.9
            with chorea (acute) (rheumatic) (Sydenham's) IØ2.Ø
        specified NEC IØ9.89
    senile — *see* Myocarditis
    syphilitic A52.Ø6
        aortic A52.Ø3
            aneurysm A52.Ø1
        congenital A5Ø.54 *[152]*
    thyrotoxic — *see also* Thyrotoxicosis EØ5.9Ø *[143]*
        with thyroid storm EØ5.91 *[143]*
    valve, valvular (obstructive) (regurgitant) — *see also* Endocarditis
        congenital NEC Q24.8
            pulmonary Q22.3
    vascular — *see* Disease, cardiovascular
heavy chain NEC C88.2
    alpha C88.3
    gamma C88.2
    mu C88.2
Hebra's
    pityriasis
        maculata et circinata L42
        rubra pilaris L44.Ø
    prurigo L28.2
hematopoietic organs D75.9
hemoglobin or Hb
    abnormal (mixed) NEC D58.2
        with thalassemia D56.9
    AS genotype D57.3
    Bart's D56.Ø
    C (Hb-C) D58.2
        with other abnormal hemoglobin NEC D58.2
        elliptocytosis D58.1
        Hb-S D57.2- ☑
        sickle-cell D57.2- ☑
        thalassemia D56.8
    Constant Spring D58.2
    D (Hb-D) D58.2
    E (Hb-E) D58.2
    E-beta thalassemia D56.5
    elliptocytosis D58.1
    H (Hb-H) (thalassemia) D56.Ø
        with other abnormal hemoglobin NEC D56.9
        Constant Spring D56.Ø
    I thalassemia D56.9
    M D74.Ø
    S or SS D57.1
    SC D57.2- ☑
    SD D57.8- ☑
    SE D57.8- ☑

Disease, diseased — *continued*

hemoglobin or Hb — *continued*
    spherocytosis D58.Ø
    unstable, hemolytic D58.2
hemolytic (newborn) P55.9
    autoimmune (cold type) (warm type) D59.1
    drug-induced D59.Ø
    due to or with
        incompatibility
            ABO (blood group) P55.1
            blood (group) (Duffy) (K) (Kell) (Kidd) (Lewis) (M) (S) NEC P55.8
            Rh (blood group) (factor) P55.Ø
            Rh negative mother P55.Ø
    specified type NEC P55.8
    unstable hemoglobin D58.2
hemorrhagic D69.9
    newborn P53
Henoch (-Schönlein) (purpura nervosa) D69.Ø
hepatic — *see* Disease, liver
hepatolenticular E83.Ø1
heredodegenerative NEC
    spinal cord G95.89
herpesviral, disseminated BØØ.7
Hers' (glycogenosis VI) E74.Ø9
Herter (-Gee) (-Heubner) (nontropical sprue) K9Ø.Ø
Heubner-Herter (nontropical sprue) K9Ø.Ø
high fetal gene or hemoglobin thalassemia D56.9
Hildenbrand's — *see* Typhus
hip (joint) M25.9
    congenital Q65.89
    suppurative MØØ.9
    tuberculous A18.Ø2
His (-Werner) (trench fever) A79.Ø
Hodgson's I71.2
    ruptured I71.1
Holla — *see* Spherocytosis
hookworm B76.9
    specified NEC B76.8
host-versus-graft D89.813
    acute D89.81Ø
    acute on chronic D89.812
    chronic D89.811
human immunodeficiency virus (HIV) B2Ø
Huntington's G1Ø
    with dementia G1Ø *[FØ2.8Ø]*
Hutchinson's (cheiropompholyx) — *see* Hutchinson's disease
hyaline (diffuse) (generalized)
    membrane (lung) (newborn) P22.Ø
        adult J8Ø
hydatid — *see* Echinococcus
hydroxyapatite deposition M11.ØØ
    ankle M11.Ø7- ☑
    elbow M11.Ø2- ☑
    foot joint M11.Ø7- ☑
    hand joint M11.Ø4- ☑
    hip M11.Ø5- ☑
    knee M11.Ø6- ☑
    multiple site M11.Ø9
    shoulder M11.Ø1- ☑
    vertebra M11.Ø8
    wrist M11.Ø3- ☑
hyperkinetic — *see* Hyperkinesia
hypertensive — *see* Hypertension
hypophysis E23.7
Iceland G93.3
I-cell E77.Ø
immune D89.9
immunoproliferative (malignant) C88.9
    small intestinal C88.3
    specified NEC C88.8
inclusion B25.9
    salivary gland B25.9
infectious, infective B99.9
    congenital P37.9
        specified NEC P37.8
        viral P35.9
            specified type NEC P35.8
    specified NEC B99.8
inflammatory
    penis N48.29
        abscess N48.21
        cellulitis N48.22
    prepuce N47.7
        balanoposthitis N47.6
    tubo-ovarian — *see* Salpingo-oophoritis
intervertebral disc — *see also* Disorder, disc

Disease, diseased — *continued*
  intervertebral disc — *see also* Disorder, disc — *continued*
    with myelopathy — *see* Disorder, disc, with, myelopathy
    cervical, cervicothoracic — *see* Disorder, disc, cervical
      with
        myelopathy — *see* Disorder, disc, cervical, with myelopathy
        neuritis, radiculitis or radiculopathy — *see* Disorder, disc, cervical, with neuritis
        specified NEC — *see* Disorder, disc, cervical, specified type NEC
    lumbar (with)
      myelopathy M51.06
      neuritis, radiculitis, radiculopathy or sciatica M51.16
      specified NEC M51.86
    lumbosacral (with)
      neuritis, radiculitis, radiculopathy or sciatica M51.17
      specified NEC M51.87
    specified NEC — *see* Disorder, disc, specified NEC
    thoracic (with)
      myelopathy M51.04
      neuritis, radiculitis or radiculopathy M51.14
      specified NEC M51.84
    thoracolumbar (with)
      myelopathy M51.05
      neuritis, radiculitis or radiculopathy M51.15
      specified NEC M51.85
  intestine K63.9
    functional K59.9
      psychogenic F45.8
      specified NEC K59.8
    organic K63.9
    protozoal A07.9
    specified NEC K63.89
  iris H21.9
    specified NEC H21.89
  iron metabolism or storage E83.10
  island (scrub typhus) A75.3
  itai-itai — *see* Poisoning, cadmium
  Jakob-Creutzfeldt — *see* Creutzfeldt-Jakob disease or syndrome
  jaw M27.9
    fibrocystic M27.49
    specified NEC M27.8
  jigger B88.1
  joint — *see also* Disorder, joint
    Charcot's — *see* Arthropathy, neuropathic (Charcot)
    degenerative — *see* Osteoarthritis
      multiple M15.9
      spine — *see* Spondylosis
    hypertrophic — *see* Osteoarthritis
    sacroiliac M53.3
    specified NEC — *see* Disorder, joint, specified type NEC
    spine NEC — *see* Dorsopathy
    suppurative — *see* Arthritis, pyogenic or pyemic
  Jourdain's (acute gingivitis) K05.00
    nonplaque induced K05.01
    plaque induced K05.00
  Kaschin-Beck (endemic polyarthritis) M12.10
    ankle M12.17- ☑
    elbow M12.12- ☑
    foot joint M12.17- ☑
    hand joint M12.14- ☑
    hip M12.15- ☑
    knee M12.16- ☑
    multiple site M12.19
    shoulder M12.11- ☑
    vertebra M12.18
    wrist M12.13- ☑
  Katayama B65.2
  Kedani (scrub typhus) A75.3
  Keshan E59
  kidney (functional) (pelvis) N28.9
    chronic N18.9
      hypertensive — *see* Hypertension, kidney
      stage 1 N18.1
      stage 2 (mild) N18.2
      stage 3 (moderate) N18.3
      stage 4 (severe) N18.4
      stage 5 N18.5
    complicating pregnancy — *see* Pregnancy, complicated by, renal disease

Disease, diseased — *continued*
  kidney — *continued*
    cystic (congenital) Q61.9
    fibrocystic (congenital) Q61.8
    hypertensive — *see* Hypertension, kidney
    in (due to)
      schistosomiasis (bilharziasis) B65.9 *[N29]*
    multicystic Q61.4
    polycystic Q61.3
      adult type Q61.2
      childhood type NEC Q61.19
        collecting duct dilatation Q61.11
  Kimmelstiel (-Wilson) (intercapillary polycystic (congenital) glomerulosclerosis) — *see* E08-E13 with .21
  Kinnier Wilson's (hepatolenticular degeneration) E83.01
  kissing — *see* Mononucleosis, infectious
  Klebs' — *see also* Glomerulonephritis N05- ☑
  Klippel-Feil (brevicollis) Q76.1
  Köhler-Pellegrini-Stieda (calcification, knee joint) — *see* Bursitis, tibial collateral
  Kok Q89.8
  König's (osteochondritis dissecans) — *see* Osteochondritis, dissecans
  Korsakoff's (nonalcoholic) F04
    alcoholic F10.96
      with dependence F10.26
  Kostmann's (infantile genetic agranulocytosis) D70.0
  kuru A81.81
  Kyasanur Forest A98.2
  labyrinth, ear — *see* Disorder, ear, inner
  lacrimal system — *see* Disorder, lacrimal system
  Lafora's — *see* Epilepsy, generalized, idiopathic
  Lancereaux-Mathieu (leptospiral jaundice) A27.0
  Landry's G61.0
  Larrey-Weil (leptospiral jaundice) A27.0
  larynx J38.7
  legionnaires' A48.1
    nonpneumonic A48.2
  Lenegre's I44.2
  lens H27.9
    specified NEC H27.8
  Lev's (acquired complete heart block) I44.2
  Lewy body (dementia) G31.83 *[F02.80]*
    with behavioral disturbance G31.83 *[F02.81]*
  Lichtheim's (subacute combined sclerosis with pernicious anemia) D51.0
  Lightwood's (renal tubular acidosis) N25.89
  Lignac's (cystinosis) E72.04
  lip K13.0
  lipid-storage E75.6
    specified NEC E75.5
  Lipschütz's N76.6
  liver (chronic) (organic) K76.9
    alcoholic (chronic) K70.9
      acute — *see* Disease, liver, alcoholic, hepatitis
      cirrhosis K70.30
        with ascites K70.31
      failure K70.40
        with coma K70.41
      fatty liver K70.0
      fibrosis K70.2
      hepatitis K70.10
        with ascites K70.11
      sclerosis K70.2
    cystic, congenital Q44.6
    drug-induced (idiosyncratic) (toxic) (predictable) (unpredictable) — *see* Disease, liver, toxic
    end stage K72.90
      due to hepatitis — *see* Hepatitis
    fatty, nonalcoholic (NAFLD) K76.0
      alcoholic K70.0
    fibrocystic (congenital) Q44.6
    fluke
      Chinese B66.1
      oriental B66.1
      sheep B66.3
    gestational alloimmune (GALD) P78.84
    glycogen storage E74.09 *[K77]*
    in (due to)
      schistosomiasis (bilharziasis) B65.9 *[K77]*
    inflammatory K75.9
      alcoholic K70.1 ☑
      specified NEC K75.89
    polycystic (congenital) Q44.6
    toxic K71.9
      with
        cholestasis K71.0
        cirrhosis (liver) K71.7

Disease, diseased — *continued*
  liver — *continued*
    toxic — *continued*
      with — *continued*
        fibrosis (liver) K71.7
        focal nodular hyperplasia K71.8
        hepatic granuloma K71.8
        hepatic necrosis K71.10
          with coma K71.11
        hepatitis NEC K71.6
          acute K71.2
          chronic
            active K71.50
              with ascites K71.51
            lobular K71.4
            persistent K71.3
          lupoid K71.50
            with ascites K71.51
        peliosis hepatis K71.8
        veno-occlusive disease (VOD) of liver K71.8
    veno-occlusive K76.5
  Lobo's (keloid blastomycosis) B48.0
  Lobstein's (brittle bones and blue sclera) Q78.0
  Ludwig's (submaxillary cellulitis) K12.2
  lumbosacral region M53.87
  lung J98.4
    black J60
    congenital Q33.9
    cystic J98.4
      congenital Q33.0
    fibroid (chronic) — *see* Fibrosis, lung
    fluke B66.4
      oriental B66.4
    in
      amyloidosis E85.4 *[J99]*
      sarcoidosis D86.0
      Sjögren's syndrome M35.02
      systemic
        lupus erythematosus M32.13
        sclerosis M34.81
    interstitial J84.9
      of childhood, specified NEC J84.848
      respiratory bronchiolitis J84.115
      specified NEC J84.89
    obstructive (chronic) J43.9
      with
        acute
          bronchitis J44.0
          exacerbation NEC J44.1
          lower respiratory infection J44.0
        alveolitis, allergic J67.9
        asthma J44.9
        bronchiectasis J47.9
          with
            exacerbation (acute) J47.1
            lower respiratory infection J47.0
        bronchitis J44.9
          with
            exacerbation (acute) J44.1
            lower respiratory infection J44.0
        emphysema J43.9
        hypersensitivity pneumonitis J67.9
      decompensated J44.1
        with
          exacerbation (acute) J44.1
    polycystic J98.4
      congenital Q33.0
    rheumatoid (diffuse) (interstitial) — *see* Rheumatoid, lung
  Lutembacher's (atrial septal defect with mitral stenosis) Q21.1
  Lyme A69.20
  lymphatic (gland) (system) (channel) (vessel) I89.9
  lymphoproliferative D47.9
    specified NEC D47.Z9 *(following* D47.4)
    T-gamma D47.Z9 *(following* D47.4)
    X-linked D82.3
  Magitot's M27.2
  malarial — *see* Malaria
  malignant — *see also* Neoplasm, malignant, by site
  Manson's B65.1
  maple bark J67.6
  maple-syrup-urine E71.0
  Marburg (virus) A98.3
  Marion's (bladder neck obstruction) N32.0
  Marsh's (exophthalmic goiter) — *see* Hyperthyroidism, with, goiter (diffuse)
  mastoid (process) — *see* Disorder, ear, middle
  Mathieu's (leptospiral jaundice) A27.0

☑ Additional Character Required — Refer to the Tabular List for Character Selection   ▽ Subterms under main terms may continue to next column or page

Disease, diseased — *continued*
- Maxcy's A75.2
- McArdle (-Schmid-Pearson) (glycogenosis V) E74.04
- mediastinum J98.59
- medullary center (idiopathic) (respiratory) G93.89
- Meige's (chronic hereditary edema) Q82.0
- meningococcal — *see* Infection, meningococcal
- mental F99
  - organic F09
- mesenchymal M35.9
- mesenteric embolic — *see also* Ischemia, intestine, acute K55.039
- metabolic, metabolism E88.9
  - bilirubin E80.7
- metal-polisher's J62.8
- metastatic — *see also* Neoplasm, secondary, by site C79.9
- microvascular - code to condition
- microvillus
  - atrophy Q43.8
  - inclusion (MVD) Q43.8
- middle ear — *see* Disorder, ear, middle
- Mikulicz' (dryness of mouth, absent or decreased lacrimation) K11.8
- Milroy's (chronic hereditary edema) Q82.0
- Minamata — *see* Poisoning, mercury
- minicore G71.2
- Minor's G95.19
- Minot's (hemorrhagic disease, newborn) P53
- Minot-von Willebrand-Jürgens (angiohemophilia) D68.0
- Mitchell's (erythromelalgia) I73.81
- mitral (valve) I05.9
  - nonrheumatic I34.9
- mixed connective tissue M35.1
- moldy hay J67.0
- Monge's T70.29 ☑
- Morgagni-Adams-Stokes (syncope with heart block) I45.9
- Morgagni's (syndrome) (hyperostosis frontalis interna) M85.2
- Morton's (with metatarsalgia) — *see* Lesion, nerve, plantar
- Morvan's G60.8
- motor neuron (bulbar) (mixed type) (spinal) G12.20
  - amyotrophic lateral sclerosis G12.21
  - familial G12.24
  - progressive bulbar palsy G12.22
  - specified NEC G12.29
- moyamoya I67.5
- mu heavy chain disease C88.2
- multicore G71.2
- muscle — *see also* Disorder, muscle
  - inflammatory — *see* Myositis
  - ocular (external) — *see* Strabismus
- musculoskeletal system, soft tissue — *see also* Disorder, soft tissue
  - specified NEC — *see* Disorder, soft tissue, specified type NEC
- mushroom workers' J67.5
- mycotic B49
- myelodysplastic, not classified C94.6
- myeloproliferative, not classified C94.6
  - chronic D47.1
- myocardium, myocardial — *see also* Degeneration, myocardial I51.5
  - primary (idiopathic) I42.9
- myoneural G70.9
- Naegeli's D69.1
- nails L60.9
  - specified NEC L60.8
- Nairobi (sheep virus) A93.8
- nasal J34.9
- nemaline body G71.2
- nerve — *see* Disorder, nerve
- nervous system G98.8
  - autonomic G90.9
  - central G96.9
    - specified NEC G96.8
  - congenital Q07.9
  - parasympathetic G90.9
  - specified NEC G98.8
  - sympathetic G90.9
  - vegetative G90.9
- neuromuscular system G70.9
- Newcastle B30.8
- Nicolas (-Durand)-Favre (climatic bubo) A55
- nipple N64.9
  - Paget's C50.01- ☑

Disease, diseased — *continued*
- nipple — *continued*
  - Paget's — *continued*
    - female C50.01- ☑
    - male C50.02- ☑
- Nishimoto (-Takeuchi) I67.5
- nonarthropod-borne NOS (viral) B34.9
  - enterovirus NEC B34.1
- nonautoimmune hemolytic D59.4
  - drug-induced D59.2
- Nonne-Milroy-Meige (chronic hereditary edema) Q82.0
- nose J34.9
- nucleus pulposus — *see* Disorder, disc
- nutritional E63.9
- oast-house-urine E72.19
- ocular
  - herpesviral B00.50
  - zoster B02.30
- obliterative vascular I77.1
- Ohara's — *see* Tularemia
- Opitz's (congestive splenomegaly) D73.2
- Oppenheim-Urbach (necrobiosis lipoidica diabetico-rum) — *see* E08-E13 with .620
- optic nerve NEC — *see* Disorder, nerve, optic
- orbit — *see* Disorder, orbit
- Oriental liver fluke B66.1
- Oriental lung fluke B66.4
- Ormond's N13.5
- Oropouche virus A93.0
- Osler-Rendu (familial hemorrhagic telangiectasia) I78.0
- osteofibrocystic E21.0
- Otto's M24.7
- outer ear — *see* Disorder, ear, external
- ovary (noninflammatory) N83.9
  - cystic N83.20- ☑
  - inflammatory — *see* Salpingo-oophoritis
  - polycystic E28.2
  - specified NEC N83.8
- Owren's (congenital) — *see* Defect, coagulation
- pancreas K86.9
  - cystic K86.2
  - fibrocystic E84.9
  - specified NEC K86.89
- panvalvular I08.9
  - specified NEC I08.8
- parametrium (noninflammatory) N83.9
- parasitic B89
  - cerebral NEC B71.9 *[G94]*
  - intestinal NOS B82.9
  - mouth B37.0
  - skin NOS B88.9
  - specified type — *see* Infestation
  - tongue B37.0
- parathyroid (gland) E21.5
  - specified NEC E21.4
- Parkinson's G20
- parodontal K05.6
- Parrot's (syphilitic osteochondritis) A50.02
- Parry's (exophthalmic goiter) — *see* Hyperthyroidism, with, goiter (diffuse)
- Parson's (exophthalmic goiter) — *see* Hyperthyroidism, with, goiter (diffuse)
- Paxton's (white piedra) B36.2
- pearl-worker's — *see* Osteomyelitis, specified type NEC
- Pellegrini-Stieda (calcification, knee joint) — *see* Bursitis, tibial collateral
- pelvis, pelvic
  - female NOS N94.9
    - specified NEC N94.89
  - gonococcal (acute) (chronic) A54.24
  - inflammatory (female) N73.9
    - acute N73.0
    - chlamydial A56.11
    - chronic N73.1
    - specified NEC N73.8
    - syphilitic (secondary) A51.42
      - late A52.76
    - tuberculous A18.17
  - organ, female N94.9
  - peritoneum, female NEC N94.89
- penis N48.9
  - inflammatory N48.29
    - abscess N48.21
    - cellulitis N48.22
  - specified NEC N48.89
- periapical tissues NOS K04.90
- periodontal K05.6
  - specified NEC K05.5

Disease, diseased — *continued*
- periosteum — *see* Disorder, bone, specified type NEC
- peripheral
  - arterial I73.9
  - autonomic nervous system G90.9
  - nerves — *see* Polyneuropathy
  - vascular NOS I73.9
- peritoneum K66.9
  - pelvic, female NEC N94.89
  - specified NEC K66.8
- persistent mucosal (middle ear) H66.20
  - left H66.22
    - with right H66.23
  - right H66.21
    - with left H66.23
- Petit's — *see* Hernia, abdomen, specified site NEC
- pharynx J39.2
  - specified NEC J39.2
- Phocas' — *see* Mastopathy, cystic
- photochromogenic (acid-fast bacilli) (pulmonary) A31.0
  - nonpulmonary A31.9
- Pick's G31.01 *[F02.80]*
  - with behavioral disturbance G31.01 *[F02.81]*
    - brain G31.01 *[F02.80]*
      - with behavioral disturbance G31.01 *[F02.81]*
  - of pericardium (pericardial pseudocirrhosis of liver) I31.1
- pigeon fancier's J67.2
- pineal gland E34.8
- pink — *see* Poisoning, mercury
- Pinkus' (lichen nitidus) L44.1
- pinworm B80
- Piry virus A93.8
- pituitary (gland) E23.7
- pituitary-snuff-taker's J67.8
- pleura (cavity) J94.9
  - specified NEC J94.8
- pneumatic drill (hammer) T75.21 ☑
- Pollitzer's (hidradenitis suppurativa) L73.2
- polycystic
  - kidney or renal Q61.3
    - adult type Q61.2
    - childhood type NEC Q61.19
      - collecting duct dilatation Q61.11
  - liver or hepatic Q44.6
  - lung or pulmonary J98.4
    - congenital Q33.0
  - ovary, ovaries E28.2
  - spleen Q89.09
- polyethylene T84.05- ☑
- Pompe's (glycogenosis II) E74.02
- Posadas-Wernicke B38.9
- Potain's (pulmonary edema) — *see* Edema, lung
- prepuce N47.8
  - inflammatory N47.7
    - balanoposthitis N47.6
- Pringle's (tuberous sclerosis) Q85.1
- prion, central nervous system A81.9
  - specified NEC A81.89
- prostate N42.9
  - specified NEC N42.89
- protozoal B64
  - acanthamebiasis — *see* Acanthamebiasis
  - African trypanosomiasis — *see* African trypanosomiasis
  - babesiosis B60.0
  - Chagas disease — *see* Chagas disease
  - intestine, intestinal A07.9
  - leishmaniasis — *see* Leishmaniasis
  - malaria — *see* Malaria
  - naegleriasis B60.2
  - pneumocystosis B59
  - specified organism NEC B60.8
  - toxoplasmosis — *see* Toxoplasmosis
- pseudo-Hurler's E77.0
- psychiatric F99
- psychotic — *see* Psychosis
- Puente's (simple glandular cheilitis) K13.0
- puerperal — *see also* Puerperal O90.89
- pulmonary — *see also* Disease, lung
  - artery I28.9
  - chronic obstructive J44.9
    - with
      - acute bronchitis J44.0
      - exacerbation (acute) J44.1
      - lower respiratory infection (acute) J44.0
    - decompensated J44.1

Disease, diseased — *continued*
pulmonary — *see also* Disease, lung — *continued*
  chronic obstructive — *continued*
    decompensated — *continued*
      with
        exacerbation (acute) J44.1
  heart I27.9
    specified NEC I27.89
  hypertensive (vascular) — *see also* Hypertension, pulmonary I27.20
    NEC I27.2 ☑
    primary (idiopathic) I27.0
  valve I37.9
    rheumatic I09.89
pulp (dental) NOS K04.90
pulseless M31.4
Putnam's (subacute combined sclerosis with pernicious anemia) D51.0
Pyle (-Cohn) (metaphyseal dysplasia) Q78.5
ragpicker's or ragsorter's A22.1
Raynaud's — *see* Raynaud's disease
reactive airway — *see* Asthma
Reclus' (cystic) — *see* Mastopathy, cystic
rectum K62.9
  specified NEC K62.89
Refsum's (heredopathia atactica polyneuritiformis) G60.1
renal (functional) (pelvis) — *see also* Disease, kidney N28.9
  with
    edema — *see* Nephrosis
    glomerular lesion — *see* Glomerulonephritis
      with edema — *see* Nephrosis
    interstitial nephritis N12
  acute N28.9
  chronic — *see also* Disease, kidney, chronic N18.9
  cystic, congenital Q61.9
  diabetic — *see* E08-E13 with .22
  end-stage (failure) N18.6
    due to hypertension I12.0
  fibrocystic (congenital) Q61.8
  hypertensive — *see* Hypertension, kidney
  lupus M32.14
  phosphate-losing (tubular) N25.0
  polycystic (congenital) Q61.3
    adult type Q61.2
    childhood type NEC Q61.19
      collecting duct dilatation Q61.11
  rapidly progressive N01.9
  subacute N01.9
Rendu-Osler-Weber (familial hemorrhagic telangiectasia) I78.0
renovascular (arteriosclerotic) — *see* Hypertension, kidney
respiratory (tract) J98.9
  acute or subacute NOS J06.9
    due to
      chemicals, gases, fumes or vapors (inhalation) J68.3
      external agent J70.9
        specified NEC J70.8
      radiation J70.0
      smoke inhalation J70.5
    noninfectious J39.8
  chronic NOS J98.9
    due to
      chemicals, gases, fumes or vapors J68.4
      external agent J70.9
        specified NEC J70.8
      radiation J70.1
    newborn P27.9
      specified NEC P27.8
  due to
    chemicals, gases, fumes or vapors J68.9
      acute or subacute NEC J68.3
      chronic J68.4
    external agent J70.9
      specified NEC J70.8
    newborn P28.9
      specified type NEC P28.89
  upper J39.9
    acute or subacute J06.9
    noninfectious NEC J39.8
    specified NEC J39.8
    streptococcal J06.9
retina, retinal H35.9
  Batten's or Batten-Mayou E75.4 *[H36]*
  specified NEC H35.89

Disease, diseased — *continued*
rheumatoid — *see* Arthritis, rheumatoid
rickettsial NOS A79.9
  specified type NEC A79.89
Riga (-Fede) (cachectic aphthae) K14.0
Riggs' (compound periodontitis) — *see* Periodontitis
Ritter's L00
Rivalta's (cervicofacial actinomycosis) A42.2
Robles' (onchocerciasis) B73.01
Roger's (congenital interventricular septal defect) Q21.0
Rosenthal's (factor XI deficiency) D68.1
Ross River B33.1
Rossbach's (hyperchlorhydria) K31.89
  psychogenic F45.8
Rotes Quérol — *see* Hyperostosis, ankylosing
Roth (-Bernhardt) — *see* Mononeuropathy, lower limb, meralgia paresthetica
Runeberg's (progressive pernicious anemia) D51.0
sacroiliac NEC M53.3
salivary gland or duct K11.9
  inclusion B25.9
  specified NEC K11.8
  virus B25.9
sandworm B76.9
Schimmelbusch's — *see* Mastopathy, cystic
Schmorl's — *see* Schmorl's disease or nodes
Schönlein (-Henoch) (purpura rheumatica) D69.0
Schottmüller's — *see* Fever, paratyphoid
Schultz's (agranulocytosis) — *see* Agranulocytosis
Schwalbe-Ziehen-Oppenheim G24.1
Schwartz-Jampel G71.13
sclera H15.9
  specified NEC H15.89
scrofulous (tuberculous) A18.2
scrotum N50.9
sebaceous glands L73.9
semilunar cartilage, cystic — *see also* Derangement, knee, meniscus, cystic
seminal vesicle N50.9
serum NEC — *see also* Reaction, serum T80.69 ☑
sexually transmitted A64
  anogenital
    herpesviral infection — *see* Herpes, anogenital
    warts A63.0
  chancroid A57
  chlamydial infection — *see* Chlamydia
  gonorrhea — *see* Gonorrhea
  granuloma inguinale A58
  specified organism NEC A63.8
  syphilis — *see* Syphilis
  trichomoniasis — *see* Trichomoniasis
Sézary C84.1- ☑
shimamushi (scrub typhus) A75.3
shipyard B30.0
sickle-cell D57.1
  with crisis (vasoocclusive pain) D57.00
    with
      acute chest syndrome D57.01
      splenic sequestration D57.02
  elliptocytosis D57.8- ☑
  Hb-C D57.20
    with crisis (vasoocclusive pain) D57.219
      with
        acute chest syndrome D57.211
        splenic sequestration D57.212
    without crisis D57.20
  Hb-SD D57.80
    with crisis D57.819
      with
        acute chest syndrome D57.811
        splenic sequestration D57.812
  Hb-SE D57.80
    with crisis D57.819
      with
        acute chest syndrome D57.811
        splenic sequestration D57.812
  specified NEC D57.80
    with crisis D57.819
      with
        acute chest syndrome D57.811
        splenic sequestration D57.812
  spherocytosis D57.80
    with crisis D57.819
      with
        acute chest syndrome D57.811
        splenic sequestration D57.812
  thalassemia D57.40
    with crisis (vasoocclusive pain) D57.419

Disease, diseased — *continued*
sickle-cell — *continued*
  thalassemia — *continued*
    with crisis — *continued*
      with
        acute chest syndrome D57.411
        splenic sequestration D57.412
    without crisis D57.40
silo-filler's J68.8
  bronchitis J68.0
  pneumonitis J68.0
  pulmonary edema J68.1
simian B B00.4
Simons' (progressive lipodystrophy) E88.1
sin nombre virus B33.4
sinus — *see* Sinusitis
Sirkari's B55.0
sixth B08.20
  due to human herpesvirus 6 B08.21
  due to human herpesvirus 7 B08.22
skin L98.9
  due to metabolic disorder NEC E88.9 *[L99]*
  specified NEC L98.8
slim (HIV) B20
small vessel I73.9
Sneddon-Wilkinson (subcorneal pustular dermatosis) L13.1
South African creeping B88.0
spinal (cord) G95.9
  congenital Q06.9
  specified NEC G95.89
spine — *see also* Spondylopathy
  joint — *see* Dorsopathy
  tuberculous A18.01
spinocerebellar (hereditary) G11.9
  specified NEC G11.8
spleen D73.9
  amyloid E85.4 *[D77]*
  organic D73.9
  polycystic Q89.09
  postinfectional D73.89
sponge-diver's — *see* Toxicity, venom, marine animal, sea anemone
Startle Q89.8
Steinert's G71.11
Sticker's (erythema infectiosum) B08.3
Stieda's (calcification, knee joint) — *see* Bursitis, tibial collateral
Stokes' (exophthalmic goiter) — *see* Hyperthyroidism, with, goiter (diffuse)
Stokes-Adams (syncope with heart block) I45.9
stomach K31.9
  functional, psychogenic F45.8
  specified NEC K31.89
stonemason's J62.8
storage
  glycogen — *see* Disease, glycogen storage
  mucopolysaccharide — *see* Mucopolysaccharidosis
striatopallidal system NEC G25.89
Stuart-Prower (congenital factor X deficiency) D68.2
Stuart's (congenital factor X deficiency) D68.2
subcutaneous tissue — *see* Disease, skin
supporting structures of teeth K08.9
  specified NEC K08.89
suprarenal (capsule) (gland) E27.9
  hyperfunction E27.0
  specified NEC E27.8
sweat glands L74.9
  specified NEC L74.8
Sweeley-Klionsky E75.21
Swift (-Feer) — *see* Poisoning, mercury
swimming-pool granuloma A31.1
Sylvest's (epidemic pleurodynia) B33.0
sympathetic nervous system G90.9
synovium — *see* Disorder, synovium
syphilitic — *see* Syphilis
systemic tissue mast cell D47.02
tanapox (virus) B08.71
Tangier E78.6
Tarral-Besnier (pityriasis rubra pilaris) L44.0
Tauri's E74.09
tear duct — *see* Disorder, lacrimal system
tendon, tendinous — *see also* Disorder, tendon
  nodular — *see* Trigger finger
terminal vessel I73.9
testis N50.9
thalassemia Hb-S — *see* Disease, sickle-cell, thalassemia
Thaysen-Gee (nontropical sprue) K90.0

☑ **Additional Character Required** — Refer to the Tabular List for Character Selection   ▽ **Subterms under main terms may continue to next column or page**

Disease, diseased — *continued*
Thomsen G71.12
throat J39.2
   septic J02.0
thromboembolic — *see* Embolism
thymus (gland) E32.9
   specified NEC E32.8
thyroid (gland) E07.9
   heart — *see also* Hyperthyroidism E05.90 *[I43]*
      with thyroid storm E05.91 *[I43]*
   specified NEC E07.89
Tietze's M94.0
tongue K14.9
   specified NEC K14.8
tonsils, tonsillar (and adenoids) J35.9
tooth, teeth K08.9
   hard tissues K03.9
      specified NEC K03.89
   pulp NEC K04.99
   specified NEC K08.89
Tourette's F95.2
trachea NEC J39.8
tricuspid I07.9
   nonrheumatic I36.9
triglyceride-storage E75.5
trophoblastic — *see* Mole, hydatidiform
tsutsugamushi A75.3
tube (fallopian) (noninflammatory) N83.9
   inflammatory — *see* Salpingitis
   specified NEC N83.8
tuberculous NEC — *see* Tuberculosis
tubo-ovarian (noninflammatory) N83.9
   inflammatory — *see* Salpingo-oophoritis
   specified NEC N83.8
tubotympanic, chronic — *see* Otitis, media, suppurative, chronic, tubotympanic
tubulo-interstitial N15.9
   specified NEC N15.8
tympanum — *see* Disorder, tympanic membrane
Uhl's Q24.8
Underwood's (sclerema neonatorum) P83.0
Unverricht (-Lundborg) — *see* Epilepsy, generalized, idiopathic
Urbach-Oppenheim (necrobiosis lipoidica diabeticorum) — *see* E08-E13 with .620
ureter N28.9
   in (due to)
      schistosomiasis (bilharziasis) B65.0 *[N29]*
urethra N36.9
   specified NEC N36.8
urinary (tract) N39.9
   bladder N32.9
      specified NEC N32.89
   specified NEC N39.8
uterus (noninflammatory) N85.9
   infective — *see* Endometritis
   inflammatory — *see* Endometritis
   specified NEC N85.8
uveal tract (anterior) H21.9
   posterior H31.9
vagabond's B85.1
vagina, vaginal (noninflammatory) N89.9
   inflammatory NEC N76.89
   specified NEC N89.8
valve, valvular I38
   multiple I08.9
      specified NEC I08.8
van Creveld-von Gierke (glycogenosis I) E74.01
vas deferens N50.9
vascular I99.9
   arteriosclerotic — *see* Arteriosclerosis
   ciliary body NEC — *see* Disorder, iris, vascular
   hypertensive — *see* Hypertension
   iris NEC — *see* Disorder, iris, vascular
   obliterative I77.1
      peripheral I73.9
   occlusive I99.8
   peripheral (occlusive) I73.9
      in diabetes mellitus — *see* E08-E13 with .51
vasomotor I73.9
vasospastic I73.9
vein I87.9
venereal — *see also* Disease, sexually transmitted A64
   chlamydial NEC A56.8
      anus A56.3
      genitourinary NOS A56.2
      pharynx A56.4
      rectum A56.3

Disease, diseased — *continued*
venereal — *see also* Disease, sexually transmitted — *continued*
   fifth A55
   sixth A55
   specified nature or type NEC A63.8
vertebra, vertebral — *see also* Spondylopathy
   disc — *see* Disorder, disc
vibration — *see* Vibration, adverse effects
viral, virus — *see also* Disease, by type of virus B34.9
   arbovirus NOS A94
   arthropod-borne NOS A94
   congenital P35.9
      specified NEC P35.8
   Hanta (with renal manifestations) (Dobrava) (Puumala) (Seoul) A98.5
      with pulmonary manifestations (Andes) (Bayou) (Bermejo) (Black Creek Canal) (Choclo) (Juquitiba) (Laguna negra) (Lechiguanas) (New York) (Oran) (Sin nombre) B33.4
   Hantaan (Korean hemorrhagic fever) A98.5
   human immunodeficiency (HIV) B20
   Kunjin A83.4
   nonarthropod-borne NOS B34.9
   Powassan A84.8
   Rocio (encephalitis) A83.6
   Sin nombre (Hantavirus) (cardio)-pulmonary syndrome) B33.4
   Tahyna B33.8
   vesicular stomatitis A93.8
vitreous H43.9
   specified NEC H43.89
vocal cord J38.3
Volkmann's, acquired T79.6 ✓
von Eulenburg's (congenital paramyotonia) G71.19
von Gierke's (glycogenosis I) E74.01
von Graefe's — *see* Strabismus, paralytic, ophthalmoplegia, progressive
von Willebrand (-Jürgens) (angiohemophilia) D68.0
Vrolik's (osteogenesis imperfecta) Q78.0
vulva (noninflammatory) N90.9
   inflammatory NEC N76.89
   specified NEC N90.89
Wallgren's (obstruction of splenic vein with collateral circulation) I87.8
Wassilieff's (leptospiral jaundice) A27.0
wasting NEC R64
   due to malnutrition E41
Waterhouse-Friderichsen A39.1
Wegner's (syphilitic osteochondritis) A50.02
Weil's (leptospiral jaundice of lung) A27.0
Weir Mitchell's (erythromelalgia) I73.81
Werdnig-Hoffmann G12.0
Wermer's E31.21
Werner-His (trench fever) A79.0
Werner-Schultz (neutropenic splenomegaly) D73.81
Wernicke-Posadas B38.9
whipworm B79
white blood cells D72.9
   specified NEC D72.89
white matter R90.82
white-spot, meaning lichen sclerosus et atrophicus L90.0
   penis N48.0
   vulva N90.4
Wilkie's K55.1
Wilkinson-Sneddon (subcorneal pustular dermatosis) L13.1
Willis' — *see* Diabetes
Wilson's (hepatolenticular degeneration) E83.01
woolsorter's A22.1
yaba monkey tumor B08.72
yaba pox (virus) B08.72
Zika virus A92.5
   congenital P35.4
zoonotic, bacterial A28.9
   specified type NEC A28.8
Disfigurement (due to scar) L90.5
Disgerminoma — *see* Dysgerminoma
DISH (diffuse idiopathic skeletal hyperostosis) — *see* Hyperostosis, ankylosing
Disinsertion, retina — *see* Detachment, retina
Dislocatable hip, congenital Q65.6
Dislocation (articular)
   with fracture — *see* Fracture
   acromioclavicular (joint) S43.10- ✓
      with displacement
         100%-200% S43.12- ✓

Dislocation — *continued*
acromioclavicular — *continued*
   with displacement — *continued*
      more than 200% S43.13- ✓
      inferior S43.14- ✓
      posterior S43.15- ✓
ankle S93.0- ✓
astragalus — *see* Dislocation, ankle
atlantoaxial S13.121 ✓
atlantooccipital S13.111 ✓
atloidooccipital S13.111 ✓
breast bone S23.29 ✓
capsule, joint — *code by* site under Dislocation
carpal (bone) — *see* Dislocation, wrist
carpometacarpal (joint) NEC S63.05- ✓
   thumb S63.04- ✓
cartilage (joint) — *code by* site under Dislocation
cervical spine (vertebra) — *see* Dislocation, vertebra, cervical
chronic — *see* Dislocation, recurrent
clavicle — *see* Dislocation, acromioclavicular joint
coccyx S33.2 ✓
congenital NEC Q68.8
coracoid — *see* Dislocation, shoulder
costal cartilage S23.29 ✓
costochondral S23.29 ✓
cricoarytenoid articulation S13.29 ✓
cricothyroid articulation S13.29 ✓
dorsal vertebra — *see* Dislocation, vertebra, thoracic
ear ossicle — *see* Discontinuity, ossicles, ear
elbow S53.10- ✓
   congenital Q68.8
   pathological — *see* Dislocation, pathological NEC, elbow
   radial head alone — *see* Dislocation, radial head
   recurrent — *see* Dislocation, recurrent, elbow
   traumatic S53.10- ✓
      anterior S53.11- ✓
      lateral S53.14- ✓
      medial S53.13- ✓
      posterior S53.12- ✓
      specified type NEC S53.19- ✓
eye, nontraumatic — *see* Luxation, globe
eyeball, nontraumatic — *see* Luxation, globe
femur
   distal end — *see* Dislocation, knee
   proximal end — *see* Dislocation, hip
fibula
   distal end — *see* Dislocation, ankle
   proximal end — *see* Dislocation, knee
finger S63.25- ✓
   index S63.25- ✓
   interphalangeal S63.27- ✓
      distal S63.29- ✓
         index S63.29- ✓
         little S63.29- ✓
         middle S63.29- ✓
         ring S63.29- ✓
      index S63.27- ✓
      little S63.27- ✓
      middle S63.27- ✓
      proximal S63.28- ✓
         index S63.28- ✓
         little S63.28- ✓
         middle S63.28- ✓
         ring S63.28- ✓
      ring S63.27- ✓
   little S63.25- ✓
   metacarpophalangeal S63.26- ✓
      index S63.26- ✓
      little S63.26- ✓
      middle S63.26- ✓
      ring S63.26- ✓
   middle S63.25- ✓
   recurrent — *see* Dislocation, recurrent, finger
   ring S63.25- ✓
   thumb — *see* Dislocation, thumb
foot S93.30- ✓
   recurrent — *see* Dislocation, recurrent, foot
   specified site NEC S93.33- ✓
   tarsal joint S93.31- ✓
   tarsometatarsal joint S93.32- ✓
   toe — *see* Dislocation, toe
fracture — *see* Fracture
glenohumeral (joint) — *see* Dislocation, shoulder
glenoid — *see* Dislocation, shoulder

Dislocation — *continued*
habitual — *see* Dislocation, recurrent
hip S73.00- ✓
  anterior S73.03- ✓
    obturator S73.02- ✓
  central S73.04- ✓
  congenital (total) Q65.2
    bilateral Q65.1
    partial Q65.5
      bilateral Q65.4
      unilateral Q65.3- ✓
    unilateral Q65.0- ✓
  developmental M24.85- ✓
  pathological — *see* Dislocation, pathological NEC, hip
  posterior S73.01- ✓
  recurrent — *see* Dislocation, recurrent, hip
humerus, proximal end — *see* Dislocation, shoulder
incomplete — *see* Subluxation, by site
incus — *see* Discontinuity, ossicles, ear
infracoracoid — *see* Dislocation, shoulder
innominate (pubic junction) (sacral junction) S33.39 ✓
  acetabulum — *see* Dislocation, hip
interphalangeal (joint(s))
  finger S63.279 ✓
    distal S63.29- ✓
      index S63.29- ✓
      little S63.29- ✓
      middle S63.29- ✓
      ring S63.29- ✓
    index S63.27- ✓
    little S63.27- ✓
    middle S63.27- ✓
    proximal S63.28- ✓
      index S63.28- ✓
      little S63.28- ✓
      middle S63.28- ✓
      ring S63.28- ✓
    ring S63.27- ✓
  foot or toe — *see* Dislocation, toe
  thumb S63.12- ✓
jaw (cartilage) (meniscus) S03.0- ✓
joint prosthesis — *see* Complications, joint prosthesis, mechanical, displacement, by site
knee S83.106 ✓
  cap — *see* Dislocation, patella
  congenital Q68.2
  old M23.8X- ✓
  patella — *see* Dislocation, patella
  pathological — *see* Dislocation, pathological NEC, knee
  proximal tibia
    anteriorly S83.11- ✓
    laterally S83.14- ✓
    medially S83.13- ✓
    posteriorly S83.12- ✓
  recurrent — *see also* Derangement, knee, specified NEC
  specified type NEC S83.19- ✓
lacrimal gland H04.16- ✓
lens (complete) H27.10
  anterior H27.12- ✓
  congenital Q12.1
  ocular implant — *see* Complications, intraocular lens
  partial H27.11- ✓
  posterior H27.13- ✓
  traumatic S05.8X- ✓
ligament — *code by* site under Dislocation
lumbar (vertebra) — *see* Dislocation, vertebra, lumbar
lumbosacral (vertebra) — *see also* Dislocation, vertebra, lumbar
  congenital Q76.49
mandible S03.0- ✓
meniscus (knee) — *see* Tear, meniscus
  other sites - code by site under Dislocation
metacarpal (bone)
  distal end — *see* Dislocation, finger
  proximal end S63.06- ✓
metacarpophalangeal (joint)
  finger S63.26- ✓
    index S63.26- ✓
    little S63.26- ✓
    middle S63.26- ✓
    ring S63.26- ✓
  thumb S63.11- ✓

Dislocation — *continued*
metatarsal (bone) — *see* Dislocation, foot
metatarsophalangeal (joint(s)) — *see* Dislocation, toe
midcarpal (joint) S63.03- ✓
midtarsal (joint) — *see* Dislocation, foot
neck S13.20 ✓
  specified site NEC S13.29 ✓
  vertebra — *see* Dislocation, vertebra, cervical
nose (septal cartilage) S03.1 ✓
occipitoatloid S13.111 ✓
old — *see* Derangement, joint, specified type NEC
ossicles, ear — *see* Discontinuity, ossicles, ear
partial — *see* Subluxation, by site
patella S83.006 ✓
  congenital Q74.1
  lateral S83.01- ✓
  recurrent (nontraumatic) M22.0- ✓
    incomplete M22.1- ✓
  specified type NEC S83.09- ✓
pathological NEC M24.30
  ankle M24.37- ✓
  elbow M24.32- ✓
  foot joint M24.37- ✓
  hand joint M24.34- ✓
  hip M24.35- ✓
  knee M24.36- ✓
  lumbosacral joint — *see* subcategory M53.2
  pelvic region — *see* Dislocation, pathological, hip
  sacroiliac — *see* subcategory M53.2 ✓
  shoulder M24.31- ✓
  wrist M24.33- ✓
pelvis NEC S33.30 ✓
  specified NEC S33.39 ✓
phalanx
  finger or hand — *see* Dislocation, finger
  foot or toe — *see* Dislocation, toe
prosthesis, internal — *see* Complications, prosthetic device, by site, mechanical
radial head S53.006 ✓
  anterior S53.01- ✓
  posterior S53.02- ✓
  specified type NEC S53.09- ✓
radiocarpal (joint) S63.02- ✓
radiohumeral (joint) — *see* Dislocation, radial head
radioulnar (joint)
  distal S63.01- ✓
  proximal — *see* Dislocation, elbow
radius
  distal end — *see* Dislocation, wrist
  proximal end — *see* Dislocation, radial head
recurrent M24.40
  ankle M24.47- ✓
  elbow M24.42- ✓
  finger M24.44- ✓
  foot joint M24.47- ✓
  hand joint M24.44- ✓
  hip M24.45- ✓
  knee M24.46- ✓
    patella — *see* Dislocation, patella, recurrent
  patella — *see* Dislocation, patella, recurrent
  sacroiliac — *see* subcategory M53.2
  shoulder M24.41- ✓
  toe M24.47- ✓
  vertebra — *see also* subcategory M43.5 ✓
    atlantoaxial M43.4
      with myelopathy M43.3
  wrist M24.43- ✓
rib (cartilage) S23.29 ✓
sacrococcygeal S33.2 ✓
sacroiliac (joint) (ligament) S33.2 ✓
  congenital Q74.2
  recurrent — *see* subcategory M53.2 ✓
sacrum S33.2 ✓
scaphoid (bone) (hand) (wrist) — *see* Dislocation, wrist
  foot — *see* Dislocation, foot
scapula — *see* Dislocation, shoulder, girdle, scapula
semilunar cartilage, knee — *see* Tear, meniscus
septal cartilage (nose) S03.1 ✓
septum (nasal) (old) J34.2
sesamoid bone — *code by* site under Dislocation
shoulder (blade) (ligament) (joint) (traumatic) S43.006 ✓
  acromioclavicular — *see* Dislocation, acromioclavicular
  chronic — *see* Dislocation, recurrent, shoulder
  congenital Q68.8

Dislocation — *continued*
shoulder — *continued*
  girdle S43.30- ✓
    scapula S43.31- ✓
    specified site NEC S43.39- ✓
  humerus S43.00- ✓
    anterior S43.01- ✓
    inferior S43.03- ✓
    posterior S43.02- ✓
  pathological — *see* Dislocation, pathological NEC, shoulder
  recurrent — *see* Dislocation, recurrent, shoulder
  specified type NEC S43.08- ✓
spine
  cervical — *see* Dislocation, vertebra, cervical
  congenital Q76.49
  due to birth trauma P11.5
  lumbar — *see* Dislocation, vertebra, lumbar
  thoracic — *see* Dislocation, vertebra, thoracic
spontaneous — *see* Dislocation, pathological
sternoclavicular (joint) S43.206 ✓
  anterior S43.21- ✓
  posterior S43.22- ✓
sternum S23.29 ✓
subglenoid — *see* Dislocation, shoulder
symphysis pubis S33.4 ✓
talus — *see* Dislocation, ankle
tarsal (bone(s)) (joint(s)) — *see* Dislocation, foot
tarsometatarsal (joint(s)) — *see* Dislocation, foot
temporomandibular (joint) S03.0- ✓
thigh, proximal end — *see* Dislocation, hip
thorax S23.20 ✓
  specified site NEC S23.29 ✓
  vertebra — *see* Dislocation, vertebra
thumb S63.10- ✓
  interphalangeal joint — *see* Dislocation, interphalangeal (joint), thumb
  metacarpophalangeal joint — *see* Dislocation, metacarpophalangeal (joint), thumb
thyroid cartilage S13.29 ✓
tibia
  distal end — *see* Dislocation, ankle
  proximal end — *see* Dislocation, knee
tibiofibular (joint)
  distal — *see* Dislocation, ankle
  superior — *see* Dislocation, knee
toe(s) S93.106 ✓
  great S93.10- ✓
    interphalangeal joint S93.11- ✓
    metatarsophalangeal joint S93.12- ✓
  interphalangeal joint S93.119 ✓
  lesser S93.106 ✓
    interphalangeal joint S93.11- ✓
    metatarsophalangeal joint S93.12- ✓
  metatarsophalangeal joint S93.12- ✓
tooth S03.2 ✓
trachea S23.29 ✓
ulna
  distal end S63.07- ✓
  proximal end — *see* Dislocation, elbow
ulnohumeral (joint) — *see* Dislocation, elbow
vertebra (articular process) (body) (traumatic)
  cervical S13.101 ✓
    atlantoaxial joint S13.121 ✓
    atlantooccipital joint S13.111 ✓
    atloidooccipital joint S13.111 ✓
    joint between
      C0 and C1 S13.111 ✓
      C1 and C2 S13.121 ✓
      C2 and C3 S13.131 ✓
      C3 and C4 S13.141 ✓
      C4 and C5 S13.151 ✓
      C5 and C6 S13.161 ✓
      C6 and C7 S13.171 ✓
      C7 and T1 S13.181 ✓
    occipitoatloid joint S13.111 ✓
  congenital Q76.49
  lumbar S33.101 ✓
    joint between
      L1 and L2 S33.111 ✓
      L2 and L3 S33.121 ✓
      L3 and L4 S33.131 ✓
      L4 and L5 S33.141 ✓
  nontraumatic — *see* Displacement, intervertebral disc
  partial — *see* Subluxation, by site

✓ Additional Character Required — Refer to the Tabular List for Character Selection   ▽ Subterms under main terms may continue to next column or page

Dislocation — *continued*
　vertebra — *continued*
　　recurrent NEC — *see* subcategory M43.5 ☑
　　thoracic S23.101 ☑
　　　joint between
　　　　T1 and T2 S23.111 ☑
　　　　T2 and T3 S23.121 ☑
　　　　T3 and T4 S23.123 ☑
　　　　T4 and T5 S23.131 ☑
　　　　T5 and T6 S23.133 ☑
　　　　T6 and T7 S23.141 ☑
　　　　T7 and T8 S23.143 ☑
　　　　T8 and T9 S23.151 ☑
　　　　T9 and T10 S23.153 ☑
　　　　T10 and T11 S23.161 ☑
　　　　T11 and T12 S23.163 ☑
　　　　T12 and L1 S23.171 ☑
　wrist (carpal bone) S63.006 ☑
　　carpometacarpal joint — *see* Dislocation, carpometacarpal (joint)
　　distal radioulnar joint — *see* Dislocation, radioulnar (joint), distal
　　metacarpal bone, proximal — *see* Dislocation, metacarpal (bone), proximal end
　　midcarpal — *see* Dislocation, midcarpal (joint)
　　radiocarpal joint — *see* Dislocation, radiocarpal (joint)
　　recurrent — *see* Dislocation, recurrent, wrist
　　specified site NEC S63.09- ☑
　　ulna — *see* Dislocation, ulna, distal end
　xiphoid cartilage S23.29 ☑
Disorder (of) — *see also* Disease
　acantholytic L11.9
　　specified NEC L11.8
　acute
　　psychotic — *see* Psychosis, acute
　　stress F43.0
　adjustment (grief) F43.20
　　with
　　　anxiety F43.22
　　　　with depressed mood F43.23
　　　conduct disturbance F43.24
　　　　with emotional disturbance F43.25
　　　depressed mood F43.21
　　　　with anxiety F43.23
　　　other specified symptom F43.29
　adrenal (capsule) (gland) (medullary) E27.9
　　specified NEC E27.8
　adrenogenital E25.9
　　drug-induced E25.8
　　iatrogenic E25.8
　　idiopathic E25.8
　adult personality (and behavior) F69
　　specified NEC F68.8
　affective (mood) — *see* Disorder, mood
　aggressive, unsocialized F91.1
　alcohol use
　　mild F10.10
　　　with
　　　　alcohol intoxication F10.129
　　　　　delirium F10.121
　　　　alcohol-induced
　　　　　anxiety disorder F10.180
　　　　　bipolar and related disorder F10.14
　　　　　depressive disorder F10.14
　　　　　psychotic disorder F10.159
　　　　　sexual dysfunction F10.181
　　　　　sleep disorder F10.182
　　　in remission (early) (sustained) F10.11
　　moderate or severe F10.20
　　　with
　　　　alcohol intoxication F10.229
　　　　　delirium F10.221
　　　　alcohol-induced
　　　　　anxiety disorder F10.280
　　　　　bipolar and related disorder F10.24
　　　　　depressive disorder F10.24
　　　　　major neurocognitive disorder, amnestic-confabulatory type F10.26
　　　　　major neurocognitive disorder, non-amnestic-confabulatory type F10.27
　　　　　mild neurocognitive disorder F10.288
　　　　　psychotic disorder F10.259
　　　　　sexual dysfunction F10.281
　　　　　sleep disorder F10.282
　　　in remission (early) (sustained) F10.21
　alcohol-related F10.99

Disorder — *continued*
　alcohol-related — *continued*
　　with
　　　amnestic disorder, persisting F10.96
　　　anxiety disorder F10.980
　　　dementia, persisting F10.97
　　　intoxication F10.929
　　　　with delirium F10.921
　　　　uncomplicated F10.920
　　　mood disorder F10.94
　　　other specified F10.988
　　　psychotic disorder F10.959
　　　　with
　　　　　delusions F10.950
　　　　　hallucinations F10.951
　　　sexual dysfunction F10.981
　　　sleep disorder F10.982
　allergic — *see* Allergy
　alveolar NEC J84.09
　amino-acid
　　cystathioninuria E72.19
　　cystinosis E72.04
　　cystinuria E72.01
　　glycinuria E72.09
　　homocystinuria E72.11
　　metabolism — *see* Disturbance, metabolism, amino-acid
　　specified NEC E72.89
　　neonatal, transitory P74.8
　　renal transport NEC E72.09
　　transport NEC E72.09
　amnesic, amnestic
　　alcohol-induced F10.96
　　　with dependence F10.26
　　due to (secondary to) general medical condition F04
　　psychoactive NEC-induced F19.96
　　　with
　　　　abuse F19.16
　　　　dependence F19.26
　　sedative, hypnotic or anxiolytic-induced F13.96
　　　with dependence F13.26
　amphetamine (or other stimulant) use
　　mild
　　　with
　　　　amphetamine, cocaine, or other stimulant intoxication
　　　　　with perceptual disturbances F15.122
　　　　　without perceptual disturbances F15.129
　　　　amphetamine (or other stimulant) -induced
　　　　　anxiety disorder F15.180
　　　　　bipolar and related disorder F15.14
　　　　　depressive disorder F15.14
　　　　　obsessive-compulsive and related disorder F15.188
　　　　　psychotic disorder F15.159
　　　　　sexual dysfunction F15.181
　　　　intoxication delirium F15.121
　　moderate or severe
　　　with
　　　　amphetamine, cocaine, or other stimulant intoxication
　　　　　with perceptual disturbances F15.222
　　　　　without perceptual disturbances F15.229
　　　　amphetamine (or other stimulant) -induced
　　　　　anxiety disorder F15.280
　　　　　bipolar and related disorder F15.24
　　　　　depressive disorder F15.24
　　　　　obsessive-compulsive and related disorder F15.288
　　　　　psychotic disorder F15.259
　　　　　sexual dysfunction F15.281
　　　　intoxication delirium F15.221
　amphetamine-type substance use
　　mild F15.10
　　　in remission (early) (sustained) F15.11
　　moderate F15.20
　　　in remission (early) (sustained) F15.21
　　severe F15.20
　　　in remission (early) (sustained) F15.21
　anaerobic glycolysis with anemia D55.2
　anxiety F41.9
　　due to (secondary to)
　　　alcohol F10.980
　　　　in
　　　　　abuse F10.180
　　　　　dependence F10.280
　　　amphetamine F15.980
　　　　in
　　　　　abuse F15.180

Disorder — *continued*
　anxiety — *continued*
　　due to — *continued*
　　　amphetamine — *continued*
　　　　in — *continued*
　　　　　dependence F15.280
　　　anxiolytic F13.980
　　　　in
　　　　　abuse F13.180
　　　　　dependence F13.280
　　　caffeine F15.980
　　　　in
　　　　　abuse F15.180
　　　　　dependence F15.280
　　　cannabis F12.980
　　　　in
　　　　　abuse F12.180
　　　　　dependence F12.280
　　　cocaine F14.980
　　　　in
　　　　　abuse F14.180
　　　　　dependence F14.180
　　　general medical condition F06.4
　　　hallucinogen F16.980
　　　　in
　　　　　abuse F16.180
　　　　　dependence F16.280
　　　hypnotic F13.980
　　　　in
　　　　　abuse F13.180
　　　　　dependence F13.280
　　　inhalant F18.980
　　　　in
　　　　　abuse F18.180
　　　　　dependence F18.280
　　　phencyclidine F16.980
　　　　in
　　　　　abuse F16.180
　　　　　dependence F16.280
　　　psychoactive substance NEC F19.980
　　　　in
　　　　　abuse F19.180
　　　　　dependence F19.280
　　　sedative F13.980
　　　　in
　　　　　abuse F13.180
　　　　　dependence F13.280
　　　volatile solvents F18.980
　　　　in
　　　　　abuse F18.180
　　　　　dependence F18.280
　　generalized F41.1
　　illness F45.21
　　mixed
　　　with depression (mild) F41.8
　　　specified NEC F41.3
　　organic F06.4
　　phobic F40.9
　　　of childhood F40.8
　　specified NEC F41.8
　aortic valve — *see* Endocarditis, aortic
　aromatic amino-acid metabolism E70.9
　　specified NEC E70.8
　arteriole NEC I77.89
　artery NEC I77.89
　articulation — *see* Disorder, joint
　attachment (childhood)
　　disinhibited F94.2
　　reactive F94.1
　attention-deficit hyperactivity (adolescent) (adult) (child) F90.9
　　combined
　　　presentation F90.2
　　　type F90.2
　　hyperactive
　　　impulsive presentation F90.1
　　　type F90.1
　　inattentive
　　　presentation F90.0
　　　type F90.0
　　specified type NEC F90.8
　attention-deficit without hyperactivity (adolescent) (adult) (child) F98.8
　auditory processing (central) H93.25
　autism spectrum F84.0
　autistic F84.0
　autoimmune D89.89
　autonomic nervous system G90.9
　　specified NEC G90.8

Dislocation — Disorder

Disorder — *continued*
  avoidant
    child or adolescent F40.10
    restrictive food intake F50.82
  balance
    acid-base E87.8
      mixed E87.4
    electrolyte E87.8
    fluid NEC E87.8
  behavioral (disruptive) — *see* Disorder, conduct
  beta-amino-acid metabolism E72.89
  bile acid and cholesterol metabolism E78.70
    Barth syndrome E78.71
    other specified E78.79
    Smith-Lemli-Opitz syndrome E78.72
  bilirubin excretion E80.6
  binge eating F50.81
  binocular
    movement H51.9
      convergence
        excess H51.12
        insufficiency H51.11
      internuclear ophthalmoplegia — *see* Ophthalmo-
        plegia, internuclear
      palsy of conjugate gaze H51.0
      specified type NEC H51.8
    vision NEC — *see* Disorder, vision, binocular
  bipolar (I) (type I) F31.9
    and related due to a known physiological condition
      with
        manic features F06.33
        manic- or hypomanic-like episodes F06.33
        mixed features F06.34
    current (or most recent) episode
      depressed F31.9
        with psychotic features F31.5
        without psychotic features F31.30
          mild F31.31
          moderate F31.32
          severe (without psychotic features) F31.4
            with psychotic features F31.5
      hypomanic F31.0
      manic F31.9
        with psychotic features F31.2
        without psychotic features F31.10
          mild F31.11
          moderate F31.12
          severe (without psychotic features)
            F31.13
            with psychotic features F31.2
      mixed F31.60
        mild F31.61
        moderate F31.62
        severe (without psychotic features) F31.63
          with psychotic features F31.64
      severe depression (without psychotic features)
        F31.4
        with psychotic features F31.5
    in remission (currently) F31.70
      in full remission
        most recent episode
          depressed F31.76
          hypomanic F31.72
          manic F31.74
          mixed F31.78
      in partial remission
        most recent episode
          depressed F31.75
          hypomanic F31.71
          manic F31.73
          mixed F31.77
    organic F06.30
    single manic episode F30.9
      mild F30.11
      moderate F30.12
      severe (without psychotic symptoms) F30.13
        with psychotic symptoms F30.2
    specified NEC F31.89
  bipolar II (type 2) F31.81
  bladder N32.9
    functional NEC N31.9
    in schistosomiasis B65.0 [N33]
    specified NEC N32.89
  bleeding D68.9
  blood D75.9
    in congenital early syphilis A50.09 [D77]
  body dysmorphic F45.22
  bone M89.9
    continuity M84.9

Disorder — *continued*
  bone — *continued*
    continuity — *continued*
      specified type NEC M84.80
        ankle M84.87- ☑
        fibula M84.86- ☑
        foot M84.87- ☑
        hand M84.84- ☑
        humerus M84.82- ☑
        neck M84.88
        pelvis M84.859
        radius M84.83- ☑
        rib M84.88
        shoulder M84.81- ☑
        skull M84.88
        thigh M84.85- ☑
        tibia M84.86- ☑
        ulna M84.83- ☑
        vertebra M84.88
    density and structure M85.9
      cyst — *see also* Cyst, bone, specified type NEC
        aneurysmal — *see* Cyst, bone, aneurysmal
        solitary — *see* Cyst, bone, solitary
      diffuse idiopathic skeletal hyperostosis — *see*
        Hyperostosis, ankylosing
      fibrous dysplasia (monostotic) — *see* Dysplasia,
        fibrous, bone
      fluorosis — *see* Fluorosis, skeletal
      hyperostosis of skull M85.2
      osteitis condensans — *see* Osteitis, condensans
      specified type NEC M85.8- ☑
        ankle M85.87- ☑
        foot M85.87- ☑
        forearm M85.83- ☑
        hand M85.84- ☑
        lower leg M85.86- ☑
        multiple sites M85.89
        neck M85.88
        rib M85.88
        shoulder M85.81- ☑
        skull M85.88
        thigh M85.85- ☑
        upper arm M85.82- ☑
        vertebra M85.88
    development and growth NEC M89.20
      carpus M89.24- ☑
      clavicle M89.21- ☑
      femur M89.25- ☑
      fibula M89.26- ☑
      finger M89.24- ☑
      humerus M89.22- ☑
      ilium M89.259
      ischium M89.259
      metacarpus M89.24- ☑
      metatarsus M89.27- ☑
      multiple sites M89.29
      neck M89.28
      radius M89.23- ☑
      rib M89.28
      scapula M89.21- ☑
      skull M89.28
      tarsus M89.27- ☑
      tibia M89.26- ☑
      toe M89.27- ☑
      ulna M89.23- ☑
      vertebra M89.28
    specified type NEC M89.8X- ☑
  brachial plexus G54.0
  branched-chain amino-acid metabolism E71.2
    specified NEC E71.19
  breast N64.9
    agalactia — *see* Agalactia
    associated with
      lactation O92.70
        specified NEC O92.79
      pregnancy O92.20
        specified NEC O92.29
      puerperium O92.20
        specified NEC O92.29
    cracked nipple — *see* Cracked nipple
    galactorrhea — *see* Galactorrhea
    hypogalactia O92.4
    lactation disorder NEC O92.79
    mastitis — *see* Mastitis
    nipple infection — *see* Infection, nipple
    retracted nipple — *see* Retraction, nipple
    specified type NEC N64.89

Disorder — *continued*
  Briquet's F45.0
  bullous, in diseases classified elsewhere L14
  caffeine use
    mild
      with
        caffeine-induced
          anxiety disorder F15.180
          sleep disorder F15.182
    moderate or severe
      with
        caffeine-induced
          anxiety disorder F15.280
          sleep disorder F15.282
  cannabis use
    mild F12.10
      with
        cannabis intoxication delirium F12.121
          with perceptual disturbances F12.122
          without perceptual disturbances F12.129
        cannabis-induced
          anxiety disorder F12.180
          psychotic disorder F12.159
          sleep disorder F12.188
      in remission (early) (sustained) F12.11
    moderate or severe F12.20
      with
        cannabis intoxication
          with perceptual disturbances F12.222
          without perceptual disturbances F12.229
        cannabis-induced
          anxiety disorder F12.280
          psychotic disorder F12.259
          sleep disorder F12.288
        delirium F12.221
      in remission (early) (sustained) F12.21
  carbohydrate
    absorption, intestinal NEC E74.39
    metabolism (congenital) E74.9
      specified NEC E74.8
  cardiac, functional I51.89
  carnitine metabolism E71.40
  cartilage M94.9
    articular NEC — *see* Derangement, joint, articular
      cartilage
    chondrocalcinosis — *see* Chondrocalcinosis
    specified type NEC M94.8X- ☑
      articular — *see* Derangement, joint, articular
        cartilage
      multiple sites M94.8X0
  catatonia (due to known physiological condition) (with
    another mental disorder) F06.1
  catatonic
    due to (secondary to) known physiological condition
      F06.1
    organic F06.1
  central auditory processing H93.25
  cervical
    region NEC M53.82
    root (nerve) NEC G54.2
  character NOS F60.9
  childhood disintegrative NEC F84.3
  cholesterol and bile acid metabolism E78.70
    Barth syndrome E78.71
    other specified E78.79
    Smith-Lemli-Opitz syndrome E78.72
  choroid H31.9
    atrophy — *see* Atrophy, choroid
    degeneration — *see* Degeneration, choroid
    detachment — *see* Detachment, choroid
    dystrophy — *see* Dystrophy, choroid
    hemorrhage — *see* Hemorrhage, choroid
    rupture — *see* Rupture, choroid
    scar — *see* Scar, chorioretinal
    solar retinopathy — *see* Retinopathy, solar
    specified type NEC H31.8
  ciliary body — *see* Disorder, iris
    degeneration — *see* Degeneration, ciliary body
  coagulation (factor) — *see also* Defect, coagulation
    D68.9
    newborn, transient P61.6
  cocaine use
    mild F14.10
      with
        amphetamine, cocaine, or other stimulant
          intoxication
          with perceptual disturbances F14.122
          without perceptual disturbances F14.129

☑ **Additional Character Required** — Refer to the Tabular List for Character Selection   ▽ **Subterms under main terms may continue to next column or page**

Disorder — *continued*
  cocaine use — *continued*
    mild — *continued*
      with — *continued*
        cocaine intoxication delirium F14.121
        cocaine-induced
          anxiety disorder F14.180
          bipolar and related disorder F14.14
          depressive disorder F14.14
          obsessive-compulsive and related disorder F14.188
          psychotic disorder F14.159
          sexual dysfunction F14.181
          sleep disorder F14.182
      in remission (early) (sustained) F14.11
    moderate or severe F14.20
      with
        amphetamine, cocaine, or other stimulant intoxication
          with perceptual disturbances F14.222
          without perceptual disturbances F14.229
        cocaine intoxication delirium F14.221
        cocaine-induced
          anxiety disorder F14.280
          bipolar and related disorder F14.24
          depressive disorder F14.24
          obsessive-compulsive and related disorder F14.288
          psychotic disorder F14.259
          sexual dysfunction F14.281
          sleep disorder F14.282
      in remission (early) (sustained) F14.21
  coccyx NEC M53.3
  cognitive F09
    due to (secondary to) general medical condition F09
    persisting R41.89
      due to
        alcohol F10.97
          with dependence F10.27
        anxiolytics F13.97
          with dependence F13.27
        hypnotics F13.97
          with dependence F13.27
        sedatives F13.97
          with dependence F13.27
        specified substance NEC F19.97
          with
            abuse F19.17
            dependence F19.27
  communication F80.9
    social pragmatic F80.82
  conduct (childhood) F91.9
    adjustment reaction — *see* Disorder, adjustment
    adolescent onset type F91.2
    childhood onset type F91.1
    compulsive F63.9
    confined to family context F91.0
    depressive F91.8
    group type F91.2
    hyperkinetic — *see* Disorder, attention-deficit hyperactivity
    oppositional defiance F91.3
    socialized F91.2
    solitary aggressive type F91.1
    specified NEC F91.8
    unsocialized (aggressive) F91.1
  conduction, heart I45.9
  congenital glycosylation (CDG) E74.8
  conjunctiva H11.9
    infection — *see* Conjunctivitis
  connective tissue, localized L94.9
    specified NEC L94.8
  conversion (functional neurological symptom disorder)
    with
      abnormal movement F44.4
      anesthesia or sensory loss F44.6
      attacks or seizures F44.5
      mixed symptoms F44.7
      special sensory symptoms F44.6
      speech symptoms F44.4
      swallowing symptoms F44.4
      weakness or paralysis F44.4
  convulsive (secondary) — *see* Convulsions
  cornea H18.9
    deformity — *see* Deformity, cornea
    degeneration — *see* Degeneration, cornea
    deposits — *see* Deposit, cornea
    due to contact lens H18.82- ☑

Disorder — *continued*
  cornea — *continued*
    due to contact lens — *continued*
      specified as edema — *see* Edema, cornea
    edema — *see* Edema, cornea
    keratitis — *see* Keratitis
    keratoconjunctivitis — *see* Keratoconjunctivitis
    membrane change — *see* Change, corneal membrane
    neovascularization — *see* Neovascularization, cornea
    scar — *see* Opacity, cornea
    specified type NEC H18.89- ☑
    ulcer — *see* Ulcer, cornea
  corpus cavernosum N48.9
  cranial nerve — *see* Disorder, nerve, cranial
  cyclothymic F34.0
  defiant oppositional F91.3
  delusional (persistent) (systematized) F22
    induced F24
  depersonalization F48.1
  depressive F32.9
    due to known physiological condition
      with
        depressive features F06.31
        major depressive-like episode F06.32
        mixed features F06.34
    major F32.9
      with psychotic symptoms F32.3
      in remission (full) F32.5
        partial F32.4
      recurrent F33.9
        with psychotic features F33.3
      single episode F32.9
        mild F32.0
        moderate F32.1
        severe (without psychotic symptoms) F32.2
          with psychotic symptoms F32.3
    organic F06.31
    persistent F34.1
    recurrent F33.9
      current episode
        mild F33.0
        moderate F33.1
        severe (without psychotic symptoms) F33.2
          with psychotic symptoms F33.3
      in remission F33.40
        full F33.42
        partial F33.41
      specified NEC F33.8
    single episode — *see* Episode, depressive
    specified NEC F32.89
  developmental F89
    arithmetical skills F81.2
    coordination (motor) F82
    expressive writing F81.81
    language F80.9
      expressive F80.1
      mixed receptive and expressive F80.2
      receptive type F80.2
      specified NEC F80.89
    learning F81.9
      arithmetical F81.2
      reading F81.0
    mixed F88
    motor coordination or function F82
    pervasive F84.9
      specified NEC F84.8
    phonological F80.0
    reading F81.0
    scholastic skills — *see also* Disorder, learning
      mixed F81.89
    specified NEC F88
    speech F80.9
      articulation F80.0
      specified NEC F80.89
    written expression F81.81
  diaphragm J98.6
  digestive (system) K92.9
    newborn P78.9
      specified NEC P78.89
    postprocedural — *see* Complication, gastrointestinal
    psychogenic F45.8
  disc (intervertebral) M51.9
    with
      myelopathy
        cervical region M50.00
        cervicothoracic region M50.03

Disorder — *continued*
  disc — *continued*
    with — *continued*
      myelopathy — *continued*
        high cervical region M50.01
        lumbar region M51.06
        mid-cervical region M50.020
        sacrococcygeal region M53.3
        thoracic region M51.04
        thoracolumbar region M51.05
      radiculopathy
        cervical region M50.10
        cervicothoracic region M50.13
        high cervical region M50.11
        lumbar region M51.16
        lumbosacral region M51.17
        mid-cervical region M50.120
        sacrococcygeal region M53.3
        thoracic region M51.14
        thoracolumbar region M51.15
    cervical M50.90
      with
        myelopathy M50.00
          C2-C3 M50.01
          C3-C4 M50.01
          C4-C5 M50.021
          C5-C6 M50.022
          C6-C7 M50.023
          C7-T1 M50.03
          cervicothoracic region M50.03
          high cervical region M50.01
          mid-cervical region M50.020
        neuritis, radiculitis or radiculopathy M50.10
          C2-C3 M50.11
          C3-C4 M50.11
          C4-C5 M50.121
          C5-C6 M50.122
          C6-C7 M50.123
          C7-T1 M50.13
          cervicothoracic region M50.13
          high cervical region M50.11
          mid-cervical region M50.120
      C2-C3 M50.91
      C3-C4 M50.91
      C4-C5 M50.921
      C5-C6 M50.922
      C6-C7 M50.923
      C7-T1 M50.93
      cervicothoracic region M50.93
      degeneration M50.30
        C2-C3 M50.31
        C3-C4 M50.31
        C4-C5 M50.321
        C5-C6 M50.322
        C6-C7 M50.323
        C7-T1 M50.33
        cervicothoracic region M50.33
        high cervical region M50.31
        mid-cervical region M50.320
      displacement M50.20
        C2-C3 M50.21
        C3-C4 M50.21
        C4-C5 M50.221
        C5-C6 M50.222
        C6-C7 M50.223
        C7-T1 M50.23
        cervicothoracic region M50.23
        high cervical region M50.21
        mid-cervical region M50.220
      high cervical region M50.91
      mid-cervical region M50.920
      specified type NEC M50.80
        C2-C3 M50.81
        C3-C4 M50.81
        C4-C5 M50.821
        C5-C6 M50.822
        C6-C7 M50.823
        C7-T1 M50.83
        cervicothoracic region M50.83
        high cervical region M50.81
        mid-cervical region M50.820
    specified NEC
      lumbar region M51.86
      lumbosacral region M51.87
      sacrococcygeal region M53.3
      thoracic region M51.84
      thoracolumbar region M51.85
  disinhibited attachment (childhood) F94.2
  disintegrative, childhood NEC F84.3

Disorder — *continued*
  disruptive F91.9
    mood dysregulation F34.81
    specified NEC F91.8
  disruptive behavior — *see* Disorder, conduct
  dissocial personality F60.2
  dissociative F44.9
    affecting
      motor function F44.4
        and sensation F44.7
      sensation F44.6
        and motor function F44.7
    brief reactive F43.0
    due to (secondary to) general medical condition F06.8
    mixed F44.7
    organic F06.8
    other specified NEC F44.89
  double heterozygous sickling — *see* Disease, sickle-cell
  dream anxiety F51.5
  drug induced hemorrhagic D68.32
  drug related F19.99
    abuse — *see* Abuse, drug
    dependence — *see* Dependence, drug
  dysmorphic body F45.22
  dysthymic F34.1
  ear H93.9- ☑
    bleeding — *see* Otorrhagia
    deafness — *see* Deafness
    degenerative H93.09- ☑
    discharge — *see* Otorrhea
    external H61.9- ☑
      auditory canal stenosis — *see* Stenosis, external ear canal
      exostosis — *see* Exostosis, external ear canal
      impacted cerumen — *see* Impaction, cerumen
      otitis — *see* Otitis, externa
      perichondritis — *see* Perichondritis, ear
      pinna — *see* Disorder, pinna
      specified type NEC H61.89- ☑
    inner H83.9- ☑
      vestibular dysfunction — *see* Disorder, vestibular function
    middle H74.9- ☑
      adhesive H74.1- ☑
      ossicle — *see* Abnormal, ear ossicles
      polyp — *see* Polyp, ear (middle)
      specified NEC, in diseases classified elsewhere H75.8- ☑
    postprocedural — *see* Complications, ear, procedure
    specified NEC, in diseases classified elsewhere H94.8- ☑
  eating (adult) (psychogenic) F50.9
    anorexia — *see* Anorexia
    binge F50.81
    bulimia F50.2
    child F98.29
      pica F98.3
      rumination disorder F98.21
    pica F50.89
      childhood F98.3
  electrolyte (balance) NEC E87.8
    with
      abortion — *see* Abortion by type complicated by specified condition NEC
      ectopic pregnancy O08.5
      molar pregnancy O08.5
    acidosis (metabolic) (respiratory) E87.2
    alkalosis (metabolic) (respiratory) E87.3
  elimination, transepidermal L87.9
    specified NEC L87.8
  emotional (persistent) F34.9
    of childhood F93.9
    specified NEC F93.8
  endocrine E34.9
    postprocedural E89.89
    specified NEC E89.89
  erectile (male) (organic) — *see also* Dysfunction, sexual, male, erectile N52.9
    nonorganic F52.21
  erythematous — *see* Erythema
  esophagus K22.9
    functional K22.4
    psychogenic F45.8
  eustachian tube H69.9- ☑
    infection — *see* Salpingitis, eustachian
    obstruction — *see* Obstruction, eustachian tube
    patulous — *see* Patulous, eustachian tube

Disorder — *continued*
  eustachian tube — *continued*
    specified NEC H69.8- ☑
  exhibitionistic F65.2
  extrapyramidal G25.9
    in deseases classified elsewhere — *see* category G26
    specified type NEC G25.89
  eye H57.9
    postprocedural — *see* Complication, postprocedural, eye
  eyelid H02.9
    cyst — *see* Cyst, eyelid
    degenerative H02.70
      chloasma — *see* Chloasma, eyelid
      madarosis — *see* Madarosis
      specified type NEC H02.79
      vitiligo — *see* Vitiligo, eyelid
      xanthelasma — *see* Xanthelasma
    dermatochalasis — *see* Dermatochalasis
    edema — *see* Edema, eyelid
    elephantiasis — *see* Elephantiasis, eyelid
    foreign body, retained — *see* Foreign body, retained, eyelid
    function H02.59
      abnormal innervation syndrome — *see* Syndrome, abnormal innervation
      blepharochalasis — *see* Blepharochalasis
      blepharoclonus — *see* Blepharoclonus
      blepharophimosis — *see* Blepharophimosis
      blepharoptosis — *see* Blepharoptosis
      lagophthalmos — *see* Lagophthalmos
      lid retraction — *see* Retraction, lid
    hypertrichosis — *see* Hypertrichosis, eyelid
    specified type NEC H02.89
    vascular H02.879
      left H02.876
        lower H02.875
        upper H02.874
      right H02.873
        lower H02.872
        upper H02.871
  factitious
    by proxy F68.A
    imposed on another F68.A
    imposed on self F68.10
      with predominantly
        psychological symptoms F68.11
          with physical symptoms F68.13
        physical symptoms F68.12
          with psychological symptoms F68.13
  factor, coagulation — *see* Defect, coagulation
  fatty acid
    metabolism E71.30
      specified NEC E71.39
    oxidation
      LCAD E71.310
      MCAD E71.311
      SCAD E71.312
      specified deficiency NEC E71.318
  feeding (infant or child) — *see also* Disorder, eating R63.3
    or eating disorder F50.9
    specified NEC F50.9
  feigned (with obvious motivation) Z76.5
    without obvious motivation — *see* Disorder, factitious
  female
    hypoactive sexual desire F52.0
    orgasmic F52.31
    sexual interest/arousal F52.22
  fetishistic F65.0
  fibroblastic M72.9
    specified NEC M72.8
  fluency
    adult onset F98.5
    childhood onset F80.81
    following
      cerebral infarction I69.323
      cerebrovascular disease I69.923
        specified disease NEC I69.823
      intracerebral hemorrhage I69.123
      nontraumatic intracranial hemorrhage NEC I69.223
      subarachnoid hemorrhage I69.023
    in conditions classified elsewhere R47.82
  fluid balance E87.8
  follicular (skin) L73.9

Disorder — *continued*
  follicular — *continued*
    specified NEC L73.8
  frotteuristic F65.81
  fructose metabolism E74.10
    essential fructosuria E74.11
    fructokinase deficiency E74.11
    fructose-1, 6-diphosphatase deficiency E74.19
    hereditary fructose intolerance E74.12
    other specified E74.19
  functional polymorphonuclear neutrophils D71
  gallbladder, biliary tract and pancreas in diseases classified elsewhere K87
  gambling F63.0
  gamma aminobutyric acid (GABA) metabolism E72.81
  gamma-glutamyl cycle E72.89
  gastric (functional) K31.9
    motility K30
    psychogenic F45.8
    secretion K30
  gastrointestinal (functional) NOS K92.9
    newborn P78.9
    psychogenic F45.8
  gender-identity or -role F64.9
    childhood F64.2
    effect on relationship F66
    of adolescence or adulthood F64.0
      nontranssexual F64.8
    specified NEC F64.8
    uncertainty F66
  genito-pelvic pain penetration F52.6
  genitourinary system
    female N94.9
    male N50.9
    psychogenic F45.8
  globe H44.9
    degenerated condition H44.50
      absolute glaucoma H44.51- ☑
      atrophy H44.52- ☑
      leucocoria H44.53- ☑
    degenerative H44.30
      chalcosis H44.31- ☑
      myopia — *see also* Myopia, degenerative H44.2- ☑
      siderosis H44.32- ☑
      specified type NEC H44.39- ☑
    endophthalmitis — *see* Endophthalmitis
    foreign body, retained — *see* Foreign body, intraocular, old, retained
    hemophthalmos — *see* Hemophthalmos
    hypotony H44.40
      due to
        ocular fistula H44.42- ☑
        specified disorder NEC H44.43- ☑
      flat anterior chamber H44.41- ☑
      primary H44.44- ☑
    luxation — *see* Luxation, globe
    specified type NEC H44.89
  glomerular (in) N05.9
    amyloidosis E85.4 [N08]
    cryoglobulinemia D89.1 [N08]
    disseminated intravascular coagulation D65 [N08]
    Fabry's disease E75.21 [N08]
    familial lecithin cholesterol acyltransferase deficiency E78.6 [N08]
    Goodpasture's syndrome M31.0
    hemolytic-uremic syndrome D59.3
    Henoch (-Schönlein) purpura D69.0 [N08]
    malariae malaria B52.0
    microscopic polyangiitis M31.7 [N08]
    multiple myeloma C90.0- ☑ [N08]
    mumps B26.83
    schistosomiasis B65.9 [N08]
    sepsis NEC A41.- ☑ [N08]
      streptococcal A40.- ☑ [N08]
    sickle-cell disorders D57.- ☑ [N08]
    strongyloidiasis B78.9 [N08]
    subacute bacterial endocarditis I33.0 [N08]
    syphilis A52.75
    systemic lupus erythematosus M32.14
    thrombotic thrombocytopenic purpura M31.1 [N08]
    Waldenström macroglobulinemia C88.0 [N08]
    Wegener's granulomatosis M31.31
  gluconeogenesis E74.4
  glucosaminoglycan metabolism — *see* Disorder, metabolism, glucosaminoglycan
  glycine metabolism E72.50
    d-glycericacidemia E72.59

112   ☑ Additional Character Required — Refer to the Tabular List for Character Selection   ▼ Subterms under main terms may continue to next column or page

Disorder — Disorder

Disorder — continued
  glycine metabolism — continued
    hyperhydroxyprolinemia E72.59
    hyperoxaluria R82.992
      primary E72.53
    hyperprolinemia E72.59
    non-ketotic hyperglycinemia E72.51
    oxalosis E72.53
    oxaluria E72.53
    sarcosinemia E72.59
    trimethylaminuria E72.52
  glycoprotein metabolism E77.9
    specified NEC E77.8
  habit (and impulse) F63.9
    involving sexual behavior NEC F65.9
    specified NEC F63.89
  hallucinogen use
    mild F16.10
      with
        hallucinogen intoxication delirium F16.121
        hallucinogen-induced
          anxiety disorder F16.180
          bipolar and related disorder F16.14
          depressive disorder F16.14
          psychotic disorder F16.159
        other hallucinogen intoxication F16.129
      in remission (early) (sustained) F16.11
    moderate or severe F16.20
      with
        hallucinogen intoxication delirium F16.221
        hallucinogen-induced
          anxiety disorder F16.280
          bipolar and related disorder F16.24
          depressive disorder F16.24
          psychotic disorder F16.259
        other hallucinogen intoxication F16.229
      in remission (early) (sustained) F16.21
  heart action I49.9
  hematological D75.9
    newborn (transient) P61.9
      specified NEC P61.8
  hematopoietic organs D75.9
  hemorrhagic NEC D69.9
    drug-induced D68.32
    due to
      extrinsic circulating anticoagulants D68.32
      increase in
        anti-IIa D68.32
        anti-Xa D68.32
      intrinsic
        circulating anticoagulants D68.318
        increase in
          anti-IXa D68.318
          antithrombin D68.318
          anti-VIIIa D68.318
          anti-XIa D68.318
    following childbirth O72.3
  hemostasis — see Defect, coagulation
  histidine metabolism E70.40
    histidinemia E70.41
    other specified E70.49
  hoarding F42.3
  hyperkinetic — see Disorder, attention-deficit hyperactivity
  hyperleucine-isoleucinemia E71.19
  hypervalinemia E71.19
  hypoactive sexual desire F52.0
  hypochondriacal F45.20
    body dysmorphic F45.22
    neurosis F45.21
    other specified F45.29
  identity
    dissociative F44.81
    illness anxiety F45.21
    of childhood F93.8
  immune mechanism (immunity) D89.9
    specified type NEC D89.89
  impaired renal tubular function N25.9
    specified NEC N25.89
  impulse (control) F63.9
  inflammatory
    pelvic, in diseases classified elsewhere — see category N74
    penis N48.29
      abscess N48.21
      cellulitis N48.22
  inhalant use
    mild F18.10

Disorder — continued
  inhalant use — continued
    mild — continued
      with
        inhalant intoxication F18.129
        inhalant intoxication delirium F18.121
        inhalant-induced
          anxiety disorder F18.180
          depressive disorder F18.14
          major neurocognitive disorder F18.17
          mild neurocognitive disorder F18.188
          psychotic disorder F18.159
      in remission (early) (sustained) F18.11
    moderate or severe F18.20
      with
        inhalant intoxication F18.229
        inhalant intoxication delirium F18.221
        inhalant-induced
          anxiety disorder F18.280
          depressive disorder F18.24
          major neurocognitive disorder F18.27
          mild neurocognitive disorder F18.288
          psychotic disorder F18.259
      in remission (early) (sustained) F18.21
  integument, newborn P83.9
    specified NEC P83.88
  intermittent explosive F63.81
  internal secretion pancreas — see Increased, secretion, pancreas, endocrine
  intestine, intestinal
    carbohydrate absorption NEC E74.39
      postoperative K91.2
    functional NEC K59.9
      postoperative K91.89
    psychogenic F45.8
    vascular K55.9
      chronic K55.1
      specified NEC K55.8
  intraoperative (intraprocedural) — see Complications, intraoperative
  involuntary emotional expression (IEED) F07.89
  iris H21.9
    adhesions — see Adhesions, iris
    atrophy — see Atrophy, iris
    chamber angle recession — see Recession, chamber angle
    cyst — see Cyst, iris
    degeneration — see Degeneration, iris
    in diseases classified elsewhere H22
    iridodialysis — see Iridodialysis
    iridoschisis — see Iridoschisis
    miotic pupillary cyst — see Cyst, pupillary
    pupillary
      abnormality — see Abnormality, pupillary
      membrane — see Membrane, pupillary
    specified type NEC H21.89
    vascular NEC H21.1X- ☑
  iron metabolism E83.10
    specified NEC E83.19
  isovaleric acidemia E71.110
  jaw, developmental M27.0
    temporomandibular — see also Anomaly, dentofacial, temporomandibular joint M26.60- ☑
  joint M25.9
    derangement — see Derangement, joint
    effusion — see Effusion, joint
    fistula — see Fistula, joint
    hemarthrosis — see Hemarthrosis
    instability — see Instability, joint
    osteophyte — see Osteophyte
    pain — see Pain, joint
    psychogenic F45.8
    specified type NEC M25.80
      ankle M25.87- ☑
      elbow M25.82- ☑
      foot joint M25.87- ☑
      hand joint M25.84- ☑
      hip M25.85- ☑
      knee M25.86- ☑
      shoulder M25.81- ☑
      wrist M25.83- ☑
    stiffness — see Stiffness, joint
  ketone metabolism E71.32
  kidney N28.9
    functional (tubular) N25.9
    in
      schistosomiasis B65.9 [N29]
    tubular function N25.9

Disorder — continued
  kidney — continued
    tubular function — continued
      specified NEC N25.89
  lacrimal system H04.9
    changes H04.69
      fistula — see Fistula, lacrimal
    gland H04.19
      atrophy — see Atrophy, lacrimal gland
      cyst — see Cyst, lacrimal, gland
      dacryops — see Dacryops
      dislocation — see Dislocation, lacrimal gland
      dry eye syndrome — see Syndrome, dry eye
      infection — see Dacryoadenitis
      granuloma — see Granuloma, lacrimal
      inflammation — see Inflammation, lacrimal
      obstruction — see Obstruction, lacrimal
      specified NEC H04.89
  lactation NEC O92.79
  language (developmental) F80.9
    expressive F80.1
    mixed receptive and expressive F80.2
    receptive F80.2
  late luteal phase dysphoric N94.89
  learning (specific) F81.9
    acalculia R48.8
    alexia R48.0
    mathematics F81.2
    reading F81.0
    specified
      with impairment in
        mathematics F81.2
        reading F81.0
        written expression F81.81
    specified NEC F81.89
    spelling F81.81
    written expression F81.81
  lens H27.9
    aphakia — see Aphakia
    cataract — see Cataract
    dislocation — see Dislocation, lens
    specified type NEC H27.8
  ligament M24.20
    ankle M24.27- ☑
    attachment, spine — see Enthesopathy, spinal
    elbow M24.22- ☑
    foot joint M24.27- ☑
    hand joint M24.24- ☑
    hip M24.25- ☑
    knee — see Derangement, knee, specified NEC
    shoulder M24.21- ☑
    vertebra M24.28
    wrist M24.23- ☑
  ligamentous attachments — see also Enthesopathy
    spine — see Enthesopathy, spinal
  lipid
    metabolism, congenital E78.9
    storage E75.6
      specified NEC E75.5
  lipoprotein
    deficiency (familial) E78.6
    metabolism E78.9
      specified NEC E78.89
  liver K76.9
    malarial B54 [K77]
  low back — see also Dorsopathy, specified NEC
  lumbosacral
    plexus G54.1
    root (nerve) NEC G54.4
  lung, interstitial, drug-induced J70.4
    acute J70.2
    chronic J70.3
  lymphoproliferative, post-transplant (PTLD) D47.Z1
    (following D47.4)
  lysine and hydroxylysine metabolism E72.3
  major neurocognitive — see Dementia, in (due to)
  male
    erectile (organic) — see also Dysfunction, sexual, male, erectile N52.9
      nonorganic F52.21
    hypoactive sexual desire F52.0
    orgasmic F52.32
  manic F30.9
    organic F06.33
  mast cell activation — see Activation, mast cell
  mastoid — see also Disorder, ear, middle
    postprocedural — see Complications, ear, procedure
  meniscus — see Derangement, knee, meniscus

Disorder — *continued*
  menopausal N95.9
    specified NEC N95.8
  menstrual N92.6
    psychogenic F45.8
    specified NEC N92.5
  mental (or behavioral) (nonpsychotic) F99
    due to (secondary to)
      amphetamine
        due to drug abuse — *see* Abuse, drug, stimulant
        due to drug dependence — *see* Dependence, drug, stimulant
      brain disease, damage and dysfunction F09
      caffeine use
        due to drug abuse — *see* Abuse, drug, stimulant
        due to drug dependence — *see* Dependence, drug, stimulant
      cannabis use
        due to drug abuse — *see* Abuse, drug, cannabis
        due to drug dependence — *see* Dependence, drug, cannabis
      general medical condition F09
      sedative or hypnotic use
        due to drug abuse — *see* Abuse, drug, sedative
        due to drug dependence — *see* Dependence, drug, sedative
      tobacco (nicotine) use — *see* Dependence, drug, nicotine
    following organic brain damage F07.9
      frontal lobe syndrome F07.0
      personality change F07.0
      postconcussional syndrome F07.81
      specified NEC F07.89
    infancy, childhood or adolescence F98.9
    neurotic — *see* Neurosis
    organic or symptomatic F09
    presenile, psychotic F03 ☑
    problem NEC
    psychoneurotic — *see* Neurosis
    psychotic — *see* Psychosis
    puerperal F53.0
    senile, psychotic NEC F03 ☑
  metabolic, amino acid, transitory, newborn P74.8
  metabolism NOS E88.9
    amino-acid E72.9
      aromatic E70.9
        albinism — *see* Albinism
        histidine E70.40
          histidinemia E70.41
          other specified E70.49
        hyperphenylalaninemia E70.1
          classical phenylketonuria E70.0
        other specified E70.8
        tryptophan E70.5
        tyrosine E70.20
          hypertyrosinemia E70.21
          other specified E70.29
      branched chain E71.2
        3-methylglutaconic aciduria E71.111
        hyperleucine-isoleucinemia E71.19
        hypervalinemia E71.19
        isovaleric acidemia E71.110
        maple syrup urine disease E71.0
        methylmalonic acidemia E71.120
        organic aciduria NEC E71.118
        other specified E71.19
        proprionate NEC E71.128
        proprionic acidemia E71.121
      glycine E72.50
        d-glycericacidemia E72.59
        hyperhydroxyprolinemia E72.59
        hyperoxaluria R82.992
          primary E72.53
        hyperprolinemia E72.59
        non-ketotic hyperglycinemia E72.51
        other specified E72.59
        sarcosinemia E72.59
        trimethylaminuria E72.52
      hydroxylysine E72.3
      lysine E72.3
      ornithine E72.4
      other specified E72.89
        beta-amino acid E72.89
        gamma-glutamyl cycle E72.89

Disorder — *continued*
  metabolism — *continued*
    amino-acid — *continued*
      straight-chain E72.89
      sulfur-bearing E72.10
        homocystinuria E72.11
        methylenetetrahydrofolate reductase deficiency E72.12
        other specified E72.19
    bile acid and cholesterol metabolism E78.70
    bilirubin E80.7
      specified NEC E80.6
    calcium E83.50
      hypercalcemia E83.52
      hypocalcemia E83.51
      other specified E83.59
    carbohydrate E74.9
      specified NEC E74.8
    cholesterol and bile acid metabolism E78.70
    congenital E88.9
    copper E83.00
      specified type NEC E83.09
      Wilson's disease E83.01
    cystinuria E72.01
    fructose E74.10
    galactose E74.20
    glucosaminoglycan E76.9
      mucopolysaccharidosis — *see* Mucopolysaccharidosis
      specified NEC E76.8
    glutamine E72.89
    glycine E72.50
    glycogen storage (hepatorenal) E74.09
    glycoprotein E77.9
      specified NEC E77.8
    glycosaminoglycan E76.9
      specified NEC E76.8
    in labor and delivery O75.89
    iron E83.10
    isoleucine E71.19
    leucine E71.19
    lipoid E78.9
    lipoprotein E78.9
      specified NEC E78.89
    magnesium E83.40
      hypermagnesemia E83.41
      hypomagnesemia E83.42
      other specified E83.49
    mineral E83.9
      specified NEC E83.89
    mitochondrial E88.40
      MELAS syndrome E88.41
      MERRF syndrome (myoclonic epilepsy associated with ragged-red fibers) E88.42
      other specified E88.49
    ornithine E72.4
    phosphatases E83.30
    phosphorus E83.30
      acid phosphatase deficiency E83.39
      hypophosphatasia E83.39
      hypophosphatemia E83.39
        familial E83.31
      other specified E83.39
      pseudovitamin D deficiency E83.32
    plasma protein NEC E88.09
    porphyrin — *see* Porphyria
    postprocedural E89.89
      specified NEC E89.89
    purine E79.9
      specified NEC E79.8
    pyrimidine E79.9
      specified NEC E79.8
    pyruvate E74.4
    serine E72.89
    sodium E87.8
    specified NEC E88.89
    threonine E72.89
    valine E71.19
    zinc E83.2
  methylmalonic acidemia E71.120
  micturition NEC — *see also* Difficulty, micturition R39.198
    feeling of incomplete emptying R39.14
    hesitancy R39.11
    poor stream R39.12
    psychogenic F45.8
    split stream R39.13
    straining R39.16
    urgency R39.15

Disorder — *continued*
  mild neurocognitive G31.84
  mitochondrial metabolism E88.40
  mitral (valve) — *see* Endocarditis, mitral
  mixed
    anxiety and depressive F41.8
    of scholastic skills (developmental) F81.89
    receptive expressive language F80.2
  mood F39
    bipolar — *see* Disorder, bipolar
    depressive — *see* Disorder, depressive
    due to (secondary to)
      alcohol F10.94
      amphetamine F15.94
        in
          abuse F15.14
          dependence F15.24
      anxiolytic F13.94
        in
          abuse F13.14
          dependence F13.24
      cocaine F14.94
        in
          abuse F14.14
          dependence F14.24
      general medical condition F06.30
      hallucinogen F16.94
        in
          abuse F16.14
          dependence F16.24
      hypnotic F13.94
        in
          abuse F13.14
          dependence F13.24
      inhalant F18.94
        in
          abuse F18.14
          dependence F18.24
      opioid F11.94
        in
          abuse F11.14
          dependence F11.24
      phencyclidine (PCP) F16.94
        in
          abuse F16.14
          dependence F16.24
      physiological condition F06.30
        with
          depressive features F06.31
          major depressive-like episode F06.32
          manic features F06.33
          mixed features F06.34
      psychoactive substance NEC F19.94
        in
          abuse F19.14
          dependence F19.24
      sedative F13.94
        in
          abuse F13.14
          dependence F13.24
      volatile solvents F18.94
        in
          abuse F18.14
          dependence F18.24
    manic episode F30.9
      with psychotic symptoms F30.2
      in remission (full) F30.4
        partial F30.3
      specified type NEC F30.8
      without psychotic symptoms F30.10
        mild F30.11
        moderate F30.12
        severe F30.13
    organic F06.30
      right hemisphere F07.89
    persistent F34.9
      cyclothymia F34.0
      dysthymia F34.1
      specified type NEC F34.89
    recurrent F39
    right hemisphere organic F07.89
  movement G25.9
    drug-induced G25.70
      akathisia G25.71
      specified NEC G25.79
    hysterical F44.4
    in diseases classified elsewhere — *see* category G26
    periodic limb G47.61
      sleep related G47.61

Disorder — *continued*
  movement — *continued*
    sleep related NEC G47.69
    specified NEC G25.89
    stereotyped F98.4
    treatment-induced G25.9
  multiple personality F44.81
  muscle M62.9
    attachment, spine — *see* Enthesopathy, spinal
    in trichinellosis — *see* Trichinellosis, with muscle disorder
    psychogenic F45.8
    specified type NEC M62.89
    tone, newborn P94.9
      specified NEC P94.8
  muscular
    attachments — *see also* Enthesopathy
      spine — *see* Enthesopathy, spinal
    urethra N36.44
  musculoskeletal system, soft tissue — *see* Disorder, soft tissue
    postprocedural M96.89
    psychogenic F45.8
  myoneural G70.9
    due to lead G70.1
    specified NEC G70.89
    toxic G70.1
  myotonic NEC G71.19
  nail, in diseases classified elsewhere L62
  neck region NEC — *see* Dorsopathy, specified NEC
  neonatal onset multisystemic inflammatory (NOMID) M04.2
  nerve G58.9
    abducent NEC — *see* Strabismus, paralytic, sixth nerve
    accessory G52.8
    acoustic — *see* subcategory H93.3 ☑
    auditory — *see* subcategory H93.3 ☑
    auriculotemporal G50.8
    axillary G54.0
    cerebral — *see* Disorder, nerve, cranial
    cranial G52.9
      eighth — *see* subcategory H93.3 ☑
      eleventh G52.8
      fifth G50.9
      first G52.0
      fourth NEC — *see* Strabismus, paralytic, fourth nerve
      multiple G52.7
      ninth G52.1
      second NEC — *see* Disorder, nerve, optic
      seventh NEC G51.8
      sixth NEC — *see* Strabismus, paralytic, sixth nerve
      specified NEC G52.8
      tenth G52.2
      third NEC — *see* Strabismus, paralytic, third nerve
      twelfth G52.3
    entrapment — *see* Neuropathy, entrapment
    facial G51.9
      specified NEC G51.8
    femoral — *see* Lesion, nerve, femoral
    glossopharyngeal NEC G52.1
    hypoglossal G52.3
    intercostal G58.0
    lateral
      cutaneous of thigh — *see* Mononeuropathy, lower limb, meralgia paresthetica
      popliteal — *see* Lesion, nerve, popliteal
    lower limb — *see* Mononeuropathy, lower limb
    medial popliteal — *see* Lesion, nerve, popliteal, medial
    median NEC — *see* Lesion, nerve, median
    multiple G58.7
    oculomotor NEC — *see* Strabismus, paralytic, third nerve
    olfactory G52.0
    optic NEC H47.09- ☑
      hemorrhage into sheath — *see* Hemorrhage, optic nerve
      ischemic H47.01- ☑
    peroneal — *see* Lesion, nerve, popliteal
    phrenic G58.8
    plantar — *see* Lesion, nerve, plantar
    pneumogastric G52.2
    posterior tibial — *see* Syndrome, tarsal tunnel
    radial — *see* Lesion, nerve, radial
    recurrent laryngeal G52.2
    root G54.9

Disorder — *continued*
  nerve — *continued*
    root — *continued*
      cervical G54.2
      lumbosacral G54.1
      specified NEC G54.8
      thoracic G54.3
    sciatic NEC — *see* Lesion, nerve, sciatic
    specified NEC G58.8
      lower limb — *see* Mononeuropathy, lower limb, specified NEC
      upper limb — *see* Mononeuropathy, upper limb, specified NEC
    sympathetic G90.9
    tibial — *see* Lesion, nerve, popliteal, medial
    trigeminal G50.9
      specified NEC G50.8
    trochlear NEC — *see* Strabismus, paralytic, fourth nerve
    ulnar — *see* Lesion, nerve, ulnar
    upper limb — *see* Mononeuropathy, upper limb
    vagus G52.2
  nervous system G98.8
    autonomic (peripheral) G90.9
      specified NEC G90.8
    central G96.9
      specified NEC G96.8
    parasympathetic G90.9
    specified NEC G98.8
    sympathetic G90.9
    vegetative G90.9
  neurocognitive R41.9
    major
      with
        aggressive behavior F01.51
        combative behavior F01.51
        violent behavior F01.51
      due to vascular disease, with behavioral disturbance F01.51
      in (due to) (other diseases classified elsewhere) — *see also* Dementia, in (due to) F02.80
        with
          aggressive behavior F02.81
          combative behavior F02.81
          violent behavior F02.81
        without behavioral disturbance F01.50
    mild G31.84
  neurodevelopmental F89
    specified NEC F88
  neurohypophysis NEC E23.3
  neurological R29.818
  neuromuscular G70.9
    hereditary NEC G71.9
    specified NEC G70.89
    toxic G70.1
  neurotic F48.9
    specified NEC F48.8
  neutrophil, polymorphonuclear D71
  nicotine use — *see* Dependence, drug, nicotine
  nightmare F51.5
  non-rapid eye movement sleep arousal
    sleep terror type F51.4
    sleepwalking type F51.3
  nose J34.9
    specified NEC J34.89
  obsessive-compulsive F42.9
    and related disorder due to a known physiological condition F06.8
  odontogenesis NOS K00.9
  opioid use
    with
      opioid-induced psychotic disorder F11.959
        with
          delusions F11.950
          hallucinations F11.951
    due to drug abuse — *see* Abuse, drug, opioid
    due to drug dependence — *see* Dependence, drug, opioid
    mild F11.10
      with
        opioid-induced
          anxiety disorder F11.188
          depressive disorder F11.14
          sexual dysfunction F11.181
        opioid intoxication
          with perceptual disturbances F11.122
          delirium F11.121
          without perceptual disturbances F11.129

Disorder — *continued*
  opioid use — *continued*
    mild — *continued*
      in remission (early) (sustained) F11.11
    moderate or severe F11.20
      with
        opioid-induced
          anxiety disorder F11.288
          anxiety disorder F11.988
          depressive disorder F11.24
          depressive disorder F11.94
          sexual dysfunction F11.281
          sexual dysfunction F11.981
        opioid intoxication
          with perceptual disturbances F11.222
          delirium F11.221
          without perceptual disturbances F11.229
      in remission (early) (sustained) F11.21
  oppositional defiant F91.3
  optic
    chiasm H47.49
      due to
        inflammatory disorder H47.41
        neoplasm H47.42
        vascular disorder H47.43
    disc H47.39- ☑
      coloboma — *see* Coloboma, optic disc
      drusen — *see* Drusen, optic disc
      pseudopapilledema — *see* Pseudopapilledema
    radiations — *see* Disorder, visual, pathway
    tracts — *see* Disorder, visual, pathway
  orbit H05.9
    cyst — *see* Cyst, orbit
    deformity — *see* Deformity, orbit
    edema — *see* Edema, orbit
    enophthalmos — *see* Enophthalmos
    exophthalmos — *see* Exophthalmos
    hemorrhage — *see* Hemorrhage, orbit
    inflammation — *see* Inflammation, orbit
    myopathy — *see* Myopathy, extraocular muscles
    retained foreign body — *see* Foreign body, orbit, old
    specified type NEC H05.89
  organic
    anxiety F06.4
    catatonic F06.1
    delusional F06.2
    dissociative F06.8
    emotionally labile (asthenic) F06.8
    mood (affective) F06.30
    schizophrenia-like F06.2
  orgasmic (female) F52.31
    male F52.32
  ornithine metabolism E72.4
  overanxious F41.1
    of childhood F93.8
  pain
    with related psychological factors F45.42
    exclusively related to psychological factors F45.41
    genito-pelvic penetration disorder F52.6
  pancreatic internal secretion E16.9
    specified NEC E16.8
  panic F41.0
    with agoraphobia F40.01
  papulosquamous L44.9
    in diseases classified elsewhere L45
    specified NEC L44.8
  paranoid F22
    induced F24
    shared F24
  paraphilic F65.9
    specified NEC F65.89
  parathyroid (gland) E21.5
    specified NEC E21.4
  parietoalveolar NEC J84.09
  paroxysmal, mixed R56.9
  patella M22.9- ☑
    chondromalacia — *see* Chondromalacia, patella
    derangement NEC M22.3X- ☑
    recurrent
      dislocation — *see* Dislocation, patella, recurrent
      subluxation — *see* Dislocation, patella, recurrent, incomplete
    specified NEC M22.8X- ☑
  patellofemoral M22.2X- ☑
  pedophilic F65.4
  pentose phosphate pathway with anemia D55.1
  perception, due to hallucinogens F16.983

Disorder — *continued*
perception, due to hallucinogens — *continued*
  in
    abuse F16.183
    dependence F16.283
peripheral nervous system NEC G64
peroxisomal E71.50
  biogenesis
    neonatal adrenoleukodystrophy E71.511
    specified disorder NEC E71.518
    Zellweger syndrome E71.510
  rhizomelic chondrodysplasia punctata E71.540
  specified form NEC E71.548
    group 1 E71.518
    group 2 E71.53
    group 3 E71.542
  X-linked adrenoleukodystrophy E71.529
    adolescent E71.521
    adrenomyeloneuropathy E71.522
    childhood E71.520
    specified form NEC E71.528
  Zellweger-like syndrome E71.541
persistent
  (somatoform) pain F45.41
  affective (mood) F34.9
personality — *see also* Personality F60.9
  affective F34.0
  aggressive F60.3
  amoral F60.2
  anankastic F60.5
  antisocial F60.2
  anxious F60.6
  asocial F60.2
  asthenic F60.7
  avoidant F60.6
  borderline F60.3
  change (secondary) due to general medical condition F07.0
  compulsive F60.5
  cyclothymic F34.0
  dependent (passive) F60.7
  depressive F34.1
  dissocial F60.2
  emotional instability F60.3
  expansive paranoid F60.0
  explosive F60.3
  following organic brain damage F07.9
  histrionic F60.4
  hyperthymic F34.0
  hypothymic F34.1
  hysterical F60.4
  immature F60.89
  inadequate F60.7
  labile F60.3
  mixed (nonspecific) F60.89
  moral deficiency F60.2
  narcissistic F60.81
  negativistic F60.89
  obsessional F60.5
  obsessive (-compulsive) F60.5
  organic F07.9
  overconscientious F60.5
  paranoid F60.0
  passive (-dependent) F60.7
  passive-aggressive F60.89
  pathological NEC F60.9
  pseudosocial F60.2
  psychopathic F60.2
  schizoid F60.1
  schizotypal F21
  self-defeating F60.7
  specified NEC F60.89
  type A F60.5
  unstable (emotional) F60.3
pervasive, developmental F84.9
phencyclidine use
  mild F16.10
    with
      phencyclidine intoxication F16.129
      phencyclidine intoxication delirium F16.121
      phencyclidine-induced
        anxiety disorder F16.180
        bipolar and related disorder F16.14
        depressive disorder F16.14
        psychotic disorder F16.159
      in remission (early) (sustained) F16.11
  moderate or severe F16.20
    with
      phencyclidine intoxication F16.229

Disorder — *continued*
phencyclidine use — *continued*
  moderate or severe — *continued*
    with — *continued*
      phencyclidine intoxication delirium F16.221
      phencyclidine-induced
        anxiety disorder F16.280
        bipolar and related disorder F16.14
        depressive disorder F16.24
        psychotic disorder F16.259
      in remission (early) (sustained) F16.21
phobic anxiety, childhood F40.8
phosphate-losing tubular N25.0
pigmentation L81.9
  choroid, congenital Q14.3
  diminished melanin formation L81.6
  iron L81.8
  specified NEC L81.8
pinna (noninfective) H61.10- ☑
  deformity, acquired H61.11- ☑
  hematoma H61.12- ☑
  perichondritis — *see* Perichondritis, ear
  specified type NEC H61.19- ☑
pituitary gland E23.7
  iatrogenic (postprocedural) E89.3
  specified NEC E23.6
platelets D69.1
plexus G54.9
  specified NEC G54.8
polymorphonuclear neutrophils D71
porphyrin metabolism — *see* Porphyria
postconcussional F07.81
posthallucinogen perception F16.983
  in
    abuse F16.183
    dependence F16.283
postmenopausal N95.9
  specified NEC N95.8
postprocedural (postoperative) — *see* Complications, postprocedural
post-transplant lymphoproliferative D47.Z1 (*following* D47.4)
post-traumatic stress (PTSD) F43.10
  acute F43.11
  chronic F43.12
premenstrual dysphoric (PMDD) F32.81
prepuce N47.8
propionic acidemia E71.121
prostate N42.9
  specified NEC N42.89
psychogenic NOS — *see also* condition F45.9
  anxiety F41.8
  appetite F50.9
  asthenic F48.8
  cardiovascular (system) F45.8
  compulsive F42.8
  cutaneous F54
  depressive F32.9
  digestive (system) F45.8
  dysmenorrheic F45.8
  dyspneic F45.8
  endocrine (system) F54
  eye NEC F45.8
  feeding — *see* Disorder, eating
  functional NEC F45.8
  gastric F45.8
  gastrointestinal (system) F45.8
  genitourinary (system) F45.8
  heart (function) (rhythm) F45.8
  hyperventilatory F45.8
  hypochondriacal — *see* Disorder, hypochondriacal
  intestinal F45.8
  joint F45.8
  learning F81.9
  limb F45.8
  lymphatic (system) F45.8
  menstrual F45.8
  micturition F45.8
  monoplegic NEC F44.4
  motor F44.4
  muscle F45.8
  musculoskeletal F45.8
  neurocirculatory F45.8
  obsessive F42.8
  occupational F48.8
  organ or part of body NEC F45.8
  paralytic NEC F44.4
  phobic F40.9

Disorder — *continued*
psychogenic — *see also* condition — *continued*
  physical NEC F45.8
  rectal F45.8
  respiratory (system) F45.8
  rheumatic F45.8
  sexual (function) F52.9
  skin (allergic) (eczematous) F54
  sleep F51.9
  specified part of body NEC F45.8
  stomach F45.8
psychological F99
  associated with
    disease classified elsewhere F54
    sexual
      development F66
      relationship F66
    uncertainty about gender identity F64.9
psychomotor NEC F44.4
  hysterical F44.4
psychoneurotic — *see also* Neurosis
  mixed NEC F48.8
psychophysiologic — *see* Disorder, somatoform
psychosexual F65.9
  development F66
  identity of childhood F64.2
psychosomatic NOS — *see* Disorder, somatoform
  multiple F45.0
  undifferentiated F45.1
psychotic — *see* Psychosis
  transient (acute) F23
puberty E30.9
  specified NEC E30.8
pulmonary (valve) — *see* Endocarditis, pulmonary
purine metabolism E79.9
pyrimidine metabolism E79.9
pyruvate metabolism E74.4
reactive attachment (childhood) F94.1
reading R48.0
  developmental (specific) F81.0
receptive language F80.2
receptor, hormonal, peripheral — *see also* Syndrome, androgen insensitivity E34.50
recurrent brief depressive F33.8
reflex R29.2
refraction H52.7
  aniseikonia H52.32
  anisometropia H52.31
  astigmatism — *see* Astigmatism
  hypermetropia — *see* Hypermetropia
  myopia — *see* Myopia
  presbyopia H52.4
  specified NEC H52.6
relationship F68.8
  due to sexual orientation F66
REM sleep behavior G47.52
renal function, impaired (tubular) N25.9
resonance R49.9
  specified NEC R49.8
respiratory function, impaired — *see also* Failure, respiration
  postprocedural — *see* Complication, postoperative, respiratory system
  psychogenic F45.8
retina H35.9
  angioid streaks H35.33
  changes in vascular appearance H35.01- ☑
  degeneration — *see* Degeneration, retina
  dystrophy (hereditary) — *see* Dystrophy, retina
  edema H35.81
  hemorrhage — *see* Hemorrhage, retina
  ischemia H35.82
  macular degeneration — *see* Degeneration, macula
  microaneurysms H35.04- ☑
  microvascular abnormality NEC H35.09
  neovascularization — *see* Neovascularization, retina
  retinopathy — *see* Retinopathy
  separation of layers H35.70
    central serous chorioretinopathy H35.71- ☑
    pigment epithelium detachment (serous) H35.72- ☑
      hemorrhagic H35.73- ☑
  specified type NEC H35.89
  telangiectasis — *see* Telangiectasis, retina
  vasculitis — *see* Vasculitis, retina
retroperitoneal K68.9
right hemisphere organic affective F07.89
rumination (infant or child) F98.21

☑ **Additional Character Required** — Refer to the Tabular List for Character Selection
▽ **Subterms under main terms may continue to next column or page**

Disorder — continued

sacrum, sacrococcygeal NEC M53.3
schizoaffective F25.9
  bipolar type F25.0
  depressive type F25.1
  manic type F25.0
  mixed type F25.0
  specified NEC F25.8
schizoid of childhood F84.5
schizophrenia spectrum and other psychotic disorder F29
  specified NEC F28
schizophreniform F20.81
  brief F23
schizotypal (personality) F21
secretion, thyrocalcitonin E07.0
sedative, hypnotic, or anxiolytic use
  mild F13.10
    with
      sedative, hypnotic, or anxiolytic intoxication F13.129
      sedative, hypnotic, or anxiolytic intoxication delirium F13.121
      sedative, hypnotic, or anxiolytic-induced
        anxiety disorder F13.180
        bipolar and related disorder F13.14
        depressive disorder F13.14
        psychotic disorder F13.159
        sexual dysfunction F13.181
    in remission (early) (sustained) F13.11
  moderate or severe F13.20
    with
      sedative, hypnotic, or anxiolytic intoxication F13.229
      sedative, hypnotic, or anxiolytic intoxication delirium F13.221
      sedative, hypnotic, or anxiolytic-induced
        anxiety disorder F13.280
        bipolar and related disorder F13.24
        depressive disorder F13.24
        major neurocognitive disorder F13.27
        mild neurocognitive disorder F13.288
        psychotic disorder F13.259
        sexual dysfunction F13.281
    in remission (early) (sustained) F13.21
seizure — see also Epilepsy G40.909
  intractable G40.919
    with status epilepticus G40.911
semantic pragmatic F80.89
  with autism F84.0
sense of smell R43.1
  psychogenic F45.8
separation anxiety, of childhood F93.0
sexual
  aversion F52.1
  function, psychogenic F52.9
  interest/arousal, female F52.22
  masochism F65.51
  maturation F66
  nonorganic F52.9
  preference — see also Deviation, sexual F65.9
    fetishistic transvestism F65.1
  relationship F66
  sadism F65.52
shyness, of childhood and adolescence F40.10
sibling rivalry F93.8
sickle-cell (sickling) (homozygous) — see Disease, sickle-cell
  heterozygous D57.3
  specified type NEC D57.8- ☑
  trait D57.3
sinus (nasal) J34.9
  specified NEC J34.89
skin L98.9
  atrophic L90.9
    specified NEC L90.8
  granulomatous L92.9
    specified NEC L92.8
  hypertrophic L91.9
    specified NEC L91.8
  infiltrative NEC L98.6
  newborn P83.9
    specified NEC P83.88
  picking F42.4
  psychogenic (allergic) (eczematous) F54
sleep G47.9
  breathing-related — see Apnea, sleep
  circadian rhythm G47.20
    advance sleep phase type G47.22

Disorder — continued

sleep — continued
  circadian rhythm — continued
    delayed sleep phase type G47.21
    due to
      alcohol
        abuse F10.182
        dependence F10.282
        use F10.982
      amphetamines
        abuse F15.182
        dependence F15.282
        use F15.982
      caffeine
        abuse F15.182
        dependence F15.282
        use F15.982
      cocaine
        abuse F14.182
        dependence F14.282
        use F14.982
      drug NEC
        abuse F19.182
        dependence F19.282
        use F19.982
      opioid
        abuse F11.182
        dependence F11.282
        use F11.982
      psychoactive substance NEC
        abuse F19.182
        dependence F19.282
        use F19.982
      sedative, hypnotic, or anxiolytic
        abuse F13.182
        dependence F13.282
        use F13.982
      stimulant NEC
        abuse F15.182
        dependence F15.282
        use F15.982
    free running type G47.24
    in conditions classified elsewhere G47.27
    irregular sleep wake type G47.23
    jet lag type G47.25
    non-24-hour sleep-wake type G47.24
    shift work type G47.26
    specified NEC G47.29
  due to
    alcohol
      abuse F10.182
      dependence F10.282
      use F10.982
    amphetamine
      abuse F15.182
      dependence F15.282
      use F15.982
    anxiolytic
      abuse F13.182
      dependence F13.282
      use F13.982
    caffeine
      abuse F15.182
      dependence F15.282
      use F15.982
    cocaine
      abuse F14.182
      dependence F14.282
      use F14.982
    drug NEC
      abuse F19.182
      dependence F19.282
      use F19.982
    hypnotic
      abuse F13.182
      dependence F13.282
      use F13.982
    opioid
      abuse F11.182
      dependence F11.282
      use F11.982
    psychoactive substance NEC
      abuse F19.182
      dependence F19.282
      use F19.982
    sedative
      abuse F13.182
      dependence F13.282
      use F13.982

Disorder — continued

sleep — continued
  due to — continued
    stimulant NEC
      abuse F15.182
      dependence F15.282
      use F15.982
  emotional F51.9
  excessive somnolence — see Hypersomnia
  hypersomnia type — see Hypersomnia
  initiating or maintaining — see Insomnia
  nightmares F51.5
  nonorganic F51.9
    specified NEC F51.8
  parasomnia type G47.50
  specified NEC G47.8
  terrors F51.4
  walking F51.3
sleep-wake pattern or schedule — see also Disorder, sleep, circadian rhythm G47.9
  specified NEC G47.8
social
  anxiety (of childhood) F40.10
    generalized F40.11
  functioning in childhood F94.9
    specified NEC F94.8
  pragmatic F80.82
soft tissue M79.9
  ankle M79.9
  due to use, overuse and pressure M70.90
    ankle M70.97- ☑
    bursitis — see Bursitis
    foot M70.97- ☑
    forearm M70.93- ☑
    hand M70.94- ☑
    lower leg M70.96- ☑
    multiple sites M70.99
    pelvic region M70.95- ☑
    shoulder region M70.91- ☑
    specified site NEC M70.98
    specified type NEC M70.80
      ankle M70.87- ☑
      foot M70.87- ☑
      forearm M70.83- ☑
      hand M70.84- ☑
      lower leg M70.86- ☑
      multiple sites M70.89
      pelvic region M70.85- ☑
      shoulder region M70.81- ☑
      specified site NEC M70.88
      thigh M70.85- ☑
      upper arm M70.82- ☑
    thigh M70.95- ☑
    upper arm M70.92- ☑
  foot M79.9
  forearm M79.9
  hand M79.9
  lower leg M79.9
  multiple sites M79.9
  occupational — see Disorder, soft tissue, due to use, overuse and pressure
  pelvic region M79.9
  shoulder region M79.9
  specified type NEC M79.89
  thigh M79.9
  upper arm M79.9
somatic symptom F45.1
somatization F45.0
somatoform F45.9
  pain (persistent) F45.41
  somatization (multiple) (long-lasting) F45.0
  specified NEC F45.8
  undifferentiated F45.1
somnolence, excessive — see Hypersomnia
specific
  arithmetical F81.2
  developmental, of motor F82
  reading F81.0
  speech and language F80.9
  spelling F81.81
  written expression F81.81
speech R47.9
  articulation (functional) (specific) F80.0
  developmental F80.9
  specified NEC R47.89
speech-sound F80.0
spelling (specific) F81.81
spine — see also Dorsopathy

Disorder — *continued*

spine — *see also* Dorsopathy — *continued*
  ligamentous or muscular attachments, peripheral — *see* Enthesopathy, spinal
  specified NEC — *see* Dorsopathy, specified NEC
stereotyped, habit or movement F98.4
stimulant use (other) (unspecified)
  mild F15.10
    in remission (early) (sustained) F15.11
  moderate or severe F15.20
    in remission (early) (sustained) F15.21
stomach (functional) — *see* Disorder, gastric
stress F43.9
  acute F43.0
  post-traumatic F43.10
    acute F43.11
    chronic F43.12
substance use (other) (unknown)
  mild F19.10
    with substance-induced
      anxiety disorder F19.180
      bipolar and related disorder F19.14
      depressive disorder F19.14
      major neurocognitive disorder F19.17
      mild neurocognitive disorder F19.188
      obsessive-compulsive and related disorder F19.188
      sexual dysfunction F19.181
    substance intoxication F19.129
    substance intoxication delirium F19.121
  moderate or severe F19.20
    with substance-induced
      anxiety disorder F19.280
      bipolar and related disorder F19.24
      depressive disorder F19.24
      major neurocognitive disorder F19.27
      mild neurocognitive disorder F19.288
      obsessive-compulsive and related disorder F19.288
      sexual dysfunction F19.281
    in remission (early) (sustained) F19.21
    substance intoxication F19.229
    substance intoxication delirium F19.221
sulfur-bearing amino-acid metabolism E72.10
sweat gland (eccrine) L74.9
  apocrine L75.9
    specified NEC L75.8
  specified NEC L74.8
synovium M67.90
  acromioclavicular M67.91- ☑
  ankle M67.97- ☑
  elbow M67.92- ☑
  foot M67.97- ☑
  forearm M67.93- ☑
  hand M67.94- ☑
  hip M67.95- ☑
  knee M67.96- ☑
  multiple sites M67.99
  rupture — *see* Rupture, synovium
  shoulder M67.91- ☑
  specified type NEC M67.80
    acromioclavicular M67.81- ☑
    ankle M67.87- ☑
    elbow M67.82- ☑
    foot M67.87- ☑
    hand M67.84- ☑
    hip M67.85- ☑
    knee M67.86- ☑
    multiple sites M67.89
    wrist M67.83- ☑
  synovitis — *see* Synovitis
  upper arm M67.92- ☑
  wrist M67.93- ☑
temperature regulation, newborn P81.9
  specified NEC P81.8
temporomandibular joint M26.60- ☑
tendon M67.90
  acromioclavicular M67.91- ☑
  ankle M67.97- ☑
  contracture — *see* Contracture, tendon
  elbow M67.92- ☑
  foot M67.97- ☑
  forearm M67.93- ☑
  hand M67.94- ☑
  hip M67.95- ☑
  knee M67.96- ☑
  multiple sites M67.99

Disorder — *continued*

tendon — *continued*
  rupture — *see* Rupture, tendon
  shoulder M67.91- ☑
  specified type NEC M67.80
    acromioclavicular M67.81- ☑
    ankle M67.87- ☑
    elbow M67.82- ☑
    foot M67.87- ☑
    hand M67.84- ☑
    hip M67.85- ☑
    knee M67.86- ☑
    multiple sites M67.89
    trunk M67.88
    wrist M67.83- ☑
  synovitis — *see* Synovitis
  tendinitis — *see* Tendinitis
  tenosynovitis — *see* Tenosynovitis
  trunk M67.98
  upper arm M67.92- ☑
  wrist M67.93- ☑
thoracic root (nerve) NEC G54.3
thyrocalcitonin hypersecretion E07.0
thyroid (gland) E07.9
  function NEC, neonatal, transitory P72.2
  iodine-deficiency related E01.8
  specified NEC E07.89
tic — *see* Tic
tobacco use
  chewing tobacco (mild) (moderate) (severe)
    in remission (early) (sustained) F17.221
  cigarettes (mild) (moderate) (severe)
    in remission (early) (sustained) F17.211
  mild F17.200
    in remission (early) (sustained) F17.201
  moderate F17.200
    in remission (early) (sustained) F17.201
  severe F17.200
    in remission (early) (sustained) F17.201
  specified product NEC (mild) (moderate) (severe)
    in remission (early) (sustained) F17.291
tooth K08.9
  development K00.9
    specified NEC K00.8
  eruption K00.6
Tourette's F95.2
trance and possession F44.89
transvestic F65.1
trauma and stressor-related F43.9
  other specified F43.8
tricuspid (valve) — *see* Endocarditis, tricuspid
tryptophan metabolism E70.5
tubular, phosphate-losing N25.0
tubulo-interstitial (in)
  brucellosis A23.9 *[N16]*
  cystinosis E72.04
  diphtheria A36.84
  glycogen storage disease E74.00 *[N16]*
  leukemia NEC C95.9- ☑ *[N16]*
  lymphoma NEC C85.9- ☑ *[N16]*
  mixed cryoglobulinemia D89.1 *[N16]*
  multiple myeloma C90.0- ☑ *[N16]*
  Salmonella infection A02.25
  sarcoidosis D86.84
  sepsis A41.9 *[N16]*
    streptococcal A40.9 *[N16]*
  systemic lupus erythematosus M32.15
  toxoplasmosis B58.83
  transplant rejection T86.91 *[N16]*
  Wilson's disease E83.01 *[N16]*
tubulo-renal function, impaired N25.9
  specified NEC N25.89
tympanic membrane H73.9- ☑
  atrophy — *see* Atrophy, tympanic membrane
  infection — *see* Myringitis
  perforation — *see* Perforation, tympanum
  specified NEC H73.89- ☑
unsocialized aggressive F91.1
urea cycle metabolism E72.20
  argininemia E72.21
  arginosuccinic aciduria E72.22
  citrullinemia E72.23
  ornithine transcarbamylase deficiency E72.4
  other specified E72.29
ureter (in) N28.9
  schistosomiasis B65.0 *[N29]*
  tuberculosis A18.11
urethra N36.9

Disorder — *continued*

urethra — *continued*
  specified NEC N36.8
urinary system N39.9
  specified NEC N39.8
valve, heart
  aortic — *see* Endocarditis, aortic
  mitral — *see* Endocarditis, mitral
  pulmonary — *see* Endocarditis, pulmonary
  rheumatic
    aortic — *see* Endocarditis, aortic, rheumatic
    mitral — *see* Endocarditis, mitral
    pulmonary — *see* Endocarditis, pulmonary, rheumatic
    tricuspid — *see* Endocarditis, tricuspid
  tricuspid — *see* Endocarditis, tricuspid
vestibular function H81.9- ☑
  specified NEC — *see* subcategory H81.8 ☑
  in diseases classified elsewhere H82.- ☑
vertigo — *see* Vertigo
vision, binocular H53.30
  abnormal retinal correspondence H53.31
  diplopia H53.2
  fusion with defective stereopsis H53.32
  simultaneous perception H53.33
  suppression H53.34
visual
  cortex
    blindness H47.619
      left brain H47.612
      right brain H47.611
    due to
      inflammatory disorder H47.629
        left brain H47.622
        right brain H47.621
      neoplasm H47.639
        left brain H47.632
        right brain H47.631
      vascular disorder H47.649
        left brain H47.642
        right brain H47.641
  pathway H47.9
    due to
      inflammatory disorder H47.51- ☑
      neoplasm H47.52- ☑
      vascular disorder H47.53- ☑
    optic chiasm — *see* Disorder, optic, chiasm
vitreous body H43.9
  crystalline deposits — *see* Deposit, crystalline
  degeneration — *see* Degeneration, vitreous
  hemorrhage — *see* Hemorrhage, vitreous
  opacities — *see* Opacity, vitreous
  prolapse — *see* Prolapse, vitreous
  specified type NEC H43.89
voice R49.9
  specified type NEC R49.8
volatile solvent use
  due to drug abuse — *see* Abuse, drug, inhalant
  due to drug dependence — *see* Dependence, drug, inhalant
voyeuristic F65.3
white blood cells D72.9
  specified NEC D72.89
withdrawing, child or adolescent F40.10
Disorientation R41.0
Displacement, displaced
acquired traumatic of bone, cartilage, joint, tendon NEC — *see* Dislocation
adrenal gland (congenital) Q89.1
appendix, retrocecal (congenital) Q43.8
auricle (congenital) Q17.4
bladder (acquired) N32.89
  congenital Q64.19
brachial plexus (congenital) Q07.8
brain stem, caudal (congenital) Q04.8
canaliculus (lacrimalis), congenital Q10.6
cardia through esophageal hiatus (congenital) Q40.1
cerebellum, caudal (congenital) Q04.8
cervix — *see* Malposition, uterus
colon (congenital) Q43.3
device, implant or graft — *see also* Complications, by site and type, mechanical T85.628 ☑
  arterial graft NEC — *see* Complication, cardiovascular device, mechanical, vascular
  breast (implant) T85.42 ☑
  catheter NEC T85.628 ☑
    dialysis (renal) T82.42 ☑
      intraperitoneal T85.621 ☑

☑ **Additional Character Required** — Refer to the Tabular List for Character Selection   ▽ **Subterms under main terms may continue to next column or page**

Displacement, displaced — *continued*
 device, implant or graft — *see also* Complications, by
  site and type, mechanical — *continued*
  catheter — *continued*
   infusion NEC T82.524 ☑
    spinal (epidural) (subdural) T85.620 ☑
   urinary
    cystostomy T83.020 ☑
    Hopkins T83.028 ☑
    ileostomy T83.028 ☑
    indwelling T83.021 ☑
    nephrostomy T83.022 ☑
    specified NEC T83.028 ☑
    urostomy T83.028 ☑
  electronic (electrode) (pulse generator) (stimulator)
   — *see* Complication, electronic stimulator
  fixation, internal (orthopedic) NEC — *see* Complication, fixation device, mechanical
  gastrointestinal — *see* Complications, prosthetic
   device, mechanical, gastrointestinal device
  genital NEC T83.428 ☑
   intrauterine contraceptive device (string)
    T83.32 ☑
   penile prosthesis (cylinder) (implanted) (pump)
    (reservoir) T83.420 ☑
   testicular prosthesis T83.421 ☑
  heart NEC — *see* Complication, cardiovascular device, mechanical
  joint prosthesis — *see* Complications, joint prosthesis, mechanical
  ocular — *see* Complications, prosthetic device,
   mechanical, ocular device
  orthopedic NEC — *see* Complication, orthopedic,
   device or graft, mechanical
  specified NEC T85.628 ☑
  urinary NEC T83.128 ☑
   graft T83.22 ☑
   sphincter, implanted T83.121 ☑
   stent (ileal conduit) (nephroureteral) T83.123 ☑
   ureteral indwelling T83.122 ☑
  vascular NEC — *see* Complication, cardiovascular
   device, mechanical
  ventricular intracranial shunt T85.02 ☑
 electronic stimulator
  bone T84.320 ☑
  cardiac — *see* Complications, cardiac device, electronic
  nervous system — *see* Complication, prosthetic
   device, mechanical, electronic nervous system
   stimulator
  urinary — *see* Complications, electronic stimulator,
   urinary
 esophageal mucosa into cardia of stomach, congenital
  Q39.8
 esophagus (acquired) K22.8
  congenital Q39.8
 eyeball (acquired) (lateral) (old) — *see* Displacement,
  globe
  congenital Q15.8
  current — *see* Avulsion, eye
 fallopian tube (acquired) N83.4- ☑
  congenital Q50.6
  opening (congenital) Q50.6
 gallbladder (congenital) Q44.1
 gastric mucosa (congenital) Q40.2
 globe (acquired) (old) (lateral) H05.21- ☑
  current — *see* Avulsion, eye
 heart (congenital) Q24.8
  acquired I51.89
 hymen (upward) (congenital) Q52.4
 intervertebral disc NEC
  with myelopathy — *see* Disorder, disc, with,
   myelopathy
  cervical, cervicothoracic (with) M50.20
   myelopathy — *see* Disorder, disc, cervical, with
    myelopathy
   neuritis, radiculitis or radiculopathy — *see* Disor-
    der, disc, cervical, with neuritis
  due to trauma — *see* Dislocation, vertebra
  lumbar region M51.26
   with
    myelopathy M51.06
    neuritis, radiculitis, radiculopathy or sciatica
     M51.16
  lumbosacral region M51.27

Displacement, displaced — *continued*
 intervertebral disc — *continued*
  lumbosacral region — *continued*
   with
    neuritis, radiculitis, radiculopathy or sciatica
     M51.17
  sacrococcygeal region M53.3
  thoracic region M51.24
   with
    myelopathy M51.04
    neuritis, radiculitis, radiculopathy M51.14
  thoracolumbar region M51.25
   with
    myelopathy M51.05
    neuritis, radiculitis, radiculopathy M51.15
 intrauterine device (string) T83.32 ☑
 kidney (acquired) N28.83
  congenital Q63.2
 lachrymal, lacrimal apparatus or duct (congenital) Q10.6
 lens, congenital Q12.1
 macula (congenital) Q14.1
 Meckel's diverticulum Q43.0
  malignant — *see* Table of Neoplasms, small intestine, malignant
 nail (congenital) Q84.6
  acquired L60.8
 opening of Wharton's duct in mouth Q38.4
 organ or site, congenital NEC — *see* Malposition, congenital
 ovary (acquired) N83.4- ☑
  congenital Q50.39
  free in peritoneal cavity (congenital) Q50.39
  into hernial sac N83.4- ☑
 oviduct (acquired) N83.4- ☑
  congenital Q50.6
 parathyroid (gland) E21.4
 parotid gland (congenital) Q38.4
 punctum lacrimale (congenital) Q10.6
 sacro-iliac (joint) (congenital) Q74.2
  current injury S33.2 ☑
  old — *see* subcategory M53.2 ☑
 salivary gland (any) (congenital) Q38.4
 spleen (congenital) Q89.09
 stomach, congenital Q40.2
 sublingual duct Q38.4
 tongue (downward) (congenital) Q38.3
 tooth, teeth, fully erupted M26.30
  horizontal M26.33
  vertical M26.34
 trachea (congenital) Q32.1
 ureter or ureteric opening or orifice (congenital) Q62.62
 uterine opening of oviducts or fallopian tubes Q50.6
 uterus, uterine — *see* Malposition, uterus
 ventricular septum Q21.0
  with rudimentary ventricle Q20.4

Disproportion
 between native and reconstructed breast N65.1
 fiber-type G71.2
Disruptio uteri — *see* Rupture, uterus
Disruption (of)
 ciliary body NEC H21.89
 closure of
  cornea T81.31 ☑
  craniotomy T81.32 ☑
  fascia (muscular) (superficial) T81.32 ☑
  internal organ or tissue T81.32 ☑
  laceration (external) (internal) T81.33 ☑
  ligament T81.32 ☑
  mucosa T81.31 ☑
  muscle or muscle flap T81.32 ☑
  ribs or rib cage T81.32 ☑
  skin and subcutaneous tissue (full-thickness) (superficial) T81.31 ☑
  skull T81.32 ☑
  sternum (sternotomy) T81.32 ☑
  tendon T81.32 ☑
  traumatic laceration (external) (internal) T81.33 ☑
 family Z63.8
  due to
   absence of family member due to military deploy-
    ment Z63.31
   absence of family member NEC Z63.32
   alcoholism and drug addiction in family Z63.72
   bereavement Z63.4
   death (assumed) or disappearance of family
    member Z63.4
   divorce or separation Z63.5
   drug addiction in family Z63.72

Disruption — *continued*
 family — *continued*
  due to — *continued*
   return of family member from military deploy-
    ment (current or past conflict) Z63.71
   stressful life events NEC Z63.79
 iris NEC H21.89
 ligament(s) — *see also* Sprain
  knee
   current injury — *see* Dislocation, knee
   old (chronic) — *see* Derangement, knee, instabil-
    ity
   spontaneous NEC — *see* Derangement, knee,
    disruption ligament
 ossicular chain — *see* Discontinuity, ossicles, ear
 pelvic ring (stable) S32.810 ☑
  unstable S32.811 ☑
 traumatic injury wound repair T81.33 ☑
 wound T81.30 ☑
  episiotomy O90.1
  operation T81.31 ☑
   cesarean O90.0
   external operation wound (superficial) T81.31 ☑
   internal operation wound (deep) T81.32 ☑
  perineal (obstetric) O90.1
  traumatic injury repair T81.33 ☑
Dissatisfaction with
 employment Z56.9
 school environment Z55.4
Dissecting — *see* condition
Dissection
 aorta I71.00
  abdominal I71.02
  thoracic I71.01
  thoracoabdominal I71.03
 artery I77.70
  basilar (trunk) I77.75
  carotid I77.71
  cerebral (nonruptured) I67.0
   ruptured — *see* Hemorrhage, intracranial, sub-
    arachnoid
  coronary I25.42
  extremity
   lower I77.77
   upper I77.76
  iliac I77.72
  precerebral
   congenital (nonruptured) Q28.1
   specified site NEC I77.75
  renal I77.73
  specified NEC I77.79
  vertebral I77.74
 precerebral artery, congenital (nonruptured) Q28.1
  Heartland A93.8
 traumatic — *see* Wound, open, by site
 vascular I99.8
 wound — *see* Wound, open
Disseminated — *see* condition
Dissociation
 auriculoventricular or atrioventricular (AV) (any degree)
  (isorhythmic) I45.89
  with heart block I44.2
 interference I45.89
Dissociative reaction, state F44.9
Dissolution, vertebra — *see* Osteoporosis
Distension, distention
 abdomen R14.0
 bladder N32.89
 cecum K63.89
 colon K63.89
 gallbladder K82.8
 intestine K63.89
 kidney N28.89
 liver K76.89
 seminal vesicle N50.89
 stomach K31.89
  acute K31.0
  psychogenic F45.8
 ureter — *see* Dilatation, ureter
 uterus N85.8
Distoma hepaticum infestation B66.3
Distomiasis B66.9
 bile passages B66.3
 hemic B65.9
 hepatic B66.3
  due to Clonorchis sinensis B66.1
 intestinal B66.5
 liver B66.3

▽ Subterms under main terms may continue to next column or page   ☑ Additional Character Required — Refer to the Tabular List for Character Selection   119

Displacement, displaced — Distomiasis

Distomiasis — *continued*
  liver — *continued*
    due to Clonorchis sinensis B66.1
  lung B66.4
  pulmonary B66.4
Distomolar (fourth molar) K00.1
Disto-occlusion (Division I) (Division II) M26.212
Distortion(s) (congenital)
  adrenal (gland) Q89.1
  arm NEC Q68.8
  bile duct or passage Q44.5
  bladder Q64.79
  brain Q04.9
  cervix (uteri) Q51.9
  chest (wall) Q67.8
    bones Q76.8
  clavicle Q74.0
  clitoris Q52.6
  coccyx Q76.49
  common duct Q44.5
  coronary Q24.5
  cystic duct Q44.5
  ear (auricle) (external) Q17.3
    inner Q16.5
    middle Q16.4
      ossicles Q16.3
  endocrine NEC Q89.2
  eustachian tube Q17.8
  eye (adnexa) Q15.8
  face bone(s) NEC Q75.8
  fallopian tube Q50.6
  femur NEC Q68.8
  fibula NEC Q68.8
  finger(s) Q68.1
  foot Q66.9- ☑
  genitalia, genital organ(s)
    female Q52.8
      external Q52.79
      internal NEC Q52.8
  gyri Q04.8
  hand bone(s) Q68.1
  heart (auricle) (ventricle) Q24.8
    valve (cusp) Q24.8
  hepatic duct Q44.5
  humerus NEC Q68.8
  hymen Q52.4
  intrafamilial communications Z63.8
  jaw NEC M26.89
  labium (majus) (minus) Q52.79
  leg NEC Q68.8
  lens Q12.8
  liver Q44.7
  lumbar spine Q76.49
    with disproportion O33.8
      causing obstructed labor O65.0
  lumbosacral (joint) (region) Q76.49
    kyphosis — *see* Kyphosis, congenital
    lordosis — *see* Lordosis, congenital
  nerve Q07.8
  nose Q30.8
  organ
    of Corti Q16.5
    or site not listed — *see* Anomaly, by site
  ossicles, ear Q16.3
  oviduct Q50.6
  pancreas Q45.3
  parathyroid (gland) Q89.2
  pituitary (gland) Q89.2
  radius NEC Q68.8
  sacroiliac joint Q74.2
  sacrum Q76.49
  scapula Q74.0
  shoulder girdle Q74.0
  skull bone(s) NEC Q75.8
    with
      anencephalus Q00.0
      encephalocele — *see* Encephalocele
      hydrocephalus Q03.9
        with spina bifida — *see* Spina bifida, with hydrocephalus
      microcephaly Q02
  spinal cord Q06.8
  spine Q76.49
    kyphosis — *see* Kyphosis, congenital
    lordosis — *see* Lordosis, congenital
  spleen Q89.09
  sternum NEC Q76.7
  thorax (wall) Q67.8

Distortion(s) — *continued*
  thorax — *continued*
    bony Q76.8
  thymus (gland) Q89.2
  thyroid (gland) Q89.2
  tibia NEC Q68.8
  toe(s) Q66.9- ☑
  tongue Q38.3
  trachea (cartilage) Q32.1
  ulna NEC Q68.8
  ureter Q62.8
  urethra Q64.79
    causing obstruction Q64.39
  uterus Q51.9
  vagina Q52.4
  vertebra Q76.49
    kyphosis — *see* Kyphosis, congenital
    lordosis — *see* Lordosis, congenital
  visual — *see also* Disturbance, vision
    shape and size H53.15
  vulva Q52.79
  wrist (bones) (joint) Q68.8
Distress
  abdomen — *see* Pain, abdominal
  acute respiratory R06.03
    syndrome (adult) (child) J80
  epigastric R10.13
  fetal P84
    complicating pregnancy — *see* Stress, fetal
  gastrointestinal (functional) K30
    psychogenic F45.8
  intestinal (functional) NOS K59.9
    psychogenic F45.8
  maternal, during labor and delivery O75.0
  relationship, with spouse or intimate partner Z63.0
  respiratory (adult) (child) R06.03
    newborn P22.9
      specified NEC P22.8
    orthopnea R06.01
    psychogenic F45.8
    shortness of breath R06.02
    specified type NEC R06.09
Distribution vessel, atypical Q27.9
  coronary artery Q24.5
  precerebral Q28.1
Distichiasis L68.8
Disturbance(s) — *see also* Disease
  absorption K90.9
    calcium E58
    carbohydrate K90.49
    fat K90.49
      pancreatic K90.3
    protein K90.49
    starch K90.49
    vitamin — *see* Deficiency, vitamin
  acid-base equilibrium E87.8
    mixed E87.4
  activity and attention (with hyperkinesis) — *see* Disorder, attention-deficit hyperactivity
  amino acid transport E72.00
  assimilation, food K90.9
  auditory nerve, except deafness — *see* subcategory H93.3 ☑
  behavior — *see* Disorder, conduct
  blood clotting (mechanism) — *see also* Defect, coagulation D68.9
  cerebral
    nerve — *see* Disorder, nerve, cranial
    status, newborn P91.9
      specified NEC P91.88
  circulatory I99.9
  conduct — *see also* Disorder, conduct F91.9
    adjustment reaction — *see* Disorder, adjustment
    compulsive F63.9
    disruptive F91.9
    hyperkinetic — *see* Disorder, attention-deficit hyperactivity
    socialized F91.2
    specified NEC F91.8
    unsocialized F91.1
  coordination R27.8
  cranial nerve — *see* Disorder, nerve, cranial
  deep sensibility — *see* Disturbance, sensation
  digestive K30
    psychogenic F45.8
  electrolyte — *see also* Imbalance, electrolyte
    newborn, transitory P74.49
      hyperammonemia P74.6

Disturbance(s) — *continued*
  electrolyte — *see also* Imbalance, electrolyte — *continued*
    newborn, transitory — *continued*
      hyperchloremia P74.421
      hyperchloremic metabolic acidosis P74.421
      hypochloremia P74.422
      potassium balance
        hyperkalemia P74.31
        hypokalemia P74.32
      sodium balance
        hypernatremia P74.21
        hyponatremia P74.22
      specified type NEC P74.49
  emotions specific to childhood and adolescence F93.9
    with
      anxiety and fearfulness NEC F93.8
      elective mutism F94.0
      oppositional disorder F91.3
      sensitivity (withdrawal) F40.10
      shyness F40.10
      social withdrawal F40.10
    involving relationship problems F93.8
    mixed F93.8
    specified NEC F93.8
  endocrine (gland) E34.9
    neonatal, transitory P72.9
      specified NEC P72.8
  equilibrium R42
  fructose metabolism E74.10
  gait — *see* Gait
    hysterical F44.4
    psychogenic F44.4
  gastrointestinal (functional) K30
    psychogenic F45.8
  habit, child F98.9
  hearing, except deafness and tinnitus — *see* Abnormal, auditory perception
  heart, functional (conditions in I44-I50)
    due to presence of (cardiac) prosthesis I97.19- ☑
    postoperative I97.89
      cardiac surgery — *see also* Infarct, myocardium, associated with revascularization procedure I97.19- ☑
  hormones E34.9
  innervation uterus (parasympathetic) (sympathetic) N85.2
  keratinization NEC
    gingiva K05.10
      nonplaque induced K05.11
      plaque induced K05.10
    lip K13.0
    oral (mucosa) (soft tissue) K13.29
    tongue K13.29
  learning (specific) — *see* Disorder, learning
  memory — *see* Amnesia
    mild, following organic brain damage F06.8
  mental F99
    associated with diseases classified elsewhere F54
  metabolism E88.9
    with
      abortion — *see* Abortion, by type with other specified complication
      ectopic pregnancy O08.5
      molar pregnancy O08.5
    amino-acid E72.9
      aromatic E70.9
      branched-chain E71.2
      straight-chain E72.89
      sulfur-bearing E72.10
    ammonia E72.20
    arginine E72.21
    arginosuccinic acid E72.22
    carbohydrate E74.9
    cholesterol E78.9
    citrulline E72.23
    cystathionine E72.19
    general E88.9
    glutamine E72.89
    histidine E70.40
    homocystine E72.19
    hydroxylysine E72.3
    in labor or delivery O75.89
    iron E83.10
    lipid E78.9
    lysine E72.3
    methionine E72.19
    neonatal, transitory P74.9

Disturbance(s) — continued

metabolism — continued
  neonatal, transitory — continued
    calcium and magnesium P71.9
      specified type NEC P71.8
    carbohydrate metabolism P70.9
      specified type NEC P70.8
    specified NEC P74.8
  ornithine E72.4
  phosphate E83.39
  sodium NEC E87.8
  threonine E72.89
  tryptophan E70.5
  tyrosine E70.20
  urea cycle E72.20
motor R29.2
nervous, functional R45.0
neuromuscular mechanism (eye), due to syphilis A52.15
nutritional E63.9
  nail L60.3
ocular motion H51.9
  psychogenic F45.8
oculogyric H51.8
  psychogenic F45.8
oculomotor H51.9
  psychogenic F45.8
olfactory nerve R43.1
optic nerve NEC — see Disorder, nerve, optic
oral epithelium, including tongue NEC K13.29
perceptual due to
  alcohol withdrawal F10.232
  amphetamine intoxication F15.922
    in
      abuse F15.122
      dependence F15.222
  anxiolytic withdrawal F13.232
  cannabis intoxication (acute) F12.922
    in
      abuse F12.122
      dependence F12.222
  cocaine intoxication (acute) F14.922
    in
      abuse F14.122
      dependence F14.222
  hypnotic withdrawal F13.232
  opioid intoxication (acute) F11.922
    in
      abuse F11.122
      dependence F11.222
  phencyclidine intoxication (acute) F16.122
  sedative withdrawal F13.232
personality (pattern) (trait) — see also Disorder, personality F60.9
  following organic brain damage F07.9
polyglandular E31.9
  specified NEC E31.8
potassium balance, newborn
  hyperkalemia P74.31
  hypokalemia P74.32
psychogenic F45.9
psychomotor F44.4
psychophysical visual H53.16
pupillary — see Anomaly, pupil, function
reflex R29.2
rhythm, heart I49.9
salivary secretion K11.7
sensation (cold) (heat) (localization) (tactile discrimination) (texture) (vibratory) NEC R20.9
  hysterical F44.6
  skin R20.9
    anesthesia R20.0
    hyperesthesia R20.3
    hypoesthesia R20.1
    paresthesia R20.2
    specified type NEC R20.8
  smell R43.9
    and taste (mixed) R43.8
    anosmia R43.0
    parosmia R43.1
    specified NEC R43.8
  taste R43.9
    and smell (mixed) R43.8
    parageusia R43.2
    specified NEC R43.8
sensory — see Disturbance, sensation
situational (transient) — see also Disorder, adjustment
  acute F43.0
sleep G47.9
  nonorganic origin F51.9

Disturbance(s) — continued

smell — see Disturbance, sensation, smell
sociopathic F60.2
sodium balance, newborn
  hypernatremia P74.21
  hyponatremia P74.22
speech R47.9
  developmental F80.9
  specified NEC R47.89
stomach (functional) K31.9
sympathetic (nerve) G90.9
taste — see Disturbance, sensation, taste
temperature
  regulation, newborn P81.9
    specified NEC P81.8
  sense R20.8
    hysterical F44.6
tooth
  eruption K00.6
  formation K00.4
  structure, hereditary NEC K00.5
touch — see Disturbance, sensation
vascular I99.9
  arteriosclerotic — see Arteriosclerosis
vasomotor I73.9
vasospastic I73.9
vision, visual H53.9
  following
    cerebral infarction I69.398
    cerebrovascular disease I69.998
      specified NEC I69.898
    intracerebral hemorrhage I69.198
    nontraumatic intracranial hemorrhage NEC I69.298
    specified disease NEC I69.898
    subarachnoid hemorrhage I69.098
  psychophysical H53.16
  specified NEC H53.8
  subjective H53.10
    day blindness H53.11
    discomfort H53.14- ☑
    distortions of shape and size H53.15
    loss
      sudden H53.13- ☑
      transient H53.12- ☑
    specified type NEC H53.19
voice R49.9
  psychogenic F44.4
  specified NEC R49.8

Diuresis R35.8
Diver's palsy, paralysis or squeeze T70.3 ☑
Diverticulitis (acute) K57.92
  bladder — see Cystitis
  ileum — see Diverticulitis, intestine, small
  intestine K57.92
    with
      abscess, perforation or peritonitis K57.80
        with bleeding K57.81
      bleeding K57.93
    congenital Q43.8
    large K57.32
      with
        abscess, perforation or peritonitis K57.20
          with bleeding K57.21
        bleeding K57.33
        small intestine K57.52
          with
            abscess, perforation or peritonitis K57.40
              with bleeding K57.41
            bleeding K57.53
    small K57.12
      with
        abscess, perforation or peritonitis K57.00
          with bleeding K57.01
        bleeding K57.13
        large intestine K57.52
          with
            abscess, perforation or peritonitis K57.40
              with bleeding K57.41
            bleeding K57.53
Diverticulosis K57.90
  with bleeding K57.91
  large intestine K57.30
    with
      bleeding K57.31
      small intestine K57.50

Diverticulosis — continued

large intestine — continued
  with — continued
    small intestine — continued
      with bleeding K57.51
  small intestine K57.10
    with
      bleeding K57.11
      large intestine K57.50
        with bleeding K57.51
Diverticulum, diverticula (multiple) K57.90
  appendix (noninflammatory) K38.2
  bladder (sphincter) N32.3
    congenital Q64.6
  bronchus (congenital) Q32.4
    acquired J98.09
  calyx, calyceal (kidney) N28.89
  cardia (stomach) K31.4
  cecum — see Diverticulosis, intestine, large
    congenital Q43.8
  colon — see Diverticulosis, intestine, large
    congenital Q43.8
  duodenum — see Diverticulosis, intestine, small
    congenital Q43.8
  epiphrenic (esophagus) K22.5
  esophagus (congenital) Q39.6
    acquired (epiphrenic) (pulsion) (traction) K22.5
  eustachian tube — see Disorder, eustachian tube, specified NEC
  fallopian tube N83.8
  gastric K31.4
  heart (congenital) Q24.8
  ileum — see Diverticulosis, intestine, small
  jejunum — see Diverticulosis, intestine, small
  kidney (pelvis) (calyces) N28.89
    with calculus — see Calculus, kidney
  Meckel's (displaced) (hypertrophic) Q43.0
    malignant — see Table of Neoplasms, small intestine, malignant
  midthoracic K22.5
  organ or site, congenital NEC — see Distortion
  pericardium (congenital) (cyst) Q24.8
    acquired I31.8
  pharyngoesophageal (congenital) Q39.6
    acquired K22.5
  pharynx (congenital) Q38.7
  rectosigmoid — see Diverticulosis, intestine, large
    congenital Q43.8
  rectum — see Diverticulosis, intestine, large
  Rokitansky's K22.5
  seminal vesicle N50.89
  sigmoid — see Diverticulosis, intestine, large
    congenital Q43.8
  stomach (acquired) K31.4
    congenital Q40.2
  trachea (acquired) J39.8
  ureter (acquired) N28.89
    congenital Q62.8
  ureterovesical orifice N28.89
  urethra (acquired) N36.1
    congenital Q64.79
  ventricle, left (congenital) Q24.8
  vesical N32.3
    congenital Q64.6
  Zenker's (esophagus) K22.5
Division
  cervix uteri (acquired) N88.8
  glans penis Q55.69
  labia minora (congenital) Q52.79
  ligament (partial or complete) (current) — see also Sprain
    with open wound — see Wound, open
  muscle (partial or complete) (current) — see also Injury, muscle
    with open wound — see Wound, open
  nerve (traumatic) — see Injury, nerve
  spinal cord — see Injury, spinal cord, by region
  vein I87.8
Divorce, causing family disruption Z63.5
Dix-Hallpike neurolabyrinthitis — see Neuronitis, vestibular
Dizziness R42
  hysterical F44.89
  psychogenic F45.8
DMAC (disseminated mycobacterium avium-intracellulare complex) A31.2
DNR (do not resuscitate) Z66

Doan-Wiseman syndrome (primary splenic neutropenia) — *see* Agranulocytosis
Doehle-Heller aortitis A52.02
Dog bite — *see* Bite
Dohle body panmyelopathic syndrome D72.0
Dolichocephaly Q67.2
Dolichocolon Q43.8
Dolichostenomelia — *see* Syndrome, Marfan's
Donohue's syndrome E34.8
Donor (organ or tissue) Z52.9
  blood (whole) Z52.000
    autologous Z52.010
    specified component (lymphocytes) (platelets) NEC Z52.008
      autologous Z52.018
      specified donor NEC Z52.098
    specified donor NEC Z52.090
    stem cells Z52.001
      autologous Z52.011
      specified donor NEC Z52.091
  bone Z52.20
    autologous Z52.21
    marrow Z52.3
    specified type NEC Z52.29
  cornea Z52.5
  egg (Oocyte) Z52.819
    age 35 and over Z52.812
      anonymous recipient Z52.812
      designated recipient Z52.813
    under age 35 Z52.810
      anonymous recipient Z52.810
      designated recipient Z52.811
  kidney Z52.4
  liver Z52.6
  lung Z52.89
  lymphocyte — *see* Donor, blood, specified components NEC
  Oocyte — *see* Donor, egg
  platelets Z52.008
  potential, examination of Z00.5
  semen Z52.89
  skin Z52.10
    autologous Z52.11
    specified type NEC Z52.19
  specified organ or tissue NEC Z52.89
  sperm Z52.89
Donovanosis A58
Dorsalgia M54.9
  psychogenic F45.41
  specified NEC M54.89
Dorsopathy M53.9
  deforming M43.9
    specified NEC — *see* subcategory M43.8 ☑
  specified NEC M53.80
    cervical region M53.82
    cervicothoracic region M53.83
    lumbar region M53.86
    lumbosacral region M53.87
    occipito-atlanto-axial region M53.81
    sacrococcygeal region M53.88
    thoracic region M53.84
    thoracolumbar region M53.85
Double
  albumin E88.09
  aortic arch Q25.45
  auditory canal Q17.8
  auricle (heart) Q20.8
  bladder Q64.79
  cervix Q51.820
    with doubling of uterus (and vagina) Q51.10
      with obstruction Q51.11
  inlet ventricle Q20.4
  kidney with double pelvis (renal) Q63.0
  meatus urinarius Q64.75
  monster Q89.4
  outlet
    left ventricle Q20.2
    right ventricle Q20.1
  pelvis (renal) with double ureter Q62.5
  tongue Q38.3
  ureter (one or both sides) Q62.5
    with double pelvis (renal) Q62.5
  urethra Q64.74
  urinary meatus Q64.75
  uterus Q51.20
    with
      doubling of cervix (and vagina) Q51.10
        with obstruction Q51.11

Double — *continued*
  uterus — *continued*
    complete Q51.21
    in pregnancy or childbirth O34.0- ☑
      causing obstructed labor O65.5
    partial Q51.22
    specified NEC Q51.28
  vagina Q52.10
    with doubling of uterus (and cervix) Q51.10
      with obstruction Q51.11
  vision H53.2
  vulva Q52.79
Douglas' pouch, cul-de-sac — *see* condition
Down syndrome Q90.9
  meiotic nondisjunction Q90.0
  mitotic nondisjunction Q90.1
  mosaicism Q90.1
  translocation Q90.2
DPD (dihydropyrimidine dehydrogenase deficiency) E88.89
Dracontiasis B72
Dracunculiasis, dracunculosis B72
Dream state, hysterical F44.89
Drepanocytic anemia — *see* Disease, sickle-cell
Dresbach's syndrome (elliptocytosis) D58.1
Dreschlera (hawaiiensis) (infection) B43.8
Dressler's syndrome I24.1
Drift, ulnar — *see* Deformity, limb, specified type NEC, forearm
Drinking (alcohol)
  excessive, to excess NEC (without dependence) F10.10
  habitual (continual) (without remission) F10.20
    with remission F10.21
Drip, postnasal (chronic) R09.82
  due to
    allergic rhinitis — *see* Rhinitis, allergic
    common cold J00
    gastroesophageal reflux — *see* Reflux, gastroe-sophageal
    nasopharyngitis — *see* Nasopharyngitis
    other known condition — *code to* condition
    sinusitis — *see* Sinusitis
Droop
  facial R29.810
    cerebrovascular disease I69.992
      cerebral infarction I69.392
      intracerebral hemorrhage I69.192
      nontraumatic intracranial hemorrhage NEC I69.292
      specified disease NEC I69.892
      subarachnoid hemorrhage I69.092
Drop (in)
  attack NEC R55
  finger — *see* Deformity, finger
  foot — *see* Deformity, limb, foot, drop
  hematocrit (precipitous) R71.0
  hemoglobin R71.0
  toe — *see* Deformity, toe, specified NEC
  wrist — *see* Deformity, limb, wrist drop
Dropped heart beats I45.9
Dropsy, dropsical — *see also* Hydrops
  abdomen R18.8
  brain — *see* Hydrocephalus
  cardiac, heart — *see* Failure, heart, congestive
  gangrenous — *see* Gangrene
  heart — *see* Failure, heart, congestive
  kidney — *see* Nephrosis
  lung — *see* Edema, lung
  newborn due to isoimmunization P56.0
  pericardium — *see* Pericarditis
Drowned, drowning (near) T75.1 ☑
Drowsiness R40.0
Drug
  abuse counseling and surveillance Z71.51
  addiction — *see* Dependence
  dependence — *see* Dependence
  habit — *see* Dependence
  harmful use — *see* Abuse, drug
  induced fever R50.2
  overdose — *see* Table of Drugs and Chemicals, by drug, poisoning
  poisoning — *see* Table of Drugs and Chemicals, by drug, poisoning
  resistant organism infection — *see also* Resistant, organism, to, drug Z16.30

Drug — *continued*
  therapy
    long term (current) (prophylactic) — *see* Therapy, drug long-term (current) (prophylactic)
    short term — *omit code*
  wrong substance given or taken in error — *see* Table of Drugs and Chemicals, by drug, poisoning
Drunkenness (without dependence) F10.129
  acute in alcoholism F10.229
  chronic (without remission) F10.20
    with remission F10.21
  pathological (without dependence) F10.129
    with dependence F10.229
  sleep F51.9
Drusen
  macula (degenerative) (retina) — *see* Degeneration, macula, drusen
  optic disc H47.32- ☑
Dry, dryness — *see also* condition
  larynx J38.7
  mouth R68.2
    due to dehydration E86.0
  nose J34.89
  socket (teeth) M27.3
  throat J39.2
DSAP L56.5
Duane's syndrome H50.81- ☑
Dubin-Johnson disease or syndrome E80.6
Dubois' disease (thymus gland) A50.59 *[E35]*
Dubowitz' syndrome Q87.19
Duchenne-Aran muscular atrophy G12.21
Duchenne-Griesinger disease G71.01
Duchenne's
  disease or syndrome
    motor neuron disease G12.22
    muscular dystrophy G71.01
  locomotor ataxia (syphilitic) A52.11
  paralysis
    birth injury P14.0
    due to or associated with
      motor neuron disease G12.22
      muscular dystrophy G71.01
Ducrey's chancre A57
Duct, ductus — *see* condition
Duhring's disease (dermatitis herpetiformis) L13.0
Dullness, cardiac (decreased) (increased) R01.2
Dumb ague — *see* Malaria
Dumbness — *see* Aphasia
Dumdum fever B55.0
Dumping syndrome (postgastrectomy) K91.1
Duodenitis (nonspecific) (peptic) K29.80
  with bleeding K29.81
Duodenocholangitis — *see* Cholangitis
Duodenum, duodenal — *see* condition
Duplay's bursitis or periarthritis — *see* Tendinitis, calcific, shoulder
Duplication, duplex — *see also* Accessory
  alimentary tract Q45.8
  anus Q43.4
  appendix (and cecum) Q43.4
  biliary duct (any) Q44.5
  bladder Q64.79
  cecum (and appendix) Q43.4
  cervix Q51.820
  chromosome NEC
    with complex rearrangements NEC Q92.5
    seen only at prometaphase Q92.8
  cystic duct Q44.5
  digestive organs Q45.8
  esophagus Q39.8
  frontonasal process Q75.8
  intestine (large) (small) Q43.4
  kidney Q63.0
  liver Q44.7
  pancreas Q45.3
  penis Q55.69
  respiratory organs NEC Q34.8
  salivary duct Q38.4
  spinal cord (incomplete) Q06.2
  stomach Q40.2
Dupré's disease (meningism) R29.1
Dupuytren's contraction or disease M72.0
Durand-Nicolas-Favre disease A55
Durotomy (inadvertent) (incidental) G97.41
Duroziez's disease (congenital mitral stenosis) Q23.2
Dutton's relapsing fever (West African) A68.1
Dwarfism E34.3
  achondroplastic Q77.4

☑ **Additional Character Required** — Refer to the Tabular List for Character Selection   ▽ Subterms under main terms may continue to next column or page

Dwarfism — *continued*
  congenital E34.3
  constitutional E34.3
  hypochondroplastic Q77.4
  hypophyseal E23.0
  infantile E34.3
  Laron-type E34.3
  Lorain (-Levi) type E23.0
  metatropic Q77.8
  nephrotic-glycosuric (with hypophosphatemic rickets)
    E72.09
  nutritional E45
  pancreatic K86.89
  pituitary E23.0
  renal N25.0
  thanatophoric Q77.1
Dyke-Young anemia (secondary) (symptomatic) D59.1
Dysacusis — *see* Abnormal, auditory perception
Dysadrenocortism E27.9
  hyperfunction E27.0
Dysarthria R47.1
  following
    cerebral infarction I69.322
    cerebrovascular disease I69.922
      specified disease NEC I69.822
    intracerebral hemorrhage I69.122
    nontraumatic intracranial hemorrhage NEC I69.222
    subarachnoid hemorrhage I69.022
Dysautonomia (familial) G90.1
Dysbarism T70.3 ☑
Dysbasia R26.2
  angiosclerotica intermittens I73.9
  hysterical F44.4
  lordotica (progressiva) G24.1
  nonorganic origin F44.4
  psychogenic F44.4
Dysbetalipoproteinemia (familial) E78.2
Dyscalculia R48.8
  developmental F81.2
Dyschezia K59.00
Dyschondroplasia (with hemangiomata) Q78.4
Dyschromia (skin) L81.9
Dyscollagenosis M35.9
Dyscranio-pygo-phalangy Q87.0
Dyscrasia
  blood (with) D75.9
    antepartum hemorrhage — *see* Hemorrhage, an-
      tepartum, with coagulation defect
    intrapartum hemorrhage O67.0
    newborn P61.9
      specified type NEC P61.8
    puerperal, postpartum O72.3
  polyglandular, pluriglandular E31.9
Dysendocrinism E34.9
Dysentery, dysenteric (catarrhal) (diarrhea) (epidemic)
  (hemorrhagic) (infectious) (sporadic) (tropical) A09
  abscess, liver A06.4
  amebic — *see also* Amebiasis A06.0
    with abscess — *see* Abscess, amebic
    acute A06.0
    chronic A06.1
  arthritis — *see also* category M01 A09
    bacillary (*see also* category M01) A03.9
  bacillary A03.9
    arthritis — *see also* category M01 A03.9
    Boyd A03.2
    Flexner A03.1
    Schmitz (-Stutzer) A03.0
    Shiga (-Kruse) A03.0
    Shigella A03.9
      boydii A03.2
      dysenteriae A03.0
      flexneri A03.1
      group A A03.0
      group B A03.1
      group C A03.2
      group D A03.3
      sonnei A03.3
      specified type NEC A03.8
    Sonne A03.3
    specified type NEC A03.8
  balantidial A07.0
  Balantidium coli A07.0
  Boyd's A03.2
  candidal B37.82
  Chilomastix A07.8
  Chinese A03.9
  coccidial A07.3

Dysentery, dysenteric — *continued*
  Dientamoeba (fragilis) A07.8
  Embadomonas A07.8
  Entamoeba, entamebic — *see* Dysentery, amebic
  Flexner-Boyd A03.2
  Flexner's A03.1
  Giardia lamblia A07.1
  Hiss-Russell A03.1
  Lamblia A07.1
  leishmanial B55.0
  malarial — *see* Malaria
  metazoal B82.0
  monilial B37.82
  protozoal A07.9
  Salmonella A02.0
  schistosomal B65.0
  Schmitz (-Stutzer) A03.0
  Shiga (-Kruse) A03.0
  Shigella NOS — *see* Dysentery, bacillary
  Sonne A03.3
  strongyloidiasis B78.0
  trichomonal A07.8
  viral — *see also* Enteritis, viral A08.4
Dysequilibrium R42
Dysesthesia R20.8
  hysterical F44.6
Dysfibrinogenemia (congenital) D68.2
Dysfunction
  adrenal E27.9
    hyperfunction E27.0
  autonomic
    due to alcohol G31.2
    somatoform F45.8
  bladder N31.9
    neurogenic NOS — *see* Dysfunction, bladder, neu-
      romuscular
    neuromuscular NOS N31.9
      atonic (motor) (sensory) N31.2
      autonomous N31.2
      flaccid N31.2
      nonreflex N31.2
      reflex N31.1
      specified NEC N31.8
      uninhibited N31.0
  bleeding, uterus N93.8
  cerebral G93.89
  colon K59.9
    psychogenic F45.8
  colostomy K94.03
  cystic duct K82.8
  cystostomy (stoma) — *see* Complications, cystostomy
  ejaculatory N53.19
    anejaculatory orgasm N53.13
    painful N53.12
    premature F52.4
    retarded N53.11
  endocrine NOS E34.9
  endometrium N85.8
  enterostomy K94.13
  erectile — *see* Dysfunction, sexual, male, erectile
  gallbladder K82.8
  gastrostomy (stoma) K94.23
  gland, glandular NOS E34.9
    meibomian, of eyelid — *see* Dysfunction, meibomi-
      an gland
  heart I51.89
  hemoglobin D75.89
  hepatic K76.89
  hypophysis E23.7
  hypothalamic NEC E23.3
  ileostomy (stoma) K94.13
  jejunostomy (stoma) K94.13
  kidney — *see* Disease, renal
  labyrinthine — *see* subcategory H83.2 ☑
  left ventricular, following sudden emotional stress
    I51.81
  liver K76.89
  male — *see* Dysfunction, sexual, male
  meibomian gland, of eyelid H02.889
    left H02.886
      lower H02.885
      upper H02.884
      upper and lower eyelids H02.88B
    right H02.883
      lower H02.882
      upper H02.881
      upper and lower eyelids H02.88A
  orgasmic (female) F52.31

Dysfunction — *continued*
  orgasmic — *continued*
    male F52.32
  ovary E28.9
    specified NEC E28.8
  papillary muscle I51.89
  parathyroid E21.4
  physiological NEC R68.89
    psychogenic F59
  pineal gland E34.8
  pituitary (gland) E23.3
  platelets D69.1
  polyglandular E31.9
    specified NEC E31.8
  psychophysiologic F59
  psychosexual F52.9
    with
      dyspareunia F52.6
      premature ejaculation F52.4
      vaginismus F52.5
  pylorus K31.9
  rectum K59.9
    psychogenic F45.8
  reflex (sympathetic) — *see* Syndrome, pain, complex
    regional I
  segmental — *see* Dysfunction, somatic
  senile R54
  sexual (due to) R37
    alcohol F10.981
    amphetamine F15.981
      in
        abuse F15.181
        dependence F15.281
    anxiolytic F13.981
      in
        abuse F13.181
        dependence F13.281
    cocaine F14.981
      in
        abuse F14.181
        dependence F14.281
    excessive sexual drive F52.8
    failure of genital response (male) F52.21
      female F52.22
    female N94.9
      aversion F52.1
      dyspareunia N94.10
        psychogenic F52.6
      frigidity F52.22
      nymphomania F52.8
      orgasmic F52.31
      psychogenic F52.9
        aversion F52.1
        dyspareunia F52.6
        frigidity F52.22
        nymphomania F52.8
        orgasmic F52.31
        vaginismus F52.5
      vaginismus N94.2
        psychogenic F52.5
    hypnotic F13.981
      in
        abuse F13.181
        dependence F13.281
    inhibited orgasm (female) F52.31
      male F52.32
    lack
      of sexual enjoyment F52.1
      or loss of sexual desire F52.0
    male N53.9
      anejaculatory orgasm N53.13
      ejaculatory N53.19
        painful N53.12
        premature F52.4
        retarded N53.11
      erectile N52.9
        drug induced N52.2
        due to
          disease classified elsewhere N52.1
          drug N52.2
        postoperative (postprocedural) N52.39
          following
            cryotherapy N52.37
            interstitial seed therapy N52.36
            prostate ablative therapy N52.37
            prostatectomy N52.34
              radical N52.31
            radiation therapy N52.35
            radical cystectomy N52.32

Dysfunction — *continued*
  sexual — *continued*
    male — *continued*
      erectile — *continued*
        postoperative — *continued*
          following — *continued*
            ultrasound ablative therapy N52.37
            urethral surgery N52.33
        psychogenic F52.21
        specified cause NEC N52.8
        vasculogenic
          arterial insufficiency N52.01
            with corporo-venous occlusive N52.03
          corporo-venous occlusive N52.02
            with arterial insufficiency N52.03
      impotence — *see* Dysfunction, sexual, male, erectile
      psychogenic F52.9
        aversion F52.1
        erectile F52.21
        orgasmic F52.32
        premature ejaculation F52.4
        satyriasis F52.8
        specified type NEC F52.8
      specified type NEC N53.8
    nonorganic F52.9
      specified NEC F52.8
    opioid F11.981
      in
        abuse F11.181
        dependence F11.281
    orgasmic dysfunction (female) F52.31
      male F52.32
    premature ejaculation F52.4
    psychoactive substances NEC F19.981
      in
        abuse F19.181
        dependence F19.281
    psychogenic F52.9
    sedative F13.981
      in
        abuse F13.181
        dependence F13.281
    sexual aversion F52.1
    vaginismus (nonorganic) (psychogenic) F52.5
  sinoatrial node I49.5
  somatic M99.09
    abdomen M99.09
    acromioclavicular M99.07
    cervical region M99.01
    cervicothoracic M99.01
    costochondral M99.08
    costovertebral M99.08
    head region M99.00
    hip M99.05
    lower extremity M99.06
    lumbar region M99.03
    lumbosacral M99.03
    occipitocervical M99.00
    pelvic region M99.05
    pubic M99.05
    rib cage M99.08
    sacral region M99.04
    sacrococcygeal M99.04
    sacroiliac M99.04
    specified NEC M99.09
    sternochondral M99.08
    sternoclavicular M99.07
    thoracic region M99.02
    thoracolumbar M99.02
    upper extremity M99.07
  somatoform autonomic F45.8
  stomach K31.89
    psychogenic F45.8
  suprarenal E27.9
    hyperfunction E27.0
  symbolic R48.9
    specified type NEC R48.8
  temporomandibular (joint) M26.69
    joint-pain syndrome M26.62- ☑
  testicular (endocrine) E29.9
    specified NEC E29.8
  thymus E32.9
  thyroid E07.9
  ureterostomy (stoma) — *see* Complications, stoma, urinary tract
  urethrostomy (stoma) — *see* Complications, stoma, urinary tract
  uterus, complicating delivery O62.9

Dysfunction — *continued*
  uterus, complicating delivery — *continued*
    hypertonic O62.4
    hypotonic O62.2
      primary O62.0
      secondary O62.1
  ventricular I51.9
    with congestive heart failure — *see also* Failure, heart I50.9
    left, reversible, following sudden emotional stress I51.81
Dysgenesis
  gonadal (due to chromosomal anomaly) Q96.9
    pure Q99.1
  renal Q60.5
    bilateral Q60.4
    unilateral Q60.3
  reticular D72.0
  tidal platelet D69.3
Dysgerminoma
  specified site — *see* Neoplasm, malignant, by site
  unspecified site
    female C56.9
    male C62.90
Dysgeusia R43.2
Dysgraphia R27.8
Dyshidrosis, dysidrosis L30.1
Dyskaryotic cervical smear R87.619
Dyskeratosis L85.8
  cervix — *see* Dysplasia, cervix
  congenital Q82.8
  uterus NEC N85.8
Dyskinesia G24.9
  biliary (cystic duct or gallbladder) K82.8
  drug induced
    orofacial G24.01
  esophagus K22.4
  hysterical F44.4
  intestinal K59.8
  nonorganic origin F44.4
  orofacial (idiopathic) G24.4
    drug induced G24.01
  psychogenic F44.4
  subacute, drug induced G24.01
  tardive G24.01
    neuroleptic induced G24.01
  trachea J39.8
  tracheobronchial J98.09
Dyslalia (developmental) F80.0
Dyslexia R48.0
  developmental F81.0
Dyslipidemia E78.5
  depressed HDL cholesterol E78.6
  elevated fasting triglycerides E78.1
Dysmaturity — *see also* Light for dates
  pulmonary (newborn) (Wilson-Mikity) P27.0
Dysmenorrhea (essential) (exfoliative) N94.6
  congestive (syndrome) N94.6
  primary N94.4
  psychogenic F45.8
  secondary N94.5
Dysmetabolic syndrome X E88.81
Dysmetria R27.8
Dysmorphism (due to)
  alcohol Q86.0
  exogenous cause NEC Q86.8
  hydantoin Q86.1
  warfarin Q86.2
Dysmorphophobia (nondelusional) F45.22
  delusional F22
Dysnomia R47.01
Dysorexia R63.0
  psychogenic F50.89
Dysostosis
  cleidocranial, cleidocranialis Q74.0
  craniofacial Q75.1
  Fairbank's (idiopathic familial generalized osteophytosis) Q78.9
  mandibulofacial (incomplete) Q75.4
  multiplex E76.01
  oculomandibular Q75.5
Dyspareunia (female) N94.10
  deep N94.12
  male N53.12
  nonorganic F52.6
  psychogenic F52.6
  secondary N94.19
  specified NEC N94.19

Dyspareunia — *continued*
  superficial (introital) N94.11
Dyspepsia R10.13
  atonic K30
  functional (allergic) (congenital) (gastrointestinal) (occupational) (reflex) K30
  intestinal K59.8
  nervous F45.8
  neurotic F45.8
  psychogenic F45.8
Dysphagia R13.10
  cervical R13.19
  following
    cerebral infarction I69.391
    cerebrovascular disease I69.991
      specified NEC I69.891
    intracerebral hemorrhage I69.191
    nontraumatic intracranial hemorrhage NEC I69.291
    specified disease NEC I69.891
    subarachnoid hemorrhage I69.091
  functional (hysterical) F45.8
  hysterical F45.8
  nervous (hysterical) F45.8
  neurogenic R13.19
  oral phase R13.11
  oropharyngeal phase R13.12
  pharyngeal phase R13.13
  pharyngoesophageal phase R13.14
  psychogenic F45.8
  sideropenic D50.1
  spastica K22.4
  specified NEC R13.19
Dysphagocytosis, congenital D71
Dysphasia R47.02
  developmental
    expressive type F80.1
    receptive type F80.2
  following
    cerebrovascular disease I69.921
      cerebral infarction I69.321
      intracerebral hemorrhage I69.121
      nontraumatic intracranial hemorrhage NEC I69.221
      specified disease NEC I69.821
      subarachnoid hemorrhage I69.021
Dysphonia R49.0
  functional F44.4
  hysterical F44.4
  psychogenic F44.4
  spastica J38.3
Dysphoria
  gender F64.9
    in
      adolescence and adulthood F64.0
      children F64.2
    specified NEC F64.8
  postpartal O90.6
Dyspituitarism E23.3
Dysplasia — *see also* Anomaly
  acetabular, congenital Q65.89
  alveolar capillary, with vein misalignment J84.843
  anus (histologically confirmed) (mild) (moderate) K62.82
    severe D01.3
  arrhythmogenic right ventricular I42.8
  arterial, fibromuscular I77.3
  asphyxiating thoracic (congenital) Q77.2
  brain Q07.9
  bronchopulmonary, perinatal P27.1
  cervix (uteri) N87.9
    mild N87.0
    moderate N87.1
    severe D06.9
  chondroectodermal Q77.6
  colon D12.6
  craniometaphyseal Q78.8
  dentinal K00.5
  diaphyseal, progressive Q78.3
  dystrophic Q77.5
  ectodermal (anhidrotic) (congenital) (hereditary) Q82.4
    hydrotic Q82.8
  epithelial, uterine cervix — *see* Dysplasia, cervix
  eye (congenital) Q11.2
  fibrous
    bone NEC (monostotic) M85.00
      ankle M85.07- ☑
      foot M85.07- ☑
      forearm M85.03- ☑

Dysplasia — *continued*
  fibrous — *continued*
    bone — *continued*
      hand M85.04- ☑
      lower leg M85.06- ☑
      multiple site M85.09
      neck M85.08
      rib M85.08
      shoulder M85.01- ☑
      skull M85.08
      specified site NEC M85.08
      thigh M85.05- ☑
      toe M85.07- ☑
      upper arm M85.02- ☑
      vertebra M85.08
    diaphyseal, progressive Q78.3
    jaw M27.8
    polyostotic Q78.1
  florid osseous — *see also* Cyst, calcifying odontogenic
  high grade, focal D12.6
  hip, congenital Q65.89
  joint, congenital Q74.8
  kidney Q61.4
    multicystic Q61.4
  leg Q74.2
  lung, congenital (not associated with short gestation) Q33.6
  mammary (gland) (benign) N60.9- ☑
    cyst (solitary) — *see* Cyst, breast
    cystic — *see* Mastopathy, cystic
    duct ectasia — *see* Ectasia, mammary duct
    fibroadenosis — *see* Fibroadenosis, breast
    fibrosclerosis — *see* Fibrosclerosis, breast
    specified type NEC N60.8- ☑
  metaphyseal Q78.5
  muscle Q79.8
  oculodentodigital Q87.0
  periapical (cemental) (cemento-osseous) — *see* Cyst, calcifying odontogenic
  periosteum — *see* Disorder, bone, specified type NEC
  polyostotic fibrous Q78.1
  prostate — *see also* Neoplasia, intraepithelial, prostate N42.30
    severe D07.5
    specified NEC N42.39
  renal Q61.4
    multicystic Q61.4
  retinal, congenital Q14.1
  right ventricular, arrhythmogenic I42.8
  septo-optic Q04.4
  skin L98.8
  spinal cord Q06.1
  spondyloepiphyseal Q77.7
  thymic, with immunodeficiency D82.1
  vagina N89.3
    mild N89.0
    moderate N89.1
    severe NEC D07.2
  vulva N90.3
    mild N90.0
    moderate N90.1
    severe NEC D07.1
Dysplasminogenemia E88.02
Dyspnea (nocturnal) (paroxysmal) R06.00
  asthmatic (bronchial) J45.909
    with
      bronchitis J45.909
        with
          exacerbation (acute) J45.901
          status asthmaticus J45.902
        chronic J44.9
      exacerbation (acute) J45.901
      status asthmaticus J45.902
    cardiac — *see* Failure, ventricular, left
  cardiac — *see* Failure, ventricular, left
  functional F45.8
  hyperventilation R06.4
  hysterical F45.8
  newborn P28.89
  orthopnea R06.01
  psychogenic F45.8
  shortness of breath R06.02
  specified type NEC R06.09
Dyspraxia R27.8
  developmental (syndrome) F82
Dysproteinemia E88.09
Dysreflexia, autonomic G90.4

Dysrhythmia
  cardiac I49.9
    newborn
      bradycardia P29.12
      occurring before birth P03.819
        before onset of labor P03.810
        during labor P03.811
      tachycardia P29.11
    postoperative I97.89
  cerebral or cortical — *see* Epilepsy
Dyssomnia — *see* Disorder, sleep
Dyssynergia
  biliary K83.8
  bladder sphincter N36.44
  cerebellaris myoclonica (Hunt's ataxia) G11.1
Dysthymia F34.1
Dysthyroidism E07.9
Dystocia O66.9
  affecting newborn P03.1
  cervical (hypotonic) O62.2
    affecting newborn P03.6
    primary O62.0
    secondary O62.1
  contraction ring O62.4
  fetal O66.9
    abnormality NEC O66.3
    conjoined twins O66.3
    oversize O66.2
  maternal O66.9
  positional O64.9 ☑
  shoulder (girdle) O66.0
    causing obstructed labor O66.0
  uterine NEC O62.4
Dystonia G24.9
  cervical G24.3
  deformans progressiva G24.1
  drug induced NEC G24.09
    acute G24.02
    specified NEC G24.09
  familial G24.1
  idiopathic G24.1
    familial G24.1
    nonfamilial G24.2
    orofacial G24.4
  lenticularis G24.8
  musculorum deformans G24.1
  neuroleptic induced (acute) G24.02
  orofacial (idiopathic) G24.4
  oromandibular G24.4
    due to drug G24.01
  specified NEC G24.8
  torsion (familial) (idiopathic) G24.1
    acquired G24.8
    genetic G24.1
    symptomatic (nonfamilial) G24.2
Dystonic movements R25.8
Dystrophy, dystrophia
  adiposogenital E23.6
  autosomal recessive, childhood type, muscular dystrophy resembling Duchenne or Becker G71.01
  Becker's type G71.01
  cervical sympathetic G90.2
  choroid (hereditary) H31.20
    central areolar H31.22
    choroideremia H31.21
    gyrate atrophy H31.23
    specified type NEC H31.29
  cornea (hereditary) H18.50
    endothelial H18.51
    epithelial H18.52
    granular H18.53
    lattice H18.54
    macular H18.55
    specified type NEC H18.59
  Duchenne's type G71.01
  due to malnutrition E45
  Erb's G71.02
  Fuchs' H18.51
  Gower's muscular G71.01
  hair L67.8
  infantile neuraxonal G31.89
  Landouzy-Déjérine G71.02
  Leyden-Möbius G71.09
  muscular G71.00
    autosomal recessive, childhood type, muscular dystrophy resembling Duchenne or Becker G71.01
    benign (Becker type) G71.01

Dystrophy, dystrophia — *continued*
  muscular — *continued*
    benign — *continued*
      scapuloperoneal with early contractures [Emery-Dreifuss] G71.09
    congenital (hereditary) (progressive) (with specific morphological abnormalities of the muscle fiber) G71.09
      myotonic G71.11
    distal G71.09
    Duchenne type G71.01
    Emery-Dreifuss G71.09
    Erb type G71.02
    facioscapulohumeral G71.02
    Gower's G71.01
    hereditary (progressive) G71.09
    Landouzy-Déjérine type G71.02
    limb-girdle G71.09
    myotonic G71.11
    progressive (hereditary) G71.09
      Charcot-Marie (-Tooth) type G60.0
    pseudohypertrophic (infantile) G71.01
    scapulohumeral G71.02
    scapuloperoneal G71.09
    severe (Duchenne type) G71.01
    specified type NEC G71.09
  myocardium, myocardial — *see* Degeneration, myocardial
  nail L60.3
    congenital Q84.6
  nutritional E45
  ocular G71.09
  oculocerebrorenal E72.03
  oculopharyngeal G71.09
  ovarian N83.8
  polyglandular E31.8
  reflex (neuromuscular) (sympathetic) — *see* Syndrome, pain, complex regional I
  retinal (hereditary) H35.50
    in
      lipid storage disorders E75.6 [H36]
      systemic lipidoses E75.6 [H36]
    involving
      pigment epithelium H35.54
      sensory area H35.53
    pigmentary H35.52
    vitreoretinal H35.51
  Salzmann's nodular — *see* Degeneration, cornea, nodular
  scapuloperoneal G71.09
  skin NEC L98.8
  sympathetic (reflex) — *see* Syndrome, pain, complex regional I
    cervical G90.2
  tapetoretinal H35.54
  thoracic, asphyxiating Q77.2
  unguium L60.3
    congenital Q84.6
  vitreoretinal H35.51
  vulva N90.4
  yellow (liver) — *see* Failure, hepatic
Dysuria R30.0
  psychogenic F45.8

E

Eales' disease H35.06- ☑
Ear — *see also* condition
  piercing Z41.3
  tropical NEC B36.9 [H62.40]
    in
      aspergillosis B44.89
      candidiasis B37.84
      moniliasis B37.84
  wax (impacted) H61.20
    left H61.22
      with right H61.23
    right H61.21
      with left H61.23
Earache — *see* subcategory H92.0 ☑
Early satiety R68.81
Eaton-Lambert syndrome — *see* Syndrome, Lambert-Eaton
Eberth's disease (typhoid fever) A01.00
Ebola virus disease A98.4
Ebstein's anomaly or syndrome (heart) Q22.5
Eccentro-osteochondrodysplasia E76.29
Ecchondroma — *see* Neoplasm, bone, benign

Ecchondrosis D48.Ø
Ecchymosis R58
  conjunctiva — *see* Hemorrhage, conjunctiva
  eye (traumatic) — *see* Contusion, eyeball
  eyelid (traumatic) — *see* Contusion, eyelid
  newborn P54.5
  spontaneous R23.3
  traumatic — *see* Contusion
Echinococciasis — *see* Echinococcus
Echinococcosis — *see* Echinococcus
Echinococcus (infection) B67.9Ø
  granulosus B67.4
    bone B67.2
    liver B67.Ø
    lung B67.1
    multiple sites B67.32
    specified site NEC B67.39
    thyroid B67.31
  liver NOS B67.8
    granulosus B67.Ø
    multilocularis B67.5
  lung NEC B67.99
    granulosus B67.1
    multilocularis B67.69
  multilocularis B67.7
    liver B67.5
    multiple sites B67.61
    specified site NEC B67.69
  specified site NEC B67.99
    granulosus B67.39
    multilocularis B67.69
  thyroid NEC B67.99
    granulosus B67.31
    multilocularis B67.69 *[E35]*
Echinorhynchiasis B83.8
Echinostomiasis B66.8
Echolalia R48.8
Echovirus, as cause of disease classified elsewhere
  B97.12
Eclampsia, eclamptic (coma) (convulsions) (delirium)
  (with hypertension) NEC O15.9
  complicating
    labor and delivery O15.1
    postpartum O15.2
    pregnancy O15.Ø- ☑
    puerperium O15.2
Economic circumstances affecting care Z59.9
Economo's disease A85.8
Ectasia, ectasis
  annuloaortic I35.8
  aorta I77.819
    with aneurysm — *see* Aneurysm, aorta
    abdominal I77.811
    thoracic I77.81Ø
    thoracoabdominal I77.812
  breast — *see* Ectasia, mammary duct
  capillary I78.8
  cornea H18.71- ☑
  gastric antral vascular (GAVE) K31.819
    with hemorrhage K31.811
    without hemorrhage K31.819
  mammary duct N60.4- ☑
  salivary gland (duct) K11.8
  sclera — *see* Sclerectasia
Ecthyma LØ8.Ø
  contagiosum BØ8.Ø2
  gangrenosum LØ8.Ø
  infectiosum BØ8.Ø2
Ectocardia Q24.8
Ectodermal dysplasia (anhidrotic) Q82.4
Ectodermosis erosiva pluriorificialis L51.1
Ectopic, ectopia (congenital)
  abdominal viscera Q45.8
    due to defect in anterior abdominal wall Q79.59
  ACTH syndrome E24.3
  adrenal gland Q89.1
  anus Q43.5
  atrial beats I49.1
  beats I49.49
    atrial I49.1
    ventricular I49.3
  bladder Q64.1Ø
  bone and cartilage in lung Q33.5
  brain Q04.8
  breast tissue Q83.8
  cardiac Q24.8
  cerebral Q04.8
  cordis Q24.8

Ectopic, ectopia — *continued*
  endometrium — *see* Endometriosis
  gastric mucosa Q4Ø.2
  gestation — *see* Pregnancy, by site
  heart Q24.8
  hormone secretion NEC E34.2
  kidney (crossed) (pelvis) Q63.2
  lens, lentis Q12.1
  mole — *see* Pregnancy, by site
  organ or site NEC — *see* Malposition, congenital
  pancreas Q45.3
  pregnancy — *see* Pregnancy, ectopic
  pupil — *see* Abnormality, pupillary
  renal Q63.2
  sebaceous glands of mouth Q38.6
  spleen Q89.Ø9
  testis Q53.ØØ
    bilateral Q53.Ø2
    unilateral Q53.Ø1
  thyroid Q89.2
  tissue in lung Q33.5
  ureter Q62.63
  ventricular beats I49.3
  vesicae Q64.1Ø
Ectromelia Q73.8
  lower limb — *see* Defect, reduction, limb, lower, specified type NEC
  upper limb — *see* Defect, reduction, limb, upper, specified type NEC
Ectropion HØ2.1Ø9
  cervix N86
    with cervicitis N72
  congenital Q1Ø.1
  eyelid HØ2.1Ø9
    cicatricial HØ2.119
      left HØ2.116
        lower HØ2.115
        upper HØ2.114
      right HØ2.113
        lower HØ2.112
        upper HØ2.111
    congenital Q1Ø.1
    left HØ2.1Ø6
      lower HØ2.1Ø5
      upper HØ2.1Ø4
    mechanical HØ2.129
      left HØ2.126
        lower HØ2.125
        upper HØ2.124
      right HØ2.123
        lower HØ2.122
        upper HØ2.121
    paralytic HØ2.159
      left HØ2.156
        lower HØ2.155
        upper HØ2.154
      right HØ2.153
        lower HØ2.152
        upper HØ2.151
    right HØ2.1Ø3
      lower HØ2.1Ø2
      upper HØ2.1Ø1
    senile HØ2.139
      left HØ2.136
        lower HØ2.135
        upper HØ2.134
      right HØ2.133
        lower HØ2.132
        upper HØ2.131
    spastic HØ2.149
      left HØ2.146
        lower HØ2.145
        upper HØ2.144
      right HØ2.143
        lower HØ2.142
        upper HØ2.141
  iris H21.89
  lip (acquired) K13.Ø
    congenital Q38.Ø
  urethra N36.8
  uvea H21.89
Eczema (acute) (chronic) (erythematous) (fissum)
  (rubrum) (squamous) — *see also* Dermatitis L30.9
  contact — *see* Dermatitis, contact
  dyshydrotic L30.1
  external ear — *see* Otitis, externa, acute, eczematoid
  flexural L20.82
  herpeticum BØØ.Ø

Eczema — *continued*
  hypertrophicum L28.Ø
  hypostatic — *see* Varix, leg, with, inflammation
  impetiginous L01.1
  infantile (due to any substance) L20.83
    intertriginous L21.1
    seborrheic L21.1
  intertriginous NEC L30.4
    infantile L21.1
  intrinsic (allergic) L20.84
  lichenified NEC L28.Ø
  marginatum (hebrae) B35.6
  pustular L30.3
  stasis I87.2
    with varicose veins — *see* Varix, leg, with, inflammation
  vaccination, vaccinatum T88.1 ☑
  varicose — *see* Varix, leg, with, inflammation
Eczematid L30.2
Eddowes (-Spurway) **syndrome** Q78.Ø
Edema, edematous (infectious) (pitting) (toxic) R60.9
  with nephritis — *see* Nephrosis
  allergic T78.3 ☑
  amputation stump (surgical) (sequelae) (late effect))
    T87.89
  angioneurotic (allergic) (any site) (with urticaria)
    T78.3 ☑
    hereditary D84.1
  angiospastic I73.9
  Berlin's (traumatic) SØ5.8X- ☑
  brain (cytotoxic) (vasogenic) G93.6
    due to birth injury P11.Ø
    newborn (anoxia or hypoxia) P52.4
      birth injury P11.Ø
    traumatic — *see* Injury, intracranial, cerebral edema
  cardiac — *see* Failure, heart, congestive
  cardiovascular — *see* Failure, heart, congestive
  cerebral — *see* Edema, brain
  cerebrospinal — *see* Edema, brain
  cervix (uteri) (acute) N88.8
    puerperal, postpartum O90.89
  chronic hereditary Q82.Ø
  circumscribed, acute T78.3 ☑
    hereditary D84.1
  conjunctiva H11.42- ☑
  cornea H18.2- ☑
    idiopathic H18.22- ☑
    secondary H18.23- ☑
      due to contact lens H18.21- ☑
  due to
    lymphatic obstruction I89.Ø
    salt retention E87.Ø
  epiglottis — *see* Edema, glottis
  essential, acute T78.3 ☑
    hereditary D84.1
  extremities, lower — *see* Edema, legs
  eyelid NEC HØ2.849
    left HØ2.846
      lower HØ2.845
      upper HØ2.844
    right HØ2.843
      lower HØ2.842
      upper HØ2.841
  familial, hereditary Q82.Ø
  famine — *see* Malnutrition, severe
  generalized R60.9
  glottis, glottic, glottidis (obstructive) (passive) J38.4
    allergic T78.3 ☑
      hereditary D84.1
  heart — *see* Failure, heart, congestive
  heat T67.7 ☑
  hereditary Q82.Ø
  inanition — *see* Malnutrition, severe
  intracranial G93.6
  iris H21.89
  joint — *see* Effusion, joint
  larynx — *see* Edema, glottis
  legs R60.Ø
    due to venous obstruction I87.1
    hereditary Q82.Ø
  localized R60.Ø
    due to venous obstruction I87.1
  lower limbs — *see* Edema, legs
  lung J81.1
    with heart condition or failure — *see* Failure, ventricular, left
    acute J81.Ø
    chemical (acute) J68.1

☑ **Additional Character Required — Refer to the Tabular List for Character Selection**   ▽ Subterms under main terms may continue to next column or page

Edema, edematous — continued
- lung — continued
  - chemical — continued
    - chronic J68.1
  - chronic J81.1
    - due to
      - chemicals, gases, fumes or vapors (inhalation) J68.1
      - external agent J70.9
        - specified NEC J70.8
      - radiation J70.1
  - due to
    - chemicals, fumes or vapors (inhalation) J68.1
    - external agent J70.9
      - specified NEC J70.8
    - high altitude T70.29 ☑
    - near drowning T75.1 ☑
    - radiation J70.0
  - meaning failure, left ventricle I50.1
- lymphatic I89.0
  - due to mastectomy I97.2
- macula H35.81
  - cystoid, following cataract surgery — see Complications, postprocedural, following cataract surgery
  - diabetic — see Diabetes, by type, with, retinopathy, with macular edema
- malignant — see Gangrene, gas
- Milroy's Q82.0
- nasopharynx J39.2
- newborn P83.30
  - hydrops fetalis — see Hydrops, fetalis
  - specified NEC P83.39
- nutritional — see also Malnutrition, severe
  - with dyspigmentation, skin and hair E40
- optic disc or nerve — see Papilledema
- orbit H05.22- ☑
- pancreas K86.89
- papilla, optic — see Papilledema
- penis N48.89
- periodic T78.3 ☑
  - hereditary D84.1
- pharynx J39.2
- pulmonary — see Edema, lung
- Quincke's T78.3 ☑
  - hereditary D84.1
- renal — see Nephrosis
- retina H35.81
  - diabetic — see Diabetes, by type, with, retinopathy, with macular edema
- salt E87.0
- scrotum N50.89
- seminal vesicle N50.89
- spermatic cord N50.89
- spinal (cord) (vascular) (nontraumatic) G95.19
- starvation — see Malnutrition, severe
- stasis — see Hypertension, venous, (chronic)
- subglottic — see Edema, glottis
- supraglottic — see Edema, glottis
- testis N44.8
- tunica vaginalis N50.89
- vas deferens N50.89
- vulva (acute) N90.89

Edentulism — see Absence, teeth, acquired
Edsall's disease T67.2 ☑
Educational handicap Z55.9
- specified NEC Z55.8
Edward's syndrome — see Trisomy, 18
Effect(s) (of) (from) — see Effect, adverse NEC
Effect, adverse
- abnormal gravitational (G) forces or states T75.81 ☑
- abuse — see Maltreatment
- air pressure T70.9 ☑
  - specified NEC T70.8 ☑
- altitude (high) — see Effect, adverse, high altitude
- anesthesia — see also Anesthesia T88.59 ☑
  - in labor and delivery O74.9
  - local, toxic
    - in labor and delivery O74.4
    - in pregnancy NEC O29.3- ☑
    - postpartum, puerperal O89.3
  - postpartum, puerperal O89.9
  - specified NEC T88.59 ☑
    - in labor and delivery O74.8
    - postpartum, puerperal O89.8
  - spinal and epidural T88.59 ☑
    - headache T88.59 ☑

Effect, adverse — continued
- anesthesia — see also Anesthesia — continued
  - spinal and epidural — continued
    - headache — continued
      - in labor and delivery O74.5
      - postpartum, puerperal O89.4
    - specified NEC
      - in labor and delivery O74.6
      - postpartum, puerperal O89.5
- antitoxin — see Complications, vaccination
- atmospheric pressure T70.9 ☑
  - due to explosion T70.8 ☑
  - high T70.3 ☑
  - low — see Effect, adverse, high altitude
  - specified effect NEC T70.8 ☑
- biological, correct substance properly administered — see Effect, adverse, drug
- blood (derivatives) (serum) (transfusion) — see Complications, transfusion
- chemical substance — see Table of Drugs and Chemicals
- cold (temperature) (weather) T69.9 ☑
  - chilblains T69.1 ☑
  - frostbite — see Frostbite
  - specified effect NEC T69.8 ☑
- drugs and medicaments T88.7 ☑
  - specified drug — see Table of Drugs and Chemicals, by drug, adverse effect
  - specified effect — code to condition
- electric current, electricity (shock) T75.4 ☑
  - burn — see Burn
- exertion (excessive) T73.3 ☑
- exposure — see Exposure
- external cause NEC T75.89 ☑
- foodstuffs T78.1 ☑
  - allergic reaction — see Allergy, food
    - causing anaphylaxis — see Shock, anaphylactic, due to food
  - noxious — see Poisoning, food, noxious
- gases, fumes, or vapors T59.9- ☑
  - specified agent — see Table of Drugs and Chemicals
- glue (airplane) sniffing
  - due to drug abuse — see Abuse, drug, inhalant
  - due to drug dependence — see Dependence, drug, inhalant
- heat — see Heat
- high altitude NEC T70.29 ☑
  - anoxia T70.29 ☑
  - on
    - ears T70.0 ☑
    - sinuses T70.1 ☑
  - polycythemia D75.1
- high pressure fluids T70.4 ☑
- hot weather — see Heat
- hunger T73.0 ☑
- immersion, foot — see Immersion
- immunization — see Complications, vaccination
- immunological agents — see Complications, vaccination
- infrared (radiation) (rays) NOS T66 ☑
  - dermatitis or eczema L59.8
- infusion — see Complications, infusion
- lack of care of infants — see Maltreatment, child
- lightning — see Lightning
- medical care T88.9 ☑
  - specified NEC T88.8 ☑
- medicinal substance, correct, properly administered — see Effect, adverse, drug
- motion T75.3 ☑
- noise, on inner ear — see subcategory H83.3 ☑
- overheated places — see Heat
- psychosocial, of work environment Z56.5
- radiation (diagnostic) (infrared) (natural source) (therapeutic) (ultraviolet) (X-ray) NOS T66 ☑
  - dermatitis or eczema — see Dermatitis, due to, radiation
  - fibrosis of lung J70.1
  - pneumonitis J70.0
  - pulmonary manifestations
    - acute J70.0
    - chronic J70.1
  - skin L59.9
- radioactive substance NOS
  - dermatitis or eczema — see Radiodermatitis
- reduced temperature T69.9 ☑
  - immersion foot or hand — see Immersion
  - specified effect NEC T69.8 ☑

Effect, adverse — continued
- serum NEC — see also Reaction, serum T80.69 ☑
- specified NEC T78.8 ☑
  - external cause NEC T75.89 ☑
- strangulation — see Asphyxia, traumatic
- submersion T75.1 ☑
- thirst T73.1 ☑
- toxic — see Toxicity
- transfusion — see Complications, transfusion
- ultraviolet (radiation) (rays) NOS T66 ☑
  - burn — see Burn
  - dermatitis or eczema — see Dermatitis, due to, ultraviolet rays
    - acute L56.8
- vaccine (any) — see Complications, vaccination
- vibration — see Vibration, adverse effects
- water pressure NEC T70.9 ☑
  - specified NEC T70.8 ☑
- weightlessness T75.82 ☑
- whole blood — see Complications, transfusion
- work environment Z56.5
Effects, late — see Sequelae
Effluvium
- anagen L65.1
- telogen L65.0
Effort syndrome (psychogenic) F45.8
Effusion
- amniotic fluid — see Pregnancy, complicated by, prematue rupture of membranes
- brain (serous) G93.6
- bronchial — see Bronchitis
- cerebral G93.6
- cerebrospinal — see also Meningitis
  - vessel G93.6
- chest — see Effusion, pleura
- chylous, chyliform (pleura) J94.0
- intracranial G93.6
- joint M25.40
  - ankle M25.47- ☑
  - elbow M25.42- ☑
  - foot joint M25.47- ☑
  - hand joint M25.44- ☑
  - hip M25.45- ☑
  - knee M25.46- ☑
  - shoulder M25.41- ☑
  - specified joint NEC M25.48
  - wrist M25.43- ☑
- malignant pleural J91.0
- meninges — see Meningitis
- pericardium, pericardial (noninflammatory) I31.3
  - acute — see Pericarditis, acute
- peritoneal (chronic) R18.8
- pleura, pleurisy, pleuritic, pleuropericardial J90
  - chylous, chyliform J94.0
  - due to systemic lupus erythematosis M32.13
  - in conditions classified elsewhere J91.8
  - influenzal — see Influenza, with, respiratory manifestations NEC
  - malignant J91.0
  - newborn P28.89
  - tuberculous NEC A15.6
    - primary (progressive) A15.7
- spinal — see Meningitis
- thorax, thoracic — see Effusion, pleura
Egg shell nails L60.3
- congenital Q84.6
Egyptian splenomegaly B65.1
Ehlers-Danlos syndrome — see also Syndrome, Ehlers-Danlos Q79.60
Ehrlichiosis A77.40
- due to
  - E. chafeensis A77.41
  - E. sennetsu A79.81
  - specified organism NEC A77.49
Eichstedt's disease B36.0
Eisenmenger's
- complex or syndrome I27.83
- defect Q21.8
Ejaculation
- delayed F52.32
- painful N53.12
- premature F52.4
- retarded N53.11
- retrograde N53.14
- semen, painful N53.12
  - psychogenic F52.6
Ekbom's syndrome (restless legs) G25.81

Ekman's syndrome (brittle bones and blue sclera) Q78.0
Elastic skin Q82.8
  acquired L57.4
Elastofibroma — *see* Neoplasm, connective tissue, benign
Elastoma (juvenile) Q82.8
  Miescher's L87.2
Elastomyofibrosis I42.4
Elastosis
  actinic, solar L57.8
  atrophicans (senile) L57.4
  perforans serpiginosa L87.2
  senilis L57.4
Elbow — *see* condition
Electric current, electricity, effects (concussion) (fatal) (nonfatal) (shock) T75.4 ☑
  burn — *see* Burn
Electric feet syndrome E53.8
Electrocution T75.4 ☑
  from electroshock gun (taser) T75.4 ☑
Electrolyte imbalance E87.8
  with
    abortion — *see* Abortion by type, complicated by, electrolyte imbalance
    ectopic pregnancy O08.5
    molar pregnancy O08.5
Elephantiasis (nonfilarial) I89.0
  arabicum — *see* Infestation, filarial
  bancroftian B74.0
  congenital (any site) (hereditary) Q82.0
  due to
    Brugia (malayi) B74.1
      timori B74.2
    mastectomy I97.2
    Wuchereria (bancrofti) B74.0
  eyelid H02.859
    left H02.856
      lower H02.855
      upper H02.854
    right H02.853
      lower H02.852
      upper H02.851
  filarial, filariensis — *see* Infestation, filarial
  glandular I89.0
  graecorum A30.9
  lymphangiectatic I89.0
  lymphatic vessel I89.0
    due to mastectomy I97.2
  scrotum (nonfilarial) I89.0
  streptococcal I89.0
  surgical I97.89
    postmastectomy I97.2
  telangiectodes I89.0
  vulva (nonfilarial) N90.89
Elevated, elevation
  antibody titer R76.0
  basal metabolic rate R94.8
  blood pressure — *see also* Hypertension
    reading (incidental) (isolated) (nonspecific), no diagnosis of hypertension R03.0
  blood sugar R73.9
  body temperature (of unknown origin) R50.9
  cancer antigen 125 [CA 125] R97.1
  carcinoembryonic antigen [CEA] R97.0
  cholesterol E78.00
    with high triglycerides E78.2
  conjugate, eye H51.0
  C-reactive protein (CRP) R79.82
  diaphragm, congenital Q79.1
  erythrocyte sedimentation rate R70.0
  fasting glucose R73.01
  fasting triglycerides E78.1
  finding on laboratory examination — *see* Findings, abnormal, inconclusive, without diagnosis, by type of exam
  GFR (glomerular filtration rate) — *see* Findings, abnormal, inconclusive, without diagnosis, by type of exam
  glucose tolerance (oral) R73.02
  immunoglobulin level R76.8
  indoleacetic acid R82.5
  lactic acid dehydrogenase (LDH) level R74.0
  leukocytes D72.829
  lipoprotein a (Lp(a)) level E78.41
  liver function
    study R94.5
    test R79.89
      alkaline phosphatase R74.8

Elevated, elevation — *continued*
  liver function — *continued*
    test — *continued*
      aminotransferase R74.0
      bilirubin R17
      hepatic enzyme R74.8
      lactate dehydrogenase R74.0
  Lp(a) (lipoprotein(a)) E78.41
  lymphocytes D72.820
  prostate specific antigen [PSA] R97.20
  Rh titer — *see* Complication(s), transfusion, incompatibility reaction, Rh (factor)
  scapula, congenital Q74.0
  sedimentation rate R70.0
  SGOT R74.0
  SGPT R74.0
  transaminase level R74.0
  triglycerides E78.1
    with high cholesterol E78.2
  tumor associated antigens [TAA] NEC R97.8
  tumor specific antigens [TSA] NEC R97.8
  urine level of
    17-ketosteroids R82.5
    catecholamine R82.5
    indoleacetic acid R82.5
    steroids R82.5
    vanillylmandelic acid (VMA) R82.5
  venous pressure I87.8
  white blood cell count D72.829
    specified NEC D72.828
Elliptocytosis (congenital) (hereditary) D58.1
  Hb C (disease) D58.1
  hemoglobin disease D58.1
  sickle-cell (disease) D57.8- ☑
    trait D57.3
Ellison-Zollinger syndrome E16.4
Ellis-van Creveld syndrome (chondroectodermal dysplasia) Q77.6
Elongated, elongation (congenital) — *see also* Distortion
  bone Q79.9
  cervix (uteri) Q51.828
    acquired N88.4
    hypertrophic N88.4
  colon Q43.8
  common bile duct Q44.5
  cystic duct Q44.5
  frenulum, penis Q55.69
  labia minora (acquired) N90.69
  ligamentum patellae Q74.1
  petiolus (epiglottidis) Q31.8
  tooth, teeth K00.2
  uvula Q38.6
Eltor cholera A00.1
Emaciation (due to malnutrition) E41
Embadomoniasis A07.8
Embedded tooth, teeth K01.0
  root only K08.3
Embolic — *see* condition
Embolism (multiple) (paradoxical) I74.9
  air (any site) (traumatic) T79.0 ☑
    following
      abortion — *see* Abortion by type complicated by embolism
      ectopic pregnancy O08.2
      infusion, therapeutic injection or transfusion T80.0 ☑
      molar pregnancy O08.2
      procedure NEC
        artery T81.719 ☑
          mesenteric T81.710 ☑
          renal T81.711 ☑
          specified NEC T81.718 ☑
        vein T81.72 ☑
    in pregnancy, childbirth or puerperium — *see* Embolism, obstetric
  amniotic fluid (pulmonary) — *see also* Embolism, obstetric
    following
      abortion — *see* Abortion by type complicated by embolism
      ectopic pregnancy O08.2
      molar pregnancy O08.2
  aorta, aortic I74.10
    abdominal I74.09
      saddle I74.01
    bifurcation I74.09
    saddle I74.01

Embolism — *continued*
  aorta, aortic — *continued*
    thoracic I74.11
  artery I74.9
    auditory, internal I65.8
    basilar — *see* Occlusion, artery, basilar
    carotid (common) (internal) — *see* Occlusion, artery, carotid
    cerebellar (anterior inferior) (posterior inferior) (superior) I66.3
    cerebral — *see* Occlusion, artery, cerebral
    choroidal (anterior) I65.8
    communicating posterior I65.8
    coronary — *see also* Infarct, myocardium
      not resulting in infarction I24.0
    extremity I74.4
      lower I74.3
      upper I74.2
    hypophyseal I65.8
    iliac I74.5
    limb I74.4
      lower I74.3
      upper I74.2
    mesenteric (with gangrene) — *see also* Ischemia, intestine, acute K55.059
    ophthalmic — *see* Occlusion, artery, retina
    peripheral I74.4
    pontine I65.8
    precerebral — *see* Occlusion, artery, precerebral
    pulmonary — *see* Embolism, pulmonary
    renal N28.0
    retinal — *see* Occlusion, artery, retina
    septic I76
    specified NEC I74.8
    vertebral — *see* Occlusion, artery, vertebral
  basilar (artery) I65.1
  blood clot
    following
      abortion — *see* Abortion by type complicated by embolism
      ectopic or molar pregnancy O08.2
      in pregnancy, childbirth or puerperium — *see* Embolism, obstetric
  brain — *see also* Occlusion, artery, cerebral
    following
      abortion — *see* Abortion by type complicated by embolism
      ectopic or molar pregnancy O08.2
    puerperal, postpartum, childbirth — *see* Embolism, obstetric
  capillary I78.8
  cardiac — *see also* Infarct, myocardium
    not resulting in infarction I51.3
  carotid (artery) (common) (internal) — *see* Occlusion, artery, carotid
  cavernous sinus (venous) — *see* Embolism, intracranial venous sinus
  cerebral — *see* Occlusion, artery, cerebral
  cholesterol — *see* Atheroembolism
  coronary (artery or vein) (systemic) — *see* Occlusion, coronary
  due to device, implant or graft — *see also* Complications, by site and type, specified NEC
    arterial graft NEC T82.818 ☑
    breast (implant) T85.818 ☑
    catheter NEC T85.818 ☑
      dialysis (renal) T82.818 ☑
        intraperitoneal T85.818 ☑
      infusion NEC T82.818 ☑
        spinal (epidural) (subdural) T85.810 ☑
      urinary (indwelling) T83.81 ☑
    electronic (electrode) (pulse generator) (stimulator)
      bone T84.81 ☑
      cardiac T82.817 ☑
      nervous system (brain) (peripheral nerve) (spinal) T85.810 ☑
      urinary T83.81 ☑
    fixation, internal (orthopedic) NEC T84.81 ☑
    gastrointestinal (bile duct) (esophagus) T85.818 ☑
    genital NEC T83.81 ☑
    heart (graft) (valve) T82.817 ☑
    joint prosthesis T84.81 ☑
    ocular (corneal graft) (orbital implant) T85.818 ☑
    orthopedic (bone graft) NEC T86.838
    specified NEC T85.818 ☑
    urinary (graft) NEC T83.81 ☑
    vascular NEC T82.818 ☑

☑ Additional Character Required — Refer to the Tabular List for Character Selection ▽ Subterms under main terms may continue to next column or page

Embolism — *continued*
    due to device, implant or graft — *see also* Complications, by site and type, specified — *continued*
        ventricular intracranial shunt T85.810 ☑
    extremities
        lower — *see* Embolism, vein, lower extremity
            arterial I74.3
        upper I74.2
    eye H34.9
    fat (cerebral) (pulmonary) (systemic) T79.1 ☑
        complicating delivery — *see* Embolism, obstetric
        following
            abortion — *see* Abortion by type complicated by embolism
            ectopic or molar pregnancy O08.2
    following
        abortion — *see* Abortion by type complicated by embolism
        ectopic or molar pregnancy O08.2
        infusion, therapeutic injection or transfusion air T80.0 ☑
    heart (fatty) — *see also* Infarct, myocardium
        not resulting in infarction I51.3
    hepatic (vein) I82.0
    in pregnancy, childbirth or puerperium — *see* Embolism, obstetric
    intestine (artery) (vein) (with gangrene) — *see also* Ischemia, intestine, acute K55.039
    intracranial — *see also* Occlusion, artery, cerebral
        venous sinus (any) G08
            nonpyogenic I67.6
    intraspinal venous sinuses or veins G08
        nonpyogenic G95.19
    kidney (artery) N28.0
    lateral sinus (venous) — *see* Embolism, intracranial, venous sinus
    leg — *see* Embolism, vein, lower extremity
        arterial I74.3
    longitudinal sinus (venous) — *see* Embolism, intracranial, venous sinus
    lung (massive) — *see* Embolism, pulmonary
    meninges I66.8
    mesenteric (artery) (vein) (with gangrene) — *see also* Ischemia, intestine, acute K55.059
    obstetric (in) (pulmonary)
        childbirth O88.22
            air O88.02
            amniotic fluid O88.12
            blood clot O88.22
            fat O88.82
            pyemic O88.32
            septic O88.32
            specified type NEC O88.82
        pregnancy O88.21- ☑
            air O88.01- ☑
            amniotic fluid O88.11- ☑
            blood clot O88.21- ☑
            fat O88.81- ☑
            pyemic O88.31- ☑
            septic O88.31- ☑
            specified type NEC O88.81- ☑
        puerperal O88.23
            air O88.03
            amniotic fluid O88.13
            blood clot O88.23
            fat O88.83
            pyemic O88.33
            septic O88.33
            specified type NEC O88.83
    ophthalmic — *see* Occlusion, artery, retina
    penis N48.81
    peripheral artery NOS I74.4
    pituitary E23.6
    popliteal (artery) I74.3
    portal (vein) I81
    postoperative, postprocedural
        artery T81.719 ☑
            mesenteric T81.710 ☑
            renal T81.711 ☑
            specified NEC T81.718 ☑
        vein T81.72 ☑
    precerebral artery — *see* Occlusion, artery, precerebral
    puerperal — *see* Embolism, obstetric
    pulmonary (acute) (artery) (vein) I26.99
        with acute cor pulmonale I26.09
        chronic I27.82

Embolism — *continued*
    pulmonary — *continued*
        following
            abortion — *see* Abortion by type complicated by embolism
            ectopic or molar pregnancy O08.2
        healed or old Z86.711
        in pregnancy, childbirth or puerperium — *see* Embolism, obstetric
        multiple subsegmental without acute cor pulmonale I26.94
        personal history of Z86.711
        saddle I26.92
            with acute cor pulmonale I26.02
        septic I26.90
            with acute cor pulmonale I26.01
        single subsegmental without acute cor pulmonale I26.93
        subsegmental NOS I26.93
    pyemic (multiple) I76
        following
            abortion — *see* Abortion by type complicated by embolism
            ectopic or molar pregnancy O08.2
        Hemophilus influenzae A41.3
        pneumococcal A40.3
            with pneumonia J13
        puerperal, postpartum, childbirth (any organism) — *see* Embolism, obstetric
        specified organism NEC A41.89
        staphylococcal A41.2
        streptococcal A40.9
    renal (artery) N28.0
        vein I82.3
    retina, retinal — *see* Occlusion, artery, retina
    saddle
        abdominal aorta I74.01
        pulmonary artery I26.92
            with acute cor pulmonale I26.02
    septic (arterial) I76
        complicating abortion — *see* Abortion, by type, complicated by, embolism
    sinus — *see* Embolism, intracranial, venous sinus
    soap complicating abortion — *see* Abortion, by type, complicated by, embolism
    spinal cord G95.19
        pyogenic origin G06.1
    spleen, splenic (artery) I74.8
    upper extremity I74.2
    vein (acute) I82.90
        antecubital I82.61- ☑
            chronic I82.71- ☑
        axillary I82.A1- ☑ (*following* I82.7)
            chronic I82.A2- ☑ (*following* I82.7)
        basilic I82.61- ☑
            chronic I82.71- ☑
        brachial I82.62- ☑
            chronic I82.72- ☑
        brachiocephalic (innominate) I82.290
            chronic I82.291
        cephalic I82.61- ☑
            chronic I82.71- ☑
        chronic I82.91
        deep (DVT) I82.40- ☑
            calf I82.4Z- ☑
                chronic I82.5Z- ☑
            lower leg I82.4Z- ☑
                chronic I82.5Z- ☑
            thigh I82.4Y- ☑
                chronic I82.5Y- ☑
            upper leg I82.4Y ☑
                chronic I82.5Y-
        femoral I82.41- ☑
            chronic I82.51- ☑
        iliac (iliofemoral) I82.42- ☑
            chronic I82.52- ☑
        innominate I82.290
            chronic I82.291
        internal jugular I82.C1- ☑ (*following* I82.7)
            chronic I82.C2- ☑ (*following* I82.7)
        lower extremity
            deep I82.40- ☑
                chronic I82.50- ☑
                specified NEC I82.49- ☑
                    chronic NEC I82.59- ☑
            distal
                deep I82.4Z- ☑

Embolism — *continued*
    vein — *continued*
        lower extremity — *continued*
            proximal
                deep I82.4Y- ☑
                    chronic I82.5Y- ☑
                superficial I82.81- ☑
        popliteal I82.43- ☑
            chronic I82.53- ☑
        radial I82.62- ☑
            chronic I82.72- ☑
        renal I82.3
        saphenous (greater) (lesser) I82.81- ☑
        specified NEC I82.890
            chronic NEC I82.891
        subclavian I82.B1- ☑ (*following* I82.7)
            chronic I82.B2- ☑ (*following* I82.7)
        thoracic NEC I82.290
            chronic I82.291
        tibial I82.44- ☑
            chronic I82.54- ☑
        ulnar I82.62- ☑
            chronic I82.72- ☑
        upper extremity I82.60- ☑
            chronic I82.70- ☑
            deep I82.62- ☑
                chronic I82.72- ☑
            superficial I82.61- ☑
                chronic I82.71- ☑
    vena cava
        inferior (acute) I82.220
            chronic I82.221
        superior (acute) I82.210
            chronic I82.211
    venous sinus G08
    vessels of brain — *see* Occlusion, artery, cerebral
Embolus — *see* Embolism
Embryoma — *see also* Neoplasm, uncertain behavior, by site
    benign — *see* Neoplasm, benign, by site
    kidney C64.- ☑
    liver C22.0
    malignant — *see also* Neoplasm, malignant, by site
        kidney C64.- ☑
        liver C22.0
        testis C62.9- ☑
            descended (scrotal) C62.1- ☑
            undescended C62.0- ☑
    testis C62.9- ☑
        descended (scrotal) C62.1- ☑
        undescended C62.0- ☑
Embryonic
    circulation Q28.9
    heart Q28.9
    vas deferens Q55.4
Embryopathia NOS Q89.9
Embryotoxon Q13.4
Emesis — *see* Vomiting
Emotional lability R45.86
Emotionality, pathological F60.3
Emotogenic disease — *see* Disorder, psychogenic
Emphysema (atrophic) (bullous) (chronic) (interlobular) (lung) (obstructive) (pulmonary) (senile) (vesicular) J43.9
    cellular tissue (traumatic) T79.7 ☑
        surgical T81.82 ☑
    centrilobular J43.2
    compensatory J98.3
    congenital (interstitial) P25.0
    conjunctiva H11.89
    connective tissue (traumatic) T79.7 ☑
        surgical T81.82 ☑
    due to chemicals, gases, fumes or vapors J68.4
    eyelid(s) — *see* Disorder, eyelid, specified type NEC
        surgical T81.82 ☑
        traumatic T79.7 ☑
    interstitial J98.2
        congenital P25.0
        perinatal period P25.0
    laminated tissue T79.7 ☑
        surgical T81.82 ☑
    mediastinal J98.2
        newborn P25.2
    orbit, orbital — *see* Disorder, orbit, specified type NEC
    panacinar J43.1
    panlobular J43.1
    specified NEC J43.8

Emphysema — *continued*
  subcutaneous (traumatic) T79.7 ☑
    nontraumatic J98.2
    postprocedural T81.82 ☑
    surgical T81.82 ☑
  surgical T81.82 ☑
  thymus (gland) (congenital) E32.8
  traumatic (subcutaneous) T79.7 ☑
  unilateral J43.0
Empty nest syndrome Z60.0
Empyema (acute) (chest) (double) (pleura) (supradiaphragmatic) (thorax) J86.9
  with fistula J86.0
  accessory sinus (chronic) — *see* Sinusitis
  antrum (chronic) — *see* Sinusitis, maxillary
  brain (any part) — *see* Abscess, brain
  ethmoidal (chronic) (sinus) — *see* Sinusitis, ethmoidal
  extradural — *see* Abscess, extradural
  frontal (chronic) (sinus) — *see* Sinusitis, frontal
  gallbladder K81.0
  mastoid (process) (acute) — *see* Mastoiditis, acute
  maxilla, maxillary M27.2
    sinus (chronic) — *see* Sinusitis, maxillary
  nasal sinus (chronic) — *see* Sinusitis
  sinus (accessory) (chronic) (nasal) — *see* Sinusitis
  sphenoidal (sinus) (chronic) — *see* Sinusitis, sphenoidal
  subarachnoid — *see* Abscess, extradural
  subdural — *see* Abscess, subdural
  tuberculous A15.6
  ureter — *see* Ureteritis
  ventricular — *see* Abscess, brain
En coup de sabre lesion L94.1
Enamel pearls K00.2
Enameloma K00.2
Enanthema, viral B09
Encephalitis (chronic) (hemorrhagic) (idiopathic) (nonepidemic) (spurious) (subacute) G04.90
  acute — *see also* Encephalitis, viral A86
    disseminated G04.00
      infectious G04.01
      noninfectious G04.81
      postimmunization (postvaccination) G04.02
      postinfectious G04.01
    inclusion body A85.8
    necrotizing hemorrhagic G04.30
      postimmunization G04.32
      postinfectious G04.31
      specified NEC G04.39
  arboviral, arbovirus NEC A85.2
  arthropod-borne NEC (viral) A85.2
  Australian A83.4
  California (virus) A83.5
  Central European (tick-borne) A84.1
  Czechoslovakian A84.1
  Dawson's (inclusion body) A81.1
  diffuse sclerosing A81.1
  disseminated, acute G04.00
  due to
    cat scratch disease A28.1
    human immunodeficiency virus (HIV) disease B20 [G05.3]
    malaria — *see* Malaria
    rickettsiosis — *see* Rickettsiosis
    smallpox inoculation G04.02
    typhus — *see* Typhus
  Eastern equine A83.2
  endemic (viral) A86
  epidemic NEC (viral) A86
  equine (acute) (infectious) (viral) A83.9
    Eastern A83.2
    Venezuelan A92.2
    Western A83.1
  Far Eastern (tick-borne) A84.0
  following vaccination or other immunization procedure G04.02
  herpes zoster B02.0
  herpesviral B00.4
    due to herpesvirus 6 B10.01
    due to herpesvirus 7 B10.09
    specified NEC B10.09
  Ilheus (virus) A83.8
  in (due to)
    actinomycosis A42.82
    adenovirus A85.1
    African trypanosomiasis B56.9 [G05.3]
    Chagas' disease (chronic) B57.42
    cytomegalovirus B25.8
    enterovirus A85.0

Encephalitis — *continued*
  in — *continued*
    herpes (simplex) virus B00.4
      due to herpesvirus 6 B10.01
      due to herpesvirus 7 B10.09
      specified NEC B10.09
    infectious disease NEC B99 ☑ [G05.3]
    influenza — *see* Influenza, with, encephalopathy
    listeriosis A32.12
    measles B05.0
    mumps B26.2
    naegleriasis B60.2
    parasitic disease NEC B89 [G05.3]
    poliovirus A80.9 [G05.3]
    rubella B06.01
    syphilis
      congenital A50.42
      late A52.14
    systemic lupus erythematosus M32.19
    toxoplasmosis (acquired) B58.2
      congenital P37.1
    tuberculosis A17.82
    zoster B02.0
  inclusion body A81.1
  infectious (acute) (virus) NEC A86
  Japanese (B type) A83.0
  La Crosse A83.5
  lead — *see* Poisoning, lead
  lethargica (acute) (infectious) A85.8
  louping ill A84.8
  lupus erythematosus, systemic M32.19
  lymphatica A87.2
  Mengo A85.8
  meningococcal A39.81
  Murray Valley A83.4
  otitic NEC H66.40 [G05.3]
  parasitic NOS B71.9
  periaxial G37.0
  periaxialis (concentrica) (diffuse) G37.5
  postchickenpox B01.11
  postexanthematous NEC B09
  postimmunization G04.02
  postinfectious NEC G04.01
  postmeasles B05.0
  postvaccinal G04.02
  postvaricella B01.11
  postviral NEC A86
  Powassan A84.8
  Rasmussen G04.81
  Rio Bravo A85.8
  Russian
    autumnal A83.0
    spring-summer (taiga) A84.0
  saturnine — *see* Poisoning, lead
  specified NEC G04.81
  St. Louis A83.3
  subacute sclerosing A81.1
  summer A83.0
  suppurative G04.81
  tick-borne A84.9
  Torula, torular (cryptococcal) B45.1
  toxic NEC G92
  trichinosis B75 [G05.3]
  type
    B A83.0
    C A83.3
  van Bogaert's A81.1
  Venezuelan equine A92.2
  Vienna A85.8
  viral, virus A86
    arthropod-borne NEC A85.2
      mosquito-borne A83.9
        Australian X disease A83.4
        California virus A83.5
        Eastern equine A83.2
        Japanese (B type) A83.0
        Murray Valley A83.4
        specified NEC A83.8
        . St. Louis A83.3
        type B A83.0
        type C A83.3
        Western equine A83.1
      tick-borne A84.9
        biundulant A84.1
        central European A84.1
        Czechoslovakian A84.1
        diphasic meningoencephalitis A84.1
        Far Eastern A84.0

Encephalitis — *continued*
  viral, virus — *continued*
    arthropod-borne — *continued*
      tick-borne — *continued*
        Russian spring-summer (taiga) A84.0
        specified NEC A84.8
      specified type NEC A85.8
    Western equine A83.1
Encephalocele Q01.9
  frontal Q01.0
  nasofrontal Q01.1
  occipital Q01.2
  specified NEC Q01.8
Encephalocystocele — *see* Encephalocele
Encephaloduroarteriomyosynangiosis (EDAMS) I67.5
Encephalomalacia (brain) (cerebellar) (cerebral) — *see* Softening, brain
Encephalomeningitis — *see* Meningoencephalitis
Encephalomeningocele — *see* Encephalocele
Encephalomeningomyelitis — *see* Meningoencephalitis
Encephalomyelitis — *see also* Encephalitis G04.90
  acute disseminated G04.00
    infectious G04.01
    noninfectious G04.81
    postimmunization G04.02
    postinfectious G04.01
  acute necrotizing hemorrhagic G04.30
    postimmunization G04.32
    postinfectious G04.31
    specified NEC G04.39
  benign myalgic G93.3
  equine A83.9
    Eastern A83.2
    Venezuelan A92.2
    Western A83.1
  in diseases classified elsewhere G05.3
  myalgic, benign G93.3
  postchickenpox B01.11
  postinfectious NEC G04.01
  postmeasles B05.0
  postvaccinal G04.02
  postvaricella B01.11
  rubella B06.01
  specified NEC G04.81
  Venezuelan equine A92.2
Encephalomyelocele — *see* Encephalocele
Encephalomyelomeningitis — *see* Meningoencephalitis
Encephalomyelopathy G96.9
Encephalomyeloradiculitis (acute) G61.0
Encephalomyeloradiculoneuritis (acute) (Guillain-Barré) G61.0
Encephalomyeloradiculopathy G96.9
Encephalopathia hyperbilirubinemica, newborn P57.9
  due to isoimmunization (conditions in P55) P57.0
Encephalopathy (acute) G93.40
  acute necrotizing hemorrhagic G04.30
    postimmunization G04.32
    postinfectious G04.31
    specified NEC G04.39
  alcoholic G31.2
  anoxic — *see* Damage, brain, anoxic
  arteriosclerotic I67.2
  centrolobar progressive (Schilder) G37.0
  congenital Q07.9
  degenerative, in specified disease NEC G32.89
  demyelinating callosal G37.1
  due to
    drugs — *see also* Table of Drugs and Chemicals G92
    hepatic — *see* Failure, hepatic
  hyperbilirubinemic, newborn P57.9
    due to isoimmunization (conditions in P55) P57.0
  hypertensive I67.4
  hypoglycemic E16.2
  hypoxic — *see* Damage, brain, anoxic
  hypoxic ischemic P91.60
    mild P91.61
    moderate P91.62
    severe P91.63
  in (due to) (with)
    birth injury P11.1
    hyperinsulinism E16.1 [G94]
    influenza — *see* Influenza, with, encephalopathy
    lack of vitamin — *see also* Deficiency, vitamin E56.9 [G32.89]
    neoplastic disease — *see also* Neoplasm D49.9 [G13.1]
    serum — *see also* Reaction, serum T80.69 ☑

Encephalopathy — *continued*
  in — *continued*
    syphilis A52.17
    trauma (postconcussional) F07.81
      current injury — *see* Injury, intracranial
    vaccination G04.02
  lead — *see* Poisoning, lead
  metabolic G93.41
    drug induced G92
    toxic G92
  myoclonic, early, symptomatic — *see* Epilepsy, generalized, specified NEC
  necrotizing, subacute (Leigh) G31.82
  neonatal P91.819
    in diseases classified elsewhere P91.811
  pellagrous E52 *[G32.89]*
  portosystemic — *see* Failure, hepatic
  postcontusional F07.81
    current injury — *see* Injury, intracranial, diffuse
  posthypoglycemic (coma) E16.1 *[G94]*
  postradiation G93.89
  saturnine — *see* Poisoning, lead
  septic G93.41
  specified NEC G93.49
  spongiform, subacute (viral) A81.09
  toxic G92
    metabolic G92
  traumatic (postconcussional) F07.81
    current injury — *see* Injury, intracranial
  vitamin B deficiency NEC E53.9 *[G32.89]*
    vitamin B1 E51.2
  Wernicke's E51.2
Encephalorrhagia — *see* Hemorrhage, intracranial, intracerebral
Encephalosis, posttraumatic F07.81
Enchondroma — *see also* Neoplasm, bone, benign
Enchondromatosis (cartilaginous) (multiple) Q78.4
Encopresis R15.9
  functional F98.1
  nonorganic origin F98.1
  psychogenic F98.1
Encounter (with health service) (for) Z76.89
  adjustment and management (of)
    breast implant Z45.81 ☑
    implanted device NEC Z45.89
    myringotomy device (stent) (tube) Z45.82
    neurostimulator (brain) (gastric) (peripheral nerve) (sacral nerve) (spinal cord) (vagus nerve) Z45.42
  administrative purpose only Z02.9
    examination for
      adoption Z02.82
      armed forces Z02.3
      disability determination Z02.71
      driving license Z02.4
      employment Z02.1
      insurance Z02.6
      medical certificate NEC Z02.79
      paternity testing Z02.81
      residential institution admission Z02.2
      school admission Z02.0
      sports Z02.5
      specified reason NEC Z02.89
  aftercare — *see* Aftercare
  antenatal screening Z36.9
    cervical length Z36.86
    chromosomal anomalies Z36.0
    congenital cardiac abnormalities Z36.83
    elevated maternal serum alphafetoprotein Z36.1
    fetal growth retardation Z36.4
    fetal lung maturity Z36.84
    fetal macrosomia Z36.88
    hydrops fetalis Z36.81
    intrauterine growth restriction (IUGR) /small-for-dates Z36.4
    isoimmunization Z36.5
    large-for-dates Z36.88
    malformations Z36.3
    non-visualized anatomy on a previous scan Z36.2
    nuchal translucency Z36.82
    raised alphafetoprotein level Z36.1
    risk of pre-term labor Z36.86
    specified follow-up NEC Z36.2
    specified genetic defects NEC Z36.8A
    specified type NEC Z36.89
    Streptococcus B Z36.85
    suspected anomaly Z36.3
    uncertain dates Z36.87

Encounter — *continued*
  assisted reproductive fertility procedure cycle Z31.83
  blood typing Z01.83
    Rh typing Z01.83
  breast augmentation or reduction Z41.1
  breast implant exchange (different material) (different size) Z45.81 ☑
  breast reconstruction following mastectomy Z42.1
  check-up — *see* Examination
  chemotherapy for neoplasm Z51.11
  colonoscopy, screening Z12.11
  counseling — *see* Counseling
  delivery, full-term, uncomplicated O80
    cesarean, without indication O82
  desensitization to allergens Z51.6
  ear piercing Z41.3
  examination — *see* Examination
  expectant parent(s) (adoptive) pre-birth pediatrician visit Z76.81
  fertility preservation procedure (prior to cancer therapy) (prior to removal of gonads) Z31.84
  fitting (of) — *see* Fitting (and adjustment) (of)
  genetic
    counseling
      nonprocreative Z71.83
      procreative Z31.5
    testing — *see* Test, genetic
  hearing conservation and treatment Z01.12
  immunotherapy for neoplasm Z51.12
  in vitro fertilization cycle Z31.83
  instruction (in)
    child care (postpartal) (prenatal) Z32.3
    childbirth Z32.2
    natural family planning
      procreative Z31.61
      to avoid pregnancy Z30.02
  insulin pump titration Z46.81
  joint prosthesis insertion following prior explantation of joint prosthesis (staged procedure)
    hip Z47.32
    knee Z47.33
    shoulder Z47.31
  laboratory (as part of a general medical examination) Z00.00
    with abnormal findings Z00.01
  mental health services (for)
    abuse NEC
      perpetrator Z69.82
      victim Z69.81
    child abuse
      nonparental
        perpetrator Z69.021
        victim Z69.020
      parental
        perpetrator Z69.011
        victim Z69.010
    child neglect
      nonparental
        perpetrator Z69.021
        victim Z69.020
      parental
        perpetrator Z69.011
        victim Z69.010
    child psychological abuse
      nonparental
        perpetrator Z69.021
        victim Z69.020
      parental
        perpetrator Z69.011
        victim Z69.010
    child sexual abuse
      nonparental
        perpetrator Z69.021
        victim Z69.020
      parental
        perpetrator Z69.011
        victim Z69.010
    non-spousal adult abuse
      perpetrator Z69.82
      victim Z69.81
    spousal or partner
      abuse
        perpetrator Z69.12
        victim Z69.11
      neglect
        perpetrator Z69.12
        victim Z69.11
      psychological abuse
        perpetrator Z69.12

Encounter — *continued*
  mental health services — *continued*
    spousal or partner — *continued*
      psychological abuse — *continued*
        victim Z69.11
      violence
        perpetrator (physical) (sexual) Z69.12
        victim (physical) Z69.11
        sexual Z69.81
  observation (for) (ruled out)
    exposure to (suspected)
      anthrax Z03.810
      biological agent NEC Z03.818
  pediatrician visit, by expectant parent(s) (adoptive) Z76.81
  placental sample (taken vaginally) — *see also* Encounter, antenatal screening Z36.9
  plastic and reconstructive surgery following medical procedure or healed injury NEC Z42.8
  pregnancy
    supervision of — *see* Pregnancy, supervision of
    test Z32.00
      result negative Z32.02
      result positive Z32.01
  procreative management and counseling for gestational carrier Z31.7
  prophylactic measures Z29.9
    antivenin Z29.12
    fluoride administration Z29.3
    immunotherapy for respiratory syncytial virus (RSV) Z29.11
    rabies immune globin Z29.14
    Rho (D) immune globulin Z29.13
    specified NEC Z29.8
  radiation therapy (antineoplastic) Z51.0
  radiological (as part of a general medical examination) Z00.00
    with abnormal findings Z00.01
  reconstructive surgery following medical procedure or healed injury NEC Z42.8
  removal (of) — *see also* Removal
    artificial
      arm Z44.00- ☑
        complete Z44.01- ☑
        partial Z44.02- ☑
      eye Z44.2- ☑
      leg Z44.10- ☑
        complete Z44.11- ☑
        partial Z44.12- ☑
    breast implant Z45.81 ☑
      tissue expander (with or without synchronous insertion of permanent implant) Z45.81 ☑
    device Z46.9
      specified NEC Z46.89
    external
      fixation device — *code to* fracture with seventh character D
      prosthesis, prosthetic device Z44.9
        breast Z44.3- ☑
        specified NEC Z44.8
    implanted device NEC Z45.89
    insulin pump Z46.81
    internal fixation device Z47.2
    myringotomy device (stent) (tube) Z45.82
    nervous system device NEC Z46.2
      brain neuropacemaker Z46.2
      visual substitution device Z46.2
        implanted Z45.31
    non-vascular catheter Z46.82
    orthodontic device Z46.4
    stent
      ureteral Z46.6
    urinary device Z46.6
  repeat cervical smear to confirm findings of recent normal smear following initial abnormal smear Z01.42
  respirator [ventilator] use during power failure Z99.12
  Rh typing Z01.83
  screening — *see* Screening
  specified NEC Z76.89
  sterilization Z30.2
  suspected condition, ruled out
    amniotic cavity and membrane Z03.71
    cervical shortening Z03.75
    fetal anomaly Z03.73
    fetal growth Z03.74
    maternal and fetal conditions NEC Z03.79
    oligohydramnios Z03.71

▽ Subterms under main terms may continue to next column or page   ☑ Additional Character Required — Refer to the Tabular List for Character Selection   131

Encephalopathy — Encounter

Encounter — *continued*
  suspected condition, ruled out — *continued*
    placental problem Z03.72
    polyhydramnios Z03.71
  suspected exposure (to), ruled out
    anthrax Z03.810
    biological agents NEC Z03.818
  termination of pregnancy, elective Z33.2
  testing — *see* Test
  therapeutic drug level monitoring Z51.81
  titration, insulin pump Z46.81
  to determine fetal viability of pregnancy O36.80 ☑
  training
    insulin pump Z46.81
  X-ray of chest (as part of a general medical examination) Z00.00
    with abnormal findings Z00.01
Encystment — *see* Cyst
Endarteritis (bacterial, subacute) (infective) I77.6
  brain I67.7
  cerebral or cerebrospinal I67.7
  deformans — *see* Arteriosclerosis
  embolic — *see* Embolism
  obliterans — *see also* Arteriosclerosis
    pulmonary I28.8
  pulmonary I28.8
  retina — *see* Vasculitis, retina
  senile — *see* Arteriosclerosis
  syphilitic A52.09
    brain or cerebral A52.04
    congenital A50.54 [I79.8]
  tuberculous A18.89
Endemic — *see* condition
Endocarditis (chronic) (marantic) (nonbacterial) (thrombotic) (valvular) I38
  with rheumatic fever (conditions in I00)
    active — *see* Endocarditis, acute, rheumatic
    inactive or quiescent (with chorea) I09.1
  acute or subacute I33.9
    infective I33.0
    rheumatic (aortic) (mitral) (pulmonary) (tricuspid) I01.1
      with chorea (acute) (rheumatic) (Sydenham's) I02.0
  aortic (heart) (nonrheumatic) (valve) I35.8
    with
      mitral disease I08.0
        with tricuspid (valve) disease I08.3
          active or acute I01.1
            with chorea (acute) (rheumatic) (Sydenham's) I02.0
      rheumatic fever (conditions in I00)
        active — *see* Endocarditis, acute, rheumatic
        inactive or quiescent (with chorea) I06.9
      tricuspid (valve) disease I08.2
        with mitral (valve) disease I08.3
    acute or subacute I33.9
    arteriosclerotic I35.8
    rheumatic I06.9
      with mitral disease I08.0
        with tricuspid (valve) disease I08.3
          active or acute I01.1
            with chorea (acute) (rheumatic) (Sydenham's) I02.0
      active or acute I01.1
        with chorea (acute) (rheumatic) (Sydenham's) I02.0
      specified NEC I06.8
    specified cause NEC I35.8
    syphilitic A52.03
  arteriosclerotic I38
  atypical verrucous (Libman-Sacks) M32.11
  bacterial (acute) (any valve) (subacute) I33.0
  candidal B37.6
  congenital Q24.8
  constrictive I33.0
  Coxiella burnetii A78 [I39]
  Coxsackie B33.21
  due to
    prosthetic cardiac valve T82.6 ☑
    Q fever A78 [I39]
    Serratia marcescens I33.0
    typhoid (fever) A01.02
  gonococcal A54.83
  infectious or infective (acute) (any valve) (subacute) I33.0
  lenta (acute) (any valve) (subacute) I33.0
  Libman-Sacks M32.11

Endocarditis — *continued*
  listerial A32.82
  Löffler's I42.3
  malignant (acute) (any valve) (subacute) I33.0
  meningococcal A39.51
  mitral (chronic) (double) (fibroid) (heart) (inactive) (valve) (with chorea) I05.9
    with
      aortic (valve) disease I08.0
        with tricuspid (valve) disease I08.3
          active or acute I01.1
            with chorea (acute) (rheumatic) (Sydenham's) I02.0
      rheumatic fever (conditions in I00)
        active — *see* Endocarditis, acute, rheumatic
        inactive or quiescent (with chorea) I05.9
      tricuspid (valve) disease I08.1
        with aortic (valve) disease I08.3
    active or acute I01.1
      with chorea (acute) (rheumatic) (Sydenham's) I02.0
    bacterial I33.0
    arteriosclerotic I34.8
    nonrheumatic I34.8
      acute or subacute I33.9
    specified NEC I05.8
  monilial B37.6
  multiple valves I08.9
    specified disorders I08.8
  mycotic (acute) (any valve) (subacute) I33.0
  pneumococcal (acute) (any valve) (subacute) I33.0
  pulmonary (chronic) (heart) (valve) I37.8
    with rheumatic fever (conditions in I00)
      active — *see* Endocarditis, acute, rheumatic
      inactive or quiescent (with chorea) I09.89
        with aortic, mitral or tricuspid disease I08.8
    acute or subacute I33.9
      rheumatic I01.1
        with chorea (acute) (rheumatic) (Sydenham's) I02.0
    arteriosclerotic I37.8
    congenital Q22.2
    rheumatic (chronic) (inactive) (with chorea) I09.89
      active or acute I01.1
        with chorea (acute) (rheumatic) (Sydenham's) I02.0
    syphilitic A52.03
  purulent (acute) (any valve) (subacute) I33.0
  Q fever A78 [I39]
  rheumatic (chronic) (inactive) (with chorea) I09.1
    active or acute (aortic) (mitral) (pulmonary) (tricuspid) I01.1
      with chorea (acute) (rheumatic) (Sydenham's) I02.0
  rheumatoid — *see* Rheumatoid, carditis
  septic (acute) (any valve) (subacute) I33.0
  streptococcal (acute) (any valve) (subacute) I33.0
  subacute — *see* Endocarditis, acute
  suppurative (acute) (any valve) (subacute) I33.0
  syphilitic A52.03
  toxic I33.9
  tricuspid (chronic) (heart) (inactive) (rheumatic) (valve) (with chorea) I07.9
    with
      aortic (valve) disease I08.2
        mitral (valve) disease I08.3
      mitral (valve) disease I08.1
        aortic (valve) disease I08.3
      rheumatic fever (conditions in I00)
        active — *see* Endocarditis, acute, rheumatic
        inactive or quiescent (with chorea) I07.8
    active or acute I01.1
      with chorea (acute) (rheumatic) (Sydenham's) I02.0
    arteriosclerotic I36.8
    nonrheumatic I36.8
      acute or subacute I33.9
    specified cause, except rheumatic I36.8
  tuberculous — *see* Tuberculosis, endocarditis
  typhoid A01.02
  ulcerative (acute) (any valve) (subacute) I33.0
  vegetative (acute) (any valve) (subacute) I33.0
  verrucous (atypical) (nonbacterial) (nonrheumatic) M32.11
Endocardium, endocardial — *see also* condition
  cushion defect Q21.2
Endocervicitis — *see also* Cervicitis
  due to intrauterine (contraceptive) device T83.69 ☑

Endocervicitis — *continued*
  hyperplastic N72
Endocrine — *see* condition
Endocrinopathy, pluriglandular E31.9
Endodontic
  overfill M27.52
  underfill M27.53
Endodontitis K04.01
  irreversible K04.02
  reversible K04.01
Endomastoiditis — *see* Mastoiditis
Endometrioma N80.9
Endometriosis N80.9
  appendix N80.5
  bladder N80.8
  bowel N80.5
  broad ligament N80.3
  cervix N80.0
  colon N80.5
  cul-de-sac (Douglas') N80.3
  exocervix N80.0
  fallopian tube N80.2
  female genital organ NEC N80.8
  gallbladder N80.8
  in scar of skin N80.6
  internal N80.0
  intestine N80.5
  lung N80.8
  myometrium N80.0
  ovary N80.1
  parametrium N80.3
  pelvic peritoneum N80.3
  peritoneal (pelvic) N80.3
  rectovaginal septum N80.4
  rectum N80.5
  round ligament N80.3
  skin (scar) N80.6
  specified site NEC N80.8
  stromal D39.0
  thorax N80.8
  umbilicus N80.8
  uterus (internal) N80.0
  vagina N80.4
  vulva N80.8
Endometritis (decidual) (nonspecific) (purulent) (senile) (atrophic) (suppurative) N71.9
  with ectopic pregnancy O08.0
  acute N71.0
  blenorrhagic (gonococcal) (acute) (chronic) A54.24
  cervix, cervical (with erosion or ectropion) — *see also* Cervicitis
    hyperplastic N72
  chlamydial A56.11
  chronic N71.1
  following
    abortion — *see* Abortion by type complicated by genital infection
    ectopic or molar pregnancy O08.0
  gonococcal, gonorrheal (acute) (chronic) A54.24
  hyperplastic — *see also* Hyperplasia, endometrial N85.00
    cervix N72
  puerperal, postpartum, childbirth O86.12
  subacute N71.0
  tuberculous A18.17
Endometrium — *see* condition
Endomyocardiopathy, South African I42.3
Endomyocarditis — *see* Endocarditis
Endomyofibrosis I42.3
Endomyometritis — *see* Endometritis
Endopericarditis — *see* Endocarditis
Endoperineuritis — *see* Disorder, nerve
Endophlebitis — *see* Phlebitis
Endophthalmia — *see* Endophthalmitis, purulent
Endophthalmitis (acute) (infective) (metastatic) (subacute) H44.009
  bleb associated — *see also* Bleb, inflamed (infected), postprocedural H59.4 ☑
  gonorrheal A54.39
  in (due to)
    cysticercosis B69.1
    onchocerciasis B73.01
    toxocariasis B83.0
  panuveitis — *see* Panuveitis
  parasitic H44.12- ☑
  purulent H44.00- ☑
    panophthalmitis — *see* Panophthalmitis
    vitreous abscess H44.02- ☑

Endophthalmitis — *continued*
  specified NEC H44.19
  sympathetic — *see* Uveitis, sympathetic
Endosalpingioma D28.2
Endosalpingiosis N94.89
Endosteitis — *see* Osteomyelitis
Endothelioma, bone — *see* Neoplasm, bone, malignant
Endotheliosis (hemorrhagic infectional) D69.8
Endotoxemia — code to condition
Endotrachelitis — *see* Cervicitis
Engelmann (-Camurati) **syndrome** Q78.3
English disease — *see* Rickets
Engman's disease L30.3
Engorgement
  breast N64.59
    newborn P83.4
    puerperal, postpartum O92.79
  lung (passive) — *see* Edema, lung
  pulmonary (passive) — *see* Edema, lung
  stomach K31.89
  venous, retina — *see* Occlusion, retina, vein, engorgement
Enlargement, enlarged — *see also* Hypertrophy
  adenoids J35.2
    with tonsils J35.3
  alveolar ridge K08.89
    congenital — *see* Anomaly, alveolar
  apertures of diaphragm (congenital) Q79.1
  gingival K06.1
  heart, cardiac — *see* Hypertrophy, cardiac
  labium majus, childhood asymmetric (CALME) N90.61
  lacrimal gland, chronic H04.03- ☑
  liver — *see* Hypertrophy, liver
  lymph gland or node R59.9
    generalized R59.1
    localized R59.0
  orbit H05.34- ☑
  organ or site, congenital NEC — *see* Anomaly, by site
  parathyroid (gland) E21.0
  pituitary fossa R93.0
  prostate N40.0
    with lower urinary tract symptoms (LUTS) N40.1
    without lower urinary tract symtpoms (LUTS) N40.0
  sella turcica R93.0
  spleen — *see* Splenomegaly
  thymus (gland) (congenital) E32.0
  thyroid (gland) — *see* Goiter
  tongue K14.8
  tonsils J35.1
    with adenoids J35.3
  uterus N85.2
  vestibular aqueduct Q16.5
Enophthalmos H05.40- ☑
  due to
    orbital tissue atrophy H05.41- ☑
    trauma or surgery H05.42- ☑
Enostosis M27.8
Entamebic, entamebiasis — *see* Amebiasis
Entanglement
  umbilical cord(s) O69.82 ☑
    with compression O69.2 ☑
    around neck (with compression) O69.81 ☑
      with compression O69.1 ☑
      without compression O69.81 ☑
    of twins in monoamniotic sac O69.2 ☑
    without compression O69.82 ☑
Enteralgia — *see* Pain, abdominal
Enteric — *see* condition
Enteritis (acute) (diarrheal) (hemorrhagic) (noninfective) K52.9
  adenovirus A08.2
  aertrycke infection A02.0
  allergic K52.29
    with
      eosinophilic gastritis or gastroenteritis K52.81
      food protein-induced enterocolitis syndrome K52.21
      food protein-induced enteropathy K52.22
      FPIES K52.21
  amebic (acute) A06.0
    with abscess — *see* Abscess, amebic
    chronic A06.1
      with abscess — *see* Abscess, amebic
      nondysenteric A06.2
    nondysenteric A06.2
  astrovirus A08.32
  bacillary NOS A03.9

Enteritis — *continued*
  bacterial A04.9
    specified NEC A04.8
  calicivirus A08.31
  candidal B37.82
  Chilomastix A07.8
  choleriformis A00.1
  chronic (noninfectious) K52.9
    ulcerative — *see* Colitis, ulcerative
  cicatrizing (chronic) — *see* Enteritis, regional, small intestine
  Clostridium
    botulinum (food poisoning) A05.1
    difficile
      not specified as recurrent A04.72
      recurrent A04.71
  coccidial A07.3
  coxsackie virus A08.39
  dietetic — *see also* Enteritis, allergic K52.29
  drug-induced K52.1
  due to
    astrovirus A08.32
    calicivirus A08.31
    coxsackie virus A08.39
    drugs K52.1
    echovirus A08.39
    enterovirus NEC A08.39
    food hypersensitivity — *see also* Enteritis, allergic K52.29
    infectious organism (bacterial) (viral) — *see* Enteritis, infectious
    torovirus A08.39
    Yersinia enterocolitica A04.6
  echovirus A08.39
  eltor A00.1
  enterovirus NEC A08.39
  eosinophilic K52.81
  epidemic (infectious) A09
  fulminant — *see also* Ischemia, intestine, acute K55.019
  gangrenous — *see* Enteritis, infectious
  giardial A07.1
  infectious NOS A09
    due to
      adenovirus A08.2
      Aerobacter aerogenes A04.8
      Arizona (bacillus) A02.0
      bacteria NOS A04.9
        specified NEC A04.8
      Campylobacter A04.5
      Clostridium difficile
        not specified as recurrent A04.72
        recurrent A04.71
      Clostridium perfringens A04.8
      Enterobacter aerogenes A04.8
      enterovirus A08.39
      Escherichia coli A04.4
        enteroaggregative A04.4
        enterohemorrhagic A04.3
        enteroinvasive A04.2
        enteropathogenic A04.0
        enterotoxigenic A04.1
        specified NEC A04.4
      specified
        bacteria NEC A04.8
        virus NEC A08.39
      Staphylococcus A04.8
      virus NEC A08.4
        specified type NEC A08.39
      Yersinia enterocolitica A04.6
    specified organism NEC A08.8
  influenzal — *see* Influenza, with, digestive manifestations
  ischemic K55.9
    acute — *see also* Ischemia, intestine, acute K55.019
    chronic K55.1
  microsporidial A07.8
  mucomembranous, myxomembranous — *see* Syndrome, irritable bowel
  mucous — *see* Syndrome, irritable bowel
  necroticans A05.2
  necrotizing of newborn — *see* Enterocolitis, necrotizing, in newborn
  neurogenic — *see* Syndrome, irritable bowel
  newborn necrotizing — *see* Enterocolitis, necrotizing, in newborn
  noninfectious K52.9
  norovirus A08.11
  parasitic NEC B82.9

Enteritis — *continued*
  paratyphoid (fever) — *see* Fever, paratyphoid
  protozoal A07.9
    specified NEC A07.8
  radiation K52.0
  regional (of) K50.90
    with
      complication K50.919
        abscess K50.914
        fistula K50.913
        intestinal obstruction K50.912
        rectal bleeding K50.911
        specified complication NEC K50.918
    colon — *see* Enteritis, regional, large intestine
    duodenum — *see* Enteritis, regional, small intestine
    ileum — *see* Enteritis, regional, small intestine
    jejunum — *see* Enteritis, regional, small intestine
    large bowel — *see* Enteritis, regional, large intestine
    large intestine (colon) (rectum) K50.10
      with
        complication K50.119
          abscess K50.114
          fistula K50.113
          intestinal obstruction K50.112
          rectal bleeding K50.111
          small intestine (duodenum) (ileum) (jejunum) involvement K50.80
            with
              complication K50.819
                abscess K50.814
                fistula K50.813
                intestinal obstruction K50.812
                rectal bleeding K50.811
                specified complication NEC K50.818
          specified complication NEC K50.118
    rectum — *see* Enteritis, regional, large intestine
    small intestine (duodenum) (ileum) (jejunum) K50.00
      with
        complication K50.019
          abscess K50.014
          fistula K50.013
          intestinal obstruction K50.012
          large intestine (colon) (rectum) involvement K50.80
            with
              complication K50.819
                abscess K50.814
                fistula K50.813
                intestinal obstruction K50.812
                rectal bleeding K50.811
                specified complication NEC K50.818
          rectal bleeding K50.011
          specified complication NEC K50.018
  rotaviral A08.0
  Salmonella, salmonellosis (arizonae) (cholerae-suis) (enteritidis) (typhimurium) A02.0
  segmental — *see* Enteritis, regional
  septic A09
  Shigella — *see* Infection, Shigella
  small round structured NEC A08.19
  spasmodic, spastic — *see* Syndrome, irritable bowel
  staphylococcal A04.8
    due to food A05.0
  torovirus A08.39
  toxic NEC K52.1
    due to Clostridium difficile
      not specified as recurrent A04.72
      recurrent A04.71
  trichomonal A07.8
  tuberculous A18.32
  typhosa A01.00
  ulcerative (chronic) — *see* Colitis, ulcerative
  viral A08.4
    adenovirus A08.2
    enterovirus A08.39
    Rotavirus A08.0
    small round structured NEC A08.19
    specified NEC A08.39
    virus specified NEC A08.39
Enterobiasis B80
Enterobius vermicularis (infection) (infestation) B80
Enterocele — *see also* Hernia, abdomen
  pelvic, pelvis (acquired) (congenital) N81.5
  vagina, vaginal (acquired) (congenital) NEC N81.5
Enterocolitis — *see also* Enteritis K52.9

Enterocolitis — *continued*
due to Clostridium difficile
not specified as recurrent A04.72
recurrent A04.71
fulminant ischemic — *see also* Ischemia, intestine,
acute K55.059
granulomatous — *see* Enteritis, regional
hemorrhagic (acute) — *see also* Ischemia, intestine,
acute K55.059
chronic K55.1
infectious NEC A09
ischemic K55.9
necrotizing K55.30
with
perforation K55.33
pneumatosis K55.32
and perforation K55.33
due to Clostridium difficile
not specified as recurrent A04.72
recurrent A04.71
in non-newborn K55.30
stage 1 (without pneumatosis, without perforation) K55.31
stage 2 (with pneumatosis, without perforation)
K55.32
stage 3 (with pneumatosis, with perforation)
K55.33
in newborn P77.9
stage 1 (without pneumatosis, without perforation) P77.1
stage 2 (with pneumatosis, without perforation)
P77.2
stage 3 (with pneumatosis, with perforation)
P77.3
without pneumatosis or perforation K55.31
noninfectious K52.9
newborn — *see* Enterocolitis, necrotizing, in newborn
pseudomembranous (newborn)
not specified as recurrent A04.72
recurrent A04.71
radiation K52.0
newborn — *see* Enterocolitis, necrotizing, in newborn
ulcerative (chronic) — *see* Pancolitis, ulcerative
(chronic)
Enterogastritis — *see* Enteritis
Enteropathy K63.9
celiac-gluten-sensitive K90.0
non-celiac K90.41
food protein-induced K52.22
hemorrhagic, terminal — *see also* Ischemia, intestine,
acute K55.059
protein-losing K90.49
Enteroperitonitis — *see* Peritonitis
Enteroptosis K63.4
Enterorrhagia K92.2
Enterospasm — *see also* Syndrome, irritable, bowel
psychogenic F45.8
Enterostenosis — *see also* Obstruction, intestine, specified NEC K56.699
Enterostomy
complication — *see* Complication, enterostomy
status Z93.4
Enterovirus, as cause of disease classified elsewhere
B97.10
coxsackievirus B97.11
echovirus B97.12
other specified B97.19
Enthesopathy (peripheral) M77.9
Achilles tendinitis — *see* Tendinitis, Achilles
ankle and tarsus M77.5- ☑
specified type NEC — *see* Enthesopathy, foot,
specified type NEC
anterior tibial syndrome M76.81- ☑
calcaneal spur — *see* Spur, bone, calcaneal
elbow region M77.8
lateral epicondylitis — *see* Epicondylitis, lateral
medial epicondylitis — *see* Epicondylitis, medial
foot NEC M77.9
metatarsalgia — *see* Metatarsalgia
specified type NEC M77.5- ☑
forearm M77.9
gluteal tendinitis — *see* Tendinitis, gluteal
hand M77.9
hip — *see* Enthesopathy, lower limb, specified type
NEC
iliac crest spur — *see* Spur, bone, iliac crest

Enthesopathy — *continued*
iliotibial band syndrome — *see* Syndrome, iliotibial
band
knee — *see* Enthesopathy, lower limb, lower leg,
specified type NEC
lateral epicondylitis — *see* Epicondylitis, lateral
lower limb (excluding foot) M76.9
Achilles tendinitis — *see* Tendinitis, Achilles
ankle and tarsus M77.5- ☑
specified type NEC — *see* Enthesopathy, foot,
specified type NEC
anterior tibial syndrome M76.81- ☑
gluteal tendinitis — *see* Tendinitis, gluteal
iliac crest spur — *see* Spur, bone, iliac crest
iliotibial band syndrome — *see* Syndrome, iliotibial
band
patellar tendinitis — *see* Tendinitis, patellar
pelvic region — *see* Enthesopathy, lower limb,
specified type NEC
peroneal tendinitis — *see* Tendinitis, peroneal
posterior tibial syndrome M76.82- ☑
psoas tendinitis — *see* Tendinitis, psoas
specified type NEC M76.89- ☑
tibial collateral bursitis — *see* Bursitis, tibial collateral
medial epicondylitis — *see* Epicondylitis, medial
metatarsalgia — *see* Metatarsalgia
multiple sites M77.9
patellar tendinitis — *see* Tendinitis, patellar
pelvis M77.9
periarthritis of wrist — *see* Periarthritis, wrist
peroneal tendinitis — *see* Tendinitis, peroneal
posterior tibial syndrome M76.82- ☑
psoas tendinitis — *see* Tendinitis, psoas
shoulder M77.9
shoulder region — *see* Lesion, shoulder
specified site NEC M77.9
specified type NEC M77.8
spinal M46.00
cervical region M46.02
cervicothoracic region M46.03
lumbar region M46.06
lumbosacral region M46.07
multiple sites M46.09
occipito-atlanto-axial region M46.01
sacrococcygeal region M46.08
thoracic region M46.04
thoracolumbar region M46.05
tibial collateral bursitis — *see* Bursitis, tibial collateral
upper arm M77.9
wrist and carpus NEC M77.8
calcaneal spur — *see* Spur, bone, calcaneal
periarthritis of wrist — *see* Periarthritis, wrist
Entomophobia F40.218
Entomophthoromycosis B46.8
Entrance, air into vein — *see* Embolism, air
Entrapment, nerve — *see* Neuropathy, entrapment
Entropion (eyelid) (paralytic) H02.009
cicatricial H02.019
left H02.016
lower H02.015
upper H02.014
right H02.013
lower H02.012
upper H02.011
congenital Q10.2
left H02.006
lower H02.005
upper H02.004
mechanical H02.029
left H02.026
lower H02.025
upper H02.024
right H02.023
lower H02.022
upper H02.021
right H02.003
lower H02.002
upper H02.001
senile H02.039
left H02.036
lower H02.035
upper H02.034
right H02.033
lower H02.032
upper H02.031
spastic H02.049
left H02.046

Entropion — *continued*
spastic — *continued*
left — *continued*
lower H02.045
upper H02.044
right H02.043
lower H02.042
upper H02.041
Enucleated eye (traumatic, current) S05.7- ☑
Enuresis R32
functional F98.0
habit disturbance F98.0
nocturnal N39.44
psychogenic F98.0
nonorganic origin F98.0
psychogenic F98.0
Eosinopenia — *see* Agranulocytosis
Eosinophilia (allergic) (hereditary) (idiopathic) (secondary) D72.1
with
angiolymphoid hyperplasia (ALHE) D18.01
infiltrative J82
Löffler's J82
peritoneal — *see* Peritonitis, eosinophilic
pulmonary NEC J82
tropical (pulmonary) J82
Eosinophilia-myalgia syndrome M35.8
Ependymitis (acute) (cerebral) (chronic) (granular) —
see Encephalomyelitis
Ependymoblastoma
specified site — *see* Neoplasm, malignant, by site
unspecified site C71.9
Ependymoma (epithelial) (malignant)
anaplastic
specified site — *see* Neoplasm, malignant, by site
unspecified site C71.9
benign
specified site — *see* Neoplasm, benign, by site
unspecified site D33.2
myxopapillary D43.2
specified site — *see* Neoplasm, uncertain behavior,
by site
unspecified site D43.2
papillary D43.2
specified site — *see* Neoplasm, uncertain behavior,
by site
unspecified site D43.2
specified site — *see* Neoplasm, malignant, by site
unspecified site C71.9
Ependymopathy G93.89
Ephelis, ephelides L81.2
Epiblepharon (congenital) Q10.3
Epicanthus, epicanthic fold (eyelid) (congenital) Q10.3
Epicondylitis (elbow)
lateral M77.1- ☑
medial M77.0- ☑
Epicystitis — *see* Cystitis
Epidemic — *see* condition
Epidermidalization, cervix — *see* Dysplasia, cervix
Epidermis, epidermal — *see* condition
Epidermodysplasia verruciformis B07.8
Epidermolysis
bullosa (congenital) Q81.9
acquired L12.30
drug-induced L12.31
specified cause NEC L12.35
dystrophica Q81.2
letalis Q81.1
simplex Q81.0
specified NEC Q81.8
necroticans combustiformis L51.2
due to drug — *see* Table of Drugs and Chemicals,
by drug
Epidermophytid — *see* Dermatophytosis
Epidermophytosis (infected) — *see* Dermatophytosis
Epididymis — *see* condition
Epididymitis (acute) (nonvenereal) (recurrent) (residual)
N45.1
with orchitis N45.3
blennorrhagic (gonococcal) A54.23
caseous (tuberculous) A18.15
chlamydial A56.19
filarial — *see also* Infestation, filarial B74.9 *[N51]*
gonococcal A54.23
syphilitic A52.76
tuberculous A18.15
Epididymo-orchitis — *see also* Epididymitis N45.3
Epidural — *see* condition

Epigastrium, epigastric — *see* condition
Epigastrocele — *see* Hernia, ventral
Epiglottis — *see* condition
Epiglottitis, epiglottiditis (acute) J05.10
  with obstruction J05.11
  chronic J37.0
Epignathus Q89.4
Epilepsia partialis continua — *see also* Kozhevnikof's epilepsy G40.1- ☑
Epilepsy, epileptic, epilepsia (attack) (cerebral) (convulsion) (fit) (seizure) G40.909

> Note: the following terms are to be considered equivalent to intractable: pharmacoresistant (pharmacologically resistant), treatment resistant, refractory (medically) and poorly controlled

with
  complex partial seizures — *see* Epilepsy, localization-related, symptomatic, with complex partial seizures
  grand mal seizures on awakening — *see* Epilepsy, generalized, specified NEC
  myoclonic absences — *see* Epilepsy, generalized, specified NEC
  myoclonic-astatic seizures — *see* Epilepsy, generalized, specified NEC
  simple partial seizures — *see* Epilepsy, localization-related, symptomatic, with simple partial seizures
akinetic — *see* Epilepsy, generalized, specified NEC
benign childhood with centrotemporal EEG spikes — *see* Epilepsy, localization-related, idiopathic
benign myoclonic in infancy G40.80- ☑
Bravais-jacksonian — *see* Epilepsy, localization-related, symptomatic, with simple partial seizures
childhood
  with occipital EEG paroxysms — *see* Epilepsy, localization-related, idiopathic
  absence G40.A09 (*following* G40.3)
    intractable G40.A19 (*following* G40.3)
      with status epilepticus G40.A11 (*following* G40.3)
      without status epilepticus G40.A19 (*following* G40.3)
    not intractable G40.A09 (*following* G40.3)
      with status epilepticus G40.A01 (*following* G40.3)
      without status epilepticus G40.A09 (*following* G40.3)
climacteric — *see* Epilepsy, specified NEC
cysticercosis B69.0
deterioration (mental) F06.8
due to syphilis A52.19
focal — *see* Epilepsy, localization-related, symptomatic, with simple partial seizures
generalized
  idiopathic G40.309
    intractable G40.319
      with status epilepticus G40.311
      without status epilepticus G40.319
    not intractable G40.309
      with status epilepticus G40.301
      without status epilepticus G40.309
  specified NEC G40.409
    intractable G40.419
      with status epilepticus G40.411
      without status epilepticus G40.419
    not intractable G40.409
      with status epilepticus G40.401
      without status epilepticus G40.409
impulsive petit mal — *see* Epilepsy, juvenile myoclonic
intractable G40.919
  with status epilepticus G40.911
  without status epilepticus G40.919
juvenile absence G40.A09 (*following* G40.3)
  intractable G40.A19 (*following* G40.3)
    with status epilepticus G40.A11 (*following* G40.3)
    without status epilepticus G40.A19 (*following* G40.3)
  not intractable G40.A09 (*following* G40.3)
    with status epilepticus G40.A01 (*following* G40.3)
    without status epilepticus G40.A09 (*following* G40.3)
juvenile myoclonic G40.B09 (*following* G40.3)
  intractable G40.B19 (*following* G40.3)
    with status epilepticus G40.B11 (*following* G40.3)
    without status epilepticus G40.B19 (*following* G40.3)

Epilepsy, epileptic, epilepsia — *continued*
juvenile myoclonic — *continued*
  not intractable G40.B09 (*following* G40.3)
    with status epilepticus G40.B01 (*following* G40.3)
    without status epilepticus G40.B09 (*following* G40.3)
localization-related (focal) (partial)
  idiopathic G40.009
    with seizures of localized onset G40.009
      intractable G40.019
        with status epilepticus G40.011
        without status epilepticus G40.019
      not intractable G40.009
        with status epilepticus G40.001
        without status epilepticus G40.009
  symptomatic
    with complex partial seizures G40.209
      intractable G40.219
        with status epilepticus G40.211
        without status epilepticus G40.219
      not intractable G40.209
        with status epilepticus G40.201
        without status epilepticus G40.209
    with simple partial seizures G40.109
      intractable G40.119
        with status epilepticus G40.111
        without status epilepticus G40.119
      not intractable G40.109
        with status epilepticus G40.101
        without status epilepticus G40.109
myoclonus, myoclonic — *see* Epilepsy, generalized, specified NEC
not intractable G40.909
  with status epilepticus G40.901
  without status epilepticus G40.909
on awakening — *see* Epilepsy, generalized, specified NEC
parasitic NOS B71.9 *[G94]*
partialis continua — *see also* Kozhevnikof's epilepsy G40.1- ☑
peripheral — *see* Epilepsy, specified NEC
procursiva — *see* Epilepsy, localization-related, symptomatic, with simple partial seizures
progressive (familial) myoclonic — *see* Epilepsy, generalized, idiopathic
reflex — *see* Epilepsy, specified NEC
related to
  alcohol G40.509
    not intractable G40.509
      with status epilepticus G40.501
      without status epliepticus G40.509
  drugs G40.509
    not intractable G40.509
      with status epilepticus G40.501
      without status epliepticus G40.509
  external causes G40.509
    not intractable G40.509
      with status epilepticus G40.501
      without status epliepticus G40.509
  hormonal changes G40.509
    not intractable G40.509
      with status epilepticus G40.501
      without status epliepticus G40.509
  sleep deprivation G40.509
    not intractable G40.509
      with status epilepticus G40.501
      without status epliepticus G40.509
  stress G40.509
    not intractable G40.509
      with status epilepticus G40.501
      without status epliepticus G40.509
somatomotor — *see* Epilepsy, localization-related, symptomatic, with simple partial seizures
somatosensory — *see* Epilepsy, localization-related, symptomatic, with simple partial seizures
spasms G40.822
  intractable G40.824
    with status epilepticus G40.823
    without status epilepticus G40.824
  not intractable G40.822
    with status epilepticus G40.821
    without status epilepticus G40.822
specified NEC G40.802
  intractable G40.804
    with status epilepticus G40.803
    without status epilepticus G40.804
  not intractable G40.802

Epilepsy, epileptic, epilepsia — *continued*
specified — *continued*
  not intractable — *continued*
    with status epilepticus G40.801
    without status epilepticus G40.802
syndromes
  generalized
    idiopathic G40.309
      intractable G40.319
        with status epilepticus G40.311
        without status epilepticus G40.319
      not intractable G40.309
        with status epilepticus G40.301
        without status epilepticus G40.309
    specified NEC G40.409
      intractable G40.419
        with status epilepticus G40.411
        without status epilepticus G40.419
      not intractable G40.409
        with status epilepticus G40.401
        without status epilepticus G40.409
  localization-related (focal) (partial)
    idiopathic G40.009
      with seizures of localized onset G40.009
        intractable G40.019
          with status epilepticus G40.011
          without status epilepticus G40.019
        not intractable G40.009
          with status epilepticus G40.001
          without status epilepticus G40.009
    symptomatic
      with complex partial seizures G40.209
        intractable G40.219
          with status epilepticus G40.211
          without status epilepticus G40.219
        not intractable G40.209
          with status epilepticus G40.201
          without status epilepticus G40.209
      with simple partial seizures G40.109
        intractable G40.119
          with status epilepticus G40.111
          without status epilepticus G40.119
        not intractable G40.109
          with status epilepticus G40.101
          without status epilepticus G40.109
  specified NEC G40.802
    intractable G40.804
      with status epilepticus G40.803
      without status epilepticus G40.804
    not intractable G40.802
      with status epilepticus G40.801
      without status epilepticus G40.802
tonic (-clonic) — *see* Epilepsy, generalized, specified NEC
twilight F05
uncinate (gyrus) — *see* Epilepsy, localization-related, symptomatic, with complex partial seizures
Unverricht (-Lundborg) (familial myoclonic) — *see* Epilepsy, generalized, idiopathic
visceral — *see* Epilepsy, specified NEC
visual — *see* Epilepsy, specified NEC
Epiloia Q85.1
Epimenorrhea N92.0
Epipharyngitis — *see* Nasopharyngitis
Epiphora H04.20- ☑
  due to
    excess lacrimation H04.21- ☑
    insufficient drainage H04.22- ☑
Epiphyseal arrest — *see* Arrest, epiphyseal
Epiphyseolysis, epiphysiolysis — *see* Osteochondropathy
Epiphysitis — *see also* Osteochondropathy
  juvenile M92.9
  syphilitic (congenital) A50.02
Epiplocele — *see* Hernia, abdomen
Epiploitis — *see* Peritonitis
Epiplosarcomphalocele — *see* Hernia, umbilicus
Episcleritis (suppurative) H15.10- ☑
  in (due to)
    syphilis A52.71
    tuberculosis A18.51
  nodular H15.12- ☑
  periodica fugax H15.11- ☑
    angioneurotic — *see* Edema, angioneurotic
  syphilitic (late) A52.71
  tuberculous A18.51
Episode
  affective, mixed F39

Episode — *continued*
  depersonalization (in neurotic state) F48.1
  depressive F32.9
    major F32.9
      mild F32.Ø
      moderate F32.1
      severe (without psychotic symptoms) F32.2
        with psychotic symptoms F32.3
    recurrent F33.9
      brief F33.8
    specified NEC F32.89
  hypomanic F3Ø.8
  manic F3Ø.9
    with
      psychotic symptoms F3Ø.2
      remission (full) F3Ø.4
        partial F3Ø.3
    other specified F3Ø.8
    recurrent F31.89
    without psychotic symptoms F3Ø.1Ø
      mild F3Ø.11
      moderate F3Ø.12
      severe (without psychotic symptoms) F3Ø.13
        with psychotic symptoms F3Ø.2
  psychotic F23
    organic FØ6.8
  schizophrenic (acute) NEC, brief F23
Epispadias (female) (male) Q64.Ø
Episplenitis D73.89
Epistaxis (multiple) RØ4.Ø
  hereditary I78.Ø
  vicarious menstruation N94.89
Epithelioma (malignant) — *see also* Neoplasm, malignant, by site
  adenoides cysticum — *see* Neoplasm, skin, benign
  basal cell — *see* Neoplasm, skin, malignant
  benign — *see* Neoplasm, benign, by site
  Bowen's — *see* Neoplasm, skin, in situ
  calcifying, of Malherbe — *see* Neoplasm, skin, benign
  external site — *see* Neoplasm, skin, malignant
  intraepidermal, Jadassohn — *see* Neoplasm, skin, benign
  squamous cell — *see* Neoplasm, malignant, by site
Epitheliomatosis pigmented Q82.1
Epitheliopathy, multifocal placoid pigment H3Ø.14- ☑
Epithelium, epithelial — *see* condition
Epituberculosis (with atelectasis) (allergic) A15.7
Eponychia Q84.6
Epstein's
  nephrosis or syndrome — *see* Nephrosis
  pearl KØ9.8
Epulis (gingiva) (fibrous) (giant cell) KØ6.8
Equinia A24.Ø
Equinovarus (congenital) (talipes) Q66.Ø- ☑
  acquired — *see* Deformity, limb, clubfoot
Equivalent
  convulsive (abdominal) — *see* Epilepsy, specified NEC
  epileptic (psychic) — *see* Epilepsy, localization-related, symptomatic, with complex partial seizures
Erb (-Duchenne) **paralysis** (birth injury) (newborn) P14.Ø
Erb-Goldflam disease or syndrome G7Ø.ØØ
  with exacerbation (acute) G7Ø.Ø1
  in crisis G7Ø.Ø1
Erb's
  disease G71.Ø2
  palsy, paralysis (brachial) (birth) (newborn) P14.Ø
    spinal (spastic) syphilitic A52.17
  pseudohypertrophic muscular dystrophy G71.Ø2
Erdheim's syndrome (acromegalic macrospondylitis) E22.Ø
Erection, painful (persistent) — *see* Priapism
Ergosterol deficiency (vitamin D) E55.9
  with
    adult osteomalacia M83.8
    rickets — *see* Rickets
Ergotism — *see also* Poisoning, food, noxious, plant
  from ergot used as drug (migraine therapy) — *see* Table of Drugs and Chemicals
Erosio interdigitalis blastomycetica B37.2
Erosion
  artery I77.2
    without rupture I77.89
  bone — *see* Disorder, bone, density and structure, specified NEC
  bronchus J98.Ø9

Erosion — *continued*
  cartilage (joint) — *see* Disorder, cartilage, specified type NEC
  cervix (uteri) (acquired) (chronic) (congenital) N86
    with cervicitis N72
  cornea (nontraumatic) — *see* Ulcer, cornea
    recurrent H18.83- ☑
    traumatic — *see* Abrasion, cornea
  dental (idiopathic) (occupational) (due to diet, drugs or vomiting) KØ3.2
  duodenum, postpyloric — *see* Ulcer, duodenum
  esophagus K22.1Ø
    with bleeding K22.11
  gastric — *see* Ulcer, stomach
  gastrojejunal — *see* Ulcer, gastrojejunal
  implanted mesh — *see* Complications, prosthetic device or implant, mesh
  intestine K63.3
  lymphatic vessel I89.8
  pylorus, pyloric (ulcer) — *see* Ulcer, stomach
  spine, aneurysmal A52.Ø9
  stomach — *see* Ulcer, stomach
  subcutaneous device pocket
    nervous system prosthetic device, implant, or graft T85.89Ø ☑
    other internal prosthetic device, implant, or graft T85.898 ☑
  teeth (idiopathic) (occupational) (due to diet, drugs or vomiting) KØ3.2
  urethra N36.8
  uterus N85.8
Erotomania F52.8
Error
  metabolism, inborn — *see* Disorder, metabolism
  refractive — *see* Disorder, refraction
Eructation R14.2
  nervous or psychogenic F45.8
Eruption
  creeping B76.9
  drug (generalized) (taken internally) L27.Ø
    fixed L27.1
    in contact with skin — *see* Dermatitis, due to drugs
    localized L27.1
  Hutchinson, summer L56.4
  Kaposi's varicelliform BØØ.Ø
  napkin L22
  polymorphous light (sun) L56.4
  recalcitrant pustular L13.8
  ringed R23.8
  skin (nonspecific) R21
    creeping (meaning hookworm) B76.9
    due to inoculation/vaccination (generalized) — *see also* Dermatitis, due to, vaccine L27.Ø
      localized L27.1
    erysipeloid A26.Ø
    feigned L98.1
    Kaposi's varicelliform BØØ.Ø
    lichenoid L28.Ø
    meaning dermatitis — *see* Dermatitis
    toxic NEC L53.Ø
  tooth, teeth, abnormal (incomplete) (late) (premature) (sequence) KØØ.6
  vesicular R23.8
Erysipelas (gangrenous) (infantile) (newborn) (phlegmonous) (suppurative) A46
  external ear A46 *[H62.4Ø]*
  puerperal, postpartum O86.89
Erysipeloid A26.9
  cutaneous (Rosenbach's) A26.Ø
  disseminated A26.8
  sepsis A26.7
  specified NEC A26.8
Erythema, erythematous (infectional) (inflammation) L53.9
  ab igne L59.Ø
  annulare (centrifugum) (rheumaticum) L53.1
  arthriticum epidemicum A25.1
  brucellum — *see* Brucellosis
  chronic figurate NEC L53.3
  chronicum migrans (Borrelia burgdorferi) A69.2Ø
  diaper L22
  due to
    chemical NEC L53.Ø
      in contact with skin L24.5
    drug (internal use) — *see* Dermatitis, due to, drugs
  elevatum diutinum L95.1
  endemic E52
  epidemic, arthritic A25.1

Erythema, erythematous — *continued*
  figuratum perstans L53.3
  gluteal L22
  heat — *code by site under* Burn, first degree
  ichthyosiforme congenitum bullous Q8Ø.3
  in diseases classified elsewhere L54
  induratum (nontuberculous) L52
    tuberculous A18.4
  infectiosum BØ8.3
  intertrigo L3Ø.4
  iris L51.9
  marginatum L53.2
    in (due to) acute rheumatic fever IØØ
  medicamentosum — *see* Dermatitis, due to, drugs
  migrans A26.Ø
    chronicum A69.2Ø
    tongue K14.1
  multiforme (major) (minor) L51.9
    bullous, bullosum L51.1
    conjunctiva L51.1
    nonbullous L51.Ø
    pemphigoides L12.Ø
    specified NEC L51.8
  napkin L22
  neonatorum P83.88
    toxic P83.1
  nodosum L52
    tuberculous A18.4
  palmar L53.8
  pernio T69.1 ☑
  rash, newborn P83.88
  scarlatiniform (recurrent) (exfoliative) L53.8
  solare L55.Ø
  specified NEC L53.8
  toxic, toxicum NEC L53.Ø
    newborn P83.1
  tuberculous (primary) A18.4
Erythematous, erythematosus — *see* condition
Erythermalgia (primary) I73.81
Erythralgia I73.81
Erythrasma LØ8.1
Erythredema (polyneuropathy) — *see* Poisoning, mercury
Erythremia (acute) C94.Ø- ☑
  chronic D45
  secondary D75.1
Erythroblastopenia — *see also* Aplasia, red cell D6Ø.9
  congenital D61.Ø1
Erythroblastophthisis D61.Ø9
Erythroblastosis (fetalis) (newborn) P55.9
  due to
    ABO (antibodies) (incompatibility) (isoimmunization) P55.1
    Rh (antibodies) (incompatibility) (isoimmunization) P55.Ø
Erythrocyanosis (crurum) I73.89
Erythrocythemia — *see* Erythremia
Erythrocytosis (megalosplenic) (secondary) D75.1
  familial D75.Ø
  oval, hereditary — *see* Elliptocytosis
  secondary D75.1
  stress D75.1
Erythroderma (secondary) — *see also* Erythema L53.9
  bullous ichthyosiform, congenital Q8Ø.3
  desquamativum L21.1
  ichthyosiform, congenital (bullous) Q8Ø.3
  neonatorum P83.88
  psoriaticum L4Ø.8
Erythrodysesthesia, palmar plantar (PPE) L27.1
Erythrogenesis imperfecta D61.Ø9
Erythroleukemia C94.Ø- ☑
Erythromelalgia I73.81
Erythrophagocytosis D75.89
Erythrophobia F4Ø.298
Erythroplakia, oral epithelium, and tongue K13.29
Erythroplasia (Queyrat) DØ7.4
  specified site — *see* Neoplasm, skin, in situ
  unspecified site DØ7.4
Escherichia coli (E. coli), **as cause of disease classified elsewhere** B96.2Ø
  non-O157 Shiga toxin-producing (with known O group) B96.22
  non-Shiga toxin-producing B96.29
  O157 with confirmation of Shiga toxin when H antigen is unknown, or is not H7 B96.21
  O157:H- (nonmotile) with confirmation of Shiga toxin B96.21

☑ **Additional Character Required** — Refer to the Tabular List for Character Selection   ⚐ Subterms under main terms may continue to next column or page

Escherichia coli (E. coli), **as cause of disease classified elsewhere** — *continued*
  O157:H7 with or without confirmation of Shiga toxin-production B96.21
   specified NEC B96.22-
  Shiga toxin-producing (with unspecified O group) (STEC) B96.23
  O157 B96.21
  specified NEC B96.29
Esophagismus K22.4
Esophagitis (acute) (alkaline) (chemical) (chronic) (infectional) (necrotic) (peptic) (postoperative) K20.9
  candidal B37.81
  due to gastrointestinal reflux disease K21.0
  eosinophilic K20.0
  reflux K21.0
  specified NEC K20.8
  tuberculous A18.83
  ulcerative K22.10
   with bleeding K22.11
Esophagocele K22.5
Esophagomalacia K22.8
Esophagospasm K22.4
Esophagostenosis K22.2
Esophagostomiasis B81.8
Esophagotracheal — *see* condition
Esophagus — *see* condition
Esophoria H50.51
  convergence, excess H51.12
  divergence, insufficiency H51.8
Esotropia — *see* Strabismus, convergent concomitant
Espundia B55.2
Essential — *see* condition
Esthesioneuroblastoma C30.0
Esthesioneurocytoma C30.0
Esthesioneuroepithelioma C30.0
Esthiomene A55
Estivo-autumnal malaria (fever) B50.9
Estrangement (marital) Z63.5
  parent-child NEC Z62.890
Estriasis — *see* Myiasis
Ethanolism — *see* Alcoholism
Etherism — *see* Dependence, drug, inhalant
Ethmoid, ethmoidal — *see* condition
Ethmoiditis (chronic) (nonpurulent) (purulent) — *see also* Sinusitis, ethmoidal
  influenzal — *see* Influenza, with, respiratory manifestations NEC
  Woakes' J33.1
Ethylism — *see* Alcoholism
Eulenburg's disease (congenital paramyotonia) G71.19
Eumycetoma B47.0
Eunuchoidism E29.1
  hypogonadotropic E23.0
European blastomycosis — *see* Cryptococcosis
Eustachian — *see* condition
Evaluation (for) (of)
  development state
   adolescent Z00.3
   period of
    delayed growth in childhood Z00.70
     with abnormal findings Z00.71
    rapid growth in childhood Z00.2
    puberty Z00.3
  growth and developmental state (period of rapid growth) Z00.2
   delayed growth Z00.70
    with abnormal findings Z00.71
  mental health (status) Z00.8
   requested by authority Z04.6
  period of
   delayed growth in childhood Z00.70
    with abnormal findings Z00.71
   rapid growth in childhood Z00.2
  suspected condition — *see* Observation
Evans syndrome D69.41
Event
  apparent life threatening in newborn and infant (ALTE) R68.13
  brief resolved unexplained event (BRUE) R68.13
Eventration — *see also* Hernia, ventral
  colon into chest — *see* Hernia, diaphragm
  diaphragm (congenital) Q79.1
Eversion
  bladder N32.89
  cervix (uteri) N86
   with cervicitis N72

Eversion — *continued*
  foot NEC — *see also* Deformity, valgus, ankle
   congenital Q66.6
  punctum lacrimale (postinfectional) (senile) H04.52- ☑
  ureter (meatus) N28.89
  urethra (meatus) N36.8
  uterus N81.4
Evidence
  cytologic
   of malignancy on anal smear R85.614
   of malignancy on cervical smear R87.614
   of malignancy on vaginal smear R87.624
Evisceration
  birth injury P15.8
  traumatic NEC
   eye — *see* Enucleated eye
Evulsion — *see* Avulsion
Ewing's sarcoma or tumor — *see* Neoplasm, bone, malignant
Examination (for) (following) (general) (of) (routine) Z00.00
  with abnormal findings Z00.01
  abuse, physical (alleged), ruled out
   adult Z04.71
   child Z04.72
  adolescent (development state) Z00.3
  alleged rape or sexual assault (victim), ruled out
   adult Z04.41
   child Z04.42
  allergy Z01.82
  annual (adult) (periodic) (physical) Z00.00
   with abnormal findings Z00.01
   gynecological Z01.419
    with abnormal findings Z01.411
  antibody response Z01.84
  blood — *see* Examination, laboratory
  blood pressure Z01.30
   with abnormal findings Z01.31
  cancer staging — *see* Neoplasm, malignant, by site
  cervical Papanicolaou smear Z12.4
   as part of routine gynecological examination Z01.419
   with abnormal findings Z01.411
  child (over 28 days old) Z00.129
   with abnormal findings Z00.121
   under 28 days old — *see* Newborn, examination
  clinical research control or normal comparison (control) (participant) Z00.6
  contraceptive (drug) maintenance (routine) Z30.8
   device (intrauterine) Z30.431
  dental Z01.20
   with abnormal findings Z01.21
  developmental — *see* Examination, child
  donor (potential) Z00.5
  ear Z01.10
   with abnormal findings NEC Z01.118
  eye Z01.00
   with abnormal findings Z01.01
   following failed vision screening Z01.020
    with abnormal findings Z01.021
  follow-up (routine) (following) Z09
   chemotherapy NEC Z09
    malignant neoplasm Z08
   fracture Z09
   malignant neoplasm Z08
   postpartum Z39.2
   psychotherapy Z09
   radiotherapy NEC Z09
    malignant neoplasm Z08
   surgery NEC Z09
    malignant neoplasm Z08
  following
   accident NEC Z04.3
    transport Z04.1
    work Z04.2
   assault, alleged, ruled out
    adult Z04.71
    child Z04.72
   motor vehicle accident Z04.1
   treatment (for) Z09
    combined NEC Z09
     fracture Z09
      malignant neoplasm Z08
     malignant neoplasm Z08
     mental disorder Z09
    specified condition NEC Z09
  forced sexual exploitation Z04.81
  forced labor exploitation Z04.82

Examination — *continued*
  gynecological Z01.419
   with abnormal findings Z01.411
   for contraceptive maintenance Z30.8
  health — *see* Examination, medical
  hearing Z01.10
   with abnormal findings NEC Z01.118
   following failed hearing screening Z01.110
   infant or child (over 28 days old) Z00.129
    with abnormal findings Z00.121
  immunity status testing Z01.84
  laboratory (as part of a general medical examination) Z00.00
   with abnormal findings Z00.01
   preprocedural Z01.812
  lactating mother Z39.1
  medical (adult) (for) (of) Z00.00
   with abnormal findings Z00.01
   administrative purpose only Z02.9
    specified NEC Z02.89
   admission to
    armed forces Z02.3
    old age home Z02.2
    prison Z02.89
    residential institution Z02.2
    school Z02.0
     following illness or medical treatment Z02.0
    summer camp Z02.89
   adoption Z02.82
   blood alcohol or drug level Z02.83
   camp (summer) Z02.89
   clinical research, normal subject (control) (participant) Z00.6
   control subject in clinical research (normal comparison) (participant) Z00.6
   donor (potential) Z00.5
   driving license Z02.4
   general (adult) Z00.00
    with abnormal findings Z00.01
   immigration Z02.89
   insurance purposes Z02.6
   marriage Z02.89
   medicolegal reasons NEC Z04.89
   naturalization Z02.89
   participation in sport Z02.5
   paternity testing Z02.81
   population survey Z00.8
   pre-employment Z02.1
   pre-operative — *see* Examination, pre-procedural
   pre-procedural
    cardiovascular Z01.810
    respiratory Z01.811
    specified NEC Z01.818
   preschool children
    for admission to school Z02.0
   prisoners
    for entrance into prison Z02.89
   recruitment for armed forces Z02.3
   specified NEC Z00.8
   sport competition Z02.5
  medicolegal reason NEC Z04.89
   following
    forced sexual exploitation Z04.81
    forced labor exploitation Z04.82
  newborn — *see* Newborn, examination
  pelvic (annual) (periodic) Z01.419
   with abnormal findings Z01.411
  period of rapid growth in childhood Z00.2
  periodic (adult) (annual) (routine) Z00.00
   with abnormal findings Z00.01
  physical (adult) — *see also* Examination, medical Z00.00
   sports Z02.5
  postpartum
   immediately after delivery Z39.0
   routine follow-up Z39.2
  pre-chemotherapy (antineoplastic) Z01.818
  prenatal (normal pregnancy) — *see also* Pregnancy, normal Z34.9- ☑
  pre-procedural (pre-operative)
   cardiovascular Z01.810
   laboratory Z01.812
   respiratory Z01.811
   specified NEC Z01.818
  prior to chemotherapy (antineoplastic) Z01.818
  psychiatric NEC Z00.8
   follow-up not needing further care Z09
   requested by authority Z04.6
  radiological (as part of a general medical examination) Z00.00

Examination — *continued*
  radiological — *continued*
    with abnormal findings Z00.01
    repeat cervical smear to confirm findings of recent
      normal smear following initial abnormal smear
      Z01.42
  skin (hypersensitivity) Z01.82
  special — *see also* Examination, by type Z01.89
    specified type NEC Z01.89
  specified type or reason NEC Z04.89
  teeth Z01.20
    with abnormal findings Z01.21
  urine — *see* Examination, laboratory
  vision Z01.00
    with abnormal findings Z01.01
    following failed vision screening Z01.020
      with abnormal findings Z01.021
    infant or child (over 28 days old) Z00.129
      with abnormal findings Z00.121
Exanthem, exanthema — *see also* Rash
  with enteroviral vesicular stomatitis B08.4
  Boston A88.0
  epidemic with meningitis A88.0 [G02]
  subitum B08.20
    due to human herpesvirus 6 B08.21
    due to human herpesvirus 7 B08.22
  viral, virus B09
    specified type NEC B08.8
Excess, excessive, excessively
  alcohol level in blood R78.0
  androgen (ovarian) E28.1
  attrition, tooth, teeth K03.0
  carotene, carotin (dietary) E67.1
  cold, effects of T69.9 ☑
    specified effect NEC T69.8 ☑
  convergence H51.12
  crying
    in child, adolescent, or adult R45.83
    in infant R68.11
  development, breast N62
  divergence H51.8
  drinking (alcohol) NEC (without dependence) F10.10
    habitual (continual) (without remission) F10.20
  eating R63.2
  estrogen E28.0
  fat — *see also* Obesity
    in heart — *see* Degeneration, myocardial
    localized E65
  foreskin N47.8
  gas R14.0
  glucagon E16.3
  heat — *see* Heat
  intermaxillary vertical dimension of fully erupted teeth
    M26.37
  interocclusal distance of fully erupted teeth M26.37
  kalium E87.5
  large
    colon K59.39
      congenital Q43.8
    infant P08.0
    organ or site, congenital NEC — *see* Anomaly, by
      site
  long
    organ or site, congenital NEC — *see* Anomaly, by
      site
  menstruation (with regular cycle) N92.0
    with irregular cycle N92.1
  napping Z72.821
  natrium E87.0
  number of teeth K00.1
  nutrient (dietary) NEC R63.2
  potassium (K) E87.5
  salivation K11.7
  secretion — *see also* Hypersecretion
    milk O92.6
    sputum R09.3
    sweat R61
  sexual drive F52.8
  short
    organ or site, congenital NEC — *see* Anomaly, by
      site
    umbilical cord in labor or delivery O69.3 ☑
  skin L98.7
    and subcutaneous tissue L98.7
    eyelid (acquired) — *see* Blepharochalasis
      congenital Q10.3
  sodium (Na) E87.0
  spacing of fully erupted teeth M26.32

Excess, excessive, excessively — *continued*
  sputum R09.3
  sweating R61
  thirst R63.1
    due to deprivation of water T73.1 ☑
  tuberosity of jaw M26.07
  vitamin
    A (dietary) E67.0
      administered as drug (prolonged intake) — *see*
        Table of Drugs and Chemicals, vitamins,
        adverse effect
      overdose or wrong substance given or taken —
        see Table of Drugs and Chemicals, vita-
        mins, poisoning
    D (dietary) E67.3
      administered as drug (prolonged intake) — *see*
        Table of Drugs and Chemicals, vitamins,
        adverse effect
      overdose or wrong substance given or taken —
        see Table of Drugs and Chemicals, vita-
        mins, poisoning
  weight
    gain R63.5
    loss R63.4
Excitability, abnormal, under minor stress (personality disorder) F60.3
Excitation
  anomalous atrioventricular I45.6
  psychogenic F30.8
  reactive (from emotional stress, psychological trauma)
    F30.8
Excitement
  hypomanic F30.8
  manic F30.9
  mental, reactive (from emotional stress, psychological
    trauma) F30.8
  state, reactive (from emotional stress, psychological
    trauma) F30.8
Excoriation (traumatic) — *see also* Abrasion
  neurotic L98.1
  skin picking disorder F42.4
Exfoliation
  due to erythematous conditions according to extent
    of body surface involved L49.0
    10-19 percent of body surface L49.1
    20-29 percent of body surface L49.2
    30-39 percent of body surface L49.3
    40-49 percent of body surface L49.4
    50-59 percent of body surface L49.5
    60-69 percent of body surface L49.6
    70-79 percent of body surface L49.7
    80-89 percent of body surface L49.8
    90-99 percent of body surface L49.9
    less than 10 percent of body surface L49.0
  teeth, due to systemic causes K08.0
Exfoliative — *see* condition
Exhaustion, exhaustive (physical NEC) R53.83
  battle F43.0
  cardiac — *see* Failure, heart
  delirium F43.0
  due to
    cold T69.8 ☑
    excessive exertion T73.3 ☑
    exposure T73.2 ☑
    neurasthenia F48.8
  heart — *see* Failure, heart
  heat — *see also* Heat, exhaustion T67.5 ☑
    due to
      salt depletion T67.4 ☑
      water depletion T67.3 ☑
  maternal, complicating delivery O75.81
  mental F48.8
  myocardium, myocardial — *see* Failure, heart
  nervous F48.8
  old age R54
  psychogenic F48.8
  psychosis F43.0
  senile R54
  vital NEC Z73.0
Exhibitionism F65.2
Exocervicitis — *see* Cervicitis
Exomphalos Q79.2
  meaning hernia — *see* Hernia, umbilicus
Exophoria H50.52
  convergence, insufficiency H51.11
  divergence, excess H51.8
Exophthalmos H05.2- ☑
  congenital Q15.8

Exophthalmos — *continued*
  constant NEC H05.24- ☑
  displacement, globe — *see* Displacement, globe
  due to thyrotoxicosis (hyperthyroidism) — *see* Hyper-
    thyroidism, with, goiter (diffuse)
  dysthyroid — *see* Hyperthyroidism, with, goiter (dif-
    fuse)
  goiter — *see* Hyperthyroidism, with, goiter (diffuse)
  intermittent NEC H05.25- ☑
  malignant — *see* Hyperthyroidism, with, goiter (diffuse)
  orbital
    edema — *see* Edema, orbit
    hemorrhage — *see* Hemorrhage, orbit
  pulsating NEC H05.26- ☑
  thyrotoxic, thyrotropic — *see* Hyperthyroidism, with,
    goiter (diffuse)
Exostosis — *see also* Disorder, bone
  cartilaginous — *see* Neoplasm, bone, benign
  congenital (multiple) Q78.6
  external ear canal H61.81- ☑
  gonococcal A54.49
  jaw (bone) M27.8
  multiple, congenital Q78.6
  orbit H05.35- ☑
  osteocartilaginous — *see* Neoplasm, bone, benign
  syphilitic A52.77
Exotropia — *see* Strabismus, divergent concomitant
Explanation of
  investigation finding Z71.2
  medication Z71.89
Exposure (to) — *see also* Contact, with T75.89 ☑
  acariasis Z20.7
  AIDS virus Z20.6
  air pollution Z77.110
  algae and algae toxins Z77.121
  algae bloom Z77.121
  anthrax Z20.810
  aromatic amines Z77.020
  aromatic (hazardous) compounds NEC Z77.028
  aromatic dyes NOS Z77.028
  arsenic Z77.010
  asbestos Z77.090
  bacterial disease NEC Z20.818
  benzene Z77.021
  blue-green algae bloom Z77.121
  body fluids (potentially hazardous) Z77.21
  brown tide Z77.121
  chemicals (chiefly nonmedicinal) (hazardous) NEC
    Z77.098
  cholera Z20.09
  chromium compounds Z77.018
  cold, effects of T69.9 ☑
    specified effect NEC T69.8 ☑
  communicable disease Z20.9
    bacterial NEC Z20.818
    specified NEC Z20.89
    viral NEC Z20.828
    Zika virus Z20.821
  cyanobacteria bloom Z77.121
  disaster Z65.5
  discrimination Z60.5
  dyes Z77.098
  effects of T73.9 ☑
  environmental tobacco smoke (acute) (chronic) Z77.22
  Escherichia coli (E. coli) Z20.01
  exhaustion due to T73.2 ☑
  fiberglass — *see* Table of Drugs and Chemicals, fiber-
    glass
  German measles Z20.4
  gonorrhea Z20.2
  hazardous metals NEC Z77.018
  hazardous substances NEC Z77.29
  hazards in the physical environment NEC Z77.128
  hazards to health NEC Z77.9
  human immunodeficiency virus (HIV) Z20.6
  human T-lymphotropic virus type-1 (HTLV-1) Z20.89
  implanted
    mesh — *see* Complications, prosthetic devise or
      implant, mesh
    prosthetic materials NEC — *see* Complications,
      prosthetic materials NEC
  infestation (parasitic) NEC Z20.7
  intestinal infectious disease NEC Z20.09
    Escherichia coli (E. coli) Z20.01
  lead Z77.011
  meningococcus Z20.811
  mold (toxic) Z77.120
  nickel dust Z77.018

☑ **Additional Character Required** — **Refer to the Tabular List for Character Selection** ☝ **Subterms under main terms may continue to next column or page**

Exposure — *continued*
  noise Z77.122
  occupational
    air contaminants NEC Z57.39
    dust Z57.2
    environmental tobacco smoke Z57.31
    extreme temperature Z57.6
    noise Z57.0
    radiation Z57.1
    risk factors Z57.9
      specified NEC Z57.8
    toxic agents (gases) (liquids) (solids) (vapors) in agriculture Z57.4
    toxic agents (gases) (liquids) (solids) (vapors) in industry NEC Z57.5
    vibration Z57.7
  parasitic disease NEC Z20.7
  pediculosis Z20.7
  persecution Z60.5
  pfiesteria piscicida Z77.121
  poliomyelitis Z20.89
  pollution
    air Z77.110
    environmental NEC Z77.118
    soil Z77.112
    water Z77.111
  polycyclic aromatic hydrocarbons Z77.028
  prenatal (drugs) (toxic chemicals) — *see* Newborn, affected by, noxious substances transmitted via placenta or breast milk
  rabies Z20.3
  radiation, naturally occurring NEC Z77.123
  radon Z77.123
  red tide (Florida) Z77.121
  rubella Z20.4
  second hand tobacco smoke (acute) (chronic) Z77.22
    in the perinatal period P96.81
  sexually-transmitted disease Z20.2
  smallpox (laboratory) Z20.89
  syphilis Z20.2
  terrorism Z65.4
  torture Z65.4
  tuberculosis Z20.1
  uranium Z77.012
  varicella Z20.820
  venereal disease Z20.2
  viral disease NEC Z20.828
  war Z65.5
  water pollution Z77.111
  Zika virus Z20.821
Exsanguination — *see* Hemorrhage
Exstrophy
  abdominal contents Q45.8
  bladder Q64.10
    cloacal Q64.12
    specified type NEC Q64.19
    supravesical fissure Q64.11
Extensive — *see* condition
Extra — *see also* Accessory
  marker chromosomes (normal individual) Q92.61
    in abnormal individual Q92.62
  rib Q76.6
    cervical Q76.5
Extrasystoles (supraventricular) I49.49
  atrial I49.1
  auricular I49.1
  junctional I49.2
  ventricular I49.3
Extrauterine gestation or pregnancy — *see* Pregnancy, by site
Extravasation
  blood R58
  chyle into mesentery I89.8
  pelvicalyceal N13.8
  pyelosinus N13.8
  urine (from ureter) R39.0
  vesicant agent
    antineoplastic chemotherapy T80.810 ☑
    other agent NEC T80.818 ☑
Extremity — *see* condition, limb
Extrophy — *see* Exstrophy
Extroversion
  bladder Q64.19
  uterus N81.4
    complicating delivery O71.2
    postpartal (old) N81.4
Extruded tooth (teeth) M26.34

Extrusion
  breast implant (prosthetic) T85.42 ☑
  eye implant (globe) (ball) T85.328 ☑
  intervertebral disc — *see* Displacement, intervertebral disc
  ocular lens implant (prosthetic) — *see* Complications, intraocular lens
  vitreous — *see* Prolapse, vitreous
Exudate
  pleural — *see* Effusion, pleura
  retina H35.89
Exudative — *see* condition
Eye, eyeball, eyelid — *see* condition
Eyestrain — *see* Disturbance, vision, subjective
Eyeworm disease of Africa B74.3

F

Faber's syndrome (achlorhydric anemia) D50.9
Fabry (-Anderson) **disease** E75.21
Faciocephalalgia, autonomic — *see also* Neuropathy, peripheral, autonomic G90.09
Factor(s)
  psychic, associated with diseases classified elsewhere F54
  psychological
    affecting physical conditions F54
    or behavioral
      affecting general medical condition F54
      associated with disorders or diseases classified elsewhere F54
Fahr disease (of brain) G23.8
Fahr Volhard disease (of kidney) I12.- ☑
Failure, failed
  abortion — *see* Abortion, attempted
  aortic (valve) I35.8
    rheumatic I06.8
  attempted abortion — *see* Abortion, attempted
  biventricular I50.82
    due to left heart failure I50.814
  bone marrow — *see* Anemia, aplastic
  cardiac — *see* Failure, heart
  cardiorenal (chronic) — *see also* Failure, renal, and Failure, heart I50.9
    hypertensive I13.2
  cardiorespiratory — *see also* Failure, heart R09.2
  cardiovascular (chronic) — *see* Failure, heart
  cerebrovascular I67.9
  cervical dilatation in labor O62.0
  circulation, circulatory (peripheral) R57.9
    newborn P29.89
  compensation — *see* Disease, heart
  compliance with medical treatment or regimen — *see* Noncompliance
  congestive — *see* Failure, heart, congestive
  dental implant (endosseous) M27.69
    due to
      failure of dental prosthesis M27.63
      lack of attached gingiva M27.62
      occlusal trauma (poor prosthetic design) M27.62
      parafunctional habits M27.62
      periodontal infection (peri-implantitis) M27.62
      poor oral hygiene M27.62
    osseointegration M27.61
      due to
        complications of systemic disease M27.61
        poor bone quality M27.61
      iatrogenic M27.61
    post-osseointegration
      biological M27.62
      due to complications of systemic disease M27.62
      iatrogenic M27.62
      mechanical M27.63
    pre-integration M27.61
    pre-osseointegration M27.61
    specified NEC M27.69
  descent of head (at term) of pregnancy (mother) O32.4 ☑
  endosseous dental implant — *see* Failure, dental implant
  engagement of head (term of pregnancy) (mother) O32.4 ☑
  erection (penile) — *see also* Dysfunction, sexual, male, erectile N52.9
    nonorganic F52.21
  examination(s), anxiety concerning Z55.2

Failure, failed — *continued*
  expansion terminal respiratory units (newborn) (primary) P28.0
  forceps NOS (with subsequent cesarean delivery) O66.5
  gain weight (child over 28 days old) R62.51
    adult R62.7
    newborn P92.6
  genital response (male) F52.21
    female F52.22
  heart (acute) (senile) (sudden) I50.9
    with
      acute pulmonary edema — *see* Failure, ventricular, left
      decompensation — *see also* Failure, heart, by type as diastolic or systolic, acute and chronic I50.9
      dilatation — *see* Disease, heart
      hypertension — *see* Hypertension, heart
      normal ejection fraction — *see* Failure, heart, diastolic
      preserved ejection fraction — *see* Failure, heart, diastolic
      reduced ejection fraction — *see* Failure, heart, systolic
    arteriosclerotic I70.90
    biventricular I50.82
      due to left heart failure I50.814
    combined left-right sided I50.82
      due to left heart failure I50.814
    compensated — *see also* Failure, heart, by type as diastolic or systolic, chronic I50.9
    complicating
      anesthesia (general) (local) or other sedation in labor and delivery O74.2
        in pregnancy O29.12- ☑
        postpartum, puerperal O89.1
      delivery (cesarean) (instrumental) O75.4
    congestive I50.9
      with rheumatic fever (conditions in I00)
        active I01.8
        inactive or quiescent (with chorea) I09.81
      newborn P29.0
      rheumatic (chronic) (inactive) (with chorea) I09.81
        active or acute I01.8
          with chorea I02.0
    decompensated — *see also* Failure, heart, by type as diastolic or systolic, acute and chronic I50.9
    degenerative — *see* Degeneration, myocardial
    diastolic (congestive) (left ventricular) I50.30
      acute (congestive) I50.31
        and (on) chronic (congestive) I50.33
      chronic (congestive) I50.32
        and (on) acute (congestive) I50.33
      combined with systolic (congestive) I50.40
        acute (congestive) I50.41
          and (on) chronic (congestive) I50.43
        chronic (congestive) I50.42
          and (on) acute (congestive) I50.43
    due to presence of cardiac prosthesis I97.13- ☑
    end stage — *see also* Failure, heart, by type as diastolic or systolic, chronic I50.84
    following cardiac surgery I97.13- ☑
    high output NOS I50.83
    hypertensive — *see* Hypertension, heart
    left (ventricular) — *see also* Failure, ventricular, left
      combined diastolic and systolic — *see* Failure, heart, diastolic, combined with systolic
      diastolic — *see* Failure, heart, diastolic
      systolic — *see* Failure, heart, systolic
    low output (syndrome) NOS I50.9
    newborn P29.0
    organic — *see* Disease, heart
    peripartum O90.3
    postprocedural I97.13- ☑
    rheumatic (chronic) (inactive) I09.9
    right (isolated) (ventricular) I50.810
      acute I50.811
        and (on) chronic I50.813
      chronic I50.812
        and acute I50.813
      secondary to left heart failure I50.814

Failure, failed — *continued*
  heart — *continued*
    specified NEC I50.89

> Note: heart failure stages A, B, C, and D are based on the American College of Cardiology and American Heart Association stages of heart failure, which complement and should not be confused with the New York Heart Association Classification of Heart Failure, into Class I, Class II, Class III, and Class IV

    stage A Z91.89
    stage B — *see also* Failure, heart, by type as diastolic or systolic I50.9
    stage C — *see also* Failure, heart, by type as diastolic or systolic I50.9
    stage D — *see also* Failure, heart, by type as diastolic or systolic, chronic I50.84
    systolic (congestive) (left ventricular) I50.20
      acute (congestive) I50.21
        and (on) chronic (congestive) I50.23
      chronic (congestive) I50.22
        and (on) acute (congestive) I50.23
      combined with diastolic (congestive) I50.40
        acute (congestive) I50.41
          and (on) chronic (congestive) I50.43
        chronic (congestive) I50.42
          and (on) acute (congestive) I50.43
    thyrotoxic — *see also* Thyrotoxicosis E05.90 *[I43]*
      with
        high output — *see also* Thyrotoxicosis I50.83
        thyroid storm E05.91 *[I43]*
          high output — *see also* Thyrotoxicosis I50.83
    valvular — *see* Endocarditis
  hepatic K72.90
    with coma K72.91
    acute or subacute K72.00
      with coma K72.01
      due to drugs K71.10
        with coma K71.11
    alcoholic (acute) (chronic) (subacute) K70.40
      with coma K70.41
    chronic K72.10
      with coma K72.11
      due to drugs (acute) (subacute) (chronic) K71.10
        with coma K71.11
    due to drugs (acute) (subacute) (chronic) K71.10
      with coma K71.11
    postprocedural K91.82
  hepatorenal K76.7
  induction (of labor) O61.9
    abortion — *see* Abortion, attempted
    by
      oxytocic drugs O61.0
      prostaglandins O61.0
    instrumental O61.1
    mechanical O61.1
    medical O61.0
    specified NEC O61.8
    surgical O61.1
  intubation during anesthesia T88.4 ☑
    in pregnancy O29.6- ☑
    labor and delivery O74.7
    postpartum, puerperal O89.6
  involution, thymus (gland) E32.0
  kidney — *see also* Disease, kidney, chronic N19
    acute — *see also* Failure, renal, acute N17.9
  lactation (complete) O92.3
    partial O92.4
  Leydig's cell, adult E29.1
  liver — *see* Failure, hepatic
  menstruation at puberty N91.0
  mitral I05.8
  myocardial, myocardium — *see also* Failure, heart I50.9
    chronic — *see also* Failure, heart, congestive I50.9
    congestive — *see also* Failure, heart, congestive I50.9
  orgasm (female) (psychogenic) F52.31
    male F52.32
  ovarian (primary) E28.39
    iatrogenic E89.40
      asymptomatic E89.40
      symptomatic E89.41
    postprocedural (postablative) (postirradiation) (postsurgical) E89.40
      asymptomatic E89.40
      symptomatic E89.41
  ovulation causing infertility N97.0

Failure, failed — *continued*
  polyglandular, autoimmune E31.0
  prosthetic joint implant — *see* Complications, joint prosthesis, mechanical, breakdown, by site
  renal N19
    with
      tubular necrosis (acute) N17.0
    acute N17.9
      with
        cortical necrosis N17.1
        medullary necrosis N17.2
        tubular necrosis N17.0
      specified NEC N17.8
    chronic N18.9
      hypertensive — *see* Hypertension, kidney
    congenital P96.0
    end stage (chronic) N18.6
      due to hypertension I12.0
    following
      abortion — *see* Abortion by type complicated by specified condition NEC
      crushing T79.5 ☑
      ectopic or molar pregnancy O08.4
      labor and delivery (acute) O90.4
    hypertensive — *see* Hypertension, kidney
    postprocedural N99.0
  respiration, respiratory J96.90
    with
      hypercapnia J96.92
      hypercarbia J96.92
      hypoxia J96.91
    acute J96.00
      with
        hypercapnia J96.02
        hypercarbia J96.02
        hypoxia J96.01
    center G93.89
    acute and (on) chronic J96.20
      with
        hypercapnia J96.22
        hypercarbia J96.22
        hypoxia J96.21
    chronic J96.10
      with
        hypercapnia J96.12
        hypercarbia J96.12
        hypoxia J96.11
    newborn P28.5
    postprocedural (acute) J95.821
      acute and chronic J95.822
  rotation
    cecum Q43.3
    colon Q43.3
    intestine Q43.3
    kidney Q63.2
  sedation (conscious) (moderate) during procedure T88.52 ☑
    history of Z92.83
  segmentation — *see also* Fusion
    fingers — *see* Syndactylism, complex, fingers
    vertebra Q76.49
      with scoliosis Q76.3
  seminiferous tubule, adult E29.1
  senile (general) R54
  sexual arousal (male) F52.21
    female F52.22
  testicular endocrine function E29.1
  to thrive (child over 28 days old) R62.51
    adult R62.7
    newborn P92.6
  transplant T86.92
    bone T86.831
      marrow T86.02
    cornea T86.841
    heart T86.22
      with lung(s) T86.32
    intestine T86.851
    kidney T86.12
    liver T86.42
    lung(s) T86.811
      with heart T86.32
    pancreas T86.891
    skin (allograft) (autograft) T86.821
    specified organ or tissue NEC T86.891
    stem cell (peripheral blood) (umbilical cord) T86.5
  trial of labor (with subsequent cesarean delivery) O66.40
    following previous cesarean delivery O66.41

Failure, failed — *continued*
  tubal ligation N99.89
  urinary — *see* Disease, kidney, chronic
  vacuum extraction NOS (with subsequent cesarean delivery) O66.5
  vasectomy N99.89
  ventouse NOS (with subsequent cesarean delivery) O66.5
  ventricular — *see also* Failure, heart I50.9
    left — *see also* Failure, heart, left I50.1
      with rheumatic fever (conditions in I00)
        active I01.8
          with chorea I02.0
        inactive or quiescent (with chorea) I09.81
      rheumatic (chronic) (inactive) (with chorea) I09.81
        active or acute I01.8
          with chorea I02.0
    right — *see* Failure, heart, right
  vital centers, newborn P91.88
Fainting (fit) R55
Fallen arches — *see* Deformity, limb, flat foot
Falling, falls (repeated) R29.6
  any organ or part — *see* Prolapse
Fallopian
  insufflation Z31.41
  tube — *see* condition
Fallot's
  pentalogy Q21.8
  tetrad or tetralogy Q21.3
  triad or trilogy Q22.3
False — *see also* condition
  croup J38.5
  joint — *see* Nonunion, fracture
  labor (pains) O47.9
    at or after 37 completed weeks of gestation O47.1
    before 37 completed weeks of gestation O47.0- ☑
  passage, urethra (prostatic) N36.5
  pregnancy F45.8
Family, familial — *see also* condition
  disruption Z63.8
    involving divorce or separation Z63.5
  Li-Fraumeni (syndrome) Z15.01
  planning advice Z30.09
  problem Z63.9
    specified NEC Z63.8
  retinoblastoma C69.2- ☑
Famine (effects of) T73.0 ☑
  edema — *see* Malnutrition, severe
Fanconi (-de Toni)(-Debré) **syndrome** E72.09
  with cystinosis E72.04
Fanconi's anemia (congenital pancytopenia) D61.09
Farber's disease or syndrome E75.29
Farcy A24.0
Farmer's
  lung J67.0
  skin L57.8
Farsightedness — *see* Hypermetropia
Fascia — *see* condition
Fasciculation R25.3
Fasciitis M72.9
  diffuse (eosinophilic) M35.4
  infective M72.8
    necrotizing M72.6
  necrotizing M72.6
  nodular M72.4
  perirenal (with ureteral obstruction) N13.5
    with infection N13.6
  plantar M72.2
  specified NEC M72.8
  traumatic (old) M72.8
    current — *code by* site under Sprain
Fascioliasis B66.3
Fasciolopsis, fasciolopsiasis (intestinal) B66.5
Fascioscapulohumeral myopathy G71.02
Fast pulse R00.0
Fat
  embolism — *see* Embolism, fat
  excessive — *see also* Obesity
    in heart — *see* Degeneration, myocardial
  in stool R19.5
  localized (pad) E65
    heart — *see* Degeneration, myocardial
    knee M79.4
    retropatellar M79.4
  necrosis
    breast N64.1
    mesentery K65.4

Fat — *continued*
  necrosis — *continued*
    omentum K65.4
  pad E65
    knee M79.4
Fatigue R53.83
  auditory deafness — *see* Deafness
  chronic R53.82
  combat F43.0
  general R53.83
    psychogenic F48.8
  heat (transient) T67.6 ☑
  muscle M62.89
  myocardium — *see* Failure, heart
  neoplasm-related R53.0
  nervous, neurosis F48.8
  operational F48.8
  psychogenic (general) F48.8
  senile R54
  voice R49.8
Fatness — *see* Obesity
Fatty — *see also* condition
  apron E65
  degeneration — *see* Degeneration, fatty
  heart (enlarged) — *see* Degeneration, myocardial
  liver NEC K76.0
    alcoholic K70.0
    nonalcoholic K76.0
  necrosis — *see* Degeneration, fatty
Fauces — *see* condition
Fauchard's disease (periodontitis) — *see* Periodontitis
Faucitis J02.9
Favism (anemia) D55.0
Favus — *see* Dermatophytosis
Fazio-Londe disease or syndrome G12.1
Fear complex or reaction F40.9
Fear of — *see* Phobia
Feared complaint unfounded Z71.1
Febris, febrile — *see also* Fever
  flava — *see also* Fever, yellow A95.9
  melitensis A23.0
  pestis — *see* Plague
  recurrens — *see* Fever, relapsing
  rubra A38.9
Fecal
  incontinence R15.9
  smearing R15.1
  soiling R15.1
  urgency R15.2
Fecalith (impaction) K56.41
  appendix K38.1
  congenital P76.8
Fede's disease K14.0
Feeble rapid pulse due to shock following injury T79.4 ☑
Feeble-minded F70
Feeding
  difficulties R63.3
  problem R63.3
    newborn P92.9
      specified NEC P92.8
    nonorganic (adult) — *see* Disorder, eating
Feeling (of)
  foreign body in throat R09.89
Feer's disease — *see* Poisoning, mercury
Feet — *see* condition
Feigned illness Z76.5
Feil-Klippel syndrome (brevicollis) Q76.1
Feinmesser's (hidrotic) **ectodermal dysplasia** Q82.4
Felinophobia F40.218
Felon — *see also* Cellulitis, digit
  with lymphangitis — *see* Lymphangitis, acute, digit
Felty's syndrome M05.00
  ankle M05.07- ☑
  elbow M05.02- ☑
  foot joint M05.07- ☑
  hand joint M05.04- ☑
  hip M05.05- ☑
  knee M05.06- ☑
  multiple site M05.09
  shoulder M05.01- ☑
  vertebra — *see* Spondylitis, ankylosing
  wrist M05.03- ☑
Female genital cutting status — *see* Female genital mutilation status (FGM)
Female genital mutilation status (FGM) N90.810
  specified NEC N90.818

Female genital mutilation status — *continued*
  type I (clitorectomy status) N90.811
  type II (clitorectomy with excision of labia minora status) N90.812
  type III (infibulation status) N90.813
  type IV N90.818
Femur, femoral — *see* condition
Fenestration, fenestrated — *see also* Imperfect, closure
  aortico-pulmonary Q21.4
  cusps, heart valve NEC Q24.8
    pulmonary Q22.3
  pulmonic cusps Q22.3
Fernell's disease (aortic aneurysm) I71.9
Fertile eunuch syndrome E23.0
Fetid
  breath R19.6
  sweat L75.0
Fetishism F65.0
  transvestic F65.1
Fetus, fetal — *see also* condition
  alcohol syndrome (dysmorphic) Q86.0
  compressus O31.0- ☑
  hydantoin syndrome Q86.1
  lung tissue P28.0
  papyraceous O31.0- ☑
Fever (inanition) (of unknown origin) (persistent) (with chills) (with rigor) R50.9
  abortus A23.1
  Aden (dengue) A90
  African tick-borne A68.1
  American
    mountain (tick) A93.2
    spotted A77.0
  aphthous B08.8
  arbovirus, arboviral A94
    hemorrhagic A94
    specified NEC A93.8
  Argentinian hemorrhagic A96.0
  Assam B55.0
  Australian Q A78
  Bangkok hemorrhagic A91
  Barmah forest A92.8
  Bartonella A44.0
  bilious, hemoglobinuric B50.8
  blackwater B50.8
  blister B00.1
  Bolivian hemorrhagic A96.1
  Bonvale dam T73.3 ☑
  boutonneuse A77.1
  brain — *see* Encephalitis
  Brazilian purpuric A48.4
  breakbone A90
  Bullis A77.0
  Bunyamwera A92.8
  Burdwan B55.0
  Bwamba A92.8
  Cameroon — *see* Malaria
  Canton A75.9
  catarrhal (acute) J00
    chronic J31.0
  cat-scratch A28.1
  Central Asian hemorrhagic A98.0
  cerebral — *see* Encephalitis
  cerebrospinal meningococcal A39.0
  Chagres B50.9
  Chandipura A92.8
  Changuinola A93.1
  Charcot's (biliary) (hepatic) (intermittent) — *see* Calculus, bile duct
  Chikungunya (viral) (hemorrhagic) A92.0
  Chitral A93.1
  Colombo — *see* Fever, paratyphoid
  Colorado tick (virus) A93.2
  congestive (remittent) — *see* Malaria
  Congo virus A98.0
  continued malarial B50.9
  Corsican — *see* Malaria
  Crimean-Congo hemorrhagic A98.0
  Cyprus — *see* Brucellosis
  dandy A90
  deer fly — *see* Tularemia
  dengue (virus) A90
    hemorrhagic A91
    sandfly A93.1
  desert B38.0
  drug induced R50.2
  due to
    conditions classified elsewhere R50.81

Fever — *continued*
  due to — *continued*
    heat T67.01 ☑
  enteric A01.00
  enteroviral exanthematous (Boston exanthem) A88.0
  ephemeral (of unknown origin) R50.9
  epidemic hemorrhagic A98.5
  erysipelatous — *see* Erysipelas
  estivo-autumnal (malarial) B50.9
  famine A75.0
  five day A79.0
  following delivery O86.4
  Fort Bragg A27.89
  gastroenteric A01.00
  gastromalarial — *see* Malaria
  Gibraltar — *see* Brucellosis
  glandular — *see* Mononucleosis, infectious
  Guama (viral) A92.8
  Haverhill A25.1
  hay (allergic) J30.1
    with asthma (bronchial) J45.909
      with
        exacerbation (acute) J45.901
        status asthmaticus J45.902
    due to
      allergen other than pollen J30.89
      pollen, any plant or tree J30.1
  heat (effects) T67.01 ☑
  hematuric, bilious B50.8
  hemoglobinuric (malarial) (bilious) B50.8
  hemorrhagic (arthropod-borne) NOS A94
    with renal syndrome A98.5
    arenaviral A96.9
      specified NEC A96.8
    Argentinian A96.0
    Bangkok A91
    Bolivian A96.1
    Central Asian A98.0
    Chikungunya A92.0
    Crimean-Congo A98.0
    dengue (virus) A91
    epidemic A98.5
    Junin (virus) A96.0
    Korean A98.5
    Kyasanur forest A98.2
    Machupo (virus) A96.1
    mite-borne A93.8
    mosquito-borne A92.8
    Omsk A98.1
    Philippine A91
    Russian A98.5
    Singapore A91
    Southeast Asia A91
    Thailand A91
    tick-borne NEC A93.8
    viral A99
      specified NEC A98.8
  hepatic — *see* Cholecystitis
  herpetic — *see* Herpes
  icterohemorrhagic A27.0
  Indiana A93.8
  infective B99.9
    specified NEC B99.8
  intermittent (bilious) — *see also* Malaria
    of unknown origin R50.9
    pernicious B50.9
  iodide R50.2
  Japanese river A75.3
  jungle — *see also* Malaria
    yellow A95.0
  Junin (virus) hemorrhagic A96.0
  Katayama B65.2
  kedani A75.3
  Kenya (tick) A77.1
  Kew Garden A79.1
  Korean hemorrhagic A98.5
  Lassa A96.2
  Lone Star A77.0
  Machupo (virus) hemorrhagic A96.1
  malaria, malarial — *see* Malaria
  Malta A23.9
  Marseilles A77.1
  marsh — *see* Malaria
  Mayaro (viral) A92.8
  Mediterranean — *see also* Brucellosis A23.9
    familial M04.1
    tick A77.1
  meningeal — *see* Meningitis

Fever — *continued*
  Meuse A79.0
  Mexican A75.2
  mianeh A68.1
  miasmatic — *see* Malaria
  mosquito-borne (viral) A92.9
    hemorrhagic A92.8
  mountain — *see also* Brucellosis
    meaning Rocky Mountain spotted fever A77.0
    tick (American) (Colorado) (viral) A93.2
  Mucambo (viral) A92.8
  mud A27.9
  Neapolitan — *see* Brucellosis
  neutropenic D70.9
  newborn P81.9
    environmental P81.0
  Nine-Mile A78
  non-exanthematous tick A93.2
  North Asian tick-borne A77.2
  Omsk hemorrhagic A98.1
  O'nyong-nyong (viral) A92.1
  Oropouche (viral) A93.0
  Oroya A44.0
  paludal — *see* Malaria
  Panama (malarial) B50.9
  Pappataci A93.1
  paratyphoid A01.4
    A A01.1
    B A01.2
    C A01.3
  parrot A70
  periodic (Mediterranean) M04.1
  persistent (of unknown origin) R50.9
  petechial A39.0
  pharyngoconjunctival B30.2
  Philippine hemorrhagic A91
  phlebotomus A93.1
  Piry (virus) A93.8
  Pixuna (viral) A92.8
  Plasmodium ovale B53.0
  polioviral (nonparalytic) A80.4
  Pontiac A48.2
  postimmunization R50.83
  postoperative R50.82
    due to infection T81.40 ☑
  posttransfusion R50.84
  postvaccination R50.83
  presenting with conditions classified elsewhere R50.81
  pretibial A27.89
  puerperal O86.4
  Q A78
  quadrilateral A78
  quartan (malaria) B52.9
  Queensland (coastal) (tick) A77.3
  quintan A79.0
  rabbit — *see* Tularemia
  rat-bite A25.9
    due to
      Spirillum A25.0
      Streptobacillus moniliformis A25.1
  recurrent — *see* Fever, relapsing
  relapsing (Borrelia) A68.9
    Carter's (Asiatic) A68.1
    Dutton's (West African) A68.1
    Koch's A68.9
    louse-borne A68.0
    Novy's
      louse-borne A68.0
      tick-borne A68.1
    Obermeyer's (European) A68.0
    tick-borne A68.1
  remittent (bilious) (congestive) (gastric) — *see* Malaria
  rheumatic (active) (acute) (chronic) (subacute) I00
    with central nervous system involvement I02.9
    active with heart involvement — *see* category I01 ☑
    inactive or quiescent with
      cardiac hypertrophy I09.89
      carditis I09.9
      endocarditis I09.1
        aortic (valve) I06.9
          with mitral (valve) disease I08.0
        mitral (valve) I05.9
          with aortic (valve) disease I08.0
        pulmonary (valve) I09.89
        tricuspid (valve) I07.8
      heart disease NEC I09.89
      heart failure (congestive) (conditions in category I50.) I09.81

Fever — *continued*
  rheumatic — *continued*
    inactive or quiescent with — *continued*
      left ventricular failure (conditions in I50.1- I50.4-) I09.81
      myocarditis, myocardial degeneration (conditions in I51.4) I09.0
      pancarditis I09.9
      pericarditis I09.2
  Rift Valley (viral) A92.4
  Rocky Mountain spotted A77.0
  rose J30.1
  Ross River B33.1
  Russian hemorrhagic A98.5
  San Joaquin (Valley) B38.0
  sandfly A93.1
  Sao Paulo A77.0
  scarlet A38.9
  seven day (leptospirosis) (autumnal) (Japanese) A27.89
    dengue A90
  shin-bone A79.0
  Singapore hemorrhagic A91
  solar A90
  Songo A98.5
  sore B00.1
  South African tick-bite A68.1
  Southeast Asia hemorrhagic A91
  spinal — *see* Meningitis
  spirillary A25.0
  splenic — *see* Anthrax
  spotted A77.9
    American A77.0
    Brazilian A77.0
    cerebrospinal meningitis A39.0
    Colombian A77.0
    due to Rickettsia
      australis A77.3
      conorii A77.1
      rickettsii A77.0
      sibirica A77.2
      specified type NEC A77.8
    Ehrlichiosis A77.40
      due to
        E. chafeensis A77.41
        specified organism NEC A77.49
    Rocky Mountain A77.0
  steroid R50.2
  streptobacillary A25.1
  subtertian B50.9
  Sumatran mite A75.3
  sun A90
  swamp A27.9
  swine A02.8
  sylvatic, yellow A95.0
  Tahyna B33.8
  tertian — *see* Malaria, tertian
  Thailand hemorrhagic A91
  thermic T67.01 ☑
  three-day A93.1
  tick
    American mountain A93.2
    Colorado A93.2
    Kemerovo A93.8
    Mediterranean A77.1
    mountain A93.2
    nonexanthematous A93.2
    Quaranfil A93.8
  tick-bite NEC A93.8
  tick-borne (hemorrhagic) NEC A93.8
  trench A79.0
  tsutsugamushi A75.3
  typhogastric A01.00
  typhoid (abortive) (hemorrhagic) (intermittent) (malignant) A01.00
    complicated by
      arthritis A01.04
      heart involvement A01.02
      meningitis A01.01
      osteomyelitis A01.05
      pneumonia A01.03
      specified NEC A01.09
  typhomalarial — *see* Malaria
  typhus — *see* Typhus (fever)
  undulant — *see* Brucellosis
  unknown origin R50.9
  uveoparotid D86.89
  valley B38.0
  Venezuelan equine A92.2

Fever — *continued*
  vesicular stomatitis A93.8
  viral hemorrhagic — *see* Fever, hemorrhagic, by type of virus
  Volhynian A79.0
  Wesselsbron (viral) A92.8
  West
    African B50.8
    Nile (viral) A92.30
      with
        complications NEC A92.39
        cranial nerve disorders A92.32
        encephalitis A92.31
        encephalomyelitis A92.31
        neurologic manifestation NEC A92.32
        optic neuritis A92.32
        polyradiculitis A92.32
  Whitmore's — *see* Melioidosis
  Wolhynian A79.0
  worm B83.9
  yellow A95.9
    jungle A95.0
    sylvatic A95.0
    urban A95.1
  Zika virus A92.5

Fibrillation
  atrial or auricular (established) I48.91
    chronic I48.20
      persistent I48.19
    paroxysmal I48.0
    permanent I48.21
    persistent (chronic) (NOS) (other) I48.19
      longstanding I48.11
  cardiac I49.8
  heart I49.8
  muscular M62.89
  ventricular I49.01

Fibrin
  ball or bodies, pleural (sac) J94.1
  chamber, anterior (eye) (gelatinous exudate) — *see* Iridocyclitis, acute

Fibrinogenolysis — *see* Fibrinolysis

Fibrinogenopenia D68.8
  acquired D65
  congenital D68.2

Fibrinolysis (hemorrhagic) (acquired) D65
  antepartum hemorrhage — *see* Hemorrhage, antepartum, with coagulation defect
  following
    abortion — *see* Abortion by type complicated by hemorrhage
    ectopic or molar pregnancy O08.1
  intrapartum O67.0
  newborn, transient P60
  postpartum O72.3

Fibrinopenia (hereditary) D68.2
  acquired D68.4

Fibrinopurulent — *see* condition

Fibrinous — *see* condition

Fibroadenoma
  cellular intracanalicular D24- ☑
  giant D24- ☑
  intracanalicular
    cellular D24- ☑
    giant D24- ☑
    specified site — *see* Neoplasm, benign, by site
    unspecified site D24- ☑
  juvenile D24- ☑
  pericanalicular
    specified site — *see* Neoplasm, benign, by site
    unspecified site D24- ☑
  phyllodes D24- ☑
  prostate D29.1
  specified site NEC — *see* Neoplasm, benign, by site
  unspecified site D24- ☑

Fibroadenosis, breast (chronic) (cystic) (diffuse) (periodic) (segmental) N60.2- ☑

Fibroangioma — *see also* Neoplasm, benign, by site
  juvenile
    specified site — *see* Neoplasm, benign, by site
    unspecified site D10.6

Fibrochondrosarcoma — *see* Neoplasm, cartilage, malignant

Fibrocystic
  disease — *see also* Fibrosis, cystic
    breast — *see* Mastopathy, cystic
    jaw M27.49
    kidney (congenital) Q61.8

Fibrocystic — *continued*
  disease — *see also* Fibrosis, cystic — *continued*
    liver Q44.6
    pancreas E84.9
  kidney (congenital) Q61.8
Fibrodysplasia ossificans progressiva — *see* Myositis,
    ossificans, progressiva
Fibroelastosis (cordis) (endocardial) (endomyocardial)
    I42.4
Fibroid (tumor) — *see also* Neoplasm, connective tissue,
    benign
  disease, lung (chronic) — *see* Fibrosis, lung
  heart (disease) — *see* Myocarditis
  in pregnancy or childbirth O34.1- ☑
    causing obstructed labor O65.5
  induration, lung (chronic) — *see* Fibrosis, lung
  lung — *see* Fibrosis, lung
  pneumonia (chronic) — *see* Fibrosis, lung
  uterus — *see also* Leiomyoma, uterus D25.9
Fibrolipoma — *see* Lipoma
Fibroliposarcoma — *see* Neoplasm, connective tissue,
    malignant
Fibroma — *see also* Neoplasm, connective tissue, benign
  ameloblastic — *see* Cyst, calcifying odontogenic
  bone (nonossifying) — *see* Disorder, bone, specified
    type NEC
    ossifying — *see* Neoplasm, bone, benign
  cementifying — *see* Neoplasm, bone, benign
  chondromyxoid — *see* Neoplasm, bone, benign
  desmoplastic — *see* Neoplasm, connective tissue, un-
    certain behavior
  durum — *see* Neoplasm, connective tissue, benign
  fascial — *see* Neoplasm, connective tissue, benign
  invasive — *see* Neoplasm, connective tissue, uncertain
    behavior
  molle — *see* Lipoma
  myxoid — *see* Neoplasm, connective tissue, benign
  nasopharynx, nasopharyngeal (juvenile) D10.6
  nonosteogenic (nonossifying) — *see* Dysplasia, fibrous
  odontogenic (central) — *see* Cyst, calcifying odonto-
    genic
  ossifying — *see* Neoplasm, bone, benign
  periosteal — *see* Neoplasm, bone, benign
  soft — *see* Lipoma
Fibromatosis M72.9
  abdominal — *see* Neoplasm, connective tissue, uncer-
    tain behavior
  aggressive — *see* Neoplasm, connective tissue, uncer-
    tain behavior
  congenital generalized — *see* Neoplasm, connective
    tissue, uncertain behavior
  Dupuytren's M72.0
  gingival K06.1
  palmar (fascial) M72.0
  plantar (fascial) M72.2
  pseudosarcomatous (proliferative) (subcutaneous)
    M72.4
  retroperitoneal D48.3
  specified NEC M72.8
Fibromyalgia M79.7
Fibromyoma — *see also* Neoplasm, connective tissue,
    benign
  uterus (corpus) — *see also* Leiomyoma, uterus
    in pregnancy or childbirth — *see* Fibroid, in preg-
      nancy or childbirth
    causing obstructed labor O65.5
Fibromyositis M79.7
Fibromyxolipoma D17.9
Fibromyxoma — *see* Neoplasm, connective tissue, be-
    nign
Fibromyxosarcoma — *see* Neoplasm, connective tissue,
    malignant
Fibro-odontoma, ameloblastic — *see* Cyst, calcifying
    odontogenic
Fibro-osteoma — *see* Neoplasm, bone, benign
Fibroplasia, retrolental H35.17- ☑
Fibropurulent — *see* condition
Fibrosarcoma — *see also* Neoplasm, connective tissue,
    malignant
  ameloblastic C41.1
    upper jaw (bone) C41.0
  congenital — *see* Neoplasm, connective tissue, malig-
    nant
  fascial — *see* Neoplasm, connective tissue, malignant
  infantile — *see* Neoplasm, connective tissue, malignant
  odontogenic C41.1
    upper jaw (bone) C41.0

Fibrosarcoma — *continued*
  periosteal — *see* Neoplasm, bone, malignant
Fibrosclerosis
  breast N60.3- ☑
  multifocal M35.5
  penis (corpora cavernosa) N48.6
Fibrosis, fibrotic
  adrenal (gland) E27.8
  amnion O41.8X- ☑
  anal papillae K62.89
  arteriocapillary — *see* Arteriosclerosis
  bladder N32.89
    interstitial — *see* Cystitis, chronic, interstitial
    localized submucosal — *see* Cystitis, chronic, inter-
      stitial
    panmural — *see* Cystitis, chronic, interstitial
  breast — *see* Fibrosclerosis, breast
  capillary — *see also* Arteriosclerosis I70.90
    lung (chronic) — *see* Fibrosis, lung
  cardiac — *see* Myocarditis
  cervix N88.8
  chorion O41.8X- ☑
  corpus cavernosum (sclerosing) N48.6
  cystic (of pancreas) E84.9
    with
      distal intestinal obstruction syndrome E84.19
      fecal impaction E84.19
      intestinal manifestations NEC E84.19
      pulmonary manifestations E84.0
      specified manifestations NEC E84.8
  due to device, implant or graft — *see also* Complica-
    tions, by site and type, specified NEC T85.828 ☑
    arterial graft NEC T82.828 ☑
    breast (implant) T85.828 ☑
    catheter NEC T85.828 ☑
      dialysis (renal) T82.828 ☑
        intraperitoneal T85.828 ☑
      infusion NEC T82.828 ☑
        spinal (epidural) (subdural) T85.820 ☑
      urinary (indwelling) T83.82 ☑
    electronic (electrode) (pulse generator) (stimulator)
      bone T84.82 ☑
      cardiac T82.827 ☑
      nervous system (brain) (peripheral nerve) (spinal)
        T85.820 ☑
      urinary T83.82 ☑
    fixation, internal (orthopedic) NEC T84.82 ☑
    gastrointestinal (bile duct) (esophagus) T85.828 ☑
    genital NEC T83.82 ☑
    heart NEC T82.827 ☑
    joint prosthesis T84.82 ☑
    ocular (corneal graft) (orbital implant) NEC
      T85.828 ☑
    orthopedic NEC T84.82 ☑
    specified NEC T85.828 ☑
    urinary NEC T83.82 ☑
    vascular NEC T82.828 ☑
    ventricular intracranial shunt T85.820 ☑
  ejaculatory duct N50.89
  endocardium — *see* Endocarditis
  endomyocardial (tropical) I42.3
  epididymis N50.89
  eye muscle — *see* Strabismus, mechanical
  heart — *see* Myocarditis
  hepatic — *see* Fibrosis, liver
  hepatolienal (portal hypertension) K76.6
  hepatosplenic (portal hypertension) K76.6
  infrapatellar fat pad M79.4
  intrascrotal N50.89
  kidney N26.9
  liver K74.0
    with sclerosis K74.2
    alcoholic K70.2
  lung (atrophic) (chronic) (confluent) (massive) (perialve-
    olar) (peribronchial) J84.10
    with
      anthracosilicosis J60
      anthracosis J60
      asbestosis J61
      bagassosis J67.1
      bauxite J63.1
      berylliosis J63.2
      byssinosis J66.0
      calcicosis J62.8
      chalicosis J62.8
      dust reticulation J64
      farmer's lung J67.0

Fibrosis, fibrotic — *continued*
  lung — *continued*
    with — *continued*
      ganister disease J62.8
      graphite J63.3
      pneumoconiosis NOS J64
      siderosis J63.4
      silicosis J62.8
    capillary J84.10
    congenital P27.8
    diffuse (idiopathic) J84.10
      chemicals, gases, fumes or vapors (inhalation)
        J68.4
    interstitial J84.10
      acute J84.114
      talc J62.0
    following radiation J70.1
    idiopathic J84.112
    postinflammatory J84.10
    silicotic J62.8
    tuberculous — *see* Tuberculosis, pulmonary
  lymphatic gland I89.8
  median bar — *see* Hyperplasia, prostate
  mediastinum (idiopathic) J98.59
  meninges G96.19
  myocardium, myocardial — *see* Myocarditis
  ovary N83.8
  oviduct N83.8
  pancreas K86.89
  penis NEC N48.6
  pericardium I31.0
  perineum, in pregnancy or childbirth O34.7- ☑
    causing obstructed labor O65.5
  pleura J94.1
  popliteal fat pad M79.4
  prostate (chronic) — *see* Hyperplasia, prostate
  pulmonary — *see also* Fibrosis, lung J84.10
    congenital P27.8
    idiopathic J84.112
  rectal sphincter K62.89
  retroperitoneal, idiopathic (with ureteral obstruction)
    N13.5
    with infection N13.6
  sclerosing mesenteric (idiopathic) K65.4
  scrotum N50.89
  seminal vesicle N50.89
  senile R54
  skin L90.5
  spermatic cord N50.89
  spleen D73.89
    in schistosomiasis (bilharziasis) B65.9 *[D77]*
  subepidermal nodular — *see* Neoplasm, skin, benign
  submucous (oral) (tongue) K13.5
  testis N44.8
    chronic, due to syphilis A52.76
  thymus (gland) E32.8
  tongue, submucous K13.5
  tunica vaginalis N50.89
  uterus (non-neoplastic) N85.8
  vagina N89.8
  valve, heart — *see* Endocarditis
  vas deferens N50.89
  vein I87.8
Fibrositis (periarticular) M79.7
  nodular, chronic (Jaccoud's) (rheumatoid) — *see*
    Arthropathy, postrheumatic, chronic
Fibrothorax J94.1
Fibrotic — *see* Fibrosis
Fibrous — *see* condition
Fibroxanthoma — *see also* Neoplasm, connective tissue,
    benign
  atypical — *see* Neoplasm, connective tissue, uncertain
    behavior
  malignant — *see* Neoplasm, connective tissue, malig-
    nant
Fibroxanthosarcoma — *see* Neoplasm, connective tis-
    sue, malignant
Fiedler's
  disease (icterohemorrhagic leptospirosis) A27.0
  myocarditis (acute) I40.1
Fifth disease B08.3
  venereal A55
Filaria, filarial, filariasis — *see* Infestation, filarial
Filatov's disease — *see* Mononucleosis, infectious
File-cutter's disease — *see* Poisoning, lead
Filling defect
  biliary tract R93.2
  bladder R93.41

Filling defect — continued
  duodenum R93.3
  gallbladder R93.2
  gastrointestinal tract R93.3
  intestine R93.3
  kidney R93.42- ☑
  stomach R93.3
  ureter R93.41
  urinary organs, specified NEC R93.49
Fimbrial cyst Q50.4
Financial problem affecting care NOS Z59.9
  bankruptcy Z59.8
  foreclosure on loan Z59.8
Findings, abnormal, inconclusive, without diagnosis
    — see also Abnormal
  17-ketosteroids, elevated R82.5
  acetonuria R82.4
  alcohol in blood R78.0
  anisocytosis R71.8
  antenatal screening of mother O28.9
    biochemical O28.1
    chromosomal O28.5
    cytological O28.2
    genetic O28.5
    hematological O28.0
    radiological O28.4
    specified NEC O28.8
    ultrasonic O28.3
  antibody titer, elevated R76.0
  anticardiolipin antibody R76.0
  antiphosphatidylglycerol antibody R76.0
  antiphosphatidylinositol antibody R76.0
  antiphosphatidylserine antibody R76.0
  antiphospholipid antibody R76.0
  bacteriuria R82.71
  bicarbonate E87.8
  bile in urine R82.2
  blood sugar R73.09
    high R73.9
    low (transient) E16.2
  body fluid or substance, specified NEC R88.8
  casts, urine R82.998
  catecholamines R82.5
  cells, urine R82.998
  chloride E87.8
  cholesterol E78.9
    high E78.00
      with high triglycerides E78.2
  chyluria R82.0
  cloudy
    dialysis effluent R88.0
    urine R82.90
  creatinine clearance R94.4
  crystals, urine R82.998
  culture
    blood R78.81
    positive — see Positive, culture
  echocardiogram R93.1
  electrolyte level, urinary R82.998
  function study NEC R94.8
    bladder R94.8
    endocrine NEC R94.7
      thyroid R94.6
    kidney R94.4
    liver R94.5
    pancreas R94.8
    placenta R94.8
    pulmonary R94.2
    spleen R94.8
  gallbladder, nonvisualization R93.2
  glucose (tolerance test) (non-fasting) R73.09
  glycosuria R81
  heart
    shadow R93.1
    sounds R01.2
  hematinuria R82.3
  hematocrit drop (precipitous) R71.0
  hemoglobinuria R82.3
  human papillomavirus (HPV) DNA test positive
    cervix
      high risk R87.810
      low risk R87.820
    vagina
      high risk R87.811
      low risk R87.821
  in blood (of substance not normally found in blood)
    R78.9
    addictive drug NEC R78.4
    alcohol (excessive level) R78.0

Findings, abnormal, inconclusive, without diagnosis
    — continued
  in blood — continued
    cocaine R78.2
    hallucinogen R78.3
    heavy metals (abnormal level) R78.79
    lead R78.71
    lithium (abnormal level) R78.89
    opiate drug R78.1
    psychotropic drug R78.5
    specified substance NEC R78.89
    steroid agent R78.6
  indoleacetic acid, elevated R82.5
  ketonuria R82.4
  lactic acid dehydrogenase (LDH) R74.0
  liver function test R79.89
  mammogram NEC R92.8
    calcification (calculus) R92.1
    inconclusive result (due to dense breasts) R92.2
    microcalcification R92.0
  mediastinal shift R93.89
  melanin, urine R82.998
  myoglobinuria R82.1
  neonatal screening P09
  nonvisualization of gallbladder R93.2
  odor of urine NOS R82.90
  Papanicolaou cervix R87.619
    non-atypical endometrial cells R87.618
  pneumoencephalogram R93.0
  poikilocytosis R71.8
  potassium (deficiency) E87.6
    excess E87.5
  PPD R76.11
  radiologic (X-ray) R93.89
    abdomen R93.5
    biliary tract R93.2
    breast R92.8
    gastrointestinal tract R93.3
    genitourinary organs R93.89
    head R93.0
    inconclusive due to excess body fat of patient R93.9
    intrathoracic organs NEC R93.1
    musculoskeletal
      limbs R93.6
      other than limb R93.7
    placenta R93.89
    retroperitoneum R93.5
    skin R93.89
    skull R93.0
    subcutaneous tissue R93.89
    testis R93.81- ☑
  red blood cell (count) (morphology) (sickling) (volume)
    R71.8
  scan NEC R94.8
    bladder R94.8
    bone R94.8
    kidney R94.4
    liver R94.2
    lung R94.2
    pancreas R94.8
    placental R94.8
    spleen R94.8
    thyroid R94.6
  sedimentation rate, elevated R70.0
  SGOT R74.0
  SGPT R74.0
  sodium (deficiency) E87.1
    excess E87.0
  specified body fluid NEC R88.8
  stress test R94.39
  testis R93.81- ☑
  thyroid (function) (metabolic rate) (scan) (uptake) R94.6
  transaminase (level) R74.0
  triglycerides E78.9
    high E78.1
      with high cholesterol E78.2
  tuberculin skin test (without active tuberculosis) R76.11
  urine R82.90
    acetone R82.4
    bacteria R82.71
    bile R82.2
    casts or cells R82.998
    chyle R82.0
    culture positive R82.79
    glucose R81
    hemoglobin R82.3
    ketone R82.4
    sugar R81
  vanillylmandelic acid (VMA), elevated R82.5

Findings, abnormal, inconclusive, without diagnosis
    — continued
  vectorcardiogram (VCG) R94.39
  ventriculogram R93.0
  white blood cell (count) (differential) (morphology)
    D72.9
  xerography R92.8
Finger — see condition
Fire, Saint Anthony's — see Erysipelas
Fire-setting
  pathological (compulsive) F63.1
Fish hook stomach K31.89
Fishmeal-worker's lung J67.8
Fissure, fissured
  anus, anal K60.2
    acute K60.0
    chronic K60.1
    congenital Q43.8
  ear, lobule, congenital Q17.8
  epiglottis (congenital) Q31.8
  larynx J38.7
    congenital Q31.8
  lip K13.0
    congenital — see Cleft, lip
  nipple N64.0
    associated with
      lactation O92.13
      pregnancy O92.11- ☑
      puerperium O92.12
  nose Q30.2
  palate (congenital) — see Cleft, palate
  skin R23.4
  spine (congenital) — see also Spina bifida
    with hydrocephalus — see Spina bifida, by site, with
      hydrocephalus
  tongue (acquired) K14.5
    congenital Q38.3
Fistula (cutaneous) L98.8
  abdomen (wall) K63.2
    bladder N32.2
    intestine NEC K63.2
    ureter N28.89
    uterus N82.5
  abdominorectal K63.2
  abdominosigmoidal K63.2
  abdominothoracic J86.0
  abdominouterine N82.5
    congenital Q51.7
  abdominovesical N32.2
  accessory sinuses — see Sinusitis
  actinomycotic — see Actinomycosis
  alveolar antrum — see Sinusitis, maxillary
  alveolar process K04.6
  anorectal K60.5
  antrobuccal — see Sinusitis, maxillary
  antrum — see Sinusitis, maxillary
  anus, anal (recurrent) (infectional) K60.3
    congenital Q43.6
      with absence, atresia and stenosis Q42.2
    tuberculous A18.32
  aorta-duodenal I77.2
  appendix, appendicular K38.3
  arteriovenous (acquired) (nonruptured) I77.0
    brain I67.1
      congenital Q28.2
        ruptured — see Fistula, arteriovenous, brain,
          ruptured
      ruptured I60.8
        intracerebral I61.8
        intraparenchymal I61.8
        intraventricular I61.5
        subarachnoid I60.8
    cerebral — see Fistula, arteriovenous, brain
    congenital (peripheral) — see also Malformation,
      arteriovenous
      brain Q28.2
        ruptured — see Fistula, arteriovenous, brain,
          ruptured
      coronary Q24.5
      pulmonary Q25.72
    coronary I25.41
      congenital Q24.5
    pulmonary I28.0
      congenital Q25.72
    surgically created (for dialysis) Z99.2
      complication — see Complication, arteriovenous,
        fistula, surgically created
    traumatic — see Injury, blood vessel

☑ Additional Character Required — Refer to the Tabular List for Character Selection   ▽ Subterms under main terms may continue to next column or page

Fistula — *continued*
artery I77.2
aural (mastoid) — *see* Mastoiditis, chronic
auricle — *see also* Disorder, pinna, specified type NEC
   congenital Q18.1
Bartholin's gland N82.8
bile duct (common) (hepatic) K83.3
   with calculus, stones — *see* Calculus, bile duct
biliary (tract) — *see* Fistula, bile duct
bladder (sphincter) NEC — *see also* Fistula, vesico-
   N32.2
   into seminal vesicle N32.2
bone — *see also* Disorder, bone, specified type NEC
   with osteomyelitis, chronic — *see* Osteomyelitis,
      chronic, with draining sinus
brain G93.89
   arteriovenous (acquired) — *see also* Fistula, arteri-
      ovenous, brain I67.1
      congenital Q28.2
branchial (cleft) Q18.0
branchiogenous Q18.0
breast N61.0
   puerperal, postpartum or gestational, due to mastitis
      (purulent) — *see* Mastitis, obstetric, purulent
bronchial J86.0
bronchocutaneous, bronchomediastinal, bronchopleural, bronchopleuromediastinal (infective) J86.0
   tuberculous NEC A15.5
bronchoesophageal J86.0
   congenital Q39.2
      with atresia of esophagus Q39.1
bronchovisceral J86.0
buccal cavity (infective) K12.2
cecosigmoidal K63.2
cecum K63.2
cerebrospinal (fluid) G96.0
cervical, lateral Q18.1
cervicoaural Q18.1
cervicosigmoidal N82.4
cervicovesical N82.1
cervix N82.8
chest (wall) J86.0
cholecystenteric — *see* Fistula, gallbladder
cholecystocolic — *see* Fistula, gallbladder
cholecystocolonic — *see* Fistula, gallbladder
cholecystoduodenal — *see* Fistula, gallbladder
cholecystogastric — *see* Fistula, gallbladder
cholecystointestinal — *see* Fistula, gallbladder
choledochoduodenal — *see* Fistula, bile duct
cholocolic K82.3
coccyx — *see* Sinus, pilonidal
colon K63.2
colostomy K94.09
colovesical N32.1
common duct — *see* Fistula, bile duct
congenital, site not listed — *see* Anomaly, by site
coronary, arteriovenous I25.41
   congenital Q24.5
costal region J86.0
cul-de-sac, Douglas' N82.8
cystic duct — *see also* Fistula, gallbladder
   congenital Q44.5
dental K04.6
diaphragm J86.0
duodenum K31.6
ear (external) (canal) — *see* Disorder, ear, external,
   specified type NEC
enterocolic K63.2
enterocutaneous K63.2
enterouterine N82.4
   congenital Q51.7
enterovaginal N82.4
   congenital Q52.2
   large intestine N82.3
   small intestine N82.2
enterovesical N32.1
epididymis N50.89
   tuberculous A18.15
esophagobronchial J86.0
   congenital Q39.2
      with atresia of esophagus Q39.1
esophagocutaneous K22.8
esophagopleural-cutaneous J86.0
esophagotracheal J86.0
   congenital Q39.2
      with atresia of esophagus Q39.1
esophagus K22.8
   congenital Q39.2

Fistula — *continued*
esophagus — *continued*
   congenital — *continued*
      with atresia of esophagus Q39.1
ethmoid — *see* Sinusitis, ethmoidal
eyeball (cornea) (sclera) — *see* Disorder, globe, hypotony
eyelid H01.8
fallopian tube, external N82.5
fecal K63.2
   congenital Q43.6
from periapical abscess K04.6
frontal sinus — *see* Sinusitis, frontal
gallbladder K82.3
   with calculus, cholelithiasis, stones — *see* Calculus,
      gallbladder
gastric K31.6
gastrocolic K31.6
   congenital Q40.2
   tuberculous A18.32
gastroenterocolic K31.6
gastroesophageal K31.6
gastrojejunal K31.6
gastrojejunocolic K31.6
genital tract (female) N82.9
   specified NEC N82.8
   to intestine NEC N82.4
   to skin N82.5
hepatic artery-portal vein, congenital Q26.6
hepatopleural J86.0
hepatopulmonary J86.0
ileorectal or ileosigmoidal K63.2
ileovaginal N82.2
ileovesical N32.1
ileum K63.2
in ano K60.3
   tuberculous A18.32
inner ear (labyrinth) — *see* subcategory H83.1 ☑
intestine NEC K63.2
intestinocolonic (abdominal) K63.2
intestinoureteral N28.89
intestinouterine N82.4
intestinovaginal N82.4
   large intestine N82.3
   small intestine N82.2
intestinovesical N32.1
ischiorectal (fossa) K61.39
jejunum K63.2
joint M25.10
   ankle M25.17- ☑
   elbow M25.12- ☑
   foot joint M25.17- ☑
   hand joint M25.14- ☑
   hip M25.15- ☑
   knee M25.16- ☑
   shoulder M25.11- ☑
   specified joint NEC M25.18
   tuberculous — *see* Tuberculosis, joint
   vertebrae M25.18
   wrist M25.13- ☑
kidney N28.89
labium (majus) (minus) N82.8
labyrinth — *see* subcategory H83.1 ☑
lacrimal (gland) (sac) H04.61-
lacrimonasal duct — *see* Fistula, lacrimal
laryngotracheal, congenital Q34.8
larynx J38.7
lip K13.0
   congenital Q38.0
lumbar, tuberculous A18.01
lung J86.0
lymphatic I89.8
mammary (gland) N61.0
mastoid (process) (region) — *see* Mastoiditis, chronic
maxillary J32.0
medial, face and neck Q18.8
mediastinal J86.0
mediastinobronchial J86.0
mediastinocutaneous J86.0
middle ear — *see* subcategory H74.8 ☑
mouth K12.2
nasal J34.89
   sinus — *see* Sinusitis
nasopharynx J39.2
nipple N64.0
nose J34.89
oral (cutaneous) K12.2
   maxillary J32.0

Fistula — *continued*
oral — *continued*
   nasal (with cleft palate) — *see* Cleft, palate
orbit, orbital — *see* Disorder, orbit, specified type NEC
oroantral J32.0
oviduct, external N82.5
palate (hard) M27.8
pancreatic K86.89
pancreaticoduodenal K86.89
parotid (gland) K11.4
   region K12.2
penis N48.89
perianal K60.3
pericardium (pleura) (sac) — *see* Pericarditis
pericecal K63.2
perineorectal K60.4
perineosigmoidal K63.2
perineum, perineal (with urethral involvement) NEC
   N36.0
   tuberculous A18.13
   ureter N28.89
perirectal K60.4
   tuberculous A18.32
peritoneum K65.9
pharyngoesophageal J39.2
pharynx J39.2
   branchial cleft (congenital) Q18.0
pilonidal (infected) (rectum) — *see* Sinus, pilonidal
pleura, pleural, pleurocutaneous, pleuroperitoneal
   J86.0
   tuberculous NEC A15.6
pleuropericardial I31.8
portal vein-hepatic artery, congenital Q26.6
postauricular H70.81-
postoperative, persistent T81.83 ☑
   specified site — *see* Fistula, by site
preauricular (congenital) Q18.1
prostate N42.89
pulmonary J86.0
   arteriovenous I28.0
      congenital Q25.72
   tuberculous — *see* Tuberculosis, pulmonary
pulmonoperitoneal J86.0
rectolabial N82.4
rectosigmoid (intercommunicating) K63.2
rectoureteral N28.89
rectourethral N36.0
   congenital Q64.73
rectouterine N82.4
   congenital Q51.7
rectovaginal N82.3
   congenital Q52.2
   tuberculous A18.18
rectovesical N32.1
   congenital Q64.79
rectovesicovaginal N82.3
rectovulval N82.4
   congenital Q52.79
rectum (to skin) K60.4
   congenital Q43.6
      with absence, atresia and stenosis Q42.0
   tuberculous A18.32
renal N28.89
retroauricular — *see* Fistula, postauricular
salivary duct or gland (any) K11.4
   congenital Q38.4
scrotum (urinary) N50.89
   tuberculous A18.15
semicircular canals — *see* subcategory H83.1 ☑
sigmoid K63.2
   to bladder N32.1
sinus — *see* Sinusitis
skin L98.8
   to genital tract (female) N82.5
splenocolic D73.89
stercoral K63.2
stomach K31.6
sublingual gland K11.4
submandibular gland K11.4
submaxillary (gland) K11.4
   region K12.2
thoracic J86.0
   duct I89.8
thoracoabdominal J86.0
thoracogastric J86.0
thoracointestinal J86.0
thorax J86.0
thyroglossal duct Q89.2

Index

Fistula — Fluctuating blood pressure

Fistula — *continued*
thyroid E07.89
trachea, congenital (external) (internal) Q32.1
tracheoesophageal J86.0
  congenital Q39.2
    with atresia of esophagus Q39.1
  following tracheostomy J95.04
traumatic arteriovenous — *see* Injury, blood vessel, by site
tuberculous — *code by* site under Tuberculosis
typhoid A01.09
umbilicourinary Q64.8
urachus, congenital Q64.4
ureter (persistent) N28.89
ureteroabdominal N28.89
ureterorectal N28.89
ureterosigmoido-abdominal N28.89
ureterovaginal N82.1
ureterovesical N32.2
urethra N36.0
  congenital Q64.79
  tuberculous A18.13
urethroperineal N36.0
urethroperineovesical N32.2
urethrorectal N36.0
  congenital Q64.73
urethroscrotal N50.89
urethrovaginal N82.1
urethrovesical N32.2
urinary (tract) (persistent) (recurrent) N36.0
uteroabdominal N82.5
  congenital Q51.7
uteroenteric, uterointestinal N82.4
  congenital Q51.7
uterorectal N82.4
  congenital Q51.7
uteroureteric N82.1
uterourethral Q51.7
uterovaginal N82.8
uterovesical N82.1
  congenital Q51.7
uterus N82.8
vagina (postpartal) (wall) N82.8
vaginocutaneous (postpartal) N82.5
vaginointestinal NEC N82.4
  large intestine N82.3
  small intestine N82.2
vaginoperineal N82.5
vasocutaneous, congenital Q55.7
vesical NEC N32.2
vesicoabdominal N32.2
vesicocervicovaginal N82.1
vesicocolic N32.1
vesicocutaneous N32.2
vesicoenteric N32.1
vesicointestinal N32.1
vesicometrorectal N82.4
vesicoperineal N32.2
vesicorectal N32.1
  congenital Q64.79
vesicosigmoidal N32.1
vesicosigmoidovaginal N82.3
vesicoureteral N82.1
vesicoureterovaginal N82.1
vesicourethral N32.2
vesicourethrorectal N32.1
vesicouterine N82.1
  congenital Q51.7
vesicovaginal N82.0
vulvorectal N82.4
  congenital Q52.79
Fit R56.9
epileptic — *see* Epilepsy
fainting R55
hysterical F44.5
newborn P90
Fitting (and adjustment) (of)
artificial
  arm — *see* Admission, adjustment, artificial, arm
  breast Z44.3 ☑
  eye Z44.2 ☑
  leg — *see* Admission, adjustment, artificial, leg
automatic implantable cardiac defibrillator (with synchronous cardiac pacemaker) Z45.02
brain neuropacemaker Z46.2
  implanted Z45.42
cardiac defibrillator — *see* Fitting (and adjustment) (of), automatic implantable cardiac defibrillator

Fitting — *continued*
catheter, non-vascular Z46.82
colostomy belt Z46.89
contact lenses Z46.0
CRT-D (resynchronization therapy defibrillator) Z45.02
CRT-P (cardiac resynchronization therapy pacemaker) Z45.018
  pulse generator Z45.010
cystostomy device Z46.6
defibrillator, cardiac — *see* Fitting (and adjustment) (of), automatic implantable cardiac defibrillator
dentures Z46.3
device NOS Z46.9
  abdominal Z46.89
  gastrointestinal NEC Z46.59
  implanted NEC Z45.89
  nervous system Z46.2
    implanted — *see* Admission, adjustment, device, implanted, nervous system
  orthodontic Z46.4
  orthoptic Z46.0
  orthotic Z46.89
  prosthetic (external) Z44.9
    breast Z44.3 ☑
    dental Z46.3
    eye Z44.2 ☑
    specified NEC Z44.8
  specified NEC Z46.89
  substitution
    auditory Z46.2
      implanted — *see* Admission, adjustment, device, implanted, hearing device
    nervous system Z46.2
      implanted — *see* Admission, adjustment, device, implanted, nervous system
    visual Z46.2
      implanted Z45.31
    urinary Z46.6
gastric lap band Z46.51
gastrointestinal appliance NEC Z46.59
glasses (reading) Z46.0
hearing aid Z46.1
ileostomy device Z46.89
insulin pump Z46.81
intestinal appliance NEC Z46.89
myringotomy device (stent) (tube) Z45.82
neuropacemaker Z46.2
  implanted Z45.42
non-vascular catheter Z46.82
orthodontic device Z46.4
orthopedic device (brace) (cast) (corset) (shoes) Z46.89
pacemaker (cardiac) (cardiac resynchronization therapy (CRT-P)) Z45.018
  nervous system (brain) (peripheral nerve) (spinal cord) Z46.2
    implanted Z45.42
  pulse generator Z45.010
portacath (port-a-cath) Z45.2
prosthesis (external) Z44.9
  arm — *see* Admission, adjustment, artificial, arm
  breast Z44.3 ☑
  dental Z46.3
  eye Z44.2 ☑
  leg — *see* Admission, adjustment, artificial, leg
  specified NEC Z44.8
spectacles Z46.0
wheelchair Z46.89
Fitzhugh-Curtis syndrome
due to
  Chlamydia trachomatis A74.81
  Neisseria gonorrhorea (gonococcal peritonitis) A54.85
Fitz's syndrome (acute hemorrhagic pancreatitis) — *see also* Pancreatitis, acute K85.80
Fixation
joint — *see* Ankylosis
larynx J38.7
stapes — *see* Ankylosis, ear ossicles
  deafness — *see* Deafness, conductive
uterus (acquired) — *see* Malposition, uterus
vocal cord J38.3
Flabby ridge K06.8
Flaccid — *see also* condition
palate, congenital Q38.5
Flail
chest S22.5 ☑
  newborn (birth injury) P13.8
joint (paralytic) M25.20

Flail — *continued*
joint — *continued*
  ankle M25.27- ☑
  elbow M25.22- ☑
  foot joint M25.27- ☑
  hand joint M25.24- ☑
  hip M25.25- ☑
  knee M25.26- ☑
  shoulder M25.21- ☑
  specified joint NEC M25.28
  wrist M25.23- ☑
Flajani's disease — *see* Hyperthyroidism, with, goiter (diffuse)
Flap, liver K71.3
Flashbacks (residual to hallucinogen use) F16.283
Flat
chamber (eye) — *see* Disorder, globe, hypotony, flat anterior chamber
chest, congenital Q67.8
foot (acquired) (fixed type) (painful) (postural) — *see also* Deformity, limb, flat foot
  congenital (rigid) (spastic (everted)) Q66.5- ☑
  rachitic sequelae (late effect) E64.3
organ or site, congenital NEC — *see* Anomaly, by site
pelvis M95.5
  with disproportion (fetopelvic) O33.0
    causing obstructed labor O65.0
  congenital Q74.2
Flatau-Schilder disease G37.0
Flatback syndrome M40.30
lumbar region M40.36
lumbosacral region M40.37
thoracolumbar region M40.35
Flattening
head, femur M89.8X5
hip — *see* Coxa, plana
lip (congenital) Q18.8
nose (congenital) Q67.4
  acquired M95.0
Flatulence R14.3
psychogenic F45.8
Flatus R14.3
vaginalis N89.8
Flax-dresser's disease J66.1
Flea bite — *see* Injury, bite, by site, superficial, insect
Flecks, glaucomatous (subcapsular) — *see* Cataract, complicated
Fleischer (-Kayser) **ring** (cornea) H18.04- ☑
Fleshy mole O02.0
Flexibilitas cerea — *see* Catalepsy
Flexion
amputation stump (surgical) T87.89
cervix — *see* Malposition, uterus
contracture, joint — *see* Contraction, joint
deformity, joint — *see also* Deformity, limb, flexion M21.20
  hip, congenital Q65.89
uterus — *see also* Malposition, uterus
  lateral — *see* Lateroversion, uterus
Flexner-Boyd dysentery A03.2
Flexner's dysentery A03.1
Flexure — *see* Flexion
Flint murmur (aortic insufficiency) I35.1
Floater, vitreous — *see* Opacity, vitreous
Floating
cartilage (joint) — *see also* Loose, body, joint
  knee — *see* Derangement, knee, loose body
gallbladder, congenital Q44.1
kidney N28.89
  congenital Q63.8
spleen D73.89
Flooding N92.0
Floor — *see* condition
Floppy
baby syndrome (nonspecific) P94.2
iris syndrome (intraoperative) (IFIS) H21.81
nonrheumatic mitral valve syndrome I34.1
Flu — *see also* Influenza
avian — *see also* Influenza, due to, identified novel influenza A virus J09.X2
bird — *see also* Influenza, due to, identified novel influenza A virus J09.X2
intestinal NEC A08.4
swine (viruses that normally cause infections in pigs) — *see also* Influenza, due to, identified novel influenza A virus J09.X2
Fluctuating blood pressure I99.8

☑ **Additional Character Required** — **Refer to the Tabular List for Character Selection**   ▽ **Subterms under main terms may continue to next column or page**

Fluid
- abdomen R18.8
- chest J94.8
- heart — *see* Failure, heart, congestive
- joint — *see* Effusion, joint
- loss (acute) E86.9
- lung — *see* Edema, lung
- overload E87.70
  - specified NEC E87.79
- peritoneal cavity R18.8
- pleural cavity J94.8
- retention R60.9

Flukes NEC — *see also* Infestation, fluke
- blood NEC — *see* Schistosomiasis
- liver B66.3

Fluor (vaginalis) N89.8
- trichomonal or due to Trichomonas (vaginalis) A59.00

Fluorosis
- dental K00.3
- skeletal M85.10
  - ankle M85.17- ☑
  - foot M85.17- ☑
  - forearm M85.13- ☑
  - hand M85.14- ☑
  - lower leg M85.16- ☑
  - multiple site M85.19
  - neck M85.18
  - rib M85.18
  - shoulder M85.11- ☑
  - skull M85.18
  - specified site NEC M85.18
  - thigh M85.15- ☑
  - toe M85.17- ☑
  - upper arm M85.12- ☑
  - vertebra M85.18

Flush syndrome E34.0

Flushing R23.2
- menopausal N95.1

Flutter
- atrial or auricular I48.92
  - atypical I48.4
  - type I I48.3
  - type II I48.4
  - typical I48.3
- heart I49.8
  - atrial or auricular I48.92
    - atypical I48.4
    - type I I48.3
    - type II I48.4
    - typical I48.3
  - ventricular I49.02
- ventricular I49.02

FNHTR (febrile nonhemolytic transfusion reaction) R50.84

Fochier's abscess — *code by* site under Abscess

Focus, Assmann's — *see* Tuberculosis, pulmonary

Fogo selvagem L10.3

Foix-Alajouanine syndrome G95.19

Fold, folds (anomalous) — *see also* Anomaly, by site
- Descemet's membrane — *see* Change, corneal membrane, Descemet's, fold
- epicanthic Q10.3
- heart Q24.8

Folie à deux F24

Follicle
- cervix (nabothian) (ruptured) N88.8
- graafian, ruptured, with hemorrhage N83.0- ☑
- nabothian N88.8

Follicular — *see* condition

Folliculitis (superficial) L73.9
- abscedens et suffodiens L66.3
- cyst N83.0- ☑
- decalvans L66.2
- deep — *see* Furuncle, by site
- gonococcal (acute) (chronic) A54.01
- keloid, keloidalis L73.0
- pustular L01.02
- ulerythematosa reticulata L66.4

Folliculome lipidique
- specified site — *see* Neoplasm, benign, by site
- unspecified site
  - female D27.9
  - male D29.20

Følling's disease E70.0

Follow-up — *see* Examination, follow-up

Fong's syndrome (hereditary osteo-onychodysplasia) Q87.2

Food
- allergy L27.2
- asphyxia (from aspiration or inhalation) — *see* Foreign body, by site
- choked on — *see* Foreign body, by site
- deprivation T73.0 ☑
  - specified kind of food NEC E63.8
- intoxication — *see* Poisoning, food
- lack of T73.0 ☑
- poisoning — *see* Poisoning, food
- rejection NEC — *see* Disorder, eating
- strangulation or suffocation — *see* Foreign body, by site
- toxemia — *see* Poisoning, food

Foot — *see* condition

Foramen ovale (nonclosure) (patent) (persistent) Q21.1

Forbes' glycogen storage disease E74.03

Fordyce-Fox disease L75.2

Fordyce's disease (mouth) Q38.6

Forearm — *see* condition

Foreign body
- with
  - laceration — *see* Laceration, by site, with foreign body
  - puncture wound — *see* Puncture, by site, with foreign body
- accidentally left following a procedure T81.509 ☑
  - aspiration T81.506 ☑
    - resulting in
      - adhesions T81.516 ☑
      - obstruction T81.526 ☑
      - perforation T81.536 ☑
      - specified complication NEC T81.596 ☑
  - cardiac catheterization T81.505 ☑
    - resulting in
      - acute reaction T81.60 ☑
        - aseptic peritonitis T81.61 ☑
        - specified NEC T81.69 ☑
      - adhesions T81.515 ☑
      - obstruction T81.525 ☑
      - perforation T81.535 ☑
      - specified complication NEC T81.595 ☑
    - causing
      - acute reaction T81.60 ☑
        - aseptic peritonitis T81.61 ☑
        - specified complication NEC T81.69 ☑
      - adhesions T81.519 ☑
      - aseptic peritonitis T81.61 ☑
      - obstruction T81.529 ☑
      - perforation T81.539 ☑
      - specified complication NEC T81.599 ☑
  - endoscopy T81.504 ☑
    - resulting in
      - adhesions T81.514 ☑
      - obstruction T81.524 ☑
      - perforation T81.534 ☑
      - specified complication NEC T81.594 ☑
  - immunization T81.503 ☑
    - resulting in
      - adhesions T81.513 ☑
      - obstruction T81.523 ☑
      - perforation T81.533 ☑
      - specified complication NEC T81.593 ☑
  - infusion T81.501 ☑
    - resulting in
      - adhesions T81.511 ☑
      - obstruction T81.521 ☑
      - perforation T81.531 ☑
      - specified complication NEC T81.591 ☑
  - injection T81.503 ☑
    - resulting in
      - adhesions T81.513 ☑
      - obstruction T81.523 ☑
      - perforation T81.533 ☑
      - specified complication NEC T81.593 ☑
  - kidney dialysis T81.502 ☑
    - resulting in
      - adhesions T81.512 ☑
      - obstruction T81.522 ☑
      - perforation T81.532 ☑
      - specified complication NEC T81.592 ☑
  - packing removal T81.507 ☑
    - resulting in
      - acute reaction T81.60 ☑
        - aseptic peritonitis T81.61 ☑
        - specified NEC T81.69 ☑

Foreign body — *continued*
- accidentally left following a procedure — *continued*
  - packing removal — *continued*
    - resulting in — *continued*
      - adhesions T81.517 ☑
      - obstruction T81.527 ☑
      - perforation T81.537 ☑
      - specified complication NEC T81.597 ☑
  - puncture T81.506 ☑
    - resulting in
      - adhesions T81.516 ☑
      - obstruction T81.526 ☑
      - perforation T81.536 ☑
      - specified complication NEC T81.596 ☑
  - specified procedure NEC T81.508 ☑
    - resulting in
      - acute reaction T81.60 ☑
        - aseptic peritonitis T81.61 ☑
        - specified NEC T81.69 ☑
      - adhesions T81.518 ☑
      - obstruction T81.528 ☑
      - perforation T81.538 ☑
      - specified complication NEC T81.598 ☑
  - surgical operation T81.500 ☑
    - resulting in
      - acute reaction T81.60 ☑
        - aseptic peritonitis T81.61 ☑
        - specified NEC T81.69 ☑
      - adhesions T81.510 ☑
      - obstruction T81.520 ☑
      - perforation T81.530 ☑
      - specified complication NEC T81.590 ☑
  - transfusion T81.501 ☑
    - resulting in
      - adhesions T81.511 ☑
      - obstruction T81.521 ☑
      - perforation T81.531 ☑
      - specified complication NEC T81.591 ☑
- alimentary tract T18.9 ☑
  - anus T18.5 ☑
  - colon T18.4 ☑
  - esophagus — *see* Foreign body, esophagus
  - mouth T18.0 ☑
  - multiple sites T18.8 ☑
  - rectosigmoid (junction) T18.5 ☑
  - rectum T18.5 ☑
  - small intestine T18.3 ☑
  - specified site NEC T18.8 ☑
  - stomach T18.2 ☑
- anterior chamber (eye) S05.5- ☑
- auditory canal — *see* Foreign body, entering through orifice, ear
- bronchus T17.508 ☑
  - causing
    - asphyxiation T17.500 ☑
      - food (bone) (seed) T17.520 ☑
      - gastric contents (vomitus) T17.510 ☑
      - specified type NEC T17.590 ☑
    - injury NEC T17.508 ☑
      - food (bone) (seed) T17.528 ☑
      - gastric contents (vomitus) T17.518 ☑
      - specified type NEC T17.598 ☑
- canthus — *see* Foreign body, conjunctival sac
- ciliary body (eye) S05.5- ☑
- conjunctival sac T15.1- ☑
- cornea T15.0- ☑
- entering through orifice
  - accessory sinus T17.0 ☑
  - alimentary canal T18.9 ☑
    - multiple parts T18.8 ☑
    - specified part NEC T18.8 ☑
  - alveolar process T18.0 ☑
  - antrum (Highmore's) T17.0 ☑
  - anus T18.5 ☑
  - appendix T18.4 ☑
  - auditory canal — *see* Foreign body, entering through orifice, ear
  - auricle — *see* Foreign body, entering through orifice, ear
  - bladder T19.1 ☑
  - bronchioles — *see* Foreign body, respiratory tract, specified site NEC
  - bronchus (main) — *see* Foreign body, bronchus
  - buccal cavity T18.0 ☑
  - canthus (inner) — *see* Foreign body, conjunctival sac

Foreign body — *continued*
  entering through orifice — *continued*
    cecum T18.4 ☑
    cervix (canal) (uteri) T19.3 ☑
    colon T18.4 ☑
    conjunctival sac — *see* Foreign body, conjunctival sac
    cornea — *see* Foreign body, cornea
    digestive organ or tract NOS T18.9 ☑
      multiple parts T18.8 ☑
      specified part NEC T18.8 ☑
    duodenum T18.3 ☑
    ear (external) T16.-
    esophagus — *see* Foreign body, esophagus
    eye (external) NOS T15.9- ☑
      conjunctival sac — *see* Foreign body, conjunctival sac
      cornea — *see* Foreign body, cornea
      specified part NEC T15.8- ☑
    eyeball — *see also* Foreign body, entering through orifice, eye, specified part NEC
      with penetrating wound — *see* Puncture, eyeball
    eyelid — *see also* Foreign body, conjunctival sac
      with
        laceration — *see* Laceration, eyelid, with foreign body
        puncture — *see* Puncture, eyelid, with foreign body
        superficial injury — *see* Foreign body, superficial, eyelid
    gastrointestinal tract T18.9 ☑
      multiple parts T18.8 ☑
      specified part NEC T18.8 ☑
    genitourinary tract T19.9 ☑
      multiple parts T19.8 ☑
      specified part NEC T19.8 ☑
    globe — *see* Foreign body, entering through orifice, eyeball
    gum T18.0 ☑
    Highmore's antrum T17.0 ☑
    hypopharynx — *see* Foreign body, pharynx
    ileum T18.3 ☑
    intestine (small) T18.3 ☑
      large T18.4 ☑
    lacrimal apparatus (punctum) — *see* Foreign body, entering through orifice, eye, specified part NEC
    large intestine T18.4 ☑
    larynx — *see* Foreign body, larynx
    lung — *see* Foreign body, respiratory tract, specified site NEC
    maxillary sinus T17.0 ☑
    mouth T18.0 ☑
    nasal sinus T17.0 ☑
    nasopharynx — *see* Foreign body, pharynx
    nose (passage) T17.1 ☑
    nostril T17.1 ☑
    oral cavity T18.0 ☑
    palate T18.0 ☑
    penis T19.4 ☑
    pharynx — *see* Foreign body, pharynx
    piriform sinus — *see* Foreign body, pharynx
    rectosigmoid (junction) T18.5 ☑
    rectum T18.5 ☑
    respiratory tract — *see* Foreign body, respiratory tract
    sinus (accessory) (frontal) (maxillary) (nasal) T17.0 ☑
      piriform — *see* Foreign body, pharynx
    small intestine T18.3 ☑
    stomach T18.2 ☑
    suffocation by — *see* Foreign body, by site
    tear ducts or glands — *see* Foreign body, entering through orifice, eye, specified part NEC
    throat — *see* Foreign body, pharynx
    tongue T18.0 ☑
    tonsil, tonsillar (fossa) — *see* Foreign body, pharynx
    trachea — *see* Foreign body, trachea
    ureter T19.8 ☑
    urethra T19.0 ☑
    uterus (any part) T19.3 ☑
    vagina T19.2 ☑
    vulva T19.2 ☑
  esophagus T18.108 ☑
    causing
      injury NEC T18.108 ☑
        food (bone) (seed) T18.128 ☑

Foreign body — *continued*
  esophagus — *continued*
    causing — *continued*
      injury — *continued*
        gastric contents (vomitus) T18.118 ☑
        specified type NEC T18.198 ☑
        tracheal compression T18.100 ☑
          food (bone) (seed) T18.120 ☑
          gastric contents (vomitus) T18.110 ☑
          specified type NEC T18.190 ☑
  feeling of, in throat R09.89
  fragment — *see* Retained, foreign body fragments (type of)
  genitourinary tract T19.9 ☑
    bladder T19.1 ☑
    multiple parts T19.8 ☑
    penis T19.4 ☑
    specified site NEC T19.8 ☑
    urethra T19.0 ☑
    uterus T19.3 ☑
      IUD Z97.5
    vagina T19.2 ☑
      contraceptive device Z97.5
    vulva T19.2 ☑
  granuloma (old) (soft tissue) — *see also* Granuloma, foreign body
    skin L92.3
  in
    laceration — *see* Laceration, by site, with foreign body
    puncture wound — *see* Puncture, by site, with foreign body
    soft tissue (residual) M79.5
  inadvertently left in operation wound — *see* Foreign body, accidentally left during a procedure
  ingestion, ingested NOS T18.9 ☑
  inhalation or inspiration — *see* Foreign body, by site
  internal organ, not entering through a natural orifice — code as specific injury with foreign body
  intraocular S05.5- ☑
    old, retained (nonmagnetic) H44.70- ☑
      anterior chamber H44.71- ☑
      ciliary body H44.72- ☑
      iris H44.72- ☑
      lens H44.73- ☑
      magnetic H44.60- ☑
        anterior chamber H44.61- ☑
        ciliary body H44.62- ☑
        iris H44.62- ☑
        lens H44.63- ☑
        posterior wall H44.64- ☑
        specified site NEC H44.69- ☑
        vitreous body H44.65- ☑
      posterior wall H44.74- ☑
      specified site NEC H44.79- ☑
      vitreous body H44.75- ☑
  iris — *see* Foreign body, intraocular
  lacrimal punctum — *see* Foreign body, entering through orifice, eye, specified part NEC
  larynx T17.308 ☑
    causing
      asphyxiation T17.300 ☑
        food (bone) (seed) T17.320 ☑
        gastric contents (vomitus) T17.310 ☑
        specified type NEC T17.390 ☑
      injury NEC T17.308 ☑
        food (bone) (seed) T17.328 ☑
        gastric contents (vomitus) T17.318 ☑
        specified type NEC T17.398 ☑
  lens — *see* Foreign body, intraocular
  ocular muscle S05.4- ☑
    old, retained — *see* Foreign body, orbit, old
  old or residual
    soft tissue (residual) M79.5
  operation wound, left accidentally — *see* Foreign body, accidentally left during a procedure
  orbit S05.4- ☑
    old, retained H05.5- ☑
  pharynx T17.208 ☑
    causing
      asphyxiation T17.200 ☑
        food (bone) (seed) T17.220 ☑
        gastric contents (vomitus) T17.210 ☑
        specified type NEC T17.290 ☑
      injury NEC T17.208 ☑
        food (bone) (seed) T17.228 ☑

Foreign body — *continued*
  pharynx — *continued*
    causing — *continued*
      injury — *continued*
        gastric contents (vomitus) T17.218 ☑
        specified type NEC T17.298 ☑
  respiratory tract T17.908 ☑
    bronchioles — *see* Foreign body, respiratory tract, specified site NEC
    bronchus — *see* Foreign body, bronchus
    causing
      asphyxiation T17.900 ☑
        food (bone) (seed) T17.920 ☑
        gastric contents (vomitus) T17.910 ☑
        specified type NEC T17.990 ☑
      injury NEC T17.908 ☑
        food (bone) (seed) T17.928 ☑
        gastric contents (vomitus) T17.918 ☑
        specified type NEC T17.998 ☑
    larynx — *see* Foreign body, larynx
    lung — *see* Foreign body, respiratory tract, specified site NEC
    multiple parts — *see* Foreign body, respiratory tract, specified site NEC
    nasal sinus T17.0 ☑
    nasopharynx — *see* Foreign body, pharynx
    nose T17.1 ☑
    nostril T17.1 ☑
    pharynx — *see* Foreign body, pharynx
    specified site NEC T17.808 ☑
      causing
        asphyxiation T17.800 ☑
          food (bone) (seed) T17.820 ☑
          gastric contents (vomitus) T17.810 ☑
          specified type NEC T17.890 ☑
        injury NEC T17.808 ☑
          food (bone) (seed) T17.828 ☑
          gastric contents (vomitus) T17.818 ☑
          specified type NEC T17.898 ☑
    throat — *see* Foreign body, pharynx
    trachea — *see* Foreign body, trachea
  retained (old) (nonmagnetic) (in)
    anterior chamber (eye) — *see* Foreign body, intraocular, old, retained, anterior chamber
      magnetic — *see* Foreign body, intraocular, old, retained, magnetic, anterior chamber
    ciliary body — *see* Foreign body, intraocular, old, retained, ciliary body
      magnetic — *see* Foreign body, intraocular, old, retained, magnetic, ciliary body
    eyelid H02.819
      left H02.816
        lower H02.815
        upper H02.814
      right H02.813
        lower H02.812
        upper H02.811
    fragments — *see* Retained, foreign body fragments (type of)
    globe — *see* Foreign body, intraocular, old, retained
      magnetic — *see* Foreign body, intraocular, old, retained, magnetic
    intraocular — *see* Foreign body, intraocular, old, retained
      magnetic — *see* Foreign body, intraocular, old, retained, magnetic
    iris — *see* Foreign body, intraocular, old, retained, iris
      magnetic — *see* Foreign body, intraocular, old, retained, magnetic, iris
    lens — *see* Foreign body, intraocular, old, retained, lens
      magnetic — *see* Foreign body, intraocular, old, retained, magnetic, lens
    muscle — *see* Foreign body, retained, soft tissue
    orbit — *see* Foreign body, orbit, old
    posterior wall of globe — *see* Foreign body, intraocular, old, retained, posterior wall
      magnetic — *see* Foreign body, intraocular, old, retained, magnetic, posterior wall
    retrobulbar — *see* Foreign body, orbit, old, retrobulbar
    soft tissue M79.5
    vitreous — *see* Foreign body, intraocular, old, retained, vitreous body
      magnetic — *see* Foreign body, intraocular, old, retained, magnetic, vitreous body

Foreign body — *continued*
  retina S05.5- ☑
  superficial, without open wound
    abdomen, abdominal (wall) S30.851 ☑
    alveolar process S00.552 ☑
    ankle S90.55- ☑
    antecubital space — *see* Foreign body, superficial, forearm
    anus S30.857 ☑
    arm (upper) S40.85- ☑
    auditory canal — *see* Foreign body, superficial, ear
    auricle — *see* Foreign body, superficial, ear
    axilla — *see* Foreign body, superficial, arm
    back, lower S30.850 ☑
    breast S20.15- ☑
    brow S00.85 ☑
    buttock S30.850 ☑
    calf — *see* Foreign body, superficial, leg
    canthus — *see* Foreign body, superficial, eyelid
    cheek S00.85 ☑
      internal S00.552 ☑
    chest wall — *see* Foreign body, superficial, thorax
    chin S00.85 ☑
    clitoris S30.854 ☑
    costal region — *see* Foreign body, superficial, thorax
    digit(s)
      foot — *see* Foreign body, superficial, toe
      hand — *see* Foreign body, superficial, finger
    ear S00.45- ☑
    elbow S50.35- ☑
    epididymis S30.853 ☑
    epigastric region S30.851 ☑
    epiglottis S10.15 ☑
    esophagus, cervical S10.15 ☑
    eyebrow — *see* Foreign body, superficial, eyelid
    eyelid S00.25- ☑
    face S00.85 ☑
    finger(s) S60.459 ☑
      index S60.45- ☑
      little S60.45- ☑
      middle S60.45- ☑
      ring S60.45- ☑
    flank S30.851 ☑
    foot (except toe(s) alone) S90.85- ☑
      toe — *see* Foreign body, superficial, toe
    forearm S50.85- ☑
      elbow only — *see* Foreign body, superficial, elbow
    forehead S00.85 ☑
    genital organs, external
      female S30.856 ☑
      male S30.855 ☑
    groin S30.851 ☑
    gum S00.552 ☑
    hand S60.55- ☑
    head S00.95 ☑
      ear — *see* Foreign body, superficial, ear
      eyelid — *see* Foreign body, superficial, eyelid
      lip S00.551 ☑
      nose S00.35 ☑
      oral cavity S00.552 ☑
      scalp S00.05 ☑
      specified site NEC S00.85 ☑
    heel — *see* Foreign body, superficial, foot
    hip S70.25- ☑
    inguinal region S30.851 ☑
    interscapular region S20.459 ☑
    jaw S00.85 ☑
    knee S80.25- ☑
    labium (majus) (minus) S30.854 ☑
    larynx S10.15 ☑
    leg (lower) S80.85- ☑
      knee — *see* Foreign body, superficial, knee
      upper — *see* Foreign body, superficial, thigh
    lip S00.551 ☑
    lower back S30.850 ☑
    lumbar region S30.850 ☑
    malar region S00.85 ☑
    mammary — *see* Foreign body, superficial, breast
    mastoid region S00.85 ☑
    mouth S00.552 ☑
    nail
      finger — *see* Foreign body, superficial, finger
      toe — *see* Foreign body, superficial, toe
    nape S10.85 ☑
    nasal S00.35 ☑

Foreign body — *continued*
  superficial, without open wound — *continued*
    neck S10.95 ☑
      specified site NEC S10.85 ☑
      throat S10.15 ☑
    nose S00.35 ☑
    occipital region S00.05 ☑
    oral cavity S00.552 ☑
    orbital region — *see* Foreign body, superficial, eyelid
    palate S00.552 ☑
    palm — *see* Foreign body, superficial, hand
    parietal region S00.05 ☑
    pelvis S30.850 ☑
    penis S30.852 ☑
    perineum
      female S30.854 ☑
      male S30.850 ☑
    periocular area — *see* Foreign body, superficial, eyelid
    phalanges
      finger — *see* Foreign body, superficial, finger
      toe — *see* Foreign body, superficial, toe
    pharynx S10.15 ☑
    pinna — *see* Foreign body, superficial, ear
    popliteal space — *see* Foreign body, superficial, knee
    prepuce S30.852 ☑
    pubic region S30.850 ☑
    pudendum
      female S30.856 ☑
      male S30.855 ☑
    sacral region S30.850 ☑
    scalp S00.05 ☑
    scapular region — *see* Foreign body, superficial, shoulder
    scrotum S30.853 ☑
    shin — *see* Foreign body, superficial, leg
    shoulder S40.25- ☑
    sternal region S20.359 ☑
    submaxillary region S00.85 ☑
    submental region S00.85 ☑
    subungual
      finger(s) — *see* Foreign body, superficial, finger
      toe(s) — *see* Foreign body, superficial, toe
    supraclavicular fossa S10.85 ☑
    supraorbital S00.85 ☑
    temple S00.85 ☑
    temporal region S00.85 ☑
    testis S30.853 ☑
    thigh S70.35- ☑
    thorax, thoracic (wall) S20.95 ☑
      back S20.45- ☑
      front S20.35- ☑
    throat S10.15 ☑
    thumb S60.35- ☑
    toe(s) (lesser) S90.456 ☑
      great S90.45- ☑
    tongue S00.552 ☑
    trachea S10.15 ☑
    tunica vaginalis S30.853 ☑
    tympanum, tympanic membrane — *see* Foreign body, superficial, ear
    uvula S00.552 ☑
    vagina S30.854 ☑
    vocal cords S10.15 ☑
    vulva S30.854 ☑
    wrist S60.85- ☑
  swallowed T18.9 ☑
  trachea T17.408 ☑
    causing
      asphyxiation T17.400 ☑
        food (bone) (seed) T17.420 ☑
        gastric contents (vomitus) T17.410 ☑
        specified type NEC T17.490 ☑
      injury NEC T17.408 ☑
        food (bone) (seed) T17.428 ☑
        gastric contents (vomitus) T17.418 ☑
        specified type NEC T17.498 ☑
  type of fragment — *see* Retained, foreign body fragments (type of)
  vitreous (humor) S05.5- ☑
Forestier's disease (rhizomelic pseudopolyarthritis) M35.3
  meaning ankylosing hyperostosis — *see* Hyperostosis, ankylosing

Formation
  hyalin in cornea — *see* Degeneration, cornea
  sequestrum in bone (due to infection) — *see* Osteomyelitis, chronic
  valve
    colon, congenital Q43.8
    ureter (congenital) Q62.39
Formication R20.2
Fort Bragg fever A27.89
Fossa — *see also* condition
  pyriform — *see* condition
Foster-Kennedy syndrome H47.14- ☑
Fothergill's
  disease (trigeminal neuralgia) — *see also* Neuralgia, trigeminal
  scarlatina anginosa A38.9
Foul breath R19.6
Foundling Z76.1
Fournier disease or gangrene N49.3
  female N76.89
Fourth
  cranial nerve — *see* condition
  molar K00.1
Foville's (peduncular) **disease or syndrome** G46.3
Fox (-Fordyce) disease (apocrine miliaria) L75.2
FPIES (food protein-induced enterocolitis syndrome) K52.21
Fracture, burst — *see* Fracture, traumatic, by site
Fracture, chronic — *see* Fracture, pathological, by site
Fracture, insufficiency — *see* Fracture, pathological, by site
Fracture, nontraumatic, NEC
  atypical
    femur M84.750- ☑
      complete
        oblique M84.759 ☑
          left side M84.758 ☑
          right side M84.757 ☑
        transverse M84.756 ☑
          left side M84.755 ☑
          right side M84.754 ☑
      incomplete M84.753 ☑
        left side M84.752 ☑
        right side M84.751 ☑
Fracture, pathological (pathologic) — *see also* Fracture, traumatic M84.40
  ankle M84.47- ☑
  carpus M84.44- ☑
  clavicle M84.41- ☑
  compression (not due to trauma) — *see also* Collapse, vertebra M48.50- ☑
  dental implant M27.63
  dental restorative material K08.539
    with loss of material K08.531
    without loss of material K08.530
  due to
    neoplastic disease NEC — *see also* Neoplasm M84.50 ☑
      ankle M84.57- ☑
      carpus M84.54- ☑
      clavicle M84.51- ☑
      femur M84.55- ☑
      fibula M84.56- ☑
      finger M84.54- ☑
      hip M84.559 ☑
      humerus M84.52- ☑
      ilium M84.550 ☑
      ischium M84.550 ☑
      metacarpus M84.54- ☑
      metatarsus M84.57- ☑
      neck M84.58 ☑
      pelvis M84.550 ☑
      radius M84.53- ☑
      rib M84.58 ☑
      scapula M84.51- ☑
      skull M84.58 ☑
      specified site NEC M84.58 ☑
      tarsus M84.57- ☑
      tibia M84.56- ☑
      toe M84.57- ☑
      ulna M84.53- ☑
      vertebra M84.58 ☑
    osteoporosis M80.00 ☑
      disuse — *see* Osteoporosis, specified type NEC, with pathological fracture

Fracture, pathological — *continued*
  due to — *continued*
    osteoporosis — *continued*
      drug-induced — *see* Osteoporosis, drug induced, with pathological fracture
      idiopathic — *see* Osteoporosis, specified type NEC, with pathological fracture
      postmenopausal — *see* Osteoporosis, postmenopausal, with pathological fracture
      postoophorectomy — *see* Osteoporosis, postoophorectomy, with pathological fracture
      postsurgical malabsorption — *see* Osteoporosis, specified type NEC, with pathological fracture
      specified cause NEC — *see* Osteoporosis, specified type NEC, with pathological fracture
    specified disease NEC M84.60 ☑
      ankle M84.67- ☑
      carpus M84.64- ☑
      clavicle M84.61- ☑
      femur M84.65- ☑
      fibula M84.66- ☑
      finger M84.64- ☑
      hip M84.65- ☑
      humerus M84.62- ☑
      ilium M84.650 ☑
      ischium M84.650 ☑
      metacarpus M84.64- ☑
      metatarsus M84.67- ☑
      neck M84.68 ☑
      radius M84.63- ☑
      rib M84.68 ☑
      scapula M84.61- ☑
      skull M84.68 ☑
      tarsus M84.67- ☑
      tibia M84.66- ☑
      toe M84.67- ☑
      ulna M84.63- ☑
      vertebra M84.68 ☑
  femur M84.45- ☑
  fibula M84.46- ☑
  finger M84.44- ☑
  hip M84.459 ☑
  humerus M84.42- ☑
  ilium M84.454 ☑
  ischium M84.454 ☑
  joint prosthesis — *see* Complications, joint prosthesis, mechanical, breakdown, by site
    periprosthetic — *see* Fracture, pathological, periprosthetic
  metacarpus M84.44- ☑
  metatarsus M84.47- ☑
  neck M84.48 ☑
  pelvis M84.454 ☑
  periprosthetic M97.9 ☑
    ankle M97.2- ☑
    elbow M97.4- ☑
    finger M97.8 ☑
    hip M97.0- ☑
    knee M97.1- ☑
    other specified joint M97.8 ☑
    shoulder M97.3- ☑
    spinal joint M97.8 ☑
    toe joint M97.8 ☑
    wrist joint M97.8 ☑
  radius M84.43- ☑
  restorative material (dental) K08.539
    with loss of material K08.531
    without loss of material K08.530
  rib M84.48 ☑
  scapula M84.41- ☑
  skull M84.48 ☑
  tarsus M84.47- ☑
  tibia M84.46- ☑
  toe M84.47- ☑
  ulna M84.43- ☑
  vertebra M84.48 ☑

Fracture, traumatic (abduction) (adduction) (separation) — *see also* Fracture, pathological T14.8 ☑
  acetabulum S32.40- ☑
    column
      anterior (displaced) (iliopubic) S32.43- ☑
        nondisplaced S32.436
      posterior (displaced) (ilioischial) S32.443 ☑
        nondisplaced S32.44- ☑
    dome (displaced) S32.48- ☑

Fracture, traumatic — *continued*
  acetabulum — *continued*
    dome — *continued*
      nondisplaced S32.48 ☑
    specified NEC S32.49- ☑
    transverse (displaced) S32.45- ☑
      with associated posterior wall fracture (displaced) S32.46- ☑
        nondisplaced S32.46- ☑
      nondisplaced S32.45- ☑
    wall
      anterior (displaced) S32.41- ☑
        nondisplaced S32.41- ☑
      medial (displaced) S32.47- ☑
        nondisplaced S32.47- ☑
      posterior (displaced) S32.42- ☑
        with associated transverse fracture (displaced) S32.46- ☑
          nondisplaced S32.46- ☑
        nondisplaced S32.42- ☑
  acromion — *see* Fracture, scapula, acromial process
  ankle S82.899 ☑
    bimalleolar (displaced) S82.84- ☑
      nondisplaced S82.84- ☑
    lateral malleolus only (displaced) S82.6- ☑
      nondisplaced S82.6- ☑
    medial malleolus (displaced) S82.5- ☑
      associated with Maisonneuve's fracture — *see* Fracture, Maisonneuve's
      nondisplaced S82.5- ☑
    talus — *see* Fracture, tarsal, talus
    trimalleolar (displaced) S82.85- ☑
      nondisplaced S82.85- ☑
  arm (upper) — *see also* Fracture, humerus, shaft
    humerus — *see* Fracture, humerus
    radius — *see* Fracture, radius
    ulna — *see* Fracture, ulna
  astragalus — *see* Fracture, tarsal, talus
  atlas — *see* Fracture, neck, cervical vertebra, first
  axis — *see* Fracture, neck, cervical vertebra, second
  back — *see* Fracture, vertebra
  Barton's — *see* Barton's fracture
  base of skull — *see* Fracture, skull, base
  basicervical (basal) (femoral) S72.0 ☑
  Bennett's — *see* Bennett's fracture
  bimalleolar — *see* Fracture, ankle, bimalleolar
  blow-out S02.3- ☑
  bone NEC T14.8 ☑
    birth injury P13.9
    following insertion of orthopedic implant, joint prosthesis or bone plate — *see* Fracture, following insertion of orthopedic implant, joint prosthesis or bone plate
    in (due to) neoplastic disease NEC — *see* Fracture, pathological, due to, neoplastic disease
    pathological (cause unknown) — *see* Fracture, pathological
  breast bone — *see* Fracture, sternum
  bucket handle (semilunar cartilage) — *see* Tear, meniscus
  burst — *see* Fracture, traumatic, by site
  calcaneus — *see* Fracture, tarsal, calcaneus
  carpal bone(s) S62.10- ☑
    capitate (displaced) S62.13- ☑
      nondisplaced S62.13- ☑
    cuneiform — *see* Fracture, carpal bone, triquetrum
    hamate (body) (displaced) S62.143 ☑
      hook process (displaced) S62.15- ☑
        nondisplaced S62.15- ☑
      nondisplaced S62.14- ☑
    larger multangular — *see* Fracture, carpal bones, trapezium
    lunate (displaced) S62.12- ☑
      nondisplaced S62.12- ☑
    navicular S62.00- ☑
      distal pole (displaced) S62.01- ☑
        nondisplaced S62.01- ☑
      middle third (displaced) S62.02- ☑
        nondisplaced S62.02- ☑
      proximal third (displaced) S62.03- ☑
        nondisplaced S62.03- ☑
      volar tuberosity — *see* Fracture, carpal bones, navicular, distal pole
    os magnum — *see* Fracture, carpal bones, capitate
    pisiform (displaced) S62.16- ☑
      nondisplaced S62.16- ☑

Fracture, traumatic — *continued*
  carpal bone(s) — *continued*
    semilunar — *see* Fracture, carpal bones, lunate
    smaller multangular — *see* Fracture, carpal bones, trapezoid
    trapezium (displaced) S62.17- ☑
      nondisplaced S62.17- ☑
    trapezoid (displaced) S62.18- ☑
      nondisplaced S62.18- ☑
    triquetrum (displaced) S62.11- ☑
      nondisplaced S62.11- ☑
    unciform — *see* Fracture, carpal bones, hamate
  cervical — *see* Fracture, vertebra, cervical
  clavicle S42.00- ☑
    acromial end (displaced) S42.03- ☑
      nondisplaced S42.03- ☑
    birth injury P13.4
    lateral end — *see* Fracture, clavicle, acromial end
    shaft (displaced) S42.02- ☑
      nondisplaced S42.02- ☑
    sternal end (anterior) (displaced) S42.01- ☑
      nondisplaced S42.01- ☑
      posterior S42.01- ☑
  coccyx S32.2 ☑
  collapsed — *see* Collapse, vertebra
  collar bone — *see* Fracture, clavicle
  Colles' — *see* Colles' fracture
  coronoid process — *see* Fracture, ulna, upper end, coronoid process
  corpus cavernosum penis S39.840 ☑
  costochondral cartilage S23.41 ☑
  costochondral, costosternal junction — *see* Fracture, rib
  cranium — *see* Fracture, skull
  cricoid cartilage S12.8 ☑
  cuboid (ankle) — *see* Fracture, tarsal, cuboid
  cuneiform
    foot — *see* Fracture, tarsal, cuneiform
    wrist — *see* Fracture, carpal, triquetrum
  delayed union — *see* Delay, union, fracture
  dental restorative material K08.539
    with loss of material K08.531
    without loss of material K08.530
  due to
    birth injury — *see* Birth, injury, fracture
    osteoporosis — *see* Osteoporosis, with fracture
  Dupuytren's — *see* Fracture, ankle, lateral malleolus
  elbow S42.40- ☑
  ethmoid (bone) (sinus) — *see* Fracture, skull, base
  face bone S02.92 ☑
  fatigue — *see also* Fracture, stress
    vertebra M48.40 ☑
      cervical region M48.42 ☑
      cervicothoracic region M48.43 ☑
      lumbar region M48.46 ☑
      lumbosacral region M48.47 ☑
      occipito-atlanto-axial region M48.41 ☑
      sacrococcygeal region M48.48 ☑
      thoracic region M48.44 ☑
      thoracolumbar region M48.45 ☑
  femur, femoral S72.9- ☑
    basicervical (basal) S72.0 ☑
    birth injury P13.2
    capital epiphyseal S79.01- ☑
    condyles, epicondyles — *see* Fracture, femur, lower end
    distal end — *see* Fracture, femur, lower end
    epiphysis
      head — *see* Fracture, femur, upper end, epiphysis
      lower — *see* Fracture, femur, lower end, epiphysis
      upper — *see* Fracture, femur, upper end, epiphysis
    following insertion of implant, prosthesis or plate M96.66- ☑
    head — *see* Fracture, femur, upper end, head
    intertrochanteric — *see* Fracture, femur, trochanteric
    intratrochanteric — *see* Fracture, femur, trochanteric
    lower end S72.40- ☑
      condyle (displaced) S72.41- ☑
      lateral (displaced) S72.42- ☑
        nondisplaced S72.42- ☑
      medial (displaced) S72.43- ☑
        nondisplaced S72.43- ☑

Fracture, traumatic — *continued*
  femur, femoral — *continued*
    lower end — *continued*
      condyle — *continued*
        nondisplaced S72.41- ☑
        epiphysis (displaced) S72.44- ☑
          nondisplaced S72.44- ☑
        physeal S79.10- ☑
          Salter-Harris
            Type I S79.11- ☑
            Type II S79.12- ☑
            Type III S79.13- ☑
            Type IV S79.14- ☑
            specified NEC S79.19- ☑
        specified NEC S72.49- ☑
        supracondylar (displaced) S72.45- ☑
          with intracondylar extension (displaced)
            S72.46- ☑
            nondisplaced S72.46- ☑
          nondisplaced S72.45- ☑
        torus S72.47- ☑
      neck — *see* Fracture, femur, upper end, neck
      pertrochanteric — *see* Fracture, femur, trochanteric
      shaft (lower third) (middle third) (upper third)
        S72.30- ☑
        comminuted (displaced) S72.35- ☑
          nondisplaced S72.35- ☑
        oblique (displaced) S72.33- ☑
          nondisplaced S72.33- ☑
        segmental (displaced) S72.36- ☑
          nondisplaced S72.36- ☑
        specified NEC S72.39- ☑
        spiral (displaced) S72.34- ☑
          nondisplaced S72.34- ☑
        transverse (displaced) S72.32- ☑
          nondisplaced S72.32- ☑
      specified site NEC — *see* subcategory S72.8 ☑
      subcapital (displaced) S72.01- ☑
      subtrochanteric (region) (section) (displaced)
        S72.2- ☑
        nondisplaced S72.2- ☑
      transcervical — *see* Fracture, femur, midcervical
      transtrochanteric — *see* Fracture, femur,
        trochanteric
      trochanteric S72.10- ☑
        apophyseal (displaced) S72.13- ☑
          nondisplaced S72.13- ☑
        greater trochanter (displaced) S72.11- ☑
          nondisplaced S72.11- ☑
        intertrochanteric (displaced) S72.14- ☑
          nondisplaced S72.14- ☑
        lesser trochanter (displaced) S72.12- ☑
          nondisplaced S72.12- ☑
      upper end S72.00- ☑
        apophyseal (displaced) S72.13- ☑
          nondisplaced S72.13- ☑
        cervicotrochanteric — *see* Fracture, femur, upper
          end, neck, base
        epiphysis (displaced) S72.02- ☑
          nondisplaced S72.02- ☑
        head S72.05- ☑
          articular (displaced) S72.06- ☑
            nondisplaced S72.06- ☑
          specified NEC S72.09- ☑
        intertrochanteric (displaced) S72.14- ☑
          nondisplaced S72.14- ☑
        intracapsular S72.01- ☑
        midcervical (displaced) S72.03- ☑
          nondisplaced S72.03- ☑
        neck S72.00- ☑
          base (displaced) S72.04- ☑
            nondisplaced S72.04- ☑
          specified NEC S72.09- ☑
        pertrochanteric — *see* Fracture, femur, upper
          end, trochanteric
        physeal S79.00- ☑
          Salter-Harris type I S79.01- ☑
          specified NEC S79.09- ☑
        subcapital (displaced) S72.01- ☑
        subtrochanteric (displaced) S72.2- ☑
          nondisplaced S72.2- ☑
        transcervical — *see* Fracture, femur, upper end,
          midcervical
        trochanteric S72.10- ☑
          greater (displaced) S72.11- ☑
            nondisplaced S72.11- ☑

Fracture, traumatic — *continued*
  femur, femoral — *continued*
    upper end — *continued*
      trochanteric — *continued*
        lesser (displaced) S72.12- ☑
          nondisplaced S72.12- ☑
  fibula (shaft) (styloid) S82.40- ☑
    comminuted (displaced) S82.45- ☑
      nondisplaced S82.45- ☑
    following insertion of implant, prosthesis or plate
      M96.67- ☑
    involving ankle or malleolus — *see* Fracture, fibula,
      lateral malleolus
    lateral malleolus (displaced) S82.6- ☑
      nondisplaced S82.6- ☑
    lower end
      physeal S89.30- ☑
        Salter-Harris
          Type I S89.31- ☑
          Type II S89.32- ☑
        specified NEC S89.39- ☑
      specified NEC S82.83- ☑
      torus S82.82- ☑
    oblique (displaced) S82.43- ☑
      nondisplaced S82.43- ☑
    segmental (displaced) S82.46- ☑
      nondisplaced S82.46- ☑
    specified NEC S82.49- ☑
    spiral (displaced) S82.44- ☑
      nondisplaced S82.44- ☑
    transverse (displaced) S82.42- ☑
      nondisplaced S82.42- ☑
    upper end
      physeal S89.20- ☑
        Salter-Harris
          Type I S89.21- ☑
          Type II S89.22- ☑
        specified NEC S89.29- ☑
      specified NEC S82.83- ☑
      torus S82.81- ☑
  finger (except thumb) S62.60- ☑
    distal phalanx (displaced) S62.63- ☑
      nondisplaced S62.66- ☑
    index S62.60- ☑
      distal phalanx (displaced) S62.63- ☑
        nondisplaced S62.66- ☑
      middle phalanx (displaced) S62.62- ☑
        nondisplaced S62.65- ☑
      proximal phalanx (displaced) S62.61- ☑
        nondisplaced S62.64- ☑
    little S62.60- ☑
      distal phalanx (displaced) S62.63- ☑
        nondisplaced S62.66- ☑
      middle phalanx (displaced) S62.62- ☑
        nondisplaced S62.65- ☑
      proximal phalanx (displaced) S62.61- ☑
        nondisplaced S62.64- ☑
    middle S62.60- ☑
      distal phalanx (displaced) S62.63- ☑
        comminuted (displaced) S62.66- ☑
      middle phalanx (displaced) S62.62- ☑
        nondisplaced S62.65- ☑
      proximal phalanx (displaced) S62.61- ☑
        nondisplaced S62.64- ☑
    middle phalanx (displaced) S62.62- ☑
      nondisplaced S62.65- ☑
    proximal phalanx (displaced) S62.61- ☑
      nondisplaced S62.64- ☑
    ring S62.60- ☑
      distal phalanx (displaced) S62.63- ☑
        nondisplaced S62.66- ☑
      middle phalanx (displaced) S62.62- ☑
        nondisplaced S62.65- ☑
      proximal phalanx (displaced) S62.61- ☑
        nondisplaced S62.64- ☑
    thumb — *see* Fracture, thumb
  following insertion (intraoperative) (postoperative) of
    orthopedic implant, joint prosthesis or bone
    plate M96.69
    femur M96.66- ☑
    fibula M96.67- ☑
    humerus M96.62- ☑
    pelvis M96.65
    radius M96.63- ☑
    specified bone NEC M96.69
    tibia M96.67- ☑

Fracture, traumatic — *continued*
  following insertion of orthopedic implant, joint pros-
    thesis or bone plate — *continued*
    ulna M96.63- ☑
  foot S92.90- ☑
    astragalus — *see* Fracture, tarsal, talus
    calcaneus — *see* Fracture, tarsal, calcaneus
    cuboid — *see* Fracture, tarsal, cuboid
    cuneiform — *see* Fracture, tarsal, cuneiform
    metatarsal — *see* Fracture, metatarsal
    navicular — *see* Fracture, tarsal, navicular
    sesamoid S92.81- ☑
    specified NEC S92.81- ☑
    talus — *see* Fracture, tarsal, talus
    tarsal — *see* Fracture, tarsal
    toe — *see* Fracture, toe
  forearm S52.9-
    radius — *see* Fracture, radius
    ulna — *see* Fracture, ulna
  fossa (anterior) (middle) (posterior) S02.19 ☑
  fragility — *see* Fracture, pathological, due to osteoporo-
    sis
  frontal (bone) (skull) S02.0 ☑
    sinus S02.19 ☑
  glenoid (cavity) (scapula) — *see* Fracture, scapula,
    glenoid cavity
  greenstick — *see* Fracture, by site
  hallux — *see* Fracture, toe, great
  hand S62.9- ☑
    carpal — *see* Fracture, carpal bone
    finger (except thumb) — *see* Fracture, finger
    metacarpal — *see* Fracture, metacarpal
    navicular (scaphoid) (hand) — *see* Fracture, carpal
      bone, navicular
    thumb — *see* Fracture, thumb
  healed or old
    with complications — *code by* Nature of the compli-
      cation
  heel bone — *see* Fracture, tarsal, calcaneus
  Hill-Sachs S42.29- ☑
  hip — *see* Fracture, femur, neck
  humerus S42.30- ☑
    anatomical neck — *see* Fracture, humerus, upper
      end
    articular process — *see* Fracture, humerus, lower
      end
    capitellum — *see* Fracture, humerus, lower end,
      condyle, lateral
    distal end — *see* Fracture, humerus, lower end
    epiphysis
      lower — *see* Fracture, humerus, lower end, phy-
        seal
      upper — *see* Fracture, humerus, upper end,
        physeal
    external condyle — *see* Fracture, humerus, lower
      end, condyle, lateral
    following insertion of implant, prosthesis or plate
      M96.62- ☑
    great tuberosity — *see* Fracture, humerus, upper
      end, greater tuberosity
    intercondylar — *see* Fracture, humerus, lower end
    internal epicondyle — *see* Fracture, humerus, lower
      end, epicondyle, medial
    lesser tuberosity — *see* Fracture, humerus, upper
      end, lesser tuberosity
    lower end S42.40- ☑
      condyle
        lateral (displaced) S42.45- ☑
          nondisplaced S42.45- ☑
        medial (displaced) S42.46- ☑
          nondisplaced S42.46- ☑
      epicondyle
        lateral (displaced) S42.43- ☑
          nondisplaced S42.43- ☑
        medial (displaced) S42.44- ☑
          incarcerated S42.44- ☑
          nondisplaced S42.44- ☑
      physeal S49.10- ☑
        Salter-Harris
          Type I S49.11- ☑
          Type II S49.12- ☑
          Type III S49.13- ☑
          Type IV S49.14- ☑
        specified NEC S49.19- ☑
      specified NEC (displaced) S42.49- ☑
        nondisplaced S42.49- ☑

Index
Fracture, traumatic — Fracture, traumatic

Fracture, traumatic — *continued*
  humerus — *continued*
    lower end — *continued*
      supracondylar (simple) (displaced) S42.41- ☑
        with intercondylar fracture — *see* Fracture, humerus, lower end
        comminuted (displaced) S42.42- ☑
          nondisplaced S42.42- ☑
        nondisplaced S42.41- ☑
      torus S42.48- ☑
      transcondylar (displaced) S42.47- ☑
        nondisplaced S42.47- ☑
    proximal end — *see* Fracture, humerus, upper end
    shaft S42.30- ☑
      comminuted (displaced) S42.35- ☑
        nondisplaced S42.35- ☑
      greenstick S42.31- ☑
      oblique (displaced) S42.33- ☑
        nondisplaced S42.33- ☑
      segmental (displaced) S42.36- ☑
        nondisplaced S42.36- ☑
      specified NEC S42.39- ☑
      spiral (displaced) S42.34- ☑
        nondisplaced S42.34- ☑
      transverse (displaced) S42.32- ☑
        nondisplaced S42.32- ☑
    supracondylar — *see* Fracture, humerus, lower end
    surgical neck — *see* Fracture, humerus, upper end, surgical neck
    trochlea — *see* Fracture, humerus, lower end, condyle, medial
    tuberosity — *see* Fracture, humerus, upper end
    upper end S42.20- ☑
      anatomical neck — *see* Fracture, humerus, upper end, specified NEC
      articular head — *see* Fracture, humerus, upper end, specified NEC
      epiphysis — *see* Fracture, humerus, upper end, physeal
      greater tuberosity (displaced) S42.25- ☑
        nondisplaced S42.25- ☑
      lesser tuberosity (displaced) S42.26- ☑
        nondisplaced S42.26- ☑
      physeal S49.00- ☑
        Salter-Harris
          Type I S49.01- ☑
          Type II S49.02- ☑
          Type III S49.03- ☑
          Type IV S49.04- ☑
        specified NEC S49.09- ☑
      specified NEC (displaced) S42.29- ☑
        nondisplaced S42.29- ☑
      surgical neck (displaced) S42.21- ☑
        four-part S42.24- ☑
        nondisplaced S42.21- ☑
        three-part S42.23- ☑
        two-part (displaced) S42.22- ☑
          nondisplaced S42.22- ☑
      torus S42.27- ☑
      transepiphyseal — *see* Fracture, humerus, upper end, physeal
  hyoid bone S12.8 ☑
  ilium S32.30- ☑
    with disruption of pelvic ring — *see* Disruption, pelvic ring
    avulsion (displaced) S32.31- ☑
      nondisplaced S32.31- ☑
    specified NEC S32.39- ☑
  impaction, impacted — *code as* Fracture, by site
  innominate bone — *see* Fracture, ilium
  instep — *see* Fracture, foot
  ischium S32.60- ☑
    with disruption of pelvic ring — *see* Disruption, pelvic ring
    avulsion (displaced) S32.61- ☑
      nondisplaced S32.61- ☑
    specified NEC S32.69- ☑
  jaw (bone) (lower) — *see* Fracture, mandible
    upper — *see* Fracture, maxilla
  joint prosthesis — *see* Complications, joint prosthesis, mechanical, breakdown, by site
    periprosthetic — *see* Fracture, traumatic, periprosthetic
  knee cap — *see* Fracture, patella
  larynx S12.8 ☑
  late effects — *see* Sequelae, fracture

Fracture, traumatic — *continued*
  leg (lower) S82.9- ☑
    ankle — *see* Fracture, ankle
    femur — *see* Fracture, femur
    fibula — *see* Fracture, fibula
    malleolus — *see* Fracture, ankle
    patella — *see* Fracture, patella
    specified site NEC S82.89- ☑
    tibia — *see* Fracture, tibia
  lumbar spine — *see* Fracture, vertebra, lumbar
  lumbosacral spine S32.9 ☑
  Maisonneuve's (displaced) S82.86- ☑
    nondisplaced S82.86- ☑
  malar bone — *see also* Fracture, maxilla S02.400 ☑
    left side S02.40B ☑
    right side S02.40A ☑
  malleolus — *see* Fracture, ankle
  malunion — *see* Fracture, by site
  mandible (lower jaw (bone)) S02.609 ☑
    alveolus S02.67- ☑
    angle (of jaw) S02.65- ☑
    body, unspecified S02.600 ☑
      left side S02.602 ☑
      right side S02.601 ☑
    condylar process S02.61- ☑
    coronoid process S02.63- ☑
    ramus, unspecified S02.64- ☑
    specified site NEC S02.69 ☑
    subcondylar process S02.62- ☑
    symphysis S02.66 ☑
  manubrium (sterni) S22.21 ☑
    dissociation from sternum S22.23 ☑
  march — *see* Fracture, traumatic, stress, by site
  maxilla, maxillary (bone) (sinus) (superior) (upper jaw) S02.401 ☑
    alveolus S02.42 ☑
    inferior — *see* Fracture, mandible
    LeFort I S02.411 ☑
    LeFort II S02.412 ☑
    LeFort III S02.413 ☑
    left side S02.40D ☑
    right side S02.40C ☑
  metacarpal S62.309 ☑
    base (displaced) S62.319 ☑
      nondisplaced S62.349 ☑
    fifth S62.30- ☑
      base (displaced) S62.31- ☑
        nondisplaced S62.34- ☑
      neck (displaced) S62.33- ☑
        nondisplaced S62.36- ☑
      shaft (displaced) S62.32- ☑
        nondisplaced S62.35- ☑
      specified NEC S62.398 ☑
    first S62.20- ☑
      base NEC (displaced) S62.23- ☑
        nondisplaced S62.23- ☑
      Bennett's — *see* Bennett's fracture
      neck (displaced) S62.25- ☑
        nondisplaced S62.25- ☑
      shaft (displaced) S62.24- ☑
        nondisplaced S62.24- ☑
      specified NEC S62.29- ☑
    fourth S62.30- ☑
      base (displaced) S62.31- ☑
        nondisplaced S62.34- ☑
      neck (displaced) S62.33- ☑
        nondisplaced S62.36- ☑
      shaft (displaced) S62.32- ☑
        nondisplaced S62.35- ☑
      specified NEC S62.39- ☑
    neck (displaced) S62.33- ☑
      nondisplaced S62.36- ☑
    Rolando's — *see* Rolando's fracture
    second S62.30- ☑
      base (displaced) S62.31- ☑
        nondisplaced S62.34- ☑
      neck (displaced) S62.33- ☑
        nondisplaced S62.36- ☑
      shaft (displaced) S62.32- ☑
        nondisplaced S62.35- ☑
      specified NEC S62.39- ☑
    shaft (displaced) S62.32- ☑
      nondisplaced S62.35- ☑
    specified NEC S62.399 ☑
    third S62.30- ☑
      base (displaced) S62.31- ☑

Fracture, traumatic — *continued*
  metacarpal — *continued*
    third — *continued*
      base — *continued*
        nondisplaced S62.34- ☑
      neck (displaced) S62.33- ☑
        nondisplaced S62.36- ☑
      shaft (displaced) S62.32- ☑
        nondisplaced S62.35- ☑
      specified NEC S62.39- ☑
  metastatic — *see* Fracture, pathological, due to, neoplastic disease — *see also* Neoplasm
  metatarsal bone S92.30- ☑
    fifth (displaced) S92.35- ☑
      nondisplaced S92.35- ☑
    first (displaced) S92.31- ☑
      nondisplaced S92.31- ☑
    fourth (displaced) S92.34- ☑
      nondisplaced S92.34- ☑
    physeal S99.10- ☑
      Salter-Harris
        Type I S99.11- ☑
        Type II S99.12- ☑
        Type III S99.13- ☑
        Type IV S99.14- ☑
      specified NEC S99.19- ☑
    second (displaced) S92.32- ☑
      nondisplaced S92.32- ☑
    third (displaced) S92.33- ☑
      nondisplaced S92.33- ☑
  Monteggia's — *see* Monteggia's fracture
  multiple
    hand (and wrist) NEC — *see* Fracture, by site
    ribs — *see* Fracture, rib, multiple
  nasal (bone(s)) S02.2 ☑
  navicular (scaphoid) (foot) — *see also* Fracture, tarsal, navicular
    hand — *see* Fracture, carpal, navicular
  neck S12.9 ☑
    cervical vertebra S12.9 ☑
      fifth (displaced) S12.400 ☑
        nondisplaced S12.401 ☑
        specified type NEC (displaced) S12.490 ☑
          nondisplaced S12.491 ☑
      first (displaced) S12.000 ☑
        burst (stable) S12.01 ☑
          unstable S12.02 ☑
        lateral mass (displaced) S12.040 ☑
          nondisplaced S12.041 ☑
        nondisplaced S12.001 ☑
        posterior arch (displaced) S12.030 ☑
          nondisplaced S12.031 ☑
        specified type NEC (displaced) S12.090 ☑
          nondisplaced S12.091 ☑
      fourth (displaced) S12.300 ☑
        nondisplaced S12.301 ☑
        specified type NEC (displaced) S12.390 ☑
          nondisplaced S12.391 ☑
      second (displaced) S12.100 ☑
        dens (anterior) (displaced) (type II) S12.110 ☑
          nondisplaced S12.112 ☑
          posterior S12.111 ☑
          specified type NEC (displaced) S12.120 ☑
            nondisplaced S12.121 ☑
        nondisplaced S12.101 ☑
        specified type NEC (displaced) S12.190 ☑
          nondisplaced S12.191 ☑
      seventh (displaced) S12.600 ☑
        nondisplaced S12.601 ☑
        specified type NEC (displaced) S12.690 ☑
          nondisplaced S12.691 ☑
      sixth (displaced) S12.500 ☑
        nondisplaced S12.501 ☑
        specified type NEC (displaced) S12.590 ☑
          nondisplaced S12.591 ☑
      third (displaced) S12.200 ☑
        nondisplaced S12.201 ☑
        specified type NEC (displaced) S12.290 ☑
          nondisplaced S12.291 ☑
    hyoid bone S12.8 ☑
    larynx S12.8 ☑
    specified site NEC S12.8 ☑
    thyroid cartilage S12.8 ☑
    trachea S12.8 ☑
  neoplastic NEC — *see* Fracture, pathological, due to, neoplastic disease

Fracture, traumatic — *continued*
neural arch — *see* Fracture, vertebra
newborn — *see* Birth, injury, fracture
nontraumatic — *see* Fracture, pathological
nonunion — *see* Nonunion, fracture
nose, nasal (bone) (septum) S02.2 ☑
occiput — *see* Fracture, skull, base, occiput
odontoid process — *see* Fracture, neck, cervical vertebra, second
olecranon (process) (ulna) — *see* Fracture, ulna, upper end, olecranon process
orbit, orbital (bone) (region) S02.85 ☑
   floor (blow-out) S02.3- ☑
   roof S02.12- ☑
   wall S02.85 ☑
      lateral S02.84- ☑
      medial S02.83- ☑
os
   calcis — *see* Fracture, tarsal, calcaneus
   magnum — *see* Fracture, carpal, capitate
   pubis — *see* Fracture, pubis
palate S02.8- ☑
parietal bone (skull) S02.0 ☑
patella S82.00- ☑
   comminuted (displaced) S82.04- ☑
      nondisplaced S82.04- ☑
   longitudinal (displaced) S82.02- ☑
      nondisplaced S82.02- ☑
   osteochondral (displaced) S82.01- ☑
      nondisplaced S82.01- ☑
   specified NEC S82.09- ☑
   transverse (displaced) S82.03- ☑
      nondisplaced S82.03- ☑
pedicle (of vertebral arch) — *see* Fracture, vertebra
pelvis, pelvic (bone) S32.9 ☑
   acetabulum — *see* Fracture, acetabulum
   circle — *see* Disruption, pelvic ring
   following insertion of implant, prosthesis or plate M96.65
   ilium — *see* Fracture, ilium
   ischium — *see* Fracture, ischium
   multiple
      with disruption of pelvic ring (circle) — *see* Disruption, pelvic ring
      without disruption of pelvic ring (circle) S32.82 ☑
   pubis — *see* Fracture, pubis
   sacrum — *see* Fracture, sacrum
   specified site NEC S32.89 ☑
periprosthetic, around internal prosthetic joint M97.9 ☑
   ankle M97.2- ☑
   elbow M97.4- ☑
   finger M97.8 ☑
   hip M97.0- ☑
   knee M97.1- ☑
   shoulder M97.3- ☑
   specified joint NEC M97.8 ☑
   spine M97.8 ☑
   toe M97.8 ☑
   wrist M97.8 ☑
phalanx
   foot — *see* Fracture, toe
   hand — *see* Fracture, finger
pisiform — *see* Fracture, carpal, pisiform
pond — *see* Fracture, skull
prosthetic device, internal — *see* Complications, prosthetic device, by site, mechanical
pubis S32.50- ☑
   with disruption of pelvic ring — *see* Disruption, pelvic ring
   specified site NEC S32.59- ☑
   superior rim S32.51- ☑
radius S52.9- ☑
   distal end — *see* Fracture, radius, lower end
   following insertion of implant, prosthesis or plate M96.63- ☑
   head — *see* Fracture, radius, upper end, head
   lower end S52.50- ☑
      Barton's — *see* Barton's fracture
      Colles' — *see* Colles' fracture
      extraarticular NEC S52.55- ☑
      intraarticular NEC S52.57- ☑
      physeal S59.20- ☑
         Salter-Harris
            Type I S59.21- ☑

Fracture, traumatic — *continued*
radius — *continued*
   lower end — *continued*
      physeal — *continued*
         Salter-Harris — *continued*
            Type II S59.22- ☑
            Type III S59.23- ☑
            Type IV S59.24- ☑
         specified NEC S59.29- ☑
      Smith's — *see* Smith's fracture
      specified NEC S52.59- ☑
      styloid process (displaced) S52.51- ☑
         nondisplaced S52.51- ☑
      torus S52.52- ☑
   neck — *see* Fracture, radius, upper end
   proximal end — *see* Fracture, radius, upper end
   shaft S52.30- ☑
      bent bone S52.38- ☑
      comminuted (displaced) S52.35- ☑
         nondisplaced S52.35- ☑
      Galeazzi's — *see* Galeazzi's fracture
      greenstick S52.31- ☑
      oblique (displaced) S52.33- ☑
         nondisplaced S52.33- ☑
      segmental (displaced) S52.36- ☑
         nondisplaced S52.36- ☑
      specified NEC S52.39- ☑
      spiral (displaced) S52.34- ☑
         nondisplaced S52.34- ☑
      transverse (displaced) S52.32- ☑
         nondisplaced S52.32- ☑
   upper end S52.10- ☑
      head (displaced) S52.12- ☑
         nondisplaced S52.12- ☑
      neck (displaced) S52.13- ☑
         nondisplaced S52.13- ☑
      physeal S59.10- ☑
         Salter-Harris
            Type I S59.11- ☑
            Type II S59.12- ☑
            Type III S59.13- ☑
            Type IV S59.14- ☑
         specified NEC S59.19- ☑
      specified NEC S52.18- ☑
      torus S52.11- ☑
ramus
   inferior or superior, pubis — *see* Fracture, pubis
   mandible — *see* Fracture, mandible
restorative material (dental) K08.539
   with loss of material K08.531
   without loss of material K08.530
rib S22.3- ☑
   with flail chest — *see* Flail, chest
   multiple S22.4- ☑
      with flail chest — *see* Flail, chest
root, tooth — *see* Fracture, tooth
sacrum S32.10 ☑
   specified NEC S32.19 ☑
   Type
      1 S32.14 ☑
      2 S32.15 ☑
      3 S32.16 ☑
      4 S32.17 ☑
   Zone
      I S32.119 ☑
         displaced (minimally) S32.111 ☑
            severely S32.112 ☑
         nondisplaced S32.110 ☑
      II S32.129 ☑
         displaced (minimally) S32.121 ☑
            severely S32.122 ☑
         nondisplaced S32.120 ☑
      III S32.139 ☑
         displaced (minimally) S32.131 ☑
            severely S32.132 ☑
         nondisplaced S32.130 ☑
scaphoid (hand) — *see also* Fracture, carpal, navicular
   foot — *see* Fracture, tarsal, navicular
scapula S42.10- ☑
   acromial process (displaced) S42.12- ☑
      nondisplaced S42.12- ☑
   body (displaced) S42.11- ☑
      nondisplaced S42.11- ☑
   coracoid process (displaced) S42.13- ☑
      nondisplaced S42.13- ☑
   glenoid cavity (displaced) S42.14- ☑

Fracture, traumatic — *continued*
scapula — *continued*
   glenoid cavity — *continued*
      nondisplaced S42.14- ☑
   neck (displaced) S42.15- ☑
      nondisplaced S42.15- ☑
   specified NEC S42.19- ☑
semilunar bone, wrist — *see* Fracture, carpal, lunate
sequelae — *see* Sequelae, fracture
sesamoid bone
   foot S92.81- ☑
   hand — *see* Fracture, carpal
   other — *see* Fracture, traumatic, by site
shepherd's — *see* Fracture, tarsal, talus
shoulder (girdle) S42.9- ☑
   blade — *see* Fracture, scapula
sinus (ethmoid) (frontal) S02.19 ☑
skull S02.91 ☑
   base S02.10- ☑
      occiput S02.119 ☑
         condyle S02.113 ☑
            specified NEC S02.118 ☑
               left side S02.11H ☑
               right side S02.11G ☑
            type I S02.110 ☑
               left side S02.11B ☑
               right side S02.11A ☑
            type II S02.111 ☑
               left side S02.11D ☑
               right side S02.11C ☑
            type III S02.112 ☑
               left side S02.11F ☑
               right side S02.11E ☑
         specified NEC S02.19 ☑
   birth injury P13.0
   frontal bone S02.0 ☑
   parietal bone S02.0 ☑
   specified site NEC S02.8- ☑
   temporal bone S02.19 ☑
   vault S02.0 ☑
Smith's — *see* Smith's fracture
sphenoid (bone) (sinus) S02.19 ☑
spine — *see* Fracture, vertebra
spinous process — *see* Fracture, vertebra
spontaneous (cause unknown) — *see* Fracture, pathological
stave (of thumb) — *see* Fracture, metacarpal, first
sternum S22.20 ☑
   with flail chest — *see* Flail, chest
   body S22.22 ☑
   manubrium S22.21 ☑
   xiphoid (process) S22.24 ☑
stress M84.30 ☑
   ankle M84.37- ☑
   carpus M84.34- ☑
   clavicle M84.31- ☑
   femoral neck M84.359 ☑
   femur M84.35- ☑
   fibula M84.36- ☑
   finger M84.34- ☑
   hip M84.359 ☑
   humerus M84.32- ☑
   ilium M84.350 ☑
   ischium M84.350 ☑
   metacarpus M84.34- ☑
   metatarsus M84.37- ☑
   neck — *see* Fracture, fatigue, vertebra
   pelvis M84.350 ☑
   radius M84.33- ☑
   rib M84.38 ☑
   scapula M84.31- ☑
   skull M84.38 ☑
   tarsus M84.37- ☑
   tibia M84.36- ☑
   toe M84.37- ☑
   ulna M84.33- ☑
   vertebra — *see* Fracture, fatigue, vertebra
supracondylar, elbow — *see* Fracture, humerus, lower end, supracondylar
symphysis pubis — *see* Fracture, pubis
talus (ankle bone) — *see* Fracture, tarsal, talus
tarsal bone(s) S92.20- ☑
   astragalus — *see* Fracture, tarsal, talus
   calcaneus S92.00- ☑
      anterior process (displaced) S92.02- ☑
         nondisplaced S92.02- ☑

▽ Subterms under main terms may continue to next column or page   ☑ Additional Character Required — Refer to the Tabular List for Character Selection   **153**

Fracture, traumatic — Fracture, traumatic

Index

Fracture, traumatic

Fracture, traumatic — *continued*
- tarsal bone(s) — *continued*
  - calcaneus — *continued*
    - body (displaced) S92.01- ☑
      - nondisplaced S92.01- ☑
    - extraarticular NEC (displaced) S92.05- ☑
      - nondisplaced S92.05- ☑
    - intraarticular (displaced) S92.06- ☑
      - nondisplaced S92.06- ☑
    - physeal S99.00- ☑
      - Salter-Harris
        - Type I S99.01- ☑
        - Type II S99.02- ☑
        - Type III S99.03- ☑
        - Type IV S99.04- ☑
      - specified NEC S99.09- ☑
    - tuberosity (displaced) S92.04- ☑
      - avulsion (displaced) S92.03- ☑
        - nondisplaced S92.03- ☑
      - nondisplaced S92.04- ☑
  - cuboid (displaced) S92.21- ☑
    - nondisplaced S92.21- ☑
  - cuneiform
    - intermediate (displaced) S92.23- ☑
      - nondisplaced S92.23- ☑
    - lateral (displaced) S92.22- ☑
      - nondisplaced S92.22- ☑
    - medial (displaced) S92.24- ☑
      - nondisplaced S92.24- ☑
  - navicular (displaced) S92.25- ☑
    - nondisplaced S92.25- ☑
  - scaphoid — *see* Fracture, tarsal, navicular
  - talus S92.10- ☑
    - avulsion (displaced) S92.15- ☑
      - nondisplaced S92.15- ☑
    - body (displaced) S92.12- ☑
      - nondisplaced S92.12- ☑
    - dome (displaced) S92.14- ☑
      - nondisplaced S92.14- ☑
    - head (displaced) S92.12- ☑
      - nondisplaced S92.12- ☑
    - lateral process (displaced) S92.14- ☑
      - nondisplaced S92.14- ☑
    - neck (displaced) S92.11- ☑
      - nondisplaced S92.11- ☑
    - posterior process (displaced) S92.13- ☑
      - nondisplaced S92.13- ☑
    - specified NEC S92.19- ☑
- temporal bone (styloid) S02.19 ☑
- thorax (bony) S22.9 ☑
  - with flail chest — *see* Flail, chest
  - rib S22.3- ☑
    - multiple S22.4- ☑
      - with flail chest — *see* Flail, chest
  - sternum S22.20 ☑
    - body S22.22 ☑
    - manubrium S22.21 ☑
    - xiphoid process S22.24 ☑
  - vertebra (displaced) S22.009 ☑
    - burst (stable) S22.001 ☑
      - unstable S22.002 ☑
    - eighth S22.069 ☑
      - burst (stable) S22.061 ☑
        - unstable S22.062 ☑
      - specified type NEC S22.068 ☑
      - wedge compression S22.060 ☑
    - eleventh S22.089 ☑
      - burst (stable) S22.081 ☑
        - unstable S22.082 ☑
      - specified type NEC S22.088 ☑
      - wedge compression S22.080 ☑
    - fifth S22.059 ☑
      - burst (stable) S22.051 ☑
        - unstable S22.052 ☑
      - specified type NEC S22.058 ☑
      - wedge compression S22.050 ☑
    - first S22.019 ☑
      - burst (stable) S22.011 ☑
        - unstable S22.012 ☑
      - specified type NEC S22.018 ☑
      - wedge compression S22.010 ☑
    - fourth S22.049 ☑
      - burst (stable) S22.041 ☑
        - unstable S22.042 ☑
      - specified type NEC S22.048 ☑
      - wedge compression S22.040 ☑

Fracture, traumatic — *continued*
- thorax — *continued*
  - vertebra — *continued*
    - ninth S22.079 ☑
      - burst (stable) S22.071 ☑
        - unstable S22.072 ☑
      - specified type NEC S22.078 ☑
      - wedge compression S22.070 ☑
    - nondisplaced S22.001 ☑
    - second S22.029 ☑
      - burst (stable) S22.021 ☑
        - unstable S22.022 ☑
      - specified type NEC S22.028 ☑
      - wedge compression S22.020 ☑
    - seventh S22.069 ☑
      - burst (stable) S22.061 ☑
        - unstable S22.062 ☑
      - specified type NEC S22.068 ☑
      - wedge compression S22.060 ☑
    - sixth S22.059 ☑
      - burst (stable) S22.051 ☑
        - unstable S22.052 ☑
      - specified type NEC S22.058 ☑
      - wedge compression S22.050 ☑
    - specified type NEC S22.008 ☑
    - tenth S22.079 ☑
      - burst (stable) S22.071 ☑
        - unstable S22.072 ☑
      - specified type NEC S22.078 ☑
      - wedge compression S22.070 ☑
    - third S22.039 ☑
      - burst (stable) S22.031 ☑
        - unstable S22.032 ☑
      - specified type NEC S22.038 ☑
      - wedge compression S22.030 ☑
    - twelfth S22.089 ☑
      - burst (stable) S22.081 ☑
        - unstable S22.082 ☑
      - specified type NEC S22.088 ☑
      - wedge compression S22.080 ☑
    - wedge compression S22.000 ☑
- thumb S62.50- ☑
  - distal phalanx (displaced) S62.52- ☑
    - nondisplaced S62.52- ☑
  - proximal phalanx (displaced) S62.51- ☑
    - nondisplaced S62.51- ☑
- thyroid cartilage S12.8 ☑
- tibia (shaft) S82.20- ☑
  - comminuted (displaced) S82.25- ☑
    - nondisplaced S82.25- ☑
  - condyles — *see* Fracture, tibia, upper end
  - distal end — *see* Fracture, tibia, lower end
  - epiphysis
    - lower — *see* Fracture, tibia, lower end
    - upper — *see* Fracture, tibia, upper end
  - following insertion of implant, prosthesis or plate M96.67- ☑
  - head (involving knee joint) — *see* Fracture, tibia, upper end
  - intercondyloid eminence — *see* Fracture, tibia, upper end
  - involving ankle or malleolus — *see* Fracture, ankle, medial malleolus
  - lower end S82.30- ☑
    - physeal S89.10- ☑
      - Salter-Harris
        - Type I S89.11- ☑
        - Type II S89.12- ☑
        - Type III S89.13- ☑
        - Type IV S89.14- ☑
      - specified NEC S89.19- ☑
    - pilon (displaced) S82.87- ☑
      - nondisplaced S82.87- ☑
    - specified NEC S82.39- ☑
    - torus S82.31- ☑
  - malleolus — *see* Fracture, ankle, medial malleolus
  - oblique (displaced) S82.23- ☑
    - nondisplaced S82.23- ☑
  - pilon — *see* Fracture, tibia, lower end, pilon
  - proximal end — *see* Fracture, tibia, upper end
  - segmental (displaced) S82.26- ☑
    - nondisplaced S82.26- ☑
  - specified NEC S82.29- ☑
  - spine — *see* Fracture, tibia, upper end, spine
  - spiral (displaced) S82.24- ☑
    - nondisplaced S82.24- ☑

Fracture, traumatic — *continued*
- tibia — *continued*
  - transverse (displaced) S82.22- ☑
    - nondisplaced S82.22- ☑
  - tuberosity — *see* Fracture, tibia, upper end, tuberosity
  - upper end S82.10- ☑
    - bicondylar (displaced) S82.14- ☑
      - nondisplaced S82.14- ☑
    - lateral condyle (displaced) S82.12- ☑
      - nondisplaced S82.12- ☑
    - medial condyle (displaced) S82.13- ☑
      - nondisplaced S82.13- ☑
    - physeal S89.00- ☑
      - Salter-Harris
        - Type I S89.01- ☑
        - Type II S89.02- ☑
        - Type III S89.03- ☑
        - Type IV S89.04- ☑
      - specified NEC S89.09- ☑
    - plateau — *see* Fracture, tibia, upper end, bicondylar
    - specified NEC S82.19- ☑
    - spine (displaced) S82.11- ☑
      - nondisplaced S82.11- ☑
    - torus S82.16- ☑
    - tuberosity (displaced) S82.15- ☑
      - nondisplaced S82.15- ☑
- toe S92.91- ☑
  - great (displaced) S92.40- ☑
    - distal phalanx (displaced) S92.42- ☑
      - nondisplaced S92.42- ☑
    - nondisplaced S92.40- ☑
    - proximal phalanx (displaced) S92.41- ☑
      - nondisplaced S92.41- ☑
    - specified NEC S92.49- ☑
  - lesser (displaced) S92.50- ☑
    - distal phalanx (displaced) S92.53- ☑
      - nondisplaced S92.53- ☑
    - middle phalanx (displaced) S92.52- ☑
      - nondisplaced S92.52- ☑
    - nondisplaced S92.50- ☑
    - proximal phalanx (displaced) S92.51- ☑
      - nondisplaced S92.51- ☑
    - specified NEC S92.59- ☑
  - physeal
    - phalanx S99.20- ☑
      - Salter-Harris
        - Type I S99.21- ☑
        - Type II S99.22- ☑
        - Type III S99.23- ☑
        - Type IV S99.24- ☑
      - specified NEC S99.29- ☑
- tooth (root) S02.5 ☑
- trachea (cartilage) S12.8 ☑
- transverse process — *see* Fracture, vertebra
- trapezium or trapezoid bone — *see* Fracture, carpal
- trimalleolar — *see* Fracture, ankle, trimalleolar
- triquetrum (cuneiform of carpus) — *see* Fracture, carpal, triquetrum
- trochanter — *see* Fracture, femur, trochanteric
- tuberosity (external) — *see* Fracture, traumatic, by site
- ulna (shaft) S52.20- ☑
  - bent bone S52.28- ☑
  - coronoid process — *see* Fracture, ulna, upper end, coronoid process
  - distal end — *see* Fracture, ulna, lower end
  - following insertion of implant, prosthesis or plate M96.63- ☑
  - head S52.60- ☑
  - lower end S52.60- ☑
    - physeal S59.00- ☑
      - Salter-Harris
        - Type I S59.01- ☑
        - Type II S59.02- ☑
        - Type III S59.03- ☑
        - Type IV S59.04- ☑
      - specified NEC S59.09- ☑
    - specified NEC S52.69- ☑
    - styloid process (displaced) S52.61- ☑
      - nondisplaced S52.61- ☑
    - torus S52.62- ☑
  - proximal end — *see* Fracture, ulna, upper end
  - shaft S52.20- ☑
    - comminuted (displaced) S52.25- ☑
      - nondisplaced S52.25- ☑

Fracture, traumatic — *continued*
  ulna — *continued*
    shaft — *continued*
      greenstick S52.21- ☑
      Monteggia's — *see* Monteggia's fracture
      oblique (displaced) S52.23- ☑
        nondisplaced S52.23- ☑
      segmental (displaced) S52.26- ☑
        nondisplaced S52.26- ☑
      specified NEC S52.29- ☑
      spiral (displaced) S52.24- ☑
        nondisplaced S52.24- ☑
      transverse (displaced) S52.22- ☑
        nondisplaced S52.22- ☑
    upper end S52.00- ☑
      coronoid process (displaced) S52.04- ☑
        nondisplaced S52.04- ☑
      olecranon process (displaced) S52.02- ☑
        with intraarticular extension S52.03- ☑
        nondisplaced S52.02- ☑
          with intraarticular extension S52.03- ☑
      specified NEC S52.09- ☑
      torus S52.01- ☑
  unciform — *see* Fracture, carpal, hamate
  vault of skull S02.0 ☑
  vertebra, vertebral (arch) (body) (column) (neural arch)
    (pedicle) (spinous process) (transverse process)
    atlas — *see* Fracture, neck, cervical vertebra, first
    axis — *see* Fracture, neck, cervical vertebra, second
    cervical (teardrop) S12.9 ☑
      axis — *see* Fracture, neck, cervical vertebra, second
      first (atlas) — *see* Fracture, neck, cervical vertebra, first
      second (axis) — *see* Fracture, neck, cervical vertebra, second
    chronic M84.48
    coccyx S32.2 ☑
    dorsal — *see* Fracture, thorax, vertebra
    lumbar S32.009 ☑
      burst (stable) S32.001 ☑
        unstable S32.002 ☑
      fifth S32.059 ☑
        burst (stable) S32.051 ☑
          unstable S32.052 ☑
        specified type NEC S32.058 ☑
        wedge compression S32.050 ☑
      first S32.019 ☑
        burst (stable) S32.011 ☑
          unstable S32.012 ☑
        specified type NEC S32.018 ☑
        wedge compression S32.010 ☑
      fourth S32.049 ☑
        burst (stable) S32.041 ☑
          unstable S32.042 ☑
        specified type NEC S32.048 ☑
        wedge compression S32.040 ☑
      second S32.029 ☑
        burst (stable) S32.021 ☑
          unstable S32.022 ☑
        specified type NEC S32.028 ☑
        wedge compression S32.020 ☑
      specified type NEC S32.008 ☑
      third S32.039 ☑
        burst (stable) S32.031 ☑
          unstable S32.032 ☑
        specified type NEC S32.038 ☑
        wedge compression S32.030 ☑
      wedge compression S32.000 ☑
    metastatic — *see* Collapse, vertebra, in, specified disease NEC — *see also* Neoplasm
    newborn (birth injury) P11.5
    sacrum S32.10 ☑
      specified NEC S32.19 ☑
      Type
        1 S32.14 ☑
        2 S32.15 ☑
        3 S32.16 ☑
        4 S32.17 ☑
      Zone
        I S32.119 ☑
          displaced (minimally) S32.111 ☑
            severely S32.112 ☑
          nondisplaced S32.110 ☑
        II S32.129 ☑
          displaced (minimally) S32.121

Fracture, traumatic — *continued*
  vertebra, vertebral — *continued*
    sacrum — *continued*
      Zone — *continued*
        II — *continued*
          displaced — *continued*
            severely S32.122 ☑
          nondisplaced S32.120 ☑
        III S32.139 ☑
          displaced (minimally) S32.131 ☑
            severely S32.132 ☑
          nondisplaced S32.130 ☑
    thoracic — *see* Fracture, thorax, vertebra
  vertex S02.0 ☑
  vomer (bone) S02.2 ☑
  wrist S62.10- ☑
    carpal — *see* Fracture, carpal bone
    navicular (scaphoid) (hand) — *see* Fracture, carpal, navicular
  xiphisternum, xiphoid (process) S22.24 ☑
  zygoma S02.402 ☑
    left side S02.40F ☑
    right side S02.40E ☑
Fragile, fragility
  autosomal site Q95.5
  bone, congenital (with blue sclera) Q78.0
  capillary (hereditary) D69.8
  hair L67.8
  nails L60.3
  non-sex chromosome site Q95.5
  X chromosome Q99.2
Fragilitas
  crinium L67.8
  ossium (with blue sclerae) (hereditary) Q78.0
  unguium L60.3
    congenital Q84.6
Fragments, cataract (lens), **following cataract surgery** H59.02- ☑
  retained foreign body — *see* Retained, foreign body fragments (type of)
Frailty (frail) R54
  mental R41.81
Frambesia, frambesial (tropica) — *see also* Yaws
  initial lesion or ulcer A66.0
  primary A66.0
Frambeside
  gummatous A66.4
  of early yaws A66.2
Frambesioma A66.1
Franceschetti-Klein (-Wildervanck) **disease or syndrome** Q75.4
Francis' disease — *see* Tularemia
Franklin disease C88.2
Frank's essential thrombocytopenia D69.3
Fraser's syndrome Q87.0
Freckle(s) L81.2
  malignant melanoma in — *see* Melanoma
  melanotic (Hutchinson's) — *see* Melanoma, in situ
  retinal D49.81
Frederickson's hyperlipoproteinemia, type
  I and V E78.3
  IIA E78.00
  IIB and III E78.2
  IV E78.1
Freeman Sheldon syndrome Q87.0
Freezing — *see also* Effect, adverse, cold T69.9 ☑
Freiberg's disease (infraction of metatarsal head or osteochondrosis) — *see* Osteochondrosis, juvenile, metatarsus
Frei's disease A55
Fremitus, friction, cardiac R01.2
Frenum, frenulum
  external os Q51.828
  tongue (shortening) (congenital) Q38.1
Frequency micturition (nocturnal) R35.0
  psychogenic F45.8
Frey's syndrome
  auriculotemporal G50.8
  hyperhidrosis L74.52
Friction
  burn — *see* Burn, by site
  fremitus, cardiac R01.2
  precordial R01.2
  sounds, chest R09.89
Friderichsen-Waterhouse syndrome or disease A39.1
Friedländer's B (bacillus) **NEC** — *see also* condition A49.8

Friedreich's
  ataxia G11.1
  combined systemic disease G11.1
  facial hemihypertrophy Q67.4
  sclerosis (cerebellum) (spinal cord) G11.1
Frigidity F52.22
Fröhlich's syndrome E23.6
Frontal — *see also* condition
  lobe syndrome F07.0
Frostbite (superficial) T33.90 ☑
  with
    partial thickness skin loss — *see* Frostbite (superficial), by site
    tissue necrosis T34.90 ☑
  abdominal wall T33.3 ☑
    with tissue necrosis T34.3 ☑
  ankle T33.81- ☑
    with tissue necrosis T34.81- ☑
  arm T33.4- ☑
    with tissue necrosis T34.4- ☑
    finger(s) — *see* Frostbite, finger
    hand — *see* Frostbite, hand
    wrist — *see* Frostbite, wrist
  ear T33.01- ☑
    with tissue necrosis T34.01- ☑
  face T33.09 ☑
    with tissue necrosis T34.09 ☑
  finger T33.53- ☑
    with tissue necrosis T34.53- ☑
  foot T33.82- ☑
    with tissue necrosis T34.82- ☑
  hand T33.52- ☑
    with tissue necrosis T34.52- ☑
  head T33.09 ☑
    with tissue necrosis T34.09 ☑
    ear — *see* Frostbite, ear
    nose — *see* Frostbite, nose
  hip (and thigh) T33.6- ☑
    with tissue necrosis T34.6- ☑
  knee T33.7- ☑
    with tissue necrosis T34.7- ☑
  leg T33.9- ☑
    with tissue necrosis T34.9- ☑
    ankle — *see* Frostbite, ankle
    foot — *see* Frostbite, foot
    knee — *see* Frostbite, knee
    lower T33.7- ☑
      with tissue necrosis T34.7- ☑
    thigh — *see* Frostbite, hip
    toe — *see* Frostbite, toe
  limb
    lower T33.99 ☑
      with tissue necrosis T34.99 ☑
    upper — *see* Frostbite, arm
  neck T33.1 ☑
    with tissue necrosis T34.1 ☑
  nose T33.02 ☑
    with tissue necrosis T34.02 ☑
  pelvis T33.3 ☑
    with tissue necrosis T34.3 ☑
  specified site NEC T33.99 ☑
    with tissue necrosis T34.99 ☑
  thigh — *see* Frostbite, hip
  thorax T33.2 ☑
    with tissue necrosis T34.2 ☑
  toes T33.83- ☑
    with tissue necrosis T34.83- ☑
  trunk T33.99 ☑
    with tissue necrosis T34.99 ☑
  wrist T33.51- ☑
    with tissue necrosis T34.51- ☑
Frotteurism F65.81
Frozen — *see also* Effect, adverse, cold T69.9 ☑
  pelvis (female) N94.89
    male K66.8
  shoulder — *see* Capsulitis, adhesive
Fructokinase deficiency E74.11
Fructose 1,6 diphosphatase deficiency E74.19
Fructosemia (benign) (essential) E74.12
Fructosuria (benign) (essential) E74.11
Fuchs'
  black spot (myopic) — *see also* Myopia, degenerative H44.2-
  dystrophy (corneal endothelium) H18.51
  heterochromic cyclitis — *see* Cyclitis, Fuchs' heterochromic

▽ Subterms under main terms may continue to next column or page   ☑ Additional Character Required — Refer to the Tabular List for Character Selection   **155**

Fracture, traumatic — Fuchs'

Fucosidosis E77.1
Fugue R68.89
  dissociative F44.1
  hysterical (dissociative) F44.1
  postictal in epilepsy — *see* Epilepsy
  reaction to exceptional stress (transient) F43.0
Fulminant, fulminating — *see* condition
Functional — *see also* condition
  bleeding (uterus) N93.8
Functioning, intellectual, borderline R41.83
Fundus — *see* condition
Fungemia NOS B49
Fungus, fungous
  cerebral G93.89
  disease NOS B49
  infection — *see* Infection, fungus
Funiculitis (acute) (chronic) (endemic) N49.1
  gonococcal (acute) (chronic) A54.23
  tuberculous A18.15
Funnel
  breast (acquired) M95.4
    congenital Q67.6
    sequelae (late effect) of rickets E64.3
  chest (acquired) M95.4
    congenital Q67.6
    sequelae (late effect) of rickets E64.3
  pelvis (acquired) M95.5
    with disproportion (fetopelvic) O33.3 ☑
      causing obstructed labor O65.3
    congenital Q74.2
FUO (fever of unknown origin) R50.9
Furfur L21.0
  microsporon B36.0
Furrier's lung J67.8
Furrowed K14.5
  nail(s) (transverse) L60.4
    congenital Q84.6
  tongue K14.5
    congenital Q38.3
Furuncle L02.92
  abdominal wall L02.221
  ankle — *see* Furuncle, lower limb
  antecubital space — *see* Furuncle, upper limb
  anus K61.0
  arm — *see* Furuncle, upper limb
  auditory canal, external — *see* Abscess, ear, external
  auricle (ear) — *see* Abscess, ear, external
  axilla (region) L02.42- ☑
  back (any part) L02.222
  breast N61.1
  buttock L02.32
  cheek (external) L02.02
  chest wall L02.223
  chin L02.02
  corpus cavernosum N48.21
  ear, external — *see* Abscess, ear, external
  external auditory canal — *see* Abscess, ear, external
  eyelid — *see* Abscess, eyelid
  face L02.02
  femoral (region) — *see* Furuncle, lower limb

Furuncle — *continued*
  finger — *see* Furuncle, hand
  flank L02.221
  foot L02.62- ☑
  forehead L02.02
  gluteal (region) L02.32
  groin L02.224
  hand L02.52- ☑
  head L02.821
    face L02.02
  hip — *see* Furuncle, lower limb
  kidney — *see* Abscess, kidney
  knee — *see* Furuncle, lower limb
  labium (majus) (minus) N76.4
  lacrimal
    gland — *see* Dacryoadenitis
    passages (duct) (sac) — *see* Inflammation, lacrimal, passages, acute
  leg (any part) — *see* Furuncle, lower limb
  lower limb L02.42- ☑
  malignant A22.0
  mouth K12.2
  navel L02.226
  neck L02.12
  nose J34.0
  orbit, orbital — *see* Abscess, orbit
  palmar (space) — *see* Furuncle, hand
  partes posteriores L02.32
  pectoral region L02.223
  penis N48.21
  perineum L02.225
  pinna — *see* Abscess, ear, external
  popliteal — *see* Furuncle, lower limb
  prepatellar — *see* Furuncle, lower limb
  scalp L02.821
  seminal vesicle N49.0
  shoulder — *see* Furuncle, upper limb
  specified site NEC L02.828
  submandibular K12.2
  temple (region) L02.02
  thumb — *see* Furuncle, hand
  toe — *see* Furuncle, foot
  trunk L02.229
    abdominal wall L02.221
    back L02.222
    chest wall L02.223
    groin L02.224
    perineum L02.225
    umbilicus L02.226
  umbilicus L02.226
  upper limb L02.42- ☑
  vulva N76.4
Furunculosis — *see* Furuncle
Fused — *see* Fusion, fused
Fusion, fused (congenital)
  astragaloscaphoid Q74.2
  atria Q21.1
  auditory canal Q16.1
  auricles, heart Q21.1
  binocular with defective stereopsis H53.32

Fusion, fused — *continued*
  bone Q79.8
  cervical spine M43.22
  choanal Q30.0
  commissure, mitral valve Q23.2
  cusps, heart valve NEC Q24.8
    mitral Q23.2
    pulmonary Q22.1
    tricuspid Q22.4
  ear ossicles Q16.3
  fingers Q70.0 ☑
  hymen Q52.3
  joint (acquired) — *see also* Ankylosis
    congenital Q74.8
  kidneys (incomplete) Q63.1
  labium (majus) (minus) Q52.5
  larynx and trachea Q34.8
  limb, congenital Q74.8
    lower Q74.2
    upper Q74.0
  lobes, lung Q33.8
  lumbosacral (acquired) M43.27
    arthrodesis status Z98.1
    congenital Q76.49
    postprocedural status Z98.1
  nares, nose, nasal, nostril(s) Q30.0
  organ or site not listed — *see* Anomaly, by site
  ossicles Q79.9
    auditory Q16.3
  pulmonic cusps Q22.1
  ribs Q76.6
  sacroiliac (joint) (acquired) M43.28
    arthrodesis status Z98.1
    congenital Q74.2
    postprocedural status Z98.1
  spine (acquired) NEC M43.20
    arthrodesis status Z98.1
    cervical region M43.22
    cervicothoracic region M43.23
    congenital Q76.49
    lumbar M43.26
    lumbosacral region M43.27
    occipito-atlanto-axial region M43.21
    postoperative status Z98.1
    sacrococcygeal region M43.28
    thoracic region M43.24
    thoracolumbar region M43.25
  sublingual duct with submaxillary duct at opening in mouth Q38.4
  testes Q55.1
  toes Q70.2- ☑
  tooth, teeth K00.2
  trachea and esophagus Q39.8
  twins Q89.4
  vagina Q52.4
  ventricles, heart Q21.0
  vertebra (arch) — *see* Fusion, spine
  vulva Q52.5
Fusospirillosis (mouth) (tongue) (tonsil) A69.1
Fussy baby R68.12

☑ **Additional Character Required** — Refer to the Tabular List for Character Selection   ▽ Subterms under main terms may continue to next column or page

G

Gain in weight (abnormal) (excessive) — *see also* Weight, gain
Gaisböck's disease (polycythemia hypertonica) D75.1
Gait abnormality R26.9
  ataxic R26.0
  falling R29.6
  hysterical (ataxic) (staggering) F44.4
  paralytic R26.1
  spastic R26.1
  specified type NEC R26.89
  staggering R26.0
  unsteadiness R26.81
  walking difficulty NEC R26.2
Galactocele (breast) N64.89
  puerperal, postpartum O92.79
Galactokinase deficiency E74.29
Galactophoritis N61.0
  gestational, puerperal, postpartum O91.2- ☑
Galactorrhea O92.6
  not associated with childbirth N64.3
Galactosemia (classic) (congenital) E74.21
Galactosuria E74.29
Galacturia R82.0
  schistosomiasis (bilharziasis) B65.0
GALD (gestational alloimmune liver disease) P78.84
Galeazzi's fracture S52.37- ☑
Galen's vein — *see* condition
Galeophobia F40.218
Gall duct — *see* condition
Gallbladder — *see also* condition
  acute K81.0
Gallop rhythm R00.8
Gallstone (colic) (cystic duct) (gallbladder) (impacted) (multiple) — *see also* Calculus, gallbladder
  with
    cholecystitis — *see* Calculus, gallbladder, with cholecystitis
  bile duct (common) (hepatic) — *see* Calculus, bile duct
  causing intestinal obstruction K56.3
  specified NEC K80.80
    with obstruction K80.81
Gambling Z72.6
  pathological (compulsive) F63.0
Gammopathy (of undetermined significance [MGUS]) D47.2
  associated with lymphoplasmacytic dyscrasia D47.2
  monoclonal D47.2
  polyclonal D89.0
Gamna's disease (siderotic splenomegaly) D73.1
Gamophobia F40.298
Gampsodactylia (congenital) Q66.7- ☑
Gamstorp's disease (adynamia episodica hereditaria) G72.3
Gandy-Nanta disease (siderotic splenomegaly) D73.1
Gang
  membership offenses Z72.810
Gangliocytoma D36.10
Ganglioglioma — *see* Neoplasm, uncertain behavior, by site
Ganglion (compound) (diffuse) (joint) (tendon (sheath)) M67.40
  ankle M67.47- ☑
  foot M67.47- ☑
  forearm M67.43- ☑
  hand M67.44- ☑
  lower leg M67.46- ☑
  multiple sites M67.49
  of yaws (early) (late) A66.6
  pelvic region M67.45- ☑
  periosteal — *see* Periostitis
  shoulder region M67.41- ☑
  specified site NEC M67.48
  thigh region M67.45- ☑
  tuberculous A18.09
  upper arm M67.42- ☑
  wrist M67.43- ☑
Ganglioneuroblastoma — *see* Neoplasm, nerve, malignant
Ganglioneuroma D36.10
  malignant — *see* Neoplasm, nerve, malignant
Ganglioneuromatosis D36.10
Ganglionitis
  fifth nerve — *see* Neuralgia, trigeminal
  gasserian (postherpetic) (postzoster) B02.21

Ganglionitis — *continued*
  geniculate G51.1
    newborn (birth injury) P11.3
    postherpetic, postzoster B02.21
  herpes zoster B02.21
  postherpetic geniculate B02.21
Gangliosidosis E75.10
  GM1 E75.19
  GM2 E75.00
    other specified E75.09
    Sandhoff disease E75.01
    Tay-Sachs disease E75.02
  GM3 E75.19
  mucolipidosis IV E75.11
Gangosa A66.5
Gangrene, gangrenous (connective tissue) (dropsical) (dry) (moist) (skin) (ulcer) — *see also* Necrosis I96
  with diabetes (mellitus) — *see* Diabetes, gangrene
  abdomen (wall) I96
  alveolar M27.3
  appendix K35.80
    with
      peritonitis, localized — *see also* Appendicitis K35.31
  arteriosclerotic (general) (senile) — *see* Arteriosclerosis, extremities, with, gangrene
  auricle I96
  Bacillus welchii A48.0
  bladder (infectious) — *see* Cystitis, specified type NEC
  bowel, cecum, or colon — *see* Gangrene, intestine
  Clostridium perfringens or welchii A48.0
  cornea H18.89- ☑
  corpora cavernosa N48.29
    noninfective N48.89
  cutaneous, spreading I96
  decubital — *see* Ulcer, pressure, by site
  diabetic (any site) — *see* Diabetes, gangrene
  emphysematous — *see* Gangrene, gas
  epidemic — *see* Poisoning, food, noxious, plant
  epididymis (infectional) N45.1
  erysipelas — *see* Erysipelas
  extremity (lower) (upper) I96
  Fournier N49.3
    female N76.89
  fusospirochetal A69.0
  gallbladder — *see* Cholecystitis, acute
  gas (bacillus) A48.0
    following
      abortion — *see* Abortion by type complicated by infection
      ectopic or molar pregnancy O08.0
  glossitis K14.0
  hernia — *see* Hernia, by site, with gangrene
  intestine, intestinal (hemorrhagic) (massive) — *see also* Infarct, intestine K55.069
    with
      mesenteric embolism — *see also* Infarct, intestine K55.069
      obstruction — *see* Obstruction, intestine
  laryngitis J04.0
  limb (lower) (upper) I96
  lung J85.0
    spirochetal A69.8
  lymphangitis I89.1
  Meleney's (synergistic) — *see* Ulcer, skin
  mesentery — *see also* Infarct, intestine K55.069
    with
      embolism — *see also* Infarct, intestine K55.069
      intestinal obstruction — *see* Obstruction, intestine
  mouth A69.0
  ovary — *see* Oophoritis
  pancreas — *see* Pancreatitis, acute
  penis N48.29
    noninfective N48.89
  perineum I96
  pharynx — *see also* Pharyngitis
    Vincent's A69.1
  presenile I73.1
  progressive synergistic — *see* Ulcer, skin
  pulmonary J85.0
  pulpal (dental) K04.1
  quinsy J36
  Raynaud's (symmetric gangrene) I73.01
  retropharyngeal J39.2
  scrotum N49.3
    noninfective N50.89

Gangrene, gangrenous — *continued*
  senile (atherosclerotic) — *see* Arteriosclerosis, extremities, with, gangrene
  spermatic cord N49.1
    noninfective N50.89
  spine I96
  spirochetal NEC A69.8
  spreading cutaneous I96
  stomatitis A69.0
  symmetrical I73.01
  testis (infectional) N45.2
    noninfective N44.8
  throat — *see also* Pharyngitis
    diphtheritic A36.0
    Vincent's A69.1
  thyroid (gland) E07.89
  tooth (pulp) K04.1
  tuberculous NEC — *see* Tuberculosis
  tunica vaginalis N49.1
    noninfective N50.89
  umbilicus I96
  uterus — *see* Endometritis
  uvulitis K12.2
  vas deferens N49.1
    noninfective N50.89
  vulva N76.89
Ganister disease J62.8
Ganser's syndrome (hysterical) F44.89
Gardner-Diamond syndrome (autoerythrocyte sensitization) D69.2
Gargoylism E76.01
Garré's disease, osteitis (sclerosing), osteomyelitis — *see* Osteomyelitis, specified type NEC
Garrod's pad, knuckle M72.1
Gartner's duct
  cyst Q52.4
  persistent Q50.6
Gas R14.3
  asphyxiation, inhalation, poisoning, suffocation NEC — *see* Table of Drugs and Chemicals
  excessive R14.0
  gangrene A48.0
    following
      abortion — *see* Abortion by type complicated by infection
      ectopic or molar pregnancy O08.0
  on stomach R14.0
  pains R14.1
Gastralgia — *see also* Pain, abdominal
Gastrectasis K31.0
  psychogenic F45.8
Gastric — *see* condition
Gastrinoma
  malignant
    pancreas C25.4
    specified site NEC — *see* Neoplasm, malignant, by site
    unspecified site C25.4
  specified site — *see* Neoplasm, uncertain behavior
  unspecified site D37.9
Gastritis (simple) K29.70
  with bleeding K29.71
  acute (erosive) K29.00
    with bleeding K29.01
  alcoholic K29.20
    with bleeding K29.21
  allergic K29.60
    with bleeding K29.61
  atrophic (chronic) K29.40
    with bleeding K29.41
  chronic (antral) (fundal) K29.50
    with bleeding K29.51
    atrophic K29.40
      with bleeding K29.41
    superficial K29.30
      with bleeding K29.31
  dietary counseling and surveillance Z71.3
  due to diet deficiency E63.9
  eosinophilic K52.81
  giant hypertrophic K29.60
    with bleeding K29.61
  granulomatous K29.60
    with bleeding K29.61
  hypertrophic (mucosa) K29.60
    with bleeding K29.61
  nervous F54
  spastic K29.60
    with bleeding K29.61

Gastritis — *continued*
specified NEC K29.60
with bleeding K29.61
superficial chronic K29.30
with bleeding K29.31
tuberculous A18.83
viral NEC A08.4
Gastrocarcinoma — *see* Neoplasm, malignant, stomach
Gastrocolic — *see* condition
Gastrodisciasis, gastrodiscoidiasis B66.8
Gastroduodenitis K29.90
with bleeding K29.91
virus, viral A08.4
specified type NEC A08.39
Gastrodynia — *see* Pain, abdominal
Gastroenteritis (acute) (chronic) (noninfectious) — *see also* Enteritis K52.9
allergic K52.29
with
eosinophilic gastritis or gastroenteritis K52.81
food protein-induced enterocolitis syndrome K52.21
food protein-induced enteropathy K52.22
dietetic — *see also* Gastroenteritis, allergic K52.29
drug-induced K52.1
due to
Cryptosporidium A07.2
drugs K52.1
food poisoning — *see* Intoxication, foodborne
radiation K52.0
eosinophilic K52.81
epidemic (infectious) A09
food hypersensitivity — *see also* Gastroenteritis, allergic K52.29
infectious — *see* Enteritis, infectious
influenzal — *see* Influenza, with gastroenteritis
noninfectious K52.9
specified NEC K52.89
rotaviral A08.0
Salmonella A02.0
toxic K52.1
viral NEC A08.4
acute infectious A08.39
type Norwalk A08.11
infantile (acute) A08.39
Norwalk agent A08.11
rotaviral A08.0
severe of infants A08.39
specified type NEC A08.39
Gastroenteropathy — *see also* Gastroenteritis K52.9
acute, due to Norovirus A08.11
acute, due to Norwalk agent A08.11
infectious A09
Gastroenteroptosis K63.4
Gastroesophageal laceration- hemorrhage syndrome K22.6
Gastrointestinal — *see* condition
Gastrojejunal — *see* condition
Gastrojejunitis — *see also* Enteritis K52.9
Gastrojejunocolic — *see* condition
Gastroliths K31.89
Gastromalacia K31.89
Gastroparalysis K31.84
diabetic — *see* Diabetes, gastroparalysis
Gastroparesis K31.84
diabetic — *see* Diabetes, by type, with gastroparesis
Gastropathy K31.9
congestive portal K31.89
erythematous K29.70
exudative K90.89
portal hypertensive K31.89
Gastroptosis K31.89
Gastrorrhagia K92.2
psychogenic F45.8
Gastroschisis (congenital) Q79.3
Gastrospasm (neurogenic) (reflex) K31.89
neurotic F45.8
psychogenic F45.8
Gastrostaxis — *see* Gastritis, with bleeding
Gastrostenosis K31.89
Gastrostomy
attention to Z43.1
status Z93.1
Gastrosuccorrhea (continuous) (intermittent) K31.89
neurotic F45.8
psychogenic F45.8
Gatophobia F40.218

Gaucher's disease or splenomegaly (adult) (infantile) E75.22
Gee (-Herter)(-Thaysen) **disease** (nontropical sprue) K90.0
Gélineau's syndrome G47.419
with cataplexy G47.411
Gemination, tooth, teeth K00.2
Gemistocytoma
specified site — *see* Neoplasm, malignant, by site
unspecified site C71.9
General, generalized — *see* condition
Genetic
carrier (status)
cystic fibrosis Z14.1
hemophilia A (asymptomatic) Z14.01
symptomatic Z14.02
specified NEC Z14.8
susceptibility to disease NEC Z15.89
malignant neoplasm Z15.09
breast Z15.01
endometrium Z15.04
ovary Z15.02
prostate Z15.03
specified NEC Z15.09
multiple endocrine neoplasia Z15.81
Genital — *see* condition
Genito-anorectal syndrome A55
Genitourinary system — *see* condition
Genu
congenital Q74.1
extrorsum (acquired) — *see also* Deformity, varus, knee
congenital Q74.1
sequelae (late effect) of rickets E64.3
introrsum (acquired) — *see also* Deformity, valgus, knee
congenital Q74.1
sequelae (late effect) of rickets E64.3
rachitic (old) E64.3
recurvatum (acquired) — *see also* Deformity, limb, specified type NEC, lower leg
congenital Q68.2
sequelae (late effect) of rickets E64.3
valgum (acquired) (knock-knee) M21.06- ☑
congenital Q74.1
sequelae (late effect) of rickets E64.3
varum (acquired) (bowleg) M21.16- ☑
congenital Q74.1
sequelae (late effect) of rickets E64.3
Geographic tongue K14.1
Geophagia — *see* Pica
Geotrichosis B48.3
stomatitis B48.3
Gephyrophobia F40.242
Gerbode defect Q21.0
GERD (gastroesophageal reflux disease) K21.9
Gerhardt's
disease (erythromelalgia) I73.81
syndrome (vocal cord paralysis) J38.00
bilateral J38.02
unilateral J38.01
German measles — *see also* Rubella
exposure to Z20.4
Germinoblastoma (diffuse) C85.9- ☑
follicular C82.9- ☑
Germinoma — *see* Neoplasm, malignant, by site
Gerontoxon — *see* Degeneration, cornea, senile
Gerstmann's syndrome R48.8
developmental F81.2
Gerstmann-Sträussler-Scheinker syndrome (GSS) A81.82
Gestation (period) — *see also* Pregnancy
ectopic — *see* Pregnancy, by site
multiple O30.9- ☑
greater than quadruplets — *see* Pregnancy, multiple (gestation), specified NEC
specified NEC — *see* Pregnancy, multiple (gestation), specified NEC
Gestational
mammary abscess O91.11- ☑
purulent mastitis O91.11- ☑
subareolar abscess O91.11- ☑
Ghon tubercle, primary infection A15.7
Ghost
teeth K00.4
vessels (cornea) H16.41- ☑
Ghoul hand A66.3
Gianotti-Crosti disease L44.4

Giant
cell
epulis K06.8
peripheral granuloma K06.8
esophagus, congenital Q39.5
kidney, congenital Q63.3
urticaria T78.3 ☑
hereditary D84.1
Giardiasis A07.1
Gibert's disease or pityriasis L42
Giddiness R42
hysterical F44.89
psychogenic F45.8
Gierke's disease (glycogenosis I) E74.01
Gigantism (cerebral) (hypophyseal) (pituitary) E22.0
constitutional E34.4
Gilbert's disease or syndrome E80.4
Gilchrist's disease B40.9
Gilford-Hutchinson disease E34.8
Gilles de la Tourette's disease or syndrome (motor-verbal tic) F95.2
Gingivitis K05.10
acute (catarrhal) K05.00
necrotizing A69.1
nonplaque induced K05.01
plaque induced K05.00
chronic (desquamative) (hyperplastic) (simple marginal) (pregnancy associated) (ulcerative) K05.10
nonplaque induced K05.11
plaque induced K05.10
expulsiva — *see* Periodontitis
necrotizing ulcerative (acute) A69.1
pellagrous E52
acute necrotizing A69.1
Vincent's A69.1
Gingivoglossitis K14.0
Gingivopericementitis — *see* Periodontitis
Gingivosis — *see* Gingivitis, chronic
Gingivostomatitis K05.10
herpesviral B00.2
necrotizing ulcerative (acute) A69.1
Gland, glandular — *see* condition
Glanders A24.0
Glanzmann (-Naegeli) **disease or thrombasthenia** D69.1
Glasgow coma scale
total score
13-15 R40.241 ☑
3-8 R40.243 ☑
9-12 R40.242 ☑
Glass-blower's disease (cataract) — *see* Cataract, specified NEC
Glaucoma H40.9
with
increased episcleral venous pressure H40.81- ☑
pseudoexfoliation of lens — *see* Glaucoma, open angle, primary, capsular
absolute H44.51- ☑
angle-closure (primary) H40.20- ☑
acute (attack) (crisis) H40.21- ☑
chronic H40.22- ☑
intermittent H40.23- ☑
residual stage H40.24- ☑
borderline H40.00- ☑
capsular (with pseudoexfoliation of lens) — *see* Glaucoma, open angle, primary, capsular
childhood Q15.0
closed angle — *see* Glaucoma, angle-closure
congenital Q15.0
corticosteroid-induced — *see* Glaucoma, secondary, drugs
hypersecretion H40.82- ☑
in (due to)
amyloidosis E85.4 [H42]
aniridia Q13.1 [H42]
concussion of globe — *see* Glaucoma, secondary, trauma
dislocation of lens — *see* Glaucoma, secondary
disorder of lens NEC — *see* Glaucoma, secondary
drugs — *see* Glaucoma, secondary, drugs
endocrine disease NOS E34.9 [H42]
eye
inflammation — *see* Glaucoma, secondary, inflammation
trauma — *see* Glaucoma, secondary, trauma
hypermature cataract — *see* Glaucoma, secondary

☑ Additional Character Required — Refer to the Tabular List for Character Selection ▽ Subterms under main terms may continue to next column or page

Glaucoma — *continued*
- in — *continued*
  - iridocyclitis — *see* Glaucoma, secondary, inflammation
  - lens disorder — *see* Glaucoma, secondary
  - Lowe's syndrome E72.03 *[H42]*
  - metabolic disease NOS E88.9 *[H42]*
  - ocular disorders NEC — *see* Glaucoma, secondary
  - onchocerciasis B73.02
  - pupillary block — *see* Glaucoma, secondary
  - retinal vein occlusion — *see* Glaucoma, secondary
  - Rieger's anomaly Q13.81 *[H42]*
  - rubeosis of iris — *see* Glaucoma, secondary
  - tumor of globe — *see* Glaucoma, secondary
  - infantile Q15.0
  - low tension — *see* Glaucoma, open angle, primary, low-tension
  - malignant H40.83- ☑
  - narrow angle — *see* Glaucoma, angle-closure
  - newborn Q15.0
  - noncongestive (chronic) — *see* Glaucoma, open angle
  - nonobstructive — *see* Glaucoma, open angle
  - obstructive — *see also* Glaucoma, angle-closure
    - due to lens changes — *see* Glaucoma, secondary
  - open angle H40.10- ☑
    - primary H40.11- ☑
      - capsular (with pseudoexfoliation of lens) H40.14- ☑
      - low-tension H40.12- ☑
      - pigmentary H40.13- ☑
      - residual stage H40.15- ☑
  - phacolytic — *see* Glaucoma, secondary
  - pigmentary — *see* Glaucoma, open angle, primary, pigmentary
  - postinfectious — *see* Glaucoma, secondary, inflammation
  - secondary (to) H40.5- ☑
    - drugs H40.6- ☑
    - inflammation H40.4- ☑
    - trauma H40.3- ☑
  - simple (chronic) H40.11- ☑
  - simplex H40.11- ☑
  - specified type NEC H40.89
  - suspect H40.00- ☑
  - syphilitic A52.71
  - traumatic — *see also* Glaucoma, secondary, trauma
    - newborn (birth injury) P15.3
  - tuberculous A18.59

Glaucomatous flecks (subcapsular) — *see* Cataract, complicated
Glazed tongue K14.4
Gleet (gonococcal) A54.01
Glénard's disease K63.4
Glioblastoma (multiforme)
- with sarcomatous component
  - specified site — *see* Neoplasm, malignant, by site
  - unspecified site C71.9
- giant cell
  - specified site — *see* Neoplasm, malignant, by site
  - unspecified site C71.9
- specified site — *see* Neoplasm, malignant, by site
- unspecified site C71.9
Glioma (malignant)
- astrocytic
  - specified site — *see* Neoplasm, malignant, by site
  - unspecified site C71.9
- mixed
  - specified site — *see* Neoplasm, malignant, by site
  - unspecified site C71.9
- nose Q30.8
- specified site NEC — *see* Neoplasm, malignant, by site
- subependymal D43.2
  - specified site — *see* Neoplasm, uncertain behavior, by site
  - unspecified site D43.2
- unspecified site C71.9
Gliomatosis cerebri C71.0
Glioneuroma — *see* Neoplasm, uncertain behavior, by site
Gliosarcoma
- specified site — *see* Neoplasm, malignant, by site
- unspecified site C71.9
Gliosis (cerebral) G93.89
- spinal G95.89
Glisson's disease — *see* Rickets
Globinuria R82.3
Globus (hystericus) F45.8

Glomangioma D18.00
- intra-abdominal D18.03
- intracranial D18.02
- skin D18.01
- specified site NEC D18.09
Glomangiomyoma D18.00
- intra-abdominal D18.03
- intracranial D18.02
- skin D18.01
- specified site NEC D18.09
Glomangiosarcoma — *see* Neoplasm, connective tissue, malignant
Glomerular
- disease in syphilis A52.75
- nephritis — *see* Glomerulonephritis
Glomerulitis — *see* Glomerulonephritis
Glomerulonephritis — *see also* Nephritis N05.9
- with
  - edema — *see* Nephrosis
  - minimal change N05.0
  - minor glomerular abnormality N05.0
- acute N00.9
- chronic N03.9
- crescentic (diffuse) NEC — *see also* N00-N07 with fourth character .7 N05.7
- dense deposit — *see also* N00-N07 with fourth character .6 N05.6
- diffuse
  - crescentic — *see also* N00-N07 with fourth character .7 N05.7
  - endocapillary proliferative — *see also* N00-N07 with fourth character .4 N05.4
  - membranous — *see also* N00-N07 with fourth character .2 N05.2
  - mesangial proliferative — *see also* N00-N07 with fourth character .3 N05.3
  - mesangiocapillary — *see also* N00-N07 with fourth character .5 N05.5
  - sclerosing N18.9
- endocapillary proliferative (diffuse) NEC — *see also* N00-N07 with fourth character .4 N05.4
- extracapillary NEC — *see also* N00-N07 with fourth character .7 N05.7
- focal (and segmental) — *see also* N00-N07 with fourth character .1 N05.1
- hypocomplementemic — *see* Glomerulonephritis, membranoproliferative
- IgA — *see* Nephropathy, IgA
- immune complex (circulating) NEC N05.8
- in (due to)
  - amyloidosis E85.4 *[N08]*
  - bilharziasis B65.9 *[N08]*
  - cryoglobulinemia D89.1 *[N08]*
  - defibrination syndrome D65 *[N08]*
  - diabetes mellitus — *see* Diabetes, glomerulosclerosis
  - disseminated intravascular coagulation D65 *[N08]*
  - Fabry (-Anderson) disease E75.21 *[N08]*
  - Goodpasture's syndrome M31.0
  - hemolytic-uremic syndrome D59.3
  - Henoch (-Schönlein) purpura D69.0 *[N08]*
  - lecithin cholesterol acyltransferase deficiency E78.6 *[N08]*
  - microscopic polyangiitis M31.7 *[N08]*
  - multiple myeloma C90.0- ☑ *[N08]*
  - Plasmodium malariae B52.0
  - schistosomiasis B65.9 *[N08]*
  - sepsis A41.9 *[N08]*
    - streptococcal A40- ☑ *[N08]*
  - sickle-cell disorders D57.- ☑ *[N08]*
  - strongyloidiasis B78.9 *[N08]*
  - subacute bacterial endocarditis I33.0 *[N08]*
  - syphilis (late) congenital A50.59 *[N08]*
  - systemic lupus erythematosus M32.14
  - thrombotic thrombocytopenic purpura M31.1 *[N08]*
  - typhoid fever A01.09
  - Waldenström macroglobulinemia C88.0 *[N08]*
  - Wegener's granulomatosis M31.31
- latent or quiescent N03.9
- lobular, lobulonodular — *see* Glomerulonephritis, membranoproliferative
- membranoproliferative (diffuse)(type 1 or 3) — *see also* N00-N07 with fourth character .5 N05.5
  - dense deposit (type 2) NEC — *see also* N00-N07 with fourth character .6 N05.6
- membranous (diffuse) NEC — *see also* N00-N07 with fourth character .2 N05.2

Glomerulonephritis — *continued*
- mesangial
  - IgA/IgG — *see* Nephropathy, IgA
  - proliferative (diffuse) NEC — *see also* N00-N07 with fourth character .3 N05.3
- mesangiocapillary (diffuse) NEC — *see also* N00-N07 with fourth character .5 N05.5
- necrotic, necrotizing NEC — *see also* N00- N07 with fourth character .8 N05.8
- nodular — *see* Glomerulonephritis, membranoproliferative
- poststreptococcal NEC N05.9
  - acute N00.9
  - chronic N03.9
  - rapidly progressive N01.9
- proliferative NEC — *see also* N00-N07 with fourth character .8 N05.8
  - diffuse (lupus) M32.14
- rapidly progressive N01.9
- sclerosing, diffuse N18.9
- specified pathology NEC — *see also* N00- N07 with fourth character .8 N05.8
- subacute N01.9
Glomerulopathy — *see* Glomerulonephritis
Glomerulosclerosis — *see also* Sclerosis, renal
- intercapillary (nodular) (with diabetes) — *see* Diabetes, glomerulosclerosis
- intracapillary — *see* Diabetes, glomerulosclerosis
Glossagra K14.6
Glossalgia K14.6
Glossitis (chronic superficial) (gangrenous) (Moeller's) K14.0
- areata exfoliativa K14.1
- atrophic K14.4
- benign migratory K14.1
- cortical superficial, sclerotic K14.0
- Hunter's D51.0
- interstitial, sclerous K14.0
- median rhomboid K14.2
- pellagrous E52
- superficial, chronic K14.0
Glossocele K14.8
Glossodynia K14.6
- exfoliativa K14.4
Glossoncus K14.8
Glossopathy K14.9
Glossophytia K14.3
Glossoplegia K14.8
Glossoptosis K14.8
Glossopyrosis K14.6
Glossotrichia K14.3
Glossy skin L90.8
Glottis — *see* condition
Glottitis — *see also* Laryngitis J04.0
Glucagonoma
- pancreas
  - benign D13.7
  - malignant C25.4
  - uncertain behavior D37.8
- specified site NEC
  - benign — *see* Neoplasm, benign, by site
  - malignant — *see* Neoplasm, malignant, by site
  - uncertain behavior — *see* Neoplasm, uncertain behavior, by site
- unspecified site
  - benign D13.7
  - malignant C25.4
  - uncertain behavior D37.8
Glucoglycinuria E72.51
Glucose-galactose malabsorption E74.39
Glue
- ear — *see* Otitis, media, nonsuppurative, chronic, mucoid
- sniffing (airplane) — *see* Abuse, drug, inhalant
- dependence — *see* Dependence, drug, inhalant
Glutaric aciduria E72.3
Glycinemia E72.51
Glycinuria (renal) (with ketosis) E72.09
Glycogen
- infiltration — *see* Disease, glycogen storage
- storage disease — *see* Disease, glycogen storage
Glycogenosis (diffuse) (generalized) — *see also* Disease, glycogen storage
- cardiac E74.02 *[I43]*
- diabetic, secondary — *see* Diabetes, glycogenosis, secondary
- pulmonary interstitial J84.842

▽ **Subterms under main terms may continue to next column or page**   ☑ **Additional Character Required — Refer to the Tabular List for Character Selection**   **159**

Glaucoma — Glycogenosis

Glycopenia E16.2
Glycosuria R81
  renal E74.8
Gnathostoma spinigerum (infection) (infestation), **gnathostomiasis** (wandering swelling) B83.1
Goiter (plunging) (substernal) E04.9
  with
    hyperthyroidism (recurrent) — *see* Hyperthyroidism, with, goiter
    thyrotoxicosis — *see* Hyperthyroidism, with, goiter
  adenomatous — *see* Goiter, nodular
  cancerous C73
  congenital (nontoxic) E03.0
    diffuse E03.0
    parenchymatous E03.0
    transitory, with normal functioning P72.0
  cystic E04.2
    due to iodine-deficiency E01.1
  due to
    enzyme defect in synthesis of thyroid hormone E07.1
    iodine-deficiency (endemic) E01.2
  dyshormonogenetic (familial) E07.1
  endemic (iodine-deficiency) E01.2
    diffuse E01.0
    multinodular E01.1
  exophthalmic — *see* Hyperthyroidism, with, goiter
  iodine-deficiency (endemic) E01.2
    diffuse E01.0
    multinodular E01.1
    nodular E01.1
  lingual Q89.2
  lymphadenoid E06.3
  malignant C73
  multinodular (cystic) (nontoxic) E04.2
    toxic or with hyperthyroidism E05.20
      with thyroid storm E05.21
  neonatal NEC P72.0
  nodular (nontoxic) (due to) E04.9
    with
      hyperthyroidism E05.20
        with thyroid storm E05.21
      thyrotoxicosis E05.20
        with thyroid storm E05.21
    endemic E01.1
    iodine-deficiency E01.1
    sporadic E04.9
    toxic E05.20
      with thyroid storm E05.21
  nontoxic E04.9
    diffuse (colloid) E04.0
    multinodular E04.2
    simple E04.0
    specified NEC E04.8
    uninodular E04.1
  simple E04.0
  toxic — *see* Hyperthyroidism, with, goiter
  uninodular (nontoxic) E04.1
    toxic or with hyperthyroidism E05.10
      with thyroid storm E05.11
Goiter-deafness syndrome E07.1
Goldberg syndrome Q89.8
Goldberg-Maxwell syndrome E34.51
Goldblatt's hypertension or kidney I70.1
Goldenhar (-Gorlin) **syndrome** Q87.0
Goldflam-Erb disease or syndrome G70.00
  with exacerbation (acute) G70.01
  in crisis G70.01
Goldscheider's disease Q81.8
Goldstein's disease (familial hemorrhagic telangiectasia) I78.0
Golfer's elbow — *see* Epicondylitis, medial
Gonadoblastoma
  specified site — *see* Neoplasm, uncertain behavior, by site
  unspecified site
    female D39.10
    male D40.10
Gonecystitis — *see* Vesiculitis
Gongylonemiasis B83.8
Goniosynechiae — *see* Adhesions, iris, goniosynechiae
Gonococcemia A54.86
Gonococcus, gonococcal (disease) (infection) — *see also* condition A54.9
  anus A54.6
  bursa, bursitis A54.49
  conjunctiva, conjunctivitis (neonatorum) A54.31
  endocardium A54.83

Gonococcus, gonococcal — *continued*
  eye A54.30
    conjunctivitis A54.31
    iridocyclitis A54.32
    keratitis A54.33
    newborn A54.31
    other specified A54.39
  fallopian tubes (acute) (chronic) A54.24
  genitourinary (organ) (system) (tract) (acute)
    lower A54.00
      with abscess (accessory gland) (periurethral) A54.1
    upper — *see also* condition A54.29
  heart A54.83
  iridocyclitis A54.32
  joint A54.42
  lymphatic (gland) (node) A54.89
  meninges, meningitis A54.81
  musculoskeletal A54.40
    arthritis A54.42
    osteomyelitis A54.43
    other specified A54.49
    spondylopathy A54.41
  pelviperitonitis A54.24
  pelvis (acute) (chronic) A54.24
  pharynx A54.5
  proctitis A54.6
  pyosalpinx (acute) (chronic) A54.24
  rectum A54.6
  skin A54.89
  specified site NEC A54.89
  tendon sheath A54.49
  throat A54.5
  urethra (acute) (chronic) A54.01
    with abscess (accessory gland) (periurethral) A54.1
  vulva (acute) (chronic) A54.02
Gonocytoma
  specified site — *see* Neoplasm, uncertain behavior, by site
  unspecified site
    female D39.10
    male D40.10
Gonorrhea (acute) (chronic) A54.9
  Bartholin's gland (acute) (chronic) (purulent) A54.02
    with abscess (accessory gland) (periurethral) A54.1
  bladder A54.01
  cervix A54.03
  conjunctiva, conjunctivitis (neonatorum) A54.31
  contact Z20.2
  Cowper's gland (with abscess) A54.1
  exposure to Z20.2
  fallopian tube (acute) (chronic) A54.24
  kidney (acute) (chronic) A54.21
  lower genitourinary tract A54.00
    with abscess (accessory gland) (periurethral) A54.1
  ovary (acute) (chronic) A54.24
  pelvis (acute) (chronic) A54.24
    female pelvic inflammatory disease A54.24
  penis A54.09
  prostate (acute) (chronic) A54.22
  seminal vesicle (acute) (chronic) A54.23
  specified site not listed — *see also* Gonococcus A54.89
  spermatic cord (acute) (chronic) A54.23
  urethra A54.01
    with abscess (accessory gland) (periurethral) A54.1
  vagina A54.02
  vas deferens (acute) (chronic) A54.23
  vulva A54.02
Goodall's disease A08.19
Goodpasture's syndrome M31.0
Gopalan's syndrome (burning feet) E53.0
Gorlin-Chaudry-Moss syndrome Q87.0
Gottron's papules L94.4
Gougerot-Blum syndrome (pigmented purpuric lichenoid dermatitis) L81.7
Gougerot-Carteaud disease or syndrome (confluent reticulate papillomatosis) L83
Gougerot's syndrome (trisymptomatic) L81.7
Gouley's syndrome (constrictive pericarditis) I31.1
Goundou A66.6
Gout, chronic — *see also* Gout, gouty M1A.9 ☑ (*following* M08)
  drug-induced M1A.20 ☑ (*following* M08)
    ankle M1A.27- ☑ (*following* M08)
    elbow M1A.22- ☑ (*following* M08)
    foot joint M1A.27- ☑ (*following* M08)
    hand joint M1A.24- ☑ (*following* M08)
    hip M1A.25- ☑ (*following* M08)

Gout, chronic — *continued*
  drug-induced — *continued*
    knee M1A.26- ☑ (*following* M08)
    multiple site M1A.29- ☑ (*following* M08)
    shoulder M1A.21- ☑ (*following* M08)
    vertebrae M1A.28 ☑ (*following* M08)
    wrist M1A.23- ☑ (*following* M08)
  idiopathic M1A.00 ☑ (*following* M08)
    ankle M1A.07- ☑ (*following* M08)
    elbow M1A.02- ☑ (*following* M08)
    foot joint M1A.07- ☑ (*following* M08)
    hand joint M1A.04- ☑ (*following* M08)
    hip M1A.05- ☑ (*following* M08)
    knee M1A.06- ☑ (*following* M08)
    multiple site M1A.09 ☑ (*following* M08)
    shoulder M1A.01- ☑ (*following* M08)
    vertebrae M1A.08 ☑ (*following* M08)
    wrist M1A.03- ☑ (*following* M08)
  in (due to) renal impairment M1A.30 ☑ (*following* M08)
    ankle M1A.37- ☑ (*following* M08)
    elbow M1A.32- ☑ (*following* M08)
    foot joint M1A.37- ☑ (*following* M08)
    hand joint M1A.34- ☑ (*following* M08)
    hip M1A.35- ☑ (*following* M08)
    knee M1A.36- ☑ (*following* M08)
    multiple site M1A.39 ☑ (*following* M08)
    shoulder M1A.31- ☑ (*following* M08)
    vertebrae M1A.38 ☑ (*following* M08)
    wrist M1A.33- ☑ (*following* M08)
  lead-induced M1A.10 ☑ (*following* M08)
    ankle M1A.17- ☑ (*following* M08)
    elbow M1A.12- ☑ (*following* M08)
    foot joint M1A.17- ☑ (*following* M08)
    hand joint M1A.14- ☑ (*following* M08)
    hip M1A.15- ☑ (*following* M08)
    knee M1A.16- ☑ (*following* M08)
    multiple site M1A.19 ☑ (*following* M08)
    shoulder M1A.11- ☑ (*following* M08)
    vertebrae M1A.18 ☑ (*following* M08)
    wrist M1A.13- ☑ (*following* M08)
  primary — *see* Gout, chronic, idiopathic
  saturnine — *see* Gout, chronic, lead-induced
  secondary NEC M1A.40 ☑ (*following* M08)
    ankle M1A.47- ☑ (*following* M08)
    elbow M1A.42- ☑ (*following* M08)
    foot joint M1A.47- ☑ (*following* M08)
    hand joint M1A.44- ☑ (*following* M08)
    hip M1A.45- ☑ (*following* M08)
    knee M1A.46- ☑ (*following* M08)
    multiple site M1A.49 ☑ (*following* M08)
    shoulder M1A.41- ☑ (*following* M08)
    vertebrae M1A.48 ☑ (*following* M08)
    wrist M1A.43- ☑ (*following* M08)
  syphilitic — *see also* subcategory M14.8- A52.77
  tophi M1A.9 ☑ (*following* M08)
Gout, gouty (acute) (attack) (flare) — *see also* Gout, chronic M10.9
  drug-induced M10.20
    ankle M10.27- ☑
    elbow M10.22- ☑
    foot joint M10.27- ☑
    hand joint M10.24- ☑
    hip M10.25- ☑
    knee M10.26- ☑
    multiple site M10.29
    shoulder M10.21- ☑
    vertebrae M10.28
    wrist M10.23- ☑
  idiopathic M10.00
    ankle M10.07- ☑
    elbow M10.02- ☑
    foot joint M10.07- ☑
    hand joint M10.04- ☑
    hip M10.05- ☑
    knee M10.06- ☑
    multiple site M10.09
    shoulder M10.01- ☑
    vertebrae M10.08
    wrist M10.03- ☑
  in (due to) renal impairment M10.30
    ankle M10.37- ☑
    elbow M10.32- ☑
    foot joint M10.37- ☑
    hand joint M10.34- ☑
    hip M10.35- ☑
    knee M10.36- ☑

160

☑ Additional Character Required — Refer to the Tabular List for Character Selection   ▽ Subterms under main terms may continue to next column or page

Gout, gouty — *continued*
  in renal impairment — *continued*
    multiple site M10.39
    shoulder M10.31- ☑
    vertebrae M10.38
    wrist M10.33- ☑
  lead-induced M10.10
    ankle M10.17- ☑
    elbow M10.12- ☑
    foot joint M10.17- ☑
    hand joint M10.14- ☑
    hip M10.15- ☑
    knee M10.16- ☑
    multiple site M10.19
    shoulder M10.11- ☑
    vertebrae M10.18
    wrist M10.13- ☑
  primary — *see* Gout, idiopathic
  saturnine — *see* Gout, lead-induced
  secondary NEC M10.40
    ankle M10.47- ☑
    elbow M10.42- ☑
    foot joint M10.47- ☑
    hand joint M10.44- ☑
    hip M10.45- ☑
    knee M10.46- ☑
    multiple site M10.49
    shoulder M10.41- ☑
    vertebrae M10.48
    wrist M10.43- ☑
  syphilitic — *see also* subcategory M14.8- A52.77
  tophi — *see* Gout, chronic
Gower's
  muscular dystrophy G71.01
  syndrome (vasovagal attack) R55
Gradenigo's syndrome — *see* Otitis, media, suppurative, acute
Graefe's disease — *see* Strabismus, paralytic, ophthalmoplegia, progressive
Graft-versus-host disease D89.813
  acute D89.810
  acute on chronic D89.812
  chronic D89.811
Grain mite (itch) B88.0
Grainhandler's disease or lung J67.8
Grand mal — *see* Epilepsy, generalized, specified NEC
Grand multipara status only (not pregnant) Z64.1
  pregnant — *see* Pregnancy, complicated by, grand multiparity
Granite worker's lung J62.8
Granular — *see also* condition
  inflammation, pharynx J31.2
  kidney (contracting) — *see* Sclerosis, renal
  liver K74.69
Granulation tissue (abnormal) (excessive) L92.9
  postmastoidectomy cavity — *see* Complications, postmastoidectomy, granulation
Granulocytopenia (primary) (malignant) — *see* Agranulocytosis
Granuloma L92.9
  abdomen K66.8
    from residual foreign body L92.3
    pyogenicum L98.0
  actinic L57.5
  annulare (perforating) L92.0
  apical K04.5
  aural — *see* Otitis, externa, specified NEC
  beryllium (skin) L92.3
  bone
    eosinophilic C96.6
    from residual foreign body — *see* Osteomyelitis, specified type NEC
    lung C96.6
  brain (any site) G06.0
    schistosomiasis B65.9 *[G07]*
  canaliculus lacrimalis — *see* Granuloma, lacrimal
  candidal (cutaneous) B37.2
  cerebral (any site) G06.0
  coccidioidal (primary) (progressive) B38.7
    lung B38.1
    meninges B38.4
  colon K63.89
  conjunctiva H11.22- ☑
  dental K04.5
  ear, middle — *see* Cholesteatoma
  eosinophilic C96.6
    bone C96.6

Granuloma — *continued*
  eosinophilic — *continued*
    lung C96.6
    oral mucosa K13.4
    skin L92.2
  eyelid H01.8
  facial (e) L92.2
  foreign body (in soft tissue) NEC M60.20
    ankle M60.27- ☑
    foot M60.27- ☑
    forearm M60.23- ☑
    hand M60.24- ☑
    in operation wound — *see* Foreign body, accidentally left during a procedure
    lower leg M60.26- ☑
    pelvic region M60.25- ☑
    shoulder region M60.21- ☑
    skin L92.3
    specified site NEC M60.28
    subcutaneous tissue L92.3
    thigh M60.25- ☑
    upper arm M60.22- ☑
  gangraenescens M31.2
  genito-inguinale A58
  giant cell (central) (reparative) (jaw) M27.1
    gingiva (peripheral) K06.8
  gland (lymph) I88.8
  hepatic NEC K75.3
    in (due to)
      berylliosis J63.2 *[K77]*
      sarcoidosis D86.89
  Hodgkin C81.9 ☑
  ileum K63.89
  infectious B99.9
    specified NEC B99.8
  inguinale (Donovan) (venereal) A58
  intestine NEC K63.89
  intracranial (any site) G06.0
  intraspinal (any part) G06.1
  iridocyclitis — *see* Iridocyclitis, chronic
  jaw (bone) (central) M27.1
    reparative giant cell M27.1
  kidney — *see also* Infection, kidney N15.8
  lacrimal H04.81- ☑
  larynx J38.7
  lethal midline (faciale(e)) M31.2
  liver NEC — *see* Granuloma, hepatic
  lung (infectious) — *see also* Fibrosis, lung
    coccidioidal B38.1
    eosinophilic C96.6
  Majocchi's B35.8
  malignant (facial(e)) M31.2
  mandible (central) M27.1
  midline (lethal) M31.2
  monilial (cutaneous) B37.2
  nasal sinus — *see* Sinusitis
  operation wound T81.89 ☑
    foreign body — *see* Foreign body, accidentally left during a procedure
    stitch T81.89 ☑
    talc — *see* Foreign body, accidentally left during a procedure
  oral mucosa K13.4
  orbit, orbital H05.11- ☑
  paracoccidioidal B41.8
  penis, venereal A58
  periapical K04.5
  peritoneum K66.8
    due to ova of helminths NOS — *see also* Helminthiasis B83.9 *[K67]*
  postmastoidectomy cavity — *see* Complications, postmastoidectomy, recurrent cholesteatoma
  prostate N42.89
  pudendi (ulcerating) A58
  pulp, internal (tooth) K03.3
  pyogenic, pyogenicum (of) (skin) L98.0
    gingiva K06.8
    maxillary alveolar ridge K04.5
    oral mucosa K13.4
  rectum K62.89
  reticulohistiocytic D76.3
  rubrum nasi L74.8
  Schistosoma — *see* Schistosomiasis
  septic (skin) L98.0
  silica (skin) L92.3
  sinus (accessory) (infective) (nasal) — *see* Sinusitis
  skin L92.9
    from residual foreign body L92.3

Granuloma — *continued*
  skin — *continued*
    pyogenicum L98.0
  spine
    syphilitic (epidural) A52.19
    tuberculous A18.01
  stitch (postoperative) T81.89 ☑
  suppurative (skin) L98.0
  swimming pool A31.1
  talc — *see also* Granuloma, foreign body
    in operation wound — *see* Foreign body, accidentally left during a procedure
  telangiectaticum (skin) L98.0
  tracheostomy J95.09
  trichophyticum B35.8
  tropicum A66.4
  umbilical P83.81
  umbilicus P83.81
  urethra N36.8
  uveitis — *see* Iridocyclitis, chronic
  vagina A58
  venereum A58
  vocal cord J38.3
Granulomatosis L92.9
  lymphoid C83.8- ☑
  miliary (listerial) A32.89
  necrotizing, respiratory M31.30
  progressive septic D71
  specified NEC L92.8
  Wegener's M31.30
    with renal involvement M31.31
Granulomatous tissue (abnormal) (excessive) L92.9
Granulosis rubra nasi L74.8
Graphite fibrosis (of lung) J63.3
Graphospasm F48.8
  organic G25.89
Grating scapula M89.8X1
Gravel (urinary) — *see* Calculus, urinary
Graves' disease — *see* Hyperthyroidism, with, goiter
Gravis — *see* condition
Grawitz tumor C64.- ☑
Gray syndrome (newborn) P93.0
Grayness, hair (premature) L67.1
  congenital Q84.2
Green sickness D50.8
Greenfield's disease
  meaning
    concentric sclerosis (encephalitis periaxialis concentrica) G37.5
    metachromatic leukodystrophy E75.25
Greenstick fracture — *code as* Fracture, by site
Grey syndrome (newborn) P93.0
Grief F43.21
  prolonged F43.29
  reaction — *see also* Disorder, adjustment F43.20
Griesinger's disease B76.0
Grinder's lung or pneumoconiosis J62.8
Grinding, teeth
  psychogenic F45.8
  sleep related G47.63
Grip
  Dabney's B33.0
  devil's B33.0
Grippe, grippal — *see also* Influenza
  Balkan A78
  summer, of Italy A93.1
Grisel's disease M43.6
Groin — *see* condition
Grooved tongue K14.5
Ground itch B76.9
Grover's disease or syndrome L11.1
Growing pains, children R29.898
Growth (fungoid) (neoplastic) (new) — *see also* Neoplasm
  adenoid (vegetative) J35.8
  benign — *see* Neoplasm, benign, by site
  malignant — *see* Neoplasm, malignant, by site
  rapid, childhood Z00.2
  secondary — *see* Neoplasm, secondary, by site
Gruby's disease B35.0
Gubler-Millard paralysis or syndrome G46.3
Guerin-Stern syndrome Q74.3
Guidance, insufficient anterior (occlusal) M26.54
Guillain-Barré disease or syndrome G61.0
  sequelae G65.0
Guinea worms (infection) (infestation) B72
Guinon's disease (motor-verbal tic) F95.2
Gull's disease E03.4

▽ Subterms under main terms may continue to next column or page   ☑ Additional Character Required — Refer to the Tabular List for Character Selection   161

Gout, gouty — Gull's disease

Gum — *see* condition
Gumboil K04.7
  with sinus K04.6
Gumma (syphilitic) A52.79
  artery A52.09
    cerebral A52.04
  bone A52.77
    of yaws (late) A66.6
  brain A52.19
  cauda equina A52.19
  central nervous system A52.3
  ciliary body A52.71
  congenital A50.59
  eyelid A52.71
  heart A52.06
  intracranial A52.19
  iris A52.71
  kidney A52.75
  larynx A52.73
  leptomeninges A52.19
  liver A52.74
  meninges A52.19
  myocardium A52.06
  nasopharynx A52.73
  neurosyphilitic A52.3
  nose A52.73
  orbit A52.71
  palate (soft) A52.79
  penis A52.76
  pericardium A52.06
  pharynx A52.73
  pituitary A52.79
  scrofulous (tuberculous) A18.4
  skin A52.79
  specified site NEC A52.79
  spinal cord A52.19
  tongue A52.79
  tonsil A52.73
  trachea A52.73
  tuberculous A18.4
  ulcerative due to yaws A66.4
  ureter A52.75
  yaws A66.4
    bone A66.6
Gunn's syndrome Q07.8
Gunshot wound — *see also* Wound, open
  fracture — *code as* Fracture, by site
  internal organs — *see* Injury, by site
Gynandrism Q56.0
Gynandroblastoma
  specified site — *see* Neoplasm, uncertain behavior, by site
  unspecified site
    female D39.10
    male D40.10
Gynecological examination (periodic) (routine) Z01.419
  with abnormal findings Z01.411
Gynecomastia N62
Gynephobia F40.291
Gyrate scalp Q82.8

H

H (Hartnup's) **disease** E72.02
Haas' disease or osteochondrosis (juvenile) (head of humerus) — *see* Osteochondrosis, juvenile, humerus
Habit, habituation
  bad sleep Z72.821
  chorea F95.8
  disturbance, child F98.9
  drug — *see* Dependence, drug
  irregular sleep Z72.821
  laxative F55.2
  spasm — *see* Tic
  tic — *see* Tic
Haemophilus (H.) **influenzae, as cause of disease classified elsewhere** B96.3
Haff disease — *see* Poisoning, mercury
Hageman's factor defect, deficiency or disease D68.2
Haglund's disease or osteochondrosis (juvenile) (os tibiale externum) — *see* Osteochondrosis, juvenile, tarsus
Hailey-Hailey disease Q82.8
Hair — *see also* condition
  plucking F63.3
    in stereotyped movement disorder F98.4
  tourniquet syndrome — *see also* Constriction, external, by site

Hair — *continued*
  tourniquet syndrome — *see also* Constriction, external, by site — *continued*
    finger S60.44- ☑
    penis S30.842 ☑
    thumb S60.34- ☑
    toe S90.44- ☑
Hairball in stomach T18.2 ☑
Hair-pulling, pathological (compulsive) F63.3
Hairy black tongue K14.3
Half vertebra Q76.49
Halitosis R19.6
Hallerman-Streiff syndrome Q87.0
Hallervorden-Spatz disease G23.0
Hallopeau's acrodermatitis or disease L40.2
Hallucination R44.3
  auditory R44.0
  gustatory R44.2
  olfactory R44.2
  specified NEC R44.2
  tactile R44.2
  visual R44.1
Hallucinosis (chronic) F28
  alcoholic (acute) F10.951
    in
      abuse F10.151
      dependence F10.251
  drug-induced F19.951
    cannabis F12.951
    cocaine F14.951
    hallucinogen F16.151
    in
      abuse F19.151
        cannabis F12.151
        cocaine F14.151
        hallucinogen F16.151
        inhalant F18.151
        opioid F11.151
        sedative, anxiolytic or hypnotic F13.151
        stimulant NEC F15.151
      dependence F19.251
        cannabis F12.251
        cocaine F14.251
        hallucinogen F16.251
        inhalant F18.251
        opioid F11.251
        sedative, anxiolytic or hypnotic F13.251
        stimulant NEC F15.251
    inhalant F18.951
    opioid F11.951
    sedative, anxiolytic or hypnotic F13.951
    stimulant NEC F15.951
  organic F06.0
Hallux
  deformity (acquired) NEC M20.5X- ☑
  limitus M20.5X- ☑
  malleus (acquired) NEC M20.3- ☑
  rigidus (acquired) M20.2- ☑
    congenital Q74.2
    sequelae (late effect) of rickets E64.3
  valgus (acquired) M20.1- ☑
    congenital Q66.6
  varus (acquired) M20.3- ☑
    congenital Q66.3- ☑
Halo, visual H53.19
Hamartoma, hamartoblastoma Q85.9
  epithelial (gingival), odontogenic, central or peripheral — *see* Cyst, calcifying odontogenic
Hamartosis Q85.9
Hamman-Rich syndrome J84.114
Hammer toe (acquired) NEC — *see also* Deformity, toe, hammer toe
  congenital Q66.89
  sequelae (late effect) of rickets E64.3
Hand — *see* condition
Hand-foot syndrome L27.1
Handicap, handicapped
  educational Z55.9
    specified NEC Z55.8
Hand-Schüller-Christian disease or syndrome C96.5
Hanging (asphyxia) (strangulation) (suffocation) — *see* Asphyxia, traumatic, due to mechanical threat
Hangnail — *see also* Cellulitis, digit
  with lymphangitis — *see* Lymphangitis, acute, digit
Hangover (alcohol) F10.129
Hanhart's syndrome Q87.0
Hanot-Chauffard (-Troisier) **syndrome** E83.19

Hanot's cirrhosis or disease K74.3
Hansen's disease — *see* Leprosy
Hantaan virus disease (Korean hemorrhagic fever) A98.5
Hantavirus disease (with renal manifestations) (Dobrava) (Puumala) (Seoul) A98.5
  with pulmonary manifestations (Andes) (Bayou) (Bermejo) (Black Creek Canal) (Choclo) (Juquitiba) (Laguna negra) (Lechiguanas) (New York) (Oran) (Sin nombre) B33.4
Happy puppet syndrome Q93.51
Harada's disease or syndrome H30.81- ☑
Hardening
  artery — *see* Arteriosclerosis
  brain G93.89
Harelip (complete) (incomplete) — *see* Cleft, lip
Harlequin (newborn) Q80.4
Harley's disease D59.6
Harmful use (of)
  alcohol F10.10
  anxiolytics — *see* Abuse, drug, sedative
  cannabinoids — *see* Abuse, drug, cannabis
  cocaine — *see* Abuse, drug, cocaine
  drug — *see* Abuse, drug
  hallucinogens — *see* Abuse, drug, hallucinogen
  hypnotics — *see* Abuse, drug, sedative
  opioids — *see* Abuse, drug, opioid
  PCP (phencyclidine) — *see* Abuse, drug, hallucinogen
  sedatives — *see* Abuse, drug, sedative
  stimulants NEC — *see* Abuse, drug, stimulant
Harris' lines — *see* Arrest, epiphyseal
Hartnup's disease E72.02
Harvester's lung J67.0
Harvesting ovum for in vitro fertilization Z31.83
Hashimoto's disease or thyroiditis E06.3
Hashitoxicosis (transient) E06.3
Hassal-Henle bodies or warts (cornea) H18.49
Haut mal — *see* Epilepsy, generalized, specified NEC
Haverhill fever A25.1
Hay fever — *see also* Fever, hay J30.1
Hayem-Widal syndrome D59.8
Haygarth's nodes M15.8
Haymaker's lung J67.0
Hb (abnormal)
  Bart's disease D56.0
  disease — *see* Disease, hemoglobin
  trait — *see* Trait
Head — *see* condition
Headache R51
  allergic NEC G44.89
  associated with sexual activity G44.82
  chronic daily R51
  cluster G44.009
    chronic G44.029
      intractable G44.021
      not intractable G44.029
    episodic G44.019
      intractable G44.011
      not intractable G44.019
    intractable G44.001
    not intractable G44.009
  cough (primary) G44.83
  daily chronic R51
  drug-induced NEC G44.40
    intractable G44.41
    not intractable G44.40
  exertional (primary) G44.84
  histamine G44.009
    intractable G44.001
    not intractable G44.009
  hypnic G44.81
  lumbar puncture G97.1
  medication overuse G44.40
    intractable G44.41
    not intractable G44.40
  menstrual — *see* Migraine, menstrual
  migraine (type) — *see also* Migraine G43.909
  nasal septum R51
  neuralgiform, short lasting unilateral, with conjunctival injection and tearing (SUNCT) G44.059
    intractable G44.051
    not intractable G44.059
  new daily persistent (NDPH) G44.52
  orgasmic G44.82
  periodic syndromes in adults and children G43.C0 (*following* G43.7)
    with refractory migraine G43.C1 (*following* G43.7)
    intractable G43.C1 (*following* G43.7)

162

☑ Additional Character Required — Refer to the Tabular List for Character Selection   ▽ Subterms under main terms may continue to next column or page

Gum — Headache

Headache — *continued*
  periodic syndromes in adults and children — *continued*
    not intractable G43.C0 (*following* G43.7)
    without refractory migraine G43.C0 (*following* G43.7)
  postspinal puncture G97.1
  post-traumatic G44.309
    acute G44.319
      intractable G44.311
      not intractable G44.319
    chronic G44.329
      intractable G44.321
      not intractable G44.329
    intractable G44.301
    not intractable G44.309
  pre-menstrual — *see* Migraine, menstrual
  preorgasmic G44.82
  primary
    cough G44.83
    exertional G44.84
    stabbing G44.85
    thunderclap G44.53
  rebound G44.40
    intractable G44.41
    not intractable G44.40
  short lasting unilateral neuralgiform, with conjunctival injection and tearing (SUNCT) G44.059
    intractable G44.051
    not intractable G44.059
  specified syndrome NEC G44.89
  spinal and epidural anesthesia - induced T88.59 ☑
    in labor and delivery O74.5
    in pregnancy O29.4- ☑
    postpartum, puerperal O89.4
  spinal fluid loss (from puncture) G97.1
  stabbing (primary) G44.85
  tension (-type) G44.209
    chronic G44.229
      intractable G44.221
      not intractable G44.229
    episodic G44.219
      intractable G44.211
      not intractable G44.219
    intractable G44.201
    not intractable G44.209
  thunderclap (primary) G44.53
  vascular NEC G44.1
Healthy
  infant
    accompanying sick mother Z76.3
    receiving care Z76.2
  person accompanying sick person Z76.3
Hearing examination Z01.10
  with abnormal findings NEC Z01.118
  following failed hearing screening Z01.110
  for hearing conservation and treatment Z01.12
  infant or child (over 28 days old) Z00.129
    with abnormal findings Z00.121
Heart — *see* condition
Heart beat
  abnormality R00.9
    specified NEC R00.8
  awareness R00.2
  rapid R00.0
  slow R00.1
Heartburn R12
  psychogenic F45.8
Heartland virus disease A93.8
Heat (effects) T67.9 ☑
  apoplexy T67.01 ☑
  burn — *see also* Burn L55.9
  collapse T67.1 ☑
  cramps T67.2 ☑
  dermatitis or eczema L59.0
  edema T67.7 ☑
  erythema — *code by site under* Burn, first degree
  excessive T67.9 ☑
    specified effect NEC T67.8 ☑
  exhaustion T67.5 ☑
    anhydrotic T67.3 ☑
    due to
      salt (and water) depletion T67.4 ☑
      water depletion T67.3 ☑
        with salt depletion T67.4 ☑
  fatigue (transient) T67.6 ☑
  fever T67.01 ☑
  hyperpyrexia T67.01 ☑
  prickly L74.0

Heat — *continued*
  prostration — *see* Heat, exhaustion
  pyrexia T67.01 ☑
  rash L74.0
  specified effect NEC T67.8 ☑
  stroke T67.01 ☑
    exertional T67.02 ☑
    specified NEC T67.09 ☑
  sunburn — *see* Sunburn
  syncope T67.01 ☑
Heavy-for-dates NEC (infant) (4000g to 4499g) P08.1
  exceptionally (4500g or more) P08.0
Hebephrenia, hebephrenic (schizophrenia) F20.1
Heberden's disease or nodes (with arthropathy) M15.1
Hebra's
  pityriasis L26
  prurigo L28.2
Heel — *see* condition
Heerfordt's disease D86.89
Hegglin's anomaly or syndrome D72.0
Heilmeyer-Schoner disease D45
Heine-Medin disease A80.0
Heinz body anemia, congenital D58.2
Heliophobia F40.228
Heller's disease or syndrome F84.3
HELLP syndrome (hemolysis, elevated liver enzymes and low platelet count) O14.2- ☑
  complicating
    childbirth O14.24
    puerperium O14.25
Helminthiasis — *see also* Infestation, helminth
  Ancylostoma B76.0
  intestinal B82.0
    mixed types (types classifiable to more than one of the titles B65.0-B81.3 and B81.8) B81.4
    specified type NEC B81.8
  mixed types (intestinal) (types classifiable to more than one of the titles B65.0-B81.3 and B81.8) B81.4
  Necator (americanus) B76.1
  specified type NEC B83.8
Heloma L84
Hemangioblastoma — *see* Neoplasm, connective tissue, uncertain behavior
  malignant — *see* Neoplasm, connective tissue, malignant
Hemangioendothelioma — *see also* Neoplasm, uncertain behavior, by site
  benign D18.00
    intra-abdominal D18.03
    intracranial D18.02
    skin D18.01
    specified site NEC D18.09
  bone (diffuse) — *see* Neoplasm, bone, malignant
  epithelioid — *see also* Neoplasm, uncertain behavior, by site
    malignant — *see* Neoplasm, malignant, by site
  malignant — *see* Neoplasm, connective tissue, malignant
Hemangiofibroma — *see* Neoplasm, benign, by site
Hemangiolipoma — *see* Lipoma
Hemangioma D18.00
  arteriovenous D18.00
    intra-abdominal D18.03
    intracranial D18.02
    skin D18.01
    specified site NEC D18.09
  capillary I78.1
    intra-abdominal D18.03
    intracranial D18.02
    skin D18.01
    specified site NEC D18.09
  cavernous D18.00
    intra-abdominal D18.03
    intracranial D18.02
    skin D18.01
    specified site NEC D18.09
  epithelioid D18.00
    intra-abdominal D18.03
    intracranial D18.02
    skin D18.01
    specified site NEC D18.09
  histiocytoid D18.00
    intra-abdominal D18.03
    intracranial D18.02
    skin D18.01
    specified site NEC D18.09
  infantile D18.00
    intra-abdominal D18.03

Hemangioma — *continued*
  infantile — *continued*
    intracranial D18.02
    skin D18.01
    specified site NEC D18.09
  intra-abdominal D18.03
  intracranial D18.02
  intramuscular D18.00
    intra-abdominal D18.03
    intracranial D18.02
    skin D18.01
    specified site NEC D18.09
  intrathoracic structures D18.09
  juvenile D18.00
  malignant — *see* Neoplasm, connective tissue, malignant
  plexiform D18.00
    intra-abdominal D18.03
    intracranial D18.02
    skin D18.01
    specified site NEC D18.09
  racemose D18.00
    intra-abdominal D18.03
    intracranial D18.02
    skin D18.01
    specified site NEC D18.09
  sclerosing — *see* Neoplasm, skin, benign
  simplex D18.00
    intra-abdominal D18.03
    intracranial D18.02
    skin D18.01
    specified site NEC D18.09
  skin D18.01
  specified site NEC D18.09
  venous D18.00
    intra-abdominal D18.03
    intracranial D18.02
    skin D18.01
    specified site NEC D18.09
  verrucous keratotic D18.00
    intra-abdominal D18.03
    intracranial D18.02
    skin D18.01
    specified site NEC D18.09
Hemangiomatosis (systemic) I78.8
  involving single site — *see* Hemangioma
Hemangiopericytoma — *see also* Neoplasm, connective tissue, uncertain behavior
  benign — *see* Neoplasm, connective tissue, benign
  malignant — *see* Neoplasm, connective tissue, malignant
Hemangiosarcoma — *see* Neoplasm, connective tissue, malignant
Hemarthrosis (nontraumatic) M25.00
  ankle M25.07- ☑
  elbow M25.02- ☑
  foot joint M25.07- ☑
  hand joint M25.04- ☑
  hip M25.05- ☑
  in hemophilic arthropathy — *see* Arthropathy, hemophilic
  knee M25.06- ☑
  shoulder M25.01- ☑
  specified joint NEC M25.08
  traumatic — *see* Sprain, by site
  vertebrae M25.08
  wrist M25.03- ☑
Hematemesis K92.0
  with ulcer — *code by site under* Ulcer, with hemorrhage K27.4
  newborn, neonatal P54.0
    due to swallowed maternal blood P78.2
Hematidrosis L74.8
Hematinuria — *see also* Hemoglobinuria
  malarial B50.8
Hematobilia K83.8
Hematocele
  female NEC N94.89
    with ectopic pregnancy O00.90
      with intrauterine pregnancy O00.91
    ovary N83.8
  male N50.1
Hematochezia — *see also* Melena K92.1
Hematochyluria — *see also* Infestation, filarial
  schistosomiasis (bilharziasis) B65.0
Hematocolpos (with hematometra or hematosalpinx) N89.7
Hematocornea — *see* Pigmentation, cornea, stromal

Hematogenous — see condition
Hematoma (traumatic) (skin surface intact) — see also
 Contusion
 with
  injury of internal organs — see Injury, by site
  open wound — see Wound, open
 amputation stump (surgical) (late) T87.89
 aorta, dissecting I71.00
  abdominal I71.02
  thoracic I71.01
  thoracoabdominal I71.03
 aortic intramural — see Dissection, aorta
 arterial (complicating trauma) — see Injury, blood
   vessel, by site
 auricle — see Contusion, ear
  nontraumatic — see Disorder, pinna, hematoma
 birth injury NEC P15.8
 brain (traumatic)
  with
   cerebral laceration or contusion (diffuse) — see
     Injury, intracranial, diffuse
    focal — see Injury, intracranial, focal
  cerebellar, traumatic S06.37- ☑
  intracerebral, traumatic — see Injury, intracranial,
    intracerebral hemorrhage
  newborn NEC P52.4
   birth injury P10.1
  nontraumatic — see Hemorrhage, intracranial
  subarachnoid, arachnoid, traumatic — see Injury,
    intracranial, subarachnoid hemorrhage
  subdural, traumatic — see Injury, intracranial, sub-
    dural hemorrhage
 breast (nontraumatic) N64.89
 broad ligament (nontraumatic) N83.7
  traumatic S37.892 ☑
 cerebellar, traumatic S06.37- ☑
 cerebral — see Hematoma, brain
 cerebrum S06.36- ☑
  left S06.35- ☑
  right S06.34- ☑
 cesarean delivery wound O90.2
 complicating delivery (perineal) (pelvic) (vagina) (vulva)
   O71.7
 corpus cavernosum (nontraumatic) N48.89
 epididymis (nontraumatic) N50.1
 epidural (traumatic) — see Injury, intracranial, epidural
   hemorrhage
  spinal — see Injury, spinal cord, by region
 episiotomy O90.2
 face, birth injury P15.4
 genital organ NEC (nontraumatic)
  female (nonobstetric) N94.89
   traumatic S30.202 ☑
  male N50.1
   traumatic S30.201 ☑
 internal organs — see Injury, by site
 intracerebral, traumatic — see Injury, intracranial, intracerebral hemorrhage
 intraoperative — see Complications, intraoperative,
   hemorrhage
 labia (nontraumatic) (nonobstetric) N90.89
 liver (subcapsular) (nontraumatic) K76.89
  birth injury P15.0
 mediastinum — see Injury, intrathoracic
 mesosalpinx (nontraumatic) N83.7
  traumatic S37.898 ☑
 muscle — code by site under Contusion
 nontraumatic
  muscle M79.81
  soft tissue M79.81
 obstetrical surgical wound O90.2
 orbit, orbital (nontraumatic) — see also Hemorrhage,
   orbit
  traumatic — see Contusion, orbit
 pelvis (female) (nontraumatic) (nonobstetric) N94.89
  obstetric O71.7
  traumatic — see Injury, by site
 penis (nontraumatic) N48.89
  birth injury P15.5
 perianal (nontraumatic) K64.5
 perineal S30.23 ☑
  complicating delivery O71.7
 perirenal — see Injury, kidney
 pinna — see Contusion, ear
  nontraumatic — see Disorder, pinna, hematoma
 placenta O43.89- ☑

Hematoma — continued
 postoperative (postprocedural) — see Complication,
   postprocedural, hematoma
 retroperitoneal (nontraumatic) K66.1
  traumatic S36.892 ☑
 scrotum, superficial S30.22 ☑
  birth injury P15.5
 seminal vesicle (nontraumatic) N50.1
  traumatic S37.892 ☑
 spermatic cord (traumatic) S37.892 ☑
  nontraumatic N50.1
 spinal (cord) (meninges) — see also Injury, spinal cord,
   by region
  newborn (birth injury) P11.5
 spleen D73.5
  intraoperative — see Complications, intraoperative,
    hemorrhage, spleen
  postprocedural (postoperative) — see Complica-
    tions, postprocedural, hemorrhage, spleen
 sternocleidomastoid, birth injury P15.2
 sternomastoid, birth injury P15.2
 subarachnoid (traumatic) — see Injury, intracranial,
   subarachnoid hemorrhage
  newborn (nontraumatic) P52.5
   due to birth injury P10.3
  nontraumatic — see Hemorrhage, intracranial,
    subarachnoid
 subdural (traumatic) — see Injury, intracranial, subdural
   hemorrhage
  newborn (localized) P52.8
   birth injury P10.0
  nontraumatic — see Hemorrhage, intracranial,
    subdural
 superficial, newborn P54.5
 testis (nontraumatic) N50.1
  birth injury P15.5
 tunica vaginalis (nontraumatic) N50.1
 umbilical cord, complicating delivery O69.5 ☑
 uterine ligament (broad) (nontraumatic) N83.7
  traumatic S37.892 ☑
 vagina (ruptured) (nontraumatic) N89.8
  complicating delivery O71.7
 vas deferens (nontraumatic) N50.1
  traumatic S37.892 ☑
 vitreous — see Hemorrhage, vitreous
 vulva (nontraumatic) (nonobstetric) N90.89
  complicating delivery O71.7
  newborn (birth injury) P15.5
Hematometra N85.7
 with hematocolpos N89.7
Hematomyelia (central) G95.19
 newborn (birth injury) P11.5
 traumatic T14.8 ☑
Hematomyelitis G04.90
Hematoperitoneum — see Hemoperitoneum
Hematophobia F40.230
Hematopneumothorax (see Hemothorax)
Hematopoiesis, cyclic D70.4
Hematoporphyria — see Porphyria
Hematorachis, hematorrhachis G95.19
 newborn (birth injury) P11.5
Hematosalpinx N83.6
 with
  hematocolpos N89.7
  hematometra N85.7
   with hematocolpos N89.7
 infectional — see Salpingitis
Hematospermia R36.1
Hematothorax (see Hemothorax)
Hematuria R31.9
 benign (familial) (of childhood) — see also Hematuria,
   idiopathic
  essential microscopic R31.1
 due to sulphonamide, sulfonamide — see Table of
   Drugs and Chemicals, by drug
 endemic — see also Schistosomiasis B65.0
 gross R31.0
 idiopathic N02.9
  with glomerular lesion
   crescentic (diffuse) glomerulonephritis N02.7
   dense deposit disease N02.6
   endocapillary proliferative glomerulonephritis
     N02.4
   focal and segmental hyalinosis or sclerosis N02.1
   membranoproliferative (diffuse) N02.5
   membranous (diffuse) N02.2
   mesangial proliferative (diffuse) N02.3
   mesangiocapillary (diffuse) N02.5

Hematuria — continued
 idiopathic — continued
  with glomerular lesion — continued
   minor abnormality N02.0
   proliferative NEC N02.8
   specified pathology NEC N02.8
 intermittent — see Hematuria, idiopathic
 malarial B50.8
 microscopic NEC (with symptoms) R31.29
  asymptomatic R31.21
  benign essential R31.1
 paroxysmal — see also Hematuria, idiopathic
  nocturnal D59.5
 persistent — see Hematuria, idiopathic
 recurrent — see Hematuria, idiopathic
 tropical — see also Schistosomiasis B65.0
 tuberculous A18.13
Hemeralopia (day blindness) H53.11
 vitamin A deficiency E50.5
Hemi-akinesia R41.4
Hemianalgesia R20.0
Hemianencephaly Q00.0
Hemianesthesia R20.0
Hemianopia, hemianopsia (heteronymous) H53.47
 homonymous H53.46- ☑
 syphilitic A52.71
Hemiathetosis R25.8
Hemiatrophy R68.89
 cerebellar G31.9
 face, facial, progressive (Romberg) G51.8
 tongue K14.8
Hemiballism (us) G25.5
Hemicardia Q24.8
Hemicephalus, hemicephaly Q00.0
Hemichorea G25.5
Hemicolitis, left — see Colitis, left sided
Hemicrania
 congenital malformation Q00.0
 continua G44.51
 meaning migraine — see also Migraine G43.909
 paroxysmal G44.039
  chronic G44.049
   intractable G44.041
   not intractable G44.049
  episodic G44.039
   intractable G44.031
   not intractable G44.039
 intractable G44.031
 not intractable G44.039
Hemidystrophy — see Hemiatrophy
Hemiectromelia Q73.8
Hemihypalgesia R20.8
Hemihypesthesia R20.1
Hemi-inattention R41.4
Hemimelia Q73.8
 lower limb — see Defect, reduction, lower limb, specified type NEC
 upper limb — see Defect, reduction, upper limb, specified type NEC
Hemiparalysis — see Hemiplegia
Hemiparesis — see Hemiplegia
Hemiparesthesia R20.2
Hemiparkinsonism G20
Hemiplegia G81.9- ☑
 alternans facialis G83.89
 ascending NEC G81.90
  spinal G95.89
 congenital (cerebral) G80.8
  spastic G80.2
 embolic (current episode) I63.4- ☑
 flaccid G81.0- ☑
 following
  cerebrovascular disease I69.959
   cerebral infarction I69.35- ☑
   intracerebral hemorrhage I69.15- ☑
   nontraumatic intracranial hemorrhage NEC
     I69.25- ☑
   specified disease NEC I69.85- ☑
   stroke NOS I69.35- ☑
   subarachnoid hemorrhage I69.05- ☑
 hysterical F44.4
 newborn NEC P91.88
  birth injury P11.9
 spastic G81.1- ☑
  congenital G80.2
 thrombotic (current episode) I63.3- ☑

Hemisection, spinal cord — *see* Injury, spinal cord, by region
Hemispasm (facial) R25.2
Hemisporosis B48.8
Hemitremor R25.1
Hemivertebra Q76.49
  failure of segmentation with scoliosis Q76.3
  fusion with scoliosis Q76.3
Hemochromatosis E83.119
  with refractory anemia D46.1
  due to repeated red blood cell transfusion E83.111
  hereditary (primary) E83.110
  neonatal P78.84
  primary E83.110
  specified NEC E83.118
Hemoglobin — *see also* condition
  abnormal (disease) — *see* Disease, hemoglobin
  AS genotype D57.3
  Constant Spring D58.2
  E-beta thalassemia D56.5
  fetal, hereditary persistence (HPFH) D56.4
  H Constant Spring D56.0
  low NOS D64.9
  S (Hb S), heterozygous D57.3
Hemoglobinemia D59.9
  due to blood transfusion T80.89 ☑
  paroxysmal D59.6
    nocturnal D59.5
Hemoglobinopathy (mixed) D58.2
  with thalassemia D56.8
  sickle-cell D57.1
    with thalassemia D57.40
      with crisis (vasoocclusive pain) D57.419
        with
          acute chest syndrome D57.411
          splenic sequestration D57.412
      without crisis D57.40
Hemoglobinuria R82.3
  with anemia, hemolytic, acquired (chronic) NEC D59.6
  cold (agglutinin) (paroxysmal) (with Raynaud's syndrome) D59.6
  due to exertion or hemolysis NEC D59.6
  intermittent D59.6
  malarial B50.8
  march D59.6
  nocturnal (paroxysmal) D59.5
  paroxysmal (cold) D59.6
    nocturnal D59.5
Hemolymphangioma D18.1
Hemolysis
  intravascular
    with
      abortion — *see* Abortion, by type, complicated by, hemorrhage
      ectopic or molar pregnancy O08.1
      hemorrhage
        antepartum — *see* Hemorrhage, antepartum, with coagulation defect
        intrapartum — *see also* Hemorrhage, complicating, delivery O67.0
      postpartum O72.3
  neonatal (excessive) P58.9
    specified NEC P58.8
Hemolytic — *see* condition
Hemopericardium I31.2
  following acute myocardial infarction (current complication) I23.0
  newborn P54.8
  traumatic — *see* Injury, heart, with hemopericardium
Hemoperitoneum K66.1
  infectional K65.9
  traumatic S36.899 ☑
    with open wound — *see* Wound, open, with penetration into peritoneal cavity
Hemophilia (classical) (familial) (hereditary) D66
  A D66
  acquired D68.311
  autoimmune D68.311
  B D67
  C D68.1
  calcipriva — *see also* Defect, coagulation D68.4
  nonfamilial — *see also* Defect, coagulation D68.4
  secondary D68.311
  vascular D68.0
Hemophthalmos H44.81- ☑
Hemopneumothorax — *see also* Hemothorax
  traumatic S27.2 ☑
Hemoptysis R04.2

Hemoptysis — *continued*
  newborn P26.9
  tuberculous — *see* Tuberculosis, pulmonary
Hemorrhage, hemorrhagic (concealed) R58
  abdomen R58
  accidental antepartum — *see* Hemorrhage, antepartum
  acute idiopathic pulmonary, in infants R04.81
  adenoid J35.8
  adrenal (capsule) (gland) E27.49
    medulla E27.8
    newborn P54.4
  after delivery — *see* Hemorrhage, postpartum
  alveolar
    lung, newborn P26.8
    process K08.89
  alveolus K08.89
  amputation stump (surgical) T87.89
  anemia (chronic) D50.0
    acute D62
  antepartum (with) O46.90
    with coagulation defect O46.00- ☑
      afibrinogenemia O46.01- ☑
      disseminated intravascular coagulation O46.02- ☑
      hypofibrinogenemia O46.01- ☑
      specified defect NEC O46.09- ☑
    before 20 weeks gestation O20.9
      specified type NEC O20.8
      threatened abortion O20.0
    due to
      abruptio placenta — *see also* Abruptio placentae O45.9- ☑
      leiomyoma, uterus — *see* Hemorrhage, antepartum, specified cause NEC
      placenta previa O44.1- ☑
    specified cause NEC — *see* subcategory O46.8X- ☑
  anus (sphincter) K62.5
  apoplexy (stroke) — *see* Hemorrhage, intracranial, intracerebral
  arachnoid — *see* Hemorrhage, intracranial, subarachnoid
  artery R58
    brain — *see* Hemorrhage, intracranial, intracerebral
  basilar (ganglion) I61.0
  bladder N32.89
  bowel K92.2
    newborn P54.3
  brain (miliary) (nontraumatic) — *see* Hemorrhage, intracranial, intracerebral
    due to
      birth injury P10.1
      syphilis A52.05
    epidural or extradural (traumatic) — *see* Injury, intracranial, epidural hemorrhage
    newborn P52.4
      birth injury P10.1
    subarachnoid — *see* Hemorrhage, intracranial, subarachnoid
    subdural — *see* Hemorrhage, intracranial, subdural
  brainstem (nontraumatic) I61.3
    traumatic S06.38- ☑
  breast N64.59
  bronchial tube — *see* Hemorrhage, lung
  bronchopulmonary — *see* Hemorrhage, lung
  bronchus — *see* Hemorrhage, lung
  bulbar I61.5
  capillary I78.8
    primary D69.8
  cecum K92.2
  cerebellar, cerebellum (nontraumatic) I61.4
    newborn P52.6
    traumatic S06.37- ☑
  cerebral, cerebrum — *see also* Hemorrhage, intracranial, intracerebral
    lobe I61.1
      newborn (anoxic) P52.4
      birth injury P10.1
  cerebromeningeal I61.8
  cerebrospinal — *see* Hemorrhage, intracranial, intracerebral
  cervix (uteri) (stump) NEC N88.8
  chamber, anterior (eye) — *see* Hyphema
  childbirth — *see* Hemorrhage, complicating, delivery
  choroid H31.30- ☑
    expulsive H31.31- ☑
  ciliary body — *see* Hyphema
  cochlea — *see* subcategory H83.8 ☑
  colon K92.2

Hemorrhage, hemorrhagic — *continued*
  complicating
    abortion — *see* Abortion, by type, complicated by, hemorrhage
    delivery O67.9
      associated with coagulation defect (afibrinogenemia) (DIC) (hyperfibrinolysis) O67.0
      specified cause NEC O67.8
    surgical procedure — *see* Hemorrhage, intraoperative
  conjunctiva H11.3- ☑
    newborn P54.8
  cord, newborn (stump) P51.9
  corpus luteum (ruptured) cyst N83.1- ☑
  cortical (brain) I61.1
  cranial — *see* Hemorrhage, intracranial
  cutaneous R23.3
    due to autosensitivity, erythrocyte D69.2
    newborn P54.5
  delayed
    following ectopic or molar pregnancy O08.1
    postpartum O72.2
  diathesis (familial) D69.9
  disease D69.9
    newborn P53
    specified type NEC D69.8
  due to or associated with
    afibrinogenemia or other coagulation defect (conditions in categories D65- D69)
      antepartum — *see* Hemorrhage, antepartum, with coagulation defect
      intrapartum O67.0
    dental implant M27.61
    device, implant or graft — *see also* Complications, by site and type, specified NEC T85.838 ☑
      arterial graft NEC T82.838 ☑
      breast T85.838 ☑
      catheter NEC T85.838 ☑
        dialysis (renal) T82.838 ☑
          intraperitoneal T85.838 ☑
        infusion NEC T82.838 ☑
          spinal (epidural) (subdural) T85.830 ☑
        urinary (indwelling) T83.83 ☑
      electronic (electrode) (pulse generator) (stimulator)
        bone T84.83 ☑
        cardiac T82.837 ☑
        nervous system (brain) (peripheral nerve) (spinal) T85.830 ☑
        urinary T83.83 ☑
      fixation, internal (orthopedic) NEC T84.83 ☑
      gastrointestinal (bile duct) (esophagus) T85.838 ☑
      genital NEC T83.83 ☑
      heart NEC T82.837 ☑
      joint prosthesis T84.83 ☑
      ocular (corneal graft) (orbital implant) NEC T85.838 ☑
      orthopedic NEC T84.83 ☑
        bone graft T86.838 ☑
      specified NEC T85.838 ☑
      urinary NEC T83.83 ☑
      vascular NEC T82.838 ☑
      ventricular intracranial shunt T85.830 ☑
    duodenum, duodenal K92.2
      ulcer — *see* Ulcer, duodenum, with hemorrhage
    dura mater — *see* Hemorrhage, intracranial, subdural
    endotracheal — *see* Hemorrhage, lung
    epicranial subaponeurotic (massive), birth injury P12.2
    epidural (traumatic) — *see also* Injury, intracranial, epidural hemorrhage
      nontraumatic I62.1
    esophagus K22.8
      varix I85.01
        secondary I85.11
    excessive, following ectopic gestation (subsequent episode) O08.1
    extradural (traumatic) — *see* Injury, intracranial, epidural hemorrhage
      birth injury P10.8
      newborn (anoxic) (nontraumatic) P52.8
      nontraumatic I62.1
    eye NEC H57.89
      fundus — *see* Hemorrhage, retina
      lid — *see* Disorder, eyelid, specified type NEC
    fallopian tube N83.6
    fibrinogenolysis — *see* Fibrinolysis

Hemorrhage, hemorrhagic — *continued*
fibrinolytic (acquired) — *see* Fibrinolysis
from
  ear (nontraumatic) — *see* Otorrhagia
  tracheostomy stoma J95.01
fundus, eye — *see* Hemorrhage, retina
funis — *see* Hemorrhage, umbilicus, cord
gastric — *see* Hemorrhage, stomach
gastroenteric K92.2
  newborn P54.3
gastrointestinal (tract) K92.2
  newborn P54.3
genital organ, male N50.1
genitourinary (tract) NOS R31.9
gingiva K06.8
globe (eye) — *see* Hemophthalmos
graafian follicle cyst (ruptured) N83.0- ☑
gum K06.8
heart I51.89
hypopharyngeal (throat) R04.1
intermenstrual (regular) N92.3
  irregular N92.1
internal (organs) NEC R58
  capsule I61.0
  ear — *see* subcategory H83.8 ☑
  newborn P54.8
intestine K92.2
  newborn P54.3
intra-abdominal R58
intra-alveolar (lung), newborn P26.8
intracerebral (nontraumatic) — *see* Hemorrhage, intracranial, intracerebral
intracranial (nontraumatic) I62.9
  birth injury P10.9
  epidural, nontraumatic I62.1
  extradural, nontraumatic I62.1
  intracerebral (nontraumatic) (in) I61.9
    brain stem I61.3
    cerebellum I61.4
    hemisphere I61.2
      cortical (superficial) I61.1
      subcortical (deep) I61.0
    intraoperative
      during a nervous system procedure G97.31
      during other procedure G97.32
    intraventricular I61.5
    multiple localized I61.6
    newborn P52.4
      birth injury P10.1
    postprocedural
      following a nervous system procedure G97.51
      following other procedure G97.52
    specified NEC I61.8
    superficial I61.1
    traumatic (diffuse) — *see* Injury, intracranial, diffuse
      focal — *see* Injury, intracranial, focal
  newborn P52.9
    specified NEC P52.8
  subarachnoid (nontraumatic) (from) I60.9
    intracranial (cerebral) artery I60.7
      anterior communicating I60.2
      basilar I60.4
      carotid siphon and bifurcation I60.0- ☑
      communicating I60.7
        anterior I60.2
        posterior I60.3- ☑
      middle cerebral I60.1- ☑
      posterior communicating I60.3- ☑
      specified artery NEC I60.6
      vertebral I60.5- ☑
    newborn P52.5
      birth injury P10.3
    specified NEC I60.8
    traumatic S06.6X- ☑
  subdural (nontraumatic) I62.00
    acute I62.01
    birth injury P10.0
    chronic I62.03
    newborn (anoxic) (hypoxic) P52.8
      birth injury P10.0
    spinal G95.19
    subacute I62.02
    traumatic — *see* Injury, intracranial, subdural hemorrhage
  traumatic — *see* Injury, intracranial, focal brain injury
intramedullary NEC G95.19

Hemorrhage, hemorrhagic — *continued*
intraocular — *see* Hemophthalmos
intraoperative, intraprocedural — *see* Complication, hemorrhage (hematoma), intraoperative (intraprocedural), by site
intrapartum — *see* Hemorrhage, complicating, delivery
intrapelvic
  female N94.89
  male K66.1
intraperitoneal K66.1
intrapontine I61.3
intraprocedural — *see* Complication, hemorrhage (hematoma), intraoperative (intraprocedural), by site
intrauterine N85.7
  complicating delivery — *see also* Hemorrhage, complicating, delivery O67.9
  postpartum — *see* Hemorrhage, postpartum
intraventricular I61.5
  newborn (nontraumatic) — *see also* Newborn, affected by, hemorrhage P52.3
    due to birth injury P10.2
    grade
      1 P52.0
      2 P52.1
      3 P52.21
      4 P52.22
intravesical N32.89
iris (postinfectional) (postinflammatory) (toxic) — *see* Hyphema
joint (nontraumatic) — *see* Hemarthrosis
kidney N28.89
knee (joint) (nontraumatic) — *see* Hemarthrosis, knee
labyrinth — *see* subcategory H83.8 ☑
lenticular striate artery I61.0
ligature, vessel — *see* Hemorrhage, postoperative
liver K76.89
lung R04.89
  newborn P26.9
    massive P26.1
    specified NEC P26.8
  tuberculous — *see* Tuberculosis, pulmonary
massive umbilical, newborn P51.0
mediastinum — *see* Hemorrhage, lung
medulla I61.3
membrane (brain) I60.8
  spinal cord — *see* Hemorrhage, spinal cord
meninges, meningeal (brain) (middle) I60.8
  spinal cord — *see* Hemorrhage, spinal cord
mesentery K66.1
metritis — *see* Endometritis
mouth K13.79
mucous membrane NEC R58
  newborn P54.8
muscle M62.89
nail (subungual) L60.8
nasal turbinate R04.0
  newborn P54.8
navel, newborn P51.9
newborn P54.9
  specified NEC P54.8
nipple N64.59
nose R04.0
  newborn P54.8
omentum K66.1
optic nerve (sheath) H47.02- ☑
orbit, orbital H05.23- ☑
ovary NEC N83.8
oviduct N83.6
pancreas K86.89
parathyroid (gland) (spontaneous) E21.4
parturition — *see* Hemorrhage, complicating, delivery
penis N48.89
pericardium, pericarditis I31.2
peritoneum, peritoneal K66.1
peritonsillar tissue J35.8
  due to infection J36
petechial R23.3
  due to autosensitivity, erythrocyte D69.2
pituitary (gland) E23.6
pleura — *see* Hemorrhage, lung
polioencephalitis, superior E51.2
polymyositis — *see* Polymyositis
pons, pontine I61.3
posterior fossa (nontraumatic) I61.8
  newborn P52.6
postmenopausal N95.0
postnasal R04.0

Hemorrhage, hemorrhagic — *continued*
postoperative — *see* Complications, postprocedural, hemorrhage, by site
postpartum NEC (following delivery of placenta) O72.1
  delayed or secondary O72.2
  retained placenta O72.0
  third stage O72.0
pregnancy — *see* Hemorrhage, antepartum
preretinal — *see* Hemorrhage, retina
prostate N42.1
puerperal — *see* Hemorrhage, postpartum
  delayed or secondary O72.2
pulmonary R04.89
  newborn P26.9
    massive P26.1
    specified NEC P26.8
  tuberculous — *see* Tuberculosis, pulmonary
purpura (primary) D69.3
rectum (sphincter) K62.5
  newborn P54.2
recurring, following initial hemorrhage at time of injury T79.2 ☑
renal N28.89
respiratory passage or tract R04.9
  specified NEC R04.89
retina, retinal (vessels) H35.6- ☑
  diabetic — *see* Diabetes, retinal, hemorrhage
retroperitoneal R58
scalp R58
scrotum N50.1
secondary (nontraumatic) R58
  following initial hemorrhage at time of injury T79.2 ☑
seminal vesicle N50.1
skin R23.3
  newborn P54.5
slipped umbilical ligature P51.8
spermatic cord N50.1
spinal (cord) G95.19
  newborn (birth injury) P11.5
spleen D73.5
  intraoperative — *see* Complications, intraoperative, hemorrhage, spleen
  postprocedural — *see* Complications, postprocedural, hemorrhage, spleen
stomach K92.2
  newborn P54.3
  ulcer — *see* Ulcer, stomach, with hemorrhage
subarachnoid (nontraumatic) — *see* Hemorrhage, intracranial, subarachnoid
subconjunctival — *see also* Hemorrhage, conjunctiva
  birth injury P15.3
subcortical (brain) I61.0
subcutaneous R23.3
subdiaphragmatic R58
subdural (acute) (nontraumatic) — *see* Hemorrhage, intracranial, subdural
subependymal
  newborn P52.0
    with intraventricular extension P52.1
      and intracerebral extension P52.22
subgaleal P12.2
subhyaloid — *see* Hemorrhage, retina
subperiosteal — *see* Disorder, bone, specified type NEC
subretinal — *see* Hemorrhage, retina
subtentorial — *see* Hemorrhage, intracranial, subdural
subungual L60.8
suprarenal (capsule) (gland) E27.49
  newborn P54.4
tentorium (traumatic) NEC — *see* Hemorrhage, brain
  newborn (birth injury) P10.4
testis N50.1
third stage (postpartum) O72.0
thorax — *see* Hemorrhage, lung
throat R04.1
thymus (gland) E32.8
thyroid (cyst) (gland) E07.89
tongue K14.8
tonsil J35.8
trachea — *see* Hemorrhage, lung
tracheobronchial R04.89
  newborn P26.0
traumatic — *code to* specific injury
  cerebellar — *see* Hemorrhage, brain
  intracranial — *see* Hemorrhage, brain
  recurring or secondary (following initial hemorrhage at time of injury) T79.2 ☑

☑ **Additional Character Required** — Refer to the Tabular List for Character Selection ▽ Subterms under main terms may continue to next column or page

Hemorrhage, hemorrhagic — *continued*
  tuberculous NEC — *see also* Tuberculosis, pulmonary
    A15.0
  tunica vaginalis N50.1
  ulcer — *code by* site under Ulcer, with hemorrhage
    K27.4
  umbilicus, umbilical
    cord
      after birth, newborn P51.9
      complicating delivery O69.5 ☑
    newborn P51.9
      massive P51.0
      slipped ligature P51.8
    stump P51.9
  urethra (idiopathic) N36.8
  uterus, uterine (abnormal) N93.9
    climacteric N92.4
    complicating delivery — *see* Hemorrhage, compli-
      cating, delivery
    dysfunctional or functional N93.8
    intermenstrual (regular) N92.3
      irregular N92.1
    postmenopausal N95.0
    postpartum — *see* Hemorrhage, postpartum
    preclimacteric or premenopausal N92.4
    prepubertal N93.8
    pubertal N92.2
  vagina (abnormal) N93.9
    newborn P54.6
  vas deferens N50.1
  vasa previa O69.4 ☑
  ventricular I61.5
  vesical N32.89
  viscera NEC R58
    newborn P54.8
  vitreous (humor) (intraocular) H43.1- ☑
  vulva N90.89
Hemorrhoids (bleeding) (without mention of degree)
  K64.9
  1st degree (grade/stage I) (without prolapse outside
    of anal canal) K64.0
  2nd degree (grade/stage II) (that prolapse with strain-
    ing but retract spontaneously) K64.1
  3rd degree (grade/stage III) (that prolapse with strain-
    ing and require manual replacement back inside
    anal canal) K64.2
  4th degree (grade/stage IV) (with prolapsed tissue that
    cannot be manually replaced) K64.3
  complicating
    pregnancy O22.4 ☑
    puerperium O87.2
  external K64.4
    with
      thrombosis K64.5
  internal (without mention of degree) K64.8
  prolapsed K64.8
  skin tags
    anus K64.4
    residual K64.4
  specified NEC K64.8
  strangulated — *see also* Hemorrhoids, by degree K64.8
  thrombosed — *see also* Hemorrhoids, by degree K64.5
  ulcerated — *see also* Hemorrhoids, by degree K64.8
Hemosalpinx N83.6
  with
    hematocolpos N89.7
    hematometra N85.7
      with hematocolpos N89.7
Hemosiderosis (dietary) E83.19
  pulmonary, idiopathic E83.1- ☑ *[J84.03]*
  transfusion T80.89 ☑
Hemothorax (bacterial) (nontuberculous) J94.2
  newborn P54.8
  traumatic S27.1 ☑
    with pneumothorax S27.2 ☑
  tuberculous NEC A15.6
Henoch (-Schönlein) **disease or syndrome** (purpura)
  D69.0
Henpue, henpuye A66.6
Hepar lobatum (syphilitic) A52.74
Hepatalgia K76.89
Hepatitis K75.9
  acute B17.9
    with coma K72.01
    with hepatic failure — *see* Failure, hepatic
    alcoholic — *see* Hepatitis, alcoholic
    infectious B17.9
    non-viral K72.0 ☑

Hepatitis — *continued*
  acute — *continued*
    viral B17.9
  alcoholic (acute) (chronic) K70.10
    with ascites K70.11
  amebic — *see* Abscess, liver, amebic
  anicteric, (viral) — *see* Hepatitis, viral
  antigen-associated (HAA) — *see* Hepatitis, B
  Australia-antigen (positive) — *see* Hepatitis, B
  autoimmune K75.4
  B B19.10
    with hepatic coma B19.11
    acute B16.9
      with
        delta-agent (coinfection) (without hepatic
          coma) B16.1
          with hepatic coma B16.0
        hepatic coma (without delta-agent coinfec-
          tion) B16.2
    chronic B18.1
      with delta-agent B18.0
  bacterial NEC K75.89
  C (viral) B19.20
    with hepatic coma B19.21
    acute B17.10
      with hepatic coma B17.11
    chronic B18.2
  catarrhal (acute) B15.9
    with hepatic coma B15.0
  cholangiolitic K75.89
  cholestatic K75.89
  chronic K73.9
    active NEC K73.2
    lobular NEC K73.1
    persistent NEC K73.0
    specified NEC K73.8
  cytomegaloviral B25.1
  due to ethanol (acute) (chronic) — *see* Hepatitis, alco-
    holic
  epidemic B15.9
    with hepatic coma B15.0
  fulminant NEC (viral) — *see* Hepatitis, viral
  granulomatous NEC K75.3
  herpesviral B00.81
  history of
    B Z86.19
    C Z86.19
  homologous serum — *see* Hepatitis, viral, type B
  in (due to)
    mumps B26.81
    toxoplasmosis (acquired) B58.1
      congenital (active) P37.1 *[K77]*
  infectious, infective B15.9
    acute (subacute) B17.9
    chronic B18.9
  inoculation — *see* Hepatitis, viral, type B
  interstitial (chronic) K74.69
  lupoid NEC K75.4
  malignant NEC (with hepatic failure) K72.90
    with coma K72.91
  neonatal (idiopathic) (toxic) P59.29
  neonatal giant cell P59.29
  newborn P59.29
  non-viral K72.0 ☑
  postimmunization — *see* Hepatitis, viral, type B
  post-transfusion — *see* Hepatitis, viral, type B
  reactive, nonspecific K75.2
  serum — *see* Hepatitis, viral, type B
  specified type NEC
    with hepatic failure — *see* Failure, hepatic
  syphilitic (late) A52.74
    congenital (early) A50.08 *[K77]*
      late A50.59 *[K77]*
    secondary A51.45
  toxic — *see also* Disease, liver, toxic K71.6
  tuberculous A18.83
  viral, virus B19.9
    with hepatic coma B19.0
    acute B17.9
    chronic B18.9
      specified NEC B18.8
      type
        B B18.1
          with delta-agent B18.0
        C B18.2
    congenital P35.3
    coxsackie B33.8 *[K77]*
    cytomegalic inclusion B25.1

Hepatitis — *continued*
  viral, virus — *continued*
    in remission, any type — *code to* Hepatitis, chronic,
      by type
    non-A, non-B B17.8
    specified type NEC (with or without coma) B17.8
    type
      A B15.9
        with hepatic coma B15.0
      B B19.10
        with hepatic coma B19.11
        acute B16.9
          with
            delta-agent (coinfection) (without
              hepatic coma) B16.1
              with hepatic coma B16.0
            hepatic coma (without delta-agent
              coinfection) B16.2
        chronic B18.1
          with delta-agent B18.0
      C B19.20
        with hepatic coma B19.21
        acute B17.10
          with hepatic coma B17.11
        chronic B18.2
      E B17.2
      non-A, non-B B17.8
Hepatization lung (acute) — *see* Pneumonia, lobar
Hepatoblastoma C22.2
Hepatocarcinoma C22.0
Hepatocholangiocarcinoma C22.0
Hepatocholangioma, benign D13.4
Hepatocholangitis K75.89
Hepatolenticular degeneration E83.01
Hepatoma (malignant) C22.0
  benign D13.4
  embryonal C22.0
Hepatomegaly — *see also* Hypertrophy, liver
  with splenomegaly R16.2
  congenital Q44.7
  in mononucleosis
    gammaherpesviral B27.09
    infectious specified NEC B27.89
Hepatoptosis K76.89
Hepatorenal syndrome following labor and delivery
  O90.4
Hepatosis K76.89
Hepatosplenomegaly R16.2
  hyperlipemic (Bürger-Grütz type) E78.3 *[K77]*
Hereditary — *see* condition
Heredodegeneration, macular — *see* Dystrophy, retina
Heredopathia atactica polyneuritiformis G60.1
Heredosyphilis — *see* Syphilis, congenital
Herlitz' syndrome Q81.1
Hermansky-Pudlak syndrome E70.331
Hermaphrodite, hermaphroditism (true) Q56.0
  46,XX with streak gonads Q99.1
  46,XX/46,XY Q99.0
  46,XY with streak gonads Q99.1
  chimera 46,XX/46,XY Q99.0
Hernia, hernial (acquired) (recurrent) K46.9
  with
    gangrene — *see* Hernia, by site, with, gangrene
    incarceration — *see* Hernia, by site, with, obstruction
    irreducible — *see* Hernia, by site, with, obstruction
    obstruction — *see* Hernia, by site, with, obstruction
    strangulation — *see* Hernia, by site, with, obstruc-
      tion
  abdomen, abdominal K46.9
    with
      gangrene (and obstruction) K46.1
      obstruction K46.0
    femoral — *see* Hernia, femoral
    incisional — *see* Hernia, incisional
    inguinal — *see* Hernia, inguinal
    specified site NEC K45.8
      with
        gangrene (and obstruction) K45.1
        obstruction K45.0
    umbilical — *see* Hernia, umbilical
    wall — *see* Hernia, ventral
  appendix — *see* Hernia, abdomen
  bladder (mucosa) (sphincter)
    congenital (female) (male) Q79.51
    female — *see* Cystocele
    male N32.89
  brain, congenital — *see* Encephalocele

Hernia, hernial — *continued*
- cartilage, vertebra — *see* Displacement, intervertebral disc
- cerebral, congenital — *see also* Encephalocele
  - endaural Q01.8
- ciliary body (traumatic) S05.2- ☑
- colon — *see* Hernia, abdomen
- Cooper's — *see* Hernia, abdomen, specified site NEC
- crural — *see* Hernia, femoral
- diaphragm, diaphragmatic K44.9
  - with
    - gangrene (and obstruction) K44.1
    - obstruction K44.0
  - congenital Q79.0
- direct (inguinal) — *see* Hernia, inguinal
- diverticulum, intestine — *see* Hernia, abdomen
- double (inguinal) — *see* Hernia, inguinal, bilateral
- due to adhesions (with obstruction) K56.50
- epigastric — *see also* Hernia, ventral K43.9
- esophageal hiatus — *see* Hernia, hiatal
- external (inguinal) — *see* Hernia, inguinal
- fallopian tube N83.4- ☑
- fascia M62.89
- femoral K41.90
  - with
    - gangrene (and obstruction) K41.40
      - not specified as recurrent K41.40
      - recurrent K41.41
    - obstruction K41.30
      - not specified as recurrent K41.30
      - recurrent K41.31
  - not specified as recurrent K41.90
  - recurrent K41.91
  - bilateral K41.20
    - with
      - gangrene (and obstruction) K41.10
        - not specified as recurrent K41.10
        - recurrent K41.11
      - obstruction K41.00
        - not specified as recurrent K41.00
        - recurrent K41.01
    - not specified as recurrent K41.20
    - recurrent K41.21
  - unilateral K41.90
    - with
      - gangrene (and obstruction) K41.40
        - not specified as recurrent K41.40
        - recurrent K41.41
      - obstruction K41.30
        - not specified as recurrent K41.30
        - recurrent K41.31
    - not specified as recurrent K41.90
    - recurrent K41.91
- foramen magnum G93.5
  - congenital Q01.8
- funicular (umbilical) — *see also* Hernia, umbilicus
  - spermatic (cord) — *see* Hernia, inguinal
- gastrointestinal tract — *see* Hernia, abdomen
- Hesselbach's — *see* Hernia, femoral, specified site NEC
- hiatal (esophageal) (sliding) K44.9
  - with
    - gangrene (and obstruction) K44.1
    - obstruction K44.0
  - congenital Q40.1
- hypogastric — *see* Hernia, ventral
- incarcerated — *see also* Hernia, by site, with obstruction
  - with gangrene — *see* Hernia, by site, with gangrene
- incisional K43.2
  - with
    - gangrene (and obstruction) K43.1
    - obstruction K43.0
- indirect (inguinal) — *see also* Hernia, inguinal
- inguinal (direct) (external) (funicular) (indirect) (internal) (oblique) (scrotal) (sliding) K40.90
  - with
    - gangrene (and obstruction) K40.40
      - not specified as recurrent K40.40
      - recurrent K40.41
    - obstruction K40.30
      - not specified as recurrent K40.30
      - recurrent K40.31
  - not specified as recurrent K40.90
  - recurrent K40.91
  - bilateral K40.20
    - with
      - gangrene (and obstruction) K40.10
        - not specified as recurrent K40.10

Hernia, hernial — *continued*
- inguinal — *continued*
  - bilateral — *continued*
    - with — *continued*
      - gangrene — *continued*
        - recurrent K40.11
      - obstruction K40.00
        - not specified as recurrent K40.00
        - recurrent K40.01
    - not specified as recurrent K40.20
    - recurrent K40.21
  - unilateral K40.90
    - with
      - gangrene (and obstruction) K40.40
        - not specified as recurrent K40.40
        - recurrent K40.41
      - obstruction K40.30
        - not specified as recurrent K40.30
        - recurrent K40.31
    - not specified as recurrent K40.90
    - recurrent K40.91
- internal — *see also* Hernia, abdomen
  - inguinal — *see* Hernia, inguinal
- interstitial — *see* Hernia, abdomen
- intervertebral cartilage or disc — *see* Displacement, intervertebral disc
- intestine, intestinal — *see* Hernia, by site
- intra-abdominal — *see* Hernia, abdomen
- iris (traumatic) S05.2- ☑
- irreducible — *see also* Hernia, by site, with obstruction
  - with gangrene — *see* Hernia, by site, with gangrene
- ischiatic — *see* Hernia, abdomen, specified site NEC
- ischiorectal — *see* Hernia, abdomen, specified site NEC
- lens (traumatic) S05.2- ☑
- linea (alba) (semilunaris) — *see* Hernia, ventral
- Littre's — *see* Hernia, abdomen
- lumbar — *see* Hernia, abdomen, specified site NEC
- lung (subcutaneous) J98.4
- mediastinum J98.59
- mesenteric (internal) — *see* Hernia, abdomen
- midline — *see* Hernia, ventral
- muscle (sheath) M62.89
- nucleus pulposus — *see* Displacement, intervertebral disc
- oblique (inguinal) — *see* Hernia, inguinal
- obstructive — *see also* Hernia, by site, with obstruction
  - with gangrene — *see* Hernia, by site, with gangrene
- obturator — *see* Hernia, abdomen, specified site NEC
- omental — *see* Hernia, abdomen
- ovary N83.4- ☑
- oviduct N83.4- ☑
- paraesophageal — *see also* Hernia, diaphragm
  - congenital Q40.1
- parastomal K43.5
  - with
    - gangrene (and obstruction) K43.4
    - obstruction K43.3
- paraumbilical — *see* Hernia, umbilicus
- perineal — *see* Hernia, abdomen, specified site NEC
- Petit's — *see* Hernia, abdomen, specified site NEC
- postoperative — *see* Hernia, incisional
- pregnant uterus — *see* Abnormal, uterus in pregnancy or childbirth
- prevesical N32.89
- properitoneal — *see* Hernia, abdomen, specified site NEC
- pudendal — *see* Hernia, abdomen, specified site NEC
- rectovaginal N81.6
- retroperitoneal — *see* Hernia, abdomen, specified site NEC
- Richter's — *see* Hernia, abdomen, with obstruction
- Rieux's, Riex's — *see* Hernia, abdomen, specified site NEC
- sac condition (adhesion) (dropsy) (inflammation) (laceration) (suppuration) — *code by site under* Hernia
- sciatic — *see* Hernia, abdomen, specified site NEC
- scrotum, scrotal — *see* Hernia, inguinal
- sliding (inguinal) — *see also* Hernia, inguinal
  - hiatus — *see* Hernia, hiatal
- spigelian — *see* Hernia, ventral
- spinal — *see* Spina bifida
- strangulated — *see also* Hernia, by site, with obstruction
  - with gangrene — *see* Hernia, by site, with gangrene
- subxiphoid — *see* Hernia, ventral
- supra-umbilicus — *see* Hernia, ventral

Hernia, hernial — *continued*
- tendon — *see* Disorder, tendon, specified type NEC
- Treitz's (fossa) — *see* Hernia, abdomen, specified site NEC
- tunica vaginalis Q55.29
- umbilicus, umbilical K42.9
  - with
    - gangrene (and obstruction) K42.1
    - obstruction K42.0
- ureter N28.89
- urethra, congenital Q64.79
- urinary meatus, congenital Q64.79
- uterus N81.4
  - pregnant — *see* Abnormal, uterus in pregnancy or childbirth
- vaginal (anterior) (wall) — *see* Cystocele
- Velpeau's — *see* Hernia, femoral
- ventral K43.9
  - with
    - gangrene (and obstruction) K43.7
    - obstruction K43.6
  - incisional K43.2
    - with
      - gangrene (and obstruction) K43.1
      - obstruction K43.0
    - recurrent — *see* Hernia, incisional
  - specified NEC K43.9
    - with
      - gangrene (and obstruction) K43.7
      - obstruction K43.6
- vesical
  - congenital (female) (male) Q79.51
  - female — *see* Cystocele
  - male N32.89
- vitreous (into wound) S05.2- ☑
  - into anterior chamber — *see* Prolapse, vitreous

Herniation — *see also* Hernia
- brain (stem) G93.5
- cerebral G93.5
- mediastinum J98.59
- nucleus pulposus — *see* Displacement, intervertebral disc

Herpangina B08.5

Herpes, herpesvirus, herpetic B00.9
- anogenital A60.9
  - perianal skin A60.1
  - rectum A60.1
  - urogenital tract A60.00
    - cervix A60.03
    - male genital organ NEC A60.02
    - penis A60.01
    - specified site NEC A60.09
    - vagina A60.04
    - vulva A60.04
- blepharitis (zoster) B02.39
  - simplex B00.59
- circinatus B35.4
  - bullosus L12.0
- conjunctivitis (simplex) B00.53
  - zoster B02.31
- cornea B02.33
- encephalitis B00.4
  - due to herpesvirus 6 B10.01
  - due to herpesvirus 7 B10.09
  - specified NEC B10.09
- eye (zoster) B02.30
  - simplex B00.50
- eyelid (zoster) B02.39
  - simplex B00.59
- facialis B00.1
- febrilis B00.1
- geniculate ganglionitis B02.21
- genital, genitalis A60.00
  - female A60.09
  - male A60.02
- gestational, gestationis O26.4- ☑
- gingivostomatitis B00.2
- human B00.9
  - 1 — *see* Herpes, simplex
  - 2 — *see* Herpes, simplex
  - 3 — *see* Varicella
  - 4 — *see* Mononucleosis, Epstein-Barr (virus)
  - 5 — *see* Disease, cytomegalic inclusion (generalized)
  - 6
    - encephalitis B10.01
    - specified NEC B10.81
  - 7
    - encephalitis B10.09

☑ **Additional Character Required** — *Refer to the Tabular List for Character Selection*   ▽ **Subterms under main terms may continue to next column or page**

Herpes, herpesvirus, herpetic — continued
  human — continued
    7 — continued
      specified NEC B10.82
      8 B10.89
    infection NEC B10.89
      Kaposi's sarcoma associated B10.89
    iridocyclitis (simplex) B00.51
      zoster B02.32
    iris (vesicular erythema multiforme) L51.9
    iritis (simplex) B00.51
    Kaposi's sarcoma associated B10.89
    keratitis (simplex) (dendritic) (disciform) (interstitial) B00.52
      zoster (interstitial) B02.33
    keratoconjunctivitis (simplex) B00.52
      zoster B02.33
    labialis B00.1
    lip B00.1
    meningitis (simplex) B00.3
      zoster B02.1
    ophthalmicus (zoster) NEC B02.30
      simplex B00.50
    penis A60.01
    perianal skin A60.1
    pharyngitis, pharyngotonsillitis B00.2
    rectum A60.1
    scrotum A60.02
    sepsis B00.7
    simplex B00.9
      complicated NEC B00.89
      congenital P35.2
      conjunctivitis B00.53
      external ear B00.1
      eyelid B00.59
      hepatitis B00.81
      keratitis (interstitial) B00.52
      myelitis B00.82
      specified complication NEC B00.89
      visceral B00.89
    stomatitis B00.2
    tonsurans B35.0
    visceral B00.89
    vulva A60.04
    whitlow B00.89
    zoster — see also condition B02.9
      auricularis B02.21
      complicated NEC B02.8
      conjunctivitis B02.31
      disseminated B02.7
      encephalitis B02.0
      eye (lid) B02.39
      geniculate ganglionitis B02.21
      keratitis (interstitial) B02.33
      meningitis B02.1
      myelitis B02.24
      neuritis, neuralgia B02.29
      ophthalmicus NEC B02.30
      oticus B02.21
      polyneuropathy B02.23
      specified complication NEC B02.8
      trigeminal neuralgia B02.22
Herpesvirus (human) — see Herpes
Herpetophobia F40.218
Herrick's anemia — see Disease, sickle-cell
Hers' disease E74.09
Herter-Gee syndrome K90.0
Herxheimer's reaction R68.89
Hesitancy
  of micturition R39.11
  urinary R39.11
Hesselbach's hernia — see Hernia, femoral, specified site NEC
Heterochromia (congenital) Q13.2
  cataract — see Cataract, complicated
  cyclitis (Fuchs) — see Cyclitis, Fuchs' heterochromic
  hair L67.1
  iritis — see Cyclitis, Fuchs' heterochromic
  retained metallic foreign body (nonmagnetic) — see Foreign body, intraocular, old, retained
    magnetic — see Foreign body, intraocular, old, retained, magnetic
  uveitis — see Cyclitis, Fuchs' heterochromic
Heterophoria — see Strabismus, heterophoria
Heterophyes, heterophyiasis (small intestine) B66.8
Heterotopia, heterotopic — see also Malposition, congenital
  cerebralis Q04.8

Heterotropia — see Strabismus
Heubner-Herter disease K90.0
Hexadactylism Q69.9
HGSIL (cytology finding) (high grade squamous intraepithelial lesion on cytologic smear) (Pap smear finding)
  anus R85.613
  cervix R87.613
    biopsy (histology) finding — see Neoplasia, intraepithelial, cervix, grade II or grade III
  vagina R87.623
    biopsy (histology) finding — see Neoplasia, intraepithelial, cervix, grade II or grade III
Hibernoma — see Lipoma
Hiccup, hiccough R06.6
  epidemic B33.0
  psychogenic F45.8
Hidden penis (congenital) Q55.64
  acquired N48.83
Hidradenitis (axillaris) (suppurative) L73.2
Hidradenoma (nodular) — see also Neoplasm, skin, benign
  clear cell — see Neoplasm, skin, benign
  papillary — see Neoplasm, skin, benign
Hidrocystoma — see Neoplasm, skin, benign
High
  altitude effects T70.20 ☑
    anoxia T70.29 ☑
    on
      ears T70.0 ☑
      sinuses T70.1 ☑
    polycythemia D75.1
  arch
    foot Q66.7- ☑
    palate, congenital Q38.5
  arterial tension — see Hypertension
  basal metabolic rate R94.8
  blood pressure — see also Hypertension
    borderline R03.0
    reading (incidental) (isolated) (nonspecific), without diagnosis of hypertension R03.0
  cholesterol E78.00
    with high triglycerides E78.2
  diaphragm (congenital) Q79.1
  expressed emotional level within family Z63.8
  head at term O32.4 ☑
  palate, congenital Q38.5
  risk
    infant NEC Z76.2
    sexual behavior (heterosexual) Z72.51
      bisexual Z72.53
      homosexual Z72.52
  scrotal testis, testes
    bilateral Q53.23
    unilateral Q53.13
  temperature (of unknown origin) R50.9
  thoracic rib Q76.6
  triglycerides E78.1
    with high cholesterol E78.2
Hildenbrand's disease A75.0
Hilum — see condition
Hip — see condition
Hippel's disease Q85.8
Hippophobia F40.218
Hippus H57.09
Hirschsprung's disease or megacolon Q43.1
Hirsutism, hirsuties L68.0
Hirudiniasis
  external B88.3
  internal B83.4
Hiss-Russell dysentery A03.1
Histidinemia, histidinuria E70.41
Histiocytoma — see also Neoplasm, skin, benign
  fibrous — see also Neoplasm, skin, benign
    atypical — see Neoplasm, connective tissue, uncertain behavior
    malignant — see Neoplasm, connective tissue, malignant
Histiocytosis D76.3
  acute differentiated progressive C96.0
  Langerhans' cell NEC C96.6
    multifocal X
      multisystemic (disseminated) C96.0
      unisystemic C96.5
    pulmonary, adult (adult PLCH) J84.82
    unifocal (X) C96.6
  lipid, lipoid D76.3

Histiocytosis — continued
  lipid, lipoid — continued
    essential E75.29
  malignant C96.A (following C96.6)
  mononuclear phagocytes NEC D76.1
    Langerhans' cells C96.6
  non-Langerhans cell D76.3
  polyostotic sclerosing D76.3
  sinus, with massive lymphadenopathy D76.3
  syndrome NEC D76.3
  X NEC C96.6
    acute (progressive) C96.0
    chronic C96.6
    multifocal C96.5
    multisystemic C96.0
    unifocal C96.6
Histoplasmosis B39.9
  with pneumonia NEC B39.2
  African B39.5
  American — see Histoplasmosis, capsulati
  capsulati B39.4
    disseminated B39.3
    generalized B39.3
    pulmonary B39.2
      acute B39.0
      chronic B39.1
  Darling's B39.4
  duboisii B39.5
  lung NEC B39.2
History
  family (of) — see also History, personal (of)
    alcohol abuse Z81.1
    allergy NEC Z84.89
    anemia Z83.2
    arthritis Z82.61
    asthma Z82.5
    blindness Z82.1
    cardiac death (sudden) Z82.41
    carrier of genetic disease Z84.81
    chromosomal anomaly Z82.79
    chronic
      disabling disease NEC Z82.8
      lower respiratory disease Z82.5
    colonic polyps Z83.71
    congenital malformations and deformations Z82.79
      polycystic kidney Z82.71
    consanguinity Z84.3
    deafness Z82.2
    diabetes mellitus Z83.3
    disability NEC Z82.8
    disease or disorder (of)
      allergic NEC Z84.89
      behavioral NEC Z81.8
      blood and blood-forming organs Z83.2
      cardiovascular NEC Z82.49
      chronic disabling NEC Z82.8
      digestive Z83.79
      ear NEC Z83.52
      elevated lipoprotein (a) (Lp(a)) Z83.430
      endocrine NEC Z83.49
      eye NEC Z83.518
        glaucoma Z83.511
      familial hypercholesterolemia Z83.42
      genitourinary NEC Z84.2
      glaucoma Z83.511
      hematological Z83.2
      immune mechanism Z83.2
      infectious NEC Z83.1
      ischemic heart Z82.49
      kidney Z84.1
      lipoprotein metabolism Z83.438
      mental NEC Z81.8
      metabolic Z83.49
      musculoskeletal NEC Z82.69
      neurological NEC Z82.0
      nutritional Z83.49
      parasitic NEC Z83.1
      psychiatric NEC Z81.8
      respiratory NEC Z83.6
      skin and subcutaneous tissue NEC Z84.0
      specified NEC Z84.89
    drug abuse NEC Z81.3
    elevated lipoprotein (a) (Lp(a)) Z83.430
    epilepsy Z82.0
    familial hypercholesterolemia Z83.42
    genetic disease carrier Z84.81
    glaucoma Z83.511
    hearing loss Z82.2
    human immunodeficiency virus (HIV) infection Z83.0

History — *continued*
 family — *see also* History, personal — *continued*
  Huntington's chorea Z82.0
  hyperlipidemia, familial combined Z83.438
  intellectual disability Z81.0
  leukemia Z80.6
  lipidemia NEC Z83.438
  malignant neoplasm (of) NOS Z80.9
   bladder Z80.52
   breast Z80.3
   bronchus Z80.1
   digestive organ Z80.0
   gastrointestinal tract Z80.0
   genital organ Z80.49
    ovary Z80.41
    prostate Z80.42
    specified organ NEC Z80.49
    testis Z80.43
   hematopoietic NEC Z80.7
   intrathoracic organ NEC Z80.2
   kidney Z80.51
   lung Z80.1
   lymphatic NEC Z80.7
   ovary Z80.41
   prostate Z80.42
   respiratory organ NEC Z80.2
   specified site NEC Z80.8
   testis Z80.43
   trachea Z80.1
   urinary organ or tract Z80.59
    bladder Z80.52
    kidney Z80.51
  mental
   disorder NEC Z81.8
  multiple endocrine neoplasia (MEN) syndrome Z83.41
  osteoporosis Z82.62
  polycystic kidney Z82.71
  polyps (colon) Z83.71
  psychiatric disorder Z81.8
  psychoactive substance abuse NEC Z81.3
  respiratory condition NEC Z83.6
   asthma and other lower respiratory conditions Z82.5
  self-harmful behavior Z81.8
  SIDS (sudden infant death syndrome) Z84.82
  skin condition Z84.0
  specified condition NEC Z84.89
  stroke (cerebrovascular) Z82.3
  substance abuse NEC Z81.4
   alcohol Z81.1
   drug NEC Z81.3
   psychoactive NEC Z81.3
   tobacco Z81.2
  sudden
   cardiac death Z82.41
   infant death syndrome (SIDS) Z84.82
  tobacco abuse Z81.2
  violence, violent behavior Z81.8
  visual loss Z82.1
 personal (of) — *see also* History, family (of)
  abuse
   adult Z91.419
    forced labor or sexual exploitation Z91.42
    physical and sexual Z91.410
    psychological Z91.411
   childhood Z62.819
    forced labor or sexual exploitation in childhood Z62.813
    physical Z62.810
    psychological Z62.811
    sexual Z62.810
  alcohol dependence F10.21
  allergy (to) Z88.9
   analgesic agent NEC Z88.6
   anesthetic Z88.4
   antibiotic agent NEC Z88.1
   anti-infective agent NEC Z88.3
   contrast media Z91.041
   drugs, medicaments and biological substances Z88.9
    specified NEC Z88.8
   food Z91.018
    additives Z91.02
    eggs Z91.012
    milk products Z91.011
    peanuts Z91.010
    seafood Z91.013
    specified food NEC Z91.018

History — *continued*
 personal — *see also* History, family — *continued*
  allergy — *continued*
   insect Z91.038
    bee Z91.030
   latex Z91.040
   medicinal agents Z88.9
    specified NEC Z88.8
   narcotic agent NEC Z88.5
   nonmedicinal agents Z91.048
   penicillin Z88.0
   serum Z88.7
   specified NEC Z91.09
   sulfonamides Z88.2
   vaccine Z88.7
  anaphylactic shock Z87.892
  anaphylaxis Z87.892
  behavioral disorders Z86.59
  benign carcinoid tumor Z86.012
  benign neoplasm Z86.018
   brain Z86.011
   carcinoid Z86.012
   colonic polyps Z86.010
  brain injury (traumatic) Z87.820
  breast implant removal Z98.86
  calculi, renal Z87.442
  cancer — *see* History, personal (of), malignant neoplasm (of)
  cardiac arrest (death), successfully resuscitated Z86.74
  cerebral infarction without residual deficit Z86.73
  cervical dysplasia Z87.410
  chemotherapy for neoplastic condition Z92.21
  childhood abuse — *see* History, personal (of), abuse
  cleft lip (corrected) Z87.730
  cleft palate (corrected) Z87.730
  collapsed vertebra (healed) Z87.311
   due to osteoporosis Z87.310
  combat and operational stress reaction Z86.51
  congenital malformation (corrected) Z87.798
   circulatory system (corrected) Z87.74
   digestive system (corrected) NEC Z87.738
   ear (corrected) Z87.721
   eye (corrected) Z87.720
   face and neck (corrected) Z87.790
   genitourinary system (corrected) NEC Z87.718
   heart (corrected) Z87.74
   integument (corrected) Z87.76
   limb(s) (corrected) Z87.76
   musculoskeletal system (corrected) Z87.76
   neck (corrected) Z87.790
   nervous system (corrected) NEC Z87.728
   respiratory system (corrected) Z87.75
   sense organs (corrected) NEC Z87.728
   specified NEC Z87.798
  contraception Z92.0
  deployment (military) Z91.82
  diabetic foot ulcer Z86.31
  disease or disorder (of) Z87.898
   anaphylaxis Z87.892
   blood and blood-forming organs Z86.2
   circulatory system Z86.79
    specified condition NEC Z86.79
   connective tissue Z87.39
   digestive system Z87.19
    colonic polyp Z86.010
    peptic ulcer disease Z87.11
    specified condition NEC Z87.19
   ear Z86.69
   endocrine Z86.39
    diabetic foot ulcer Z86.31
    gestational diabetes Z86.32
    specified type NEC Z86.39
   eye Z86.69
   genital (track) system NEC
    female Z87.42
    male Z87.438
   hematological Z86.2
   Hodgkin Z85.71
   immune mechanism Z86.2
   infectious Z86.19
    malaria Z86.13
    Methicillin resistant Staphylococcus aureus (MRSA) Z86.14
    poliomyelitis Z86.12
    specified NEC Z86.19
    tuberculosis Z86.11
   mental NEC Z86.59
   metabolic Z86.39

History — *continued*
 personal — *see also* History, family — *continued*
  disease or disorder — *continued*
   metabolic — *continued*
    diabetic foot ulcer Z86.31
    gestational diabetes Z86.32
    specified type NEC Z86.39
   musculoskeletal NEC Z87.39
   nervous system Z86.69
   nutritional Z86.39
   parasitic Z86.19
   respiratory system NEC Z87.09
   sense organs Z86.69
   skin Z87.2
   specified site or type NEC Z87.898
   subcutaneous tissue Z87.2
   trophoblastic Z87.59
   urinary system NEC Z87.448
  drug dependence — *see* Dependence, drug, by type, in remission
  drug therapy
   antineoplastic chemotherapy Z92.21
   estrogen Z92.23
   immunosupression Z92.25
   inhaled steroids Z92.240
   monoclonal drug Z92.22
   specified NEC Z92.29
   steroid Z92.241
   systemic steroids Z92.241
  dysplasia
   cervical (mild) (moderate) Z87.410
    severe (grade III) Z86.001
   prostatic Z87.430
   vaginal (mild) (moderate) Z87.411
    severe (grade III) Z86.002
   vulvar (mild) (moderate) Z87.412
    severe (grade III) Z86.002
  embolism (venous) Z86.718
   pulmonary Z86.711
  encephalitis Z86.61
  estrogen therapy Z92.23
  extracorporeal membrane oxygenation (ECMO) Z92.81
  failed conscious sedation Z92.83
  failed moderate sedation Z92.83
  fall, falling Z91.81
  forced labor or sexual exploitation Z91.42
   in childhood Z62.813
  fracture (healed)
   fatigue Z87.312
   fragility Z87.310
   osteoporosis Z87.310
   pathological NEC Z87.311
   stress Z87.312
   traumatic Z87.81
  gestational diabetes Z86.32
  hepatitis
   B Z86.19
   C Z86.19
  Hodgkin disease Z85.71
  hyperthermia, malignant Z88.4
  hypospadias (corrected) Z87.710
  hysterectomy Z90.710
  immunosuppression therapy Z92.25
  in situ neoplasm
   breast Z86.000
   cervix uteri Z86.001
   digestive organs, specified NEC Z86.004
   esophagus Z86.003
   genital organs, specified NEC Z86.002
   melanoma Z86.006
   middle ear Z86.005
   oral cavity Z86.003
   respiratory system Z86.005
   skin Z86.007
   specified NEC Z86.008
   stomach Z86.003
  in utero procedure during pregnancy Z98.870
  in utero procedure while a fetus Z98.871
  infection NEC Z86.19
   central nervous system Z86.61
   latent tuberculosis Z86.15
   Methicillin resistant Staphylococcus aureus (MRSA) Z86.14
   urinary (recurrent) (tract) Z87.440
  injury NEC Z87.828
  irradiation Z92.3
  kidney stones Z87.442
  latent tuberculosis infection Z86.15

☑ **Additional Character Required** — Refer to the Tabular List for Character Selection   ▽ **Subterms under main terms may continue to next column or page**

History — *continued*
  personal — *see also* History, family — *continued*
    leukemia Z85.6
    lymphoma (non-Hodgkin) Z85.72
    malignant melanoma (skin) Z85.820
    malignant neoplasm (of) Z85.9
      accessory sinuses Z85.22
      anus NEC Z85.048
        carcinoid Z85.040
      bladder Z85.51
      bone Z85.830
      brain Z85.841
      breast Z85.3
      bronchus NEC Z85.118
        carcinoid Z85.110
      carcinoid — *see* History, personal (of), malignant neoplasm, by site, carcinioid
      cervix Z85.41
      colon NEC Z85.038
        carcinoid Z85.030
      digestive organ Z85.00
        specified NEC Z85.09
      endocrine gland NEC Z85.858
      epididymis Z85.48
      esophagus Z85.01
      eye Z85.840
      gastrointestinal tract — *see* History, malignant neoplasm, digestive organ
      genital organ
        female Z85.40
          specified NEC Z85.44
        male Z85.45
          specified NEC Z85.49
      hematopoietic NEC Z85.79
      intrathoracic organ Z85.20
      kidney NEC Z85.528
        carcinoid Z85.520
      large intestine NEC Z85.038
        carcinoid Z85.030
      larynx Z85.21
      liver Z85.05
      lung NEC Z85.118
        carcinoid Z85.110
      mediastinum Z85.29
      Merkel cell Z85.821
      middle ear Z85.22
      nasal cavities Z85.22
      nervous system NEC Z85.848
      oral cavity Z85.819
        specified site NEC Z85.818
      ovary Z85.43
      pancreas Z85.07
      pelvis Z85.53
      pharynx Z85.819
        specified site NEC Z85.818
      pleura Z85.29
      prostate Z85.46
      rectosigmoid junction NEC Z85.048
        carcinoid Z85.040
      rectum NEC Z85.048
        carcinoid Z85.040
      respiratory organ Z85.20
      sinuses, accessory Z85.22
      skin NEC Z85.828
        melanoma Z85.820
        Merkel cell Z85.821
      small intestine NEC Z85.068
        carcinoid Z85.060
      soft tissue Z85.831
      specified site NEC Z85.89
      stomach NEC Z85.028
        carcinoid Z85.020
      testis Z85.47
      thymus NEC Z85.238
        carcinoid Z85.230
      thyroid Z85.850
      tongue Z85.810
      trachea Z85.12
      urinary organ or tract Z85.50
        specified NEC Z85.59
      uterus Z85.42
    maltreatment Z91.89
    medical treatment NEC Z92.89
    melanoma Z85.820
      in situ Z86.006
      malignant (skin) Z85.820
    meningitis Z86.61
    mental disorder Z86.59
    Merkel cell carcinoma (skin) Z85.821

History — *continued*
  personal — *see also* History, family — *continued*
    Methicillin resistant Staphylococcus aureus (MRSA) Z86.14
    military deployment Z91.82
    military war, peacekeeping and humanitarian deployment (current or past conflict) Z91.82
    myocardial infarction (old) I25.2
    neglect (in)
      adult Z91.412
      childhood Z62.812
    neoplasia
      anal intraepithelial, III [AIN III] Z86.004
      high-grade prostatic intraepithelial, III [HGPIN III] Z86.002
      vaginal intraepithelial, III [VAIN III] Z86.002
      vulvar intraepithelial, III [VIN III] Z86.002
    neoplasm
      benign Z86.018
        brain Z86.011
        colon polyp Z86.010
      in situ
        breast Z86.000
        cervix uteri Z86.001
        digestive organs, specified NEC Z86.004
        esophagus Z86.003
        genital organs, specified NEC Z86.002
        melanoma Z86.006
        middle ear Z86.005
        oral cavity Z86.003
        respiratory system Z86.005
        skin Z86.007
        specified NEC Z86.008
        stomach Z86.003
      malignant — *see* History of, malignant neoplasm
      uncertain behavior Z86.03
    nephrotic syndrome Z87.441
    nicotine dependence Z87.891
    noncompliance with medical treatment or regimen — *see* Noncompliance
    nutritional deficiency Z86.39
    obstetric complications Z87.59
      childbirth Z87.59
      pregnancy Z87.59
      pre-term labor Z87.51
      puerperium Z87.59
    osteoporosis fractures Z87.31 ☑
    parasuicide (attempt) Z91.5
    physical trauma NEC Z87.828
      self-harm or suicide attempt Z91.5
    pneumonia (recurrent) Z87.01
    poisoning NEC Z91.89
      self-harm or suicide attempt Z91.5
    poor personal hygiene Z91.89
    preterm labor Z87.51
    procedure during pregnancy Z98.870
    procedure while a fetus Z98.871
    prolonged reversible ischemic neurologic deficit (PRIND) Z86.73
    prostatic dysplasia Z87.430
    psychological
      abuse
        adult Z91.411
        child Z62.811
      trauma, specified NEC Z91.49
    radiation therapy Z92.3
    removal
      implant
        breast Z98.86
    renal calculi Z87.442
    respiratory condition NEC Z87.09
    retained foreign body fully removed Z87.821
    risk factors NEC Z91.89
    self-harm Z91.5
    self-poisoning attempt Z91.5
    sex reassignment Z87.890
    sleep-wake cycle problem Z72.821
    specified NEC Z87.898
    steroid therapy (systemic) Z92.241
      inhaled Z92.240
    stroke without residual deficits Z86.73
    substance abuse NEC F10-F19
    sudden cardiac arrest Z86.74
    sudden cardiac death successfully resuscitated Z86.74
    suicide attempt Z91.5
    surgery NEC Z98.890
      with uterine scar Z98.891
      sex reassignment Z87.890

History — *continued*
  personal — *see also* History, family — *continued*
    surgery — *continued*
      transplant — *see* Transplant
    thrombophlebitis Z86.72
    thrombosis (venous) Z86.718
      pulmonary Z86.711
    tobacco dependence Z87.891
    transient ischemic attack (TIA) without residual deficits Z86.73
    trauma (physical) NEC Z87.828
      psychological NEC Z91.49
      self-harm Z91.5
    traumatic brain injury Z87.820
    tuberculosis, latent infection Z86.15
    unhealthy sleep-wake cycle Z72.821
    unintended awareness under general anesthesia Z92.84
    urinary calculi Z87.442
    urinary (recurrent) (tract) infection(s) Z87.440
    uterine scar from previous surgery Z98.891
    vaginal dysplasia Z87.411
    venous thrombosis or embolism Z86.718
      pulmonary Z86.711
    vulvar dysplasia Z87.412
His-Werner disease A79.0
HIV — *see also* Human, immunodeficiency virus B20
  laboratory evidence (nonconclusive) R75
  nonconclusive test (in infants) R75
  positive, seropositive Z21
Hives (bold) — *see* Urticaria
Hoarseness R49.0
Hobo Z59.0
Hodgkin disease — *see* Lymphoma, Hodgkin
Hodgson's disease I71.2
  ruptured I71.1
Hoffa-Kastert disease E88.89
Hoffa's disease E88.89
Hoffmann-Bouveret syndrome I47.9
Hoffmann's syndrome E03.9 *[G73.7]*
Hole (round)
  macula H35.34- ☑
  retina (without detachment) — *see* Break, retina, round hole
    with detachment — *see* Detachment, retina, with retinal, break
Holiday relief care Z75.5
Hollenhorst's plaque — *see* Occlusion, artery, retina
Hollow foot (congenital) Q66.7- ☑
  acquired — *see* Deformity, limb, foot, specified NEC
Holoprosencephaly Q04.2
Holt-Oram syndrome Q87.2
Homelessness Z59.0
Homesickness — *see* Disorder, adjustment
Homocystinemia, homocystinuria E72.11
Homogentisate 1,2-dioxygenase deficiency E70.29
Homologous serum hepatitis (prophylactic) (therapeutic) — *see* Hepatitis, viral, type B
Honeycomb lung J98.4
  congenital Q33.0
Hooded
  clitoris Q52.6
  penis Q55.69
Hookworm (disease) (infection) (infestation) B76.9
  with anemia B76.9 *[D63.8]*
  specified NEC B76.8
Hordeolum (eyelid) (externum) (recurrent) H00.019
  internum H00.029
    left H00.026
      lower H00.025
      upper H00.024
    right H00.023
      lower H00.022
      upper H00.021
  left H00.016
    lower H00.015
    upper H00.014
  right H00.013
    lower H00.012
    upper H00.011
Horn
  cutaneous L85.8
  nail L60.2
    congenital Q84.6
Horner (-Claude Bernard) **syndrome** G90.2
  traumatic — *see* Injury, nerve, cervical sympathetic
Horseshoe kidney (congenital) Q63.1

Horton's headache or neuralgia G44.Ø99
  intractable G44.Ø91
  not intractable G44.Ø99
Hospital hopper syndrome — *see* Disorder, factitious
Hospitalism in children — *see* Disorder, adjustment
Hostility R45.5
  towards child Z62.3
Hot flashes
  menopausal N95.1
Hourglass (contracture) — *see also* Contraction, hourglass
  stomach K31.89
    congenital Q4Ø.2
    stricture K31.2
Household, housing circumstance affecting care Z59.9
  specified NEC Z59.8
Housemaid's knee — *see* Bursitis, prepatellar
Hudson (-Stähli) **line** (cornea) — *see* Pigmentation, cornea, anterior
Human
  bite (open wound) — *see also* Bite
    intact skin surface — *see* Bite, superficial
  herpesvirus — *see* Herpes
  immunodeficiency virus (HIV) disease (infection) B2Ø
    asymptomatic status Z21
    contact Z2Ø.6
    counseling Z71.7
    dementia B2Ø [FØ2.8Ø]
      with behavioral disturbance B2Ø [FØ2.81]
    exposure to Z2Ø.6
    laboratory evidence R75
    type-2 (HIV 2) as cause of disease classified elsewhere B97.35
  papillomavirus (HPV)
    DNA test positive
      high risk
        cervix R87.81Ø
        vagina R87.811
      low risk
        cervix R87.82Ø
        vagina R87.821
    screening for Z11.51
  T-cell lymphotropic virus
    type-1 (HTLV-I) infection B33.3
      as cause of disease classified elsewhere B97.33
      carrier Z22.6
    type-2 (HTLV-II) as cause of disease classified elsewhere B97.34
Humidifier lung or pneumonitis J67.7
Humiliation (experience) **in childhood** Z62.898
Humpback (acquired) — *see* Kyphosis
Hunchback (acquired) — *see* Kyphosis
Hunger T73.Ø ☑
  air, psychogenic F45.8
Hungry bone syndrome E83.81
Hunner's ulcer — *see* Cystitis, chronic, interstitial
Hunter's
  glossitis D51.Ø
  syndrome E76.1
Huntington's disease or chorea G1Ø
  with dementia G1Ø [FØ2.8Ø]
    with behavioral disturbance G1Ø [FØ2.81]
Hunt's
  disease or syndrome (herpetic geniculate ganglionitis) BØ2.21
    dyssynergia cerebellaris myoclonica G11.1
  neuralgia BØ2.21
Hurler (-Scheie) **disease or syndrome** E76.Ø2
Hurst's disease G36.1
Hurthle cell
  adenocarcinoma C73
  adenoma D34
  carcinoma C73
  tumor D34
Hutchinson-Boeck disease or syndrome — *see* Sarcoidosis
Hutchinson-Gilford disease or syndrome E34.8
Hutchinson's
  disease, meaning
    angioma serpiginosum L81.7
    pompholyx (cheiropompholyx) L3Ø.1
    prurigo estivalis L56.4
    summer eruption or summer prurigo L56.4
  melanotic freckle — *see* Melanoma, in situ
    malignant melanoma in — *see* Melanoma
  teeth or incisors (congenital syphilis) A5Ø.52
  triad (congenital syphilis) A5Ø.53

Hyalin plaque, sclera, senile H15.89
Hyaline membrane (disease) (lung) (pulmonary) (newborn) P22.Ø
Hyalinosis
  cutis (et mucosae) E78.89
  focal and segmental (glomerular) — *see also* NØØ-NØ7
    with fourth character .1 NØ5.1
Hyalitis, hyalosis, asteroid — *see also* Deposit, crystalline
  syphilitic (late) A52.71
Hydatid
  cyst or tumor — *see* Echinococcus
  mole — *see* Hydatidiform mole
  Morgagni
    female Q5Ø.5
    male (epididymal) Q55.4
    testicular Q55.29
Hydatidiform mole (benign) (complicating pregnancy) (delivered) (undelivered) OØ1.9
  classical OØ1.Ø
  complete OØ1.Ø
  incomplete OØ1.1
  invasive D39.2
  malignant D39.2
  partial OØ1.1
Hydatidosis — *see* Echinococcus
Hydradenitis (axillaris) (suppurative) L73.2
Hydradenoma — *see* Hidradenoma
Hydramnios O4Ø.- ☑
Hydrancephaly, hydranencephaly QØ4.3
  with spina bifida — *see* Spina bifida, with hydrocephalus
Hydrargyrism NEC — *see* Poisoning, mercury
Hydrarthrosis — *see also* Effusion, joint
  gonococcal A54.42
  intermittent M12.4Ø
    ankle M12.47- ☑
    elbow M12.42- ☑
    foot joint M12.47- ☑
    hand joint M12.44- ☑
    hip M12.45- ☑
    knee M12.46- ☑
    multiple site M12.49
    shoulder M12.41- ☑
    specified joint NEC M12.48
    wrist M12.43- ☑
  of yaws (early) (late) — *see also* subcategory M14.8- A66.6
  syphilitic (late) A52.77
    congenital A5Ø.55 [M12.8Ø]
Hydremia D64.89
Hydrencephalocele (congenital) — *see* Encephalocele
Hydrencephalomeningocele (congenital) — *see* Encephalocele
Hydroa R23.8
  aestivale L56.4
  vacciniforme L56.4
Hydroadenitis (axillaris) (suppurative) L73.2
Hydrocalycosis — *see* Hydronephrosis
Hydrocele (spermatic cord) (testis) (tunica vaginalis) N43.3
  canal of Nuck N94.89
  communicating N43.2
    congenital P83.5
  congenital P83.5
  encysted N43.Ø
  female NEC N94.89
  infected N43.1
  newborn P83.5
  round ligament N94.89
  specified NEC N43.2
  spinalis — *see* Spina bifida
  vulva N9Ø.89
Hydrocephalus (acquired) (external) (internal) (malignant) (recurrent) G91.9
  aqueduct Sylvius stricture QØ3.Ø
  causing disproportion O33.6 ☑
    with obstructed labor O66.3
  communicating G91.Ø
  congenital (external) (internal) QØ3.9
    with spina bifida QØ5.4
      cervical QØ5.Ø
      dorsal QØ5.1
      lumbar QØ5.2
      lumbosacral QØ5.2
      sacral QØ5.3
      thoracic QØ5.1

Hydrocephalus — *continued*
  congenital — *continued*
    with spina bifida — *continued*
      thoracolumbar QØ5.1
    specified NEC QØ3.8
  due to toxoplasmosis (congenital) P37.1
  foramen Magendie block (acquired) G91.1
    congenital — *see also* Hydrocephalus, congenital QØ3.1
  in (due to)
    infectious disease NEC B89 [G91.4]
    neoplastic disease NEC — *see also* Neoplasm G91.4
    parasitic disease B89 [G91.4]
  newborn QØ3.9
    with spina bifida — *see* Spina bifida, with hydrocephalus
  noncommunicating G91.1
  normal pressure G91.2
    secondary G91.Ø
  obstructive G91.1
  otitic G93.2
  post-traumatic NEC G91.3
  secondary G91.4
    post-traumatic G91.3
  specified NEC G91.8
  syphilitic, congenital A5Ø.49
Hydrocolpos (congenital) N89.8
Hydrocystoma — *see* Neoplasm, skin, benign
Hydroencephalocele (congenital) — *see* Encephalocele
Hydroencephalomeningocele (congenital) — *see* Encephalocele
Hydrohematopneumothorax — *see* Hemothorax
Hydromeningitis — *see* Meningitis
Hydromeningocele (spinal) — *see also* Spina bifida
  cranial — *see* Encephalocele
Hydrometra N85.8
Hydrometrocolpos N89.8
Hydromicrocephaly QØ2
Hydromphalos (since birth) Q45.8
Hydromyelia QØ6.4
Hydromyelocele — *see* Spina bifida
Hydronephrosis (atrophic) (early) (functionless) (intermittent) (primary) (secondary) NEC N13.3Ø
  with
    infection N13.6
    obstruction (by) (of)
      renal calculus N13.2
        with infection N13.6
      ureteral NEC N13.1
        with infection N13.6
        calculus N13.2
          with infection N13.6
      ureteropelvic junction (congenital) Q62.11
        acquired N13.Ø
          with infection N13.6
    ureteral stricture NEC N13.1
      with infection N13.6
  congenital Q62.Ø
    due to acquired occlusion of ureteropelvic junction N13.Ø
  specified type NEC N13.39
  tuberculous A18.11
Hydropericarditis — *see* Pericarditis
Hydropericardium — *see* Pericarditis
Hydroperitoneum R18.8
Hydrophobia — *see* Rabies
Hydrophthalmos Q15.Ø
Hydropneumohemothorax — *see* Hemothorax
Hydropneumopericarditis — *see* Pericarditis
Hydropneumopericardium — *see* Pericarditis
Hydropneumothorax J94.8
  traumatic — *see* Injury, intrathoracic, lung
  tuberculous NEC A15.6
Hydrops R6Ø.9
  abdominis R18.8
  articulorum intermittens — *see* Hydrarthrosis, intermittent
  cardiac — *see* Failure, heart, congestive
  causing obstructed labor (mother) O66.3
  endolymphatic H81.Ø- ☑
  fetal — *see* Pregnancy, complicated by, hydrops, fetalis
  fetalis P83.2
    due to
      ABO isoimmunization P56.Ø
      alpha thalassemia D56.Ø
      hemolytic disease P56.9Ø
        specified NEC P56.99
      isoimmunization (ABO) (Rh) P56.Ø

☑ **Additional Character Required** — Refer to the Tabular List for Character Selection ▽ **Subterms under main terms may continue to next column or page**

Index

Hydrops — *continued*
　fetalis — *continued*
　　due to — *continued*
　　　other specified nonhemolytic disease NEC P83.2
　　　Rh incompatibility P56.0
　　during pregnancy — *see* Pregnancy, complicated
　　　by, hydrops, fetalis
　gallbladder K82.1
　joint — *see* Effusion, joint
　labyrinth H81.0- ☑
　newborn (idiopathic) P83.2
　　due to
　　　ABO isoimmunization P56.0
　　　alpha thalassemia D56.0
　　　hemolytic disease P56.90
　　　　specified NEC P56.99
　　　isoimmunization (ABO) (Rh) P56.0
　　　Rh incompatibility P56.0
　nutritional — *see* Malnutrition, severe
　pericardium — *see* Pericarditis
　pleura — *see* Hydrothorax
　spermatic cord — *see* Hydrocele
Hydropyonephrosis N13.6
Hydrorachis Q06.4
Hydrorrhea (nasal) J34.89
　pregnancy — *see* Rupture, membranes, premature
Hydrosadenitis (axillaris) (suppurative) L73.2
Hydrosalpinx (fallopian tube) (follicularis) N70.11
Hydrothorax (double) (pleura) J94.8
　chylous (nonfilarial) I89.8
　　filarial — *see also* Infestation, filarial B74.9 *[J91.8]*
　traumatic — *see* Injury, intrathoracic
　tuberculous NEC (non primary) A15.6
Hydroureter — *see also* Hydronephrosis N13.4
　with infection N13.6
　congenital Q62.39
Hydroureteronephrosis — *see* Hydronephrosis
Hydrourethra N36.8
Hydroxykynureninuria E70.8
Hydroxylysinemia E72.3
Hydroxyprolinemia E72.59
Hygiene, sleep
　abuse Z72.821
　inadequate Z72.821
　poor Z72.821
Hygroma (congenital) (cystic) D18.1
　praepatellare, prepatellar — *see* Bursitis, prepatellar
Hymen — *see* condition
Hymenolepis, hymenolepiasis (diminuta) (infection)
　　(infestation) (nana) B71.0
Hypalgesia R20.8
Hyperacidity (gastric) K31.89
　psychogenic F45.8
Hyperactive, hyperactivity F90.9
　basal cell, uterine cervix — *see* Dysplasia, cervix
　bowel sounds R19.12
　cervix epithelial (basal) — *see* Dysplasia, cervix
　child F90.9
　　attention deficit — *see* Disorder, attention-deficit
　　　hyperactivity
　detrusor muscle N32.81
　gastrointestinal K31.89
　　psychogenic F45.8
　nasal mucous membrane J34.3
　stomach K31.89
　thyroid (gland) — *see* Hyperthyroidism
Hyperacusis H93.23- ☑
Hyperadrenalism E27.5
Hyperadrenocorticism E24.9
　congenital E25.0
　iatrogenic E24.2
　　correct substance properly administered — *see* Table of Drugs and Chemicals, by drug, adverse effect
　　overdose or wrong substance given or taken — *see* Table of Drugs and Chemicals, by drug, poisoning
　not associated with Cushing's syndrome E27.0
　pituitary-dependent E24.0
Hyperaldosteronism E26.9
　familial (type I) E26.02
　glucocorticoid-remediable E26.02
　primary (due to (bilateral) adrenal hyperplasia) E26.09
　primary NEC E26.09
　secondary E26.1
　specified NEC E26.89
Hyperalgesia R20.8

Hyperalimentation R63.2
　carotene, carotin E67.1
　specified NEC E67.8
　vitamin
　　A E67.0
　　D E67.3
Hyperaminoaciduria
　arginine E72.21
　cystine E72.01
　lysine E72.3
　ornithine E72.4
Hyperammonemia (congenital) E72.20
Hyperazotemia — *see* Uremia
Hyperbetalipoproteinemia (familial) E78.00
　with prebetalipoproteinemia E78.2
Hyperbicarbonatemia P74.41
Hyperbilirubinemia
　constitutional E80.6
　familial conjugated E80.6
　neonatal (transient) — *see* Jaundice, newborn
Hypercalcemia, hypocalciuric, familial E83.52
Hypercalciuria, idiopathic R82.994
Hypercapnia R06.89
　newborn P84
Hypercarotenemia (dietary) E67.1
Hypercementosis K03.4
Hyperchloremia E87.8
Hyperchlorhydria K31.89
　neurotic F45.8
　psychogenic F45.8
Hypercholesterinemia — *see* Hypercholesterolemia
Hypercholesterolemia (essential) (primary) (pure) E78.00
　with hyperglyceridemia, endogenous E78.2
　dietary counseling and surveillance Z71.3
　familial E78.01
　hereditary E78.01
Hyperchylia gastrica, psychogenic F45.8
Hyperchylomicronemia (familial) (primary) E78.3
　with hyperbetalipoproteinemia E78.3
Hypercoagulable (state) D68.59
　activated protein C resistance D68.51
　antithrombin (III) deficiency D68.59
　factor V Leiden mutation D68.51
　primary NEC D68.59
　protein C deficiency D68.59
　protein S deficiency D68.59
　prothrombin gene mutation D68.52
　secondary D68.69
　specified NEC D68.69
Hypercoagulation (state) D68.59
Hypercorticalism, pituitary-dependent E24.0
Hypercorticosolism — *see* Cushing's, syndrome
Hypercorticosteronism E24.2
　correct substance properly administered — *see* Table of Drugs and Chemicals, by drug, adverse effect
　overdose or wrong substance given or taken — *see* Table of Drugs and Chemicals, by drug, poisoning
Hypercortisonism E24.2
　correct substance properly administered — *see* Table of Drugs and Chemicals, by drug, adverse effect
　overdose or wrong substance given or taken — *see* Table of Drugs and Chemicals, by drug, poisoning
Hyperekplexia Q89.8
Hyperelectrolytemia E87.8
Hyperemesis R11.10
　with nausea R11.2
　gravidarum (mild) O21.0
　　with
　　　carbohydrate depletion O21.1
　　　dehydration O21.1
　　　electrolyte imbalance O21.1
　　　metabolic disturbance O21.1
　　severe (with metabolic disturbance) O21.1
　projectile R11.12
　psychogenic F45.8
Hyperemia (acute) (passive) R68.89
　anal mucosa K62.89
　bladder N32.89
　cerebral I67.89
　conjunctiva H11.43- ☑
　ear internal, acute — *see* subcategory H83.0 ☑
　enteric K59.8
　eye — *see* Hyperemia, conjunctiva
　eyelid (active) (passive) — *see* Disorder, eyelid, specified type NEC
　intestine K59.8
　iris — *see* Disorder, iris, vascular
　kidney N28.89

Hyperemia — *continued*
　labyrinth — *see* subcategory H83.0 ☑
　liver (active) K76.89
　lung (passive) — *see* Edema, lung
　pulmonary (passive) — *see* Edema, lung
　renal N28.89
　retina H35.89
　stomach K31.89
Hyperesthesia (body surface) R20.3
　larynx (reflex) J38.7
　　hysterical F44.89
　pharynx (reflex) J39.2
　　hysterical F44.89
Hyperestrogenism (drug-induced) (iatrogenic) E28.0
Hyperexplexia Q89.8
Hyperfibrinolysis — *see* Fibrinolysis
Hyperfructosemia E74.19
Hyperfunction
　adrenal cortex, not associated with Cushing's syndrome E27.0
　　medulla E27.5
　　　adrenomedullary E27.5
　　virilism E25.9
　　　congenital E25.0
　ovarian E28.8
　pancreas K86.89
　parathyroid (gland) E21.3
　pituitary (gland) (anterior) E22.9
　　specified NEC E22.8
　polyglandular E31.1
　testicular E29.0
Hypergammaglobulinemia D89.2
　polyclonal D89.0
　Waldenström D89.0
Hypergastrinemia E16.4
Hyperglobulinemia R77.1
Hyperglycemia, hyperglycemic (transient) R73.9
　coma — *see* Diabetes, by type, with coma
　postpancreatectomy E89.1
Hyperglyceridemia (endogenous) (essential) (familial) (hereditary) (pure) E78.1
　mixed E78.3
Hyperglycinemia (non-ketotic) E72.51
Hypergonadism
　ovarian E28.8
　testicular (primary) (infantile) E29.0
Hyperheparinemia D68.32
Hyperhidrosis, hyperidrosis R61
　focal
　　primary L74.519
　　　axilla L74.510
　　　face L74.511
　　　palms L74.512
　　　soles L74.513
　　secondary L74.52
　generalized R61
　localized
　　primary L74.519
　　　axilla L74.510
　　　face L74.511
　　　palms L74.512
　　　soles L74.513
　　secondary L74.52
　psychogenic F45.8
　secondary R61
　　focal L74.52
Hyperhistidinemia E70.41
Hyperhomocysteinemia E72.11
Hyperhydroxyprolinemia E72.59
Hyperinsulinism (functional) E16.1
　with
　　coma (hypoglycemic) E15
　　encephalopathy E16.1 *[G94]*
　ectopic E16.1
　therapeutic misadventure (from administration of insulin) — *see* subcategory T38.3 ☑
Hyperkalemia E87.5
Hyperkeratosis — *see also* Keratosis L85.9
　cervix N88.0
　due to yaws (early) (late) (palmar or plantar) A66.3
　follicularis Q82.8
　　penetrans (in cutem) L87.0
　palmoplantaris climacterica L85.1
　pinta A67.1
　senile (with pruritus) L57.0
　universalis congenita Q80.8
　vocal cord J38.3
　vulva N90.4

Hydrops — Hyperkeratosis

Hyperkinesia, hyperkinetic (disease) (reaction) (syndrome) (childhood) (adolescence) — see also Disorder, attention-deficit hyperactivity
  heart I51.89
Hyperleucine-isoleucinemia E71.19
Hyperlipemia, hyperlipidemia E78.5
  combined E78.2
    familial E78.49
  group
    A E78.00
    B E78.1
    C E78.2
    D E78.3
  mixed E78.2
  specified NEC E78.49
Hyperlipidosis E75.6
  hereditary NEC E75.5
Hyperlipoproteinemia E78.5
  Fredrickson's type
    I E78.3
    IIa E78.00
    IIb E78.2
    III E78.2
    IV E78.1
    V E78.3
  low-density-lipoprotein-type (LDL) E78.00
  very-low-density-lipoprotein-type (VLDL) E78.1
Hyperlucent lung, unilateral J43.0
Hyperlysinemia E72.3
Hypermagnesemia E83.41
  neonatal P71.8
Hypermenorrhea N92.0
Hypermethioninemia E72.19
Hypermetropia (congenital) H52.0- ☑
Hypermobility, hypermotility
  cecum — see Syndrome, irritable bowel
  coccyx — see subcategory M53.2 ☑
  colon — see Syndrome, irritable bowel
    psychogenic F45.8
  ileum K58.9
  intestine — see also Syndrome, irritable bowel K58.9
    psychogenic F45.8
  meniscus (knee) — see Derangement, knee, meniscus
  scapula — see Instability, joint, shoulder
  stomach K31.89
    psychogenic F45.8
  syndrome M35.7
  urethra N36.41
    with intrinsic sphincter deficiency N36.43
Hypernasality R49.21
Hypernatremia E87.0
Hypernephroma C64.- ☑
Hyperopia — see Hypermetropia
Hyperorexia nervosa F50.2
Hyperornithinemia E72.4
Hyperosmia R43.1
Hyperosmolality E87.0
Hyperostosis (monomelic) — see also Disorder, bone, density and structure, specified NEC
  ankylosing (spine) M48.10
    cervical region M48.12
    cervicothoracic region M48.13
    lumbar region M48.16
    lumbosacral region M48.17
    multiple sites M48.19
    occipito-atlanto-axial region M48.11
    sacrococcygeal region M48.18
    thoracic region M48.14
    thoracolumbar region M48.15
  cortical (skull) M85.2
    infantile M89.8X- ☑
  frontal, internal of skull M85.2
  interna frontalis M85.2
  skeletal, diffuse idiopathic — see Hyperostosis, ankylosing
  skull M85.2
    congenital Q75.8
  vertebral, ankylosing — see Hyperostosis, ankylosing
Hyperovarism E28.8
Hyperoxaluria R82.992
  primary E72.53
Hyperparathyroidism E21.3
  primary E21.0
  secondary (renal) N25.81
    non-renal E21.1
  specified NEC E21.2
  tertiary E21.2
Hyperpathia R20.8

Hyperperistalsis R19.2
  psychogenic F45.8
Hyperpermeability, capillary I78.8
Hyperphagia R63.2
Hyperphenylalaninemia NEC E70.1
Hyperphoria (alternating) H50.53
Hyperphosphatemia E83.39
Hyperpiesis, hyperpiesia — see Hypertension
Hyperpigmentation — see also Pigmentation
  melanin NEC L81.4
  postinflammatory L81.0
Hyperpinealism E34.8
Hyperpituitarism E22.9
Hyperplasia, hyperplastic
  adenoids J35.2
  adrenal (capsule) (cortex) (gland) E27.8
    with
      sexual precocity (male) E25.9
        congenital E25.0
      virilism, adrenal E25.9
        congenital E25.0
      virilization (female) E25.9
        congenital E25.0
    congenital E25.0
    salt-losing E25.0
  adrenomedullary E27.5
  angiolymphoid, eosinophilia (ALHE) D18.01
  appendix (lymphoid) K38.0
  artery, fibromuscular I77.3
  bone — see also Hypertrophy, bone
    marrow D75.89
  breast — see also Hypertrophy, breast
    atypical, atypia N60.9- ☑
      ductal N60.9- ☑
      lobular N60.9- ☑
  C-cell, thyroid E07.0
  cementation (tooth) (teeth) K03.4
  cervical gland R59.0
  cervix (uteri) (basal cell) (endometrium) (polypoid) — see also Dysplasia, cervix
    congenital Q51.828
  clitoris, congenital Q52.6
  denture K06.2
  endocervicitis N72
  endometrium, endometrial (adenomatous) (cystic) (glandular) (glandular-cystic) (polypoid) N85.00
    with atypia N85.02
    benign N85.01
    cervix — see Dysplasia, cervix
    complex (without atypia) N85.01
    simple (without atypia) N85.01
  epithelial L85.9
    focal, oral, including tongue K13.29
    nipple N62
    skin L85.9
    tongue K13.29
    vaginal wall N89.3
  erythroid D75.89
  fibromuscular of artery (carotid) (renal) I77.3
  genital
    female NEC N94.89
    male N50.89
  gingiva K06.1
  glandularis cystica uteri (interstitialis) — see also Hyperplasia, endometrial N85.00
  gum K06.1
  hymen, congenital Q52.4
  irritative, edentulous (alveolar) K06.2
  jaw M26.09
    alveolar M26.79
    lower M26.03
      alveolar M26.72
    upper M26.01
      alveolar M26.71
  kidney (congenital) Q63.3
  labia N90.69
    epithelial N90.3
  liver (congenital) Q44.7
    nodular, focal K76.89
  lymph gland or node R59.9
  mandible, mandibular M26.03
    alveolar M26.72
    unilateral condylar M27.8
  maxilla, maxillary M26.01
    alveolar M26.71
  myometrium, myometrial N85.2
  neuroendocrine cell, of infancy J84.841

Hyperplasia, hyperplastic — continued
  nose
    lymphoid J34.89
    polypoid J33.9
  oral mucosa (irritative) K13.6
  organ or site, congenital NEC — see Anomaly, by site
  ovary N83.8
  palate, papillary (irritative) K13.6
  pancreatic islet cells E16.9
    alpha E16.8
      with excess
        gastrin E16.4
        glucagon E16.3
    beta E16.1
  parathyroid (gland) E21.0
  pharynx (lymphoid) J39.2
  prostate (adenofibromatous) (nodular) N40.0
    with lower urinary tract symptoms (LUTS) N40.1
    without lower urinary tract symtpoms (LUTS) N40.0
  renal artery I77.89
  reticulo-endothelial (cell) D75.89
  salivary gland (any) K11.1
  Schimmelbusch's — see Mastopathy, cystic
  suprarenal capsule (gland) E27.8
  thymus (gland) (persistent) E32.0
  thyroid (gland) — see Goiter
  tonsils (faucial) (infective) (lingual) (lymphoid) J35.1
    with adenoids J35.3
  unilateral condylar M27.8
  uterus, uterine N85.2
    endometrium (glandular) — see also Hyperplasia, endometrial N85.00
  vulva N90.69
    epithelial N90.3
Hyperpnea — see Hyperventilation
Hyperpotassemia E87.5
Hyperprebetalipoproteinemia (familial) E78.1
Hyperprolactinemia E22.1
Hyperprolinemia (type I) (type II) E72.59
Hyperproteinemia E88.09
Hyperprothrombinemia, causing coagulation factor deficiency D68.4
Hyperpyrexia R50.9
  heat (effects) T67.01 ☑
  malignant, due to anesthetic T88.3 ☑
  rheumatic — see Fever, rheumatic
  unknown origin R50.9
Hyper-reflexia R29.2
Hypersalivation K11.7
Hypersecretion
  ACTH (not associated with Cushing's syndrome) E27.0
    pituitary E24.0
  adrenaline E27.5
  adrenomedullary E27.5
  androgen (testicular) E29.0
    ovarian (drug-induced) (iatrogenic) E28.1
  calcitonin E07.0
  catecholamine E27.5
  corticoadrenal E24.9
  cortisol E24.9
  epinephrine E27.5
  estrogen E28.0
  gastric K31.89
    psychogenic F45.8
  gastrin E16.4
  glucagon E16.3
  hormone(s)
    ACTH (not associated with Cushing's syndrome) E27.0
      pituitary E24.0
    antidiuretic E22.2
    growth E22.0
    intestinal NEC E34.1
    ovarian androgen E28.1
    pituitary E22.9
    testicular E29.0
    thyroid stimulating E05.80
      with thyroid storm E05.81
  insulin — see Hyperinsulinism
  lacrimal glands — see Epiphora
  medulloadrenal E27.5
  milk O92.6
  ovarian androgens E28.1
  salivary gland (any) K11.7
  thyrocalcitonin E07.0
  upper respiratory J39.8
Hypersegmentation, leukocytic, hereditary D72.0

☑ Additional Character Required — Refer to the Tabular List for Character Selection   ▽ Subterms under main terms may continue to next column or page

Hypersensitive, hypersensitiveness, hypersensitivity
— *see also* Allergy
carotid sinus G90.01
colon — *see* Irritable, colon
drug T88.7 ☑
gastrointestinal K52.29
    immediate K52.29
    psychogenic F45.8
labyrinth — *see* subcategory H83.2 ☑
pain R20.8
pneumonitis — *see* Pneumonitis, allergic
reaction T78.40 ☑
    upper respiratory tract NEC J39.3
Hypersomnia (organic) G47.10
due to
    alcohol
        abuse F10.182
        dependence F10.282
        use F10.982
    amphetamines
        abuse F15.182
        dependence F15.282
        use F15.982
    caffeine
        abuse F15.182
        dependence F15.282
        use F15.982
    cocaine
        abuse F14.182
        dependence F14.282
        use F14.982
    drug NEC
        abuse F19.182
        dependence F19.282
        use F19.982
    medical condition G47.14
    mental disorder F51.13
    opioid
        abuse F11.182
        dependence F11.282
        use F11.982
    psychoactive substance NEC
        abuse F19.182
        dependence F19.282
        use F19.982
    sedative, hypnotic, or anxiolytic
        abuse F13.182
        dependence F13.282
        use F13.982
    stimulant NEC
        abuse F15.182
        dependence F15.282
        use F15.982
idiopathic G47.11
    with long sleep time G47.11
    without long sleep time G47.12
menstrual related G47.13
nonorganic origin F51.11
    specified NEC F51.19
not due to a substance or known physiological condition F51.11
    specified NEC F51.19
primary F51.11
recurrent G47.13
specified NEC G47.19
Hypersplenia, hypersplenism D73.1
Hyperstimulation, ovaries (associated with induced ovulation) N98.1
Hypersusceptibility — *see* Allergy
Hypertelorism (ocular) (orbital) Q75.2
Hypertension, hypertensive (accelerated) (benign) (essential) (idiopathic) (malignant) (systemic) I10
with
    heart failure (congestive) I11.0
    heart involvement (conditions in I50.-, I51.4- I51.9 due to hypertension) — *see* Hypertension, heart
    kidney involvement — *see* Hypertension, kidney
benign, intracranial G93.2
borderline R03.0
cardiorenal (disease) I13.10
    with heart failure I13.0
        with stage 1 through stage 4 chronic kidney disease I13.0
        with stage 5 or end stage renal disease I13.2
    without heart failure I13.10
        with stage 1 through stage 4 chronic kidney disease I13.10

Hypertension, hypertensive — *continued*
cardiorenal — *continued*
    without heart failure — *continued*
        with stage 5 or end stage renal disease I13.11
cardiovascular
    disease (arteriosclerotic) (sclerotic) — *see* Hypertension, heart
    renal (disease) — *see* Hypertension, cardiorenal
chronic venous — *see* Hypertension, venous (chronic)
complicating
    childbirth (labor) O16.4
        pre-existing O10.92
        with
            heart disease O10.12
                with renal disease O10.32
            pre-eclampsia O11.4
            renal disease O10.22
                with heart disease O10.32
            essential O10.02
        secondary O10.42
    pregnancy O16.- ☑
        with edema — *see also* Pre-eclampsia O14.9- ☑
        gestational (pregnancy induced) (without proteinuria) O13.- ☑
            with proteinuria O14.9- ☑
                mild pre-eclampsia O14.0- ☑
                moderate pre-eclampsia O14.0- ☑
                severe pre-eclampsia O14.1- ☑
                    with hemolysis, elevated liver enzymes and low platelet count (HELLP) O14.2- ☑
        pre-existing O10.91- ☑
            with
                heart disease O10.11- ☑
                    with renal disease O10.31- ☑
                pre-eclampsia — *see* category O11
                renal disease O10.21- ☑
                    with heart disease O10.31- ☑
            essential O10.01- ☑
            secondary O10.41- ☑
        transient O13- ☑
    puerperium, pre-existing O16.5
        pre-existing
            with
                heart disease O10.13
                    with renal disease O10.33
                pre-eclampsia O11.5
                renal disease O10.23
                    with heart disease O10.33
            essential O10.03
        pregnancy-induced O13.9
        secondary O10.43
crisis I16.9
due to
    endocrine disorders I15.2
    pheochromocytoma I15.2
    renal disorders NEC I15.1
        arterial I15.0
    renovascular disorders I15.0
    specified disease NEC I15.8
emergency I16.1
encephalopathy I67.4
gestational (without significant proteinuria) (pregnancy-induced) (transient) O13.- ☑
with significant proteinuria — *see* Pre-eclampsia
complicating
    delivery O13.4
    puerperium O13.5
Goldblatt's I70.1
heart (disease) (conditions in I51.4-I51.9 due to hypertension) I11.9
with
    heart failure (congestive) I11.0
    kidney disease (chronic) — *see* Hypertension, cardiorenal
intracranial (benign) G93.2
kidney I12.9
with
    heart disease — *see* Hypertension, cardiorenal
    stage 1 through stage 4 chronic kidney disease I12.9
    stage 5 chronic kidney disease (CKD) or end stage renal disease (ESRD) I12.0
lesser circulation I27.0
maternal O16- ☑
newborn P29.2
    pulmonary (persistent) P29.30
ocular H40.05- ☑

Hypertension, hypertensive — *continued*
pancreatic duct — *code to* underlying condition
    with chronic pancreatitis K86.1
portal (due to chronic liver disease) (idiopathic) K76.6
    gastropathy K31.89
    in (due to) schistosomiasis (bilharziasis) B65.9 *[K77]*
postoperative I97.3
psychogenic F45.8
pulmonary I27.20
    with
        cor pulmonale (chronic) I27.29
            acute I26.09
        right heart ventricular strain/failure I27.29
            acute I26.09
        right to left shunt related to congenital heart disease I27.83
        unclear multifactorial mechanisms I27.29
    arterial (associated) (drug-induced) (toxin-induced) I27.21
    chronic thromboembolic I27.24
    due to
        hematologic disorders I27.29
        left heart disease I27.22
        lung diseases and hypoxia I27.23
        metabolic disorders I27.29
        specified systemic disorders I27.29
    group 1 (associated) (drug-induced) (toxin-induced) I27.21
    group 2 I27.22
    group 3 I27.23
    group 4 I27.24
    group 5 I27.29
    of newborn (persistent) P29.30
    primary (idiopathic) I27.0
    secondary
        arterial I27.21
        specified NEC I27.29
renal — *see* Hypertension, kidney
renovascular I15.0
secondary NEC I15.9
    due to
        endocrine disorders I15.2
        pheochromocytoma I15.2
        renal disorders NEC I15.1
            arterial I15.0
        renovascular disorders I15.0
    specified NEC I15.8
transient R03.0
    of pregnancy O13.- ☑
urgency I16.0
venous (chronic)
    due to
        deep vein thrombosis — *see* Syndrome, post-thrombotic
    idiopathic I87.309
        with
            inflammation I87.32- ☑
                with ulcer I87.33- ☑
            specified complication NEC I87.39- ☑
            ulcer I87.31- ☑
                with inflammation I87.33- ☑
        asymptomatic I87.30- ☑
Hypertensive urgency — *see* Hypertension
Hyperthecosis ovary E28.8
Hyperthermia (of unknown origin) — *see also* Hyperpyrexia
malignant, due to anesthesia T88.3 ☑
newborn P81.9
    environmental P81.0
Hyperthyroid (recurrent) — *see* Hyperthyroidism
Hyperthyroidism (latent) (pre-adult) (recurrent) E05.90
with
    goiter (diffuse) E05.00
        with thyroid storm E05.01
        nodular (multinodular) E05.20
            with thyroid storm E05.21
            uninodular E05.10
                with thyroid storm E05.11
    storm E05.91
due to ectopic thyroid tissue E05.30
    with thyroid storm E05.31
neonatal, transitory P72.1
specified NEC E05.80
    with thyroid storm E05.81
Hypertony, hypertonia, hypertonicity
bladder N31.8
congenital P94.1
stomach K31.89

Hypertony, hypertonia, hypertonicity — *continued*
  stomach — *continued*
    psychogenic F45.8
  uterus, uterine (contractions) (complicating delivery) O62.4

Hypertrichosis L68.9
  congenital Q84.2
  eyelid H02.869
    left H02.866
      lower H02.865
      upper H02.864
    right H02.863
      lower H02.862
      upper H02.861
  lanuginosa Q84.2
    acquired L68.1
  localized L68.2
  specified NEC L68.8

Hypertriglyceridemia, essential E78.1

Hypertrophy, hypertrophic
  adenofibromatous, prostate — *see* Enlargement, enlarged, prostate
  adenoids (infective) J35.2
    with tonsils J35.3
  adrenal cortex E27.8
  alveolar process or ridge — *see* Anomaly, alveolar
  anal papillae K62.89
  artery I77.89
    congenital NEC Q27.8
      digestive system Q27.8
      lower limb Q27.8
      specified site NEC Q27.8
      upper limb Q27.8
  auricular — *see* Hypertrophy, cardiac
  Bartholin's gland N75.8
  bile duct (common) (hepatic) K83.8
  bladder (sphincter) (trigone) N32.89
  bone M89.30
    carpus M89.34- ☑
    clavicle M89.31- ☑
    femur M89.35- ☑
    fibula M89.36- ☑
    finger M89.34- ☑
    humerus M89.32- ☑
    ilium M89.359
    ischium M89.359
    metacarpus M89.34- ☑
    metatarsus M89.37- ☑
    multiple sites M89.39
    neck M89.38
    radius M89.33- ☑
    rib M89.38
    scapula M89.31- ☑
    skull M89.38
    tarsus M89.37- ☑
    tibia M89.36- ☑
    toe M89.37- ☑
    ulna M89.33- ☑
    vertebra M89.38
  brain G93.89
  breast N62
    cystic — *see* Mastopathy, cystic
    newborn P83.4
    pubertal, massive N62
    puerperal, postpartum — *see* Disorder, breast, specified type NEC
    senile (parenchymatous) N62
  cardiac (chronic) (idiopathic) I51.7
    with rheumatic fever (conditions in I00)
      active I01.8
      inactive or quiescent (with chorea) I09.89
    congenital NEC Q24.8
    fatty — *see* Degeneration, myocardial
    hypertensive — *see* Hypertension, heart
    rheumatic (with chorea) I09.89
      active or acute I01.8
        with chorea I02.0
    valve — *see* Endocarditis
  cartilage — *see* Disorder, cartilage, specified type NEC
  cecum — *see* Megacolon
  cervix (uteri) N88.8
    congenital Q51.828
    elongation N88.4
  clitoris (cirrhotic) N90.89
    congenital Q52.6
  colon — *see also* Megacolon
    congenital Q43.2

Hypertrophy, hypertrophic — *continued*
  conjunctiva, lymphoid H11.89
  corpora cavernosa N48.89
  cystic duct K82.8
  duodenum K31.89
  endometrium (glandular) — *see also* Hyperplasia, endometrial N85.00
    cervix N88.8
  epididymis N50.89
  esophageal hiatus (congenital) Q79.1
    with hernia — *see* Hernia, hiatal
  eyelid — *see* Disorder, eyelid, specified type NEC
  fat pad E65
    knee (infrapatellar) (popliteal) (prepatellar) (retropatellar) M79.4
  foot (congenital) Q74.2
  frenulum, frenum (tongue) K14.8
    lip K13.0
  gallbladder K82.8
  gastric mucosa K29.60
    with bleeding K29.61
  gland, glandular R59.9
    generalized R59.1
    localized R59.0
  gum (mucous membrane) K06.1
  heart (idiopathic) — *see also* Hypertrophy, cardiac
    valve — *see also* Endocarditis I38
  hemifacial Q67.4
  hepatic — *see* Hypertrophy, liver
  hiatus (esophageal) Q79.1
  hilus gland R59.0
  hymen, congenital Q52.4
  ileum K63.89
  intestine NEC K63.89
  jejunum K63.89
  kidney (compensatory) N28.81
    congenital Q63.3
  labium (majus) (minus) N90.60
  ligament — *see* Disorder, ligament
  lingual tonsil (infective) J35.1
    with adenoids J35.3
  lip K13.0
    congenital Q18.6
  liver R16.0
    acute K76.89
    cirrhotic — *see* Cirrhosis, liver
    congenital Q44.7
    fatty — *see* Fatty, liver
  lymph, lymphatic gland R59.9
    generalized R59.1
    localized R59.0
    tuberculous — *see* Tuberculosis, lymph gland
  mammary gland — *see* Hypertrophy, breast
  Meckel's diverticulum (congenital) Q43.0
    malignant — *see* Table of Neoplasms, small intestine, malignant
  median bar — *see* Hyperplasia, prostate
  meibomian gland — *see* Chalazion
  meniscus, knee, congenital Q74.1
  metatarsal head — *see* Hypertrophy, bone, metatarsus
  metatarsus — *see* Hypertrophy, bone, metatarsus
  mucous membrane
    alveolar ridge K06.2
    gum K06.1
    nose (turbinate) J34.3
  muscle M62.89
  muscular coat, artery I77.89
  myocardium — *see also* Hypertrophy, cardiac
    idiopathic I42.2
  myometrium N85.2
  nail L60.2
    congenital Q84.5
  nasal J34.89
    alae J34.89
    bone J34.89
    cartilage J34.89
    mucous membrane (septum) J34.3
    sinus J34.89
    turbinate J34.3
  nasopharynx, lymphoid (infectional) (tissue) (wall) J35.2
  nipple N62
  organ or site, congenital NEC — *see* Anomaly, by site
  ovary N83.8
  palate (hard) M27.8
    soft K13.79
  pancreas, congenital Q45.3
  parathyroid (gland) E21.0
  parotid gland K11.1

Hypertrophy, hypertrophic — *continued*
  penis N48.89
  pharyngeal tonsil J35.2
  pharynx J39.2
    lymphoid (infectional) (tissue) (wall) J35.2
  pituitary (anterior) (fossa) (gland) E23.6
  prepuce (congenital) N47.8
    female N90.89
  prostate — *see* Enlargement, enlarged, prostate
    congenital Q55.4
  pseudomuscular G71.09
  pylorus (adult) (muscle) (sphincter) K31.1
    congenital or infantile Q40.0
  rectal, rectum (sphincter) K62.89
  rhinitis (turbinate) J31.0
  salivary gland (any) K11.1
    congenital Q38.4
  scaphoid (tarsal) — *see* Hypertrophy, bone, tarsus
  scar L91.0
  scrotum N50.89
  seminal vesicle N50.89
  sigmoid — *see* Megacolon
  skin L91.9
    specified NEC L91.8
  spermatic cord N50.89
  spleen — *see* Splenomegaly
  spondylitis — *see* Spondylosis
  stomach K31.89
  sublingual gland K11.1
  submandibular gland K11.1
  suprarenal cortex (gland) E27.8
  synovial NEC M67.20
    acromioclavicular M67.21- ☑
    ankle M67.27- ☑
    elbow M67.22- ☑
    foot M67.27- ☑
    hand M67.24- ☑
    hip M67.25- ☑
    knee M67.26- ☑
    multiple sites M67.29
    specified site NEC M67.28
    wrist M67.23- ☑
  tendon — *see* Disorder, tendon, specified type NEC
  testis N44.8
    congenital Q55.29
  thymic, thymus (gland) (congenital) E32.0
  thyroid (gland) — *see* Goiter
  toe (congenital) Q74.2
    acquired — *see also* Deformity, toe, specified NEC
  tongue K14.8
    congenital Q38.2
    papillae (foliate) K14.3
  tonsils (faucial) (infective) (lingual) (lymphoid) J35.1
    with adenoids J35.3
  tunica vaginalis N50.89
  ureter N28.89
  urethra N36.8
  uterus N85.2
    neck (with elongation) N88.4
    puerperal O90.89
  uvula K13.79
  vagina N89.8
  vas deferens N50.89
  vein I87.8
  ventricle, ventricular (heart) — *see also* Hypertrophy, cardiac
    congenital Q24.8
    in tetralogy of Fallot Q21.3
  verumontanum N36.8
  vocal cord J38.3
  vulva N90.60
    stasis (nonfilarial) N90.69

Hypertropia H50.2- ☑
Hypertyrosinemia E70.21
Hyperuricemia (asymptomatic) E79.0
Hyperuricosuria R82.993
Hypervalinemia E71.19
Hyperventilation (tetany) R06.4
  hysterical F45.8
  psychogenic F45.8
  syndrome F45.8
Hypervitaminosis (dietary) NEC E67.8
  A E67.0
    administered as drug (prolonged intake) — *see* Table of Drugs and Chemicals, vitamins, adverse effect

☑ **Additional Character Required** — Refer to the Tabular List for Character Selection   🔻 **Subterms under main terms may continue to next column or page**

Hypervitaminosis — *continued*
  A — *continued*
    overdose or wrong substance given or taken — *see* Table of Drugs and Chemicals, vitamins, poisoning
  B6 E67.2
  D E67.3
    administered as drug (prolonged intake) — *see* Table of Drugs and Chemicals, vitamins, adverse effect
    overdose or wrong substance given or taken — *see* Table of Drugs and Chemicals, vitamins, poisoning
  K E67.8
    administered as drug (prolonged intake) — *see* Table of Drugs and Chemicals, vitamins, adverse effect
    overdose or wrong substance given or taken — *see* Table of Drugs and Chemicals, vitamins, poisoning
Hypervolemia E87.70
  specified NEC E87.79
Hypesthesia R20.1
  cornea — *see* Anesthesia, cornea
Hyphema H21.0- ☑
  traumatic S05.1- ☑
Hypoacidity, gastric K31.89
  psychogenic F45.8
Hypoadrenalism, hypoadrenia E27.40
  primary E27.1
  tuberculous A18.7
Hypoadrenocorticism E27.40
  pituitary E23.0
  primary E27.1
Hypoalbuminemia E88.09
Hypoaldosteronism E27.40
Hypoalphalipoproteinemia E78.6
Hypobarism T70.29 ☑
Hypobaropathy T70.29 ☑
Hypobetalipoproteinemia (familial) E78.6
Hypocalcemia E83.51
  dietary E58
  neonatal P71.1
    due to cow's milk P71.0
  phosphate-loading (newborn) P71.1
Hypochloremia E87.8
Hypochlorhydria K31.89
  neurotic F45.8
  psychogenic F45.8
Hypochondria, hypochondriac, hypochondriasis (reaction) F45.21
  sleep F51.03
Hypochondrogenesis Q77.0
Hypochondroplasia Q77.4
Hypochromasia, blood cells D50.8
Hypocitraturia R82.991
Hypodontia — *see* Anodontia
Hypoeosinophilia D72.89
Hypoesthesia R20.1
Hypofibrinogenemia D68.8
  acquired D65
  congenital (hereditary) D68.2
Hypofunction
  adrenocortical E27.40
    drug-induced E27.3
    postprocedural E89.6
    primary E27.1
  adrenomedullary, postprocedural E89.6
  cerebral R29.818
  corticoadrenal NEC E27.40
  intestinal K59.8
  labyrinth — *see* subcategory H83.2 ☑
  ovary E28.39
  pituitary (gland) (anterior) E23.0
  testicular E29.1
    postprocedural (postsurgical) (postirradiation) (iatrogenic) E89.5
Hypogalactia O92.4
Hypogammaglobulinemia — *see also* Agammaglobulinemia D80.1
  hereditary D80.0
  nonfamilial D80.1
  transient, of infancy D80.7
Hypogenitalism (congenital) — *see* Hypogonadism
Hypoglossia Q38.3
Hypoglycemia (spontaneous) E16.2
  coma E15

Hypoglycemia — *continued*
  coma — *continued*
    diabetic — *see* Diabetes, by type, with hypoglycemia, with coma
  diabetic — *see* Diabetes, hypoglycemia
  dietary counseling and surveillance Z71.3
  drug-induced E16.0
    with coma (nondiabetic) E15
  due to insulin E16.0
    with coma (nondiabetic) E15
    therapeutic misadventure — *see* subcategory T38.3 ☑
  functional, nonhyperinsulinemic E16.1
  iatrogenic E16.0
    with coma (nondiabetic) E15
  in infant of diabetic mother P70.1
    gestational diabetes P70.0
  infantile E16.1
  leucine-induced E71.19
  neonatal (transitory) P70.4
    iatrogenic P70.3
  reactive (not drug-induced) E16.1
  transitory neonatal P70.4
Hypogonadism
  female E28.39
  hypogonadotropic E23.0
  male E29.1
  ovarian (primary) E28.39
  pituitary E23.0
  testicular (primary) E29.1
Hypohidrosis, hypoidrosis L74.4
Hypoinsulinemia, postprocedural E89.1
Hypokalemia E87.6
Hypoleukocytosis — *see* Agranulocytosis
Hypolipoproteinemia (alpha) (beta) E78.6
Hypomagnesemia E83.42
  neonatal P71.2
Hypomania, hypomanic reaction F30.8
Hypomenorrhea — *see* Oligomenorrhea
Hypometabolism R63.8
Hypomotility
  gastrointestinal (tract) K31.89
    psychogenic F45.8
  intestine K59.8
    psychogenic F45.8
  stomach K31.89
    psychogenic F45.8
Hyponasality R49.22
Hyponatremia E87.1
Hypo-osmolality E87.1
Hypo-ovarianism, hypo-ovarism E28.39
Hypoparathyroidism E20.9
  familial E20.8
  idiopathic E20.0
  neonatal, transitory P71.4
  postprocedural E89.2
  specified NEC E20.8
Hypoperfusion (in)
  newborn P96.89
Hypopharyngitis — *see* Laryngopharyngitis
Hypophoria H50.53
Hypophosphatemia, hypophosphatasia (acquired) (congenital) (renal) E83.39
  familial E83.31
Hypophyseal, hypophysis — *see also* condition
  dwarfism E23.0
  gigantism E22.0
Hypopiesis — *see* Hypotension
Hypopinealism E34.8
Hypopituitarism (juvenile) E23.0
  drug-induced E23.1
  due to
    hypophysectomy E89.3
    radiotherapy E89.3
  iatrogenic NEC E23.1
  postirradiation E89.3
  postpartum O99.285
  postprocedural E89.3
Hypoplasia, hypoplastic
  adrenal (gland), congenital Q89.1
  alimentary tract, congenital Q45.8
    upper Q40.8
  anus, anal (canal) Q42.3
    with fistula Q42.2
  aorta, aortic Q25.42
    ascending, in hypoplastic left heart syndrome Q23.4
    valve Q23.1
      in hypoplastic left heart syndrome Q23.4

Hypoplasia, hypoplastic — *continued*
  areola, congenital Q83.8
  arm (congenital) — *see* Defect, reduction, upper limb
  artery (peripheral) Q27.8
    brain (congenital) Q28.3
    coronary Q24.5
    digestive system Q27.8
    lower limb Q27.8
    pulmonary Q25.79
      functional, unilateral J43.0
    retinal (congenital) Q14.1
    specified site NEC Q27.8
    umbilical Q27.0
    upper limb Q27.8
  auditory canal Q17.8
    causing impairment of hearing Q16.9
  biliary duct or passage Q44.5
  bone NOS Q79.9
    face Q75.8
    marrow D61.9
      megakaryocytic D69.49
    skull — *see* Hypoplasia, skull
  brain Q02
    gyri Q04.3
    part of Q04.3
  breast (areola) N64.82
  bronchus Q32.4
  cardiac Q24.8
  carpus — *see* Defect, reduction, upper limb, specified type NEC
  cartilage hair Q78.8
  cecum Q42.8
  cementum K00.4
  cephalic Q02
  cerebellum Q04.3
  cervix (uteri), congenital Q51.821
  clavicle (congenital) Q74.0
  coccyx Q76.49
  colon Q42.9
    specified NEC Q42.8
  corpus callosum Q04.0
  cricoid cartilage Q31.2
  digestive organ(s) or tract NEC Q45.8
    upper (congenital) Q40.8
  ear (auricle) (lobe) Q17.2
    middle Q16.4
  enamel of teeth (neonatal) (postnatal) (prenatal) K00.4
  endocrine (gland) NEC Q89.2
  endometrium N85.8
  epididymis (congenital) Q55.4
  epiglottis Q31.2
  erythroid, congenital D61.01
  esophagus (congenital) Q39.8
  eustachian tube Q17.8
  eye Q11.2
  eyelid (congenital) Q10.3
  face Q18.8
    bone(s) Q75.8
  femur (congenital) — *see* Defect, reduction, lower limb, specified type NEC
  fibula (congenital) — *see* Defect, reduction, lower limb, specified type NEC
  finger (congenital) — *see* Defect, reduction, upper limb, specified type NEC
  focal dermal Q82.8
  foot — *see* Defect, reduction, lower limb, specified type NEC
  gallbladder Q44.0
  genitalia, genital organ(s)
    female, congenital Q52.8
      external Q52.79
      internal NEC Q52.8
    in adiposogenital dystrophy E23.6
  glottis Q31.2
  hair Q84.2
  hand (congenital) — *see* Defect, reduction, upper limb, specified type NEC
  heart Q24.8
  humerus (congenital) — *see* Defect, reduction, upper limb, specified type NEC
  intestine Q41.9
    large Q42.9
      specified NEC Q42.8
  jaw M26.09
    alveolar M26.79
    lower M26.04
      alveolar M26.74
    upper M26.02

Hypoplasia, hypoplastic — *continued*
 jaw — *continued*
  upper — *continued*
   alveolar M26.73
 kidney(s) Q60.5
  bilateral Q60.4
  unilateral Q60.3
 labium (majus) (minus), congenital Q52.79
 larynx Q31.2
 left heart syndrome Q23.4
 leg (congenital) — *see* Defect, reduction, lower limb
 limb Q73.8
  lower (congenital) — *see* Defect, reduction, lower limb
  upper (congenital) — *see* Defect, reduction, upper limb
 liver Q44.7
 lung (lobe) (not associated with short gestation) Q33.6
  associated with immaturity, low birth weight, prematurity, or short gestation P28.0
 mammary (areola), congenital Q83.8
 mandible, mandibular M26.04
  alveolar M26.74
  unilateral condylar M27.8
 maxillary M26.02
  alveolar M26.73
 medullary D61.9
 megakaryocytic D69.49
 metacarpus — *see* Defect, reduction, upper limb, specified type NEC
 metatarsus — *see* Defect, reduction, lower limb, specified type NEC
 muscle Q79.8
 nail(s) Q84.6
 nose, nasal Q30.1
 optic nerve H47.03- ☑
 osseous meatus (ear) Q17.8
 ovary, congenital Q50.39
 pancreas Q45.0
 parathyroid (gland) Q89.2
 parotid gland Q38.4
 patella Q74.1
 pelvis, pelvic girdle Q74.2
 penis (congenital) Q55.62
 peripheral vascular system Q27.8
  digestive system Q27.8
  lower limb Q27.8
  specified site NEC Q27.8
  upper limb Q27.8
 pituitary (gland) (congenital) Q89.2
 pulmonary (not associated with short gestation) Q33.6
  artery, functional J43.0
  associated with short gestation P28.0
 radioulnar — *see* Defect, reduction, upper limb, specified type NEC
 radius — *see* Defect, reduction, upper limb
 rectum Q42.1
  with fistula Q42.0
 respiratory system NEC Q34.8
 rib Q76.6
 right heart syndrome Q22.6
 sacrum Q76.49
 scapula Q74.0
 scrotum Q55.1
 shoulder girdle Q74.0
 skin Q82.8
 skull (bone) Q75.8
  with
   anencephaly Q00.0
   encephalocele — *see* Encephalocele
   hydrocephalus Q03.9
    with spina bifida — *see* Spina bifida, by site, with hydrocephalus
   microcephaly Q02
 spinal (cord) (ventral horn cell) Q06.1
 spine Q76.49
 sternum Q76.7
 tarsus — *see* Defect, reduction, lower limb, specified type NEC
 testis Q55.1
 thymic, with immunodeficiency D82.1
 thymus (gland) Q89.2
  with immunodeficiency D82.1
 thyroid (gland) E03.1
  cartilage Q31.2
 tibiofibular (congenital) — *see* Defect, reduction, lower limb, specified type NEC

Hypoplasia, hypoplastic — *continued*
 toe — *see* Defect, reduction, lower limb, specified type NEC
 tongue Q38.3
 Turner's K00.4
 ulna (congenital) — *see* Defect, reduction, upper limb
 umbilical artery Q27.0
 unilateral condylar M27.8
 ureter Q62.8
 uterus, congenital Q51.811
 vagina Q52.4
 vascular NEC peripheral Q27.8
  brain Q28.3
  digestive system Q27.8
  lower limb Q27.8
  specified site NEC Q27.8
  upper limb Q27.8
  vein(s) (peripheral) Q27.8
   brain Q28.3
   digestive system Q27.8
   great Q26.8
   lower limb Q27.8
   specified site NEC Q27.8
   upper limb Q27.8
  vena cava (inferior) (superior) Q26.8
  vertebra Q76.49
 vulva, congenital Q52.79
 zonule (ciliary) Q12.8
Hypoplasminogenemia E88.02
Hypopnea, obstructive sleep apnea G47.33
Hypopotassemia E87.6
Hypoproconvertinemia, congenital (hereditary) D68.2
Hypoproteinemia E77.8
Hypoprothrombinemia (congenital) (hereditary) (idiopathic) D68.2
 acquired D68.4
 newborn, transient P61.6
Hypoptyalism K11.7
Hypopyon (eye) (anterior chamber) — *see* Iridocyclitis, acute, hypopyon
Hypopyrexia R68.0
Hyporeflexia R29.2
Hyposecretion
 ACTH E23.0
 antidiuretic hormone E23.2
 ovary E28.39
 salivary gland (any) K11.7
 vasopressin E23.2
Hyposegmentation, leukocytic, hereditary D72.0
Hyposiderinemia D50.9
Hypospadias Q54.9
 balanic Q54.0
 coronal Q54.0
 glandular Q54.0
 penile Q54.1
 penoscrotal Q54.2
 perineal Q54.3
 specified NEC Q54.8
Hypospermatogenesis — *see* Oligospermia
Hyposplenism D73.0
Hypostasis pulmonary, passive — *see* Edema, lung
Hypostatic — *see* condition
Hyposthenuria N28.89
Hypotension (arterial) (constitutional) I95.9
 chronic I95.89
 due to (of) hemodialysis I95.3
 drug-induced I95.2
 iatrogenic I95.89
 idiopathic (permanent) I95.0
 intracranial, following ventricular shunting (ventriculostomy) G97.2
 intra-dialytic I95.3
 maternal, syndrome (following labor and delivery) O26.5- ☑
 neurogenic, orthostatic G90.3
 orthostatic (chronic) I95.1
  due to drugs I95.2
  neurogenic G90.3
 postoperative I95.81
 postural I95.1
 specified NEC I95.89
Hypothermia (accidental) T68 ☑
 due to anesthesia, anesthetic T88.51 ☑
 low environmental temperature T68 ☑
 neonatal P80.9
  environmental (mild) NEC P80.8
  mild P80.8
  severe (chronic) (cold injury syndrome) P80.0

Hypothermia — *continued*
 neonatal — *continued*
  specified NEC P80.8
 not associated with low environmental temperature R68.0
Hypothyroidism (acquired) E03.9
 autoimmune — *see* Thyroiditis, autoimmune
 congenital (without goiter) E03.1
  with goiter (diffuse) E03.0
 due to
  exogenous substance NEC E03.2
  iodine-deficiency, acquired E01.8
   subclinical E02
  irradiation therapy E89.0
  medicament NEC E03.2
  P-aminosalicylic acid (PAS) E03.2
  phenylbutazone E03.2
  resorcinol E03.2
  sulfonamide E03.2
  surgery E89.0
  thiourea group drugs E03.2
 iatrogenic NEC E03.2
 iodine-deficiency (acquired) E01.8
  congenital — *see* Syndrome, iodine- deficiency, congenital
  subclinical E02
 neonatal, transitory P72.2
 postinfectious E03.3
 postirradiation E89.0
 postprocedural E89.0
 postsurgical E89.0
 specified NEC E03.8
 subclinical, iodine-deficiency related E02
Hypotonia, hypotonicity, hypotony
 bladder N31.2
 congenital (benign) P94.2
 eye — *see* Disorder, globe, hypotony
Hypotrichosis — *see* Alopecia
Hypotropia H50.2- ☑
Hypoventilation R06.89
 congenital central alveolar G47.35
 sleep related
  idiopathic nonobstructive alveolar G47.34
  in conditions classified elsewhere G47.36
Hypovitaminosis — *see* Deficiency, vitamin
Hypovolemia E86.1
 surgical shock T81.19 ☑
 traumatic (shock) T79.4 ☑
Hypoxemia R09.02
 newborn P84
 sleep related, in conditions classified elsewhere G47.36
Hypoxia — *see also* Anoxia R09.02
 cerebral, during a procedure NEC G97.81
  postprocedural NEC G97.82
 intrauterine P84
 myocardial — *see* Insufficiency, coronary
 newborn P84
 sleep-related G47.34
Hypsarhythmia — *see* Epilepsy, generalized, specified NEC
Hysteralgia, pregnant uterus O26.89- ☑
Hysteria, hysterical (conversion) (dissociative state) F44.9
 anxiety F41.8
 convulsions F44.5
 psychosis, acute F44.9
Hysteroepilepsy F44.5

I

IBDU (colonic inflammatory bowel dissease unclassified) K52.3
Ichthyoparasitism due to Vandellia cirrhosa B88.8
Ichthyosis (congenital) Q80.9
 acquired L85.0
 fetalis Q80.4
 hystrix Q80.8
 lamellar Q80.2
 lingual K13.29
 palmaris and plantaris Q82.8
 simplex Q80.0
 vera Q80.8
 vulgaris Q80.0
 X-linked Q80.1
Ichthyotoxism — *see* Poisoning, fish
 bacterial — *see* Intoxication, foodborne
Icteroanemia, hemolytic (acquired) D59.9
 congenital — *see* Spherocytosis

☑ Additional Character Required — Refer to the Tabular List for Character Selection · Subterms under main terms may continue to next column or page

Icterus — *see also* Jaundice
  conjunctiva R17
  gravis, newborn P55.0
  hematogenous (acquired) D59.9
  hemolytic (acquired) D59.9
    congenital — *see* Spherocytosis
  hemorrhagic (acute) (leptospiral) (spirochetal) A27.0
    newborn P53
  infectious B15.9
    with hepatic coma B15.0
    leptospiral A27.0
    spirochetal A27.0
  neonatorum — *see* Jaundice, newborn
  newborn P59.9
  spirochetal A27.0
Ictus solaris, solis T67.01 ☑
Id reaction (due to bacteria) L30.2
Ideation
  homicidal R45.850
  suicidal R45.851
Identity disorder (child) F64.9
  gender role F64.2
  psychosexual F64.2
Idioglossia F80.0
Idiopathic — *see* condition
Idiot, idiocy (congenital) F73
  amaurotic (Bielschowsky(-Jansky)) (family) (infantile (late)) (juvenile (late)) (Vogt-Spielmeyer) E75.4
  microcephalic Q02
IgE asthma J45.909
IIAC (idiopathic infantile arterial calcification) Q28.8
Ileitis (chronic) (noninfectious) — *see also* Enteritis K52.9
  backwash — *see* Pancolitis, ulcerative (chronic)
  infectious A09
  regional (ulcerative) — *see* Enteritis, regional, small intestine
  segmental — *see* Enteritis, regional
  terminal (ulcerative) — *see* Enteritis, regional, small intestine
Ileocolitis — *see also* Enteritis K52.9
  infectious A09
  regional — *see* Enteritis, regional
  ulcerative K51.0- ☑
Ileostomy
  attention to Z43.2
  malfunctioning K94.13
  status Z93.2
    with complication — *see* Complications, enterostomy
Ileotyphus — *see* Typhoid
Ileum — *see* condition
Ileus (bowel) (colon) (inhibitory) (intestine) K56.7
  adynamic K56.0
  due to gallstone (in intestine) K56.3
  duodenal (chronic) K31.5
  gallstone K56.3
  mechanical NEC — *see also* Obstruction, intestine, specified NEC K56.699
  meconium P76.0
    in cystic fibrosis E84.11
    meaning meconium plug (without cystic fibrosis) P76.0
  myxedema K59.8
  neurogenic K56.0
    Hirschsprung's disease or megacolon Q43.1
  newborn
    due to meconium P76.0
      in cystic fibrosis E84.11
      meaning meconium plug (without cystic fibrosis) P76.0
    transitory P76.1
  obstructive — *see also* Obstruction, intestine, specified NEC K56.699
  paralytic K56.0
  postoperative K91.89
Iliac — *see* condition
Iliotibial band syndrome M76.3- ☑
Illiteracy Z55.0
Illness — *see also* Disease R69
  manic-depressive — *see* Disorder, bipolar
Imbalance R26.89
  autonomic G90.8
  constituents of food intake E63.1
  electrolyte E87.8
    with
      abortion — *see* Abortion by type, complicated by, electrolyte imbalance
      molar pregnancy O08.5

Imbalance — *continued*
  electrolyte — *continued*
    due to hyperemesis gravidarum O21.1
    following ectopic or molar pregnancy O08.5
    neonatal, transitory NEC P74.49
      potassium
        hyperkalemia P74.31
        hypokalemia P74.32
      sodium
        hypernatremia P74.21
        hyponatremia P74.22
  endocrine E34.9
  eye muscle NOS H50.9
  hormone E34.9
  hysterical F44.4
  labyrinth — *see* subcategory H83.2 ☑
  posture R29.3
  protein-energy — *see* Malnutrition
  sympathetic G90.8
Imbecile, imbecility (I.Q. 35-49) F71
Imbedding, intrauterine device T83.39 ☑
Imbibition, cholesterol (gallbladder) K82.4
Imbrication, teeth,, fully erupted M26.30
Imerslund (-Gräsbeck) **syndrome** D51.1
Immature — *see also* Immaturity
  birth (less than 37 completed weeks) — *see* Preterm, newborn
    extremely (less than 28 completed weeks) — *see* Immaturity, extreme
  personality F60.89
Immaturity (less than 37 completed weeks) — *see also* Preterm, newborn
  extreme of newborn (less than 28 completed weeks of gestation) (less than 196 completed days of gestation) (unspecified weeks of gestation) P07.20
    gestational age
      23 completed weeks (23 weeks, 0 days through 23 weeks, 6 days) P07.22
      24 completed weeks (24 weeks, 0 days through 24 weeks, 6 days) P07.23
      25 completed weeks (25 weeks, 0 days through 25 weeks, 6 days) P07.24
      26 completed weeks (26 weeks, 0 days through 26 weeks, 6 days) P07.25
      27 completed weeks (27 weeks, 0 days through 27 weeks, 6 days) P07.26
      less than 23 completed weeks P07.21
  fetus or infant light-for-dates — *see* Light-for-dates
  lung, newborn P28.0
  organ or site NEC — *see* Hypoplasia
  pulmonary, newborn P28.0
  reaction F60.89
  sexual (female) (male), after puberty E30.0
Immersion T75.1 ☑
  foot T69.02- ☑
  hand T69.01- ☑
Immobile, immobility
  complete, due to severe physical disability or frailty R53.2
  intestine K59.8
  syndrome (paraplegic) M62.3
Immune reconstitution (inflammatory) syndrome [IRIS] D89.3
Immunization — *see also* Vaccination
  ABO — *see* Incompatibility, ABO
    in newborn P55.1
  appropriate for age
    child (over 28 days old) Z00.129
      with abnormal findings Z00.121
  complication — *see* Complications, vaccination
  encounter for Z23
  not done (not carried out) Z28.9
    because (of)
      acute illness of patient Z28.01
      allergy to vaccine (or component) Z28.04
      caregiver refusal Z28.82
      chronic illness of patient Z28.02
      contraindication NEC Z28.09
      delay in delivery of vaccine Z28.83
      group pressure Z28.1
      guardian refusal Z28.82
      immune compromised state of patient Z28.03
      lack of availability of vaccine Z28.83
      manufacturer delay of vaccine Z28.83
      parent refusal Z28.82
      patient had disease being vaccinated against Z28.81

Immunization — *continued*
  not done — *continued*
    because — *continued*
      patient refusal Z28.21
      patient's belief Z28.1
      religious beliefs of patient Z28.1
      specified reason NEC Z28.89
        of patient Z28.29
      unavailability of vaccine Z28.83
      unspecified patient reason Z28.20
  Rh factor
    affecting management of pregnancy NEC O36.09- ☑
      anti-D antibody O36.01- ☑
    from transfusion — *see* Complication(s), transfusion, incompatibility reaction, Rh (factor)
Immunocytoma C83.0- ☑
Immunodeficiency D84.9
  with
    adenosine-deaminase deficiency — *see also* Deficiency, adenosine deaminase D81.30
    antibody defects D80.9
      specified type NEC D80.8
    hyperimmunoglobulinemia D80.6
    increased immunoglobulin M (IgM) D80.5
    major defect D82.9
      specified type NEC D82.8
    partial albinism D82.8
    short-limbed stature D82.2
    thrombocytopenia and eczema D82.0
  antibody with
    hyperimmunoglobulinemia D80.6
    near-normal immunoglobulins D80.6
  autosomal recessive, Swiss type D80.0
  combined D81.9
    biotin-dependent carboxylase D81.819
      biotinidase D81.810
      holocarboxylase synthetase D81.818
      specified type NEC D81.818
    severe (SCID) D81.9
      with
        low or normal B-cell numbers D81.2
        low T- and B-cell numbers D81.1
        reticular dysgenesis D81.0
    specified type NEC D81.89
  common variable D83.9
    with
      abnormalities of B-cell numbers and function D83.0
      autoantibodies to B- or T-cells D83.2
      immunoregulatory T-cell disorders D83.1
    specified type NEC D83.8
  following hereditary defective response to Epstein-Barr virus (EBV) D82.3
  selective, immunoglobulin
    A (IgA) D80.2
    G (IgG) (subclasses) D80.3
    M (IgM) D80.4
  severe combined (SCID) D81.9
    due to adenosine deaminase deficiency D81.31
  specified type NEC D84.8
  X-linked, with increased IgM D80.5
Immunotherapy (encounter for)
  antineoplastic Z51.12
Impaction, impacted
  bowel, colon, rectum — *see also* Impaction, fecal K56.49
    by gallstone K56.3
  calculus — *see* Calculus
  cerumen (ear) (external) H61.2- ☑
  cuspid — *see* Impaction, tooth
  dental (same or adjacent tooth) K01.1
  fecal, feces K56.41
  fracture — *see* Fracture, by site
  gallbladder — *see* Calculus, gallbladder
  gallstone(s) — *see* Calculus, gallbladder
    bile duct (common) (hepatic) — *see* Calculus, bile duct
    cystic duct — *see* Calculus, gallbladder
    in intestine, with obstruction (any part) K56.3
  intestine (calculous) NEC — *see also* Impaction, fecal K56.49
    gallstone, with ileus K56.3
  intrauterine device (IUD) T83.39 ☑
  molar — *see* Impaction, tooth
  shoulder, causing obstructed labor O66.0
  tooth, teeth K01.1
  turbinate J34.89

▽ **Subterms under main terms may continue to next column or page**   ☑ **Additional Character Required — Refer to the Tabular List for Character Selection**   **179**

Icterus — Impaction, impacted

Impaired, impairment (function)
auditory discrimination — *see* Abnormal, auditory
    perception
cognitive, mild, so stated G31.84
dual sensory Z73.82
fasting glucose R73.01
glucose tolerance (oral) R73.02
hearing — *see* Deafness
heart — *see* Disease, heart
kidney N28.9
    disorder resulting from N25.9
        specified NEC N25.89
liver K72.90
    with coma K72.91
mastication K08.89
mild cognitive, so stated G31.84
mobility
    ear ossicles — *see* Ankylosis, ear ossicles
    requiring care provider Z74.09
myocardium, myocardial — *see* Insufficiency, myocar-
    dial
rectal sphincter R19.8
renal (acute) (chronic) N28.9
    disorder resulting from N25.9
        specified NEC N25.89
vision NEC H54.7
    both eyes H54.3
Impediment, speech R47.9
psychogenic (childhood) F98.8
slurring R47.81
specified NEC R47.89
Impending
coronary syndrome I20.0
delirium tremens F10.239
myocardial infarction I20.0
Imperception auditory (acquired) — *see also* Deafness
congenital H93.25
Imperfect
aeration, lung (newborn) NEC — *see* Atelectasis
closure (congenital)
    alimentary tract NEC Q45.8
        lower Q43.8
        upper Q40.8
    atrioventricular ostium Q21.2
    atrium (secundum) Q21.1
    branchial cleft NOS Q18.2
        cyst Q18.0
        fistula Q18.0
        sinus Q18.0
    choroid Q14.3
    cricoid cartilage Q31.8
    cusps, heart valve NEC Q24.8
        pulmonary Q22.3
    ductus
        arteriosus Q25.0
        Botalli Q25.0
    ear drum (causing impairment of hearing) Q16.4
    esophagus with communication to bronchus or
        trachea Q39.1
    eyelid Q10.3
    foramen
        botalli Q21.1
        ovale Q21.1
    genitalia, genital organ(s) or system
        female Q52.8
            external Q52.79
            internal NEC Q52.8
        male Q55.8
    glottis Q31.8
    interatrial ostium or septum Q21.1
    interauricular ostium or septum Q21.1
    interventricular ostium or septum Q21.0
    larynx Q31.8
    lip — *see* Cleft, lip
    nasal septum Q30.3
    nose Q30.2
    omphalomesenteric duct Q43.0
    optic nerve entry Q14.2
    organ or site not listed — *see* Anomaly, by site
    ostium
        interatrial Q21.1
        interauricular Q21.1
        interventricular Q21.0
    palate — *see* Cleft, palate
    preauricular sinus Q18.1
    retina Q14.1
    roof of orbit Q75.8
    sclera Q13.5

Imperfect — *continued*
closure — *continued*
    septum
        aorticopulmonary Q21.4
        atrial (secundum) Q21.1
        between aorta and pulmonary artery Q21.4
        heart Q21.9
        interatrial (secundum) Q21.1
        interauricular (secundum) Q21.1
        interventricular Q21.0
            in tetralogy of Fallot Q21.3
        nasal Q30.3
        ventricular Q21.0
            with pulmonary stenosis or atresia, dextrapo-
                sition of aorta, and hypertrophy of right
                ventricle Q21.3
            in tetralogy of Fallot Q21.3
    skull Q75.0
        with
            anencephaly Q00.0
            encephalocele — *see* Encephalocele
            hydrocephalus Q03.9
                with spina bifida — *see* Spina bifida, by
                    site, with hydrocephalus
            microcephaly Q02
    spine (with meningocele) — *see* Spina bifida
    trachea Q32.1
    tympanic membrane (causing impairment of hear-
        ing) Q16.4
    uterus Q51.818
    vitelline duct Q43.0
erection — *see* Dysfunction, sexual, male, erectile
fusion — *see* Imperfect, closure
inflation, lung (newborn) — *see* Atelectasis
posture R29.3
rotation, intestine Q43.3
septum, ventricular Q21.0
Imperfectly descended testis — *see* Cryptorchid
Imperforate (congenital) — *see also* Atresia
anus Q42.3
    with fistula Q42.2
cervix (uteri) Q51.828
esophagus Q39.0
    with tracheoesophageal fistula Q39.1
hymen Q52.3
jejunum Q41.1
pharynx Q38.8
rectum Q42.1
    with fistula Q42.0
urethra Q64.39
vagina Q52.4
Impervious (congenital) — *see also* Atresia
anus Q42.3
    with fistula Q42.2
bile duct Q44.2
esophagus Q39.0
    with tracheoesophageal fistula Q39.1
intestine (small) Q41.9
    large Q42.9
        specified NEC Q42.8
rectum Q42.1
    with fistula Q42.0
ureter — *see* Atresia, ureter
urethra Q64.39
Impetiginization of dermatoses L01.1
Impetigo (any organism) (any site) (circinate) (contagiosa)
    (simplex) (vulgaris) L01.00
Bockhart's L01.02
bullous, bullosa L01.03
external ear L01.00 [H62.40]
follicularis L01.02
furfuracea L30.5
herpetiformis L40.1
    nonobstetrical L40.1
neonatorum L01.03
nonbullous L01.01
specified type NEC L01.09
ulcerative L01.09
Impingement (on teeth)
joint — *see* Disorder, joint, specified type NEC
soft tissue
    anterior M26.81
    posterior M26.82
Implant, endometrial N80.9
Implantation
anomalous — *see* Anomaly, by site
    ureter Q62.63

Implantation — *continued*
cyst
    external area or site (skin) NEC L72.0
    iris — *see* Cyst, iris, implantation
    vagina N89.8
    vulva N90.7
dermoid (cyst) — *see* Implantation, cyst
Impotence (sexual) N52.9
counseling Z70.1
organic origin — *see also* Dysfunction, sexual, male,
    erectile N52.9
psychogenic F52.21
Impression, basilar Q75.8
Imprisonment, anxiety concerning Z65.1
Improper care (child) (newborn) — *see* Maltreatment
Improperly tied umbilical cord (causing hemorrhage)
    P51.8
Impulsiveness (impulsive) R45.87
Inability to swallow — *see* Aphagia
Inaccessible, inaccessibility
health care NEC Z75.3
    due to
        waiting period Z75.2
            for admission to facility elsewhere Z75.1
    other helping agencies Z75.4
Inactive — *see* condition
Inadequate, inadequacy
aesthetics of dental restoration K08.56
biologic, constitutional, functional, or social F60.7
development
    child R62.50
    genitalia
        after puberty NEC E30.0
        congenital
            female Q52.8
                external Q52.79
                internal Q52.8
            male Q55.8
    lungs Q33.6
        associated with short gestation P28.0
    organ or site not listed — *see* Anomaly, by site
diet (causing nutritional deficiency) E63.9
eating habits Z72.4
environment, household Z59.1
family support Z63.8
food (supply) NEC Z59.4
    hunger effects T73.0 ☑
functional F60.7
household care, due to
    family member
        handicapped or ill Z74.2
        on vacation Z75.5
        temporarily away from home Z74.2
    technical defects in home Z59.1
    temporary absence from home of person rendering
        care Z74.2
housing (heating) (space) Z59.1
income (financial) Z59.6
intrafamilial communication Z63.8
material resources Z59.9
mental — *see* Disability, intellectual
parental supervision or control of child Z62.0
personality F60.7
pulmonary
    function R06.89
        newborn P28.5
    ventilation, newborn P28.5
sample of cytologic smear
    anus R85.615
    cervix R87.615
    vagina R87.625
social F60.7
    insurance Z59.7
    skills NEC Z73.4
supervision of child by parent Z62.0
teaching affecting education Z55.8
welfare support Z59.7
Inanition R64
with edema — *see* Malnutrition, severe
due to
    deprivation of food T73.0 ☑
    malnutrition — *see* Malnutrition
fever R50.9
Inappropriate
change in quantitative human chorionic gonadotropin
    (hCG) in early pregnancy O02.81
diet or eating habits Z72.4

☑ Additional Character Required — Refer to the Tabular List for Character Selection   ▽ Subterms under main terms may continue to next column or page

Index

Inappropriate — *continued*
  level of quantitative human chorionic gonadotropin (hCG) for gestational age in early pregnancy O02.81
  secretion
    antidiuretic hormone (ADH) (excessive) E22.2
      deficiency E23.2
    pituitary (posterior) E22.2
Inattention at or after birth — *see* Neglect
Incarceration, incarcerated
  enterocele K46.0
    gangrenous K46.1
  epiplocele K46.0
    gangrenous K46.1
  exomphalos K42.0
    gangrenous K42.1
  hernia — *see also* Hernia, by site, with obstruction
    with gangrene — *see* Hernia, by site, with gangrene
  iris, in wound — *see* Injury, eye, laceration, with prolapse
  lens, in wound — *see* Injury, eye, laceration, with prolapse
  omphalocele K42.0
  prison, anxiety concerning Z65.1
  rupture — *see* Hernia, by site
  sarcoepiplocele K46.0
    gangrenous K46.1
  sarcoepiplomphalocele K42.0
    with gangrene K42.1
  uterus N85.8
    gravid O34.51- ☑
      causing obstructed labor O65.5
Incised wound
  external — *see* Laceration
  internal organs — *see* Injury, by site
Incision, incisional
  hernia K43.2
    with
      gangrene (and obstruction) K43.1
      obstruction K43.0
  surgical, complication — *see* Complications, surgical procedure
  traumatic
    external — *see* Laceration
    internal organs — *see* Injury, by site
Inclusion
  azurophilic leukocytic D72.0
  blennorrhea (neonatal) (newborn) P39.1
  gallbladder in liver (congenital) Q44.1
Incompatibility
  ABO
    affecting management of pregnancy O36.11- ☑
      anti-A sensitization O36.11- ☑
      anti-B sensitization O36.19- ☑
      specified NEC O36.19- ☑
    infusion or transfusion reaction — *see* Complication(s), transfusion, incompatibility reaction, ABO
    newborn P55.1
  blood (group) (Duffy) (K) (Kell) (Kidd) (Lewis) (M) (S) NEC
    affecting management of pregnancy O36.11- ☑
      anti-A sensitization O36.11- ☑
      anti-B sensitization O36.19- ☑
    infusion or transfusion reaction T80.89 ☑
    newborn P55.8
  divorce or estrangement Z63.5
  Rh (blood group) (factor) Z31.82
    affecting management of pregnancy NEC O36.09- ☑
      anti-D antibody O36.01- ☑
    infusion or transfusion reaction — *see* Complication(s), transfusion, incompatibility reaction, Rh (factor)
    newborn P55.0
  rhesus — *see* Incompatibility, Rh
Incompetency, incompetent, incompetence
  annular
    aortic (valve) — *see* Insufficiency, aortic
    mitral (valve) I34.0
    pulmonary valve (heart) I37.1
  aortic (valve) — *see* Insufficiency, aortic
  cardiac valve — *see* Endocarditis
  cervix, cervical (os) N88.3
    in pregnancy O34.3- ☑
  chronotropic I45.89
    with
      autonomic dysfunction G90.8
      ischemic heart disease I25.89

Incompetency, incompetent, incompetence — *continued*
  chronotropic — *continued*
    with — *continued*
      left ventricular dysfunction I51.89
      sinus node dysfunction I49.8
  esophagogastric (junction) (sphincter) K22.0
  mitral (valve) — *see* Insufficiency, mitral
  pelvic fundus N81.89
  pubocervical tissue N81.82
  pulmonary valve (heart) I37.1
    congenital Q22.3
  rectovaginal tissue N81.83
  tricuspid (annular) (valve) — *see* Insufficiency, tricuspid
  valvular — *see* Endocarditis
    congenital Q24.8
  vein, venous (saphenous) (varicose) — *see* Varix, leg
Incomplete — *see also* condition
  bladder, emptying R33.9
  defecation R15.0
  expansion lungs (newborn) NEC — *see* Atelectasis
  rotation, intestine Q43.3
Inconclusive
  diagnostic imaging due to excess body fat of patient R93.9
  findings on diagnostic imaging of breast NEC R92.8
  mammogram (due to dense breasts) R92.2
Incontinence R32
  anal sphincter R15.9
  coital N39.491
  feces R15.9
    nonorganic origin F98.1
  insensible (urinary) N39.42
  overflow N39.490
  postural (urinary) N39.492
  psychogenic F45.8
  rectal R15.9
  reflex N39.498
  stress (female) (male) N39.3
    and urge N39.46
  urethral sphincter R32
  urge N39.41
    and stress (female) (male) N39.46
  urine (urinary) R32
    continuous N39.45
    due to cognitive impairment, or severe physical disability or immobility R39.81
    functional R39.81
    insensible N39.42
    mixed (stress and urge) N39.46
    nocturnal N39.44
    nonorganic origin F98.0
    overflow N39.490
    post dribbling N39.43
    postural N39.492
    reflex N39.498
    specified NEC N39.498
    stress (female) (male) N39.3
      and urge N39.46
    total N39.498
    unaware N39.42
    urge N39.41
      and stress (female) (male) N39.46
Incontinentia pigmenti Q82.3
Incoordinate, incoordination
  esophageal-pharyngeal (newborn) — *see* Dysphagia
  muscular R27.8
  uterus (action) (contractions) (complicating delivery) O62.4
Increase, increased
  abnormal, in development R63.8
  androgens (ovarian) E28.1
  anticoagulants (antithrombin) (anti-VIIIa) (anti-IXa) (anti-Xa) (anti-XIa) — *see* Circulating anticoagulants
  cold sense R20.8
  estrogen E28.0
  function
    adrenal
      cortex — *see* Cushing's, syndrome
      medulla E27.5
    pituitary (gland) (anterior) (lobe) E22.9
      posterior E22.2
  heat sense R20.8
  intracranial pressure (benign) G93.2
  permeability, capillaries I78.8
  pressure, intracranial G93.2

Increase, increased — *continued*
  secretion
    gastrin E16.4
    glucagon E16.3
    pancreas, endocrine E16.9
      growth hormone-releasing hormone E16.8
      pancreatic polypeptide E16.8
      somatostatin E16.8
      vasoactive-intestinal polypeptide E16.8
  sphericity, lens Q12.4
  splenic activity D73.1
  venous pressure I87.8
    portal K76.6
Increta placenta O43.22- ☑
Incrustation, cornea, foreign body (lead)(zinc) — *see* Foreign body, cornea
Incyclophoria H50.54
Incyclotropia — *see* Cyclotropia
Indeterminate sex Q56.4
India rubber skin Q82.8
Indigestion (acid) (bilious) (functional) K30
  catarrhal K31.89
  due to decomposed food NOS A05.9
  nervous F45.8
  psychogenic F45.8
Indirect — *see* condition
Induratio penis plastica N48.6
Induration, indurated
  brain G93.89
  breast (fibrous) N64.51
    puerperal, postpartum O92.29
  broad ligament N83.8
  chancre
    anus A51.1
    congenital A50.07
    extragenital NEC A51.2
  corpora cavernosa (penis) (plastic) N48.6
  liver (chronic) K76.89
  lung (black) (chronic) (fibroid) — *see also* Fibrosis, lung J84.10
    essential brown J84.03
  penile (plastic) N48.6
  phlebitic — *see* Phlebitis
  skin R23.4
Inebriety (without dependence) — *see* Alcohol, intoxication
Inefficiency, kidney N28.9
Inelasticity, skin R23.4
Inequality, leg (length) (acquired) — *see also* Deformity, limb, unequal length
  congenital — *see* Defect, reduction, lower limb
  lower leg — *see* Deformity, limb, unequal length
Inertia
  bladder (neurogenic) N31.2
  stomach K31.89
    psychogenic F45.8
  uterus, uterine during labor O62.2
    during latent phase of labor O62.0
    primary O62.0
    secondary O62.1
  vesical (neurogenic) N31.2
Infancy, infantile, infantilism — *see also* condition
  celiac K90.0
  genitalia, genitals (after puberty) E30.0
  Herter's (nontropical sprue) K90.0
  intestinal K90.0
  Lorain E23.0
  pancreatic K86.89
  pelvis M95.5
    with disproportion (fetopelvic) O33.1
      causing obstructed labor O65.1
  pituitary E23.0
  renal N25.0
  uterus — *see* Infantile, genitalia
Infant(s) — *see also* Infancy
  excessive crying R68.11
  irritable child R68.12
  lack of care — *see* Neglect
  liveborn (singleton) Z38.2
    born in hospital Z38.00
      by cesarean Z38.01
    born outside hospital Z38.1
    multiple NEC Z38.8
      born in hospital Z38.68
        by cesarean Z38.69
      born outside hospital Z38.7
    quadruplet Z38.8
      born in hospital Z38.63

Infant(s) — *continued*
  liveborn — *continued*
    quadruplet — *continued*
      born in hospital — *continued*
        by cesarean Z38.64
      born outside hospital Z38.7
    quintuplet Z38.8
      born in hospital Z38.65
        by cesarean Z38.66
      born outside hospital Z38.7
    triplet Z38.8
      born in hospital Z38.61
        by cesarean Z38.62
      born outside hospital Z38.7
    twin Z38.5
      born in hospital Z38.30
        by cesarean Z38.31
      born outside hospital Z38.4
  of diabetic mother (syndrome of) P70.1
    gestational diabetes P70.0
Infantile — *see also* condition
  genitalia, genitals E30.0
  os, uterine E30.0
  penis E30.0
  testis E29.1
  uterus E30.0
Infantilism — *see* Infancy
Infarct, infarction
  adrenal (capsule) (gland) E27.49
  appendices epiploicae — *see also* Infarct, intestine K55.069
  bowel — *see also* Infarct, intestine K55.069
  brain (stem) — *see* Infarct, cerebral
  breast N64.89
  brewer's (kidney) N28.0
  cardiac — *see* Infarct, myocardium
  cerebellar — *see* Infarct, cerebral
  cerebral (acute) (chronic) — *see also* Occlusion, artery, cerebral or precerebral, with infarction I63.9
    aborted I63.9
    cortical I63.9
    due to
      cerebral venous thrombosis, nonpyogenic I63.6
      embolism
        cerebral arteries I63.4- ☑
        precerebral arteries I63.1- ☑
      occlusion NEC
        cerebral arteries I63.5- ☑
        precerebral arteries I63.2- ☑
        small artery I63.81
      stenosis NEC
        cerebral arteries I63.5- ☑
        precerebral arteries I63.2- ☑
        small artery I63.81
      thrombosis
        cerebral artery I63.3- ☑
        precerebral artery I63.0- ☑
    intraoperative
      during cardiac surgery I97.810
      during other surgery I97.811
    postprocedural
      following cardiac surgery I97.820
      following other surgery I97.821
    specified NEC I63.89
  colon (acute) (agnogenic) (embolic) (hemorrhagic) (nonocclusive) (nonthrombotic) (occlusive) (segmental) (thrombotic) (with gangrene) — *see also* Infarct, intestine K55.049
  coronary artery — *see* Infarct, myocardium
  embolic — *see* Embolism
  fallopian tube N83.8
  gallbladder K82.8
  heart — *see* Infarct, myocardium
  hepatic K76.3
  hypophysis (anterior lobe) E23.6
  impending (myocardium) I20.0
  intestine (acute) (agnogenic) (embolic) (hemorrhagic) (nonocclusive) (nonthrombotic) (occlusive) (thrombotic) (with gangrene) K55.069
    diffuse K55.062
    focal K55.061
    large K55.049
      diffuse K55.042
      focal K55.041
    small K55.029
      diffuse K55.022
      focal K55.021
  kidney N28.0

Infarct, infarction — *continued*
  lacunar I63.81
  liver K76.3
  lung (embolic) (thrombotic) — *see* Embolism, pulmonary
  lymph node I89.8
  mesentery, mesenteric (embolic) (thrombotic) (with gangrene) — *see also* Infarct, intestine K55.069
  muscle (ischemic) M62.20
    ankle M62.27- ☑
    foot M62.27- ☑
    forearm M62.23- ☑
    hand M62.24- ☑
    lower leg M62.26- ☑
    pelvic region M62.25- ☑
    shoulder region M62.21- ☑
    specified site NEC M62.28
    thigh M62.25- ☑
    upper arm M62.22- ☑
  myocardium, myocardial (acute) (with stated duration of 4 weeks or less) I21.9
    associated with revascularization procedure I21.A9
    diagnosed on ECG, but presenting no symptoms I25.2
    due to
      demand ischemia I21.A1
      ischemic imbalance I21.A1
    healed or old I25.2
    intraoperative — *see also* Infarct, myocardium, associated with revascularization procedure
      during cardiac surgery I97.790
      during other surgery I97.791
    non-Q wave I21.4
    non-ST elevation (NSTEMI) I21.4
      subsequent I22.2
    nontransmural I21.4
    past (diagnosed on ECG or other investigation, but currently presenting no symptoms) I25.2
    postprocedural — *see also* Infarct, myocardium, associated with revascularization procedure
      following cardiac surgery — *see also* Infarct, myocardium, type 4 or type 5 I97.190
      following other surgery I97.191
    Q wave (*see also* Infarct, myocardium, by site) I21.3
    secondary to
      demand ischemia I21.A1
      ischemic imbalance I21.A1
    ST elevation (STEMI) I21.3
      anterior (anteroapical) (anterolateral) (anteroseptal) (Q wave) (wall) I21.09
        subsequent I22.0
      inferior (diaphragmatic) (inferolateral) (inferoposterior) (wall) NEC I21.19
        subsequent I22.1
      inferoposterior transmural (Q wave) I21.11
      involving
        coronary artery of anterior wall NEC I21.09
        coronary artery of inferior wall NEC I21.19
        diagonal coronary artery I21.02
        left anterior descending coronary artery I21.02
        left circumflex coronary artery I21.21
        left main coronary artery I21.01
        oblique marginal coronary artery I21.21
        right coronary artery I21.11
      lateral (apical-lateral) (basal-lateral) (high) I21.29
        subsequent I22.8
      posterior (posterobasal) (posterolateral) (posteroseptal) (true) I21.29
        subsequent I22.8
      septal I21.29
        subsequent I22.8
      specified NEC I21.29
        subsequent I22.8
      subsequent I22.9
    subsequent (recurrent) (reinfarction) I22.9
      anterior (anteroapical) (anterolateral) (anteroseptal) (wall) I22.0
      diaphragmatic (wall) I22.1
      inferior (diaphragmatic) (inferolateral) (inferoposterior) (wall) I22.1
      lateral (apical-lateral) (basal-lateral) (high) I22.8
      non-ST elevation (NSTEMI) I22.2
      posterior (posterobasal) (posterolateral) (posteroseptal) (true) I22.8
      septal I22.8
      specified NEC I22.8
      ST elevation I22.9

Infarct, infarction — *continued*
  myocardium, myocardial — *continued*
    subsequent — *continued*
      ST elevation — *continued*
        anterior (anteroapical) (anterolateral) (anteroseptal) (wall) I22.0
        inferior (diaphragmatic) (inferolateral) (inferoposterior) (wall) I22.1
        specified NEC I22.8
      subendocardial I22.2
      transmural I22.9
        anterior (anteroapical) (anterolateral) (anteroseptal) (wall) I22.0
        diaphragmatic (wall) I22.1
        inferior (diaphragmatic) (inferolateral) (inferoposterior) (wall) I22.1
        lateral (apical-lateral) (basal-lateral) (high) I22.8
        posterior (posterobasal) (posterolateral) (posteroseptal) (true) I22.8
        specified NEC I22.8
      type 1 — *see also* Infarction, myocardial, subsequent, by site, or by ST elevation or non-ST elevation I22.9
      type 2 I21.A1
      type 3 I21.A9
      type 4 I21.A9
      type 5 I21.A9
    syphilitic A52.06
    transmural I21.9
      anterior (anteroapical) (anterolateral) (anteroseptal) (Q wave) (wall) NEC I21.09
      inferior (diaphragmatic) (inferolateral) (inferoposterior) (Q wave) (wall) NEC I21.19
      inferoposterior (Q wave) I21.11
      lateral (apical-lateral) (basal-lateral) (high) NEC I21.29
      posterior (posterobasal) (posterolateral) (posteroseptal) (true) NEC I21.29
      septal NEC I21.29
      specified NEC I21.29
    type 1 — *see also* Infarction, myocardial, by site, or by ST elevation or non-ST elevation I21.9
    type 2 I21.A1
    type 3 I21.A9
    type 4 (a) (b) (c) I21.A9
    type 5 I21.A9
  nontransmural I21.4
  omentum — *see also* Infarct, intestine K55.069
  ovary N83.8
  pancreas K86.89
  papillary muscle — *see* Infarct, myocardium
  parathyroid gland E21.4
  pituitary (gland) E23.6
  placenta O43.81- ☑
  prostate N42.89
  pulmonary (artery) (vein) (hemorrhagic) — *see* Embolism, pulmonary
  renal (embolic) (thrombotic) N28.0
  retina, retinal (artery) — *see* Occlusion, artery, retina
  spinal (cord) (acute) (embolic) (nonembolic) G95.11
  spleen D73.5
    embolic or thrombotic I74.8
  subendocardial (acute) (nontransmural) I21.4
  suprarenal (capsule) (gland) E27.49
  testis N50.1
  thrombotic — *see also* Thrombosis
    artery, arterial — *see* Embolism
  thyroid (gland) E07.89
  ventricle (heart) — *see* Infarct, myocardium
Infecting — *see* condition
Infection, infected, infective (opportunistic) B99.9
  with
    drug resistant organism — *see* Resistance (to), drug — *see also* specific organism
    lymphangitis — *see* Lymphangitis
    organ dysfunction (acute) R65.20
      with septic shock R65.21
  abscess (skin) — *code by* site under Abscess
  Absidia — *see* Mucormycosis
  Acanthamoeba — *see* Acanthamebiasis
  Acanthocheilonema (perstans) (streptocerca) B74.4
  accessory sinus (chronic) — *see* Sinusitis
  achorion — *see* Dermatophytosis
  Acremonium falciforme B47.0
  acromioclavicular M00.9
  Actinobacillus (actinomycetem-comitans) A28.8
    mallei A24.0

☑ **Additional Character Required** — Refer to the Tabular List for Character Selection   ▽ **Subterms under main terms may continue to next column or page**

Infection, infected, infective — *continued*
  Actinobacillus — *continued*
    muris A25.1
  Actinomadura B47.1
  Actinomyces (israelii) — *see also* Actinomycosis A42.9
  Actinomycetales — *see* Actinomycosis
  actinomycotic NOS — *see* Actinomycosis
  adenoid (and tonsil) J03.90
    chronic J35.02
  adenovirus NEC
    as cause of disease classified elsewhere B97.0
    unspecified nature or site B34.0
  aerogenes capsulatus A48.0
  aertrycke — *see* Infection, salmonella
  alimentary canal NOS — *see* Enteritis, infectious
  Allescheria boydii B48.2
  Alternaria B48.8
  alveolus, alveolar (process) K04.7
  Ameba, amebic (histolytica) — *see* Amebiasis
  amniotic fluid, sac or cavity O41.10- ☑
    chorioamnionitis O41.12- ☑
    placentitis O41.14- ☑
  amputation stump (surgical) — *see* Complication,
      amputation stump, infection
  Ancylostoma (duodenalis) B76.0
  Anisakiasis, Anisakis larvae B81.0
  anthrax — *see* Anthrax
  antrum (chronic) — *see* Sinusitis, maxillary
  anus, anal (papillae) (sphincter) K62.89
  arbovirus (arbor virus) A94
    specified type NEC A93.8
  artificial insemination N98.0
  Ascaris lumbricoides — *see* Ascariasis
  Ascomycetes B47.0
  Aspergillus (flavus) (fumigatus) (terreus) — *see* As-
      pergillosis
  atypical
    acid-fast (bacilli) — *see* Mycobacterium, atypical
    mycobacteria — *see* Mycobacterium, atypical
    virus A81.9
      specified type NEC A81.89
  auditory meatus (external) — *see* Otitis, externa, infec-
      tive
  auricle (ear) — *see* Otitis, externa, infective
  axillary gland (lymph) L04.2
  Bacillus A49.9
    abortus A23.1
    anthracis — *see* Anthrax
    Ducrey's (any location) A57
    Flexner's A03.1
    Friedländer's NEC A49.8
    gas (gangrene) A48.0
    mallei A24.0
    melitensis A23.0
    paratyphoid, paratyphosus A01.4
      A A01.1
      B A01.2
      C A01.3
    Shiga (-Kruse) A03.0
    suipestifer — *see* Infection, salmonella
    swimming pool A31.1
    typhosa A01.00
    welchii — *see* Gangrene, gas
  bacterial NOS A49.9
    as cause of disease classified elsewhere B96.89
      Bacteroides fragilis [B. fragilis] B96.6
      Clostridium perfringens [C. perfringens] B96.7
      Enterobacter sakazakii B96.89
      Enterococcus B95.2
      Escherichia coli [E. coli] — *see also* Escherichia
        coli B96.20
      Helicobacter pylori [H.pylori] B96.81
      Hemophilus influenzae [H. influenzae] B96.3
      Klebsiella pneumoniae [K. pneumoniae] B96.1
      Mycoplasma pneumoniae [M. pneumoniae]
        B96.0
      Proteus (mirabilis) (morganii) B96.4
      Pseudomonas (aeruginosa) (mallei) (pseudoma-
        llei) B96.5
      Staphylococcus B95.8
        aureus (methicillin susceptible) (MSSA) B95.61
          methicillin resistant (MRSA) B95.62
        specified NEC B95.7
      Streptococcus B95.5
        group A B95.0
        group B B95.1
        pneumoniae B95.3
        specified NEC B95.4

Infection, infected, infective — *continued*
  bacterial — *continued*
    as cause of disease classified elsewhere — *contin-
        ued*
      Vibrio vulnificus B96.82
    specified NEC A48.8
  Bacterium
    paratyphosum A01.4
      A A01.1
      B A01.2
      C A01.3
    typhosum A01.00
  Bacteroides NEC A49.8
    fragilis, as cause of disease classified elsewhere
        B96.6
  Balantidium coli A07.0
  Bartholin's gland N75.8
  Basidiobolus B46.8
  bile duct (common) (hepatic) — *see* Cholangitis
  bladder — *see* Cystitis
  Blastomyces, blastomycotic — *see also* Blastomycosis
    brasiliensis — *see* Paracoccidioidomycosis
    dermatitidis — *see* Blastomycosis
    European — *see* Cryptococcosis
    Loboi B48.0
    North American B40.9
    South American — *see* Paracoccidioidomycosis
  bleb, postprocedure — *see* Blebitis
  bone — *see* Osteomyelitis
  Bordetella — *see* Whooping cough
  Borrelia bergdorfi A69.20
  brain — *see also* Encephalitis G04.90
    membranes — *see* Meningitis
    septic G06.0
      meninges — *see* Meningitis, bacterial
  branchial cyst Q18.0
  breast — *see* Mastitis
  bronchus — *see* Bronchitis
  Brucella A23.9
    abortus A23.1
    canis A23.3
    melitensis A23.0
    mixed A23.8
    specified NEC A23.8
    suis A23.2
  Brugia (malayi) B74.1
    timori B74.2
  bursa — *see* Bursitis, infective
  buttocks (skin) L08.9
  Campylobacter, intestinal A04.5
    as cause of disease classified elsewhere B96.81
  Candida (albicans) (tropicalis) — *see* Candidiasis
  candiru B88.8
  Capillaria (intestinal) B81.1
    hepatica B83.8
    philippinensis B81.1
  cartilage — *see* Disorder, cartilage, specified type NEC
  cat liver fluke B66.0
  catheter-related bloodstream (CRBSI) T80.211 ☑
  cellulitis — *code by* site under Cellulitis
  central line-associated T80.219 ☑
    bloodstream (CLABSI) T80.211 ☑
    specified NEC T80.218 ☑
  Cephalosporium falciforme B47.0
  cerebrospinal — *see* Meningitis
  cervical gland (lymph) L04.0
  cervix — *see* Cervicitis
  cesarean delivery wound (puerperal) O86.00
  cestodes — *see* Infestation, cestodes
  chest J22
  Chilomastix (intestinal) A07.8
  Chlamydia, chlamydial A74.9
    anus A56.3
    genitourinary tract A56.2
      lower A56.00
      specified NEC A56.19
    lymphogranuloma A55
    pharynx A56.4
    psittaci A70
    rectum A56.3
    sexually transmitted NEC A56.8
  cholera — *see* Cholera
  Cladosporium
    bantianum (brain abscess) B43.1
    carrionii B43.0
    castellanii B36.1
    trichoides (brain abscess) B43.1
    werneckii B36.1

Infection, infected, infective — *continued*
  Clonorchis (sinensis) (liver) B66.1
  Clostridium NEC
    bifermentans A48.0
    botulinum (food poisoning) A05.1
      infant A48.51
      wound A48.52
    difficile
      as cause of disease classified elsewhere B96.89
      foodborne (disease)
        not specified as recurrent A04.72
        recurrent A04.71
      gas gangrene A48.0
      necrotizing enterocolitis
        not specified as recurrent A04.72
        recurrent A04.71
      sepsis A41.4
    gas-forming NEC A48.0
    histolyticum A48.0
    novyi, causing gas gangrene A48.0
    oedematiens A48.0
    perfringens
      as cause of disease classified elsewhere B96.7
      due to food A05.2
      foodborne (disease) A05.2
      gas gangrene A48.0
      sepsis A41.4
    septicum, causing gas gangrene A48.0
    sordellii, causing gas gangrene A48.0
    welchii
      as cause of disease classified elsewhere B96.7
      foodborne (disease) A05.2
      gas gangrene A48.0
      necrotizing enteritis A05.2
      sepsis A41.4
  Coccidioides (immitis) — *see* Coccidioidomycosis
  colon — *see* Enteritis, infectious
  colostomy K94.02
  common duct — *see* Cholangitis
  congenital P39.9
    Candida (albicans) P37.5
    cytomegalovirus P35.1
    hepatitis, viral P35.3
    herpes simplex P35.2
    infectious or parasitic disease P37.9
      specified NEC P37.8
    listeriosis (disseminated) P37.2
    malaria NEC P37.4
      falciparum P37.3
    Plasmodium falciparum P37.3
    poliomyelitis P35.8
    rubella P35.0
    skin P39.4
    toxoplasmosis (acute) (subacute) (chronic) P37.1
    tuberculosis P37.0
    urinary (tract) P39.3
    vaccinia P35.8
    virus P35.9
      specified type NEC P35.8
  Conidiobolus B46.8
  coronavirus NEC B34.2
    as cause of disease classified elsewhere B97.29
    severe acute respiratory syndrome (SARS associated)
        B97.21
  corpus luteum — *see* Salpingo-oophoritis
  Corynebacterium diphtheriae — *see* Diphtheria
  cotia virus B08.8
  Coxiella burnetii A78
  coxsackie — *see* Coxsackie
  Cryptococcus neoformans — *see* Cryptococcosis
  Cryptosporidium A07.2
  Cunninghamella — *see* Mucormycosis
  cyst — *see* Cyst
  cystic duct — *see also* Cholecystitis K81.9
  Cysticercus cellulosae — *see* Cysticercosis
  cytomegalovirus, cytomegaloviral B25.9
    congenital P35.1
    maternal, maternal care for (suspected) damage to
        fetus O35.3 ☑
    mononucleosis B27.10
      with
        complication NEC B27.19
        meningitis B27.12
        polyneuropathy B27.11
  delta-agent (acute), in hepatitis B carrier B17.0
  dental (pulpal origin) K04.7
  Deuteromycetes B47.0
  Dicrocoelium dendriticum B66.2

Index

Infection, infected, infective — *continued*
Dipetalonema (perstans) (streptocerca) B74.4
diphtherial — *see* Diphtheria
Diphyllobothrium (adult) (latum) (pacificum) B70.0
   larval B70.1
Diplogonoporus (grandis) B71.8
Dipylidium caninum B67.4
Dirofilaria B74.8
Dracunculus medinensis B72
Drechslera (hawaiiensis) B43.8
Ducrey Haemophilus (any location) A57
due to or resulting from
   artificial insemination N98.0
   central venous catheter T80.219 ☑
      bloodstream T80.211 ☑
      exit or insertion site T80.212 ☑
      localized T80.212 ☑
      port or reservoir T80.212 ☑
      specified NEC T80.218 ☑
      tunnel T80.212 ☑
   device, implant or graft — *see also* Complications,
      by site and type, infection or inflammation
      T85.79 ☑
      arterial graft NEC T82.7 ☑
      breast (implant) T85.79 ☑
      catheter NEC T85.79 ☑
         dialysis (renal) T82.7 ☑
            intraperitoneal T85.71 ☑
         infusion NEC T82.7 ☑
            cranial T85.735 ☑
            intrathecal T85.735 ☑
            spinal (epidural) (subdural) T85.735 ☑
            subarachnoid T85.735 ☑
         urinary T83.518 ☑
            cystostomy T83.510 ☑
            Hopkins T83.518 ☑
            ileostomy T83.518 ☑
            nephrostomy T83.512 ☑
            specified NEC T83.518 ☑
            urethral indwelling T83.511 ☑
            urostomy T83.518 ☑
      electronic (electrode) (pulse generator) (stimula-
         tor)
         bone T84.7 ☑
         cardiac T82.7 ☑
         nervous system T85.738 ☑
            brain T85.731 ☑
            cranial nerve T85.732 ☑
            gastric nerve T85.732 ☑
            generator pocket T85.734 ☑
            neurostimulator generator T85.734 ☑
            peripheral nerve T85.732 ☑
            sacral nerve T85.732 ☑
            spinal cord T85.733 ☑
            vagal nerve T85.732 ☑
         urinary (indwelling) T83.51 ☑
      fixation, internal (orthopedic) NEC — *see* Compli-
         cation, fixation device, infection
      gastrointestinal (bile duct) (esophagus) T85.79 ☑
         neurostimulator electrode (lead) T85.732 ☑
      genital NEC T83.69 ☑
      heart NEC T82.7 ☑
         valve (prosthesis) T82.6 ☑
            graft T82.7 ☑
      joint prosthesis — *see* Complication, joint pros-
         thesis, infection
      ocular (corneal graft) (orbital implant) NEC
         T85.79 ☑
      orthopedic NEC T84.7 ☑
      penile (cylinder) (pump) (resevoir) T83.61 ☑
      specified NEC T85.79 ☑
      testicular T83.62 ☑
      urinary NEC T83.598 ☑
         ileal conduit stent T83.593 ☑
         implanted neurostimulation T83.590 ☑
         implanted sphincter T83.591 ☑
         indwelling ureteral stent T83.592 ☑
         nephroureteral stent T83.593 ☑
         specified stent NEC T83.593 ☑
      vascular NEC T82.7 ☑
      ventricular intracranial (communicating) shunt
         T85.730 ☑
   Hickman catheter T80.219 ☑
      bloodstream T80.211 ☑
      localized T80.212 ☑
      specified NEC T80.218 ☑

Infection, infected, infective — *continued*
due to or resulting from — *continued*
   immunization or vaccination T88.0 ☑
   infusion, injection or transfusion NEC T80.29 ☑
   injury NEC — *code by* site under Wound, open
   peripherally inserted central catheter (PICC)
      T80.219 ☑
      bloodstream T80.211 ☑
      localized T80.212 ☑
      specified NEC T80.218 ☑
   portacath (port-a-cath) T80.219 ☑
      bloodstream T80.211 ☑
      localized T80.212 ☑
      specified NEC T80.218 ☑
   pulmonary artery catheter — *see* Infection, due to
      or resulting from, central venous catheter
   surgery T81.40 ☑
   Swan Ganz catheter — *see* Infection, due to or re-
      sulting from, central venous catheter
   triple lumen catheter T80.219 ☑
      bloodstream T80.211 ☑
      localized T80.212 ☑
      specified NEC T80.218 ☑
   umbilical venous catheter T80.219 ☑
      bloodstream T80.211 ☑
      localized T80.212 ☑
      specified NEC T80.218 ☑
during labor NEC O75.3
ear (middle) — *see also* Otitis media
   external — *see* Otitis, externa, infective
   inner — *see* subcategory H83.0 ☑
Eberthella typhosa A01.00
Echinococcus — *see* Echinococcus
echovirus
   as cause of disease classified elsewhere B97.12
   unspecified nature or site B34.1
endocardium I33.0
endocervix — *see* Cervicitis
Entamoeba — *see* Amebiasis
enteric — *see* Enteritis, infectious
Enterobacter sakazakii B96.89
Enterobius vermicularis B80
enterostomy K94.12
enterovirus B34.1
   as cause of disease classified elsewhere B97.10
      coxsackievirus B97.11
      echovirus B97.12
      specified NEC B97.19
Entomophthora B46.8
Epidermophyton — *see* Dermatophytosis
epididymis — *see* Epididymitis
episiotomy (puerperal) O86.09
Erysipelothrix (insidiosa) (rhusiopathiae) — *see*
   Erysipeloid
erythema infectiosum B08.3
Escherichia (E.) coli NEC A49.8
   as cause of disease classified elsewhere — *see also*
      Escherichia coli B96.20
   congenital P39.8
      sepsis P36.4
   generalized A41.51
   intestinal — *see* Enteritis, infectious, due to, Es-
      cherichia coli
ethmoidal (chronic) (sinus) — *see* Sinusitis, ethmoidal
eustachian tube (ear) — *see* Salpingitis, eustachian
external auditory canal (meatus) NEC — *see* Otitis, externa, infective
eye (purulent) — *see* Endophthalmitis, purulent
eyelid — *see* Inflammation, eyelid
fallopian tube — *see* Salpingo-oophoritis
Fasciola (gigantica) (hepatica) (indica) B66.3
Fasciolopsis (buski) B66.5
filarial — *see* Infestation, filarial
finger (skin) L08.9
   nail L03.01- ☑
      fungus B35.1
fish tapeworm B70.0
   larval B70.1
flagellate, intestinal A07.9
fluke — *see* Infestation, fluke
focal
   teeth (pulpal origin) K04.7
   tonsils J35.01
Fonsecaea (compactum) (pedrosoi) B43.0
food — *see* Intoxication, foodborne
foot (skin) L08.9
   dermatophytic fungus B35.3

Infection, infected, infective — *continued*
Francisella tularensis — *see* Tularemia
frontal (sinus) (chronic) — *see* Sinusitis, frontal
fungus NOS B49
   beard B35.0
   dermatophytic — *see* Dermatophytosis
   foot B35.3
   groin B35.6
   hand B35.2
   nail B35.1
   pathogenic to compromised host only B48.8
   perianal (area) B35.6
   scalp B35.0
   skin B36.9
      foot B35.3
      hand B35.2
      toenails B35.1
Fusarium B48.8
gallbladder — *see* Cholecystitis
gas bacillus — *see* Gangrene, gas
gastrointestinal — *see* Enteritis, infectious
generalized NEC — *see* Sepsis
generator pocket, implanted electronic neurostimulator
   T85.734 ☑
genital organ or tract
   female — *see* Disease, pelvis, inflammatory
   male N49.9
      multiple sites N49.8
      specified NEC N49.8
Ghon tubercle, primary A15.7
Giardia lamblia A07.1
gingiva (chronic) K05.10
   acute K05.00
      nonplaque induced K05.01
      plaque induced K05.00
   nonplaque induced K05.11
   plaque induced K05.10
glanders A24.0
glenosporopsis B48.0
Gnathostoma (spinigerum) B83.1
Gongylonema B83.8
gonococcal — *see* Gonococcus
gram-negative bacilli NOS A49.9
guinea worm B72
gum (chronic) K05.10
   acute K05.00
      nonplaque induced K05.01
      plaque induced K05.00
   nonplaque induced K05.11
   plaque induced K05.10
Haemophilus — *see* Infection, Hemophilus
heart — *see* Carditis
Helicobacter pylori A04.8
   as cause of disease classified elsewhere B96.81
helminths B83.9
   intestinal B82.0
      mixed (types classifiable to more than one of the
         titles B65.0-B81.3 and B81.8) B81.4
      specified type NEC B81.8
   specified type NEC B83.8
Hemophilus
   aegyptius, systemic A48.4
   ducrey (any location) A57
   generalized A41.3
   influenzae NEC A49.2
      as cause of disease classified elsewhere B96.3
   herpes (simplex) — *see also* Herpes
      congenital P35.2
      disseminated B00.7
      zoster B02.9
herpesvirus, herpesviral — *see* Herpes
Heterophyes (heterophyes) B66.8
hip (joint) NEC M00.9
   due to internal joint prosthesis
      left T84.52 ☑
      right T84.51 ☑
   skin NEC L08.9
Histoplasma — *see* Histoplasmosis
   American B39.4
   capsulatum B39.4
hookworm B76.9
human
   papilloma virus A63.0
   T-cell lymphotropic virus type-1 (HTLV-1) B33.3
hydrocele N43.0
Hymenolepis B71.0
hypopharynx — *see* Pharyngitis
inguinal (lymph) glands L04.1

Infection, infected, infective — *continued*
  inguinal glands — *continued*
    due to soft chancre A57
  intervertebral disc, pyogenic M46.30
    cervical region M46.32
    cervicothoracic region M46.33
    lumbar region M46.36
    lumbosacral region M46.37
    multiple sites M46.39
    occipito-atlanto-axial region M46.31
    sacrococcygeal region M46.38
    thoracic region M46.34
    thoracolumbar region M46.35
  intestine, intestinal — *see* Enteritis, infectious
    specified NEC A08.8
  intra-amniotic affecting newborn NEC P39.2
  Isospora belli or hominis A07.3
  Japanese B encephalitis A83.0
  jaw (bone) (lower) (upper) M27.2
  joint NEC M00.9
    due to internal joint prosthesis T84.50 ☑
  kidney (cortex) (hematogenous) N15.9
    with calculus N20.0
      with hydronephrosis N13.6
    following ectopic gestation O08.83
    pelvis and ureter (cystic) N28.85
    puerperal (postpartum) O86.21
    specified NEC N15.8
  Klebsiella (K.) pneumoniae NEC A49.8
    as cause of disease classified elsewhere B96.1
  knee (joint) NEC M00.9
    joint M00.9
    due to internal joint prosthesis
      left T84.54 ☑
      right T84.53 ☑
    skin L08.9
  Koch's — *see* Tuberculosis
  labia (majora) (minora) (acute) — *see* Vulvitis
  lacrimal
    gland — *see* Dacryoadenitis
    passages (duct) (sac) — *see* Inflammation, lacrimal,
      passages
  lancet fluke B66.2
  larynx NEC J38.7
  leg (skin) NOS L08.9
  Legionella pneumophila A48.1
    nonpneumonic A48.2
  Leishmania — *see also* Leishmaniasis
    aethiopica B55.1
    braziliensis B55.2
    chagasi B55.0
    donovani B55.0
    infantum B55.0
    major B55.1
    mexicana B55.1
    tropica B55.1
  lentivirus, as cause of disease classified elsewhere
    B97.31
  Leptosphaeria senegalensis B47.0
  Leptospira interrogans A27.9
    autumnalis A27.89
    canicola A27.89
    hebdomadis A27.89
    icterohaemorrhagiae A27.0
    pomona A27.89
    specified type NEC A27.89
  leptospirochetal NEC — *see* Leptospirosis
  Listeria monocytogenes — *see also* Listeriosis
    congenital P37.2
  Loa loa B74.3
    with conjunctival infestation B74.3
    eyelid B74.3
  Loboa loboi B48.0
  local, skin (staphylococcal) (streptococcal) L08.9
    abscess — *code by* site under Abscess
    cellulitis — *code by* site under Cellulitis
    specified NEC L08.89
    ulcer — *see* Ulcer, skin
  Loefflerella mallei A24.0
  lung — *see also* Pneumonia J18.9
    atypical Mycobacterium A31.0
    spirochetal A69.8
    tuberculous — *see* Tuberculosis, pulmonary
    virus — *see* Pneumonia, viral
  lymph gland — *see also* Lymphadenitis, acute
    mesenteric I88.0
  lymphoid tissue, base of tongue or posterior pharynx,
    NEC (chronic) J35.03

Infection, infected, infective — *continued*
  Madurella (grisea) (mycetomii) B47.0
  major
    following ectopic or molar pregnancy O08.0
    puerperal, postpartum, childbirth O85
  Malassezia furfur B36.0
  Malleomyces
    mallei A24.0
    pseudomallei (whitmori) — *see* Melioidosis
  mammary gland N61.0
  Mansonella (ozzardi) (perstans) (streptocerca) B74.4
  mastoid — *see* Mastoiditis
  maxilla, maxillary M27.2
    sinus (chronic) — *see* Sinusitis, maxillary
  mediastinum J98.51
  Medina (worm) B72
  meibomian cyst or gland — *see* Hordeolum
  meninges — *see* Meningitis, bacterial
  meningococcal — *see also* condition A39.9
    adrenals A39.1
    brain A39.81
    cerebrospinal A39.0
    conjunctiva A39.89
    endocardium A39.51
    heart A39.50
      endocardium A39.51
      myocardium A39.52
      pericardium A39.53
    joint A39.83
    meninges A39.0
    meningococcemia A39.4
      acute A39.2
      chronic A39.3
    myocardium A39.52
    pericardium A39.53
    retrobulbar neuritis A39.82
    specified site NEC A39.89
  mesenteric lymph nodes or glands NEC I88.0
  Metagonimus B66.8
  metatarsophalangeal M00.9
  methicillin
    resistant Staphylococcus aureus (MRSA) A49.02
    susceptible Staphylococcus aureus (MSSA) A49.01
  Microsporum, microsporic — *see* Dermatophytosis
  mixed flora (bacterial) NEC A49.8
  Monilia — *see* Candidiasis
  Monosporium apiospermum B48.2
  mouth, parasitic B37.0
  Mucor — *see* Mucormycosis
  muscle NEC — *see* Myositis, infective
  mycelium NOS B49
  mycetoma B47.9
    actinomycotic NEC B47.1
    mycotic NEC B47.0
  Mycobacterium, mycobacterial — *see* Mycobacterium
  Mycoplasma NEC A49.3
    pneumoniae, as cause of disease classified else-
      where B96.0
  mycotic NOS B49
    pathogenic to compromised host only B48.8
    skin NOS B36.9
  myocardium NEC I40.0
  nail (chronic)
    with lymphangitis — *see* Lymphangitis, acute, digit
    finger L03.01- ☑
      fungus B35.1
    ingrowing L60.0
    toe L03.03- ☑
      fungus B35.1
  nasal sinus (chronic) — *see* Sinusitis
  nasopharynx — *see* Nasopharyngitis
  navel L08.82
  Necator americanus B76.1
  Neisseria — *see* Gonococcus
  Neotestudina rosatii B47.0
  newborn P39.9
    intra-amniotic NEC P39.2
    skin P39.4
    specified type NEC P39.8
  nipple N61.0
    associated with
      lactation O91.03
      pregnancy O91.01- ☑
      puerperium O91.02
  Nocardia — *see* Nocardiosis
  obstetrical surgical wound (puerperal) O86.00
    incisional site
      deep O86.02

Infection, infected, infective — *continued*
  obstetrical surgical wound — *continued*
    incisional site — *continued*
      superficial O86.01
    organ and space site O86.03
    surgical site specified NEC O86.09
  Oesophagostomum (apiostomum) B81.8
  Oestrus ovis — *see* Myiasis
  Oidium albicans B37.9
  Onchocerca (volvulus) — *see* Onchocerciasis
  oncovirus, as cause of disease classified elsewhere
    B97.32
  operation wound T81.49 ☑
  Opisthorchis (felineus) (viverrini) B66.0
  orbit, orbital — *see* Inflammation, orbit
  orthopoxvirus NEC B08.09
  ovary — *see* Salpingo-oophoritis
  Oxyuris vermicularis B80
  pancreas (acute) — *see* Pancreatitis, acute
    abscess — *see* Pancreatitis, acute
    specified NEC — *see also* Pancreatitis, acute K85.80
  papillomavirus, as cause of disease classified elsewhere
    B97.7
  papovavirus NEC B34.4
  Paracoccidioides brasiliensis — *see* Paracoccidioidomy-
    cosis
  Paragonimus (westermani) B66.4
  parainfluenza virus B34.8
  parameningococcus NOS A39.9
  parapoxvirus B08.60
    specified NEC B08.69
  parasitic B89
  Parastrongylus
    cantonensis B83.2
    costaricensis B81.3
    paratyphoid A01.4
      Type A A01.1
      Type B A01.2
      Type C A01.3
  paraurethral ducts N34.2
  parotid gland — *see* Sialoadenitis
  parvovirus NEC B34.3
    as cause of disease classified elsewhere B97.6
  Pasteurella NEC A28.0
    multocida A28.0
    pestis — *see* Plague
    pseudotuberculosis A28.0
    septica (cat bite) (dog bite) A28.0
    tularensis — *see* Tularemia
  pelvic, female — *see* Disease, pelvis, inflammatory
  Penicillium (marneffei) B48.4
  penis (glans) (retention) NEC N48.29
  periapical K04.5
  peridental, periodontal K05.20
    generalized — *see* Periodontitis, aggressive, gener-
      alized
    localized — *see* Periodontitis, aggressive, localized
  perinatal period P39.9
    specified type NEC P39.8
  perineal repair (puerperal) O86.09
  periorbital — *see* Inflammation, orbit
  perirectal K62.89
  perirenal — *see* Infection, kidney
  peritoneal — *see* Peritonitis
  periureteral N28.89
  Petriellidium boydii B48.2
  pharynx — *see also* Pharyngitis
    coxsackievirus B08.5
    posterior, lymphoid (chronic) J35.03
  Phialophora
    gougerotii (subcutaneous abscess or cyst) B43.2
    jeanselmei (subcutaneous abscess or cyst) B43.2
    verrucosa (skin) B43.0
  Piedraia hortae B36.3
  pinta A67.9
    intermediate A67.1
    late A67.2
    mixed A67.3
    primary A67.0
  pinworm B80
  pityrosporum furfur B36.0
  pleuro-pneumonia-like organism (PPLO) NEC A49.3
    as cause of disease classified elsewhere B96.0
  pneumococcus, pneumococcal NEC A49.1
    as cause of disease classified elsewhere B95.3
    generalized (purulent) A40.3
      with pneumonia J13
  Pneumocystis carinii (pneumonia) B59

Infection, infected, infective — *continued*
Pneumocystis jiroveci (pneumonia) B59
port or reservoir T80.212 ☑
postoperative T81.40 ☑
postoperative wound T81.49 ☑
  surgical site
    deep incisional T81.42 ☑
    organ and space T81.43 ☑
    specified NEC T81.49 ☑
    superficial incisional T81.41 ☑
postprocedural T81.40 ☑
postvaccinal T88.0 ☑
prepuce NEC N47.7
  with penile inflammation N47.6
prion — *see* Disease, prion, central nervous system
prostate (capsule) — *see* Prostatitis
Proteus (mirabilis) (morganii) (vulgaris) NEC A49.8
  as cause of disease classified elsewhere B96.4
protozoal NEC B64
  intestinal A07.9
    specified NEC A07.8
  specified NEC B60.8
Pseudoallescheria boydii B48.2
Pseudomonas NEC A49.8
  as cause of disease classified elsewhere B96.5
  mallei A24.0
  pneumonia J15.1
  pseudomallei — *see* Melioidosis
puerperal O86.4
  genitourinary tract NEC O86.89
  major or generalized O85
  minor O86.4
  specified NEC O86.89
pulmonary — *see* Infection, lung
purulent — *see* Abscess
Pyrenochaeta romeroi B47.0
Q fever A78
rectum (sphincter) K62.89
renal — *see also* Infection, kidney
  pelvis and ureter (cystic) N28.85
reovirus, as cause of disease classified elsewhere B97.5
respiratory (tract) NEC J98.8
  acute J22
  chronic J98.8
  influenzal (upper) (acute) — *see* Influenza, with, respiratory manifestations NEC
  lower (acute) J22
    chronic — *see* Bronchitis, chronic
  rhinovirus J00
  syncytial virus (RSV) — *see* Infection, virus, respiratory syncytial (RSV)
  upper (acute) NOS J06.9
    chronic J39.8
    streptococcal J06.9
    viral NOS J06.9
      due to respiratory syncytial virus (RSV) J06.9 [B97.4]
resulting from
  presence of internal prosthesis, implant, graft — *see* Complications, by site and type, infection
retortamoniasis A07.8
retroperitoneal NEC K68.9
retrovirus B33.3
  as cause of disease classified elsewhere B97.30
    human
      immunodeficiency, type 2 (HIV 2) B97.35
      T-cell lymphotropic
        type I (HTLV-I) B97.33
        type II (HTLV-II) B97.34
    lentivirus B97.31
    oncovirus B97.32
    specified NEC B97.39
Rhinosporidium (seeberi) B48.1
rhinovirus
  as cause of disease classified elsewhere B97.89
  unspecified nature or site B34.8
Rhizopus — *see* Mucormycosis
rickettsial NOS A79.9
roundworm (large) NEC B82.0
  Ascariasis — *see also* Ascariasis B77.9
rubella — *see* Rubella
Saccharomyces — *see* Candidiasis
salivary duct or gland (any) — *see* Sialoadenitis
Salmonella (aertrycke) (arizonae) (callinarum) (choleraesuis) (enteritidis) (suipestifer) (typhimurium) A02.9
  with
    (gastro)enteritis A02.0

Infection, infected, infective — *continued*
Salmonella — *continued*
  with — *continued*
    sepsis A02.1
    specified manifestation NEC A02.8
  due to food (poisoning) A02.9
  hirschfeldii A01.3
  localized A02.20
    arthritis A02.23
    meningitis A02.21
    osteomyelitis A02.24
    pneumonia A02.22
    pyelonephritis A02.25
    specified NEC A02.29
  paratyphi A01.4
    A A01.1
    B A01.2
    C A01.3
  schottmuelleri A01.2
  typhi, typhosa — *see* Typhoid
Sarcocystis A07.8
scabies B86
Schistosoma — *see* Infestation, Schistosoma
scrotum (acute) NEC N49.2
seminal vesicle — *see* Vesiculitis
septic
  localized, skin — *see* Abscess
sheep liver fluke B66.3
Shigella A03.9
  boydii A03.2
  dysenteriae A03.0
  flexneri A03.1
  group
    A A03.0
    B A03.1
    C A03.2
    D A03.3
  Schmitz (-Stutzer) A03.0
  schmitzii A03.0
  shigae A03.0
  sonnei A03.3
  specified NEC A03.8
shoulder (joint) NEC M00.9
  due to internal joint prosthesis T84.59 ☑
  skin NEC L08.9
sinus (accessory) (chronic) (nasal) — *see also* Sinusitis
  pilonidal — *see* Sinus, pilonidal
  skin NEC L08.89
Skene's duct or gland — *see* Urethritis
skin (local) (staphylococcal) (streptococcal) L08.9
  abscess — *code by* site under Abscess
  cellulitis — *code by* site under Cellulitis
  due to fungus B36.9
    specified type NEC B36.8
  mycotic B36.9
    specified type NEC B36.8
  newborn P39.4
  ulcer — *see* Ulcer, skin
slow virus A81.9
  specified NEC A81.89
Sparganum (mansoni) (proliferum) (baxteri) B70.1
specific — *see also* Syphilis
  to perinatal period — *see* Infection, congenital
specified NEC B99.8
spermatic cord NEC N49.1
sphenoidal (sinus) — *see* Sinusitis, sphenoidal
spinal cord NOS — *see also* Myelitis G04.91
  abscess G06.1
  meninges — *see* Meningitis
  streptococcal G04.89
Spirillum A25.0
spirochetal NOS A69.9
  lung A69.8
  specified NEC A69.8
Spirometra larvae B70.1
spleen D73.89
Sporotrichum, Sporothrix (schenckii) — *see* Sporotrichosis
staphylococcal, unspecified site
  as cause of disease classified elsewhere B95.8
    aureus (methicillin susceptible) (MSSA) B95.61
      methicillin resistant (MRSA) B95.62
    specified NEC B95.7
  aureus (methicillin susceptible) (MSSA) A49.01
    methicillin resistant (MRSA) A49.02
  food poisoning A05.0
  generalized (purulent) A41.2
  pneumonia — *see* Pneumonia, staphylococcal

Infection, infected, infective — *continued*
Stellantchasmus falcatus B66.8
streptobacillus moniliformis A25.1
streptococcal NEC A49.1
  as cause of disease classified elsewhere B95.5
  B genitourinary complicating
    childbirth O98.82
    pregnancy O98.81- ☑
    puerperium O98.83
  congenital
    sepsis P36.10
      group B P36.0
      specified NEC P36.19
  generalized (purulent) A40.9
Streptomyces B47.1
Strongyloides (stercoralis) — *see* Strongyloidiasis
stump (amputation) (surgical) — *see* Complication, amputation stump, infection
subcutaneous tissue, local L08.9
suipestifer — *see* Infection, salmonella
swimming pool bacillus A31.1
Taenia — *see* Infestation, Taenia
Taeniarhynchus saginatus B68.1
tapeworm — *see* Infestation, tapeworm
tendon (sheath) — *see* Tenosynovitis, infective NEC
Ternidens diminutus B81.8
testis — *see* Orchitis
threadworm B80
throat — *see* Pharyngitis
thyroglossal duct K14.8
toe (skin) L08.9
  cellulitis L03.03- ☑
    fungus B35.1
  nail L03.03- ☑
    fungus B35.1
tongue NEC K14.0
  parasitic B37.0
tonsil (and adenoid) (faucial) (lingual) (pharyngeal) — *see* Tonsillitis
tooth, teeth K04.7
  periapical K04.7
  peridental, periodontal K05.20
    generalized — *see* Periodontitis, aggressive, generalized
    localized — *see* Periodontitis, aggressive, localized
  pulp K04.01
    irreversible K04.02
    reversible K04.01
  socket M27.3
TORCH — *see* Infection, congenital
  without active infection P00.2
Torula histolytica — *see* Cryptococcosis
Toxocara (canis) (cati) (felis) B83.0
Toxoplasma gondii — *see* Toxoplasma
trachea, chronic J42
trematode NEC — *see* Infestation, fluke
trench fever A79.0
Treponema pallidum — *see* Syphilis
Trichinella (spiralis) B75
Trichomonas A59.9
  cervix A59.09
  intestine A07.8
  prostate A59.02
  specified site NEC A59.8
  urethra A59.03
  urogenitalis A59.00
  vagina A59.01
  vulva A59.01
Trichophyton, trichophytic — *see* Dermatophytosis
Trichosporon (beigelii) cutaneum B36.2
Trichostrongylus B81.2
Trichuris (trichiura) B79
Trombicula (irritans) B88.0
Trypanosoma
  brucei
    gambiense B56.0
    rhodesiense B56.1
  cruzi — *see* Chagas' disease
tubal — *see* Salpingo-oophoritis
tuberculous
  latent (LTBI) Z22.7
  NEC — *see* Tuberculosis
tubo-ovarian — *see* Salpingo-oophoritis
tunica vaginalis N49.1
tunnel T80.212 ☑
tympanic membrane NEC — *see* Myringitis
typhoid (abortive) (ambulant) (bacillus) — *see* Typhoid

☑ **Additional Character Required** — Refer to the Tabular List for Character Selection ▽ Subterms under main terms may continue to next column or page

Infection, infected, infective — *continued*
- typhus A75.9
  - flea-borne A75.2
  - mite-borne A75.3
  - recrudescent A75.1
  - tick-borne A77.9
    - African A77.1
    - North Asian A77.2
- umbilicus L08.82
- ureter — *see* Ureteritis
- urethra — *see* Urethritis
- urinary (tract) N39.0
  - bladder — *see* Cystitis
  - complicating
    - pregnancy O23.4- ☑
      - specified type NEC O23.3- ☑
  - kidney — *see* Infection, kidney
  - newborn P39.3
  - puerperal (postpartum) O86.20
  - tuberculous A18.13
  - urethra — *see* Urethritis
- uterus, uterine — *see* Endometritis
- vaccination T88.0 ☑
- vaccinia not from vaccination B08.011
- vagina (acute) — *see* Vaginitis
- varicella B01.9
- varicose veins — *see* Varix
- vas deferens NEC N49.1
- vesical — *see* Cystitis
- Vibrio
  - cholerae A00.0
    - El Tor A00.1
  - parahaemolyticus (food poisoning) A05.3
  - vulnificus
    - as cause of disease classified elsewhere B96.82
    - foodborne intoxication A05.5
- Vincent's (gum) (mouth) (tonsil) A69.1
- virus, viral NOS B34.9
  - adenovirus
    - as cause of disease classified elsewhere B97.0
    - unspecified nature or site B34.0
  - arborvirus, arbovirus arthropod-borne A94
  - as cause of disease classified elsewhere B97.89
    - adenovirus B97.0
    - coronavirus B97.29
      - SARS-associated B97.21
    - coxsackievirus B97.11
    - echovirus B97.12
    - enterovirus B97.10
      - coxsackievirus B97.11
      - echovirus B97.12
      - specified NEC B97.19
    - human
      - immunodeficiency, type 2 (HIV 2) B97.35
      - metapneumovirus B97.81
      - T-cell lymphotropic,
        - type I (HTLV-I) B97.33
        - type II (HTLV-II) B97.34
    - papillomavirus B97.7
    - parvovirus B97.6
    - reovirus B97.5
    - respiratory syncytial (RSV) — *see* Infection, virus, respiratory syncytial (RSV)
    - retrovirus B97.30
      - human
        - immunodeficiency, type 2 (HIV 2) B97.35
        - T-cell lymphotropic,
          - type I (HTLV-I) B97.33
          - type II (HTLV-II) B97.34
      - lentivirus B97.31
      - oncovirus B97.32
      - specified NEC B97.39
    - specified NEC B97.89
  - central nervous system A89
    - atypical A81.9
      - specified NEC A81.89
    - enterovirus NEC A88.8
      - meningitis A87.0
    - slow virus A81.9
      - specified NEC A81.89
    - specified NEC A88.8
  - chest J98.8
  - cotia B08.8
  - coxsackie — *see also* Infection, coxsackie B34.1
    - as cause of disease classified elsewhere B97.11
  - ECHO
    - as cause of disease classified elsewhere B97.12
    - unspecified nature or site B34.1

Infection, infected, infective — *continued*
- virus, viral — *continued*
  - encephalitis, tick-borne A84.9
  - enterovirus, as cause of disease classified elsewhere B97.10
    - coxsackievirus B97.11
    - echovirus B97.12
    - specified NEC B97.19
  - exanthem NOS B09
  - human metapneumovirus as cause of disease classified elsewhere B97.81
  - human papilloma as cause of disease classified elsewhere B97.7
  - intestine — *see* Enteritis, viral
  - respiratory syncytial (RSV)
    - as cause of disease classified elsewhere B97.4
    - bronchiolitis J21.0
    - bronchitis J20.5
    - bronchopneumonia J12.1
    - otitis media H65- ☑ *[B97.4]*
    - pneumonia J12.1
    - upper respiratory infection J06.9 *[B97.4]*
  - rhinovirus
    - as cause of disease classified elsewhere B97.89
    - unspecified nature or site B34.8
  - slow A81.9
    - specified NEC A81.89
  - specified type NEC B33.8
    - as cause of disease classified elsewhere B97.89
    - unspecified nature or site B34.8
  - unspecified nature or site B34.9
  - West Nile — *see* Virus, West Nile
  - vulva (acute) — *see* Vulvitis
  - West Nile — *see* Virus, West Nile
  - whipworm B79
  - worms B83.9
    - specified type NEC B83.8
  - Wuchereria (bancrofti) B74.0
    - malayi B74.1
  - yatapoxvirus B08.70
    - specified NEC B08.79
  - yeast — *see also* Candidiasis B37.9
  - yellow fever — *see* Fever, yellow
  - Yersinia
    - enterocolitica (intestinal) A04.6
    - pestis — *see* Plague
    - pseudotuberculosis A28.2
  - Zeis' gland — *see* Hordeolum
  - Zika virus A92.5
    - congenital P35.4
  - zoonotic bacterial NOS A28.9
  - Zopfia senegalensis B47.0

Infective, infectious — *see* condition

Infertility
- female N97.9
  - age-related N97.8
  - associated with
    - anovulation N97.0
    - cervical (mucus) disease or anomaly N88.3
    - congenital anomaly
      - cervix N88.3
      - fallopian tube N97.1
      - uterus N97.2
      - vagina N97.8
    - dysmucorrhea N88.3
    - fallopian tube disease or anomaly N97.1
    - pituitary-hypothalamic origin E23.0
    - specified origin NEC N97.8
    - Stein-Leventhal syndrome E28.2
    - uterine disease or anomaly N97.2
    - vaginal disease or anomaly N97.8
  - due to
    - cervical anomaly N88.3
    - fallopian tube anomaly N97.1
    - ovarian failure E28.39
    - Stein-Leventhal syndrome E28.2
    - uterine anomaly N97.2
    - vaginal anomaly N97.8
  - nonimplantation N97.2
  - origin
    - cervical N88.3
    - tubal (block) (occlusion) (stenosis) N97.1
    - uterine N97.2
    - vaginal N97.8
- male N46.9
  - azoospermia N46.01
    - extratesticular cause N46.029
      - drug therapy N46.021

Infertility — *continued*
- male — *continued*
  - azoospermia — *continued*
    - extratesticular cause — *continued*
      - efferent duct obstruction N46.023
      - infection N46.022
      - radiation N46.024
      - specified cause NEC N46.029
      - systemic disease N46.025
  - oligospermia N46.11
    - extratesticular cause N46.129
      - drug therapy N46.121
      - efferent duct obstruction N46.123
      - infection N46.122
      - radiation N46.124
      - specified cause NEC N46.129
      - systemic disease N46.125
  - specified type NEC N46.8

Infestation B88.9
- Acanthocheilonema (perstans) (streptocerca) B74.4
- Acariasis B88.0
  - demodex folliculorum B88.0
  - sarcoptes scabiei B86
  - trombiculae B88.0
- Agamofilaria streptocerca B74.4
- Ancylostoma, ankylostoma (braziliense) (caninum) (ceylanicum) (duodenale) B76.0
  - americanum B76.1
  - new world B76.1
- Anisakis larvae, anisakiasis B81.0
- arthropod NEC B88.2
- Ascaris lumbricoides — *see* Ascariasis
- Balantidium coli A07.0
- beef tapeworm B68.1
- Bothriocephalus (latus) B70.0
  - larval B70.1
- broad tapeworm B70.0
  - larval B70.1
- Brugia (malayi) B74.1
  - timori B74.2
- candiru B88.8
- Capillaria
  - hepatica B83.8
  - philippinensis B81.1
- cat liver fluke B66.0
- cestodes B71.9
  - diphyllobothrium — *see* Infestation, diphyllobothrium
  - dipylidiasis B71.1
  - hymenolepiasis B71.0
  - specified type NEC B71.8
- chigger B88.0
- chigo, chigoe B88.1
- Clonorchis (sinensis) (liver) B66.1
- coccidial A07.3
- crab-lice B85.3
- Cysticercus cellulosae — *see* Cysticercosis
- Demodex (folliculorum) B88.0
- Dermanyssus gallinae B88.0
- Dermatobia (hominis) — *see* Myiasis
- Dibothriocephalus (latus) B70.0
  - larval B70.1
- Dicrocoelium dendriticum B66.2
- Diphyllobothrium (adult) (latum) (intestinal) (pacificum) B70.0
  - larval B70.1
- Diplogonoporus (grandis) B71.8
- Dipylidium caninum B67.4
- Distoma hepaticum B66.3
- dog tapeworm B67.4
- Dracunculus medinensis B72
- dragon worm B72
- dwarf tapeworm B71.0
- Echinococcus — *see* Echinococcus
- Echinostomum ilocanum B66.8
- Entamoeba (histolytica) — *see* Infection, Ameba
- Enterobius vermicularis B80
- eyelid
  - in (due to)
    - leishmaniasis B55.1
    - loiasis B74.3
    - onchocerciasis B73.09
    - phthiriasis B85.3
    - parasitic NOS B89
- eyeworm B74.3
- Fasciola (gigantica) (hepatica) (indica) B66.3
- Fasciolopsis (buski) (intestine) B66.5
- filarial B74.9

Index — Infestation — Inflammation, inflamed, inflammatory

Infestation — continued
  filarial — continued
    bancroftian B74.0
    conjunctiva B74.9
    due to
      Acanthocheilonema (perstans) (streptocerca)
        B74.4
      Brugia (malayi) B74.1
        timori B74.2
      Dracunculus medinensis B72
      guinea worm B72
      loa loa B74.3
      Mansonella (ozzardi) (perstans) (streptocerca)
        B74.4
      Onchocerca volvulus B73.00
        eye B73.00
        eyelid B73.09
      Wuchereria (bancrofti) B74.0
    Malayan B74.1
    ozzardi B74.4
    specified type NEC B74.8
  fish tapeworm B70.0
    larval B70.1
  fluke B66.9
    blood NOS — see Schistosomiasis
    cat liver B66.0
    intestinal B66.5
    lancet B66.2
    liver (sheep) B66.3
      cat B66.0
      Chinese B66.1
      due to clonorchiasis B66.1
      oriental B66.1
    lung (oriental) B66.4
    sheep liver B66.3
    specified type NEC B66.8
  fly larvae — see Myiasis
  Gasterophilus (intestinalis) — see Myiasis
  Gastrodiscoides hominis B66.8
  Giardia lamblia A07.1
  Gnathostoma (spinigerum) B83.1
  Gongylonema B83.8
  guinea worm B72
  helminth B83.9
    angiostrongyliasis B83.2
      intestinal B81.3
    gnathostomiasis B83.1
    hirudiniasis, internal B83.4
    intestinal B82.0
      angiostrongyliasis B81.3
      anisakiasis B81.0
      ascariasis — see Ascariasis
      capillariasis B81.1
      cysticercosis — see Cysticercosis
      diphyllobothriasis — see Infestation, diphyl-
        lobothriasis
      dracunculiasis B72
      echinococcus — see Echinococcosis
      enterobiasis B80
      filariasis — see Infestation, filarial
      fluke — see Infestation, fluke
      hookworm — see Infestation, hookworm
      mixed (types classifiable to more than one of the
        titles B65.0-B81.3 and B81.8) B81.4
      onchocerciasis — see Onchocerciasis
      schistosomiasis — see Infestation, schistosoma
      specified
        cestode NEC — see Infestation, cestode
        type NEC B81.8
      strongyloidiasis — see Strongyloidiasis
      taenia — see Infestation, taenia
      trichinellosis B75
      trichostrongyliasis B81.2
      trichuriasis B79
    specified type NEC B83.8
    syngamiasis B83.3
    visceral larva migrans B83.0
  Heterophyes (heterophyes) B66.8
  hookworm B76.9
    ancylostomiasis B76.0
    necatoriasis B76.1
    specified type NEC B76.8
  Hymenolepis (diminuta) (nana) B71.0
  intestinal NEC B82.9
  leeches (aquatic) (land) — see Hirudiniasis
  Leishmania — see Leishmaniasis
  lice, louse — see Infestation, Pediculus
  Linguatula B88.8

Infestation — continued
  Liponyssoides sanguineus B88.0
  Loa loa B74.3
    conjunctiva B74.3
    eyelid B74.3
  louse — see Infestation, Pediculus
  maggots — see Myiasis
  Mansonella (ozzardi) (perstans) (streptocerca) B74.4
  Medina (worm) B72
  Metagonimus (yokogawai) B66.8
  microfilaria streptocerca — see Onchocerciasis
    eye B73.00
    eyelid B73.09
  mites B88.9
    scabic B86
  Monilia (albicans) — see Candidiasis
  mouth B37.0
  Necator americanus B76.1
  nematode NEC (intestinal) B82.0
    Ancylostoma B76.0
    conjunctiva NEC B83.9
    Enterobius vermicularis B80
    Gnathostoma spinigerum B83.1
    physaloptera B80
    specified NEC B81.8
    trichostrongylus B81.2
    trichuris (trichuria) B79
  Oesophagostomum (apiostomum) B81.8
  Oestrus ovis — see also Myiasis B87.9
  Onchocerca (volvulus) — see Onchocerciasis
  Opisthorchis (felineus) (viverrini) B66.0
  orbit, parasitic NOS B89
  Oxyuris vermicularis B80
  Paragonimus (westermani) B66.4
  parasite, parasitic B89
    eyelid B89
    intestinal NOS B82.9
    mouth B37.0
    skin B88.9
    tongue B37.0
  Parastrongylus
    cantonensis B83.2
    costaricensis B81.3
  Pediculus B85.2
    body B85.1
    capitis (humanus) (any site) B85.0
    corporis (humanus) (any site) B85.1
    head B85.0
    mixed (classifiable to more than one of the titles
      B85.0 - B85.3) B85.4
    pubis (any site) B85.3
  Pentastoma B88.8
  Phthirus (pubis) (any site) B85.3
    with any infestation classifiable to B85.0 - B85.2
      B85.4
  pinworm B80
  pork tapeworm (adult) B68.0
  protozoal NEC B64
    intestinal A07.9
      specified NEC A07.8
    specified NEC B60.8
  pubic, louse B85.3
  rat tapeworm B71.0
  red bug B88.0
  roundworm (large) NEC B82.0
    Ascariasis — see also Ascariasis B77.9
  sandflea B88.1
  Sarcoptes scabiei B86
  scabies B86
  Schistosoma B65.9
    bovis B65.8
    cercariae B65.3
    haematobium B65.0
    intercalatum B65.8
    japonicum B65.2
    mansoni B65.1
    mattheei B65.8
    mekongi B65.8
    specified type NEC B65.8
    spindale B65.8
  screw worms — see Myiasis
  skin NOS B88.9
  Sparganum (mansoni) (proliferum) (baxteri) B70.1
    larval B70.1
  specified type NEC B88.8
  Spirometra larvae B70.1
  Stellantchasmus falcatus B66.8
  Strongyloides stercoralis — see Strongyloidiasis

Infestation — continued
  Taenia B68.9
    diminuta B71.0
    echinococcus — see Echinococcus
    mediocanellata B68.1
    nana B71.0
    saginata B68.1
    solium (intestinal form) B68.0
      larval form — see Cysticercosis
  Taeniarhynchus saginatus B68.1
  tapeworm B71.9
    beef B68.1
    broad B70.0
      larval B70.1
    dog B67.4
    dwarf B71.0
    fish B70.0
      larval B70.1
    pork B68.0
    rat B71.0
  Ternidens diminutus B81.8
  Tetranychus molestissimus B88.0
  threadworm B80
  tongue B37.0
  Toxocara (canis) (cati) (felis) B83.0
  trematode(s) NEC — see Infestation, fluke
  Trichinella (spiralis) B75
  Trichocephalus B79
  Trichomonas — see Trichomoniasis
  Trichostrongylus B81.2
  Trichuris (trichiura) B79
  Trombicula (irritans) B88.0
  Tunga penetrans B88.1
  Uncinaria americana B76.1
  Vandellia cirrhosa B88.8
  whipworm B79
  worms B83.9
    intestinal B82.0
  Wuchereria (bancrofti) B74.0
Infiltrate, infiltration
  amyloid (generalized) (localized) — see Amyloidosis
  calcareous NEC R89.7
    localized — see Degeneration, by site
  calcium salt R89.7
  cardiac
    fatty — see Degeneration, myocardial
    glycogenic E74.02 [I43]
  corneal — see Edema, cornea
  eyelid — see Inflammation, eyelid
  glycogen, glycogenic — see Disease, glycogen storage
  heart, cardiac
    fatty — see Degeneration, myocardial
    glycogenic E74.02 [I43]
  inflammatory in vitreous H43.89
  kidney N28.89
  leukemic — see Leukemia
  liver K76.89
    fatty — see Fatty, liver NEC
    glycogen — see also Disease, glycogen storage
      E74.03 [K77]
  lung R91.8
    eosinophilic J82
  lymphatic — see also Leukemia, lymphatic C91.9- ☑
    gland I88.9
  muscle, fatty M62.89
  myocardium, myocardial
    fatty — see Degeneration, myocardial
    glycogenic E74.02 [I43]
  on chest x-ray R91.8
  pulmonary R91.8
    with eosinophilia J82
  skin (lymphocytic) L98.6
  thymus (gland) (fatty) E32.8
  urine R39.0
  vesicant agent
    antineoplastic chemotherapy T80.810 ☑
    other agent NEC T80.818 ☑
  vitreous body H43.89
Infirmity R68.89
  senile R54
Inflammation, inflamed, inflammatory (with exuda-
    tion)
  abducent (nerve) — see Strabismus, paralytic, sixth
    nerve
  accessory sinus (chronic) — see Sinusitis
  adrenal (gland) E27.8
  alveoli, teeth M27.3
    scorbutic E54

Inflammation, inflamed, inflammatory —
continued
- anal canal, anus K62.89
- antrum (chronic) — *see* Sinusitis, maxillary
- appendix — *see* Appendicitis
- arachnoid — *see* Meningitis
- areola N61.0
  - puerperal, postpartum or gestational — *see* Infection, nipple
- areolar tissue NOS L08.9
- artery — *see* Arteritis
- auditory meatus (external) — *see* Otitis, externa
- Bartholin's gland N75.8
- bile duct (common) (hepatic) or passage — *see* Cholangitis
- bladder — *see* Cystitis
- bone — *see* Osteomyelitis
- brain — *see also* Encephalitis
  - membrane — *see* Meningitis
- breast N61.0
  - puerperal, postpartum, gestational — *see* Mastitis, obstetric
- broad ligament — *see* Disease, pelvis, inflammatory
- bronchi — *see* Bronchitis
- catarrhal J00
- cecum — *see* Appendicitis
- cerebral — *see also* Encephalitis
  - membrane — *see* Meningitis
- cerebrospinal
  - meningococcal A39.0
- cervix (uteri) — *see* Cervicitis
- chest J98.8
- chorioretinal H30.9- ☑
  - cyclitis — *see* Cyclitis
  - disseminated H30.10- ☑
    - generalized H30.13- ☑
    - peripheral H30.12- ☑
    - posterior pole H30.11- ☑
  - epitheliopathy — *see* Epitheliopathy
  - focal H30.00- ☑
    - juxtapapillary H30.01- ☑
    - macular H30.04- ☑
    - paramacular — *see* Inflammation, chorioretinal, focal, macular
    - peripheral H30.03- ☑
    - posterior pole H30.02- ☑
  - specified type NEC H30.89- ☑
- choroid — *see* Inflammation, chorioretinal
- chronic, postmastoidectomy cavity — *see* Complications, postmastoidectomy, inflammation
- colon — *see* Enteritis
- connective tissue (diffuse) NEC — *see* Disorder, soft tissue, specified type NEC
- cornea — *see* Keratitis
- corpora cavernosa N48.29
- cranial nerve — *see* Disorder, nerve, cranial
- Douglas' cul-de-sac or pouch (chronic) N73.0
- due to device, implant or graft — *see also* Complications, by site and type, infection or inflammation
  - arterial graft T82.7 ☑
  - breast (implant) T85.79 ☑
  - catheter T85.79 ☑
    - dialysis (renal) T82.7 ☑
      - intraperitoneal T85.71 ☑
    - infusion T82.7 ☑
      - cranial T85.735 ☑
      - intrathecal T85.735 ☑
      - spinal (epidural) (subdural) T85.735 ☑
      - subarachnoid T85.735 ☑
    - urinary T83.518 ☑
      - cystostomy T83.510 ☑
      - Hopkins T83.518 ☑
      - ileostomy T83.518 ☑
      - nephrostomy T83.512 ☑
      - specified NEC T83.518 ☑
      - urethral indwelling T83.511 ☑
      - urostomy T83.518 ☑
  - electronic (electrode) (pulse generator) (stimulator)
    - bone T84.7 ☑
    - cardiac T82.7 ☑
    - nervous system T85.738 ☑
      - brain T85.731 ☑
      - cranial nerve T85.732 ☑
      - gastric nerve T85.732 ☑
      - neurostimulator generator T85.734 ☑
      - peripheral nerve T85.732 ☑

Inflammation, inflamed, inflammatory —
continued
- due to device, implant or graft — *see also* Complications, by site and type, infection or inflammation — *continued*
  - electronic — *continued*
    - nervous system — *continued*
      - sacral nerve T85.732 ☑
      - spinal cord T85.733 ☑
      - vagal nerve T85.732 ☑
    - urinary T83.590 ☑
  - fixation, internal (orthopedic) NEC — *see* Complication, fixation device, infection
  - gastrointestinal (bile duct) (esophagus) T85.79 ☑
    - neurostimulator electrode (lead) T85.732 ☑
  - genital NEC T83.69 ☑
  - heart NEC T82.7 ☑
    - valve (prosthesis) T82.6 ☑
      - graft T82.7 ☑
  - joint prosthesis — *see* Complication, joint prosthesis, infection
  - ocular (corneal graft) (orbital implant) NEC T85.79 ☑
  - orthopedic NEC T84.7 ☑
  - penile (cylinder) (pump) (resevoir) T83.61 ☑
  - specified NEC T85.79 ☑
  - testicular T83.62 ☑
  - urinary NEC T83.598 ☑
    - ileal conduit stent T83.593 ☑
    - implanted neurostimulation T83.590 ☑
    - implanted sphincter T83.591 ☑
    - indwelling ureteral stent T83.592 ☑
    - nephroureteral stent T83.593 ☑
    - specified stent NEC T83.593 ☑
  - vascular NEC T82.7 ☑
  - ventricular intracranial (communicating) shunt T85.730 ☑
- duodenum K29.80
  - with bleeding K29.81
- dura mater — *see* Meningitis
- ear (middle) — *see also* Otitis, media
  - external — *see* Otitis, externa
  - inner — *see* subcategory H83.0 ☑
- epididymis — *see* Epididymitis
- esophagus K20.9
- ethmoidal (sinus) (chronic) — *see* Sinusitis, ethmoidal
- eustachian tube (catarrhal) — *see* Salpingitis, eustachian
- eyelid H01.9
  - abscess — *see* Abscess, eyelid
  - blepharitis — *see* Blepharitis
  - chalazion — *see* Chalazion
  - dermatosis (noninfectious) — *see* Dermatosis, eyelid
  - hordeolum — *see* Hordeolum
  - specified NEC H01.8
- fallopian tube — *see* Salpingo-oophoritis
- fascia — *see* Myositis
- follicular, pharynx J31.2
- frontal (sinus) (chronic) — *see* Sinusitis, frontal
- gallbladder — *see* Cholecystitis
- gastric — *see* Gastritis
- gastrointestinal — *see* Enteritis
- genital organ (internal) (diffuse)
  - female — *see* Disease, pelvis, inflammatory
  - male N49.9
    - multiple sites N49.8
    - specified NEC N49.8
- gland (lymph) — *see* Lymphadenitis
- glottis — *see* Laryngitis
- granular, pharynx J31.2
- gum K05.10
  - nonplaque induced K05.11
  - plaque induced K05.10
- heart — *see* Carditis
- hepatic duct — *see* Cholangitis
- ileoanal (internal) pouch K91.850
- ileum — *see also* Enteritis
  - regional or terminal — *see* Enteritis, regional
- intestinal pouch K91.850
- intestine (any part) — *see* Enteritis
- jaw (acute) (bone) (chronic) (lower) (suppurative) (upper) M27.2
- joint NEC — *see* Arthritis
  - sacroiliac M46.1
- kidney — *see* Nephritis
- knee (joint) M13.169
  - tuberculous A18.02
- labium (majus) (minus) — *see* Vulvitis

Inflammation, inflamed, inflammatory —
continued
- lacrimal
  - gland — *see* Dacryoadenitis
  - passages (duct) (sac) — *see also* Dacryocystitis
    - canaliculitis — *see* Canaliculitis, lacrimal
- larynx — *see* Laryngitis
- leg NOS L08.9
- lip K13.0
- liver (capsule) — *see also* Hepatitis
  - chronic K73.9
  - suppurative K75.0
- lung (acute) — *see also* Pneumonia
  - chronic J98.4
- lymph gland or node — *see* Lymphadenitis
- lymphatic vessel — *see* Lymphangitis
- maxilla, maxillary M27.2
  - sinus (chronic) — *see* Sinusitis, maxillary
- membranes of brain or spinal cord — *see* Meningitis
- meninges — *see* Meningitis
- mouth K12.1
- muscle — *see* Myositis
- myocardium — *see* Myocarditis
- nasal sinus (chronic) — *see* Sinusitis
- nasopharynx — *see* Nasopharyngitis
- navel L08.82
- nerve NEC — *see* Neuralgia
- nipple N61.0
  - puerperal, postpartum or gestational — *see* Infection, nipple
- nose — *see* Rhinitis
- oculomotor (nerve) — *see* Strabismus, paralytic, third nerve
- optic nerve — *see* Neuritis, optic
- orbit (chronic) H05.10
  - acute H05.00
    - abscess — *see* Abscess, orbit
    - cellulitis — *see* Cellulitis, orbit
    - osteomyelitis — *see* Osteomyelitis, orbit
    - periostitis — *see* Periostitis, orbital
    - tenonitis — *see* Tenonitis, eye
  - granuloma — *see* Granuloma, orbit
  - myositis — *see* Myositis, orbital
- ovary — *see* Salpingo-oophoritis
- oviduct — *see* Salpingo-oophoritis
- pancreas (acute) — *see* Pancreatitis
- parametrium N73.0
- parotid region L08.9
- pelvis, female — *see* Disease, pelvis, inflammatory
- penis (corpora cavernosa) N48.29
- perianal K62.89
- pericardium — *see* Pericarditis
- perineum (female) (male) L08.9
- perirectal K62.89
- peritoneum — *see* Peritonitis
- periuterine — *see* Disease, pelvis, inflammatory
- perivesical — *see* Cystitis
- petrous bone (acute) (chronic) — *see* Petrositis
- pharynx (acute) — *see* Pharyngitis
- pia mater — *see* Meningitis
- pleura — *see* Pleurisy
- polyp, colon — *see also* Polyp, colon, inflammatory K51.40
- prostate — *see also* Prostatitis
  - specified type NEC N41.8
- rectosigmoid — *see* Rectosigmoiditis
- rectum — *see also* Proctitis K62.89
- respiratory, upper — *see also* Infection, respiratory, upper J06.9
  - acute, due to radiation J70.0
  - chronic, due to external agent — *see* condition, respiratory, chronic, due to
  - due to
    - chemicals, gases, fumes or vapors (inhalation) J68.2
    - radiation J70.1
- retina — *see* Chorioretinitis
- retrocecal — *see* Appendicitis
- retroperitoneal — *see* Peritonitis
- salivary duct or gland (any) (suppurative) — *see* Sialoadenitis
- scorbutic, alveoli, teeth E54
- scrotum N49.2
- seminal vesicle — *see* Vesiculitis
- sigmoid — *see* Enteritis
- sinus — *see* Sinusitis
- Skene's duct or gland — *see* Urethritis

Inflammation, inflamed, inflammatory —
continued
skin L08.9
spermatic cord N49.1
sphenoidal (sinus) — *see* Sinusitis, sphenoidal
spinal
cord — *see* Encephalitis
membrane — *see* Meningitis
nerve — *see* Disorder, nerve
spine — *see* Spondylopathy, inflammatory
spleen (capsule) D73.89
stomach — *see* Gastritis
subcutaneous tissue L08.9
suprarenal (gland) E27.8
synovial — *see* Tenosynovitis
tendon (sheath) NEC — *see* Tenosynovitis
testis — *see* Orchitis
throat (acute) — *see* Pharyngitis
thymus (gland) E32.8
thyroid (gland) — *see* Thyroiditis
tongue K14.0
tonsil — *see* Tonsillitis
trachea — *see* Tracheitis
trochlear (nerve) — *see* Strabismus, paralytic, fourth
nerve
tubal — *see* Salpingo-oophoritis
tuberculous NEC — *see* Tuberculosis
tubo-ovarian — *see* Salpingo-oophoritis
tunica vaginalis N49.1
tympanic membrane — *see* Tympanitis
umbilicus, umbilical L08.82
uterine ligament — *see* Disease, pelvis, inflammatory
uterus (catarrhal) — *see* Endometritis
uveal tract (anterior) NOS — *see also* Iridocyclitis
posterior — *see* Chorioretinitis
vagina — *see* Vaginitis
vas deferens N49.1
vein — *see also* Phlebitis
intracranial or intraspinal (septic) G08
thrombotic I80.9
leg — *see* Phlebitis, leg
lower extremity — *see* Phlebitis, leg
vocal cord J38.3
vulva — *see* Vulvitis
Wharton's duct (suppurative) — *see* Sialoadenitis
Inflation, lung, imperfect (newborn) — *see* Atelectasis
Influenza (bronchial) (epidemic) (respiratory (upper))
(unidentified influenza virus) J11.1
with
digestive manifestations J11.2
encephalopathy J11.81
enteritis J11.2
gastroenteritis J11.2
gastrointestinal manifestations J11.2
laryngitis J11.1
myocarditis J11.82
otitis media J11.83
pharyngitis J11.1
pneumonia J11.00
specified type J11.08
respiratory manifestations NEC J11.1
specified manifestation NEC J11.89
A/H5N1 — *see also* Influenza, due to, identified novel
influenza A virus J09.X2
avian — *see also* Influenza, due to, identified novel influenza A virus J09.X2
bird — *see also* Influenza, due to, identified novel influenza A virus J09.X2
novel (2009) H1N1 influenza — *see also* Influenza, due
to, identified influenza virus NEC J10.1
novel influenza A/H1N1 — *see also* Influenza, due to,
identified influenza virus NEC J10.1
due to
avian — *see also* Influenza, due to, identified novel
influenza A virus J09.X2
identified influenza virus NEC J10.1
with
digestive manifestations J10.2
encephalopathy J10.81
enteritis J10.2
gastroenteritis J10.2
gastrointestinal manifestations J10.2
laryngitis J10.1
myocarditis J10.82
otitis media J10.83
pharyngitis J10.1
pneumonia (unspecified type) J10.00

Influenza — *continued*
due to — *continued*
identified influenza virus — *continued*
with — *continued*
pneumonia — *continued*
with same identified influenza virus
J10.01
specified type NEC J10.08
respiratory manifestations NEC J10.1
specified manifestation NEC J10.89
identified novel influenza A virus J09.X2
with
digestive manifestations J09.X3
encephalopathy J09.X9
enteritis J09.X3
gastroenteritis J09.X3
gastrointestinal manifestations J09.X3
laryngitis J09.X2
myocarditis J09.X9
otitis media J09.X9
pharyngitis J09.X2
pneumonia J09.X1
respiratory manifestations NEC J09.X2
specified manifestation NEC J09.X9
upper respiratory symptoms J09.X2
of other animal origin, not bird or swine — *see also*
Influenza, due to, identified novel influenza A
virus J09.X2
swine (viruses that normally cause infections in pigs)
— *see also* Influenza, due to, identified novel
influenza A virus J09.X2
Influenzal — *see* Influenza
Influenza-like disease — *see* Influenza
Infraction, Freiberg's (metatarsal head) — *see* Osteochondrosis, juvenile, metatarsus
Infraeruption of tooth (teeth) M26.34
Infusion complication, misadventure, or reaction —
see Complications, infusion
Ingestion
chemical — *see* Table of Drugs and Chemicals, by
substance, poisoning
drug or medicament
correct substance properly administered — *see* Table of Drugs and Chemicals, by drug, adverse
effect
overdose or wrong substance given or taken — *see*
Table of Drugs and Chemicals, by drug, poisoning
foreign body — *see* Foreign body, alimentary tract
multiple drug — *see* Table of Drugs and Chemicals,
multiple
tularemia A21.3
Ingrowing
hair (beard) L73.1
nail (finger) (toe) L60.0
Inguinal — *see also* condition
testicle Q53.9
bilateral Q53.212
unilateral Q53.112
Inhalant-induced
anxiety disorder F18.980
depressive disorder F18.94
major neurocognitive disorder F18.97
mild neurocognitive disorder F18.988
psychotic disorder F18.959
Inhalation
anthrax A22.1
flame T27.3 ☑
food or foreign body — *see* Foreign body, by site
gases, fumes, or vapors NEC T59.9- ☑
specified agent — *see* Table of Drugs and Chemicals,
by substance
liquid or vomitus — *see* Asphyxia
meconium (newborn) P24.00
with
with respiratory symptoms P24.01
pneumonia (pneumonitis) P24.01
mucus — *see* Asphyxia, mucus
oil or gasoline (causing suffocation) — *see* Foreign
body, by site
smoke J70.5
due to chemicals, gases, fumes and vapors J68.9
steam — *see* Toxicity, vapors
stomach contents or secretions — *see* Foreign body,
by site
due to anesthesia (general) (local) or other sedation
T88.59 ☑
in labor and delivery O74.0

Inhalation — *continued*
stomach contents or secretions — *see* Foreign body,
by site — *continued*
due to anesthesia or other sedation — *continued*
in pregnancy O29.01- ☑
postpartum, puerperal O89.01
Inhibition, orgasm
female F52.31
male F52.32
Inhibitor, systemic lupus erythematosus (presence
of) D68.62
Iniencephalus, iniencephaly Q00.2
Injection, traumatic jet (air) (industrial) (water) (paint
or dye) T70.4 ☑
Injury — *see also* specified injury type T14.90 ☑
abdomen, abdominal S39.91 ☑
blood vessel — *see* Injury, blood vessel, abdomen
cavity — *see* Injury, intra-abdominal
contusion S30.1 ☑
internal — *see* Injury, intra-abdominal
intra-abdominal organ — *see* Injury, intra-abdominal
nerve — *see* Injury, nerve, abdomen
open — *see* Wound, open, abdomen
specified NEC S39.81 ☑
superficial — *see* Injury, superficial, abdomen
Achilles tendon S86.00- ☑
laceration S86.02- ☑
specified type NEC S86.09- ☑
strain S86.01- ☑
acoustic, resulting in deafness — *see* Injury, nerve,
acoustic
adrenal (gland) S37.819 ☑
contusion S37.812 ☑
laceration S37.813 ☑
specified type NEC S37.818 ☑
alveolar (process) S09.93 ☑
ankle S99.91- ☑
contusion — *see* Contusion, ankle
dislocation — *see* Dislocation, ankle
fracture — *see* Fracture, ankle
nerve — *see* Injury, nerve, ankle
open — *see* Wound, open, ankle
specified type NEC S99.81- ☑
sprain — *see* Sprain, ankle
superficial — *see* Injury, superficial, ankle
anterior chamber, eye — *see* Injury, eye, specified site
NEC
anus — *see* Injury, abdomen
aorta (thoracic) S25.00 ☑
abdominal S35.00 ☑
laceration (minor) (superficial) S35.01 ☑
major S35.02 ☑
specified type NEC S35.09 ☑
laceration (minor) (superficial) S25.01 ☑
major S25.02 ☑
specified type NEC S25.09 ☑
arm (upper) S49.9- ☑
blood vessel — *see* Injury, blood vessel, arm
contusion — *see* Contusion, arm, upper
fracture — *see* Fracture, humerus
lower — *see* Injury, forearm
muscle — *see* Injury, muscle, shoulder
nerve — *see* Injury, nerve, arm
open — *see* Wound, open, arm
specified type NEC S49.8- ☑
superficial — *see* Injury, superficial, arm
artery (complicating trauma) — *see also* Injury, blood
vessel, by site
cerebral or meningeal — *see* Injury, intracranial
auditory canal (external) (meatus) S09.91 ☑
auricle, auris, ear S09.91 ☑
axilla — *see* Injury, shoulder
back — *see* Injury, back, lower
bile duct S36.13 ☑
birth — *see also* Birth, injury P15.9
bladder (sphincter) S37.20 ☑
at delivery O71.5
contusion S37.22 ☑
laceration S37.23 ☑
obstetrical trauma O71.5
specified type NEC S37.29 ☑
blast (air) (hydraulic) (immersion) (underwater) NEC
T14.8 ☑
acoustic nerve trauma — *see* Injury, nerve, acoustic
bladder — *see* Injury, bladder

Injury — *continued*
  blast — *continued*
    brain — *see* Concussion
    colon — *see* Injury, intestine, large
    ear (primary) S09.31- ☑
      secondary S09.39- ☑
    generalized T70.8 ☑
    lung — *see* Injury, intrathoracic, lung
    multiple body organs T70.8 ☑
    peritoneum S36.81 ☑
    rectum S36.61 ☑
    retroperitoneum S36.898 ☑
    small intestine S36.419 ☑
      duodenum S36.410 ☑
      specified site NEC S36.418 ☑
    specified
      intra-abdominal organ NEC S36.898 ☑
      pelvic organ NEC S37.899 ☑
  blood vessel NEC T14.8 ☑
    abdomen S35.9 ☑
      aorta — *see* Injury, aorta, abdominal
      celiac artery — *see* Injury, blood vessel, celiac
        artery
      iliac vessel — *see* Injury, blood vessel, iliac
      laceration S35.91 ☑
      mesenteric vessel — *see* Injury, mesenteric
      portal vein — *see* Injury, blood vessel, portal vein
      renal vessel — *see* Injury, blood vessel, renal
      specified vessel NEC S35.8X- ☑
      splenic vessel — *see* Injury, blood vessel, splenic
      vena cava — *see* Injury, vena cava, inferior
    ankle — *see* Injury, blood vessel, foot
    aorta (abdominal) (thoracic) — *see* Injury, aorta
    arm (upper) NEC S45.90- ☑
      forearm — *see* Injury, blood vessel, forearm
      laceration S45.91- ☑
      specified
        site NEC S45.80- ☑
          laceration S45.81- ☑
          specified type NEC S45.89- ☑
        type NEC S45.99- ☑
      superficial vein S45.30- ☑
        laceration S45.31- ☑
        specified type NEC S45.39- ☑
    axillary
      artery S45.00- ☑
        laceration S45.01- ☑
        specified type NEC S45.09- ☑
      vein S45.20- ☑
        laceration S45.21- ☑
        specified type NEC S45.29- ☑
    azygos vein — *see* Injury, blood vessel, thoracic,
      specified site NEC
    brachial
      artery S45.10- ☑
        laceration S45.11- ☑
        specified type NEC S45.19- ☑
      vein S45.20- ☑
        laceration S45.219 ☑
        specified type NEC S45.29- ☑
    carotid artery (common) (external) (internal, extracra-
      nial) S15.00- ☑
      internal, intracranial S06.8- ☑
      laceration (minor) (superficial) S15.01- ☑
        major S15.02- ☑
      specified type NEC S15.09- ☑
    celiac artery S35.219 ☑
      branch S35.299 ☑
        laceration (minor) (superficial) S35.291 ☑
          major S35.292 ☑
        specified NEC S35.298 ☑
      laceration (minor) (superficial) S35.211 ☑
        major S35.212 ☑
      specified type NEC S35.218 ☑
    cerebral — *see* Injury, intracranial
    deep plantar — *see* Injury, blood vessel, plantar
      artery
    digital (hand) — *see* Injury, blood vessel, finger
    dorsal
      artery (foot) S95.00- ☑
        laceration S95.01- ☑
        specified type NEC S95.09- ☑
      vein (foot) S95.20- ☑
        laceration S95.21- ☑
        specified type NEC S95.29- ☑

Injury — *continued*
  blood vessel — *continued*
    due to accidental laceration during procedure —
      see Laceration, accidental complicating
      surgery
    extremity — *see* Injury, blood vessel, limb
    femoral
      artery (common) (superficial) S75.00- ☑
        laceration (minor) (superficial) S75.01- ☑
          major S75.02- ☑
        specified type NEC S75.09- ☑
      vein (hip level) (thigh level) S75.10- ☑
        laceration (minor) (superficial) S75.11- ☑
          major S75.12- ☑
        specified type NEC S75.19- ☑
    finger S65.50- ☑
      index S65.50- ☑
        laceration S65.51- ☑
        specified type NEC S65.59- ☑
      laceration S65.51- ☑
      little S65.50- ☑
        laceration S65.51- ☑
        specified type NEC S65.59- ☑
      middle S65.50- ☑
        laceration S65.51- ☑
        specified type NEC S65.59- ☑
      specified type NEC S65.59- ☑
      thumb — *see* Injury, blood vessel, thumb
    foot S95.90- ☑
      dorsal
        artery — *see* Injury, blood vessel, dorsal,
          artery
        vein — *see* Injury, blood vessel, dorsal, vein
      laceration S95.91- ☑
      plantar artery — *see* Injury, blood vessel, plantar
        artery
      specified
        site NEC S95.80- ☑
          laceration S95.81- ☑
          specified type NEC S95.89- ☑
        specified type NEC S95.99- ☑
    forearm S55.90- ☑
      laceration S55.91- ☑
      radial artery — *see* Injury, blood vessel, radial
        artery
      specified
        site NEC S55.80- ☑
          laceration S55.81- ☑
          specified type NEC S55.89- ☑
        type NEC S55.99- ☑
      ulnar artery — *see* Injury, blood vessel, ulnar
        artery
      vein S55.20- ☑
        laceration S55.21- ☑
        specified type NEC S55.29- ☑
    gastric
      artery — *see* Injury, mesenteric, artery, branch
      vein — *see* Injury, blood vessel, abdomen
    gastroduodenal artery — *see* Injury, mesenteric,
      artery, branch
    greater saphenous vein (lower leg level) S85.30- ☑
      hip (and thigh) level S75.20- ☑
        laceration (minor) (superficial) S75.21- ☑
          major S75.22- ☑
        specified type NEC S75.29- ☑
      laceration S85.31- ☑
      specified type NEC S85.39- ☑
    hand (level) S65.90- ☑
      finger — *see* Injury, blood vessel, finger
      laceration S65.91- ☑
      palmar arch — *see* Injury, blood vessel, palmar
        arch
      radial artery — *see* Injury, blood vessel, radial
        artery, hand
      specified
        site NEC S65.80- ☑
          laceration S65.81- ☑
          specified type NEC S65.89- ☑
        type NEC S65.99- ☑
      thumb — *see* Injury, blood vessel, thumb
      ulnar artery — *see* Injury, blood vessel, ulnar
        artery, hand
    head S09.0 ☑
      intracranial — *see* Injury, intracranial
      multiple S09.0 ☑

Injury — *continued*
  blood vessel — *continued*
    hepatic
      artery — *see* Injury, mesenteric, artery
      vein — *see* Injury, vena cava, inferior
    hip S75.90- ☑
      femoral artery — *see* Injury, blood vessel,
        femoral, artery
      femoral vein — *see* Injury, blood vessel, femoral,
        vein
      greater saphenous vein — *see* Injury, blood ves-
        sel, greater saphenous, hip level
      laceration S75.91- ☑
      specified
        site NEC S75.80- ☑
          laceration S75.81- ☑
          specified type NEC S75.89- ☑
        type NEC S75.99- ☑
    hypogastric (artery) (vein) — *see* Injury, blood ves-
      sel, iliac
    iliac S35.5- ☑
      artery S35.51- ☑
      specified vessel NEC S35.5- ☑
      uterine vessel — *see* Injury, blood vessel, uterine
      vein S35.51- ☑
    innominate — *see* Injury, blood vessel, thoracic, in-
      nominate
    intercostal (artery) (vein) — *see* Injury, blood vessel,
      thoracic, intercostal
    jugular vein (external) S15.20- ☑
      internal S15.30- ☑
        laceration (minor) (superficial) S15.31- ☑
          major S15.32- ☑
        specified type NEC S15.39- ☑
      laceration (minor) (superficial) S15.21- ☑
        major S15.22- ☑
      specified type NEC S15.29- ☑
    leg (level) (lower) S85.90- ☑
      greater saphenous — *see* Injury, blood vessel,
        greater saphenous
      laceration S85.91- ☑
      lesser saphenous — *see* Injury, blood vessel,
        lesser saphenous
      peroneal artery — *see* Injury, blood vessel, per-
        oneal artery
      popliteal
        artery — *see* Injury, blood vessel, popliteal,
          artery
        vein — *see* Injury, blood vessel, popliteal, vein
      specified
        site NEC S85.80- ☑
          laceration S85.81- ☑
          specified type NEC S85.89- ☑
        type NEC S85.99- ☑
      thigh — *see* Injury, blood vessel, hip
      tibial artery — *see* Injury, blood vessel, tibial
        artery
    lesser saphenous vein (lower leg level) S85.40- ☑
      laceration S85.41- ☑
      specified type NEC S85.49- ☑
    limb
      lower — *see* Injury, blood vessel, leg
      upper — *see* Injury, blood vessel, arm
    lower back — *see* Injury, blood vessel, abdomen
      specified NEC — *see* Injury, blood vessel, ab-
        domen, specified, site NEC
    mammary (artery) (vein) — *see* Injury, blood vessel,
      thoracic, specified site NEC
    mesenteric (inferior) (superior)
      artery — *see* Injury, mesenteric, artery
      vein — *see* Injury, blood vessel, mesenteric, vein
    neck S15.9 ☑
      specified site NEC S15.8 ☑
    ovarian (artery) (vein) — *see* subcategory S35.8 ☑
    palmar arch (superficial) S65.20- ☑
      deep S65.30- ☑
        laceration S65.31- ☑
        specified type NEC S65.39- ☑
      laceration S65.21- ☑
      specified type NEC S65.29- ☑
    pelvis — *see* Injury, blood vessel, abdomen
      specified NEC — *see* Injury, blood vessel, ab-
        domen, specified, site NEC
    peroneal artery S85.20- ☑
      laceration S85.21- ☑
      specified type NEC S85.29- ☑

Index

Injury — Injury

Injury — *continued*
- blood vessel — *continued*
  - plantar artery (deep) (foot) S95.10- ☑
    - laceration S95.11- ☑
    - specified type NEC S95.19- ☑
  - popliteal
    - artery S85.00- ☑
      - laceration S85.01- ☑
      - specified type NEC S85.09- ☑
    - vein S85.50- ☑
      - laceration S85.51- ☑
      - specified type NEC S85.59- ☑
  - portal vein S35.319
    - laceration S35.311 ☑
    - specified type NEC S35.318 ☑
  - precerebral — *see* Injury, blood vessel, neck
  - pulmonary (artery) (vein) — *see* Injury, blood vessel, thoracic, pulmonary
  - radial artery (forearm level) S55.10- ☑
    - hand and wrist (level) S65.10- ☑
      - laceration S65.11- ☑
      - specified type NEC S65.19- ☑
    - laceration S55.11- ☑
    - specified type NEC S55.19- ☑
  - renal
    - artery S35.40- ☑
      - laceration S35.41- ☑
      - specified NEC S35.49- ☑
    - vein S35.40- ☑
      - laceration S35.41- ☑
      - specified NEC S35.49- ☑
  - saphenous vein (greater) (lower leg level) — *see* Injury, blood vessel, greater saphenous
    - hip and thigh level — *see* Injury, blood vessel, greater saphenous, hip level
    - lesser — *see* Injury, blood vessel, lesser saphenous
  - shoulder
    - specified NEC — *see* Injury, blood vessel, arm, specified site NEC
    - superficial vein — *see* Injury, blood vessel, arm, superficial vein
  - specified NEC T14.8 ☑
  - splenic
    - artery — *see* Injury, blood vessel, celiac artery, branch
    - vein S35.329 ☑
      - laceration S35.321 ☑
      - specified NEC S35.328 ☑
  - subclavian — *see* Injury, blood vessel, thoracic, innominate
  - thigh — *see* Injury, blood vessel, hip
  - thoracic S25.90 ☑
    - aorta S25.00 ☑
      - laceration (minor) (superficial) S25.01 ☑
        - major S25.02 ☑
      - specified type NEC S25.09 ☑
    - azygos vein — *see* Injury, blood vessel, thoracic, specified, site NEC
    - innominate
      - artery S25.10- ☑
        - laceration (minor) (superficial) S25.11- ☑
          - major S25.12- ☑
        - specified type NEC S25.19- ☑
      - vein S25.30- ☑
        - laceration (minor) (superficial) S25.31- ☑
          - major S25.32- ☑
        - specified type NEC S25.39- ☑
    - intercostal S25.50- ☑
      - laceration S25.51- ☑
      - specified type NEC S25.59- ☑
    - laceration S25.91 ☑
    - mammary vessel — *see* Injury, blood vessel, thoracic, specified, site NEC
    - pulmonary S25.40- ☑
      - laceration (minor) (superficial) S25.41- ☑
        - major S25.42- ☑
      - specified type NEC S25.49- ☑
    - specified
      - site NEC S25.80- ☑
        - laceration S25.81- ☑
        - specified type NEC S25.89- ☑
      - type NEC S25.99 ☑
    - subclavian — *see* Injury, blood vessel, thoracic, innominate
    - vena cava (superior) S25.20 ☑

Injury — *continued*
- blood vessel — *continued*
  - thoracic — *continued*
    - vena cava — *continued*
      - laceration (minor) (superficial) S25.21 ☑
        - major S25.22 ☑
      - specified type NEC S25.29 ☑
  - thumb S65.40- ☑
    - laceration S65.41- ☑
    - specified type NEC S65.49- ☑
  - tibial artery S85.10- ☑
    - anterior S85.13- ☑
      - laceration S85.14- ☑
      - specified injury NEC S85.15- ☑
    - laceration S85.11- ☑
    - posterior S85.16- ☑
      - laceration S85.17- ☑
      - specified injury NEC S85.18- ☑
    - specified injury NEC S85.12- ☑
  - ulnar artery (forearm level) S55.00- ☑
    - hand and wrist (level) S65.00- ☑
      - laceration S65.01- ☑
      - specified type NEC S65.09- ☑
    - laceration S55.01- ☑
    - specified type NEC S55.09- ☑
  - upper arm (level) — *see* Injury, blood vessel, arm
    - superficial vein — *see* Injury, blood vessel, arm, superficial vein
  - uterine S35.5- ☑
    - artery S35.53- ☑
    - vein S35.53- ☑
  - vena cava — *see* Injury, vena cava
  - vertebral artery S15.10- ☑
    - laceration (minor) (superficial) S15.11- ☑
      - major S15.12- ☑
    - specified type NEC S15.19- ☑
  - wrist (level) — *see* Injury, blood vessel, hand
- brachial plexus S14.3 ☑
  - newborn P14.3
- brain (traumatic) S06.9- ☑
  - diffuse (axonal) S06.2X- ☑
  - focal S06.30- ☑
- brainstem S06.38- ☑
- breast NOS S29.9 ☑
- broad ligament — *see* Injury, pelvic organ, specified site NEC
- bronchus, bronchi — *see* Injury, intrathoracic, bronchus
- brow S09.90 ☑
- buttock S39.92 ☑
- canthus, eye S05.90 ☑
- cardiac plexus — *see* Injury, nerve, thorax, sympathetic
- cauda equina S34.3 ☑
- cavernous sinus — *see* Injury, intracranial
- cecum — *see* Injury, colon
- celiac ganglion or plexus — *see* Injury, nerve, lumbosacral, sympathetic
- cerebellum — *see* Injury, intracranial
- cerebral — *see* Injury, intracranial
- cervix (uteri) — *see* Injury, uterus
- cheek (wall) S09.93 ☑
- chest — *see* Injury, thorax
- childbirth (newborn) — *see also* Birth, injury
  - maternal NEC O71.9
- chin S09.93 ☑
- choroid (eye) — *see* Injury, eye, specified site NEC
- clitoris S39.94 ☑
- coccyx — *see also* Injury, back, lower
  - complicating delivery O71.6
- colon — *see* Injury, intestine, large
- common bile duct — *see* Injury, liver
- conjunctiva (superficial) — *see* Injury, eye, conjunctiva
- conus medullaris — *see* Injury, spinal, sacral
- cord
  - spermatic (pelvic region) S37.898 ☑
    - scrotal region S39.848 ☑
  - spinal — *see* Injury, spinal cord, by region
- cornea — *see* Injury, eye, specified site NEC
  - abrasion — *see* Injury, eye, cornea, abrasion
- cortex (cerebral) — *see also* Injury, intracranial
  - visual — *see* Injury, nerve, optic
- costal region NEC S29.9 ☑
- costochondral NEC S29.9 ☑
- cranial
  - cavity — *see* Injury, intracranial
  - nerve — *see* Injury, nerve, cranial
- crushing — *see* Crush

Injury — *continued*
- cutaneous sensory nerve
- cystic duct — *see* Injury, liver
- deep tissue — *see* Contusion, by site
  - meaning pressure ulcer — *see* Ulcer, pressure, unstageable, by site
- delivery (newborn) P15.9
  - maternal NEC O71.9
- Descemet's membrane — *see* Injury, eyeball, penetrating
- diaphragm — *see* Injury, intrathoracic, diaphragm
- duodenum — *see* Injury, intestine, small, duodenum
- ear (auricle) (external) (canal) S09.91 ☑
  - abrasion — *see* Abrasion, ear
  - bite — *see* Bite, ear
  - blister — *see* Blister, ear
  - bruise — *see* Contusion, ear
  - contusion — *see* Contusion, ear
  - external constriction — *see* Constriction, external, ear
  - hematoma — *see* Hematoma, ear
  - inner — *see* Injury, ear, middle
  - laceration — *see* Laceration, ear
  - middle S09.30- ☑
    - blast — *see* Injury, blast, ear
    - specified NEC S09.39- ☑
  - puncture — *see* Puncture, ear
  - superficial — *see* Injury, superficial, ear
- eighth cranial nerve (acoustic or auditory) — *see* Injury, nerve, acoustic
- elbow S59.90- ☑
  - contusion — *see* Contusion, elbow
  - dislocation — *see* Dislocation, elbow
  - fracture — *see* Fracture, ulna, upper end
  - open — *see* Wound, open, elbow
  - specified NEC S59.80- ☑
  - sprain — *see* Sprain, elbow
  - superficial — *see* Injury, superficial, elbow
- eleventh cranial nerve (accessory) — *see* Injury, nerve, accessory
- epididymis S39.94 ☑
- epigastric region S39.91 ☑
- epiglottis NEC S19.89 ☑
- esophageal plexus — *see* Injury, nerve, thorax, sympathetic
- esophagus (thoracic part) — *see also* Injury, intrathoracic, esophagus
  - cervical NEC S19.85 ☑
- eustachian tube S09.30 ☑
- eye S05.9- ☑
  - avulsion S05.7- ☑
  - ball — *see* Injury, eyeball
  - conjunctiva S05.0- ☑
  - cornea
    - abrasion S05.0- ☑
    - laceration S05.3- ☑
      - with prolapse S05.2- ☑
  - lacrimal apparatus S05.8X- ☑
  - orbit penetration S05.4- ☑
  - specified site NEC S05.8X- ☑
- eyeball S05.8X- ☑
  - contusion S05.1- ☑
  - penetrating S05.6- ☑
    - with
      - foreign body S05.5- ☑
      - prolapse or loss of intraocular tissue S05.2- ☑
      - without prolapse or loss of intraocular tissue S05.3- ☑
  - specified type NEC S05.8- ☑
- eyebrow S09.93 ☑
- eyelid S09.93 ☑
  - abrasion — *see* Abrasion, eyelid
  - contusion — *see* Contusion, eyelid
  - open — *see* Wound, open, eyelid
- face S09.93 ☑
- fallopian tube S37.509 ☑
  - bilateral S37.502 ☑
    - blast injury S37.512 ☑
    - contusion S37.522 ☑
    - laceration S37.532 ☑
    - specified type NEC S37.592 ☑
  - blast injury (primary) S37.519 ☑
    - bilateral S37.512 ☑
    - secondary — *see* Injury, fallopian tube, specified type NEC
    - unilateral S37.511 ☑

Injury — *continued*
　fallopian tube — *continued*
　　contusion S37.529 ☑
　　　bilateral S37.522 ☑
　　　unilateral S37.521 ☑
　　laceration S37.539 ☑
　　　bilateral S37.532 ☑
　　　unilateral S37.531 ☑
　　specified type NEC S37.599 ☑
　　　bilateral S37.592 ☑
　　　unilateral S37.591 ☑
　　unilateral S37.501 ☑
　　　blast injury S37.511 ☑
　　　contusion S37.521 ☑
　　　laceration S37.531 ☑
　　　specified type NEC S37.591 ☑
　fascia — *see* Injury, muscle
　fifth cranial nerve (trigeminal) — *see* Injury, nerve, trigeminal
　finger (nail) S69.9- ☑
　　blood vessel — *see* Injury, blood vessel, finger
　　contusion — *see* Contusion, finger
　　dislocation — *see* Dislocation, finger
　　fracture — *see* Fracture, finger
　　muscle — *see* Injury, muscle, finger
　　nerve — *see* Injury, nerve, digital, finger
　　open — *see* Wound, open, finger
　　specified NEC S69.8- ☑
　　sprain — *see* Sprain, finger
　　superficial — *see* Injury, superficial, finger
　first cranial nerve (olfactory) — *see* Injury, nerve, olfactory
　flank — *see* Injury, abdomen
　foot S99.92- ☑
　　blood vessel — *see* Injury, blood vessel, foot
　　contusion — *see* Contusion, foot
　　dislocation — *see* Dislocation, foot
　　fracture — *see* Fracture, foot
　　muscle — *see* Injury, muscle, foot
　　open — *see* Wound, open, foot
　　specified type NEC S99.82- ☑
　　sprain — *see* Sprain, foot
　　superficial — *see* Injury, superficial, foot
　forceps NOS P15.9
　forearm S59.91- ☑
　　blood vessel — *see* Injury, blood vessel, forearm
　　contusion — *see* Contusion, forearm
　　fracture — *see* Fracture, forearm
　　muscle — *see* Injury, muscle, forearm
　　nerve — *see* Injury, nerve, forearm
　　open — *see* Wound, open, forearm
　　specified NEC S59.81- ☑
　　superficial — *see* Injury, superficial, forearm
　forehead S09.90 ☑
　fourth cranial nerve (trochlear) — *see* Injury, nerve, trochlear
　gallbladder S36.129 ☑
　　contusion S36.122 ☑
　　laceration S36.123 ☑
　　specified NEC S36.128 ☑
　ganglion
　　celiac, coeliac — *see* Injury, nerve, lumbosacral, sympathetic
　　gasserian — *see* Injury, nerve, trigeminal
　　stellate — *see* Injury, nerve, thorax, sympathetic
　　thoracic sympathetic — *see* Injury, nerve, thorax, sympathetic
　gasserian ganglion — *see* Injury, nerve, trigeminal
　gastric artery — *see* Injury, blood vessel, celiac artery, branch
　gastroduodenal artery — *see* Injury, blood vessel, celiac artery, branch
　gastrointestinal tract — *see* Injury, intra-abdominal
　　with open wound into abdominal cavity — *see* Wound, open, with penetration into peritoneal cavity
　　colon — *see* Injury, intestine, large
　　rectum — *see* Injury, intestine, large, rectum
　　　with open wound into abdominal cavity S36.61 ☑
　　small intestine — *see* Injury, intestine, small
　　specified site NEC — *see* Injury, intra-abdominal, specified, site NEC
　　stomach — *see* Injury, stomach
　genital organ(s)
　　external S39.94 ☑

Injury — *continued*
　genital organ(s) — *continued*
　　external — *continued*
　　　specified NEC S39.848 ☑
　　internal S37.90 ☑
　　　fallopian tube — *see* Injury, fallopian tube
　　　ovary — *see* Injury, ovary
　　　prostate — *see* Injury, prostate
　　　seminal vesicle — *see* Injury, pelvis, organ, specified site NEC
　　　uterus — *see* Injury, uterus
　　　vas deferens — *see* Injury, pelvis, organ, specified site NEC
　　obstetrical trauma O71.9
　gland
　　lacrimal laceration — *see* Injury, eye, specified site NEC
　　salivary S09.93 ☑
　　thyroid NEC S19.84 ☑
　globe (eye) S05.90 ☑
　　specified NEC S05.8X- ☑
　groin — *see* Injury, abdomen
　gum S09.90 ☑
　hand S69.9- ☑
　　blood vessel — *see* Injury, blood vessel, hand
　　contusion — *see* Contusion, hand
　　fracture — *see* Fracture, hand
　　muscle — *see* Injury, muscle, hand
　　nerve — *see* Injury, nerve, hand
　　open — *see* Wound, open, hand
　　specified NEC S69.8- ☑
　　sprain — *see* Sprain, hand
　　superficial — *see* Injury, superficial, hand
　head S09.90 ☑
　　with loss of consciousness S06.9- ☑
　　specified NEC S09.8 ☑
　heart S26.90 ☑
　　with hemopericardium S26.00 ☑
　　　contusion S26.01 ☑
　　　laceration (mild) S26.020 ☑
　　　　major S26.022 ☑
　　　　moderate S26.021 ☑
　　　specified type NEC S26.09 ☑
　　contusion S26.91 ☑
　　laceration S26.92 ☑
　　specified type NEC S26.99 ☑
　　without hemopericardium S26.10 ☑
　　　contusion S26.11 ☑
　　　laceration S26.12 ☑
　　　specified type NEC S26.19 ☑
　heel — *see* Injury, foot
　hepatic
　　artery — *see* Injury, blood vessel, celiac artery, branch
　　duct — *see* Injury, liver
　　vein — *see* Injury, vena cava, inferior
　hip S79.91- ☑
　　blood vessel — *see* Injury, blood vessel, hip
　　contusion — *see* Contusion, hip
　　dislocation — *see* Dislocation, hip
　　fracture — *see* Fracture, femur, neck
　　muscle — *see* Injury, muscle, hip
　　nerve — *see* Injury, nerve, hip
　　open — *see* Wound, open, hip
　　specified NEC S79.81- ☑
　　sprain — *see* Sprain, hip
　　superficial — *see* Injury, superficial, hip
　hymen S39.94 ☑
　hypogastric
　　blood vessel — *see* Injury, blood vessel, iliac
　　plexus — *see* Injury, nerve, lumbosacral, sympathetic
　ileum — *see* Injury, intestine, small
　iliac region S39.91 ☑
　instrumental (during surgery) — *see* Laceration, accidental complicating surgery
　　birth injury — *see* Birth, injury
　　nonsurgical — *see* Injury, by site
　　obstetrical O71.9
　　　bladder O71.5
　　　cervix O71.3
　　　high vaginal O71.4
　　　perineal NOS O70.9
　　　urethra O71.5
　　　uterus O71.5
　　　　with rupture or perforation O71.1

Injury — *continued*
　internal T14.8 ☑
　　aorta — *see* Injury, aorta
　　bladder (sphincter) — *see* Injury, bladder
　　　with
　　　　ectopic or molar pregnancy O08.6
　　　　following ectopic or molar pregnancy O08.6
　　　　obstetrical trauma O71.5
　　bronchus, bronchi — *see* Injury, intrathoracic, bronchus
　　cecum — *see* Injury, intestine, large
　　cervix (uteri) — *see also* Injury, uterus
　　　with ectopic or molar pregnancy O08.6
　　　following ectopic or molar pregnancy O08.6
　　　obstetrical trauma O71.3
　　chest — *see* Injury, intrathoracic
　　gastrointestinal tract — *see* Injury, intra-abdominal
　　heart — *see* Injury, heart
　　intestine NEC — *see* Injury, intestine
　　intrauterine — *see* Injury, uterus
　　mesentery — *see* Injury, intra-abdominal, specified, site NEC
　　pelvis, pelvic (organ) S37.90 ☑
　　　following ectopic or molar pregnancy (subsequent episode) O08.6
　　　obstetrical trauma NEC O71.5
　　　　rupture or perforation O71.1
　　　specified NEC S39.83 ☑
　　rectum — *see* Injury, intestine, large, rectum
　　stomach — *see* Injury, stomach
　　ureter — *see* Injury, ureter
　　urethra (sphincter) following ectopic or molar pregnancy O08.6
　　uterus — *see* Injury, uterus
　interscapular area — *see* Injury, thorax
　intestine
　　large S36.509 ☑
　　　ascending (right) S36.500 ☑
　　　　blast injury (primary) S36.510 ☑
　　　　　secondary S36.590 ☑
　　　　contusion S36.520 ☑
　　　　laceration S36.530 ☑
　　　　specified type NEC S36.590 ☑
　　　blast injury (primary) S36.519 ☑
　　　　ascending (right) S36.510 ☑
　　　　descending (left) S36.512 ☑
　　　　rectum S36.61 ☑
　　　　sigmoid S36.513 ☑
　　　　specified site NEC S36.518 ☑
　　　　transverse S36.511 ☑
　　　contusion S36.529 ☑
　　　　ascending (right) S36.520 ☑
　　　　descending (left) S36.522 ☑
　　　　rectum S36.62 ☑
　　　　sigmoid S36.523 ☑
　　　　specified site NEC S36.528 ☑
　　　　transverse S36.521 ☑
　　　descending (left) S36.502 ☑
　　　　blast injury (primary) S36.512 ☑
　　　　　secondary S36.592 ☑
　　　　contusion S36.522 ☑
　　　　laceration S36.532 ☑
　　　　specified type NEC S36.592 ☑
　　　laceration S36.539 ☑
　　　　ascending (right) S36.530 ☑
　　　　descending (left) S36.532 ☑
　　　　rectum S36.63 ☑
　　　　sigmoid S36.533 ☑
　　　　specified site NEC S36.538 ☑
　　　　transverse S36.531 ☑
　　　rectum S36.60 ☑
　　　　blast injury (primary) S36.61 ☑
　　　　　secondary S36.69 ☑
　　　　contusion S36.62 ☑
　　　　laceration S36.63 ☑
　　　　specified type NEC S36.69 ☑
　　　sigmoid S36.503 ☑
　　　　blast injury (primary) S36.513 ☑
　　　　　secondary S36.593 ☑
　　　　contusion S36.523 ☑
　　　　laceration S36.533 ☑
　　　　specified type NEC S36.593 ☑
　　　specified
　　　　site NEC S36.508 ☑
　　　　　blast injury (primary) S36.518 ☑
　　　　　　secondary S36.598 ☑

▽ Subtterms under main terms may continue to next column or page　　　☑ Additional Character Required — Refer to the Tabular List for Character Selection　　　**193**

Injury — Injury

Injury — *continued*
  intestine — *continued*
    large — *continued*
      specified — *continued*
        site — *continued*
          contusion S36.528 ✓
          laceration S36.538 ✓
          specified type NEC S36.598 ✓
        type NEC S36.599 ✓
          ascending (right) S36.590 ✓
          descending (left) S36.592 ✓
          rectum S36.69 ✓
          sigmoid S36.593 ✓
          specified site NEC S36.598 ✓
          transverse S36.591 ✓
      transverse S36.501 ✓
        blast injury (primary) S36.511 ✓
          secondary S36.591 ✓
        contusion S36.521 ✓
        laceration S36.531 ✓
        specified type NEC S36.591 ✓
    small S36.409 ✓
      blast injury (primary) S36.419 ✓
        duodenum S36.410 ✓
        secondary S36.499 ✓
          duodenum S36.490 ✓
          specified site NEC S36.498 ✓
        specified site NEC S36.418 ✓
      contusion S36.429 ✓
        duodenum S36.420 ✓
        specified site NEC S36.428 ✓
      duodenum S36.400 ✓
        blast injury (primary) S36.410 ✓
          secondary S36.490 ✓
        contusion S36.420 ✓
        laceration S36.430 ✓
        specified NEC S36.490 ✓
      laceration S36.439 ✓
        duodenum S36.430 ✓
        specified site NEC S36.438 ✓
      specified
        site NEC S36.408 ✓
        type NEC S36.499 ✓
          duodenum S36.490 ✓
          specified site NEC S36.498 ✓
  intra-abdominal S36.90 ✓
    adrenal gland — *see* Injury, adrenal gland
    bladder — *see* Injury, bladder
    colon — *see* Injury, intestine, large
    contusion S36.92 ✓
    fallopian tube — *see* Injury, fallopian tube
    gallbladder — *see* Injury, gallbladder
    intestine — *see* Injury, intestine
    kidney — *see* Injury, kidney
    laceration S36.93 ✓
    liver — *see* Injury, liver
    ovary — *see* Injury, ovary
    pancreas — *see* Injury, pancreas
    pelvic NOS S37.90 ✓
    peritoneum — *see* Injury, Intra-abdominal, specified, site NEC
    prostate — *see* Injury, prostate
    rectum — *see* Injury, intestine, large, rectum
    retroperitoneum — *see* Injury, intra-abdominal, specified, site NEC
    seminal vesicle — *see* Injury, pelvis, organ, specified site NEC
    small intestine — *see* Injury, intestine, small
    specified
      pelvic S37.90 ✓
        specified
          site NEC S37.899 ✓
            specified type NEC S37.898 ✓
          type NEC S37.99 ✓
      site NEC S36.899 ✓
        contusion S36.892 ✓
        laceration S36.893 ✓
        specified type NEC S36.898 ✓
      type NEC S36.99 ✓
    spleen — *see* Injury, spleen
    stomach — *see* Injury, stomach
    ureter — *see* Injury, ureter
    urethra — *see* Injury, urethra
    uterus — *see* Injury, uterus
    vas deferens — *see* Injury, pelvis, organ, specified site NEC

Injury — *continued*
  intracranial (traumatic) S06.9- ✓
    cerebellar hemorrhage, traumatic — *see* Injury, intracranial, focal
    cerebral edema, traumatic S06.1X- ✓
      diffuse S06.1X- ✓
      focal S06.1X- ✓
    diffuse (axonal) S06.2X- ✓
    epidural hemorrhage (traumatic) S06.4X- ✓
    focal brain injury S06.30- ✓
      contusion — *see* Contusion, cerebral
      laceration — *see* Laceration, cerebral
      intracerebral hemorrhage, traumatic S06.36- ✓
        left side S06.35- ✓
        right side S06.34- ✓
    subarachnoid hemorrhage, traumatic S06.6X- ✓
    subdural hemorrhage, traumatic S06.5X- ✓
  intraocular — *see* Injury, eyeball, penetrating
  intrathoracic S27.9 ✓
    bronchus S27.409 ✓
      bilateral S27.402 ✓
      blast injury (primary) S27.419 ✓
        bilateral S27.412 ✓
        secondary — *see* Injury, intrathoracic, bronchus, specified type NEC
        unilateral S27.411 ✓
      contusion S27.429 ✓
        bilateral S27.422 ✓
        unilateral S27.421 ✓
      laceration S27.439 ✓
        bilateral S27.432 ✓
        unilateral S27.431 ✓
      specified type NEC S27.499 ✓
        bilateral S27.492 ✓
        unilateral S27.491 ✓
      unilateral S27.401 ✓
    diaphragm S27.809 ✓
      contusion S27.802 ✓
      laceration S27.803 ✓
      specified type NEC S27.808 ✓
    esophagus (thoracic) S27.819 ✓
      contusion S27.812 ✓
      laceration S27.813 ✓
      specified type NEC S27.818 ✓
    heart — *see* Injury, heart
    hemopneumothorax S27.2 ✓
    hemothorax S27.1 ✓
    lung S27.309 ✓
      aspiration J69.0
      bilateral S27.302 ✓
      blast injury (primary) S27.319 ✓
        bilateral S27.312 ✓
        secondary — *see* Injury, intrathoracic, lung, specified type NEC
        unilateral S27.311 ✓
      contusion S27.329 ✓
        bilateral S27.322 ✓
        unilateral S27.321 ✓
      laceration S27.339 ✓
        bilateral S27.332 ✓
        unilateral S27.331 ✓
      specified type NEC S27.399 ✓
        bilateral S27.392 ✓
        unilateral S27.391 ✓
      unilateral S27.301 ✓
    pleura S27.60 ✓
      laceration S27.63 ✓
      specified type NEC S27.69 ✓
    pneumothorax S27.0 ✓
    specified organ NEC S27.899 ✓
      contusion S27.892 ✓
      laceration S27.893 ✓
      specified type NEC S27.898 ✓
    thoracic duct — *see* Injury, intrathoracic, specified organ NEC
    thymus gland — *see* Injury, intrathoracic, specified organ NEC
    trachea, thoracic S27.50 ✓
      blast (primary) S27.51 ✓
      contusion S27.52 ✓
      laceration S27.53 ✓
      specified type NEC S27.59 ✓
  iris — *see* Injury, eye, specified site NEC
    penetrating — *see* Injury, eyeball, penetrating
  jaw S09.93 ✓
  jejunum — *see* Injury, intestine, small

Injury — *continued*
  joint NOS T14.8 ✓
    old or residual — *see* Disorder, joint, specified type NEC
  kidney S37.00- ✓
    acute (nontraumatic) N17.9
    contusion — *see* Contusion, kidney
    laceration — *see* Laceration, kidney
    specified NEC S37.09- ✓
  knee S89.9- ✓
    contusion — *see* Contusion, knee
    dislocation — *see* Dislocation, knee
    meniscus (lateral) (medial) — *see* Sprain, knee, specified site NEC
      old injury or tear — *see* Derangement, knee, meniscus, due to old injury
    open — *see* Wound, open, knee
    specified NEC S89.8- ✓
    sprain — *see* Sprain, knee
    superficial — *see* Injury, superficial, knee
  labium (majus) (minus) S39.94 ✓
  labyrinth, ear S09.30- ✓
  lacrimal apparatus, duct, gland, or sac — *see* Injury, eye, specified site NEC
  larynx NEC S19.81 ✓
  leg (lower) S89.9- ✓
    blood vessel — *see* Injury, blood vessel, leg
    contusion — *see* Contusion, leg
    fracture — *see* Fracture, leg
    muscle — *see* Injury, muscle, leg
    nerve — *see* Injury, nerve, leg
    open — *see* Wound, open, leg
    specified NEC S89.8- ✓
    superficial — *see* Injury, superficial, leg
  lens, eye — *see* Injury, eye, specified site NEC
    penetrating — *see* Injury, eyeball, penetrating
  limb NEC T14.8 ✓
  lip S09.93 ✓
  liver S36.119 ✓
    contusion S36.112 ✓
    laceration S36.113 ✓
      major (stellate) S36.116 ✓
      minor S36.114 ✓
      moderate S36.115 ✓
    specified NEC S36.118 ✓
  lower back S39.92 ✓
    specified NEC S39.82 ✓
  lumbar, lumbosacral (region) S39.92 ✓
    plexus — *see* Injury, lumbosacral plexus
  lumbosacral plexus S34.4 ✓
  lung — *see also* Injury, intrathoracic, lung
    aspiration J69.0
    transfusion-related (TRALI) J95.84
  lymphatic thoracic duct — *see* Injury, intrathoracic, specified organ NEC
  malar region S09.93 ✓
  mastoid region S09.90 ✓
  maxilla S09.93 ✓
  mediastinum — *see* Injury, intrathoracic, specified organ NEC
  membrane, brain — *see* Injury, intracranial
  meningeal artery — *see* Injury, intracranial, subdural hemorrhage
  meninges (cerebral) — *see* Injury, intracranial
  mesenteric
    artery
      branch S35.299 ✓
        laceration (minor) (superficial) S35.291 ✓
          major S35.292 ✓
        specified NEC S35.298 ✓
      inferior S35.239 ✓
        laceration (minor) (superficial) S35.231 ✓
          major S35.232 ✓
        specified NEC S35.238 ✓
      superior S35.229 ✓
        laceration (minor) (superficial) S35.221 ✓
          major S35.222 ✓
        specified NEC S35.228 ✓
    plexus (inferior) (superior) — *see* Injury, nerve, lumbosacral, sympathetic
    vein
      inferior S35.349 ✓
        laceration S35.341 ✓
        specified NEC S35.348 ✓
      superior S35.339 ✓
        laceration S35.331 ✓

✓ **Additional Character Required** — Refer to the Tabular List for Character Selection ▽ Subterms under main terms may continue to next column or page

Injury — *continued*
- mesenteric — *continued*
  - vein — *continued*
    - superior — *continued*
      - specified NEC S35.338 ☑
- mesentery — *see* Injury, intra-abdominal, specified site NEC
- mesosalpinx — *see* Injury, pelvic organ, specified site NEC
- middle ear S09.30- ☑
- midthoracic region NOS S29.9 ☑
- mouth S09.93 ☑
- multiple NOS T07 ☑
- muscle (and fascia) (and tendon)
  - abdomen S39.001 ☑
    - laceration S39.021 ☑
    - specified type NEC S39.091 ☑
    - strain S39.011 ☑
  - abductor
    - thumb, forearm level — *see* Injury, muscle, thumb, abductor
  - adductor
    - thigh S76.20- ☑
      - laceration S76.22- ☑
      - specified type NEC S76.29- ☑
      - strain S76.21- ☑
  - ankle — *see* Injury, muscle, foot
  - anterior muscle group, at leg level (lower) S86.20- ☑
    - laceration S86.22- ☑
    - specified type NEC S86.29- ☑
    - strain S86.21- ☑
  - arm (upper) — *see* Injury, muscle, shoulder
  - biceps (parts NEC) S46.20- ☑
    - laceration S46.22- ☑
    - long head S46.10- ☑
      - laceration S46.12- ☑
      - specified type NEC S46.19- ☑
      - strain S46.11- ☑
    - specified type NEC S46.29- ☑
    - strain S46.21- ☑
  - extensor
    - finger(s) (other than thumb) — *see* Injury, muscle, finger by site, extensor
    - forearm level, specified NEC — *see* Injury, muscle, forearm, extensor
    - thumb — *see* Injury, muscle, thumb, extensor
    - toe (large) (ankle level) (foot level) — *see* Injury, muscle, toe, extensor
  - finger
    - extensor (forearm level) S56.40- ☑
      - hand level S66.309 ☑
        - laceration S66.329 ☑
        - specified type NEC S66.399 ☑
        - strain S66.319 ☑
      - laceration S56.429 ☑
      - specified type NEC S56.499 ☑
      - strain S56.419 ☑
    - flexor (forearm level) S56.10- ☑
      - hand level S66.109 ☑
        - laceration S66.129 ☑
        - specified type NEC S66.199 ☑
        - strain S66.119 ☑
      - laceration S56.129 ☑
      - specified type NEC S56.199 ☑
      - strain S56.119 ☑
    - index
      - extensor (forearm level)
        - hand level S66.308 ☑
          - laceration S66.32- ☑
          - specified type NEC S66.39- ☑
          - strain S66.31- ☑
        - specified type NEC S56.492- ☑
      - flexor (forearm level)
        - hand level S66.108 ☑
          - laceration S66.12- ☑
          - specified type NEC S66.19- ☑
          - strain S66.11- ☑
        - specified type NEC S56.19- ☑
        - strain S56.11- ☑
      - intrinsic S66.50- ☑
        - laceration S66.52- ☑
        - specified type NEC S66.59- ☑
        - strain S66.51- ☑
    - intrinsic S66.509 ☑
      - laceration S66.529 ☑
      - specified type NEC S66.599 ☑

Injury — *continued*
- muscle — *continued*
  - finger — *continued*
    - intrinsic — *continued*
      - strain S66.519 ☑
    - little
      - extensor (forearm level)
        - hand level S66.30- ☑
          - laceration S66.32- ☑
          - specified type NEC S66.39- ☑
          - strain S66.31- ☑
        - laceration S56.42- ☑
        - specified type NEC S56.49- ☑
        - strain S56.41- ☑
      - flexor (forearm level)
        - hand level S66.10- ☑
          - laceration S66.12- ☑
          - specified type NEC S66.19- ☑
          - strain S66.11- ☑
        - laceration S56.12- ☑
        - specified type NEC S56.19- ☑
        - strain S56.11- ☑
      - intrinsic S66.50- ☑
        - laceration S66.52- ☑
        - specified type NEC S66.59- ☑
        - strain S66.51- ☑
    - middle
      - extensor (forearm level)
        - hand level S66.30- ☑
          - laceration S66.32- ☑
          - specified type NEC S66.39- ☑
          - strain S66.31- ☑
        - laceration S56.42- ☑
        - specified type NEC S56.49- ☑
        - strain S56.41- ☑
      - flexor (forearm level)
        - hand level S66.10- ☑
          - laceration S66.12- ☑
          - specified type NEC S66.19- ☑
          - strain S66.11- ☑
        - laceration S56.12- ☑
        - specified type NEC S56.19- ☑
        - strain S56.11- ☑
      - intrinsic S66.50- ☑
        - laceration S66.52- ☑
        - specified type NEC S66.59- ☑
        - strain S66.51- ☑
    - ring
      - extensor (forearm level)
        - hand level S66.30- ☑
          - laceration S66.32- ☑
          - specified type NEC S66.39- ☑
          - strain S66.31- ☑
        - laceration S56.42- ☑
        - specified type NEC S56.49- ☑
        - strain S56.41- ☑
      - flexor (forearm level)
        - hand level S66.10- ☑
          - laceration S66.12- ☑
          - specified type NEC S66.19- ☑
          - strain S66.11- ☑
        - laceration S56.12- ☑
        - specified type NEC S56.19- ☑
        - strain S56.11- ☑
      - intrinsic S66.50- ☑
        - laceration S66.52- ☑
        - specified type NEC S66.59- ☑
        - strain S66.51- ☑
  - flexor
    - finger(s) (other than thumb) — *see* Injury, muscle, finger
    - forearm level, specified NEC — *see* Injury, muscle, forearm, flexor
    - thumb — *see* Injury, muscle, thumb, flexor
    - toe (long) (ankle level) (foot level) — *see* Injury, muscle, toe, flexor
  - foot S96.90- ☑
    - intrinsic S96.20- ☑
      - laceration S96.22- ☑
      - specified type NEC S96.29- ☑
      - strain S96.21- ☑
    - laceration S96.92- ☑
    - long extensor, toe — *see* Injury, muscle, toe, extensor
    - long flexor, toe — *see* Injury, muscle, toe, flexor

Injury — *continued*
- muscle — *continued*
  - foot — *continued*
    - specified
      - site NEC S96.80- ☑
        - laceration S96.82- ☑
        - specified type NEC S96.89- ☑
        - strain S96.81- ☑
      - type S96.99- ☑
    - strain S96.91- ☑
  - forearm (level) S56.90- ☑
    - extensor S56.50- ☑
      - laceration S56.52- ☑
      - specified type NEC S56.59- ☑
      - strain S56.51- ☑
    - flexor S56.20- ☑
      - laceration S56.22- ☑
      - specified type NEC S56.29- ☑
      - strain S56.21- ☑
    - laceration S56.92- ☑
    - specified S56.99- ☑
      - site NEC S56.80- ☑
        - laceration S56.82- ☑
        - strain S56.81- ☑
        - type NEC S56.89- ☑
    - strain S56.91- ☑
  - hand (level) S66.90- ☑
    - laceration S66.92- ☑
    - specified
      - site NEC S66.80- ☑
        - laceration S66.82- ☑
        - specified type NEC S66.89- ☑
        - strain S66.81- ☑
      - type NEC S66.99- ☑
    - strain S66.91- ☑
  - head S09.10 ☑
    - laceration S09.12 ☑
    - specified type NEC S09.19 ☑
    - strain S09.11 ☑
  - hip NEC S76.00- ☑
    - laceration S76.02- ☑
    - specified type NEC S76.09- ☑
    - strain S76.01- ☑
  - intrinsic
    - ankle and foot level — *see* Injury, muscle, foot, intrinsic
    - finger (other than thumb) — *see* Injury, muscle, finger by site, intrinsic
    - foot (level) — *see* Injury, muscle, foot, intrinsic
    - thumb — *see* Injury, muscle, thumb, intrinsic
  - leg (level) (lower) S86.90- ☑
    - Achilles tendon — *see* Injury, Achilles tendon
    - anterior muscle group — *see* Injury, muscle, anterior muscle group
    - laceration S86.92- ☑
    - peroneal muscle group — *see* Injury, muscle, peroneal muscle group
    - posterior muscle group — *see* Injury, muscle, posterior muscle group, leg level
    - specified
      - site NEC S86.80- ☑
        - laceration S86.82- ☑
        - specified type NEC S86.89- ☑
        - strain S86.81- ☑
      - type NEC S86.99- ☑
    - strain S86.91- ☑
  - long
    - extensor toe, at ankle and foot level — *see* Injury, muscle, toe, extensor
    - flexor, toe, at ankle and foot level — *see* Injury, muscle, toe, flexor
    - head, biceps — *see* Injury, muscle, biceps, long head
  - lower back S39.002 ☑
    - laceration S39.022 ☑
    - specified type NEC S39.092 ☑
    - strain S39.012 ☑
  - neck (level) S16.9 ☑
    - laceration S16.2 ☑
    - specified type NEC S16.8 ☑
    - strain S16.1 ☑
  - pelvis S39.003 ☑
    - laceration S39.023 ☑
    - specified type NEC S39.093 ☑
    - strain S39.013 ☑

◺ Subterms under main terms may continue to next column or page   ☑ Additional Character Required — Refer to the Tabular List for Character Selection   **195**

Injury — Injury

Injury — *continued*
  muscle — *continued*
    peroneal muscle group, at leg level (lower)
        S86.30- ☑
      laceration S86.32- ☑
      specified type NEC S86.39- ☑
      strain S86.31- ☑
    posterior muscle (group)
      leg level (lower) S86.10- ☑
        laceration S86.12- ☑
        specified type NEC S86.19- ☑
        strain S86.11- ☑
      thigh level S76.30- ☑
        laceration S76.32- ☑
        specified type NEC S76.39- ☑
        strain S76.31- ☑
    quadriceps (thigh) S76.10- ☑
      laceration S76.12- ☑
      specified type NEC S76.19- ☑
      strain S76.11- ☑
    shoulder S46.90- ☑
      laceration S46.92- ☑
      rotator cuff — *see* Injury, rotator cuff
      specified site NEC S46.80- ☑
        laceration S46.82- ☑
        specified type NEC S46.89- ☑
        strain S46.81- ☑
      specified type NEC S46.99- ☑
      strain S46.91- ☑
    thigh NEC (level) S76.90- ☑
      adductor — *see* Injury, muscle, adductor, thigh
      laceration S76.92- ☑
      posterior muscle (group) — *see* Injury, muscle, posterior muscle, thigh level
      quadriceps — *see* Injury, muscle, quadriceps
      specified
        site NEC S76.80- ☑
          laceration S76.82- ☑
          specified type NEC S76.89- ☑
          strain S76.81- ☑
        type NEC S76.99- ☑
      strain S76.91- ☑
    thorax (level) S29.009 ☑
      back wall S29.002 ☑
      front wall S29.001 ☑
      laceration S29.029 ☑
        back wall S29.022 ☑
        front wall S29.021 ☑
      specified type NEC S29.099 ☑
        back wall S29.092 ☑
        front wall S29.091 ☑
      strain S29.019 ☑
        back wall S29.012 ☑
        front wall S29.011 ☑
    thumb
      abductor (forearm level) S56.30- ☑
        laceration S56.32- ☑
        specified type NEC S56.39- ☑
        strain S56.31- ☑
      extensor (forearm level) S56.30- ☑
        hand level S66.20- ☑
          laceration S66.22- ☑
          specified type NEC S66.29- ☑
          strain S66.21- ☑
        laceration S56.32- ☑
        specified type NEC S56.39- ☑
        strain S56.31- ☑
      flexor (forearm level) S56.00- ☑
        hand level S66.00- ☑
          laceration S66.02- ☑
          specified type NEC S66.09- ☑
          strain S66.01- ☑
        laceration S56.02- ☑
        specified type NEC S56.09- ☑
        strain S56.01- ☑
        wrist level — *see* Injury, muscle, thumb, flexor, hand level
      intrinsic S66.40- ☑
        laceration S66.42- ☑
        specified type NEC S66.49- ☑
        strain S66.41- ☑
    toe — *see also* Injury, muscle, foot
      extensor, long S96.10- ☑
        laceration S96.12- ☑
        specified type NEC S96.19- ☑
        strain S96.11- ☑

Injury — *continued*
  muscle — *continued*
    toe — *see also* Injury, muscle, foot — *continued*
      flexor, long S96.00- ☑
        laceration S96.02- ☑
        specified type NEC S96.09- ☑
        strain S96.01- ☑
      triceps S46.30- ☑
        laceration S46.32- ☑
        specified type NEC S46.39- ☑
        strain S46.31- ☑
    wrist (and hand) level — *see* Injury, muscle, hand
  musculocutaneous nerve — *see* Injury, nerve, musculocutaneous
  myocardium — *see* Injury, heart
  nape — *see* Injury, neck
  nasal (septum) (sinus) S09.92 ☑
  nasopharynx S09.92 ☑
  neck S19.9 ☑
    specified NEC S19.80 ☑
      specified site NEC S19.89 ☑
  nerve NEC T14.8 ☑
    abdomen S34.9 ☑
      peripheral S34.6 ☑
      specified site NEC S34.8 ☑
    abducens S04.4- ☑
      contusion S04.4- ☑
      laceration S04.4- ☑
      specified type NEC S04.4- ☑
    abducent — *see* Injury, nerve, abducens
    accessory S04.7- ☑
      contusion S04.7- ☑
      laceration S04.7- ☑
      specified type NEC S04.7- ☑
    acoustic S04.6- ☑
      contusion S04.6- ☑
      laceration S04.6- ☑
      specified type NEC S04.6- ☑
    ankle S94.9- ☑
      cutaneous sensory S94.3- ☑
      specified site NEC — *see* subcategory S94.8 ☑
    anterior crural, femoral — *see* Injury, nerve, femoral
    arm (upper) S44.9- ☑
      axillary — *see* Injury, nerve, axillary
      cutaneous — *see* Injury, nerve, cutaneous, arm
      median — *see* Injury, nerve, median, upper arm
      musculocutaneous — *see* Injury, nerve, musculocutaneous
      radial — *see* Injury, nerve, radial, upper arm
      specified site NEC — *see* subcategory S44.8 ☑
      ulnar — *see* Injury, nerve, ulnar, arm
    auditory — *see* Injury, nerve, acoustic
    axillary S44.3- ☑
    brachial plexus — *see* Injury, brachial plexus
    cervical sympathetic S14.5 ☑
    cranial S04.9 ☑
      contusion S04.9 ☑
      eighth (acoustic or auditory) — *see* Injury, nerve, acoustic
      eleventh (accessory) — *see* Injury, nerve, accessory
      fifth (trigeminal) — *see* Injury, nerve, trigeminal
      first (olfactory) — *see* Injury, nerve, olfactory
      fourth (trochlear) — *see* Injury, nerve, trochlear
      laceration S04.9 ☑
      ninth (glossopharyngeal) — *see* Injury, nerve, glossopharyngeal
      second (optic) — *see* Injury, nerve, optic
      seventh (facial) — *see* Injury, nerve, facial
      sixth (abducent) — *see* Injury, nerve, abducens
      specified
        nerve NEC S04.89- ☑
          contusion S04.89- ☑
          laceration S04.89- ☑
          specified type NEC S04.89- ☑
        type NEC S04.9 ☑
      tenth (pneumogastric or vagus) — *see* Injury, nerve, vagus
      third (oculomotor) — *see* Injury, nerve, oculomotor
      twelfth (hypoglossal) — *see* Injury, nerve, hypoglossal
    cutaneous sensory
      ankle (level) S94.3- ☑
      arm (upper) (level) S44.5- ☑

Injury — *continued*
  nerve — *continued*
    cutaneous sensory — *continued*
      foot (level) — *see* Injury, nerve, cutaneous sensory, ankle
      forearm (level) S54.3- ☑
      hip (level) S74.2- ☑
      leg (lower level) S84.2- ☑
      shoulder (level) — *see* Injury, nerve, cutaneous sensory, arm
      thigh (level) — *see* Injury, nerve, cutaneous sensory, hip
    deep peroneal — *see* Injury, nerve, peroneal, foot
    digital
      finger S64.4- ☑
        index S64.49- ☑
        little S64.49- ☑
        middle S64.49- ☑
        ring S64.49- ☑
      thumb S64.3- ☑
      toe — *see* Injury, nerve, ankle, specified site NEC
    eighth cranial (acoustic or auditory) — *see* Injury, nerve, acoustic
    eleventh cranial (accessory) — *see* Injury, nerve, accessory
    facial S04.5- ☑
      contusion S04.5- ☑
      laceration S04.5- ☑
      newborn P11.3
      specified type NEC S04.5- ☑
    femoral (hip level) (thigh level) S74.1- ☑
    fifth cranial (trigeminal) — *see* Injury, nerve, trigeminal
    finger (digital) — *see* Injury, nerve, digital, finger
    first cranial (olfactory) — *see* Injury, nerve, olfactory
    foot S94.9- ☑
      cutaneous sensory S94.3- ☑
      deep peroneal S94.2- ☑
      lateral plantar S94.0- ☑
      medial plantar S94.1- ☑
      specified site NEC — *see* subcategory S94.8 ☑
    forearm (level) S54.9- ☑
      cutaneous sensory — *see* Injury, nerve, cutaneous sensory, forearm
      median — *see* Injury, nerve, median
      radial — *see* Injury, nerve, radial
      specified site NEC — *see* subcategory S54.8 ☑
      ulnar — *see* Injury, nerve, ulnar
    fourth cranial (trochlear) — *see* Injury, nerve, trochlear
    glossopharyngeal S04.89- ☑
      specified type NEC S04.89- ☑
    hand S64.9- ☑
      median — *see* Injury, nerve, median, hand
      radial — *see* Injury, nerve, radial, hand
      specified NEC — *see* subcategory S64.8 ☑
      ulnar — *see* Injury, nerve, ulnar, hand
    hip (level) S74.9- ☑
      cutaneous sensory — *see* Injury, nerve, cutaneous sensory, hip
      femoral — *see* Injury, nerve, femoral
      sciatic — *see* Injury, nerve, sciatic
      specified site NEC — *see* subcategory S74.8 ☑
    hypoglossal S04.89- ☑
      specified type NEC S04.89- ☑
    lateral plantar S94.0- ☑
    leg (lower) S84.9- ☑
      cutaneous sensory — *see* Injury, nerve, cutaneous sensory, leg
      peroneal — *see* Injury, nerve, peroneal
      specified site NEC — *see* subcategory S84.8 ☑
      tibial — *see* Injury, nerve, tibial
      upper — *see* Injury, nerve, thigh
    lower
      back — *see* Injury, nerve, abdomen, specified site NEC
        peripheral — *see* Injury, nerve, abdomen, peripheral
      limb — *see* Injury, nerve, leg
    lumbar plexus — *see* Injury, nerve, lumbosacral, sympathetic
    lumbar spinal — *see* Injury, nerve, spinal, lumbar
    lumbosacral
      plexus — *see* Injury, nerve, lumbosacral, sympathetic
      sympathetic S34.5 ☑

☑ Additional Character Required — Refer to the Tabular List for Character Selection   ▽ Subterms under main terms may continue to next column or page

Injury — *continued*
 nerve — *continued*
  medial plantar S94.1- ☑
  median (forearm level) S54.1- ☑
   hand (level) S64.1- ☑
   upper arm (level) S44.1- ☑
   wrist (level) — *see* Injury, nerve, median, hand
  musculocutaneous S44.4- ☑
  musculospiral (upper arm level) — *see* Injury, nerve, radial, upper arm
  neck S14.9 ☑
   peripheral S14.4 ☑
   specified site NEC S14.8 ☑
   sympathetic S14.5 ☑
  ninth cranial (glossopharyngeal) — *see* Injury, nerve, glossopharyngeal
  oculomotor S04.1- ☑
   contusion S04.1- ☑
   laceration S04.1- ☑
   specified type NEC S04.1- ☑
  olfactory S04.81- ☑
   specified type NEC S04.81- ☑
  optic S04.01- ☑
   contusion S04.01- ☑
   laceration S04.01- ☑
   specified type NEC S04.01- ☑
  pelvic girdle — *see* Injury, nerve, hip
  pelvis — *see* Injury, nerve, abdomen, specified site NEC
   peripheral — *see* Injury, nerve, abdomen, peripheral
  peripheral NEC T14.8 ☑
   abdomen — *see* Injury, nerve, abdomen, peripheral
   lower back — *see* Injury, nerve, abdomen, peripheral
   neck — *see* Injury, nerve, neck, peripheral
   pelvis — *see* Injury, nerve, abdomen, peripheral
   specified NEC T14.8 ☑
  peroneal (lower leg level) S84.1- ☑
   foot S94.2- ☑
  plexus
   brachial — *see* Injury, brachial plexus
   celiac, coeliac — *see* Injury, nerve, lumbosacral, sympathetic
   mesenteric, inferior — *see* Injury, nerve, lumbosacral, sympathetic
   sacral — *see* Injury, lumbosacral plexus
   spinal
    brachial — *see* Injury, brachial plexus
    lumbosacral — *see* Injury, lumbosacral plexus
  pneumogastric — *see* Injury, nerve, vagus
  radial (forearm level) S54.2- ☑
   hand (level) S64.2- ☑
   upper arm (level) S44.2- ☑
   wrist (level) — *see* Injury, nerve, radial, hand
  root — *see* Injury, nerve, spinal, root
  sacral plexus — *see* Injury, lumbosacral plexus
  sacral spinal — *see* Injury, nerve, spinal, sacral
  sciatic (hip level) (thigh level) S74.0- ☑
  second cranial (optic) — *see* Injury, nerve, optic
  seventh cranial (facial) — *see* Injury, nerve, facial
  shoulder — *see* Injury, nerve, arm
  sixth cranial (abducent) — *see* Injury, nerve, abducens
  spinal
   plexus — *see* Injury, nerve, plexus, spinal
   root
    cervical S14.2 ☑
    dorsal S24.2 ☑
    lumbar S34.21 ☑
    sacral S34.22 ☑
    thoracic — *see* Injury, nerve, spinal, root, dorsal
  splanchnic — *see* Injury, nerve, lumbosacral, sympathetic
  sympathetic NEC — *see* Injury, nerve, lumbosacral, sympathetic
   cervical — *see* Injury, nerve, cervical sympathetic
  tenth cranial (pneumogastric or vagus) — *see* Injury, nerve, vagus
  thigh (level) — *see* Injury, nerve, hip
   cutaneous sensory — *see* Injury, nerve, cutaneous sensory, hip
   femoral — *see* Injury, nerve, femoral
   sciatic — *see* Injury, nerve, sciatic

Injury — *continued*
 nerve — *continued*
  thigh — *see* Injury, nerve, hip — *continued*
   specified NEC — *see* Injury, nerve, hip
  third cranial (oculomotor) — *see* Injury, nerve, oculomotor
  thorax S24.9 ☑
   peripheral S24.3 ☑
   specified site NEC S24.8 ☑
   sympathetic S24.4 ☑
  thumb, digital — *see* Injury, nerve, digital, thumb
  tibial (lower leg level) (posterior) S84.0- ☑
  toe — *see* Injury, nerve, ankle
  trigeminal S04.3- ☑
   contusion S04.3- ☑
   laceration S04.3- ☑
   specified type NEC S04.3- ☑
  trochlear S04.2- ☑
   contusion S04.2- ☑
   laceration S04.2- ☑
   specified type NEC S04.2- ☑
  twelfth cranial (hypoglossal) — *see* Injury, nerve, hypoglossal
  ulnar (forearm level) S54.0- ☑
   arm (upper) (level) S44.0- ☑
   hand (level) S64.0- ☑
   wrist (level) — *see* Injury, nerve, ulnar, hand
  vagus S04.89- ☑
   specified type NEC S04.89- ☑
  wrist (level) — *see* Injury, nerve, hand
 ninth cranial nerve (glossopharyngeal) — *see* Injury, nerve, glossopharyngeal
 nose (septum) S09.92 ☑
 obstetrical O71.9
  specified NEC O71.89
 occipital (region) (scalp) S09.90 ☑
  lobe — *see* Injury, intracranial
 optic chiasm S04.02 ☑
 optic radiation S04.03- ☑
 optic tract and pathways S04.03- ☑
 orbit, orbital (region) — *see* Injury, eye
  penetrating (with foreign body) — *see* Injury, eye, orbit, penetrating
  specified NEC — *see* Injury, eye, specified site NEC
 ovary, ovarian S37.409 ☑
  bilateral S37.402 ☑
   contusion S37.422 ☑
   laceration S37.432 ☑
   specified type NEC S37.492 ☑
  blood vessel — *see* Injury, blood vessel, ovarian
  contusion S37.429 ☑
   bilateral S37.422 ☑
   unilateral S37.421 ☑
  laceration S37.439 ☑
   bilateral S37.432 ☑
   unilateral S37.431 ☑
  specified type NEC S37.499 ☑
   bilateral S37.492 ☑
   unilateral S37.491 ☑
  unilateral S37.401 ☑
   contusion S37.421 ☑
   laceration S37.431 ☑
   specified type NEC S37.491 ☑
 palate (hard) (soft) S09.93 ☑
 pancreas S36.209 ☑
  body S36.201 ☑
   contusion S36.221 ☑
   laceration S36.231 ☑
    major S36.261 ☑
    minor S36.241 ☑
    moderate S36.251 ☑
   specified type NEC S36.291 ☑
  contusion S36.229 ☑
  head S36.200 ☑
   contusion S36.220 ☑
   laceration S36.230 ☑
    major S36.260 ☑
    minor S36.240 ☑
    moderate S36.250 ☑
   specified type NEC S36.290 ☑
  laceration S36.239 ☑
   major S36.269 ☑
   minor S36.249 ☑
   moderate S36.259 ☑
  specified type NEC S36.299 ☑
  tail S36.202 ☑

Injury — *continued*
 pancreas — *continued*
  tail — *continued*
   contusion S36.222 ☑
   laceration S36.232 ☑
    major S36.262 ☑
    minor S36.242 ☑
    moderate S36.252 ☑
   specified type NEC S36.292 ☑
 parietal (region) (scalp) S09.90 ☑
  lobe — *see* Injury, intracranial
 patellar ligament (tendon) S76.10- ☑
  laceration S76.12- ☑
  specified NEC S76.19- ☑
  strain S76.11- ☑
 pelvis, pelvic (floor) S39.93 ☑
  complicating delivery O70.1
  joint or ligament, complicating delivery O71.6
  organ S37.90 ☑
   with ectopic or molar pregnancy O08.6
   complication of abortion — *see* Abortion
   contusion S37.92 ☑
   following ectopic or molar pregnancy O08.6
   laceration S37.93 ☑
   obstetrical trauma NEC O71.5
   specified
    site NEC S37.899 ☑
     contusion S37.892 ☑
     laceration S37.893 ☑
     specified type NEC S37.898 ☑
    type NEC S37.99 ☑
  specified NEC S39.83 ☑
 penis S39.94 ☑
 perineum S39.94 ☑
 peritoneum S36.81 ☑
  laceration S36.893 ☑
 periurethral tissue — *see* Injury, urethra
  complicating delivery O71.82
 phalanges
  foot — *see* Injury, foot
  hand — *see* Injury, hand
 pharynx NEC S19.85 ☑
 pleura — *see* Injury, intrathoracic, pleura
 plexus
  brachial — *see* Injury, brachial plexus
  cardiac — *see* Injury, nerve, thorax, sympathetic
  celiac, coeliac — *see* Injury, nerve, lumbosacral, sympathetic
  esophageal — *see* Injury, nerve, thorax, sympathetic
  hypogastric — *see* Injury, nerve, lumbosacral, sympathetic
  lumbar, lumbosacral — *see* Injury, lumbosacral plexus
  mesenteric — *see* Injury, nerve, lumbosacral, sympathetic
  pulmonary — *see* Injury, nerve, thorax, sympathetic
 postcardiac surgery (syndrome) I97.0
 prepuce S39.94 ☑
 pressure
  injury — *see* Ulcer, pressure, by site
 prostate S37.829 ☑
  contusion S37.822 ☑
  laceration S37.823 ☑
  specified type NEC S37.828 ☑
 pubic region S39.94 ☑
 pudendum S39.94 ☑
 pulmonary plexus — *see* Injury, nerve, thorax, sympathetic
 rectovaginal septum NEC S39.83 ☑
 rectum — *see* Injury, intestine, large, rectum
 retina — *see* Injury, eye, specified site NEC
  penetrating — *see* Injury, eyeball, penetrating
 retroperitoneal — *see* Injury, intra-abdominal, specified site NEC
 rotator cuff (muscle(s)) (tendon(s)) S46.00- ☑
  laceration S46.02- ☑
  specified type NEC S46.09- ☑
  strain S46.01- ☑
 round ligament — *see* Injury, pelvic organ, specified site NEC
 sacral plexus — *see* Injury, lumbosacral plexus
 salivary duct or gland S09.93 ☑
 scalp S09.90 ☑
  newborn (birth injury) P12.9
   due to monitoring (electrode) (sampling incision) P12.4

🐦 Subterms under main terms may continue to next column or page   ☑ **Additional Character Required** — Refer to the Tabular List for Character Selection   **197**

Injury — Injury

Injury — *continued*
  scalp — *continued*
    newborn — *continued*
      specified NEC P12.89
        caput succedaneum P12.81
  scapular region — *see* Injury, shoulder
  sclera — *see* Injury, eye, specified site NEC
    penetrating — *see* Injury, eyeball, penetrating
  scrotum S39.94 ☑
  second cranial nerve (optic) — *see* Injury, nerve, optic
  seminal vesicle — *see* Injury, pelvic organ, specified
    site NEC
  seventh cranial nerve (facial) — *see* Injury, nerve, facial
  shoulder S49.9- ☑
    blood vessel — *see* Injury, blood vessel, arm
    contusion — *see* Contusion, shoulder
    dislocation — *see* Dislocation, shoulder
    fracture — *see* Fracture, shoulder
    muscle — *see* Injury, muscle, shoulder
    nerve — *see* Injury, nerve, shoulder
    open — *see* Wound, open, shoulder
    specified type NEC S49.8- ☑
    sprain — *see* Sprain, shoulder girdle
    superficial — *see* Injury, superficial, shoulder
  sinus
    cavernous — *see* Injury, intracranial
    nasal S09.92 ☑
  sixth cranial nerve (abducent) — *see* Injury, nerve, abducens
  skeleton, birth injury P13.9
    specified part NEC P13.8
  skin NEC T14.8 ☑
    surface intact — *see* Injury, superficial
  skull NEC S09.90 ☑
  specified NEC T14.8 ☑
  spermatic cord (pelvic region) S37.898 ☑
    scrotal region S39.848 ☑
  spinal (cord)
    cervical (neck) S14.109 ☑
      anterior cord syndrome S14.139 ☑
        C1 level S14.131 ☑
        C2 level S14.132 ☑
        C3 level S14.133 ☑
        C4 level S14.134 ☑
        C5 level S14.135 ☑
        C6 level S14.136 ☑
        C7 level S14.137 ☑
        C8 level S14.138 ☑
      Brown-Séquard syndrome S14.149 ☑
        C1 level S14.141 ☑
        C2 level S14.142 ☑
        C3 level S14.143 ☑
        C4 level S14.144 ☑
        C5 level S14.145 ☑
        C6 level S14.146 ☑
        C7 level S14.147 ☑
        C8 level S14.148 ☑
      C1 level S14.101 ☑
      C2 level S14.102 ☑
      C3 level S14.103 ☑
      C4 level S14.104 ☑
      C5 level S14.105 ☑
      C6 level S14.106 ☑
      C7 level S14.107 ☑
      C8 level S14.108 ☑
      central cord syndrome S14.129 ☑
        C1 level S14.121 ☑
        C2 level S14.122 ☑
        C3 level S14.123 ☑
        C4 level S14.124 ☑
        C5 level S14.125 ☑
        C6 level S14.126 ☑
        C7 level S14.127 ☑
        C8 level S14.128 ☑
      complete lesion S14.119 ☑
        C1 level S14.111 ☑
        C2 level S14.112 ☑
        C3 level S14.113 ☑
        C4 level S14.114 ☑
        C5 level S14.115 ☑
        C6 level S14.116 ☑
        C7 level S14.117 ☑
        C8 level S14.118 ☑
      concussion S14.0 ☑
      edema S14.0 ☑
      incomplete lesion specified NEC S14.159 ☑

Injury — *continued*
  spinal — *continued*
    cervical — *continued*
      incomplete lesion specified — *continued*
        C1 level S14.151 ☑
        C2 level S14.152 ☑
        C3 level S14.153 ☑
        C4 level S14.154 ☑
        C5 level S14.155 ☑
        C6 level S14.156 ☑
        C7 level S14.157 ☑
        C8 level S14.158 ☑
      posterior cord syndrome S14.159 ☑
        C1 level S14.151 ☑
        C2 level S14.152 ☑
        C3 level S14.153 ☑
        C4 level S14.154 ☑
        C5 level S14.155 ☑
        C6 level S14.156 ☑
        C7 level S14.157 ☑
        C8 level S14.158 ☑
    dorsal — *see* Injury, spinal, thoracic
    lumbar S34.109 ☑
      complete lesion S34.119 ☑
        L1 level S34.111 ☑
        L2 level S34.112 ☑
        L3 level S34.113 ☑
        L4 level S34.114 ☑
        L5 level S34.115 ☑
      concussion S34.01 ☑
      edema S34.01 ☑
      incomplete lesion S34.129 ☑
        L1 level S34.121 ☑
        L2 level S34.122 ☑
        L3 level S34.123 ☑
        L4 level S34.124 ☑
        L5 level S34.125 ☑
      L1 level S34.101 ☑
      L2 level S34.102 ☑
      L3 level S34.103 ☑
      L4 level S34.104 ☑
      L5 level S34.105 ☑
    nerve root NEC
      cervical — *see* Injury, nerve, spinal, root, cervical
      dorsal — *see* Injury, nerve, spinal, root, dorsal
      lumbar S34.21 ☑
      sacral S34.22 ☑
      thoracic — *see* Injury, nerve, spinal, root, dorsal
    plexus
      brachial — *see* Injury, brachial plexus
      lumbosacral — *see* Injury, lumbosacral plexus
    sacral S34.139 ☑
      complete lesion S34.131 ☑
      incomplete lesion S34.132 ☑
    thoracic S24.109 ☑
      anterior cord syndrome S24.139 ☑
        T1 level S24.131 ☑
        T2-T6 level S24.132 ☑
        T7-T10 level S24.133 ☑
        T11-T12 level S24.134 ☑
      Brown-Séquard syndrome S24.149 ☑
        T1 level S24.141 ☑
        T2-T6 level S24.142 ☑
        T7-T10 level S24.143 ☑
        T11-T12 level S24.144 ☑
      complete lesion S24.119 ☑
        T1 level S24.111 ☑
        T2-T6 level S24.112 ☑
        T7-T10 level S24.113 ☑
        T11-T12 level S24.114 ☑
      concussion S24.0 ☑
      edema S24.0 ☑
      incomplete lesion specified NEC S24.159 ☑
        T1 level S24.151 ☑
        T2-T6 level S24.152 ☑
        T7-T10 level S24.153 ☑
        T11-T12 level S24.154 ☑
      posterior cord syndrome S24.159 ☑
        T1 level S24.151 ☑
        T2-T6 level S24.152 ☑
        T7-T10 level S24.153 ☑
        T11-T12 level S24.154 ☑
      T1 level S24.101 ☑
      T2-T6 level S24.102 ☑
      T7-T10 level S24.103 ☑
      T11-T12 level S24.104 ☑

Injury — *continued*
  splanchnic nerve — *see* Injury, nerve, lumbosacral, sympathetic
  spleen S36.00 ☑
    contusion S36.029 ☑
      major S36.021 ☑
      minor S36.020 ☑
    laceration S36.039 ☑
      major (massive) (stellate) S36.032 ☑
      moderate S36.031 ☑
      superficial (capsular) (minor) S36.030 ☑
    specified type NEC S36.09 ☑
  splenic artery — *see* Injury, blood vessel, celiac artery, branch
  stellate ganglion — *see* Injury, nerve, thorax, sympathetic
  sternal region S29.9 ☑
  stomach S36.30 ☑
    contusion S36.32 ☑
    laceration S36.33 ☑
    specified type NEC S36.39 ☑
  subconjunctival — *see* Injury, eye, conjunctiva
  subcutaneous NEC T14.8 ☑
  submaxillary region S09.93 ☑
  submental region S09.93 ☑
  subungual
    fingers — *see* Injury, hand
    toes — *see* Injury, foot
  superficial NEC T14.8 ☑
    abdomen, abdominal (wall) S30.92 ☑
      abrasion S30.811 ☑
      bite S30.871 ☑
        insect S30.861 ☑
      contusion S30.1 ☑
      external constriction S30.841 ☑
      foreign body S30.851 ☑
    abrasion — *see* Abrasion, by site
    adnexa, eye NEC — *see* Injury, eye, specified site NEC
    alveolar process — *see* Injury, superficial, oral cavity
    ankle S90.91- ☑
      abrasion — *see* Abrasion, ankle
      bite — *see* Bite, ankle
      blister — *see* Blister, ankle
      contusion — *see* Contusion, ankle
      external constriction — *see* Constriction, external, ankle
      foreign body — *see* Foreign body, superficial, ankle
    anus S30.98 ☑
    arm (upper) S40.92- ☑
      abrasion — *see* Abrasion, arm
      bite — *see* Bite, superficial, arm
      blister — *see* Blister, arm (upper)
      contusion — *see* Contusion, arm
      external constriction — *see* Constriction, external, arm
      foreign body — *see* Foreign body, superficial, arm
    auditory canal (external) (meatus) — *see* Injury, superficial, ear
    auricle — *see* Injury, superficial, ear
    axilla — *see* Injury, superficial, arm
    back — *see also* Injury, superficial, thorax, back
      lower S30.91 ☑
        abrasion S30.810 ☑
        contusion S30.0 ☑
        external constriction S30.840 ☑
        superficial
          bite NEC S30.870 ☑
            insect S30.860 ☑
          foreign body S30.850 ☑
    bite NEC — *see* Bite, superficial NEC, by site
    blister — *see* Blister, by site
    breast S20.10- ☑
      abrasion — *see* Abrasion, breast
      bite — *see* Bite, superficial, breast
      contusion — *see* Contusion, breast
      external constriction — *see* Constriction, external, breast
      foreign body — *see* Foreign body, superficial, breast
    brow — *see* Injury, superficial, head, specified NEC
    buttock S30.91 ☑
    calf — *see* Injury, superficial, leg

Injury — *continued*
  superficial — *continued*
    canthus, eye — *see* Injury, superficial, periocular area
    cheek (external) — *see* Injury, superficial, head, specified NEC
      internal — *see* Injury, superficial, oral cavity
    chest wall — *see* Injury, superficial, thorax
    chin — *see* Injury, superficial, head NEC
    clitoris S30.95 ☑
    conjunctiva — *see* Injury, eye, conjunctiva
      with foreign body (in conjunctival sac) — *see* Foreign body, conjunctival sac
    contusion — *see* Contusion, by site
    costal region — *see* Injury, superficial, thorax
    digit(s)
      hand — *see* Injury, superficial, finger
    ear (auricle) (canal) (external) S00.40- ☑
      abrasion — *see* Abrasion, ear
      bite — *see* Bite, superficial, ear
      contusion — *see* Contusion, ear
      external constriction — *see* Constriction, external, ear
      foreign body — *see* Foreign body, superficial, ear
    elbow S50.90- ☑
      abrasion — *see* Abrasion, elbow
      bite — *see* Bite, superficial, elbow
      blister — *see* Blister, elbow
      contusion — *see* Contusion, elbow
      external constriction — *see* Constriction, external, elbow
      foreign body — *see* Foreign body, superficial, elbow
    epididymis S30.94 ☑
    epigastric region S30.92 ☑
    epiglottis — *see* Injury, superficial, throat
    esophagus
      cervical — *see* Injury, superficial, throat
    external constriction — *see* Constriction, external, by site
    extremity NEC T14.8 ☑
    eyeball NEC — *see* Injury, eye, specified site NEC
    eyebrow — *see* Injury, superficial, periocular area
    eyelid S00.20- ☑
      abrasion — *see* Abrasion, eyelid
      bite — *see* Bite, superficial, eyelid
      contusion — *see* Contusion, eyelid
      external constriction — *see* Constriction, external, eyelid
      foreign body — *see* Foreign body, superficial, eyelid
    face NEC — *see* Injury, superficial, head, specified NEC
    finger(s) S60.949 ☑
      abrasion — *see* Abrasion, finger
      bite — *see* Bite, superficial, finger
      blister — *see* Blister, finger
      contusion — *see* Contusion, finger
      external constriction — *see* Constriction, external, finger
      foreign body — *see* Foreign body, superficial, finger
      index S60.94- ☑
      insect bite — *see* Bite, by site, superficial, insect
      little S60.94- ☑
      middle S60.94- ☑
      ring S60.94- ☑
    flank S30.92 ☑
    foot S90.92- ☑
      abrasion — *see* Abrasion, foot
      bite — *see* Bite, foot
      blister — *see* Blister, foot
      contusion — *see* Contusion, foot
      external constriction — *see* Constriction, external, foot
      foreign body — *see* Foreign body, superficial, foot
    forearm S50.91- ☑
      abrasion — *see* Abrasion, forearm
      bite — *see* Bite, forearm, superficial
      blister — *see* Blister, forearm
      contusion — *see* Contusion, forearm
      elbow only — *see* Injury, superficial, elbow
      external constriction — *see* Constriction, external, forearm

Injury — *continued*
  superficial — *continued*
    forearm — *continued*
      foreign body — *see* Foreign body, superficial, forearm
    forehead — *see* Injury, superficial, head NEC
    foreign body — *see* Foreign body, superficial
    genital organs, external
      female S30.97 ☑
      male S30.96 ☑
    globe (eye) — *see* Injury, eye, specified site NEC
    groin S30.92 ☑
    gum — *see* Injury, superficial, oral cavity
    hand S60.92- ☑
      abrasion — *see* Abrasion, hand
      bite — *see* Bite, superficial, hand
      contusion — *see* Contusion, hand
      external constriction — *see* Constriction, external, hand
      foreign body — *see* Foreign body, superficial, hand
    head S00.90 ☑
      ear — *see* Injury, superficial, ear
      eyelid — *see* Injury, superficial, eyelid
      nose S00.30 ☑
      oral cavity S00.502 ☑
      scalp S00.00 ☑
      specified site NEC S00.80 ☑
    heel — *see* Injury, superficial, foot
    hip S70.91- ☑
      abrasion — *see* Abrasion, hip
      bite — *see* Bite, superficial, hip
      blister — *see* Blister, hip
      contusion — *see* Contusion, hip
      external constriction — *see* Constriction, external, hip
      foreign body — *see* Foreign body, superficial, hip
    iliac region — *see* Injury, superficial, abdomen
    inguinal region — *see* Injury, superficial, abdomen
    insect bite — *see* Bite, by site, superficial, insect
    interscapular region — *see* Injury, superficial, thorax, back
    jaw — *see* Injury, superficial, head, specified NEC
    knee S80.91- ☑
      abrasion — *see* Abrasion, knee
      bite — *see* Bite, superficial, knee
      blister — *see* Blister, knee
      contusion — *see* Contusion, knee
      external constriction — *see* Constriction, external, knee
      foreign body — *see* Foreign body, superficial, knee
    labium (majus) (minus) S30.95 ☑
    lacrimal (apparatus) (gland) (sac) — *see* Injury, eye, specified site NEC
    larynx — *see* Injury, superficial, throat
    leg (lower) S80.92- ☑
      abrasion — *see* Abrasion, leg
      bite — *see* Bite, superficial, leg
      contusion — *see* Contusion, leg
      external constriction — *see* Constriction, external, leg
      foreign body — *see* Foreign body, superficial, leg
      knee — *see* Injury, superficial, knee
    limb NEC T14.8 ☑
    lip S00.501 ☑
    lower back S30.91 ☑
    lumbar region S30.91 ☑
    malar region — *see* Injury, superficial, head, specified NEC
    mammary — *see* Injury, superficial, breast
    mastoid region — *see* Injury, superficial, head, specified NEC
    mouth — *see* Injury, superficial, oral cavity
    muscle NEC T14.8 ☑
    nail NEC T14.8 ☑
      finger — *see* Injury, superficial, finger
      toe — *see* Injury, superficial, toe
    nasal (septum) — *see* Injury, superficial, nose
    neck S10.90 ☑
      specified site NEC S10.80 ☑
    nose (septum) S00.30 ☑
    occipital region — *see* Injury, superficial, scalp
    oral cavity S00.502 ☑

Injury — *continued*
  superficial — *continued*
    orbital region — *see* Injury, superficial, periocular area
    palate — *see* Injury, superficial, oral cavity
    palm — *see* Injury, superficial, hand
    parietal region — *see* Injury, superficial, scalp
    pelvis S30.91 ☑
      girdle — *see* Injury, superficial, hip
    penis S30.93 ☑
    perineum
      female S30.95 ☑
      male S30.91 ☑
    periocular area S00.20- ☑
      abrasion — *see* Abrasion, eyelid
      bite — *see* Bite, superficial, eyelid
      contusion — *see* Contusion, eyelid
      external constriction — *see* Constriction, external, eyelid
      foreign body — *see* Foreign body, superficial, eyelid
    phalanges
      finger — *see* Injury, superficial, finger
      toe — *see* Injury, superficial, toe
    pharynx — *see* Injury, superficial, throat
    pinna — *see* Injury, superficial, ear
    popliteal space — *see* Injury, superficial, knee
    prepuce S30.93 ☑
    pubic region S30.91 ☑
    pudendum
      female S30.97 ☑
      male S30.96 ☑
    sacral region S30.91 ☑
    scalp S00.00 ☑
    scapular region — *see* Injury, superficial, shoulder
    sclera — *see* Injury, eye, specified site NEC
    scrotum S30.94 ☑
    shin — *see* Injury, superficial, leg
    shoulder S40.91- ☑
      abrasion — *see* Abrasion, shoulder
      bite — *see* Bite, superficial, shoulder
      blister — *see* Blister, shoulder
      contusion — *see* Contusion, shoulder
      external constriction — *see* Constriction, external, shoulder
      foreign body — *see* Foreign body, superficial, shoulder
    skin NEC T14.8 ☑
    sternal region — *see* Injury, superficial, thorax, front
    subconjunctival — *see* Injury, eye, specified site NEC
    subcutaneous NEC T14.8 ☑
    submaxillary region — *see* Injury, superficial, head, specified NEC
    submental region — *see* Injury, superficial, head, specified NEC
    subungual
      finger(s) — *see* Injury, superficial, finger
      toe(s) — *see* Injury, superficial, toe
    supraclavicular fossa — *see* Injury, superficial, neck
    supraorbital — *see* Injury, superficial, head, specified NEC
    temple — *see* Injury, superficial, head, specified NEC
    temporal region — *see* Injury, superficial, head, specified NEC
    testis S30.94 ☑
    thigh S70.92- ☑
      abrasion — *see* Abrasion, thigh
      bite — *see* Bite, superficial, thigh
      blister — *see* Blister, thigh
      contusion — *see* Contusion, thigh
      external constriction — *see* Constriction, external, thigh
      foreign body — *see* Foreign body, superficial, thigh
    thorax, thoracic (wall) S20.90 ☑
      abrasion — *see* Abrasion, thorax
      back S20.40- ☑
      bite — *see* Bite, thorax, superficial
      blister — *see* Blister, thorax
      contusion — *see* Contusion, thorax
      external constriction — *see* Constriction, external, thorax
      foreign body — *see* Foreign body, superficial, thorax
      front S20.30- ☑
    throat S10.10 ☑

Injury — *continued*
  superficial — *continued*
    throat — *continued*
      abrasion S10.11 ☑
      bite S10.17 ☑
        insect S10.16 ☑
      blister S10.12 ☑
      contusion S10.0 ☑
      external constriction S10.14 ☑
      foreign body S10.15 ☑
    thumb S60.93- ☑
      abrasion — *see* Abrasion, thumb
      bite — *see* Bite, superficial, thumb
      blister — *see* Blister, thumb
      contusion — *see* Contusion, thumb
      external constriction — *see* Constriction, external, thumb
      foreign body — *see* Foreign body, superficial, thumb
      insect bite — *see* Bite, by site, superficial, insect
      specified type NEC S60.39 ☑
    toe(s) S90.93- ☑
      abrasion — *see* Abrasion, toe
      bite — *see* Bite, toe
      blister — *see* Blister, toe
      contusion — *see* Contusion, toe
      external constriction — *see* Constriction, external, toe
      foreign body — *see* Foreign body, superficial, toe
      great S90.93- ☑
    tongue — *see* Injury, superficial, oral cavity
    tooth, teeth — *see* Injury, superficial, oral cavity
    trachea S10.10 ☑
    tunica vaginalis S30.94 ☑
    tympanum, tympanic membrane — *see* Injury, superficial, ear
    uvula — *see* Injury, superficial, oral cavity
    vagina S30.95 ☑
    vocal cords — *see* Injury, superficial, throat
    vulva S30.95 ☑
    wrist S60.91- ☑
  supraclavicular region — *see* Injury, neck
  supraorbital S09.93 ☑
  suprarenal gland (multiple) — *see* Injury, adrenal
  surgical complication (external or internal site) — *see* Laceration, accidental complicating surgery
  temple S09.90 ☑
  temporal region S09.90 ☑
  tendon — *see also* Injury, muscle, by site
    abdomen — *see* Injury, muscle, abdomen
    Achilles — *see* Injury, Achilles tendon
    lower back — *see* Injury, muscle, lower back
    pelvic organs — *see* Injury, muscle, pelvis
  tenth cranial nerve (pneumogastric or vagus) — *see* Injury, nerve, vagus
  testis S39.94 ☑
  thigh S79.92- ☑
    blood vessel — *see* Injury, blood vessel, hip
    contusion — *see* Contusion, thigh
    fracture — *see* Fracture, femur
    muscle — *see* Injury, muscle, thigh
    nerve — *see* Injury, nerve, thigh
    open — *see* Wound, open, thigh
    specified NEC S79.82- ☑
    superficial — *see* Injury, superficial, thigh
  third cranial nerve (oculomotor) — *see* Injury, nerve, oculomotor
  thorax, thoracic S29.9 ☑
    blood vessel — *see* Injury, blood vessel, thorax
    cavity — *see* Injury, intrathoracic
    dislocation — *see* Dislocation, thorax
    external (wall) S29.9 ☑
      contusion — *see* Contusion, thorax
      nerve — *see* Injury, nerve, thorax
      open — *see* Wound, open, thorax
      specified NEC S29.8 ☑
    sprain — *see* Sprain, thorax
    superficial — *see* Injury, superficial, thorax
    fracture — *see* Fracture, thorax
    internal — *see* Injury, intrathoracic
    intrathoracic organ — *see* Injury, intrathoracic
    sympathetic ganglion — *see* Injury, nerve, thorax, sympathetic
  throat — *see also* Injury, neck S19.9 ☑
  thumb S69.9- ☑

Injury — *continued*
  thumb — *continued*
    blood vessel — *see* Injury, blood vessel, thumb
    contusion — *see* Contusion, thumb
    dislocation — *see* Dislocation, thumb
    fracture — *see* Fracture, thumb
    muscle — *see* Injury, muscle, thumb
    nerve — *see* Injury, nerve, digital, thumb
    open — *see* Wound, open, thumb
    specified NEC S69.8- ☑
    sprain — *see* Sprain, thumb
    superficial — *see* Injury, superficial, thumb
  thymus (gland) — *see* Injury, intrathoracic, specified organ NEC
  thyroid (gland) NEC S19.84 ☑
  toe S99.92- ☑
    contusion — *see* Contusion, toe
    dislocation — *see* Dislocation, toe
    fracture — *see* Fracture, toe
    muscle — *see* Injury, muscle, toe
    open — *see* Wound, open, toe
    specified type NEC S99.82- ☑
    sprain — *see* Sprain, toe
    superficial — *see* Injury, superficial, toe
  tongue S09.93 ☑
  tonsil S09.93 ☑
  tooth S09.93 ☑
  trachea (cervical) NEC S19.82 ☑
    thoracic — *see* Injury, intrathoracic, trachea, thoracic
  transfusion-related acute lung (TRALI) J95.84
  tunica vaginalis S39.94 ☑
  twelfth cranial nerve (hypoglossal) — *see* Injury, nerve, hypoglossal
  ureter S37.10 ☑
    contusion S37.12 ☑
    laceration S37.13 ☑
    specified type NEC S37.19 ☑
  urethra (sphincter) S37.30 ☑
    at delivery O71.5
    contusion S37.32 ☑
    laceration S37.33 ☑
    specified type NEC S37.39 ☑
  urinary organ S37.90 ☑
    contusion S37.92 ☑
    laceration S37.93 ☑
    specified
      site NEC S37.899 ☑
        contusion S37.892 ☑
        laceration S37.893 ☑
        specified type NEC S37.898 ☑
      type NEC S37.99 ☑
  uterus, uterine S37.60 ☑
    with ectopic or molar pregnancy O08.6
    blood vessel — *see* Injury, blood vessel, iliac
    contusion S37.62 ☑
    laceration S37.63 ☑
      cervix at delivery O71.3
    rupture associated with obstetrics — *see* Rupture, uterus
    specified type NEC S37.69 ☑
  uvula S09.93 ☑
  vagina S39.93 ☑
    abrasion S30.814 ☑
    bite S31.45 ☑
      insect S30.864 ☑
      superficial NEC S30.874 ☑
    contusion S30.23 ☑
    crush S38.03 ☑
    during delivery — *see* Laceration, vagina, during delivery
    external constriction S30.844 ☑
    insect bite S30.864 ☑
    laceration S31.41 ☑
      with foreign body S31.42 ☑
    open wound S31.40 ☑
    puncture S31.43 ☑
      with foreign body S31.44 ☑
    superficial S30.95 ☑
      foreign body S30.854 ☑
  vas deferens — *see* Injury, pelvic organ, specified site NEC
  vascular NEC T14.8 ☑
  vein — *see* Injury, blood vessel
  vena cava (superior) S25.20 ☑
    inferior S35.10 ☑
      laceration (minor) (superficial) S35.11 ☑

Injury — *continued*
  vena cava — *continued*
    inferior — *continued*
      laceration — *continued*
        major S35.12 ☑
        specified type NEC S35.19 ☑
      laceration (minor) (superficial) S25.21 ☑
        major S25.22 ☑
        specified type NEC S25.29 ☑
  vesical (sphincter) — *see* Injury, bladder
  visual cortex S04.04- ☑
  vitreous (humor) S05.90 ☑
    specified NEC S05.8X- ☑
  vocal cord NEC S19.83 ☑
  vulva S39.94 ☑
    abrasion S30.814 ☑
    bite S31.45 ☑
      insect S30.864 ☑
      superficial NEC S30.874 ☑
    contusion S30.23 ☑
    crush S38.03 ☑
    during delivery — *see* Laceration, perineum, female, during delivery
    external constriction S30.844 ☑
    insect bite S30.864 ☑
    laceration S31.41 ☑
      with foreign body S31.42 ☑
    open wound S31.40 ☑
    puncture S31.43 ☑
      with foreign body S31.44 ☑
    superficial S30.95 ☑
      foreign body S30.854 ☑
  whiplash (cervical spine) S13.4 ☑
  wrist S69.9- ☑
    blood vessel — *see* Injury, blood vessel, hand
    contusion — *see* Contusion, wrist
    dislocation — *see* Dislocation, wrist
    fracture — *see* Fracture, wrist
    muscle — *see* Injury, muscle, hand
    nerve — *see* Injury, nerve, hand
    open — *see* Wound, open, wrist
    specified NEC S69.8- ☑
    sprain — *see* Sprain, wrist
    superficial — *see* Injury, superficial, wrist
Inoculation — *see also* Vaccination
  complication or reaction — *see* Complications, vaccination
Insanity, insane — *see also* Psychosis
  adolescent — *see* Schizophrenia
  confusional F28
    acute or subacute F05
  delusional F22
  senile F03 ☑
Insect
  bite — *see* Bite, by site, superficial, insect
  venomous, poisoning NEC (by) — *see* Venom, arthropod
Insensitivity
  adrenocorticotropin hormone (ACTH) E27.49
  androgen E34.50
    complete E34.51
    partial E34.52
Insertion
  cord (umbilical) lateral or velamentous O43.12- ☑
  intrauterine contraceptive device (encounter for) — *see* Intrauterine contraceptive device
Insolation (sunstroke) T67.01 ☑
Insomnia (organic) G47.00
  adjustment F51.02
  adjustment disorder F51.02
  behavioral, of childhood Z73.819
    combined type Z73.812
    limit setting type Z73.811
    sleep-onset association type Z73.810
  childhood Z73.819
  chronic F51.04
    somatized tension F51.04
  conditioned F51.04
  due to
    alcohol
      abuse F10.182
      dependence F10.282
      use F10.982
    amphetamines
      abuse F15.182
      dependence F15.282
      use F15.982

☑ **Additional Character Required — Refer to the Tabular List for Character Selection**   ▼ **Subterms under main terms may continue to next column or page**

Insomnia — *continued*
  due to — *continued*
    anxiety disorder F51.05
    caffeine
      abuse F15.182
      dependence F15.282
      use F15.982
    cocaine
      abuse F14.182
      dependence F14.282
      use F14.982
    depression F51.05
    drug NEC
      abuse F19.182
      dependence F19.282
      use F19.982
    medical condition G47.01
    mental disorder NEC F51.05
    opioid
      abuse F11.182
      dependence F11.282
      use F11.982
    psychoactive substance NEC
      abuse F19.182
      dependence F19.182
      use F19.982
    sedative, hypnotic, or anxiolytic
      abuse F13.182
      dependence F13.282
      use F13.982
    stimulant NEC
      abuse F15.182
      dependence F15.282
      use F15.982
  fatal familial (FFI) A81.83
  idiopathic F51.01
  learned F51.3
  nonorganic origin F51.01
  not due to a substance or known physiological condition F51.01
    specified NEC F51.09
  paradoxical F51.03
  primary F51.01
  psychiatric F51.05
  psychophysiologic F51.04
  related to psychopathology F51.05
  short-term F51.02
  specified NEC G47.09
  stress-related F51.02
  transient F51.02
  without objective findings F51.02
Inspiration
  food or foreign body — *see* Foreign body, by site
  mucus — *see* Asphyxia, mucus
Inspissated bile syndrome (newborn) P59.1
Instability
  emotional (excessive) F60.3
  joint (post-traumatic) M25.30
    ankle M25.37- ☑
    due to old ligament injury — *see* Disorder, ligament
    elbow M25.32- ☑
    flail — *see* Flail, joint
    foot M25.37- ☑
    hand M25.34- ☑
    hip M25.35- ☑
    knee M25.36- ☑
    lumbosacral — *see* subcategory M53.2 ☑
    prosthesis — *see* Complications, joint prosthesis, mechanical, displacement, by site
    sacroiliac — *see* subcategory M53.2 ☑
    secondary to
      old ligament injury — *see* Disorder, ligament
      removal of joint prosthesis M96.89
    shoulder (region) M25.31- ☑
    spine — *see* subcategory M53.2 ☑
    wrist M25.33- ☑
  knee (chronic) M23.5- ☑
  lumbosacral — *see* subcategory M53.2 ☑
  nervous F48.8
  personality (emotional) F60.3
  spine — *see* Instability, joint, spine
  vasomotor R55
Institutional syndrome (childhood) F94.2
Institutionalization, affecting child Z62.22
  disinhibited attachment F94.2
Insufficiency, insufficient
  accommodation, old age H52.4
  adrenal (gland) E27.40

Insufficiency, insufficient — *continued*
  adrenal — *continued*
    primary E27.1
  adrenocortical E27.40
    drug-induced E27.3
    iatrogenic E27.3
    primary E27.1
  anatomic crown height K08.89
  anterior (occlusal) guidance M26.54
  anus K62.89
  aortic (valve) I35.1
    with
      mitral (valve) disease I08.0
        with tricuspid (valve) disease I08.3
      stenosis I35.2
      tricuspid (valve) disease I08.2
        with mitral (valve) disease I08.3
    congenital Q23.1
    rheumatic I06.1
      with
        mitral (valve) disease I08.0
          with tricuspid (valve) disease I08.3
        stenosis I06.2
          with mitral (valve) disease I08.0
            with tricuspid (valve) disease I08.3
        tricuspid (valve) disease I08.2
          with mitral (valve) disease I08.3
    specified cause NEC I35.1
    syphilitic A52.03
  arterial I77.1
    basilar G45.0
    carotid (hemispheric) G45.1
    cerebral I67.81
    coronary (acute or subacute) I24.8
    mesenteric K55.1
    peripheral I73.9
    precerebral (multiple) (bilateral) G45.2
    vertebral G45.0
  arteriovenous I99.8
  biliary K83.8
  cardiac — *see also* Insufficiency, myocardial
    due to presence of (cardiac) prosthesis I97.11- ☑
    postprocedural I97.11- ☑
  cardiorenal, hypertensive I13.2
  cardiovascular — *see* Disease, cardiovascular
  cerebrovascular (acute) I67.81
    with transient focal neurological signs and symptoms G45.8
  circulatory NEC I99.8
    newborn P29.89
  clinical crown length K08.89
  convergence H51.11
  coronary (acute or subacute) I24.8
    chronic or with a stated duration of over 4 weeks I25.89
  corticoadrenal E27.40
    primary E27.1
  dietary E63.9
  divergence H51.8
  food T73.0 ☑
  gastroesophageal K22.8
  gonadal
    ovary E28.39
    testis E29.1
  heart — *see also* Insufficiency, myocardial
    newborn P29.0
    valve — *see* Endocarditis
  hepatic — *see* Failure, hepatic
  idiopathic autonomic G90.09
  interocclusal distance of fully erupted teeth (ridge) M26.36
  kidney N28.9
    acute N28.9
    chronic N18.9
  lacrimal (secretion) H04.12- ☑
    passages — *see* Stenosis, lacrimal
  liver — *see* Failure, hepatic
  lung — *see* Insufficiency, pulmonary
  mental (congenital) — *see* Disability, intellectual
  mesenteric K55.1
  mitral (valve) I34.0
    with
      aortic valve disease I08.0
        with tricuspid (valve) disease I08.3
      obstruction or stenosis I05.2
        with aortic valve disease I08.0
      tricuspid (valve) disease I08.1
        with aortic (valve) disease I08.3

Insufficiency, insufficient — *continued*
  mitral — *continued*
    congenital Q23.3
    rheumatic I05.1
      with
        aortic valve disease I08.0
          with tricuspid (valve) disease I08.3
        obstruction or stenosis I05.2
          with aortic valve disease I08.0
            with tricuspid (valve) disease I08.3
        tricuspid (valve) disease I08.1
          with aortic (valve) disease I08.3
    active or acute I01.1
      with chorea, rheumatic (Sydenham's) I02.0
    specified cause, except rheumatic I34.0
  muscle — *see also* Disease, muscle
    heart — *see* Insufficiency, myocardial
  ocular NEC H50.9
  myocardial, myocardium (with arteriosclerosis) — *see also* Failure, heart I50.9
    with
      rheumatic fever (conditions in I00) I09.0
        active, acute or subacute I01.2
          with chorea I02.0
        inactive or quiescent (with chorea) I09.0
    congenital Q24.8
    hypertensive — *see* Hypertension, heart
    newborn P29.0
    rheumatic I09.0
      active, acute, or subacute I01.2
    syphilitic A52.06
  nourishment T73.0 ☑
  pancreatic K86.89
    exocrine K86.81
  parathyroid (gland) E20.9
  peripheral vascular (arterial) I73.9
  pituitary E23.0
  placental (mother) O36.51- ☑
  platelets D69.6
  prenatal care affecting management of pregnancy O09.3- ☑
  progressive pluriglandular E31.0
  pulmonary J98.4
    acute, following surgery (nonthoracic) J95.2
      thoracic J95.1
    chronic, following surgery J95.3
    following
      shock J98.4
      trauma J98.4
    newborn P28.89
    valve I37.1
      with stenosis I37.2
      congenital Q22.2
      rheumatic I09.89
        with aortic, mitral or tricuspid (valve) disease I08.8
  pyloric K31.89
  renal (acute) N28.9
    chronic N18.9
  respiratory R06.89
    newborn P28.5
  rotation — *see* Malrotation
  sleep syndrome F51.12
  social insurance Z59.7
  suprarenal E27.40
    primary E27.1
  tarso-orbital fascia, congenital Q10.3
  testis E29.1
  thyroid (gland) (acquired) E03.9
    congenital E03.1
  tricuspid (valve) (rheumatic) I07.1
    with
      aortic (valve) disease I08.2
        with mitral (valve) disease I08.3
      mitral (valve) disease I08.1
        with aortic (valve) disease I08.3
      obstruction or stenosis I07.2
        with aortic (valve) disease I08.2
          with mitral (valve) disease I08.3
    congenital Q22.8
    nonrheumatic I36.1
      with stenosis I36.2
  urethral sphincter R32
  valve, valvular (heart) I38
    aortic — *see* Insufficiency, aortic (valve)
    congenital Q24.8
    mitral — *see* Insufficiency, mitral (valve)
    pulmonary — *see* Insufficiency, pulmonary, valve

Insufficiency, insufficient — *continued*
 valve, valvular — *continued*
  tricuspid — *see* Insufficiency, tricuspid (valve)
 vascular I99.8
  intestine K55.9
   acute — *see also* Ischemia, intestine, acute K55.059
  mesenteric K55.1
  peripheral I73.9
  renal — *see* Hypertension, kidney
 velopharyngeal
  acquired K13.79
  congenital Q38.8
 venous (chronic) (peripheral) I87.2
 ventricular — *see* Insufficiency, myocardial
 welfare support Z59.7
Insufflation, fallopian Z31.41
Insular — *see* condition
Insulinoma
 pancreas
  benign D13.7
  malignant C25.4
  uncertain behavior D37.8
 specified site
  benign — *see* Neoplasm, by site, benign
  malignant — *see* Neoplasm, by site, malignant
  uncertain behavior — *see* Neoplasm, by site, uncertain behavior
 unspecified site
  benign D13.7
  malignant C25.4
  uncertain behavior D37.8
Insuloma — *see* Insulinoma
Interference
 balancing side M26.56
 non-working side M26.56
Intermenstrual — *see* condition
Intermittent — *see* condition
Internal — *see* condition
Interrogation
 cardiac defibrillator (automatic) (implantable) Z45.02
 cardiac pacemaker Z45.018
 cardiac (event) (loop) recorder Z45.09
 infusion pump (implanted) (intrathecal) Z45.1
 neurostimulator Z46.2
Interruption
 aortic arch Q25.21
 bundle of His I44.30
 phase-shift, sleep cycle — *see* Disorder, sleep, circadian rhythm
 sleep phase-shift, or 24 hour sleep-wake cycle — *see* Disorder, sleep, circadian rhythm
Interstitial — *see* condition
Intertrigo L30.4
 labialis K13.0
Intervertebral disc — *see* condition
Intestine, intestinal — *see* condition
Intolerance
 carbohydrate K90.49
 disaccharide, hereditary E73.0
 fat NEC K90.49
  pancreatic K90.3
 food K90.49
  dietary counseling and surveillance Z71.3
 fructose E74.10
  hereditary E74.12
 glucose (-galactose) E74.39
 gluten K90.41
 lactose E73.9
  specified NEC E73.8
 lysine E72.3
 milk NEC K90.49
  lactose E73.9
 protein K90.49
 starch NEC K90.49
 sucrose (-isomaltose) E74.31
Intoxicated NEC (without dependence) — *see* Alcohol, intoxication
Intoxication
 acid E87.2
 alcoholic (acute) (without dependence) — *see* Alcohol, intoxication
 alimentary canal K52.1
 amphetamine (without dependence) — *see also* Abuse, drug, stimulant, with intoxication
  with dependence — *see* Dependence, drug, stimulant, with intoxication
  stimulant NEC F15.10

Intoxication — *continued*
 amphetamine — *see also* Abuse, drug, stimulant, with intoxication — *continued*
  stimulant — *continued*
   with
    anxiety disorder F15.180
    intoxication F15.129
     with
      delirium F15.121
      perceptual disturbance F15.122
 anxiolytic (acute) (without dependence) — *see* Abuse, drug, sedative, with intoxication
  with dependence — *see* Dependence, drug, sedative, with intoxication
 caffeine F15.929
  with dependence — *see* Dependence, drug, stimulant, with intoxication
 cannabinoids (acute) (without dependence) — *see* Use, cannabis, with intoxication
  with
   abuse — *see* Abuse, drug, cannabis, with intoxication
   dependence — *see* Dependence, drug, cannabis, with intoxication
 chemical — *see* Table of Drugs and Chemicals
  via placenta or breast milk — *see* - Absorption, chemical, through placenta
 cocaine (acute) (without dependence) — *see* Abuse, drug, cocaine, with intoxication
  with dependence — *see* Dependence, drug, cocaine, with intoxication
 drug
  acute (without dependence) — *see* Abuse, drug, by type with intoxication
   with dependence — *see* Dependence, drug, by type with intoxication
  addictive
   via placenta or breast milk — *see* Absorption, drug, addictive, through placenta
  newborn P93.8
   gray baby syndrome P93.0
  overdose or wrong substance given or taken — *see* Table of Drugs and Chemicals, by drug, poisoning
 enteric K52.1
 foodborne A05.9
  bacterial A05.9
  classical (Clostridium botulinum) A05.1
  due to
   Bacillus cereus A05.4
   bacterium A05.9
    specified NEC A05.8
   Clostridium
    botulinum A05.1
    perfringens A05.2
    welchii A05.2
   Salmonella A02.9
    with
     (gastro)enteritis A02.0
     localized infection(s) A02.20
      arthritis A02.23
      meningitis A02.21
      osteomyelitis A02.24
      pneumonia A02.22
      pyelonephritis A02.25
      specified NEC A02.29
     sepsis A02.1
     specified manifestation NEC A02.8
   Staphylococcus A05.0
   Vibrio
    parahaemolyticus A05.3
    vulnificus A05.5
  enterotoxin, staphylococcal A05.0
  noxious — *see* Poisoning, food, noxious
 gastrointestinal K52.1
 hallucinogenic (without dependence) — *see* Abuse, drug, hallucinogen, with intoxication
  with dependence — *see* Dependence, drug, hallucinogen, with intoxication
 hypnotic (acute) (without dependence) — *see* Abuse, drug, sedative, with intoxication
  with dependence — *see* Dependence, drug, sedative, with intoxication
 inhalant (acute) (without dependence) — *see* Abuse, drug, inhalant, with intoxication
  with dependence — *see* Dependence, drug, inhalant, with intoxication

Intoxication — *continued*
 meaning
  inebriation — *see* category F10 ☑
  poisoning — *see* Table of Drugs and Chemicals
 methyl alcohol (acute) (without dependence) — *see* Alcohol, intoxication
 opioid (acute) (without dependence) — *see* Abuse, drug, opioid, with intoxication
  with dependence — *see* Dependence, drug, opioid, with intoxication
 pathologic NEC (without dependence) — *see* Alcohol, intoxication
 phencyclidine (without dependence) — *see* Abuse, drug, hallucinogen, with intoxication
  with dependence — *see* Dependence, drug, hallucinogen, with intoxication
 potassium (K) E87.5
 psychoactive substance NEC (without dependence) — *see* Abuse, drug, psychoactive NEC, with intoxication
  with dependence — *see* Dependence, drug, psychoactive NEC, with intoxication
 sedative (acute) (without dependence) — *see* Abuse, drug, sedative, with intoxication
  with dependence — *see* Dependence, drug, sedative, with intoxication
 serum — *see also* Reaction, serum T80.69 ☑
 uremic — *see* Uremia
 volatile solvents (acute) (without dependence) — *see* Abuse, drug, inhalant, with intoxication
  with dependence — *see* Dependence, drug, inhalant, with intoxication
 water E87.79
Intraabdominal testis, testes
 bilateral Q53.211
 unilateral Q53.111
Intracranial — *see* condition
Intrahepatic gallbladder Q44.1
Intraligamentous — *see* condition
Intrathoracic — *see also* condition
 kidney Q63.2
Intrauterine contraceptive device
 checking Z30.431
 in situ Z97.5
 insertion Z30.430
  immediately following removal Z30.433
 management Z30.431
 reinsertion Z30.433
 removal Z30.432
 replacement Z30.433
 retention in pregnancy O26.3- ☑
Intraventricular — *see* condition
Intrinsic deformity — *see* Deformity
Intubation, difficult or failed T88.4 ☑
Intumescence, lens (eye) (cataract) — *see* Cataract
Intussusception (bowel) (colon) (enteric) (ileocecal) (ileocolic) (intestine) (rectum) K56.1
 appendix K38.8
 congenital Q43.8
 ureter (with obstruction) N13.5
Invagination (bowel, colon, intestine or rectum) K56.1
Inversion
 albumin-globulin (A-G) ratio E88.09
 bladder N32.89
 cecum — *see* Intussusception
 cervix N88.8
 chromosome in normal individual Q95.1
 circadian rhythm — *see* Disorder, sleep, circadian rhythm
 nipple N64.59
  congenital Q83.8
  gestational — *see* Retraction, nipple
  puerperal, postpartum — *see* Retraction, nipple
 nyctohemeral rhythm — *see* Disorder, sleep, circadian rhythm
 optic papilla Q14.2
 organ or site, congenital NEC — *see* Anomaly, by site
 sleep rhythm — *see* Disorder, sleep, circadian rhythm
 testis (congenital) Q55.29
 uterus (chronic) (postinfectional) (postpartal, old) N85.5
  postpartum O71.2
 vagina (posthysterectomy) N99.3
 ventricular Q20.5
Investigation — *see also* Examination Z04.9
 clinical research subject (control) (normal comparison) (participant) Z00.6
Involuntary movement, abnormal R25.9

Involution, involutional — *see also* condition
  breast, cystic — *see* Dysplasia, mammary, specified
    type NEC
  depression (single episode) F32.89
    recurrent episode F33.9
  melancholia (single episode) F32.89
    recurrent episode F33.8
  ovary, senile — *see* Atrophy, ovary
  thymus failure E32.8
I.Q.
  20-34 F72
  35-49 F71
  50-69 F70
  under 20 F73
IRDS (type I) P22.0
  type II P22.1
Irideremia Q13.1
Iridis rubeosis — *see* Disorder, iris, vascular
Iridochoroiditis (panuveitis) — *see* Panuveitis
Iridocyclitis H20.9
  acute H20.0- ☑
    hypopyon H20.05- ☑
    primary H20.01- ☑
    recurrent H20.02- ☑
    secondary (noninfectious) H20.04- ☑
      infectious H20.03- ☑
  chronic H20.1- ☑
  due to allergy — *see* Iridocyclitis, acute, secondary
  endogenous — *see* Iridocyclitis, acute, primary
  Fuchs' — *see* Cyclitis, Fuchs' heterochromic
  gonococcal A54.32
  granulomatous — *see* Iridocyclitis, chronic
  herpes, herpetic (simplex) B00.51
    zoster B02.32
  hypopyon — *see* Iridocyclitis, acute, hypopyon
  in (due to)
    ankylosing spondylitis M45.9
    gonococcal infection A54.32
    herpes (simplex) virus B00.51
      zoster B02.32
    infectious disease NOS B99 ☑
    parasitic disease NOS B89 *[H22]*
    sarcoidosis D86.83
    syphilis A51.43
    tuberculosis A18.54
    zoster B02.32
  lens-induced H20.2- ☑
  nongranulomatous — *see* Iridocyclitis, acute
  recurrent — *see* Iridocyclitis, acute, recurrent
  rheumatic — *see* Iridocyclitis, chronic
  subacute — *see* Iridocyclitis, acute
  sympathetic — *see* Uveitis, sympathetic
  syphilitic (secondary) A51.43
  tuberculous (chronic) A18.54
  Vogt-Koyanagi H20.82- ☑
Iridocyclochoroiditis (panuveitis) — *see* Panuveitis
Iridodialysis H21.53- ☑
Iridodonesis H21.89
Iridoplegia (complete) (partial) (reflex) H57.09
Iridoschisis H21.25- ☑
Iris — *see also* condition
  bombé — *see* Membrane, pupillary
Iritis — *see also* Iridocyclitis
  chronic — *see* Iridocyclitis, chronic
  diabetic — *see* E08-E13 with .39
  due to
    herpes simplex B00.51
    leprosy A30.9 *[H22]*
  gonococcal A54.32
  gouty — *see also* Gout, by type M10.9 *[H22]*
  granulomatous — *see* Iridocyclitis, chronic
  lens induced — *see* Iridocyclitis, lens-induced
  papulosa (syphilitic) A52.71
  rheumatic — *see* Iridocyclitis, chronic
  syphilitic (secondary) A51.43
    congenital (early) A50.01
    late A52.71
  tuberculous A18.54
Iron — *see* condition
Iron-miner's lung J63.4
Irradiated enamel (tooth, teeth) K03.89
Irradiation effects, adverse T66 ☑
Irreducible, irreducibility — *see* condition
Irregular, irregularity
  action, heart I49.9
  alveolar process K08.89
  bleeding N92.6

Irregular, irregularity — *continued*
  breathing R06.89
  contour of cornea (acquired) — *see* Deformity, cornea
    congenital Q13.4
  contour, reconstructed breast N65.0
  dentin (in pulp) K04.3
  eye movements H55.89
    nystagmus — *see* Nystagmus
    saccadic H55.81
  labor O62.2
  menstruation (cause unknown) N92.6
  periods N92.6
  prostate N42.9
  pupil — *see* Abnormality, pupillary
  reconstructed breast N65.0
  respiratory R06.89
  septum (nasal) J34.2
  shape, organ or site, congenital NEC — *see* Distortion
  sleep-wake pattern (rhythm) G47.23
Irritable, irritability R45.4
  bladder N32.89
  bowel (syndrome) K58.9
    with
      constipation K58.1
      diarrhea K58.0
    mixed K58.2
    psychogenic F45.8
    specified NEC K58.8
  bronchial — *see* Bronchitis
  cerebral, in newborn P91.3
  colon — *see also* Irritable, bowel K58.9
    with diarrhea K58.0
    psychogenic F45.8
  duodenum K59.8
  heart (psychogenic) F45.8
  hip — *see* Derangement, joint, specified type NEC, hip
  ileum K59.8
  infant R68.12
  jejunum K59.8
  rectum K59.8
  stomach K31.89
    psychogenic F45.8
  sympathetic G90.8
  urethra N36.8
Irritation
  anus K62.89
  axillary nerve G54.0
  bladder N32.89
  brachial plexus G54.0
  bronchial — *see* Bronchitis
  cervical plexus G54.2
  cervix — *see* Cervicitis
  choroid, sympathetic — *see* Endophthalmitis
  cranial nerve — *see* Disorder, nerve, cranial
  gastric K31.89
    psychogenic F45.8
  globe, sympathetic — *see* Uveitis, sympathetic
  labyrinth — *see* subcategory H83.2 ☑
  lumbosacral plexus G54.1
  meninges (traumatic) — *see* Injury, intracranial
    nontraumatic — *see* Meningismus
  nerve — *see* Disorder, nerve
  nervous R45.0
  penis N48.89
  perineum NEC L29.3
  peripheral autonomic nervous system G90.8
  peritoneum — *see* Peritonitis
  pharynx J39.2
  plantar nerve — *see* Lesion, nerve, plantar
  spinal (cord) (traumatic) — *see also* Injury, spinal cord,
    by region
    nerve G58.9
      root NEC — *see* Radiculopathy
    nontraumatic — *see* Myelopathy
  stomach K31.89
    psychogenic F45.8
  sympathetic nerve NEC G90.8
  ulnar nerve — *see* Lesion, nerve, ulnar
  vagina N89.8
Ischemia, ischemic I99.8
  bowel (transient)
    acute — *see also* Ischemia, intestine, acute K55.059
    chronic K55.1
    due to mesenteric artery insufficiency K55.1
  brain — *see* Ischemia, cerebral
  cardiac (see Disease, heart, ischemic)
  cardiomyopathy I25.5
  cerebral (chronic) (generalized) I67.82

Ischemia, ischemic — *continued*
  cerebral — *continued*
    arteriosclerotic I67.2
    intermittent G45.9
    newborn P91.0
    recurrent focal G45.8
    transient G45.9
  colon chronic (due to mesenteric artery insufficiency)
    K55.1
  coronary — *see* Disease, heart, ischemic
  demand (coronary) — *see also* Angina I24.8
    with myocardial infarction I21.A1
    resulting in myocardial infarction I21.A1
  heart (chronic or with a stated duration of over 4 weeks)
    I25.9
    acute or with a stated duration of 4 weeks or less
      I24.9
    subacute I24.9
  infarction, muscle — *see* Infarct, muscle
  intestine (large) (small) (transient) K55.9
    acute K55.059
      diffuse K55.052
      focal K55.051
      large K55.039
        diffuse K55.032
        focal K55.031
      small K55.019
        diffuse K55.012
        focal K55.011
    chronic K55.1
    due to mesenteric artery insufficiency K55.1
  kidney N28.0
  mesenteric, acute — *see also* Ischemia, intestine, acute
    K55.059
  muscle, traumatic T79.6 ☑
  myocardium, myocardial (chronic or with a stated du-
    ration of over 4 weeks) I25.9
    acute, without myocardial infarction I51.3
    silent (asymptomatic) I25.6
    transient of newborn P29.4
  renal N28.0
  retina, retinal — *see* Occlusion, artery, retina
  small bowel
    acute K55.019
      diffuse K55.012
      focal K55.011
    chronic K55.1
    due to mesenteric artery insufficiency K55.1
  spinal cord G95.11
  subendocardial — *see* Insufficiency, coronary
  supply (coronary) — *see also* Angina I25.9
    due to vasospasm I20.1
Ischial spine — *see* condition
Ischialgia — *see* Sciatica
Ischiopagus Q89.4
Ischium, ischial — *see* condition
Ischuria R34
Iselin's disease or osteochondrosis — *see* Osteochon-
  drosis, juvenile, metatarsus
Islands of
  parotid tissue in
    lymph nodes Q38.6
    neck structures Q38.6
  submaxillary glands in
    fascia Q38.6
    lymph nodes Q38.6
    neck muscles Q38.6
Islet cell tumor, pancreas D13.7
Isoimmunization NEC — *see also* Incompatibility
  affecting management of pregnancy (ABO) (with hy-
    drops fetalis) O36.11- ☑
    anti-A sensitization O36.11- ☑
    anti-B sensitization O36.19- ☑
    anti-c sensitization O36.09- ☑
    anti-C sensitization O36.09- ☑
    anti-e sensitization O36.09- ☑
    anti-E sensitization O36.09- ☑
    Rh NEC O36.09- ☑
      anti-D antibody O36.01- ☑
    specified NEC O36.19- ☑
  newborn P55.9
    with
      hydrops fetalis P56.0
      kernicterus P57.0
    ABO (blood groups) P55.1
    Rhesus (Rh) factor P55.0
    specified type NEC P55.8

Isolation, isolated
  dwelling Z59.8
  family Z63.79
  social Z60.4
Isoleucinosis E71.19
Isomerism atrial appendages (with asplenia or
    polysplenia) Q20.6
Isosporiasis, isosporosis A07.3
Isovaleric acidemia E71.110
Issue of
  medical certificate Z02.79
    for disability determination Z02.71
  repeat prescription (appliance) (glasses) (medicinal
      substance, medicament, medicine) Z76.0
    contraception — see Contraception
Itch, itching — see also Pruritus
  baker's L23.6
  barber's B35.0
  bricklayer's L24.5
  cheese B88.0
  clam digger's B65.3
  coolie B76.9
  copra B88.0
  dew B76.9
  dhobi B35.6
  filarial — see Infestation, filarial
  grain B88.0
  grocer's B88.0
  ground B76.9
  harvest B88.0
  jock B35.6
  Malabar B35.5
    beard B35.0
    foot B35.3
    scalp B35.0
  meaning scabies B86
  Norwegian B86
  perianal L29.0
  poultrymen's B88.0
  sarcoptic B86
  scabies B86
  scrub B88.0
  straw B88.0
  swimmer's B65.3
  water B76.9
  winter L29.8
Ivemark's syndrome (asplenia with congenital heart
    disease) Q89.01
Ivory bones Q78.2
Ixodiasis NEC B88.8

J

Jaccoud's syndrome — see Arthropathy, postrheumatic,
    chronic
Jackson's
  membrane Q43.3
  paralysis or syndrome G83.89
  veil Q43.3
Jacquet's dermatitis (diaper dermatitis) L22
Jadassohn-Pellizari's disease or anetoderma L90.2
Jadassohn's
  blue nevus — see Nevus
  intraepidermal epithelioma — see Neoplasm, skin,
    benign
Jaffe-Lichtenstein (-Uehlinger) **syndrome** — see Dys-
    plasia, fibrous, bone NEC
Jakob-Creutzfeldt disease or syndrome — see
    Creutzfeldt-Jakob disease or syndrome
Jaksch-Luzet disease D64.89
Jamaican
  neuropathy G92
  paraplegic tropical ataxic-spastic syndrome G92
Janet's disease F48.8
Janiceps Q89.4
Jansky-Bielschowsky amaurotic idiocy E75.4
Japanese
  B-type encephalitis A83.0
  river fever A75.3
Jaundice (yellow) R17
  acholuric (familial) (splenomegalic) — see also Sphero-
    cytosis
    acquired D59.8
  breast-milk (inhibitor) P59.3
  catarrhal (acute) B15.9
    with hepatic coma B15.0
  cholestatic (benign) R17

Jaundice — continued
  due to or associated with
    delayed conjugation P59.8
      associated with (due to) preterm delivery P59.0
    preterm delivery P59.0
  epidemic (catarrhal) B15.9
    with hepatic coma B15.0
    leptospiral A27.0
    spirochetal A27.0
  familial nonhemolytic (congenital) (Gilbert) E80.4
    Crigler-Najjar E80.5
  febrile (acute) B15.9
    with hepatic coma B15.0
    leptospiral A27.0
    spirochetal A27.0
  hematogenous D59.9
  hemolytic (acquired) D59.9
    congenital — see Spherocytosis
  hemorrhagic (acute) (leptospiral) (spirochetal) A27.0
  infectious (acute) (subacute) B15.9
    with hepatic coma B15.0
    leptospiral A27.0
    spirochetal A27.0
  leptospiral (hemorrhagic) A27.0
  malignant (without coma) K72.90
    with coma K72.91
  neonatal — see Jaundice, newborn
  newborn P59.9
    due to or associated with
      ABO
        antibodies P55.1
        incompatibility, maternal/fetal P55.1
        isoimmunization P55.1
      absence or deficiency of enzyme system for
        bilirubin conjugation (congenital) P59.8
      bleeding P58.1
      breast milk inhibitors to conjugation P59.3
        associated with preterm delivery P59.0
      bruising P58.0
      Crigler-Najjar syndrome E80.5
      delayed conjugation P59.8
        associated with preterm delivery P59.0
      drugs or toxins
        given to newborn P58.42
        transmitted from mother P58.41
      excessive hemolysis P58.9
        due to
          bleeding P58.1
          bruising P58.0
          drugs or toxins
            given to newborn P58.42
            transmitted from mother P58.41
          infection P58.2
          polycythemia P58.3
          swallowed maternal blood P58.5
        specified type NEC P58.8
      galactosemia E74.21
      Gilbert syndrome E80.4
      hemolytic disease P55.9
        ABO isoimmunization P55.1
        Rh isoimmunization P55.0
        specified NEC P55.8
      hepatocellular damage P59.20
        specified NEC P59.29
      hereditary hemolytic anemia P58.8
      hypothyroidism, congenital E03.1
      incompatibility, maternal/fetal NOS P55.9
      infection P58.2
      inspissated bile syndrome P59.1
      isoimmunization NOS P55.9
      mucoviscidosis E84.9
      polycythemia P58.3
      preterm delivery P59.0
      Rh
        antibodies P55.0
        incompatibility, maternal/fetal P55.0
        isoimmunization P55.0
      specified cause NEC P59.8
      swallowed maternal blood P58.5
      spherocytosis (congenital) D58.0
  nonhemolytic congenital familial (Gilbert) E80.4
  nuclear, newborn — see also Kernicterus of newborn
    P57.9
  obstructive — see also Obstruction, bile duct K83.1
  post-immunization — see Hepatitis, viral, type, B
  post-transfusion — see Hepatitis, viral, type, B
  regurgitation — see also Obstruction, bile duct K83.1

Jaundice — continued
  serum (homologous) (prophylactic) (therapeutic) —
    see Hepatitis, viral, type, B
  spirochetal (hemorrhagic) A27.0
  symptomatic R17
    newborn P59.9
Jaw — see condition
Jaw-winking phenomenon or syndrome Q07.8
Jealousy
  alcoholic F10.988
  childhood F93.8
  sibling F93.8
Jejunitis — see Enteritis
Jejunostomy status Z93.4
Jejunum, jejunal — see condition
Jensen's disease — see Inflammation, chorioretinal, fo-
    cal, juxtapapillary
Jerks, myoclonic G25.3
Jervell-Lange-Nielsen syndrome I45.81
Jeune's disease Q77.2
Jigger disease B88.1
Job's syndrome (chronic granulomatous disease) D71
Joint — see also condition
  mice — see Loose, body, joint
    knee M23.4- ☑
Jordan's anomaly or syndrome D72.0
Joseph-Diamond-Blackfan anemia (congenital hy-
    poplastic) D61.01
Jungle yellow fever A95.0
Jüngling's disease — see Sarcoidosis
Juvenile — see condition

K

Kahler's disease C90.0- ☑
Kakke E51.11
Kala-azar B55.0
Kallmann's syndrome E23.0
Kanner's syndrome (autism) — see Psychosis, childhood
Kaposi's
  dermatosis (xeroderma pigmentosum) Q82.1
  lichen ruber L44.0
    acuminatus L44.0
  sarcoma
    colon C46.4
    connective tissue C46.1
    gastrointestinal organ C46.4
    lung C46.5- ☑
    lymph node (multiple) C46.3
    palate (hard) (soft) C46.2
    rectum C46.4
    skin (multiple sites) C46.0
    specified site NEC C46.7
    stomach C46.4
    unspecified site C46.9
  varicelliform eruption B00.0
    vaccinia T88.1 ☑
Kartagener's syndrome or triad (sinusitis, bronchiecta-
    sis, situs inversus) Q89.3
Karyotype
  with abnormality except iso (Xq) Q96.2
  45,X Q96.0
  46,X
    iso (Xq) Q96.1
  46,XX Q98.3
    with streak gonads Q50.32
    hermaphrodite (true) Q99.1
    male Q98.3
  46,XY
    with streak gonads Q56.1
    female Q97.3
    hermaphrodite (true) Q99.1
  47,XXX Q97.0
  47,XXY Q98.0
  47,XYY Q98.5
Kaschin-Beck disease — see Disease, Kaschin-Beck
Katayama's disease or fever B65.2
Kawasaki's syndrome M30.3
Kayser-Fleischer ring (cornea) (pseudosclerosis)
    H18.04- ☑
Kaznelson's syndrome (congenital hypoplastic anemia)
    D61.01
Kearns-Sayre syndrome H49.81- ☑
Kedani fever A75.3
Kelis L91.0
Kelly (-Patterson) **syndrome** (sideropenic dysphagia)
    D50.1

☑ **Additional Character Required — Refer to the Tabular List for Character Selection**   ▼ Subterms under main terms may continue to next column or page

Keloid, cheloid L91.0
  acne L73.0
  Addison's L94.0
  cornea — *see* Opacity, cornea
  Hawkin's L91.0
  scar L91.0
Keloma L91.0
Kenya fever A77.1
Keratectasia — *see also* Ectasia, cornea
  congenital Q13.4
Keratinization of alveolar ridge mucosa
  excessive K13.23
  minimal K13.22
Keratinized residual ridge mucosa
  excessive K13.23
  minimal K13.22
Keratitis (nodular) (nonulcerative) (simple) (zonular)
    H16.9
  with ulceration (central) (marginal) (perforated) (ring)
    — *see* Ulcer, cornea
  actinic — *see* Photokeratitis
  arborescens (herpes simplex) B00.52
  areolar H16.11- ☑
  bullosa H16.8
  deep H16.309
    specified type NEC H16.399
  dendritic (a) (herpes simplex) B00.52
  disciform (is) (herpes simplex) B00.52
    varicella B01.81
  filamentary H16.12- ☑
  gonococcal (congenital or prenatal) A54.33
  herpes, herpetic (simplex) B00.52
    zoster B02.33
  in (due to)
    acanthamebiasis B60.13
    adenovirus B30.0
    exanthema — *see also* Exanthem B09
    herpes (simplex) virus B00.52
    measles B05.81
    syphilis A50.31
    tuberculosis A18.52
    zoster B02.33
  interstitial (nonsyphilitic) H16.30- ☑
    diffuse H16.32- ☑
    herpes, herpetic (simplex) B00.52
      zoster B02.33
    sclerosing H16.33- ☑
    specified type NEC H16.39- ☑
    syphilitic (congenital) (late) A50.31
    tuberculous A18.52
  macular H16.11- ☑
  nummular H16.11- ☑
  oyster shuckers' H16.8
  parenchymatous — *see* Keratitis, interstitial
  petrificans H16.8
  postmeasles B05.81
  punctata
    leprosa A30.9 [H16.14-] ☑
    syphilitic (profunda) A50.31
  punctate H16.14- ☑
  purulent H16.8
  rosacea L71.8
  sclerosing H16.33- ☑
  specified type NEC H16.8
  stellate H16.11- ☑
  striate H16.11- ☑
  superficial H16.10- ☑
    with conjunctivitis — *see* Keratoconjunctivitis
    due to light — *see* Photokeratitis
  suppurative H16.8
  syphilitic (congenital) (prenatal) A50.31
  trachomatous A71.1
    sequelae B94.0
  tuberculous A18.52
  vesicular H16.8
  xerotic — *see also* Keratomalacia H16.8
    vitamin A deficiency E50.4
Keratoacanthoma L85.8
Keratocele — *see* Descemetocele
Keratoconjunctivitis H16.20- ☑
  Acanthamoeba B60.13
  adenoviral B30.0
  epidemic B30.0
  exposure H16.21- ☑
  herpes, herpetic (simplex) B00.52
    zoster B02.33
  in exanthema — *see also* Exanthem B09
  infectious B30.0

Keratoconjunctivitis — *continued*
  lagophthalmic — *see* Keratoconjunctivitis, specified
    type NEC
  neurotrophic H16.23- ☑
  phlyctenular H16.25- ☑
  postmeasles B05.81
  shipyard B30.0
  sicca (Sjogren's) M35.0- ☑
    not Sjogren's H16.22- ☑
  specified type NEC H16.29- ☑
  tuberculous (phlyctenular) A18.52
  vernal H16.26- ☑
Keratoconus H18.60- ☑
  congenital Q13.4
  stable H18.61- ☑
  unstable H18.62- ☑
Keratocyst (dental) (odontogenic) — *see* Cyst, calcifying
    odontogenic
Keratoderma, keratodermia (congenital) (palmaris et
    plantaris) (symmetrical) Q82.8
  acquired L85.1
    in diseases classified elsewhere L86
  climactericum L85.1
  gonococcal A54.89
  gonorrheal A54.89
  punctata L85.2
  Reiter's — *see* Reiter's disease
Keratodermatocele — *see* Descemetocele
Keratoglobus H18.79 ☑
  congenital Q15.8
    with glaucoma Q15.0
Keratohemia — *see* Pigmentation, cornea, stromal
Keratoiritis — *see also* Iridocyclitis
  syphilitic A50.39
  tuberculous A18.54
Keratoma L57.0
  palmaris and plantaris hereditarium Q82.8
  senile L57.0
Keratomalacia H18.44- ☑
  vitamin A deficiency E50.4
Keratomegaly Q13.4
Keratomycosis B49
  nigrans, nigricans (palmaris) B36.1
Keratopathy H18.9
  band H18.42- ☑
  bullous (aphakic), following cataract surgery H59.01- ☑
  bullous H18.1- ☑
Keratoscleritis, tuberculous A18.52
Keratosis L57.0
  actinic L57.0
  arsenical L85.8
  congenital, specified NEC Q80.8
  female genital NEC N94.89
  follicularis Q82.8
    acquired L11.0
    congenita Q82.8
    et parafollicularis in cutem penetrans L87.0
    spinulosa (decalvans) Q82.8
    vitamin A deficiency E50.8
  gonococcal A54.89
  male genital (external) N50.89
  nigricans L83
  obturans, external ear (canal) — *see* Cholesteatoma,
    external ear
  palmaris et plantaris (inherited) (symmetrical) Q82.8
    acquired L85.1
  penile N48.89
  pharynx J39.2
  pilaris, acquired L85.8
  punctata (palmaris et plantaris) L85.2
  scrotal N50.89
  seborrheic L82.1
    inflamed L82.0
  senile L57.0
  solar L57.0
  tonsillaris J35.8
  vagina N89.4
  vegetans Q82.8
  vitamin A deficiency E50.8
  vocal cord J38.3
Kerato-uveitis — *see* Iridocyclitis
Kerion (celsi) B35.0
Kernicterus of newborn (not due to isoimmunization)
    P57.9
  due to isoimmunization (conditions in P55.0-P55.9)
    P57.0
  specified type NEC P57.8
Kerunoparalysis T75.09 ☑

Keshan disease E59
Ketoacidosis E87.2
  diabetic — *see* Diabetes, by type, with ketoacidosis
Ketonuria R82.4
Ketosis NEC E88.89
  diabetic — *see* Diabetes, by type, with ketoacidosis
Kew Garden fever A79.1
Kidney — *see* condition
Kienböck's disease — *see also* Osteochondrosis, juvenile,
    hand, carpal lunate
  adult M93.1
Kimmelstiel (-Wilson) disease — *see* Diabetes, Kimmel-
    stiel (-Wilson) disease
Kink, kinking
  artery I77.1
  hair (acquired) L67.8
  ileum or intestine — *see* Obstruction, intestine
  Lane's — *see* Obstruction, intestine
  organ or site, congenital NEC — *see* Anomaly, by site
  ureter (pelvic junction) N13.5
    with
      hydronephrosis N13.1
        with infection N13.6
      pyelonephritis (chronic) N11.1
    congenital Q62.39
  vein(s) I87.8
    caval I87.1
    peripheral I87.1
Kinnier Wilson's disease (hepatolenticular degenera-
    tion) E83.01
Kissing spine M48.20
  cervical region M48.22
  cervicothoracic region M48.23
  lumbar region M48.26
  lumbosacral region M48.27
  occipito-atlanto-axial region M48.21
  thoracic region M48.24
  thoracolumbar region M48.25
Klatskin's tumor C22.1
Klauder's disease A26.8
Klebs' disease — *see also* Glomerulonephritis N05- ☑
**Klebsiella (K.) pneumoniae, as cause of disease clas-
    sified elsewhere** B96.1
Klein (e)-Levin syndrome G47.13
Kleptomania F63.2
Klinefelter's syndrome Q98.4
  karyotype 47,XXY Q98.0
  male with more than two X chromosomes Q98.1
Klippel-Feil deficiency, disease, or syndrome (brevi-
    collis) Q76.1
Klippel's disease I67.2
Klippel-Trenaunay (-Weber) syndrome Q87.2
Klumpke (-Déjerine) palsy, paralysis (birth) (newborn)
    P14.1
Knee — *see* condition
Knock knee (acquired) M21.06- ☑
  congenital Q74.1
Knot
  intestinal, syndrome (volvulus) K56.2
  surfer S89.8- ☑
  umbilical cord (true) O69.2 ☑
Knotting (of)
  hair L67.8
  intestine K56.2
Knuckle pad (Garrod's) M72.1
Koch's
  infection — *see* Tuberculosis
  relapsing fever A68.9
Koch-Weeks' conjunctivitis — *see* Conjunctivitis, acute,
    mucopurulent
Köebner's syndrome Q81.8
Köenig's disease (osteochondritis dissecans) — *see* Os-
    teochondritis, dissecans
Köhler-Pellegrini-Steida disease or syndrome (calci-
    fication, knee joint) — *see* Bursitis, tibial collateral
Köhler's disease
  patellar — *see* Osteochondrosis, juvenile, patella
  tarsal navicular — *see* Osteochondrosis, juvenile, tarsus
Koilonychia L60.3
  congenital Q84.6
Kojevnikov's, epilepsy — *see* Kozhevnikof's epilepsy
Koplik's spots B05.9
Kopp's asthma E32.8
Korsakoff's (Wernicke) **disease, psychosis or syn-
    drome** (alcoholic) F10.96
  with dependence F10.26

Keloid, cheloid — Korsakoff's

▽ Subterms under main terms may continue to next column or page   ☑ Additional Character Required — Refer to the Tabular List for Character Selection   **205**

Korsakoff's (Wernicke) **disease, psychosis or syndrome** — *continued*
  drug-induced
    due to drug abuse — *see* Abuse, drug, by type, with amnestic disorder
    due to drug dependence — *see* Dependence, drug, by type, with amnestic disorder
    nonalcoholic F04
Korsakov's disease, psychosis or syndrome — *see* Korsakoff's disease
Korsakow's disease, psychosis or syndrome — *see* Korsakoff's disease
Kostmann's disease or syndrome (infantile genetic agranulocytosis) — *see* Agranulocytosis
Kozhevnikof's epilepsy G40.109
  intractable G40.119
    with status epilepticus G40.111
    without status epilepticus G40.119
  not intractable G40.109
    with status epilepticus G40.101
    without status epilepticus G40.109
Krabbe's
  disease E75.23
  syndrome, congenital muscle hypoplasia Q79.8
Kraepelin-Morel disease — *see* Schizophrenia
Kraft-Weber-Dimitri disease Q85.8
Kraurosis
  ani K62.89
  penis N48.0
  vagina N89.8
  vulva N90.4
Kreotoxism A05.9
Krukenberg's
  spindle — *see* Pigmentation, cornea, posterior
  tumor C79.6- ☑
Kufs' disease E75.4
Kugelberg-Welander disease G12.1
Kuhnt-Junius degeneration — *see also* Degeneration, macula H35.32- ☑
Kümmell's disease or spondylitis — *see* Spondylopathy, traumatic
Kupffer cell sarcoma C22.3
Kuru A81.81
Kussmaul's
  disease M30.0
  respiration E87.2
    in diabetic acidosis — *see* Diabetes, by type, with ketoacidosis
Kwashiorkor E40
  marasmic, marasmus type E42
Kyasanur Forest disease A98.2
Kyphoscoliosis, kyphoscoliotic (acquired) — *see also* Scoliosis M41.9
  congenital Q67.5
  heart (disease) I27.1
  sequelae of rickets E64.3
  tuberculous A18.01
Kyphosis, kyphotic (acquired) M40.209
  cervical region M40.202
  cervicothoracic region M40.203
  congenital Q76.419
    cervical region Q76.412
    cervicothoracic region Q76.413
    occipito-atlanto-axial region Q76.411
    thoracic region Q76.414
    thoracolumbar region Q76.415
  Morquio-Brailsford type (spinal) — *see also* subcategory M49.8 E76.219
  postlaminectomy M96.3
  postradiation therapy M96.2
  postural (adolescent) M40.00
    cervicothoracic region M40.03
    thoracic region M40.04
    thoracolumbar region M40.05
  secondary NEC M40.10
    cervical region M40.12
    cervicothoracic region M40.13
    thoracic region M40.14
    thoracolumbar region M40.15
  sequelae of rickets E64.3
  specified type NEC M40.299
    cervical region M40.292
    cervicothoracic region M40.293
    thoracic region M40.294
    thoracolumbar region M40.295
  syphilitic, congenital A50.56
  thoracic region M40.204
  thoracolumbar region M40.205

Kyphosis, kyphotic — *continued*
  tuberculous A18.01
Kyrle disease L87.0

L

Labia, labium — *see* condition
Labile
  blood pressure R09.89
  vasomotor system I73.9
Labioglossal paralysis G12.29
Labium leporinum — *see* Cleft, lip
Labor — *see* Delivery
Labored breathing — *see* Hyperventilation
Labyrinthitis (circumscribed) (destructive) (diffuse) (inner ear) (latent) (purulent) (suppurative) — *see also* subcategory H83.0 ☑
  syphilitic A52.79
Laceration
  with abortion — *see* Abortion, by type, complicated by laceration of pelvic organs
  abdomen, abdominal
    wall S31.119 ☑
      with
        foreign body S31.129 ☑
        penetration into peritoneal cavity S31.619 ☑
          with foreign body S31.629 ☑
      epigastric region S31.112 ☑
        with
          foreign body S31.122 ☑
          penetration into peritoneal cavity S31.612 ☑
            with foreign body S31.622 ☑
      left
        lower quadrant S31.114 ☑
          with
            foreign body S31.124 ☑
            penetration into peritoneal cavity S31.614 ☑
              with foreign body S31.624 ☑
        upper quadrant S31.111 ☑
          with
            foreign body S31.121 ☑
            penetration into peritoneal cavity S31.611 ☑
              with foreign body S31.621 ☑
      periumbilic region S31.115 ☑
        with
          foreign body S31.125 ☑
          penetration into peritoneal cavity S31.615 ☑
            with foreign body S31.625 ☑
      right
        lower quadrant S31.113 ☑
          with
            foreign body S31.123 ☑
            penetration into peritoneal cavity S31.613 ☑
              with foreign body S31.623 ☑
        upper quadrant S31.110 ☑
          with
            foreign body S31.120 ☑
            penetration into peritoneal cavity S31.610 ☑
              with foreign body S31.620 ☑
  accidental, complicating surgery — *see* Complications, surgical, accidental puncture or laceration
  Achilles tendon S86.02- ☑
  adrenal gland S37.813 ☑
  alveolar (process) — *see* Laceration, oral cavity
  ankle S91.01- ☑
    with
      foreign body S91.02- ☑
  antecubital space — *see* Laceration, elbow
  anus (sphincter) S31.831 ☑
    with
      ectopic or molar pregnancy O08.6
      foreign body S31.832 ☑
    complicating delivery — *see* Delivery, complicated, by, laceration, anus (sphincter)
    following ectopic or molar pregnancy O08.6
    nontraumatic, nonpuerperal — *see* Fissure, anus
  arm (upper) S41.11- ☑
    with foreign body S41.12- ☑
    lower — *see* Laceration, forearm

Laceration — *continued*
  auditory canal (external) (meatus) — *see* Laceration, ear
  auricle, ear — *see* Laceration, ear
  axilla — *see* Laceration, arm
  back — *see also* Laceration, thorax, back
    lower S31.010 ☑
      with
        foreign body S31.020 ☑
          with penetration into retroperitoneal space S31.021 ☑
        penetration into retroperitoneal space S31.011 ☑
  bile duct S36.13 ☑
  bladder S37.23 ☑
    with ectopic or molar pregnancy O08.6
    following ectopic or molar pregnancy O08.6
    obstetrical trauma O71.5
  blood vessel — *see* Injury, blood vessel
  bowel — *see also* Laceration, intestine
    with ectopic or molar pregnancy O08.6
    complicating abortion — *see* Abortion, by type, complicated by, specified condition NEC
    following ectopic or molar pregnancy O08.6
    obstetrical trauma O71.5
  brain (any part) (cortex) (diffuse) (membrane) — *see also* Injury, intracranial, diffuse
    during birth P10.8
      with hemorrhage P10.1
    focal — *see* Injury, intracranial, focal brain injury
  brainstem S06.38- ☑
  breast S21.01- ☑
    with foreign body S21.02- ☑
  broad ligament S37.893 ☑
    with ectopic or molar pregnancy O08.6
    following ectopic or molar pregnancy O08.6
    laceration syndrome N83.8
    obstetrical trauma O71.6
    syndrome (laceration) N83.8
  buttock S31.801 ☑
    with foreign body S31.802 ☑
    left S31.821 ☑
      with foreign body S31.822 ☑
    right S31.811 ☑
      with foreign body S31.812 ☑
  calf — *see* Laceration, leg
  canaliculus lacrimalis — *see* Laceration, eyelid
  canthus, eye — *see* Laceration, eyelid
  capsule, joint — *see* Sprain
  causing eversion of cervix uteri (old) N86
  central (perineal), complicating delivery O70.9
  cerebellum, traumatic S06.37- ☑
  cerebral S06.33- ☑
    during birth P10.8
      with hemorrhage P10.1
    left side S06.32- ☑
    right side S06.31- ☑
  cervix (uteri)
    with ectopic or molar pregnancy O08.6
    following ectopic or molar pregnancy O08.6
    nonpuerperal, nontraumatic N88.1
    obstetrical trauma (current) O71.3
    old (postpartal) N88.1
    traumatic S37.63 ☑
  cheek (external) S01.41- ☑
    with foreign body S01.42- ☑
    internal — *see* Laceration, oral cavity
  chest wall — *see* Laceration, thorax
  chin — *see* Laceration, head, specified site NEC
  chordae tendinae NEC I51.1
    concurrent with acute myocardial infarction — *see* Infarct, myocardium
    following acute myocardial infarction (current complication) I23.4
  clitoris — *see* Laceration, vulva
  colon — *see* Laceration, intestine, large, colon
  common bile duct S36.13 ☑
  cortex (cerebral) — *see* Injury, intracranial, diffuse
  costal region — *see* Laceration, thorax
  cystic duct S36.13 ☑
  diaphragm S27.803 ☑
  digit(s)
    foot — *see* Laceration, toe
    hand — *see* Laceration, finger
  duodenum S36.430 ☑
  ear (canal) (external) S01.31- ☑
    with foreign body S01.32- ☑

☑ **Additional Character Required** — Refer to the Tabular List for Character Selection   ▽ **Subterms under main terms may continue to next column or page**

Laceration — *continued*
ear — *continued*
  drum S09.2- ☑
 elbow S51.01- ☑
  with
   foreign body S51.02- ☑
 epididymis — *see* Laceration, testis
 epigastric region — *see* Laceration, abdomen, wall, epigastric region
 esophagus K22.8
  traumatic
   cervical S11.21 ☑
    with foreign body S11.22 ☑
   thoracic S27.813 ☑
 eye (ball) S05.3- ☑
  with prolapse or loss of intraocular tissue S05.2- ☑
  penetrating S05.6- ☑
 eyebrow — *see* Laceration, eyelid
 eyelid S01.11- ☑
  with foreign body S01.12- ☑
 face NEC — *see* Laceration, head, specified site NEC
 fallopian tube S37.539 ☑
  bilateral S37.532 ☑
  unilateral S37.531 ☑
 finger(s) S61.219 ☑
  with
   damage to nail S61.319 ☑
    with
     foreign body S61.329 ☑
   foreign body S61.229 ☑
  index S61.218 ☑
   with
    damage to nail S61.318 ☑
     with
      foreign body S61.328 ☑
    foreign body S61.228 ☑
   left S61.211 ☑
    with
     damage to nail S61.311 ☑
      with
       foreign body S61.321 ☑
     foreign body S61.221 ☑
   right S61.210 ☑
    with
     damage to nail S61.310 ☑
      with
       foreign body S61.320 ☑
     foreign body S61.220 ☑
  little S61.218 ☑
   with
    damage to nail S61.318 ☑
     with
      foreign body S61.328 ☑
    foreign body S61.228 ☑
   left S61.217 ☑
    with
     damage to nail S61.317 ☑
      with
       foreign body S61.327 ☑
     foreign body S61.227 ☑
   right S61.216 ☑
    with
     damage to nail S61.316 ☑
      with
       foreign body S61.326 ☑
     foreign body S61.226 ☑
  middle S61.218 ☑
   with
    damage to nail S61.318 ☑
     with
      foreign body S61.328 ☑
    foreign body S61.228 ☑
   left S61.213 ☑
    with
     damage to nail S61.313 ☑
      with
       foreign body S61.323 ☑
     foreign body S61.223 ☑
   right S61.212 ☑
    with
     damage to nail S61.312 ☑
      with
       foreign body S61.322 ☑
     foreign body S61.222 ☑
  ring S61.218 ☑

Laceration — *continued*
finger(s) — *continued*
 ring — *continued*
  with
   damage to nail S61.318 ☑
    with
     foreign body S61.328 ☑
   foreign body S61.228 ☑
  left S61.215 ☑
   with
    damage to nail S61.315 ☑
     with
      foreign body S61.325 ☑
    foreign body S61.225 ☑
  right S61.214 ☑
   with
    damage to nail S61.314 ☑
     with
      foreign body S61.324 ☑
    foreign body S61.224 ☑
 flank S31.119 ☑
  with foreign body S31.129 ☑
 foot (except toe(s) alone) S91.319 ☑
  with foreign body S91.329 ☑
  left S91.312 ☑
   with foreign body S91.322 ☑
  right S91.311 ☑
   with foreign body S91.321 ☑
  toe — *see* Laceration, toe
 forearm S51.819 ☑
  with
   foreign body S51.829 ☑
  elbow only — *see* Laceration, elbow
  left S51.812 ☑
   with
    foreign body S51.822 ☑
  right S51.811 ☑
   with
    foreign body S51.821 ☑
 forehead S01.81 ☑
  with foreign body S01.82 ☑
 fourchette O70.0
  with ectopic or molar pregnancy O08.6
  complicating delivery O70.0
  following ectopic or molar pregnancy O08.6
 gallbladder S36.123 ☑
 genital organs, external
  female S31.512 ☑
   with foreign body S31.522 ☑
   vagina — *see* Laceration, vagina
   vulva — *see* Laceration, vulva
  male S31.511 ☑
   with foreign body S31.521 ☑
   penis — *see* Laceration, penis
   scrotum — *see* Laceration, scrotum
   testis — *see* Laceration, testis
 groin — *see* Laceration, abdomen, wall
 gum — *see* Laceration, oral cavity
 hand S61.419 ☑
  with
   foreign body S61.429 ☑
  finger — *see* Laceration, finger
  left S61.412 ☑
   with
    foreign body S61.422 ☑
  right S61.411 ☑
   with
    foreign body S61.421 ☑
  thumb — *see* Laceration, thumb
 head S01.91 ☑
  with foreign body S01.92 ☑
  cheek — *see* Laceration, cheek
  ear — *see* Laceration, ear
  eyelid — *see* Laceration, eyelid
  lip — *see* Laceration, lip
  nose — *see* Laceration, nose
  oral cavity — *see* Laceration, oral cavity
  scalp S01.01 ☑
   with foreign body S01.02 ☑
  specified site NEC S01.81 ☑
   with foreign body S01.82 ☑
  temporomandibular area — *see* Laceration, cheek
 heart — *see* Injury, heart, laceration
 heel — *see* Laceration, foot
 hepatic duct S36.13 ☑
 hip S71.019 ☑

Laceration — *continued*
hip — *continued*
 with foreign body S71.029 ☑
 left S71.012 ☑
  with foreign body S71.022 ☑
 right S71.011 ☑
  with foreign body S71.021 ☑
 hymen — *see* Laceration, vagina
 hypochondrium — *see* Laceration, abdomen, wall
 hypogastric region — *see* Laceration, abdomen, wall
 ileum S36.438 ☑
 inguinal region — *see* Laceration, abdomen, wall
 instep — *see* Laceration, foot
 internal organ — *see* Injury, by site
 interscapular region — *see* Laceration, thorax, back
 intestine
  large
   colon S36.539 ☑
    ascending S36.530 ☑
    descending S36.532 ☑
    sigmoid S36.533 ☑
    specified site NEC S36.538 ☑
   rectum S36.63 ☑
   transverse S36.531 ☑
  small S36.439 ☑
   duodenum S36.430 ☑
   specified site NEC S36.438 ☑
 intra-abdominal organ S36.93 ☑
  intestine — *see* Laceration, intestine
  liver — *see* Laceration, liver
  pancreas — *see* Laceration, pancreas
  peritoneum S36.81 ☑
  specified site NEC S36.893 ☑
  spleen — *see* Laceration, spleen
  stomach — *see* Laceration, stomach
 intracranial NEC — *see also* Injury, intracranial, diffuse
  birth injury P10.9
 jaw — *see* Laceration, head, specified site NEC
 jejunum S36.438 ☑
 joint capsule — *see* Sprain, by site
 kidney S37.03- ☑
  major (greater than 3 cm) (massive) (stellate) S37.06- ☑
  minor (less than 1 cm) S37.04- ☑
  moderate (1 to 3 cm) S37.05- ☑
  multiple S37.06- ☑
 knee S81.01- ☑
  with foreign body S81.02- ☑
 labium (majus) (minus) — *see* Laceration, vulva
 lacrimal duct — *see* Laceration, eyelid
 large intestine — *see* Laceration, intestine, large
 larynx S11.011 ☑
  with foreign body S11.012 ☑
 leg (lower) S81.819 ☑
  with foreign body S81.829 ☑
  foot — *see* Laceration, foot
  knee — *see* Laceration, knee
  left S81.812 ☑
   with foreign body S81.822 ☑
  right S81.811 ☑
   with foreign body S81.821 ☑
  upper — *see* Laceration, thigh
 ligament — *see* Sprain
 lip S01.511 ☑
  with foreign body S01.521 ☑
 liver S36.113 ☑
  major (stellate) S36.116 ☑
  minor S36.114 ☑
  moderate S36.115 ☑
 loin — *see* Laceration, abdomen, wall
 lower back — *see* Laceration, back, lower
 lumbar region — *see* Laceration, back, lower
 lung S27.339 ☑
  bilateral S27.332 ☑
  unilateral S27.331 ☑
 malar region — *see* Laceration, head, specified site NEC
 mammary — *see* Laceration, breast
 mastoid region — *see* Laceration, head, specified site NEC
 meninges — *see* Injury, intracranial, diffuse
 meniscus — *see* Tear, meniscus
 mesentery S36.893 ☑
 mesosalpinx S37.893 ☑
 mouth — *see* Laceration, oral cavity
 muscle — *see* Injury, muscle, by site, laceration

Laceration — *continued*

nail
  finger — *see* Laceration, finger, with damage to nail
  toe — *see* Laceration, toe, with damage to nail
nasal (septum) (sinus) — *see* Laceration, nose
nasopharynx — *see* Laceration, head, specified site NEC
neck S11.91 ☑
  with foreign body S11.92 ☑
  involving
    cervical esophagus S11.21 ☑
      with foreign body S11.22 ☑
    larynx — *see* Laceration, larynx
    pharynx — *see* Laceration, pharynx
    thyroid gland — *see* Laceration, thyroid gland
    trachea — *see* Laceration, trachea
  specified site NEC S11.81 ☑
    with foreign body S11.82 ☑
nerve — *see* Injury, nerve
nose (septum) (sinus) S01.21 ☑
  with foreign body S01.22 ☑
ocular NOS S05.3-
  adnexa NOS S01.11- ☑
oral cavity S01.512 ☑
  with foreign body S01.522 ☑
orbit (eye) — *see* Wound, open, ocular, orbit
ovary S37.439 ☑
  bilateral S37.432 ☑
  unilateral S37.431 ☑
palate — *see* Laceration, oral cavity
palm — *see* Laceration, hand
pancreas S36.239 ☑
pelvic S31.010 ☑
  with
    foreign body S31.020 ☑
      penetration into retroperitoneal cavity S31.021 ☑
    penetration into retroperitoneal cavity S31.011 ☑
  floor — *see also* Laceration, back, lower
    with ectopic or molar pregnancy O08.6
    complicating delivery O70.1
    following ectopic or molar pregnancy O08.6
    old (postpartal) N81.89
  organ S37.93 ☑
penis S31.21 ☑
  with foreign body S31.22 ☑
perineum
  female S31.41 ☑
    with
      ectopic or molar pregnancy O08.6
      foreign body S31.42 ☑
    during delivery O70.9
      first degree O70.0
      fourth degree O70.3
      second degree O70.1
      third degree — *see also* Delivery, complicated, by, laceration, perineum, third degree O70.20
    old (postpartal) N81.89
    postpartal N81.89
    secondary (postpartal) O90.1
  male S31.119 ☑
    with foreign body S31.129 ☑
periocular area (with or without lacrimal passages) — *see* Laceration, eyelid
peritoneum S36.893 ☑
periumbilic region — *see* Laceration, abdomen, wall, periumbilic
periurethral tissue — *see* Laceration, urethra
phalanges
  finger — *see* Laceration, finger
  toe — *see* Laceration, toe
pharynx S11.21 ☑
  with foreign body S11.22 ☑
pinna — *see* Laceration, ear
popliteal space — *see* Laceration, knee
prepuce — *see* Laceration, penis
prostate S37.823 ☑
pubic region S31.119 ☑
  with foreign body S31.129 ☑
pudendum — *see* Laceration, genital organs, external
rectovaginal septum — *see* Laceration, vagina
rectum S36.63 ☑
retroperitoneum S36.893 ☑
round ligament S37.893 ☑
sacral region — *see* Laceration, back, lower

Laceration — *continued*

sacroiliac region — *see* Laceration, back, lower
salivary gland — *see* Laceration, oral cavity
scalp S01.01 ☑
  with foreign body S01.02 ☑
scapular region — *see* Laceration, shoulder
scrotum S31.31 ☑
  with foreign body S31.32 ☑
seminal vesicle S37.893 ☑
shin — *see* Laceration, leg
shoulder S41.019 ☑
  with foreign body S41.029 ☑
  left S41.012 ☑
    with foreign body S41.022 ☑
  right S41.011 ☑
    with foreign body S41.021 ☑
small intestine — *see* Laceration, intestine, small
spermatic cord — *see* Laceration, testis
spinal cord (meninges) — *see also* Injury, spinal cord, by region
  due to injury at birth P11.5
  newborn (birth injury) P11.5
spleen S36.039 ☑
  major (massive) (stellate) S36.032 ☑
  moderate S36.031 ☑
  superficial (minor) S36.030 ☑
sternal region — *see* Laceration, thorax, front
stomach S36.33 ☑
submaxillary region — *see* Laceration, head, specified site NEC
submental region — *see* Laceration, head, specified site NEC
subungual
  finger(s) — *see* Laceration, finger, with damage to nail
  toe(s) — *see* Laceration, toe, with damage to nail
suprarenal gland — *see* Laceration, adrenal gland
temple, temporal region — *see* Laceration, head, specified site NEC
temporomandibular area — *see* Laceration, cheek
tendon — *see* Injury, muscle, by site, laceration
  Achilles S86.02- ☑
tentorium cerebelli — *see* Injury, intracranial, diffuse
testis S31.31 ☑
  with foreign body S31.32 ☑
thigh S71.11- ☑
  with foreign body S71.12- ☑
thorax, thoracic (wall) S21.91 ☑
  with foreign body S21.92 ☑
    back S21.22- ☑
      with penetration into thoracic cavity S21.42- ☑
    front S21.12- ☑
      with penetration into thoracic cavity S21.32- ☑
  back S21.21- ☑
    with
      foreign body S21.22- ☑
        with penetration into thoracic cavity S21.42- ☑
      penetration into thoracic cavity S21.41- ☑
  breast — *see* Laceration, breast
  front S21.11- ☑
    with
      foreign body S21.12- ☑
        with penetration into thoracic cavity S21.32- ☑
      penetration into thoracic cavity S21.31- ☑
thumb S61.019 ☑
  with
    damage to nail S61.119 ☑
      with
        foreign body S61.129 ☑
    foreign body S61.029 ☑
  left S61.012 ☑
    with
      damage to nail S61.112 ☑
        with
          foreign body S61.122 ☑
      foreign body S61.022 ☑
  right S61.011 ☑
    with
      damage to nail S61.111 ☑
        with
          foreign body S61.121 ☑
      foreign body S61.021 ☑

Laceration — *continued*

thyroid gland S11.11 ☑
  with foreign body S11.12 ☑
toe(s) S91.119 ☑
  with
    damage to nail S91.219 ☑
      with
        foreign body S91.229 ☑
    foreign body S91.129 ☑
  great S91.113 ☑
    with
      damage to nail S91.213 ☑
        with
          foreign body S91.223 ☑
      foreign body S91.123 ☑
    left S91.112 ☑
      with
        damage to nail S91.212 ☑
          with
            foreign body S91.222 ☑
        foreign body S91.122 ☑
    right S91.111 ☑
      with
        damage to nail S91.211 ☑
          with
            foreign body S91.221 ☑
        foreign body S91.121 ☑
  lesser S91.116 ☑
    with
      damage to nail S91.216 ☑
        with
          foreign body S91.226 ☑
      foreign body S91.126 ☑
    left S91.115 ☑
      with
        damage to nail S91.215 ☑
          with
            foreign body S91.225 ☑
        foreign body S91.125 ☑
    right S91.114 ☑
      with
        damage to nail S91.214 ☑
          with
            foreign body S91.224 ☑
        foreign body S91.124 ☑
tongue — *see* Laceration, oral cavity
trachea S11.021 ☑
  with foreign body S11.022 ☑
tunica vaginalis — *see* Laceration, testis
tympanum, tympanic membrane — *see* Laceration, ear, drum
umbilical region S31.115 ☑
  with foreign body S31.125 ☑
ureter S37.13 ☑
urethra S37.33 ☑
  with or following ectopic or molar pregnancy O08.6
  obstetrical trauma O71.5
urinary organ NEC S37.893 ☑
uterus S37.63 ☑
  with ectopic or molar pregnancy O08.6
  following ectopic or molar pregnancy O08.6
  nonpuerperal, nontraumatic N85.8
  obstetrical trauma NEC O71.81
  old (postpartal) N85.8
uvula — *see* Laceration, oral cavity
vagina S31.41 ☑
  with
    ectopic or molar pregnancy O08.6
    foreign body S31.42 ☑
  during delivery O71.4
    with perineal laceration — *see* Laceration, perineum, female, during delivery
  following ectopic or molar pregnancy O08.6
  nonpuerperal, nontraumatic N89.8
  old (postpartal) N89.8
vas deferens S37.893 ☑
vesical — *see* Laceration, bladder
vocal cords S11.031 ☑
  with foreign body S11.032 ☑
vulva S31.41 ☑
  with
    ectopic or molar pregnancy O08.6
    foreign body S31.42 ☑
  complicating delivery O70.0
  following ectopic or molar pregnancy O08.6
  nonpuerperal, nontraumatic N90.89
  old (postpartal) N90.89

Laceration — *continued*
  wrist S61.519 ☑
    with
      foreign body S61.529 ☑
    left S61.512 ☑
      with
        foreign body S61.522 ☑
    right S61.511 ☑
      with
        foreign body S61.521 ☑
Lack of
  achievement in school Z55.3
  adequate
    food Z59.4
    intermaxillary vertical dimension of fully erupted
      teeth M26.36
    sleep Z72.820
  appetite (see Anorexia) R63.0
  awareness R41.9
  care
    in home Z74.2
    of infant (at or after birth) T76.02 ☑
      confirmed T74.02 ☑
  cognitive functions R41.9
  coordination R27.9
    ataxia R27.0
    specified type NEC R27.8
  development (physiological) R62.50
    failure to thrive (child over 28 days old) R62.51
      adult R62.7
      newborn P92.6
    short stature R62.52
    specified type NEC R62.59
  energy R53.83
  financial resources Z59.6
  food T73.0 ☑
  growth R62.52
  heating Z59.1
  housing (permanent) (temporary) Z59.0
    adequate Z59.1
  learning experiences in childhood Z62.898
  leisure time (affecting life-style) Z73.2
  material resources Z59.9
  memory — *see also* Amnesia
    mild, following organic brain damage F06.8
  ovulation N97.0
  parental supervision or control of child Z62.0
  person able to render necessary care Z74.2
  physical exercise Z72.3
  play experience in childhood Z62.898
  posterior occlusal support M26.57
  relaxation (affecting life-style) Z73.2
  sexual
    desire F52.0
    enjoyment F52.1
  shelter Z59.0
  sleep (adequate) Z72.820
  supervision of child by parent Z62.0
  support, posterior occlusal M26.57
  water T73.1 ☑
Lacrimal — *see* condition
Lacrimation, abnormal — *see* Epiphora
Lacrimonasal duct — *see* condition
Lactation, lactating (breast) (puerperal, postpartum)
  associated
    cracked nipple O92.13
    retracted nipple O92.03
  defective O92.4
  disorder NEC O92.79
  excessive O92.6
  failed (complete) O92.3
    partial O92.4
  mastitis NEC — *see* Mastitis, obstetric
  mother (care and/or examination) Z39.1
  nonpuerperal N64.3
Lacticemia, excessive E87.2
Lacunar skull Q75.8
Laennec's cirrhosis K70.30
  with ascites K70.31
  nonalcoholic K74.69
Lafora's disease — *see* Epilepsy, generalized, idiopathic
Lag, lid (nervous) — *see* Retraction, lid
Lagophthalmos (eyelid) (nervous) H02.209
  bilateral, upper and lower eyelids H02.20C
  cicatricial H02.219
    bilateral, upper and lower eyelids H02.21C
    left H02.216
      lower H02.215

Lagophthalmos — *continued*
  cicatricial — *continued*
    left — *continued*
      upper H02.214
      upper and lower eyelids H02.21B
    right H02.213
      lower H02.212
      upper H02.211
      upper and lower eyelids H02.21A
  keratoconjunctivitis — *see* Keratoconjunctivitis
  left H02.206
    lower H02.205
    upper H02.204
    upper and lower eyelids H02.20B
  mechanical H02.229
    bilateral, upper and lower eyelids H02.22C
    left H02.226
      lower H02.225
      upper H02.224
      upper and lower eyelids H02.22B
    right H02.223
      lower H02.222
      upper H02.221
      upper and lower eyelids H02.22A
  paralytic H02.239
    bilateral, upper and lower eyelids H02.23C
    left H02.236
      lower H02.235
      upper H02.234
      upper and lower eyelids H02.23B
    right H02.233
      lower H02.232
      upper H02.231
      upper and lower eyelids H02.23A
  right H02.203
    lower H02.202
    upper H02.201
    upper and lower eyelids H02.20A
Laki-Lorand factor deficiency — *see* Defect, coagulation, specified type NEC
Lalling F80.0
Lambert-Eaton syndrome — *see* Syndrome, Lambert-Eaton
Lambliasis, lambliosis A07.1
Landau-Kleffner syndrome — *see* Epilepsy, specified NEC
Landouzy-Déjérine dystrophy or facioscapulohumeral atrophy G71.02
Landouzy's disease (icterohemorrhagic leptospirosis) A27.0
Landry-Guillain-Barré, syndrome or paralysis G61.0
Landry's disease or paralysis G61.0
Lane's
  band Q43.3
  kink — *see* Obstruction, intestine
  syndrome K90.2
Langdon Down syndrome — *see* Trisomy, 21
Lapsed immunization schedule status Z28.3
Large
  baby (regardless of gestational age) (4000g to 4499g) P08.1
  ear, congenital Q17.1
  physiological cup Q14.2
  stature R68.89
Large-for-dates NEC (infant) (4000g to 4499g) P08.1
  affecting management of pregnancy O36.6- ☑
  exceptionally (4500g or more) P08.0
Larsen-Johansson disease orosteochondrosis — *see* Osteochondrosis, juvenile, patella
Larsen's syndrome (flattened facies and multiple congenital dislocations) Q74.8
Larva migrans
  cutaneous B76.9
    Ancylostoma B76.0
  visceral B83.0
Laryngeal — *see* condition
Laryngismus (stridulus) J38.5
  congenital P28.89
  diphtheritic A36.2
Laryngitis (acute) (edematous) (fibrinous) (infective) (infiltrative) (malignant) (membranous) (phlegmonous) (pneumococcal) (pseudomembranous) (septic) (subglottic) (suppurative) (ulcerative) J04.0
  with
    influenza, flu, or grippe — *see* Influenza, with, laryngitis
    tracheitis (acute) — *see* Laryngotracheitis
  atrophic J37.0

Laryngitis — *continued*
  catarrhal J37.0
  chronic J37.0
    with tracheitis (chronic) J37.1
  diphtheritic A36.2
  due to external agent — *see* Inflammation, respiratory, upper, due to
  H. influenzae J04.0
  Hemophilus influenzae J04.0
  hypertrophic J37.0
  influenzal — *see* Influenza, with, respiratory manifestations NEC
  obstructive J05.0
  sicca J37.0
  spasmodic J05.0
    acute J04.0
  streptococcal J04.0
  stridulous J05.0
  syphilitic (late) A52.73
    congenital A50.59 [J99]
      early A50.03 [J99]
  tuberculous A15.5
  Vincent's A69.1
Laryngocele (congenital) (ventricular) Q31.3
Laryngofissure J38.7
  congenital Q31.8
Laryngomalacia (congenital) Q31.5
Laryngopharyngitis (acute) J06.0
  chronic J37.0
  due to external agent — *see* Inflammation, respiratory, upper, due to
Laryngoplegia J38.00
  bilateral J38.02
  unilateral J38.01
Laryngoptosis J38.7
Laryngospasm J38.5
Laryngostenosis J38.6
Laryngotracheitis (acute) (Infectional) (infective) (viral) J04.2
  atrophic J37.1
  catarrhal J37.1
  chronic J37.1
  diphtheritic A36.2
  due to external agent — *see* Inflammation, respiratory, upper, due to
  Hemophilus influenzae J04.2
  hypertrophic J37.1
  influenzal — *see* Influenza, with, respiratory manifestations NEC
  pachydermic J38.7
  sicca J37.1
  spasmodic J38.5
    acute J05.0
  streptococcal J04.2
  stridulous J38.5
  syphilitic (late) A52.73
    congenital A50.59 [J99]
      early A50.03 [J99]
  tuberculous A15.5
  Vincent's A69.1
Laryngotracheobronchitis — *see* Bronchitis
Larynx, laryngeal — *see* condition
Lassa fever A96.2
Lassitude — *see* Weakness
Late
  talker R62.0
  walker R62.0
Late effect(s) — *see* Sequelae
Latent — *see* condition
Laterocession — *see* Lateroversion
Lateroflexion — *see* Lateroversion
Lateroversion
  cervix — *see* Lateroversion, uterus
  uterus, uterine (cervix) (postinfectional) (postpartal, old) N85.4
    congenital Q51.818
    in pregnancy or childbirth O34.59- ☑
Lathyrism — *see* Poisoning, food, noxious, plant
Launois' syndrome (pituitary gigantism) E22.0
Launois-Bensaude adenolipomatosis E88.89
Laurence-Moon (-Bardet)-**Biedl syndrome** Q87.89
Lax, laxity — *see also* Relaxation
  ligament (ous) — *see also* Disorder, ligament
    familial M35.7
    knee — *see* Derangement, knee
  skin (acquired) L57.4
    congenital Q82.8
Laxative habit F55.2

Lazy leukocyte syndrome D70.8
Lead miner's lung J63.6
Leak, leakage
  air NEC J93.82
    postprocedural J95.812
  amniotic fluid — *see* Rupture, membranes, premature
  blood (microscopic), fetal, into maternal circulation
    affecting management of pregnancy — *see*
    Pregnancy, complicated by
  cerebrospinal fluid G96.0
    from spinal (lumbar) puncture G97.0
  device, implant or graft — *see also* Complications, by
    site and type, mechanical
    arterial graft NEC — *see* Complication, cardiovascu-
      lar device, mechanical, vascular
    breast (implant) T85.43 ☑
    catheter NEC T85.638 ☑
      dialysis (renal) T82.43 ☑
        intraperitoneal T85.631 ☑
      infusion NEC T82.534 ☑
        spinal (epidural) (subdural) T85.630 ☑
      urinary T83.038 ☑
        cystostomy T83.030 ☑
        Hopkins T83.038 ☑
        ileostomy T83.038 ☑
        indwelling T83.031 ☑
        nephrostomy T83.032 ☑
        specified T83.038 ☑
        urostomy T83.038 ☑
    gastrointestinal — *see* Complications, prosthetic
      device, mechanical, gastrointestinal device
    genital NEC T83.498 ☑
      penile prosthesis (cylinder) (implanted) (pump)
        (reservoir) T83.490 ☑
      testicular prosthesis T83.491 ☑
    heart NEC — *see* Complication, cardiovascular de-
      vice, mechanical
    joint prosthesis — *see* Complications, joint prosthe-
      sis, mechanical, specified NEC, by site
    ocular NEC — *see* Complications, prosthetic device,
      mechanical, ocular device
    orthopedic NEC — *see* Complication, orthopedic,
      device, mechanical
    persistent air J93.82
    specified NEC T85.638 ☑
    urinary NEC — *see also* Complication, genitourinary,
      device, urinary, mechanical
      graft T83.23 ☑
    vascular NEC — *see* Complication, cardiovascular
      device, mechanical
    ventricular intracranial shunt T85.03 ☑
  urine — *see* Incontinence
Leaky heart — *see* Endocarditis
Learning defect (specific) F81.9
Leather bottle stomach C16.9
Leber's
  congenital amaurosis H35.50
  optic atrophy (hereditary) H47.22
Lederer's anemia D59.1
Leeches (external) — *see* Hirudiniasis
Leg — *see* condition
Legg (-Calvé)-**Perthes disease, syndrome or osteo-**
  chondrosis M91.1- ☑
Legionellosis A48.1
  nonpneumonic A48.2
Legionnaires'
  disease A48.1
    nonpneumonic A48.2
    pneumonia A48.1
Leigh's disease G31.82
Leiner's disease L21.1
Leiofibromyoma — *see* Leiomyoma
Leiomyoblastoma — *see* Neoplasm, connective tissue,
  benign
Leiomyofibroma — *see also* Neoplasm, connective tissue, benign
  uterus (cervix) (corpus) D25.9
Leiomyoma — *see also* Neoplasm, connective tissue,
  benign
  bizarre — *see* Neoplasm, connective tissue, benign
  cellular — *see* Neoplasm, connective tissue, benign
  epithelioid — *see* Neoplasm, connective tissue, benign
  uterus (cervix) (corpus) D25.9
    intramural D25.1
    submucous D25.0
    subserosal D25.2
  vascular — *see* Neoplasm, connective tissue, benign

Leiomyoma, leiomyomatosis (intravascular) — *see*
  Neoplasm, connective tissue, uncertain behavior
Leiomyosarcoma — *see also* Neoplasm, connective tissue, malignant
  epithelioid — *see* Neoplasm, connective tissue, malig-
    nant
  myxoid — *see* Neoplasm, connective tissue, malignant
Leishmaniasis B55.9
  American (mucocutaneous) B55.2
    cutaneous B55.1
  Asian Desert B55.1
  Brazilian B55.2
  cutaneous (any type) B55.1
  dermal — *see also* Leishmaniasis, cutaneous
    post-kala-azar B55.0
  eyelid B55.1
  infantile B55.0
  Mediterranean B55.0
  mucocutaneous (American) (New World) B55.2
  naso-oral B55.2
  nasopharyngeal B55.2
  old world B55.1
  tegumentaria diffusa B55.1
  visceral B55.0
Leishmanoid, dermal — *see also* Leishmaniasis, cutaneous
  post-kala-azar B55.0
Lenegre's disease I44.2
Lengthening, leg — *see* Deformity, limb, unequal length
Lennert's lymphoma — *see* Lymphoma, Lennert's
Lennox-Gastaut syndrome G40.812
  intractable G40.814
    with status epilepticus G40.813
    without status epilepticus G40.814
  not intractable G40.812
    with status epilepticus G40.811
    without status epilepticus G40.812
Lens — *see* condition
Lenticonus (anterior) (posterior) (congenital) Q12.8
Lenticular degeneration, progressive E83.01
Lentiglobus (posterior) (congenital) Q12.8
Lentigo (congenital) L81.4
  maligna — *see also* Melanoma, in situ
    melanoma — *see* Melanoma
Lentivirus, as cause of disease classified elsewhere
  B97.31
Leontiasis
  ossium M85.2
  syphilitic (late) A52.78
    congenital A50.59
Lepothrix A48.8
Lepra — *see* Leprosy
Leprechaunism E34.8
Leprosy A30.- ☑
  with muscle disorder A30.9 *[M63.80]*
    ankle A30.9 *[M63.87-]* ☑
    foot A30.9 *[M63.87-]* ☑
    forearm A30.9 *[M63.83-]* ☑
    hand A30.9 *[M63.84-]* ☑
    lower leg A30.9 *[M63.86-]* ☑
    multiple sites A30.9 *[M63.89]*
    pelvic region A30.9 *[M63.85-]* ☑
    shoulder region A30.9 *[M63.81-]* ☑
    specified site NEC A30.9 *[M63.88]*
    thigh A30.9 *[M63.85-]* ☑
    upper arm A30.9 *[M63.82-]* ☑
  anesthetic A30.9
  BB A30.3
  BL A30.4
  borderline (infiltrated) (neuritic) A30.3
    lepromatous A30.4
    tuberculoid A30.2
  BT A30.2
  dimorphous (infiltrated) (neuritic) A30.3
  I A30.0
  indeterminate (macular) (neuritic) A30.0
  lepromatous (diffuse) (infiltrated) (macular) (neuritic)
    (nodular) A30.5
  LL A30.5
  macular (early) (neuritic) (simple) A30.9
  maculoanesthetic A30.9
  mixed A30.3
  neural A30.9
  nodular A30.5
  primary neuritic A30.3
  specified type NEC A30.8
  TT A30.1

Leprosy — *continued*
  tuberculoid (major) (minor) A30.1
Leptocytosis, hereditary D56.9
Leptomeningitis (chronic) (circumscribed) (hemorrhagic)
  (nonsuppurative) — *see* Meningitis
Leptomeningopathy G96.19
Leptospiral — *see* condition
Leptospirochetal — *see* condition
Leptospirosis A27.9
  canicola A27.89
  due to Leptospira interrogans serovar icterohaemorrha-
    giae A27.0
  icterohemorrhagica A27.0
  pomona A27.89
  Weil's disease A27.0
Leptus dermatitis B88.0
Leriche's syndrome (aortic bifurcation occlusion) I74.09
Leri's pleonosteosis Q78.8
Leri-Weill syndrome Q77.8
Lermoyez' syndrome — *see* Vertigo, peripheral NEC
Lesch-Nyhan syndrome E79.1
Leser-Trélat disease L82.1
  inflamed L82.0
Lesion(s) (nontraumatic)
  abducens nerve — *see* Strabismus, paralytic, sixth nerve
  alveolar process K08.9
  angiocentric immunoproliferative D47.Z9 (*following*
    D47.4)
  anorectal K62.9
  aortic (valve) I35.9
  auditory nerve — *see* subcategory H93.3 ☑
  basal ganglion G25.9
  bile duct — *see* Disease, bile duct
  biomechanical M99.9
    specified type NEC M99.89
      abdomen M99.89
      acromioclavicular M99.87
      cervical region M99.81
      cervicothoracic M99.81
      costochondral M99.88
      costovertebral M99.88
      head region M99.80
      hip M99.85
      lower extremity M99.86
      lumbar region M99.83
      lumbosacral M99.83
      occipitocervical M99.80
      pelvic region M99.85
      pubic M99.85
      rib cage M99.88
      sacral region M99.84
      sacrococcygeal M99.84
      sacroiliac M99.84
      specified NEC M99.89
      sternochondral M99.88
      sternoclavicular M99.87
      thoracic region M99.82
      thoracolumbar M99.82
      upper extremity M99.87
  bladder N32.9
  bone — *see* Disorder, bone
  brachial plexus G54.0
  brain G93.9
    congenital Q04.9
    vascular I67.9
      degenerative I67.9
      hypertensive I67.4
  buccal cavity K13.79
  calcified — *see* Calcification
  canthus — *see* Disorder, eyelid
  carate — *see* Pinta, lesions
  cardia K31.9
  cardiac — *see also* Disease, heart I51.9
    congenital Q24.9
    valvular — *see* Endocarditis
  cauda equina G83.4
  cecum K63.9
  cerebral — *see* Lesion, brain
  cerebrovascular I67.9
    degenerative I67.9
    hypertensive I67.4
  cervical (nerve) root NEC G54.2
  chiasmal — *see* Disorder, optic, chiasm
  chorda tympani G51.8
  coin, lung R91.1
  colon K63.9
  combined periodontic - endodontic K05.5
  congenital — *see* Anomaly, by site

Lesion(s) — *continued*
conjunctiva H11.9
conus medullaris — *see* Injury, conus medullaris
coronary artery — *see* Ischemia, heart
cranial nerve G52.9
  eighth — *see* Disorder, ear
  eleventh G52.9
  fifth G50.9
  first G52.0
  fourth — *see* Strabismus, paralytic, fourth nerve
  seventh G51.9
  sixth — *see* Strabismus, paralytic, sixth nerve
  tenth G52.2
  twelfth G52.3
cystic — *see* Cyst
degenerative — *see* Degeneration
duodenum K31.9
edentulous (alveolar) ridge, associated with trauma, due to traumatic occlusion K06.2
en coup de sabre L94.1
eyelid — *see* Disorder, eyelid
gasserian ganglion G50.8
gastric K31.9
gastroduodenal K31.9
gastrointestinal K63.9
gingiva, associated with trauma K06.2
glomerular
  focal and segmental — *see also* N00-N07 with fourth character .1 N05.1
  minimal change — *see also* N00-N07 with fourth character .0 N05.0
heart (organic) — *see* Disease, heart
hyperchromic, due to pinta (carate) A67.1
hyperkeratotic — *see* Hyperkeratosis
hypothalamic E23.7
ileocecal K63.9
ileum K63.9
iliohypogastric nerve G57.8- ☑
inflammatory — *see* Inflammation
intestine K63.9
intracerebral — *see* Lesion, brain
intrachiasmal (optic) — *see* Disorder, optic, chiasm
intracranial, space-occupying R90.0
joint — *see* Disorder, joint
  sacroiliac (old) M53.3
keratotic — *see* Keratosis
kidney — *see* Disease, renal
laryngeal nerve (recurrent) G52.2
lip K13.0
liver K76.9
lumbosacral
  plexus G54.1
  root (nerve) NEC G54.4
lung (coin) R91.1
maxillary sinus J32.0
mitral I05.9
Morel-Lavallée — *see* Hematoma, by site
motor cortex NEC G93.89
mouth K13.79
nerve G58.9
  femoral G57.2- ☑
  median G56.1- ☑
    carpal tunnel syndrome — *see* Syndrome, carpal tunnel
  plantar G57.6- ☑
  popliteal (lateral) G57.3- ☑
    medial G57.4- ☑
  radial G56.3- ☑
  sciatic G57.0- ☑
  spinal — *see* Injury, nerve, spinal
  ulnar G56.2- ☑
nervous system, congenital Q07.9
nonallopathic — *see* Lesion, biomechanical
nose (internal) J34.89
obstructive — *see* Obstruction
obturator nerve G57.8- ☑
oral mucosa K13.70
organ or site NEC — *see* Disease, by site
osteolytic — *see* Osteolysis
peptic K27.9
periodontal, due to traumatic occlusion K05.5
pharynx J39.2
pigment, pigmented (skin) L81.9
pinta — *see* Pinta, lesions
polypoid — *see* Polyp
prechiasmal (optic) — *see* Disorder, optic, chiasm
primary — *see also* Syphilis, primary A51.0

Lesion(s) — *continued*
primary — *see also* Syphilis, primary — *continued*
  carate A67.0
  pinta A67.0
  yaws A66.0
pulmonary J98.4
  valve I37.9
pylorus K31.9
rectosigmoid K63.9
retina, retinal H35.9
sacroiliac (joint) (old) M53.3
salivary gland K11.9
  benign lymphoepithelial K11.8
saphenous nerve G57.8- ☑
sciatic nerve G57.0- ☑
secondary — *see* Syphilis, secondary
shoulder (region) M75.9-
  specified NEC M75.8-
sigmoid K63.9
sinus (accessory) (nasal) J34.89
skin L98.9
  suppurative L08.0
SLAP S43.43-
spinal cord G95.9
  congenital Q06.9
spleen D73.89
stomach K31.9
superior glenoid labrum S43.43- ☑
syphilitic — *see* Syphilis
tertiary — *see* Syphilis, tertiary
thoracic root (nerve) NEC G54.3
tonsillar fossa J35.9
tooth, teeth K08.9
  white spot
    chewing surface K02.51
    pit and fissure surface K02.51
    smooth surface K02.61
traumatic — *see* specific type of injury by site
tricuspid (valve) I07.9
  nonrheumatic I36.9
trigeminal nerve G50.9
ulcerated or ulcerative — *see* Ulcer, skin
uterus N85.9
vagina N89.8
vagus nerve G52.2
valvular — *see* Endocarditis
vascular I99.9
  affecting central nervous system I67.9
  following trauma NEC T14.8 ☑
  umbilical cord, complicating delivery O69.5 ☑
vulva N90.89
warty — *see* Verruca
white spot (tooth)
  chewing surface K02.51
  pit and fissure surface K02.51
  smooth surface K02.61
Lethargic — *see* condition
Lethargy R53.83
Letterer-Siwe's disease C96.0
Leukemia, leukemic C95.9- ☑
acute basophilic C94.8- ☑
acute bilineal C95.0- ☑
acute erythroid C94.0- ☑
acute lymphoblastic C91.0- ☑
acute megakaryoblastic C94.2- ☑
acute megakaryocytic C94.2- ☑
acute mixed lineage C95.0- ☑
acute monoblastic (monoblastic/monocytic) C93.0- ☑
acute monocytic (monoblastic/monocytic) C93.0- ☑
acute myeloblastic (minimal differentiation) (with maturation) C92.0- ☑
acute myeloid, NOS C92.0- ☑
  with
    11q23-abnormality C92.6- ☑
    dysplasia of remaining hematopoesis and/or myelodysplastic disease in its history C92.A- ☑ (*following* C92.6)
    multilineage dysplasia C92.A- ☑ (*following* C92.6)
    variation of MLL-gene C92.6- ☑
  M6 (a)(b) C94.0- ☑
  M7 C94.2- ☑
acute myelomonocytic C92.5- ☑
acute promyelocytic C92.4- ☑
adult T-cell (HTLV-1-associated) (acute variant) (chronic variant) (lymphomatoid variant) (smouldering variant) C91.5- ☑

Leukemia, leukemic — *continued*
aggressive NK-cell C94.8- ☑
AML (1/ETO) (M0) (M1) (M2) (without a FAB classification) C92.0- ☑
AML M3 C92.4-
AML M4 (Eo with inv(16) or t(16;16)) C92.5- ☑
AML M5 C93.0- ☑
AML M5a C93.0- ☑
AML M5b C93.0- ☑
AML Me with t (15;17) and variants C92.4- ☑
atypical chronic myeloid, BCR/ABL-negative C92.2- ☑
biphenotypic acute C95.0- ☑
blast cell C95.0- ☑
Burkitt-type, mature B-cell C91.A- ☑ (*following* C91.6)
chronic lymphocytic, of B-cell type C91.1- ☑
chronic monocytic C93.1- ☑
chronic myelogenous (Philadelphia chromosome (Ph1) positive) (t(9;22)) (q34;q11) (with crisis of blast cells) C92.1- ☑
chronic myeloid, BCR/ABL-positive C92.1- ☑
  atypical, BCR/ABL-negative C92.2- ☑
chronic myelomonocytic C93.1- ☑
chronic neutrophilic D47.1
CMML (-1) (-2) (with eosinophilia) C93.1- ☑
granulocytic — *see also* Category C92 C92.9- ☑
hairy cell C91.4- ☑
juvenile myelomonocytic C93.3- ☑
lymphoid C91.9- ☑
  specified NEC C91.Z- ☑ (*following* C91.6)
mast cell C94.3- ☑
mature B-cell, Burkitt-type C91.A- ☑ (*following* C91.6)
monocytic (subacute) C93.9- ☑
  specified NEC C93.Z- ☑ (*following* C93.3)
myelogenous — *see also* Category C92 C92.9- ☑
myeloid C92.9- ☑
  specified NEC C92.Z- ☑ (*following* C92.6)
plasma cell C90.1- ☑
plasmacytic C90.1- ☑
prolymphocytic
  of B-cell type C91.3- ☑
  of T-cell type C91.6- ☑
specified NEC C94.8- ☑
stem cell, of unclear lineage C95.0- ☑
subacute lymphocytic C91.9- ☑
T-cell large granular lymphocytic C91.Z- ☑ (*following* C91.6)
unspecified cell type C95.9- ☑
  acute C95.0- ☑
  chronic C95.1- ☑
Leukemoid reaction — *see also* Reaction, leukemoid D72.823
Leukoaraiosis (hypertensive) I67.81
Leukoariosis — *see* Leukoaraiosis
Leukocoria — *see* Disorder, globe, degenerated condition, leucocoria
Leukocytopenia D72.819
Leukocytosis D72.829
eosinophilic D72.1
Leukoderma, leukodermia NEC L81.5
syphilitic A51.39
  late A52.79
Leukodystrophy E75.29
Leukoedema, oral epithelium K13.29
Leukoencephalitis G04.81
acute (subacute) hemorrhagic G36.1
  postimmunization or postvaccinal G04.02
postinfectious G04.01
subacute sclerosing A81.1
van Bogaert's (sclerosing) A81.1
Leukoencephalopathy — *see also* Encephalopathy G93.49
Binswanger's I67.3
heroin vapor G92
metachromatic E75.25
multifocal (progressive) A81.2
postimmunization and postvaccinal G04.02
progressive multifocal A81.2
reversible, posterior G93.6
van Bogaert's (sclerosing) A81.1
vascular, progressive I67.3
Leukoerythroblastosis D75.9
Leukokeratosis — *see also* Leukoplakia
mouth K13.21
nicotina palati K13.24
oral mucosa K13.21
tongue K13.21
vocal cord J38.3

Leukokraurosis vulva (e) N90.4
Leukoma (cornea) — *see also* Opacity, cornea
  adherent H17.0- ☑
  interfering with central vision — *see* Opacity, cornea, central
Leukomalacia, cerebral, newborn P91.2
  periventricular P91.2
Leukomelanopathy, hereditary D72.0
Leukonychia (punctata) (striata) L60.8
  congenital Q84.4
Leukopathia unguium L60.8
  congenital Q84.4
Leukopenia D72.819
  basophilic D72.818
  chemotherapy (cancer) induced D70.1
  congenital D70.0
  cyclic D70.0
  drug induced NEC D70.2
    due to cytoreductive cancer chemotherapy D70.1
  eosinophilic D72.818
  familial D70.0
  infantile genetic D70.0
  malignant D70.9
  periodic D70.0
  transitory neonatal P61.5
Leukopenic — *see* condition
Leukoplakia
  anus K62.89
  bladder (postinfectional) N32.89
  buccal K13.21
  cervix (uteri) N88.0
  esophagus K22.8
  gingiva K13.21
  hairy (oral mucosa) (tongue) K13.3
  kidney (pelvis) N28.89
  larynx J38.7
  lip K13.21
  mouth K13.21
  oral epithelium, including tongue (mucosa) K13.21
  palate K13.21
  pelvis (kidney) N28.89
  penis (infectional) N48.0
  rectum K62.89
  syphilitic (late) A52.79
  tongue K13.21
  ureter (postinfectional) N28.89
  urethra (postinfectional) N36.8
  uterus N85.8
  vagina N89.4
  vocal cord J38.3
  vulva N90.4
Leukorrhea N89.8
  due to Trichomonas (vaginalis) A59.00
  trichomonal A59.00
Leukosarcoma C85.9- ☑
Levocardia (isolated) Q24.1
  with situs inversus Q89.3
Levotransposition Q20.5
Lev's disease or syndrome (acquired complete heart block) I44.2
Levulosuria — *see* Fructosuria
Levurid L30.2
Lewy body (ies) (dementia) (disease) G31.83
Leyden-Moebius dystrophy G71.09
Leydig cell
  carcinoma
    specified site — *see* Neoplasm, malignant, by site
    unspecified site
      female C56.9
      male C62.9- ☑
  tumor
    benign
      specified site — *see* Neoplasm, benign, by site
      unspecified site
        female D27.- ☑
        male D29.2- ☑
    malignant
      specified site — *see* Neoplasm, malignant, by site
      unspecified site
        female C56.- ☑
        male C62.9- ☑
    specified site — *see* Neoplasm, uncertain behavior, by site
    unspecified site
      female D39.1- ☑
      male D40.1- ☑

Leydig-Sertoli cell tumor
  specified site — *see* Neoplasm, benign, by site
  unspecified site
    female D27.- ☑
    male D29.2- ☑
LGSIL (Low grade squamous intraepithelial lesion on cytologic smear of)
  anus R85.612
  cervix R87.612
  vagina R87.622
Liar, pathologic F60.2
Libido
  decreased R68.82
Libman-Sacks disease M32.11
Lice (infestation) B85.2
  body (Pediculus corporis) B85.1
  crab B85.3
  head (Pediculus capitis) B85.0
  mixed (classifiable to more than one of the titles B85.0-B85.3) B85.4
  pubic (Phthirus pubis) B85.3
Lichen L28.0
  albus L90.0
    penis N48.0
    vulva N90.4
  amyloidosis E85.4 *[L99]*
  atrophicus L90.0
    penis N48.0
    vulva N90.4
  congenital Q82.8
  myxedematosus L98.5
  nitidus L44.1
  pilaris Q82.8
    acquired L85.8
  planopilaris L66.1
  planus (chronicus) L43.9
    annularis L43.8
    bullous L43.1
    follicular L66.1
    hypertrophic L43.0
    moniliformis L44.3
    of Wilson L43.9
    specified NEC L43.8
    subacute (active) L43.3
    tropicus L43.3
  ruber
    acuminatus L44.0
    moniliformis L44.3
    planus L43.9
  sclerosus (et atrophicus) L90.0
    penis N48.0
    vulva N90.4
  scrofulosus (primary) (tuberculous) A18.4
  simplex (chronicus) (circumscriptus) L28.0
  striatus L44.2
  urticatus L28.2
Lichenification L28.0
Lichenoides tuberculosis (primary) A18.4
Lichtheim's disease or syndrome D51.0
Lien migrans D73.89
Ligament — *see* condition
Light
  for gestational age — *see* Light for dates
  headedness R42
Light-for-dates (infant) P05.00
  with weight of
    499 grams or less P05.01
    500-749 grams P05.02
    750-999 grams P05.03
    1000-1249 grams P05.04
    1250-1499 grams P05.05
    1500-1749 grams P05.06
    1750-1999 grams P05.07
    2000-2499 grams P05.08
    2500 grams and over P05.09
  affecting management of pregnancy O36.59- ☑
  and small-for-dates — *see* Small for dates
  specified NEC P05.09
Lightning (effects) (stroke) (struck by) T75.00 ☑
  burn — *see* Burn
  foot E53.8
  shock T75.01 ☑
  specified effect NEC T75.09 ☑
Lightwood-Albright syndrome N25.89
Lightwood's disease or syndrome (renal tubular acidosis) N25.89
Lignac (-de Toni) (-Fanconi) (-Debré) **disease or syndrome** E72.09

Lignac (-de Toni) (-Fanconi) (-Debré) **disease or syndrome** — *continued*
  with cystinosis E72.04
Ligneous thyroiditis E06.5
Likoff's syndrome I20.8
Limb — *see* condition
Limbic epilepsy personality syndrome F07.0
Limitation, limited
  activities due to disability Z73.6
  cardiac reserve — *see* Disease, heart
  eye muscle duction, traumatic — *see* Strabismus, mechanical
  mandibular range of motion M26.52
Lindau (-von Hippel) **disease** Q85.8
Line(s)
  Beau's L60.4
  Harris' — *see* Arrest, epiphyseal
  Hudson's (cornea) — *see* Pigmentation, cornea, anterior
  Stähli's (cornea) — *see* Pigmentation, cornea, anterior
Linea corneae senilis — *see* Change, cornea, senile
Lingua
  geographica K14.1
  nigra (villosa) K14.3
  plicata K14.5
  tylosis K13.29
Lingual — *see* condition
Linguatulosis B88.8
Linitis (gastric) **plastica** C16.9
Lip — *see* condition
Lipedema — *see* Edema
Lipemia — *see also* Hyperlipidemia
  retina, retinalis E78.3
Lipidosis E75.6
  cerebral (infantile) (juvenile) (late) E75.4
  cerebroretinal E75.4
  cerebroside E75.22
  cholesterol (cerebral) E75.5
  glycolipid E75.21
  hepatosplenomegalic E78.3
  sphingomyelin — *see* Niemann-Pick disease or syndrome
  sulfatide E75.29
Lipoadenoma — *see* Neoplasm, benign, by site
Lipoblastoma — *see* Lipoma
Lipoblastomatosis — *see* Lipoma
Lipochondrodystrophy E76.01
Lipochrome histiocytosis (familial) D71
Lipodermatosclerosis — *see* Varix, leg, with, inflammation
  ulcerated — *see* Varix, leg, with, ulcer, with inflammation by site
Lipodystrophia progressiva E88.1
Lipodystrophy (progressive) E88.1
  insulin E88.1
  intestinal K90.81
  mesenteric K65.4
Lipofibroma — *see* Lipoma
Lipofuscinosis, neuronal (with ceroidosis) E75.4
Lipogranuloma, sclerosing L92.8
Lipogranulomatosis E78.89
Lipoid — *see also* condition
  histiocytosis D76.3
    essential E75.29
  nephrosis N04.9
  proteinosis of Urbach E78.89
Lipoidemia — *see* Hyperlipidemia
Lipoidosis — *see* Lipidosis
Lipoma D17.9
  fetal D17.9
    fat cell D17.9
  infiltrating D17.9
  intramuscular D17.9
  pleomorphic D17.9
  site classification
    arms (skin) (subcutaneous) D17.2- ☑
    connective tissue D17.30
      intra-abdominal D17.5
      intrathoracic D17.4
      peritoneum D17.79
      retroperitoneum D17.79
      specified site NEC D17.39
      spermatic cord D17.6
    face (skin) (subcutaneous) D17.0
    genitourinary organ NEC D17.72
    head (skin) (subcutaneous) D17.0
    intra-abdominal D17.5
    intrathoracic D17.4

Lipoma — *continued*
  site classification — *continued*
    kidney D17.71
    legs (skin) (subcutaneous) D17.2- ☑
    neck (skin) (subcutaneous) D17.0
    peritoneum D17.79
    retroperitoneum D17.79
    skin D17.30
      specified site NEC D17.39
    specified site NEC D17.79
    spermatic cord D17.6
    subcutaneous D17.30
      specified site NEC D17.39
    trunk (skin) (subcutaneous) D17.1
    unspecified D17.9
  spindle cell D17.9
Lipomatosis E88.2
  dolorosa (Dercum) E88.2
  fetal — *see* Lipoma
  Launois-Bensaude E88.89
Lipomyoma — *see* Lipoma
Lipomyxoma — *see* Lipoma
Lipomyxosarcoma — *see* Neoplasm, connective tissue, malignant
Lipoprotein metabolism disorder E78.9
Lipoproteinemia E78.5
  broad-beta E78.2
  floating-beta E78.2
  hyper-pre-beta E78.1
Liposarcoma — *see also* Neoplasm, connective tissue, malignant
  dedifferentiated — *see* Neoplasm, connective tissue, malignant
  differentiated type — *see* Neoplasm, connective tissue, malignant
  embryonal — *see* Neoplasm, connective tissue, malignant
  mixed type — *see* Neoplasm, connective tissue, malignant
  myxoid — *see* Neoplasm, connective tissue, malignant
  pleomorphic — *see* Neoplasm, connective tissue, malignant
  round cell — *see* Neoplasm, connective tissue, malignant
  well differentiated type — *see* Neoplasm, connective tissue, malignant
Liposynovitis prepatellaris E88.89
Lipping, cervix N86
Lipschütz disease or ulcer N76.6
Lipuria R82.0
  schistosomiasis (bilharziasis) B65.0
Lisping F80.0
Lissauer's paralysis A52.17
Lissencephalia, lissencephaly Q04.3
Listeriosis, listerellosis A32.9
  congenital (disseminated) P37.2
  cutaneous A32.0
  neonatal, newborn (disseminated) P37.2
  oculoglandular A32.81
  specified NEC A32.89
Lithemia E79.0
Lithiasis — *see* Calculus
Lithosis J62.8
Lithuria R82.998
Litigation, anxiety concerning Z65.3
Little leaguer's elbow — *see* Epicondylitis, medial
Little's disease G80.9
Littre's
  gland — *see* condition
  hernia — *see* Hernia, abdomen
Littritis — *see* Urethritis
Livedo (annularis) (racemosa) (reticularis) R23.1
Liver — *see* condition
Living alone (problems with) Z60.2
  with handicapped person Z74.2
Lloyd's syndrome — *see* Adenomatosis, endocrine
Loa loa, loaiasis, loasis B74.3
Lobar — *see* condition
Lobomycosis B48.0
Lobo's disease B48.0
Lobotomy syndrome F07.0
Lobstein (-Ekman) **disease or syndrome** Q78.0
Lobster-claw hand Q71.6- ☑
Lobulation (congenital) — *see also* Anomaly, by site
  kidney, Q63.1
  liver, abnormal Q44.7
  spleen Q89.09

Lobule, lobular — *see* condition
Local, localized — *see* condition
Locked twins causing obstructed labor O66.1
Locked-in state G83.5
Locking
  joint — *see* Derangement, joint, specified type NEC
  knee — *see* Derangement, knee
Lockjaw — *see* Tetanus
Löffler's
  endocarditis I42.3
  eosinophilia J82
  pneumonia J82
  syndrome (eosinophilic pneumonitis) J82
Loiasis (with conjunctival infestation) (eyelid) B74.3
Lone Star fever A77.0
Long
  labor O63.9
    first stage O63.0
    second stage O63.1
  QT syndrome I45.81
Longitudinal stripes or grooves, nails L60.8
  congenital Q84.6
Long-term (current) (prophylactic) **drug therapy** (use of)
  agents affecting estrogen receptors and estrogen levels NEC Z79.818
  anastrozole (Arimidex) Z79.811
  antibiotics Z79.2
    short-term use — *omit code*
  anticoagulants Z79.01
  anti-inflammatory, non-steroidal (NSAID) Z79.1
  antiplatelet Z79.02
  antithrombotics Z79.02
  aromatase inhibitors Z79.811
  aspirin Z79.82
  birth control pill or patch Z79.3
  bisphosphonates Z79.83
  contraceptive, oral Z79.3
  drug, specified NEC Z79.899
  estrogen receptor downregulators Z79.818
  Evista Z79.810
  exemestane (Aromasin) Z79.811
  Fareston Z79.810
  fulvestrant (Faslodex) Z79.818
  gonadotropin-releasing hormone (GnRH) agonist Z79.818
  goserelin acetate (Zoladex) Z79.818
  hormone replacement Z79.890
  insulin Z79.4
  letrozole (Femara) Z79.811
  leuprolide acetate (leuprorelin) (Lupron) Z79.818
  megestrol acetate (Megace) Z79.818
  methadone for pain management Z79.891
  Nolvadex Z79.810
  non-steroidal anti-inflammatories (NSAID) Z79.1
  opiate analgesic Z79.891
  oral
    antidiabetic Z79.84
    contraceptive Z79.3
    hypoglycemic Z79.84
  raloxifene (Evista) Z79.810
  selective estrogen receptor modulators (SERMs) Z79.810
  steroids
    inhaled Z79.51
    systemic Z79.52
  tamoxifen (Nolvadex) Z79.810
  toremifene (Fareston) Z79.810
Loop
  intestine — *see* Volvulus
  vascular on papilla (optic) Q14.2
Loose — *see also* condition
  body
    joint M24.00
      ankle M24.07- ☑
      elbow M24.02- ☑
      hand M24.04- ☑
      hip M24.05- ☑
      knee M23.4- ☑
      shoulder (region) M24.01- ☑
      specified site NEC M24.08
      toe M24.07- ☑
      vertebra M24.08
      wrist M24.03- ☑
    knee M23.4- ☑
  sheath, tendon — *see* Disorder, tendon, specified type NEC
  cartilage — *see* Loose, body, joint

Loose — *continued*
  skin and subcutaneous tissue (following bariatric surgery weight loss) (following dietary weight loss) L98.7
  tooth, teeth K08.89
Loosening
  aseptic
    joint prosthesis — *see* Complications, joint prosthesis, mechanical, loosening, by site
  epiphysis — *see* Osteochondropathy
  mechanical
    joint prosthesis — *see* Complications, joint prosthesis, mechanical, loosening, by site
Looser-Milkman (-Debray) **syndrome** M83.8
Lop ear (deformity) Q17.3
Lorain (-Levi) **short stature syndrome** E23.0
Lordosis M40.50
  acquired — *see* Lordosis, specified type NEC
  congenital Q76.429
    lumbar region Q76.426
    lumbosacral region Q76.427
    sacral region Q76.428
    sacrococcygeal region Q76.428
    thoracolumbar region Q76.425
  lumbar region M40.56
  lumbosacral region M40.57
  postsurgical M96.4
  postural — *see* Lordosis, specified type NEC
  rachitic (late effect) (sequelae) E64.3
  sequelae of rickets E64.3
  specified type NEC M40.40
    lumbar region M40.46
    lumbosacral region M40.47
    thoracolumbar region M40.45
  thoracolumbar region M40.55
  tuberculous A18.01
Loss (of)
  appetite — *see also* Anorexia R63.0
    hysterical F50.89
    nonorganic origin F50.89
    psychogenic F50.89
  blood — *see* Hemorrhage
  bone — *see* Loss, substance of, bone
  consciousness, transient R55
    traumatic — *see* Injury, intracranial
  control, sphincter, rectum R15.9
    nonorganic origin F98.1
  elasticity, skin R23.4
  family (member) in childhood Z62.898
  fluid (acute) E86.9
  function of labyrinth — *see* subcategory H83.2 ☑
  hair, nonscarring — *see* Alopecia
  hearing — *see also* Deafness
    central NOS H90.5
    conductive H90.2
      bilateral H90.0
      unilateral
        with
          restricted hearing on the contralateral side H90.A1- ☑
          unrestricted hearing on the contralateral side H90.1- ☑
    mixed conductive and sensorineural hearing loss H90.8
      bilateral H90.6
      unilateral
        with
          restricted hearing on the contralateral side H90.A3- ☑
          unrestricted hearing on the contralateral side H90.7- ☑
    neural NOS H90.5
    perceptive NOS H90.5
    sensorineural NOS H90.5
      bilateral H90.3
      unilateral
        with
          restricted hearing onthe contralateral side H90.A2- ☑
          unrestricted hearing on the contralateral side H90.4- ☑
    sensory NOS H90.5
  height R29.890
  limb or member, traumatic, current — *see* Amputation, traumatic
  love relationship in childhood Z62.898
  memory — *see also* Amnesia
    mild, following organic brain damage F06.8

Loss — *continued*
mind — *see* Psychosis
occlusal vertical dimension of fully erupted teeth M26.37
organ or part — *see* Absence, by site, acquired
ossicles, ear (partial) H74.32- ☑
parent in childhood Z63.4
pregnancy, recurrent N96
 care in current pregnancy O26.2- ☑
 without current pregnancy N96
recurrent pregnancy — *see* Loss, pregnancy, recurrent
self-esteem, in childhood Z62.898
sense of
 smell — *see* Disturbance, sensation, smell
 taste — *see* Disturbance, sensation, taste
 touch R20.8
sensory R44.9
 dissociative F44.6
sexual desire F52.0
sight (acquired) (complete) (congenital) — *see* Blindness
substance of
 bone — *see* Disorder, bone, density and structure, specified NEC
 horizontal alveolar K06.3
 cartilage — *see* Disorder, cartilage, specified type NEC
 auricle (ear) — *see* Disorder, pinna, specified type NEC
 vitreous (humor) H15.89
tooth, teeth — *see* Absence, teeth, acquired
vision, visual H54.7
 both eyes H54.3
 one eye H54.60
 left (normal vision on right) H54.62
 right (normal vision on left) H54.61
 specified as blindness — *see* Blindness
 subjective
 sudden H53.13- ☑
 transient H53.12- ☑
vitreous — *see* Prolapse, vitreous
voice — *see* Aphonia
weight (abnormal) (cause unknown) R63.4
Louis-Bar syndrome (ataxia-telangiectasia) G11.3
Louping ill (encephalitis) A84.8
Louse, lousiness — *see* Lice
Low
achiever, school Z55.3
back syndrome M54.5
basal metabolic rate R94.8
birthweight (2499 grams or less) P07.10
 with weight of
 1000-1249 grams P07.14
 1250-1499 grams P07.15
 1500-1749 grams P07.16
 1750-1999 grams P07.17
 2000-2499 grams P07.18
 extreme (999 grams or less) P07.00
 with weight of
 499 grams or less P07.01
 500-749 grams P07.02
 750-999 grams P07.03
 for gestational age — *see* Light for dates
blood pressure — *see also* Hypotension
 reading (incidental) (isolated) (nonspecific) R03.1
cardiac reserve — *see* Disease, heart
function — *see also* Hypofunction
 kidney N28.9
hematocrit D64.9
hemoglobin D64.9
income Z59.6
level of literacy Z55.0
lying
 kidney N28.89
 organ or site, congenital — *see* Malposition, congenital
output syndrome (cardiac) — *see* Failure, heart
platelets (blood) — *see* Thrombocytopenia
reserve, kidney N28.89
salt syndrome E87.1
self esteem R45.81
set ears Q17.4
vision H54.2X- ☑
 one eye (other eye normal) H54.50
 left (normal vision on right) H54.52A- ☑
 other eye blind — *see* Blindness
 right (normal vision on left) H54.511- ☑

Low-density-lipoprotein-type (LDL) **hyperlipoproteinemia** E78.00
Lowe's syndrome E72.03
Lown-Ganong-Levine syndrome I45.6
LSD reaction (acute) (without dependence) F16.90
 with dependence F16.20
L-shaped kidney Q63.8
LTBI (latent tuberculosis infection) Z22.7
Ludwig's angina or disease K12.2
Lues (venerea), **luetic** — *see* Syphilis
Luetscher's syndrome (dehydration) E86.0
Lumbago, lumbalgia M54.5
 with sciatica M54.4- ☑
 due to intervertebral disc disorder M51.17
 due to displacement, intervertebral disc M51.27
 with sciatica M51.17
Lumbar — *see* condition
Lumbarization, vertebra, congenital Q76.49
Lumbermen's itch B88.0
Lump — *see also* Mass
 breast N63.0
 axillary tail
 left N63.32
 right N63.31
 left
 lower inner quadrant N63.24
 lower outer quadrant N63.23
 overlapping quadrants N63.25
 unspecified quadrant N63.20
 upper inner quadrant N63.22
 upper outer quadrant N63.21
 right
 lower inner quadrant N63.14
 lower outer quadrant N63.13
 overlapping quadrants N63.15
 unspecified quadrant N63.10
 upper inner quadrant N63.12
 upper outer quadrant N63.11
 subareolar
 left N63.42
 right N63.41
Lunacy — *see* Psychosis
Lung — *see* condition
Lupoid (miliary) **of Boeck** D86.3
Lupus
anticoagulant D68.62
 with
 hemorrhagic disorder D68.312
 hypercoagulable state D68.62
 finding without diagnosis R76.0
discoid (local) L93.0
erythematosus (discoid) (local) L93.0
 disseminated — *see* Lupus, erythematosus, systemic
 eyelid H01.129
 left H01.126
 lower H01.125
 upper H01.124
 right H01.123
 lower H01.122
 upper H01.121
 profundus L93.2
 specified NEC L93.2
 subacute cutaneous L93.1
 systemic M32.9
 with organ or system involvement M32.10
 endocarditis M32.11
 lung M32.13
 pericarditis M32.12
 renal (glomerular) M32.14
 tubulo-interstitial M32.15
 specified organ or system NEC M32.19
 drug-induced M32.0
 inhibitor (presence of) D68.62
 with
 hemorrhagic disorder D68.312
 hypercoagulable state D68.62
 finding without diagnosis R76.0
 specified NEC M32.8
exedens A18.4
hydralazine M32.0
 correct substance properly administered — *see* Table of Drugs and Chemicals, by drug, adverse effect
 overdose or wrong substance given or taken — *see* Table of Drugs and Chemicals, by drug, poisoning
nephritis (chronic) M32.14
nontuberculous, not disseminated L93.0

Lupus — *continued*
panniculitis L93.2
pernio (Besnier) D86.3
systemic — *see* Lupus, erythematosus, systemic
tuberculous A18.4
 eyelid A18.4
 vulgaris A18.4
 eyelid A18.4
Luteinoma D27.- ☑
Lutembacher's disease or syndrome (atrial septal defect with mitral stenosis) Q21.1
Luteoma D27.- ☑
Lutz (-Splendore-de Almeida) **disease** — *see* Paracoccidioidomycosis
Luxation — *see also* Dislocation
eyeball (nontraumatic) — *see* Luxation, globe
 birth injury P15.3
globe, nontraumatic H44.82- ☑
lacrimal gland — *see* Dislocation, lacrimal gland
lens (old) (partial) (spontaneous)
 congenital Q12.1
 syphilitic A50.39
Lycanthropy F22
Lyell's syndrome L51.2
 due to drug L51.2
 correct substance properly administered — *see* Table of Drugs and Chemicals, by drug, adverse effect
 overdose or wrong substance given or taken — *see* Table of Drugs and Chemicals, by drug, poisoning
Lyme disease A69.20
Lymph
gland or node — *see* condition
scrotum — *see* Infestation, filarial
Lymphadenitis I88.9
with ectopic or molar pregnancy O08.0
acute L04.9
 axilla L04.2
 face L04.0
 head L04.0
 hip L04.3
 limb
 lower L04.3
 upper L04.2
 neck L04.0
 shoulder L04.2
 specified site NEC L04.8
 trunk L04.1
anthracosis (occupational) J60
any site, except mesenteric I88.9
 chronic I88.1
 subacute I88.1
breast
 gestational — *see* Mastitis, obstetric
 puerperal, postpartum (nonpurulent) O91.22
chancroidal (congenital) A57
chronic I88.1
 mesenteric I88.0
due to
 Brugia (malayi) B74.1
 timori B74.2
 chlamydial lymphogranuloma A55
 diphtheria (toxin) A36.89
 lymphogranuloma venereum A55
 Wuchereria bancrofti B74.0
following ectopic or molar pregnancy O08.0
gonorrheal A54.89
infective — *see* Lymphadenitis, acute
mesenteric (acute) (chronic) (nonspecific) (subacute) I88.0
 due to Salmonella typhi A01.09
 tuberculous A18.39
mycobacterial A31.8
purulent — *see* Lymphadenitis, acute
pyogenic — *see* Lymphadenitis, acute
regional, nonbacterial I88.8
septic — *see* Lymphadenitis, acute
subacute, unspecified site I88.1
suppurative — *see* Lymphadenitis, acute
syphilitic (early) (secondary) A51.49
 late A52.79
tuberculous — *see* Tuberculosis, lymph gland
venereal (chlamydial) A55
Lymphadenoid goiter E06.3
Lymphadenopathy (generalized) R59.1
angioimmunoblastic, with dysproteinemia (AILD) C86.5
due to toxoplasmosis (acquired) B58.89

☑ **Additional Character Required** — Refer to the Tabular List for Character Selection ▽ **Subterms under main terms may continue to next column or page**

Lymphadenopathy — *continued*
  due to toxoplasmosis — *continued*
    congenital (acute) (subacute) (chronic) P37.1
  localized R59.0
  syphilitic (early) (secondary) A51.49
Lymphadenosis R59.1
Lymphangiectasis I89.0
  conjunctiva H11.89
  postinfectional I89.0
  scrotum I89.0
Lymphangiectatic elephantiasis, nonfilarial I89.0
Lymphangioendothelioma D18.1
  malignant — *see* Neoplasm, connective tissue, malignant
Lymphangioleiomyomatosis J84.81
Lymphangioma D18.1
  capillary D18.1
  cavernous D18.1
  cystic D18.1
  malignant — *see* Neoplasm, connective tissue, malignant
Lymphangiomyoma D18.1
Lymphangiomyomatosis J84.81
Lymphangiosarcoma — *see* Neoplasm, connective tissue, malignant
Lymphangitis I89.1
  with
    abscess — *code by* site under Abscess
    cellulitis — *code by* site under Cellulitis
    ectopic or molar pregnancy O08.0
  acute L03.91
    abdominal wall L03.321
    ankle — *see* Lymphangitis, acute, lower limb
    arm — *see* Lymphangitis, acute, upper limb
    auricle (ear) — *see* Lymphangitis, acute, ear
    axilla L03.12- ☑
    back (any part) L03.322
    buttock L03.327
    cervical (meaning neck) L03.222
    cheek (external) L03.212
    chest wall L03.323
    digit
      finger — *see* Lymphangitis, acute, finger
      toe — *see* Lymphangitis, acute, toe
    ear (external) H60.1- ☑
    external auditory canal — *see* Lymphangitis, acute, ear
    eyelid — *see* Abscess, eyelid
    face NEC L03.212
    finger (intrathecal) (periosteal) (subcutaneous) (subcuticular) L03.02- ☑
    foot — *see* Lymphangitis, acute, lower limb
    gluteal (region) L03.327
    groin L03.324
    hand — *see* Lymphangitis, acute, upper limb
    head NEC L03.891
      face (any part, except ear, eye and nose) L03.212
    heel — *see* Lymphangitis, acute, lower limb
    hip — *see* Lymphangitis, acute, lower limb
    jaw (region) L03.212
    knee — *see* Lymphangitis, acute, lower limb
    leg — *see* Lymphangitis, acute, lower limb
    lower limb L03.12- ☑
      toe — *see* Lymphangitis, acute, toe
    navel L03.326
    neck (region) L03.222
    orbit, orbital — *see* Cellulitis, orbit
    pectoral (region) L03.323
    perineal, perineum L03.325
    scalp (any part) L03.891
    shoulder — *see* Lymphangitis, acute, upper limb
    specified site NEC L03.898
    thigh — *see* Lymphangitis, acute, lower limb
    thumb (intrathecal) (periosteal) (subcutaneous) (subcuticular) — *see* Lymphangitis, acute, finger
    toe (intrathecal) (periosteal) (subcutaneous) (subcuticular) L03.04- ☑
    trunk L03.329
      abdominal wall L03.321
      back (any part) L03.322
      buttock L03.327
      chest wall L03.323
      groin L03.324
      perineal, perineum L03.325
      umbilicus L03.326
    umbilicus L03.326

Lymphangitis — *continued*
  acute — *continued*
    upper limb L03.12- ☑
      axilla — *see* Lymphangitis, acute, axilla
      finger — *see* Lymphangitis, acute, finger
      thumb — *see* Lymphangitis, acute, finger
      wrist — *see* Lymphangitis, acute, upper limb
  breast
    gestational — *see* Mastitis, obstetric
  chancroidal A57
  chronic (any site) I89.1
  due to
    Brugia (malayi) B74.1
      timori B74.2
    Wuchereria bancrofti B74.0
  following ectopic or molar pregnancy O08.89
  penis
    acute N48.29
    gonococcal (acute) (chronic) A54.09
  puerperal, postpartum, childbirth O86.89
  strumous, tuberculous A18.2
  subacute (any site) I89.1
  tuberculous — *see* Tuberculosis, lymph gland
Lymphatic (vessel) — *see* condition
Lymphatism E32.8
Lymphectasia I89.0
Lymphedema (acquired) — *see also* Elephantiasis
  congenital Q82.0
  hereditary (chronic) (idiopathic) Q82.0
  postmastectomy I97.2
  praecox I89.0
  secondary I89.0
  surgical NEC I97.89
    postmastectomy (syndrome) I97.2
Lymphoblastic — *see* condition
Lymphoblastoma (diffuse) — *see* Lymphoma, lymphoblastic (diffuse)
  giant follicular — *see* Lymphoma, lymphoblastic (diffuse)
  macrofollicular — *see* Lymphoma, lymphoblastic (diffuse)
Lymphocele I89.8
Lymphocytic
  chorioencephalitis (acute) (serous) A87.2
  choriomeningitis (acute) (serous) A87.2
  meningoencephalitis A87.2
Lymphocytoma, benign cutis L98.8
Lymphocytopenia D72.810
Lymphocytosis (symptomatic) D72.820
  infectious (acute) B33.8
Lymphoepithelioma — *see* Neoplasm, malignant, by site
Lymphogranuloma (malignant) — *see also* Lymphoma, Hodgkin
  chlamydial A55
  inguinale A55
  venereum (any site) (chlamydial) (with stricture of rectum) A55
Lymphogranulomatosis (malignant) — *see also* Lymphoma, Hodgkin
  benign (Boeck's sarcoid) (Schaumann's) D86.1
Lymphohistiocytosis, hemophagocytic (familial) D76.1
Lymphoid — *see* condition
Lymphoma (of) (malignant) C85.90
  adult T-cell (HTLV-1-associated) (acute variant) (chronic variant) (lymphomatoid variant) (smouldering variant) C91.5- ☑
  anaplastic large cell
    ALK-negative C84.7- ☑
    ALK-positive C84.6- ☑
    CD30-positive C84.6- ☑
    primary cutaneous C86.6
  angioimmunoblastic T-cell C86.5
  BALT C88.4
  B-cell C85.1- ☑
  blastic NK-cell C86.4
  blastic plasmacytoid dendritic cell neoplasm (BPDCN) C86.4
  B-precursor C83.5- ☑
  bronchial-associated lymphoid tissue [BALT-lymphoma] C88.4
  Burkitt (atypical) C83.7- ☑
  Burkitt-like C83.7- ☑
  centrocytic C83.1- ☑
  cutaneous follicle center C82.6- ☑
  cutaneous T-cell C84.A- ☑ (*following* C84.7)
  diffuse follicle center C82.5- ☑

Lymphoma — *continued*
  diffuse large cell C83.3- ☑
    anaplastic C83.3- ☑
    B-cell C83.3- ☑
    CD30-positive C83.3- ☑
    centroblastic C83.3- ☑
    immunoblastic C83.3- ☑
    plasmablastic C83.3- ☑
    subtype not specified C83.3- ☑
    T-cell rich C83.3- ☑
  enteropathy-type (associated) (intestinal) T-cell C86.2
  extranodal marginal zone B-cell lymphoma of mucosa-associated lymphoid tissue [MALT-lymphoma] C88.4
  extranodal NK/T-cell, nasal type C86.0
  follicular C82.9- ☑
    grade
      I C82.0- ☑
      II C82.1- ☑
      III C82.2- ☑
      IIIa C82.3- ☑
      IIIb C82.4- ☑
    specified NEC C82.8- ☑
  hepatosplenic T-cell (alpha-beta) (gamma-delta) C86.1
  histiocytic C85.9- ☑
    true C96.A (*following* C96.6)
  Hodgkin C81.9 ☑
    lymphocyte depleted (classical) C81.3- ☑
    lymphocyte-rich (classical) C81.4- ☑
    mixed cellularity (classical) C81.2- ☑
    nodular
      lymphocyte predominant C81.0- ☑
      sclerosis (classical) C81.1- ☑
    nodular sclerosis (classical) C81.1- ☑
    specified NEC (classical) C81.7- ☑
  intravascular large B-cell C83.8- ☑
  Lennert's C84.4- ☑
  lymphoblastic (diffuse) C83.5- ☑
  lymphoblastic B-cell C83.5- ☑
  lymphoblastic T-cell C83.5- ☑
  lymphoepithelioid C84.4- ☑
  lymphoplasmacytic C83.0- ☑
    with IgM-production C88.0
  MALT C88.4
  mantle cell C83.1- ☑
  mature T-cell NEC C84.4- ☑
  mature T/NK-cell C84.9- ☑
    specified NEC C84.Z- ☑ (*following* C84.7)
  mediastinal (thymic) large B-cell C85.2- ☑
  Mediterranean C88.3
  mucosa-associated lymphoid tissue [MALT-lymphoma] C88.4
  NK/T cell C84.9- ☑
  nodal marginal zone C83.0- ☑
  non-follicular (diffuse) C83.9- ☑
    specified NEC C83.8- ☑
  non-Hodgkin — *see also* Lymphoma, by type C85.9- ☑
    specified NEC C85.8- ☑
  non-leukemic variant of B-CLL C83.0- ☑
  peripheral T-cell, not classified C84.4- ☑
  primary cutaneous
    anaplastic large cell C86.6
    CD30-positive large T-cell C86.6
  primary effusion B-cell C83.8- ☑
  SALT C88.4
  skin-associated lymphoid tissue [SALT-lymphoma] C88.4
  small cell B-cell C83.0- ☑
  splenic marginal zone C83.0- ☑
  subcutaneous panniculitis-like T-cell C86.3
  T-precursor C83.5- ☑
  true histiocytic C96.A (*following* C96.6)
Lymphomatosis — *see* Lymphoma
Lymphopathia venereum, veneris A55
Lymphopenia D72.810
Lymphoplasmacytic leukemia — *see* Leukemia, chronic lymphocytic, B-cell type
Lymphoproliferation, X-linked disease D82.3
Lymphoreticulosis, benign (of inoculation) A28.1
Lymphorrhea I89.8
Lymphosarcoma (diffuse) — *see also* Lymphoma C85.9- ☑
Lymphostasis I89.8
Lypemania — *see* Melancholia
Lysine and hydroxylysine metabolism disorder E72.3
Lyssa — *see* Rabies

M

Macacus ear Q17.3
Maceration, wet feet, tropical (syndrome) T69.02- ☑
MacLeod's syndrome J43.0
Macrocephalia, macrocephaly Q75.3
Macrocheilia, macrochilia (congenital) Q18.6
Macrocolon — see also Megacolon Q43.1
Macrocornea Q15.8
  with glaucoma Q15.0
Macrocytic — see condition
Macrocytosis D75.89
Macrodactylia, macrodactylism (fingers) (thumbs) Q74.0
  toes Q74.2
Macrodontia K00.2
Macrogenia M26.05
Macrogenitosomia (adrenal) (male) (praecox) E25.9
  congenital E25.0
Macroglobulinemia (idiopathic) (primary) C88.0
  monoclonal (essential) D47.2
  Waldenström C88.0
Macroglossia (congenital) Q38.2
  acquired K14.8
Macrognathia, macrognathism (congenital) (mandibular) (maxillary) M26.09
Macrogyria (congenital) Q04.8
Macrohydrocephalus — see Hydrocephalus
Macromastia — see Hypertrophy, breast
Macrophthalmos Q11.3
  in congenital glaucoma Q15.0
Macropsia H53.15
Macrosigmoid K59.39
  congenital Q43.2
Macrospondylitis , acromegalic E22.0
Macrostomia (congenital) Q18.4
Macrotia (external ear) (congenital) Q17.1
Macula
  cornea, corneal — see Opacity, cornea
  degeneration (atrophic) (exudative) (senile) — see also Degeneration, macula
    hereditary — see Dystrophy, retina
Maculae ceruleae B85.1
Maculopathy, toxic — see Degeneration, macula, toxic
Madarosis (eyelid) H02.729
  left H02.726
    lower H02.725
    upper H02.724
  right H02.723
    lower H02.722
    upper H02.721
Madelung's
  deformity (radius) Q74.0
  disease
    radial deformity Q74.0
    symmetrical lipomas, neck E88.89
Madness — see Psychosis
Madura
  foot B47.9
    actinomycotic B47.1
    mycotic B47.0
Maduromycosis B47.0
Maffucci's syndrome Q78.4
Magnesium metabolism disorder — see Disorder, metabolism, magnesium
Main en griffe (acquired) — see also Deformity, limb, clawhand
  congenital Q74.0
Maintenance (encounter for)
  antineoplastic chemotherapy Z51.11
  antineoplastic radiation therapy Z51.0
  methadone F11.20
Majocchi's
  disease L81.7
  granuloma B35.8
Major — see condition
Mal de los pintos — see Pinta
Mal de mer T75.3 ☑
Malabar itch (any site) B35.5
Malabsorption K90.9
  calcium K90.89
  carbohydrate K90.49
  disaccharide E73.9
  fat K90.49
  galactose E74.20
  glucose (-galactose) E74.39

Malabsorption — continued
  intestinal K90.9
    specified NEC K90.89
  isomaltose E74.31
  lactose E73.9
  methionine E72.19
  monosaccharide E74.39
  postgastrectomy K91.2
  postsurgical K91.2
  protein K90.49
  starch K90.49
  sucrose E74.39
  syndrome K90.9
    postsurgical K91.2
Malacia, bone (adult) M83.9
  juvenile — see Rickets
Malacoplakia
  bladder N32.89
  pelvis (kidney) N28.89
  ureter N28.89
  urethra N36.8
Malacosteon, juvenile — see Rickets
Maladaptation — see Maladjustment
Maladie de Roger Q21.0
Maladjustment
  conjugal Z63.0
    involving divorce or estrangement Z63.5
  educational Z55.4
  family Z63.9
  marital Z63.0
    involving divorce or estrangement Z63.5
  occupational NEC Z56.89
  simple, adult — see Disorder, adjustment
  situational — see Disorder, adjustment
  social Z60.9
    due to
      acculturation difficulty Z60.3
      discrimination and persecution (perceived) Z60.5
      exclusion and isolation Z60.4
      life-cycle (phase of life) transition Z60.0
      rejection Z60.4
      specified reason NEC Z60.8
Malaise R53.81
Malakoplakia — see Malacoplakia
Malaria, malarial (fever) B54
  with
    blackwater fever B50.8
      hemoglobinuric (bilious) B50.8
    hemoglobinuria B50.8
  accidentally induced (therapeutically) — code by type under Malaria
  algid B50.9
  cerebral B50.0 *[G94]*
  clinically diagnosed (without parasitological confirmation) B54
  congenital NEC P37.4
    falciparum P37.3
  congestion, congestive B54
  continued (fever) B50.9
  estivo-autumnal B50.9
  falciparum B50.9
    with complications NEC B50.8
      cerebral B50.0 *[G94]*
      severe B50.8
  hemorrhagic B54
  malariae B52.9
    with
      complications NEC B52.8
      glomerular disorder B52.0
  malignant (tertian) — see Malaria, falciparum
  mixed infections — code to first listed type in B50-B53
  ovale B53.0
  parasitologically confirmed NEC B53.8
  pernicious, acute — see Malaria, falciparum
  Plasmodium (P.)
    falciparum NEC — see Malaria, falciparum
    malariae NEC B52.9
      with Plasmodium
        falciparum (and or vivax) — see Malaria, falciparum
        vivax — see also Malaria, vivax
          and falciparum — see Malaria, falciparum
    ovale B53.0
      with Plasmodium malariae — see also Malaria, malariae
        and vivax — see also Malaria, vivax
          and falciparum — see Malaria, falciparum
    simian B53.1

Malaria, malarial — continued
  Plasmodium — continued
    simian — continued
      with Plasmodium malariae — see also Malaria, malariae
        and vivax — see also Malaria, vivax
          and falciparum — see Malaria, falciparum
    vivax NEC B51.9
      with Plasmodium falciparum — see Malaria, falciparum
  quartan — see Malaria, malariae
  quotidian — see Malaria, falciparum
  recurrent B54
  remittent B54
  specified type NEC (parasitologically confirmed) B53.8
  spleen B54
  subtertian (fever) — see Malaria, falciparum
  tertian (benign) — see also Malaria, vivax
    malignant B50.9
  tropical B50.9
  typhoid B54
  vivax B51.9
    with
      complications NEC B51.8
      ruptured spleen B51.0
Malassez's disease (cystic) N50.89
Malassimilation K90.9
Maldescent, testis Q53.9
  bilateral Q53.20
    abdominal Q53.211
    perineal Q53.22
  unilateral Q53.10
    abdominal Q53.111
    perineal Q53.12
Maldevelopment — see also Anomaly
  brain Q07.9
  colon Q43.9
  hip Q74.2
    congenital dislocation Q65.2
      bilateral Q65.1
      unilateral Q65.0- ☑
  mastoid process Q75.8
  middle ear Q16.4
    except ossicles Q16.4
    ossicles Q16.3
  ossicles Q16.3
  spine Q76.49
  toe Q74.2
Male type pelvis Q74.2
  with disproportion (fetopelvic) O33.3 ☑
    causing obstructed labor O65.3
Malformation (congenital) — see also Anomaly
  adrenal gland Q89.1
  affecting multiple systems with skeletal changes NEC Q87.5
  alimentary tract Q45.9
    specified type NEC Q45.8
    upper Q40.9
      specified type NEC Q40.8
  aorta Q25.40
    absence Q25.41
    aneurysm, congenital Q25.43
    aplasia Q25.41
    atresia Q25.29
      aortic arch Q25.21
    coarctation (preductal) (postductal) Q25.1
    dilatation, congenital Q25.44
    hypoplasia Q25.42
    patent ductus arteriosus Q25.0
    specified type NEC Q25.49
    stenosis Q25.1
      supravalvular Q25.3
  aortic valve Q23.9
    specified NEC Q23.8
  arteriovenous, aneurysmatic (congenital) Q27.30
    brain Q28.2
      ruptured I60.8
        intracerebral I61.8
        intraparenchymal I61.8
        intraventricular I61.5
        subarachnoid I60.8
    cerebral — see also Malformation, arteriovenous, brain Q28.2
    peripheral Q27.30
      digestive system — see Angiodysplasia
        congenital Q27.33
      lower limb Q27.32
      other specified site Q27.39

☑ **Additional Character Required** — Refer to the Tabular List for Character Selection   ▽ **Subterms under main terms may continue to next column or page**

Malformation — *continued*
　arteriovenous, aneurysmatic — *continued*
　　peripheral — *continued*
　　　renal vessel Q27.34
　　　upper limb Q27.31
　　precerebral vessels (nonruptured) Q28.0
　auricle
　　ear (congenital) Q17.3
　　　acquired H61.119
　　　　left H61.112
　　　　　with right H61.113
　　　　right H61.111
　　　　　with left H61.113
　bile duct Q44.5
　bladder Q64.79
　　aplasia Q64.5
　　diverticulum Q64.6
　　exstrophy — *see* Exstrophy, bladder
　　neck obstruction Q64.31
　bone Q79.9
　　face Q75.9
　　　specified type NEC Q75.8
　　skull Q75.9
　　　specified type NEC Q75.8
　brain (multiple) Q04.9
　　arteriovenous Q28.2
　　specified type NEC Q04.8
　branchial cleft Q18.2
　breast Q83.9
　　specified type NEC Q83.8
　broad ligament Q50.6
　bronchus Q32.4
　bursa Q79.9
　cardiac
　　chambers Q20.9
　　　specified type NEC Q20.8
　　septum Q21.9
　　　specified type NEC Q21.8
　cerebral Q04.9
　　vessels Q28.3
　cervix uteri Q51.9
　　specified type NEC Q51.828
　Chiari
　　Type I G93.5
　　Type II Q07.01
　choroid (congenital) Q14.3
　　plexus Q07.8
　circulatory system Q28.9
　cochlea Q16.5
　cornea Q13.4
　coronary vessels Q24.5
　corpus callosum (congenital) Q04.0
　diaphragm Q79.1
　digestive system NEC, specified type NEC Q45.8
　dura Q07.9
　　brain Q04.9
　　spinal Q06.9
　ear Q17.9
　　causing impairment of hearing Q16.9
　　external Q17.9
　　　accessory auricle Q17.0
　　　causing impairment of hearing Q16.9
　　　　absence of
　　　　　auditory canal Q16.1
　　　　　auricle Q16.0
　　　macrotia Q17.1
　　　microtia Q17.2
　　　misplacement Q17.4
　　　misshapen NEC Q17.3
　　　prominence Q17.5
　　　specified type NEC Q17.8
　　inner Q16.5
　　middle Q16.4
　　　absence of eustachian tube Q16.2
　　　ossicles (fusion) Q16.3
　　ossicles Q16.3
　　specified type NEC Q17.8
　epididymis Q55.4
　esophagus Q39.9
　　specified type NEC Q39.8
　eye Q15.9
　　lid Q10.3
　　specified NEC Q15.8
　fallopian tube Q50.6
　genital organ — *see* Anomaly, genitalia
　great
　　artery Q25.9
　　　aorta — *see* Malformation, aorta

Malformation — *continued*
　great — *continued*
　　artery — *continued*
　　　pulmonary artery — *see* Malformation, pul-
　　　　monary, artery
　　　specified type NEC Q25.8
　　vein Q26.9
　　　anomalous
　　　　portal venous connection Q26.5
　　　　pulmonary venous connection Q26.4
　　　　　partial Q26.3
　　　　　total Q26.2
　　　persistent left superior vena cava Q26.1
　　　portal vein-hepatic artery fistula Q26.6
　　　specified type NEC Q26.8
　　　vena cava stenosis, congenital Q26.0
　gum Q38.6
　hair Q84.2
　heart Q24.9
　　specified type NEC Q24.8
　integument Q84.9
　　specified type NEC Q84.8
　internal ear Q16.5
　intestine Q43.9
　　specified type NEC Q43.8
　iris Q13.2
　joint Q74.9
　　ankle Q74.2
　　lumbosacral Q76.49
　　sacroiliac Q74.2
　　specified type NEC Q74.8
　kidney Q63.9
　　accessory Q63.0
　　giant Q63.3
　　horseshoe Q63.1
　　hydronephrosis Q62.0
　　malposition Q63.2
　　specified type NEC Q63.8
　lacrimal apparatus Q10.6
　lingual Q38.3
　lip Q38.0
　liver Q44.7
　lung Q33.9
　meninges or membrane (congenital) Q07.9
　　cerebral Q04.8
　　spinal (cord) Q06.9
　middle ear Q16.4
　　ossicles Q16.3
　mitral valve Q23.9
　　specified NEC Q23.8
　Mondini's (congenital) (malformation, cochlea) Q16.5
　mouth (congenital) Q38.6
　multiple types NEC Q89.7
　musculoskeletal system Q79.9
　myocardium Q24.8
　nail Q84.6
　nervous system (central) Q07.9
　nose Q30.9
　　specified type NEC Q30.8
　optic disc Q14.2
　orbit Q10.7
　ovary Q50.39
　palate Q38.5
　parathyroid gland Q89.2
　pelvic organs or tissues NEC
　　in pregnancy or childbirth O34.8- ☑
　　　causing obstructed labor O65.5
　penis Q55.69
　　aplasia Q55.5
　　curvature (lateral) Q55.61
　　hypoplasia Q55.62
　pericardium Q24.8
　peripheral vascular system Q27.9
　　specified type NEC Q27.8
　pharynx Q38.8
　precerebral vessels Q28.1
　prostate Q55.4
　pulmonary
　　arteriovenous Q25.72
　　artery Q25.9
　　　atresia Q25.5
　　　specified type NEC Q25.79
　　　stenosis Q25.6
　　valve Q22.3
　renal artery Q27.2
　respiratory system Q34.9
　retina Q14.1
　scrotum — *see* Malformation, testis and scrotum
　seminal vesicles Q55.4

Malformation — *continued*
　sense organs NEC Q07.9
　skin Q82.9
　specified NEC Q89.8
　spinal
　　cord Q06.9
　　nerve root Q07.8
　spine Q76.49
　　kyphosis — *see* Kyphosis, congenital
　　lordosis — *see* Lordosis, congenital
　spleen Q89.09
　stomach Q40.3
　　specified type NEC Q40.2
　teeth, tooth K00.9
　tendon Q79.9
　testis and scrotum Q55.20
　　aplasia Q55.0
　　hypoplasia Q55.1
　　polyorchism Q55.21
　　retractile testis Q55.22
　　scrotal transposition Q55.23
　　specified NEC Q55.29
　thorax, bony Q76.9
　throat Q38.8
　thyroid gland Q89.2
　tongue (congenital) Q38.3
　　hypertrophy Q38.2
　　tie Q38.1
　trachea Q32.1
　tricuspid valve Q22.9
　　specified type NEC Q22.8
　umbilical cord NEC (complicating delivery) O69.89 ☑
　umbilicus Q89.9
　ureter Q62.8
　　agenesis Q62.4
　　duplication Q62.5
　　malposition — *see* Malposition, congenital, ureter
　　obstructive defect — *see* Defect, obstructive, ureter
　　vesico-uretero-renal reflux Q62.7
　urethra Q64.79
　　aplasia Q64.5
　　duplication Q64.74
　　posterior valves Q64.2
　　prolapse Q64.71
　　stricture Q64.32
　urinary system Q64.9
　uterus Q51.9
　　specified type NEC Q51.818
　vagina Q52.4
　vas deferens Q55.4
　　atresia Q55.3
　vascular system, peripheral Q27.9
　venous — *see* Anomaly, vein(s)
　vulva Q52.70
Malfunction — *see also* Dysfunction
　cardiac electronic device T82.119 ☑
　　electrode T82.110 ☑
　　pulse generator T82.111 ☑
　　specified type NEC T82.118 ☑
　catheter device NEC T85.618 ☑
　　cystostomy T83.010 ☑
　　dialysis (renal) (vascular) T82.41 ☑
　　　intraperitoneal T85.611 ☑
　　infusion NEC T82.514 ☑
　　　cranial T85.610 ☑
　　　epidural T85.610 ☑
　　　intrathecal T85.610 ☑
　　　spinal T85.610 ☑
　　　subarachnoid T85.610 ☑
　　　subdural T85.610 ☑
　　urinary — *see also* Breakdown, device, catheter
　　　T83.018 ☑
　colostomy K94.03
　　valve K94.03
　cystostomy (stoma) N99.512
　　catheter T83.010 ☑
　enteric stoma K94.13
　enterostomy K94.13
　esophagostomy K94.33
　gastroenteric K31.89
　gastrostomy K94.23
　ileostomy K94.13
　　valve K94.13
　intrathecal infusion pump T85.615 ☑
　jejunostomy K94.13
　nervous system device, implant or graft, specified NEC
　　T85.615 ☑

▽ Subterms under main terms may continue to next column or page　　☑ Additional Character Required — Refer to the Tabular List for Character Selection　　**217**

Malformation — Malfunction

Malfunction — *continued*
- pacemaker — *see* Malfunction, cardiac electronic device
- prosthetic device, internal — *see* Complications, prosthetic device, by site, mechanical
- tracheostomy J95.03
- urinary device NEC — *see* Complication, genitourinary, device, urinary, mechanical
- valve
  - colostomy K94.03
  - heart T82.09 ☑
  - ileostomy K94.13
- vascular graft or shunt NEC — *see* Complication, cardiovascular device, mechanical, vascular
- ventricular (communicating shunt) T85.01 ☑

Malherbe's tumor — *see* Neoplasm, skin, benign
Malibu disease L98.8
Malignancy — *see also* Neoplasm, malignant, by site
- unspecified site (primary) C80.1

Malignant — *see* condition
Malingerer, malingering Z76.5
Mallet finger (acquired) — *see* Deformity, finger, mallet finger
- congenital Q74.0
- sequelae of rickets E64.3

Malleus A24.0
Mallory's bodies R89.7
Mallory-Weiss syndrome K22.6
Malnutrition E46
- degree
  - first E44.1
  - mild (protein) E44.1
  - moderate (protein) E44.0
  - second E44.0
  - severe (protein-energy) E43
    - intermediate form E42
      - with
        - kwashiorkor (and marasmus) E42
        - marasmus E41
  - third E43
- following gastrointestinal surgery K91.2
- intrauterine
  - light-for-dates — *see* Light for dates
  - small-for-dates — *see* Small for dates
- lack of care, or neglect (child) (infant) T76.02 ☑
  - confirmed T74.02 ☑
- malignant E40
- protein E46
  - calorie E46
    - mild E44.1
    - moderate E44.0
    - severe E43
      - intermediate form E42
        - with
          - kwashiorkor (and marasmus) E42
          - marasmus E41
  - energy E46
    - mild E44.1
    - moderate E44.0
    - severe E43
      - intermediate form E42
        - with
          - kwashiorkor (and marasmus) E42
          - marasmus E41
  - severe (protein-energy) E43
    - with
      - kwashiorkor (and marasmus) E42
      - marasmus E41

Malocclusion (teeth) M26.4
- Angle's M26.219
  - class I M26.211
  - class II M26.212
  - class III M26.213
- due to
  - abnormal swallowing M26.59
  - mouth breathing M26.59
  - tongue, lip or finger habits M26.59
- temporomandibular (joint) M26.69

Malposition
- cervix — *see* Malposition, uterus
- congenital
  - adrenal (gland) Q89.1
  - alimentary tract Q45.8
    - lower Q43.8
    - upper Q40.8
  - aorta Q25.49
  - appendix Q43.8
  - arterial trunk Q20.0

Malposition — *continued*
- congenital — *continued*
  - artery (peripheral) Q27.8
    - coronary Q24.5
    - digestive system Q27.8
    - lower limb Q27.8
    - pulmonary Q25.79
    - specified site NEC Q27.8
    - upper limb Q27.8
  - auditory canal Q17.8
    - causing impairment of hearing Q16.9
  - auricle (ear) Q17.4
    - causing impairment of hearing Q16.9
    - cervical Q18.2
  - biliary duct or passage Q44.5
  - bladder (mucosa) — *see* Exstrophy, bladder
  - brachial plexus Q07.8
  - brain tissue Q04.8
  - breast Q83.8
  - bronchus Q32.4
  - cecum Q43.8
  - clavicle Q74.0
  - colon Q43.8
  - digestive organ or tract NEC Q45.8
    - lower Q43.8
    - upper Q40.8
  - ear (auricle) (external) Q17.4
    - ossicles Q16.3
  - endocrine (gland) NEC Q89.2
  - epiglottis Q31.8
  - eustachian tube Q17.8
  - eye Q15.8
  - facial features Q18.8
  - fallopian tube Q50.6
  - finger(s) Q68.1
    - supernumerary Q69.0
  - foot Q66.9-
  - gallbladder Q44.1
  - gastrointestinal tract Q45.8
  - genitalia, genital organ(s) or tract Q52.8
    - female Q52.8
      - external Q52.79
      - internal NEC Q52.8
    - male Q55.8
  - glottis Q31.8
  - hand Q68.1
  - heart Q24.8
    - dextrocardia Q24.0
      - with complete transposition of viscera Q89.3
  - hepatic duct Q44.5
  - hip (joint) Q65.89
  - intestine (large) (small) Q43.8
    - with anomalous adhesions, fixation or malrotation Q43.3
  - joint NEC Q68.8
  - kidney Q63.2
  - larynx Q31.8
  - limb Q68.8
    - lower Q68.8
    - upper Q68.8
  - liver Q44.7
  - lung (lobe) Q33.8
  - nail(s) Q84.6
  - nerve Q07.8
  - nervous system NEC Q07.8
  - nose, nasal (septum) Q30.8
  - organ or site not listed — *see* Anomaly, by site
  - ovary Q50.39
  - pancreas Q45.3
  - parathyroid (gland) Q89.2
  - patella Q74.1
  - peripheral vascular system Q27.8
  - pituitary (gland) Q89.2
  - respiratory organ or system NEC Q34.8
  - rib (cage) Q76.6
    - supernumerary in cervical region Q76.5
  - scapula Q74.0
  - shoulder Q74.0
  - spinal cord Q06.8
  - spleen Q89.09
  - sternum NEC Q76.7
  - stomach Q40.2
  - symphysis pubis Q74.2
  - thymus (gland) Q89.2
  - thyroid (gland) (tissue) Q89.2
    - cartilage Q31.8
  - toe(s) Q66.9- ☑
    - supernumerary Q69.2
  - tongue Q38.3

Malposition — *continued*
- congenital — *continued*
  - trachea Q32.1
  - ureter Q62.60
    - deviation Q62.61
    - displacement Q62.62
    - ectopia Q62.63
    - specified type NEC Q62.69
  - uterus Q51.818
  - vein(s) (peripheral) Q27.8
    - great Q26.8
  - vena cava (inferior) (superior) Q26.8
- device, implant or graft — *see also* Complications, by site and type, mechanical T85.628 ☑
  - arterial graft NEC — *see* Complication, cardiovascular device, mechanical, vascular
  - breast (implant) T85.42 ☑
  - catheter NEC T85.628 ☑
    - cystostomy T83.020 ☑
    - dialysis (renal) T82.42 ☑
      - intraperitoneal T85.621 ☑
    - infusion NEC T82.524 ☑
      - spinal (epidural) (subdural) T85.620 ☑
    - urinary — *see also* Displacement, device, catheter, urinary T83.028 ☑
  - electronic (electrode) (pulse generator) (stimulator)
    - bone T84.320 ☑
    - cardiac T82.129 ☑
      - electrode T82.120 ☑
      - pulse generator T82.121 ☑
      - specified type NEC T82.128 ☑
    - nervous system — *see* Complication, prosthetic device, mechanical, electronic nervous system stimulator
    - urinary — *see* Complication, genitourinary, device, urinary, mechanical
  - fixation, internal (orthopedic) NEC — *see* Complication, fixation device, mechanical
  - gastrointestinal — *see* Complications, prosthetic device, mechanical, gastrointestinal device
  - genital NEC T83.428 ☑
    - intrauterine contraceptive device (string) T83.32 ☑
    - penile prosthesis (cylinder) (implanted) (pump) (reservoir) T83.420 ☑
    - testicular prosthesis T83.421 ☑
  - heart NEC — *see* Complication, cardiovascular device, mechanical
  - joint prosthesis — *see* Complication, joint prosthesis, mechanical
  - ocular NEC — *see* Complications, prosthetic device, mechanical, ocular device
  - orthopedic NEC — *see* Complication, orthopedic, device, mechanical
  - specified NEC T85.628 ☑
  - urinary NEC — *see also* Complication, genitourinary, device, urinary, mechanical
    - graft T83.22 ☑
  - vascular NEC — *see* Complication, cardiovascular device, mechanical
  - ventricular intracranial shunt T85.02 ☑
- fetus — *see* Pregnancy, complicated by (management affected by), presentation, fetal
- gallbladder K82.8
- gastrointestinal tract, congenital Q45.8
- heart, congenital NEC Q24.8
- joint prosthesis — *see* Complications, joint prosthesis, mechanical, displacement, by site
- stomach K31.89
  - congenital Q40.2
- tooth, teeth, fully erupted M26.30
- uterus (acute) (acquired) (adherent) (asymptomatic) (postinfectional) (postpartal) (old) N85.4
  - anteflexion or anteversion N85.4
    - congenital Q51.818
  - flexion N85.4
    - lateral — *see* Lateroversion, uterus
  - inversion N85.5
  - lateral (flexion) (version) — *see* Lateroversion, uterus
    - in pregnancy or childbirth — *see* subcategory O34.5 ☑
  - retroflexion or retroversion — *see* Retroversion, uterus

Malposture R29.3
Malrotation
- cecum Q43.3
- colon Q43.3

     ☑ **Additional Character Required** — **Refer to the Tabular List for Character Selection**   ▽ **Subterms under main terms may continue to next column or page**

Malrotation — *continued*
　intestine Q43.3
　kidney Q63.2
Malta fever — *see* Brucellosis
Maltreatment
　adult
　　abandonment
　　　confirmed T74.01 ☑
　　　suspected T76.01 ☑
　　bullying
　　　confirmed T74.31 ☑
　　　suspected T76.31 ☑
　　confirmed T74.91 ☑
　　history of Z91.419
　　intimidation (through social media)
　　　confirmed T74.31 ☑
　　　suspected T76.31 ☑
　　neglect
　　　confirmed T74.01 ☑
　　　suspected T76.01 ☑
　　physical abuse
　　　confirmed T74.11 ☑
　　　suspected T76.11 ☑
　　psychological abuse
　　　confirmed T74.31 ☑
　　　history of Z91.411
　　　suspected T76.31 ☑
　　sexual abuse
　　　confirmed T74.21 ☑
　　　suspected T76.21 ☑
　　suspected T76.91 ☑
　child
　　abandonment
　　　confirmed T74.02 ☑
　　　suspected T76.02 ☑
　　bullying
　　　confirmed T74.32 ☑
　　　suspected T76.32 ☑
　　confirmed T74.92 ☑
　　history of — *see* History, personal (of), abuse
　　intimidation (through social media)
　　　confirmed T74.32 ☑
　　　suspected T76.32 ☑
　　neglect
　　　confirmed T74.02 ☑
　　　history of — *see* History, personal (of), abuse
　　　suspected T76.02 ☑
　　physical abuse
　　　confirmed T74.12 ☑
　　　history of — *see* History, personal (of), abuse
　　　suspected T76.12 ☑
　　psychological abuse
　　　confirmed T74.32 ☑
　　　history of — *see* History, personal (of), abuse
　　　suspected T76.32 ☑
　　sexual abuse
　　　confirmed T74.22 ☑
　　　history of — *see* History, personal (of), abuse
　　　suspected T76.22 ☑
　　suspected T76.92 ☑
　personal history of Z91.89
Maltworker's lung J67.4
Malunion, fracture — *see* Fracture, by site
Mammillitis N61.0
　puerperal, postpartum O91.02
Mammitis — *see* Mastitis
Mammogram (examination) Z12.39
　routine Z12.31
Mammoplasia N62
Management (of)
　bone conduction hearing device (implanted) Z45.320
　cardiac pacemaker NEC Z45.018
　cerebrospinal fluid drainage device Z45.41
　cochlear device (implanted) Z45.321
　contraceptive Z30.9
　　specified NEC Z30.8
　implanted device Z45.9
　　specified NEC Z45.89
　infusion pump Z45.1
　procreative Z31.9
　　male factor infertility in female Z31.81
　　specified NEC Z31.89
　prosthesis (external) — *see also* Fitting Z44.9
　　implanted Z45.9
　　　specified NEC Z45.89
　renal dialysis catheter Z49.01
　vascular access device Z45.2

Mangled — *see* specified injury by site
Mania (monopolar) — *see also* Disorder, mood, manic
　　episode
　with psychotic symptoms F30.2
　without psychotic symptoms F30.10
　　mild F30.11
　　moderate F30.12
　　severe F30.13
　Bell's F30.8
　chronic (recurrent) F31.89
　hysterical F44.89
　puerperal F30.8
　recurrent F31.89
Manic depression F31.9
Manic-depressive insanity, psychosis, or syndrome
　— *see* Disorder, bipolar
Mannosidosis E77.1
Mansonelliasis, mansonellosis B74.4
Manson's
　disease B65.1
　schistosomiasis B65.1
Manual — *see* condition
Maple-bark-stripper's lung (disease) J67.6
Maple-syrup-urine disease E71.0
Marable's syndrome (celiac artery compression) I77.4
Marasmus E41
　due to malnutrition E41
　intestinal E41
　nutritional E41
　senile R54
　tuberculous NEC — *see* Tuberculosis
Marble
　bones Q78.2
　skin R23.8
Marburg virus disease A98.3
March
　fracture — *see* Fracture, traumatic, stress, by site
　hemoglobinuria D59.6
Marchesani (-Weill) **syndrome** Q87.0
Marchiafava (-Bignami) **syndrome or disease** G37.1
Marchiafava-Micheli syndrome D59.5
Marcus Gunn's syndrome Q07.8
Marfan's syndrome — *see* Syndrome, Marfan's
Marie-Bamberger disease — *see* Osteoarthropathy,
　　hypertrophic, specified NEC
Marie-Charcot-Tooth neuropathic muscular atrophy
　G60.0
Marie's
　cerebellar ataxia (late-onset) G11.2
　disease or syndrome (acromegaly) E22.0
Marie-Strümpell arthritis, disease or spondylitis —
　　see Spondylitis, ankylosing
Marion's disease (bladder neck obstruction) N32.0
Marital conflict Z63.0
Mark
　port wine Q82.5
　raspberry Q82.5
　strawberry Q82.5
　stretch L90.6
　tattoo L81.8
Marker heterochromatin — *see* Extra, marker chromo-
　　somes
Maroteaux-Lamy syndrome (mild) (severe) E76.29
Marrow (bone)
　arrest D61.9
　poor function D75.89
Marseilles fever A77.1
Marsh fever — *see* Malaria
Marshall's (hidrotic) **ectodermal dysplasia** Q82.4
Marsh's disease (exophthalmic goiter) E05.00
　with storm E05.01
Masculinization (female) **with adrenal hyperplasia**
　E25.9
　congenital E25.0
Masculinovoblastoma D27.- ☑
Masochism (sexual) F65.51
Mason's lung J62.8
Mass
　abdominal R19.00
　　epigastric R19.06
　　generalized R19.07
　　left lower quadrant R19.04
　　left upper quadrant R19.02
　　periumbilic R19.05
　　right lower quadrant R19.03
　　right upper quadrant R19.01
　　specified site NEC R19.09

Mass — *continued*
　breast — *see also* Lump, breast N63.0
　chest R22.2
　cystic — *see* Cyst
　ear H93.8- ☑
　head R22.0
　intra-abdominal (diffuse) (generalized) — *see* Mass,
　　abdominal
　kidney N28.89
　liver R16.0
　localized (skin) R22.9
　　chest R22.2
　　head R22.0
　　limb
　　　lower R22.4- ☑
　　　upper R22.3- ☑
　　neck R22.1
　　trunk R22.2
　lung R91.8
　malignant — *see* Neoplasm, malignant, by site
　neck R22.1
　pelvic (diffuse) (generalized) — *see* Mass, abdominal
　specified organ NEC — *see* Disease, by site
　splenic R16.1
　substernal thyroid — *see* Goiter
　superficial (localized) R22.9
　umbilical (diffuse) (generalized) R19.09
Massive — *see* condition
Mast cell
　disease, systemic tissue D47.02
　leukemia C94.3- ☑
　neoplasm
　　malignant C96.20
　　　specified type NEC C96.29
　　of uncertain behavior NEC D47.09
　sarcoma C96.22
　tumor D47.09
Mastalgia N64.4
Masters-Allen syndrome N83.8
Mastitis (acute) (diffuse) (nonpuerperal) (subacute) N61.0
　with abscess N61.1
　chronic (cystic) — *see* Mastopathy, cystic
　cystic (Schimmelbusch's type) — *see* Mastopathy, cystic
　fibrocystic — *see* Mastopathy, cystic
　infective N61.0
　　newborn P39.0
　interstitial, gestational or puerperal — *see* Mastitis,
　　obstetric
　neonatal (noninfective) P83.4
　　infective P39.0
　obstetric (interstitial) (nonpurulent)
　　associated with
　　　lactation O91.23
　　　pregnancy O91.21- ☑
　　　puerperium O91.22
　　purulent
　　　associated with
　　　　lactation O91.13
　　　　pregnancy O91.11- ☑
　　　　puerperium O91.12
　periductal — *see* Ectasia, mammary duct
　phlegmonous — *see* Mastopathy, cystic
　plasma cell — *see* Ectasia, mammary duct
　without abscess N61.0
Mastocytoma (extracutaneous) D47.09
　malignant C96.29
　solitary D47.01
Mastocytosis D47.09
　aggressive systemic C96.21
　cutaneous (diffuse) (maculopapular) D47.01
　　congenital Q82.2
　　of neonatal onset Q82.2
　　of newborn onset Q82.2
　indolent systemic D47.02
　isolated bone marrow D47.02
　malignant C96.29
　systemic (indolent) (smoldering)
　　with an associated hematological non-mast cell
　　　lineage disease (SM-AHNMD) D47.02
Mastodynia N64.4
Mastoid — *see* condition
Mastoidalgia — *see* subcategory H92.0 ☑
Mastoiditis (coalescent) (hemorrhagic) (suppurative)
　H70.9- ☑
　acute, subacute H70.00- ☑
　　complicated NEC H70.09- ☑
　　subperiosteal H70.01- ☑

Mastoiditis — continued
chronic (necrotic) (recurrent) H70.1- ☑
in (due to)
infectious disease NEC B99 ☑ [H75.0-] ☑
parasitic disease NEC B89 [H75.0-] ☑
tuberculosis A18.03
petrositis — see Petrositis
postauricular fistula — see Fistula, postauricular
specified NEC H70.89- ☑
tuberculous A18.03
Mastopathy, mastopathia N64.9
chronica cystica — see Mastopathy, cystic
cystic (chronic) (diffuse) N60.1- ☑
with epithelial proliferation N60.3- ☑
diffuse cystic — see Mastopathy, cystic
estrogenic, oestrogenica N64.89
ovarian origin N64.89
Mastoplasia, mastoplastia N62
Masturbation (excessive) F98.8
Maternal care (for) — see Pregnancy (complicated by)
(management affected by)
Mathieu's disease (leptospiral jaundice) A27.0
Mauclaire's disease or osteochondrosis — see Osteochondrosis, juvenile, hand, metacarpal
Maxcy's disease A75.2
Maxilla, maxillary — see condition
May (-Hegglin) **anomaly or syndrome** D72.0
McArdle (-Schmid)(-Pearson) **disease** (glycogen storage)
E74.04
McCune-Albright syndrome Q78.1
McQuarrie's syndrome (idiopathic familial hypo-
glycemia) E16.2
Meadow's syndrome Q86.1
Measles (black) (hemorrhagic) (suppressed) B05.9
with
complications NEC B05.89
encephalitis B05.0
intestinal complications B05.4
keratitis (keratoconjunctivitis) B05.81
meningitis B05.1
otitis media B05.3
pneumonia B05.2
French — see Rubella
German — see Rubella
Liberty — see Rubella
Meatitis, urethral — see Urethritis
Meatus, meatal — see condition
Meat-wrappers' asthma J68.9
Meckel-Gruber syndrome Q61.9
Meckel's diverticulitis, diverticulum (displaced) (hypertrophic) Q43.0
· malignant — see Table of Neoplasms, small intestine,
malignant
Meconium
ileus, newborn P76.0
in cystic fibrosis E84.11
meaning meconium plug (without cystic fibrosis)
P76.0
obstruction, newborn P76.0
due to fecaliths P76.0
in mucoviscidosis E84.11
peritonitis P78.0
plug syndrome (newborn) NEC P76.0
Median — see also condition
arcuate ligament syndrome I77.4
bar (prostate) (vesical orifice) — see Hyperplasia,
prostate
rhomboid glossitis K14.2
Mediastinal shift R93.89
Mediastinitis (acute) (chronic) J98.51
syphilitic A52.73
tuberculous A15.8
Mediastinopericarditis — see also Pericarditis
acute I30.9
adhesive I31.0
chronic I31.8
rheumatic I09.2
Mediastinum, mediastinal — see condition
Medicine poisoning — see Table of Drugs and Chemicals, by drug, poisoning
Mediterranean
fever — see Brucellosis
familial M04.1
tick A77.1
kala-azar B55.0
leishmaniasis B55.0
tick fever A77.1

Medulla — see condition
Medullary cystic kidney Q61.5
Medullated fibers
optic (nerve) Q14.8
retina Q14.1
Medulloblastoma
desmoplastic C71.6
specified site — see Neoplasm, malignant, by site
unspecified site C71.6
Medulloepithelioma — see also Neoplasm, malignant,
by site
teratoid — see Neoplasm, malignant, by site
Medullomyoblastoma
specified site — see Neoplasm, malignant, by site
unspecified site C71.6
Meekeren-Ehlers-Danlos syndrome — see also Syndrome, Ehlers-Danlos Q79.69
Megacolon (acquired) (functional) (not Hirschsprung's
disease) (in) K59.39
Chagas' disease B57.32
congenital, congenitum (aganglionic) Q43.1
Hirschsprung's (disease) Q43.1
toxic NEC K59.31
due to Clostridium difficile
not specified as recurrent A04.72
recurrent A04.71
Megaesophagus (functional) K22.0
congenital Q39.5
in (due to) Chagas' disease B57.31
Megalencephaly Q04.5
Megalerythema (epidemic) B08.3
Megaloappendix Q43.8
Megalocephalus, megalocephaly NEC Q75.3
Megalocornea Q15.8
with glaucoma Q15.0
Megalocytic anemia D53.1
Megalodactylia (fingers) (thumbs) (congenital) Q74.0
toes Q74.2
Megaloduodenum Q43.8
Megaloesophagus (functional) K22.0
congenital Q39.5
Megalogastria (acquired) K31.89
congenital Q40.2
Megalophthalmos Q11.3
Megalopsia H53.15
Megalosplenia — see Splenomegaly
Megaloureter N28.82
congenital Q62.2
Megarectum K62.89
Megasigmoid K59.39
congenital Q43.2
Megaureter N28.82
congenital Q62.2
Megavitamin-B6 syndrome E67.2
Megrim — see Migraine
Meibomian
cyst, infected — see Hordeolum
gland — see condition
sty, stye — see Hordeolum
Meibomitis — see Hordeolum
Meige-Milroy disease (chronic hereditary edema) Q82.0
Meige's syndrome Q82.0
Melalgia, nutritional E53.8
Melancholia F32.9
climacteric (single episode) F32.89
recurrent episode F33.8
hypochondriac F45.29
intermittent (single episode) F32.89
recurrent episode F33.8
involutional (single episode) F32.89
recurrent episode F33.8
menopausal (single episode) F32.89
recurrent episode F33.8
puerperal F32.89
reactive (emotional stress or trauma) F32.3
recurrent F33.9
senile F03 ☑
stuporous (single episode) F32.89
recurrent episode F33.8
Melanemia R79.89
Melanoameloblastoma — see Neoplasm, bone, benign
Melanoblastoma — see Melanoma
Melanocarcinoma — see Melanoma
Melanocytoma, eyeball D31.9- ☑
Melanocytosis, neurocutaneous Q82.8
Melanoderma, melanodermia L81.4
Melanodontia, infantile K03.89

Melanodontoclasia K03.89
Melanoepithelioma — see Melanoma
Melanoma (malignant) C43.9
acral lentiginous, malignant — see Melanoma, skin, by
site
amelanotic — see Melanoma, skin, by site
balloon cell — see Melanoma, skin, by site
benign — see Nevus
desmoplastic, malignant — see Melanoma, skin, by
site
epithelioid cell — see Melanoma, skin, by site
with spindle cell, mixed — see Melanoma, skin, by
site
in
giant pigmented nevus — see Melanoma, skin, by
site
Hutchinson's melanotic freckle — see Melanoma,
skin, by site
junctional nevus — see Melanoma, skin, by site
precancerous melanosis — see Melanoma, skin, by
site
in situ D03.9
abdominal wall D03.59
ala nasi D03.39
ankle D03.7- ☑
anus, anal (margin) (skin) D03.51
arm D03.6- ☑
auditory canal D03.2- ☑
auricle (ear) D03.2- ☑
auricular canal (external) D03.2- ☑
axilla, axillary fold D03.59
back D03.59
breast D03.52
brow D03.39
buttock D03.59
canthus (eye) D03.1- ☑
cheek (external) D03.39
chest wall D03.59
chin D03.39
choroid D03.8
conjunctiva D03.8
ear (external) D03.2- ☑
external meatus (ear) D03.2- ☑
eye D03.8
eyebrow D03.39
eyelid (lower) (upper) D03.1- ☑
face D03.30
specified NEC D03.39
female genital organ (external) NEC D03.8
finger D03.6- ☑
flank D03.59
foot D03.7- ☑
forearm D03.6- ☑
forehead D03.39
foreskin D03.8
gluteal region D03.59
groin D03.59
hand D03.6- ☑
heel D03.7- ☑
helix D03.2- ☑
hip D03.7 ☑
interscapular region D03.59
iris D03.8
jaw D03.39
knee D03.7- ☑
labium (majus) (minus) D03.8
lacrimal gland D03.8
leg D03.7- ☑
lip (lower) (upper) D03.0
lower limb NEC D03.7- ☑
male genital organ (external) NEC D03.8
nail D03.9
finger D03.6- ☑
toe D03.7- ☑
neck D03.4
nose (external) D03.39
orbit D03.8
penis D03.8
perianal skin D03.51
perineum D03.51
pinna D03.2- ☑
popliteal fossa or space D03.7- ☑
prepuce D03.8
pudendum D03.8
retina D03.8
retrobulbar D03.8
scalp D03.4

☑ Additional Character Required — Refer to the Tabular List for Character Selection   ▽ Subterms under main terms may continue to next column or page

Melanoma — *continued*
  in situ — *continued*
    scrotum D03.8
    shoulder D03.6- ☑
    specified site NEC D03.8
    submammary fold D03.52
    temple D03.39
    thigh D03.7- ☑
    toe D03.7- ☑
    trunk NEC D03.59
    umbilicus D03.59
    upper limb NEC D03.6- ☑
    vulva D03.8
  juvenile — *see* Nevus
  malignant, of soft parts except skin — *see* Neoplasm,
    connective tissue, malignant
  metastatic
    breast C79.81
    genital organ C79.82
    specified site NEC C79.89
  neurotropic, malignant — *see* Melanoma, skin, by site
  nodular — *see* Melanoma, skin, by site
  regressing, malignant — *see* Melanoma, skin, by site
  skin C43.9
    abdominal wall C43.59
    ala nasi C43.31
    ankle C43.7- ☑
    anus, anal (skin) C43.51
    arm C43.6- ☑
    auditory canal (external) C43.2- ☑
    auricle (ear) C43.2- ☑
    auricular canal (external) C43.2- ☑
    axilla, axillary fold C43.59
    back C43.59
    breast (female) (male) C43.52
    brow C43.39
    buttock C43.59
    canthus (eye) C43.1- ☑
    cheek (external) C43.39
    chest wall C43.59
    chin C43.39
    ear (external) C43.2- ☑
    elbow C43.6- ☑
    external meatus (ear) C43.2- ☑
    eyebrow C43.39
    eyelid (lower) (upper) C43.1- ☑
    face C43.30
      specified NEC C43.39
    female genital organ (external) NEC C51.9
    finger C43.6- ☑
    flank C43.59
    foot C43.7- ☑
    forearm C43.6- ☑
    forehead C43.39
    foreskin C60.0
    glabella C43.39
    gluteal region C43.59
    groin C43.59
    hand C43.6- ☑
    heel C43.7- ☑
    helix C43.2- ☑
    hip C43.7- ☑
    interscapular region C43.59
    jaw (external) C43.39
    knee C43.7- ☑
    labium C51.9
      majus C51.0
      minus C51.1
    leg C43.7- ☑
    lip (lower) (upper) C43.0
    lower limb NEC C43.7- ☑
    male genital organ (external) NEC C63.9
    nail
      finger C43.6- ☑
      toe C43.7- ☑
    nasolabial groove C43.39
    nates C43.59
    neck C43.4
    nose (external) C43.31
    overlapping site C43.8
    palpebra C43.1- ☑
    penis C60.9
    perianal skin C43.51
    perineum C43.51
    pinna C43.2- ☑
    popliteal fossa or space C43.7- ☑
    prepuce C60.0

Melanoma — *continued*
  skin — *continued*
    pudendum C51.9
    scalp C43.4
    scrotum C63.2
    shoulder C43.6- ☑
    skin NEC C43.9
    submammary fold C43.52
    temple C43.39
    thigh C43.7- ☑
    toe C43.7- ☑
    trunk NEC C43.59
    umbilicus C43.59
    upper limb NEC C43.6- ☑
    vulva C51.9
      overlapping sites C51.8
  spindle cell
    with epithelioid, mixed — *see* Melanoma, skin, by
      site
    type A C69.4- ☑
    type B C69.4- ☑
  superficial spreading — *see* Melanoma, skin, by site
Melanosarcoma — *see also* Melanoma
  epithelioid cell — *see* Melanoma
Melanosis L81.4
  addisonian E27.1
    tuberculous A18.7
  adrenal E27.1
  colon K63.89
  conjunctiva — *see* Pigmentation, conjunctiva
    congenital Q13.89
  cornea (presenile) (senile) — *see also* Pigmentation,
    cornea
    congenital Q13.4
  eye NEC H57.89
    congenital Q15.8
  lenticularis progressiva Q82.1
  liver K76.89
  precancerous — *see also* Melanoma, in situ
    malignant melanoma in — *see* Melanoma
  Riehl's L81.4
  sclera H15.89
    congenital Q13.89
  suprarenal E27.1
  tar L81.4
  toxic L81.4
Melanuria R82.998
MELAS syndrome E88.41
Melasma L81.1
  adrenal (gland) E27.1
  suprarenal (gland) E27.1
Melena K92.1
  with ulcer — *code by* site under Ulcer, with hemorrhage
    K27.4
  due to swallowed maternal blood P78.2
  newborn, neonatal P54.1
    due to swallowed maternal blood P78.2
Meleney's
  gangrene (cutaneous) — *see* Ulcer, skin
  ulcer (chronic undermining) — *see* Ulcer, skin
Melioidosis A24.9
  acute A24.1
  chronic A24.2
  fulminating A24.1
  pneumonia A24.1
  pulmonary (chronic) A24.2
    acute A24.1
    subacute A24.2
  sepsis A24.1
  specified NEC A24.3
  subacute A24.2
Melitensis, febris A23.0
Melkersson (-Rosenthal) **syndrome** G51.2
Mellitus, diabetes — *see* Diabetes
Melorheostosis (bone) — *see* Disorder, bone, density
  and structure, specified NEC
Meloschisis Q18.4
Melotia Q17.4
Membrana
  capsularis lentis posterior Q13.89
  epipapillaris Q14.2
Membranacea placenta O43.19- ☑
Membranaceous uterus N85.8
Membrane(s), membranous — *see also* condition
  cyclitic — *see* Membrane, pupillary
  folds, congenital — *see* Web
  Jackson's Q43.3
  over face of newborn P28.9

Membrane(s), membranous — *continued*
  premature rupture — *see* Rupture, membranes, prema-
    ture
  pupillary H21.4- ☑
    persistent Q13.89
  retained (with hemorrhage) (complicating delivery)
    O72.2
    without hemorrhage O73.1
  secondary cataract — *see* Cataract, secondary
  unruptured (causing asphyxia) — *see* Asphyxia, new-
    born
  vitreous — *see* Opacity, vitreous, membranes and
    strands
Membranitis — *see* Chorioamnionitis
Memory disturbance, lack or loss — *see also* Amnesia
  mild, following organic brain damage F06.8
Menadione deficiency E56.1
Menarche
  delayed E30.0
  precocious E30.1
Mendacity, pathologic F60.2
Mendelson's syndrome (due to anesthesia) J95.4
  in labor and delivery O74.0
  in pregnancy O29.01- ☑
  obstetric O74.0
  postpartum, puerperal O89.01
Ménétrier's disease or syndrome K29.60
  with bleeding K29.61
Ménière's disease, syndrome or vertigo H81.0- ☑
Meninges, meningeal — *see* condition
Meningioma — *see also* Neoplasm, meninges, benign
  angioblastic — *see* Neoplasm, meninges, benign
  angiomatous — *see* Neoplasm, meninges, benign
  endotheliomatous — *see* Neoplasm, meninges, benign
  fibroblastic — *see* Neoplasm, meninges, benign
  fibrous — *see* Neoplasm, meninges, benign
  hemangioblastic — *see* Neoplasm, meninges, benign
  hemangiopericytic — *see* Neoplasm, meninges, benign
  malignant — *see* Neoplasm, meninges, malignant
  meningiothelial — *see* Neoplasm, meninges, benign
  meningotheliomatous — *see* Neoplasm, meninges,
    benign
  mixed — *see* Neoplasm, meninges, benign
  multiple — *see* Neoplasm, meninges, uncertain behav-
    ior
  papillary — *see* Neoplasm, meninges, uncertain behav-
    ior
  psammomatous — *see* Neoplasm, meninges, benign
  syncytial — *see* Neoplasm, meninges, benign
  transitional — *see* Neoplasm, meninges, benign
Meningiomatosis (diffuse) — *see* Neoplasm, meninges,
  uncertain behavior
Meningism — *see* Meningismus
Meningismus (infectional) (pneumococcal) R29.1
  due to serum or vaccine R29.1
  influenzal — *see* Influenza, with, manifestations NEC
Meningitis (basal) (basic) (brain) (cerebral) (cervical)
    (congestive) (diffuse) (hemorrhagic) (infantile)
    (membranous) (metastatic) (nonspecific) (pontine)
    (progressive) (simple) (spinal) (subacute) (sympa-
    thetic) (toxic) G03.9
  abacterial G03.0
  actinomycotic A42.81
  adenoviral A87.1
  arbovirus A87.8
  aseptic (acute) G03.0
  bacterial G00.9
    Escherichia coli (E. coli) G00.8
    Friedländer (bacillus) G00.8
    gram-negative G00.9
    H. influenzae G00.0
    Klebsiella G00.8
    pneumococcal G00.1
    specified organism NEC G00.8
    staphylococcal G00.3
    streptococcal (acute) G00.2
  benign recurrent (Mollaret) G03.2
  candidal B37.5
  caseous (tuberculous) A17.0
  cerebrospinal A39.0
  chronic NEC G03.1
  clear cerebrospinal fluid NEC G03.0
  coxsackievirus A87.0
  cryptococcal B45.1
  diplococcal (gram positive) A39.0
  echovirus A87.0
  enteroviral A87.0
  eosinophilic B83.2

Meningitis — *continued*
epidemic NEC A39.0
Escherichia coli (E. coli) G00.8
fibrinopurulent G00.9
  specified organism NEC G00.8
Friedländer (bacillus) G00.8
gonococcal A54.81
gram-negative cocci G00.9
gram-positive cocci G00.9
H. influenzae G00.0
Haemophilus (influenzae) G00.0
in (due to)
  adenovirus A87.1
  African trypanosomiasis B56.9 [G02]
  anthrax A22.8
  bacterial disease NEC A48.8 [G01]
  Chagas' disease (chronic) B57.41
  chickenpox B01.0
  coccidioidomycosis B38.4
  Diplococcus pneumoniae G00.1
  enterovirus A87.0
  herpes (simplex) virus B00.3
    zoster B02.1
  infectious mononucleosis B27.92
  leptospirosis A27.81
  Listeria monocytogenes A32.11
  Lyme disease A69.21
  measles B05.1
  mumps (virus) B26.1
  neurosyphilis (late) A52.13
  parasitic disease NEC B89 [G02]
  poliovirus A80.9 [G02]
  preventive immunization, inoculation or vaccination G03.8
  rubella B06.02
  Salmonella infection A02.21
  specified cause NEC G03.8
  Streptococcal pneumoniae G00.1
  typhoid fever A01.01
  varicella B01.0
  viral disease NEC A87.8
  whooping cough A37.90
  zoster B02.1
infectious G00.9
influenzal (H. influenzae) G00.0
Klebsiella G00.8
leptospiral (aseptic) A27.81
lymphocytic (acute) (benign) (serous) A87.2
meningococcal A39.0
Mima polymorpha G00.8
Mollaret (benign recurrent) G03.2
monilial B37.5
mycotic NEC B49 [G02]
Neisseria A39.0
nonbacterial G03.0
nonpyogenic NEC G03.0
ossificans G96.19
pneumococcal streptococcus pneumoniae G00.1
poliovirus A80.9 [G02]
postmeasles B05.1
purulent G00.9
  specified organism NEC G00.8
pyogenic G00.9
  specified organism NEC G00.8
Salmonella (arizonae) (Cholerae-Suis) (enteritidis) (typhimurium) A02.21
septic G00.9
  specified organism NEC G00.8
serosa circumscripta NEC G03.0
serous NEC G93.2
specified organism NEC G00.8
sporotrichosis B42.81
staphylococcal G00.3
sterile G03.0
Streptococcal (acute) G00.2
  pneumoniae G00.1
suppurative G00.9
  specified organism NEC G00.8
syphilitic (late) (tertiary) A52.13
  acute A51.41
  congenital A50.41
  secondary A51.41
Torula histolytica (cryptococcal) B45.1
traumatic (complication of injury) T79.8 ☑
tuberculous A17.0
typhoid A01.01
viral NEC A87.9
Yersinia pestis A20.3

Meningocele (spinal) — *see also* Spina bifida
  with hydrocephalus — *see* Spina bifida, by site, with hydrocephalus
  acquired (traumatic) G96.19
  cerebral — *see* Encephalocele
Meningocerebritis — *see* Meningoencephalitis
Meningococcemia A39.4
  acute A39.2
  chronic A39.3
Meningococcus, meningococcal — *see also* condition A39.9
  adrenalitis, hemorrhagic A39.1
  carrier (suspected) of Z22.31
  meningitis (cerebrospinal) A39.0
Meningoencephalitis — *see also* Encephalitis G04.90
  acute NEC — *see also* Encephalitis, viral A86
  bacterial NEC G04.2
  California A83.5
  diphasic A84.1
  eosinophilic B83.2
  epidemic A39.81
  herpesviral, herpetic B00.4
    due to herpesvirus 6 B10.01
    due to herpesvirus 7 B10.09
    specified NEC B10.09
  in (due to)
    blastomycosis NEC B40.81
    diseases classified elsewhere G05.3
    free-living amebae B60.2
    H. influenzae G00.0
    Hemophilus influenzae (H .influenzae) G00.0
    herpes B00.4
      due to herpesvirus 6 B10.01
      due to herpesvirus 7 B10.09
      specified NEC B10.09
    Lyme disease A69.22
    mercury — *see* subcategory T56.1 ☑
    mumps B26.2
    Naegleria (amebae) (organisms) (fowleri) B60.2
    Parastrongylus cantonensis B83.2
    toxoplasmosis (acquired) B58.2
      congenital P37.1
  infectious (acute) (viral) A86
  influenzal (H. influenzae) G00.0
  Listeria monocytogenes A32.12
  lymphocytic (serous) A87.2
  mumps B26.2
  parasitic NEC B89 [G05.3]
  pneumococcal G04.2
  primary amebic B60.2
  specific (syphilitic) A52.14
  specified organism NEC G04.81
  staphylococcal G04.2
  streptococcal G04.2
  syphilitic A52.14
  toxic NEC G92
    due to mercury — *see* subcategory T56.1 ☑
  tuberculous A17.82
  virus NEC A86
Meningoencephalocele — *see also* Encephalocele
  syphilitic A52.19
    congenital A50.49
Meningoencephalomyelitis — *see also* Meningoencephalitis
  acute NEC (viral) A86
    disseminated G04.00
      postimmunization or postvaccination G04.02
      postinfectious G04.01
    due to
      actinomycosis A42.82
      Torula B45.1
      Toxoplasma or toxoplasmosis (acquired) B58.2
        congenital P37.1
    postimmunization or postvaccination G04.02
Meningoencephalomyelopathy G96.9
Meningoencephalopathy G96.9
Meningomyelitis — *see also* Meningoencephalitis
  bacterial NEC G04.2
  blastomycotic NEC B40.81
  cryptococcal B45.1
  in diseases classified elsewhere G05.4
  meningococcal A39.81
  syphilitic A52.14
  tuberculous A17.82
Meningomyelocele — *see also* Spina bifida
  syphilitic A52.19
Meningomyeloneuritis — *see* Meningoencephalitis
Meningoradiculitis — *see* Meningitis

Meningovascular — *see* condition
Menkes' disease or syndrome E83.09
  meaning maple-syrup-urine disease E71.0
Menometrorrhagia N92.1
Menopause, menopausal (asymptomatic) (state) Z78.0
  arthritis (any site) NEC — *see* Arthritis, specified form NEC
  bleeding N92.4
  depression (single episode) F32.89
    agitated (single episode) F32.2
      recurrent episode F33.9
    psychotic (single episode) F32.89
      recurrent episode F33.9
    recurrent episode F33.8
  melancholia (single episode) F32.89
    recurrent episode F33.8
  paranoid state F22
  premature E28.319
    asymptomatic E28.319
      postirradiation E89.40
      postsurgical E89.40
    symptomatic E28.310
      postirradiation E89.41
      postsurgical E89.41
  psychosis NEC F28
  symptomatic N95.1
  toxic polyarthritis NEC — *see* Arthritis, specified form NEC
Menorrhagia (primary) N92.0
  climacteric N92.4
    menopausal N92.4
  menopausal N92.4
  perimenopausal N92.4
  postclimacteric N95.0
  postmenopausal N95.0
  preclimacteric or premenopausal N92.4
  pubertal (menses retained) N92.2
Menostaxis N92.0
Menses, retention N94.89
Menstrual — *see* Menstruation
Menstruation
  absent — *see* Amenorrhea
  anovulatory N97.0
  cycle, irregular N92.6
  delayed N91.0
  disorder N93.9
    psychogenic F45.8
  during pregnancy O20.8
  excessive (with regular cycle) N92.0
    with irregular cycle N92.1
      at puberty N92.2
  frequent N92.0
  infrequent — *see* Oligomenorrhea
  irregular N92.6
    specified NEC N92.5
  latent N92.5
  membranous N92.5
  painful — *see also* Dysmenorrhea N94.6
    primary N94.4
    psychogenic F45.8
    secondary N94.5
  passage of clots N92.0
  precocious E30.1
  protracted N92.5
  rare — *see* Oligomenorrhea
  retained N94.89
  retrograde N92.5
  scanty — *see* Oligomenorrhea
  suppression N94.89
  vicarious (nasal) N94.89
Mental — *see also* condition
  deficiency — *see* Disability, intellectual
  deterioration — *see* Psychosis
  disorder — *see* Disorder, mental
  exhaustion F48.8
  insufficiency (congenital) — *see* Disability, intellectual
  observation without need for further medical care Z03.89
  retardation — *see* Disability, intellectual
  subnormality — *see* Disability, intellectuall
  upset — *see* Disorder, mental
Meralgia paresthetica G57.1- ☑
Mercurial — *see* condition
Mercurialism — *see* subcategory T56.1 ☑
Merkel cell tumor — *see* Carcinoma, Merkel cell
Merocele — *see* Hernia, femoral
Meromelia
  lower limb — *see* Defect, reduction, lower limb

☑ Additional Character Required — Refer to the Tabular List for Character Selection

⬇ Subterms under main terms may continue to next column or page

Meromelia — *continued*
 lower limb — *see* Defect, reduction, lower limb — *continued*
  intercalary
   femur — *see* Defect, reduction, lower limb, specified type NEC
    tibiofibular (complete) (incomplete) — *see* Defect, reduction, lower limb
  upper limb — *see* Defect, reduction, upper limb
   intercalary, humeral, radioulnar — *see* Agenesis, arm, with hand present
MERRF syndrome (myoclonic epilepsy associated with ragged-red fiber) E88.42
Merzbacher-Pelizaeus disease E75.29
Mesaortitis — *see* Aortitis
Mesarteritis — *see* Arteritis
Mesencephalitis — *see* Encephalitis
Mesenchymoma — *see also* Neoplasm, connective tissue, uncertain behavior
 benign — *see* Neoplasm, connective tissue, benign
 malignant — *see* Neoplasm, connective tissue, malignant
Mesenteritis
 retractile K65.4
 sclerosing K65.4
Mesentery, mesenteric — *see* condition
Mesiodens, mesiodentes K00.1
Mesio-occlusion M26.213
Mesocolon — *see* condition
Mesonephroma (malignant) — *see* Neoplasm, malignant, by site
 benign — *see* Neoplasm, benign, by site
Mesophlebitis — *see* Phlebitis
Mesostromal dysgenesis Q13.89
Mesothelioma (malignant) C45.9
 benign
  mesentery D19.1
  mesocolon D19.1
  omentum D19.1
  peritoneum D19.1
  pleura D19.0
  specified site NEC D19.7
  unspecified site D19.9
 biphasic C45.9
  benign
   mesentery D19.1
   mesocolon D19.1
   omentum D19.1
   peritoneum D19.1
   pleura D19.0
   specified site NEC D19.7
   unspecified site D19.9
 cystic D48.4
 epithelioid C45.9
  benign
   mesentery D19.1
   mesocolon D19.1
   omentum D19.1
   peritoneum D19.1
   pleura D19.0
   specified site NEC D19.7
   unspecified site D19.9
 fibrous C45.9
  benign
   mesentery D19.1
   mesocolon D19.1
   omentum D19.1
   peritoneum D19.1
   pleura D19.0
   specified site NEC D19.7
   unspecified site D19.9
 site classification
  liver C45.7
  lung C45.7
  mediastinum C45.7
  mesentery C45.1
  mesocolon C45.1
  omentum C45.1
  pericardium C45.2
  peritoneum C45.1
  pleura C45.0
   parietal C45.0
  retroperitoneum C45.7
  specified site NEC C45.7
  unspecified C45.9
Metabolic syndrome E88.81
Metagonimiasis B66.8
Metagonimus infestation (intestine) B66.8

Metal
 pigmentation L81.8
 polisher's disease J62.8
Metamorphopsia H53.15
Metaplasia
 apocrine (breast) — *see* Dysplasia, mammary, specified type NEC
 cervix (squamous) — *see* Dysplasia, cervix
 endometrium (squamous) (uterus) N85.8
 esophagus K22.7- ☑
 kidney (pelvis) (squamous) N28.89
 myelogenous D73.1
 myeloid (agnogenic) (megakaryocytic) D73.1
 spleen D73.1
 squamous cell, bladder N32.89
Metastasis, metastatic
 abscess — *see* Abscess
 calcification E83.59
 cancer
  from specified site — *see* Neoplasm, malignant, by site
  to specified site — *see* Neoplasm, secondary, by site
 deposits (in) — *see* Neoplasm, secondary, by site
 disease — *see also* Neoplasm, secondary, by site C79.9
 spread (to) — *see* Neoplasm, secondary, by site
Metastrongyliasis B83.8
Metatarsalgia M77.4- ☑
 anterior G57.6- ☑
 Morton's G57.6- ☑
Metatarsus, metatarsal — *see also* condition
 adductus, congenital Q66.22- ☑
 valgus (abductus), congenital Q66.6
 varus (congenital) Q66.22- ☑
  primus Q66.21- ☑
Methadone use — *see* Use, opioid
Methemoglobinemia D74.9
 acquired (with sulfhemoglobinemia) D74.8
 congenital D74.0
 enzymatic (congenital) D74.0
 Hb M disease D74.0
 hereditary D74.0
 toxic D74.8
Methemoglobinuria — *see* Hemoglobinuria
Methioninemia E72.19
Methylmalonic acidemia E71.120
Metritis (catarrhal) (hemorrhagic) (septic) (suppurative) — *see also* Endometritis
 cervical — *see* Cervicitis
Metropathia hemorrhagica N93.8
Metroperitonitis — *see* Peritonitis, pelvic, female
Metrorrhagia N92.1
 climacteric N92.4
 menopausal N92.4
 perimenopausal N92.4
 postpartum NEC (atonic) (following delivery of placenta) O72.1
  delayed or secondary O72.2
 preclimacteric or premenopausal N92.4
 psychogenic F45.8
Metrorrhexis — *see* Rupture, uterus
Metrosalpingitis N70.91
Metrostaxis N93.8
Metrovaginitis — *see* Endometritis
Meyer-Schwickerath and Weyers syndrome Q87.0
Meynert's amentia (nonalcoholic) F04
 alcoholic F10.96
  with dependence F10.26
Mibelli's disease (porokeratosis) Q82.8
Mice, joint — *see* Loose, body, joint
 knee M23.4- ☑
Micrencephalon, micrencephaly Q02
Microalbuminuria R80.9
Microaneurysm, retinal — *see also* Disorder, retina, microaneurysms
 diabetic — *see* E08-E13 with .31
Microangiopathy (peripheral) I73.9
 thrombotic M31.1
Microcalcifications, breast R92.0
Microcephalus, microcephalic, microcephaly Q02
 due to toxoplasmosis (congenital) P37.1
Microcheilia Q18.7
Microcolon (congenital) Q43.8
Microcornea (congenital) Q13.4
Microcytic — *see* condition
Microdeletions NEC Q93.88
Microdontia K00.2
Microdrepanocytosis D57.40

Microdrepanocytosis — *continued*
 with crisis (vasoocclusive pain) D57.419
  with
   acute chest syndrome D57.411
   splenic sequestration D57.412
Microembolism
 atherothrombotic — *see* Atheroembolism
 retinal — *see* Occlusion, artery, retina
Microencephalon Q02
Microfilaria streptocerca infestation — *see* Onchocerciasis
Microgastria (congenital) Q40.2
Microgenia M26.06
Microgenitalia, congenital
 female Q52.8
 male Q55.8
Microglioma — *see* Lymphoma, non-Hodgkin, specified NEC
Microglossia (congenital) Q38.3
Micrognathia, micrognathism (congenital) (mandibular) (maxillary) M26.09
Microgyria (congenital) Q04.3
Microinfarct of heart — *see* Insufficiency, coronary
Microlentia (congenital) Q12.8
Microlithiasis, alveolar, pulmonary J84.02
Micromastia N64.82
Micromyelia (congenital) Q06.8
Micropenis Q55.62
Microphakia (congenital) Q12.8
Microphthalmos, microphthalmia (congenital) Q11.2
 due to toxoplasmosis P37.1
Micropsia H53.15
Microscopic polyangiitis (polyarteritis) M31.7
Microsporidiosis B60.8
 intestinal A07.8
Microsporon furfur infestation B36.0
Microsporosis — *see also* Dermatophytosis
 nigra B36.1
Microstomia (congenital) Q18.5
Microtia (congenital) (external ear) Q17.2
Microtropia H50.40
Microvillus inclusion disease (MVD) (MVID) Q43.8
Micturition
 disorder NEC — *see also* Difficulty, micturition R39.198
  psychogenic F45.8
 frequency R35.0
  psychogenic F45.8
 hesitancy R39.11
 incomplete emptying R39.14
 nocturnal R35.1
 painful R30.9
  dysuria R30.0
  psychogenic F45.8
  tenesmus R30.1
 poor stream R39.12
 position dependent R39.192
 split stream R39.13
 straining R39.16
 urgency R39.15
Mid plane — *see* condition
Middle
 ear — *see* condition
 lobe (right) syndrome J98.19
Miescher's elastoma L87.2
Mietens' syndrome Q87.2
Migraine (idiopathic) G43.909
 with refractory migraine G43.919
  with status migrainosus G43.911
  without status migrainosus G43.919
 with aura (acute-onset) (prolonged) (typical) (without headache) G43.109
  with refractory migraine G43.119
   with status migrainosus G43.111
   without status migrainosus G43.119
  intractable G43.119
   with status migrainosus G43.111
   without status migrainosus G43.119
  not intractable G43.109
   with status migrainosus G43.101
   without status migrainosus G43.109
  persistent G43.509
   with cerebral infarction G43.609
    with refractory migraine G43.619
     with status migrainosus G43.611
     without status migrainosus G43.619
    intractable G43.619
     with status migrainosus G43.611
     without status migrainosus G43.619

Migraine — *continued*
with aura — *continued*
  persistent — *continued*
    with cerebral infarction — *continued*
      not intractable G43.609
        with status migrainosus G43.601
        without status migrainosus G43.609
      without refractory migraine G43.609
        with status migrainosus G43.601
        without status migrainosus G43.609
    without cerebral infarction G43.509
      with refractory migraine G43.519
        with status migrainosus G43.511
        without status migrainosus G43.519
      intractable G43.519
        with status migrainosus G43.511
        without status migrainosus G43.519
      not intractable G43.509
        with status migrainosus G43.501
        without status migrainosus G43.509
      without refractory migraine G43.509
        with status migrainosus G43.501
        without status migrainosus G43.509
  without mention of refractory migraine G43.109
    with status migrainosus G43.101
    without status migrainosus G43.109
abdominal G43.D0 (*following* G43.7)
  with refractory migraine G43.D1 (*following* G43.7)
  intractable G43.D1 (*following* G43.7)
  not intractable G43.D0 (*following* G43.7)
  without refractory migraine G43.D0 (*following* G43.7)
basilar — *see* Migraine, with aura
classical — *see* Migraine, with aura
common — *see* Migraine, without aura
complicated G43.109
equivalents — *see* Migraine, with aura
familiar — *see* Migraine, hemiplegic
hemiplegic G43.409
  with refractory migraine G43.419
    with status migrainosus G43.411
    without status migrainosus G43.419
  intractable G43.419
    with status migrainosus G43.411
    without status migrainosus G43.419
  not intractable G43.409
    with status migrainosus G43.401
    without status migrainosus G43.409
  without refractory migraine G43.409
    with status migrainosus G43.401
    without status migrainosus G43.409
intractable G43.919
  with status migrainosus G43.911
  without status migrainosus G43.919
menstrual G43.829
  with refractory migraine G43.839
    with status migrainosus G43.831
    without status migrainosus G43.839
  intractable G43.839
    with status migrainosus G43.831
    without status migrainosus G43.839
  not intractable 4G43.829
    with status migrainosus G43.821
    without status migrainosus G43.829
  without refractory migraine G43.829
    with status migrainosus G43.821
    without status migrainosus G43.829
menstrually related — *see* Migraine, menstrual
not intractable G43.909
  with status migrainosus G43.901
  without status migrainosus G43.919
ophthalmoplegic G43.B0 (*following* G43.7)
  with refractory migraine G43.B1 (*following* G43.7)
  intractable G43.B1 (*following* G43.7)
  not intractable G43.B0 (*following* G43.7)
  without refractory migraine G43.B0 (*following* G43.7)
persistent aura (with, without) cerebral infarction —
    see Migraine, with aura, persistent
preceded or accompanied by transient focal neurolog-
    ical phenomena — *see* Migraine, with aura
pre-menstrual — *see* Migraine, menstrual
pure menstrual — *see* Migraine, menstrual
retinal — *see* Migraine, with aura
specified NEC G43.809
  intractable G43.819
    with status migrainosus G43.811
    without status migrainosus G43.819
  not intractable G43.809
    with status migrainosus G43.801

Migraine — *continued*
specified — *continued*
  not intractable — *continued*
    without status migrainosus G43.809
sporadic — *see* Migraine, hemiplegic
transformed — *see* Migraine, without aura, chronic
triggered seizures — *see* Migraine, with aura
without aura G43.009
  with refractory migraine G43.019
    with status migrainosus G43.011
    without status migrainosus G43.019
  chronic G43.709
    with refractory migraine G43.719
      with status migrainosus G43.711
      without status migrainosus G43.719
    intractable
      with status migrainosus G43.711
      without status migrainosus G43.719
    not intractable
      with status migrainosus G43.701
      without status migrainosus G43.709
    without refractory migraine G43.709
      with status migrainosus G43.701
      without status migrainosus G43.709
  intractable
    with status migrainosus G43.011
    without status migrainosus G43.019
  not intractable
    with status migrainosus G43.001
    without status migrainosus G43.009
  without mention of refractory migraine G43.009
    with status migrainosus G43.001
    without status migrainosus G43.009
without refractory migraine G43.909
  wIth status migrainosus G43.901
  without status migrainosus G43.919

Migrant, social Z59.0
Migration, anxiety concerning Z60.3
Migratory, migrating — *see also* condition
  person Z59.0
  testis Q55.29
Mikity-Wilson disease or syndrome P27.0
Mikulicz' disease or syndrome K11.8
Miliaria L74.3
  alba L74.1
  apocrine L75.2
  crystallina L74.1
  profunda L74.2
  rubra L74.0
  tropicalis L74.2
Miliary — *see* condition
Milium L72.0
  colloid L57.8
Milk
  crust L21.0
  excessive secretion O92.6
  poisoning — *see* Poisoning, food, noxious
  retention O92.79
  sickness — *see* Poisoning, food, noxious
  spots I31.0
Milk-alkali disease or syndrome E83.52
Milk-leg (deep vessels) (nonpuerperal) — *see* Embolism,
  vein, lower extremity
  complicating pregnancy O22.3- ☑
  puerperal, postpartum, childbirth O87.1
Milkman's disease or syndrome M83.8
Milky urine — *see* Chyluria
Millard-Gubler (-Foville) **paralysis or syndrome** G46.3
Millar's asthma J38.5
Miller Fisher syndrome G61.0
Mills' disease — *see* Hemiplegia
Millstone maker's pneumoconiosis J62.8
Milroy's disease (chronic hereditary edema) Q82.0
Minamata disease T56.1 ☑
Miners' asthma or lung J60
Minkowski-Chauffard syndrome — *see* Spherocytosis
Minor — *see* condition
Minor's disease (hematomyelia) G95.19
Minot's disease (hemorrhagic disease), newborn P53
Minot-von Willebrand-Jurgens disease or syndrome
  (angiohemophilia) D68.0
Minus (and plus) **hand** (intrinsic) — *see* Deformity, limb,
  specified type NEC, forearm
Miosis (pupil) H57.03
Mirizzi's syndrome (hepatic duct stenosis) K83.1
Mirror writing F81.0

Misadventure (of) (prophylactic) (therapeutic) — *see
  also* Complications T88.9 ☑
administration of insulin (by accident) — *see* subcategory T38.3 ☑
infusion — *see* Complications, infusion
local applications (of fomentations, plasters, etc.)
  T88.9 ☑
  burn or scald — *see* Burn
  specified NEC T88.8 ☑
medical care (early) (late) T88.9 ☑
  adverse effect of drugs or chemicals — *see* Table of
    Drugs and Chemicals
  burn or scald — *see* Burn
  specified NEC T88.8 ☑
specified NEC T88.8 ☑
surgical procedure (early) (late) — *see* Complications,
  surgical procedure
transfusion — *see* Complications, transfusion
vaccination or other immunological procedure — *see*
  Complications, vaccination
Miscarriage O03.9
Misdirection, aqueous H40.83- ☑
Misperception, sleep state F51.02
Misplaced, misplacement
  ear Q17.4
  kidney (acquired) N28.89
    congenital Q63.2
  organ or site, congenital NEC — *see* Malposition, con-
    genital
Missed
  abortion O02.1
  delivery O36.4 ☑
Missing — *see also* Absence
  string of intrauterine contraceptive device T83.32- ☑
Misuse of drugs F19.99
Mitchell's disease (erythromelalgia) I73.81
Mite(s) (infestation) B88.9
  diarrhea B88.0
  grain (itch) B88.0
  hair follicle (itch) B88.0
  in sputum B88.0
Mitral — *see* condition
Mittelschmerz N94.0
Mixed — *see* condition
MMN (multifocal motor neuropathy) G61.82
MNGIE (Mitochondrial Neurogastrointestinal Encephalopathy) **syndrome** E88.49
Mobile, mobility
  cecum Q43.3
  excessive — *see* Hypermobility
  gallbladder, congenital Q44.1
  kidney N28.89
  organ or site, congenital NEC — *see* Malposition, con-
    genital
Mobitz heart block (atrioventricular) I44.1
Moebius, Möbius
  disease (ophthalmoplegic migraine) — *see* Migraine,
    ophthalmoplegic
  syndrome Q87.0
    congenital oculofacial paralysis (with other anoma-
      lies) Q87.0
    ophthalmoplegic migraine — *see* Migraine, ophthal-
      moplegic
Moeller's glossitis K14.0
Mohr's syndrome (Types I and II) Q87.0
Mola destruens D39.2
Molar pregnancy O02.0
Molarization of premolars K00.2
Molding, head (during birth) — *omit code*
Mole (pigmented) — *see also* Nevus
  blood O02.0
  Breus' O02.0
  cancerous — *see* Melanoma
  carneous O02.0
  destructive D39.2
  fleshy O02.0
  hydatid, hydatidiform (benign) (complicating pregnan-
    cy) (delivered) (undelivered) O01.9
    classical O01.0
    complete O01.0
    incomplete O01.1
    invasive D39.2
    malignant D39.2
    partial O01.1
  intrauterine O02.0
  invasive (hydatidiform) D39.2

Mole — *continued*
  malignant
    meaning
      malignant hydatidiform mole D39.2
      melanoma — *see* Melanoma
  nonhydatidiform O02.0
  nonpigmented — *see* Nevus
  pregnancy NEC O02.0
  skin — *see* Nevus
  tubal O00.10- ☑
    with intrauterine pregnancy O00.11- ☑
  vesicular — *see* Mole, hydatidiform
Molimen, molimina (menstrual) N94.3
Molluscum contagiosum (epitheliale) B08.1
Mönckeberg's arteriosclerosis, disease, or sclerosis
  — *see* Arteriosclerosis, extremities
Mondini's malformation (cochlea) Q16.5
Mondor's disease I80.8
Monge's disease T70.29 ☑
Monilethrix (congenital) Q84.1
Moniliasis — *see also* Candidiasis B37.9
  neonatal P37.5
Monitoring (encounter for)
  therapeutic drug level Z51.81
Monkey malaria B53.1
Monkeypox B04
Monoarthritis M13.10
  ankle M13.17- ☑
  elbow M13.12- ☑
  foot joint M13.17- ☑
  hand joint M13.14- ☑
  hip M13.15- ☑
  knee M13.16- ☑
  shoulder M13.11- ☑
  wrist M13.13- ☑
Monoblastic — *see* condition
Monochromat (ism), monochromatopsia (acquired)
  (congenital) H53.51
Monocytic — *see* condition
Monocytopenia D72.818
Monocytosis (symptomatic) D72.821
Monomania — *see* Psychosis
Mononeuritis G58.9
  cranial nerve — *see* Disorder, nerve, cranial
  femoral nerve G57.2-
  lateral
    cutaneous nerve of thigh G57.1- ☑
    popliteal nerve G57.3- ☑
  lower limb G57.9- ☑
    specified nerve NEC G57.8- ☑
  medial popliteal nerve G57.4- ☑
  median nerve G56.1- ☑
  multiplex G58.7
  plantar nerve G57.6- ☑
  posterior tibial nerve G57.5- ☑
  radial nerve G56.3- ☑
  sciatic nerve G57.0- ☑
  specified NEC G58.8
  tibial nerve G57.4- ☑
  ulnar nerve G56.2- ☑
  upper limb G56.9- ☑
    specified nerve NEC G56.8- ☑
  vestibular — *see* subcategory H93.3
Mononeuropathy G58.9
  carpal tunnel syndrome — *see* Syndrome, carpal tunnel
  diabetic NEC — *see* E08-E13 with .41
  femoral nerve — *see* Lesion, nerve, femoral
  ilioinguinal nerve G57.8- ☑
  in diseases classified elsewhere — *see* category G59
  intercostal G58.0
  lower limb G57.9- ☑
    causalgia — *see* Causalgia, lower limb
    femoral nerve — *see* Lesion, nerve, femoral
    meralgia paresthetica G57.1- ☑
    plantar nerve — *see* Lesion, nerve, plantar
    popliteal nerve — *see* Lesion, nerve, popliteal
    sciatic nerve — *see* Lesion, nerve, sciatic
    specified NEC G57.8- ☑
    tarsal tunnel syndrome — *see* Syndrome, tarsal
      tunnel
  median nerve — *see* Lesion, nerve, median
  multiplex G58.7
  obturator nerve G57.8- ☑
  popliteal nerve — *see* Lesion, nerve, popliteal
  radial nerve — *see* Lesion, nerve, radial
  saphenous nerve G57.8- ☑

Mononeuropathy — *continued*
  specified NEC G58.8
  tarsal tunnel syndrome — *see* Syndrome, tarsal tunnel
  tuberculous A17.83
  ulnar nerve — *see* Lesion, nerve, ulnar
  upper limb G56.9- ☑
    carpal tunnel syndrome — *see* Syndrome, carpal
      tunnel
    causalgia — *see* Causalgia
    median nerve — *see* Lesion, nerve, median
    radial nerve — *see* Lesion, nerve, radial
    specified site NEC G56.8- ☑
    ulnar nerve — *see* Lesion, nerve, ulnar
Mononucleosis, infectious B27.90
  with
    complication NEC B27.99
    meningitis B27.92
    polyneuropathy B27.91
  cytomegaloviral B27.10
    with
      complication NEC B27.19
      meningitis B27.12
      polyneuropathy B27.11
  Epstein-Barr (virus) B27.00
    with
      complication NEC B27.09
      meningitis B27.02
      polyneuropathy B27.01
  gammaherpesviral B27.00
    with
      complication NEC B27.09
      meningitis B27.02
      polyneuropathy B27.01
  specified NEC B27.80
    with
      complication NEC B27.89
      meningitis B27.82
      polyneuropathy B27.81
Monoplegia G83.3- ☑
  congenital (cerebral) G80.8
    spastic G80.1
  embolic (current episode) I63.4- ☑
  following
    cerebrovascular disease
      cerebral infarction
        lower limb I69.34- ☑
        upper limb I69.33- ☑
      intracerebral hemorrhage
        lower limb I69.14- ☑
        upper limb I69.13- ☑
      lower limb I69.94- ☑
      nontraumatic intracranial hemorrhage NEC
        lower limb I69.24- ☑
        upper limb I69.23- ☑
      specified disease NEC
        lower limb I69.84- ☑
        upper limb I69.83- ☑
      stroke NOS
        lower limb I69.34- ☑
        upper limb I69.33- ☑
      subarachnoid hemorrhage
        lower limb I69.04- ☑
        upper limb I69.03- ☑
      upper limb I69.93- ☑
  hysterical (transient) F44.4
  lower limb G83.1- ☑
  psychogenic (conversion reaction) F44.4
  thrombotic (current episode) I63.3- ☑
  transient R29.818
  upper limb G83.2- ☑
Monorchism, monorchidism Q55.0
Monosomy — *see also* Deletion, chromosome Q93.9
  specified NEC Q93.89
  whole chromosome
    meiotic nondisjunction Q93.0
    mitotic nondisjunction Q93.1
    mosaicism Q93.1
  X Q96.9
Monster, monstrosity (single) Q89.7
  acephalic Q00.0
  twin Q89.4
Monteggia's fracture (-dislocation) S52.27- ☑
Mooren's ulcer (cornea) — *see* Ulcer, cornea, Mooren's
Moore's syndrome — *see* Epilepsy, specified NEC
Mooser-Neill reaction A75.2
Mooser's bodies A75.2
Morbidity not stated or unknown R69

Morbilli — *see* Measles
Morbus — *see also* Disease
  angelicus, anglorum E55.0
  Beigel B36.2
  caducus — *see* Epilepsy
  celiacus K90.0
  comitialis — *see* Epilepsy
  cordis — *see also* Disease, heart I51.9
    valvulorum — *see* Endocarditis
  coxae senilis M16.9
    tuberculous A18.02
  hemorrhagicus neonatorum P53
  maculosus neonatorum P54.5
Morel (-Stewart)(-Morgagni) **syndrome** M85.2
Morel-Kraepelin disease — *see* Schizophrenia
Morel-Moore syndrome M85.2
Morgagni's
  cyst, organ, hydatid, or appendage
    female Q50.5
    male (epididymal) Q55.4
      testicular Q55.29
  syndrome M85.2
Morgagni-Stewart-Morel syndrome M85.2
Morgagni-Stokes-Adams syndrome I45.9
Morgagni-Turner (-Albright) **syndrome** Q96.9
Moria F07.0
Moron (I.Q. 50-69) F70
Morphea L94.0
Morphinism (without remission) F11.20
  with remission F11.21
Morphinomania (without remission) F11.20
  with remission F11.21
Morquio (-Ullrich)(-Brailsford) **disease or syndrome** —
  see Mucopolysaccharidosis
Mortification (dry) (moist) — *see* Gangrene
Morton's metatarsalgia (neuralgia)(neuroma) (syn-
  drome) G57.6- ☑
Morvan's disease or syndrome G60.8
Mosaicism, mosaic (autosomal) (chromosomal)
  45,X/46,XX Q96.3
  45,X/other cell lines NEC with abnormal sex chromo-
    some Q96.4
  sex chromosome
    female Q97.8
    lines with various numbers of X chromosomes Q97.2
    male Q98.7
  XY Q96.3
Moschowitz' disease M31.1
Mother yaw A66.0
Motion sickness (from travel, any vehicle) (from round-
  abouts or swings) T75.3 ☑
Mottled, mottling, teeth (enamel) (endemic) (nonen-
  demic) K00.3
Mounier-Kuhn syndrome Q32.4
  with bronchiectasis J47.9
    exacerbation (acute) J47.1
    lower respiratory infection J47.0
  acquired J98.09
    with bronchiectasis J47.9
      with
        exacerbation (acute) J47.1
        lower respiratory infection J47.0
Mountain
  sickness T70.29 ☑
    with polycythemia , acquired (acute) D75.1
  tick fever A93.2
Mouse, joint — *see* Loose, body, joint
  knee M23.4- ☑
Mouth — *see* condition
Movable
  coccyx — *see* subcategory M53.2 ☑
  kidney N28.89
    congenital Q63.8
  spleen D73.89
Movements, dystonic R25.8
Moyamoya disease I67.5
MRSA (Methicillin resistant Staphylococcus aureus)
  infection A49.02
    as the cause of diseases classified elsewhere B95.62
  sepsis A41.02
MSD (multiple sulfatase deficiency) E75.26
MSSA (Methicillin susceptible Staphylococcus aureus)
  infection A49.01
    as the cause of diseases classified elsewhere B95.61
  sepsis A41.01
Mucha-Habermann disease L41.0
Mucinosis (cutaneous) (focal) (papular) (skin) L98.5

Mucinosis — *continued*
  oral K13.79
Mucocele
  appendix K38.8
  buccal cavity K13.79
  gallbladder K82.1
  lacrimal sac, chronic H04.43- ☑
  nasal sinus J34.1
  nose J34.1
  salivary gland (any) K11.6
  sinus (accessory) (nasal) J34.1
  turbinate (bone) (middle) (nasal) J34.1
  uterus N85.8
Mucolipidosis
  I E77.1
  II, III E77.0
  IV E75.11
Mucopolysaccharidosis E76.3
  beta-gluduronidase deficiency E76.29
  cardiopathy E76.3 *[I52]*
  Hunter's syndrome E76.1
  Hurler's syndrome E76.01
  Hurler-Scheie syndrome E76.02
  Maroteaux-Lamy syndrome E76.29
  Morquio syndrome E76.219
    A E76.210
    B E76.211
    classic E76.210
  Sanfilippo syndrome E76.22
  Scheie's syndrome E76.03
  specified NEC E76.29
  type
    I
      Hurler's syndrome E76.01
      Hurler-Scheie syndrome E76.02
      Scheie's syndrome E76.03
    II E76.1
    III E76.22
    IV E76.219
    IVA E76.210
    IVB E76.211
    VI E76.29
    VII E76.29
Mucormycosis B46.5
  cutaneous B46.3
  disseminated B46.4
  gastrointestinal B46.2
  generalized B46.4
  pulmonary B46.0
  rhinocerebral B46.1
  skin B46.3
  subcutaneous B46.3
Mucositis (ulcerative) K12.30
  due to drugs NEC K12.32
  gastrointestinal K92.81
  mouth (oral) (oropharyngeal) K12.30
    due to antineoplastic therapy K12.31
    due to drugs NEC K12.32
    due to radiation K12.33
    specified NEC K12.39
    viral K12.39
  nasal J34.81
  oral cavity — *see* Mucositis, mouth
  oral soft tissues — *see* Mucositis, mouth
  vagina and vulva N76.81
Mucositis necroticans agranulocytica — *see* Agranulocytosis
Mucous — *see also* condition
  patches (syphilitic) A51.39
    congenital A50 07
Mucoviscidosis E84.9
  with meconium obstruction E84.11
Mucus
  asphyxia or suffocation — *see* Asphyxia, mucus
  in stool R19.5
  plug — *see* Asphyxia, mucus
Muguet B37.0
Mulberry molars (congenital syphilis) A50.52
Müllerian mixed tumor
  specified site — *see* Neoplasm, malignant, by site
  unspecified site C54.9
Multicystic kidney (development) Q61.4
Multiparity (grand) Z64.1
  affecting management of pregnancy, labor and delivery
    (supervision only) O09.4- ☑
  requiring contraceptive management — *see* Contra-
    ception
Multipartita placenta O43.19- ☑

Multiple, multiplex — *see also* condition
  digits (congenital) Q69.9
  endocrine neoplasia — *see* Neoplasia, endocrine,
    multiple (MEN)
  personality F44.81
Mumps B26.9
  arthritis B26.85
  complication NEC B26.89
  encephalitis B26.2
  hepatitis B26.81
  meningitis (aseptic) B26.1
  meningoencephalitis B26.2
  myocarditis B26.82
  oophoritis B26.89
  orchitis B26.0
  pancreatitis B26.3
  polyneuropathy B26.84
Mumu — *see also* Infestation, filarial B74.9 *[N51]*
Münchhausen's syndrome — *see* Disorder, factitious
Münchmeyer's syndrome — *see* Myositis, ossificans,
  progressiva
Mural — *see* condition
Murmur (cardiac) (heart) (organic) R01.1
  abdominal R19.15
  aortic (valve) — *see* Endocarditis, aortic
  benign R01.0
  diastolic — *see* Endocarditis
  Flint I35.1
  functional R01.0
  Graham Steell I37.1
  innocent R01.0
  mitral (valve) — *see* Insufficiency, mitral
  nonorganic R01.0
  presystolic, mitral — *see* Insufficiency, mitral
  pulmonic (valve) I37.8
  systolic R01.1
  tricuspid (valve) I07.9
  valvular — *see* Endocarditis
Murri's disease (intermittent hemoglobinuria) D59.6
Muscle, muscular — *see also* condition
  carnitine (palmityltransferase) deficiency E71.314
Musculoneuralgia — *see* Neuralgia
Mushrooming hip — *see* Derangement, joint, specified
  NEC, hip
Mushroom-workers' (pickers') **disease or lung** J67.5
Mutation(s)
  factor V Leiden D68.51
  prothrombin gene D68.52
  surfactant, of lung J84.83
Mutism — *see also* Aphasia
  deaf (acquired) (congenital) NEC H91.3
  elective (adjustment reaction) (childhood) F94.0
  hysterical F44.4
  selective (childhood) F94.0
MVD (microvillus inclusion disease) Q43.8
MVID (microvillus inclusion disease) Q43.8
Myalgia M79.10
  auxiliary muscles, head and neck M79.12
  epidemic (cervical) B33.0
  mastication muscle M79.11
  site specified NEC M79.18
  traumatic NEC T14.8 ☑
Myasthenia G70.9
  congenital G70.2
  cordis — *see* Failure, heart
  developmental G70.2
  gravis G70.00
    with exacerbation (acute) G70.01
    in crisis G70.01
    neonatal, transient P94.0
    pseudoparalytica G70.00
      with exacerbation (acute) G70.01
      in crisis G70.01
  stomach, psychogenic F45.8
  syndrome
    in
      diabetes mellitus — *see* E08-E13 with .44
      neoplastic disease — *see also* Neoplasm
        D49.9 *[G73.3]*
      pernicious anemia D51.0 *[G73.3]*
      thyrotoxicosis E05.90 *[G73.3]*
        with thyroid storm E05.91 *[G73.3]*
Myasthenic M62.81
Mycelium infection B49
Mycetismus — *see* Poisoning, food, noxious, mushroom
Mycetoma B47.9
  actinomycotic B47.1
  bone (mycotic) B47.9 *[M90.80]*

Mycetoma — *continued*
  eumycotic B47.0
  foot B47.9
    actinomycotic B47.1
    mycotic B47.0
  madurae NEC B47.9
    mycotic B47.0
  maduromycotic B47.0
  mycotic B47.0
  nocardial B47.1
Mycobacteriosis — *see* Mycobacterium
Mycobacterium, mycobacterial (infection) A31.9
  anonymous A31.9
  atypical A31.9
    cutaneous A31.1
    pulmonary A31.0
      tuberculous — *see* Tuberculosis, pulmonary
    specified site NEC A31.8
  avium (intracellulare complex) A31.0
  balnei A31.1
  Battey A31.0
  chelonei A31.8
  cutaneous A31.1
  extrapulmonary systemic A31.8
  fortuitum A31.8
  intracellulare (Battey bacillus) A31.0
  kakaferifu A31.8
  kansasii (yellow bacillus) A31.0
  kasongo A31.8
  leprae — *see also* Leprosy A30.9
  luciflavum A31.1
  marinum (M. balnei) A31.1
  nonspecific — *see* Mycobacterium, atypical
  pulmonary (atypical) A31.0
    tuberculous — *see* Tuberculosis, pulmonary
  scrofulaceum A31.8
  simiae A31.8
  systemic, extrapulmonary A31.8
  szulgai A31.8
  terrae A31.8
  triviale A31.8
  tuberculosis (human, bovine) — *see* Tuberculosis
  ulcerans A31.1
  xenopi A31.8
Mycoplasma (M.) **pneumoniae, as cause of disease
  classified elsewhere** B96.0
Mycosis, mycotic B49
  cutaneous NEC B36.9
  ear B36.9
    in
      aspergillosis B44.89
      candidiasis B37.84
      moniliasis B37.84
  fungoides (extranodal) (solid organ) C84.0- ☑
  mouth B37.0
  nails B35.1
  opportunistic B48.8
  skin NEC B36.9
  specified NEC B48.8
  stomatitis B37.0
  vagina, vaginitis (candidal) B37.3
Mydriasis (pupil) H57.04
Myelatelia Q06.1
Myelinolysis, pontine, central G37.2
Myelitis (acute) (ascending) (childhood) (chronic) (descending) (diffuse) (disseminated) (idiopathic)
  (pressure) (progressive) (spinal cord) (subacute) —
  see also Encephalitis G04.91
  herpes simplex B00.82
  herpes zoster B02.24
  in diseases classified elsewhere G05.4
  necrotizing, subacute G37.4
  optic neuritis in G36.0
  postchickenpox B01.12
  postherpetic B02.24
  postimmunization G04.02
  postinfectious NEC G04.89
  postvaccinal G04.02
  specified NEC G04.89
  syphilitic (transverse) A52.14
  toxic G92
  transverse (in demyelinating diseases of central nervous
    system) G37.3
  tuberculous A17.82
  varicella B01.12
Myeloblastic — *see* condition
Myeloblastoma
  granular cell — *see also* Neoplasm, connective tissue

Myeloblastoma — *continued*
  granular cell — *see also* Neoplasm, connective tissue
    — *continued*
      malignant — *see* Neoplasm, connective tissue, malignant
      tongue D10.1
Myelocele — *see* Spina bifida
Myelocystocele — *see* Spina bifida
Myelocytic — *see* condition
Myelodysplasia D46.9
  specified NEC D46.Z (*following* D46.4)
  spinal cord (congenital) Q06.1
Myelodysplastic syndrome D46.9
  with
    5q deletion D46.C (*following* D46.2)
    isolated del (5q) chromosomal abnormality D46.C
      (*following* D46.2)
  specified NEC D46.Z (*following* D46.4)
Myeloencephalitis — *see* Encephalitis
Myelofibrosis D75.81
  with myeloid metaplasia D47.4
  acute C94.4- ☑
  idiopathic (chronic) D47.4
  primary D47.1
  secondary D75.81
    in myeloproliferative disease D47.4
Myelogenous — *see* condition
Myeloid — *see* condition
Myelokathexis D70.9
Myeloleukodystrophy E75.29
Myelolipoma — *see* Lipoma
Myeloma (multiple) C90.0- ☑
  monostotic C90.3 ☑
    plasma cell C90.0- ☑
  plasma cell C90.0- ☑
  solitary — *see also* Plasmacytoma, solitary C90.3- ☑
Myelomalacia G95.89
Myelomatosis C90.0- ☑
Myelomeningitis — *see* Meningoencephalitis
Myelomeningocele (spinal cord) — *see* Spina bifida
Myelo-osteo-musculodysplasia hereditaria Q79.8
Myelopathic
  anemia D64.89
  muscle atrophy — *see* Atrophy, muscle, spinal
  pain syndrome G89.0
Myelopathy (spinal cord) G95.9
  drug-induced G95.89
  in (due to)
    degeneration or displacement, intervertebral disc
      NEC — *see* Disorder, disc, with, myelopathy
    infection — *see* Encephalitis
    intervertebral disc disorder — *see also* Disorder,
      disc, with, myelopathy
    mercury — *see* subcategory T56.1 ☑
    neoplastic disease — *see also* Neoplasm
      D49.9 [G99.2]
    pernicious anemia D51.0 [G99.2]
    spondylosis — *see* Spondylosis, with myelopathy
      NEC
  necrotic (subacute) (vascular) G95.19
  radiation-induced G95.89
  spondylogenic NEC — *see* Spondylosis, with
    myelopathy NEC
  toxic G95.89
  transverse, acute G37.3
  vascular G95.19
  vitamin B12 E53.8 [G32.0]
Myelophthisis D61.82
Myeloradiculitis G04.91
Myeloradiculodysplasia (spinal) Q06.1
Myelosarcoma C92.3- ☑
Myelosclerosis D75.89
  with myeloid metaplasia D47.4
  disseminated, of nervous system G35
  megakaryocytic D47.4
    with myeloid metaplasia D47.4
Myelosis
  acute C92.0- ☑
  aleukemic C92.9- ☑
  chronic D47.1
  erythremic (acute) C94.0- ☑
  megakaryocytic C94.2- ☑
  nonleukemic D72.828
  subacute C92.9- ☑
Myiasis (cavernous) B87.9
  aural B87.4
  creeping B87.0

Myiasis — *continued*
  cutaneous B87.0
  dermal B87.0
  ear (external) (middle) B87.4
  eye B87.2
  genitourinary B87.81
  intestinal B87.82
  laryngeal B87.3
  nasopharyngeal B87.3
  ocular B87.2
  orbit B87.2
  skin B87.0
  specified site NEC B87.89
  traumatic B87.1
  wound B87.1
Myoadenoma, prostate — *see* Hyperplasia, prostate
Myoblastoma
  granular cell — *see also* Neoplasm, connective tissue,
    benign
      malignant — *see* Neoplasm, connective tissue, malignant
  tongue D10.1
Myocardial — *see* condition
Myocardiopathy (congestive) (constrictive) (familial)
    (hypertrophic nonobstructive) (idiopathic) (infiltrative) (obstructive) (primary) (restrictive) (sporadic)
    — *see also* Cardiomyopathy I42.9
  alcoholic I42.6
  cobalt-beer I42.6
  glycogen storage E74.02 [I43]
  hypertrophic obstructive I42.1
  in (due to)
    beriberi E51.12
    cardiac glycogenosis E74.02 [I43]
    Friedreich's ataxia G11.1 [I43]
    myotonia atrophica G71.11 [I43]
    progressive muscular dystrophy G71.09 [I43]
  obscure (African) I42.8
  secondary I42.9
  thyrotoxic E05.90 [I43]
    with storm E05.91 [I43]
  toxic NEC I42.7
Myocarditis (with arteriosclerosis)(chronic)(fibroid) (interstitial) (old) (progressive) (senile) I51.4
  with
    rheumatic fever (conditions in I00) I09.0
      active — *see* Myocarditis, acute, rheumatic
      inactive or quiescent (with chorea) I09.0
  active I40.9
    rheumatic I01.2
      with chorea (acute) (rheumatic) (Sydenham's)
        I02.0
  acute or subacute (interstitial) I40.9
    due to
      streptococcus (beta-hemolytic) I01.2
    idiopathic I40.1
    rheumatic I01.2
      with chorea (acute) (rheumatic) (Sydenham's)
        I02.0
    specified NEC I40.8
  aseptic of newborn B33.22
  bacterial (acute) I40.0
  Coxsackie (virus) B33.22
  diphtheritic A36.81
  eosinophilic I40.1
  epidemic of newborn (Coxsackie) B33.22
  Fiedler's (acute) (isolated) I40.1
  giant cell (acute) (subacute) I40.1
  gonococcal A54.83
  granulomatous (idiopathic) (isolated) (nonspecific) I40.1
  hypertensive — *see* Hypertension, heart
  idiopathic (granulomatous) I40.1
  in (due to)
    diphtheria A36.81
    epidemic louse-borne typhus A75.0 [I41]
    Lyme disease A69.29
    sarcoidosis D86.85
    scarlet fever A38.1
    toxoplasmosis (acquired) B58.81
    typhoid A01.02
    typhus NEC A75.9 [I41]
  infective I40.0
  influenzal — *see* Influenza, with, myocarditis
  isolated (acute) I40.1
  meningococcal A39.52
  mumps B26.82
  nonrheumatic, active I40.9
  parenchymatous I40.9

Myocarditis — *continued*
  pneumococcal I40.0
  rheumatic (chronic) (inactive) (with chorea) I09.0
    active or acute I01.2
      with chorea (acute) (rheumatic) (Sydenham's)
        I02.0
  rheumatoid — *see* Rheumatoid, carditis
  septic I40.0
  staphylococcal I40.0
  suppurative I40.0
  syphilitic (chronic) A52.06
  toxic I40.8
    rheumatic — *see* Myocarditis, acute, rheumatic
  tuberculous A18.84
  typhoid A01.02
  valvular — *see* Endocarditis
  virus, viral I40.0
    of newborn (Coxsackie) B33.22
Myocardium, myocardial — *see* condition
Myocardosis — *see* Cardiomyopathy
Myoclonus, myoclonic, myoclonia (familial) (essential)
    (multifocal) (simplex) G25.3
  drug-induced G25.3
  epilepsy — *see also* Epilepsy, generalized, specified
    NEC G40.4- ☑
  familial (progressive) G25.3
  epileptica G40.409
    with status epilepticus G40.401
  facial G51.3- ☑
  familial progressive G25.3
  Friedreich's G25.3
  jerks G25.3
  massive G25.3
  palatal G25.3
  pharyngeal G25.3
Myocytolysis I51.5
Myodiastasis — *see* Diastasis, muscle
Myoendocarditis — *see* Endocarditis
Myoepithelioma — *see* Neoplasm, benign, by site
Myofasciitis (acute) — *see* Myositis
Myofibroma — *see also* Neoplasm, connective tissue,
    benign
  uterus (cervix) (corpus) — *see* Leiomyoma
Myofibromatosis D48.1
  infantile Q89.8
Myofibrosis M62.89
  heart — *see* Myocarditis
  scapulohumeral — *see* Lesion, shoulder, specified NEC
Myofibrositis M79.7
  scapulohumeral — *see* Lesion, shoulder, specified NEC
Myoglobulinuria, myoglobinuria (primary) R82.1
Myokymia, facial G51.4
Myolipoma — *see* Lipoma
Myoma — *see also* Neoplasm, connective tissue, benign
  malignant — *see* Neoplasm, connective tissue, malignant
  prostate D29.1
  uterus (cervix) (corpus) — *see* Leiomyoma
Myomalacia M62.89
Myometritis — *see* Endometritis
Myometrium — *see* condition
Myonecrosis, clostridial A48.0
Myopathy G72.9
  acute
    necrotizing G72.81
    quadriplegic G72.81
  alcoholic G72.1
  benign congenital G71.2
  central core G71.2
  centronuclear G71.2
  congenital (benign) G71.2
  critical illness G72.81
  distal G71.09
  drug-induced G72.0
  endocrine NEC E34.9 [G73.7]
  extraocular muscles H05.82- ☑
  facioscapulohumeral G71.02
  hereditary G71.9
    specified NEC G71.8
  immune NEC G72.49
  in (due to)
    Addison's disease E27.1 [G73.7]
    alcohol G72.1
    amyloidosis E85.0 [G73.7]
    cretinism E00.9 [G73.7]
    Cushing's syndrome E24.9 [G73.7]
    drugs G72.0

Index

Myopathy — Myxosarcoma

Myopathy — *continued*
  in — *continued*
    endocrine disease NEC E34.9 *[G73.7]*
    giant cell arteritis M31.6 *[G73.7]*
    glycogen storage disease E74.00 *[G73.7]*
    hyperadrenocorticism E24.9 *[G73.7]*
    hyperparathyroidism NEC E21.3 *[G73.7]*
    hypoparathyroidism E20.9 *[G73.7]*
    hypopituitarism E23.0 *[G73.7]*
    hypothyroidism E03.9 *[G73.7]*
    infectious disease NEC B99 ☑ *[G73.7]*
    lipid storage disease E75.6 *[G73.7]*
    metabolic disease NEC E88.9 *[G73.7]*
    myxedema E03.9 *[G73.7]*
    parasitic disease NEC B89 *[G73.7]*
    polyarteritis nodosa M30.0 *[G73.7]*
    rheumatoid arthritis — *see* Rheumatoid, myopathy
    sarcoidosis D86.87
    scleroderma M34.82
    sicca syndrome M35.03
    Sjögren's syndrome M35.03
    systemic lupus erythematosus M32.19
    thyrotoxicosis (hyperthyroidism) E05.90 *[G73.7]*
      with thyroid storm E05.91 *[G73.7]*
    toxic agent NEC G72.2
  inflammatory NEC G72.49
  intensive care (ICU) G72.81
  limb-girdle G71.09
  mitochondrial NEC G71.3
  myotubular G71.2
  mytonic, proximal (PROMM) G71.11
  nemaline G71.2
  ocular G71.09
  oculopharyngeal G71.09
  of critical illness G72.81
  primary G71.9
    specified NEC G71.8
  progressive NEC G72.89
  proximal myotonic (PROMM) G71.11
  rod G71.2
  scapulohumeral G71.02
  specified NEC G72.89
  toxic G72.2
Myopericarditis — *see also* Pericarditis
  chronic rheumatic I09.2
Myopia (axial) (congenital) H52.1- ☑
  degenerative (malignant) H44.20
    with
      choroidal neovascularization H44.2A- ☑
      foveoschisis H44.2D- ☑
      macular hole H44.2B- ☑
      retinal detachment H44.2C- ☑
      specified maculopathy NEC H44.2E- ☑
    bilateral H44.23
    left eye H44.22
    right eye H44.21
  malignant — *see also* Myopia, degenerative H44.2- ☑
  pernicious — *see also* Myopia, degenerative H44.2- ☑
  progressive high (degenerative) — *see also* Myopia, degenerative H44.2- ☑
Myosarcoma — *see* Neoplasm, connective tissue, malignant
Myosis (pupil) H57.03
  stromal (endolymphatic) D39.0
Myositis M60.9
  clostridial A48.0
  due to posture — *see* Myositis, specified type NEC
  epidemic B33.0
  fibrosa or fibrous (chronic), Volkmann's T79.6
  foreign body granuloma — *see* Granuloma, foreign body
  in (due to)
    bilharziasis B65.9 *[M63.8-]* ☑
    cysticercosis B69.81
    leprosy A30.9 *[M63.8-]* ☑
    mycosis B49 *[M63.8-]* ☑
    sarcoidosis D86.87
    schistosomiasis B65.9 *[M63.8-]* ☑
    syphilis
      late A52.78
      secondary A51.49
    toxoplasmosis (acquired) B58.82

Myositis — *continued*
  in — *continued*
    trichinellosis B75 *[M63.8-]* ☑
    tuberculosis A18.09
  inclusion body [IBM] G72.41
  infective M60.009
    arm M60.002
      left M60.001
      right M60.000
    leg M60.005
      left M60.004
      right M60.003
    lower limb M60.005
      ankle M60.07- ☑
      foot M60.07- ☑
      lower leg M60.06- ☑
      thigh M60.05- ☑
      toe M60.07- ☑
    multiple sites M60.09
    specified site NEC M60.08
    upper limb M60.002
      finger M60.04- ☑
      forearm M60.03- ☑
      hand M60.04- ☑
      shoulder region M60.01- ☑
      upper arm M60.02- ☑
  interstitial M60.10
    ankle M60.17- ☑
    foot M60.17- ☑
    forearm M60.13- ☑
    hand M60.14- ☑
    lower leg M60.16- ☑
    multiple sites M60.19
    shoulder region M60.11- ☑
    specified site NEC M60.18
    thigh M60.15- ☑
    upper arm M60.12- ☑
  mycotic B49 *[M63.8-]* ☑
  orbital, chronic H05.12- ☑
  ossificans or ossifying (circumscripta) — *see also* Ossification, muscle, specified NEC
    in (due to)
      burns M61.30
        ankle M61.37- ☑
        foot M61.37- ☑
        forearm M61.33- ☑
        hand M61.34- ☑
        lower leg M61.36- ☑
        multiple sites M61.39
        pelvic region M61.35- ☑
        shoulder region M61.31- ☑
        specified site NEC M61.38
        thigh M61.35- ☑
        upper arm M61.32- ☑
      quadriplegia or paraplegia M61.20
        ankle M61.27- ☑
        foot M61.27- ☑
        forearm M61.23- ☑
        hand M61.24- ☑
        lower leg M61.26- ☑
        multiple sites M61.29
        pelvic region M61.25- ☑
        shoulder region M61.21- ☑
        specified site NEC M61.28
        thigh M61.25- ☑
        upper arm M61.22- ☑
    progressiva M61.10
      ankle M61.17- ☑
      finger M61.14- ☑
      foot M61.17- ☑
      forearm M61.13- ☑
      hand M61.14- ☑
      lower leg M61.16- ☑
      multiple sites M61.19
      pelvic region M61.15- ☑
      shoulder region M61.11- ☑
      specified site NEC M61.18
      thigh M61.15- ☑
      toe M61.17- ☑
      upper arm M61.12- ☑
    traumatica M61.00

Myositis — *continued*
  ossificans or ossifying — *see also* Ossification, muscle, specified — *continued*
    traumatica — *continued*
      ankle M61.07- ☑
      foot M61.07- ☑
      forearm M61.03- ☑
      hand M61.04- ☑
      lower leg M61.06- ☑
      multiple sites M61.09
      pelvic region M61.05- ☑
      shoulder region M61.01- ☑
      specified site NEC M61.08
      thigh M61.05- ☑
      upper arm M61.02- ☑
  purulent — *see* Myositis, infective
  specified type NEC M60.80
    ankle M60.87- ☑
    foot M60.87- ☑
    forearm M60.83- ☑
    hand M60.84- ☑
    lower leg M60.86- ☑
    multiple sites M60.89
    pelvic region M60.85- ☑
    shoulder region M60.81- ☑
    specified site NEC M60.88
    thigh M60.85- ☑
    upper arm M60.82- ☑
  suppurative — *see* Myositis, infective
  traumatic (old) — *see* Myositis, specified type NEC
Myospasia impulsiva F95.2
Myotonia (acquisita) (intermittens) M62.89
  atrophica G71.11
  chondrodystrophic G71.13
  congenita (acetazolamide responsive) (dominant) (recessive) G71.12
  drug-induced G71.14
  dystrophica G71.11
  fluctuans G71.19
  levior G71.12
  permanens G71.19
  symptomatic G71.19
Myotonic pupil — *see* Anomaly, pupil, function, tonic pupil
Myriapodiasis B88.2
Myringitis H73.2- ☑
  with otitis media — *see* Otitis, media
  acute H73.00- ☑
    bullous H73.01- ☑
    specified NEC H73.09- ☑
  bullous — *see* Myringitis, acute, bullous
  chronic H73.1- ☑
Mysophobia F40.228
Mytilotoxism — *see* Poisoning, fish
Myxadenitis labialis K13.0
Myxedema (adult) (idiocy) (infantile) (juvenile) — *see also* Hypothyroidism E03.9
  circumscribed E05.90
    with storm E05.91
  coma E03.5
  congenital E00.1
  cutis L98.5
  localized (pretibial) E05.90
    with storm E05.91
  papular L98.5
Myxochondrosarcoma — *see* Neoplasm, cartilage, malignant
Myxofibroma — *see* Neoplasm, connective tissue, benign
  odontogenic — *see* Cyst, calcifying odontogenic
Myxofibrosarcoma — *see* Neoplasm, connective tissue, malignant
Myxolipoma D17.9
Myxoliposarcoma — *see* Neoplasm, connective tissue, malignant
Myxoma — *see also* Neoplasm, connective tissue, benign
  nerve sheath — *see* Neoplasm, nerve, benign
  odontogenic — *see* Cyst, calcifying odontogenic
Myxosarcoma — *see* Neoplasm, connective tissue, malignant

228

☑ **Additional Character Required** — Refer to the Tabular List for Character Selection   ▽ **Subterms under main terms may continue to next column or page**

N

Naegeli's
  disease Q82.8
  leukemia, monocytic C93.1- ☑
Naegleriasis (with meningoencephalitis) B60.2
Naffziger's syndrome G54.0
Naga sore — *see* Ulcer, skin
Nägele's pelvis M95.5
  with disproportion (fetopelvic) O33.0
    causing obstructed labor O65.0
Nail — *see also* condition
  biting F98.8
  patella syndrome Q87.2
Nanism, nanosomia — *see* Dwarfism
Nanophyetiasis B66.8
Nanukayami A27.89
Napkin rash L22
Narcolepsy G47.419
  with cataplexy G47.411
  in conditions classified elsewhere G47.429
    with cataplexy G47.421
Narcosis R06.89
Narcotism — *see* Dependence
NARP (Neuropathy, Ataxia and Retinitis pigmentosa)
  syndrome E88.49
Narrow
  anterior chamber angle H40.03- ☑
  gingival width (of periodontal soft tissue) K05.5
  pelvis — *see* Contraction, pelvis
Narrowing — *see also* Stenosis
  artery I77.1
    auditory, internal I65.8
    basilar — *see* Occlusion, artery, basilar
    carotid — *see* Occlusion, artery, carotid
    cerebellar — *see* Occlusion, artery, cerebellar
    cerebral — *see* Occlusion artery, cerebral
    choroidal — *see* Occlusion, artery, precerebral,
      specified NEC
    communicating posterior — *see* Occlusion, artery,
      precerebral, specified NEC
    coronary — *see also* Disease, heart, ischemic,
      atherosclerotic
      congenital Q24.5
        syphilitic A50.54 [I52]
      due to syphilis NEC A52.06
    hypophyseal — *see* Occlusion, artery, precerebral,
      specified NEC
    pontine — *see* Occlusion, artery, precerebral, spec-
      ified NEC
    precerebral — *see* Occlusion, artery, precerebral
    vertebral — *see* Occlusion, artery, vertebral
  auditory canal (external) — *see* Stenosis, external ear
    canal
  eustachian tube — *see* Obstruction, eustachian tube
  eyelid — *see* Disorder, eyelid function
  larynx J38.6
  mesenteric artery — *see also* Ischemia, intestine, acute
    K55.059
  palate M26.89
  palpebral fissure — *see* Disorder, eyelid function
  ureter N13.5
    with infection N13.6
  urethra — *see* Stricture, urethra
Narrowness, abnormal, eyelid Q10.3
Nasal — *see* condition
Nasolachrymal, nasolacrimal — *see* condition
Nasopharyngeal — *see also* condition
  pituitary gland Q89.2
  torticollis M43.6
Nasopharyngitis (acute) (infective) (streptococcal)
    (subacute) J00
  chronic (suppurative) (ulcerative) J31.1
Nasopharynx, nasopharyngeal — *see* condition
Natal tooth, teeth K00.6
Nausea (without vomiting) R11.0
  with vomiting R11.2
  gravidarum — *see* Hyperemesis, gravidarum
  marina T75.3 ☑
  navalis T75.3 ☑
Navel — *see* condition
Neapolitan fever — *see* Brucellosis
Near drowning T75.1 ☑
Nearsightedness — *see* Myopia
Near-syncope R55
Nebula, cornea — *see* Opacity, cornea

Necator americanus infestation B76.1
Necatoriasis B76.1
Neck — *see* condition
Necrobiosis R68.89
  lipoidica NEC L92.1
    with diabetes — *see* E08-E13 with .620
Necrolysis, toxic epidermal L51.2
  due to drug
    correct substance properly administered — *see* Ta-
      ble of Drugs and Chemicals, by drug, adverse
      effect
    overdose or wrong substance given or taken — *see*
      Table of Drugs and Chemicals, by drug, poi-
      soning
Necrophilia F65.89
Necrosis, necrotic (ischemic) — *see also* Gangrene
  adrenal (capsule) (gland) E27.49
  amputation stump (surgical) (late) T87.50
    arm T87.5- ☑
    leg T87.5- ☑
  antrum J32.0
  aorta (hyaline) — *see also* Aneurysm, aorta
    cystic medial — *see* Dissection, aorta
  artery I77.5
  bladder (aseptic) (sphincter) N32.89
  bone — *see also* Osteonecrosis M87.9
    aseptic or avascular — *see* Osteonecrosis
      idiopathic M87.00
    ethmoid J32.2
    jaw M27.2
    tuberculous — *see* Tuberculosis, bone
  brain I67.89
  breast (aseptic) (fat) (segmental) N64.1
  bronchus J98.09
  central nervous system NEC I67.89
  cerebellar I67.89
  cerebral I67.89
  colon — *see also* Infarct, intestine K55.049
  cornea H18.89- ☑
  cortical (acute) (renal) N17.1
  cystic medial (aorta) — *see* Dissection, aorta
  dental pulp K04.1
  esophagus K22.8
  ethmoid (bone) J32.2
  eyelid — *see* Disorder, eyelid, degenerative
  fat, fatty (generalized) — *see also* Disorder, soft tissue,
      specified type NEC)
    abdominal wall K65.4
    breast (aseptic) (segmental) N64.1
    localized — *see* Degeneration, by site, fatty
    mesentery K65.4
    omentum K65.4
    pancreas K86.89
    peritoneum K65.4
    skin (subcutaneous), newborn P83.0
    subcutaneous, due to birth injury P15.6
  gallbladder — *see* Cholecystitis, acute
  heart — *see* Infarct, myocardium
  hip, aseptic or avascular — *see* Osteonecrosis, by type,
      femur
  intestine (acute) (hemorrhagic) (massive) — *see also*
      Infarct, intestine K55.069
  jaw M27.2
  kidney (bilateral) N28.0
    acute N17.9
    cortical (acute) (bilateral) N17.1
      with ectopic or molar pregnancy O08.4
    medullary (bilateral) (in acute renal failure) (papil-
      lary) N17.2
    papillary (bilateral) (in acute renal failure) N17.2
    tubular N17.0
      with ectopic or molar pregnancy O08.4
      complicating
        abortion — *see* Abortion, by type, complicat-
          ed by, tubular necrosis
        ectopic or molar pregnancy O08.4
        pregnancy — *see* Pregnancy, complicated by,
          diseases of, specified type or system
          NEC
      following ectopic or molar pregnancy O08.4
      traumatic T79.5 ☑
  larynx J38.7
  liver (with hepatic failure) (cell) — *see* Failure, hepatic
    hemorrhagic, central K76.2
  lung J85.0
  lymphatic gland — *see* Lymphadenitis, acute
  mammary gland (fat) (segmental) N64.1
  mastoid (chronic) — *see* Mastoiditis, chronic

Necrosis, necrotic — *continued*
  medullary (acute) (renal) N17.2
  mesentery — *see also* Infarct, intestine K55.069
    fat K65.4
  mitral valve — *see* Insufficiency, mitral
  myocardium, myocardial — *see* Infarct, myocardium
  nose J34.0
  omentum (with mesenteric infarction) — *see also* In-
      farct, intestine K55.069
    fat K65.4
  orbit, orbital — *see* Osteomyelitis, orbit
  ossicles, ear — *see* Abnormal, ear ossicles
  ovary N70.92
  pancreas (aseptic) (duct) (fat) K86.89
    acute (infective) — *see* Pancreatitis, acute
    infective — *see* Pancreatitis, acute
  papillary (acute) (renal) N17.2
  perineum N90.89
  peritoneum (with mesenteric infarction) — *see also*
      Infarct, intestine K55.069
    fat K65.4
  pharynx J02.9
    in granulocytopenia — *see* Neutropenia
    Vincent's A69.1
  phosphorus — *see* subcategory T54.2 ☑
  pituitary (gland) E23.0
    postpartum O99.285
    Sheehan O99.285
  pressure — *see* Ulcer, pressure, by site
  pulmonary J85.0
  pulp (dental) K04.1
  radiation — *see* Necrosis, by site
  radium — *see* Necrosis, by site
  renal — *see* Necrosis, kidney
  sclera H15.89
  scrotum N50.89
  skin or subcutaneous tissue NEC I96
  spine, spinal (column) — *see also* Osteonecrosis, by
      type, vertebra
    cord G95.19
  spleen D73.5
  stomach K31.89
  stomatitis (ulcerative) A69.0
  subcutaneous fat, newborn P83.88
  subendocardial (acute) I21.4
    chronic I25.89
  suprarenal (capsule) (gland) E27.49
  testis N50.89
  thymus (gland) E32.8
  tonsil J35.8
  trachea J39.8
  tuberculous NEC — *see* Tuberculosis
  tubular (acute) (anoxic) (renal) (toxic) N17.0
    postprocedural N99.0
  vagina N89.8
  vertebra — *see also* Osteonecrosis, by type, vertebra
    tuberculous A18.01
  vulva N90.89
  X-ray — *see* Necrosis, by site
Necrospermia — *see* Infertility, male
Need (for)
  care provider because (of)
    assistance with personal care Z74.1
    continuous supervision required Z74.3
    impaired mobility Z74.09
    no other household member able to render care
      Z74.2
    specified reason NEC Z74.8
  immunization — *see* Vaccination
  vaccination — *see* Vaccination
Neglect
  adult
    confirmed T74.01 ☑
    history of Z91.412
    suspected T76.01 ☑
  child (childhood)
    confirmed T74.02 ☑
    history of Z62.812
    suspected T76.02 ☑
  emotional, in childhood Z62.898
  hemispatial R41.4
  left-sided R41.4
  sensory R41.4
  visuospatial R41.4
Neisserian infection NEC — *see* Gonococcus
Nelaton's syndrome G60.8
Nelson's syndrome E24.1
Nematodiasis (intestinal) B82.0

Nematodiasis — *continued*
Ancylostoma B76.0
Neonatal — *see also* Newborn
acne L70.4
bradycardia P29.12
screening, abnormal findings on P09
tachycardia P29.11
tooth, teeth K00.6
Neonatorum — *see* condition
Neoplasia
endocrine, multiple (MEN) E31.20
type I E31.21
type IIA E31.22
type IIB E31.23
intraepithelial (histologically confirmed)
anal (AIN) (histologically confirmed) K62.82
grade I K62.82
grade II K62.82
severe D01.3
cervical glandular (histologically confirmed) D06.9
cervix (uteri) (CIN) (histologically confirmed) N87.9
glandular D06.9
grade I N87.0
grade II N87.1
grade III (severe dysplasia) — *see also* Carcinoma, cervix uteri, in situ D06.9
prostate (histologically confirmed) (PIN) N42.31
grade I N42.31
grade II N42.31
grade III (severe dysplasia) D07.5
vagina (histologically confirmed) (VAIN) N89.3
grade I N89.0
grade II N89.1
grade III (severe dysplasia) D07.2
vulva (histologically confirmed) (VIN) N90.3
grade I N90.0
grade II N90.1
grade III (severe dysplasia) D07.1
Neoplasm, neoplastic — *see also* Table of Neoplasms
lipomatous, benign — *see* Lipoma
malignant mast cell C96.20
specified type NEC C96.29
mast cell, of uncertain behavior NEC D47.09
Neovascularization
ciliary body — *see* Disorder, iris, vascular
cornea H16.40- ☑
deep H16.44- ☑
ghost vessels — *see* Ghost, vessels
localized H16.43- ☑
pannus — *see* Pannus
iris — *see* Disorder, iris, vascular
retina H35.05- ☑
Nephralgia N23
Nephritis, nephritic (albuminuric) (azotemic) (congenital) (disseminated) (epithelial) (familial) (focal) (granulomatous) (hemorrhagic) (infantile) (nonsuppurative, excretory) (uremic) N05.9
with
dense deposit disease N05.6
diffuse
crescentic glomerulonephritis N05.7
endocapillary proliferative glomerulonephritis N05.4
membranous glomerulonephritis N05.2
mesangial proliferative glomerulonephritis N05.3
mesangiocapillary glomerulonephritis N05.5
edema — *see* Nephrosis
focal and segmental glomerular lesions N05.1
foot process disease N04.9
glomerular lesion
diffuse sclerosing N05.8
hypocomplementemic — *see* Nephritis, membranoproliferative
IgA — *see* Nephropathy, IgA
lobular, lobulonodular — *see* Nephritis, membranoproliferative
nodular — *see* Nephritis, membranoproliferative
lesion of
glomerulonephritis, proliferative N05.8
renal necrosis N05.9
minor glomerular abnormality N05.0
specified morphological changes NEC N05.8
acute N00.9
with
dense deposit disease N00.6
diffuse
crescentic glomerulonephritis N00.7

Nephritis, nephritic — *continued*
acute — *continued*
with — *continued*
diffuse — *continued*
endocapillary proliferative glomerulonephritis N00.4
membranous glomerulonephritis N00.2
mesangial proliferative glomerulonephritis N00.3
mesangiocapillary glomerulonephritis N00.5
focal and segmental glomerular lesions N00.1
minor glomerular abnormality N00.0
specified morphological changes NEC N00.8
amyloid E85.4 *[N08]*
antiglomerular basement membrane (anti-GBM) antibody NEC
in Goodpasture's syndrome M31.0
antitubular basement membrane (tubulo-interstitial) NEC N12
toxic — *see* Nephropathy, toxic
arteriolar — *see* Hypertension, kidney
arteriosclerotic — *see* Hypertension, kidney
ascending — *see* Nephritis, tubulo-interstitial
atrophic N03.9
Balkan (endemic) N15.0
calculous, calculus — *see* Calculus, kidney
cardiac — *see* Hypertension, kidney
cardiovascular — *see* Hypertension, kidney
chronic N03.9
with
dense deposit disease N03.6
diffuse
crescentic glomerulonephritis N03.7
endocapillary proliferative glomerulonephritis N03.4
membranous glomerulonephritis N03.2
mesangial proliferative glomerulonephritis N03.3
mesangiocapillary glomerulonephritis N03.5
focal and segmental glomerular lesions N03.1
minor glomerular abnormality N03.0
specified morphological changes NEC N03.8
arteriosclerotic — *see* Hypertension, kidney
cirrhotic N26.9
complicating pregnancy O26.83- ☑
croupous N00.9
degenerative — *see* Nephrosis
diffuse sclerosing N05.8
due to
diabetes mellitus — *see* E08-E13 with .21
subacute bacterial endocarditis I33.0
systemic lupus erythematosus (chronic) M32.14
typhoid fever A01.09
gonococcal (acute) (chronic) A54.21
hypocomplementemic — *see* Nephritis, membranoproliferative
IgA — *see* Nephropathy, IgA
immune complex (circulating) NEC N05.8
infective — *see* Nephritis, tubulo-interstitial
interstitial — *see* Nephritis, tubulo-interstitial
lead N14.3
membranoproliferative (diffuse) (type 1 or 3) — *see also* N00-N07 with fourth character .5 N05.5
type 2 — *see also* N00-N07 with fourth character .6 N05.6
minimal change N05.0
necrotic, necrotizing NEC — *see also* N00-N07 with fourth character .8 N05.8
nephrotic — *see* Nephrosis
nodular — *see* Nephritis, membranoproliferative
polycystic Q61.3
adult type Q61.2
autosomal
dominant Q61.2
recessive NEC Q61.19
childhood type NEC Q61.19
infantile type NEC Q61.19
poststreptococcal N05.9
acute N00.9
chronic N03.9
rapidly progressive N01.9
proliferative NEC — *see also* N00-N07 with fourth character .8 N05.8
purulent — *see* Nephritis, tubulo-interstitial
rapidly progressive N01.9
with
dense deposit disease N01.6

Nephritis, nephritic — *continued*
rapidly progressive — *continued*
with — *continued*
diffuse
crescentic glomerulonephritis N01.7
endocapillary proliferative glomerulonephritis N01.4
membranous glomerulonephritis N01.2
mesangial proliferative glomerulonephritis N01.3
mesangiocapillary glomerulonephritis N01.5
focal and segmental glomerular lesions N01.1
minor glomerular abnormality N01.0
specified morphological changes NEC N01.8
salt losing or wasting NEC N28.89
saturnine N14.3
sclerosing, diffuse N05.8
septic — *see* Nephritis, tubulo-interstitial
specified pathology NEC — *see also* N00-N07 with fourth character .8 N05.8
subacute N01.9
suppurative — *see* Nephritis, tubulo-interstitial
syphilitic (late) A52.75
congenital A50.59 *[N08]*
early (secondary) A51.44
toxic — *see* Nephropathy, toxic
tubal, tubular — *see* Nephritis, tubulo-interstitial
tuberculous A18.11
tubulo-interstitial (in) N12
acute (infectious) N10
chronic (infectious) N11.9
nonobstructive N11.8
reflux-associated N11.0
obstructive N11.1
specified NEC N11.8
due to
brucellosis A23.9 *[N16]*
cryoglobulinemia D89.1 *[N16]*
glycogen storage disease E74.00 *[N16]*
Sjögren's syndrome M35.04
vascular — *see* Hypertension, kidney
war N00.9
Nephroblastoma (epithelial) (mesenchymal) C64- ☑
Nephrocalcinosis E83.59 *[N29]*
Nephrocystitis, pustular — *see* Nephritis, tubulo-interstitial
Nephrolithiasis (congenital) (pelvis) (recurrent) — *see also* Calculus, kidney
Nephroma C64- ☑
mesoblastic D41.0- ☑
Nephronephritis — *see* Nephrosis
Nephronophthisis Q61.5
Nephropathia epidemica A98.5
Nephropathy — *see also* Nephritis N28.9
with
edema — *see* Nephrosis
glomerular lesion — *see* Glomerulonephritis
amyloid, hereditary E85.0
analgesic N14.0
with medullary necrosis, acute N17.2
Balkan (endemic) N15.0
chemical — *see* Nephropathy, toxic
diabetic — *see* E08-E13 with .21
drug-induced N14.2
specified NEC N14.1
focal and segmental hyalinosis or sclerosis N02.1
heavy metal-induced N14.3
hereditary NEC N07.9
with
dense deposit disease N07.6
diffuse
crescentic glomerulonephritis N07.7
endocapillary proliferative glomerulonephritis N07.4
membranous glomerulonephritis N07.2
mesangial proliferative glomerulonephritis N07.3
mesangiocapillary glomerulonephritis N07.5
focal and segmental glomerular lesions N07.1
minor glomerular abnormality N07.0
specified morphological changes NEC N07.8
hypercalcemic N25.89
hypertensive — *see* Hypertension, kidney
hypokalemic (vacuolar) N25.89
IgA N02.8
with glomerular lesion N02.9
focal and segmental hyalinosis or sclerosis N02.1
membranoproliferative (diffuse) N02.5

Nephropathy — continued
　IgA — continued
　　with glomerular lesion — continued
　　　membranous (diffuse) N02.2
　　　mesangial proliferative (diffuse) N02.3
　　　mesangiocapillary (diffuse) N02.5
　　　proliferative NEC N02.8
　　　specified pathology NEC N02.8
　lead N14.3
　membranoproliferative (diffuse) N02.5
　membranous (diffuse) N02.2
　mesangial (IgA/IgG) — see Nephropathy, IgA
　　proliferative (diffuse) N02.3
　mesangiocapillary (diffuse) N02.5
　obstructive N13.8
　phenacetin N17.2
　phosphate-losing N25.0
　potassium depletion N25.89
　pregnancy-related O26.83- ☑
　proliferative NEC — see also N00-N07 with fourth
　　character .8 N05.8
　protein-losing N25.89
　saturnine N14.3
　sickle-cell D57.- ☑ [N08]
　toxic NEC N14.4
　　due to
　　　drugs N14.2
　　　　analgesic N14.0
　　　　specified NEC N14.1
　　　heavy metals N14.3
　vasomotor N17.0
　water-losing N25.89
Nephroptosis N28.83
Nephropyosis — see Abscess, kidney
Nephrorrhagia N28.89
Nephrosclerosis (arteriolar)(arteriosclerotic) (chronic)
　(hyaline) — see also Hypertension, kidney
　hyperplastic — see Hypertension, kidney
　senile N26.9
Nephrosis, nephrotic (Epstein's) (syndrome) (congenital)
　N04.9
　with
　　foot process disease N04.9
　　glomerular lesion N04.1
　　hypocomplementemic N04.5
　acute N04.9
　anoxic — see Nephrosis, tubular
　chemical — see Nephrosis, tubular
　cholemic K76.7
　diabetic — see E08-E13 with .21
　Finnish type (congenital) Q89.8
　hemoglobin N10
　hemoglobinuric — see Nephrosis, tubular
　in
　　amyloidosis E85.4 [N08]
　　diabetes mellitus — see E08-E13 with .21
　　epidemic hemorrhagic fever A98.5
　　malaria (malariae) B52.0
　ischemic — see Nephrosis, tubular
　lipoid N04.9
　lower nephron — see Nephrosis, tubular
　malarial (malariae) B52.0
　minimal change N04.0
　myoglobin N10
　necrotizing — see Nephrosis, tubular
　osmotic (sucrose) N25.89
　radiation N04.9
　syphilitic (late) A52.75
　toxic — see Nephrosis, tubular
　tubular (acute) N17.0
　　postprocedural N99.0
　　radiation N04.9
Nephrosonephritis, hemorrhagic (endemic) A98.5
Nephrostomy
　attention to Z43.6
　status Z93.6
Nerve — see also condition
　injury — see Injury, nerve, by body site
Nerves R45.0
Nervous — see also condition R45.0
　heart F45.8
　stomach F45.8
　tension R45.0
Nervousness R45.0
Nesidioblastoma
　pancreas D13.7
　specified site NEC — see Neoplasm, benign, by site
　unspecified site D13.7

Nettleship's syndrome — see Urticaria pigmentosa
Neumann's disease or syndrome L10.1
Neuralgia, neuralgic (acute) M79.2
　accessory (nerve) G52.8
　acoustic (nerve) — see subcategory H93.3 ☑
　auditory (nerve) — see subcategory H93.3 ☑
　ciliary G44.009
　　intractable G44.001
　　not intractable G44.009
　cranial
　　nerve — see also Disorder, nerve, cranial
　　　fifth or trigeminal — see Neuralgia, trigeminal
　　postherpetic, postzoster B02.29
　ear — see subcategory H92.0 ☑
　facialis vera G51.1
　Fothergill's — see Neuralgia, trigeminal
　glossopharyngeal (nerve) G52.1
　Horton's G44.099
　　intractable G44.091
　　not intractable G44.099
　Hunt's B02.21
　hypoglossal (nerve) G52.3
　infraorbital — see Neuralgia, trigeminal
　malarial — see Malaria
　migrainous G44.009
　　intractable G44.001
　　not intractable G44.009
　Morton's G57.6- ☑
　nerve, cranial — see Disorder, nerve, cranial
　nose G52.0
　occipital M54.81
　olfactory G52.0
　penis N48.9
　perineum R10.2
　postherpetic NEC B02.29
　　trigeminal B02.22
　pubic region R10.2
　scrotum R10.2
　Sluder's G44.89
　specified nerve NEC G58.8
　spermatic cord R10.2
　sphenopalatine (ganglion) G90.09
　trifacial — see Neuralgia, trigeminal
　trigeminal G50.0
　　postherpetic, postzoster B02.22
　vagus (nerve) G52.2
　writer's F48.8
　　organic G25.89
Neurapraxia — see Injury, nerve
Neurasthenia F48.8
　cardiac F45.8
　gastric F45.8
　heart F45.8
Neurilemmoma — see also Neoplasm, nerve, benign
　acoustic (nerve) D33.3
　malignant — see also Neoplasm, nerve, malignant
　　acoustic (nerve) C72.4- ☑
Neurilemmosarcoma — see Neoplasm, nerve, malignant
Neurinoma — see Neoplasm, nerve, benign
Neurinomatosis — see Neoplasm, nerve, uncertain be-
　havior
Neuritis (rheumatoid) M79.2
　abducens (nerve) — see Strabismus, paralytic, sixth
　　nerve
　accessory (nerve) G52.8
　acoustic (nerve) — see also subcategory H93.3 ☑
　　in (due to)
　　　infectious disease NEC B99 ☑ [H94.0-] ☑
　　　parasitic disease NEC B89 [H94.0-] ☑
　　syphilitic A52.15
　alcoholic G62.1
　　with psychosis — see Psychosis, alcoholic
　amyloid, any site E85.4 [G63]
　auditory (nerve) — see subcategory H93.3 ☑
　brachial — see Radiculopathy
　　due to displacement, intervertebral disc — see Dis-
　　　order, disc, cervical, with neuritis
　cranial nerve
　　due to Lyme disease A69.22
　　eighth or acoustic or auditory — see subcategory
　　　H93.3 ☑
　　eleventh or accessory G52.8
　　fifth or trigeminal G51.0
　　first or olfactory G52.0
　　fourth or trochlear — see Strabismus, paralytic,
　　　fourth nerve
　　second or optic — see Neuritis, optic

Neuritis — continued
　cranial nerve — continued
　　seventh or facial G51.8
　　　newborn (birth injury) P11.3
　　sixth or abducent — see Strabismus, paralytic, sixth
　　　nerve
　　tenth or vagus G52.2
　　third or oculomotor — see Strabismus, paralytic,
　　　third nerve
　　twelfth or hypoglossal G52.3
　Déjérine-Sottas G60.0
　diabetic (mononeuropathy) — see E08-E13 with .41
　　polyneuropathy — see E08-E13 with .42
　due to
　　beriberi E51.11
　　displacement, prolapse or rupture, intervertebral
　　　disc — see Disorder, disc, with, radiculopathy
　　herniation, nucleus pulposus M51.9 [G55]
　endemic E51.11
　facial G51.8
　　newborn (birth injury) P11.3
　general — see Polyneuropathy
　geniculate ganglion G51.1
　　due to herpes (zoster) B02.21
　gouty — see also Gout, by type M10.9 [G63]
　hypoglossal (nerve) G52.3
　ilioinguinal (nerve) G57.9- ☑
　infectious (multiple) NEC G61.0
　interstitial hypertrophic progressive G60.0
　lumbar M54.16
　lumbosacral M54.17
　multiple — see also Polyneuropathy
　　endemic E51.11
　　infective, acute G61.0
　multiplex endemica E51.11
　nerve root — see Radiculopathy
　oculomotor (nerve) — see Strabismus, paralytic, third
　　nerve
　olfactory nerve G52.0
　optic (nerve) (hereditary) (sympathetic) H46.9
　　with demyelination G36.0
　　in myelitis G36.0
　　nutritional H46.2
　　papillitis — see Papillitis, optic
　　retrobulbar H46.1- ☑
　　specified type NEC H46.8
　　toxic H46.3
　peripheral (nerve) G62.9
　　multiple — see Polyneuropathy
　　single — see Mononeuritis
　pneumogastric (nerve) G52.2
　postherpetic, postzoster B02.29
　progressive hypertrophic interstitial G60.0
　retrobulbar — see also Neuritis, optic, retrobulbar
　　in (due to)
　　　late syphilis A52.15
　　　meningococcal infection A39.82
　　meningococcal A39.82
　　syphilitic A52.15
　sciatic (nerve) — see also Sciatica
　　due to displacement of intervertebral disc — see
　　　Disorder, disc, with, radiculopathy
　serum — see also Reaction, serum T80.69 ☑
　shoulder-girdle G54.5
　specified nerve NEC G58.8
　spinal (nerve) root — see Radiculopathy
　syphilitic A52.15
　thenar (median) G56.1- ☑
　thoracic M54.14
　toxic NEC G62.2
　trochlear (nerve) — see Strabismus, paralytic, fourth
　　nerve
　vagus (nerve) G52.2
Neuroastrocytoma — see Neoplasm, uncertain behavior,
　by site
Neuroavitaminosis E56.9 [G99.8]
Neuroblastoma
　olfactory C30.0
　specified site — see Neoplasm, malignant, by site
　unspecified site C74.90
Neurochorioretinitis — see Chorioretinitis
Neurocirculatory asthenia F45.8
Neurocysticercosis B69.0
Neurocytoma — see Neoplasm, benign, by site
Neurodermatitis (circumscribed) (circumscripta) (local)
　L28.0
　atopic L20.81
　diffuse (Brocq) L20.81

Neurodermatitis — continued
  disseminated L20.81
Neuroencephalomyelopathy, optic G36.0
Neuroepithelioma — see also Neoplasm, malignant, by site
  olfactory C30.0
Neurofibroma — see also Neoplasm, nerve, benign
  melanotic — see Neoplasm, nerve, benign
  multiple — see Neurofibromatosis
  plexiform — see Neoplasm, nerve, benign
Neurofibromatosis (multiple) (nonmalignant) Q85.00
  acoustic Q85.02
  malignant — see Neoplasm, nerve, malignant
  specified NEC Q85.09
  type 1 (von Recklinghausen) Q85.01
  type 2 Q85.02
Neurofibrosarcoma — see Neoplasm, nerve, malignant
Neurogenic — see also condition
  bladder — see also Dysfunction, bladder, neuromuscular N31.9
    cauda equina syndrome G83.4
  bowel NEC K59.2
  heart F45.8
Neuroglioma — see Neoplasm, uncertain behavior, by site
Neurolabyrinthitis (of Dix and Hallpike) — see Neuronitis, vestibular
Neurolathyrism — see Poisoning, food, noxious, plant
Neuroleprosy A30.9
Neuroma — see also Neoplasm, nerve, benign
  acoustic (nerve) D33.3
  amputation (stump) (traumatic) (surgical complication) (late) T87.3- ☑
    arm T87.3- ☑
    leg T87.3- ☑
  digital (toe) G57.6- ☑
  interdigital G58.8
    lower limb (toe) G57.8- ☑
    upper limb G56.8- ☑
  intermetatarsal G57.8- ☑
  Morton's G57.6- ☑
  nonneoplastic
    arm G56.9- ☑
    leg G57.9- ☑
    lower extremity G57.9- ☑
    upper extremity G56.9- ☑
  optic (nerve) D33.3
  plantar G57.6- ☑
  plexiform — see Neoplasm, nerve, benign
  surgical (nonneoplastic)
    arm G56.9- ☑
    leg G57.9- ☑
    lower extremity G57.9- ☑
    upper extremity G56.9- ☑
Neuromyalgia — see Neuralgia
Neuromyasthenia (epidemic) (postinfectious) G93.3
Neuromyelitis G36.9
  ascending G61.0
  optica G36.0
Neuromyopathy G70.9
  paraneoplastic D49.9 [G13.0]
Neuromyotonia (Isaacs) G71.19
Neuronevus — see Nevus
Neuronitis G58.9
  ascending (acute) G57.2- ☑
  vestibular H81.2- ☑
Neuroparalytic — see condition
Neuropathy, neuropathic G62.9
  acute motor G62.81
  alcoholic G62.1
    with psychosis — see Psychosis, alcoholic
  arm G56.9- ☑
  autonomic, peripheral — see Neuropathy, peripheral, autonomic
  axillary G56.9- ☑
  bladder N31.9
    atonic (motor) (sensory) N31.2
    autonomous N31.2
    flaccid N31.2
    nonreflex N31.2
    reflex N31.1
    uninhibited N31.0
  brachial plexus G54.0
  cervical plexus G54.2
  chronic
    progressive segmentally demyelinating G62.89
    relapsing demyelinating G62.89

Neuropathy, neuropathic — continued
  Déjérine-Sottas G60.0
  diabetic — see E08-E13 with .40
    mononeuropathy — see E08-E13 with .41
    polyneuropathy — see E08-E13 with .42
  entrapment G58.9
    iliohypogastric nerve G57.8- ☑
    ilioinguinal nerve G57.8- ☑
    lateral cutaneous nerve of thigh G57.1- ☑
    median nerve G56.0- ☑
    obturator nerve G57.8- ☑
    peroneal nerve G57.3- ☑
    posterior tibial nerve G57.5- ☑
    saphenous nerve G57.8- ☑
    ulnar nerve G56.2- ☑
  facial nerve G51.9
  hereditary G60.9
    motor and sensory (types I-IV) G60.0
    sensory G60.8
    specified NEC G60.8
  hypertrophic G60.0
    Charcot-Marie-Tooth G60.0
    Déjérine-Sottas G60.0
    interstitial progressive G60.0
    of infancy G60.0
    Refsum G60.1
  idiopathic G60.9
    progressive G60.3
    specified NEC G60.8
  in association with hereditary ataxia G60.2
  intercostal G58.0
  ischemic — see Disorder, nerve
  Jamaica (ginger) G62.2
  leg NEC G57.9- ☑
  lower extremity G57.9- ☑
  lumbar plexus G54.1
  median nerve G56.1- ☑
  motor and sensory — see also Polyneuropathy
    hereditary (types I-IV) G60.0
  multifocal motor (MMN) G61.82
  multiple (acute) (chronic) — see Polyneuropathy
  optic (nerve) — see also Neuritis, optic
    ischemic H47.01- ☑
  paraneoplastic (sensorial) (Denny Brown) D49.9 [G13.0]
  peripheral (nerve) — see also Polyneuropathy G62.9
    autonomic G90.9
      idiopathic G90.09
      in (due to)
        amyloidosis E85.4 [G99.0]
        diabetes mellitus — see E08-E13 with .43
        endocrine disease NEC E34.9 [G99.0]
        gout M10.00 [G99.0]
        hyperthyroidism E05.90 [G99.0]
          with thyroid storm E05.91 [G99.0]
        metabolic disease NEC E88.9 [G99.0]
    idiopathic G60.9
      progressive G60.3
    in (due to)
      antitetanus serum G62.0
      arsenic G62.2
      drugs NEC G62.0
      lead G62.2
      organophosphate compounds G62.2
      toxic agent NEC G62.2
  plantar nerves G57.6- ☑
  progressive
    hypertrophic interstitial G60.0
    inflammatory G62.81
  radicular NEC — see Radiculopathy
  sacral plexus G54.1
  sciatic G57.0- ☑
  serum G61.1
  toxic NEC G62.2
  trigeminal sensory G50.8
  ulnar nerve G56.2- ☑
  uremic N18.9 [G63]
  vitamin B12 E53.8 [G63]
    with anemia (pernicious) D51.0 [G63]
      due to dietary deficiency D51.3 [G63]
Neurophthisis — see also Disorder, nerve
  peripheral, diabetic — see E08-E13 with .42
Neuroretinitis — see Chorioretinitis
Neuroretinopathy, hereditary optic H47.22
Neurosarcoma — see Neoplasm, nerve, malignant
Neurosclerosis — see Disorder, nerve
Neurosis, neurotic F48.9
  anankastic F42.8

Neurosis, neurotic — continued
  anxiety (state) F41.1
    panic type F41.0
  asthenic F48.8
  bladder F45.8
  cardiac (reflex) F45.8
  cardiovascular F45.8
  character F60.9
  colon F45.8
  compensation F68.10
  compulsive, compulsion F42.8
  conversion F44.9
  craft F48.8
  cutaneous F45.8
  depersonalization F48.1
  depressive (reaction) (type) F34.1
  environmental F48.8
  excoriation L98.1
  fatigue F48.8
  functional — see Disorder, somatoform
  gastric F45.8
  gastrointestinal F45.8
  heart F45.8
  hypochondriacal F45.21
  hysterical F44.9
  incoordination F45.8
    larynx F45.8
    vocal cord F45.8
  intestine F45.8
  larynx (sensory) F45.8
    hysterical F44.4
  mixed NEC F48.8
  musculoskeletal F45.8
  obsessional F42.8
  obsessive-compulsive F42.8
  occupational F48.8
  ocular NEC F45.8
  organ — see Disorder, somatoform
  pharynx F45.8
  phobic F40.9
  posttraumatic (situational) F43.10
    acute F43.11
    chronic F43.12
  psychasthenic (type) F48.8
  railroad F48.8
  rectum F45.8
  respiratory F45.8
  rumination F45.8
  sexual F65.9
  situational F48.8
  social F40.10
    generalized F40.11
    specified type NEC F48.8
  state F48.9
    with depersonalization episode F48.1
  stomach F45.8
  traumatic F43.10
    acute F43.11
    chronic F43.12
  vasomotor F45.8
  visceral F45.8
  war F48.8
Neurospongioblastosis diffusa Q85.1
Neurosyphilis (arrested) (early) (gumma) (late) (latent) (recurrent) (relapse) A52.3
  with ataxia (cerebellar) (locomotor) (spastic) (spinal) A52.19
  aneurysm (cerebral) A52.05
  arachnoid (adhesive) A52.13
  arteritis (any artery) (cerebral) A52.04
  asymptomatic A52.2
  congenital A50.40
  dura (mater) A52.13
  general paresis A52.17
  hemorrhagic A52.05
  juvenile (asymptomatic) (meningeal) A50.40
  leptomeninges (aseptic) A52.13
  meningeal, meninges (adhesive) A52.13
  meningitis A52.13
  meningovascular (diffuse) A52.13
  optic atrophy A52.15
  parenchymatous (degenerative) A52.19
  paresis, paretic A52.17
    juvenile A50.45
  remission in (sustained) A52.3
  serological (without symptoms) A52.2
  specified nature or site NEC A52.19
  tabes, tabetic (dorsalis) A52.11
    juvenile A50.45

Neurosyphilis — *continued*
  taboparesis A52.17
    juvenile A50.45
  thrombosis (cerebral) A52.05
  vascular (cerebral) NEC A52.05
Neurothekeoma — *see* Neoplasm, nerve, benign
Neurotic — *see* Neurosis
Neurotoxemia — *see* Toxemia
Neutroclusion M26.211
Neutropenia, neutropenic (chronic) (genetic) (idiopathic) (immune) (infantile) (malignant) (pernicious) (splenic) D70.9
  congenital (primary) D70.0
  cyclic D70.4
  cytoreductive cancer chemotherapy sequela D70.1
  drug-induced D70.2
    due to cytoreductive cancer chemotherapy D70.1
  due to infection D70.3
  fever D70.9
  neonatal, transitory (isoimmune) (maternal transfer) P61.5
  periodic D70.4
  secondary (cyclic) (periodic) (splenic) D70.4
    drug-induced D70.2
      due to cytoreductive cancer chemotherapy D70.1
  toxic D70.8
Neutrophilia, hereditary giant D72.0
Nevocarcinoma — *see* Melanoma
Nevus D22.9
  achromic — *see* Neoplasm, skin, benign
  amelanotic — *see* Neoplasm, skin, benign
  angiomatous D18.00
    intra-abdominal D18.03
    intracranial D18.02
    skin D18.01
    specified site NEC D18.09
  araneus I78.1
  balloon cell — *see* Neoplasm, skin, benign
  bathing trunk D48.5
  blue — *see* Neoplasm, skin, benign
    cellular — *see* Neoplasm, skin, benign
    giant — *see* Neoplasm, skin, benign
    Jadassohn's — *see* Neoplasm, skin, benign
    malignant — *see* Melanoma
  capillary D18.00
    intra-abdominal D18.03
    intracranial D18.02
    skin D18.01
    specified site NEC D18.09
  cavernous D18.00
    intra-abdominal D18.03
    intracranial D18.02
    skin D18.01
    specified site NEC D18.09
  cellular — *see* Neoplasm, skin, benign
    blue — *see* Neoplasm, skin, benign
  choroid D31.3- ☑
  comedonicus Q82.5
  conjunctiva D31.0- ☑
  dermal — *see* Neoplasm, skin, benign
    with epidermal nevus — *see* Neoplasm, skin, benign
  dysplastic — *see* Neoplasm, skin, benign
  eye D31.9- ☑
  flammeus Q82.5
  hemangiomatous D18.00
    intra-abdominal D18.03
    intracranial D18.02
    skin D18.01
    specified site NEC D18.09
  iris D31.4- ☑
  lacrimal gland D31.5- ☑
  lymphatic D18.1
  magnocellular
    specified site — *see* Neoplasm, benign, by site
    unspecified site D31.40
  malignant — *see* Melanoma
  meaning hemangioma D18.00
    intra-abdominal D18.03
    intracranial D18.02
    skin D18.01
    specified site NEC D18.09
  mouth (mucosa) D10.30
    specified site NEC D10.39
    white sponge Q38.6
  multiplex Q85.1
  non-neoplastic I78.1
  oral mucosa D10.30
    specified site NEC D10.39

Nevus — *continued*
  oral mucosa — *continued*
    white sponge Q38.6
  orbit D31.6- ☑
  pigmented
    giant — *see also* Neoplasm, skin, uncertain behavior D48.5
    malignant melanoma in — *see* Melanoma
  portwine Q82.5
  retina D31.2- ☑
  retrobulbar D31.6- ☑
  sanguineous Q82.5
  senile I78.1
  skin D22.9
    abdominal wall D22.5
    ala nasi D22.39
    ankle D22.7- ☑
    anus, anal D22.5
    arm D22.6- ☑
    auditory canal (external) D22.2- ☑
    auricle (ear) D22.2- ☑
    auricular canal (external) D22.2- ☑
    axilla, axillary fold D22.5
    back D22.5
    breast D22.5
    brow D22.39
    buttock D22.5
    canthus (eye) D22.1- ☑
    cheek (external) D22.39
    chest wall D22.5
    chin D22.39
    ear (external) D22.2- ☑
    external meatus (ear) D22.2- ☑
    eyebrow D22.39
    eyelid (lower) (upper) D22.1- ☑
    face D22.30
      specified NEC D22.39
    female genital organ (external) NEC D28.0
    finger D22.6- ☑
    flank D22.5
    foot D22.7- ☑
    forearm D22.6- ☑
    forehead D22.39
    foreskin D29.0
    genital organ (external) NEC
      female D28.0
      male D29.9
    gluteal region D22.5
    groin D22.5
    hand D22.6- ☑
    heel D22.7- ☑
    helix D22.2- ☑
    hip D22.7- ☑
    interscapular region D22.5
    jaw D22.39
    knee D22.7- ☑
    labium (majus) (minus) D28.0
    leg D22.7- ☑
    lip (lower) (upper) D22.0
    lower limb D22.7- ☑
    male genital organ (external) D29.9
    nail D22.9
      finger D22.6- ☑
      toe D22.7- ☑
    nasolabial groove D22.39
    nates D22.5
    neck D22.4
    nose (external) D22.39
    palpebra D22.1- ☑
    penis D29.0
    perianal skin D22.5
    perineum D22.5
    pinna D22.2- ☑
    popliteal fossa or space D22.7- ☑
    prepuce D29.0
    pudendum D28.0
    scalp D22.4
    scrotum D29.4
    shoulder D22.6- ☑
    submammary fold D22.5
    temple D22.39
    thigh D22.7- ☑
    toe D22.7- ☑
    trunk NEC D22.5
    umbilicus D22.5
    upper limb D22.6- ☑
    vulva D28.0

Nevus — *continued*
  specified site NEC — *see* Neoplasm, by site, benign
  spider I78.1
  stellar I78.1
  strawberry Q82.5
  Sutton's benign D22.9
  unius lateris Q82.5
  Unna's Q82.5
  vascular Q82.5
  verrucous Q82.5
Newborn (infant) (liveborn) (singleton) Z38.2
  abstinence syndrome P96.1
  acne L70.4
  affected by
    abnormalities of membranes P02.9
      specified NEC P02.8
    abruptio placenta P02.1
    amino-acid metabolic disorder, transitory P74.8
    amniocentesis (while in utero) P00.6
    amnionitis P02.78
    apparent life threatening event (ALTE) R68.13
    bleeding (into)
      cerebral cortex P52.22
      germinal matrix P52.0
      ventricles P52.1
    breech delivery P03.0
    cardiac arrest P29.81
    cardiomyopathy I42.8
      congenital I42.4
    cerebral ischemia P91.0
    Cesarean delivery P03.4
    chemotherapy agents P04.11
    chorioamnionitis P02.78
    cocaine (crack) P04.41
    complications of labor and delivery P03.9
      specified NEC P03.89
    compression of umbilical cord NEC P02.5
    contracted pelvis P03.1
    cyanosis P28.2
    delivery P03.9
      Cesarean P03.4
      forceps P03.2
      vacuum extractor P03.3
    drugs of addiction P04.40
      cocaine P04.41
      hallucinogens P04.42
      specified drug NEC P04.49
    entanglement (knot) in umbilical cord P02.5
    environmental chemicals P04.6
    fetal (intrauterine)
      growth retardation P05.9
      inflammatory response syndrome (FIRS) P02.70
      malnutrition not light or small for gestational age P05.2
    FIRS (fetal inflammatory response syndrome) P02.70
    forceps delivery P03.2
    heart rate abnormalities
      bradycardia P29.12
      intrauterine P03.819
        before onset of labor P03.810
        during labor P03.811
      tachycardia P29.11
    hemorrhage (antepartum) P02.1
      cerebellar (nontraumatic) P52.6
      intracerebral (nontraumatic) P52.4
      intracranial (nontraumatic) P52.9
        specified NEC P52.8
      intraventricular (nontraumatic) P52.3
        grade 1 P52.0
        grade 2 P52.1
        grade 3 P52.21
        grade 4 P52.22
      posterior fossa (nontraumatic) P52.6
      subarachnoid (nontraumatic) P52.5
      subependymal P52.0
        with intracerebral extension P52.22
        with intraventricular extension P52.1
          with enlargment of ventricles P52.21
        without intraventricular extension P52.0
    hypoxic ischemic encephalopathy [HIE] P91.60
      mild P91.61
      moderate P91.62
      severe P91.63
    induction of labor P03.89
    intestinal perforation P78.0
    intrauterine (fetal) blood loss P50.9
      due to (from)
        cut end of co-twin cord P50.5

⚐ Subterms under main terms may continue to next column or page   ☑ **Additional Character Required — Refer to the Tabular List for Character Selection**   **233**

Neurosyphilis — Newborn

Newborn — *continued*
affected by — *continued*
  intrauterine blood loss — *continued*
    due to — *continued*
      hemorrhage into
        co-twin P50.3
          maternal circulation P50.4
        placenta P50.2
        ruptured cord blood P50.1
        vasa previa P50.0
      specified NEC P50.8
  intrauterine (fetal) hemorrhage P50.9
  intrauterine (in utero) procedure P96.5
  malpresentation (malposition) NEC P03.1
  maternal (complication of) (use of)
    alcohol P04.3
    amphetamines P04.16
    analgesia (maternal) P04.0
    anesthesia (maternal) P04.0
    anticonvulsants P04.13
    antidepressants P04.15
    antineoplastic chemotherapy P04.11
    anxiolytics P04.1A
    blood loss P02.1
    cannabis P04.81
    circulatory disease P00.3
    condition P00.9
      specified NEC P00.89
    cytotoxic drugs P04.12
    delivery P03.9
      Cesarean P03.4
      forceps P03.2
      vacuum extractor P03.3
    diabetes mellitus (pre-existing) P70.1
    disorder P00.9
      specified NEC P00.89
    drugs (addictive) (illegal) NEC P04.49
    ectopic pregnancy P01.4
    gestational diabetes P70.0
    hemorrhage P02.1
    hypertensive disorder P00.0
    incompetent cervix P01.0
    infectious disease P00.2
    injury P00.5
    labor and delivery P03.9
    malpresentation before labor P01.7
    maternal death P01.6
    medical procedure P00.7
    medication P04.19
      specified type NEC P04.18
    multiple pregnancy P01.5
    nutritional disorder P00.4
    oligohydramnios P01.2
    opiates P04.14
      administered for procedures during pregnancy or labor and delivery P04.0
    parasitic disease P00.2
    periodontal disease P00.81
    placenta previa P02.0
    polyhydramnios P01.3
    precipitate delivery P03.5
    pregnancy P01.9
      specified P01.8
    premature rupture of membranes P01.1
    renal disease P00.1
    respiratory disease P00.3
    sedative-hypnotics P04.17
    surgical procedure P00.6
    tranquilizers administered for procedures during pregnancy or labor and delivery P04.0
    urinary tract disease P00.1
    uterine contraction (abnormal) P03.6
  meconium peritonitis P78.0
  medication (legal) (maternal use) (prescribed) P04.19
  membrane abnormalities P02.9
    specified NEC P02.8
  membranitis P02.78
  methamphetamine(s) P04.49
  mixed metabolic and respiratory acidosis P84
  neonatal abstinence syndrome P96.1
  noxious substances transmitted via placenta or breast milk P04.9
    cannabis P04.81
    specified NEC P04.89
  nutritional supplements P04.5
  placenta previa P02.0
  placental
    abnormality (functional) (morphological) P02.20

Newborn — *continued*
affected by — *continued*
  placental — *continued*
    abnormality — *continued*
      specified NEC P02.29
    dysfunction P02.29
    infarction P02.29
    insufficiency P02.29
    separation NEC P02.1
    transfusion syndromes P02.3
  placentitis P02.78
  precipitate delivery P03.5
  prolapsed cord P02.4
  respiratory arrest P28.81
  slow intrauterine growth P05.9
  tobacco P04.2
  twin to twin transplacental transfusion P02.3
  umbilical cord (tightly) around neck P02.5
  umbilical cord condition P02.60
    short cord P02.69
    specified NEC P02.69
  uterine contractions (abnormal) P03.6
  vasa previa P02.69
    from intrauterine blood loss P50.0
apnea P28.4
  obstructive P28.4
  primary P28.3
  sleep (central) (obstructive) (primary) P28.3
born in hospital Z38.00
  by cesarean Z38.01
born outside hospital Z38.1
breast buds P96.89
breast engorgement P83.4
check-up — *see* Newborn, examination
convulsion P90
dehydration P74.1
examination
  8 to 28 days old Z00.111
  under 8 days old Z00.110
fever P81.9
  environmentally-induced P81.0
hyperbilirubinemia P59.9
  of prematurity P59.0
hypernatremia P74.21
hyponatremia P74.22
infection P39.9
  candidal P37.5
  specified NEC P39.8
  urinary tract P39.3
jaundice P59.9
  due to
    breast milk inhibitor P59.3
    hepatocellular damage P59.20
      specified NEC P59.29
    preterm delivery P59.0
  of prematurity P59.0
  specified NEC P59.8
late metabolic acidosis P74.0
mastitis P39.0
  infective P39.0
  noninfective P83.4
multiple born NEC Z38.8
  born in hospital Z38.68
    by cesarean Z38.69
  born outside hospital Z38.7
omphalitis P38.9
  with mild hemorrhage P38.1
  without hemorrhage P38.9
post-term P08.21
prolonged gestation (over 42 completed weeks) P08.22
quadruplet Z38.8
  born in hospital Z38.63
    by cesarean Z38.64
  born outside hospital Z38.7
quintuplet Z38.8
  born in hospital Z38.65
    by cesarean Z38.66
  born outside hospital Z38.7
seizure P90
sepsis (congenital) P36.9
  due to
    anaerobes NEC P36.5
    Escherichia coli P36.4
    Staphylococcus P36.30
      aureus P36.2
      specified NEC P36.39
    Streptococcus P36.10
      group B P36.0
      specified NEC P36.19

Newborn — *continued*
sepsis — *continued*
  specified NEC P36.8
triplet Z38.8
  born in hospital Z38.61
    by cesarean Z38.62
  born outside hospital Z38.7
twin Z38.5
  born in hospital Z38.30
    by cesarean Z38.31
  born outside hospital Z38.4
vomiting P92.09
  bilious P92.01
weight check Z00.111
Newcastle conjunctivitis or disease B30.8
Nezelof's syndrome (pure alymphocytosis) D81.4
Niacin (amide) **deficiency** E52
Nicolas (-Durand)-**Favre disease** A55
Nicotine — *see* Tobacco
Nicotinic acid deficiency E52
Niemann-Pick disease or syndrome E75.249
  specified NEC E75.248
  type
    A E75.240
    B E75.241
    C E75.242
    D E75.243
Night
  blindness — *see* Blindness, night
  sweats R61
  terrors (child) F51.4
Nightmares (REM sleep type) F51.5
NIHSS (National Institutes of Health Stroke Scale) **score** R29.7- ☑
Nipple — *see* condition
Nisbet's chancre A57
Nishimoto (-Takeuchi) **disease** I67.5
Nitritoid crisis or reaction — *see* Crisis, nitritoid
Nitrosohemoglobinemia D74.8
Njovera A65
Nocardiosis, nocardiasis A43.9
  cutaneous A43.1
  lung A43.0
  pneumonia A43.0
  pulmonary A43.0
  specified site NEC A43.8
Nocturia R35.1
  psychogenic F45.8
Nocturnal — *see* condition
Nodal rhythm I49.8
Node(s) — *see also* Nodule
  Bouchard's (with arthropathy) M15.2
  Haygarth's M15.8
  Heberden's (with arthropathy) M15.1
  larynx J38.7
  lymph — *see* condition
  milker's B08.03
  Osler's I33.0
  Schmorl's — *see* Schmorl's disease
  singer's J38.2
  teacher's J38.2
  tuberculous — *see* Tuberculosis, lymph gland
  vocal cord J38.2
Nodule(s), **nodular**
  actinomycotic — *see* Actinomycosis
  breast NEC — *see also* Lump, breast N63.0
  colloid (cystic), thyroid E04.1
  cutaneous — *see* Swelling, localized
  endometrial (stromal) D26.1
  Haygarth's M15.8
  inflammatory — *see* Inflammation
  juxta-articular
    syphilitic A52.77
    yaws A66.7
  larynx J38.7
  lung, solitary (subsegmental branch of the bronchial tree) R91.1
    multiple R91.8
  milker's B08.03
  prostate N40.2
    with lower urinary tract symptoms (LUTS) N40.3
    without lower urinary tract symptoms (LUTS) N40.2
  pulmonary, solitary (subsegmental branch of the bronchial tree) R91.1
  retrocardiac R09.89
  rheumatoid M06.30
    ankle M06.37- ☑
    elbow M06.32- ☑

Nodule(s), **nodular** — *continued*
  rheumatoid — *continued*
    foot joint M06.37- ☑
    hand joint M06.34- ☑
    hip M06.35- ☑
    knee M06.36- ☑
    multiple site M06.39
    shoulder M06.31- ☑
    vertebra M06.38
    wrist M06.33- ☑
  scrotum (inflammatory) N49.2
  singer's J38.2
  solitary, lung (subsegmental branch of the bronchial tree) R91.1
    multiple R91.8
  subcutaneous — *see* Swelling, localized
  teacher's J38.2
  thyroid (cold) (gland) (nontoxic) E04.1
    with thyrotoxicosis E05.20
      with thyroid storm E05.21
    toxic or with hyperthyroidism E05.20
      with thyroid storm E05.21
  vocal cord J38.2
Noma (gangrenous) (hospital) (infective) A69.0
  auricle I96
  mouth A69.0
  pudendi N76.89
  vulvae N76.89
Nomad, nomadism Z59.0
NOMID (neonatal onset multisystemic inflammatory disorder) M04.2
Nonadherence to medical treatment Z91.19
Nonautoimmune hemolytic anemia D59.4
  drug-induced D59.2
Nonclosure — *see also* Imperfect, closure
  ductus arteriosus (Botallo's) Q25.0
  foramen
    botalli Q21.1
    ovale Q21.1
Noncompliance Z91.19
  with
    dialysis Z91.15
    dietary regimen Z91.11
    medical treatment Z91.19
    medication regimen NEC Z91.14
      underdosing — *see also* Table of Drugs and Chemicals, categories T36-T50, with final character 6 Z91.14
        intentional NEC Z91.128
          due to financial hardship of patient Z91.120
        unintentional NEC Z91.138
          due to patient's age related debility Z91.130
    renal dialysis Z91.15
Nondescent (congenital) — *see also* Malposition, congenital
  cecum Q43.3
  colon Q43.3
  testicle Q53.9
    bilateral Q53.20
      abdominal Q53.211
      perineal Q53.22
    unilateral Q53.10
      abdominal Q53.111
      perineal Q53.12
Nondevelopment
  brain Q02
    part of Q04.3
  heart Q24.8
  organ or site, congenital NEC — *see* Hypoplasia
Nonengagement
  head NEC O32.4 ☑
    in labor, causing obstructed labor O64.8 ☑
Nonexanthematous tick fever A93.2
Nonexpansion, lung (newborn) P28.0
Nonfunctioning
  cystic duct — *see also* Disease, gallbladder K82.8
  gallbladder — *see also* Disease, gallbladder K82.8
  kidney N28.9
  labyrinth — *see* subcategory H83.2 ☑
Non-Hodgkin lymphoma NEC — *see* Lymphoma, non-Hodgkin
Nonimplantation, ovum N97.2
Noninsufflation, fallopian tube N97.1
Non-ketotic hyperglycinemia E72.51
Nonne-Milroy syndrome Q82.0
Nonovulation N97.0

Non-palpable testicle(s)
  bilateral R39.84
  unilateral R39.83
Nonpatent fallopian tube N97.1
Nonpneumatization, lung NEC P28.0
Nonrotation — *see* Malrotation
Nonsecretion, urine — *see* Anuria
Nonunion
  fracture — *see* Fracture, by site
  joint, following fusion or arthrodesis M96.0
  organ or site, congenital NEC — *see* Imperfect, closure
  symphysis pubis, congenital Q74.2
Nonvisualization, gallbladder R93.2
Nonvital, nonvitalized tooth K04.99
Non-working side interference M26.56
Noonan's syndrome Q87.19
Normocytic anemia (infectional) due to blood loss (chronic) D50.0
  acute D62
Norrie's disease (congenital) Q15.8
North American blastomycosis B40.9
Norwegian itch B86
Nose, nasal — *see* condition
Nosebleed R04.0
Nose-picking F98.8
Nosomania F45.21
Nosophobia F45.22
Nostalgia F43.20
Notch of iris Q13.2
Notching nose, congenital (tip) Q30.2
Nothnagel's
  syndrome — *see* Strabismus, paralytic, third nerve
  vasomotor acroparesthesia I73.89
Novy's relapsing fever A68.9
  louse-borne A68.0
  tick-borne A68.1
Noxious
  foodstuffs, poisoning by — *see* Poisoning, food, noxious, plant
  substances transmitted through placenta or breast milk P04.9
Nucleus pulposus — *see* condition
Numbness R20.0
Nuns' knee — *see* Bursitis, prepatellar
Nursemaid's elbow S53.03- ☑
Nutcracker esophagus K22.4
Nutmeg liver K76.1
Nutrient element deficiency E61.9
  specified NEC E61.8
Nutrition deficient or insufficient — *see also* Malnutrition E46
  due to
    insufficient food T73.0 ☑
    lack of
      care (child) T76.02 ☑
        adult T76.01 ☑
      food T73.0 ☑
Nutritional stunting E45
Nyctalopia (night blindness) — *see* Blindness, night
Nycturia R35.1
  psychogenic F45.8
Nymphomania F52.8
Nystagmus H55.00
  benign paroxysmal — *see* Vertigo, benign paroxysmal
  central positional H81.4
  congenital H55.01
  dissociated H55.04
  latent H55.02
  miners' H55.09
  positional
    benign paroxysmal H81.4
    central H81.4
  specified form NEC H55.09
  visual deprivation H55.03

O

Obermeyer's relapsing fever (European) A68.9
Obesity E66.9
  with alveolar hypoventilation E66.2
  adrenal E27.8
  complicating
    childbirth O99.214
    pregnancy O99.21- ☑
    puerperium O99.215
  constitutional E66.8
  dietary counseling and surveillance Z71.3

Obesity — *continued*
  drug-induced E66.1
  due to
    drug E66.1
    excess calories E66.09
      morbid E66.01
      severe E66.01
  endocrine E66.8
  endogenous E66.8
  exogenous E66.09
  familial E66.8
  glandular E66.8
  hypothyroid — *see* Hypothyroidism
  hypoventilation syndrome (OHS) E66.2
  morbid E66.01
    with
      alveolar hypoventilation E66.2
      obesity hypoventilation syndrome (OHS) E66.2
    due to excess calories E66.01
  nutritional E66.09
  pituitary E23.6
  severe E66.01
  specified type NEC E66.8
Oblique — *see* condition
Obliteration
  appendix (lumen) K38.8
  artery I77.1
  bile duct (noncalculous) K83.1
  common duct (noncalculous) K83.1
  cystic duct — *see* Obstruction, gallbladder
  disease, arteriolar I77.1
  endometrium N85.8
  eye, anterior chamber — *see* Disorder, globe, hypotony
  fallopian tube N97.1
  lymphatic vessel I89.0
    due to mastectomy I97.2
  organ or site, congenital NEC — *see* Atresia, by site
  ureter N13.5
    with infection N13.6
  urethra — *see* Stricture, urethra
  vein I87.8
  vestibule (oral) K08.89
Observation (following) (for) (without need for further medical care) Z04.9
  accident NEC Z04.3
    at work Z04.2
    transport Z04.1
  adverse effect of drug Z03.6
  alleged rape or sexual assault (victim), ruled out
    adult Z04.41
    child Z04.42
  criminal assault Z04.89
  development state
    adolescent Z00.3
    period of rapid growth in childhood Z00.2
    puberty Z00.3
  disease, specified NEC Z03.89
  following work accident Z04.2
  forced sexual exploitation Z04.81
  forced labor exploitation Z04.82
  growth and development state — *see* Observation, development state
  injuries (accidental) NEC — *see also* Observation, accident
  newborn (for)
    suspected condition, related to exposure from the mother or birth process — *see* Newborn, affected by, maternal
    ruled out Z05.9
      cardiac Z05.0
      connective tissue Z05.73
      gastrointestinal Z05.5
      genetic Z05.41
      genitourinary Z05.6
      immunologic Z05.43
      infectious Z05.11
      metabolic Z05.42
      musculoskeletal Z05.72
      neurological Z05.2
      respiratory Z05.3
      skin and subcutaneous tissue Z05.71
      specified condition NEC Z05.8
  postpartum
    immediately after delivery Z39.0
    routine follow-up Z39.2
  pregnancy (normal) (without complication) Z34.9- ☑
    high risk O09.9- ☑
  suicide attempt, alleged NEC Z03.89

Observation — *continued*
  suicide attempt, alleged — *continued*
    self-poisoning Z03.6
  suspected, ruled out — *see also* Suspected condition, ruled out
    abuse, physical
      adult Z04.71
      child Z04.72
    accident at work Z04.2
    adult battering victim Z04.71
    child battering victim Z04.72
    condition NEC Z03.89
      newborn — *see also* Observation, newborn (for), suspected condition, ruled out Z05.9
    drug poisoning or adverse effect Z03.6
    exposure (to)
      anthrax Z03.810
      biological agent NEC Z03.818
    inflicted injury NEC Z04.89
    suicide attempt, alleged Z03.89
      self-poisoning Z03.6
    toxic effects from ingested substance (drug) (poison) Z03.6
  toxic effects from ingested substance (drug) (poison) Z03.6
Obsession, obsessional state F42.8
  mixed thoughts and acts F42.2
Obsessive-compulsive neurosis or reaction F42.8
Obstetric embolism, septic — *see* Embolism, obstetric, septic
Obstetrical trauma (complicating delivery) O71.9
  with or following ectopic or molar pregnancy O08.6
  specified type NEC O71.89
Obstipation — *see* Constipation
Obstruction, obstructed, obstructive
  airway J98.8
    with
      allergic alveolitis J67.9
      asthma J45.909
        with
          exacerbation (acute) J45.901
          status asthmaticus J45.902
      bronchiectasis J47.9
        with
          exacerbation (acute) J47.1
          lower respiratory infection J47.0
      bronchitis (chronic) J44.9
      emphysema J43.9
    chronic J44.9
      with
        allergic alveolitis — *see* Pneumonitis, hypersensitivity
        bronchiectasis J47.9
          with
            exacerbation (acute) J47.1
            lower respiratory infection J47.0
    due to
      foreign body — *see* Foreign body, by site, causing asphyxia
      inhalation of fumes or vapors J68.9
      laryngospasm J38.5
  ampulla of Vater K83.1
  aortic (heart) (valve) — *see* Stenosis, aortic
  aortoiliac I74.09
  aqueduct of Sylvius G91.1
    congenital Q03.0
      with spina bifida — *see* Spina bifida, by site, with hydrocephalus
  Arnold-Chiari — *see* Arnold-Chiari disease
  artery — *see also* Atherosclerosis, artery I70.9
    basilar (complete) (partial) — *see* Occlusion, artery, basilar
    carotid (complete) (partial) — *see* Occlusion, artery, carotid
    cerebellar — *see* Occlusion, artery, cerebellar
    cerebral (anterior) (middle) (posterior) — *see* Occlusion, artery, cerebral
    precerebral — *see* Occlusion, artery, precerebral
    renal N28.0
    retinal NEC — *see* Occlusion, artery, retina
    stent — *see* Restenosis, stent
    vertebral (complete) (partial) — *see* Occlusion, artery, vertebral
  band (intestinal) — *see also* Obstruction, intestine, specified NEC K56.699
  bile duct or passage (common) (hepatic) (noncalculous) K83.1
    with calculus K80.51

Obstruction, obstructed, obstructive — *continued*
  bile duct or passage — *continued*
    congenital (causing jaundice) Q44.3
  biliary (duct) (tract) K83.1
    gallbladder K82.0
  bladder-neck (acquired) N32.0
    congenital Q64.31
    due to hyperplasia (hypertrophy) of prostate — *see* Hyperplasia, prostate
  bowel — *see* Obstruction, intestine
  bronchus J98.09
  canal, ear — *see* Stenosis, external ear canal
  cardia K22.2
  caval veins (inferior) (superior) I87.1
  cecum — *see* Obstruction, intestine
  circulatory I99.8
  colon — *see* Obstruction, intestine
  common duct (noncalculous) K83.1
  coronary (artery) — *see* Occlusion, coronary
  cystic duct — *see* Obstruction, gallbladder
    with calculus K80.21
  device, implant or graft — *see also* Complications, by site and type, mechanical T85.698 ☑
    arterial graft NEC — *see* Complication, cardiovascular device, mechanical, vascular
    catheter NEC T85.628 ☑
      cystostomy T83.090 ☑
      dialysis (renal) T82.49 ☑
        intraperitoneal T85.691 ☑
      Hopkins T83.098 ☑
      ileostomy T83.098 ☑
      infusion NEC T82.594 ☑
        spinal (epidural) (subdural) T85.690 ☑
      nephrostomy T83.092 ☑
      urethral indwelling T83.091 ☑
      urinary T83.098 ☑
      urostomy T83.098 ☑
    due to infection T85.79 ☑
    gastrointestinal — *see* Complications, prosthetic device, mechanical, gastrointestinal device
    genital NEC T83.498 ☑
      intrauterine contraceptive device T83.39 ☑
      penile prosthesis (cylinder) (implanted) (pump) (resevoir) T83.490 ☑
      testicular prosthesis T83.491 ☑
    heart NEC — *see* Complication, cardiovascular device, mechanical
    joint prosthesis — *see* Complications, joint prosthesis, mechanical, specified NEC, by site
    orthopedic NEC — *see* Complication, orthopedic, device, mechanical
    specified NEC T85.628 ☑
    urinary NEC — *see* Complication, genitourinary, device, urinary, mechanical
      graft T83.29 ☑
    vascular NEC — *see* Complication, cardiovascular device, mechanical
    ventricular intracranial shunt T85.09 ☑
  due to foreign body accidentally left in operative wound T81.529 ☑
  duodenum K31.5
  ejaculatory duct N50.89
  esophagus K22.2
  eustachian tube (complete) (partial) H68.10- ☑
    cartilagenous (extrinsic) H68.13- ☑
    intrinsic H68.12- ☑
    osseous H68.11- ☑
  fallopian tube (bilateral) N97.1
  fecal K56.41
    with hernia — *see* Hernia, by site, with obstruction
  foramen of Monro (congenital) Q03.8
    with spina bifida — *see* Spina bifida, by site, with hydrocephalus
  foreign body — *see* Foreign body
  gallbladder K82.0
    with calculus, stones K80.21
    congenital Q44.1
  gastric outlet K31.1
  gastrointestinal — *see* Obstruction, intestine
  hepatic K76.89
    duct (noncalculous) K83.1
  ileum — *see* Obstruction, intestine
  iliofemoral (artery) I74.5
  intestine K56.609
    with
      adhesions (intestinal) (peritoneal) K56.50
        complete K56.52

Obstruction, obstructed, obstructive — *continued*
  intestine — *continued*
    with — *continued*
      adhesions — *continued*
        incomplete K56.51
        partial K56.51
      adynamic K56.0
      by gallstone K56.3
      complete K56.601
      congenital (small) Q41.9
        large Q42.9
          specified part NEC Q42.8
      incomplete K56.600
      neurogenic K56.0
        Hirschsprung's disease or megacolon Q43.1
      newborn P76.9
        due to
          fecaliths P76.8
          inspissated milk P76.2
          meconium (plug) P76.0
            in mucoviscidosis E84.11
        specified NEC P76.8
      partial K56.600
      postoperative K91.30
        complete K91.32
        incomplete K91.31
        partial K91.31
      reflex K56.0
      specified NEC K56.699
        complete K56.691
        incomplete K56.690
        partial K56.690
      volvulus K56.2
  intracardiac ball valve prosthesis T82.09 ☑
  jejunum — *see* Obstruction, intestine
  joint prosthesis — *see* Complications, joint prosthesis, mechanical, specified NEC, by site
  kidney (calices) N28.89
  labor — *see* Delivery
  lacrimal (passages) (duct)
    by
      dacryolith — *see* Dacryolith
      stenosis — *see* Stenosis, lacrimal
    congenital Q10.5
    neonatal H04.53- ☑
  lacrimonasal duct — *see* Obstruction, lacrimal
  lacteal, with steatorrhea K90.2
  laryngitis — *see* Laryngitis
  larynx NEC J38.6
    congenital Q31.8
  lung J98.4
    disease, chronic J44.9
  lymphatic I89.0
  meconium (plug)
    newborn P76.0
      due to fecaliths P76.0
        in mucoviscidosis E84.11
  mitral — *see* Stenosis, mitral
  nasal J34.89
  nasolacrimal duct — *see also* Obstruction, lacrimal
    congenital Q10.5
  nasopharynx J39.2
  nose J34.89
  organ or site, congenital NEC — *see* Atresia, by site
  pancreatic duct K86.89
  parotid duct or gland K11.8
  pelviureteral junction N13.5
    with hydronephrosis N13.0
    congenital Q62.39
  pharynx J39.2
  portal (circulation) (vein) I81
  prostate — *see also* Hyperplasia, prostate
    valve (urinary) N32.0
  pulmonary valve (heart) I37.0
  pyelonephritis (chronic) N11.1
  pylorus
    adult K31.1
    congenital or infantile Q40.0
  rectosigmoid — *see* Obstruction, intestine
  rectum K62.4
  renal N28.89
    outflow N13.8
    pelvis, congenital Q62.39
  respiratory J98.8
    chronic J44.9
  retinal (vessels) H34.9
  salivary duct (any) K11.8
    with calculus K11.5

Obstruction, obstructed, obstructive — *continued*
sigmoid — *see* Obstruction, intestine
sinus (accessory) (nasal) J34.89
Stensen's duct K11.8
stomach NEC K31.89
  acute K31.0
  congenital Q40.2
  due to pylorospasm K31.3
submandibular duct K11.8
submaxillary gland K11.8
  with calculus K11.5
thoracic duct I89.0
thrombotic — *see* Thrombosis
trachea J39.8
tracheostomy airway J95.03
tricuspid (valve) — *see* Stenosis, tricuspid
upper respiratory, congenital Q34.8
ureter (functional) (pelvic junction) NEC N13.5
  with
      hydronephrosis N13.1
        with infection N13.6
      pyelonephritis (chronic) N11.1
  congenital Q62.39
  due to calculus — *see* Calculus, ureter
urethra NEC N36.8
  congenital Q64.39
urinary (moderate) N13.9
  due to hyperplasia (hypertrophy) of prostate — *see*
      Hyperplasia, prostate
  organ or tract (lower) N13.9
  prostatic valve N32.0
  specified NEC N13.8
uropathy N13.9
uterus N85.8
vagina N89.5
valvular — *see* Endocarditis
vein, venous I87.1
  caval (inferior) (superior) I87.1
  thrombotic — *see* Thrombosis
vena cava (inferior) (superior) I87.1
vesical NEC N32.0
vesicourethral orifice N32.0
  congenital Q64.31
vessel NEC I99.8
  stent — *see* Restenosis, stent
Obturator — *see* condition
Occlusal wear, teeth K03.0
Occlusio pupillae — *see* Membrane, pupillary
Occlusion, occluded
anus K62.4
  congenital Q42.3
    with fistula Q42.2
aortoiliac (chronic) I74.09
aqueduct of Sylvius G91.1
  congenital Q03.0
    with spina bifida — *see* Spina bifida, by site, with
      hydrocephalus
artery — *see also* Atherosclerosis, artery I70.9 ☑
  auditory, internal I65.8
  basilar I65.1
    with
      infarction I63.22
        due to
          embolism I63.12
          thrombosis I63.02
  brain or cerebral I66.9
    with infarction (due to) I63.5- ☑
      embolism I63.4- ☑
      thrombosis I63.3- ☑
  carotid I65.2- ☑
    with
      infarction I63.23- ☑
        due to
          embolism I63.13- ☑
          thrombosis I63.03- ☑
  cerebellar (anterior inferior) (posterior inferior) (superior) I66.3
    with infarction I63.54- ☑
      due to
        embolism I63.44- ☑
        thrombosis I63.34- ☑
  cerebral I66.9
    with infarction I63.50
      due to
        embolism I63.40
          specified NEC I63.49
        thrombosis I63.30
          specified NEC I63.39

Occlusion, occluded — *continued*
artery — *see also* Atherosclerosis, artery — *continued*
  cerebral — *continued*
    anterior I66.1- ☑
      with infarction I63.52- ☑
        due to
          embolism I63.42- ☑
          thrombosis I63.32- ☑
    middle I66.0- ☑
      with infarction I63.51- ☑
        due to
          embolism I63.41- ☑
          thrombosis I63.31- ☑
    posterior I66.2- ☑
      with infarction I63.53- ☑
        due to
          embolism I63.43- ☑
          thrombosis I63.33- ☑
    specified NEC I66.8
      with infarction I63.59
        due to
          embolism I63.4- ☑
          thrombosis I63.3- ☑
  choroidal (anterior) — *see* Occlusion, artery, precerebral, specified NEC
  communicating posterior — *see* Occlusion, artery, precerebral, specified NEC
  complete
    coronary I25.82
    extremities I70.92
  coronary (acute) (thrombotic) (without myocardial infarction) I24.0
    with myocardial infarction — *see* Infarction, myocardium
    chronic total I25.82
    complete I25.82
    healed or old I25.2
    total (chronic) I25.82
  hypophyseal — *see* Occlusion, artery, precerebral, specified NEC
  iliac I74.5
  lower extremities due to stenosis or stricture I77.1
  mesenteric (embolic) (thrombotic) — *see also* Infarct, intestine K55.069
  perforating — *see* Occlusion, artery, cerebral, specified NEC
  peripheral I77.9
    thrombotic or embolic I74.4
  pontine — *see* Occlusion, artery, precerebral, specified NEC
  precerebral I65.9
    with infarction I63.20
      specified NEC I63.29
      due to
        embolism I63.10
          specified NEC I63.19
        thrombosis I63.00
          specified NEC I63.09
    basilar — *see* Occlusion, artery, basilar
    carotid — *see* Occlusion, artery, carotid
    puerperal O88.23
    specified NEC I65.8
      with infarction I63.29
        due to
          embolism I63.19
          thrombosis I63.09
    vertebral — *see* Occlusion, artery, vertebral
  renal N28.0
  retinal
    branch H34.23- ☑
    central H34.1- ☑
    partial H34.21- ☑
    transient H34.0- ☑
  spinal — *see* Occlusion, artery, precerebral, vertebral
  total (chronic)
    coronary I25.82
    extremities I70.92
  vertebral I65.0- ☑
    with
      infarction I63.21- ☑
        due to
          embolism I63.11- ☑
          thrombosis I63.01- ☑
basilar artery — *see* Occlusion, artery, basilar
bile duct (common) (hepatic) (noncalculous) K83.1
bowel — *see* Obstruction, intestine

Occlusion, occluded — *continued*
carotid (artery) (common) (internal) — *see* Occlusion, artery, carotid
centric (of teeth) M26.59
  maximum intercuspation discrepancy M26.55
cerebellar (artery) — *see* Occlusion, artery, cerebellar
cerebral (artery) — *see* Occlusion, artery, cerebral
cerebrovascular — *see also* Occlusion, artery, cerebral
  with infarction I63.5- ☑
cervical canal — *see* Stricture, cervix
cervix (uteri) — *see* Stricture, cervix
choanal Q30.0
choroidal (artery) — *see* Occlusion, artery, precerebral, specified NEC
colon — *see* Obstruction, intestine
communicating posterior artery — *see* Occlusion, artery, precerebral, specified NEC
coronary (artery) (vein) (thrombotic) — *see also* Infarct, myocardium
  chronic total I25.82
  healed or old I25.2
  not resulting in infarction I24.0
  total (chronic) I25.82
cystic duct — *see* Obstruction, gallbladder
embolic — *see* Embolism
fallopian tube N97.1
  congenital Q50.6
gallbladder — *see also* Obstruction, gallbladder
  congenital (causing jaundice) Q44.1
gingiva, traumatic K06.2
hymen N89.6
  congenital Q52.3
hypophyseal (artery) — *see* Occlusion, artery, precerebral, specified NEC
iliac artery I74.5
intestine — *see* Obstruction, intestine
lacrimal passages — *see* Obstruction, lacrimal
lung J98.4
lymph or lymphatic channel I89.0
mammary duct N64.89
mesenteric artery (embolic) (thrombotic) — *see also* Infarct, intestine K55.069
nose J34.89
  congenital Q30.0
organ or site, congenital NEC — *see* Atresia, by site
oviduct N97.1
  congenital Q50.6
peripheral arteries
  due to stricture or stenosis I77.1
  upper extremity I74.2
pontine (artery) — *see* Occlusion, artery, precerebral, specified NEC
posterior lingual, of mandibular teeth M26.29
precerebral artery — *see* Occlusion, artery, precerebral
punctum lacrimale — *see* Obstruction, lacrimal
pupil — *see* Membrane, pupillary
pylorus, adult — *see also* Stricture, pylorus K31.1
renal artery N28.0
retina, retinal
  artery — *see* Occlusion, artery, retinal
  vein (central) H34.81- ☑
    engorgement H34.82- ☑
    tributary H34.83- ☑
  vessels H34.9
spinal artery — *see* Occlusion, artery, precerebral, vertebral
teeth (mandibular) (posterior lingual) M26.29
thoracic duct I89.0
thrombotic — *see* Thrombosis, artery
traumatic
  edentulous (alveolar) ridge K06.2
  gingiva K06.2
  periodontal K05.5
tubal N97.1
ureter (complete) (partial) N13.5
  congenital Q62.10
ureteropelvic junction N13.5
  congenital Q62.11
ureterovesical orifice N13.5
  congenital Q62.12
urethra — *see* Stricture, urethra
uterus N85.8
vagina N89.5
vascular NEC I99.8
vein — *see* Thrombosis
  retinal — *see* Occlusion, retinal, vein
vena cava (inferior) (superior) — *see* Embolism, vena cava

Occlusion, occluded — *continued*
  ventricle (brain) NEC G91.1
  vertebral (artery) — *see* Occlusion, artery, vertebral
  vessel (blood) I99.8
  vulva N90.5
Occult
  blood in feces (stools) R19.5
Occupational
  problems NEC Z56.89
Ochlophobia — *see* Agoraphobia
Ochronosis (endogenous) E70.29
Ocular muscle — *see* condition
Oculogyric crisis or disturbance H51.8
  psychogenic F45.8
Oculomotor syndrome H51.9
Oculopathy
  syphilitic NEC A52.71
    congenital
      early A50.01
      late A50.30
    early (secondary) A51.43
    late A52.71
Oddi's sphincter spasm K83.4
Odontalgia K08.89
Odontoameloblastoma — *see* Cyst, calcifying odontogenic
Odontoclasia K03.89
Odontodysplasia, regional K00.4
Odontogenesis imperfecta K00.5
Odontoma (ameloblastic) (complex) (compound) (fibroameloblastic) — *see* Cyst, calcifying odontogenic
Odontomyelitis (closed) (open) K04.01
  irreversible K04.02
  reversible K04.01
Odontorrhagia K08.89
Odontosarcoma, ameloblastic C41.1
  upper jaw (bone) C41.0
Oestriasis — *see* Myiasis
Oguchi's disease H53.63
Ohara's disease — *see* Tularemia
OHS (obesity hypoventilation syndrome) E66.2
Oidiomycosis — *see* Candidiasis
Oidium albicans infection — *see* Candidiasis
Old age (without mention of debility) R54
  dementia F03 ☑
Old (previous) **myocardial infarction** I25.2
Olfactory — *see* condition
Oligemia — *see* Anemia
Oligoastrocytoma
  specified site — *see* Neoplasm, malignant, by site
  unspecified site C71.9
Oligocythemia D64.9
Oligodendroblastoma
  specified site — *see* Neoplasm, malignant
  unspecified site C71.9
Oligodendroglioma
  anaplastic type
    specified site — *see* Neoplasm, malignant, by site
    unspecified site C71.9
  specified site — *see* Neoplasm, malignant, by site
  unspecified site C71.9
Oligodontia — *see* Anodontia
Oligoencephalon Q02
Oligohidrosis L74.4
Oligohydramnios O41.0- ☑
Oligohydrosis L74.4
Oligomenorrhea N91.5
  primary N91.3
  secondary N91.4
Oligophrenia — *see also* Disability, intellectual
  phenylpyruvic E70.0
Oligospermia N46.11
  due to
    drug therapy N46.121
    efferent duct obstruction N46.123
    infection N46.122
    radiation N46.124
    specified cause NEC N46.129
    systemic disease N46.125
Oligotrichia — *see* Alopecia
Oliguria R34
  with, complicating or following ectopic or molar pregnancy O08.4
  postprocedural N99.0
Ollier's disease Q78.4
Omenotocele — *see* Hernia, abdomen, specified site NEC
Omentitis — *see* Peritonitis

Omentum, omental — *see* condition
Omphalitis (congenital) (newborn) P38.9
  with mild hemorrhage P38.1
  without hemorrhage P38.9
  not of newborn L08.82
  tetanus A33
Omphalocele Q79.2
Omphalomesenteric duct, persistent Q43.0
Omphalorrhagia, newborn P51.9
Omsk hemorrhagic fever A98.1
Onanism (excessive) F98.8
Onchocerciasis, onchocercosis B73.1
  with
    eye disease B73.00
      endophthalmitis B73.01
      eyelid B73.09
      glaucoma B73.02
      specified NEC B73.09
    eyelid B73.09
    eye NEC B73.00
Oncocytoma — *see* Neoplasm, benign, by site
Oncovirus, as cause of disease classified elsewhere B97.32
Ondine's curse — *see* Apnea, sleep
Oneirophrenia F23
Onychauxis L60.2
  congenital Q84.5
Onychia — *see also* Cellulitis, digit
  with lymphangitis — *see* Lymphangitis, acute, digit
  candidal B37.2
  dermatophytic B35.1
Onychitis — *see also* Cellulitis, digit
  with lymphangitis — *see* Lymphangitis, acute, digit
Onychocryptosis L60.0
Onychodystrophy L60.3
  congenital Q84.6
Onychogryphosis, onychogryposis L60.2
Onycholysis L60.1
Onychomadesis L60.8
Onychomalacia L60.3
Onychomycosis (finger) (toe) B35.1
Onycho-osteodysplasia Q87.2
Onychophagia F98.8
Onychophosis L60.8
Onychoptosis L60.8
Onychorrhexis L60.3
  congenital Q84.6
Onychoschizia L60.3
Onyxis (finger) (toe) L60.0
Onyxitis — *see also* Cellulitis, digit
  with lymphangitis — *see* Lymphangitis, acute, digit
Oophoritis (cystic) (infectional) (interstitial) N70.92
  with salpingitis N70.93
  acute N70.02
    with salpingitis N70.03
  chronic N70.12
    with salpingitis N70.13
  complicating abortion — *see* Abortion, by type, complicated by, oophoritis
Oophorocele N83.4- ☑
Opacity, opacities
  cornea H17.- ☑
    central H17.1- ☑
    congenital Q13.3
    degenerative — *see* Degeneration, cornea
    hereditary — *see* Dystrophy, cornea
    inflammatory — *see* Keratitis
    minor H17.81- ☑
    peripheral H17.82- ☑
    sequelae of trachoma (healed) B94.0
    specified NEC H17.89
  enamel (teeth) (fluoride) (nonfluoride) K00.3
  lens — *see* Cataract
  snowball — *see* Deposit, crystalline
  vitreous (humor) NEC H43.39- ☑
    congenital Q14.0
    membranes and strands H43.31- ☑
Opalescent dentin (hereditary) K00.5
Open, opening
  abnormal, organ or site, congenital — *see* Imperfect, closure
  angle with
    borderline
      findings
        high risk H40.02- ☑
        low risk H40.01- ☑
      intraocular pressure H40.00- ☑

Open, opening — *continued*
  angle with — *continued*
    cupping of discs H40.01- ☑
    glaucoma (primary) — *see* Glaucoma, open angle
  bite
    anterior M26.220
    posterior M26.221
  false — *see* Imperfect, closure
  margin on tooth restoration K08.51
  restoration margins of tooth K08.51
  wound — *see* Wound, open
Operational fatigue F48.8
Operative — *see* condition
Operculitis — *see* Periodontitis
Operculum — *see* Break, retina
Ophiasis L63.2
Ophthalmia — *see also* Conjunctivitis H10.9
  actinic rays — *see* Photokeratitis
  allergic (acute) — *see* Conjunctivitis, acute, atopic
  blennorrhagic (gonococcal) (neonatorum) A54.31
  diphtheritic A36.86
  Egyptian A71.1
  electrica — *see* Photokeratitis
  gonococcal (neonatorum) A54.31
  metastatic — *see* Endophthalmitis, purulent
  migraine — *see* Migraine, ophthalmoplegic
  neonatorum, newborn P39.1
    gonococcal A54.31
  nodosa H16.24- ☑
  purulent — *see* Conjunctivitis, acute, mucopurulent
  spring — *see* Conjunctivitis, acute, atopic
  sympathetic — *see* Uveitis, sympathetic
Ophthalmitis — *see* Ophthalmia
Ophthalmocele (congenital) Q15.8
Ophthalmoneuromyelitis G36.0
Ophthalmoplegia — *see also* Strabismus, paralytic
  anterior internuclear — *see* Ophthalmoplegia, internuclear
  ataxia-areflexia G61.0
  diabetic — *see* E08-E13 with .39
  exophthalmic E05.00
    with thyroid storm E05.01
  external H49.88- ☑
    progressive H49.4- ☑
      with pigmentary retinopathy — *see* Kearns-Sayre syndrome
    total H49.3- ☑
  internal (complete) (total) H52.51- ☑
  internuclear H51.2- ☑
  migraine — *see* Migraine, ophthalmoplegic
  Parinaud's H49.88- ☑
  progressive external — *see* Ophthalmoplegia, external, progressive
  supranuclear, progressive G23.1
  total (external) — *see* Ophthalmoplegia, external, total
Opioid(s)
  abuse — *see* Abuse, drug, opioids
  dependence — *see* Dependence, drug, opioids
  induced, without use disorder
    anxiety disorder F11.988
    delirium F11.921
    depressive disorder F11.94
    sexual dysfunction F11.981
    sleep disorder F11.982
Opisthognathism M26.09
Opisthorchiasis (felineus) (viverrini) B66.0
Opitz' disease D73.2
Opiumism — *see* Dependence, drug, opioid
Oppenheim's disease G70.2
Oppenheim-Urbach disease (necrobiosis lipoidica diabeticorum) — *see* E08-E13 with .620
Optic nerve — *see* condition
Orbit — *see* condition
Orchioblastoma C62.9- ☑
Orchitis (gangrenous) (nonspecific) (septic) (suppurative) N45.2
  blennorrhagic (gonococcal) (acute) (chronic) A54.23
  chlamydial A56.19
  filarial — *see also* Infestation, filarial B74.9 *[N51]*
  gonococcal (acute) (chronic) A54.23
  mumps B26.0
  syphilitic A52.76
  tuberculous A18.15
Orf (virus disease) B08.02
Organic — *see also* condition
  brain syndrome F09
  heart — *see* Disease, heart

Organic — *continued*
  mental disorder F09
  psychosis F09
Orgasm
  anejaculatory N53.13
Oriental
  bilharziasis B65.2
  schistosomiasis B65.2
Orifice — *see* condition
Origin of both great vessels from right ventricle
  Q20.1
Ormond's disease (with ureteral obstruction) N13.5
  with infection N13.6
Ornithine metabolism disorder E72.4
Ornithinemia (Type I) (Type II) E72.4
Ornithosis A70
Orotaciduria, oroticaciduria (congenital) (hereditary)
    (pyrimidine deficiency) E79.8
  anemia D53.0
Orthodontics
  adjustment Z46.4
  fitting Z46.4
Orthopnea R06.01
Orthopoxvirus B08.09
Os, uterus — *see* condition
Osgood-Schlatter disease or osteochondrosis — *see*
    Osteochondrosis, juvenile, tibia
Osler (-Weber)-**Rendu disease** I78.0
Osler's nodes I33.0
Osmidrosis L75.0
Osseous — *see* condition
Ossification
  artery — *see* Arteriosclerosis
  auricle (ear) — *see* Disorder, pinna, specified type NEC
  bronchial J98.09
  cardiac — *see* Degeneration, myocardial
  cartilage (senile) — *see* Disorder, cartilage, specified
      type NEC
  coronary (artery) — *see* Disease, heart, ischemic,
      atherosclerotic
  diaphragm J98.6
  ear, middle — *see* Otosclerosis
  falx cerebri G96.19
  fontanel, premature Q75.0
  heart — *see also* Degeneration, myocardial
    valve — *see* Endocarditis
  larynx J38.7
  ligament — *see* Disorder, tendon, specified type NEC
    posterior longitudinal — *see* Spondylopathy, spec-
        ified NEC
  meninges (cerebral) (spinal) G96.19
  multiple, eccentric centers — *see* Disorder, bone, de-
      velopment or growth
  muscle — *see also* Calcification, muscle
    due to burns — *see* Myositis, ossificans, in, burns
    paralytic — *see* Myositis, ossificans, in, quadriplegia
    progressive — *see* Myositis, ossificans, progressiva
    specified NEC M61.50
      ankle M61.57- ☑
      foot M61.57- ☑
      forearm M61.53- ☑
      hand M61.54- ☑
      lower leg M61.56- ☑
      multiple sites M61.59
      pelvic region M61.55- ☑
      shoulder region M61.51- ☑
      specified site NEC M61.58
      thigh M61.55- ☑
      upper arm M61.52- ☑
    traumatic — *see* Myositis, ossificans, traumatica
  myocardium, myocardial — *see* Degeneration, myocar-
      dial
  penis N48.89
  periarticular — *see* Disorder, joint, specified type NEC
  pinna — *see* Disorder, pinna, specified type NEC
  rider's bone — *see* Ossification, muscle, specified NEC
  sclera H15.89
  subperiosteal, post-traumatic M89.8X- ☑
  tendon — *see* Disorder, tendon, specified type NEC
  trachea J39.8
  tympanic membrane — *see* Disorder, tympanic mem-
      brane, specified NEC
  vitreous (humor) — *see* Deposit, crystalline
Osteitis — *see also* Osteomyelitis
  alveolar M27.3
  condensans M85.30
    ankle M85.37- ☑

Osteitis — *continued*
  condensans — *continued*
    foot M85.37- ☑
    forearm M85.33- ☑
    hand M85.34- ☑
    lower leg M85.36- ☑
    multiple site M85.39
    neck M85.38
    rib M85.38
    shoulder M85.31- ☑
    skull M85.38
    specified site NEC M85.38
    thigh M85.35- ☑
    toe M85.37- ☑
    upper arm M85.32- ☑
    vertebra M85.38
  deformans M88.9
    in (due to)
      malignant neoplasm of bone C41.9 *[M90.60]*
      neoplastic disease — *see also* Neoplasm
          D49.9 *[M90.60]*
        carpus D49.9 *[M90.64-]* ☑
        clavicle D49.9 *[M90.61-]* ☑
        femur D49.9 *[M90.65-]* ☑
        fibula D49.9 *[M90.66-]* ☑
        finger D49.9 *[M90.64-]* ☑
        humerus D49.9 *[M90.62-]* ☑
        ilium D49.9 *[M90.65-]* ☑
        ischium D49.9 *[M90.65-]* ☑
        metacarpus D49.9 *[M90.64-]* ☑
        metatarsus D49.9 *[M90.67-]* ☑
        multiple sites D49.9 *[M90.69]*
        neck D49.9 *[M90.68]*
        radius D49.9 *[M90.63-]* ☑
        rib D49.9 *[M90.68]*
        scapula D49.9 *[M90.61-]* ☑
        skull D49.9 *[M90.68]*
        tarsus D49.9 *[M90.67-]* ☑
        tibia D49.9 *[M90.66-]* ☑
        toe D49.9 *[M90.67-]* ☑
        ulna D49.9 *[M90.63-]* ☑
        vertebra D49.9 *[M90.68]*
    skull M88.0
    specified NEC — *see* Paget's disease, bone, by site
    vertebra M88.1
  due to yaws A66.6
  fibrosa NEC — *see* Cyst, bone, by site
    circumscripta — *see* Dysplasia, fibrous, bone NEC
    cystica (generalisata) E21.0
    disseminata Q78.1
    osteoplastica E21.0
  fragilitans Q78.0
  Garr's (sclerosing) — *see* Osteomyelitis, specified type
      NEC
  jaw (acute) (chronic) (lower) (suppurative) (upper)
      M27.2
  parathyroid E21.0
  petrous bone (acute) (chronic) — *see* Petrositis
  sclerotic, nonsuppurative — *see* Osteomyelitis, speci-
      fied type NEC
  tuberculosa A18.09
    cystica D86.89
    multiplex cystoides D86.89
Osteoarthritis M19.90
  ankle M19.07- ☑
  elbow M19.02- ☑
  foot joint M19.07- ☑
  generalized M15.9
    erosive M15.4
    primary M15.0
    specified NEC M15.8
  hand joint M19.04- ☑
    first carpometacarpal joint M18.9
  hip M16.1- ☑
    bilateral M16.0
    due to hip dysplasia (unilateral) M16.3- ☑
      bilateral M16.2
  interphalangeal
    distal (Heberden) M15.1
    proximal (Bouchard) M15.2
  knee M17.1- ☑
    bilateral M17.0
  post-traumatic NEC M19.92
    ankle M19.17- ☑
    elbow M19.12- ☑
    foot joint M19.17- ☑
    hand joint M19.14- ☑

Osteoarthritis — *continued*
  post-traumatic — *continued*
    hand joint — *continued*
      first carpometacarpal joint M18.3- ☑
        bilateral M18.2
    hip M16.5- ☑
      bilateral M16.4
    knee M17.3- ☑
      bilateral M17.2
    shoulder M19.11- ☑
    wrist M19.13- ☑
  primary M19.91
    ankle M19.07- ☑
    elbow M19.02- ☑
    foot joint M19.07- ☑
    hand joint M19.04- ☑
      first carpometacarpal joint M18.1- ☑
        bilateral M18.0
    hip M16.1- ☑
      bilateral M16.0
    knee M17.1- ☑
      bilateral M17.0
    multiple sites M89.49
    shoulder M19.01- ☑
    spine — *see* Spondylosis
    wrist M19.03- ☑
  secondary M19.93
    ankle M19.27- ☑
    elbow M19.22- ☑
    foot joint M19.27- ☑
    hand joint M19.24- ☑
      first carpometacarpal joint M18.5- ☑
        bilateral M18.4
    hip M16.7
      bilateral M16.6
    knee M17.5
      bilateral M17.4
    multiple M15.3
    shoulder M19.21- ☑
    spine — *see* Spondylosis
    wrist M19.23- ☑
  shoulder M19.01- ☑
  spine — *see* Spondylosis
  wrist M19.03- ☑
Osteoarthropathy (hypertrophic) M19.90
  ankle — *see* Osteoarthritis, primary, ankle
  elbow — *see* Osteoarthritis, primary, elbow
  foot joint — *see* Osteoarthritis, primary, foot
  hand joint — *see* Osteoarthritis, primary, hand joint
  knee joint — *see* Osteoarthritis, primary, knee
  multiple site — *see* Osteoarthritis, primary, multiple
      joint
  pulmonary — *see also* Osteoarthropathy, specified
      type NEC
    hypertrophic — *see* Osteoarthropathy, hypertrophic,
        specified type NEC
  secondary — *see* Osteoarthropathy, specified type NEC
  secondary hypertrophic — *see* Osteoarthropathy,
      specified type NEC
  shoulder — *see* Osteoarthritis, primary, shoulder
  specified joint NEC — *see* Osteoarthritis, primary,
      specified joint NEC
  specified type NEC M89.40
    carpus M89.44- ☑
    clavicle M89.41- ☑
    femur M89.45- ☑
    fibula M89.46- ☑
    finger M89.44- ☑
    humerus M89.42- ☑
    ilium M89.459
    ischium M89.459
    metacarpus M89.44- ☑
    metatarsus M89.47- ☑
    multiple sites M89.49
    neck M89.48
    radius M89.43- ☑
    rib M89.48
    scapula M89.41- ☑
    skull M89.48
    tarsus M89.47- ☑
    tibia M89.46- ☑
    toe M89.47- ☑
    ulna M89.43- ☑
    vertebra M89.48
  spine — *see* Spondylosis
  wrist — *see* Osteoarthritis, primary, wrist

Osteoarthrosis (degenerative) (hypertrophic) (joint) — *see also* Osteoarthritis
deformans alkaptonurica E70.29 *[M36.8]*
erosive M15.4
generalized M15.9
primary M15.0
polyarticular M15.9
spine — *see* Spondylosis
Osteoblastoma — *see* Neoplasm, bone, benign
aggressive — *see* Neoplasm, bone, uncertain behavior
Osteochondritis — *see also* Osteochondropathy, by site
Brailsford's — *see* Osteochondrosis, juvenile, radius
dissecans M93.20
ankle M93.27- ☑
elbow M93.22- ☑
foot M93.27- ☑
hand M93.24- ☑
hip M93.25- ☑
knee M93.26- ☑
multiple sites M93.29
shoulder joint M93.21- ☑
specified site NEC M93.28
wrist M93.23- ☑
juvenile M92.9
patellar — *see* Osteochondrosis, juvenile, patella
syphilitic (congenital) (early) A50.02 *[M90.80]*
ankle A50.02 *[M90.87-]* ☑
elbow A50.02 *[M90.82-]* ☑
foot A50.02 *[M90.87-]* ☑
forearm A50.02 *[M90.83-]* ☑
hand A50.02 *[M90.84-]* ☑
hip A50.02 *[M90.85-]* ☑
knee A50.02 *[M90.86-]* ☑
multiple sites A50.02 *[M90.89]*
shoulder joint A50.02 *[M90.81-]* ☑
specified site NEC A50.02 *[M90.88]*
Osteochondroarthrosis deformans endemica — *see* Disease, Kaschin-Beck
Osteochondrodysplasia Q78.9
with defects of growth of tubular bones and spine Q77.9
specified NEC Q77.8
specified NEC Q78.8
Osteochondrodystrophy E78.9
Osteochondrolysis — *see* Osteochondritis, dissecans
Osteochondroma — *see* Neoplasm, bone, benign
Osteochondromatosis D48.0
syndrome Q78.4
Osteochondromyxosarcoma — *see* Neoplasm, bone, malignant
Osteochondropathy M93.90
ankle M93.97- ☑
elbow M93.92- ☑
foot M93.97- ☑
hand M93.94- ☑
hip M93.95- ☑
Kienböck's disease of adults M93.1
knee M93.96- ☑
multiple joints M93.99
osteochondritis dissecans — *see* Osteochondritis, dissecans
osteochondrosis — *see* Osteochondrosis
shoulder region M93.91- ☑
slipped upper femoral epiphysis — *see* Slipped, epiphysis, upper femoral
specified joint NEC M93.98
specified type NEC M93.80
ankle M93.87- ☑
elbow M93.82- ☑
foot M93.87- ☑
hand M93.84- ☑
hip M93.85- ☑
knee M93.86- ☑
multiple joints M93.89
shoulder region M93.81- ☑
specified joint NEC M93.88
wrist M93.83- ☑
syphilitic, congenital
early A50.02 *[M90.80]*
late A50.56 *[M90.80]*
wrist M93.93- ☑
Osteochondrosarcoma — *see* Neoplasm, bone, malignant
Osteochondrosis — *see also* Osteochondropathy, by site
acetabulum (juvenile) M91.0

Osteochondrosis — *continued*
adult — *see* Osteochondropathy, specified type NEC, by site
astragalus (juvenile) — *see* Osteochondrosis, juvenile, tarsus
Blount's — *see* Osteochondrosis, juvenile, tibia
Buchanan's M91.0
Burns' — *see* Osteochondrosis, juvenile, ulna
calcaneus (juvenile) — *see* Osteochondrosis, juvenile, tarsus
capitular epiphysis (femur) (juvenile) — *see* Legg-Calvé-Perthes disease
carpal (juvenile) (lunate) (scaphoid) — *see* Osteochondrosis, juvenile, hand, carpal lunate
adult M93.1
coxae juvenilis — *see* Legg-Calvé-Perthes disease
deformans juvenilis, coxae — *see* Legg-Calvé-Perthes disease
Diaz's — *see* Osteochondrosis, juvenile, tarsus
dissecans (knee) (shoulder) — *see* Osteochondritis, dissecans
femoral capital epiphysis (juvenile) — *see* Legg-Calvé-Perthes disease
femur (head), juvenile — *see* Legg-Calvé-Perthes disease
fibula (juvenile) — *see* Osteochondrosis, juvenile, fibula
foot NEC (juvenile) M92.8
Freiberg's — *see* Osteochondrosis, juvenile, metatarsus
Haas' (juvenile) — *see* Osteochondrosis, juvenile, humerus
Haglund's — *see* Osteochondrosis, juvenile, tarsus
hip (juvenile) — *see* Legg-Calvé-Perthes disease
humerus (capitulum) (head) (juvenile) — *see* Osteochondrosis, juvenile, humerus
ilium, iliac crest (juvenile) M91.0
ischiopubic synchondrosis M91.0
Iselin's — *see* Osteochondrosis, juvenile, metatarsus
juvenile, juvenilis M92.9
after congenital dislocation of hip reduction — *see* Osteochondrosis, juvenile, hip, specified NEC
arm — *see* Osteochondrosis, juvenile, upper limb NEC
capitular epiphysis (femur) — *see* Legg-Calvé-Perthes disease
clavicle, sternal epiphysis — *see* Osteochondrosis, juvenile, upper limb NEC
coxae — *see* Legg-Calvé-Perthes disease
deformans M92.9
fibula M92.5- ☑
foot NEC M92.8
hand M92.20- ☑
carpal lunate M92.21- ☑
metacarpal head M92.22- ☑
specified site NEC M92.29- ☑
head of femur — *see* Legg-Calvé-Perthes disease
hip and pelvis M91.9- ☑
coxa plana — *see* Coxa, plana
femoral head — *see* Legg-Calvé-Perthes disease
pelvis M91.0
pseudocoxalgia — *see* Pseudocoxalgia
specified NEC M91.8- ☑
humerus M92.0- ☑
limb
lower NEC M92.8
upper NEC — *see* Osteochondrosis, juvenile, upper limb NEC
medial cuneiform bone — *see* Osteochondrosis, juvenile, tarsus
metatarsus M92.7- ☑
patella M92.4- ☑
radius M92.1- ☑
specified site NEC M92.8
spine M42.00
cervical region M42.02
cervicothoracic region M42.03
lumbar region M42.06
lumbosacral region M42.07
multiple sites M42.09
occipito-atlanto-axial region M42.01
sacrococcygeal region M42.08
thoracic region M42.04
thoracolumbar region M42.05
tarsus M92.6- ☑
tibia M92.5- ☑
ulna M92.1- ☑
upper limb NEC M92.3- ☑

Osteochondrosis — *continued*
juvenile, juvenilis — *continued*
vertebra (body) (epiphyseal plates) (Calvé's) (Scheuermann's) — *see* Osteochondrosis, juvenile, spine
Kienböck's — *see* Osteochondrosis, juvenile, hand, carpal lunate
adult M93.1
Köhler's
patellar — *see* Osteochondrosis, juvenile, patella
tarsal navicular — *see* Osteochondrosis, juvenile, tarsus
Legg-Perthes (-Calvé)(-Waldenström) — *see* Legg-Calvé-Perthes disease
limb
lower NEC (juvenile) M92.8
upper NEC (juvenile) — *see* Osteochondrosis, juvenile, upper limb NEC
lunate bone (carpal) (juvenile) — *see also* Osteochondrosis, juvenile, hand, carpal lunate
adult M93.1
Mauclaire's — *see* Osteochondrosis, juvenile, hand, metacarpal
metacarpal (head) (juvenile) — *see* Osteochondrosis, juvenile, hand, metacarpal
metatarsus (fifth) (head) (juvenile) (second) — *see* Osteochondrosis, juvenile, metatarsus
navicular (juvenile) — *see* Osteochondrosis, juvenile, tarsus
os
calcis (juvenile) — *see* Osteochondrosis, juvenile, tarsus
tibiale externum (juvenile) — *see* Osteochondrosis, juvenile, tarsus
Osgood-Schlatter — *see* Osteochondrosis, juvenile, tibia
Panner's — *see* Osteochondrosis, juvenile, humerus
patellar center (juvenile) (primary) (secondary) — *see* Osteochondrosis, juvenile, patella
pelvis (juvenile) M91.0
Pierson's M91.0
radius (head) (juvenile) — *see* Osteochondrosis, juvenile, radius
Scheuermann's — *see* Osteochondrosis, juvenile, spine
Sever's — *see* Osteochondrosis, juvenile, tarsus
Sinding-Larsen — *see* Osteochondrosis, juvenile, patella
spine M42.9
adult M42.10
cervical region M42.12
cervicothoracic region M42.13
lumbar region M42.16
lumbosacral region M42.17
multiple sites M42.19
occipito-atlanto-axial region M42.11
sacrococcygeal region M42.18
thoracic region M42.14
thoracolumbar region M42.15
juvenile — *see* Osteochondrosis, juvenile, spine
symphysis pubis (juvenile) M91.0
syphilitic (congenital) A50.02
talus (juvenile) — *see* Osteochondrosis, juvenile, tarsus
tarsus (navicular) (juvenile) — *see* Osteochondrosis, juvenile, tarsus
tibia (proximal) (tubercle) (juvenile) — *see* Osteochondrosis, juvenile, tibia
tuberculous — *see* Tuberculosis, bone
ulna (lower) (juvenile) — *see* Osteochondrosis, juvenile, ulna
van Neck's M91.0
vertebral — *see* Osteochondrosis, spine
Osteoclastoma D48.0
malignant — *see* Neoplasm, bone, malignant
Osteodynia — *see* Disorder, bone, specified type NEC
Osteodystrophy Q78.9
azotemic N25.0
congenital Q78.9
parathyroid, secondary E21.1
renal N25.0
Osteofibroma — *see* Neoplasm, bone, benign
Osteofibrosarcoma — *see* Neoplasm, bone, malignant
Osteogenesis imperfecta Q78.0
Osteogenic — *see* condition
Osteolysis M89.50
carpus M89.54- ☑
clavicle M89.51- ☑
femur M89.55- ☑

☑ Additional Character Required — Refer to the Tabular List for Character Selection
Ⓥ Subterms under main terms may continue to next column or page

Osteolysis — continued
- fibula M89.56- ☑
- finger M89.54- ☑
- humerus M89.52- ☑
- ilium M89.559
- ischium M89.559
- joint prosthesis (periprosthetic) — see Complications, joint prosthesis, mechanical, periprosthetic, osteolysis, by site
- metacarpus M89.54- ☑
- metatarsus M89.57- ☑
- multiple sites M89.59
- neck M89.58
- periprosthetic — see Complications, joint prosthesis, mechanical, periprosthetic, osteolysis, by site
- radius M89.53- ☑
- rib M89.58
- scapula M89.51- ☑
- skull M89.58
- tarsus M89.57- ☑
- tibia M89.56- ☑
- toe M89.57- ☑
- ulna M89.53- ☑
- vertebra M89.58

Osteoma — see also Neoplasm, bone, benign
- osteoid — see also Neoplasm, bone, benign
  - giant — see Neoplasm, bone, benign

Osteomalacia M83.9
- adult M83.9
  - drug-induced NEC M83.5
  - due to
    - malabsorption (postsurgical) M83.2
    - malnutrition M83.3
  - specified NEC M83.8
- aluminium-induced M83.4
- infantile — see Rickets
- juvenile — see Rickets
- oncogenic E83.89
- pelvis M83.8
- puerperal M83.0
- senile M83.1
- vitamin-D-resistant in adults E83.31 [M90.8-] ☑
  - carpus E83.31 [M90.84-] ☑
  - clavicle E83.31 [M90.81-] ☑
  - femur E83.31 [M90.85-] ☑
  - fibula E83.31 [M90.86-] ☑
  - finger E83.31 [M90.84-] ☑
  - humerus E83.31 [M90.82-] ☑
  - ilium E83.31 [M90.859]
  - ischium E83.31 [M90.859]
  - metacarpus E83.31 [M90.84-] ☑
  - metatarsus E83.31 [M90.87-] ☑
  - multiple sites E83.31 [M90.89]
  - neck E83.31 [M90.88]
  - radius E83.31 [M90.83-] ☑
  - rib E83.31 [M90.88]
  - scapula E83.31 [M90.819]
  - skull E83.31 [M90.88]
  - tarsus E83.31 [M90.879]
  - tibia E83.31 [M90.869]
  - toe E83.31 [M90.879]
  - ulna E83.31 [M90.839]
  - vertebra E83.31 [M90.88]

Osteomyelitis (general) (infective) (localized) (neonatal) (purulent) (septic) (staphylococcal) (streptococcal) (suppurative) (with periostitis) M86.9
- acute M86.10
  - carpus M86.14- ☑
  - clavicle M86.11- ☑
  - femur M86.15- ☑
  - fibula M86.16- ☑
  - finger M86.14- ☑
  - hematogenous M86.00
    - carpus M86.04- ☑
    - clavicle M86.01- ☑
    - femur M86.05- ☑
    - fibula M86.06- ☑
    - finger M86.04- ☑
    - humerus M86.02- ☑
    - ilium M86.059
    - ischium M86.059
    - mandible M27.2
    - metacarpus M86.04- ☑
    - metatarsus M86.07- ☑
    - multiple sites M86.09
    - neck M86.08
    - orbit H05.02- ☑

Osteomyelitis — continued
- acute — continued
  - hematogenous — continued
    - petrous bone — see Petrositis
    - radius M86.03- ☑
    - rib M86.08
    - scapula M86.01- ☑
    - skull M86.08
    - tarsus M86.07- ☑
    - tibia M86.06- ☑
    - toe M86.07- ☑
    - ulna M86.03- ☑
    - vertebra — see Osteomyelitis, vertebra
  - humerus M86.12- ☑
  - ilium M86.18
  - ischium M86.18
  - mandible M27.2
  - metacarpus M86.14- ☑
  - metatarsus M86.17- ☑
  - multiple sites M86.19
  - neck M86.18
  - orbit H05.02- ☑
  - petrous bone — see Petrositis
  - radius M86.13- ☑
  - rib M86.18
  - scapula M86.11- ☑
  - skull M86.18
  - tarsus M86.17- ☑
  - tibia M86.16- ☑
  - toe M86.17- ☑
  - ulna M86.13- ☑
  - vertebra — see Osteomyelitis, vertebra
- chronic (or old) M86.60
  - with draining sinus M86.40
    - carpus M86.44- ☑
    - clavicle M86.41- ☑
    - femur M86.45- ☑
    - fibula M86.46- ☑
    - finger M86.44- ☑
    - humerus M86.42- ☑
    - ilium M86.459
    - ischium M86.459
    - mandible M27.2
    - metacarpus M86.44- ☑
    - metatarsus M86.47- ☑
    - multiple sites M86.49
    - neck M86.48
    - orbit H05.01- ☑
    - petrous bone — see Petrositis
    - radius M86.43- ☑
    - rib M86.48
    - scapula M86.41- ☑
    - skull M86.48
    - tarsus M86.47- ☑
    - tibia M86.46- ☑
    - toe M86.47- ☑
    - ulna M86.43- ☑
    - vertebra — see Osteomyelitis, vertebra
  - carpus M86.64- ☑
  - clavicle M86.61- ☑
  - femur M86.65- ☑
  - fibula M86.66- ☑
  - finger M86.64- ☑
  - hematogenous NEC M86.50
    - carpus M86.54- ☑
    - clavicle M86.51- ☑
    - femur M86.55- ☑
    - fibula M86.56- ☑
    - finger M86.54- ☑
    - humerus M86.52- ☑
    - ilium M86.559
    - ischium M86.559
    - mandible M27.2
    - metacarpus M86.54- ☑
    - metatarsus M86.57- ☑
    - multifocal M86.30
      - carpus M86.34- ☑
      - clavicle M86.31- ☑
      - femur M86.35- ☑
      - fibula M86.36- ☑
      - finger M86.34- ☑
      - humerus M86.32- ☑
      - ilium M86.359
      - ischium M86.359
      - metacarpus M86.34- ☑
      - metatarsus M86.37- ☑

Osteomyelitis — continued
- chronic — continued
  - hematogenous — continued
    - multifocal — continued
      - multiple sites M86.39
      - neck M86.38
      - radius M86.33- ☑
      - rib M86.38
      - scapula M86.31- ☑
      - skull M86.38
      - tarsus M86.37- ☑
      - tibia M86.36- ☑
      - toe M86.37- ☑
      - ulna M86.33- ☑
      - vertebra — see Osteomyelitis, vertebra
    - multiple sites M86.59
    - neck M86.58
    - orbit H05.02- ☑
    - petrous bone — see Petrositis
    - radius M86.53- ☑
    - rib M86.58
    - scapula M86.51- ☑
    - skull M86.58
    - tarsus M86.57- ☑
    - tibia M86.56- ☑
    - toe M86.57- ☑
    - ulna M86.53- ☑
    - vertebra — see Osteomyelitis, vertebra
  - humerus M86.62- ☑
  - ilium M86.659
  - ischium M86.659
  - mandible M27.2
  - metacarpus M86.64- ☑
  - metatarsus M86.67- ☑
  - multifocal — see Osteomyelitis, chronic, hematogenous, multifocal
  - multiple sites M86.69
  - neck M86.68
  - orbit H05.02- ☑
  - petrous bone — see Petrositis
  - radius M86.63- ☑
  - rib M86.68
  - scapula M86.61- ☑
  - skull M86.68
  - tarsus M86.67- ☑
  - tibia M86.66- ☑
  - toe M86.67- ☑
  - ulna M86.63- ☑
  - vertebra — see Osteomyelitis, vertebra
- echinococcal B67.2
- Garr's — see Osteomyelitis, specified type NEC
- in diabetes mellitus — see E08-E13 with .69
- jaw (acute) (chronic) (lower) (neonatal) (suppurative) (upper) M27.2
- nonsuppurating — see Osteomyelitis, specified type NEC
- orbit H05.02- ☑
- petrous bone — see Petrositis
- Salmonella (arizonae) (cholerae-suis) (enteritidis) (typhimurium) A02.24
- sclerosing, nonsuppurative — see Osteomyelitis, specified type NEC
- specified type NEC — see also subcategory M86.8X- ☑
  - mandible M27.2
  - orbit H05.02- ☑
  - petrous bone — see Petrositis
  - vertebra — see Osteomyelitis, vertebra
- subacute M86.20
  - carpus M86.24- ☑
  - clavicle M86.21- ☑
  - femur M86.25- ☑
  - fibula M86.26- ☑
  - finger M86.24- ☑
  - humerus M86.22- ☑
  - mandible M27.2
  - metacarpus M86.24- ☑
  - metatarsus M86.27- ☑
  - multiple sites M86.29
  - neck M86.28
  - orbit H05.02- ☑
  - petrous bone — see Petrositis
  - radius M86.23- ☑
  - rib M86.28
  - scapula M86.21- ☑
  - skull M86.28
  - tarsus M86.27- ☑
  - tibia M86.26- ☑

Osteomyelitis — *continued*
  subacute — *continued*
    toe M86.27- ☑
    ulna M86.23- ☑
    vertebra — *see* Osteomyelitis, vertebra
  syphilitic A52.77
    congenital (early) A50.02 *[M90.80]*
  tuberculous — *see* Tuberculosis, bone
  typhoid A01.05
  vertebra M46.20
    cervical region M46.22
    cervicothoracic region M46.23
    lumbar region M46.26
    lumbosacral region M46.27
    occipito-atlanto-axial region M46.21
    sacrococcygeal region M46.28
    thoracic region M46.24
    thoracolumbar region M46.25
Osteomyelofibrosis D47.4
Osteomyelosclerosis D75.89
Osteonecrosis M87.9
  due to
    drugs — *see* Osteonecrosis, secondary, due to, drugs
    trauma — *see* Osteonecrosis, secondary, due to, trauma
  idiopathic aseptic M87.00
    ankle M87.07- ☑
    carpus M87.03- ☑
    clavicle M87.01- ☑
    femur M87.05- ☑
    fibula M87.06- ☑
    finger M87.04- ☑
    humerus M87.02- ☑
    ilium M87.050
    ischium M87.050
    metacarpus M87.04- ☑
    metatarsus M87.07- ☑
    multiple sites M87.09
    neck M87.08
    pelvis M87.050
    radius M87.03- ☑
    rib M87.08
    scapula M87.01- ☑
    skull M87.08
    tarsus M87.07- ☑
    tibia M87.06- ☑
    toe M87.07- ☑
    ulna M87.03- ☑
    vertebra M87.08
  secondary NEC M87.30
    carpus M87.33- ☑
    clavicle M87.31- ☑
    due to
      drugs M87.10
        carpus M87.13- ☑
        clavicle M87.11- ☑
        femur M87.15- ☑
        fibula M87.16- ☑
        finger M87.14- ☑
        humerus M87.12- ☑
        ilium M87.159
        ischium M87.159
        jaw M87.180
        metacarpus M87.14- ☑
        metatarsus M87.17- ☑
        multiple sites M87.19
        neck M87.18
        radius M87.13- ☑
        rib M87.18 ☑
        scapula M87.11- ☑
        skull M87.18 ☑
        tarsus M87.17- ☑
        tibia M87.16- ☑
        toe M87.17- ☑
        ulna M87.13- ☑
        vertebra M87.18 ☑
      hemoglobinopathy NEC D58.2 *[M90.50]*
        carpus D58.2 *[M90.54-]* ☑
        clavicle D58.2 *[M90.51-]* ☑
        femur D58.2 *[M90.55-]* ☑
        fibula D58.2 *[M90.56-]* ☑
        finger D58.2 *[M90.54-]* ☑
        humerus D58.2 *[M90.52-]* ☑
        ilium D58.2 *[M90.55-]* ☑
        ischium D58.2 *[M90.55-]* ☑
        metacarpus D58.2 *[M90.54-]* ☑
        metatarsus D58.2 *[M90.57-]* ☑

Osteonecrosis — *continued*
  secondary — *continued*
    due to — *continued*
      hemoglobinopathy — *continued*
        multiple sites D58.2 *[M90.58]*
        neck D58.2 *[M90.58]*
        radius D58.2 *[M90.53-]* ☑
        rib D58.2 *[M90.58]*
        scapula D58.2 *[M90.51-]* ☑
        skull D58.2 *[M90.58]*
        tarsus D58.2 *[M90.57-]* ☑
        tibia D58.2 *[M90.56-]* ☑
        toe D58.2 *[M90.57-]* ☑
        ulna D58.2 *[M90.53-]* ☑
        vertebra D58.2 *[M90.58]*
      trauma (previous) M87.20
        carpus M87.23- ☑
        clavicle M87.21- ☑
        femur M87.25- ☑
        fibula M87.26- ☑
        finger M87.24- ☑
        humerus M87.22- ☑
        ilium M87.25- ☑
        ischium M87.25- ☑
        metacarpus M87.24- ☑
        metatarsus M87.27- ☑
        multiple sites M87.29
        neck M87.28
        radius M87.23- ☑
        rib M87.28
        scapula M87.21- ☑
        skull M87.28
        tarsus M87.27- ☑
        tibia M87.26- ☑
        toe M87.27- ☑
        ulna M87.23- ☑
        vertebra M87.28
    femur M87.35- ☑
    fibula M87.36- ☑
    finger M87.34- ☑
    humerus M87.32- ☑
    ilium M87.350
    in
      caisson disease T70.3 ☑ *[M90.50]*
        carpus T70.3 ☑ *[M90.54-]* ☑
        clavicle T70.3 ☑ *[M90.51-]* ☑
        femur T70.3 ☑ *[M90.55-]* ☑
        fibula T70.3 ☑ *[M90.56-]* ☑
        finger T70.3 ☑ *[M90.54-]* ☑
        humerus T70.3 ☑ *[M90.52-]* ☑
        ilium T70.3 ☑ *[M90.55-]* ☑
        ischium T70.3 ☑ *[M90.55-]* ☑
        metacarpus T70.3 ☑ *[M90.54-]* ☑
        metatarsus T70.3 ☑ *[M90.57-]* ☑
        multiple sites T70.3 ☑ *[M90.59]*
        neck T70.3 ☑ *[M90.58]*
        radius T70.3 ☑ *[M90.53-]* ☑
        rib T70.3 ☑ *[M90.58]*
        scapula T70.3 ☑ *[M90.51-]* ☑
        skull T70.3 ☑ *[M90.58]*
        tarsus T70.3 ☑ *[M90.57-]* ☑
        tibia T70.3 ☑ *[M90.56-]* ☑
        toe T70.3 ☑ *[M90.57-]* ☑
        ulna T70.3 ☑ *[M90.53-]* ☑
        vertebra T70.3 ☑ *[M90.58]*
    ischium M87.350
    metacarpus M87.34- ☑
    metatarsus M87.37- ☑
    multiple site M87.39
    neck M87.38
    radius M87.33- ☑
    rib M87.38
    scapula M87.319
    skull M87.38
    tarsus M87.379
    tibia M87.366
    toe M87.379
    ulna M87.33- ☑
    vertebra M87.38
  specified type NEC M87.80
    carpus M87.83- ☑
    clavicle M87.81- ☑
    femur M87.85- ☑
    fibula M87.86- ☑
    finger M87.84- ☑
    humerus M87.82- ☑

Osteonecrosis — *continued*
  specified type — *continued*
    ilium M87.85- ☑
    ischium M87.85- ☑
    metacarpus M87.84- ☑
    metatarsus M87.87- ☑
    multiple sites M87.89
    neck M87.88
    radius M87.83- ☑
    rib M87.88
    scapula M87.81- ☑
    skull M87.88
    tarsus M87.87- ☑
    tibia M87.86- ☑
    toe M87.87- ☑
    ulna M87.83- ☑
    vertebra M87.88
Osteo-onycho-arthro-dysplasia Q87.2
Osteo-onychodysplasia, hereditary Q87.2
Osteopathia condensans disseminata Q78.8
Osteopathy — *see also* Osteomyelitis, Osteonecrosis, Osteoporosis
  after poliomyelitis M89.60
    carpus M89.64- ☑
    clavicle M89.61- ☑
    femur M89.65- ☑
    fibula M89.66- ☑
    finger M89.64- ☑
    humerus M89.62- ☑
    ilium M89.659
    ischium M89.659
    metacarpus M89.64- ☑
    metatarsus M89.67- ☑
    multiple sites M89.69
    neck M89.68
    radius M89.63- ☑
    rib M89.68
    scapula M89.61- ☑
    skull M89.68
    tarsus M89.67- ☑
    tibia M89.66- ☑
    toe M89.67- ☑
    ulna M89.63- ☑
    vertebra M89.68
  in (due to)
    renal osteodystrophy N25.0
    specified diseases classified elsewhere — *see* sub-category M90.8 ☑
Osteopenia M85.8- ☑
  borderline M85.8- ☑
Osteoperiostitis — *see* Osteomyelitis, specified type NEC
Osteopetrosis (familial) Q78.2
Osteophyte M25.70
  ankle M25.77- ☑
  elbow M25.72- ☑
  foot joint M25.77- ☑
  hand joint M25.74- ☑
  hip M25.75- ☑
  knee M25.76- ☑
  shoulder M25.71- ☑
  spine M25.78
  vertebrae M25.78
  wrist M25.73- ☑
Osteopoikilosis Q78.8
Osteoporosis (female) (male) M81.0
  with current pathological fracture M80.00 ☑
  age-related M81.0
    with current pathologic fracture M80.00 ☑
      carpus M80.04- ☑
      clavicle M80.01- ☑
      fibula M80.06- ☑
      finger M80.04- ☑
      humerus M80.02- ☑
      ilium M80.05- ☑
      ischium M80.05- ☑
      metacarpus M80.04- ☑
      metatarsus M80.07- ☑
      pelvis M80.05- ☑
      radius M80.03- ☑
      scapula M80.01- ☑
      tarsus M80.07- ☑
      tibia M80.06- ☑
      toe M80.07- ☑
      ulna M80.03- ☑
      vertebra M80.08

☑ **Additional Character Required** — **Refer to the Tabular List for Character Selection**

☲ Subterms under main terms may continue to next column or page

Osteoporosis — *continued*
- disuse M81.8
  - with current pathological fracture M80.80 ☑
    - carpus M80.84- ☑
    - clavicle M80.81- ☑
    - fibula M80.86- ☑
    - finger M80.84- ☑
    - humerus M80.82- ☑
    - ilium M80.85- ☑
    - ischium M80.85- ☑
    - metacarpus M80.84- ☑
    - metatarsus M80.87- ☑
    - pelvis M80.85- ☑
    - radius M80.83- ☑
    - scapula M80.81- ☑
    - tarsus M80.87- ☑
    - tibia M80.86- ☑
    - toe M80.87- ☑
    - ulna M80.83- ☑
    - vertebra M80.88 ☑
- drug-induced — *see* Osteoporosis, specified type NEC
- idiopathic — *see* Osteoporosis, specified type NEC
- involutional — *see* Osteoporosis, age-related
- Lequesne M81.6
- localized M81.6
- postmenopausal M81.0
  - with pathological fracture M80.00 ☑
    - carpus M80.04- ☑
    - clavicle M80.01- ☑
    - fibula M80.06- ☑
    - finger M80.04- ☑
    - humerus M80.02- ☑
    - ilium M80.05- ☑
    - ischium M80.05- ☑
    - metacarpus M80.04- ☑
    - metatarsus M80.07- ☑
    - pelvis M80.05- ☑
    - radius M80.03- ☑
    - scapula M80.01- ☑
    - tarsus M80.07- ☑
    - tibia M80.06- ☑
    - toe M80.07- ☑
    - ulna M80.03- ☑
    - vertebra M80.08 ☑
- postoophorectomy — *see* Osteoporosis, specified type NEC
- postsurgical malabsorption — *see* Osteoporosis, specified type NEC
- post-traumatic — *see* Osteoporosis, specified type NEC
- senile — *see* Osteoporosis, age-related
- specified type NEC M81.8
  - with pathological fracture M80.80 ☑
    - carpus M80.84- ☑
    - clavicle M80.81- ☑·
    - fibula M80.86- ☑
    - finger M80.84- ☑
    - humerus M80.82- ☑
    - ilium M80.85- ☑
    - ischium M80.85- ☑
    - metacarpus M80.84- ☑
    - metatarsus M80.87- ☑
    - pelvis M80.85- ☑
    - radius M80.83- ☑
    - scapula M80.81- ☑
    - tarsus M80.87- ☑
    - tibia M80.86- ☑
    - toe M80.87- ☑
    - ulna M80.83- ☑
    - vertebra M80.88 ☑

Osteopsathyrosis (idiopathica) Q78.0
Osteoradionecrosis, jaw (acute) (chronic) (lower) (suppurative) (upper) M27.2
Osteosarcoma (any form) — *see* Neoplasm, bone, malignant
Osteosclerosis Q78.2
- acquired M85.8- ☑
- congenita Q77.4
- fragilitas (generalisata) Q78.2
- myelofibrosis D75.81

Osteosclerotic anemia D64.89
Osteosis
- cutis L94.2
- renal fibrocystic N25.0

Österreicher-Turner syndrome Q87.2
Ostium
- atrioventriculare commune Q21.2

Ostium — *continued*
- primum (arteriosum) (defect) (persistent) Q21.2
- secundum (arteriosum) (defect) (patent) (persistent) Q21.1

Ostrum-Furst syndrome Q75.8
Otalgia H92.0 ☑
Otitis (acute) H66.90
- with effusion — *see also* Otitis, media, nonsuppurative
  - purulent — *see* Otitis, media, suppurative
- adhesive — *see* subcategory H74.1 ☑
- chronic — *see also* Otitis, media, chronic
  - with effusion — *see also* Otitis, media, nonsuppurative, chronic
- externa H60.9- ☑
  - abscess — *see* Abscess, ear, external
  - acute (noninfective) H60.50- ☑
    - actinic H60.51- ☑
    - chemical H60.52- ☑
    - contact H60.53- ☑
    - eczematoid H60.54- ☑
    - infective — *see* Otitis, externa, infective
    - reactive H60.55- ☑
    - specified NEC H60.59- ☑
  - cellulitis — *see* Cellulitis, ear
  - chronic H60.6- ☑
  - diffuse — *see* Otitis, externa, infective, diffuse
  - hemorrhagic — *see* Otitis, externa, infective, hemorrhagic
  - in (due to)
    - aspergillosis B44.89
    - candidiasis B37.84
    - erysipelas A46 *[H62.40]*
    - herpes (simplex) virus infection B00.1
      - zoster B02.8
    - impetigo L01.00 *[H62.40]*
    - infectious disease NEC B99 ☑ *[H62.4-]*
    - mycosis NEC B36.9 *[H62.40]*
    - parasitic disease NEC B89 *[H62.40]*
    - viral disease NEC B34.9 *[H62.40]*
    - zoster B02.8
  - infective NEC H60.39- ☑
    - abscess — *see* Abscess, ear, external
    - cellulitis — *see* Cellulitis, ear
    - diffuse H60.31- ☑
    - hemorrhagic H60.32- ☑
    - swimmer's ear — *see* Swimmer's, ear
  - malignant H60.2- ☑
  - mycotic NEC B36.9 *[H62.40]*
    - in
      - aspergillosis B44.89
      - candidiasis B37.84
      - moniliasis B37.84
  - necrotizing — *see* Otitis, externa, malignant
  - Pseudomonas aeruginosa — *see* Otitis, externa, malignant
  - reactive — *see* Otitis, externa, acute, reactive
  - specified NEC — *see* subcategory H60.8 ☑
  - tropical NEC B36.9 *[H62.40]*
    - in
      - aspergillosis B44.89
      - candidiasis B37.84
      - moniliasis B37.84
- insidiosa — *see* Otosclerosis
- interna H83.0 ☑
- media (hemorrhagic) (staphylococcal) (streptococcal) H66.9- ☑
  - with effusion (nonpurulent) — *see* Otitis, media, nonsuppurative
  - acute, subacute H66.90
    - allergic — *see* Otitis, media, nonsuppurative, acute, allergic
    - exudative — *see* Otitis, media, suppurative, acute
    - mucoid — *see* Otitis, media, nonsuppurative, acute
    - necrotizing — *see also* Otitis, media, suppurative, acute
      - in
        - measles B05.3
        - scarlet fever A38.0
    - nonsuppurative NEC — *see* Otitis, media, nonsuppurative, acute
    - purulent — *see* Otitis, media, suppurative, acute
    - sanguinous — *see* Otitis, media, nonsuppurative, acute
    - secretory — *see* Otitis, media, nonsuppurative, acute, serous

Otitis — *continued*
- media — *continued*
  - acute, subacute — *continued*
    - seromucinous — *see* Otitis, media, nonsuppurative, acute
    - serous — *see* Otitis, media, nonsuppurative, acute, serous
    - suppurative — *see* Otitis, media, suppurative, acute
  - allergic — *see* Otitis, media, nonsuppurative
  - catarrhal — *see* Otitis, media, nonsuppurative
  - chronic H66.90
    - with effusion (nonpurulent) — *see* Otitis, media, nonsuppurative, chronic
    - allergic — *see* Otitis, media, nonsuppurative, chronic, allergic
    - benign suppurative — *see* Otitis, media, suppurative, chronic, tubotympanic
    - catarrhal — *see* Otitis, media, nonsuppurative, chronic, serous
    - exudative — *see* Otitis, media, nonsuppurative, chronic
    - mucinous — *see* Otitis, media, nonsuppurative, chronic, mucoid
    - mucoid — *see* Otitis, media, nonsuppurative, chronic, mucoid
    - nonsuppurative NEC — *see* Otitis, media, nonsuppurative, chronic
    - purulent — *see* Otitis, media, suppurative, chronic
    - secretory — *see* Otitis, media, nonsuppurative, chronic, mucoid
    - seromucinous — *see* Otitis, media, nonsuppurative, chronic
    - serous — *see* Otitis, media, nonsuppurative, chronic, serous
    - suppurative — *see* Otitis, media, suppurative, chronic
    - transudative — *see* Otitis, media, nonsuppurative, chronic, mucoid
  - exudative — *see* Otitis, media, suppurative
  - in (due to) (with)
    - influenza — *see* Influenza, with, otitis media
    - measles B05.3
    - scarlet fever A38.0
    - tuberculosis A18.6
    - viral disease NEC B34.- ☑ *[H67.-]*
  - mucoid — *see* Otitis, media, nonsuppurative
  - nonsuppurative H65.9- ☑
    - acute or subacute NEC H65.19- ☑
      - allergic H65.11- ☑
        - recurrent H65.11- ☑
      - recurrent H65.19- ☑
      - secretory — *see* Otitis, media, nonsuppurative, serous
      - serous H65.0- ☑
        - recurrent H65.0- ☑
    - chronic H65.49- ☑
      - allergic H65.41- ☑
      - mucoid H65.3- ☑
      - serous H65.2- ☑
  - postmeasles B05.3
  - purulent — *see* Otitis, media, suppurative
  - secretory — *see* Otitis, media, nonsuppurative
  - seromucinous — *see* Otitis, media, nonsuppurative
  - serous — *see* Otitis, media, nonsuppurative
  - suppurative H66.4- ☑
    - acute H66.00- ☑
      - with rupture of ear drum H66.01- ☑
      - recurrent H66.00- ☑
        - with rupture of ear drum H66.01- ☑
    - chronic — *see also* subcategory H66.3 ☑
      - atticoantral H66.2- ☑
      - benign — *see* Otitis, media, suppurative, chronic, tubotympanic
      - tubotympanic H66.1- ☑
  - transudative — *see* Otitis, media, nonsuppurative
  - tuberculous A18.6

Otocephaly Q18.2
Otolith syndrome — *see* subcategory H81.8 ☑
Otomycosis (diffuse) **NEC** B36.9 *[H62.40]*
- in
  - aspergillosis B44.89
  - candidiasis B37.84
  - moniliasis B37.84

Otoporosis — *see* Otosclerosis
Otorrhagia (nontraumatic) H92.2- ☑

Otorrhagia — *continued*
traumatic — *code by* Type of injury
Otorrhea H92.1- ☑
cerebrospinal G96.0
Otosclerosis (general) H80.9- ☑
cochlear (endosteal) H80.2- ☑
involving
otic capsule — *see* Otosclerosis, cochlear
oval window
nonobliterative H80.0- ☑
obliterative H80.1- ☑
round window — *see* Otosclerosis, cochlear
nonobliterative — *see* Otosclerosis, involving, oval
window, nonobliterative
obliterative — *see* Otosclerosis, involving, oval window,
obliterative
specified NEC H80.8- ☑
Otospongiosis — *see* Otosclerosis
Otto's disease or pelvis M24.7
Outcome of delivery Z37.9
multiple births Z37.9
all liveborn Z37.50
quadruplets Z37.52
quintuplets Z37.53
sextuplets Z37.54
specified number NEC Z37.59
triplets Z37.51
all stillborn Z37.7
some liveborn Z37.60
quadruplets Z37.62
quintuplets Z37.63
sextuplets Z37.64
specified number NEC Z37.69
triplets Z37.61
single NEC Z37.9
liveborn Z37.0
stillborn Z37.1
twins NEC Z37.9
both liveborn Z37.2
both stillborn Z37.4
one liveborn, one stillborn Z37.3
Outlet — *see* condition
Ovalocytosis (congenital) (hereditary) — *see* Elliptocytosis
Ovarian — *see* Condition
Ovariocele N83.4- ☑
Ovaritis (cystic) — *see* Oophoritis
Ovary, ovarian — *see also* condition
resistant syndrome E28.39
vein syndrome N13.8
Overactive — *see also* Hyperfunction
adrenal cortex NEC E27.0
bladder N32.81
hypothalamus E23.3
thyroid — *see* Hyperthyroidism
Overactivity R46.3
child — *see* Disorder, attention-deficit hyperactivity
Overbite (deep) (excessive) (horizontal) (vertical) M26.29
Overbreathing — *see* Hyperventilation
Overconscientious personality F60.5
Overdevelopment — *see* Hypertrophy
Overdistension — *see* Distension
Overdose, overdosage (drug) — *see* Table of Drugs and
Chemicals, by drug, poisoning
Overeating R63.2
nonorganic origin F50.89
psychogenic F50.89
Overexertion (effects) (exhaustion) T73.3 ☑
Overexposure (effects) T73.9 ☑
exhaustion T73.2 ☑
Overfeeding — *see* Overeating
newborn P92.4
Overfill, endodontic M27.52
Overgrowth, bone — *see* Hypertrophy, bone
Overhanging of dental restorative material (unrepairable) K08.52
Overheated (places) (effects) — *see* Heat
Overjet (excessive horizontal) M26.23
Overlaid, overlying (suffocation) — *see* Asphyxia, traumatic, due to mechanical threat
Overlap, excessive horizontal (teeth) M26.23
Overlapping toe (acquired) — *see also* Deformity, toe,
specified NEC
congenital (fifth toe) Q66.89
Overload
circulatory, due to transfusion (blood) (blood components) (TACO) E87.71

Overload — *continued*
fluid E87.70
due to transfusion (blood) (blood components)
E87.71
specified NEC E87.79
iron, due to repeated red blood cell transfusions
E83.111
potassium (K) E87.5
sodium (Na) E87.0
Overnutrition — *see* Hyperalimentation
Overproduction — *see also* Hypersecretion
ACTH E27.0
catecholamine E27.5
growth hormone E22.0
Overprotection, child by parent Z62.1
Overriding
aorta Q25.49
finger (acquired) — *see* Deformity, finger
congenital Q68.1
toe (acquired) — *see also* Deformity, toe, specified NEC
congenital Q66.89
Overstrained R53.83
heart — *see* Hypertrophy, cardiac
Overuse, muscle NEC M70.8- ☑
Overweight E66.3
Overworked R53.83
Oviduct — *see* condition
Ovotestis Q56.0
Ovulation (cycle)
failure or lack of N97.0
pain N94.0
Ovum — *see* condition
Owren's disease or syndrome (parahemophilia) D68.2
Ox heart — *see* Hypertrophy, cardiac
Oxalosis E72.53
Oxaluria E72.53
Oxycephaly, oxycephalic Q75.0
syphilitic, congenital A50.02
Oxyuriasis B80
Oxyuris vermicularis (infestation) B80
Ozena J31.0

P

Pachyderma, pachydermia L85.9
larynx (verrucosa) J38.7
Pachydermatocele (congenital) Q82.8
Pachydermoperiostosis — *see also* Osteoarthropathy,
hypertrophic, specified type NEC
clubbed nail M89.40 *[L62]*
Pachygyria Q04.3
Pachymeningitis (adhesive) (basal) (brain) (cervical)
(chronic)(circumscribed) (external) (fibrous) (hemorrhagic) (hypertrophic) (internal) (purulent) (spinal)
(suppurative) — *see* Meningitis
Pachyonychia (congenital) Q84.5
Pacinian tumor — *see* Neoplasm, skin, benign
Pad, knuckle or Garrod's M72.1
Paget's disease
with infiltrating duct carcinoma — *see* Neoplasm,
breast, malignant
bone M88.9
carpus M88.84- ☑
clavicle M88.81- ☑
femur M88.85- ☑
fibula M88.86- ☑
finger M88.84- ☑
humerus M88.82- ☑
ilium M88.85- ☑
in neoplastic disease — *see* Osteitis, deformans, in
neoplastic disease
ischium M88.85- ☑
metacarpus M88.84- ☑
metatarsus M88.87- ☑
multiple sites M88.89
neck M88.88
radius M88.83- ☑
rib M88.88
scapula M88.81- ☑
skull M88.0
specified NEC M88.88
tarsus M88.87- ☑
tibia M88.86- ☑
toe M88.87- ☑
ulna M88.83- ☑
vertebra M88.1
breast (female) C50.01- ☑

Paget's disease — *continued*
breast — *continued*
male C50.02- ☑
extramammary — *see also* Neoplasm, skin, malignant
anus C21.0
margin C44.590
skin C44.590
intraductal carcinoma — *see* Neoplasm, breast, malignant
malignant — *see* Neoplasm, skin, malignant
breast (female) C50.01- ☑
male C50.02- ☑
unspecified site (female) C50.01- ☑
male C50.02- ☑
mammary — *see* Paget's disease, breast
nipple — *see* Paget's disease, breast
osteitis deformans — *see* Paget's disease, bone
Paget-Schroetter syndrome I82.890
Pain(s) — *see also* Painful R52
abdominal R10.9
colic R10.83
generalized R10.84
with acute abdomen R10.0
lower R10.30
left quadrant R10.32
pelvic or perineal R10.2
periumbilical R10.33
right quadrant R10.31
rebound — *see* Tenderness, abdominal, rebound
severe with abdominal rigidity R10.0
tenderness — *see* Tenderness, abdominal
upper R10.10
epigastric R10.13
left quadrant R10.12
right quadrant R10.11
acute R52
due to trauma G89.11
neoplasm related G89.3
postprocedural NEC G89.18
post-thoracotomy G89.12
specified by site — *code to* Pain, by site
adnexa (uteri) R10.2
anginoid — *see* Pain, precordial
anus K62.89
arm — *see* Pain, limb, upper
axillary (axilla) M79.62- ☑
back (postural) M54.9
bladder R39.89
associated with micturition — *see* Micturition,
painful
chronic R39.82
bone — *see* Disorder, bone, specified type NEC
breast N64.4
broad ligament R10.2
cancer associated (acute) (chronic) G89.3
cecum — *see* Pain, abdominal
cervicobrachial M53.1
chest (central) R07.9
anterior wall R07.89
atypical R07.89
ischemic I20.9
musculoskeletal R07.89
non-cardiac R07.89
on breathing R07.1
pleurodynia R07.81
precordial R07.2
wall (anterior) R07.89
chronic G89.29
associated with significant psychosocial dysfunction
G89.4
due to trauma G89.21
neoplasm related G89.3
postoperative NEC G89.28
postprocedural NEC G89.28
post-thoracotomy G89.22
specified NEC G89.29
coccyx M53.3
colon — *see* Pain, abdominal
coronary — *see* Angina
costochondral R07.1
diaphragm R07.1
due to cancer G89.3
due to device, implant or graft — *see also* Complications, by site and type, specified NEC T85.848 ☑
arterial graft NEC T82.848 ☑
breast (implant) T85.848 ☑
catheter NEC T85.848 ☑
dialysis (renal) T82.848 ☑

Pain(s) — *continued*
  due to device, implant or graft — *see also* Complications, by site and type, specified — *continued*
      catheter — *continued*
        dialysis — *continued*
            intraperitoneal T85.848 ☑
          infusion NEC T82.848 ☑
              spinal (epidural) (subdural) T85.840 ☑
          urinary (indwelling) T83.84 ☑
        electronic (electrode) (pulse generator) (stimulator)
            bone T85.840 ☑
            cardiac T82.847 ☑
            nervous system (brain) (peripheral nerve) (spinal)
                T85.84 ☑
            urinary T83.84 ☑
      fixation, internal (orthopedic) NEC T84.84 ☑
      gastrointestinal (bile duct) (esophagus) T85.848 ☑
      genital NEC T83.84 ☑
      heart NEC T82.847 ☑
      infusion NEC T85.848 ☑
      joint prosthesis T84.84 ☑
      ocular (corneal graft) (orbital implant) NEC
          T85.848 ☑
      orthopedic NEC T84.84 ☑
      specified NEC T85.848 ☑
      urinary NEC T83.84 ☑
      vascular NEC T82.848 ☑
      ventricular intracranial shunt T85.840 ☑
  due to malignancy (primary) (secondary) G89.3
  ear — *see* subcategory H92.0 ☑
  epigastric, epigastrium R10.13
  eye — *see* Pain, ocular
  face, facial R51
    atypical G50.1
  female genital organs NEC N94.89
  finger — *see* Pain, limb, upper
  flank — *see* Pain, abdominal
  foot — *see* Pain, limb, lower
  gallbladder K82.9
  gas (intestinal) R14.1
  gastric — *see* Pain, abdominal
  generalized NOS R52
  genital organ
    female N94.89
    male N50.89
  groin — *see* Pain, abdominal, lower
  hand — *see* Pain, limb, upper
  head — *see* Headache
  heart — *see* Pain, precordial
  infra-orbital — *see* Neuralgia, trigeminal
  intercostal R07.82
  intermenstrual N94.0
  jaw R68.84
  joint M25.50
    ankle M25.57- ☑
    elbow M25.52- ☑
    finger M25.54- ☑
    foot M25.57- ☑
    hand M25.54- ☑
    hip M25.55- ☑
    knee M25.56- ☑
    shoulder M25.51- ☑
    toe M25.57- ☑
    wrist M25.53- ☑
  kidney N23
  laryngeal R07.0
  leg — *see* Pain, limb, lower
  limb M79.609
    lower M79.60- ☑
      foot M79.67- ☑
      lower leg M79.66- ☑
      thigh M79.65- ☑
      toe M79.67- ☑
    upper M79.60- ☑
      axilla M79.62- ☑
      finger M79.64- ☑
      forearm M79.63- ☑
      hand M79.64- ☑
      upper arm M79.62- ☑
  loin M54.5
  low back M54.5
  lumbar region M54.5
  mandibular R68.84
  mastoid — *see* subcategory H92.0 ☑
  maxilla R68.84
  menstrual — *see also* Dysmenorrhea N94.6
  metacarpophalangeal (joint) — *see* Pain, joint, hand

Pain(s) — *continued*
  metatarsophalangeal (joint) — *see* Pain, joint, foot
  mouth K13.79
  muscle — *see* Myalgia
  musculoskeletal — *see also* Pain, by site M79.18
  myofascial M79.18
  nasal J34.89
  nasopharynx J39.2
  neck NEC M54.2
  nerve NEC — *see* Neuralgia
  neuromuscular — *see* Neuralgia
  nose J34.89
  ocular H57.1- ☑
  ophthalmic — *see* Pain, ocular
  orbital region — *see* Pain, ocular
  ovary N94.89
  over heart — *see* Pain, precordial
  ovulation N94.0
  pelvic (female) R10.2
  penis N48.89
  pericardial — *see* Pain, precordial
  perineal, perineum R10.2
  pharynx J39.2
  pleura, pleural, pleuritic R07.81
  postoperative NOS G89.18
  postprocedural NOS G89.18
  post-thoracotomy G89.12
  precordial (region) R07.2
  premenstrual N94.3
  psychogenic (persistent) (any site) F45.41
  radicular (spinal) — *see* Radiculopathy
  rectum K62.89
  respiration R07.1
  retrosternal R07.2
  rheumatoid, muscular — *see* Myalgia
  rib R07.81
  root (spinal) — *see* Radiculopathy
  round ligament (stretch) R10.2
  sacroiliac M53.3
  sciatic — *see* Sciatica
  scrotum N50.82
  seminal vesicle N50.89
  shoulder M25.51- ☑
  spermatic cord N50.89
  spinal root — *see* Radiculopathy
  spine M54.9
    cervical M54.2
    low back M54.5
      with sciatica M54.4- ☑
    thoracic M54.6
  stomach — *see* Pain, abdominal
  substernal R07.2
  temporomandibular (joint) M26.62- ☑
  testis N50.81- ☑
  thoracic spine M54.6
    with radicular and visceral pain M54.14
  throat R07.0
  tibia — *see* Pain, limb, lower
  toe — *see* Pain, limb, lower
  tongue K14.6
  tooth K08.89
  trigeminal — *see* Neuralgia, trigeminal
  tumor associated G89.3
  ureter N23
  urinary (organ) (system) N23
  uterus NEC N94.89
  vagina R10.2
  vertebrogenic (syndrome) M54.89
  vesical R39.89
    associated with micturition — *see* Micturition, painful
  vulva R10.2
Painful — *see also* Pain
  coitus
    female N94.10
    male N53.12
      psychogenic F52.6
  ejaculation (semen) N53.12
      psychogenic F52.6
  erection — *see* Priapism
  feet syndrome E53.8
  joint replacement (hip) (knee) T84.84 ☑
  menstruation — *see* Dysmenorrhea
      psychogenic F45.8
  micturition — *see* Micturition, painful
  respiration R07.1
  scar NEC L90.5
  wire sutures T81.89 ☑

Painter's colic — *see* subcategory T56.0 ☑
Palate — *see* condition
Palatoplegia K13.79
Palatoschisis — *see* Cleft, palate
Palilalia R48.8
Palliative care Z51.5
Pallor R23.1
  optic disc, temporal — *see* Atrophy, optic
Palmar — *see also* condition
  fascia — *see* condition
Palpable
  cecum K63.89
  kidney N28.89
  ovary N83.8
  prostate N42.9
  spleen — *see* Splenomegaly
Palpitations (heart) R00.2
  psychogenic F45.8
Palsy — *see also* Paralysis G83.9
  atrophic diffuse (progressive) G12.22
  Bell's — *see also* Palsy, facial
    newborn P11.3
  brachial plexus NEC G54.0
    newborn (birth injury) P14.3
  brain — *see* Palsy, cerebral
  bulbar (progressive) (chronic) G12.22
    of childhood (Fazio-Londe) G12.1
    pseudo NEC G12.29
    supranuclear (progressive) G23.1
  cerebral (congenital) G80.9
    ataxic G80.4
    athetoid G80.3
    choreathetoid G80.3
    diplegic G80.8
      spastic G80.1
    dyskinetic G80.3
      athetoid G80.3
      choreathetoid G80.3
      distonic G80.3
    dystonic G80.3
    hemiplegic G80.8
      spastic G80.2
    mixed G80.8
    monoplegic G80.8
      spastic G80.1
    paraplegic G80.8
      spastic G80.1
    quadriplegic G80.8
      spastic G80.0
    spastic G80.1
      diplegic G80.1
      hemiplegic G80.2
      monoplegic G80.1
      quadriplegic G80.0
      specified NEC G80.1
      tetrapelgic G80.0
    specified NEC G80.8
    syphilitic A52.12
      congenital A50.49
    tetraplegic G80.8
      spastic G80.0
  cranial nerve — *see also* Disorder, nerve, cranial
    multiple G52.7
      in
        infectious disease B99 ☑ *[G53]*
        neoplastic disease — *see also* Neoplasm
            D49.9 *[G53]*
        parasitic disease B89 *[G53]*
        sarcoidosis D86.82
  creeping G12.22
  diver's T70.3 ☑
  Erb's P14.0
  facial G51.0
    newborn (birth injury) P11.3
  glossopharyngeal G52.1
  Klumpke (-Déjérine) P14.1
  lead — *see* subcategory T56.0 ☑
  median nerve (tardy) G56.1- ☑
  nerve G58.9
    specified NEC G58.8
  peroneal nerve (acute) (tardy) G57.3- ☑
  progressive supranuclear G23.1
  pseudobulbar NEC G12.29
  radial nerve (acute) G56.3- ☑
  seventh nerve — *see also* Palsy, facial
    newborn P11.3
  shaking — *see* Parkinsonism
  spastic (cerebral) (spinal) G80.1

Palsy — continued
  ulnar nerve (tardy) G56.2- ☑
  wasting G12.29
Paludism — see Malaria
Panangiitis M30.0
Panaris, panaritium — see also Cellulitis, digit
  with lymphangitis — see Lymphangitis, acute, digit
Panarteritis nodosa M30.0
  brain or cerebral I67.7
Pancake heart R93.1
  with cor pulmonale (chronic) I27.81
Pancarditis (acute) (chronic) I51.89
  rheumatic I09.89
    active or acute I01.8
Pancoast's syndrome or tumor C34.1- ☑
Pancolitis, ulcerative (chronic) K51.00
  with
    abscess K51.014
    complication K51.019
    fistula K51.013
    obstruction K51.012
    rectal bleeding K51.011
    specified complication NEC K51.018
Pancreas, pancreatic — see condition
Pancreatitis (annular) (apoplectic) (calcareous) (edematous) (hemorrhagic) (malignant) (recurrent) (subacute) (suppurative) K85.90
  with necrosis (uninfected) K85.91
    infected K85.92
  acute (without necrosis or infection) K85.90
    with necrosis (uninfected) K85.91
      infected K85.92
    alcohol induced (without necrosis or infection) K85.20
      with necrosis (uninfected) K85.21
        infected K85.22
    biliary (without necrosis or infection) K85.10
      with necrosis (uninfected) K85.11
        infected K85.12
    drug induced (without necrosis or infection) K85.30
      with necrosis (uninfected) K85.31
        infected K85.32
    gallstone (without necrosis or infection) K85.10
      with necrosis (uninfected) K85.11
        infected K85.12
    idiopathic (without necrosis or infection) K85.00
      with necrosis (uninfected) K85.01
        infected K85.02
    specified NEC (without necrosis or infection) K85.80
      with necrosis (uninfected) K85.81
        infected K85.82
  chronic (infectious) K86.1
    alcohol-induced K86.0
    recurrent K86.1
    relapsing K86.1
  cystic (chronic) K86.1
  cytomegaloviral B25.2
  fibrous (chronic) K86.1
  gallstone (without necrosis or infection) K85.10
    with necrosis (uninfected) K85.11
      infected K85.12
  gangrenous — see Pancreatitis, acute
  interstitial (chronic) K86.1
    acute — see also Pancreatitis, acute K85.80
  mumps B26.3
  recurrent (chronic) K86.1
  relapsing, chronic K86.1
  syphilitic A52.74
Pancreatoblastoma — see Neoplasm, pancreas, malignant
Pancreolithiasis K86.89
Pancytolysis D75.89
Pancytopenia (acquired) D61.818
  with
    malformations D61.09
    myelodysplastic syndrome — see Syndrome, myelodysplastic
  antineoplastic chemotherapy induced D61.810
  congenital D61.09
  drug-induced NEC D61.811
PANDAS (pediatric autoimmune neuropsychiatric disorders associated with streptococcal infections syndrome) D89.89
Panencephalitis, subacute, sclerosing A81.1
Panhematopenia D61.9
  congenital D61.09
  constitutional D61.09
  splenic, primary D73.1

Panhemocytopenia D61.9
  congenital D61.09
  constitutional D61.09
Panhypogonadism E29.1
Panhypopituitarism E23.0
  prepubertal E23.0
Panic (attack) (state) F41.0
  reaction to exceptional stress (transient) F43.0
Panmyelopathy, familial, constitutional D61.09
Panmyelophthisis D61.82
  congenital D61.09
Panmyelosis (acute) (with myelofibrosis) C94.4- ☑
Panner's disease — see Osteochondrosis, juvenile, humerus
Panneuritis endemica E51.11
Panniculitis (nodular) (nonsuppurative) M79.3
  back M54.00
    cervical region M54.02
    cervicothoracic region M54.03
    lumbar region M54.06
    lumbosacral region M54.07
    multiple sites M54.09
    occipito-atlanto-axial region M54.01
    sacrococcygeal region M54.08
    thoracic region M54.04
    thoracolumbar region M54.05
  lupus L93.2
  mesenteric K65.4
  neck M54.02
    cervicothoracic region M54.03
    occipito-atlanto-axial region M54.01
  relapsing M35.6
Panniculus adiposus (abdominal) E65
Pannus (allergic) (cornea) (degenerativus) (keratic) H16.42- ☑
  abdominal (symptomatic) E65
  trachomatosus, trachomatous (active) A71.1
Panophthalmitis H44.01- ☑
Pansinusitis (chronic) (hyperplastic) (nonpurulent) (purulent) J32.4
  acute J01.40
    recurrent J01.41
  tuberculous A15.8
Panuveitis (sympathetic) H44.11- ☑
Panvalvular disease I08.9
  specified NEC I08.8
PAPA (pyogenic arthritis, pyoderma gangrenosum, and acne syndrome) M04.8
Papanicolaou smear, cervix Z12.4
  as part of routine gynecological examination Z01.419
    with abnormal findings Z01.411
  for suspected neoplasm Z12.4
  nonspecific abnormal finding R87.619
  routine Z01.419
    with abnormal findings Z01.411
Papilledema (choked disc) H47.10
  associated with
    decreased ocular pressure H47.12
    increased intracranial pressure H47.11
    retinal disorder H47.13
  Foster-Kennedy syndrome H47.14- ☑
Papillitis H46.00
  anus K62.89
  chronic lingual K14.4
  necrotizing, kidney N17.2
  optic H46.0- ☑
  rectum K62.89
  renal, necrotizing N17.2
  tongue K14.0
Papilloma — see also Neoplasm, benign, by site
  acuminatum (female) (male) (anogenital) A63.0
  basal cell L82.1
    inflamed L82.0
  benign pinta (primary) A67.0
  bladder (urinary) (transitional cell) D41.4
  choroid plexus (lateral ventricle) (third ventricle) D33.0
    anaplastic C71.5
    fourth ventricle D33.1
    malignant C71.5
  renal pelvis (transitional cell) D41.1- ☑
    benign D30.1- ☑
  Schneiderian
    specified site — see Neoplasm, benign, by site
    unspecified site D14.0
  serous surface
    borderline malignancy
      specified site — see Neoplasm, uncertain behavior, by site

Papilloma — continued
  serous surface — continued
    borderline malignancy — continued
      unspecified site D39.10
    specified site — see Neoplasm, benign, by site
    unspecified site D27.9
  transitional (cell)
    bladder (urinary) D41.4
    inverted type — see Neoplasm, uncertain behavior, by site
    renal pelvis D41.1- ☑
    ureter D41.2- ☑
  ureter (transitional cell) D41.2- ☑
    benign D30.2- ☑
  urothelial — see Neoplasm, uncertain behavior, by site
  villous — see Neoplasm, uncertain behavior, by site
    adenocarcinoma in — see Neoplasm, malignant, by site
    in situ — see Neoplasm, in situ
  yaws, plantar or palmar A66.1
Papillomata, multiple, of yaws A66.1
Papillomatosis — see also Neoplasm, benign, by site
  confluent and reticulated L83
  cystic, breast — see Mastopathy, cystic
  ductal, breast — see Mastopathy, cystic
  intraductal (diffuse) — see Neoplasm, benign, by site
  subareolar duct D24- ☑
Papillomavirus, as cause of disease classified elsewhere B97.7
Papillon-Léage and Psaume syndrome Q87.0
Papule(s) R23.8
  carate (primary) A67.0
  fibrous, of nose D22.39
  Gottron's L94.4
  pinta (primary) A67.0
Papulosis
  lymphomatoid C86.6
  malignant I77.89
Papyraceous fetus O31.0- ☑
Para-albuminemia E88.09
Paracephalus Q89.7
Parachute mitral valve Q23.2
Paracoccidioidomycosis B41.9
  disseminated B41.7
  generalized B41.7
  mucocutaneous-lymphangitic B41.8
  pulmonary B41.0
  specified NEC B41.8
  visceral B41.8
Paradentosis K05.4
Paraffinoma T88.8 ☑
Paraganglioma D44.7
  adrenal D35.0- ☑
    malignant C74.1- ☑
  aortic body D44.7
    malignant C75.5
  carotid body D44.6
    malignant C75.4
  chromaffin — see also Neoplasm, benign, by site
    malignant — see Neoplasm, malignant, by site
  extra-adrenal D44.7
    malignant C75.5
      specified site — see Neoplasm, malignant, by site
      unspecified site C75.5
    specified site — see Neoplasm, uncertain behavior, by site
    unspecified site D44.7
  gangliocytic D13.2
    specified site — see Neoplasm, benign, by site
    unspecified site D13.2
  glomus jugulare D44.7
    malignant C75.5
  jugular D44.7
  malignant C75.5
    specified site — see Neoplasm, malignant, by site
    unspecified site C75.5
  nonchromaffin D44.7
    malignant C75.5
      specified site — see Neoplasm, malignant, by site
      unspecified site C75.5
    specified site — see Neoplasm, uncertain behavior, by site
    unspecified site D44.7
  parasympathetic D44.7

Paraganglioma — *continued*
  parasympathetic — *continued*
    specified site — *see* Neoplasm, uncertain behavior,
      by site
    unspecified site D44.7
  specified site — *see* Neoplasm, uncertain behavior, by
    site
  sympathetic D44.7
    specified site — *see* Neoplasm, uncertain behavior,
      by site
    unspecified site D44.7
  unspecified site D44.7
Parageusia R43.2
  psychogenic F45.8
Paragonimiasis B66.4
Paragranuloma, Hodgkin — *see* Lymphoma, Hodgkin,
  specified NEC
Parahemophilia — *see also* Defect, coagulation D68.2
Parakeratosis R23.4
  variegata L41.0
Paralysis, paralytic (complete) (incomplete) G83.9
  with
    syphilis A52.17
  abducens, abducent (nerve) — *see* Strabismus, paralyt-
    ic, sixth nerve
  abductor, lower extremity G57.9- ☑
  accessory nerve G52.8
  accommodation — *see also* Paresis, of accommodation
    hysterical F44.89
  acoustic nerve (except Deafness) H93.3 ☑
  agitans — *see also* Parkinsonism G20
    arteriosclerotic G21.4
  alternating (oculomotor) G83.89
  amyotrophic G12.21
  ankle G57.9- ☑
  anus (sphincter) K62.89
  arm — *see* Monoplegia, upper limb
  ascending (spinal), acute G61.0
  association G12.29
  asthenic bulbar G70.00
    with exacerbation (acute) G70.01
    in crisis G70.01
  ataxic (hereditary) G11.9
    general (syphilitic) A52.17
  atrophic G58.9
    infantile, acute — *see* Poliomyelitis, paralytic
    progressive G12.22
    spinal (acute) — *see* Poliomyelitis, paralytic
  axillary G54.0
  Babinski-Nageotte's G83.89
  Bell's G51.0
    newborn P11.3
  Benedikt's G46.3
  birth injury P14.9
    spinal cord P11.5
  bladder (neurogenic) (sphincter) N31.2
  bowel, colon or intestine K56.0
  brachial plexus G54.0
    birth injury P14.3
    newborn (birth injury) P14.3
  brain G83.9
    diplegia G83.0
    triplegia G83.89
  bronchial J98.09
  Brown-Séquard G83.81
  bulbar (chronic) (progressive) G12.22
    infantile — *see* Poliomyelitis, paralytic
    poliomyelitic — *see* Poliomyelitis, paralytic
    pseudo G12.29
  bulbospinal G70.00
    with exacerbation (acute) G70.01
    in crisis G70.01
  cardiac — *see also* Failure, heart I50.9
  cerebrocerebellar, diplegic G80.1
  cervical
    plexus G54.2
    sympathetic G90.09
  Céstan-Chenais G46.3
  Charcot-Marie-Tooth type G60.0
  Clark's G80.9
  colon K56.0
  compressed air T70.3 ☑
  compression
    arm G56.9- ☑
    leg G57.9- ☑
    lower extremity G57.9- ☑
    upper extremity G56.9- ☑
  congenital (cerebral) — *see* Palsy, cerebral

Paralysis, paralytic — *continued*
  conjugate movement (gaze) (of eye) H51.0
    cortical (nuclear) (supranuclear) H51.0
  cordis — *see* Failure, heart
  cranial or cerebral nerve G52.9
  creeping G12.22
  crossed leg G83.89
  crutch — *see* Injury, brachial plexus
  deglutition R13.0
    hysterical F44.4
  dementia A52.17
  descending (spinal) NEC G12.29
  diaphragm (flaccid) J98.6
    due to accidental dissection of phrenic nerve during
      procedure — *see* Puncture, accidental compli-
      cating surgery
  digestive organs NEC K59.8
  diplegic — *see* Diplegia
  divergence (nuclear) H51.8
  diver's T70.3 ☑
  Duchenne's
    birth injury P14.0
    due to or associated with
      motor neuron disease G12.22
      muscular dystrophy G71.02
  due to intracranial or spinal birth injury — *see* Palsy,
    cerebral
  embolic (current episode) I63.4- ☑
  Erb (-Duchenne) (birth) (newborn) P14.0
  Erb's syphilitic spastic spinal A52.17
  esophagus K22.8
  eye muscle (extrinsic) H49.9
    intrinsic — *see also* Paresis, of accommodation
  facial (nerve) G51.0
    birth injury P11.3
    congenital P11.3
    following operation NEC — *see* Puncture, accidental
      complicating surgery
    newborn (birth injury) P11.3
  familial (recurrent) (periodic) G72.3
    spastic G11.4
  fauces J39.2
  finger G56.9- ☑
  gait R26.1
  gastric nerve (nondiabetic) G52.2
  gaze, conjugate H51.0
  general (progressive) (syphilitic) A52.17
    juvenile A50.45
  glottis J38.00
    bilateral J38.02
    unilateral J38.01
  gluteal G54.1
  Gubler (-Millard) G46.3
  hand — *see* Monoplegia, upper limb
  heart — *see* Arrest, cardiac
  hemiplegic — *see* Hemiplegia
  hyperkalemic periodic (familial) G72.3
  hypoglossal (nerve) G52.3
  hypokalemic periodic G72.3
  hysterical F44.4
  ileus K56.0
  infantile — *see also* Poliomyelitis, paralytic A80.30
    bulbar — *see* Poliomyelitis, paralytic
    cerebral — *see* Palsy, cerebral
    spastic — *see* Palsy, cerebral, spastic
  infective — *see* Poliomyelitis, paralytic
  inferior nuclear G83.9
  internuclear — *see* Ophthalmoplegia, internuclear
  intestine K56.0
  iris H57.09
    due to diphtheria (toxin) A36.89
  ischemic, Volkmann's (complicating trauma) T79.6 ☑
  Jackson's G83.89
  jake — *see* Poisoning, food, noxious, plant
  Jamaica ginger (jake) G62.2
  juvenile general A50.45
  Klumpke (-Déjérine) (birth) (newborn) P14.1
  labioglossal (laryngeal) (pharyngeal) G12.29
  Landry's G61.0
  laryngeal nerve (recurrent) (superior) (unilateral) J38.00
    bilateral J38.02
    unilateral J38.01
  larynx J38.00
    bilateral J38.02
    due to diphtheria (toxin) A36.2
    unilateral J38.01
  lateral G12.23
  lead T56.0 ☑

Paralysis, paralytic — *continued*
  left side — *see* Hemiplegia
  leg G83.1- ☑
    both — *see* Paraplegia
    crossed G83.89
    hysterical F44.4
    psychogenic F44.4
    transient or transitory R29.818
      traumatic NEC — *see* Injury, nerve, leg
  levator palpebrae superioris — *see* Blepharoptosis,
    paralytic
  limb — *see* Monoplegia
  lip K13.0
  Lissauer's A52.17
  lower limb — *see* Monoplegia, lower limb
    both — *see* Paraplegia
  lung J98.4
  median nerve G56.1- ☑
  medullary (tegmental) G83.89
  mesencephalic NEC G83.89
    tegmental G83.89
  middle alternating G83.89
  Millard-Gubler-Foville G46.3
  monoplegic — *see* Monoplegia
  motor G83.9
  muscle, muscular NEC G72.89
    due to nerve lesion G58.9
    eye (extrinsic) H49.9
      intrinsic — *see* Paresis, of accommodation
      oblique — *see* Strabismus, paralytic, fourth nerve
    iris sphincter H21.9
    ischemic (Volkmann's) (complicating trauma)
      T79.6 ☑
    progressive G12.21
    progressive, spinal G12.25
    pseudohypertrophic G71.02
    spinal progressive G12.25
  musculocutaneous nerve G56.9- ☑
  musculospiral G56.9- ☑
  nerve — *see also* Disorder, nerve
    abducent — *see* Strabismus, paralytic, sixth nerve
    accessory G52.8
    auditory (except Deafness) H93.3 ☑
    birth injury P14.9
    cranial or cerebral G52.9
    facial G51.0
      birth injury P11.3
      congenital P11.3
      newborn (birth injury) P11.3
    fourth or trochlear — *see* Strabismus, paralytic,
      fourth nerve
    newborn (birth injury) P14.9
    oculomotor — *see* Strabismus, paralytic, third nerve
    phrenic (birth injury) P14.2
    radial G56.3- ☑
    seventh or facial G51.0
      newborn (birth injury) P11.3
    sixth or abducent — *see* Strabismus, paralytic, sixth
      nerve
    syphilitic A52.15
    third or oculomotor — *see* Strabismus, paralytic,
      third nerve
    trigeminal G50.9
    trochlear — *see* Strabismus, paralytic, fourth nerve
    ulnar G56.2- ☑
  normokalemic periodic G72.3
  ocular H49.9
    alternating G83.89
  oculofacial, congenital (Moebius) Q87.0
  oculomotor (external bilateral) (nerve) — *see* Strabis-
    mus, paralytic, third nerve
  palate (soft) K13.79
  paratrigeminal G50.9
  periodic (familial) (hyperkalemic) (hypokalemic) (my-
    otonic) (normokalemic) (potassium sensitive)
    (secondary) G72.3
  peripheral autonomic nervous system — *see* Neuropa-
    thy, peripheral, autonomic
  peroneal (nerve) G57.3- ☑
  pharynx J39.2
  phrenic nerve G56.8- ☑
  plantar nerve(s) G57.6- ☑
  pneumogastric nerve G52.2
  poliomyelitis (current) — *see* Poliomyelitis, paralytic
  popliteal nerve G57.3- ☑
  postepileptic transitory G83.84
  progressive (atrophic) (bulbar) (spinal) G12.22
    general A52.17

▽ **Subterms under main terms may continue to next column or page**   ☑ **Additional Character Required — Refer to the Tabular List for Character Selection**   **247**

Paraganglioma — Paralysis, paralytic

Paralysis, paralytic — *continued*
  progressive — *continued*
    infantile acute — *see* Poliomyelitis, paralytic
    supranuclear G23.1
  pseudobulbar G12.29
  pseudohypertrophic (muscle) G71.09
  psychogenic F44.4
  quadriceps G57.9- ☑
  quadriplegic — *see* Tetraplegia
  radial nerve G56.3- ☑
  rectus muscle (eye) H49.9
  recurrent isolated sleep G47.53
  respiratory (muscle) (system) (tract) R06.81
    center NEC G93.89
    congenital P28.89
    newborn P28.89
  right side — *see* Hemiplegia
  saturnine T56.0 ☑
  sciatic nerve G57.0- ☑
  senile G83.9
  shaking — *see* Parkinsonism
  shoulder G56.9- ☑
  sleep, recurrent isolated G47.53
  spastic G83.9
    cerebral — *see* Palsy, cerebral, spastic
    congenital (cerebral) — *see* Palsy, cerebral, spastic
    familial G11.4
    hereditary G11.4
    quadriplegic G80.0
    syphilitic (spinal) A52.17
  sphincter, bladder — *see* Paralysis, bladder
  spinal (cord) G83.9
    accessory nerve G52.8
    acute — *see* Poliomyelitis, paralytic
    ascending acute G61.0
    atrophic (acute) — *see also* Poliomyelitis, paralytic
      spastic, syphilitic A52.17
    congenital NEC — *see* Palsy, cerebral
    hereditary G95.89
    infantile — *see* Poliomyelitis, paralytic
    progressive G12.21
      muscle G12.25
    sequelae NEC G83.89
  sternomastoid G52.8
  stomach K31.84
    diabetic — *see* Diabetes, by type, with gastroparesis
    nerve G52.2
      diabetic — *see* Diabetes, by type, with gastroparesis
  stroke — *see* Infarct, brain
  subcapsularis G56.8- ☑
  supranuclear (progressive) G23.1
  sympathetic G90.8
    cervical G90.09
    nervous system — *see* Neuropathy, peripheral, autonomic
  syndrome G83.9
    specified NEC G83.89
  syphilitic spastic spinal (Erb's) A52.17
  thigh G57.9- ☑
  throat J39.2
    diphtheritic A36.0
    muscle J39.2
  thrombotic (current episode) I63.3- ☑
  thumb G56.9- ☑
  tick — *see* Toxicity, venom, arthropod, specified NEC
  Todd's (postepileptic transitory paralysis) G83.84
  toe G57.6- ☑
  tongue K14.8
  transient R29.5
    arm or leg NEC R29.818
    traumatic NEC — *see* Injury, nerve
  trapezius G52.8
  traumatic, transient NEC — *see* Injury, nerve
  trembling — *see* Parkinsonism
  triceps brachii G56.9- ☑
  trigeminal nerve G50.9
  trochlear (nerve) — *see* Strabismus, paralytic, fourth nerve
  ulnar nerve G56.2- ☑
  upper limb — *see* Monoplegia, upper limb
  uremic N18.9 *[G99.8]*
  uveoparotitic D86.89
  uvula K13.79
    postdiphtheritic A36.0
  vagus nerve G52.2
  vasomotor NEC G90.8
  velum palati K13.79

Paralysis, paralytic — *continued*
  vesical — *see* Paralysis, bladder
  vestibular nerve (except Vertigo) H93.3 ☑
  vocal cords J38.00
    bilateral J38.02
    unilateral J38.01
  Volkmann's (complicating trauma) T79.6 ☑
  wasting G12.29
  Weber's G46.3
  wrist G56.9- ☑
Paramedial urethrovesical orifice Q64.79
Paramenia N92.6
Parametritis — *see also* Disease, pelvis, inflammatory N73.2
  acute N73.0
  complicating abortion — *see* Abortion, by type, complicated by, parametritis
Parametrium, parametric — *see* condition
Paramnesia — *see* Amnesia
Paramolar K00.1
Paramyloidosis E85.89
Paramyoclonus multiplex G25.3
Paramyotonia (congenita) G71.19
Parangi — *see* Yaws
Paranoia (querulans) F22
  senile F03 ☑
Paranoid
  dementia (senile) F03 ☑
    praecox — *see* Schizophrenia
  personality F60.0
  psychosis (climacteric) (involutional) (menopausal) F22
    psychogenic (acute) F23
    senile F03 ☑
  reaction (acute) F23
    chronic F22
  schizophrenia F20.0
  state (climacteric) (involutional) (menopausal) (simple) F22
    senile F03 ☑
  tendencies F60.0
  traits F60.0
  trends F60.0
  type, psychopathic personality F60.0
Paraparesis — *see* Paraplegia
Paraphasia R47.02
Paraphilia F65.9
Paraphimosis (congenital) N47.2
  chancroidal A57
Paraphrenia, paraphrenic (late) F22
  schizophrenia F20.0
Paraplegia (lower) G82.20
  ataxic — *see* Degeneration, combined, spinal cord
  complete G82.21
  congenital (cerebral) G80.8
    spastic G80.1
  familial spastic G11.4
  functional (hysterical) F44.4
  hereditary, spastic G11.4
  hysterical F44.4
  incomplete G82.22
  Pott's A18.01
  psychogenic F44.4
  spastic
    Erb's spinal, syphilitic A52.17
    hereditary G11.4
    tropical G04.1
  syphilitic (spastic) A52.17
  traumatic
    current injury — code to injury with seventh character A
    sequela of previous injury — code to injury with seventh character S
  tropical spastic G04.1
Parapoxvirus B08.60
  specified NEC B08.69
Paraproteinemia D89.2
  benign (familial) D89.2
  monoclonal D47.2
  secondary to malignant disease D47.2
Parapsoriasis L41.9
  en plaques L41.4
  guttata L41.1
  large plaque L41.4
  retiform, retiformis L41.5
  small plaque L41.3
  specified NEC L41.8
  varioliformis (acuta) L41.0
Parasitic — *see also* condition

Parasitic — *continued*
  disease NEC B89
  stomatitis B37.0
  sycosis (beard) (scalp) B35.0
  twin Q89.4
Parasitism B89
  intestinal B82.9
  skin B88.9
  specified — *see* Infestation
Parasitophobia F40.218
Parasomnia G47.50
  due to
    alcohol
      abuse F10.182
      dependence F10.282
      use F10.982
    amphetamines
      abuse F15.182
      dependence F15.282
      use F15.982
    caffeine
      abuse F15.182
      dependence F15.282
      use F15.982
    cocaine
      abuse F14.182
      dependence F14.282
      use F14.982
    drug NEC
      abuse F19.182
      dependence F19.282
      use F19.982
    opioid
      abuse F11.182
      dependence F11.282
      use F11.982
    psychoactive substance NEC
      abuse F19.182
      dependence F19.282
      use F19.982
    sedative, hypnotic, or anxiolytic
      abuse F13.182
      dependence F13.282
      use F13.982
    stimulant NEC
      abuse F15.182
      dependence F15.282
      use F15.982
  in conditions classified elsewhere G47.54
  nonorganic origin F51.8
  organic G47.50
  specified NEC G47.59
Paraspadias Q54.9
Paraspasmus facialis G51.8
Parasuicide (attempt)
  history of (personal) Z91.5
    in family Z81.8
Parathyroid gland — *see* condition
Parathyroid tetany E20.9
Paratrachoma A74.0
Paratyphlitis — *see* Appendicitis
Paratyphoid (fever) — *see* Fever, paratyphoid
Paratyphus — *see* Fever, paratyphoid
Paraurethral duct Q64.79
Paraurethritis — *see also* Urethritis
  gonococcal (acute) (chronic) (with abscess) A54.1
Paravaccinia NEC B08.04
Paravaginitis — *see* Vaginitis
Parencephalitis — *see also* Encephalitis
  sequelae G09
Parent-child conflict — *see* Conflict, parent-child
  estrangement NEC Z62.890
Paresis — *see also* Paralysis
  accommodation — *see* Paresis, of accommodation
  Bernhardt's G57.1- ☑
  bladder (sphincter) — *see also* Paralysis, bladder
    tabetic A52.17
  bowel, colon or intestine K56.0
  extrinsic muscle, eye H49.9
  general (progressive) (syphilitic) A52.17
    juvenile A50.45
  heart — *see* Failure, heart
  insane (syphilitic) A52.17
  juvenile (general) A50.45
  of accommodation H52.52- ☑
  peripheral progressive (idiopathic) G60.3
  pseudohypertrophic G71.09
  senile G83.9

Paresis — *continued*
 syphilitic (general) A52.17
  congenital A50.45
 vesical NEC N31.2
Paresthesia — *see also* Disturbance, sensation, skin R20.2
 Bernhardt G57.1- ☑
Paretic — *see* condition
Parinaud's
 conjunctivitis H10.89
 oculoglandular syndrome H10.89
 ophthalmoplegia H49.88- ☑
Parkinsonism (idiopathic) (primary) G20
 with neurogenic orthostatic hypotension (symptomatic) G90.3
 arteriosclerotic G21.4
 dementia G31.83 *[F02.80]*
  with behavioral disturbance G31.83 *[F02.81]*
 due to
  drugs NEC G21.19
   neuroleptic G21.11
  medication-induced NEC G21.19
 neuroleptic induced G21.11
 postencephalitic G21.3
 secondary G21.9
  due to
   arteriosclerosis G21.4
   drugs NEC G21.19
    neuroleptic G21.11
   encephalitis G21.3
   external agents NEC G21.2
   syphilis A52.19
  specified NEC G21.8
 syphilitic A52.19
 treatment-induced NEC G21.19
 vascular G21.4
Parkinson's disease, syndrome or tremor — *see* Parkinsonism
Parodontitis — *see* Periodontitis
Parodontosis K05.4
Paronychia — *see also* Cellulitis, digit
 with lymphangitis — *see* Lymphangitis, acute, digit
 candidal (chronic) B37.2
 tuberculous (primary) A18.4
Parorexia (psychogenic) F50.89
Parosmia R43.1
 psychogenic F45.8
Parotid gland — *see* condition
Parotitis, parotiditis (allergic)(nonspecific toxic) (purulent) (septic) (suppurative) — *see also* Sialoadenitis
 epidemic — *see* Mumps
 infectious — *see* Mumps
 postoperative K91.89
 surgical K91.89
Parrot fever A70
Parrot's disease (early congenital syphilitic pseudoparalysis) A50.02
Parry-Romberg syndrome G51.8
Parry's disease or syndrome E05.00
 with thyroid storm E05.01
Pars planitis — *see* Cyclitis
Parsonage (-Aldren)-**Turner syndrome** G54.5
Parson's disease (exophthalmic goiter) E05.00
 with thyroid storm E05.01
Particolored infant Q82.8
Parturition — *see* Delivery
Parulis K04.7
 with sinus K04.6
Parvovirus, as cause of disease classified elsewhere B97.6
Pasini and Pierini's atrophoderma L90.3
Passage
 false, urethra N36.5
 meconium (newborn) during delivery P03.82
 of sounds or bougies — *see* Attention to, artificial, opening
Passive — *see* condition
 smoking Z77.22
Pasteurella septica A28.0
Pasteurellosis — *see* Infection, Pasteurella
PAT (paroxysmal atrial tachycardia) I47.1
Patau's syndrome — *see* Trisomy, 13
Patches
 mucous (syphilitic) A51.39
  congenital A50.07
 smokers' (mouth) K13.24
Patellar — *see* condition
Patent — *see also* Imperfect, closure

Patent — *continued*
 canal of Nuck Q52.4
 cervix N88.3
 ductus arteriosus or Botallo's Q25.0
 foramen
  botalli Q21.1
  ovale Q21.1
 interauricular septum Q21.1
 interventricular septum Q21.0
 omphalomesenteric duct Q43.0
 os (uteri) — *see* Patent, cervix
 ostium secundum Q21.1
 urachus Q64.4
 vitelline duct Q43.0
Paterson (-Brown)(-Kelly) **syndrome or web** D50.1
Pathologic, pathological — *see also* condition
 asphyxia R09.01
 fire-setting F63.1
 gambling F63.0
 ovum O02.0
 resorption, tooth K03.3
 stealing F63.2
Pathology (of) — *see* Disease
 periradicular, associated with previous endodontic treatment NEC M27.59
Pattern, sleep-wake, irregular G47.23
Patulous — *see also* Imperfect, closure (congenital)
 alimentary tract Q45.8
  lower Q43.8
  upper Q40.8
 eustachian tube H69.0- ☑
Pause, sinoatrial I49.5
Paxton's disease B36.2
Pearl(s)
 enamel K00.2
 Epstein's K09.8
Pearl-worker's disease — *see* Osteomyelitis, specified type NEC
Pectenosis K62.4
Pectoral — *see* condition
Pectus
 carinatum (congenital) Q67.7
  acquired M95.4
  rachitic sequelae (late effect) E64.3
 excavatum (congenital) Q67.6
  acquired M95.4
  rachitic sequelae (late effect) E64.3
 recurvatum (congenital) Q67.6
Pedatrophia E41
Pederosis F65.4
Pediculosis (infestation) B85.2
 capitis (head-louse) (any site) B85.0
 corporis (body-louse) (any site) B85.1
 eyelid B85.0
 mixed (classifiable to more than one of the titles B85.0-B85.3) B85.4
 pubis (pubic louse) (any site) B85.3
 vestimenti B85.1
 vulvae B85.3
Pediculus (infestation) — *see* Pediculosis
Pedophilia F65.4
Peg-shaped teeth K00.2
Pelade — *see* Alopecia, areata
Pelger-Huët anomaly or syndrome D72.0
Peliosis (rheumatica) D69.0
 hepatis K76.4
  with toxic liver disease K71.8
Pelizaeus-Merzbacher disease E75.29
Pellagra (alcoholic) (with polyneuropathy) E52
Pellagra-cerebellar-ataxia-renal aminoaciduria syndrome E72.02
Pellegrini (-Stieda) **disease or syndrome** — *see* Bursitis, tibial collateral
Pellizzi's syndrome E34.8
Pel's crisis A52.11
Pelvic — *see also* condition
 examination (periodic) (routine) Z01.419
  with abnormal findings Z01.411
 kidney, congenital Q63.2
Pelviolithiasis — *see* Calculus, kidney
Pelviperitonitis — *see also* Peritonitis, pelvic
 gonococcal A54.24
 puerperal O85
Pelvis — *see* condition or type
Pemphigoid L12.9
 benign, mucous membrane L12.1
 bullous L12.0
 cicatricial L12.1

Pemphigoid — *continued*
 juvenile L12.2
 ocular L12.1
 specified NEC L12.8
Pemphigus L10.9
 benign familial (chronic) Q82.8
 Brazilian L10.3
 circinatus L13.0
 conjunctiva L12.1
 drug-induced L10.5
 erythematosus L10.4
 foliaceus L10.2
 gangrenous — *see* Gangrene
 neonatorum L01.03
 ocular L12.1
 paraneoplastic L10.81
 specified NEC L10.89
 syphilitic (congenital) A50.06
 vegetans L10.1
 vulgaris L10.0
 wildfire L10.3
Pendred's syndrome E07.1
Pendulous
 abdomen, in pregnancy — *see* Pregnancy, complicated
  by, abnormal, pelvic organs or tissues NEC
 breast N64.89
Penetrating wound — *see also* Puncture
 with internal injury — *see* Injury, by site
 eyeball — *see* Puncture, eyeball
 orbit (with or without foreign body) — *see* Puncture, orbit
 uterus by instrument with or following ectopic or molar pregnancy O08.6
Penicillosis B48.4
Penis — *see* condition
Penitis N48.29
Pentalogy of Fallot Q21.8
Pentasomy X syndrome Q97.1
Pentosuria (essential) E74.8
Percreta placenta - O43.23 ☑
Peregrinating patient — *see* Disorder, factitious
Perforation, perforated (nontraumatic) (of)
 accidental during procedure (blood vessel) (nerve) (organ) — *see* Complication, accidental puncture or laceration
 antrum — *see* Sinusitis, maxillary
 appendix K35.32
  with localized peritonitis K35.32
 atrial septum, multiple Q21.1
 attic, ear — *see* Perforation, tympanum, attic
 bile duct (common) (hepatic) K83.2
  cystic K82.2
 bladder (urinary)
  with or following ectopic or molar pregnancy O08.6
  obstetrical trauma O71.5
  traumatic S37.29 ☑
   at delivery O71.5
 bowel K63.1
  with or following ectopic or molar pregnancy O08.6
  newborn P78.0
  obstetrical trauma O71.5
  traumatic — *see* Laceration, intestine
 broad ligament N83.8
  with or following ectopic or molar pregnancy O08.6
  obstetrical trauma O71.6
 by
  device, implant or graft — *see also* Complications, by site and type, mechanical T85.628 ☑
   arterial graft NEC — *see* Complication, cardiovascular device, mechanical, vascular
   breast (implant) T85.49 ☑
   catheter NEC T85.698 ☑
    cystostomy T83.090 ☑
    dialysis (renal) T82.49 ☑
     intraperitoneal T85.691 ☑
    infusion NEC T82.594 ☑
     spinal (epidural) (subdural) T85.690 ☑
    urinary — *see also* Complications, catheter, urinary T83.098 ☑
   electronic (electrode) (pulse generator) (stimulator)
    bone T84.390 ☑
    cardiac T82.199 ☑
     electrode T82.190 ☑
     pulse generator T82.191 ☑
     specified type NEC T82.198 ☑

Perforation, perforated — *continued*
　by — *continued*
　　device, implant or graft — *see also* Complications,
　　　by site and type, mechanical — *continued*
　　　electronic — *continued*
　　　　nervous system — *see* Complication, prosthet-
　　　　　ic device, mechanical, electronic ner-
　　　　　vous system stimulator
　　　　urinary — *see* Complication, genitourinary,
　　　　　device, urinary, mechanical
　　　fixation, internal (orthopedic) NEC — *see* Compli-
　　　　cation, fixation device, mechanical
　　　gastrointestinal — *see* Complications, prosthetic
　　　　device, mechanical, gastrointestinal device
　　　genital NEC T83.498 ☑
　　　　intrauterine contraceptive device T83.39 ☑
　　　　penile prosthesis T83.490 ☑
　　　heart NEC — *see* Complication, cardiovascular
　　　　device, mechanical
　　　joint prosthesis — *see* Complications, joint
　　　　prosthesis, mechanical, specified NEC, by
　　　　site
　　　ocular NEC — *see* Complications, prosthetic de-
　　　　vice, mechanical, ocular device
　　　orthopedic NEC — *see* Complication, orthopedic,
　　　　device, mechanical
　　　specified NEC T85.628 ☑
　　　urinary NEC — *see also* Complication, genitouri-
　　　　nary, device, urinary, mechanical
　　　　graft T83.29 ☑
　　　vascular NEC — *see* Complication, cardiovascular
　　　　device, mechanical
　　　ventricular intracranial shunt T85.09 ☑
　　foreign body left accidentally in operative wound
　　　T81.539 ☑
　　instrument (any) during a procedure, accidental —
　　　see Puncture, accidental complicating surgery
　cecum K35.32
　　with localized peritonitis K35.32
　cervix (uteri) N88.8
　　with or following ectopic or molar pregnancy O08.6
　　obstetrical trauma O71.3
　colon K63.1
　　newborn P78.0
　　obstetrical trauma O71.5
　　traumatic — *see* Laceration, intestine, large
　common duct (bile) K83.2
　cornea (due to ulceration) — *see* Ulcer, cornea, perfo-
　　rated
　cystic duct K82.2
　diverticulum (intestine) K57.80
　　with bleeding K57.81
　　large intestine K57.20
　　　with
　　　　bleeding K57.21
　　　　small intestine K57.40
　　　　　with bleeding K57.41
　　small intestine K57.00
　　　with
　　　　bleeding K57.01
　　　　large intestine K57.40
　　　　　with bleeding K57.41
　ear drum — *see* Perforation, tympanum
　esophagus K22.3
　ethmoidal sinus — *see* Sinusitis, ethmoidal
　frontal sinus — *see* Sinusitis, frontal
　gallbladder K82.2
　heart valve — *see* Endocarditis
　ileum K63.1
　　newborn P78.0
　　obstetrical trauma O71.5
　　traumatic — *see* Laceration, intestine, small
　instrumental, surgical (accidental) (blood vessel) (nerve)
　　(organ) — *see* Puncture, accidental complicating
　　surgery
　intestine NEC K63.1
　　with ectopic or molar pregnancy O08.6
　　newborn P78.0
　　obstetrical trauma O71.5
　　traumatic — *see* Laceration, intestine
　　ulcerative NEC K63.1
　　　newborn P78.0
　jejunum, jejunal K63.1
　　obstetrical trauma O71.5
　　traumatic — *see* Laceration, intestine, small
　　ulcer — *see* Ulcer, gastrojejunal, with perforation
　joint prosthesis — *see* Complications, joint prosthesis,
　　mechanical, specified NEC, by site

Perforation, perforated — *continued*
　mastoid (antrum) (cell) — *see* Disorder, mastoid,
　　specified NEC
　maxillary sinus — *see* Sinusitis, maxillary
　membrana tympani — *see* Perforation, tympanum
　nasal
　　septum J34.89
　　　congenital Q30.3
　　　syphilitic A52.73
　　sinus J34.89
　　　congenital Q30.8
　　　due to sinusitis — *see* Sinusitis
　palate — *see also* Cleft, palate Q35.9
　　syphilitic A52.79
　palatine vault — *see also* Cleft, palate, hard Q35.1
　　syphilitic A52.79
　　congenital A50.59
　pars flaccida (ear drum) — *see* Perforation, tympanum,
　　attic
　pelvic
　　floor S31.030 ☑
　　　with
　　　　ectopic or molar pregnancy O08.6
　　　　penetration into retroperitoneal space
　　　　　S31.031 ☑
　　　　retained foreign body S31.040 ☑
　　　　　with penetration into retroperitoneal
　　　　　　space S31.041 ☑
　　　following ectopic or molar pregnancy O08.6
　　　obstetrical trauma O70.1
　　organ S37.99 ☑
　　　adrenal gland S37.818 ☑
　　　bladder — *see* Perforation, bladder
　　　fallopian tube S37.599 ☑
　　　　bilateral S37.592 ☑
　　　　unilateral S37.591 ☑
　　　kidney S37.09- ☑
　　　obstetrical trauma O71.5
　　　ovary S37.499 ☑
　　　　bilateral S37.492 ☑
　　　　unilateral S37.491 ☑
　　　prostate S37.828 ☑
　　　specified organ NEC S37.898 ☑
　　　ureter — *see* Perforation, ureter
　　　urethra — *see* Perforation, urethra
　　　uterus — *see* Perforation, uterus
　perineum — *see* Laceration, perineum
　pharynx J39.2
　rectum K63.1
　　newborn P78.0
　　obstetrical trauma O71.5
　　traumatic S36.63 ☑
　root canal space due to endodontic treatment M27.51
　sigmoid K63.1
　　newborn P78.0
　　obstetrical trauma O71.5
　　traumatic S36.533 ☑
　sinus (accessory) (chronic) (nasal) J34.89
　sphenoidal sinus — *see* Sinusitis, sphenoidal
　surgical (accidental) (by instrument) (blood vessel)
　　(nerve) (organ) — *see* Puncture, accidental
　　complicating surgery
　traumatic
　　external — *see* Puncture
　　eye — *see* Puncture, eyeball
　　internal organ — *see* Injury, by site
　tympanum, tympanic (membrane) (persistent post-
　　traumatic) (postinflammatory) H72.9- ☑
　　attic H72.1- ☑
　　　multiple — *see* Perforation, tympanum, multiple
　　　total — *see* Perforation, tympanum, total
　　central H72.0- ☑
　　　multiple — *see* Perforation, tympanum, multiple
　　　total — *see* Perforation, tympanum, total
　　marginal NEC — *see* subcategory H72.2 ☑
　　multiple H72.81- ☑
　　pars flaccida — *see* Perforation, tympanum, attic
　　total H72.82- ☑
　　traumatic, current episode S09.2- ☑
　typhoid, gastrointestinal — *see* Typhoid
　ulcer — *see* Ulcer, by site, with perforation
　ureter N28.89
　　traumatic S37.19 ☑
　urethra N36.8
　　with ectopic or molar pregnancy O08.6
　　following ectopic or molar pregnancy O08.6
　　obstetrical trauma O71.5

Perforation, perforated — *continued*
　urethra — *continued*
　　traumatic S37.39 ☑
　　　at delivery O71.5
　uterus
　　with ectopic or molar pregnancy O08.6
　　by intrauterine contraceptive device T83.39 ☑
　　following ectopic or molar pregnancy O08.6
　　obstetrical trauma O71.1
　　traumatic S37.69 ☑
　　　obstetric O71.1
　uvula K13.79
　　syphilitic A52.79
　vagina O71.4
　　obstetrical trauma O71.4
　　other trauma — *see* Puncture, vagina

Periadenitis mucosa necrotica recurrens K12.0
Periappendicitis (acute) — *see* Appendicitis
Periarteritis nodosa (disseminated) (infectious) (necro-
　tizing) M30.0
Periarthritis (joint) — *see also* Enthesopathy
　Duplay's M75.0- ☑
　gonococcal A54.42
　humeroscapularis — *see* Capsulitis, adhesive
　scapulohumeral — *see* Capsulitis, adhesive
　shoulder — *see* Capsulitis, adhesive
　wrist M77.2- ☑
Periarthrosis (angioneural) — *see* Enthesopathy
Pericapsulitis, adhesive (shoulder) — *see* Capsulitis,
　adhesive
Pericarditis (with decompensation) (with effusion) I31.9
　with rheumatic fever (conditions in I00)
　　active — *see* Pericarditis, rheumatic
　　inactive or quiescent I09.2
　acute (hemorrhagic) (nonrheumatic) (Sicca) I30.9
　　with chorea (acute) (rheumatic) (Sydenham's) I02.0
　　benign I30.8
　　nonspecific I30.0
　　rheumatic I01.0
　　　with chorea (acute) (Sydenham's) I02.0
　adhesive or adherent (chronic) (external) (internal) I31.0
　　acute — *see* Pericarditis, acute
　　rheumatic I09.2
　bacterial (acute) (subacute) (with serous or seropuru-
　　lent effusion) I30.1
　calcareous I31.1
　cholesterol (chronic) I31.8
　　acute I30.9
　chronic (nonrheumatic) I31.9
　　rheumatic I09.2
　constrictive (chronic) I31.1
　coxsackie B33.23
　fibrinocaseous (tuberculous) A18.84
　fibrinopurulent I30.1
　fibrinous I30.8
　fibrous I31.0
　gonococcal A54.83
　idiopathic I30.0
　in systemic lupus erythematosus M32.12
　infective I30.1
　meningococcal A39.53
　neoplastic (chronic) I31.8
　　acute I30.9
　obliterans, obliterating I31.0
　plastic I31.0
　pneumococcal I30.1
　postinfarction I24.1
　purulent I30.1
　rheumatic (active) (acute) (with effusion) (with pneu-
　　monia) I01.0
　　with chorea (acute) (rheumatic) (Sydenham's) I02.0
　　chronic or inactive (with chorea) I09.2
　rheumatoid — *see* Rheumatoid, carditis
　septic I30.1
　serofibrinous I30.8
　staphylococcal I30.1
　streptococcal I30.1
　suppurative I30.1
　syphilitic A52.06
　tuberculous A18.84
　uremic N18.9 *[I32]*
　viral I30.1
Pericardium, pericardial — *see* condition
Pericellulitis — *see* Cellulitis
Pericementitis (chronic) (suppurative) — *see also* Peri-
　odontitis
　acute K05.20

Pericementitis — *continued*
  acute — *continued*
    generalized — *see* Periodontitis, aggressive, generalized
    localized — *see* Periodontitis, aggressive, localized
Perichondritis
  auricle — *see* Perichondritis, ear
  bronchus J98.09
  ear (external) H61.00- ☑
    acute H61.01- ☑
    chronic H61.02- ☑
  external auditory canal — *see* Perichondritis, ear
  larynx J38.7
    syphilitic A52.73
    typhoid A01.09
  nose J34.89
  pinna — *see* Perichondritis, ear
  trachea J39.8
Periclasia K05.4
Pericoronitis — *see* Periodontitis
Pericystitis N30.90
  with hematuria N30.91
Peridiverticulitis (intestine) K57.92
  cecum — *see* Diverticulitis, intestine, large
  colon — *see* Diverticulitis, intestine, large
  duodenum — *see* Diverticulitis, intestine, small
  intestine — *see* Diverticulitis, intestine
  jejunum — *see* Diverticulitis, intestine, small
  rectosigmoid — *see* Diverticulitis, intestine, large
  rectum — *see* Diverticulitis, intestine, large
  sigmoid — *see* Diverticulitis, intestine, large
Periendocarditis — *see* Endocarditis
Periepididymitis N45.1
Perifolliculitis L01.02
  abscedens, caput, scalp L66.3
  capitis, abscedens (et suffodiens) L66.3
  superficial pustular L01.02
Perihepatitis K65.8
Perilabyrinthitis (acute) — *see* subcategory H83.0 ☑
Perimeningitis — *see* Meningitis
Perimetritis — *see* Endometritis
Perimetrosalpingitis — *see* Salpingo-oophoritis
Perineocele N81.81
Perinephric, perinephritic — *see* condition
Perinephritis — *see also* Infection, kidney
  purulent — *see* Abscess, kidney
Perineum, perineal — *see* condition
Perineuritis NEC — *see* Neuralgia
Periodic — *see* condition
Periodontitis (chronic) (complex) (compound) (local)
    (simplex) K05.30
  acute K05.20
    generalized K05.229
      moderate K05.222
      severe K05.223
      slight K05.221
    localized K05.219
      moderate K05.212
      severe K05.213
      slight K05.211
  apical K04.5
    acute (pulpal origin) K04.4
  generalized K05.329
    moderate K05.322
    severe K05.323
    slight K05.321
  localized K05.319
    moderate K05.312
    severe K05.313
    slight K05.311
Periodontoclasia K05.4
Periodontosis (juvenile) K05.4
Periods — *see also* Menstruation
  heavy N92.0
  irregular N92.6
  shortened intervals (irregular) N92.1
Perionychia — *see also* Cellulitis, digit
  with lymphangitis — *see* Lymphangitis, acute, digit
Perioophoritis — *see* Salpingo-oophoritis
Periorchitis N45.2
Periosteum, periosteal — *see* condition
Periostitis (albuminosa) (circumscribed) (diffuse) (infective) (monomelic) — *see also* Osteomyelitis
  alveolar M27.3
  alveolodental M27.3
  dental M27.3
  gonorrheal A54.43

Periostitis — *continued*
  jaw (lower) (upper) M27.2
  orbit H05.03- ☑
  syphilitic A52.77
    congenital (early) A50.02 *[M90.80]*
    secondary A51.46
  tuberculous — *see* Tuberculosis, bone
  yaws (hypertrophic) (early) (late) A66.6 *[M90.80]*
Periostosis (hyperplastic) — *see also* Disorder, bone, specified type NEC
  with osteomyelitis — *see* Osteomyelitis, specified type NEC
Peripartum
  cardiomyopathy O90.3
Periphlebitis — *see* Phlebitis
Periproctitis K62.89
Periprostatitis — *see* Prostatitis
Perirectal — *see* condition
Perirenal — *see* condition
Perisalpingitis — *see* Salpingo-oophoritis
Perisplenitis (infectional) D73.89
Peristalsis, visible or reversed R19.2
Peritendinitis — *see* Enthesopathy
Peritoneum, peritoneal — *see* condition
Peritonitis (adhesive) (bacterial) (fibrinous) (hemorrhagic) (idiopathic) (localized) (perforative) (primary) (with adhesions) (with effusion) K65.9
  with or following
    abscess K65.1
    appendicitis
      with perforation or rupture K35.32
      generalized — *see also* Appendicitis K35.20
      localized — *see also* Appendicitis K35.30
    diverticular disease (intestine) K57.80
      with bleeding K57.81
      ectopic or molar pregnancy O08.0
      large intestine K57.20
        with
          bleeding K57.21
          small intestine K57.40
            with bleeding K57.41
      small intestine K57.00
        with
          bleeding K57.01
          large intestine K57.40
            with bleeding K57.41
  acute (generalized) K65.0
  aseptic T81.61 ☑
  bile, biliary K65.3
  chemical T81.61 ☑
  chlamydial A74.81
  chronic proliferative K65.8
  complicating abortion — *see* Abortion, by type, complicated by, pelvic peritonitis
  congenital P78.1
  diaphragmatic K65.0
  diffuse K65.0
  diphtheritic A36.89
  disseminated K65.0
  due to
    bile K65.3
    foreign
      body or object accidentally left during a procedure (instrument) (sponge) (swab) T81.599 ☑
      substance accidentally left during a procedure (chemical) (powder) (talc) T81.61 ☑
    talc T81.61 ☑
    urine K65.8
  eosinophilic K65.8
    acute K65.0
  fibrocaseous (tuberculous) A18.31
  fibropurulent K65.0
  following ectopic or molar pregnancy O08.0
  general (ized) K65.0
  gonococcal A54.85
  meconium (newborn) P78.0
  neonatal P78.1
    meconium P78.0
  pancreatic K65.0
  paroxysmal, familial E85.0
    benign E85.0
  pelvic
    female N73.5
      acute N73.3
      chronic N73.4
        with adhesions N73.6
    male K65.0

Peritonitis — *continued*
  periodic, familial E85.0
  proliferative, chronic K65.8
  puerperal, postpartum, childbirth O85
  purulent K65.0
  septic K65.0
  specified NEC K65.8
  spontaneous bacterial K65.2
  subdiaphragmatic K65.0
  subphrenic K65.0
  suppurative K65.0
  syphilitic A52.74
    congenital (early) A50.08 *[K67]*
  talc T81.61 ☑
  tuberculous A18.31
  urine K65.8
Peritonsillar — *see* condition
Peritonsillitis J36
Perityphlitis K37
Periureteritis N28.89
Periurethral — *see* condition
Periurethritis (gangrenous) — *see* Urethritis
Periuterine — *see* condition
Perivaginitis — *see* Vaginitis
Perivasculitis, retinal H35.06- ☑
Perivasitis (chronic) N49.1
Perivesiculitis (seminal) — *see* Vesiculitis
Perlèche NEC K13.0
  due to
    candidiasis B37.83
    moniliasis B37.83
    riboflavin deficiency E53.0
    vitamin B2 (riboflavin) deficiency E53.0
Pernicious — *see* condition
Pernio, perniosis T69.1 ☑
Perpetrator (of abuse) — *see* Index to External Causes of Injury, Perpetrator
Persecution
  delusion F22
  social Z60.5
Perseveration (tonic) R48.8
Persistence, persistent (congenital)
  anal membrane Q42.3
    with fistula Q42.2
  arteria stapedia Q16.3
  atrioventricular canal Q21.2
  branchial cleft NOS Q18.2
    cyst Q18.0
    fistula Q18.0
    sinus Q18.0
  bulbus cordis in left ventricle Q21.8
  canal of Cloquet Q14.0
  capsule (opaque) Q12.8
  cilioretinal artery or vein Q14.8
  cloaca Q43.7
  communication — *see* Fistula, congenital
  convolutions
    aortic arch Q25.46
    fallopian tube Q50.6
    oviduct Q50.6
    uterine tube Q50.6
  double aortic arch Q25.45
  ductus arteriosus (Botalli) Q25.0
  fetal
    circulation P29.38
    form of cervix (uteri) Q51.828
    hemoglobin, hereditary (HPFH) D56.4
  foramen
    Botalli Q21.1
    ovale Q21.1
  Gartner's duct Q52.4
  hemoglobin, fetal (hereditary) (HPFH) D56.4
  hyaloid
    artery (generally incomplete) Q14.0
    system Q14.8
  hymen, in pregnancy or childbirth — *see* Pregnancy, complicated by, abnormal, vulva
  lanugo Q84.2
  left
    posterior cardinal vein Q26.8
    root with right arch of aorta Q25.49
    superior vena cava Q26.1
  Meckel's diverticulum Q43.0
    malignant — *see* Table of Neoplasms, small intestine, malignant
  mucosal disease (middle ear) — *see* Otitis, media, suppurative, chronic, tubotympanic
  nail(s), anomalous Q84.6

▽ Subterms under main terms may continue to next column or page   ☑ Additional Character Required — Refer to the Tabular List for Character Selection   **251**

Pericementitis — Persistence, persistent

Persistence, persistent — *continued*
  omphalomesenteric duct Q43.0
  organ or site not listed — *see* Anomaly, by site
  ostium
    atrioventriculare commune Q21.2
    primum Q21.2
    secundum Q21.1
  ovarian rests in fallopian tube Q50.6
  pancreatic tissue in intestinal tract Q43.8
  primary (deciduous)
    teeth K00.6
    vitreous hyperplasia Q14.0
  pupillary membrane Q13.89
  rhesus (Rh) titer — *see* Complication(s), transfusion, incompatibility reaction, Rh (factor)
  right aortic arch Q25.47
  sinus
    urogenitalis
      female Q52.8
      male Q55.8
    venosus with imperfect incorporation in right auricle Q26.8
  thymus (gland) (hyperplasia) E32.0
  thyroglossal duct Q89.2
  thyrolingual duct Q89.2
  truncus arteriosus or communis Q20.0
  tunica vasculosa lentis Q12.2
  umbilical sinus Q64.4
  urachus Q64.4
  vitelline duct Q43.0
Person (with)
  admitted for clinical research, as a control subject (normal comparison) (participant) Z00.6
  awaiting admission to adequate facility elsewhere Z75.1
  concern (normal) about sick person in family Z63.6
  consulting on behalf of another Z71.0
  feigning illness Z76.5
  living (in)
    alone Z60.2
    boarding school Z59.3
    residential institution Z59.3
    without
      adequate housing (heating) (space) Z59.1
      housing (permanent) (temporary) Z59.0
      person able to render necessary care Z74.2
      shelter Z59.0
  on waiting list Z75.1
  sick or handicapped in family Z63.6
Personality (disorder) F60.9
  accentuation of traits (type A pattern) Z73.1
  affective F34.0
  aggressive F60.3
  amoral F60.2
  anacastic, anankastic F60.5
  antisocial F60.2
  anxious F60.6
  asocial F60.2
  asthenic F60.7
  avoidant F60.6
  borderline F60.3
  change due to organic condition (enduring) F07.0
  compulsive F60.5
  cycloid F34.0
  cyclothymic F34.0
  dependent F60.7
  depressive F34.1
  dissocial F60.2
  dual F44.81
  eccentric F60.89
  emotionally unstable F60.3
  expansive paranoid F60.0
  explosive F60.3
  fanatic F60.0
  haltlose type F60.89
  histrionic F60.4
  hyperthymic F34.0
  hypothymic F34.1
  hysterical F60.4
  immature F60.89
  inadequate F60.7
  labile (emotional) F60.3
  mixed (nonspecific) F60.89
  morally defective F60.2
  multiple F44.81
  narcissistic F60.81
  obsessional F60.5
  obsessive (-compulsive) F60.5
  organic F07.0

Personality — *continued*
  overconscientious F60.5
  paranoid F60.0
  passive (-dependent) F60.7
  passive-aggressive F60.89
  pathologic F60.9
  pattern defect or disturbance F60.9
  pseudopsychopathic (organic) F07.0
  pseudoretarded (organic) F07.0
  psychoinfantile F60.4
  psychoneurotic NEC F60.89
  psychopathic F60.2
  querulant F60.0
  sadistic F60.89
  schizoid F60.1
  self-defeating F60.89
  sensitive paranoid F60.0
  sociopathic (amoral) (antisocial) (asocial) (dissocial) F60.2
  specified NEC F60.89
  type A Z73.1
  unstable (emotional) F60.3
Perthes' disease — *see* Legg-Calvé-Perthes disease
Pertussis — *see also* Whooping cough A37.90
Perversion, perverted
  appetite F50.89
    psychogenic F50.89
  function
    pituitary gland E23.2
      posterior lobe E22.2
  sense of smell and taste R43.8
    psychogenic F45.8
  sexual — *see* Deviation, sexual
Pervious, congenital — *see also* Imperfect, closure
  ductus arteriosus Q25.0
Pes (congenital) — *see also* Talipes
  acquired — *see also* Deformity, limb, foot, specified NEC
    planus — *see* Deformity, limb, flat foot
  adductus Q66.89
  cavus Q66.7- ☑
  deformity NEC, acquired — *see* Deformity, limb, foot, specified NEC
  planus (acquired) (any degree) — *see also* Deformity, limb, flat foot
    rachitic sequelae (late effect) E64.3
  valgus Q66.6
Pest, pestis — *see* Plague
Petechia, petechiae R23.3
  newborn P54.5
Petechial typhus A75.9
Peter's anomaly Q13.4
Petit mal seizure — *see* Epilepsy, childhood, absence
Petit's hernia — *see* Hernia, abdomen, specified site NEC
Petrellidosis B48.2
Petrositis H70.20- ☑
  acute H70.21- ☑
  chronic H70.22- ☑
Peutz-Jeghers disease or syndrome Q85.8
Peyronie's disease N48.6
PFAPA (periodic fever, aphthous stomatitis, pharyngitis, and adenopathy syndrome) M04.8
Pfeiffer's disease — *see* Mononucleosis, infectious
Phagedena (dry) (moist) (sloughing) — *see also* Gangrene
  geometric L88
  penis N48.29
  tropical — *see* Ulcer, skin
  vulva N76.6
Phagedenic — *see* condition
Phakoma H35.89
Phakomatosis — *see also* specific eponymous syndromes Q85.9
  Bourneville's Q85.1
  specified NEC Q85.8
Phantom limb syndrome (without pain) G54.7
  with pain G54.7
Pharyngeal pouch syndrome D82.1
Pharyngitis (acute) (catarrhal) (gangrenous) (infective) (malignant) (membranous) (phlegmonous) (pseudomembranous) (simple) (subacute) (suppurative) (ulcerative) (viral) J02.9
  with influenza, flu, or grippe — *see* Influenza, with, pharyngitis
  aphthous B08.5
  atrophic J31.2
  chlamydial A56.4
  chronic (atrophic) (granular) (hypertrophic) J31.2

Pharyngitis — *continued*
  coxsackievirus B08.5
  diphtheritic A36.0
  enteroviral vesicular B08.5
  follicular (chronic) J31.2
  fusospirochetal A69.1
  gonococcal A54.5
  granular (chronic) J31.2
  herpesviral B00.2
  hypertrophic J31.2
  infectional, chronic J31.2
  influenzal — *see* Influenza, with, respiratory manifestations NEC
  lymphonodular, acute (enteroviral) B08.8
  pneumococcal J02.8
  purulent J02.9
  putrid J02.9
  septic J02.0
  sicca J31.2
  specified organism NEC J02.8
  staphylococcal J02.8
  streptococcal J02.0
  syphilitic, congenital (early) A50.03
  tuberculous A15.8
  vesicular, enteroviral B08.5
  viral NEC J02.8
Pharyngoconjunctivitis, viral B30.2
Pharyngolaryngitis (acute) J06.0
  chronic J37.0
Pharyngoplegia J39.2
Pharyngotonsillitis, herpesviral B00.2
Pharyngotracheitis, chronic J42
Pharynx, pharyngeal — *see* condition
Phencyclidine-induced
  anxiety disorder F16.980
  bipolar and related disorder F16.94
  depressive disorder F16.94
  psychotic disorder F16.959
Phenomenon
  Arthus' — *see* Arthus' phenomenon
  jaw-winking Q07.8
  lupus erythematosus (LE) cell M32.9
  Raynaud's (secondary) I73.00
    with gangrene I73.01
  vasomotor R55
  vasospastic I73.9
  vasovagal R55
  Wenckebach's I44.1
Phenylketonuria E70.1
  classical E70.0
  maternal E70.1
Pheochromoblastoma
  specified site — *see* Neoplasm, malignant, by site
  unspecified site C74.10
Pheochromocytoma
  malignant
    specified site — *see* Neoplasm, malignant, by site
    unspecified site C74.10
  specified site — *see* Neoplasm, benign, by site
  unspecified site D35.00
Pheohyphomycosis — *see* Chromomycosis
Pheomycosis — *see* Chromomycosis
Phimosis (congenital) (due to infection) N47.1
  chancroidal A57
Phlebectasia — *see also* Varix
  congenital Q27.4
Phlebitis (infective) (pyemic) (septic) (suppurative) I80.9
  antepartum — *see* Thrombophlebitis, antepartum
  blue — *see* Phlebitis, leg, deep
  breast, superficial I80.8
  calf muscular vein (NOS) I80.25- ☑
  cavernous (venous) sinus — *see* Phlebitis, intracranial (venous) sinus
  cerebral (venous) sinus — *see* Phlebitis, intracranial (venous) sinus
  chest wall, superficial I80.8
  cranial (venous) sinus — *see* Phlebitis, intracranial (venous) sinus
  deep (vessels) — *see* Phlebitis, leg, deep
  due to implanted device — *see* Complications, by site and type, specified NEC
  during or resulting from a procedure T81.72 ☑
  femoral vein (superficial) I80.1- ☑
  femoropopliteal vein I80.0- ☑
  gastrocnemial vein I80.25- ☑
  gestational — *see* Phlebopathy, gestational
  hepatic veins I80.8
  iliac vein (common) (external) (internal) I80.21- ☑

☑ **Additional Character Required** — Refer to the Tabular List for Character Selection   ▽ **Subterms under main terms may continue to next column or page**

Phlebitis — *continued*
 iliofemoral — *see* Phlebitis, femoral vein
 intracranial (venous) sinus (any) G08
  nonpyogenic I67.6
 intraspinal venous sinuses and veins G08
  nonpyogenic G95.19
 lateral (venous) sinus — *see* Phlebitis, intracranial (venous) sinus
 leg I80.3
  antepartum — *see* Thrombophlebitis, antepartum
  deep (vessels) NEC I80.20- ☑
   iliac I80.21- ☑
   popliteal vein I80.22- ☑
   specified vessel NEC I80.29- ☑
   tibial vein (anterior) (posterior) I80.23- ☑
  femoral vein (superficial) I80.1- ☑
  superficial (vessels) I80.0- ☑
 longitudinal sinus — *see* Phlebitis, intracranial (venous) sinus
 lower limb — *see* Phlebitis, leg
 migrans, migrating (superficial) I82.1
 pelvic
  with ectopic or molar pregnancy O08.0
  following ectopic or molar pregnancy O08.0
  puerperal, postpartum O87.1
 peroneal vein I80.24- ☑
 popliteal vein — *see* Phlebitis, leg, deep, popliteal
 portal (vein) K75.1
 postoperative T81.72 ☑
 pregnancy — *see* Thrombophlebitis, antepartum
 puerperal, postpartum, childbirth O87.0
  deep O87.1
  pelvic O87.1
  superficial O87.0
 retina — *see* Vasculitis, retina
 saphenous (accessory) (great) (long) (small) — *see* Phlebitis, leg, superficial
 sinus (meninges) — *see* Phlebitis, intracranial (venous) sinus
 soleal vein I80.25- ☑
 specified site NEC I80.8
 syphilitic A52.09
 tibial vein — *see* Phlebitis, leg, deep, tibial
 ulcerative I80.9
  leg — *see* Phlebitis, leg
 umbilicus I80.8
 uterus (septic) — *see* Endometritis
 varicose (leg) (lower limb) — *see* Varix, leg, with, inflammation
Phlebofibrosis I87.8
Phleboliths I87.8
Phlebopathy,
 gestational O22.9- ☑
 puerperal O87.9
Phlebosclerosis I87.8
Phlebothrombosis — *see also* Thrombosis
 antepartum — *see* Thrombophlebitis, antepartum
 pregnancy — *see* Thrombophlebitis, antepartum
 puerperal — *see* Thrombophlebitis, puerperal
Phlebotomus fever A93.1
Phlegmasia
 alba dolens O87.1
  nonpuerperal — *see* Phlebitis, femoral vein
 cerulea dolens — *see* Phlebitis, leg, deep
Phlegmon — *see* Abscess
Phlegmonous — *see* condition
Phlyctenulosis (allergic) (keratoconjunctivitis) (nontuberculous) — *see also* Keratoconjunctivitis
 cornea — *see* Keratoconjunctivitis
 tuberculous A18.52
Phobia, phobic F40.9
 animal F40.218
  spiders F40.210
 examination F40.298
 reaction F40.9
 simple F40.298
 social F40.10
  generalized F40.11
 specific (isolated) F40.298
  animal F40.218
   spiders F40.210
  blood F40.230
  injection F40.231
  injury F40.233
  men F40.290
  natural environment F40.228
   thunderstorms F40.220

Phobia, phobic — *continued*
 specific — *continued*
  situational F40.248
   bridges F40.242
   closed in spaces F40.240
   flying F40.243
   heights F40.241
  specified focus NEC F40.298
  transfusion F40.231
  women F40.291
 specified NEC F40.8
  medical care NEC F40.232
 state F40.9
Phocas' disease — *see* Mastopathy, cystic
Phocomelia Q73.1
 lower limb — *see* Agenesis, leg, with foot present
 upper limb — *see* Agenesis, arm, with hand present
Phoria H50.50
Phosphate-losing tubular disorder N25.0
Phosphatemia E83.39
Phosphaturia E83.39
Photodermatitis (sun) L56.8
 chronic L57.8
 due to drug L56.8
 light other than sun L59.8
Photokeratitis H16.13- ☑
Photophobia H53.14- ☑
Photophthalmia — *see* Photokeratitis
Photopsia H53.19
Photoretinitis — *see* Retinopathy, solar
Photosensitivity, photosensitization (sun) skin L56.8
 light other than sun L59.8
Phrenitis — *see* Encephalitis
Phrynoderma (vitamin A deficiency) E50.8
Phthiriasis (pubis) B85.3
 with any infestation classifiable to B85.0-B85.2 B85.4
Phthirus infestation — *see* Phthiriasis
Phthisis — *see also* Tuberculosis
 bulbi (infectional) — *see* Disorder, globe, degenerated condition, atrophy
 eyeball (due to infection) — *see* Disorder, globe, degenerated condition, atrophy
Phycomycosis — *see* Zygomycosis
Physalopteriasis B81.8
Physical restraint status Z78.1
Phytobezoar T18.9 ☑
 intestine T18.3 ☑
 stomach T18.2 ☑
Pian — *see* Yaws
Pianoma A66.1
Pica F50.89
 in adults F50.89
 infant or child F98.3
Picking, nose F98.8
Pick-Niemann disease — *see* Niemann-Pick disease or syndrome
Pick's
 cerebral atrophy G31.01 *[F02.80]*
  with behavioral disturbance G31.01 *[F02.81]*
 disease or syndrome (brain) G31.01 *[F02.80]*
  with behavioral disturbance G31.01 *[F02.81]*
   brain G31.01 *[F02.80]*
    with behavioral disturbance G31.01 *[F02.81]*
   pericardium (pericardial pseudocirrhosis of liver) I31.1
 syndrome
  brain G31.01 *[F02.80]*
   with behavioral disturbance G31.01 *[F02.81]*
  of heart (pericardial pseudocirrhosis of liver) I31.1
Pickwickian syndrome E66.2
Piebaldism E70.39
Piedra (beard) (scalp) B36.8
 black B36.3
 white B36.2
Pierre Robin deformity or syndrome Q87.0
Pierson's disease or osteochondrosis M91.0
Pig-bel A05.2
Pigeon
 breast or chest (acquired) M95.4
  congenital Q67.7
  rachitic sequelae (late effect) E64.3
 breeder's disease or lung J67.2
 fancier's disease or lung J67.2
 toe — *see* Deformity, toe, specified NEC
Pigmentation (abnormal) (anomaly) L81.9
 conjunctiva H11.13- ☑
 cornea (anterior) H18.01- ☑

Pigmentation — *continued*
 cornea — *continued*
  posterior H18.05- ☑
  stromal H18.06- ☑
 diminished melanin formation NEC L81.6
 iron L81.8
 lids, congenital Q82.8
 limbus corneae — *see* Pigmentation, cornea
 metals L81.8
 optic papilla, congenital Q14.2
 retina, congenital (grouped) (nevoid) Q14.1
 scrotum, congenital Q82.8
 tattoo L81.8
Piles — *see also* Hemorrhoids K64.9
Pili
 annulati or torti (congenital) Q84.1
 incarnati L73.1
Pill roller hand (intrinsic) — *see* Parkinsonism
Pilomatrixoma — *see* Neoplasm, skin, benign
 malignant — *see* Neoplasm, skin, malignant
Pilonidal — *see* condition
Pimple R23.8
PIN — *see* Neoplasia, intraepithelial, prostate
Pinched nerve — *see* Neuropathy, entrapment
Pindborg tumor — *see* Cyst, calcifying odontogenic
Pineal body or gland — *see* condition
Pinealoblastoma C75.3
Pinealoma D44.5
 malignant C75.3
Pineoblastoma C75.3
Pineocytoma D44.5
Pinguecula H11.15- ☑
Pingueculitis H10.81- ☑
Pinhole meatus — *see also* Stricture, urethra N35.919
Pink
 disease — *see* subcategory T56.1 ☑
 eye — *see* Conjunctivitis, acute, mucopurulent
Pinkus' disease (lichen nitidus) L44.1
Pinpoint
 meatus — *see* Stricture, urethra
 os (uteri) — *see* Stricture, cervix
Pins and needles R20.2
Pinta A67.9
 cardiovascular lesions A67.2
 chancre (primary) A67.0
 erythematous plaques A67.1
 hyperchromic lesions A67.1
 hyperkeratosis A67.1
 lesions A67.9
  cardiovascular A67.2
  hyperchromic A67.1
  intermediate A67.1
  late A67.2
  mixed A67.3
  primary A67.0
  skin (achromic) (cicatricial) (dyschromic) A67.2
   hyperchromic A67.1
   mixed (achromic and hyperchromic) A67.3
 papule (primary) A67.0
 skin lesions (achromic) (cicatricial) (dyschromic) A67.2
  hyperchromic A67.1
  mixed (achromic and hyperchromic) A67.3
 vitiligo A67.2
Pintids A67.1
Pinworm (disease) (infection) (infestation) B80.0
Piroplasmosis B60.0
Pistol wound — *see* Gunshot wound
Pitchers' elbow — *see* Derangement, joint, specified type NEC, elbow
Pithecoid pelvis Q74.2
 with disproportion (fetopelvic) O33.0
  causing obstructed labor O65.0
Pithiatism F48.8
Pitted — *see* Pitting
Pitting — *see also* Edema R60.9
 lip R60.0
 nail L60.8
 teeth K00.4
Pituitary gland — *see* condition
Pituitary-snuff-taker's disease J67.8
Pityriasis (capitis) L21.0
 alba L30.5
 circinata (et maculata) L42
 furfuracea L21.0
 Hebra's L26
 lichenoides L41.0
  chronica L41.1

Pityriasis — *continued*
  lichenoides — *continued*
    et varioliformis (acuta) L41.0
  maculata (et circinata) L30.5
  nigra B36.1
  pilaris, Hebra's L44.0
  rosea L42
  rotunda L44.8
  rubra (Hebra) pilaris L44.0
  simplex L30.5
  specified type NEC L30.5
  streptogenes L30.5
  versicolor (scrotal) B36.0
Placenta, placental — *see* Pregnancy, complicated by (care of) (management affected by), specified condition
Placentitis O41.14- ☑
Plagiocephaly Q67.3
Plague A20.9
  abortive A20.8
  ambulatory A20.8
  asymptomatic A20.8
  bubonic A20.0
  cellulocutaneous A20.1
  cutaneobubonic A20.1
  lymphatic gland A20.0
  meningitis A20.3
  pharyngeal A20.8
  pneumonic (primary) (secondary) A20.2
  pulmonary, pulmonic A20.2
  septicemic A20.7
  tonsillar A20.8
    septicemic A20.7
Planning, family
  contraception Z30.9
  procreation Z31.69
Plaque(s)
  artery, arterial — *see* Arteriosclerosis
  calcareous — *see* Calcification
  coronary, lipid rich I25.83
  epicardial I31.8
  erythematous, of pinta A67.1
  Hollenhorst's — *see* Occlusion, artery, retina
  lipid rich, coronary I25.83
  pleural (without asbestos) J92.9
    with asbestos J92.0
  tongue K13.29
Plasmacytoma C90.3- ☑
  extramedullary C90.2- ☑
  medullary C90.0- ☑
  solitary C90.3- ☑
Plasmacytopenia D72.818
Plasmacytosis D72.822
Plaster ulcer — *see* Ulcer, pressure, by site
Plateau iris syndrome (post-iridectomy) (postprocedural) (without glaucoma) H21.82
  with glaucoma H40.22- ☑
Platybasia Q75.8
Platyonychia (congenital) Q84.6
  acquired L60.8
Platypelloid pelvis M95.5
  with disproportion (fetopelvic) O33.0
    causing obstructed labor O65.0
  congenital Q74.2
Platyspondylisis Q76.49
Plaut (-Vincent) **disease** — *see also* Vincent's A69.1
Plethora R23.2
  newborn P61.1
Pleura, pleural — *see* condition
Pleuralgia R07.81
Pleurisy (acute) (adhesive) (chronic) (costal) (diaphragmatic) (double) (dry) (fibrinous) (fibrous) (interlobar) (latent) (plastic) (primary) (residual) (sicca) (sterile) (subacute) (unresolved) R09.1
  with
    adherent pleura J86.0
    effusion J90
      chylous, chyliform J94.0
      tuberculous (non primary) A15.6
        primary (progressive) A15.7
    tuberculosis — *see* Pleurisy, tuberculous (non primary)
  encysted — *see* Pleurisy, with effusion
  exudative — *see* Pleurisy, with effusion
  fibrinopurulent, fibropurulent — *see* Pyothorax
  hemorrhagic — *see* Hemothorax
  pneumococcal J90
  purulent — *see* Pyothorax

Pleurisy — *continued*
  septic — *see* Pyothorax
  serofibrinous — *see* Pleurisy, with effusion
  seropurulent — *see* Pyothorax
  serous — *see* Pleurisy, with effusion
  staphylococcal J86.9
  streptococcal J90
  suppurative — *see* Pyothorax
  traumatic (post) (current) — *see* Injury, intrathoracic, pleura
  tuberculous (with effusion) (non primary) A15.6
    primary (progressive) A15.7
Pleuritis sicca — *see* Pleurisy
Pleurobronchopneumonia — *see* Pneumonia, broncho-
Pleurodynia R07.81
  epidemic B33.0
  viral B33.0
Pleuropericarditis — *see also* Pericarditis
  acute I30.9
Pleuropneumonia (acute) (bilateral) (double) (septic) — *see also* Pneumonia J18.8
  chronic — *see* Fibrosis, lung
Pleuro-pneumonia-like-organism (PPLO), as cause of disease classified elsewhere B96.0
Pleurorrhea — *see* Pleurisy, with effusion
Plexitis, brachial G54.0
Plica
  polonica B85.0
  syndrome, knee M67.5- ☑
  tonsil J35.8
Plicated tongue K14.5
Plug
  bronchus NEC J98.09
  meconium (newborn) NEC syndrome P76.0
  mucus — *see* Asphyxia, mucus
Plumbism — *see* subcategory T56.0 ☑
Plummer's disease E05.20
  with thyroid storm E05.21
Plummer-Vinson syndrome D50.1
Pluricarential syndrome of infancy E40
Plus (and minus) **hand** (intrinsic) — *see* Deformity, limb, specified type NEC, forearm
Pneumathemia — *see* Air, embolism
Pneumatic hammer (drill) syndrome T75.21 ☑
Pneumatocele (lung) J98.4
  intracranial G93.89
  tension J44.9
Pneumatosis
  cystoides intestinalis K63.89
  intestinalis K63.89
  peritonei K66.8
Pneumaturia R39.89
Pneumoblastoma — *see* Neoplasm, lung, malignant
Pneumocephalus G93.89
Pneumococcemia A40.3
Pneumococcus, pneumococcal — *see* condition
Pneumoconiosis (due to) (inhalation of) J64
  with tuberculosis (any type in A15) J65
  aluminum J63.0
  asbestos J61
  bagasse, bagassosis J67.1
  bauxite J63.1
  beryllium J63.2
  coal miners' (simple) J60
  coalworkers' (simple) J60
  collier's J60
  cotton dust J66.0
  diatomite (diatomaceous earth) J62.8
  dust
    inorganic NEC J63.6
    lime J62.8
    marble J62.8
    organic NEC J66.8
  fumes or vapors (from silo) J68.9
  graphite J63.3
  grinder's J62.8
  kaolin J62.8
  mica J62.8
  millstone maker's J62.8
  mineral fibers NEC J61
  miner's J60
  moldy hay J67.0
  potter's J62.8
  rheumatoid — *see* Rheumatoid, lung
  sandblaster's J62.8
  silica, silicate NEC J62.8
    with carbon J60
  stonemason's J62.8

Pneumoconiosis — *continued*
  talc (dust) J62.0
Pneumocystis carinii pneumonia B59
Pneumocystis jiroveci (pneumonia) B59
Pneumocystosis (with pneumonia) B59
Pneumohemopericardium I31.2
Pneumohemothorax J94.2
  traumatic S27.2 ☑
Pneumohydropericardium — *see* Pericarditis
Pneumohydrothorax — *see* Hydrothorax
Pneumomediastinum J98.2
  congenital or perinatal P25.2
Pneumomycosis B49 *[J99]*
Pneumonia (acute) (double) (migratory) (purulent) (septic) (unresolved) J18.9
  with
    influenza — *see* Influenza, with, pneumonia
    lung abscess J85.1
      due to specified organism — *see* Pneumonia, in (due to)
  adenoviral J12.0
  adynamic J18.2
  alba A50.04
  allergic (eosinophilic) J82
  alveolar — *see* Pneumonia, lobar
  anaerobes J15.8
  anthrax A22.1
  apex, apical — *see* Pneumonia, lobar
  Ascaris B77.81
  aspiration J69.0
    due to
      aspiration of microorganisms
        bacterial J15.9
        viral J12.9
      food (regurgitated) J69.0
      gastric secretions J69.0
      milk (regurgitated) J69.0
      oils, essences J69.1
      solids, liquids NEC J69.8
      vomitus J69.0
    newborn P24.81
      amniotic fluid (clear) P24.11
      blood P24.21
      food (regurgitated) P24.31
      liquor (amnii) P24.11
      meconium P24.01
      milk P24.31
      mucus P24.11
      specified NEC P24.81
      stomach contents P24.31
    postprocedural J95.4
  atypical NEC J18.9
  bacillus J15.9
    specified NEC J15.8
  bacterial J15.9
    specified NEC J15.8
  Bacteroides (fragilis) (oralis) (melaninogenicus) J15.8
  basal, basic, basilar — *see* Pneumonia, by type
  bronchiolitis obliterans organized (BOOP) J84.89
  broncho-, bronchial (confluent) (croupous) (diffuse) (disseminated) (hemorrhagic) (involving lobes) (lobar) (terminal) J18.0
    allergic (eosinophilic) J82
    aspiration — *see* Pneumonia, aspiration
    bacterial J15.9
      specified NEC J15.8
    chronic — *see* Fibrosis, lung
    diplococcal J13
    Eaton's agent J15.7
    Escherichia coli (E. coli) J15.5
    Friedländer's bacillus J15.0
    Hemophilus influenzae J14
    hypostatic J18.2
    inhalation — *see also* Pneumonia, aspiration
      due to fumes or vapors (chemical) J68.0
      of oils or essences J69.1
    Klebsiella (pneumoniae) J15.0
    lipid, lipoid J69.1
      endogenous J84.89
    Mycoplasma (pneumoniae) J15.7
    pleuro-pneumonia-like-organisms (PPLO) J15.7
    pneumococcal J13
    Proteus J15.6
    Pseudomonas J15.1
    Serratia marcescens J15.6
    specified organism NEC J16.8
    staphylococcal — *see* Pneumonia, staphylococcal
    streptococcal NEC J15.4

☑ Additional Character Required — Refer to the Tabular List for Character Selection
▽ Subterms under main terms may continue to next column or page

Pneumonia — *continued*
  broncho-, bronchial — *continued*
    streptococcal — *continued*
      group B J15.3
      pneumoniae J13
    viral, virus — *see* Pneumonia, viral
  Butyrivibrio (fibriosolvens) J15.8
  Candida B37.1
  caseous — *see* Tuberculosis, pulmonary
  catarrhal — *see* Pneumonia, broncho
  chlamydial J16.0
    congenital P23.1
  cholesterol J84.89
  cirrhotic (chronic) — *see* Fibrosis, lung
  Clostridium (haemolyticum) (novyi) J15.8
  confluent — *see* Pneumonia, broncho
  congenital (infective) P23.9
    due to
      bacterium NEC P23.6
      Chlamydia P23.1
      Escherichia coli P23.4
      Haemophilus influenzae P23.6
      infective organism NEC P23.8
      Klebsiella pneumoniae P23.6
      Mycoplasma P23.6
      Pseudomonas P23.5
      Staphylococcus P23.2
      Streptococcus (except group B) P23.6
        group B P23.3
      viral agent P23.0
    specified NEC P23.8
  croupous — *see* Pneumonia, lobar
  cryptogenic organizing J84.116
  cytomegalic inclusion B25.0
  cytomegaloviral B25.0
  deglutition — *see* Pneumonia, aspiration
  desquamative interstitial J84.117
  diffuse — *see* Pneumonia, broncho
  diplococcal, diplococcus (broncho-) (lobar) J13
  disseminated (focal) — *see* Pneumonia, broncho
  Eaton's agent J15.7
  embolic, embolism — *see* Embolism, pulmonary
  Enterobacter J15.6
  eosinophilic J82
  Escherichia coli (E. coli) J15.5
  Eubacterium J15.8
  fibrinous — *see* Pneumonia, lobar
  fibroid, fibrous (chronic) — *see* Fibrosis, lung
  Friedländer's bacillus J15.0
  Fusobacterium (nucleatum) J15.8
  gangrenous J85.0
  giant cell (measles) B05.2
  gonococcal A54.84
  gram-negative bacteria NEC J15.6
    anaerobic J15.8
  Hemophilus influenzae (broncho) (lobar) J14
  human metapneumovirus J12.3
  hypostatic (broncho) (lobar) J18.2
  in (due to)
    actinomycosis A42.0
    adenovirus J12.0
    anthrax A22.1
    ascariasis B77.81
    aspergillosis B44.9
    Bacillus anthracis A22.1
    Bacterium anitratum J15.6
    candidiasis B37.1
    chickenpox B01.2
    Chlamydia J16.0
      neonatal P23.1
    coccidioidomycosis B38.2
      acute B38.0
      chronic B38.1
    cytomegalovirus disease B25.0
    Diplococcus (pneumoniae) J13
    Eaton's agent J15.7
    Enterobacter J15.6
    Escherichia coli (E. coli) J15.5
    Friedländer's bacillus J15.0
    fumes and vapors (chemical) (inhalation) J68.0
    gonorrhea A54.84
    Hemophilus influenzae (H. influenzae) J14
    Herellea J15.6
    histoplasmosis B39.2
      acute B39.0
      chronic B39.1
    human metapneumovirus J12.3
    Klebsiella (pneumoniae) J15.0

Pneumonia — *continued*
  in — *continued*
    measles B05.2
    Mycoplasma (pneumoniae) J15.7
    nocardiosis, nocardiasis A43.0
    ornithosis A70
    parainfluenza virus J12.2
    pleuro-pneumonia-like-organism (PPLO) J15.7
    pneumococcus J13
    pneumocystosis (Pneumocystis carinii) (Pneumocystis jiroveci) B59
    Proteus J15.6
    Pseudomonas NEC J15.1
      pseudomallei A24.1
    psittacosis A70
    Q fever A78
    respiratory syncytial virus (RSV) J12.1
    rheumatic fever I00 *[J17]*
    rubella B06.81
    Salmonella (infection) A02.22
      typhi A01.03
    schistosomiasis B65.9 *[J17]*
    Serratia marcescens J15.6
    specified
      bacterium NEC J15.8
      organism NEC J16.8
    spirochetal NEC A69.8
    Staphylococcus J15.20
      aureus (methicillin susceptible) (MSSA) J15.211
        methicillin resistant (MRSA) J15.212
      specified NEC J15.29
    Streptococcus J15.4
      group B J15.3
      pneumoniae J13
      specified NEC J15.4
    toxoplasmosis B58.3
    tularemia A21.2
    typhoid (fever) A01.03
    varicella B01.2
    virus — *see* Pneumonia, viral
    whooping cough A37.91
      due to
        Bordetella parapertussis A37.11
        Bordetella pertussis A37.01
        specified NEC A37.81
    Yersinia pestis A20.2
  inhalation of food or vomit — *see* Pneumonia, aspiration
  interstitial J84.9
    chronic J84.111
    desquamative J84.117
    due to
      collagen vascular disease J84.17
      known underlying cause J84.17
    idiopathic NOS J84.111
    in disease classified elsewhere J84.17
    lymphocytic (due to collagen vascular disease) (in diseases classified elsewhere) J84.17
    lymphoid J84.2
    non-specific J84.89
      due to
        collagen vascular disease J84.17
        known underlying cause J84.17
      idiopathic J84.113
      in diseases classified elsewhere J84.17
    plasma cell B59
    pseudomonas J15.1
    usual J84.112
      due to collagen vascular disease J84.17
      idiopathic J84.112
      in diseases classified elsewhere J84.17
  Klebsiella (pneumoniae) J15.0
  lipid, lipoid (exogenous) J69.1
    endogenous J84.89
  lobar (disseminated) (double) (interstitial) J18.1
    bacterial J15.9
      specified NEC J15.8
    chronic — *see* Fibrosis, lung
    Escherichia coli (E. coli) J15.5
    Friedländer's bacillus J15.0
    Hemophilus influenzae J14
    hypostatic J18.2
    Klebsiella (pneumoniae) J15.0
    pneumococcal J13
    Proteus J15.6
    Pseudomonas J15.1
    specified organism NEC J16.8
    staphylococcal — *see* Pneumonia, staphylococcal
    streptococcal NEC J15.4

Pneumonia — *continued*
  lobar — *continued*
    Streptococcus pneumoniae J13
    viral, virus — *see* Pneumonia, viral
  lobular — *see* Pneumonia, broncho
  Löffler's J82
  lymphoid interstitial J84.2
  massive — *see* Pneumonia, lobar
  meconium P24.01
  MRSA (methicillin resistant Staphylococcus aureus) J15.212
  MSSA (methicillin susceptible Staphylococcus aureus) J15.211
  multilobar — *see* Pneumonia, by type
  Mycoplasma (pneumoniae) J15.7
  necrotic J85.0
  neonatal P23.9
    aspiration — *see* Aspiration, by substance, with pneumonia
  nitrogen dioxide J68.0
  organizing J84.89
    due to
      collagen vascular disease J84.17
      known underlying cause J84.17
    in diseases classified elsewhere J84.17
  orthostatic J18.2
  parainfluenza virus J12.2
  parenchymatous — *see* Fibrosis, lung
  passive J18.2
  patchy — *see* Pneumonia, broncho
  Peptococcus J15.8
  Peptostreptococcus J15.8
  plasma cell (of infants) B59
  pleurolobar — *see* Pneumonia, lobar
  pleuro-pneumonia-like organism (PPLO) J15.7
  pneumococcal (broncho) (lobar) J13
  Pneumocystis (carinii) (jiroveci) B59
  postinfectional NEC B99 ☑ *[J17]*
  postmeasles B05.2
  Proteus J15.6
  Pseudomonas J15.1
  psittacosis A70
  radiation J70.0
  respiratory syncytial virus (RSV) J12.1
  resulting from a procedure J95.89
  rheumatic I00 *[J17]*
  Salmonella (arizonae) (cholerae-suis) (enteritidis) (typhimurium) A02.22
    typhi A01.03
    typhoid fever A01.03
  SARS-associated coronavirus J12.81
  segmented, segmental — *see* Pneumonia, broncho-
  Serratia marcescens J15.6
  specified NEC J18.8
    bacterium NEC J15.8
    organism NEC J16.8
    virus NEC J12.89
  spirochetal NEC A69.8
  staphylococcal (broncho) (lobar) J15.20
    aureus (methicillin susceptible) (MSSA) J15.211
      methicillin resistant (MRSA) J15.212
    specified NEC J15.29
  static, stasis J18.2
  streptococcal NEC (broncho) (lobar) J15.4
    group
      A J15.4
      B J15.3
      specified NEC J15.4
  Streptococcus pneumoniae J13
  syphilitic, congenital (early) A50.04
  traumatic (complication) (early) (secondary) T79.8 ☑
  tuberculous (any) — *see* Tuberculosis, pulmonary
  tularemic A21.2
  varicella B01.2
  Veillonella J15.8
  ventilator associated J95.851
  viral, virus (broncho) (interstitial) (lobar) J12.9
    adenoviral J12.0
    congenital P23.0
    human metapneumovirus J12.3
    parainfluenza J12.2
    respiratory syncytial (RSV) J12.1
    SARS-associated coronavirus J12.81
    specified NEC J12.89
  white (congenital) A50.04
Pneumonic — *see* condition
Pneumonitis (acute) (primary) — *see also* Pneumonia
  air-conditioner J67.7

Pneumonitis — continued
  allergic (due to) J67.9
    organic dust NEC J67.8
    red cedar dust J67.8
    sequoiosis J67.8
    wood dust J67.8
  aspiration J69.0
    due to
      anesthesia J95.4
        during
          labor and delivery O74.0
          pregnancy O29.01- ☑
          puerperium O89.01
      fumes or gases J68.0
      obstetric O74.0
  chemical (due to gases, fumes or vapors) (inhalation) J68.0
    due to anesthesia J95.4
  cholesterol J84.89
  chronic — see Fibrosis, lung
  congenital rubella P35.0
  crack (cocaine) J68.0
  due to
    beryllium J68.0
    cadmium J68.0
    crack (cocaine) J68.0
    detergent J69.8
    fluorocarbon-polymer J68.0
    food, vomit (aspiration) J69.0
    fumes or vapors J68.0
    gases, fumes or vapors (inhalation) J68.0
    inhalation
      blood J69.8
      essences J69.1
      food (regurgitated), milk, vomit J69.0
      oils, essences J69.1
      saliva J69.0
      solids, liquids NEC J69.8
    manganese J68.0
    nitrogen dioxide J68.0
    oils, essences J69.1
    solids, liquids NEC J69.8
    toxoplasmosis (acquired) B58.3
      congenital P37.1
    vanadium J68.0
    ventilator J95.851
  eosinophilic J82
  hypersensitivity J67.9
    air conditioner lung J67.7
    bagassosis J67.1
    bird fancier's lung J67.2
    farmer's lung J67.0
    maltworker's lung J67.4
    maple bark-stripper's lung J67.6
    mushroom worker's lung J67.5
    specified organic dust NEC J67.8
    suberosis J67.3
  interstitial (chronic) J84.89
    acute J84.114
    lymphoid J84.2
    non-specific J84.89
      idiopathic J84.113
  lymphoid, interstitial J84.2
  meconium P24.01
  postanesthetic J95.4
    correct substance properly administered — see Table of Drugs and Chemicals, by drug, adverse effect
    in labor and delivery O74.0
    in pregnancy O29.01- ☑
    obstetric O74.0
    overdose or wrong substance given or taken (by accident) — see Table of Drugs and Chemicals, by drug, poisoning
    postpartum, puerperal O89.01
  postoperative J95.4
    obstetric O74.0
  radiation J70.0
  rubella, congenital P35.0
  ventilation (air-conditioning) J67.7
  ventilator associated J95.851
  wood-dust J67.8
Pneumoconiosis — see Pneumoconiosis
Pneumoparotid K11.8
Pneumopathy NEC J98.4
  alveolar J84.09
  due to organic dust NEC J66.8
  parietoalveolar J84.09

Pneumopericarditis — see also Pericarditis
  acute I30.9
Pneumopericardium — see also Pericarditis
  congenital P25.3
  newborn P25.3
  traumatic (post) — see Injury, heart
Pneumophagia (psychogenic) F45.8
Pneumopleurisy, pneumopleuritis — see also Pneumonia J18.8
Pneumopyopericardium I30.1
Pneumopyothorax — see Pyopneumothorax
  with fistula J86.0
Pneumorrhagia — see also Hemorrhage, lung
  tuberculous — see Tuberculosis, pulmonary
Pneumothorax NOS J93.9
  acute J93.83
  chronic J93.81
  congenital P25.1
  perinatal period P25.1
  postprocedural J95.811
  specified NEC J93.83
  spontaneous NOS J93.83
    newborn P25.1
    primary J93.11
    secondary J93.12
    tension J93.0
  tense valvular, infectional J93.0
  tension (spontaneous) J93.0
  traumatic S27.0 ☑
    with hemothorax S27.2 ☑
  tuberculous — see Tuberculosis, pulmonary
Podagra — see also Gout M10.9
Podencephalus Q01.9
Poikilocytosis R71.8
Poikiloderma L81.6
  Civatte's L57.3
  congenital Q82.8
  vasculare atrophicans L94.5
Poikilodermatomyositis M33.10
  with
    myopathy M33.12
    respiratory involvement M33.11
    specified organ involvement NEC M33.19
Pointed ear (congenital) Q17.3
Poison ivy, oak, sumac or other plant dermatitis (allergic) (contact) L23.7
Poisoning (acute) — see also Table of Drugs and Chemicals
  algae and toxins T65.82- ☑
  Bacillus B (aertrycke) (cholerae (suis)) (paratyphosus) (suipestifer) A02.9
    botulinus A05.1
  bacterial toxins A05.9
  berries, noxious — see Poisoning, food, noxious, berries
  botulism A05.1
  ciguatera fish T61.0- ☑
  Clostridium botulinum A05.1
  death-cap (Amanita phalloides) (Amanita verna) — see Poisoning, food, noxious, mushrooms
  drug — see Table of Drugs and Chemicals, by drug, poisoning
  epidemic, fish (noxious) — see Poisoning, seafood
    bacterial A05.9
  fava bean D55.0
  fish (noxious) T61.9- ☑
    bacterial — see Intoxication, foodborne, by agent
    ciguatera fish — see Poisoning, ciguatera fish
    scombroid fish — see Poisoning, scombroid fish
    specified type NEC T61.77- ☑
  food NEC A05.9
    bacterial — see Intoxication, foodborne, by agent
    due to
      Bacillus (aertrycke) (choleraesuis) (paratyphosus) (suipestifer) A02.9
        botulinus A05.1
      Clostridium (perfringens) (Welchii) A05.2
      salmonella (aertrycke) (callinarum) (choleraesuis) (enteritidis) (paratyphi) (suipestifer) A02.9
        with
          gastroenteritis A02.0
          sepsis A02.1
      staphylococcus A05.0
      Vibrio
        parahaemolyticus A05.3
        vulnificus A05.5
    noxious or naturally toxic T62.9- ☑
      berries — see subcategory T62.1 ☑
      fish — see Poisoning, seafood

Poisoning — continued
  food — continued
    noxious or naturally toxic — continued
      mushrooms — see subcategory T62.0X ☑
      plants NEC — see subcategory T62.2X ☑
      seafood — see Poisoning, seafood
      specified NEC — see subcategory T62.8X ☑
    ichthyotoxism — see Poisoning, seafood
    kreotoxism, food A05.9
    latex T65.81- ☑
    lead T56.0- ☑
    mushroom — see Poisoning, food, noxious, mushroom
    mussels — see Poisoning, shellfish
      bacterial — see Intoxication, foodborne, by agent
    nicotine (tobacco) T65.2- ☑
    noxious foodstuffs — see Poisoning, food, noxious
    plants, noxious — see Poisoning, food, noxious, plants NEC
    ptomaine — see Poisoning, food
    radiation J70.0
    Salmonella (arizonae) (cholerae-suis) (enteritidis) (typhimurium) A02.9
    scombroid fish T61.1- ☑
    seafood (noxious) T61.9- ☑
      bacterial — see Intoxication, foodborne, by agent
      fish — see Poisoning, fish
      shellfish — see Poisoning, shellfish
      specified NEC — see subcategory T61.8X ☑
    shellfish (amnesic) (azaspiracid) (diarrheic) (neurotoxic) (noxious) (paralytic) T61.78- ☑
      bacterial — see Intoxication, foodborne, by agent
      ciguatera mollusk — see Poisoning, ciguatera fish
    specified substance NEC T65.891 ☑
    Staphylococcus, food A05.0
    tobacco (nicotine) T65.2- ☑
    water E87.79
Poker spine — see Spondylitis, ankylosing
Poland syndrome Q79.8
Polioencephalitis (acute) (bulbar) A80.9
  inferior G12.22
  influenzal — see Influenza, with, encephalopathy
  superior hemorrhagic (acute) (Wernicke's) E51.2
  Wernicke's E51.2
Polioencephalomyelitis (acute) (anterior) A80.9
  with beriberi E51.2
Polioencephalopathy, superior hemorrhagic E51.2
  with
    beriberi E51.11
    pellagra E52
Poliomeningoencephalitis — see Meningoencephalitis
Poliomyelitis (acute) (anterior) (epidemic) A80.9
  with paralysis (bulbar) — see Poliomyelitis, paralytic
  abortive A80.4
  ascending (progressive) — see Poliomyelitis, paralytic
  bulbar (paralytic) — see Poliomyelitis, paralytic
  congenital P35.8
  nonepidemic A80.9
  nonparalytic A80.4
  paralytic A80.30
    specified NEC A80.39
    vaccine-associated A80.0
    wild virus
      imported A80.1
      indigenous A80.2
  spinal, acute A80.9
Poliosis (eyebrow) (eyelashes) L67.1
  circumscripta, acquired L67.1
Pollakiuria R35.0
  psychogenic F45.8
Pollinosis J30.1
Pollitzer's disease L73.2
Polyadenitis — see also Lymphadenitis
  malignant A20.0
Polyalgia M79.89
Polyangiitis M30.0
  microscopic M31.7
  overlap syndrome M30.8
Polyarteritis
  microscopic M31.7
  nodosa M30.0
    with lung involvement M30.1
    juvenile M30.2
    related condition NEC M30.8
Polyarthralgia — see Pain, joint
Polyarthritis, polyarthropathy — see also Arthritis M13.0

Polyarthritis, polyarthropathy — *continued*
  due to or associated with other specified conditions — *see* Arthritis
  epidemic (Australian) (with exanthema) B33.1
  infective — *see* Arthritis, pyogenic or pyemic
  inflammatory M06.4
  juvenile (chronic) (seronegative) M08.3
  migratory M13.8- ☑
  rheumatic, acute — *see* Fever, rheumatic
Polyarthrosis M15.9
  post-traumatic M15.3
  primary M15.0
  specified NEC M15.8
Polycarential syndrome of infancy E40
Polychondritis (atrophic) (chronic) — *see also* Disorder, cartilage, specified type NEC
  relapsing M94.1
Polycoria Q13.2
Polycystic (disease)
  degeneration, kidney Q61.3
    autosomal dominant (adult type) Q61.2
    autosomal recessive (infantile type) NEC Q61.19
  kidney Q61.3
    autosomal
      dominant Q61.2
      recessive NEC Q61.19
    autosomal dominant (adult type) Q61.2
    autosomal recessive (childhood type) NEC Q61.19
    infantile type NEC Q61.19
  liver Q44.6
  lung J98.4
    congenital Q33.0
  ovary, ovaries E28.2
  spleen Q89.09
Polycythemia (secondary) D75.1
  acquired D75.1
  benign (familial) D75.0
  due to
    donor twin P61.1
    erythropoietin D75.1
    fall in plasma volume D75.1
    high altitude D75.1
    maternal-fetal transfusion P61.1
    stress D75.1
  emotional D75.1
  erythropoietin D75.1
  familial (benign) D75.0
  Gaisböck's (hypertonica) D75.1
  high altitude D75.1
  hypertonica D75.1
  hypoxemic D75.1
  neonatorum P61.1
  nephrogenous D75.1
  relative D75.1
  secondary D75.1
  spurious D75.1
  stress D75.1
  vera D45
Polycytosis cryptogenica D75.1
Polydactylism, polydactyly Q69.9
  toes Q69.2
Polydipsia R63.1
Polydystrophy, pseudo-Hurler E77.0
Polyembryoma — *see* Neoplasm, malignant, by site
Polyglandular
  deficiency E31.0
  dyscrasia E31.9
  dysfunction E31.9
  syndrome E31.8
Polyhydramnios O40.- ☑
Polymastia Q83.1
Polymenorrhea N92.0
Polymyalgia M35.3
  arteritica, giant cell M31.5
  rheumatica M35.3
    with giant cell arteritis M31.5
Polymyositis (acute) (chronic) (hemorrhagic) M33.20
  with
    myopathy M33.22
    respiratory involvement M33.21
    skin involvement — *see* Dermatopolymyositis
    specified organ involvement NEC M33.29
  ossificans (generalisata) (progressiva) — *see* Myositis, ossificans, progressiva
Polyneuritis, polyneuritic — *see also* Polyneuropathy
  acute (post-)infective G61.0
  alcoholic G62.1
  cranialis G52.7

Polyneuritis, polyneuritic — *continued*
  demyelinating, chronic inflammatory (CIDP) G61.81
  diabetic — *see* Diabetes, polyneuropathy
  diphtheritic A36.83
  due to lack of vitamin NEC E56.9 *[G63]*
  endemic E51.11
  erythredema — *see* subcategory T56.1 ☑
  febrile, acute G61.0
  hereditary ataxic G60.1
  idiopathic, acute G61.0
  infective (acute) G61.0
  inflammatory, chronic demyelinating (CIDP) G61.81
  nutritional E63.9 *[G63]*
  postinfective (acute) G61.0
  specified NEC G62.89
Polyneuropathy (peripheral) G62.9
  alcoholic G62.1
  amyloid (Portuguese) E85.1 *[G63]*
    transthyretin-related (ATTR) familial E85.1 *[G63]*
  arsenical G62.2
  critical illness G62.81
  demyelinating, chronic inflammatory (CIDP) G61.81
  diabetic — *see* Diabetes, polyneuropathy
  drug-induced G62.0
  hereditary G60.9
    specified NEC G60.8
  idiopathic G60.9
    progressive G60.3
  in (due to)
    alcohol G62.1
      sequelae G65.2
    amyloidosis, familial (Portuguese) E85.1 *[G63]*
    antitetanus serum G61.1
    arsenic G62.2
      sequelae G65.2
    avitaminosis NEC E56.9 *[G63]*
    beriberi E51.11
    collagen vascular disease NEC M35.9 *[G63]*
    deficiency (of)
      B (-complex) vitamins E53.9 *[G63]*
      vitamin B6 E53.1 *[G63]*
    diabetes — *see* Diabetes, polyneuropathy
    diphtheria A36.83
    drug or medicament G62.0
      correct substance properly administered — *see* Table of Drugs and Chemicals, by drug, adverse effect
      overdose or wrong substance given or taken — *see* Table of Drugs and Chemicals, by drug, poisoning
    endocrine disease NEC E34.9 *[G63]*
    herpes zoster B02.23
    hypoglycemia E16.2 *[G63]*
    infectious
      disease NEC B99 ☑ *[G63]*
      mononucleosis B27.91
    lack of vitamin NEC E56.9 *[G63]*
    lead G62.2
      sequelae G65.2
    leprosy A30.9 *[G63]*
    Lyme disease A69.22
    metabolic disease NEC E88.9 *[G63]*
    microscopic polyangiitis M31.7 *[G63]*
    mumps B26.84
    neoplastic disease — *see also* Neoplasm D49.9 *[G63]*
    nutritional deficiency NEC E63.9 *[G63]*
    organophosphate compounds G62.2
      sequelae G65.2
    parasitic disease NEC B89 *[G63]*
    pellagra E52 *[G63]*
    polyarteritis nodosa M30.0
    porphyria E80.20 *[G63]*
    radiation G62.82
    rheumatoid arthritis — *see* Rheumatoid, polyneuropathy
    sarcoidosis D86.89
    serum G61.1
    syphilis (late) A52.15
      congenital A50.43
    systemic
      connective tissue disorder M35.9 *[G63]*
      lupus erythematosus M32.19
    toxic agent NEC G62.2
      sequelae G65.2
  inflammatory G61.9
    chronic demyelinating (CIDP) G61.81
    sequelae G65.1
    specified NEC G61.89

Polyneuropathy — *continued*
  lead G62.2
    sequelae G65.2
  nutritional NEC E63.9 *[G63]*
  postherpetic (zoster) B02.23
  progressive G60.3
  radiation-induced G62.82
  sensory (hereditary) (idiopathic) G60.8
  specified NEC G62.89
  syphilitic (late) A52.15
    congenital A50.43
  transthyretin-related (ATTR) familial amyloid E85.1
    triorthocresyl phosphate G62.2
      sequelae G65.2
    tuberculosis A17.89
    uremia N18.9 *[G63]*
    vitamin B12 deficiency E53.8 *[G63]*
      with anemia (pernicious) D51.0 *[G63]*
        due to dietary deficiency D51.3 *[G63]*
    zoster B02.23
Polyopia H53.8
Polyorchism, polyorchidism Q55.21
Polyosteoarthritis — *see also* Osteoarthritis, generalized M15.9
  post-traumatic M15.3
  specified NEC M15.8
Polyostotic fibrous dysplasia Q78.1
Polyotia Q17.0
Polyp, polypus
  accessory sinus J33.8
  adenocarcinoma in — *see* Neoplasm, malignant, by site
  adenocarcinoma in situ in — *see* Neoplasm, in situ, by site
  adenoid tissue J33.0
  adenomatous — *see also* Neoplasm, benign, by site
    adenocarcinoma in — *see* Neoplasm, malignant, by site
    adenocarcinoma in situ in — *see* Neoplasm, in situ, by site
    carcinoma in — *see* Neoplasm, malignant, by site
    carcinoma in situ in — *see* Neoplasm, in situ, by site
    multiple — *see* Neoplasm, benign
      adenocarcinoma in — *see* Neoplasm, malignant, by site
      adenocarcinoma in situ in — *see* Neoplasm, in situ, by site
  antrum J33.8
  anus, anal (canal) K62.0
  Bartholin's gland N84.3
  bladder D41.4
  carcinoma in — *see* Neoplasm, malignant, by site
  carcinoma in situ in — *see* Neoplasm, in situ, by site
  cecum D12.0
  cervix (uteri) N84.1
    in pregnancy or childbirth — *see* Pregnancy, complicated by, abnormal, cervix
    mucous N84.1
    nonneoplastic N84.1
  choanal J33.0
  cholesterol K82.4
  clitoris N84.3
  colon K63.5
    adenomatous D12.6
      ascending D12.2
      cecum D12.0
      descending D12.4
    hyperplastic, (any site) K63.5
    inflammatory K51.40
      with
        abscess K51.414
        complication K51.419
          specified NEC K51.418
        fistula K51.413
        intestinal obstruction K51.412
        rectal bleeding K51.411
    sigmoid D12.5
    transverse D12.3
  corpus uteri N84.0
  dental K04.01
    irreversible K04.02
    reversible K04.01
  duodenum K31.7
  ear (middle) H74.4- ☑
  endometrium N84.0
  ethmoidal (sinus) J33.8
  fallopian tube N84.8
  female genital tract N84.9

Polyp, polypus — *continued*
  female genital tract — *continued*
    specified NEC N84.8
  frontal (sinus) J33.8
  gallbladder K82.4
  gingiva, gum K06.8
  labia, labium (majus) (minus) N84.3
  larynx (mucous) J38.1
    adenomatous D14.1
  malignant — *see* Neoplasm, malignant, by site
  maxillary (sinus) J33.8
  middle ear — *see* Polyp, ear (middle)
  myometrium N84.0
  nares
    anterior J33.9
    posterior J33.0
  nasal (mucous) J33.9
    cavity J33.0
    septum J33.0
  nasopharyngeal J33.0
  nose (mucous) J33.9
  oviduct N84.8
  pharynx J39.2
  placenta O90.89
  prostate — *see* Enlargement, enlarged, prostate
  pudenda, pudendum N84.3
  pulpal (dental) K04.01
    irreversible K04.02
    reversible K04.01
  rectum (nonadenomatous) K62.1
    adenomatous — *see* Polyp, adenomatous
  septum (nasal) J33.0
  sinus (accessory) (ethmoidal) (frontal) (maxillary)
    (sphenoidal) J33.8
  sphenoidal (sinus) J33.8
  stomach K31.7
    adenomatous D13.1
  tube, fallopian N84.8
  turbinate, mucous membrane J33.8
  umbilical, newborn P83.6
  ureter N28.89
  urethra N36.2
  uterus (body) (corpus) (mucous) N84.0
    cervix N84.1
    in pregnancy or childbirth — *see* Pregnancy, com-
      plicated by, tumor, uterus
  vagina N84.2
  vocal cord (mucous) J38.1
  vulva N84.3
Polyphagia R63.2
Polyploidy Q92.7
Polypoid — *see* condition
Polyposis — *see also* Polyp
  coli (adenomatous) D12.6
    adenocarcinoma in C18.9
    adenocarcinoma in situ in — *see* Neoplasm, in situ,
      by site
    carcinoma in C18.9
  colon (adenomatous) D12.6
  familial D12.6
    adenocarcinoma in situ in — *see* Neoplasm, in situ,
      by site
  intestinal (adenomatous) D12.6
  malignant lymphomatous C83.1- ☑
  multiple, adenomatous — *see also* Neoplasm, benign
    D36.9
Polyradiculitis — *see* Polyneuropathy
Polyradiculoneuropathy (acute) (postinfective) (seg-
  mentally demyelinating) G61.0
Polyserositis
  due to pericarditis I31.1
  pericardial I31.1
  periodic, familial E85.0
  tuberculous A19.9
    acute A19.1
    chronic A19.9
Polysplenia syndrome Q89.09
Polysyndactyly — *see also* Syndactylism, syndactyly
  Q70.4
Polytrichia L68.3
Polyunguia Q84.6
Polyuria R35.8
  nocturnal R35.1
  psychogenic F45.8
Pompe's disease (glycogen storage) E74.02
Pompholyx L30.1
Poncet's disease (tuberculous rheumatism) A18.09
Pond fracture — *see* Fracture, skull

Ponos B55.0
Pons, pontine — *see* condition
Poor
  aesthetic of existing restoration of tooth K08.56
  contractions, labor O62.2
  gingival margin to tooth restoration K08.51
  personal hygiene R46.0
  prenatal care, affecting management of pregnancy —
    see Pregnancy, complicated by, insufficient,
    prenatal care
  sucking reflex (newborn) R29.2
  urinary stream R39.12
  vision NEC H54.7
Poradenitis, nostras inguinalis or venerea A55
Porencephaly (congenital) (developmental) (true) Q04.6
  acquired G93.0
  nondevelopmental G93.0
  traumatic (post) F07.89
Porocephaliasis B88.8
Porokeratosis Q82.8
Poroma, eccrine — *see* Neoplasm, skin, benign
Porphyria (South African) E80.20
  acquired E80.20
  acute intermittent (hepatic) (Swedish) E80.21
  cutanea tarda (hereditary) (symptomatic) E80.1
  due to drugs E80.20
    correct substance properly administered — *see* Ta-
      ble of Drugs and Chemicals, by drug, adverse
      effect
    overdose or wrong substance given or taken — *see*
      Table of Drugs and Chemicals, by drug, poi-
      soning
  erythropoietic (congenital) (hereditary) E80.0
  hepatocutaneous type E80.1
  secondary E80.20
  toxic NEC E80.20
  variegata E80.20
Porphyrinuria — *see* Porphyria
Porphyruria — *see* Porphyria
Port wine nevus, mark, or stain Q82.5
Portal — *see* condition
Posadas-Wernicke disease B38.9
Positive
  culture (nonspecific)
    blood R78.81
    bronchial washings R84.5
    cerebrospinal fluid R83.5
    cervix uteri R87.5
    nasal secretions R84.5
    nipple discharge R89.5
    nose R84.5
      staphylococcus (Methicillin susceptible) Z22.321
        Methicillin resistant Z22.322
    peritoneal fluid R85.5
    pleural fluid R84.5
    prostatic secretions R86.5
    saliva R85.5
    seminal fluid R86.5
    sputum R84.5
    synovial fluid R89.5
    throat scrapings R84.5
    urine R82.79
    vagina R87.5
    vulva R87.5
    wound secretions R89.5
  PPD (skin test) R76.11
  serology for syphilis A53.0
    false R76.8
    with signs or symptoms — *code as* Syphilis, by site
      and stage
  skin test, tuberculin (without active tuberculosis) R76.11
  test, human immunodeficiency virus (HIV) R75
  VDRL A53.0
    with signs or symptoms — *code by* site and stage
      under Syphilis A53.9
  Wassermann reaction A53.0
Postcardiotomy syndrome I97.0
Postcaval ureter Q62.62
Postcholecystectomy syndrome K91.5
Postclimacteric bleeding N95.0
Postcommissurotomy syndrome I97.0
Postconcussional syndrome F07.81
Postcontusional syndrome F07.81
Postcricoid region — *see* condition
Post-dates (40-42 weeks) (pregnancy) (mother) O48.0
  more than 42 weeks gestation O48.1
Postencephalitic syndrome F07.89
Posterior — *see* condition

Posterolateral sclerosis (spinal cord) — *see* Degenera-
  tion, combined
Postexanthematous — *see* condition
Postfebrile — *see* condition
Postgastrectomy dumping syndrome K91.1
Posthemiplegic chorea — *see* Monoplegia
Posthemorrhagic anemia (chronic) D50.0
  acute D62
  newborn P61.3
Postherpetic neuralgia (zoster) B02.29
  trigeminal B02.22
Posthitis N47.7
Postimmunization complication or reaction — *see*
  Complications, vaccination
Postinfectious — *see* condition
Postlaminectomy syndrome NEC M96.1
Postleukotomy syndrome F07.0
Postmastectomy lymphedema (syndrome) I97.2
Postmaturity, postmature (over 42 weeks)
  maternal (over 42 weeks gestation) O48.1
  newborn P08.22
Postmeasles complication NEC — *see also* condition
  B05.89
Postmenopausal
  endometrium (atrophic) N95.8
    suppurative — *see also* Endometritis N71.9
  osteoporosis — *see* Osteoporosis, postmenopausal
Postnasal drip R09.82
  due to
    allergic rhinitis — *see* Rhinitis, allergic
    common cold J00
    gastroesophageal reflux — *see* Reflux, gastroe-
      sophageal
    nasopharyngitis — *see* Nasopharyngitis
    other known condition — *code to* condition
    sinusitis — *see* Sinusitis
Postnatal — *see* condition
Postoperative (postprocedural) — *see* Complication,
  postoperative
  pneumothorax, therapeutic Z98.3
  state NEC Z98.890
Postpancreatectomy hyperglycemia E89.1
Postpartum — *see* Puerperal
Postphlebitic syndrome — *see* Syndrome, postthrom-
  botic
Postpolio (myelitic) **syndrome** G14
Postpoliomyelitic — *see also* condition
  osteopathy — *see* Osteopathy, after poliomyelitis
Postprocedural — *see also* Postoperative
  hypoinsulinemia E89.1
Postschizophrenic depression F32.89
Postsurgery status — *see also* Status (post)
  pneumothorax, therapeutic Z98.3
Post-term (40-42 weeks) (pregnancy) (mother) O48.0
  infant P08.21
  more than 42 weeks gestation (mother) O48.1
Post-traumatic brain syndrome, nonpsychotic F07.81
Post-typhoid abscess A01.09
Postures, hysterical F44.2
Postvaccinal reaction or complication — *see* Complications, vaccination
Postvalvulotomy syndrome I97.0
Potain's
  disease (pulmonary edema) — *see* Edema, lung
  syndrome (gastrectasis with dyspepsia) K31.0
Potter's
  asthma J62.8
  facies Q60.6
  lung J62.8
  syndrome (with renal agenesis) Q60.6
Pott's
  curvature (spinal) A18.01
  disease or paraplegia A18.01
  spinal curvature A18.01
  tumor, puffy — *see* Osteomyelitis, specified type NEC
Pouch
  bronchus Q32.4
  Douglas' — *see* condition
  esophagus, esophageal, congenital Q39.6
    acquired K22.5
  gastric K31.4
  Hartmann's K82.8
  pharynx, pharyngeal (congenital) Q38.7
Pouchitis K91.850
Poultrymen's itch B88.0
Poverty NEC Z59.6
  extreme Z59.5

Poxvirus NEC B08.8
Prader-Willi syndrome Q87.11
Prader-Willi-like syndrome Q87.19
Preauricular appendage or tag Q17.0
Prebetalipoproteinemia (acquired) (essential) (familial) (hereditary) (primary) (secondary) E78.1
   with chylomicronemia E78.3
Precipitate labor or delivery O62.3
Preclimacteric bleeding (menorrhagia) N92.4
Precocious
   adrenarche E30.1
   menarche E30.1
   menstruation E30.1
   pubarche E30.1
   puberty E30.1
     central E22.8
   sexual development NEC E30.1
   thelarche E30.8
Precocity, sexual (constitutional) (cryptogenic) (female) (idiopathic) (male) E30.1
   with adrenal hyperplasia E25.9
     congenital E25.0
Precordial pain R07.2
Predeciduous teeth K00.2
Prediabetes, prediabetic R73.03
   complicating
     pregnancy — see Pregnancy, complicated by, diseases of, specified type or system NEC
     puerperium O99.89
Predislocation status of hip at birth Q65.6
Pre-eclampsia O14.9- ☑
   with pre-existing hypertension — see Hypertension, complicating pregnancy, pre-existing, with, pre-eclampsia
   complicating
     childbirth O14.94
     puerperium O14.95
   mild O14.0- ☑
     complicating
       childbirth O14.04
       puerperium O14.05
   moderate O14.0- ☑
     complicating
       childbirth O14.04
       puerperium O14.05
   severe O14.1- ☑
     with hemolysis, elevated liver enzymes and low platelet count (HELLP) O14.2- ☑
     complicating
       childbirth O14.24
       puerperium O14.25
     complicating
       childbirth O14.14
       puerperium O14.15
Pre-eruptive color change, teeth, tooth K00.8
Pre-excitation atrioventricular conduction I45.6
Preglaucoma H40.00- ☑
Pregnancy (single) (uterine) — see also Delivery and Puerperal

Note: The Tabular must be reviewed for assignment of appropriate seventh character for multiple gestation codes in Chapter 15

Note: The Tabular must be reviewed for assignment of the appropriate character indicating the trimester of the pregnancy

   abdominal (ectopic) O00.00
     with intrauterine pregnancy O00.01
     with viable fetus O36.7- ☑
   ampullar O00.10- ☑
     with intrauterine pregnancy O00.11- ☑
   biochemical O02.81
   broad ligament O00.80
     with intrauterine pregnancy O00.81
   cervical O00.8
     with intrauterine pregnancy O00.81
   chemical O02.81
   complicated by (care of) (management affected by)
     abnormal, abnormality
       cervix O34.4- ☑
         causing obstructed labor O65.5
       cord (umbilical) O69.9 ☑
       fetal heart rate or rhythm O36.83- ☑
       findings on antenatal screening of mother O28.9
         biochemical O28.1
         chromosomal O28.5

Pregnancy — continued
   complicated by — continued
     abnormal, abnormality — continued
       findings on antenatal screening of mother — continued
         cytological O28.2
         genetic O28.5
         hematological O28.0
         radiological O28.4
         specified NEC O28.8
         ultrasonic O28.3
       glucose (tolerance) NEC O99.810
       pelvic organs O34.9-
         specified NEC O34.8- ☑
           causing obstructed labor O65.5
       pelvis (bony) (major) NEC O33.0
       perineum O34.7- ☑
       position
         placenta O44.0- ☑
           with hemorrhage O44.1- ☑
         uterus O34.59-
       uterus O34.59- ☑
         causing obstructed labor O65.5
         congenital O34.0- ☑
       vagina O34.6- ☑
         causing obstructed labor O65.5
       vulva O34.7- ☑
         causing obstructed labor O65.5
     abruptio placentae — see Abruptio placentae
     abscess or cellulitis
       bladder O23.1-
       breast O91.11- ☑
       genital organ or tract O23.9- ☑
     abuse
       physical O9A.31 ☑ (following O99)
       psychological O9A.51 ☑ (following O99)
       sexual O9A.41 ☑ (following O99)
     adverse effect anesthesia O29.9- ☑
       aspiration pneumonitis O29.01- ☑
       cardiac arrest O29.11- ☑
       cardiac complication NEC O29.19- ☑
       cardiac failure O29.12- ☑
       central nervous system complication NEC O29.29- ☑
       cerebral anoxia O29.21- ☑
       failed or difficult intubation O29.6- ☑
       inhalation of stomach contents or secretions NOS O29.01- ☑
       local, toxic reaction O29.3X ☑
       Mendelson's syndrome O29.01- ☑
       pressure collapse of lung O29.02- ☑
       pulmonary complications NEC O29.09- ☑
       specified NEC O29.8X- ☑
       spinal and epidural type NEC O29.5X ☑
         induced headache O29.4- ☑
     albuminuria — see also Proteinuria, gestational O12.1- ☑
     alcohol use O99.31- ☑
     amnionitis O41.12- ☑
     anaphylactoid syndrome of pregnancy O88.01- ☑
     anemia (conditions in D50-D64) (pre-existing) O99.01- ☑
       complicating the puerperium O99.03
     antepartum hemorrhage O46.9- ☑
       with coagulation defect — see Hemorrhage, antepartum, with coagulation defect
       specified NEC O46.8X- ☑
     appendicitis O99.61- ☑
     atrophy (yellow) (acute) liver (subacute) O26.61- ☑
     bariatric surgery status O99.84- ☑
     bicornis or bicornuate uterus O34.0- ☑
     biliary tract problems O26.61- ☑
     breech presentation O32.1 ☑
     cardiovascular diseases (conditions in I00-I09, I20-I52, I70-I99) O99.41- ☑
     cerebrovascular disorders (conditions in I60-I69) O99.41- ☑
     cervical shortening O26.87- ☑
     cervicitis O23.51- ☑
     chloasma (gravidarum) O26.89- ☑
     cholecystitis O99.61- ☑
     cholestasis (intrahepatic) O26.61- ☑
     chorioamnionitis O41.12- ☑
     circulatory system disorder (conditions in I00-I09, I20-I99, O99.41-)
     compound presentation O32.6 ☑

Pregnancy — continued
   complicated by — continued
     conjoined twins O30.02- ☑
     connective system disorders (conditions in M00-M99) O99.89
     contracted pelvis (general) O33.1
       inlet O33.2
       outlet O33.3 ☑
     convulsions (eclamptic) (uremic) — see also Eclampsia O15.9
     cracked nipple O92.11- ☑
     cystitis O23.1- ☑
     cystocele O34.8- ☑
     death of fetus (near term) O36.4 ☑
       early pregnancy O02.1
       of one fetus or more in multiple gestation O31.2- ☑
     deciduitis O41.14- ☑
     decreased fetal movement O36.81- ☑
     dental problems O99.61- ☑
     diabetes (mellitus) O24.91- ☑
       gestational (pregnancy induced) — see Diabetes, gestational
       pre-existing O24.31- ☑
         specified NEC O24.81- ☑
         type 1 O24.01- ☑
         type 2 O24.11- ☑
     digestive system disorders (conditions in K00-K93) O99.61- ☑
     diseases of — see Pregnancy, complicated by, specified body system disease
       biliary tract O26.61- ☑
       blood NEC (conditions in D65-D77) O99.11- ☑
       liver O26.61- ☑
       specified NEC O99.89
     disorders of — see Pregnancy, complicated by, specified body system disorder
       amniotic fluid and membranes O41.9- ☑
         specified NEC O41.8X- ☑
       biliary tract O26.61- ☑
       ear and mastoid process (conditions in H60-H95) O99.89
       eye and adnexa (conditions in H00-H59) O99.89
       liver O26.61- ☑
       skin (conditions in L00-L99) O99.71- ☑
       specified NEC O99.89
     displacement, uterus NEC O34.59- ☑
       causing obstructed labor O65.5
     disproportion (due to) O33.9
       fetal (ascites) (hydrops) (meningomyelocele) (sacral teratoma) (tumor) deformities NEC O33.7
       generally contracted pelvis O33.1
       hydrocephalic fetus O33.6 ☑
       inlet contraction of pelvis O33.2
       mixed maternal and fetal origin O33.4 ☑
       specified NEC O33.8
     double uterus O34.0- ☑
       causing obstructed labor O65.5
     drug use (conditions in F11-F19) O99.32- ☑
     eclampsia, eclamptic (coma) (convulsions) (delirium) (nephritis) (uremia) — see also Eclampsia O15.- ☑
     ectopic pregnancy — see Pregnancy, ectopic
     edema O12.0- ☑
       with
         gestational hypertension, mild — see also Pre-eclampsia O14.0- ☑
         proteinuria O12.2- ☑
     effusion, amniotic fluid — see Pregnancy, complicated by, premature rupture of membranes
     elderly
       multigravida O09.52- ☑
       primigravida O09.51- ☑
     embolism — see also Embolism, obstetric, pregnancy O88.- ☑
     endocrine diseases NEC O99.28- ☑
     endometritis O86.12
     excessive weight gain O26.0- ☑
     exhaustion O26.81- ☑
       during labor and delivery O75.81
     face presentation O32.3 ☑
     failed induction of labor O61.9
       instrumental O61.1
       mechanical O61.1
       medical O61.0
       specified NEC O61.8

Pregnancy — *continued*
  complicated by — *continued*
    failed induction of labor — *continued*
      surgical O61.1
    failed or difficult intubation for anesthesia O29.6- ☑
    false labor (pains) O47.9
      at or after 37 completed weeks of pregnancy O47.1
      before 37 completed weeks of pregnancy O47.0- ☑
    fatigue O26.81- ☑
      during labor and delivery O75.81
    fatty metamorphosis of liver O26.61- ☑
    female genital mutilation O34.8- ☑ *[N90.81-]* ☑
    fetal (maternal care for)
      abnormality or damage O35.9 ☑
        acid-base balance O68
        specified type NEC O35.8 ☑
      acidemia O68
      acidosis O68
      alkalosis O68
      anemia and thrombocytopenia O36.82- ☑
      anencephaly O35.0 ☑
      bradycardia O36.83- ☑
      chromosomal abnormality (conditions in Q90-Q99) O35.1 ☑
      conjoined twins O30.02- ☑
      damage from
        amniocentesis O35.7 ☑
        biopsy procedures O35.7 ☑
        drug addiction O35.5 ☑
        hematological investigation O35.7 ☑
        intrauterine contraceptive device O35.7 ☑
        maternal
          alcohol addiction O35.4 ☑
          cytomegalovirus infection O35.3 ☑
          disease NEC O35.8 ☑
          drug addiction O35.5 ☑
          listeriosis O35.8 ☑
          rubella O35.3 ☑
          toxoplasmosis O35.8 ☑
          viral infection O35.3 ☑
        medical procedure NEC O35.7 ☑
        radiation O35.6 ☑
      death (near term) O36.4 ☑
        early pregnancy O02.1
      decreased movement O36.81- ☑
      depressed heart rate tones O36.83- ☑
      disproportion due to deformity (fetal) O33.7 ☑
      excessive growth (large for dates) O36.6- ☑
      growth retardation O36.59- ☑
        light for dates O36.59- ☑
        small for dates O36.59- ☑
      heart rate irregularity (abnormal variability) (bradycardia) (decelerations) (tachycardia) O36.83- ☑
      hereditary disease O35.2 ☑
      hydrocephalus O35.0 ☑
      intrauterine death O36.4 ☑
      non-reassuring heart rate or rhythm O36.83- ☑
      poor growth O36.59- ☑
        light for dates O36.59- ☑
        small for dates O36.59- ☑
      problem O36.9- ☑
        specified NEC O36.89- ☑
      reduction (elective) O31.3- ☑
      selective termination O31.3- ☑
      spina bifida O35.0 ☑
      thrombocytopenia O36.82- ☑
    fibroid (tumor) (uterus) O34.1- ☑
    fissure of nipple O92.11- ☑
    gallstones O99.61- ☑
    gastric banding status O99.84- ☑
    gastric bypass status O99.84- ☑
    genital herpes (asymptomatic) (history of) (inactive) O98.3- ☑
    genital tract infection O23.9- ☑
    glomerular diseases (conditions in N00-N07) O26.83- ☑
      with hypertension, pre-existing — *see* Hypertension, complicating, pregnancy, pre-existing, with, renal disease
    gonorrhea O98.21- ☑
    grand multiparity O09.4 ☑
    habitual aborter — *see* Pregnancy, complicated by, recurrent pregnancy loss

Pregnancy — *continued*
  complicated by — *continued*
    HELLP syndrome (hemolysis, elevated liver enzymes and low platelet count) O14.2- ☑
    hemorrhage
      antepartum — *see* Hemorrhage, antepartum
      before 20 completed weeks gestation O20.9
        specified NEC O20.8
      due to premature separation, placenta — *see also* Abruptio placentae O45.9- ☑
      early O20.9
        specified NEC O20.8
      threatened abortion O20.0
    hemorrhoids O22.4- ☑
    hepatitis (viral) O98.41- ☑
    herniation of uterus O34.59- ☑
    high
      head at term O32.4 ☑
      risk — *see* Supervision (of) (for), high-risk
    history of in utero procedure during previous pregnancy O09.82- ☑
    HIV O98.71- ☑
    human immunodeficiency virus (HIV) disease O98.71- ☑
    hydatidiform mole — *see also* Mole, hydatidiform O01.9
    hydramnios O40.- ☑
    hydrocephalic fetus (disproportion) O33.6 ☑
    hydrops
      amnii O40.- ☑
      fetalis O36.2- ☑
        associated with isoimmunization — *see also* Pregnancy, complicated by, isoimmunization O36.11- ☑
    hydrorrhea O42.90
    hyperemesis (gravidarum) (mild) — *see also* Hyperemesis, gravidarum O21.0
    hypertension — *see* Hypertension, complicating pregnancy
    hypertensive
      heart and renal disease, pre-existing — *see* Hypertension, complicating, pregnancy, pre-existing, with, heart disease, with renal disease
      heart disease, pre-existing — *see* Hypertension, complicating, pregnancy, pre-existing, with, heart disease
      renal disease, pre-existing — *see* Hypertension, complicating, pregnancy, pre-existing, with, renal disease
    hypotension O26.5- ☑
    immune disorders NEC (conditions in D80-D89) O99.11- ☑
    incarceration, uterus O34.51- ☑
    incompetent cervix O34.3- ☑
    inconclusive fetal viability O36.80 ☑
    infection(s) O98.91- ☑
      amniotic fluid or sac O41.10- ☑
      bladder O23.1- ☑
      carrier state NEC O99.830
        streptococcus B O99.820
      genital organ or tract O23.9- ☑
        specified NEC O23.59- ☑
      genitourinary tract O23.9- ☑
      gonorrhea O98.21- ☑
      hepatitis (viral) O98.41- ☑
      HIV O98.71- ☑
      human immunodeficiency virus (HIV) O98.71- ☑
      kidney O23.0- ☑
      nipple O91.01- ☑
      parasitic disease O98.91- ☑
        specified NEC O98.81- ☑
      protozoal disease O98.61- ☑
      sexually transmitted NEC O98.31- ☑
      specified type NEC O98.81- ☑
      syphilis O98.11- ☑
      tuberculosis O98.01- ☑
      urethra O23.2- ☑
      urinary (tract) O23.4- ☑
        specified NEC O23.3- ☑
      viral disease O98.51- ☑
    injury or poisoning (conditions in S00-T88) O9A.21- ☑ *(following O99)*
      due to abuse
        physical O9A.31- ☑ *(following O99)*
        psychological O9A.51- ☑ *(following O99)*
        sexual O9A.41- ☑ *(following O99)*

Pregnancy — *continued*
  complicated by — *continued*
    insufficient
      prenatal care O09.3- ☑
      weight gain O26.1- ☑
    insulin resistance O26.89 ☑
    intrauterine fetal death (near term) O36.4 ☑
      early pregnancy O02.1
      multiple gestation (one fetus or more) O31.2- ☑
    isoimmunization O36.11- ☑
      anti-A sensitization O36.11- ☑
      anti-B sensitization O36.19- ☑
      Rh O36.09- ☑
        anti-D antibody O36.01- ☑
      specified NEC O36.19- ☑
    laceration of uterus NEC O71.81
    malformation
      placenta, placental (vessel) O43.10- ☑
        specified NEC O43.19- ☑
      uterus (congenital) O34.0- ☑
    malnutrition (conditions in E40-E46) O25.1- ☑
    maternal hypotension syndrome O26.5- ☑
    mental disorders (conditions in F01-F09, F20-F99) O99.34- ☑
      alcohol use O99.31- ☑
      drug use O99.32- ☑
      smoking O99.33- ☑
    mentum presentation O32.3 ☑
    metabolic disorders O99.28- ☑
    missed
      abortion O02.1
      delivery O36.4 ☑
    multiple gestations O30.9- ☑
      conjoined twins O30.02 ☑
      quadruplet — *see* Pregnancy, quadruplet
      specified complication NEC O31.8X- ☑
      specified number of multiples NEC — *see* Pregnancy, multiple (gestation), specified NEC
      triplet — *see* Pregnancy, triplet
      twin — *see* Pregnancy, twin
    musculoskeletal condition (conditions is M00-M99) O99.89
    necrosis, liver (conditions in K72) O26.61- ☑
    neoplasm
      benign
        cervix O34.4- ☑
        corpus uteri O34.1- ☑
        uterus O34.1- ☑
      malignant O9A.11- ☑ *(following O99)*
    nephropathy NEC O26.83- ☑
    nervous system condition (conditions in G00-G99) O99.35- ☑
    nutritional diseases NEC O99.28- ☑
    obesity (pre-existing) O99.21- ☑
    obesity surgery status O99.84- ☑
    oblique lie or presentation O32.2 ☑
    older mother — *see* Pregnancy, complicated by, elderly
    oligohydramnios O41.0- ☑
      with premature rupture of membranes — *see also* Pregnancy, complicated by, premature rupture of membranes O42.- ☑
    onset (spontaneous) of labor after 37 completed weeks of gestation but before 39 completed weeks gestation, with delivery by (planned) cesarean section O75.82
    oophoritis O23.52- ☑
    overdose, drug — *see also* Table of Drugs and Chemicals, by drug, poisoning O9A.21- ☑ *(following O99)*
    oversize fetus O33.5 ☑
    papyraceous fetus O31.0- ☑
    pelvic inflammatory disease O99.89
    periodontal disease O99.61- ☑
    peripheral neuritis O26.82- ☑
    peritoneal (pelvic) adhesions O99.89
    phlebitis O22.9- ☑
    phlebopathy O22.9- ☑
    phlebothrombosis (superficial) O22.2- ☑
      deep O22.3- ☑
    placenta accreta O43.21- ☑
    placenta increta O43.22- ☑
    placenta percreta O43.23- ☑
    placenta previa O44.0- ☑
      complete O44.0- ☑
        with hemorrhage O44.1- ☑

☑ **Additional Character Required** — Refer to the Tabular List for Character Selection   ▽ **Subterms under main terms may continue to next column or page**

Pregnancy — *continued*
  complicated by — *continued*
    placenta previa — *continued*
      marginal O44.2- ☑
        with hemorrhage O44.3- ☑
      partial O44.2- ☑
        with hemorrhage O44.3- ☑
    placental disorder O43.9- ☑
      specified NEC O43.89- ☑
    placental dysfunction O43.89- ☑
    placental infarction O43.81- ☑
    placental insufficiency O36.51- ☑
    placental transfusion syndromes
      fetomaternal O43.01- ☑
      fetus to fetus O43.02- ☑
      maternofetal O43.01- ☑
    placentitis O41.14- ☑
    pneumonia O99.51- ☑
    poisoning — *see also* Table of Drugs and Chemicals
      O9A.21 ☑ (*following* O99)
    polyhydramnios O40- ☑
    polymorphic eruption of pregnancy O26.86
    poor obstetric history NEC O09.29- ☑
    postmaturity (post-term) (40 to 42 weeks) O48.0
      more than 42 completed weeks gestation (pro-
        longed) O48.1
    pre-eclampsia O14.9- ☑
      mild O14.0- ☑
      moderate O14.0- ☑
      severe O14.1- ☑
        with hemolysis, elevated liver enzymes and
          low platelet count (HELLP) O14.2- ☑
    premature labor — *see* Pregnancy, complicated by,
      preterm labor
    premature rupture of membranes O42.90
      with onset of labor
        within 24 hours O42.00
          at or after 37 weeks gestation, onset of
            labor within 24 hours of rupture
            O42.02
          pre-term (before 37 completed weeks of
            gestation) O42.01- ☑
        after 24 hours O42.10
          at or after 37 weeks gestation, onset of
            labor more than 24 hours following
            rupture O42.12
          pre-term (before 37 completed weeks of
            gestation) O42.11- ☑
      at or after 37 weeks gestation, unspecified as to
        length of time between rupture and onset
        of labor O42.92
      full-term, unspecified as to length of time be-
        tween rupture and onset of labor O42.92
      pre-term (before 37 completed weeks of gesta-
        tion) O42.91- ☑
    premature separation of placenta — *see also*
      Abruptio placentae O45.9- ☑
    presentation, fetal — *see* Delivery, complicated by,
      malposition
    preterm delivery O60.10 ☑
    preterm labor
      with delivery O60.10 ☑
        preterm O60.10 ☑
        term O60.20 ☑
      second trimester
        with term delivery O60.22 ☑
        without delivery O60.02
        with preterm delivery
          second trimester O60.12 ☑
          third trimester O60.13 ☑
      third trimester
        with term delivery O60.23 ☑
        without delivery O60.03
        with third trimester preterm delivery
          O60.14 ☑
      without delivery O60.00
        second trimester O60.02
        third trimester O60.03
    previous history of — *see* Pregnancy, supervision
      of, high-risk
    prolapse, uterus O34.52- ☑
    proteinuria (gestational) — *see also* Proteinuria,
      gestational O12.1- ☑
      with edema O12.2- ☑
    pruritic urticarial papules and plaques of pregnancy
      (PUPPP) O26.86
    pruritus (neurogenic) O26.89- ☑

Pregnancy — *continued*
  complicated by — *continued*
    psychosis or psychoneurosis (puerperal) F53.1
    ptyalism O26.89- ☑
    PUPPP (pruritic urticarial papules and plaques of
      pregnancy) O26.86
    pyelitis O23.0- ☑
    recurrent pregnancy loss O26.2- ☑
    renal disease or failure NEC O26.83- ☑
      with secondary hypertension, pre-existing —
        see Hypertension, complicating, pregnan-
        cy, pre-existing, secondary
      hypertensive, pre-existing — *see* Hypertension,
        complicating, pregnancy, pre-existing,
        with, renal disease
    respiratory condition (conditions in J00-J99)
      O99.51- ☑
    retained, retention
      dead ovum O02.0
      intrauterine contraceptive device O26.3- ☑
    retroversion, uterus O34.53- ☑
    Rh immunization, incompatibility or sensitization
      NEC O36.09- ☑
      anti-D antibody O36.01- ☑
    rupture
      amnion (premature) — *see also* Pregnancy,
        complicated by, premature rupture of
        membranes O42- ☑
      membranes (premature) — *see also* Pregnancy,
        complicated by, premature rupture of
        membranes O42- ☑
      uterus (during labor) O71.1
        before onset of labor O71.0- ☑
    salivation (excessive) O26.89- ☑
    salpingitis O23.52- ☑
    salpingo-oophoritis O23.52- ☑
    sepsis (conditions in A40, A41) O98.81- ☑
    size date discrepancy (uterine) O26.84- ☑
    skin condition (conditions in L00-L99) O99.71- ☑
    smoking (tobacco) O99.33- ☑
    social problem O09.7- ☑
    specified condition NEC O26.89- ☑
    spotting O26.85- ☑
    streptococcus group B (GBS) carrier state O99.820
    subluxation of symphysis (pubis) O26.71- ☑
    syphilis (conditions in A50-A53) O98.11- ☑
    threatened
      abortion O20.0
      labor O47.9
        at or after 37 completed weeks of gestation
          O47.1
        before 37 completed weeks of gestation
          O47.0- ☑
    thrombophlebitis (superficial) O22.2- ☑
    thrombosis O22.9- ☑
      cerebral venous O22.5- ☑
      cerebrovenous sinus O22.5- ☑
      deep O22.3- ☑
    tobacco use disorder (smoking) O99.33- ☑
    torsion of uterus O34.59- ☑
    toxemia O14.9- ☑
    transverse lie or presentation O32.2 ☑
    tuberculosis (conditions in A15-A19) O98.01- ☑
    tumor (benign)
      cervix O34.4- ☑
      malignant O9A.11- ☑ (*following* O99)
      uterus O34.1- ☑
    unstable lie O32.0
    upper respiratory infection O99.51- ☑
    urethritis O23.2- ☑
    uterine size date discrepancy O26.84- ☑
    vaginitis or vulvitis O23.59- ☑
    varicose veins (lower extremities) O22.0- ☑
      genitals O22.1- ☑
      legs O22.0- ☑
      perineal O22.1- ☑
      vaginal or vulval O22.1- ☑
    venereal disease NEC (conditions in A63.8)
      O98.31- ☑
    venous disorders O22.9- ☑
      specified NEC O22.8X- ☑
    very young mother — *see* Pregnancy, complicated
      by, young mother
    viral diseases (conditions in A80-B09, B25-B34)
      O98.51- ☑
    vomiting O21.9
      due to diseases classified elsewhere O21.8

Pregnancy — *continued*
  complicated by — *continued*
    vomiting — *continued*
      hyperemesis gravidarum (mild) — *see also* Hy-
        peremesis, gravidarum O21.0
      late (occurring after 20 weeks of gestation) O21.2
    young mother
      multigravida O09.62- ☑
      primigravida O09.61- ☑
  complicated NOS O26.9- ☑
  concealed O09.3- ☑
  continuing following
    elective fetal reduction of one or more fetus
      O31.3- ☑
    intrauterine death of one or more fetus O31.2- ☑
    spontaneous abortion of one or more fetus
      O31.1- ☑
  cornual O00.80
    with intrauterine pregnancy O00.81
  ectopic (ruptured) O00.90
    with intrauterine pregnancy O00.91
    abdominal O00.00
      with
        intrauterine pregnancy O00.01
        viable fetus O36.7- ☑
    cervical O00.80
      with intrauterine pregnancy O00.81
    complicated (by) O08.9
      afibrinogenemia O08.1
      cardiac arrest O08.81
      chemical damage of pelvic organ(s) O08.6
      circulatory collapse O08.3
      defibrination syndrome O08.1
      electrolyte imbalance O08.5
      embolism (amniotic fluid) (blood clot) (pul-
        monary) (septic) O08.2
      endometritis O08.0
      genital tract and pelvic infection O08.0
      hemorrhage (delayed) (excessive) O08.1
      infection
        genital tract or pelvic O08.0
        kidney O08.83
        urinary tract O08.3
      intravascular coagulation O08.1
      laceration of pelvic organ(s) O08.6
      metabolic disorder O08.5
      oliguria O08.4
      oophoritis O08.0
      parametritis O08.0
      pelvic peritonitis O08.0
      perforation of pelvic organ(s) O08.6
      renal failure or shutdown O08.4
      salpingitis or salpingo-oophoritis O08.0
      sepsis O08.82
      shock O08.83
        septic O08.82
      specified condition NEC O08.89
      tubular necrosis (renal) O08.4
      uremia O08.4
      urinary infection O08.83
      venous complication NEC O08.7
        embolism O08.2
    cornual O00.80
      with intrauterine pregnancy O00.81
    intraligamentous O00.80
      with intrauterine pregnancy O00.81
    mural O00.80
      with intrauterine pregnancy O00.81
    ovarian O00.20- ☑
      with intrauterine pregnancy O00.21- ☑
    specified site NEC O00.80
      with intrauterine pregnancy O00.81
    tubal (ruptured) O00.10- ☑
      with intrauterine pregnancy O00.11- ☑
  examination (normal) Z34.9- ☑
    first Z34.0- ☑
    high-risk — *see* Pregnancy, supervision of, high-risk
    specified Z34.8- ☑
  extrauterine — *see* Pregnancy, ectopic
  fallopian O00.10- ☑
    with intrauterine pregnancy O00.11- ☑
  false F45.8
  gestational carrier Z33.3
  heptachorionic, hepta-amniotic (septuplets) O30.83- ☑
  hexachorionic, hexa-amniotic (sextuplets) O30.83- ☑
  hidden O09.3- ☑
  high-risk — *see* Pregnancy, supervision of, high-risk
  incidental finding Z33.1

Pregnancy — *continued*
  interstitial O00.80
    with intrauterine pregnancy O00.81
  intraligamentous O00.80
    with intrauterine pregnancy O00.81
  intramural O00.80
    with intrauterine pregnancy O00.81
  intraperitoneal O00.00
    with intrauterine pregnancy O00.01
  isthmian O00.10- ☑
    with intrauterine pregnancy O00.11- ☑
  mesometric (mural) O00.80
    with intrauterine pregnancy O00.81
  molar NEC O02.0
    complicated (by) O08.9
      afibrinogenemia O08.1
      cardiac arrest O08.81
      chemical damage of pelvic organ(s) O08.6
      circulatory collapse O08.3
      defibrination syndrome O08.1
      electrolyte imbalance O08.5
      embolism (amniotic fluid) (blood clot) (pul-
          monary) (septic) O08.2
      endometritis O08.0
      genital tract and pelvic infection O08.0
      hemorrhage (delayed) (excessive) O08.1
      infection
        genital tract or pelvic O08.0
        kidney O08.83
        urinary tract O08.83
      intravascular coagulation O08.1
      laceration of pelvic organ(s) O08.6
      metabolic disorder O08.5
      oliguria O08.4
      oophoritis O08.0
      parametritis O08.0
      pelvic peritonitis O08.0
      perforation of pelvic organ(s) O08.6
      renal failure or shutdown O08.4
      salpingitis or salpingo-oophoritis O08.0
      sepsis O08.82
      shock O08.3
        septic O08.82
      specified condition NEC O08.89
      tubular necrosis (renal) O08.4
      uremia O08.4
      urinary infection O08.83
      venous complication NEC O08.7
        embolism O08.2
    hydatidiform — *see also* Mole, hydatidiform O01.9
  multiple (gestation) O30.9-
    greater than quadruplets — *see* Pregnancy, multiple
        (gestation), specified NEC
    specified NEC O30.80- ☑
      with
        two or more monoamniotic fetuses
            O30.82- ☑
        two or more monochorionic fetuses
            O30.81- ☑
        number of chorions and amnions are both equal
            to the number of fetuses O30.83- ☑
      two or more monoamniotic fetuses O30.82- ☑
      two or more monochorionic fetuses O30.81- ☑
      unable to determine number of placenta and
          number of amniotic sacs O30.89- ☑
      unspecified number of placenta and unspecified
          number of amniotic sacs O30.80- ☑
  mural O00.80
    with intrauterine pregnancy O00.81
  normal (supervision of) Z34.9- ☑
    first Z34.0- ☑
    high-risk — *see* Pregnancy, supervision of, high-risk
    specified Z34.8- ☑
  ovarian O00.20- ☑
    with intrauterine pregnancy O00.21- ☑
  pentachorionic, penta-amniotic (quintuplets)
      O30.83- ☑
  postmature (40 to 42 weeks) O48.0
    more than 42 weeks gestation O48.1
  post-term (40 to 42 weeks) O48.0
  prenatal care only Z34.9- ☑
    first Z34.0- ☑
    high-risk — *see* Pregnancy, supervision of, high-risk
    specified Z34.8- ☑
  prolonged (more than 42 weeks gestation) O48.1
  quadruplet O30.20- ☑
    with
      two or more monoamniotic fetuses O30.22- ☑

Pregnancy — *continued*
  quadruplet — *continued*
    with — *continued*
      two or more monochorionic fetuses O30.21- ☑
      quadrachorionic/quadra-amniotic O30.23- ☑
    two or more monoamniotic fetuses O30.22- ☑
    two or more monochorionic fetuses O30.21- ☑
    unable to determine number of placenta and num-
        ber of amniotic sacs O30.29- ☑
    unspecified number of placenta and unspecified
        number of amniotic sacs O30.20- ☑
  quintuplet — *see* Pregnancy, multiple (gestation),
      specified NEC
  sextuplet — *see* Pregnancy, multiple (gestation),
      specified NEC
  supervision of
    concealed pregnancy O09.3- ☑
    elderly mother
      multigravida O09.52- ☑
      primigravida O09.51- ☑
    hidden pregnancy O09.3- ☑
    high-risk O09.9- ☑
      due to (history of)
        ectopic pregnancy O09.1- ☑
        elderly — *see* Pregnancy, supervision, elderly
            mother
        grand multiparity O09.4 ☑
        in utero procedure during previous pregnancy
            O09.82- ☑
        in vitro fertilization O09.81- ☑
        infertility O09.0- ☑
        insufficient prenatal care O09.3- ☑
        molar pregnancy O09.A- ☑
        multiple previous pregnancies O09.4- ☑
        older mother — *see* Pregnancy, supervision
            of, elderly mother
        poor reproductive or obstetric history NEC
            O09.29- ☑
        pre-term labor O09.21- ☑
        previous
          neonatal death O09.29- ☑
        social problems O09.7- ☑
        specified NEC O09.89- ☑
        very young mother — *see* Pregnancy, super-
            vision, young mother
      resulting from in vitro fertilization O09.81- ☑
    normal Z34.9- ☑
      first Z34.0- ☑
      specified NEC Z34.8- ☑
    young mother
      multigravida O09.62- ☑
      primigravida O09.61- ☑
  triplet O30.10- ☑
    with
      two or more monoamniotic fetuses O30.12- ☑
      two or more monochorionic fetuses O30.11- ☑
    trichorionic/triamniotic O30.13- ☑
    two or more monoamniotic fetuses O30.12- ☑
    two or more monochorionic fetuses O30.11- ☑
    unable to determine number of placenta and num-
        ber of amniotic sacs O30.19- ☑
    unspecified number of placenta and unspecified
        number of amniotic sacs O30.10- ☑
  tubal (with abortion) (with rupture) O00.10- ☑
    with intrauterine pregnancy O00.11- ☑
  twin O30.00- ☑
    conjoined O30.02- ☑
    dichorionic/diamniotic (two placenta, two amniotic
        sacs) O30.04- ☑
    monochorionic/diamniotic (one placenta, two am-
        niotic sacs) O30.03- ☑
    monochorionic/monoamniotic (one placenta, one
        amniotic sac) O30.01- ☑
    unable to determine number of placenta and num-
        ber of amniotic sacs O30.09- ☑
    unspecified number of placenta and unspecified
        number of amniotic sacs O30.00- ☑
  unwanted Z64.0
  weeks of gestation
    8 weeks Z3A.08 (*following* Z36)
    9 weeks Z3A.09 (*following* Z36)
    10 weeks Z3A.10 (*following* Z36)
    11 weeks Z3A.11 (*following* Z36)
    12 weeks Z3A.12 (*following* Z36)
    13 weeks Z3A.13 (*following* Z36)
    14 weeks Z3A.14 (*following* Z36)
    15 weeks Z3A.15 (*following* Z36)

Pregnancy — *continued*
  weeks of gestation — *continued*
    16 weeks Z3A.16 (*following* Z36)
    17 weeks Z3A.17 (*following* Z36)
    18 weeks Z3A.18 (*following* Z36)
    19 weeks Z3A.19 (*following* Z36)
    20 weeks Z3A.20 (*following* Z36)
    21 weeks Z3A.21 (*following* Z36)
    22 weeks Z3A.22 (*following* Z36)
    23 weeks Z3A.23 (*following* Z36)
    24 weeks Z3A.24 (*following* Z36)
    25 weeks Z3A.25 (*following* Z36)
    26 weeks Z3A.26 (*following* Z36)
    27 weeks Z3A.27 (*following* Z36)
    28 weeks Z3A.28 (*following* Z36)
    29 weeks Z3A.29 (*following* Z36)
    30 weeks Z3A.30 (*following* Z36)
    31 weeks Z3A.31 (*following* Z36)
    32 weeks Z3A.32 (*following* Z36)
    33 weeks Z3A.33 (*following* Z36)
    34 weeks Z3A.34 (*following* Z36)
    35 weeks Z3A.35 (*following* Z36)
    36 weeks Z3A.36 (*following* Z36)
    37 weeks Z3A.37 (*following* Z36)
    38 weeks Z3A.38 (*following* Z36)
    39 weeks Z3A.39 (*following* Z36)
    40 weeks Z3A.40 (*following* Z36)
    41 weeks Z3A.41 (*following* Z36)
    42 weeks Z3A.42 (*following* Z36)
    greater than 42 weeks Z3A.49 (*following* Z36)
    less than 8 weeks Z3A.01 (*following* Z36)
    not specified Z3A.00 (*following* Z36)
Preiser's disease — *see* Osteonecrosis, secondary, due
    to, trauma, metacarpus
Pre-kwashiorkor — *see* Malnutrition, severe
Preleukemia (syndrome) D46.9
Preluxation, hip, congenital Q65.6
Premature — *see also* condition
  adrenarche E27.0
  aging E34.8
  beats I49.40
    atrial I49.1
    auricular I49.1
    supraventricular I49.1
  birth NEC — *see* Preterm, newborn
  closure, foramen ovale Q21.8
  contraction
    atrial I49.1
    atrioventricular I49.2
    auricular I49.1
    auriculoventricular I49.49
    heart (extrasystole) I49.49
    junctional I49.2
    ventricular I49.3
  delivery — *see also* Pregnancy, complicated by,
      preterm labor O60.10 ☑
  ejaculation F52.4
  infant NEC — *see* Preterm, newborn
    light-for-dates — *see* Light for dates
  labor — *see* Pregnancy, complicated by, preterm labor
  lungs P28.0
  menopause E28.319
    asymptomatic E28.319
    symptomatic E28.310
  newborn
    extreme (less than 28 completed weeks) — *see* Im-
        maturity, extreme
    less than 37 completed weeks — *see* Preterm,
        newborn
  puberty E30.1
  rupture membranes or amnion — *see* Pregnancy,
      complicated by, premature rupture of mem-
      branes
  senility E34.8
  thelarche E30.8
  ventricular systole I49.3
Prematurity NEC (less than 37 completed weeks) — *see*
    Preterm, newborn
  extreme (less than 28 completed weeks) — *see* Imma-
      turity, extreme
Premenstrual
  dysphoric disorder (PMDD) F32.81
  tension (syndrome) N94.3
Premolarization, cuspids K00.2
Prenatal
  care, normal pregnancy — *see* Pregnancy, normal
  screening of mother — *see also* Encounter, antenatal
      screening Z36.9

☑ **Additional Character Required** — Refer to the Tabular List for Character Selection   ▽ **Subterms under main terms may continue to next column or page**

Prenatal — *continued*
  teeth K00.6
Preparatory care for subsequent treatment NEC
  for dialysis Z49.01
    peritoneal Z49.02
Prepartum — *see* condition
Preponderance, left or right ventricular I51.7
Prepuce — *see* condition
PRES (posterior reversible encephalopathy syndrome) I67.83
Presbycardia R54
Presbycusis, presbyacusia H91.1-
Presbyesophagus K22.8
Presbyophrenia F03 ☑
Presbyopia H52.4
Prescription of contraceptives (initial) Z30.019
  barrier Z30.018
  diaphragm Z30.018
  emergency (postcoital) Z30.012
  implantable subdermal Z30.017
  injectable Z30.013
  intrauterine contraceptive device Z30.014
  pills Z30.011
  postcoital (emergency) Z30.012
  repeat Z30.40
    barrier Z30.49
    diaphragm Z30.49
    implantable subdermal Z30.46
    injectable Z30.42
    pills Z30.41
    specified type NEC Z30.49
    transdermal patch hormonal Z30.45
    vaginal ring hormonal Z30.44
  specified type NEC Z30.018
    transdermal patch hormonal Z30.016
    vaginal ring hormonal Z30.015
Presence (of)
  ankle-joint implant (functional) (prosthesis) Z96.66- ☑
  aortocoronary (bypass) graft Z95.1
  arterial-venous shunt (dialysis) Z99.2
  artificial
    eye (globe) Z97.0
    heart (fully implantable) (mechanical) Z95.812
      valve Z95.2
    larynx Z96.3
    lens (intraocular) Z96.1
    limb (complete) (partial) Z97.1- ☑
      arm Z97.1- ☑
        bilateral Z97.15
      leg Z97.1- ☑
        bilateral Z97.16
  audiological implant (functional) Z96.29
  bladder implant (functional) Z96.0
  bone
    conduction hearing device Z96.29
    implant (functional) NEC Z96.7
    joint (prosthesis) — *see* Presence, joint implant
  cardiac
    defibrillator (functional) (with synchronous cardiac pacemaker) Z95.810
    implant or graft Z95.9
      specified type NEC Z95.818
    pacemaker Z95.0
    resynchronization therapy
      defibrillator Z95.810
      pacemaker Z95.0
  cardioverter-defibrillator (ICD) Z95.810
  cerebrospinal fluid drainage device Z98.2
  cochlear implant (functional) Z96.21
  contact lens (es) Z97.3
  coronary artery graft or prosthesis Z95.5
  CRT-D (cardiac resynchronization therapy defibrillator) Z95.810
  CRT-P (cardiac resynchronization therapy pacemaker) Z95.0
  CSF shunt Z98.2
  dental prosthesis device Z97.2
  dentures Z97.2
  device (external) NEC Z97.8
    cardiac NEC Z95.818
    heart assist Z95.811
    implanted (functional) Z96.9
      specified NEC Z96.89
    prosthetic Z97.8
  ear implant Z96.20
    cochlear implant Z96.21
    myringotomy tube Z96.22
    specified type NEC Z96.29

Presence — *continued*
  elbow-joint implant (functional) (prosthesis) Z96.62- ☑
  endocrine implant (functional) NEC Z96.49
  eustachian tube stent or device (functional) Z96.29
  external hearing-aid or device Z97.4
  finger-joint implant (functional) (prosthetic) Z96.69- ☑
  functional implant Z96.9
    specified NEC Z96.89
  graft
    cardiac NEC Z95.818
    vascular NEC Z95.828
  hearing-aid or device (external) Z97.4
    implant (bone) (cochlear) (functional) Z96.21
  heart assist device Z95.811
  heart valve implant (functional) Z95.2
    prosthetic Z95.2
    specified type NEC Z95.4
    xenogenic Z95.3
  hip-joint implant (functional) (prosthesis) Z96.64- ☑
  ICD (cardioverter-defibrillator) Z95.810
  implanted device (artificial) (functional) (prosthetic) Z96.9
    automatic cardiac defibrillator (with synchronous cardiac pacemaker) Z95.810
    cardiac pacemaker Z95.0
    cochlear Z96.21
    dental Z96.5
    heart Z95.812
    heart valve Z95.2
      prosthetic Z95.2
      specified NEC Z95.4
      xenogenic Z95.3
    insulin pump Z96.41
    intraocular lens Z96.1
    joint Z96.60
      ankle Z96.66- ☑
      elbow Z96.62- ☑
      finger Z96.69- ☑
      hip Z96.64- ☑
      knee Z96.65- ☑
      shoulder Z96.61- ☑
      specified NEC Z96.698
      wrist Z96.63- ☑
    larynx Z96.3
    myringotomy tube Z96.22
    otological Z96.20
      cochlear Z96.21
      eustachian stent Z96.29
      myringotomy Z96.22
      specified NEC Z96.29
      stapes Z96.29
    skin Z96.81
    skull plate Z96.7
    specified NEC Z96.89
    urogenital Z96.0
  insulin pump (functional) Z96.41
  intestinal bypass or anastomosis Z98.0
  intraocular lens (functional) Z96.1
  intrauterine contraceptive device (IUD) Z97.5
  intravascular implant (functional) (prosthetic) NEC Z95.9
    coronary artery Z95.5
    defibrillator (with synchronous cardiac pacemaker) Z95.810
    peripheral vessel (with angioplasty) Z95.820
  joint implant (prosthetic) (any) Z96.60
    ankle — *see* Presence, ankle joint implant
    elbow — *see* Presence, elbow joint implant
    finger — *see* Presence, finger joint implant
    hip — *see* Presence, hip joint implant
    knee — *see* Presence, knee joint implant
    shoulder — *see* Presence, shoulder joint implant
    specified joint NEC Z96.698
    wrist — *see* Presence, wrist joint implant
  knee-joint implant (functional) (prosthesis) Z96.65- ☑
  laryngeal implant (functional) Z96.3
  mandibular implant (dental) Z96.5
  myringotomy tube(s) Z96.22
  neurostimulator (brain) (gastric) (peripheral nerve) (sacral nerve) (spinal cord) (vagus nerve) Z96.82
  orthopedic-joint implant (prosthetic) (any) — *see* Presence, joint implant
  otological implant (functional) Z96.29
  shoulder-joint implant (functional) (prosthesis) Z96.61- ☑
  skull-plate implant Z96.7
  spectacles Z97.3
  stapes implant (functional) Z96.29

Presence — *continued*
  systemic lupus erythematosus [SLE] inhibitor D68.62
  tendon implant (functional) (graft) Z96.7
  tooth root(s) implant Z96.5
  ureteral stent Z96.0
  urethral stent Z96.0
  urogenital implant (functional) Z96.0
  vascular implant or device Z95.9
    access port device Z95.828
    specified type NEC Z95.828
  wrist-joint implant (functional) (prosthesis) Z96.63- ☑
Presenile — *see also* condition
  dementia F03 ☑
  premature aging E34.8
Presentation, fetal — *see* Delivery, complicated by, malposition
Prespondylolisthesis (congenital) Q76.2
Pressure
  area, skin — *see* Ulcer, pressure, by site
  brachial plexus G54.0
  brain G93.5
    injury at birth NEC P11.1
  cerebral — *see* Pressure, brain
  chest R07.89
  cone, tentorial G93.5
  hyposystolic — *see also* Hypotension
    incidental reading, without diagnosis of hypotension R03.1
  increased
    intracranial (benign) G93.2
      injury at birth P11.0
    intraocular H40.05- ☑
  injury — *see* Ulcer, pressure, by site
  lumbosacral plexus G54.1
  mediastinum J98.59
  necrosis (chronic) — *see* Ulcer, pressure, by site
  parental, inappropriate (excessive) Z62.6
  sore (chronic) — *see* Ulcer, pressure, by site
  spinal cord G95.20
  ulcer (chronic) — *see* Ulcer, pressure, by site
  venous, increased I87.8
Pre-syncope R55
Preterm
  delivery — *see also* Pregnancy, complicated by, preterm labor O60.10 ☑
  labor — *see* Pregnancy, complicated by, preterm labor
  newborn (infant) P07.30
    gestational age
      28 completed weeks (28 weeks, 0 days through 28 weeks, 6 days) P07.31
      29 completed weeks (29 weeks, 0 days through 29 weeks, 6 days) P07.32
      30 completed weeks (30 weeks, 0 days through 30 weeks, 6 days) P07.33
      31 completed weeks (31 weeks, 0 days through 31 weeks, 6 days) P07.34
      32 completed weeks (32 weeks, 0 days through 32 weeks, 6 days) P07.35
      33 completed weeks (33 weeks, 0 days through 33 weeks, 6 days) P07.36
      34 completed weeks (34 weeks, 0 days through 34 weeks, 6 days) P07.37
      35 completed weeks (35 weeks, 0 days through 35 weeks, 6 days) P07.38
      36 completed weeks (36 weeks, 0 days through 36 weeks, 6 days) P07.39
Previa
  placenta (total) (without hemorrhage) O44.0- ☑
    with hemorrhage O44.1- ☑
    complete O44.0- ☑
      with hemorrhage O44.1- ☑
    low — *see also* Delivery, complicated, by, placenta, low O44.4- ☑
      with hemorrhage O44.5- ☑
    marginal O44.2- ☑
      with hemorrhage O44.3- ☑
    partial O44.2- ☑
      with hemorrhage O44.3- ☑
  vasa O69.4 ☑
Priapism N48.30
  due to
    disease classified elsewhere N48.32
    drug N48.33
    specified cause NEC N48.39
    trauma N48.31
Prickling sensation (skin) R20.2
Prickly heat L74.0

▽ Subterms under main terms may continue to next column or page   ☑ Additional Character Required — Refer to the Tabular List for Character Selection   263

Prenatal — Prickly heat

Primary — see condition
Primigravida
elderly, affecting management of pregnancy, labor and delivery (supervision only) — see Pregnancy, complicated by, elderly, primigravida
older, affecting management of pregnancy, labor and delivery (supervision only) — see Pregnancy, complicated by, elderly, primigravida
very young, affecting management of pregnancy, labor and delivery (supervision only) — see Pregnancy, complicated by, young mother, primigravida
Primipara
elderly, affecting management of pregnancy, labor and delivery (supervision only) — see Pregnancy, complicated by, elderly, primigravida
older, affecting management of pregnancy, labor and delivery (supervision only) — see Pregnancy, complicated by, elderly, primigravida
very young, affecting management of pregnancy, labor and delivery (supervision only) — see Pregnancy, complicated by, young mother, primigravida
Primus varus Q66.21- ☑
PRIND (Prolonged reversible ischemic neurologic deficit) I63.9
Pringle's disease (tuberous sclerosis) Q85.1
Prinzmetal angina I20.1
Prizefighter ear — see Cauliflower ear
Problem (with) (related to)
academic Z55.8
acculturation Z60.3
adjustment (to)
change of job Z56.1
life-cycle transition Z60.0
pension Z60.0
retirement Z60.0
adopted child Z62.821
alcoholism in family Z63.72
atypical parenting situation Z62.9
bankruptcy Z59.8
behavioral (adult) F69
drug seeking Z76.5
birth of sibling affecting child Z62.898
care (of)
provider dependency Z74.9
specified NEC Z74.8
sick or handicapped person in family or household Z63.6
child
abuse (affecting the child) — see Maltreatment, child
custody or support proceedings Z65.3
in care of non-parental family member Z62.21
in foster care Z62.21
in welfare custody Z62.21
living in orphanage or group home Z62.22
child-rearing Z62.9
specified NEC Z62.898
communication (developmental) F80.9
conflict or discord (with)
boss Z56.4
classmates Z55.4
counselor Z64.4
employer Z56.4
family Z63.9
specified NEC Z63.8
probation officer Z64.4
social worker Z64.4
teachers Z55.4
workmates Z56.4
conviction in legal proceedings Z65.0
with imprisonment Z65.1
counselor Z64.4
creditors Z59.8
digestive K92.9
drug addict in family Z63.72
ear — see Disorder, ear
economic Z59.9
affecting care Z59.9
specified NEC Z59.8
education Z55.9
specified NEC Z55.8
employment Z56.9
change of job Z56.1
discord Z56.4
environment Z56.5
sexual harassment Z56.81
specified NEC Z56.89
stressful schedule Z56.3

Problem — continued
employment — continued
stress NEC Z56.6
threat of job loss Z56.2
unemployment Z56.0
enuresis, child F98.0
eye H57.9
failed examinations (school) Z55.2
falling Z91.81
family — see also Disruption, family Z63.9
specified NEC Z63.8
feeding (elderly) (infant) R63.3
newborn P92.9
breast P92.5
overfeeding P92.4
slow P92.2
specified NEC P92.8
underfeeding P92.3
nonorganic F50.89
finance Z59.9
specified NEC Z59.8
foreclosure on loan Z59.8
foster child Z62.822
frightening experience(s) in childhood Z62.898
genital NEC
female N94.9
male N50.9
health care Z75.9
specified NEC Z75.8
hearing — see Deafness
homelessness Z59.0
housing Z59.9
inadequate Z59.1
isolated Z59.8
specified NEC Z59.8
identity (of childhood) F93.8
illegitimate pregnancy (unwanted) Z64.0
illiteracy Z55.0
impaired mobility Z74.09
imprisonment or incarceration Z65.1
inadequate teaching affecting education Z55.8
inappropriate (excessive) parental pressure Z62.6
influencing health status NEC Z78.9
in-law Z63.1
institutionalization, affecting child Z62.22
intrafamilial communication Z63.8
jealousy, child F93.8
landlord Z59.2
language (developmental) F80.9
learning (developmental) F81.9
legal Z65.3
conviction without imprisonment Z65.0
imprisonment Z65.1
release from prison Z65.2
life-management Z73.9
specified NEC Z73.89
life-style Z72.9
gambling Z72.6
high-risk sexual behavior (heterosexual) Z72.51
bisexual Z72.53
homosexual Z72.52
inappropriate eating habits Z72.4
self-damaging behavior NEC Z72.89
specified NEC Z72.89
tobacco use Z72.0
literacy Z55.9
low level Z55.0
specified NEC Z55.8
living alone Z60.2
lodgers Z59.2
loss of love relationship in childhood Z62.898
marital Z63.0
involving
divorce Z63.5
estrangement Z63.5
gender identity F66
mastication K08.89
medical
care, within family Z63.6
facilities Z75.9
specified NEC Z75.8
mental F48.9
multiparity Z64.1
negative life events in childhood Z62.9
altered pattern of family relationships Z62.898
frightening experience Z62.898
loss of
love relationship Z62.898
self-esteem Z62.898

Problem — continued
negative life events in childhood — continued
physical abuse (alleged) — see Maltreatment, child
removal from home Z62.29
specified event NEC Z62.898
neighbor Z59.2
neurological NEC R29.818
new step-parent affecting child Z62.898
none (feared complaint unfounded) Z71.1
occupational NEC Z56.89
parent-child — see Conflict, parent-child
personal hygiene Z91.89
personality F69
phase-of-life transition, adjustment Z60.0
presence of sick or disabled person in family or household Z63.79
needing care Z63.6
primary support group (family) Z63.9
specified NEC Z63.8
probation officer Z64.4
psychiatric F99
psychosexual (development) F66
psychosocial Z65.9
religious or spiritual Z65.8
specified NEC Z65.8
relationship Z63.9
childhood F93.8
release from prison Z65.2
religious or spiritual Z65.8
removal from home affecting child Z62.29
seeking and accepting known hazardous and harmful behavioral or psychological interventions Z65.8
chemical, nutritional or physical interventions Z65.8
sexual function (nonorganic) F52.9
sight H54.7
sleep disorder, child F51.9
smell — see Disturbance, sensation, smell
social
environment Z60.9
specified NEC Z60.8
exclusion and rejection Z60.4
worker Z64.4
speech R47.9
developmental F80.9
specified NEC R47.89
swallowing — see Dysphagia
taste — see Disturbance, sensation, taste
tic, child F95.0
underachievement in school Z55.3
unemployment Z56.0
threatened Z56.2
unwanted pregnancy Z64.0
upbringing Z62.9
specified NEC Z62.898
urinary N39.9
voice production R47.89
work schedule (stressful) Z56.3
Procedure (surgical)
converted
arthroscopic to open Z53.33
laparoscopic to open Z53.31
specified procedure NEC to open Z53.39
thoracoscopic to open Z53.32
for purpose other than remedying health state Z41.9
specified NEC Z41.8
not done Z53.9
because of
administrative reasons Z53.8
contraindication Z53.09
smoking Z53.01
patient's decision Z53.20
for reasons of belief or group pressure Z53.1
left against medical advice (AMA) Z53.21
specified reason NEC Z53.29
specified reason NEC Z53.8
Procidentia (uteri) N81.3
Proctalgia K62.89
fugax K59.4
spasmodic K59.4
Proctitis K62.89
amebic (acute) A06.0
chlamydial A56.3
gonococcal A54.6
granulomatous — see Enteritis, regional, large intestine
herpetic A60.1
radiation K62.7
tuberculous A18.32
ulcerative (chronic) K51.20

Proctitis — *continued*
 ulcerative — *continued*
  with
   complication K51.219
    abscess K51.214
    fistula K51.213
    obstruction K51.212
    rectal bleeding K51.211
    specified NEC K51.218
Proctocele
 female (without uterine prolapse) N81.6
  with uterine prolapse N81.2
   complete N81.3
 male K62.3
Proctocolitis
 food protein-induced K52.82
 food-induced eosinophilic K52.82
 milk protein-induced K52.82
 mucosal — *see* Rectosigmoiditis, ulcerative
Proctoptosis K62.3
Proctorrhagia K62.5
Proctosigmoiditis K63.89
 ulcerative (chronic) — *see* Rectosigmoiditis, ulcerative
Proctospasm K59.4
 psychogenic F45.8
Profichet's disease — *see* Disorder, soft tissue, specified type NEC
Progeria E34.8
Prognathism (mandibular) (maxillary) M26.19
Progonoma (melanotic) — *see* Neoplasm, benign, by site
Progressive — *see* condition
Prolactinoma
 specified site — *see* Neoplasm, benign, by site
 unspecified site D35.2
Prolapse, prolapsed
 anus, anal (canal) (sphincter) K62.2
 arm or hand O32.2 ☑
  causing obstructed labor O64.4 ☑
 bladder (mucosa) (sphincter) (acquired)
  congenital Q79.4
  female — *see* Cystocele
  male N32.89
 breast implant (prosthetic) T85.49 ☑
 cecostomy K94.09
 cecum K63.4
 cervix, cervical (hypertrophied) N81.2
  anterior lip, obstructing labor O65.5
  congenital Q51.828
  postpartal, old N81.2
  stump N81.85
 ciliary body (traumatic) — *see* Laceration, eye(ball), with prolapse or loss of interocular tissue
 colon (pedunculated) K63.4
 colostomy K94.09
 disc (intervertebral) — *see* Displacement, intervertebral disc
 eye implant (orbital) T85.398 ☑
  lens (ocular) — *see* Complications, intraocular lens
 fallopian tube N83.4- ☑
 gastric (mucosa) K31.89
 genital, female N81.9
  specified NEC N81.89
 globe, nontraumatic — *see* Luxation, globe
 ileostomy bud K94.19
 intervertebral disc — *see* Displacement, intervertebral disc
 intestine (small) K63.4
 iris (traumatic) — *see* Laceration, eye(ball), with prolapse or loss of interocular tissue
  nontraumatic H21.89
 kidney N28.83
  congenital Q63.2
 laryngeal muscles or ventricle J38.7
 liver K76.89
 meatus urinarius N36.8
 mitral (valve) I34.1
 ocular lens implant — *see* Complications, intraocular lens
 organ or site, congenital NEC — *see* Malposition, congenital
 ovary N83.4- ☑
 pelvic floor, female N81.89
 perineum, female N81.89
 rectum (mucosa) (sphincter) K62.3
  due to trichuris trichuria B79
 spleen D73.89
 stomach K31.89

Prolapse, prolapsed — *continued*
 umbilical cord
  complicating delivery O69.0 ☑
 urachus, congenital Q64.4
 ureter N28.89
  with obstruction N13.5
   with infection N13.6
 ureterovesical orifice N28.89
 urethra (acquired) (infected) (mucosa) N36.8
  congenital Q64.71
 urinary meatus N36.8
  congenital Q64.72
 uterovaginal N81.4
  complete N81.3
  incomplete N81.2
 uterus (with prolapse of vagina) N81.4
  complete N81.3
  congenital Q51.818
  first degree N81.2
  in pregnancy or childbirth — *see* Pregnancy, complicated by, abnormal, uterus
  incomplete N81.2
  postpartal (old) N81.4
  second degree N81.2
  third degree N81.3
 uveal (traumatic) — *see* Laceration, eye(ball), with prolapse or loss of interocular tissue
 vagina (anterior) (wall) — *see* Cystocele
  with prolapse of uterus N81.4
   complete N81.3
   incomplete N81.2
  posterior wall N81.6
  posthysterectomy N99.3
 vitreous (humor) H43.0- ☑
  in wound — *see* Laceration, eye(ball), with prolapse or loss of interocular tissue
 womb — *see* Prolapse, uterus
Prolapsus, female N81.9
 specified NEC N81.89
Proliferation(s)
 primary cutaneous CD30-positive large T-cell C86.6
 prostate, atypical small acinar N42.32
Proliferative — *see* condition
Prolonged, prolongation (of)
 bleeding (time) (idiopathic) R79.1
 coagulation (time) R79.1
 gestation (over 42 completed weeks)
  mother O48.1
  newborn P08.22
 interval I44.0
 labor O63.9
  first stage O63.0
  second stage O63.1
 partial thromboplastin time (PTT) R79.1
 pregnancy (more than 42 weeks gestation) O48.1
 prothrombin time R79.1
 QT interval R94.31
 uterine contractions in labor O62.4
Prominence, prominent
 auricle (congenital) (ear) Q17.5
 ischial spine or sacral promontory with disproportion (fetopelvic)
  with disproportion (fetopelvic) O33.0
   causing obstructed labor O65.0-
 nose (congenital) acquired M95.0
Promiscuity — *see* High, risk, sexual behavior
Pronation
 ankle — *see* Deformity, limb, foot, specified NEC
 foot — *see also* Deformity, limb, foot, specified NEC
  congenital Q74.2
Prophylactic
 administration of
  antibiotics, long-term Z79.2
   short-term use — *omit code*
  drug — *see also* Long-term (current) drug therapy (use of) Z79.899
 medication Z79.899
 organ removal (for neoplasia management) Z40.00
  breast Z40.01
  fallopian tube(s) Z40.03
   with ovary(s) Z40.02
  ovary(s) Z40.02
  specified site NEC Z40.09
 surgery Z40.9
  for risk factors related to malignant neoplasm — *see* Prophylactic, organ removal
  specified NEC Z40.8
 vaccination Z23

Propionic acidemia E71.121
Proptosis (ocular) — *see also* Exophthalmos
 thyroid — *see* Hyperthyroidism, with goiter
Prosecution, anxiety concerning Z65.3
Prosopagnosia R48.3
Prostadynia N42.81
Prostate, prostatic — *see* condition
Prostatism — *see* Hyperplasia, prostate
Prostatitis (congestive) (suppurative) (with cystitis) N41.9
 acute N41.0
 cavitary N41.8
 chronic N41.1
 diverticular N41.8
 due to Trichomonas (vaginalis) A59.02
 fibrous N41.1
 gonococcal (acute) (chronic) A54.22
 granulomatous N41.4
 hypertrophic N41.1
 subacute N41.1
 trichomonal A59.02
 tuberculous A18.14
Prostatocystitis N41.3
Prostatorrhea N42.89
Prostatosis N42.82
Prostration R53.83
 heat — *see also* Heat, exhaustion
  anhydrotic T67.3 ☑
  due to
   salt (and water) depletion T67.4 ☑
   water depletion T67.3 ☑
 nervous F48.8
 senile R54
Protanomaly (anomalous trichromat) H53.54
Protanopia (complete) (incomplete) H53.54
Protection (against) (from) — *see* Prophylactic
Protein
 deficiency NEC — *see* Malnutrition
 malnutrition — *see* Malnutrition
 sickness — *see also* Reaction, serum T80.69 ☑
Proteinemia R77.9
Proteinosis
 alveolar (pulmonary) J84.01
 lipid or lipoid (of Urbach) E78.89
Proteinuria R80.9
 Bence Jones R80.3
 complicating pregnancy — *see* Proteinuria, gestational
 gestational
  complicating
   childbirth O12.14
   pregnancy O12.1- ☑
    with edema O12.2- ☑
   puerperium O12.15
 idiopathic R80.0
 isolated R80.0
  with glomerular lesion N06.9
   dense deposit disease N06.6
   diffuse
    crescentic glomerulonephritis N06.7
    endocapillary proliferative glomerulonephritis N06.4
    mesangiocapillary glomerulonephritis N06.5
   focal and segmental hyalinosis or sclerosis N06.1
   membranous (diffuse) N06.2
   mesangial proliferative (diffuse) N06.3
   minimal change N06.0
   specified pathology NEC N06.8
 orthostatic R80.2
  with glomerular lesion — *see* Proteinuria, isolated, with glomerular lesion
 persistent R80.1
  with glomerular lesion — *see* Proteinuria, isolated, with glomerular lesion
 postural R80.2
  with glomerular lesion — *see* Proteinuria, isolated, with glomerular lesion
 pre-eclamptic — *see* Pre-eclampsia
 puerperal O12.15
 specified type NEC R80.8
Proteolysis, pathologic D65
Proteus (mirabilis) (morganii), **as cause of disease classified elsewhere** B96.4
Prothrombin gene mutation D68.52
Protoporphyria, erythropoietic E80.0
Protozoal — *see also* condition
 disease B64
  specified NEC B60.8

☝ **Subterms under main terms may continue to next column or page** ☑ **Additional Character Required — Refer to the Tabular List for Character Selection** **265**

Proctitis — Protozoal

Protrusion, protrusio
acetabuli M24.7
acetabulum (into pelvis) M24.7
device, implant or graft — see also Complications, by site and type, mechanical T85.698 ☑
arterial graft NEC — see Complication, cardiovascular device, mechanical, vascular
breast (implant) T85.49 ☑
catheter NEC T85.698 ☑
cystostomy T83.090 ☑
dialysis (renal) T82.49 ☑
intraperitoneal T85.691 ☑
infusion NEC T82.594 ☑
spinal (epidural) (subdural) T85.690 ☑
urinary — see also Complications, catheter, urinary T83.098 ☑
electronic (electrode) (pulse generator) (stimulator) bone T84.390 ☑
nervous system — see Complication, prosthetic device, mechanical, electronic nervous system stimulator
fixation, internal (orthopedic) NEC — see Complication, fixation device, mechanical
gastrointestinal — see Complications, prosthetic device, mechanical, gastrointestinal device
genital NEC T83.498 ☑
intrauterine contraceptive device T83.39 ☑
penile prosthesis (cylinder) (implanted) (pump) (resevoir) T83.490 ☑
testicular prosthesis T83.491 ☑
heart NEC — see Complication, cardiovascular device, mechanical
joint prosthesis — see Complications, joint prosthesis, mechanical, specified NEC, by site
ocular NEC — see Complications, prosthetic device, mechanical, ocular device
orthopedic NEC — see Complication, orthopedic, device, mechanical
specified NEC T85.628 ☑
urinary — see also Complication, genitourinary, device, urinary, mechanical
graft T83.29 ☑
vascular NEC — see Complication, cardiovascular device, mechanical
ventricular intracranial shunt T85.09 ☑
intervertebral disc — see Displacement, intervertebral disc
joint prosthesis — see Complications, joint prosthesis, mechanical, specified NEC, by site
nucleus pulposus — see Displacement, intervertebral disc
Prune belly (syndrome) Q79.4
Prurigo (ferox) (gravis) (Hebrae) (Hebra's) (mitis) (simplex) L28.2
Besnier's L20.0
estivalis L56.4
nodularis L28.1
psychogenic F45.8
Pruritus, pruritic (essential) L29.9
ani, anus L29.0
psychogenic F45.8
anogenital L29.3
psychogenic F45.8
due to onchocerca volvulus B73.1
gravidarum — see Pregnancy, complicated by, specified pregnancy-related condition NEC
hiemalis L29.8
neurogenic (any site) F45.8
perianal L29.0
psychogenic (any site) F45.8
scroti, scrotum L29.1
psychogenic F45.8
senile, senilis L29.8
specified NEC L29.8
psychogenic F45.8
Trichomonas A59.9
vulva, vulvae L29.2
psychogenic F45.8
Pseudarthrosis, pseudoarthrosis (bone) — see Nonunion, fracture
clavicle, congenital Q74.0
joint, following fusion or arthrodesis M96.0
Pseudoaneurysm — see Aneurysm
Pseudoangina (pectoris) — see Angina
Pseudoangioma I81
Pseudoarteriosus Q28.8
Pseudoarthrosis — see Pseudarthrosis

Pseudobulbar affect (PBA) F48.2
Pseudochromhidrosis L67.8
Pseudocirrhosis, liver, pericardial I31.1
Pseudocowpox B08.03
Pseudocoxalgia M91.3- ☑
Pseudocroup J38.5
Pseudo-Cushing's syndrome, alcohol-induced E24.4
Pseudocyesis F45.8
Pseudocyst
lung J98.4
pancreas K86.3
retina — see Cyst, retina
Pseudoelephantiasis neuroarthritica Q82.0
Pseudoexfoliation, capsule (lens) — see Cataract, specified NEC
Pseudofolliculitis barbae L73.1
Pseudoglioma H44.89
Pseudohemophilia (Bernuth's) (hereditary) (type B) D68.0
Type A D69.8
vascular D69.8
Pseudohermaphroditism Q56.3
adrenal E25.8
female Q56.2
with adrenocortical disorder E25.8
without adrenocortical disorder Q56.2
adrenal (congenital) E25.0
unspecified E25.9
male Q56.1
with
5-alpha-reductase deficiency E29.1
adrenocortical disorder E25.8
androgen resistance E34.51
cleft scrotum Q56.1
feminizing testis E34.51
without gonadal disorder Q56.1
adrenal E25.8
unspecified E25.9
Pseudo-Hurler's polydystrophy E77.0
Pseudohydrocephalus G93.2
Pseudohypertrophic muscular dystrophy (Erb's) G71.02
Pseudohypertrophy, muscle G71.09
Pseudohypoparathyroidism E20.1
Pseudoinsomnia F51.03
Pseudoleukemia, infantile D64.89
Pseudomembranous — see condition
Pseudomeningocele (cerebral) (infective) (post-traumatic) G96.19
postprocedural (spinal) G97.82
Pseudomenses (newborn) P54.6
Pseudomenstruation (newborn) P54.6
Pseudomonas
aeruginosa, as cause of disease classified elsewhere B96.5
mallei infection A24.0
as cause of disease classified elsewhere B96.5
pseudomallei, as cause of disease classified elsewhere B96.5
Pseudomyotonia G71.19
Pseudomyxoma peritonei C78.6
Pseudoneuritis, optic (nerve) (disc) (papilla), **congenital** Q14.2
Pseudo-obstruction intestine (acute) (chronic) (idiopathic) (intermittent secondary) (primary) K59.8
Pseudopapilledema H47.33- ☑
congenital Q14.2
Pseudoparalysis
arm or leg R29.818
atonic, congenital P94.2
Pseudopelade L66.0
Pseudophakia Z96.1
Pseudopolyarthritis, rhizomelic M35.3
Pseudopolycythemia D75.1
Pseudopseudohypoparathyroidism E20.1
Pseudopterygium H11.81- ☑
Pseudoptosis (eyelid) — see Blepharochalasis
Pseudopuberty, precocious
female heterosexual E25.8
male isosexual E25.8
Pseudorickets (renal) N25.0
Pseudorubella B08.20
Pseudosclerema, newborn P83.88
Pseudosclerosis (brain)
Jakob's — see Creutzfeldt-Jakob disease or syndrome of Westphal (Strümpell) E83.01
spastic — see Creutzfeldt-Jakob disease or syndrome

Pseudotetanus — see Convulsions
Pseudotetany R29.0
hysterical F44.5
Pseudotruncus arteriosus Q25.49
Pseudotuberculosis A28.2
enterocolitis A04.8
pasteurella (infection) A28.0
Pseudotumor
cerebri G93.2
orbital H05.11 ☑
Pseudoxanthoma elasticum Q82.8
Psilosis (sprue) (tropical) K90.1
nontropical K90.0
Psittacosis A70
Psoitis M60.88
Psoriasis L40.9
arthropathic L40.50
arthritis mutilans L40.52
distal interphalangeal L40.51
juvenile L40.54
other specified L40.59
spondylitis L40.53
buccal K13.29
flexural L40.8
guttate L40.4
mouth K13.29
nummular L40.0
plaque L40.0
psychogenic F54
pustular (generalized) L40.1
palmaris et plantaris L40.3
specified NEC L40.8
vulgaris L40.0
Psychasthenia F48.8
Psychiatric disorder or problem F99
Psychogenic — see also condition
factors associated with physical conditions F54
Psychological and behavioral factors affecting medical condition F59
Psychoneurosis, psychoneurotic — see also Neurosis
anxiety (state) F41.1
depersonalization F48.1
hypochondriacal F45.21
hysteria F44.9
neurasthenic F48.8
personality NEC F60.89
Psychopathy, psychopathic
affectionless F94.2
autistic F84.5
constitution, post-traumatic F07.81
personality — see Disorder, personality
sexual — see Deviation, sexual
state F60.2
Psychosexual identity disorder of childhood F64.2
Psychosis, psychotic F29
acute (transient) F23
hysterical F44.9
affective — see Disorder, mood
alcoholic F10.959
with
abuse F10.159
anxiety disorder F10.980
with
abuse F10.180
dependence F10.280
delirium tremens F10.231
delusions F10.950
with
abuse F10.150
dependence F10.250
dementia F10.97
with dependence F10.27
dependence F10.259
hallucinosis F10.951
with
abuse F10.151
dependence F10.251
mood disorder F10.94
with
abuse F10.14
dependence F10.24
paranoia F10.950
with
abuse F10.150
dependence F10.250
persisting amnesia F10.96
with dependence F10.26
amnestic confabulatory F10.96

Psychosis, psychotic — *continued*
  alcoholic — *continued*
    amnestic confabulatory — *continued*
      with dependence F10.26
    delirium tremens F10.231
    Korsakoff's, Korsakov's, Korsakow's F10.26
    paranoid type F10.950
      with
        abuse F10.150
        dependence F10.250
  anergastic — *see* Psychosis, organic
  arteriosclerotic (simple type) (uncomplicated) F01.50
    with behavioral disturbance F01.51
  childhood F84.0
    atypical F84.8
  climacteric — *see* Psychosis, involutional
  confusional F29
    acute or subacute F05
    reactive F23
  cycloid F23
  depressive — *see* Disorder, depressive
  disintegrative (childhood) F84.3
  drug-induced — *see* F11-F19 with .X59
    paranoid and hallucinatory states — *see* F11-F19
      with .X50 or .X51
  due to or associated with
    addiction, drug — *see* F11-F19 with .X59
    dependence
      alcohol F10.259
      drug — *see* F11-F19 with .X59
    epilepsy F06.8
    Huntington's chorea F06.8
    ischemia, cerebrovascular (generalized) F06.8
    multiple sclerosis F06.8
    physical disease F06.8
    presenile dementia F03 ☑
    senile dementia F03 ☑
    vascular disease (arteriosclerotic) (cerebral) F01.50
      with behavioral disturbance F01.51
  epileptic F06.8
  episode F23
    due to or associated with physical condition F06.8
  exhaustive F43.0
  hallucinatory, chronic F28
  hypomanic F30.8
  hysterical (acute) F44.9
  induced F24
  infantile F84.0
    atypical F84.8
  infective (acute) (subacute) F05
  involutional F28
    depressive — *see* Disorder, depressive
    melancholic — *see* Disorder, depressive
    paranoid (state) F22
  Korsakoff's, Korsakov's, Korsakow's (nonalcoholic) F04
    alcoholic F10.96
      in dependence F10.26
    induced by other psychoactive substance — *see*
      categories F11-F19 with .X5X
  mania, manic (single episode) F30.2
    recurrent type F31.89
  manic-depressive — *see* Disorder, bipolar
  menopausal — *see* Psychosis, involutional
  mixed schizophrenic and affective F25.8
  multi-infarct (cerebrovascular) F01.50
    with behavioral disturbance F01.51
  nonorganic F29
    specified NEC F28
  organic F09
    due to or associated with
      arteriosclerosis (cerebral) — *see* Psychosis, arte-
        riosclerotic
      cerebrovascular disease, arteriosclerotic — *see*
        Psychosis, arteriosclerotic
      childbirth — *see* Psychosis, puerperal
      Creutzfeldt-Jakob disease or syndrome — *see*
        Creutzfeldt-Jakob disease or syndrome
      dependence, alcohol F10.259
      disease
        alcoholic liver F10.259
        brain, arteriosclerotic — *see* Psychosis, arte-
          riosclerotic
        cerebrovascular F01.50
          with behavioral disturbance F01.51
        Creutzfeldt-Jakob — *see* Creutzfeldt-Jakob
          disease or syndrome
        endocrine or metabolic F06.8
          acute or subacute F05

Psychosis, psychotic — *continued*
  organic — *continued*
    due to or associated with — *continued*
      disease — *continued*
        liver, alcoholic F10.259
      epilepsy transient (acute) F05
      infection
        brain (intracranial) F06.8
          acute or subacute F05
      intoxication
        alcoholic (acute) F10.259
        drug F11-F19 with .x59
      ischemia, cerebrovascular (generalized) — *see*
        Psychosis, arteriosclerotic
      puerperium — *see* Psychosis, puerperal
      trauma, brain (birth) (from electric current) (sur-
        gical) F06.8
        acute or subacute F05
    infective F06.8
      acute or subacute F05
    post-traumatic F06.8
      acute or subacute F05
  paranoiac F22
  paranoid (climacteric) (involutional) (menopausal) F22
    psychogenic (acute) F23
    schizophrenic F20.0
    senile F03 ☑
  postpartum (NOS) F53.1
  presbyophrenic (type) F03 ☑
  presenile F03 ☑
  psychogenic (paranoid) F23
    depressive F32.3
  puerperal (NOS) F53.1
    specified type — *see* Psychosis, by type
  reactive (brief) (transient) (emotional stress) (psycho-
    logical trauma) F23
    depressive F32.3
      recurrent F33.3
    excitative type F30.8
  schizoaffective F25.9
    depressive type F25.1
    manic type F25.0
  schizophrenia, schizophrenic — *see* Schizophrenia
  schizophrenia-like, in epilepsy F06.2
  schizophreniform F20.81
    affective type F25.9
    brief F23
    confusional type F23
    mixed type F25.0
  senile NEC F03 ☑
    depressed or paranoid type F03 ☑
    simple deterioration F03 ☑
    specified type — *code to* condition
  shared F24
  situational (reactive) F23
  symbiotic (childhood) F84.3
  symptomatic F09
Psychosomatic — *see* Disorder, psychosomatic
Psychosyndrome, organic F07.9
Psychotic episode due to or associated with physical
  condition F06.8
Pterygium (eye) H11.00- ☑
  amyloid H11.01- ☑
  central H11.02- ☑
  colli Q18.3
  double H11.03- ☑
  peripheral
    progressive H11.05- ☑
    stationary H11.04- ☑
  recurrent H11.06- ☑
Ptilosis (eyelid) — *see* Madarosis
Ptomaine (poisoning) — *see* Poisoning, food
Ptosis — *see also* Blepharoptosis
  adiposa (false) — *see* Blepharoptosis
  breast N64.81-
  brow H57.81- ☑
  cecum K63.4
  colon K63.4
  congenital (eyelid) Q10.0
    specified site NEC — *see* Anomaly, by site
  eyebrow H57.81- ☑
  eyelid — *see* Blepharoptosis
    congenital Q10.0
  gastric K31.89
  intestine K63.4
  kidney N28.83
  liver K76.89
  renal N28.83

Ptosis — *continued*
  splanchnic K63.4
  spleen D73.89
  stomach K31.89
  viscera K63.4
PTP D69.51
Ptyalism (periodic) K11.7
  hysterical F45.8
  pregnancy — *see* Pregnancy, complicated by, specified
    pregnancy-related condition NEC
  psychogenic F45.8
Ptyalolithiasis K11.5
Pubarche, precocious E30.1
Pubertas praecox E30.1
Puberty (development state) Z00.3
  bleeding (excessive) N92.2
  delayed E30.0
  precocious (constitutional) (cryptogenic) (idiopathic)
    E30.1
    central E22.8
    due to
      ovarian hyperfunction E28.1
        estrogen E28.0
      testicular hyperfunction E29.0
  premature E30.1
    due to
      adrenal cortical hyperfunction E25.8
      pineal tumor E34.8
      pituitary (anterior) hyperfunction E22.8
Puckering, macula — *see* Degeneration, macula, puckering
Pudenda, pudendum — *see* condition
Puente's disease (simple glandular cheilitis) K13.0
Puerperal, puerperium (complicated by, complications)
  abnormal glucose (tolerance test) O99.815
  abscess
    areola O91.02
      associated with lactation O91.03
    Bartholin's gland O86.19
    breast O91.12
      associated with lactation O91.13
    cervix (uteri) O86.11
    genital organ NEC O86.19
    kidney O86.21
    mammary O91.12
      associated with lactation O91.13
    nipple O91.02
      associated with lactation O91.03
    peritoneum O85
    subareolar O91.12
      associated with lactation O91.13
    urinary tract — *see* Puerperal, infection, urinary
    uterus O86.12
    vagina (wall) O86.13
    vaginorectal O86.13
    vulvovaginal gland O86.13
  adnexitis O86.19
  afibrinogenemia, or other coagulation defect O72.3
  albuminuria (acute) (subacute) — *see* Proteinuria,
    gestational
  alcohol use O99.315
  anemia O90.81
    pre-existing (pre-pregnancy) O99.03
  anesthetic death O89.8
  apoplexy O99.43
  bariatric surgery status O99.845
  blood disorder NEC O99.13
  blood dyscrasia O72.3
  cardiomyopathy O90.3
  cerebrovascular disorder (conditions in I60-I69) O99.43
  cervicitis O86.11
  circulatory system disorder O99.43
  coagulopathy (any) O99.13
    with hemorrhage O72.3
  complications O90.9
    specified NEC O90.89
  convulsions — *see* Eclampsia
  cystitis O86.22
  cystopyelitis O86.29
  delirium NEC F05
  diabetes O24.93
    gestational — *see* Puerperal, gestational diabetes
    pre-existing O24.33
      specified NEC O24.83
      type 1 O24.03
      type 2 O24.13
  digestive system disorder O99.63
  disease O90.9

▽ **Subterms under main terms may continue to next column or page**   ☑ **Additional Character Required — Refer to the Tabular List for Character Selection**   **267**

Psychosis, psychotic — Puerperal, puerperium

Puerperal, puerperium — *continued*
  disease — *continued*
    breast NEC O92.29
    cerebrovascular (acute) O99.43
    nonobstetric NEC O99.89
    tubo-ovarian O86.19
    Valsuani's O99.03
  disorder O90.9
    biliary tract O26.63
    lactation O92.70
    liver O26.63
    nonobstetric NEC O99.89
  disruption
    cesarean wound O90.0
    episiotomy wound O90.1
    perineal laceration wound O90.1
  drug use O99.325
  eclampsia (with pre-existing hypertension) O15.2
  embolism (pulmonary) (blood clot) — *see* Embolism, obstetric, puerperal
  endocrine, nutritional or metabolic disease NEC O99.285
  endophlebitis — *see* Puerperal, phlebitis
  endotrachelitis O86.11
  failure
    lactation (complete) O92.3
      partial O92.4
    renal, acute O90.4
  fever (of unknown origin) O86.4
    septic O85
  fissure, nipple O92.12
    associated with lactation O92.13
  fistula
    breast (due to mastitis) O91.12
      associated with lactation O91.13
    nipple O91.02
      associated with lactation O91.03
  galactophoritis O91.22
    associated with lactation O91.23
  galactorrhea O92.6
  gastric banding status O99.845
  gastric bypass status O99.845
  gastrointestinal disease NEC O99.63
  gestational
    diabetes O24.439
      diet controlled O24.430
      insulin (and diet) controlled O24.434
      oral drug controlled (antidiabetic) (hypoglycemic) O24.435
    edema O12.05
      with proteinuria O12.25
    proteinuria O12.15
  gonorrhea O98.23
  hematoma, subdural O99.43
  hemiplegia, cerebral O99.355
    due to cerbrovascular disorder O99.43
  hemorrhage O72.1
    brain O99.43
    bulbar O99.43
    cerebellar O99.43
    cerebral O99.43
    cortical O99.43
    delayed or secondary O72.2
    extradural O99.43
    internal capsule O99.43
    intracranial O99.43
    intrapontine O99.43
    meningeal O99.43
    pontine O99.43
    retained placenta O72.0
    subarachnoid O99.43
    subcortical O99.43
    subdural O99.43
    third stage O72.0
    uterine, delayed O72.2
    ventricular O99.43
  hemorrhoids O87.2
  hepatorenal syndrome O90.4
  hypertension — *see* Hypertension, complicating, puerperium
  hypertrophy, breast O92.29
  induration breast (fibrous) O92.29
  infection O86.4
    cervix O86.11
    generalized O85
    genital tract NEC O86.19
      obstetric surgical wound O86.09
    kidney (bacillus coli) O86.21
    maternal O98.93

Puerperal, puerperium — *continued*
  infection — *continued*
    maternal — *continued*
      carrier state NEC O99.835
      gonorrhea O98.23
      human immunodeficiency virus (HIV) O98.73
      protozoal O98.63
      sexually transmitted NEC O98.33
      specified NEC O98.83
      streptococcus group B (GBS) carrier state O99.825
      syphilis O98.13
      tuberculosis O98.03
      viral hepatitis O98.43
      viral NEC O98.53
    nipple O91.02
      associated with lactation O91.03
    peritoneum O85
    renal O86.21
    specified NEC O86.89
    urinary (asymptomatic) (tract) NEC O86.20
      bladder O86.22
      kidney O86.21
      specified site NEC O86.29
      urethra O86.22
    vagina O86.13
    vein — *see* Puerperal, phlebitis
  ischemia, cerebral O99.43
  lymphangitis O86.89
    breast O91.22
      associated with lactation O91.23
  malignancy O9A.13 (*following* O99)
  malnutrition O25.3
  mammillitis O91.02
    associated with lactation O91.03
  mammitis O91.22
    associated with lactation O91.23
  mania F30.8
  mastitis O91.22
    associated with lactation O91.23
    purulent O91.12
      associated with lactation O91.13
  melancholia — *see* Disorder, depressive
  mental disorder NEC O99.345
  metroperitonitis O85
  metrorrhagia — *see* Hemorrhage, postpartum
  metrosalpingitis O86.19
  metrovaginitis O86.13
  milk leg O87.1
  monoplegia, cerebral O99.43
  mood disturbance O90.6
  necrosis, liver (acute) (subacute) (conditions in subcategory K72.0) O26.63
    with renal failure O90.4
  nervous system disorder O99.355
  obesity (pre-existing prior to pregnancy) O99.215
  obesity surgery status O99.845
  occlusion, precerebral artery O99.43
  paralysis
    bladder (sphincter) O90.89
    cerebral O99.43
  paralytic stroke O99.43
  parametritis O85
  paravaginitis O86.13
  pelviperitonitis O85
  perimetritis O86.12
  perimetrosalpingitis O86.19
  perinephritis O86.21
  periphlebitis — *see* Puerperal phlebitis
  peritoneal infection O85
  peritonitis (pelvic) O85
  perivaginitis O86.13
  phlebitis O87.0
    deep O87.1
    pelvic O87.1
    superficial O87.0
  phlebothrombosis, deep O87.1
  phlegmasia alba dolens O87.1
  placental polyp O90.89
  pneumonia, embolic — *see* Embolism, obstetric, puerperal
  pre-eclampsia — *see* Pre-eclampsia
  psychosis (NOS) F53.1
  pyelitis O86.21
  pyelocystitis O86.29
  pyelonephritis O86.21
  pyelonephrosis O86.21
  pyemia O85
  pyocystitis O86.29
  pyohemia O85

Puerperal, puerperium — *continued*
  pyometra O86.12
  pyonephritis O86.21
  pyosalpingitis O86.19
  pyrexia (of unknown origin) O86.4
  renal
    disease NEC O90.89
    failure O90.4
  respiratory disease NEC O99.53
  retention
    decidua — *see* Retention, decidua
    placenta O72.0
    secundines — *see* Retention, secundines
  retrated nipple O92.02
  salpingo-ovaritis O86.19
  salpingoperitonitis O85
  secondary perineal tear O90.1
  sepsis (pelvic) O85
  sepsis O85
  septic thrombophlebitis O86.81
  skin disorder NEC O99.73
  specified condition NEC O99.89
  stroke O99.43
  subinvolution (uterus) O90.89
  subluxation of symphysis (pubis) O26.73
  suppuration — *see* Puerperal, abscess
  tetanus A34
  thelitis O91.02
    associated with lactation O91.03
  thrombocytopenia O72.3
  thrombophlebitis (superficial) O87.0
    deep O87.1
    pelvic O87.1
    septic O86.81
  thrombosis (venous) — *see* Thrombosis, puerperal
  thyroiditis O90.5
  toxemia (eclamptic) (pre-eclamptic) (with convulsions) O15.2
  trauma, non-obstetric O9A.23 (*following* O99)
    caused by abuse (physical) (suspected) O9A.33 (*following* O99)
      confirmed O9A.33 (*following* O99)
      psychological (suspected) O9A.53 (*following* O99)
        confirmed O9A.53 (*following* O99)
      sexual (suspected) O9A.43 (*following* O99)
        confirmed O9A.43 (*following* O99)
  uremia (due to renal failure) O90.4
  urethritis O86.22
  vaginitis O86.13
  varicose veins (legs) O87.4
    vulva or perineum O87.8
  venous O87.9
  vulvitis O86.19
  vulvovaginitis O86.13
  white leg O87.1
Puerperium — *see* Puerperal
Pulmolithiasis J98.4
Pulmonary — *see* condition
Pulpitis (acute) (anachoretic) (chronic) (hyperplastic) (putrescent) (suppurative) (ulcerative) K04.01
  irreversible K04.02
  reversible K04.01
Pulpless tooth K04.99
Pulse
  alternating R00.8
  bigeminal R00.8
  fast R00.0
  feeble, rapid due to shock following injury T79.4 ☑
  rapid R00.0
  weak R09.89
Pulsus alternans or trigeminus R00.8
Punch drunk F07.81
Punctum lacrimale occlusion — *see* Obstruction, lacrimal
Puncture
  abdomen, abdominal
    wall S31.139 ☑
      with
        foreign body S31.149 ☑
        penetration into peritoneal cavity S31.639 ☑
          with foreign body S31.649 ☑
        epigastric region S31.132 ☑
          with
            foreign body S31.142 ☑
            penetration into peritoneal cavity S31.632 ☑
              with foreign body S31.642 ☑

☑ **Additional Character Required** — Refer to the Tabular List for Character Selection   ⬐ Subterms under main terms may continue to next column or page

Puncture — continued
　abdomen, abdominal — continued
　　wall — continued
　　　left
　　　　lower quadrant S31.134 ☑
　　　　　with
　　　　　　foreign body S31.144 ☑
　　　　　　penetration into peritoneal cavity
　　　　　　　S31.634 ☑
　　　　　　　with foreign body S31.644 ☑
　　　　upper quadrant S31.131 ☑
　　　　　with
　　　　　　foreign body S31.141 ☑
　　　　　　penetration into peritoneal cavity
　　　　　　　S31.631 ☑
　　　　　　　with foreign body S31.641 ☑
　　　periumbilic region S31.135 ☑
　　　　with
　　　　　foreign body S31.145 ☑
　　　　　penetration into peritoneal cavity
　　　　　　S31.635 ☑
　　　　　　with foreign body S31.645 ☑
　　　right
　　　　lower quadrant S31.133 ☑
　　　　　with
　　　　　　foreign body S31.143 ☑
　　　　　　penetration into peritoneal cavity
　　　　　　　S31.633 ☑
　　　　　　　with foreign body S31.643 ☑
　　　　upper quadrant S31.130 ☑
　　　　　with
　　　　　　foreign body S31.140 ☑
　　　　　　penetration into peritoneal cavity
　　　　　　　S31.630 ☑
　　　　　　　with foreign body S31.640 ☑
　accidental, complicating surgery — see Complication,
　　accidental puncture or laceration
　alveolar (process) — see Puncture, oral cavity
　ankle S91.039 ☑
　　with
　　　foreign body S91.049 ☑
　　left S91.032 ☑
　　　with
　　　　foreign body S91.042 ☑
　　right S91.031 ☑
　　　with
　　　　foreign body S91.041 ☑
　anus S31.833 ☑
　　with foreign body S31.834 ☑
　arm (upper) S41.139 ☑
　　with foreign body S41.149 ☑
　　left S41.132 ☑
　　　with foreign body S41.142 ☑
　　lower — see Puncture, forearm
　　right S41.131 ☑
　　　with foreign body S41.141 ☑
　auditory canal (external) (meatus) — see Puncture, ear
　auricle, ear — see Puncture, ear
　axilla — see Puncture, arm
　back — see also Puncture, thorax, back
　　lower S31.030 ☑
　　　with
　　　　foreign body S31.040 ☑
　　　　　with penetration into retroperitoneal
　　　　　　space S31.041 ☑
　　　　penetration into retroperitoneal space
　　　　　S31.031 ☑
　bladder (traumatic) S37.29 ☑
　　nontraumatic N32.89
　breast S21.039 ☑
　　with foreign body S21.049 ☑
　　left S21.032 ☑
　　　with foreign body S21.042 ☑
　　right S21.031 ☑
　　　with foreign body S21.041 ☑
　buttock S31.803 ☑
　　with foreign body S31.804 ☑
　　left S31.823 ☑
　　　with foreign body S31.824 ☑
　　right S31.813 ☑
　　　with foreign body S31.814 ☑
　by
　　device, implant or graft — see Complications, by
　　　site and type, mechanical
　　foreign body left accidentally in operative wound
　　　T81.539 ☑

Puncture — continued
　by — continued
　　instrument (any) during a procedure, accidental —
　　　see Puncture, accidental complicating surgery
　calf — see Puncture, leg
　canaliculus lacrimalis — see Puncture, eyelid
　canthus, eye — see Puncture, eyelid
　cervical esophagus S11.23 ☑
　　with foreign body S11.24 ☑
　cheek (external) S01.439 ☑
　　with foreign body S01.449 ☑
　　internal — see Puncture, oral cavity
　　left S01.432 ☑
　　　with foreign body S01.442 ☑
　　right S01.431 ☑
　　　with foreign body S01.441 ☑
　chest wall — see Puncture, thorax
　chin — see Puncture, head, specified site NEC
　clitoris — see Puncture, vulva
　costal region — see Puncture, thorax
　digit(s)
　　foot — see Puncture, toe
　　hand — see Puncture, finger
　ear (canal) (external) S01.339 ☑
　　with foreign body S01.349 ☑
　　drum S09.2- ☑
　　left S01.332 ☑
　　　with foreign body S01.342 ☑
　　right S01.331 ☑
　　　with foreign body S01.341 ☑
　elbow S51.039 ☑
　　with
　　　foreign body S51.049 ☑
　　left S51.032 ☑
　　　with
　　　　foreign body S51.042 ☑
　　right S51.031 ☑
　　　with
　　　　foreign body S51.041 ☑
　epididymis — see Puncture, testis
　epigastric region — see Puncture, abdomen, wall, epi-
　　gastric
　epiglottis S11.83 ☑
　　with foreign body S11.84 ☑
　esophagus
　　cervical S11.23 ☑
　　　with foreign body S11.24 ☑
　　thoracic S27.818 ☑
　eyeball S05.6- ☑
　　with foreign body S05.5- ☑
　eyebrow — see Puncture, eyelid
　eyelid S01.13- ☑
　　with foreign body S01.14- ☑
　　left S01.132 ☑
　　　with foreign body S01.142 ☑
　　right S01.131 ☑
　　　with foreign body S01.141 ☑
　face NEC — see Puncture, head, specified site NEC
　finger(s) S61.239 ☑
　　with
　　　damage to nail S61.339 ☑
　　　　with
　　　　　foreign body S61.349 ☑
　　　foreign body S61.249 ☑
　　index S61.238 ☑
　　　with
　　　　damage to nail S61.338 ☑
　　　　　with
　　　　　　foreign body S61.348 ☑
　　　　foreign body S61.248 ☑
　　　left S61.231 ☑
　　　　with
　　　　　damage to nail S61.331 ☑
　　　　　　with
　　　　　　　foreign body S61.341 ☑
　　　　　foreign body S61.241 ☑
　　　right S61.230 ☑
　　　　with
　　　　　damage to nail S61.330 ☑
　　　　　　with
　　　　　　　foreign body S61.340 ☑
　　　　　foreign body S61.240 ☑
　　little S61.238 ☑
　　　with
　　　　damage to nail S61.338 ☑

Puncture — continued
　finger(s) — continued
　　little — continued
　　　with — continued
　　　　damage to nail — continued
　　　　　with
　　　　　　foreign body S61.348 ☑
　　　　foreign body S61.248 ☑
　　　left S61.237 ☑
　　　　with
　　　　　damage to nail S61.337 ☑
　　　　　　with
　　　　　　　foreign body S61.347 ☑
　　　　　foreign body S61.247 ☑
　　　right S61.236 ☑
　　　　with
　　　　　damage to nail S61.336 ☑
　　　　　　with
　　　　　　　foreign body S61.346 ☑
　　　　　foreign body S61.246 ☑
　　middle S61.238 ☑
　　　with
　　　　damage to nail S61.338 ☑
　　　　　with
　　　　　　foreign body S61.348 ☑
　　　　foreign body S61.248 ☑
　　　left S61.233 ☑
　　　　with
　　　　　damage to nail S61.333 ☑
　　　　　　with
　　　　　　　foreign body S61.343 ☑
　　　　　foreign body S61.243 ☑
　　　right S61.232 ☑
　　　　with
　　　　　damage to nail S61.332 ☑
　　　　　　with
　　　　　　　foreign body S61.342 ☑
　　　　　foreign body S61.242 ☑
　　ring S61.238 ☑
　　　with
　　　　damage to nail S61.338 ☑
　　　　　with
　　　　　　foreign body S61.348 ☑
　　　　foreign body S61.248 ☑
　　　left S61.235 ☑
　　　　with
　　　　　damage to nail S61.335 ☑
　　　　　　with
　　　　　　　foreign body S61.345 ☑
　　　　　foreign body S61.245 ☑
　　　right S61.234 ☑
　　　　with
　　　　　damage to nail S61.334 ☑
　　　　　　with
　　　　　　　foreign body S61.344 ☑
　　　　　foreign body S61.244 ☑
　flank S31.139 ☑
　　with foreign body S31.149 ☑
　foot (except toe(s) alone) S91.339 ☑
　　with foreign body S91.349 ☑
　　left S91.332 ☑
　　　with foreign body S91.342 ☑
　　right S91.331 ☑
　　　with foreign body S91.341 ☑
　　toe — see Puncture, toe
　forearm S51.839 ☑
　　with
　　　foreign body S51.849 ☑
　　elbow only — see Puncture, elbow
　　left S51.832 ☑
　　　with
　　　　foreign body S51.842 ☑
　　right S51.831 ☑
　　　with
　　　　foreign body S51.841 ☑
　forehead — see Puncture, head, specified site NEC
　genital organs, external
　　female S31.532 ☑
　　　with foreign body S31.542 ☑
　　　vagina — see Puncture, vagina
　　　vulva — see Puncture, vulva
　　male S31.531 ☑
　　　with foreign body S31.541 ☑
　　　penis — see Puncture, penis
　　　scrotum — see Puncture, scrotum
　　　testis — see Puncture, testis

▽ **Subterms under main terms may continue to next column or page**　　☑ **Additional Character Required — Refer to the Tabular List for Character Selection**　　269

Puncture — Puncture

Puncture — *continued*
  groin — *see* Puncture, abdomen, wall
  gum — *see* Puncture, oral cavity
  hand S61.439 ✓
    with
      foreign body S61.449 ✓
    finger — *see* Puncture, finger
    left S61.432 ✓
      with
        foreign body S61.442 ✓
    right S61.431 ✓
      with
        foreign body S61.441 ✓
    thumb — *see* Puncture, thumb
  head S01.93 ✓
    with foreign body S01.94 ✓
    cheek — *see* Puncture, cheek
    ear — *see* Puncture, ear
    eyelid — *see* Puncture, eyelid
    lip — *see* Puncture, oral cavity
    nose — *see* Puncture, nose
    oral cavity — *see* Puncture, oral cavity
    scalp S01.03 ✓
      with foreign body S01.04 ✓
    specified site NEC S01.83 ✓
      with foreign body S01.84 ✓
    temporomandibular area — *see* Puncture, cheek
  heart S26.99 ✓
    with hemopericardium S26.09 ✓
    without hemopericardium S26.19 ✓
  heel — *see* Puncture, foot
  hip S71.039 ✓
    with foreign body S71.049 ✓
    left S71.032 ✓
      with foreign body S71.042 ✓
    right S71.031 ✓
      with foreign body S71.041 ✓
  hymen — *see* Puncture, vagina
  hypochondrium — *see* Puncture, abdomen, wall
  hypogastric region — *see* Puncture, abdomen, wall
  inguinal region — *see* Puncture, abdomen, wall
  instep — *see* Puncture, foot
  internal organs — *see* Injury, by site
  interscapular region — *see* Puncture, thorax, back
  intestine
    large
      colon S36.599 ✓
        ascending S36.590 ✓
        descending S36.592 ✓
        sigmoid S36.593 ✓
        specified site NEC S36.598 ✓
        transverse S36.591 ✓
      rectum S36.69 ✓
    small S36.499 ✓
      duodenum S36.490 ✓
      specified site NEC S36.498 ✓
  intra-abdominal organ S36.99 ✓
    gallbladder S36.128 ✓
    intestine — *see* Puncture, intestine
    liver S36.118 ✓
    pancreas — *see* Puncture, pancreas
    peritoneum S36.81 ✓
    specified site NEC S36.898 ✓
    spleen S36.09 ✓
    stomach S36.39 ✓
  jaw — *see* Puncture, head, specified site NEC
  knee S81.039 ✓
    with foreign body S81.049 ✓
    left S81.032 ✓
      with foreign body S81.042 ✓
    right S81.031 ✓
      with foreign body S81.041 ✓
  labium (majus) (minus) — *see* Puncture, vulva
  lacrimal duct — *see* Puncture, eyelid
  larynx S11.013 ✓
    with foreign body S11.014 ✓
  leg (lower) S81.839 ✓
    with foreign body S81.849 ✓
    foot — *see* Puncture, foot
    knee — *see* Puncture, knee
    left S81.832 ✓
      with foreign body S81.842 ✓
    right S81.831 ✓
      with foreign body S81.841 ✓
    upper — *see* Puncture, thigh
  lip S01.531 ✓

Puncture — *continued*
  lip — *continued*
    with foreign body S01.541 ✓
  loin — *see* Puncture, abdomen, wall
  lower back — *see* Puncture, back, lower
  lumbar region — *see* Puncture, back, lower
  malar region — *see* Puncture, head, specified site NEC
  mammary — *see* Puncture, breast
  mastoid region — *see* Puncture, head, specified site NEC
  mouth — *see* Puncture, oral cavity
  nail
    finger — *see* Puncture, finger, with damage to nail
    toe — *see* Puncture, toe, with damage to nail
  nasal (septum) (sinus) — *see* Puncture, nose
  nasopharynx — *see* Puncture, head, specified site NEC
  neck S11.93 ✓
    with foreign body S11.94 ✓
    involving
      cervical esophagus — *see* Puncture, cervical esophagus
      larynx — *see* Puncture, larynx
      pharynx — *see* Puncture, pharynx
      thyroid gland — *see* Puncture, thyroid gland
      trachea — *see* Puncture, trachea
    specified site NEC S11.83 ✓
      with foreign body S11.84 ✓
  nose (septum) (sinus) S01.23 ✓
    with foreign body S01.24 ✓
  ocular — *see* Puncture, eyeball
  oral cavity S01.532 ✓
    with foreign body S01.542 ✓
  orbit S05.4- ✓
  palate — *see* Puncture, oral cavity
  palm — *see* Puncture, hand
  pancreas S36.299 ✓
    body S36.291 ✓
    head S36.290 ✓
    tail S36.292 ✓
  pelvis — *see* Puncture, back, lower
  penis S31.23 ✓
    with foreign body S31.24 ✓
  perineum
    female S31.43 ✓
      with foreign body S31.44 ✓
    male S31.139 ✓
      with foreign body S31.149 ✓
  periocular area (with or without lacrimal passages) — *see* Puncture, eyelid
  phalanges
    finger — *see* Puncture, finger
    toe — *see* Puncture, toe
  pharynx S11.23 ✓
    with foreign body S11.24 ✓
  pinna — *see* Puncture, ear
  popliteal space — *see* Puncture, knee
  prepuce — *see* Puncture, penis
  pubic region S31.139 ✓
    with foreign body S31.149 ✓
  pudendum — *see* Puncture, genital organs, external
  rectovaginal septum — *see* Puncture, vagina
  sacral region — *see* Puncture, back, lower
  sacroiliac region — *see* Puncture, back, lower
  salivary gland — *see* Puncture, oral cavity
  scalp S01.03 ✓
    with foreign body S01.04 ✓
  scapular region — *see* Puncture, shoulder
  scrotum S31.33 ✓
    with foreign body S31.34 ✓
  shin — *see* Puncture, leg
  shoulder S41.039 ✓
    with foreign body S41.049 ✓
    left S41.032 ✓
      with foreign body S41.042 ✓
    right S41.031 ✓
      with foreign body S41.041 ✓
  spermatic cord — *see* Puncture, testis
  sternal region — *see* Puncture, thorax, front
  submaxillary region — *see* Puncture, head, specified site NEC
  submental region — *see* Puncture, head, specified site NEC
  subungual
    finger(s) — *see* Puncture, finger, with damage to nail
    toe — *see* Puncture, toe, with damage to nail

Puncture — *continued*
  supraclavicular fossa — *see* Puncture, neck, specified site NEC
  temple, temporal region — *see* Puncture, head, specified site NEC
  temporomandibular area — *see* Puncture, cheek
  testis S31.33 ✓
    with foreign body S31.34 ✓
  thigh S71.139 ✓
    with foreign body S71.149 ✓
    left S71.132 ✓
      with foreign body S71.142 ✓
    right S71.131 ✓
      with foreign body S71.141 ✓
  thorax, thoracic (wall) S21.93 ✓
    with foreign body S21.94 ✓
    back S21.23- ✓
      with
        foreign body S21.24- ✓
          with penetration S21.44 ✓
        penetration S21.43 ✓
    breast — *see* Puncture, breast
    front S21.13- ✓
      with
        foreign body S21.14- ✓
          with penetration S21.34 ✓
        penetration S21.33 ✓
  throat — *see* Puncture, neck
  thumb S61.039 ✓
    with
      damage to nail S61.139 ✓
        with
          foreign body S61.149 ✓
      foreign body S61.049 ✓
    left S61.032 ✓
      with
        damage to nail S61.132 ✓
          with
            foreign body S61.142 ✓
        foreign body S61.042 ✓
    right S61.031 ✓
      with
        damage to nail S61.131 ✓
          with
            foreign body S61.141 ✓
        foreign body S61.041 ✓
  thyroid gland S11.13 ✓
    with foreign body S11.14 ✓
  toe(s) S91.139 ✓
    with
      damage to nail S91.239 ✓
        with
          foreign body S91.249 ✓
      foreign body S91.149 ✓
    great S91.133 ✓
      with
        damage to nail S91.233 ✓
          with
            foreign body S91.243 ✓
        foreign body S91.143 ✓
      left S91.132 ✓
        with
          damage to nail S91.232 ✓
            with
              foreign body S91.242 ✓
          foreign body S91.142 ✓
      right S91.131 ✓
        with
          damage to nail S91.231 ✓
            with
              foreign body S91.241 ✓
          foreign body S91.141 ✓
    lesser S91.136 ✓
      with
        damage to nail S91.236 ✓
          with
            foreign body S91.246 ✓
        foreign body S91.146 ✓
      left S91.135 ✓
        with
          damage to nail S91.235 ✓
            with
              foreign body S91.245 ✓
          foreign body S91.145 ✓
      right S91.134 ✓

✓ Additional Character Required — Refer to the Tabular List for Character Selection ▽ Subterms under main terms may continue to next column or page

Puncture — *continued*
  toe(s) — *continued*
    lesser — *continued*
      right — *continued*
        with
          damage to nail S91.234 ☑
            with
              foreign body S91.244 ☑
          foreign body S91.144 ☑
  tongue — *see* Puncture, oral cavity
  trachea S11.023 ☑
    with foreign body S11.024 ☑
  tunica vaginalis — *see* Puncture, testis
  tympanum, tympanic membrane S09.2- ☑
  umbilical region S31.135 ☑
    with foreign body S31.145 ☑
  uvula — *see* Puncture, oral cavity
  vagina S31.43 ☑
    with foreign body S31.44 ☑
  vocal cords S11.033 ☑
    with foreign body S11.034 ☑
  vulva S31.43 ☑
    with foreign body S31.44 ☑
  wrist S61.539 ☑
    with
      foreign body S61.549 ☑
    left S61.532 ☑
      with
        foreign body S61.542 ☑
    right S61.531 ☑
      with
        foreign body S61.541 ☑
PUO (pyrexia of unknown origin) R50.9
Pupillary membrane (persistent) Q13.89
Pupillotonia — *see* Anomaly, pupil, function, tonic pupil
Purpura D69.2
  abdominal D69.0
  allergic D69.0
  anaphylactoid D69.0
  annularis telangiectodes L81.7
  arthritic D69.0
  autoerythrocyte sensitization D69.2
  autoimmune D69.0
  bacterial D69.0
  Bateman's (senile) D69.2
  capillary fragility (hereditary) (idiopathic) D69.8
  cryoglobulinemic D89.1
  Devil's pinches D69.2
  fibrinolytic — *see* Fibrinolysis
  fulminans, fulminous D65
  gangrenous D65
  hemorrhagic, hemorrhagica D69.3
    not due to thrombocytopenia D69.0
  Henoch (-Schönlein) (allergic) D69.0
  hypergammaglobulinemic (benign) (Waldenström)
    D89.0
  idiopathic (thrombocytopenic) D69.3
    nonthrombocytopenic D69.0
  immune thrombocytopenic D69.3
  infectious D69.0
  malignant D69.0
  neonatorum P54.5
  nervosa D69.0
  newborn P54.5
  nonthrombocytopenic D69.2
    hemorrhagic D69.0
    idiopathic D69.0
  nonthrombopenic D69.2
  peliosis rheumatica D69.0
  posttransfusion (post-transfusion) (from (fresh) whole
    blood or blood products) D69.51
  primary D69.49
  red cell membrane sensitivity D69.2
  rheumatica D69.0
  Schönlein (-Henoch) (allergic) D69.0
  scorbutic E54 *[D77]*
  senile D69.2
  simplex D69.2
  symptomatica D69.0
  telangiectasia annularis L81.7
  thrombocytopenic D69.49
    congenital D69.42
    hemorrhagic D69.3
    hereditary D69.42
    idiopathic D69.3
    immune D69.3
    neonatal, transitory P61.0
    thrombotic M31.1

Purpura — *continued*
  thrombohemolytic — *see* Fibrinolysis
  thrombolytic — *see* Fibrinolysis
  thrombopenic D69.49
  thrombotic, thrombocytopenic M31.1
  toxic D69.0
  vascular D69.0
  visceral symptoms D69.0
Purpuric spots R23.3
Purulent — *see* condition
Pus
  in
    stool R19.5
    urine N39.0
  tube (rupture) — *see* Salpingo-oophoritis
Pustular rash L08.0
Pustule (nonmalignant) L08.9
  malignant A22.0
Pustulosis palmaris et plantaris L40.3
Putnam (-Dana) **disease or syndrome** — *see* Degeneration, combined
Putrescent pulp (dental) K04.1
Pyarthritis, pyarthrosis — *see* Arthritis, pyogenic or pyemic
  tuberculous — *see* Tuberculosis, joint
Pyelectasis — *see* Hydronephrosis
Pyelitis (congenital) (uremic) — *see also* Pyelonephritis
  with
    calculus — *see* category N20 ☑
      with hydronephrosis N13.6
    contracted kidney N11.9
  acute N10
  chronic N11.9
    with calculus — *see* category N20 ☑
      with hydronephrosis N13.6
  cystica N28.84
  puerperal (postpartum) O86.21
  tuberculous A18.11
Pyelocystitis — *see* Pyelonephritis
Pyelonephritis — *see also* Nephritis, tubulo-interstitial
  with
    calculus — *see* category N20 ☑
      with hydronephrosis N13.6
    contracted kidney N11.9
  acute N10
  calculous — *see* category N20 ☑
    with hydronephrosis N13.6
  chronic N11.9
    with calculus — *see* category N20 ☑
      with hydronephrosis N13.6
    associated with ureteral obstruction or stricture
      N11.1
    nonobstructive N11.8
      with reflux (vesicoureteral) N11.0
    obstructive N11.1
    specified NEC N11.8
  in (due to)
    brucellosis A23.9 *[N16]*
    cryoglobulinemia (mixed) D89.1 *[N16]*
    cystinosis E72.04
    diphtheria A36.84
    glycogen storage disease E74.09 *[N16]*
    leukemia NEC C95.9- ☑ *[N16]*
    lymphoma NEC C85.90 *[N16]*
    multiple myeloma C90.0- ☑ *[N16]*
    obstruction N11.1
    Salmonella infection A02.25
    sarcoidosis D86.84
    sepsis A41.9 *[N16]*
    Sjögren's disease M35.04
    toxoplasmosis B58.83
    transplant rejection T86.91 *[N16]*
    Wilson's disease E83.01 *[N16]*
  nonobstructive N12
    with reflux (vesicoureteral) N11.0
    chronic N11.8
  syphilitic A52.75
Pyelonephrosis (obstructive) N11.1
  chronic N11.9
Pyelophlebitis I80.8
Pyeloureteritis cystica N28.85
Pyemia, pyemic (fever) (infection) (purulent) — *see also* Sepsis
  joint — *see* Arthritis, pyogenic or pyemic
  liver K75.1
  pneumococcal A40.3
  portal K75.1

Pyemia, pyemic — *continued*
  postvaccinal T88.0 ☑
  puerperal, postpartum, childbirth O85
  specified organism NEC A41.89
  tuberculous — *see* Tuberculosis, miliary
Pygopagus Q89.4
Pyknoepilepsy (idiopathic) — *see* Pyknolepsy
Pyknolepsy G40.A09 (*following* G40.3)
  intractable G40.A19 (*following* G40.3)
    with status epilepticus G40.A11 (*following* G40.3)
    without status epilepticus G40.A19 (*following* G40.3)
  not intractable G40.A09 (*following* G40.3)
    with status epilepticus G40.A01 (*following* G40.3)
    without status epilepticus G40.A09 (*following* G40.3)
Pylephlebitis K75.1
Pyle's syndrome Q78.5
Pylethrombophlebitis K75.1
Pylethrombosis K75.1
Pyloritis K29.90
  with bleeding K29.91
Pylorospasm (reflex) **NEC** K31.3
  congenital or infantile Q40.0
  neurotic F45.8
  newborn Q40.0
  psychogenic F45.8
Pylorus, pyloric — *see* condition
Pyoarthrosis — *see* Arthritis, pyogenic or pyemic
Pyocele
  mastoid — *see* Mastoiditis, acute
  sinus (accessory) — *see* Sinusitis
  turbinate (bone) J32.9
  urethra — *see also* Urethritis N34.0
Pyocolpos — *see* Vaginitis
Pyocystitis N30.80
  with hematuria N30.81
Pyoderma, pyodermia L08.0
  gangrenosum L88
  newborn P39.4
  phagedenic L88
  vegetans L08.81
Pyodermatitis L08.0
  vegetans L08.81
Pyogenic — *see* condition
Pyohydronephrosis N13.6
Pyometra, pyometrium, pyometritis — *see* Endometritis
Pyomyositis (tropical) — *see* Myositis, infective
Pyonephritis N12
Pyonephrosis N13.6
  tuberculous A18.11
Pyo-oophoritis — *see* Salpingo-oophoritis
Pyo-ovarium — *see* Salpingo-oophoritis
Pyopericarditis, pyopericardium I30.1
Pyophlebitis — *see* Phlebitis
Pyopneumopericardium I30.1
Pyopneumothorax (infective) J86.9
  with fistula J86.0
  tuberculous NEC A15.6
Pyosalpinx, pyosalpingitis — *see also* Salpingo-oophoritis
Pyothorax J86.9
  with fistula J86.0
  tuberculous NEC A15.6
Pyoureter N28.89
  tuberculous A18.11
Pyramidopallidonigral syndrome G20
Pyrexia (of unknown origin) R50.9
  atmospheric T67.01 ☑
  during labor NEC O75.2
  heat T67.01 ☑
  newborn P81.9
    environmentally-induced P81.0
  persistent R50.9
  puerperal O86.4
Pyroglobulinemia NEC E88.09
Pyromania F63.1
Pyrosis R12
Pyuria (bacterial) (sterile) R82.81

Q

Q fever A78
  with pneumonia A78
Quadricuspid aortic valve Q23.8
Quadrilateral fever A78
Quadriparesis — *see* Quadriplegia
  meaning muscle weakness M62.81

Subterms under main terms may continue to next column or page   ☑ Additional Character Required — Refer to the Tabular List for Character Selection   271

Puncture — Quadriparesis

Quadriplegia G82.50
  complete
    C1-C4 level G82.51
    C5-C7 level G82.53
  congenital (cerebral) (spinal) G80.8
    spastic G80.0
  embolic (current episode) I63.4- ☑
  functional R53.2
  incomplete
    C1-C4 level G82.52
    C5-C7 level G82.54
  thrombotic (current episode) I63.3- ☑
  traumatic — *code to* injury with seventh character S
    current episode — *see* Injury, spinal (cord), cervical
Quadruplet, pregnancy — *see* Pregnancy, quadruplet
Quarrelsomeness F60.3
Queensland fever A77.3
Quervain's disease M65.4
  thyroid E06.1
Queyrat's erythroplasia D07.4
  penis D07.4
  specified site — *see* Neoplasm, skin, in situ
  unspecified site D07.4
Quincke's disease or edema T78.3 ☑
  hereditary D84.1
Quinsy (gangrenous) J36
Quintan fever A79.0
Quintuplet, pregnancy — *see* Pregnancy, quintuplet

R

Rabbit fever — *see* Tularemia
Rabies A82.9
  contact Z20.3
  exposure to Z20.3
  inoculation reaction — *see* Complications, vaccination
  sylvatic A82.0
  urban A82.1
Rachischisis — *see* Spina bifida
Rachitic — *see also* condition
  deformities of spine (late effect) (sequelae) E64.3
  pelvis (late effect) (sequelae) E64.3
    with disproportion (fetopelvic) O33.0
      causing obstructed labor O65.0
Rachitis, rachitism (acute) (tarda) — *see also* Rickets
  renalis N25.0
  sequelae E64.3
Radial nerve — *see* condition
Radiation
  burn — *see* Burn
  effects NOS T66 ☑
  sickness NOS T66 ☑
  therapy, encounter for Z51.0
Radiculitis (pressure) (vertebrogenic) — *see* Radiculopathy
Radiculomyelitis — *see also* Encephalitis
  toxic, due to
    Clostridium tetani A35
    Corynebacterium diphtheriae A36.82
Radiculopathy M54.10
  cervical region M54.12
  cervicothoracic region M54.13
  due to
    disc disorder
      C3 M50.11
      C4 M50.11
      C5 M50.121
      C6 M50.122
      C7 M50.123
    displacement of intervertebral disc — *see* Disorder, disc, with, radiculopathy
  leg M54.1- ☑
  lumbar region M54.16
  lumbosacral region M54.17
  occipito-atlanto-axial region M54.11
  postherpetic B02.29
  sacrococcygeal region M54.18
  syphilitic A52.11
  thoracic region (with visceral pain) M54.14
  thoracolumbar region M54.15
Radiodermal burns (acute, chronic, or occupational) — *see* Burn
Radiodermatitis L58.9
  acute L58.0
  chronic L58.1
Radiotherapy session Z51.0
RAEB (refractory anemia with excess blasts) D46.2- ☑

Rage, meaning rabies — *see* Rabies
Ragpicker's disease A22.1
Ragsorter's disease A22.1
Raillietiniasis B71.8
Railroad neurosis F48.8
Railway spine F48.8
Raised — *see also* Elevated
  antibody titer R76.0
Rake teeth, tooth M26.39
Rales R09.89
Ramifying renal pelvis Q63.8
Ramsay-Hunt disease or syndrome — *see also* Hunt's disease B02.21
  meaning dyssynergia cerebellaris myoclonica G11.1
Ranula K11.6
  congenital Q38.4
Rape
  adult
    confirmed T74.21 ☑
    suspected T76.21 ☑
  alleged, observation or examination, ruled out
    adult Z04.41
    child Z04.42
  child
    confirmed T74.22 ☑
    suspected T76.22 ☑
Rapid
  feeble pulse, due to shock, following injury T79.4 ☑
  heart (beat) R00.0
    psychogenic F45.8
  second stage (delivery) O62.3
  time-zone change syndrome G47.25
Rarefaction, bone — *see* Disorder, bone, density and structure, specified NEC
Rash (toxic) R21
  canker A38.9
  diaper L22
  drug (internal use) L27.0
    contact — *see also* Dermatitis, due to, drugs, external L25.1
  following immunization T88.1 ☑
  food — *see* Dermatitis, due to, food
  heat L74.0
  napkin (psoriasiform) L22
  nettle — *see* Urticaria
  pustular L08.0
  rose R21
    epidemic B06.9
  scarlet A38.9
  serum — *see also* Reaction, serum T80.69 ☑
  wandering tongue K14.1
Rasmussen aneurysm — *see* Tuberculosis, pulmonary
Rasmussen encephalitis G04.81
Rat-bite fever A25.9
  due to Streptobacillus moniliformis A25.1
  spirochetal (morsus muris) A25.0
Rathke's pouch tumor D44.3
Raymond (-Céstan) **syndrome** I65.8
Raynaud's disease, phenomenon or syndrome (secondary) I73.00
  with gangrene (symmetric) I73.01
RDS (newborn) (type I) P22.0
  type II P22.1
Reaction — *see also* Disorder
  withdrawing, child or adolescent F93.8
  adaptation — *see* Disorder, adjustment
  adjustment (anxiety) (conduct disorder) (depressiveness) (distress) — *see* Disorder, adjustment
    with
      mutism, elective (child) (adolescent) F94.0
  adverse
    food (any) (ingested) NEC T78.1 ☑
      anaphylactic — *see* Shock, anaphylactic, due to food
  affective — *see* Disorder, mood
  allergic — *see* Allergy
  anaphylactic — *see* Shock, anaphylactic
  anaphylactoid — *see* Shock, anaphylactic
  anesthesia — *see* Anesthesia, complication
  antitoxin (prophylactic) (therapeutic) — *see* Complications, vaccination
  anxiety F41.1
  Arthus — *see* Arthus' phenomenon
  asthenic F48.8
  combat and operational stress F43.0
  compulsive F42.8
  conversion F44.9

Reaction — *continued*
  crisis, acute F43.0
  deoxyribonuclease (DNA) (DNase) hypersensitivity D69.2
  depressive (single episode) F32.9
    affective (single episode) F31.4
      recurrent episode F33.9
    neurotic F34.1
    psychoneurotic F34.1
    psychotic F32.3
    recurrent — *see* Disorder, depressive, recurrent
  dissociative F44.9
  drug NEC T88.7 ☑
    addictive — *see* Dependence, drug
      transmitted via placenta or breast milk — *see* Absorption, drug, addictive, through placenta
    allergic — *see* Allergy, drug
    lichenoid L43.2
    newborn P93.8
      gray baby syndrome P93.0
    overdose or poisoning (by accident) — *see* Table of Drugs and Chemicals, by drug, poisoning
    photoallergic L56.1
    phototoxic L56.0
    withdrawal — *see* Dependence, by drug, with, withdrawal
      infant of dependent mother P96.1
      newborn P96.1
    wrong substance given or taken (by accident) — *see* Table of Drugs and Chemicals, by drug, poisoning
  fear F40.9
    child (abnormal) F93.8
  febrile nonhemolytic transfusion (FNHTR) R50.84
  fluid loss, cerebrospinal G97.1
  foreign
    body NEC — *see* Granuloma, foreign body
      in operative wound (inadvertently left) — *see* Foreign body, accidentally left during a procedure
    substance accidentally left during a procedure (chemical) (powder) (talc) T81.60 ☑
      aseptic peritonitis T81.61 ☑
      body or object (instrument) (sponge) (swab) — *see* Foreign body, accidentally left during a procedure
    specified reaction NEC T81.69 ☑
  grief — *see* Disorder, adjustment
  Herxheimer's R68.89
  hyperkinetic — *see* Hyperkinesia
  hypochondriacal F45.20
  hypoglycemic, due to insulin E16.0
    with coma (diabetic) — *see* Diabetes, coma
      nondiabetic E15
    therapeutic misadventure — *see* subcategory T38.3 ☑
  hypomanic F30.8
  hysterical F44.9
  immunization — *see* Complications, vaccination
  incompatibility
    ABO blood group (infusion) (transfusion) — *see* Complication(s), transfusion, incompatibility reaction, ABO
      delayed serologic T80.39 ☑
    minor blood group (Duffy) (E) (K) (Kell) (Kidd) (Lewis) (M) (N) (P) (S) T80.89 ☑
    Rh (factor) (infusion) (transfusion) — *see* Complication(s), transfusion, incompatibility reaction, Rh (factor)
  inflammatory — *see* Infection
  infusion — *see* Complications, infusion
  inoculation (immune serum) — *see* Complications, vaccination
  insulin T38.3- ☑
  involutional psychotic — *see* Disorder, depressive
  leukemoid D72.823
    basophilic D72.823
    lymphocytic D72.823
    monocytic D72.823
    myelocytic D72.823
    neutrophilic D72.823
  LSD (acute)
    due to drug abuse — *see* Abuse, drug, hallucinogen
    due to drug dependence — *see* Dependence, drug, hallucinogen
  lumbar puncture G97.1
  manic-depressive — *see* Disorder, bipolar

☑ **Additional Character Required** — Refer to the Tabular List for Character Selection   ▽ **Subterms under main terms may continue to next column or page**

Reaction — *continued*
  neurasthenic F48.8
  neurogenic — *see* Neurosis
  neurotic F48.9
  neurotic-depressive F34.1
  nitritoid — *see* Crisis, nitritoid
  nonspecific
    to
      cell mediated immunity measurement of gamma interferon antigen response without active tuberculosis R76.12
      QuantiFERON-TB test (QFT) without active tuberculosis R76.12
      tuberculin test — *see also* Reaction, tuberculin skin test R76.11
  obsessive-compulsive F42.8
  organic, acute or subacute — *see* Delirium
  paranoid (acute) F23
    chronic F22
    senile F03 ☑
  passive dependency F60.7
  phobic F40.9
  post-traumatic stress, uncomplicated Z73.3
  psychogenic F99
  psychoneurotic — *see also* Neurosis
    compulsive F42.8
    depersonalization F48.1
    depressive F34.1
    hypochondriacal F45.20
    neurasthenic F48.8
    obsessive F42.8
  psychophysiologic — *see* Disorder, somatoform
  psychosomatic — *see* Disorder, somatoform
  psychotic — *see* Psychosis
  scarlet fever toxin — *see* Complications, vaccination
  schizophrenic F23
    acute (brief) (undifferentiated) F23
    latent F21
    undifferentiated (acute) (brief) F23
  serological for syphilis — *see* Serology for syphilis
  serum T80.69 ☑
    anaphylactic (immediate) — *see also* Shock, anaphylactic T80.59 ☑
    specified reaction NEC
      due to
        administration of blood and blood products T80.61 ☑
        immunization T80.62 ☑
        serum specified NEC T80.69 ☑
        vaccination T80.62 ☑
  situational — *see* Disorder, adjustment
  somatization — *see* Disorder, somatoform
  spinal puncture G97.1
  stress (severe) F43.9
    acute (agitation) ("daze") (disorientation) (disturbance of consciousness) (flight reaction) (fugue) F43.0
    specified NEC F43.8
  surgical procedure — *see* Complications, surgical procedure
  tetanus antitoxin — *see* Complications, vaccination
  toxic, to local anesthesia T88.59 ☑
    in labor and delivery O74.4
    in pregnancy O29.3X- ☑
    postpartum, puerperal O89.3
  toxin-antitoxin — *see* Complications, vaccination
  transfusion (blood) (bone marrow) (lymphocytes) (allergic) — *see* Complications, transfusion
  tuberculin skin test, abnormal R76.11
  vaccination (any) — *see* Complications, vaccination
Reactive airway disease — *see* Asthma
Reactive depression — *see* Reaction, depressive
Rearrangement
  chromosomal
    balanced (in) Q95.9
      abnormal individual (autosomal) Q95.2
        non-sex (autosomal) chromosomes Q95.2
        sex/non-sex chromosomes Q95.3
      specified NEC Q95.8
Recalcitrant patient — *see* Noncompliance
Recanalization, thrombus — *see* Thrombosis
Recession, receding
  chamber angle (eye) H21.55- ☑
  chin M26.09
  gingival (postinfective) (postoperative)
    generalized K06.020
      minimal K06.021
      moderate K06.022

Recession, receding — *continued*
  gingival — *continued*
    generalized — *continued*
      severe K06.023
    localized K06.010
      minimal K06.011
      moderate K06.012
      severe K06.013
Recklinghausen disease Q85.01
  bones E21.0
Reclus' disease (cystic) — *see* Mastopathy, cystic
Recrudescent typhus (fever) A75.1
Recruitment, auditory H93.21- ☑
Rectalgia K62.89
Rectitis K62.89
Rectocele
  female (without uterine prolapse) N81.6
    with uterine prolapse N81.4
      incomplete N81.2
  in pregnancy — *see* Pregnancy, complicated by, abnormal, pelvic organs or tissues NEC
  male K62.3
Rectosigmoid junction — *see* condition
Rectosigmoiditis K63.89
  ulcerative (chronic) K51.30
    with
      complication K51.319
        abscess K51.314
        fistula K51.313
        obstruction K51.312
        rectal bleeding K51.311
        specified NEC K51.318
Rectourethral — *see* condition
Rectovaginal — *see* condition
Rectovesical — *see* condition
Rectum, rectal — *see* condition
Recurrent — *see* condition
  pregnancy loss — *see* Loss (of), pregnancy, recurrent
Red bugs B88.0
Red tide — *see also* Table of Drugs and Chemicals T65.82- ☑
Red-cedar lung or pneumonitis J67.8
Reduced
  mobility Z74.09
  ventilatory or vital capacity R94.2
Redundant, redundancy
  anus (congenital) Q43.8
  clitoris N90.89
  colon (congenital) Q43.8
  foreskin (congenital) N47.8
  intestine (congenital) Q43.8
  labia N90.69
  organ or site, congenital NEC — *see* Accessory
  panniculus (abdominal) E65
  prepuce (congenital) N47.8
  pylorus K31.89
  rectum (congenital) Q43.8
  scrotum N50.89
  sigmoid (congenital) Q43.8
  skin L98.7
    and subcutaneous tissue L98.7
    of face L57.4
      eyelids — *see* Blepharochalasis
  stomach K31.89
Reduplication — *see* Duplication
Reflex R29.2
  hyperactive gag J39.2
  pupillary, abnormal — *see* Anomaly, pupil, function
  vasoconstriction I73.9
  vasovagal R55
Reflux K21.9
  acid K21.9
  esophageal K21.9
    with esophagitis K21.0
    newborn P78.83
  gastroesophageal K21.9
    with esophagitis K21.0
  mitral — *see* Insufficiency, mitral
  ureteral — *see* Reflux, vesicoureteral
  vesicoureteral (with scarring) N13.70
    with
      nephropathy N13.729
        with hydroureter N13.739
          bilateral N13.732
          unilateral N13.731
        bilateral N13.722
        unilateral N13.721
        without hydroureter N13.729

Reflux — *continued*
  vesicoureteral — *continued*
    with — *continued*
      nephropathy — *continued*
        without hydroureter — *continued*
          bilateral N13.722
          unilateral N13.721
      pyelonephritis (chronic) N11.0
    congenital Q62.7
    without nephropathy N13.71
Reforming, artificial openings — *see* Attention to, artificial, opening
Refractive error — *see* Disorder, refraction
Refsum's disease or syndrome G60.1
Refusal of
  food, psychogenic F50.89
  treatment (because of) Z53.20
    left against medical advice (AMA) Z53.21
    patient's decision NEC Z53.29
    reasons of belief or group pressure Z53.1
Regional — *see* condition
Regurgitation R11.10
  aortic (valve) — *see* Insufficiency, aortic
  food — *see also* Vomiting
    with reswallowing — *see* Rumination
    newborn P92.1
  gastric contents — *see* Vomiting
  heart — *see* Endocarditis
  mitral (valve) — *see* Insufficiency, mitral
    congenital Q23.3
  myocardial — *see* Endocarditis
  pulmonary (valve) (heart) I37.1
    congenital Q22.2
    syphilitic A52.03
  tricuspid — *see* Insufficiency, tricuspid
  valve, valvular — *see* Endocarditis
    congenital Q24.8
  vesicoureteral — *see* Reflux, vesicoureteral
Reichmann's disease or syndrome K31.89
Reichmann's disease or syndrome K31.89
Reifenstein syndrome E34.52
Reinsertion
  implantable subdermal contraceptive Z30.46
  intrauterine contraceptive device Z30.433
Reiter's disease, syndrome, or urethritis M02.30
  ankle M02.37- ☑
  elbow M02.32- ☑
  foot joint M02.37- ☑
  hand joint M02.34- ☑
  hip M02.35- ☑
  knee M02.36- ☑
  multiple site M02.39
  shoulder M02.31- ☑
  vertebra M02.38
  wrist M02.33- ☑
Rejection
  food, psychogenic F50.89
  transplant T86.91
    bone T86.830
      marrow T86.01
    cornea T86.840
    heart T86.21
      with lung(s) T86.31
    intestine T86.850
    kidney T86.11
    liver T86.41
    lung(s) T86.810
      with heart T86.31
    organ (immune or nonimmune cause) T86.91
    pancreas T86.890
    skin (allograft) (autograft) T86.820
    specified NEC T86.890
    stem cell (peripheral blood) (umbilical cord) T86.5
Relapsing fever A68.9
  Carter's (Asiatic) A68.1
  Dutton's (West African) A68.1
  Koch's A68.9
  louse-borne (epidemic) A68.0
  Novy's (American) A68.1
  Obermeyers's (European) A68.0
  Spirillum A68.9
  tick-borne (endemic) A68.1
Relationship
  occlusal
    open anterior M26.220
    open posterior M26.221
Relaxation
  anus (sphincter) K62.89
    psychogenic F45.8

Relaxation — *continued*
  arch (foot) — *see also* Deformity, limb, flat foot
  back ligaments — *see* Instability, joint, spine
  bladder (sphincter) N31.2
  cardioesophageal K21.9
  cervix — *see* Incompetency, cervix
  diaphragm J98.6
  joint (capsule) (ligament) (paralytic) — *see* Flail, joint
    congenital NEC Q74.8
  lumbosacral (joint) — *see* subcategory M53.2 ☑
  pelvic floor N81.89
  perineum N81.89
  posture R29.3
  rectum (sphincter) K62.89
  sacroiliac (joint) — *see* subcategory M53.2 ☑
  scrotum N50.89
  urethra (sphincter) N36.44
  vesical N31.2
Release from prison, anxiety concerning Z65.2
Remains
  canal of Cloquet Q14.0
  capsule (opaque) Q14.8
Remittent fever (malarial) B54
Remnant
  canal of Cloquet Q14.0
  capsule (opaque) Q14.8
  cervix, cervical stump (acquired) (postoperative) N88.8
  cystic duct, postcholecystectomy K91.5
  fingernail L60.8
    congenital Q84.6
  meniscus, knee — *see* Derangement, knee, meniscus,
    specified NEC
  thyroglossal duct Q89.2
  tonsil J35.8
    infected (chronic) J35.01
  urachus Q64.4
Removal (from) (of)
  artificial
    arm Z44.00- ☑
      complete Z44.01- ☑
      partial Z44.02- ☑
    eye Z44.2- ☑
    leg Z44.10- ☑
      complete Z44.11- ☑
      partial Z44.12- ☑
  breast implant Z45.81 ☑
  cardiac pulse generator (battery) (end-of-life) Z45.010
  catheter (urinary) (indwelling) Z46.6
    from artificial opening — *see* Attention to, artificial,
      opening
    non-vascular Z46.82
    vascular NEC Z45.2
  device Z46.9
    contraceptive Z30.432
      implantable subdermal Z30.46
    implanted NEC Z45.89
    specified NEC Z46.89
  drains Z48.03
  dressing (nonsurgical) Z48.00
    surgical Z48.01
  external
    fixation device — *code to* fracture with seventh
      character D
    prosthesis, prosthetic device Z44.9
      breast Z44.3- ☑
      specified NEC Z44.8
  home in childhood (to foster home or institution)
    Z62.29
  ileostomy Z43.2
  insulin pump Z46.81
  myringotomy device (stent) (tube) Z45.82
  nervous system device NEC Z46.2
    brain neuropacemaker Z46.2
    visual substitution device Z46.2
      implanted Z45.31
  non-vascular catheter Z46.82
  organ, prophylactic (for neoplasia management) —
    see Prophylactic, organ removal
  orthodontic device Z46.4
  staples Z48.02
  stent
    ureteral Z46.6
  suture Z48.02
  urinary device Z46.6
  vascular access device or catheter Z45.2
Ren
  arcuatus Q63.1
  mobile, mobilis N28.89

Ren — *continued*
  mobile, mobilis — *continued*
    congenital Q63.8
  unguliformis Q63.1
Renal — *see* condition
Rendu-Osler-Weber disease or syndrome I78.0
Reninoma D41.0- ☑
Renon-Delille syndrome E23.3
Reovirus, as cause of disease classified elsewhere
  B97.5
Repeated falls NEC R29.6
Replaced chromosome by dicentric ring Q93.2
Replacement by artificial or mechanical device or
  prosthesis of
  bladder Z96.0
  blood vessel NEC Z95.828
  bone NEC Z96.7
  cochlea Z96.21
  coronary artery Z95.5
  eustachian tube Z96.29
  eye globe Z97.0
  heart Z95.812
    valve Z95.2
      prosthetic Z95.2
      specified NEC Z95.4
      xenogenic Z95.3
  intestine Z96.89
  joint Z96.60
    hip — *see* Presence, hip joint implant
    knee — *see* Presence, knee joint implant
    specified site NEC Z96.698
  larynx Z96.3
  lens Z96.1
  limb(s) — *see* Presence, artificial, limb
  mandible NEC (for tooth root implant(s)) Z96.5
  organ NEC Z96.89
  peripheral vessel NEC Z95.828
  stapes Z96.29
  teeth Z97.2
  tendon Z96.7
  tissue NEC Z96.89
  tooth root(s) Z96.5
  vessel NEC Z95.828
    coronary (artery) Z95.5
Request for expert evidence Z04.89
Reserve, decreased or low
  cardiac — *see* Disease, heart
  kidney N28.89
Residual — *see also* condition
  ovary syndrome N99.83
  state, schizophrenic F20.5
  urine R39.198
Resistance, resistant (to)
  activated protein C D68.51
  complicating pregnancy O26.89 ☑
  insulin E88.81
  organism(s)
    to
      drug Z16.30
        aminoglycosides Z16.29
        amoxicillin Z16.11
        ampicillin Z16.11
        antibiotic(s) Z16.20
          multiple Z16.24
          specified NEC Z16.29
        antifungal Z16.32
        antimicrobial (single) Z16.30
          multiple Z16.35
          specified NEC Z16.39
        antimycobacterial (single) Z16.341
          multiple Z16.342
        antiparasitic Z16.31
        antiviral Z16.33
        beta lactam antibiotics Z16.10
          specified NEC Z16.19
        cephalosporins Z16.19
        extended beta lactamase (ESBL) Z16.12
        fluoroquinolones Z16.23
        macrolides Z16.29
        methicillin — *see* MRSA
        multiple drugs (MDRO)
          antibiotics Z16.24
          antimicrobial Z16.35
          antimycobacterials Z16.342
        penicillins Z16.11
        quinine (and related compounds) Z16.31
        quinolones Z16.23
        sulfonamides Z16.29

Resistance, resistant — *continued*
  organism(s) — *continued*
    to — *continued*
      drug — *continued*
        tetracyclines Z16.29
        tuberculostatics (single) Z16.341
          multiple Z16.342
        vancomycin Z16.21
          related antibiotics Z16.22
  thyroid hormone E07.89
Resorption
  dental (roots) K03.3
    alveoli M26.79
  teeth (external) (internal) (pathological) (roots) K03.3
Respiration
  Cheyne-Stokes R06.3
  decreased due to shock, following injury T79.4 ☑
  disorder of, psychogenic F45.8
  insufficient, or poor R06.89
    newborn P28.5
  painful R07.1
  sighing, psychogenic F45.8
Respiratory — *see also* condition
  distress syndrome (newborn) (type I) P22.0
    type II P22.1
  syncytial virus, as cause of disease classified elsewhere
    — *see also* Virus, respiratory syncytial (RSV) B97.4
Respite care Z75.5
Response (drug)
  photoallergic L56.1
  phototoxic L56.0
Restenosis
  stent
    vascular
      end stent
        adjacent to stent — *see* Arteriosclerosis
        within the stent
          coronary T82.855 ☑
          peripheral T82.856 ☑
      in stent
        coronary vessel T82.855 ☑
        peripheral vessel T82.856 ☑
Restless legs (syndrome) G25.81
Restlessness R45.1
Restoration (of)
  dental
    aesthetically inadequate or displeasing K08.56
    defective K08.50
      specified NEC K08.59
    failure of marginal integrity K08.51
    failure of periodontal anatomical intergrity K08.54
  organ continuity from previous sterilization (tuboplas-
    ty) (vasoplasty) Z31.0
    aftercare Z31.42
  tooth (existing)
    contours biologically incompatible with oral health
      K08.54
    open margins K08.51
    overhanging K08.52
    poor aesthetic K08.56
    poor gingival margins K08.51
    unsatisfactory, of tooth K08.50
      specified NEC K08.59
Restorative material (dental)
  allergy to K08.55
  fractured K08.539
    with loss of material K08.531
    without loss of material K08.530
  unrepairable overhanging of K08.52
Restriction of housing space Z59.1
Rests, ovarian, in fallopian tube Q50.6
Restzustand (schizophrenic) F20.5
Retained — *see also* Retention
  cholelithiasis following cholecystectomy K91.86
  foreign body fragments (type of) Z18.9
    acrylics Z18.2
    animal quill(s) or spines Z18.31
    cement Z18.83
    concrete Z18.83
    crystalline Z18.83
    depleted isotope Z18.09
    depleted uranium Z18.01
    diethylhexyl phthalates Z18.2
    glass Z18.81
    isocyanate Z18.2
    magnetic metal Z18.11
    metal Z18.10
    nonmagnectic metal Z18.12

☑ **Additional Character Required** — **Refer to the Tabular List for Character Selection**   🚩 **Subterms under main terms may continue to next column or page**

Retained — *continued*
  foreign body fragments — *continued*
    nontherapeutic radioactive Z18.09
    organic NEC Z18.39
    plastic Z18.2
    quill(s) (animal) Z18.31
    radioactive (nontherapeutic) NEC Z18.09
    specified NEC Z18.89
    spine(s) (animal) Z18.31
    stone Z18.83
    tooth (teeth) Z18.32
    wood Z18.33
  fragments (type of) Z18.9
    acrylics Z18.2
    animal quill(s) or spines Z18.31
    cement Z18.83
    concrete Z18.83
    crystalline Z18.83
    depleted isotope Z18.09
    depleted uranium Z18.01
    diethylhexyl phthalates Z18.2
    glass Z18.81
    isocyanate Z18.2
    magnetic metal Z18.11
    metal Z18.10
    nonmagnectic metal Z18.12
    nontherapeutic radioactive Z18.09
    organic NEC Z18.39
    plastic Z18.2
    quill(s) (animal) Z18.31
    radioactive (nontherapeutic) NEC Z18.09
    specified NEC Z18.89
    spine(s) (animal) Z18.31
    stone Z18.83
    tooth (teeth) Z18.32
    wood Z18.33
  gallstones, following cholecystectomy K91.86
Retardation
  development, developmental, specific — *see* Disorder, developmental
  endochondral bone growth — *see* Disorder, bone, development or growth
  growth R62.50
    due to malnutrition E45
  mental — *see* Disability, intellectual
  motor function, specific F82
  physical (child) R62.52
    due to malnutrition E45
  reading (specific) F81.0
  spelling (specific) (without reading disorder) F81.81
Retching — *see* Vomiting
Retention — *see also* Retained
  bladder — *see* Retention, urine
  carbon dioxide E87.2
  cholelithiasis following cholecystectomy K91.86
  cyst — *see* Cyst
  dead
    fetus (at or near term) (mother) O36.4 ☑
      early fetal death O02.1
    ovum O02.0
  decidua (fragments) (following delivery) (with hemorrhage) O72.2
    without hemorrhage O73.1
  deciduous tooth K00.6
  dental root K08.3
  fecal — *see* Constipation
  fetus
    dead O36.4 ☑
      early O02.1
  fluid R60.9
  foreign body — *see also* Foreign body, retained
    current trauma — *code as* Foreign body, by site or type
  gallstones, following cholecystectomy K91.86
  gastric K31.89
  intrauterine contraceptive device, in pregnancy — *see* Pregnancy, complicated by, retention, intrauterine device
  membranes (complicating delivery) (with hemorrhage) O72.2
    with abortion — *see* Abortion, by type
    without hemorrhage O73.1
  meniscus — *see* Derangement, meniscus
  menses N94.89
  milk (puerperal, postpartum) O92.79
  nitrogen, extrarenal R39.2
  ovary syndrome N99.83
  placenta (total) (with hemorrhage) O72.0

Retention — *continued*
  placenta — *continued*
    without hemorrhage O73.0
    portions or fragments (with hemorrhage) O72.2
      without hemorrhage O73.1
  products of conception
    early pregnancy (dead fetus) O02.1
    following
      delivery (with hemorrhage) O72.2
        without hemorrhage O73.1
  secundines (following delivery) (with hemorrhage) O72.0
    without hemorrhage O73.0
    complicating puerperium (delayed hemorrhage) O72.2
    partial O72.2
      without hemorrhage O73.1
  smegma, clitoris N90.89
  urine R33.9
    due to hyperplasia (hypertrophy) of prostate — *see* Hyperplasia, prostate
    drug-induced R33.0
    organic R33.8
      drug-induced R33.0
    psychogenic F45.8
    specified NEC R33.8
  water (in tissues) — *see* Edema
Reticulation, dust — *see* Pneumoconiosis
Reticulocytosis R70.1
Reticuloendotheliosis
  acute infantile C96.0
  leukemic C91.4- ☑
  nonlipid C96.0
Reticulohistiocytoma (giant-cell) D76.3
Reticuloid, actinic L57.1
Reticulosis (skin)
  acute of infancy C96.0
  hemophagocytic, familial D76.1
  histiocytic medullary C96.A (*following* C96.6)
  lipomelanotic I89.8
  malignant (midline) C86.0
  polymorphic C83.8- ☑
  Sézary — *see* Sézary disease
Retina, retinal — *see also* condition
  dark area D49.81
Retinitis — *see also* Inflammation, chorioretinal
  albuminurica N18.9 *[H32]*
  diabetic — *see* Diabetes, retinitis
  disciformis — *see* Degeneration, macula
  focal — *see* Inflammation, chorioretinal, focal
  gravidarum — *see* Pregnancy, complicated by, specified pregnancy-related condition NEC
  juxtapapillaris — *see* Inflammation, chorioretinal, focal, juxtapapillary
  luetic — *see* Retinitis, syphilitic
  pigmentosa H35.52
  proliferans — *see* Disorder, globe, degenerative, specified type NEC
  proliferating — *see* Disorder, globe, degenerative, specified type NEC
  renal N18.9 *[H32]*
  syphilitic (early) (secondary) A51.43
    central, recurrent A52.71
    congenital (early) A50.01 *[H32]*
    late A52.71
  tuberculous A18.53
Retinoblastoma C69.2- ☑
  differentiated C69.2- ☑
  undifferentiated C69.2- ☑
Retinochoroiditis — *see also* Inflammation, chorioretinal
  disseminated — *see* Inflammation, chorioretinal, disseminated
    syphilitic A52.71
  focal — *see* Inflammation, chorioretinal
  juxtapapillaris — *see* Inflammation, chorioretinal, focal, juxtapapillary
Retinopathy (background) H35.00
  arteriosclerotic I70.8 *[H35.0-]* ☑
  atherosclerotic I70.8 *[H35.0-]* ☑
  central serous — *see* Chorioretinopathy, central serous
  Coats H35.02- ☑
  diabetic — *see* Diabetes, retinopathy
  exudative H35.02- ☑
  hypertensive H35.03- ☑
  in (due to)
    diabetes — *see* Diabetes, retinopathy
    sickle-cell disorders D57.- ☑ *[H36]*

Retinopathy — *continued*
  of prematurity H35.10- ☑
    stage 0 H35.11- ☑
    stage 1 H35.12- ☑
    stage 2 H35.13- ☑
    stage 3 H35.14- ☑
    stage 4 H35.15- ☑
    stage 5 H35.16- ☑
  pigmentary, congenital — *see* Dystrophy, retina
  proliferative NEC H35.2- ☑
    diabetic — *see* Diabetes, retinopathy, proliferative
    sickle-cell D57.- ☑ *[H36]*
  solar H31.02- ☑
Retinoschisis H33.10- ☑
  congenital Q14.1
  specified type NEC H33.19- ☑
Retortamoniasis A07.8
Retractile testis Q55.22
Retraction
  cervix — *see* Retroversion, uterus
  drum (membrane) — *see* Disorder, tympanic membrane, specified NEC
  finger — *see* Deformity, finger
  lid H02.539
    left H02.536
      lower H02.535
      upper H02.534
    right H02.533
      lower H02.532
      upper H02.531
  lung J98.4
  mediastinum J98.59
  nipple N64.53
    associated with
      lactation O92.03
      pregnancy O92.01- ☑
      puerperium O92.02
    congenital Q83.8
  palmar fascia M72.0
  pleura — *see* Pleurisy
  ring, uterus (Bandl's) (pathological) O62.4
  sternum (congenital) Q76.7
    acquired M95.4
  uterus — *see* Retroversion, uterus
  valve (heart) — *see* Endocarditis
Retrobulbar — *see* condition
Retrocecal — *see* condition
Retrocession — *see* Retroversion
Retrodisplacement — *see* Retroversion
Retroflection, retroflexion — *see* Retroversion
Retrognathia, retrognathism (mandibular) (maxillary) M26.19
Retrograde menstruation N92.5
Retroperineal — *see* condition
Retroperitoneal — *see* condition
Retroperitonitis K68.9
Retropharyngeal — *see* condition
Retroplacental — *see* condition
Retroposition — *see* Retroversion
Retroprosthetic membrane T85.398 ☑
Retrosternal thyroid (congenital) Q89.2
Retroversion, retroverted
  cervix — *see* Retroversion, uterus
  female NEC — *see* Retroversion, uterus
  iris H21.89
  testis (congenital) Q55.29
  uterus (acquired) (acute) (any degree) (asymptomatic) (cervix) (postinfectional) (postpartal, old) N85.4
    congenital Q51.818
    in pregnancy O34.53- ☑
Retrovirus, as cause of disease classified elsewhere B97.30
  human
    immunodeficiency, type 2 (HIV 2) B97.35
    T-cell lymphotropic
      type I (HTLV-I) B97.33
      type II (HTLV-II) B97.34
  lentivirus B97.31
  oncovirus B97.32
  specified NEC B97.39
Retrusion, premaxilla (developmental) M26.09
Rett's disease or syndrome F84.2
Reverse peristalsis R19.2
Reye's syndrome G93.7
Rh (factor)
  hemolytic disease (newborn) P55.0

Rh — continued
  incompatibility, immunization or sensitization
      affecting management of pregnancy NEC O36.09- ☑
        anti-D antibody O36.01- ☑
      newborn P55.0
      transfusion reaction — see Complication(s), transfusion, incompatibility reaction, Rh (factor)
    negative mother affecting newborn P55.0
    titer elevated — see Complication(s), transfusion, incompatibility reaction, Rh (factor)
    transfusion reaction — see Complication(s), transfusion, incompatibility reaction, Rh (factor)
Rhabdomyolysis (idiopathic) NEC M62.82
  traumatic T79.6 ☑
Rhabdomyoma — see also Neoplasm, connective tissue, benign
  adult — see Neoplasm, connective tissue, benign
  fetal — see Neoplasm, connective tissue, benign
  glycogenic — see Neoplasm, connective tissue, benign
Rhabdomyosarcoma (any type) — see Neoplasm, connective tissue, malignant
Rhabdosarcoma — see Rhabdomyosarcoma
Rhesus (factor) **incompatibility** — see Rh, incompatibility
Rheumatic (acute) (subacute)
  adherent pericardium I09.2
  chronic I09.89
  coronary arteritis I01.8
  degeneration, myocardium I09.0
  fever (acute) — see Fever, rheumatic
  heart — see Disease, heart, rheumatic
  myocardial degeneration — see Degeneration, myocardium
  myocarditis (chronic) (inactive) (with chorea) I09.0
    active or acute I01.2
    with chorea (acute) (rheumatic) (Sydenham's) I02.0
  pancarditis, acute I01.8
    with chorea (acute (rheumatic) Sydenham's) I02.0
  pericarditis (active) (acute) (with effusion) (with pneumonia) I01.0
    with chorea (acute) (rheumatic) (Sydenham's) I02.0
    chronic or inactive I09.2
  pneumonia I00 [J17]
  torticollis M43.6
  typhoid fever A01.09
Rheumatism (articular) (neuralgic) (nonarticular) M79.0
  gout — see Arthritis, rheumatoid
  intercostal, meaning Tietze's disease M94.0
  palindromic (any site) M12.30
    ankle M12.37- ☑
    elbow M12.32- ☑
    foot joint M12.37- ☑
    hand joint M12.34- ☑
    hip M12.35- ☑
    knee M12.36- ☑
    multiple site M12.39
    shoulder M12.31- ☑
    specified joint NEC M12.38
    vertebrae M12.38
    wrist M12.33- ☑
  sciatic M54.4- ☑
Rheumatoid — see also condition
  arthritis — see also Arthritis, rheumatoid
    with involvement of organs NEC M05.60
      ankle M05.67- ☑
      elbow M05.62- ☑
      foot joint M05.67- ☑
      hand joint M05.64- ☑
      hip M05.65- ☑
      knee M05.66- ☑
      multiple site M05.69
      shoulder M05.61- ☑
      vertebra — see Spondylitis, ankylosing
      wrist M05.63- ☑
    seronegative — see Arthritis, rheumatoid, seronegative
    seropositive — see Arthritis, rheumatoid, seropositive
  carditis M05.30
    ankle M05.37- ☑
    elbow M05.32- ☑
    foot joint M05.37- ☑
    hand joint M05.34- ☑
    hip M05.35- ☑
    knee M05.36- ☑
    multiple site M05.39
    shoulder M05.31- ☑

Rheumatoid — continued
  carditis — continued
    vertebra — see Spondylitis, ankylosing
    wrist M05.33- ☑
  endocarditis — see Rheumatoid, carditis
  lung (disease) M05.10
    ankle M05.17- ☑
    elbow M05.12- ☑
    foot joint M05.17- ☑
    hand joint M05.14- ☑
    hip M05.15- ☑
    knee M05.16- ☑
    multiple site M05.19
    shoulder M05.11- ☑
    vertebra — see Spondylitis, ankylosing
    wrist M05.13- ☑
  myocarditis — see Rheumatoid, carditis
  myopathy M05.40
    ankle M05.47- ☑
    elbow M05.42- ☑
    foot joint M05.47- ☑
    hand joint M05.44- ☑
    hip M05.45- ☑
    knee M05.46- ☑
    multiple site M05.49
    shoulder M05.41- ☑
    vertebra — see Spondylitis, ankylosing
    wrist M05.43- ☑
  pericarditis — see Rheumatoid, carditis
  polyarthritis — see Arthritis, rheumatoid
  polyneuropathy M05.50
    ankle M05.57- ☑
    elbow M05.52- ☑
    foot joint M05.57- ☑
    hand joint M05.54- ☑
    hip M05.55- ☑
    knee M05.56- ☑
    multiple site M05.59
    shoulder M05.51- ☑
    vertebra — see Spondylitis, ankylosing
    wrist M05.53- ☑
  vasculitis M05.20
    ankle M05.27- ☑
    elbow M05.22- ☑
    foot joint M05.27- ☑
    hand joint M05.24- ☑
    hip M05.25- ☑
    knee M05.26- ☑
    multiple site M05.29
    shoulder M05.21- ☑
    vertebra — see Spondylitis, ankylosing
    wrist M05.23- ☑
Rhinitis (atrophic) (catarrhal) (chronic) (croupous) (fibrinous) (granulomatous) (hyperplastic) (hypertrophic) (membranous) (obstructive) (purulent) (suppurative) (ulcerative) J31.0
  with
    sore throat — see Nasopharyngitis
  acute J00
  allergic J30.9
    with asthma J45.909
      with
        exacerbation (acute) J45.901
        status asthmaticus J45.902
    due to
      food J30.5
      pollen J30.1
    nonseasonal J30.89
    perennial J30.89
    seasonal NEC J30.2
    specified NEC J30.89
  infective J00
  pneumococcal J00
  syphilitic A52.73
    congenital A50.05 [J99]
  tuberculous A15.8
  vasomotor J30.0
Rhinoantritis (chronic) — see Sinusitis, maxillary
Rhinodacryolith — see Dacryolith
Rhinolith (nasal sinus) J34.89
Rhinomegaly J34.89
Rhinopharyngitis (acute) (subacute) — see also Nasopharyngitis
  chronic J31.1
  destructive ulcerating A66.5
  mutilans A66.5
Rhinophyma L71.1

Rhinorrhea J34.89
  cerebrospinal (fluid) G96.0
  paroxysmal — see Rhinitis, allergic
  spasmodic — see Rhinitis, allergic
Rhinosalpingitis — see Salpingitis, eustachian
Rhinoscleroma A48.8
Rhinosporidiosis B48.1
Rhinovirus infection NEC B34.8
Rhizomelic chondrodysplasia punctata E71.540
Rhythm
  atrioventricular nodal I49.8
  disorder I49.9
    coronary sinus I49.8
    ectopic I49.8
    nodal I49.8
  escape I49.9
  heart, abnormal I49.9
  idioventricular I44.2
  nodal I49.8
  sleep, inversion G47.2- ☑
    nonorganic origin — see Disorder, sleep, circadian rhythm, psychogenic
Rhytidosis facialis L98.8
Rib — see also condition
  cervical Q76.5
Riboflavin deficiency E53.0
Rice bodies — see also Loose, body, joint
  knee M23.4- ☑
Richter syndrome — see Leukemia, chronic lymphocytic, B-cell type
Richter's hernia — see Hernia, abdomen, with obstruction
Ricinism — see Poisoning, food, noxious, plant
Rickets (active) (acute) (adolescent) (chest wall) (congenital) (current) (infantile) (intestinal) E55.0
  adult — see Osteomalacia
  celiac K90.0
  hypophosphatemic with nephrotic-glycosuric dwarfism E72.09
  inactive E64.3
  kidney N25.0
  renal N25.0
  sequelae, any E64.3
  vitamin-D-resistant E83.31 [M90.80]
Rickettsial disease A79.9
  specified type NEC A79.89
Rickettsialpox (Rickettsia akari) A79.1
Rickettsiosis A79.9
  due to
    Ehrlichia sennetsu A79.81
    Rickettsia akari (rickettsialpox) A79.1
  specified type NEC A79.89
  tick-borne A77.9
  vesicular A79.1
Rider's bone — see Ossification, muscle, specified NEC
Ridge, alveolus — see also condition
  flabby K06.8
Ridged ear, congenital Q17.3
Riedel's
  lobe, liver Q44.7
  struma, thyroiditis or disease E06.5
Rieger's anomaly or syndrome Q13.81
Riehl's melanosis L81.4
Rietti-Greppi-Micheli anemia D56.9
Rieux's hernia — see Hernia, abdomen, specified site NEC
Riga (-Fede) **disease** K14.0
Riggs' disease — see Periodontitis
Right aortic arch Q25.47
Right middle lobe syndrome J98.11
Rigid, rigidity — see also condition
  abdominal R19.30
    with severe abdominal pain R10.0
    epigastric R19.36
    generalized R19.37
    left lower quadrant R19.34
    left upper quadrant R19.32
    periumbilic R19.35
    right lower quadrant R19.33
    right upper quadrant R19.31
  articular, multiple, congenital Q68.8
  cervix (uteri) in pregnancy — see Pregnancy, complicated by, abnormal, cervix
  hymen (acquired) (congenital) N89.6
  nuchal R29.1
  pelvic floor in pregnancy — see Pregnancy, complicated by, abnormal, pelvic organs or tissues NEC

Rigid, rigidity — *continued*
  perineum or vulva in pregnancy — *see* Pregnancy, complicated by, abnormal, vulva
  spine — *see* Dorsopathy, specified NEC
  vagina in pregnancy — *see* Pregnancy, complicated by, abnormal, vagina
Rigors R68.89
  with fever R50.9
Riley-Day syndrome G90.1
RIND (reversible ischemic neurologic deficit) I63.9
Ring(s)
  aorta (vascular) Q25.45
  Bandl's O62.4
  contraction, complicating delivery O62.4
  esophageal, lower (muscular) K22.2
  Fleischer's (cornea) H18.04- ☑
  hymenal, tight (acquired) (congenital) N89.6
  Kayser-Fleischer (cornea) H18.04- ☑
  retraction, uterus, pathological O62.4
  Schatzki's (esophagus) (lower) K22.2
    congenital Q39.3
  Soemmerring's — *see* Cataract, secondary
  vascular (congenital) Q25.8
    aorta Q25.45
Ringed hair (congenital) Q84.1
Ringworm B35.9
  beard B35.0
  black dot B35.0
  body B35.4
  Burmese B35.5
  corporeal B35.4
  foot B35.3
  groin B35.6
  hand B35.2
  honeycomb B35.0
  nails B35.1
  perianal (area) B35.6
  scalp B35.0
  specified NEC B35.8
  Tokelau B35.5
Rise, venous pressure I87.8
Rising, PSA following treatment for malignant neoplasm of prostate R97.21
Risk
  for
    dental caries Z91.849
      high Z91.843
      low Z91.841
      moderate Z91.842
  suicidal
    meaning personal history of attempted suicide Z91.5
    meaning suicidal ideation — *see* Ideation, suicidal
Ritter's disease L00
Rivalry, sibling Z62.891
Rivalta's disease A42.2
River blindness B73.01
Robert's pelvis Q74.2
  with disproportion (fetopelvic) O33.0
    causing obstructed labor O65.0
Robin (-Pierre) **syndrome** Q87.0
Robinow-Silvermann-Smith syndrome Q87.19
Robinson's (hidrotic) **ectodermal dysplasia or syndrome** Q82.4
Robles' disease B73.01
Rocky Mountain (spotted) **fever** A77.0
Roetheln — *see* Rubella
Roger's disease Q21.0
Rokitansky-Aschoff sinuses (gallbladder) K82.8
Rolando's fracture (displaced) S62.22- ☑
  nondisplaced S62.22- ☑
Romano-Ward (prolonged QT interval) **syndrome** I45.81
Romberg's disease or syndrome G51.8
Roof, mouth — *see* condition
Rosacea L71.9
  acne L71.9
  keratitis L71.8
  specified NEC L71.8
Rosary, rachitic E55.0
Rose
  cold J30.1
  fever J30.1
  rash R21
    epidemic B06.9
Rosenbach's erysipeloid A26.0
Rosenthal's disease or syndrome D68.1
Roseola B09
  infantum B08.20

Roseola — *continued*
  infantum — *continued*
    due to human herpesvirus 6 B08.21
    due to human herpesvirus 7 B08.22
Ross River disease or fever B33.1
Rossbach's disease K31.89
  psychogenic F45.8
Rostan's asthma (cardiac) — *see* Failure, ventricular, left
Rotation
  anomalous, incomplete or insufficient, intestine Q43.3
  cecum (congenital) Q43.3
  colon (congenital) Q43.3
  spine, incomplete or insufficient — *see* Dorsopathy, deforming, specified NEC
  tooth, teeth, fully erupted M26.35
  vertebra, incomplete or insufficient — *see* Dorsopathy, deforming, specified NEC
Rotes Quérol disease or syndrome — *see* Hyperostosis, ankylosing
Roth (-Bernhardt) **disease or syndrome** — *see* Meralgia paraesthetica
Rothmund (-Thomson) **syndrome** Q82.8
Rotor's disease or syndrome E80.6
Round
  back (with wedging of vertebrae) — *see* Kyphosis
    sequelae (late effect) of rickets E64.3
  worms (large) (infestation) NEC B82.0
    Ascariasis — *see also* Ascariasis B77.9
Roussy-Lévy syndrome G60.0
Rubella (German measles) B06.9
  complication NEC B06.09
    neurological B06.00
  congenital P35.0
  contact Z20.4
  exposure to Z20.4
  maternal
    care for (suspected) damage to fetus O35.3 ☑
    manifest rubella in infant P35.0
    suspected damage to fetus affecting management of pregnancy O35.3 ☑
  specified complications NEC B06.89
Rubeola (meaning measles) — *see* Measles
  meaning rubella — *see* Rubella
Rubeosis, iris — *see* Disorder, iris, vascular
Rubinstein-Taybi syndrome Q87.2
Rudimentary (congenital) — *see also* Agenesis
  arm — *see* Defect, reduction, upper limb
  bone Q79.9
  cervix uteri Q51.828
  eye Q11.2
  lobule of ear Q17.3
  patella Q74.1
  respiratory organs in thoracopagus Q89.4
  tracheal bronchus Q32.4
  uterus Q51.818
    in male Q56.1
  vagina Q52.0
Ruled out condition — *see* Observation, suspected
Rumination R11.10
  with nausea R11.2
  disorder of infancy F98.21
  neurotic F42.8
  newborn P92.1
  obsessional F42.8
  psychogenic F42.8
Runeberg's disease D51.0
Runny nose R09.89
Rupia (syphilitic) A51.39
  congenital A50.06
  tertiary A52.79
Rupture, ruptured
  abscess (spontaneous) — *code by* site under Abscess
  aneurysm — *see* Aneurysm
  anus (sphincter) — *see* Laceration, anus
  aorta, aortic I71.8
    abdominal I71.3
    arch I71.1
    ascending I71.1
    descending I71.8
      abdominal I71.3
      thoracic I71.1
    syphilitic A52.01
    thoracoabdominal I71.5
    thorax, thoracic I71.1
    transverse I71.1
    traumatic — *see* Injury, aorta, laceration, major
    valve or cusp — *see also* Endocarditis, aortic I35.8

Rupture, ruptured — *continued*
  appendix (with peritonitis) — *see also* Appendicitis K35.32
    with localized peritonitis — *see also* Appendicitis K35.32
  arteriovenous fistula, brain — *see* Fistula, arteriovenous, brain, ruptured
  artery I77.2
    brain — *see* Hemorrhage, intracranial, intracerebral
    coronary — *see* Infarct, myocardium
    heart — *see* Infarct, myocardium
    pulmonary I28.8
    traumatic (complication) — *see* Injury, blood vessel
  bile duct (common) (hepatic) K83.2
    cystic K82.2
  bladder (sphincter) (nontraumatic) (spontaneous) N32.89
    following ectopic or molar pregnancy O08.6
    obstetrical trauma O71.5
    traumatic S37.29 ☑
  blood vessel — *see also* Hemorrhage
    brain — *see* Hemorrhage, intracranial, intracerebral
    heart — *see* Infarct, myocardium
    traumatic (complication) — *see* Injury, blood vessel, laceration, major, by site
  bone — *see* Fracture
  bowel (nontraumatic) K63.1
  brain
    aneurysm (congenital) — *see also* Hemorrhage, intracranial, subarachnoid
      syphilitic A52.05
    hemorrhagic — *see* Hemorrhage, intracranial, intracerebral
  capillaries I78.8
  cardiac (auricle) (ventricle) (wall) I23.3
    with hemopericardium I23.0
    infectional I40.9
    traumatic — *see* Injury, heart
  cartilage (articular) (current) — *see also* Sprain
    knee S83.3- ☑
    semilunar — *see* Tear, meniscus
  cecum (with peritonitis) K65.0
    with peritoneal abscess K35.33
    traumatic S36.598 ☑
  celiac artery, traumatic — *see* Injury, blood vessel, celiac artery, laceration, major
  cerebral aneurysm (congenital) (see Hemorrhage, intracranial, subarachnoid)
  cervix (uteri)
    with ectopic or molar pregnancy O08.6
    following ectopic or molar pregnancy O08.6
    obstetrical trauma O71.3
    traumatic S37.69 ☑
  chordae tendineae NEC I51.1
    concurrent with acute myocardial infarction — *see* Infarct, myocardium
    following acute myocardial infarction (current complication) I23.4
  choroid (direct) (indirect) (traumatic) H31.32- ☑
  circle of Willis I60.6
  colon (nontraumatic) K63.1
    traumatic — *see* Injury, intestine, large
  cornea (traumatic) — *see* Injury, eye, laceration
  coronary (artery) (thrombotic) — *see* Infarct, myocardium
  corpus luteum (infected) (ovary) N83.1- ☑
  cyst — *see* Cyst
  cystic duct K82.2
  Descemet's membrane — *see* Change, corneal membrane, Descemet's, rupture
    traumatic — *see* Injury, eye, laceration
  diaphragm, traumatic — *see* Injury, intrathoracic, diaphragm
  disc — *see* Rupture, intervertebral disc
  diverticulum (intestine) K57.80
    with bleeding K57.81
    bladder N32.3
    large intestine K57.20
      with
        bleeding K57.21
        small intestine K57.40
          with bleeding K57.41
    small intestine K57.00
      with
        bleeding K57.01
        large intestine K57.40
          with bleeding K57.41
  duodenal stump K31.89

Rupture, ruptured — *continued*
- ear drum (nontraumatic) — *see also* Perforation, tympanum
  - traumatic S09.2- ☑
    - due to blast injury — *see* Injury, blast, ear
- esophagus K22.3
- eye (without prolapse or loss of intraocular tissue) — *see* Injury, eye, laceration
- fallopian tube NEC (nonobstetric) (nontraumatic) N83.8
  - due to pregnancy O00.10- ☑
    - with intrauterine pregnancy O00.11- ☑
- fontanel P13.1
- gallbladder K82.2
  - traumatic S36.128 ☑
- gastric — *see also* Rupture, stomach
  - vessel K92.2
- globe (eye) (traumatic) — *see* Injury, eye, laceration
- graafian follicle (hematoma) N83.0- ☑
- heart — *see* Rupture, cardiac
- hymen (nontraumatic) (nonintentional) N89.8
- internal organ, traumatic — *see* Injury, by site
- intervertebral disc — *see* Displacement, intervertebral disc
  - traumatic — *see* Rupture, traumatic, intervertebral disc
- intestine NEC (nontraumatic) K63.1
  - traumatic — *see* Injury, intestine
- iris — *see also* Abnormality, pupillary
  - traumatic — *see* Injury, eye, laceration
- joint capsule, traumatic — *see* Sprain
- kidney (traumatic) S37.06- ☑
  - birth injury P15.8
  - nontraumatic N28.89
- lacrimal duct (traumatic) — *see* Injury, eye, specified site NEC
- lens (cataract) (traumatic) — *see* Cataract, traumatic
- ligament, traumatic — *see* Rupture, traumatic, ligament, by site
- liver S36.116 ☑
  - birth injury P15.0
- lymphatic vessel I89.8
- marginal sinus (placental) (with hemorrhage) — *see* Hemorrhage, antepartum, specified cause NEC
- membrana tympani (nontraumatic) — *see* Perforation, tympanum
- membranes (spontaneous)
  - artificial
    - delayed delivery following O75.5
  - delayed delivery following — *see* Pregnancy, complicated by, premature rupture of membranes
- meningeal artery I60.8
- meniscus (knee) — *see also* Tear, meniscus
  - old — *see* Derangement, meniscus
  - site other than knee — *code as* Sprain
- mesenteric artery, traumatic — *see* Injury, mesenteric, artery, laceration, major
- mesentery (nontraumatic) K66.8
  - traumatic — *see* Injury, intra-abdominal, specified, site NEC
- mitral (valve) I34.8
- muscle (traumatic) — *see also* Strain
  - diastasis — *see* Diastasis, muscle
  - nontraumatic M62.10
    - ankle M62.17- ☑
    - foot M62.17- ☑
    - forearm M62.13- ☑
    - hand M62.14- ☑
    - lower leg M62.16- ☑
    - pelvic region M62.15- ☑
    - shoulder region M62.11- ☑
    - specified site NEC M62.18
    - thigh M62.15- ☑
    - upper arm M62.12- ☑
  - traumatic — *see* Strain, by site
- musculotendinous junction NEC, nontraumatic — *see* Rupture, tendon, spontaneous
- mycotic aneurysm causing cerebral hemorrhage — *see* Hemorrhage, intracranial, subarachnoid
- myocardium, myocardial — *see* Rupture, cardiac
  - traumatic — *see* Injury, heart
- nontraumatic, meaning hernia — *see* Hernia
- obstructed — *see* Hernia, by site, obstructed
- operation wound — *see* Disruption, wound, operation
- ovary, ovarian N83.8
  - corpus luteum cyst N83.1- ☑
  - follicle (graafian) N83.0- ☑
- oviduct (nonobstetric) (nontraumatic) N83.8

Rupture, ruptured — *continued*
- oviduct — *continued*
  - due to pregnancy O00.10- ☑
    - with intrauterine pregnancy O00.11- ☑
- pancreas (nontraumatic) K86.89
  - traumatic S36.299 ☑
- papillary muscle NEC I51.2
  - following acute myocardial infarction (current complication) I23.5
- pelvic
  - floor, complicating delivery O70.1
  - organ NEC, obstetrical trauma O71.5
- perineum (nonobstetric) (nontraumatic) N90.89
  - complicating delivery — *see* Delivery, complicated, by, laceration, anus (sphincter)
- postoperative wound — *see* Disruption, wound, operation
- prostate (traumatic) S37.828 ☑
- pulmonary
  - artery I28.8
  - valve (heart) I37.8
  - vein I28.8
  - vessel I28.8
- pus tube — *see* Salpingitis
- pyosalpinx — *see* Salpingitis
- rectum (nontraumatic) K63.1
  - traumatic S36.69 ☑
- retina, retinal (traumatic) (without detachment) — *see also* Break, retina
  - with detachment — *see* Detachment, retina, with retinal, break
- rotator cuff (nontraumatic) M75.10- ☑
  - complete M75.12- ☑
  - incomplete M75.11- ☑
- sclera — *see* Injury, eye, laceration
- sigmoid (nontraumatic) K63.1
  - traumatic S36.593 ☑
- spinal cord — *see also* Injury, spinal cord, by region
  - due to injury at birth P11.5
  - newborn (birth injury) P11.5
- spleen (traumatic) S36.09 ☑
  - birth injury P15.1
  - congenital (birth injury) P15.1
  - due to P. vivax malaria B51.0
  - nontraumatic D73.5
  - spontaneous D73.5
- splenic vein R58
  - traumatic — *see* Injury, blood vessel, splenic vein
- stomach (nontraumatic) (spontaneous) K31.89
  - traumatic S36.39 ☑
- supraspinatus (complete) (incomplete) (nontraumatic) — *see* Tear, rotator cuff
- symphysis pubis
  - obstetric O71.6
  - traumatic S33.4 ☑
- synovium (cyst) M66.10
  - ankle M66.17- ☑
  - elbow M66.12- ☑
  - finger M66.14- ☑
  - foot M66.17- ☑
  - forearm M66.13
  - hand M66.14- ☑
  - pelvic region M66.15- ☑
  - shoulder region M66.11- ☑
  - specified site NEC M66.18
  - thigh M66.15- ☑
  - toe M66.17- ☑
  - upper arm M66.12- ☑
  - wrist M66.13- ☑
- tendon (traumatic) — *see* Strain
  - nontraumatic (spontaneous) M66.9
    - ankle M66.87- ☑
    - extensor M66.20
      - ankle M66.27- ☑
      - foot M66.27- ☑
      - forearm M66.23- ☑
      - hand M66.24- ☑
      - lower leg M66.26- ☑
      - multiple sites M66.29
      - pelvic region M66.25- ☑
      - shoulder region M66.21- ☑
      - specified site NEC M66.28
      - thigh M66.25- ☑
      - upper arm M66.22- ☑
    - flexor M66.30
      - ankle M66.37- ☑
      - foot M66.37- ☑

Rupture, ruptured — *continued*
- tendon — *see* Strain — *continued*
  - nontraumatic — *continued*
    - flexor — *continued*
      - forearm M66.33- ☑
      - hand M66.34- ☑
      - lower leg M66.36- ☑
      - multiple sites M66.39
      - pelvic region M66.35- ☑
      - shoulder region M66.31- ☑
      - specified site NEC M66.38
      - thigh M66.35- ☑
      - upper arm M66.32- ☑
    - foot M66.87- ☑
    - forearm M66.83- ☑
    - hand M66.84- ☑
    - lower leg M66.86- ☑
    - multiple sites M66.89
    - pelvic region M66.85- ☑
    - shoulder region M66.81- ☑
    - specified
      - site NEC M66.88
      - tendon M66.80
    - thigh M66.85- ☑
    - upper arm M66.82- ☑
- thoracic duct I89.8
- tonsil J35.8
- traumatic
  - aorta — *see* Injury, aorta, laceration, major
  - diaphragm — *see* Injury, intrathoracic, diaphragm
  - external site — *see* Wound, open, by site
  - eye — *see* Injury, eye, laceration
  - internal organ — *see* Injury, by site
  - intervertebral disc
    - cervical S13.0 ☑
    - lumbar S33.0 ☑
    - thoracic S23.0 ☑
  - kidney S37.06- ☑
  - ligament — *see also* Sprain
    - ankle — *see* Sprain, ankle
    - carpus — *see* Rupture, traumatic, ligament, wrist
    - collateral (hand) — *see* Rupture, traumatic, ligament, finger, collateral
    - finger (metacarpophalangeal) (interphalangeal) S63.40- ☑
      - collateral S63.41- ☑
        - index S63.41- ☑
        - little S63.41- ☑
        - middle S63.41- ☑
        - ring S63.41- ☑
      - index S63.40- ☑
      - little S63.40- ☑
      - middle S63.40- ☑
      - palmar S63.42- ☑
        - index S63.42- ☑
        - little S63.42- ☑
        - middle S63.42- ☑
        - ring S63.42- ☑
      - ring S63.40- ☑
      - specified site NEC S63.499 ☑
        - index S63.49- ☑
        - little S63.49- ☑
        - middle S63.49- ☑
        - ring S63.49- ☑
      - volar plate S63.43- ☑
        - index S63.43- ☑
        - little S63.43- ☑
        - middle S63.43- ☑
        - ring S63.43- ☑
    - foot — *see* Sprain, foot
    - radial collateral S53.2- ☑
    - radiocarpal — *see* Rupture, traumatic, ligament, wrist, radiocarpal
    - ulnar collateral S53.3- ☑
    - ulnocarpal — *see* Rupture, traumatic, ligament, wrist, ulnocarpal
    - wrist S63.30- ☑
      - collateral S63.31- ☑
      - radiocarpal S63.32- ☑
      - specified site NEC S63.39- ☑
      - ulnocarpal (palmar) S63.33- ☑
  - liver S36.116 ☑
  - membrana tympani — *see* Rupture, ear drum, traumatic
  - muscle or tendon — *see* Strain
  - myocardium — *see* Injury, heart

☑ **Additional Character Required** — **Refer to the Tabular List for Character Selection**   ▽ **Subterms under main terms may continue to next column or page**

Rupture, ruptured — continued
  traumatic — continued
    pancreas S36.299 ☑
    rectum S36.69 ☑
    sigmoid S36.593 ☑
    spleen S36.09 ☑
    stomach S36.39 ☑
    symphysis pubis S33.4 ☑
    tympanum, tympanic (membrane) — see Rupture,
      ear drum, traumatic
    ureter S37.19 ☑
    uterus S37.69 ☑
    vagina — see Injury, vagina
    vena cava — see Injury, vena cava, laceration, major
  tricuspid (heart) (valve) I07.8
  tube, tubal (nonobstetric) (nontraumatic) N83.8
    abscess — see Salpingitis
    due to pregnancy O00.10- ☑
      with intrauterine pregnancy O00.11- ☑
  tympanum, tympanic (membrane) (nontraumatic) —
      see also Perforation, tympanic membrane
      H72.9- ☑
    traumatic — see Rupture, ear drum, traumatic
  umbilical cord, complicating delivery O69.89 ☑
  ureter (traumatic) S37.19 ☑
    nontraumatic N28.89
  urethra (nontraumatic) N36.8
    with ectopic or molar pregnancy O08.6
    following ectopic or molar pregnancy O08.6
    obstetrical trauma O71.5
    traumatic S37.39 ☑
  uterosacral ligament (nonobstetric) (nontraumatic)
      N83.8
  uterus (traumatic) S37.69 ☑
    before labor O71.0- ☑
    during or after labor O71.1
    nonpuerperal, nontraumatic N85.8
    pregnant (during labor) O71.1
      before labor O71.0- ☑
  vagina — see Injury, vagina
  valve, valvular (heart) — see Endocarditis
  varicose vein — see Varix
  varix — see Varix
  vena cava R58
    traumatic — see Injury, vena cava, laceration, major
  vesical (urinary) N32.89
  vessel (blood) R58
    pulmonary I28.8
    traumatic — see Injury, blood vessel
  viscus R19.8
  vulva complicating delivery O70.0
Russell-Silver syndrome Q87.19
Russian spring-summer type encephalitis A84.0
Rust's disease (tuberculous cervical spondylitis) A18.01
Ruvalcaba-Myhre-Smith syndrome E71.440
Rytand-Lipsitch syndrome I44.2

S

Saber, sabre shin or tibia (syphilitic) A50.56 [M90.8-] ☑
Sac lacrimal — see condition
Saccharomyces infection B37.9
Saccharopinuria E72.3
Saccular — see condition
Sacculation
  aorta (nonsyphilitic) — see Aneurysm, aorta
  bladder N32.3
  intralaryngeal (congenital) (ventricular) Q31.3
  larynx (congenital) (ventricular) Q31.3
  organ or site, congenital — see Distortion
  pregnant uterus — see Pregnancy, complicated by,
    abnormal, uterus
  ureter N28.89
  urethra N36.1
  vesical N32.3
Sachs' amaurotic familial idiocy or disease E75.02
Sachs-Tay disease E75.02
Sacks-Libman disease M32.11
Sacralgia M53.3
Sacralization Q76.49
Sacrodynia M53.3
Sacroiliac joint — see condition
Sacroiliitis NEC M46.1
Sacrum — see condition
Saddle
  back — see Lordosis

Saddle — continued
  embolus
    abdominal aorta I74.01
    pulmonary artery I26.92
      with acute cor pulmonale I26.02
  injury — code to condition
  nose M95.0
    due to syphilis A50.57
Sadism (sexual) F65.52
Sadness, postpartal O90.6
Sadomasochism F65.50
Saemisch's ulcer (cornea) — see Ulcer, cornea, central
Sagging
  skin and subcutaneous tissue (following bariatric
    surgery weight loss) (following dietary weight
    loss) L98.7
Sahib disease B55.0
Sailors' skin L57.8
Saint
  Anthony's fire — see Erysipelas
  triad — see Hernia, diaphragm
  Vitus' dance — see Chorea, Sydenham's
Salaam
  attack(s) — see Epilepsy, spasms
  tic R25.8
Salicylism
  abuse F55.8
  overdose or wrong substance given — see Table of
    Drugs and Chemicals, by drug, poisoning
Salivary duct or gland — see condition
Salivation, excessive K11.7
Salmonella — see Infection, Salmonella
Salmonellosis A02.0
Salpingitis (catarrhal) (fallopian tube) (nodular) (pseud-
    ofollicular) (purulent) (septic) N70.91
  with oophoritis N70.93
  acute N70.01
    with oophoritis N70.03
  chlamydial A56.11
  chronic N70.11
    with oophoritis N70.13
  complicating abortion — see Abortion, by type, com-
    plicated by, salpingitis
  ear — see Salpingitis, eustachian
  eustachian (tube) H68.00- ☑
    acute H68.01- ☑
    chronic H68.02- ☑
  follicularis N70.11
    with oophoritis N70.13
  gonococcal (acute) (chronic) A54.24
  interstitial, chronic N70.11
    with oophoritis N70.13
  isthmica nodosa N70.11
    with oophoritis N70.13
  specific (gonococcal) (acute) (chronic) A54.24
  tuberculous (acute) (chronic) A18.17
  venereal (gonococcal) (acute) (chronic) A54.24
Salpingocele N83.4- ☑
Salpingo-oophoritis (catarrhal) (purulent) (ruptured)
    (septic) (suppurative) N70.93
  acute N70.03
    with ectopic or molar pregnancy O08.0
    following ectopic or molar pregnancy O08.0
    gonococcal A54.24
  chronic N70.13
  following ectopic or molar pregnancy O08.0
  gonococcal (acute) (chronic) A54.24
  puerperal O86.19
  specific (gonococcal) (acute) (chronic) A54.24
  subacute N70.03
  tuberculous (acute) (chronic) A18.17
  venereal (gonococcal) (acute) (chronic) A54.24
Salpingo-ovaritis — see Salpingo-oophoritis
Salpingoperitonitis — see Salpingo-oophoritis
Salzmann's nodular dystrophy — see Degeneration,
    cornea, nodular
Sampson's cyst or tumor N80.1
San Joaquin (Valley) **fever** B38.0
Sandblaster's asthma, lung or pneumoconiosis J62.8
Sander's disease (paranoia) F22
Sandfly fever A93.1
Sandhoff's disease E75.01
Sanfilippo (Type B) (Type C) (Type D) **syndrome** E76.22
Sanger-Brown ataxia G11.2
Sao Paulo fever or typhus A77.0
Saponification, mesenteric K65.8

Sarcocele (benign)
  syphilitic A52.76
    congenital A50.59
Sarcocystosis A07.8
Sarcoepiplocele — see Hernia
Sarcoepiplomphalocele Q79.2
Sarcoid — see also Sarcoidosis
  arthropathy D86.86
  Boeck's D86.9
  Darier-Roussy D86.3
  iridocyclitis D86.83
  meningitis D86.81
  myocarditis D86.85
  myositis D86.87
  pyelonephritis D86.84
  Spiegler-Fendt L08.89
Sarcoidosis D86.9
  with
    cranial nerve palsies D86.82
    hepatic granuloma D86.89
    polyarthritis D86.86
    tubulo-interstitial nephropathy D86.84
  combined sites NEC D86.89
  lung D86.0
    and lymph nodes D86.2
  lymph nodes D86.1
    and lung D86.2
  meninges D86.81
  skin D86.3
  specified type NEC D86.89
Sarcoma (of) — see also Neoplasm, connective tissue,
    malignant
  alveolar soft part — see Neoplasm, connective tissue,
    malignant
  ameloblastic C41.1
    upper jaw (bone) C41.0
  botryoid — see Neoplasm, connective tissue, malignant
  botryoides — see Neoplasm, connective tissue, malig-
    nant
  cerebellar C71.6
    circumscribed (arachnoidal) C71.6
  circumscribed (arachnoidal) cerebellar C71.6
  clear cell — see also Neoplasm, connective tissue, ma-
    lignant
    kidney C64.- ☑
  dendritic cells (accessory cells) C96.4
  embryonal — see Neoplasm, connective tissue, malig-
    nant
  endometrial (stromal) C54.1
    isthmus C54.0
  epithelioid (cell) — see Neoplasm, connective tissue,
    malignant
  Ewing's — see Neoplasm, bone, malignant
  follicular dendritic cell C96.4
  germinoblastic (diffuse) — see Lymphoma, diffuse
    large cell
    follicular — see Lymphoma, follicular, specified NEC
  giant cell (except of bone) — see also Neoplasm, con-
    nective tissue, malignant
    bone — see Neoplasm, bone, malignant
  glomoid — see Neoplasm, connective tissue, malignant
  granulocytic C92.3- ☑
  hemangioendothelial — see Neoplasm, connective
    tissue, malignant
  hemorrhagic, multiple — see Sarcoma, Kaposi's
  histiocytic C96.A (following C96.6)
  Hodgkin — see Lymphoma, Hodgkin
  immunoblastic (diffuse) — see Lymphoma, diffuse
    large cell
  interdigitating dendritic cell C96.4
  Kaposi's
    colon C46.4
    connective tissue C46.1
    gastrointestinal organ C46.4
    lung C46.5- ☑
    lymph node(s) C46.3
    palate (hard) (soft) C46.2
    rectum C46.4
    skin C46.0
    specified site NEC C46.7
    stomach C46.4
    unspecified site C46.9
  Kupffer cell C22.3
  Langerhans cell C96.4
  leptomeningeal — see Neoplasm, meninges, malignant
  liver NEC C22.4
  lymphangioendothelial — see Neoplasm, connective
    tissue, malignant

Sarcoma — continued
  lymphoblastic — see Lymphoma, lymphoblastic (diffuse)
  lymphocytic — see Lymphoma, small cell B-cell
  mast cell C96.22
  melanotic — see Melanoma
  meningeal — see Neoplasm, meninges, malignant
  meningothelial — see Neoplasm, meninges, malignant
  mesenchymal — see also Neoplasm, connective tissue, malignant
    mixed — see Neoplasm, connective tissue, malignant
  mesothelial — see Mesothelioma
  monstrocellular
    specified site — see Neoplasm, malignant, by site
    unspecified site C71.9
  myeloid C92.3- ☑
  neurogenic — see Neoplasm, nerve, malignant
  odontogenic C41.1
    upper jaw (bone) C41.0
  osteoblastic — see Neoplasm, bone, malignant
  osteogenic — see also Neoplasm, bone, malignant
    juxtacortical — see Neoplasm, bone, malignant
    periosteal — see Neoplasm, bone, malignant
  periosteal — see also Neoplasm, bone, malignant
    osteogenic — see Neoplasm, bone, malignant
  pleomorphic cell — see Neoplasm, connective tissue, malignant
  reticulum cell (diffuse) — see Lymphoma, diffuse large cell
    nodular — see Lymphoma, follicular
    pleomorphic cell type — see Lymphoma, diffuse large cell
  rhabdoid — see Neoplasm, malignant, by site
  round cell — see Neoplasm, connective tissue, malignant
  small cell — see Neoplasm, connective tissue, malignant
  soft tissue — see Neoplasm, connective tissue, malignant
  spindle cell — see Neoplasm, connective tissue, malignant
  stromal (endometrial) C54.1
    isthmus C54.0
  synovial — see also Neoplasm, connective tissue, malignant
    biphasic — see Neoplasm, connective tissue, malignant
    epithelioid cell — see Neoplasm, connective tissue, malignant
    spindle cell — see Neoplasm, connective tissue, malignant

Sarcomatosis
  meningeal — see Neoplasm, meninges, malignant
  specified site NEC — see Neoplasm, connective tissue, malignant
  unspecified site C80.1
Sarcopenia (age-related) M62.84
Sarcosinemia E72.59
Sarcosporidiosis (intestinal) A07.8
Satiety, early R68.81
Saturnine — see condition
Saturnism
  overdose or wrong substance given or taken — see Table of Drugs and Chemicals, by drug, poisoning
Satyriasis F52.8
Sauriasis — see Ichthyosis
SBE (subacute bacterial endocarditis) I33.0
Scabies (any site) B86
Scabs R23.4
Scaglietti-Dagnini syndrome E22.0
Scald — see Burn
Scalenus anticus (anterior) **syndrome** G54.0
Scales R23.4
Scaling, skin R23.4
Scalp — see condition
Scapegoating affecting child Z62.3
Scaphocephaly Q75.0
Scapulalgia M89.8X1
Scapulohumeral myopathy G71.02
Scar, scarring — see also Cicatrix L90.5
  adherent L90.5
  atrophic L90.5
  cervix
    in pregnancy or childbirth — see Pregnancy, complicated by, abnormal cervix
  cheloid L91.0

Scar, scarring — continued
  chorioretinal H31.00- ☑
    posterior pole macula H31.01- ☑
    postsurgical H59.81- ☑
    solar retinopathy H31.02- ☑
    specified type NEC H31.09- ☑
  choroid — see Scar, chorioretinal
  conjunctiva H11.24- ☑
  cornea H17.9
    xerophthalmic — see also Opacity, cornea
      vitamin A deficiency E50.6
  duodenum, obstructive K31.5
  hypertrophic L91.0
  keloid L91.0
  labia N90.89
  lung (base) J98.4
  macula — see Scar, chorioretinal, posterior pole
  muscle M62.89
  myocardium, myocardial I25.2
  painful L90.5
  posterior pole (eye) — see Scar, chorioretinal, posterior pole
  retina — see Scar, chorioretinal
  trachea J39.8
  transmural uterine, in pregnancy O34.29
  uterus N85.8
    in pregnancy O34.29
  vagina N89.8
    postoperative N99.2
  vulva N90.89
Scarabiasis B88.2
Scarlatina (anginosa) (maligna) A38.9
  myocarditis (acute) A38.1
    old — see Myocarditis
  otitis media A38.0
  ulcerosa A38.8
Scarlet fever (albuminuria) (angina) A38.9
Schamberg's disease (progressive pigmentary dermatosis) L81.7
Schatzki's ring (acquired) (esophagus) (lower) K22.2
  congenital Q39.3
Schaufenster krankheit I20.8
Schaumann's
  benign lymphogranulomatosis D86.1
  disease or syndrome — see Sarcoidosis
Scheie's syndrome E76.03
Schenck's disease B42.1
Scheuermann's disease or osteochondrosis — see Osteochondrosis, juvenile, spine
Schilder (-Flatau) **disease** G37.0
Schilling-type monocytic leukemia C93.0- ☑
Schimmelbusch's disease, cystic mastitis, or hyperplasia — see Mastopathy, cystic
Schistosoma infestation — see Infestation, Schistosoma
Schistosomiasis B65.9
  with muscle disorder B65.9 [M63.80]
    ankle B65.9 [M63.87-] ☑
    foot B65.9 [M63.87-] ☑
    forearm B65.9 [M63.83-] ☑
    hand B65.9 [M63.84-] ☑
    lower leg B65.9 [M63.86-] ☑
    multiple sites B65.9 [M63.89]
    pelvic region B65.9 [M63.85-] ☑
    shoulder region B65.9 [M63.81-] ☑
    specified site NEC B65.9 [M63.88]
    thigh B65.9 [M63.85-] ☑
    upper arm B65.9 [M63.82-] ☑
  Asiatic B65.2
  bladder B65.0
  chestermani B65.8
  colon B65.1
  cutaneous B65.3
  due to
    S. haematobium B65.0
    S. japonicum B65.2
    S. mansoni B65.1
    S. mattheii B65.8
  Eastern B65.2
  genitourinary tract B65.0
  intestinal B65.1
  lung NEC B65.9 [J99]
    pneumonia B65.9 [J17]
  Manson's (intestinal) B65.1
  oriental B65.2
  pulmonary NEC B65.9 [J99]
    pneumonia B65.9

Schistosomiasis — continued
  Schistosoma
    haematobium B65.0
    japonicum B65.2
    mansoni B65.1
  specified type NEC B65.8
  urinary B65.0
  vesical B65.0
Schizencephaly Q04.6
Schizoaffective psychosis F25.9
Schizodontia K00.2
Schizoid personality F60.1
Schizophrenia, schizophrenic F20.9
  acute (brief) (undifferentiated) F23
  atypical (form) F20.3
  borderline F21
  catalepsy F20.2
  catatonic (type) (excited) (withdrawn) F20.2
  cenesthopathic, cenesthesiopathic F20.89
  childhood type F84.5
  chronic undifferentiated F20.5
  cyclic F25.0
  disorganized (type) F20.1
  flexibilitas cerea F20.2
  hebephrenic (type) F20.1
  incipient F21
  latent F21
  negative type F20.5
  paranoid (type) F20.0
  paraphrenic F20.0
  post-psychotic depression F32.89
  prepsychotic F21
  prodromal F21
  pseudoneurotic F21
  pseudopsychopathic F21
  reaction F23
  residual (state) (type) F20.5
  restzustand F20.5
  schizoaffective (type) — see Psychosis, schizoaffective
  simple (type) F20.89
  simplex F20.89
  specified type NEC F20.89
  spectrum and other psychotic disorder F29
    specified NEC F28
  stupor F20.2
  syndrome of childhood F84.5
  undifferentiated (type) F20.3
    chronic F20.5
Schizothymia (persistent) F60.1
Schlatter-Osgood disease or osteochondrosis — see Osteochondrosis, juvenile, tibia
Schlatter's tibia — see Osteochondrosis, juvenile, tibia
Schmidt's syndrome (polyglandular, autoimmune) E31.0
Schmincke's carcinoma or tumor — see Neoplasm, nasopharynx, malignant
Schmitz (-Stutzer) **dysentery** A03.0
Schmorl's disease or nodes
  lumbar region M51.46
  lumbosacral region M51.47
  sacrococcygeal region M53.3
  thoracic region M51.44
  thoracolumbar region M51.45
Schneiderian
  papilloma — see Neoplasm, nasopharynx, benign
    specified site — see Neoplasm, benign, by site
    unspecified site D14.0
    specified site — see Neoplasm, malignant, by site
    unspecified site C30.0
Scholte's syndrome (malignant carcinoid) E34.0
Scholz (-Bielchowsky-Henneberg) **disease or syndrome** E75.25
Schönlein (-Henoch) disease or purpura (primary) (rheumatic) D69.0
Schottmuller's disease A01.4
Schroeder's syndrome (endocrine hypertensive) E27.0
Schüller-Christian disease or syndrome C96.5
Schultze's type acroparesthesia, simple I73.89
Schultz's disease or syndrome — see Agranulocytosis
Schwalbe-Ziehen-Oppenheim disease G24.1
Schwannoma — see also Neoplasm, nerve, benign
  malignant — see also Neoplasm, nerve, malignant
    with rhabdomyoblastic differentiation — see Neoplasm, nerve, malignant
  melanocytic — see Neoplasm, nerve, benign
  pigmented — see Neoplasm, nerve, benign
Schwannomatosis Q85.03
Schwartz (-Jampel) **syndrome** G71.13
Schwartz-Bartter syndrome E22.2

☑ **Additional Character Required** — Refer to the Tabular List for Character Selection   📖 **Subterms under main terms may continue to next column or page**

Schweniger-Buzzi anetoderma L90.1
Sciatic — *see* condition
Sciatica (infective)
  with lumbago M54.4- ☑
    due to intervertebral disc disorder — *see* Disorder, disc, with, radiculopathy
  due to displacement of intervertebral disc (with lumbago) — *see* Disorder, disc, with, radiculopathy
  wallet M54.3- ☑
Scimitar syndrome Q26.8
Sclera — *see* condition
Sclerectasia H15.84- ☑
Scleredema
  adultorum — *see* Sclerosis, systemic
  Buschke's — *see* Sclerosis, systemic
  newborn P83.0
Sclerema (adiposum) (edematosum) (neonatorum) (newborn) P83.0
  adultorum — *see* Sclerosis, systemic
Scleriasis — *see* Scleroderma
Scleritis H15.00- ☑
  with corneal involvement H15.04- ☑
  anterior H15.01- ☑
  brawny H15.02- ☑
  in (due to) zoster B02.34
  posterior H15.03- ☑
  specified type NEC H15.09- ☑
  syphilitic A52.71
  tuberculous (nodular) A18.51
Sclerochoroiditis H31.8
Scleroconjunctivitis — *see* Scleritis
Sclerocystic ovary syndrome E28.2
Sclerodactyly, sclerodactylia L94.3
Scleroderma, sclerodermia (acrosclerotic) (diffuse) (generalized) (progressive) (pulmonary) — *see also* Sclerosis, systemic M34.9
  circumscribed L94.0
  linear L94.1
  localized L94.0
  newborn P83.88
  systemic M34.9
Sclerokeratitis H16.8
  tuberculous A18.52
Scleroma nasi A48.8
Scleromalacia (perforans) H15.05- ☑
Scleromyxedema L98.5
Sclérose en plaques G35
Sclerosis, sclerotic
  adrenal (gland) E27.8
  Alzheimer's — *see* Disease, Alzheimer's
  amyotrophic (lateral) G12.21
  aorta, aortic I70.0
    valve — *see* Endocarditis, aortic
  artery, arterial, arteriolar, arteriovascular — *see* Arteriosclerosis
  ascending multiple G35
  brain (generalized) (lobular) G37.9
    artery, arterial I67.2
    diffuse G37.0
    disseminated G35
    insular G35
    Krabbe's E75.23
    miliary G35
    multiple G35
    presenile (Alzheimer's) — *see* Disease, Alzheimer's, early onset
    senile (arteriosclerotic) I67.2
    stem, multiple G35
    tuberous Q85.1
  bulbar, multiple G35
  bundle of His I44.39
  cardiac — *see* Disease, heart, ischemic, atherosclerotic
  cardiorenal — *see* Hypertension, cardiorenal
  cardiovascular — *see also* Disease, cardiovascular
    renal — *see* Hypertension, cardiorenal
  cerebellar — *see* Sclerosis, brain
  cerebral — *see* Sclerosis, brain
  cerebrospinal (disseminated) (multiple) G35
  cerebrovascular I67.2
  choroid — *see* Degeneration, choroid
  combined (spinal cord) — *see also* Degeneration, combined
    multiple G35
  concentric (Balo) G37.5
  cornea — *see* Opacity, cornea
  coronary (artery) I25.10

Sclerosis, sclerotic — *continued*
  coronary — *continued*
    with angina pectoris — *see* Arteriosclerosis, coronary (artery)
  corpus cavernosum
    female N90.89
    male N48.6
  diffuse (brain) (spinal cord) G37.0
  disseminated G35
  dorsal G35
  dorsolateral (spinal cord) — *see* Degeneration, combined
  endometrium N85.5
  extrapyramidal G25.9
  eye, nuclear (senile) — *see* Cataract, senile, nuclear
  focal and segmental (glomerular) — *see also* N00-N07
    with fourth character .1 N05.1
  Friedreich's (spinal cord) G11.1
  funicular (spermatic cord) N50.89
  general (vascular) — *see* Arteriosclerosis
  gland (lymphatic) I89.8
  hepatic K74.1
    alcoholic K70.2
  hereditary
    cerebellar G11.9
    spinal (Friedreich's ataxia) G11.1
  hippocampal G93.81
  insular G35
  kidney — *see* Sclerosis, renal
  larynx J38.7
  lateral (amyotrophic) (descending) (spinal) G12.21
    primary G12.23
  lens, senile nuclear — *see* Cataract, senile, nuclear
  liver K74.1
    with fibrosis K74.2
      alcoholic K70.2
    alcoholic K70.2
    cardiac K76.1
  lung — *see* Fibrosis, lung
  mastoid — *see* Mastoiditis, chronic
  mesial temporal G93.81
  mitral I05.8
  Mönckeberg's (medial) — *see* Arteriosclerosis, extremities
  multiple (brain stem) (cerebral) (generalized) (spinal cord) G35
  myocardium, myocardial — *see* Disease, heart, ischemic, atherosclerotic
  nuclear (senile), eye — *see* Cataract, senile, nuclear
  ovary N83.8
  pancreas K86.89
  penis N48.6
  peripheral arteries — *see* Arteriosclerosis, extremities
  plaques G35
  pluriglandular E31.8
  polyglandular E31.8
  posterolateral (spinal cord) — *see* Degeneration, combined
  presenile (Alzheimer's) — *see* Disease, Alzheimer's, early onset
  primary, lateral G12.23
  progressive, systemic M34.0
  pulmonary — *see* Fibrosis, lung
    artery I27.0
    valve (heart) — *see* Endocarditis, pulmonary
  renal N26.9
    with
      cystine storage disease E72.09
      hypertensive heart disease (conditions in I11) — *see* Hypertension, cardiorenal
      arteriolar (hyaline) (hyperplastic) — *see* Hypertension, kidney
  retina (senile) (vascular) H35.00
  senile (vascular) — *see* Arteriosclerosis
  spinal (cord) (progressive) G95.89
    ascending G61.0
    combined — *see also* Degeneration, combined
      multiple G35
      syphilitic A52.11
    disseminated G35
    dorsolateral — *see* Degeneration, combined
    hereditary (Friedreich's) (mixed form) G11.1
    lateral (amyotrophic) G12.21
      progressive G12.23
    multiple G35
    posterior (syphilitic) A52.11
  stomach K31.89
  subendocardial, congenital I42.4

Sclerosis, sclerotic — *continued*
  systemic M34.9
    with
      lung involvement M34.81
      myopathy M34.82
      polyneuropathy M34.83
    drug-induced M34.2
    due to chemicals NEC M34.2
    progressive M34.0
    specified NEC M34.89
  temporal (mesial) G93.81
  tricuspid (heart) (valve) I07.8
  tuberous (brain) Q85.1
  tympanic membrane — *see* Disorder, tympanic membrane, specified NEC
  valve, valvular (heart) — *see* Endocarditis
  vascular — *see* Arteriosclerosis
  vein I87.8
Scoliosis (acquired) (postural) M41.9
  adolescent (idiopathic) — *see* Scoliosis, idiopathic, adolescent
  congenital Q67.5
    due to bony malformation Q76.3
    failure of segmentation (hemivertebra) Q76.3
    hemivertebra fusion Q76.3
    postural Q67.5
  idiopathic M41.20
    adolescent M41.129
      cervical region M41.122
      cervicothoracic region M41.123
      lumbar region M41.126
      lumbosacral region M41.127
      thoracic region M41.124
      thoracolumbar region M41.125
    cervical region M41.22
    cervicothoracic region M41.23
    infantile M41.00
      cervical region M41.02
      cervicothoracic region M41.03
      lumbar region M41.06
      lumbosacral region M41.07
      sacrococcygeal region M41.08
      thoracic region M41.04
      thoracolumbar region M41.05
    juvenile M41.119
      cervical region M41.112
      cervicothoracic region M41.113
      lumbar region M41.116
      lumbosacral region M41.117
      thoracic region M41.114
      thoracolumbar region M41.115
    lumbar region M41.26
    lumbosacral region M41.27
    thoracic region M41.24
    thoracolumbar region M41.25
  infantile — *see* Scoliosis, idiopathic, infantile
  neuromuscular M41.40
    cervical region M41.42
    cervicothoracic region M41.43
    lumbar region M41.46
    lumbosacral region M41.47
    occipito-atlanto-axial region M41.41
    thoracic region M41.44
    thoracolumbar region M41.45
  paralytic — *see* Scoliosis, neuromuscular
  postradiation therapy M96.5
  rachitic (late effect or sequelae) E64.3 *[M49.80]*
    cervical region E64.3 *[M49.82]*
    cervicothoracic region E64.3 *[M49.83]*
    lumbar region E64.3 *[M49.86]*
    lumbosacral region E64.3 *[M49.87]*
    multiple sites E64.3 *[M49.89]*
    occipito-atlanto-axial region E64.3 *[M49.81]*
    sacrococcygeal region E64.3 *[M49.88]*
    thoracic region E64.3 *[M49.84]*
    thoracolumbar region E64.3 *[M49.85]*
  sciatic M54.4- ☑
  secondary (to) NEC M41.50
    cerebral palsy, Friedreich's ataxia, poliomyelitis, neuromuscular disorders — *see* Scoliosis, neuromuscular
    cervical region M41.52
    cervicothoracic region M41.53
    lumbar region M41.56
    lumbosacral region M41.57
    thoracic region M41.54
    thoracolumbar region M41.55
  specified form NEC M41.80

Scoliosis — continued
 specified form — continued
  cervical region M41.82
  cervicothoracic region M41.83
  lumbar region M41.86
  lumbosacral region M41.87
  thoracic region M41.84
  thoracolumbar region M41.85
 thoracogenic M41.30
  thoracic region M41.34
  thoracolumbar region M41.35
 tuberculous A18.01
Scoliotic pelvis
 with disproportion (fetopelvic) O33.0
  causing obstructed labor O65.0
Scorbutus, scorbutic — see also Scurvy
 anemia D53.2
Score, NIHSS (National Institutes of Health Stroke Scale)
 R29.7- ☑
Scotoma (arcuate) (Bjerrum) (central) (ring) — see also
  Defect, visual field, localized, scotoma
 scintillating H53.19
Scratch — see Abrasion
Scratchy throat R09.89
Screening (for) Z13.9
 alcoholism Z13.39
 anemia Z13.0
 anomaly, congenital Z13.89
 antenatal, of mother — see also Encounter, antenatal
  screening Z36.9
 arterial hypertension Z13.6
 arthropod-borne viral disease NEC Z11.59
 autism Z13.41
 bacteriuria, asymptomatic Z13.89
 behavioral disorder Z13.30
  specified NEC Z13.39
 brain injury, traumatic Z13.850
 bronchitis, chronic Z13.83
 brucellosis Z11.2
 cardiovascular disorder Z13.6
 cataract Z13.5
 chlamydial diseases Z11.8
 cholera Z11.0
 chromosomal abnormalities (nonprocreative) NEC
  Z13.79
 colonoscopy Z12.11
 congenital
  dislocation of hip Z13.89
  eye disorder Z13.5
  malformation or deformation Z13.89
 contamination NEC Z13.88
 cystic fibrosis Z13.228
 dengue fever Z11.59
 dental disorder Z13.84
 depression (adult) (adolescent) (child) Z13.31
  maternal Z13.32
  perinatal Z13.32
 developmental
  delays Z13.40
   global (milestones) Z13.42
   specified NEC Z13.49
  handicap Z13.42
   in early childhood Z13.42
 diabetes mellitus Z13.1
 diphtheria Z11.2
 disability, intellectual Z13.39
 disease or disorder Z13.9
  bacterial NEC Z11.2
   intestinal infectious Z11.0
   respiratory tuberculosis Z11.1
  behavioral Z13.30
   specified NEC Z13.39
  blood or blood-forming organ Z13.0
  cardiovascular Z13.6
  Chagas' Z11.6
  chlamydial Z11.8
  dental Z13.89
  developmental delays Z13.40
   global (milestones) Z13.42
   specified NEC Z13.49
  digestive tract NEC Z13.818
   lower GI Z13.811
   upper GI Z13.810
  ear Z13.5
  endocrine Z13.29
  eye Z13.5
  genitourinary Z13.89
  heart Z13.6

Screening — continued
 disease or disorder — continued
  human immunodeficiency virus (HIV) infection Z11.4
  immunity Z13.0
  infection
   intestinal Z11.0
    specified NEC Z11.6
  infectious Z11.9
  mental health and behavioral Z13.30
   specified NEC Z13.39
  metabolic Z13.228
  neurological Z13.89
  nutritional Z13.21
   metabolic Z13.228
    lipoid disorders Z13.220
  protozoal Z11.6
   intestinal Z11.0
  respiratory Z13.83
  rheumatic Z13.828
  rickettsial Z11.8
  sexually-transmitted NEC Z11.3
   human immunodeficiency virus (HIV) Z11.4
  sickle-cell (trait) Z13.0
  skin Z13.89
  specified NEC Z13.89
  spirochetal Z11.8
  thyroid Z13.29
  vascular Z13.6
  venereal Z11.3
  viral NEC Z11.59
   human immunodeficiency virus (HIV) Z11.4
   intestinal Z11.0
 elevated titer Z13.89
 emphysema Z13.83
 encephalitis, viral (mosquito or tick borne) Z11.59
 exposure to contaminants (toxic) Z13.88
 fever
  dengue Z11.59
  hemorrhagic Z11.59
  yellow Z11.59
 filariasis Z11.6
 galactosemia Z13.228
 gastrointestinal condition Z13.818
 genetic (nonprocreative) - for procreative management
   — see Testing, genetic, for procreative management
  disease carrier status (nonprocreative) Z13.71
  specified NEC (nonprocreative) Z13.79
 genitourinary condition Z13.89
 glaucoma Z13.5
 gonorrhea Z11.3
 gout Z13.89
 helminthiasis (intestinal) Z11.6
 hematopoietic malignancy Z12.89
 hemoglobinopathies NEC Z13.0
 hemorrhagic fever Z11.59
 Hodgkin disease Z12.89
 human immunodeficiency virus (HIV) Z11.4
 human papillomavirus Z11.51
 hypertension Z13.6
 immunity disorders Z13.0
 infant or child (over 28 days old) Z00.129
  with abnormal findings Z00.121
 infection
  mycotic Z11.8
  parasitic Z11.8
 ingestion of radioactive substance Z13.88
 intellectual disability Z13.39
 intestinal
  helminthiasis Z11.6
  infectious disease Z11.0
 leishmaniasis Z11.6
 leprosy Z11.2
 leptospirosis Z11.8
 leukemia Z12.89
 lymphoma Z12.89
 malaria Z11.6
 malnutrition Z13.29
  metabolic Z13.228
  nutritional Z13.21
 measles Z11.59
 mental health disorder Z13.30
  specified NEC Z13.39
 metabolic errors, inborn Z13.228
 multiphasic Z13.89
 musculoskeletal disorder Z13.828
  osteoporosis Z13.820
 mycoses Z11.8
 myocardial infarction (acute) Z13.6

Screening — continued
 neoplasm (malignant) (of) Z12.9
  bladder Z12.6
  blood Z12.89
  breast Z12.39
   routine mammogram Z12.31
  cervix Z12.4
  colon Z12.11
  genitourinary organs NEC Z12.79
   bladder Z12.6
   cervix Z12.4
   ovary Z12.73
   prostate Z12.5
   testis Z12.71
   vagina Z12.72
  hematopoietic system Z12.89
  intestinal tract Z12.10
   colon Z12.11
   rectum Z12.12
   small intestine Z12.13
  lung Z12.2
  lymph (glands) Z12.89
  nervous system Z12.82
  oral cavity Z12.81
  prostate Z12.5
  rectum Z12.12
  respiratory organs Z12.2
  skin Z12.83
  small intestine Z12.13
  specified site NEC Z12.89
  stomach Z12.0
 nephropathy Z13.89
 nervous system disorders NEC Z13.858
 neurological condition Z13.89
 osteoporosis Z13.820
 parasitic infestation Z11.9
  specified NEC Z11.8
 phenylketonuria Z13.228
 plague Z11.2
 poisoning (chemical) (heavy metal) Z13.88
 poliomyelitis Z11.59
 postnatal, chromosomal abnormalities Z13.89
 prenatal, of mother — see also Encounter, antenatal
  screening Z36.9
 protozoal disease Z11.6
  intestinal Z11.0
 pulmonary tuberculosis Z11.1
 radiation exposure Z13.88
 respiratory condition Z13.83
 respiratory tuberculosis Z11.1
 rheumatoid arthritis Z13.828
 rubella Z11.59
 schistosomiasis Z11.6
 sexually-transmitted disease NEC Z11.3
  human immunodeficiency virus (HIV) Z11.4
 sickle-cell disease or trait Z13.0
 skin condition Z13.89
 sleeping sickness Z11.6
 special Z13.9
  specified NEC Z13.89
 syphilis Z11.3
 tetanus Z11.2
 trachoma Z11.8
 traumatic brain injury Z13.850
 trypanosomiasis Z11.6
 tuberculosis, respiratory Z11.1
  active Z11.1
  latent Z11.7
 venereal disease Z11.3
 viral encephalitis (mosquito- or tick-borne) Z11.59
 whooping cough Z11.2
 worms, intestinal Z11.6
 yaws Z11.8
 yellow fever Z11.59
Scrofula, scrofulosis (tuberculosis of cervical lymph
  glands) A18.2
Scrofulide (primary) (tuberculous) A18.4
Scrofuloderma, scrofulodermia (any site) (primary)
  A18.4
Scrofulosus lichen (primary) (tuberculous) A18.4
Scrofulous — see condition
Scrotal tongue K14.5
Scrotum — see condition
Scurvy, scorbutic E54
 anemia D53.2
 gum E54
 infantile E54
 rickets E55.0 [M90.80]

☑ Additional Character Required — Refer to the Tabular List for Character Selection   ▽ Subterms under main terms may continue to next column or page

Sealpox B08.62
Seasickness T75.3 ☑
Seatworm (infection) (infestation) B80
Sebaceous — *see also* condition
  cyst — *see* Cyst, sebaceous
Seborrhea, seborrheic L21.9
  capillitii R23.8
  capitis L21.0
  dermatitis L21.9
    infantile L21.1
  eczema L21.9
    infantile L21.1
  sicca L21.0
Seckel's syndrome Q87.19
Seclusion, pupil — *see* Membrane, pupillary
Second hand tobacco smoke exposure (acute)
  (chronic) Z77.22
  in the perinatal period P96.81
Secondary
  dentin (in pulp) K04.3
  neoplasm, secondaries — *see* Table of Neoplasms,
    secondary
Secretion
  antidiuretic hormone, inappropriate E22.2
  catecholamine, by pheochromocytoma E27.5
  hormone
    antidiuretic, inappropriate (syndrome) E22.2
    by
      carcinoid tumor E34.0
      pheochromocytoma E27.5
    ectopic NEC E34.2
  urinary
    excessive R35.8
    suppression R34
Section
  nerve, traumatic — *see* Injury, nerve
Sedative, hypnotic, or anxiolytic-induced
  anxiety disorder F13.980
  bipolar and related disorder F13.94
  delirium F13.921
  depressive disorder F13.94
  major neurocognitive disorder F13.97
  mild neurocognitive disorder F13.988
  psychotic disorder F13.959
  sexual dysfunction F13.981
  sleep disorder F13.982
Segmentation, incomplete (congenital) — *see also*
  Fusion
  bone NEC Q78.8
  lumbosacral (joint) (vertebra) Q76.49
Seitelberger's syndrome (infantile neuraxonal dystrophy) G31.89
Seizure(s) — *see also* Convulsions R56.9
  absence G40.A- ☑ (*following* G40.3)
  akinetic — *see* Epilepsy, generalized, specified NEC
  atonic — *see* Epilepsy, generalized, specified NEC
  autonomic (hysterical) F44.5
  convulsive — *see* Convulsions
  cortical (focal) (motor) — *see* Epilepsy, localization-re-
    lated, symptomatic, with simple partial seizures
  disorder — *see also* Epilepsy G40.909
  due to stroke — *see* Sequelae (of), disease, cerebrovas-
    cular, by type, specified NEC
  epileptic — *see* Epilepsy
  febrile (simple) R56.00
    with status epilepticus G40.901
    complex (atypical) (complicated) R56.01
      with status epilepticus G40.901
  grand mal G40.409
    intractable G40.419
      with status epilepticus G40.411
      without status epilepticus G40.419
    not intractable G40.409
      with status epilepticus G40.401
      without status epilepticus G40.409
  heart — *see* Disease, heart
  hysterical F44.5
  intractable G40.919
    with status epilepticus G40.911
  Jacksonian (focal) (motor type) (sensory type) — *see*
    Epilepsy, localization-related, symptomatic, with
    simple partial seizures
  newborn P90
  nonspecific epileptic
    atonic — *see* Epilepsy, generalized, specified NEC
    clonic — *see* Epilepsy, generalized, specified NEC
    myoclonic — *see* Epilepsy, generalized, specified
      NEC

Seizure(s) — *continued*
  nonspecific epileptic — *continued*
    tonic — *see* Epilepsy, generalized, specified NEC
    tonic-clonic — *see* Epilepsy, generalized, specified
      NEC
  partial, developing into secondarily generalized
    seizures
    complex — *see* Epilepsy, localization-related,
      symptomatic, with complex partial seizures
    simple — *see* Epilepsy, localization-related, symp-
      tomatic, with simple partial seizures
  petit mal G40.A- ☑ (*following* G40.3)
    intractable G40.419
      with status epilepticus G40.411
      without status epilepticus G40.419
    not intractable G40.409
      with status epilepticus G40.401
      without status epilepticus G40.409
  post traumatic R56.1
  recurrent G40.909
  specified NEC G40.89
  uncinate — *see* Epilepsy, localization-related, symp-
    tomatic, with complex partial seizures
Selenium deficiency, dietary E59
Self-damaging behavior (life-style) Z72.89
Self-harm (attempted)
  history (personal) Z91.5
    in family Z81.8
Self-mutilation (attempted)
  history (personal) Z91.5
    in family Z81.8
Self-poisoning
  history (personal) Z91.5
    in family Z81.8
  observation following (alleged) attempt Z03.6
Semicoma R40.1
Seminal vesiculitis N49.0
Seminoma C62.9- ☑
  specified site — *see* Neoplasm, malignant, by site
Senear-Usher disease or syndrome L10.4
Senectus R54
Senescence (without mention of psychosis) R54
Senile, senility — *see also* condition R41.81
  with
    acute confusional state F05
    mental changes NOS F03 ☑
    psychosis NEC — *see* Psychosis, senile
  asthenia R54
  cervix (atrophic) N88.8
  debility R54
  endometrium (atrophic) N85.8
  fallopian tube (atrophic) — *see* Atrophy, fallopian tube
  heart (failure) R54
  ovary (atrophic) — *see* Atrophy, ovary
  premature E34.8
  vagina, vaginitis (atrophic) N95.2
  wart L82.1
Sensation
  burning (skin) R20.8
    tongue K14.6
  loss of R20.8
  prickling (skin) R20.2
  tingling (skin) R20.2
Sense loss
  smell — *see* Disturbance, sensation, smell
  taste — *see* Disturbance, sensation, taste
  touch R20.8
Sensibility disturbance (cortical) (deep) (vibratory) R20.9
Sensitive, sensitivity — *see also* Allergy
  carotid sinus G90.01
  child (excessive) F93.8
  cold, autoimmune D59.1
  dentin K03.89
  gluten (non-celiac) K90.41
  latex Z91.040
  methemoglobin D74.8
  tuberculin, without clinical or radiological symptoms
    R76.11
  visual
    glare H53.71
    impaired contrast H53.72
Sensitiver Beziehungswahn F22
Sensitization, auto-erythrocytic D69.2
Separation
  anxiety, abnormal (of childhood) F93.0
  apophysis, traumatic — *code as* Fracture, by site
  choroid — *see* Detachment, choroid

Separation — *continued*
  epiphysis, epiphyseal
    nontraumatic — *see also* Osteochondropathy,
      specified type NEC
      upper femoral — *see* Slipped, epiphysis, upper
        femoral
    traumatic — *code as* Fracture, by site
  fracture — *see* Fracture
  infundibulum cardiac from right ventricle by a partition
    Q24.3
  joint (traumatic) (current) — *code by* site under Dislo-
    cation
  muscle (nontraumatic) — *see* Diastasis, muscle
  pubic bone, obstetrical trauma O71.6
  retina, retinal — *see* Detachment, retina
  symphysis pubis, obstetrical trauma O71.6
  tracheal ring, incomplete, congenital Q32.1
Sepsis (generalized) (unspecified organism) A41.9
  with
    organ dysfunction (acute) (multiple) R65.20
      with septic shock R65.21
  actinomycotic A42.7
  adrenal hemorrhage syndrome (meningococcal) A39.1
  anaerobic A41.4
  Bacillus anthracis A22.7
  Brucella — *see also* Brucellosis A23.9
  candidal B37.7
  cryptogenic A41.9
  due to device, implant or graft T85.79 ☑
    arterial graft NEC T82.7 ☑
    breast (implant) T85.79 ☑
    catheter NEC T85.79 ☑
      dialysis (renal) T82.7 ☑
        intraperitoneal T85.71 ☑
      infusion NEC T82.7 ☑
        spinal (cranial) (epidural) (intrathecal) (spinal)
          (subarachnoid) (subdural) T85.735 ☑
      urethral indwelling T83.511 ☑
      urinary T83.518 ☑
    ectopic or molar pregnancy O08.82
    electronic (electrode) (pulse generator) (stimulator)
      bone T84.7 ☑
      cardiac T82.7 ☑
      nervous system T85.738 ☑
        brain T85.731 ☑
        neurostimulator generator T85.734 ☑
        peripheral nerve T85.732 ☑
        spinal cord T85.733 ☑
      urinary T83.590 ☑
    fixation, internal (orthopedic) — *see* Complication,
      fixation device, infection
    gastrointestinal (bile duct) (esophagus) T85.79 ☑
      neurostimulator electrode (lead) T85.732 ☑
    genital T83.69 ☑
    heart NEC T82.7 ☑
      valve (prosthesis) T82.6 ☑
        graft T82.7 ☑
    joint prosthesis — *see* Complication, joint prosthe-
      sis, infection
    ocular (corneal graft) (orbital implant) T85.79 ☑
    orthopedic NEC T84.7 ☑
      fixation device, internal — *see* Complication,
        fixation device, infection
    specified NEC T85.79 ☑
    vascular T82.7 ☑
    ventricular intracranial (communicating) shunt
      T85.730 ☑
  during labor O75.3
  Enterococcus A41.81
  Erysipelothrix (rhusiopathiae) (erysipeloid) A26.7
  Escherichia coli (E. coli) A41.5 ☑
  extraintestinal yersiniosis A28.2
  following
    abortion (subsequent episode) O08.0
      current episode — *see* Abortion
    ectopic or molar pregnancy O08.82
    immunization T88.0 ☑
    infusion, therapeutic injection or transfusion NEC
      T80.29 ☑
    obstetrical procedure O86.04
  gangrenous A41.9
  gonococcal A54.86
  Gram-negative (organism) A41.5 ☑
    anaerobic A41.4
  Haemophilus influenzae A41.3
  herpesviral B00.7
  intra-abdominal K65.1

☝ Subterms under main terms may continue to next column or page   ☑ Additional Character Required — Refer to the Tabular List for Character Selection   **283**

Sealpox — Sepsis

Sepsis — *continued*
  intraocular — *see* Endophthalmitis, purulent
  Listeria monocytogenes A32.7
  localized — *code to* specific localized infection
    in operation wound T81.49 ☑
    skin — *see* Abscess
  malleus A24.0
  melioidosis A24.1
  meningeal — *see* Meningitis
  meningococcal A39.4
    acute A39.2
    chronic A39.3
  MSSA (Methicillin susceptible Staphylococcus aureus) A41.01
  newborn P36.9
    due to
      anaerobes NEC P36.5
      Escherichia coli P36.4
      Staphylococcus P36.30
        aureus P36.2
        specified NEC P36.39
      Streptococcus P36.10
        group B P36.0
        specified NEC P36.19
      specified NEC P36.8
  Pasteurella multocida A28.0
  pelvic, puerperal, postpartum, childbirth O85
  pneumococcal A40.3
  postprocedural T81.44 ☑
  puerperal, postpartum, childbirth (pelvic) O85
  Salmonella (arizonae) (cholerae-suis) (enteritidis) (typhimurium) A02.1
  severe R65.20
    with septic shock R65.21
  Shigella — *see also* Dysentery, bacillary A03.9
  skin, localized — *see* Abscess
  specified organism NEC A41.89
  Staphylococcus, staphylococcal A41.2
    aureus (methicillin susceptible) (MSSA) A41.01
      methicillin resistant (MRSA) A41.02
    coagulase-negative A41.1
    specified NEC A41.1
  Streptococcus, streptococcal A40.9
    agalactiae A40.1
    group
      A A40.0
      B A40.1
      D A41.81
    neonatal P36.10
      group B P36.0
      specified NEC P36.19
    pneumoniae A40.3
    pyogenes A40.0
    specified NEC A40.8
  tracheostomy stoma J95.02
  tularemic A21.7
  umbilical, umbilical cord (newborn) — *see* Sepsis, newborn
  Yersinia pestis A20.7
Septate — *see* Septum
Septic — *see* condition
  arm — *see* Cellulitis, upper limb
    with lymphangitis — *see* Lymphangitis, acute, upper limb
  embolus — *see* Embolism
  finger — *see* Cellulitis, digit
    with lymphangitis — *see* Lymphangitis, acute, digit
  foot — *see* Cellulitis, lower limb
    with lymphangitis — *see* Lymphangitis, acute, lower limb
  gallbladder (acute) K81.0
  hand — *see* Cellulitis, upper limb
    with lymphangitis — *see* Lymphangitis, acute, upper limb
  joint — *see* Arthritis, pyogenic or pyemic
  leg — *see* Cellulitis, lower limb
    with lymphangitis — *see* Lymphangitis, acute, lower limb
  nail — *see also* Cellulitis, digit
    with lymphangitis — *see* Lymphangitis, acute, digit
  sore — *see also* Abscess
    throat J02.0
      streptococcal J02.0
  spleen (acute) D73.89
  teeth, tooth (pulpal origin) K04.4
  throat — *see* Pharyngitis
  thrombus — *see* Thrombosis
  toe — *see* Cellulitis, digit

Septic — *continued*
  toe — *see* Cellulitis, digit — *continued*
    with lymphangitis — *see* Lymphangitis, acute, digit
  tonsils, chronic J35.01
    with adenoiditis J35.03
  uterus — *see* Endometritis
Septicemia A41.9
  meaning sepsis — *see* Sepsis
Septum, septate (congenital) — *see also* Anomaly, by site
  anal Q42.3
    with fistula Q42.2
  aqueduct of Sylvius Q03.0
    with spina bifida — *see* Spina bifida, by site, with hydrocephalus
  uterus Q51.20
    complete Q51.21
    partial Q51.22
    specified NEC Q51.28
  vagina Q52.10
    in pregnancy — *see* Pregnancy, complicated by, abnormal vagina
      causing obstructed labor O65.5
    longitudinal Q52.129
      microperforate
        left side Q52.124
        right side Q52.123
      nonobstruction Q52.120
      obstructing Q52.129
        left side Q52.122
        right side Q52.121
    transverse Q52.11
Sequelae (of) — *see also* condition
  abscess, intracranial or intraspinal (conditions in G06) G09
  amputation — *code to* injury with seventh character S
  burn and corrosion — *code to* injury with seventh character S
  calcium deficiency E64.8
  cerebrovascular disease — *see* Sequelae, disease, cerebrovascular
  childbirth O94
  contusion — *code to* injury with seventh character S
  corrosion — *see* Sequelae, burn and corrosion
  crushing injury — *code to* injury with seventh character S
  disease
    cerebrovascular I69.90
      alteration of sensation I69.998
      aphasia I69.920
      apraxia I69.990
      ataxia I69.993
      cognitive deficits I69.91 ☑
      disturbance of vision I69.998
      dysarthria I69.922
      dysphagia I69.991
      dysphasia I69.921
      facial droop I69.992
      facial weakness I69.992
      fluency disorder I69.923
      hemiplegia I69.95- ☑
      hemorrhage
        intracerebral — *see* Sequelae, hemorrhage, intracerebral
        intracranial, nontraumatic NEC — *see* Sequelae, hemorrhage, intracranial, nontraumatic
        subarachnoid — *see* Sequelae, hemorrhage, subarachnoid
      language deficit I69.928
      monoplegia
        lower limb I69.94- ☑
        upper limb I69.93- ☑
      paralytic syndrome I69.96- ☑
      specified effect NEC I69.998
      specified type NEC I69.80
        alteration of sensation I69.898
        aphasia I69.820
        apraxia I69.890
        ataxia I69.893
        cognitive deficits I69.81 ☑
        disturbance of vision I69.898
        dysarthria I69.822
        dysphagia I69.891
        dysphasia I69.821
        facial droop I69.892
        facial weakness I69.892

Sequelae — *continued*
  disease — *continued*
    cerebrovascular — *continued*
      specified type — *continued*
        fluency disorder I69.823
        hemiplegia I69.85- ☑
        language deficit I69.828
        monoplegia
          lower limb I69.84- ☑
          upper limb I69.83- ☑
        paralytic syndrome I69.86- ☑
        specified effect NEC I69.898
      speech deficit I69.928
        speech deficit I69.828
      stroke NOS — *see* Sequelae, stroke NOS
  dislocation — *code to* injury with seventh character S
  encephalitis or encephalomyelitis (conditions in G04) G09
    in infectious disease NEC B94.8
    viral B94.1
  external cause — *code to* injury with seventh character S
  foreign body entering natural orifice — *code to* injury with seventh character S
  fracture — *code to* injury with seventh character S
  frostbite — *code to* injury with seventh character S
  Hansen's disease B92
  hemorrhage
    intracerebral I69.10
      alteration of sensation I69.198
      aphasia I69.120
      apraxia I69.190
      ataxia I69.193
      cognitive deficits I69.11 ☑
      disturbance of vision I69.198
      dysarthria I69.122
      dysphagia I69.191
      dysphasia I69.121
      facial droop I69.192
      facial weakness I69.192
      fluency disorder I69.123
      hemiplegia I69.15- ☑
      language deficit NEC I69.128
      monoplegia
        lower limb I69.14- ☑
        upper limb I69.13- ☑
      paralytic syndrome I69.16- ☑
      specified effect NEC I69.198
      speech deficit NEC I69.128
    intracranial, nontraumatic NEC I69.20
      alteration of sensation I69.298
      aphasia I69.220
      apraxia I69.290
      ataxia I69.293
      cognitive deficits I69.21 ☑
      disturbance of vision I69.298
      dysarthria I69.222
      dysphagia I69.291
      dysphasia I69.221
      facial droop I69.292
      facial weakness I69.292
      fluency disorder I69.223
      hemiplegia I69.25- ☑
      language deficit NEC I69.228
      monoplegia
        lower limb I69.24- ☑
        upper limb I69.23- ☑
      paralytic syndrome I69.26- ☑
      specified effect NEC I69.298
      speech deficit NEC I69.228
    subarachnoid I69.00
      alteration of sensation I69.098
      aphasia I69.020
      apraxia I69.090
      ataxia I69.093
      cognitive deficits — *see* subcategory I69.01- ☑
      disturbance of vision I69.098
      dysarthria I69.022
      dysphagia I69.091
      dysphasia I69.021
      facial droop I69.092
      facial weakness I69.092
      fluency disorder I69.023
      hemiplegia I69.05- ☑
      language deficit NEC I69.028
      monoplegia
        lower limb I69.04- ☑
        upper limb I69.03- ☑

Sequelae — *continued*
  hemorrhage — *continued*
    subarachnoid — *continued*
      paralytic syndrome I69.06- ☑
      specified effect NEC I69.098
      speech deficit NEC I69.028
  hepatitis, viral B94.2
  hyperalimentation E68
  infarction
    cerebral I69.30
      alteration of sensation I69.398
      aphasia I69.320
      apraxia I69.390
      ataxia I69.393
      cognitive deficits I69.31 ☑
      disturbance of vision I69.398
      dysarthria I69.322
      dysphagia I69.391
      dysphasia I69.321
      facial droop I69.392
      facial weakness I69.392
      fluency disorder I69.323
      hemiplegia I69.35- ☑
      language deficit NEC I69.328
      monoplegia
        lower limb I69.34- ☑
        upper limb I69.33- ☑
      paralytic syndrome I69.36- ☑
      specified effect NEC I69.398
      speech deficit NEC I69.328
  infection, pyogenic, intracranial or intraspinal G09
  infectious disease B94.9
    specified NEC B94.8
  injury — *code to* injury with seventh character S
  leprosy B92
  meningitis
    bacterial (conditions in G00) G09
    other or unspecified cause (conditions in G03) G09
  muscle (and tendon) injury — *code to* injury with seventh character S
  myelitis — *see* Sequelae, encephalitis
  niacin deficiency E64.8
  nutritional deficiency E64.9
    specified NEC E64.8
  obstetrical condition O94
  parasitic disease B94.9
  phlebitis or thrombophlebitis of intracranial or intraspinal venous sinuses and veins (conditions in G08) G09
  poisoning — *code to* poisoning with seventh character S
    nonmedicinal substance — *see* Sequelae, toxic effect, nonmedicinal substance
  poliomyelitis (acute) B91
  pregnancy O94
  protein-energy malnutrition E64.0
  puerperium O94
  rickets E64.3
  selenium deficiency E64.8
  sprain and strain — *code to* injury with seventh character S
  stroke NOS I69.30
    alteration in sensation I69.398
    aphasia I69.320
    apraxia I69.390
    ataxia I69.393
    cognitive deficits I69.31 ☑
    disturbance of vision I69.398
    dysarthria I69.322
    dysphagia I69.391
    dysphasia I69.321
    facial droop I69.392
    facial weakness I69.392
    hemiplegia I69.35- ☑
    language deficit NEC I69.328
    monoplegia
      lower limb I69.34- ☑
      upper limb I69.33- ☑
    paralytic syndrome I69.36- ☑
    specified effect NEC I69.398
    speech deficit NEC I69.328
  tendon and muscle injury — *code to* injury with seventh character S
  thiamine deficiency E64.8
  trachoma B94.0
  tuberculosis B90.9
    bones and joints B90.2
    central nervous system B90.0

Sequelae — *continued*
  tuberculosis — *continued*
    genitourinary B90.1
    pulmonary (respiratory) B90.9
    specified organs NEC B90.8
  viral
    encephalitis B94.1
    hepatitis B94.2
  vitamin deficiency NEC E64.8
    A E64.1
    B E64.8
    C E64.2
  wound, open — *code to* injury with seventh character S
Sequestration — *see also* Sequestrum
  disk — *see* Displacement, intervertebral disk
  lung, congenital Q33.2
Sequestrum
  bone — *see* Osteomyelitis, chronic
  dental M27.2
  jaw bone M27.2
  orbit — *see* Osteomyelitis, orbit
  sinus (accessory) (nasal) — *see* Sinusitis
Sequoiosis lung or pneumonitis J67.8
Serology for syphilis
  doubtful
    with signs or symptoms — *code by* site and stage under Syphilis
    follow-up of latent syphilis — *see* Syphilis, latent
  negative, with signs or symptoms — *code by* site and stage under Syphilis
  positive A53.0
    with signs or symptoms — *code by* site and stage under Syphilis
  reactivated A53.0
Seroma — *see also* Hematoma
  postprocedural — *see* Complication, postprocedural, seroma
  traumatic, secondary and recurrent T79.2 ☑
Seropurulent — *see* condition
Serositis, multiple K65.8
  pericardial I31.1
  peritoneal K65.8
Serous — *see* condition
Sertoli cell
  adenoma
    specified site — *see* Neoplasm, benign, by site
    unspecified site
      female D27.9
      male D29.20
  carcinoma
    specified site — *see* Neoplasm, malignant, by site
    unspecified site (male) C62.9- ☑
      female C56.9
  tumor
    with lipid storage
      specified site — *see* Neoplasm, benign, by site
      unspecified site
        female D27.9
        male D29.20
    specified site — *see* Neoplasm, benign, by site
    unspecified site
      female D27.9
      male D29.20
Sertoli-Leydig cell tumor — *see* Neoplasm, benign, by site
  specified site — *see* Neoplasm, benign, by site
  unspecified site
    female D27.9
    male D29.20
Serum
  allergy, allergic reaction — *see also* Reaction, serum T80.69 ☑
    shock — *see also* Shock, anaphylactic T80.59 ☑
  arthritis — *see also* Reaction, serum T80.69 ☑
  complication or reaction NEC — *see also* Reaction, serum T80.69 ☑
  disease NEC — *see also* Reaction, serum T80.69 ☑
  hepatitis — *see also* Hepatitis, viral, type B
    carrier (suspected) of B18.1
  intoxication — *see also* Reaction, serum T80.69 ☑
  neuritis — *see also* Reaction, serum T80.69 ☑
  neuropathy G61.1
  poisoning NEC — *see also* Reaction, serum T80.69 ☑
  rash NEC — *see also* Reaction, serum T80.69 ☑
  reaction NEC — *see also* Reaction, serum T80.69 ☑
  sickness NEC — *see also* Reaction, serum T80.69 ☑

Serum — *continued*
  urticaria — *see also* Reaction, serum T80.69 ☑
Sesamoiditis M25.8- ☑
Severe sepsis R65.20
  with septic shock R65.21
Sever's disease or osteochondrosis — *see* Osteochondrosis, juvenile, tarsus
Sex
  chromosome mosaics Q97.8
    lines with various numbers of X chromosomes Q97.2
  education Z70.8
  reassignment surgery status Z87.890
Sextuplet pregnancy — *see* Pregnancy, sextuplet
Sexual
  function, disorder of (psychogenic) F52.9
  immaturity (female) (male) E30.0
  impotence (psychogenic) organic origin NEC — *see* Dysfunction, sexual, male
  precocity (constitutional) (cryptogenic)(female) (idiopathic) (male) E30.1
Sexuality, pathologic — *see* Deviation, sexual
Sézary disease C84.1- ☑
Shadow, lung R91.8
Shaking palsy or paralysis — *see* Parkinsonism
Shallowness, acetabulum — *see* Derangement, joint, specified type NEC, hip
Shaver's disease J63.1
Sheath (tendon) — *see* condition
Sheathing, retinal vessels H35.01- ☑
Shedding
  nail L60.8
  premature, primary (deciduous) teeth K00.6
Sheehan's disease or syndrome E23.0
Shelf, rectal K62.89
Shell teeth K00.5
Shellshock (current) F43.0
  lasting state — *see* Disorder, post-traumatic stress
Shield kidney Q63.1
Shift
  auditory threshold (temporary) H93.24- ☑
  mediastinal R93.89
Shifting sleep-work schedule (affecting sleep) G47.26
Shiga (-Kruse) **dysentery** A03.0
Shiga's bacillus A03.0
Shigella (dysentery) — *see* Dysentery, bacillary
Shigellosis A03.9
  Group A A03.0
  Group B A03.1
  Group C A03.2
  Group D A03.3
Shin splints S86.89- ☑
Shingles — *see* Herpes, zoster
Shipyard disease or eye B30.0
Shirodkar suture, in pregnancy — *see* Pregnancy, complicated by, incompetent cervix
Shock R57.9
  with ectopic or molar pregnancy O08.3
  adrenal (cortical) (Addisonian) E27.2
  adverse food reaction (anaphylactic) — *see* Shock, anaphylactic, due to food
  allergic — *see* Shock, anaphylactic
  anaphylactic T78.2 ☑
    chemical — *see* Table of Drugs and Chemicals
    due to drug or medicinal substance
      correct substance properly administered T88.6 ☑
      overdose or wrong substance given or taken (by accident) — *see* Table of Drugs and Chemicals, by drug, poisoning
    due to food (nonpoisonous) T78.00 ☑
      additives T78.06 ☑
      dairy products T78.07 ☑
      eggs T78.08 ☑
      fish T78.03 ☑
        shellfish T78.02 ☑
      fruit T78.04 ☑
      milk T78.07 ☑
      nuts T78.05 ☑
        multiple types T78.05 ☑
        peanuts T78.01 ☑
      peanuts T78.01 ☑
      seeds T78.05 ☑
      specified type NEC T78.09 ☑
      vegetable T78.04 ☑
    following sting(s) — *see* Venom
    immunization T80.52 ☑
    serum T80.59 ☑
      blood and blood products T80.51 ☑

Index | **Shock — Simulation, conscious**

Shock — *continued*
anaphylactic — *continued*
  serum — *continued*
    immunization T80.52 ☑
    specified NEC T80.59 ☑
    vaccination T80.52 ☑
anaphylactoid — *see* Shock, anaphylactic
anesthetic
  correct substance properly administered T88.2 ☑
  overdose or wrong substance given or taken — *see* Table of Drugs and Chemicals, by drug, poisoning
  specified anesthetic — *see* Table of Drugs and Chemicals, by drug, poisoning
cardiogenic R57.0
chemical substance — *see* Table of Drugs and Chemicals
complicating ectopic or molar pregnancy O08.3
culture — *see* Disorder, adjustment
drug
  due to correct substance properly administered T88.6 ☑
  overdose or wrong substance given or taken (by accident) — *see* Table of Drugs and Chemicals, by drug, poisoning
during or after labor and delivery O75.1
electric T75.4 ☑
  (taser) T75.4 ☑
endotoxic R65.21
  postprocedural (resulting from a procedure, not elsewhere classified) T81.12 ☑
following
  ectopic or molar pregnancy O08.3
  injury (immediate) (delayed) T79.4 ☑
  labor and delivery O75.1
food (anaphylactic) — *see* Shock, anaphylactic, due to food
from electroshock gun (taser) T75.4 ☑
gram-negative R65.21
  postprocedural (resulting from a procedure, not elsewhere classified) T81.12 ☑
hematologic R57.8
hemorrhagic R57.8
  surgery (intraoperative) (postoperative) T81.19 ☑
  trauma T79.4 ☑
hypovolemic R57.1
  surgical T81.19 ☑
  traumatic T79.4 ☑
insulin E15
  therapeutic misadventure — *see* subcategory T38.3 ☑
kidney N17.0
  traumatic (following crushing) T79.5 ☑
lightning T75.01 ☑
liver K72.00
lung J80
obstetric O75.1
  with ectopic or molar pregnancy O08.3
  following ectopic or molar pregnancy O08.3
pleural (surgical) T81.19 ☑
  due to trauma T79.4 ☑
postprocedural (postoperative) T81.10 ☑
  with ectopic or molar pregnancy O08.3
  cardiogenic T81.11 ☑
  endotoxic T81.12 ☑
  following ectopic or molar pregnancy O08.3
  gram-negative T81.12 ☑
  hypovolemic T81.19 ☑
  septic T81.12 ☑
  specified type NEC T81.19 ☑
psychic F43.0
septic (due to severe sepsis) R65.21
specified NEC R57.8
surgical T81.10 ☑
taser gun (taser) T75.4 ☑
therapeutic misadventure NEC T81.10 ☑
thyroxin
  overdose or wrong substance given or taken — *see* Table of Drugs and Chemicals, by drug, poisoning
toxic, syndrome A48.3
transfusion — *see* Complications, transfusion
traumatic (immediate) (delayed) T79.4 ☑
Shoemaker's chest M95.4
Short, shortening, shortness
arm (acquired) — *see also* Deformity, limb, unequal length

Short, shortening, shortness — *continued*
arm — *see also* Deformity, limb, unequal length — *continued*
  congenital Q71.81- ☑
  forearm — *see* Deformity, limb, unequal length
bowel syndrome K91.2
breath R06.02
cervical (complicating pregnancy) O26.87- ☑
  non-gravid uterus N88.3
common bile duct, congenital Q44.5
cord (umbilical), complicating delivery O69.3 ☑
cystic duct, congenital Q44.5
esophagus (congenital) Q39.8
femur (acquired) — *see* Deformity, limb, unequal length, femur
  congenital — *see* Defect, reduction, lower limb, longitudinal, femur
frenum, frenulum, linguae (congenital) Q38.1
hip (acquired) — *see also* Deformity, limb, unequal length
  congenital Q65.89
leg (acquired) — *see also* Deformity, limb, unequal length
  congenital Q72.81- ☑
  lower leg — *see also* Deformity, limb, unequal length
limbed stature, with immunodeficiency D82.2
lower limb (acquired) — *see also* Deformity, limb, unequal length
  congenital Q72.81- ☑
organ or site, congenital NEC — *see* Distortion
palate, congenital Q38.5
radius (acquired) — *see also* Deformity, limb, unequal length
  congenital — *see* Defect, reduction, upper limb, longitudinal, radius
rib syndrome Q77.2
stature (child) (hereditary) (idiopathic) NEC R62.52
  constitutional E34.3
  due to endocrine disorder E34.3
  Laron-type E34.3
tendon — *see also* Contraction, tendon
  with contracture of joint — *see* Contraction, joint
  Achilles (acquired) M67.0- ☑
    congenital Q66.89
  congenital Q79.8
thigh (acquired) — *see also* Deformity, limb, unequal length, femur
  congenital — *see* Defect, reduction, lower limb, longitudinal, femur
tibialis anterior (tendon) — *see* Contraction, tendon
umbilical cord
  complicating delivery O69.3 ☑
upper limb, congenital — *see* Defect, reduction, upper limb, specified type NEC
urethra N36.8
uvula, congenital Q38.5
vagina (congenital) Q52.4
Shortsightedness — *see* Myopia
Shoshin (acute fulminating beriberi) E51.11
Shoulder — *see* condition
Shovel-shaped incisors K00.2
Shower, thromboembolic — *see* Embolism
Shunt
arterial-venous (dialysis) Z99.2
arteriovenous, pulmonary (acquired) I28.0
  congenital Q25.72
cerebral ventricle (communicating) in situ Z98.2
surgical, prosthetic, with complications — *see* Complications, cardiovascular, device or implant
Shutdown, renal N28.9
Shy-Drager syndrome G90.3
Sialadenitis, sialadenosis (any gland) (chronic) (periodic) (suppurative) — *see* Sialoadenitis
Sialectasia K11.8
Sialidosis E77.1
Sialitis, silitis (any gland) (chronic) (suppurative) — *see* Sialoadenitis
Sialoadenitis (any gland) (periodic) (suppurative) K11.20
acute K11.21
  recurrent K11.22
chronic K11.23
Sialoadenopathy K11.9
Sialoangitis — *see* Sialoadenitis
Sialodochitis (fibrinosa) — *see* Sialoadenitis
Sialodocholithiasis K11.5
Sialolithiasis K11.5 ·

Sialometaplasia, necrotizing K11.8
Sialorrhea — *see also* Ptyalism
periodic — *see* Sialoadenitis
Sialosis K11.7
Siamese twin Q89.4
Sibling rivalry Z62.891
Sicard's syndrome G52.7
Sicca syndrome M35.00
with
  keratoconjunctivitis M35.01
  lung involvement M35.02
  myopathy M35.03
  renal tubulo-interstitial disorders M35.04
specified organ involvement NEC M35.09
Sick R69
or handicapped person in family Z63.79
  needing care at home Z63.6
sinus (syndrome) I49.5
Sick-euthyroid syndrome E07.81
Sickle-cell
anemia — *see* Disease, sickle-cell
trait D57.3
Sicklemia — *see also* Disease, sickle-cell
trait D57.3
Sickness
air (travel) T75.3 ☑
airplane T75.3 ☑
alpine T70.29 ☑
altitude T70.20 ☑
Andes T70.29 ☑
aviator's T70.29 ☑
balloon T70.29 ☑
car T75.3 ☑
compressed air T70.3 ☑
decompression T70.3 ☑
green D50.8
milk — *see* Poisoning, food, noxious
motion T75.3 ☑
mountain T70.29 ☑
  acute D75.1
protein — *see also* Reaction, serum T80.69 ☑
radiation T66 ☑
roundabout (motion) T75.3 ☑
sea T75.3 ☑
serum NEC — *see also* Reaction, serum T80.69 ☑
sleeping (African) B56.9
  by Trypanosoma B56.9
    brucei
      gambiense B56.0
      rhodesiense B56.1
    East African B56.1
    Gambian B56.0
    Rhodesian B56.1
    West African B56.0
swing (motion) T75.3 ☑
train (railway) (travel) T75.3 ☑
travel (any vehicle) T75.3 ☑
Sideropenia — *see* Anemia, iron deficiency
Siderosilicosis J62.8
Siderosis (lung) J63.4
eye (globe) — *see* Disorder, globe, degenerative, siderosis
Siemens' syndrome (ectodermal dysplasia) Q82.8
Sighing R06.89
psychogenic F45.8
Sigmoid — *see also* condition
flexure — *see* condition
kidney Q63.1
Sigmoiditis — *see also* Enteritis K52.9
infectious A09
noninfectious K52.9
Silfversköld's syndrome Q78.9
Silicosiderosis J62.8
Silicosis, silicotic (simple) (complicated) J62.8
with tuberculosis J65
Silicotuberculosis J65
Silo-fillers' disease J68.8
bronchitis J68.0
pneumonitis J68.0
pulmonary edema J68.1
Silver's syndrome Q87.19
Simian malaria B53.1
Simmonds' cachexia or disease E23.0
Simons' disease or syndrome (progressive lipodystrophy) E88.1
Simple, simplex — *see* condition
Simulation, conscious (of illness) Z76.5

Simultanagnosia (asimultagnosia) R48.3
Sin Nombre virus disease (Hantavirus) (cardio)-pulmonary syndrome) B33.4
Sinding-Larsen disease or osteochondrosis — *see* Osteochondrosis, juvenile, patella
Singapore hemorrhagic fever A91
Singer's node or nodule J38.2
Single
  atrium Q21.2
  coronary artery Q24.5
  umbilical artery Q27.0
  ventricle Q20.4
Singultus R06.6
  epidemicus B33.0
Sinus — *see also* Fistula
  abdominal K63.89
  arrest I45.5
  arrhythmia I49.8
  bradycardia R00.1
  branchial cleft (internal) (external) Q18.0
  coccygeal — *see* Sinus, pilonidal
  dental K04.6
  dermal (congenital) Q06.8
    with abscess Q06.8
    coccygeal, pilonidal — *see* Sinus, coccygeal
  infected, skin NEC L08.89
  marginal, ruptured or bleeding — *see* Hemorrhage, antepartum, specified cause NEC
  medial, face and neck Q18.8
  pause I45.5
  pericranii Q01.9
  pilonidal (infected) (rectum) L05.92
    with abscess L05.02
  preauricular Q18.1
  rectovaginal N82.3
  Rokitansky-Aschoff (gallbladder) K82.8
  sacrococcygeal (dermoid) (infected) — *see* Sinus, pilonidal
  tachycardia R00.0
    paroxysmal I47.1
  tarsi syndrome M25.57- ☑
  testis N50.89
  tract (postinfective) — *see* Fistula
  urachus Q64.4
Sinusitis (accessory) (chronic) (hyperplastic) (nasal) (nonpurulent) (purulent) J32.9
  acute J01.90
    ethmoidal J01.20
      recurrent J01.21
    frontal J01.10
      recurrent J01.11
    involving more than one sinus, other than pansinusitis J01.80
      recurrent J01.81
    maxillary J01.00
      recurrent J01.01
    pansinusitis J01.40
      recurrent J01.41
    recurrent J01.91
    specified NEC J01.80
      recurrent J01.81
    sphenoidal J01.30
      recurrent J01.31
  allergic — *see* Rhinitis, allergic
  due to high altitude T70.1 ☑
  ethmoidal J32.2
    acute J01.20
      recurrent J01.21
  frontal J32.1
    acute J01.10
      recurrent J01.11
  influenzal — *see* Influenza, with, respiratory manifestations NEC
  involving more than one sinus but not pansinusitis J32.8
    acute J01.80
      recurrent J01.81
  maxillary J32.0
    acute J01.00
      recurrent J01.01
  sphenoidal J32.3
    acute J01.30
      recurrent J01.31
  tuberculous, any sinus A15.8
Sinusitis-bronchiectasis-situs inversus (syndrome) (triad) Q89.3
Sipple's syndrome E31.22
Sirenomelia (syndrome) Q87.2

Siriasis T67.01 ☑
Sirkari's disease B55.0
Siti A65
Situation, psychiatric F99
Situational
  disturbance (transient) — *see* Disorder, adjustment
    acute F43.0
  maladjustment — *see* Disorder, adjustment
  reaction — *see* Disorder, adjustment
    acute F43.0
Situs inversus or transversus (abdominalis) (thoracis) Q89.3
Sixth disease B08.20
  due to human herpesvirus 6 B08.21
  due to human herpesvirus 7 B08.22
Sjögren-Larsson syndrome Q87.19
Sjögren's syndrome or disease — *see* Sicca syndrome
Skeletal — *see* condition
Skene's gland — *see* condition
Skenitis — *see* Urethritis
Skerljevo A65
Skevas-Zerfus disease — *see* Toxicity, venom, marine animal, sea anemone
Skin — *see also* condition
  clammy R23.1
  donor — *see* Donor, skin
  hidebound M35.9
Slate-dressers' or slate-miners' lung J62.8
Sleep
  apnea — *see* Apnea, sleep
  deprivation Z72.820
  disorder or disturbance G47.9
    child F51.9
      nonorganic origin F51.9
      specified NEC G47.8
  disturbance G47.9
    nonorganic origin F51.9
  drunkenness F51.9
  rhythm inversion G47.2- ☑
  terrors F51.4
  walking F51.3
    hysterical F44.89
Sleep hygiene
  abuse Z72.821
  inadequate Z72.821
  poor Z72.821
Sleeping sickness — *see* Sickness, sleeping
Sleeplessness — *see* Insomnia
  menopausal N95.1
Sleep-wake schedule disorder G47.20
Slim disease (in HIV infection) B20
Slipped, slipping
  epiphysis (traumatic) — *see also* Osteochondropathy, specified type NEC
    capital femoral (traumatic)
      acute (on chronic) S79.01- ☑
    current traumatic — *code as* Fracture, by site
    upper femoral (nontraumatic) M93.00- ☑
      acute M93.01- ☑
        on chronic M93.03- ☑
      chronic M93.02- ☑
  intervertebral disc — *see* Displacement, intervertebral disc
  ligature, umbilical P51.8
  patella — *see* Disorder, patella, derangement NEC
  rib M89.8X8
  sacroiliac joint — *see* subcategory M53.2 ☑
  tendon — *see* Disorder, tendon
  ulnar nerve, nontraumatic — *see* Lesion, nerve, ulnar
  vertebra NEC — *see* Spondylolisthesis
Slocumb's syndrome E27.0
Sloughing (multiple) (phagedena) (skin) — *see also* Gangrene
  abscess — *see* Abscess
  appendix K38.8
  fascia — *see* Disorder, soft tissue, specified type NEC
  scrotum N50.89
  tendon — *see* Disorder, tendon
  transplanted organ — *see* Rejection, transplant
  ulcer — *see* Ulcer, skin
Slow
  feeding, newborn P92.2
  flow syndrome, coronary I20.8
  heart (beat) R00.1
Slowing, urinary stream R39.198
Sluder's neuralgia (syndrome) G44.89
Slurred, slurring speech R47.81

Small (ness)
  for gestational age — *see* Small for dates
  introitus, vagina N89.6
  kidney (unknown cause) N27.9
    bilateral N27.1
    unilateral N27.0
  ovary (congenital) Q50.39
  pelvis
    with disproportion (fetopelvic) O33.1
      causing obstructed labor O65.1
  uterus N85.8
  white kidney N03.9
Small-and-light-for-dates — *see* Small for dates
Small-for-dates (infant) P05.10
  with weight of
    499 grams or less P05.11
    500-749 grams P05.12
    750-999 grams P05.13
    1000-1249 grams P05.14
    1250-1499 grams P05.15
    1500-1749 grams P05.16
    1750-1999 grams P05.17
    2000-2499 grams P05.18
    2500 grams and over P05.19
  specified NEC P05.19
Smallpox B03
Smearing, fecal R15.1
Smith-Lemli-Opitz syndrome E78.72
Smith's fracture S52.54- ☑
Smoker — *see* Dependence, drug, nicotine
Smoker's
  bronchitis J41.0
  cough J41.0
  palate K13.24
  throat J31.2
  tongue K13.24
Smoking
  passive Z77.22
Smothering spells R06.81
Snaggle teeth, tooth M26.39
Snapping
  finger — *see* Trigger finger
  hip — *see* Derangement, joint, specified type NEC, hip
    involving the iliotibial band M76.3- ☑
  knee — *see* Derangement, knee
    involving the iliotibial band M76.3- ☑
Sneddon-Wilkinson disease or syndrome (sub-corneal pustular dermatosis) L13.1
Sneezing (intractable) R06.7
Sniffing
  cocaine
    abuse — *see* Abuse, drug, cocaine
    dependence — *see* Dependence, drug, cocaine
  gasoline
    abuse — *see* Abuse, drug, inhalant
    dependence — *see* Dependence, drug, inhalant
  glue (airplane)
    abuse — *see* Abuse, drug, inhalant
    drug dependence — *see* Dependence, drug, inhalant
Sniffles
  newborn P28.89
Snoring R06.83
Snow blindness — *see* Photokeratitis
Snuffles (non-syphilitic) R06.5
  newborn P28.89
  syphilitic (infant) A50.05 *[J99]*
Social
  exclusion Z60.4
    due to discrimination or persecution (perceived) Z60.5
  migrant Z59.0
    acculturation difficulty Z60.3
  rejection Z60.4
    due to discrimination or persecution Z60.5
  role conflict NEC Z73.5
  skills inadequacy NEC Z73.4
  transplantation Z60.3
Sodoku A25.0
Soemmerring's ring — *see* Cataract, secondary
Soft — *see also* condition
  nails L60.3
Softening
  bone — *see* Osteomalacia
  brain (necrotic) (progressive) G93.89
    congenital Q04.8
    embolic I63.4- ☑

Softening — *continued*
  brain — *continued*
    hemorrhagic — *see* Hemorrhage, intracranial, intracerebral
      occlusive I63.5- ☑
      thrombotic I63.3- ☑
  cartilage M94.2- ☑
    patella M22.4- ☑
  cerebellar — *see* Softening, brain
  cerebral — *see* Softening, brain
  cerebrospinal — *see* Softening, brain
  myocardial, heart — *see* Degeneration, myocardial
  spinal cord G95.89
  stomach K31.89
Soldier's
  heart F45.8
  patches I31.0
Solitary
  cyst, kidney N28.1
  kidney, congenital Q60.0
Solvent abuse — *see* Abuse, drug, inhalant
  dependence — *see* Dependence, drug, inhalant
Somatization reaction, somatic reaction — *see* Disorder, somatoform
Somnambulism F51.3
  hysterical F44.89
Somnolence R40.0
  nonorganic origin F51.11
Sonne dysentery A03.3
Soor B37.0
Sore
  bed — *see* Ulcer, pressure, by site
  chiclero B55.1
  Delhi B55.1
  desert — *see* Ulcer, skin
  eye H57.1- ☑
  Lahore B55.1
  mouth K13.79
    canker K12.0
  muscle M79.10
  Naga — *see* Ulcer, skin
  of skin — *see* Ulcer, skin
  oriental B55.1
  pressure — *see* Ulcer, pressure, by site
  skin L98.9
  soft A57
  throat (acute) — *see also* Pharyngitis
    with influenza, flu, or grippe — *see* Influenza, with, respiratory manifestations NEC
    chronic J31.2
    coxsackie (virus) B08.5
    diphtheritic A36.0
    herpesviral B00.2
    influenzal — *see* Influenza, with, respiratory manifestations NEC
    septic J02.0
    streptococcal (ulcerative) J02.0
    viral NEC J02.8
      coxsackie B08.5
    tropical — *see* Ulcer, skin
    veldt — *see* Ulcer, skin
Soto's syndrome (cerebral gigantism) Q87.3
South African cardiomyopathy syndrome I42.8
Southeast Asian hemorrhagic fever A91
Spacing
  abnormal, tooth, teeth, fully erupted M26.30
  excessive, tooth, fully erupted M26.32
Spade-like hand (congenital) Q68.1
Spading nail L60.8
  congenital Q84.6
Spanish collar N47.1
Sparganosis B70.1
Spasm(s), **spastic, spasticity** — *see also* condition R25.2
  accommodation — *see* Spasm, of accommodation
  ampulla of Vater K83.4
  anus, ani (sphincter) (reflex) K59.4
    psychogenic F45.8
  artery I73.9
    cerebral G45.9
  Bell's G51.3- ☑
  bladder (sphincter, external or internal) N32.89
    psychogenic F45.8
  bronchus, bronchiole J98.01
  cardia K22.0
  cardiac I20.1
  carpopedal — *see* Tetany
  cerebral (arteries) (vascular) G45.9

Spasm(s), spastic, spasticity — *continued*
  cervix, complicating delivery O62.4
  ciliary body (of accommodation) — *see* Spasm, of accommodation
  colon — *see also* Irritable, bowel K58.9
    with diarrhea K58.0
    psychogenic F45.8
  common duct K83.8
  compulsive — *see* Tic
  conjugate H51.8
  coronary (artery) I20.1
  diaphragm (reflex) R06.6
    epidemic B33.0
    psychogenic F45.8
  duodenum K59.8
  epidemic diaphragmatic (transient) B33.0
  esophagus (diffuse) K22.4
    psychogenic F45.8
  facial G51.3- ☑
  fallopian tube N83.8
  gastrointestinal (tract) K31.89
    psychogenic F45.8
  glottis J38.5
    hysterical F44.4
    psychogenic F45.8
      conversion reaction F44.4
    reflex through recurrent laryngeal nerve J38.5
  habit — *see* Tic
  heart I20.1
  hemifacial (clonic) G51.3- ☑
  hourglass — *see* Contraction, hourglass
  hysterical F44.4
  infantile — *see* Epilepsy, spasms
  inferior oblique, eye H51.8
  intestinal — *see also* Syndrome, irritable bowel K58.9
    psychogenic F45.8
  larynx, laryngeal J38.5
    hysterical F44.4
    psychogenic F45.8
      conversion reaction F44.4
  levator palpebrae superioris — *see* Disorder, eyelid function
  muscle NEC M62.838
    back M62.830
  nerve, trigeminal G51.0
  nervous F45.8
  nodding F98.4
  occupational F48.8
  oculogyric H51.8
    psychogenic F45.8
  of accommodation H52.53- ☑
  ophthalmic artery — *see* Occlusion, artery, retina
  perineal, female N94.89
  peroneo-extensor — *see also* Deformity, limb, flat foot
  pharynx (reflex) J39.2
    hysterical F45.8
    psychogenic F45.8
  psychogenic F45.8
  pylorus NEC K31.3
    adult hypertrophic K31.89
    congenital or infantile Q40.0
    psychogenic F45.8
  rectum (sphincter) K59.4
    psychogenic F45.8
  retinal (artery) — *see* Occlusion, artery, retina
  sigmoid — *see also* Syndrome, irritable bowel K58.9
    psychogenic F45.8
  sphincter of Oddi K83.4
  stomach K31.89
    neurotic F45.8
  throat J39.2
    hysterical F45.8
    psychogenic F45.8
  tic F95.9
    chronic F95.1
    transient of childhood F95.0
  tongue K14.8
  torsion (progressive) G24.1
  trigeminal nerve — *see* Neuralgia, trigeminal
  ureter N13.5
  urethra (sphincter) N35.919
  uterus N85.8
    complicating labor O62.4
  vagina N94.2
    psychogenic F52.5
  vascular I73.9
  vasomotor I73.9
  vein NEC I87.8

Spasm(s), spastic, spasticity — *continued*
  viscera — *see* Pain, abdominal
Spasmodic — *see* condition
Spasmophilia — *see* Tetany
Spasmus nutans F98.4
Spastic, spasticity — *see also* Spasm
  child (cerebral) (congenital) (paralysis) G80.1
Speaker's throat R49.8
Specific, specified — *see* condition
Speech
  defect, disorder, disturbance, impediment R47.9
    psychogenic, in childhood and adolescence F98.8
    slurring R47.81
    specified NEC R47.89
Spencer's disease A08.19
Spens' syndrome (syncope with heart block) I45.9
Sperm counts (fertility testing) Z31.41
  postvasectomy Z30.8
  reversal Z31.42
Spermatic cord — *see* condition
Spermatocele N43.40
  congenital Q55.4
  multiple N43.42
  single N43.41
Spermatocystitis N49.0
Spermatocytoma C62.9- ☑
  specified site — *see* Neoplasm, malignant, by site
Spermatorrhea N50.89
Sphacelus — *see* Gangrene
Sphenoidal — *see* condition
Sphenoiditis (chronic) — *see* Sinusitis, sphenoidal
Sphenopalatine ganglion neuralgia G90.09
Sphericity, increased, lens (congenital) Q12.4
Spherocytosis (congenital) (familial) (hereditary) D58.0
  hemoglobin disease D58.0
  sickle-cell (disease) D57.8- ☑
Spherophakia Q12.4
Sphincter — *see* condition
Sphincteritis, sphincter of Oddi — *see* Cholangitis
Sphingolipidosis E75.3
  specified NEC E75.29
Sphingomyelinosis E75.3
Spicule tooth K00.2
Spider
  bite — *see* Toxicity, venom, spider
  fingers — *see* Syndrome, Marfan's
  nevus I78.1
  toes — *see* Syndrome, Marfan's
  vascular I78.1
Spiegler-Fendt
  benign lymphocytoma L98.8
  sarcoid L08.89
Spielmeyer-Vogt disease E75.4
Spina bifida (aperta) Q05.9
  with hydrocephalus NEC Q05.4
  cervical Q05.5
    with hydrocephalus Q05.0
  dorsal Q05.6
    with hydrocephalus Q05.1
  lumbar Q05.7
    with hydrocephalus Q05.2
  lumbosacral Q05.7
    with hydrocephalus Q05.2
  occulta Q76.0
  sacral Q05.8
    with hydrocephalus Q05.3
  thoracic Q05.6
    with hydrocephalus Q05.1
  thoracolumbar Q05.6
    with hydrocephalus Q05.1
Spindle, Krukenberg's — *see* Pigmentation, cornea, posterior
Spine, spinal — *see* condition
Spiradenoma (eccrine) — *see* Neoplasm, skin, benign
Spirillosis A25.0
Spirillum
  minus A25.0
  obermeieri infection A68.0
Spirochetal — *see* condition
Spirochetosis A69.9
  arthritic, arthritica A69.9
  bronchopulmonary A69.8
  icterohemorrhagic A27.0
  lung A69.8
Spirometrosis B70.1
Spitting blood — *see* Hemoptysis
Splanchnoptosis K63.4

Spleen, splenic — *see* condition
Splenectasis — *see* Splenomegaly
Splenitis (interstitial) (malignant) (nonspecific) D73.89
  malarial — *see also* Malaria B54 *[D77]*
  tuberculous A18.85
Splenocele D73.89
Splenomegaly, splenomegalia (Bengal) (cryptogenic)
    (idiopathic) (tropical) R16.1
  with hepatomegaly R16.2
  cirrhotic D73.2
  congenital Q89.09
  congestive, chronic D73.2
  Egyptian B65.1
  Gaucher's E75.22
  malarial — *see also* Malaria B54 *[D77]*
  neutropenic D73.81
  Niemann-Pick — *see* Niemann-Pick disease or syn-
    drome
  siderotic D73.2
  syphilitic A52.79
    congenital (early) A50.08 *[D77]*
Splenopathy D73.9
Splenoptosis D73.89
Splenosis D73.89
Splinter — *see* Foreign body, superficial, by site
Split, splitting
  foot Q72.7- ☑
  hand Q71.6 ☑
  heart sounds R01.2
  lip, congenital — *see* Cleft, lip
  nails L60.3
  urinary stream R39.13
Spondylarthrosis — *see* Spondylosis
Spondylitis (chronic) — *see also* Spondylopathy, inflam-
    matory
  ankylopoietica — *see* Spondylitis, ankylosing
  ankylosing (chronic) M45.9
    with lung involvement M45.9 *[J99]*
    cervical region M45.2
    cervicothoracic region M45.3
    juvenile M08.1
    lumbar region M45.6
    lumbosacral region M45.7
    multiple sites M45.0
    occipito-atlanto-axial region M45.1
    sacrococcygeal region M45.8
    thoracic region M45.4
    thoracolumbar region M45.5
  atrophic (ligamentous) — *see* Spondylitis, ankylosing
  deformans (chronic) — *see* Spondylosis
  gonococcal A54.41
  gouty — *see also* Gout, by type, vertebrae M10.08
  in (due to)
    brucellosis A23.9 *[M49.80]*
      cervical region A23.9 *[M49.82]*
      cervicothoracic region A23.9 *[M49.83]*
      lumbar region A23.9 *[M49.86]*
      lumbosacral region A23.9 *[M49.87]*
      multiple sites A23.9 *[M49.89]*
      occipito-atlanto-axial region A23.9 *[M49.81]*
      sacrococcygeal region A23.9 *[M49.88]*
      thoracic region A23.9 *[M49.84]*
      thoracolumbar region A23.9 *[M49.85]*
    enterobacteria — *see also* subcategory M49.8 A04.9
    tuberculosis A18.01
  infectious NEC — *see* Spondylopathy, infective
  juvenile ankylosing (chronic) M08.1
  Kümmell's — *see* Spondylopathy, traumatic
  Marie-Strümpell — *see* Spondylitis, ankylosing
  muscularis — *see* Spondylopathy, specified NEC
  psoriatic L40.53
  rheumatoid — *see* Spondylitis, ankylosing
  rhizomelica — *see* Spondylitis, ankylosing
  sacroiliac NEC M46.1
  senescent, senile — *see* Spondylosis
  traumatic (chronic) or post-traumatic — *see* Spondy-
    lopathy, traumatic
  tuberculous A18.01
  typhosa A01.05
Spondylolisthesis (acquired) (degenerative) M43.10
  with disproportion (fetopelvic) O33.0
    causing obstructed labor O65.0
  cervical region M43.12
  cervicothoracic region M43.13
  congenital Q76.2
  lumbar region M43.16
  lumbosacral region M43.17

Spondylolisthesis — *continued*
  multiple sites M43.19
  occipito-atlanto-axial region M43.11
  sacrococcygeal region M43.18
  thoracic region M43.14
  thoracolumbar region M43.15
  traumatic (old) M43.10
    acute
      fifth cervical (displaced) S12.430 ☑
        nondisplaced S12.431 ☑
        specified type NEC (displaced) S12.450 ☑
          nondisplaced S12.451 ☑
        type III S12.44 ☑
      fourth cervical (displaced) S12.330 ☑
        nondisplaced S12.331 ☑
        specified type NEC (displaced) S12.350 ☑
          nondisplaced S12.351 ☑
        type III S12.34 ☑
      second cervical (displaced) S12.130 ☑
        nondisplaced S12.131 ☑
        specified type NEC (displaced) S12.150 ☑
          nondisplaced S12.151 ☑
        type III S12.14 ☑
      seventh cervical (displaced) S12.630 ☑
        nondisplaced S12.631 ☑
        specified type NEC (displaced) S12.650 ☑
          nondisplaced S12.651 ☑
        type III S12.64 ☑
      sixth cervical (displaced) S12.530 ☑
        nondisplaced S12.531 ☑
        specified type NEC (displaced) S12.550 ☑
          nondisplaced S12.551 ☑
        type III S12.54 ☑
      third cervical (displaced) S12.230 ☑
        nondisplaced S12.231 ☑
        specified type NEC (displaced) S12.250 ☑
          nondisplaced S12.251 ☑
        type III S12.24 ☑
Spondylolysis (acquired) M43.00
  cervical region M43.02
  cervicothoracic region M43.03
  congenital Q76.2
  lumbar region M43.06
  lumbosacral region M43.07
    with disproportion (fetopelvic) O33.0
      causing obstructed labor O65.8
  multiple sites M43.09
  occipito-atlanto-axial region M43.01
  sacrococcygeal region M43.08
  thoracic region M43.04
  thoracolumbar region M43.05
Spondylopathy M48.9
  infective NEC M46.50
    cervical region M46.52
    cervicothoracic region M46.53
    lumbar region M46.56
    lumbosacral region M46.57
    multiple sites M46.59
    occipito-atlanto-axial region M46.51
    sacrococcygeal region M46.58
    thoracic region M46.54
    thoracolumbar region M46.55
  inflammatory M46.90
    cervical region M46.92
    cervicothoracic region M46.93
    lumbar region M46.96
    lumbosacral region M46.97
    multiple sites M46.99
    occipito-atlanto-axial region M46.91
    sacrococcygeal region M46.98
    specified type NEC M46.80
      cervical region M46.82
      cervicothoracic region M46.83
      lumbar region M46.86
      lumbosacral region M46.87
      multiple sites M46.89
      occipito-atlanto-axial region M46.81
      sacrococcygeal region M46.88
      thoracic region M46.84
      thoracolumbar region M46.85
    thoracic region M46.94
    thoracolumbar region M46.95
  neuropathic, in
    syringomyelia and syringobulbia G95.0
    tabes dorsalis A52.11
  specified NEC — *see* subcategory M48.8 ☑
  traumatic M48.30

Spondylopathy — *continued*
  traumatic — *continued*
    cervical region M48.32
    cervicothoracic region M48.33
    lumbar region M48.36
    lumbosacral region M48.37
    occipito-atlanto-axial region M48.31
    sacrococcygeal region M48.38
    thoracic region M48.34
    thoracolumbar region M48.35
Spondylosis M47.9
  with
    disproportion (fetopelvic) O33.0
      causing obstructed labor O65.0
    myelopathy NEC M47.10
      cervical region M47.12
      cervicothoracic region M47.13
      lumbar region M47.16
      occipito-atlanto-axial region M47.11
      thoracic region M47.14
      thoracolumbar region M47.15
    radiculopathy M47.20
      cervical region M47.22
      cervicothoracic region M47.23
      lumbar region M47.26
      lumbosacral region M47.27
      occipito-atlanto-axial region M47.21
      sacrococcygeal region M47.28
      thoracic region M47.24
      thoracolumbar region M47.25
  specified NEC M47.899
    cervical region M47.892
    cervicothoracic region M47.893
    lumbar region M47.896
    lumbosacral region M47.897
    occipito-atlanto-axial region M47.891
    sacrococcygeal region M47.898
    thoracic region M47.894
    thoracolumbar region M47.895
  traumatic — *see* Spondylopathy, traumatic
  without myelopathy or radiculopathy M47.819
    cervical region M47.812
    cervicothoracic region M47.813
    lumbar region M47.816
    lumbosacral region M47.817
    occipito-atlanto-axial region M47.811
    sacrococcygeal region M47.818
    thoracic region M47.814
    thoracolumbar region M47.815
Sponge
  inadvertently left in operation wound — *see* Foreign
    body, accidentally left during a procedure
  kidney (medullary) Q61.5
Sponge-diver's disease — *see* Toxicity, venom, marine
    animal, sea anemone
Spongioblastoma (any type) — *see* Neoplasm, malig-
    nant, by site
  specified site — *see* Neoplasm, malignant, by site
  unspecified site C71.9
Spongioneuroblastoma — *see* Neoplasm, malignant,
    by site
Spontaneous — *see also* condition
  fracture (cause unknown) — *see* Fracture, pathological
Spoon nail L60.3
  congenital Q84.6
Sporadic — *see* condition
Sporothrix schenckii infection — *see* Sporotrichosis
Sporotrichosis B42.9
  arthritis B42.82
  disseminated B42.7
  generalized B42.7
  lymphocutaneous (fixed) (progressive) B42.1
  pulmonary B42.0
  specified NEC B42.89
Spots, spotting (in) (of)
  Bitot's — *see also* Pigmentation, conjunctiva
    in the young child E50.1
    vitamin A deficiency E50.1
  café, au lait L81.3
  Cayenne pepper I78.1
  cotton wool, retina — *see* Occlusion, artery, retina
  de Morgan's (senile angiomas) I78.1
  Fuchs' black (myopic) — *see also* Myopia, degenerative
    H44.2- ☑
  intermenstrual (regular) N92.0
    irregular N92.1
  Koplik's B05.9
  liver L81.4

Spots, spotting — *continued*
  pregnancy O26.85- ☑
  purpuric R23.3
  ruby I78.1
Spotted fever — *see* Fever, spotted N92.3
Sprain (joint) (ligament)
  acromioclavicular joint or ligament S43.5- ☑
  ankle S93.40- ☑
    calcaneofibular ligament S93.41- ☑
    deltoid ligament S93.42- ☑
    internal collateral ligament — *see* Sprain, ankle, specified ligament NEC
    specified ligament NEC S93.49- ☑
    talofibular ligament — *see* Sprain, ankle, specified ligament NEC
    tibiofibular ligament S93.43- ☑
  anterior longitudinal, cervical S13.4 ☑
  atlas, atlanto-axial, atlanto-occipital S13.4 ☑
  breast bone — *see* Sprain, sternum
  calcaneofibular — *see* Sprain, ankle
  carpal — *see* Sprain, wrist
  carpometacarpal — *see* Sprain, hand, specified site NEC
  cartilage
    costal S23.41 ☑
    semilunar (knee) — *see* Sprain, knee, specified site NEC
      with current tear — *see* Tear, meniscus
    thyroid region S13.5 ☑
    xiphoid — *see* Sprain, sternum
  cervical, cervicodorsal, cervicothoracic S13.4 ☑
  chondrosternal S23.421 ☑
  coracoclavicular S43.8- ☑
  coracohumeral S43.41- ☑
  coronary, knee — *see* Sprain, knee, specified site NEC
  costal cartilage S23.41 ☑
  cricoarytenoid articulation or ligament S13.5 ☑
  cricothyroid articulation S13.5 ☑
  cruciate, knee — *see* Sprain, knee, cruciate
  deltoid, ankle — *see* Sprain, ankle
  dorsal (spine) S23.3 ☑
  elbow S53.40- ☑
    radial collateral ligament S53.43- ☑
    radiohumeral S53.41- ☑
    rupture
      radial collateral ligament — *see* Rupture, traumatic, ligament, radial collateral
      ulnar collateral ligament — *see* Rupture, traumatic, ligament, ulnar collateral
    specified type NEC S53.49- ☑
    ulnar collateral ligament S53.44- ☑
    ulnohumeral S53.42- ☑
  femur, head — *see* Sprain, hip
  fibular collateral, knee — *see* Sprain, knee, collateral
  fibulocalcaneal — *see* Sprain, ankle
  finger(s) S63.61- ☑
    index S63.61- ☑
    interphalangeal (joint) S63.63- ☑
      index S63.63- ☑
      little S63.63- ☑
      middle S63.63- ☑
      ring S63.63- ☑
    little S63.61- ☑
    metacarpophalangeal (joint) S63.65- ☑
    middle S63.61- ☑
    ring S63.61- ☑
    specified site NEC S63.69- ☑
      index S63.69- ☑
      little S63.69- ☑
      middle S63.69- ☑
      ring S63.69- ☑
  foot S93.60- ☑
    specified ligament NEC S93.69- ☑
    tarsal ligament S93.61- ☑
    tarsometatarsal ligament S93.62- ☑
    toe — *see* Sprain, toe
  hand S63.9- ☑
    finger — *see* Sprain, finger
    specified site NEC — *see* subcategory S63.8 ☑
    thumb — *see* Sprain, thumb
  head S03.9 ☑
  hip S73.10- ☑
    iliofemoral ligament S73.11- ☑
    ischiocapsular (ligament) S73.12- ☑
    specified NEC S73.19- ☑
  iliofemoral — *see* Sprain, hip

Sprain — *continued*
  innominate
    acetabulum — *see* Sprain, hip
    sacral junction S33.6 ☑
  internal
    collateral, ankle — *see* Sprain, ankle
    semilunar cartilage — *see* Sprain, knee, specified site NEC
  interphalangeal
    finger — *see* Sprain, finger, interphalangeal (joint)
    toe — *see* Sprain, toe, interphalangeal joint
  ischiocapsular — *see* Sprain, hip
  ischiofemoral — *see* Sprain, hip
  jaw (articular disc) (cartilage) (meniscus) S03.4- ☑
    old M26.69
  knee S83.9- ☑
    collateral ligament S83.40- ☑
      lateral (fibular) S83.42- ☑
      medial (tibial) S83.41- ☑
    cruciate ligament S83.50- ☑
      anterior S83.51- ☑
      posterior S83.52- ☑
    lateral (fibular) collateral ligament S83.42- ☑
    medial (tibial) collateral ligament S83.41- ☑
    patellar ligament S76.11- ☑
    specified site NEC S83.8X- ☑
    superior tibiofibular joint (ligament) S83.6- ☑
  lateral collateral, knee — *see* Sprain, knee, collateral
  lumbar (spine) S33.5 ☑
  lumbosacral S33.9 ☑
  mandible (articular disc) S03.4- ☑
    old M26.69
  medial collateral, knee — *see* Sprain, knee, collateral
  meniscus
    jaw S03.4- ☑
      old M26.69
    knee — *see* Sprain, knee, specified site NEC
      with current tear — *see* Tear, meniscus
        old — *see* Derangement, knee, meniscus, due to old tear
    mandible S03.4- ☑
      old M26.69
  metacarpal (distal) (proximal) — *see* Sprain, hand, specified site NEC
  metacarpophalangeal — *see* Sprain, finger, metacarpophalangeal (joint)
  metatarsophalangeal — *see* Sprain, toe, metatarsophalangeal joint
  midcarpal — *see* Sprain, hand, specified site NEC
  midtarsal — *see* Sprain, foot, specified site NEC
  neck S13.9 ☑
    anterior longitudinal cervical ligament S13.4 ☑
    atlanto-axial joint S13.4 ☑
    atlanto-occipital joint S13.4 ☑
    cervical spine S13.4 ☑
    cricoarytenoid ligament S13.5 ☑
    cricothyroid ligament S13.5 ☑
    specified site NEC S13.8 ☑
    thyroid region (cartilage) S13.5 ☑
  nose S03.8 ☑
  orbicular, hip — *see* Sprain, hip
  patella — *see* Sprain, knee, specified site NEC
  patellar ligament S76.11- ☑
  pelvis NEC S33.8 ☑
  phalanx
    finger — *see* Sprain, finger
    toe — *see* Sprain, toe
  pubofemoral — *see* Sprain, hip
  radiocarpal — *see* Sprain, wrist
  radiohumeral — *see* Sprain, elbow
  radius, collateral — *see* Rupture, traumatic, ligament, radial collateral
  rib (cage) S23.41 ☑
  rotator cuff (capsule) S43.42- ☑
  sacroiliac (region)
    chronic or old — *see* subcategory M53.2 ☑
    joint S33.6 ☑
  scaphoid (hand) — *see* Sprain, hand, specified site NEC
  scapula (r) — *see* Sprain, shoulder girdle, specified site NEC
  semilunar cartilage (knee) — *see* Sprain, knee, specified site NEC
    with current tear — *see* Tear, meniscus
      old — *see* Derangement, knee, meniscus, due to old tear
  shoulder joint S43.40- ☑

Sprain — *continued*
  shoulder joint — *continued*
    acromioclavicular joint (ligament) — *see* Sprain, acromioclavicular joint
    blade — *see* Sprain, shoulder, girdle, specified site NEC
    coracoclavicular joint (ligament) — *see* Sprain, coracoclavicular joint
    coracohumeral ligament — *see* Sprain, coracohumeral joint
    girdle S43.9- ☑
      specified site NEC S43.8- ☑
    rotator cuff — *see* Sprain, rotator cuff
    specified site NEC S43.49- ☑
    sternoclavicular joint (ligament) — *see* Sprain, sternoclavicular joint
  spine
    cervical S13.4 ☑
    lumbar S33.5 ☑
    thoracic S23.3 ☑
  sternoclavicular joint S43.6- ☑
  sternum S23.429 ☑
    chondrosternal joint S23.421 ☑
    specified site NEC S23.428 ☑
    sternoclavicular (joint) (ligament) S23.420 ☑
  symphysis
    jaw S03.4- ☑
      old M26.69
    mandibular S03.4- ☑
      old M26.69
  talofibular — *see* Sprain, ankle
  tarsal — *see* Sprain, foot, specified site NEC
  tarsometatarsal — *see* Sprain, foot, specified site NEC
  temporomandibular S03.4- ☑
    old M26.69
  thorax S23.9 ☑
    ribs S23.41 ☑
    specified site NEC S23.8 ☑
    spine S23.3 ☑
    sternum — *see* Sprain, sternum
  thumb S63.60- ☑
    interphalangeal (joint) S63.62- ☑
    metacarpophalangeal (joint) S63.64- ☑
    specified site NEC S63.68- ☑
  thyroid cartilage or region S13.5 ☑
  tibia (proximal end) — *see* Sprain, knee, specified site NEC
  tibial collateral, knee — *see* Sprain, knee, collateral
  tibiofibular
    distal — *see* Sprain, ankle
    superior — *see* Sprain, knee, specified site NEC
  toe(s) S93.50- ☑
    great S93.50- ☑
    interphalangeal joint S93.51- ☑
      great S93.51- ☑
      lesser S93.51- ☑
    lesser S93.50- ☑
    metatarsophalangeal joint S93.52- ☑
      great S93.52- ☑
      lesser S93.52- ☑
  ulna, collateral — *see* Rupture, traumatic, ligament, ulnar collateral
  ulnohumeral — *see* Sprain, elbow
  wrist S63.50- ☑
    carpal S63.51- ☑
    radiocarpal S63.52- ☑
    specified site NEC S63.59- ☑
  xiphoid cartilage — *see* Sprain, sternum
Sprengel's deformity (congenital) Q74.0
Sprue (tropical) K90.1
  celiac K90.0
  idiopathic K90.49
  meaning thrush B37.0
  nontropical K90.0
Spur, bone — *see also* Enthesopathy
  calcaneal M77.3- ☑
  iliac crest M76.2- ☑
  nose (septum) J34.89
Spurway's syndrome Q78.0
Sputum
  abnormal (amount) (color) (odor) (purulent) R09.3
  blood-stained R04.2
  excessive (cause unknown) R09.3
Squamous — *see also* condition
  epithelium in
    cervical canal (congenital) Q51.828

☑ Additional Character Required — Refer to the Tabular List for Character Selection   ▽ Subterms under main terms may continue to next column or page

Squamous — *continued*
  epithelium in — *continued*
    uterine mucosa (congenital) Q51.818
Squashed nose M95.0
  congenital Q67.4
Squeeze, diver's T70.3 ☑
Squint — *see also* Strabismus
  accommodative — *see* Strabismus, convergent concomitant
SSADHD (succinic semialdehyde dehydrogenase deficiency) E72.81
St. Hubert's disease A82.9
Stab — *see also* Laceration
  internal organs — *see* Injury, by site
Stafne's cyst or cavity M27.0
Staggering gait R26.0
  hysterical F44.4
Staghorn calculus — *see* Calculus, kidney
Stähli's line (cornea) (pigment) — *see* Pigmentation, cornea, anterior
Stain, staining
  meconium (newborn) P96.83
  port wine Q82.5
  tooth, teeth (hard tissues) (extrinsic) K03.6
    due to
      accretions K03.6
      deposits (betel) (black) (green) (materia alba) (orange) (soft) (tobacco) K03.6
      metals (copper) (silver) K03.7
      nicotine K03.6
      pulpal bleeding K03.7
      tobacco K03.6
    intrinsic K00.8
Stammering — *see also* Disorder, fluency F80.81
Standstill
  auricular I45.5
  cardiac — *see* Arrest, cardiac
  sinoatrial I45.5
  ventricular — *see* Arrest, cardiac
Stannosis J63.5
Stanton's disease — *see* Melioidosis
Staphylitis (acute) (catarrhal) (chronic) (gangrenous) (membranous) (suppurative) (ulcerative) K12.2
Staphylococcal scalded skin syndrome L00
Staphylococcemia A41.2
Staphylococcus, staphylococcal — *see also* condition
  as cause of disease classified elsewhere B95.8
    aureus (methicillin susceptible) (MSSA) B95.61
      methicillin resistant (MRSA) B95.62
    specified NEC, as cause of disease classified elsewhere B95.7
Staphyloma (sclera)
  cornea H18.72- ☑
  equatorial H15.81- ☑
  localized (anterior) H15.82- ☑
  posticum H15.83- ☑
  ring H15.85- ☑
Stargardt's disease — *see* Dystrophy, retina
Starvation (inanition) (due to lack of food) T73.0 ☑
  edema — *see* Malnutrition, severe
Stasis
  bile (noncalculous) K83.1
  bronchus J98.09
    with infection — *see* Bronchitis
  cardiac — *see* Failure, heart, congestive
  cecum K59.8
  colon K59.8
  dermatitis I87.2
    with
      varicose ulcer — *see* Varix, leg, with ulcer, with inflammation
      varicose veins — *see* Varix, leg, with, inflammation
    due to postthrombotic syndrome — *see* Syndrome, postthrombotic
  duodenal K31.5
  eczema — *see* Varix, leg, with, inflammation
  edema — *see* Hypertension, venous (chronic), idiopathic
  foot T69.0- ☑
  ileocecal coil K59.8
  ileum K59.8
  intestinal K59.8
  jejunum K59.8
  kidney N19
  liver (cirrhotic) K76.1
  lymphatic I89.8

Stasis — *continued*
  pneumonia J18.2
  pulmonary — *see* Edema, lung
  rectal K59.8
  renal N19
    tubular N17.0
  ulcer — *see* Varix, leg, with, with ulcer
    without varicose veins I87.2
  urine — *see* Retention, urine
  venous I87.8
State (of)
  affective and paranoid, mixed, organic psychotic F06.8
  agitated R45.1
    acute reaction to stress F43.0
  anxiety (neurotic) F41.1
  apprehension F41.1
  burn-out Z73.0
  climacteric, female Z78.0
    symptomatic N95.1
  compulsive F42.8
    mixed with obsessional thoughts F42.2
  confusional (psychogenic) F44.89
    acute — *see also* Delirium
      with
        arteriosclerotic dementia F01.50
          with behavioral disturbance F01.51
        senility or dementia F05
      alcoholic F10.231
    epileptic F05
    reactive (from emotional stress, psychological trauma) F44.89
    subacute — *see* Delirium
  convulsive — *see* Convulsions
  crisis F43.0
  depressive F32.9
    neurotic F34.1
  dissociative F44.9
  emotional shock (stress) R45.7
  hypercoagulation — *see* Hypercoagulable
  locked-in G83.5
  menopausal Z78.0
    symptomatic N95.1
  neurotic F48.9
    with depersonalization F48.1
  obsessional F42.8
  oneiroid (schizophrenia-like) F23
  organic
    hallucinatory (nonalcoholic) F06.0
    paranoid (-hallucinatory) F06.2
  panic F41.0
  paranoid F22
    climacteric F22
    involutional F22
    menopausal F22
    organic F06.2
    senile F03 ☑
    simple F22
  persistent vegetative R40.3
  phobic F40.9
  postleukotomy F07.0
  pregnant
    gestational carrier Z33.3
    incidental Z33.1
  psychogenic, twilight F44.89
  psychopathic (constitutional) F60.2
  psychotic, organic — *see also* Psychosis, organic
    mixed paranoid and affective F06.8
    senile or presenile F03 ☑
    transient NEC F06.8
      with
        depression F06.31
        hallucinations F06.0
  residual schizophrenic F20.5
  restlessness R45.1
  stress (emotional) R45.7
  tension (mental) F48.9
    specified NEC F48.8
  transient organic psychotic NEC F06.8
    depressive type F06.31
    hallucinatory type F06.0
  twilight
    epileptic F05
    psychogenic F44.89
  vegetative, persistent R40.3
  vital exhaustion Z73.0
  withdrawal, — *see* Withdrawal, state
Status (post) — *see also* Presence (of)

Status — *continued*
  absence, epileptic — *see* Epilepsy, by type, with status epilepticus
  administration of tPA (rtPA) in a different facility within the last 24 hours prior to admission to current facility Z92.82
  adrenalectomy (unilateral) (bilateral) E89.6
  anastomosis Z98.0
  anginosus I20.9
  angioplasty (peripheral) Z98.62
    with implant Z95.820
    coronary artery Z98.61
      with implant Z95.5
  aortocoronary bypass Z95.1
  arthrodesis Z98.1
  artificial opening (of) Z93.9
    gastrointestinal tract Z93.4
    specified NEC Z93.8
    urinary tract Z93.6
    vagina Z93.8
  asthmaticus — *see* Asthma, by type, with status asthmaticus
  awaiting organ transplant Z76.82
  bariatric surgery Z98.84
  bed confinement Z74.01
  bleb, filtering (vitreous), after glaucoma surgery Z98.83
  breast implant Z98.82
    removal Z98.86
  cataract extraction Z98.4- ☑
  cholecystectomy Z90.49
  clitorectomy N90.811
    with excision of labia minora N90.812
  colectomy (complete) (partial) Z90.49
  colonization — *see* Carrier (suspected) of
  colostomy Z93.3
  convulsivus idiopathicus — *see* Epilepsy, by type, with status epilepticus
  coronary artery angioplasty — *see* Status, angioplasty, coronary artery
  coronary artery bypass graft Z95.1
  cystectomy (urinary bladder) Z90.6
  cystostomy Z93.50
    appendico-vesicostomy Z93.52
    cutaneous Z93.51
    specified NEC Z93.59
  delinquent immunization Z28.3
  dental Z98.818
    crown Z98.811
    fillings Z98.811
    restoration Z98.811
    sealant Z98.810
    specified NEC Z98.818
  deployment (current) (military) Z56.82
  dialysis (hemodialysis) (peritoneal) Z99.2
  do not resuscitate (DNR) Z66
  donor — *see* Donor
  embedded fragments — *see* Retained, foreign body fragments (type of)
  embedded splinter — *see* Retained, foreign body fragments (type of)
  enterostomy Z93.4
  epileptic, epilepticus — *see also* Epilepsy, by type, with status epilepticus G40.901
  estrogen receptor
    negative Z17.1
    positive Z17.0
  female genital cutting — *see* Female genital mutilation status
  female genital mutilation — *see* Female genital mutilation status
  filtering (vitreous) bleb after glaucoma surgery Z98.83
  gastrectomy (complete) (partial) Z90.3
  gastric banding Z98.84
  gastric bypass for obesity Z98.84
  gastrostomy Z93.1
  human immunodeficiency virus (HIV) infection, asymptomatic Z21
  hysterectomy (complete) (total) Z90.710
    partial (with remaining cervial stump) Z90.711
  ileostomy Z93.2
  implant
    breast Z98.82
  infibulation N90.813
  intestinal bypass Z98.0
  jejunostomy Z93.4
  lapsed immunization schedule Z28.3
  laryngectomy Z90.02
  lymphaticus E32.8

Status — *continued*
  malignancy
    castrate resistant prostate Z19.2
    hormone resistant Z19.2
    hormone sensitive Z19.1
  marmoratus G80.3
  mastectomy (unilateral) (bilateral) Z90.1- ☑
  military deployment status (current) Z56.82
    in theater or in support of military war, peacekeeping and humanitarian operations Z56.82
  nephrectomy (unilateral) (bilateral) Z90.5
  nephrostomy Z93.6
  obesity surgery Z98.84
  oophorectomy
    bilateral Z90.722
    unilateral Z90.721
  organ replacement
    by artificial or mechanical device or prosthesis of
      artery Z95.828
      bladder Z96.0
      blood vessel Z95.828
      breast Z97.8
      eye globe Z97.0
      heart Z95.812
        valve Z95.2
      intestine Z97.8
      joint Z96.60
        hip — *see* Presence, hip joint implant
        knee — *see* Presence, knee joint implant
        specified site NEC Z96.698
      kidney Z97.8
      larynx Z96.3
      lens Z96.1
      limbs — *see* Presence, artificial, limb
      liver Z97.8
      lung Z97.8
      pancreas Z97.8
    by organ transplant (heterologous)(homologous) — *see* Transplant
  pacemaker
    brain Z96.89
    cardiac Z95.0
    specified NEC Z96.89
  pancreatectomy Z90.410
    complete Z90.410
    partial Z90.411
    total Z90.410
  physical restraint Z78.1
  pneumonectomy (complete) (partial) Z90.2
  pneumothorax, therapeutic Z98.3
  postcommotio cerebri F07.81
  postoperative (postprocedural) NEC Z98.890
    breast implant Z98.82
    dental Z98.818
      crown Z98.811
      fillings Z98.811
      restoration Z98.811
      sealant Z98.810
      specified NEC Z98.818
    pneumothorax, therapeutic Z98.3
    uterine scar Z98.891
  postpartum (routine follow-up) Z39.2
    care immediately after delivery Z39.0
  postsurgical (postprocedural) NEC Z98.890
    pneumothorax, therapeutic Z98.3
  pregnancy, incidental Z33.1
  prosthesis coronary angioplasty Z95.5
  pseudophakia Z96.1
  renal dialysis (hemodialysis) (peritoneal) Z99.2
  retained foreign body — *see* Retained, foreign body fragments (type of)
  reversed jejunal transposition (for bypass) Z98.0
  salpingo-oophorectomy
    bilateral Z90.722
    unilateral Z90.721
  sex reassignment surgery status Z87.890
  shunt
    arteriovenous (for dialysis) Z99.2
    cerebrospinal fluid Z98.2
    ventricular (communicating) (for drainage) Z98.2
  splenectomy Z90.81
  thymicolymphaticus E32.8
  thymicus E32.8
  thymolymphaticus E32.8
  thyroidectomy (hypothyroidism) E89.0
  tooth (teeth) extraction — *see also* Absence, teeth, acquired K08.409

Status — *continued*
  tPA (rtPA) administration in a different facility within the last 24 hours prior to admission to current facility Z92.82
  tracheostomy Z93.0
  transplant — *see* Transplant
    organ removed Z98.85
  tubal ligation Z98.51
  underimmunization Z28.3
  ureterostomy Z93.6
  urethrostomy Z93.6
  vagina, artificial Z93.8
  vasectomy Z98.52
  wheelchair confinement Z99.3
Stealing
  child problem F91.8
    in company with others Z72.810
  pathological (compulsive) F63.2
Steam burn — *see* Burn
Steatocystoma multiplex L72.2
Steatohepatitis (nonalcoholic) (NASH) K75.81
Steatoma L72.3
  eyelid (cystic) — *see* Dermatosis, eyelid
    infected — *see* Hordeolum
Steatorrhea (chronic) K90.9
  with lacteal obstruction K90.2
  idiopathic (adult) (infantile) K90.9
  pancreatic K90.3
  primary K90.0
  tropical K90.1
Steatosis E88.89
  heart — *see* Degeneration, myocardial
  kidney N28.89
  liver NEC K76.0
Steele-Richardson-Olszewski disease or syndrome G23.1
Steinbrocker's syndrome G90.8
Steinert's disease G71.11
Stein-Leventhal syndrome E28.2
Stein's syndrome E28.2
STEMI — *see also* Infarct, myocardium, ST elevation I21.3
Stenocardia I20.8
Stenocephaly Q75.8
Stenosis, stenotic (cicatricial) — *see also* Stricture
  ampulla of Vater K83.1
  anus, anal (canal) (sphincter) K62.4
    and rectum K62.4
    congenital Q42.3
      with fistula Q42.2
  aorta (ascending) (supraventricular) (congenital) Q25.1
    arteriosclerotic I70.0
    calcified I70.0
    supravalvular Q25.3
  aortic (valve) I35.0
    with insufficiency I35.2
    congenital Q23.0
    rheumatic I06.0
      with
        incompetency, insufficiency or regurgitation I06.2
          with mitral (valve) disease I08.0
            with tricuspid (valve) disease I08.3
        mitral (valve) disease I08.0
          with tricuspid (valve) disease I08.3
        tricuspid (valve) disease I08.2
          with mitral (valve) disease I08.3
    specified cause NEC I35.0
    syphilitic A52.03
  aqueduct of Sylvius (congenital) Q03.0
    with spina bifida — *see* Spina bifida, by site, with hydrocephalus
    acquired G91.1
  artery NEC — *see also* Arteriosclerosis I77.1
    celiac I77.4
    cerebral — *see* Occlusion, artery, cerebral
    extremities — *see* Arteriosclerosis, extremities
    precerebral — *see* Occlusion, artery, precerebral
    pulmonary (congenital) Q25.6
      acquired I28.8
    renal I70.1
    stent
      coronary T82.855 ☑
      peripheral T82.856 ☑
  bile duct (common) (hepatic) K83.1
    congenital Q44.3
  bladder-neck (acquired) N32.0
    congenital Q64.31
  brain G93.89

Stenosis, stenotic — *continued*
  bronchus J98.09
    congenital Q32.3
    syphilitic A52.72
  cardia (stomach) K22.2
    congenital Q39.3
  cardiovascular — *see* Disease, cardiovascular
  caudal M48.08
  cervix, cervical (canal) N88.2
    congenital Q51.828
    in pregnancy or childbirth — *see* Pregnancy, complicated by, abnormal cervix
  colon — *see also* Obstruction, intestine
    congenital Q42.9
      specified NEC Q42.8
  colostomy K94.03
  common (bile) duct K83.1
    congenital Q44.3
  coronary (artery) — *see* Disease, heart, ischemic, atherosclerotic
  cystic duct — *see* Obstruction, gallbladder
  due to presence of device, implant or graft — *see also* Complications, by site and type, specified NEC T85.858 ☑
    arterial graft NEC T82.858 ☑
    breast (implant) T85.858 ☑
    catheter T85.858 ☑
      dialysis (renal) T82.858 ☑
        intraperitoneal T85.858 ☑
      infusion NEC T82.858 ☑
        spinal (epidural) (subdural) T85.850 ☑
      urinary (indwelling) T83.85 ☑
    fixation, internal (orthopedic) NEC T84.85 ☑
    gastrointestinal (bile duct) (esophagus) T85.858 ☑
    genital NEC T83.85 ☑
    heart NEC T82.857 ☑
    joint prosthesis T84.85 ☑
    ocular (corneal graft) (orbital implant) NEC T85.858 ☑
    orthopedic NEC T84.85 ☑
    specified NEC T85.858 ☑
    urinary NEC T83.85 ☑
    vascular NEC T82.858 ☑
    ventricular intracranial shunt T85.850 ☑
  duodenum K31.5
    congenital Q41.0
  ejaculatory duct NEC N50.89
    stent
      vascular
        end stent
          adjacent to stent — *see* Arteriosclerosis
          within the stent
            coronary T82.855 ☑
            peripheral T82.856 ☑
        in stent
          coronary vessel T82.855 ☑
          peripheral vessel T82.856 ☑
  endocervical os — *see* Stenosis, cervix
  enterostomy K94.13
  esophagus K22.2
    congenital Q39.3
    syphilitic A52.79
      congenital A50.59 *[K23]*
  eustachian tube — *see* Obstruction, eustachian tube
  external ear canal (acquired) H61.30- ☑
    congenital Q16.1
    due to
      inflammation H61.32- ☑
      trauma H61.31- ☑
    postprocedural H95.81- ☑
    specified cause NEC H61.39- ☑
  gallbladder — *see* Obstruction, gallbladder
  glottis J38.6
  heart valve (congenital) Q24.8
    aortic Q23.0
    mitral Q23.2
    pulmonary Q22.1
    tricuspid Q22.4
  hepatic duct K83.1
  hymen N89.6
  hypertrophic subaortic (idiopathic) I42.1
  ileum — *see also* Obstruction, intestine, specified NEC K56.699
    congenital Q41.2
  infundibulum cardia Q24.3
  intervertebral foramina — *see also* Lesion, biomechanical, specified NEC

☑ **Additional Character Required** — Refer to the Tabular List for Character Selection   ▽ **Subterms under main terms may continue to next column or page**

Stenosis, stenotic — *continued*
  intervertebral foramina — *see also* Lesion, biomechan-
    ical, specified — *continued*
    connective tissue M99.79
      abdomen M99.79
      cervical region M99.71
      cervicothoracic M99.71
      head region M99.70
      lumbar region M99.73
      lumbosacral M99.73
      occipitocervical M99.70
      sacral region M99.74
      sacrococcygeal M99.74
      sacroiliac M99.74
      specified NEC M99.79
      thoracic region M99.72
      thoracolumbar M99.72
    disc M99.79
      abdomen M99.79
      cervical region M99.71
      cervicothoracic M99.71
      head region M99.70
      lower extremity M99.76
      lumbar region M99.73
      lumbosacral M99.73
      occipitocervical M99.70
      pelvic M99.75
      rib cage M99.78
      sacral region M99.74
      sacrococcygeal M99.74
      sacroiliac M99.74
      specified NEC M99.79
      thoracic region M99.72
      thoracolumbar M99.72
      upper extremity M99.77
    osseous M99.69
      abdomen M99.69
      cervical region M99.61
      cervicothoracic M99.61
      head region M99.60
      lower extremity M99.66
      lumbar region M99.63
      lumbosacral M99.63
      occipitocervical M99.60
      pelvic M99.65
      rib cage M99.68
      sacral region M99.64
      sacrococcygeal M99.64
      sacroiliac M99.64
      specified NEC M99.69
      thoracic region M99.62
      thoracolumbar M99.62
      upper extremity M99.67
    subluxation — *see* Stenosis, intervertebral foramina,
      osseous
  intestine — *see also* Obstruction, intestine
    congenital (small) Q41.9
      large Q42.9
        specified NEC Q42.8
      specified NEC Q41.8
    jejunum — *see also* Obstruction, intestine, specified
      NEC K56.699
    congenital Q41.1
  lacrimal (passage)
    canaliculi H04.54- ☑
    congenital Q10.5
    duct H04.55- ☑
    punctum H04.56- ☑
    sac H04.57- ☑
  lacrimonasal duct — *see* Stenosis, lacrimal, duct
    congenital Q10.5
  larynx J38.6
    congenital NEC Q31.8
      subglottic Q31.1
    syphilitic A52.73
      congenital A50.59 [J99]
  mitral (chronic) (inactive) (valve) I05.0
    with
      aortic valve disease I08.0
      incompetency, insufficiency or regurgitation
        I05.2
    active or acute I01.1
      with rheumatic or Sydenham's chorea I02.0
    congenital Q23.2
    specified cause, except rheumatic I34.2
    syphilitic A52.03
  myocardium, myocardial — *see also* Degeneration,
    myocardial

Stenosis, stenotic — *continued*
  myocardium, myocardial — *see also* Degeneration,
    myocardial
    hypertrophic subaortic (idiopathic) I42.1
  nares (anterior) (posterior) J34.89
    congenital Q30.0
  nasal duct — *see* Stenosis, lacrimal, duct
    congenital Q10.5
  nasolacrimal duct — *see also* Stenosis, lacrimal, duct
    congenital Q10.5
  neural canal — *see also* Lesion, biomechanical, speci-
    fied NEC
    connective tissue M99.49
      abdomen M99.49
      cervical region M99.41
      cervicothoracic M99.41
      head region M99.40
      lower extremity M99.46
      lumbar region M99.43
      lumbosacral M99.43
      occipitocervical M99.40
      pelvic M99.45
      rib cage M99.48
      sacral region M99.44
      sacrococcygeal M99.44
      sacroiliac M99.44
      specified NEC M99.49
      thoracic region M99.42
      thoracolumbar M99.42
      upper extremity M99.47
    intervertebral disc M99.59
      abdomen M99.59
      cervical region M99.51
      cervicothoracic M99.51
      head region M99.50
      lower extremity M99.56
      lumbar region M99.53
      lumbosacral M99.53
      occipitocervical M99.50
      pelvic M99.55
      rib cage M99.58
      sacral region M99.54
      sacrococcygeal M99.54
      sacroiliac M99.54
      specified NEC M99.59
      thoracic region M99.52
      thoracolumbar M99.52
      upper extremity M99.57
    osseous M99.39
      abdomen M99.39
      cervical region M99.31
      cervicothoracic M99.31
      head region M99.30
      lower extremity M99.36
      lumbar region M99.33
      lumbosacral M99.33
      occipitocervical M99.30
      pelvic M99.35
      rib cage M99.38
      sacral region M99.34
      sacrococcygeal M99.34
      sacroiliac M99.34
      specified NEC M99.39
      thoracic region M99.32
      thoracolumbar M99.32
      upper extremity M99.37
    subluxation M99.29
      cervical region M99.21
      cervicothoracic M99.21
      head region M99.20
      lower extremity M99.26
      lumbar region M99.23
      lumbosacral M99.23
      occipitocervical M99.20
      pelvic M99.25
      rib cage M99.28
      sacral region M99.24
      sacrococcygeal M99.24
      sacroiliac M99.24
      specified NEC M99.29
      thoracic region M99.22
      thoracolumbar M99.22
      upper extremity M99.27
  organ or site, congenital NEC — *see* Atresia, by site
  papilla of Vater K83.1
  pulmonary (artery) (congenital) Q25.6
    with ventricular septal defect, transposition of aorta,
      and hypertrophy of right ventricle Q21.3
    acquired I28.8

Stenosis, stenotic — *continued*
  pulmonary — *continued*
    in tetralogy of Fallot Q21.3
    infundibular Q24.3
    subvalvular Q24.3
    supravalvular Q25.6
    valve I37.0
      with insufficiency I37.2
      congenital Q22.1
      rheumatic I09.89
        with aortic, mitral or tricuspid (valve) disease
          I08.8
    vein, acquired I28.8
    vessel NEC I28.8
  pulmonic (congenital) Q22.1
    infundibular Q24.3
    subvalvular Q24.3
  pylorus (hypertrophic) (acquired) K31.1
    adult K31.1
    congenital Q40.0
    infantile Q40.0
  rectum (sphincter) — *see* Stricture, rectum
  renal artery I70.1
    congenital Q27.1
  salivary duct (any) K11.8
  sphincter of Oddi K83.1
  spinal M48.00
    cervical region M48.02
    cervicothoracic region M48.03
    lumbar region (NOS) (without neurogenic claudica-
      tion) M48.061
      with neurogenic claudication M48.062
    lumbosacral region M48.07
    occipito-atlanto-axial region M48.01
    sacrococcygeal region M48.08
    thoracic region M48.04
    thoracolumbar region M48.05
  stomach, hourglass K31.2
  subaortic (congenital) Q24.4
    hypertrophic (idiopathic) I42.1
  subglottic J38.6
    congenital Q31.1
    postprocedural J95.5
  trachea J39.8
    congenital Q32.1
    syphilitic A52.73
    tuberculous NEC A15.5
  tracheostomy J95.03
  tricuspid (valve) I07.0
    with
      aortic (valve) disease I08.2
      incompetency, insufficiency or regurgitation
        I07.2
        with aortic (valve) disease I08.2
          with mitral (valve) disease I08.3
        mitral (valve) disease I08.1
          with aortic (valve) disease I08.3
    congenital Q22.4
    nonrheumatic I36.0
      with insufficiency I36.2
  tubal N97.1
  ureter — *see* Atresia, ureter
  ureteropelvic junction, congenital Q62.11
  ureterovesical orifice, congenital Q62.12
  urethra (valve) *see also* Stricture, urethra
    congenital Q64.32
  urinary meatus, congenital Q64.33
  vagina N89.5
    congenital Q52.4
    in pregnancy — *see* Pregnancy, complicated by,
      abnormal vagina
      causing obstructed labor O65.5
  valve (cardiac) (heart) — *see also* Endocarditis I38
    congenital Q24.8
      aortic Q23.0
      mitral Q23.2
      pulmonary Q22.1
      tricuspid Q22.4
  vena cava (inferior) (superior) I87.1
    congenital Q26.0
  vesicourethral orifice Q64.31
  vulva N90.5
Stent jail T82.897 ☑
Stercolith (impaction) K56.41
  appendix K38.1
Stercoraceous, stercoral ulcer K63.3
  anus or rectum K62.6
Stereotypies NEC F98.4

Sterility — *see* Infertility
Sterilization — *see* Encounter (for), sterilization
Sternalgia — *see* Angina
Sternopagus Q89.4
Sternum bifidum Q76.7
Steroid
  effects (adverse) (adrenocortical) (iatrogenic)
    cushingoid E24.2
      correct substance properly administered — *see* Table of Drugs and Chemicals, by drug, adverse effect
      overdose or wrong substance given or taken — *see* Table of Drugs and Chemicals, by drug, poisoning
    diabetes — *see* subcategory E09 ☑
      correct substance properly administered — *see* Table of Drugs and Chemicals, by drug, adverse effect
      overdose or wrong substance given or taken — *see* Table of Drugs and Chemicals, by drug, poisoning
    fever R50.2
    insufficiency E27.3
      correct substance properly administered — *see* Table of Drugs and Chemicals, by drug, adverse effect
      overdose or wrong substance given or taken — *see* Table of Drugs and Chemicals, by drug, poisoning
    responder H40.04- ☑
Stevens-Johnson disease or syndrome L51.1
  toxic epidermal necrolysis overlap L51.3
Stewart-Morel syndrome M85.2
Sticker's disease B08.3
Sticky eye — *see* Conjunctivitis, acute, mucopurulent
Stieda's disease — *see* Bursitis, tibial collateral
Stiff neck — *see* Torticollis
Stiff-man syndrome G25.82
Stiffness, joint NEC M25.60
  ankle M25.67- ☑
  ankylosis — *see* Ankylosis, joint
  contracture — *see* Contraction, joint
  elbow M25.62- ☑
  foot M25.67- ☑
  hand M25.64- ☑
  hip M25.65- ☑
  knee M25.66- ☑
  shoulder M25.61- ☑
  wrist M25.63- ☑
Stigmata congenital syphilis A50.59
Stillbirth P95
Still-Felty syndrome — *see* Felty's syndrome
Still's disease or syndrome (juvenile) M08.20
  adult-onset M06.1
  ankle M08.27- ☑
  elbow M08.22- ☑
  foot joint M08.27- ☑
  hand joint M08.24- ☑
  hip M08.25- ☑
  knee M08.26- ☑
  multiple site M08.29
  shoulder M08.21- ☑
  vertebra M08.28
  wrist M08.23- ☑
Stimulation, ovary E28.1
Sting (venomous) (with allergic or anaphylactic shock) — *see* Table of Drugs and Chemicals, by animal or substance, poisoning
Stippled epiphyses Q78.8
Stitch
  abscess T81.41 ☑
  burst (in operation wound) — *see* Disruption, wound, operation
Stokes' disease E05.00
  with thyroid storm E05.01
Stokes-Adams disease or syndrome I45.9
Stokvis (-Talma) **disease** D74.8
Stoma malfunction
  colostomy K94.03
  enterostomy K94.13
  gastrostomy K94.23
  ileostomy K94.13
  tracheostomy J95.03
Stomach — *see* condition
Stomatitis (denture) (ulcerative) K12.1
  angular K13.0
    due to dietary or vitamin deficiency E53.0

Stomatitis — *continued*
  aphthous K12.0
  bovine B08.61
  candidal B37.0
  catarrhal K12.1
  diphtheritic A36.89
  due to
    dietary deficiency E53.0
    thrush B37.0
    vitamin deficiency
      B group NEC E53.9
      B2 (riboflavin) E53.0
  epidemic B08.8
  epizootic B08.8
  follicular K12.1
  gangrenous A69.0
  Geotrichum B48.3
  herpesviral, herpetic B00.2
  herpetiformis K12.0
  malignant K12.1
  membranous acute K12.1
  monilial B37.0
  mycotic B37.0
  necrotizing ulcerative A69.0
  parasitic B37.0
  septic K12.1
  spirochetal A69.1
  suppurative (acute) K12.2
  ulceromembranous A69.1
  vesicular K12.1
    with exanthem (enteroviral) B08.4
    virus disease A93.8
  Vincent's A69.1
Stomatocytosis D58.8
Stomatomycosis B37.0
Stomatorrhagia K13.79
Stone(s) — *see also* Calculus
  bladder (diverticulum) N21.0
  cystine E72.09
  heart syndrome I50.1
  kidney N20.0
  prostate N42.0
  pulpal (dental) K04.2
  renal N20.0
  salivary gland or duct (any) K11.5
  urethra (impacted) N21.1
  urinary (duct) (impacted) (passage) N20.9
    bladder (diverticulum) N21.0
    lower tract N21.9
    specified NEC N21.8
  xanthine E79.8 *[N22]*
Stonecutter's lung J62.8
Stonemason's asthma, disease, lung or pneumoconiosis J62.8
Stoppage
  heart — *see* Arrest, cardiac
  urine — *see* Retention, urine
Storm, thyroid — *see* Thyrotoxicosis
Strabismus (congenital) (nonparalytic) H50.9
  concomitant H50.40
    convergent — *see* Strabismus, convergent concomitant
    divergent — *see* Strabismus, divergent concomitant
  convergent concomitant H50.00
    accommodative component H50.43
    alternating H50.05
      with
        A pattern H50.06
        specified nonconcomitances NEC H50.08
        V pattern H50.07
    monocular H50.01- ☑
      with
        A pattern H50.02- ☑
        specified nonconcomitances NEC H50.04- ☑
        V pattern H50.03- ☑
      intermittent H50.31- ☑
        alternating H50.32
  cyclotropia H50.41 ☑
  divergent concomitant H50.10
    alternating H50.15
      with
        A pattern H50.16
        specified noncomitances NEC H50.18
        V pattern H50.17
    monocular H50.11- ☑
      with
        A pattern H50.12- ☑
        specified noncomitances NEC H50.14- ☑

Strabismus — *continued*
  divergent concomitant — *continued*
    monocular — *continued*
      with — *continued*
        V pattern H50.13- ☑
      intermittent H50.33 ☑
        alternating H50.34
  Duane's syndrome H50.81- ☑
  due to adhesions, scars H50.69
  heterophoria H50.50
    alternating H50.55
    cyclophoria H50.54
    esophoria H50.51
    exophoria H50.52
    vertical H50.53
  heterotropia H50.40
    intermittent H50.30
  hypertropia H50.2- ☑
  hypotropia — *see* Hypertropia
  latent H50.50
  mechanical H50.60
    Brown's sheath syndrome H50.61- ☑
    specified type NEC H50.69
  monofixation syndrome H50.42
  paralytic H49.9
    abducens nerve H49.2- ☑
    fourth nerve H49.1- ☑
    Kearns-Sayre syndrome H49.81- ☑
    ophthalmoplegia (external)
      progressive H49.4- ☑
        with pigmentary retinopathy H49.81- ☑
      total H49.3- ☑
    sixth nerve H49.2- ☑
    specified type NEC H49.88- ☑
    third nerve H49.0- ☑
    trochlear nerve H49.1- ☑
  specified type NEC H50.89
  vertical H50.2- ☑
Strain
  back S39.012 ☑
  cervical S16.1 ☑
  eye NEC — *see* Disturbance, vision, subjective
  heart — *see* Disease, heart
  low back S39.012 ☑
  mental NOS Z73.3
    work-related Z56.6
  muscle (tendon) — *see* Injury, muscle, by site, strain
  neck S16.1 ☑
  physical NOS Z73.3
    work-related Z56.6
  postural — *see also* Disorder, soft tissue, due to use
  psychological NEC Z73.3
  tendon — *see* Injury, muscle, by site, strain
Straining, on urination R39.16
Strand, vitreous — *see* Opacity, vitreous, membranes and strands
Strangulation, strangulated — *see also* Asphyxia, traumatic
  appendix K38.8
  bladder-neck N32.0
  bowel or colon K56.2
  food or foreign body — *see* Foreign body, by site
  hemorrhoids — *see* Hemorrhoids, with complication
  hernia — *see also* Hernia, by site, with obstruction
    with gangrene — *see* Hernia, by site, with gangrene
  intestine (large) (small) K56.2
    with hernia — *see also* Hernia, by site, with obstruction
      with gangrene — *see* Hernia, by site, with gangrene
  mesentery K56.2
  mucus — *see* Asphyxia, mucus
  omentum K56.2
  organ or site, congenital NEC — *see* Atresia, by site
  ovary — *see* Torsion, ovary
  penis N48.89
    foreign body T19.4 ☑
  rupture — *see* Hernia, by site, with obstruction
  stomach due to hernia — *see also* Hernia, by site, with obstruction
    with gangrene — *see* Hernia, by site, with gangrene
  vesicourethral orifice N32.0
Strangury R30.0
Straw itch B88.0
Strawberry
  gallbladder K82.4
  mark Q82.5

☑ **Additional Character Required** — **Refer to the Tabular List for Character Selection**　　▼ **Subterms under main terms may continue to next column or page**

Strawberry — *continued*
  tongue (red) (white) K14.3
Streak(s)
  macula, angioid H35.33
  ovarian Q50.32
Strephosymbolia F81.0
  secondary to organic lesion R48.8
Streptobacillary fever A25.1
Streptobacillosis A25.1
Streptobacillus moniliformis A25.1
Streptococcus, streptococcal — *see also* condition
  as cause of disease classified elsewhere B95.5
  group
      A, as cause of disease classified elsewhere B95.0
      B, as cause of disease classified elsewhere B95.1
      D, as cause of disease classified elsewhere B95.2
  pneumoniae, as cause of disease classified elsewhere
      B95.3
  specified NEC, as cause of disease classified elsewhere
      B95.4
Streptomycosis B47.1
Streptotrichosis A48.8
Stress F43.9
  family — *see* Disruption, family
  fetal P84
      complicating pregnancy O77.9
          due to drug administration O77.1
  mental NEC Z73.3
      work-related Z56.6
  physical NEC Z73.3
      work-related Z56.6
  polycythemia D75.1
  reaction — *see also* Reaction, stress F43.9
  work schedule Z56.3
Stretching, nerve — *see* Injury, nerve
Striae albicantes, atrophicae or distensae (cutis) L90.6
Stricture — *see also* Stenosis
  ampulla of Vater K83.1
  anus (sphincter) K62.4
      congenital Q42.3
          with fistula Q42.2
      infantile Q42.3
          with fistula Q42.2
  aorta (ascending) (congenital) Q25.1
      arteriosclerotic I70.0
      calcified I70.0
      supravalvular, congenital Q25.3
  aortic (valve) — *see* Stenosis, aortic
  aqueduct of Sylvius (congenital) Q03.0
      with spina bifida — *see* Spina bifida, by site, with
          hydrocephalus
      acquired G91.1
  artery I77.1
      basilar — *see* Occlusion, artery, basilar
      carotid — *see* Occlusion, artery, carotid
      celiac I77.4
      congenital (peripheral) Q27.8
          cerebral Q28.3
          coronary Q24.5
          digestive system Q27.8
          lower limb Q27.8
          retinal Q14.1
          specified site NEC Q27.8
          umbilical Q27.0
          upper limb Q27.8
      coronary — *see* Disease, heart, ischemic,
          atherosclerotic
          congenital Q24.5
      precerebral — *see* Occlusion, artery, precerebral
      pulmonary (congenital) Q25.6
          acquired I28.8
      renal I70.1
      vertebral — *see* Occlusion, artery, vertebral
  auditory canal (external) (congenital)
      acquired — *see* Stenosis, external ear canal
  bile duct (common) (hepatic) K83.1
      congenital Q44.3
      postoperative K91.89
  bladder N32.89
      neck N32.0
  bowel — *see* Obstruction, intestine
  brain G93.89
  bronchus J98.09
      congenital Q32.3
      syphilitic A52.72
  cardia (stomach) K22.2
      congenital Q39.3
  cardiac — *see also* Disease, heart

Stricture — *continued*
  cardiac — *see also* Disease, heart — *continued*
      orifice (stomach) K22.2
  cecum — *see* Obstruction, intestine
  cervix, cervical (canal) N88.2
      congenital Q51.828
      in pregnancy — *see* Pregnancy, complicated by,
          abnormal cervix
          causing obstructed labor O65.5
  colon — *see also* Obstruction, intestine
      congenital Q42.9
      specified NEC Q42.8
  colostomy K94.03
  common (bile) duct K83.1
  coronary (artery) — *see* Disease, heart, ischemic,
      atherosclerotic
  cystic duct — *see* Obstruction, gallbladder
  digestive organs NEC, congenital Q45.8
  duodenum K31.5
      congenital Q41.0
  ear canal (external) (congenital) Q16.1
      acquired — *see* Stricture, auditory canal, acquired
  ejaculatory duct N50.89
  enterostomy K94.13
  esophagus K22.2
      congenital Q39.3
      syphilitic A52.79
          congenital A50.59 *[K23]*
  eustachian tube — *see also* Obstruction, eustachian
      tube
      congenital Q17.8
  fallopian tube N97.1
      gonococcal A54.24
      tuberculous A18.17
  gallbladder — *see* Obstruction, gallbladder
  glottis J38.6
  heart — *see also* Disease, heart
      valve — *see also* Endocarditis I38
          aortic Q23.0
          mitral Q23.2
          pulmonary Q22.1
          tricuspid Q22.4
  hepatic duct K83.1
  hourglass, of stomach K31.2
  hymen N89.6
  hypopharynx J39.2
  ileum — *see also* Obstruction, intestine, specified NEC
      K56.699
      congenital Q41.2
  intestine — *see also* Obstruction, intestine
      congenital (small) Q41.9
          large Q42.9
              specified NEC Q42.8
          specified NEC Q41.8
      ischemic K55.1
  jejunum — *see also* Obstruction, intestine, specified
      NEC K56.699
      congenital Q41.1
  lacrimal passages — *see also* Stenosis, lacrimal
      congenital Q10.5
  larynx J38.6
      congenital NEC Q31.8
          subglottic Q31.1
      syphilitic A52.73
          congenital A50.59 *[J99]*
  meatus
      ear (congenital) Q16.1
          acquired — *see* Stricture, auditory canal, ac-
              quired
      osseous (ear) (congenital) Q16.1
          acquired — *see* Stricture, auditory canal, ac-
              quired
      urinarius — *see also* Stricture, urethra
          congenital Q64.33
  mitral (valve) — *see* Stenosis, mitral
  myocardium, myocardial I51.5
      hypertrophic subaortic (idiopathic) I42.1
  nares (anterior) (posterior) J34.89
      congenital Q30.0
  nasal duct — *see also* Stenosis, lacrimal, duct
      congenital Q10.5
  nasolacrimal duct — *see also* Stenosis, lacrimal, duct
      congenital Q10.5
  nasopharynx J39.2
      syphilitic A52.73
  nose J34.89
      congenital Q30.0
  nostril (anterior) (posterior) J34.89

Stricture — *continued*
  nostril — *continued*
      congenital Q30.0
      syphilitic A52.73
          congenital A50.59 *[J99]*
  organ or site, congenital NEC — *see* Atresia, by site
  os uteri — *see* Stricture, cervix
  osseous meatus (ear) (congenital) Q16.1
      acquired — *see* Stricture, auditory canal, acquired
  oviduct — *see* Stricture, fallopian tube
  pelviureteric junction Q62.11
      acquired, with hydronephrosis N13.0
  penis, by foreign body T19.4 ☑
  pharynx J39.2
  prostate N42.89
  pulmonary, pulmonic
      artery (congenital) Q25.6
          acquired I28.8
          noncongenital I28.8
      infundibulum (congenital) Q24.3
      valve I37.0
          congenital Q22.1
      vein, acquired I28.8
      vessel NEC I28.8
  punctum lacrimale — *see also* Stenosis, lacrimal,
      punctum
      congenital Q10.5
  pylorus (hypertrophic) K31.1
      adult K31.1
      congenital Q40.0
      infantile Q40.0
  rectosigmoid — *see also* Obstruction, intestine, speci-
      fied NEC K56.699
  rectum (sphincter) K62.4
      congenital Q42.1
          with fistula Q42.0
      due to
          chlamydial lymphogranuloma A55
          irradiation K91.89
          lymphogranuloma venereum A55
      gonococcal A54.6
      inflammatory (chlamydial) A55
      syphilitic A52.74
      tuberculous A18.32
  renal artery I70.1
      congenital Q27.1
  salivary duct or gland (any) K11.8
  sigmoid (flexure) — *see* Obstruction, intestine
  spermatic cord N50.89
  stoma (following) (of)
      colostomy K94.03
      enterostomy K94.13
      gastrostomy K94.23
      ileostomy K94.13
      tracheostomy J95.03
  stomach K31.89
      congenital Q40.2
      hourglass K31.2
  subaortic Q24.4
      hypertrophic (acquired) (idiopathic) I42.1
  subglottic J38.6
  syphilitic NEC A52.79
  trachea J39.8
      congenital Q32.1
      syphilitic A52.73
      tuberculous NEC A15.5
  tracheostomy J95.03
  tricuspid (valve) — *see* Stenosis, tricuspid
  tunica vaginalis N50.89
  ureter (postoperative) N13.5
      with
          hydronephrosis N13.1
              with infection N13.6
          pyelonephritis (chronic) N11.1
      congenital — *see* Atresia, ureter
      tuberculous A18.11
  ureteropelvic junction (congenital) Q62.11
      acquired, with hydronephrosis N13.0
  ureterovesical orifice N13.5
      with infection N13.6
  urethra (organic) (spasmodic) — *see also* Stricture,
      urethra, male N35.919
      associated with schistosomiasis B65.0 *[N37]*
      congenital Q64.39
          valvular (posterior) Q64.2
      due to
          infection — *see* Stricture, urethra, postinfective
          trauma — *see* Stricture, urethra, post-traumatic

▽ Subterms under main terms may continue to next column or page   ☑ Additional Character Required — Refer to the Tabular List for Character Selection   **295**

Strawberry — Stricture

Stricture — continued
  urethra — see also Stricture, urethra, male — continued
    female N35.92
    gonococcal, gonorrheal A54.01
    infective NEC — see Stricture, urethra, postinfective
    late effect (sequelae) of injury — see Stricture, urethra, post-traumatic
    male N35.919
      anterior urethra N35.914
      bulbous urethra N35.912
      meatal N35.911
      membranous urethra N35.913
      overlapping sites N35.916
    postcatheterization — see Stricture, urethra, postprocedural
    postinfective NEC
      female N35.12
      male N35.119
        anterior urethra N35.114
        bulbous urethra N35.112
        meatal N35.111
        membranous urethra N35.113
        overlapping sites N35.116
    postobstetric N35.021
    postoperative — see Stricture, urethra, postprocedural
    postprocedural
      female N99.12
      male N99.114
        anterior bulbous urethra N99.113
        bulbous urethra N99.111
        fossa navicularis N99.115
        meatal N99.110
        membranous urethra N99.112
        overlapping sites N99.116
    post-traumatic
      female N35.028
        due to childbirth N35.021
      male N35.014
        anterior urethra N35.013
        bulbous urethra N35.011
        meatal N35.010
        membranous urethra N35.012
        overlapping sites N35.016
    sequela (late effect) of
      childbirth N35.021
      injury — see Stricture, urethra, post-traumatic
    specified cause NEC
      female N35.82
      male N35.819
        anterior urethra N35.814
        bulbous urethra N35.812
        meatal N35.811
        membranous urethra N35.813
        overlapping sites N35.816
    syphilitic A52.76
    traumatic — see Stricture, urethra, post-traumatic
    valvular (posterior), congenital Q64.2
  urinary meatus — see Stricture, urethra
  uterus, uterine (synechiae) N85.6
    os (external) (internal) — see Stricture, cervix
  vagina (outlet) — see Stenosis, vagina
  valve (cardiac) (heart) — see also Endocarditis
    congenital
      aortic Q23.0
      mitral Q23.2
      pulmonary Q22.1
      tricuspid Q22.4
  vas deferens N50.89
    congenital Q55.4
  vein I87.1
  vena cava (inferior) (superior) NEC I87.1
    congenital Q26.0
  vesicourethral orifice N32.0
    congenital Q64.31
  vulva (acquired) N90.5
Stridor R06.1
  congenital (larynx) P28.89
Stridulous — see condition
Stroke (apoplectic) (brain) (embolic) (ischemic) (paralytic) (thrombotic) I63.9
  cryptogenic — see also infarction, cerebral I63.9
  epileptic — see Epilepsy
  heat T67.01 ☑
    exertional T67.02 ☑
    specified NEC T67.09 ☑
  in evolution I63.9

Stroke — continued
  intraoperative
    during cardiac surgery I97.810
    during other surgery I97.811
  lightning — see Lightning
  meaning
    cerebral hemorrhage — code to Hemorrhage, intracranial
    cerebral infarction — code to Infarction, cerebral
  postprocedural
    following cardiac surgery I97.820
    following other surgery I97.821
  sun T67.01 ☑
    specified NEC T67.09 ☑
  unspecified (NOS) I63.9
Stromatosis, endometrial D39.0
Strongyloidiasis, strongyloidosis B78.9
  cutaneous B78.1
  disseminated B78.7
  intestinal B78.0
Strophulus pruriginosus L28.2
Struck by lightning — see Lightning
Struma — see also Goiter
  Hashimoto E06.3
  lymphomatosa E06.3
  nodosa (simplex) E04.9
    endemic E01.2
      multinodular E01.1
    multinodular E04.2
      iodine-deficiency related E01.1
    toxic or with hyperthyroidism E05.20
      with thyroid storm E05.21
      multinodular E05.20
        with thyroid storm E05.21
      uninodular E05.10
        with thyroid storm E05.11
    toxicosa E05.20
      with thyroid storm E05.21
      multinodular E05.20
        with thyroid storm E05.21
      uninodular E05.10
        with thyroid storm E05.11
    uninodular E04.1
  ovarii D27.- ☑
  Riedel's E06.5
Strumipriva cachexia E03.4
Strümpell-Marie spine — see Spondylitis, ankylosing
Strümpell-Westphal pseudosclerosis E83.01
Stuart deficiency disease (factor X) D68.2
Stuart-Prower factor deficiency (factor X) D68.2
Student's elbow — see Bursitis, elbow, olecranon
Stump — see Amputation
Stunting, nutritional E45
Stupor (catatonic) R40.1
  depressive (single episode) F32.89
    recurrent episode F33.8
  dissociative F44.2
  manic F30.2
  manic-depressive F31.89
  psychogenic (anergic) F44.2
  reaction to exceptional stress (transient) F43.0
Sturge (-Weber) (-Dimitri) (-Kalischer) **disease or syndrome** Q85.8
Stuttering F80.81
  adult onset F98.5
  childhood onset F80.81
  following cerebrovascular disease — see Disorder, fluency. following cerebrovascular disease
  in conditions classified elsewhere R47.82
Sty, stye (external) (internal) (meibomian) (zeisian) — see Hordeolum
Subacidity, gastric K31.89
  psychogenic F45.8
Subacute — see condition
Subarachnoid — see condition
Subcortical — see condition
Subcostal syndrome, nerve compression — see Mononeuropathy, upper limb, specified site NEC
Subcutaneous, subcuticular — see condition
Subdural — see condition
Subendocardium — see condition
Subependymoma
  specified site — see Neoplasm, uncertain behavior, by site
  unspecified site D43.2
Suberosis J67.3
Subglossitis — see Glossitis

Subhemophilia D66
Subinvolution
  breast (postlactational) (postpuerperal) N64.89
  puerperal O90.89
  uterus (chronic) (nonpuerperal) N85.3
    puerperal O90.89
Sublingual — see condition
Sublinguitis — see Sialoadenitis
Subluxatable hip Q65.6
Subluxation — see also Dislocation
  acromioclavicular S43.11- ☑
  ankle S93.0- ☑
  atlantoaxial, recurrent M43.4
    with myelopathy M43.3
  carpometacarpal (joint) NEC S63.05- ☑
    thumb S63.04- ☑
  complex, vertebral — see Complex, subluxation
  congenital — see also Malposition, congenital
    hip — see Dislocation, hip, congenital, partial
    joint (excluding hip)
      lower limb Q68.8
      shoulder Q68.8
      upper limb Q68.8
  elbow (traumatic) S53.10- ☑
    anterior S53.11- ☑
    lateral S53.14- ☑
    medial S53.13- ☑
    posterior S53.12- ☑
    specified type NEC S53.19- ☑
  finger S63.20- ☑
    index S63.20- ☑
    interphalangeal S63.22- ☑
      distal S63.24- ☑
        index S63.24- ☑
        little S63.24- ☑
        middle S63.24- ☑
        ring S63.24- ☑
      index S63.22- ☑
      little S63.22- ☑
      middle S63.22- ☑
      proximal S63.23- ☑
        index S63.23- ☑
        little S63.23- ☑
        middle S63.23- ☑
        ring S63.23- ☑
      ring S63.22- ☑
    little S63.20- ☑
    metacarpophalangeal S63.21- ☑
      index S63.21- ☑
      little S63.21- ☑
      middle S63.21- ☑
      ring S63.21- ☑
    middle S63.20- ☑
    ring S63.20- ☑
  foot S93.30- ☑
    specified site NEC S93.33- ☑
    tarsal joint S93.31- ☑
    tarsometatarsal joint S93.32- ☑
    toe — see Subluxation, toe
  hip S73.00- ☑
    anterior S73.03- ☑
      obturator S73.02- ☑
    central S73.04- ☑
    posterior S73.01- ☑
  interphalangeal (joint)
    finger S63.22- ☑
      distal joint S63.24- ☑
        thumb S63.24- ☑
        little S63.24- ☑
        middle S63.24- ☑
        ring S63.24- ☑
      index S63.22- ☑
      little S63.22- ☑
      middle S63.22- ☑
      proximal joint S63.23- ☑
        index S63.23- ☑
        little S63.23- ☑
        middle S63.23- ☑
        ring S63.23- ☑
      ring S63.22- ☑
      thumb S63.12- ☑
    toe S93.13- ☑
      great S93.13- ☑
      lesser S93.13- ☑
  joint prosthesis — see Complications, joint prosthesis, mechanical, displacement, by site

☑ Additional Character Required — Refer to the Tabular List for Character Selection   ▽ Subterms under main terms may continue to next column or page

Subluxation — *continued*
  knee S83.10- ☑
    cap — *see* Subluxation, patella
    patella — *see* Subluxation, patella
    proximal tibia
      anteriorly S83.11- ☑
      laterally S83.14- ☑
      medially S83.13- ☑
      posteriorly S83.12- ☑
      specified type NEC S83.19- ☑
  lens — *see* Dislocation, lens, partial
  ligament, traumatic — *see* Sprain, by site
  metacarpal (bone)
    proximal end S63.06- ☑
  metacarpophalangeal (joint)
    finger S63.21- ☑
      index S63.21- ☑
      little S63.21- ☑
      middle S63.21- ☑
      ring S63.21- ☑
      thumb S63.11- ☑
  metatarsophalangeal joint S93.14- ☑
    great toe S93.14- ☑
    lesser toe S93.14- ☑
  midcarpal (joint) S63.03- ☑
  patella S83.00- ☑
    lateral S83.01- ☑
    recurrent (nontraumatic) — *see* Dislocation, patella,
      recurrent, incomplete
    specified type NEC S83.09- ☑
  pathological — *see* Dislocation, pathological
  radial head S53.00- ☑
    anterior S53.01- ☑
    nursemaid's elbow S53.03- ☑
    posterior S53.02- ☑
    specified type NEC S53.09- ☑
  radiocarpal (joint) S63.02- ☑
  radioulnar (joint)
    distal S63.01- ☑
    proximal — *see* Subluxation, elbow
  shoulder
    congenital Q68.8
    girdle S43.30- ☑
      scapula S43.31- ☑
      specified site NEC S43.39- ☑
    traumatic S43.00- ☑
      anterior S43.01- ☑
      inferior S43.03- ☑
      posterior S43.02- ☑
      specified type NEC S43.08- ☑
  sternoclavicular (joint) S43.20- ☑
    anterior S43.21- ☑
    posterior S43.22- ☑
  symphysis (pubis)
  thumb S63.103 ☑
    interphalangeal joint — *see* Subluxation, interpha-
      langeal (joint), thumb
    metacarpophalangeal joint — *see* Subluxation,
      metacarpophalangeal (joint), thumb
  toe(s) S93.10- ☑
    great S93.10- ☑
      interphalangeal joint S93.13- ☑
      metatarsophalangeal joint S93.14- ☑
    interphalangeal joint S93.13- ☑
    lesser S93.10- ☑
      interphalangeal joint S93.13- ☑
      metatarsophalangeal joint S93.14- ☑
    metatarsophalangeal joint S93.149 ☑
  ulna
    distal end S63.07- ☑
    proximal end — *see* Subluxation, elbow
  ulnohumeral joint — *see* Subluxation, elbow
  vertebral
    recurrent NEC — *see* subcategory M43.5 ☑
    traumatic
      cervical S13.100 ☑
        atlantoaxial joint S13.120 ☑
        atlantooccipital joint S13.110 ☑
        atloidooccipital joint S13.110 ☑
        joint between
          C0 and C1 S13.110 ☑
          C1 and C2 S13.120 ☑
          C2 and C3 S13.130 ☑
          C3 and C4 S13.140 ☑
          C4 and C5 S13.150 ☑
          C5 and C6 S13.160 ☑

Subluxation — *continued*
  vertebral — *continued*
    traumatic — *continued*
      cervical — *continued*
        joint between — *continued*
          C6 and C7 S13.170 ☑
          C7 and T1 S13.180 ☑
          occipitoatloid joint S13.110 ☑
      lumbar S33.100 ☑
        joint between
          L1 and L2 S33.110 ☑
          L2 and L3 S33.120 ☑
          L3 and L4 S33.130 ☑
          L4 and L5 S33.140 ☑
      thoracic S23.100 ☑
        joint between
          T1 and T2 S23.110 ☑
          T2 and T3 S23.120 ☑
          T3 and T4 S23.122 ☑
          T4 and T5 S23.130 ☑
          T5 and T6 S23.132 ☑
          T6 and T7 S23.140 ☑
          T7 and T8 S23.142 ☑
          T8 and T9 S23.150 ☑
          T9 and T10 S23.152 ☑
          T10 and T11 S23.160 ☑
          T11 and T12 S23.162 ☑
          T12 and L1 S23.170 ☑
    wrist (carpal bone) S63.00- ☑
      carpometacarpal joint — *see* Subluxation, car-
        pometacarpal (joint)
      distal radioulnar joint — *see* Subluxation, radioulnar
        (joint), distal
      metacarpal bone, proximal — *see* Subluxation,
        metacarpal (bone), proximal end
      midcarpal — *see* Subluxation, midcarpal (joint)
      radiocarpal joint — *see* Subluxation, radiocarpal
        (joint)
      recurrent — *see* Dislocation, recurrent, wrist
      specified site NEC S63.09- ☑
      ulna — *see* Subluxation, ulna, distal end
Submaxillary — *see* condition
Submersion (fatal) (nonfatal) T75.1 ☑
Submucous — *see* condition
Subnormal, subnormality
  accommodation (old age) H52.4
  mental — *see* Disability, intellectual
  temperature (accidental) T68 ☑
Subphrenic — *see* condition
Subscapular nerve — *see* condition
Subseptus uterus Q51.28
Subsiding appendicitis K36
Substance (other psychoactive) **-induced**
  anxiety disorder F19.980
  bipolar and related disorder F19.94
  delirium F19.921
  depressive disorder F19.94
  major neurocognitive disorder F19.97
  mild neurocognitive disorder F19.988
  obsessive-compulsive and related disorder F19.988
  psychotic disorder F19.959
  sexual dysfunction F19.981
  sleep disorder F19.982
Substernal thyroid E04.9
  congenital Q89.2
Substitution disorder F44.9
Subtentorial — *see* condition
Subthyroidism (acquired) — *see also* Hypothyroidism
  congenital E03.1
Succenturiate placenta O43.19- ☑
Sucking thumb, child (excessive) F98.8
Sudamen, sudamina L74.1
Sudanese kala-azar B55.0
Sudden
  hearing loss — *see* Deafness, sudden
  heart failure — *see* Failure, heart
Sudeck's atrophy, disease, or syndrome — *see* Algo-
  neurodystrophy
Suffocation — *see* Asphyxia, traumatic
Sugar
  blood
    high (transient) R73.9
    low (transient) E16.2
  in urine R81
Suicide, suicidal (attempted) T14.91 ☑
  by poisoning — *see* Table of Drugs and Chemicals
  history of (personal) Z91.5

Suicide, suicidal — *continued*
  history of — *continued*
    in family Z81.8
  ideation — *see* Ideation, suicidal
  risk
    meaning personal history of attempted suicide Z91.5
    meaning suicidal ideation — *see* Ideation, suicidal
  tendencies
    meaning personal history of attempted suicide Z91.5
    meaning suicidal ideation — *see* Ideation, suicidal
  trauma — *see* nature of injury by site
Suipestifer infection — *see* Infection, salmonella
Sulfhemoglobinemia, sulphemoglobinemia (acquired) (with methemoglobinemia) D74.8
Sumatran mite fever A75.3
Summer — *see* condition
Sunburn L55.9
  due to
    tanning bed (acute) L56.8
      chronic L57.8
    ultraviolet radiation (acute) L56.8
      chronic L57.8
  first degree L55.0
  second degree L55.1
  third degree L55.2
SUNCT (short lasting unilateral neuralgiform headache
  with conjunctival injection and tearing) G44.059
  intractable G44.051
  not intractable G44.059
Sundowning F05
Sunken acetabulum — *see* Derangement, joint, specified type NEC, hip
Sunstroke T67.01 ☑
  specified NEC T67.09 ☑
Superfecundation — *see* Pregnancy, multiple
Superfetation — *see* Pregnancy, multiple
Superinvolution (uterus) N85.8
Supernumerary (congenital)
  aortic cusps Q23.8
  auditory ossicles Q16.3
  bone Q79.8
  breast Q83.1
  carpal bones Q74.0
  cusps, heart valve NEC Q24.8
    aortic Q23.8
    mitral Q23.2
    pulmonary Q22.3
  digit(s) Q69.9
  ear (lobule) Q17.0
  fallopian tube Q50.6
  finger Q69.0
  hymen Q52.4
  kidney Q63.0
  lacrimonasal duct Q10.6
  lobule (ear) Q17.0
  mitral cusps Q23.2
  muscle Q79.8
  nipple(s) Q83.3
  organ or site not listed — *see* Accessory
  ossicles, auditory Q16.3
  ovary Q50.31
  oviduct Q50.6
  pulmonary, pulmonic cusps Q22.3
  rib Q76.6
    cervical or first (syndrome) Q76.5
  roots (of teeth) K00.2
  spleen Q89.09
  tarsal bones Q74.2
  teeth K00.1
  testis Q55.29
  thumb Q69.1
  toe Q69.2
  uterus Q51.28
  vagina Q52.1 ☑
  vertebra Q76.49
Supervision (of)
  contraceptive — *see* Prescription, contraceptives
  dietary (for) Z71.3
    allergy (food) Z71.3
    colitis Z71.3
    diabetes mellitus Z71.3
    food allergy or intolerance Z71.3
    gastritis Z71.3
    hypercholesterolemia Z71.3
    hypoglycemia Z71.3
    intolerance (food) Z71.3
    obesity Z71.3
    specified NEC Z71.3

Supervision — *continued*
healthy infant or child Z76.2
  foundling Z76.1
high-risk pregnancy — *see* Pregnancy, complicated by, high, risk
lactation Z39.1
pregnancy — *see* Pregnancy, supervision of
Supplemental teeth K00.1
Suppression
binocular vision H53.34
lactation O92.5
menstruation N94.89
ovarian secretion E28.39
renal N28.9
urine, urinary secretion R34
Suppuration, suppurative — *see also* condition
accessory sinus (chronic) — *see* Sinusitis
adrenal gland
antrum (chronic) — *see* Sinusitis, maxillary
bladder — *see* Cystitis
brain G06.0
  sequelae G09
breast N61.1
  puerperal, postpartum or gestational — *see* Mastitis, obstetric, purulent
dental periosteum M27.3
ear (middle) — *see also* Otitis, media
  external NEC — *see* Otitis, externa, infective
  internal — *see* subcategory H83.0 ☑
ethmoidal (chronic) (sinus) — *see* Sinusitis, ethmoidal
fallopian tube — *see* Salpingo-oophoritis
frontal (chronic) (sinus) — *see* Sinusitis, frontal
gallbladder (acute) K81.0
gum K05.20
  generalized — *see* Periodontitis, aggressive, generalized
  localized — *see* Periodontitis, aggressive, localized
intracranial G06.0
joint — *see* Arthritis, pyogenic or pyemic
labyrinthine — *see* subcategory H83.0 ☑
lung — *see* Abscess, lung
mammary gland N61.1
  puerperal, postpartum O91.12
    associated with lactation O91.13
maxilla, maxillary M27.2
  sinus (chronic) — *see* Sinusitis, maxillary
muscle — *see* Myositis, infective
nasal sinus (chronic) — *see* Sinusitis
pancreas, acute — *see also* Pancreatitis, acute K85.80
parotid gland — *see* Sialoadenitis
pelvis, pelvic
  female — *see* Disease, pelvis, inflammatory
  male K65.0
pericranial — *see* Osteomyelitis
salivary duct or gland (any) — *see* Sialoadenitis
sinus (accessory) (chronic) (nasal) — *see* Sinusitis
sphenoidal sinus (chronic) — *see* Sinusitis, sphenoidal
thymus (gland) E32.1
thyroid (gland) E06.0
tonsil — *see* Tonsillitis
uterus — *see* Endometritis
Supraeruption of tooth (teeth) M26.34
Supraglottitis J04.30
with obstruction J04.31
Suprarenal (gland) — *see* condition
Suprascapular nerve — *see* condition
Suprasellar — *see* condition
Surfer's knots or nodules S89.8- ☑
Surgical
emphysema T81.82 ☑
procedures, complication or misadventure — *see* Complications, surgical procedures
shock T81.10 ☑
Surveillance (of) (for) — *see also* Observation
alcohol abuse Z71.41
contraceptive — *see* Prescription, contraceptives
dietary Z71.3
drug abuse Z71.51
Susceptibility to disease, genetic Z15.89
malignant neoplasm Z15.09
  breast Z15.01
  endometrium Z15.04
  ovary Z15.02
  prostate Z15.03
  specified NEC Z15.09
multiple endocrine neoplasia Z15.81

Suspected condition, ruled out — *see also* Observation, suspected
amniotic cavity and membrane Z03.71
cervical shortening Z03.75
fetal anomaly Z03.73
fetal growth Z03.74
maternal and fetal conditions NEC Z03.79
newborn — *see also* Observation, newborn, suspected condition ruled out Z05.9
oligohydramnios Z03.71
placental problem Z03.72
polyhydramnios Z03.71
Suspended uterus
in pregnancy or childbirth — *see* Pregnancy, complicated by, abnormal uterus
Sutton's nevus D22.9
Suture
burst (in operation wound) T81.31 ☑
  external operation wound T81.31 ☑
  internal operation wound T81.32 ☑
inadvertently left in operation wound — *see* Foreign body, accidentally left during a procedure
removal Z48.02
Swab inadvertently left in operation wound — *see* Foreign body, accidentally left during a procedure
Swallowed, swallowing
difficulty — *see* Dysphagia
foreign body — *see* Foreign body, alimentary tract
Swan-neck deformity (finger) — *see* Deformity, finger, swan-neck
Swearing, compulsive F42.8
in Gilles de la Tourette's syndrome F95.2
Sweat, sweats
fetid L75.0
night R61
Sweating, excessive R61
Sweeley-Klionsky disease E75.21
Sweet's disease or dermatosis L98.2
Swelling (of) R60.9
abdomen, abdominal (not referable to any particular organ) — *see* Mass, abdominal
ankle — *see* Effusion, joint, ankle
arm M79.89
  forearm M79.89
breast — *see also* Lump, breast N63.0
Calabar B74.3
cervical gland R59.0
chest, localized R22.2
ear H93.8- ☑
extremity (lower) (upper) — *see* Disorder, soft tissue, specified type NEC
finger M79.89
foot M79.89
glands R59.9
  generalized R59.1
  localized R59.0
hand M79.89
head (localized) R22.0
inflammatory — *see* Inflammation
intra-abdominal — *see* Mass, abdominal
joint — *see* Effusion, joint
leg M79.89
  lower M79.89
limb — *see* Disorder, soft tissue, specified type NEC
localized (skin) R22.9
  chest R22.2
  head R22.0
  limb
    lower — *see* Mass, localized, limb, lower
    upper — *see* Mass, localized, limb, upper
  neck R22.1
  trunk R22.2
neck (localized) R22.1
pelvic — *see* Mass, abdominal
scrotum N50.89
splenic — *see* Splenomegaly
testis N50.89
toe M79.89
umbilical R19.09
wandering, due to Gnathostoma (spinigerum) B83.1
white — *see* Tuberculosis, arthritis
Swift (-Feer) disease
overdose or wrong substance given or taken — *see* Table of Drugs and Chemicals, by drug, poisoning
Swimmer's
cramp T75.1 ☑
ear H60.33- ☑

Swimmer's — *continued*
itch B65.3
Swimming in the head R42
Swollen — *see* Swelling
Swyer syndrome Q99.1
Sycosis L73.8
barbae (not parasitic) L73.8
contagiosa (mycotic) B35.0
lupoides L73.8
mycotic B35.0
parasitic B35.0
vulgaris L73.8
Sydenham's chorea — *see* Chorea, Sydenham's
Sylvatic yellow fever A95.0
Sylvest's disease B33.0
Symblepharon H11.23- ☑
congenital Q10.3
Symond's syndrome G93.2
Sympathetic — *see* condition
Sympatheticotonia G90.8
Sympathicoblastoma
specified site — *see* Neoplasm, malignant, by site
unspecified site C74.90
Sympathogonioma — *see* Sympathicoblastoma
Symphalangy (fingers) (toes) Q70.9
Symptoms NEC R68.89
breast NEC N64.59
cold J00
development NEC R63.8
factitious, self-induced — *see* Disorder, factitious
genital organs, female R10.2
involving
  abdomen NEC R19.8
  appearance NEC R46.89
  awareness R41.9
    altered mental status R41.82
    amnesia — *see* Amnesia
    borderline intellectual functioning R41.83
    coma — *see* Coma
    disorientation R41.0
    neurologic neglect syndrome R41.4
    senile cognitive decline R41.81
    specified symptom NEC R41.89
  behavior NEC R46.89
  cardiovascular system NEC R09.89
  chest NEC R09.89
  circulatory system NEC R09.89
  cognitive functions R41.9
    altered mental status R41.82
    amnesia — *see* Amnesia
    borderline intellectual functioning R41.83
    coma — *see* Coma
    disorientation R41.0
    neurologic neglect syndrome R41.4
    senile cognitive decline R41.81
    specified symptom NEC R41.89
  development NEC R62.50
  digestive system NEC R19.8
  emotional state NEC R45.89
    emotional lability R45.86
  food and fluid intake R63.8
  general perceptions and sensations R44.9
    specified NEC R44.8
  musculoskeletal system R29.91
    specified NEC R29.898
  nervous system R29.90
    specified NEC R29.818
  pelvis NEC R19.8
  respiratory system NEC R09.89
  skin and integument R23.9
  urinary system R39.9
menopausal N95.1
metabolism NEC R63.8
neurotic F48.8
of infancy R68.19
pelvis NEC, female R10.2
skin and integument NEC R23.9
subcutaneous tissue NEC R23.9
viral cold J00
Sympus Q74.2
Syncephalus Q89.4
Synchondrosis
abnormal (congenital) Q78.8
ischiopubic M91.0
Synchysis (scintillans) (senile) (vitreous body) H43.89
Syncope (near) (pre-) R55
anginosa I20.8
bradycardia R00.1

☑ Additional Character Required — Refer to the Tabular List for Character Selection   ▼ Subterms under main terms may continue to next column or page

Syncope — *continued*
   cardiac R55
   carotid sinus G90.01
   due to spinal (lumbar) puncture G97.1
   heart R55
   heat T67.1 ☑
   laryngeal R05
   psychogenic F48.8
   tussive R05
   vasoconstriction R55
   vasodepressor R55
   vasomotor R55
   vasovagal R55
Syndactylism, syndactyly Q70.9
   complex (with synostosis)
      fingers Q70.0- ☑
      toes Q70.2- ☑
   simple (without synostosis)
      fingers Q70.1- ☑
      toes Q70.3- ☑
Syndrome — *see also* Disease
   5q minus NOS D46.C (*following* D46.2)
   48,XXXX Q97.1
   49,XXXXX Q97.1
   abdominal
      acute R10.0
      muscle deficiency Q79.4
   abnormal innervation H02.519
      left H02.516
         lower H02.515
         upper H02.514
      right H02.513
         lower H02.512
         upper H02.511
   abstinence, neonatal P96.1
   acid pulmonary aspiration, obstetric O74.0
   acquired immunodeficiency — *see* Human, immunod-
         eficiency virus (HIV) disease
   acute abdominal R10.0
   acute respiratory distress (adult) (child) J80
      idiopathic J84.114
   Adair-Dighton Q78.0
   Adams-Stokes (-Morgagni) I45.9
   adiposogenital E23.6
   adrenal
      hemorrhage (meningococcal) A39.1
      meningococcic A39.1
   adrenocortical — *see* Cushing's, syndrome
   adrenogenital E25.9
      congenital, associated with enzyme deficiency E25.0
   afferent loop NEC K91.89
   Alagille's Q44.7
   alcohol withdrawal (without convulsions) — *see* De-
         pendence, alcohol, with, withdrawal
   Alder's D72.0
   Aldrich (-Wiskott) D82.0
   alien hand R41.4
   Alport Q87.81
   alveolar hypoventilation E66.2
   alveolocapillary block J84.10
   amnesic, amnestic (confabulatory) (due to) — *see* Dis-
         order, amnesic
   amyostatic (Wilson's disease) E83.01
   androgen insensitivity E34.50
      complete E34.51
      partial E34.52
   androgen resistance — *see also* Syndrome, androgen
         insensitivity E34.50
   Angelman Q93.51
   anginal — *see* Angina
   ankyloglossia superior Q38.1
   anterior
      chest wall R07.89
      cord G83.82
      spinal artery G95.19
         compression M47.019
            cervical region M47.012
            cervicothoracic region M47.013
            lumbar region M47.016
            occipito-atlanto-axial region M47.011
            thoracic region M47.014
            thoracolumbar region M47.015
      tibial M76.81- ☑
   antibody deficiency D80.9
      agammaglobulinemic D80.1
         hereditary D80.0
      congenital D80.0
      hypogammaglobulinemic D80.1

Syndrome — *continued*
   antibody deficiency — *continued*
      hypogammaglobulinemic — *continued*
         hereditary D80.0
   anticardiolipin (-antibody) D68.61
   antidepressant discontinuation T43.205 ☑
   antiphospholipid (-antibody) D68.61
   aortic
      arch M31.4
      bifurcation I74.09
   aortomesenteric duodenum occlusion K31.5
   apical ballooning (transient left ventricular) I51.81
   arcuate ligament I77.4
   argentaffin, argintaffinoma E34.0
   Arnold-Chiari — *see* Arnold-Chiari disease
   Arrillaga-Ayerza I27.0
   arterial tortuosity Q87.82
   arteriovenous steal T82.898- ☑
   Asherman's N85.6
   aspiration, of newborn — *see* Aspiration, by substance,
         with pneumonia
      meconium P24.01
   ataxia-telangiectasia G11.3
   auriculotemporal G50.8
   autoerythrocyte sensitization (Gardner-Diamond) D69.2
   autoimmune lymphoproliferative [ALPS] D89.82
   autoimmune polyglandular E31.0
   autoinflammatory M04.9
      specified type NEC M04.8
   autosomal — *see* Abnormal, autosomes
   Avellis' G46.8
   Ayerza (-Arrillaga) I27.0
   Babinski-Nageotte G83.89
   Bakwin-Krida Q78.5
   bare lymphocyte D81.6
   Barré-Guillain G61.0
   Barré-Liéou M53.0
   Barrett's — *see* Barrett's, esophagus
   Barsony-Polgar K22.4
   Bársony-Teschendorf K22.4
   Barth E78.71
   Bartter's E26.81
   basal cell nevus Q87.89
   Basedow's E05.00
      with thyroid storm E05.01
   basilar artery G45.0
   Batten-Steinert G71.11
   battered
      baby or child — *see* Maltreatment, child, physical
            abuse
      spouse — *see* Maltreatment, adult, physical abuse
   Beals Q87.40
   Beau's I51.5
   Beck's I65.8
   Benedikt's G46.3
   Béquez César (-Steinbrinck-Chédiak-Higashi) E70.330
   Bernhardt-Roth — *see* Meralgia paresthetica
   Bernheim's — *see* Failure, heart, right
   big spleen D73.1
   Bing-Horton's — *see* Horton's headache
   Birt-Hogg-Dube syndrome Q87.89
   Björck (-Thorsen) E34.0
   black
      lung J60
      widow spider bite — *see* Toxicity, venom, spider,
            black widow
   Blackfan-Diamond D61.01
   Blau M04.8
   blind loop K90.2
      congenital Q43.8
      postsurgical K91.2
   blue sclera Q78.0
   blue toe I75.02- ☑
   Boder-Sedgewick G11.3
   Boerhaave's K22.3
   Borjeson Forssman Lehmann Q89.8
   Bouillaud's I01.9
   Bourneville (-Pringle) Q85.1
   Bouveret (-Hoffman) I47.9
   brachial plexus G54.0
   bradycardia-tachycardia I49.5
   brain (nonpsychotic) F09
      with psychosis, psychotic reaction F09
         acute or subacute — *see* Delirium
      congenital — *see* Disability, intellectual
      organic F09
         post-traumatic (nonpsychotic) F07.81

Syndrome — *continued*
   brain — *continued*
      organic — *continued*
         post-traumatic — *continued*
            psychotic F09
      personality change F07.0
      postcontusional F07.81
      post-traumatic, nonpsychotic F07.81
      psycho-organic F09
      psychotic F06.8
   brain stem stroke G46.3
   Brandt's (acrodermatitis enteropathica) E83.2
   broad ligament laceration N83.8
   Brock's J98.11
   bronze baby P83.88
   Brown-Sequard G83.81
   Brugada I49.8
   bubbly lung P27.0
   Buchem's M85.2
   Budd-Chiari I82.0
   bulbar (progressive) G12.22
   Bürger-Grütz E78.3
   Burke's K86.89
   Burnett's (milk-alkali) E83.52
   burning feet E53.9
   Bywaters' T79.5 ☑
   Call-Fleming I67.841
   carbohydrate-deficient glycoprotein (CDGS) E77.8
   carcinogenic thrombophlebitis I82.1
   carcinoid E34.0
   cardiac asthma I50.1
   cardiacos negros I27.0
   cardiofaciocutaneous Q87.89
   cardiopulmonary-obesity E66.2
   cardiorenal — *see* Hypertension, cardiorenal
   cardiorespiratory distress (idiopathic), newborn P22.0
   cardiovascular renal — *see* Hypertension, cardiorenal
   carotid
      artery (hemispheric) (internal) G45.1
      body G90.01
      sinus G90.01
   carpal tunnel G56.0- ☑
   Cassidy (-Scholte) E34.0
   cat cry Q93.4
   cat eye Q92.8
   cauda equina G83.4
   causalgia — *see* Causalgia
   celiac K90.0
      artery compression I77.4
      axis I77.4
   central pain G89.0
   cerebellar
      hereditary G11.9
      stroke G46.4
   cerebellomedullary malformation — *see* Spina bifida
   cerebral
      artery
         anterior G46.1
         middle G46.0
         posterior G46.2
      gigantism E22.0
   cervical (root) M53.1
      disc — *see* Disorder, disc, cervical, with neuritis
      fusion Q76.1
      posterior, sympathicus M53.0
      rib Q76.5
      sympathetic paralysis G90.2
   cervicobrachial (diffuse) M53.1
   cervicocranial M53.0
   cervicodorsal outlet G54.2
   cervicothoracic outlet G54.0
   Céstan (-Raymond) I65.8
   Charcot's (angina cruris) (intermittent claudication)
         I73.9
   Charcot-Weiss-Baker G90.09
   CHARGE Q89.8
   Chédiak-Higashi (-Steinbrinck) E70.330
   chest wall R07.1
   Chiari's (hepatic vein thrombosis) I82.0
   Chilaiditi's Q43.3
   child maltreatment — *see* Maltreatment, child
   chondrocostal junction M94.0
   chondroectodermal dysplasia Q77.6
   chromosome 4 short arm deletion Q93.3
   chromosome 5 short arm deletion Q93.4
   chronic
      infantile neurological, cutaneous and articular
         (CINCA) M04.2

Syndrome — *continued*
- chronic — *continued*
  - pain G89.4
    - personality F68.8
- Churg-Strauss M30.1
- Clarke-Hadfield K86.89
- Clerambault's automatism G93.89
- Clouston's (hidrotic ectodermal dysplasia) Q82.4
- clumsiness, clumsy child F82
- cluster headache G44.009
  - intractable G44.001
  - not intractable G44.009
- Coffin-Lowry Q89.8
- cold injury (newborn) P80.0
- combined immunity deficiency D81.9
- compartment (deep) (posterior) (traumatic) T79.A0 ☑ (*following* T79.7)
  - abdomen T79.A3 ☑ (*following* T79.7)
  - lower extremity (hip, buttock, thigh, leg, foot, toes) T79.A2 ☑ (*following* T79.7)
  - nontraumatic
    - abdomen M79.A3 (*following* M79.7)
    - lower extremity (hip, buttock, thigh, leg, foot, toes) M79.A2- (*following* M79.7)
    - specified site NEC M79.A9 (*following* M79.7)
    - upper extremity (shoulder, arm, forearm, wrist, hand, fingers) M79.A1- ☑ (*following* M79.7)
  - postprocedural — *see* Syndrome, compartment, nontraumatic
  - specified site NEC T79.A9 ☑ (*following* T79.7)
  - upper extremity (shoulder, arm, forearm, wrist, hand, fingers) T79.A1 ☑ (*following* T79.7)
- complex regional pain — *see* Syndrome, pain, complex regional
- compression T79.5 ☑
  - anterior spinal — *see* Syndrome, anterior, spinal artery, compression
  - cauda equina G83.4
  - celiac artery I77.4
  - vertebral artery M47.029
    - cervical region M47.022
    - occipito-atlanto-axial region M47.021
- concussion F07.81
- congenital
  - affecting multiple systems NEC Q87.89
  - central alveolar hypoventilation G47.35
  - facial diplegia Q87.0
  - muscular hypertrophy-cerebral Q87.89
  - oculo-auriculovertebral Q87.0
  - oculofacial diplegia (Moebius) Q87.0
  - rubella (manifest) P35.0
- congestion-fibrosis (pelvic), female N94.89
- congestive dysmenorrhea N94.6
- connective tissue M35.9
  - overlap NEC M35.1
- Conn's E26.01
- conus medullaris G95.81
- cord
  - anterior G83.82
  - posterior G83.83
- coronary
  - acute NEC I24.9
  - insufficiency or intermediate I20.0
  - slow flow I20.8
- Costen's (complex) M26.69
- costochondral junction M94.0
- costoclavicular G54.0
- costovertebral E22.0
- Cowden Q85.8
- craniovertebral M53.0
- Creutzfeldt-Jakob — *see* Creutzfeldt-Jakob disease or syndrome
- crib death R99
- cricopharyngeal — *see* Dysphagia
- cri-du-chat Q93.4
- croup J05.0
- CRPS I — *see* Syndrome, pain, complex regional I
- crush T79.5 ☑
- cryopyrin-associated perodic M04.2
- cryptophthalmos Q87.0
- cubital tunnel — *see* Lesion, nerve, ulnar
- Curschmann (-Batten) (-Steinert) G71.11
- Cushing's E24.9
  - alcohol-induced E24.4
  - due to
    - alcohol
      - drugs E24.2

Syndrome — *continued*
- Cushing's — *continued*
  - due to — *continued*
    - ectopic ACTH E24.3
    - overproduction of pituitary ACTH E24.0
  - drug-induced E24.2
  - overdose or wrong substance given or taken — *see* Table of Drugs and Chemicals, by drug, poisoning
  - pituitary-dependent E24.0
  - specified type NEC E24.8
- cystic duct stump K91.5
- Dana-Putnam D51.0
- Danbolt (-Cross) (acrodermatitis enteropathica) E83.2
- Dandy-Walker Q03.1
  - with spina bifida Q07.01
- Danlos' — *see also* Syndrome, Ehlers-Danlos Q79.60
- De Quervain E34.51
- de Toni-Fanconi (-Debré) E72.09
  - with cystinosis E72.04
- defibrination — *see also* Fibrinolysis
  - with
    - antepartum hemorrhage — *see* Hemorrhage, antepartum, with coagulation defect
    - intrapartum hemorrhage — *see* Hemorrhage, complicating, delivery
  - newborn P60
  - postpartum O72.3
- Degos' I77.89
- Déjérine-Roussy G89.0
- delayed sleep phase G47.21
- demyelinating G37.9
- dependence — *see* F10-F19 with fourth character .2
- depersonalization (-derealization) F48.1
- di George's D82.1
- diabetes mellitus in newborn infant P70.2
- diabetes mellitus-hypertension-nephrosis — *see* Diabetes, nephrosis
- diabetes-nephrosis — *see* Diabetes, nephrosis
- diabetic amyotrophy — *see* Diabetes, amyotrophy
- dialysis associated steal T82.898- ☑
- Diamond-Blackfan D61.01
- Diamond-Gardener D69.2
- DIC (diffuse or disseminated intravascular coagulopathy) D65
- Dighton's Q78.0
- disequilibrium E87.8
- Döhle body-panmyelopathic D72.0
- dorsolateral medullary G46.4
- double athetosis G80.3
- Down — *see also* Down syndrome Q90.9
- Dresbach's (elliptocytosis) D58.1
- Dressler's (postmyocardial infarction) I24.1
  - postcardiotomy I97.0
- drug withdrawal, infant of dependent mother P96.1
- dry eye H04.12- ☑
- due to abnormality
  - chromosomal Q99.9
    - sex
      - female phenotype Q97.9
      - male phenotype Q98.9
    - specified NEC Q99.8
- dumping (postgastrectomy) K91.1
  - nonsurgical K31.89
- Dupré's (meningism) R29.1
- dysmetabolic X E88.81
- dyspraxia, developmental F82
- Eagle-Barrett Q79.4
- Eaton-Lambert — *see* Syndrome, Lambert-Eaton
- Ebstein's Q22.5
- ectopic ACTH E24.3
- eczema-thrombocytopenia D82.0
- Eddowes' Q78.0
- effort (psychogenic) F45.8
- Ehlers-Danlos Q79.60
  - classical (cEDS) (classical EDS) Q79.61
  - hypermobile (hEDS) (hypermobile EDS) Q79.62
  - specified NEC Q79.69
  - vascular (vascular EDS) (vEDS) Q79.63
- Eisenmenger's I27.83
- Ekman's Q78.0
- electric feet E53.8
- Ellis-van Creveld Q77.6
- empty nest Z60.0
- endocrine-hypertensive E27.0
- entrapment — *see* Neuropathy, entrapment
- eosinophilia-myalgia M35.8
- epileptic — *see also* Epilepsy, by type

Syndrome — *continued*
- epileptic — *see also* Epilepsy, by type — *continued*
  - absence G40.A09 (*following* G40.3)
    - intractable G40.A19 (*following* G40.3)
      - with status epilepticus G40.A11 (*following* G40.3)
      - without status epilepticus G40.A19 (*following* G40.3)
    - not intractable G40.A09 (*following* G40.3)
      - with status epilepticus G40.A01 (*following* G40.3)
      - without status epilepticus G40.A09 (*following* G40.3)
- Erdheim-Chester (ECD) E88.89
- Erdheim's E22.0
- erythrocyte fragmentation D59.4
- Evans D69.41
- exhaustion F48.8
- extrapyramidal G25.9
  - specified NEC G25.89
- eye retraction — *see* Strabismus
- eyelid-malar-mandible Q87.0
- Faber's D50.9
- facial pain, paroxysmal G50.0
- Fallot's Q21.3
- familial cold autoinflammatory M04.2
- familial eczema-thrombocytopenia (Wiskott-Aldrich) D82.0
- Fanconi (-de Toni) (-Debré) E72.09
  - with cystinosis E72.04
- Fanconi's (anemia) (congenital pancytopenia) D61.09
- fatigue
  - chronic R53.82
  - psychogenic F48.8
- faulty bowel habit K59.39
- Feil-Klippel (brevicollis) Q76.1
- Felty's — *see* Felty's syndrome
- fertile eunuch E23.0
- fetal
  - alcohol (dysmorphic) Q86.0
  - hydantoin Q86.1
- Fiedler's I40.1
- first arch Q87.0
- fish odor E72.89
- Fisher's G61.0
- Fitzhugh-Curtis
  - due to
    - Chlamydia trachomatis A74.81
    - Neisseria gonorrhorea (gonococcal peritonitis) A54.85
- Fitz's — *see also* Pancreatitis, acute K85.80
- Flajani (-Basedow) E05.00
  - with thyroid storm E05.01
- flatback — *see* Flatback syndrome
- floppy
  - baby P94.2
  - iris (intraoeprative) (IFIS) H21.81
  - mitral valve I34.1
- flush E34.0
- Foix-Alajouanine G95.19
- Fong's Q87.2
- food protein-induced enterocolitis (FPIES) K52.21
- foramen magnum G93.5
- Foster-Kennedy H47.14- ☑
- Foville's (peduncular) G46.3
- fragile X Q99.2
- Franceschetti Q75.4
- Frey's
  - auriculotemporal G50.8
  - hyperhidrosis L74.52
- Friderichsen-Waterhouse A39.1
- Froin's G95.89
- frontal lobe F07.0
- Fukuhara E88.49
- functional
  - bowel K59.9
  - prepubertal castrate E29.1
- Gaisböck's D75.1
- ganglion (basal ganglia brain) G25.9
  - geniculi G51.1
- Gardner-Diamond D69.2
- gastroesophageal
  - junction K22.0
  - laceration-hemorrhage K22.6
- gastrojejunal loop obstruction K91.89
- Gee-Herter-Heubner K90.0
- Gelineau's G47.419
  - with cataplexy G47.411
- genito-anorectal A55

☑ **Additional Character Required** — Refer to the Tabular List for Character Selection ▽ **Subterms under main terms may continue to next column or page**

Syndrome — *continued*
    Gerstmann-Sträussler-Scheinker (GSS) A81.82
    Gianotti-Crosti L44.4
    giant platelet (Bernard-Soulier) D69.1
    Gilles de la Tourette's F95.2
    Glass Q87.89
    goiter-deafness E07.1
    Goldberg Q89.8
    Goldberg-Maxwell E34.51
    Good's D83.8
    Gopalan' (burning feet) E53.8
    Gorlin's Q87.89
    Gougerot-Blum L81.7
    Gouley's I31.1
    Gower's R55
    gray or grey (newborn) P93.0
        platelet D69.1
    Gubler-Millard G46.3
    Guillain-Barré (-Strohl) G61.0
    gustatory sweating G50.8
    Hadfield-Clarke K86.89
    hair tourniquet — *see* Constriction, external, by site
    Hamman's J98.19
    hand-foot L27.1
    hand-shoulder G90.8
    hantavirus (cardio)-pulmonary (HPS) (HCPS) B33.4
    happy puppet Q93.51
    Harada's H30.81- ☑
    Hayem-Faber D50.9
    headache NEC G44.89
        complicated NEC G44.59
    Heberden's I20.8
    Hedinger's E34.0
    Hegglin's D72.0
    HELLP (hemolysis, elevated liver enzymes and low
        platelet count) O14.2- ☑
        complicating
            childbirth O14.24
            puerperium O14.25
    hemolytic-uremic D59.3
    hemophagocytic, infection-associated D76.2
    Henoch-Schönlein D69.0
    hepatic flexure K59.8
    hepatopulmonary K76.81
    hepatorenal K76.7
        following delivery O90.4
        postoperative or postprocedural K91.83
        postpartum, puerperal O90.4
    hepatourologic K76.7
    Herter (-Gee) (nontropical sprue) K90.0
    Heubner-Herter K90.0
    Heyd's K76.7
    Hilger's G90.09
    histamine-like (fish poisoning) — *see* Poisoning, fish
    histiocytic D76.3
    histiocytosis NEC D76.3
    HIV infection, acute B20
    Hoffmann-Werdnig G12.0
    Hollander-Simons E88.1
    Hoppe-Goldflam G70.00
        with exacerbation (acute) G70.01
        in crisis G70.01
    Horner's G90.2
    hungry bone E83.81
    hunterian glossitis D51.0
    Hutchinson's triad A50.53
    hyperabduction G54.0
    hyperammonemia-hyperornithinemia-homocitrulline-
        mia E72.4
    hypereosinophilic (idiopathic) D72.1
    hyperimmunoglobulin D M04.1
    hyperimmunoglobulin E (IgE) D82.4
    hyperkalemic E87.5
    hyperkinetic — *see* Hyperkinesia
    hypermobility M35.7
    hypernatremia E87.0
    hyperosmolarity E87.0
    hyperperfusion G97.82
    hypersplenic D73.1
    hypertransfusion, newborn P61.1
    hyperventilation F45.8
    hyperviscosity (of serum)
        polycythemic D75.1
        sclerothymic D58.8
    hypoglycemic (familial) (neonatal) E16.2
    hypokalemic E87.6
    hyponatremic E87.1
    hypopituitarism E23.0
    hypoplastic left-heart Q23.4

Syndrome — *continued*
    hypopotassemia E87.6
    hyposmolality E87.1
    hypotension, maternal O26.5- ☑
    hypothenar hammer I73.89
    hypoventilation, obesity (OHS) E66.2
    ICF (intravascular coagulation-fibrinolysis) D65
    idiopathic
        cardiorespiratory distress, newborn P22.0
        nephrotic (infantile) N04.9
    iliotibial band M76.3- ☑
    immobility, immobilization (paraplegic) M62.3
    immune reconstitution D89.3
    immune reconstitution inflammatory [IRIS] D89.3
    immunity deficiency, combined D81.9
    immunodeficiency
        acquired — *see* Human, immunodeficiency virus
            (HIV) disease
        combined D81.9
    impending coronary I20.0
    impingement, shoulder M75.4- ☑
    inappropriate secretion of antidiuretic hormone E22.2
    infant
        gestational diabetes P70.0
        of diabetic mother P70.1
    infantilism (pituitary) E23.0
    inferior vena cava I87.1
    inspissated bile (newborn) P59.1
    institutional (childhood) F94.2
    insufficient sleep F51.12
    intermediate coronary (artery) I20.0
    interspinous ligament — *see* Spondylopathy, specified
        NEC
    intestinal
        carcinoid E34.0
        knot K56.2
    intravascular coagulation-fibrinolysis (ICF) D65
    iodine-deficiency, congenital E00.9
        type
            mixed E00.2
            myxedematous E00.1
            neurological E00.0
    IRDS (idiopathic respiratory distress, newborn) P22.0
    irritable
        bowel K58.9
            with
                constipation K58.1
                diarrhea K58.0
            mixed K58.2
            psychogenic F45.8
            specified NEC K58.8
        heart (psychogenic) F45.8
        weakness F48.8
    ischemic
        bowel (transient) K55.9
            chronic K55.1
            due to mesenteric artery insufficiency K55.1
        steal T82.898 ☑
    IVC (intravascular coagulopathy) D65
    Ivemark's Q89.01
    Jaccoud's — *see* Arthropathy, postrheumatic, chronic
    Jackson's G83.89
    Jakob-Creutzfeldt — *see* Creutzfeldt-Jakob disease or
        syndrome
    jaw-winking Q07.8
    Jervell-Lange-Nielsen I45.81
    jet lag G47.25
    Job's D71
    Joseph-Diamond-Blackfan D61.01
    jugular foramen G52.7
    Kabuki Q89.8
    Kanner's (autism) F84.0
    Kartagener's Q89.3
    Kelly's D50.1
    Kimmelstiel-Wilson — *see* Diabetes, specified type,
        with Kimmelstiel-Wilson disease
    Klein (e)-Levine G47.13
    Klippel-Feil (brevicollis) Q76.1
    Köhler-Pellegrini-Steida — *see* Bursitis, tibial collateral
    König's K59.8
    Korsakoff (-Wernicke) (nonalcoholic) F04
        alcoholic F10.26
    Kostmann's D70.0
    Krabbe's congenital muscle hypoplasia Q79.8
    labyrinthine — *see* subcategory H83.2 ☑
    lacunar NEC G46.7
    Lambert-Eaton G70.80

Syndrome — *continued*
    Lambert-Eaton — *continued*
        in
            neoplastic disease G73.1
            specified disease NEC G70.81
    Landau-Kleffner — *see* Epilepsy, specified NEC
    Larsen's Q74.8
    lateral
        cutaneous nerve of thigh G57.1- ☑
        medullary G46.4
    Launois' E22.0
    lazy
        leukocyte D70.8
        posture M62.3
    Lemiere I80.8
    Lennox-Gastaut G40.812
        intractable G40.814
            with status epilepticus G40.813
            without status epilepticus G40.814
        not intractable G40.812
            with status epilepticus G40.811
            without status epilepticus G40.812
    lenticular, progressive E83.01
    Leopold-Levi's E05.90
    Lev's I44.2
    Lichtheim's D51.0
    Li-Fraumeni Z15.01
    Lightwood's N25.89
    Lignac (de Toni) (-Fanconi) (-Debré) E72.09
        with cystinosis E72.04
    Likoff's I20.8
    limbic epilepsy personality F07.0
    liver-kidney K76.7
    lobotomy F07.0
    Loffler's J82
    long arm 18 or 21 deletion Q93.89
    long QT I45.81
    Louis-Barré G11.3
    low
        atmospheric pressure T70.29 ☑
        back M54.5
        output (cardiac) I50.9
    lower radicular, newborn (birth injury) P14.8
    Luetscher's (dehydration) E86.0
    Lupus anticoagulant D68.62
    Lutembacher's Q21.1
    macrophage activation D76.1
        due to infection D76.2
    magnesium-deficiency R29.0
    Majeed M04.8
    Mal de Debarquement R42
    malabsorption K90.9
        postsurgical K91.2
    malformation, congenital, due to
        alcohol Q86.0
        exogenous cause NEC Q86.8
        hydantoin Q86.1
        warfarin Q86.2
    malignant
        carcinoid E34.0
        neuroleptic G21.0
    Mallory-Weiss K22.6
    mandibulofacial dysostosis Q75.4
    manic-depressive — *see* Disorder, bipolar
    maple-syrup-urine E71.0
    Marable's I77.4
    Marfan's Q87.40
        with
            cardiovascular manifestations Q87.418
                aortic dilation Q87.410
            ocular manifestations Q87.42
            skeletal manifestations Q87.43
    Marie's (acromegaly) E22.0
    mast cell activation — *see* Activation, mast cell
    maternal hypotension — *see* Syndrome, hypotension,
        maternal
    May (-Hegglin) D72.0
    McArdle (-Schmidt) (-Pearson) E74.04
    McQuarrie's E16.2
    meconium plug (newborn) P76.0
    median arcuate ligament I77.4
    Meekeren-Ehlers-Danlos Q79.6 ☑
    megavitamin-B6 E67.2
    Meige G24.4
    MELAS E88.41
    Mendelson's O74.0
    MERRF (myoclonic epilepsy associated with ragged-
        red fibers) E88.42

Syndrome — *continued*

mesenteric
artery (superior) K55.1
vascular insufficiency K55.1
metabolic E88.81
metastatic carcinoid E34.0
micrognathia-glossoptosis Q87.0
midbrain NEC G93.89
middle lobe (lung) J98.19
middle radicular G54.0
migraine — *see also* Migraine G43.909
Mikulicz' K11.8
milk-alkali E83.52
Millard-Gubler G46.3
Miller-Dieker Q93.88
Miller-Fisher G61.0
Minkowski-Chauffard D58.0
Mirizzi's K83.1
MNGIE (Mitochondrial Neurogastrointestinal Encephalopathy) E88.49
Möbius, ophthalmoplegic migraine — *see* Migraine, ophthalmoplegic
monofixation H50.42
Morel-Moore M85.2
Morel-Morgagni M85.2
Morgagni (-Morel) (-Stewart) M85.2
Morgagni-Adams-Stokes I45.9
Mounier-Kuhn Q32.4
with bronchiectasis J47.9
with
exacerbation (acute) J47.1
lower respiratory infection J47.0
acquired J98.09
with bronchiectasis J47.9
with
exacerbation (acute) J47.1
lower respiratory infection J47.0
Muckle-Wells M04.2
mucocutaneous lymph node (acute febrile) (MCLS) M30.3
multiple endocrine neoplasia (MEN) — *see* Neoplasia, endocrine, multiple (MEN)
multiple operations — *see* Disorder, factitious
myasthenic G70.9
in
diabetes mellitus — *see* Diabetes, amyotrophy
endocrine disease NEC E34.9 *[G73.3]*
neoplastic disease — *see also* Neoplasm D49.9 *[G73.3]*
thyrotoxicosis (hyperthyroidism) E05.90 *[G73.3]*
with thyroid storm E05.91 *[G73.3]*
myelodysplastic D46.9
with
5q deletion D46.C *(following* D46.2)
isolated del (5q) chromosomal abnormality D46.C *(following* D46.2)
lesions, low grade D46.20
specified NEC D46.Z *(following* D46.4)
myelopathic pain G89.0
myeloproliferative (chronic) D47.1
myofascial pain M79.18
Naffziger's G54.0
nail patella Q87.2
NARP (Neuropathy, Ataxia and Retinitis pigmentosa) E88.49
neonatal abstinence P96.1
nephritic — *see also* Nephritis
with edema — *see* Nephrosis
acute N00.9
chronic N03.9
rapidly progressive N01.9
nephrotic (congenital) — *see also* Nephrosis N04.9
with
dense deposit disease N04.6
diffuse
crescentic glomerulonephritis N04.7
endocapillary proliferative glomerulonephritis N04.4
membranous glomerulonephritis N04.2
mesangial proliferative glomerulonephritis N04.3
mesangiocapillary glomerulonephritis N04.5
focal and segmental glomerular lesions N04.1
minor glomerular abnormality N04.0
specified morphological changes NEC N04.8
diabetic — *see* Diabetes, nephrosis
neurologic neglect R41.4
Nezelof's D81.4

Syndrome — *continued*

Nonne-Milroy-Meige Q82.0
Nothnagel's vasomotor acroparesthesia I73.89
obesity hypoventilation (OHS) E66.2
oculomotor H51.9
ophthalmoplegia-cerebellar ataxia — *see* Strabismus, paralytic, third nerve
oral allergy T78.1 ☑
oral-facial-digital Q87.0
organic
affective F06.30
amnesic (not alcohol- or drug-induced) F04
brain F09
depressive F06.31
hallucinosis F06.0
personality F07.0
Ormond's N13.5
oro-facial-digital Q87.0
os trigonum Q68.8
Osler-Weber-Rendu I78.0
osteoporosis-osteomalacia M83.8
Osterreicher-Turner Q87.2
otolith — *see* subcategory H81.8 ☑
oto-palatal-digital Q87.0
outlet (thoracic) G54.0
ovary
polycystic E28.2
resistant E28.39
sclerocystic E28.2
Owren's D68.2
Paget-Schroetter I82.890
pain — *see also* Pain
complex regional I G90.50
lower limb G90.52- ☑
specified site NEC G90.59
upper limb G90.51- ☑
complex regional II — *see* Causalgia
painful
bruising D69.2
feet E53.8
prostate N42.81
paralysis agitans — *see* Parkinsonism
paralytic G83.9
specified NEC G83.89
Parinaud's H51.0
parkinsonian — *see* Parkinsonism
Parkinson's — *see* Parkinsonism
paroxysmal facial pain G50.0
Parry's E05.00
with thyroid storm E05.01
Parsonage (-Aldren)-Turner G54.5
patella clunk M25.86- ☑
Paterson (-Brown) (-Kelly) D50.1
pectoral girdle I77.89
pectoralis minor I77.89
pediatric autoimmune neuropsychiatric disorders associated with streptococcal infections (PANDAS) D89.89
Pelger-Huet D72.0
pellagra-cerebellar ataxia-renal aminoaciduria E72.02
pellagroid E52
Pellegrini-Stieda — *see* Bursitis, tibial collateral
pelvic congestion-fibrosis, female N94.89
penta X Q97.1
peptic ulcer — *see* Ulcer, peptic
perabduction I77.89
periodic fever M04.1
periodic fever, aphthous stomatitis, pharyngitis, and adenopathy [PFAPA] M04.8
periodic headache, in adults and children — *see* Headache, periodic syndromes in adults and children
periurethral fibrosis N13.5
phantom limb (without pain) G54.7
with pain G54.6
pharyngeal pouch D82.1
Pick's — *see* Disease, Pick's
Pickwickian E66.2
PIE (pulmonary infiltration with eosinophilia) J82
pigmentary pallidal degeneration (progressive) G23.0
pineal E34.8
pituitary E22.0
placental transfusion — *see* Pregnancy, complicated by, placental transfusion syndromes
plantar fascia M72.2
plateau iris (post-iridectomy) (postprocedural) H21.82
Plummer-Vinson D50.1
pluricarential of infancy E40

Syndrome — *continued*

plurideficiency E40
pluriglandular (compensatory) E31.8
autoimmune E31.0
pneumatic hammer T75.21 ☑
polyangiitis overlap M30.8
polycarential of infancy E40
polyglandular E31.8
autoimmune E31.0
polysplenia Q89.09
pontine NEC G93.89
popliteal
artery entrapment I77.89
post endometrial ablation N99.85
web Q87.89
post chemoembolization — *code to* associated conditions
postcardiac injury
postcardiotomy I97.0
postmyocardial infarction I24.1
postcardiotomy I97.0
postcholecystectomy K91.5
postcommissurotomy I97.0
postconcussional F07.81
postcontusional F07.81
postencephalitic F07.89
posterior
cervical sympathetic M53.0
cord G83.83
fossa compression G93.5
reversible encephalopathy (PRES) I67.83
postgastrectomy (dumping) K91.1
postgastric surgery K91.1
postinfarction I24.1
postlaminectomy NEC M96.1
postleukotomy F07.0
postmastectomy lymphedema I97.2
postmyocardial infarction I24.1
postoperative NEC T81.9 ☑
blind loop K90.2
postpartum panhypopituitary (Sheehan) E23.0
postpolio (myelitic) G14
postthrombotic I87.009
with
inflammation I87.02- ☑
with ulcer I87.03- ☑
specified complication NEC I87.09- ☑
ulcer I87.01- ☑
with inflammation I87.03- ☑
asymptomatic I87.00- ☑
postvagotomy K91.1
postvalvulotomy I97.0
postviral NEC G93.3
fatigue G93.3
Potain's K31.0
potassium intoxication E87.5
Prader-Willi Q87.11
Prader-Willi-like Q87.19
precerebral artery (multiple) (bilateral) G45.2
preinfarction I20.0
preleukemic D46.9
premature senility E34.8
premenstrual dysphoric F32.81
premenstrual tension N94.3
Prinzmetal-Massumi R07.1
prune belly Q79.4
pseudo -Turner's Q87.19
pseudocarpal tunnel (sublimis) — *see* Syndrome, carpal tunnel
pseudoparalytica G70.00
with exacerbation (acute) G70.01
in crisis G70.01
psycho-organic (nonpsychotic severity) F07.9
acute or subacute F05
depressive type F06.31
hallucinatory type F06.0
nonpsychotic severity F07.0
specified NEC F07.89
pulmonary
arteriosclerosis I27.0
dysmaturity (Wilson-Mikity) P27.0
hypoperfusion (idiopathic) P22.0
renal (hemorrhagic) (Goodpasture's) M31.0
pure
motor lacunar G46.5
sensory lacunar G46.6
Putnam-Dana D51.0

☑ **Additional Character Required — Refer to the Tabular List for Character Selection**   ▽ **Subterms under main terms may continue to next column or page**

Syndrome — *continued*
- pyogenic arthritis, pyoderma gangrenosum, and acne [PAPA] M04.8
- pyramidopallidonigral G20
- pyriformis — *see* Lesion, nerve, sciatic
- QT interval prolongation I45.81
- radicular NEC — *see* Radiculopathy
  - upper limbs, newborn (birth injury) P14.3
- rapid time-zone change G47.25
- Rasmussen G04.81
- Raymond (-Céstan) I65.8
- Raynaud's I73.00
  - with gangrene I73.01
- RDS (respiratory distress syndrome, newborn) P22.0
- reactive airways dysfunction J68.3
- Refsum's G60.1
- Reifenstein E34.52
- renal glomerulohyalinosis-diabetic — *see* Diabetes, nephrosis
- Rendu-Osler-Weber I78.0
- residual ovary N99.83
- resistant ovary E28.39
- respiratory
  - distress
    - acute J80
      - adult J80
      - child J80
      - idiopathic J84.114
    - newborn (idiopathic) (type I) P22.0
      - type II P22.1
- restless legs G25.81
- retinoblastoma (familial) C69.2 ☑
- retroperitoneal fibrosis N13.5
- retroviral seroconversion (acute) Z21
- Reye's G93.7
- Richter — *see* Leukemia, chronic lymphocytic, B-cell type
- Ridley's I50.1
- right
  - heart, hypoplastic Q22.6
  - ventricular obstruction — *see* Failure, heart, right
- Romano-Ward (prolonged QT interval) I45.81
- rotator cuff, shoulder — *see also* Tear, rotator cuff M75.10- ☑
- Rotes Quérol — *see* Hyperostosis, ankylosing
- Roth — *see* Meralgia paresthetica
- rubella (congenital) P35.0
- Ruvalcaba-Myhre-Smith E71.440
- Rytand-Lipsitch I44.2
- salt
  - depletion E87.1
    - due to heat NEC T67.8 ☑
      - causing heat exhaustion or prostration T67.4 ☑
  - low E87.1
- salt-losing N28.89
- SATB2-associated Q87.89
- Scaglietti-Dagnini E22.0
- scalenus anticus (anterior) G54.0
- scapulocostal — *see* Mononeuropathy, upper limb, specified site NEC
- scapuloperoneal G71.09
- schizophrenic, of childhood NEC F84.5
- Schnitzler D47.2
- Scholte's E34.0
- Schroeder's E27.0
- Schüller-Christian C96.5
- Schwachman's — *see* Syndrome, Shwachman's
- Schwartz (-Jampel) G71.13
- Schwartz-Bartter E22.2
- scimitar Q26.8
- sclerocystic ovary E28.2
- Seitelberger's G31.89
- septicemic adrenal hemorrhage A39.1
- seroconversion, retroviral (acute) Z21
- serous meningitis G93.2
- severe acute respiratory (SARS) J12.81
- shaken infant T74.4 ☑
- shock (traumatic) T79.4 ☑
  - kidney N17.0
    - following crush injury T79.5 ☑
  - toxic A48.3
- shock-lung J80
- Shone's — *code to* specific anomalies
- short
  - bowel K91.2
  - rib Q77.2
- shoulder-hand — *see* Algoneurodystrophy

Syndrome — *continued*
- Shwachman's D70.4
- sicca — *see* Sicca syndrome
- sick
  - cell E87.1
  - sinus I49.5
- sick-euthyroid E07.81
- sideropenic D50.1
- Siemens' ectodermal dysplasia Q82.4
- Silfversköld's Q78.9
- Simons' E88.1
- sinus tarsi M25.57- ☑
- sinusitis-bronchiectasis-situs inversus Q89.3
- Sipple's E31.22
- sirenomelia Q87.2
- Slocumb's E27.0
- slow flow, coronary I20.8
- Sluder's G44.89
- Smith-Magenis Q93.88
- Sneddon-Wilkinson L13.1
- Sotos' Q87.3
- South African cardiomyopathy I42.8
- spasmodic
  - upward movement, eyes H51.8
  - winking F95.8
- Spen's I45.9
- splenic
  - agenesis Q89.01
  - flexure K59.8
  - neutropenia D73.81
- Spurway's Q78.0
- staphylococcal scalded skin L00
- steal
  - arteriovenous T82.898- ☑
  - ischemic T82.898- ☑
  - subclavian G45.8
- Stein-Leventhal E28.2
- Stein's E28.2
- Stevens-Johnson syndrome L51.1
  - toxic epidermal necrolysis overlap L51.3
- Stewart-Morel M85.2
- Stickler Q89.8
- stiff baby Q89.8
- stiff man G25.82
- Still-Felty — *see* Felty's syndrome
- Stokes (-Adams) I45.9
- stone heart I50.1
- straight back, congenital Q76.49
- subclavian steal G45.8
- subcoracoid-pectoralis minor G54.0
- subcostal nerve compression I77.89
- subphrenic interposition Q43.3
- superior
  - cerebellar artery I63.89
  - mesenteric artery K55.1
  - semi-circular canal dehiscence H83.8X- ☑
  - vena cava I87.1
- supine hypotensive (maternal) — *see* Syndrome, hypotension, maternal
- suprarenal cortical E27.0
- supraspinatus — *see also* Tear, rotator cuff M75.10- ☑
- Susac G93.49
- swallowed blood P78.2
- sweat retention L74.0
- Swyer Q99.1
- Symond's G93.2
- sympathetic
  - cervical paralysis G90.2
  - pelvic, female N94.89
- systemic inflammatory response (SIRS), of non-infectious origin (without organ dysfunction) R65.10
  - with acute organ dysfunction R65.11
- tachycardia-bradycardia I49.5
- takotsubo I51.81
- TAR (thrombocytopenia with absent radius) Q87.2
- tarsal tunnel G57.5- ☑
- teething K00.7
- tegmental G93.89
- telangiectasic-pigmentation-cataract Q82.8
- temporal pyramidal apex — *see* Otitis, media, suppurative, acute
- temporomandibular joint-pain-dysfunction M26.62- ☑
- Terry's — *see also* Myopia, degenerative H44.2- ☑
- testicular feminization — *see also* Syndrome, androgen insensitivity E34.51
- thalamic pain (hyperesthetic) G89.0
- thoracic outlet (compression) G54.0
- Thorson-Björck E34.0

Syndrome — *continued*
- thrombocytopenia with absent radius (TAR) Q87.2
- thyroid-adrenocortical insufficiency E31.0
- tibial
  - anterior M76.81- ☑
  - posterior M76.82- ☑
- Tietze's M94.0
- time-zone (rapid) G47.25
- Toni-Fanconi E72.09
  - with cystinosis E72.04
- Touraine's Q79.8
- tourniquet — *see* Constriction, external, by site
- toxic shock A48.3
- transient left ventricular apical ballooning I51.81
- traumatic vasospastic T75.22 ☑
- Treacher Collins Q75.4
- triple X, female Q97.0
- trisomy Q92.9
  - 13 Q91.7
    - meiotic nondisjunction Q91.4
    - mitotic nondisjunction Q91.5
    - mosaicism Q91.5
    - translocation Q91.6
  - 18 Q91.3
    - meiotic nondisjunction Q91.0
    - mitotic nondisjunction Q91.1
    - mosaicism Q91.1
    - translocation Q91.2
  - 20 (q)(p) Q92.8
  - 21 Q90.9
    - meiotic nondisjunction Q90.0
    - mitotic nondisjunction Q90.1
    - mosaicism Q90.1
    - translocation Q90.2
  - 22 Q92.8
- tropical wet feet T69.0- ☑
- Trousseau's I82.1
- tumor lysis (following antineoplastic chemotherapy) (spontaneous) NEC E88.3
- tumor necrosis factor receptor associated periodic (TRAPS) M04.1
- Twiddler's (due to)
  - automatic implantable defibrillator T82.198 ☑
  - cardiac pacemaker T82.198 ☑
- Unverricht (-Lundborg) — *see* Epilepsy, generalized, idiopathic
- upward gaze H51.8
- uremia, chronic — *see also* Disease, kidney, chronic N18.9
- urethral N34.3
- urethro-oculo-articular — *see* Reiter's disease
- urohepatic K76.7
- vago-hypoglossal G52.7
- van Buchem's M85.2
- van der Hoeve's Q78.0
- vascular NEC in cerebrovascular disease G46.8
- vasoconstriction, reversible cerebrovascular I67.841
- vasomotor I73.9
- vasospastic (traumatic) T75.22 ☑
- vasovagal R55
- VATER Q87.2
- velo-cardio-facial Q93.81
- vena cava (inferior) (superior) (obstruction) I87.1
- vertebral
  - artery G45.0
    - compression — *see* Syndrome, anterior, spinal artery, compression
  - steal G45.0
- vertebro-basilar artery G45.0
- vertebrogenic (pain) M54.89
- vertiginous — *see* Disorder, vestibular function
- Vinson-Plummer D50.1
- virus B34.9
- visceral larva migrans B83.0
- visual disorientation H53.8
- vitamin B6 deficiency E53.1
- vitreal corneal H59.01- ☑
- vitreous (touch) H59.01- ☑
- Vogt-Koyanagi H20.82- ☑
- Volkmann's T79.6 ☑
- von Schroetter's I82.890
- von Willebrand (-Jürgen) D68.0
- Waldenström-Kjellberg D50.1
- Wallenberg's G46.3
- water retention E87.79
- Waterhouse (-Friderichsen) A39.1
- Weber-Gubler G46.3
- Weber-Leyden G46.3

▼ **Subterms under main terms may continue to next column or page**   ☑ **Additional Character Required — Refer to the Tabular List for Character Selection**   **303**

Syndrome — Syndrome

Syndrome — *continued*
 Weber's G46.3
 Wegener's M31.3Ø
  with
    kidney involvement M31.31
    lung involvement M31.3Ø
     with kidney involvement M31.31
 Weingarten's (tropical eosinophilia) J82
 Weiss-Baker G9Ø.Ø9
 Werdnig-Hoffman G12.Ø
 Wermer's E31.21
 Werner's E34.8
 Wernicke-Korsakoff (nonalcoholic) FØ4
  alcoholic F1Ø.26
 Westphal-Strümpell E83.Ø1
 West's — *see* Epilepsy, spasms
 wet
  feet (maceration) (tropical) T69.Ø- ☑
  lung, newborn P22.1
 whiplash S13.4 ☑
 whistling face Q87.Ø
 Wilkie's K55.1
 Wilkinson-Sneddon L13.1
 Willebrand (-Jürgens) D68.Ø
 Williams Q93.82
 Wilson's (hepatolenticular degeneration) E83.Ø1
 Wiskott-Aldrich D82.Ø
 withdrawal — *see* Withdrawal, state
  drug
    infant of dependent mother P96.1
    therapeutic use, newborn P96.2
 Woakes' (ethmoiditis) J33.1
 Wright's (hyperabduction) G54.Ø
 X I2Ø.9
 XXXX Q97.1
 XXXXX Q97.1
 XXXXY Q98.1
 XXY Q98.Ø
 Yao MØ4.8
 yellow nail L6Ø.5
 Zahorsky's BØ8.5
 Zellweger syndrome E71.51Ø
 Zellweger-like syndrome E71.541
Synechia (anterior) (iris) (posterior) (pupil) — *see also*
  Adhesions, iris
 intra-uterine (traumatic) N85.6
Synesthesia R2Ø.8
Syngamiasis, syngamosis B83.3
Synodontia KØØ.2
Synorchidism, synorchism Q55.1
Synostosis (congenital) Q78.8
 astragalo-scaphoid Q74.2
 radioulnar Q74.Ø
Synovial sarcoma — *see* Neoplasm, connective tissue,
  malignant
Synovioma (malignant) — *see also* Neoplasm, connective
  tissue, malignant
 benign — *see* Neoplasm, connective tissue, benign
Synoviosarcoma — *see* Neoplasm, connective tissue,
  malignant
Synovitis — *see also* Tenosynovitis M65.9
 crepitant
  hand M7Ø.Ø- ☑
  wrist M7Ø.Ø3- ☑
 gonococcal A54.49
 gouty — *see* Gout
 in (due to)
  crystals M65.8- ☑
  gonorrhea A54.49
  syphilis (late) A52.78
  use, overuse, pressure — *see* Disorder, soft tissue,
   due to use
 infective NEC — *see* Tenosynovitis, infective NEC
 specified NEC — *see* Tenosynovitis, specified type NEC
 syphilitic A52.78
  congenital (early) A5Ø.Ø2
 toxic — *see* Synovitis, transient
 transient M67.3- ☑
  ankle M67.37- ☑
  elbow M67.32- ☑
  foot joint M67.37- ☑
  hand joint M67.34- ☑
  hip M67.35- ☑
  knee M67.36- ☑
  multiple site M67.39
  pelvic region M67.35- ☑
  shoulder M67.31- ☑
  specified joint NEC M67.38

Synovitis — *continued*
 transient — *continued*
  wrist M67.33- ☑
 traumatic, current — *see* Sprain
 tuberculous — *see* Tuberculosis, synovitis
 villonodular (pigmented) M12.2- ☑
  ankle M12.27- ☑
  elbow M12.22- ☑
  foot joint M12.27- ☑
  hand joint M12.24- ☑
  hip M12.25- ☑
  knee M12.26- ☑
  multiple site M12.29
  pelvic region M12.25- ☑
  shoulder M12.21- ☑
  specified joint NEC M12.28
  vertebrae M12.28
  wrist M12.23- ☑
Syphilid A51.39
 congenital A5Ø.Ø6
 newborn A5Ø.Ø6
 tubercular (late) A52.79
Syphilis, syphilitic (acquired) A53.9
 abdomen (late) A52.79
 acoustic nerve A52.15
 adenopathy (secondary) A51.49
 adrenal (gland) (with cortical hypofunction) A52.79
 age under 2 years NOS — *see also* Syphilis, congenital,
   early
  acquired A51.9
 alopecia (secondary) A51.32
 anemia (late) A52.79 *[D63.8]*
 aneurysm (aorta) (ruptured) A52.Ø1
  central nervous system A52.Ø5
  congenital A5Ø.54 *[I79.Ø]*
 anus (late) A52.74
  primary A51.1
  secondary A51.39
 aorta (arch) (abdominal) (thoracic) A52.Ø2
  aneurysm A52.Ø1
 aortic (insufficiency) (regurgitation) (stenosis) A52.Ø3
  aneurysm A52.Ø1
 arachnoid (adhesive) (cerebral) (spinal) A52.13
 asymptomatic — *see* Syphilis, latent
 ataxia (locomotor) A52.11
 atrophoderma maculatum A51.39
 auricular fibrillation A52.Ø6
 bladder (late) A52.76
 bone A52.77
  secondary A51.46
 brain A52.17
 breast (late) A52.79
 bronchus (late) A52.72
 bubo (primary) A51.Ø
 bulbar palsy A52.19
 bursa (late) A52.78
 cardiac decompensation A52.Ø6
 cardiovascular A52.ØØ
 central nervous system (late) (recurrent) (relapse) (tertiary) A52.3
  with
    ataxia A52.11
    general paralysis A52.17
     juvenile A5Ø.45
    paresis (general) A52.17
     juvenile A5Ø.45
    tabes (dorsalis) A52.11
     juvenile A5Ø.45
    taboparesis A52.17
     juvenile A5Ø.45
  aneurysm A52.Ø5
  congenital A5Ø.4Ø
  juvenile A5Ø.4Ø
  remission in (sustained) A52.3
  serology doubtful, negative, or positive A52.3
  specified nature or site NEC A52.19
  vascular A52.Ø5
 cerebral A52.17
  meningovascular A52.13
  nerves (multiple palsies) A52.15
  sclerosis A52.17
  thrombosis A52.Ø5
 cerebrospinal (tabetic type) A52.12
 cerebrovascular A52.Ø5
 cervix (late) A52.76
 chancre (multiple) A51.Ø
  extragenital A51.2
  Rollet's A51.Ø

Syphilis, syphilitic — *continued*
 Charcot's joint A52.16
 chorioretinitis A51.43
  congenital A5Ø.Ø1
  late A52.71
  prenatal A5Ø.Ø1
 choroiditis — *see* Syphilitic chorioretinitis
 choroidoretinitis — *see* Syphilitic chorioretinitis
 ciliary body (secondary) A51.43
  late A52.71
 colon (late) A52.74
 combined spinal sclerosis A52.11
 condyloma (latum) A51.31
 congenital A5Ø.9
  with
    paresis (general) A5Ø.45
    tabes (dorsalis) A5Ø.45
    taboparesis A5Ø.45
  chorioretinitis, choroiditis A5Ø.Ø1 *[H32]*
  early, or less than 2 years after birth NEC A5Ø.2
    with manifestations — *see* Syphilis, congenital,
     early, symptomatic
    latent (without manifestations) A5Ø.1
     negative spinal fluid test A5Ø.1
     serology positive A5Ø.1
    symptomatic A5Ø.Ø9
     cutaneous A5Ø.Ø6
     mucocutaneous A5Ø.Ø7
     oculopathy A5Ø.Ø1
     osteochondropathy A5Ø.Ø2
     pharyngitis A5Ø.Ø3
     pneumonia A5Ø.Ø4
     rhinitis A5Ø.Ø5
     visceral A5Ø.Ø8
  interstitial keratitis A5Ø.31
  juvenile neurosyphilis A5Ø.45
  late, or 2 years or more after birth NEC A5Ø.7
    chorioretinitis, choroiditis A5Ø.32
    interstitial keratitis A5Ø.31
    juvenile neurosyphilis A5Ø.45
    latent (without manifestations) A5Ø.6
     negative spinal fluid test A5Ø.6
     serology positive A5Ø.6
    symptomatic or with manifestations NEC A5Ø.59
     arthropathy A5Ø.55
     cardiovascular A5Ø.54
     Clutton's joints A5Ø.51
     Hutchinson's teeth A5Ø.52
     Hutchinson's triad A5Ø.53
     osteochondropathy A5Ø.56
     saddle nose A5Ø.57
 conjugal A53.9
  tabes A52.11
 conjunctiva (late) A52.71
 contact Z2Ø.2
 cord bladder A52.19
 cornea, late A52.71
 coronary (artery) (sclerosis) A52.Ø6
 coryza, congenital A5Ø.Ø5
 cranial nerve A52.15
  multiple palsies A52.15
 cutaneous — *see* Syphilis, skin
 dacryocystitis (late) A52.71
 degeneration, spinal cord A52.12
 dementia paralytica A52.17
  juvenilis A5Ø.45
 destruction of bone A52.77
 dilatation, aorta A52.Ø1
 due to blood transfusion A53.9
 dura mater A52.13
 ear A52.79
  inner A52.79
    nerve (eighth) A52.15
    neurorecurrence A52.15
 early A51.9
  cardiovascular A52.ØØ
  central nervous system A52.3
  latent (without manifestations) (less than 2 years
   after infection) A51.5
    negative spinal fluid test A51.5
    serological relapse after treatment A51.5
    serology positive A51.5
  relapse (treated, untreated) A51.9
  skin A51.39
  symptomatic A51.9
    extragenital chancre A51.2
    primary, except extragenital chancre A51.Ø
    secondary — *see also* Syphilis, secondary A51.39
     relapse (treated, untreated) A51.49

☑ **Additional Character Required** — Refer to the Tabular List for Character Selection ▽ **Subterms under main terms may continue to next column or page**

Syphilis, syphilitic — *continued*
- early — *continued*
  - ulcer A51.39
- eighth nerve (neuritis) A52.15
- endemic A65
- endocarditis A52.03
  - aortic A52.03
  - pulmonary A52.03
- epididymis (late) A52.76
- epiglottis (late) A52.73
- epiphysitis (congenital) (early) A50.02
- episcleritis (late) A52.71
- esophagus A52.79
- eustachian tube A52.73
- exposure to Z20.2
- eye A52.71
- eyelid (late) (with gumma) A52.71
- fallopian tube (late) A52.76
- fracture A52.77
- gallbladder (late) A52.74
- gastric (polyposis) (late) A52.74
- general A53.9
  - paralysis A52.17
    - juvenile A50.45
- genital (primary) A51.0
- glaucoma A52.71
- gumma NEC A52.79
  - cardiovascular system A52.00
  - central nervous system A52.3
  - congenital A50.59
- heart (block) (decompensation) (disease) (failure) A52.06 [I52]
  - valve NEC A52.03
- hemianesthesia A52.19
- hemianopsia A52.71
- hemiparesis A52.17
- hemiplegia A52.17
- hepatic artery A52.09
- hepatis A52.74
- hepatomegaly, congenital A50.08
- hereditaria tarda — *see* Syphilis, congenital, late
- hereditary — *see* Syphilis, congenital
- Hutchinson's teeth A50.52
- hyalitis A52.71
- inactive — *see* Syphilis, latent
- infantum — *see* Syphilis, congenital
- inherited — *see* Syphilis, congenital
- internal ear A52.79
- intestine (late) A52.74
- iris, iritis (secondary) A51.43
  - late A52.71
- joint (late) A52.77
- keratitis (congenital) (interstitial) (late) A50.31
- kidney (late) A52.75
- lacrimal passages (late) A52.71
- larynx (late) A52.73
- late A52.9
  - cardiovascular A52.00
  - central nervous system A52.3
  - kidney A52.75
  - latent or 2 years or more after infection (without manifestations) A52.8
    - negative spinal fluid test A52.8
    - serology positive A52.8
  - paresis A52.17
  - specified site NEC A52.79
  - symptomatic or with manifestations A52.79
  - tabes A52.11
- latent A53.0
  - with signs or symptoms — *code by* site and stage under Syphilis
  - central nervous system A52.2
  - date of infection unspecified A53.0
  - early, or less than 2 years after infection A51.5
  - follow-up of latent syphilis A53.0
    - date of infection unspecified A53.0
    - late, or 2 years or more after infection A52.8
  - late, or 2 years or more after infection A52.8
  - positive serology (only finding) A53.0
    - date of infection unspecified A53.0
    - early, or less than 2 years after infection A51.5
    - late, or 2 years or more after infection A52.8
- lens (late) A52.71
- leukoderma A51.39
  - late A52.79
- lienitis A52.79
- lip A51.39
  - chancre (primary) A51.2

Syphilis, syphilitic — *continued*
- lip — *continued*
  - late A52.79
- Lissauer's paralysis A52.17
- liver A52.74
- locomotor ataxia A52.11
- lung A52.72
- lymph gland (early) (secondary) A51.49
  - late A52.79
- lymphadenitis (secondary) A51.49
- macular atrophy of skin A51.39
  - striated A52.79
- mediastinum (late) A52.73
- meninges (adhesive) (brain) (spinal cord) A52.13
- meningitis A52.13
  - acute (secondary) A51.41
  - congenital A50.41
- meningoencephalitis A52.14
- meningovascular A52.13
  - congenital A50.41
- mesarteritis A52.09
  - brain A52.04
- middle ear A52.77
- mitral stenosis A52.03
- monoplegia A52.17
- mouth (secondary) A51.39
  - late A52.79
- mucocutaneous (secondary) A51.39
  - late A52.79
- mucous
  - membrane (secondary) A51.39
    - late A52.79
  - patches A51.39
    - congenital A50.07
- mulberry molars A50.52
- muscle A52.78
- myocardium A52.06
- nasal sinus (late) A52.73
- neonatorum — *see* Syphilis, congenital
- nephrotic syndrome (secondary) A51.44
- nerve palsy (any cranial nerve) A52.15
  - multiple A52.15
- nervous system, central A52.3
- neuritis A52.15
  - acoustic A52.15
- neurorecidive of retina A52.19
- neuroretinitis A52.19
- newborn — *see* Syphilis, congenital
- nodular superficial (late) A52.79
- nonvenereal A65
- nose (late) A52.73
  - saddle back deformity A50.57
- occlusive arterial disease A52.09
- oculopathy A52.71
- ophthalmic (late) A52.71
- optic nerve (atrophy) (neuritis) (papilla) A52.15
- orbit (late) A52.71
- organic A53.9
- osseous (late) A52.77
- osteochondritis (congenital) (early) A50.02 [M90.80]
- osteoporosis A52.77
- ovary (late) A52.76
- oviduct (late) A52.76
- palate (late) A52.79
- pancreas (late) A52.74
- paralysis A52.17
  - general A52.17
    - juvenile A50.45
- paresis (general) A52.17
  - juvenile A50.45
- paresthesia A52.19
- Parkinson's disease or syndrome A52.19
- paroxysmal tachycardia A52.06
- pemphigus (congenital) A50.06
- penis (chancre) A51.0
  - late A52.76
- pericardium A52.06
- perichondritis, larynx (late) A52.73
- periosteum (late) A52.77
  - congenital (early) A50.02 [M90.80]
  - early (secondary) A51.46
- peripheral nerve A52.79
- petrous bone (late) A52.77
- pharynx (late) A52.73
  - secondary A51.39
- pituitary (gland) A52.79
- pleura (late) A52.73
- pneumonia, white A50.04
- pontine lesion A52.17

Syphilis, syphilitic — *continued*
- portal vein A52.09
- primary A51.0
  - anal A51.1
  - and secondary — *see* Syphilis, secondary
  - central nervous system A52.3
  - extragenital chancre NEC A51.2
  - fingers A51.2
  - genital A51.0
  - lip A51.2
  - specified site NEC A51.2
  - tonsils A51.2
- prostate (late) A52.76
- ptosis (eyelid) A52.71
- pulmonary (late) A52.72
  - artery A52.09
- pyelonephritis (late) A52.75
- recently acquired, symptomatic A51.9
- rectum (late) A52.74
- respiratory tract (late) A52.73
- retina, late A52.71
- retrobulbar neuritis A52.15
- salpingitis A52.76
- sclera (late) A52.71
- sclerosis
  - cerebral A52.17
  - coronary A52.06
  - multiple A52.11
- scotoma (central) A52.71
- scrotum (late) A52.76
- secondary (and primary) A51.49
  - adenopathy A51.49
  - anus A51.39
  - bone A51.46
  - chorioretinitis, choroiditis A51.43
  - hepatitis A51.45
  - liver A51.45
  - lymphadenitis A51.49
  - meningitis (acute) A51.41
  - mouth A51.39
  - mucous membranes A51.39
  - periosteum, periostitis A51.46
  - pharynx A51.39
  - relapse (treated, untreated) A51.49
  - skin A51.39
  - specified form NEC A51.49
  - tonsil A51.39
  - ulcer A51.39
  - viscera NEC A51.49
  - vulva A51.39
- seminal vesicle (late) A52.76
- seronegative with signs or symptoms — *code by* site and stage under Syphilis
- seropositive
  - with signs or symptoms — *code by* site and stage under Syphilis
  - follow-up of latent syphilis — *see* Syphilis, latent
  - only finding — *see* Syphilis, latent
- seventh nerve (paralysis) A52.15
- sinus, sinusitis (late) A52.73
- skeletal system A52.77
- skin (with ulceration) (early) (secondary) A51.39
  - late or tertiary A52.79
- small intestine A52.74
- spastic spinal paralysis A52.17
- spermatic cord (late) A52.76
- spinal (cord) A52.12
- spleen A52.79
- splenomegaly A52.79
- spondylitis A52.77
- staphyloma A52.71
- stigmata (congenital) A50.59
- stomach A52.74
- synovium A52.78
- tabes dorsalis (late) A52.11
  - juvenile A50.45
- tabetic type A52.11
  - juvenile A50.45
- taboparesis A52.17
  - juvenile A50.45
- tachycardia A52.06
- tendon (late) A52.78
- tertiary A52.9
  - with symptoms NEC A52.79
  - cardiovascular A52.00
  - central nervous system A52.3
  - multiple NEC A52.79
  - specified site NEC A52.79
- testis A52.76

Syphilis, syphilitic — *continued*
thorax A52.73
throat A52.73
thymus (gland) (late) A52.79
thyroid (late) A52.79
tongue (late) A52.79
tonsil (lingual) (late) A52.73
primary A51.2
secondary A51.39
trachea (late) A52.73
tunica vaginalis (late) A52.76
ulcer (any site) (early) (secondary) A51.39
late A52.79
perforating A52.79
foot A52.11
urethra (late) A52.76
urogenital (late) A52.76
uterus (late) A52.76
uveal tract (secondary) A51.43
late A52.71
uveitis (secondary) A51.43
late A52.71

Syphilis, syphilitic — *continued*
uvula (late) (perforated) A52.79
vagina A51.0
late A52.76
valvulitis NEC A52.03
vascular A52.00
brain (cerebral) A52.05
ventriculi A52.74
vesicae urinariae (late) A52.76
viscera (abdominal) (late) A52.74
secondary A51.49
vitreous (opacities) (late) A52.71
hemorrhage A52.71
vulva A51.0
late A52.76
secondary A51.39
Syphiloma A52.79
cardiovascular system A52.00
central nervous system A52.3
circulatory system A52.00
congenital A50.59
Syphilophobia F45.29

Syringadenoma — *see also* Neoplasm, skin, benign
papillary — *see* Neoplasm, skin, benign
Syringobulbia G95.0
Syringocystadenoma — *see* Neoplasm, skin, benign
papillary — *see* Neoplasm, skin, benign
Syringoma — *see also* Neoplasm, skin, benign
chondroid — *see* Neoplasm, skin, benign
Syringomyelia G95.0
Syringomyelitis — *see* Encephalitis
Syringomyelocele — *see* Spina bifida
Syringopontia G95.0
System, systemic — *see also* condition
disease, combined — *see* Degeneration, combined
inflammatory response syndrome (SIRS) of non-infectious origin (without organ dysfunction) R65.10
with acute organ dysfunction R65.11
lupus erythematosus M32.9
inhibitor present D68.62

☑ **Additional Character Required — Refer to the Tabular List for Character Selection** ▽ **Subterms under main terms may continue to next column or page**

T

Tabacism, tabacosis, tabagism — *see also* Poisoning, tobacco
  meaning dependence (without remission) F17.200
    with
      disorder F17.299
        in remission F17.211
        specified disorder NEC F17.298
        withdrawal F17.203
Tabardillo A75.9
  flea-borne A75.2
  louse-borne A75.0
Tabes, tabetic A52.10
  with
    central nervous system syphilis A52.10
    Charcot's joint A52.16
    cord bladder A52.19
    crisis, viscera (any) A52.19
    paralysis, general A52.17
    paresis (general) A52.17
    perforating ulcer (foot) A52.19
  arthropathy (Charcot) A52.16
  bladder A52.19
  bone A52.11
  cerebrospinal A52.12
  congenital A50.45
  conjugal A52.10
  dorsalis A52.11
    juvenile A50.49
  juvenile A50.49
  latent A52.19
  mesenterica A18.39
  paralysis, insane, general A52.17
  spasmodic A52.17
  syphilis (cerebrospinal) A52.12
Taboparalysis A52.17
Taboparesis (remission) A52.17
  juvenile A50.45
TAC (trigeminal autonomic cephalgia) **NEC** G44.099
  intractable G44.091
  not intractable G44.099
Tache noir S60.22- ☑
Tachyalimentation K91.2
Tachyarrhythmia, tachyrhythmia — *see* Tachycardia
Tachycardia R00.0
  atrial (paroxysmal) I47.1
  auricular I47.1
  AV nodal re-entry (re-entrant) I47.1
  junctional (paroxysmal) I47.1
  newborn P29.11
  nodal (paroxysmal) I47.1
  non-paroxysmal AV nodal I45.89
  paroxysmal (sustained) (nonsustained) I47.9
    with sinus bradycardia I49.5
    atrial (PAT) I47.1
    atrioventricular (AV) (re-entrant) I47.1
      psychogenic F54
    junctional I47.1
      ectopic I47.1
    nodal I47.1
    psychogenic (atrial) (supraventricular) (ventricular) F54
    supraventricular (sustained) I47.1
      psychogenic F54
    ventricular I47.1
      psychogenic F54
  psychogenic F45.8
  sick sinus I49.5
  sinoauricular NOS R00.0
    paroxysmal I47.1
  sinus [sinusal] NOS R00.0
    paroxysmal I47.1
  supraventricular I47.1
  ventricular (paroxysmal) (sustained) I47.2
    psychogenic F54
Tachygastria K31.89
Tachypnea R06.82
  hysterical F45.8
  newborn (idiopathic) (transitory) P22.1
  psychogenic F45.8
  transitory, of newborn P22.1
TACO (transfusion associated circulatory overload) E87.71
Taenia (infection) (infestation) B68.9
  diminuta B71.0
  echinococcal infestation B67.90
  mediocanellata B68.1

Taenia — *continued*
  nana B71.0
  saginata B68.1
  solium (intestinal form) B68.0
    larval form — *see* Cysticercosis
Taeniasis (intestine) — *see* Taenia
Tag (hypertrophied skin) (infected) L91.8
  adenoid J35.8
  anus K64.4
  hemorrhoidal K64.4
  hymen N89.8
  perineal N90.89
  preauricular Q17.0
  sentinel K64.4
  skin L91.8
    accessory (congenital) Q82.8
    anus K64.4
    congenital Q82.8
    preauricular Q17.0
  tonsil J35.8
  urethra, urethral N36.8
  vulva N90.89
Tahyna fever B33.8
Takahara's disease E80.3
Takayasu's disease or syndrome M31.4
Talcosis (pulmonary) J62.0
Talipes (congenital) Q66.89
  acquired, planus — *see* Deformity, limb, flat foot
  asymmetric Q66.89
  calcaneovalgus Q66.4- ☑
  calcaneovarus Q66.1- ☑
  calcaneus Q66.89
  cavus Q66.7- ☑
  equinovalgus Q66.6
  equinovarus Q66.0- ☑
  equinus Q66.89
  percavus Q66.7- ☑
  planovalgus Q66.6
  planus (acquired) (any degree) — *see also* Deformity, limb, flat foot
    congenital Q66.5- ☑
    due to rickets (sequelae) E64.3
  valgus Q66.6
  varus Q66.3- ☑
Tall stature, constitutional E34.4
Talma's disease M62.89
Talon noir S90.3- ☑
  hand S60.22- ☑
  heel S90.3- ☑
  toe S90.1- ☑
Tamponade, heart I31.4
Tanapox (virus disease) B08.71
Tangier disease E78.6
Tantrum, child problem F91.8
Tapeworm (infection) (infestation) — *see* Infestation, tapeworm
Tapia's syndrome G52.7
TAR (thrombocytopenia with absent radius) **syndrome** Q87.2
Tarral-Besnier disease L44.0
Tarsal tunnel syndrome — *see* Syndrome, tarsal tunnel
Tarsalgia — *see* Pain, limb, lower
Tarsitis (eyelid) H01.8
  syphilitic A52.71
  tuberculous A18.4
Tartar (teeth) (dental calculus) K03.6
Tattoo (mark) L81.8
Tauri's disease E74.09
Taurodontism K00.2
Taussig-Bing syndrome Q20.1
Taybi's syndrome Q87.2
Tay-Sachs amaurotic familial idiocy or disease E75.02
TBI (traumatic brain injury) S06.9 ☑
Teacher's node or nodule J38.2
Tear, torn (traumatic) — *see also* Laceration
  with abortion — *see* Abortion
  annular fibrosis M51.35
  anus, anal (sphincter) S31.831 ☑
    complicating delivery
      with third degree perineal laceration — *see also* Delivery, complicated, by, laceration, perineum, third degree O70.20
        with mucosa O70.3
      without third degree perineal laceration O70.4
    nontraumatic (healed) (old) K62.81
  articular cartilage, old — *see* Derangement, joint, articular cartilage, by site

Tear, torn — *continued*
  bladder
    with ectopic or molar pregnancy O08.6
    following ectopic or molar pregnancy O08.6
    obstetrical O71.5
    traumatic — *see* Injury, bladder
  bowel
    with ectopic or molar pregnancy O08.6
    following ectopic or molar pregnancy O08.6
    obstetrical trauma O71.5
  broad ligament
    with ectopic or molar pregnancy O08.6
    following ectopic or molar pregnancy O08.6
    obstetrical trauma O71.6
  bucket handle (knee) (meniscus) — *see* Tear, meniscus
  capsule, joint — *see* Sprain
  cartilage — *see also* Sprain
    articular, old — *see* Derangement, joint, articular cartilage, by site
  cervix
    with ectopic or molar pregnancy O08.6
    following ectopic or molar pregnancy O08.6
    obstetrical trauma (current) O71.3
    old N88.1
    traumatic — *see* Injury, uterus
  dural G97.41
    nontraumatic G96.11
  internal organ — *see* Injury, by site
  knee cartilage
    articular (current) S83.3- ☑
    old — *see* Derangement, knee, meniscus, due to old tear
  ligament — *see* Sprain
  meniscus (knee) (current injury) S83.209 ☑
    bucket-handle S83.20- ☑
    lateral
      bucket-handle S83.25- ☑
      complex S83.27- ☑
      peripheral S83.26- ☑
      specified type NEC S83.28- ☑
    medial
      bucket-handle S83.21- ☑
      complex S83.23- ☑
      peripheral S83.22- ☑
      specified type NEC S83.24- ☑
    old — *see* Derangement, knee, meniscus, due to old tear
    site other than knee — *code as* Sprain
    specified type NEC S83.20- ☑
  muscle — *see* Strain
  pelvic
    floor, complicating delivery O70.1
    organ NEC, obstetrical trauma O71.5
      with ectopic or molar pregnancy O08.6
      following ectopic or molar pregnancy O08.6
  perineal, secondary O90.1
  periurethral tissue, obstetrical trauma O71.82
    with ectopic or molar pregnancy O08.6
    following ectopic or molar pregnancy O08.6
  rectovaginal septum — *see* Laceration, vagina
  retina, retinal (without detachment) (horseshoe) — *see also* Break, retina, horseshoe
    with detachment — *see* Detachment, retina, with retinal, break
  rotator cuff (nontraumatic) M75.10- ☑
    complete M75.12- ☑
    incomplete M75.11- ☑
    traumatic S46.01- ☑
      capsule S43.42- ☑
  semilunar cartilage, knee — *see* Tear, meniscus
  supraspinatus (complete) (incomplete) (nontraumatic) — *see also* Tear, rotator cuff M75.10- ☑
  tendon — *see* Strain
  tentorial, at birth P10.4
  umbilical cord
    complicating delivery O69.89 ☑
  urethra
    with ectopic or molar pregnancy O08.6
    following ectopic or molar pregnancy O08.6
    obstetrical trauma O71.5
  uterus — *see* Injury, uterus
  vagina — *see* Laceration, vagina
  vessel, from catheter — *see* Puncture, accidental complicating surgery
  vulva, complicating delivery O70.0
Tear-stone — *see* Dacryolith
Teeth — *see also* condition

Teeth — *continued*
- grinding
  - psychogenic F45.8
  - sleep related G47.63
Teething (syndrome) K00.7
Telangiectasia, telangiectasis (verrucous) I78.1
- ataxic (cerebellar) (Louis-Bar) G11.3
- familial I78.0
- hemorrhagic, hereditary (congenital) (senile) I78.0
- hereditary, hemorrhagic (congenital) (senile) I78.0
- juxtafoveal H35.07- ☑
- macular H35.07- ☑
- macularis eruptiva perstans D47.01
- parafoveal H35.07- ☑
- retinal (idiopathic) (juxtafoveal) (macular) (parafoveal) H35.07- ☑
- spider I78.1
Telephone scatologia F65.89
Telescoped bowel or intestine K56.1
- congenital Q43.8
Temperature
- body, high (of unknown origin) R50.9
- cold, trauma from T69.9 ☑
  - newborn P80.0
  - specified effect NEC T69.8 ☑
Temple — *see* condition
Temporal — *see* condition
Temporomandibular joint pain-dysfunction syndrome M26.62- ☑
Temporosphenoidal — *see* condition
Tendency
- bleeding — *see* Defect, coagulation
- suicide
  - meaning personal history of attempted suicide Z91.5
  - meaning suicidal ideation — *see* Ideation, suicidal
- to fall R29.6
Tenderness, abdominal R10.819
- epigastric R10.816
- generalized R10.817
- left lower quadrant R10.814
- left upper quadrant R10.812
- periumbilic R10.815
- rebound R10.829
  - epigastric R10.826
  - generalized R10.827
  - left lower quadrant R10.824
  - left upper quadrant R10.822
  - periumbilic R10.825
  - right lower quadrant R10.823
  - right upper quadrant R10.821
- right lower quadrant R10.813
- right upper quadrant R10.811
Tendinitis, tendonitis — *see also* Enthesopathy
- Achilles M76.6- ☑
- adhesive — *see* Tenosynovitis, specified type NEC
  - shoulder — *see* Capsulitis, adhesive
- bicipital M75.2- ☑
- calcific M65.2- ☑
  - ankle M65.27- ☑
  - foot M65.27- ☑
  - forearm M65.23- ☑
  - hand M65.24- ☑
  - lower leg M65.26- ☑
  - multiple sites M65.29
  - pelvic region M65.25- ☑
  - shoulder M75.3- ☑
  - specified site NEC M65.28
  - thigh M65.25- ☑
  - upper arm M65.22- ☑
- due to use, overuse, pressure — *see also* Disorder, soft tissue, due to use
  - specified NEC — *see* Disorder, soft tissue, due to use, specified NEC
- gluteal M76.0- ☑
- patellar M76.5- ☑
- peroneal M76.7- ☑
- psoas M76.1- ☑
- tibial (posterior) M76.82- ☑
  - anterior M76.81- ☑
- trochanteric — *see* Bursitis, hip, trochanteric
Tendon — *see* condition
Tendosynovitis — *see* Tenosynovitis
Tenesmus (rectal) R19.8
- vesical R30.1
Tennis elbow — *see* Epicondylitis, lateral
Tenonitis — *see also* Tenosynovitis
- eye (capsule) H05.04- ☑

Tenontosynovitis — *see* Tenosynovitis
Tenontothecitis — *see* Tenosynovitis
Tenophyte — *see* Disorder, synovium, specified type NEC
Tenosynovitis — *see also* Synovitis M65.9
- adhesive — *see* Tenosynovitis, specified type NEC
  - shoulder — *see* Capsulitis, adhesive
- bicipital (calcifying) — *see* Tendinitis, bicipital
- gonococcal A54.49
- in (due to)
  - crystals M65.8- ☑
  - gonorrhea A54.49
  - syphilis (late) A52.78
  - use, overuse, pressure — *see also* Disorder, soft tissue, due to use
    - specified NEC — *see* Disorder, soft tissue, due to use, specified NEC
- infective NEC M65.1- ☑
  - ankle M65.17- ☑
  - foot M65.17- ☑
  - forearm M65.13- ☑
  - hand M65.14- ☑
  - lower leg M65.16- ☑
  - multiple sites M65.19
  - pelvic region M65.15- ☑
  - shoulder region M65.11- ☑
  - specified site NEC M65.18
  - thigh M65.15- ☑
  - upper arm M65.12- ☑
- radial styloid M65.4
- shoulder region M65.81- ☑
  - adhesive — *see* Capsulitis, adhesive
- specified type NEC M65.88
  - ankle M65.87- ☑
  - foot M65.87- ☑
  - forearm M65.83- ☑
  - hand M65.84- ☑
  - lower leg M65.86- ☑
  - multiple sites M65.89
  - pelvic region M65.85- ☑
  - shoulder region M65.81- ☑
  - specified site NEC M65.88
  - thigh M65.85- ☑
  - upper arm M65.82- ☑
- tuberculous — *see* Tuberculosis, tenosynovitis
Tenovaginitis — *see* Tenosynovitis
Tension
- arterial, high — *see also* Hypertension
  - without diagnosis of hypertension R03.0
- headache G44.209
  - intractable G44.201
  - not intractable G44.209
- nervous R45.0
- pneumothorax J93.0
- premenstrual N94.3
- state (mental) F48.9
Tentorium — *see* condition
Teratencephalus Q89.8
Teratism Q89.7
Teratoblastoma (malignant) — *see* Neoplasm, malignant, by site
Teratocarcinoma — *see also* Neoplasm, malignant, by site
- liver C22.7
Teratoma (solid) — *see also* Neoplasm, uncertain behavior, by site
- with embryonal carcinoma, mixed — *see* Neoplasm, malignant, by site
- with malignant transformation — *see* Neoplasm, malignant, by site
- adult (cystic) — *see* Neoplasm, benign, by site
- benign — *see* Neoplasm, benign, by site
- combined with choriocarcinoma — *see* Neoplasm, malignant, by site
- cystic (adult) — *see* Neoplasm, benign, by site
- differentiated — *see* Neoplasm, benign, by site
- embryonal — *see also* Neoplasm, malignant, by site
  - liver C22.7
- immature — *see* Neoplasm, malignant, by site
- liver C22.7
  - adult, benign, cystic, differentiated type or mature D13.4
- malignant — *see also* Neoplasm, malignant, by site
  - anaplastic — *see* Neoplasm, malignant, by site
  - intermediate — *see* Neoplasm, malignant, by site
    - specified site — *see* Neoplasm, malignant, by site
    - unspecified site C62.90

Teratoma — *continued*
- malignant — *see also* Neoplasm, malignant, by site — *continued*
  - undifferentiated — *see* Neoplasm, malignant, by site
  - mature — *see* Neoplasm, uncertain behavior, by site
    - malignant — *see* Neoplasm, by site, malignant, by site
- ovary D27.- ☑
  - embryonal, immature or malignant C56- ☑
- solid — *see* Neoplasm, uncertain behavior, by site
- testis C62.9- ☑
  - adult, benign, cystic, differentiated type or mature D29.2- ☑
  - scrotal C62.1- ☑
  - undescended C62.0- ☑
Termination
- anomalous — *see also* Malposition, congenital
  - right pulmonary vein Q26.3
- pregnancy, elective Z33.2
Ternidens diminutus infestation B81.8
Ternidensiasis B81.8
Terror(s) night (child) F51.4
Terrorism, victim of Z65.4
Terry's syndrome — *see also* Myopia, degenerative H44.2- ☑
Tertiary — *see* condition
Test, tests, testing (for)
- adequacy (for dialysis)
  - hemodialysis Z49.31
  - peritoneal Z49.32
- blood pressure Z01.30
  - abnormal reading — *see* Blood, pressure
- blood typing Z01.83
  - Rh typing Z01.83
- blood-alcohol Z04.89
  - positive — *see* Findings, abnormal, in blood
- blood-drug Z04.89
  - positive — *see* Findings, abnormal, in blood
- cardiac pulse generator (battery) Z45.010
- fertility Z31.41
- genetic
  - disease carrier status for procreative management
    - female Z31.430
    - male Z31.440
  - male partner of patient with recurrent pregnancy loss Z31.441
  - procreative management NEC
    - female Z31.438
    - male Z31.448
- hearing Z01.10
  - with abnormal findings NEC Z01.118
  - infant or child (over 28 days old) Z00.129
    - with abnormal findings Z00.121
- HIV (human immunodeficiency virus)
  - nonconclusive (in infants) R75
  - positive Z21
  - seropositive Z21
- immunity status Z01.84
- intelligence NEC Z01.89
- laboratory (as part of a general medical examination) Z00.00
  - with abnormal finding Z00.01
  - for medicolegal reason NEC Z04.89
- male partner of patient with recurrent pregnancy loss Z31.441
- Mantoux (for tuberculosis) Z11.1
  - abnormal result R76.11
- pregnancy, positive first pregnancy — *see* Pregnancy, normal, first
- procreative Z31.49
  - fertility Z31.41
- skin, diagnostic
  - allergy Z01.82
    - special screening examination — *see* Screening, by name of disease
  - Mantoux Z11.1
  - tuberculin Z11.1
- specified NEC Z01.89
- tuberculin Z11.1
  - abnormal result R76.11
- vision Z01.00
  - with abnormal findings Z01.01
  - following failed vision screening Z01.020
    - with abnormal findings Z01.021
  - infant or child (over 28 days old) Z00.129
    - with abnormal findings Z00.121
- Wassermann Z11.3

Test, tests, testing — *continued*
  Wassermann — *continued*
    positive — *see* Serology for syphilis, positive
Testicle, testicular, testis — *see also* condition
  feminization syndrome — *see also* Syndrome, androgen insensitivity E34.51
  migrans Q55.29
Tetanus, tetanic (cephalic) (convulsions) A35
  with
    abortion A34
    ectopic or molar pregnancy O08.0
  following ectopic or molar pregnancy O08.0
  inoculation reaction (due to serum) — *see* Complications, vaccination
  neonatorum A33
  obstetrical A34
  puerperal, postpartum, childbirth A34
Tetany (due to) R29.0
  alkalosis E87.3
  associated with rickets E55.0
  convulsions R29.0
    hysterical F44.5
  functional (hysterical) F44.5
  hyperkinetic R29.0
    hysterical F44.5
  hyperpnea R06.4
    hysterical F44.5
    psychogenic F45.8
  hyperventilation — *see also* Hyperventilation R06.4
    hysterical F44.5
  neonatal (without calcium or magnesium deficiency) P71.3
  parathyroid (gland) E20.9
  parathyroprival E89.2
  post- (para)thyroidectomy E89.2
  postoperative E89.2
  pseudotetany R29.0
  psychogenic (conversion reaction) F44.5
Tetralogy of Fallot Q21.3
Tetraplegia (chronic) — *see also* Quadriplegia G82.50
Thailand hemorrhagic fever A91
Thalassanemia — *see* Thalassemia
Thalassemia (anemia) (disease) D56.9
  with other hemoglobinopathy D56.8
  alpha (major) (severe) (triple gene defect) D56.0
    minor D56.3
    silent carrier D56.3
    trait D56.3
  beta (severe) D56.1
    homozygous D56.1
    major D56.1
    minor D56.3
    trait D56.3
  delta-beta (homozygous) D56.2
    minor D56.3
    trait D56.3
  dominant D56.8
  hemoglobin
    C D56.8
    E-beta D56.5
  intermedia D56.1
  major D56.1
  minor D56.3
  mixed D56.8
  sickle-cell — *see* Disease, sickle-cell, thalassemia
  specified type NEC D56.8
  trait D56.3
  variants D56.8
Thanatophoric dwarfism or short stature Q77.1
Thaysen-Gee disease (nontropical sprue) K90.0
Thaysen's disease K90.0
Thecoma D27- ☑
  luteinized D27- ☑
  malignant C56- ☑
Thelarche, premature E30.8
Thelaziasis B83.8
Thelitis N61.0
  puerperal, postpartum or gestational — *see* Infection, nipple
Therapeutic — *see* condition
Therapy
  drug, long-term (current) (prophylactic)
    agents affecting estrogen receptors and estrogen levels NEC Z79.818
    anastrozole (Arimidex) Z79.811
    antibiotics Z79.2
      short-term use — *omit code*
    anticoagulants Z79.01

Therapy — *continued*
  drug, long-term — *continued*
    anti-inflammatory Z79.1
    antiplatelet Z79.02
    antithrombotics Z79.02
    aromatase inhibitors Z79.811
    aspirin Z79.82
    birth control pill or patch Z79.3
    bisphosphonates Z79.83
    contraceptive, oral Z79.3
    drug, specified NEC Z79.899
    estrogen receptor downregulators Z79.818
    Evista Z79.810
    exemestane (Aromasin) Z79.811
    Fareston Z79.810
    fulvestrant (Faslodex) Z79.818
    gonadotropin-releasing hormone (GnRH) agonist Z79.818
    goserelin acetate (Zoladex) Z79.818
    hormone replacement Z79.890
    insulin Z79.4
    letrozole (Femara) Z79.811
    leuprolide acetate (leuprorelin) (Lupron) Z79.818
    megestrol acetate (Megace) Z79.818
    methadone
      for pain management Z79.891
      maintenance therapy F11.20
    Nolvadex Z79.810
    opiate analgesic Z79.891
    oral contraceptive Z79.3
    raloxifene (Evista) Z79.810
    selective estrogen receptor modulators (SERMs) Z79.810
    short term — *omit code*
    steroids
      inhaled Z79.51
      systemic Z79.52
    tamoxifen (Nolvadex) Z79.810
    toremifene (Fareston) Z79.810
Thermic — *see* condition
Thermography (abnormal) — *see also* Abnormal, diagnostic imaging R93.89
  breast R92.8
Thermoplegia T67.01 ☑
Thesaurismosis, glycogen — *see* Disease, glycogen storage
Thiamin deficiency E51.9
  specified NEC E51.8
Thiaminic deficiency with beriberi E51.11
Thibierge-Weissenbach syndrome — *see* Sclerosis, systemic
Thickening
  bone — *see* Hypertrophy, bone
  breast N64.59
  endometrium R93.89
  epidermal L85.9
    specified NEC L85.8
  hymen N89.6
  larynx J38.7
  nail L60.2
    congenital Q84.5
  periosteal — *see* Hypertrophy, bone
  pleura J92.9
    with asbestos J92.0
  skin R23.4
  subepiglottic J38.7
  tongue K14.8
  valve, heart — *see* Endocarditis
Thigh — *see* condition
Thinning vertebra — *see* Spondylopathy, specified NEC
Thirst, excessive R63.1
  due to deprivation of water T73.1 ☑
Thomsen disease G71.12
Thoracic — *see also* condition
  kidney Q63.2
  outlet syndrome G54.0
Thoracogastroschisis (congenital) Q79.8
Thoracopagus Q89.4
Thorax — *see* condition
Thorn's syndrome N28.89
Thorson-Björck syndrome E34.0
Threadworm (infection) (infestation) B80
Threatened
  abortion O20.0
    with subsequent abortion O03.9
  job loss, anxiety concerning Z56.2
  labor (without delivery) O47.9
    at or after 37 completed weeks of gestation O47.1

Threatened — *continued*
  labor — *continued*
    before 37 completed weeks of gestation O47.0- ☑
  loss of job, anxiety concerning Z56.2
  miscarriage O20.0
  unemployment, anxiety concerning Z56.2
Three-day fever A93.1
Threshers' lung J67.0
Thrix annulata (congenital) Q84.1
Throat — *see* condition
Thrombasthenia (Glanzmann) (hemorrhagic) (hereditary) D69.1
Thromboangiitis I73.1
  obliterans (general) I73.1
    cerebral I67.89
    vessels
      brain I67.89
      spinal cord I67.89
Thromboarteritis — *see* Arteritis
Thromboasthenia (Glanzmann) (hemorrhagic) (hereditary) D69.1
Thrombocytasthenia (Glanzmann) D69.1
Thrombocythemia (essential) (hemorrhagic) (idiopathic) (primary) D47.3
Thrombocytopathy (dystrophic) (granulopenic) D69.1
Thrombocytopenia, thrombocytopenic D69.6
  with absent radius (TAR) Q87.2
  congenital D69.42
  dilutional D69.59
  due to
    (massive) blood transfusion D69.59
    drugs D69.59
    extracorporeal circulation of blood D69.59
    platelet alloimmunization D69.59
  essential D69.3
  heparin induced (HIT) D75.82
  hereditary D69.42
  idiopathic D69.3
  neonatal, transitory P61.0
    due to
      exchange transfusion P61.0
      idiopathic maternal thrombocytopenia P61.0
      isoimmunization P61.0
  primary NEC D69.49
    idiopathic D69.3
  puerperal, postpartum O72.3
  secondary D69.59
  transient neonatal P61.0
Thrombocytosis, essential D47.3
  primary D47.3
Thromboembolism — *see* Embolism
Thrombopathy (Bernard-Soulier) D69.1
  constitutional D68.0
  Willebrand-Jürgens D68.0
Thrombopenia — *see* Thrombocytopenia
Thrombophilia D68.59
  primary NEC D68.59
  secondary NEC D68.69
  specified NEC D68.69
Thrombophlebitis I80.9
  antepartum O22.2- ☑
    deep O22.3- ☑
    superficial O22.2- ☑
  calf muscular vein (NOS) I80.25- ☑
  cavernous (venous) sinus G08
    complicating pregnancy O22.5- ☑
    nonpyogenic I67.6
  cerebral (sinus) (vein) G08
    nonpyogenic I67.6
    sequelae G09
  due to implanted device — *see* Complications, by site and type, specified NEC
  during or resulting from a procedure NEC T81.72 ☑
  femoral vein (superficial) I80.1- ☑
  femoropopliteal vein I80.0- ☑
  gastrocnemial vein I80.25- ☑
  hepatic (vein) I80.8
  idiopathic, recurrent I82.1
  iliac vein (common) (external) (internal) I80.21- ☑
  iliofemoral I80.1- ☑
  intracranial venous sinus (any) G08
    nonpyogenic I67.6
    sequelae G09
  intraspinal venous sinuses and veins G08
    nonpyogenic G95.19
  lateral (venous) sinus G08
    nonpyogenic I67.6
  leg I80.3

Thrombophlebitis — *continued*
 leg — *continued*
  superficial I80.0- ☑
 longitudinal (venous) sinus G08
  nonpyogenic I67.6
 lower extremity I80.299
 migrans, migrating I82.1
 pelvic
  with ectopic or molar pregnancy O08.0
  following ectopic or molar pregnancy O08.0
  puerperal O87.1
 peroneal vein I80.24- ☑
 popliteal vein — *see* Phlebitis, leg, deep, popliteal
 portal (vein) K75.1
 postoperative T81.72 ☑
 pregnancy — *see* Thrombophlebitis, antepartum
 puerperal, postpartum, childbirth O87.0
  deep O87.1
  pelvic O87.1
  septic O86.81
  superficial O87.0
 saphenous (greater) (lesser) I80.0- ☑
 sinus (intracranial) G08
  nonpyogenic I67.6
 soleal vein I80.25- ☑
 specified site NEC I80.8
 tibial vein (anterior) (posterior) I80.23- ☑
Thrombosis, thrombotic (bland) (multiple) (progressive) (silent) (vessel) I82.90
 anal K64.5
 antepartum — *see* Thrombophlebitis, antepartum
 aorta, aortic I74.10
  abdominal I74.09
   saddle I74.01
  bifurcation I74.09
  saddle I74.01
  specified site NEC I74.19
  terminal I74.09
  thoracic I74.11
  valve — *see* Endocarditis, aortic
 apoplexy I63.3- ☑
 artery, arteries (postinfectional) I74.9
  auditory, internal — *see* Occlusion, artery, precerebral, specified NEC
  basilar — *see* Occlusion, artery, basilar
  carotid (common) (internal) — *see* Occlusion, artery, carotid
  cerebellar (anterior inferior) (posterior inferior) (superior) — *see* Occlusion, artery, cerebellar
  cerebral — *see* Occlusion, artery, cerebral
  choroidal (anterior) — *see* Occlusion, artery, precerebral, specified NEC
  communicating, posterior — *see* Occlusion, artery, precerebral, specified NEC
  coronary — *see also* Infarct, myocardium
   not resulting in infarction I24.0
  hepatic I74.8
  hypophyseal — *see* Occlusion, artery, precerebral, specified NEC
  iliac I74.5
  limb I74.4
   lower I74.3
   upper I74.2
  meningeal, anterior or posterior — *see* Occlusion, artery, cerebral, specified NEC
  mesenteric (with gangrene) — *see also* Infarct, intestine K55.069
  ophthalmic — *see* Occlusion, artery, retina
  pontine — *see* Occlusion, artery, precerebral, specified NEC
  precerebral — *see* Occlusion, artery, precerebral
  pulmonary (iatrogenic) — *see* Embolism, pulmonary
  renal N28.0
  retinal — *see* Occlusion, artery, retina
  spinal, anterior or posterior G95.11
  traumatic NEC T14.8 ☑
  vertebral — *see* Occlusion, artery, vertebral
 atrium, auricular — *see also* Infarct, myocardium
  following acute myocardial infarction (current complication) I23.6
  not resulting in infarction I51.3
  old I51.3
 basilar (artery) — *see* Occlusion, artery, basilar
 brain (artery) (stem) — *see also* Occlusion, artery, cerebral
  due to syphilis A52.05
  puerperal O99.43
  sinus — *see* Thrombosis, intracranial venous sinus

Thrombosis, thrombotic — *continued*
 capillary I78.8
 cardiac — *see also* Infarct, myocardium
  not resulting in infarction I51.3
  old I51.3
  valve — *see* Endocarditis
 carotid (artery) (common) (internal) — *see* Occlusion, artery, carotid
 cavernous (venous) sinus — *see* Thrombosis, intracranial venous sinus
 cerebellar artery (anterior inferior) (posterior inferior) (superior) I66.3
 cerebral (artery) — *see* Occlusion, artery, cerebral
 cerebrovenous sinus — *see also* Thrombosis, intracranial venous sinus
  puerperium O87.3
 chronic I82.91
 coronary (artery) (vein) — *see also* Infarct, myocardium
  not resulting in infarction I24.0
 corpus cavernosum N48.89
 cortical I66.9
 deep — *see* Embolism, vein, lower extremity
 due to device, implant or graft — *see also* Complications, by site and type, specified NEC T85.868 ☑
  arterial graft NEC T82.868 ☑
  breast (implant) T85.868 ☑
  catheter NEC T85.868 ☑
   dialysis (renal) T82.868 ☑
    intraperitoneal T85.868 ☑
   infusion NEC T82.868 ☑
    spinal (epidural) (subdural) T85.860 ☑
   urinary (indwelling) T83.86 ☑
  electronic (electrode) (pulse generator) (stimulator)
   bone T84.86 ☑
   cardiac T82.867 ☑
   nervous system (brain) (peripheral nerve) (spinal) T85.860 ☑
   urinary T83.86 ☑
  fixation, internal (orthopedic) NEC T84.86 ☑
  gastrointestinal (bile duct) (esophagus) T85.868 ☑
  genital NEC T83.86 ☑
  heart T82.867 ☑
  joint prosthesis T84.86 ☑
  ocular (corneal graft) (orbital implant) NEC T85.868 ☑
  orthopedic NEC T84.86 ☑
  specified NEC T85.868 ☑
  urinary NEC T83.86 ☑
  vascular NEC T82.868 ☑
  ventricular intracranial shunt T85.860 ☑
 during the puerperium — *see* Thrombosis, puerperal
 endocardial — *see also* Infarct, myocardium
  not resulting in infarction I51.3
 eye — *see* Occlusion, retina
 genital organ
  female NEC N94.89
   pregnancy — *see* Thrombophlebitis, antepartum
  male N50.1
 gestational — *see* Phlebopathy, gestational
 heart (chamber) — *see also* Infarct, myocardium
  not resulting in infarction I51.3
  old I51.3
 hepatic (vein) I82.0
  artery I74.8
 history (of) Z86.718
 intestine (with gangrene) — *see also* Infarct, intestine K55.069
 intracardiac NEC (apical) (atrial) (auricular) (ventricular) (old) I51.3
 intracranial (arterial) I66.9
  venous sinus (any) G08
   nonpyogenic origin I67.6
   puerperium O87.3
 intramural — *see also* Infarct, myocardium
  not resulting in infarction I51.3
  old I51.3
 intraspinal venous sinuses and veins G08
  nonpyogenic G95.19
 kidney (artery) N28.0
 lateral (venous) sinus — *see* Thrombosis, intracranial venous sinus
 leg — *see* Thrombosis, vein, lower extremity
  arterial I74.3
 liver (venous) I82.0
  artery I74.8
  portal vein I81

Thrombosis, thrombotic — *continued*
 longitudinal (venous) sinus — *see* Thrombosis, intracranial venous sinus
 lower limb — *see* Thrombosis, vein, lower extremity
 lung (iatrogenic) (postoperative) — *see* Embolism, pulmonary
 meninges (brain) (arterial) I66.8
 mesenteric (artery) (with gangrene) — *see also* Infarct, intestine K55.069
  vein (inferior) (superior) K55.0 ☑
 mitral I34.8
 mural — *see also* Infarct, myocardium
  due to syphilis A52.06
  not resulting in infarction I51.3
  old I51.3
 omentum (with gangrene) — *see also* Infarct, intestine K55.069
 ophthalmic — *see* Occlusion, retina
 pampiniform plexus (male) N50.1
 parietal — *see also* Infarct, myocardium
  not resulting in infarction I24.0
 penis, superficial vein N48.81
 perianal venous K64.5
 peripheral arteries I74.4
  upper I74.2
 personal history (of) Z86.718
 portal I81
  due to syphilis A52.09
 precerebral artery — *see* Occlusion, artery, precerebral
 puerperal, postpartum O87.0
  brain (artery) O99.43
   venous (sinus) O87.3
  cardiac O99.43
  cerebral (artery) O99.43
   venous (sinus) O87.3
  superficial O87.0
 pulmonary (artery) (iatrogenic) (postoperative) (vein) — *see* Embolism, pulmonary
 renal (artery) N28.0
  vein I82.3
 resulting from presence of device, implant or graft — *see* Complications, by site and type, specified NEC
 retina, retinal — *see* Occlusion, retina
 scrotum N50.1
 seminal vesicle N50.1
 sigmoid (venous) sinus — *see* Thrombosis, intracranial venous sinus
 sinus, intracranial (any) — *see* Thrombosis, intracranial venous sinus
 specified site NEC I82.890
  chronic I82.891
 spermatic cord N50.1
 spinal cord (arterial) G95.11
  due to syphilis A52.09
  pyogenic origin G06.1
 spleen, splenic D73.5
  artery I74.8
 testis N50.1
 traumatic NEC T14.8 ☑
 tricuspid I07.8
 tumor — *see* Neoplasm, unspecified behavior, by site
 tunica vaginalis N50.1
 umbilical cord (vessels), complicating delivery O69.5 ☑
 vas deferens N50.1
 vein (acute) I82.90
  antecubital I82.61- ☑
   chronic I82.71- ☑
  axillary I82.A1- ☑ (*following* I82.7)
   chronic I82.A2- ☑ (*following* I82.7)
  basilic I82.61- ☑
   chronic I82.71- ☑
  brachial I82.62- ☑
   chronic I82.72- ☑
  brachiocephalic (innominate) I82.290
   chronic I82.291
  cephalic I82.61- ☑
   chronic I82.71- ☑
  cerebral, nonpyogenic I67.6
  chronic I82.91
  deep (DVT) I82.40- ☑
   calf I82.4Z- ☑
    chronic I82.5Z- ☑
   lower leg I82.4Z- ☑
    chronic I82.5Z- ☑
   thigh I82.4Y- ☑
    chronic I82.5Y- ☑

☑ **Additional Character Required** — **Refer to the Tabular List for Character Selection**   ▽ Subterms under main terms may continue to next column or page

Thrombosis, thrombotic — *continued*
  vein — *continued*
    deep — *continued*
      upper leg I82.4Y ☑
        chronic I82.5Y- ☑
      femoral I82.41- ☑
        chronic I82.51- ☑
      iliac (iliofemoral) I82.42- ☑
        chronic I82.52- ☑
      innominate I82.290
        chronic I82.291
      internal jugular I82.C1- ☑ (*following* I82.7)
        chronic I82.C2- ☑ (*following* I82.7)
      lower extremity
        deep I82.40- ☑
          chronic I82.50- ☑
          specified NEC I82.49- ☑
            chronic NEC I82.59- ☑
        distal
          deep I82.4Z- ☑
        proximal
          deep I82.4Y- ☑
            chronic I82.5Y- ☑
      superficial I82.81- ☑
    perianal K64.5
    popliteal I82.43- ☑
      chronic I82.53- ☑
    radial I82.62- ☑
      chronic I82.72- ☑
    renal I82.3
    saphenous (greater) (lesser) I82.81- ☑
    specified NEC I82.890
      chronic NEC I82.891
    subclavian I82.B1- ☑ (*following* I82.7)
      chronic I82.B2- ☑ (*following* I82.7)
    thoracic NEC I82.290
      chronic I82.291
    tibial I82.44- ☑
      chronic I82.54- ☑
    ulnar I82.62- ☑
      chronic I82.72- ☑
    upper extremity I82.60- ☑
      chronic I82.70- ☑
      deep I82.62- ☑
        chronic I82.72- ☑
      superficial I82.61- ☑
        chronic I82.71- ☑
    vena cava
      inferior I82.220
        chronic I82.221
      superior I82.210
        chronic I82.211
    venous, perianal K64.5
    ventricle — *see also* Infarct, myocardium
      following acute myocardial infarction (current complication) I23.6
      not resulting in infarction I24.0
      old I51.3
Thrombus — *see* Thrombosis
Thrush — *see also* Candidiasis
  newborn P37.5
  oral B37.0
  vaginal B37.3
Thumb — *see also* condition
  sucking (child problem) F98.8
Thymitis E32.8
Thymoma (benign) D15.0
  malignant C37
Thymus, thymic (gland) — *see* condition
Thyrocele — *see* Goiter
Thyroglossal — *see also* condition
  cyst Q89.2
  duct, persistent Q89.2
Thyroid (gland) (body) — *see also* condition
  hormone resistance E07.89
  lingual Q89.2
  nodule (cystic) (nontoxic) (single) E04.1
Thyroiditis E06.9
  acute (nonsuppurative) (pyogenic) (suppurative) E06.0
  autoimmune E06.3
  chronic (nonspecific) (sclerosing) E06.5
    with thyrotoxicosis, transient E06.2
    fibrous E06.5
    lymphadenoid E06.3
    lymphocytic E06.3
    lymphoid E06.3
  de Quervain's E06.1

Thyroiditis — *continued*
  drug-induced E06.4
  fibrous (chronic) E06.5
  giant-cell (follicular) E06.1
  granulomatous (de Quervain) (subacute) E06.1
  Hashimoto's (struma lymphomatosa) E06.3
  iatrogenic E06.4
  ligneous E06.5
  lymphocytic (chronic) E06.3
  lymphoid E06.3
  lymphomatous E06.3
  nonsuppurative E06.1
  postpartum, puerperal O90.5
  pseudotuberculous E06.1
  pyogenic E06.0
  radiation E06.4
  Riedel's E06.5
  subacute (granulomatous) E06.1
  suppurative E06.0
  tuberculous A18.81
  viral E06.1
  woody E06.5
Thyrolingual duct, persistent Q89.2
Thyromegaly E01.0
Thyrotoxic
  crisis — *see* Thyrotoxicosis
  heart disease or failure — *see also* Thyrotoxicosis E05.90 [I43]
    with thyroid storm E05.91 [I43]
  storm — *see* Thyrotoxicosis
Thyrotoxicosis (recurrent) E05.90
  with
    goiter (diffuse) E05.00
      with thyroid storm E05.01
      adenomatous uninodular E05.10
        with thyroid storm E05.11
      multinodular E05.20
        with thyroid storm E05.21
      nodular E05.20
        with thyroid storm E05.21
      uninodular E05.10
        with thyroid storm E05.11
    infiltrative
      dermopathy E05.00
        with thyroid storm E05.01
      ophthalmopathy E05.00
        with thyroid storm E05.01
    single thyroid nodule E05.10
      with thyroid storm E05.11
    thyroid storm E05.91
  due to
    ectopic thyroid nodule or tissue E05.30
      with thyroid storm E05.31
    ingestion of (excessive) thyroid material E05.40
      with thyroid storm E05.41
    overproduction of thyroid-stimulating hormone E05.80
      with thyroid storm E05.81
    specified cause NEC E05.80
      with thyroid storm E05.81
  factitia E05.40
    with thyroid storm E05.41
  heart — *see also* Failure, heart, high-output E05.90 [I43]
    with thyroid storm — *see also* Failure, heart, high-output E05.91 [I43]
    failure — *see also* Failure, heart, high-output E05.90 [I43]
  neonatal (transient) P72.1
  transient with chronic thyroiditis E06.2
Tibia vara — *see* Osteochondrosis, juvenile, tibia
Tic (disorder) F95.9
  breathing F95.8
  child problem F95.0
  compulsive F95.1
  de la Tourette F95.2
  degenerative (generalized) (localized) G25.69
    facial G25.69
  disorder
    chronic
      motor F95.1
      vocal F95.1
    combined vocal and multiple motor F95.2
    transient F95.0
  douloureux F95.9
    atypical G50.1
    postherpetic, postzoster B02.22
  drug-induced G25.61
  eyelid F95.8

Tic — *continued*
  habit F95.9
    chronic F95.1
    transient of childhood F95.0
  lid, transient of childhood F95.0
  motor-verbal F95.2
  occupational F48.8
  orbicularis F95.8
    transient of childhood F95.0
  organic origin G25.69
  postchoreic G25.69
  provisional F95.0
  psychogenic, compulsive F95.1
  salaam R25.8
  spasm (motor or vocal) F95.9
    chronic F95.1
    transient of childhood F95.0
  specified NEC F95.8
Tick-borne — *see* condition
Tietze's disease or syndrome M94.0
Tight, tightness
  anus K62.89
  chest R07.89
  fascia (lata) M62.89
  foreskin (congenital) N47.1
  hymen, hymenal ring N89.6
  introitus (acquired) (congenital) N89.6
  rectal sphincter K62.89
  tendon — *see* Short, tendon
  urethral sphincter N35.919
Tilting vertebra — *see* Dorsopathy, deforming, specified NEC
Timidity, child F93.8
Tinea (intersecta) (tarsi) B35.9
  amiantacea L44.8
  asbestina B35.0
  barbae B35.0
  beard B35.0
  black dot B35.0
  blanca B36.2
  capitis B35.0
  corporis B35.4
  cruris B35.6
  flava B36.0
  foot B35.3
  furfuracea B36.0
  imbricata (Tokelau) B35.5
  kerion B35.0
  manuum B35.2
  microsporic — *see* Dermatophytosis
  nigra B36.1
  nodosa — *see* Piedra
  pedis B35.3
  scalp B35.0
  specified NEC B35.8
  sycosis B35.0
  tonsurans B35.0
  trichophytic — *see* Dermatophytosis
  unguium B35.1
  versicolor B36.0
Tingling sensation (skin) R20.2
Tin-miner's lung J63.5
Tinnitus NOS H93.1- ☑
  audible H93.1- ☑
  aurium H93.1- ☑
  pulsatile H93.A- ☑
  subjective H93.1- ☑
Tipped tooth (teeth) M26.33
Tipping
  pelvis M95.5
    with disproportion (fetopelvic) O33.0
      causing obstructed labor O65.0
  tooth (teeth), fully erupted M26.33
Tiredness R53.83
Tissue — *see* condition
Tobacco (nicotine)
  abuse — *see* Tobacco, use
  dependence — *see* Dependence, drug, nicotine
  harmful use Z72.0
  heart — *see* Tobacco, toxic effect
  maternal use, affecting newborn P04.2
  toxic effect — *see* Table of Drugs and Chemicals, by substance, poisoning
    chewing tobacco — *see* Table of Drugs and Chemicals, by substance, poisoning
    cigarettes — *see* Table of Drugs and Chemicals, by substance, poisoning
  use Z72.0

Tobacco — *continued*
use — *continued*
complicating
childbirth O99.334
pregnancy O99.33- ☑
puerperium O99.335
counseling and surveillance Z71.6
history Z87.891
withdrawal state — *see also* Dependence, drug, nicotine F17.203
Tocopherol deficiency E56.0
Todd's
cirrhosis K74.3
paralysis (postepileptic) (transitory) G83.84
Toe — *see* condition
Toilet, artificial opening — *see* Attention to, artificial, opening
Tokelau (ringworm) B35.5
Tollwut — *see* Rabies
Tommaselli's disease R31.9
correct substance properly administered — *see* Table of Drugs and Chemicals, by drug, adverse effect
overdose or wrong substance given or taken — *see* Table of Drugs and Chemicals, by drug, poisoning
Tongue — *see also* condition
tie Q38.1
Tonic pupil — *see* Anomaly, pupil, function, tonic pupil
Toni-Fanconi syndrome (cystinosis) E72.09
with cystinosis E72.04
Tonsil — *see* condition
Tonsillitis (acute) (catarrhal) (croupous) (follicular) (gangrenous) (infective) (lacunar) (lingual) (malignant) (membranous) (parenchymatous) (phlegmonous) (pseudomembranous) (purulent) (septic) (subacute) (suppurative) (toxic) (ulcerative) (vesicular) (viral) J03.90
chronic J35.01
with adenoiditis J35.03
diphtheritic A36.0
hypertrophic J35.01
with adenoiditis J35.03
recurrent J03.91
specified organism NEC J03.80
recurrent J03.81
staphylococcal J03.80
recurrent J03.81
streptococcal J03.00
recurrent J03.01
tuberculous A15.8
Vincent's A69.1
Tooth, teeth — *see* condition
Toothache K08.89
Topagnosis R20.8
Tophi — *see* Gout, chronic
TORCH infection — *see* Infection, congenital
without active infection P00.2
Torn — *see* Tear
Tornwaldt's cyst or disease J39.2
Torsion
accessory tube — *see* Torsion, fallopian tube
adnexa (female) — *see* Torsion, fallopian tube
aorta, acquired I77.1
appendix epididymis N44.04
appendix testis N44.03
bile duct (common) (hepatic) K83.8
congenital Q44.5
bowel, colon or intestine K56.2
cervix — *see* Malposition, uterus
cystic duct K82.8
dystonia — *see* Dystonia, torsion
epididymis (appendix) N44.04
fallopian tube N83.52- ☑
with ovary N83.53
gallbladder K82.8
congenital Q44.1
hydatid of Morgagni
female N83.52- ☑
male N44.03
kidney (pedicle) (leading to infarction) N28.0
Meckel's diverticulum (congenital) Q43.0
malignant — *see* Table of Neoplasms, small intestine, malignant
mesentery K56.2
omentum K56.2
organ or site, congenital NEC — *see* Anomaly, by site
ovary (pedicle) N83.51- ☑
with fallopian tube N83.53
congenital Q50.2

Torsion — *continued*
oviduct — *see* Torsion, fallopian tube
penis (acquired) N48.82
congenital Q55.63
spasm — *see* Dystonia, torsion
spermatic cord N44.02
extravaginal N44.01
intravaginal N44.02
spleen D73.5
testis, testicle N44.00
appendix N44.03
tibia — *see* Deformity, limb, specified type NEC, lower leg
uterus — *see* Malposition, uterus
Torticollis (intermittent) (spastic) M43.6
congenital (sternomastoid) Q68.0
due to birth injury P15.8
hysterical F44.4
ocular R29.891
psychogenic F45.8
conversion reaction F44.4
rheumatic M43.6
rheumatoid M06.88
spasmodic G24.3
traumatic, current S13.4 ☑
Tortipelvis G24.1
Tortuous
aortic arch Q25.46
artery I77.1
organ or site, congenital NEC — *see* Distortion
retinal vessel, congenital Q14.1
ureter N13.8
urethra N36.8
vein — *see* Varix
Torture, victim of Z65.4
Torula, torular (histolytica) (infection) — *see* Cryptococcosis
Torulosis — *see* Cryptococcosis
Torus (mandibularis) (palatinus) M27.0
fracture — *see* Fracture, by site, torus
Touraine's syndrome Q79.8
Tourette's syndrome F95.2
Tourniquet syndrome — *see* Constriction, external, by site
Tower skull Q75.0
with exophthalmos Q87.0
Toxemia R68.89
bacterial — *see* Sepsis
burn — *see* Burn
eclamptic (with pre-existing hypertension) — *see* Eclampsia
erysipelatous — *see* Erysipelas
fatigue R68.89
food — *see* Poisoning, food
gastrointestinal K52.1
intestinal K52.1
kidney — *see* Uremia
malarial — *see* Malaria
myocardial — *see* Myocarditis, toxic
of pregnancy — *see* Pre-eclampsia
pre-eclamptic — *see* Pre-eclampsia
small intestine K52.1
staphylococcal, due to food A05.0
stasis R68.89
uremic — *see* Uremia
urinary — *see* Uremia
Toxemica cerebropathia psychica (nonalcoholic) F04
alcoholic — *see* Alcohol, amnestic disorder
Toxic (poisoning) — *see also* condition T65.91 ☑
effect — *see* Table of Drugs and Chemicals, by substance, poisoning
shock syndrome A48.3
thyroid (gland) — *see* Thyrotoxicosis
Toxicemia — *see* Toxemia
Toxicity — *see* Table of Drugs and Chemicals, by substance, poisoning
fava bean D55.0
food, noxious — *see* Poisoning, food
from drug or nonmedicinal substance — *see* Table of Drugs and Chemicals, by drug
Toxicosis — *see also* Toxemia
capillary, hemorrhagic D69.0
Toxinfection, gastrointestinal K52.1
Toxocariasis B83.0
Toxoplasma, toxoplasmosis (acquired) B58.9
with
hepatitis B58.1

Toxoplasma, toxoplasmosis — *continued*
with — *continued*
meningoencephalitis B58.2
ocular involvement B58.00
other organ involvement B58.89
pneumonia, pneumonitis B58.3
congenital (acute) (subacute) (chronic) P37.1
maternal, manifest toxoplasmosis in infant (acute) (subacute) (chronic) P37.1
tPA (rtPA) **administration in a different facility within the last 24 hours prior to admission to current facility** Z92.82
Trabeculation, bladder N32.89
Trachea — *see* condition
Tracheitis (catarrhal) (infantile) (membranous) (plastic) (septal) (suppurative) (viral) J04.10
with
bronchitis (15 years of age and above) J40
acute or subacute — *see* Bronchitis, acute
chronic J42
tuberculous NEC A15.5
under 15 years of age J20.9
laryngitis (acute) J04.2
chronic J37.1
tuberculous NEC A15.5
acute J04.10
with obstruction J04.11
chronic J42
with
bronchitis (chronic) J42
laryngitis (chronic) J37.1
diphtheritic (membranous) A36.89
due to external agent — *see* Inflammation, respiratory, upper, due to
syphilitic A52.73
tuberculous A15.5
Trachelitis (nonvenereal) — *see* Cervicitis
Tracheobronchial — *see* condition
Tracheobronchitis (15 years of age and above) — *see also* Bronchitis
due to
Bordetella bronchiseptica A37.80
with pneumonia A37.81
Francisella tularensis A21.8
Tracheobronchomegaly Q32.4
with bronchiectasis J47.9
with
exacerbation (acute) J47.1
lower respiratory infection J47.0
acquired J98.09
with bronchiectasis J47.9
with
exacerbation (acute) J47.1
lower respiratory infection J47.0
Tracheobronchopneumonitis — *see* Pneumonia, broncho-
Tracheocele (external) (internal) J39.8
congenital Q32.1
Tracheomalacia J39.8
congenital Q32.0
Tracheopharyngitis (acute) J06.9
chronic J42
due to external agent — *see* Inflammation, respiratory, upper, due to
Tracheostenosis J39.8
Tracheostomy
complication — *see* Complication, tracheostomy
status Z93.0
attention to Z43.0
malfunctioning J95.03
Trachoma, trachomatous A71.9
active (stage) A71.1
contraction of conjunctiva A71.1
dubium A71.0
healed or sequelae B94.0
initial (stage) A71.0
pannus A71.1
Türck's J37.0
Traction, vitreomacular H43.82- ☑
Train sickness T75.3 ☑
Trait(s)
Hb-S D57.3
hemoglobin
abnormal NEC D58.2
with thalassemia D56.3
C — *see* Disease, hemoglobin C
S (Hb-S) D57.3
Lepore D56.3

☑ Additional Character Required — Refer to the Tabular List for Character Selection   ▽ Subterms under main terms may continue to next column or page

Trait(s) — *continued*
   personality, accentuated Z73.1
   sickle-cell D57.3
      with elliptocytosis or spherocytosis D57.3
   type A personality Z73.1
Tramp Z59.0
Trance R41.89
   hysterical F44.89
Transaminasemia R74.0
Transection
   abdomen (partial) S38.3 ☑
   aorta (incomplete) — *see also* Injury, aorta
      complete — *see* Injury, aorta, laceration, major
   carotid artery (incomplete) — *see also* Injury, blood
      vessel, carotid, laceration
      complete — *see* Injury, blood vessel, carotid, lacer-
         ation, major
   celiac artery (incomplete) S35.211 ☑
      branch (incomplete) S35.291 ☑
         complete S35.292 ☑
      complete S35.212 ☑
   innominate
      artery (incomplete) — *see also* Injury, blood vessel,
         thoracic, innominate, artery, laceration
         complete — *see* Injury, blood vessel, thoracic,
            innominate, artery, laceration, major
      vein (incomplete) — *see also* Injury, blood vessel,
         thoracic, innominate, vein, laceration
         complete — *see* Injury, blood vessel, thoracic,
            innominate, vein, laceration, major
   jugular vein (external) (incomplete) — *see also* Injury,
      blood vessel, jugular vein, laceration
      complete — *see* Injury, blood vessel, jugular vein,
         laceration, major
      internal (incomplete) — *see also* Injury, blood vessel,
         jugular vein, internal, laceration
         complete — *see* Injury, blood vessel, jugular vein,
            internal, laceration, major
   mesenteric artery (incomplete) — *see also* Injury,
      mesenteric, artery, laceration
      complete — *see* Injury, mesenteric artery, laceration,
         major
   pulmonary vessel (incomplete) — *see also* Injury, blood
      vessel, thoracic, pulmonary, laceration
      complete — *see* Injury, blood vessel, thoracic, pul-
         monary, laceration, major
   subclavian — *see* Transection, innominate
   vena cava (incomplete) — *see also* Injury, vena cava
      complete — *see* Injury, vena cava, laceration, major
   vertebral artery (incomplete) — *see also* Injury, blood
      vessel, vertebral, laceration
      complete — *see* Injury, blood vessel, vertebral, lac-
         eration, major
Transfusion
   associated (red blood cell) hemochromatosis E83.111
   blood
      ABO incompatible — *see* Complication(s), transfu-
         sion, incompatibility reaction, ABO
      minor blood group (Duffy) (E) (K) (Kell) (Kidd) (Lewis)
         (M) (N) (P) (S) T80.89 ☑
      reaction or complication — *see* Complications,
         transfusion
   fetomaternal (mother) — *see* Pregnancy, complicated
      by, placenta, transfusion syndrome
   maternofetal (mother) — *see* Pregnancy, complicated
      by, placenta, transfusion syndrome
   placental (syndrome) (mother) — *see* Pregnancy,
      complicated by, placenta, transfusion syndrome
   reaction (adverse) — *see* Complications, transfusion
   related acute lung injury (TRALI) J95.84
   twin-to-twin — *see* Pregnancy, complicated by, placen-
      ta, transfusion syndrome, fetus to fetus
Transient (meaning homeless) — *see also* condition Z59.0
Translocation
   balanced autosomal Q95.9
      in normal individual Q95.0
   chromosomes NEC Q99.8
      balanced and insertion in normal individual Q95.0
   Down syndrome Q90.2
   trisomy
      13 Q91.6
      18 Q91.2
      21 Q90.2
Translucency, iris — *see* Degeneration, iris
**Transmission of chemical substances through the
      placenta** — *see* Absorption, chemical, through
      placenta

Transparency, lung, unilateral J43.0
Transplant (ed) (status) Z94.9
   awaiting organ Z76.82
   bone Z94.6
      marrow Z94.81
   candidate Z76.82
   complication — *see* Complication, transplant
   cornea Z94.7
   heart Z94.1
      and lung(s) Z94.3
      valve Z95.2
         prosthetic Z95.2
         specified NEC Z95.4
         xenogenic Z95.3
   intestine Z94.82
   kidney Z94.0
   liver Z94.4
   lung(s) Z94.2
      and heart Z94.3
   organ (failure) (infection) (rejection) Z94.9
      removal status Z98.85
   pancreas Z94.83
   skin Z94.5
   social Z60.3
   specified organ or tissue NEC Z94.89
   stem cells Z94.84
   tissue Z94.9
Transplants, ovarian, endometrial N80.1
Transposed — *see* Transposition
Transposition (congenital) — *see also* Malposition,
      congenital
   abdominal viscera Q89.3
   aorta (dextra) Q20.3
   appendix Q43.8
   colon Q43.8
   corrected Q20.5
   great vessels (complete) (partial) Q20.3
   heart Q24.0
      with complete transposition of viscera Q89.3
   intestine (large) (small) Q43.8
   reversed jejunal (for bypass) (status) Z98.0
   scrotum Q55.23
   stomach Q40.2
      with general transposition of viscera Q89.3
   tooth, teeth, fully erupted M26.30
   vessels, great (complete) (partial) Q20.3
   viscera (abdominal) (thoracic) Q89.3
Transsexualism F64.0
Transverse — *see also* condition
   arrest (deep), in labor O64.0 ☑
   lie (mother) O32.2 ☑
      causing obstructed labor O64.8 ☑
Transvestism, transvestitism (dual-role) F64.1
   fetishistic F65.1
Trapped placenta (with hemorrhage) O72.0
   without hemorrhage O73.0
TRAPS (tumor necrosis factor receptor associated periodic
      syndrome) M04.1
Trauma, traumatism — *see also* Injury
   acoustic — *see* subcategory H83.3 ☑
   birth — *see* Birth, injury
   complicating ectopic or molar pregnancy O08.6
   during delivery O71.9
   following ectopic or molar pregnancy O08.6
   obstetric O71.9
      specified NEC O71.89
   occusal
      primary K08.81
      secondary K08.82
Traumatic — *see also* condition
   brain injury S06.9 ☑
Treacher Collins syndrome Q75.4
Treitz's hernia — *see* Hernia, abdomen, specified site
      NEC
Trematode infestation — *see* Infestation, fluke
Trematodiasis — *see* Infestation, fluke
Trembling paralysis — *see* Parkinsonism
Tremor(s) R25.1
   drug induced G25.1
   essential (benign) G25.0
   familial G25.0
   hereditary G25.0
   hysterical F44.4
   intention G25.2
   medication induced postural G25.1
   mercurial — *see* subcategory T56.1 ☑
   Parkinson's — *see* Parkinsonism
   psychogenic (conversion reaction) F44.4

Tremor(s) — *continued*
   senilis R54
   specified type NEC G25.2
Trench
   fever A79.0
   foot — *see* Immersion, foot
   mouth A69.1
Treponema pallidum infection — *see* Syphilis
Treponematosis
   due to
      T. pallidum — *see* Syphilis
      T. pertenue — *see* Yaws
Triad
   Hutchinson's (congenital syphilis) A50.53
   Kartagener's Q89.3
   Saint's — *see* Hernia, diaphragm
Trichiasis (eyelid) H02.059
   with entropion — *see* Entropion
   left H02.056
      lower H02.055
      upper H02.054
   right H02.053
      lower H02.052
      upper H02.051
Trichinella spiralis (infection) (infestation) B75
Trichinellosis, trichiniasis, trichinelliasis, trichinosis
   B75
   with muscle disorder B75 *[M63.80]*
      ankle B75 *[M63.87-]* ☑
      foot B75 *[M63.87-]* ☑
      forearm B75 *[M63.83-]* ☑
      hand B75 *[M63.84-]* ☑
      lower leg B75 *[M63.86-]* ☑
      multiple sites B75 *[M63.89]*
      pelvic region B75 *[M63.85-]* ☑
      shoulder region B75 *[M63.81-]* ☑
      specified site NEC B75 *[M63.88]*
      thigh B75 *[M63.85-]* ☑
      upper arm B75 *[M63.82-]* ☑
Trichobezoar T18.9 ☑
   intestine T18.3 ☑
   stomach T18.2 ☑
Trichocephaliasis, trichocephalosis B79
Trichocephalus infestation B79
Trichoclasis L67.8
Trichoepithelioma — *see also* Neoplasm, skin, benign
   malignant — *see* Neoplasm, skin, malignant
Trichofolliculoma — *see* Neoplasm, skin, benign
Tricholemmoma — *see* Neoplasm, skin, benign
Trichomoniasis A59.9
   bladder A59.03
   cervix A59.09
   intestinal A07.8
   prostate A59.02
   seminal vesicles A59.09
   specified site NEC A59.8
   urethra A59.03
   urogenitalis A59.00
   vagina A59.01
   vulva A59.01
Trichomycosis
   axillaris A48.8
   nodosa, nodularis B36.8
Trichonodosis L67.8
Trichophytid, trichophyton infection — *see* Dermato-
      phytosis
Trichophytobezoar T18.9 ☑
   intestine T18.3 ☑
   stomach T18.2 ☑
Trichophytosis — *see* Dermatophytosis
Trichoptilosis L67.8
Trichorrhexis (nodosa) (invaginata) L67.0
Trichosis axillaris A48.8
Trichosporosis nodosa B36.2
Trichostasis spinulosa (congenital) Q84.1
Trichostrongyliasis, trichostrongylosis (small intes-
      tine) B81.2
Trichostrongylus infection B81.2
Trichotillomania F63.3
Trichromat, trichromatopsia, anomalous (congenital)
   H53.55
Trichuriasis B79
Trichuris trichiura (infection) (infestation) (any site) B79
Tricuspid (valve) — *see* condition
Trifid — *see also* Accessory
   kidney (pelvis) Q63.8
   tongue Q38.3

▽ **Subterms under main terms may continue to next column or page**   ☑ **Additional Character Required — Refer to the Tabular List for Character Selection**   **313**

Trait — Trifid

Trigeminal neuralgia — *see* Neuralgia, trigeminal
Trigeminy R00.8
Trigger finger (acquired) M65.30
   congenital Q74.0
   index finger M65.32- ☑
   little finger M65.35- ☑
   middle finger M65.33- ☑
   ring finger M65.34- ☑
   thumb M65.31- ☑
Trigonitis (bladder) (chronic) (pseudomembranous)
   N30.30
   with hematuria N30.31
Trigonocephaly Q75.0
Trilocular heart — *see* Cor triloculare
Trimethylaminuria E72.52
Tripartite placenta O43.19- ☑
Triphalangeal thumb Q74.0
Triple — *see also* Accessory
   kidneys Q63.0
   uteri Q51.818
   X, female Q97.0
Triplegia G83.89
   congenital G80.8
Triplet (newborn) — *see also* Newborn, triplet
   complicating pregnancy — *see* Pregnancy, triplet
Triplication — *see* Accessory
Triploidy Q92.7
Trismus R25.2
   neonatorum A33
   newborn A33
Trisomy (syndrome) Q92.9
   13 (partial) Q91.7
     meiotic nondisjunction Q91.4
     mitotic nondisjunction Q91.5
     mosaicism Q91.5
     translocation Q91.6
   18 (partial) Q91.3
     meiotic nondisjunction Q91.0
     mitotic nondisjunction Q91.1
     mosaicism Q91.1
     translocation Q91.2
   20 Q92.8
   21 (partial) Q90.9
     meiotic nondisjunction Q90.0
     mitotic nondisjunction Q90.1
     mosaicism Q90.1
     translocation Q90.2
   22 Q92.8
   autosomes Q92.9
   chromosome specified NEC Q92.8
     partial Q92.2
       due to unbalanced translocation Q92.5
     specified NEC Q92.8
     whole (nonsex chromosome)
       meiotic nondisjunction Q92.0
       mitotic nondisjunction Q92.1
       mosaicism Q92.1
   due to
     dicentrics — *see* Extra, marker chromosomes
     extra rings — *see* Extra, marker chromosomes
     isochromosomes — *see* Extra, marker chromosomes
   specified NEC Q92.8
   whole chromosome Q92.9
     meiotic nondisjunction Q92.0
     mitotic nondisjunction Q92.1
     mosaicism Q92.1
     partial Q92.9
     specified NEC Q92.8
Tritanomaly, tritanopia H53.55
Trombiculosis, trombiculiasis, trombidiosis B88.0
Trophedema (congenital) (hereditary) Q82.0
Trophoblastic disease — *see also* Mole, hydatidiform
   O01.9
Tropholymphedema Q82.0
Trophoneurosis NEC G96.8
   disseminated M34.9
Tropical — *see* condition
Trouble — *see also* Disease
   heart — *see* Disease, heart
   kidney — *see* Disease, renal
   nervous R45.0
   sinus — *see* Sinusitis
Trousseau's syndrome (thrombophlebitis migrans) I82.1
Truancy, childhood
   from school Z72.810
Truncus
   arteriosus (persistent) Q20.0

Truncus — *continued*
   communis Q20.0
Trunk — *see* condition
Trypanosomiasis
   African B56.9
     by Trypanosoma brucei
       gambiense B56.0
       rhodesiense B56.1
   American — *see* Chagas' disease
   Brazilian — *see* Chagas' disease
   by Trypanosoma
     brucei gambiense B56.0
     brucei rhodesiense B56.1
     cruzi — *see* Chagas' disease
   gambiensis, Gambian B56.0
   rhodesiensis, Rhodesian B56.1
   South American — *see* Chagas' disease
   where
     African trypanosomiasis is prevalent B56.9
     Chagas' disease is prevalent B57.2
T-shaped incisors K00.2
Tsutsugamushi (disease) (fever) A75.3
Tube, tubal, tubular — *see* condition
Tubercle — *see also* Tuberculosis
   brain, solitary A17.81
   Darwin's Q17.8
   Ghon, primary infection A15.7
Tuberculid, tuberculide (indurating, subcutaneous)
   (lichenoid) (miliary) (papulonecrotic) (primary) (skin)
   A18.4
Tuberculoma — *see also* Tuberculosis
   brain A17.81
   meninges (cerebral) (spinal) A17.1
   spinal cord A17.81
Tuberculosis, tubercular, tuberculous (calcification)
   (calcified) (caseous) (chromogenic acid-fast bacilli)
   (degeneration) (fibrocaseous) (fistula) (interstitial)
   (isolated circumscribed lesions) (necrosis)
   (parenchymatous) (ulcerative) A15.9
   with pneumoconiosis (any condition in J60-J64) J65
   abdomen (lymph gland) A18.39
   abscess (respiratory) A15.9
     bone A18.03
       hip A18.02
       knee A18.02
       sacrum A18.01
       specified site NEC A18.03
       spinal A18.01
       vertebra A18.01
     brain A17.81
     breast A18.89
     Cowper's gland A18.15
     dura (mater) (cerebral) (spinal) A17.81
     epidural (cerebral) (spinal) A17.81
     female pelvis A18.17
     frontal sinus A15.8
     genital organs NEC A18.10
     genitourinary A18.10
     gland (lymphatic) — *see* Tuberculosis, lymph gland
     hip A18.02
     intestine A18.32
     ischiorectal A18.32
     joint NEC A18.02
       hip A18.02
       knee A18.02
       specified NEC A18.02
       vertebral A18.01
     kidney A18.11
     knee A18.02
     latent Z22.7
     lumbar (spine) A18.01
     lung — *see* Tuberculosis, pulmonary
     meninges (cerebral) (spinal) A17.0
     muscle A18.09
     perianal (fistula) A18.32
     perinephritic A18.11
     perirectal A18.32
     rectum A18.32
     retropharyngeal A15.8
     sacrum A18.01
     scrofulous A18.2
     scrotum A18.15
     skin (primary) A18.4
     spinal cord A17.81
     spine or vertebra (column) A18.01
     subdiaphragmatic A18.31
     testis A18.15
     urinary A18.13

Tuberculosis, tubercular, tuberculous — *continued*
   abscess — *continued*
     uterus A18.17
   accessory sinus — *see* Tuberculosis, sinus
   Addison's disease A18.7
   adenitis — *see* Tuberculosis, lymph gland
   adenoids A15.8
   adenopathy — *see* Tuberculosis, lymph gland
   adherent pericardium A18.84
   adnexa (uteri) A18.17
   adrenal (capsule) (gland) A18.7
   alimentary canal A18.32
   anemia A18.89
   ankle (joint) (bone) A18.02
   anus A18.32
   apex, apical — *see* Tuberculosis, pulmonary
   appendicitis, appendix A18.32
   arachnoid A17.0
   artery, arteritis A18.89
     cerebral A18.89
   arthritis (chronic) (synovial) A18.02
     spine or vertebra (column) A18.01
   articular — *see* Tuberculosis, joint
   ascites A18.31
   asthma — *see* Tuberculosis, pulmonary
   axilla, axillary (gland) A18.2
   bladder A18.12
   bone A18.03
     hip A18.02
     knee A18.02
     limb NEC A18.03
     sacrum A18.01
     spine or vertebral column A18.01
   bowel (miliary) A18.32
   brain A17.81
   breast A18.89
   broad ligament A18.17
   bronchi, bronchial, bronchus A15.5
     ectasia, ectasis (bronchiectasis) — *see* Tuberculosis,
       pulmonary
     fistula A15.5
       primary (progressive) A15.7
     gland or node A15.4
       primary (progressive) A15.7
     lymph gland or node A15.4
       primary (progressive) A15.7
   bronchiectasis — *see* Tuberculosis, pulmonary
   bronchitis A15.5
   bronchopleural A15.6
   bronchopneumonia, bronchopneumonic — *see* Tuber-
     culosis, pulmonary
   bronchorrhagia A15.5
   bronchotracheal A15.5
   bronze disease A18.7
   buccal cavity A18.83
   bulbourethral gland A18.15
   bursa A18.09
   cachexia A15.9
   cardiomyopathy A18.84
   caries — *see* Tuberculosis, bone
   cartilage A18.02
     intervertebral A18.01
   catarrhal — *see* Tuberculosis, respiratory
   cecum A18.32
   cellulitis (primary) A18.4
   cerebellum A17.81
   cerebral, cerebrum A17.81
   cerebrospinal A17.81
     meninges A17.0
   cervical (lymph gland or node) A18.2
   cervicitis, cervix (uteri) A18.16
   chest — *see* Tuberculosis, respiratory
   chorioretinitis A18.53
   choroid, choroiditis A18.53
   ciliary body A18.54
   colitis A18.32
   collier's J65
   colliquativa (primary) A18.4
   colon A18.32
   complex, primary A15.7
   congenital P37.0
   conjunctiva A18.59
   connective tissue (systemic) A18.89
   contact Z20.1
   cornea (ulcer) A18.52
   Cowper's gland A18.15
   coxae A18.02
   coxalgia A18.02

☑ **Additional Character Required** — **Refer to the Tabular List for Character Selection**   ▽ **Subterms under main terms may continue to next column or page**

Tuberculosis, tubercular, tuberculous — *continued*
  cul-de-sac of Douglas A18.17
  curvature, spine A18.Ø1
  cutis (colliquativa) (primary) A18.4
  cyst, ovary A18.18
  cystitis A18.12
  dactylitis A18.Ø3
  diarrhea A18.32
  diffuse — *see* Tuberculosis, miliary
  digestive tract A18.32
  disseminated — *see* Tuberculosis, miliary
  duodenum A18.32
  dura (mater) (cerebral) (spinal) A17.Ø
    abscess (cerebral) (spinal) A17.81
  dysentery A18.32
  ear (inner) (middle) A18.6
    bone A18.Ø3
    external (primary) A18.4
    skin (primary) A18.4
  elbow A18.Ø2
  emphysema — *see* Tuberculosis, pulmonary
  empyema A15.6
  encephalitis A17.82
  endarteritis A18.89
  endocarditis A18.84
    aortic A18.84
    mitral A18.84
    pulmonary A18.84
    tricuspid A18.84
  endocrine glands NEC A18.82
  endometrium A18.17
  enteric, enterica, enteritis A18.32
  enterocolitis A18.32
  epididymis, epididymitis A18.15
  epidural abscess (cerebral) (spinal) A17.81
  epiglottis A15.5
  episcleritis A18.51
  erythema (induratum) (nodosum) (primary) A18.4
  esophagus A18.83
  eustachian tube A18.6
  exposure (to) Z20.1
  exudative — *see* Tuberculosis, pulmonary
  eye A18.5Ø
  eyelid (primary) (lupus) A18.4
  fallopian tube (acute) (chronic) A18.17
  fascia A18.Ø9
  fauces A15.8
  female pelvic inflammatory disease A18.17
  finger A18.Ø3
  first infection A15.7
  gallbladder A18.83
  ganglion A18.Ø9
  gastritis A18.83
  gastrocolic fistula A18.32
  gastroenteritis A18.32
  gastrointestinal tract A18.32
  general, generalized — *see* Tuberculosis, miliary
  genital organs A18.1Ø
  genitourinary A18.1Ø
  genu A18.Ø2
  glandula suprarenalis A18.7
  glandular, general A18.2
  glottis A15.5
  grinder's J65
  gum A18.83
  hand A18.Ø3
  heart A18.84
  hematogenous — *see* Tuberculosis, miliary
  hemoptysis — *see* Tuberculosis, pulmonary
  hemorrhage NEC — *see* Tuberculosis, pulmonary
  hemothorax A15.6
  hepatitis A18.83
  hilar lymph nodes A15.4
    primary (progressive) A15.7
  hip (joint) (disease) (bone) A18.Ø2
  hydropneumothorax A15.6
  hydrothorax A15.6
  hypoadrenalism A18.7
  hypopharynx A15.8
  ileocecal (hyperplastic) A18.32
  ileocolitis A18.32
  ileum A18.32
  iliac spine (superior) A18.Ø3
  immunological findings only A15.7
  indurativa (primary) A18.4
  infantile A15.7
  infection A15.9
    without clinical manifestations A15.7

Tuberculosis, tubercular, tuberculous — *continued*
  infraclavicular gland A18.2
  inguinal gland A18.2
  inguinalis A18.2
  intestine (any part) A18.32
  iridocyclitis A18.54
  iris, iritis A18.54
  ischiorectal A18.32
  jaw A18.Ø3
  jejunum A18.32
  joint A18.Ø2
    vertebral A18.Ø1
  keratitis (interstitial) A18.52
  keratoconjunctivitis A18.52
  kidney A18.11
  knee (joint) A18.Ø2
  kyphosis, kyphoscoliosis A18.Ø1
  laryngitis A15.5
  larynx A15.5
  latent Z22.7
  leptomeninges, leptomeningitis (cerebral) (spinal)
    A17.Ø
  lichenoides (primary) A18.4
  linguae A18.83
  lip A18.83
  liver A18.83
  lordosis A18.Ø1
  lung — *see* Tuberculosis, pulmonary
  lupus vulgaris A18.4
  lymph gland or node (peripheral) A18.2
    abdomen A18.39
    bronchial A15.4
      primary (progressive) A15.7
    cervical A18.2
    hilar A15.4
      primary (progressive) A15.7
    intrathoracic A15.4
      primary (progressive) A15.7
    mediastinal A15.4
      primary (progressive) A15.7
    mesenteric A18.39
    retroperitoneal A18.39
    tracheobronchial A15.4
      primary (progressive) A15.7
  lymphadenitis — *see* Tuberculosis, lymph gland
  lymphangitis — *see* Tuberculosis, lymph gland
  lymphatic (gland) (vessel) — *see* Tuberculosis, lymph
    gland
  mammary gland A18.89
  marasmus A15.9
  mastoiditis A18.Ø3
  mediastinal lymph gland or node A15.4
    primary (progressive) A15.7
  mediastinitis A15.8
    primary (progressive) A15.7
  mediastinum A15.8
    primary (progressive) A15.7
  medulla A17.81
  melanosis, Addisonian A18.7
  meninges, meningitis (basilar) (cerebral) (cerebrospinal)
    (spinal) A17.Ø
  meningoencephalitis A17.82
  mesentery, mesenteric (gland or node) A18.39
  miliary A19.9
    acute A19.2
      multiple sites A19.1
      single specified site A19.Ø
    chronic A19.8
    specified NEC A19.8
  millstone makers' J65
  miner's J65
  molder's J65
  mouth A18.83
  multiple A19.9
    acute A19.1
    chronic A19.8
  muscle A18.Ø9
  myelitis A17.82
  myocardium, myocarditis A18.84
  nasal (passage) (sinus) A15.8
  nasopharynx A15.8
  neck gland A18.2
  nephritis A18.11
  nerve (mononeuropathy) A17.83
  nervous system A17.9
  nose (septum) A15.8
  ocular A18.5Ø
  omentum A18.31
  oophoritis (acute) (chronic) A18.17

Tuberculosis, tubercular, tuberculous — *continued*
  optic (nerve trunk) (papilla) A18.59
  orbit A18.59
  orchitis A18.15
  organ, specified NEC A18.89
  osseous — *see* Tuberculosis, bone
  osteitis — *see* Tuberculosis, bone
  osteomyelitis — *see* Tuberculosis, bone
  otitis media A18.6
  ovary, ovaritis (acute) (chronic) A18.17
  oviduct (acute) (chronic) A18.17
  pachymeningitis A17.Ø
  palate (soft) A18.83
  pancreas A18.83
  papulonecrotic (a) (primary) A18.4
  parathyroid glands A18.82
  paronychia (primary) A18.4
  parotid gland or region A18.83
  pelvis (bony) A18.Ø3
  penis A18.15
  peribronchitis A15.5
  pericardium, pericarditis A18.84
  perichondritis, larynx A15.5
  periostitis — *see* Tuberculosis, bone
  perirectal fistula A18.32
  peritoneum NEC A18.31
  peritonitis A18.31
  pharynx, pharyngitis A15.8
  phlyctenulosis (keratoconjunctivitis) A18.52
  phthisis NEC — *see* Tuberculosis, pulmonary
  pituitary gland A18.82
  pleura, pleural, pleurisy, pleuritis (fibrinous) (oblitera-
    tive) (purulent) (simple plastic) (with effusion)
    A15.6
    primary (progressive) A15.7
  pneumonia, pneumonic — *see* Tuberculosis, pul-
    monary
  pneumothorax (spontaneous) (tense valvular) — *see*
    Tuberculosis, pulmonary
  polyneuropathy A17.89
  polyserositis A19.9
    acute A19.1
    chronic A19.8
  potter's J65
  prepuce A18.15
  primary (complex) A15.7
  proctitis A18.32
  prostate, prostatitis A18.14
  pulmonalis — *see* Tuberculosis, pulmonary
  pulmonary (cavitated) (fibrotic) (infiltrative) (nodular)
    A15.Ø
    childhood type or first infection A15.7
    primary (complex) A15.7
  pyelitis A18.11
  pyelonephritis A18.11
  pyemia — *see* Tuberculosis, miliary
  pyonephrosis A18.11
  pyopneumothorax A15.6
  pyothorax A15.6
  rectum (fistula) (with abscess) A18.32
  reinfection stage — *see* Tuberculosis, pulmonary
  renal A18.11
  renis A18.11
  respiratory A15.9
    primary A15.7
    specified site NEC A15.8
  retina, retinitis A18.53
  retroperitoneal (lymph gland or node) A18.39
  rheumatism NEC A18.Ø9
  rhinitis A15.8
  sacroiliac (joint) A18.Ø1
  sacrum A18.Ø1
  salivary gland A18.83
  salpingitis (acute) (chronic) A18.17
  sandblaster's J65
  sclera A18.51
  scoliosis A18.Ø1
  scrofulous A18.2
  scrotum A18.15
  seminal tract or vesicle A18.15
  senile A15.9
  septic — *see* Tuberculosis, miliary
  shoulder (joint) A18.Ø2
    blade A18.Ø3
  sigmoid A18.32
  sinus (any nasal) A15.8
    bone A18.Ø3
    epididymis A18.15

Tuberculosis, tubercular, tuberculous — *continued*
skeletal NEC A18.03
skin (any site) (primary) A18.4
small intestine A18.32
soft palate A18.83
spermatic cord A18.15
spine, spinal (column) A18.01
   cord A17.81
   medulla A17.81
   membrane A17.0
   meninges A17.0
spleen, splenitis A18.85
spondylitis A18.01
sternoclavicular joint A18.02
stomach A18.83
stonemason's J65
subcutaneous tissue (cellular) (primary) A18.4
subcutis (primary) A18.4
subdeltoid bursa A18.83
submaxillary (region) A18.83
supraclavicular gland A18.2
suprarenal (capsule) (gland) A18.7
swelling, joint (*see also* category M01) — *see also* Tuberculosis, joint A18.02
symphysis pubis A18.02
synovitis A18.09
   articular A18.02
   spine or vertebra A18.01
systemic — *see* Tuberculosis, miliary
tarsitis A18.4
tendon (sheath) — *see* Tuberculosis, tenosynovitis
tenosynovitis A18.09
   spine or vertebra A18.01
testis A18.15
throat A15.8
thymus gland A18.82
thyroid gland A18.81
tongue A18.83
tonsil, tonsillitis A15.8
trachea, tracheal A15.5
   lymph gland or node A15.4
      primary (progressive) A15.7
tracheobronchial A15.5
   lymph gland or node A15.4
      primary (progressive) A15.7
tubal (acute) (chronic) A18.17
tunica vaginalis A18.15
ulcer (skin) (primary) A18.4
   bowel or intestine A18.32
   specified NEC — *see* Tuberculosis, by site
unspecified site A15.9
ureter A18.11
urethra, urethral (gland) A18.13
urinary organ or tract A18.13
uterus A18.17
uveal tract A18.54
uvula A18.83
vagina A18.18
vas deferens A18.15
verruca, verrucosa (cutis) (primary) A18.4
vertebra (column) A18.01
vesiculitis A18.15
vulva A18.18
wrist (joint) A18.02
Tuberculum
Carabelli — *see* Excludes Note at K00.2
occlusal — *see* Excludes Note at K00.2
paramolare K00.2
Tuberosity, enitre maxillary M26.07
Tuberous sclerosis (brain) Q85.1
Tubo-ovarian — *see* condition
Tuboplasty, after previous sterilization Z31.0
aftercare Z31.42
Tubotympanitis, catarrhal (chronic) — *see* Otitis, media,
   nonsuppurative, chronic, serous
Tularemia A21.9
with
   conjunctivitis A21.1
   pneumonia A21.2
abdominal A21.3
bronchopneumonic A21.2
conjunctivitis A21.1
cryptogenic A21.3
enteric A21.3
gastrointestinal A21.3
generalized A21.7
ingestion A21.3
intestinal A21.3

Tularemia — *continued*
oculoglandular A21.1
ophthalmic A21.1
pneumonia (any), pneumonic A21.2
pulmonary A21.2
sepsis A21.7
specified NEC A21.8
typhoidal A21.7
ulceroglandular A21.0
Tularensis conjunctivitis A21.1
Tumefaction — *see also* Swelling
liver — *see* Hypertrophy, liver
Tumor — *see also* Neoplasm, unspecified behavior, by
   site
acinar cell — *see* Neoplasm, uncertain behavior, by site
acinic cell — *see* Neoplasm, uncertain behavior, by site
adenocarcinoid — *see* Neoplasm, malignant, by site
adenomatoid — *see also* Neoplasm, benign, by site
   odontogenic — *see* Cyst, calcifying odontogenic
adnexal (skin) — *see* Neoplasm, skin, benign, by site
adrenal
   cortical (benign) D35.0- ☑
      malignant C74.0- ☑
   rest — *see* Neoplasm, benign, by site
alpha-cell
   malignant
      pancreas C25.4
      specified site NEC — *see* Neoplasm, malignant,
         by site
      unspecified site C25.4
   pancreas D13.7
   specified site NEC — *see* Neoplasm, benign, by site
   unspecified site D13.7
aneurysmal — *see* Aneurysm
aortic body D44.7
   malignant C75.5
Askin's — *see* Neoplasm, connective tissue, malignant
basal cell — *see also* Neoplasm, skin, uncertain behavior D48.5
Bednar — *see* Neoplasm, skin, malignant
benign (unclassified) — *see* Neoplasm, benign, by site
beta-cell
   malignant
      pancreas C25.4
      specified site NEC — *see* Neoplasm, malignant,
         by site
      unspecified site C25.4
   pancreas D13.7
   specified site NEC — *see* Neoplasm, benign, by site
   unspecified site D13.7
Brenner D27.9
   borderline malignancy D39.1- ☑
   malignant C56- ☑
   proliferating D39.1- ☑
bronchial alveolar, intravascular D38.1
Brooke's — *see* Neoplasm, skin, benign
brown fat — *see* Lipoma
Burkitt — *see* Lymphoma, Burkitt
calcifying epithelial odontogenic — *see* Cyst, calcifying
   odontogenic
carcinoid D3A.00 (*following* D36)
   benign D3A.00 (*following* D36)
      appendix D3A.020 (*following* D36)
      ascending colon D3A.022 (*following* D36)
      bronchus (lung) D3A.090 (*following* D36)
      cecum D3A.021 (*following* D36)
      colon D3A.029 (*following* D36)
      descending colon D3A.024 (*following* D36)
      duodenum D3A.010 (*following* D36)
      foregut NOS D3A.094 (*following* D36)
      hindgut NOS D3A.096 (*following* D36)
      ileum D3A.012 (*following* D36)
      jejunum D3A.011 (*following* D36)
      kidney D3A.093 (*following* D36)
      large intestine D3A.029 (*following* D36)
      lung (bronchus) D3A.090 (*following* D36)
      midgut NOS D3A.095 (*following* D36)
      rectum D3A.026 (*following* D36)
      sigmoid colon D3A.025 (*following* D36)
      small intestine D3A.019 (*following* D36)
      specified NEC D3A.098 (*following* D36)
      stomach D3A.092 (*following* D36)
      thymus D3A.091 (*following* D36)
      transverse colon D3A.023 (*following* D36)
   malignant C7A.00 (*following* C75)
      appendix C7A.020 (*following* C75)
      ascending colon C7A.022 (*following* C75)
      bronchus (lung) C7A.090 (*following* C75)

Tumor — *continued*
carcinoid — *continued*
   malignant — *continued*
      cecum C7A.021 (*following* C75)
      colon C7A.029 (*following* C75)
      descending colon C7A.024 (*following* C75)
      duodenum C7A.010 (*following* C75)
      foregut NOS C7A.094 (*following* C75)
      hindgut NOS C7A.096 (*following* C75)
      ileum C7A.012 (*following* C75)
      jejunum C7A.011 (*following* C75)
      kidney C7A.093 (*following* C75)
      large intestine C7A.029 (*following* C75)
      lung (bronchus) C7A.090 (*following* C75)
      midgut NOS C7A.095 (*following* C75)
      rectum C7A.026 (*following* C75)
      sigmoid colon C7A.025 (*following* C75)
      small intestine C7A.019 (*following* C75)
      specified NEC C7A.098 (*following* C75)
      stomach C7A.092 (*following* C75)
      thymus C7A.091 (*following* C75)
      transverse colon C7A.023 (*following* C75)
   mesentary metastasis C7B.04 (*following* C75)
   secondary C7B.00 (*following* C75)
      bone C7B.03 (*following* C75)
      distant lymph nodes C7B.01 (*following* C75)
      liver C7B.02 (*following* C75)
      peritoneum C7B.04 (*following* C75)
      specified NEC C7B.09 (*following* C75)
carotid body D44.6
   malignant C75.4
cells — *see also* Neoplasm, unspecified behavior, by
   site
   benign — *see* Neoplasm, benign, by site
   malignant — *see* Neoplasm, malignant, by site
   uncertain whether benign or malignant — *see*
      Neoplasm, uncertain behavior, by site
cervix, in pregnancy or childbirth — *see* Pregnancy,
   complicated by, tumor, cervix
chondromatous giant cell — *see* Neoplasm, bone, benign
chromaffin — *see also* Neoplasm, benign, by site
   malignant — *see* Neoplasm, malignant, by site
Cock's peculiar L72.3
Codman's — *see* Neoplasm, bone, benign
dentigerous, mixed — *see* Cyst, calcifying odontogenic
dermoid — *see* Neoplasm, benign, by site
   with malignant transformation C56- ☑
desmoid (extra-abdominal) — *see also* Neoplasm,
   connective tissue, uncertain behavior
   abdominal — *see* Neoplasm, connective tissue, un-
      certain behavior
embolus — *see* Neoplasm, secondary, by site
embryonal (mixed) — *see also* Neoplasm, uncertain
   behavior, by site
   liver C22.7
endodermal sinus
   specified site — *see* Neoplasm, malignant, by site
   unspecified site
      female C56.- ☑
      male C62.90
epithelial
   benign — *see* Neoplasm, benign, by site
   malignant — *see* Neoplasm, malignant, by site
Ewing's — *see* Neoplasm, bone, malignant, by site
fatty — *see* Lipoma
fibroid — *see* Leiomyoma
G cell
   malignant
      pancreas C25.4
      specified site NEC — *see* Neoplasm, malignant,
         by site
      unspecified site C25.4
   specified site — *see* Neoplasm, uncertain behavior,
      by site
   unspecified site D37.8
germ cell — *see also* Neoplasm, malignant, by site
   mixed — *see* Neoplasm, malignant, by site
ghost cell, odontogenic — *see* Cyst, calcifying odontogenic
giant cell — *see also* Neoplasm, uncertain behavior,
   by site
   bone D48.0
      malignant — *see* Neoplasm, bone, malignant
   chondromatous — *see* Neoplasm, bone, benign
   malignant — *see* Neoplasm, malignant, by site
   soft parts — *see* Neoplasm, connective tissue, un-
      certain behavior

☑ Additional Character Required — Refer to the Tabular List for Character Selection   Ⓦ Subterms under main terms may continue to next column or page

Tumor — *continued*

giant cell — *see also* Neoplasm, uncertain behavior, by site — *continued*
  soft parts — *see* Neoplasm, connective tissue, uncertain behavior — *continued*
    malignant — *see* Neoplasm, connective tissue, malignant
glomus D18.00
  intra-abdominal D18.03
  intracranial D18.02
  jugulare D44.7
    malignant C75.5
  skin D18.01
  specified site NEC D18.09
gonadal stromal — *see* Neoplasm, uncertain behavior, by site
granular cell — *see also* Neoplasm, connective tissue, benign
  malignant — *see* Neoplasm, connective tissue, malignant
granulosa cell D39.1- ☑
  juvenile D39.1- ☑
  malignant C56- ☑
granulosa cell-theca cell D39.1- ☑
  malignant C56- ☑
Grawitz's C64- ☑
hemorrhoidal — *see* Hemorrhoids
hilar cell D27- ☑
hilus cell D27- ☑
Hurthle cell (benign) D34
  malignant C73
hydatid — *see* Echinococcus
hypernephroid — *see also* Neoplasm, uncertain behavior, by site
interstitial cell — *see also* Neoplasm, uncertain behavior, by site
  benign — *see* Neoplasm, benign, by site
  malignant — *see* Neoplasm, malignant, by site
intravascular bronchial alveolar D38.1
islet cell — *see* Neoplasm, benign, by site
  malignant — *see* Neoplasm, malignant, by site
    pancreas C25.4
    specified site NEC — *see* Neoplasm, malignant, by site
    unspecified site C25.4
  pancreas D13.7
  specified site NEC — *see* Neoplasm, benign, by site
  unspecified site D13.7
juxtaglomerular D41.0- ☑
Klatskin's C22.1
Krukenberg's C79.6- ☑
Leydig cell — *see* Neoplasm, uncertain behavior, by site
  benign — *see* Neoplasm, benign, by site
    specified site — *see* Neoplasm, benign, by site
    unspecified site
      female D27.9
      male D29.20
  malignant — *see* Neoplasm, malignant, by site
    specified site — *see* Neoplasm, malignant, by site
    unspecified site
      female C56.9
      male C62.90
  specified site — *see* Neoplasm, uncertain behavior, by site
  unspecified site
    female D39.10
    male D40.10
lipid cell, ovary D27- ☑
lipoid cell, ovary D27- ☑
malignant — *see also* Neoplasm, malignant, by site C80.1
  fusiform cell (type) C80.1
  giant cell (type) C80.1
  localized, plasma cell — *see* Plasmacytoma, solitary
  mixed NEC C80.1
  small cell (type) C80.1
  spindle cell (type) C80.1
  unclassified C80.1
mast cell D47.09
melanotic, neuroectodermal — *see* Neoplasm, benign, by site
Merkel cell — *see* Carcinoma, Merkel cell
mesenchymal
  malignant — *see* Neoplasm, connective tissue, malignant

Tumor — *continued*

mesenchymal — *continued*
  mixed — *see* Neoplasm, connective tissue, uncertain behavior
mesodermal, mixed — *see also* Neoplasm, malignant, by site
  liver C22.4
mesonephric — *see also* Neoplasm, uncertain behavior, by site
  malignant — *see* Neoplasm, malignant, by site
metastatic
  from specified site — *see* Neoplasm, malignant, by site
  of specified site — *see* Neoplasm, malignant, by site
  to specified site — *see* Neoplasm, secondary, by site
mixed NEC — *see also* Neoplasm, benign, by site
  malignant — *see* Neoplasm, malignant, by site
mucinous of low malignant potential
  specified site — *see* Neoplasm, malignant, by site
  unspecified site C56.9
mucocarcinoid
  specified site — *see* Neoplasm, malignant, by site
  unspecified site C18.1
mucoepidermoid — *see* Neoplasm, uncertain behavior, by site
Müllerian, mixed
  specified site — *see* Neoplasm, malignant, by site
  unspecified site C54.9
myoepithelial — *see* Neoplasm, benign, by site
neuroectodermal (peripheral) — *see* Neoplasm, malignant, by site
  primitive
    specified site — *see* Neoplasm, malignant, by site
    unspecified site C71.9
neuroendocrine D3A.8 (*following* D36)
  malignant poorly differentiated C7A.1 (*following* C75)
  secondary NEC C7B.8 (*following* C75)
  specified NEC C7A.8 (*following* C75)
neurogenic olfactory C30.0
nonencapsulated sclerosing C73
odontogenic (adenomatoid) (benign) (calcifying epithelial) (keratocystic) (squamous) — *see* Cyst, calcifying odontogenic
  malignant C41.1
    upper jaw (bone) C41.0
ovarian stromal D39.1- ☑
ovary, in pregnancy — *see* Pregnancy, complicated by
pacinian — *see* Neoplasm, skin, benign
Pancoast's — *see* Pancoast's syndrome
papillary — *see also* Papilloma
  cystic D37.9
  mucinous of low malignant potential C56- ☑
    specified site — *see* Neoplasm, malignant, by site
    unspecified site C56.9
  serous of low malignant potential
    specified site — *see* Neoplasm, malignant, by site
    unspecified site C56.9
pelvic, in pregnancy or childbirth — *see* Pregnancy, complicated by
phantom F45.8
phyllodes D48.6- ☑
  benign D24- ☑
  malignant — *see* Neoplasm, breast, malignant
Pindborg — *see* Cyst, calcifying odontogenic
placental site trophoblastic D39.2
plasma cell (malignant) (localized) — *see* Plasmacytoma, solitary
polyvesicular vitelline
  specified site — *see* Neoplasm, malignant, by site
  unspecified site
    female C56.9
    male C62.90
Pott's puffy — *see* Osteomyelitis, specified NEC
Rathke's pouch D44.3
retinal anlage — *see* Neoplasm, benign, by site
salivary gland type, mixed — *see* Neoplasm, salivary gland, benign
  malignant — *see* Neoplasm, salivary gland, malignant
Sampson's N80.1
Schmincke's — *see* Neoplasm, nasopharynx, malignant
sclerosing stromal D27- ☑
sebaceous — *see* Cyst, sebaceous

Tumor — *continued*

secondary — *see* Neoplasm, secondary, by site
  carcinoid C7B.00 (*following* C75)
    bone C7B.03 (*following* C75)
    distant lymph nodes C7B.01 (*following* C75)
    liver C7B.02 (*following* C75)
    peritoneum C7B.04 (*following* C75)
    specified NEC C7B.09 (*following* C75)
  neuroendocrine NEC C7B.8 (*following* C75)
serous of low malignant potential
  specified site — *see* Neoplasm, malignant, by site
  unspecified site C56.9
Sertoli cell — *see* Neoplasm, benign, by site
  with lipid storage
    specified site — *see* Neoplasm, benign, by site
    unspecified site
      female D27.9
      male D29.20
  specified site — *see* Neoplasm, benign, by site
  unspecified site
    female D27.9
    male D29.20
Sertoli-Leydig cell — *see* Neoplasm, benign, by site
  specified site — *see* Neoplasm, benign, by site
  unspecified site
    female D27.9
    male D29.20
sex cord (-stromal) — *see* Neoplasm, uncertain behavior, by site
  with annular tubules D39.1- ☑
skin appendage — *see* Neoplasm, skin, benign
smooth muscle — *see* Neoplasm, connective tissue, uncertain behavior
soft tissue
  benign — *see* Neoplasm, connective tissue, benign
  malignant — *see* Neoplasm, connective tissue, malignant
sternomastoid (congenital) Q68.0
stromal
  endometrial D39.0
  gastric D48.1
    benign D21.4
    malignant C16.9
    uncertain behavior D48.1
  gastrointestinal C49.A- ☑
    benign D21.4
    esophagus C49.A1
    malignant C49.A0
      colon C49.A4
      duodenum C49.A3
      esophagus C49.A1
      ileum C49.A3
      jejunum C49.A3
      large intestine C49.A4
      Meckel diverticulum C49.A3
      omentum C49.A9
      peritoneum C49.A9
      rectum C49.A5
      small intestine C49.A3
      specified site NEC C49.A9
      stomach C49.A2
    rectum C49.A5
    small intestine C49.A3
    specified site NEC C49.A9
    stomach C49.A2
    uncertain behavior D48.1
  intestine
    benign D21.4
    malignant
      large C49.A4
      small C49.A3
    uncertain behavior D48.1
  ovarian D39.1- ☑
  stomach C49.A2
    benign D21.4
    malignant C49.A2
    uncertain behavior D48.1
sweat gland — *see also* Neoplasm, skin, uncertain behavior
  benign — *see* Neoplasm, skin, benign
  malignant — *see* Neoplasm, skin, malignant
syphilitic, brain A52.17
testicular D40.10
testicular stromal D40.1- ☑
theca cell D27.- ☑
theca cell-granulosa cell D39.1- ☑
Triton, malignant — *see* Neoplasm, nerve, malignant
trophoblastic, placental site D39.2

Tumor — *continued*
  turban D23.4
  uterus (body), in pregnancy or childbirth — *see* Pregnancy, complicated by, tumor, uterus
  vagina, in pregnancy or childbirth — *see* Pregnancy, complicated by
  varicose — *see* Varix
  von Recklinghausen's — *see* Neurofibromatosis
  vulva or perineum, in pregnancy or childbirth — *see* Pregnancy, complicated by
    causing obstructed labor O65.5
  Warthin's — *see* Neoplasm, salivary gland, benign
  Wilms' C64- ☑
  yolk sac — *see* Neoplasm, malignant, by site
    specified site — *see* Neoplasm, malignant, by site
    unspecified site
      female C56.9
      male C62.90
Tumor lysis syndrome (following antineoplastic chemotherapy) (spontaneous) NEC E88.3
Tumorlet — *see* Neoplasm, uncertain behavior, by site
Tungiasis B88.1
Tunica vasculosa lentis Q12.2
Turban tumor D23.4
Türck's trachoma J37.0
Turner-Kieser syndrome Q87.2
Turner-like syndrome Q87.19
Turner's
  hypoplasia (tooth) K00.4
  syndrome Q96.9
    specified NEC Q96.8
  tooth K00.4
Turner-Ullrich syndrome Q96.9
Tussis convulsiva — *see* Whooping cough
Twiddler's syndrome (due to)
  automatic implantable defibrillator T82.198
  cardiac pacemaker T82.198 ☑
Twilight state
  epileptic F05
  psychogenic F44.89
Twin (newborn) — *see also* Newborn, twin
  conjoined Q89.4
  pregnancy — *see* Pregnancy, twin
Twinning, teeth K00.2
Twist, twisted
  bowel, colon or intestine K56.2
  hair (congenital) Q84.1
  mesentery K56.2
  omentum K56.2
  organ or site, congenital NEC — *see* Anomaly, by site
  ovarian pedicle — *see* Torsion, ovary
Twitching R25.3
Tylosis (acquired) L84
  buccalis K13.29
  linguae K13.29
  palmaris et plantaris (congenital) (inherited) Q82.8
    acquired L85.1
Tympanism R14.0
Tympanites (abdominal) (intestinal) R14.0
Tympanitis — *see* Myringitis
Tympanosclerosis H74.0 ☑
Tympanum — *see* condition
Tympany
  abdomen R14.0
  chest R09.89
Type A behavior pattern Z73.1
Typhlitis — *see* Appendicitis
Typhoenteritis — *see* Typhoid
Typhoid (abortive) (ambulant) (any site) (clinical) (fever) (hemorrhagic) (infection) (intermittent) (malignant) (rheumatic) (Widal negative) A01.00
  with pneumonia A01.03
  abdominal A01.09
  arthritis A01.04
  carrier (suspected) of Z22.0
  cholecystitis (current) A01.09
  endocarditis A01.02
  heart involvement A01.02
  inoculation reaction — *see* Complications, vaccination
  meningitis A01.01
  mesenteric lymph nodes A01.09
  myocarditis A01.02
  osteomyelitis A01.05
  perichondritis, larynx A01.09
  pneumonia A01.03
  specified NEC A01.09
  spine A01.05

Typhoid — *continued*
  ulcer (perforating) A01.09
Typhomalaria (fever) — *see* Malaria
Typhomania A01.00
Typhoperitonitis A01.09
Typhus (fever) A75.9
  abdominal, abdominalis — *see* Typhoid
  African tick A77.1
  amarillic A95.9
  brain A75.9 *[G94]*
  cerebral A75.9 *[G94]*
  classical A75.0
  due to Rickettsia
    prowazekii A75.0
      recrudescent A75.1
    tsutsugamushi A75.3
    typhi A75.2
  endemic (flea-borne) A75.2
  epidemic (louse-borne) A75.0
  exanthematicus SAI A75.0
    brillii SAI A75.1
    mexicanus SAI A75.2
    typhus murinus A75.2
  exanthematic NEC A75.0
  flea-borne A75.2
  India tick A77.1
  Kenya (tick) A77.1
  louse-borne A75.0
  Mexican A75.2
  mite-borne A75.3
  murine A75.2
  North Asian tick-borne A77.2
  petechial A75.9
  Queensland tick A77.3
  rat A75.2
  recrudescent A75.1
  recurrens — *see* Fever, relapsing
  Sao Paulo A77.0
  scrub (China) (India) (Malaysia) (New Guinea) A75.3
  shop (of Malaysia) A75.2
  Siberian tick A77.2
  tick-borne A77.9
  tropical (mite-borne) A75.3
Tyrosinemia E70.21
  newborn, transitory P74.5
Tyrosinosis E70.21
Tyrosinuria E70.29

U

Uhl's anomaly or disease Q24.8
Ulcer, ulcerated, ulcerating, ulceration, ulcerative
  alveolar process M27.3
  amebic (intestine) A06.1
    skin A06.7
  anastomotic — *see* Ulcer, gastrojejunal
  anorectal K62.6
  antral — *see* Ulcer, stomach
  anus (sphincter) (solitary) K62.6
  aorta — *see* Aneurysm
  aphthous (oral) (recurrent) K12.0
    genital organ(s)
      female N76.6
      male N50.89
  artery I77.2
  atrophic — *see* Ulcer, skin
    decubitus — *see* Ulcer, pressure, by site
  back L98.429
    with
      bone involvement without evidence of necrosis L98.426
      bone necrosis L98.424
      exposed fat layer L98.422
      muscle involvement without evidence of necrosis L98.425
      muscle necrosis L98.423
      skin breakdown only L98.421
      specified severity NEC L98.428
  Barrett's (esophagus) K22.10
    with bleeding K22.11
  bile duct (common) (hepatic) K83.8
  bladder (solitary) (sphincter) NEC N32.89
    bilharzial B65.9 *[N33]*
    in schistosomiasis (bilharzial) B65.9 *[N33]*
    submucosal — *see* Cystitis, interstitial
    tuberculous A18.12
  bleeding K27.4
  bone — *see* Osteomyelitis, specified type NEC

Ulcer, ulcerated, ulcerating, ulceration, ulcerative — *continued*
  bowel — *see* Ulcer, intestine
  breast N61.1
  bronchus J98.09
  buccal (cavity) (traumatic) K12.1
  Buruli A31.1
  buttock L98.419
    with
      bone involvement without evidence of necrosis L98.416
      bone necrosis L98.414
      exposed fat layer L98.412
      muscle involvement without evidence of necrosis L98.415
      muscle necrosis L98.413
      skin breakdown only L98.411
      specified severity NEC L98.418
  cancerous — *see* Neoplasm, malignant, by site
  cardia K22.10
    with bleeding K22.11
  cardioesophageal (peptic) K22.10
    with bleeding K22.11
  cecum — *see* Ulcer, intestine
  cervix (uteri) (decubitus) (trophic) N86
    with cervicitis N72
  chancroidal A57
  chiclero B55.1
  chronic (cause unknown) — *see* Ulcer, skin
  Cochin-China B55.1
  colon — *see* Ulcer, intestine
  conjunctiva H10.89
  cornea H16.00- ☑
    with hypopyon H16.03- ☑
      central I116.01- ☑
    dendritic (herpes simplex) B00.52
    marginal H16.04- ☑
    Mooren's H16.05- ☑
    mycotic H16.06- ☑
    perforated H16.07- ☑
    ring H16.02- ☑
    tuberculous (phlyctenular) A18.52
  corpus cavernosum (chronic) N48.5
  crural — *see* Ulcer, lower limb
  Curling's — *see* Ulcer, peptic, acute
  Cushing's — *see* Ulcer, peptic, acute
  cystic duct K82.8
  cystitis (interstitial) — *see* Cystitis, interstitial
  decubitus — *see* Ulcer, pressure, by site
  dendritic, cornea (herpes simplex) B00.52
  diabetes, diabetic — *see* Diabetes, ulcer
  Dieulafoy's K25.0
  due to
    infection NEC — *see* Ulcer, skin
    radiation NEC L59.8
    trophic disturbance (any region) — *see* Ulcer, skin
    X-ray L58.1
  duodenum, duodenal (eroded) (peptic) K26.9
    with
      hemorrhage K26.4
        and perforation K26.6
      perforation K26.5
    acute K26.3
      with
        hemorrhage K26.0
          and perforation K26.2
        perforation K26.1
    chronic K26.7
      with
        hemorrhage K26.4
          and perforation K26.6
        perforation K26.5
  dysenteric A09
  elusive — *see* Cystitis, interstitial
  endocarditis (acute) (chronic) (subacute) I28.8
  epiglottis J38.7
  esophagus (peptic) K22.10
    with bleeding K22.11
    due to
      aspirin K22.10
        with bleeding K22.11
      gastrointestinal reflux disease K21.0
      ingestion of chemical or medicament K22.10
        with bleeding K22.11
    fungal K22.10
      with bleeding K22.11
    infective K22.10
      with bleeding K22.11

Ulcer, ulcerated, ulcerating, ulceration, ulcerative
— *continued*
  esophagus — *continued*
    varicose — *see* Varix, esophagus
  eyelid (region) H01.8
  fauces J39.2
  Fenwick (-Hunner) (solitary) — *see* Cystitis, interstitial
  fistulous — *see* Ulcer, skin
  foot (indolent) (trophic) — *see* Ulcer, lower limb
  frambesial, initial A66.0
  frenum (tongue) K14.0
  gallbladder or duct K82.8
  gangrenous — *see* Gangrene
  gastric — *see* Ulcer, stomach
  gastrocolic — *see* Ulcer, gastrojejunal
  gastroduodenal — *see* Ulcer, peptic
  gastroesophageal — *see* Ulcer, stomach
  gastrointestinal — *see* Ulcer, gastrojejunal
  gastrojejunal (peptic) K28.9
    with
      hemorrhage K28.4
        and perforation K28.6
      perforation K28.5
    acute K28.3
      with
        hemorrhage K28.0
          and perforation K28.2
        perforation K28.1
    chronic K28.7
      with
        hemorrhage K28.4
          and perforation K28.6
        perforation K28.5
  gastrojejunocolic — *see* Ulcer, gastrojejunal
  gingiva K06.8
  gingivitis K05.10
    nonplaque induced K05.11
    plaque induced K05.10
  glottis J38.7
  granuloma of pudenda A58
  gum K06.8
  gumma, due to yaws A66.4
  heel — *see* Ulcer, lower limb
  hemorrhoid — *see also* Hemorrhoids, by degree K64.8
  Hunner's — *see* Cystitis, interstitial
  hypopharynx J39.2
  hypopyon (chronic) (subacute) — *see* Ulcer, cornea, with hypopyon
  hypostaticum — *see* Ulcer, varicose
  ileum — *see* Ulcer, intestine
  intestine, intestinal K63.3
    with perforation K63.1
    amebic A06.1
    duodenal — *see* Ulcer, duodenum
    granulocytopenic (with hemorrhage) — *see* Neutropenia
    marginal — *see* Ulcer, gastrojejunal
    perforating K63.1
      newborn P78.0
    primary, small intestine K63.3
    rectum K62.6
    stercoraceous, stercoral K63.3
    tuberculous A18.32
    typhoid (fever) — *see* Typhoid
    varicose I86.8
  jejunum, jejunal — *see* Ulcer, gastrojejunal
  keratitis — *see* Ulcer, cornea
  knee — *see* Ulcer, lower limb
  labium (majus) (minus) N76.6
  laryngitis — *see* Laryngitis
  larynx (aphthous) (contact) J38.7
    diphtheritic A36.2
  leg — *see* Ulcer, lower limb
  lip K13.0
  Lipschütz's N76.6
  lower limb (atrophic) (chronic) (neurogenic) (perforating) (pyogenic) (trophic) (tropical) L97.909
    with
      bone involvement without evidence of necrosis L97.906
      bone necrosis L97.904
      exposed fat layer L97.902
      muscle involvement without evidence of necrosis L97.905
      muscle necrosis L97.903
      skin breakdown only L97.901
      specified severity NEC L97.908
    ankle L97.309

Ulcer, ulcerated, ulcerating, ulceration, ulcerative
— *continued*
  lower limb — *continued*
    ankle — *continued*
      with
        bone involvement without evidence of necrosis L97.306
        bone necrosis L97.304
        exposed fat layer L97.302
        muscle involvement without evidence of necrosis L97.305
        muscle necrosis L97.303
        skin breakdown only L97.301
        specified severity NEC L97.308
      left L97.329
        with
          bone involvement without evidence of necrosis L97.326
          bone necrosis L97.324
          exposed fat layer L97.322
          muscle involvement without evidence of necrosis L97.325
          muscle necrosis L97.323
          skin breakdown only L97.321
          specified severity NEC L97.328
      right L97.319
        with
          bone involvement without evidence of necrosis L97.316
          bone necrosis L97.314
          exposed fat layer L97.312
          muscle involvement without evidence of necrosis L97.315
          muscle necrosis L97.313
          skin breakdown only L97.311
          specified severity NEC L97.318
    calf L97.209
      with
        bone involvement without evidence of necrosis L97.206
        bone necrosis L97.204
        exposed fat layer L97.202
        muscle involvement without evidence of necrosis L97.205
        muscle necrosis L97.203
        skin breakdown only L97.201
        specified severity NEC L97.208
      left L97.229
        with
          bone involvement without evidence of necrosis L97.226
          bone necrosis L97.224
          exposed fat layer L97.222
          muscle involvement without evidence of necrosis L97.225
          muscle necrosis L97.223
          skin breakdown only L97.221
          specified severity NEC L97.228
      right L97.219
        with
          bone involvement without evidence of necrosis L97.216
          bone necrosis L97.214
          exposed fat layer L97.212
          muscle involvement without evidence of necrosis L97.215
          muscle necrosis L97.213
          skin breakdown only L97.211
          specified severity NEC L97.218
    decubitus — *see* Ulcer, pressure, by site
    foot specified NEC L97.509
      with
        bone involvement without evidence of necrosis L97.506
        bone necrosis L97.504
        exposed fat layer L97.502
        muscle involvement without evidence of necrosis L97.505
        muscle necrosis L97.503
        skin breakdown only L97.501
        specified severity NEC L97.508
      left L97.529
        with
          bone involvement without evidence of necrosis L97.526
          bone necrosis L97.524
          exposed fat layer L97.522
          muscle involvement without evidence of necrosis L97.525

Ulcer, ulcerated, ulcerating, ulceration, ulcerative
— *continued*
  lower limb — *continued*
    foot specified — *continued*
      left — *continued*
        with — *continued*
          muscle necrosis L97.523
          skin breakdown only L97.521
          specified severity NEC L97.528
      right L97.519
        with
          bone involvement without evidence of necrosis L97.516
          bone necrosis L97.514
          exposed fat layer L97.512
          muscle involvement without evidence of necrosis L97.515
          muscle necrosis L97.513
          skin breakdown only L97.511
          specified severity NEC L97.518
    heel L97.409
      with
        bone involvement without evidence of necrosis L97.406
        bone necrosis L97.404
        exposed fat layer L97.402
        muscle involvement without evidence of necrosis L97.405
        muscle necrosis L97.403
        skin breakdown only L97.401
        specified severity NEC L97.408
      left L97.429
        with
          bone involvement without evidence of necrosis L97.426
          bone necrosis L97.424
          exposed fat layer L97.422
          muscle involvement without evidence of necrosis L97.425
          muscle necrosis L97.423
          skin breakdown only L97.421
          specified severity NEC L97.428
      right L97.419
        with
          bone involvement without evidence of necrosis L97.416
          bone necrosis L97.414
          exposed fat layer L97.412
          muscle involvement without evidence of necrosis L97.415
          muscle necrosis L97.413
          skin breakdown only L97.411
          specified severity NEC L97.418
    left L97.929
      with
        bone involvement without evidence of necrosis L97.926
        bone necrosis L97.924
        exposed fat layer L97.922
        muscle involvement without evidence of necrosis L97.925
        muscle necrosis L97.923
        skin breakdown only L97.921
        specified severity NEC L97.928
    leprous A30.1
    lower leg NOS L97.909
      with
        bone involvement without evidence of necrosis L97.906
        bone necrosis L97.904
        exposed fat layer L97.902
        muscle involvement without evidence of necrosis L97.905
        muscle necrosis L97.903
        skin breakdown only L97.901
        specified severity NEC L97.908
      left L97.929
        with
          bone involvement without evidence of necrosis L97.926
          bone necrosis L97.924
          exposed fat layer L97.922
          muscle involvement without evidence of necrosis L97.925
          muscle necrosis L97.923
          skin breakdown only L97.921
          specified severity NEC L97.928
      right L97.919

Ulcer, ulcerated, ulcerating, ulceration, ulcerative
— continued
    lower limb — continued
        lower leg — continued
            right — continued
                with
                    bone involvement without evidence of
                        necrosis L97.916
                    bone necrosis L97.914
                    exposed fat layer L97.912
                    muscle involvement without evidence of
                        necrosis L97.915
                    muscle necrosis L97.913
                    skin breakdown only L97.911
                    specified severity NEC L97.918
            specified site NEC L97.809
                with
                    bone involvement without evidence of
                        necrosis L97.806
                    bone necrosis L97.804
                    exposed fat layer L97.802
                    muscle involvement without evidence of
                        necrosis L97.805
                    muscle necrosis L97.803
                    skin breakdown only L97.801
                    specified severity NEC L97.808
                left L97.829
                    with
                        bone involvement without evidence
                            of necrosis L97.826
                        bone necrosis L97.824
                        exposed fat layer L97.822
                        muscle involvement without evidence
                            of necrosis L97.825
                        muscle necrosis L97.823
                        skin breakdown only L97.821
                        specified severity NEC L97.828
                right L97.819
                    with
                        bone involvement without evidence
                            of necrosis L97.816
                        bone necrosis L97.814
                        exposed fat layer L97.812
                        muscle involvement without evidence
                            of necrosis L97.815
                        muscle necrosis L97.813
                        skin breakdown only L97.811
                        specified severity NEC L97.818
            midfoot L97.409
                with
                    bone involvement without evidence of
                        necrosis L97.406
                    bone necrosis L97.404
                    exposed fat layer L97.402
                    muscle involvement without evidence of
                        necrosis L97.405
                    muscle necrosis L97.403
                    skin breakdown only L97.401
                    specified severity NEC L97.408
                left L97.429
                    with
                        bone involvement without evidence of
                            necrosis L97.426
                        bone necrosis L97.424
                        exposed fat layer L97.422
                        muscle involvement without evidence of
                            necrosis L97.425
                        muscle necrosis L97.423
                        skin breakdown only L97.421
                        specified severity NEC L97.428
                right L97.419
                    with
                        bone involvement without evidence of
                            necrosis L97.416
                        bone necrosis L97.414
                        exposed fat layer L97.412
                        muscle involvement without evidence of
                            necrosis L97.415
                        muscle necrosis L97.413
                        skin breakdown only L97.411
                        specified severity NEC L97.418
            right L97.919
                with
                    bone involvement without evidence of
                        necrosis L97.916
                    bone necrosis L97.914
                    exposed fat layer L97.912
                    muscle involvement without evidence of
                        necrosis L97.915

Ulcer, ulcerated, ulcerating, ulceration, ulcerative
— continued
    lower limb — continued
        right — continued
            with — continued
                muscle necrosis L97.913
                skin breakdown only L97.911
                specified severity NEC L97.918
        syphilitic A52.19
        thigh L97.109
            with
                bone involvement without evidence of
                    necrosis L97.106
                bone necrosis L97.104
                exposed fat layer L97.102
                muscle involvement without evidence of
                    necrosis L97.105
                muscle necrosis L97.103
                skin breakdown only L97.101
                specified severity NEC L97.108
            left L97.129
                with
                    bone involvement without evidence of
                        necrosis L97.126
                    bone necrosis L97.124
                    exposed fat layer L97.122
                    muscle involvement without evidence of
                        necrosis L97.125
                    muscle necrosis L97.123
                    skin breakdown only L97.121
                    specified severity NEC L97.128
            right L97.119
                with
                    bone involvement without evidence of
                        necrosis L97.116
                    bone necrosis L97.114
                    exposed fat layer L97.112
                    muscle involvement without evidence of
                        necrosis L97.115
                    muscle necrosis L97.113
                    skin breakdown only L97.111
                    specified severity NEC L97.118
        toe L97.509
            with
                bone involvement without evidence of
                    necrosis L97.506
                bone necrosis L97.504
                exposed fat layer L97.502
                muscle involvement without evidence of
                    necrosis L97.505
                muscle necrosis L97.503
                skin breakdown only L97.501
                specified severity NEC L97.508
            left L97.529
                with
                    bone involvement without evidence of
                        necrosis L97.526
                    bone necrosis L97.524
                    exposed fat layer L97.522
                    muscle involvement without evidence of
                        necrosis L97.525
                    muscle necrosis L97.523
                    skin breakdown only L97.521
                    specified severity NEC L97.528
            right L97.519
                with
                    bone involvement without evidence of
                        necrosis L97.516
                    bone necrosis L97.514
                    exposed fat layer L97.512
                    muscle involvement without evidence of
                        necrosis L97.515
                    muscle necrosis L97.513
                    skin breakdown only L97.511
                    specified severity NEC L97.518
        varicose — see Varix, leg, with, ulcer
    luetic — see Ulcer, syphilitic
    lung J98.4
        tuberculous — see Tuberculosis, pulmonary
    malignant — see Neoplasm, malignant, by site
    marginal NEC — see Ulcer, gastrojejunal
    meatus (urinarius) N34.2
    Meckel's diverticulum Q43.0
        malignant — see Table of Neoplasms, small intes-
            tine, malignant
    Meleney's (chronic undermining) — see Ulcer, skin
    Mooren's (cornea) — see Ulcer, cornea, Mooren's
    mycobacterial (skin) A31.1

Ulcer, ulcerated, ulcerating, ulceration, ulcerative
— continued
    nasopharynx J39.2
    neck, uterus N86
    neurogenic NEC — see Ulcer, skin
    nose, nasal (passage) (infective) (septum) J34.0
        skin — see Ulcer, skin
        spirochetal A69.8
        varicose (bleeding) I86.8
    oral mucosa (traumatic) K12.1
    palate (soft) K12.1
    penis (chronic) N48.5
    peptic (site unspecified) K27.9
        with
            hemorrhage K27.4
                and perforation K27.6
            perforation K27.5
        acute K27.3
            with
                hemorrhage K27.0
                    and perforation K27.2
                perforation K27.1
        chronic K27.7
            with
                hemorrhage K27.4
                    and perforation K27.6
                perforation K27.5
        esophagus K22.10
            with bleeding K22.11
        newborn P78.82
    perforating K27.5
        skin — see Ulcer, skin
    peritonsillar J35.8
    phagedenic (tropical) — see Ulcer, skin
    pharynx J39.2
    phlebitis — see Phlebitis
    plaster — see Ulcer, pressure, by site
    popliteal space — see Ulcer, lower limb
    postpyloric — see Ulcer, duodenum
    prepuce N47.7
    prepyloric — see Ulcer, stomach
    pressure (pressure area) L89.9- ☑
        ankle L89.5- ☑
        back L89.1- ☑
        buttock L89.3- ☑
        coccyx L89.15- ☑
        contiguous site of back, buttock, hip L89.4- ☑
        elbow L89.0- ☑
        face L89.81- ☑
        head L89.81- ☑
        heel L89.6- ☑
        hip L89.2- ☑
        sacral region (tailbone) L89.15- ☑
        specified site NEC L89.89- ☑
        stage 1 (healing) (pre-ulcer skin changes limited to
            persistent focal edema)
            ankle L89.5- ☑
            back L89.1- ☑
            buttock L89.3- ☑
            coccyx L89.15- ☑
            contiguous site of back, buttock, hip L89.4- ☑
            elbow L89.0- ☑
            face L89.81- ☑
            head L89.81- ☑
            heel L89.6- ☑
            hip L89.2- ☑
            sacral region (tailbone) L89.15- ☑
            specified site NEC L89.89- ☑
        stage 2 (healing) (abrasion, blister, partial thickness
            skin loss involving epidermis and/or dermis)
            ankle L89.5- ☑
            back L89.1- ☑
            buttock L89.3- ☑
            coccyx L89.15- ☑
            contiguous site of back, buttock, hip L89.4- ☑
            elbow L89.0- ☑
            face L89.81- ☑
            head L89.81- ☑
            heel L89.6- ☑
            hip L89.2- ☑
            sacral region (tailbone) L89.15- ☑
            specified site NEC L89.89- ☑
        stage 3 (healing) (full thickness skin loss involving
            damage or necrosis of subcutaneous tissue)
            ankle L89.5- ☑
            back L89.1- ☑
            buttock L89.3- ☑

Ulcer, ulcerated, ulcerating, ulceration, ulcerative
— continued
  pressure — continued
    stage 3 — continued
      coccyx L89.15- ☑
      contiguous site of back, buttock, hip L89.4- ☑
      elbow L89.0- ☑
      face L89.81- ☑
      head L89.81- ☑
      heel L89.6- ☑
      hip L89.2- ☑
      sacral region (tailbone) L89.15- ☑
      specified site NEC L89.89- ☑
    stage 4 (healing) (necrosis of soft tissues through to underlying muscle, tendon, or bone)
      ankle L89.5- ☑
      back L89.1- ☑
      buttock L89.3- ☑
      coccyx L89.15- ☑
      contiguous site of back, buttock, hip L89.4- ☑
      elbow L89.0- ☑
      face L89.81- ☑
      head L89.81- ☑
      heel L89.6- ☑
      hip L89.2- ☑
      sacral region (tailbone) L89.15- ☑
      specified site NEC L89.89- ☑
    unspecified stage
      ankle L89.5- ☑
      back L89.1- ☑
      buttock L89.3- ☑
      coccyx L89.15- ☑
      contiguous site of back, buttock, hip L89.4- ☑
      elbow L89.0- ☑
      face L89.81- ☑
      head L89.81- ☑
      heel L89.6- ☑
      hip L89.2- ☑
      sacral region (tailbone) L89.15- ☑
      specified site NEC L89.89- ☑
    unstageable
      ankle L89.5- ☑
      back L89.1- ☑
      buttock L89.3- ☑
      coccyx L89.15- ☑
      contiguous site of back, buttock, hip L89.4- ☑
      elbow L89.0- ☑
      face L89.81- ☑
      head L89.81- ☑
      heel L89.6- ☑
      hip L89.2- ☑
      sacral region (tailbone) L89.15- ☑
      specified site NEC L89.89- ☑
  primary of intestine K63.3
    with perforation K63.1
  prostate N41.9
  pyloric — see Ulcer, stomach
  rectosigmoid K63.3
    with perforation K63.1
  rectum (sphincter) (solitary) K62.6
    stercoraceous, stercoral K62.6
  retina — see Inflammation, chorioretinal
  rodent — see also Neoplasm, skin, malignant
  sclera — see Scleritis
  scrofulous (tuberculous) A18.2
  scrotum N50.89
    tuberculous A18.15
    varicose I86.1
  seminal vesicle N50.89
  sigmoid — see Ulcer, intestine
  skin (atrophic) (chronic) (neurogenic) (non-healing) (perforating) (pyogenic) (trophic) (tropical) L98.499
    with gangrene — see Gangrene
    amebic A06.7
    back — see Ulcer, back
    buttock — see Ulcer, buttock
    decubitus — see Ulcer, pressure
    lower limb — see Ulcer, lower limb
    mycobacterial A31.1
    specified site NEC L98.499
      with
        bone involvement without evidence of necrosis L98.496
        bone necrosis L98.494
        exposed fat layer L98.492

Ulcer, ulcerated, ulcerating, ulceration, ulcerative
— continued
  skin — continued
    specified site — continued
      with — continued
        muscle involvement without evidence of necrosis L98.495
        muscle necrosis L98.493
        skin breakdown only L98.491
        specified severity NEC L98.498
    tuberculous (primary) A18.4
    varicose — see Ulcer, varicose
  sloughing — see Ulcer, skin
  solitary, anus or rectum (sphincter) K62.6
  sore throat J02.9
    streptococcal J02.0
  spermatic cord N50.89
  spine (tuberculous) A18.01
  stasis (venous) — see Varix, leg, with, ulcer
    without varicose veins I87.2
  stercoraceous, stercoral K63.3
    with perforation K63.1
    anus or rectum K62.6
  stoma, stomal — see Ulcer, gastrojejunal
  stomach (eroded) (peptic) (round) K25.9
    with
      hemorrhage K25.4
        and perforation K25.6
      perforation K25.5
    acute K25.3
      with
        hemorrhage K25.0
          and perforation K25.2
        perforation K25.1
    chronic K25.7
      with
        hemorrhage K25.4
          and perforation K25.6
        perforation K25.5
  stomal — see Ulcer, gastrojejunal
  stomatitis K12.1
  stress — see Ulcer, peptic
  strumous (tuberculous) A18.2
  submucosal, bladder — see Cystitis, interstitial
  syphilitic (any site) (early) (secondary) A51.39
    late A52.79
    perforating A52.79
      foot A52.11
  testis N50.89
  thigh — see Ulcer, lower limb
  throat J39.2
    diphtheritic A36.0
  toe — see Ulcer, lower limb
  tongue (traumatic) K14.0
  tonsil J35.8
    diphtheritic A36.0
  trachea J39.8
  trophic — see Ulcer, skin
  tropical — see Ulcer, skin
  tuberculous — see Tuberculosis, ulcer
  tunica vaginalis N50.89
  turbinate J34.89
  typhoid (perforating) — see Typhoid
  unspecified site — see Ulcer, skin
  urethra (meatus) — see Urethritis
  uterus N85.8
    cervix N86
      with cervicitis N72
    neck N86
      with cervicitis N72
  vagina N76.5
    in Behçet's disease M35.2 [N77.0]
    pessary N89.8
  valve, heart I33.0
  varicose (lower limb, any part) — see also Varix, leg, with, ulcer
    broad ligament I86.2
    esophagus — see Varix, esophagus
    inflamed or infected — see Varix, leg, with ulcer, with inflammation
    nasal septum I86.8
    perineum I86.3
    scrotum I86.1
    specified site NEC I86.8
    sublingual I86.0
    vulva I86.3
  vas deferens N50.89
  vulva (acute) (infectional) N76.6

Ulcer, ulcerated, ulcerating, ulceration, ulcerative
— continued
  vulva — continued
    in (due to)
      Behçet's disease M35.2 [N77.0]
      herpesviral (herpes simplex) infection A60.04
      tuberculosis A18.18
  vulvobuccal, recurring N76.6
  X-ray L58.1
  yaws A66.4
Ulcerosa scarlatina A38.8
Ulcus — see also Ulcer
  cutis tuberculosum A18.4
  duodeni — see Ulcer, duodenum
  durum (syphilitic) A51.0
    extragenital A51.2
  gastrojejunale — see Ulcer, gastrojejunal
  hypostaticum — see Ulcer, varicose
  molle (cutis) (skin) A57
  serpens corneae — see Ulcer, cornea, central
  ventriculi — see Ulcer, stomach
Ulegyria Q04.8
Ulerythema
  ophryogenes, congenital Q84.2
  sycosiforme L73.8
Ullrich (-Bonnevie)(-Turner) **syndrome** — see also Turner's syndrome Q87.19
Ullrich-Feichtiger syndrome Q87.0
Ulnar — see condition
Ulorrhagia, ulorrhea K06.8
Umbilicus, umbilical — see condition
Unacceptable
  contours of tooth K08.54
  morphology of tooth K08.54
Unavailability (of)
  bed at medical facility Z75.1
  health service-related agencies Z75.4
  medical facilities (at) Z75.3
    due to
      investigation by social service agency Z75.2
      lack of services at home Z75.0
      remoteness from facility Z75.3
      waiting list Z75.1
    home Z75.0
    outpatient clinic Z75.3
  schooling Z55.1
  social service agencies Z75.4
Uncinaria americana infestation B76.1
Uncinariasis B76.9
Uncongenial work Z56.5
Unconscious (ness) — see Coma
Under observation — see Observation
Underachievement in school Z55.3
Underdevelopment — see also Undeveloped
  nose Q30.1
  sexual E30.0
Underdosing — see also Table of Drugs and Chemicals, categories T36-T50, with final character 6 Z91.14
  intentional NEC Z91.128
    due to financial hardship of patient Z91.120
  unintentional NEC Z91.138
    due to patient's age related debility Z91.130
Underfeeding, newborn P92.3
Underfill, endodontic M27.53
Underimmunization status Z28.3
Undernourishment — see Malnutrition
Undernutrition — see Malnutrition
Underweight R63.6
  for gestational age — see Light for dates
Underwood's disease P83.0
Undescended — see also Malposition, congenital
  cecum Q43.3
  colon Q43.3
  testicle — see Cryptorchid
Undeveloped, undevelopment — see also Hypoplasia
  brain (congenital) Q02
  cerebral (congenital) Q02
  heart Q24.8
  lung Q33.6
  testis E29.1
  uterus E30.0
Undiagnosed (disease) R69
Undulant fever — see Brucellosis
Unemployment, anxiety concerning Z56.0
  threatened Z56.2
Unequal length (acquired) (limb) — see also Deformity, limb, unequal length

Index

Unequal length — Use

Unequal length — *continued*
  leg — *see also* Deformity, limb, unequal length
    congenital Q72.9- ☑
Unextracted dental root K08.3
Unguis incarnatus L60.0
Unhappiness R45.2
Unicornate uterus Q51.4
  in pregnancy or childbirth O34.00
Unilateral — *see also* condition
  development, breast N64.89
  organ or site, congenital NEC — *see* Agenesis, by site
Unilocular heart Q20.8
Union, abnormal — *see also* Fusion
  larynx and trachea Q34.8
Universal mesentery Q43.3
Unrepairable overhanging of dental restorative materials K08.52
Unsatisfactory
  restoration of tooth K08.50
    specified NEC K08.59
  sample of cytologic smear
    anus R85.615
    cervix R87.615
    vagina R87.625
  surroundings Z59.1
  work Z56.5
Unsoundness of mind — *see* Psychosis
Unstable
  back NEC — *see* Instability, joint, spine
  hip (congenital) Q65.6
    acquired — *see* Derangement, joint, specified type NEC, hip
  joint — *see* Instability, joint
  secondary to removal of joint prosthesis M96.89
  lie (mother) O32.0 ☑
  lumbosacral joint (congenital) — *see* subcategory M53.2
  sacroiliac — *see* subcategory M53.2 ☑
  spine NEC — *see* Instability, joint, spine
Unsteadiness on feet R26.81
Untruthfulness, child problem F91.8
Unverricht (-Lundborg) **disease or epilepsy** — *see* Epilepsy, generalized, idiopathic
Unwanted pregnancy Z64.0
Upbringing, institutional Z62.22
  away from parents NEC Z62.29
  in care of non-parental family member Z62.21
  in foster care Z62.21
  in orphanage or group home Z62.22
  in welfare custody Z62.21
Upper respiratory — *see* condition
Upset
  gastric K30
  gastrointestinal K30
    psychogenic F45.8
  intestinal (large) (small) K59.9
    psychogenic F45.8
  menstruation N93.9
  mental F48.9
  stomach K30
    psychogenic F45.8
Urachus — *see also* condition
  patent or persistent Q64.4
Urbach-Oppenheim disease (necrobiosis lipoidica diabeticorum) — *see* E08-E13 with .620
Urbach's lipoid proteinosis E78.89
Urbach-Wiethe disease E78.89
Urban yellow fever A95.1
Urea
  blood, high — *see* Uremia
  cycle metabolism disorder — *see* Disorder, urea cycle metabolism
Uremia, uremic N19
  with
    ectopic or molar pregnancy O08.4
    polyneuropathy N18.9 *[G63]*
  chronic NOS — *see also* Disease, kidney, chronic N18.9
    due to hypertension — *see* Hypertensive, kidney
  complicating
    ectopic or molar pregnancy O08.4
  congenital P96.0
  extrarenal R39.2
  following ectopic or molar pregnancy O08.4
  newborn P96.0
  prerenal R39.2
Ureter, ureteral — *see* condition
Ureteralgia N23

Ureterectasis — *see* Hydroureter
Ureteritis N28.89
  cystica N28.86
  due to calculus N20.1
    with calculus, kidney N20.2
      with hydronephrosis N13.2
  gonococcal (acute) (chronic) A54.21
  nonspecific N28.89
Ureterocele N28.89
  congenital (orthotopic) Q62.31
  ectopic Q62.32
Ureterolith, ureterolithiasis — *see* Calculus, ureter
Ureterostomy
  attention to Z43.6
  status Z93.6
Urethra, urethral — *see* condition
Urethralgia R39.89
Urethritis (anterior) (posterior) N34.2
  calculus N21.1
  candidal B37.41
  chlamydial A56.01
  diplococcal (gonococcal) A54.01
    with abscess (accessory gland) (periurethral) A54.1
  gonococcal A54.01
    with abscess (accessory gland) (periurethral) A54.1
  nongonococcal N34.1
    Reiter's — *see* Reiter's disease
  nonspecific N34.1
  nonvenereal N34.1
  postmenopausal N34.2
  puerperal O86.22
  Reiter's — *see* Reiter's disease
  specified NEC N34.2
  trichomonal or due to Trichomonas (vaginalis) A59.03
Urethrocele N81.0
  with
    cystocele — *see* Cystocele
    prolapse of uterus — *see* Prolapse, uterus
Urethrolithiasis (with colic or infection) N21.1
Urethrorectal — *see* condition
Urethrorrhagia N36.8
Urethrorrhea R36.9
Urethrostomy
  attention to Z43.6
  status Z93.6
Urethrotrigonitis — *see* Trigonitis
Urethrovaginal — *see* condition
Urgency
  fecal R15.2
  hypertensive — *see* Hypertension
  urinary R39.15
Urhidrosis, uridrosis L74.8
Uric acid in blood (increased) E79.0
Uricacidemia (asymptomatic) E79.0
Uricemia (asymptomatic) E79.0
Uricosuria R82.998
Urinary — *see* condition
Urination
  frequent R35.0
  painful R30.9
Urine
  blood in — *see* Hematuria
  discharge, excessive R35.8
  enuresis, nonorganic origin F98.0
  extravasation R39.0
  frequency R35.0
  incontinence R32
    nonorganic origin F98.0
  intermittent stream R39.198
  pus in N39.0
  retention or stasis R33.9
    organic R33.8
      drug-induced R33.0
    psychogenic F45.8
  secretion
    deficient R34
    excessive R35.8
    frequency R35.0
  stream
    intermittent R39.198
    slowing R39.198
    splitting R39.13
    weak R39.12
Urinemia — *see* Uremia
Urinoma, urethra N36.8
Uroarthritis, infectious (Reiter's) — *see* Reiter's disease
Urodialysis R34
Urolithiasis — *see* Calculus, urinary

Uronephrosis — *see* Hydronephrosis
Uropathy N39.9
  obstructive N13.9
    specified NEC N13.8
  reflux N13.9
    specified NEC N13.8
  vesicoureteral reflux-associated — *see* Reflux, vesicoureteral
Urosepsis — *code to* condition
Urticaria L50.9
  with angioneurotic edema T78.3 ☑
    hereditary D84.1
  allergic L50.0
  cholinergic L50.5
  chronic L50.8
  cold, familial L50.2
  contact L50.6
  dermatographic L50.3
  due to
    cold or heat L50.2
    drugs L50.0
    food L50.0
    inhalants L50.0
    plants L50.6
    serum — *see also* Reaction, serum T80.69 ☑
  factitial L50.3
  familial cold M04.2
  giant T78.3 ☑
    hereditary D84.1
  gigantea T78.3 ☑
  idiopathic L50.1
  larynx T78.3 ☑
    hereditary D84.1
  neonatorum P83.88
  nonallergic L50.1
  papulosa (Hebra) L28.2
  pigmentosa D47.01
    congenital Q82.2
    of neonatal onset Q82.2
    of newborn onset Q82.2
  recurrent periodic L50.8
  serum — *see also* Reaction, serum T80.69 ☑
  solar L56.3
  specified type NEC L50.8
  thermal (cold) (heat) L50.2
  vibratory L50.4
  xanthelasmoidea — *see* Urticaria pigmentosa
Use (of)
  alcohol Z72.89
    with
      intoxication F10.929
      sleep disorder F10.982
    harmful — *see* Abuse, alcohol
  amphetamines — *see* Use, stimulant NEC
  caffeine — *see* Use, stimulant NEC
  cannabis F12.90
    with
      anxiety disorder F12.980
      intoxication F12.929
        with
          delirium F12.921
          perceptual disturbance F12.922
        uncomplicated F12.920
      other specified disorder F12.988
      psychosis F12.959
        delusions F12.950
        hallucinations F12.951
      unspecified disorder F12.99
      withdrawal F12.93
  cocaine F14.90
    with
      anxiety disorder F14.980
      intoxication F14.929
        with
          delirium F14.921
          perceptual disturbance F14.922
        uncomplicated F14.920
      other specified disorder F14.988
      psychosis F14.959
        delusions F14.950
        hallucinations F14.951
      sexual dysfunction F14.981
      sleep disorder F14.982
      unspecified disorder F14.99
    harmful — *see* Abuse, drug, cocaine
  drug(s) NEC F19.90
    with sleep disorder F19.982
    harmful — *see* Abuse, drug, by type

Use — *continued*
hallucinogen NEC F16.90
  with
    anxiety disorder F16.980
    intoxication F16.929
      with
        delirium F16.921
      uncomplicated F16.920
    mood disorder F16.94
    other specified disorder F16.988
    perception disorder (flashbacks) F16.983
    psychosis F16.959
      delusions F16.950
      hallucinations F16.951
    unspecified disorder F16.99
  harmful — *see* Abuse, drug, hallucinogen NEC
inhalants F18.90
  with
    anxiety disorder F18.980
    intoxication F18.929
      with delirium F18.921
      uncomplicated F18.920
    mood disorder F18.94
    other specified disorder F18.988
    persisting dementia F18.97
    psychosis F18.959
      delusions F18.950
      hallucinations F18.951
    unspecified disorder F18.99
  harmful — *see* Abuse, drug, inhalant
methadone — *see* Use, opioid
nonprescribed drugs F19.90
  harmful — *see* Abuse, non-psychoactive substance
opioid F11.90
  with
    disorder F11.99
      mood F11.94
      sleep F11.982
      specified type NEC F11.988
    intoxication F11.929
      with
        delirium F11.921
        perceptual disturbance F11.922
      uncomplicated F11.920
    withdrawal F11.93
  harmful — *see* Abuse, drug, opioid
patent medicines F19.90
  harmful — *see* Abuse, non-psychoactive substance
psychoactive drug NEC F19.90
  with
    anxiety disorder F19.980
    intoxication F19.929
      with
        delirium F19.921
        perceptual disturbance F19.922
      uncomplicated F19.920
    mood disorder F19.94
    other specified disorder F19.988
    persisting
      amnestic disorder F19.96
      dementia F19.97
    psychosis F19.959
      delusions F19.950
      hallucinations F19.951
    sexual dysfunction F19.981
    sleep disorder F19.982
    unspecified disorder F19.99
    withdrawal F19.939
      with
        delirium F19.931
        perceptual disturbance F19.932
      uncomplicated F19.930
  harmful — *see* Abuse, drug NEC, psychoactive NEC
sedative, hypnotic, or anxiolytic F13.90
  with
    anxiety disorder F13.980
    intoxication F13.929
      with
        delirium F13.921
      uncomplicated F13.920
    other specified disorder F13.988
    persisting
      amnestic disorder F13.96
      dementia F13.97
    psychosis F13.959
      delusions F13.950
      hallucinations F13.951
    sexual dysfunction F13.981

Use — *continued*
sedative, hypnotic, or anxiolytic — *continued*
  with — *continued*
    sleep disorder F13.982
    unspecified disorder F13.99
  harmful — *see* Abuse, drug, sedative, hypnotic, or anxiolytic
stimulant NEC F15.90
  with
    anxiety disorder F15.980
    intoxication F15.929
      with
        delirium F15.921
        perceptual disturbance F15.922
      uncomplicated F15.920
    mood disorder F15.94
    other specified disorder F15.988
    psychosis F15.959
      delusions F15.950
      hallucinations F15.951
    sexual dysfunction F15.981
    sleep disorder F15.982
    unspecified disorder F15.99
    withdrawal F15.93
  harmful — *see* Abuse, drug, stimulant NEC
tobacco Z72.0
  with dependence — *see* Dependence, drug, nicotine
volatile solvents — *see also* Use, inhalant F18.90
  harmful — *see* Abuse, drug, inhalant
Usher-Senear disease or syndrome L10.4
Uta B55.1
Uteromegaly N85.2
Uterovaginal — *see* condition
Uterovesical — *see* condition
Uveal — *see* condition
Uveitis (anterior) — *see also* Iridocyclitis
  acute — *see* Iridocyclitis, acute
  chronic — *see* Iridocyclitis, chronic
  due to toxoplasmosis (acquired) B58.09
    congenital P37.1
  granulomatous — *see* Iridocyclitis, chronic
  heterochromic — *see* Cyclitis, Fuchs' heterochromic
  lens-induced — *see* Iridocyclitis, lens-induced
  posterior — *see* Chorioretinitis
  sympathetic H44.13- ☑
  syphilitic (secondary) A51.43
    congenital (early) A50.01
    late A52.71
  tuberculous A18.54
Uveoencephalitis — *see* Inflammation, chorioretinal
Uveokeratitis — *see* Iridocyclitis
Uveoparotitis D86.89
Uvula — *see* condition
Uvulitis (acute) (catarrhal) (chronic) (membranous) (suppurative) (ulcerative) K12.2

V

Vaccination (prophylactic)
  complication or reaction — *see* Complications, vaccination
  delayed Z28.9
  encounter for Z23
  not done — *see* Immunization, not done, because (of)
Vaccinia (generalized) (localized) T88.1 ☑
  congenital P35.8
  without vaccination B08.011
Vacuum, in sinus (accessory) (nasal) J34.89
Vagabond, vagabondage Z59.0
Vagabond's disease B85.1
Vagina, vaginal — *see* condition
Vaginalitis (tunica) (testis) N49.1
Vaginismus (reflex) N94.2
  functional F52.5
  nonorganic F52.5
  psychogenic F52.5
  secondary N94.2
Vaginitis (acute) (circumscribed) (diffuse) (emphysematous) (nonvenereal) (ulcerative) N76.0
  with ectopic or molar pregnancy O08.0
  amebic A06.82
  atrophic, postmenopausal N95.2
  bacterial N76.0
  blennorrhagic (gonococcal) A54.02
  candidal B37.3
  chlamydial A56.02
  chronic N76.1

Vaginitis — *continued*
  due to Trichomonas (vaginalis) A59.01
  following ectopic or molar pregnancy O08.0
  gonococcal A54.02
    with abscess (accessory gland) (periurethral) A54.1
  granuloma A58
  in (due to)
    candidiasis B37.3
    herpesviral (herpes simplex) infection A60.04
    pinworm infection B80 *[N77.1]*
  monilial B37.3
  mycotic (candidal) B37.3
  postmenopausal atrophic N95.2
  puerperal (postpartum) O86.13
  senile (atrophic) N95.2
  subacute or chronic N76.1
  syphilitic (early) A51.0
    late A52.76
  trichomonal A59.01
  tuberculous A18.18
Vaginosis — *see* Vaginitis
Vagotonia G52.2
Vagrancy Z59.0
VAIN — *see* Neoplasia, intraepithelial, vagina
Vallecula — *see* condition
Valley fever B38.0
Valsuani's disease — *see* Anemia, obstetric
Valve, valvular (formation) — *see also* condition
  cerebral ventricle (communicating) in situ Z98.2
  cervix, internal os Q51.828
  congenital NEC — *see* Atresia, by site
  ureter (pelvic junction) (vesical orifice) Q62.39
  urethra (congenital) (posterior) Q64.2
Valvulitis (chronic) — *see* Endocarditis
Valvulopathy — *see* Endocarditis
Van Bogaert's leukoencephalopathy (sclerosing) (subacute) A81.1
Van Bogaert-Scherer-Epstein disease or syndrome E75.5
Van Buchem's syndrome M85.2
Van Creveld-von Gierke disease E74.01
Van der Hoeve (-de Kleyn) **syndrome** Q78.0
Van der Woude's syndrome Q38.0
Van Neck's disease or osteochondrosis M91.0
Vanishing lung J44.9
Vapor asphyxia or suffocation T59.9 ☑
  specified agent — *see* Table of Drugs and Chemicals
Variance, lethal ball, prosthetic heart valve T82.09 ☑
Variants, thalassemic D56.8
Variations in hair color L67.1
Varicella B01.9
  with
    complications NEC B01.89
    encephalitis B01.11
    encephalomyelitis B01.11
    meningitis B01.0
    myelitis B01.12
    pneumonia B01.2
  congenital P35.8
Varices — *see* Varix
Varicocele (scrotum) (thrombosed) I86.1
  ovary I86.2
  perineum I86.3
  spermatic cord (ulcerated) I86.1
Varicose
  aneurysm (ruptured) I77.0
  dermatitis — *see* Varix, leg, with, inflammation
  eczema — *see* Varix, leg, with, inflammation
  phlebitis — *see* Varix, with, inflammation
  tumor — *see* Varix
  ulcer (lower limb, any part) — *see also* Varix, leg, with, ulcer
    anus — *see also* Hemorrhoids K64.8
    esophagus — *see* Varix, esophagus
    inflamed or infected — *see* Varix, leg, with ulcer, with inflammation
    nasal septum I86.8
    perineum I86.3
    scrotum I86.1
    specified site NEC I86.8
  vein — *see* Varix
  vessel — *see* Varix, leg
Varicosis, varicosities, varicosity — *see* Varix
Variola (major) (minor) B03
Varioloid B03
Varix (lower limb) I83.90

▽ **Subterms under main terms may continue to next column or page**   ☑ **Additional Character Required — Refer to the Tabular List for Character Selection**   **323**

Use — Varix

Varix — *continued*
with
bleeding I83.899
edema I83.899
inflammation I83.10
with ulcer (venous) I83.209
pain I83.819
rupture I83.899
specified complication NEC I83.899
stasis dermatitis I83.10
with ulcer (venous) I83.209
swelling I83.899
ulcer I83.009
with inflammation I83.209
aneurysmal I77.0
asymptomatic I83.9- ☑
bladder I86.2
broad ligament I86.2
complicating
childbirth (lower extremity) O87.4
anus or rectum O87.2
genital (vagina, vulva or perineum) O87.8
pregnancy (lower extremity) O22.0- ☑
anus or rectum O22.4- ☑
genital (vagina, vulva or perineum) O22.1- ☑
puerperium (lower extremity) O87.4
anus or rectum O87.2
genital (vagina, vulva, perineum) O87.8
congenital (any site) Q27.8
esophagus (idiopathic) (primary) (ulcerated) I85.00
bleeding I85.01
congenital Q27.8
in (due to)
alcoholic liver disease I85.10
bleeding I85.11
cirrhosis of liver I85.10
bleeding I85.11
portal hypertension I85.10
bleeding I85.11
schistosomiasis I85.10
bleeding I85.11
toxic liver disease I85.10
bleeding I85.11
secondary I85.10
bleeding I85.11
gastric I86.4
inflamed or infected I83.10
ulcerated I83.209
labia (majora) I86.3
leg (asymptomatic) I83.90
with
edema I83.899
inflammation I83.10
with ulcer — *see* Varix, leg, with, ulcer, with inflammation by site
pain I83.819
specified complication NEC I83.899
swelling I83.899
ulcer I83.009
with inflammation I83.209
ankle I83.003
with inflammation I83.203
calf I83.002
with inflammation I83.202
foot NEC I83.005
with inflammation I83.205
heel I83.004
with inflammation I83.204
lower leg NEC I83.008
with inflammation I83.208
midfoot I83.004
with inflammation I83.204
thigh I83.001
with inflammation I83.201
bilateral (asymptomatic) I83.93
with
edema I83.893
pain I83.813
specified complication NEC I83.893
swelling I83.893
ulcer I83.0- ☑
with inflammation I83.209
left (asymptomatic) I83.92
with
edema I83.892
inflammation I83.12
with ulcer — *see* Varix, leg, with, ulcer, with inflammation by site

Varix — *continued*
leg — *continued*
left — *continued*
with — *continued*
pain I83.812
specified complication NEC I83.892
swelling I83.892
ulcer I83.029
with inflammation I83.229
ankle I83.023
with inflammation I83.223
calf I83.022
with inflammation I83.222
foot NEC I83.025
with inflammation I83.225
heel I83.024
with inflammation I83.224
lower leg NEC I83.028
with inflammation I83.228
midfoot I83.024
with inflammation I83.224
thigh I83.021
with inflammation I83.221
right (asymptomatic) I83.91
with
edema I83.891
inflammation I83.11
with ulcer — *see* Varix, leg, with, ulcer, with inflammation by site
pain I83.811
specified complication NEC I83.891
swelling I83.891
ulcer I83.019
with inflammation I83.219
ankle I83.013
with inflammation I83.213
calf I83.012
with inflammation I83.212
foot NEC I83.015
with inflammation I83.215
heel I83.014
with inflammation I83.214
lower leg NEC I83.018
with inflammation I83.218
midfoot I83.014
with inflammation I83.214
thigh I83.011
with inflammation I83.211
nasal septum I86.8
orbit I86.8
congenital Q27.8
ovary I86.2
papillary I78.1
pelvis I86.2
perineum I86.3
pharynx I86.8
placenta O43.89- ☑
renal papilla I86.8
retina H35.09
scrotum (ulcerated) I86.1
sigmoid colon I86.8
specified site NEC I86.8
spinal (cord) (vessels) I86.8
spleen, splenic (vein) (with phlebolith) I86.8
stomach I86.4
sublingual I86.0
ulcerated I83.009
inflamed or infected I83.209
uterine ligament I86.2
vagina I86.8
vocal cord I86.8
vulva I86.3
Vas deferens — *see* condition
Vas deferentitis N49.1
Vasa previa O69.4 ☑
hemorrhage from, affecting newborn P50.0
Vascular — *see also* condition
loop on optic papilla Q14.2
spasm I73.9
spider I78.1
Vascularization, cornea — *see* Neovascularization, cornea
Vasculitis I77.6
allergic D69.0
cryoglobulinemic D89.1
disseminated I77.6
hypocomplementemic M31.8
kidney I77.89

Vasculitis — *continued*
livedoid L95.0
nodular L95.8
retina H35.06- ☑
rheumatic — *see* Fever, rheumatic
rheumatoid — *see* Rheumatoid, vasculitis
skin (limited to) L95.9
specified NEC L95.8
systemic M31.8
Vasculopathy, necrotizing M31.9
cardiac allograft T86.290
specified NEC M31.8
Vasitis (nodosa) N49.1
tuberculous A18.15
Vasodilation I73.9
Vasomotor — *see* condition
Vasoplasty, after previous sterilization Z31.0
aftercare Z31.42
Vasospasm (vasoconstriction) I73.9
cerebral (cerebrovascular) (artery) I67.848
reversible I67.841
coronary I20.1
nerve
arm — *see* Mononeuropathy, upper limb
brachial plexus G54.0
cervical plexus G54.2
leg — *see* Mononeuropathy, lower limb
peripheral NOS I73.9
retina (artery) — *see* Occlusion, artery, retina
Vasospastic — *see* condition
Vasovagal attack (paroxysmal) R55
psychogenic F45.8
VATER syndrome Q87.2
Vater's ampulla — *see* condition
Vegetation, vegetative
adenoid (nasal fossa) J35.8
endocarditis (acute) (any valve) (subacute) I33.0
heart (mycotic) (valve) I33.0
Veil
Jackson's Q43.3
Vein, venous — *see* condition
Veldt sore — *see* Ulcer, skin
Velpeau's hernia — *see* Hernia, femoral
Venereal
bubo A55
disease A64
granuloma inguinale A58
lymphogranuloma (Durand-Nicolas-Favre) A55
Venofibrosis I87.8
Venom, venomous — *see* Table of Drugs and Chemicals, by animal or substance, poisoning
Venous — *see* condition
Ventilator lung, newborn P27.8
Ventral — *see* condition
Ventricle, ventricular — *see also* condition
escape I49.3
inversion Q20.5
Ventriculitis (cerebral) — *see also* Encephalitis G04.90
Ventriculostomy status Z98.2
Vernet's syndrome G52.7
Verneuil's disease (syphilitic bursitis) A52.78
Verruca (due to HPV) (filiformis) (simplex) (viral) (vulgaris) B07.9
acuminata A63.0
necrogenica (primary) (tuberculosa) A18.4
plana B07.8
plantaris B07.0
seborrheica L82.1
inflamed L82.0
senile (seborrheic) L82.1
inflamed L82.0
tuberculosa (primary) A18.4
venereal A63.0
Verrucosities — *see* Verruca
Verruga peruana, peruviana A44.1
Version
with extraction
cervix — *see* Malposition, uterus
uterus (postinfectional) (postpartal, old) — *see* Malposition, uterus
Vertebra, vertebral — *see* condition
Vertical talus (congenital) Q66.80
left foot Q66.82
right foot Q66.81
Vertigo R42
auditory — *see* Vertigo, aural
aural H81.31- ☑

☑ **Additional Character Required** — Refer to the Tabular List for Character Selection   �声 **Subterms under main terms may continue to next column or page**

Vertigo — *continued*
   benign paroxysmal (positional) H81.1- ☑
   central (origin) H81.4
   cerebral H81.4
   Dix and Hallpike (epidemic) — *see* Neuronitis,
      vestibular
   due to infrasound T75.23 ☑
   epidemic A88.1
      Dix and Hallpike — *see* Neuronitis, vestibular
      Pedersen's — *see* Neuronitis, vestibular
      vestibular neuronitis — *see* Neuronitis, vestibular
   hysterical F44.89
   infrasound T75.23 ☑
   labyrinthine — *see* subcategory H81.0 ☑
   laryngeal R05
   malignant positional H81.4
   Ménière's — *see* subcategory H81.0 ☑
   menopausal N95.1
   otogenic — *see* Vertigo, aural
   paroxysmal positional, benign — *see* Vertigo, benign
      paroxysmal
   Pedersen's (epidemic) — *see* Neuronitis, vestibular
   peripheral NEC H81.39- ☑
   positional
      benign paroxysmal — *see* Vertigo, benign paroxys-
         mal
      malignant H81.4
Very-low-density-lipoprotein-type (VLDL) **hyper-**
   lipoproteinemia E78.1
Vesania — *see* Psychosis
Vesical — *see* condition
Vesicle
   cutaneous R23.8
   seminal — *see* condition
   skin R23.8
Vesicocolic — *see* condition
Vesicoperineal — *see* condition
Vesicorectal — *see* condition
Vesicourethrorectal — *see* condition
Vesicovaginal — *see* condition
Vesicular — *see* condition
Vesiculitis (seminal) N49.0
   amebic A06.82
   gonorrheal (acute) (chronic) A54.23
   trichomonal A59.09
   tuberculous A18.15
Vestibulitis (ear) — *see also* subcategory H83.0 ☑
   nose (external) J34.89
   vulvar N94.810
Vestibulopathy , acute peripheral (recurrent) — *see*
   Neuronitis, vestibular
Vestige, vestigial — *see also* Persistence
   branchial Q18.0
   structures in vitreous Q14.0
Vibration
   adverse effects T75.20 ☑
      pneumatic hammer syndrome T75.21 ☑
      specified effect NEC T75.29 ☑
      vasospastic syndrome T75.22 ☑
      vertigo from infrasound T75.23 ☑
   exposure (occupational) Z57.7
   vertigo T75.23 ☑
Vibriosis A28.9
Victim (of)
   crime Z65.4
   disaster Z65.5
   terrorism Z65.4
   torture Z65.4
   war Z65.5
Vidal's disease L28.0
Villaret's syndrome G52.7
Villous — *see* condition
VIN — *see* Neoplasia, intraepithelial, vulva
Vincent's infection (angina) (gingivitis) A69.1
   stomatitis NEC A69.1
Vinson-Plummer syndrome D50.1
Violence, physical R45.6
Viosterol deficiency — *see* Deficiency, calciferol
Vipoma — *see* Neoplasm, malignant, by site
Viremia B34.9
Virilism (adrenal) E25.9
   congenital E25.0
Virilization (female) (suprarenal) E25.9
   congenital E25.0
   isosexual E28.2
Virulent bubo A57
Virus, viral — *see also* condition

Virus, viral — *continued*
   as cause of disease classified elsewhere B97.89
      respiratory syncytial virus (RSV) — *see* Virus, infec-
        tion, respiratory syncytial (RSV)
   cytomegalovirus B25.9
   human immunodeficiency (HIV) — *see* Human, immun-
      odeficiency virus (HIV) disease
   infection — *see* Infection, virus
   respiratory syncytial (RSV)
      as cause of disease classified elsewhere B97.4
      bronchiolitis J21.0
      bronchitis J20.5
      bronchopneumonia J12.1
      otitis media H65.- ☑ *[B97.4]*
      pneumonia J12.1
      upper respiratory infection J06.9 *[B97.4]*
   specified NEC B34.8
   swine influenza (viruses that normally cause infections
      in pigs) — *see also* Influenza, due to, identified
      novel influenza A virus J09.X2
   West Nile (fever) A92.30
      with
         complications NEC A92.39
         cranial nerve disorders A92.32
         encephalitis A92.31
         encephalomyelitis A92.31
         neurologic manifestation NEC A92.32
         optic neuritis A92.32
         polyradiculitis A92.32
Viscera, visceral — *see* condition
Visceroptosis K63.4
Visible peristalsis R19.2
Vision, visual
   binocular, suppression H53.34
   blurred, blurring H53.8
      hysterical F44.6
   defect, defective NEC H54.7
   disorientation (syndrome) H53.8
   disturbance H53.9
      hysterical F44.6
   double H53.2
   examination Z01.00
      with abnormal findings Z01.01
      following failed vision screening Z01.020
         with abnormal findings Z01.021
   field, limitation (defect) — *see* Defect, visual field
   hallucinations R44.1
   halos H53.19
   loss — *see* Loss, vision
      sudden — *see* Disturbance, vision, subjective, loss,
         sudden
   low (both eyes) — *see* Low, vision
   perception, simultaneous without fusion H53.33
Vitality, lack or want of R53.83
   newborn P96.89
Vitamin deficiency — *see* Deficiency, vitamin
Vitelline duct, persistent Q43.0
Vitiligo L80
   eyelid H02.739
      left H02.736
         lower H02.735
         upper H02.734
      right H02.733
         lower H02.732
         upper H02.731
   pinta A67.2
   vulva N90.89
Vitreal corneal syndrome H59.01- ☑
Vitreoretinopathy, proliferative — *see also*
   Retinopathy, proliferative
   with retinal detachment — *see* Detachment, retina,
      traction
Vitreous — *see also* condition
   touch syndrome — *see* Complication, postprocedural,
      following cataract surgery
Vocal cord — *see* condition
Vogt-Koyanagi syndrome H20.82- ☑
Vogt's disease or syndrome G80.3
Vogt-Spielmeyer amaurotic idiocy or disease E75.4
Voice
   change R49.9
      specified NEC R49.8
   loss — *see* Aphonia
Volhynian fever A79.0
Volkmann's ischemic contracture or paralysis (com-
   plicating trauma) T79.6
Volvulus (bowel) (colon) (intestine) K56.2
   with perforation K56.2

Volvulus — *continued*
   congenital Q43.8
   duodenum K31.5
   fallopian tube — *see* Torsion, fallopian tube
   oviduct — *see* Torsion, fallopian tube
   stomach (due to absence of gastrocolic ligament)
      K31.89
Vomiting R11.10
   with nausea R11.2
   asphyxia — *see* Foreign body, by site, causing asphyxia,
      gastric contents
   bilious (cause unknown) R11.14
      following gastro-intestinal surgery K91.0
      in newborn P92.01
   blood — *see* Hematemesis
   causing asphyxia, choking, or suffocation — *see* For-
      eign body, by site
   cyclical, in migraine G43.A0 (*following* G43.7)
      with refractory migraine G43.A1 (*following* G43.7)
      intractable G43.A1 (*following* G43.7)
      not intractable G43.A0 (*following* G43.7)
      psychogenic F50.89
      without refractory migraine G43.A0 (*following* G43.7)
   cyclical syndrome NOS (unrelated to migraine) R11.15
   fecal mater R11.13
   following gastrointestinal surgery K91.0
      psychogenic F50.89
   functional K31.89
   hysterical F50.89
   nervous F50.89
   neurotic F50.89
   newborn NEC P92.09
      bilious P92.01
   periodic R11.10
      psychogenic F50.89
   persistent R11.15
   projectile R11.12
   psychogenic F50.89
   uremic — *see* Uremia
   without nausea R11.11
Vomito negro — *see* Fever, yellow
Von Bezold's abscess — *see* Mastoiditis, acute
Von Economo-Cruchet disease A85.8
Von Eulenburg's disease G71.19
Von Gierke's disease E74.01
Von Hippel (-Lindau) **disease or syndrome** Q85.8
Von Jaksch's anemia or disease D64.89
Von Recklinghausen
   disease (neurofibromatosis) Q85.01
      bones E21.0
Von Schroetter's syndrome I82.890
Von Willebrand (-Jurgens)(-Minot) **disease or syn-**
   drome D68.0
Von Zumbusch's disease L40.1
Voyeurism F65.3
Vrolik's disease Q78.0
Vulva — *see* condition
Vulvismus N94.2
Vulvitis (acute) (allergic) (atrophic) (hypertrophic) (intertriginous) (senile) N76.2
   with ectopic or molar pregnancy O08.0
   adhesive, congenital Q52.79
   blennorrhagic (gonococcal) A54.02
   candidal B37.3
   chlamydial A56.02
   due to Haemophilus ducreyi A57
   following ectopic or molar pregnancy O08.0
   gonococcal A54.02
      with abscess (accessory gland) (periurethral) A54.1
   herpesviral A60.04
   leukoplakic N90.4
   monilial B37.3
   puerperal (postpartum) O86.19
   subacute or chronic N76.3
   syphilitic (early) A51.0
      late A52.76
   trichomonal A59.01
   tuberculous A18.18
Vulvodynia N94.819
   specified NEC N94.818
Vulvorectal — *see* condition
Vulvovaginitis (acute) — *see* Vaginitis

W

Waiting list, person on Z75.1
   for organ transplant Z76.82
   undergoing social agency investigation Z75.2

Waldenström
  hypergammaglobulinemia D89.0
  syndrome or macroglobulinemia C88.0
Waldenström-Kjellberg syndrome D50.1
Walking
  difficulty R26.2
    psychogenic F44.4
  sleep F51.3
    hysterical F44.89
Wall, abdominal — see condition
Wallenberg's disease or syndrome G46.3
Wallgren's disease I87.8
Wandering
  gallbladder, congenital Q44.1
  in diseases classified elsewhere Z91.83
  kidney, congenital Q63.8
  organ or site, congenital NEC — see Malposition, congenital, by site
  pacemaker (heart) I49.8
  spleen D73.89
War neurosis F48.8
Wart (due to HPV) (filiform) (infectious) (viral) B07.9
  anogenital region (venereal) A63.0
  common B07.8
  external genital organs (venereal) A63.0
  flat B07.8
  Hassal-Henle's (of cornea) H18.49
  Peruvian A44.1
  plantar B07.0
  prosector (tuberculous) A18.4
  seborrheic L82.1
    inflamed L82.0
  senile (seborrheic) L82.1
    inflamed L82.0
  tuberculous A18.4
  venereal A63.0
Warthin's tumor — see Neoplasm, salivary gland, benign
Wassilieff's disease A27.0
Wasting
  disease R64
    due to malnutrition E41
  extreme (due to malnutrition) E41
  muscle NEC — see Atrophy, muscle
Water
  clefts (senile cataract) — see Cataract, senile, incipient
  deprivation of T73.1 ☑
  intoxication E87.79
  itch B76.9
  lack of T73.1 ☑
  loading E87.70
  on
    brain — see Hydrocephalus
    chest J94.8
  poisoning E87.79
Waterbrash R12
Waterhouse (-Friderichsen) **syndrome or disease** (meningococcal) A39.1
Water-losing nephritis N25.89
Watermelon stomach K31.819
  with hemorrhage K31.811
  without hemorrhage K31.819
Watsoniasis B66.8
Wax in ear — see Impaction, cerumen
Weak, weakening, weakness (generalized) R53.1
  arches (acquired) — see also Deformity, limb, flat foot
  bladder (sphincter) R32
  facial R29.810
    following
      cerebrovascular disease I69.992
        cerebral infarction I69.392
        intracerebral hemorrhage I69.192
        nontraumatic intracranial hemorrhage NEC I69.292
        specified disease NEC I69.892
        stroke I69.392
        subarachnoid hemorrhage I69.092
  foot (double) — see also Weak, arches
  heart, cardiac — see Failure, heart
  mind F70
  muscle M62.81
  myocardium — see Failure, heart
  newborn P96.89
  pelvic fundus N81.89
  pubocervical tissue N81.82
  rectovaginal tissue N81.83
  senile R54
  urinary stream R39.12
  valvular — see Endocarditis

Wear, worn (with normal or routine use)
  articular bearing surface of internal joint prosthesis — see Complications, joint prosthesis, mechanical, wear of articular bearing surfaces, by site
  device, implant or graft — see Complications, by site, mechanical complication
  tooth, teeth (approximal) (hard tissues) (interproximal) (occlusal) K03.0
Weather, weathered
  effects of
    cold T69.9 ☑
      specified effect NEC T69.8 ☑
    hot — see Heat
  skin L57.8
Weaver's syndrome Q87.3
Web, webbed (congenital)
  duodenal Q43.8
  esophagus Q39.4
  fingers Q70.1- ☑
  larynx (glottic) (subglottic) Q31.0
  neck (pterygium colli) Q18.3
  Paterson-Kelly D50.1
  popliteal syndrome Q87.89
  toes Q70.3- ☑
Weber-Christian disease M35.6
Weber-Cockayne syndrome (epidermolysis bullosa) Q81.8
Weber-Gubler syndrome G46.3
Weber-Leyden syndrome G46.3
Weber-Osler syndrome I78.0
Weber's paralysis or syndrome G46.3
Wedge-shaped or wedging vertebra — see Collapse, vertebra NEC
Wegener's granulomatosis or syndrome M31.30
  with
    kidney involvement M31.31
    lung involvement M31.30
      with kidney involvement M31.31
Wegner's disease A50.02
Weight
  1000-2499 grams at birth (low) — see Low, birthweight
  999 grams or less at birth (extremely low) — see Low, birthweight, extreme
  and length below 10th percentile for gestational age P05.1- ☑
  below but length above 10th percentile for gestational age P05.0- ☑
  gain (abnormal) (excessive) R63.5
    in pregnancy — see Pregnancy, complicated by, excessive weight gain
      low — see Pregnancy, complicated by, insufficient, weight gain
  loss (abnormal) (cause unknown) R63.4
Weightlessness (effect of) T75.82 ☑
Weil (I)-**Marchesani syndrome** Q87.19
Weil's disease A27.0
Weingarten's syndrome J82
Weir Mitchell's disease I73.81
Weiss-Baker syndrome G90.09
Wells' disease L98.3
Wen — see Cyst, sebaceous
Wenckebach's block or phenomenon I44.1
Werdnig-Hoffmann syndrome (muscular atrophy) G12.0
Werlhof's disease D69.3
Wermer's disease or syndrome E31.21
Werner-His disease A79.0
Werner's disease or syndrome E34.8
Wernicke-Korsakoff's syndrome or psychosis (alcoholic) F10.96
  with dependence F10.26
  drug-induced
    due to drug abuse — see Abuse, drug, by type, with amnestic disorder
    due to drug dependence — see Dependence, drug, by type, with amnestic disorder
  nonalcoholic F04
Wernicke-Posadas disease B38.9
Wernicke's
  developmental aphasia F80.2
  disease or syndrome E51.2
  encephalopathy E51.2
  polioencephalitis, superior E51.2
West African fever B50.8
Westphal-Strümpell syndrome E83.01
West's syndrome — see Epilepsy, spasms

Wet
  feet, tropical (maceration) (syndrome) — see Immersion, foot
  lung (syndrome), newborn P22.1
Wharton's duct — see condition
Wheal — see Urticaria
Wheezing R06.2
Whiplash injury S13.4 ☑
Whipple's disease — see also subcategory M14.8- K90.81
Whipworm (disease) (infection) (infestation) B79
Whistling face Q87.0
White — see also condition
  kidney, small N03.9
  leg, puerperal, postpartum, childbirth O87.1
  mouth B37.0
  patches of mouth K13.29
  spot lesions, teeth
    chewing surface K02.51
    pit and fissure surface K02.51
    smooth surface K02.61
Whitehead L70.0
Whitlow — see also Cellulitis, digit
  with lymphangitis — see Lymphangitis, acute, digit
  herpesviral B00.89
Whitmore's disease or fever — see Melioidosis
Whooping cough A37.90
  with pneumonia A37.91
    due to Bordetella
      bronchiseptica A37.81
      parapertussis A37.11
      pertussis A37.01
    specified organism NEC A37.81
  due to
    Bordetella
      bronchiseptica A37.80
        with pneumonia A37.81
      parapertussis A37.10
        with pneumonia A37.11
      pertussis A37.00
        with pneumonia A37.01
    specified NEC A37.80
      with pneumonia A37.81
Wichman's asthma J38.5
Wide cranial sutures, newborn P96.3
Widening aorta — see Ectasia, aorta
  with aneurysm — see Aneurysm, aorta
Wilkie's disease or syndrome K55.1
Wilkinson-Sneddon disease or syndrome L13.1
Willebrand (-Jürgens) **thrombopathy** D68.0
Williams syndrome Q93.82
Willige-Hunt disease or syndrome G23.1
Wilms' tumor C64- ☑
Wilson-Mikity syndrome P27.0
Wilson's
  disease or syndrome E83.01
  hepatolenticular degeneration E83.01
  lichen ruber L43.9
Window — see also Imperfect, closure
  aorticopulmonary Q21.4
Winter — see condition
Wiskott-Aldrich syndrome D82.0
Withdrawal state — see also Dependence, drug by type, with withdrawal
  alcohol
    with perceptual disturbances F10.232
    without perceptual disturbances F10.239
  caffeine F15.93
  cannabis F12.23
  newborn
    correct therapeutic substance properly administered P96.2
    infant of dependent mother P96.1
    therapeutic substance, neonatal P96.2
Witts' anemia D50.8
Witzelsucht F07.0
Woakes' ethmoiditis or syndrome J33.1
Wolff-Hirschorn syndrome Q93.3
Wolff-Parkinson-White syndrome I45.6
Wolhynian fever A79.0
Wolman's disease E75.5
Woolly, wooly hair (congenital) (nevus) Q84.1
Woolsorter's disease A22.1
Word
  blindness (congenital) (developmental) F81.0
  deafness (congenital) (developmental) H93.25

☑ **Additional Character Required — Refer to the Tabular List for Character Selection**   ⬇ **Subterms under main terms may continue to next column or page**

Worm(s) (infection) (infestation) — *see also* Infestation, helminth
  guinea B72
  in intestine NEC B82.0
Worm-eaten soles A66.3
Worn out — *see* Exhaustion
  cardiac
    defibrillator (with synchronous cardiac pacemaker) Z45.02
    pacemaker
      battery Z45.010
      lead Z45.018
  device, implant or graft — *see* Complications, by site, mechanical
Worried well Z71.1
Worries R45.82
Wound check Z48.0- ☑
  due to injury — *code to* Injury, by site, using appropriate seventh character for subsequent encounter
Wound, open T14.8- ☑
  abdomen, abdominal
    wall S31.109 ☑
      with penetration into peritoneal cavity S31.609 ☑
      bite — *see* Bite, abdomen, wall
      epigastric region S31.102 ☑
        with penetration into peritoneal cavity S31.602 ☑
        bite — *see* Bite, abdomen, wall, epigastric region
        laceration — *see* Laceration, abdomen, wall, epigastric region
        puncture — *see* Puncture, abdomen, wall, epigastric region
      laceration — *see* Laceration, abdomen, wall
      left
        lower quadrant S31.104 ☑
          with penetration into peritoneal cavity S31.604 ☑
          bite — *see* Bite, abdomen, wall, left, lower quadrant
          laceration — *see* Laceration, abdomen, wall, left, lower quadrant
          puncture — *see* Puncture, abdomen, wall, left, lower quadrant
        upper quadrant S31.101 ☑
          with penetration into peritoneal cavity S31.601 ☑
          bite — *see* Bite, abdomen, wall, left, upper quadrant
          laceration — *see* Laceration, abdomen, wall, left, upper quadrant
          puncture — *see* Puncture, abdomen, wall, left, upper quadrant
      periumbilic region S31.105 ☑
        with penetration into peritoneal cavity S31.605 ☑
        bite — *see* Bite, abdomen, wall, periumbilic region
        laceration — *see* Laceration, abdomen, wall, periumbilic region
        puncture — *see* Puncture, abdomen, wall, periumbilic region
      puncture — *see* Puncture, abdomen, wall
      right
        lower quadrant S31.103 ☑
          with penetration into peritoneal cavity S31.603 ☑
          bite — *see* Bite, abdomen, wall, right, lower quadrant
          laceration — *see* Laceration, abdomen, wall, right, lower quadrant
          puncture — *see* Puncture, abdomen, wall, right, lower quadrant
        upper quadrant S31.100 ☑
          with penetration into peritoneal cavity S31.600 ☑
          bite — *see* Bite, abdomen, wall, right, upper quadrant
          laceration — *see* Laceration, abdomen, wall, right, upper quadrant
          puncture — *see* Puncture, abdomen, wall, right, upper quadrant
  alveolar (process) — *see* Wound, open, oral cavity
  ankle S91.00- ☑
    bite — *see* Bite, ankle
    laceration — *see* Laceration, ankle

Wound, open — *continued*
  ankle — *continued*
    puncture — *see* Puncture, ankle
  antecubital space — *see* Wound, open, elbow
  anterior chamber, eye — *see* Wound, open, ocular
  anus S31.839 ☑
    bite S31.835 ☑
    laceration — *see* Laceration, anus
    puncture — *see* Puncture, anus
  arm (upper) S41.10- ☑
    with amputation — *see* Amputation, traumatic, arm
    bite — *see* Bite, arm
    forearm — *see* Wound, open, forearm
    laceration — *see* Laceration, arm
    puncture — *see* Puncture, arm
  auditory canal (external) (meatus) — *see* Wound, open, ear
  auricle, ear — *see* Wound, open, ear
  axilla — *see* Wound, open, arm
  back — *see also* Wound, open, thorax, back
    lower S31.000 ☑
      with penetration into retroperitoneal space S31.001 ☑
      bite — *see* Bite, back, lower
      laceration — *see* Laceration, back, lower
      puncture — *see* Puncture, back, lower
  bite — *see* Bite
  blood vessel — *see* Injury, blood vessel
  breast S21.00- ☑
    with amputation — *see* Amputation, traumatic, breast
    bite — *see* Bite, breast
    laceration — *see* Laceration, breast
    puncture — *see* Puncture, breast
  buttock S31.809 ☑
    bite — *see* Bite, buttock
    laceration — *see* Laceration, buttock
    left S31.829 ☑
    puncture — *see* Puncture, buttock
    right S31.819 ☑
  calf — *see* Wound, open, leg
  canaliculus lacrimalis — *see* Wound, open, eyelid
  canthus, eye — *see* Wound, open, eyelid
  cervical esophagus S11.20 ☑
    bite S11.25 ☑
    laceration — *see* Laceration, esophagus, traumatic, cervical
    puncture — *see* Puncture, cervical esophagus
  cheek (external) S01.40- ☑
    bite — *see* Bite, cheek
    internal — *see* Wound, open, oral cavity
    laceration — *see* Laceration, cheek
    puncture — *see* Puncture, cheek
  chest wall — *see* Wound, open, thorax
  chin — *see* Wound, open, head, specified site NEC
  choroid — *see* Wound, open, ocular
  ciliary body (eye) — *see* Wound, open, ocular
  clitoris S31.40 ☑
    with amputation — *see* Amputation, traumatic, clitoris
    bite S31.45 ☑
    laceration — *see* Laceration, vulva
    puncture — *see* Puncture, vulva
  conjunctiva — *see* Wound, open, ocular
  cornea — *see* Wound, open, ocular
  costal region — *see* Wound, open, thorax
  Descemet's membrane — *see* Wound, open, ocular
  digit(s)
    foot — *see* Wound, open, toe
    hand — *see* Wound, open, finger
  ear (canal) (external) S01.30- ☑
    with amputation — *see* Amputation, traumatic, ear
    bite — *see* Bite, ear
    drum S09.2- ☑
    laceration — *see* Laceration, ear
    puncture — *see* Puncture, ear
  elbow S51.00- ☑
    bite — *see* Bite, elbow
    laceration — *see* Laceration, elbow
    puncture — *see* Puncture, elbow
  epididymis — *see* Wound, open, testis
  epigastric region S31.102 ☑
    with penetration into peritoneal cavity S31.602 ☑
    bite — *see* Bite, abdomen, wall, epigastric region
    laceration — *see* Laceration, abdomen, wall, epigastric region

Wound, open — *continued*
  epigastric region — *continued*
    puncture — *see* Puncture, abdomen, wall, epigastric region
  epiglottis — *see* Wound, open, neck, specified site NEC
  esophagus (thoracic) S27.819 ☑
    cervical — *see* Wound, open, cervical esophagus
    laceration S27.813 ☑
    specified type NEC S27.818 ☑
  eye — *see* Wound, open, ocular
  eyeball — *see* Wound, open, ocular
  eyebrow — *see* Wound, open, eyelid
  eyelid S01.10- ☑
    bite — *see* Bite, eyelid
    laceration — *see* Laceration, eyelid
    puncture — *see* Puncture, eyelid
  face NEC — *see* Wound, open, head, specified site NEC
  finger(s) S61.209 ☑
    with
      amputation — *see* Amputation, traumatic, finger
      damage to nail S61.309 ☑
    bite — *see* Bite, finger
    index S61.208 ☑
      with
        damage to nail S61.308 ☑
      left S61.201 ☑
        with
          damage to nail S61.301 ☑
      right S61.200 ☑
        with
          damage to nail S61.300 ☑
    laceration — *see* Laceration, finger
    little S61.208 ☑
      with
        damage to nail S61.308 ☑
      left S61.207 ☑
        with damage to nail S61.307 ☑
      right S61.206 ☑
        with damage to nail S61.306 ☑
    middle S61.208 ☑
      with
        damage to nail S61.308 ☑
      left S61.203 ☑
        with damage to nail S61.303 ☑
      right S61.202 ☑
        with damage to nail S61.302 ☑
    puncture — *see* Puncture, finger
    ring S61.208 ☑
      with
        damage to nail S61.308 ☑
      left S61.205 ☑
        with damage to nail S61.305 ☑
      right S61.204 ☑
        with damage to nail S61.304 ☑
  flank — *see* Wound, open, abdomen, wall
  foot (except toe(s) alone) S91.30- ☑
    with amputation — *see* Amputation, traumatic, foot
    bite — *see* Bite, foot
    laceration — *see* Laceration, foot
    puncture — *see* Puncture, foot
    toe — *see* Wound, open, toe
  forearm S51.80- ☑
    with
      amputation — *see* Amputation, traumatic, forearm
    bite — *see* Bite, forearm
    elbow only — *see* Wound, open, elbow
    laceration — *see* Laceration, forearm
    puncture — *see* Puncture, forearm
  forehead — *see* Wound, open, head, specified site NEC
  genital organs, external
    with amputation — *see* Amputation, traumatic, genital organs
    bite — *see* Bite, genital organ
    female S31.502 ☑
      vagina S31.40 ☑
      vulva S31.40 ☑
    laceration — *see* Laceration, genital organ
    male S31.501 ☑
      penis S31.20 ☑
      scrotum S31.30 ☑
      testes S31.30 ☑
    puncture — *see* Puncture, genital organ
  globe (eye) — *see* Wound, open, ocular
  groin — *see* Wound, open, abdomen, wall
  gum — *see* Wound, open, oral cavity

Wound, open — *continued*
  hand S61.40- ☑
    with
      amputation — *see* Amputation, traumatic, hand
    bite — *see* Bite, hand
    finger(s) — *see* Wound, open, finger
    laceration — *see* Laceration, hand
    puncture — *see* Puncture, hand
    thumb — *see* Wound, open, thumb
  head S01.90 ☑
    bite — *see* Bite, head
    cheek — *see* Wound, open, cheek
    ear — *see* Wound, open, ear
    eyelid — *see* Wound, open, eyelid
    laceration — *see* Laceration, head
    lip — *see* Wound, open, lip
    nose S01.20 ☑
    oral cavity — *see* Wound, open, oral cavity
    puncture — *see* Puncture, head
    scalp — *see* Wound, open, scalp
    specified site NEC S01.80 ☑
    temporomandibular area — *see* Wound, open, cheek
  heel — *see* Wound, open, foot
  hip S71.00- ☑
    with amputation — *see* Amputation, traumatic, hip
    bite — *see* Bite, hip
    laceration — *see* Laceration, hip
    puncture — *see* Puncture, hip
  hymen S31.40 ☑
    bite — *see* Bite, vulva
    laceration — *see* Laceration, vagina
    puncture — *see* Puncture, vagina
  hypochondrium S31.109 ☑
    bite — *see* Bite, hypochondrium
    laceration — *see* Laceration, hypochondrium
    puncture — *see* Puncture, hypochondrium
  hypogastric region S31.109 ☑
    bite — *see* Bite, hypogastric region
    laceration — *see* Laceration, hypogastric region
    puncture — *see* Puncture, hypogastric region
  iliac (region) — *see* Wound, open, inguinal region
  inguinal region S31.109 ☑
    bite — *see* Bite, abdomen, wall, lower quadrant
    laceration — *see* Laceration, inguinal region
    puncture — *see* Puncture, inguinal region
  instep — *see* Wound, open, foot
  interscapular region — *see* Wound, open, thorax, back
  intraocular — *see* Wound, open, ocular
  iris — *see* Wound, open, ocular
  jaw — *see* Wound, open, head, specified site NEC
  knee S81.00- ☑
    bite — *see* Bite, knee
    laceration — *see* Laceration, knee
    puncture — *see* Puncture, knee
  left
    lower quadrant S31.104 ☑
      with penetration into peritoneal cavity S31.604 ☑
      bite — *see* Bite, abdomen, wall, left, lower quadrant
      laceration — *see* Laceration, abdomen, wall, left, lower quadrant
      puncture — *see* Puncture, abdomen, wall, left, lower quadrant
    upper quadrant S31.101 ☑
      with penetration into peritoneal cavity S31.601 ☑
      bite — *see* Bite, abdomen, wall, left, upper quadrant
      laceration — *see* Laceration, abdomen, wall, left, upper quadrant
      puncture — *see* Puncture, abdomen, wall, left, upper quadrant
  leg (lower) S81.80- ☑
    with amputation — *see* Amputation, traumatic, leg
    ankle — *see* Wound, open, ankle
    bite — *see* Bite, leg
    foot — *see* Wound, open, foot

leg — *continued*
    knee — *see* Wound, open, knee
    laceration — *see* Laceration, leg
    puncture — *see* Puncture, leg
    toe — *see* Wound, open, toe
    upper — *see* Wound, open, thigh
  lip S01.501 ☑
    bite — *see* Bite, lip
    laceration — *see* Laceration, lip
    puncture — *see* Puncture, lip
  loin S31.109 ☑
    bite — *see* Bite, abdomen, wall
    laceration — *see* Laceration, loin
    puncture — *see* Puncture, loin
  lower back — *see* Wound, open, back, lower
  lumbar region — *see* Wound, open, back, lower
  malar region — *see* Wound, open, head, specified site NEC
  mammary — *see* Wound, open, breast
  mastoid region — *see* Wound, open, head, specified site NEC
  mouth — *see* Wound, open, oral cavity
  nail
    finger — *see* Wound, open, finger, with damage to nail
    toe — *see* Wound, open, toe, with damage to nail
  nape (neck) — *see* Wound, open, neck
  nasal (septum) (sinus) — *see* Wound, open, nose
  nasopharynx — *see* Wound, open, head, specified site NEC
  neck S11.90 ☑
    bite — *see* Bite, neck
    involving
      cervical esophagus S11.20 ☑
      larynx — *see* Wound, open, larynx
      pharynx S11.20 ☑
      thyroid S11.10 ☑
      trachea (cervical) S11.029 ☑
        bite — *see* Bite, trachea
        laceration S11.021 ☑
          with foreign body S11.022 ☑
        puncture S11.023 ☑
          with foreign body S11.024 ☑
    laceration — *see* Laceration, neck
    puncture — *see* Puncture, neck
    specified site NEC S11.80 ☑
      specified type NEC S11.89 ☑
  nose (septum) (sinus) S01.20 ☑
    with amputation — *see* Amputation, traumatic, nose
    bite — *see* Bite, nose
    laceration — *see* Laceration, nose
    puncture — *see* Puncture, nose
  ocular S05.90 ☑
    avulsion (traumatic enucleation) S05.7- ☑
    eyeball S05.6- ☑
      with foreign body S05.5- ☑
    eyelid — *see* Wound, open, eyelid
    laceration and rupture S05.3- ☑
      with prolapse or loss of intraocular tissue S05.2- ☑
    orbit (penetrating) (with or without foreign body) S05.4- ☑
    periocular area — *see* Wound, open, eyelid
    specified NEC S05.8X- ☑
  oral cavity S01.502 ☑
    bite S01.552 ☑
    laceration — *see* Laceration, oral cavity
    puncture — *see* Puncture, oral cavity
  orbit — *see* Wound, open, ocular, orbit
  palate — *see* Wound, open, oral cavity
  palm — *see* Wound, open, hand
  pelvis, pelvic — *see also* Wound, open, back, lower
    girdle — *see* Wound, open, hip
  penetrating — *see* Puncture, by site
  penis S31.20 ☑
    with amputation — *see* Amputation, traumatic, penis
    bite S31.25 ☑
    laceration — *see* Laceration, penis
    puncture — *see* Puncture, penis
  perineum
    bite — *see* Bite, perineum
    female S31.502 ☑
    laceration — *see* Laceration, perineum

perineum — *continued*
    male S31.501 ☑
    puncture — *see* Puncture, perineum
  periocular area (with or without lacrimal passages) — *see* Wound, open, eyelid
  periumbilic region S31.105 ☑
    with penetration into peritoneal cavity S31.605 ☑
    bite — *see* Bite, abdomen, wall, periumbilic region
    laceration — *see* Laceration, abdomen, wall, periumbilic region
    puncture — *see* Puncture, abdomen, wall, periumbilic region
  phalanges
    finger — *see* Wound, open, finger
    toe — *see* Wound, open, toe
  pharynx S11.20 ☑
  pinna — *see* Wound, open, ear
  popliteal space — *see* Wound, open, knee
  prepuce — *see* Wound, open, penis
  pubic region — *see* Wound, open, back, lower
  pudendum — *see* Wound, open, genital organs, external
  puncture wound — *see* Puncture
  rectovaginal septum — *see* Wound, open, vagina
  right
    lower quadrant S31.103 ☑
      with penetration into peritoneal cavity S31.603 ☑
      bite — *see* Bite, abdomen, wall, right, lower quadrant
      laceration — *see* Laceration, abdomen, wall, right, lower quadrant
      puncture — *see* Puncture, abdomen, wall, right, lower quadrant
    upper quadrant S31.100 ☑
      with penetration into peritoneal cavity S31.600 ☑
      bite — *see* Bite, abdomen, wall, right, upper quadrant
      laceration — *see* Laceration, abdomen, wall, right, upper quadrant
      puncture — *see* Puncture, abdomen, wall, right, upper quadrant
  sacral region — *see* Wound, open, back, lower
  sacroiliac region — *see* Wound, open, back, lower
  salivary gland — *see* Wound, open, oral cavity
  scalp S01.00 ☑
    bite S01.05 ☑
    laceration — *see* Laceration, scalp
    puncture — *see* Puncture, scalp
  scalpel, newborn (birth injury) P15.8
  scapular region — *see* Wound, open, shoulder
  sclera — *see* Wound, open, ocular
  scrotum S31.30 ☑
    with amputation — *see* Amputation, traumatic, scrotum
    bite S31.35 ☑
    laceration — *see* Laceration, scrotum
    puncture — *see* Puncture, scrotum
  shin — *see* Wound, open, leg
  shoulder S41.00- ☑
    with amputation — *see* Amputation, traumatic, arm
    bite — *see* Bite, shoulder
    laceration — *see* Laceration, shoulder
    puncture — *see* Puncture, shoulder
  skin NOS T14.8 ☑
  spermatic cord — *see* Wound, open, testis
  sternal region — *see* Wound, open, thorax, front wall
  submaxillary region — *see* Wound, open, head, specified site NEC
  submental region — *see* Wound, open, head, specified site NEC
  subungual
    finger(s) — *see* Wound, open, finger
    toe(s) — *see* Wound, open, toe
  supraclavicular region — *see* Wound, open, neck, specified site NEC
  temple, temporal region — *see* Wound, open, head, specified site NEC
  temporomandibular area — *see* Wound, open, cheek
  testis S31.30 ☑
    with amputation — *see* Amputation, traumatic, testes
    bite S31.35 ☑
    laceration — *see* Laceration, testis
    puncture — *see* Puncture, testis

☑ **Additional Character Required** — **Refer to the Tabular List for Character Selection**   ▽ **Subterms under main terms may continue to next column or page**

Wound, open — *continued*
    thigh S71.1Ø- ☑
        with amputation — *see* Amputation, traumatic, hip
        bite — *see* Bite, thigh
        laceration — *see* Laceration, thigh
        puncture — *see* Puncture, thigh
    thorax, thoracic (wall) S21.9Ø ☑
        back S21.2Ø-
            with penetration S21.4Ø ☑
        bite — *see* Bite, thorax
        breast — *see* Wound, open, breast
        front S21.1Ø-
            with penetration S21.3Ø ☑
        laceration — *see* Laceration, thorax
        puncture — *see* Puncture, thorax
    throat — *see* Wound, open, neck
    thumb S61.ØØ9 ☑
        with
            amputation — *see* Amputation, traumatic, thumb
            damage to nail S61.1Ø9 ☑
        bite — *see* Bite, thumb
        laceration — *see* Laceration, thumb
        left S61.ØØ2 ☑
            with
                damage to nail S61.1Ø2 ☑
        puncture — *see* Puncture, thumb
        right S61.ØØ1 ☑
            with
                damage to nail S61.1Ø1 ☑
    thyroid (gland) — *see* Wound, open, neck, thyroid
    toe(s) S91.1Ø9 ☑
        with
            amputation — *see* Amputation, traumatic, toe
            damage to nail S91.2Ø9 ☑
        bite — *see* Bite, toe
        great S91.1Ø3 ☑
            with
                damage to nail S91.2Ø3 ☑
            left S91.1Ø2 ☑
                with
                    damage to nail S91.2Ø2 ☑
            right S91.1Ø1 ☑
                with
                    damage to nail S91.2Ø1 ☑
        laceration — *see* Laceration, toe
        lesser S91.1Ø6 ☑
            with
                damage to nail S91.2Ø6 ☑
            left S91.1Ø5 ☑
                with
                    damage to nail S91.2Ø5 ☑
            right S91.1Ø4 ☑
                with
                    damage to nail S91.2Ø4 ☑
        puncture — *see* Puncture, toe
    tongue — *see* Wound, open, oral cavity
    trachea (cervical region) — *see* Wound, open, neck, trachea
    tunica vaginalis — *see* Wound, open, testis
    tympanum, tympanic membrane SØ9.2- ☑
        laceration — *see* Laceration, ear, drum
        puncture — *see* Puncture, tympanum
    umbilical region — *see* Wound, open, abdomen, wall, periumbilic region
    uvula — *see* Wound, open, oral cavity
    vagina S31.4Ø ☑
        bite S31.45 ☑
        laceration — *see* Laceration, vagina
        puncture — *see* Puncture, vagina
    vitreous (humor) — *see* Wound, open, ocular
    vocal cord S11.Ø39 ☑
        bite — *see* Bite, vocal cord
        laceration S11.Ø31 ☑
            with foreign body S11.Ø32 ☑
        puncture S11.Ø33 ☑
            with foreign body S11.Ø34 ☑
    vulva S31.4Ø ☑
        with amputation — *see* Amputation, traumatic, vulva
        bite S31.45 ☑
        laceration — *see* Laceration, vulva
        puncture — *see* Puncture, vulva
    wrist S61.5Ø- ☑
        bite — *see* Bite, wrist

Wound, open — *continued*
    wrist — *continued*
        laceration — *see* Laceration, wrist
        puncture — *see* Puncture, wrist
Wound, superficial — *see* Injury — *see also* specified injury type
Wright's syndrome G54.Ø
Wrist — *see* condition
Wrong drug (by accident) (given in error) — *see* Table of Drugs and Chemicals, by drug, poisoning
Wry neck — *see* Torticollis
Wuchereria (bancrofti) **infestation** B74.Ø
Wuchereriasis B74.Ø
Wuchernde Struma Langhans C73

X

Xanthelasma (eyelid) (palpebrarum) HØ2.6Ø
    left HØ2.66
        lower HØ2.65
        upper HØ2.64
    right HØ2.63
        lower HØ2.62
        upper HØ2.61
Xanthelasmatosis (essential) E78.2
Xanthinuria, hereditary E79.8
Xanthoastrocytoma
    specified site — *see* Neoplasm, malignant, by site
    unspecified site C71.9
Xanthofibroma — *see* Neoplasm, connective tissue, benign
Xanthogranuloma D76.3
Xanthoma(s), xanthomatosis (primary) (familial) (hereditary) E75.5
    with
        hyperlipoproteinemia
            Type I E78.3
            Type III E78.2
            Type IV E78.1
            Type V E78.3
    bone (generalisata) C96.5
    cerebrotendinous E75.5
    cutaneotendinous E75.5
    disseminatum (skin) E78.2
    eruptive E78.2
    hypercholesterinemic E78.ØØ
    hypercholesterolemic E78.ØØ
    hyperlipidemic E78.5
    joint E75.5
    multiple (skin) E78.2
    tendon (sheath) E75.5
    tuberosum E78.2
    tuberous E78.2
    tubo-eruptive E78.2
    verrucous, oral mucosa K13.4
Xanthosis R23.8
Xenophobia F4Ø.1Ø
Xeroderma — *see also* Ichthyosis
    acquired L85.Ø
        eyelid HØ1.149
            left HØ1.146
                lower HØ1.145
                upper HØ1.144
            right HØ1.143
                lower HØ1.142
                upper HØ1.141
    pigmentosum Q82.1
    vitamin A deficiency E5Ø.8
Xerophthalmia (vitamin A deficiency) E5Ø.7
    unrelated to vitamin A deficiency — *see* Keratoconjunctivitis
Xerosis
    conjunctiva H11.14- ☑
        with Bitot's spots — *see also* Pigmentation, conjunctiva
            vitamin A deficiency E5Ø.1
        vitamin A deficiency E5Ø.Ø
    cornea H18.89- ☑
        with ulceration — *see* Ulcer, cornea
            vitamin A deficiency E5Ø.3
        vitamin A deficiency E5Ø.2
    cutis L85.3
    skin L85.3
Xerostomia K11.7
Xiphopagus Q89.4
XO syndrome Q96.9

X-ray (of)
    abnormal findings — *see* Abnormal, diagnostic imaging
    breast (mammogram) (routine) Z12.31
    chest
        routine (as part of a general medical examination) ZØØ.ØØ
            with abnormal findings ZØØ.Ø1
        routine (as part of a general medical examination) ZØØ.ØØ
            with abnormal findings ZØØ.Ø1
XXXXY syndrome Q98.1
XXY syndrome Q98.Ø

Y

Yaba pox (virus disease) BØ8.72
Yatapoxvirus BØ8.7Ø
    specified NEC BØ8.79
Yawning RØ6.89
    psychogenic F45.8
Yaws A66.9
    bone lesions A66.6
    butter A66.1
    chancre A66.Ø
    cutaneous, less than five years after infection A66.2
    early (cutaneous) (macular) (maculopapular) (micropapular) (papular) A66.2
        frambeside A66.2
        skin lesions NEC A66.2
    eyelid A66.2
    ganglion A66.6
    gangosis, gangosa A66.5
    gumma, gummata A66.4
        bone A66.6
    gummatous
        frambeside A66.4
        osteitis A66.6
        periostitis A66.6
    hydrarthrosis — *see also* subcategory M14.8- A66.6
    hyperkeratosis (early) (late) A66.3
    initial lesions A66.Ø
    joint lesions — *see also* subcategory M14.8- A66.6
    juxta-articular nodules A66.7
    late nodular (ulcerated) A66.4
    latent (without clinical manifestations) (with positive serology) A66.8
    mother A66.Ø
    mucosal A66.7
    multiple papillomata A66.1
    nodular, late (ulcerated) A66.4
    osteitis A66.6
    papilloma, plantar or palmar A66.1
    periostitis (hypertrophic) A66.6
    specified NEC A66.7
    ulcers A66.4
    wet crab A66.1
Yeast infection — *see also* Candidiasis B37.9
Yellow
    atrophy (liver) — *see* Failure, hepatic
    fever — *see* Fever, yellow
    jack — *see* Fever, yellow
    jaundice — *see* Jaundice
    nail syndrome L6Ø.5
Yersiniosis — *see also* Infection, Yersinia
    extraintestinal A28.2
    intestinal AØ4.6

Z

Zahorsky's syndrome (herpangina) BØ8.5
Zellweger's syndrome E71.51Ø
Zenker's diverticulum (esophagus) K22.5
Ziehen-Oppenheim disease G24.1
Zieve's syndrome K7Ø.Ø
Zika NOS A92.5
    congenital P35.4
Zinc
    deficiency, dietary E6Ø
    metabolism disorder E83.2
Zollinger-Ellison syndrome E16.4
Zona — *see* Herpes, zoster
Zoophobia F4Ø.218
Zoster (herpes) — *see* Herpes, zoster
Zygomycosis B46.9
    specified NEC B46.8
Zymotic — *see* condition

(left margin, vertical) Neoplasm Table

(left margin, vertical) Neoplasm, abdomen, abdominal — Neoplasm, bile or biliary

Note: The list below gives the code number for neoplasms by anatomical site. For each site there are six possible code numbers according to whether the neoplasm in question is malignant, benign, in situ, of uncertain behavior, or of unspecified nature. The description of the neoplasm will often indicate which of the six columns is appropriate; e.g., malignant melanoma of skin, benign fibroadenoma of breast, carcinoma in situ of cervix uteri. Where such descriptors are not present, the remainder of the Index should be consulted where guidance is given to the appropriate column for each morphological (histological) variety listed; e.g., Mesonephroma – see Neoplasm, malignant; Embryoma — see also Neoplasm, uncertain behavior; Disease, Bowen's – see Neoplasm, skin, in situ. However, the guidance in the Index can be overridden if one of the descriptors mentioned above is present; e.g., malignant adenoma of colon is coded to C18.9 and not to D12.6 as the adjective "malignant" overrides the Index entry "Adenoma — see also Neoplasm, benign, by site." Codes listed with a dash -, following the code have a required additional character for laterality. The tabular list must be reviewed for the complete code.

	Malignant Primary	Malignant Secondary	Ca in situ	Benign	Uncertain Behavior	Unspecified Behavior
Neoplasm, neoplastic	C80.1	C79.9	D09.9	D36.9	D48.9	D49.9
abdomen, abdominal	C76.2	C79.8-☑	D09.8	D36.7	D48.7	D49.89
cavity	C76.2	C79.8-☑	D09.8	D36.7	D48.7	D49.89
organ	C76.2	C79.8-☑	D09.8	D36.7	D48.7	D49.89
viscera	C76.2	C79.8-☑	D09.8	D36.7	D48.7	D49.89
wall — see also Neoplasm, abdomen, wall, skin	C44.509	C79.2	D04.5	D23.5	D48.5	D49.2
connective tissue	C49.4	C79.8-☑	—	D21.4	D48.1	D49.2
skin	C44.509	—	—	—	—	—
basal cell carcinoma	C44.519					
specified type NEC	C44.599					
squamous cell carcinoma	C44.529					
abdominopelvic	C76.8	C79.8-☑	—	D36.7	D48.7	D49.89
accessory sinus — see Neoplasm, sinus						
acoustic nerve	C72.4-☑	C79.49		D33.3	D43.3	D49.7
adenoid (pharynx) (tissue)	C11.1	C79.89	D00.08	D10.6	D37.05	D49.0
adipose tissue — see also Neoplasm, connective tissue	C49.4	C79.89	—	D21.9	D48.1	D49.2
adnexa (uterine)	C57.4	C79.89	D07.39	D28.7	D39.8	D49.59
adrenal	C74.9-☑	C79.7-☑	D09.3	D35.0-☑	D44.1-☑	D49.7
capsule	C74.9-☑	C79.7-☑	D09.3	D35.0-☑	D44.1-☑	D49.7
cortex	C74.0-☑	C79.7-☑	D09.3	D35.0-☑	D44.1-☑	D49.7
gland	C74.9-☑	C79.7-☑	D09.3	D35.0-☑	D44.1-☑	D49.7
medulla	C74.1-☑	C79.7-☑	D09.3	D35.0-☑	D44.1-☑	D49.7
ala nasi (external) — see also Neoplasm, skin, nose	C44.301	C79.2	D04.39	D23.39	D48.5	D49.2
alimentary canal or tract NEC	C26.9	C78.80	D01.9	D13.9	D37.9	D49.0
alveolar	C03.9	C79.89	D00.03	D10.39	D37.09	D49.0
mucosa	C03.9	C79.89	D00.03	D10.39	D37.09	D49.0
lower	C03.1	C79.89	D00.03	D10.39	D37.09	D49.0
upper	C03.0	C79.89	D00.03	D10.39	D37.09	D49.0
ridge or process	C41.1	C79.51	—	D16.5	D48.0	D49.2
carcinoma	C03.9	C79.8-☑	—	—	—	—
lower	C03.1	C79.8-☑	—	—	—	—
upper	C03.0	C79.8-☑	—	—	—	—
lower	C41.1	C79.51	—	D16.5	D48.0	D49.2
mucosa	C03.9	C79.89	D00.03	D10.39	D37.09	D49.0
lower	C03.1	C79.89	D00.03	D10.39	D37.09	D49.0
upper	C03.0	C79.89	D00.03	D10.39	D37.09	D49.0
upper	C41.0	C79.51	—	D16.4	D48.0	D49.2
sulcus	C06.1	C79.89	D00.02	D10.39	D37.09	D49.0
alveolus	C03.9	C79.89	D00.03	D10.39	D37.09	D49.0
lower	C03.1	C79.89	D00.03	D10.39	D37.09	D49.0
upper	C03.0	C79.89	D00.03	D10.39	D37.09	D49.0
ampulla of Vater	C24.1	C78.89	D01.5	D13.5	D37.6	D49.0
ankle NEC	C76.5-☑	C79.89	D04.7-☑	D36.7	D48.7	D49.89
anorectum, anorectal (junction)	C21.8	C78.5	D01.3	D12.9	D37.8	D49.0
antecubital fossa or space	C76.4-☑	C79.89	D04.6-☑	D36.7	D48.7	D49.89

	Malignant Primary	Malignant Secondary	Ca in situ	Benign	Uncertain Behavior	Unspecified Behavior
Neoplasm, neoplastic *— continued*						
antrum (Highmore) (maxillary)	C31.0	C78.39	D02.3	D14.0	D38.5	D49.1
pyloric	C16.3	C78.89	D00.2	D13.1	D37.1	D49.0
tympanicum	C30.1	C78.39	D02.3	D14.0	D38.5	D49.1
anus, anal	C21.0	C78.5	D01.3	D12.9	D37.8	D49.0
canal	C21.1	C78.5	D01.3	D12.9	D37.8	D49.0
cloacogenic zone	C21.2	C78.5	D01.3	D12.9	D37.8	D49.0
margin — see also Neoplasm, anus, skin	C44.500	C79.2	D04.5	D23.5	D48.5	D49.2
overlapping lesion with rectosigmoid junction or rectum	C21.8	—	—	—	—	—
skin	C44.500	C79.2	D04.5	D23.5	D48.5	D49.2
basal cell carcinoma	C44.510	—	—	—	—	—
specified type NEC	C44.590	—	—	—	—	—
squamous cell carcinoma	C44.520	—	—	—	—	—
sphincter	C21.1	C78.5	D01.3	D12.9	D37.8	D49.0
aorta (thoracic)	C49.3	C79.89	—	D21.3	D48.1	D49.2
abdominal	C49.4	C79.89	—	D21.4	D48.1	D49.2
aortic body	C75.5	C79.89	—	D35.6	D44.7	D49.7
aponeurosis	C49.9	C79.89	—	D21.9	D48.1	D49.2
palmar	C49.1-☑	C79.89	—	D21.1-☑	D48.1	D49.2
plantar	C49.2-☑	C79.89	—	D21.2-☑	D48.1	D49.2
appendix	C18.1	C78.5	D01.0	D12.1	D37.3	D49.0
arachnoid	C70.9	C79.49	—	D32.9	D42.9	D49.7
cerebral	C70.0	C79.32	—	D32.0	D42.0	D49.7
spinal	C70.1	C79.49	—	D32.1	D42.1	D49.7
areola	C50.0-☑	C79.81	D05-☑	D24-☑	D48.6-☑	D49.3
arm NEC	C76.4-☑	C79.89	D04.6-☑	D36.7	D48.7	D49.89
artery — see Neoplasm, connective tissue						
aryepiglottic fold	C13.1	C79.89	D00.08	D10.7	D37.05	D49.0
hypopharyngeal aspect	C13.1	C79.89	D00.08	D10.7	D37.05	D49.0
laryngeal aspect	C32.1	C78.39	D02.0	D14.1	D38.0	D49.1
marginal zone	C13.1	C79.89	D00.08	D10.7	D37.05	D49.0
arytenoid (cartilage)	C32.3	C78.39	D02.0	D14.1	D38.0	D49.1
fold — see Neoplasm, aryepiglottic						
associated with transplanted organ	C80.2	—	—	—	—	—
atlas	C41.2	C79.51	—	D16.6	D48.0	D49.2
atrium, cardiac	C38.0	C79.89	—	D15.1	D48.7	D49.89
auditory canal (external) (skin)	C44.20-☑	C79.2	D04.2-☑	D23.2-☑	D48.5	D49.2
internal	C30.1	C78.39	D02.3	D14.0	D38.5	D49.1
nerve	C72.4-☑	C79.49	—	D33.3	D43.3	D49.7
tube	C30.1	C78.39	D02.3	D14.0	D38.5	D49.1
opening	C11.2	C79.89	D00.08	D10.6	D37.05	D49.0
auricle, ear — see also Neoplasm, skin, ear	C44.20-☑	C79.2	D04.2-☑	D23.2-☑	D48.5	D49.2
auricular canal (external) — see also Neoplasm, skin, ear	C44.20-☑	C79.2	D04.2-☑	D23.2-☑	D48.5	D49.2
internal	C30.1	C78.39	D02.3	D14.0	D38.5	D49.2
autonomic nerve or nervous system NEC (see Neoplasm, nerve, peripheral)						
axilla, axillary	C76.1	C79.89	D09.8	D36.7	D48.7	D49.89
fold — see also Neoplasm, skin, trunk	C44.509	C79.2	D04.5	D23.5	D48.5	D49.2
back NEC	C76.8	C79.89	D04.5	D36.7	D48.7	D49.89
Bartholin's gland	C51.0	C79.82	D07.1	D28.0	D39.8	D49.59
basal ganglia	C71.0	C79.31	—	D33.0	D43.0	D49.6
basis pedunculi	C71.7	C79.31	—	D33.1	D43.1	D49.6
bile or biliary (tract)	C24.9	C78.89	D01.5	D13.5	D37.6	D49.0

☑ **Additional Character Required — Refer to the Tabular List for Character Selection**   🔺 **Subterms under main terms may continue to next column or page**

Neoplasm, neoplastic

	Malignant Primary	Malignant Secondary	Ca in situ	Benign	Uncertain Behavior	Unspecified Behavior
— *continued*						
bile or biliary —						
continued						
canaliculi (biliferi) (intrahepatic)	C22.1	C78.7	D01.5	D13.4	D37.6	D49.0
canals, interlobular	C22.1	C78.89	D01.5	D13.4	D37.6	D49.0
duct or passage (common) (cystic) (extrahepatic)	C24.0	C78.89	D01.5	D13.5	D37.6	D49.0
interlobular	C22.1	C78.89	D01.5	D13.4	D37.6	D49.0
intrahepatic	C22.1	C78.7	D01.5	D13.4	D37.6	D49.0
and extrahepatic	C24.8	C78.89	D01.5	D13.5	D37.6	D49.0
bladder (urinary)	C67.9	C79.11	D09.0	D30.3	D41.4	D49.4
dome	C67.1	C79.11	D09.0	D30.3	D41.4	D49.4
neck	C67.5	C79.11	D09.0	D30.3	D41.4	D49.4
orifice	C67.9	C79.11	D09.0	D30.3	D41.4	D49.4
ureteric	C67.6	C79.11	D09.0	D30.3	D41.4	D49.4
urethral	C67.5	C79.11	D09.0	D30.3	D41.4	D49.4
overlapping lesion	C67.8	—	—	—	—	—
sphincter	C67.8	C79.11	D09.0	D30.3	D41.4	D49.4
trigone	C67.0	C79.11	D09.0	D30.3	D41.4	D49.4
urachus	C67.7	C79.11	D09.0	D30.3	D41.4	D49.4
wall	C67.9	C79.11	D09.0	D30.3	D41.4	D49.4
anterior	C67.3	C79.11	D09.0	D30.3	D41.4	D49.4
lateral	C67.2	C79.11	D09.0	D30.3	D41.4	D49.4
posterior	C67.4	C79.11	D09.0	D30.3	D41.4	D49.4
blood vessel — *see* Neoplasm, connective tissue						
bone (periosteum)	C41.9	C79.51	—	D16.9-	D48.0	D49.2
acetabulum						
ankle	C40.3-✓	C79.51	—	D16.3-✓	—	—
arm NEC	C40.0-✓	C79.51	—	D16.0-✓	—	—
astragalus	C40.3-✓	C79.51	—	D16.3-✓	—	—
atlas	C41.2	C79.51	—	D16.6	D48.0	D49.2
axis	C41.2	C79.51	—	D16.6	D48.0	D49.2
back NEC	C41.2	C79.51	—	D16.6	D48.0	D49.2
calcaneus	C40.3-✓	C79.51	—	D16.3-✓	—	—
calvarium	C41.0	C79.51	—	D16.4	D48.0	D49.2
carpus (any)	C40.1-✓	C79.51	—	D16.1-✓	—	—
cartilage NEC	C41.9	C79.51	—	D16.9	D48.0	D49.2
clavicle	C41.3	C79.51	—	D16.7	D48.0	D49.2
clivus	C41.0	C79.51	—	D16.4	D48.0	D49.2
coccygeal vertebra	C41.4	C79.51	—	D16.8	D48.0	D49.2
coccyx	C41.4	C79.51	—	D16.8	D48.0	D49.2
costal cartilage	C41.3	C79.51	—	D16.7	D48.0	D49.2
costovertebral joint	C41.3	C79.51	—	D16.7	D48.0	D49.2
cranial	C41.0	C79.51	—	D16.4	D48.0	D49.2
cuboid	C40.3-✓	C79.51	—	D16.3-✓	—	—
cuneiform	C41.9	C79.51	—	D16.9	D48.0	D49.2
elbow	C40.0-✓	C79.51	—	D16.0-✓	—	—
ethmoid (labyrinth)	C41.0	C79.51	—	D16.4	D48.0	D49.2
face	C41.0	C79.51	—	D16.4	D48.0	D49.2
femur (any part)	C40.2-✓	C79.51	—	D16.2-✓	—	—
fibula (any part)	C40.2-✓	C79.51	—	D16.2-✓	—	—
finger (any)	C40.1-✓	C79.51	—	D16.1-✓	—	—
foot	C40.3-✓	C79.51	—	D16.3-✓	—	—
forearm	C40.0-✓	C79.51	—	D16.0-✓	—	—
frontal	C41.0	C79.51	—	D16.4	D48.0	D49.2
hand	C40.1-✓	C79.51	—	D16.1-✓	—	—
heel	C40.3-✓	C79.51	—	D16.3-✓	—	—
hip	C41.4	C79.51	—	D16.8	D48.0	D49.2
humerus (any part)	C40.0-✓	C79.51	—	D16.0-✓	—	—
hyoid	C41.0	C79.51	—	D16.4	D48.0	D49.2
ilium	C41.4	C79.51	—	D16.8	D48.0	D49.2
innominate	C41.4	C79.51	—	D16.8	D48.0	D49.2
intervertebral cartilage or disc	C41.2	C79.51	—	D16.6	D48.0	D49.2
ischium	C41.4	C79.51	—	D16.8	D48.0	D49.2
jaw (lower)	C41.1	C79.51	—	D16.5	D48.0	D49.2
knee	C40.2-✓	C79.51	—	D16.2-✓	—	—
leg NEC	C40.2-✓	C79.51	—	D16.2-✓	—	—
limb NEC	C40.9-✓	C79.51	—	D16.9	—	—

Neoplasm, neoplastic

	Malignant Primary	Malignant Secondary	Ca in situ	Benign	Uncertain Behavior	Unspecified Behavior
— *continued*						
bone — *continued*						
limb — *continued*						
lower (long bones)	C40.2-✓	C79.51	—	D16.2-✓	—	—
short bones	C40.3-✓	C79.51	—	D16.3-✓	—	—
upper (long bones)	C40.0-✓	C79.51	—	D16.0-✓	—	—
short bones	C40.1-✓	C79.51	—	D16.1-✓	—	—
malar	C41.0	C79.51	—	D16.4	D48.0	D49.2
mandible	C41.1	C79.51	—	D16.5	D48.0	D49.2
marrow NEC (any bone)	C96.9	C79.52	—	—	D47.9	D49.89
mastoid	C41.0	C79.51	—	D16.4	D48.0	D49.2
maxilla, maxillary (superior)	C41.0	C79.51	—	D16.4	D48.0	D49.2
inferior	C41.1	C79.51	—	D16.5	D48.0	D49.2
metacarpus (any)	C40.1-✓	C79.51	—	D16.1-✓	—	—
metatarsus (any)	C40.3-✓	C79.51	—	D16.3-✓	—	—
navicular ankle	C40.3-✓	C79.51	—	—	—	—
hand	C40.1-✓	C79.51	—	—	—	—
nose, nasal	C41.0	C79.51	—	D16.4	D48.0	D49.2
occipital	C41.0	C79.51	—	D16.4	D48.0	D49.2
orbit	C41.0	C79.51	—	D16.4	D48.0	D49.2
overlapping sites	C40.8-✓	—	—	—	—	—
parietal	C41.0	C79.51	—	D16.4	D48.0	D49.2
patella	C40.2-✓	C79.51	—	—	—	—
pelvic	C41.4	C79.51	—	D16.8	D48.0	D49.2
phalanges foot	C40.3-✓	C79.51	—	—	—	—
hand	C40.1-✓	C79.51	—	—	—	—
pubic	C41.4	C79.51	—	D16.8	D48.0	D49.2
radius (any part)	C40.0-✓	C79.51	—	D16.0-✓	—	—
rib	C41.3	C79.51	—	D16.7	D48.0	D49.2
sacral vertebra	C41.4	C79.51	—	D16.8	D48.0	D49.2
sacrum	C41.4	C79.51	—	D16.8	D48.0	D49.2
scaphoid of ankle	C40.3-✓	C79.51	—	—	—	—
of hand	C40.1-✓	C79.51	—	—	—	—
scapula (any part)	C40.0-✓	C79.51	—	D16.0-✓	—	—
sella turcica	C41.0	C79.51	—	D16.4	D48.0	D49.2
shoulder	C40.0-✓	C79.51	—	D16.0-✓	—	—
skull	C41.0	C79.51	—	D16.4	D48.0	D49.2
sphenoid	C41.0	C79.51	—	D16.4	D48.0	D49.2
spine, spinal (column)	C41.2	C79.51	—	D16.6	D48.0	D49.2
coccyx	C41.4	C79.51	—	D16.8	D48.0	D49.2
sacrum	C41.4	C79.51	—	D16.8	D48.0	D49.2
sternum	C41.3	C79.51	—	D16.7	D48.0	D49.2
tarsus (any)	C40.3-✓	C79.51	—	—	—	—
temporal	C41.0	C79.51	—	D16.4	D48.0	D49.2
thumb	C40.1-✓	C79.51	—	—	—	—
tibia (any part)	C40.2-✓	C79.51	—	—	—	—
toe (any)	C40.3-✓	C79.51	—	—	—	—
trapezium	C40.1-✓	C79.51	—	—	—	—
trapezoid	C40.1-✓	C79.51	—	—	—	—
turbinate	C41.0	C79.51	—	D16.4	D48.0	D49.2
ulna (any part)	C40.0-✓	C79.51	—	D16.0-✓	—	—
unciform	C40.1-✓	C79.51	—	—	—	—
vertebra (column)	C41.2	C79.51	—	D16.6	D48.0	D49.2
coccyx	C41.4	C79.51	—	D16.8	D48.0	D49.2
sacrum	C41.4	C79.51	—	D16.8	D48.0	D49.2
vomer	C41.0	C79.51	—	D16.4	D48.0	D49.2
wrist	C40.1-✓	C79.51	—	—	—	—
xiphoid process	C41.3	C79.51	—	D16.7	D48.0	D49.2
zygomatic	C41.0	C79.51	—	D16.4	D48.0	D49.2
book-leaf (mouth) — *ventral surface of tongue and floor of mouth*	C06.89	C79.89	D00.00	D10.39	D37.09	D49.0
bowel — *see* Neoplasm, intestine						
brachial plexus	C47.1-✓	C79.89	—	D36.12	D48.2	D49.2
brain NEC	C71.9	C79.31	—	D33.2	D43.2	D49.6

▽ **Subterms under main terms may continue to next column or page**   ☑ **Additional Character Required — Refer to the Tabular List for Character Selection**

Neoplasm, neoplastic — continued

	Malignant Primary	Malignant Secondary	Ca in situ	Benign	Uncertain Behavior	Unspecified Behavior
brain — continued						
basal ganglia	C71.0	C79.31	—	D33.0	D43.0	D49.6
cerebellopontine angle	C71.6	C79.31	—	D33.1	D43.1	D49.6
cerebellum NOS	C71.6	C79.31	—	D33.1	D43.1	D49.6
cerebrum	C71.0	C79.31	—	D33.0	D43.0	D49.6
choroid plexus	C71.7	C79.31	—	D33.1	D43.1	D49.6
corpus callosum	C71.8	C79.31	—	D33.2	D43.2	D49.6
corpus striatum	C71.0	C79.31	—	D33.0	D43.0	D49.6
cortex (cerebral)	C71.0	C79.31	—	D33.0	D43.0	D49.6
frontal lobe	C71.1	C79.31	—	D33.0	D43.0	D49.6
globus pallidus	C71.0	C79.31	—	D33.0	D43.0	D49.6
hippocampus	C71.2	C79.31	—	D33.0	D43.0	D49.6
hypothalamus	C71.0	C79.31	—	D33.0	D43.0	D49.6
internal capsule	C71.0	C79.31	—	D33.0	D43.0	D49.6
medulla oblongata	C71.7	C79.31	—	D33.1	D43.1	D49.6
meninges	C70.0	C79.32	—	D32.0	D42.0	D49.7
midbrain	C71.7	C79.31	—	D33.1	D43.1	D49.6
occipital lobe	C71.4	C79.31	—	D33.0	D43.0	D49.6
overlapping lesion	C71.8	C79.31	—	—	—	—
parietal lobe	C71.3	C79.31	—	D33.0	D43.0	D49.6
peduncle	C71.7	C79.31	—	D33.1	D43.1	D49.6
pons	C71.7	C79.31	—	D33.1	D43.1	D49.6
stem	C71.7	C79.31	—	D33.1	D43.1	D49.6
tapetum	C71.8	C79.31	—	D33.2	D43.2	D49.6
temporal lobe	C71.2	C79.31	—	D33.0	D43.0	D49.6
thalamus	C71.0	C79.31	—	D33.0	D43.0	D49.6
uncus	C71.2	C79.31	—	D33.0	D43.0	D49.6
ventricle (floor)	C71.5	C79.31	—	D33.0	D43.0	D49.6
fourth	C71.7	C79.31	—	D33.1	D43.1	D49.6
branchial (cleft) (cyst) (vestiges)	C10.4	C79.89	D00.08	D10.5	D37.05	D49.0
breast (connective tissue) (glandular tissue) (soft parts)	C50.9-✓	C79.81	D05.-✓	D24.-✓	D48.6-✓	D49.3
areola	C50.0-✓	C79.81	D05.-✓	D24.-✓	D48.6-✓	D49.3
axillary tail	C50.6-✓	C79.81	D05.-✓	D24.-✓	D48.6-✓	D49.3
central portion	C50.1-✓	C79.81	D05.-✓	D24.-✓	D48.6-✓	D49.3
inner	C50.8-✓	C79.81	D05.-✓	D24.-✓	D48.6-✓	D49.3
lower	C50.8-✓	C79.81	D05.-✓	D24.-✓	D48.6-✓	D49.3
lower-inner quadrant	C50.3-✓	C79.81	D05.-✓	D24.-✓	D48.6-✓	D49.3
lower-outer quadrant	C50.5-✓	C79.81	D05.-✓	D24.-✓	D48.6-✓	D49.3
mastectomy site (skin) — see also Neoplasm, breast, skin	C44.501	C79.2	—	—	—	—
specified as breast tissue	C50.8-✓	C79.81	—	—	—	—
midline	C50.8-✓	C79.81	D05.-✓	D24.-✓	D48.6-✓	D49.3
nipple	C50.0-✓	C79.81	D05.-✓	D24.-✓	D48.6-✓	D49.3
outer	C50.8-✓	C79.81	D05.-✓	D24.-✓	D48.6-✓	D49.3
overlapping lesion	C50.8-✓	—	—	—	—	—
skin	C44.501	C79.2	D04.5	D23.5	D48.5	D49.2
basal cell carcinoma	C44.511	—	—	—	—	—
specified type NEC	C44.591	—	—	—	—	—
squamous cell carcinoma	C44.521	—	—	—	—	—
tail (axillary)	C50.6-✓	C79.81	D05.-✓	D24.-✓	D48.6-✓	D49.3
upper	C50.8-✓	C79.81	D05.-✓	D24.-✓	D48.6-✓	D49.3
upper-inner quadrant	C50.2-✓	C79.81	D05.-✓	D24.-✓	D48.6-✓	D49.3
upper-outer quadrant	C50.4-✓	C79.81	D05.-✓	D24.-✓	D48.6-✓	D49.3
broad ligament	C57.1-✓	C79.82	D07.39	D28.2	D39.8	D49.59
bronchiogenic, bronchogenic (lung)	C34.9-✓	C78.0-✓	D02.2-✓	D14.3-✓	D38.1	D49.1
bronchiole	C34.9-✓	C78.0-✓	D02.2-✓	D14.3-✓	D38.1	D49.1
bronchus	C34.9-✓	C78.0-✓	D02.2-✓	D14.3-✓	D38.1	D49.1
carina	C34.0-✓	C78.0-✓	D02.2-✓	D14.3-✓	D38.1	D49.1
lower lobe of lung	C34.3-✓	C78.0-✓	D02.2-✓	D14.3-✓	D38.1	D49.1

Neoplasm, neoplastic — continued

	Malignant Primary	Malignant Secondary	Ca in situ	Benign	Uncertain Behavior	Unspecified Behavior
bronchus — continued						
main	C34.0-✓	C78.0-✓	D02.2-✓	D14.3-✓	D38.1	D49.1
middle lobe of lung	C34.2	C78.0-✓	D02.21	D14.31	D38.1	D49.1
overlapping lesion	C34.8-✓	—	—	—	—	—
upper lobe of lung	C34.1-✓	C78.0-✓	D02.2-✓	D14.3-✓	D38.1	D49.1
brow	C44.309	C79.2	D04.39	D23.39	D48.5	D49.2
basal cell carcinoma	C44.319	—	—	—	—	—
specified type NEC	C44.399	—	—	—	—	—
squamous cell carcinoma	C44.329	—	—	—	—	—
buccal (cavity)	C06.9	C79.89	D00.00	D10.39	D37.09	D49.0
commissure	C06.0	C79.89	D00.02	D10.39	D37.09	D49.0
groove (lower) (upper)	C06.1	C79.89	D00.02	D10.39	D37.09	D49.0
mucosa	C06.0	C79.89	D00.02	D10.39	D37.09	D49.0
sulcus (lower) (upper)	C06.1	C79.89	D00.02	D10.39	D37.09	D49.0
bulbourethral gland	C68.0	C79.19	D09.19	D30.4	D41.3	D49.59
bursa — see Neoplasm, connective tissue						
buttock NEC	C76.3	C79.89	D04.5	D36.7	D48.7	D49.89
calf	C76.5-✓	C79.89	D04.7-✓	D36.7	D48.7	D49.89
calvarium	C41.0	C79.51	—	D16.4	D48.0	D49.2
calyx, renal	C65.-✓	C79.0-✓	D09.19	D30.1-✓	D41.1-✓	D49.51-✓
canal anal	C21.1	C78.5	D01.3	D12.9	D37.8	D49.0
auditory (external) — see also Neoplasm, skin, ear	C44.20-✓	C79.2	D04.2-✓	D23.2-✓	D48.5	D49.2
auricular (external) — see also Neoplasm, skin, ear	C44.20-✓	C79.2	D04.2-✓	D23.2-✓	D48.5	D49.2
canaliculi, biliary (biliferi) (intrahepatic)	C22.1	C78.7	D01.5	D13.4	D37.6	D49.0
canthus (eye) (inner) (outer)	C44.10-✓	C79.2	D04.1-✓	D23.1-✓	D48.5	D49.2
basal cell carcinoma	C44.11-✓	—	—	—	—	—
sebaceous cell	C44.13-✓	—	—	—	—	—
specified type NEC	C44.19-✓	—	—	—	—	—
squamous cell carcinoma	C44.12-✓	—	—	—	—	—
capillary — see Neoplasm, connective tissue						
caput coli	C18.0	C78.5	D01.0	D12.0	D37.4	D49.0
carcinoid — see Tumor, carcinoid						
cardia (gastric)	C16.0	C78.89	D00.2	D13.1	D37.1	D49.0
cardiac orifice (stomach)	C16.0	C78.89	D00.2	D13.1	D37.1	D49.0
cardio-esophageal junction	C16.0	C78.89	D00.2	D13.1	D37.1	D49.0
cardio-esophagus	C16.0	C78.89	D00.2	D13.1	D37.1	D49.0
carina (bronchus)	C34.0-✓	C78.0-✓	D02.2-✓	D14.3-✓	D38.1	D49.1
carotid (artery)	C49.0	C79.89	—	D21.0	D48.1	D49.2
body	C75.4	C79.89	—	D35.5	D44.6	D49.7
carpus (any bone)	C40.1-✓	C79.51	—	D16.1-✓	—	—
cartilage (articular) (joint) NEC — see also Neoplasm, bone	C41.9	C79.51	—	D16.9	D48.0	D49.2
arytenoid	C32.3	C78.39	D02.0	D14.1	D38.0	D49.1
auricular	C49.0	C79.89	—	D21.0	D48.1	D49.2
bronchi	C34.0-✓	C78.39	—	D14.3-✓	D38.1	D49.1
costal	C41.3	C79.51	—	D16.7	D48.0	D49.2
cricoid	C32.3	C78.39	D02.0	D14.1	D38.0	D49.1
cuneiform	C32.3	C78.39	D02.0	D14.1	D38.0	D49.1
ear (external)	C49.0	C79.89	—	D21.0	D48.1	D49.2
ensiform	C41.3	C79.51	—	D16.7	D48.0	D49.2
epiglottis	C32.1	C78.39	D02.0	D14.1	D38.0	D49.1

✓ **Additional Character Required — Refer to the Tabular List for Character Selection** ▽ **Subterms under main terms may continue to next column or page**

Neoplasm, neoplastic	Malignant Primary	Malignant Secondary	Ca in situ	Benign	Uncertain Behavior	Unspecified Behavior
— *continued*						
cartilage — *see also*						
Neoplasm, bone —						
continued						
epiglottis —						
continued						
anterior						
surface	C10.1	C79.89	D00.08	D10.5	D37.05	D49.0
eyelid	C49.0	C79.89	—	D21.0	D48.1	D49.2
intervertebral	C41.2	C79.51	—	D16.6	D48.0	D49.2
larynx, laryngeal	C32.3	C78.39	D02.0	D14.1	D38.0	D49.1
nose, nasal	C30.0	C78.39	D02.3	D14.0	D38.5	D49.1
pinna	C49.0	C79.89	—	D21.0	D48.1	D49.2
rib	C41.3	C79.51	—	D16.7	D48.0	D49.2
semilunar						
(knee)	C40.2-☑	C79.51	—	D16.2-☑	D48.0	D49.2
thyroid	C32.3	C78.39	D02.0	D14.1	D38.0	D49.1
trachea	C33	C78.39	D02.1	D14.2	D38.1	D49.1
cauda equina	C72.1	C79.49	—	D33.4	D43.4	D49.7
cavity						
buccal	C06.9	C79.89	D00.00	D10.30	D37.09	D49.0
nasal	C30.0	C78.39	D02.3	D14.0	D38.5	D49.1
oral	C06.9	C79.89	D00.00	D10.30	D37.09	D49.0
peritoneal	C48.2	C78.6	—	D20.1	D48.4	D49.0
tympanic	C30.1	C78.39	D02.3	D14.0	D38.5	D49.1
cecum	C18.0	C78.5	D01.0	D12.0	D37.4	D49.0
central nervous						
system	C72.9	C79.40	—	—	—	—
cerebellopontine						
(angle)	C71.6	C79.31	—	D33.1	D43.1	D49.6
cerebellum,						
cerebellar	C71.6	C79.31	—	D33.1	D43.1	D49.6
cerebrum, cerebra						
(cortex)						
(hemisphere)						
(white matter)	C71.0	C79.31	—	D33.0	D43.0	D49.6
meninges	C70.0	C79.32	—	D32.0	D42.0	D49.7
peduncle	C71.7	C79.31	—	D33.1	D43.1	D49.6
ventricle	C71.5	C79.31	—	D33.0	D43.0	D49.6
fourth	C71.7	C79.31	—	D33.1	D43.1	D49.6
cervical region	C76.0	C79.89	D09.8	D36.7	D48.7	D49.89
cervix (cervical) (uteri)						
(uterus)	C53.9	C79.82	D06.9	D26.0	D39.0	D49.59
canal	C53.0	C79.82	D06.0	D26.0	D39.0	D49.59
endocervix (canal)						
(gland)	C53.0	C79.82	D06.0	D26.0	D39.0	D49.59
exocervix	C53.1	C79.82	D06.1	D26.0	D39.0	D49.59
external os	C53.1	C79.82	D06.1	D26.0	D39.0	D49.59
internal os	C53.0	C79.82	D06.0	D26.0	D39.0	D49.59
nabothian gland	C53.0	C79.82	D06.0	D26.0	D39.0	D49.59
overlapping						
lesion	C53.8	—	—	—	—	—
squamocolumnar						
junction	C53.8	C79.82	D06.7	D26.0	D39.0	D49.59
stump	C53.8	C79.82	D06.7	D26.0	D39.0	D49.59
cheek	C76.0	C79.89	D09.8	D36.7	D48.7	D49.89
external	C44.309	C79.2	D04.39	D23.39	D48.5	D49.2
basal cell						
carcinoma	C44.319	—	—	—	—	—
specified type						
NEC	C44.399	—	—	—	—	—
squamous cell						
carcinoma	C44.329	—	—	—	—	—
inner aspect	C06.0	C79.89	D00.02	D10.39	D37.09	D49.0
internal	C06.0	C79.89	D00.02	D10.39	D37.09	D49.0
mucosa	C06.0	C79.89	D00.02	D10.39	D37.09	D49.0
chest (wall) NEC	C76.1	C79.89	D09.8	D36.7	D48.7	D49.89
chiasma opticum	C72.3-☑	C79.49	—	D33.3	D43.3	D49.7
chin	C44.309	C79.2	D04.39	D23.39	D48.5	D49.2
basal cell						
carcinoma	C44.319	—	—	—	—	—
specified type						
NEC	C44.399	—	—	—	—	—
squamous cell						
carcinoma	C44.329	—	—	—	—	—
choana	C11.3	C79.89	D00.08	D10.6	D37.05	D49.0
cholangiole	C22.1	C78.89	D01.5	D13.4	D37.6	D49.0
choledochal duct	C24.0	C78.89	D01.5	D13.5	D37.6	D49.0
choroid	C69.3-☑	C79.49	D09.2-☑	D31.3-☑	D48.7	D49.81
plexus	C71.5	C79.31	—	D33.0	D43.0	D49.6
ciliary body	C69.4-☑	C79.49	D09.2-☑	D31.4-☑	D48.7	D49.89
clavicle	C41.3	C79.51	—	D16.7	D48.0	D49.2

Neoplasm, neoplastic	Malignant Primary	Malignant Secondary	Ca in situ	Benign	Uncertain Behavior	Unspecified Behavior
— *continued*						
clitoris	C51.2	C79.82	D07.1	D28.0	D39.8	D49.59
clivus	C41.0	C79.51	—	D16.4	D48.0	D49.2
cloacogenic zone	C21.2	C78.5	D01.3	D12.9	D37.8	D49.0
coccygeal						
body or glomus	C49.5	C79.89	—	D21.5	D48.1	D49.2
vertebra	C41.4	C79.51	—	D16.8	D48.0	D49.2
coccyx	C41.4	C79.51	—	D16.8	D48.0	D49.2
colon — *see also*						
Neoplasm,						
intestine,						
large	C18.9	C78.5	—	—	—	—
with rectum	C19	C78.5	D01.1	D12.7	D37.5	D49.0
columnella — *see also*						
Neoplasm, skin,						
face	C44.390	C79.2	D04.39	D23.39	D48.5	D49.2
column, spinal — *see*						
Neoplasm, spine						
commissure						
labial, lip	C00.6	C79.89	D00.01	D10.39	D37.01	D49.0
laryngeal	C32.0	C78.39	D02.0	D14.1	D38.0	D49.1
common (bile)						
duct	C24.0	C78.89	D01.5	D13.5	D37.6	D49.0
concha — *see also*						
Neoplasm, skin,						
ear	C44.20-☑	C79.2	D04.2-☑	D23.2-☑	D48.5	D49.2
nose	C30.0	C78.39	D02.3	D14.0	D38.5	D49.1
conjunctiva	C69.0-☑	C79.49	D09.2-☑	D31.0-☑	D48.7	D49.89
connective tissue						
NEC	C49.9	C79.89	—	D21.9	D48.1	D49.2

Note: For neoplasms of connective tissue (blood vessel, bursa, fascia, ligament, muscle, peripheral nerves, sympathetic and parasympathetic nerves and ganglia, synovia, tendon, etc.) or of morphological types that indicate connective tissue, code according to the list under "Neoplasm, connective tissue". For sites that do not appear in this list, code to neoplasm of that site; e.g., fibrosarcoma, pancreas (C25.9)

Note: Morphological types that indicate connective tissue appear in their proper place in the alphabetic index with the instruction "see Neoplasm, connective tissue ...."

	Malignant Primary	Malignant Secondary	Ca in situ	Benign	Uncertain Behavior	Unspecified Behavior
abdomen	C49.4	C79.89	—	D21.4	D48.1	D49.2
abdominal wall	C49.4	C79.89	—	D21.4	D48.1	D49.2
ankle	C49.2-☑	C79.89	—	D21.2-☑	D48.1	D49.2
antecubital fossa or						
space	C49.1-☑	C79.89	—	D21.1-☑	D48.1	D49.2
arm	C49.1-☑	C79.89	—	D21.1-☑	D48.1	D49.2
auricle (ear)	C49.0	C79.89	—	D21.0	D48.1	D49.2
axilla	C49.3	C79.89	—	D21.3	D48.1	D49.2
back	C49.6	C79.89	—	D21.6	D48.1	D49.2
breast — *see*						
Neoplasm,						
breast						
buttock	C49.5	C79.89	—	D21.5	D48.1	D49.2
calf	C49.2-☑	C79.89	—	D21.2-☑	D48.1	D49.2
cervical region	C49.0	C79.89	—	D21.0	D48.1	D49.2
cheek	C49.0	C79.89	—	D21.0	D48.1	D49.2
chest (wall)	C49.3	C79.89	—	D21.3	D48.1	D49.2
chin	C49.0	C79.89	—	D21.0	D48.1	D49.2
diaphragm	C49.3	C79.89	—	D21.3	D48.1	D49.2
ear (external)	C49.0	C79.89	—	D21.0	D48.1	D49.2
elbow	C49.1-☑	C79.89	—	D21.1-☑	D48.1	D49.2
extrarectal	C49.5	C79.89	—	D21.5	D48.1	D49.2
extremity	C49.9	C79.89	—	D21.9	D48.1	D49.2
lower	C49.2-☑	C79.89	—	D21.2-☑	D48.1	D49.2
upper	C49.1-☑	C79.89	—	D21.1-☑	D48.1	D49.2
eyelid	C49.0	C79.89	—	D21.0	D48.1	D49.2
face	C49.0	C79.89	—	D21.0	D48.1	D49.2
finger	C49.1-☑	C79.89	—	D21.1-☑	D48.1	D49.2
flank	C49.6	C79.89	—	D21.6	D48.1	D49.2
foot	C49.2-☑	C79.89	—	D21.2-☑	D48.1	D49.2
forearm	C49.1-☑	C79.89	—	D21.1-☑	D48.1	D49.2
forehead	C49.0	C79.89	—	D21.0	D48.1	D49.2
gastric	C49.4	C79.89	—	D21.4	D48.1	D49.2
gastrointestinal	C49.4	C79.89	—	D21.4	D48.1	D49.2
gluteal region	C49.5	C79.89	—	D21.5	D48.1	D49.2
great vessels						
NEC	C49.3	C79.89	—	D21.3	D48.1	D49.2
groin	C49.5	C79.89	—	D21.5	D48.1	D49.2
hand	C49.1-☑	C79.89	—	D21.1-☑	D48.1	D49.2
head	C49.0	C79.89	—	D21.0	D48.1	D49.2

Neoplasm Table

Neoplasm, connective tissue NEC — Neoplasm, ear

Neoplasm, neoplastic — continued	Malignant Primary	Malignant Secondary	Ca in situ	Benign	Uncertain Behavior	Unspecified Behavior
connective tissue — *continued*						
heel	C49.2-✓	C79.89	—	D21.2-✓	D48.1	D49.2
hip	C49.2-✓	C79.89	—	D21.2-✓	D48.1	D49.2
hypochondrium	C49.4	C79.89	—	D21.4	D48.1	D49.2
iliopsoas muscle	C49.5	C79.89	—	D21.5	D48.1	D49.2
infraclavicular region	C49.3	C79.89	—	D21.3	D48.1	D49.2
inguinal (canal) (region)	C49.5	C79.89	—	D21.5	D48.1	D49.2
intestinal	C49.4	C79.89	—	D21.4	D48.1	D49.2
intrathoracic	C49.3	C79.89	—	D21.3	D48.1	D49.2
ischiorectal fossa	C49.5	C79.89	—	D21.5	D48.1	D49.2
jaw	C03.9	C79.89	D00.03	D10.39	D48.1	D49.0
knee	C49.2-✓	C79.89	—	D21.2-✓	D48.1	D49.2
leg	C49.2-✓	C79.89	—	D21.2-✓	D48.1	D49.2
limb NEC	C49.9	C79.89	—	D21.9	D48.1	D49.2
lower	C49.2-✓	C79.89	—	D21.2-✓	D48.1	D49.2
upper	C49.1-✓	C79.89	—	D21.1-✓	D48.1	D49.2
nates	C49.5	C79.89	—	D21.5	D48.1	D49.2
neck	C49.0	C79.89	—	D21.0	D48.1	D49.2
orbit	C69.6-✓	C79.49	D09.2-✓	D31.6-✓	D48.1	D49.89
overlapping lesion	C49.8	—	—	—	—	—
pararectal	C49.5	C79.89	—	D21.5	D48.1	D49.2
para-urethral	C49.5	C79.89	—	D21.5	D48.1	D49.2
paravaginal	C49.5	C79.89	—	D21.5	D48.1	D49.2
pelvis (floor)	C49.5	C79.89	—	D21.5	D48.1	D49.2
pelvo-abdominal	C49.8	C79.89	—	D21.6	D48.1	D49.2
perineum	C49.5	C79.89	—	D21.5	D48.1	D49.2
perirectal (tissue)	C49.5	C79.89	—	D21.5	D48.1	D49.2
periurethral (tissue)	C49.5	C79.89	—	D21.5	D48.1	D49.2
popliteal fossa or space	C49.2-✓	C79.89	—	D21.2-✓	D48.1	D49.2
presacral	C49.5	C79.89	—	D21.5	D48.1	D49.2
psoas muscle	C49.4	C79.89	—	D21.4	D48.1	D49.2
pterygoid fossa	C49.0	C79.89	—	D21.0	D48.1	D49.2
rectovaginal septum or wall	C49.5	C79.89	—	D21.5	D48.1	D49.2
rectovesical	C49.5	C79.89	—	D21.5	D48.1	D49.2
retroperitoneum	C48.0	C78.6	—	D20.0	D48.3	D49.0
sacrococcygeal region	C49.5	C79.89	—	D21.5	D48.1	D49.2
scalp	C49.0	C79.89	—	D21.0	D48.1	D49.2
scapular region	C49.3	C79.89	—	D21.3	D48.1	D49.2
shoulder	C49.1-✓	C79.89	—	D21.1-✓	D48.1	D49.2
skin (dermis) NEC — *see also* Neoplasm, skin, by site	C44.90	C79.2	D04.9	D23.9	D48.5	D49.2
stomach	C49.4	C79.89	—	D21.4	D48.1	D49.2
submental	C49.0	C79.89	—	D21.0	D48.1	D49.2
supraclavicular region	C49.0	C79.89	—	D21.0	D48.1	D49.2
temple	C49.0	C79.89	—	D21.0	D48.1	D49.2
temporal region	C49.0	C79.89	—	D21.0	D48.1	D49.2
thigh	C49.2-✓	C79.89	—	D21.2-✓	D48.1	D49.2
thoracic (duct) (wall)	C49.3	C79.89	—	D21.3	D48.1	D49.2
thorax	C49.3	C79.89	—	D21.3	D48.1	D49.2
thumb	C49.1-✓	C79.89	—	D21.1-✓	D48.1	D49.2
toe	C49.2-✓	C79.89	—	D21.2-✓	D48.1	D49.2
trunk	C49.6	C79.89	—	D21.6	D48.1	D49.2
umbilicus	C49.4	C79.89	—	D21.4	D48.1	D49.2
vesicorectal	C49.5	C79.89	—	D21.5	D48.1	D49.2
wrist	C49.1-✓	C79.89	—	D21.1-✓	D48.1	D49.2
conus medullaris	C72.0	C79.49	—	D33.4	D43.4	D49.7
cord (true) (vocal)	C32.0	C78.39	D02.0	D14.1	D38.0	D49.1
false	C32.1	C78.39	D02.0	D14.1	D38.0	D49.1
spermatic	C63.1-✓	C79.82	D07.69	D29.8	D40.8	D49.59
spinal (cervical) (lumbar) (thoracic)	C72.0	C79.49	—	D33.4	D43.4	D49.7
cornea (limbus)	C69.1-✓	C79.49	D09.2-✓	D31.1-✓	D48.7	D49.89
corpus						
albicans	C56.-✓	C79.6-✓	D07.39	D27.-✓	D39.1-✓	D49.59
callosum, brain	C71.0	C79.31	—	D33.2	D43.2	D49.6

Neoplasm, neoplastic — continued	Malignant Primary	Malignant Secondary	Ca in situ	Benign	Uncertain Behavior	Unspecified Behavior
corpus — *continued*						
cavernosum	C60.2	C79.82	D07.4	D29.0	D40.8	D49.59
gastric	C16.2	C78.89	D00.2	D13.1	D37.1	D49.0
overlapping sites	C54.8	—	—	—	—	—
penis	C60.2	C79.82	D07.4	D29.0	D40.8	D49.59
striatum, cerebrum	C71.0	C79.31	—	D33.0	D43.0	D49.6
uteri	C54.9	C79.82	D07.0	D26.1	D39.0	D49.59
isthmus	C54.0	C79.82	D07.0	D26.1	D39.0	D49.59
cortex						
adrenal	C74.0-✓	C79.7-✓	D09.3	D35.0-✓	D44.1-✓	D49.7
cerebral	C71.0	C79.31	—	D33.0	D43.0	D49.6
costal cartilage	C41.3	C79.51	—	D16.7	D48.0	D49.2
costovertebral joint	C41.3	C79.51	—	D16.7	D48.0	D49.2
Cowper's gland	C68.0	C79.19	D09.19	D30.4	D41.3	D49.59
cranial (fossa, any)	C71.9	C79.31	—	D33.2	D43.2	D49.6
meninges	C70.0	C79.32	—	D32.0	D42.0	D49.7
nerve	C72.50	C79.49	—	D33.3	D43.3	D49.7
specified NEC	C72.59	C79.49	—	D33.3	D43.3	D49.7
craniobuccal pouch	C75.2	C79.89	D09.3	D35.2	D44.3	D49.7
craniopharyngeal (duct) (pouch)	C75.2	C79.89	D09.3	D35.3	D44.4	D49.7
cricoid	C13.0	C79.89	D00.08	D10.7	D37.05	D49.0
cartilage	C32.3	C78.39	D02.0	D14.1	D38.0	D49.1
cricopharynx	C13.0	C79.89	D00.08	D10.7	D37.05	D49.0
crypt of Morgagni	C21.8	C78.5	D01.3	D12.9	D37.8	D49.0
crystalline lens	C69.4-✓	C79.49	D09.2-✓	D31.4-✓	D48.7	D49.89
cul-de-sac (Douglas')	C48.1	C78.6	—	D20.1	D48.4	D49.0
cuneiform cartilage	C32.3	C78.39	D02.0	D14.1	D38.0	D49.1
cutaneous — *see* Neoplasm, skin						
cutis — *see* Neoplasm, skin						
cystic (bile) duct (common)	C24.0	C78.89	D01.5	D13.5	D37.6	D49.0
dermis — *see* Neoplasm, skin						
diaphragm	C49.3	C79.89	—	D21.3	D48.1	D49.2
digestive organs, system, tube, or tract NEC	C26.9	C78.89	D01.9	D13.9	D37.9	D49.0
disc, intervertebral	C41.2	C79.51	—	D16.6	D48.0	D49.2
disease, generalized	C80.0	—	—	—	—	—
disseminated	C80.0	—	—	—	—	—
Douglas' cul-de-sac or pouch	C48.1	C78.6	—	D20.1	D48.4	D49.0
duodenojejunal junction	C17.8	C78.4	D01.49	D13.39	D37.2	D49.0
duodenum	C17.0	C78.4	D01.49	D13.2	D37.2	D49.0
dura (cranial) (mater)	C70.9	C79.49	—	D32.9	D42.9	D49.7
cerebral	C70.0	C79.32	—	D32.0	D42.0	D49.7
spinal	C70.1	C79.49	—	D32.1	D42.1	D49.7
ear (external) — *see also* Neoplasm, skin, ear	C44.20-✓	C79.2	D04.2-✓	D23.2-✓	D48.5	D49.2
auricle or auris — *see also* Neoplasm, skin, ear	C44.20-✓	C79.2	D04.2-✓	D23.2-✓	D48.5	D49.2
canal, external — *see also* Neoplasm, skin, ear	C44.20-✓	C79.2	D04.2-✓	D23.2-✓	D48.5	D49.2
cartilage	C49.0	C79.89	—	D21.0	D48.1	D49.2
external meatus — *see also* Neoplasm, skin, ear	C44.20-✓	C79.2	D04.2-✓	D23.2-✓	D48.5	D49.2
inner	C30.1	C78.39	D02.3	D14.0	D38.5	D49.1
lobule — *see also* Neoplasm, skin, ear	C44.20-✓	C79.2	D04.2-✓	D23.2-✓	D48.5	D49.2
middle	C30.1	C78.39	D02.3	D14.0	D38.5	D49.1
overlapping lesion with accessory sinuses	C31.8	—	—	—	—	—

Neoplasm, neoplastic	Malignant Primary	Malignant Secondary	Ca in situ	Benign	Uncertain Behavior	Unspecified Behavior
— continued						
ear — see also						
Neoplasm, skin, ear						
— continued						
skin	C44.20-☑	C79.2	D04.2-☑	D23.2-☑	D48.5	D49.2
basal cell						
carcinoma	C44.21-☑	—	—	—	—	—
specified type NEC	C44.29-☑	—	—	—	—	—
squamous cell						
carcinoma	C44.22-☑	—	—	—	—	—
earlobe	C44.20-☑	C79.2	D04.2-☑	D23.2-☑	D48.5	D49.2
basal cell						
carcinoma	C44.21-☑	—	—	—	—	—
specified type NEC	C44.29-☑	—	—	—	—	—
squamous cell						
carcinoma	C44.22-☑	—	—	—	—	—
ejaculatory duct	C63.7	C79.82	D07.69	D29.8	D40.8	D49.59
elbow NEC	C76.4-☑	C79.89	D04.6-☑	D36.7	D48.7	D49.89
endocardium	C38.0	C79.89	—	D15.1	D48.7	D49.89
endocervix (canal) (gland)	C53.0	C79.82	D06.0	D26.0	D39.0	D49.59
endocrine gland NEC	C75.9	C79.89	D09.3	D35.9	D44.9	D49.7
pluriglandular	C75.8	C79.89	D09.3	D35.7	D44.9	D49.7
endometrium (gland) (stroma)	C54.1	C79.82	D07.0	D26.1	D39.0	D49.59
ensiform cartilage	C41.3	C79.51	—	D16.7	D48.0	D49.2
enteric — see Neoplasm, intestine						
ependyma (brain)	C71.5	C79.31	—	D33.0	D43.0	D49.6
fourth ventricle	C71.7	C79.31	—	D33.1	D43.1	D49.6
epicardium	C38.0	C79.89	—	D15.1	D48.7	D49.89
epididymis	C63.0-☑	C79.82	D07.69	D29.3-☑	D40.8	D49.59
epidural	C72.9	C79.49	—	D33.9	D43.9	D49.7
epiglottis	C32.1	C78.39	D02.0	D14.1	D38.0	D49.1
anterior aspect or surface	C10.1	C79.89	D00.08	D10.5	D37.05	D49.0
cartilage	C32.3	C78.39	D02.0	D14.1	D38.0	D49.1
free border (margin)	C10.1	C79.89	D00.08	D10.5	D37.05	D49.0
junctional region	C10.8	C79.89	D00.08	D10.5	D37.05	D49.0
posterior (laryngeal) surface	C32.1	C78.39	D02.0	D14.1	D38.0	D49.1
suprahyoid portion	C32.1	C78.39	D02.0	D14.1	D38.0	D49.1
esophagogastric junction	C16.0	C78.89	D00.2	D13.1	D37.1	D49.0
esophagus	C15.9	C78.89	D00.1	D13.0	D37.8	D49.0
abdominal	C15.5	C78.89	D00.1	D13.0	D37.8	D49.0
cervical	C15.3	C78.89	D00.1	D13.0	D37.8	D49.0
distal (third)	C15.5	C78.89	D00.1	D13.0	D37.8	D49.0
lower (third)	C15.5	C78.89	D00.1	D13.0	D37.8	D49.0
middle (third)	C15.4	C78.89	D00.1	D13.0	D37.8	D49.0
overlapping lesion	C15.8	—	—	—	—	—
proximal (third)	C15.3	C78.89	D00.1	D13.0	D37.8	D49.0
thoracic	C15.4	C78.89	D00.1	D13.0	D37.8	D49.0
upper (third)	C15.3	C78.89	D00.1	D13.0	D37.8	D49.0
ethmoid (sinus)	C31.1	C78.39	D02.3	D14.0	D38.5	D49.1
bone or labyrinth	C41.0	C79.51	—	D16.4	D48.0	D49.2
eustachian tube	C30.1	C78.39	D02.3	D14.0	D38.5	D49.1
exocervix	C53.1	C79.82	D06.1	D26.0	D39.0	D49.59
external						
meatus (ear) — see also Neoplasm, skin, ear	C44.20-☑	C79.2	D04.2-☑	D23.2-☑	D48.5	D49.2
os, cervix uteri	C53.1	C79.82	D06.1	D26.0	D39.0	D49.59
extradural	C72.9	C79.49	—	D33.9	D43.9	D49.7
extrahepatic (bile) duct	C24.0	C78.89	D01.5	D13.5	D37.6	D49.0
overlapping lesion with gallbladder	C24.8	—	—	—	—	—
extraocular muscle	C69.6-☑	C79.49	D09.2-☑	D31.6-☑	D48.7	D49.89
extrarectal	C76.3	C79.89	D09.8	D36.7	D48.7	D49.89
extremity	C76.8	C79.89	D04.8	D36.7	D48.7	D49.89

Neoplasm, neoplastic	Malignant Primary	Malignant Secondary	Ca in situ	Benign	Uncertain Behavior	Unspecified Behavior
— continued						
extremity — continued						
lower	C76.5-☑	C79.89	D04.7-☑	D36.7	D48.7	D49.89
upper	C76.4-☑	C79.89	D04.6-☑	D36.7	D48.7	D49.89
eyeball	C69.9-☑	C79.49	D09.2-☑	D31.9-☑	D48.7	D49.89
eyebrow	C44.309	C79.2	D04.39	D23.39	D48.5	D49.2
basal cell carcinoma	C44.319	—				
specified type NEC	C44.399	—				
squamous cell carcinoma	C44.329	—				
eyelid (lower) (skin) (upper)	C44.10-☑	—				
basal cell carcinoma	C44.11-☑	—				
cartilage	C49.0	C79.89	—	D21.0	D48.1	D49.2
sebaceous cell	C44.13-☑	—				
specified type NEC	C44.19-☑	—				
squamous cell carcinoma	C44.12-☑	—				
eye NEC	C69.9-☑	C79.49	D09.2-☑	D31.9-☑	D48.7	D49.89
overlapping sites	C69.8-☑	—	—	—	—	—
face NEC	C76.0	C79.89	D04.39	D36.7	D48.7	D49.89
fallopian tube (accessory)	C57.0-☑	C79.82	D07.39	D28.2	D39.8	D49.59
falx (cerebella) (cerebri)	C70.0	C79.32	—	D32.0	D42.0	D49.7
fascia — see also Neoplasm, connective tissue						
palmar	C49.1-☑	C79.89	—	D21.1-☑	D48.1	D49.2
plantar	C49.2-☑	C79.89	—	D21.2-☑	D48.1	D49.2
fatty tissue — see Neoplasm, connective tissue						
fauces, faucial NEC	C10.9	C79.89	D00.08	D10.5	D37.05	D49.0
pillars	C09.1	C79.89	D00.08	D10.5	D37.05	D49.0
tonsil	C09.9	C79.89	D00.08	D10.4	D37.05	D49.0
femur (any part)	C40.2-☑			D16.2-☑		
fetal membrane	C58	C79.82	D07.0	D26.7	D39.2	D49.59
fibrous tissue — see Neoplasm, connective tissue						
fibula (any part)	C40.2-☑	C79.51	—	D16.2-☑	—	—
filum terminale	C72.0	C79.49	—	D33.4	D43.4	D49.7
finger NEC	C76.4-☑	C79.89	D04.6-☑	D36.7	D48.7	D49.89
flank NEC	C76.8	C79.89	D04.5	D36.7	D48.7	D49.89
follicle, nabothian	C53.0	C79.82	D06.0	D26.0	D39.0	D49.59
foot NEC	C76.5-☑	C79.89	D04.7-☑	D36.7	D48.7	D49.89
forearm NEC	C76.4-☑	C79.89	D04.6-☑	D36.7	D48.7	D49.89
forehead (skin)	C44.309	C79.2	D04.39	D23.39	D48.5	D49.2
basal cell carcinoma	C44.319	—				
specified type NEC	C44.399	—				
squamous cell carcinoma	C44.329	—				
foreskin	C60.0	C79.82	D07.4	D29.0	D40.8	D49.59
fornix						
pharyngeal	C11.3	C79.89	D00.08	D10.6	D37.05	D49.0
vagina	C52	C79.82	D07.2	D28.1	D39.8	D49.59
fossa (of)						
anterior (cranial)	C71.9	C79.31	—	D33.2	D43.2	D49.6
cranial	C71.9	C79.31	—	D33.2	D43.2	D49.6
ischiorectal	C76.3	C79.89	D09.8	D36.7	D48.7	D49.89
middle (cranial)	C71.9	C79.31	—	D33.2	D43.2	D49.6
piriform	C12	C79.89	D00.08	D10.7	D37.05	D49.0
pituitary	C75.1	C79.89	D09.3	D35.2	D44.3	D49.7
posterior (cranial)	C71.9	C79.31	—	D33.2	D43.2	D49.6
pterygoid	C49.0	C79.89	—	D21.0	D48.1	D49.2
pyriform	C12	C79.89	D00.08	D10.7	D37.05	D49.0
Rosenmuller	C11.2	C79.89	D00.08	D10.6	D37.05	D49.0
tonsillar	C09.0	C79.89	D00.08	D10.5	D37.05	D49.0
fourchette	C51.9	C79.82	D07.1	D28.0	D39.8	D49.59
frenulum						
labii — see Neoplasm, lip, internal						

Neoplasm, neoplastic
— *continued*

	Malignant Primary	Malignant Secondary	Ca in situ	Benign	Uncertain Behavior	Unspecified Behavior
frenulum — *continued*						
linguae	C02.2	C79.89	D00.07	D10.1	D37.02	D49.0
frontal						
bone	C41.0	C79.51	—	D16.4	D48.0	D49.2
lobe, brain	C71.1	C79.31	—	D33.0	D43.0	D49.6
pole	C71.1	C79.31	—	D33.0	D43.0	D49.6
sinus	C31.2	C78.39	D02.3	D14.0	D38.5	D49.1
fundus						
stomach	C16.1	C78.89	D00.2	D13.1	D37.1	D49.0
uterus	C54.3	C79.82	D07.0	D26.1	D39.0	D49.59
gallbladder	C23	C78.89	D01.5	D13.5	D37.6	D49.0
overlapping lesion with extrahepatic bile ducts	C24.8	—	—	—	—	—
gall duct						
(extrahepatic)	C24.0	C78.89	D01.5	D13.5	D37.6	D49.0
intrahepatic	C22.1	C78.7	D01.5	D13.4	D37.6	D49.0
ganglia — *see also* Neoplasm, nerve,						
peripheral	C47.9	C79.89	—	D36.10	D48.2	D49.2
basal	C71.0	C79.31	—	D33.0	D43.0	D49.6
cranial nerve	C72.50	C79.49	—	D33.3	D43.3	D49.7
Gartner's duct	C52	C79.82	D07.2	D28.1	D39.8	D49.59
gastric — *see* Neoplasm, stomach						
gastrocolic	C26.9	C78.89	D01.9	D13.9	D37.9	D49.0
gastroesophageal junction	C16.0	C78.89	D00.2	D13.1	D37.1	D49.0
gastrointestinal (tract) NEC	C26.9	C78.89	D01.9	D13.9	D37.9	D49.0
generalized	C80.0	—	—	—	—	—
genital organ or tract						
female NEC	C57.9	C79.82	D07.30	D28.9	D39.9	D49.59
overlapping lesion	C57.8	—	—	—	—	—
specified site NEC	C57.7	C79.82	D07.39	D28.7	D39.8	D49.59
male NEC	C63.9	C79.82	D07.60	D29.9	D40.9	D49.59
overlapping lesion	C63.8	—	—	—	—	—
specified site NEC	C63.7	C79.82	D07.69	D29.8	D40.8	D49.59
genitourinary tract						
female	C57.9	C79.82	D07.30	D28.9	D39.9	D49.59
male	C63.9	C79.82	D07.60	D29.9	D40.9	D49.59
gingiva (alveolar) (marginal)	C03.9	C79.89	D00.03	D10.39	D37.09	D49.0
lower	C03.1	C79.89	D00.03	D10.39	D37.09	D49.0
mandibular	C03.1	C79.89	D00.03	D10.39	D37.09	D49.0
maxillary	C03.0	C79.89	D00.03	D10.39	D37.09	D49.0
upper	C03.0	C79.89	D00.03	D10.39	D37.09	D49.0
gland, glandular (lymphatic) (system) — *see also* Neoplasm, lymph gland						
endocrine NEC	C75.9	C79.89	D09.3	D35.9	D44.9	D49.7
salivary — *see* Neoplasm, salivary gland						
glans penis	C60.1	C79.82	D07.4	D29.0	D40.8	D49.59
globus pallidus	C71.0	C79.31	—	D33.0	D43.0	D49.6
glomus						
coccygeal	C49.5	C79.89	—	D21.5	D48.1	D49.2
jugularis	C75.5	C79.89	—	D35.6	D44.7	D49.7
glosso-epiglottic fold(s)	C10.1	C79.89	D00.08	D10.5	D37.05	D49.0
glossopalatine fold	C09.1	C79.89	D00.08	D10.5	D37.05	D49.0
glossopharyngeal sulcus	C09.0	C79.89	D00.08	D10.5	D37.05	D49.0
glottis	C32.0	C78.39	D02.0	D14.1	D38.0	D49.1
gluteal region	C76.3	C79.89	D04.5	D36.7	D48.7	D49.89
great vessels NEC	C49.3	C79.89	—	D21.3	D48.1	D49.2
groin NEC	C76.3	C79.89	D04.5	D36.7	D48.7	D49.89
gum	C03.9	C79.89	D00.03	D10.39	D37.09	D49.0
lower	C03.1	C79.89	D00.03	D10.39	D37.09	D49.0
upper	C03.0	C79.89	D00.03	D10.39	D37.09	D49.0
hand NEC	C76.4-☑	C79.89	D04.6-☑	D36.7	D48.7	D49.89
head NEC	C76.0	C79.89	D04.4	D36.7	D48.7	D49.89
heart	C38.0	C79.89	—	D15.1	D48.7	D49.89

Neoplasm, neoplastic
— *continued*

	Malignant Primary	Malignant Secondary	Ca in situ	Benign	Uncertain Behavior	Unspecified Behavior
heel NEC	C76.5-☑	C79.89	D04.7-☑	D36.7	D48.7	D49.89
helix — *see also* Neoplasm, skin,						
ear	C44.20-☑	C79.2	D04.2-☑	D23.2-☑	D48.5	D49.2
hematopoietic, hemopoietic tissue						
NEC	C96.9	—	—	—	—	—
specified NEC	C96.Z	—	—	—	—	—
hemisphere, cerebral	C71.0	C79.31		D33.0	D43.0	D49.6
hemorrhoidal zone	C21.1	C78.5	D01.3	D12.9	D37.8	D49.0
hepatic — *see also* Index to disease, by histology	C22.9	C78.7	D01.5	D13.4	D37.6	D49.0
duct (bile)	C24.0	C78.89	D01.5	D13.5	D37.6	D49.0
flexure (colon)	C18.3	C78.5	D01.0	D12.3	D37.4	D49.0
primary	C22.8	C78.7	D01.5	D13.4	D37.6	D49.0
hepatobiliary	C24.9	C78.89	D01.5	D13.5	D37.6	D49.0
hepatoblastoma	C22.2	C78.7	D01.5	D13.4	D37.6	D49.0
hepatoma	C22.0	C78.7	D01.5	D13.4	D37.6	D49.0
hilus of lung	C34.0-☑	C78.0-☑	D02.2-☑	D14.3-☑	D38.1	D49.1
hippocampus, brain	C71.2	C79.31	—	D33.0	D43.0	D49.6
hip NEC	C76.5-☑	C79.89	D04.7-☑	D36.7	D48.7	D49.89
humerus (any part)	C40.0-☑	C79.51	D16.0-☑	—	—	
hymen	C52	C79.82	D07.2	D28.1	D39.8	D49.59
hypopharynx, hypopharyngeal NEC	C13.9	C79.89	D00.08	D10.7	D37.05	D49.0
overlapping lesion	C13.8	—	—	—	—	—
postcricoid region	C13.0	C79.89	D00.08	D10.7	D37.05	D49.0
posterior wall	C13.2	C79.89	D00.08	D10.7	D37.05	D49.0
pyriform fossa (sinus)	C12	C79.89	D00.08	D10.7	D37.05	D49.0
hypophysis	C75.1	C79.89	D09.3	D35.2	D44.3	D49.7
hypothalamus	C71.0	C79.31		D33.0	D43.0	D49.6
ileocecum, ileocecal (coil) (junction) (valve)	C18.0	C78.5	D01.0	D12.0	D37.4	D49.0
ileum	C17.2	C78.4	D01.49	D13.39	D37.2	D49.0
ilium	C41.4	C79.51		D16.8	D48.0	D49.2
immunoproliferative NEC	C88.9	—	—	—	—	—
infraclavicular (region)	C76.1	C79.89	D04.5	D36.7	D48.7	D49.89
inguinal (region)	C76.3	C79.89	D04.5	D36.7	D48.7	D49.89
insula	C71.0	C79.31		D33.0	D43.0	D49.6
insular tissue (pancreas)	C25.4	C78.89	D01.7	D13.7	D37.8	D49.0
brain	C71.0	C79.31	—	D33.0	D43.0	D49.6
interarytenoid fold	C13.1	C78.39	D00.08	D10.7	D37.05	D49.0
hypopharyngeal aspect	C13.1	C79.89	D00.08	D10.7	D37.05	D49.0
laryngeal aspect	C32.1	C78.39	D02.0	D14.1	D38.0	D49.1
marginal zone	C13.1	C79.89	D00.08	D10.7	D37.05	D49.0
interdental papillae	C03.9	C79.89	D00.03	D10.39	D37.09	D49.0
lower	C03.1	C79.89	D00.03	D10.39	D37.09	D49.0
upper	C03.0	C79.89	D00.03	D10.39	D37.09	D49.0
internal						
capsule	C71.0	C79.31	—	D33.0	D43.0	D49.6
os (cervix)	C53.0	C79.82	D06.0	D26.0	D39.0	D49.59
intervertebral cartilage or disc	C41.2	C79.51		D16.6	D48.0	D49.2
intestine, intestinal	C26.0	C78.80	D01.40	D13.9	D37.8	D49.0
large	C18.9	C78.5	D01.0	D12.6	D37.4	D49.0
appendix	C18.1	C78.5	D01.0	D12.1	D37.3	D49.0
caput coli	C18.0	C78.5	D01.0	D12.0	D37.4	D49.0
cecum	C18.0	C78.5	D01.0	D12.0	D37.4	D49.0
colon	C18.9	C78.5	D01.0	D12.6	D37.4	D49.0
and rectum	C19	C78.5	D01.1	D12.7	D37.5	D49.0
ascending	C18.2	C78.5	D01.0	D12.2	D37.4	D49.0
caput	C18.0	C78.5	D01.0	D12.0	D37.4	D49.0
descending	C18.6	C78.5	D01.0	D12.4	D37.4	D49.0
distal	C18.6	C78.5	D01.0	D12.4	D37.4	D49.0

☑ Additional Character Required — Refer to the Tabular List for Character Selection　　　 Subterms under main terms may continue to next column or page

Neoplasm, neoplastic	Malignant Primary	Malignant Secondary	Ca in situ	Benign	Uncertain Behavior	Unspecified Behavior
— continued						
intestine, intestinal — continued						
large — continued						
colon — continued						
left	C18.6	C78.5	D01.0	D12.4	D37.4	D49.0
overlapping lesion	C18.8	—	—	—	—	—
pelvic	C18.7	C78.5	D01.0	D12.5	D37.4	D49.0
right	C18.2	C78.5	D01.0	D12.2	D37.4	D49.0
sigmoid (flexure)	C18.7	C78.5	D01.0	D12.5	D37.4	D49.0
transverse	C18.4	C78.5	D01.0	D12.3	D37.4	D49.0
hepatic flexure	C18.3	C78.5	D01.0	D12.3	D37.4	D49.0
ileocecum, ileocecal (coil) (valve)	C18.0	C78.5	D01.0	D12.0	D37.4	D49.0
overlapping lesion	C18.8	—	—	—	—	—
sigmoid flexure (lower)						
(upper)	C18.7	C78.5	D01.0	D12.5	D37.4	D49.0
splenic flexure	C18.5	C78.5	D01.0	D12.3	D37.4	D49.0
small	C17.9	C78.4	D01.40	D13.30	D37.2	D49.0
duodenum	C17.0	C78.4	D01.49	D13.2	D37.2	D49.0
ileum	C17.2	C78.4	D01.49	D13.39	D37.2	D49.0
jejunum	C17.1	C78.4	D01.49	D13.39	D37.2	D49.0
overlapping lesion	C17.8	—	—	—	—	—
tract NEC	C26.0	C78.89	D01.40	D13.9	D37.8	D49.0
intra-abdominal	C76.2	C79.89	D09.8	D36.7	D48.7	D49.89
intracranial NEC	C71.9	C79.31	—	D33.2	D43.2	D49.6
intrahepatic (bile) duct	C22.1	C78.7	D01.5	D13.4	D37.6	D49.0
intraocular	C69.9-☑	C79.49	D09.2-☑	D31.9-☑	D48.7	D49.89
intraorbital	C69.6-☑	C79.49	D09.2-☑	D31.6-☑	D48.7	D49.89
intrasellar	C75.1	C79.89	D09.3	D35.2	D44.3	D49.7
intrathoracic (cavity) (organs)	C76.1	C79.89	D09.8	D15.9	D48.7	D49.89
specified NEC	C76.1	C79.89	D09.8	D15.7	—	—
iris	C69.4-☑	C79.49	D09.2-☑	D31.4-☑	D48.7	D49.89
ischiorectal (fossa)	C76.3	C79.89	D09.8	D36.7	D48.7	D49.89
ischium	C41.4	C79.51	—	D16.8	D48.0	D49.2
island of Reil	C71.0	C79.31	—	D33.0	D43.0	D49.6
islands or islets of Langerhans	C25.4	C78.89	D01.7	D13.7	D37.8	D49.0
isthmus uteri	C54.0	C79.82	D07.0	D26.1	D39.0	D49.59
jaw	C76.0	C79.89	D09.8	D36.7	D48.7	D49.89
bone	C41.1	C79.51	—	D16.5	D48.0	D49.2
lower	C41.1	C79.51	—	D16.5	—	—
upper	C41.0	C79.51	—	D16.4	—	—
carcinoma (any type) (lower) (upper)	C76.0	C79.89				
skin — see also Neoplasm, skin, face	C44.309	C79.2	D04.39	D23.39	D48.5	D49.2
soft tissues	C03.9	C79.89	D00.03	D10.39	D37.09	D49.0
lower	C03.1	C79.89	D00.03	D10.39	D37.09	D49.0
upper	C03.0	C79.89	D00.03	D10.39	D37.09	D49.0
jejunum	C17.1	C78.4	D01.49	D13.39	D37.2	D49.0
joint NEC — see also Neoplasm, bone	C41.9	C79.51	—	D16.9	D48.0	D49.2
acromioclavicular	C40.0-☑	C79.51	—	D16.0-☑	—	—
bursa or synovial membrane — see Neoplasm, connective tissue						
costovertebral	C41.3	C79.51	—	D16.7	D48.0	D49.2
sternocostal	C41.3	C79.51	—	D16.7	D48.0	D49.2
temporomandibular	C41.1	C79.51	—	D16.5	D48.0	D49.2
junction						
anorectal	C21.8	C78.5	D01.3	D12.9	D37.8	D49.0
cardioesophageal	C16.0	C78.89	D00.2	D13.1	D37.1	D49.0
esophagogastric	C16.0	C78.89	D00.2	D13.1	D37.1	D49.0
gastroesophageal	C16.0	C78.89	D00.2	D13.1	D37.1	D49.0
hard and soft palate	C05.9	C79.89	D00.00	D10.39	D37.09	D49.0
ileocecal	C18.0	C78.5	D01.0	D12.0	D37.4	D49.0

Neoplasm, neoplastic	Malignant Primary	Malignant Secondary	Ca in situ	Benign	Uncertain Behavior	Unspecified Behavior
— continued						
junction — continued						
pelvirectal	C19	C78.5	D01.1	D12.7	D37.5	D49.0
pelviureteric	C65.-☑	C79.0-☑	D09.19	D30.1-☑	D41.1-☑	D49.59
rectosigmoid	C19	C78.5	D01.1	D12.7	D37.5	D49.0
squamocolumnar, of cervix	C53.8	C79.82	D06.7	D26.0	D39.0	D49.59
Kaposi's sarcoma — see Kaposi's, sarcoma						
kidney (parenchymal)	C64.-☑	C79.0-☑	D09.19	D30.0-☑	D41.0-☑	D49.51-☑
calyx	C65.-☑	C79.0-☑	D09.19	D30.1-☑	D41.1-☑	D49.51-☑
hilus	C65.-☑	C79.0-☑	D09.19	D30.1-☑	D41.1-☑	D49.51-☑
pelvis	C65.-☑	C79.0-☑	D09.19	D30.1-☑	D41.1-☑	D49.51-☑
knee NEC	C76.5-☑	C79.89	D04.7-☑	D36.7	D48.7	D49.89
labia (skin)	C51.9	C79.82	D07.1	D28.0	D39.8	D49.59
majora	C51.0	C79.82	D07.1	D28.0	D39.8	D49.59
minora	C51.1	C79.82	D07.1	D28.0	D39.8	D49.59
labial — see also Neoplasm, lip	C00.9	C79.89	D00.01	D10.0	D37.01	D49.0
sulcus (lower)						
(upper)	C06.1	C79.89	D00.02	D10.39	D37.09	D49.0
labium (skin)	C51.9	C79.82	D07.1	D28.0	D39.8	D49.59
majus	C51.0	C79.82	D07.1	D28.0	D39.8	D49.59
minus	C51.1	C79.82	D07.1	D28.0	D39.8	D49.59
lacrimal						
canaliculi	C69.5-☑	C79.49	D09.2-☑	D31.5-☑	D48.7	D49.89
duct (nasal)	C69.5-☑	C79.49	D09.2-☑	D31.5-☑	D48.7	D49.89
gland	C69.5-☑	C79.49	D09.2-☑	D31.5-☑	D48.7	D49.89
punctum	C69.5-☑	C79.49	D09.2-☑	D31.5-☑	D48.7	D49.89
sac	C69.5-☑	C79.49	D09.2-☑	D31.5-☑	D48.7	D49.89
Langerhans, islands or islets	C25.4	C78.89	D01.7	D13.7	D37.8	D49.0
laryngopharynx	C13.9	C79.89	D00.08	D10.7	D37.05	D49.0
larynx, laryngeal NEC	C32.9	C78.39	D02.0	D14.1	D38.0	D49.1
aryepiglottic fold	C32.1	C78.39	D02.0	D14.1	D38.0	D49.1
cartilage (arytenoid) (cricoid) (cuneiform) (thyroid)	C32.3	C78.39	D02.0	D14.1	D38.0	D49.1
commissure (anterior) (posterior)	C32.0	C78.39	D02.0	D14.1	D38.0	D49.1
extrinsic NEC	C32.1	C78.39	D02.0	D14.1	D38.0	D49.1
meaning hypopharynx	C13.9	C79.89	D00.08	D10.7	D37.05	D49.0
interarytenoid fold	C32.1	C78.39	D02.0	D14.1	D38.0	D49.1
intrinsic	C32.0	C78.39	D02.0	D14.1	D38.0	D49.1
overlapping lesion	C32.8	—	—	—	—	—
ventricular band	C32.1	C78.39	D02.0	D14.1	D38.0	D49.1
leg NEC	C76.5-☑	C79.89	D04.7-☑	D36.7	D48.7	D49.89
lens, crystalline	C69.4-☑	C79.49	D09.2-☑	D31.4-☑	D48.7	D49.89
lid (lower) (upper)	C44.10-☑	C79.2	D04.1-☑	D23.1-☑	D48.5	D49.2
basal cell carcinoma	C44.11-☑	—	—	—	—	—
sebaceous cell	C44.13-☑	—	—	—	—	—
specified type NEC	C44.19-☑	—	—	—	—	—
squamous cell carcinoma	C44.12-☑	—	—	—	—	—
ligament — see also Neoplasm, connective tissue						
broad	C57.1-☑	C79.82	D07.39	D28.2	D39.8	D49.59
Mackenrodt's	C57.7	C79.82	D07.39	D28.7	D39.8	D49.59
non-uterine — see Neoplasm, connective tissue						
round	C57.2-☑	C79.82	—	D28.2	D39.8	D49.59
sacro-uterine	C57.3	C79.82	—	D28.2	D39.8	D49.59
uterine	C57.3	C79.82	—	D28.2	D39.8	D49.59
utero-ovarian	C57.7	C79.82	D07.39	D28.2	D39.8	D49.59
uterosacral	C57.3	C79.82	—	D28.2	D39.8	D49.59
limb	C76.8	C79.89	D04.8	D36.7	D48.7	D49.89
lower	C76.5-☑	C79.89	D04.7-☑	D36.7	D48.7	D49.89
upper	C76.4-☑	C79.89	D04.6-☑	D36.7	D48.7	D49.89
limbus of cornea	C69.1-☑	C79.49	D09.2-☑	D31.1-☑	D48.7	D49.89

Neoplasm, neoplastic — continued

	Malignant Primary	Malignant Secondary	Ca in situ	Benign	Uncertain Behavior	Unspecified Behavior
lingual NEC — see also Neoplasm, tongue	C02.9	C79.89	D00.07	D10.1	D37.02	D49.0
lingula, lung	C34.1-☑	C78.0-☑	D02.2-☑	D14.3-☑	D38.1	D49.1
lip	C00.9	C79.89	D00.01	D10.0	D37.01	D49.0
buccal aspect — see Neoplasm, lip, internal						
commissure	C00.6	C79.89	D00.01	D10.0	D37.01	D49.0
external	C00.2	C79.89	D00.01	D10.0	D37.01	D49.0
lower	C00.1	C79.89	D00.01	D10.0	D37.01	D49.0
upper	C00.0	C79.89	D00.01	D10.0	D37.01	D49.0
frenulum — see Neoplasm, lip, internal						
inner aspect — see Neoplasm, lip, internal						
internal	C00.5	C79.89	D00.01	D10.0	D37.01	D49.0
lower	C00.4	C79.89	D00.01	D10.0	D37.01	D49.0
upper	C00.3	C79.89	D00.01	D10.0	D37.01	D49.0
lipstick area	C00.2	C79.89	D00.01	D10.0	D37.01	D49.0
lower	C00.1	C79.89	D00.01	D10.0	D37.01	D49.0
upper	C00.0	C79.89	D00.01	D10.0	D37.01	D49.0
lower	C00.1	C79.89	D00.01	D10.0	D37.01	D49.0
internal	C00.4	C79.89	D00.01	D10.0	D37.01	D49.0
mucosa — see Neoplasm, lip, internal						
oral aspect — see Neoplasm, lip, internal						
overlapping lesion	C00.8	—	—	—	—	—
with oral cavity or pharynx	C14.8	—	—	—	—	—
skin (commissure) (lower) (upper)	C44.00	C79.2	D04.0	D23.0	D48.5	D49.2
basal cell carcinoma	C44.01	—	—	—	—	—
specified type NEC	C44.09	—	—	—	—	—
squamous cell carcinoma	C44.02	—	—	—	—	—
upper	C00.0	C79.89	D00.01	D10.0	D37.01	D49.0
internal	C00.3	C79.89	D00.01	D10.0	D37.01	D49.0
vermilion border	C00.2	C79.89	D00.01	D10.0	D37.01	D49.0
lower	C00.1	C79.89	D00.01	D10.0	D37.01	D49.0
upper	C00.0	C79.89	D00.01	D10.0	D37.01	D49.0
lipomatous — see Lipoma, by site						
liver — see also Index to disease, by histology	C22.9	C78.7	D01.5	D13.4	D37.6	D49.0
• primary	C22.8	C78.7	D01.5	D13.4	D37.6	D49.0
lumbosacral plexus	C47.5	C79.89	—	D36.16	D48.2	D49.2
lung	C34.9-☑	C78.0-☑	D02.2-☑	D14.3-☑	D38.1	D49.1
azygos lobe	C34.1-☑	C78.0-☑	D02.2-☑	D14.3-☑	D38.1	D49.1
carina	C34.0-☑	C78.0-☑	D02.2-☑	D14.3-☑	D38.1	D49.1
hilus	C34.0-☑	C78.0-☑	D02.2-☑	D14.3-☑	D38.1	D49.1
lingula	C34.1-☑	C78.0-☑	D02.2-☑	D14.3-☑	D38.1	D49.1
lobe NEC	C34.9-☑	C78.0-☑	D02.2-☑	D14.3-☑	D38.1	D49.1
lower lobe	C34.3-☑	C78.0-☑	D02.2-☑	D14.3-☑	D38.1	D49.1
main bronchus	C34.0-☑	C78.0-☑	D02.2-☑	D14.3-☑	D38.1	D49.1
mesothelioma — see Mesothelioma						
middle lobe	C34.2	C78.0-☑	D02.21	D14.31	D38.1	D49.1
overlapping lesion	C34.8-☑	*	—	—	—	—
upper lobe	C34.1-☑	C78.0-☑	D02.2-☑	D14.3-☑	D38.1	D49.1
lymph, lymphatic channel NEC	C49.9	C79.89	—	D21.9	D48.1	D49.2
gland (secondary)	—	C77.9	—	D36.0	D48.7	D49.89
abdominal	—	C77.2	—	D36.0	D48.7	D49.89
aortic	—	C77.2	—	D36.0	D48.7	D49.89
arm	—	C77.3	—	D36.0	D48.7	D49.89

Neoplasm, neoplastic — continued

lymph, lymphatic channel — continued
gland — continued

	Malignant Primary	Malignant Secondary	Ca in situ	Benign	Uncertain Behavior	Unspecified Behavior
auricular (anterior) (posterior)	—	C77.0	—	D36.0	D48.7	D49.89
axilla, axillary	—	C77.3	—	D36.0	D48.7	D49.89
brachial	—	C77.3	—	D36.0	D48.7	D49.89
bronchial	—	C77.1	—	D36.0	D48.7	D49.89
bronchopulmonary	—	C77.1	—	D36.0	D48.7	D49.89
celiac	—	C77.2	—	D36.0	D48.7	D49.89
cervical	—	C77.0	—	D36.0	D48.7	D49.89
cervicofacial	—	C77.0	—	D36.0	D48.7	D49.89
Cloquet	—	C77.4	—	D36.0	D48.7	D49.89
colic	—	C77.2	—	D36.0	D48.7	D49.89
common duct	—	C77.2	—	D36.0	D48.7	D49.89
cubital	—	C77.3	—	D36.0	D48.7	D49.89
diaphragmatic	—	C77.1	—	D36.0	D48.7	D49.89
epigastric, inferior	—	C77.1	—	D36.0	D48.7	D49.89
epitrochlear	—	C77.3	—	D36.0	D48.7	D49.89
esophageal	—	C77.1	—	D36.0	D48.7	D49.89
face	—	C77.0	—	D36.0	D48.7	D49.89
femoral	—	C77.4	—	D36.0	D48.7	D49.89
gastric	—	C77.2	—	D36.0	D48.7	D49.89
groin	—	C77.4	—	D36.0	D48.7	D49.89
head	—	C77.0	—	D36.0	D48.7	D49.89
hepatic	—	C77.2	—	D36.0	D48.7	D49.89
hilar (pulmonary)	—	C77.1	—	D36.0	D48.7	D49.89
splenic	—	C77.2	—	D36.0	D48.7	D49.89
hypogastric	—	C77.5	—	D36.0	D48.7	D49.89
ileocolic	—	C77.2	—	D36.0	D48.7	D49.89
iliac	—	C77.5	—	D36.0	D48.7	D49.89
infraclavicular	—	C77.3	—	D36.0	D48.7	D49.89
inguina, inguinal	—	C77.4	—	D36.0	D48.7	D49.89
innominate	—	C77.1	—	D36.0	D48.7	D49.89
intercostal	—	C77.1	—	D36.0	D48.7	D49.89
intestinal	—	C77.2	—	D36.0	D48.7	D49.89
intrabdominal	—	C77.2	—	D36.0	D48.7	D49.89
intrapelvic	—	C77.5	—	D36.0	D48.7	D49.89
intrathoracic	—	C77.1	—	D36.0	D48.7	D49.89
jugular	—	C77.0	—	D36.0	D48.7	D49.89
leg	—	C77.4	—	D36.0	D48.7	D49.89
limb						
lower	—	C77.4	—	D36.0	D48.7	D49.89
upper	—	C77.3	—	D36.0	D48.7	D49.89
lower limb	—	C77.4	—	D36.0	D48.7	D49.89
lumbar	—	C77.2	—	D36.0	D48.7	D49.89
mandibular	—	C77.0	—	D36.0	D48.7	D49.89
mediastinal	—	C77.1	—	D36.0	D48.7	D49.89
mesenteric (inferior) (superior)	—	C77.2	—	D36.0	D48.7	D49.89
midcolic	—	C77.2	—	D36.0	D48.7	D49.89
multiple sites in categories C77.0 - C77.5	—	C77.8	—	D36.0	D48.7	D49.89
neck	—	C77.0	—	D36.0	D48.7	D49.89
obturator	—	C77.5	—	D36.0	D48.7	D49.89
occipital	—	C77.0	—	D36.0	D48.7	D49.89
pancreatic	—	C77.2	—	D36.0	D48.7	D49.89
para-aortic	—	C77.2	—	D36.0	D48.7	D49.89
paracervical	—	C77.5	—	D36.0	D48.7	D49.89
parametrial	—	C77.5	—	D36.0	D48.7	D49.89
parasternal	—	C77.1	—	D36.0	D48.7	D49.89
parotid	—	C77.0	—	D36.0	D48.7	D49.89
pectoral	—	C77.3	—	D36.0	D48.7	D49.89
pelvic	—	C77.5	—	D36.0	D48.7	D49.89
peri-aortic	—	C77.2	—	D36.0	D48.7	D49.89
peripancreatic	—	C77.2	—	D36.0	D48.7	D49.89
popliteal	—	C77.4	—	D36.0	D48.7	D49.89
porta hepatis	—	C77.2	—	D36.0	D48.7	D49.89
portal	—	C77.2	—	D36.0	D48.7	D49.89
preauricular	—	C77.0	—	D36.0	D48.7	D49.89
prelaryngeal	—	C77.0	—	D36.0	D48.7	D49.89
presymphysial	—	C77.5	—	D36.0	D48.7	D49.89
pretracheal	—	C77.0	—	D36.0	D48.7	D49.89
primary (any site) NEC	C96.9	—	—	—	—	—

☑ Additional Character Required — Refer to the Tabular List for Character Selection   Subterms under main terms may continue to next column or page

	Malignant Primary	Malignant Secondary	Ca in situ	Benign	Uncertain Behavior	Unspecified Behavior
Neoplasm, neoplastic						
— continued						
lymph, lymphatic						
channel —						
continued						
gland — *continued*						
pulmonary						
(hiler)	—	C77.1	—	D36.0	D48.7	D49.89
pyloric	—	C77.2	—	D36.0	D48.7	D49.89
retroperitoneal	—	C77.2	—	D36.0	D48.7	D49.89
retropharyngeal	—	C77.0	—	D36.0	D48.7	D49.89
Rosenmuller's	—	C77.4	—	D36.0	D48.7	D49.89
sacral	—	C77.5	—	D36.0	D48.7	D49.89
scalene	—	C77.0	—	D36.0	D48.7	D49.89
site NEC	—	C77.9	—	D36.0	D48.7	D49.89
splenic (hilar)	—	C77.2	—	D36.0	D48.7	D49.89
subclavicular	—	C77.3	—	D36.0	D48.7	D49.89
subinguinal	—	C77.4	—	D36.0	D48.7	D49.89
sublingual	—	C77.0	—	D36.0	D48.7	D49.89
submandibular	—	C77.0	—	D36.0	D48.7	D49.89
submaxillary	—	C77.0	—	D36.0	D48.7	D49.89
submental	—	C77.0	—	D36.0	D48.7	D49.89
subscapular	—	C77.3	—	D36.0	D48.7	D49.89
supraclavicular	—	C77.0	—	D36.0	D48.7	D49.89
thoracic	—	C77.1	—	D36.0	D48.7	D49.89
tibial	—	C77.4	—	D36.0	D48.7	D49.89
tracheal	—	C77.1	—	D36.0	D48.7	D49.89
tracheobronchial	—	C77.1	—	D36.0	D48.7	D49.89
upper limb	—	C77.3	—	D36.0	D48.7	D49.89
Virchow's	—	C77.0	—	D36.0	D48.7	D49.89
node — *see also*						
Neoplasm, lymph						
gland						
primary NEC	C96.9	—	—	—	—	—
vessel — *see also*						
Neoplasm,						
connective						
tissue	C49.9	C79.89	—	D21.9	D48.1	D49.2
Mackenrodt's						
ligament	C57.7	C79.82	D07.39	D28.7	D39.8	D49.59
malar	C41.0	C79.51	—	D16.4	D48.0	D49.2
region — *see*						
Neoplasm, cheek						
mammary gland — *see*						
Neoplasm, breast						
mandible	C41.1	C79.51	—	D16.5	D48.0	D49.2
alveolar						
mucosa						
(carcinoma)	C03.1	C79.89	D00.03	D10.39	D37.09	D49.0
ridge or						
process	C41.1	C79.51	—	D16.5	D48.0	D49.2
marrow (bone)						
NEC	C96.9	C79.52	—	—	D47.9	D49.89
mastectomy site (skin)						
— *see also*						
Neoplasm, breast,						
skin	C44.501	C79.2	—	—	—	—
specified as breast						
tissue	C50.8-☑	C79.81	—	—	—	—
mastoid (air cells)						
(antrum)						
(cavity)	C30.1	C78.39	D02.3	D14.0	D38.5	D49.1
bone or process	C41.0	C79.51	—	D16.4	D48.0	D49.2
maxilla, maxillary						
(superior)	C41.0	C79.51	—	D16.4	D48.0	D49.2
alveolar						
mucosa	C03.0	C79.89	D00.03	D10.39	D37.09	D49.0
ridge or process						
(carcinoma)	C41.0	C79.51	—	D16.4	D48.0	D49.2
antrum	C31.0	C78.39	D02.3	D14.0	D38.5	D49.1
carcinoma	C03.0	C79.51	—	—	—	—
inferior — *see*						
Neoplasm,						
mandible						
sinus	C31.0	C78.39	D02.3	D14.0	D38.5	D49.1
meatus external (ear)						
— *see also*						
Neoplasm, skin,						
ear	C44.20-☑	C79.2	D04.2-☑	D23.2-☑	D48.5	D49.2
Meckel diverticulum,						
malignant	C17.3	C78.4	D01.49	D13.39	D37.2	D49.0
mediastinum,						
mediastinal	C38.3	C78.1	—	D15.2	D38.3	D49.89
anterior	C38.1	C78.1	—	D15.2	D38.3	D49.89

	Malignant Primary	Malignant Secondary	Ca in situ	Benign	Uncertain Behavior	Unspecified Behavior
Neoplasm, neoplastic						
— continued						
mediastinum,						
mediastinal —						
continued						
posterior	C38.2	C78.1	—	D15.2	D38.3	D49.89
medulla						
adrenal	C74.1-☑	C79.7-☑	D09.3	D35.0-☑	D44.1-☑	D49.7
oblongata	C71.7	C79.31	—	D33.1	D43.1	D49.6
meibomian gland	C44.10-☑	C79.2	D04.1-☑	D23.1-☑	D48.5	D49.2
basal cell						
carcinoma	C44.11-☑	—	—	—	—	—
sebaceous cell	C44.13-☑	—	—	—	—	—
specified type						
NEC	C44.19-☑	—	—	—	—	—
squamous cell						
carcinoma	C44.12-☑	—	—	—	—	—
melanoma — *see*						
Melanoma						
meninges	C70.9	C79.49	—	D32.9	D42.9	D49.7
brain	C70.0	C79.32	—	D32.0	D42.0	D49.7
cerebral	C70.0	C79.32	—	D32.0	D42.0	D49.7
crainial	C70.0	C79.32	—	D32.0	D42.0	D49.7
intracranial	C70.0	C79.32	—	D32.0	D42.0	D49.7
spinal (cord)	C70.1	C79.49	—	D32.1	D42.1	D49.7
meniscus, knee joint						
(lateral)						
(medial)	C40.2-☑	C79.51	—	D16.2-☑	D48.0	D49.2
Merkel cell — *see*						
Carcinoma, Merkel						
cell						
mesentery,						
mesenteric	C48.1	C78.6	—	D20.1	D48.4	D49.0
mesoappendix	C48.1	C78.6	—	D20.1	D48.4	D49.0
mesocolon	C48.1	C78.6	—	D20.1	D48.4	D49.0
mesopharynx — *see*						
Neoplasm,						
oropharynx						
mesosalpinx	C57.1-☑	C79.82	D07.39	D28.2	D39.8	D49.59
mesothelial tissue —						
see Mesothelioma						
mesothelioma — *see*						
Mesothelioma						
mesovarium	C57.1-☑	C79.82	D07.39	D28.2	D39.8	D49.59
metacarpus (any						
bone)	C40.1-☑	C79.51	—	D16.1-☑	—	—
metastatic NEC — *see*						
also Neoplasm, by						
site,						
secondary	—	C79.9	—	—	—	—
metatarsus (any						
bone)	C40.3-☑	C79.51	—	D16.3-☑	—	—
midbrain	C71.7	C79.31	—	D33.1	D43.1	D49.6
milk duct — *see*						
Neoplasm, breast						
mons						
pubis	C51.9	C79.82	D07.1	D28.0	D39.8	D49.59
veneris	C51.9	C79.82	D07.1	D28.0	D39.8	D49.59
motor tract	C72.9	C79.49	—	D33.9	D43.9	D49.7
brain	C71.9	C79.31	—	D33.2	D43.2	D49.6
cauda equina	C72.1	C79.49	—	D33.4	D43.4	D49.7
spinal	C72.0	C79.49	—	D33.4	D43.4	D49.7
mouth	C06.9	C79.89	D00.00	D10.30	D37.09	D49.0
book-leaf	C06.89	C79.89	—	—	—	—
floor	C04.9	C79.89	D00.06	D10.2	D37.09	D49.0
anterior						
portion	C04.0	C79.89	D00.06	D10.2	D37.09	D49.0
lateral portion	C04.1	C79.89	D00.06	D10.2	D37.09	D49.0
overlapping						
lesion	C04.8	—	—	—	—	—
overlapping						
NEC	C06.80	—	—	—	—	—
roof	C05.9	C79.89	D00.00	D10.39	D37.09	D49.0
specified part						
NEC	C06.89	C79.89	D00.00	D10.39	D37.09	D49.0
vestibule	C06.1	C79.89	D00.00	D10.39	D37.09	D49.0
mucosa						
alveolar (ridge or						
process)	C03.9	C79.89	D00.03	D10.39	D37.09	D49.0
lower	C03.1	C79.89	D00.03	D10.39	D37.09	D49.0
upper	C03.0	C79.89	D00.03	D10.39	D37.09	D49.0
buccal	C06.0	C79.89	D00.02	D10.39	D37.09	D49.0
cheek	C06.0	C79.89	D00.02	D10.39	D37.09	D49.0

Neoplasm, mucosa — Neoplasm, nerve

Neoplasm, neoplastic — continued	Malignant Primary	Malignant Secondary	Ca in situ	Benign	Uncertain Behavior	Unspecified Behavior
mucosa — continued						
lip — see Neoplasm, lip, internal						
nasal	C30.0	C78.39	D02.3	D14.0	D38.5	D49.1
oral	C06.0	C79.89	D00.02	D10.39	D37.09	D49.0
Mullerian duct						
female	C57.7	C79.82	D07.39	D28.7	D39.8	D49.59
male	C63.7	C79.82	D07.69	D29.8	D40.8	D49.59
muscle — see also Neoplasm, connective tissue						
extraocular	C69.6-☑	C79.49	D09.2-☑	D31.6-☑	D48.7	D49.89
myocardium	C38.0	C79.89	—	D15.1	D48.7	D49.89
myometrium	C54.2	C79.82	D07.0	D26.1	D39.0	D49.59
myopericardium	C38.0	C79.89	—	D15.1	D48.7	D49.89
nabothian gland (follicle)	C53.0	C79.82	D06.0	D26.0	D39.0	D49.59
nail — see also Neoplasm, skin, limb	C44.90	C79.2	D04.9	D23.9	D48.5	D49.2
finger — see also Neoplasm, skin, limb, upper	C44.60-☑	C79.2	D04.6-☑	D23.6-☑	D48.5	D49.2
toe — see also Neoplasm, skin, limb, lower	C44.70-☑	C79.2	D04.7-☑	D23.7-☑	D48.5	D49.2
nares, naris (anterior) (posterior)	C30.0	C78.39	D02.3	D14.0	D38.5	D49.1
nasal — see Neoplasm, nose						
nasolabial groove — see also Neoplasm, skin, face	C44.309	C79.2	D04.39	D23.39	D48.5	D49.2
nasolacrimal duct	C69.5-☑	C79.49	D09.2-☑	D31.5-☑	D48.7	D49.89
nasopharynx, nasopharyngeal	C11.9	C79.89	D00.08	D10.6	D37.05	D49.0
floor	C11.3	C79.89	D00.08	D10.6	D37.05	D49.0
overlapping lesion	C11.8	—	—	—	—	—
roof	C11.0	C79.89	D00.08	D10.6	D37.05	D49.0
wall	C11.9	C79.89	D00.08	D10.6	D37.05	D49.0
anterior	C11.3	C79.89	D00.08	D10.6	D37.05	D49.0
lateral	C11.2	C79.89	D00.08	D10.6	D37.05	D49.0
posterior	C11.1	C79.89	D00.08	D10.6	D37.05	D49.0
superior	C11.0	C79.89	D00.08	D10.6	D37.05	D49.0
nates — see also Neoplasm, skin, trunk	C44.509	C79.2	D04.5	D23.5	D48.5	D49.2
neck NEC	C76.0	C79.89	D09.8	D36.7	D48.7	D49.89
skin	C44.40	—	—	—	—	—
basal cell carcinoma	C44.41	—	—	—	—	—
specified type NEC	C44.49	—	—	—	—	—
squamous cell carcinoma	C44.42	—	—	—	—	—
nerve (ganglion)	C47.9	C79.89	—	D36.10	D48.2	D49.2
abducens	C72.59	C79.49	—	D33.3	D43.3	D49.7
accessory (spinal)	C72.59	C79.49	—	D33.3	D43.3	D49.7
acoustic	C72.4-☑	C79.49	—	D33.3	D43.3	D49.7
auditory	C72.4-☑	C79.49	—	D33.3	D43.3	D49.7
autonomic NEC — see also Neoplasm, nerve, peripheral	C47.9	C79.89	—	D36.10	D48.2	D49.2
brachial	C47.1-☑	C79.89	—	D36.12	D48.2	D49.2
cranial	C72.50	C79.49	—	D33.3	D43.3	D49.7
specified NEC	C72.59	C79.49	—	D33.3	D43.3	D49.7
facial	C72.59	C79.49	—	D33.3	D43.3	D49.7
femoral	C47.2-☑	C79.89	—	D36.13	D48.2	D49.2
ganglion NEC — see also Neoplasm, nerve, peripheral	C47.9	C79.89	—	D36.10	D48.2	D49.2
glossopharyngeal	C72.59	C79.49	—	D33.3	D43.3	D49.7
hypoglossal	C72.59	C79.49	—	D33.3	D43.3	D49.7
intercostal	C47.3	C79.89	—	D36.14	D48.2	D49.2
lumbar	C47.6	C79.89	—	D36.17	D48.2	D49.2
median	C47.1-☑	C79.89	—	D36.12	D48.2	D49.2
obturator	C47.2-☑	C79.89	—	D36.13	D48.2	D49.2

Neoplasm, neoplastic — continued	Malignant Primary	Malignant Secondary	Ca in situ	Benign	Uncertain Behavior	Unspecified Behavior
nerve — continued						
oculomotor	C72.59	C79.49	—	D33.3	D43.3	D49.7
olfactory	C47.2-☑	C79.49	—	D33.3	D43.3	D49.7
optic	C72.3-☑	C79.49	—	D33.3	D43.3	D49.7
parasympathetic NEC	C47.9	C79.89	—	D36.10	D48.2	D49.2
peripheral NEC	C47.9	C79.89	—	D36.10	D48.2	D49.2
abdomen	C47.4	C79.89	—	D36.15	D48.2	D49.2
abdominal wall	C47.4	C79.89	—	D36.15	D48.2	D49.2
ankle	C47.2-☑	C79.89	—	D36.13	D48.2	D49.2
antecubital fossa or space	C47.1-☑	C79.89	—	D36.12	D48.2	D49.2
arm	C47.1-☑	C79.89	—	D36.12	D48.2	D49.2
auricle (ear)	C47.0	C79.89	—	D36.11	D48.2	D49.2
axilla	C47.3	C79.89	—	D36.12	D48.2	D49.2
back	C47.6	C79.89	—	D36.17	D48.2	D49.2
buttock	C47.5	C79.89	—	D36.16	D48.2	D49.2
calf	C47.2-☑	C79.89	—	D36.13	D48.2	D49.2
cervical region	C47.0	C79.89	—	D36.11	D48.2	D49.2
cheek	C47.0	C79.89	—	D36.11	D48.2	D49.2
chest (wall)	C47.3	C79.89	—	D36.14	D48.2	D49.2
chin	C47.0	C79.89	—	D36.11	D48.2	D49.2
ear (external)	C47.0	C79.89	—	D36.11	D48.2	D49.2
elbow	C47.1-☑	C79.89	—	D36.12	D48.2	D49.2
extrarectal	C47.5	C79.89	—	D36.16	D48.2	D49.2
extremity	C47.9	C79.89	—	D36.10	D48.2	D49.2
lower	C47.2-☑	C79.89	—	D36.13	D48.2	D49.2
upper	C47.1-☑	C79.89	—	D36.12	D48.2	D49.2
eyelid	C47.0	C79.89	—	D36.11	D48.2	D49.2
face	C47.0	C79.89	—	D36.11	D48.2	D49.2
finger	C47.1-☑	C79.89	—	D36.12	D48.2	D49.2
flank	C47.6	C79.89	—	D36.17	D48.2	D49.2
foot	C47.2-☑	C79.89	—	D36.13	D48.2	D49.2
forearm	C47.1-☑	C79.89	—	D36.12	D48.2	D49.2
forehead	C47.0	C79.89	—	D36.11	D48.2	D49.2
gluteal region	C47.5	C79.89	—	D36.16	D48.2	D49.2
groin	C47.5	C79.89	—	D36.16	D48.2	D49.2
hand	C47.1-☑	C79.89	—	D36.12	D48.2	D49.2
head	C47.0	C79.89	—	D36.11	D48.2	D49.2
heel	C47.2-☑	C79.89	—	D36.13	D48.2	D49.2
hip	C47.2-☑	C79.89	—	D36.13	D48.2	D49.2
infraclavicular region	C47.3	C79.89	—	D36.14	D48.2	D49.2
inguinal (canal) (region)	C47.5	C79.89	—	D36.16	D48.2	D49.2
intrathoracic	C47.3	C79.89	—	D36.14	D48.2	D49.2
ischiorectal fossa	C47.5	C79.89	—	D36.16	D48.2	D49.2
knee	C47.2-☑	C79.89	—	D36.13	D48.2	D49.2
leg	C47.2-☑	C79.89	—	D36.13	D48.2	D49.2
limb NEC	C47.9	C79.89	—	D36.10	D48.2	D49.2
lower	C47.2-☑	C79.89	—	D36.13	D48.2	D49.2
upper	C47.1-☑	C79.89	—	D36.12	D48.2	D49.2
nates	C47.5	C79.89	—	D36.16	D48.2	D49.2
neck	C47.0	C79.89	—	D36.11	D48.2	D49.2
orbit	C69.6-☑	C79.49	—	D31.6-☑	D48.7	D49.2
pararectal	C47.5	C79.89	—	D36.16	D48.2	D49.2
paraurethral	C47.5	C79.89	—	D36.16	D48.2	D49.2
paravaginal	C47.5	C79.89	—	D36.16	D48.2	D49.2
pelvis (floor)	C47.5	C79.89	—	D36.16	D48.2	D49.2
pelvoabdominal	C47.8	C79.89	—	D36.17	D48.2	D49.2
perineum	C47.5	C79.89	—	D36.16	D48.2	D49.2
perirectal (tissue)	C47.5	C79.89	—	D36.16	D48.2	D49.2
periurethral (tissue)	C47.5	C79.89	—	D36.16	D48.2	D49.2
popliteal fossa or space	C47.2-☑	C79.89	—	D36.13	D48.2	D49.2
presacral	C47.5	C79.89	—	D36.16	D48.2	D49.2
pterygoid fossa	C47.0	C79.89	—	D36.11	D48.2	D49.2
rectovaginal septum or wall	C47.5	C79.89	—	D36.16	D48.2	D49.2
rectovesical	C47.5	C79.89	—	D36.16	D48.2	D49.2
sacrococcygeal region	C47.5	C79.89	—	D36.16	D48.2	D49.2
scalp	C47.0	C79.89	—	D36.11	D48.2	D49.2

☑ Additional Character Required — Refer to the Tabular List for Character Selection ▽ Subterms under main terms may continue to next column or page

Neoplasm, neoplastic — continued	Malignant Primary	Malignant Secondary	Ca in situ	Benign	Uncertain Behavior	Unspecified Behavior
nerve — continued						
peripheral — continued						
scapular region	C47.3	C79.89	—	D36.14	D48.2	D49.2
shoulder	C47.1-☑	C79.89	—	D36.12	D48.2	D49.2
submental	C47.0	C79.89	—	D36.11	D48.2	D49.2
supraclavicular region	C47.0	C79.89	—	D36.11	D48.2	D49.2
temple	C47.0	C79.89	—	D36.11	D48.2	D49.2
temporal region	C47.0	C79.89	—	D36.11	D48.2	D49.2
thigh	C47.2-☑	C79.89	—	D36.13	D48.2	D49.2
thoracic (duct) (wall)	C47.3	C79.89	—	D36.14	D48.2	D49.2
thorax	C47.3	C79.89	—	D36.14	D48.2	D49.2
thumb	C47.1-☑	C79.89	—	D36.12	D48.2	D49.2
toe	C47.2-☑	C79.89	—	D36.13	D48.2	D49.2
trunk	C47.6	C79.89	—	D36.17	D48.2	D49.2
umbilicus	C47.4	C79.89	—	D36.15	D48.2	D49.2
vesicorectal	C47.5	C79.89	—	D36.16	D48.2	D49.2
wrist	C47.1-☑	C79.89	—	D36.12	D48.2	D49.2
radial	C47.1-☑	C79.89	—	D36.12	D48.2	D49.2
sacral	C47.5	C79.89	—	D36.16	D48.2	D49.2
sciatic	C47.2-☑	C79.89	—	D36.13	D48.2	D49.2
spinal NEC	C47.9	C79.89	—	D36.10	D48.2	D49.2
accessory	C72.59	C79.49	—	D33.3	D43.3	D49.7
sympathetic NEC — see also Neoplasm, nerve, peripheral	C47.9	C79.89	—	D36.10	D48.2	D49.2
trigeminal	C72.59	C79.49	—	D33.3	D43.3	D49.7
trochlear	C72.59	C79.49	—	D33.3	D43.3	D49.7
ulnar	C47.1-☑	C79.89	—	D36.12	D48.2	D49.2
vagus	C72.59	C79.49	—	D33.3	D43.3	D49.7
nervous system (central)	C72.9	C79.40	—	D33.9	D43.9	D49.7
autonomic — see Neoplasm, nerve, peripheral						
parasympathetic — see Neoplasm, nerve, peripheral						
specified site NEC	—	C79.49	—	D33.7	D43.8	—
sympathetic — see Neoplasm, nerve, peripheral						
nevus — see Nevus						
nipple	C50.0-☑	C79.81	D05.-☑	D24.-☑	—	—
nose, nasal	C76.0	C79.89	D09.8	D36.7	D48.7	D49.89
ala (external) (nasi) — see also Neoplasm, nose, skin	C44.301	C79.2	D04.39	D23.39	D48.5	D49.2
bone	C41.0	C79.51	—	D16.4	D48.0	D49.2
cartilage	C30.0	C78.39	D02.3	D14.0	D38.5	D49.1
cavity	C30.0	C78.39	D02.3	D14.0	D38.5	D49.1
choana	C11.3	C79.89	D00.08	D10.6	D37.05	D49.0
external (skin) — see also Neoplasm, nose, skin	C44.301	C79.2	D04.39	D23.39	D48.5	D49.2
fossa	C30.0	C78.39	D02.3	D14.0	D38.5	D49.1
internal	C30.0	C78.39	D02.3	D14.0	D38.5	D49.1
mucosa	C30.0	C78.39	D02.3	D14.0	D38.5	D49.1
septum	C30.0	C78.39	D02.3	D14.0	D38.5	D49.1
posterior margin	C11.3	C79.89	D00.08	D10.6	D37.05	D49.0
sinus — see Neoplasm, sinus						
skin	C44.301	C79.2	D04.39	D23.39	D48.5	D49.2
basal cell carcinoma	C44.311	—	—	—	—	—
specified type NEC	C44.391	—	—	—	—	—
squamous cell carcinoma	C44.321	—	—	—	—	—
turbinate (mucosa)	C30.0	C78.39	D02.3	D14.0	D38.5	D49.1
bone	C41.0	C79.51	—	D16.4	D48.0	D49.2
vestibule	C30.0	C78.39	D02.3	D14.0	D38.5	D49.1

Neoplasm, neoplastic — continued	Malignant Primary	Malignant Secondary	Ca in situ	Benign	Uncertain Behavior	Unspecified Behavior
nostril	C30.0	C78.39	D02.3	D14.0	D38.5	D49.1
nucleus pulposus	C41.2	C79.51	—	D16.6	D48.0	D49.2
occipital bone	C41.0	C79.51	—	D16.4	D48.0	D49.2
lobe or pole, brain	C71.4	C79.31	—	D33.0	D43.0	D49.6
odontogenic — see Neoplasm, jaw bone						
olfactory nerve or bulb	C72.2-☑	C79.49	—	D33.3	D43.3	D49.7
olive (brain)	C71.7	C79.31	—	D33.1	D43.1	D49.6
omentum	C48.1	C78.6	—	D20.1	D48.4	D49.0
operculum (brain)	C71.0	C79.31	—	D33.0	D43.0	D49.6
optic nerve, chiasm, or tract	C72.3-☑	C79.49	—	D33.3	D43.3	D49.7
oral (cavity)	C06.9	C79.89	D00.00	D10.30	D37.09	D49.0
ill-defined	C14.8	C79.89	D00.00	D10.30	D37.09	D49.0
mucosa	C06.0	C79.89	D00.02	D10.39	D37.09	D49.0
orbit	C69.6-☑	C79.49	D09.2-☑	D31.6-☑	D48.7	D49.89
autonomic nerve	C69.6-☑	C79.49	—	D31.6-☑	D48.7	D49.2
bone	C41.0	C79.51	—	D16.4	D48.0	D49.2
eye	C69.6-☑	C79.49	D09.2-☑	D31.6-☑	D48.7	D49.89
peripheral nerves	C69.6-☑	C79.49	—	D31.6-☑	D48.7	D49.2
soft parts	C69.6-☑	C79.49	D09.2-☑	D31.6-☑	D48.7	D49.89
organ of Zuckerkandl	C75.5	C79.89	—	D35.6	D44.7	D49.7
oropharynx	C10.9	C79.89	D00.08	D10.5	D37.05	D49.0
branchial cleft (vestige)	C10.4	C79.89	D00.08	D10.5	D37.05	D49.0
junctional region	C10.8	C79.89	D00.08	D10.5	D37.05	D49.0
lateral wall	C10.2	C79.89	D00.08	D10.5	D37.05	D49.0
overlapping lesion	C10.8	—	—	—	—	—
pillars or fauces	C09.1	C79.89	D00.08	D10.5	D37.05	D49.0
posterior wall	C10.3	C79.89	D00.08	D10.5	D37.05	D49.0
vallecula	C10.0	C79.89	D00.08	D10.5	D37.05	D49.0
os external	C53.1	C79.82	D06.1	D26.0	D39.0	D49.59
internal	C53.0	C79.82	D06.0	D26.0	D39.0	D49.59
ovary	C56.-☑	C79.6-☑	D07.39	D27.-☑	D39.1-☑	D49.59
oviduct	C57.0-☑	C79.82	D07.39	D28.2	D39.8	D49.59
palate	C05.9	C79.89	D00.00	D10.39	D37.09	D49.0
hard	C05.0	C79.89	D00.05	D10.39	D37.09	D49.0
junction of hard and soft palate	C05.9	C79.89	D00.00	D10.39	D37.09	D49.0
overlapping lesions	C05.8	—	—	—	—	—
soft	C05.1	C79.89	D00.04	D10.39	D37.09	D49.0
nasopharyngeal surface	C11.3	C79.89	D00.08	D10.6	D37.05	D49.0
posterior surface	C11.3	C79.89	D00.08	D10.6	D37.05	D49.0
superior surface	C11.3	C79.89	D00.08	D10.6	D37.05	D49.0
palatoglossal arch	C09.1	C79.89	D00.00	D10.5	D37.09	D49.0
palatopharyngeal arch	C09.1	C79.89	D00.00	D10.5	D37.09	D49.0
pallium	C71.0	C79.31	—	D33.0	D43.0	D49.6
palpebra	C44.10-☑	C79.2	D04.1-☑	D23.1-☑	D48.5	D49.2
basal cell carcinoma	C44.11-☑	—	—	—	—	—
sebaceous cell	C44.13-☑	—	—	—	—	—
specified type NEC	C44.19-☑	—	—	—	—	—
squamous cell carcinoma	C44.12-☑	—	—	—	—	—
pancreas	C25.9	C78.89	D01.7	D13.6	D37.8	D49.0
body	C25.1	C78.89	D01.7	D13.6	D37.8	D49.0
duct (of Santorini) (of Wirsung)	C25.3	C78.89	D01.7	D13.6	D37.8	D49.0
ectopic tissue	C25.7	C78.89	—	D13.6	D37.8	D49.0
head	C25.0	C78.89	D01.7	D13.6	D37.8	D49.0
islet cells	C25.4	C78.89	D01.7	D13.7	D37.8	D49.0
neck	C25.7	C78.89	D01.7	D13.6	D37.8	D49.0
overlapping lesion	C25.8	—	—	—	—	—
tail	C25.2	C78.89	D01.7	D13.6	D37.8	D49.0

Neoplasm Table

Neoplasm, nerve — Neoplasm, pancreas

Neoplasm, neoplastic — continued	Malignant Primary	Malignant Secondary	Ca in situ	Benign	Uncertain Behavior	Unspecified Behavior
para-aortic body	C75.5	C79.89	—	D35.6	D44.7	D49.7
paraganglion NEC	C75.5	C79.89	—	D35.6	D44.7	D49.7
parametrium	C57.3	C79.82	—	D28.2	D39.8	D49.59
paranephric	C48.0	C78.6	—	D20.0	D48.3	D49.0
pararectal	C76.3	C79.89	—	D36.7	D48.7	D49.89
parasagittal (region)	C76.0	C79.89	D09.8	D36.7	D48.7	D49.89
parasellar	C72.9	C79.49	—	D33.9	D43.8	D49.7
parathyroid (gland)	C75.0	C79.89	D09.3	D35.1	D44.2	D49.7
paraurethral	C76.3	C79.89	—	D36.7	D48.7	D49.89
gland	C68.1	C79.19	D09.19	D30.8	D41.8	D49.59
paravaginal	C76.3	C79.89	—	D36.7	D48.7	D49.89
parenchyma, kidney	C64.-✓	C79.0-✓	D09.19	D30.0-✓	D41.0-✓	D49.51-✓
parietal bone	C41.0	C79.51	—	D16.4	D48.0	D49.2
lobe, brain	C71.3	C79.31	—	D33.0	D43.0	D49.6
paroophoron	C57.1-✓	C79.82	D07.39	D28.2	D39.8	D49.59
parotid (duct) (gland)	C07	C79.89	D00.00	D11.0	D37.030	D49.0
parovarium	C57.1-✓	C79.82	D07.39	D28.2	D39.8	D49.59
patella	C40.20	C79.51	—			
peduncle, cerebral	C71.7	C79.31	—	D33.1	D43.1	D49.6
pelvirectal junction	C19	C78.5	D01.1	D12.7	D37.5	D49.0
pelvis, pelvic	C76.3	C79.89	D09.8	D36.7	D48.7	D49.89
bone	C41.4	C79.51	—	D16.8	D48.0	D49.2
floor	C76.3	C79.89	D09.8	D36.7	D48.7	D49.89
renal	C65.-✓	C79.0-✓	D09.19	D30.1-✓	D41.1-✓	D49.51-✓
viscera	C76.3	C79.89	D09.8	D36.7	D48.7	D49.89
wall	C76.3	C79.89	D09.8	D36.7	D48.7	D49.89
pelvo-abdominal	C76.8	C79.89	D09.8	D36.7	D48.7	D49.89
penis	C60.9	C79.82	D07.4	D29.0	D40.8	D49.59
body	C60.2	C79.82	D07.4	D29.0	D40.8	D49.59
corpus (cavernosum)	C60.2	C79.82	D07.4	D29.0	D40.8	D49.59
glans	C60.1	C79.82	D07.4	D29.0	D40.8	D49.59
overlapping sites	C60.8	—	—	—	—	—
skin NEC	C60.9	C79.82	D07.4	D29.0	D40.8	D49.59
periadrenal (tissue)	C48.0	C78.6	—	D20.0	D48.3	D49.0
perianal (skin) — see also Neoplasm, anus, skin	C44.500	C79.2	D04.5	D23.5	D48.5	D49.2
pericardium	C38.0	C79.89	—	D15.1	D48.7	D49.89
perinephric	C48.0	C78.6	—	D20.0	D48.3	D49.0
perineum	C76.3	C79.89	D09.8	D36.7	D48.7	D49.89
periodontal tissue NEC	C03.9	C79.89	D00.03	D10.39	D37.09	D49.0
periosteum — see Neoplasm, bone						
peripancreatic	C48.0	C78.6	—	D20.0	D48.3	D49.0
peripheral nerve NEC	C47.9	C79.89	—	D36.10	D48.2	D49.2
perirectal (tissue)	C76.3	C79.89	—	D36.7	D48.7	D49.89
perirenal (tissue)	C48.0	C78.6	—	D20.0	D48.3	D49.0
peritoneum, peritoneal (cavity)	C48.2	C78.6	—	D20.1	D48.4	D49.0
benign mesothelial tissue — see Mesothelioma, benign						
overlapping lesion with digestive organs	C48.8	—	—	—	—	—
	C26.9	—	—	—	—	—
parietal	C48.1	C78.6	—	D20.1	D48.4	D49.0
pelvic	C48.1	C78.6	—	D20.1	D48.4	D49.0
specified part NEC	C48.1	C78.6	—	D20.1	D48.4	D49.0
peritonsillar (tissue)	C76.0	C79.89	D09.8	D36.7	D48.7	D49.89
periurethral tissue	C76.3	C79.89	—	D36.7	D48.7	D49.89
phalanges foot	C40.3-✓	C79.51	—	D16.3-✓	—	—
hand	C40.1-✓	C79.51	—	D16.1-✓	—	—
pharynx, pharyngeal	C14.0	C79.89	D00.08	D10.9	D37.05	D49.0
bursa	C11.1	C79.89	D00.08	D10.6	D37.05	D49.0

Neoplasm, neoplastic — continued	Malignant Primary	Malignant Secondary	Ca in situ	Benign	Uncertain Behavior	Unspecified Behavior
pharynx, pharyngeal — continued						
fornix	C11.3	C79.89	D00.08	D10.6	D37.05	D49.0
recess	C11.2	C79.89	D00.08	D10.6	D37.05	D49.0
region	C14.0	C79.89	D00.08	D10.9	D37.05	D49.0
tonsil	C11.1	C79.89	D00.08	D10.6	D37.05	D49.0
wall (lateral) (posterior)	C14.0	C79.89	D00.08	D10.9	D37.05	D49.0
pia mater	C70.9	C79.40	—	D32.9	D42.9	D49.7
cerebral	C70.0	C79.32	—	D32.0	D42.0	D49.7
cranial	C70.0	C79.32	—	D32.0	D42.0	D49.7
spinal	C70.1	C79.49	—	D32.1	D42.1	D49.7
pillars of fauces	C09.1	C79.89	D00.08	D10.5	D37.05	D49.0
pineal (body) (gland)	C75.3	C79.89	D09.3	D35.4	D44.5	D49.7
pinna (ear) NEC — see also Neoplasm, skin, ear	C44.20-✓	C79.2	D04.2-✓	D23.2-✓	D48.5	D49.2
piriform fossa or sinus	C12	C79.89	D00.08	D10.7	D37.05	D49.0
pituitary (body) (fossa) (gland) (lobe)	C75.1	C79.89	D09.3	D35.2	D44.3	D49.7
placenta	C58	C79.82	D07.0	D26.7	D39.2	D49.59
pleura, pleural (cavity)	C38.4	C78.2	—	D19.0	D38.2	D49.1
overlapping lesion with heart or mediastinum	C38.8	—	—	—	—	—
parietal	C38.4	C78.2	—	D19.0	D38.2	D49.1
visceral	C38.4	C78.2	—	D19.0	D38.2	D49.1
plexus brachial	C47.1-✓	C79.89	—	D36.12	D48.2	D49.2
cervical	C47.0	C79.89	—	D36.11	D48.2	D49.2
choroid	C71.5	C79.31	—	D33.0	D43.0	D49.6
lumbosacral	C47.5	C79.89	—	D36.16	D48.2	D49.2
sacral	C47.5	C79.89	—	D36.16	D48.2	D49.2
pluriendocrine	C75.8	C79.89	D09.3	D35.7	D44.9	D49.7
pole frontal	C71.1	C79.31	—	D33.0	D43.0	D49.6
occipital	C71.4	C79.31	—	D33.0	D43.0	D49.6
pons (varolii)	C71.7	C79.31	—	D33.1	D43.1	D49.6
popliteal fossa or space	C76.5-✓	C79.89	D04.7-✓	D36.7	D48.7	D49.89
postcricoid (region)	C13.0	C79.89	D00.08	D10.7	D37.05	D49.0
posterior fossa (cranial)	C71.9	C79.31	—	D33.2	D43.2	D49.6
postnasal space	C11.9	C79.89	D00.08	D10.6	D37.05	D49.0
prepuce	C60.0	C79.82	D07.4	D29.0	D40.8	D49.59
prepylorus	C16.4	C78.89	D00.2	D13.1	D37.1	D49.0
presacral (region)	C76.3	C79.89	—	D36.7	D48.7	D49.89
prostate (gland)	C61	C79.82	D07.5	D29.1	D40.0	D49.59
utricle	C68.0	C79.19	D09.19	D30.4	D41.3	D49.59
pterygoid fossa	C49.0	C79.89	—	D21.0	D48.1	D49.2
pubic bone	C41.4	C79.51	—	D16.8	D48.0	D49.2
pudenda, pudendum (female)	C51.9	C79.82	D07.1	D28.0	D39.8	D49.59
pulmonary — see also Neoplasm, lung	C34.9-✓	C78.0-✓	D02.2-✓	D14.3-✓	D38.1	D49.1
putamen	C71.0	C79.31	—	D33.0	D43.0	D49.6
pyloric antrum	C16.3	C78.89	D00.2	D13.1	D37.1	D49.0
canal	C16.4	C78.89	D00.2	D13.1	D37.1	D49.0
pylorus	C16.4	C78.89	D00.2	D13.1	D37.1	D49.0
pyramid (brain)	C71.7	C79.31	—	D33.1	D43.1	D49.6
pyriform fossa or sinus	C12	C79.89	D00.08	D10.7	D37.05	D49.0
radius (any part)	C40.0-✓	C79.51	—	D16.0-✓	—	—
Rathke's pouch	C75.1	C79.89	D09.3	D35.2	D44.3	D49.7
rectosigmoid (junction)	C19	C78.5	D01.1	D12.7	D37.5	D49.0
overlapping lesion with anus or rectum	C21.8	—	—	—	—	—
rectouterine pouch	C48.1	C78.6	—	D20.1	D48.4	D49.0
rectovaginal septum or wall	C76.3	C79.89	D09.8	D36.7	D48.7	D49.89
rectovesical septum	C76.3	C79.89	D09.8	D36.7	D48.7	D49.89
rectum (ampulla)	C20	C78.5	D01.2	D12.8	D37.5	D49.0

Neoplasm, neoplastic — continued	Malignant Primary	Malignant Secondary	Ca in situ	Benign	Uncertain Behavior	Unspecified Behavior
rectum — continued						
and colon	C19	C78.5	D01.1	D12.7	D37.5	D49.0
overlapping lesion with anus or rectosigmoid junction	C21.8	—	—	—	—	—
renal	C64.-☑	C79.0-☑	D09.19	D30.0-☑	D41.0-☑	D49.51-☑
calyx	C65.-☑	C79.0-☑	D09.19	D30.1-☑	D41.1-☑	D49.51-☑
hilus	C65.-☑	C79.0-☑	D09.19	D30.1-☑	D41.1-☑	D49.51-☑
parenchyma	C64.-☑	C79.0-☑	D09.19	D30.0-☑	D41.0-☑	D49.51-☑
pelvis	C65.-☑	C79.0-☑	D09.19	D30.1-☑	D41.1-☑	D49.51-☑
respiratory						
organs or system NEC	C39.9	C78.30	D02.4	D14.4	D38.6	D49.1
tract NEC	C39.9	C78.30	D02.4	D14.4	D38.5	D49.1
upper	C39.0	C78.30	D02.4	D14.4	D38.5	D49.1
retina	C69.2-☑	C79.49	D09.2-☑	D31.2-☑	D48.7	D49.81
retrobulbar	C69.6-☑	C79.49	—	D31.6-☑	D48.7	D49.89
retrocecal	C48.0	C78.6	—	D20.0	D48.3	D49.0
retromolar (area) (triangle) (trigone)	C06.2	C79.89	D00.00	D10.39	D37.09	D49.0
retro-orbital	C76.0	C79.89	D09.8	D36.7	D48.7	D49.89
retroperitoneal (space) (tissue)	C48.0	C78.6	—	D20.0	D48.3	D49.0
retroperitoneum	C48.0	C78.6	—	D20.0	D48.3	D49.0
retropharyngeal	C14.0	C79.89	D00.08	D10.9	D37.05	D49.0
retrovesical (septum)	C76.3	C79.89	D09.8	D36.7	D48.7	D49.89
rhinencephalon	C71.0	C79.31	—	D33.0	D43.0	D49.6
rib	C41.3	C79.51	—	D16.7	D48.0	D49.2
Rosenmuller's fossa	C11.2	C79.89	D00.08	D10.6	D37.05	D49.0
round ligament	C57.2-☑	C79.82	—	D28.2	D39.8	D49.59
sacrococcyx, sacrococcygeal	C41.4	C79.51	—	D16.8	D48.0	D49.2
region	C76.3	C79.89	D09.8	D36.7	D48.7	D49.89
sacrouterine ligament	C57.3	C79.82	—	D28.2	D39.8	D49.59
sacrum, sacral (vertebra)	C41.4	C79.51	—	D16.8	D48.0	D49.2
salivary gland or duct (major)	C08.9	C79.89	D00.00	D11.9	D37.039	D49.0
minor NEC	C06.9	C79.89	D00.00	D10.39	D37.04	D49.0
overlapping lesion	C08.9	—	—	—	—	—
parotid	C07	C79.89	D00.00	D11.0	D37.030	D49.0
pluriglandular	C08.9	C79.89	D00.00	D11.9	D37.039	D49.0
sublingual	C08.1	C79.89	D00.00	D11.7	D37.031	D49.0
submandibular	C08.0	C79.89	D00.00	D11.7	D37.032	D49.0
submaxillary	C08.0	C79.89	D00.00	D11.7	D37.032	D49.0
salpinx (uterine)	C57.0-☑	C79.82	D07.39	D28.2	D39.8	D49.59
Santorini's duct	C25.3	C78.89	D01.7	D13.6	D37.8	D49.0
scalp	C44.40	C79.2	D04.4	D23.4	D48.5	D49.2
basal cell carcinoma	C44.41	—	—	—	—	—
specified type NEC	C44.49	—	—	—	—	—
squamous cell carcinoma	C44.42	—	—	—	—	—
scapula (any part)	C40.0-☑	C79.51	—	D16.0-☑	—	—
scapular region	C76.1	C79.89	D09.8	D36.7	D48.7	D49.89
scar NEC — see also Neoplasm, skin, by site	C44.90	C79.2	D04.9	D23.9	D48.5	D49.2
sciatic nerve	C47.2-☑	C79.89	—	D36.13	D48.2	D49.2
sclera	C69.4-☑	C79.49	D09.2-☑	D31.4-☑	D48.7	D49.89
scrotum (skin)	C63.2	C79.82	D07.61	D29.4	D40.8	D49.59
sebaceous gland — see Neoplasm, skin						
sella turcica	C75.1	C79.89	D09.3	D35.2	D44.3	D49.7
bone	C41.0	C79.51	—	D16.4	D48.0	D49.2
semilunar cartilage (knee)	C40.2-☑	C79.51	—	D16.2-☑	D48.0	D49.2
seminal vesicle	C63.7	C79.82	D07.69	D29.8	D40.8	D49.59
septum						
nasal	C30.0	C78.39	D02.3	D14.0	D38.5	D49.1
posterior margin	C11.3	C79.89	D00.08	D10.6	D37.05	D49.0
rectovaginal	C76.3	C79.89	D09.8	D36.7	D48.7	D49.89
rectovesical	C76.3	C79.89	D09.8	D36.7	D48.7	D49.89

Neoplasm, neoplastic — continued	Malignant Primary	Malignant Secondary	Ca in situ	Benign	Uncertain Behavior	Unspecified Behavior
septum — continued						
urethrovaginal	C57.9	C79.82	D07.30	D28.9	D39.9	D49.59
vesicovaginal	C57.9	C79.82	D07.30	D28.9	D39.9	D49.59
shoulder NEC	C76.4-☑	C79.89	D04.6-☑	D36.7	D48.7	D49.89
sigmoid flexure (lower) (upper)	C18.7	C78.5	D01.0	D12.5	D37.4	D49.0
sinus (accessory)	C31.9	C78.39	D02.3	D14.0	D38.5	D49.1
bone (any)	C41.0	C79.51	—	D16.4	D48.0	D49.2
ethmoidal	C31.1	C78.39	D02.3	D14.0	D38.5	D49.1
frontal	C31.2	C78.39	D02.3	D14.0	D38.5	D49.1
maxillary	C31.0	C78.39	D02.3	D14.0	D38.5	D49.1
nasal, paranasal NEC	C31.9	C78.39	D02.3	D14.0	D38.5	D49.1
overlapping lesion	C31.8	—	—	—	—	—
pyriform	C12	C79.89	D00.08	D10.7	D37.05	D49.0
sphenoid	C31.3	C78.39	D02.3	D14.0	D38.5	D49.1
skeleton, skeletal NEC	C41.9	C79.51	—	D16.9	D48.0	D49.2
Skene's gland	C68.1	C79.19	D09.19	D30.8	D41.8	D49.59
skin NOS	C44.90	C79.2	D04.9	D23.9	D48.5	D49.2
abdominal wall	C44.509	C79.2	D04.5	D23.5	D48.5	D49.2
basal cell carcinoma	C44.519	—	—	—	—	—
specified type NEC	C44.599	—	—	—	—	—
squamous cell carcinoma	C44.529	—	—	—	—	—
ala nasi — see also Neoplasm, nose, skin	C44.301	C79.2	D04.39	D23.39	D48.5	D49.2
ankle — see also Neoplasm, skin, limb, lower	C44.70-☑	C79.2	D04.7-☑	D23.7-☑	D48.5	D49.2
antecubital space — see also Neoplasm, skin, limb, upper	C44.60-☑	C79.2	D04.6-☑	D23.6-☑	D48.5	D49.2
anus	C44.500	C79.2	D04.5	D23.5	D48.5	D49.2
basal cell carcinoma	C44.510	—	—	—	—	—
specified type NEC	C44.590	—	—	—	—	—
squamous cell carcinoma	C44.520	—	—	—	—	—
arm — see also Neoplasm, skin, limb, upper	C44.60-☑	C79.2	D04.6-☑	D23.6-☑	D48.5	D49.2
auditory canal (external) — see also Neoplasm, skin, ear	C44.20-☑	C79.2	D04.2-☑	D23.2-☑	D48.5	D49.2
auricle (ear) — see also Neoplasm, skin, ear	C44.20-☑	C79.2	D04.2-☑	D23.2-☑	D48.5	D49.2
auricular canal (external) — see also Neoplasm, skin, ear	C44.20-☑	C79.2	D04.2-☑	D23.2-☑	D48.5	D49.2
axilla, axillary fold — see also Neoplasm, skin, trunk	C44.509	C79.2	D04.5	D23.5	D48.5	D49.2
back — see also Neoplasm, skin, trunk	C44.509	C79.2	D04.5	D23.5	D48.5	D49.2
basal cell carcinoma	C44.91	—	—	—	—	—
breast	C44.501	C79.2	D04.5	D23.5	D48.5	D49.2
basal cell carcinoma	C44.511	—	—	—	—	—
specified type NEC	C44.591	—	—	—	—	—
squamous cell carcinoma	C44.521	—	—	—	—	—
brow — see also Neoplasm, skin, face	C44.309	C79.2	D04.39	D23.39	D48.5	D49.2
buttock — see also Neoplasm, skin, trunk	C44.509	C79.2	D04.5	D23.5	D48.5	D49.2

Neoplasm Table

Neoplasm, rectum — Neoplasm, skin NOS

Neoplasm Table

Neoplasm, skin NOS — Neoplasm, skin NOS

Neoplasm, neoplastic	Malignant Primary	Malignant Secondary	Ca in situ	Benign	Uncertain Behavior	Unspecified Behavior
— continued						
skin — continued						
calf — see also						
Neoplasm, skin, limb, lower	C44.70-☑	C79.2	D04.7-☑	D23.7-☑	D48.5	D49.2
canthus (eye) (inner) (outer)	C44.10-☑	C79.2	D04.1-☑	D23.1-☑	D48.5	D49.2
basal cell carcinoma	C44.11-☑	—	—	—	—	—
sebaceous cell	C44.13-☑	—	—	—	—	—
specified type NEC	C44.19-☑	—	—	—	—	—
squamous cell carcinoma	C44.12-☑	—	—	—	—	—
cervical region — see also Neoplasm, skin, neck	C44.40	C79.2	D04.4	D23.4	D48.5	D49.2
cheek (external) — see also Neoplasm, skin, face	C44.309	C79.2	D04.39	D23.39	D48.5	D49.2
chest (wall) — see also Neoplasm, skin, trunk	C44.509	C79.2	D04.5	D23.5	D48.5	D49.2
chin — see also Neoplasm, skin, face	C44.309	C79.2	D04.39	D23.39	D48.5	D49.2
clavicular area — see also Neoplasm, skin, trunk	C44.509	C79.2	D04.5	D23.5	D48.5	D49.2
clitoris	C51.2	C79.82	D07.1	D28.0	D39.8	D49.59
columnella — see also Neoplasm, skin, face	C44.309	C79.2	D04.39	D23.39	D48.5	D49.2
concha — see also Neoplasm, skin, ear	C44.20-☑	C79.2	D04.2-☑	D23.2-☑	D48.5	D49.2
ear (external)	C44.20-☑	C79.2	D04.2-☑	D23.2-☑	D48.5	D49.2
basal cell carcinoma	C44.21-☑	—	—	—	—	—
specified type NEC	C44.29-☑	—	—	—	—	—
squamous cell carcinoma	C44.22-☑	—	—	—	—	—
elbow — see also Neoplasm, skin, limb, upper	C44.60-☑	C79.2	D04.6-☑	D23.6-☑	D48.5	D49.2
eyebrow — see also Neoplasm, skin, face	C44.309	C79.2	D04.39	D23.39	D48.5	D49.2
eyelid	C44.10-☑	C79.2	D04.1-☑	D23.1-☑	D48.5	D49.2
basal cell carcinoma	C44.11-☑	—	—	—	—	—
sebaceous cell	C44.13-☑	—	—	—	—	—
specified type NEC	C44.19-☑	—	—	—	—	—
squamous cell carcinoma	C44.12-☑	—	—	—	—	—
face NOS	C44.300	C79.2	D04.30	D23.30	D48.5	D49.2
basal cell carcinoma	C44.310	—	—	—	—	—
specified type NEC	C44.390	—	—	—	—	—
squamous cell carcinoma	C44.320	—	—	—	—	—
female genital organs (external)	C51.9	C79.82	D07.1	D28.0	D39.8	D49.59
clitoris	C51.2	C79.82	D07.1	D28.0	D39.8	D49.59
labium NEC	C51.9	C79.82	D07.1	D28.0	D39.8	D49.59
majus	C51.0	C79.82	D07.1	D28.0	D39.8	D49.59
minus	C51.1	C79.82	D07.1	D28.0	D39.8	D49.59
pudendum	C51.9	C79.82	D07.1	D28.0	D39.8	D49.59
vulva	C51.9	C79.82	D07.1	D28.0	D39.8	D49.59
finger — see also Neoplasm, skin, limb, upper	C44.60-☑	C79.2	D04.6-☑	D23.6-☑	D48.5	D49.2
flank — see also Neoplasm, skin, trunk	C44.509	C79.2	D04.5	D23.5	D48.5	D49.2
foot — see also Neoplasm, skin, limb, lower	C44.70-☑	C79.2	D04.7-☑	D23.7-☑	D48.5	D49.2

Neoplasm, neoplastic	Malignant Primary	Malignant Secondary	Ca in situ	Benign	Uncertain Behavior	Unspecified Behavior
— continued						
skin — continued						
forearm — see also Neoplasm, skin, limb, upper	C44.60-☑	C79.2	D04.6-☑	D23.6-☑	D48.5	D49.2
forehead — see also Neoplasm, skin, face	C44.309	C79.2	D04.39	D23.39	D48.5	D49.2
glabella — see also Neoplasm, skin, face	C44.309	C79.2	D04.39	D23.39	D48.5	D49.2
gluteal region — see also Neoplasm, skin, trunk	C44.509	C79.2	D04.5	D23.5	D48.5	D49.2
groin — see also Neoplasm, skin, trunk	C44.509	C79.2	D04.5	D23.5	D48.5	D49.2
hand — see also Neoplasm, skin, limb, upper	C44.60-☑	C79.2	D04.6-☑	D23.6-☑	D48.5	D49.2
head NEC — see also Neoplasm, skin, scalp	C44.40	C79.2	D04.4	D23.4	D48.5	D49.2
heel — see also Neoplasm, skin, limb, lower	C44.70-☑	C79.2	D04.7-☑	D23.7-☑	D48.5	D49.2
helix — see also Neoplasm, skin, ear	C44.20-☑	C79.2	D04.2-☑	D23.2-☑	D48.5	D49.2
hip — see also Neoplasm, skin, limb, lower	C44.70-☑	C79.2	D04.7-☑	D23.7-☑	D48.5	D49.2
infraclavicular region — see also Neoplasm, skin, trunk	C44.509	C79.2	D04.5	D23.5	D48.5	D49.2
inguinal region — see also Neoplasm, skin, trunk	C44.509	C79.2	D04.5	D23.5	D48.5	D49.2
jaw — see also Neoplasm, skin, face	C44.309	C79.2	D04.39	D23.39	D48.5	D49.2
Kaposi's sarcoma — see Kaposi's, sarcoma, skin						
knee — see also Neoplasm, skin, limb, lower	C44.70-☑	C79.2	D04.7-☑	D23.7-☑	D48.5	D49.2
labia						
majora	C51.0	C79.82	D07.1	D28.0	D39.8	D49.59
minora	C51.1	C79.82	D07.1	D28.0	D39.8	D49.59
leg — see also Neoplasm, skin, limb, lower	C44.70-☑	C79.2	D04.7-☑	D23.7-☑	D48.5	D49.2
lid (lower) (upper)	C44.10-☑	C79.2	D04.1-☑	D23.1-☑	D48.5	D49.2
basal cell carcinoma	C44.11-☑	—	—	—	—	—
sebaceous cell	C44.13-☑	—	—	—	—	—
specified type NEC	C44.19-☑	—	—	—	—	—
squamous cell carcinoma	C44.12-☑	—	—	—	—	—
limb NEC	C44.90	C79.2	D04.9	D23.9	D48.5	D49.2
basal cell carcinoma	C44.91	—	—	—	—	—
lower	C44.70-☑	C79.2	D04.7-☑	D23.7-☑	D48.5	D49.2
basal cell carcinoma	C44.71-☑	—	—	—	—	—
specified type NEC	C44.79-☑	—	—	—	—	—
squamous cell carcinoma	C44.72-☑	—	—	—	—	—
upper	C44.60-☑	C79.2	D04.6-☑	D23.6-☑	D48.5	D49.2
basal cell carcinoma	C44.61-☑	—	—	—	—	—
specified type NEC	C44.69-☑	—	—	—	—	—
squamous cell carcinoma	C44.62-☑	—	—	—	—	—
lip (lower) (upper)	C44.00	C79.2	D04.0	D23.0	D48.5	D49.2

	Malignant Primary	Malignant Secondary	Ca in situ	Benign	Uncertain Behavior	Unspecified Behavior
Neoplasm, neoplastic						
— *continued*						
skin — *continued*						
lip — *continued*						
basal cell						
carcinoma	C44.01	—	—	—	—	—
specified type NEC	C44.09	—	—	—	—	—
squamous cell carcinoma	C44.02	—	—	—	—	—
male genital organs	C63.9	C79.82	D07.60	D29.9	D40.8	D49.59
penis	C60.9	C79.82	D07.4	D29.0	D40.8	D49.59
prepuce	C60.0	C79.82	D07.4	D29.0	D40.8	D49.59
scrotum	C63.2	C79.82	D07.61	D29.4	D40.8	D49.59
mastectomy site (skin) — *see also* Neoplasm, skin, breast	C44.501	C79.2	—	—	—	—
specified as breast tissue	C50.8-✓	C79.81	—	—	—	—
meatus, acoustic (external) — *see also* Neoplasm, skin, ear	C44.20-✓	C79.2	D04.2-✓	D23.2-✓	D48.5	D49.2
melanotic — *see* Melanoma						
Merkel cell — *see* Carcinoma, Merkel cell						
nates — *see also* Neoplasm, skin, trunk	C44.509	C79.2	D04.5	D23.5	D48.5	D49.2
neck	C44.40	C79.2	D04.4	D23.4	D48.5	D49.2
basal cell carcinoma	C44.41	—	—	—	—	—
specified type NEC	C44.49	—	—	—	—	—
squamous cell carcinoma	C44.42	—	—	—	—	—
nevus — *see* Nevus, skin						
nose (external) — *see also* Neoplasm, nose, skin	C44.301	C79.2	D04.39	D23.39	D48.5	D49.2
overlapping lesion	C44.80	—	—	—	—	—
basal cell carcinoma	C44.81	—	—	—	—	—
specified type NEC	C44.89	—	—	—	—	—
squamous cell carcinoma	C44.82	—	—	—	—	—
palm — *see also* Neoplasm, skin, limb, upper	C44.60-✓	C79.2	D04.6-✓	D23.6-✓	D48.5	D49.2
palpebra	C44.10-✓	C79.2	D04.1-✓	D23.1-✓	D48.5	D49.2
basal cell carcinoma	C44.11-✓	—	—	—	—	—
sebaceous cell	C44.13-✓	—	—	—	—	—
specified type NEC	C44.19-✓	—	—	—	—	—
squamous cell carcinoma	C44.12-✓	—	—	—	—	—
penis NEC	C60.9	C79.82	D07.4	D29.0	D40.8	D49.59
perianal — *see also* Neoplasm, skin, anus	C44.500	C79.2	D04.5	D23.5	D48.5	D49.2
perineum — *see also* Neoplasm, skin, anus	C44.500	C79.2	D04.5	D23.5	D48.5	D49.2
pinna — *see also* Neoplasm, skin, ear	C44.20-✓	C79.2	D04.2-✓	D23.2-✓	D48.5	D49.2
plantar — *see also* Neoplasm, skin, limb, lower	C44.70-✓	C79.2	D04.7-✓	D23.7-✓	D48.5	D49.2
popliteal fossa or space — *see also* Neoplasm, skin, limb, lower	C44.70-✓	C79.2	D04.7-✓	D23.7-✓	D48.5	D49.2
prepuce	C60.0	C79.82	D07.4	D29.0	D40.8	D49.59
Neoplasm, neoplastic						
— *continued*						
skin — *continued*						
pubes — *see also* Neoplasm, skin, trunk	C44.509	C79.2	D04.5	D23.5	D48.5	D49.2
sacrococcygeal region — *see also* Neoplasm, skin, trunk	C44.509	C79.2	D04.5	D23.5	D48.5	D49.2
scalp	C44.40	C79.2	D04.4	D23.4	D48.5	D49.2
basal cell carcinoma	C44.41	—	—	—	—	—
specified type NEC	C44.49	—	—	—	—	—
squamous cell carcinoma	C44.42	—	—	—	—	—
scapular region — *see also* Neoplasm, skin, trunk	C44.509	C79.2	D04.5	D23.5	D48.5	D49.2
scrotum	C63.2	C79.82	D07.61	D29.4	D40.8	D49.59
shoulder — *see also* Neoplasm, skin, limb, upper	C44.60-✓	C79.2	D04.6-✓	D23.6-✓	D48.5	D49.2
sole (foot) — *see also* Neoplasm, skin, limb, lower	C44.70-✓	C79.2	D04.7-✓	D23.7-✓	D48.5	D49.2
specified sites NEC	C44.80	C79.2	D04.8	D23.9	D48.5	D49.2
basal cell carcinoma	C44.81	—	—	—	—	—
specified type NEC	C44.89	—	—	—	—	—
squamous cell carcinoma	C44.82	—	—	—	—	—
specified type NEC	C44.99	—	—	—	—	—
squamous cell carcinoma	C44.92	—	—	—	—	—
submammary fold — *see also* Neoplasm, skin, trunk	C44.509	C79.2	D04.5	D23.5	D48.5	D49.2
supraclavicular region — *see also* Neoplasm, skin, neck	C44.40	C79.2	D04.4	D23.4	D48.5	D49.2
temple — *see also* Neoplasm, skin, face	C44.309	C79.2	D04.39	D23.39	D48.5	D49.2
thigh — *see also* Neoplasm, skin, limb, lower	C44.70-✓	C79.2	D04.7-✓	D23.7-✓	D48.5	D49.2
thoracic wall — *see also* Neoplasm, skin, trunk	C44.509	C79.2	D04.5	D23.5	D48.5	D49.2
thumb — *see also* Neoplasm, skin, limb, upper	C44.60-✓	C79.2	D04.6-✓	D23.6-✓	D48.5	D49.2
toe — *see also* Neoplasm, skin, limb, lower	C44.70-✓	C79.2	D04.7-✓	D23.7-✓	D48.5	D49.2
tragus — *see also* Neoplasm, skin, ear	C44.20-✓	C79.2	D04.2-✓	D23.2-✓	D48.5	D49.2
trunk	C44.509	C79.2	D04.5	D23.5	D48.5	D49.2
basal cell carcinoma	C44.519	—	—	—	—	—
specified type NEC	C44.599	—	—	—	—	—
squamous cell carcinoma	C44.529	—	—	—	—	—
umbilicus — *see also* Neoplasm, skin, trunk	C44.509	C79.2	D04.5	D23.5	D48.5	D49.2
vulva	C51.9	C79.82	D07.1	D28.0	D39.8	D49.59
overlapping lesion	C51.8					
wrist — *see also* Neoplasm, skin, limb, upper	C44.60-✓	C79.2	D04.6-✓	D23.6-✓	D48.5	D49.2
skull	C41.0	C79.51		D16.4	D48.0	D49.2

Neoplasm, neoplastic — continued	Malignant Primary	Malignant Secondary	Ca in situ	Benign	Uncertain Behavior	Unspecified Behavior
soft parts or tissues — see Neoplasm, connective tissue						
specified site NEC	C76.8	C79.89	D09.8	D36.7	D48.7	D49.89
spermatic cord	C63.1-☑	C79.82	D07.69	D29.8	D40.8	D49.59
sphenoid	C31.3	C78.39	D02.3	D14.0	D38.5	D49.1
bone	C41.0	C79.51	—	D16.4	D48.0	D49.2
sinus	C31.3	C78.39	D02.3	D14.0	D38.5	D49.1
sphincter						
anal	C21.1	C78.5	D01.3	D12.9	D37.8	D49.0
of Oddi	C24.0	C78.89	D01.5	D13.5	D37.6	D49.0
spine, spinal						
(column)	C41.2	C79.51	—	D16.6	D48.0	D49.2
bulb	C71.7	C79.31	—	D33.1	D43.1	D49.6
coccyx	C41.4	C79.51	—	D16.8	D48.0	D49.2
cord (cervical) (lumbar) (sacral) (thoracic)	C72.0	C79.49	—	D33.4	D43.4	D49.7
dura mater	C70.1	C79.49	—	D32.1	D42.1	D49.7
lumbosacral	C41.2	C79.51	—	D16.6	D48.0	D49.2
marrow NEC	C96.9	C79.52	—	—	D47.9	D49.89
membrane	C70.1	C79.49	—	D32.1	D42.1	D49.7
meninges	C70.1	C79.49	—	D32.1	D42.1	D49.7
nerve (root)	C47.9	C79.89	—	D36.10	D48.2	D49.2
pia mater	C70.1	C79.49	—	D32.1	D42.1	D49.7
root	C47.9	C79.89	—	D36.10	D48.2	D49.2
sacrum	C41.4	C79.51	—	D16.8	D48.0	D49.2
spleen, splenic NEC	C26.1	C78.89	D01.7	D13.9	D37.8	D49.0
flexure (colon)	C18.5	C78.5	D01.0	D12.3	D37.4	D49.0
stem, brain	C71.7	C79.31	—	D33.1	D43.1	D49.6
Stensen's duct	C07	C79.89	D00.00	D11.0	D37.030	D49.0
sternum	C41.3	C79.51	—	D16.7	D48.0	D49.2
stomach	C16.9	C78.89	D00.2	D13.1	D37.1	D49.0
antrum (pyloric)	C16.3	C78.89	D00.2	D13.1	D37.1	D49.0
body	C16.2	C78.89	D00.2	D13.1	D37.1	D49.0
cardia	C16.0	C78.89	D00.2	D13.1	D37.1	D49.0
cardiac orifice	C16.0	C78.89	D00.2	D13.1	D37.1	D49.0
corpus	C16.2	C78.89	D00.2	D13.1	D37.1	D49.0
fundus	C16.1	C78.89	D00.2	D13.1	D37.1	D49.0
greater curvature NEC	C16.6	C78.89	D00.2	D13.1	D37.1	D49.0
lesser curvature NEC	C16.5	C78.89	D00.2	D13.1	D37.1	D49.0
overlapping lesion	C16.8	—	—	—	—	—
prepylorus	C16.4	C78.89	D00.2	D13.1	D37.1	D49.0
pylorus	C16.4	C78.89	D00.2	D13.1	D37.1	D49.0
wall NEC	C16.9	C78.89	D00.2	D13.1	D37.1	D49.0
anterior NEC	C16.8	C78.89	D00.2	D13.1	D37.1	D49.0
posterior NEC	C16.8	C78.89	D00.2	D13.1	D37.1	D49.0
stroma, endometrial	C54.1	C79.82	D07.0	D26.1	D39.0	D49.59
stump, cervical	C53.8	C79.82	D06.7	D26.0	D39.0	D49.59
subcutaneous (nodule) (tissue) NEC — see Neoplasm, connective tissue						
subdural	C70.9	C79.32	—	D32.9	D42.9	D49.7
subglottis, subglottic	C32.2	C78.39	D02.0	D14.1	D38.0	D49.1
sublingual	C04.9	C79.89	D00.06	D10.2	D37.09	D49.0
gland or duct	C08.1	C79.89	D00.00	D11.7	D37.031	D49.0
submandibular gland	C08.0	C79.89	D00.00	D11.7	D37.032	D49.0
submaxillary gland or duct	C08.0	C79.89	D00.00	D11.7	D37.032	D49.0
submental	C76.0	C79.89	D09.8	D36.7	D48.7	D49.89
subpleural	C34.9-☑	C78.0-☑	D02.2-☑	D14.3-☑	D38.1	D49.1
substernal	C38.1	C78.1	—	D15.2	D38.3	D49.89
sudoriferous, sudoriparous gland, site unspecified	C44.90	C79.2	D04.9	D23.9	D48.5	D49.2
specified site — see Neoplasm, skin						
supraclavicular region	C76.0	C79.89	D09.8	D36.7	D48.7	D49.89
supraglottis	C32.1	C78.39	D02.0	D14.1	D38.0	D49.1
suprarenal	C74.9-☑	C79.7-☑	D09.3	D35.0-☑	D44.1-☑	D49.7
capsule	C74.9-☑	C79.7-☑	D09.3	D35.0-☑	D44.1-☑	D49.7

Neoplasm, neoplastic — continued	Malignant Primary	Malignant Secondary	Ca in situ	Benign	Uncertain Behavior	Unspecified Behavior
suprarenal — continued						
cortex	C74.0-☑	C79.7-☑	D09.3	D35.0-☑	D44.1-☑	D49.7
gland	C74.9-☑	C79.7-☑	D09.3	D35.0-☑	D44.1-☑	D49.7
medulla	C74.1-☑	C79.7-☑	D09.3	D35.0-☑	D44.1-☑	D49.7
suprasellar (region)	C71.9	C79.31	—	D33.2	D43.2	D49.6
supratentorial (brain) NEC	C71.0	C79.31	—	D33.0	D43.0	D49.6
sweat gland (apocrine) (eccrine), site unspecified	C44.90	C79.2	D04.9	D23.9	D48.5	D49.2
specified site — see Neoplasm, skin						
sympathetic nerve or nervous system NEC	C47.9	C79.89	—	D36.10	D48.2	D49.2
symphysis pubis	C41.4	C79.51	—	D16.8	D48.0	D49.2
synovial membrane — see Neoplasm, connective tissue						
tapetum, brain	C71.8	C79.31	—	D33.2	D43.2	D49.6
tarsus (any bone)	C40.3-☑	C79.51	—	D16.3-☑	—	—
temple (skin) — see also Neoplasm, skin, face	C44.309	C79.2	D04.39	D23.39	D48.5	D49.2
temporal						
bone	C41.0	C79.51	—	D16.4	D48.0	D49.2
lobe or pole	C71.2	C79.31	—	D33.0	D43.0	D49.6
region	C76.0	C79.89	D09.8	D36.7	D48.7	D49.89
skin — see also Neoplasm, skin, face	C44.309	C79.2	D04.39	D23.39	D48.5	D49.2
tendon (sheath) — see Neoplasm, connective tissue						
tentorium (cerebelli)	C70.0	C79.32	—	D32.0	D42.0	D49.7
testis, testes	C62.9-☑	C79.82	D07.69	D29.2-☑	D40.1-☑	D49.59
descended	C62.1-☑	C79.82	D07.69	D29.2-☑	D40.1-☑	D49.59
ectopic	C62.0-☑	C79.82	D07.69	D29.2-☑	D40.1-☑	D49.59
retained	C62.0-☑	C79.82	D07.69	D29.2-☑	D40.1-☑	D49.59
scrotal	C62.1-☑	C79.82	D07.69	D29.2-☑	D40.1-☑	D49.59
undescended	C62.0-☑	C79.82	D07.69	D29.2-☑	D40.1-☑	D49.59
unspecified whether descended or undescended	C62.9-☑	C79.82	D07.69	D29.2-☑	D40.1-☑	D49.59
thalamus	C71.0	C79.31	—	D33.0	D43.0	D49.6
thigh NEC	C76.5-☑	C79.89	D04.7-☑	D36.7	D48.7	D49.89
thorax, thoracic (cavity) (organs NEC)	C76.1	C79.89	D09.8	D36.7	D48.7	D49.89
duct	C49.3	C79.89		D21.3	D48.1	D49.2
wall NEC	C76.1	C79.89	D09.8	D36.7	D48.7	D49.89
throat	C14.0	C79.89	D00.08	D10.9	D37.05	D49.0
thumb NEC	C76.4-☑	C79.89	D04.6-☑	D36.7	D48.7	D49.89
thymus (gland)	C37	C79.89	D09.3	D15.0	D38.4	D49.89
thyroglossal duct	C73	C79.89	D09.3	D34	D44.0	D49.7
thyroid (gland)	C73	C79.89	D09.3	D34	D44.0	D49.7
cartilage	C32.3	C78.39	D02.0	D14.1	D38.0	D49.1
tibia (any part)	C40.2-☑	C79.51	—	D16.2-☑	—	—
toe NEC	C76.5-☑	C79.89	D04.7-☑	D36.7	D48.7	D49.89
tongue	C02.9	C79.89	D00.07	D10.1	D37.02	D49.0
anterior (two-thirds) NEC	C02.3	C79.89	D00.07	D10.1	D37.02	D49.0
dorsal surface	C02.0	C79.89	D00.07	D10.1	D37.02	D49.0
ventral surface	C02.2	C79.89	D00.07	D10.1	D37.02	D49.0
base (dorsal surface)	C01	C79.89	D00.07	D10.1	D37.02	D49.0
border (lateral)	C02.1	C79.89	D00.07	D10.1	D37.02	D49.0
dorsal surface NEC	C02.0	C79.89	D00.07	D10.1	D37.02	D49.0
fixed part NEC	C01	C79.89	D00.07	D10.1	D37.02	D49.0
foreamen cecum	C02.0	C79.89	D00.07	D10.1	D37.02	D49.0
frenulum linguae	C02.2	C79.89	D00.07	D10.1	D37.02	D49.0
junctional zone	C02.8	C79.89	D00.07	D10.1	D37.02	D49.0
margin (lateral)	C02.1	C79.89	D00.07	D10.1	D37.02	D49.0
midline NEC	C02.0	C79.89	D00.07	D10.1	D37.02	D49.0
mobile part NEC	C02.3	C79.89	D00.07	D10.1	D37.02	D49.0

☑ Additional Character Required — Refer to the Tabular List for Character Selection ▽ Subterms under main terms may continue to next column or page

Neoplasm Table

Neoplasm, neoplastic — continued	Malignant Primary	Malignant Secondary	Ca in situ	Benign	Uncertain Behavior	Unspecified Behavior
tongue — continued						
overlapping lesion	C02.8	—	—	—	—	—
posterior (third)	C01	C79.89	D00.07	D10.1	D37.02	D49.0
root	C01	C79.89	D00.07	D10.1	D37.02	D49.0
surface (dorsal)	C02.0	C79.89	D00.07	D10.1	D37.02	D49.0
base	C01	C79.89	D00.07	D10.1	D37.02	D49.0
ventral	C02.2	C79.89	D00.07	D10.1	D37.02	D49.0
tip	C02.1	C79.89	D00.07	D10.1	D37.02	D49.0
tonsil	C02.4	C79.89	D00.07	D10.1	D37.02	D49.0
tonsil	C09.9	C79.89	D00.08	D10.4	D37.05	D49.0
fauces, faucial	C09.9	C79.89	D00.08	D10.4	D37.05	D49.0
lingual	C02.4	C79.89	D00.07	D10.1	D37.02	D49.0
overlapping sites	C09.8	—	—	—	—	—
palatine	C09.9	C79.89	D00.08	D10.4	D37.05	D49.0
pharyngeal	C11.1	C79.89	D00.08	D10.6	D37.05	D49.0
pillar (anterior) (posterior)	C09.1	C79.89	D00.08	D10.5	D37.05	D49.0
tonsillar fossa	C09.0	C79.89	D00.08	D10.5	D37.05	D49.0
tooth socket NEC	C03.9	C79.89	D00.03	D10.39	D37.09	D49.0
trachea (cartilage) (mucosa)	C33	C78.39	D02.1	D14.2	D38.1	D49.1
overlapping lesion with bronchus or lung	C34.8-☑	—	—	—	—	—
tracheobronchial	C34.8-☑	C78.39	D02.1	D14.2	D38.1	D49.1
overlapping lesion with lung	C34.8-☑	—	—	—	—	—
tragus — see also Neoplasm, skin, ear	C44.20-☑	C79.2	D04.2-☑	D23.2-☑	D48.5	D49.2
trunk NEC	C76.8	C79.89	D04.5	D36.7	D48.7	D49.89
tubo-ovarian	C57.8	C79.82	D07.39	D28.7	D39.8	D49.59
tunica vaginalis	C63.7	C79.82	D07.69	D29.8	D40.8	D49.59
turbinate (bone)	C41.0	C79.51	—	D16.4	D48.0	D49.2
nasal	C30.0	C78.39	D02.3	D14.0	D38.5	D49.1
tympanic cavity	C30.1	C78.39	D02.3	D14.0	D38.5	D49.1
ulna (any part)	C40.0-☑	C79.51	—	D16.0-☑	—	—
umbilicus, umbilical — see also Neoplasm, skin, trunk	C44.509	C79.2	D04.5	D23.5	D48.5	D49.2
uncus, brain	C71.2	C79.31	—	D33.0	D43.0	D49.6
unknown site or unspecified	C80.1	C79.9	D09.9	D36.9	D48.9	D49.9
urachus	C67.7	C79.11	D09.0	D30.3	D41.4	D49.4
ureter-bladder (junction)	C67.6	C79.11	D09.0	D30.3	D41.4	D49.4
ureter, ureteral	C66.-☑	C79.19	D09.19	D30.2-☑	D41.2-☑	D49.59
orifice (bladder)	C67.6	C79.11	D09.0	D30.3	D41.4	D49.4
urethra, urethral (gland)	C68.0	C79.19	D09.19	D30.4	D41.3	D49.59
orifice, internal	C67.5	C79.11	D09.0	D30.3	D41.4	D49.4
urethrovaginal (septum)	C57.9	C79.82	D07.30	D28.9	D39.8	D49.59
urinary organ or system	C68.9	C79.10	D09.10	D30.9	D41.9	D49.59
bladder — see Neoplasm, bladder						
overlapping lesion	C68.8	—	—	—	—	—
specified sites NEC	C68.8	C79.19	D09.19	D30.8	D41.8	D49.59
utero-ovarian	C57.8	C79.82	D07.39	D28.7	D39.8	D49.59
ligament	C57.1-☑	C79.82	D07.39	D28.2	D39.8	D49.59
uterosacral ligament	C57.3	C79.82	—	D28.2	D39.8	D49.59
uterus, uteri, uterine	C55	C79.82	D07.0	D26.9	D39.0	D49.59
adnexa NEC	C57.4	C79.82	D07.39	D28.7	D39.8	D49.59
body	C54.9	C79.82	D07.0	D26.1	D39.0	D49.59
cervix	C53.9	C79.82	D06.9	D26.0	D39.0	D49.59
cornu	C54.9	C79.82	D07.0	D26.1	D39.0	D49.59
corpus	C54.9	C79.82	D07.0	D26.1	D39.0	D49.59
endocervix (canal) (gland)	C53.0	C79.82	D06.0	D26.0	D39.0	D49.59
endometrium	C54.1	C79.82	D07.0	D26.1	D39.0	D49.59
exocervix	C53.1	C79.82	D06.1	D26.0	D39.0	D49.59
external os	C53.1	C79.82	D06.1	D26.0	D39.0	D49.59
fundus	C54.3	C79.82	D07.0	D26.1	D39.0	D49.59

Neoplasm, neoplastic — continued	Malignant Primary	Malignant Secondary	Ca in situ	Benign	Uncertain Behavior	Unspecified Behavior
uterus, uteri, uterine — continued						
internal os	C53.0	C79.82	D06.0	D26.0	D39.0	D49.59
isthmus	C54.0	C79.82	D07.0	D26.1	D39.0	D49.59
ligament	C57.3	C79.82	—	D28.2	D39.8	D49.59
broad	C57.1-☑	C79.82	D07.39	D28.2	D39.8	D49.59
round	C57.2-☑	C79.82	—	D28.2	D39.8	D49.59
lower segment	C54.0	C79.82	D07.0	D26.1	D39.0	D49.59
myometrium	C54.2	C79.82	D07.0	D26.1	D39.0	D49.59
overlapping sites	C54.8	—	—	—	—	—
squamocolumnar junction	C53.8	C79.82	D06.7	D26.0	D39.0	D49.59
tube	C57.0-☑	C79.82	D07.39	D28.2	D39.8	D49.59
utricle, prostatic	C68.0	C79.19	D09.19	D30.4	D41.3	D49.59
uveal tract	C69.4-☑	C79.49	D09.2-☑	D31.4-☑	D48.7	D49.89
uvula	C05.2	C79.89	D00.04	D10.39	D37.09	D49.0
vagina, vaginal (fornix) (vault) (wall)	C52	C79.82	D07.2	D28.1	D39.8	D49.59
vaginovesical	C57.9	C79.82	D07.30	D28.9	D39.9	D49.59
septum	C57.9	C79.82	D07.30	D28.9	D39.9	D49.59
vallecula (epigiottis)	C10.0	C79.89	D00.08	D10.5	D37.05	D49.0
vascular — see Neoplasm, connective tissue						
vas deferens	C63.1-☑	C79.82	D07.69	D29.8	D40.8	D49.59
Vater's ampulla	C24.1	C78.89	D01.5	D13.5	D37.6	D49.0
vein, venous — see Neoplasm, connective tissue						
vena cava (abdominal) (inferior)	C49.4	C79.89	—	D21.4	D48.1	D49.2
superior	C49.3	C79.89	—	D21.3	D48.1	D49.2
ventricle (cerebral) (floor) (lateral) (third)	C71.5	C79.31	—	D33.0	D43.0	D49.6
cardiac (left) (right)	C38.0	C79.89	—	D15.1	D48.7	D49.89
fourth	C71.7	C79.31	—	D33.1	D43.1	D49.6
ventricular band of larynx	C32.1	C78.39	D02.0	D14.1	D38.0	D49.1
ventriculus — see Neoplasm, stomach						
vermillion border — see Neoplasm, lip						
vermis, cerebellum	C71.6	C79.31	—	D33.1	D43.1	D49.6
vertebra (column)	C41.2	C79.51	—	D16.6	D48.0	D49.2
coccyx	C41.4	C79.51	—	D16.8	D48.0	D49.2
marrow NEC	C96.9	C79.52	—	—	D47.9	D49.89
sacrum	C41.4	C79.51	—	D16.8	D48.0	D49.2
vesical — see Neoplasm, bladder						
vesicle, seminal	C63.7	C79.82	D07.69	D29.8	D40.8	D49.59
vesicocervical tissue	C57.9	C79.82	D07.30	D28.9	D39.9	D49.59
vesicorectal	C76.3	C79.82	D09.8	D36.7	D48.7	D49.89
vesicovaginal	C57.9	C79.82	D07.30	D28.9	D39.9	D49.59
septum	C57.9	C79.82	D07.30	D28.9	D39.8	D49.59
vessel (blood) — see Neoplasm, connective tissue						
vestibular gland, greater	C51.0	C79.82	D07.1	D28.0	D39.8	D49.59
vestibule						
mouth	C06.1	C79.89	D00.00	D10.39	D37.09	D49.0
nose	C30.0	C78.39	D02.3	D14.0	D38.5	D49.1
Virchow's gland	C77.0	C77.0	—	D36.0	D48.7	D49.89
viscera NEC	C76.8	C79.89	D09.8	D36.7	D48.7	D49.89
vocal cords (true)	C32.0	C78.39	D02.0	D14.1	D38.0	D49.1
false	C32.1	C78.39	D02.0	D14.1	D38.0	D49.1
vomer	C41.0	C79.51	—	D16.4	D48.0	D49.2
vulva	C51.9	C79.82	D07.1	D28.0	D39.8	D49.59
vulvovaginal gland	C51.0	C79.82	D07.1	D28.0	D39.8	D49.59
Waldeyer's ring	C14.2	C79.89	D00.08	D10.9	D37.05	D49.0
Wharton's duct	C08.0	C79.89	D00.00	D11.7	D37.032	D49.0
white matter (central) (cerebral)	C71.0	C79.31	—	D33.0	D43.0	D49.6

	Malignant Primary	Malignant Secondary	Ca in situ	Benign	Uncertain Behavior	Unspecified Behavior
Neoplasm, neoplastic						
— *continued*						
windpipe	C33	C78.39	D02.1	D14.2	D38.1	D49.1
Wirsung's duct	C25.3	C78.89	D01.7	D13.6	D37.8	D49.0
wolffian (body) (duct)						
female	C57.7	C79.82	D07.39	D28.7	D39.8	D49.59
male	C63.7	C79.82	D07.69	D29.8	D40.8	D49.59
womb — *see*						
Neoplasm, uterus						
wrist NEC	C76.4-☑	C79.89	D04.6-☑	D36.7	D48.7	D49.89
xiphoid process	C41.3	C79.51	—	D16.7	D48.0	D49.2
Zuckerkandl						
organ	C75.5	C79.89	—	D35.6	D44.7	D49.7

☑ **Additional Character Required — Refer to the Tabular List for Character Selection**   ▽ **Subterms under main terms may continue to next column or page**

Substance	Poisoning, Accidental (unintentional)	Poisoning, Intentional Self-harm	Poisoning, Assault	Poisoning, Undetermined	Adverse Effect	Under-dosing
14-Hydroxydihydromorphinone	T40.2X1	T40.2X2	T40.2X3	T40.2X4	T40.2X5	T40.2X6
1-Propanol	T51.3X1	T51.3X2	T51.3X3	T51.3X4	—	—
2,3,7,8-Tetrachlorodibenzo-p-dioxin	T53.7X1	T53.7X2	T53.7X3	T53.7X4	—	—
2,4,5-T (trichlorophenoxyacetic acid)	T60.1X1	T60.1X2	T60.1X3	T60.1X4	—	—
2,4,5-Trichlorophenoxyacetic acid	T60.3X1	T60.3X2	T60.3X3	T60.3X4	—	—
2,4-D (dichlorophenoxyacetic acid)	T60.3X1	T60.3X2	T60.3X3	T60.3X4	—	—
2,4-Toluene diisocyanate	T65.0X1	T65.0X2	T65.0X3	T65.0X4	—	—
2-Deoxy-5-fluorouridine	T45.1X1	T45.1X2	T45.1X3	T45.1X4	T45.1X5	T45.1X6
2-Ethoxyethanol	T52.3X1	T52.3X2	T52.3X3	T52.3X4	—	—
2-Methoxyethanol	T52.3X1	T52.3X2	T52.3X3	T52.3X4	—	—
2-Propanol	T51.2X1	T51.2X2	T51.2X3	T51.2X4	—	—
3,4-methylenedioxymeth-amphetamine	T43.641	T43.642	T43.643	T43.644	—	—
4-Aminobutyric acid	T43.8X1	T43.8X2	T43.8X3	T43.8X4	T43.8X5	T43.8X6
4-Aminophenol derivatives	T39.1X1	T39.1X2	T39.1X3	T39.1X4	T39.1X5	T39.1X6
5-Deoxy-5-fluorouridine	T45.1X1	T45.1X2	T45.1X3	T45.1X4	T45.1X5	T45.1X6
5-Methoxypsoralen (5-MOP)	T50.991	T50.992	T50.993	T50.994	T50.995	T50.996
8-Aminoquinoline drugs	T37.2X1	T37.2X2	T37.2X3	T37.2X4	T37.2X5	T37.2X6
8-Methoxypsoralen (8-MOP)	T50.991	T50.992	T50.993	T50.994	T50.995	T50.996
ABOB	T37.5X1	T37.5X2	T37.5X3	T37.5X4	T37.5X5	T37.5X6
Abrine	T62.2X1	T62.2X2	T62.2X3	T62.2X4	—	—
Abrus (seed)	T62.2X1	T62.2X2	T62.2X3	T62.2X4	—	—
Absinthe	T51.0X1	T51.0X2	T51.0X3	T51.0X4	—	—
beverage	T51.0X1	T51.0X2	T51.0X3	T51.0X4	—	—
Acaricide	T60.8X1	T60.8X2	T60.8X3	T60.8X4	—	—
Acebutolol	T44.7X1	T44.7X2	T44.7X3	T44.7X4	T44.7X5	T44.7X6
Acecarbromal	T42.6X1	T42.6X2	T42.6X3	T42.6X4	T42.6X5	T42.6X6
Aceclidine	T44.1X1	T44.1X2	T44.1X3	T44.1X4	T44.1X5	T44.1X6
Acedapsone	T37.0X1	T37.0X2	T37.0X3	T37.0X4	T37.0X5	T37.0X6
Acefylline piperazine	T48.6X1	T48.6X2	T48.6X3	T48.6X4	T48.6X5	T48.6X6
Acemorphan	T40.2X1	T40.2X2	T40.2X3	T40.2X4	T40.2X5	T40.2X6
Acenocoumarin	T45.511	T45.512	T45.513	T45.514	T45.515	T45.516
Acenocoumarol	T45.511	T45.512	T45.513	T45.514	T45.515	T45.516
Acepifylline	T48.6X1	T48.6X2	T48.6X3	T48.6X4	T48.6X5	T48.6X6
Acepromazine	T43.3X1	T43.3X2	T43.3X3	T43.3X4	T43.3X5	T43.3X6
Acesulfamethoxypyridazine	T37.0X1	T37.0X2	T37.0X3	T37.0X4	T37.0X5	T37.0X6
Acetal	T52.8X1	T52.8X2	T52.8X3	T52.8X4	—	—
Acetaldehyde (vapor)	T52.8X1	T52.8X2	T52.8X3	T52.8X4	—	—
liquid	T65.891	T65.892	T65.893	T65.894	—	—
Acetaminophen	T39.1X1	T39.1X2	T39.1X3	T39.1X4	T39.1X5	T39.1X6
Acetaminosalol	T39.1X1	T39.1X2	T39.1X3	T39.1X4	T39.1X5	T39.1X6
Acetanilide	T39.1X1	T39.1X2	T39.1X3	T39.1X4	T39.1X5	T39.1X6
Acetarsol	T37.3X1	T37.3X2	T37.3X3	T37.3X4	T37.3X5	T37.3X6
Acetazolamide	T50.2X1	T50.2X2	T50.2X3	T50.2X4	T50.2X5	T50.2X6
Acetiamine	T45.2X1	T45.2X2	T45.2X3	T45.2X4	T45.2X5	T45.2X6
Acetic						
acid	T54.2X1	T54.2X2	T54.2X3	T54.2X4	—	—
with sodium acetate (ointment)	T49.3X1	T49.3X2	T49.3X3	T49.3X4	T49.3X5	T49.3X6
ester (solvent)(vapor)	T52.8X1	T52.8X2	T52.8X3	T52.8X4	—	—
irrigating solution	T50.3X1	T50.3X2	T50.3X3	T50.3X4	T50.3X5	T50.3X6
medicinal (lotion)	T49.2X1	T49.2X2	T49.2X3	T49.2X4	T49.2X5	T49.2X6
anhydride	T65.891	T65.892	T65.893	T65.894	—	—
ether (vapor)	T52.8X1	T52.8X2	T52.8X3	T52.8X4	—	—
Acetohexamide	T38.3X1	T38.3X2	T38.3X3	T38.3X4	T38.3X5	T38.3X6
Acetohydroxamic acid	T50.991	T50.992	T50.993	T50.994	T50.995	T50.996
Acetomenaphthone	T45.7X1	T45.7X2	T45.7X3	T45.7X4	T45.7X5	T45.7X6
Acetomorphine	T40.1X1	T40.1X2	T40.1X3	T40.1X4	—	—
Acetone (oils)	T52.4X1	T52.4X2	T52.4X3	T52.4X4	—	—
chlorinated	T52.4X1	T52.4X2	T52.4X3	T52.4X4	—	—
vapor	T52.4X1	T52.4X2	T52.4X3	T52.4X4	—	—
Acetonitrile	T52.8X1	T52.8X2	T52.8X3	T52.8X4	—	—
Acetophenazine	T43.3X1	T43.3X2	T43.3X3	T43.3X4	T43.3X5	T43.3X6
Acetophenetedin	T39.1X1	T39.1X2	T39.1X3	T39.1X4	T39.1X5	T39.1X6
Acetophenone	T52.4X1	T52.4X2	T52.4X3	T52.4X4	—	—
Acetorphine	T40.2X1	T40.2X2	T40.2X3	T40.2X4	—	—
Acetosulfone (sodium)	T37.1X1	T37.1X2	T37.1X3	T37.1X4	T37.1X5	T37.1X6
Acetrizoate (sodium)	T50.8X1	T50.8X2	T50.8X3	T50.8X4	T50.8X5	T50.8X6
Acetrizoic acid	T50.8X1	T50.8X2	T50.8X3	T50.8X4	T50.8X5	T50.8X6
Acetyl						
bromide	T53.6X1	T53.6X2	T53.6X3	T53.6X4	—	—
chloride	T53.6X1	T53.6X2	T53.6X3	T53.6X4	—	—
Acetylcarbromal	T42.6X1	T42.6X2	T42.6X3	T42.6X4	T42.6X5	T42.6X6
Acetylcholine						
chloride	T44.1X1	T44.1X2	T44.1X3	T44.1X4	T44.1X5	T44.1X6
derivative	T44.1X1	T44.1X2	T44.1X3	T44.1X4	T44.1X5	T44.1X6

Substance	Poisoning, Accidental (unintentional)	Poisoning, Intentional Self-harm	Poisoning, Assault	Poisoning, Undetermined	Adverse Effect	Under-dosing
Acetylcysteine	T48.4X1	T48.4X2	T48.4X3	T48.4X4	T48.4X5	T48.4X6
Acetyldigitoxin	T46.0X1	T46.0X2	T46.0X3	T46.0X4	T46.0X5	T46.0X6
Acetyldigoxin	T46.0X1	T46.0X2	T46.0X3	T46.0X4	T46.0X5	T46.0X6
Acetyldihydrocodeine	T40.2X1	T40.2X2	T40.2X3	T40.2X4	—	—
Acetyldihydrocodeinone	T40.2X1	T40.2X2	T40.2X3	T40.2X4	—	—
Acetylene (gas)	T59.891	T59.892	T59.893	T59.894	—	—
dichloride	T53.6X1	T53.6X2	T53.6X3	T53.6X4	—	—
incomplete combustion of	T58.11	T58.12	T58.13	T58.14	—	—
industrial	T59.891	T59.892	T59.893	T59.894	—	—
tetrachloride	T53.6X1	T53.6X2	T53.6X3	T53.6X4	—	—
vapor	T53.6X1	T53.6X2	T53.6X3	T53.6X4	—	—
Acetylpheneturide	T42.6X1	T42.6X2	T42.6X3	T42.6X4	T42.6X5	T42.6X6
Acetylphenylhydrazine	T39.8X1	T39.8X2	T39.8X3	T39.8X4	T39.8X5	T39.8X6
Acetylsalicylic acid (salts)	T39.011	T39.012	T39.013	T39.014	T39.015	T39.016
enteric coated	T39.011	T39.012	T39.013	T39.014	T39.015	T39.016
Acetylsulfamethoxypyridazine	T37.0X1	T37.0X2	T37.0X3	T37.0X4	T37.0X5	T37.0X6
Achromycin	T36.4X1	T36.4X2	T36.4X3	T36.4X4	T36.4X5	T36.4X6
ophthalmic preparation	T49.5X1	T49.5X2	T49.5X3	T49.5X4	T49.5X5	T49.5X6
topical NEC	T49.0X1	T49.0X2	T49.0X3	T49.0X4	T49.0X5	T49.0X6
Aciclovir	T37.5X1	T37.5X2	T37.5X3	T37.5X4	T37.5X5	T37.5X6
Acidifying agent NEC	T50.901	T50.902	T50.903	T50.904	T50.905	T50.906
Acid (corrosive) NEC	T54.2X1	T54.2X2	T54.2X3	T54.2X4	—	—
Acipimox	T46.6X1	T46.6X2	T46.6X3	T46.6X4	T46.6X5	T46.6X6
Acitretin	T50.991	T50.992	T50.993	T50.994	T50.995	T50.996
Aclarubicin	T45.1X1	T45.1X2	T45.1X3	T45.1X4	T45.1X5	T45.1X6
Aclatonium napadisilate	T48.1X1	T48.1X2	T48.1X3	T48.1X4	T48.1X5	T48.1X6
Aconite (wild)	T46.991	T46.992	T46.993	T46.994	T46.995	T46.996
Aconitine	T46.991	T46.992	T46.993	T46.994	T46.995	T46.996
Aconitum ferox	T46.991	T46.992	T46.993	T46.994	T46.995	T46.996
Acridine	T65.6X1	T65.6X2	T65.6X3	T65.6X4	—	—
vapor	T59.891	T59.892	T59.893	T59.894	—	—
Acriflavine	T37.91	T37.92	T37.93	T37.94	T37.95	T37.96
Acriflavinium chloride	T49.0X1	T49.0X2	T49.0X3	T49.0X4	T49.0X5	T49.0X6
Acrinol	T49.0X1	T49.0X2	T49.0X3	T49.0X4	T49.0X5	T49.0X6
Acrisorcin	T49.0X1	T49.0X2	T49.0X3	T49.0X4	T49.0X5	T49.0X6
Acrivastine	T45.0X1	T45.0X2	T45.0X3	T45.0X4	T45.0X5	T45.0X6
Acrolein (gas)	T59.891	T59.892	T59.893	T59.894	—	—
liquid	T54.1X1	T54.1X2	T54.1X3	T54.1X4	—	—
Acrylamide	T65.891	T65.892	T65.893	T65.894	—	—
Acrylic resin	T49.3X1	T49.3X2	T49.3X3	T49.3X4	T49.3X5	T49.3X6
Acrylonitrile	T65.891	T65.892	T65.893	T65.894	—	—
Actaea spicata	T62.2X1	T62.2X2	T62.2X3	T62.2X4	—	—
berry	T62.1X1	T62.1X2	T62.1X3	T62.1X4	—	—
Acterol	T37.3X1	T37.3X2	T37.3X3	T37.3X4	T37.3X5	T37.3X6
ACTH	T38.811	T38.812	T38.813	T38.814	T38.815	T38.816
Actinomycin C	T45.1X1	T45.1X2	T45.1X3	T45.1X4	T45.1X5	T45.1X6
Actinomycin D	T45.1X1	T45.1X2	T45.1X3	T45.1X4	T45.1X5	T45.1X6
Activated charcoal — see also Charcoal, medicinal	T47.6X1	T47.6X2	T47.6X3	T47.6X4	T47.6X5	T47.6X6
Acyclovir	T37.5X1	T37.5X2	T37.5X3	T37.5X4	T37.5X5	T37.5X6
Adenine	T45.2X1	T45.2X2	T45.2X3	T45.2X4	T45.2X5	T45.2X6
arabinoside	T37.5X1	T37.5X2	T37.5X3	T37.5X4	T37.5X5	T37.5X6
Adenosine (phosphate)	T46.2X1	T46.2X2	T46.2X3	T46.2X4	T46.2X5	T46.2X6
ADH	T38.891	T38.892	T38.893	T38.894	T38.895	T38.896
Adhesive NEC	T65.891	T65.892	T65.893	T65.894	—	—
Adicillin	T36.0X1	T36.0X2	T36.0X3	T36.0X4	T36.0X5	T36.0X6
Adiphenine	T44.3X1	T44.3X2	T44.3X3	T44.3X4	T44.3X5	T44.3X6
Adipiodone	T50.8X1	T50.8X2	T50.8X3	T50.8X4	T50.8X5	T50.8X6
Adjunct, pharmaceutical	T50.901	T50.902	T50.903	T50.904	T50.905	T50.906
Adrenal (extract, cortex or medulla) (glucocorticoids) (hormones) (mineralocorticoids)	T38.0X1	T38.0X2	T38.0X3	T38.0X4	T38.0X5	T38.0X6
ENT agent	T49.6X1	T49.6X2	T49.6X3	T49.6X4	T49.6X5	T49.6X6
ophthalmic preparation	T49.5X1	T49.5X2	T49.5X3	T49.5X4	T49.5X5	T49.5X6
topical NEC	T49.0X1	T49.0X2	T49.0X3	T49.0X4	T49.0X5	T49.0X6
Adrenalin — see Adrenaline						
Adrenaline	T44.5X1	T44.5X2	T44.5X3	T44.5X4	T44.5X5	T44.5X6
Adrenergic NEC	T44.901	T44.902	T44.903	T44.904	T44.905	T44.906
blocking agent NEC	T44.8X1	T44.8X2	T44.8X3	T44.8X4	T44.8X5	T44.8X6
beta, heart	T44.7X1	T44.7X2	T44.7X3	T44.7X4	T44.7X5	T44.7X6
specified NEC	T44.991	T44.992	T44.993	T44.994	T44.995	T44.996
Adrenochrome						
derivative	T46.991	T46.992	T46.993	T46.994	T46.995	T46.996
(mono) semicarbazone	T46.991	T46.992	T46.993	T46.994	T46.995	T46.996
Adrenocorticotrophic hormone	T38.811	T38.812	T38.813	T38.814	T38.815	T38.816
Adrenocorticotrophin	T38.811	T38.812	T38.813	T38.814	T38.815	T38.816
Adriamycin	T45.1X1	T45.1X2	T45.1X3	T45.1X4	T45.1X5	T45.1X6
Aerosol spray NEC	T65.91	T65.92	T65.93	T65.94	—	—
Aerosporin	T36.8X1	T36.8X2	T36.8X3	T36.8X4	T36.8X5	T36.8X6
ENT agent	T49.6X1	T49.6X2	T49.6X3	T49.6X4	T49.6X5	T49.6X6
ophthalmic preparation	T49.5X1	T49.5X2	T49.5X3	T49.5X4	T49.5X5	T49.5X6

Substance	Poisoning, Accidental (unintentional)	Poisoning, Intentional Self-harm	Poisoning, Assault	Poisoning, Undetermined	Adverse Effect	Under-dosing
Aerosporin — continued						
topical NEC	T49.0X1	T49.0X2	T49.0X3	T49.0X4	T49.0X5	T49.0X6
Aethusa cynapium	T62.2X1	T62.2X2	T62.2X3	T62.2X4	—	—
Afghanistan black	T40.7X1	T40.7X2	T40.7X3	T40.7X4	T40.7X5	T40.7X6
Aflatoxin	T64.01	T64.02	T64.03	T64.04		
Afloqualone	T42.8X1	T42.8X2	T42.8X3	T42.8X4	T42.8X5	T42.8X6
African boxwood	T62.2X1	T62.2X2	T62.2X3	T62.2X4	—	—
Agar	T47.4X1	T47.4X2	T47.4X3	T47.4X4	T47.4X5	T47.4X6
Agonist						
predominantly						
alpha-adrenoreceptor	T44.4X1	T44.4X2	T44.4X3	T44.4X4	T44.4X5	T44.4X6
beta-adrenoreceptor	T44.5X1	T44.5X2	T44.5X3	T44.5X4	T44.5X5	T44.5X6
Agricultural agent NEC	T65.91	T65.92	T65.93	T65.94		
Agrypnal	T42.3X1	T42.3X2	T42.3X3	T42.3X4	T42.3X5	T42.3X6
AHLG	T50.Z11	T50.Z12	T50.Z13	T50.Z14	T50.Z15	T50.Z16
Air contaminant(s), source/type NOS	T65.91	T65.92	T65.93	T65.94	—	—
Ajmaline	T46.2X1	T46.2X2	T46.2X3	T46.2X4	T46.2X5	T46.2X6
Akee	T62.1X1	T62.1X2	T62.1X3	T62.1X4	—	—
Akrinol	T49.0X1	T49.0X2	T49.0X3	T49.0X4	T49.0X5	T49.0X6
Akritoin	T37.8X1	T37.8X2	T37.8X3	T37.8X4	T37.8X5	T37.8X6
Alacepril	T46.4X1	T46.4X2	T46.4X3	T46.4X4	T46.4X5	T46.4X6
Alantolactone	T37.4X1	T37.4X2	T37.4X3	T37.4X4	T37.4X5	T37.4X6
Albamycin	T36.8X1	T36.8X2	T36.8X3	T36.8X4	T36.8X5	T36.8X6
Albendazole	T37.4X1	T37.4X2	T37.4X3	T37.4X4	T37.4X5	T37.4X6
Albumin						
bovine	T45.8X1	T45.8X2	T45.8X3	T45.8X4	T45.8X5	T45.8X6
human serum	T45.8X1	T45.8X2	T45.8X3	T45.8X4	T45.8X5	T45.8X6
salt-poor	T45.8X1	T45.8X2	T45.8X3	T45.8X4	T45.8X5	T45.8X6
normal human serum	T45.8X1	T45.8X2	T45.8X3	T45.8X4	T45.8X5	T45.8X6
Albuterol	T48.6X1	T48.6X2	T48.6X3	T48.6X4	T48.6X5	T48.6X6
Albutoin	T42.0X1	T42.0X2	T42.0X3	T42.0X4	T42.0X5	T42.0X6
Alclometasone	T49.0X1	T49.0X2	T49.0X3	T49.0X4	T49.0X5	T49.0X6
Alcohol	T51.91	T51.92	T51.93	T51.94	—	—
absolute	T51.0X1	T51.0X2	T51.0X3	T51.0X4	—	—
beverage	T51.0X1	T51.0X2	T51.0X3	T51.0X4	—	—
allyl	T51.8X1	T51.8X2	T51.8X3	T51.8X4	—	—
amyl	T51.3X1	T51.3X2	T51.3X3	T51.3X4	—	—
antifreeze	T51.1X1	T51.1X2	T51.1X3	T51.1X4	—	—
beverage	T51.0X1	T51.0X2	T51.0X3	T51.0X4	—	—
butyl	T51.3X1	T51.3X2	T51.3X3	T51.3X4	—	—
dehydrated	T51.0X1	T51.0X2	T51.0X3	T51.0X4	—	—
beverage	T51.0X1	T51.0X2	T51.0X3	T51.0X4	—	—
denatured	T51.0X1	T51.0X2	T51.0X3	T51.0X4	—	—
deterrent NEC	T50.6X1	T50.6X2	T50.6X3	T50.6X4	T50.6X5	T50.6X6
diagnostic (gastric function)	T50.8X1	T50.8X2	T50.8X3	T50.8X4	T50.8X5	T50.8X6
ethyl	T51.0X1	T51.0X2	T51.0X3	T51.0X4	—	—
beverage	T51.0X1	T51.0X2	T51.0X3	T51.0X4	—	—
grain	T51.0X1	T51.0X2	T51.0X3	T51.0X4	—	—
beverage	T51.0X1	T51.0X2	T51.0X3	T51.0X4	—	—
industrial	T51.0X1	T51.0X2	T51.0X3	T51.0X4	—	—
isopropyl	T51.2X1	T51.2X2	T51.2X3	T51.2X4	—	—
methyl	T51.1X1	T51.1X2	T51.1X3	T51.1X4	—	—
preparation for consumption	T51.0X1	T51.0X2	T51.0X3	T51.0X4	—	—
propyl	T51.3X1	T51.3X2	T51.3X3	T51.3X4	—	—
secondary	T51.2X1	T51.2X2	T51.2X3	T51.2X4	—	—
radiator	T51.1X1	T51.1X2	T51.1X3	T51.1X4	—	—
rubbing	T51.2X1	T51.2X2	T51.2X3	T51.2X4	—	—
specified type NEC	T51.8X1	T51.8X2	T51.8X3	T51.8X4	—	—
surgical	T51.0X1	T51.0X2	T51.0X3	T51.0X4	—	—
vapor (from any type of Alcohol)	T59.891	T59.892	T59.893	T59.894	—	—
wood	T51.1X1	T51.1X2	T51.1X3	T51.1X4	—	—
Alcuronium (chloride)	T48.1X1	T48.1X2	T48.1X3	T48.1X4	T48.1X5	T48.1X6
Aldactone	T50.0X1	T50.0X2	T50.0X3	T50.0X4	T50.0X5	T50.0X6
Aldesulfone sodium	T37.1X1	T37.1X2	T37.1X3	T37.1X4	T37.1X5	T37.1X6
Aldicarb	T60.0X1	T60.0X2	T60.0X3	T60.0X4		
Aldomet	T46.5X1	T46.5X2	T46.5X3	T46.5X4	T46.5X5	T46.5X6
Aldosterone	T50.0X1	T50.0X2	T50.0X3	T50.0X4	T50.0X5	T50.0X6
Aldrin (dust)	T60.1X1	T60.1X2	T60.1X3	T60.1X4		
Aleve — see Naproxen						
Alexitol sodium	T47.1X1	T47.1X2	T47.1X3	T47.1X4	T47.1X5	T47.1X6
Alfacalcidol	T45.2X1	T45.2X2	T45.2X3	T45.2X4	T45.2X5	T45.2X6
Alfadolone	T41.1X1	T41.1X2	T41.1X3	T41.1X4	T41.1X5	T41.1X6
Alfaxalone	T41.1X1	T41.1X2	T41.1X3	T41.1X4	T41.1X5	T41.1X6
Alfentanil	T40.4X1	T40.4X2	T40.4X3	T40.4X4	T40.4X5	T40.4X6
Alfuzosin (hydrochloride)	T44.8X1	T44.8X2	T44.8X3	T44.8X4	T44.8X5	T44.8X6
Algae (harmful) (toxin)	T65.821	T65.822	T65.823	T65.824		
Algeldrate	T47.1X1	T47.1X2	T47.1X3	T47.1X4	T47.1X5	T47.1X6
Algin	T47.8X1	T47.8X2	T47.8X3	T47.8X4	T47.8X5	T47.8X6
Alglucerase	T45.3X1	T45.3X2	T45.3X3	T45.3X4	T45.3X5	T45.3X6
Alidase	T45.3X1	T45.3X2	T45.3X3	T45.3X4	T45.3X5	T45.3X6
Alimemazine	T43.3X1	T43.3X2	T43.3X3	T43.3X4	T43.3X5	T43.3X6
Aliphatic thiocyanates	T65.0X1	T65.0X2	T65.0X3	T65.0X4	—	—
Alizapride	T45.0X1	T45.0X2	T45.0X3	T45.0X4	T45.0X5	T45.0X6
Alkali (caustic)	T54.3X1	T54.3X2	T54.3X3	T54.3X4		
Alkaline antiseptic solution (aromatic)	T49.6X1	T49.6X2	T49.6X3	T49.6X4	T49.6X5	T49.6X6
Alkalinizing agents (medicinal)	T50.901	T50.902	T50.903	T50.904	T50.905	T50.906
Alkalizing agent NEC	T50.901	T50.902	T50.903	T50.904	T50.905	T50.906
Alka-seltzer	T39.011	T39.012	T39.013	T39.014	T39.015	T39.016
Alkavervir	T46.5X1	T46.5X2	T46.5X3	T46.5X4	T46.5X5	T46.5X6
Alkonium (bromide)	T49.0X1	T49.0X2	T49.0X3	T49.0X4	T49.0X5	T49.0X6
Alkylating drug NEC	T45.1X1	T45.1X2	T45.1X3	T45.1X4	T45.1X5	T45.1X6
antimyeloproliferative	T45.1X1	T45.1X2	T45.1X3	T45.1X4	T45.1X5	T45.1X6
lymphatic	T45.1X1	T45.1X2	T45.1X3	T45.1X4	T45.1X5	T45.1X6
Alkylisocyanate	T65.0X1	T65.0X2	T65.0X3	T65.0X4	—	—
Allantoin	T49.4X1	T49.4X2	T49.4X3	T49.4X4	T49.4X5	T49.4X6
Allegron	T43.011	T43.012	T43.013	T43.014	T43.015	T43.016
Allethrin	T49.0X1	T49.0X2	T49.0X3	T49.0X4	T49.0X5	T49.0X6
Allobarbital	T42.3X1	T42.3X2	T42.3X3	T42.3X4	T42.3X5	T42.3X6
Allopurinol	T50.4X1	T50.4X2	T50.4X3	T50.4X4	T50.4X5	T50.4X6
Allyl						
alcohol	T51.8X1	T51.8X2	T51.8X3	T51.8X4		
disulfide	T46.6X1	T46.6X2	T46.6X3	T46.6X4	T46.6X5	T46.6X6
Allylestrenol	T38.5X1	T38.5X2	T38.5X3	T38.5X4	T38.5X5	T38.5X6
Allylisopropylacetylurea	T42.6X1	T42.6X2	T42.6X3	T42.6X4	T42.6X5	T42.6X6
Allylisopropylmalonylurea	T42.3X1	T42.3X2	T42.3X3	T42.3X4	T42.3X5	T42.3X6
Allylthiourea	T49.3X1	T49.3X2	T49.3X3	T49.3X4	T49.3X5	T49.3X6
Allyltribromide	T42.6X1	T42.6X2	T42.6X3	T42.6X4	T42.6X5	T42.6X6
Allypropymal	T42.3X1	T42.3X2	T42.3X3	T42.3X4	T42.3X5	T42.3X6
Almagate	T47.1X1	T47.1X2	T47.1X3	T47.1X4	T47.1X5	T47.1X6
Almasilate	T47.1X1	T47.1X2	T47.1X3	T47.1X4	T47.1X5	T47.1X6
Almitrine	T50.7X1	T50.7X2	T50.7X3	T50.7X4	T50.7X5	T50.7X6
Aloes	T47.2X1	T47.2X2	T47.2X3	T47.2X4	T47.2X5	T47.2X6
Aloglutamol	T47.1X1	T47.1X2	T47.1X3	T47.1X4	T47.1X5	T47.1X6
Aloin	T47.2X1	T47.2X2	T47.2X3	T47.2X4	T47.2X5	T47.2X6
Aloxidone	T42.2X1	T42.2X2	T42.2X3	T42.2X4	T42.2X5	T42.2X6
Alpha						
acetyldigoxin	T46.0X1	T46.0X2	T46.0X3	T46.0X4	T46.0X5	T46.0X6
adrenergic blocking drug	T44.6X1	T44.6X2	T44.6X3	T44.6X4	T44.6X5	T44.6X6
amylase	T45.3X1	T45.3X2	T45.3X3	T45.3X4	T45.3X5	T45.3X6
tocoferol (acetate)	T45.2X1	T45.2X2	T45.2X3	T45.2X4	T45.2X5	T45.2X6
tocopherol	T45.2X1	T45.2X2	T45.2X3	T45.2X4	T45.2X5	T45.2X6
Alphadolone	T41.1X1	T41.1X2	T41.1X3	T41.1X4	T41.1X5	T41.1X6
Alphaprodine	T40.4X1	T40.4X2	T40.4X3	T40.4X4	T40.4X5	T40.4X6
Alphaxalone	T41.1X1	T41.1X2	T41.1X3	T41.1X4	T41.1X5	T41.1X6
Alprazolam	T42.4X1	T42.4X2	T42.4X3	T42.4X4	T42.4X5	T42.4X6
Alprenolol	T44.7X1	T44.7X2	T44.7X3	T44.7X4	T44.7X5	T44.7X6
Alprostadil	T46.7X1	T46.7X2	T46.7X3	T46.7X4	T46.7X5	T46.7X6
Alsactide	T38.811	T38.812	T38.813	T38.814	T38.815	T38.816
Alseroxylon	T46.5X1	T46.5X2	T46.5X3	T46.5X4	T46.5X5	T46.5X6
Alteplase	T45.611	T45.612	T45.613	T45.614	T45.615	T45.616
Altizide	T50.2X1	T50.2X2	T50.2X3	T50.2X4	T50.2X5	T50.2X6
Altretamine	T45.1X1	T45.1X2	T45.1X3	T45.1X4	T45.1X5	T45.1X6
Alum (medicinal)	T49.4X1	T49.4X2	T49.4X3	T49.4X4	T49.4X5	T49.4X6
nonmedicinal (ammonium) (potassium)	T56.891	T56.892	T56.893	T56.894	—	—
Aluminium, aluminum						
acetate	T49.2X1	T49.2X2	T49.2X3	T49.2X4	T49.2X5	T49.2X6
solution	T49.0X1	T49.0X2	T49.0X3	T49.0X4	T49.0X5	T49.0X6
aspirin	T39.011	T39.012	T39.013	T39.014	T39.015	T39.016
bis (acetylsalicylate)	T39.011	T39.012	T39.013	T39.014	T39.015	T39.016
carbonate (gel, basic)	T47.1X1	T47.1X2	T47.1X3	T47.1X4	T47.1X5	T47.1X6
chlorhydroxide-complex	T47.1X1	T47.1X2	T47.1X3	T47.1X4	T47.1X5	T47.1X6
chloride	T49.2X1	T49.2X2	T49.2X3	T49.2X4	T49.2X5	T49.2X6
clofibrate	T46.6X1	T46.6X2	T46.6X3	T46.6X4	T46.6X5	T46.6X6
diacetate	T49.2X1	T49.2X2	T49.2X3	T49.2X4	T49.2X5	T49.2X6
glycinate	T47.1X1	T47.1X2	T47.1X3	T47.1X4	T47.1X5	T47.1X6
hydroxide (gel)	T47.1X1	T47.1X2	T47.1X3	T47.1X4	T47.1X5	T47.1X6
hydroxide-magnesium carb. gel	T47.1X1	T47.1X2	T47.1X3	T47.1X4	T47.1X5	T47.1X6
magnesium silicate	T47.1X1	T47.1X2	T47.1X3	T47.1X4	T47.1X5	T47.1X6
nicotinate	T46.7X1	T46.7X2	T46.7X3	T46.7X4	T46.7X5	T46.7X6
ointment (surgical) (topical)	T49.3X1	T49.3X2	T49.3X3	T49.3X4	T49.3X5	T49.3X6
phosphate	T47.1X1	T47.1X2	T47.1X3	T47.1X4	T47.1X5	T47.1X6
salicylate	T39.091	T39.092	T39.093	T39.094	T39.095	T39.096
silicate	T47.1X1	T47.1X2	T47.1X3	T47.1X4	T47.1X5	T47.1X6
sodium silicate	T47.1X1	T47.1X2	T47.1X3	T47.1X4	T47.1X5	T47.1X6
subacetate	T49.2X1	T49.2X2	T49.2X3	T49.2X4	T49.2X5	T49.2X6
sulfate	T49.0X1	T49.0X2	T49.0X3	T49.0X4	T49.0X5	T49.0X6
tannate	T47.6X1	T47.6X2	T47.6X3	T47.6X4	T47.6X5	T47.6X6

Additional Character May Be Required — Refer to the Tabular List for Character Selection   Subterms under main terms may continue to next column or page

Substance	Poisoning, Accidental (unintentional)	Poisoning, Intentional Self-harm	Poisoning, Assault	Poisoning, Undetermined	Adverse Effect	Under-dosing
Aluminium, aluminum — continued						
topical NEC	T49.3X1	T49.3X2	T49.3X3	T49.3X4	T49.3X5	T49.3X6
Alurate	T42.3X1	T42.3X2	T42.3X3	T42.3X4	T42.3X5	T42.3X6
Alverine	T44.3X1	T44.3X2	T44.3X3	T44.3X4	T44.3X5	T44.3X6
Alvodine	T40.2X1	T40.2X2	T40.2X3	T40.2X4	T40.2X5	T40.2X6
Amanita phalloides	T62.0X1	T62.0X2	T62.0X3	T62.0X4	—	—
Amanitine	T62.0X1	T62.0X2	T62.0X3	T62.0X4	—	—
Amantadine	T42.8X1	T42.8X2	T42.8X3	T42.8X4	T42.8X5	T42.8X6
Ambazone	T49.6X1	T49.6X2	T49.6X3	T49.6X4	T49.6X5	T49.6X6
Ambenonium (chloride)	T44.0X1	T44.0X2	T44.0X3	T44.0X4	T44.0X5	T44.0X6
Ambroxol	T48.4X1	T48.4X2	T48.4X3	T48.4X4	T48.4X5	T48.4X6
Ambuphylline	T48.6X1	T48.6X2	T48.6X3	T48.6X4	T48.6X5	T48.6X6
Ambutonium bromide	T44.3X1	T44.3X2	T44.3X3	T44.3X4	T44.3X5	T44.3X6
Amcinonide	T49.0X1	T49.0X2	T49.0X3	T49.0X4	T49.0X5	T49.0X6
Amdinocilline	T36.0X1	T36.0X2	T36.0X3	T36.0X4	T36.0X5	T36.0X6
Ametazole	T50.8X1	T50.8X2	T50.8X3	T50.8X4	T50.8X5	T50.8X6
Amethocaine	T41.3X1	T41.3X2	T41.3X3	T41.3X4	T41.3X5	T41.3X6
regional	T41.3X1	T41.3X2	T41.3X3	T41.3X4	T41.3X5	T41.3X6
spinal	T41.3X1	T41.3X2	T41.3X3	T41.3X4	T41.3X5	T41.3X6
Amethopterin	T45.1X1	T45.1X2	T45.1X3	T45.1X4	T45.1X5	T45.1X6
Amezinium metilsulfate	T44.991	T44.992	T44.993	T44.994	T44.995	T44.996
Amfebutamone	T43.291	T43.292	T43.293	T43.294	T43.295	T43.296
Amfepramone	T50.5X1	T50.5X2	T50.5X3	T50.5X4	T50.5X5	T50.5X6
Amfetamine	T43.621	T43.622	T43.623	T43.624	T43.625	T43.626
Amfetaminil	T43.621	T43.622	T43.623	T43.624	T43.625	T43.626
Amfomycin	T36.8X1	T36.8X2	T36.8X3	T36.8X4	T36.8X5	T36.8X6
Amidefrine mesilate	T48.5X1	T48.5X2	T48.5X3	T48.5X4	T48.5X5	T48.5X6
Amidone	T40.3X1	T40.3X2	T40.3X3	T40.3X4	T40.3X5	T40.3X6
Amidopyrine	T39.2X1	T39.2X2	T39.2X3	T39.2X4	T39.2X5	T39.2X6
Amidotrizoate	T50.8X1	T50.8X2	T50.8X3	T50.8X4	T50.8X5	T50.8X6
Amiflamine	T43.1X1	T43.1X2	T43.1X3	T43.1X4	T43.1X5	T43.1X6
Amikacin	T36.5X1	T36.5X2	T36.5X3	T36.5X4	T36.5X5	T36.5X6
Amikhelline	T46.3X1	T46.3X2	T46.3X3	T46.3X4	T46.3X5	T46.3X6
Amiloride	T50.2X1	T50.2X2	T50.2X3	T50.2X4	T50.2X5	T50.2X6
Aminacrine	T49.0X1	T49.0X2	T49.0X3	T49.0X4	T49.0X5	T49.0X6
Amineptine	T43.011	T43.012	T43.013	T43.014	T43.015	T43.016
Aminitrozole	T37.3X1	T37.3X2	T37.3X3	T37.3X4	T37.3X5	T37.3X6
Aminoacetic acid (derivatives)	T50.3X1	T50.3X2	T50.3X3	T50.3X4	T50.3X5	T50.3X6
Amino acids	T50.3X1	T50.3X2	T50.3X3	T50.3X4	T50.3X5	T50.3X6
Aminoacridine	T49.0X1	T49.0X2	T49.0X3	T49.0X4	T49.0X5	T49.0X6
Aminobenzoic acid (-p)	T49.3X1	T49.3X2	T49.3X3	T49.3X4	T49.3X5	T49.3X6
Aminocaproic acid	T45.621	T45.622	T45.623	T45.624	T45.625	T45.626
Aminoethylisothiourium	T45.8X1	T45.8X2	T45.8X3	T45.8X4	T45.8X5	T45.8X6
Aminofenazone	T39.2X1	T39.2X2	T39.2X3	T39.2X4	T39.2X5	T39.2X6
Aminoglutethimide	T45.1X1	T45.1X2	T45.1X3	T45.1X4	T45.1X5	T45.1X6
Aminohippuric acid	T50.8X1	T50.8X2	T50.8X3	T50.8X4	T50.8X5	T50.8X6
Aminomethylbenzoic acid	T45.691	T45.692	T45.693	T45.694	T45.695	T45.696
Aminometradine	T50.2X1	T50.2X2	T50.2X3	T50.2X4	T50.2X5	T50.2X6
Aminopentamide	T44.3X1	T44.3X2	T44.3X3	T44.3X4	T44.3X5	T44.3X6
Aminophenazone	T39.2X1	T39.2X2	T39.2X3	T39.2X4	T39.2X5	T39.2X6
Aminophenol	T54.0X1	T54.0X2	T54.0X3	T54.0X4	—	—
Aminophenylpyridone	T43.591	T43.592	T43.593	T43.594	T43.595	T43.596
Aminophylline	T48.6X1	T48.6X2	T48.6X3	T48.6X4	T48.6X5	T48.6X6
Aminopterin sodium	T45.1X1	T45.1X2	T45.1X3	T45.1X4	T45.1X5	T45.1X6
Aminopyrine	T39.2X1	T39.2X2	T39.2X3	T39.2X4	T39.2X5	T39.2X6
Aminorex	T50.5X1	T50.5X2	T50.5X3	T50.5X4	T50.5X5	T50.5X6
Aminosalicylic acid	T37.1X1	T37.1X2	T37.1X3	T37.1X4	T37.1X5	T37.1X6
Aminosalylum	T37.1X1	T37.1X2	T37.1X3	T37.1X4	T37.1X5	T37.1X6
Amiodarone	T46.2X1	T46.2X2	T46.2X3	T46.2X4	T46.2X5	T46.2X6
Amiphenazole	T50.7X1	T50.7X2	T50.7X3	T50.7X4	T50.7X5	T50.7X6
Amiquinsin	T46.5X1	T46.5X2	T46.5X3	T46.5X4	T46.5X5	T46.5X6
Amisometradine	T50.2X1	T50.2X2	T50.2X3	T50.2X4	T50.2X5	T50.2X6
Amisulpride	T43.591	T43.592	T43.593	T43.594	T43.595	T43.596
Amitriptyline	T43.011	T43.012	T43.013	T43.014	T43.015	T43.016
Amitriptylinoxide	T43.011	T43.012	T43.013	T43.014	T43.015	T43.016
Amlexanox	T48.6X1	T48.6X2	T48.6X3	T48.6X4	T48.6X5	T48.6X6
Ammonia (fumes) (gas) (vapor)	T59.891	T59.892	T59.893	T59.894	—	—
aromatic spirit	T48.991	T48.992	T48.993	T48.994	T48.995	T48.996
liquid (household)	T54.3X1	T54.3X2	T54.3X3	T54.3X4	—	—
Ammoniated mercury	T49.0X1	T49.0X2	T49.0X3	T49.0X4	T49.0X5	T49.0X6
Ammonium						
acid tartrate	T49.5X1	T49.5X2	T49.5X3	T49.5X4	T49.5X5	T49.5X6
bromide	T42.6X1	T42.6X2	T42.6X3	T42.6X4	T42.6X5	T42.6X6
carbonate	T54.3X1	T54.3X2	T54.3X3	T54.3X4	—	—
chloride	T50.991	T50.992	T50.993	T50.994	T50.995	T50.996
expectorant	T48.4X1	T48.4X2	T48.4X3	T48.4X4	T48.4X5	T48.4X6
compounds (household) NEC	T54.3X1	T54.3X2	T54.3X3	T54.3X4	—	—
fumes (any usage)	T59.891	T59.892	T59.893	T59.894	—	—
industrial	T54.3X1	T54.3X2	T54.3X3	T54.3X4	—	—

Substance	Poisoning, Accidental (unintentional)	Poisoning, Intentional Self-harm	Poisoning, Assault	Poisoning, Undetermined	Adverse Effect	Under-dosing
Ammonium — continued						
ichthyosulronate	T49.4X1	T49.4X2	T49.4X3	T49.4X4	T49.4X5	T49.4X6
mandelate	T37.91	T37.92	T37.93	T37.94	T37.95	T37.96
sulfamate	T60.3X1	T60.3X2	T60.3X3	T60.3X4	—	—
sulfonate resin	T47.8X1	T47.8X2	T47.8X3	T47.8X4	T47.8X5	T47.8X6
Amobarbital (sodium)	T42.3X1	T42.3X2	T42.3X3	T42.3X4	T42.3X5	T42.3X6
Amodiaquine	T37.2X1	T37.2X2	T37.2X3	T37.2X4	T37.2X5	T37.2X6
Amopyroquin (e)	T37.2X1	T37.2X2	T37.2X3	T37.2X4	T37.2X5	T37.2X6
Amoxapine	T43.011	T43.012	T43.013	T43.014	T43.015	T43.016
Amoxicillin	T36.0X1	T36.0X2	T36.0X3	T36.0X4	T36.0X5	T36.0X6
Amperozide	T43.591	T43.592	T43.593	T43.594	T43.595	T43.596
Amphenidone	T43.591	T43.592	T43.593	T43.594	T43.595	T43.596
Amphetamine NEC	T43.621	T43.622	T43.623	T43.624	T43.625	T43.626
Amphomycin	T36.8X1	T36.8X2	T36.8X3	T36.8X4	T36.8X5	T36.8X6
Amphotalide	T37.4X1	T37.4X2	T37.4X3	T37.4X4	T37.4X5	T37.4X6
Amphotericin B	T36.7X1	T36.7X2	T36.7X3	T36.7X4	T36.7X5	T36.7X6
topical	T49.0X1	T49.0X2	T49.0X3	T49.0X4	T49.0X5	T49.0X6
Ampicillin	T36.0X1	T36.0X2	T36.0X3	T36.0X4	T36.0X5	T36.0X6
Amprotropine	T44.3X1	T44.3X2	T44.3X3	T44.3X4	T44.3X5	T44.3X6
Amsacrine	T45.1X1	T45.1X2	T45.1X3	T45.1X4	T45.1X5	T45.1X6
Amygdaline	T62.2X1	T62.2X2	T62.2X3	T62.2X4	—	—
Amyl						
acetate	T52.8X1	T52.8X2	T52.8X3	T52.8X4	—	—
vapor	T59.891	T59.892	T59.893	T59.894	—	—
alcohol	T51.3X1	T51.3X2	T51.3X3	T51.3X4	—	—
chloride	T53.6X1	T53.6X2	T53.6X3	T53.6X4	—	—
formate	T52.8X1	T52.8X2	T52.8X3	T52.8X4	—	—
nitrite	T46.3X1	T46.3X2	T46.3X3	T46.3X4	T46.3X5	T46.3X6
propionate	T65.891	T65.892	T65.893	T65.894	—	—
Amylase	T47.5X1	T47.5X2	T47.5X3	T47.5X4	T47.5X5	T47.5X6
Amyleine, regional	T41.3X1	T41.3X2	T41.3X3	T41.3X4	T41.3X5	T41.3X6
Amylene						
dichloride	T53.6X1	T53.6X2	T53.6X3	T53.6X4	—	—
hydrate	T51.3X1	T51.3X2	T51.3X3	T51.3X4	—	—
Amylmetacresol	T49.6X1	T49.6X2	T49.6X3	T49.6X4	T49.6X5	T49.6X6
Amylobarbitone	T42.3X1	T42.3X2	T42.3X3	T42.3X4	T42.3X5	T42.3X6
Amylocaine, regional	T41.3X1	T41.3X2	T41.3X3	T41.3X4	T41.3X5	T41.3X6
infiltration (subcutaneous)	T41.3X1	T41.3X2	T41.3X3	T41.3X4	T41.3X5	T41.3X6
nerve block (peripheral) (plexus)	T41.3X1	T41.3X2	T41.3X3	T41.3X4	T41.3X5	T41.3X6
spinal	T41.3X1	T41.3X2	T41.3X3	T41.3X4	T41.3X5	T41.3X6
topical (surface)	T41.3X1	T41.3X2	T41.3X3	T41.3X4	T41.3X5	T41.3X6
Amylopectin	T47.6X1	T47.6X2	T47.6X3	T47.6X4	T47.6X5	T47.6X6
Amytal (sodium)	T42.3X1	T42.3X2	T42.3X3	T42.3X4	T42.3X5	T42.3X6
Anabolic steroid	T38.7X1	T38.7X2	T38.7X3	T38.7X4	T38.7X5	T38.7X6
Analeptic NEC	T50.7X1	T50.7X2	T50.7X3	T50.7X4	T50.7X5	T50.7X6
Analgesic	T39.91	T39.92	T39.93	T39.94	T39.95	T39.96
anti-inflammatory NEC	T39.91	T39.92	T39.93	T39.94	T39.95	T39.96
propionic acid derivative	T39.311	T39.312	T39.313	T39.314	T39.315	T39.316
antirheumatic NEC	T39.4X1	T39.4X2	T39.4X3	T39.4X4	T39.4X5	T39.4X6
aromatic NEC	T39.1X1	T39.1X2	T39.1X3	T39.1X4	T39.1X5	T39.1X6
narcotic NEC	T40.601	T40.602	T40.603	T40.604	T40.605	T40.606
combination	T40.601	T40.602	T40.603	T40.604	T40.605	T40.606
obstetric	T40.601	T40.602	T40.603	T40.604	T40.605	T40.606
non-narcotic NEC	T39.91	T39.92	T39.93	T39.94	T39.95	T39.96
combination	T39.91	T39.92	T39.93	T39.94	T39.95	T39.96
pyrazole	T39.2X1	T39.2X2	T39.2X3	T39.2X4	T39.2X5	T39.2X6
specified NEC	T39.8X1	T39.8X2	T39.8X3	T39.8X4	T39.8X5	T39.8X6
Analgin	T39.2X1	T39.2X2	T39.2X3	T39.2X4	T39.2X5	T39.2X6
Anamirta cocculus	T62.1X1	T62.1X2	T62.1X3	T62.1X4	—	—
Ancillin	T36.0X1	T36.0X2	T36.0X3	T36.0X4	T36.0X5	T36.0X6
Ancrod	T45.691	T45.692	T45.693	T45.694	T45.695	T45.696
Androgen	T38.7X1	T38.7X2	T38.7X3	T38.7X4	T38.7X5	T38.7X6
Androgen-estrogen mixture	T38.7X1	T38.7X2	T38.7X3	T38.7X4	T38.7X5	T38.7X6
Androstalone	T38.7X1	T38.7X2	T38.7X3	T38.7X4	T38.7X5	T38.7X6
Androstanolone	T38.7X1	T38.7X2	T38.7X3	T38.7X4	T38.7X5	T38.7X6
Androsterone	T38.7X1	T38.7X2	T38.7X3	T38.7X4	T38.7X5	T38.7X6
Anemone pulsatilla	T62.2X1	T62.2X2	T62.2X3	T62.2X4	—	—
Anesthesia						
caudal	T41.3X1	T41.3X2	T41.3X3	T41.3X4	T41.3X5	T41.3X6
endotracheal	T41.0X1	T41.0X2	T41.0X3	T41.0X4	T41.0X5	T41.0X6
epidural	T41.3X1	T41.3X2	T41.3X3	T41.3X4	T41.3X5	T41.3X6
inhalation	T41.0X1	T41.0X2	T41.0X3	T41.0X4	T41.0X5	T41.0X6
local	T41.3X1	T41.3X2	T41.3X3	T41.3X4	T41.3X5	T41.3X6
mucosal	T41.3X1	T41.3X2	T41.3X3	T41.3X4	T41.3X5	T41.3X6
muscle relaxation	T48.1X1	T48.1X2	T48.1X3	T48.1X4	T48.1X5	T48.1X6
nerve blocking	T41.3X1	T41.3X2	T41.3X3	T41.3X4	T41.3X5	T41.3X6
plexus blocking	T41.3X1	T41.3X2	T41.3X3	T41.3X4	T41.3X5	T41.3X6
potentiated	T41.201	T41.202	T41.203	T41.204	T41.205	T41.206
rectal	T41.201	T41.202	T41.203	T41.204	T41.205	T41.206
general	T41.201	T41.202	T41.203	T41.204	T41.205	T41.206
local	T41.3X1	T41.3X2	T41.3X3	T41.3X4	T41.3X5	T41.3X6

Table of Drugs and Chemicals

Substance	Poisoning, Accidental (unintentional)	Poisoning, Intentional Self-harm	Poisoning, Assault	Poisoning, Undetermined	Adverse Effect	Under-dosing
Anesthesia — continued						
regional	T41.3X1	T41.3X2	T41.3X3	T41.3X4	T41.3X5	T41.3X6
surface	T41.3X1	T41.3X2	T41.3X3	T41.3X4	T41.3X5	T41.3X6
Anesthetic NEC — see also	T41.41	T41.42	T41.43	T41.44	T41.45	T41.46
Anesthesia						
with muscle relaxant	T41.201	T41.202	T41.203	T41.204	T41.205	T41.206
general	T41.201	T41.202	T41.203	T41.204	T41.205	T41.206
local	T41.3X1	T41.3X2	T41.3X3	T41.3X4	T41.3X5	T41.3X6
gaseous NEC	T41.0X1	T41.0X2	T41.0X3	T41.0X4	T41.0X5	T41.0X6
general NEC	T41.201	T41.202	T41.203	T41.204	T41.205	T41.206
halogenated hydrocarbon derivatives NEC	T41.0X1	T41.0X2	T41.0X3	T41.0X4	T41.0X5	T41.0X6
infiltration NEC	T41.3X1	T41.3X2	T41.3X3	T41.3X4	T41.3X5	T41.3X6
intravenous NEC	T41.1X1	T41.1X2	T41.1X3	T41.1X4	T41.1X5	T41.1X6
local NEC	T41.3X1	T41.3X2	T41.3X3	T41.3X4	T41.3X5	T41.3X6
rectal	T41.201	T41.202	T41.203	T41.204	T41.205	T41.206
general	T41.201	T41.202	T41.203	T41.204	T41.205	T41.206
local	T41.3X1	T41.3X2	T41.3X3	T41.3X4	T41.3X5	T41.3X6
regional NEC	T41.3X1	T41.3X2	T41.3X3	T41.3X4	T41.3X5	T41.3X6
spinal NEC	T41.3X1	T41.3X2	T41.3X3	T41.3X4	T41.3X5	T41.3X6
thiobarbiturate	T41.1X1	T41.1X2	T41.1X3	T41.1X4	T41.1X5	T41.1X6
topical	T41.3X1	T41.3X2	T41.3X3	T41.3X4	T41.3X5	T41.3X6
Aneurine	T45.2X1	T45.2X2	T45.2X3	T45.2X4	T45.2X5	T45.2X6
Angio-Conray	T50.8X1	T50.8X2	T50.8X3	T50.8X4	T50.8X5	T50.8X6
Angiotensin	T44.5X1	T44.5X2	T44.5X3	T44.5X4	T44.5X5	T44.5X6
Angiotensinamide	T44.991	T44.992	T44.993	T44.994	T44.995	T44.996
Anhydrohydroxy-progesterone	T38.5X1	T38.5X2	T38.5X3	T38.5X4	T38.5X5	T38.5X6
Anhydron	T50.2X1	T50.2X2	T50.2X3	T50.2X4	T50.2X5	T50.2X6
Anileridine	T40.4X1	T40.4X2	T40.4X3	T40.4X4	T40.4X5	T40.4X6
Aniline (dye) (liquid)	T65.3X1	T65.3X2	T65.3X3	T65.3X4	—	—
analgesic	T39.1X1	T39.1X2	T39.1X3	T39.1X4	T39.1X5	T39.1X6
derivatives, therapeutic NEC	T39.1X1	T39.1X2	T39.1X3	T39.1X4	T39.1X5	T39.1X6
vapor	T65.3X1	T65.3X2	T65.3X3	T65.3X4	—	—
Aniscoropine	T44.3X1	T44.3X2	T44.3X3	T44.3X4	T44.3X5	T44.3X6
Anise oil	T47.5X1	T47.5X2	T47.5X3	T47.5X4	T47.5X5	T47.5X6
Anisidine	T65.3X1	T65.3X2	T65.3X3	T65.3X4	—	—
Anisindione	T45.511	T45.512	T45.513	T45.514	T45.515	T45.516
Anisotropine methyl-bromide	T44.3X1	T44.3X2	T44.3X3	T44.3X4	T44.3X5	T44.3X6
Anistreplase	T45.611	T45.612	T45.613	T45.614	T45.615	T45.616
Anorexiant (central)	T50.5X1	T50.5X2	T50.5X3	T50.5X4	T50.5X5	T50.5X6
Anorexic agents	T50.5X1	T50.5X2	T50.5X3	T50.5X4	T50.5X5	T50.5X6
Ansamycin	T36.6X1	T36.6X2	T36.6X3	T36.6X4	T36.6X5	T36.6X6
Ant (bite) (sting)	T63.421	T63.422	T63.423	T63.424	—	—
Antabuse	T50.6X1	T50.6X2	T50.6X3	T50.6X4	T50.6X5	T50.6X6
Antacid NEC	T47.1X1	T47.1X2	T47.1X3	T47.1X4	T47.1X5	T47.1X6
Antagonist						
Aldosterone	T50.0X1	T50.0X2	T50.0X3	T50.0X4	T50.0X5	T50.0X6
alpha-adrenoreceptor	T44.6X1	T44.6X2	T44.6X3	T44.6X4	T44.6X5	T44.6X6
anticoagulant	T45.7X1	T45.7X2	T45.7X3	T45.7X4	T45.7X5	T45.7X6
beta-adrenoreceptor	T44.7X1	T44.7X2	T44.7X3	T44.7X4	T44.7X5	T44.7X6
extrapyramidal NEC	T44.3X1	T44.3X2	T44.3X3	T44.3X4	T44.3X5	T44.3X6
folic acid	T45.1X1	T45.1X2	T45.1X3	T45.1X4	T45.1X5	T45.1X6
H2 receptor	T47.0X1	T47.0X2	T47.0X3	T47.0X4	T47.0X5	T47.0X6
heavy metal	T45.8X1	T45.8X2	T45.8X3	T45.8X4	T45.8X5	T45.8X6
narcotic analgesic	T50.7X1	T50.7X2	T50.7X3	T50.7X4	T50.7X5	T50.7X6
opiate	T50.7X1	T50.7X2	T50.7X3	T50.7X4	T50.7X5	T50.7X6
pyrimidine	T45.1X1	T45.1X2	T45.1X3	T45.1X4	T45.1X5	T45.1X6
serotonin	T46.5X1	T46.5X2	T46.5X3	T46.5X4	T46.5X5	T46.5X6
Antazolin (e)	T45.0X1	T45.0X2	T45.0X3	T45.0X4	T45.0X5	T45.0X6
Anterior pituitary hormone NEC	T38.811	T38.812	T38.813	T38.814	T38.815	T38.816
Anthelmintic NEC	T37.4X1	T37.4X2	T37.4X3	T37.4X4	T37.4X5	T37.4X6
Anthiolimine	T37.4X1	T37.4X2	T37.4X3	T37.4X4	T37.4X5	T37.4X6
Anthralin	T49.4X1	T49.4X2	T49.4X3	T49.4X4	T49.4X5	T49.4X6
Anthramycin	T45.1X1	T45.1X2	T45.1X3	T45.1X4	T45.1X5	T45.1X6
Antiadrenergic NEC	T44.8X1	T44.8X2	T44.8X3	T44.8X4	T44.8X5	T44.8X6
Antiallergic NEC	T45.0X1	T45.0X2	T45.0X3	T45.0X4	T45.0X5	T45.0X6
Antiandrogen NEC	T38.6X1	T38.6X2	T38.6X3	T38.6X4	T38.6X5	T38.6X6
Anti-anemic (drug) (preparation)	T45.8X1	T45.8X2	T45.8X3	T45.8X4	T45.8X5	T45.8X6
Antianxiety drug NEC	T43.501	T43.502	T43.503	T43.504	T43.505	T43.506
Antiaris toxicaria	T65.891	T65.892	T65.893	T65.894	—	—
Antiarteriosclerotic drug	T46.6X1	T46.6X2	T46.6X3	T46.6X4	T46.6X5	T46.6X6
Antiasthmatic drug NEC	T48.6X1	T48.6X2	T48.6X3	T48.6X4	T48.6X5	T48.6X6
Antibiotic NEC	T36.91	T36.92	T36.93	T36.94	T36.95	T36.96
aminoglycoside	T36.5X1	T36.5X2	T36.5X3	T36.5X4	T36.5X5	T36.5X6
anticancer	T45.1X1	T45.1X2	T45.1X3	T45.1X4	T45.1X5	T45.1X6
antifungal	T36.7X1	T36.7X2	T36.7X3	T36.7X4	T36.7X5	T36.7X6
antimycobacterial	T36.5X1	T36.5X2	T36.5X3	T36.5X4	T36.5X5	T36.5X6
antineoplastic	T45.1X1	T45.1X2	T45.1X3	T45.1X4	T45.1X5	T45.1X6
b-lactam NEC	T36.1X1	T36.1X2	T36.1X3	T36.1X4	T36.1X5	T36.1X6

Substance	Poisoning, Accidental (unintentional)	Poisoning, Intentional Self-harm	Poisoning, Assault	Poisoning, Undetermined	Adverse Effect	Under-dosing
Antibiotic — continued						
cephalosporin (group)	T36.1X1	T36.1X2	T36.1X3	T36.1X4	T36.1X5	T36.1X6
chloramphenicol (group)	T36.2X1	T36.2X2	T36.2X3	T36.2X4	T36.2X5	T36.2X6
ENT	T49.6X1	T49.6X2	T49.6X3	T49.6X4	T49.6X5	T49.6X6
eye	T49.5X1	T49.5X2	T49.5X3	T49.5X4	T49.5X5	T49.5X6
fungicidal (local)	T49.0X1	T49.0X2	T49.0X3	T49.0X4	T49.0X5	T49.0X6
intestinal	T36.8X1	T36.8X2	T36.8X3	T36.8X4	T36.8X5	T36.8X6
local	T49.0X1	T49.0X2	T49.0X3	T49.0X4	T49.0X5	T49.0X6
macrolides	T36.3X1	T36.3X2	T36.3X3	T36.3X4	T36.3X5	T36.3X6
polypeptide	T36.8X1	T36.8X2	T36.8X3	T36.8X4	T36.8X5	T36.8X6
specified NEC	T36.8X1	T36.8X2	T36.8X3	T36.8X4	T36.8X5	T36.8X6
tetracycline (group)	T36.4X1	T36.4X2	T36.4X3	T36.4X4	T36.4X5	T36.4X6
throat	T49.6X1	T49.6X2	T49.6X3	T49.6X4	T49.6X5	T49.6X6
Anticancer agents NEC	T45.1X1	T45.1X2	T45.1X3	T45.1X4	T45.1X5	T45.1X6
Anticholesterolemic drug NEC	T46.6X1	T46.6X2	T46.6X3	T46.6X4	T46.6X5	T46.6X6
Anticholinergic NEC	T44.3X1	T44.3X2	T44.3X3	T44.3X4	T44.3X5	T44.3X6
Anticholinesterase	T44.0X1	T44.0X2	T44.0X3	T44.0X4	T44.0X5	T44.0X6
organophosphorus	T44.0X1	T44.0X2	T44.0X3	T44.0X4	T44.0X5	T44.0X6
insecticide	T60.0X1	T60.0X2	T60.0X3	T60.0X4	—	—
nerve gas	T59.891	T59.892	T59.893	T59.894	—	—
reversible	T44.0X1	T44.0X2	T44.0X3	T44.0X4	T44.0X5	T44.0X6
ophthalmological	T49.5X1	T49.5X2	T49.5X3	T49.5X4	T49.5X5	T49.5X6
Anticoagulant NEC	T45.511	T45.512	T45.513	T45.514	T45.515	T45.516
Antagonist	T45.7X1	T45.7X2	T45.7X3	T45.7X4	T45.7X5	T45.7X6
Anti-common-cold drug NEC	T48.5X1	T48.5X2	T48.5X3	T48.5X4	T48.5X5	T48.5X6
Anticonvulsant	T42.71	T42.72	T42.73	T42.74	T42.75	T42.76
barbiturate	T42.3X1	T42.3X2	T42.3X3	T42.3X4	T42.3X5	T42.3X6
combination (with barbiturate)	T42.3X1	T42.3X2	T42.3X3	T42.3X4	T42.3X5	T42.3X6
hydantoin	T42.0X1	T42.0X2	T42.0X3	T42.0X4	T42.0X5	T42.0X6
hypnotic NEC	T42.6X1	T42.6X2	T42.6X3	T42.6X4	T42.6X5	T42.6X6
oxazolidinedione	T42.2X1	T42.2X2	T42.2X3	T42.2X4	T42.2X5	T42.2X6
pyrimidinedione	T42.6X1	T42.6X2	T42.6X3	T42.6X4	T42.6X5	T42.6X6
specified NEC	T42.6X1	T42.6X2	T42.6X3	T42.6X4	T42.6X5	T42.6X6
succinimide	T42.2X1	T42.2X2	T42.2X3	T42.2X4	T42.2X5	T42.2X6
Antidepressant	T43.201	T43.202	T43.203	T43.204	T43.205	T43.206
monoamine oxidase inhibitor	T43.1X1	T43.1X2	T43.1X3	T43.1X4	T43.1X5	T43.1X6
selective serotonin norepinephrine reuptake inhibitor	T43.211	T43.212	T43.213	T43.214	T43.215	T43.216
selective serotonin reuptake inhibitor	T43.221	T43.222	T43.223	T43.224	T43.225	T43.226
specified NEC	T43.291	T43.292	T43.293	T43.294	T43.295	T43.296
tetracyclic	T43.021	T43.022	T43.023	T43.024	T43.025	T43.026
triazolopyridine	T43.211	T43.212	T43.213	T43.214	T43.215	T43.216
tricyclic	T43.011	T43.012	T43.013	T43.014	T43.015	T43.016
Antidiabetic NEC	T38.3X1	T38.3X2	T38.3X3	T38.3X4	T38.3X5	T38.3X6
biguanide	T38.3X1	T38.3X2	T38.3X3	T38.3X4	T38.3X5	T38.3X6
and sulfonyl combined	T38.3X1	T38.3X2	T38.3X3	T38.3X4	T38.3X5	T38.3X6
combined	T38.3X1	T38.3X2	T38.3X3	T38.3X4	T38.3X5	T38.3X6
sulfonylurea	T38.3X1	T38.3X2	T38.3X3	T38.3X4	T38.3X5	T38.3X6
Antidiarrheal drug NEC	T47.6X1	T47.6X2	T47.6X3	T47.6X4	T47.6X5	T47.6X6
absorbent	T47.6X1	T47.6X2	T47.6X3	T47.6X4	T47.6X5	T47.6X6
Anti-D immunoglobulin (human)	T50.Z11	T50.Z12	T50.Z13	T50.Z14	T50.Z15	T50.Z16
Antidiphtheria serum	T50.Z11	T50.Z12	T50.Z13	T50.Z14	T50.Z15	T50.Z16
Antidiuretic hormone	T38.891	T38.892	T38.893	T38.894	T38.895	T38.896
Antidote NEC	T50.6X1	T50.6X2	T50.6X3	T50.6X4	T50.6X5	T50.6X6
heavy metal	T45.8X1	T45.8X2	T45.8X3	T45.8X4	T45.8X5	T45.8X6
Antidysrhythmic NEC	T46.2X1	T46.2X2	T46.2X3	T46.2X4	T46.2X5	T46.2X6
Antiemetic drug	T45.0X1	T45.0X2	T45.0X3	T45.0X4	T45.0X5	T45.0X6
Antiepilepsy agent	T42.71	T42.72	T42.73	T42.74	T42.75	T42.76
combination	T42.5X1	T42.5X2	T42.5X3	T42.5X4	T42.5X5	T42.5X6
mixed	T42.5X1	T42.5X2	T42.5X3	T42.5X4	T42.5X5	T42.5X6
specified, NEC	T42.6X1	T42.6X2	T42.6X3	T42.6X4	T42.6X5	T42.6X6
Antiestrogen NEC	T38.6X1	T38.6X2	T38.6X3	T38.6X4	T38.6X5	T38.6X6
Antifertility pill	T38.4X1	T38.4X2	T38.4X3	T38.4X4	T38.4X5	T38.4X6
Antifibrinolytic drug	T45.621	T45.622	T45.623	T45.624	T45.625	T45.626
Antifilarial drug	T37.4X1	T37.4X2	T37.4X3	T37.4X4	T37.4X5	T37.4X6
Antiflatulent	T47.5X1	T47.5X2	T47.5X3	T47.5X4	T47.5X5	T47.5X6
Antifreeze	T65.91	T65.92	T65.93	T65.94	—	—
alcohol	T51.1X1	T51.1X2	T51.1X3	T51.1X4	—	—
ethylene glycol	T51.8X1	T51.8X2	T51.8X3	T51.8X4	—	—
Antifungal						
antibiotic (systemic)	T36.7X1	T36.7X2	T36.7X3	T36.7X4	T36.7X5	T36.7X6
anti-infective NEC	T37.91	T37.92	T37.93	T37.94	T37.95	T37.96
disinfectant, local	T49.0X1	T49.0X2	T49.0X3	T49.0X4	T49.0X5	T49.0X6
nonmedicinal (spray)	T60.3X1	T60.3X2	T60.3X3	T60.3X4	—	—
topical	T49.0X1	T49.0X2	T49.0X3	T49.0X4	T49.0X5	T49.0X6

Additional Character May Be Required — Refer to the Tabular List for Character Selection Subterms under main terms may continue to next column or page

Substance	Poisoning, Accidental (unintentional)	Poisoning, Intentional Self-harm	Poisoning, Assault	Poisoning, Undetermined	Adverse Effect	Under-dosing
Anti-gastric-secretion drug NEC	T47.1X1	T47.1X2	T47.1X3	T47.1X4	T47.1X5	T47.1X6
Antigonadotrophin NEC	T38.6X1	T38.6X2	T38.6X3	T38.6X4	T38.6X5	T38.6X6
Antihallucinogen	T43.501	T43.502	T43.503	T43.504	T43.505	T43.506
Antihelmintics	T37.4X1	T37.4X2	T37.4X3	T37.4X4	T37.4X5	T37.4X6
Antihemophilic						
factor	T45.8X1	T45.8X2	T45.8X3	T45.8X4	T45.8X5	T45.8X6
fraction	T45.8X1	T45.8X2	T45.8X3	T45.8X4	T45.8X5	T45.8X6
globulin concentrate	T45.7X1	T45.7X2	T45.7X3	T45.7X4	T45.7X5	T45.7X6
human plasma	T45.8X1	T45.8X2	T45.8X3	T45.8X4	T45.8X5	T45.8X6
plasma, dried	T45.7X1	T45.7X2	T45.7X3	T45.7X4	T45.7X5	T45.7X6
Antihemorrhoidal preparation	T49.2X1	T49.2X2	T49.2X3	T49.2X4	T49.2X5	T49.2X6
Antiheparin drug	T45.7X1	T45.7X2	T45.7X3	T45.7X4	T45.7X5	T45.7X6
Antihistamine	T45.0X1	T45.0X2	T45.0X3	T45.0X4	T45.0X5	T45.0X6
Antihookworm drug	T37.4X1	T37.4X2	T37.4X3	T37.4X4	T37.4X5	T37.4X6
Anti-human lymphocytic globulin	T50.Z11	T50.Z12	T50.Z13	T50.Z14	T50.Z15	T50.Z16
Antihyperlipidemic drug	T46.6X1	T46.6X2	T46.6X3	T46.6X4	T46.6X5	T46.6X6
Antihypertensive drug NEC	T46.5X1	T46.5X2	T46.5X3	T46.5X4	T46.5X5	T46.5X6
Anti-infective NEC	T37.91	T37.92	T37.93	T37.94	T37.95	T37.96
anthelmintic	T37.4X1	T37.4X2	T37.4X3	T37.4X4	T37.4X5	T37.4X6
antibiotics	T36.91	T36.92	T36.93	T36.94	T36.95	T36.96
specified NEC	T36.8X1	T36.8X2	T36.8X3	T36.8X4	T36.8X5	T36.8X6
antimalarial	T37.2X1	T37.2X2	T37.2X3	T37.2X4	T37.2X5	T37.2X6
antimycobacterial NEC	T37.1X1	T37.1X2	T37.1X3	T37.1X4	T37.1X5	T37.1X6
antibiotics	T36.5X1	T36.5X2	T36.5X3	T36.5X4	T36.5X5	T36.5X6
antiprotozoal NEC	T37.3X1	T37.3X2	T37.3X3	T37.3X4	T37.3X5	T37.3X6
blood	T37.2X1	T37.2X2	T37.2X3	T37.2X4	T37.2X5	T37.2X6
antiviral	T37.5X1	T37.5X2	T37.5X3	T37.5X4	T37.5X5	T37.5X6
arsenical	T37.8X1	T37.8X2	T37.8X3	T37.8X4	T37.8X5	T37.8X6
bismuth, local	T49.0X1	T49.0X2	T49.0X3	T49.0X4	T49.0X5	T49.0X6
ENT	T49.6X1	T49.6X2	T49.6X3	T49.6X4	T49.6X5	T49.6X6
eye NEC	T49.5X1	T49.5X2	T49.5X3	T49.5X4	T49.5X5	T49.5X6
heavy metals NEC	T37.8X1	T37.8X2	T37.8X3	T37.8X4	T37.8X5	T37.8X6
local NEC	T49.0X1	T49.0X2	T49.0X3	T49.0X4	T49.0X5	T49.0X6
specified NEC	T49.0X1	T49.0X2	T49.0X3	T49.0X4	T49.0X5	T49.0X6
mixed	T37.91	T37.92	T37.93	T37.94	T37.95	T37.96
ophthalmic preparation	T49.5X1	T49.5X2	T49.5X3	T49.5X4	T49.5X5	T49.5X6
topical NEC	T49.0X1	T49.0X2	T49.0X3	T49.0X4	T49.0X5	T49.0X6
Anti-inflammatory drug NEC	T39.391	T39.392	T39.393	T39.394	T39.395	T39.396
local	T49.0X1	T49.0X2	T49.0X3	T49.0X4	T49.0X5	T49.0X6
nonsteroidal NEC	T39.391	T39.392	T39.393	T39.394	T39.395	T39.396
propionic acid derivative	T39.311	T39.312	T39.313	T39.314	T39.315	T39.316
specified NEC	T39.391	T39.392	T39.393	T39.394	T39.395	T39.396
Antikaluretic	T50.3X1	T50.3X2	T50.3X3	T50.3X4	T50.3X5	T50.3X6
Antiknock (tetraethyl lead)	T56.0X1	T56.0X2	T56.0X3	T56.0X4	—	—
Antilipemic drug NEC	T46.6X1	T46.6X2	T46.6X3	T46.6X4	T46.6X5	T46.6X6
Antimalarial	T37.2X1	T37.2X2	T37.2X3	T37.2X4	T37.2X5	T37.2X6
prophylactic NEC	T37.2X1	T37.2X2	T37.2X3	T37.2X4	T37.2X5	T37.2X6
pyrimidine derivative	T37.2X1	T37.2X2	T37.2X3	T37.2X4	T37.2X5	T37.2X6
Antimetabolite	T45.1X1	T45.1X2	T45.1X3	T45.1X4	T45.1X5	T45.1X6
Antimitotic agent	T45.1X1	T45.1X2	T45.1X3	T45.1X4	T45.1X5	T45.1X6
Antimony (compounds) (vapor) NEC	T56.891	T56.892	T56.893	T56.894	—	—
anti-infectives	T37.8X1	T37.8X2	T37.8X3	T37.8X4	T37.8X5	T37.8X6
dimercaptosuccinate	T37.3X1	T37.3X2	T37.3X3	T37.3X4	T37.3X5	T37.3X6
hydride	T56.891	T56.892	T56.893	T56.894	—	—
pesticide (vapor)	T60.8X1	T60.8X2	T60.8X3	T60.8X4	—	—
potassium (sodium) tartrate	T37.8X1	T37.8X2	T37.8X3	T37.8X4	T37.8X5	T37.8X6
sodium dimercaptosuccinate	T37.3X1	T37.3X2	T37.3X3	T37.3X4	T37.3X5	T37.3X6
tartrated	T37.8X1	T37.8X2	T37.8X3	T37.8X4	T37.8X5	T37.8X6
Antimuscarinic NEC	T44.3X1	T44.3X2	T44.3X3	T44.3X4	T44.3X5	T44.3X6
Antimycobacterial drug NEC	T37.1X1	T37.1X2	T37.1X3	T37.1X4	T37.1X5	T37.1X6
antibiotics	T36.5X1	T36.5X2	T36.5X3	T36.5X4	T36.5X5	T36.5X6
combination	T37.1X1	T37.1X2	T37.1X3	T37.1X4	T37.1X5	T37.1X6
Antinausea drug	T45.0X1	T45.0X2	T45.0X3	T45.0X4	T45.0X5	T45.0X6
Antinematode drug	T37.4X1	T37.4X2	T37.4X3	T37.4X4	T37.4X5	T37.4X6
Antineoplastic NEC	T45.1X1	T45.1X2	T45.1X3	T45.1X4	T45.1X5	T45.1X6
alkaloidal	T45.1X1	T45.1X2	T45.1X3	T45.1X4	T45.1X5	T45.1X6
antibiotics	T45.1X1	T45.1X2	T45.1X3	T45.1X4	T45.1X5	T45.1X6
combination	T45.1X1	T45.1X2	T45.1X3	T45.1X4	T45.1X5	T45.1X6
estrogen	T38.5X1	T38.5X2	T38.5X3	T38.5X4	T38.5X5	T38.5X6
steroid	T38.7X1	T38.7X2	T38.7X3	T38.7X4	T38.7X5	T38.7X6
Antiparasitic drug (systemic)	T37.91	T37.92	T37.93	T37.94	T37.95	T37.96
local	T49.0X1	T49.0X2	T49.0X3	T49.0X4	T49.0X5	T49.0X6
specified NEC	T37.8X1	T37.8X2	T37.8X3	T37.8X4	T37.8X5	T37.8X6

Substance	Poisoning, Accidental (unintentional)	Poisoning, Intentional Self-harm	Poisoning, Assault	Poisoning, Undetermined	Adverse Effect	Under-dosing
Antiparkinsonism drug NEC	T42.8X1	T42.8X2	T42.8X3	T42.8X4	T42.8X5	T42.8X6
Antiperspirant NEC	T49.2X1	T49.2X2	T49.2X3	T49.2X4	T49.2X5	T49.2X6
Antiphlogistic NEC	T39.4X1	T39.4X2	T39.4X3	T39.4X4	T39.4X5	T39.4X6
Antiplatyhelmintic drug	T37.4X1	T37.4X2	T37.4X3	T37.4X4	T37.4X5	T37.4X6
Antiprotozoal drug NEC	T37.3X1	T37.3X2	T37.3X3	T37.3X4	T37.3X5	T37.3X6
blood	T37.2X1	T37.2X2	T37.2X3	T37.2X4	T37.2X5	T37.2X6
local	T49.0X1	T49.0X2	T49.0X3	T49.0X4	T49.0X5	T49.0X6
Antipruritic drug NEC	T49.1X1	T49.1X2	T49.1X3	T49.1X4	T49.1X5	T49.1X6
Antipsychotic drug	T43.501	T43.502	T43.503	T43.504	T43.505	T43.506
specified NEC	T43.591	T43.592	T43.593	T43.594	T43.595	T43.596
Antipyretic	T39.91	T39.92	T39.93	T39.94	T39.95	T39.96
specified NEC	T39.8X1	T39.8X2	T39.8X3	T39.8X4	T39.8X5	T39.8X6
Antipyrine	T39.2X1	T39.2X2	T39.2X3	T39.2X4	T39.2X5	T39.2X6
Antirabies hyperimmune serum	T50.Z11	T50.Z12	T50.Z13	T50.Z14	T50.Z15	T50.Z16
Antirheumatic NEC	T39.4X1	T39.4X2	T39.4X3	T39.4X4	T39.4X5	T39.4X6
Antirigidity drug NEC	T42.8X1	T42.8X2	T42.8X3	T42.8X4	T42.8X5	T42.8X6
Antischistosomal drug	T37.4X1	T37.4X2	T37.4X3	T37.4X4	T37.4X5	T37.4X6
Antiscorpion sera	T50.Z11	T50.Z12	T50.Z13	T50.Z14	T50.Z15	T50.Z16
Antiseborrheics	T49.4X1	T49.4X2	T49.4X3	T49.4X4	T49.4X5	T49.4X6
Antiseptics (external) (medicinal)	T49.0X1	T49.0X2	T49.0X3	T49.0X4	T49.0X5	T49.0X6
Antistine	T45.0X1	T45.0X2	T45.0X3	T45.0X4	T45.0X5	T45.0X6
Antitapeworm drug	T37.4X1	T37.4X2	T37.4X3	T37.4X4	T37.4X5	T37.4X6
Antitetanus immunoglobulin	T50.Z11	T50.Z12	T50.Z13	T50.Z14	T50.Z15	T50.Z16
Antithrombotic	T45.521	T45.522	T45.523	T45.524	T45.525	T45.526
Antithyroid drug NEC	T38.2X1	T38.2X2	T38.2X3	T38.2X4	T38.2X5	T38.2X6
Antitoxin	T50.Z11	T50.Z12	T50.Z13	T50.Z14	T50.Z15	T50.Z16
diphtheria	T50.Z11	T50.Z12	T50.Z13	T50.Z14	T50.Z15	T50.Z16
gas gangrene	T50.Z11	T50.Z12	T50.Z13	T50.Z14	T50.Z15	T50.Z16
tetanus	T50.Z11	T50.Z12	T50.Z13	T50.Z14	T50.Z15	T50.Z16
Antitrichomonal drug	T37.3X1	T37.3X2	T37.3X3	T37.3X4	T37.3X5	T37.3X6
Antituberculars	T37.1X1	T37.1X2	T37.1X3	T37.1X4	T37.1X5	T37.1X6
antibiotics	T36.5X1	T36.5X2	T36.5X3	T36.5X4	T36.5X5	T36.5X6
Antitussive NEC	T48.3X1	T48.3X2	T48.3X3	T48.3X4	T48.3X5	T48.3X6
codeine mixture	T40.2X1	T40.2X2	T40.2X3	T40.2X4	T40.2X5	T40.2X6
opiate	T40.2X1	T40.2X2	T40.2X3	T40.2X4	T40.2X5	T40.2X6
Antivaricose drug	T46.8X1	T46.8X2	T46.8X3	T46.8X4	T46.8X5	T46.8X6
Antivenin, antivenom (sera)	T50.Z11	T50.Z12	T50.Z13	T50.Z14	T50.Z15	T50.Z16
crotaline	T50.Z11	T50.Z12	T50.Z13	T50.Z14	T50.Z15	T50.Z16
spider bite	T50.Z11	T50.Z12	T50.Z13	T50.Z14	T50.Z15	T50.Z16
Antivertigo drug	T45.0X1	T45.0X2	T45.0X3	T45.0X4	T45.0X5	T45.0X6
Antiviral drug NEC	T37.5X1	T37.5X2	T37.5X3	T37.5X4	T37.5X5	T37.5X6
eye	T49.5X1	T49.5X2	T49.5X3	T49.5X4	T49.5X5	T49.5X6
Antiwhipworm drug	T37.4X1	T37.4X2	T37.4X3	T37.4X4	T37.4X5	T37.4X6
Ant poison — see Insecticide						
Antrol — see also by specific chemical substance	T60.91	T60.92	T60.93	T60.94	—	—
fungicide	T60.91	T60.92	T60.93	T60.94	—	—
ANTU (alpha naphthylthiourea)	T60.4X1	T60.4X2	T60.4X3	T60.4X4	—	—
Apalcillin	T36.0X1	T36.0X2	T36.0X3	T36.0X4	T36.0X5	T36.0X6
APC	T48.5X1	T48.5X2	T48.5X3	T48.5X4	T48.5X5	T48.5X6
Aplonidine	T44.4X1	T44.4X2	T44.4X3	T44.4X4	T44.4X5	T44.4X6
Apomorphine	T47.7X1	T47.7X2	T47.7X3	T47.7X4	T47.7X5	T47.7X6
Appetite depressants, central	T50.5X1	T50.5X2	T50.5X3	T50.5X4	T50.5X5	T50.5X6
Apraclonidine (hydrochloride)	T44.4X1	T44.4X2	T44.4X3	T44.4X4	T44.4X5	T44.4X6
Apresoline	T46.5X1	T46.5X2	T46.5X3	T46.5X4	T46.5X5	T46.5X6
Aprindine	T46.2X1	T46.2X2	T46.2X3	T46.2X4	T46.2X5	T46.2X6
Aprobarbital	T42.3X1	T42.3X2	T42.3X3	T42.3X4	T42.3X5	T42.3X6
Apronalide	T42.6X1	T42.6X2	T42.6X3	T42.6X4	T42.6X5	T42.6X6
Aprotinin	T45.621	T45.622	T45.623	T45.624	T45.625	T45.626
Aptocaine	T41.3X1	T41.3X2	T41.3X3	T41.3X4	T41.3X5	T41.3X6
Aqua fortis	T54.2X1	T54.2X2	T54.2X3	T54.2X4	—	—
Ara-A	T37.5X1	T37.5X2	T37.5X3	T37.5X4	T37.5X5	T37.5X6
Ara-C	T45.1X1	T45.1X2	T45.1X3	T45.1X4	T45.1X5	T45.1X6
Arachis oil	T49.3X1	T49.3X2	T49.3X3	T49.3X4	T49.3X5	T49.3X6
cathartic	T47.4X1	T47.4X2	T47.4X3	T47.4X4	T47.4X5	T47.4X6
Aralen	T37.2X1	T37.2X2	T37.2X3	T37.2X4	T37.2X5	T37.2X6
Arecoline	T44.1X1	T44.1X2	T44.1X3	T44.1X4	T44.1X5	T44.1X6
Arginine	T50.991	T50.992	T50.993	T50.994	T50.995	T50.996
glutamate	T50.991	T50.992	T50.993	T50.994	T50.995	T50.996
Argyrol	T49.0X1	T49.0X2	T49.0X3	T49.0X4	T49.0X5	T49.0X6
ENT agent	T49.6X1	T49.6X2	T49.6X3	T49.6X4	T49.6X5	T49.6X6
ophthalmic preparation	T49.5X1	T49.5X2	T49.5X3	T49.5X4	T49.5X5	T49.5X6
Aristocort	T38.0X1	T38.0X2	T38.0X3	T38.0X4	T38.0X5	T38.0X6
ENT agent	T49.6X1	T49.6X2	T49.6X3	T49.6X4	T49.6X5	T49.6X6
ophthalmic preparation	T49.5X1	T49.5X2	T49.5X3	T49.5X4	T49.5X5	T49.5X6

▼ Subterms under main terms may continue to next column or page   Additional Character May Be Required — Refer to the Tabular List for Character Selection   353

Anti-gastric-secretion drug NEC — Aristocort

Table of Drugs and Chemicals

Aristocort — Benzamine

Substance	Poisoning, Accidental (unintentional)	Poisoning, Intentional Self-harm	Poisoning, Assault	Poisoning, Undetermined	Adverse Effect	Under-dosing
Aristocort — *continued*						
topical NEC	T49.0X1	T49.0X2	T49.0X3	T49.0X4	T49.0X5	T49.0X6
Aromatics, corrosive	T54.1X1	T54.1X2	T54.1X3	T54.1X4	—	—
disinfectants	T54.1X1	T54.1X2	T54.1X3	T54.1X4	—	—
Arsenate of lead	T57.0X1	T57.0X2	T57.0X3	T57.0X4	—	—
herbicide	T57.0X1	T57.0X2	T57.0X3	T57.0X4	—	—
Arsenic, arsenicals (compounds) (dust) (vapor) **NEC**	T57.0X1	T57.0X2	T57.0X3	T57.0X4	—	—
anti-infectives	T37.8X1	T37.8X2	T37.8X3	T37.8X4	T37.8X5	T37.8X6
pesticide (dust) (fumes)	T57.0X1	T57.0X2	T57.0X3	T57.0X4	—	—
Arsine (gas)	T57.0X1	T57.0X2	T57.0X3	T57.0X4	—	—
Arsphenamine (silver)	T37.8X1	T37.8X2	T37.8X3	T37.8X4	T37.8X5	T37.8X6
Arsthinol	T37.3X1	T37.3X2	T37.3X3	T37.3X4	T37.3X5	T37.3X6
Artane	T44.3X1	T44.3X2	T44.3X3	T44.3X4	T44.3X5	T44.3X6
Arthropod (venomous) **NEC**	T63.481	T63.482	T63.483	T63.484	—	—
Articaine	T41.3X1	T41.3X2	T41.3X3	T41.3X4	T41.3X5	T41.3X6
Asbestos	T57.8X1	T57.8X2	T57.8X3	T57.8X4	—	—
Ascaridole	T37.4X1	T37.4X2	T37.4X3	T37.4X4	T37.4X5	T37.4X6
Ascorbic acid	T45.2X1	T45.2X2	T45.2X3	T45.2X4	T45.2X5	T45.2X6
Asiaticoside	T49.0X1	T49.0X2	T49.0X3	T49.0X4	T49.0X5	T49.0X6
Asparaginase	T45.1X1	T45.1X2	T45.1X3	T45.1X4	T45.1X5	T45.1X6
Aspidium (oleoresin)	T37.4X1	T37.4X2	T37.4X3	T37.4X4	T37.4X5	T37.4X6
Aspirin (aluminum)	T39.011	T39.012	T39.013	T39.014	T39.015	T39.016
(soluble)	T36.0X1	T36.0X2	T36.0X3	T36.0X4	T36.0X5	T36.0X6
Aspoxicillin	T36.0X1	T36.0X2	T36.0X3	T36.0X4	T36.0X5	T36.0X6
Astemizole	T45.0X1	T45.0X2	T45.0X3	T45.0X4	T45.0X5	T45.0X6
Astringent (local)	T49.2X1	T49.2X2	T49.2X3	T49.2X4	T49.2X5	T49.2X6
specified NEC	T49.2X1	T49.2X2	T49.2X3	T49.2X4	T49.2X5	T49.2X6
Astromicin	T36.5X1	T36.5X2	T36.5X3	T36.5X4	T36.5X5	T36.5X6
Ataractic drug NEC	T43.501	T43.502	T43.503	T43.504	T43.505	T43.506
Atenolol	T44.7X1	T44.7X2	T44.7X3	T44.7X4	T44.7X5	T44.7X6
Atonia drug, intestinal	T47.4X1	T47.4X2	T47.4X3	T47.4X4	T47.4X5	T47.4X6
Atophan	T50.4X1	T50.4X2	T50.4X3	T50.4X4	T50.4X5	T50.4X6
Atracurium besilate	T48.1X1	T48.1X2	T48.1X3	T48.1X4	T48.1X5	T48.1X6
Atropine	T44.3X1	T44.3X2	T44.3X3	T44.3X4	T44.3X5	T44.3X6
derivative	T44.3X1	T44.3X2	T44.3X3	T44.3X4	T44.3X5	T44.3X6
methonitrate	T44.3X1	T44.3X2	T44.3X3	T44.3X4	T44.3X5	T44.3X6
Attapulgite	T47.6X1	T47.6X2	T47.6X3	T47.6X4	T47.6X5	T47.6X6
Auramine	T65.891	T65.892	T65.893	T65.894	—	—
dye	T65.6X1	T65.6X2	T65.6X3	T65.6X4	—	—
fungicide	T60.3X1	T60.3X2	T60.3X3	T60.3X4	—	—
Auranofin	T39.4X1	T39.4X2	T39.4X3	T39.4X4	T39.4X5	T39.4X6
Aurantiin	T46.991	T46.992	T46.993	T46.994	T46.995	T46.996
Aureomycin	T36.4X1	T36.4X2	T36.4X3	T36.4X4	T36.4X5	T36.4X6
ophthalmic preparation	T49.5X1	T49.5X2	T49.5X3	T49.5X4	T49.5X5	T49.5X6
topical NEC	T49.0X1	T49.0X2	T49.0X3	T49.0X4	T49.0X5	T49.0X6
Aurothioglucose	T39.4X1	T39.4X2	T39.4X3	T39.4X4	T39.4X5	T39.4X6
Aurothioglycanide	T39.4X1	T39.4X2	T39.4X3	T39.4X4	T39.4X5	T39.4X6
Aurothiomalate sodium	T39.4X1	T39.4X2	T39.4X3	T39.4X4	T39.4X5	T39.4X6
Aurotioprol	T39.4X1	T39.4X2	T39.4X3	T39.4X4	T39.4X5	T39.4X6
Automobile fuel	T52.0X1	T52.0X2	T52.0X3	T52.0X4	—	—
Autonomic nervous system agent NEC	T44.901	T44.902	T44.903	T44.904	T44.905	T44.906
Avlosulfon	T37.1X1	T37.1X2	T37.1X3	T37.1X4	T37.1X5	T37.1X6
Avomine	T42.6X1	T42.6X2	T42.6X3	T42.6X4	T42.6X5	T42.6X6
Axerophthol	T45.2X1	T45.2X2	T45.2X3	T45.2X4	T45.2X5	T45.2X6
Azacitidine	T45.1X1	T45.1X2	T45.1X3	T45.1X4	T45.1X5	T45.1X6
Azacyclonol	T43.591	T43.592	T43.593	T43.594	T43.595	T43.596
Azadirachta	T60.2X1	T60.2X2	T60.2X3	T60.2X4	—	—
Azanidazole	T37.3X1	T37.3X2	T37.3X3	T37.3X4	T37.3X5	T37.3X6
Azapetine	T46.7X1	T46.7X2	T46.7X3	T46.7X4	T46.7X5	T46.7X6
Azapropazone	T39.2X1	T39.2X2	T39.2X3	T39.2X4	T39.2X5	T39.2X6
Azaribine	T45.1X1	T45.1X2	T45.1X3	T45.1X4	T45.1X5	T45.1X6
Azaserine	T45.1X1	T45.1X2	T45.1X3	T45.1X4	T45.1X5	T45.1X6
Azatadine	T45.0X1	T45.0X2	T45.0X3	T45.0X4	T45.0X5	T45.0X6
Azatepa	T45.1X1	T45.1X2	T45.1X3	T45.1X4	T45.1X5	T45.1X6
Azathioprine	T45.1X1	T45.1X2	T45.1X3	T45.1X4	T45.1X5	T45.1X6
Azelaic acid	T49.0X1	T49.0X2	T49.0X3	T49.0X4	T49.0X5	T49.0X6
Azelastine	T45.0X1	T45.0X2	T45.0X3	T45.0X4	T45.0X5	T45.0X6
Azidocillin	T36.0X1	T36.0X2	T36.0X3	T36.0X4	T36.0X5	T36.0X6
Azidothymidine	T37.5X1	T37.5X2	T37.5X3	T37.5X4	T37.5X5	T37.5X6
Azinphos (ethyl) (methyl)	T60.0X1	T60.0X2	T60.0X3	T60.0X4	—	—
Aziridine (chelating)	T54.1X1	T54.1X2	T54.1X3	T54.1X4	—	—
Azithromycin	T36.3X1	T36.3X2	T36.3X3	T36.3X4	T36.3X5	T36.3X6
Azlocillin	T36.0X1	T36.0X2	T36.0X3	T36.0X4	T36.0X5	T36.0X6
Azobenzene smoke	T65.3X1	T65.3X2	T65.3X3	T65.3X4	—	—
acaricide	T60.8X1	T60.8X2	T60.8X3	T60.8X4	—	—
Azosulfamide	T37.0X1	T37.0X2	T37.0X3	T37.0X4	T37.0X5	T37.0X6
AZT	T37.5X1	T37.5X2	T37.5X3	T37.5X4	T37.5X5	T37.5X6
Aztreonam	T36.1X1	T36.1X2	T36.1X3	T36.1X4	T36.1X5	T36.1X6
Azulfidine	T37.0X1	T37.0X2	T37.0X3	T37.0X4	T37.0X5	T37.0X6
Azuresin	T50.8X1	T50.8X2	T50.8X3	T50.8X4	T50.8X5	T50.8X6
b-acetyldigoxin	T46.0X1	T46.0X2	T46.0X3	T46.0X4	T46.0X5	T46.0X6
P-Acetamidophenol	T39.1X1	T39.1X2	T39.1X3	T39.1X4	T39.1X5	T39.1X6
Bacampicillin	T36.0X1	T36.0X2	T36.0X3	T36.0X4	T36.0X5	T36.0X6
Bacillus						
lactobacillus	T47.8X1	T47.8X2	T47.8X3	T47.8X4	T47.8X5	T47.8X6
subtilis	T47.6X1	T47.6X2	T47.6X3	T47.6X4	T47.6X5	T47.6X6
Bacimycin	T49.0X1	T49.0X2	T49.0X3	T49.0X4	T49.0X5	T49.0X6
ophthalmic preparation	T49.5X1	T49.5X2	T49.5X3	T49.5X4	T49.5X5	T49.5X6
Bacitracin zinc	T49.0X1	T49.0X2	T49.0X3	T49.0X4	T49.0X5	T49.0X6
with neomycin	T49.0X1	T49.0X2	T49.0X3	T49.0X4	T49.0X5	T49.0X6
ENT agent	T49.6X1	T49.6X2	T49.6X3	T49.6X4	T49.6X5	T49.6X6
ophthalmic preparation	T49.5X1	T49.5X2	T49.5X3	T49.5X4	T49.5X5	T49.5X6
topical NEC	T49.0X1	T49.0X2	T49.0X3	T49.0X4	T49.0X5	T49.0X6
Baclofen	T42.8X1	T42.8X2	T42.8X3	T42.8X4	T42.8X5	T42.8X6
Baking soda	T50.991	T50.992	T50.993	T50.994	T50.995	T50.996
BAL	T45.8X1	T45.8X2	T45.8X3	T45.8X4	T45.8X5	T45.8X6
Bambuterol	T48.6X1	T48.6X2	T48.6X3	T48.6X4	T48.6X5	T48.6X6
Bamethan (sulfate)	T46.7X1	T46.7X2	T46.7X3	T46.7X4	T46.7X5	T46.7X6
Bamifylline	T48.6X1	T48.6X2	T48.6X3	T48.6X4	T48.6X5	T48.6X6
Bamipine	T45.0X1	T45.0X2	T45.0X3	T45.0X4	T45.0X5	T45.0X6
Baneberry — *see* Actaea spicata						
Banewort — *see* Belladonna						
Barbenyl	T42.3X1	T42.3X2	T42.3X3	T42.3X4	T42.3X5	T42.3X6
Barbexaclone	T42.6X1	T42.6X2	T42.6X3	T42.6X4	T42.6X5	T42.6X6
Barbital	T42.3X1	T42.3X2	T42.3X3	T42.3X4	T42.3X5	T42.3X6
sodium	T42.3X1	T42.3X2	T42.3X3	T42.3X4	T42.3X5	T42.3X6
Barbitone	T42.3X1	T42.3X2	T42.3X3	T42.3X4	T42.3X5	T42.3X6
Barbiturate NEC	T42.3X1	T42.3X2	T42.3X3	T42.3X4	T42.3X5	T42.3X6
with tranquilizer	T42.3X1	T42.3X2	T42.3X3	T42.3X4	T42.3X5	T42.3X6
anesthetic (intravenous)	T41.1X1	T41.1X2	T41.1X3	T41.1X4	T41.1X5	T41.1X6
Barium (carbonate) (chloride) (sulfite)	T57.8X1	T57.8X2	T57.8X3	T57.8X4	—	—
diagnostic agent	T50.8X1	T50.8X2	T50.8X3	T50.8X4	T50.8X5	T50.8X6
pesticide	T60.4X1	T60.4X2	T60.4X3	T60.4X4	—	—
rodenticide	T60.4X1	T60.4X2	T60.4X3	T60.4X4	—	—
sulfate (medicinal)	T50.8X1	T50.8X2	T50.8X3	T50.8X4	T50.8X5	T50.8X6
Barrier cream	T49.3X1	T49.3X2	T49.3X3	T49.3X4	T49.3X5	T49.3X6
Basic fuchsin	T49.0X1	T49.0X2	T49.0X3	T49.0X4	T49.0X5	T49.0X6
Battery acid or fluid	T54.2X1	T54.2X2	T54.2X3	T54.2X4	—	—
Bay rum	T51.8X1	T51.8X2	T51.8X3	T51.8X4	—	—
b-benzalbutyramide	T46.6X1	T46.6X2	T46.6X3	T46.6X4	T46.6X5	T46.6X6
BCG (vaccine)	T50.A91	T50.A92	T50.A93	T50.A94	T50.A95	T50.A96
BCNU	T45.1X1	T45.1X2	T45.1X3	T45.1X4	T45.1X5	T45.1X6
Bearsfoot	T62.2X1	T62.2X2	T62.2X3	T62.2X4	—	—
Beclamide	T42.6X1	T42.6X2	T42.6X3	T42.6X4	T42.6X5	T42.6X6
Beclomethasone	T44.5X1	T44.5X2	T44.5X3	T44.5X4	T44.5X5	T44.5X6
Bee (sting) (venom)	T63.441	T63.442	T63.443	T63.444	—	—
Befunolol	T49.5X1	T49.5X2	T49.5X3	T49.5X4	T49.5X5	T49.5X6
Bekanamycin	T36.5X1	T36.5X2	T36.5X3	T36.5X4	T36.5X5	T36.5X6
Belladonna — *see also* Nightshade						
alkaloids	T44.3X1	T44.3X2	T44.3X3	T44.3X4	T44.3X5	T44.3X6
extract	T44.3X1	T44.3X2	T44.3X3	T44.3X4	T44.3X5	T44.3X6
herb	T44.3X1	T44.3X2	T44.3X3	T44.3X4	T44.3X5	T44.3X6
Bemegride	T50.7X1	T50.7X2	T50.7X3	T50.7X4	T50.7X5	T50.7X6
Benactyzine	T44.3X1	T44.3X2	T44.3X3	T44.3X4	T44.3X5	T44.3X6
Benadryl	T45.0X1	T45.0X2	T45.0X3	T45.0X4	T45.0X5	T45.0X6
Benaprizine	T44.3X1	T44.3X2	T44.3X3	T44.3X4	T44.3X5	T44.3X6
Benazepril	T46.4X1	T46.4X2	T46.4X3	T46.4X4	T46.4X5	T46.4X6
Bencyclane	T46.7X1	T46.7X2	T46.7X3	T46.7X4	T46.7X5	T46.7X6
Bendazol	T46.3X1	T46.3X2	T46.3X3	T46.3X4	T46.3X5	T46.3X6
Bendrofluazide	T50.2X1	T50.2X2	T50.2X3	T50.2X4	T50.2X5	T50.2X6
Bendroflumethiazide	T50.2X1	T50.2X2	T50.2X3	T50.2X4	T50.2X5	T50.2X6
Benemid	T50.4X1	T50.4X2	T50.4X3	T50.4X4	T50.4X5	T50.4X6
Benethamine penicillin	T36.0X1	T36.0X2	T36.0X3	T36.0X4	T36.0X5	T36.0X6
Benexate	T47.1X1	T47.1X2	T47.1X3	T47.1X4	T47.1X5	T47.1X6
Benfluorex	T46.6X1	T46.6X2	T46.6X3	T46.6X4	T46.6X5	T46.6X6
Benfotiamine	T45.2X1	T45.2X2	T45.2X3	T45.2X4	T45.2X5	T45.2X6
Benisone	T49.0X1	T49.0X2	T49.0X3	T49.0X4	T49.0X5	T49.0X6
Benomyl	T60.0X1	T60.0X2	T60.0X3	T60.0X4	—	—
Benoquin	T49.8X1	T49.8X2	T49.8X3	T49.8X4	T49.8X5	T49.8X6
Benoxinate	T41.3X1	T41.3X2	T41.3X3	T41.3X4	T41.3X5	T41.3X6
Benperidol	T43.4X1	T43.4X2	T43.4X3	T43.4X4	T43.4X5	T43.4X6
Benproperine	T48.3X1	T48.3X2	T48.3X3	T48.3X4	T48.3X5	T48.3X6
Benserazide	T42.8X1	T42.8X2	T42.8X3	T42.8X4	T42.8X5	T42.8X6
Bentazepam	T42.4X1	T42.4X2	T42.4X3	T42.4X4	T42.4X5	T42.4X6
Bentiromide	T50.8X1	T50.8X2	T50.8X3	T50.8X4	T50.8X5	T50.8X6
Bentonite	T49.3X1	T49.3X2	T49.3X3	T49.3X4	T49.3X5	T49.3X6
Benzalbutyramide	T46.6X1	T46.6X2	T46.6X3	T46.6X4	T46.6X5	T46.6X6
Benzalkonium (chloride)	T49.0X1	T49.0X2	T49.0X3	T49.0X4	T49.0X5	T49.0X6
ophthalmic preparation	T49.5X1	T49.5X2	T49.5X3	T49.5X4	T49.5X5	T49.5X6
Benzamidosalicylate (calcium)	T37.1X1	T37.1X2	T37.1X3	T37.1X4	T37.1X5	T37.1X6
Benzamine	T41.3X1	T41.3X2	T41.3X3	T41.3X4	T41.3X5	T41.3X6

Substance	Poisoning, Accidental (unintentional)	Poisoning, Intentional Self-harm	Poisoning, Assault	Poisoning, Undetermined	Adverse Effect	Under-dosing
Benzamine — *continued*						
lactate	T49.1X1	T49.1X2	T49.1X3	T49.1X4	T49.1X5	T49.1X6
Benzamphetamine	T50.5X1	T50.5X2	T50.5X3	T50.5X4	T50.5X5	T50.5X6
Benzapril hydrochloride	T46.5X1	T46.5X2	T46.5X3	T46.5X4	T46.5X5	T46.5X6
Benzathine	T36.0X1	T36.0X2	T36.0X3	T36.0X4	T36.0X5	T36.0X6
benzylpenicillin						
Benzathine penicillin	T36.0X1	T36.0X2	T36.0X3	T36.0X4	T36.0X5	T36.0X6
Benzatropine	T42.8X1	T42.8X2	T42.8X3	T42.8X4	T42.8X5	T42.8X6
Benzbromarone	T50.4X1	T50.4X2	T50.4X3	T50.4X4	T50.4X5	T50.4X6
Benzcarbimine	T45.1X1	T45.1X2	T45.1X3	T45.1X4	T45.1X5	T45.1X6
Benzedrex	T44.991	T44.992	T44.993	T44.994	T44.995	T44.996
Benzedrine (amphetamine)	T43.621	T43.622	T43.623	T43.624	T43.625	T43.626
Benzenamine	T65.3X1	T65.3X2	T65.3X3	T65.3X4	—	—
Benzene	T52.1X1	T52.1X2	T52.1X3	T52.1X4	—	—
homologues (acetyl) (dimethyl) (methyl) (solvent)	T52.2X1	T52.2X2	T52.2X3	T52.2X4	—	—
Benzethonium (chloride)	T49.0X1	T49.0X2	T49.0X3	T49.0X4	T49.0X5	T49.0X6
Benzfetamine	T50.5X1	T50.5X2	T50.5X3	T50.5X4	T50.5X5	T50.5X6
Benzhexol	T44.3X1	T44.3X2	T44.3X3	T44.3X4	T44.3X5	T44.3X6
Benzhydramine (chloride)	T45.0X1	T45.0X2	T45.0X3	T45.0X4	T45.0X5	T45.0X6
Benzidine	T65.891	T65.892	T65.893	T65.894		
Benzilonium bromide	T44.3X1	T44.3X2	T44.3X3	T44.3X4	T44.3X5	T44.3X6
Benzimidazole	T60.3X1	T60.3X2	T60.3X3	T60.3X4		
Benzin (e) — *see* Ligroin						
Benziodarone	T46.3X1	T46.3X2	T46.3X3	T46.3X4	T46.3X5	T46.3X6
Benznidazole	T37.3X1	T37.3X2	T37.3X3	T37.3X4	T37.3X5	T37.3X6
Benzocaine	T41.3X1	T41.3X2	T41.3X3	T41.3X4	T41.3X5	T41.3X6
Benzodiapin	T42.4X1	T42.4X2	T42.4X3	T42.4X4	T42.4X5	T42.4X6
Benzodiazepine NEC	T42.4X1	T42.4X2	T42.4X3	T42.4X4	T42.4X5	T42.4X6
Benzoic acid	T49.0X1	T49.0X2	T49.0X3	T49.0X4	T49.0X5	T49.0X6
with salicylic acid	T49.0X1	T49.0X2	T49.0X3	T49.0X4	T49.0X5	T49.0X6
Benzoin (tincture)	T48.5X1	T48.5X2	T48.5X3	T48.5X4	T48.5X5	T48.5X6
Benzol (benzene)	T52.1X1	T52.1X2	T52.1X3	T52.1X4	—	—
vapor	T52.0X1	T52.0X2	T52.0X3	T52.0X4	—	—
Benzomorphan	T40.2X1	T40.2X2	T40.2X3	T40.2X4	T40.2X5	T40.2X6
Benzonatate	T48.3X1	T48.3X2	T48.3X3	T48.3X4	T48.3X5	T48.3X6
Benzophenones	T49.3X1	T49.3X2	T49.3X3	T49.3X4	T49.3X5	T49.3X6
Benzopyrone	T46.991	T46.992	T46.993	T46.994	T46.995	T46.996
Benzothiadiazides	T50.2X1	T50.2X2	T50.2X3	T50.2X4	T50.2X5	T50.2X6
Benzoxonium chloride	T49.0X1	T49.0X2	T49.0X3	T49.0X4	T49.0X5	T49.0X6
Benzoylpas calcium	T37.1X1	T37.1X2	T37.1X3	T37.1X4	T37.1X5	T37.1X6
Benzoyl peroxide	T49.0X1	T49.0X2	T49.0X3	T49.0X4	T49.0X5	T49.0X6
Benzperidin	T43.591	T43.592	T43.593	T43.594	T43.595	T43.596
Benzperidol	T43.591	T43.592	T43.593	T43.594	T43.595	T43.596
Benzphetamine	T50.5X1	T50.5X2	T50.5X3	T50.5X4	T50.5X5	T50.5X6
Benzpyrinium bromide	T44.1X1	T44.1X2	T44.1X3	T44.1X4	T44.1X5	T44.1X6
Benzquinamide	T45.0X1	T45.0X2	T45.0X3	T45.0X4	T45.0X5	T45.0X6
Benzthiazide	T50.2X1	T50.2X2	T50.2X3	T50.2X4	T50.2X5	T50.2X6
Benztropine						
anticholinergic	T44.3X1	T44.3X2	T44.3X3	T44.3X4	T44.3X5	T44.3X6
antiparkinson	T42.8X1	T42.8X2	T42.8X3	T42.8X4	T42.8X5	T42.8X6
Benzydamine	T49.0X1	T49.0X2	T49.0X3	T49.0X4	T49.0X5	T49.0X6
Benzyl						
acetate	T52.8X1	T52.8X2	T52.8X3	T52.8X4	—	—
alcohol	T49.0X1	T49.0X2	T49.0X3	T49.0X4	T49.0X5	T49.0X6
benzoate	T49.0X1	T49.0X2	T49.0X3	T49.0X4	T49.0X5	T49.0X6
Benzoic acid	T49.0X1	T49.0X2	T49.0X3	T49.0X4	T49.0X5	T49.0X6
morphine	T40.2X1	T40.2X2	T40.2X3	T40.2X4	—	—
nicotinate	T46.6X1	T46.6X2	T46.6X3	T46.6X4	T46.6X5	T46.6X6
penicillin	T36.0X1	T36.0X2	T36.0X3	T36.0X4	T36.0X5	T36.0X6
Benzylhydrochlorthiazide	T50.2X1	T50.2X2	T50.2X3	T50.2X4	T50.2X5	T50.2X6
Benzylpenicillin	T36.0X1	T36.0X2	T36.0X3	T36.0X4	T36.0X5	T36.0X6
Benzylthiouracil	T38.2X1	T38.2X2	T38.2X3	T38.2X4	T38.2X5	T38.2X6
Bephenium	T37.4X1	T37.4X2	T37.4X3	T37.4X4	T37.4X5	T37.4X6
hydroxynaphthoate						
Bepridil	T46.1X1	T46.1X2	T46.1X3	T46.1X4	T46.1X5	T46.1X6
Bergamot oil	T65.891	T65.892	T65.893	T65.894		
Bergapten	T50.991	T50.992	T50.993	T50.994	T50.995	T50.996
Berries, poisonous	T62.1X1	T62.1X2	T62.1X3	T62.1X4	—	—
Beryllium (compounds)	T56.7X1	T56.7X2	T56.7X3	T56.7X4	—	—
beta adrenergic blocking agent, heart	T44.7X1	T44.7X2	T44.7X3	T44.7X4	T44.7X5	T44.7X6
Betacarotene	T45.2X1	T45.2X2	T45.2X3	T45.2X4	T45.2X5	T45.2X6
Beta-Chlor	T42.6X1	T42.6X2	T42.6X3	T42.6X4	T42.6X5	T42.6X6
Betahistine	T46.7X1	T46.7X2	T46.7X3	T46.7X4	T46.7X5	T46.7X6
Betaine	T47.5X1	T47.5X2	T47.5X3	T47.5X4	T47.5X5	T47.5X6
Betamethasone	T49.0X1	T49.0X2	T49.0X3	T49.0X4	T49.0X5	T49.0X6
topical	T49.0X1	T49.0X2	T49.0X3	T49.0X4	T49.0X5	T49.0X6
Betamicin	T36.8X1	T36.8X2	T36.8X3	T36.8X4	T36.8X5	T36.8X6
Betanidine	T46.5X1	T46.5X2	T46.5X3	T46.5X4	T46.5X5	T46.5X6
Betaxolol	T44.7X1	T44.7X2	T44.7X3	T44.7X4	T44.7X5	T44.7X6
Betazole	T50.8X1	T50.8X2	T50.8X3	T50.8X4	T50.8X5	T50.8X6
Bethanechol	T44.1X1	T44.1X2	T44.1X3	T44.1X4	T44.1X5	T44.1X6

Substance	Poisoning, Accidental (unintentional)	Poisoning, Intentional Self-harm	Poisoning, Assault	Poisoning, Undetermined	Adverse Effect	Under-dosing
Bethanechol — *continued*						
chloride	T44.1X1	T44.1X2	T44.1X3	T44.1X4	T44.1X5	T44.1X6
Bethanidine	T46.5X1	T46.5X2	T46.5X3	T46.5X4	T46.5X5	T46.5X6
Betoxycaine	T41.3X1	T41.3X2	T41.3X3	T41.3X4	T41.3X5	T41.3X6
Betula oil	T49.3X1	T49.3X2	T49.3X3	T49.3X4	T49.3X5	T49.3X6
Bevantolol	T44.7X1	T44.7X2	T44.7X3	T44.7X4	T44.7X5	T44.7X6
Bevonium metilsulfate	T44.3X1	T44.3X2	T44.3X3	T44.3X4	T44.3X5	T44.3X6
Bezafibrate	T46.6X1	T46.6X2	T46.6X3	T46.6X4	T46.6X5	T46.6X6
Bezitramide	T40.4X1	T40.4X2	T40.4X3	T40.4X4	T40.4X5	T40.4X6
BHA	T50.991	T50.992	T50.993	T50.994	T50.995	T50.996
Bhang	T40.7X1	T40.7X2	T40.7X3	T40.7X4	T40.7X5	T40.7X6
BHC (medicinal)	T49.0X1	T49.0X2	T49.0X3	T49.0X4	T49.0X5	T49.0X6
nonmedicinal (vapor)	T53.6X1	T53.6X2	T53.6X3	T53.6X4		
Bialamicol	T37.3X1	T37.3X2	T37.3X3	T37.3X4	T37.3X5	T37.3X6
Bibenzonium bromide	T48.3X1	T48.3X2	T48.3X3	T48.3X4	T48.3X5	T48.3X6
Bibrocathol	T49.5X1	T49.5X2	T49.5X3	T49.5X4	T49.5X5	T49.5X6
Bichloride of mercury — *see* Mercury, chloride						
Bichromates (calcium) (potassium)(sodium) (crystals)	T57.8X1	T57.8X2	T57.8X3	T57.8X4	—	—
fumes	T56.2X1	T56.2X2	T56.2X3	T56.2X4	—	—
Biclotymol	T49.6X1	T49.6X2	T49.6X3	T49.6X4	T49.6X5	T49.6X6
Bicucculine	T50.7X1	T50.7X2	T50.7X3	T50.7X4	T50.7X5	T50.7X6
Bifemelane	T43.291	T43.292	T43.293	T43.294	T43.295	T43.296
Biguanide derivatives, oral	T38.3X1	T38.3X2	T38.3X3	T38.3X4	T38.3X5	T38.3X6
Bile salts	T47.5X1	T47.5X2	T47.5X3	T47.5X4	T47.5X5	T47.5X6
Biligrafin	T50.8X1	T50.8X2	T50.8X3	T50.8X4	T50.8X5	T50.8X6
Bilopaque	T50.8X1	T50.8X2	T50.8X3	T50.8X4	T50.8X5	T50.8X6
Binifibrate	T46.6X1	T46.6X2	T46.6X3	T46.6X4	T46.6X5	T46.6X6
Binitrobenzol	T65.3X1	T65.3X2	T65.3X3	T65.3X4	—	—
Bioflavonoid(s)	T46.991	T46.992	T46.993	T46.994	T46.995	T46.996
Biological substance NEC	T50.901	T50.902	T50.903	T50.904	T50.905	T50.906
Biotin	T45.2X1	T45.2X2	T45.2X3	T45.2X4	T45.2X5	T45.2X6
Biperiden	T44.3X1	T44.3X2	T44.3X3	T44.3X4	T44.3X5	T44.3X6
Bisacodyl	T47.2X1	T47.2X2	T47.2X3	T47.2X4	T47.2X5	T47.2X6
Bisbentiamine	T45.2X1	T45.2X2	T45.2X3	T45.2X4	T45.2X5	T45.2X6
Bisbutiamine	T45.2X1	T45.2X2	T45.2X3	T45.2X4	T45.2X5	T45.2X6
Bisdequalinium (salts) (diacetate)	T49.6X1	T49.6X2	T49.6X3	T49.6X4	T49.6X5	T49.6X6
Bishydroxycoumarin	T45.511	T45.512	T45.513	T45.514	T45.515	T45.516
Bismarsen	T37.8X1	T37.8X2	T37.8X3	T37.8X4	T37.8X5	T37.8X6
Bismuth salts	T47.6X1	T47.6X2	T47.6X3	T47.6X4	T47.6X5	T47.6X6
aluminate	T47.1X1	T47.1X2	T47.1X3	T47.1X4	T47.1X5	T47.1X6
anti-infectives	T37.8X1	T37.8X2	T37.8X3	T37.8X4	T37.8X5	T37.8X6
formic iodide	T49.0X1	T49.0X2	T49.0X3	T49.0X4	T49.0X5	T49.0X6
glycolylarsenate	T49.0X1	T49.0X2	T49.0X3	T49.0X4	T49.0X5	T49.0X6
nonmedicinal (compounds) NEC	T65.91	T65.92	T65.93	T65.94	—	—
subcarbonate	T47.6X1	T47.6X2	T47.6X3	T47.6X4	T47.6X5	T47.6X6
subsalicylate	T37.8X1	T37.8X2	T37.8X3	T37.8X4	T37.8X5	T37.8X6
sulfarsphenamine	T37.8X1	T37.8X2	T37.8X3	T37.8X4	T37.8X5	T37.8X6
Bisoprolol	T44.7X1	T44.7X2	T44.7X3	T44.7X4	T44.7X5	T44.7X6
Bisoxatin	T47.2X1	T47.2X2	T47.2X3	T47.2X4	T47.2X5	T47.2X6
Bisulepin (hydrochloride)	T45.0X1	T45.0X2	T45.0X3	T45.0X4	T45.0X5	T45.0X6
Bithionol	T37.8X1	T37.8X2	T37.8X3	T37.8X4	T37.8X5	T37.8X6
anthelminthic	T37.4X1	T37.4X2	T37.4X3	T37.4X4	T37.4X5	T37.4X6
Bitolterol	T48.6X1	T48.6X2	T48.6X3	T48.6X4	T48.6X5	T48.6X6
Bitoscanate	T37.4X1	T37.4X2	T37.4X3	T37.4X4	T37.4X5	T37.4X6
Bitter almond oil	T62.8X1	T62.8X2	T62.8X3	T62.8X4	—	—
Bittersweet	T62.2X1	T62.2X2	T62.2X3	T62.2X4	—	—
Black						
flag	T60.91	T60.92	T60.93	T60.94		
henbane	T62.2X1	T62.2X2	T62.2X3	T62.2X4		
leaf (40)	T60.91	T60.92	T60.93	T60.94		
widow spider (bite)	T63.311	T63.312	T63.313	T63.314		
antivenin	T50.Z11	T50.Z12	T50.Z13	T50.Z14	T50.Z15	T50.Z16
Blast furnace gas (carbon monoxide from)	T58.8X1	T58.8X2	T58.8X3	T58.8X4		
Bleach	T54.91	T54.92	T54.93	T54.94		
Bleaching agent (medicinal)	T49.4X1	T49.4X2	T49.4X3	T49.4X4	T49.4X5	T49.4X6
Bleomycin	T45.1X1	T45.1X2	T45.1X3	T45.1X4	T45.1X5	T45.1X6
Blockain	T41.3X1	T41.3X2	T41.3X3	T41.3X4	T41.3X5	T41.3X6
infiltration (subcutaneous)	T41.3X1	T41.3X2	T41.3X3	T41.3X4	T41.3X5	T41.3X6
nerve block (peripheral) (plexus)	T41.3X1	T41.3X2	T41.3X3	T41.3X4	T41.3X5	T41.3X6
topical (surface)	T41.3X1	T41.3X2	T41.3X3	T41.3X4	T41.3X5	T41.3X6
Blockers, calcium channel	T46.1X1	T46.1X2	T46.1X3	T46.1X4	T46.1X5	T46.1X6
Blood (derivatives) (natural) (plasma) (whole)	T45.8X1	T45.8X2	T45.8X3	T45.8X4	T45.8X5	T45.8X6
dried	T45.8X1	T45.8X2	T45.8X3	T45.8X4	T45.8X5	T45.8X6

▽ Subterms under main terms may continue to next column or page   Additional Character May Be Required — Refer to the Tabular List for Character Selection   **355**

Benzamine — Blood

Substance	Poisoning, Accidental (unintentional)	Poisoning, Intentional Self-harm	Poisoning, Assault	Poisoning, Undetermined	Adverse Effect	Under-dosing
Blood — continued						
drug affecting NEC	T45.91	T45.92	T45.93	T45.94	T45.95	T45.96
expander NEC	T45.8X1	T45.8X2	T45.8X3	T45.8X4	T45.8X5	T45.8X6
fraction NEC	T45.8X1	T45.8X2	T45.8X3	T45.8X4	T45.8X5	T45.8X6
substitute (macromolecular)	T45.8X1	T45.8X2	T45.8X3	T45.8X4	T45.8X5	T45.8X6
Blue velvet	T40.2X1	T40.2X2	T40.2X3	T40.2X4	—	—
Bone meal	T62.8X1	T62.8X2	T62.8X3	T62.8X4	—	—
Bonine	T45.0X1	T45.0X2	T45.0X3	T45.0X4	T45.0X5	T45.0X6
Bopindolol	T44.7X1	T44.7X2	T44.7X3	T44.7X4	T44.7X5	T44.7X6
Boracic acid	T49.0X1	T49.0X2	T49.0X3	T49.0X4	T49.0X5	T49.0X6
ENT agent	T49.6X1	T49.6X2	T49.6X3	T49.6X4	T49.6X5	T49.6X6
ophthalmic preparation	T49.5X1	T49.5X2	T49.5X3	T49.5X4	T49.5X5	T49.5X6
Borane complex	T57.8X1	T57.8X2	T57.8X3	T57.8X4	—	—
Borate(s)	T57.8X1	T57.8X2	T57.8X3	T57.8X4	—	—
buffer	T50.991	T50.992	T50.993	T50.994	T50.995	T50.996
cleanser	T54.91	T54.92	T54.93	T54.94	—	—
sodium	T57.8X1	T57.8X2	T57.8X3	T57.8X4	—	—
Borax (cleanser)	T54.91	T54.92	T54.93	T54.94	—	—
Bordeaux mixture	T60.3X1	T60.3X2	T60.3X3	T60.3X4	—	—
Boric acid	T49.0X1	T49.0X2	T49.0X3	T49.0X4	T49.0X5	T49.0X6
ENT agent	T49.6X1	T49.6X2	T49.6X3	T49.6X4	T49.6X5	T49.6X6
ophthalmic preparation	T49.5X1	T49.5X2	T49.5X3	T49.5X4	T49.5X5	T49.5X6
Bornaprine	T44.3X1	T44.3X2	T44.3X3	T44.3X4	T44.3X5	T44.3X6
Boron	T57.8X1	T57.8X2	T57.8X3	T57.8X4	—	—
hydride NEC	T57.8X1	T57.8X2	T57.8X3	T57.8X4	—	—
fumes or gas	T57.8X1	T57.8X2	T57.8X3	T57.8X4	—	—
trifluoride	T59.891	T59.892	T59.893	T59.894	—	—
Botox	T48.291	T48.292	T48.293	T48.294	T48.295	T48.296
Botulinus anti-toxin (type A, B)	T50.Z11	T50.Z12	T50.Z13	T50.Z14	T50.Z15	T50.Z16
Brake fluid vapor	T59.891	T59.892	T59.893	T59.894	—	—
Brallobarbital	T42.3X1	T42.3X2	T42.3X3	T42.3X4	T42.3X5	T42.3X6
Bran (wheat)	T47.4X1	T47.4X2	T47.4X3	T47.4X4	T47.4X5	T47.4X6
Brass (fumes)	T56.891	T56.892	T56.893	T56.894	—	—
Brasso	T52.0X1	T52.0X2	T52.0X3	T52.0X4	—	—
Bretylium tosilate	T46.2X1	T46.2X2	T46.2X3	T46.2X4	T46.2X5	T46.2X6
Brevital (sodium)	T41.1X1	T41.1X2	T41.1X3	T41.1X4	T41.1X5	T41.1X6
Brinase	T45.3X1	T45.3X2	T45.3X3	T45.3X4	T45.3X5	T45.3X6
British antilewisite	T45.8X1	T45.8X2	T45.8X3	T45.8X4	T45.8X5	T45.8X6
Brodifacoum	T60.4X1	T60.4X2	T60.4X3	T60.4X4	—	—
Bromal (hydrate)	T42.6X1	T42.6X2	T42.6X3	T42.6X4	T42.6X5	T42.6X6
Bromazepam	T42.4X1	T42.4X2	T42.4X3	T42.4X4	T42.4X5	T42.4X6
Bromazine	T45.0X1	T45.0X2	T45.0X3	T45.0X4	T45.0X5	T45.0X6
Brombenzylcyanide	T59.3X1	T59.3X2	T59.3X3	T59.3X4	—	—
Bromelains	T45.3X1	T45.3X2	T45.3X3	T45.3X4	T45.3X5	T45.3X6
Bromethalin	T60.4X1	T60.4X2	T60.4X3	T60.4X4	—	—
Bromhexine	T48.4X1	T48.4X2	T48.4X3	T48.4X4	T48.4X5	T48.4X6
Bromide salts	T42.6X1	T42.6X2	T42.6X3	T42.6X4	T42.6X5	T42.6X6
Bromindione	T45.511	T45.512	T45.513	T45.514	T45.515	T45.516
Bromine						
compounds (medicinal)	T42.6X1	T42.6X2	T42.6X3	T42.6X4	T42.6X5	T42.6X6
sedative	T42.6X1	T42.6X2	T42.6X3	T42.6X4	T42.6X5	T42.6X6
vapor	T59.891	T59.892	T59.893	T59.894	—	—
Bromisoval	T42.6X1	T42.6X2	T42.6X3	T42.6X4	T42.6X5	T42.6X6
Bromisovalum	T42.6X1	T42.6X2	T42.6X3	T42.6X4	T42.6X5	T42.6X6
Bromobenzylcyanide	T59.3X1	T59.3X2	T59.3X3	T59.3X4	—	—
Bromochlorosalicylani-lide	T49.0X1	T49.0X2	T49.0X3	T49.0X4	T49.0X5	T49.0X6
Bromocriptine	T42.8X1	T42.8X2	T42.8X3	T42.8X4	T42.8X5	T42.8X6
Bromodiphenhydramine	T45.0X1	T45.0X2	T45.0X3	T45.0X4	T45.0X5	T45.0X6
Bromoform	T42.6X1	T42.6X2	T42.6X3	T42.6X4	T42.6X5	T42.6X6
Bromophenol blue reagent	T50.991	T50.992	T50.993	T50.994	T50.995	T50.996
Bromopride	T47.8X1	T47.8X2	T47.8X3	T47.8X4	T47.8X5	T47.8X6
Bromosalicylchloranitide	T49.0X1	T49.0X2	T49.0X3	T49.0X4	T49.0X5	T49.0X6
Bromosalicylhydroxamic acid	T37.1X1	T37.1X2	T37.1X3	T37.1X4	T37.1X5	T37.1X6
Bromo-seltzer	T39.1X1	T39.1X2	T39.1X3	T39.1X4	T39.1X5	T39.1X6
Bromoxynil	T60.3X1	T60.3X2	T60.3X3	T60.3X4	—	—
Bromperidol	T43.4X1	T43.4X2	T43.4X3	T43.4X4	T43.4X5	T43.4X6
Brompheniramine	T45.0X1	T45.0X2	T45.0X3	T45.0X4	T45.0X5	T45.0X6
Bromsulfophthalein	T50.8X1	T50.8X2	T50.8X3	T50.8X4	T50.8X5	T50.8X6
Bromural	T42.6X1	T42.6X2	T42.6X3	T42.6X4	T42.6X5	T42.6X6
Bromvaletone	T42.6X1	T42.6X2	T42.6X3	T42.6X4	T42.6X5	T42.6X6
Bronchodilator NEC	T48.6X1	T48.6X2	T48.6X3	T48.6X4	T48.6X5	T48.6X6
Brotizolam	T42.4X1	T42.4X2	T42.4X3	T42.4X4	T42.4X5	T42.4X6
Brovincamine	T46.7X1	T46.7X2	T46.7X3	T46.7X4	T46.7X5	T46.7X6
Brown recluse spider (bite) (venom)	T63.331	T63.332	T63.333	T63.334	—	—
Brown spider (bite) (venom)	T63.391	T63.392	T63.393	T63.394	—	—
Broxaterol	T48.6X1	T48.6X2	T48.6X3	T48.6X4	T48.6X5	T48.6X6
Broxuridine	T45.1X1	T45.1X2	T45.1X3	T45.1X4	T45.1X5	T45.1X6

Substance	Poisoning, Accidental (unintentional)	Poisoning, Intentional Self-harm	Poisoning, Assault	Poisoning, Undetermined	Adverse Effect	Under-dosing
Broxyquinoline	T37.8X1	T37.8X2	T37.8X3	T37.8X4	T37.8X5	T37.8X6
Bruceine	T48.291	T48.292	T48.293	T48.294	T48.295	T48.296
Brucia	T62.2X1	T62.2X2	T62.2X3	T62.2X4	—	—
Brucine	T65.1X1	T65.1X2	T65.1X3	T65.1X4	—	—
Brunswick green — *see* Copper						
Bruten — *see* Ibuprofen						
Bryonia	T47.2X1	T47.2X2	T47.2X3	T47.2X4	T47.2X5	T47.2X6
Buclizine	T45.0X1	T45.0X2	T45.0X3	T45.0X4	T45.0X5	T45.0X6
Buclosamide	T49.0X1	T49.0X2	T49.0X3	T49.0X4	T49.0X5	T49.0X6
Budesonide	T44.5X1	T44.5X2	T44.5X3	T44.5X4	T44.5X5	T44.5X6
Budralazine	T46.5X1	T46.5X2	T46.5X3	T46.5X4	T46.5X5	T46.5X6
Bufferin	T39.011	T39.012	T39.013	T39.014	T39.015	T39.016
Buflomedil	T46.7X1	T46.7X2	T46.7X3	T46.7X4	T46.7X5	T46.7X6
Buformin	T38.3X1	T38.3X2	T38.3X3	T38.3X4	T38.3X5	T38.3X6
Bufotenine	T40.991	T40.992	T40.993	T40.994	—	—
Bufrolin	T48.6X1	T48.6X2	T48.6X3	T48.6X4	T48.6X5	T48.6X6
Bufylline	T48.6X1	T48.6X2	T48.6X3	T48.6X4	T48.6X5	T48.6X6
Bulk filler	T50.5X1	T50.5X2	T50.5X3	T50.5X4	T50.5X5	T50.5X6
cathartic	T47.4X1	T47.4X2	T47.4X3	T47.4X4	T47.4X5	T47.4X6
Bumetanide	T50.1X1	T50.1X2	T50.1X3	T50.1X4	T50.1X5	T50.1X6
Bunaftine	T46.2X1	T46.2X2	T46.2X3	T46.2X4	T46.2X5	T46.2X6
Bunamiodyl	T50.8X1	T50.8X2	T50.8X3	T50.8X4	T50.8X5	T50.8X6
Bunazosin	T44.6X1	T44.6X2	T44.6X3	T44.6X4	T44.6X5	T44.6X6
Bunitrolol	T44.7X1	T44.7X2	T44.7X3	T44.7X4	T44.7X5	T44.7X6
Buphenine	T46.7X1	T46.7X2	T46.7X3	T46.7X4	T46.7X5	T46.7X6
Bupivacaine	T41.3X1	T41.3X2	T41.3X3	T41.3X4	T41.3X5	T41.3X6
infiltration (subcutaneous)	T41.3X1	T41.3X2	T41.3X3	T41.3X4	T41.3X5	T41.3X6
nerve block (peripheral) (plexus)	T41.3X1	T41.3X2	T41.3X3	T41.3X4	T41.3X5	T41.3X6
spinal	T41.3X1	T41.3X2	T41.3X3	T41.3X4	T41.3X5	T41.3X6
Bupranolol	T44.7X1	T44.7X2	T44.7X3	T44.7X4	T44.7X5	T44.7X6
Buprenorphine	T40.4X1	T40.4X2	T40.4X3	T40.4X4	T40.4X5	T40.4X6
Bupropion	T43.291	T43.292	T43.293	T43.294	T43.295	T43.296
Burimamide	T47.1X1	T47.1X2	T47.1X3	T47.1X4	T47.1X5	T47.1X6
Buserelin	T38.891	T38.892	T38.893	T38.894	T38.895	T38.896
Buspirone	T43.591	T43.592	T43.593	T43.594	T43.595	T43.596
Busulfan, busulphan	T45.1X1	T45.1X2	T45.1X3	T45.1X4	T45.1X5	T45.1X6
Butabarbital (sodium)	T42.3X1	T42.3X2	T42.3X3	T42.3X4	T42.3X5	T42.3X6
Butabarbitone	T42.3X1	T42.3X2	T42.3X3	T42.3X4	T42.3X5	T42.3X6
Butabarpal	T42.3X1	T42.3X2	T42.3X3	T42.3X4	T42.3X5	T42.3X6
Butacaine	T41.3X1	T41.3X2	T41.3X3	T41.3X4	T41.3X5	T41.3X6
Butalamine	T46.7X1	T46.7X2	T46.7X3	T46.7X4	T46.7X5	T46.7X6
Butalbital	T42.3X1	T42.3X2	T42.3X3	T42.3X4	T42.3X5	T42.3X6
Butallylonal	T42.3X1	T42.3X2	T42.3X3	T42.3X4	T42.3X5	T42.3X6
Butamben	T41.3X1	T41.3X2	T41.3X3	T41.3X4	T41.3X5	T41.3X6
Butamirate	T48.3X1	T48.3X2	T48.3X3	T48.3X4	T48.3X5	T48.3X6
Butane (distributed in mobile container)	T59.891	T59.892	T59.893	T59.894	—	—
distributed through pipes	T59.891	T59.892	T59.893	T59.894	—	—
incomplete combustion	T58.11	T58.12	T58.13	T58.14	—	—
Butanilicaine	T41.3X1	T41.3X2	T41.3X3	T41.3X4	T41.3X5	T41.3X6
Butanol	T51.3X1	T51.3X2	T51.3X3	T51.3X4	—	—
Butanone, 2-butanone	T52.4X1	T52.4X2	T52.4X3	T52.4X4	—	—
Butantrone	T49.4X1	T49.4X2	T49.4X3	T49.4X4	T49.4X5	T49.4X6
Butaperazine	T43.3X1	T43.3X2	T43.3X3	T43.3X4	T43.3X5	T43.3X6
Butazolidin	T39.2X1	T39.2X2	T39.2X3	T39.2X4	T39.2X5	T39.2X6
Butetamate	T48.6X1	T48.6X2	T48.6X3	T48.6X4	T48.6X5	T48.6X6
Butethal	T42.3X1	T42.3X2	T42.3X3	T42.3X4	T42.3X5	T42.3X6
Butethamate	T44.3X1	T44.3X2	T44.3X3	T44.3X4	T44.3X5	T44.3X6
Buthalitone (sodium)	T41.1X1	T41.1X2	T41.1X3	T41.1X4	T41.1X5	T41.1X6
Butisol (sodium)	T42.3X1	T42.3X2	T42.3X3	T42.3X4	T42.3X5	T42.3X6
Butizide	T50.2X1	T50.2X2	T50.2X3	T50.2X4	T50.2X5	T50.2X6
Butobarbital	T42.3X1	T42.3X2	T42.3X3	T42.3X4	T42.3X5	T42.3X6
sodium	T42.3X1	T42.3X2	T42.3X3	T42.3X4	T42.3X5	T42.3X6
Butobarbitone	T42.3X1	T42.3X2	T42.3X3	T42.3X4	T42.3X5	T42.3X6
Butoconazole (nitrate)	T49.0X1	T49.0X2	T49.0X3	T49.0X4	T49.0X5	T49.0X6
Butorphanol	T40.4X1	T40.4X2	T40.4X3	T40.4X4	T40.4X5	T40.4X6
Butriptyline	T43.011	T43.012	T43.013	T43.014	T43.015	T43.016
Butropium bromide	T44.3X1	T44.3X2	T44.3X3	T44.3X4	T44.3X5	T44.3X6
Buttercups	T62.2X1	T62.2X2	T62.2X3	T62.2X4	—	—
Butter of antimony — *see* Antimony						
Butyl						
acetate (secondary)	T52.8X1	T52.8X2	T52.8X3	T52.8X4	—	—
alcohol	T51.3X1	T51.3X2	T51.3X3	T51.3X4	—	—
aminobenzoate	T41.3X1	T41.3X2	T41.3X3	T41.3X4	T41.3X5	T41.3X6
butyrate	T52.8X1	T52.8X2	T52.8X3	T52.8X4	—	—
carbinol	T51.3X1	T51.3X2	T51.3X3	T51.3X4	—	—
carbitol	T52.3X1	T52.3X2	T52.3X3	T52.3X4	—	—
cellosolve	T52.3X1	T52.3X2	T52.3X3	T52.3X4	—	—
chloral (hydrate)	T42.6X1	T42.6X2	T42.6X3	T42.6X4	T42.6X5	T42.6X6
formate	T52.8X1	T52.8X2	T52.8X3	T52.8X4	—	—
lactate	T52.8X1	T52.8X2	T52.8X3	T52.8X4	—	—

Substance	Poisoning, Accidental (unintentional)	Poisoning, Intentional Self-harm	Poisoning, Assault	Poisoning, Undetermined	Adverse Effect	Under-dosing
Butyl — *continued*						
propionate	T52.8X1	T52.8X2	T52.8X3	T52.8X4	—	—
scopolamine bromide	T44.3X1	T44.3X2	T44.3X3	T44.3X4	T44.3X5	T44.3X6
thiobarbital sodium	T41.1X1	T41.1X2	T41.1X3	T41.1X4	T41.1X5	T41.1X6
Butylated hydroxyanisole	T50.991	T50.992	T50.993	T50.994	T50.995	T50.996
Butylchloral hydrate	T42.6X1	T42.6X2	T42.6X3	T42.6X4	T42.6X5	T42.6X6
Butyltoluene	T52.2X1	T52.2X2	T52.2X3	T52.2X4	—	—
Butyn	T41.3X1	T41.3X2	T41.3X3	T41.3X4	T41.3X5	T41.3X6
Butyrophenone (-based tranquilizers)	T43.4X1	T43.4X2	T43.4X3	T43.4X4	T43.4X5	T43.4X6
Cabergoline	T42.8X1	T42.8X2	T42.8X3	T42.8X4	T42.8X5	T42.8X6
Cacodyl, cacodylic acid	T57.0X1	T57.0X2	T57.0X3	T57.0X4	—	—
Cactinomycin	T45.1X1	T45.1X2	T45.1X3	T45.1X4	T45.1X5	T45.1X6
Cade oil	T49.4X1	T49.4X2	T49.4X3	T49.4X4	T49.4X5	T49.4X6
Cadexomer iodine	T49.0X1	T49.0X2	T49.0X3	T49.0X4	T49.0X5	T49.0X6
Cadmium (chloride) (fumes) (oxide)	T56.3X1	T56.3X2	T56.3X3	T56.3X4		
sulfide (medicinal) NEC	T49.4X1	T49.4X2	T49.4X3	T49.4X4	T49.4X5	T49.4X6
Cadralazine	T46.5X1	T46.5X2	T46.5X3	T46.5X4	T46.5X5	T46.5X6
Caffeine	T43.611	T43.612	T43.613	T43.614	T43.615	T43.616
Calabar bean	T62.2X1	T62.2X2	T62.2X3	T62.2X4	—	—
Caladium seguinum	T62.2X1	T62.2X2	T62.2X3	T62.2X4	—	—
Calamine (lotion)	T49.3X1	T49.3X2	T49.3X3	T49.3X4	T49.3X5	T49.3X6
Calcifediol	T45.2X1	T45.2X2	T45.2X3	T45.2X4	T45.2X5	T45.2X6
Calciferol	T45.2X1	T45.2X2	T45.2X3	T45.2X4	T45.2X5	T45.2X6
Calcitonin	T50.991	T50.992	T50.993	T50.994	T50.995	T50.996
Calcitriol	T45.2X1	T45.2X2	T45.2X3	T45.2X4	T45.2X5	T45.2X6
Calcium	T50.3X1	T50.3X2	T50.3X3	T50.3X4	T50.3X5	T50.3X6
actylsalicylate	T39.011	T39.012	T39.013	T39.014	T39.015	T39.016
benzamidosalicylate	T37.1X1	T37.1X2	T37.1X3	T37.1X4	T37.1X5	T37.1X6
bromide	T42.6X1	T42.6X2	T42.6X3	T42.6X4	T42.6X5	T42.6X6
bromolactobionate	T42.6X1	T42.6X2	T42.6X3	T42.6X4	T42.6X5	T42.6X6
carbaspirin	T39.011	T39.012	T39.013	T39.014	T39.015	T39.016
carbimide	T50.6X1	T50.6X2	T50.6X3	T50.6X4	T50.6X5	T50.6X6
carbonate	T47.1X1	T47.1X2	T47.1X3	T47.1X4	T47.1X5	T47.1X6
chloride	T50.991	T50.992	T50.993	T50.994	T50.995	T50.996
anhydrous	T50.991	T50.992	T50.993	T50.994	T50.995	T50.996
cyanide	T57.8X1	T57.8X2	T57.8X3	T57.8X4	—	—
dioctyl sulfosuccinate	T47.4X1	T47.4X2	T47.4X3	T47.4X4	T47.4X5	T47.4X6
disodium edathamil	T45.8X1	T45.8X2	T45.8X3	T45.8X4	T45.8X5	T45.8X6
disodium edetate	T45.8X1	T45.8X2	T45.8X3	T45.8X4	T45.8X5	T45.8X6
dobesilate	T46.991	T46.992	T46.993	T46.994	T46.995	T46.996
EDTA	T45.8X1	T45.8X2	T45.8X3	T45.8X4	T45.8X5	T45.8X6
ferrous citrate	T45.4X1	T45.4X2	T45.4X3	T45.4X4	T45.4X5	T45.4X6
folinate	T45.8X1	T45.8X2	T45.8X3	T45.8X4	T45.8X5	T45.8X6
glubionate	T50.3X1	T50.3X2	T50.3X3	T50.3X4	T50.3X5	T50.3X6
gluconate	T50.3X1	T50.3X2	T50.3X3	T50.3X4	T50.3X5	T50.3X6
gluconogalactogluconate	T50.3X1	T50.3X2	T50.3X3	T50.3X4	T50.3X5	T50.3X6
hydrate, hydroxide	T54.3X1	T54.3X2	T54.3X3	T54.3X4	—	—
hypochlorite	T54.3X1	T54.3X2	T54.3X3	T54.3X4	—	—
iodide	T48.4X1	T48.4X2	T48.4X3	T48.4X4	T48.4X5	T48.4X6
ipodate	T50.8X1	T50.8X2	T50.8X3	T50.8X4	T50.8X5	T50.8X6
lactate	T50.3X1	T50.3X2	T50.3X3	T50.3X4	T50.3X5	T50.3X6
leucovorin	T45.8X1	T45.8X2	T45.8X3	T45.8X4	T45.8X5	T45.8X6
mandelate	T37.91	T37.92	T37.93	T37.94	T37.95	T37.96
oxide	T54.3X1	T54.3X2	T54.3X3	T54.3X4	—	—
pantothenate	T45.2X1	T45.2X2	T45.2X3	T45.2X4	T45.2X5	T45.2X6
phosphate	T50.3X1	T50.3X2	T50.3X3	T50.3X4	T50.3X5	T50.3X6
salicylate	T39.091	T39.092	T39.093	T39.094	T39.095	T39.096
salts	T50.3X1	T50.3X2	T50.3X3	T50.3X4	T50.3X5	T50.3X6
Calculus-dissolving drug	T50.991	T50.992	T50.993	T50.994	T50.995	T50.996
Calomel	T49.0X1	T49.0X2	T49.0X3	T49.0X4	T49.0X5	T49.0X6
Caloric agent	T50.3X1	T50.3X2	T50.3X3	T50.3X4	T50.3X5	T50.3X6
Calusterone	T38.7X1	T38.7X2	T38.7X3	T38.7X4	T38.7X5	T38.7X6
Camazepam	T42.4X1	T42.4X2	T42.4X3	T42.4X4	T42.4X5	T42.4X6
Camomile	T49.0X1	T49.0X2	T49.0X3	T49.0X4	T49.0X5	T49.0X6
Camoquin	T37.2X1	T37.2X2	T37.2X3	T37.2X4	T37.2X5	T37.2X6
Camphor						
insecticide	T60.2X1	T60.2X2	T60.2X3	T60.2X4	—	—
medicinal	T49.8X1	T49.8X2	T49.8X3	T49.8X4	T49.8X5	T49.8X6
Camylofin	T44.3X1	T44.3X2	T44.3X3	T44.3X4	T44.3X5	T44.3X6
Cancer chemotherapy drug regimen	T45.1X1	T45.1X2	T45.1X3	T45.1X4	T45.1X5	T45.1X6
Candeptin	T49.0X1	T49.0X2	T49.0X3	T49.0X4	T49.0X5	T49.0X6
Candicidin	T49.0X1	T49.0X2	T49.0X3	T49.0X4	T49.0X5	T49.0X6
Cannabinol	T40.7X1	T40.7X2	T40.7X3	T40.7X4	T40.7X5	T40.7X6
Cannabis (derivatives)	T40.7X1	T40.7X2	T40.7X3	T40.7X4	T40.7X5	T40.7X6
Canned heat	T51.1X1	T51.1X2	T51.1X3	T51.1X4	—	—
Canrenoic acid	T50.0X1	T50.0X2	T50.0X3	T50.0X4	T50.0X5	T50.0X6
Canrenone	T50.0X1	T50.0X2	T50.0X3	T50.0X4	T50.0X5	T50.0X6
Cantharides, cantharidin, cantharis	T49.8X1	T49.8X2	T49.8X3	T49.8X4	T49.8X5	T49.8X6
Canthaxanthin	T50.991	T50.992	T50.993	T50.994	T50.995	T50.996

Substance	Poisoning, Accidental (unintentional)	Poisoning, Intentional Self-harm	Poisoning, Assault	Poisoning, Undetermined	Adverse Effect	Under-dosing
Capillary-active drug NEC	T46.901	T46.902	T46.903	T46.904	T46.905	T46.906
Capreomycin	T36.8X1	T36.8X2	T36.8X3	T36.8X4	T36.8X5	T36.8X6
Capsicum	T49.4X1	T49.4X2	T49.4X3	T49.4X4	T49.4X5	T49.4X6
Captafol	T60.3X1	T60.3X2	T60.3X3	T60.3X4	—	—
Captan	T60.3X1	T60.3X2	T60.3X3	T60.3X4	—	—
Captodiame, captodiamine	T43.591	T43.592	T43.593	T43.594	T43.595	T43.596
Captopril	T46.4X1	T46.4X2	T46.4X3	T46.4X4	T46.4X5	T46.4X6
Caramiphen	T44.3X1	T44.3X2	T44.3X3	T44.3X4	T44.3X5	T44.3X6
Carazolol	T44.7X1	T44.7X2	T44.7X3	T44.7X4	T44.7X5	T44.7X6
Carbachol	T44.1X1	T44.1X2	T44.1X3	T44.1X4	T44.1X5	T44.1X6
Carbacrylamine (resin)	T50.3X1	T50.3X2	T50.3X3	T50.3X4	T50.3X5	T50.3X6
Carbamate (insecticide)	T60.0X1	T60.0X2	T60.0X3	T60.0X4	—	—
Carbamate (sedative)	T42.6X1	T42.6X2	T42.6X3	T42.6X4	T42.6X5	T42.6X6
herbicide	T60.0X1	T60.0X2	T60.0X3	T60.0X4	—	—
insecticide	T60.0X1	T60.0X2	T60.0X3	T60.0X4	—	—
Carbamazepine	T42.1X1	T42.1X2	T42.1X3	T42.1X4	T42.1X5	T42.1X6
Carbamide	T47.3X1	T47.3X2	T47.3X3	T47.3X4	T47.3X5	T47.3X6
peroxide	T49.0X1	T49.0X2	T49.0X3	T49.0X4	T49.0X5	T49.0X6
topical	T49.8X1	T49.8X2	T49.8X3	T49.8X4	T49.8X5	T49.8X6
Carbamylcholine chloride	T44.1X1	T44.1X2	T44.1X3	T44.1X4	T44.1X5	T44.1X6
Carbaril	T60.0X1	T60.0X2	T60.0X3	T60.0X4	—	—
Carbarsone	T37.3X1	T37.3X2	T37.3X3	T37.3X4	T37.3X5	T37.3X6
Carbaryl	T60.0X1	T60.0X2	T60.0X3	T60.0X4	—	—
Carbaspirin	T39.011	T39.012	T39.013	T39.014	T39.015	T39.016
Carbazochrome (salicylate) (sodium sulfonate)	T49.4X1	T49.4X2	T49.4X3	T49.4X4	T49.4X5	T49.4X6
Carbenicillin	T36.0X1	T36.0X2	T36.0X3	T36.0X4	T36.0X5	T36.0X6
Carbenoxolone	T47.1X1	T47.1X2	T47.1X3	T47.1X4	T47.1X5	T47.1X6
Carbetapentane	T48.3X1	T48.3X2	T48.3X3	T48.3X4	T48.3X5	T48.3X6
Carbethyl salicylate	T39.091	T39.092	T39.093	T39.094	T39.095	T39.096
Carbidopa (with levodopa)	T42.8X1	T42.8X2	T42.8X3	T42.8X4	T42.8X5	T42.8X6
Carbimazole	T38.2X1	T38.2X2	T38.2X3	T38.2X4	T38.2X5	T38.2X6
Carbinol	T51.1X1	T51.1X2	T51.1X3	T51.1X4	—	—
Carbinoxamine	T45.0X1	T45.0X2	T45.0X3	T45.0X4	T45.0X5	T45.0X6
Carbiphene	T39.8X1	T39.8X2	T39.8X3	T39.8X4	T39.8X5	T39.8X6
Carbitol	T52.3X1	T52.3X2	T52.3X3	T52.3X4	—	—
Carbocaine	T41.3X1	T41.3X2	T41.3X3	T41.3X4	T41.3X5	T41.3X6
infiltration (subcutaneous)	T41.3X1	T41.3X2	T41.3X3	T41.3X4	T41.3X5	T41.3X6
nerve block (peripheral) (plexus)	T41.3X1	T41.3X2	T41.3X3	T41.3X4	T41.3X5	T41.3X6
topical (surface)	T41.3X1	T41.3X2	T41.3X3	T41.3X4	T41.3X5	T41.3X6
Carbocisteine	T48.4X1	T48.4X2	T48.4X3	T48.4X4	T48.4X5	T48.4X6
Carbocromen	T46.3X1	T46.3X2	T46.3X3	T46.3X4	T46.3X5	T46.3X6
Carbol fuchsin	T49.0X1	T49.0X2	T49.0X3	T49.0X4	T49.0X5	T49.0X6
Carbolic acid — *see also* Phenol	T54.0X1	T54.0X2	T54.0X3	T54.0X4	—	—
Carbolonium (bromide)	T48.1X1	T48.1X2	T48.1X3	T48.1X4	T48.1X5	T48.1X6
Carbo medicinalis	T47.6X1	T47.6X2	T47.6X3	T47.6X4	T47.6X5	T47.6X6
Carbomycin	T36.8X1	T36.8X2	T36.8X3	T36.8X4	T36.8X5	T36.8X6
Carbon						
bisulfide (liquid)	T65.4X1	T65.4X2	T65.4X3	T65.4X4	—	—
vapor	T65.4X1	T65.4X2	T65.4X3	T65.4X4	—	—
dioxide (gas)	T59.7X1	T59.7X2	T59.7X3	T59.7X4	—	—
medicinal	T41.5X1	T41.5X2	T41.5X3	T41.5X4	T41.5X5	T41.5X6
nonmedicinal	T59.7X1	T59.7X2	T59.7X3	T59.7X4	—	—
snow	T49.4X1	T49.4X2	T49.4X3	T49.4X4	T49.4X5	T49.4X6
disulfide (liquid)	T65.4X1	T65.4X2	T65.4X3	T65.4X4	—	—
vapor	T65.4X1	T65.4X2	T65.4X3	T65.4X4	—	—
monoxide (from incomplete combustion)	T58.91	T58.92	T58.93	T58.94	—	—
blast furnace gas	T58.8X1	T58.8X2	T58.8X3	T58.8X4	—	—
butane (distributed in mobile container)	T58.11	T58.12	T58.13	T58.14	—	—
distributed through pipes	T58.11	T58.12	T58.13	T58.14	—	—
charcoal fumes	T58.2X1	T58.2X2	T58.2X3	T58.2X4	—	—
coal	T58.2X1	T58.2X2	T58.2X3	T58.2X4	—	—
coke (in domestic stoves, fireplaces)	T58.2X1	T58.2X2	T58.2X3	T58.2X4	—	—
exhaust gas (motor) not in transit	T58.01	T58.02	T58.03	T58.04	—	—
combustion engine, any not in watercraft	T58.01	T58.02	T58.03	T58.04	—	—
farm tractor, not in transit	T58.01	T58.02	T58.03	T58.04	—	—
gas engine	T58.01	T58.02	T58.03	T58.04	—	—
motor pump	T58.01	T58.02	T58.03	T58.04	—	—
motor vehicle, not in transit	T58.01	T58.02	T58.03	T58.04	—	—
fuel (in domestic use)	T58.2X1	T58.2X2	T58.2X3	T58.2X4	—	—
gas (piped)	T58.11	T58.12	T58.13	T58.14	—	—
in mobile container	T58.11	T58.12	T58.13	T58.14	—	—

Table of Drugs and Chemicals

Carbon — Central nervous system

Substance	Poisoning, Accidental (unintentional)	Poisoning, Intentional Self-harm	Poisoning, Assault	Poisoning, Undetermined	Adverse Effect	Under-dosing
Carbon — *continued*						
monoxide — *continued*						
fuel — *continued*						
piped (natural)	T58.11	T58.12	T58.13	T58.14	—	—
utility	T58.11	T58.12	T58.13	T58.14	—	—
in mobile container	T58.11	T58.12	T58.13	T58.14	—	—
gas (piped)	T58.11	T58.12	T58.13	T58.14	—	—
illuminating gas	T58.11	T58.12	T58.13	T58.14	—	—
industrial fuels or gases, any	T58.8X1	T58.8X2	T58.8X3	T58.8X4	—	—
kerosene (in domestic stoves, fireplaces)	T58.2X1	T58.2X2	T58.2X3	T58.2X4	—	—
kiln gas or vapor	T58.8X1	T58.8X2	T58.8X3	T58.8X4	—	—
motor exhaust gas, not in transit	T58.01	T58.02	T58.03	T58.04	—	—
piped gas (manufactured) (natural)	T58.11	T58.12	T58.13	T58.14	—	—
producer gas	T58.8X1	T58.8X2	T58.8X3	T58.8X4	—	—
propane (distributed in mobile container)	T58.11	T58.12	T58.13	T58.14	—	—
distributed through pipes	T58.11	T58.12	T58.13	T58.14	—	—
solid (in domestic stoves, fireplaces)	T58.2X1	T58.2X2	T58.2X3	T58.2X4	—	—
specified source NEC	T58.8X1	T58.8X2	T58.8X3	T58.8X4	—	—
stove gas	T58.11	T58.12	T58.13	T58.14	—	—
piped	T58.11	T58.12	T58.13	T58.14	—	—
utility gas	T58.11	T58.12	T58.13	T58.14	—	—
piped	T58.11	T58.12	T58.13	T58.14	—	—
water gas	T58.11	T58.12	T58.13	T58.14	—	—
wood (in domestic stoves, fireplaces)	T58.2X1	T58.2X2	T58.2X3	T58.2X4	—	—
tetrachloride (vapor) NEC	T53.0X1	T53.0X2	T53.0X3	T53.0X4	—	—
liquid (cleansing agent) NEC	T53.0X1	T53.0X2	T53.0X3	T53.0X4	—	—
solvent	T53.0X1	T53.0X2	T53.0X3	T53.0X4	—	—
Carbonic acid gas	T59.7X1	T59.7X2	T59.7X3	T59.7X4	—	—
anhydrase inhibitor NEC	T50.2X1	T50.2X2	T50.2X3	T50.2X4	T50.2X5	T50.2X6
Carbophenothion	T60.0X1	T60.0X2	T60.0X3	T60.0X4	—	—
Carboplatin	T45.1X1	T45.1X2	T45.1X3	T45.1X4	T45.1X5	T45.1X6
Carboprost	T48.0X1	T48.0X2	T48.0X3	T48.0X4	T48.0X5	T48.0X6
Carboquone	T45.1X1	T45.1X2	T45.1X3	T45.1X4	T45.1X5	T45.1X6
Carbowax	T49.3X1	T49.3X2	T49.3X3	T49.3X4	T49.3X5	T49.3X6
Carboxymethylcellulose	T47.4X1	T47.4X2	T47.4X3	T47.4X4	T47.4X5	T47.4X6
Carbrital	T42.3X1	T42.3X2	T42.3X3	T42.3X4	T42.3X5	T42.3X6
Carbromal	T42.6X1	T42.6X2	T42.6X3	T42.6X4	T42.6X5	T42.6X6
Carbutamide	T38.3X1	T38.3X2	T38.3X3	T38.3X4	T38.3X5	T38.3X6
Carbuterol	T48.6X1	T48.6X2	T48.6X3	T48.6X4	T48.6X5	T48.6X6
Cardiac						
depressants	T46.2X1	T46.2X2	T46.2X3	T46.2X4	T46.2X5	T46.2X6
rhythm regulator	T46.2X1	T46.2X2	T46.2X3	T46.2X4	T46.2X5	T46.2X6
specified NEC	T46.2X1	T46.2X2	T46.2X3	T46.2X4	T46.2X5	T46.2X6
Cardiografin	T50.8X1	T50.8X2	T50.8X3	T50.8X4	T50.8X5	T50.8X6
Cardiogreen	T50.8X1	T50.8X2	T50.8X3	T50.8X4	T50.8X5	T50.8X6
Cardiotonic (glycoside) **NEC**	T46.0X1	T46.0X2	T46.0X3	T46.0X4	T46.0X5	T46.0X6
Cardiovascular drug NEC	T46.901	T46.902	T46.903	T46.904	T46.905	T46.906
Cardrase	T50.2X1	T50.2X2	T50.2X3	T50.2X4	T50.2X5	T50.2X6
Carfecillin	T36.0X1	T36.0X2	T36.0X3	T36.0X4	T36.0X5	T36.0X6
Carfenazine	T43.3X1	T43.3X2	T43.3X3	T43.3X4	T43.3X5	T43.3X6
Carfusin	T49.0X1	T49.0X2	T49.0X3	T49.0X4	T49.0X5	T49.0X6
Carindacillin	T36.0X1	T36.0X2	T36.0X3	T36.0X4	T36.0X5	T36.0X6
Carisoprodol	T42.8X1	T42.8X2	T42.8X3	T42.8X4	T42.8X5	T42.8X6
Carmellose	T47.4X1	T47.4X2	T47.4X3	T47.4X4	T47.4X5	T47.4X6
Carminative	T47.5X1	T47.5X2	T47.5X3	T47.5X4	T47.5X5	T47.5X6
Carmofur	T45.1X1	T45.1X2	T45.1X3	T45.1X4	T45.1X5	T45.1X6
Carmustine	T45.1X1	T45.1X2	T45.1X3	T45.1X4	T45.1X5	T45.1X6
Carotene	T45.2X1	T45.2X2	T45.2X3	T45.2X4	T45.2X5	T45.2X6
Carphenazine	T43.3X1	T43.3X2	T43.3X3	T43.3X4	T43.3X5	T43.3X6
Carpipramine	T42.4X1	T42.4X2	T42.4X3	T42.4X4	T42.4X5	T42.4X6
Carprofen	T39.311	T39.312	T39.313	T39.314	T39.315	T39.316
Carpronium chloride	T44.3X1	T44.3X2	T44.3X3	T44.3X4	T44.3X5	T44.3X6
Carrageenan	T47.8X1	T47.8X2	T47.8X3	T47.8X4	T47.8X5	T47.8X6
Carteolol	T44.7X1	T44.7X2	T44.7X3	T44.7X4	T44.7X5	T44.7X6
Carter's Little Pills	T47.2X1	T47.2X2	T47.2X3	T47.2X4	T47.2X5	T47.2X6
Cascara (sagrada)	T47.2X1	T47.2X2	T47.2X3	T47.2X4	T47.2X5	T47.2X6
Cassava	T62.2X1	T62.2X2	T62.2X3	T62.2X4	—	—
Castellani's paint	T49.0X1	T49.0X2	T49.0X3	T49.0X4	T49.0X5	T49.0X6
Castor						
bean	T62.2X1	T62.2X2	T62.2X3	T62.2X4	—	—
oil	T47.2X1	T47.2X2	T47.2X3	T47.2X4	T47.2X5	T47.2X6
Catalase	T45.3X1	T45.3X2	T45.3X3	T45.3X4	T45.3X5	T45.3X6
Caterpillar (sting)	T63.431	T63.432	T63.433	T63.434	—	—
Catha (edulis) (tea)	T43.691	T43.692	T43.693	T43.694	—	—

Substance	Poisoning, Accidental (unintentional)	Poisoning, Intentional Self-harm	Poisoning, Assault	Poisoning, Undetermined	Adverse Effect	Under-dosing
Cathartic NEC	T47.4X1	T47.4X2	T47.4X3	T47.4X4	T47.4X5	T47.4X6
anthracene derivative	T47.2X1	T47.2X2	T47.2X3	T47.2X4	T47.2X5	T47.2X6
bulk	T47.4X1	T47.4X2	T47.4X3	T47.4X4	T47.4X5	T47.4X6
contact	T47.2X1	T47.2X2	T47.2X3	T47.2X4	T47.2X5	T47.2X6
emollient NEC	T47.4X1	T47.4X2	T47.4X3	T47.4X4	T47.4X5	T47.4X6
irritant NEC	T47.2X1	T47.2X2	T47.2X3	T47.2X4	T47.2X5	T47.2X6
mucilage	T47.4X1	T47.4X2	T47.4X3	T47.4X4	T47.4X5	T47.4X6
saline	T47.3X1	T47.3X2	T47.3X3	T47.3X4	T47.3X5	T47.3X6
vegetable	T47.2X1	T47.2X2	T47.2X3	T47.2X4	T47.2X5	T47.2X6
Cathine	T50.5X1	T50.5X2	T50.5X3	T50.5X4	T50.5X5	T50.5X6
Cathomycin	T36.8X1	T36.8X2	T36.8X3	T36.8X4	T36.8X5	T36.8X6
Cation exchange resin	T50.3X1	T50.3X2	T50.3X3	T50.3X4	T50.3X5	T50.3X6
Caustic(s) NEC	T54.91	T54.92	T54.93	T54.94	—	—
alkali	T54.3X1	T54.3X2	T54.3X3	T54.3X4	—	—
hydroxide	T54.3X1	T54.3X2	T54.3X3	T54.3X4	—	—
potash	T54.3X1	T54.3X2	T54.3X3	T54.3X4	—	—
soda	T54.3X1	T54.3X2	T54.3X3	T54.3X4	—	—
specified NEC	T54.91	T54.92	T54.93	T54.94	—	—
Ceepryn	T49.0X1	T49.0X2	T49.0X3	T49.0X4	T49.0X5	T49.0X6
ENT agent	T49.6X1	T49.6X2	T49.6X3	T49.6X4	T49.6X5	T49.6X6
lozenges	T49.6X1	T49.6X2	T49.6X3	T49.6X4	T49.6X5	T49.6X6
Cefacetrile	T36.1X1	T36.1X2	T36.1X3	T36.1X4	T36.1X5	T36.1X6
Cefaclor	T36.1X1	T36.1X2	T36.1X3	T36.1X4	T36.1X5	T36.1X6
Cefadroxil	T36.1X1	T36.1X2	T36.1X3	T36.1X4	T36.1X5	T36.1X6
Cefalexin	T36.1X1	T36.1X2	T36.1X3	T36.1X4	T36.1X5	T36.1X6
Cefaloglycin	T36.1X1	T36.1X2	T36.1X3	T36.1X4	T36.1X5	T36.1X6
Cefaloridine	T36.1X1	T36.1X2	T36.1X3	T36.1X4	T36.1X5	T36.1X6
Cefalosporins	T36.1X1	T36.1X2	T36.1X3	T36.1X4	T36.1X5	T36.1X6
Cefalotin	T36.1X1	T36.1X2	T36.1X3	T36.1X4	T36.1X5	T36.1X6
Cefamandole	T36.1X1	T36.1X2	T36.1X3	T36.1X4	T36.1X5	T36.1X6
Cefamycin antibiotic	T36.1X1	T36.1X2	T36.1X3	T36.1X4	T36.1X5	T36.1X6
Cefapirin	T36.1X1	T36.1X2	T36.1X3	T36.1X4	T36.1X5	T36.1X6
Cefatrizine	T36.1X1	T36.1X2	T36.1X3	T36.1X4	T36.1X5	T36.1X6
Cefazedone	T36.1X1	T36.1X2	T36.1X3	T36.1X4	T36.1X5	T36.1X6
Cefazolin	T36.1X1	T36.1X2	T36.1X3	T36.1X4	T36.1X5	T36.1X6
Cefbuperazone	T36.1X1	T36.1X2	T36.1X3	T36.1X4	T36.1X5	T36.1X6
Cefetamet	T36.1X1	T36.1X2	T36.1X3	T36.1X4	T36.1X5	T36.1X6
Cefixime	T36.1X1	T36.1X2	T36.1X3	T36.1X4	T36.1X5	T36.1X6
Cefmenoxime	T36.1X1	T36.1X2	T36.1X3	T36.1X4	T36.1X5	T36.1X6
Cefmetazole	T36.1X1	T36.1X2	T36.1X3	T36.1X4	T36.1X5	T36.1X6
Cefminox	T36.1X1	T36.1X2	T36.1X3	T36.1X4	T36.1X5	T36.1X6
Cefonicid	T36.1X1	T36.1X2	T36.1X3	T36.1X4	T36.1X5	T36.1X6
Cefoperazone	T36.1X1	T36.1X2	T36.1X3	T36.1X4	T36.1X5	T36.1X6
Ceforanide	T36.1X1	T36.1X2	T36.1X3	T36.1X4	T36.1X5	T36.1X6
Cefotaxime	T36.1X1	T36.1X2	T36.1X3	T36.1X4	T36.1X5	T36.1X6
Cefotetan	T36.1X1	T36.1X2	T36.1X3	T36.1X4	T36.1X5	T36.1X6
Cefotiam	T36.1X1	T36.1X2	T36.1X3	T36.1X4	T36.1X5	T36.1X6
Cefoxitin	T36.1X1	T36.1X2	T36.1X3	T36.1X4	T36.1X5	T36.1X6
Cefpimizole	T36.1X1	T36.1X2	T36.1X3	T36.1X4	T36.1X5	T36.1X6
Cefpiramide	T36.1X1	T36.1X2	T36.1X3	T36.1X4	T36.1X5	T36.1X6
Cefradine	T36.1X1	T36.1X2	T36.1X3	T36.1X4	T36.1X5	T36.1X6
Cefroxadine	T36.1X1	T36.1X2	T36.1X3	T36.1X4	T36.1X5	T36.1X6
Cefsulodin	T36.1X1	T36.1X2	T36.1X3	T36.1X4	T36.1X5	T36.1X6
Ceftazidime	T36.1X1	T36.1X2	T36.1X3	T36.1X4	T36.1X5	T36.1X6
Cefteram	T36.1X1	T36.1X2	T36.1X3	T36.1X4	T36.1X5	T36.1X6
Ceftezole	T36.1X1	T36.1X2	T36.1X3	T36.1X4	T36.1X5	T36.1X6
Ceftizoxime	T36.1X1	T36.1X2	T36.1X3	T36.1X4	T36.1X5	T36.1X6
Ceftriaxone	T36.1X1	T36.1X2	T36.1X3	T36.1X4	T36.1X5	T36.1X6
Cefuroxime	T36.1X1	T36.1X2	T36.1X3	T36.1X4	T36.1X5	T36.1X6
Cefuzonam	T36.1X1	T36.1X2	T36.1X3	T36.1X4	T36.1X5	T36.1X6
Celestone	T38.0X1	T38.0X2	T38.0X3	T38.0X4	T38.0X5	T38.0X6
topical	T49.0X1	T49.0X2	T49.0X3	T49.0X4	T49.0X5	T49.0X6
Celiprolol	T44.7X1	T44.7X2	T44.7X3	T44.7X4	T44.7X5	T44.7X6
Cellosolve	T52.91	T52.92	T52.93	T52.94	—	—
Cell stimulants and proliferants	T49.8X1	T49.8X2	T49.8X3	T49.8X4	T49.8X5	T49.8X6
Cellulose						
cathartic	T47.4X1	T47.4X2	T47.4X3	T47.4X4	T47.4X5	T47.4X6
hydroxyethyl	T47.4X1	T47.4X2	T47.4X3	T47.4X4	T47.4X5	T47.4X6
nitrates (topical)	T49.3X1	T49.3X2	T49.3X3	T49.3X4	T49.3X5	T49.3X6
oxidized	T49.4X1	T49.4X2	T49.4X3	T49.4X4	T49.4X5	T49.4X6
Centipede (bite)	T63.411	T63.412	T63.413	T63.414	—	—
Central nervous system						
depressants	T42.71	T42.72	T42.73	T42.74	T42.75	T42.76
anesthetic (general) NEC	T41.201	T41.202	T41.203	T41.204	T41.205	T41.206
gases NEC	T41.0X1	T41.0X2	T41.0X3	T41.0X4	T41.0X5	T41.0X6
intravenous	T41.1X1	T41.1X2	T41.1X3	T41.1X4	T41.1X5	T41.1X6
barbiturates	T42.3X1	T42.3X2	T42.3X3	T42.3X4	T42.3X5	T42.3X6
benzodiazepines	T42.4X1	T42.4X2	T42.4X3	T42.4X4	T42.4X5	T42.4X6
bromides	T42.6X1	T42.6X2	T42.6X3	T42.6X4	T42.6X5	T42.6X6
cannabis sativa	T40.7X1	T40.7X2	T40.7X3	T40.7X4	T40.7X5	T40.7X6
chloral hydrate	T42.6X1	T42.6X2	T42.6X3	T42.6X4	T42.6X5	T42.6X6
ethanol	T51.0X1	T51.0X2	T51.0X3	T51.0X4	—	—

Additional Character May Be Required — Refer to the Tabular List for Character Selection

Subterms under main terms may continue to next column or page

Substance	Poisoning, Accidental (unintentional)	Poisoning, Intentional Self-harm	Poisoning, Assault	Poisoning, Undetermined	Adverse Effect	Underdosing
Central nervous system — continued						
depressants — continued						
hallucinogenics	T40.901	T40.902	T40.903	T40.904	T40.905	T40.906
hypnotics	T42.71	T42.72	T42.73	T42.74	T42.75	T42.76
specified NEC	T42.6X1	T42.6X2	T42.6X3	T42.6X4	T42.6X5	T42.6X6
muscle relaxants	T42.8X1	T42.8X2	T42.8X3	T42.8X4	T42.8X5	T42.8X6
paraldehyde	T42.6X1	T42.6X2	T42.6X3	T42.6X4	T42.6X5	T42.6X6
sedatives;	T42.71	T42.72	T42.73	T42.74	T42.75	T42.76
sedative-hypnotics						
mixed NEC	T42.6X1	T42.6X2	T42.6X3	T42.6X4	T42.6X5	T42.6X6
specified NEC	T42.6X1	T42.6X2	T42.6X3	T42.6X4	T42.6X5	T42.6X6
muscle-tone depressants	T42.8X1	T42.8X2	T42.8X3	T42.8X4	T42.8X5	T42.8X6
stimulants	T43.601	T43.602	T43.603	T43.604	T43.605	T43.606
amphetamines	T43.621	T43.622	T43.623	T43.624	T43.625	T43.626
analeptics	T50.7X1	T50.7X2	T50.7X3	T50.7X4	T50.7X5	T50.7X6
antidepressants	T43.201	T43.202	T43.203	T43.204	T43.205	T43.206
opiate antagonists	T50.7X1	T50.7X2	T50.7X3	T50.7X4	T50.7X5	T50.7X6
specified NEC	T43.691	T43.692	T43.693	T43.694	T43.695	T43.696
Cephalexin	T36.1X1	T36.1X2	T36.1X3	T36.1X4	T36.1X5	T36.1X6
Cephaloglycin	T36.1X1	T36.1X2	T36.1X3	T36.1X4	T36.1X5	T36.1X6
Cephaloridine	T36.1X1	T36.1X2	T36.1X3	T36.1X4	T36.1X5	T36.1X6
Cephalosporins	T36.1X1	T36.1X2	T36.1X3	T36.1X4	T36.1X5	T36.1X6
N (adicillin)	T36.0X1	T36.0X2	T36.0X3	T36.0X4	T36.0X5	T36.0X6
Cephalothin	T36.1X1	T36.1X2	T36.1X3	T36.1X4	T36.1X5	T36.1X6
Cephalotin	T36.1X1	T36.1X2	T36.1X3	T36.1X4	T36.1X5	T36.1X6
Cephradine	T36.1X1	T36.1X2	T36.1X3	T36.1X4	T36.1X5	T36.1X6
Cerbera (odallam)	T62.2X1	T62.2X2	T62.2X3	T62.2X4	—	—
Cerberin	T46.0X1	T46.0X2	T46.0X3	T46.0X4	T46.0X5	T46.0X6
Cerebral stimulants	T43.601	T43.602	T43.603	T43.604	T43.605	T43.606
psychotherapeutic	T43.601	T43.602	T43.603	T43.604	T43.605	T43.606
specified NEC	T43.691	T43.692	T43.693	T43.694	T43.695	T43.696
Cerium oxalate	T45.0X1	T45.0X2	T45.0X3	T45.0X4	T45.0X5	T45.0X6
Cerous oxalate	T45.0X1	T45.0X2	T45.0X3	T45.0X4	T45.0X5	T45.0X6
Ceruletide	T50.8X1	T50.8X2	T50.8X3	T50.8X4	T50.8X5	T50.8X6
Cetalkonium (chloride)	T49.0X1	T49.0X2	T49.0X3	T49.0X4	T49.0X5	T49.0X6
Cethexonium chloride	T49.0X1	T49.0X2	T49.0X3	T49.0X4	T49.0X5	T49.0X6
Cetiedil	T46.7X1	T46.7X2	T46.7X3	T46.7X4	T46.7X5	T46.7X6
Cetirizine	T45.0X1	T45.0X2	T45.0X3	T45.0X4	T45.0X5	T45.0X6
Cetomacrogol	T50.991	T50.992	T50.993	T50.994	T50.995	T50.996
Cetotiamine	T45.2X1	T45.2X2	T45.2X3	T45.2X4	T45.2X5	T45.2X6
Cetoxime	T45.0X1	T45.0X2	T45.0X3	T45.0X4	T45.0X5	T45.0X6
Cetraxate	T47.1X1	T47.1X2	T47.1X3	T47.1X4	T47.1X5	T47.1X6
Cetrimide	T49.0X1	T49.0X2	T49.0X3	T49.0X4	T49.0X5	T49.0X6
Cetrimonium (bromide)	T49.0X1	T49.0X2	T49.0X3	T49.0X4	T49.0X5	T49.0X6
Cetylpyridinium chloride	T49.0X1	T49.0X2	T49.0X3	T49.0X4	T49.0X5	T49.0X6
ENT agent	T49.6X1	T49.6X2	T49.6X3	T49.6X4	T49.6X5	T49.6X6
lozenges	T49.6X1	T49.6X2	T49.6X3	T49.6X4	T49.6X5	T49.6X6
Cevadilla — see Sabadilla						
Cevitamic acid	T45.2X1	T45.2X2	T45.2X3	T45.2X4	T45.2X5	T45.2X6
Chalk, precipitated	T47.1X1	T47.1X2	T47.1X3	T47.1X4	T47.1X5	T47.1X6
Chamomile	T49.0X1	T49.0X2	T49.0X3	T49.0X4	T49.0X5	T49.0X6
Ch'an su	T46.0X1	T46.0X2	T46.0X3	T46.0X4	T46.0X5	T46.0X6
Charcoal	T47.6X1	T47.6X2	T47.6X3	T47.6X4	T47.6X5	T47.6X6
activated — see also Charcoal, medicinal						
fumes (Carbon monoxide)	T58.2X1	T58.2X2	T58.2X3	T58.2X4	—	—
industrial	T58.8X1	T58.8X2	T58.8X3	T58.8X4	—	—
medicinal (activated)	T47.6X1	T47.6X2	T47.6X3	T47.6X4	T47.6X5	T47.6X6
antidiarrheal	T47.6X1	T47.6X2	T47.6X3	T47.6X4	T47.6X5	T47.6X6
poison control	T47.8X1	T47.8X2	T47.8X3	T47.8X4	T47.8X5	T47.8X6
specified use other than for diarrhea	T47.8X1	T47.8X2	T47.8X3	T47.8X4	T47.8X5	T47.8X6
topical	T49.8X1	T49.8X2	T49.8X3	T49.8X4	T49.8X5	T49.8X6
Chaulmosulfone	T37.1X1	T37.1X2	T37.1X3	T37.1X4	T37.1X5	T37.1X6
Chelating agent NEC	T50.6X1	T50.6X2	T50.6X3	T50.6X4	T50.6X5	T50.6X6
Chelidonium majus	T62.2X1	T62.2X2	T62.2X3	T62.2X4	—	—
Chemical substance NEC	T65.91	T65.92	T65.93	T65.94	—	—
Chenodeoxycholic acid	T47.5X1	T47.5X2	T47.5X3	T47.5X4	T47.5X5	T47.5X6
Chenodiol	T47.5X1	T47.5X2	T47.5X3	T47.5X4	T47.5X5	T47.5X6
Chenopodium	T37.4X1	T37.4X2	T37.4X3	T37.4X4	T37.4X5	T37.4X6
Cherry laurel	T62.2X1	T62.2X2	T62.2X3	T62.2X4	—	—
Chinidin (e)	T46.2X1	T46.2X2	T46.2X3	T46.2X4	T46.2X5	T46.2X6
Chiniofon	T37.8X1	T37.8X2	T37.8X3	T37.8X4	T37.8X5	T37.8X6
Chlophedianol	T48.3X1	T48.3X2	T48.3X3	T48.3X4	T48.3X5	T48.3X6
Chloral	T42.6X1	T42.6X2	T42.6X3	T42.6X4	T42.6X5	T42.6X6
derivative	T42.6X1	T42.6X2	T42.6X3	T42.6X4	T42.6X5	T42.6X6
hydrate	T42.6X1	T42.6X2	T42.6X3	T42.6X4	T42.6X5	T42.6X6
Chloralamide	T42.6X1	T42.6X2	T42.6X3	T42.6X4	T42.6X5	T42.6X6
Chloralodol	T42.6X1	T42.6X2	T42.6X3	T42.6X4	T42.6X5	T42.6X6
Chloralose	T60.4X1	T60.4X2	T60.4X3	T60.4X4	—	—
Chlorambucil	T45.1X1	T45.1X2	T45.1X3	T45.1X4	T45.1X5	T45.1X6
Chloramine	T57.8X1	T57.8X2	T57.8X3	T57.8X4	—	—

Substance	Poisoning, Accidental (unintentional)	Poisoning, Intentional Self-harm	Poisoning, Assault	Poisoning, Undetermined	Adverse Effect	Underdosing
Chloramine — continued						
T	T49.0X1	T49.0X2	T49.0X3	T49.0X4	T49.0X5	T49.0X6
topical	T49.0X1	T49.0X2	T49.0X3	T49.0X4	T49.0X5	T49.0X6
Chloramphenicol	T36.2X1	T36.2X2	T36.2X3	T36.2X4	T36.2X5	T36.2X6
ENT agent	T49.6X1	T49.6X2	T49.6X3	T49.6X4	T49.6X5	T49.6X6
ophthalmic preparation	T49.5X1	T49.5X2	T49.5X3	T49.5X4	T49.5X5	T49.5X6
topical NEC	T49.0X1	T49.0X2	T49.0X3	T49.0X4	T49.0X5	T49.0X6
Chlorate (potassium) (sodium) NEC	T60.3X1	T60.3X2	T60.3X3	T60.3X4	—	—
herbicide	T60.3X1	T60.3X2	T60.3X3	T60.3X4	—	—
Chlorazanil	T50.2X1	T50.2X2	T50.2X3	T50.2X4	T50.2X5	T50.2X6
Chlorbenzene, chlorbenzol	T53.7X1	T53.7X2	T53.7X3	T53.7X4	—	—
Chlorbenzoxamine	T44.3X1	T44.3X2	T44.3X3	T44.3X4	T44.3X5	T44.3X6
Chlorbutol	T42.6X1	T42.6X2	T42.6X3	T42.6X4	T42.6X5	T42.6X6
Chlorcyclizine	T45.0X1	T45.0X2	T45.0X3	T45.0X4	T45.0X5	T45.0X6
Chlordan (e) (dust)	T60.1X1	T60.1X2	T60.1X3	T60.1X4	—	—
Chlordantoin	T49.0X1	T49.0X2	T49.0X3	T49.0X4	T49.0X5	T49.0X6
Chlordiazepoxide	T42.4X1	T42.4X2	T42.4X3	T42.4X4	T42.4X5	T42.4X6
Chlordiethyl benzamide	T49.3X1	T49.3X2	T49.3X3	T49.3X4	T49.3X5	T49.3X6
Chloresium	T49.8X1	T49.8X2	T49.8X3	T49.8X4	T49.8X5	T49.8X6
Chlorethiazol	T42.6X1	T42.6X2	T42.6X3	T42.6X4	T42.6X5	T42.6X6
Chlorethyl — see Ethyl chloride						
Chloretone	T42.6X1	T42.6X2	T42.6X3	T42.6X4	T42.6X5	T42.6X6
Chlorex	T53.6X1	T53.6X2	T53.6X3	T53.6X4	—	—
insecticide	T60.1X1	T60.1X2	T60.1X3	T60.1X4	—	—
Chlorfenvinphos	T60.0X1	T60.0X2	T60.0X3	T60.0X4	—	—
Chlorhexadol	T42.6X1	T42.6X2	T42.6X3	T42.6X4	T42.6X5	T42.6X6
Chlorhexamide	T45.1X1	T45.1X2	T45.1X3	T45.1X4	T45.1X5	T45.1X6
Chlorhexidine	T49.0X1	T49.0X2	T49.0X3	T49.0X4	T49.0X5	T49.0X6
Chlorhydroxyquinolin	T49.0X1	T49.0X2	T49.0X3	T49.0X4	T49.0X5	T49.0X6
Chloride of lime (bleach)	T54.3X1	T54.3X2	T54.3X3	T54.3X4	—	—
Chlorimipramine	T43.011	T43.012	T43.013	T43.014	T43.015	T43.016
Chlorinated						
camphene	T53.6X1	T53.6X2	T53.6X3	T53.6X4	—	—
diphenyl	T53.7X1	T53.7X2	T53.7X3	T53.7X4	—	—
hydrocarbons NEC	T53.91	T53.92	T53.93	T53.94	—	—
solvents	T53.91	T53.92	T53.93	T53.94	—	—
lime (bleach)	T54.3X1	T54.3X2	T54.3X3	T54.3X4	—	—
and boric acid solution	T49.0X1	T49.0X2	T49.0X3	T49.0X4	T49.0X5	T49.0X6
naphthalene (insecticide)	T60.1X1	T60.1X2	T60.1X3	T60.1X4	—	—
industrial (non-pesticide)	T53.7X1	T53.7X2	T53.7X3	T53.7X4	—	—
pesticide NEC	T60.8X1	T60.8X2	T60.8X3	T60.8X4	—	—
soda — see also sodium hypochlorite						
solution	T49.0X1	T49.0X2	T49.0X3	T49.0X4	T49.0X5	T49.0X6
Chlorine (fumes) (gas)	T59.4X1	T59.4X2	T59.4X3	T59.4X4	—	—
bleach	T54.3X1	T54.3X2	T54.3X3	T54.3X4	—	—
compound gas NEC	T59.4X1	T59.4X2	T59.4X3	T59.4X4	—	—
disinfectant	T59.4X1	T59.4X2	T59.4X3	T59.4X4	—	—
releasing agents NEC	T59.4X1	T59.4X2	T59.4X3	T59.4X4	—	—
Chlorisondamine chloride	T46.991	T46.992	T46.993	T46.994	T46.995	T46.996
Chlormadinone	T38.5X1	T38.5X2	T38.5X3	T38.5X4	T38.5X5	T38.5X6
Chlormephos	T60.0X1	T60.0X2	T60.0X3	T60.0X4	—	—
Chlormerodrin	T50.2X1	T50.2X2	T50.2X3	T50.2X4	T50.2X5	T50.2X6
Chlormethiazole	T42.6X1	T42.6X2	T42.6X3	T42.6X4	T42.6X5	T42.6X6
Chlormethine	T45.1X1	T45.1X2	T45.1X3	T45.1X4	T45.1X5	T45.1X6
Chlormethylenecycline	T36.4X1	T36.4X2	T36.4X3	T36.4X4	T36.4X5	T36.4X6
Chlormezanone	T42.6X1	T42.6X2	T42.6X3	T42.6X4	T42.6X5	T42.6X6
Chloroacetic acid	T60.3X1	T60.3X2	T60.3X3	T60.3X4	—	—
Chloroacetone	T59.3X1	T59.3X2	T59.3X3	T59.3X4	—	—
Chloroacetophenone	T59.3X1	T59.3X2	T59.3X3	T59.3X4	—	—
Chloroaniline	T53.7X1	T53.7X2	T53.7X3	T53.7X4	—	—
Chlorobenzene, chlorobenzol	T53.7X1	T53.7X2	T53.7X3	T53.7X4	—	—
Chlorobromomethane (fire extinguisher)	T53.6X1	T53.6X2	T53.6X3	T53.6X4	—	—
Chlorobutanol	T49.0X1	T49.0X2	T49.0X3	T49.0X4	T49.0X5	T49.0X6
Chlorocresol	T49.0X1	T49.0X2	T49.0X3	T49.0X4	T49.0X5	T49.0X6
Chlorodehydromethyltestosterone	T38.7X1	T38.7X2	T38.7X3	T38.7X4	T38.7X5	T38.7X6
Chlorodinitrobenzene	T53.7X1	T53.7X2	T53.7X3	T53.7X4	—	—
dust or vapor	T53.7X1	T53.7X2	T53.7X3	T53.7X4	—	—
Chlorodiphenyl	T53.7X1	T53.7X2	T53.7X3	T53.7X4	—	—
Chloroethane — see Ethyl chloride						
Chloroethylene	T53.6X1	T53.6X2	T53.6X3	T53.6X4	—	—
Chlorofluorocarbons	T53.5X1	T53.5X2	T53.5X3	T53.5X4	—	—
Chloroform (fumes) (vapor)	T53.1X1	T53.1X2	T53.1X3	T53.1X4	—	—
anesthetic	T41.0X1	T41.0X2	T41.0X3	T41.0X4	T41.0X5	T41.0X6
solvent	T53.1X1	T53.1X2	T53.1X3	T53.1X4	—	—
water, concentrated	T41.0X1	T41.0X2	T41.0X3	T41.0X4	T41.0X5	T41.0X6
Chloroguanide	T37.2X1	T37.2X2	T37.2X3	T37.2X4	T37.2X5	T37.2X6

Table of Drugs and Chemicals

Substance	Poisoning, Accidental (unintentional)	Poisoning, Intentional Self-harm	Poisoning, Assault	Poisoning, Undetermined	Adverse Effect	Under-dosing
Chloromycetin	T36.2X1	T36.2X2	T36.2X3	T36.2X4	T36.2X5	T36.2X6
ENT agent	T49.6X1	T49.6X2	T49.6X3	T49.6X4	T49.6X5	T49.6X6
ophthalmic preparation	T49.5X1	T49.5X2	T49.5X3	T49.5X4	T49.5X5	T49.5X6
otic solution	T49.6X1	T49.6X2	T49.6X3	T49.6X4	T49.6X5	T49.6X6
topical NEC	T49.0X1	T49.0X2	T49.0X3	T49.0X4	T49.0X5	T49.0X6
Chloronitrobenzene	T53.7X1	T53.7X2	T53.7X3	T53.7X4	—	—
dust or vapor	T53.7X1	T53.7X2	T53.7X3	T53.7X4	—	—
Chlorophacinone	T60.4X1	T60.4X2	T60.4X3	T60.4X4	—	—
Chlorophenol	T53.7X1	T53.7X2	T53.7X3	T53.7X4	—	—
Chlorophenothane	T60.1X1	T60.1X2	T60.1X3	T60.1X4	—	—
Chlorophyll	T50.991	T50.992	T50.993	T50.994	T50.995	T50.996
Chloropicrin (fumes)	T53.6X1	T53.6X2	T53.6X3	T53.6X4	—	—
fumigant	T60.8X1	T60.8X2	T60.8X3	T60.8X4	—	—
fungicide	T60.3X1	T60.3X2	T60.3X3	T60.3X4	—	—
pesticide	T60.8X1	T60.8X2	T60.8X3	T60.8X4	—	—
Chloroprocaine	T41.3X1	T41.3X2	T41.3X3	T41.3X4	T41.3X5	T41.3X6
infiltration (subcutaneous)	T41.3X1	T41.3X2	T41.3X3	T41.3X4	T41.3X5	T41.3X6
nerve block (peripheral) (plexus)	T41.3X1	T41.3X2	T41.3X3	T41.3X4	T41.3X5	T41.3X6
spinal	T41.3X1	T41.3X2	T41.3X3	T41.3X4	T41.3X5	T41.3X6
Chloroptic	T49.5X1	T49.5X2	T49.5X3	T49.5X4	T49.5X5	T49.5X6
Chloropurine	T45.1X1	T45.1X2	T45.1X3	T45.1X4	T45.1X5	T45.1X6
Chloropyramine	T45.0X1	T45.0X2	T45.0X3	T45.0X4	T45.0X5	T45.0X6
Chloropyrifos	T60.0X1	T60.0X2	T60.0X3	T60.0X4	—	—
Chloropyrilene	T45.0X1	T45.0X2	T45.0X3	T45.0X4	T45.0X5	T45.0X6
Chloroquine	T37.2X1	T37.2X2	T37.2X3	T37.2X4	T37.2X5	T37.2X6
Chlorothalonil	T60.3X1	T60.3X2	T60.3X3	T60.3X4	—	—
Chlorothen	T45.0X1	T45.0X2	T45.0X3	T45.0X4	T45.0X5	T45.0X6
Chlorothiazide	T50.2X1	T50.2X2	T50.2X3	T50.2X4	T50.2X5	T50.2X6
Chlorothymol	T49.4X1	T49.4X2	T49.4X3	T49.4X4	T49.4X5	T49.4X6
Chlorotrianisene	T38.5X1	T38.5X2	T38.5X3	T38.5X4	T38.5X5	T38.5X6
Chlorovinyldichloroarsine, not in war	T57.0X1	T57.0X2	T57.0X3	T57.0X4		
Chloroxine	T49.4X1	T49.4X2	T49.4X3	T49.4X4	T49.4X5	T49.4X6
Chloroxylenol	T49.0X1	T49.0X2	T49.0X3	T49.0X4	T49.0X5	T49.0X6
Chlorphenamine	T45.0X1	T45.0X2	T45.0X3	T45.0X4	T45.0X5	T45.0X6
Chlorphenesin	T42.8X1	T42.8X2	T42.8X3	T42.8X4	T42.8X5	T42.8X6
topical (antifungal)	T49.0X1	T49.0X2	T49.0X3	T49.0X4	T49.0X5	T49.0X6
Chlorpheniramine	T45.0X1	T45.0X2	T45.0X3	T45.0X4	T45.0X5	T45.0X6
Chlorphenoxamine	T45.0X1	T45.0X2	T45.0X3	T45.0X4	T45.0X5	T45.0X6
Chlorphentermine	T50.5X1	T50.5X2	T50.5X3	T50.5X4	T50.5X5	T50.5X6
Chlorprocaine — see Chloroprocaine						
Chlorproguanil	T37.2X1	T37.2X2	T37.2X3	T37.2X4	T37.2X5	T37.2X6
Chlorpromazine	T43.3X1	T43.3X2	T43.3X3	T43.3X4	T43.3X5	T43.3X6
Chlorpropamide	T38.3X1	T38.3X2	T38.3X3	T38.3X4	T38.3X5	T38.3X6
Chlorprothixene	T43.4X1	T43.4X2	T43.4X3	T43.4X4	T43.4X5	T43.4X6
Chlorquinaldol	T49.0X1	T49.0X2	T49.0X3	T49.0X4	T49.0X5	T49.0X6
Chlorquinol	T49.0X1	T49.0X2	T49.0X3	T49.0X4	T49.0X5	T49.0X6
Chlortalidone	T50.2X1	T50.2X2	T50.2X3	T50.2X4	T50.2X5	T50.2X6
Chlortetracycline	T36.4X1	T36.4X2	T36.4X3	T36.4X4	T36.4X5	T36.4X6
Chlorthalidone	T50.2X1	T50.2X2	T50.2X3	T50.2X4	T50.2X5	T50.2X6
Chlorthion	T60.0X1	T60.0X2	T60.0X3	T60.0X4	—	—
Chlorthiophos	T60.0X1	T60.0X2	T60.0X3	T60.0X4	—	—
Chlortrianisene	T38.5X1	T38.5X2	T38.5X3	T38.5X4	T38.5X5	T38.5X6
Chlor-Trimeton	T45.0X1	T45.0X2	T45.0X3	T45.0X4	T45.0X5	T45.0X6
Chlorzoxazone	T42.8X1	T42.8X2	T42.8X3	T42.8X4	T42.8X5	T42.8X6
Choke damp	T59.7X1	T59.7X2	T59.7X3	T59.7X4	—	—
Cholagogues	T47.5X1	T47.5X2	T47.5X3	T47.5X4	T47.5X5	T47.5X6
Cholebrine	T50.8X1	T50.8X2	T50.8X3	T50.8X4	T50.8X5	T50.8X6
Cholecalciferol	T45.2X1	T45.2X2	T45.2X3	T45.2X4	T45.2X5	T45.2X6
Cholecystokinin	T50.8X1	T50.8X2	T50.8X3	T50.8X4	T50.8X5	T50.8X6
Cholera vaccine	T50.A91	T50.A92	T50.A93	T50.A94	T50.A95	T50.A96
Choleretic	T47.5X1	T47.5X2	T47.5X3	T47.5X4	T47.5X5	T47.5X6
Cholesterol-lowering agents	T46.6X1	T46.6X2	T46.6X3	T46.6X4	T46.6X5	T46.6X6
Cholestyramine (resin)	T46.6X1	T46.6X2	T46.6X3	T46.6X4	T46.6X5	T46.6X6
Cholic acid	T47.5X1	T47.5X2	T47.5X3	T47.5X4	T47.5X5	T47.5X6
Choline	T48.6X1	T48.6X2	T48.6X3	T48.6X4	T48.6X5	T48.6X6
chloride	T50.991	T50.992	T50.993	T50.994	T50.995	T50.996
dihydrogen citrate	T50.991	T50.992	T50.993	T50.994	T50.995	T50.996
salicylate	T39.091	T39.092	T39.093	T39.094	T39.095	T39.096
theophyllinate	T48.6X1	T48.6X2	T48.6X3	T48.6X4	T48.6X5	T48.6X6
Cholinergic (drug) **NEC**	T44.1X1	T44.1X2	T44.1X3	T44.1X4	T44.1X5	T44.1X6
muscle tone enhancer	T44.1X1	T44.1X2	T44.1X3	T44.1X4	T44.1X5	T44.1X6
organophosphorus	T44.0X1	T44.0X2	T44.0X3	T44.0X4	T44.0X5	T44.0X6
insecticide	T60.0X1	T60.0X2	T60.0X3	T60.0X4	—	—
nerve gas	T59.891	T59.892	T59.893	T59.894	—	—
trimethyl ammonium propanediol	T44.1X1	T44.1X2	T44.1X3	T44.1X4	T44.1X5	T44.1X6
Cholinesterase reactivator	T50.6X1	T50.6X2	T50.6X3	T50.6X4	T50.6X5	T50.6X6
Cholografin	T50.8X1	T50.8X2	T50.8X3	T50.8X4	T50.8X5	T50.8X6
Chorionic gonadotropin	T38.891	T38.892	T38.893	T38.894	T38.895	T38.896

Substance	Poisoning, Accidental (unintentional)	Poisoning, Intentional Self-harm	Poisoning, Assault	Poisoning, Undetermined	Adverse Effect	Under-dosing
Chromate	T56.2X1	T56.2X2	T56.2X3	T56.2X4	—	—
dust or mist	T56.2X1	T56.2X2	T56.2X3	T56.2X4	—	—
lead — see also lead	T56.0X1	T56.0X2	T56.0X3	T56.0X4	—	—
paint	T56.0X1	T56.0X2	T56.0X3	T56.0X4	—	—
Chromic						
acid	T56.2X1	T56.2X2	T56.2X3	T56.2X4	—	—
dust or mist	T56.2X1	T56.2X2	T56.2X3	T56.2X4	—	—
phosphate 32P	T45.1X1	T45.1X2	T45.1X3	T45.1X4	T45.1X5	T45.1X6
Chromium	T56.2X1	T56.2X2	T56.2X3	T56.2X4	—	—
compounds — see Chromate						
sesquioxide	T50.8X1	T50.8X2	T50.8X3	T50.8X4	T50.8X5	T50.8X6
Chromomycin A3	T45.1X1	T45.1X2	T45.1X3	T45.1X4	T45.1X5	T45.1X6
Chromonar	T46.3X1	T46.3X2	T46.3X3	T46.3X4	T46.3X5	T46.3X6
Chromyl chloride	T56.2X1	T56.2X2	T56.2X3	T56.2X4	—	—
Chrysarobin	T49.4X1	T49.4X2	T49.4X3	T49.4X4	T49.4X5	T49.4X6
Chrysazin	T47.2X1	T47.2X2	T47.2X3	T47.2X4	T47.2X5	T47.2X6
Chymar	T45.3X1	T45.3X2	T45.3X3	T45.3X4	T45.3X5	T45.3X6
ophthalmic preparation	T49.5X1	T49.5X2	T49.5X3	T49.5X4	T49.5X5	T49.5X6
Chymopapain	T45.3X1	T45.3X2	T45.3X3	T45.3X4	T45.3X5	T45.3X6
Chymotrypsin	T45.3X1	T45.3X2	T45.3X3	T45.3X4	T45.3X5	T45.3X6
ophthalmic preparation	T49.5X1	T49.5X2	T49.5X3	T49.5X4	T49.5X5	T49.5X6
Cianidanol	T50.991	T50.992	T50.993	T50.994	T50.995	T50.996
Cianopramine	T43.011	T43.012	T43.013	T43.014	T43.015	T43.016
Cibenzoline	T46.2X1	T46.2X2	T46.2X3	T46.2X4	T46.2X5	T46.2X6
Ciclacillin	T36.0X1	T36.0X2	T36.0X3	T36.0X4	T36.0X5	T36.0X6
Ciclobarbital — see Hexobarbital						
Ciclonicate	T46.7X1	T46.7X2	T46.7X3	T46.7X4	T46.7X5	T46.7X6
Ciclopirox (olamine)	T49.0X1	T49.0X2	T49.0X3	T49.0X4	T49.0X5	T49.0X6
Ciclosporin	T45.1X1	T45.1X2	T45.1X3	T45.1X4	T45.1X5	T45.1X6
Cicuta maculata or virosa	T62.2X1	T62.2X2	T62.2X3	T62.2X4	—	—
Cicutoxin	T62.2X1	T62.2X2	T62.2X3	T62.2X4	—	—
Cigarette lighter fluid	T52.0X1	T52.0X2	T52.0X3	T52.0X4	—	—
Cigarettes (tobacco)	T65.221	T65.222	T65.223	T65.224	—	—
Ciguatoxin	T61.01	T61.02	T61.03	T61.04	—	—
Cilazapril	T46.4X1	T46.4X2	T46.4X3	T46.4X4	T46.4X5	T46.4X6
Cimetidine	T47.0X1	T47.0X2	T47.0X3	T47.0X4	T47.0X5	T47.0X6
Cimetropium bromide	T44.3X1	T44.3X2	T44.3X3	T44.3X4	T44.3X5	T44.3X6
Cinchocaine	T41.3X1	T41.3X2	T41.3X3	T41.3X4	T41.3X5	T41.3X6
topical (surface)	T41.3X1	T41.3X2	T41.3X3	T41.3X4	T41.3X5	T41.3X6
Cinchona	T37.2X1	T37.2X2	T37.2X3	T37.2X4	T37.2X5	T37.2X6
Cinchonine alkaloids	T37.2X1	T37.2X2	T37.2X3	T37.2X4	T37.2X5	T37.2X6
Cinchophen	T50.4X1	T50.4X2	T50.4X3	T50.4X4	T50.4X5	T50.4X6
Cinepazide	T46.7X1	T46.7X2	T46.7X3	T46.7X4	T46.7X5	T46.7X6
Cinnamedrine	T48.5X1	T48.5X2	T48.5X3	T48.5X4	T48.5X5	T48.5X6
Cinnarizine	T45.0X1	T45.0X2	T45.0X3	T45.0X4	T45.0X5	T45.0X6
Cinoxacin	T37.8X1	T37.8X2	T37.8X3	T37.8X4	T37.8X5	T37.8X6
Ciprofibrate	T46.6X1	T46.6X2	T46.6X3	T46.6X4	T46.6X5	T46.6X6
Ciprofloxacin	T36.8X1	T36.8X2	T36.8X3	T36.8X4	T36.8X5	T36.8X6
Cisapride	T47.8X1	T47.8X2	T47.8X3	T47.8X4	T47.8X5	T47.8X6
Cisplatin	T45.1X1	T45.1X2	T45.1X3	T45.1X4	T45.1X5	T45.1X6
Citalopram	T43.221	T43.222	T43.223	T43.224	T43.225	T43.226
Citanest	T41.3X1	T41.3X2	T41.3X3	T41.3X4	T41.3X5	T41.3X6
infiltration (subcutaneous)	T41.3X1	T41.3X2	T41.3X3	T41.3X4	T41.3X5	T41.3X6
nerve block (peripheral) (plexus)	T41.3X1	T41.3X2	T41.3X3	T41.3X4	T41.3X5	T41.3X6
Citric acid	T47.5X1	T47.5X2	T47.5X3	T47.5X4	T47.5X5	T47.5X6
Citrovorum (factor)	T45.8X1	T45.8X2	T45.8X3	T45.8X4	T45.8X5	T45.8X6
Claviceps purpurea	T62.2X1	T62.2X2	T62.2X3	T62.2X4	—	—
Clavulanic acid	T36.1X1	T36.1X2	T36.1X3	T36.1X4	T36.1X5	T36.1X6
Cleaner, cleansing agent, type not specified	T65.891	T65.892	T65.893	T65.894	—	—
of paint or varnish	T52.91	T52.92	T52.93	T52.94	—	—
specified type NEC	T65.891	T65.892	T65.893	T65.894	—	—
Clebopride	T47.8X1	T47.8X2	T47.8X3	T47.8X4	T47.8X5	T47.8X6
Clefamide	T37.3X1	T37.3X2	T37.3X3	T37.3X4	T37.3X5	T37.3X6
Clemastine	T45.0X1	T45.0X2	T45.0X3	T45.0X4	T45.0X5	T45.0X6
Clematis vitalba	T62.2X1	T62.2X2	T62.2X3	T62.2X4	—	—
Clemizole	T45.0X1	T45.0X2	T45.0X3	T45.0X4	T45.0X5	T45.0X6
penicillin	T36.0X1	T36.0X2	T36.0X3	T36.0X4	T36.0X5	T36.0X6
Clenbuterol	T48.6X1	T48.6X2	T48.6X3	T48.6X4	T48.6X5	T48.6X6
Clidinium bromide	T44.3X1	T44.3X2	T44.3X3	T44.3X4	T44.3X5	T44.3X6
Clindamycin	T36.8X1	T36.8X2	T36.8X3	T36.8X4	T36.8X5	T36.8X6
Clinofibrate	T46.6X1	T46.6X2	T46.6X3	T46.6X4	T46.6X5	T46.6X6
Clioquinol	T37.8X1	T37.8X2	T37.8X3	T37.8X4	T37.8X5	T37.8X6
Cliradon	T40.2X1	T40.2X2	T40.2X3	T40.2X4		
Clobazam	T42.4X1	T42.4X2	T42.4X3	T42.4X4	T42.4X5	T42.4X6
Clobenzorex	T50.5X1	T50.5X2	T50.5X3	T50.5X4	T50.5X5	T50.5X6
Clobetasol	T49.0X1	T49.0X2	T49.0X3	T49.0X4	T49.0X5	T49.0X6
Clobetasone	T49.0X1	T49.0X2	T49.0X3	T49.0X4	T49.0X5	T49.0X6
Clobutinol	T48.3X1	T48.3X2	T48.3X3	T48.3X4	T48.3X5	T48.3X6
Clocortolone	T38.0X1	T38.0X2	T38.0X3	T38.0X4	T38.0X5	T38.0X6
Clodantoin	T49.0X1	T49.0X2	T49.0X3	T49.0X4	T49.0X5	T49.0X6

Additional Character May Be Required — Refer to the Tabular List for Character Selection

☞ Subterms under main terms may continue to next column or page

Chloromycetin — Clodantoin

Substance	Poisoning, Accidental (unintentional)	Poisoning, Intentional Self-harm	Poisoning, Assault	Poisoning, Undetermined	Adverse Effect	Under-dosing
Clodronic acid	T50.991	T50.992	T50.993	T50.994	T50.995	T50.996
Clofazimine	T37.1X1	T37.1X2	T37.1X3	T37.1X4	T37.1X5	T37.1X6
Clofedanol	T48.3X1	T48.3X2	T48.3X3	T48.3X4	T48.3X5	T48.3X6
Clofenamide	T50.2X1	T50.2X2	T50.2X3	T50.2X4	T50.2X5	T50.2X6
Clofenotane	T49.0X1	T49.0X2	T49.0X3	T49.0X4	T49.0X5	T49.0X6
Clofezone	T39.2X1	T39.2X2	T39.2X3	T39.2X4	T39.2X5	T39.2X6
Clofibrate	T46.6X1	T46.6X2	T46.6X3	T46.6X4	T46.6X5	T46.6X6
Clofibride	T46.6X1	T46.6X2	T46.6X3	T46.6X4	T46.6X5	T46.6X6
Cloforex	T50.5X1	T50.5X2	T50.5X3	T50.5X4	T50.5X5	T50.5X6
Clomethiazole	T42.6X1	T42.6X2	T42.6X3	T42.6X4	T42.6X5	T42.6X6
Clometocillin	T36.0X1	T36.0X2	T36.0X3	T36.0X4	T36.0X5	T36.0X6
Clomifene	T38.5X1	T38.5X2	T38.5X3	T38.5X4	T38.5X5	T38.5X6
Clomiphene	T38.5X1	T38.5X2	T38.5X3	T38.5X4	T38.5X5	T38.5X6
Clomipramine	T43.011	T43.012	T43.013	T43.014	T43.015	T43.016
Clomocycline	T36.4X1	T36.4X2	T36.4X3	T36.4X4	T36.4X5	T36.4X6
Clonazepam	T42.4X1	T42.4X2	T42.4X3	T42.4X4	T42.4X5	T42.4X6
Clonidine	T46.5X1	T46.5X2	T46.5X3	T46.5X4	T46.5X5	T46.5X6
Clonixin	T39.8X1	T39.8X2	T39.8X3	T39.8X4	T39.8X5	T39.8X6
Clopamide	T50.2X1	T50.2X2	T50.2X3	T50.2X4	T50.2X5	T50.2X6
Clopenthixol	T43.4X1	T43.4X2	T43.4X3	T43.4X4	T43.4X5	T43.4X6
Cloperastine	T48.3X1	T48.3X2	T48.3X3	T48.3X4	T48.3X5	T48.3X6
Clophedianol	T48.3X1	T48.3X2	T48.3X3	T48.3X4	T48.3X5	T48.3X6
Cloponone	T36.2X1	T36.2X2	T36.2X3	T36.2X4	T36.2X5	T36.2X6
Cloprednol	T38.0X1	T38.0X2	T38.0X3	T38.0X4	T38.0X5	T38.0X6
Cloral betaine	T42.6X1	T42.6X2	T42.6X3	T42.6X4	T42.6X5	T42.6X6
Cloramfenicol	T36.2X1	T36.2X2	T36.2X3	T36.2X4	T36.2X5	T36.2X6
Clorazepate (dipotassium)	T42.4X1	T42.4X2	T42.4X3	T42.4X4	T42.4X5	T42.4X6
Clorexolone	T50.2X1	T50.2X2	T50.2X3	T50.2X4	T50.2X5	T50.2X6
Clorfenamine	T45.0X1	T45.0X2	T45.0X3	T45.0X4	T45.0X5	T45.0X6
Clorgiline	T43.1X1	T43.1X2	T43.1X3	T43.1X4	T43.1X5	T43.1X6
Clorotepine	T44.3X1	T44.3X2	T44.3X3	T44.3X4	T44.3X5	T44.3X6
Clorox (bleach)	T54.91	T54.92	T54.93	T54.94	—	—
Clorprenaline	T48.6X1	T48.6X2	T48.6X3	T48.6X4	T48.6X5	T48.6X6
Clortermine	T50.5X1	T50.5X2	T50.5X3	T50.5X4	T50.5X5	T50.5X6
Clotiapine	T43.591	T43.592	T43.593	T43.594	T43.595	T43.596
Clotiazepam	T42.4X1	T42.4X2	T42.4X3	T42.4X4	T42.4X5	T42.4X6
Clotibric acid	T46.6X1	T46.6X2	T46.6X3	T46.6X4	T46.6X5	T46.6X6
Clotrimazole	T49.0X1	T49.0X2	T49.0X3	T49.0X4	T49.0X5	T49.0X6
Cloxacillin	T36.0X1	T36.0X2	T36.0X3	T36.0X4	T36.0X5	T36.0X6
Cloxazolam	T42.4X1	T42.4X2	T42.4X3	T42.4X4	T42.4X5	T42.4X6
Cloxiquine	T49.0X1	T49.0X2	T49.0X3	T49.0X4	T49.0X5	T49.0X6
Clozapine	T42.4X1	T42.4X2	T42.4X3	T42.4X4	T42.4X5	T42.4X6
Coagulant NEC	T45.7X1	T45.7X2	T45.7X3	T45.7X4	T45.7X5	T45.7X6
Coal (carbon monoxide from) — see also Carbon, monoxide, coal	T58.2X1	T58.2X2	T58.2X3	T58.2X4		
oil — see Kerosene						
tar	T49.1X1	T49.1X2	T49.1X3	T49.1X4	T49.1X5	T49.1X6
fumes	T59.891	T59.892	T59.893	T59.894	—	—
medicinal (ointment)	T49.4X1	T49.4X2	T49.4X3	T49.4X4	T49.4X5	T49.4X6
analgesics NEC	T39.2X1	T39.2X2	T39.2X3	T39.2X4	T39.2X5	T39.2X6
naphtha (solvent)	T52.0X1	T52.0X2	T52.0X3	T52.0X4	—	—
Cobalamine	T45.2X1	T45.2X2	T45.2X3	T45.2X4	T45.2X5	T45.2X6
Cobalt (nonmedicinal) (fumes) (industrial)	T56.891	T56.892	T56.893	T56.894	—	—
medicinal (trace) (chloride)	T45.8X1	T45.8X2	T45.8X3	T45.8X4	T45.8X5	T45.8X6
Cobra (venom)	T63.041	T63.042	T63.043	T63.044	—	—
Coca (leaf)	T40.5X1	T40.5X2	T40.5X3	T40.5X4	T40.5X5	T40.5X6
Cocaine	T40.5X1	T40.5X2	T40.5X3	T40.5X4	T40.5X5	T40.5X6
topical anesthetic	T41.3X1	T41.3X2	T41.3X3	T41.3X4	T41.3X5	T41.3X6
Cocarboxylase	T45.3X1	T45.3X2	T45.3X3	T45.3X4	T45.3X5	T45.3X6
Coccidioidin	T50.8X1	T50.8X2	T50.8X3	T50.8X4	T50.8X5	T50.8X6
Cocculus indicus	T62.1X1	T62.1X2	T62.1X3	T62.1X4	—	—
Cochineal	T65.6X1	T65.6X2	T65.6X3	T65.6X4	—	—
medicinal products	T50.991	T50.992	T50.993	T50.994	T50.995	T50.996
Codeine	T40.2X1	T40.2X2	T40.2X3	T40.2X4	T40.2X5	T40.2X6
Cod-liver oil	T45.2X1	T45.2X2	T45.2X3	T45.2X4	T45.2X5	T45.2X6
Coenzyme A	T50.991	T50.992	T50.993	T50.994	T50.995	T50.996
Coffee	T62.8X1	T62.8X2	T62.8X3	T62.8X4	—	—
Cogalactoisomerase	T50.991	T50.992	T50.993	T50.994	T50.995	T50.996
Cogentin	T44.3X1	T44.3X2	T44.3X3	T44.3X4	T44.3X5	T44.3X6
Coke fumes or gas (carbon monoxide)	T58.2X1	T58.2X2	T58.2X3	T58.2X4		
industrial use	T58.8X1	T58.8X2	T58.8X3	T58.8X4	—	—
Colace	T47.4X1	T47.4X2	T47.4X3	T47.4X4	T47.4X5	T47.4X6
Colaspase	T45.1X1	T45.1X2	T45.1X3	T45.1X4	T45.1X5	T45.1X6
Colchicine	T50.4X1	T50.4X2	T50.4X3	T50.4X4	T50.4X5	T50.4X6
Colchicum	T62.2X1	T62.2X2	T62.2X3	T62.2X4	—	—
Cold cream	T49.3X1	T49.3X2	T49.3X3	T49.3X4	T49.3X5	T49.3X6
Colecalciferol	T45.2X1	T45.2X2	T45.2X3	T45.2X4	T45.2X5	T45.2X6
Colestipol	T46.6X1	T46.6X2	T46.6X3	T46.6X4	T46.6X5	T46.6X6
Colestyramine	T46.6X1	T46.6X2	T46.6X3	T46.6X4	T46.6X5	T46.6X6
Colimycin	T36.8X1	T36.8X2	T36.8X3	T36.8X4	T36.8X5	T36.8X6

Substance	Poisoning, Accidental (unintentional)	Poisoning, Intentional Self-harm	Poisoning, Assault	Poisoning, Undetermined	Adverse Effect	Under-dosing
Colistimethate	T36.8X1	T36.8X2	T36.8X3	T36.8X4	T36.8X5	T36.8X6
Colistin	T36.8X1	T36.8X2	T36.8X3	T36.8X4	T36.8X5	T36.8X6
sulfate (eye preparation)	T49.5X1	T49.5X2	T49.5X3	T49.5X4	T49.5X5	T49.5X6
Collagen	T50.991	T50.992	T50.993	T50.994	T50.995	T50.996
Collagenase	T49.4X1	T49.4X2	T49.4X3	T49.4X4	T49.4X5	T49.4X6
Collodion	T49.3X1	T49.3X2	T49.3X3	T49.3X4	T49.3X5	T49.3X6
Colocynth	T47.2X1	T47.2X2	T47.2X3	T47.2X4	T47.2X5	T47.2X6
Colophony adhesive	T49.3X1	T49.3X2	T49.3X3	T49.3X4	T49.3X5	T49.3X6
Colorant — see also Dye	T50.991	T50.992	T50.993	T50.994	T50.995	T50.996
Coloring matter — see Dye(s)						
Combustion gas (after combustion) — see Carbon, monoxide						
prior to combustion	T59.891	T59.892	T59.893	T59.894	—	—
Compazine	T43.3X1	T43.3X2	T43.3X3	T43.3X4	T43.3X5	T43.3X6
Compound						
1080 (sodium fluoroacetate)	T60.4X1	T60.4X2	T60.4X3	T60.4X4		
269 (endrin)	T60.1X1	T60.1X2	T60.1X3	T60.1X4		
3422 (parathion)	T60.0X1	T60.0X2	T60.0X3	T60.0X4		
3911 (phorate)	T60.0X1	T60.0X2	T60.0X3	T60.0X4		
3956 (toxaphene)	T60.1X1	T60.1X2	T60.1X3	T60.1X4		
4049 (malathion)	T60.0X1	T60.0X2	T60.0X3	T60.0X4		
4069 (malathion)	T60.0X1	T60.0X2	T60.0X3	T60.0X4		
4124 (dicapthon)	T60.0X1	T60.0X2	T60.0X3	T60.0X4		
42 (warfarin)	T60.4X1	T60.4X2	T60.4X3	T60.4X4		
497 (dieldrin)	T60.1X1	T60.1X2	T60.1X3	T60.1X4		
E (cortisone)	T38.0X1	T38.0X2	T38.0X3	T38.0X4	T38.0X5	T38.0X6
F (hydrocortisone)	T38.0X1	T38.0X2	T38.0X3	T38.0X4	T38.0X5	T38.0X6
Congener, anabolic	T38.7X1	T38.7X2	T38.7X3	T38.7X4	T38.7X5	T38.7X6
Congo red	T50.8X1	T50.8X2	T50.8X3	T50.8X4	T50.8X5	T50.8X6
Coniine, conine	T62.2X1	T62.2X2	T62.2X3	T62.2X4		
Conium (maculatum)	T62.2X1	T62.2X2	T62.2X3	T62.2X4		
Conjugated estrogenic substances	T38.5X1	T38.5X2	T38.5X3	T38.5X4	T38.5X5	T38.5X6
Contac	T48.5X1	T48.5X2	T48.5X3	T48.5X4	T48.5X5	T48.5X6
Contact lens solution	T49.5X1	T49.5X2	T49.5X3	T49.5X4	T49.5X5	T49.5X6
Contraceptive (oral)	T38.4X1	T38.4X2	T38.4X3	T38.4X4	T38.4X5	T38.4X6
vaginal	T49.8X1	T49.8X2	T49.8X3	T49.8X4	T49.8X5	T49.8X6
Contrast medium, radiography	T50.8X1	T50.8X2	T50.8X3	T50.8X4	T50.8X5	T50.8X6
Convallaria glycosides	T46.0X1	T46.0X2	T46.0X3	T46.0X4	T46.0X5	T46.0X6
Convallaria majalis	T62.2X1	T62.2X2	T62.2X3	T62.2X4	—	—
berry	T62.1X1	T62.1X2	T62.1X3	T62.1X4	—	—
Copperhead snake (bite) (venom)	T63.061	T63.062	T63.063	T63.064		
Copper (dust) (fumes) (nonmedicinal) NEC	T56.4X1	T56.4X2	T56.4X3	T56.4X4		
arsenate, arsenite	T57.0X1	T57.0X2	T57.0X3	T57.0X4	—	—
insecticide	T60.2X1	T60.2X2	T60.2X3	T60.2X4	—	—
emetic	T47.7X1	T47.7X2	T47.7X3	T47.7X4	T47.7X5	T47.7X6
fungicide	T60.3X1	T60.3X2	T60.3X3	T60.3X4	—	—
gluconate	T49.0X1	T49.0X2	T49.0X3	T49.0X4	T49.0X5	T49.0X6
insecticide	T60.2X1	T60.2X2	T60.2X3	T60.2X4	—	—
medicinal (trace)	T45.8X1	T45.8X2	T45.8X3	T45.8X4	T45.8X5	T45.8X6
oleate	T49.0X1	T49.0X2	T49.0X3	T49.0X4	T49.0X5	T49.0X6
sulfate	T56.4X1	T56.4X2	T56.4X3	T56.4X4	—	—
cupric	T56.4X1	T56.4X2	T56.4X3	T56.4X4	—	—
fungicide	T60.3X1	T60.3X2	T60.3X3	T60.3X4	—	—
medicinal						
ear	T49.6X1	T49.6X2	T49.6X3	T49.6X4	T49.6X5	T49.6X6
emetic	T47.7X1	T47.7X2	T47.7X3	T47.7X4	T47.7X5	T47.7X6
eye	T49.5X1	T49.5X2	T49.5X3	T49.5X4	T49.5X5	T49.5X6
cuprous	T56.4X1	T56.4X2	T56.4X3	T56.4X4	—	—
fungicide	T60.3X1	T60.3X2	T60.3X3	T60.3X4	—	—
medicinal						
ear	T49.6X1	T49.6X2	T49.6X3	T49.6X4	T49.6X5	T49.6X6
emetic	T47.7X1	T47.7X2	T47.7X3	T47.7X4	T47.7X5	T47.7X6
eye	T49.5X1	T49.5X2	T49.5X3	T49.5X4	T49.5X5	T49.5X6
Coral (sting)	T63.691	T63.692	T63.693	T63.694	—	—
snake (bite) (venom)	T63.021	T63.022	T63.023	T63.024	—	—
Corbadrine	T49.6X1	T49.6X2	T49.6X3	T49.6X4	T49.6X5	T49.6X6
Cordite	T65.891	T65.892	T65.893	T65.894	—	—
vapor	T59.891	T59.892	T59.893	T59.894		
Cordran	T49.0X1	T49.0X2	T49.0X3	T49.0X4	T49.0X5	T49.0X6
Corn cures	T49.4X1	T49.4X2	T49.4X3	T49.4X4	T49.4X5	T49.4X6
Cornhusker's lotion	T49.3X1	T49.3X2	T49.3X3	T49.3X4	T49.3X5	T49.3X6
Corn starch	T49.3X1	T49.3X2	T49.3X3	T49.3X4	T49.3X5	T49.3X6
Coronary vasodilator NEC	T46.3X1	T46.3X2	T46.3X3	T46.3X4	T46.3X5	T46.3X6
Corrosive NEC	T54.91	T54.92	T54.93	T54.94	—	—
acid NEC	T54.2X1	T54.2X2	T54.2X3	T54.2X4	—	—
aromatics	T54.1X1	T54.1X2	T54.1X3	T54.1X4	—	—
disinfectant	T54.1X1	T54.1X2	T54.1X3	T54.1X4	—	—

Substance	Poisoning, Accidental (unintentional)	Poisoning, Intentional Self-harm	Poisoning, Assault	Poisoning, Undetermined	Adverse Effect	Under-dosing
Corrosive — *continued*						
fumes NEC	T54.91	T54.92	T54.93	T54.94	—	—
specified NEC	T54.91	T54.92	T54.93	T54.94	—	—
sublimate	T56.1X1	T56.1X2	T56.1X3	T56.1X4	—	—
Cortate	T38.0X1	T38.0X2	T38.0X3	T38.0X4	T38.0X5	T38.0X6
Cort-Dome	T38.0X1	T38.0X2	T38.0X3	T38.0X4	T38.0X5	T38.0X6
ENT agent	T49.6X1	T49.6X2	T49.6X3	T49.6X4	T49.6X5	T49.6X6
ophthalmic preparation	T49.5X1	T49.5X2	T49.5X3	T49.5X4	T49.5X5	T49.5X6
topical NEC	T49.0X1	T49.0X2	T49.0X3	T49.0X4	T49.0X5	T49.0X6
Cortef	T38.0X1	T38.0X2	T38.0X3	T38.0X4	T38.0X5	T38.0X6
ENT agent	T49.6X1	T49.6X2	T49.6X3	T49.6X4	T49.6X5	T49.6X6
ophthalmic preparation	T49.5X1	T49.5X2	T49.5X3	T49.5X4	T49.5X5	T49.5X6
topical NEC	T49.0X1	T49.0X2	T49.0X3	T49.0X4	T49.0X5	T49.0X6
Corticosteroid	T38.0X1	T38.0X2	T38.0X3	T38.0X4	T38.0X5	T38.0X6
ENT agent	T49.6X1	T49.6X2	T49.6X3	T49.6X4	T49.6X5	T49.6X6
mineral	T50.0X1	T50.0X2	T50.0X3	T50.0X4	T50.0X5	T50.0X6
ophthalmic	T49.5X1	T49.5X2	T49.5X3	T49.5X4	T49.5X5	T49.5X6
topical NEC	T49.0X1	T49.0X2	T49.0X3	T49.0X4	T49.0X5	T49.0X6
Corticotropin	T38.811	T38.812	T38.813	T38.814	T38.815	T38.816
Cortisol	T49.0X1	T49.0X2	T49.0X3	T49.0X4	T49.0X5	T49.0X6
ENT agent	T49.6X1	T49.6X2	T49.6X3	T49.6X4	T49.6X5	T49.6X6
ophthalmic preparation	T49.5X1	T49.5X2	T49.5X3	T49.5X4	T49.5X5	T49.5X6
topical NEC	T49.0X1	T49.0X2	T49.0X3	T49.0X4	T49.0X5	T49.0X6
Cortisone (acetate)	T38.0X1	T38.0X2	T38.0X3	T38.0X4	T38.0X5	T38.0X6
ENT agent	T49.6X1	T49.6X2	T49.6X3	T49.6X4	T49.6X5	T49.6X6
ophthalmic preparation	T49.5X1	T49.5X2	T49.5X3	T49.5X4	T49.5X5	T49.5X6
topical NEC	T49.0X1	T49.0X2	T49.0X3	T49.0X4	T49.0X5	T49.0X6
Cortivazol	T38.0X1	T38.0X2	T38.0X3	T38.0X4	T38.0X5	T38.0X6
Cortogen	T38.0X1	T38.0X2	T38.0X3	T38.0X4	T38.0X5	T38.0X6
ENT agent	T49.6X1	T49.6X2	T49.6X3	T49.6X4	T49.6X5	T49.6X6
ophthalmic preparation	T49.5X1	T49.5X2	T49.5X3	T49.5X4	T49.5X5	T49.5X6
Cortone	T38.0X1	T38.0X2	T38.0X3	T38.0X4	T38.0X5	T38.0X6
ENT agent	T49.6X1	T49.6X2	T49.6X3	T49.6X4	T49.6X5	T49.6X6
ophthalmic preparation	T49.5X1	T49.5X2	T49.5X3	T49.5X4	T49.5X5	T49.5X6
Cortril	T38.0X1	T38.0X2	T38.0X3	T38.0X4	T38.0X5	T38.0X6
ENT agent	T49.6X1	T49.6X2	T49.6X3	T49.6X4	T49.6X5	T49.6X6
ophthalmic preparation	T49.5X1	T49.5X2	T49.5X3	T49.5X4	T49.5X5	T49.5X6
topical NEC	T49.0X1	T49.0X2	T49.0X3	T49.0X4	T49.0X5	T49.0X6
Corynebacterium parvum	T45.1X1	T45.1X2	T45.1X3	T45.1X4	T45.1X5	T45.1X6
Cosmetic preparation	T49.8X1	T49.8X2	T49.8X3	T49.8X4	T49.8X5	T49.8X6
Cosmetics	T49.8X1	T49.8X2	T49.8X3	T49.8X4	T49.8X5	T49.8X6
Cosyntropin	T38.811	T38.812	T38.813	T38.814	T38.815	T38.816
Cotarnine	T45.7X1	T45.7X2	T45.7X3	T45.7X4	T45.7X5	T45.7X6
Co-trimoxazole	T36.8X1	T36.8X2	T36.8X3	T36.8X4	T36.8X5	T36.8X6
Cottonseed oil	T49.3X1	T49.3X2	T49.3X3	T49.3X4	T49.3X5	T49.3X6
Cough mixture (syrup)	T48.4X1	T48.4X2	T48.4X3	T48.4X4	T48.4X5	T48.4X6
containing opiates	T40.2X1	T40.2X2	T40.2X3	T40.2X4	T40.2X5	T40.2X6
expectorants	T48.4X1	T48.4X2	T48.4X3	T48.4X4	T48.4X5	T48.4X6
Coumadin	T45.511	T45.512	T45.513	T45.514	T45.515	T45.516
rodenticide	T60.4X1	T60.4X2	T60.4X3	T60.4X4	—	—
Coumaphos	T60.0X1	T60.0X2	T60.0X3	T60.0X4	—	—
Coumarin	T45.511	T45.512	T45.513	T45.514	T45.515	T45.516
Coumetarol	T45.511	T45.512	T45.513	T45.514	T45.515	T45.516
Cowbane	T62.2X1	T62.2X2	T62.2X3	T62.2X4	—	—
Cozyme	T45.2X1	T45.2X2	T45.2X3	T45.2X4	T45.2X5	T45.2X6
Crack	T40.5X1	T40.5X2	T40.5X3	T40.5X4	—	—
Crataegus extract	T46.0X1	T46.0X2	T46.0X3	T46.0X4	T46.0X5	T46.0X6
Creolin	T54.1X1	T54.1X2	T54.1X3	T54.1X4	—	—
disinfectant	T54.1X1	T54.1X2	T54.1X3	T54.1X4	—	—
Creosol (compound)	T49.0X1	T49.0X2	T49.0X3	T49.0X4	T49.0X5	T49.0X6
Creosote (coal tar)	T49.0X1	T49.0X2	T49.0X3	T49.0X4	T49.0X5	T49.0X6
(beechwood)						
medicinal (expectorant)	T48.4X1	T48.4X2	T48.4X3	T48.4X4	T48.4X5	T48.4X6
syrup	T48.4X1	T48.4X2	T48.4X3	T48.4X4	T48.4X5	T48.4X6
Cresol(s)	T49.0X1	T49.0X2	T49.0X3	T49.0X4	T49.0X5	T49.0X6
and soap solution	T49.0X1	T49.0X2	T49.0X3	T49.0X4	T49.0X5	T49.0X6
Cresyl acetate	T49.0X1	T49.0X2	T49.0X3	T49.0X4	T49.0X5	T49.0X6
Cresylic acid	T49.0X1	T49.0X2	T49.0X3	T49.0X4	T49.0X5	T49.0X6
Crimidine	T60.4X1	T60.4X2	T60.4X3	T60.4X4	—	—
Croconazole	T37.8X1	T37.8X2	T37.8X3	T37.8X4	T37.8X5	T37.8X6
Cromoglicic acid	T48.6X1	T48.6X2	T48.6X3	T48.6X4	T48.6X5	T48.6X6
Cromolyn	T48.6X1	T48.6X2	T48.6X3	T48.6X4	T48.6X5	T48.6X6
Cromonar	T46.3X1	T46.3X2	T46.3X3	T46.3X4	T46.3X5	T46.3X6
Cropropamide	T39.8X1	T39.8X2	T39.8X3	T39.8X4	T39.8X5	T39.8X6
with crotethamide	T50.7X1	T50.7X2	T50.7X3	T50.7X4	T50.7X5	T50.7X6
Crotamiton	T49.0X1	T49.0X2	T49.0X3	T49.0X4	T49.0X5	T49.0X6
Crotethamide	T39.8X1	T39.8X2	T39.8X3	T39.8X4	T39.8X5	T39.8X6
with cropropamide	T50.7X1	T50.7X2	T50.7X3	T50.7X4	T50.7X5	T50.7X6
Croton (oil)	T47.2X1	T47.2X2	T47.2X3	T47.2X4	T47.2X5	T47.2X6
chloral	T42.6X1	T42.6X2	T42.6X3	T42.6X4	T42.6X5	T42.6X6
Crude oil	T52.0X1	T52.0X2	T52.0X3	T52.0X4	—	—
Cryogenine	T39.8X1	T39.8X2	T39.8X3	T39.8X4	T39.8X5	T39.8X6
Cryolite (vapor)	T60.1X1	T60.1X2	T60.1X3	T60.1X4	—	—

Substance	Poisoning, Accidental (unintentional)	Poisoning, Intentional Self-harm	Poisoning, Assault	Poisoning, Undetermined	Adverse Effect	Under-dosing
Cryolite — *continued*						
insecticide	T60.1X1	T60.1X2	T60.1X3	T60.1X4	—	—
Cryptenamine (tannates)	T46.5X1	T46.5X2	T46.5X3	T46.5X4	T46.5X5	T46.5X6
Crystal violet	T49.0X1	T49.0X2	T49.0X3	T49.0X4	T49.0X5	T49.0X6
Cuckoopint	T62.2X1	T62.2X2	T62.2X3	T62.2X4	—	—
Cumetharol	T45.511	T45.512	T45.513	T45.514	T45.515	T45.516
Cupric						
acetate	T60.3X1	T60.3X2	T60.3X3	T60.3X4	—	—
acetoarsenite	T57.0X1	T57.0X2	T57.0X3	T57.0X4	—	—
arsenate	T57.0X1	T57.0X2	T57.0X3	T57.0X4	—	—
gluconate	T49.0X1	T49.0X2	T49.0X3	T49.0X4	T49.0X5	T49.0X6
oleate	T49.0X1	T49.0X2	T49.0X3	T49.0X4	T49.0X5	T49.0X6
sulfate	T56.4X1	T56.4X2	T56.4X3	T56.4X4	—	—
Cuprous sulfate — *see also*	T56.4X1	T56.4X2	T56.4X3	T56.4X4	—	—
Copper sulfate						
Curare, curarine	T48.1X1	T48.1X2	T48.1X3	T48.1X4	T48.1X5	T48.1X6
Cyamemazine	T43.3X1	T43.3X2	T43.3X3	T43.3X4	T43.3X5	T43.3X6
Cyamopsis tetragonoloba	T46.6X1	T46.6X2	T46.6X3	T46.6X4	T46.6X5	T46.6X6
Cyanacetyl hydrazide	T37.1X1	T37.1X2	T37.1X3	T37.1X4	T37.1X5	T37.1X6
Cyanic acid (gas)	T59.891	T59.892	T59.893	T59.894	—	—
Cyanide(s) (compounds)	T65.0X1	T65.0X2	T65.0X3	T65.0X4	—	—
(potassium) (sodium)						
NEC						
dust or gas (inhalation)	T57.3X1	T57.3X2	T57.3X3	T57.3X4		
NEC						
fumigant	T65.0X1	T65.0X2	T65.0X3	T65.0X4		
hydrogen	T57.3X1	T57.3X2	T57.3X3	T57.3X4		
mercuric — *see* Mercury						
pesticide (dust) (fumes)	T65.0X1	T65.0X2	T65.0X3	T65.0X4	—	—
Cyanoacrylate adhesive	T49.3X1	T49.3X2	T49.3X3	T49.3X4	T49.3X5	T49.3X6
Cyanocobalamin	T45.8X1	T45.8X2	T45.8X3	T45.8X4	T45.8X5	T45.8X6
Cyanogen (chloride) (gas)	T59.891	T59.892	T59.893	T59.894		
NEC						
Cyclacillin	T36.0X1	T36.0X2	T36.0X3	T36.0X4	T36.0X5	T36.0X6
Cyclaine	T41.3X1	T41.3X2	T41.3X3	T41.3X4	T41.3X5	T41.3X6
Cyclamate	T50.991	T50.992	T50.993	T50.994	T50.995	T50.996
Cyclamen europaeum	T62.2X1	T62.2X2	T62.2X3	T62.2X4	—	—
Cyclandelate	T46.7X1	T46.7X2	T46.7X3	T46.7X4	T46.7X5	T46.7X6
Cyclazocine	T50.7X1	T50.7X2	T50.7X3	T50.7X4	T50.7X5	T50.7X6
Cyclizine	T45.0X1	T45.0X2	T45.0X3	T45.0X4	T45.0X5	T45.0X6
Cyclobarbital	T42.3X1	T42.3X2	T42.3X3	T42.3X4	T42.3X5	T42.3X6
Cyclobarbitone	T42.3X1	T42.3X2	T42.3X3	T42.3X4	T42.3X5	T42.3X6
Cyclobenzaprine	T48.1X1	T48.1X2	T48.1X3	T48.1X4	T48.1X5	T48.1X6
Cyclodrine	T44.3X1	T44.3X2	T44.3X3	T44.3X4	T44.3X5	T44.3X6
Cycloguanil embonate	T37.2X1	T37.2X2	T37.2X3	T37.2X4	T37.2X5	T37.2X6
Cyclohexane	T52.8X1	T52.8X2	T52.8X3	T52.8X4	—	—
Cyclohexanol	T51.8X1	T51.8X2	T51.8X3	T51.8X4	—	—
Cyclohexanone	T52.4X1	T52.4X2	T52.4X3	T52.4X4	—	—
Cycloheximide	T60.3X1	T60.3X2	T60.3X3	T60.3X4	—	—
Cyclohexyl acetate	T52.8X1	T52.8X2	T52.8X3	T52.8X4	—	—
Cycloleucin	T45.1X1	T45.1X2	T45.1X3	T45.1X4	T45.1X5	T45.1X6
Cyclomethycaine	T41.3X1	T41.3X2	T41.3X3	T41.3X4	T41.3X5	T41.3X6
Cyclopentamine	T44.4X1	T44.4X2	T44.4X3	T44.4X4	T44.4X5	T44.4X6
Cyclopenthiazide	T50.2X1	T50.2X2	T50.2X3	T50.2X4	T50.2X5	T50.2X6
Cyclopentolate	T44.3X1	T44.3X2	T44.3X3	T44.3X4	T44.3X5	T44.3X6
Cyclophosphamide	T45.1X1	T45.1X2	T45.1X3	T45.1X4	T45.1X5	T45.1X6
Cycloplegic drug	T49.5X1	T49.5X2	T49.5X3	T49.5X4	T49.5X5	T49.5X6
Cyclopropane	T41.291	T41.292	T41.293	T41.294	T41.295	T41.296
Cyclopyrabital	T39.8X1	T39.8X2	T39.8X3	T39.8X4	T39.8X5	T39.8X6
Cycloserine	T37.1X1	T37.1X2	T37.1X3	T37.1X4	T37.1X5	T37.1X6
Cyclosporin	T45.1X1	T45.1X2	T45.1X3	T45.1X4	T45.1X5	T45.1X6
Cyclothiazide	T50.2X1	T50.2X2	T50.2X3	T50.2X4	T50.2X5	T50.2X6
Cycrimine	T44.3X1	T44.3X2	T44.3X3	T44.3X4	T44.3X5	T44.3X6
Cyhalothrin	T60.1X1	T60.1X2	T60.1X3	T60.1X4	—	—
Cymarin	T46.0X1	T46.0X2	T46.0X3	T46.0X4	T46.0X5	T46.0X6
Cypermethrin	T60.1X1	T60.1X2	T60.1X3	T60.1X4	—	—
Cyphenothrin	T60.2X1	T60.2X2	T60.2X3	T60.2X4	—	—
Cyproheptadine	T45.0X1	T45.0X2	T45.0X3	T45.0X4	T45.0X5	T45.0X6
Cyproterone	T38.6X1	T38.6X2	T38.6X3	T38.6X4	T38.6X5	T38.6X6
Cysteamine	T50.6X1	T50.6X2	T50.6X3	T50.6X4	T50.6X5	T50.6X6
Cytarabine	T45.1X1	T45.1X2	T45.1X3	T45.1X4	T45.1X5	T45.1X6
Cytisus						
laburnum	T62.2X1	T62.2X2	T62.2X3	T62.2X4	—	—
scoparius	T62.2X1	T62.2X2	T62.2X3	T62.2X4	—	—
Cytochrome C	T47.5X1	T47.5X2	T47.5X3	T47.5X4	T47.5X5	T47.5X6
Cytomel	T38.1X1	T38.1X2	T38.1X3	T38.1X4	T38.1X5	T38.1X6
Cytosine arabinoside	T45.1X1	T45.1X2	T45.1X3	T45.1X4	T45.1X5	T45.1X6
Cytoxan	T45.1X1	T45.1X2	T45.1X3	T45.1X4	T45.1X5	T45.1X6
Cytozyme	T45.7X1	T45.7X2	T45.7X3	T45.7X4	T45.7X5	T45.7X6
S-Carboxymethylcysteine	T48.4X1	T48.4X2	T48.4X3	T48.4X4	T48.4X5	T48.4X6
Dacarbazine	T45.1X1	T45.1X2	T45.1X3	T45.1X4	T45.1X5	T45.1X6
Dactinomycin	T45.1X1	T45.1X2	T45.1X3	T45.1X4	T45.1X5	T45.1X6
DADPS	T37.1X1	T37.1X2	T37.1X3	T37.1X4	T37.1X5	T37.1X6

Additional Character May Be Required — Refer to the Tabular List for Character Selection   Subterms under main terms may continue to next column or page

Substance	Poisoning, Accidental (unintentional)	Poisoning, Intentional Self-harm	Poisoning, Assault	Poisoning, Undetermined	Adverse Effect	Under-dosing
Dakin's solution	T49.0X1	T49.0X2	T49.0X3	T49.0X4	T49.0X5	T49.0X6
Dalapon (sodium)	T60.3X1	T60.3X2	T60.3X3	T60.3X4	—	—
Dalmane	T42.4X1	T42.4X2	T42.4X3	T42.4X4	T42.4X5	T42.4X6
Danazol	T38.6X1	T38.6X2	T38.6X3	T38.6X4	T38.6X5	T38.6X6
Danilone	T45.511	T45.512	T45.513	T45.514	T45.515	T45.516
Danthron	T47.2X1	T47.2X2	T47.2X3	T47.2X4	T47.2X5	T47.2X6
Dantrolene	T42.8X1	T42.8X2	T42.8X3	T42.8X4	T42.8X5	T42.8X6
Dantron	T47.2X1	T47.2X2	T47.2X3	T47.2X4	T47.2X5	T47.2X6
Daphne (gnidium) (mezereum)	T62.2X1	T62.2X2	T62.2X3	T62.2X4	—	—
berry	T62.1X1	T62.1X2	T62.1X3	T62.1X4	—	—
Dapsone	T37.1X1	T37.1X2	T37.1X3	T37.1X4	T37.1X5	T37.1X6
Daraprim	T37.2X1	T37.2X2	T37.2X3	T37.2X4	T37.2X5	T37.2X6
Darnel	T62.2X1	T62.2X2	T62.2X3	T62.2X4	—	—
Darvon	T39.8X1	T39.8X2	T39.8X3	T39.8X4	T39.8X5	T39.8X6
Daunomycin	T45.1X1	T45.1X2	T45.1X3	T45.1X4	T45.1X5	T45.1X6
Daunorubicin	T45.1X1	T45.1X2	T45.1X3	T45.1X4	T45.1X5	T45.1X6
DBI	T38.3X1	T38.3X2	T38.3X3	T38.3X4	T38.3X5	T38.3X6
D-Con	T60.91	T60.92	T60.93	T60.94	—	—
insecticide	T60.2X1	T60.2X2	T60.2X3	T60.2X4	—	—
rodenticide	T60.4X1	T60.4X2	T60.4X3	T60.4X4	—	—
DDAVP	T38.891	T38.892	T38.893	T38.894	T38.895	T38.896
DDE (bis(chlorophenyl)-dichloroethylene)	T60.2X1	T60.2X2	T60.2X3	T60.2X4	—	—
DDS	T37.1X1	T37.1X2	T37.1X3	T37.1X4	T37.1X5	T37.1X6
DDT (dust)	T60.1X1	T60.1X2	T60.1X3	T60.1X4	—	—
Deadly nightshade — *see also* Belladonna	T62.2X1	T62.2X2	T62.2X3	T62.2X4	—	—
berry	T62.1X1	T62.1X2	T62.1X3	T62.1X4	—	—
Deamino-D-arginine vasopressin	T38.891	T38.892	T38.893	T38.894	T38.895	T38.896
Deanol (aceglumate)	T50.991	T50.992	T50.993	T50.994	T50.995	T50.996
Debrisoquine	T46.5X1	T46.5X2	T46.5X3	T46.5X4	T46.5X5	T46.5X6
Decaborane	T57.8X1	T57.8X2	T57.8X3	T57.8X4	—	—
fumes	T59.891	T59.892	T59.893	T59.894	—	—
Decadron	T38.0X1	T38.0X2	T38.0X3	T38.0X4	T38.0X5	T38.0X6
ENT agent	T49.6X1	T49.6X2	T49.6X3	T49.6X4	T49.6X5	T49.6X6
ophthalmic preparation	T49.5X1	T49.5X2	T49.5X3	T49.5X4	T49.5X5	T49.5X6
topical NEC	T49.0X1	T49.0X2	T49.0X3	T49.0X4	T49.0X5	T49.0X6
Decahydronaphthalene	T52.8X1	T52.8X2	T52.8X3	T52.8X4	—	—
Decalin	T52.8X1	T52.8X2	T52.8X3	T52.8X4	—	—
Decamethonium (bromide)	T48.1X1	T48.1X2	T48.1X3	T48.1X4	T48.1X5	T48.1X6
Decholin	T47.5X1	T47.5X2	T47.5X3	T47.5X4	T47.5X5	T47.5X6
Declomycin	T36.4X1	T36.4X2	T36.4X3	T36.4X4	T36.4X5	T36.4X6
Decongestant, nasal (mucosa)	T48.5X1	T48.5X2	T48.5X3	T48.5X4	T48.5X5	T48.5X6
combination	T48.5X1	T48.5X2	T48.5X3	T48.5X4	T48.5X5	T48.5X6
Deet	T60.8X1	T60.8X2	T60.8X3	T60.8X4	—	—
Deferoxamine	T45.8X1	T45.8X2	T45.8X3	T45.8X4	T45.8X5	T45.8X6
Deflazacort	T38.0X1	T38.0X2	T38.0X3	T38.0X4	T38.0X5	T38.0X6
Deglycyrrhizinized extract of licorice	T48.4X1	T48.4X2	T48.4X3	T48.4X4	T48.4X5	T48.4X6
Dehydrocholic acid	T47.5X1	T47.5X2	T47.5X3	T47.5X4	T47.5X5	T47.5X6
Dehydroemetine	T37.3X1	T37.3X2	T37.3X3	T37.3X4	T37.3X5	T37.3X6
Dekalin	T52.8X1	T52.8X2	T52.8X3	T52.8X4	—	—
Delalutin	T38.5X1	T38.5X2	T38.5X3	T38.5X4	T38.5X5	T38.5X6
Delorazepam	T42.4X1	T42.4X2	T42.4X3	T42.4X4	T42.4X5	T42.4X6
Delphinium	T62.2X1	T62.2X2	T62.2X3	T62.2X4	—	—
Deltamethrin	T60.1X1	T60.1X2	T60.1X3	T60.1X4	—	—
Deltasone	T38.0X1	T38.0X2	T38.0X3	T38.0X4	T38.0X5	T38.0X6
Deltra	T38.0X1	T38.0X2	T38.0X3	T38.0X4	T38.0X5	T38.0X6
Delvinal	T42.3X1	T42.3X2	T42.3X3	T42.3X4	T42.3X5	T42.3X6
Demecarium (bromide)	T49.5X1	T49.5X2	T49.5X3	T49.5X4	T49.5X5	T49.5X6
Demeclocycline	T36.4X1	T36.4X2	T36.4X3	T36.4X4	T36.4X5	T36.4X6
Demecolcine	T45.1X1	T45.1X2	T45.1X3	T45.1X4	T45.1X5	T45.1X6
Demegestone	T38.5X1	T38.5X2	T38.5X3	T38.5X4	T38.5X5	T38.5X6
Demelanizing agents	T49.8X1	T49.8X2	T49.8X3	T49.8X4	T49.8X5	T49.8X6
Demephion -O and -S	T60.0X1	T60.0X2	T60.0X3	T60.0X4	—	—
Demerol	T40.2X1	T40.2X2	T40.2X3	T40.2X4	T40.2X5	T40.2X6
Demethylchlortetracycline	T36.4X1	T36.4X2	T36.4X3	T36.4X4	T36.4X5	T36.4X6
Demethyltetracycline	T36.4X1	T36.4X2	T36.4X3	T36.4X4	T36.4X5	T36.4X6
Demeton -O and -S	T60.0X1	T60.0X2	T60.0X3	T60.0X4	—	—
Demulcent (external)	T49.3X1	T49.3X2	T49.3X3	T49.3X4	T49.3X5	T49.3X6
specified NEC	T49.3X1	T49.3X2	T49.3X3	T49.3X4	T49.3X5	T49.3X6
Demulen	T38.4X1	T38.4X2	T38.4X3	T38.4X4	T38.4X5	T38.4X6
Denatured alcohol	T51.0X1	T51.0X2	T51.0X3	T51.0X4	—	—
Dendrid	T49.5X1	T49.5X2	T49.5X3	T49.5X4	T49.5X5	T49.5X6
Dental drug, topical application NEC	T49.7X1	T49.7X2	T49.7X3	T49.7X4	T49.7X5	T49.7X6
Dentifrice	T49.7X1	T49.7X2	T49.7X3	T49.7X4	T49.7X5	T49.7X6
Deodorant spray (feminine hygiene)	T49.8X1	T49.8X2	T49.8X3	T49.8X4	T49.8X5	T49.8X6
Deoxycortone	T50.0X1	T50.0X2	T50.0X3	T50.0X4	T50.0X5	T50.0X6
Deoxyribonuclease (pancreatic)	T45.3X1	T45.3X2	T45.3X3	T45.3X4	T45.3X5	T45.3X6
Depilatory	T49.4X1	T49.4X2	T49.4X3	T49.4X4	T49.4X5	T49.4X6
Deprenalin	T42.8X1	T42.8X2	T42.8X3	T42.8X4	T42.8X5	T42.8X6
Deprenyl	T42.8X1	T42.8X2	T42.8X3	T42.8X4	T42.8X5	T42.8X6
Depressant						
appetite (central)	T50.5X1	T50.5X2	T50.5X3	T50.5X4	T50.5X5	T50.5X6
cardiac	T46.2X1	T46.2X2	T46.2X3	T46.2X4	T46.2X5	T46.2X6
central nervous system (anesthetic) — *see also* Central nervous system, depressants	T42.71	T42.72	T42.73	T42.74	T42.75	T42.76
general anesthetic	T41.201	T41.202	T41.203	T41.204	T41.205	T41.206
muscle tone	T42.8X1	T42.8X2	T42.8X3	T42.8X4	T42.8X5	T42.8X6
muscle tone, central	T42.8X1	T42.8X2	T42.8X3	T42.8X4	T42.8X5	T42.8X6
psychotherapeutic	T43.501	T43.502	T43.503	T43.504	T43.505	T43.506
Depressant, appetite	T50.5X1	T50.5X2	T50.5X3	T50.5X4	T50.5X5	T50.5X6
Deptropine	T45.0X1	T45.0X2	T45.0X3	T45.0X4	T45.0X5	T45.0X6
Dequalinium (chloride)	T49.0X1	T49.0X2	T49.0X3	T49.0X4	T49.0X5	T49.0X6
Derris root	T60.2X1	T60.2X2	T60.2X3	T60.2X4	—	—
Deserpidine	T46.5X1	T46.5X2	T46.5X3	T46.5X4	T46.5X5	T46.5X6
Desferrioxamine	T45.8X1	T45.8X2	T45.8X3	T45.8X4	T45.8X5	T45.8X6
Desipramine	T43.011	T43.012	T43.013	T43.014	T43.015	T43.016
Deslanoside	T46.0X1	T46.0X2	T46.0X3	T46.0X4	T46.0X5	T46.0X6
Desloughing agent	T49.4X1	T49.4X2	T49.4X3	T49.4X4	T49.4X5	T49.4X6
Desmethylimipramine	T43.011	T43.012	T43.013	T43.014	T43.015	T43.016
Desmopressin	T38.891	T38.892	T38.893	T38.894	T38.895	T38.896
Desocodeine	T40.2X1	T40.2X2	T40.2X3	T40.2X4	T40.2X5	T40.2X6
Desogestrel	T38.5X1	T38.5X2	T38.5X3	T38.5X4	T38.5X5	T38.5X6
Desomorphine	T40.2X1	T40.2X2	T40.2X3	T40.2X4	—	—
Desonide	T49.0X1	T49.0X2	T49.0X3	T49.0X4	T49.0X5	T49.0X6
Desoximetasone	T49.0X1	T49.0X2	T49.0X3	T49.0X4	T49.0X5	T49.0X6
Desoxycorticosteroid	T50.0X1	T50.0X2	T50.0X3	T50.0X4	T50.0X5	T50.0X6
Desoxycortone	T50.0X1	T50.0X2	T50.0X3	T50.0X4	T50.0X5	T50.0X6
Desoxyephedrine	T43.621	T43.622	T43.623	T43.624	T43.625	T43.626
Detaxtran	T46.6X1	T46.6X2	T46.6X3	T46.6X4	T46.6X5	T46.6X6
Detergent	T49.2X1	T49.2X2	T49.2X3	T49.2X4	T49.2X5	T49.2X6
external medication	T49.2X1	T49.2X2	T49.2X3	T49.2X4	T49.2X5	T49.2X6
local	T49.2X1	T49.2X2	T49.2X3	T49.2X4	T49.2X5	T49.2X6
medicinal	T49.2X1	T49.2X2	T49.2X3	T49.2X4	T49.2X5	T49.2X6
nonmedicinal	T55.1X1	T55.1X2	T55.1X3	T55.1X4	—	—
specified NEC	T55.1X1	T55.1X2	T55.1X3	T55.1X4	—	—
Deterrent, alcohol	T50.6X1	T50.6X2	T50.6X3	T50.6X4	T50.6X5	T50.6X6
Detoxifying agent	T50.6X1	T50.6X2	T50.6X3	T50.6X4	T50.6X5	T50.6X6
Detrothyronine	T38.1X1	T38.1X2	T38.1X3	T38.1X4	T38.1X5	T38.1X6
Dettol (external medication)	T49.0X1	T49.0X2	T49.0X3	T49.0X4	T49.0X5	T49.0X6
Dexamethasone	T38.0X1	T38.0X2	T38.0X3	T38.0X4	T38.0X5	T38.0X6
ENT agent	T49.6X1	T49.6X2	T49.6X3	T49.6X4	T49.6X5	T49.6X6
ophthalmic preparation	T49.5X1	T49.5X2	T49.5X3	T49.5X4	T49.5X5	T49.5X6
topical NEC	T49.0X1	T49.0X2	T49.0X3	T49.0X4	T49.0X5	T49.0X6
Dexamfetamine	T43.621	T43.622	T43.623	T43.624	T43.625	T43.626
Dexamphetamine	T43.621	T43.622	T43.623	T43.624	T43.625	T43.626
Dexbrompheniramine	T45.0X1	T45.0X2	T45.0X3	T45.0X4	T45.0X5	T45.0X6
Dexchlorpheniramine	T45.0X1	T45.0X2	T45.0X3	T45.0X4	T45.0X5	T45.0X6
Dexedrine	T43.621	T43.622	T43.623	T43.624	T43.625	T43.626
Dexetimide	T44.3X1	T44.3X2	T44.3X3	T44.3X4	T44.3X5	T44.3X6
Dexfenfluramine	T50.5X1	T50.5X2	T50.5X3	T50.5X4	T50.5X5	T50.5X6
Dexpanthenol	T45.2X1	T45.2X2	T45.2X3	T45.2X4	T45.2X5	T45.2X6
Dextran (40) (70) (150)	T45.8X1	T45.8X2	T45.8X3	T45.8X4	T45.8X5	T45.8X6
Dextriferron	T45.4X1	T45.4X2	T45.4X3	T45.4X4	T45.4X5	T45.4X6
Dextroamphetamine	T43.621	T43.622	T43.623	T43.624	T43.625	T43.626
Dextro calcium pantothenate	T45.2X1	T45.2X2	T45.2X3	T45.2X4	T45.2X5	T45.2X6
Dextromethorphan	T48.3X1	T48.3X2	T48.3X3	T48.3X4	T48.3X5	T48.3X6
Dextromoramide	T40.4X1	T40.4X2	T40.4X3	T40.4X4	—	—
topical	T49.8X1	T49.8X2	T49.8X3	T49.8X4	T49.8X5	T49.8X6
Dextro pantothenyl alcohol	T45.2X1	T45.2X2	T45.2X3	T45.2X4	T45.2X5	T45.2X6
Dextropropoxyphene	T40.4X1	T40.4X2	T40.4X3	T40.4X4	T40.4X5	T40.4X6
Dextrorphan	T40.2X1	T40.2X2	T40.2X3	T40.2X4	T40.2X5	T40.2X6
Dextrose	T50.3X1	T50.3X2	T50.3X3	T50.3X4	T50.3X5	T50.3X6
concentrated solution, intravenous	T46.8X1	T46.8X2	T46.8X3	T46.8X4	T46.8X5	T46.8X6
Dextrothyroxin	T38.1X1	T38.1X2	T38.1X3	T38.1X4	T38.1X5	T38.1X6
Dextrothyroxine sodium	T38.1X1	T38.1X2	T38.1X3	T38.1X4	T38.1X5	T38.1X6
DFP	T44.0X1	T44.0X2	T44.0X3	T44.0X4	T44.0X5	T44.0X6
DHE	T37.3X1	T37.3X2	T37.3X3	T37.3X4	T37.3X5	T37.3X6
45	T46.5X1	T46.5X2	T46.5X3	T46.5X4	T46.5X5	T46.5X6
Diabinese	T38.3X1	T38.3X2	T38.3X3	T38.3X4	T38.3X5	T38.3X6
Diacetone alcohol	T52.4X1	T52.4X2	T52.4X3	T52.4X4	—	—
Diacetyl monoxime	T50.991	T50.992	T50.993	T50.994	—	—
Diacetylmorphine	T40.1X1	T40.1X2	T40.1X3	T40.1X4	—	—
Diachylon plaster	T49.4X1	T49.4X2	T49.4X3	T49.4X4	T49.4X5	T49.4X6

Substance	Poisoning, Accidental (unintentional)	Poisoning, Intentional Self-harm	Poisoning, Assault	Poisoning, Undetermined	Adverse Effect	Under-dosing
Diaethylstilboestrolum	T38.5X1	T38.5X2	T38.5X3	T38.5X4	T38.5X5	T38.5X6
Diagnostic agent NEC	T50.8X1	T50.8X2	T50.8X3	T50.8X4	T50.8X5	T50.8X6
Dial (soap)	T49.2X1	T49.2X2	T49.2X3	T49.2X4	T49.2X5	T49.2X6
sedative	T42.3X1	T42.3X2	T42.3X3	T42.3X4	T42.3X5	T42.3X6
Dialkyl carbonate	T52.91	T52.92	T52.93	T52.94		
Diallylbarbituric acid	T42.3X1	T42.3X2	T42.3X3	T42.3X4	T42.3X5	T42.3X6
Diallymal	T42.3X1	T42.3X2	T42.3X3	T42.3X4	T42.3X5	T42.3X6
Dialysis solution (intraperitoneal)	T50.3X1	T50.3X2	T50.3X3	T50.3X4	T50.3X5	T50.3X6
Diaminodiphenylsulfone	T37.1X1	T37.1X2	T37.1X3	T37.1X4	T37.1X5	T37.1X6
Diamorphine	T40.1X1	T40.1X2	T40.1X3	T40.1X4	—	—
Diamox	T50.2X1	T50.2X2	T50.2X3	T50.2X4	T50.2X5	T50.2X6
Diamthazole	T49.0X1	T49.0X2	T49.0X3	T49.0X4	T49.0X5	T49.0X6
Dianthone	T47.2X1	T47.2X2	T47.2X3	T47.2X4	T47.2X5	T47.2X6
Diaphenylsulfone	T37.0X1	T37.0X2	T37.0X3	T37.0X4	T37.0X5	T37.0X6
Diasone (sodium)	T37.1X1	T37.1X2	T37.1X3	T37.1X4	T37.1X5	T37.1X6
Diastase	T47.5X1	T47.5X2	T47.5X3	T47.5X4	T47.5X5	T47.5X6
Diatrizoate	T50.8X1	T50.8X2	T50.8X3	T50.8X4	T50.8X5	T50.8X6
Diazepam	T42.4X1	T42.4X2	T42.4X3	T42.4X4	T42.4X5	T42.4X6
Diazinon	T60.0X1	T60.0X2	T60.0X3	T60.0X4	—	—
Diazomethane (gas)	T59.891	T59.892	T59.893	T59.894		
Diazoxide	T46.5X1	T46.5X2	T46.5X3	T46.5X4	T46.5X5	T46.5X6
Dibekacin	T36.5X1	T36.5X2	T36.5X3	T36.5X4	T36.5X5	T36.5X6
Dibenamine	T44.6X1	T44.6X2	T44.6X3	T44.6X4	T44.6X5	T44.6X6
Dibenzepin	T43.011	T43.012	T43.013	T43.014	T43.015	T43.016
Dibenzheptropine	T45.0X1	T45.0X2	T45.0X3	T45.0X4	T45.0X5	T45.0X6
Dibenzyline	T44.6X1	T44.6X2	T44.6X3	T44.6X4	T44.6X5	T44.6X6
Diborane (gas)	T59.891	T59.892	T59.893	T59.894		
Dibromochloropropane	T60.8X1	T60.8X2	T60.8X3	T60.8X4	—	—
Dibromodulcitol	T45.1X1	T45.1X2	T45.1X3	T45.1X4	T45.1X5	T45.1X6
Dibromoethane	T53.6X1	T53.6X2	T53.6X3	T53.6X4	—	—
Dibromomannitol	T45.1X1	T45.1X2	T45.1X3	T45.1X4	T45.1X5	T45.1X6
Dibromopropamidine isethionate	T49.0X1	T49.0X2	T49.0X3	T49.0X4	T49.0X5	T49.0X6
Dibrompropamidine	T49.0X1	T49.0X2	T49.0X3	T49.0X4	T49.0X5	T49.0X6
Dibucaine	T41.3X1	T41.3X2	T41.3X3	T41.3X4	T41.3X5	T41.3X6
topical (surface)	T41.3X1	T41.3X2	T41.3X3	T41.3X4	T41.3X5	T41.3X6
Dibunate sodium	T48.3X1	T48.3X2	T48.3X3	T48.3X4	T48.3X5	T48.3X6
Dibutoline sulfate	T44.3X1	T44.3X2	T44.3X3	T44.3X4	T44.3X5	T44.3X6
Dicamba	T60.3X1	T60.3X2	T60.3X3	T60.3X4	—	—
Dicapthon	T60.0X1	T60.0X2	T60.0X3	T60.0X4	—	—
Dichlobenil	T60.3X1	T60.3X2	T60.3X3	T60.3X4	—	—
Dichlone	T60.3X1	T60.3X2	T60.3X3	T60.3X4	—	—
Dichloralphenozone	T42.6X1	T42.6X2	T42.6X3	T42.6X4	T42.6X5	T42.6X6
Dichlorbenzidine	T65.3X1	T65.3X2	T65.3X3	T65.3X4		
Dichlorhydrin	T52.8X1	T52.8X2	T52.8X3	T52.8X4		
Dichlorhydroxyquinoline	T37.8X1	T37.8X2	T37.8X3	T37.8X4	T37.8X5	T37.8X6
Dichlorobenzene	T53.7X1	T53.7X2	T53.7X3	T53.7X4		
Dichlorobenzyl alcohol	T49.6X1	T49.6X2	T49.6X3	T49.6X4	T49.6X5	T49.6X6
Dichlorodifluoromethane	T53.5X1	T53.5X2	T53.5X3	T53.5X4		
Dichloroethane	T52.8X1	T52.8X2	T52.8X3	T52.8X4		
Dichloroethylene	T53.6X1	T53.6X2	T53.6X3	T53.6X4		
Dichloroethyl sulfide, not in war	T59.891	T59.892	T59.893	T59.894		
Dichloroformoxine, not in war	T59.891	T59.892	T59.893	T59.894		
Dichlorohydrin, alpha-dichlorohydrin	T52.8X1	T52.8X2	T52.8X3	T52.8X4		
Dichloromethane (solvent)	T53.4X1	T53.4X2	T53.4X3	T53.4X4		
vapor	T53.4X1	T53.4X2	T53.4X3	T53.4X4		
Dichloronaphthoquinone	T60.3X1	T60.3X2	T60.3X3	T60.3X4		
Dichlorophen	T37.4X1	T37.4X2	T37.4X3	T37.4X4	T37.4X5	T37.4X6
Dichloropropene	T60.3X1	T60.3X2	T60.3X3	T60.3X4	—	—
Dichloropropionic acid	T60.3X1	T60.3X2	T60.3X3	T60.3X4	—	—
Dichlorphenamide	T50.2X1	T50.2X2	T50.2X3	T50.2X4	T50.2X5	T50.2X6
Dichlorvos	T60.0X1	T60.0X2	T60.0X3	T60.0X4	—	—
Diclofenac	T39.391	T39.392	T39.393	T39.394	T39.395	T39.396
Diclofenamide	T50.2X1	T50.2X2	T50.2X3	T50.2X4	T50.2X5	T50.2X6
Diclofensine	T43.291	T43.292	T43.293	T43.294	T43.295	T43.296
Diclonixine	T39.8X1	T39.8X2	T39.8X3	T39.8X4	T39.8X5	T39.8X6
Dicloxacillin	T36.0X1	T36.0X2	T36.0X3	T36.0X4	T36.0X5	T36.0X6
Dicophane	T49.0X1	T49.0X2	T49.0X3	T49.0X4	T49.0X5	T49.0X6
Dicoumarol, dicoumarin, dicumarol	T45.511	T45.512	T45.513	T45.514	T45.515	T45.516
Dicrotophos	T60.0X1	T60.0X2	T60.0X3	T60.0X4	—	—
Dicyanogen (gas)	T65.0X1	T65.0X2	T65.0X3	T65.0X4	—	—
Dicyclomine	T44.3X1	T44.3X2	T44.3X3	T44.3X4	T44.3X5	T44.3X6
Dicycloverine	T44.3X1	T44.3X2	T44.3X3	T44.3X4	T44.3X5	T44.3X6
Dideoxycytidine	T37.5X1	T37.5X2	T37.5X3	T37.5X4	T37.5X5	T37.5X6
Dideoxyinosine	T37.5X1	T37.5X2	T37.5X3	T37.5X4	T37.5X5	T37.5X6
Dieldrin (vapor)	T60.1X1	T60.1X2	T60.1X3	T60.1X4	—	—
Diemal	T42.3X1	T42.3X2	T42.3X3	T42.3X4	T42.3X5	T42.3X6
Dienestrol	T38.5X1	T38.5X2	T38.5X3	T38.5X4	T38.5X5	T38.5X6

Substance	Poisoning, Accidental (unintentional)	Poisoning, Intentional Self-harm	Poisoning, Assault	Poisoning, Undetermined	Adverse Effect	Under-dosing
Dienoestrol	T38.5X1	T38.5X2	T38.5X3	T38.5X4	T38.5X5	T38.5X6
Dietetic drug NEC	T50.901	T50.902	T50.903	T50.904	T50.905	T50.906
Diethazine	T42.8X1	T42.8X2	T42.8X3	T42.8X4	T42.8X5	T42.8X6
Diethyl						
barbituric acid	T42.3X1	T42.3X2	T42.3X3	T42.3X4	T42.3X5	T42.3X6
carbamazine	T37.4X1	T37.4X2	T37.4X3	T37.4X4	T37.4X5	T37.4X6
carbinol	T51.3X1	T51.3X2	T51.3X3	T51.3X4	—	—
carbonate	T52.8X1	T52.8X2	T52.8X3	T52.8X4		
ether (vapor) — see also ether	T41.0X1	T41.0X2	T41.0X3	T41.0X4	T41.0X5	T41.0X6
oxide	T52.8X1	T52.8X2	T52.8X3	T52.8X4		
propion	T50.5X1	T50.5X2	T50.5X3	T50.5X4	T50.5X5	T50.5X6
stilbestrol	T38.5X1	T38.5X2	T38.5X3	T38.5X4	T38.5X5	T38.5X6
toluamide (nonmedicinal)	T60.8X1	T60.8X2	T60.8X3	T60.8X4		
medicinal	T49.3X1	T49.3X2	T49.3X3	T49.3X4	T49.3X5	T49.3X6
Diethylcarbamazine	T37.4X1	T37.4X2	T37.4X3	T37.4X4	T37.4X5	T37.4X6
Diethylene						
dioxide	T52.8X1	T52.8X2	T52.8X3	T52.8X4		
glycol (monoacetate) (monobutyl ether) (monoethyl ether)	T52.3X1	T52.3X2	T52.3X3	T52.3X4		
Diethylhexylphthalate	T65.891	T65.892	T65.893	T65.894	—	—
Diethylpropion	T50.5X1	T50.5X2	T50.5X3	T50.5X4	T50.5X5	T50.5X6
Diethylstilbestrol	T38.5X1	T38.5X2	T38.5X3	T38.5X4	T38.5X5	T38.5X6
Diethylstilboestrol	T38.5X1	T38.5X2	T38.5X3	T38.5X4	T38.5X5	T38.5X6
Diethylsulfone-diethylmethane	T42.6X1	T42.6X2	T42.6X3	T42.6X4	T42.6X5	T42.6X6
Diethyltoluamide	T49.0X1	T49.0X2	T49.0X3	T49.0X4	T49.0X5	T49.0X6
Diethyltryptamine (DET)	T40.991	T40.992	T40.993	T40.994	—	—
Difebarbamate	T42.3X1	T42.3X2	T42.3X3	T42.3X4	T42.3X5	T42.3X6
Difencloxazine	T40.2X1	T40.2X2	T40.2X3	T40.2X4	T40.2X5	T40.2X6
Difenidol	T45.0X1	T45.0X2	T45.0X3	T45.0X4	T45.0X5	T45.0X6
Difenoxin	T47.6X1	T47.6X2	T47.6X3	T47.6X4	T47.6X5	T47.6X6
Difetarsone	T37.3X1	T37.3X2	T37.3X3	T37.3X4	T37.3X5	T37.3X6
Diffusin	T45.3X1	T45.3X2	T45.3X3	T45.3X4	T45.3X5	T45.3X6
Diflorasone	T49.0X1	T49.0X2	T49.0X3	T49.0X4	T49.0X5	T49.0X6
Diflos	T44.0X1	T44.0X2	T44.0X3	T44.0X4	T44.0X5	T44.0X6
Diflubenzuron	T60.1X1	T60.1X2	T60.1X3	T60.1X4	—	—
Diflucortolone	T49.0X1	T49.0X2	T49.0X3	T49.0X4	T49.0X5	T49.0X6
Diflunisal	T39.091	T39.092	T39.093	T39.094	T39.095	T39.096
Difluoromethyldopa	T42.8X1	T42.8X2	T42.8X3	T42.8X4	T42.8X5	T42.8X6
Difluorophate	T44.0X1	T44.0X2	T44.0X3	T44.0X4	T44.0X5	T44.0X6
Digestant NEC	T47.5X1	T47.5X2	T47.5X3	T47.5X4	T47.5X5	T47.5X6
Digitalin (e)	T46.0X1	T46.0X2	T46.0X3	T46.0X4	T46.0X5	T46.0X6
Digitalis (leaf)(glycoside)	T46.0X1	T46.0X2	T46.0X3	T46.0X4	T46.0X5	T46.0X6
lanata	T46.0X1	T46.0X2	T46.0X3	T46.0X4	T46.0X5	T46.0X6
purpurea	T46.0X1	T46.0X2	T46.0X3	T46.0X4	T46.0X5	T46.0X6
Digitoxin	T46.0X1	T46.0X2	T46.0X3	T46.0X4	T46.0X5	T46.0X6
Digitoxose	T46.0X1	T46.0X2	T46.0X3	T46.0X4	T46.0X5	T46.0X6
Digoxin	T46.0X1	T46.0X2	T46.0X3	T46.0X4	T46.0X5	T46.0X6
Digoxine	T46.0X1	T46.0X2	T46.0X3	T46.0X4	T46.0X5	T46.0X6
Dihydralazine	T46.5X1	T46.5X2	T46.5X3	T46.5X4	T46.5X5	T46.5X6
Dihydrazine	T46.5X1	T46.5X2	T46.5X3	T46.5X4	T46.5X5	T46.5X6
Dihydrocodeine	T40.2X1	T40.2X2	T40.2X3	T40.2X4	T40.2X5	T40.2X6
Dihydrocodeinone	T40.2X1	T40.2X2	T40.2X3	T40.2X4	T40.2X5	T40.2X6
Dihydroergocornine	T46.7X1	T46.7X2	T46.7X3	T46.7X4	T46.7X5	T46.7X6
Dihydroergocristine (mesilate)	T46.7X1	T46.7X2	T46.7X3	T46.7X4	T46./X5	T46.7X6
Dihydroergokryptine	T46.7X1	T46.7X2	T46.7X3	T46.7X4	T46.7X5	T46.7X6
Dihydroergotamine	T46.5X1	T46.5X2	T46.5X3	T46.5X4	T46.5X5	T46.5X6
Dihydroergotoxine	T46.7X1	T46.7X2	T46.7X3	T46.7X4	T46.7X5	T46.7X6
mesilate	T46.7X1	T46.7X2	T46.7X3	T46.7X4	T46.7X5	T46.7X6
Dihydrohydroxycodeinone	T40.2X1	T40.2X2	T40.2X3	T40.2X4	T40.2X5	T40.2X6
Dihydrohydroxymorphinone	T40.2X1	T40.2X2	T40.2X3	T40.2X4	T40.2X5	T40.2X6
Dihydroisocodeine	T40.2X1	T40.2X2	T40.2X3	T40.2X4	T40.2X5	T40.2X6
Dihydromorphine	T40.2X1	T40.2X2	T40.2X3	T40.2X4	—	—
Dihydromorphinone	T40.2X1	T40.2X2	T40.2X3	T40.2X4	T40.2X5	T40.2X6
Dihydrostreptomycin	T36.5X1	T36.5X2	T36.5X3	T36.5X4	T36.5X5	T36.5X6
Dihydrotachysterol	T45.2X1	T45.2X2	T45.2X3	T45.2X4	T45.2X5	T45.2X6
Dihydroxyaluminum aminoacetate	T47.1X1	T47.1X2	T47.1X3	T47.1X4	T47.1X5	T47.1X6
Dihydroxyaluminum sodium carbonate	T47.1X1	T47.1X2	T47.1X3	T47.1X4	T47.1X5	T47.1X6
Dihydroxyanthraquinone	T47.2X1	T47.2X2	T47.2X3	T47.2X4	T47.2X5	T47.2X6
Dihydroxycodeinone	T40.2X1	T40.2X2	T40.2X3	T40.2X4	T40.2X5	T40.2X6
Dihydroxypropyl theophylline	T50.2X1	T50.2X2	T50.2X3	T50.2X4	T50.2X5	T50.2X6
Diiodohydroxyquin	T37.8X1	T37.8X2	T37.8X3	T37.8X4	T37.8X5	T37.8X6
topical	T49.0X1	T49.0X2	T49.0X3	T49.0X4	T49.0X5	T49.0X6
Diiodohydroxyquinoline	T37.8X1	T37.8X2	T37.8X3	T37.8X4	T37.8X5	T37.8X6
Diiodotyrosine	T38.2X1	T38.2X2	T38.2X3	T38.2X4	T38.2X5	T38.2X6
Diisopromine	T44.3X1	T44.3X2	T44.3X3	T44.3X4	T44.3X5	T44.3X6
Diisopropylamine	T46.3X1	T46.3X2	T46.3X3	T46.3X4	T46.3X5	T46.3X6
Diisopropylfluorophosphonate	T44.0X1	T44.0X2	T44.0X3	T44.0X4	T44.0X5	T44.0X6

Additional Character May Be Required — Refer to the Tabular List for Character Selection   ▽ Subterms under main terms may continue to next column or page

Substance	Poisoning, Accidental (unintentional)	Poisoning, Intentional Self-harm	Poisoning, Assault	Poisoning, Undetermined	Adverse Effect	Under-dosing
Dilantin	T42.0X1	T42.0X2	T42.0X3	T42.0X4	T42.0X5	T42.0X6
Dilaudid	T40.2X1	T40.2X2	T40.2X3	T40.2X4	T40.2X5	T40.2X6
Dilazep	T46.3X1	T46.3X2	T46.3X3	T46.3X4	T46.3X5	T46.3X6
Dill	T47.5X1	T47.5X2	T47.5X3	T47.5X4	T47.5X5	T47.5X6
Diloxanide	T37.3X1	T37.3X2	T37.3X3	T37.3X4	T37.3X5	T37.3X6
Diltiazem	T46.1X1	T46.1X2	T46.1X3	T46.1X4	T46.1X5	T46.1X6
Dimazole	T49.0X1	T49.0X2	T49.0X3	T49.0X4	T49.0X5	T49.0X6
Dimefline	T50.7X2	T50.7X2	T50.7X3	T50.7X4	T50.7X5	T50.7X6
Dimefox	T60.0X1	T60.0X2	T60.0X3	T60.0X4	—	—
Dimemorfan	T48.3X1	T48.3X2	T48.3X3	T48.3X4	T48.3X5	T48.3X6
Dimenhydrinate	T45.0X1	T45.0X2	T45.0X3	T45.0X4	T45.0X5	T45.0X6
Dimercaprol (British anti-lewisite)	T45.8X1	T45.8X2	T45.8X3	T45.8X4	T45.8X5	T45.8X6
Dimercaptopropanol	T45.8X1	T45.8X2	T45.8X3	T45.8X4	T45.8X5	T45.8X6
Dimestrol	T38.5X1	T38.5X2	T38.5X3	T38.5X4	T38.5X5	T38.5X6
Dimetane	T45.0X1	T45.0X2	T45.0X3	T45.0X4	T45.0X5	T45.0X6
Dimethicone	T47.1X1	T47.1X2	T47.1X3	T47.1X4	T47.1X5	T47.1X6
Dimethindene	T45.0X1	T45.0X2	T45.0X3	T45.0X4	T45.0X5	T45.0X6
Dimethisoquin	T49.1X1	T49.1X2	T49.1X3	T49.1X4	T49.1X5	T49.1X6
Dimethisterone	T38.5X1	T38.5X2	T38.5X3	T38.5X4	T38.5X5	T38.5X6
Dimethoate	T60.0X1	T60.0X2	T60.0X3	T60.0X4	—	—
Dimethocaine	T41.3X1	T41.3X2	T41.3X3	T41.3X4	T41.3X5	T41.3X6
Dimethoxanate	T48.3X1	T48.3X2	T48.3X3	T48.3X4	T48.3X5	T48.3X6
Dimethyl						
arsine, arsinic acid	T57.0X1	T57.0X2	T57.0X3	T57.0X4	—	—
carbinol	T51.2X1	T51.2X2	T51.2X3	T51.2X4	—	—
carbonate	T52.8X1	T52.8X2	T52.8X3	T52.8X4	—	—
diguanide	T38.3X1	T38.3X2	T38.3X3	T38.3X4	T38.3X5	T38.3X6
ketone	T52.4X1	T52.4X2	T52.4X3	T52.4X4	—	—
vapor	T52.4X1	T52.4X2	T52.4X3	T52.4X4	—	—
meperidine	T40.2X1	T40.2X2	T40.2X3	T40.2X4	T40.2X5	T40.2X6
parathion	T60.0X1	T60.0X2	T60.0X3	T60.0X4	—	—
phthlate	T49.3X1	T49.3X2	T49.3X3	T49.3X4	T49.3X5	T49.3X6
polysiloxane	T47.8X1	T47.8X2	T47.8X3	T47.8X4	T47.8X5	T47.8X6
sulfate (fumes)	T59.891	T59.892	T59.893	T59.894	—	—
liquid	T65.891	T65.892	T65.893	T65.894	—	—
sulfoxide (nonmedicinal)	T52.8X1	T52.8X2	T52.8X3	T52.8X4	—	—
medicinal	T49.4X1	T49.4X2	T49.4X3	T49.4X4	T49.4X5	T49.4X6
tryptamine	T40.991	T40.992	T40.993	T40.994	—	—
tubocurarine	T48.1X1	T48.1X2	T48.1X3	T48.1X4	T48.1X5	T48.1X6
Dimethylamine sulfate	T49.4X1	T49.4X2	T49.4X3	T49.4X4	T49.4X5	T49.4X6
Dimethylformamide	T52.8X1	T52.8X2	T52.8X3	T52.8X4	—	—
Dimethyltubocurarinium chloride	T48.1X1	T48.1X2	T48.1X3	T48.1X4	T48.1X5	T48.1X6
Dimeticone	T47.1X1	T47.1X2	T47.1X3	T47.1X4	T47.1X5	T47.1X6
Dimetilan	T60.0X1	T60.0X2	T60.0X3	T60.0X4	—	—
Dimetindene	T45.0X1	T45.0X2	T45.0X3	T45.0X4	T45.0X5	T45.0X6
Dimetotiazine	T43.3X1	T43.3X2	T43.3X3	T43.3X4	T43.3X5	T43.3X6
Dimorpholamine	T50.7X1	T50.7X2	T50.7X3	T50.7X4	T50.7X5	T50.7X6
Dimoxyline	T46.3X1	T46.3X2	T46.3X3	T46.3X4	T46.3X5	T46.3X6
Dinitrobenzene	T65.3X1	T65.3X2	T65.3X3	T65.3X4	—	—
vapor	T59.891	T59.892	T59.893	T59.894	—	—
Dinitrobenzol	T65.3X1	T65.3X2	T65.3X3	T65.3X4	—	—
vapor	T59.891	T59.892	T59.893	T59.894	—	—
Dinitrobutylphenol	T65.3X1	T65.3X2	T65.3X3	T65.3X4	—	—
Dinitro (-ortho-)cresol (pesticide) (spray)	T65.3X1	T65.3X2	T65.3X3	T65.3X4	—	—
Dinitrocyclohexylphenol	T65.3X1	T65.3X2	T65.3X3	T65.3X4	—	—
Dinitrophenol	T65.3X1	T65.3X2	T65.3X3	T65.3X4	—	—
Dinoprost	T48.0X1	T48.0X2	T48.0X3	T48.0X4	T48.0X5	T48.0X6
Dinoprostone	T48.0X1	T48.0X2	T48.0X3	T48.0X4	T48.0X5	T48.0X6
Dinoseb	T60.3X1	T60.3X2	T60.3X3	T60.3X4	—	—
Dioctyl sulfosuccinate (calcium)	T47.4X1	T47.4X2	T47.4X3	T47.4X4	T47.4X5	T47.4X6
(sodium)	T50.8X1	T50.8X2	T50.8X3	T50.8X4	T50.8X5	T50.8X6
Diodone	T50.8X1	T50.8X2	T50.8X3	T50.8X4	T50.8X5	T50.8X6
Diodoquin	T37.8X1	T37.8X2	T37.8X3	T37.8X4	T37.8X5	T37.8X6
Dionin	T40.2X1	T40.2X2	T40.2X3	T40.2X4	T40.2X5	T40.2X6
Diosmin	T46.991	T46.992	T46.993	T46.994	T46.995	T46.996
Dioxane	T52.8X1	T52.8X2	T52.8X3	T52.8X4	—	—
Dioxathion	T60.0X1	T60.0X2	T60.0X3	T60.0X4	—	—
Dioxin	T53.7X1	T53.7X2	T53.7X3	T53.7X4	—	—
Dioxopromethazine	T43.3X1	T43.3X2	T43.3X3	T43.3X4	T43.3X5	T43.3X6
Dioxyline	T46.3X1	T46.3X2	T46.3X3	T46.3X4	T46.3X5	T46.3X6
Dipentene	T52.8X1	T52.8X2	T52.8X3	T52.8X4	—	—
Diperodon	T41.3X1	T41.3X2	T41.3X3	T41.3X4	T41.3X5	T41.3X6
Diphacinone	T60.4X1	T60.4X2	T60.4X3	T60.4X4	—	—
Diphemanil	T44.3X1	T44.3X2	T44.3X3	T44.3X4	T44.3X5	T44.3X6
metilsulfate	T44.3X1	T44.3X2	T44.3X3	T44.3X4	T44.3X5	T44.3X6
Diphenadione	T45.511	T45.512	T45.513	T45.514	T45.515	T45.516
rodenticide	T60.4X1	T60.4X2	T60.4X3	T60.4X4	—	—
Diphenhydramine	T45.0X1	T45.0X2	T45.0X3	T45.0X4	T45.0X5	T45.0X6
Diphenidol	T45.0X1	T45.0X2	T45.0X3	T45.0X4	T45.0X5	T45.0X6
Diphenoxylate	T47.6X1	T47.6X2	T47.6X3	T47.6X4	T47.6X5	T47.6X6

Substance	Poisoning, Accidental (unintentional)	Poisoning, Intentional Self-harm	Poisoning, Assault	Poisoning, Undetermined	Adverse Effect	Under-dosing
Diphenylamine	T65.3X1	T65.3X2	T65.3X3	T65.3X4	—	—
Diphenylbutazone	T39.2X1	T39.2X2	T39.2X3	T39.2X4	T39.2X5	T39.2X6
Diphenylchloroarsine, not in war	T57.0X1	T57.0X2	T57.0X3	T57.0X4	—	—
Diphenylhydantoin	T42.0X1	T42.0X2	T42.0X3	T42.0X4	T42.0X5	T42.0X6
Diphenylmethane dye	T52.1X1	T52.1X2	T52.1X3	T52.1X4	—	—
Diphenylpyraline	T45.0X1	T45.0X2	T45.0X3	T45.0X4	T45.0X5	T45.0X6
Diphtheria						
antitoxin	T50.Z11	T50.Z12	T50.Z13	T50.Z14	T50.Z15	T50.Z16
toxoid	T50.A91	T50.A92	T50.A93	T50.A94	T50.A95	T50.A96
with tetanus toxoid	T50.A21	T50.A22	T50.A23	T50.A24	T50.A25	T50.A26
with pertussis component	T50.A11	T50.A12	T50.A13	T50.A14	T50.A15	T50.A16
vaccine	T50.A91	T50.A92	T50.A93	T50.A94	T50.A95	T50.A96
combination						
without pertussis	T50.A21	T50.A22	T50.A23	T50.A24	T50.A25	T50.A26
including pertussis	T50.A11	T50.A12	T50.A13	T50.A14	T50.A15	T50.A16
Diphylline	T50.2X1	T50.2X2	T50.2X3	T50.2X4	T50.2X5	T50.2X6
Dipipanone	T40.4X1	T40.4X2	T40.4X3	T40.4X4	—	—
Dipivefrine	T49.5X1	T49.5X2	T49.5X3	T49.5X4	T49.5X5	T49.5X6
Diplovax	T50.B91	T50.B92	T50.B93	T50.B94	T50.B95	T50.B96
Diprophylline	T50.2X1	T50.2X2	T50.2X3	T50.2X4	T50.2X5	T50.2X6
Dipropyline	T48.291	T48.292	T48.293	T48.294	T48.295	T48.296
Dipyridamole	T46.3X1	T46.3X2	T46.3X3	T46.3X4	T46.3X5	T46.3X6
Dipyrone	T39.2X1	T39.2X2	T39.2X3	T39.2X4	T39.2X5	T39.2X6
Diquat (dibromide)	T60.3X1	T60.3X2	T60.3X3	T60.3X4	—	—
Disinfectant	T65.891	T65.892	T65.893	T65.894	—	—
alkaline	T54.3X1	T54.3X2	T54.3X3	T54.3X4	—	—
aromatic	T54.1X1	T54.1X2	T54.1X3	T54.1X4	—	—
intestinal	T37.8X1	T37.8X2	T37.8X3	T37.8X4	T37.8X5	T37.8X6
Disipal	T42.8X1	T42.8X2	T42.8X3	T42.8X4	T42.8X5	T42.8X6
Disodium edetate	T50.6X1	T50.6X2	T50.6X3	T50.6X4	T50.6X5	T50.6X6
Disoprofol	T41.291	T41.292	T41.293	T41.294	T41.295	T41.296
Disopyramide	T46.2X1	T46.2X2	T46.2X3	T46.2X4	T46.2X5	T46.2X6
Distigmine (bromide)	T44.0X1	T44.0X2	T44.0X3	T44.0X4	T44.0X5	T44.0X6
Disulfamide	T50.2X1	T50.2X2	T50.2X3	T50.2X4	T50.2X5	T50.2X6
Disulfanilamide	T37.0X1	T37.0X2	T37.0X3	T37.0X4	T37.0X5	T37.0X6
Disulfiram	T50.6X1	T50.6X2	T50.6X3	T50.6X4	T50.6X5	T50.6X6
Disulfoton	T60.0X1	T60.0X2	T60.0X3	T60.0X4	—	—
Dithiazanine iodide	T37.4X1	T37.4X2	T37.4X3	T37.4X4	T37.4X5	T37.4X6
Dithiocarbamate	T60.0X1	T60.0X2	T60.0X3	T60.0X4	—	—
Dithranol	T49.4X1	T49.4X2	T49.4X3	T49.4X4	T49.4X5	T49.4X6
Diucardin	T50.2X1	T50.2X2	T50.2X3	T50.2X4	T50.2X5	T50.2X6
Diupres	T50.2X1	T50.2X2	T50.2X3	T50.2X4	T50.2X5	T50.2X6
Diuretic NEC	T50.2X1	T50.2X2	T50.2X3	T50.2X4	T50.2X5	T50.2X6
benzothiadiazine	T50.2X1	T50.2X2	T50.2X3	T50.2X4	T50.2X5	T50.2X6
carbonic acid anhydrase inhibitors	T50.2X1	T50.2X2	T50.2X3	T50.2X4	T50.2X5	T50.2X6
furfuryl NEC	T50.2X1	T50.2X2	T50.2X3	T50.2X4	T50.2X5	T50.2X6
loop (high-ceiling)	T50.1X1	T50.1X2	T50.1X3	T50.1X4	T50.1X5	T50.1X6
mercurial NEC	T50.2X1	T50.2X2	T50.2X3	T50.2X4	T50.2X5	T50.2X6
osmotic	T50.2X1	T50.2X2	T50.2X3	T50.2X4	T50.2X5	T50.2X6
purine NEC	T50.2X1	T50.2X2	T50.2X3	T50.2X4	T50.2X5	T50.2X6
saluretic NEC	T50.2X1	T50.2X2	T50.2X3	T50.2X4	T50.2X5	T50.2X6
sulfonamide	T50.2X1	T50.2X2	T50.2X3	T50.2X4	T50.2X5	T50.2X6
thiazide NEC	T50.2X1	T50.2X2	T50.2X3	T50.2X4	T50.2X5	T50.2X6
xanthine	T50.2X1	T50.2X2	T50.2X3	T50.2X4	T50.2X5	T50.2X6
Diurgin	T50.2X1	T50.2X2	T50.2X3	T50.2X4	T50.2X5	T50.2X6
Diuril	T50.2X1	T50.2X2	T50.2X3	T50.2X4	T50.2X5	T50.2X6
Diuron	T60.3X1	T60.3X2	T60.3X3	T60.3X4	—	—
Divalproex	T42.6X1	T42.6X2	T42.6X3	T42.6X4	T42.6X5	T42.6X6
Divinyl ether	T41.0X1	T41.0X2	T41.0X3	T41.0X4	T41.0X5	T41.0X6
Dixanthogen	T49.0X1	T49.0X2	T49.0X3	T49.0X4	T49.0X5	T49.0X6
Dixyrazine	T43.3X1	T43.3X2	T43.3X3	T43.3X4	T43.3X5	T43.3X6
D-lysergic acid diethylamide	T40.8X1	T40.8X2	T40.8X3	T40.8X4	—	—
DMCT	T36.4X1	T36.4X2	T36.4X3	T36.4X4	T36.4X5	T36.4X6
DMSO — see Dimethyl sulfoxide						
DNBP	T60.3X1	T60.3X2	T60.3X3	T60.3X4	—	—
DNOC	T65.3X1	T65.3X2	T65.3X3	T65.3X4	—	—
Dobutamine	T44.5X1	T44.5X2	T44.5X3	T44.5X4	T44.5X5	T44.5X6
DOCA	T38.0X1	T38.0X2	T38.0X3	T38.0X4	T38.0X5	T38.0X6
Docusate sodium	T47.4X1	T47.4X2	T47.4X3	T47.4X4	T47.4X5	T47.4X6
Dodicin	T49.0X1	T49.0X2	T49.0X3	T49.0X4	T49.0X5	T49.0X6
Dofamium chloride	T49.0X1	T49.0X2	T49.0X3	T49.0X4	T49.0X5	T49.0X6
Dolophine	T40.3X1	T40.3X2	T40.3X3	T40.3X4	T40.3X5	T40.3X6
Doloxene	T39.8X1	T39.8X2	T39.8X3	T39.8X4	T39.8X5	T39.8X6
Domestic gas (after combustion) — see Gas, utility						
prior to combustion	T59.891	T59.892	T59.893	T59.894	—	—
Domiodol	T48.4X1	T48.4X2	T48.4X3	T48.4X4	T48.4X5	T48.4X6
Domiphen (bromide)	T49.0X1	T49.0X2	T49.0X3	T49.0X4	T49.0X5	T49.0X6
Domperidone	T45.0X1	T45.0X2	T45.0X3	T45.0X4	T45.0X5	T45.0X6

Subterms under main terms may continue to next column or page   Additional Character May Be Required — Refer to the Tabular List for Character Selection   365

Dilantin — Domperidone

Table of Drugs and Chemicals

Dopa — Esculoside

Substance	Poisoning, Accidental (unintentional)	Poisoning, Intentional Self-harm	Poisoning, Assault	Poisoning, Undetermined	Adverse Effect	Under-dosing
Dopa	T42.8X1	T42.8X2	T42.8X3	T42.8X4	T42.8X5	T42.8X6
Dopamine	T44.991	T44.992	T44.993	T44.994	T44.995	T44.996
Doriden	T42.6X1	T42.6X2	T42.6X3	T42.6X4	T42.6X5	T42.6X6
Dormiral	T42.3X1	T42.3X2	T42.3X3	T42.3X4	T42.3X5	T42.3X6
Dormison	T42.6X1	T42.6X2	T42.6X3	T42.6X4	T42.6X5	T42.6X6
Dornase	T48.4X1	T48.4X2	T48.4X3	T48.4X4	T48.4X5	T48.4X6
Dorsacaine	T41.3X1	T41.3X2	T41.3X3	T41.3X4	T41.3X5	T41.3X6
Dosulepin	T43.011	T43.012	T43.013	T43.014	T43.015	T43.016
Dothiepin	T43.011	T43.012	T43.013	T43.014	T43.015	T43.016
Doxantrazole	T48.6X1	T48.6X2	T48.6X3	T48.6X4	T48.6X5	T48.6X6
Doxapram	T50.7X1	T50.7X2	T50.7X3	T50.7X4	T50.7X5	T50.7X6
Doxazosin	T44.6X1	T44.6X2	T44.6X3	T44.6X4	T44.6X5	T44.6X6
Doxepin	T43.011	T43.012	T43.013	T43.014	T43.015	T43.016
Doxifluridine	T45.1X1	T45.1X2	T45.1X3	T45.1X4	T45.1X5	T45.1X6
Doxorubicin	T45.1X1	T45.1X2	T45.1X3	T45.1X4	T45.1X5	T45.1X6
Doxycycline	T36.4X1	T36.4X2	T36.4X3	T36.4X4	T36.4X5	T36.4X6
Doxylamine	T45.0X1	T45.0X2	T45.0X3	T45.0X4	T45.0X5	T45.0X6
Dramamine	T45.0X1	T45.0X2	T45.0X3	T45.0X4	T45.0X5	T45.0X6
Drano (drain cleaner)	T54.3X1	T54.3X2	T54.3X3	T54.3X4	—	—
Dressing, live pulp	T49.7X1	T49.7X2	T49.7X3	T49.7X4	T49.7X5	T49.7X6
Drocode	T40.2X1	T40.2X2	T40.2X3	T40.2X4	T40.2X5	T40.2X6
Dromoran	T40.2X1	T40.2X2	T40.2X3	T40.2X4	T40.2X5	T40.2X6
Dromostanolone	T38.7X1	T38.7X2	T38.7X3	T38.7X4	T38.7X5	T38.7X6
Dronabinol	T40.7X1	T40.7X2	T40.7X3	T40.7X4	T40.7X5	T40.7X6
Droperidol	T43.591	T43.592	T43.593	T43.594	T43.595	T43.596
Dropropizine	T48.3X1	T48.3X2	T48.3X3	T48.3X4	T48.3X5	T48.3X6
Drostanolone	T38.7X1	T38.7X2	T38.7X3	T38.7X4	T38.7X5	T38.7X6
Drotaverine	T44.3X1	T44.3X2	T44.3X3	T44.3X4	T44.3X5	T44.3X6
Drotrecogin alfa	T45.511	T45.512	T45.513	T45.514	T45.515	T45.516
Drug NEC	T50.901	T50.902	T50.903	T50.904	T50.905	T50.906
specified NEC	T50.991	T50.992	T50.993	T50.994	T50.995	T50.996
DTIC	T45.1X1	T45.1X2	T45.1X3	T45.1X4	T45.1X5	T45.1X6
Duboisine	T44.3X1	T44.3X2	T44.3X3	T44.3X4	T44.3X5	T44.3X6
Dulcolax	T47.2X1	T47.2X2	T47.2X3	T47.2X4	T47.2X5	T47.2X6
Duponol (C) (EP)	T49.2X1	T49.2X2	T49.2X3	T49.2X4	T49.2X5	T49.2X6
Durabolin	T38.7X1	T38.7X2	T38.7X3	T38.7X4	T38.7X5	T38.7X6
Dyclone	T41.3X1	T41.3X2	T41.3X3	T41.3X4	T41.3X5	T41.3X6
Dyclonine	T41.3X1	T41.3X2	T41.3X3	T41.3X4	T41.3X5	T41.3X6
Dydrogesterone	T38.5X1	T38.5X2	T38.5X3	T38.5X4	T38.5X5	T38.5X6
Dye NEC	T65.6X1	T65.6X2	T65.6X3	T65.6X4	—	—
antiseptic	T49.0X1	T49.0X2	T49.0X3	T49.0X4	T49.0X5	T49.0X6
diagnostic agents	T50.8X1	T50.8X2	T50.8X3	T50.8X4	T50.8X5	T50.8X6
pharmaceutical NEC	T50.901	T50.902	T50.903	T50.904	T50.905	T50.906
Dyflos	T44.0X1	T44.0X2	T44.0X3	T44.0X4	T44.0X5	T44.0X6
Dymelor	T38.3X1	T38.3X2	T38.3X3	T38.3X4	T38.3X5	T38.3X6
Dynamite	T65.3X1	T65.3X2	T65.3X3	T65.3X4	—	—
fumes	T59.891	T59.892	T59.893	T59.894	—	—
Dyphylline	T44.3X1	T44.3X2	T44.3X3	T44.3X4	T44.3X5	T44.3X6
b-eucaine	T49.1X1	T49.1X2	T49.1X3	T49.1X4	T49.1X5	T49.1X6
Ear drug NEC	T49.6X1	T49.6X2	T49.6X3	T49.6X4	T49.6X5	T49.6X6
Ear preparations	T49.6X1	T49.6X2	T49.6X3	T49.6X4	T49.6X5	T49.6X6
Echothiophate, echothiophate, ecothiophate	T49.5X1	T49.5X2	T49.5X3	T49.5X4	T49.5X5	T49.5X6
Econazole	T49.0X1	T49.0X2	T49.0X3	T49.0X4	T49.0X5	T49.0X6
Ecothiopate iodide	T49.5X1	T49.5X2	T49.5X3	T49.5X4	T49.5X5	T49.5X6
Ecstasy	T43.641	T43.642	T43.643	T43.644	—	—
Ectylurea	T42.6X1	T42.6X2	T42.6X3	T42.6X4	T42.6X5	T42.6X6
Edathamil disodium	T45.8X1	T45.8X2	T45.8X3	T45.8X4	T45.8X5	T45.8X6
Edecrin	T50.1X1	T50.1X2	T50.1X3	T50.1X4	T50.1X5	T50.1X6
Edetate, disodium (calcium)	T45.8X1	T45.8X2	T45.8X3	T45.8X4	T45.8X5	T45.8X6
Edoxudine	T49.5X1	T49.5X2	T49.5X3	T49.5X4	T49.5X5	T49.5X6
Edrophonium	T44.0X1	T44.0X2	T44.0X3	T44.0X4	T44.0X5	T44.0X6
chloride	T44.0X1	T44.0X2	T44.0X3	T44.0X4	T44.0X5	T44.0X6
EDTA	T50.6X1	T50.6X2	T50.6X3	T50.6X4	T50.6X5	T50.6X6
Eflornithine	T37.2X1	T37.2X2	T37.2X3	T37.2X4	T37.2X5	T37.2X6
Efloxate	T46.3X1	T46.3X2	T46.3X3	T46.3X4	T46.3X5	T46.3X6
Elase	T49.8X1	T49.8X2	T49.8X3	T49.8X4	T49.8X5	T49.8X6
Elastase	T47.5X1	T47.5X2	T47.5X3	T47.5X4	T47.5X5	T47.5X6
Elaterium	T47.2X1	T47.2X2	T47.2X3	T47.2X4	T47.2X5	T47.2X6
Elcatonin	T50.991	T50.992	T50.993	T50.994	T50.995	T50.996
Elder	T62.2X1	T62.2X2	T62.2X3	T62.2X4	—	—
berry, (unripe)	T62.1X1	T62.1X2	T62.1X3	T62.1X4	—	—
Electrolyte balance drug	T50.3X1	T50.3X2	T50.3X3	T50.3X4	T50.3X5	T50.3X6
Electrolytes NEC	T50.3X1	T50.3X2	T50.3X3	T50.3X4	T50.3X5	T50.3X6
Electrolytic agent NEC	T50.3X1	T50.3X2	T50.3X3	T50.3X4	T50.3X5	T50.3X6
Elemental diet	T50.901	T50.902	T50.903	T50.904	T50.905	T50.906
Elliptinium acetate	T45.1X1	T45.1X2	T45.1X3	T45.1X4	T45.1X5	T45.1X6
Embramine	T45.0X1	T45.0X2	T45.0X3	T45.0X4	T45.0X5	T45.0X6
Emepronium (salts)	T44.3X1	T44.3X2	T44.3X3	T44.3X4	T44.3X5	T44.3X6
bromide	T44.3X1	T44.3X2	T44.3X3	T44.3X4	T44.3X5	T44.3X6
Emetic NEC	T47.7X1	T47.7X2	T47.7X3	T47.7X4	T47.7X5	T47.7X6
Emetine	T37.3X1	T37.3X2	T37.3X3	T37.3X4	T37.3X5	T37.3X6
Emollient NEC	T49.3X1	T49.3X2	T49.3X3	T49.3X4	T49.3X5	T49.3X6
Emorfazone	T39.8X1	T39.8X2	T39.8X3	T39.8X4	T39.8X5	T39.8X6
Emylcamate	T43.591	T43.592	T43.593	T43.594	T43.595	T43.596
Enalapril	T46.4X1	T46.4X2	T46.4X3	T46.4X4	T46.4X5	T46.4X6
Enalaprilat	T46.4X1	T46.4X2	T46.4X3	T46.4X4	T46.4X5	T46.4X6
Encainide	T46.2X1	T46.2X2	T46.2X3	T46.2X4	T46.2X5	T46.2X6
Endocaine	T41.3X1	T41.3X2	T41.3X3	T41.3X4	T41.3X5	T41.3X6
Endosulfan	T60.2X1	T60.2X2	T60.2X3	T60.2X4	—	—
Endothall	T60.3X1	T60.3X2	T60.3X3	T60.3X4	—	—
Endralazine	T46.5X1	T46.5X2	T46.5X3	T46.5X4	T46.5X5	T46.5X6
Endrin	T60.1X1	T60.1X2	T60.1X3	T60.1X4	—	—
Enflurane	T41.0X1	T41.0X2	T41.0X3	T41.0X4	T41.0X5	T41.0X6
Enhexymal	T42.3X1	T42.3X2	T42.3X3	T42.3X4	T42.3X5	T42.3X6
Enocitabine	T45.1X1	T45.1X2	T45.1X3	T45.1X4	T45.1X5	T45.1X6
Enovid	T38.4X1	T38.4X2	T38.4X3	T38.4X4	T38.4X5	T38.4X6
Enoxacin	T36.8X1	T36.8X2	T36.8X3	T36.8X4	T36.8X5	T36.8X6
Enoxaparin (sodium)	T45.511	T45.512	T45.513	T45.514	T45.515	T45.516
Enpiprazole	T43.591	T43.592	T43.593	T43.594	T43.595	T43.596
Enprofylline	T48.6X1	T48.6X2	T48.6X3	T48.6X4	T48.6X5	T48.6X6
Enprostil	T47.1X1	T47.1X2	T47.1X3	T47.1X4	T47.1X5	T47.1X6
Enterogastrone	T38.891	T38.892	T38.893	T38.894	T38.895	T38.896
ENT preparations (anti-infectives)	T49.6X1	T49.6X2	T49.6X3	T49.6X4	T49.6X5	T49.6X6
Enviomycin	T36.8X1	T36.8X2	T36.8X3	T36.8X4	T36.8X5	T36.8X6
Enzodase	T45.3X1	T45.3X2	T45.3X3	T45.3X4	T45.3X5	T45.3X6
Enzyme NEC	T45.3X1	T45.3X2	T45.3X3	T45.3X4	T45.3X5	T45.3X6
depolymerizing	T49.8X1	T49.8X2	T49.8X3	T49.8X4	T49.8X5	T49.8X6
fibrolytic	T45.3X1	T45.3X2	T45.3X3	T45.3X4	T45.3X5	T45.3X6
gastric	T47.5X1	T47.5X2	T47.5X3	T47.5X4	T47.5X5	T47.5X6
intestinal	T47.5X1	T47.5X2	T47.5X3	T47.5X4	T47.5X5	T47.5X6
local action	T49.4X1	T49.4X2	T49.4X3	T49.4X4	T49.4X5	T49.4X6
proteolytic	T49.4X1	T49.4X2	T49.4X3	T49.4X4	T49.4X5	T49.4X6
thrombolytic	T45.3X1	T45.3X2	T45.3X3	T45.3X4	T45.3X5	T45.3X6
EPAB	T41.3X1	T41.3X2	T41.3X3	T41.3X4	T41.3X5	T41.3X6
Epanutin	T42.0X1	T42.0X2	T42.0X3	T42.0X4	T42.0X5	T42.0X6
Ephedra	T44.991	T44.992	T44.993	T44.994	T44.995	T44.996
Ephedrine	T44.991	T44.992	T44.993	T44.994	T44.995	T44.996
Epichlorhydrin, epichlorohydrin	T52.8X1	T52.8X2	T52.8X3	T52.8X4		
Epicillin	T36.0X1	T36.0X2	T36.0X3	T36.0X4	T36.0X5	T36.0X6
Epiestriol	T38.5X1	T38.5X2	T38.5X3	T38.5X4	T38.5X5	T38.5X6
Epilim — see Sodium valproate						
Epimestrol	T38.5X1	T38.5X2	T38.5X3	T38.5X4	T38.5X5	T38.5X6
Epinephrine	T44.5X1	T44.5X2	T44.5X3	T44.5X4	T44.5X5	T44.5X6
Epirubicin	T45.1X1	T45.1X2	T45.1X3	T45.1X4	T45.1X5	T45.1X6
Epitiostanol	T38.7X1	T38.7X2	T38.7X3	T38.7X4	T38.7X5	T38.7X6
Epitizide	T50.2X1	T50.2X2	T50.2X3	T50.2X4	T50.2X5	T50.2X6
EPN	T60.0X1	T60.0X2	T60.0X3	T60.0X4	—	—
EPO	T45.8X1	T45.8X2	T45.8X3	T45.8X4	T45.8X5	T45.8X6
Epoetin alpha	T45.8X1	T45.8X2	T45.8X3	T45.8X4	T45.8X5	T45.8X6
Epomediol	T50.991	T50.992	T50.993	T50.994	T50.995	T50.996
Epoprostenol	T45.521	T45.522	T45.523	T45.524	T45.525	T45.526
Epoxy resin	T65.891	T65.892	T65.893	T65.894	—	—
Eprazinone	T48.4X1	T48.4X2	T48.4X3	T48.4X4	T48.4X5	T48.4X6
Epsilon aminocaproic acid	T45.621	T45.622	T45.623	T45.624	T45.625	T45.626
Epsom salt	T47.3X1	T47.3X2	T47.3X3	T47.3X4	T47.3X5	T47.3X6
Eptazocine	T40.4X1	T40.4X2	T40.4X3	T40.4X4	T40.4X5	T40.4X6
Equanil	T43.591	T43.592	T43.593	T43.594	T43.595	T43.596
Equisetum	T62.2X1	T62.2X2	T62.2X3	T62.2X4	—	—
diuretic	T50.2X1	T50.2X2	T50.2X3	T50.2X4	T50.2X5	T50.2X6
Ergobasine	T48.0X1	T48.0X2	T48.0X3	T48.0X4	T48.0X5	T48.0X6
Ergocalciferol	T45.2X1	T45.2X2	T45.2X3	T45.2X4	T45.2X5	T45.2X6
Ergoloid mesylates	T46.7X1	T46.7X2	T46.7X3	T46.7X4	T46.7X5	T46.7X6
Ergometrine	T48.0X1	T48.0X2	T48.0X3	T48.0X4	T48.0X5	T48.0X6
Ergonovine	T48.0X1	T48.0X2	T48.0X3	T48.0X4	T48.0X5	T48.0X6
Ergotamine	T46.5X1	T46.5X2	T46.5X3	T46.5X4	T46.5X5	T46.5X6
Ergotocine	T48.0X1	T48.0X2	T48.0X3	T48.0X4	T48.0X5	T48.0X6
Ergotrate	T48.0X1	T48.0X2	T48.0X3	T48.0X4	T48.0X5	T48.0X6
Ergot NEC	T64.81	T64.82	T64.83	T64.84	—	—
derivative	T48.0X1	T48.0X2	T48.0X3	T48.0X4	T48.0X5	T48.0X6
medicinal (alkaloids)	T48.0X1	T48.0X2	T48.0X3	T48.0X4	T48.0X5	T48.0X6
prepared	T48.0X1	T48.0X2	T48.0X3	T48.0X4	T48.0X5	T48.0X6
Erithrityl tetranitrate	T46.3X1	T46.3X2	T46.3X3	T46.3X4	T46.3X5	T46.3X6
Erythrityl tetranitrate	T46.3X1	T46.3X2	T46.3X3	T46.3X4	T46.3X5	T46.3X6
Erythrol tetranitrate	T46.3X1	T46.3X2	T46.3X3	T46.3X4	T46.3X5	T46.3X6
Erythromycin (salts)	T36.3X1	T36.3X2	T36.3X3	T36.3X4	T36.3X5	T36.3X6
ophthalmic preparation	T49.5X1	T49.5X2	T49.5X3	T49.5X4	T49.5X5	T49.5X6
topical NEC	T49.0X1	T49.0X2	T49.0X3	T49.0X4	T49.0X5	T49.0X6
Erythropoietin	T45.8X1	T45.8X2	T45.8X3	T45.8X4	T45.8X5	T45.8X6
human	T45.8X1	T45.8X2	T45.8X3	T45.8X4	T45.8X5	T45.8X6
Escin	T46.991	T46.992	T46.993	T46.994	T46.995	T46.996
Esculin	T45.2X1	T45.2X2	T45.2X3	T45.2X4	T45.2X5	T45.2X6
Esculoside	T45.2X1	T45.2X2	T45.2X3	T45.2X4	T45.2X5	T45.2X6

Additional Character May Be Required — Refer to the Tabular List for Character Selection   ▽ Subterms under main terms may continue to next column or page

Substance	Poisoning, Accidental (unintentional)	Poisoning, Intentional Self-harm	Poisoning, Assault	Poisoning, Undetermined	Adverse Effect	Under-dosing
ESDT (ether-soluble tar distillate)	T49.1X1	T49.1X2	T49.1X3	T49.1X4	T49.1X5	T49.1X6
Eserine	T49.5X1	T49.5X2	T49.5X3	T49.5X4	T49.5X5	T49.5X6
Esflurbiprofen	T39.311	T39.312	T39.313	T39.314	T39.315	T39.316
Eskabarb	T42.3X1	T42.3X2	T42.3X3	T42.3X4	T42.3X5	T42.3X6
Eskalith	T43.8X1	T43.8X2	T43.8X3	T43.8X4	T43.8X5	T43.8X6
Esmolol	T44.7X1	T44.7X2	T44.7X3	T44.7X4	T44.7X5	T44.7X6
Estanozolol	T38.7X1	T38.7X2	T38.7X3	T38.7X4	T38.7X5	T38.7X6
Estazolam	T42.4X1	T42.4X2	T42.4X3	T42.4X4	T42.4X5	T42.4X6
Estradiol	T38.5X1	T38.5X2	T38.5X3	T38.5X4	T38.5X5	T38.5X6
with testosterone	T38.7X1	T38.7X2	T38.7X3	T38.7X4	T38.7X5	T38.7X6
benzoate	T38.5X1	T38.5X2	T38.5X3	T38.5X4	T38.5X5	T38.5X6
Estramustine	T45.1X1	T45.1X2	T45.1X3	T45.1X4	T45.1X5	T45.1X6
Estriol	T38.5X1	T38.5X2	T38.5X3	T38.5X4	T38.5X5	T38.5X6
Estrogen	T38.5X1	T38.5X2	T38.5X3	T38.5X4	T38.5X5	T38.5X6
with progesterone	T38.5X1	T38.5X2	T38.5X3	T38.5X4	T38.5X5	T38.5X6
conjugated	T38.5X1	T38.5X2	T38.5X3	T38.5X4	T38.5X5	T38.5X6
Estrone	T38.5X1	T38.5X2	T38.5X3	T38.5X4	T38.5X5	T38.5X6
Estropipate	T38.5X1	T38.5X2	T38.5X3	T38.5X4	T38.5X5	T38.5X6
Etacrynate sodium	T50.1X1	T50.1X2	T50.1X3	T50.1X4	T50.1X5	T50.1X6
Etacrynic acid	T50.1X1	T50.1X2	T50.1X3	T50.1X4	T50.1X5	T50.1X6
Etafedrine	T48.6X1	T48.6X2	T48.6X3	T48.6X4	T48.6X5	T48.6X6
Etafenone	T46.3X1	T46.3X2	T46.3X3	T46.3X4	T46.3X5	T46.3X6
Etambutol	T37.1X1	T37.1X2	T37.1X3	T37.1X4	T37.1X5	T37.1X6
Etamiphyllin	T48.6X1	T48.6X2	T48.6X3	T48.6X4	T48.6X5	T48.6X6
Etamivan	T50.7X1	T50.7X2	T50.7X3	T50.7X4	T50.7X5	T50.7X6
Etamsylate	T45.7X1	T45.7X2	T45.7X3	T45.7X4	T45.7X5	T45.7X6
Etebenecid	T50.4X1	T50.4X2	T50.4X3	T50.4X4	T50.4X5	T50.4X6
Ethacridine	T49.0X1	T49.0X2	T49.0X3	T49.0X4	T49.0X5	T49.0X6
Ethacrynic acid	T50.1X1	T50.1X2	T50.1X3	T50.1X4	T50.1X5	T50.1X6
Ethadione	T42.2X1	T42.2X2	T42.2X3	T42.2X4	T42.2X5	T42.2X6
Ethambutol	T37.1X1	T37.1X2	T37.1X3	T37.1X4	T37.1X5	T37.1X6
Ethamide	T50.2X1	T50.2X2	T50.2X3	T50.2X4	T50.2X5	T50.2X6
Ethamivan	T50.7X1	T50.7X2	T50.7X3	T50.7X4	T50.7X5	T50.7X6
Ethamsylate	T45.7X1	T45.7X2	T45.7X3	T45.7X4	T45.7X5	T45.7X6
Ethanol	T51.0X1	T51.0X2	T51.0X3	T51.0X4	—	—
beverage	T51.0X1	T51.0X2	T51.0X3	T51.0X4	—	—
Ethanolamine oleate	T46.8X1	T46.8X2	T46.8X3	T46.8X4	T46.8X5	T46.8X6
Ethaverine	T44.3X1	T44.3X2	T44.3X3	T44.3X4	T44.3X5	T44.3X6
Ethchlorvynol	T42.6X1	T42.6X2	T42.6X3	T42.6X4	T42.6X5	T42.6X6
Ethebenecid	T50.4X1	T50.4X2	T50.4X3	T50.4X4	T50.4X5	T50.4X6
Ether (vapor)	T41.0X1	T41.0X2	T41.0X3	T41.0X4	T41.0X5	T41.0X6
anesthetic	T41.0X1	T41.0X2	T41.0X3	T41.0X4	T41.0X5	T41.0X6
divinyl	T41.0X1	T41.0X2	T41.0X3	T41.0X4	T41.0X5	T41.0X6
ethyl (medicinal)	T41.0X1	T41.0X2	T41.0X3	T41.0X4	T41.0X5	T41.0X6
nonmedicinal	T52.8X1	T52.8X2	T52.8X3	T52.8X4	—	—
petroleum — see Ligroin						
solvent	T52.8X1	T52.8X2	T52.8X3	T52.8X4	—	—
Ethiazide	T50.2X1	T50.2X2	T50.2X3	T50.2X4	T50.2X5	T50.2X6
Ethidium chloride (vapor)	T59.891	T59.892	T59.893	T59.894	—	—
Ethinamate	T42.6X1	T42.6X2	T42.6X3	T42.6X4	T42.6X5	T42.6X6
Ethinylestradiol, ethinyloestradiol	T38.5X1	T38.5X2	T38.5X3	T38.5X4	T38.5X5	T38.5X6
with						
levonorgestrel	T38.4X1	T38.4X2	T38.4X3	T38.4X4	T38.4X5	T38.4X6
norethisterone	T38.4X1	T38.4X2	T38.4X3	T38.4X4	T38.4X5	T38.4X6
Ethiodized oil (131 I)	T50.8X1	T50.8X2	T50.8X3	T50.8X4	T50.8X5	T50.8X6
Ethion	T60.0X1	T60.0X2	T60.0X3	T60.0X4	—	—
Ethionamide	T37.1X1	T37.1X2	T37.1X3	T37.1X4	T37.1X5	T37.1X6
Ethioniamide	T37.1X1	T37.1X2	T37.1X3	T37.1X4	T37.1X5	T37.1X6
Ethisterone	T38.5X1	T38.5X2	T38.5X3	T38.5X4	T38.5X5	T38.5X6
Ethobral	T42.3X1	T42.3X2	T42.3X3	T42.3X4	T42.3X5	T42.3X6
Ethocaine (infiltration)	T41.3X1	T41.3X2	T41.3X3	T41.3X4	T41.3X5	T41.3X6
(topical)	T41.3X1	T41.3X2	T41.3X3	T41.3X4	T41.3X5	T41.3X6
nerve block (peripheral) (plexus)	T41.3X1	T41.3X2	T41.3X3	T41.3X4	T41.3X5	T41.3X6
spinal	T41.3X1	T41.3X2	T41.3X3	T41.3X4	T41.3X5	T41.3X6
Ethoheptazine	T40.4X1	T40.4X2	T40.4X3	T40.4X4	T40.4X5	T40.4X6
Ethopropazine	T44.3X1	T44.3X2	T44.3X3	T44.3X4	T44.3X5	T44.3X6
Ethosuximide	T42.2X1	T42.2X2	T42.2X3	T42.2X4	T42.2X5	T42.2X6
Ethotoin	T42.0X1	T42.0X2	T42.0X3	T42.0X4	T42.0X5	T42.0X6
Ethoxazene	T37.91	T37.92	T37.93	T37.94	T37.95	T37.96
Ethoxazorutoside	T46.991	T46.992	T46.993	T46.994	T46.995	T46.996
Ethoxzolamide	T50.2X1	T50.2X2	T50.2X3	T50.2X4	T50.2X5	T50.2X6
Ethyl						
acetate	T52.8X1	T52.8X2	T52.8X3	T52.8X4	—	—
alcohol	T51.0X1	T51.0X2	T51.0X3	T51.0X4	—	—
beverage	T51.0X1	T51.0X2	T51.0X3	T51.0X4	—	—
aldehyde (vapor)	T59.891	T59.892	T59.893	T59.894	—	—
liquid	T52.8X1	T52.8X2	T52.8X3	T52.8X4	—	—
aminobenzoate	T41.3X1	T41.3X2	T41.3X3	T41.3X4	T41.3X5	T41.3X6
aminophenothiazine	T43.3X1	T43.3X2	T43.3X3	T43.3X4	T43.3X5	T43.3X6
benzoate	T52.8X1	T52.8X2	T52.8X3	T52.8X4	—	—

Substance	Poisoning, Accidental (unintentional)	Poisoning, Intentional Self-harm	Poisoning, Assault	Poisoning, Undetermined	Adverse Effect	Under-dosing
Ethyl — continued						
biscoumacetate	T45.511	T45.512	T45.513	T45.514	T45.515	T45.516
bromide (anesthetic)	T41.0X1	T41.0X2	T41.0X3	T41.0X4	T41.0X5	T41.0X6
carbamate	T45.1X1	T45.1X2	T45.1X3	T45.1X4	T45.1X5	T45.1X6
carbinol	T51.3X1	T51.3X2	T51.3X3	T51.3X4	—	—
carbonate	T52.8X1	T52.8X2	T52.8X3	T52.8X4	—	—
chaulmoograte	T37.1X1	T37.1X2	T37.1X3	T37.1X4	T37.1X5	T37.1X6
chloride (anesthetic)	T41.0X1	T41.0X2	T41.0X3	T41.0X4	T41.0X5	T41.0X6
anesthetic (local)	T41.3X1	T41.3X2	T41.3X3	T41.3X4	T41.3X5	T41.3X6
inhaled	T41.0X1	T41.0X2	T41.0X3	T41.0X4	T41.0X5	T41.0X6
local	T49.4X1	T49.4X2	T49.4X3	T49.4X4	T49.4X5	T49.4X6
solvent	T53.6X1	T53.6X2	T53.6X3	T53.6X4	—	—
dibunate	T48.3X1	T48.3X2	T48.3X3	T48.3X4	T48.3X5	T48.3X6
dichloroarsine (vapor)	T57.0X1	T57.0X2	T57.0X3	T57.0X4	—	—
estranol	T38.7X1	T38.7X2	T38.7X3	T38.7X4	T38.7X5	T38.7X6
ether — see also ether						
formate NEC (solvent)	T52.8X1	T52.8X2	T52.8X3	T52.8X4	—	—
fumarate	T49.4X1	T49.4X2	T49.4X3	T49.4X4	T49.4X5	T49.4X6
hydroxyisobutyrate NEC (solvent)	T52.8X1	T52.8X2	T52.8X3	T52.8X4	—	—
iodoacetate	T59.3X1	T59.3X2	T59.3X3	T59.3X4	—	—
lactate NEC (solvent)	T52.8X1	T52.8X2	T52.8X3	T52.8X4	—	—
loflazepate	T42.4X1	T42.4X2	T42.4X3	T42.4X4	T42.4X5	T42.4X6
mercuric chloride	T56.1X1	T56.1X2	T56.1X3	T56.1X4	—	—
methylcarbinol	T51.8X1	T51.8X2	T51.8X3	T51.8X4	—	—
morphine	T40.2X1	T40.2X2	T40.2X3	T40.2X4	T40.2X5	T40.2X6
noradrenaline	T48.6X1	T48.6X2	T48.6X3	T48.6X4	T48.6X5	T48.6X6
oxybutyrate NEC (solvent)	T52.8X1	T52.8X2	T52.8X3	T52.8X4	—	—
Ethylene (gas)	T59.891	T59.892	T59.893	T59.894	—	—
anesthetic (general)	T41.0X1	T41.0X2	T41.0X3	T41.0X4	T41.0X5	T41.0X6
chlorohydrin	T52.8X1	T52.8X2	T52.8X3	T52.8X4	—	—
vapor	T53.6X1	T53.6X2	T53.6X3	T53.6X4	—	—
dichloride	T52.8X1	T52.8X2	T52.8X3	T52.8X4	—	—
vapor	T53.6X1	T53.6X2	T53.6X3	T53.6X4	—	—
dinitrate	T52.3X1	T52.3X2	T52.3X3	T52.3X4	—	—
glycol(s)	T52.8X1	T52.8X2	T52.8X3	T52.8X4	—	—
dinitrate	T52.3X1	T52.3X2	T52.3X3	T52.3X4	—	—
monobutyl ether	T52.3X1	T52.3X2	T52.3X3	T52.3X4	—	—
imine	T54.1X1	T54.1X2	T54.1X3	T54.1X4	—	—
oxide (fumigant) (nonmedicinal)	T59.891	T59.892	T59.893	T59.894	—	—
medicinal	T49.0X1	T49.0X2	T49.0X3	T49.0X4	T49.0X5	T49.0X6
Ethylenediaminetetra-acetic acid	T50.6X1	T50.6X2	T50.6X3	T50.6X4	T50.6X5	T50.6X6
Ethylenediamine theophylline	T48.6X1	T48.6X2	T48.6X3	T48.6X4	T48.6X5	T48.6X6
Ethylenedinitrilotetra-acetate	T50.6X1	T50.6X2	T50.6X3	T50.6X4	T50.6X5	T50.6X6
Ethylestrenol	T38.7X1	T38.7X2	T38.7X3	T38.7X4	T38.7X5	T38.7X6
Ethylhydroxycellulose	T47.4X1	T47.4X2	T47.4X3	T47.4X4	T47.4X5	T47.4X6
Ethylidene						
chloride NEC	T53.6X1	T53.6X2	T53.6X3	T53.6X4	—	—
diacetate	T60.3X1	T60.3X2	T60.3X3	T60.3X4	—	—
dicoumarin	T45.511	T45.512	T45.513	T45.514	T45.515	T45.516
dicoumarol	T45.511	T45.512	T45.513	T45.514	T45.515	T45.516
diethyl ether	T52.0X1	T52.0X2	T52.0X3	T52.0X4	—	—
Ethylmorphine	T40.2X1	T40.2X2	T40.2X3	T40.2X4	T40.2X5	T40.2X6
Ethylnorepinephrine	T48.6X1	T48.6X2	T48.6X3	T48.6X4	T48.6X5	T48.6X6
Ethylparachlorophen-oxyisobutyrate	T46.6X1	T46.6X2	T46.6X3	T46.6X4	T46.6X5	T46.6X6
Ethynodiol	T38.4X1	T38.4X2	T38.4X3	T38.4X4	T38.4X5	T38.4X6
with mestranol diacetate	T38.4X1	T38.4X2	T38.4X3	T38.4X4	T38.4X5	T38.4X6
Etidocaine	T41.3X1	T41.3X2	T41.3X3	T41.3X4	T41.3X5	T41.3X6
infiltration (subcutaneous)	T41.3X1	T41.3X2	T41.3X3	T41.3X4	T41.3X5	T41.3X6
nerve (peripheral) (plexus)	T41.3X1	T41.3X2	T41.3X3	T41.3X4	T41.3X5	T41.3X6
Etidronate	T50.991	T50.992	T50.993	T50.994	T50.995	T50.996
Etidronic acid (disodium salt)	T50.991	T50.992	T50.993	T50.994	T50.995	T50.996
Etifoxine	T42.6X1	T42.6X2	T42.6X3	T42.6X4	T42.6X5	T42.6X6
Etilefrine	T44.4X1	T44.4X2	T44.4X3	T44.4X4	T44.4X5	T44.4X6
Etilfen	T42.3X1	T42.3X2	T42.3X3	T42.3X4	T42.3X5	T42.3X6
Etinodiol	T38.4X1	T38.4X2	T38.4X3	T38.4X4	T38.4X5	T38.4X6
Etiroxate	T46.6X1	T46.6X2	T46.6X3	T46.6X4	T46.6X5	T46.6X6
Etizolam	T42.4X1	T42.4X2	T42.4X3	T42.4X4	T42.4X5	T42.4X6
Etodolac	T39.391	T39.392	T39.393	T39.394	T39.395	T39.396
Etofamide	T37.3X1	T37.3X2	T37.3X3	T37.3X4	T37.3X5	T37.3X6
Etofibrate	T46.6X1	T46.6X2	T46.6X3	T46.6X4	T46.6X5	T46.6X6
Etofylline	T46.7X1	T46.7X2	T46.7X3	T46.7X4	T46.7X5	T46.7X6
clofibrate	T46.6X1	T46.6X2	T46.6X3	T46.6X4	T46.6X5	T46.6X6
Etoglucid	T45.1X1	T45.1X2	T45.1X3	T45.1X4	T45.1X5	T45.1X6
Etomidate	T41.1X1	T41.1X2	T41.1X3	T41.1X4	T41.1X5	T41.1X6
Etomide	T39.8X1	T39.8X2	T39.8X3	T39.8X4	T39.8X5	T39.8X6
Etomidoline	T44.3X1	T44.3X2	T44.3X3	T44.3X4	T44.3X5	T44.3X6
Etoposide	T45.1X1	T45.1X2	T45.1X3	T45.1X4	T45.1X5	T45.1X6

Substance	Poisoning, Accidental (unintentional)	Poisoning, Intentional Self-harm	Poisoning, Assault	Poisoning, Undetermined	Adverse Effect	Under-dosing
Etorphine	T40.2X1	T40.2X2	T40.2X3	T40.2X4	T40.2X5	T40.2X6
Etoval	T42.3X1	T42.3X2	T42.3X3	T42.3X4	T42.3X5	T42.3X6
Etozolin	T50.1X1	T50.1X2	T50.1X3	T50.1X4	T50.1X5	T50.1X6
Etretinate	T50.991	T50.992	T50.993	T50.994	T50.995	T50.996
Etryptamine	T43.691	T43.692	T43.693	T43.694	T43.695	T43.696
Etybenzatropine	T44.3X1	T44.3X2	T44.3X3	T44.3X4	T44.3X5	T44.3X6
Etynodiol	T38.4X1	T38.4X2	T38.4X3	T38.4X4	T38.4X5	T38.4X6
Eucaine	T41.3X1	T41.3X2	T41.3X3	T41.3X4	T41.3X5	T41.3X6
Eucalyptus oil	T49.7X1	T49.7X2	T49.7X3	T49.7X4	T49.7X5	T49.7X6
Eucatropine	T49.5X1	T49.5X2	T49.5X3	T49.5X4	T49.5X5	T49.5X6
Eucodal	T40.2X1	T40.2X2	T40.2X3	T40.2X4	T40.2X5	T40.2X6
Euneryl	T42.3X1	T42.3X2	T42.3X3	T42.3X4	T42.3X5	T42.3X6
Euphthalmine	T44.3X1	T44.3X2	T44.3X3	T44.3X4	T44.3X5	T44.3X6
Eurax	T49.0X1	T49.0X2	T49.0X3	T49.0X4	T49.0X5	T49.0X6
Euresol	T49.4X1	T49.4X2	T49.4X3	T49.4X4	T49.4X5	T49.4X6
Euthroid	T38.1X1	T38.1X2	T38.1X3	T38.1X4	T38.1X5	T38.1X6
Evans blue	T50.8X1	T50.8X2	T50.8X3	T50.8X4	T50.8X5	T50.8X6
Evipal	T42.3X1	T42.3X2	T42.3X3	T42.3X4	T42.3X5	T42.3X6
sodium	T41.1X1	T41.1X2	T41.1X3	T41.1X4	T41.1X5	T41.1X6
Evipan	T42.3X1	T42.3X2	T42.3X3	T42.3X4	T42.3X5	T42.3X6
sodium	T41.1X1	T41.1X2	T41.1X3	T41.1X4	T41.1X5	T41.1X6
Exalamide	T49.0X1	T49.0X2	T49.0X3	T49.0X4	T49.0X5	T49.0X6
Exalgin	T39.1X1	T39.1X2	T39.1X3	T39.1X4	T39.1X5	T39.1X6
Excipients, pharmaceutical	T50.901	T50.902	T50.903	T50.904	T50.905	T50.906
Exhaust gas (engine) (motor vehicle)	T58.01	T58.02	T58.03	T58.04	—	—
Ex-Lax (phenolphthalein)	T47.2X1	T47.2X2	T47.2X3	T47.2X4	T47.2X5	T47.2X6
Expectorant NEC	T48.4X1	T48.4X2	T48.4X3	T48.4X4	T48.4X5	T48.4X6
Extended insulin zinc suspension	T38.3X1	T38.3X2	T38.3X3	T38.3X4	T38.3X5	T38.3X6
External medications (skin) (mucous membrane)	T49.91	T49.92	T49.93	T49.94	T49.95	T49.96
dental agent	T49.7X1	T49.7X2	T49.7X3	T49.7X4	T49.7X5	T49.7X6
ENT agent	T49.6X1	T49.6X2	T49.6X3	T49.6X4	T49.6X5	T49.6X6
ophthalmic preparation	T49.5X1	T49.5X2	T49.5X3	T49.5X4	T49.5X5	T49.5X6
specified NEC	T49.8X1	T49.8X2	T49.8X3	T49.8X4	T49.8X5	T49.8X6
Extrapyramidal antagonist NEC	T44.3X1	T44.3X2	T44.3X3	T44.3X4	T44.3X5	T44.3X6
Eye agents (anti-infective)	T49.5X1	T49.5X2	T49.5X3	T49.5X4	T49.5X5	T49.5X6
Eye drug NEC	T49.5X1	T49.5X2	T49.5X3	T49.5X4	T49.5X5	T49.5X6
FAC (fluorouracil + doxorubicin + cyclophosphamide)	T45.1X1	T45.1X2	T45.1X3	T45.1X4	T45.1X5	T45.1X6
Factor						
I (fibrinogen)	T45.8X1	T45.8X2	T45.8X3	T45.8X4	T45.8X5	T45.8X6
III (thromboplastin)	T45.8X1	T45.8X2	T45.8X3	T45.8X4	T45.8X5	T45.8X6
IX complex	T45.7X1	T45.7X2	T45.7X3	T45.7X4	T45.7X5	T45.7X6
human	T45.8X1	T45.8X2	T45.8X3	T45.8X4	T45.8X5	T45.8X6
VIII (antihemophilic Factor) (concentrate)	T45.8X1	T45.8X2	T45.8X3	T45.8X4	T45.8X5	T45.8X6
Famotidine	T47.0X1	T47.0X2	T47.0X3	T47.0X4	T47.0X5	T47.0X6
Fat suspension, intravenous	T50.991	T50.992	T50.993	T50.994	T50.995	T50.996
Fazadinium bromide	T48.1X1	T48.1X2	T48.1X3	T48.1X4	T48.1X5	T48.1X6
Febarbamate	T42.3X1	T42.3X2	T42.3X3	T42.3X4	T42.3X5	T42.3X6
Fecal softener	T47.4X1	T47.4X2	T47.4X3	T47.4X4	T47.4X5	T47.4X6
Fedrilate	T48.3X1	T48.3X2	T48.3X3	T48.3X4	T48.3X5	T48.3X6
Felodipine	T46.1X1	T46.1X2	T46.1X3	T46.1X4	T46.1X5	T46.1X6
Felypressin	T38.891	T38.892	T38.893	T38.894	T38.895	T38.896
Femoxetine	T43.221	T43.222	T43.223	T43.224	T43.225	T43.226
Fenalcomine	T46.3X1	T46.3X2	T46.3X3	T46.3X4	T46.3X5	T46.3X6
Fenamisal	T37.1X1	T37.1X2	T37.1X3	T37.1X4	T37.1X5	T37.1X6
Fenazone	T39.2X1	T39.2X2	T39.2X3	T39.2X4	T39.2X5	T39.2X6
Fenbendazole	T37.4X1	T37.4X2	T37.4X3	T37.4X4	T37.4X5	T37.4X6
Fenbutrazate	T50.5X1	T50.5X2	T50.5X3	T50.5X4	T50.5X5	T50.5X6
Fencamfamine	T43.691	T43.692	T43.693	T43.694	T43.695	T43.696
Fendiline	T46.1X1	T46.1X2	T46.1X3	T46.1X4	T46.1X5	T46.1X6
Fenetylline	T43.691	T43.692	T43.693	T43.694	T43.695	T43.696
Fenflumizole	T39.391	T39.392	T39.393	T39.394	T39.395	T39.396
Fenfluramine	T50.5X1	T50.5X2	T50.5X3	T50.5X4	T50.5X5	T50.5X6
Fenobarbital	T42.3X1	T42.3X2	T42.3X3	T42.3X4	T42.3X5	T42.3X6
Fenofibrate	T46.6X1	T46.6X2	T46.6X3	T46.6X4	T46.6X5	T46.6X6
Fenoprofen	T39.311	T39.312	T39.313	T39.314	T39.315	T39.316
Fenoterol	T48.6X1	T48.6X2	T48.6X3	T48.6X4	T48.6X5	T48.6X6
Fenoverine	T44.3X1	T44.3X2	T44.3X3	T44.3X4	T44.3X5	T44.3X6
Fenoxazoline	T48.5X1	T48.5X2	T48.5X3	T48.5X4	T48.5X5	T48.5X6
Fenproporex	T50.5X1	T50.5X2	T50.5X3	T50.5X4	T50.5X5	T50.5X6
Fenquizone	T50.2X1	T50.2X2	T50.2X3	T50.2X4	T50.2X5	T50.2X6
Fentanyl	T40.4X1	T40.4X2	T40.4X3	T40.4X4	T40.4X5	T40.4X6
Fentazin	T43.3X1	T43.3X2	T43.3X3	T43.3X4	T43.3X5	T43.3X6
Fenthion	T60.0X1	T60.0X2	T60.0X3	T60.0X4	—	—
Fenticlor	T49.0X1	T49.0X2	T49.0X3	T49.0X4	T49.0X5	T49.0X6
Fenylbutazone	T39.2X1	T39.2X2	T39.2X3	T39.2X4	T39.2X5	T39.2X6

Substance	Poisoning, Accidental (unintentional)	Poisoning, Intentional Self-harm	Poisoning, Assault	Poisoning, Undetermined	Adverse Effect	Under-dosing
Feprazone	T39.2X1	T39.2X2	T39.2X3	T39.2X4	T39.2X5	T39.2X6
Fer de lance (bite) (venom)	T63.061	T63.062	T63.063	T63.064	—	—
Ferric — see also Iron						
chloride	T45.4X1	T45.4X2	T45.4X3	T45.4X4	T45.4X5	T45.4X6
citrate	T45.4X1	T45.4X2	T45.4X3	T45.4X4	T45.4X5	T45.4X6
hydroxide						
colloidal	T45.4X1	T45.4X2	T45.4X3	T45.4X4	T45.4X5	T45.4X6
polymaltose	T45.4X1	T45.4X2	T45.4X3	T45.4X4	T45.4X5	T45.4X6
pyrophosphate	T45.4X1	T45.4X2	T45.4X3	T45.4X4	T45.4X5	T45.4X6
Ferritin	T45.4X1	T45.4X2	T45.4X3	T45.4X4	T45.4X5	T45.4X6
Ferrocholinate	T45.4X1	T45.4X2	T45.4X3	T45.4X4	T45.4X5	T45.4X6
Ferrodextrane	T45.4X1	T45.4X2	T45.4X3	T45.4X4	T45.4X5	T45.4X6
Ferropolimaler	T45.4X1	T45.4X2	T45.4X3	T45.4X4	T45.4X5	T45.4X6
Ferrous — see also Iron						
phosphate	T45.4X1	T45.4X2	T45.4X3	T45.4X4	T45.4X5	T45.4X6
salt	T45.4X1	T45.4X2	T45.4X3	T45.4X4	T45.4X5	T45.4X6
with folic acid	T45.4X1	T45.4X2	T45.4X3	T45.4X4	T45.4X5	T45.4X6
Ferrous fumerate, gluconate, lactate, salt NEC, sulfate (medicinal)	T45.4X1	T45.4X2	T45.4X3	T45.4X4	T45.4X5	T45.4X6
Ferrovanadium (fumes)	T59.891	T59.892	T59.893	T59.894	—	—
Ferrum — see Iron						
Fertilizers NEC	T65.891	T65.892	T65.893	T65.894	—	—
with herbicide mixture	T60.3X1	T60.3X2	T60.3X3	T60.3X4	—	—
Fetoxilate	T47.6X1	T47.6X2	T47.6X3	T47.6X4	T47.6X5	T47.6X6
Fiber, dietary	T47.4X1	T47.4X2	T47.4X3	T47.4X4	T47.4X5	T47.4X6
Fiberglass	T65.831	T65.832	T65.833	T65.834	—	—
Fibrinogen (human)	T45.8X1	T45.8X2	T45.8X3	T45.8X4	T45.8X5	T45.8X6
Fibrinolysin (human)	T45.691	T45.692	T45.693	T45.694	T45.695	T45.696
Fibrinolysis						
affecting drug	T45.601	T45.602	T45.603	T45.604	T45.605	T45.606
inhibitor NEC	T45.621	T45.622	T45.623	T45.624	T45.625	T45.626
Fibrinolytic drug	T45.611	T45.612	T45.613	T45.614	T45.615	T45.616
Filix mas	T37.4X1	T37.4X2	T37.4X3	T37.4X4	T37.4X5	T37.4X6
Filtering cream	T49.3X1	T49.3X2	T49.3X3	T49.3X4	T49.3X5	T49.3X6
Fiorinal	T39.011	T39.012	T39.013	T39.014	T39.015	T39.016
Firedamp	T59.891	T59.892	T59.893	T59.894	—	—
Fish, noxious, nonbacterial	T61.91	T61.92	T61.93	T61.94	—	—
ciguatera	T61.01	T61.02	T61.03	T61.04	—	—
scombroid	T61.11	T61.12	T61.13	T61.14	—	—
shell	T61.781	T61.782	T61.783	T61.784	—	—
specified NEC	T61.771	T61.772	T61.773	T61.774	—	—
Flagyl	T37.3X1	T37.3X2	T37.3X3	T37.3X4	T37.3X5	T37.3X6
Flavine adenine dinucleotide	T45.2X1	T45.2X2	T45.2X3	T45.2X4	T45.2X5	T45.2X6
Flavodic acid	T46.991	T46.992	T46.993	T46.994	T46.995	T46.996
Flavoxate	T44.3X1	T44.3X2	T44.3X3	T44.3X4	T44.3X5	T44.3X6
Flaxedil	T48.1X1	T48.1X2	T48.1X3	T48.1X4	T48.1X5	T48.1X6
Flaxseed (medicinal)	T49.3X1	T49.3X2	T49.3X3	T49.3X4	T49.3X5	T49.3X6
Flecainide	T46.2X1	T46.2X2	T46.2X3	T46.2X4	T46.2X5	T46.2X6
Fleroxacin	T36.8X1	T36.8X2	T36.8X3	T36.8X4	T36.8X5	T36.8X6
Floctafenine	T39.8X1	T39.8X2	T39.8X3	T39.8X4	T39.8X5	T39.8X6
Flomax	T44.6X1	T44.6X2	T44.6X3	T44.6X4	T44.6X5	T44.6X6
Flomoxef	T36.1X1	T36.1X2	T36.1X3	T36.1X4	T36.1X5	T36.1X6
Flopropione	T44.3X1	T44.3X2	T44.3X3	T44.3X4	T44.3X5	T44.3X6
Florantyrone	T47.5X1	T47.5X2	T47.5X3	T47.5X4	T47.5X5	T47.5X6
Floraquin	T37.8X1	T37.8X2	T37.8X3	T37.8X4	T37.8X5	T37.8X6
Florinef	T38.0X1	T38.0X2	T38.0X3	T38.0X4	T38.0X5	T38.0X6
ENT agent	T49.6X1	T49.6X2	T49.6X3	T49.6X4	T49.6X5	T49.6X6
ophthalmic preparation	T49.5X1	T49.5X2	T49.5X3	T49.5X4	T49.5X5	T49.5X6
topical NEC	T49.0X1	T49.0X2	T49.0X3	T49.0X4	T49.0X5	T49.0X6
Flowers of sulfur	T49.4X1	T49.4X2	T49.4X3	T49.4X4	T49.4X5	T49.4X6
Floxuridine	T45.1X1	T45.1X2	T45.1X3	T45.1X4	T45.1X5	T45.1X6
Fluanisone	T43.4X1	T43.4X2	T43.4X3	T43.4X4	T43.4X5	T43.4X6
Flubendazole	T37.4X1	T37.4X2	T37.4X3	T37.4X4	T37.4X5	T37.4X6
Fluclorolone acetonide	T49.0X1	T49.0X2	T49.0X3	T49.0X4	T49.0X5	T49.0X6
Flucloxacillin	T36.0X1	T36.0X2	T36.0X3	T36.0X4	T36.0X5	T36.0X6
Fluconazole	T37.8X1	T37.8X2	T37.8X3	T37.8X4	T37.8X5	T37.8X6
Flucytosine	T37.8X1	T37.8X2	T37.8X3	T37.8X4	T37.8X5	T37.8X6
Fludeoxyglucose (18F)	T50.8X1	T50.8X2	T50.8X3	T50.8X4	T50.8X5	T50.8X6
Fludiazepam	T42.4X1	T42.4X2	T42.4X3	T42.4X4	T42.4X5	T42.4X6
Fludrocortisone	T50.0X1	T50.0X2	T50.0X3	T50.0X4	T50.0X5	T50.0X6
ENT agent	T49.6X1	T49.6X2	T49.6X3	T49.6X4	T49.6X5	T49.6X6
ophthalmic preparation	T49.5X1	T49.5X2	T49.5X3	T49.5X4	T49.5X5	T49.5X6
topical NEC	T49.0X1	T49.0X2	T49.0X3	T49.0X4	T49.0X5	T49.0X6
Fludroxycortide	T49.0X1	T49.0X2	T49.0X3	T49.0X4	T49.0X5	T49.0X6
Flufenamic acid	T39.391	T39.392	T39.393	T39.394	T39.395	T39.396
Fluindione	T45.511	T45.512	T45.513	T45.514	T45.515	T45.516
Flumequine	T37.8X1	T37.8X2	T37.8X3	T37.8X4	T37.8X5	T37.8X6
Flumethasone	T49.0X1	T49.0X2	T49.0X3	T49.0X4	T49.0X5	T49.0X6
Flumethiazide	T50.2X1	T50.2X2	T50.2X3	T50.2X4	T50.2X5	T50.2X6
Flumidin	T37.5X1	T37.5X2	T37.5X3	T37.5X4	T37.5X5	T37.5X6

Additional Character May Be Required — Refer to the Tabular List for Character Selection   ▽ Subterms under main terms may continue to next column or page

Substance	Poisoning, Accidental (unintentional)	Poisoning, Intentional Self-harm	Poisoning, Assault	Poisoning, Undetermined	Adverse Effect	Under-dosing
Flunarizine	T46.7X1	T46.7X2	T46.7X3	T46.7X4	T46.7X5	T46.7X6
Flunidazole	T37.8X1	T37.8X2	T37.8X3	T37.8X4	T37.8X5	T37.8X6
Flunisolide	T48.6X1	T48.6X2	T48.6X3	T48.6X4	T48.6X5	T48.6X6
Flunitrazepam	T42.4X1	T42.4X2	T42.4X3	T42.4X4	T42.4X5	T42.4X6
Fluocinolone (acetonide)	T49.0X1	T49.0X2	T49.0X3	T49.0X4	T49.0X5	T49.0X6
Fluocinonide	T49.0X1	T49.0X2	T49.0X3	T49.0X4	T49.0X5	T49.0X6
Fluocortin (butyl)	T49.0X1	T49.0X2	T49.0X3	T49.0X4	T49.0X5	T49.0X6
Fluocortolone	T49.0X1	T49.0X2	T49.0X3	T49.0X4	T49.0X5	T49.0X6
Fluohydrocortisone	T38.0X1	T38.0X2	T38.0X3	T38.0X4	T38.0X5	T38.0X6
ENT agent	T49.6X1	T49.6X2	T49.6X3	T49.6X4	T49.6X5	T49.6X6
ophthalmic preparation	T49.5X1	T49.5X2	T49.5X3	T49.5X4	T49.5X5	T49.5X6
topical NEC	T49.0X1	T49.0X2	T49.0X3	T49.0X4	T49.0X5	T49.0X6
Fluonid	T49.0X1	T49.0X2	T49.0X3	T49.0X4	T49.0X5	T49.0X6
Fluopromazine	T43.3X1	T43.3X2	T43.3X3	T43.3X4	T43.3X5	T43.3X6
Fluoracetate	T60.8X1	T60.8X2	T60.8X3	T60.8X4	—	—
Fluorescein	T50.8X1	T50.8X2	T50.8X3	T50.8X4	T50.8X5	T50.8X6
Fluorhydrocortisone	T50.0X1	T50.0X2	T50.0X3	T50.0X4	T50.0X5	T50.0X6
Fluoride (nonmedicinal) (pesticide) (sodium) NEC	T60.8X1	T60.8X2	T60.8X3	T60.8X4	—	—
hydrogen — see Hydrofluoric acid						
medicinal NEC	T50.991	T50.992	T50.993	T50.994	T50.995	T50.996
dental use	T49.7X1	T49.7X2	T49.7X3	T49.7X4	T49.7X5	T49.7X6
not pesticide NEC	T54.91	T54.92	T54.93	T54.94	—	—
stannous	T49.7X1	T49.7X2	T49.7X3	T49.7X4	T49.7X5	T49.7X6
Fluorinated corticosteroids	T38.0X1	T38.0X2	T38.0X3	T38.0X4	T38.0X5	T38.0X6
Fluorine (gas)	T59.5X1	T59.5X2	T59.5X3	T59.5X4	—	—
salt — see Fluoride(s)						
Fluoristan	T49.7X1	T49.7X2	T49.7X3	T49.7X4	T49.7X5	T49.7X6
Fluormetholone	T49.0X1	T49.0X2	T49.0X3	T49.0X4	T49.0X5	T49.0X6
Fluoroacetate	T60.8X1	T60.8X2	T60.8X3	T60.8X4	—	—
Fluorocarbon monomer	T53.6X1	T53.6X2	T53.6X3	T53.6X4	—	—
Fluorocytosine	T37.8X1	T37.8X2	T37.8X3	T37.8X4	T37.8X5	T37.8X6
Fluorodeoxyuridine	T45.1X1	T45.1X2	T45.1X3	T45.1X4	T45.1X5	T45.1X6
Fluorometholone	T49.0X1	T49.0X2	T49.0X3	T49.0X4	T49.0X5	T49.0X6
ophthalmic preparation	T49.5X1	T49.5X2	T49.5X3	T49.5X4	T49.5X5	T49.5X6
Fluorophosphate insecticide	T60.0X1	T60.0X2	T60.0X3	T60.0X4	—	—
Fluorosol	T46.3X1	T46.3X2	T46.3X3	T46.3X4	T46.3X5	T46.3X6
Fluorouracil	T45.1X1	T45.1X2	T45.1X3	T45.1X4	T45.1X5	T45.1X6
Fluorphenylalanine	T49.5X1	T49.5X2	T49.5X3	T49.5X4	T49.5X5	T49.5X6
Fluothane	T41.0X1	T41.0X2	T41.0X3	T41.0X4	T41.0X5	T41.0X6
Fluoxetine	T43.221	T43.222	T43.223	T43.224	T43.225	T43.226
Fluoxymesterone	T38.7X1	T38.7X2	T38.7X3	T38.7X4	T38.7X5	T38.7X6
Flupenthixol	T43.4X1	T43.4X2	T43.4X3	T43.4X4	T43.4X5	T43.4X6
Flupentixol	T43.4X1	T43.4X2	T43.4X3	T43.4X4	T43.4X5	T43.4X6
Fluphenazine	T43.3X1	T43.3X2	T43.3X3	T43.3X4	T43.3X5	T43.3X6
Fluprednidene	T49.0X1	T49.0X2	T49.0X3	T49.0X4	T49.0X5	T49.0X6
Fluprednisolone	T38.0X1	T38.0X2	T38.0X3	T38.0X4	T38.0X5	T38.0X6
Fluradoline	T39.8X1	T39.8X2	T39.8X3	T39.8X4	T39.8X5	T39.8X6
Flurandrenolide	T49.0X1	T49.0X2	T49.0X3	T49.0X4	T49.0X5	T49.0X6
Flurandrenolone	T49.0X1	T49.0X2	T49.0X3	T49.0X4	T49.0X5	T49.0X6
Flurazepam	T42.4X1	T42.4X2	T42.4X3	T42.4X4	T42.4X5	T42.4X6
Flurbiprofen	T39.311	T39.312	T39.313	T39.314	T39.315	T39.316
Flurobate	T49.0X1	T49.0X2	T49.0X3	T49.0X4	T49.0X5	T49.0X6
Fluroxene	T41.0X1	T41.0X2	T41.0X3	T41.0X4	T41.0X5	T41.0X6
Fluspirilene	T43.591	T43.592	T43.593	T43.594	T43.595	T43.596
Flutamide	T38.6X1	T38.6X2	T38.6X3	T38.6X4	T38.6X5	T38.6X6
Flutazolam	T38.0X1	T38.0X2	T38.0X3	T38.0X4	T38.0X5	T38.0X6
Fluticasone propionate	T38.0X1	T38.0X2	T38.0X3	T38.0X4	T38.0X5	T38.0X6
Flutoprazepam	T42.4X1	T42.4X2	T42.4X3	T42.4X4	T42.4X5	T42.4X6
Flutropium bromide	T48.6X1	T48.6X2	T48.6X3	T48.6X4	T48.6X5	T48.6X6
Fluvoxamine	T43.221	T43.222	T43.223	T43.224	T43.225	T43.226
Folacin	T45.8X1	T45.8X2	T45.8X3	T45.8X4	T45.8X5	T45.8X6
Folic acid	T45.8X1	T45.8X2	T45.8X3	T45.8X4	T45.8X5	T45.8X6
with ferrous salt	T45.2X1	T45.2X2	T45.2X3	T45.2X4	T45.2X5	T45.2X6
antagonist	T45.1X1	T45.1X2	T45.1X3	T45.1X4	T45.1X5	T45.1X6
Folinic acid	T45.8X1	T45.8X2	T45.8X3	T45.8X4	T45.8X5	T45.8X6
Folium stramoniae	T48.6X1	T48.6X2	T48.6X3	T48.6X4	T48.6X5	T48.6X6
Follicle-stimulating hormone, human	T38.811	T38.812	T38.813	T38.814	T38.815	T38.816
Folpet	T60.3X1	T60.3X2	T60.3X3	T60.3X4	—	—
Fominoben	T48.3X1	T48.3X2	T48.3X3	T48.3X4	T48.3X5	T48.3X6
Food, foodstuffs, noxious, nonbacterial, NEC	T62.91	T62.92	T62.93	T62.94	—	—
berries	T62.1X1	T62.1X2	T62.1X3	T62.1X4	—	—
fish — see also Fish	T61.91	T61.92	T61.93	T61.94	—	—
mushrooms	T62.0X1	T62.0X2	T62.0X3	T62.0X4	—	—
plants	T62.2X1	T62.2X2	T62.2X3	T62.2X4	—	—
seafood	T61.91	T61.92	T61.93	T61.94	—	—
specified NEC	T61.8X1	T61.8X2	T61.8X3	T61.8X4	—	—
seeds	T62.2X1	T62.2X2	T62.2X3	T62.2X4	—	—

Substance	Poisoning, Accidental (unintentional)	Poisoning, Intentional Self-harm	Poisoning, Assault	Poisoning, Undetermined	Adverse Effect	Under-dosing
Food, foodstuffs, noxious, nonbacterial, — continued						
shellfish	T61.781	T61.782	T61.783	T61.784	—	—
specified NEC	T62.8X1	T62.8X2	T62.8X3	T62.8X4	—	—
Fool's parsley	T62.2X1	T62.2X2	T62.2X3	T62.2X4	—	—
Formaldehyde (solution), gas or vapor	T59.2X1	T59.2X2	T59.2X3	T59.2X4	—	—
fungicide	T60.3X1	T60.3X2	T60.3X3	T60.3X4	—	—
Formalin	T59.2X1	T59.2X2	T59.2X3	T59.2X4	—	—
fungicide	T60.3X1	T60.3X2	T60.3X3	T60.3X4	—	—
vapor	T59.2X1	T59.2X2	T59.2X3	T59.2X4	—	—
Formic acid	T54.2X1	T54.2X2	T54.2X3	T54.2X4	—	—
vapor	T59.891	T59.892	T59.893	T59.894	—	—
Foscarnet sodium	T37.5X1	T37.5X2	T37.5X3	T37.5X4	T37.5X5	T37.5X6
Fosfestrol	T38.5X1	T38.5X2	T38.5X3	T38.5X4	T38.5X5	T38.5X6
Fosfomycin	T36.8X1	T36.8X2	T36.8X3	T36.8X4	T36.8X5	T36.8X6
Fosfonet sodium	T37.5X1	T37.5X2	T37.5X3	T37.5X4	T37.5X5	T37.5X6
Fosinopril	T46.4X1	T46.4X2	T46.4X3	T46.4X4	T46.4X5	T46.4X6
sodium	T46.4X1	T46.4X2	T46.4X3	T46.4X4	T46.4X5	T46.4X6
Fowler's solution	T57.0X1	T57.0X2	T57.0X3	T57.0X4	—	—
Foxglove	T62.2X1	T62.2X2	T62.2X3	T62.2X4	—	—
Framycetin	T36.5X1	T36.5X2	T36.5X3	T36.5X4	T36.5X5	T36.5X6
Frangula	T47.2X1	T47.2X2	T47.2X3	T47.2X4	T47.2X5	T47.2X6
extract	T47.2X1	T47.2X2	T47.2X3	T47.2X4	T47.2X5	T47.2X6
Frei antigen	T50.8X1	T50.8X2	T50.8X3	T50.8X4	T50.8X5	T50.8X6
Freon	T53.5X1	T53.5X2	T53.5X3	T53.5X4	—	—
Fructose	T50.3X1	T50.3X2	T50.3X3	T50.3X4	T50.3X5	T50.3X6
Frusemide	T50.1X1	T50.1X2	T50.1X3	T50.1X4	T50.1X5	T50.1X6
FSH	T38.811	T38.812	T38.813	T38.814	T38.815	T38.816
Ftorafur	T45.1X1	T45.1X2	T45.1X3	T45.1X4	T45.1X5	T45.1X6
Fuel						
automobile	T52.0X1	T52.0X2	T52.0X3	T52.0X4	—	—
exhaust gas, not in transit	T58.01	T58.02	T58.03	T58.04	—	—
vapor NEC	T52.0X1	T52.0X2	T52.0X3	T52.0X4	—	—
gas (domestic use) — see also Carbon, monoxide, fuel, utility	T59.891	T59.892	T59.893	T59.894	—	—
utility	T59.891	T59.892	T59.893	T59.894	—	—
incomplete combustion of — see Carbon, monoxide, fuel, utility						
in mobile container	T59.891	T59.892	T59.893	T59.894	—	—
piped (natural)	T59.891	T59.892	T59.893	T59.894	—	—
industrial, incomplete combustion	T58.8X1	T58.8X2	T58.8X3	T58.8X4	—	—
Fugillin	T36.8X1	T36.8X2	T36.8X3	T36.8X4	T36.8X5	T36.8X6
Fulminate of mercury	T56.1X1	T56.1X2	T56.1X3	T56.1X4	—	—
Fulvicin	T36.7X1	T36.7X2	T36.7X3	T36.7X4	T36.7X5	T36.7X6
Fumadil	T36.8X1	T36.8X2	T36.8X3	T36.8X4	T36.8X5	T36.8X6
Fumagillin	T36.8X1	T36.8X2	T36.8X3	T36.8X4	T36.8X5	T36.8X6
Fumaric acid	T49.4X1	T49.4X2	T49.4X3	T49.4X4	T49.4X5	T49.4X6
Fumes (from)	T59.91	T59.92	T59.93	T59.94	—	—
carbon monoxide — see Carbon, monoxide						
charcoal (domestic use) — see Charcoal, fumes						
chloroform — see Chloroform						
coke (in domestic stoves, fireplaces) — see Coke fumes						
corrosive NEC	T54.91	T54.92	T54.93	T54.94	—	—
ether — see ether						
freons	T53.5X1	T53.5X2	T53.5X3	T53.5X4	—	—
hydrocarbons	T59.891	T59.892	T59.893	T59.894	—	—
petroleum (liquefied)	T59.891	T59.892	T59.893	T59.894	—	—
distributed through pipes (pure or mixed with air)	T59.891	T59.892	T59.893	T59.894	—	—
lead — see lead						
metal — see Metals, or the specified metal						
nitrogen dioxide	T59.0X1	T59.0X2	T59.0X3	T59.0X4	—	—
pesticides — see Pesticides						
petroleum (liquefied)	T59.891	T59.892	T59.893	T59.894	—	—
distributed through pipes (pure or mixed with air)	T59.891	T59.892	T59.893	T59.894	—	—
polyester	T59.891	T59.892	T59.893	T59.894	—	—
specified source NEC — see also substance specified	T59.891	T59.892	T59.893	T59.894	—	—
sulfur dioxide	T59.1X1	T59.1X2	T59.1X3	T59.1X4	—	—
Fumigant NEC	T60.91	T60.92	T60.93	T60.94	—	—

▽ Subterms under main terms may continue to next column or page   Additional Character May Be Required — Refer to the Tabular List for Character Selection   **369**

Flunarizine — Fumigant NEC

Table of Drugs and Chemicals

Fungicide NEC — Gentamicin

Substance	Poisoning, Accidental (unintentional)	Poisoning, Intentional Self-harm	Poisoning, Assault	Poisoning, Undetermined	Adverse Effect	Under-dosing
Fungicide NEC	T60.3X1	T60.3X2	T60.3X3	T60.3X4	—	—
(nonmedicinal)						
Fungi, noxious, used as food	T62.0X1	T62.0X2	T62.0X3	T62.0X4	—	—
Fungizone	T36.7X1	T36.7X2	T36.7X3	T36.7X4	T36.7X5	T36.7X6
topical	T49.0X1	T49.0X2	T49.0X3	T49.0X4	T49.0X5	T49.0X6
Furacin	T49.0X1	T49.0X2	T49.0X3	T49.0X4	T49.0X5	T49.0X6
Furadantin	T37.91	T37.92	T37.93	T37.94	T37.95	T37.96
Furazolidone	T37.8X1	T37.8X2	T37.8X3	T37.8X4	T37.8X5	T37.8X6
Furazolium chloride	T49.0X1	T49.0X2	T49.0X3	T49.0X4	T49.0X5	T49.0X6
Furfural	T52.8X1	T52.8X2	T52.8X3	T52.8X4	—	—
Furnace (coal burning) (domestic), gas from	T58.2X1	T58.2X2	T58.2X3	T58.2X4	—	—
industrial	T58.8X1	T58.8X2	T58.8X3	T58.8X4	—	—
Furniture polish	T65.891	T65.892	T65.893	T65.894	—	—
Furosemide	T50.1X1	T50.1X2	T50.1X3	T50.1X4	T50.1X5	T50.1X6
Furoxone	T37.91	T37.92	T37.93	T37.94	T37.95	T37.96
Fursultiamine	T45.2X1	T45.2X2	T45.2X3	T45.2X4	T45.2X5	T45.2X6
Fusafungine	T36.8X1	T36.8X2	T36.8X3	T36.8X4	T36.8X5	T36.8X6
Fusel oil (any) (amyl) (butyl) (propyl), vapor	T51.3X1	T51.3X2	T51.3X3	T51.3X4	—	—
Fusidate (ethanolamine) (sodium)	T36.8X1	T36.8X2	T36.8X3	T36.8X4	T36.8X5	T36.8X6
Fusidic acid	T36.8X1	T36.8X2	T36.8X3	T36.8X4	T36.8X5	T36.8X6
Fytic acid, nonasodium	T50.6X1	T50.6X2	T50.6X3	T50.6X4	T50.6X5	T50.6X6
b-Galactosidase	T47.5X1	T47.5X2	T47.5X3	T47.5X4	T47.5X5	T47.5X6
GABA	T43.8X1	T43.8X2	T43.8X3	T43.8X4	T43.8X5	T43.8X6
Gadopentetic acid	T50.8X1	T50.8X2	T50.8X3	T50.8X4	T50.8X5	T50.8X6
Galactose	T50.3X1	T50.3X2	T50.3X3	T50.3X4	T50.3X5	T50.3X6
Galantamine	T44.0X1	T44.0X2	T44.0X3	T44.0X4	T44.0X5	T44.0X6
Gallamine (triethiodide)	T48.1X1	T48.1X2	T48.1X3	T48.1X4	T48.1X5	T48.1X6
Gallium citrate	T50.991	T50.992	T50.993	T50.994	T50.995	T50.996
Gallopamil	T46.1X1	T46.1X2	T46.1X3	T46.1X4	T46.1X5	T46.1X6
Gamboge	T47.2X1	T47.2X2	T47.2X3	T47.2X4	T47.2X5	T47.2X6
Gamimune	T50.Z11	T50.Z12	T50.Z13	T50.Z14	T50.Z15	T50.Z16
Gamma-aminobutyric acid	T43.8X1	T43.8X2	T43.8X3	T43.8X4	T43.8X5	T43.8X6
Gamma-benzene hexachloride (medicinal)	T49.0X1	T49.0X2	T49.0X3	T49.0X4	T49.0X5	T49.0X6
nonmedicinal, vapor	T53.6X1	T53.6X2	T53.6X3	T53.6X4	—	—
Gamma-BHC (medicinal) — see also Gamma-benzene hexachloride	T49.0X1	T49.0X2	T49.0X3	T49.0X4	T49.0X5	T49.0X6
Gamma globulin	T50.Z11	T50.Z12	T50.Z13	T50.Z14	T50.Z15	T50.Z16
Gamulin	T50.Z11	T50.Z12	T50.Z13	T50.Z14	T50.Z15	T50.Z16
Ganciclovir (sodium)	T37.5X1	T37.5X2	T37.5X3	T37.5X4	T37.5X5	T37.5X6
Ganglionic blocking drug NEC	T44.2X1	T44.2X2	T44.2X3	T44.2X4	T44.2X5	T44.2X6
specified NEC	T44.2X1	T44.2X2	T44.2X3	T44.2X4	T44.2X5	T44.2X6
Ganja	T40.7X1	T40.7X2	T40.7X3	T40.7X4	T40.7X5	T40.7X6
Garamycin	T36.5X1	T36.5X2	T36.5X3	T36.5X4	T36.5X5	T36.5X6
ophthalmic preparation	T49.5X1	T49.5X2	T49.5X3	T49.5X4	T49.5X5	T49.5X6
topical NEC	T49.0X1	T49.0X2	T49.0X3	T49.0X4	T49.0X5	T49.0X6
Gardenal	T42.3X1	T42.3X2	T42.3X3	T42.3X4	T42.3X5	T42.3X6
Gardepanyl	T42.3X1	T42.3X2	T42.3X3	T42.3X4	T42.3X5	T42.3X6
Gaseous substance — see Gas						
Gasoline	T52.0X1	T52.0X2	T52.0X3	T52.0X4	—	—
vapor	T52.0X1	T52.0X2	T52.0X3	T52.0X4	—	—
Gastric enzymes	T47.5X1	T47.5X2	T47.5X3	T47.5X4	T47.5X5	T47.5X6
Gastrografin	T50.8X1	T50.8X2	T50.8X3	T50.8X4	T50.8X5	T50.8X6
Gastrointestinal drug	T47.91	T47.92	T47.93	T47.94	T47.95	T47.96
biological	T47.8X1	T47.8X2	T47.8X3	T47.8X4	T47.8X5	T47.8X6
specified NEC	T47.8X1	T47.8X2	T47.8X3	T47.8X4	T47.8X5	T47.8X6
Gas NEC	T59.91	T59.92	T59.93	T59.94	—	—
acetylene	T59.891	T59.892	T59.893	T59.894	—	—
incomplete combustion of	T58.11	T58.12	T58.13	T58.14	—	—
air contaminants, source or type not specified	T59.91	T59.92	T59.93	T59.94	—	—
anesthetic	T41.0X1	T41.0X2	T41.0X3	T41.0X4	T41.0X5	T41.0X6
blast furnace	T58.8X1	T58.8X2	T58.8X3	T58.8X4	—	—
butane — see butane						
carbon monoxide — see Carbon, monoxide						
chlorine	T59.4X1	T59.4X2	T59.4X3	T59.4X4	—	—
coal	T58.2X1	T58.2X2	T58.2X3	T58.2X4	—	—
cyanide	T57.3X1	T57.3X2	T57.3X3	T57.3X4	—	—
dicyanogen	T65.0X1	T65.0X2	T65.0X3	T65.0X4	—	—
domestic — see Domestic gas						
exhaust	T58.01	T58.02	T58.03	T58.04	—	—
from utility (for cooking, heating, or lighting) (after combustion) — see Carbon, monoxide, fuel, utility						

Substance	Poisoning, Accidental (unintentional)	Poisoning, Intentional Self-harm	Poisoning, Assault	Poisoning, Undetermined	Adverse Effect	Under-dosing
Gas — continued						
from utility — see Carbon, monoxide, fuel, utility — continued						
prior to combustion	T59.891	T59.892	T59.893	T59.894	—	—
from wood- or coal-burning stove or fireplace	T58.2X1	T58.2X2	T58.2X3	T58.2X4	—	—
fuel (domestic use) (after combustion) — see also Carbon, monoxide, fuel						
industrial use	T58.8X1	T58.8X2	T58.8X3	T58.8X4	—	—
prior to combustion	T59.891	T59.892	T59.893	T59.894	—	—
utility	T59.891	T59.892	T59.893	T59.894	—	—
incomplete combustion of — see Carbon, monoxide, fuel, utility						
in mobile container	T59.891	T59.892	T59.893	T59.894	—	—
piped (natural)	T59.891	T59.892	T59.893	T59.894	—	—
garage	T58.01	T58.02	T58.03	T58.04	—	—
hydrocarbon NEC	T59.891	T59.892	T59.893	T59.894	—	—
incomplete combustion of — see Carbon, monoxide, fuel, utility						
liquefied — see butane						
piped	T59.891	T59.892	T59.893	T59.894	—	—
hydrocyanic acid	T65.0X1	T65.0X2	T65.0X3	T65.0X4	—	—
illuminating (after combustion)	T58.11	T58.12	T58.13	T58.14	—	—
prior to combustion	T59.891	T59.892	T59.893	T59.894	—	—
incomplete combustion, any — see Carbon, monoxide						
kiln	T58.8X1	T58.8X2	T58.8X3	T58.8X4	—	—
lacrimogenic	T59.3X1	T59.3X2	T59.3X3	T59.3X4	—	—
liquefied petroleum — see butane						
marsh	T59.891	T59.892	T59.893	T59.894	—	—
motor exhaust, not in transit	T58.01	T58.02	T58.03	T58.04	—	—
mustard, not in war	T59.891	T59.892	T59.893	T59.894	—	—
natural	T59.891	T59.892	T59.893	T59.894	—	—
nerve, not in war	T59.91	T59.92	T59.93	T59.94	—	—
oil	T52.0X1	T52.0X2	T52.0X3	T52.0X4	—	—
petroleum (liquefied) (distributed in mobile containers)	T59.891	T59.892	T59.893	T59.894	—	—
piped (pure or mixed with air)	T59.891	T59.892	T59.893	T59.894	—	—
piped (manufactured) (natural) NEC	T59.891	T59.892	T59.893	T59.894	—	—
producer	T58.8X1	T58.8X2	T58.8X3	T58.8X4	—	—
propane — see propane						
refrigerant (chlorofluoro-carbon)	T53.5X1	T53.5X2	T53.5X3	T53.5X4	—	—
not chlorofluoro-carbon	T59.891	T59.892	T59.893	T59.894	—	—
sewer	T59.91	T59.92	T59.93	T59.94	—	—
specified source NEC	T59.91	T59.92	T59.93	T59.94	—	—
stove (after combustion)	T58.11	T58.12	T58.13	T58.14	—	—
prior to combustion	T59.891	T59.892	T59.893	T59.894	—	—
tear	T59.3X1	T59.3X2	T59.3X3	T59.3X4	—	—
therapeutic	T41.5X1	T41.5X2	T41.5X3	T41.5X4	T41.5X5	T41.5X6
utility (for cooking, heating, or lighting) (piped) NEC	T59.891	T59.892	T59.893	T59.894	—	—
incomplete combustion of — see Carbon, monoxide, fuel, utilty						
in mobile container	T59.891	T59.892	T59.893	T59.894	—	—
piped (natural)	T59.891	T59.892	T59.893	T59.894	—	—
water	T58.11	T58.12	T58.13	T58.14	—	—
incomplete combustion of — see Carbon, monoxide, fuel, utility						
Gaultheria procumbens	T62.2X1	T62.2X2	T62.2X3	T62.2X4	—	—
Gefarnate	T44.3X1	T44.3X2	T44.3X3	T44.3X4	T44.3X5	T44.3X6
Gelatin (intravenous)	T45.8X1	T45.8X2	T45.8X3	T45.8X4	T45.8X5	T45.8X6
absorbable (sponge)	T45.7X1	T45.7X2	T45.7X3	T45.7X4	T45.7X5	T45.7X6
Gelfilm	T49.8X1	T49.8X2	T49.8X3	T49.8X4	T49.8X5	T49.8X6
Gelfoam	T45.7X1	T45.7X2	T45.7X3	T45.7X4	T45.7X5	T45.7X6
Gelsemine	T50.991	T50.992	T50.993	T50.994	T50.995	T50.996
Gelsemium (sempervirens)	T62.2X1	T62.2X2	T62.2X3	T62.2X4	—	—
Gemeprost	T48.0X1	T48.0X2	T48.0X3	T48.0X4	T48.0X5	T48.0X6
Gemfibrozil	T46.6X1	T46.6X2	T46.6X3	T46.6X4	T46.6X5	T46.6X6
Gemonil	T42.3X1	T42.3X2	T42.3X3	T42.3X4	T42.3X5	T42.3X6
Gentamicin	T36.5X1	T36.5X2	T36.5X3	T36.5X4	T36.5X5	T36.5X6

Substance	Poisoning, Accidental (unintentional)	Poisoning, Intentional Self-harm	Poisoning, Assault	Poisoning, Undetermined	Adverse Effect	Under-dosing
Gentamicin — *continued*						
ophthalmic preparation	T49.5X1	T49.5X2	T49.5X3	T49.5X4	T49.5X5	T49.5X6
topical NEC	T49.0X1	T49.0X2	T49.0X3	T49.0X4	T49.0X5	T49.0X6
Gentian	T47.5X1	T47.5X2	T47.5X3	T47.5X4	T47.5X5	T47.5X6
violet	T49.0X1	T49.0X2	T49.0X3	T49.0X4	T49.0X5	T49.0X6
Gepefrine	T44.4X1	T44.4X2	T44.4X3	T44.4X4	T44.4X5	T44.4X6
Gestonorone caproate	T38.5X1	T38.5X2	T38.5X3	T38.5X4	T38.5X5	T38.5X6
Gexane	T49.0X1	T49.0X2	T49.0X3	T49.0X4	T49.0X5	T49.0X6
Gila monster (venom)	T63.111	T63.112	T63.113	T63.114	—	—
Ginger	T47.5X1	T47.5X2	T47.5X3	T47.5X4	T47.5X5	T47.5X6
Jamaica — *see* Jamaica, ginger						
Gitalin	T46.0X1	T46.0X2	T46.0X3	T46.0X4	T46.0X5	T46.0X6
amorphous	T46.0X1	T46.0X2	T46.0X3	T46.0X4	T46.0X5	T46.0X6
Gitaloxin	T46.0X1	T46.0X2	T46.0X3	T46.0X4	T46.0X5	T46.0X6
Gitoxin	T46.0X1	T46.0X2	T46.0X3	T46.0X4	T46.0X5	T46.0X6
Glafenine	T39.8X1	T39.8X2	T39.8X3	T39.8X4	T39.8X5	T39.8X6
Glandular extract (medicinal) NEC	T50.Z91	T50.Z92	T50.Z93	T50.Z94	T50.Z95	T50.Z96
Glaucarubin	T37.3X1	T37.3X2	T37.3X3	T37.3X4	T37.3X5	T37.3X6
Glibenclamide	T38.3X1	T38.3X2	T38.3X3	T38.3X4	T38.3X5	T38.3X6
Glibornuride	T38.3X1	T38.3X2	T38.3X3	T38.3X4	T38.3X5	T38.3X6
Gliclazide	T38.3X1	T38.3X2	T38.3X3	T38.3X4	T38.3X5	T38.3X6
Glimidine	T38.3X1	T38.3X2	T38.3X3	T38.3X4	T38.3X5	T38.3X6
Glipizide	T38.3X1	T38.3X2	T38.3X3	T38.3X4	T38.3X5	T38.3X6
Gliquidone	T38.3X1	T38.3X2	T38.3X3	T38.3X4	T38.3X5	T38.3X6
Glisolamide	T38.3X1	T38.3X2	T38.3X3	T38.3X4	T38.3X5	T38.3X6
Glisoxepide	T38.3X1	T38.3X2	T38.3X3	T38.3X4	T38.3X5	T38.3X6
Globin zinc insulin	T38.3X1	T38.3X2	T38.3X3	T38.3X4	T38.3X5	T38.3X6
Globulin						
antilymphocytic	T50.Z11	T50.Z12	T50.Z13	T50.Z14	T50.Z15	T50.Z16
antirhesus	T50.Z11	T50.Z12	T50.Z13	T50.Z14	T50.Z15	T50.Z16
antivenin	T50.Z11	T50.Z12	T50.Z13	T50.Z14	T50.Z15	T50.Z16
antiviral	T50.Z11	T50.Z12	T50.Z13	T50.Z14	T50.Z15	T50.Z16
Glucagon	T38.3X1	T38.3X2	T38.3X3	T38.3X4	T38.3X5	T38.3X6
Glucocorticoids	T38.0X1	T38.0X2	T38.0X3	T38.0X4	T38.0X5	T38.0X6
Glucocorticosteroid	T38.0X1	T38.0X2	T38.0X3	T38.0X4	T38.0X5	T38.0X6
Gluconic acid	T50.991	T50.992	T50.993	T50.994	T50.995	T50.996
Glucosamine sulfate	T39.4X1	T39.4X2	T39.4X3	T39.4X4	T39.4X5	T39.4X6
Glucose	T50.3X1	T50.3X2	T50.3X3	T50.3X4	T50.3X5	T50.3X6
with sodium chloride	T50.3X1	T50.3X2	T50.3X3	T50.3X4	T50.3X5	T50.3X6
Glucosulfone sodium	T37.1X1	T37.1X2	T37.1X3	T37.1X4	T37.1X5	T37.1X6
Glucurolactone	T47.8X1	T47.8X2	T47.8X3	T47.8X4	T47.8X5	T47.8X6
Glue NEC	T52.8X1	T52.8X2	T52.8X3	T52.8X4	—	—
Glutamic acid	T47.5X1	T47.5X2	T47.5X3	T47.5X4	T47.5X5	T47.5X6
Glutaral (medicinal)	T49.0X1	T49.0X2	T49.0X3	T49.0X4	T49.0X5	T49.0X6
nonmedicinal	T65.891	T65.892	T65.893	T65.894	—	—
Glutaraldehyde (nonmedicinal)	T65.891	T65.892	T65.893	T65.894		
medicinal	T49.0X1	T49.0X2	T49.0X3	T49.0X4	T49.0X5	T49.0X6
Glutathione	T50.6X1	T50.6X2	T50.6X3	T50.6X4	T50.6X5	T50.6X6
Glutethimide	T42.6X1	T42.6X2	T42.6X3	T42.6X4	T42.6X5	T42.6X6
Glyburide	T38.3X1	T38.3X2	T38.3X3	T38.3X4	T38.3X5	T38.3X6
Glycerin	T47.4X1	T47.4X2	T47.4X3	T47.4X4	T47.4X5	T47.4X6
Glycerol	T47.4X1	T47.4X2	T47.4X3	T47.4X4	T47.4X5	T47.4X6
borax	T49.6X1	T49.6X2	T49.6X3	T49.6X4	T49.6X5	T49.6X6
intravenous	T50.3X1	T50.3X2	T50.3X3	T50.3X4	T50.3X5	T50.3X6
iodinated	T48.4X1	T48.4X2	T48.4X3	T48.4X4	T48.4X5	T48.4X6
Glycerophosphate	T50.991	T50.992	T50.993	T50.994	T50.995	T50.996
Glyceryl						
gualacolate	T48.4X1	T48.4X2	T48.4X3	T48.4X4	T48.4X5	T48.4X6
nitrate	T46.3X1	T46.3X2	T46.3X3	T46.3X4	T46.3X5	T46.3X6
triacetate (topical)	T49.0X1	T49.0X2	T49.0X3	T49.0X4	T49.0X5	T49.0X6
trinitrate	T46.3X1	T46.3X2	T46.3X3	T46.3X4	T46.3X5	T46.3X6
Glycine	T50.3X1	T50.3X2	T50.3X3	T50.3X4	T50.3X5	T50.3X6
Glyclopyramide	T38.3X1	T38.3X2	T38.3X3	T38.3X4	T38.3X5	T38.3X6
Glycobiarsol	T37.3X1	T37.3X2	T37.3X3	T37.3X4	T37.3X5	T37.3X6
Glycols (ether)	T52.3X1	T52.3X2	T52.3X3	T52.3X4	—	—
Glyconiazide	T37.1X1	T37.1X2	T37.1X3	T37.1X4	T37.1X5	T37.1X6
Glycopyrrolate	T44.3X1	T44.3X2	T44.3X3	T44.3X4	T44.3X5	T44.3X6
Glycopyrronium	T44.3X1	T44.3X2	T44.3X3	T44.3X4	T44.3X5	T44.3X6
bromide	T44.3X1	T44.3X2	T44.3X3	T44.3X4	T44.3X5	T44.3X6
Glycoside, cardiac (stimulant)	T46.0X1	T46.0X2	T46.0X3	T46.0X4	T46.0X5	T46.0X6
Glycyclamide	T38.3X1	T38.3X2	T38.3X3	T38.3X4	T38.3X5	T38.3X6
Glycyrrhiza extract	T48.4X1	T48.4X2	T48.4X3	T48.4X4	T48.4X5	T48.4X6
Glycyrrhizic acid	T48.4X1	T48.4X2	T48.4X3	T48.4X4	T48.4X5	T48.4X6
Glycyrrhizinate potassium	T48.4X1	T48.4X2	T48.4X3	T48.4X4	T48.4X5	T48.4X6
Glymidine sodium	T38.3X1	T38.3X2	T38.3X3	T38.3X4	T38.3X5	T38.3X6
Glyphosate	T60.3X1	T60.3X2	T60.3X3	T60.3X4	—	—
Glyphylline	T48.6X1	T48.6X2	T48.6X3	T48.6X4	T48.6X5	T48.6X6
Gold						
colloidal (I98Au)	T45.1X1	T45.1X2	T45.1X3	T45.1X4	T45.1X5	T45.1X6
salts	T39.4X1	T39.4X2	T39.4X3	T39.4X4	T39.4X5	T39.4X6

Substance	Poisoning, Accidental (unintentional)	Poisoning, Intentional Self-harm	Poisoning, Assault	Poisoning, Undetermined	Adverse Effect	Under-dosing
Golden sulfide of antimony	T56.891	T56.892	T56.893	T56.894	—	—
Goldylocks	T62.2X1	T62.2X2	T62.2X3	T62.2X4	—	—
Gonadal tissue extract	T38.902	T38.902	T38.903	T38.904	T38.905	T38.906
female	T38.5X1	T38.5X2	T38.5X3	T38.5X4	T38.5X5	T38.5X6
male	T38.7X1	T38.7X2	T38.7X3	T38.7X4	T38.7X5	T38.7X6
Gonadorelin	T38.891	T38.892	T38.893	T38.894	T38.895	T38.896
Gonadotropin	T38.891	T38.892	T38.893	T38.894	T38.895	T38.896
chorionic	T38.891	T38.892	T38.893	T38.894	T38.895	T38.896
pituitary	T38.811	T38.812	T38.813	T38.814	T38.815	T38.816
Goserelin	T45.1X1	T45.1X2	T45.1X3	T45.1X4	T45.1X5	T45.1X6
Grain alcohol	T51.0X1	T51.0X2	T51.0X3	T51.0X4	—	—
Gramicidin	T49.0X1	T49.0X2	T49.0X3	T49.0X4	T49.0X5	T49.0X6
Granisetron	T45.0X1	T45.0X2	T45.0X3	T45.0X4	T45.0X5	T45.0X6
Gratiola officinalis	T62.2X1	T62.2X2	T62.2X3	T62.2X4	—	—
Grease	T65.891	T65.892	T65.893	T65.894	—	—
Green hellebore	T62.2X1	T62.2X2	T62.2X3	T62.2X4	—	—
Green soap	T49.2X1	T49.2X2	T49.2X3	T49.2X4	T49.2X5	T49.2X6
Grifulvin	T36.7X1	T36.7X2	T36.7X3	T36.7X4	T36.7X5	T36.7X6
Griseofulvin	T36.7X1	T36.7X2	T36.7X3	T36.7X4	T36.7X5	T36.7X6
Growth hormone	T38.811	T38.812	T38.813	T38.814	T38.815	T38.816
Guaiacol derivatives	T48.4X1	T48.4X2	T48.4X3	T48.4X4	T48.4X5	T48.4X6
Guaiac reagent	T50.991	T50.992	T50.993	T50.994	T50.995	T50.996
Guaifenesin	T48.4X1	T48.4X2	T48.4X3	T48.4X4	T48.4X5	T48.4X6
Guaimesal	T48.4X1	T48.4X2	T48.4X3	T48.4X4	T48.4X5	T48.4X6
Guaiphenesin	T48.4X1	T48.4X2	T48.4X3	T48.4X4	T48.4X5	T48.4X6
Guamecycline	T36.4X1	T36.4X2	T36.4X3	T36.4X4	T36.4X5	T36.4X6
Guanabenz	T46.5X1	T46.5X2	T46.5X3	T46.5X4	T46.5X5	T46.5X6
Guanacline	T46.5X1	T46.5X2	T46.5X3	T46.5X4	T46.5X5	T46.5X6
Guanadrel	T46.5X1	T46.5X2	T46.5X3	T46.5X4	T46.5X5	T46.5X6
Guanatol	T37.2X1	T37.2X2	T37.2X3	T37.2X4	T37.2X5	T37.2X6
Guanethidine	T46.5X1	T46.5X2	T46.5X3	T46.5X4	T46.5X5	T46.5X6
Guanfacine	T46.5X1	T46.5X2	T46.5X3	T46.5X4	T46.5X5	T46.5X6
Guano	T65.891	T65.892	T65.893	T65.894	—	—
Guanochlor	T46.5X1	T46.5X2	T46.5X3	T46.5X4	T46.5X5	T46.5X6
Guanoclor	T46.5X1	T46.5X2	T46.5X3	T46.5X4	T46.5X5	T46.5X6
Guanoctine	T46.5X1	T46.5X2	T46.5X3	T46.5X4	T46.5X5	T46.5X6
Guanoxabenz	T46.5X1	T46.5X2	T46.5X3	T46.5X4	T46.5X5	T46.5X6
Guanoxan	T46.5X1	T46.5X2	T46.5X3	T46.5X4	T46.5X5	T46.5X6
Guar gum (medicinal)	T46.6X1	T46.6X2	T46.6X3	T46.6X4	T46.6X5	T46.6X6
Hachimycin	T36.7X1	T36.7X2	T36.7X3	T36.7X4	T36.7X5	T36.7X6
Hair						
dye	T49.4X1	T49.4X2	T49.4X3	T49.4X4	T49.4X5	T49.4X6
preparation NEC	T49.4X1	T49.4X2	T49.4X3	T49.4X4	T49.4X5	T49.4X6
Halazepam	T42.4X1	T42.4X2	T42.4X3	T42.4X4	T42.4X5	T42.4X6
Halcinolone	T49.0X1	T49.0X2	T49.0X3	T49.0X4	T49.0X5	T49.0X6
Halcinonide	T49.0X1	T49.0X2	T49.0X3	T49.0X4	T49.0X5	T49.0X6
Halethazole	T49.0X1	T49.0X2	T49.0X3	T49.0X4	T49.0X5	T49.0X6
Hallucinogen NOS	T40.901	T40.902	T40.903	T40.904	T40.905	T40.906
specified NEC	T40.991	T40.992	T40.993	T40.994	T40.995	T40.996
Halofantrine	T37.2X1	T37.2X2	T37.2X3	T37.2X4	T37.2X5	T37.2X6
Halofenate	T46.6X1	T46.6X2	T46.6X3	T46.6X4	T46.6X5	T46.6X6
Halometasone	T49.0X1	T49.0X2	T49.0X3	T49.0X4	T49.0X5	T49.0X6
Haloperidol	T43.4X1	T43.4X2	T43.4X3	T43.4X4	T43.4X5	T43.4X6
Haloprogin	T49.0X1	T49.0X2	T49.0X3	T49.0X4	T49.0X5	T49.0X6
Halotex	T49.0X1	T49.0X2	T49.0X3	T49.0X4	T49.0X5	T49.0X6
Halothane	T41.0X1	T41.0X2	T41.0X3	T41.0X4	T41.0X5	T41.0X6
Haloxazolam	T42.4X1	T42.4X2	T42.4X3	T42.4X4	T42.4X5	T42.4X6
Halquinols	T49.0X1	T49.0X2	T49.0X3	T49.0X4	T49.0X5	T49.0X6
Hamamelis	T49.2X1	T49.2X2	T49.2X3	T49.2X4	T49.2X5	T49.2X6
Haptendextran	T45.8X1	T45.8X2	T45.8X3	T45.8X4	T45.8X5	T45.8X6
Harmonyl	T46.5X1	T46.5X2	T46.5X3	T46.5X4	T46.5X5	T46.5X6
Hartman's solution	T50.3X1	T50.3X2	T50.3X3	T50.3X4	T50.3X5	T50.3X6
Hashish	T40.7X1	T40.7X2	T40.7X3	T40.7X4	T40.7X5	T40.7X6
Hawaiian Woodrose seeds	T40.991	T40.992	T40.993	T40.994	—	—
HCB	T60.3X1	T60.3X2	T60.3X3	T60.3X4	—	—
HCH	T53.6X1	T53.6X2	T53.6X3	T53.6X4	—	—
medicinal	T49.0X1	T49.0X2	T49.0X3	T49.0X4	T49.0X5	T49.0X6
HCN	T57.3X1	T57.3X2	T57.3X3	T57.3X4	—	—
Headache cures, drugs, powders NEC	T50.901	T50.902	T50.903	T50.904	T50.905	T50.906
Heavenly Blue (morning glory)	T40.991	T40.992	T40.993	T40.994	—	—
Heavy metal antidote	T45.8X1	T45.8X2	T45.8X3	T45.8X4	T45.8X5	T45.8X6
Hedaquinium	T49.0X1	T49.0X2	T49.0X3	T49.0X4	T49.0X5	T49.0X6
Hedge hyssop	T62.2X1	T62.2X2	T62.2X3	T62.2X4	—	—
Heet	T49.8X1	T49.8X2	T49.8X3	T49.8X4	T49.8X5	T49.8X6
Helenin	T37.4X1	T37.4X2	T37.4X3	T37.4X4	T37.4X5	T37.4X6
Helium (nonmedicinal) NEC	T59.891	T59.892	T59.893	T59.894	—	—
medicinal	T48.991	T48.992	T48.993	T48.994	T48.995	T48.996
Hellebore (black) (green) (white)	T62.2X1	T62.2X2	T62.2X3	T62.2X4	—	—
Hematin	T45.8X1	T45.8X2	T45.8X3	T45.8X4	T45.8X5	T45.8X6

Substance	Poisoning, Accidental (unintentional)	Poisoning, Intentional Self-harm	Poisoning, Assault	Poisoning, Undetermined	Adverse Effect	Under-dosing
Hematinic preparation	T45.8X1	T45.8X2	T45.8X3	T45.8X4	T45.8X5	T45.8X6
Hematological agent	T45.91	T45.92	T45.93	T45.94	T45.95	T45.96
specified NEC	T45.8X1	T45.8X2	T45.8X3	T45.8X4	T45.8X5	T45.8X6
Hemlock	T62.2X1	T62.2X2	T62.2X3	T62.2X4	—	—
Hemostatic	T45.621	T45.622	T45.623	T45.624	T45.625	T45.626
drug, systemic	T45.621	T45.622	T45.623	T45.624	T45.625	T45.626
Hemostyptic	T49.4X1	T49.4X2	T49.4X3	T49.4X4	T49.4X5	T49.4X6
Henbane	T62.2X1	T62.2X2	T62.2X3	T62.2X4	—	—
Heparin (sodium)	T45.511	T45.512	T45.513	T45.514	T45.515	T45.516
action reverser	T45.7X1	T45.7X2	T45.7X3	T45.7X4	T45.7X5	T45.7X6
Heparin-fraction	T45.511	T45.512	T45.513	T45.514	T45.515	T45.516
Heparinoid (systemic)	T45.511	T45.512	T45.513	T45.514	T45.515	T45.516
Hepatic secretion stimulant	T47.8X1	T47.8X2	T47.8X3	T47.8X4	T47.8X5	T47.8X6
Hepatitis B						
immune globulin	T50.Z11	T50.Z12	T50.Z13	T50.Z14	T50.Z15	T50.Z16
vaccine	T50.B91	T50.B92	T50.B93	T50.B94	T50.B95	T50.B96
Hepronicate	T46.7X1	T46.7X2	T46.7X3	T46.7X4	T46.7X5	T46.7X6
Heptabarb	T42.3X1	T42.3X2	T42.3X3	T42.3X4	T42.3X5	T42.3X6
Heptabarbital	T42.3X1	T42.3X2	T42.3X3	T42.3X4	T42.3X5	T42.3X6
Heptabarbitone	T42.3X1	T42.3X2	T42.3X3	T42.3X4	T42.3X5	T42.3X6
Heptachlor	T60.1X1	T60.1X2	T60.1X3	T60.1X4	—	—
Heptalgin	T40.2X1	T40.2X2	T40.2X3	T40.2X4	T40.2X5	T40.2X6
Heptaminol	T46.3X1	T46.3X2	T46.3X3	T46.3X4	T46.3X5	T46.3X6
Herbicide NEC	T60.3X1	T60.3X2	T60.3X3	T60.3X4	—	—
Heroin	T40.1X1	T40.1X2	T40.1X3	T40.1X4	—	—
Herplex	T49.5X1	T49.5X2	T49.5X3	T49.5X4	T49.5X5	T49.5X6
HES	T45.8X1	T45.8X2	T45.8X3	T45.8X4	T45.8X5	T45.8X6
Hesperidin	T46.991	T46.992	T46.993	T46.994	T46.995	T46.996
Hetacillin	T36.0X1	T36.0X2	T36.0X3	T36.0X4	T36.0X5	T36.0X6
Hetastarch	T45.8X1	T45.8X2	T45.8X3	T45.8X4	T45.8X5	T45.8X6
HETP	T60.0X1	T60.0X2	T60.0X3	T60.0X4	—	—
Hexachlorobenzene (vapor)	T60.3X1	T60.3X2	T60.3X3	T60.3X4	—	—
Hexachlorocyclohexane	T53.6X1	T53.6X2	T53.6X3	T53.6X4	—	—
Hexachlorophene	T49.0X1	T49.0X2	T49.0X3	T49.0X4	T49.0X5	T49.0X6
Hexadiline	T46.3X1	T46.3X2	T46.3X3	T46.3X4	T46.3X5	T46.3X6
Hexadimethrine (bromide)	T45.7X1	T45.7X2	T45.7X3	T45.7X4	T45.7X5	T45.7X6
Hexadylamine	T46.3X1	T46.3X2	T46.3X3	T46.3X4	T46.3X5	T46.3X6
Hexaethyl tetraphosphate	T60.0X1	T60.0X2	T60.0X3	T60.0X4	—	—
Hexafluorenium bromide	T48.1X1	T48.1X2	T48.1X3	T48.1X4	T48.1X5	T48.1X6
Hexafluronium (bromide)	T48.1X1	T48.1X2	T48.1X3	T48.1X4	T48.1X5	T48.1X6
Hexa-germ	T49.2X1	T49.2X2	T49.2X3	T49.2X4	T49.2X5	T49.2X6
Hexahydrobenzol	T52.8X1	T52.8X2	T52.8X3	T52.8X4	—	—
Hexahydrocresol(s)	T51.8X1	T51.8X2	T51.8X3	T51.8X4	—	—
arsenide	T57.0X1	T57.0X2	T57.0X3	T57.0X4	—	—
arseniurated	T57.0X1	T57.0X2	T57.0X3	T57.0X4	—	—
cyanide	T57.3X1	T57.3X2	T57.3X3	T57.3X4	—	—
gas	T59.891	T59.892	T59.893	T59.894	—	—
Fluoride (liquid)	T57.8X1	T57.8X2	T57.8X3	T57.8X4	—	—
vapor	T59.891	T59.892	T59.893	T59.894	—	—
phophorated	T60.0X1	T60.0X2	T60.0X3	T60.0X4	—	—
sulfate	T57.8X1	T57.8X2	T57.8X3	T57.8X4	—	—
sulfide (gas)	T59.6X1	T59.6X2	T59.6X3	T59.6X4	—	—
arseniurated	T57.0X1	T57.0X2	T57.0X3	T57.0X4	—	—
sulfurated	T57.8X1	T57.8X2	T57.8X3	T57.8X4	—	—
Hexahydrophenol	T51.8X1	T51.8X2	T51.8X3	T51.8X4	—	—
Hexalen	T51.8X1	T51.8X2	T51.8X3	T51.8X4	—	—
Hexamethonium bromide	T44.2X1	T44.2X2	T44.2X3	T44.2X4	T44.2X5	T44.2X6
Hexamethylene	T52.8X1	T52.8X2	T52.8X3	T52.8X4	—	—
Hexamethylmelamine	T45.1X1	T45.1X2	T45.1X3	T45.1X4	T45.1X5	T45.1X6
Hexamidine	T49.0X1	T49.0X2	T49.0X3	T49.0X4	T49.0X5	T49.0X6
Hexamine (mandelate)	T37.8X1	T37.8X2	T37.8X3	T37.8X4	T37.8X5	T37.8X6
Hexanone, 2-hexanone	T52.4X1	T52.4X2	T52.4X3	T52.4X4	—	—
Hexanuorenium	T48.1X1	T48.1X2	T48.1X3	T48.1X4	T48.1X5	T48.1X6
Hexapropymate	T42.6X1	T42.6X2	T42.6X3	T42.6X4	T42.6X5	T42.6X6
Hexasonium iodide	T44.3X1	T44.3X2	T44.3X3	T44.3X4	T44.3X5	T44.3X6
Hexcarbacholine bromide	T48.1X1	T48.1X2	T48.1X3	T48.1X4	T48.1X5	T48.1X6
Hexemal	T42.3X1	T42.3X2	T42.3X3	T42.3X4	T42.3X5	T42.3X6
Hexestrol	T38.5X1	T38.5X2	T38.5X3	T38.5X4	T38.5X5	T38.5X6
Hexethal (sodium)	T42.3X1	T42.3X2	T42.3X3	T42.3X4	T42.3X5	T42.3X6
Hexetidine	T37.8X1	T37.8X2	T37.8X3	T37.8X4	T37.8X5	T37.8X6
Hexobarbital	T42.3X1	T42.3X2	T42.3X3	T42.3X4	T42.3X5	T42.3X6
rectal	T41.291	T41.292	T41.293	T41.294	T41.295	T41.296
sodium	T41.1X1	T41.1X2	T41.1X3	T41.1X4	T41.1X5	T41.1X6
Hexobendine	T46.3X1	T46.3X2	T46.3X3	T46.3X4	T46.3X5	T46.3X6
Hexocyclium	T44.3X1	T44.3X2	T44.3X3	T44.3X4	T44.3X5	T44.3X6
metilsulfate	T44.3X1	T44.3X2	T44.3X3	T44.3X4	T44.3X5	T44.3X6
Hexoestrol	T38.5X1	T38.5X2	T38.5X3	T38.5X4	T38.5X5	T38.5X6
Hexone	T52.4X1	T52.4X2	T52.4X3	T52.4X4	—	—
Hexoprenaline	T48.6X1	T48.6X2	T48.6X3	T48.6X4	T48.6X5	T48.6X6
Hexylcaine	T41.3X1	T41.3X2	T41.3X3	T41.3X4	T41.3X5	T41.3X6
Hexylresorcinol	T52.2X1	T52.2X2	T52.2X3	T52.2X4	—	—

Substance	Poisoning, Accidental (unintentional)	Poisoning, Intentional Self-harm	Poisoning, Assault	Poisoning, Undetermined	Adverse Effect	Under-dosing
HGH (human growth hormone)	T38.811	T38.812	T38.813	T38.814	T38.815	T38.816
Hinkle's pills	T47.2X1	T47.2X2	T47.2X3	T47.2X4	T47.2X5	T47.2X6
Histalog	T50.8X1	T50.8X2	T50.8X3	T50.8X4	T50.8X5	T50.8X6
Histamine (phosphate)	T50.8X1	T50.8X2	T50.8X3	T50.8X4	T50.8X5	T50.8X6
Histoplasmin	T50.8X1	T50.8X2	T50.8X3	T50.8X4	T50.8X5	T50.8X6
Holly berries	T62.2X1	T62.2X2	T62.2X3	T62.2X4	—	—
Homatropine	T44.3X1	T44.3X2	T44.3X3	T44.3X4	T44.3X5	T44.3X6
methylbromide	T44.3X1	T44.3X2	T44.3X3	T44.3X4	T44.3X5	T44.3X6
Homochlorcyclizine	T45.0X1	T45.0X2	T45.0X3	T45.0X4	T45.0X5	T45.0X6
Homosalate	T49.3X1	T49.3X2	T49.3X3	T49.3X4	T49.3X5	T49.3X6
Homo-tet	T50.Z11	T50.Z12	T50.Z13	T50.Z14	T50.Z15	T50.Z16
Hormone	T38.801	T38.802	T38.803	T38.804	T38.805	T38.806
adrenal cortical steroids	T38.0X1	T38.0X2	T38.0X3	T38.0X4	T38.0X5	T38.0X6
androgenic	T38.7X1	T38.7X2	T38.7X3	T38.7X4	T38.7X5	T38.7X6
anterior pituitary NEC	T38.811	T38.812	T38.813	T38.814	T38.815	T38.816
antidiabetic agents	T38.3X1	T38.3X2	T38.3X3	T38.3X4	T38.3X5	T38.3X6
antidiuretic	T38.891	T38.892	T38.893	T38.894	T38.895	T38.896
cancer therapy	T45.1X1	T45.1X2	T45.1X3	T45.1X4	T45.1X5	T45.1X6
follicle stimulating	T38.811	T38.812	T38.813	T38.814	T38.815	T38.816
gonadotropic	T38.891	T38.892	T38.893	T38.894	T38.895	T38.896
pituitary	T38.811	T38.812	T38.813	T38.814	T38.815	T38.816
growth	T38.811	T38.812	T38.813	T38.814	T38.815	T38.816
luteinizing	T38.811	T38.812	T38.813	T38.814	T38.815	T38.816
ovarian	T38.5X1	T38.5X2	T38.5X3	T38.5X4	T38.5X5	T38.5X6
oxytocic	T48.0X1	T48.0X2	T48.0X3	T48.0X4	T48.0X5	T48.0X6
parathyroid (derivatives)	T50.991	T50.992	T50.993	T50.994	T50.995	T50.996
pituitary (posterior) NEC	T38.891	T38.892	T38.893	T38.894	T38.895	T38.896
anterior	T38.811	T38.812	T38.813	T38.814	T38.815	T38.816
specified, NEC	T38.891	T38.892	T38.893	T38.894	T38.895	T38.896
thyroid	T38.1X1	T38.1X2	T38.1X3	T38.1X4	T38.1X5	T38.1X6
Hornet (sting)	T63.451	T63.452	T63.453	T63.454	—	—
Horse anti-human lymphocytic serum	T50.Z11	T50.Z12	T50.Z13	T50.Z14	T50.Z15	T50.Z16
Horticulture agent NEC	T65.91	T65.92	T65.93	T65.94	—	—
with pesticide	T60.91	T60.92	T60.93	T60.94	—	—
Human						
albumin	T45.8X1	T45.8X2	T45.8X3	T45.8X4	T45.8X5	T45.8X6
growth hormone (HGH)	T38.811	T38.812	T38.813	T38.814	T38.815	T38.816
immune serum	T50.Z11	T50.Z12	T50.Z13	T50.Z14	T50.Z15	T50.Z16
Hyaluronidase	T45.3X1	T45.3X2	T45.3X3	T45.3X4	T45.3X5	T45.3X6
Hyazyme	T45.3X1	T45.3X2	T45.3X3	T45.3X4	T45.3X5	T45.3X6
Hycodan	T40.2X1	T40.2X2	T40.2X3	T40.2X4	T40.2X5	T40.2X6
Hydantoin derivative NEC	T42.0X1	T42.0X2	T42.0X3	T42.0X4	T42.0X5	T42.0X6
Hydeltra	T38.0X1	T38.0X2	T38.0X3	T38.0X4	T38.0X5	T38.0X6
Hydergine	T44.6X1	T44.6X2	T44.6X3	T44.6X4	T44.6X5	T44.6X6
Hydrabamine penicillin	T36.0X1	T36.0X2	T36.0X3	T36.0X4	T36.0X5	T36.0X6
Hydralazine	T46.5X1	T46.5X2	T46.5X3	T46.5X4	T46.5X5	T46.5X6
Hydrargaphen	T49.0X1	T49.0X2	T49.0X3	T49.0X4	T49.0X5	T49.0X6
Hydrargyri aminochloridum	T49.0X1	T49.0X2	T49.0X3	T49.0X4	T49.0X5	T49.0X6
Hydrastine	T48.291	T48.292	T48.293	T48.294	T48.295	T48.296
Hydrazine	T54.1X1	T54.1X2	T54.1X3	T54.1X4	—	—
monoamine oxidase inhibitors	T43.1X1	T43.1X2	T43.1X3	T43.1X4	T43.1X5	T43.1X6
Hydrazoic acid, azides	T54.2X1	T54.2X2	T54.2X3	T54.2X4	—	—
Hydriodic acid	T48.4X1	T48.4X2	T48.4X3	T48.4X4	T48.4X5	T48.4X6
Hydrocarbon gas	T59.891	T59.892	T59.893	T59.894	—	—
incomplete combustion of — see Carbon, monoxide, fuel, utility						
liquefied (mobile container)	T59.891	T59.892	T59.893	T59.894	—	—
piped (natural)	T59.891	T59.892	T59.893	T59.894	—	—
Hydrochloric acid (liquid)	T54.2X1	T54.2X2	T54.2X3	T54.2X4	—	—
medicinal (digestant)	T47.5X1	T47.5X2	T47.5X3	T47.5X4	T47.5X5	T47.5X6
vapor	T59.891	T59.892	T59.893	T59.894	—	—
Hydrochlorothiazide	T50.2X1	T50.2X2	T50.2X3	T50.2X4	T50.2X5	T50.2X6
Hydrocodone	T40.2X1	T40.2X2	T40.2X3	T40.2X4	T40.2X5	T40.2X6
Hydrocortisone (derivatives)	T38.0X1	T38.0X2	T38.0X3	T38.0X4	T38.0X5	—
aceponate	T49.0X1	T49.0X2	T49.0X3	T49.0X4	T49.0X5	T49.0X6
ENT agent	T49.6X1	T49.6X2	T49.6X3	T49.6X4	T49.6X5	T49.6X6
ophthalmic preparation	T49.5X1	T49.5X2	T49.5X3	T49.5X4	T49.5X5	T49.5X6
topical NEC	T49.0X1	T49.0X2	T49.0X3	T49.0X4	T49.0X5	T49.0X6
Hydrocortone	T38.0X1	T38.0X2	T38.0X3	T38.0X4	T38.0X5	T38.0X6
ENT agent	T49.6X1	T49.6X2	T49.6X3	T49.6X4	T49.6X5	T49.6X6
ophthalmic preparation	T49.5X1	T49.5X2	T49.5X3	T49.5X4	T49.5X5	T49.5X6
topical NEC	T49.0X1	T49.0X2	T49.0X3	T49.0X4	T49.0X5	T49.0X6
Hydrocyanic acid (liquid)	T57.3X1	T57.3X2	T57.3X3	T57.3X4	—	—
gas	T65.0X1	T65.0X2	T65.0X3	T65.0X4	—	—
Hydroflumethiazide	T50.2X1	T50.2X2	T50.2X3	T50.2X4	T50.2X5	T50.2X6
Hydrofluoric acid (liquid)	T54.2X1	T54.2X2	T54.2X3	T54.2X4	—	—

Substance	Poisoning, Accidental (unintentional)	Poisoning, Intentional Self-harm	Poisoning, Assault	Poisoning, Undetermined	Adverse Effect	Under-dosing
Hydrofluoric acid — *continued*						
vapor	T59.891	T59.892	T59.893	T59.894	—	—
Hydrogen						
arsenide	T57.0X1	T57.0X2	T57.0X3	T57.0X4	—	—
arseniureted	T57.0X1	T57.0X2	T57.0X3	T57.0X4	—	—
chloride	T57.8X1	T57.8X2	T57.8X3	T57.8X4	—	—
cyanide (salts)	T57.3X1	T57.3X2	T57.3X3	T57.3X4	—	—
gas	T57.3X1	T57.3X2	T57.3X3	T57.3X4	—	—
Fluoride	T59.5X1	T59.5X2	T59.5X3	T59.5X4	—	—
vapor	T59.5X1	T59.5X2	T59.5X3	T59.5X4	—	—
peroxide	T49.0X1	T49.0X2	T49.0X3	T49.0X4	T49.0X5	T49.0X6
phosphureted	T57.1X1	T57.1X2	T57.1X3	T57.1X4	—	—
sulfide	T59.6X1	T59.6X2	T59.6X3	T59.6X4	—	—
arseniureted	T57.0X1	T57.0X2	T57.0X3	T57.0X4	—	—
sulfureted	T59.6X1	T59.6X2	T59.6X3	T59.6X4	—	—
Hydromethylpyridine	T46.7X1	T46.7X2	T46.7X3	T46.7X4	T46.7X5	T46.7X6
Hydromorphinol	T40.2X1	T40.2X2	T40.2X3	T40.2X4	—	—
Hydromorphinone	T40.2X1	T40.2X2	T40.2X3	T40.2X4	T40.2X5	T40.2X6
Hydromorphone	T40.2X1	T40.2X2	T40.2X3	T40.2X4	T40.2X5	T40.2X6
Hydromox	T50.2X1	T50.2X2	T50.2X3	T50.2X4	T50.2X5	T50.2X6
Hydrophilic lotion	T49.3X1	T49.3X2	T49.3X3	T49.3X4	T49.3X5	T49.3X6
Hydroquinidine	T46.2X1	T46.2X2	T46.2X3	T46.2X4	T46.2X5	T46.2X6
Hydroquinone	T52.2X1	T52.2X2	T52.2X3	T52.2X4	—	—
vapor	T59.891	T59.892	T59.893	T59.894	—	—
Hydrosulfuric acid (gas)	T59.6X1	T59.6X2	T59.6X3	T59.6X4	—	—
Hydrotalcite	T47.1X1	T47.1X2	T47.1X3	T47.1X4	T47.1X5	T47.1X6
Hydrous wool fat	T49.3X1	T49.3X2	T49.3X3	T49.3X4	T49.3X5	T49.3X6
Hydroxide, caustic	T54.3X1	T54.3X2	T54.3X3	T54.3X4	—	—
Hydroxocobalamin	T45.8X1	T45.8X2	T45.8X3	T45.8X4	T45.8X5	T45.8X6
Hydroxyamphetamine	T49.5X1	T49.5X2	T49.5X3	T49.5X4	T49.5X5	T49.5X6
Hydroxycarbamide	T45.1X1	T45.1X2	T45.1X3	T45.1X4	T45.1X5	T45.1X6
Hydroxychloroquine	T37.8X1	T37.8X2	T37.8X3	T37.8X4	T37.8X5	T37.8X6
Hydroxydihydrocodeinone	T40.2X1	T40.2X2	T40.2X3	T40.2X4	T40.2X5	T40.2X6
Hydroxyestrone	T38.5X1	T38.5X2	T38.5X3	T38.5X4	T38.5X5	T38.5X6
Hydroxyethyl starch	T45.8X1	T45.8X2	T45.8X3	T45.8X4	T45.8X5	T45.8X6
Hydroxymethylpentanone	T52.4X1	T52.4X2	T52.4X3	T52.4X4	—	—
Hydroxyphenamate	T43.591	T43.592	T43.593	T43.594	T43.595	T43.596
Hydroxyphenylbutazone	T39.2X1	T39.2X2	T39.2X3	T39.2X4	T39.2X5	T39.2X6
Hydroxyprogesterone	T38.5X1	T38.5X2	T38.5X3	T38.5X4	T38.5X5	T38.5X6
caproate	T38.5X1	T38.5X2	T38.5X3	T38.5X4	T38.5X5	T38.5X6
Hydroxyquinoline (derivatives) NEC	T37.8X1	T37.8X2	T37.8X3	T37.8X4	T37.8X5	T37.8X6
Hydroxystilbamidine	T37.3X1	T37.3X2	T37.3X3	T37.3X4	T37.3X5	T37.3X6
Hydroxytoluene (nonmedicinal)	T54.0X1	T54.0X2	T54.0X3	T54.0X4	—	—
medicinal	T49.0X1	T49.0X2	T49.0X3	T49.0X4	T49.0X5	T49.0X6
Hydroxyurea	T45.1X1	T45.1X2	T45.1X3	T45.1X4	T45.1X5	T45.1X6
Hydroxyzine	T43.591	T43.592	T43.593	T43.594	T43.595	T43.596
Hyoscine	T44.3X1	T44.3X2	T44.3X3	T44.3X4	T44.3X5	T44.3X6
Hyoscyamine	T44.3X1	T44.3X2	T44.3X3	T44.3X4	T44.3X5	T44.3X6
Hyoscyamus	T44.3X1	T44.3X2	T44.3X3	T44.3X4	T44.3X5	T44.3X6
dry extract	T44.3X1	T44.3X2	T44.3X3	T44.3X4	T44.3X5	T44.3X6
Hypaque	T50.8X1	T50.8X2	T50.8X3	T50.8X4	T50.8X5	T50.8X6
Hypertussis	T50.Z11	T50.Z12	T50.Z13	T50.Z14	T50.Z15	T50.Z16
Hypnotic	T42.71	T42.72	T42.73	T42.74	T42.75	T42.76
anticonvulsant	T42.71	T42.72	T42.73	T42.74	T42.75	T42.76
specified NEC	T42.6X1	T42.6X2	T42.6X3	T42.6X4	T42.6X5	T42.6X6
Hypochlorite	T49.0X1	T49.0X2	T49.0X3	T49.0X4	T49.0X5	T49.0X6
Hypophysis, posterior	T38.891	T38.892	T38.893	T38.894	T38.895	T38.896
Hypotensive NEC	T46.5X1	T46.5X2	T46.5X3	T46.5X4	T46.5X5	T46.5X6
Hypromellose	T49.5X1	T49.5X2	T49.5X3	T49.5X4	T49.5X5	T49.5X6
Ibacitabine	T37.5X1	T37.5X2	T37.5X3	T37.5X4	T37.5X5	T37.5X6
Ibopamine	T44.991	T44.992	T44.993	T44.994	T44.995	T44.996
Ibufenac	T39.311	T39.312	T39.313	T39.314	T39.315	T39.316
Ibuprofen	T39.311	T39.312	T39.313	T39.314	T39.315	T39.316
Ibuproxam	T39.311	T39.312	T39.313	T39.314	T39.315	T39.316
Ibuterol	T48.6X1	T48.6X2	T48.6X3	T48.6X4	T48.6X5	T48.6X6
Ichthammol	T49.0X1	T49.0X2	T49.0X3	T49.0X4	T49.0X5	T49.0X6
Ichthyol	T49.4X1	T49.4X2	T49.4X3	T49.4X4	T49.4X5	T49.4X6
Idarubicin	T45.1X1	T45.1X2	T45.1X3	T45.1X4	T45.1X5	T45.1X6
Idrocilamide	T42.8X1	T42.8X2	T42.8X3	T42.8X4	T42.8X5	T42.8X6
Ifenprodil	T46.7X1	T46.7X2	T46.7X3	T46.7X4	T46.7X5	T46.7X6
Ifosfamide	T45.1X1	T45.1X2	T45.1X3	T45.1X4	T45.1X5	T45.1X6
Iletin	T38.3X1	T38.3X2	T38.3X3	T38.3X4	T38.3X5	T38.3X6
Ilex	T62.2X1	T62.2X2	T62.2X3	T62.2X4	—	—
Illuminating gas (after combustion)	T58.11	T58.12	T58.13	T58.14	—	—
prior to combustion	T59.891	T59.892	T59.893	T59.894	—	—
Ilopan	T45.2X1	T45.2X2	T45.2X3	T45.2X4	T45.2X5	T45.2X6
Iloprost	T46.7X1	T46.7X2	T46.7X3	T46.7X4	T46.7X5	T46.7X6
Ilotycin	T36.3X1	T36.3X2	T36.3X3	T36.3X4	T36.3X5	T36.3X6
ophthalmic preparation	T49.5X1	T49.5X2	T49.5X3	T49.5X4	T49.5X5	T49.5X6
topical NEC	T49.0X1	T49.0X2	T49.0X3	T49.0X4	T49.0X5	T49.0X6

Substance	Poisoning, Accidental (unintentional)	Poisoning, Intentional Self-harm	Poisoning, Assault	Poisoning, Undetermined	Adverse Effect	Under-dosing
Imidazole-4-carboxamide	T45.1X1	T45.1X2	T45.1X3	T45.1X4	T45.1X5	T45.1X6
Iminostilbene	T42.1X1	T42.1X2	T42.1X3	T42.1X4	T42.1X5	T42.1X6
Imipenem	T36.0X1	T36.0X2	T36.0X3	T36.0X4	T36.0X5	T36.0X6
Imipramine	T43.011	T43.012	T43.013	T43.014	T43.015	T43.016
Immu-G	T50.Z11	T50.Z12	T50.Z13	T50.Z14	T50.Z15	T50.Z16
Immuglobin	T50.Z11	T50.Z12	T50.Z13	T50.Z14	T50.Z15	T50.Z16
Immune						
globulin	T50.Z11	T50.Z12	T50.Z13	T50.Z14	T50.Z15	T50.Z16
serum globulin	T50.Z11	T50.Z12	T50.Z13	T50.Z14	T50.Z15	T50.Z16
Immunoglobin human (intravenous) (normal) unmodified	T50.Z11	T50.Z12	T50.Z13	T50.Z14	T50.Z15	T50.Z16
Immunosuppressive drug	T45.1X1	T45.1X2	T45.1X3	T45.1X4	T45.1X5	T45.1X6
Immu-tetanus	T50.Z11	T50.Z12	T50.Z13	T50.Z14	T50.Z15	T50.Z16
Indalpine	T43.221	T43.222	T43.223	T43.224	T43.225	T43.226
Indanazoline	T48.5X1	T48.5X2	T48.5X3	T48.5X4	T48.5X5	T48.5X6
Indandione (derivatives)	T45.511	T45.512	T45.513	T45.514	T45.515	T45.516
Indapamide	T46.5X1	T46.5X2	T46.5X3	T46.5X4	T46.5X5	T46.5X6
Indendione (derivatives)	T45.511	T45.512	T45.513	T45.514	T45.515	T45.516
Indenolol	T44.7X1	T44.7X2	T44.7X3	T44.7X4	T44.7X5	T44.7X6
Inderal	T44.7X1	T44.7X2	T44.7X3	T44.7X4	T44.7X5	T44.7X6
Indian						
hemp	T40.7X1	T40.7X2	T40.7X3	T40.7X4	T40.7X5	T40.7X6
tobacco	T62.2X1	T62.2X2	T62.2X3	T62.2X4	—	—
Indigo carmine	T50.8X1	T50.8X2	T50.8X3	T50.8X4	T50.8X5	T50.8X6
Indobufen	T45.521	T45.522	T45.523	T45.524	T45.525	T45.526
Indocin	T39.2X1	T39.2X2	T39.2X3	T39.2X4	T39.2X5	T39.2X6
Indocyanine green	T50.8X1	T50.8X2	T50.8X3	T50.8X4	T50.8X5	T50.8X6
Indometacin	T39.391	T39.392	T39.393	T39.394	T39.395	T39.396
Indomethacin	T39.391	T39.392	T39.393	T39.394	T39.395	T39.396
farnesil	T39.4X1	T39.4X2	T39.4X3	T39.4X4	T39.4X5	T39.4X6
Indoramin	T44.6X1	T44.6X2	T44.6X3	T44.6X4	T44.6X5	T44.6X6
Industrial						
alcohol	T51.0X1	T51.0X2	T51.0X3	T51.0X4	—	—
fumes	T59.891	T59.892	T59.893	T59.894	—	—
solvents (fumes) (vapors)	T52.91	T52.92	T52.93	T52.94	—	—
Influenza vaccine	T50.B91	T50.B92	T50.B93	T50.B94	T50.B95	T50.B96
Ingested substance NEC	T65.91	T65.92	T65.93	T65.94	—	—
INH	T37.1X1	T37.1X2	T37.1X3	T37.1X4	T37.1X5	T37.1X6
Inhalation, gas (noxious) — *see* Gas						
Inhibitor						
angiotensin-converting enzyme	T46.4X1	T46.4X2	T46.4X3	T46.4X4	T46.4X5	T46.4X6
carbonic anhydrase	T50.2X1	T50.2X2	T50.2X3	T50.2X4	T50.2X5	T50.2X6
fibrinolysis	T45.621	T45.622	T45.623	T45.624	T45.625	T45.626
monoamine oxidase NEC	T43.1X1	T43.1X2	T43.1X3	T43.1X4	T43.1X5	T43.1X6
hydrazine	T43.1X1	T43.1X2	T43.1X3	T43.1X4	T43.1X5	T43.1X6
postsynaptic	T43.8X1	T43.8X2	T43.8X3	T43.8X4	T43.8X5	T43.8X6
prothrombin synthesis	T45.511	T45.512	T45.513	T45.514	T45.515	T45.516
Ink	T65.891	T65.892	T65.893	T65.894	—	—
Inorganic substance NEC	T57.91	T57.92	T57.93	T57.94	—	—
Inosine pranobex	T37.5X1	T37.5X2	T37.5X3	T37.5X4	T37.5X5	T37.5X6
Inositol	T50.991	T50.992	T50.993	T50.994	T50.995	T50.996
nicotinate	T46.7X1	T46.7X2	T46.7X3	T46.7X4	T46.7X5	T46.7X6
Inproquone	T45.1X1	T45.1X2	T45.1X3	T45.1X4	T45.1X5	T45.1X6
Insecticide NEC	T60.91	T60.92	T60.93	T60.94	—	—
carbamate	T60.0X1	T60.0X2	T60.0X3	T60.0X4	—	—
chlorinated	T60.1X1	T60.1X2	T60.1X3	T60.1X4	—	—
mixed	T60.91	T60.92	T60.93	T60.94	—	—
organochlorine	T60.1X1	T60.1X2	T60.1X3	T60.1X4	—	—
organophosphorus	T60.0X1	T60.0X2	T60.0X3	T60.0X4	—	—
Insect (sting), venomous	T63.481	T63.482	T63.483	T63.484	—	—
ant	T63.421	T63.422	T63.423	T63.424	—	—
bee	T63.441	T63.442	T63.443	T63.444	—	—
caterpillar	T63.431	T63.432	T63.433	T63.434	—	—
hornet	T63.451	T63.452	T63.453	T63.454	—	—
wasp	T63.461	T63.462	T63.463	T63.464	—	—
Insular tissue extract	T38.3X1	T38.3X2	T38.3X3	T38.3X4	T38.3X5	T38.3X6
Insulin (amorphous) (globin) (isophane) (Lente) (NPH) (Semilente) (Ultralente)	T38.3X1	T38.3X2	T38.3X3	T38.3X4	T38.3X5	T38.3X6
defalan	T38.3X1	T38.3X2	T38.3X3	T38.3X4	T38.3X5	T38.3X6
human	T38.3X1	T38.3X2	T38.3X3	T38.3X4	T38.3X5	T38.3X6
injection, soluble	T38.3X1	T38.3X2	T38.3X3	T38.3X4	T38.3X5	T38.3X6
biphasic	T38.3X1	T38.3X2	T38.3X3	T38.3X4	T38.3X5	T38.3X6
intermediate acting	T38.3X1	T38.3X2	T38.3X3	T38.3X4	T38.3X5	T38.3X6
protamine zinc	T38.3X1	T38.3X2	T38.3X3	T38.3X4	T38.3X5	T38.3X6
slow acting	T38.3X1	T38.3X2	T38.3X3	T38.3X4	T38.3X5	T38.3X6
zinc						
protamine injection	T38.3X1	T38.3X2	T38.3X3	T38.3X4	T38.3X5	T38.3X6
suspension (amorphous) (crystalline)	T38.3X1	T38.3X2	T38.3X3	T38.3X4	T38.3X5	T38.3X6

Table of Drugs and Chemicals

Hydrofluoric acid — Insulin

Substance	Poisoning, Accidental (unintentional)	Poisoning, Intentional Self-harm	Poisoning, Assault	Poisoning, Undetermined	Adverse Effect	Under-dosing
Interferon (alpha) (beta) (gamma)	T37.5X1	T37.5X2	T37.5X3	T37.5X4	T37.5X5	T37.5X6
Intestinal motility control drug	T47.6X1	T47.6X2	T47.6X3	T47.6X4	T47.6X5	T47.6X6
biological	T47.8X1	T47.8X2	T47.8X3	T47.8X4	T47.8X5	T47.8X6
Intranarcon	T41.1X1	T41.1X2	T41.1X3	T41.1X4	T41.1X5	T41.1X6
Intravenous						
amino acids	T50.991	T50.992	T50.993	T50.994	T50.995	T50.996
fat suspension	T50.991	T50.992	T50.993	T50.994	T50.995	T50.996
Inulin	T50.8X1	T50.8X2	T50.8X3	T50.8X4	T50.8X5	T50.8X6
Invert sugar	T50.3X1	T50.3X2	T50.3X3	T50.3X4	T50.3X5	T50.3X6
Inza — *see* Naproxen						
Iobenzamic acid	T50.8X1	T50.8X2	T50.8X3	T50.8X4	T50.8X5	T50.8X6
Iocarmic acid	T50.8X1	T50.8X2	T50.8X3	T50.8X4	T50.8X5	T50.8X6
Iocetamic acid	T50.8X1	T50.8X2	T50.8X3	T50.8X4	T50.8X5	T50.8X6
Iodamide	T50.8X1	T50.8X2	T50.8X3	T50.8X4	T50.8X5	T50.8X6
Iodide NEC — *see also*	T49.0X1	T49.0X2	T49.0X3	T49.0X4	T49.0X5	T49.0X6
Iodine						
mercury (ointment)	T49.0X1	T49.0X2	T49.0X3	T49.0X4	T49.0X5	T49.0X6
methylate	T49.0X1	T49.0X2	T49.0X3	T49.0X4	T49.0X5	T49.0X6
potassium (expectorant) NEC	T48.4X1	T48.4X2	T48.4X3	T48.4X4	T48.4X5	T48.4X6
Iodinated						
contrast medium	T50.8X1	T50.8X2	T50.8X3	T50.8X4	T50.8X5	T50.8X6
glycerol	T48.4X1	T48.4X2	T48.4X3	T48.4X4	T48.4X5	T48.4X6
human serum albumin (131I)	T50.8X1	T50.8X2	T50.8X3	T50.8X4	T50.8X5	T50.8X6
Iodine (antiseptic, external) (tincture) **NEC**	T49.0X1	T49.0X2	T49.0X3	T49.0X4	T49.0X5	T49.0X6
125 — *see also* Radiation sickness, and Exposure to radioactivce isotopes						
therapeutic	T50.991	T50.992	T50.993	T50.994	T50.995	T50.996
131 — *see also* Radiation sickness, and Exposure to radioactivce isotopes						
therapeutic	T38.2X1	T38.2X2	T38.2X3	T38.2X4	T38.2X5	T38.2X6
diagnostic	T50.8X1	T50.8X2	T50.8X3	T50.8X4	T50.8X5	T50.8X6
for thyroid conditions (antithyroid)	T38.2X1	T38.2X2	T38.2X3	T38.2X4	T38.2X5	T38.2X6
solution	T49.0X1	T49.0X2	T49.0X3	T49.0X4	T49.0X5	T49.0X6
vapor	T59.891	T59.892	T59.893	T59.894	—	—
Iodipamide	T50.8X1	T50.8X2	T50.8X3	T50.8X4	T50.8X5	T50.8X6
Iodized (poppy seed) oil	T50.8X1	T50.8X2	T50.8X3	T50.8X4	T50.8X5	T50.8X6
Iodobismitol	T37.8X1	T37.8X2	T37.8X3	T37.8X4	T37.8X5	T37.8X6
Iodochlorhydroxyquin	T37.8X1	T37.8X2	T37.8X3	T37.8X4	T37.8X5	T37.8X6
topical	T49.0X1	T49.0X2	T49.0X3	T49.0X4	T49.0X5	T49.0X6
Iodochlorhydroxyquinoline	T37.8X1	T37.8X2	T37.8X3	T37.8X4	T37.8X5	T37.8X6
Iodocholesterol (131I)	T50.8X1	T50.8X2	T50.8X3	T50.8X4	T50.8X5	T50.8X6
Iodoform	T49.0X1	T49.0X2	T49.0X3	T49.0X4	T49.0X5	T49.0X6
Iodohippuric acid	T50.8X1	T50.8X2	T50.8X3	T50.8X4	T50.8X5	T50.8X6
Iodopanoic acid	T50.8X1	T50.8X2	T50.8X3	T50.8X4	T50.8X5	T50.8X6
Iodophthalein (sodium)	T50.8X1	T50.8X2	T50.8X3	T50.8X4	T50.8X5	T50.8X6
Iodopyracet	T50.8X1	T50.8X2	T50.8X3	T50.8X4	T50.8X5	T50.8X6
Iodoquinol	T37.8X1	T37.8X2	T37.8X3	T37.8X4	T37.8X5	T37.8X6
Iodoxamic acid	T50.8X1	T50.8X2	T50.8X3	T50.8X4	T50.8X5	T50.8X6
Iofendylate	T50.8X1	T50.8X2	T50.8X3	T50.8X4	T50.8X5	T50.8X6
Ioglycamic acid	T50.8X1	T50.8X2	T50.8X3	T50.8X4	T50.8X5	T50.8X6
Iohexol	T50.8X1	T50.8X2	T50.8X3	T50.8X4	T50.8X5	T50.8X6
Ion exchange resin						
anion	T47.8X1	T47.8X2	T47.8X3	T47.8X4	T47.8X5	T47.8X6
cation	T50.3X1	T50.3X2	T50.3X3	T50.3X4	T50.3X5	T50.3X6
cholestyramine	T46.6X1	T46.6X2	T46.6X3	T46.6X4	T46.6X5	T46.6X6
intestinal	T47.8X1	T47.8X2	T47.8X3	T47.8X4	T47.8X5	T47.8X6
Iopamidol	T50.8X1	T50.8X2	T50.8X3	T50.8X4	T50.8X5	T50.8X6
Iopanoic acid	T50.8X1	T50.8X2	T50.8X3	T50.8X4	T50.8X5	T50.8X6
Iophenoic acid	T50.8X1	T50.8X2	T50.8X3	T50.8X4	T50.8X5	T50.8X6
Iopodate, sodium	T50.8X1	T50.8X2	T50.8X3	T50.8X4	T50.8X5	T50.8X6
Iopodic acid	T50.8X1	T50.8X2	T50.8X3	T50.8X4	T50.8X5	T50.8X6
Iopromide	T50.8X1	T50.8X2	T50.8X3	T50.8X4	T50.8X5	T50.8X6
Iopydol	T50.8X1	T50.8X2	T50.8X3	T50.8X4	T50.8X5	T50.8X6
Iotalamic acid	T50.8X1	T50.8X2	T50.8X3	T50.8X4	T50.8X5	T50.8X6
Iothalamate	T50.8X1	T50.8X2	T50.8X3	T50.8X4	T50.8X5	T50.8X6
Iothiouracil	T38.2X1	T38.2X2	T38.2X3	T38.2X4	T38.2X5	T38.2X6
Iotrol	T50.8X1	T50.8X2	T50.8X3	T50.8X4	T50.8X5	T50.8X6
Iotrolan	T50.8X1	T50.8X2	T50.8X3	T50.8X4	T50.8X5	T50.8X6
Iotroxate	T50.8X1	T50.8X2	T50.8X3	T50.8X4	T50.8X5	T50.8X6
Iotroxic acid	T50.8X1	T50.8X2	T50.8X3	T50.8X4	T50.8X5	T50.8X6
Ioversol	T50.8X1	T50.8X2	T50.8X3	T50.8X4	T50.8X5	T50.8X6
Ioxaglate	T50.8X1	T50.8X2	T50.8X3	T50.8X4	T50.8X5	T50.8X6
Ioxaglic acid	T50.8X1	T50.8X2	T50.8X3	T50.8X4	T50.8X5	T50.8X6
Ioxitalamic acid	T50.8X1	T50.8X2	T50.8X3	T50.8X4	T50.8X5	T50.8X6
Ipecac	T47.7X1	T47.7X2	T47.7X3	T47.7X4	T47.7X5	T47.7X6

Substance	Poisoning, Accidental (unintentional)	Poisoning, Intentional Self-harm	Poisoning, Assault	Poisoning, Undetermined	Adverse Effect	Under-dosing
Ipecacuanha	T48.4X1	T48.4X2	T48.4X3	T48.4X4	T48.4X5	T48.4X6
Ipodate, calcium	T50.8X1	T50.8X2	T50.8X3	T50.8X4	T50.8X5	T50.8X6
Ipral	T42.3X1	T42.3X2	T42.3X3	T42.3X4	T42.3X5	T42.3X6
Ipratropium (bromide)	T48.6X1	T48.6X2	T48.6X3	T48.6X4	T48.6X5	T48.6X6
Ipriflavone	T46.3X1	T46.3X2	T46.3X3	T46.3X4	T46.3X5	T46.3X6
Iprindole	T43.011	T43.012	T43.013	T43.014	T43.015	T43.016
Iproclozide	T43.1X1	T43.1X2	T43.1X3	T43.1X4	T43.1X5	T43.1X6
Iprofenin	T50.8X1	T50.8X2	T50.8X3	T50.8X4	T50.8X5	T50.8X6
Iproheptine	T49.2X1	T49.2X2	T49.2X3	T49.2X4	T49.2X5	T49.2X6
Iproniazid	T43.1X1	T43.1X2	T43.1X3	T43.1X4	T43.1X5	T43.1X6
Iproplatin	T45.1X1	T45.1X2	T45.1X3	T45.1X4	T45.1X5	T45.1X6
Iproveratril	T46.1X1	T46.1X2	T46.1X3	T46.1X4	T46.1X5	T46.1X6
Iron (compounds) (medicinal) **NEC**	T45.4X1	T45.4X2	T45.4X3	T45.4X4	T45.4X5	T45.4X6
ammonium	T45.4X1	T45.4X2	T45.4X3	T45.4X4	T45.4X5	T45.4X6
dextran injection	T45.4X1	T45.4X2	T45.4X3	T45.4X4	T45.4X5	T45.4X6
nonmedicinal	T56.891	T56.892	T56.893	T56.894	—	—
salts	T45.4X1	T45.4X2	T45.4X3	T45.4X4	T45.4X5	T45.4X6
sorbitex	T45.4X1	T45.4X2	T45.4X3	T45.4X4	T45.4X5	T45.4X6
sorbitol citric acid complex	T45.4X1	T45.4X2	T45.4X3	T45.4X4	T45.4X5	T45.4X6
Irrigating fluid (vaginal)	T49.8X1	T49.8X2	T49.8X3	T49.8X4	T49.8X5	T49.8X6
eye	T49.5X1	T49.5X2	T49.5X3	T49.5X4	T49.5X5	T49.5X6
Isepamicin	T36.5X1	T36.5X2	T36.5X3	T36.5X4	T36.5X5	T36.5X6
Isoaminile (citrate)	T48.3X1	T48.3X2	T48.3X3	T48.3X4	T48.3X5	T48.3X6
Isoamyl nitrite	T46.3X1	T46.3X2	T46.3X3	T46.3X4	T46.3X5	T46.3X6
Isobenzan	T60.1X1	T60.1X2	T60.1X3	T60.1X4	—	—
Isobutyl acetate	T52.8X1	T52.8X2	T52.8X3	T52.8X4	—	—
Isocarboxazid	T43.1X1	T43.1X2	T43.1X3	T43.1X4	T43.1X5	T43.1X6
Isoconazole	T49.0X1	T49.0X2	T49.0X3	T49.0X4	T49.0X5	T49.0X6
Isocyanate	T65.0X1	T65.0X2	T65.0X3	T65.0X4	—	—
Isoephedrine	T44.991	T44.992	T44.993	T44.994	T44.995	T44.996
Isoetarine	T48.6X1	T48.6X2	T48.6X3	T48.6X4	T48.6X5	T48.6X6
Isoethadione	T42.2X1	T42.2X2	T42.2X3	T42.2X4	T42.2X5	T42.2X6
Isoetharine	T44.5X1	T44.5X2	T44.5X3	T44.5X4	T44.5X5	T44.5X6
Isoflurane	T41.0X1	T41.0X2	T41.0X3	T41.0X4	T41.0X5	T41.0X6
Isoflurophate	T44.0X1	T44.0X2	T44.0X3	T44.0X4	T44.0X5	T44.0X6
Isomaltose, ferric complex	T45.4X1	T45.4X2	T45.4X3	T45.4X4	T45.4X5	T45.4X6
Isometheptene	T44.3X1	T44.3X2	T44.3X3	T44.3X4	T44.3X5	T44.3X6
Isoniazid	T37.1X1	T37.1X2	T37.1X3	T37.1X4	T37.1X5	T37.1X6
with						
rifampicin	T36.6X1	T36.6X2	T36.6X3	T36.6X4	T36.6X5	T36.6X6
thioacetazone	T37.1X1	T37.1X2	T37.1X3	T37.1X4	T37.1X5	T37.1X6
Isonicotinic acid hydrazide	T37.1X1	T37.1X2	T37.1X3	T37.1X4	T37.1X5	T37.1X6
Isonipecaine	T40.4X1	T40.4X2	T40.4X3	T40.4X4	T40.4X5	T40.4X6
Isopentaquine	T37.2X1	T37.2X2	T37.2X3	T37.2X4	T37.2X5	T37.2X6
Isophane insulin	T38.3X1	T38.3X2	T38.3X3	T38.3X4	T38.3X5	T38.3X6
Isophorone	T65.891	T65.892	T65.893	T65.894	—	—
Isophosphamide	T45.1X1	T45.1X2	T45.1X3	T45.1X4	T45.1X5	T45.1X6
Isopregnenone	T38.5X1	T38.5X2	T38.5X3	T38.5X4	T38.5X5	T38.5X6
Isoprenaline	T48.6X1	T48.6X2	T48.6X3	T48.6X4	T48.6X5	T48.6X6
Isopromethazine	T43.3X1	T43.3X2	T43.3X3	T43.3X4	T43.3X5	T43.3X6
Isopropamide	T44.3X1	T44.3X2	T44.3X3	T44.3X4	T44.3X5	T44.3X6
iodide	T44.3X1	T44.3X2	T44.3X3	T44.3X4	T44.3X5	T44.3X6
Isopropanol	T51.2X1	T51.2X2	T51.2X3	T51.2X4	—	—
Isopropyl						
acetate	T52.8X1	T52.8X2	T52.8X3	T52.8X4	—	—
alcohol	T51.2X1	T51.2X2	T51.2X3	T51.2X4	—	—
medicinal	T49.4X1	T49.4X2	T49.4X3	T49.4X4	T49.4X5	T49.4X6
ether	T52.8X1	T52.8X2	T52.8X3	T52.8X4	—	—
Isopropylaminophenazone	T39.2X1	T39.2X2	T39.2X3	T39.2X4	T39.2X5	T39.2X6
Isoproterenol	T48.6X1	T48.6X2	T48.6X3	T48.6X4	T48.6X5	T48.6X6
Isosorbide dinitrate	T46.3X1	T46.3X2	T46.3X3	T46.3X4	T46.3X5	T46.3X6
Isothipendyl	T45.0X1	T45.0X2	T45.0X3	T45.0X4	T45.0X5	T45.0X6
Isotretinoin	T50.991	T50.992	T50.993	T50.994	T50.995	T50.996
Isoxazolyl penicillin	T36.0X1	T36.0X2	T36.0X3	T36.0X4	T36.0X5	T36.0X6
Isoxicam	T39.391	T39.392	T39.393	T39.394	T39.395	T39.396
Isoxsuprine	T46.7X1	T46.7X2	T46.7X3	T46.7X4	T46.7X5	T46.7X6
Ispagula	T47.4X1	T47.4X2	T47.4X3	T47.4X4	T47.4X5	T47.4X6
husk	T47.4X1	T47.4X2	T47.4X3	T47.4X4	T47.4X5	T47.4X6
Isradipine	T46.1X1	T46.1X2	T46.1X3	T46.1X4	T46.1X5	T46.1X6
I-thyroxine sodium	T38.1X1	T38.1X2	T38.1X3	T38.1X4	T38.1X5	T38.1X6
Itraconazole	T37.8X1	T37.8X2	T37.8X3	T37.8X4	T37.8X5	T37.8X6
Itramin tosilate	T46.3X1	T46.3X2	T46.3X3	T46.3X4	T46.3X5	T46.3X6
Ivermectin	T37.4X1	T37.4X2	T37.4X3	T37.4X4	T37.4X5	T37.4X6
Izoniazid	T37.1X1	T37.1X2	T37.1X3	T37.1X4	T37.1X5	T37.1X6
with thioacetazone	T37.1X1	T37.1X2	T37.1X3	T37.1X4	T37.1X5	T37.1X6
Jalap	T47.2X1	T47.2X2	T47.2X3	T47.2X4	T47.2X5	T47.2X6
Jamaica						
dogwood (bark)	T39.8X1	T39.8X2	T39.8X3	T39.8X4	T39.8X5	T39.8X6
ginger	T65.891	T65.892	T65.893	T65.894	—	—
root	T62.2X1	T62.2X2	T62.2X3	T62.2X4	—	—
Jatropha	T62.2X1	T62.2X2	T62.2X3	T62.2X4	—	—
curcas	T62.2X1	T62.2X2	T62.2X3	T62.2X4	—	—

Additional Character May Be Required — Refer to the Tabular List for Character Selection ▽ Subterms under main terms may continue to next column or page

Substance	Poisoning, Accidental (unintentional)	Poisoning, Intentional Self-harm	Poisoning, Assault	Poisoning, Undetermined	Adverse Effect	Underdosing
Jectofer	T45.4X1	T45.4X2	T45.4X3	T45.4X4	T45.4X5	T45.4X6
Jellyfish (sting)	T63.621	T63.622	T63.623	T63.624	—	—
Jequirity (bean)	T62.2X1	T62.2X2	T62.2X3	T62.2X4	—	—
Jimson weed (stramonium)	T62.2X1	T62.2X2	T62.2X3	T62.2X4	—	—
seeds	T62.2X1	T62.2X2	T62.2X3	T62.2X4	—	—
Josamycin	T36.3X1	T36.3X2	T36.3X3	T36.3X4	T36.3X5	T36.3X6
Juniper tar	T49.1X1	T49.1X2	T49.1X3	T49.1X4	T49.1X5	T49.1X6
Kallidinogenase	T46.7X1	T46.7X2	T46.7X3	T46.7X4	T46.7X5	T46.7X6
Kallikrein	T46.7X1	T46.7X2	T46.7X3	T46.7X4	T46.7X5	T46.7X6
Kanamycin	T36.5X1	T36.5X2	T36.5X3	T36.5X4	T36.5X5	T36.5X6
Kantrex	T36.5X1	T36.5X2	T36.5X3	T36.5X4	T36.5X5	T36.5X6
Kaolin	T47.6X1	T47.6X2	T47.6X3	T47.6X4	T47.6X5	T47.6X6
light	T47.6X1	T47.6X2	T47.6X3	T47.6X4	T47.6X5	T47.6X6
Karaya (gum)	T47.4X1	T47.4X2	T47.4X3	T47.4X4	T47.4X5	T47.4X6
Kebuzone	T39.2X1	T39.2X2	T39.2X3	T39.2X4	T39.2X5	T39.2X6
Kelevan	T60.1X1	T60.1X2	T60.1X3	T60.1X4	—	—
Kemithal	T41.1X1	T41.1X2	T41.1X3	T41.1X4	T41.1X5	T41.1X6
Kenacort	T38.0X1	T38.0X2	T38.0X3	T38.0X4	T38.0X5	T38.0X6
Keratolytic drug NEC	T49.4X1	T49.4X2	T49.4X3	T49.4X4	T49.4X5	T49.4X6
anthracene	T49.4X1	T49.4X2	T49.4X3	T49.4X4	T49.4X5	T49.4X6
Keratoplastic NEC	T49.4X1	T49.4X2	T49.4X3	T49.4X4	T49.4X5	T49.4X6
Kerosene, kerosine (fuel) (solvent) NEC	T52.0X1	T52.0X2	T52.0X3	T52.0X4	—	—
insecticide	T52.0X1	T52.0X2	T52.0X3	T52.0X4	—	—
vapor	T52.0X1	T52.0X2	T52.0X3	T52.0X4	—	—
Ketamine	T41.291	T41.292	T41.293	T41.294	T41.295	T41.296
Ketazolam	T42.4X1	T42.4X2	T42.4X3	T42.4X4	T42.4X5	T42.4X6
Ketazon	T39.2X1	T39.2X2	T39.2X3	T39.2X4	T39.2X5	T39.2X6
Ketobemidone	T40.4X1	T40.4X2	T40.4X3	T40.4X4	—	—
Ketoconazole	T49.0X1	T49.0X2	T49.0X3	T49.0X4	T49.0X5	T49.0X6
Ketols	T52.4X1	T52.4X2	T52.4X3	T52.4X4	—	—
Ketone oils	T52.4X1	T52.4X2	T52.4X3	T52.4X4	—	—
Ketoprofen	T39.311	T39.312	T39.313	T39.314	T39.315	T39.316
Ketorolac	T39.8X1	T39.8X2	T39.8X3	T39.8X4	T39.8X5	T39.8X6
Ketotifen	T45.0X1	T45.0X2	T45.0X3	T45.0X4	T45.0X5	T45.0X6
Khat	T43.691	T43.692	T43.693	T43.694	—	—
Khellin	T46.3X1	T46.3X2	T46.3X3	T46.3X4	T46.3X5	T46.3X6
Khelloside	T46.3X1	T46.3X2	T46.3X3	T46.3X4	T46.3X5	T46.3X6
Kiln gas or vapor (carbon monoxide)	T58.8X1	T58.8X2	T58.8X3	T58.8X4	—	—
Kitasamycin	T36.3X1	T36.3X2	T36.3X3	T36.3X4	T36.3X5	T36.3X6
Konsyl	T47.4X1	T47.4X2	T47.4X3	T47.4X4	T47.4X5	T47.4X6
Kosam seed	T62.2X1	T62.2X2	T62.2X3	T62.2X4	—	—
Krait (venom)	T63.091	T63.092	T63.093	T63.094	—	—
Kwell (insecticide)	T60.1X1	T60.1X2	T60.1X3	T60.1X4	—	—
anti-infective (topical)	T49.0X1	T49.0X2	T49.0X3	T49.0X4	T49.0X5	T49.0X6
Labetalol	T44.8X1	T44.8X2	T44.8X3	T44.8X4	T44.8X5	T44.8X6
Laburnum (seeds)	T62.2X1	T62.2X2	T62.2X3	T62.2X4	—	—
leaves	T62.2X1	T62.2X2	T62.2X3	T62.2X4	—	—
Lachesine	T49.5X1	T49.5X2	T49.5X3	T49.5X4	T49.5X5	T49.5X6
Lacidipine	T46.5X1	T46.5X2	T46.5X3	T46.5X4	T46.5X5	T46.5X6
Lacquer	T65.6X1	T65.6X2	T65.6X3	T65.6X4	—	—
Lacrimogenic gas	T59.3X1	T59.3X2	T59.3X3	T59.3X4	—	—
Lactated potassic saline	T50.3X1	T50.3X2	T50.3X3	T50.3X4	T50.3X5	T50.3X6
Lactic acid	T49.8X1	T49.8X2	T49.8X3	T49.8X4	T49.8X5	T49.8X6
Lactobacillus						
acidophilus	T47.6X1	T47.6X2	T47.6X3	T47.6X4	T47.6X5	T47.6X6
compound	T47.6X1	T47.6X2	T47.6X3	T47.6X4	T47.6X5	T47.6X6
bifidus, lyophilized	T47.6X1	T47.6X2	T47.6X3	T47.6X4	T47.6X5	T47.6X6
bulgaricus	T47.6X1	T47.6X2	T47.6X3	T47.6X4	T47.6X5	T47.6X6
sporogenes	T47.6X1	T47.6X2	T47.6X3	T47.6X4	T47.6X5	T47.6X6
Lactoflavin	T45.2X1	T45.2X2	T45.2X3	T45.2X4	T45.2X5	T45.2X6
Lactose (as excipient)	T50.901	T50.902	T50.903	T50.904	T50.905	T50.906
Lactuca (virosa) (extract)	T42.6X1	T42.6X2	T42.6X3	T42.6X4	T42.6X5	T42.6X6
Lactucarium	T42.6X1	T42.6X2	T42.6X3	T42.6X4	T42.6X5	T42.6X6
Lactulose	T47.3X1	T47.3X2	T47.3X3	T47.3X4	T47.3X5	T47.3X6
Laevo — see Levo-						
Lanatosides	T46.0X1	T46.0X2	T46.0X3	T46.0X4	T46.0X5	T46.0X6
Lanolin	T49.3X1	T49.3X2	T49.3X3	T49.3X4	T49.3X5	T49.3X6
Largactil	T43.3X1	T43.3X2	T43.3X3	T43.3X4	T43.3X5	T43.3X6
Larkspur	T62.2X1	T62.2X2	T62.2X3	T62.2X4	—	—
Laroxyl	T43.011	T43.012	T43.013	T43.014	T43.015	T43.016
Lasix	T50.1X1	T50.1X2	T50.1X3	T50.1X4	T50.1X5	T50.1X6
Lassar's paste	T49.4X1	T49.4X2	T49.4X3	T49.4X4	T49.4X5	T49.4X6
Latamoxef	T36.1X1	T36.1X2	T36.1X3	T36.1X4	T36.1X5	T36.1X6
Latex	T65.811	T65.812	T65.813	T65.814	—	—
Lathyrus (seed)	T62.2X1	T62.2X2	T62.2X3	T62.2X4	—	—
Laudanum	T40.0X1	T40.0X2	T40.0X3	T40.0X4	T40.0X5	T40.0X6
Laudexium	T48.1X1	T48.1X2	T48.1X3	T48.1X4	T48.1X5	T48.1X6
Laughing gas	T41.0X1	T41.0X2	T41.0X3	T41.0X4	T41.0X5	T41.0X6
Laurel, black or cherry	T62.2X1	T62.2X2	T62.2X3	T62.2X4	—	—
Laurolinium	T49.0X1	T49.0X2	T49.0X3	T49.0X4	T49.0X5	T49.0X6
Lauryl sulfoacetate	T49.2X1	T49.2X2	T49.2X3	T49.2X4	T49.2X5	T49.2X6
Laxative NEC	T47.4X1	T47.4X2	T47.4X3	T47.4X4	T47.4X5	T47.4X6
osmotic	T47.3X1	T47.3X2	T47.3X3	T47.3X4	T47.3X5	T47.3X6
saline	T47.3X1	T47.3X2	T47.3X3	T47.3X4	T47.3X5	T47.3X6
stimulant	T47.2X1	T47.2X2	T47.2X3	T47.2X4	T47.2X5	T47.2X6
L-dopa	T42.8X1	T42.8X2	T42.8X3	T42.8X4	T42.8X5	T42.8X6
Lead (dust) (fumes) (vapor)	T56.0X1	T56.0X2	T56.0X3	T56.0X4	—	—
NEC						
acetate	T49.2X1	T49.2X2	T49.2X3	T49.2X4	T49.2X5	T49.2X6
alkyl (fuel additive)	T56.0X1	T56.0X2	T56.0X3	T56.0X4	—	—
anti-infectives	T37.8X1	T37.8X2	T37.8X3	T37.8X4	T37.8X5	T37.8X6
antiknock compound (tetraethyl)	T56.0X1	T56.0X2	T56.0X3	T56.0X4	—	—
arsenate, arsenite (dust)(herbicide) (insecticide) (vapor)	T57.0X1	T57.0X2	T57.0X3	T57.0X4	—	—
carbonate	T56.0X1	T56.0X2	T56.0X3	T56.0X4	—	—
paint	T56.0X1	T56.0X2	T56.0X3	T56.0X4	—	—
chromate	T56.0X1	T56.0X2	T56.0X3	T56.0X4	—	—
paint	T56.0X1	T56.0X2	T56.0X3	T56.0X4	—	—
dioxide	T56.0X1	T56.0X2	T56.0X3	T56.0X4	—	—
inorganic	T56.0X1	T56.0X2	T56.0X3	T56.0X4	—	—
iodide	T56.0X1	T56.0X2	T56.0X3	T56.0X4	—	—
pigment (paint)	T56.0X1	T56.0X2	T56.0X3	T56.0X4	—	—
monoxide (dust)	T56.0X1	T56.0X2	T56.0X3	T56.0X4	—	—
paint	T56.0X1	T56.0X2	T56.0X3	T56.0X4	—	—
organic	T56.0X1	T56.0X2	T56.0X3	T56.0X4	—	—
oxide	T56.0X1	T56.0X2	T56.0X3	T56.0X4	—	—
paint	T56.0X1	T56.0X2	T56.0X3	T56.0X4	—	—
paint	T56.0X1	T56.0X2	T56.0X3	T56.0X4	—	—
salts	T56.0X1	T56.0X2	T56.0X3	T56.0X4	—	—
specified compound NEC	T56.0X1	T56.0X2	T56.0X3	T56.0X4	—	—
tetra-ethyl	T56.0X1	T56.0X2	T56.0X3	T56.0X4	—	—
Lebanese red	T40.7X1	T40.7X2	T40.7X3	T40.7X4	T40.7X5	T40.7X6
Lefetamine	T39.8X1	T39.8X2	T39.8X3	T39.8X4	T39.8X5	T39.8X6
Lenperone	T43.4X1	T43.4X2	T43.4X3	T43.4X4	T43.4X5	T43.4X6
Lente lietin (insulin)	T38.3X1	T38.3X2	T38.3X3	T38.3X4	T38.3X5	T38.3X6
Leptazol	T50.7X1	T50.7X2	T50.7X3	T50.7X4	T50.7X5	T50.7X6
Leptophos	T60.0X1	T60.0X2	T60.0X3	T60.0X4	—	—
Leritine	T40.2X1	T40.2X2	T40.2X3	T40.2X4	T40.2X5	T40.2X6
Letosteine	T48.4X1	T48.4X2	T48.4X3	T48.4X4	T48.4X5	T48.4X6
Letter	T38.1X1	T38.1X2	T38.1X3	T38.1X4	T38.1X5	T38.1X6
Lettuce opium	T42.6X1	T42.6X2	T42.6X3	T42.6X4	T42.6X5	T42.6X6
Leucinocaine	T41.3X1	T41.3X2	T41.3X3	T41.3X4	—	—
Leucocianidol	T46.991	T46.992	T46.993	T46.994	T46.995	T46.996
Leucovorin (factor)	T45.8X1	T45.8X2	T45.8X3	T45.8X4	T45.8X5	T45.8X6
Leukeran	T45.1X1	T45.1X2	T45.1X3	T45.1X4	T45.1X5	T45.1X6
Leuprolide	T38.891	T38.892	T38.893	T38.894	T38.895	T38.896
Levalbuterol	T48.6X1	T48.6X2	T48.6X3	T48.6X4	T48.6X5	T48.6X6
Levallorphan	T50.7X1	T50.7X2	T50.7X3	T50.7X4	T50.7X5	T50.7X6
Levamisole	T37.4X1	T37.4X2	T37.4X3	T37.4X4	T37.4X5	T37.4X6
Levanil	T42.6X1	T42.6X2	T42.6X3	T42.6X4	T42.6X5	T42.6X6
Levarterenol	T44.4X1	T44.4X2	T44.4X3	T44.4X4	T44.4X5	T44.4X6
Levdropropizine	T48.3X1	T48.3X2	T48.3X3	T48.3X4	T48.3X5	T48.3X6
Levobunolol	T49.5X1	T49.5X2	T49.5X3	T49.5X4	T49.5X5	T49.5X6
Levocabastine (hydrochloride)	T45.0X1	T45.0X2	T45.0X3	T45.0X4	T45.0X5	T45.0X6
Levocarnitine	T50.991	T50.992	T50.993	T50.994	T50.995	T50.996
Levodopa	T42.8X1	T42.8X2	T42.8X3	T42.8X4	T42.8X5	T42.8X6
with carbidopa	T42.8X1	T42.8X2	T42.8X3	T42.8X4	T42.8X5	T42.8X6
Levo-dromoran	T40.2X1	T40.2X2	T40.2X3	T40.2X4	T40.2X5	T40.2X6
Levoglutamide	T50.991	T50.992	T50.993	T50.994	T50.995	T50.996
Levoid	T38.1X1	T38.1X2	T38.1X3	T38.1X4	T38.1X5	T38.1X6
Levo-isomethadone	T40.3X1	T40.3X2	T40.3X3	T40.3X4	T40.3X5	T40.3X6
Levomepromazine	T43.3X1	T43.3X2	T43.3X3	T43.3X4	T43.3X5	T43.3X6
Levonordefrin	T49.6X1	T49.6X2	T49.6X3	T49.6X4	T49.6X5	T49.6X6
Levonorgestrel	T38.4X1	T38.4X2	T38.4X3	T38.4X4	T38.4X5	T38.4X6
with ethinylestradiol	T38.5X1	T38.5X2	T38.5X3	T38.5X4	T38.5X5	T38.5X6
Levopromazine	T43.3X1	T43.3X2	T43.3X3	T43.3X4	T43.3X5	T43.3X6
Levoprome	T42.6X1	T42.6X2	T42.6X3	T42.6X4	T42.6X5	T42.6X6
Levopropoxyphene	T40.4X1	T40.4X2	T40.4X3	T40.4X4	T40.4X5	T40.4X6
Levopropylhexedrine	T50.5X1	T50.5X2	T50.5X3	T50.5X4	T50.5X5	T50.5X6
Levoproxyphylline	T48.6X1	T48.6X2	T48.6X3	T48.6X4	T48.6X5	T48.6X6
Levorphanol	T40.4X1	T40.4X2	T40.4X3	T40.4X4	T40.4X5	T40.4X6
Levothyroxine	T38.1X1	T38.1X2	T38.1X3	T38.1X4	T38.1X5	T38.1X6
sodium	T38.1X1	T38.1X2	T38.1X3	T38.1X4	T38.1X5	T38.1X6
Levsin	T44.3X1	T44.3X2	T44.3X3	T44.3X4	T44.3X5	T44.3X6
Levulose	T50.3X1	T50.3X2	T50.3X3	T50.3X4	T50.3X5	T50.3X6
Lewisite (gas), not in war	T57.0X1	T57.0X2	T57.0X3	T57.0X4	—	—
Librium	T42.4X1	T42.4X2	T42.4X3	T42.4X4	T42.4X5	T42.4X6
Lidex	T49.0X1	T49.0X2	T49.0X3	T49.0X4	T49.0X5	T49.0X6
Lidocaine	T41.3X1	T41.3X2	T41.3X3	T41.3X4	T41.3X5	T41.3X6
regional	T41.3X1	T41.3X2	T41.3X3	T41.3X4	T41.3X5	T41.3X6
spinal	T41.3X1	T41.3X2	T41.3X3	T41.3X4	T41.3X5	T41.3X6

▽ Subterms under main terms may continue to next column or page   Additional Character May Be Required — Refer to the Tabular List for Character Selection   375

Jectofer — Lidocaine

Table of Drugs and Chemicals

Lidofenin — Mecamylamine

Substance	Poisoning, Accidental (unintentional)	Poisoning, Intentional Self-harm	Poisoning, Assault	Poisoning, Undetermined	Adverse Effect	Under-dosing
Lidofenin	T50.8X1	T50.8X2	T50.8X3	T50.8X4	T50.8X5	T50.8X6
Lidoflazine	T46.1X1	T46.1X2	T46.1X3	T46.1X4	T46.1X5	T46.1X6
Lighter fluid	T52.0X1	T52.0X2	T52.0X3	T52.0X4	—	—
Lignin hemicellulose	T47.6X1	T47.6X2	T47.6X3	T47.6X4	T47.6X5	T47.6X6
Lignocaine	T41.3X1	T41.3X2	T41.3X3	T41.3X4	T41.3X5	T41.3X6
regional	T41.3X1	T41.3X2	T41.3X3	T41.3X4	T41.3X5	T41.3X6
spinal	T41.3X1	T41.3X2	T41.3X3	T41.3X4	T41.3X5	T41.3X6
Ligroin (e) (solvent)	T52.0X1	T52.0X2	T52.0X3	T52.0X4	—	—
vapor	T59.891	T59.892	T59.893	T59.894	—	—
Ligustrum vulgare	T62.2X1	T62.2X2	T62.2X3	T62.2X4	—	—
Lily of the valley	T62.2X1	T62.2X2	T62.2X3	T62.2X4	—	—
Lime (chloride)	T54.3X1	T54.3X2	T54.3X3	T54.3X4	—	—
Limonene	T52.8X1	T52.8X2	T52.8X3	T52.8X4	—	—
Lincomycin	T36.8X1	T36.8X2	T36.8X3	T36.8X4	T36.8X5	T36.8X6
Lindane (insecticide) (nonmedicinal) (vapor)	T53.6X1	T53.6X2	T53.6X3	T53.6X4	—	—
medicinal	T49.0X1	T49.0X2	T49.0X3	T49.0X4	T49.0X5	T49.0X6
Liniments NEC	T49.91	T49.92	T49.93	T49.94	T49.95	T49.96
Linoleic acid	T46.6X1	T46.6X2	T46.6X3	T46.6X4	T46.6X5	T46.6X6
Linolenic acid	T46.6X1	T46.6X2	T46.6X3	T46.6X4	T46.6X5	T46.6X6
Linseed	T47.4X1	T47.4X2	T47.4X3	T47.4X4	T47.4X5	T47.4X6
Liothyronine	T38.1X1	T38.1X2	T38.1X3	T38.1X4	T38.1X5	T38.1X6
Liotrix	T38.1X1	T38.1X2	T38.1X3	T38.1X4	T38.1X5	T38.1X6
Lipancreatin	T47.5X1	T47.5X2	T47.5X3	T47.5X4	T47.5X5	T47.5X6
Lipo-alprostadil	T46.7X1	T46.7X2	T46.7X3	T46.7X4	T46.7X5	T46.7X6
Lipo-Lutin	T38.5X1	T38.5X2	T38.5X3	T38.5X4	T38.5X5	T38.5X6
Lipotropic drug NEC	T50.901	T50.902	T50.903	T50.904	T50.905	T50.906
Liquefied petroleum gases	T59.891	T59.892	T59.893	T59.894	—	—
piped (pure or mixed with air)	T59.891	T59.892	T59.893	T59.894	—	—
Liquid						
paraffin	T47.4X1	T47.4X2	T47.4X3	T47.4X4	T47.4X5	T47.4X6
petrolatum	T47.4X1	T47.4X2	T47.4X3	T47.4X4	T47.4X5	T47.4X6
topical	T49.3X1	T49.3X2	T49.3X3	T49.3X4	T49.3X5	T49.3X6
specified NEC	T65.891	T65.892	T65.893	T65.894	—	—
substance	T65.91	T65.92	T65.93	T65.94	—	—
Liquor creosolis compositus	T65.891	T65.892	T65.893	T65.894	—	—
Liquorice	T48.4X1	T48.4X2	T48.4X3	T48.4X4	T48.4X5	T48.4X6
extract	T47.8X1	T47.8X2	T47.8X3	T47.8X4	T47.8X5	T47.8X6
Lisinopril	T46.4X1	T46.4X2	T46.4X3	T46.4X4	T46.4X5	T46.4X6
Lisuride	T42.8X1	T42.8X2	T42.8X3	T42.8X4	T42.8X5	T42.8X6
Lithane	T43.8X1	T43.8X2	T43.8X3	T43.8X4	T43.8X5	T43.8X6
Lithium	T56.891	T56.892	T56.893	T56.894	—	—
gluconate	T43.591	T43.592	T43.593	T43.594	T43.595	T43.596
salts (carbonate)	T43.591	T43.592	T43.593	T43.594	T43.595	T43.596
Lithonate	T43.8X1	T43.8X2	T43.8X3	T43.8X4	T43.8X5	T43.8X6
Liver						
extract	T45.8X1	T45.8X2	T45.8X3	T45.8X4	T45.8X5	T45.8X6
for parenteral use	T45.8X1	T45.8X2	T45.8X3	T45.8X4	T45.8X5	T45.8X6
fraction 1	T45.8X1	T45.8X2	T45.8X3	T45.8X4	T45.8X5	T45.8X6
hydrolysate	T45.8X1	T45.8X2	T45.8X3	T45.8X4	T45.8X5	T45.8X6
Lizard (bite) (venom)	T63.121	T63.122	T63.123	T63.124	—	—
LMD	T45.8X1	T45.8X2	T45.8X3	T45.8X4	T45.8X5	T45.8X6
Lobelia	T62.2X1	T62.2X2	T62.2X3	T62.2X4	—	—
Lobeline	T50.7X1	T50.7X2	T50.7X3	T50.7X4	T50.7X5	T50.7X6
Local action drug NEC	T49.8X1	T49.8X2	T49.8X3	T49.8X4	T49.8X5	T49.8X6
Locorten	T49.0X1	T49.0X2	T49.0X3	T49.0X4	T49.0X5	T49.0X6
Lofepramine	T43.011	T43.012	T43.013	T43.014	T43.015	T43.016
Lolium temulentum	T62.2X1	T62.2X2	T62.2X3	T62.2X4	—	—
Lomotil	T47.6X1	T47.6X2	T47.6X3	T47.6X4	T47.6X5	T47.6X6
Lomustine	T45.1X1	T45.1X2	T45.1X3	T45.1X4	T45.1X5	T45.1X6
Lonidamine	T45.1X1	T45.1X2	T45.1X3	T45.1X5	I45.1X5	T45.1X6
Loperamide	T47.6X1	T47.6X2	T47.6X3	T47.6X4	T47.6X5	T47.6X6
Loprazolam	T42.4X1	T42.4X2	T42.4X3	T42.4X4	T42.4X5	T42.4X6
Lorajmine	T46.2X1	T46.2X2	T46.2X3	T46.2X4	T46.2X5	T46.2X6
Loratidine	T45.0X1	T45.0X2	T45.0X3	T45.0X4	T45.0X5	T45.0X6
Lorazepam	T42.4X1	T42.4X2	T42.4X3	T42.4X4	T42.4X5	T42.4X6
Lorcainide	T46.2X1	T46.2X2	T46.2X3	T46.2X4	T46.2X5	T46.2X6
Lormetazepam	T42.4X1	T42.4X2	T42.4X3	T42.4X4	T42.4X5	T42.4X6
Lotions NEC	T49.91	T49.92	T49.93	T49.94	T49.95	T49.96
Lotusate	T42.3X1	T42.3X2	T42.3X3	T42.3X4	T42.3X5	T42.3X6
Lovastatin	T46.6X1	T46.6X2	T46.6X3	T46.6X4	T46.6X5	T46.6X6
Lowila	T49.2X1	T49.2X2	T49.2X3	T49.2X4	T49.2X5	T49.2X6
Loxapine	T43.591	T43.592	T43.593	T43.594	T43.595	T43.596
Lozenges (throat)	T49.6X1	T49.6X2	T49.6X3	T49.6X4	T49.6X5	T49.6X6
LSD	T40.8X1	T40.8X2	T40.8X3	T40.8X4	—	—
L-Tryptophan — *see* amino acid						
Lubricant, eye	T49.5X1	T49.5X2	T49.5X3	T49.5X4	T49.5X5	T49.5X6
Lubricating oil NEC	T52.0X1	T52.0X2	T52.0X3	T52.0X4	—	—
Lucanthone	T37.4X1	T37.4X2	T37.4X3	T37.4X4	T37.4X5	T37.4X6
Luminal	T42.3X1	T42.3X2	T42.3X3	T42.3X4	T42.3X5	T42.3X6
Lung irritant (gas) NEC	T59.91	T59.92	T59.93	T59.94	—	—

Substance	Poisoning, Accidental (unintentional)	Poisoning, Intentional Self-harm	Poisoning, Assault	Poisoning, Undetermined	Adverse Effect	Under-dosing
Luteinizing hormone	T38.811	T38.812	T38.813	T38.814	T38.815	T38.816
Lutocylol	T38.5X1	T38.5X2	T38.5X3	T38.5X4	T38.5X5	T38.5X6
Lutromone	T38.5X1	T38.5X2	T38.5X3	T38.5X4	T38.5X5	T38.5X6
Lututrin	T48.291	T48.292	T48.293	T48.294	T48.295	T48.296
Lye (concentrated)	T54.3X1	T54.3X2	T54.3X3	T54.3X4	—	—
Lygranum (skin test)	T50.8X1	T50.8X2	T50.8X3	T50.8X4	T50.8X5	T50.8X6
Lymecycline	T36.4X1	T36.4X2	T36.4X3	T36.4X4	T36.4X5	T36.4X6
Lymphogranuloma venereum antigen	T50.8X1	T50.8X2	T50.8X3	T50.8X4	T50.8X5	T50.8X6
Lynestrenol	T38.4X1	T38.4X2	T38.4X3	T38.4X4	T38.4X5	T38.4X6
Lyovac Sodium Edecrin	T50.1X1	T50.1X2	T50.1X3	T50.1X4	T50.1X5	T50.1X6
Lypressin	T38.891	T38.892	T38.893	T38.894	T38.895	T38.896
Lysergic acid diethylamide	T40.8X1	T40.8X2	T40.8X3	T40.8X4	—	—
Lysergide	T40.8X1	T40.8X2	T40.8X3	T40.8X4	—	—
Lysine vasopressin	T38.891	T38.892	T38.893	T38.894	T38.895	T38.896
Lysol	T54.1X1	T54.1X2	T54.1X3	T54.1X4	—	—
Lysozyme	T49.0X1	T49.0X2	T49.0X3	T49.0X4	T49.0X5	T49.0X6
Lytta (vitatta)	T49.8X1	T49.8X2	T49.8X3	T49.8X4	T49.8X5	T49.8X6
Mace	T59.3X1	T59.3X2	T59.3X3	T59.3X4	—	—
Macrogol	T50.991	T50.992	T50.993	T50.994	T50.995	T50.996
Macrolide						
anabolic drug	T38.7X1	T38.7X2	T38.7X3	T38.7X4	T38.7X5	T38.7X6
antibiotic	T36.3X1	T36.3X2	T36.3X3	T36.3X4	T36.3X5	T36.3X6
Mafenide	T49.0X1	T49.0X2	T49.0X3	T49.0X4	T49.0X5	T49.0X6
Magaldrate	T47.1X1	T47.1X2	T47.1X3	T47.1X4	T47.1X5	T47.1X6
Magic mushroom	T40.991	T40.992	T40.993	T40.994	—	—
Magnamycin	T36.8X1	T36.8X2	T36.8X3	T36.8X4	T36.8X5	T36.8X6
Magnesia magma	T47.1X1	T47.1X2	T47.1X3	T47.1X4	T47.1X5	T47.1X6
Magnesium NEC	T56.891	T56.892	T56.893	T56.894	—	—
carbonate	T47.1X1	T47.1X2	T47.1X3	T47.1X4	T47.1X5	T47.1X6
citrate	T47.4X1	T47.4X2	T47.4X3	T47.4X4	T47.4X5	T47.4X6
hydroxide	T47.1X1	T47.1X2	T47.1X3	T47.1X4	T47.1X5	T47.1X6
oxide	T47.1X1	T47.1X2	T47.1X3	T47.1X4	T47.1X5	T47.1X6
peroxide	T49.0X1	T49.0X2	T49.0X3	T49.0X4	T49.0X5	T49.0X6
salicylate	T39.091	T39.092	T39.093	T39.094	T39.095	T39.096
silicofluoride	T50.3X1	T50.3X2	T50.3X3	T50.3X4	T50.3X5	T50.3X6
sulfate	T47.4X1	T47.4X2	T47.4X3	T47.4X4	T47.4X5	T47.4X6
thiosulfate	T45.0X1	T45.0X2	T45.0X3	T45.0X4	T45.0X5	T45.0X6
trisilicate	T47.1X1	T47.1X2	T47.1X3	T47.1X4	T47.1X5	T47.1X6
Malathion (medicinal)	T49.0X1	T49.0X2	T49.0X3	T49.0X4	T49.0X5	T49.0X6
insecticide	T60.0X1	T60.0X2	T60.0X3	T60.0X4	—	—
Male fern extract	T37.4X1	T37.4X2	T37.4X3	T37.4X4	T37.4X5	T37.4X6
M-AMSA	T45.1X1	T45.1X2	T45.1X3	T45.1X4	T45.1X5	T45.1X6
Mandelic acid	T37.8X1	T37.8X2	T37.8X3	T37.8X4	T37.8X5	T37.8X6
Manganese (dioxide) (salts)	T57.2X1	T57.2X2	T57.2X3	T57.2X4	—	—
medicinal	T50.991	T50.992	T50.993	T50.994	T50.995	T50.996
Mannitol	T47.3X1	T47.3X2	T47.3X3	T47.3X4	T47.3X5	T47.3X6
hexanitrate	T46.3X1	T46.3X2	T46.3X3	T46.3X4	T46.3X5	T46.3X6
Mannomustine	T45.1X1	T45.1X2	T45.1X3	T45.1X4	T45.1X5	T45.1X6
MAO inhibitors	T43.1X1	T43.1X2	T43.1X3	T43.1X4	T43.1X5	T43.1X6
Mapharsen	T37.8X1	T37.8X2	T37.8X3	T37.8X4	T37.8X5	T37.8X6
Maphenide	T49.0X1	T49.0X2	T49.0X3	T49.0X4	T49.0X5	T49.0X6
Maprotiline	T43.021	T43.022	T43.023	T43.024	T43.025	T43.026
Marcaine	T41.3X1	T41.3X2	T41.3X3	T41.3X4	T41.3X5	T41.3X6
infiltration (subcutaneous)	T41.3X1	T41.3X2	T41.3X3	T41.3X4	T41.3X5	T41.3X6
nerve block (peripheral) (plexus)	T41.3X1	T41.3X2	T41.3X3	T41.3X4	T41.3X5	T41.3X6
Marezine	T45.0X1	T45.0X2	T45.0X3	T45.0X4	T45.0X5	T45.0X6
Marihuana	T40.7X1	T40.7X2	T40.7X3	T40.7X4	T40.7X5	T40.7X6
Marijuana	T40.7X1	T40.7X2	T40.7X3	T40.7X4	T40.7X5	T40.7X6
Marine (sting)	T63.691	T63.692	T63.693	T63.694	—	—
animals (sting)	T63.691	T63.692	T63.693	T63.694	—	—
plants (sting)	T63.711	T63.712	T63.713	T63.714	—	—
Marplan	T43.1X1	T43.1X2	T43.1X3	T43.1X4	T43.1X5	T43.1X6
Marsh gas	T59.891	T59.892	T59.893	T59.894	—	—
Marsilid	T43.1X1	T43.1X2	T43.1X3	T43.1X4	T43.1X5	T43.1X6
Matulane	T45.1X1	T45.1X2	T45.1X3	T45.1X4	T45.1X5	T45.1X6
Mazindol	T50.5X1	T50.5X2	T50.5X3	T50.5X4	T50.5X5	T50.5X6
MCPA	T60.3X1	T60.3X2	T60.3X3	T60.3X4	—	—
MDMA	T43.641	T43.642	T43.643	T43.644	—	—
Meadow saffron	T62.2X1	T62.2X2	T62.2X3	T62.2X4	—	—
Measles virus vaccine (attenuated)	T50.B91	T50.B92	T50.B93	T50.B94	T50.B95	T50.B96
Meat, noxious	T62.8X1	T62.8X2	T62.8X3	T62.8X4	—	—
Meballymal	T42.3X1	T42.3X2	T42.3X3	T42.3X4	T42.3X5	T42.3X6
Mebanazine	T43.1X1	T43.1X2	T43.1X3	T43.1X4	T43.1X5	T43.1X6
Mebaral	T42.3X1	T42.3X2	T42.3X3	T42.3X4	T42.3X5	T42.3X6
Mebendazole	T37.4X1	T37.4X2	T37.4X3	T37.4X4	T37.4X5	T37.4X6
Mebeverine	T44.3X1	T44.3X2	T44.3X3	T44.3X4	T44.3X5	T44.3X6
Mebhydrolin	T45.0X1	T45.0X2	T45.0X3	T45.0X4	T45.0X5	T45.0X6
Mebumal	T42.3X1	T42.3X2	T42.3X3	T42.3X4	T42.3X5	T42.3X6
Mebutamate	T43.591	T43.592	T43.593	T43.594	T43.595	T43.596
Mecamylamine	T44.2X1	T44.2X2	T44.2X3	T44.2X4	T44.2X5	T44.2X6

Additional Character May Be Required — Refer to the Tabular List for Character Selection — Subterms under main terms may continue to next column or page

Substance	Poisoning, Accidental (unintentional)	Poisoning, Intentional Self-harm	Poisoning, Assault	Poisoning, Undetermined	Adverse Effect	Under-dosing
Mechlorethamine	T45.1X1	T45.1X2	T45.1X3	T45.1X4	T45.1X5	T45.1X6
Mecillinam	T36.0X1	T36.0X2	T36.0X3	T36.0X4	T36.0X5	T36.0X6
Meclizine (hydrochloride)	T45.0X1	T45.0X2	T45.0X3	T45.0X4	T45.0X5	T45.0X6
Meclocycline	T36.4X1	T36.4X2	T36.4X3	T36.4X4	T36.4X5	T36.4X6
Meclofenamate	T39.391	T39.392	T39.393	T39.394	T39.395	T39.396
Meclofenamic acid	T39.391	T39.392	T39.393	T39.394	T39.395	T39.396
Meclofenoxate	T43.691	T43.692	T43.693	T43.694	T43.695	T43.696
Meclozine	T45.0X1	T45.0X2	T45.0X3	T45.0X4	T45.0X5	T45.0X6
Mecobalamin	T45.8X1	T45.8X2	T45.8X3	T45.8X4	T45.8X5	T45.8X6
Mecoprop	T60.3X1	T60.3X2	T60.3X3	T60.3X4	—	—
Mecrilate	T49.3X1	T49.3X2	T49.3X3	T49.3X4	T49.3X5	T49.3X6
Mecysteine	T48.4X1	T48.4X2	T48.4X3	T48.4X4	T48.4X5	T48.4X6
Medazepam	T42.4X1	T42.4X2	T42.4X3	T42.4X4	T42.4X5	T42.4X6
Medicament NEC	T50.901	T50.902	T50.903	T50.904	T50.905	T50.906
Medinal	T42.3X1	T42.3X2	T42.3X3	T42.3X4	T42.3X5	T42.3X6
Medomin	T42.3X1	T42.3X2	T42.3X3	T42.3X4	T42.3X5	T42.3X6
Medrogestone	T38.5X1	T38.5X2	T38.5X3	T38.5X4	T38.5X5	T38.5X6
Medroxalol	T44.8X1	T44.8X2	T44.8X3	T44.8X4	T44.8X5	T44.8X6
Medroxyprogesterone acetate (depot)	T38.5X1	T38.5X2	T38.5X3	T38.5X4	T38.5X5	T38.5X6
Medrysone	T49.0X1	T49.0X2	T49.0X3	T49.0X4	T49.0X5	T49.0X6
Mefenamic acid	T39.391	T39.392	T39.393	T39.394	T39.395	T39.396
Mefenorex	T50.5X1	T50.5X2	T50.5X3	T50.5X4	T50.5X5	T50.5X6
Mefloquine	T37.2X1	T37.2X2	T37.2X3	T37.2X4	T37.2X5	T37.2X6
Mefruside	T50.2X1	T50.2X2	T50.2X3	T50.2X4	T50.2X5	T50.2X6
Megahallucinogen	T40.901	T40.902	T40.903	T40.904	T40.905	T40.906
Megestrol	T38.5X1	T38.5X2	T38.5X3	T38.5X4	T38.5X5	T38.5X6
Meglumine						
antimoniate	T37.8X1	T37.8X2	T37.8X3	T37.8X4	T37.8X5	T37.8X6
diatrizoate	T50.8X1	T50.8X2	T50.8X3	T50.8X4	T50.8X5	T50.8X6
iodipamide	T50.8X1	T50.8X2	T50.8X3	T50.8X4	T50.8X5	T50.8X6
iotroxate	T50.8X1	T50.8X2	T50.8X3	T50.8X4	T50.8X5	T50.8X6
MEK (methyl ethyl ketone)	T52.4X1	T52.4X2	T52.4X3	T52.4X4	—	—
Meladinin	T49.3X1	T49.3X2	T49.3X3	T49.3X4	T49.3X5	T49.3X6
Meladrazine	T44.3X1	T44.3X2	T44.3X3	T44.3X4	T44.3X5	T44.3X6
Melaleuca alternifolia oil	T49.0X1	T49.0X2	T49.0X3	T49.0X4	T49.0X5	T49.0X6
Melanizing agents	T49.3X1	T49.3X2	T49.3X3	T49.3X4	T49.3X5	T49.3X6
Melanocyte-stimulating hormone	T38.891	T38.892	T38.893	T38.894	T38.895	T38.896
Melarsonyl potassium	T37.3X1	T37.3X2	T37.3X3	T37.3X4	T37.3X5	T37.3X6
Melarsoprol	T37.3X1	T37.3X2	T37.3X3	T37.3X4	T37.3X5	T37.3X6
Melia azedarach	T62.2X1	T62.2X2	T62.2X3	T62.2X4	—	—
Melitracen	T43.011	T43.012	T43.013	T43.014	T43.015	T43.016
Mellaril	T43.3X1	T43.3X2	T43.3X3	T43.3X4	T43.3X5	T43.3X6
Meloxine	T49.3X1	T49.3X2	T49.3X3	T49.3X4	T49.3X5	T49.3X6
Melperone	T43.4X1	T43.4X2	T43.4X3	T43.4X4	T43.4X5	T43.4X6
Melphalan	T45.1X1	T45.1X2	T45.1X3	T45.1X4	T45.1X5	T45.1X6
Memantine	T43.8X1	T43.8X2	T43.8X3	T43.8X4	T43.8X5	T43.8X6
Menadiol	T45.7X1	T45.7X2	T45.7X3	T45.7X4	T45.7X5	T45.7X6
sodium sulfate	T45.7X1	T45.7X2	T45.7X3	T45.7X4	T45.7X5	T45.7X6
Menadione	T45.7X1	T45.7X2	T45.7X3	T45.7X4	T45.7X5	T45.7X6
sodium bisulfite	T45.7X1	T45.7X2	T45.7X3	T45.7X4	T45.7X5	T45.7X6
Menaphthone	T45.7X1	T45.7X2	T45.7X3	T45.7X4	T45.7X5	T45.7X6
Menaquinone	T45.7X1	T45.7X2	T45.7X3	T45.7X4	T45.7X5	T45.7X6
Menatetrenone	T45.7X1	T45.7X2	T45.7X3	T45.7X4	T45.7X5	T45.7X6
Meningococcal vaccine	T50.A91	T50.A92	T50.A93	T50.A94	T50.A95	T50.A96
Menningovax (-AC) (-C)	T50.A91	T50.A92	T50.A93	T50.A94	T50.A95	T50.A96
Menotropins	T38.811	T38.812	T38.813	T38.814	T38.815	T38.816
Menthol	T48.5X1	T48.5X2	T48.5X3	T48.5X4	T48.5X5	T48.5X6
Mepacrine	T37.2X1	T37.2X2	T37.2X3	T37.2X4	T37.2X5	T37.2X6
Meparfynol	T42.6X1	T42.6X2	T42.6X3	T42.6X4	T42.6X5	T42.6X6
Mepartricin	T36.7X1	T36.7X2	T36.7X3	T36.7X4	T36.7X5	T36.7X6
Mepazine	T43.3X1	T43.3X2	T43.3X3	T43.3X4	T43.3X5	T43.3X6
Mepenzolate	T44.3X1	T44.3X2	T44.3X3	T44.3X4	T44.3X5	T44.3X6
bromide	T44.3X1	T44.3X2	T44.3X3	T44.3X4	T44.3X5	T44.3X6
Meperidine	T40.4X1	T40.4X2	T40.4X3	T40.4X4	T40.4X5	T40.4X6
Mephebarbital	T42.3X1	T42.3X2	T42.3X3	T42.3X4	T42.3X5	T42.3X6
Mephenamin (e)	T42.8X1	T42.8X2	T42.8X3	T42.8X4	T42.8X5	T42.8X6
Mephenesin	T42.8X1	T42.8X2	T42.8X3	T42.8X4	T42.8X5	T42.8X6
Mephenhydramine	T45.0X1	T45.0X2	T45.0X3	T45.0X4	T45.0X5	T45.0X6
Mephenoxalone	T42.8X1	T42.8X2	T42.8X3	T42.8X4	T42.8X5	T42.8X6
Mephentermine	T44.991	T44.992	T44.993	T44.994	T44.995	T44.996
Mephenytoin	T42.0X1	T42.0X2	T42.0X3	T42.0X4	T42.0X5	T42.0X6
with phenobarbital	T42.3X1	T42.3X2	T42.3X3	T42.3X4	T42.3X5	T42.3X6
Mephobarbital	T42.3X1	T42.3X2	T42.3X3	T42.3X4	T42.3X5	T42.3X6
Mephosfolan	T60.0X1	T60.0X2	T60.0X3	T60.0X4	—	—
Mepindolol	T44.7X1	T44.7X2	T44.7X3	T44.7X4	T44.7X5	T44.7X6
Mepiperphenidol	T44.3X1	T44.3X2	T44.3X3	T44.3X4	T44.3X5	T44.3X6
Mepitiostane	T38.7X1	T38.7X2	T38.7X3	T38.7X4	T38.7X5	T38.7X6
Mepivacaine	T41.3X1	T41.3X2	T41.3X3	T41.3X4	T41.3X5	T41.3X6
epidural	T41.3X1	T41.3X2	T41.3X3	T41.3X4	T41.3X5	T41.3X6
Meprednisone	T38.0X1	T38.0X2	T38.0X3	T38.0X4	T38.0X5	T38.0X6
Meprobam	T43.591	T43.592	T43.593	T43.594	T43.595	T43.596

Substance	Poisoning, Accidental (unintentional)	Poisoning, Intentional Self-harm	Poisoning, Assault	Poisoning, Undetermined	Adverse Effect	Under-dosing
Meprobamate	T43.591	T43.592	T43.593	T43.594	T43.595	T43.596
Meproscillarin	T46.0X1	T46.0X2	T46.0X3	T46.0X4	T46.0X5	T46.0X6
Meprylcaine	T41.3X1	T41.3X2	T41.3X3	T41.3X4	T41.3X5	T41.3X6
Meptazinol	T39.8X1	T39.8X2	T39.8X3	T39.8X4	T39.8X5	T39.8X6
Mepyramine	T45.0X1	T45.0X2	T45.0X3	T45.0X4	T45.0X5	T45.0X6
Mequitazine	T43.3X1	T43.3X2	T43.3X3	T43.3X4	T43.3X5	T43.3X6
Meralluride	T50.2X1	T50.2X2	T50.2X3	T50.2X4	T50.2X5	T50.2X6
Merbaphen	T50.2X1	T50.2X2	T50.2X3	T50.2X4	T50.2X5	T50.2X6
Merbromin	T49.0X1	T49.0X2	T49.0X3	T49.0X4	T49.0X5	T49.0X6
Mercaptobenzothiazole salts	T49.0X1	T49.0X2	T49.0X3	T49.0X4	T49.0X5	T49.0X6
Mercaptomerin	T50.2X1	T50.2X2	T50.2X3	T50.2X4	T50.2X5	T50.2X6
Mercaptopurine	T45.1X1	T45.1X2	T45.1X3	T45.1X4	T45.1X5	T45.1X6
Mercumatilin	T50.2X1	T50.2X2	T50.2X3	T50.2X4	T50.2X5	T50.2X6
Mercuramide	T50.2X1	T50.2X2	T50.2X3	T50.2X4	T50.2X5	T50.2X6
Mercurochrome	T49.0X1	T49.0X2	T49.0X3	T49.0X4	T49.0X5	T49.0X6
Mercurophylline	T50.2X1	T50.2X2	T50.2X3	T50.2X4	T50.2X5	T50.2X6
Mercury, mercurial, mercuric, mercurous (compounds) (cyanide) (fumes) (nonmedicinal) (vapor)	T56.1X1	T56.1X2	T56.1X3	T56.1X4	—	—
NEC						
ammoniated	T49.0X1	T49.0X2	T49.0X3	T49.0X4	T49.0X5	T49.0X6
anti-infective						
local	T49.0X1	T49.0X2	T49.0X3	T49.0X4	T49.0X5	T49.0X6
systemic	T37.8X1	T37.8X2	T37.8X3	T37.8X4	T37.8X5	T37.8X6
topical	T49.0X1	T49.0X2	T49.0X3	T49.0X4	T49.0X5	T49.0X6
chloride (ammoniated)	T49.0X1	T49.0X2	T49.0X3	T49.0X4	T49.0X5	T49.0X6
fungicide	T56.1X1	T56.1X2	T56.1X3	T56.1X4	—	—
diuretic NEC	T50.2X1	T50.2X2	T50.2X3	T50.2X4	T50.2X5	T50.2X6
fungicide	T56.1X1	T56.1X2	T56.1X3	T56.1X4	—	—
organic (fungicide)	T56.1X1	T56.1X2	T56.1X3	T56.1X4	—	—
oxide, yellow	T49.0X1	T49.0X2	T49.0X3	T49.0X4	T49.0X5	T49.0X6
Mersalyl	T50.2X1	T50.2X2	T50.2X3	T50.2X4	T50.2X5	T50.2X6
Merthiolate	T49.0X1	T49.0X2	T49.0X3	T49.0X4	T49.0X5	T49.0X6
ophthalmic preparation	T49.5X1	T49.5X2	T49.5X3	T49.5X4	T49.5X5	T49.5X6
Meruvax	T50.B91	T50.B92	T50.B93	T50.B94	T50.B95	T50.B96
Mesalazine	T47.8X1	T47.8X2	T47.8X3	T47.8X4	T47.8X5	T47.8X6
Mescal buttons	T40.991	T40.992	T40.993	T40.994	—	—
Mescaline	T40.991	T40.992	T40.993	T40.994	—	—
Mesna	T48.4X1	T48.4X2	T48.4X3	T48.4X4	T48.4X5	T48.4X6
Mesoglycan	T46.6X1	T46.6X2	T46.6X3	T46.6X4	T46.6X5	T46.6X6
Mesoridazine	T43.3X1	T43.3X2	T43.3X3	T43.3X4	T43.3X5	T43.3X6
Mestanolone	T38.7X1	T38.7X2	T38.7X3	T38.7X4	T38.7X5	T38.7X6
Mesterolone	T38.7X1	T38.7X2	T38.7X3	T38.7X4	T38.7X5	T38.7X6
Mestranol	T38.5X1	T38.5X2	T38.5X3	T38.5X4	T38.5X5	T38.5X6
Mesulergine	T42.8X1	T42.8X2	T42.8X3	T42.8X4	T42.8X5	T42.8X6
Mesulfen	T49.0X1	T49.0X2	T49.0X3	T49.0X4	T49.0X5	T49.0X6
Mesuximide	T42.2X1	T42.2X2	T42.2X3	T42.2X4	T42.2X5	T42.2X6
Metabutethamine	T41.3X1	T41.3X2	T41.3X3	T41.3X4	T41.3X5	T41.3X6
Metactesylacetate	T49.0X1	T49.0X2	T49.0X3	T49.0X4	T49.0X5	T49.0X6
Metacycline	T36.4X1	T36.4X2	T36.4X3	T36.4X4	T36.4X5	T36.4X6
Metaldehyde (snail killer)	T60.8X1	T60.8X2	T60.8X3	T60.8X4	—	—
NEC						
Metals (heavy) (nonmedicinal)	T56.91	T56.92	T56.93	T56.94	—	—
dust, fumes, or vapor NEC	T56.91	T56.92	T56.93	T56.94	—	—
light NEC	T56.91	T56.92	T56.93	T56.94	—	—
dust, fumes, or vapor NEC	T56.91	T56.92	T56.93	T56.94	—	—
specified NEC	T56.891	T56.892	T56.893	T56.894	—	—
thallium	T56.811	T56.812	T56.813	T56.814	—	—
Metamfetamine	T43.621	T43.622	T43.623	T43.624	T43.625	T43.626
Metamizole sodium	T39.2X1	T39.2X2	T39.2X3	T39.2X4	T39.2X5	T39.2X6
Metampicillin	T36.0X1	T36.0X2	T36.0X3	T36.0X4	T36.0X5	T36.0X6
Metamucil	T47.4X1	T47.4X2	T47.4X3	T47.4X4	T47.4X5	T47.4X6
Metandienone	T38.7X1	T38.7X2	T38.7X3	T38.7X4	T38.7X5	T38.7X6
Metandrostenolone	T38.7X1	T38.7X2	T38.7X3	T38.7X4	T38.7X5	T38.7X6
Metaphen	T49.0X1	T49.0X2	T49.0X3	T49.0X4	T49.0X5	T49.0X6
Metaphos	T60.0X1	T60.0X2	T60.0X3	T60.0X4	—	—
Metapramine	T43.011	T43.012	T43.013	T43.014	T43.015	T43.016
Metaproterenol	T48.291	T48.292	T48.293	T48.294	T48.295	T48.296
Metaraminol	T44.4X1	T44.4X2	T44.4X3	T44.4X4	T44.4X5	T44.4X6
Metaxalone	T42.8X1	T42.8X2	T42.8X3	T42.8X4	T42.8X5	T42.8X6
Metenolone	T38.7X1	T38.7X2	T38.7X3	T38.7X4	T38.7X5	T38.7X6
Metergoline	T42.8X1	T42.8X2	T42.8X3	T42.8X4	T42.8X5	T42.8X6
Metescufylline	T46.991	T46.992	T46.993	T46.994	T46.995	T46.996
Metetoin	T42.0X1	T42.0X2	T42.0X3	T42.0X4	T42.0X5	T42.0X6
Metformin	T38.3X1	T38.3X2	T38.3X3	T38.3X4	T38.3X5	T38.3X6
Methacholine	T44.1X1	T44.1X2	T44.1X3	T44.1X4	T44.1X5	T44.1X6
Methacycline	T36.4X1	T36.4X2	T36.4X3	T36.4X4	T36.4X5	T36.4X6
Methadone	T40.3X1	T40.3X2	T40.3X3	T40.3X4	T40.3X5	T40.3X6
Methallenestril	T38.5X1	T38.5X2	T38.5X3	T38.5X4	T38.5X5	T38.5X6

Substance	Poisoning, Accidental (unintentional)	Poisoning, Intentional Self-harm	Poisoning, Assault	Poisoning, Undetermined	Adverse Effect	Under-dosing
Methallenoestril	T38.5X1	T38.5X2	T38.5X3	T38.5X4	T38.5X5	T38.5X6
Methamphetamine	T43.621	T43.622	T43.623	T43.624	T43.625	T43.626
Methampyrone	T39.2X1	T39.2X2	T39.2X3	T39.2X4	T39.2X5	T39.2X6
Methandienone	T38.7X1	T38.7X2	T38.7X3	T38.7X4	T38.7X5	T38.7X6
Methandriol	T38.7X1	T38.7X2	T38.7X3	T38.7X4	T38.7X5	T38.7X6
Methandrostenolone	T38.7X1	T38.7X2	T38.7X3	T38.7X4	T38.7X5	T38.7X6
Methane	T59.891	T59.892	T59.893	T59.894	—	—
Methanethiol	T59.891	T59.892	T59.893	T59.894	—	—
Methaniazide	T37.1X1	T37.1X2	T37.1X3	T37.1X4	T37.1X5	T37.1X6
Methanol (vapor)	T51.1X1	T51.1X2	T51.1X3	T51.1X4	—	—
Methantheline	T44.3X1	T44.3X2	T44.3X3	T44.3X4	T44.3X5	T44.3X6
Methanthelinium bromide	T44.3X1	T44.3X2	T44.3X3	T44.3X4	T44.3X5	T44.3X6
Methaphenilene	T45.0X1	T45.0X2	T45.0X3	T45.0X4	T45.0X5	T45.0X6
Methapyrilene	T45.0X1	T45.0X2	T45.0X3	T45.0X4	T45.0X5	T45.0X6
Methaqualone (compound)	T42.6X1	T42.6X2	T42.6X3	T42.6X4	T42.6X5	T42.6X6
Metharbital	T42.3X1	T42.3X2	T42.3X3	T42.3X4	T42.3X5	T42.3X6
Methazolamide	T50.2X1	T50.2X2	T50.2X3	T50.2X4	T50.2X5	T50.2X6
Methdilazine	T43.3X1	T43.3X2	T43.3X3	T43.3X4	T43.3X5	T43.3X6
Methedrine	T43.621	T43.622	T43.623	T43.624	T43.625	T43.626
Methenamine (mandelate)	T37.8X1	T37.8X2	T37.8X3	T37.8X4	T37.8X5	T37.8X6
Methenolone	T38.7X1	T38.7X2	T38.7X3	T38.7X4	T38.7X5	T38.7X6
Methergine	T48.0X1	T48.0X2	T48.0X3	T48.0X4	T48.0X5	T48.0X6
Methetoin	T42.0X1	T42.0X2	T42.0X3	T42.0X4	T42.0X5	T42.0X6
Methiacil	T38.2X1	T38.2X2	T38.2X3	T38.2X4	T38.2X5	T38.2X6
Methicillin	T36.0X1	T36.0X2	T36.0X3	T36.0X4	T36.0X5	T36.0X6
Methimazole	T38.2X1	T38.2X2	T38.2X3	T38.2X4	T38.2X5	T38.2X6
Methiodal sodium	T50.8X1	T50.8X2	T50.8X3	T50.8X4	T50.8X5	T50.8X6
Methionine	T50.991	T50.992	T50.993	T50.994	T50.995	T50.996
Methisazone	T37.5X1	T37.5X2	T37.5X3	T37.5X4	T37.5X5	T37.5X6
Methisoprinol	T37.5X1	T37.5X2	T37.5X3	T37.5X4	T37.5X5	T37.5X6
Methitural	T42.3X1	T42.3X2	T42.3X3	T42.3X4	T42.3X5	T42.3X6
Methixene	T44.3X1	T44.3X2	T44.3X3	T44.3X4	T44.3X5	T44.3X6
Methobarbital, methobarbitone	T42.3X1	T42.3X2	T42.3X3	T42.3X4	T42.3X5	T42.3X6
Methocarbamol	T42.8X1	T42.8X2	T42.8X3	T42.8X4	T42.8X5	T42.8X6
skeletal muscle relaxant	T48.1X1	T48.1X2	T48.1X3	T48.1X4	T48.1X5	T48.1X6
Methohexital	T41.1X1	T41.1X2	T41.1X3	T41.1X4	T41.1X5	T41.1X6
Methohexitone	T41.1X1	T41.1X2	T41.1X3	T41.1X4	T41.1X5	T41.1X6
Methoin	T42.0X1	T42.0X2	T42.0X3	T42.0X4	T42.0X5	T42.0X6
Methopholine	T39.8X1	T39.8X2	T39.8X3	T39.8X4	T39.8X5	T39.8X6
Methopromazine	T43.3X1	T43.3X2	T43.3X3	T43.3X4	T43.3X5	T43.3X6
Methorate	T48.3X1	T48.3X2	T48.3X3	T48.3X4	T48.3X5	T48.3X6
Methoserpidine	T46.5X1	T46.5X2	T46.5X3	T46.5X4	T46.5X5	T46.5X6
Methotrexate	T45.1X1	T45.1X2	T45.1X3	T45.1X4	T45.1X5	T45.1X6
Methotrimeprazine	T43.3X1	T43.3X2	T43.3X3	T43.3X4	T43.3X5	T43.3X6
Methoxa-Dome	T49.3X1	T49.3X2	T49.3X3	T49.3X4	T49.3X5	T49.3X6
Methoxamine	T44.4X1	T44.4X2	T44.4X3	T44.4X4	T44.4X5	T44.4X6
Methoxsalen	T50.991	T50.992	T50.993	T50.994	T50.995	T50.996
Methoxyaniline	T65.3X1	T65.3X2	T65.3X3	T65.3X4	—	—
Methoxybenzyl penicillin	T36.0X1	T36.0X2	T36.0X3	T36.0X4	T36.0X5	T36.0X6
Methoxychlor	T53.7X1	T53.7X2	T53.7X3	T53.7X4	—	—
Methoxy-DDT	T53.7X1	T53.7X2	T53.7X3	T53.7X4	—	—
Methoxyflurane	T41.0X1	T41.0X2	T41.0X3	T41.0X4	T41.0X5	T41.0X6
Methoxyphenamine	T48.6X1	T48.6X2	T48.6X3	T48.6X4	T48.6X5	T48.6X6
Methoxypromazine	T43.3X1	T43.3X2	T43.3X3	T43.3X4	T43.3X5	T43.3X6
Methscopolamine bromide	T44.3X1	T44.3X2	T44.3X3	T44.3X4	T44.3X5	T44.3X6
Methsuximide	T42.2X1	T42.2X2	T42.2X3	T42.2X4	T42.2X5	T42.2X6
Methyclothiazide	T50.2X1	T50.2X2	T50.2X3	T50.2X4	T50.2X5	T50.2X6
Methyl						
acetate	T52.4X1	T52.4X2	T52.4X3	T52.4X4	—	—
acetone	T52.4X1	T52.4X2	T52.4X3	T52.4X4	—	—
acrylate	165.891	165.892	T65.893	T65.894	—	—
alcohol	T51.1X1	T51.1X2	T51.1X3	T51.1X4	—	—
aminophenol	T65.3X1	T65.3X2	T65.3X3	T65.3X4	—	—
amphetamine	T43.621	T43.622	T43.623	T43.624	T43.625	T43.626
androstanolone	T38.7X1	T38.7X2	T38.7X3	T38.7X4	T38.7X5	T38.7X6
atropine	T44.3X1	T44.3X2	T44.3X3	T44.3X4	T44.3X5	T44.3X6
benzene	T52.2X1	T52.2X2	T52.2X3	T52.2X4	—	—
benzoate	T52.8X1	T52.8X2	T52.8X3	T52.8X4	—	—
benzol	T52.2X1	T52.2X2	T52.2X3	T52.2X4	—	—
bromide (gas)	T59.891	T59.892	T59.893	T59.894	—	—
fumigant	T60.8X1	T60.8X2	T60.8X3	T60.8X4	—	—
butanol	T51.3X1	T51.3X2	T51.3X3	T51.3X4	—	—
carbinol	T51.1X1	T51.1X2	T51.1X3	T51.1X4	—	—
carbonate	T52.8X1	T52.8X2	T52.8X3	T52.8X4	—	—
CCNU	T45.1X1	T45.1X2	T45.1X3	T45.1X4	T45.1X5	T45.1X6
cellosolve	T52.91	T52.92	T52.93	T52.94	—	—
cellulose	T47.4X1	T47.4X2	T47.4X3	T47.4X4	T47.4X5	T47.4X6
chloride (gas)	T59.891	T59.892	T59.893	T59.894	—	—
chloroformate	T59.3X1	T59.3X2	T59.3X3	T59.3X4	—	—
cyclohexane	T52.8X1	T52.8X2	T52.8X3	T52.8X4	—	—
cyclohexanol	T51.8X1	T51.8X2	T51.8X3	T51.8X4	—	—

Substance	Poisoning, Accidental (unintentional)	Poisoning, Intentional Self-harm	Poisoning, Assault	Poisoning, Undetermined	Adverse Effect	Under-dosing
Methyl — *continued*						
cyclohexanone	T52.8X1	T52.8X2	T52.8X3	T52.8X4	—	—
cyclohexyl acetate	T52.8X1	T52.8X2	T52.8X3	T52.8X4	—	—
demeton	T60.0X1	T60.0X2	T60.0X3	T60.0X4	—	—
dihydromorphinone	T40.2X1	T40.2X2	T40.2X3	T40.2X4	T40.2X5	T40.2X6
ergometrine	T48.0X1	T48.0X2	T48.0X3	T48.0X4	T48.0X5	T48.0X6
ergonovine	T48.0X1	T48.0X2	T48.0X3	T48.0X4	T48.0X5	T48.0X6
ethyl ketone	T52.4X1	T52.4X2	T52.4X3	T52.4X4	—	—
glucamine antimonate	T37.8X1	T37.8X2	T37.8X3	T37.8X4	T37.8X5	T37.8X6
hydrazine	T65.891	T65.892	T65.893	T65.894	—	—
iodide	T65.891	T65.892	T65.893	T65.894	—	—
isobutyl ketone	T52.4X1	T52.4X2	T52.4X3	T52.4X4	—	—
isothiocyanate	T60.3X1	T60.3X2	T60.3X3	T60.3X4	—	—
mercaptan	T59.891	T59.892	T59.893	T59.894	—	—
morphine NEC	T40.2X1	T40.2X2	T40.2X3	T40.2X4	T40.2X5	T40.2X6
nicotinate	T49.4X1	T49.4X2	T49.4X3	T49.4X4	T49.4X5	T49.4X6
paraben	T49.0X1	T49.0X2	T49.0X3	T49.0X4	T49.0X5	T49.0X6
parafynol	T42.6X1	T42.6X2	T42.6X3	T42.6X4	T42.6X5	T42.6X6
parathion	T60.0X1	T60.0X2	T60.0X3	T60.0X4	—	—
peridol	T43.4X1	T43.4X2	T43.4X3	T43.4X4	T43.4X5	T43.4X6
phenidate	T43.631	T43.632	T43.633	T43.634	T43.635	T43.636
prednisolone	T38.0X1	T38.0X2	T38.0X3	T38.0X4	T38.0X5	T38.0X6
ENT agent	T49.6X1	T49.6X2	T49.6X3	T49.6X4	T49.6X5	T49.6X6
ophthalmic preparation	T49.5X1	T49.5X2	T49.5X3	T49.5X4	T49.5X5	T49.5X6
topical NEC	T49.0X1	T49.0X2	T49.0X3	T49.0X4	T49.0X5	T49.0X6
propylcarbinol	T51.3X1	T51.3X2	T51.3X3	T51.3X4	—	—
rosaniline NEC	T49.0X1	T49.0X2	T49.0X3	T49.0X4	T49.0X5	T49.0X6
salicylate	T49.2X1	T49.2X2	T49.2X3	T49.2X4	T49.2X5	T49.2X6
sulfate (fumes)	T59.891	T59.892	T59.893	T59.894	—	—
liquid	T52.8X1	T52.8X2	T52.8X3	T52.8X4	—	—
sulfonal	T42.6X1	T42.6X2	T42.6X3	T42.6X4	T42.6X5	T42.6X6
testosterone	T38.7X1	T38.7X2	T38.7X3	T38.7X4	T38.7X5	T38.7X6
thiouracil	T38.2X1	T38.2X2	T38.2X3	T38.2X4	T38.2X5	T38.2X6
Methylamphetamine	T43.621	T43.622	T43.623	T43.624	T43.625	T43.626
Methylated spirit	T51.1X1	T51.1X2	T51.1X3	T51.1X4	—	—
Methylatropine nitrate	T44.3X1	T44.3X2	T44.3X3	T44.3X4	T44.3X5	T44.3X6
Methylbenactyzium bromide	T44.3X1	T44.3X2	T44.3X3	T44.3X4	T44.3X5	T44.3X6
Methylbenzethonium chloride	T49.0X1	T49.0X2	T49.0X3	T49.0X4	T49.0X5	T49.0X6
Methylcellulose	T47.4X1	T47.4X2	T47.4X3	T47.4X4	T47.4X5	T47.4X6
laxative	T47.4X1	T47.4X2	T47.4X3	T47.4X4	T47.4X5	T47.4X6
Methylchlorophenoxyacetic acid	T60.3X1	T60.3X2	T60.3X3	T60.3X4	—	—
Methyldopa	T46.5X1	T46.5X2	T46.5X3	T46.5X4	T46.5X5	T46.5X6
Methyldopate	T46.5X1	T46.5X2	T46.5X3	T46.5X4	T46.5X5	T46.5X6
Methylene						
blue	T50.6X1	T50.6X2	T50.6X3	T50.6X4	T50.6X5	T50.6X6
chloride or dichloride (solvent) NEC	T53.4X1	T53.4X2	T53.4X3	T53.4X4	—	—
Methylenedioxyamphetamine	T43.621	T43.622	T43.623	T43.624	T43.625	T43.626
Methylenedioxymeth-amphetamine	T43.641	T43.642	T43.643	T43.644	—	—
Methylergometrine	T48.0X1	T48.0X2	T48.0X3	T48.0X4	T48.0X5	T48.0X6
Methylergonovine	T48.0X1	T48.0X2	T48.0X3	T48.0X4	T48.0X5	T48.0X6
Methylestrenolone	T38.5X1	T38.5X2	T38.5X3	T38.5X4	T38.5X5	T38.5X6
Methylethyl cellulose	T50.991	T50.992	T50.993	T50.994	T50.995	T50.996
Methylhexabital	T42.3X1	T42.3X2	T42.3X3	T42.3X4	T42.3X5	T42.3X6
Methylmorphine	T40.2X1	T40.2X2	T40.2X3	T40.2X4	T40.2X5	T40.2X6
Methylparaben (ophthalmic)	T49.5X1	T49.5X2	T49.5X3	T49.5X4	T49.5X5	T49.5X6
Methylparafynol	T42.6X1	T42.6X2	T42.6X3	T42.6X4	T42.6X5	T42.6X6
Methylpentynol, methylpenthynol	T42.6X1	T42.6X2	T42.6X3	T42.6X4	T42.6X5	T42.6X6
Methylphenidate	T43.631	T43.632	T43.633	T43.634	T43.635	T43.636
Methylphenobarbital	T42.3X1	T42.3X2	T42.3X3	T42.3X4	T42.3X5	T42.3X6
Methylpolysiloxane	T47.1X1	T47.1X2	T47.1X3	T47.1X4	T47.1X5	T47.1X6
Methylprednisolone — *see Methyl, prednisolone*						
Methylrosaniline	T49.0X1	T49.0X2	T49.0X3	T49.0X4	T49.0X5	T49.0X6
Methylrosanilinium chloride	T49.0X1	T49.0X2	T49.0X3	T49.0X4	T49.0X5	T49.0X6
Methyltestosterone	T38.7X1	T38.7X2	T38.7X3	T38.7X4	T38.7X5	T38.7X6
Methylthionine chloride	T50.6X1	T50.6X2	T50.6X3	T50.6X4	T50.6X5	T50.6X6
Methylthioninium chloride	T50.6X1	T50.6X2	T50.6X3	T50.6X4	T50.6X5	T50.6X6
Methylthiouracil	T38.2X1	T38.2X2	T38.2X3	T38.2X4	T38.2X5	T38.2X6
Methyprylon	T42.6X1	T42.6X2	T42.6X3	T42.6X4	T42.6X5	T42.6X6
Methysergide	T46.5X1	T46.5X2	T46.5X3	T46.5X4	T46.5X5	T46.5X6
Metiamide	T47.1X1	T47.1X2	T47.1X3	T47.1X4	T47.1X5	T47.1X6
Meticillin	T36.0X1	T36.0X2	T36.0X3	T36.0X4	T36.0X5	T36.0X6
Meticrane	T50.2X1	T50.2X2	T50.2X3	T50.2X4	T50.2X5	T50.2X6
Metildigoxin	T46.0X1	T46.0X2	T46.0X3	T46.0X4	T46.0X5	T46.0X6

Substance	Poisoning, Accidental (unintentional)	Poisoning, Intentional Self-harm	Poisoning, Assault	Poisoning, Undetermined	Adverse Effect	Under-dosing
Metipranolol	T49.5X1	T49.5X2	T49.5X3	T49.5X4	T49.5X5	T49.5X6
Metirosine	T46.5X1	T46.5X2	T46.5X3	T46.5X4	T46.5X5	T46.5X6
Metisazone	T37.5X1	T37.5X2	T37.5X3	T37.5X4	T37.5X5	T37.5X6
Metixene	T44.3X1	T44.3X2	T44.3X3	T44.3X4	T44.3X5	T44.3X6
Metizoline	T48.5X1	T48.5X2	T48.5X3	T48.5X4	T48.5X5	T48.5X6
Metoclopramide	T45.0X1	T45.0X2	T45.0X3	T45.0X4	T45.0X5	T45.0X6
Metofenazate	T43.3X1	T43.3X2	T43.3X3	T43.3X4	T43.3X5	T43.3X6
Metofoline	T39.8X1	T39.8X2	T39.8X3	T39.8X4	T39.8X5	T39.8X6
Metolazone	T50.2X1	T50.2X2	T50.2X3	T50.2X4	T50.2X5	T50.2X6
Metopon	T40.2X1	T40.2X2	T40.2X3	T40.2X4	T40.2X5	T40.2X6
Metoprine	T45.1X1	T45.1X2	T45.1X3	T45.1X4	T45.1X5	T45.1X6
Metoprolol	T44.7X1	T44.7X2	T44.7X3	T44.7X4	T44.7X5	T44.7X6
Metrifonate	T60.0X1	T60.0X2	T60.0X3	T60.0X4	—	—
Metrizamide	T50.8X1	T50.8X2	T50.8X3	T50.8X4	T50.8X5	T50.8X6
Metrizoic acid	T50.8X1	T50.8X2	T50.8X3	T50.8X4	T50.8X5	T50.8X6
Metronidazole	T37.8X1	T37.8X2	T37.8X3	T37.8X4	T37.8X5	T37.8X6
Metycaine	T41.3X1	T41.3X2	T41.3X3	T41.3X4	T41.3X5	T41.3X6
infiltration (subcutaneous)	T41.3X1	T41.3X2	T41.3X3	T41.3X4	T41.3X5	T41.3X6
nerve block (peripheral) (plexus)	T41.3X1	T41.3X2	T41.3X3	T41.3X4	T41.3X5	T41.3X6
topical (surface)	T41.3X1	T41.3X2	T41.3X3	T41.3X4	T41.3X5	T41.3X6
Metyrapone	T50.8X1	T50.8X2	T50.8X3	T50.8X4	T50.8X5	T50.8X6
Mevinphos	T60.0X1	T60.0X2	T60.0X3	T60.0X4	—	—
Mexazolam	T42.4X1	T42.4X2	T42.4X3	T42.4X4	T42.4X5	T42.4X6
Mexenone	T49.3X1	T49.3X2	T49.3X3	T49.3X4	T49.3X5	T49.3X6
Mexiletine	T46.2X1	T46.2X2	T46.2X3	T46.2X4	T46.2X5	T46.2X6
Mezereon	T62.2X1	T62.2X2	T62.2X3	T62.2X4	—	—
berries	T62.1X1	T62.1X2	T62.1X3	T62.1X4	—	—
Mezlocillin	T36.0X1	T36.0X2	T36.0X3	T36.0X4	T36.0X5	T36.0X6
Mianserin	T43.021	T43.022	T43.023	T43.024	T43.025	T43.026
Micatin	T49.0X1	T49.0X2	T49.0X3	T49.0X4	T49.0X5	T49.0X6
Miconazole	T49.0X1	T49.0X2	T49.0X3	T49.0X4	T49.0X5	T49.0X6
Micronomicin	T36.5X1	T36.5X2	T36.5X3	T36.5X4	T36.5X5	T36.5X6
Midazolam	T42.4X1	T42.4X2	T42.4X3	T42.4X4	T42.4X5	T42.4X6
Midecamycin	T36.3X1	T36.3X2	T36.3X3	T36.3X4	T36.3X5	T36.3X6
Mifepristone	T38.6X1	T38.6X2	T38.6X3	T38.6X4	T38.6X5	T38.6X6
Milk of magnesia	T47.1X1	T47.1X2	T47.1X3	T47.1X4	T47.1X5	T47.1X6
Millipede (tropical)	T63.411	T63.412	T63.413	T63.414	—	—
(venomous)						
Miltown	T43.591	T43.592	T43.593	T43.594	T43.595	T43.596
Milverine	T44.3X1	T44.3X2	T44.3X3	T44.3X4	T44.3X5	T44.3X6
Minaprine	T43.291	T43.292	T43.293	T43.294	T43.295	T43.296
Minaxolone	T41.291	T41.292	T41.293	T41.294	T41.295	T41.296
Mineral						
acids	T54.2X1	T54.2X2	T54.2X3	T54.2X4	—	—
oil (laxative)(medicinal)	T47.4X1	T47.4X2	T47.4X3	T47.4X4	T47.4X5	T47.4X6
emulsion	T47.2X1	T47.2X2	T47.2X3	T47.2X4	T47.2X5	T47.2X6
nonmedicinal	T52.0X1	T52.0X2	T52.0X3	T52.0X4	—	—
topical	T49.3X1	T49.3X2	T49.3X3	T49.3X4	T49.3X5	T49.3X6
salt NEC	T50.3X1	T50.3X2	T50.3X3	T50.3X4	T50.3X5	T50.3X6
spirits	T52.0X1	T52.0X2	T52.0X3	T52.0X4	—	—
Mineralocorticosteroid	T50.0X1	T50.0X2	T50.0X3	T50.0X4	T50.0X5	T50.0X6
Minocycline	T36.4X1	T36.4X2	T36.4X3	T36.4X4	T36.4X5	T36.4X6
Minoxidil	T46.7X1	T46.7X2	T46.7X3	T46.7X4	T46.7X5	T46.7X6
Miokamycin	T36.3X1	T36.3X2	T36.3X3	T36.3X4	T36.3X5	T36.3X6
Miotic drug	T49.5X1	T49.5X2	T49.5X3	T49.5X4	T49.5X5	T49.5X6
Mipafox	T60.0X1	T60.0X2	T60.0X3	T60.0X4	—	—
Mirex	T60.1X1	T60.1X2	T60.1X3	T60.1X4	—	—
Mirtazapine	T43.021	T43.022	T43.023	T43.024	T43.025	T43.026
Misonidazole	T37.3X1	T37.3X2	T37.3X3	T37.3X4	T37.3X5	T37.3X6
Misoprostol	T47.1X1	T47.1X2	T47.1X3	T47.1X4	T47.1X5	T47.1X6
Mithramycin	T45.1X1	T45.1X2	T45.1X3	T45.1X4	T45.1X5	T45.1X6
Mitobronitol	T45.1X1	T45.1X2	T45.1X3	T45.1X4	T45.1X5	T45.1X6
Mitoguazone	T45.1X1	T45.1X2	T45.1X3	T45.1X4	T45.1X5	T45.1X6
Mitolactol	T45.1X1	T45.1X2	T45.1X3	T45.1X4	T45.1X5	T45.1X6
Mitomycin	T45.1X1	T45.1X2	T45.1X3	T45.1X4	T45.1X5	T45.1X6
Mitopodozide	T45.1X1	T45.1X2	T45.1X3	T45.1X4	T45.1X5	T45.1X6
Mitotane	T45.1X1	T45.1X2	T45.1X3	T45.1X4	T45.1X5	T45.1X6
Mitoxantrone	T45.1X1	T45.1X2	T45.1X3	T45.1X4	T45.1X5	T45.1X6
Mivacurium chloride	T48.1X1	T48.1X2	T48.1X3	T48.1X4	T48.1X5	T48.1X6
Miyari bacteria	T47.6X1	T47.6X2	T47.6X3	T47.6X4	T47.6X5	T47.6X6
Moclobemide	T43.1X1	T43.1X2	T43.1X3	T43.1X4	T43.1X5	T43.1X6
Moderil	T46.5X1	T46.5X2	T46.5X3	T46.5X4	T46.5X5	T46.5X6
Mofebutazone	T39.2X1	T39.2X2	T39.2X3	T39.2X4	T39.2X5	T39.2X6
Mogadon — see Nitrazepam						
Molindone	T43.591	T43.592	T43.593	T43.594	T43.595	T43.596
Molsidomine	T46.3X1	T46.3X2	T46.3X3	T46.3X4	T46.3X5	T46.3X6
Mometasone	T49.0X1	T49.0X2	T49.0X3	T49.0X4	T49.0X5	T49.0X6
Monistat	T49.0X1	T49.0X2	T49.0X3	T49.0X4	T49.0X5	T49.0X6
Monkshood	T62.2X1	T62.2X2	T62.2X3	T62.2X4	—	—
Monoamine oxidase inhibitor NEC	T43.1X1	T43.1X2	T43.1X3	T43.1X4	T43.1X5	T43.1X6
hydrazine	T43.1X1	T43.1X2	T43.1X3	T43.1X4	T43.1X5	T43.1X6
Monobenzone	T49.4X1	T49.4X2	T49.4X3	T49.4X4	T49.4X5	T49.4X6
Monochloroacetic acid	T60.3X1	T60.3X2	T60.3X3	T60.3X4	—	—
Monochlorobenzene	T53.7X1	T53.7X2	T53.7X3	T53.7X4	—	—
Monoethanolamine	T46.8X1	T46.8X2	T46.8X3	T46.8X4	T46.8X5	T46.8X6
oleate	T46.8X1	T46.8X2	T46.8X3	T46.8X4	T46.8X5	T46.8X6
Monooctanoin	T50.991	T50.992	T50.993	T50.994	T50.995	T50.996
Monophenylbutazone	T39.2X1	T39.2X2	T39.2X3	T39.2X4	T39.2X5	T39.2X6
Monosodium glutamate	T65.891	T65.892	T65.893	T65.894	—	—
Monosulfiram	T49.0X1	T49.0X2	T49.0X3	T49.0X4	T49.0X5	T49.0X6
Monoxide, carbon — see Carbon, monoxide						
Monoxidine hydrochloride	T46.1X1	T46.1X2	T46.1X3	T46.1X4	T46.1X5	T46.1X6
Monuron	T60.3X1	T60.3X2	T60.3X3	T60.3X4	—	—
Moperone	T43.4X1	T43.4X2	T43.4X3	T43.4X4	T43.4X5	T43.4X6
Mopidamol	T45.1X1	T45.1X2	T45.1X3	T45.1X4	T45.1X5	T45.1X6
MOPP (mechloreth-amine + vincristine + prednisone + procarba-zine)	T45.1X1	T45.1X2	T45.1X3	T45.1X4	T45.1X5	T45.1X6
Morfin	T40.2X1	T40.2X2	T40.2X3	T40.2X4	T40.2X5	T40.2X6
Morinamide	T37.1X1	T37.1X2	T37.1X3	T37.1X4	T37.1X5	T37.1X6
Morning glory seeds	T40.991	T40.992	T40.993	T40.994		
Moroxydine	T37.5X1	T37.5X2	T37.5X3	T37.5X4	T37.5X5	T37.5X6
Morphazinamide	T37.1X1	T37.1X2	T37.1X3	T37.1X4	T37.1X5	T37.1X6
Morphine	T40.2X1	T40.2X2	T40.2X3	T40.2X4	T40.2X5	T40.2X6
antagonist	T50.7X1	T50.7X2	T50.7X3	T50.7X4	T50.7X5	T50.7X6
Morpholinylethylmorphine	T40.2X1	T40.2X2	T40.2X3	T40.2X4	—	—
Morsuximide	T42.2X1	T42.2X2	T42.2X3	T42.2X4	T42.2X5	T42.2X6
Mosapramine	T43.591	T43.592	T43.593	T43.594	T43.595	T43.596
Moth balls — see also Pesticides	T60.2X1	T60.2X2	T60.2X3	T60.2X4	—	—
naphthalene	T60.2X1	T60.2X2	T60.2X3	T60.2X4	—	—
paradichlorobenzene	T60.1X1	T60.1X2	T60.1X3	T60.1X4	—	—
Motor exhaust gas	T58.01	T58.02	T58.03	T58.04	—	—
Mouthwash (antiseptic) (zinc chloride)	T49.6X1	T49.6X2	T49.6X3	T49.6X4	T49.6X5	T49.6X6
Moxastine	T45.0X1	T45.0X2	T45.0X3	T45.0X4	T45.0X5	T45.0X6
Moxaverine	T44.3X1	T44.3X2	T44.3X3	T44.3X4	T44.3X5	T44.3X6
Moxisylyte	T46.7X1	T46.7X2	T46.7X3	T46.7X4	T46.7X5	T46.7X6
Mucilage, plant	T47.4X1	T47.4X2	T47.4X3	T47.4X4	T47.4X5	T47.4X6
Mucolytic drug	T48.4X1	T48.4X2	T48.4X3	T48.4X4	T48.4X5	T48.4X6
Mucomyst	T48.4X1	T48.4X2	T48.4X3	T48.4X4	T48.4X5	T48.4X6
Mucous membrane agents (external)	T49.91	T49.92	T49.93	T49.94	T49.95	T49.96
specified NEC	T49.8X1	T49.8X2	T49.8X3	T49.8X4	T49.8X5	T49.8X6
Multiple unspecified drugs, medicaments and biological substances	T50.911	T50.912	T50.913	T50.914	T50.915	T50.916
Mumps						
immune globulin (human)	T50.Z11	T50.Z12	T50.Z13	T50.Z14	T50.Z15	T50.Z16
skin test antigen	T50.8X1	T50.8X2	T50.8X3	T50.8X4	T50.8X5	T50.8X6
vaccine	T50.B91	T50.B92	T50.B93	T50.B94	T50.B95	T50.B96
Mumpsvax	T50.B91	T50.B92	T50.B93	T50.B94	T50.B95	T50.B96
Mupirocin	T49.0X1	T49.0X2	T49.0X3	T49.0X4	T49.0X5	T49.0X6
Muriatic acid — see Hydrochloric acid						
Muromonab-CD3	T45.1X1	T45.1X2	T45.1X3	T45.1X4	T45.1X5	T45.1X6
Muscle-action drug NEC	T48.201	T48.202	T48.203	T48.204	T48.205	T48.206
Muscle affecting agents NEC	T48.201	T48.202	T48.203	T48.204	T48.205	T48.206
oxytocic	T48.0X1	T48.0X2	T48.0X3	T48.0X4	T48.0X5	T48.0X6
relaxants	T48.201	T48.202	T48.203	T48.204	T48.205	T48.206
central nervous system	T42.8X1	T42.8X2	T42.8X3	T42.8X4	T42.8X5	T42.8X6
skeletal	T48.1X1	T48.1X2	T48.1X3	T48.1X4	T48.1X5	T48.1X6
smooth	T44.3X1	T44.3X2	T44.3X3	T44.3X4	T44.3X5	T44.3X6
Muscle relaxant — see Relaxant, muscle						
Muscle-tone depressant, central NEC	T42.8X1	T42.8X2	T42.8X3	T42.8X4	T42.8X5	T42.8X6
specified NEC	T42.8X1	T42.8X2	T42.8X3	T42.8X4	T42.8X5	T42.8X6
Mushroom, noxious	T62.0X1	T62.0X2	T62.0X3	T62.0X4	—	—
Mussel, noxious	T61.781	T61.782	T61.783	T61.784	—	—
Mustard (emetic)	T47.7X1	T47.7X2	T47.7X3	T47.7X4	T47.7X5	T47.7X6
black	T47.7X1	T47.7X2	T47.7X3	T47.7X4	T47.7X5	T47.7X6
gas, not in war	T59.91	T59.92	T59.93	T59.94	—	—
nitrogen	T45.1X1	T45.1X2	T45.1X3	T45.1X4	T45.1X5	T45.1X6
Mustine	T45.1X1	T45.1X2	T45.1X3	T45.1X4	T45.1X5	T45.1X6
M-vac	T45.1X1	T45.1X2	T45.1X3	T45.1X4	T45.1X5	T45.1X6
Mycifradin	T36.5X1	T36.5X2	T36.5X3	T36.5X4	T36.5X5	T36.5X6
topical	T49.0X1	T49.0X2	T49.0X3	T49.0X4	T49.0X5	T49.0X6
Mycitracin	T36.8X1	T36.8X2	T36.8X3	T36.8X4	T36.8X5	T36.8X6
ophthalmic preparation	T49.5X1	T49.5X2	T49.5X3	T49.5X4	T49.5X5	T49.5X6
Mycostatin	T36.7X1	T36.7X2	T36.7X3	T36.7X4	T36.7X5	T36.7X6
topical	T49.0X1	T49.0X2	T49.0X3	T49.0X4	T49.0X5	T49.0X6

Table of Drugs and Chemicals

Substance	Poisoning, Accidental (unintentional)	Poisoning, Intentional Self-harm	Poisoning, Assault	Poisoning, Undetermined	Adverse Effect	Under-dosing
Mycotoxins	T64.81	T64.82	T64.83	T64.84	—	—
aflatoxin	T64.01	T64.02	T64.03	T64.04	—	—
specified NEC	T64.81	T64.82	T64.83	T64.84	—	—
Mydriacyl	T44.3X1	T44.3X2	T44.3X3	T44.3X4	T44.3X5	T44.3X6
Mydriatic drug	T49.5X1	T49.5X2	T49.5X3	T49.5X4	T49.5X5	T49.5X6
Myelobromal	T45.1X1	T45.1X2	T45.1X3	T45.1X4	T45.1X5	T45.1X6
Myleran	T45.1X1	T45.1X2	T45.1X3	T45.1X4	T45.1X5	T45.1X6
Myochrysin (e)	T39.2X1	T39.2X2	T39.2X3	T39.2X4	T39.2X5	T39.2X6
Myoneural blocking agents	T48.1X1	T48.1X2	T48.1X3	T48.1X4	T48.1X5	T48.1X6
Myralact	T49.0X1	T49.0X2	T49.0X3	T49.0X4	T49.0X5	T49.0X6
Myristica fragrans	T62.2X1	T62.2X2	T62.2X3	T62.2X4	—	—
Myristicin	T65.891	T65.892	T65.893	T65.894	—	—
Mysoline	T42.3X1	T42.3X2	T42.3X3	T42.3X4	T42.3X5	T42.3X6
Nabilone	T40.7X1	T40.7X2	T40.7X3	T40.7X4	T40.7X5	T40.7X6
Nabumetone	T39.391	T39.392	T39.393	T39.394	T39.395	T39.396
Nadolol	T44.7X1	T44.7X2	T44.7X3	T44.7X4	T44.7X5	T44.7X6
Nafcillin	T36.0X1	T36.0X2	T36.0X3	T36.0X4	T36.0X5	T36.0X6
Nafoxidine	T38.6X1	T38.6X2	T38.6X3	T38.6X4	T38.6X5	T38.6X6
Naftazone	T46.991	T46.992	T46.993	T46.994	T46.995	T46.996
Naftidrofuryl (oxalate)	T46.7X1	T46.7X2	T46.7X3	T46.7X4	T46.7X5	T46.7X6
Naftifine	T49.0X1	T49.0X2	T49.0X3	T49.0X4	T49.0X5	T49.0X6
Nail polish remover	T52.91	T52.92	T52.93	T52.94	—	—
Nalbuphine	T40.4X1	T40.4X2	T40.4X3	T40.4X4	T40.4X5	T40.4X6
Naled	T60.0X1	T60.0X2	T60.0X3	T60.0X4	—	—
Nalidixic acid	T37.8X1	T37.8X2	T37.8X3	T37.8X4	T37.8X5	T37.8X6
Nalorphine	T50.7X1	T50.7X2	T50.7X3	T50.7X4	T50.7X5	T50.7X6
Naloxone	T50.7X1	T50.7X2	T50.7X3	T50.7X4	T50.7X5	T50.7X6
Naltrexone	T50.7X1	T50.7X2	T50.7X3	T50.7X4	T50.7X5	T50.7X6
Namenda	T43.8X1	T43.8X2	T43.8X3	T43.8X4	T43.8X5	T43.8X6
Nandrolone	T38.7X1	T38.7X2	T38.7X3	T38.7X4	T38.7X5	T38.7X6
Naphazoline	T48.5X1	T48.5X2	T48.5X3	T48.5X4	T48.5X5	T48.5X6
Naphtha (painters') (petroleum)	T52.0X1	T52.0X2	T52.0X3	T52.0X4	—	—
solvent	T52.0X1	T52.0X2	T52.0X3	T52.0X4	—	—
vapor	T52.0X1	T52.0X2	T52.0X3	T52.0X4	—	—
Naphthalene (non-chlorinated)	T60.2X1	T60.2X2	T60.2X3	T60.2X4	—	—
chlorinated	T60.1X1	T60.1X2	T60.1X3	T60.1X4	—	—
vapor	T60.1X1	T60.1X2	T60.1X3	T60.1X4	—	—
insecticide or moth repellent	T60.2X1	T60.2X2	T60.2X3	T60.2X4	—	—
chlorinated	T60.1X1	T60.1X2	T60.1X3	T60.1X4	—	—
vapor	T60.2X1	T60.2X2	T60.2X3	T60.2X4	—	—
chlorinated	T60.1X1	T60.1X2	T60.1X3	T60.1X4	—	—
Naphthol	T65.891	T65.892	T65.893	T65.894	—	—
Naphthylamine	T65.891	T65.892	T65.893	T65.894	—	—
Naphthylthiourea (ANTU)	T60.4X1	T60.4X2	T60.4X3	T60.4X4	—	—
Naprosyn — *see* Naproxen						
Naproxen	T39.311	T39.312	T39.313	T39.314	T39.315	T39.316
Narcotic (drug)	T40.601	T40.602	T40.603	T40.604	T40.605	T40.606
analgesic NEC	T40.601	T40.602	T40.603	T40.604	T40.605	T40.606
antagonist	T50.7X1	T50.7X2	T50.7X3	T50.7X4	T50.7X5	T50.7X6
specified NEC	T40.691	T40.692	T40.693	T40.694	T40.695	T40.696
synthetic	T40.4X1	T40.4X2	T40.4X3	T40.4X4	T40.4X5	T40.4X6
Narcotine	T48.3X1	T48.3X2	T48.3X3	T48.3X4	T48.3X5	T48.3X6
Nardil	T43.1X1	T43.1X2	T43.1X3	T43.1X4	T43.1X5	T43.1X6
Nasal drug NEC	T49.6X1	T49.6X2	T49.6X3	T49.6X4	T49.6X5	T49.6X6
Natamycin	T49.0X1	T49.0X2	T49.0X3	T49.0X4	T49.0X5	T49.0X6
Natrium cyanide — *see* Cyanide(s)						
Natural						
blood (product)	T45.8X1	T45.8X2	T45.8X3	T45.8X4	T45.8X5	T45.8X6
gas (piped)	T59.891	T59.892	T59.893	T59.894	—	—
incomplete combustion	T58.11	T58.12	T58.13	T58.14	—	—
Nealbarbital	T42.3X1	T42.3X2	T42.3X3	T42.3X4	T42.3X5	T42.3X6
Nectadon	T48.3X1	T48.3X2	T48.3X3	T48.3X4	T48.3X5	T48.3X6
Nedocromil	T48.6X1	T48.6X2	T48.6X3	T48.6X4	T48.6X5	T48.6X6
Nefopam	T39.8X1	T39.8X2	T39.8X3	T39.8X4	T39.8X5	T39.8X6
Nematocyst (sting)	T63.691	T63.692	T63.693	T63.694	—	—
Nembutal	T42.3X1	T42.3X2	T42.3X3	T42.3X4	T42.3X5	T42.3X6
Nemonapride	T43.591	T43.592	T43.593	T43.594	T43.595	T43.596
Neoarsphenamine	T37.8X1	T37.8X2	T37.8X3	T37.8X4	T37.8X5	T37.8X6
Neocinchophen	T50.4X1	T50.4X2	T50.4X3	T50.4X4	T50.4X5	T50.4X6
Neomycin (derivatives)	T36.5X1	T36.5X2	T36.5X3	T36.5X4	T36.5X5	T36.5X6
with						
bacitracin	T49.0X1	T49.0X2	T49.0X3	T49.0X4	T49.0X5	T49.0X6
neostigmine	T44.0X1	T44.0X2	T44.0X3	T44.0X4	T44.0X5	T44.0X6
ENT agent	T49.6X1	T49.6X2	T49.6X3	T49.6X4	T49.6X5	T49.6X6
ophthalmic preparation	T49.5X1	T49.5X2	T49.5X3	T49.5X4	T49.5X5	T49.5X6
topical NEC	T49.0X1	T49.0X2	T49.0X3	T49.0X4	T49.0X5	T49.0X6
Neonal	T42.3X1	T42.3X2	T42.3X3	T42.3X4	T42.3X5	T42.3X6
Neoprontosil	T37.0X1	T37.0X2	T37.0X3	T37.0X4	T37.0X5	T37.0X6

Substance	Poisoning, Accidental (unintentional)	Poisoning, Intentional Self-harm	Poisoning, Assault	Poisoning, Undetermined	Adverse Effect	Under-dosing
Neosalvarsan	T37.8X1	T37.8X2	T37.8X3	T37.8X4	T37.8X5	T37.8X6
Neosilversalvarsan	T37.8X1	T37.8X2	T37.8X3	T37.8X4	T37.8X5	T37.8X6
Neosporin	T36.8X1	T36.8X2	T36.8X3	T36.8X4	T36.8X5	T36.8X6
ENT agent	T49.6X1	T49.6X2	T49.6X3	T49.6X4	T49.6X5	T49.6X6
opthalmic preparation	T49.5X1	T49.5X2	T49.5X3	T49.5X4	T49.5X5	T49.5X6
topical NEC	T49.0X1	T49.0X2	T49.0X3	T49.0X4	T49.0X5	T49.0X6
Neostigmine bromide	T44.0X1	T44.0X2	T44.0X3	T44.0X4	T44.0X5	T44.0X6
Neraval	T42.3X1	T42.3X2	T42.3X3	T42.3X4	T42.3X5	T42.3X6
Neravan	T42.3X1	T42.3X2	T42.3X3	T42.3X4	T42.3X5	T42.3X6
Nerium oleander	T62.2X1	T62.2X2	T62.2X3	T62.2X4	—	—
Nerve gas, not in war	T59.91	T59.92	T59.93	T59.94	—	—
Nesacaine	T41.3X1	T41.3X2	T41.3X3	T41.3X4	T41.3X5	T41.3X6
infiltration (subcutaneous)	T41.3X1	T41.3X2	T41.3X3	T41.3X4	T41.3X5	T41.3X6
nerve block (peripheral) (plexus)	T41.3X1	T41.3X2	T41.3X3	T41.3X4	T41.3X5	T41.3X6
Netilmicin	T36.5X1	T36.5X2	T36.5X3	T36.5X4	T36.5X5	T36.5X6
Neurobarb	T42.3X1	T42.3X2	T42.3X3	T42.3X4	T42.3X5	T42.3X6
Neuroleptic drug NEC	T43.501	T43.502	T43.503	T43.504	T43.505	T43.506
Neuromuscular blocking drug	T48.1X1	T48.1X2	T48.1X3	T48.1X4	T48.1X5	T48.1X6
Neutral insulin injection	T38.3X1	T38.3X2	T38.3X3	T38.3X4	T38.3X5	T38.3X6
Neutral spirits	T51.0X1	T51.0X2	T51.0X3	T51.0X4	—	—
beverage	T51.0X1	T51.0X2	T51.0X3	T51.0X4	—	—
Niacin	T46.7X1	T46.7X2	T46.7X3	T46.7X4	T46.7X5	T46.7X6
Niacinamide	T45.2X1	T45.2X2	T45.2X3	T45.2X4	T45.2X5	T45.2X6
Nialamide	T43.1X1	T43.1X2	T43.1X3	T43.1X4	T43.1X5	T43.1X6
Niaprazine	T42.6X1	T42.6X2	T42.6X3	T42.6X4	T42.6X5	T42.6X6
Nicametate	T46.7X1	T46.7X2	T46.7X3	T46.7X4	T46.7X5	T46.7X6
Nicardipine	T46.1X1	T46.1X2	T46.1X3	T46.1X4	T46.1X5	T46.1X6
Nicergoline	T46.7X1	T46.7X2	T46.7X3	T46.7X4	T46.7X5	T46.7X6
Nickel (carbonyl) (tetra-carbonyl) (fumes) (vapor)	T56.891	T56.892	T56.893	T56.894	—	—
Nickelocene	T56.891	T56.892	T56.893	T56.894	—	—
Niclosamide	T37.4X1	T37.4X2	T37.4X3	T37.4X4	T37.4X5	T37.4X6
Nicofuranose	T46.7X1	T46.7X2	T46.7X3	T46.7X4	T46.7X5	T46.7X6
Nicomorphine	T40.2X1	T40.2X2	T40.2X3	T40.2X4	—	—
Nicorandil	T46.3X1	T46.3X2	T46.3X3	T46.3X4	T46.3X5	T46.3X6
Nicotiana (plant)	T62.2X1	T62.2X2	T62.2X3	T62.2X4	—	—
Nicotinamide	T45.2X1	T45.2X2	T45.2X3	T45.2X4	T45.2X5	T45.2X6
Nicotine (insecticide) (spray) (sulfate) NEC	T60.2X1	T60.2X2	T60.2X3	T60.2X4	—	—
from tobacco	T65.291	T65.292	T65.293	T65.294	—	—
cigarettes	T65.221	T65.222	T65.223	T65.224	—	—
not insecticide	T65.291	T65.292	T65.293	T65.294	—	—
Nicotinic acid	T46.7X1	T46.7X2	T46.7X3	T46.7X4	T46.7X5	T46.7X6
Nicotinyl alcohol	T46.7X1	T46.7X2	T46.7X3	T46.7X4	T46.7X5	T46.7X6
Nicoumalone	T45.511	T45.512	T45.513	T45.514	T45.515	T45.516
Nifedipine	T46.1X1	T46.1X2	T46.1X3	T46.1X4	T46.1X5	T46.1X6
Nifenazone	T39.2X1	T39.2X2	T39.2X3	T39.2X4	T39.2X5	T39.2X6
Nifuraldezone	T37.91	T37.92	T37.93	T37.94	T37.95	T37.96
Nifuratel	T37.8X1	T37.8X2	T37.8X3	T37.8X4	T37.8X5	T37.8X6
Nifurtimox	T37.3X1	T37.3X2	T37.3X3	T37.3X4	T37.3X5	T37.3X6
Nifurtoinol	T37.8X1	T37.8X2	T37.8X3	T37.8X4	T37.8X5	T37.8X6
Nightshade, deadly (solanum) — *see also* Belladonna	T62.2X1	T62.2X2	T62.2X3	T62.2X4		
berry	T62.1X1	T62.1X2	T62.1X3	T62.1X4	—	—
Nikethamide	T50.7X1	T50.7X2	T50.7X3	T50.7X4	T50.7X5	T50.7X6
Nilstat	T36.7X1	T36.7X2	T36.7X3	T36.7X4	T36.7X5	T36.7X6
topical	T49.0X1	T49.0X2	T49.0X3	T49.0X4	T49.0X5	T49.0X6
Nilutamide	T38.6X1	T38.6X2	T38.6X3	T38.6X4	T38.6X5	T38.6X6
Nimesulide	T39.391	T39.392	T39.393	T39.394	T39.395	T39.396
Nimetazepam	T42.4X1	T42.4X2	T42.4X3	T42.4X4	T42.4X5	T42.4X6
Nimodipine	T46.1X1	T46.1X2	T46.1X3	T46.1X4	T46.1X5	T46.1X6
Nimorazole	T37.3X1	T37.3X2	T37.3X3	T37.3X4	T37.3X5	T37.3X6
Nimustine	T45.1X1	T45.1X2	T45.1X3	T45.1X4	T45.1X5	T45.1X6
Niridazole	T37.4X1	T37.4X2	T37.4X3	T37.4X4	T37.4X5	T37.4X6
Nisentil	T40.2X1	T40.2X2	T40.2X3	T40.2X4	T40.2X5	T40.2X6
Nisoldipine	T46.1X1	T46.1X2	T46.1X3	T46.1X4	T46.1X5	T46.1X6
Nitramine	T65.3X1	T65.3X2	T65.3X3	T65.3X4	—	—
Nitrate, organic	T46.3X1	T46.3X2	T46.3X3	T46.3X4	T46.3X5	T46.3X6
Nitrazepam	T42.4X1	T42.4X2	T42.4X3	T42.4X4	T42.4X5	T42.4X6
Nitrefazole	T50.6X1	T50.6X2	T50.6X3	T50.6X4	T50.6X5	T50.6X6
Nitrendipine	T46.1X1	T46.1X2	T46.1X3	T46.1X4	T46.1X5	T46.1X6
Nitric						
acid (liquid)	T54.2X1	T54.2X2	T54.2X3	T54.2X4	—	—
vapor	T59.891	T59.892	T59.893	T59.894	—	—
oxide (gas)	T59.0X1	T59.0X2	T59.0X3	T59.0X4	—	—
Nitrimidazine	T37.3X1	T37.3X2	T37.3X3	T37.3X4	T37.3X5	T37.3X6
Nitrite, amyl (medicinal) (vapor)	T46.3X1	T46.3X2	T46.3X3	T46.3X4	T46.3X5	T46.3X6
Nitroaniline	T65.3X1	T65.3X2	T65.3X3	T65.3X4	—	—
vapor	T59.891	T59.892	T59.893	T59.894	—	—
Nitrobenzene, nitrobenzol	T65.3X1	T65.3X2	T65.3X3	T65.3X4	—	—

Additional Character May Be Required — Refer to the Tabular List for Character Selection ▽ Subterms under main terms may continue to next column or page

Substance	Poisoning, Accidental (unintentional)	Poisoning, Intentional Self-harm	Poisoning, Assault	Poisoning, Undetermined	Adverse Effect	Under-dosing
Nitrobenzene, nitrobenzol — continued						
vapor	T65.3X1	T65.3X2	T65.3X3	T65.3X4	—	—
Nitrocellulose	T65.891	T65.892	T65.893	T65.894	—	—
lacquer	T65.891	T65.892	T65.893	T65.894	—	—
Nitrodiphenyl	T65.3X1	T65.3X2	T65.3X3	T65.3X4	—	—
Nitrofural	T49.0X1	T49.0X2	T49.0X3	T49.0X4	T49.0X5	T49.0X6
Nitrofurantoin	T37.8X1	T37.8X2	T37.8X3	T37.8X4	T37.8X5	T37.8X6
Nitrofurazone	T49.0X1	T49.0X2	T49.0X3	T49.0X4	T49.0X5	T49.0X6
Nitrogen	T59.0X1	T59.0X2	T59.0X3	T59.0X4	—	—
mustard	T45.1X1	T45.1X2	T45.1X3	T45.1X4	T45.1X5	T45.1X6
Nitroglycerin, nitroglycerol (medicinal)	T46.3X1	T46.3X2	T46.3X3	T46.3X4	T46.3X5	T46.3X6
nonmedicinal	T65.5X1	T65.5X2	T65.5X3	T65.5X4	—	—
fumes	T65.5X1	T65.5X2	T65.5X3	T65.5X4	—	—
Nitroglycol	T52.3X1	T52.3X2	T52.3X3	T52.3X4	—	—
Nitrohydrochloric acid	T54.2X1	T54.2X2	T54.2X3	T54.2X4	—	—
Nitromersol	T49.0X1	T49.0X2	T49.0X3	T49.0X4	T49.0X5	T49.0X6
Nitronaphthalene	T65.891	T65.892	T65.893	T65.894	—	—
Nitrophenol	T54.0X1	T54.0X2	T54.0X3	T54.0X4	—	—
Nitropropane	T52.8X1	T52.8X2	T52.8X3	T52.8X4	—	—
Nitroprusside	T46.5X1	T46.5X2	T46.5X3	T46.5X4	T46.5X5	T46.5X6
Nitrosodimethylamine	T65.3X1	T65.3X2	T65.3X3	T65.3X4	—	—
Nitrothiazol	T37.4X1	T37.4X2	T37.4X3	T37.4X4	T37.4X5	T37.4X6
Nitrotoluene, nitrotoluol	T65.3X1	T65.3X2	T65.3X3	T65.3X4	—	—
vapor	T65.3X1	T65.3X2	T65.3X3	T65.3X4	—	—
Nitrous						
acid (liquid)	T54.2X1	T54.2X2	T54.2X3	T54.2X4	—	—
fumes	T59.891	T59.892	T59.893	T59.894	—	—
ether spirit	T46.3X1	T46.3X2	T46.3X3	T46.3X4	T46.3X5	T46.3X6
oxide	T41.0X1	T41.0X2	T41.0X3	T41.0X4	T41.0X5	T41.0X6
Nitroxoline	T37.8X1	T37.8X2	T37.8X3	T37.8X4	T37.8X5	T37.8X6
Nitrozone	T49.0X1	T49.0X2	T49.0X3	T49.0X4	T49.0X5	T49.0X6
Nizatidine	T47.0X1	T47.0X2	T47.0X3	T47.0X4	T47.0X5	T47.0X6
Nizofenone	T43.8X1	T43.8X2	T43.8X3	T43.8X4	T43.8X5	T43.8X6
Noctec	T42.6X1	T42.6X2	T42.6X3	T42.6X4	T42.6X5	T42.6X6
Noludar	T42.6X1	T42.6X2	T42.6X3	T42.6X4	T42.6X5	T42.6X6
Nomegestrol	T38.5X1	T38.5X2	T38.5X3	T38.5X4	T38.5X5	T38.5X6
Nomifensine	T43.291	T43.292	T43.293	T43.294	T43.295	T43.296
Nonoxinol	T49.8X1	T49.8X2	T49.8X3	T49.8X4	T49.8X5	T49.8X6
Nonylphenoxy (polyethoxyethanol)	T49.8X1	T49.8X2	T49.8X3	T49.8X4	T49.8X5	T49.8X6
Noptil	T42.3X1	T42.3X2	T42.3X3	T42.3X4	T42.3X5	T42.3X6
Noradrenaline	T44.4X1	T44.4X2	T44.4X3	T44.4X4	T44.4X5	T44.4X6
Noramidopyrine	T39.2X1	T39.2X2	T39.2X3	T39.2X4	T39.2X5	T39.2X6
methanesulfonate sodium	T39.2X1	T39.2X2	T39.2X3	T39.2X4	T39.2X5	T39.2X6
Norbormide	T60.4X1	T60.4X2	T60.4X3	T60.4X4		
Nordazepam	T42.4X1	T42.4X2	T42.4X3	T42.4X4	T42.4X5	T42.4X6
Norepinephrine	T44.4X1	T44.4X2	T44.4X3	T44.4X4	T44.4X5	T44.4X6
Norethandrolone	T38.7X1	T38.7X2	T38.7X3	T38.7X4	T38.7X5	T38.7X6
Norethindrone	T38.4X1	T38.4X2	T38.4X3	T38.4X4	T38.4X5	T38.4X6
Norethisterone (acetate) (enantate)	T38.4X1	T38.4X2	T38.4X3	T38.4X4	T38.4X5	T38.4X6
with ethinylestradiol	T38.5X1	T38.5X2	T38.5X3	T38.5X4	T38.5X5	T38.5X6
Noretynodrel	T38.5X1	T38.5X2	T38.5X3	T38.5X4	T38.5X5	T38.5X6
Norfenefrine	T44.4X1	T44.4X2	T44.4X3	T44.4X4	T44.4X5	T44.4X6
Norfloxacin	T36.8X1	T36.8X2	T36.8X3	T36.8X4	T36.8X5	T36.8X6
Norgestrel	T38.4X1	T38.4X2	T38.4X3	T38.4X4	T38.4X5	T38.4X6
Norgestrienone	T38.4X1	T38.4X2	T38.4X3	T38.4X4	T38.4X5	T38.4X6
Norlestrin	T38.4X1	T38.4X2	T38.4X3	T38.4X4	T38.4X5	T38.4X6
Norlutin	T38.4X1	T38.4X2	T38.4X3	T38.4X4	T38.4X5	T38.4X6
Normal serum albumin (human), salt-poor	T45.8X1	T45.8X2	T45.8X3	T45.8X4	T45.8X5	T45.8X6
Normethandrone	T38.5X1	T38.5X2	T38.5X3	T38.5X4	T38.5X5	T38.5X6
Normison — see Benzodiazepines						
Normorphine	T40.2X1	T40.2X2	T40.2X3	T40.2X4	—	—
Norpseudoephedrine	T50.5X1	T50.5X2	T50.5X3	T50.5X4	T50.5X5	T50.5X6
Nortestosterone (furanpropionate)	T38.7X1	T38.7X2	T38.7X3	T38.7X4	T38.7X5	T38.7X6
Nortriptyline	T43.011	T43.012	T43.013	T43.014	T43.015	T43.016
Noscapine	T48.3X1	T48.3X2	T48.3X3	T48.3X4	T48.3X5	T48.3X6
Nose preparations	T49.6X1	T49.6X2	T49.6X3	T49.6X4	T49.6X5	T49.6X6
Novobiocin	T36.5X1	T36.5X2	T36.5X3	T36.5X4	T36.5X5	T36.5X6
Novocain (infiltration)	T41.3X1	T41.3X2	T41.3X3	T41.3X4	T41.3X5	T41.3X6
(topical)	T41.3X1	T41.3X2	T41.3X3	T41.3X4	T41.3X5	T41.3X6
nerve block (peripheral) (plexus)	T41.3X1	T41.3X2	T41.3X3	T41.3X4	T41.3X5	T41.3X6
spinal	T41.3X1	T41.3X2	T41.3X3	T41.3X4	T41.3X5	T41.3X6
Noxious foodstuff	T62.91	T62.92	T62.93	T62.94	—	—
specified NEC	T62.8X1	T62.8X2	T62.8X3	T62.8X4	—	—
Noxiptiline	T43.011	T43.012	T43.013	T43.014	T43.015	T43.016
Noxytiolin	T49.0X1	T49.0X2	T49.0X3	T49.0X4	T49.0X5	T49.0X6

Substance	Poisoning, Accidental (unintentional)	Poisoning, Intentional Self-harm	Poisoning, Assault	Poisoning, Undetermined	Adverse Effect	Under-dosing
NPH Iletin (insulin)	T38.3X1	T38.3X2	T38.3X3	T38.3X4	T38.3X5	T38.3X6
Numorphan	T40.2X1	T40.2X2	T40.2X3	T40.2X4	T40.2X5	T40.2X6
Nunol	T42.3X1	T42.3X2	T42.3X3	T42.3X4	T42.3X5	T42.3X6
Nupercaine (spinal anesthetic)	T41.3X1	T41.3X2	T41.3X3	T41.3X4	T41.3X5	T41.3X6
topical (surface)	T41.3X1	T41.3X2	T41.3X3	T41.3X4	T41.3X5	T41.3X6
Nutmeg oil (liniment)	T49.3X1	T49.3X2	T49.3X3	T49.3X4	T49.3X5	T49.3X6
Nutritional supplement	T50.901	T50.902	T50.903	T50.904	T50.905	T50.906
Nux vomica	T65.1X1	T65.1X2	T65.1X3	T65.1X4	—	—
Nydrazid	T37.1X1	T37.1X2	T37.1X3	T37.1X4	T37.1X5	T37.1X6
Nylidrin	T46.7X1	T46.7X2	T46.7X3	T46.7X4	T46.7X5	T46.7X6
Nystatin	T36.7X1	T36.7X2	T36.7X3	T36.7X4	T36.7X5	T36.7X6
topical	T49.0X1	T49.0X2	T49.0X3	T49.0X4	T49.0X5	T49.0X6
Nytol	T45.0X1	T45.0X2	T45.0X3	T45.0X4	T45.0X5	T45.0X6
Obidoxime chloride	T50.6X1	T50.6X2	T50.6X3	T50.6X4	T50.6X5	T50.6X6
Octafonium (chloride)	T49.3X1	T49.3X2	T49.3X3	T49.3X4	T49.3X5	T49.3X6
Octamethyl pyrophosphoramide	T60.0X1	T60.0X2	T60.0X3	T60.0X4	—	—
Octanoin	T50.991	T50.992	T50.993	T50.994	T50.995	T50.996
Octatropine methylbromide	T44.3X1	T44.3X2	T44.3X3	T44.3X4	T44.3X5	T44.3X6
Octotiamine	T45.2X1	T45.2X2	T45.2X3	T45.2X4	T45.2X5	T45.2X6
Octoxinol (9)	T49.8X1	T49.8X2	T49.8X3	T49.8X4	T49.8X5	T49.8X6
Octreotide	T38.991	T38.992	T38.993	T38.994	T38.995	T38.996
Octyl nitrite	T46.3X1	T46.3X2	T46.3X3	T46.3X4	T46.3X5	T46.3X6
Oestradiol	T38.5X1	T38.5X2	T38.5X3	T38.5X4	T38.5X5	T38.5X6
Oestriol	T38.5X1	T38.5X2	T38.5X3	T38.5X4	T38.5X5	T38.5X6
Oestrogen	T38.5X1	T38.5X2	T38.5X3	T38.5X4	T38.5X5	T38.5X6
Oestrone	T38.5X1	T38.5X2	T38.5X3	T38.5X4	T38.5X5	T38.5X6
Ofloxacin	T36.8X1	T36.8X2	T36.8X3	T36.8X4	T36.8X5	T36.8X6
Oil (of)	T65.891	T65.892	T65.893	T65.894	—	—
bitter almond	T62.8X1	T62.8X2	T62.8X3	T62.8X4	—	—
cloves	T49.7X1	T49.7X2	T49.7X3	T49.7X4	T49.7X5	T49.7X6
colors	T65.6X1	T65.6X2	T65.6X3	T65.6X4	—	—
fumes	T59.891	T59.892	T59.893	T59.894	—	—
lubricating	T52.0X1	T52.0X2	T52.0X3	T52.0X4	—	—
Niobe	T52.8X1	T52.8X2	T52.8X3	T52.8X4	—	—
vitriol (liquid)	T54.2X1	T54.2X2	T54.2X3	T54.2X4	—	—
fumes	T54.2X1	T54.2X2	T54.2X3	T54.2X4	—	—
wintergreen (bitter) NEC	T49.3X1	T49.3X2	T49.3X3	T49.3X4	T49.3X5	T49.3X6
Oily preparation (for skin)	T49.3X1	T49.3X2	T49.3X3	T49.3X4	T49.3X5	T49.3X6
Ointment NEC	T49.3X1	T49.3X2	T49.3X3	T49.3X4	T49.3X5	T49.3X6
Olanzapine	T43.591	T43.592	T43.593	T43.594	T43.595	T43.596
Oleander	T62.2X1	T62.2X2	T62.2X3	T62.2X4	—	—
Oleandomycin	T36.3X1	T36.3X2	T36.3X3	T36.3X4	T36.3X5	T36.3X6
Oleandrin	T46.0X1	T46.0X2	T46.0X3	T46.0X4	T46.0X5	T46.0X6
Oleic acid	T46.6X1	T46.6X2	T46.6X3	T46.6X4	T46.6X5	T46.6X6
Oleovitamin A	T45.2X1	T45.2X2	T45.2X3	T45.2X4	T45.2X5	T45.2X6
Oleum ricini	T47.2X1	T47.2X2	T47.2X3	T47.2X4	T47.2X5	T47.2X6
Olive oil (medicinal) NEC	T47.4X1	T47.4X2	T47.4X3	T47.4X4	T47.4X5	T47.4X6
Olivomycin	T45.1X1	T45.1X2	T45.1X3	T45.1X4	T45.1X5	T45.1X6
Olsalazine	T47.8X1	T47.8X2	T47.8X3	T47.8X4	T47.8X5	T47.8X6
Omeprazole	T47.1X1	T47.1X2	T47.1X3	T47.1X4	T47.1X5	T47.1X6
OMPA	T60.0X1	T60.0X2	T60.0X3	T60.0X4	—	—
Oncovin	T45.1X1	T45.1X2	T45.1X3	T45.1X4	T45.1X5	T45.1X6
Ondansetron	T45.0X1	T45.0X2	T45.0X3	T45.0X4	T45.0X5	T45.0X6
Ophthaine	T41.3X1	T41.3X2	T41.3X3	T41.3X4	T41.3X5	T41.3X6
Ophthetic	T41.3X1	T41.3X2	T41.3X3	T41.3X4	T41.3X5	T41.3X6
Opiate NEC	T40.601	T40.602	T40.603	T40.604	T40.605	T40.606
antagonists	T50.7X1	T50.7X2	T50.7X3	T50.7X4	T50.7X5	T50.7X6
Opioid NEC	T40.2X1	T40.2X2	T40.2X3	T40.2X4	T40.2X5	T40.2X6
Opipramol	T43.011	T43.012	T43.013	T43.014	T43.015	T43.016
Opium alkaloids (total)	T40.0X1	T40.0X2	T40.0X3	T40.0X4	T40.0X5	T40.0X6
standardized powdered	T40.0X1	T40.0X2	T40.0X3	T40.0X4	T40.0X5	T40.0X6
tincture (camphorated)	T40.0X1	T40.0X2	T40.0X3	T40.0X4	T40.0X5	T40.0X6
Oracon	T38.4X1	T38.4X2	T38.4X3	T38.4X4	T38.4X5	T38.4X6
Oragrafin	T50.8X1	T50.8X2	T50.8X3	T50.8X4	T50.8X5	T50.8X6
Oral contraceptives	T38.4X1	T38.4X2	T38.4X3	T38.4X4	T38.4X5	T38.4X6
Oral rehydration salts	T50.3X1	T50.3X2	T50.3X3	T50.3X4	T50.3X5	T50.3X6
Orazamide	T50.991	T50.992	T50.993	T50.994	T50.995	T50.996
Orciprenaline	T48.291	T48.292	T48.293	T48.294	T48.295	T48.296
Organidin	T48.4X1	T48.4X2	T48.4X3	T48.4X4	T48.4X5	T48.4X6
Organonitrate NEC	T46.3X1	T46.3X2	T46.3X3	T46.3X4	T46.3X5	T46.3X6
Organophosphates	T60.0X1	T60.0X2	T60.0X3	T60.0X4	—	—
Orimune	T50.B91	T50.B92	T50.B93	T50.B94	T50.B95	T50.B96
Orinase	T38.3X1	T38.3X2	T38.3X3	T38.3X4	T38.3X5	T38.3X6
Ormeloxifene	T38.6X1	T38.6X2	T38.6X3	T38.6X4	T38.6X5	T38.6X6
Ornidazole	T37.3X1	T37.3X2	T37.3X3	T37.3X4	T37.3X5	T37.3X6
Ornithine aspartate	T50.991	T50.992	T50.993	T50.994	T50.995	T50.996
Ornoprostil	T47.1X1	T47.1X2	T47.1X3	T47.1X4	T47.1X5	T47.1X6
Orphenadrine (hydrochloride)	T42.8X1	T42.8X2	T42.8X3	T42.8X4	T42.8X5	T42.8X6
Ortal (sodium)	T42.3X1	T42.3X2	T42.3X3	T42.3X4	T42.3X5	T42.3X6

▽ Subterms under main terms may continue to next column or page　　Additional Character May Be Required — Refer to the Tabular List for Character Selection　　381

Nitrobenzene, nitrobenzol — Ortal

Table of Drugs and Chemicals

Orthoboric acid — Peanut oil

Substance	Poisoning, Accidental (unintentional)	Poisoning, Intentional Self-harm	Poisoning, Assault	Poisoning, Undetermined	Adverse Effect	Under-dosing
Orthoboric acid	T49.0X1	T49.0X2	T49.0X3	T49.0X4	T49.0X5	T49.0X6
ENT agent	T49.6X1	T49.6X2	T49.6X3	T49.6X4	T49.6X5	T49.6X6
ophthalmic preparation	T49.5X1	T49.5X2	T49.5X3	T49.5X4	T49.5X5	T49.5X6
Orthocaine	T41.3X1	T41.3X2	T41.3X3	T41.3X4	T41.3X5	T41.3X6
Orthodichlorobenzene	T53.7X1	T53.7X2	T53.7X3	T53.7X4	—	—
Ortho-Novum	T38.4X1	T38.4X2	T38.4X3	T38.4X4	T38.4X5	T38.4X6
Orthotolidine (reagent)	T54.2X1	T54.2X2	T54.2X3	T54.2X4	—	—
Osmic acid (liquid)	T54.2X1	T54.2X2	T54.2X3	T54.2X4	—	—
fumes	T54.2X1	T54.2X2	T54.2X3	T54.2X4	—	—
Osmotic diuretics	T50.2X1	T50.2X2	T50.2X3	T50.2X4	T50.2X5	T50.2X6
Otilonium bromide	T44.3X1	T44.3X2	T44.3X3	T44.3X4	T44.3X5	T44.3X6
Otorhinolaryngological drug NEC	T49.6X1	T49.6X2	T49.6X3	T49.6X4	T49.6X5	T49.6X6
Ouabain (e)	T46.0X1	T46.0X2	T46.0X3	T46.0X4	T46.0X5	T46.0X6
Ovarian						
hormone	T38.5X1	T38.5X2	T38.5X3	T38.5X4	T38.5X5	T38.5X6
stimulant	T38.5X1	T38.5X2	T38.5X3	T38.5X4	T38.5X5	T38.5X6
Ovral	T38.4X1	T38.4X2	T38.4X3	T38.4X4	T38.4X5	T38.4X6
Ovulen	T38.4X1	T38.4X2	T38.4X3	T38.4X4	T38.4X5	T38.4X6
Oxacillin	T36.0X1	T36.0X2	T36.0X3	T36.0X4	T36.0X5	T36.0X6
Oxalic acid	T54.2X1	T54.2X2	T54.2X3	T54.2X4	—	—
ammonium salt	T50.991	T50.992	T50.993	T50.994	T50.995	T50.996
Oxamniquine	T37.4X1	T37.4X2	T37.4X3	T37.4X4	T37.4X5	T37.4X6
Oxanamide	T43.591	T43.592	T43.593	T43.594	T43.595	T43.596
Oxandrolone	T38.7X1	T38.7X2	T38.7X3	T38.7X4	T38.7X5	T38.7X6
Oxantel	T37.4X1	T37.4X2	T37.4X3	T37.4X4	T37.4X5	T37.4X6
Oxapium iodide	T44.3X1	T44.3X2	T44.3X3	T44.3X4	T44.3X5	T44.3X6
Oxaprotiline	T43.021	T43.022	T43.023	T43.024	T43.025	T43.026
Oxaprozin	T39.311	T39.312	T39.313	T39.314	T39.315	T39.316
Oxatomide	T45.0X1	T45.0X2	T45.0X3	T45.0X4	T45.0X5	T45.0X6
Oxazepam	T42.4X1	T42.4X2	T42.4X3	T42.4X4	T42.4X5	T42.4X6
Oxazimedrine	T50.5X1	T50.5X2	T50.5X3	T50.5X4	T50.5X5	T50.5X6
Oxazolam	T42.4X1	T42.4X2	T42.4X3	T42.4X4	T42.4X5	T42.4X6
Oxazolidine derivatives	T42.2X1	T42.2X2	T42.2X3	T42.2X4	T42.2X5	T42.2X6
Oxazolidinedione (derivative)	T42.2X1	T42.2X2	T42.2X3	T42.2X4	T42.2X5	T42.2X6
Ox bile extract	T47.5X1	T47.5X2	T47.5X3	T47.5X4	T47.5X5	T47.5X6
Oxcarbazepine	T42.1X1	T42.1X2	T42.1X3	T42.1X4	T42.1X5	T42.1X6
Oxedrine	T44.4X1	T44.4X2	T44.4X3	T44.4X4	T44.4X5	T44.4X6
Oxeladin (citrate)	T48.3X1	T48.3X2	T48.3X3	T48.3X4	T48.3X5	T48.3X6
Oxendolone	T38.5X1	T38.5X2	T38.5X3	T38.5X4	T38.5X5	T38.5X6
Oxetacaine	T41.3X1	T41.3X2	T41.3X3	T41.3X4	T41.3X5	T41.3X6
Oxethazine	T41.3X1	T41.3X2	T41.3X3	T41.3X4	T41.3X5	T41.3X6
Oxetorone	T39.8X1	T39.8X2	T39.8X3	T39.8X4	T39.8X5	T39.8X6
Oxiconazole	T49.0X1	T49.0X2	T49.0X3	T49.0X4	T49.0X5	T49.0X6
Oxidizing agent NEC	T54.91	T54.92	T54.93	T54.94	—	—
Oxipurinol	T50.4X1	T50.4X2	T50.4X3	T50.4X4	T50.4X5	T50.4X6
Oxitriptan	T43.291	T43.292	T43.293	T43.294	T43.295	T43.296
Oxitropium bromide	T48.6X1	T48.6X2	T48.6X3	T48.6X4	T48.6X5	T48.6X6
Oxodipine	T46.1X1	T46.1X2	T46.1X3	T46.1X4	T46.1X5	T46.1X6
Oxolamine	T48.3X1	T48.3X2	T48.3X3	T48.3X4	T48.3X5	T48.3X6
Oxolinic acid	T37.8X1	T37.8X2	T37.8X3	T37.8X4	T37.8X5	T37.8X6
Oxomemazine	T43.3X1	T43.3X2	T43.3X3	T43.3X4	T43.3X5	T43.3X6
Oxophenarsine	T37.3X1	T37.3X2	T37.3X3	T37.3X4	T37.3X5	T37.3X6
Oxprenolol	T44.7X1	T44.7X2	T44.7X3	T44.7X4	T44.7X5	T44.7X6
Oxsoralen	T49.3X1	T49.3X2	T49.3X3	T49.3X4	T49.3X5	T49.3X6
Oxtriphylline	T48.6X1	T48.6X2	T48.6X3	T48.6X4	T48.6X5	T48.6X6
Oxybate sodium	T41.291	T41.292	T41.293	T41.294	T41.295	T41.296
Oxybuprocaine	T41.3X1	T41.3X2	T41.3X3	T41.3X4	T41.3X5	T41.3X6
Oxybutynin	T44.3X1	T44.3X2	T44.3X3	T44.3X4	T44.3X5	T44.3X6
Oxychlorosene	T49.0X1	T49.0X2	T49.0X3	T49.0X4	T49.0X5	T49.0X6
Oxycodone	T40.2X1	T40.2X2	T40.2X3	T40.2X4	T40.2X5	T40.2X6
Oxyfedrine	T46.3X1	T46.3X2	T46.3X3	T46.3X4	T46.3X5	T46.3X6
Oxygen	T41.5X1	T41.5X2	T41.5X3	T41.5X4	T41.5X5	T41.5X6
Oxylone	T49.0X1	T49.0X2	T49.0X3	T49.0X4	T49.0X5	T49.0X6
ophthalmic preparation	T49.5X1	T49.5X2	T49.5X3	T49.5X4	T49.5X5	T49.5X6
Oxymesterone	T38.7X1	T38.7X2	T38.7X3	T38.7X4	T38.7X5	T38.7X6
Oxymetazoline	T48.5X1	T48.5X2	T48.5X3	T48.5X4	T48.5X5	T48.5X6
Oxymetholone	T38.7X1	T38.7X2	T38.7X3	T38.7X4	T38.7X5	T38.7X6
Oxymorphone	T40.2X1	T40.2X2	T40.2X3	T40.2X4	T40.2X5	T40.2X6
Oxypertine	T43.591	T43.592	T43.593	T43.594	T43.595	T43.596
Oxyphenbutazone	T39.2X1	T39.2X2	T39.2X3	T39.2X4	T39.2X5	T39.2X6
Oxyphencyclimine	T44.3X1	T44.3X2	T44.3X3	T44.3X4	T44.3X5	T44.3X6
Oxyphenisatine	T47.2X1	T47.2X2	T47.2X3	T47.2X4	T47.2X5	T47.2X6
Oxyphenonium bromide	T44.3X1	T44.3X2	T44.3X3	T44.3X4	T44.3X5	T44.3X6
Oxypolygelatin	T45.8X1	T45.8X2	T45.8X3	T45.8X4	T45.8X5	T45.8X6
Oxyquinoline (derivatives)	T37.8X1	T37.8X2	T37.8X3	T37.8X4	T37.8X5	T37.8X6
Oxytetracycline	T36.4X1	T36.4X2	T36.4X3	T36.4X4	T36.4X5	T36.4X6
Oxytocic drug NEC	T48.0X1	T48.0X2	T48.0X3	T48.0X4	T48.0X5	T48.0X6
Oxytocin (synthetic)	T48.0X1	T48.0X2	T48.0X3	T48.0X4	T48.0X5	T48.0X6
Ozone	T59.891	T59.892	T59.893	T59.894	—	—
PABA	T49.3X1	T49.3X2	T49.3X3	T49.3X4	T49.3X5	T49.3X6
Packed red cells	T45.8X1	T45.8X2	T45.8X3	T45.8X4	T45.8X5	T45.8X6
Padimate	T49.3X1	T49.3X2	T49.3X3	T49.3X4	T49.3X5	T49.3X6
Paint NEC	T65.6X1	T65.6X2	T65.6X3	T65.6X4	—	—
cleaner	T52.91	T52.92	T52.93	T52.94	—	—
fumes NEC	T59.891	T59.892	T59.893	T59.894	—	—
lead (fumes)	T56.0X1	T56.0X2	T56.0X3	T56.0X4	—	—
solvent NEC	T52.8X1	T52.8X2	T52.8X3	T52.8X4	—	—
stripper	T52.8X1	T52.8X2	T52.8X3	T52.8X4	—	—
Palfium	T40.2X1	T40.2X2	T40.2X3	T40.2X4	—	—
Palm kernel oil	T50.991	T50.992	T50.993	T50.994	T50.995	T50.996
Paludrine	T37.2X1	T37.2X2	T37.2X3	T37.2X4	T37.2X5	T37.2X6
PAM (pralidoxime)	T50.6X1	T50.6X2	T50.6X3	T50.6X4	T50.6X5	T50.6X6
Pamaquine (naphthoute)	T37.2X1	T37.2X2	T37.2X3	T37.2X4	T37.2X5	T37.2X6
Panadol	T39.1X1	T39.1X2	T39.1X3	T39.1X4	T39.1X5	T39.1X6
Pancreatic						
digestive secretion stimulant	T47.8X1	T47.8X2	T47.8X3	T47.8X4	T47.8X5	T47.8X6
dornase	T45.3X1	T45.3X2	T45.3X3	T45.3X4	T45.3X5	T45.3X6
Pancreatin	T47.5X1	T47.5X2	T47.5X3	T47.5X4	T47.5X5	T47.5X6
Pancrelipase	T47.5X1	T47.5X2	T47.5X3	T47.5X4	T47.5X5	T47.5X6
Pancuronium (bromide)	T48.1X1	T48.1X2	T48.1X3	T48.1X4	T48.1X5	T48.1X6
Pangamic acid	T45.2X1	T45.2X2	T45.2X3	T45.2X4	T45.2X5	T45.2X6
Panthenol	T45.2X1	T45.2X2	T45.2X3	T45.2X4	T45.2X5	T45.2X6
topical	T49.8X1	T49.8X2	T49.8X3	T49.8X4	T49.8X5	T49.8X6
Pantopon	T40.0X1	T40.0X2	T40.0X3	T40.0X4	T40.0X5	T40.0X6
Pantothenic acid	T45.2X1	T45.2X2	T45.2X3	T45.2X4	T45.2X5	T45.2X6
Panwarfin	T45.511	T45.512	T45.513	T45.514	T45.515	T45.516
Papain	T47.5X1	T47.5X2	T47.5X3	T47.5X4	T47.5X5	T47.5X6
digestant	T47.5X1	T47.5X2	T47.5X3	T47.5X4	T47.5X5	T47.5X6
Papaveretum	T40.0X1	T40.0X2	T40.0X3	T40.0X4	T40.0X5	T40.0X6
Papaverine	T44.3X1	T44.3X2	T44.3X3	T44.3X4	T44.3X5	T44.3X6
Para-acetamidophenol	T39.1X1	T39.1X2	T39.1X3	T39.1X4	T39.1X5	T39.1X6
Para-aminobenzoic acid	T49.3X1	T49.3X2	T49.3X3	T49.3X4	T49.3X5	T49.3X6
Para-aminophenol derivatives	T39.1X1	T39.1X2	T39.1X3	T39.1X4	T39.1X5	T39.1X6
Para-aminosalicylic acid	T37.1X1	T37.1X2	T37.1X3	T37.1X4	T37.1X5	T37.1X6
Paracetaldehyde	T42.6X1	T42.6X2	T42.6X3	T42.6X4	T42.6X5	T42.6X6
Paracetamol	T39.1X1	T39.1X2	T39.1X3	T39.1X4	T39.1X5	T39.1X6
Parachlorophenol (camphorated)	T49.0X1	T49.0X2	T49.0X3	T49.0X4	T49.0X5	T49.0X6
Paracodin	T40.2X1	T40.2X2	T40.2X3	T40.2X4	T40.2X5	T40.2X6
Paradione	T42.2X1	T42.2X2	T42.2X3	T42.2X4	T42.2X5	T42.2X6
Paraffin(s) (wax)	T52.0X1	T52.0X2	T52.0X3	T52.0X4	—	—
liquid (medicinal)	T47.4X1	T47.4X2	T47.4X3	T47.4X4	T47.4X5	T47.4X6
nonmedicinal	T52.0X1	T52.0X2	T52.0X3	T52.0X4	—	—
Paraformaldehyde	T60.3X1	T60.3X2	T60.3X3	T60.3X4	—	—
Paraldehyde	T42.6X1	T42.6X2	T42.6X3	T42.6X4	T42.6X5	T42.6X6
Paramethadione	T42.2X1	T42.2X2	T42.2X3	T42.2X4	T42.2X5	T42.2X6
Paramethasone	T38.0X1	T38.0X2	T38.0X3	T38.0X4	T38.0X5	T38.0X6
acetate	T49.0X1	T49.0X2	T49.0X3	T49.0X4	T49.0X5	T49.0X6
Paraoxon	T60.0X1	T60.0X2	T60.0X3	T60.0X4	—	—
Paraquat	T60.3X1	T60.3X2	T60.3X3	T60.3X4	—	—
Parasympatholytic NEC	T44.3X1	T44.3X2	T44.3X3	T44.3X4	T44.3X5	T44.3X6
Parasympathomimetic drug NEC	T44.1X1	T44.1X2	T44.1X3	T44.1X4	T44.1X5	T44.1X6
Parathion	T60.0X1	T60.0X2	T60.0X3	T60.0X4	—	—
Parathormone	T50.991	T50.992	T50.993	T50.994	T50.995	T50.996
Parathyroid extract	T50.991	T50.992	T50.993	T50.994	T50.995	T50.996
Paratyphoid vaccine	T50.A91	T50.A92	T50.A93	T50.A94	T50.A95	T50.A96
Paredrine	T44.4X1	T44.4X2	T44.4X3	T44.4X4	T44.4X5	T44.4X6
Paregoric	T40.0X1	T40.0X2	T40.0X3	T40.0X4	T40.0X5	T40.0X6
Pargyline	T46.5X1	T46.5X2	T46.5X3	T46.5X4	T46.5X5	T46.5X6
Paris green	T57.0X1	T57.0X2	T57.0X3	T57.0X4	—	—
insecticide	T57.0X1	T57.0X2	T57.0X3	T57.0X4	—	—
Parnate	T43.1X1	T43.1X2	T43.1X3	T43.1X4	T43.1X5	T43.1X6
Paromomycin	T36.5X1	T36.5X2	T36.5X3	T36.5X4	T36.5X5	T36.5X6
Paroxypropione	T45.1X1	T45.1X2	T45.1X3	T45.1X4	T45.1X5	T45.1X6
Parzone	T40.2X1	T40.2X2	T40.2X3	T40.2X4	T40.2X5	T40.2X6
PAS	T37.1X1	T37.1X2	T37.1X3	T37.1X4	T37.1X5	T37.1X6
Pasiniazid	T37.1X1	T37.1X2	T37.1X3	T37.1X4	T37.1X5	T37.1X6
PBB (polybrominated biphenyls)	T65.891	T65.892	T65.893	T65.894	—	—
PCB	T65.891	T65.892	T65.893	T65.894	—	—
PCP						
meaning pentachlorophenol	T60.1X1	T60.1X2	T60.1X3	T60.1X4	—	—
fungicide	T60.3X1	T60.3X2	T60.3X3	T60.3X4	—	—
herbicide	T60.3X1	T60.3X2	T60.3X3	T60.3X4	—	—
insecticide	T60.1X1	T60.1X2	T60.1X3	T60.1X4	—	—
meaning phencyclidine	T40.991	T40.992	T40.993	T40.994	—	—
Peach kernel oil (emulsion)	T47.4X1	T47.4X2	T47.4X3	T47.4X4	T47.4X5	T47.4X6
Peanut oil (emulsion) NEC	T47.4X1	T47.4X2	T47.4X3	T47.4X4	T47.4X5	T47.4X6
topical	T49.3X1	T49.3X2	T49.3X3	T49.3X4	T49.3X5	T49.3X6

Table of Drugs and Chemicals

Substance	Poisoning, Accidental (unintentional)	Poisoning, Intentional Self-harm	Poisoning, Assault	Poisoning, Undetermined	Adverse Effect	Under-dosing
Pearly Gates (morning glory seeds)	T40.991	T40.992	T40.993	T40.994	—	—
Pecazine	T43.3X1	T43.3X2	T43.3X3	T43.3X4	T43.3X5	T43.3X6
Pectin	T47.6X1	T47.6X2	T47.6X3	T47.6X4	T47.6X5	T47.6X6
Pefloxacin	T37.8X1	T37.8X2	T37.8X3	T37.8X4	T37.8X5	T37.8X6
Pegademase, bovine	T50.Z91	T50.Z92	T50.Z93	T50.Z94	T50.Z95	T50.Z96
Pelletierine tannate	T37.4X1	T37.4X2	T37.4X3	T37.4X4	T37.4X5	T37.4X6
Pemirolast (potassium)	T48.6X1	T48.6X2	T48.6X3	T48.6X4	T48.6X5	T48.6X6
Pemoline	T50.7X1	T50.7X2	T50.7X3	T50.7X4	T50.7X5	T50.7X6
Pempidine	T44.2X1	T44.2X2	T44.2X3	T44.2X4	T44.2X5	T44.2X6
Penamecillin	T36.0X1	T36.0X2	T36.0X3	T36.0X4	T36.0X5	T36.0X6
Penbutolol	T44.7X1	T44.7X2	T44.7X3	T44.7X4	T44.7X5	T44.7X6
Penethamate	T36.0X1	T36.0X2	T36.0X3	T36.0X4	T36.0X5	T36.0X6
Penfluridol	T43.591	T43.592	T43.593	T43.594	T43.595	T43.596
Penflutizide	T50.2X1	T50.2X2	T50.2X3	T50.2X4	T50.2X5	T50.2X6
Pengitoxin	T46.0X1	T46.0X2	T46.0X3	T46.0X4	T46.0X5	T46.0X6
Penicillamine	T50.6X1	T50.6X2	T50.6X3	T50.6X4	T50.6X5	T50.6X6
Penicillin (any)	T36.0X1	T36.0X2	T36.0X3	T36.0X4	T36.0X5	T36.0X6
Penicillinase	T45.3X1	T45.3X2	T45.3X3	T45.3X4	T45.3X5	T45.3X6
Penicilloyl polylysine	T50.8X1	T50.8X2	T50.8X3	T50.8X4	T50.8X5	T50.8X6
Penimepicycline	T36.4X1	T36.4X2	T36.4X3	T36.4X4	T36.4X5	T36.4X6
Pentachloroethane	T53.6X1	T53.6X2	T53.6X3	T53.6X4	—	—
Pentachloronaphthalene	T53.7X1	T53.7X2	T53.7X3	T53.7X4	—	—
Pentachlorophenol (pesticide)	T60.1X1	T60.1X2	T60.1X3	T60.1X4	—	—
fungicide	T60.3X1	T60.3X2	T60.3X3	T60.3X4	—	—
herbicide	T60.3X1	T60.3X2	T60.3X3	T60.3X4	—	—
insecticide	T60.1X1	T60.1X2	T60.1X3	T60.1X4	—	—
Pentaerythritol	T46.3X1	T46.3X2	T46.3X3	T46.3X4	T46.3X5	T46.3X6
chloral	T42.6X1	T42.6X2	T42.6X3	T42.6X4	T42.6X5	T42.6X6
tetranitrate NEC	T46.3X1	T46.3X2	T46.3X3	T46.3X4	T46.3X5	T46.3X6
Pentaerythrityl tetranitrate	T46.3X1	T46.3X2	T46.3X3	T46.3X4	T46.3X5	T46.3X6
Pentagastrin	T50.8X1	T50.8X2	T50.8X3	T50.8X4	—	T50.8X6
Pentalin	T53.6X1	T53.6X2	T53.6X3	T53.6X4	—	—
Pentamethonium bromide	T44.2X1	T44.2X2	T44.2X3	T44.2X4	T44.2X5	T44.2X6
Pentamidine	T37.3X1	T37.3X2	T37.3X3	T37.3X4	T37.3X5	T37.3X6
Pentanol	T51.3X1	T51.3X2	T51.3X3	T51.3X4	—	—
Pentapyrrolinium (bitartrate)	T44.2X1	T44.2X2	T44.2X3	T44.2X4	T44.2X5	T44.2X6
Pentaquine	T37.2X1	T37.2X2	T37.2X3	T37.2X4	T37.2X5	T37.2X6
Pentazocine	T40.4X1	T40.4X2	T40.4X3	T40.4X4	T40.4X5	T40.4X6
Pentetrazole	T50.7X1	T50.7X2	T50.7X3	T50.7X4	T50.7X5	T50.7X6
Penthienate bromide	T44.3X1	T44.3X2	T44.3X3	T44.3X4	T44.3X5	T44.3X6
Pentifylline	T46.7X1	T46.7X2	T46.7X3	T46.7X4	T46.7X5	T46.7X6
Pentobarbital	T42.3X1	T42.3X2	T42.3X3	T42.3X4	T42.3X5	T42.3X6
sodium	T42.3X1	T42.3X2	T42.3X3	T42.3X4	T42.3X5	T42.3X6
Pentobarbitone	T42.3X1	T42.3X2	T42.3X3	T42.3X4	T42.3X5	T42.3X6
Pentolonium tartrate	T44.2X1	T44.2X2	T44.2X3	T44.2X4	T44.2X5	T44.2X6
Pentosan polysulfate (sodium)	T39.8X1	T39.8X2	T39.8X3	T39.8X4	T39.8X5	T39.8X6
Pentostatin	T45.1X1	T45.1X2	T45.1X3	T45.1X4	T45.1X5	T45.1X6
Pentothal	T41.1X1	T41.1X2	T41.1X3	T41.1X4	T41.1X5	T41.1X6
Pentoxifylline	T46.7X1	T46.7X2	T46.7X3	T46.7X4	T46.7X5	T46.7X6
Pentoxyverine	T48.3X1	T48.3X2	T48.3X3	T48.3X4	T48.3X5	T48.3X6
Pentrinat	T46.3X1	T46.3X2	T46.3X3	T46.3X4	T46.3X5	T46.3X6
Pentylenetetrazole	T50.7X1	T50.7X2	T50.7X3	T50.7X4	T50.7X5	T50.7X6
Pentylsalicylamide	T37.1X1	T37.1X2	T37.1X3	T37.1X4	T37.1X5	T37.1X6
Pentymal	T42.3X1	T42.3X2	T42.3X3	T42.3X4	T42.3X5	T42.3X6
Peplomycin	T45.1X1	T45.1X2	T45.1X3	T45.1X4	T45.1X5	T45.1X6
Peppermint (oil)	T47.5X1	T47.5X2	T47.5X3	T47.5X4	T47.5X5	T47.5X6
Pepsin	T47.5X1	T47.5X2	T47.5X3	T47.5X4	T47.5X5	T47.5X6
digestant	T47.5X1	T47.5X2	T47.5X3	T47.5X4	T47.5X5	T47.5X6
Pepstatin	T47.1X1	T47.1X2	T47.1X3	T47.1X4	T47.1X5	T47.1X6
Peptavlon	T50.8X1	T50.8X2	T50.8X3	T50.8X4	T50.8X5	T50.8X6
Perazine	T43.3X1	T43.3X2	T43.3X3	T43.3X4	T43.3X5	T43.3X6
Percaine (spinal)	T41.3X1	T41.3X2	T41.3X3	T41.3X4	T41.3X5	T41.3X6
topical (surface)	T41.3X1	T41.3X2	T41.3X3	T41.3X4	T41.3X5	T41.3X6
Perchloroethylene	T53.3X1	T53.3X2	T53.3X3	T53.3X4	—	—
medicinal	T37.4X1	T37.4X2	T37.4X3	T37.4X4	T37.4X5	T37.4X6
vapor	T53.3X1	T53.3X2	T53.3X3	T53.3X4	—	—
Percodan	T40.2X1	T40.2X2	T40.2X3	T40.2X4	T40.2X5	T40.2X6
Percogesic — see also acetaminophen	T45.0X1	T45.0X2	T45.0X3	T45.0X4	T45.0X5	T45.0X6
Percorten	T38.0X1	T38.0X2	T38.0X3	T38.0X4	T38.0X5	T38.0X6
Pergolide	T42.8X1	T42.8X2	T42.8X3	T42.8X4	T42.8X5	T42.8X6
Pergonal	T38.811	T38.812	T38.813	T38.814	T38.815	T38.816
Perhexilene	T46.3X1	T46.3X2	T46.3X3	T46.3X4	T46.3X5	T46.3X6
Perhexiline (maleate)	T46.3X1	T46.3X2	T46.3X3	T46.3X4	T46.3X5	T46.3X6
Periactin	T45.0X1	T45.0X2	T45.0X3	T45.0X4	T45.0X5	T45.0X6
Periciazine	T43.3X1	T43.3X2	T43.3X3	T43.3X4	T43.3X5	T43.3X6
Periclor	T42.6X1	T42.6X2	T42.6X3	T42.6X4	T42.6X5	T42.6X6
Perindopril	T46.4X1	T46.4X2	T46.4X3	T46.4X4	T46.4X5	T46.4X6
Perisoxal	T39.8X1	T39.8X2	T39.8X3	T39.8X4	T39.8X5	T39.8X6
Peritoneal dialysis solution	T50.3X1	T50.3X2	T50.3X3	T50.3X4	T50.3X5	T50.3X6
Peritrate	T46.3X1	T46.3X2	T46.3X3	T46.3X4	T46.3X5	T46.3X6
Perlapine	T42.4X1	T42.4X2	T42.4X3	T42.4X4	T42.4X5	T42.4X6
Permanganate	T65.891	T65.892	T65.893	T65.894	—	—
Permethrin	T60.1X1	T60.1X2	T60.1X3	T60.1X4	—	—
Pernocton	T42.3X1	T42.3X2	T42.3X3	T42.3X4	T42.3X5	T42.3X6
Pernoston	T42.3X1	T42.3X2	T42.3X3	T42.3X4	T42.3X5	T42.3X6
Peronine	T40.2X1	T40.2X2	T40.2X3	T40.2X4	—	—
Perphenazine	T43.3X1	T43.3X2	T43.3X3	T43.3X4	T43.3X5	T43.3X6
Pertofrane	T43.011	T43.012	T43.013	T43.014	T43.015	T43.016
Pertussis						
immune serum (human)	T50.Z11	T50.Z12	T50.Z13	T50.Z14	T50.Z15	T50.Z16
vaccine (with diphtheria toxoid) (with tetanus toxoid)	T50.A11	T50.A12	T50.A13	T50.A14	T50.A15	T50.A16
Peruvian balsam	T49.0X1	T49.0X2	T49.0X3	T49.0X4	T49.0X5	T49.0X6
Peruvoside	T46.0X1	T46.0X2	T46.0X3	T46.0X4	T46.0X5	T46.0X6
Pesticide (dust) (fumes) (vapor) NEC	T60.91	T60.92	T60.93	T60.94	—	—
arsenic	T57.0X1	T57.0X2	T57.0X3	T57.0X4	—	—
chlorinated	T60.1X1	T60.1X2	T60.1X3	T60.1X4	—	—
cyanide	T65.0X1	T65.0X2	T65.0X3	T65.0X4	—	—
kerosene	T52.0X1	T52.0X2	T52.0X3	T52.0X4	—	—
mixture (of compounds)	T60.91	T60.92	T60.93	T60.94	—	—
naphthalene	T60.2X1	T60.2X2	T60.2X3	T60.2X4	—	—
organochlorine (compounds)	T60.1X1	T60.1X2	T60.1X3	T60.1X4	—	—
petroleum (distillate) (products) NEC	T60.8X1	T60.8X2	T60.8X3	T60.8X4	—	—
specified ingredient NEC	T60.8X1	T60.8X2	T60.8X3	T60.8X4	—	—
strychnine	T65.1X1	T65.1X2	T65.1X3	T65.1X4	—	—
thallium	T60.4X1	T60.4X2	T60.4X3	T60.4X4	—	—
Pethidine	T40.4X1	T40.4X2	T40.4X3	T40.4X4	T40.4X5	T40.4X6
Petrichloral	T42.6X1	T42.6X2	T42.6X3	T42.6X4	T42.6X5	T42.6X6
Petrol	T52.0X1	T52.0X2	T52.0X3	T52.0X4	—	—
vapor	T52.0X1	T52.0X2	T52.0X3	T52.0X4	—	—
Petrolatum	T49.3X1	T49.3X2	T49.3X3	T49.3X4	T49.3X5	T49.3X6
hydrophilic	T49.3X1	T49.3X2	T49.3X3	T49.3X4	T49.3X5	T49.3X6
liquid	T47.4X1	T47.4X2	T47.4X3	T47.4X4	T47.4X5	T47.4X6
topical	T49.3X1	T49.3X2	T49.3X3	T49.3X4	T49.3X5	T49.3X6
nonmedicinal	T52.0X1	T52.0X2	T52.0X3	T52.0X4	—	—
red veterinary	T49.3X1	T49.3X2	T49.3X3	T49.3X4	T49.3X5	T49.3X6
white	T49.3X1	T49.3X2	T49.3X3	T49.3X4	T49.3X5	T49.3X6
Petroleum (products) NEC	T52.0X1	T52.0X2	T52.0X3	T52.0X4	—	—
benzine(s) — see Ligroin						
ether — see Ligroin						
jelly — see Petrolatum						
naphtha — see Ligroin						
pesticide	T60.8X1	T60.8X2	T60.8X3	T60.8X4	—	—
solids	T52.0X1	T52.0X2	T52.0X3	T52.0X4	—	—
solvents	T52.0X1	T52.0X2	T52.0X3	T52.0X4	—	—
vapor	T52.0X1	T52.0X2	T52.0X3	T52.0X4	—	—
Peyote	T40.991	T40.992	T40.993	T40.994	—	—
Phanodorm, phanodorn	T42.3X1	T42.3X2	T42.3X3	T42.3X4	T42.3X5	T42.3X6
Phanquinone	T37.3X1	T37.3X2	T37.3X3	T37.3X4	T37.3X5	T37.3X6
Phanquone	T37.3X1	T37.3X2	T37.3X3	T37.3X4	T37.3X5	T37.3X6
Pharmaceutical						
adjunct NEC	T50.901	T50.902	T50.903	T50.904	T50.905	T50.906
excipient NEC	T50.901	T50.902	T50.903	T50.904	T50.905	T50.906
sweetener	T50.901	T50.902	T50.903	T50.904	T50.905	T50.906
viscous agent	T50.901	T50.902	T50.903	T50.904	T50.905	T50.906
Phemitone	T42.3X1	T42.3X2	T42.3X3	T42.3X4	T42.3X5	T42.3X6
Phenacaine	T41.3X1	T41.3X2	T41.3X3	T41.3X4	T41.3X5	T41.3X6
Phenacemide	T42.6X1	T42.6X2	T42.6X3	T42.6X4	T42.6X5	T42.6X6
Phenacetin	T39.1X1	T39.1X2	T39.1X3	T39.1X4	T39.1X5	T39.1X6
Phenadoxone	T40.2X1	T40.2X2	T40.2X3	T40.2X4	—	—
Phenaglycodol	T43.591	T43.592	T43.593	T43.594	T43.595	T43.596
Phenantoin	T42.0X1	T42.0X2	T42.0X3	T42.0X4	T42.0X5	T42.0X6
Phenaphthazine reagent	T50.991	T50.992	T50.993	T50.994	T50.995	T50.996
Phenazocine	T40.4X1	T40.4X2	T40.4X3	T40.4X4	T40.4X5	T40.4X6
Phenazone	T39.2X1	T39.2X2	T39.2X3	T39.2X4	T39.2X5	T39.2X6
Phenazopyridine	T39.8X1	T39.8X2	T39.8X3	T39.8X4	T39.8X5	T39.8X6
Phenbenicillin	T36.0X1	T36.0X2	T36.0X3	T36.0X4	T36.0X5	T36.0X6
Phenbutrazate	T50.5X1	T50.5X2	T50.5X3	T50.5X4	T50.5X5	T50.5X6
Phencyclidine	T40.991	T40.992	T40.993	T40.994	T40.995	T40.996
Phendimetrazine	T50.5X1	T50.5X2	T50.5X3	T50.5X4	T50.5X5	T50.5X6
Phenelzine	T43.1X1	T43.1X2	T43.1X3	T43.1X4	T43.1X5	T43.1X6
Phenemal	T42.3X1	T42.3X2	T42.3X3	T42.3X4	T42.3X5	T42.3X6
Phenergan	T42.6X1	T42.6X2	T42.6X3	T42.6X4	T42.6X5	T42.6X6
Pheneticillin	T36.0X1	T36.0X2	T36.0X3	T36.0X4	T36.0X5	T36.0X6
Pheneturide	T42.6X1	T42.6X2	T42.6X3	T42.6X4	T42.6X5	T42.6X6
Phenformin	T38.3X1	T38.3X2	T38.3X3	T38.3X4	T38.3X5	T38.3X6

Table of Drugs and Chemicals

Phenglutarimide — Pitkin's solution

Substance	Poisoning, Accidental (unintentional)	Poisoning, Intentional Self-harm	Poisoning, Assault	Poisoning, Undetermined	Adverse Effect	Under-dosing
Phenglutarimide	T44.3X1	T44.3X2	T44.3X3	T44.3X4	T44.3X5	T44.3X6
Phenicarbazide	T39.8X1	T39.8X2	T39.8X3	T39.8X4	T39.8X5	T39.8X6
Phenindamine	T45.0X1	T45.0X2	T45.0X3	T45.0X4	T45.0X5	T45.0X6
Phenindione	T45.511	T45.512	T45.513	T45.514	T45.515	T45.516
Pheniprazine	T43.1X1	T43.1X2	T43.1X3	T43.1X4	T43.1X5	T43.1X6
Pheniramine	T45.0X1	T45.0X2	T45.0X3	T45.0X4	T45.0X5	T45.0X6
Phenisatin	T47.2X1	T47.2X2	T47.2X3	T47.2X4	T47.2X5	T47.2X6
Phenmetrazine	T50.5X1	T50.5X2	T50.5X3	T50.5X4	T50.5X5	T50.5X6
Phenobal	T42.3X1	T42.3X2	T42.3X3	T42.3X4	T42.3X5	T42.3X6
Phenobarbital	T42.3X1	T42.3X2	T42.3X3	T42.3X4	T42.3X5	T42.3X6
with						
mephenytoin	T42.3X1	T42.3X2	T42.3X3	T42.3X4	T42.3X5	T42.3X6
phenytoin	T42.3X1	T42.3X2	T42.3X3	T42.3X4	T42.3X5	T42.3X6
sodium	T42.3X1	T42.3X2	T42.3X3	T42.3X4	T42.3X5	T42.3X6
Phenobarbitone	T42.3X1	T42.3X2	T42.3X3	T42.3X4	T42.3X5	T42.3X6
Phenobutiodil	T50.8X1	T50.8X2	T50.8X3	T50.8X4	T50.8X5	T50.8X6
Phenoctide	T49.0X1	T49.0X2	T49.0X3	T49.0X4	T49.0X5	T49.0X6
Phenol	T49.0X1	T49.0X2	T49.0X3	T49.0X4	T49.0X5	T49.0X6
disinfectant	T54.0X1	T54.0X2	T54.0X3	T54.0X4	—	—
in oil injection	T46.8X1	T46.8X2	T46.8X3	T46.8X4	T46.8X5	T46.8X6
medicinal	T49.1X1	T49.1X2	T49.1X3	T49.1X4	T49.1X5	T49.1X6
nonmedicinal NEC	T54.0X1	T54.0X2	T54.0X3	T54.0X4	—	—
pesticide	T60.8X1	T60.8X2	T60.8X3	T60.8X4	—	—
red	T50.8X1	T50.8X2	T50.8X3	T50.8X4	T50.8X5	T50.8X6
Phenolic preparation	T49.1X1	T49.1X2	T49.1X3	T49.1X4	T49.1X5	T49.1X6
Phenolphthalein	T47.2X1	T47.2X2	T47.2X3	T47.2X4	T47.2X5	T47.2X6
Phenolsulfonphthalein	T50.8X1	T50.8X2	T50.8X3	T50.8X4	T50.8X5	T50.8X6
Phenomorphan	T40.2X1	T40.2X2	T40.2X3	T40.2X4	—	—
Phenonyl	T42.3X1	T42.3X2	T42.3X3	T42.3X4	T42.3X5	T42.3X6
Phenoperidine	T40.4X1	T40.4X2	T40.4X3	T40.4X4	—	—
Phenopyrazone	T46.991	T46.992	T46.993	T46.994	T46.995	T46.996
Phenoquin	T50.4X1	T50.4X2	T50.4X3	T50.4X4	T50.4X5	T50.4X6
Phenothiazine (psychotropic) NEC	T43.3X1	T43.3X2	T43.3X3	T43.3X4	T43.3X5	T43.3X6
insecticide	T60.2X1	T60.2X2	T60.2X3	T60.2X4	—	—
Phenothrin	T49.0X1	T49.0X2	T49.0X3	T49.0X4	T49.0X5	T49.0X6
Phenoxybenzamine	T46.7X1	T46.7X2	T46.7X3	T46.7X4	T46.7X5	T46.7X6
Phenoxyethanol	T49.0X1	T49.0X2	T49.0X3	T49.0X4	T49.0X5	T49.0X6
Phenoxymethyl penicillin	T36.0X1	T36.0X2	T36.0X3	T36.0X4	T36.0X5	T36.0X6
Phenprobamate	T42.8X1	T42.8X2	T42.8X3	T42.8X4	T42.8X5	T42.8X6
Phenprocoumon	T45.511	T45.512	T45.513	T45.514	T45.515	T45.516
Phensuximide	T42.2X1	T42.2X2	T42.2X3	T42.2X4	T42.2X5	T42.2X6
Phentermine	T50.5X1	T50.5X2	T50.5X3	T50.5X4	T50.5X5	T50.5X6
Phenthicillin	T36.0X1	T36.0X2	T36.0X3	T36.0X4	T36.0X5	T36.0X6
Phentolamine	T46.7X1	T46.7X2	T46.7X3	T46.7X4	T46.7X5	T46.7X6
Phenyl						
butazone	T39.2X1	T39.2X2	T39.2X3	T39.2X4	T39.2X5	T39.2X6
enediamine	T65.3X1	T65.3X2	T65.3X3	T65.3X4	—	—
hydrazine	T65.3X1	T65.3X2	T65.3X3	T65.3X4	—	—
antineoplastic	T45.1X1	T45.1X2	T45.1X3	T45.1X4	T45.1X5	T45.1X6
mercuric compounds — see Mercury						
salicylate	T49.3X1	T49.3X2	T49.3X3	T49.3X4	T49.3X5	T49.3X6
Phenylalanine mustard	T45.1X1	T45.1X2	T45.1X3	T45.1X4	T45.1X5	T45.1X6
Phenylbutazone	T39.2X1	T39.2X2	T39.2X3	T39.2X4	T39.2X5	T39.2X6
Phenylenediamine	T65.3X1	T65.3X2	T65.3X3	T65.3X4	—	—
Phenylephrine	T44.4X1	T44.4X2	T44.4X3	T44.4X4	T44.4X5	T44.4X6
Phenylethylbiguanide	T38.3X1	T38.3X2	T38.3X3	T38.3X4	T38.3X5	T38.3X6
Phenylmercuric						
acetate	T49.0X1	T49.0X2	T49.0X3	T49.0X4	T49.0X5	T49.0X6
borate	T49.0X1	T49.0X2	T49.0X3	T49.0X4	T49.0X5	T49.0X6
nitrate	T49.0X1	T49.0X2	T49.0X3	T49.0X4	T49.0X5	T49.0X6
Phenylmethylbarbitone	T42.3X1	T42.3X2	T42.3X3	T42.3X4	T42.3X5	T42.3X6
Phenylpropanol	T47.5X1	T47.5X2	T47.5X3	T47.5X4	T47.5X5	T47.5X6
Phenylpropanolamine	T44.991	T44.992	T44.993	T44.994	T44.995	T44.996
Phenylsulfthion	T60.0X1	T60.0X2	T60.0X3	T60.0X4	—	—
Phenyltoloxamine	T45.0X1	T45.0X2	T45.0X3	T45.0X4	T45.0X5	T45.0X6
Phenyramidol, phenyramidon	T39.8X1	T39.8X2	T39.8X3	T39.8X4	T39.8X5	T39.8X6
Phenytoin	T42.0X1	T42.0X2	T42.0X3	T42.0X4	T42.0X5	T42.0X6
with Phenobarbital	T42.3X1	T42.3X2	T42.3X3	T42.3X4	T42.3X5	T42.3X6
pHisoHex	T49.2X1	T49.2X2	T49.2X3	T49.2X4	T49.2X5	T49.2X6
Pholcodine	T48.3X1	T48.3X2	T48.3X3	T48.3X4	T48.3X5	T48.3X6
Pholedrine	T46.991	T46.992	T46.993	T46.994	T46.995	T46.996
Phorate	T60.0X1	T60.0X2	T60.0X3	T60.0X4	—	—
Phosdrin	T60.0X1	T60.0X2	T60.0X3	T60.0X4	—	—
Phosfolan	T60.0X1	T60.0X2	T60.0X3	T60.0X4	—	—
Phosgene (gas)	T59.891	T59.892	T59.893	T59.894	—	—
Phosphamidon	T60.0X1	T60.0X2	T60.0X3	T60.0X4	—	—
Phosphate	T65.891	T65.892	T65.893	T65.894	—	—
laxative	T47.4X1	T47.4X2	T47.4X3	T47.4X4	T47.4X5	T47.4X6
organic	T60.0X1	T60.0X2	T60.0X3	T60.0X4	—	—
solvent	T52.91	T52.92	T52.93	T52.94	—	—
Phosphate — continued						
tricresyl	T65.891	T65.892	T65.893	T65.894	—	—
Phosphine	T57.1X1	T57.1X2	T57.1X3	T57.1X4	—	—
fumigant	T57.1X1	T57.1X2	T57.1X3	T57.1X4	—	—
Phospholine	T49.5X1	T49.5X2	T49.5X3	T49.5X4	T49.5X5	T49.5X6
Phosphoric acid	T54.2X1	T54.2X2	T54.2X3	T54.2X4	—	—
Phosphorus (compound) NEC	T57.1X1	T57.1X2	T57.1X3	T57.1X4	—	—
pesticide	T60.0X1	T60.0X2	T60.0X3	T60.0X4	—	—
Phthalates	T65.891	T65.892	T65.893	T65.894	—	—
Phthalic anhydride	T65.891	T65.892	T65.893	T65.894	—	—
Phthalimidoglutarimide	T42.6X1	T42.6X2	T42.6X3	T42.6X4	T42.6X5	T42.6X6
Phthalylsulfathiazole	T37.0X1	T37.0X2	T37.0X3	T37.0X4	T37.0X5	T37.0X6
Phylloquinone	T45.7X1	T45.7X2	T45.7X3	T45.7X4	T45.7X5	T45.7X6
Physeptone	T40.3X1	T40.3X2	T40.3X3	T40.3X4	T40.3X5	T40.3X6
Physostigma venenosum	T62.2X1	T62.2X2	T62.2X3	T62.2X4	—	—
Physostigmine	T49.5X1	T49.5X2	T49.5X3	T49.5X4	T49.5X5	T49.5X6
Phytolacca decandra	T62.2X1	T62.2X2	T62.2X3	T62.2X4	—	—
berries	T62.1X1	T62.1X2	T62.1X3	T62.1X4	—	—
Phytomenadione	T45.7X1	T45.7X2	T45.7X3	T45.7X4	T45.7X5	T45.7X6
Phytonadione	T45.7X1	T45.7X2	T45.7X3	T45.7X4	T45.7X5	T45.7X6
Picoperine	T48.3X1	T48.3X2	T48.3X3	T48.3X4	T48.3X5	T48.3X6
Picosulfate (sodium)	T47.2X1	T47.2X2	T47.2X3	T47.2X4	T47.2X5	T47.2X6
Picric (acid)	T54.2X1	T54.2X2	T54.2X3	T54.2X4	—	—
Picrotoxin	T50.7X1	T50.7X2	T50.7X3	T50.7X4	T50.7X5	T50.7X6
Piketoprofen	T49.0X1	T49.0X2	T49.0X3	T49.0X4	T49.0X5	T49.0X6
Pilocarpine	T44.1X1	T44.1X2	T44.1X3	T44.1X4	T44.1X5	T44.1X6
Pilocarpus (jaborandi) extract	T44.1X1	T44.1X2	T44.1X3	T44.1X4	T44.1X5	T44.1X6
Pilsicainide (hydrochloride)	T46.2X1	T46.2X2	T46.2X3	T46.2X4	T46.2X5	T46.2X6
Pimaricin	T36.7X1	T36.7X2	T36.7X3	T36.7X4	T36.7X5	T36.7X6
Pimeclone	T50.7X1	T50.7X2	T50.7X3	T50.7X4	T50.7X5	T50.7X6
Pimelic ketone	T52.8X1	T52.8X2	T52.8X3	T52.8X4	—	—
Pimethixene	T45.0X1	T45.0X2	T45.0X3	T45.0X4	T45.0X5	T45.0X6
Piminodine	T40.2X1	T40.2X2	T40.2X3	T40.2X4	T40.2X5	T40.2X6
Pimozide	T43.591	T43.592	T43.593	T43.594	T43.595	T43.596
Pinacidil	T46.5X1	T46.5X2	T46.5X3	T46.5X4	T46.5X5	T46.5X6
Pinaverium bromide	T44.3X1	T44.3X2	T44.3X3	T44.3X4	T44.3X5	T44.3X6
Pinazepam	T42.4X1	T42.4X2	T42.4X3	T42.4X4	T42.4X5	T42.4X6
Pindolol	T44.7X1	T44.7X2	T44.7X3	T44.7X4	T44.7X5	T44.7X6
Pindone	T60.4X1	T60.4X2	T60.4X3	T60.4X4	—	—
Pine oil (disinfectant)	T65.891	T65.892	T65.893	T65.894	—	—
Pinkroot	T37.4X1	T37.4X2	T37.4X3	T37.4X4	T37.4X5	T37.4X6
Pipadone	T40.2X1	T40.2X2	T40.2X3	T40.2X4	—	—
Pipamazine	T45.0X1	T45.0X2	T45.0X3	T45.0X4	T45.0X5	T45.0X6
Pipamperone	T43.4X1	T43.4X2	T43.4X3	T43.4X4	T43.4X5	T43.4X6
Pipazetate	T48.3X1	T48.3X2	T48.3X3	T48.3X4	T48.3X5	T48.3X6
Pipemidic acid	T37.8X1	T37.8X2	T37.8X3	T37.8X4	T37.8X5	T37.8X6
Pipenzolate bromide	T44.3X1	T44.3X2	T44.3X3	T44.3X4	T44.3X5	T44.3X6
Piperacetazine	T43.3X1	T43.3X2	T43.3X3	T43.3X4	T43.3X5	T43.3X6
Piperacillin	T36.0X1	T36.0X2	T36.0X3	T36.0X4	T36.0X5	T36.0X6
Piperazine	T37.4X1	T37.4X2	T37.4X3	T37.4X4	T37.4X5	T37.4X6
estrone sulfate	T38.5X1	T38.5X2	T38.5X3	T38.5X4	T38.5X5	T38.5X6
Piper cubeba	T62.2X1	T62.2X2	T62.2X3	T62.2X4	—	—
Piperidine	T48.3X1	T48.3X2	T48.3X3	T48.3X4	T48.3X5	T48.3X6
Piperidolate	T44.3X1	T44.3X2	T44.3X3	T44.3X4	T44.3X5	T44.3X6
Piperocaine	T41.3X1	T41.3X2	T41.3X3	T41.3X4	T41.3X5	T41.3X6
infiltration (subcutaneous)	T41.3X1	T41.3X2	T41.3X3	T41.3X4	T41.3X5	T41.3X6
nerve block (peripheral) (plexus)	T41.3X1	T41.3X2	T41.3X3	T41.3X4	T41.3X5	T41.3X6
topical (surface)	T41.3X1	T41.3X2	T41.3X3	T41.3X4	T41.3X5	T41.3X6
Piperonyl butoxide	T60.8X1	T60.8X2	T60.8X3	T60.8X4	—	—
Pipethanate	T44.3X1	T44.3X2	T44.3X3	T44.3X4	T44.3X5	T44.3X6
Pipobroman	T45.1X1	T45.1X2	T45.1X3	T45.1X4	T45.1X5	T45.1X6
Pipotiazine	T43.3X1	T43.3X2	T43.3X3	T43.3X4	T43.3X5	T43.3X6
Pipoxizine	T45.0X1	T45.0X2	T45.0X3	T45.0X4	T45.0X5	T45.0X6
Pipradrol	T43.691	T43.692	T43.693	T43.694	T43.695	T43.696
Piprinhydrinate	T45.0X1	T45.0X2	T45.0X3	T45.0X4	T45.0X5	T45.0X6
Pirarubicin	T45.1X1	T45.1X2	T45.1X3	T45.1X4	T45.1X5	T45.1X6
Pirazinamide	T37.1X1	T37.1X2	T37.1X3	T37.1X4	T37.1X5	T37.1X6
Pirbuterol	T48.6X1	T48.6X2	T48.6X3	T48.6X4	T48.6X5	T48.6X6
Pirenzepine	T47.1X1	T47.1X2	T47.1X3	T47.1X4	T47.1X5	T47.1X6
Piretanide	T50.1X1	T50.1X2	T50.1X3	T50.1X4	T50.1X5	T50.1X6
Piribedil	T42.8X1	T42.8X2	T42.8X3	T42.8X4	T42.8X5	T42.8X6
Piridoxilate	T46.3X1	T46.3X2	T46.3X3	T46.3X4	T46.3X5	T46.3X6
Piritramide	T40.4X1	T40.4X2	T40.4X3	T40.4X4	—	—
Piromidic acid	T37.8X1	T37.8X2	T37.8X3	T37.8X4	T37.8X5	T37.8X6
Piroxicam	T39.391	T39.392	T39.393	T39.394	T39.395	T39.396
beta-cyclodextrin complex	T39.8X1	T39.8X2	T39.8X3	T39.8X4	T39.8X5	T39.8X6
Pirozadil	T46.6X1	T46.6X2	T46.6X3	T46.6X4	T46.6X5	T46.6X6
Piscidia (bark) (erythrina)	T39.8X1	T39.8X2	T39.8X3	T39.8X4	T39.8X5	T39.8X6
Pitch	T65.891	T65.892	T65.893	T65.894	—	—
Pitkin's solution	T41.3X1	T41.3X2	T41.3X3	T41.3X4	T41.3X5	T41.3X6

Table of Drugs and Chemicals

Substance	Poisoning, Accidental (unintentional)	Poisoning, Intentional Self-harm	Poisoning, Assault	Poisoning, Undetermined	Adverse Effect	Under-dosing
Pitocin	T48.0X1	T48.0X2	T48.0X3	T48.0X4	T48.0X5	T48.0X6
Pitressin (tannate)	T38.891	T38.892	T38.893	T38.894	T38.895	T38.896
Pituitary extracts	T38.891	T38.892	T38.893	T38.894	T38.895	T38.896
(posterior)						
anterior	T38.811	T38.812	T38.813	T38.814	T38.815	T38.816
Pituitrin	T38.891	T38.892	T38.893	T38.894	T38.895	T38.896
Pivampicillin	T36.0X1	T36.0X2	T36.0X3	T36.0X4	T36.0X5	T36.0X6
Pivmecillinam	T36.0X1	T36.0X2	T36.0X3	T36.0X4	T36.0X5	T36.0X6
Placental hormone	T38.891	T38.892	T38.893	T38.894	T38.895	T38.896
Placidyl	T42.6X1	T42.6X2	T42.6X3	T42.6X4	T42.6X5	T42.6X6
Plague vaccine	T50.A91	T50.A92	T50.A93	T50.A94	T50.A95	T50.A96
Plant						
food or fertilizer NEC	T65.891	T65.892	T65.893	T65.894	—	—
containing herbicide	T60.3X1	T60.3X2	T60.3X3	T60.3X4	—	—
noxious, used as food	T62.2X1	T62.2X2	T62.2X3	T62.2X4	—	—
berries	T62.1X1	T62.1X2	T62.1X3	T62.1X4	—	—
seeds	T62.2X1	T62.2X2	T62.2X3	T62.2X4	—	—
specified type NEC	T62.2X1	T62.2X2	T62.2X3	T62.2X4	—	—
Plasma	T45.8X1	T45.8X2	T45.8X3	T45.8X4	T45.8X5	T45.8X6
expander NEC	T45.8X1	T45.8X2	T45.8X3	T45.8X4	T45.8X5	T45.8X6
protein fraction (human)	T45.8X1	T45.8X2	T45.8X3	T45.8X4	T45.8X5	T45.8X6
Plasmanate	T45.8X1	T45.8X2	T45.8X3	T45.8X4	T45.8X5	T45.8X6
Plasminogen (tissue)	T45.611	T45.612	T45.613	T45.614	T45.615	T45.616
activator						
Plaster dressing	T49.3X1	T49.3X2	T49.3X3	T49.3X4	T49.3X5	T49.3X6
Plastic dressing	T49.3X1	T49.3X2	T49.3X3	T49.3X4	T49.3X5	T49.3X6
Plegicil	T43.3X1	T43.3X2	T43.3X3	T43.3X4	T43.3X5	T43.3X6
Plicamycin	T45.1X1	T45.1X2	T45.1X3	T45.1X4	T45.1X5	T45.1X6
Podophyllotoxin	T49.8X1	T49.8X2	T49.8X3	T49.8X4	T49.8X5	T49.8X6
Podophyllum (resin)	T49.4X1	T49.4X2	T49.4X3	T49.4X4	T49.4X5	T49.4X6
Poisonous berries	T62.1X1	T62.1X2	T62.1X3	T62.1X4	—	—
Poison NEC	T65.91	T65.92	T65.93	T65.94	—	—
Pokeweed (any part)	T62.2X1	T62.2X2	T62.2X3	T62.2X4	—	—
Poldine metilsulfate	T44.3X1	T44.3X2	T44.3X3	T44.3X4	T44.3X5	T44.3X6
Polidexide (sulfate)	T46.6X1	T46.6X2	T46.6X3	T46.6X4	T46.6X5	T46.6X6
Polidocanol	T46.8X1	T46.8X2	T46.8X3	T46.8X4	T46.8X5	T46.8X6
Poliomyelitis vaccine	T50.B91	T50.B92	T50.B93	T50.B94	T50.B95	T50.B96
Polish (car) (floor) (furniture)	T65.891	T65.892	T65.893	T65.894	—	—
(metal) (porcelain)						
(silver)						
abrasive	T65.891	T65.892	T65.893	T65.894	—	—
porcelain	T65.891	T65.892	T65.893	T65.894	—	—
Poloxalkol	T47.4X1	T47.4X2	T47.4X3	T47.4X4	T47.4X5	T47.4X6
Poloxamer	T47.4X1	T47.4X2	T47.4X3	T47.4X4	T47.4X5	T47.4X6
Polyaminostyrene resins	T50.3X1	T50.3X2	T50.3X3	T50.3X4	T50.3X5	T50.3X6
Polycarbophil	T47.4X1	T47.4X2	T47.4X3	T47.4X4	T47.4X5	T47.4X6
Polychlorinated biphenyl	T65.891	T65.892	T65.893	T65.894	—	—
Polycycline	T36.4X1	T36.4X2	T36.4X3	T36.4X4	T36.4X5	T36.4X6
Polyester fumes	T59.891	T59.892	T59.893	T59.894	—	—
Polyester resin hardener	T52.91	T52.92	T52.93	T52.94	—	—
fumes	T59.891	T59.892	T59.893	T59.894	—	—
Polyestradiol phosphate	T38.5X1	T38.5X2	T38.5X3	T38.5X4	T38.5X5	T38.5X6
Polyethanolamine alkyl sulfate	T49.2X1	T49.2X2	T49.2X3	T49.2X4	T49.2X5	T49.2X6
Polyethylene adhesive	T49.3X1	T49.3X2	T49.3X3	T49.3X4	T49.3X5	T49.3X6
Polyferose	T45.4X1	T45.4X2	T45.4X3	T45.4X4	T45.4X5	T45.4X6
Polygeline	T45.8X1	T45.8X2	T45.8X3	T45.8X4	T45.8X5	T45.8X6
Polymyxin	T36.8X1	T36.8X2	T36.8X3	T36.8X4	T36.8X5	T36.8X6
B	T36.8X1	T36.8X2	T36.8X3	T36.8X4	T36.8X5	T36.8X6
ENT agent	T49.6X1	T49.6X2	T49.6X3	T49.6X4	T49.6X5	T49.6X6
ophthalmic preparation	T49.5X1	T49.5X2	T49.5X3	T49.5X4	T49.5X5	T49.5X6
topical NEC	T49.0X1	T49.0X2	T49.0X3	T49.0X4	T49.0X5	T49.0X6
E sulfate (eye preparation)	T49.5X1	T49.5X2	T49.5X3	T49.5X4	T49.5X5	T49.5X6
Polynoxylin	T49.0X1	T49.0X2	T49.0X3	T49.0X4	T49.0X5	T49.0X6
Polyoestradiol phosphate	T38.5X1	T38.5X2	T38.5X3	T38.5X4	T38.5X5	T38.5X6
Polyoxymethyleneurea	T49.0X1	T49.0X2	T49.0X3	T49.0X4	T49.0X5	T49.0X6
Polysilane	T47.8X1	T47.8X2	T47.8X3	T47.8X4	T47.8X5	T47.8X6
Polytetrafluoroethylene (inhaled)	T59.891	T59.892	T59.893	T59.894	—	—
Polythiazide	T50.2X1	T50.2X2	T50.2X3	T50.2X4	T50.2X5	T50.2X6
Polyvidone	T45.8X1	T45.8X2	T45.8X3	T45.8X4	T45.8X5	T45.8X6
Polyvinylpyrrolidone	T45.8X1	T45.8X2	T45.8X3	T45.8X4	T45.8X5	T45.8X6
Pontocaine (hydrochloride) (infiltration) (topical)	T41.3X1	T41.3X2	T41.3X3	T41.3X4	T41.3X5	T41.3X6
nerve block (peripheral) (plexus)	T41.3X1	T41.3X2	T41.3X3	T41.3X4	T41.3X5	T41.3X6
spinal	T41.3X1	T41.3X2	T41.3X3	T41.3X4	T41.3X5	T41.3X6
Porfiromycin	T45.1X1	T45.1X2	T45.1X3	T45.1X4	T45.1X5	T45.1X6
Posterior pituitary hormone NEC	T38.891	T38.892	T38.893	T38.894	T38.895	T38.896
Pot	T40.7X1	T40.7X2	T40.7X3	T40.7X4	T40.7X5	T40.7X6
Potash (caustic)	T54.3X1	T54.3X2	T54.3X3	T54.3X4	—	—
Potassic saline injection (lactated)	T50.3X1	T50.3X2	T50.3X3	T50.3X4	T50.3X5	T50.3X6
Potassium (salts) NEC	T50.3X1	T50.3X2	T50.3X3	T50.3X4	T50.3X5	T50.3X6
aminobenzoate	T45.8X1	T45.8X2	T45.8X3	T45.8X4	T45.8X5	T45.8X6
aminosalicylate	T37.1X1	T37.1X2	T37.1X3	T37.1X4	T37.1X5	T37.1X6
antimony ' tartrate'	T37.8X1	T37.8X2	T37.8X3	T37.8X4	T37.8X5	T37.8X6
arsenite (solution)	T57.0X1	T57.0X2	T57.0X3	T57.0X4	—	—
bichromate	T56.2X1	T56.2X2	T56.2X3	T56.2X4	—	—
bisulfate	T47.3X1	T47.3X2	T47.3X3	T47.3X4	T47.3X5	T47.3X6
bromide	T42.6X1	T42.6X2	T42.6X3	T42.6X4	T42.6X5	T42.6X6
canrenoate	T50.0X1	T50.0X2	T50.0X3	T50.0X4	T50.0X5	T50.0X6
carbonate	T54.3X1	T54.3X2	T54.3X3	T54.3X4	—	—
chlorate NEC	T65.891	T65.892	T65.893	T65.894	—	—
chloride	T50.3X1	T50.3X2	T50.3X3	T50.3X4	T50.3X5	T50.3X6
citrate	T50.991	T50.992	T50.993	T50.994	T50.995	T50.996
cyanide	T65.0X1	T65.0X2	T65.0X3	T65.0X4	—	—
ferric hexacyanoferrate (medicinal)	T50.6X1	T50.6X2	T50.6X3	T50.6X4	T50.6X5	T50.6X6
nonmedicinal	T65.891	T65.892	T65.893	T65.894	—	—
Fluoride	T57.8X1	T57.8X2	T57.8X3	T57.8X4	—	—
glucaldrate	T47.1X1	T47.1X2	T47.1X3	T47.1X4	T47.1X5	T47.1X6
hydroxide	T54.3X1	T54.3X2	T54.3X3	T54.3X4	—	—
iodate	T49.0X1	T49.0X2	T49.0X3	T49.0X4	T49.0X5	T49.0X6
iodide	T48.4X1	T48.4X2	T48.4X3	T48.4X4	T48.4X5	T48.4X6
nitrate	T57.8X1	T57.8X2	T57.8X3	T57.8X4	—	—
oxalate	T65.891	T65.892	T65.893	T65.894	—	—
perchlorate (nonmedicinal) NEC	T65.891	T65.892	T65.893	T65.894	—	—
antithyroid	T38.2X1	T38.2X2	T38.2X3	T38.2X4	T38.2X5	T38.2X6
medicinal	T38.2X1	T38.2X2	T38.2X3	T38.2X4	T38.2X5	T38.2X6
Permanganate (nonmedicinal)	T65.891	T65.892	T65.893	T65.894	—	—
medicinal	T49.0X1	T49.0X2	T49.0X3	T49.0X4	T49.0X5	T49.0X6
sulfate	T47.2X1	T47.2X2	T47.2X3	T47.2X4	T47.2X5	T47.2X6
Potassium-removing resin	T50.3X1	T50.3X2	T50.3X3	T50.3X4	T50.3X5	T50.3X6
Potassium-retaining drug	T50.3X1	T50.3X2	T50.3X3	T50.3X4	T50.3X5	T50.3X6
Povidone	T45.8X1	T45.8X2	T45.8X3	T45.8X4	T45.8X5	T45.8X6
iodine	T49.0X1	T49.0X2	T49.0X3	T49.0X4	T49.0X5	T49.0X6
Practolol	T44.7X1	T44.7X2	T44.7X3	T44.7X4	T44.7X5	T44.7X6
Prajmalium bitartrate	T46.2X1	T46.2X2	T46.2X3	T46.2X4	T46.2X5	T46.2X6
Pralidoxime (iodide)	T50.6X1	T50.6X2	T50.6X3	T50.6X4	T50.6X5	T50.6X6
chloride	T50.6X1	T50.6X2	T50.6X3	T50.6X4	T50.6X5	T50.6X6
Pramiverine	T44.3X1	T44.3X2	T44.3X3	T44.3X4	T44.3X5	T44.3X6
Pramocaine	T49.1X1	T49.1X2	T49.1X3	T49.1X4	T49.1X5	T49.1X6
Pramoxine	T49.1X1	T49.1X2	T49.1X3	T49.1X4	T49.1X5	T49.1X6
Prasterone	T38.7X1	T38.7X2	T38.7X3	T38.7X4	T38.7X5	T38.7X6
Pravastatin	T46.6X1	T46.6X2	T46.6X3	T46.6X4	T46.6X5	T46.6X6
Prazepam	T42.4X1	T42.4X2	T42.4X3	T42.4X4	T42.4X5	T42.4X6
Praziquantel	T37.4X1	T37.4X2	T37.4X3	T37.4X4	T37.4X5	T37.4X6
Prazitone	T43.291	T43.292	T43.293	T43.294	T43.295	T43.296
Prazosin	T44.6X1	T44.6X2	T44.6X3	T44.6X4	T44.6X5	T44.6X6
Prednicarbate	T49.0X1	T49.0X2	T49.0X3	T49.0X4	T49.0X5	T49.0X6
Prednimustine	T45.1X1	T45.1X2	T45.1X3	T45.1X4	T45.1X5	T45.1X6
Prednisolone	T38.0X1	T38.0X2	T38.0X3	T38.0X4	T38.0X5	T38.0X6
ENT agent	T49.6X1	T49.6X2	T49.6X3	T49.6X4	T49.6X5	T49.6X6
ophthalmic preparation	T49.5X1	T49.5X2	T49.5X3	T49.5X4	T49.5X5	T49.5X6
steaglate	T49.0X1	T49.0X2	T49.0X3	T49.0X4	T49.0X5	T49.0X6
topical NEC	T49.0X1	T49.0X2	T49.0X3	T49.0X4	T49.0X5	T49.0X6
Prednisone	T38.0X1	T38.0X2	T38.0X3	T38.0X4	T38.0X5	T38.0X6
Prednylidene	T38.0X1	T38.0X2	T38.0X3	T38.0X4	T38.0X5	T38.0X6
Pregnandiol	T38.5X1	T38.5X2	T38.5X3	T38.5X4	T38.5X5	T38.5X6
Pregneninolone	T38.5X1	T38.5X2	T38.5X3	T38.5X4	T38.5X5	T38.5X6
Preludin	T43.691	T43.692	T43.693	T43.694	T43.695	T43.696
Premarin	T38.5X1	T38.5X2	T38.5X3	T38.5X4	T38.5X5	T38.5X6
Premedication anesthetic	T41.201	T41.202	T41.203	T41.204	T41.205	T41.206
Prenalterol	T44.5X1	T44.5X2	T44.5X3	T44.5X4	T44.5X5	T44.5X6
Prenoxdiazine	T48.3X1	T48.3X2	T48.3X3	T48.3X4	T48.3X5	T48.3X6
Prenylamine	T46.3X1	T46.3X2	T46.3X3	T46.3X4	T46.3X5	T46.3X6
Preparation H	T49.8X1	T49.8X2	T49.8X3	T49.8X4	T49.8X5	T49.8X6
Preparation, local	T49.4X1	T49.4X2	T49.4X3	T49.4X4	T49.4X5	T49.4X6
Preservative (nonmedicinal)	T65.891	T65.892	T65.893	T65.894	—	—
medicinal	T50.901	T50.902	T50.903	T50.904	T50.905	T50.906
wood	T60.91	T60.92	T60.93	T60.94	—	—
Prethcamide	T50.7X1	T50.7X2	T50.7X3	T50.7X4	T50.7X5	T50.7X6
Pride of China	T62.2X1	T62.2X2	T62.2X3	T62.2X4	—	—
Pridinol	T44.3X1	T44.3X2	T44.3X3	T44.3X4	T44.3X5	T44.3X6
Prifinium bromide	T44.3X1	T44.3X2	T44.3X3	T44.3X4	T44.3X5	T44.3X6
Prilocaine	T41.3X1	T41.3X2	T41.3X3	T41.3X4	T41.3X5	T41.3X6
infiltration (subcutaneous)	T41.3X1	T41.3X2	T41.3X3	T41.3X4	T41.3X5	T41.3X6
nerve block (peripheral) (plexus)	T41.3X1	T41.3X2	T41.3X3	T41.3X4	T41.3X5	T41.3X6
regional	T41.3X1	T41.3X2	T41.3X3	T41.3X4	T41.3X5	T41.3X6

Pitocin — Prilocaine

Table of Drugs and Chemicals

Primaquine — Psychotherapeutic drug NEC

Substance	Poisoning, Accidental (unintentional)	Poisoning, Intentional Self-harm	Poisoning, Assault	Poisoning, Undetermined	Adverse Effect	Under-dosing
Primaquine	T37.2X1	T37.2X2	T37.2X3	T37.2X4	T37.2X5	T37.2X6
Primidone	T42.6X1	T42.6X2	T42.6X3	T42.6X4	T42.6X5	T42.6X6
Primula (veris)	T62.2X1	T62.2X2	T62.2X3	T62.2X4	—	—
Prinadol	T40.2X1	T40.2X2	T40.2X3	T40.2X4	T40.2X5	T40.2X6
Priscol, Priscoline	T44.6X1	T44.6X2	T44.6X3	T44.6X4	T44.6X5	T44.6X6
Pristinamycin	T36.3X1	T36.3X2	T36.3X3	T36.3X4	T36.3X5	T36.3X6
Privet	T62.2X1	T62.2X2	T62.2X3	T62.2X4	—	—
berries	T62.1X1	T62.1X2	T62.1X3	T62.1X4	—	—
Privine	T44.4X1	T44.4X2	T44.4X3	T44.4X4	T44.4X5	T44.4X6
Pro-Banthine	T44.3X1	T44.3X2	T44.3X3	T44.3X4	T44.3X5	T44.3X6
Probarbital	T42.3X1	T42.3X2	T42.3X3	T42.3X4	T42.3X5	T42.3X6
Probenecid	T50.4X1	T50.4X2	T50.4X3	T50.4X4	T50.4X5	T50.4X6
Probucol	T46.6X1	T46.6X2	T46.6X3	T46.6X4	T46.6X5	T46.6X6
Procainamide	T46.2X1	T46.2X2	T46.2X3	T46.2X4	T46.2X5	T46.2X6
Procaine	T41.3X1	T41.3X2	T41.3X3	T41.3X4	T41.3X5	T41.3X6
benzylpenicillin	T36.0X1	T36.0X2	T36.0X3	T36.0X4	T36.0X5	T36.0X6
nerve block (peripheral) (plexus)	T41.3X1	T41.3X2	T41.3X3	T41.3X4	T41.3X5	T41.3X6
penicillin G	T36.0X1	T36.0X2	T36.0X3	T36.0X4	T36.0X5	T36.0X6
regional	T41.3X1	T41.3X2	T41.3X3	T41.3X4	T41.3X5	T41.3X6
spinal	T41.3X1	T41.3X2	T41.3X3	T41.3X4	T41.3X5	T41.3X6
Procalmidol	T43.591	T43.592	T43.593	T43.594	T43.595	T43.596
Procarbazine	T45.1X1	T45.1X2	T45.1X3	T45.1X4	T45.1X5	T45.1X6
Procaterol	T44.5X1	T44.5X2	T44.5X3	T44.5X4	T44.5X5	T44.5X6
Prochlorperazine	T43.3X1	T43.3X2	T43.3X3	T43.3X4	T43.3X5	T43.3X6
Procyclidine	T44.3X1	T44.3X2	T44.3X3	T44.3X4	T44.3X5	T44.3X6
Producer gas	T58.8X1	T58.8X2	T58.8X3	T58.8X4	—	—
Profadol	T40.4X1	T40.4X2	T40.4X3	T40.4X4	T40.4X5	T40.4X6
Profenamine	T44.3X1	T44.3X2	T44.3X3	T44.3X4	T44.3X5	T44.3X6
Profenil	T44.3X1	T44.3X2	T44.3X3	T44.3X4	T44.3X5	T44.3X6
Proflavine	T49.0X1	T49.0X2	T49.0X3	T49.0X4	T49.0X5	T49.0X6
Progabide	T42.6X1	T42.6X2	T42.6X3	T42.6X4	T42.6X5	T42.6X6
Progesterone	T38.5X1	T38.5X2	T38.5X3	T38.5X4	T38.5X5	T38.5X6
Progestin	T38.5X1	T38.5X2	T38.5X3	T38.5X4	T38.5X5	T38.5X6
oral contraceptive	T38.4X1	T38.4X2	T38.4X3	T38.4X4	T38.4X5	T38.4X6
Progestogen NEC	T38.5X1	T38.5X2	T38.5X3	T38.5X4	T38.5X5	T38.5X6
Progestone	T38.5X1	T38.5X2	T38.5X3	T38.5X4	T38.5X5	T38.5X6
Proglumide	T47.1X1	T47.1X2	T47.1X3	T47.1X4	T47.1X5	T47.1X6
Proguanil	T37.2X1	T37.2X2	T37.2X3	T37.2X4	T37.2X5	T37.2X6
Prolactin	T38.811	T38.812	T38.813	T38.814	T38.815	T38.816
Prolintane	T43.691	T43.692	T43.693	T43.694	T43.695	T43.696
Proloid	T38.1X1	T38.1X2	T38.1X3	T38.1X4	T38.1X5	T38.1X6
Proluton	T38.5X1	T38.5X2	T38.5X3	T38.5X4	T38.5X5	T38.5X6
Promacetin	T37.1X1	T37.1X2	T37.1X3	T37.1X4	T37.1X5	T37.1X6
Promazine	T43.3X1	T43.3X2	T43.3X3	T43.3X4	T43.3X5	T43.3X6
Promedol	T40.2X1	T40.2X2	T40.2X3	T40.2X4	—	—
Promegestone	T38.5X1	T38.5X2	T38.5X3	T38.5X4	T38.5X5	T38.5X6
Promethazine (teoclate)	T43.3X1	T43.3X2	T43.3X3	T43.3X4	T43.3X5	T43.3X6
Promin	T37.1X1	T37.1X2	T37.1X3	T37.1X4	T37.1X5	T37.1X6
Pronase	T45.3X1	T45.3X2	T45.3X3	T45.3X4	T45.3X5	T45.3X6
Pronestyl (hydrochloride)	T46.2X1	T46.2X2	T46.2X3	T46.2X4	T46.2X5	T46.2X6
Pronetalol	T44.7X1	T44.7X2	T44.7X3	T44.7X4	T44.7X5	T44.7X6
Prontosil	T37.0X1	T37.0X2	T37.0X3	T37.0X4	T37.0X5	T37.0X6
Propachlor	T60.3X1	T60.3X2	T60.3X3	T60.3X4	—	—
Propafenone	T46.2X1	T46.2X2	T46.2X3	T46.2X4	T46.2X5	T46.2X6
Propallylonal	T42.3X1	T42.3X2	T42.3X3	T42.3X4	T42.3X5	T42.3X6
Propamidine	T49.0X1	T49.0X2	T49.0X3	T49.0X4	T49.0X5	T49.0X6
Propane (distributed in mobile container)	T59.891	T59.892	T59.893	T59.894	—	—
distributed through pipes	T59.891	T59.892	T59.893	T59.894	—	—
incomplete combustion	T58.11	T58.12	T58.13	T58.14	—	—
Propanidid	T41.291	T41.292	T41.293	T41.294	T41.295	T41.296
Propanil	T60.3X1	T60.3X2	T60.3X3	T60.3X4	—	—
Propantheline	T44.3X1	T44.3X2	T44.3X3	T44.3X4	T44.3X5	T44.3X6
bromide	T44.3X1	T44.3X2	T44.3X3	T44.3X4	T44.3X5	T44.3X6
Proparacaine	T41.3X1	T41.3X2	T41.3X3	T41.3X4	T41.3X5	T41.3X6
Propatylnitrate	T46.3X1	T46.3X2	T46.3X3	T46.3X4	T46.3X5	T46.3X6
Propicillin	T36.0X1	T36.0X2	T36.0X3	T36.0X4	T36.0X5	T36.0X6
Propiolactone	T49.0X1	T49.0X2	T49.0X3	T49.0X4	T49.0X5	T49.0X6
Propiomazine	T45.0X1	T45.0X2	T45.0X3	T45.0X4	T45.0X5	T45.0X6
Propionaldehyde (medicinal)	T42.6X1	T42.6X2	T42.6X3	T42.6X4	T42.6X5	T42.6X6
Propionate (calcium) (sodium)	T49.0X1	T49.0X2	T49.0X3	T49.0X4	T49.0X5	T49.0X6
Propion gel	T49.0X1	T49.0X2	T49.0X3	T49.0X4	T49.0X5	T49.0X6
Propitocaine	T41.3X1	T41.3X2	T41.3X3	T41.3X4	T41.3X5	T41.3X6
infiltration (subcutaneous)	T41.3X1	T41.3X2	T41.3X3	T41.3X4	T41.3X5	T41.3X6
nerve block (peripheral) (plexus)	T41.3X1	T41.3X2	T41.3X3	T41.3X4	T41.3X5	T41.3X6
Propofol	T41.291	T41.292	T41.293	T41.294	T41.295	T41.296
Propoxur	T60.0X1	T60.0X2	T60.0X3	T60.0X4	—	—
Propoxycaine	T41.3X1	T41.3X2	T41.3X3	T41.3X4	T41.3X5	T41.3X6
infiltration (subcutaneous)	T41.3X1	T41.3X2	T41.3X3	T41.3X4	T41.3X5	T41.3X6
Propoxycaine — *continued*						
nerve block (peripheral) (plexus)	T41.3X1	T41.3X2	T41.3X3	T41.3X4	T41.3X5	T41.3X6
topical (surface)	T41.3X1	T41.3X2	T41.3X3	T41.3X4	T41.3X5	T41.3X6
Propoxyphene	T40.4X1	T40.4X2	T40.4X3	T40.4X4	T40.4X5	T40.4X6
Propranolol	T44.7X1	T44.7X2	T44.7X3	T44.7X4	T44.7X5	T44.7X6
Propyl						
alcohol	T51.3X1	T51.3X2	T51.3X3	T51.3X4	—	—
carbinol	T51.3X1	T51.3X2	T51.3X3	T51.3X4	—	—
hexadrine	T44.4X1	T44.4X2	T44.4X3	T44.4X4	T44.4X5	T44.4X6
iodone	T50.8X1	T50.8X2	T50.8X3	T50.8X4	T50.8X5	T50.8X6
thiouracil	T38.2X1	T38.2X2	T38.2X3	T38.2X4	T38.2X5	T38.2X6
Propylaminophenothiazine	T43.3X1	T43.3X2	T43.3X3	T43.3X4	T43.3X5	T43.3X6
Propylene	T59.891	T59.892	T59.893	T59.894	—	—
Propylhexedrine	T48.5X1	T48.5X2	T48.5X3	T48.5X4	T48.5X5	T48.5X6
Propyliodone	T50.8X1	T50.8X2	T50.8X3	T50.8X4	T50.8X5	T50.8X6
Propylparaben (ophthalmic)	T49.5X1	T49.5X2	T49.5X3	T49.5X4	T49.5X5	T49.5X6
Propylthiouracil	T38.2X1	T38.2X2	T38.2X3	T38.2X4	T38.2X5	T38.2X6
Propyphenazone	T39.2X1	T39.2X2	T39.2X3	T39.2X4	T39.2X5	T39.2X6
Proquazone	T39.391	T39.392	T39.393	T39.394	T39.395	T39.396
Proscillaridin	T46.0X1	T46.0X2	T46.0X3	T46.0X4	T46.0X5	T46.0X6
Prostacyclin	T45.521	T45.522	T45.523	T45.524	T45.525	T45.526
Prostaglandin (I2)	T45.521	T45.522	T45.523	T45.524	T45.525	T45.526
E1	T46.7X1	T46.7X2	T46.7X3	T46.7X4	T46.7X5	T46.7X6
E2	T48.0X1	T48.0X2	T48.0X3	T48.0X4	T48.0X5	T48.0X6
F2 alpha	T48.0X1	T48.0X2	T48.0X3	T48.0X4	T48.0X5	T48.0X6
Prostigmin	T44.0X1	T44.0X2	T44.0X3	T44.0X4	T44.0X5	T44.0X6
Prosultiamine	T45.2X1	T45.2X2	T45.2X3	T45.2X4	T45.2X5	T45.2X6
Protamine sulfate	T45.7X1	T45.7X2	T45.7X3	T45.7X4	T45.7X5	T45.7X6
zinc insulin	T38.3X1	T38.3X2	T38.3X3	T38.3X4	T38.3X5	T38.3X6
Protease	T47.5X1	T47.5X2	T47.5X3	T47.5X4	T47.5X5	T47.5X6
Protectant, skin NEC	T49.3X1	T49.3X2	T49.3X3	T49.3X4	T49.3X5	T49.3X6
Protein hydrolysate	T50.991	T50.992	T50.993	T50.994	T50.995	T50.996
Prothiaden — *see* Dothiepin hydrochloride						
Prothionamide	T37.1X1	T37.1X2	T37.1X3	T37.1X4	T37.1X5	T37.1X6
Prothipendyl	T43.591	T43.592	T43.593	T43.594	T43.595	T43.596
Prothoate	T60.0X1	T60.0X2	T60.0X3	T60.0X4	—	—
Prothrombin						
activator	T45.7X1	T45.7X2	T45.7X3	T45.7X4	T45.7X5	T45.7X6
synthesis inhibitor	T45.511	T45.512	T45.513	T45.514	T45.515	T45.516
Protionamide	T37.1X1	T37.1X2	T37.1X3	T37.1X4	T37.1X5	T37.1X6
Protirelin	T38.891	T38.892	T38.893	T38.894	T38.895	T38.896
Protokylol	T48.6X1	T48.6X2	T48.6X3	T48.6X4	T48.6X5	T48.6X6
Protopam	T50.6X1	T50.6X2	T50.6X3	T50.6X4	T50.6X5	T50.6X6
Protoveratrine(s) (A) (B)	T46.5X1	T46.5X2	T46.5X3	T46.5X4	T46.5X5	T46.5X6
Protriptyline	T43.011	T43.012	T43.013	T43.014	T43.015	T43.016
Provera	T38.5X1	T38.5X2	T38.5X3	T38.5X4	T38.5X5	T38.5X6
Provitamin A	T45.2X1	T45.2X2	T45.2X3	T45.2X4	T45.2X5	T45.2X6
Proxibarbal	T42.3X1	T42.3X2	T42.3X3	T42.3X4	T42.3X5	T42.3X6
Proxymetacaine	T41.3X1	T41.3X2	T41.3X3	T41.3X4	T41.3X5	T41.3X6
Proxyphylline	T48.6X1	T48.6X2	T48.6X3	T48.6X4	T48.6X5	T48.6X6
Prozac — *see* Fluoxetine hydrochloride						
Prunus						
laurocerasus	T62.2X1	T62.2X2	T62.2X3	T62.2X4	—	—
virginiana	T62.2X1	T62.2X2	T62.2X3	T62.2X4	—	—
Prussian blue						
commercial	T65.891	T65.892	T65.893	T65.894	—	—
therapeutic	T50.6X1	T50.6X2	T50.6X3	T50.6X4	T50.6X5	T50.6X6
Prussic acid	T65.0X1	T65.0X2	T65.0X3	T65.0X4	—	—
vapor	T57.3X1	T57.3X2	T57.3X3	T57.3X4	—	—
Pseudoephedrine	T44.991	T44.992	T44.993	T44.994	T44.995	T44.996
Psilocin	T40.991	T40.992	T40.993	T40.994	—	—
Psilocybin	T40.991	T40.992	T40.993	T40.994	—	—
Psilocybine	T40.991	T40.992	T40.993	T40.994	—	—
Psoralene (nonmedicinal)	T65.891	T65.892	T65.893	T65.894	—	—
Psoralens (medicinal)	T50.991	T50.992	T50.993	T50.994	T50.995	T50.996
PSP (phenolsulfonphthalein)	T50.8X1	T50.8X2	T50.8X3	T50.8X4	T50.8X5	T50.8X6
Psychodysleptic drug NOS	T40.901	T40.902	T40.903	T40.904	T40.905	T40.906
specified NEC	T40.991	T40.992	T40.993	T40.994	T40.995	T40.996
Psychostimulant	T43.601	T43.602	T43.603	T43.604	T43.605	T43.606
amphetamine	T43.621	T43.622	T43.623	T43.624	T43.625	T43.626
caffeine	T43.611	T43.612	T43.613	T43.614	T43.615	T43.616
methylphenidate	T43.631	T43.632	T43.633	T43.634	T43.635	T43.636
specified NEC	T43.691	T43.692	T43.693	T43.694	T43.695	T43.696
Psychotherapeutic drug NEC	T43.91	T43.92	T43.93	T43.94	T43.95	T43.96
antidepressants — *see also* Antidepressant	T43.201	T43.202	T43.203	T43.204	T43.205	T43.206
specified NEC	T43.8X1	T43.8X2	T43.8X3	T43.8X4	T43.8X5	T43.8X6

Additional Character May Be Required — Refer to the Tabular List for Character Selection   ▽ Subterms under main terms may continue to next column or page

Substance	Poisoning, Accidental (unintentional)	Poisoning, Intentional Self-harm	Poisoning, Assault	Poisoning, Undetermined	Adverse Effect	Under-dosing
Psychotherapeutic drug — continued						
tranquilizers NEC	T43.501	T43.502	T43.503	T43.504	T43.505	T43.506
Psychotomimetic agents	T40.901	T40.902	T40.903	T40.904	T40.905	T40.906
Psychotropic drug NEC	T43.91	T43.92	T43.93	T43.94	T43.95	T43.96
specified NEC	T43.8X1	T43.8X2	T43.8X3	T43.8X4	T43.8X5	T43.8X6
Psyllium hydrophilic mucilloid	T47.4X1	T47.4X2	T47.4X3	T47.4X4	T47.4X5	T47.4X6
Pteroylglutamic acid	T45.8X1	T45.8X2	T45.8X3	T45.8X4	T45.8X5	T45.8X6
Pteroyltriglutamate	T45.1X1	T45.1X2	T45.1X3	T45.1X4	T45.1X5	T45.1X6
PTFE — see Polytetrafluoroethylene						
Pulp						
devitalizing paste	T49.7X1	T49.7X2	T49.7X3	T49.7X4	T49.7X5	T49.7X6
dressing	T49.7X1	T49.7X2	T49.7X3	T49.7X4	T49.7X5	T49.7X6
Pulsatilla	T62.2X1	T62.2X2	T62.2X3	T62.2X4	—	—
Pumpkin seed extract	T37.4X1	T37.4X2	T37.4X3	T37.4X4	T37.4X5	T37.4X6
Purex (bleach)	T54.91	T54.92	T54.93	T54.94	—	—
Purgative NEC — see also Cathartic	T47.4X1	T47.4X2	T47.4X3	T47.4X4	T47.4X5	T47.4X6
Purine analogue (antineoplastic)	T45.1X1	T45.1X2	T45.1X3	T45.1X4	T45.1X5	T45.1X6
Purine diuretics	T50.2X1	T50.2X2	T50.2X3	T50.2X4	T50.2X5	T50.2X6
Purinethol	T45.1X1	T45.1X2	T45.1X3	T45.1X4	T45.1X5	T45.1X6
PVP	T45.8X1	T45.8X2	T45.8X3	T45.8X4	T45.8X5	T45.8X6
Pyrabital	T39.8X1	T39.8X2	T39.8X3	T39.8X4	T39.8X5	T39.8X6
Pyramidon	T39.2X1	T39.2X2	T39.2X3	T39.2X4	T39.2X5	T39.2X6
Pyrantel	T37.4X1	T37.4X2	T37.4X3	T37.4X4	T37.4X5	T37.4X6
Pyrathiazine	T45.0X1	T45.0X2	T45.0X3	T45.0X4	T45.0X5	T45.0X6
Pyrazinamide	T37.1X1	T37.1X2	T37.1X3	T37.1X4	T37.1X5	T37.1X6
Pyrazinoic acid (amide)	T37.1X1	T37.1X2	T37.1X3	T37.1X4	T37.1X5	T37.1X6
Pyrazole (derivatives)	T39.2X1	T39.2X2	T39.2X3	T39.2X4	T39.2X5	T39.2X6
Pyrazolone analgesic NEC	T39.2X1	T39.2X2	T39.2X3	T39.2X4	T39.2X5	T39.2X6
Pyrethrin, pyrethrum (nonmedicinal)	T60.2X1	T60.2X2	T60.2X3	T60.2X4	—	—
Pyrethrum extract	T49.0X1	T49.0X2	T49.0X3	T49.0X4	T49.0X5	T49.0X6
Pyribenzamine	T45.0X1	T45.0X2	T45.0X3	T45.0X4	T45.0X5	T45.0X6
Pyridine	T52.8X1	T52.8X2	T52.8X3	T52.8X4	—	—
aldoxime methiodide	T50.6X1	T50.6X2	T50.6X3	T50.6X4	T50.6X5	T50.6X6
aldoxime methyl chloride	T50.6X1	T50.6X2	T50.6X3	T50.6X4	T50.6X5	T50.6X6
vapor	T59.891	T59.892	T59.893	T59.894	—	—
Pyridium	T39.8X1	T39.8X2	T39.8X3	T39.8X4	T39.8X5	T39.8X6
Pyridostigmine bromide	T44.0X1	T44.0X2	T44.0X3	T44.0X4	T44.0X5	T44.0X6
Pyridoxal phosphate	T45.2X1	T45.2X2	T45.2X3	T45.2X4	T45.2X5	T45.2X6
Pyridoxine	T45.2X1	T45.2X2	T45.2X3	T45.2X4	T45.2X5	T45.2X6
Pyrilamine	T45.0X1	T45.0X2	T45.0X3	T45.0X4	T45.0X5	T45.0X6
Pyrimethamine	T37.2X1	T37.2X2	T37.2X3	T37.2X4	T37.2X5	T37.2X6
with sulfadoxine	T37.2X1	T37.2X2	T37.2X3	T37.2X4	T37.2X5	T37.2X6
Pyrimidine antagonist	T45.1X1	T45.1X2	T45.1X3	T45.1X4	T45.1X5	T45.1X6
Pyriminil	T60.4X1	T60.4X2	T60.4X3	T60.4X4	—	—
Pyrithione zinc	T49.4X1	T49.4X2	T49.4X3	T49.4X4	T49.4X5	T49.4X6
Pyrithyldione	T42.6X1	T42.6X2	T42.6X3	T42.6X4	T42.6X5	T42.6X6
Pyrogallic acid	T49.0X1	T49.0X2	T49.0X3	T49.0X4	T49.0X5	T49.0X6
Pyrogallol	T49.0X1	T49.0X2	T49.0X3	T49.0X4	T49.0X5	T49.0X6
Pyroxylin	T49.3X1	T49.3X2	T49.3X3	T49.3X4	T49.3X5	T49.3X6
Pyrrobutamine	T45.0X1	T45.0X2	T45.0X3	T45.0X4	T45.0X5	T45.0X6
Pyrrolizidine alkaloids	T62.8X1	T62.8X2	T62.8X3	T62.8X4	—	—
Pyrvinium chloride	T37.4X1	T37.4X2	T37.4X3	T37.4X4	T37.4X5	T37.4X6
PZI	T38.3X1	T38.3X2	T38.3X3	T38.3X4	T38.3X5	T38.3X6
Quaalude	T42.6X1	T42.6X2	T42.6X3	T42.6X4	T42.6X5	T42.6X6
Quarternary ammonium						
anti-infective	T49.0X1	T49.0X2	T49.0X3	T49.0X4	T49.0X5	T49.0X6
ganglion blocking	T44.2X1	T44.2X2	T44.2X3	T44.2X4	T44.2X5	T44.2X6
parasympatholytic	T44.3X1	T44.3X2	T44.3X3	T44.3X4	T44.3X5	T44.3X6
Quazepam	T42.4X1	T42.4X2	T42.4X3	T42.4X4	T42.4X5	T42.4X6
Quicklime	T54.3X1	T54.3X2	T54.3X3	T54.3X4	—	—
Quillaja extract	T48.4X1	T48.4X2	T48.4X3	T48.4X4	T48.4X5	T48.4X6
Quinacrine	T37.2X1	T37.2X2	T37.2X3	T37.2X4	T37.2X5	T37.2X6
Quinaglute	T46.2X1	T46.2X2	T46.2X3	T46.2X4	T46.2X5	T46.2X6
Quinalbarbital	T42.3X1	T42.3X2	T42.3X3	T42.3X4	T42.3X5	T42.3X6
Quinalbarbitone sodium	T42.3X1	T42.3X2	T42.3X3	T42.3X4	T42.3X5	T42.3X6
Quinalphos	T60.0X1	T60.0X2	T60.0X3	T60.0X4	—	—
Quinapril	T46.4X1	T46.4X2	T46.4X3	T46.4X4	T46.4X5	T46.4X6
Quinestradiol	T38.5X1	T38.5X2	T38.5X3	T38.5X4	T38.5X5	T38.5X6
Quinestradol	T38.5X1	T38.5X2	T38.5X3	T38.5X4	T38.5X5	T38.5X6
Quinestrol	T38.5X1	T38.5X2	T38.5X3	T38.5X4	T38.5X5	T38.5X6
Quinethazone	T50.2X1	T50.2X2	T50.2X3	T50.2X4	T50.2X5	T50.2X6
Quingestanol	T38.4X1	T38.4X2	T38.4X3	T38.4X4	T38.4X5	T38.4X6
Quinidine	T46.2X1	T46.2X2	T46.2X3	T46.2X4	T46.2X5	T46.2X6
Quinine	T37.2X1	T37.2X2	T37.2X3	T37.2X4	T37.2X5	T37.2X6
Quiniobine	T37.8X1	T37.8X2	T37.8X3	T37.8X4	T37.8X5	T37.8X6
Quinisocaine	T49.1X1	T49.1X2	T49.1X3	T49.1X4	T49.1X5	T49.1X6
Quinocide	T37.2X1	T37.2X2	T37.2X3	T37.2X4	T37.2X5	T37.2X6

Substance	Poisoning, Accidental (unintentional)	Poisoning, Intentional Self-harm	Poisoning, Assault	Poisoning, Undetermined	Adverse Effect	Under-dosing
Quinoline (derivatives) NEC	T37.8X1	T37.8X2	T37.8X3	T37.8X4	T37.8X5	T37.8X6
Quinupramine	T43.011	T43.012	T43.013	T43.014	T43.015	T43.016
Quotane	T41.3X1	T41.3X2	T41.3X3	T41.3X4	T41.3X5	T41.3X6
Rabies						
immune globulin (human)	T50.Z11	T50.Z12	T50.Z13	T50.Z14	T50.Z15	T50.Z16
vaccine	T50.B91	T50.B92	T50.B93	T50.B94	T50.B95	T50.B96
Racemoramide	T40.2X1	T40.2X2	T40.2X3	T40.2X4	—	—
Racemorphan	T40.2X1	T40.2X2	T40.2X3	T40.2X4	T40.2X5	T40.2X6
Racepinefrin	T44.5X1	T44.5X2	T44.5X3	T44.5X4	T44.5X5	T44.5X6
Raclopride	T43.591	T43.592	T43.593	T43.594	T43.595	T43.596
Radiator alcohol	T51.1X1	T51.1X2	T51.1X3	T51.1X4	—	—
Radioactive drug NEC	T50.8X1	T50.8X2	T50.8X3	T50.8X4	T50.8X5	T50.8X6
Radio-opaque (drugs) (materials)	T50.8X1	T50.8X2	T50.8X3	T50.8X4	T50.8X5	T50.8X6
Ramifenazone	T39.2X1	T39.2X2	T39.2X3	T39.2X4	T39.2X5	T39.2X6
Ramipril	T46.4X1	T46.4X2	T46.4X3	T46.4X4	T46.4X5	T46.4X6
Ranitidine	T47.0X1	T47.0X2	T47.0X3	T47.0X4	T47.0X5	T47.0X6
Ranunculus	T62.2X1	T62.2X2	T62.2X3	T62.2X4	—	—
Rat poison NEC	T60.4X1	T60.4X2	T60.4X3	T60.4X4	—	—
Rattlesnake (venom)	T63.011	T63.012	T63.013	T63.014	—	—
Raubasine	T46.7X1	T46.7X2	T46.7X3	T46.7X4	T46.7X5	T46.7X6
Raudixin	T46.5X1	T46.5X2	T46.5X3	T46.5X4	T46.5X5	T46.5X6
Rautensin	T46.5X1	T46.5X2	T46.5X3	T46.5X4	T46.5X5	T46.5X6
Rautina	T46.5X1	T46.5X2	T46.5X3	T46.5X4	T46.5X5	T46.5X6
Rautotal	T46.5X1	T46.5X2	T46.5X3	T46.5X4	T46.5X5	T46.5X6
Rauwiloid	T46.5X1	T46.5X2	T46.5X3	T46.5X4	T46.5X5	T46.5X6
Rauwoldin	T46.5X1	T46.5X2	T46.5X3	T46.5X4	T46.5X5	T46.5X6
Rauwolfia (alkaloids)	T46.5X1	T46.5X2	T46.5X3	T46.5X4	T46.5X5	T46.5X6
Razoxane	T45.1X1	T45.1X2	T45.1X3	T45.1X4	T45.1X5	T45.1X6
Realgar	T57.0X1	T57.0X2	T57.0X3	T57.0X4	—	—
Recombinant (R) — see specific protein						
Red blood cells, packed	T45.8X1	T45.8X2	T45.8X3	T45.8X4	T45.8X5	T45.8X6
Red squill (scilliroside)	T60.4X1	T60.4X2	T60.4X3	T60.4X4	—	—
Reducing agent, industrial NEC	T65.891	T65.892	T65.893	T65.894	—	—
Refrigerant gas (chlorofluorocarbon)	T53.5X1	T53.5X2	T53.5X3	T53.5X4	—	—
not chlorofluorocarbon	T59.891	T59.892	T59.893	T59.894	—	—
Regroton	T50.2X1	T50.2X2	T50.2X3	T50.2X4	T50.2X5	T50.2X6
Rehydration salts (oral)	T50.3X1	T50.3X2	T50.3X3	T50.3X4	T50.3X5	T50.3X6
Rela	T42.8X1	T42.8X2	T42.8X3	T42.8X4	T42.8X5	T42.8X6
Relaxant, muscle						
anesthetic	T48.1X1	T48.1X2	T48.1X3	T48.1X4	T48.1X5	T48.1X6
central nervous system	T42.8X1	T42.8X2	T42.8X3	T42.8X4	T42.8X5	T42.8X6
skeletal NEC	T48.1X1	T48.1X2	T48.1X3	T48.1X4	T48.1X5	T48.1X6
smooth NEC	T44.3X1	T44.3X2	T44.3X3	T44.3X4	T44.3X5	T44.3X6
Remoxipride	T43.591	T43.592	T43.593	T43.594	T43.595	T43.596
Renese	T50.2X1	T50.2X2	T50.2X3	T50.2X4	T50.2X5	T50.2X6
Renografin	T50.8X1	T50.8X2	T50.8X3	T50.8X4	T50.8X5	T50.8X6
Replacement solution	T50.3X1	T50.3X2	T50.3X3	T50.3X4	T50.3X5	T50.3X6
Reproterol	T48.6X1	T48.6X2	T48.6X3	T48.6X4	T48.6X5	T48.6X6
Rescinnamine	T46.5X1	T46.5X2	T46.5X3	T46.5X4	T46.5X5	T46.5X6
Reserpin (e)	T46.5X1	T46.5X2	T46.5X3	T46.5X4	T46.5X5	T46.5X6
Resorcin, resorcinol (nonmedicinal)	T65.891	T65.892	T65.893	T65.894	—	—
medicinal	T49.4X1	T49.4X2	T49.4X3	T49.4X4	T49.4X5	T49.4X6
Respaire	T48.4X1	T48.4X2	T48.4X3	T48.4X4	T48.4X5	T48.4X6
Respiratory drug NEC	T48.901	T48.902	T48.903	T48.904	T48.905	T48.906
antiasthmatic NEC	T48.6X1	T48.6X2	T48.6X3	T48.6X4	T48.6X5	T48.6X6
anti-common-cold NEC	T48.5X1	T48.5X2	T48.5X3	T48.5X4	T48.5X5	T48.5X6
expectorant NEC	T48.4X1	T48.4X2	T48.4X3	T48.4X4	T48.4X5	T48.4X6
stimulant	T48.901	T48.902	T48.903	T48.904	T48.905	T48.906
Retinoic acid	T49.0X1	T49.0X2	T49.0X3	T49.0X4	T49.0X5	T49.0X6
Retinol	T45.2X1	T45.2X2	T45.2X3	T45.2X4	T45.2X5	T45.2X6
Rh (D) immune globulin (human)	T50.Z11	T50.Z12	T50.Z13	T50.Z14	T50.Z15	T50.Z16
Rhodine	T39.011	T39.012	T39.013	T39.014	T39.015	T39.016
RhoGAM	T50.Z11	T50.Z12	T50.Z13	T50.Z14	T50.Z15	T50.Z16
Rhubarb						
dry extract	T47.2X1	T47.2X2	T47.2X3	T47.2X4	T47.2X5	T47.2X6
tincture, compound	T47.2X1	T47.2X2	T47.2X3	T47.2X4	T47.2X5	T47.2X6
Ribavirin	T37.5X1	T37.5X2	T37.5X3	T37.5X4	T37.5X5	T37.5X6
Riboflavin	T45.2X1	T45.2X2	T45.2X3	T45.2X4	T45.2X5	T45.2X6
Ribostamycin	T36.5X1	T36.5X2	T36.5X3	T36.5X4	T36.5X5	T36.5X6
Ricin	T62.2X1	T62.2X2	T62.2X3	T62.2X4	—	—
Ricinus communis	T62.2X1	T62.2X2	T62.2X3	T62.2X4	—	—
Rickettsial vaccine NEC	T50.A91	T50.A92	T50.A93	T50.A94	T50.A95	T50.A96
Rifabutin	T36.6X1	T36.6X2	T36.6X3	T36.6X4	T36.6X5	T36.6X6
Rifamide	T36.6X1	T36.6X2	T36.6X3	T36.6X4	T36.6X5	T36.6X6
Rifampicin	T36.6X1	T36.6X2	T36.6X3	T36.6X4	T36.6X5	T36.6X6
with isoniazid	T37.1X1	T37.1X2	T37.1X3	T37.1X4	T37.1X5	T37.1X6
Rifampin	T36.6X1	T36.6X2	T36.6X3	T36.6X4	T36.6X5	T36.6X6

Substance	Poisoning, Accidental (unintentional)	Poisoning, Intentional Self-harm	Poisoning, Assault	Poisoning, Undetermined	Adverse Effect	Under-dosing
Rifamycin	T36.6X1	T36.6X2	T36.6X3	T36.6X4	T36.6X5	T36.6X6
Rifaximin	T36.6X1	T36.6X2	T36.6X3	T36.6X4	T36.6X5	T36.6X6
Rimantadine	T37.5X1	T37.5X2	T37.5X3	T37.5X4	T37.5X5	T37.5X6
Rimazolium metilsulfate	T39.8X1	T39.8X2	T39.8X3	T39.8X4	T39.8X5	T39.8X6
Rimifon	T37.1X1	T37.1X2	T37.1X3	T37.1X4	T37.1X5	T37.1X6
Rimiterol	T48.6X1	T48.6X2	T48.6X3	T48.6X4	T48.6X5	T48.6X6
Ringer (lactate) **solution**	T50.3X1	T50.3X2	T50.3X3	T50.3X4	T50.3X5	T50.3X6
Ristocetin	T36.8X1	T36.8X2	T36.8X3	T36.8X4	T36.8X5	T36.8X6
Ritalin	T43.631	T43.632	T43.633	T43.634	T43.635	T43.636
Ritodrine	T44.5X1	T44.5X2	T44.5X3	T44.5X4	T44.5X5	T44.5X6
Roach killer — see Insecticide						
Rociverine	T44.3X1	T44.3X2	T44.3X3	T44.3X4	T44.3X5	T44.3X6
Rocky Mountain spotted fever vaccine	T50.A91	T50.A92	T50.A93	T50.A94	T50.A95	T50.A96
Rodenticide NEC	T60.4X1	T60.4X2	T60.4X3	T60.4X4	—	—
Rohypnol	T42.4X1	T42.4X2	T42.4X3	T42.4X4	T42.4X5	T42.4X6
Rokitamycin	T36.3X1	T36.3X2	T36.3X3	T36.3X4	T36.3X5	T36.3X6
Rolaids	T47.1X1	T47.1X2	T47.1X3	T47.1X4	T47.1X5	T47.1X6
Rolitetracycline	T36.4X1	T36.4X2	T36.4X3	T36.4X4	T36.4X5	T36.4X6
Romilar	T48.3X1	T48.3X2	T48.3X3	T48.3X4	T48.3X5	T48.3X6
Ronifibrate	T46.6X1	T46.6X2	T46.6X3	T46.6X4	T46.6X5	T46.6X6
Rosaprostol	T47.1X1	T47.1X2	T47.1X3	T47.1X4	T47.1X5	T47.1X6
Rose bengal sodium (131I)	T50.8X1	T50.8X2	T50.8X3	T50.8X4	T50.8X5	T50.8X6
Rose water ointment	T49.3X1	T49.3X2	T49.3X3	T49.3X4	T49.3X5	T49.3X6
Rosoxacin	T37.8X1	T37.8X2	T37.8X3	T37.8X4	T37.8X5	T37.8X6
Rotenone	T60.2X1	T60.2X2	T60.2X3	T60.2X4	—	—
Rotoxamine	T45.0X1	T45.0X2	T45.0X3	T45.0X4	T45.0X5	T45.0X6
Rough-on-rats	T60.4X1	T60.4X2	T60.4X3	T60.4X4	—	—
Roxatidine	T47.0X1	T47.0X2	T47.0X3	T47.0X4	T47.0X5	T47.0X6
Roxithromycin	T36.3X1	T36.3X2	T36.3X3	T36.3X4	T36.3X5	T36.3X6
Rt-PA	T45.611	T45.612	T45.613	T45.614	T45.615	T45.616
Rubbing alcohol	T51.2X1	T51.2X2	T51.2X3	T51.2X4	—	—
Rubefacient	T49.4X1	T49.4X2	T49.4X3	T49.4X4	T49.4X5	T49.4X6
Rubella vaccine	T50.B91	T50.B92	T50.B93	T50.B94	T50.B95	T50.B96
Rubeola vaccine	T50.B91	T50.B92	T50.B93	T50.B94	T50.B95	T50.B96
Rubidium chloride Rb82	T50.8X1	T50.8X2	T50.8X3	T50.8X4	T50.8X5	T50.8X6
Rubidomycin	T45.1X1	T45.1X2	T45.1X3	T45.1X4	T45.1X5	T45.1X6
Rue	T62.2X1	T62.2X2	T62.2X3	T62.2X4	—	—
Rufocromomycin	T45.1X1	T45.1X2	T45.1X3	T45.1X4	T45.1X5	T45.1X6
Russel's viper venin	T45.7X1	T45.7X2	T45.7X3	T45.7X4	T45.7X5	T45.7X6
Ruta (graveolens)	T62.2X1	T62.2X2	T62.2X3	T62.2X4	—	—
Rutinum	T46.991	T46.992	T46.993	T46.994	T46.995	T46.996
Rutoside	T46.991	T46.992	T46.993	T46.994	T46.995	T46.996
b-sitosterol(s)	T46.6X1	T46.6X2	T46.6X3	T46.6X4	T46.6X5	T46.6X6
Sabadilla (plant)	T62.2X1	T62.2X2	T62.2X3	T62.2X4	—	—
pesticide	T60.2X1	T60.2X2	T60.2X3	T60.2X4	—	—
Saccharated iron oxide	T45.8X1	T45.8X2	T45.8X3	T45.8X4	T45.8X5	T45.8X6
Saccharin	T50.901	T50.902	T50.903	T50.904	T50.905	T50.906
Saccharomyces boulardii	T47.6X1	T47.6X2	T47.6X3	T47.6X4	T47.6X5	T47.6X6
Safflower oil	T46.6X1	T46.6X2	T46.6X3	T46.6X4	T46.6X5	T46.6X6
Safrazine	T43.1X1	T43.1X2	T43.1X3	T43.1X4	T43.1X5	T43.1X6
Salazosulfapyridine	T37.0X1	T37.0X2	T37.0X3	T37.0X4	T37.0X5	T37.0X6
Salbutamol	T48.6X1	T48.6X2	T48.6X3	T48.6X4	T48.6X5	T48.6X6
Salicylamide	T39.091	T39.092	T39.093	T39.094	T39.095	T39.096
Salicylate NEC	T39.091	T39.092	T39.093	T39.094	T39.095	T39.096
methyl	T49.3X1	T49.3X2	T49.3X3	T49.3X4	T49.3X5	T49.3X6
theobromine calcium	T50.2X1	T50.2X2	T50.2X3	T50.2X4	T50.2X5	T50.2X6
Salicylazosulfapyridine	T37.0X1	T37.0X2	T37.0X3	T37.0X4	T37.0X5	T37.0X6
Salicylhydroxamic acid	T49.0X1	T49.0X2	T49.0X3	T49.0X4	T49.0X5	T49.0X6
Salicylic acid	T49.4X1	T49.4X2	T49.4X3	T49.4X4	T49.4X5	T49.4X6
with benzoic acid	T49.4X1	T49.4X2	T49.4X3	T49.4X4	T49.4X5	T49.4X6
congeners	T39.091	T39.092	T39.093	T39.094	T39.095	T39.096
derivative	T39.091	T39.092	T39.093	T39.094	T39.095	T39.096
salts	T39.091	T39.092	T39.093	T39.094	T39.095	T39.096
Salinazid	T37.1X1	T37.1X2	T37.1X3	T37.1X4	T37.1X5	T37.1X6
Salmeterol	T48.6X1	T48.6X2	T48.6X3	T48.6X4	T48.6X5	T48.6X6
Salol	T49.3X1	T49.3X2	T49.3X3	T49.3X4	T49.3X5	T49.3X6
Salsalate	T39.091	T39.092	T39.093	T39.094	T39.095	T39.096
Salt-replacing drug	T50.901	T50.902	T50.903	T50.904	T50.905	T50.906
Salt-retaining mineralocorticoid	T50.0X1	T50.0X2	T50.0X3	T50.0X4	T50.0X5	T50.0X6
Salt substitute	T50.901	T50.902	T50.903	T50.904	T50.905	T50.906
Saluretic NEC	T50.2X1	T50.2X2	T50.2X3	T50.2X4	T50.2X5	T50.2X6
Saluron	T50.2X1	T50.2X2	T50.2X3	T50.2X4	T50.2X5	T50.2X6
Salvarsan 606 (neosilver) (silver)	T37.8X1	T37.8X2	T37.8X3	T37.8X4	T37.8X5	T37.8X6
Sambucus canadensis	T62.2X1	T62.2X2	T62.2X3	T62.2X4	—	—
berry	T62.1X1	T62.1X2	T62.1X3	T62.1X4	—	—
Sandril	T46.5X1	T46.5X2	T46.5X3	T46.5X4	T46.5X5	T46.5X6
Sanguinaria canadensis	T62.2X1	T62.2X2	T62.2X3	T62.2X4	—	—
Saniflush (cleaner)	T54.2X1	T54.2X2	T54.2X3	T54.2X4	—	—
Santonin	T37.4X1	T37.4X2	T37.4X3	T37.4X4	T37.4X5	T37.4X6
Santyl	T49.8X1	T49.8X2	T49.8X3	T49.8X4	T49.8X5	T49.8X6

Substance	Poisoning, Accidental (unintentional)	Poisoning, Intentional Self-harm	Poisoning, Assault	Poisoning, Undetermined	Adverse Effect	Under-dosing
Saralasin	T46.5X1	T46.5X2	T46.5X3	T46.5X4	T46.5X5	T46.5X6
Sarcolysin	T45.1X1	T45.1X2	T45.1X3	T45.1X4	T45.1X5	T45.1X6
Sarkomycin	T45.1X1	T45.1X2	T45.1X3	T45.1X4	T45.1X5	T45.1X6
Saroten	T43.011	T43.012	T43.013	T43.014	T43.015	T43.016
Saturnine — see Lead						
Savin (oil)	T49.4X1	T49.4X2	T49.4X3	T49.4X4	T49.4X5	T49.4X6
Scammony	T47.2X1	T47.2X2	T47.2X3	T47.2X4	T47.2X5	T47.2X6
Scarlet red	T49.8X1	T49.8X2	T49.8X3	T49.8X4	T49.8X5	T49.8X6
Scheele's green	T57.0X1	T57.0X2	T57.0X3	T57.0X4	—	—
insecticide	T57.0X1	T57.0X2	T57.0X3	T57.0X4	—	—
Schizontozide (blood)	T37.2X1	T37.2X2	T37.2X3	T37.2X4	T37.2X5	T37.2X6
(tissue)						
Schradan	T60.0X1	T60.0X2	T60.0X3	T60.0X4	—	—
Schweinfurth green	T57.0X1	T57.0X2	T57.0X3	T57.0X4	—	—
insecticide	T57.0X1	T57.0X2	T57.0X3	T57.0X4	—	—
Scilla, rat poison	T60.4X1	T60.4X2	T60.4X3	T60.4X4	—	—
Scillaren	T60.4X1	T60.4X2	T60.4X3	T60.4X4	—	—
Sclerosing agent	T46.8X1	T46.8X2	T46.8X3	T46.8X4	T46.8X5	T46.8X6
Scombrotoxin	T61.11	T61.12	T61.13	T61.14	—	—
Scopolamine	T44.3X1	T44.3X2	T44.3X3	T44.3X4	T44.3X5	T44.3X6
Scopolia extract	T44.3X1	T44.3X2	T44.3X3	T44.3X4	T44.3X5	T44.3X6
Scouring powder	T65.891	T65.892	T65.893	T65.894	—	—
Sea						
anemone (sting)	T63.631	T63.632	T63.633	T63.634	—	—
cucumber (sting)	T63.691	T63.692	T63.693	T63.694	—	—
snake (bite) (venom)	T63.091	T63.092	T63.093	T63.094	—	—
urchin spine (puncture)	T63.691	T63.692	T63.693	T63.694	—	—
Seafood	T61.91	T61.92	T61.93	T61.94	—	—
specified NEC	T61.8X1	T61.8X2	T61.8X3	T61.8X4	—	—
Secbutabarbital	T42.3X1	T42.3X2	T42.3X3	T42.3X4	T42.3X5	T42.3X6
Secbutabarbitone	T42.3X1	T42.3X2	T42.3X3	T42.3X4	T42.3X5	T42.3X6
Secnidazole	T37.3X1	T37.3X2	T37.3X3	T37.3X4	T37.3X5	T37.3X6
Secobarbital	T42.3X1	T42.3X2	T42.3X3	T42.3X4	T42.3X5	T42.3X6
Seconal	T42.3X1	T42.3X2	T42.3X3	T42.3X4	T42.3X5	T42.3X6
Secretin	T50.8X1	T50.8X2	T50.8X3	T50.8X4	T50.8X5	T50.8X6
Sedative NEC	T42.71	T42.72	T42.73	T42.74	T42.75	T42.76
mixed NEC	T42.6X1	T42.6X2	T42.6X3	T42.6X4	T42.6X5	T42.6X6
Sedormid	T42.6X1	T42.6X2	T42.6X3	T42.6X4	T42.6X5	T42.6X6
Seed disinfectant or dressing	T60.8X1	T60.8X2	T60.8X3	T60.8X4	—	—
Seeds (poisonous)	T62.2X1	T62.2X2	T62.2X3	T62.2X4	—	—
Selegiline	T42.8X1	T42.8X2	T42.8X3	T42.8X4	T42.8X5	T42.8X6
Selenium NEC	T56.891	T56.892	T56.893	T56.894	—	—
disulfide or sulfide	T49.4X1	T49.4X2	T49.4X3	T49.4X4	T49.4X5	T49.4X6
fumes	T59.891	T59.892	T59.893	T59.894	—	—
sulfide	T49.4X1	T49.4X2	T49.4X3	T49.4X4	T49.4X5	T49.4X6
Selenomethionine (75Se)	T50.8X1	T50.8X2	T50.8X3	T50.8X4	T50.8X5	T50.8X6
Selsun	T49.4X1	T49.4X2	T49.4X3	T49.4X4	T49.4X5	T49.4X6
Semustine	T45.1X1	T45.1X2	T45.1X3	T45.1X4	T45.1X5	T45.1X6
Senega syrup	T48.4X1	T48.4X2	T48.4X3	T48.4X4	T48.4X5	T48.4X6
Senna	T47.2X1	T47.2X2	T47.2X3	T47.2X4	T47.2X5	T47.2X6
Sennoside A+B	T47.2X1	T47.2X2	T47.2X3	T47.2X4	T47.2X5	T47.2X6
Septisol	T49.2X1	T49.2X2	T49.2X3	T49.2X4	T49.2X5	T49.2X6
Seractide	T38.811	T38.812	T38.813	T38.814	T38.815	T38.816
Serax	T42.4X1	T42.4X2	T42.4X3	T42.4X4	T42.4X5	T42.4X6
Serenesil	T42.6X1	T42.6X2	T42.6X3	T42.6X4	T42.6X5	T42.6X6
Serenium (hydrochloride)	T37.91	T37.92	T37.93	T37.94	T37.95	T37.96
Serepax — see Oxazepam						
Sermorelin	T38.891	T38.892	T38.893	T38.894	T38.895	T38.896
Sernyl	T41.1X1	T41.1X2	T41.1X3	T41.1X4	T41.1X5	T41.1X6
Serotonin	T50.991	T50.992	T50.993	T50.994	T50.995	T50.996
Serpasil	T46.5X1	T46.5X2	T46.5X3	T46.5X4	T46.5X5	T46.5X6
Serrapeptase	T45.3X1	T45.3X2	T45.3X3	T45.3X4	T45.3X5	T45.3X6
Serum						
antibotulinus	T50.Z11	T50.Z12	T50.Z13	T50.Z14	T50.Z15	T50.Z16
anticytotoxic	T50.Z11	T50.Z12	T50.Z13	T50.Z14	T50.Z15	T50.Z16
antidiphtheria	T50.Z11	T50.Z12	T50.Z13	T50.Z14	T50.Z15	T50.Z16
antimeningococcus	T50.Z11	T50.Z12	T50.Z13	T50.Z14	T50.Z15	T50.Z16
anti-Rh	T50.Z11	T50.Z12	T50.Z13	T50.Z14	T50.Z15	T50.Z16
anti-snake-bite	T50.Z11	T50.Z12	T50.Z13	T50.Z14	T50.Z15	T50.Z16
antitetanic	T50.Z11	T50.Z12	T50.Z13	T50.Z14	T50.Z15	T50.Z16
antitoxic	T50.Z11	T50.Z12	T50.Z13	T50.Z14	T50.Z15	T50.Z16
complement (inhibitor)	T45.8X1	T45.8X2	T45.8X3	T45.8X4	T45.8X5	T45.8X6
convalescent	T50.Z11	T50.Z12	T50.Z13	T50.Z14	T50.Z15	T50.Z16
hemolytic complement	T45.8X1	T45.8X2	T45.8X3	T45.8X4	T45.8X5	T45.8X6
immune (human)	T50.Z11	T50.Z12	T50.Z13	T50.Z14	T50.Z15	T50.Z16
protective NEC	T50.Z11	T50.Z12	T50.Z13	T50.Z14	T50.Z15	T50.Z16
Setastine	T45.0X1	T45.0X2	T45.0X3	T45.0X4	T45.0X5	T45.0X6
Setoperone	T43.591	T43.592	T43.593	T43.594	T43.595	T43.596
Sewer gas	T59.91	T59.92	T59.93	T59.94	—	—
Shampoo	T55.0X1	T55.0X2	T55.0X3	T55.0X4	—	—
Shellfish, noxious, nonbacterial	T61.781	T61.782	T61.783	T61.784	—	—

Substance	Poisoning, Accidental (unintentional)	Poisoning, Intentional Self-harm	Poisoning, Assault	Poisoning, Undetermined	Adverse Effect	Under-dosing
Sildenafil	T46.7X1	T46.7X2	T46.7X3	T46.7X4	T46.7X5	T46.7X6
Silibinin	T50.991	T50.992	T50.993	T50.994	T50.995	T50.996
Silicone NEC	T65.891	T65.892	T65.893	T65.894	—	—
medicinal	T49.3X1	T49.3X2	T49.3X3	T49.3X4	T49.3X5	T49.3X6
Silvadene	T49.0X1	T49.0X2	T49.0X3	T49.0X4	T49.0X5	T49.0X6
Silver	T49.0X1	T49.0X2	T49.0X3	T49.0X4	T49.0X5	T49.0X6
anti-infectives	T49.0X1	T49.0X2	T49.0X3	T49.0X4	T49.0X5	T49.0X6
arsphenamine	T37.8X1	T37.8X2	T37.8X3	T37.8X4	T37.8X5	T37.8X6
colloidal	T49.0X1	T49.0X2	T49.0X3	T49.0X4	T49.0X5	T49.0X6
nitrate	T49.0X1	T49.0X2	T49.0X3	T49.0X4	T49.0X5	T49.0X6
ophthalmic preparation	T49.5X1	T49.5X2	T49.5X3	T49.5X4	T49.5X5	T49.5X6
toughened (keratolytic)	T49.4X1	T49.4X2	T49.4X3	T49.4X4	T49.4X5	T49.4X6
nonmedicinal (dust)	T56.891	T56.892	T56.893	T56.894	—	—
protein	T49.5X1	T49.5X2	T49.5X3	T49.5X4	T49.5X5	T49.5X6
salvarsan	T37.8X1	T37.8X2	T37.8X3	T37.8X4	T37.8X5	T37.8X6
sulfadiazine	T49.4X1	T49.4X2	T49.4X3	T49.4X4	T49.4X5	T49.4X6
Silymarin	T50.991	T50.992	T50.993	T50.994	T50.995	T50.996
Simaldrate	T47.1X1	T47.1X2	T47.1X3	T47.1X4	T47.1X5	T47.1X6
Simazine	T60.3X1	T60.3X2	T60.3X3	T60.3X4	—	—
Simethicone	T47.1X1	T47.1X2	T47.1X3	T47.1X4	T47.1X5	T47.1X6
Simfibrate	T46.6X1	T46.6X2	T46.6X3	T46.6X4	T46.6X5	T46.6X6
Simvastatin	T46.6X1	T46.6X2	T46.6X3	T46.6X4	T46.6X5	T46.6X6
Sincalide	T50.8X1	T50.8X2	T50.8X3	T50.8X4	T50.8X5	T50.8X6
Sinequan	T43.011	T43.012	T43.013	T43.014	T43.015	T43.016
Singoserp	T46.5X1	T46.5X2	T46.5X3	T46.5X4	T46.5X5	T46.5X6
Sintrom	T45.511	T45.512	T45.513	T45.514	T45.515	T45.516
Sisomicin	T36.5X1	T36.5X2	T36.5X3	T36.5X4	T36.5X5	T36.5X6
Sitosterols	T46.6X1	T46.6X2	T46.6X3	T46.6X4	T46.6X5	T46.6X6
Skeletal muscle relaxants	T48.1X1	T48.1X2	T48.1X3	T48.1X4	T48.1X5	T48.1X6
Skin						
agents (external)	T49.91	T49.92	T49.93	T49.94	T49.95	T49.96
specified NEC	T49.8X1	T49.8X2	T49.8X3	T49.8X4	T49.8X5	T49.8X6
test antigen	T50.8X1	T50.8X2	T50.8X3	T50.8X4	T50.8X5	T50.8X6
Sleep-eze	T45.0X1	T45.0X2	T45.0X3	T45.0X4	T45.0X5	T45.0X6
Sleeping draught, pill	T42.71	T42.72	T42.73	T42.74	T42.75	T42.76
Smallpox vaccine	T50.B11	T50.B12	T50.B13	T50.B14	T50.B15	T50.B16
Smelter fumes NEC	T56.91	T56.92	T56.93	T56.94	—	—
Smog	T59.1X1	T59.1X2	T59.1X3	T59.1X4	—	—
Smoke NEC	T59.811	T59.812	T59.813	T59.814	—	—
Smooth muscle relaxant	T44.3X1	T44.3X2	T44.3X3	T44.3X4	T44.3X5	T44.3X6
Snail killer NEC	T60.8X1	T60.8X2	T60.8X3	T60.8X4	—	—
Snake venom or bite	T63.001	T63.002	T63.003	T63.004	—	—
hemocoagulase	T45.7X1	T45.7X2	T45.7X3	T45.7X4	T45.7X5	T45.7X6
Snuff	T65.211	T65.212	T65.213	T65.214	—	—
Soap (powder) (product)	T55.0X1	T55.0X2	T55.0X3	T55.0X4	—	—
enema	T47.4X1	T47.4X2	T47.4X3	T47.4X4	T47.4X5	T47.4X6
medicinal, soft	T49.2X1	T49.2X2	T49.2X3	T49.2X4	T49.2X5	T49.2X6
superfatted	T49.2X1	T49.2X2	T49.2X3	T49.2X4	T49.2X5	T49.2X6
Sobrerol	T48.4X1	T48.4X2	T48.4X3	T48.4X4	T48.4X5	T48.4X6
Soda (caustic)	T54.3X1	T54.3X2	T54.3X3	T54.3X4	—	—
bicarb	T47.1X1	T47.1X2	T47.1X3	T47.1X4	T47.1X5	T47.1X6
chlorinated — see Sodium, hypochlorite						
Sodium						
acetosulfone	T37.1X1	T37.1X2	T37.1X3	T37.1X4	T37.1X5	T37.1X6
acetrizoate	T50.8X1	T50.8X2	T50.8X3	T50.8X4	T50.8X5	T50.8X6
acid phosphate	T50.3X1	T50.3X2	T50.3X3	T50.3X4	T50.3X5	T50.3X6
alginate	T47.8X1	T47.8X2	T47.8X3	T47.8X4	T47.8X5	T47.8X6
amidotrizoate	T50.8X1	T50.8X2	T50.8X3	T50.8X4	T50.8X5	T50.8X6
aminopterin	T45.1X1	T45.1X2	T45.1X3	T45.1X4	T45.1X5	T45.1X6
amylosulfate	T47.8X1	T47.8X2	T47.8X3	T47.8X4	T47.8X5	T47.8X6
amytal	T42.3X1	T42.3X2	T42.3X3	T42.3X4	T42.3X5	T42.3X6
antimony gluconate	T37.3X1	T37.3X2	T37.3X3	T37.3X4	T37.3X5	T37.3X6
arsenate	T57.0X1	T57.0X2	T57.0X3	T57.0X4	—	—
aurothiomalate	T39.4X1	T39.4X2	T39.4X3	T39.4X4	T39.4X5	T39.4X6
aurothiosulfate	T39.4X1	T39.4X2	T39.4X3	T39.4X4	T39.4X5	T39.4X6
barbiturate	T42.3X1	T42.3X2	T42.3X3	T42.3X4	T42.3X5	T42.3X6
basic phosphate	T47.4X1	T47.4X2	T47.4X3	T47.4X4	T47.4X5	T47.4X6
bicarbonate	T47.1X1	T47.1X2	T47.1X3	T47.1X4	T47.1X5	T47.1X6
bichromate	T57.8X1	T57.8X2	T57.8X3	T57.8X4	—	—
biphosphate	T50.3X1	T50.3X2	T50.3X3	T50.3X4	T50.3X5	T50.3X6
bisulfate	T65.891	T65.892	T65.893	T65.894	—	—
borate						
cleanser	T57.8X1	T57.8X2	T57.8X3	T57.8X4	—	—
eye	T49.5X1	T49.5X2	T49.5X3	T49.5X4	T49.5X5	T49.5X6
therapeutic	T49.8X1	T49.8X2	T49.8X3	T49.8X4	T49.8X5	T49.8X6
bromide	T42.6X1	T42.6X2	T42.6X3	T42.6X4	T42.6X5	T42.6X6
cacodylate (nonmedicinal) NEC	T50.8X1	T50.8X2	T50.8X3	T50.8X4	T50.8X5	T50.8X6
anti-infective	T37.8X1	T37.8X2	T37.8X3	T37.8X4	T37.8X5	T37.8X6
herbicide	T60.3X1	T60.3X2	T60.3X3	T60.3X4	—	—
calcium edetate	T45.8X1	T45.8X2	T45.8X3	T45.8X4	T45.8X5	T45.8X6
carbonate NEC	T54.3X1	T54.3X2	T54.3X3	T54.3X4	—	—
Sodium — continued						
chlorate NEC	T65.891	T65.892	T65.893	T65.894	—	—
herbicide	T54.91	T54.92	T54.93	T54.94	—	—
chloride	T50.3X1	T50.3X2	T50.3X3	T50.3X4	T50.3X5	T50.3X6
with glucose	T50.3X1	T50.3X2	T50.3X3	T50.3X4	T50.3X5	T50.3X6
chromate	T65.891	T65.892	T65.893	T65.894	—	—
citrate	T50.991	T50.992	T50.993	T50.994	T50.995	T50.996
cromoglicate	T48.6X1	T48.6X2	T48.6X3	T48.6X4	T48.6X5	T48.6X6
cyanide	T65.0X1	T65.0X2	T65.0X3	T65.0X4	—	—
cyclamate	T50.3X1	T50.3X2	T50.3X3	T50.3X4	T50.3X5	T50.3X6
dehydrocholate	T45.8X1	T45.8X2	T45.8X3	T45.8X4	T45.8X5	T45.8X6
diatrizoate	T50.8X1	T50.8X2	T50.8X3	T50.8X4	T50.8X5	T50.8X6
dibunate	T48.4X1	T48.4X2	T48.4X3	T48.4X4	T48.4X5	T48.4X6
dioctyl sulfosuccinate	T47.4X1	T47.4X2	T47.4X3	T47.4X4	T47.4X5	T47.4X6
dipantoyl ferrate	T45.8X1	T45.8X2	T45.8X3	T45.8X4	T45.8X5	T45.8X6
edetate	T45.8X1	T45.8X2	T45.8X3	T45.8X4	T45.8X5	T45.8X6
ethacrynate	T50.1X1	T50.1X2	T50.1X3	T50.1X4	T50.1X5	T50.1X6
feredetate	T45.8X1	T45.8X2	T45.8X3	T45.8X4	T45.8X5	T45.8X6
Fluoride — see Fluoride						
fluoroacetate (dust) (pesticide)	T60.4X1	T60.4X2	T60.4X3	T60.4X4	—	—
free salt	T50.3X1	T50.3X2	T50.3X3	T50.3X4	T50.3X5	T50.3X6
fusidate	T36.8X1	T36.8X2	T36.8X3	T36.8X4	T36.8X5	T36.8X6
glucaldrate	T47.1X1	T47.1X2	T47.1X3	T47.1X4	T47.1X5	T47.1X6
glucosulfone	T37.1X1	T37.1X2	T37.1X3	T37.1X4	T37.1X5	T37.1X6
glutamate	T45.8X1	T45.8X2	T45.8X3	T45.8X4	T45.8X5	T45.8X6
hydrogen carbonate	T50.3X1	T50.3X2	T50.3X3	T50.3X4	T50.3X5	T50.3X6
hydroxide	T54.3X1	T54.3X2	T54.3X3	T54.3X4	—	—
hypochlorite (bleach) NEC	T54.3X1	T54.3X2	T54.3X3	T54.3X4	—	—
disinfectant	T54.3X1	T54.3X2	T54.3X3	T54.3X4	—	—
medicinal (anti-infective) (external)	T49.0X1	T49.0X2	T49.0X3	T49.0X4	T49.0X5	T49.0X6
vapor	T54.3X1	T54.3X2	T54.3X3	T54.3X4	—	—
hyposulfite	T49.0X1	T49.0X2	T49.0X3	T49.0X4	T49.0X5	T49.0X6
indigotin disulfonate	T50.8X1	T50.8X2	T50.8X3	T50.8X4	T50.8X5	T50.8X6
iodide	T50.991	T50.992	T50.993	T50.994	T50.995	T50.996
I-131	T50.8X1	T50.8X2	T50.8X3	T50.8X4	T50.8X5	T50.8X6
therapeutic	T38.2X1	T38.2X2	T38.2X3	T38.2X4	T38.2X5	T38.2X6
iodohippurate (131I)	T50.8X1	T50.8X2	T50.8X3	T50.8X4	T50.8X5	T50.8X6
iopodate	T50.8X1	T50.8X2	T50.8X3	T50.8X4	T50.8X5	T50.8X6
iothalamate	T50.8X1	T50.8X2	T50.8X3	T50.8X4	T50.8X5	T50.8X6
iron edetate	T45.4X1	T45.4X2	T45.4X3	T45.4X4	T45.4X5	T45.4X6
lactate (compound solution)	T45.8X1	T45.8X2	T45.8X3	T45.8X4	T45.8X5	T45.8X6
lauryl (sulfate)	T49.2X1	T49.2X2	T49.2X3	T49.2X4	T49.2X5	T49.2X6
L-triiodothyronine	T38.1X1	T38.1X2	T38.1X3	T38.1X4	T38.1X5	T38.1X6
magnesium citrate	T50.991	T50.992	T50.993	T50.994	T50.995	T50.996
mersalate	T50.2X1	T50.2X2	T50.2X3	T50.2X4	T50.2X5	T50.2X6
metasilicate	T65.891	T65.892	T65.893	T65.894	—	—
metrizoate	T50.8X1	T50.8X2	T50.8X3	T50.8X4	T50.8X5	T50.8X6
monofluoroacetate (pesticide)	T60.1X1	T60.1X2	T60.1X3	T60.1X4	—	—
morrhuate	T46.8X1	T46.8X2	T46.8X3	T46.8X4	T46.8X5	T46.8X6
nafcillin	T36.0X1	T36.0X2	T36.0X3	T36.0X4	T36.0X5	T36.0X6
nitrate (oxidizing agent)	T65.891	T65.892	T65.893	T65.894	—	—
nitrite	T50.6X1	T50.6X2	T50.6X3	T50.6X4	T50.6X5	T50.6X6
nitroferricyanide	T46.5X1	T46.5X2	T46.5X3	T46.5X4	T46.5X5	T46.5X6
nitroprusside	T46.5X1	T46.5X2	T46.5X3	T46.5X4	T46.5X5	T46.5X6
oxalate	T65.891	T65.892	T65.893	T65.894	—	—
oxide/peroxide	T65.891	T65.892	T65.893	T65.894	—	—
oxybate	T41.291	T41.292	T41.293	T41.294	T41.295	T41.296
para-aminohippurate	T50.8X1	T50.8X2	T50.8X3	T50.8X4	T50.8X5	T50.8X6
perborate (nonmedicinal) NEC	T65.891	T65.892	T65.893	T65.894	—	—
medicinal	T49.0X1	T49.0X2	T49.0X3	T49.0X4	T49.0X5	T49.0X6
soap	T55.0X1	T55.0X2	T55.0X3	T55.0X4	—	—
percarbonate — see Sodium, perborate						
pertechnetate Tc99m	T50.8X1	T50.8X2	T50.8X3	T50.8X4	T50.8X5	T50.8X6
phosphate						
cellulose	T45.8X1	T45.8X2	T45.8X3	T45.8X4	T45.8X5	T45.8X6
dibasic	T47.2X1	T47.2X2	T47.2X3	T47.2X4	T47.2X5	T47.2X6
monobasic	T47.2X1	T47.2X2	T47.2X3	T47.2X4	T47.2X5	T47.2X6
phytate	T50.6X1	T50.6X2	T50.6X3	T50.6X4	T50.6X5	T50.6X6
picosulfate	T47.2X1	T47.2X2	T47.2X3	T47.2X4	T47.2X5	T47.2X6
polyhydroxyaluminium monocarbonate	T47.1X1	T47.1X2	T47.1X3	T47.1X4	T47.1X5	T47.1X6
polystyrene sulfonate	T50.3X1	T50.3X2	T50.3X3	T50.3X4	T50.3X5	T50.3X6
propionate	T49.0X1	T49.0X2	T49.0X3	T49.0X4	T49.0X5	T49.0X6
propyl hydroxybenzoate	T50.991	T50.992	T50.993	T50.994	T50.995	T50.996
psylliate	T46.8X1	T46.8X2	T46.8X3	T46.8X4	T46.8X5	T46.8X6
removing resins	T50.3X1	T50.3X2	T50.3X3	T50.3X4	T50.3X5	T50.3X6
salicylate	T39.091	T39.092	T39.093	T39.094	T39.095	T39.096

▽ Subterms under main terms may continue to next column or page　　Additional Character May Be Required — Refer to the Tabular List for Character Selection　　389

Sildenafil — Sodium

Table of Drugs and Chemicals — Sodium — Strychnine

Substance	Poisoning, Accidental (unintentional)	Poisoning, Intentional Self-harm	Poisoning, Assault	Poisoning, Undetermined	Adverse Effect	Under-dosing
Sodium — continued						
salt NEC	T50.3X1	T50.3X2	T50.3X3	T50.3X4	T50.3X5	T50.3X6
selenate	T60.2X1	T60.2X2	T60.2X3	T60.2X4	—	—
stibogluconate	T37.3X1	T37.3X2	T37.3X3	T37.3X4	T37.3X5	T37.3X6
sulfate	T47.4X1	T47.4X2	T47.4X3	T47.4X4	T47.4X5	T47.4X6
sulfoxone	T37.1X1	T37.1X2	T37.1X3	T37.1X4	T37.1X5	T37.1X6
tetradecyl sulfate	T46.8X1	T46.8X2	T46.8X3	T46.8X4	T46.8X5	T46.8X6
thiopental	T41.1X1	T41.1X2	T41.1X3	T41.1X4	T41.1X5	T41.1X6
thiosalicylate	T39.091	T39.092	T39.093	T39.094	T39.095	T39.096
thiosulfate	T50.6X1	T50.6X2	T50.6X3	T50.6X4	T50.6X5	T50.6X6
tolbutamide	T38.3X1	T38.3X2	T38.3X3	T38.3X4	T38.3X5	T38.3X6
(L)-triiodothyronine	T38.1X1	T38.1X2	T38.1X3	T38.1X4	T38.1X5	T38.1X6
tyropanoate	T50.8X1	T50.8X2	T50.8X3	T50.8X4	T50.8X5	T50.8X6
valproate	T42.6X1	T42.6X2	T42.6X3	T42.6X4	T42.6X5	T42.6X6
versenate	T50.6X1	T50.6X2	T50.6X3	T50.6X4	T50.6X5	T50.6X6
Sodium-free salt	T50.901	T50.902	T50.903	T50.904	T50.905	T50.906
Sodium-removing resin	T50.3X1	T50.3X2	T50.3X3	T50.3X4	T50.3X5	T50.3X6
Soft soap	T55.0X1	T55.0X2	T55.0X3	T55.0X4	—	—
Solanine	T62.2X1	T62.2X2	T62.2X3	T62.2X4	—	—
berries	T62.1X1	T62.1X2	T62.1X3	T62.1X4	—	—
Solanum dulcamara	T62.2X1	T62.2X2	T62.2X3	T62.2X4	—	—
berries	T62.1X1	T62.1X2	T62.1X3	T62.1X4	—	—
Solapsone	T37.1X1	T37.1X2	T37.1X3	T37.1X4	T37.1X5	T37.1X6
Solar lotion	T49.3X1	T49.3X2	T49.3X3	T49.3X4	T49.3X5	T49.3X6
Solasulfone	T37.1X1	T37.1X2	T37.1X3	T37.1X4	T37.1X5	T37.1X6
Soldering fluid	T65.891	T65.892	T65.893	T65.894	—	—
Solid substance	T65.91	T65.92	T65.93	T65.94	—	—
specified NEC	T65.891	T65.892	T65.893	T65.894	—	—
Solvent, industrial NEC	T52.91	T52.92	T52.93	T52.94	—	—
naphtha	T52.0X1	T52.0X2	T52.0X3	T52.0X4	—	—
petroleum	T52.0X1	T52.0X2	T52.0X3	T52.0X4	—	—
specified NEC	T52.8X1	T52.8X2	T52.8X3	T52.8X4	—	—
Soma	T42.8X1	T42.8X2	T42.8X3	T42.8X4	T42.8X5	T42.8X6
Somatorelin	T38.891	T38.892	T38.893	T38.894	T38.895	T38.896
Somatostatin	T38.991	T38.992	T38.993	T38.994	T38.995	T38.996
Somatotropin	T38.811	T38.812	T38.813	T38.814	T38.815	T38.816
Somatrem	T38.811	T38.812	T38.813	T38.814	T38.815	T38.816
Somatropin	T38.811	T38.812	T38.813	T38.814	T38.815	T38.816
Sominex	T45.0X1	T45.0X2	T45.0X3	T45.0X4	T45.0X5	T45.0X6
Somnos	T42.6X1	T42.6X2	T42.6X3	T42.6X4	T42.6X5	T42.6X6
Somonal	T42.3X1	T42.3X2	T42.3X3	T42.3X4	T42.3X5	T42.3X6
Soneryl	T42.3X1	T42.3X2	T42.3X3	T42.3X4	T42.3X5	T42.3X6
Soothing syrup	T50.901	T50.902	T50.903	T50.904	T50.905	T50.906
Sopor	T42.6X1	T42.6X2	T42.6X3	T42.6X4	T42.6X5	T42.6X6
Soporific	T42.71	T42.72	T42.73	T42.74	T42.75	T42.76
Soporific drug	T42.71	T42.72	T42.73	T42.74	T42.75	T42.76
specified type NEC	T42.6X1	T42.6X2	T42.6X3	T42.6X4	T42.6X5	T42.6X6
Sorbide nitrate	T46.3X1	T46.3X2	T46.3X3	T46.3X4	T46.3X5	T46.3X6
Sorbitol	T47.4X1	T47.4X2	T47.4X3	T47.4X4	T47.4X5	T47.4X6
Sotalol	T44.7X1	T44.7X2	T44.7X3	T44.7X4	T44.7X5	T44.7X6
Sotradecol	T46.8X1	T46.8X2	T46.8X3	T46.8X4	T46.8X5	T46.8X6
Soysterol	T46.6X1	T46.6X2	T46.6X3	T46.6X4	T46.6X5	T46.6X6
Spacoline	T44.3X1	T44.3X2	T44.3X3	T44.3X4	T44.3X5	T44.3X6
Spanish fly	T49.8X1	T49.8X2	T49.8X3	T49.8X4	T49.8X5	T49.8X6
Sparine	T43.3X1	T43.3X2	T43.3X3	T43.3X4	T43.3X5	T43.3X6
Sparteine	T48.0X1	T48.0X2	T48.0X3	T48.0X4	T48.0X5	T48.0X6
Spasmolytic						
anticholinergics	T44.3X1	T44.3X2	T44.3X3	T44.3X4	T44.3X5	T44.3X6
autonomic	T44.3X1	T44.3X2	T44.3X3	T44.3X4	T44.3X5	T44.3X6
bronchial NEC	T48.6X1	T48.6X2	T48.6X3	T48.6X4	T48.6X5	T48.6X6
quaternary ammonium	T44.3X1	T44.3X2	T44.3X3	T44.3X4	T44.3X5	T44.3X6
skeletal muscle NEC	T48.1X1	T48.1X2	T48.1X3	T48.1X4	T48.1X5	T48.1X6
Spectinomycin	T36.5X1	T36.5X2	T36.5X3	T36.5X4	T36.5X5	T36.5X6
Speed	T43.621	T43.622	T43.623	T43.624	T43.625	T43.626
Spermicide	T49.8X1	T49.8X2	T49.8X3	T49.8X4	T49.8X5	T49.8X6
Spider (bite) (venom)	T63.391	T63.392	T63.393	T63.394	—	—
antivenin	T50.Z11	T50.Z12	T50.Z13	T50.Z14	T50.Z15	T50.Z16
Spigelia (root)	T37.4X1	T37.4X2	T37.4X3	T37.4X4	T37.4X5	T37.4X6
Spindle inactivator	T50.4X1	T50.4X2	T50.4X3	T50.4X4	T50.4X5	T50.4X6
Spiperone	T43.4X1	T43.4X2	T43.4X3	T43.4X4	T43.4X5	T43.4X6
Spiramycin	T36.3X1	T36.3X2	T36.3X3	T36.3X4	T36.3X5	T36.3X6
Spirapril	T46.4X1	T46.4X2	T46.4X3	T46.4X4	T46.4X5	T46.4X6
Spirilene	T43.591	T43.592	T43.593	T43.594	T43.595	T43.596
Spirit(s) (neutral) NEC	T51.0X1	T51.0X2	T51.0X3	T51.0X4	—	—
beverage	T51.0X1	T51.0X2	T51.0X3	T51.0X4	—	—
industrial	T51.0X1	T51.0X2	T51.0X3	T51.0X4	—	—
mineral	T52.0X1	T52.0X2	T52.0X3	T52.0X4	—	—
of salt — see Hydrochloric acid						
surgical	T51.0X1	T51.0X2	T51.0X3	T51.0X4	—	—
Spironolactone	T50.0X1	T50.0X2	T50.0X3	T50.0X4	T50.0X5	T50.0X6
Spiroperidol	T43.4X1	T43.4X2	T43.4X3	T43.4X4	T43.4X5	T43.4X6
Sponge, absorbable (gelatin)	T45.7X1	T45.7X2	T45.7X3	T45.7X4	T45.7X5	T45.7X6
Sporostacin	T49.0X1	T49.0X2	T49.0X3	T49.0X4	T49.0X5	T49.0X6
Spray (aerosol)	T65.91	T65.92	T65.93	T65.94	—	—
cosmetic	T65.891	T65.892	T65.893	T65.894	—	—
medicinal NEC	T50.901	T50.902	T50.903	T50.904	T50.905	T50.906
pesticides — see Pesticides						
specified content — see specific substance						
Spurge flax	T62.2X1	T62.2X2	T62.2X3	T62.2X4	—	—
Spurges	T62.2X1	T62.2X2	T62.2X3	T62.2X4	—	—
Sputum viscosity-lowering drug	T48.4X1	T48.4X2	T48.4X3	T48.4X4	T48.4X5	T48.4X6
Squill	T46.0X1	T46.0X2	T46.0X3	T46.0X4	T46.0X5	T46.0X6
rat poison	T60.4X1	T60.4X2	T60.4X3	T60.4X4	—	—
Squirting cucumber (cathartic)	T47.2X1	T47.2X2	T47.2X3	T47.2X4	T47.2X5	T47.2X6
Stains	T65.6X1	T65.6X2	T65.6X3	T65.6X4	—	—
Stannous fluoride	T49.7X1	T49.7X2	T49.7X3	T49.7X4	T49.7X5	T49.7X6
Stanolone	T38.7X1	T38.7X2	T38.7X3	T38.7X4	T38.7X5	T38.7X6
Stanozolol	T38.7X1	T38.7X2	T38.7X3	T38.7X4	T38.7X5	T38.7X6
Staphisagria or stavesacre (pediculicide)	T49.0X1	T49.0X2	T49.0X3	T49.0X4	T49.0X5	T49.0X6
Starch	T50.901	T50.902	T50.903	T50.904	T50.905	T50.906
Stelazine	T43.3X1	T43.3X2	T43.3X3	T43.3X4	T43.3X5	T43.3X6
Stemetil	T43.3X1	T43.3X2	T43.3X3	T43.3X4	T43.3X5	T43.3X6
Stepronin	T48.4X1	T48.4X2	T48.4X3	T48.4X4	T48.4X5	T48.4X6
Sterculia	T47.4X1	T47.4X2	T47.4X3	T47.4X4	T47.4X5	T47.4X6
Sternutator gas	T59.891	T59.892	T59.893	T59.894	—	—
Steroid	T38.0X1	T38.0X2	T38.0X3	T38.0X4	T38.0X5	T38.0X6
anabolic	T38.7X1	T38.7X2	T38.7X3	T38.7X4	T38.7X5	T38.7X6
androgenic	T38.7X1	T38.7X2	T38.7X3	T38.7X4	T38.7X5	T38.7X6
antineoplastic, hormone	T38.7X1	T38.7X2	T38.7X3	T38.7X4	T38.7X5	T38.7X6
estrogen	T38.5X1	T38.5X2	T38.5X3	T38.5X4	T38.5X5	T38.5X6
ENT agent	T49.6X1	T49.6X2	T49.6X3	T49.6X4	T49.6X5	T49.6X6
ophthalmic preparation	T49.5X1	T49.5X2	T49.5X3	T49.5X4	T49.5X5	T49.5X6
topical NEC	T49.0X1	T49.0X2	T49.0X3	T49.0X4	T49.0X5	T49.0X6
Stibine	T56.891	T56.892	T56.893	T56.894	—	—
Stibogluconate	T37.3X1	T37.3X2	T37.3X3	T37.3X4	T37.3X5	T37.3X6
Stibophen	T37.4X1	T37.4X2	T37.4X3	T37.4X4	T37.4X5	T37.4X6
Stilbamidine (isetionate)	T37.3X1	T37.3X2	T37.3X3	T37.3X4	T37.3X5	T37.3X6
Stilbestrol	T38.5X1	T38.5X2	T38.5X3	T38.5X4	T38.5X5	T38.5X6
Stilboestrol	T38.5X1	T38.5X2	T38.5X3	T38.5X4	T38.5X5	T38.5X6
Stimulant						
central nervous system — see also Psychostimulant	T43.601	T43.602	T43.603	T43.604	T43.605	T43.606
analeptics	T50.7X1	T50.7X2	T50.7X3	T50.7X4	T50.7X5	T50.7X6
opiate antagonist	T50.7X1	T50.7X2	T50.7X3	T50.7X4	T50.7X5	T50.7X6
psychotherapeutic NEC — see also Psychotherapeutic drug	T43.601	T43.602	T43.603	T43.604	T43.605	T43.606
specified NEC	T43.691	T43.692	T43.693	T43.694	T43.695	T43.696
respiratory	T48.901	T48.902	T48.903	T48.904	T48.905	T48.906
Stone-dissolving drug	T50.901	T50.902	T50.903	T50.904	T50.905	T50.906
Storage battery (cells) (acid)	T54.2X1	T54.2X2	T54.2X3	T54.2X4	—	—
Stovaine	T41.3X1	T41.3X2	T41.3X3	T41.3X4	T41.3X5	T41.3X6
infiltration (subcutaneous)	T41.3X1	T41.3X2	T41.3X3	T41.3X4	T41.3X5	T41.3X6
nerve block (peripheral) (plexus)	T41.3X1	T41.3X2	T41.3X3	T41.3X4	T41.3X5	T41.3X6
spinal	T41.3X1	T41.3X2	T41.3X3	T41.3X4	T41.3X5	T41.3X6
topical (surface)	T41.3X1	T41.3X2	T41.3X3	T41.3X4	T41.3X5	T41.3X6
Stovarsal	T37.8X1	T37.8X2	T37.8X3	T37.8X4	T37.8X5	T37.8X6
Stove gas — see Gas, stove						
Stoxil	T49.5X1	T49.5X2	T49.5X3	T49.5X4	T49.5X5	T49.5X6
Stramonium	T48.6X1	T48.6X2	T48.6X3	T48.6X4	T48.6X5	T48.6X6
natural state	T62.2X1	T62.2X2	T62.2X3	T62.2X4	—	—
Streptodornase	T45.3X1	T45.3X2	T45.3X3	T45.3X4	T45.3X5	T45.3X6
Streptoduocin	T36.5X1	T36.5X2	T36.5X3	T36.5X4	T36.5X5	T36.5X6
Streptokinase	T45.611	T45.612	T45.613	T45.614	T45.615	T45.616
Streptomycin (derivative)	T36.5X1	T36.5X2	T36.5X3	T36.5X4	T36.5X5	T36.5X6
Streptonivicin	T36.5X1	T36.5X2	T36.5X3	T36.5X4	T36.5X5	T36.5X6
Streptovarycin	T36.5X1	T36.5X2	T36.5X3	T36.5X4	T36.5X5	T36.5X6
Streptozocin	T45.1X1	T45.1X2	T45.1X3	T45.1X4	T45.1X5	T45.1X6
Streptozotocin	T45.1X1	T45.1X2	T45.1X3	T45.1X4	T45.1X5	T45.1X6
Stripper (paint) (solvent)	T52.8X1	T52.8X2	T52.8X3	T52.8X4	—	—
Strobane	T60.1X1	T60.1X2	T60.1X3	T60.1X4	—	—
Strofantina	T46.0X1	T46.0X2	T46.0X3	T46.0X4	T46.0X5	T46.0X6
Strophanthin (g) (k)	T46.0X1	T46.0X2	T46.0X3	T46.0X4	T46.0X5	T46.0X6
Strophanthus	T46.0X1	T46.0X2	T46.0X3	T46.0X4	T46.0X5	T46.0X6
Strophanthin	T46.0X1	T46.0X2	T46.0X3	T46.0X4	T46.0X5	T46.0X6
Strophantin-g	T46.0X1	T46.0X2	T46.0X3	T46.0X4	T46.0X5	T46.0X6
Strychnine (nonmedicinal) (pesticide) (salts)	T65.1X1	T65.1X2	T65.1X3	T65.1X4	—	—
medicinal	T48.291	T48.292	T48.293	T48.294	T48.295	T48.296

Additional Character May Be Required — Refer to the Tabular List for Character Selection   ▽ Subterms under main terms may continue to next column or page

Substance	Poisoning, Accidental (unintentional)	Poisoning, Intentional Self-harm	Poisoning, Assault	Poisoning, Undetermined	Adverse Effect	Under-dosing
Strychnos (ignatii) — see Strychnine						
Styramate	T42.8X1	T42.8X2	T42.8X3	T42.8X4	T42.8X5	T42.8X6
Styrene	T65.891	T65.892	T65.893	T65.894	—	—
Succinimide, antiepileptic or anticonvulsant	T42.2X1	T42.2X2	T42.2X3	T42.2X4	T42.2X5	T42.2X6
mercuric — see Mercury						
Succinylcholine	T48.1X1	T48.1X2	T48.1X3	T48.1X4	T48.1X5	T48.1X6
Succinylsulfathiazole	T37.0X1	T37.0X2	T37.0X3	T37.0X4	T37.0X5	T37.0X6
Sucralfate	T47.1X1	T47.1X2	T47.1X3	T47.1X4	T47.1X5	T47.1X6
Sucrose	T50.3X1	T50.3X2	T50.3X3	T50.3X4	T50.3X5	T50.3X6
Sufentanil	T40.4X1	T40.4X2	T40.4X3	T40.4X4	T40.4X5	T40.4X6
Sulbactam	T36.0X1	T36.0X2	T36.0X3	T36.0X4	T36.0X5	T36.0X6
Sulbenicillin	T36.0X1	T36.0X2	T36.0X3	T36.0X4	T36.0X5	T36.0X6
Sulbentine	T49.0X1	T49.0X2	T49.0X3	T49.0X4	T49.0X5	T49.0X6
Sulfacetamide	T49.0X1	T49.0X2	T49.0X3	T49.0X4	T49.0X5	T49.0X6
ophthalmic preparation	T49.5X1	T49.5X2	T49.5X3	T49.5X4	T49.5X5	T49.5X6
Sulfachlorpyridazine	T37.0X1	T37.0X2	T37.0X3	T37.0X4	T37.0X5	T37.0X6
Sulfacitine	T37.0X1	T37.0X2	T37.0X3	T37.0X4	T37.0X5	T37.0X6
Sulfadiasulfone sodium	T37.0X1	T37.0X2	T37.0X3	T37.0X4	T37.0X5	T37.0X6
Sulfadiazine	T37.0X1	T37.0X2	T37.0X3	T37.0X4	T37.0X5	T37.0X6
silver (topical)	T49.0X1	T49.0X2	T49.0X3	T49.0X4	T49.0X5	T49.0X6
Sulfadimethoxine	T37.0X1	T37.0X2	T37.0X3	T37.0X4	T37.0X5	T37.0X6
Sulfadimidine	T37.0X1	T37.0X2	T37.0X3	T37.0X4	T37.0X5	T37.0X6
Sulfadoxine	T37.0X1	T37.0X2	T37.0X3	T37.0X4	T37.0X5	T37.0X6
with pyrimethamine	T37.2X1	T37.2X2	T37.2X3	T37.2X4	T37.2X5	T37.2X6
Sulfaethidole	T37.0X1	T37.0X2	T37.0X3	T37.0X4	T37.0X5	T37.0X6
Sulfafurazole	T37.0X1	T37.0X2	T37.0X3	T37.0X4	T37.0X5	T37.0X6
Sulfaguanidine	T37.0X1	T37.0X2	T37.0X3	T37.0X4	T37.0X5	T37.0X6
Sulfalene	T37.0X1	T37.0X2	T37.0X3	T37.0X4	T37.0X5	T37.0X6
Sulfaloxate	T37.0X1	T37.0X2	T37.0X3	T37.0X4	T37.0X5	T37.0X6
Sulfaloxic acid	T37.0X1	T37.0X2	T37.0X3	T37.0X4	T37.0X5	T37.0X6
Sulfamazone	T39.2X1	T39.2X2	T39.2X3	T39.2X4	T39.2X5	T39.2X6
Sulfamerazine	T37.0X1	T37.0X2	T37.0X3	T37.0X4	T37.0X5	T37.0X6
Sulfameter	T37.0X1	T37.0X2	T37.0X3	T37.0X4	T37.0X5	T37.0X6
Sulfamethazine	T37.0X1	T37.0X2	T37.0X3	T37.0X4	T37.0X5	T37.0X6
Sulfamethizole	T37.0X1	T37.0X2	T37.0X3	T37.0X4	T37.0X5	T37.0X6
Sulfamethoxazole	T37.0X1	T37.0X2	T37.0X3	T37.0X4	T37.0X5	T37.0X6
with trimethoprim	T36.8X1	T36.8X2	T36.8X3	T36.8X4	T36.8X5	T36.8X6
Sulfamethoxydiazine	T37.0X1	T37.0X2	T37.0X3	T37.0X4	T37.0X5	T37.0X6
Sulfamethoxypyridazine	T37.0X1	T37.0X2	T37.0X3	T37.0X4	T37.0X5	T37.0X6
Sulfamethylthiazole	T37.0X1	T37.0X2	T37.0X3	T37.0X4	T37.0X5	T37.0X6
Sulfametoxydiazine	T37.0X1	T37.0X2	T37.0X3	T37.0X4	T37.0X5	T37.0X6
Sulfamidopyrine	T39.2X1	T39.2X2	T39.2X3	T39.2X4	T39.2X5	T39.2X6
Sulfamonomethoxine	T37.0X1	T37.0X2	T37.0X3	T37.0X4	T37.0X5	T37.0X6
Sulfamoxole	T37.0X1	T37.0X2	T37.0X3	T37.0X4	T37.0X5	T37.0X6
Sulfamylon	T49.0X1	T49.0X2	T49.0X3	T49.0X4	T49.0X5	T49.0X6
Sulfan blue (diagnostic dye)	T50.8X1	T50.8X2	T50.8X3	T50.8X4	T50.8X5	T50.8X6
Sulfanilamide	T37.0X1	T37.0X2	T37.0X3	T37.0X4	T37.0X5	T37.0X6
Sulfanilylguanidine	T37.0X1	T37.0X2	T37.0X3	T37.0X4	T37.0X5	T37.0X6
Sulfaperin	T37.0X1	T37.0X2	T37.0X3	T37.0X4	T37.0X5	T37.0X6
Sulfaphenazole	T37.0X1	T37.0X2	T37.0X3	T37.0X4	T37.0X5	T37.0X6
Sulfaphenylthiazole	T37.0X1	T37.0X2	T37.0X3	T37.0X4	T37.0X5	T37.0X6
Sulfaproxyline	T37.0X1	T37.0X2	T37.0X3	T37.0X4	T37.0X5	T37.0X6
Sulfapyridine	T37.0X1	T37.0X2	T37.0X3	T37.0X4	T37.0X5	T37.0X6
Sulfapyrimidine	T37.0X1	T37.0X2	T37.0X3	T37.0X4	T37.0X5	T37.0X6
Sulfarsphenamine	T37.8X1	T37.8X2	T37.8X3	T37.8X4	T37.8X5	T37.8X6
Sulfasalazine	T37.0X1	T37.0X2	T37.0X3	T37.0X4	T37.0X5	T37.0X6
Sulfasuxidine	T37.0X1	T37.0X2	T37.0X3	T37.0X4	T37.0X5	T37.0X6
Sulfasymazine	T37.0X1	T37.0X2	T37.0X3	T37.0X4	T37.0X5	T37.0X6
Sulfated amylopectin	T47.8X1	T47.8X2	T47.8X3	T47.8X4	T47.8X5	T47.8X6
Sulfathiazole	T37.0X1	T37.0X2	T37.0X3	T37.0X4	T37.0X5	T37.0X6
Sulfatostearate	T49.2X1	T49.2X2	T49.2X3	T49.2X4	T49.2X5	T49.2X6
Sulfinpyrazone	T50.4X1	T50.4X2	T50.4X3	T50.4X4	T50.4X5	T50.4X6
Sulfiram	T49.0X1	T49.0X2	T49.0X3	T49.0X4	T49.0X5	T49.0X6
Sulfisomidine	T37.0X1	T37.0X2	T37.0X3	T37.0X4	T37.0X5	T37.0X6
Sulfisoxazole	T37.0X1	T37.0X2	T37.0X3	T37.0X4	T37.0X5	T37.0X6
ophthalmic preparation	T49.5X1	T49.5X2	T49.5X3	T49.5X4	T49.5X5	T49.5X6
Sulfobromophthalein (sodium)	T50.8X1	T50.8X2	T50.8X3	T50.8X4	T50.8X5	T50.8X6
Sulfobromphthalein	T50.8X1	T50.8X2	T50.8X3	T50.8X4	T50.8X5	T50.8X6
Sulfogaiacol	T48.4X1	T48.4X2	T48.4X3	T48.4X4	T48.4X5	T48.4X6
Sulfomyxin	T36.8X1	T36.8X2	T36.8X3	T36.8X4	T36.8X5	T36.8X6
Sulfonal	T42.6X1	T42.6X2	T42.6X3	T42.6X4	T42.6X5	T42.6X6
Sulfonamide NEC	T37.0X1	T37.0X2	T37.0X3	T37.0X4	T37.0X5	T37.0X6
eye	T49.5X1	T49.5X2	T49.5X3	T49.5X4	T49.5X5	T49.5X6
Sulfonazide	T37.1X1	T37.1X2	T37.1X3	T37.1X4	T37.1X5	T37.1X6
Sulfones	T37.1X1	T37.1X2	T37.1X3	T37.1X4	T37.1X5	T37.1X6
Sulfonethylmethane	T42.6X1	T42.6X2	T42.6X3	T42.6X4	T42.6X5	T42.6X6
Sulfonmethane	T42.6X1	T42.6X2	T42.6X3	T42.6X4	T42.6X5	T42.6X6
Sulfonphthal, sulfonphthol	T50.8X1	T50.8X2	T50.8X3	T50.8X4	T50.8X5	T50.8X6

Substance	Poisoning, Accidental (unintentional)	Poisoning, Intentional Self-harm	Poisoning, Assault	Poisoning, Undetermined	Adverse Effect	Under-dosing
Sulfonylurea derivatives, oral	T38.3X1	T38.3X2	T38.3X3	T38.3X4	T38.3X5	T38.3X6
Sulforidazine	T43.3X1	T43.3X2	T43.3X3	T43.3X4	T43.3X5	T43.3X6
Sulfoxone	T37.1X1	T37.1X2	T37.1X3	T37.1X4	T37.1X5	T37.1X6
Sulfuric acid	T54.2X1	T54.2X2	T54.2X3	T54.2X4	—	—
Sulfur, sulfurated, sulfuric, sulfurous, sulfuryl (compounds NEC) (medicinal)	T49.4X1	T49.4X2	T49.4X3	T49.4X4	T49.4X5	T49.4X6
acid	T54.2X1	T54.2X2	T54.2X3	T54.2X4	—	—
dioxide (gas)	T59.1X1	T59.1X2	T59.1X3	T59.1X4	—	—
ether — see Ether(s)						
hydrogen	T59.6X1	T59.6X2	T59.6X3	T59.6X4	—	—
medicinal (keratolytic) (ointment) NEC	T49.4X1	T49.4X2	T49.4X3	T49.4X4	T49.4X5	T49.4X6
ointment	T49.0X1	T49.0X2	T49.0X3	T49.0X4	T49.0X5	T49.0X6
pesticide (vapor)	T60.91	T60.92	T60.93	T60.94	—	—
vapor NEC	T59.891	T59.892	T59.893	T59.894	—	—
Sulglicotide	T47.1X1	T47.1X2	T47.1X3	T47.1X4	T47.1X5	T47.1X6
Sulindac	T39.391	T39.392	T39.393	T39.394	T39.395	T39.396
Sulisatin	T47.2X1	T47.2X2	T47.2X3	T47.2X4	T47.2X5	T47.2X6
Sulisobenzone	T49.3X1	T49.3X2	T49.3X3	T49.3X4	T49.3X5	T49.3X6
Sulkowitch's reagent	T50.8X1	T50.8X2	T50.8X3	T50.8X4	T50.8X5	T50.8X6
Sulmetozine	T44.3X1	T44.3X2	T44.3X3	T44.3X4	T44.3X5	T44.3X6
Suloctidil	T46.7X1	T46.7X2	T46.7X3	T46.7X4	T46.7X5	T46.7X6
Sulph- — see also Sulf-						
Sulphadiazine	T37.0X1	T37.0X2	T37.0X3	T37.0X4	T37.0X5	T37.0X6
Sulphadimethoxine	T37.0X1	T37.0X2	T37.0X3	T37.0X4	T37.0X5	T37.0X6
Sulphadimidine	T37.0X1	T37.0X2	T37.0X3	T37.0X4	T37.0X5	T37.0X6
Sulphadione	T37.1X1	T37.1X2	T37.1X3	T37.1X4	T37.1X5	T37.1X6
Sulphafurazole	T37.0X1	T37.0X2	T37.0X3	T37.0X4	T37.0X5	T37.0X6
Sulphamethizole	T37.0X1	T37.0X2	T37.0X3	T37.0X4	T37.0X5	T37.0X6
Sulphamethoxazole	T37.0X1	T37.0X2	T37.0X3	T37.0X4	T37.0X5	T37.0X6
Sulphan blue	T50.8X1	T50.8X2	T50.8X3	T50.8X4	T50.8X5	T50.8X6
Sulphaphenazole	T37.0X1	T37.0X2	T37.0X3	T37.0X4	T37.0X5	T37.0X6
Sulphapyridine	T37.0X1	T37.0X2	T37.0X3	T37.0X4	T37.0X5	T37.0X6
Sulphasalazine	T37.0X1	T37.0X2	T37.0X3	T37.0X4	T37.0X5	T37.0X6
Sulphinpyrazone	T50.4X1	T50.4X2	T50.4X3	T50.4X4	T50.4X5	T50.4X6
Sulpiride	T43.591	T43.592	T43.593	T43.594	T43.595	T43.596
Sulprostone	T48.0X1	T48.0X2	T48.0X3	T48.0X4	T48.0X5	T48.0X6
Sulpyrine	T39.2X1	T39.2X2	T39.2X3	T39.2X4	T39.2X5	T39.2X6
Sultamicillin	T36.0X1	T36.0X2	T36.0X3	T36.0X4	T36.0X5	T36.0X6
Sulthiame	T42.6X1	T42.6X2	T42.6X3	T42.6X4	T42.6X5	T42.6X6
Sultiame	T42.6X1	T42.6X2	T42.6X3	T42.6X4	T42.6X5	T42.6X6
Sultopride	T43.591	T43.592	T43.593	T43.594	T43.595	T43.596
Sumatriptan	T39.8X1	T39.8X2	T39.8X3	T39.8X4	T39.8X5	T39.8X6
Sunflower seed oil	T46.6X1	T46.6X2	T46.6X3	T46.6X4	T46.6X5	T46.6X6
Superinone	T48.4X1	T48.4X2	T48.4X3	T48.4X4	T48.4X5	T48.4X6
Suprofen	T39.311	T39.312	T39.313	T39.314	T39.315	T39.316
Suramin (sodium)	T37.4X1	T37.4X2	T37.4X3	T37.4X4	T37.4X5	T37.4X6
Surfacaine	T41.3X1	T41.3X2	T41.3X3	T41.3X4	T41.3X5	T41.3X6
Surital	T41.1X1	T41.1X2	T41.1X3	T41.1X4	T41.1X5	T41.1X6
Sutilains	T45.3X1	T45.3X2	T45.3X3	T45.3X4	T45.3X5	T45.3X6
Suxamethonium (chloride)	T48.1X1	T48.1X2	T48.1X3	T48.1X4	T48.1X5	T48.1X6
Suxethonium (chloride)	T48.1X1	T48.1X2	T48.1X3	T48.1X4	T48.1X5	T48.1X6
Suxibuzone	T39.2X1	T39.2X2	T39.2X3	T39.2X4	T39.2X5	T39.2X6
Sweetener	T50.901	T50.902	T50.903	T50.904	T50.905	T50.906
Sweet niter spirit	T46.3X1	T46.3X2	T46.3X3	T46.3X4	T46.3X5	T46.3X6
Sweet oil (birch)	T49.3X1	T49.3X2	T49.3X3	T49.3X4	T49.3X5	T49.3X6
Sym-dichloroethyl ether	T53.6X1	T53.6X2	T53.6X3	T53.6X4	—	—
Sympatholytic NEC	T44.8X1	T44.8X2	T44.8X3	T44.8X4	T44.8X5	T44.8X6
haloalkylamine	T44.8X1	T44.8X2	T44.8X3	T44.8X4	T44.8X5	T44.8X6
Sympathomimetic NEC	T44.901	T44.902	T44.903	T44.904	T44.905	T44.906
anti-common-cold	T48.5X1	T48.5X2	T48.5X3	T48.5X4	T48.5X5	T48.5X6
bronchodilator	T48.6X1	T48.6X2	T48.6X3	T48.6X4	T48.6X5	T48.6X6
specified NEC	T44.991	T44.992	T44.993	T44.994	T44.995	T44.996
Synagis	T50.B91	T50.B92	T50.B93	T50.B94	T50.B95	T50.B96
Synalar	T49.0X1	T49.0X2	T49.0X3	T49.0X4	T49.0X5	T49.0X6
Synthroid	T38.1X1	T38.1X2	T38.1X3	T38.1X4	T38.1X5	T38.1X6
Syntocinon	T48.0X1	T48.0X2	T48.0X3	T48.0X4	T48.0X5	T48.0X6
Syrosingopine	T46.5X1	T46.5X2	T46.5X3	T46.5X4	T46.5X5	T46.5X6
Systemic drug	T45.91	T45.92	T45.93	T45.94	T45.95	T45.96
specified NEC	T45.8X1	T45.8X2	T45.8X3	T45.8X4	T45.8X5	T45.8X6
Tablets — see also specified substance	T50.901	T50.902	T50.903	T50.904	T50.905	T50.906
Tace	T38.5X1	T38.5X2	T38.5X3	T38.5X4	T38.5X5	T38.5X6
Tacrine	T44.0X1	T44.0X2	T44.0X3	T44.0X4	T44.0X5	T44.0X6
Tadalafil	T46.7X1	T46.7X2	T46.7X3	T46.7X4	T46.7X5	T46.7X6
Talampicillin	T36.0X1	T36.0X2	T36.0X3	T36.0X4	T36.0X5	T36.0X6
Talbutal	T42.3X1	T42.3X2	T42.3X3	T42.3X4	T42.3X5	T42.3X6
Talc powder	T49.3X1	T49.3X2	T49.3X3	T49.3X4	T49.3X5	T49.3X6
Talcum	T49.3X1	T49.3X2	T49.3X3	T49.3X4	T49.3X5	T49.3X6
Taleranol	T38.6X1	T38.6X2	T38.6X3	T38.6X4	T38.6X5	T38.6X6

Substance	Poisoning, Accidental (unintentional)	Poisoning, Intentional Self-harm	Poisoning, Assault	Poisoning, Undetermined	Adverse Effect	Under-dosing
Tamoxifen	T38.6X1	T38.6X2	T38.6X3	T38.6X4	T38.6X5	T38.6X6
Tamsulosin	T44.6X1	T44.6X2	T44.6X3	T44.6X4	T44.6X5	T44.6X6
Tandearil, tanderil	T39.2X1	T39.2X2	T39.2X3	T39.2X4	T39.2X5	T39.2X6
Tannic acid	T49.2X1	T49.2X2	T49.2X3	T49.2X4	T49.2X5	T49.2X6
medicinal (astringent)	T49.2X1	T49.2X2	T49.2X3	T49.2X4	T49.2X5	T49.2X6
Tannin — *see* Tannic acid						
Tansy	T62.2X1	T62.2X2	T62.2X3	T62.2X4	—	—
TAO	T36.3X1	T36.3X2	T36.3X3	T36.3X4	T36.3X5	T36.3X6
Tapazole	T38.2X1	T38.2X2	T38.2X3	T38.2X4	T38.2X5	T38.2X6
Taractan	T43.591	T43.592	T43.593	T43.594	T43.595	T43.596
Tarantula (venomous)	T63.321	T63.322	T63.323	T63.324	—	—
Tartar emetic	T37.8X1	T37.8X2	T37.8X3	T37.8X4	T37.8X5	T37.8X6
Tartaric acid	T65.891	T65.892	T65.893	T65.894	—	—
Tartrated antimony (anti-infective)	T37.8X1	T37.8X2	T37.8X3	T37.8X4	T37.8X5	T37.8X6
Tartrate, laxative	T47.4X1	T47.4X2	T47.4X3	T47.4X4	T47.4X5	T47.4X6
Tar NEC	T52.0X1	T52.0X2	T52.0X3	T52.0X4	—	—
camphor	T60.1X1	T60.1X2	T60.1X3	T60.1X4	—	—
distillate	T49.1X1	T49.1X2	T49.1X3	T49.1X4	T49.1X5	T49.1X6
fumes	T59.891	T59.892	T59.893	T59.894	—	—
medicinal	T49.1X1	T49.1X2	T49.1X3	T49.1X4	T49.1X5	T49.1X6
ointment	T49.1X1	T49.1X2	T49.1X3	T49.1X4	T49.1X5	T49.1X6
Tauromustine	T45.1X1	T45.1X2	T45.1X3	T45.1X4	T45.1X5	T45.1X6
TCA — *see* Trichloroacetic acid						
TCDD	T53.7X1	T53.7X2	T53.7X3	T53.7X4	—	—
TDI (vapor)	T65.0X1	T65.0X2	T65.0X3	T65.0X4	—	—
Tear						
gas	T59.3X1	T59.3X2	T59.3X3	T59.3X4	—	—
solution	T49.5X1	T49.5X2	T49.5X3	T49.5X4	T49.5X5	T49.5X6
Teclothiazide	T50.2X1	T50.2X2	T50.2X3	T50.2X4	T50.2X5	T50.2X6
Teclozan	T37.3X1	T37.3X2	T37.3X3	T37.3X4	T37.3X5	T37.3X6
Tegafur	T45.1X1	T45.1X2	T45.1X3	T45.1X4	T45.1X5	T45.1X6
Tegretol	T42.1X1	T42.1X2	T42.1X3	T42.1X4	T42.1X5	T42.1X6
Teicoplanin	T36.8X1	T36.8X2	T36.8X3	T36.8X4	T36.8X5	T36.8X6
Telepaque	T50.8X1	T50.8X2	T50.8X3	T50.8X4	T50.8X5	T50.8X6
Tellurium	T56.891	T56.892	T56.893	T56.894	—	—
fumes	T56.891	T56.892	T56.893	T56.894	—	—
TEM	T45.1X1	T45.1X2	T45.1X3	T45.1X4	T45.1X5	T45.1X6
Temazepam	T42.4X1	T42.4X2	T42.4X3	T42.4X4	T42.4X5	T42.4X6
Temocillin	T36.0X1	T36.0X2	T36.0X3	T36.0X4	T36.0X5	T36.0X6
Tenamfetamine	T43.621	T43.622	T43.623	T43.624	T43.625	T43.626
Teniposide	T45.1X1	T45.1X2	T45.1X3	T45.1X4	T45.1X5	T45.1X6
Tenitramine	T46.3X1	T46.3X2	T46.3X3	T46.3X4	T46.3X5	T46.3X6
Tenoglicin	T48.4X1	T48.4X2	T48.4X3	T48.4X4	T48.4X5	T48.4X6
Tenonitrozole	T37.3X1	T37.3X2	T37.3X3	T37.3X4	T37.3X5	T37.3X6
Tenoxicam	T39.391	T39.392	T39.393	T39.394	T39.395	T39.396
TEPA	T45.1X1	T45.1X2	T45.1X3	T45.1X4	T45.1X5	T45.1X6
TEPP	T60.0X1	T60.0X2	T60.0X3	T60.0X4	—	—
Teprotide	T46.5X1	T46.5X2	T46.5X3	T46.5X4	T46.5X5	T46.5X6
Terazosin	T44.6X1	T44.6X2	T44.6X3	T44.6X4	T44.6X5	T44.6X6
Terbufos	T60.0X1	T60.0X2	T60.0X3	T60.0X4	—	—
Terbutaline	T48.6X1	T48.6X2	T48.6X3	T48.6X4	T48.6X5	T48.6X6
Terconazole	T49.0X1	T49.0X2	T49.0X3	T49.0X4	T49.0X5	T49.0X6
Terfenadine	T45.0X1	T45.0X2	T45.0X3	T45.0X4	T45.0X5	T45.0X6
Teriparatide (acetate)	T50.991	T50.992	T50.993	T50.994	T50.995	T50.996
Terizidone	T37.1X1	T37.1X2	T37.1X3	T37.1X4	T37.1X5	T37.1X6
Terlipressin	T38.891	T38.892	T38.893	T38.894	T38.895	T38.896
Terodiline	T46.3X1	T46.3X2	T46.3X3	T46.3X4	T46.3X5	T46.3X6
Teroxalene	T37.4X1	T37.4X2	T37.4X3	T37.4X4	T37.4X5	T37.4X6
Terpin (cis) **hydrate**	T48.4X1	T48.4X2	T48.4X3	T48.4X4	T48.4X5	T48.4X6
Terramycin	T36.4X1	T36.4X2	T36.4X3	T36.4X4	T36.4X5	T36.4X6
Tertatolol	T44.7X1	T44.7X2	T44.7X3	T44.7X4	T44.7X5	T44.7X6
Tessalon	T48.3X1	T48.3X2	T48.3X3	T48.3X4		T48.3X6
Testolactone	T38.7X1	T38.7X2	T38.7X3	T38.7X4	T38.7X5	T38.7X6
Testosterone	T38.7X1	T38.7X2	T38.7X3	T38.7X4	T38.7X5	T38.7X6
Tetanus toxoid or vaccine	T50.A91	T50.A92	T50.A93	T50.A94	T50.A95	T50.A96
antitoxin	T50.Z11	T50.Z12	T50.Z13	T50.Z14	T50.Z15	T50.Z16
immune globulin (human)	T50.Z11	T50.Z12	T50.Z13	T50.Z14	T50.Z15	T50.Z16
toxoid	T50.A91	T50.A92	T50.A93	T50.A94	T50.A95	T50.A96
with diphtheria toxoid	T50.A21	T50.A22	T50.A23	T50.A24	T50.A25	T50.A26
with pertussis	T50.A11	T50.A12	T50.A13	T50.A14	T50.A15	T50.A16
Tetrabenazine	T43.591	T43.592	T43.593	T43.594	T43.595	T43.596
Tetracaine	T41.3X1	T41.3X2	T41.3X3	T41.3X4	T41.3X5	T41.3X6
nerve block (peripheral) (plexus)	T41.3X1	T41.3X2	T41.3X3	T41.3X4	T41.3X5	T41.3X6
regional	T41.3X1	T41.3X2	T41.3X3	T41.3X4	T41.3X5	T41.3X6
spinal	T41.3X1	T41.3X2	T41.3X3	T41.3X4	T41.3X5	T41.3X6
Tetrachlorethylene — *see* Tetrachloroethylene						
Tetrachlormethiazide	T50.2X1	T50.2X2	T50.2X3	T50.2X4	T50.2X5	T50.2X6
Tetrachloroethane	T53.6X1	T53.6X2	T53.6X3	T53.6X4	—	—
vapor	T53.6X1	T53.6X2	T53.6X3	T53.6X4	—	—
paint or varnish	T53.6X1	T53.6X2	T53.6X3	T53.6X4	—	—

Substance	Poisoning, Accidental (unintentional)	Poisoning, Intentional Self-harm	Poisoning, Assault	Poisoning, Undetermined	Adverse Effect	Under-dosing
Tetrachloroethylene (liquid)	T53.3X1	T53.3X2	T53.3X3	T53.3X4	—	—
medicinal	T37.4X1	T37.4X2	T37.4X3	T37.4X4	T37.4X5	T37.4X6
vapor	T53.3X1	T53.3X2	T53.3X3	T53.3X4	—	—
Tetrachloromethane — *see* Carbon tetrachloride						
Tetracosactide	T38.811	T38.812	T38.813	T38.814	T38.815	T38.816
Tetracosactrin	T38.811	T38.812	T38.813	T38.814	T38.815	T38.816
Tetracycline	T36.4X1	T36.4X2	T36.4X3	T36.4X4	T36.4X5	T36.4X6
ophthalmic preparation	T49.5X1	T49.5X2	T49.5X3	T49.5X4	T49.5X5	T49.5X6
topical NEC	T49.0X1	T49.0X2	T49.0X3	T49.0X4	T49.0X5	T49.0X6
Tetradifon	T60.8X1	T60.8X2	T60.8X3	T60.8X4	—	—
Tetradotoxin	T61.771	T61.772	T61.773	T61.774	—	—
Tetraethyl						
lead	T56.0X1	T56.0X2	T56.0X3	T56.0X4	—	—
pyrophosphate	T60.0X1	T60.0X2	T60.0X3	T60.0X4	—	—
Tetraethylammonium chloride	T44.2X1	T44.2X2	T44.2X3	T44.2X4	T44.2X5	T44.2X6
Tetraethylthiuram disulfide	T50.6X1	T50.6X2	T50.6X3	T50.6X4	T50.6X5	T50.6X6
Tetrahydroaminoacridine	T44.0X1	T44.0X2	T44.0X3	T44.0X4	T44.0X5	T44.0X6
Tetrahydrocannabinol	T40.7X1	T40.7X2	T40.7X3	T40.7X4	T40.7X5	T40.7X6
Tetrahydrofuran	T52.8X1	T52.8X2	T52.8X3	T52.8X4	—	—
Tetrahydronaphthalene	T52.8X1	T52.8X2	T52.8X3	T52.8X4	—	—
Tetrahydrozoline	T49.5X1	T49.5X2	T49.5X3	T49.5X4	T49.5X5	T49.5X6
Tetralin	T52.8X1	T52.8X2	T52.8X3	T52.8X4	—	—
Tetramethrin	T60.2X1	T60.2X2	T60.2X3	T60.2X4	—	—
Tetramethylthiuram (disulfide) **NEC**	T60.3X1	T60.3X2	T60.3X3	T60.3X4	—	—
medicinal	T49.0X1	T49.0X2	T49.0X3	T49.0X4	T49.0X5	T49.0X6
Tetramisole	T37.4X1	T37.4X2	T37.4X3	T37.4X4	T37.4X5	T37.4X6
Tetranicotinoyl fructose	T46.7X1	T46.7X2	T46.7X3	T46.7X4	T46.7X5	T46.7X6
Tetrazepam	T42.4X1	T42.4X2	T42.4X3	T42.4X4	T42.4X5	T42.4X6
Tetronal	T42.6X1	T42.6X2	T42.6X3	T42.6X4	T42.6X5	T42.6X6
Tetryl	T65.3X1	T65.3X2	T65.3X3	T65.3X4	—	—
Tetrylammonium chloride	T44.2X1	T44.2X2	T44.2X3	T44.2X4	T44.2X5	T44.2X6
Tetryzoline	T49.5X1	T49.5X2	T49.5X3	T49.5X4	T49.5X5	T49.5X6
Thalidomide	T45.1X1	T45.1X2	T45.1X3	T45.1X4	—	T45.1X6
Thallium (compounds) (dust)	T56.811	T56.812	T56.813	T56.814	—	—
NEC						
pesticide	T60.4X1	T60.4X2	T60.4X3	T60.4X4	—	—
THC	T40.7X1	T40.7X2	T40.7X3	T40.7X4	T40.7X5	T40.7X6
Thebacon	T48.3X1	T48.3X2	T48.3X3	T48.3X4	T48.3X5	T48.3X6
Thebaine	T40.2X1	T40.2X2	T40.2X3	T40.2X4	T40.2X5	T40.2X6
Thenoic acid	T49.6X1	T49.6X2	T49.6X3	T49.6X4	T49.6X5	T49.6X6
Thenyldiamine	T45.0X1	T45.0X2	T45.0X3	T45.0X4	T45.0X5	T45.0X6
Theobromine (calcium salicylate)	T48.6X1	T48.6X2	T48.6X3	T48.6X4	T48.6X5	T48.6X6
sodium salicylate	T48.6X1	T48.6X2	T48.6X3	T48.6X4	T48.6X5	T48.6X6
Theophyllamine	T48.6X1	T48.6X2	T48.6X3	T48.6X4	T48.6X5	T48.6X6
Theophylline	T48.6X1	T48.6X2	T48.6X3	T48.6X4	T48.6X5	T48.6X6
aminobenzoic acid	T48.6X1	T48.6X2	T48.6X3	T48.6X4	T48.6X5	T48.6X6
ethylenediamine	T48.6X1	T48.6X2	T48.6X3	T48.6X4	T48.6X5	T48.6X6
piperazine	T48.6X1	T48.6X2	T48.6X3	T48.6X4	T48.6X5	T48.6X6
p-amino-benzoate						
Thiabendazole	T37.4X1	T37.4X2	T37.4X3	T37.4X4	T37.4X5	T37.4X6
Thialbarbital	T41.1X1	T41.1X2	T41.1X3	T41.1X4	T41.1X5	T41.1X6
Thiamazole	T38.2X1	T38.2X2	T38.2X3	T38.2X4	T38.2X5	T38.2X6
Thiambutosine	T37.1X1	T37.1X2	T37.1X3	T37.1X4	T37.1X5	T37.1X6
Thiamine	T45.2X1	T45.2X2	T45.2X3	T45.2X4	T45.2X5	T45.2X6
Thiamphenicol	T36.2X1	T36.2X2	T36.2X3	T36.2X4	T36.2X5	T36.2X6
Thiamylal	T41.1X1	T41.1X2	T41.1X3	T41.1X4	T41.1X5	T41.1X6
sodium	T41.1X1	T41.1X2	T41.1X3	T41.1X4	T41.1X5	T41.1X6
Thiazesim	T43.291	T43.292	T43.293	T43.294	T43.295	T43.296
Thiazides (diuretics)	T50.2X1	T50.2X2	T50.2X3	T50.2X4	T50.2X5	T50.2X6
Thiazinamium metilsulfate	T43.3X1	T43.3X2	T43.3X3	T43.3X4	T43.3X5	T43.3X6
Thiethylperazine	T43.3X1	T43.3X2	T43.3X3	T43.3X4	T43.3X5	T43.3X6
Thimerosal	T49.0X1	T49.0X2	T49.0X3	T49.0X4	T49.0X5	T49.0X6
ophthalmic preparation	T49.5X1	T49.5X2	T49.5X3	T49.5X4	T49.5X5	T49.5X6
Thioacetazone	T37.1X1	T37.1X2	T37.1X3	T37.1X4	T37.1X5	T37.1X6
with isoniazid	T37.1X1	T37.1X2	T37.1X3	T37.1X4	T37.1X5	T37.1X6
Thiobarbital sodium	T41.1X1	T41.1X2	T41.1X3	T41.1X4	T41.1X5	T41.1X6
Thiobarbiturate anesthetic	T41.1X1	T41.1X2	T41.1X3	T41.1X4	T41.1X5	T41.1X6
Thiobismol	T37.8X1	T37.8X2	T37.8X3	T37.8X4	T37.8X5	T37.8X6
Thiobutabarbital sodium	T41.1X1	T41.1X2	T41.1X3	T41.1X4	T41.1X5	T41.1X6
Thiocarbamate (insecticide)	T60.0X1	T60.0X2	T60.0X3	T60.0X4	—	—
Thiocarbamide	T38.2X1	T38.2X2	T38.2X3	T38.2X4	T38.2X5	T38.2X6
Thiocarbarsone	T37.8X1	T37.8X2	T37.8X3	T37.8X4	T37.8X5	T37.8X6
Thiocarlide	T37.1X1	T37.1X2	T37.1X3	T37.1X4	T37.1X5	T37.1X6
Thioctamide	T50.991	T50.992	T50.993	T50.994	T50.995	T50.996

Substance	Poisoning, Accidental (unintentional)	Poisoning, Intentional Self-harm	Poisoning, Assault	Poisoning, Undetermined	Adverse Effect	Under-dosing
Thioctic acid	T50.991	T50.992	T50.993	T50.994	T50.995	T50.996
Thiofos	T60.0X1	T60.0X2	T60.0X3	T60.0X4	—	—
Thioglycolate	T49.4X1	T49.4X2	T49.4X3	T49.4X4	T49.4X5	T49.4X6
Thioglycolic acid	T65.891	T65.892	T65.893	T65.894	—	—
Thioguanine	T45.1X1	T45.1X2	T45.1X3	T45.1X4	T45.1X5	T45.1X6
Thiomercaptomerin	T50.2X1	T50.2X2	T50.2X3	T50.2X4	T50.2X5	T50.2X6
Thiomerin	T50.2X1	T50.2X2	T50.2X3	T50.2X4	T50.2X5	T50.2X6
Thiomersal	T49.0X1	T49.0X2	T49.0X3	T49.0X4	T49.0X5	T49.0X6
Thionazin	T60.0X1	T60.0X2	T60.0X3	T60.0X4	—	—
Thiopental (sodium)	T41.1X1	T41.1X2	T41.1X3	T41.1X4	T41.1X5	T41.1X6
Thiopentone (sodium)	T41.1X1	T41.1X2	T41.1X3	T41.1X4	T41.1X5	T41.1X6
Thiopropazate	T43.3X1	T43.3X2	T43.3X3	T43.3X4	T43.3X5	T43.3X6
Thioproperazine	T43.3X1	T43.3X2	T43.3X3	T43.3X4	T43.3X5	T43.3X6
Thioridazine	T43.3X1	T43.3X2	T43.3X3	T43.3X4	T43.3X5	T43.3X6
Thiosinamine	T49.3X1	T49.3X2	T49.3X3	T49.3X4	T49.3X5	T49.3X6
Thiotepa	T45.1X1	T45.1X2	T45.1X3	T45.1X4	T45.1X5	T45.1X6
Thiothixene	T43.4X1	T43.4X2	T43.4X3	T43.4X4	T43.4X5	T43.4X6
Thiouracil (benzyl) (methyl) (propyl)	T38.2X1	T38.2X2	T38.2X3	T38.2X4	T38.2X5	T38.2X6
Thiourea	T38.2X1	T38.2X2	T38.2X3	T38.2X4	T38.2X5	T38.2X6
Thiphenamil	T44.3X1	T44.3X2	T44.3X3	T44.3X4	T44.3X5	T44.3X6
Thiram	T60.3X1	T60.3X2	T60.3X3	T60.3X4	—	—
medicinal	T49.2X1	T49.2X2	T49.2X3	T49.2X4	T49.2X5	T49.2X6
Thonzylamine (systemic)	T45.0X1	T45.0X2	T45.0X3	T45.0X4	T45.0X5	T45.0X6
mucosal decongestant	T48.5X1	T48.5X2	T48.5X3	T48.5X4	T48.5X5	T48.5X6
Thorazine	T43.3X1	T43.3X2	T43.3X3	T43.3X4	T43.3X5	T43.3X6
Thorium dioxide	T50.8X1	T50.8X2	T50.8X3	T50.8X4	T50.8X5	T50.8X6
suspension						
Thornapple	T62.2X1	T62.2X2	T62.2X3	T62.2X4	—	—
Throat drug NEC	T49.6X1	T49.6X2	T49.6X3	T49.6X4	T49.6X5	T49.6X6
Thrombin	T45.7X1	T45.7X2	T45.7X3	T45.7X4	T45.7X5	T45.7X6
Thrombolysin	T45.611	T45.612	T45.613	T45.614	T45.615	T45.616
Thromboplastin	T45.7X1	T45.7X2	T45.7X3	T45.7X4	T45.7X5	T45.7X6
Thurfyl nicotinate	T46.7X1	T46.7X2	T46.7X3	T46.7X4	T46.7X5	T46.7X6
Thymol	T49.0X1	T49.0X2	T49.0X3	T49.0X4	T49.0X5	T49.0X6
Thymopentin	T37.5X1	T37.5X2	T37.5X3	T37.5X4	T37.5X5	T37.5X6
Thymoxamine	T46.7X1	T46.7X2	T46.7X3	T46.7X4	T46.7X5	T46.7X6
Thymus extract	T38.891	T38.892	T38.893	T38.894	T38.895	T38.896
Thyreotrophic hormone	T38.811	T38.812	T38.813	T38.814	T38.815	T38.816
Thyroglobulin	T38.1X1	T38.1X2	T38.1X3	T38.1X4	T38.1X5	T38.1X6
Thyroid (hormone)	T38.1X1	T38.1X2	T38.1X3	T38.1X4	T38.1X5	T38.1X6
Thyrolar	T38.1X1	T38.1X2	T38.1X3	T38.1X4	T38.1X5	T38.1X6
Thyrotrophin	T38.811	T38.812	T38.813	T38.814	T38.815	T38.816
Thyrotropic hormone	T38.811	T38.812	T38.813	T38.814	T38.815	T38.816
Thyroxine	T38.1X1	T38.1X2	T38.1X3	T38.1X4	T38.1X5	T38.1X6
Tiabendazole	T37.4X1	T37.4X2	T37.4X3	T37.4X4	T37.4X5	T37.4X6
Tiamizide	T50.2X1	T50.2X2	T50.2X3	T50.2X4	T50.2X5	T50.2X6
Tianeptine	T43.291	T43.292	T43.293	T43.294	T43.295	T43.296
Tiapamil	T46.1X1	T46.1X2	T46.1X3	T46.1X4	T46.1X5	T46.1X6
Tiapride	T43.591	T43.592	T43.593	T43.594	T43.595	T43.596
Tiaprofenic acid	T39.311	T39.312	T39.313	T39.314	T39.315	T39.316
Tiaramide	T39.8X1	T39.8X2	T39.8X3	T39.8X4	T39.8X5	T39.8X6
Ticarcillin	T36.0X1	T36.0X2	T36.0X3	T36.0X4	T36.0X5	T36.0X6
Ticlatone	T49.0X1	T49.0X2	T49.0X3	T49.0X4	T49.0X5	T49.0X6
Ticlopidine	T45.521	T45.522	T45.523	T45.524	T45.525	T45.526
Ticrynafen	T50.1X1	T50.1X2	T50.1X3	T50.1X4	T50.1X5	T50.1X6
Tidiacic	T50.991	T50.992	T50.993	T50.994	T50.995	T50.996
Tiemonium	T44.3X1	T44.3X2	T44.3X3	T44.3X4	T44.3X5	T44.3X6
iodide	T44.3X1	T44.3X2	T44.3X3	T44.3X4	T44.3X5	T44.3X6
Tienilic acid	T50.1X1	T50.1X2	T50.1X3	T50.1X4	T50.1X5	T50.1X6
Tifenamil	T44.3X1	T44.3X2	T44.3X3	T44.3X4	T44.3X5	T44.3X6
Tigan	T45.0X1	T45.0X2	T45.0X3	T45.0X4	T45.0X5	T45.0X6
Tigloidine	T44.3X1	T44.3X2	T44.3X3	T44.3X4	T44.3X5	T44.3X6
Tilactase	T47.5X1	T47.5X2	T47.5X3	T47.5X4	T47.5X5	T47.5X6
Tiletamine	T41.291	T41.292	T41.293	T41.294	T41.295	T41.296
Tilidine	T40.4X1	T40.4X2	T40.4X3	T40.4X4	—	—
Timepidium bromide	T44.3X1	T44.3X2	T44.3X3	T44.3X4	T44.3X5	T44.3X6
Timiperone	T43.4X1	T43.4X2	T43.4X3	T43.4X4	T43.4X5	T43.4X6
Timolol	T44.7X1	T44.7X2	T44.7X3	T44.7X4	T44.7X5	T44.7X6
Tincture, iodine — see Iodine						
Tindal	T43.3X1	T43.3X2	T43.3X3	T43.3X4	T43.3X5	T43.3X6
Tinidazole	T37.3X1	T37.3X2	T37.3X3	T37.3X4	T37.3X5	T37.3X6
Tin (chloride) (dust) (oxide)	T56.6X1	T56.6X2	T56.6X3	T56.6X4	—	—
NEC						
anti-infectives	T37.8X1	T37.8X2	T37.8X3	T37.8X4	T37.8X5	T37.8X6
Tinoridine	T39.8X1	T39.8X2	T39.8X3	T39.8X4	T39.8X5	T39.8X6
Tiocarlide	T37.1X1	T37.1X2	T37.1X3	T37.1X4	T37.1X5	T37.1X6
Tioclomarol	T45.511	T45.512	T45.513	T45.514	T45.515	T45.516
Tioconazole	T49.0X1	T49.0X2	T49.0X3	T49.0X4	T49.0X5	T49.0X6
Tioguanine	T45.1X1	T45.1X2	T45.1X3	T45.1X4	T45.1X5	T45.1X6
Tiopronin	T50.991	T50.992	T50.993	T50.994	T50.995	T50.996
Tiotixene	T43.4X1	T43.4X2	T43.4X3	T43.4X4	T43.4X5	T43.4X6
Tioxolone	T49.4X1	T49.4X2	T49.4X3	T49.4X4	T49.4X5	T49.4X6

Substance	Poisoning, Accidental (unintentional)	Poisoning, Intentional Self-harm	Poisoning, Assault	Poisoning, Undetermined	Adverse Effect	Under-dosing
Tipepidine	T48.3X1	T48.3X2	T48.3X3	T48.3X4	T48.3X5	T48.3X6
Tiquizium bromide	T44.3X1	T44.3X2	T44.3X3	T44.3X4	T44.3X5	T44.3X6
Tiratricol	T38.1X1	T38.1X2	T38.1X3	T38.1X4	T38.1X5	T38.1X6
Tisopurine	T50.4X1	T50.4X2	T50.4X3	T50.4X4	T50.4X5	T50.4X6
Titanium (compounds) (vapor)	T56.891	T56.892	T56.893	T56.894	—	—
dioxide	T49.3X1	T49.3X2	T49.3X3	T49.3X4	T49.3X5	T49.3X6
ointment	T49.3X1	T49.3X2	T49.3X3	T49.3X4	T49.3X5	T49.3X6
oxide	T49.3X1	T49.3X2	T49.3X3	T49.3X4	T49.3X5	T49.3X6
tetrachloride	T56.891	T56.892	T56.893	T56.894	—	—
Titanocene	T56.891	T56.892	T56.893	T56.894	—	—
Titroid	T38.1X1	T38.1X2	T38.1X3	T38.1X4	T38.1X5	T38.1X6
Tizanidine	T42.8X1	T42.8X2	T42.8X3	T42.8X4	T42.8X5	T42.8X6
TMTD	T60.3X1	T60.3X2	T60.3X3	T60.3X4	—	—
TNT (fumes)	T65.3X1	T65.3X2	T65.3X3	T65.3X4	—	—
Toadstool	T62.0X1	T62.0X2	T62.0X3	T62.0X4	—	—
Tobacco NEC	T65.291	T65.292	T65.293	T65.294	—	—
cigarettes	T65.221	T65.222	T65.223	T65.224	—	—
Indian	T62.2X1	T62.2X2	T62.2X3	T62.2X4	—	—
smoke, second-hand	T65.221	T65.222	T65.223	T65.224	—	—
Tobramycin	T36.5X1	T36.5X2	T36.5X3	T36.5X4	T36.5X5	T36.5X6
Tocainide	T46.2X1	T46.2X2	T46.2X3	T46.2X4	T46.2X5	T46.2X6
Tocoferol	T45.2X1	T45.2X2	T45.2X3	T45.2X4	T45.2X5	T45.2X6
Tocopherol	T45.2X1	T45.2X2	T45.2X3	T45.2X4	T45.2X5	T45.2X6
acetate	T45.2X1	T45.2X2	T45.2X3	T45.2X4	T45.2X5	T45.2X6
Tocosamine	T48.0X1	T48.0X2	T48.0X3	T48.0X4	T48.0X5	T48.0X6
Todralazine	T46.5X1	T46.5X2	T46.5X3	T46.5X4	T46.5X5	T46.5X6
Tofisopam	T42.4X1	T42.4X2	T42.4X3	T42.4X4	T42.4X5	T42.4X6
Tofranil	T43.011	T43.012	T43.013	T43.014	T43.015	T43.016
Toilet deodorizer	T65.891	T65.892	T65.893	T65.894	—	—
Tolamolol	T44.7X1	T44.7X2	T44.7X3	T44.7X4	T44.7X5	T44.7X6
Tolazamide	T38.3X1	T38.3X2	T38.3X3	T38.3X4	T38.3X5	T38.3X6
Tolazoline	T46.7X1	T46.7X2	T46.7X3	T46.7X4	T46.7X5	T46.7X6
Tolbutamide (sodium)	T38.3X1	T38.3X2	T38.3X3	T38.3X4	T38.3X5	T38.3X6
Tolciclate	T49.0X1	T49.0X2	T49.0X3	T49.0X4	T49.0X5	T49.0X6
Tolmetin	T39.391	T39.392	T39.393	T39.394	T39.395	T39.396
Tolnaftate	T49.0X1	T49.0X2	T49.0X3	T49.0X4	T49.0X5	T49.0X6
Tolonidine	T46.5X1	T46.5X2	T46.5X3	T46.5X4	T46.5X5	T46.5X6
Toloxatone	T42.6X1	T42.6X2	T42.6X3	T42.6X4	T42.6X5	T42.6X6
Tolperisone	T44.3X1	T44.3X2	T44.3X3	T44.3X4	T44.3X5	T44.3X6
Tolserol	T42.8X1	T42.8X2	T42.8X3	T42.8X4	T42.8X5	T42.8X6
Toluene (liquid)	T52.2X1	T52.2X2	T52.2X3	T52.2X4	—	—
diisocyanate	T65.0X1	T65.0X2	T65.0X3	T65.0X4	—	—
Toluidine	T65.891	T65.892	T65.893	T65.894	—	—
vapor	T59.891	T59.892	T59.893	T59.894	—	—
Toluol (liquid)	T52.2X1	T52.2X2	T52.2X3	T52.2X4	—	—
vapor	T52.2X1	T52.2X2	T52.2X3	T52.2X4	—	—
Toluylenediamine	T65.3X1	T65.3X2	T65.3X3	T65.3X4	—	—
Tolylene-2,4-diisocyanate	T65.0X1	T65.0X2	T65.0X3	T65.0X4	—	—
Tonic NEC	T50.901	T50.902	T50.903	T50.904	T50.905	T50.906
Topical action drug NEC	T49.91	T49.92	T49.93	T49.94	T49.95	T49.96
ear, nose or throat	T49.6X1	T49.6X2	T49.6X3	T49.6X4	T49.6X5	T49.6X6
eye	T49.5X1	T49.5X2	T49.5X3	T49.5X4	T49.5X5	T49.5X6
skin	T49.91	T49.92	T49.93	T49.94	T49.95	T49.96
specified NEC	T49.8X1	T49.8X2	T49.8X3	T49.8X4	T49.8X5	T49.8X6
Toquizine	T44.3X1	T44.3X2	T44.3X3	T44.3X4	T44.3X5	T44.3X6
Toremifene	T38.6X1	T38.6X2	T38.6X3	T38.6X4	T38.6X5	T38.6X6
Tosylchloramide sodium	T49.8X1	T49.8X2	T49.8X3	T49.8X4	T49.8X5	T49.8X6
Toxaphene (dust) (spray)	T60.1X1	T60.1X2	T60.1X3	T60.1X4	—	—
Toxin, diphtheria (Schick Test)	T50.8X1	T50.8X2	T50.8X3	T50.8X4	T50.8X5	T50.8X6
Toxoid						
combined	T50.A21	T50.A22	T50.A23	T50.A24	T50.A25	T50.A26
diphtheria	T50.A91	T50.A92	T50.A93	T50.A94	T50.A95	T50.A96
tetanus	T50.A91	T50.A92	T50.A93	T50.A94	T50.A95	T50.A96
Trace element NEC	T45.8X1	T45.8X2	T45.8X3	T45.8X4	T45.8X5	T45.8X6
Tractor fuel NEC	T52.0X1	T52.0X2	T52.0X3	T52.0X4	—	—
Tragacanth	T50.991	T50.992	T50.993	T50.994	T50.995	T50.996
Tramadol	T40.4X1	T40.4X2	T40.4X3	T40.4X4	T40.4X5	T40.4X6
Tramazoline	T48.5X1	T48.5X2	T48.5X3	T48.5X4	T48.5X5	T48.5X6
Tranexamic acid	T45.621	T45.622	T45.623	T45.624	T45.625	T45.626
Tranilast	T45.0X1	T45.0X2	T45.0X3	T45.0X4	T45.0X5	T45.0X6
Tranquilizer NEC	T43.501	T43.502	T43.503	T43.504	T43.505	T43.506
with hypnotic or sedative	T42.6X1	T42.6X2	T42.6X3	T42.6X4	T42.6X5	T42.6X6
benzodiazepine NEC	T42.4X1	T42.4X2	T42.4X3	T42.4X4	T42.4X5	T42.4X6
butyrophenone NEC	T43.4X1	T43.4X2	T43.4X3	T43.4X4	T43.4X5	T43.4X6
carbamate	T43.591	T43.592	T43.593	T43.594	T43.595	T43.596
dimethylamine	T43.3X1	T43.3X2	T43.3X3	T43.3X4	T43.3X5	T43.3X6
ethylamine	T43.3X1	T43.3X2	T43.3X3	T43.3X4	T43.3X5	T43.3X6
hydroxyzine	T43.591	T43.592	T43.593	T43.594	T43.595	T43.596
major NEC	T43.501	T43.502	T43.503	T43.504	T43.505	T43.506
penothiazine NEC	T43.3X1	T43.3X2	T43.3X3	T43.3X4	T43.3X5	T43.3X6
phenothiazine-based	T43.3X1	T43.3X2	T43.3X3	T43.3X4	T43.3X5	T43.3X6

Substance	Poisoning, Accidental (unintentional)	Poisoning, Intentional Self-harm	Poisoning, Assault	Poisoning, Undetermined	Adverse Effect	Under-dosing
Tranquilizer — continued						
piperazine NEC	T43.3X1	T43.3X2	T43.3X3	T43.3X4	T43.3X5	T43.3X6
piperidine	T43.3X1	T43.3X2	T43.3X3	T43.3X4	T43.3X5	T43.3X6
propylamine	T43.3X1	T43.3X2	T43.3X3	T43.3X4	T43.3X5	T43.3X6
specified NEC	T43.591	T43.592	T43.593	T43.594	T43.595	T43.596
thioxanthene NEC	T43.591	T43.592	T43.593	T43.594	T43.595	T43.596
Tranxene	T42.4X1	T42.4X2	T42.4X3	T42.4X4	T42.4X5	T42.4X6
Tranylcypromine	T43.1X1	T43.1X2	T43.1X3	T43.1X4	T43.1X5	T43.1X6
Trapidil	T46.3X1	T46.3X2	T46.3X3	T46.3X4	T46.3X5	T46.3X6
Trasentine	T44.3X1	T44.3X2	T44.3X3	T44.3X4	T44.3X5	T44.3X6
Travert	T50.3X1	T50.3X2	T50.3X3	T50.3X4	T50.3X5	T50.3X6
Trazodone	T43.211	T43.212	T43.213	T43.214	T43.215	T43.216
Trecator	T37.1X1	T37.1X2	T37.1X3	T37.1X4	T37.1X5	T37.1X6
Treosulfan	T45.1X1	T45.1X2	T45.1X3	T45.1X4	T45.1X5	T45.1X6
Tretamine	T45.1X1	T45.1X2	T45.1X3	T45.1X4	T45.1X5	T45.1X6
Tretinoin	T49.0X1	T49.0X2	T49.0X3	T49.0X4	T49.0X5	T49.0X6
Tretoquinol	T48.6X1	T48.6X2	T48.6X3	T48.6X4	T48.6X5	T48.6X6
Triacetin	T49.0X1	T49.0X2	T49.0X3	T49.0X4	T49.0X5	T49.0X6
Triacetoxyanthracene	T49.4X1	T49.4X2	T49.4X3	T49.4X4	T49.4X5	T49.4X6
Triacetyloleandomycin	T36.3X1	T36.3X2	T36.3X3	T36.3X4	T36.3X5	T36.3X6
Triamcinolone	T38.0X1	T38.0X2	T38.0X3	T38.0X4	T38.0X5	T38.0X6
ENT agent	T49.6X1	T49.6X2	T49.6X3	T49.6X4	T49.6X5	T49.6X6
hexacetonide	T49.0X1	T49.0X2	T49.0X3	T49.0X4	T49.0X5	T49.0X6
ophthalmic preparation	T49.5X1	T49.5X2	T49.5X3	T49.5X4	T49.5X5	T49.5X6
topical NEC	T49.0X1	T49.0X2	T49.0X3	T49.0X4	T49.0X5	T49.0X6
Triampyzine	T44.3X1	T44.3X2	T44.3X3	T44.3X4	T44.3X5	T44.3X6
Triamterene	T50.2X1	T50.2X2	T50.2X3	T50.2X4	T50.2X5	T50.2X6
Triazine (herbicide)	T60.3X1	T60.3X2	T60.3X3	T60.3X4	—	—
Triaziquone	T45.1X1	T45.1X2	T45.1X3	T45.1X4	T45.1X5	T45.1X6
Triazolam	T42.4X1	T42.4X2	T42.4X3	T42.4X4	T42.4X5	T42.4X6
Triazole (herbicide)	T60.3X1	T60.3X2	T60.3X3	T60.3X4	—	—
Tribenoside	T46.991	T46.992	T46.993	T46.994	T46.995	T46.996
Tribromacetaldehyde	T42.6X1	T42.6X2	T42.6X3	T42.6X4	T42.6X5	T42.6X6
Tribromoethanol, rectal	T41.291	T41.292	T41.293	T41.294	T41.295	T41.296
Tribromomethane	T42.6X1	T42.6X2	T42.6X3	T42.6X4	T42.6X5	T42.6X6
Trichlorethane	T53.2X1	T53.2X2	T53.2X3	T53.2X4	—	—
Trichlorethylene	T53.2X1	T53.2X2	T53.2X3	T53.2X4	—	—
Trichlorfon	T60.0X1	T60.0X2	T60.0X3	T60.0X4	—	—
Trichlormethiazide	T50.2X1	T50.2X2	T50.2X3	T50.2X4	T50.2X5	T50.2X6
Trichlormethine	T45.1X1	T45.1X2	T45.1X3	T45.1X4	T45.1X5	T45.1X6
Trichloroacetic acid, Trichloracetic acid	T54.2X1	T54.2X2	T54.2X3	T54.2X4	—	—
medicinal	T49.4X1	T49.4X2	T49.4X3	T49.4X4	T49.4X5	T49.4X6
Trichloroethane	T53.2X1	T53.2X2	T53.2X3	T53.2X4	—	—
Trichloroethanol	T42.6X1	T42.6X2	T42.6X3	T42.6X4	T42.6X5	T42.6X6
Trichloroethylene (liquid)	T53.2X1	T53.2X2	T53.2X3	T53.2X4	—	—
(vapor)						
anesthetic (gas)	T41.0X1	T41.0X2	T41.0X3	T41.0X4	T41.0X5	T41.0X6
vapor NEC	T53.2X1	T53.2X2	T53.2X3	T53.2X4	—	—
Trichloroethyl phosphate	T42.6X1	T42.6X2	T42.6X3	T42.6X4	T42.6X5	T42.6X6
Trichlorofluoromethane NEC	T53.5X1	T53.5X2	T53.5X3	T53.5X4	—	—
Trichloronate	T60.0X1	T60.0X2	T60.0X3	T60.0X4	—	—
Trichloropropane	T53.6X1	T53.6X2	T53.6X3	T53.6X4	—	—
Trichlorotriethylamine	T45.1X1	T45.1X2	T45.1X3	T45.1X4	T45.1X5	T45.1X6
Trichomonacides NEC	T37.3X1	T37.3X2	T37.3X3	T37.3X4	T37.3X5	T37.3X6
Trichomycin	T36.7X1	T36.7X2	T36.7X3	T36.7X4	T36.7X5	T36.7X6
Triclobisonium chloride	T49.0X1	T49.0X2	T49.0X3	T49.0X4	T49.0X5	T49.0X6
Triclocarban	T49.0X1	T49.0X2	T49.0X3	T49.0X4	T49.0X5	T49.0X6
Triclofos	T42.6X1	T42.6X2	T42.6X3	T42.6X4	T42.6X5	T42.6X6
Triclosan	T49.0X1	T49.0X2	T49.0X3	T49.0X4	T49.0X5	T49.0X6
Tricresyl phosphate	T65.891	T65.892	T65.893	T65.894	—	—
solvent	T52.91	T52.92	T52.93	T52.94	—	—
Tricyclamol chloride	T44.3X1	T44.3X2	T44.3X3	T44.3X4	T44.3X5	T44.3X6
Tridesilon	T49.0X1	T49.0X2	T49.0X3	T49.0X4	T49.0X5	T49.0X6
Tridihexethyl iodide	T44.3X1	T44.3X2	T44.3X3	T44.3X4	T44.3X5	T44.3X6
Tridione	T42.2X1	T42.2X2	T42.2X3	T42.2X4	T42.2X5	T42.2X6
Trientine	T45.8X1	T45.8X2	T45.8X3	T45.8X4	T45.8X5	T45.8X6
Triethanolamine NEC	T54.3X1	T54.3X2	T54.3X3	T54.3X4	—	—
detergent	T54.3X1	T54.3X2	T54.3X3	T54.3X4	—	—
trinitrate (biphosphate)	T46.3X1	T46.3X2	T46.3X3	T46.3X4	T46.3X5	T46.3X6
Triethanomelamine	T45.1X1	T45.1X2	T45.1X3	T45.1X4	T45.1X5	T45.1X6
Triethylenemelamine	T45.1X1	T45.1X2	T45.1X3	T45.1X4	T45.1X5	T45.1X6
Triethylenephosphoramide	T45.1X1	T45.1X2	T45.1X3	T45.1X4	T45.1X5	T45.1X6
Triethylenethiophosphoramide	T45.1X1	T45.1X2	T45.1X3	T45.1X4	T45.1X5	T45.1X6
Trifluoperazine	T43.3X1	T43.3X2	T43.3X3	T43.3X4	T43.3X5	T43.3X6
Trifluoroethyl vinyl ether	T41.0X1	T41.0X2	T41.0X3	T41.0X4	T41.0X5	T41.0X6
Trifluperidol	T43.4X1	T43.4X2	T43.4X3	T43.4X4	T43.4X5	T43.4X6
Triflupromazine	T43.3X1	T43.3X2	T43.3X3	T43.3X4	T43.3X5	T43.3X6
Trifluridine	T37.5X1	T37.5X2	T37.5X3	T37.5X4	T37.5X5	T37.5X6
Triflusal	T45.521	T45.522	T45.523	T45.524	T45.525	T45.526
Trihexyphenidyl	T44.3X1	T44.3X2	T44.3X3	T44.3X4	T44.3X5	T44.3X6
Triiodothyronine	T38.1X1	T38.1X2	T38.1X3	T38.1X4	T38.1X5	T38.1X6
Trilene	T41.0X1	T41.0X2	T41.0X3	T41.0X4	T41.0X5	T41.0X6
Trilostane	T38.991	T38.992	T38.993	T38.994	T38.995	T38.996
Trimebutine	T44.3X1	T44.3X2	T44.3X3	T44.3X4	T44.3X5	T44.3X6
Trimecaine	T41.3X1	T41.3X2	T41.3X3	T41.3X4	T41.3X5	T41.3X6
Trimeprazine (tartrate)	T44.3X1	T44.3X2	T44.3X3	T44.3X4	T44.3X5	T44.3X6
Trimetaphan camsilate	T44.2X1	T44.2X2	T44.2X3	T44.2X4	T44.2X5	T44.2X6
Trimetazidine	T46.7X1	T46.7X2	T46.7X3	T46.7X4	T46.7X5	T46.7X6
Trimethadione	T42.2X1	T42.2X2	T42.2X3	T42.2X4	T42.2X5	T42.2X6
Trimethaphan	T44.2X1	T44.2X2	T44.2X3	T44.2X4	T44.2X5	T44.2X6
Trimethidinium	T44.2X1	T44.2X2	T44.2X3	T44.2X4	T44.2X5	T44.2X6
Trimethobenzamide	T45.0X1	T45.0X2	T45.0X3	T45.0X4	T45.0X5	T45.0X6
Trimethoprim	T37.8X1	T37.8X2	T37.8X3	T37.8X4	T37.8X5	T37.8X6
with sulfamethoxazole	T36.8X1	T36.8X2	T36.8X3	T36.8X4	T36.8X5	T36.8X6
Trimethylcarbinol	T51.3X1	T51.3X2	T51.3X3	T51.3X4	—	—
Trimethylpsoralen	T49.3X1	T49.3X2	T49.3X3	T49.3X4	T49.3X5	T49.3X6
Trimeton	T45.0X1	T45.0X2	T45.0X3	T45.0X4	T45.0X5	T45.0X6
Trimetrexate	T45.1X1	T45.1X2	T45.1X3	T45.1X4	T45.1X5	T45.1X6
Trimipramine	T43.011	T43.012	T43.013	T43.014	T43.015	T43.016
Trimustine	T45.1X1	T45.1X2	T45.1X3	T45.1X4	T45.1X5	T45.1X6
Trinitrine	T46.3X1	T46.3X2	T46.3X3	T46.3X4	T46.3X5	T46.3X6
Trinitrobenzol	T65.3X1	T65.3X2	T65.3X3	T65.3X4	—	—
Trinitrophenol	T65.3X1	T65.3X2	T65.3X3	T65.3X4	—	—
Trinitrotoluene (fumes)	T65.3X1	T65.3X2	T65.3X3	T65.3X4	—	—
Trional	T42.6X1	T42.6X2	T42.6X3	T42.6X4	T42.6X5	T42.6X6
Triorthocresyl phosphate	T65.891	T65.892	T65.893	T65.894	—	—
Trioxide of arsenic	T57.0X1	T57.0X2	T57.0X3	T57.0X4	—	—
Trioxysalen	T49.4X1	T49.4X2	T49.4X3	T49.4X4	T49.4X5	T49.4X6
Tripamide	T50.2X1	T50.2X2	T50.2X3	T50.2X4	T50.2X5	T50.2X6
Triparanol	T46.6X1	T46.6X2	T46.6X3	T46.6X4	T46.6X5	T46.6X6
Tripelennamine	T45.0X1	T45.0X2	T45.0X3	T45.0X4	T45.0X5	T45.0X6
Triperiden	T44.3X1	T44.3X2	T44.3X3	T44.3X4	T44.3X5	T44.3X6
Triperidol	T43.4X1	T43.4X2	T43.4X3	T43.4X4	T43.4X5	T43.4X6
Triphenylphosphate	T65.891	T65.892	T65.893	T65.894	—	—
Triple						
bromides	T42.6X1	T42.6X2	T42.6X3	T42.6X4	T42.6X5	T42.6X6
carbonate	T47.1X1	T47.1X2	T47.1X3	T47.1X4	T47.1X5	T47.1X6
vaccine						
DPT	T50.A11	T50.A12	T50.A13	T50.A14	T50.A15	T50.A16
including pertussis	T50.A11	T50.A12	T50.A13	T50.A14	T50.A15	T50.A16
MMR	T50.B91	T50.B92	T50.B93	T50.B94	T50.B95	T50.B96
Triprolidine	T45.0X1	T45.0X2	T45.0X3	T45.0X4	T45.0X5	T45.0X6
Trisodium hydrogen edetate	T50.6X1	T50.6X2	T50.6X3	T50.6X4	T50.6X5	T50.6X6
Trisoralen	T49.3X1	T49.3X2	T49.3X3	T49.3X4	T49.3X5	T49.3X6
Trisulfapyrimidines	T37.0X1	T37.0X2	T37.0X3	T37.0X4	T37.0X5	T37.0X6
Trithiozine	T44.3X1	T44.3X2	T44.3X3	T44.3X4	T44.3X5	T44.3X6
Tritiozine	T44.3X1	T44.3X2	T44.3X3	T44.3X4	T44.3X5	T44.3X6
Tritoqualine	T45.0X1	T45.0X2	T45.0X3	T45.0X4	T45.0X5	T45.0X6
Trofosfamide	T45.1X1	T45.1X2	T45.1X3	T45.1X4	T45.1X5	T45.1X6
Troleandomycin	T36.3X1	T36.3X2	T36.3X3	T36.3X4	T36.3X5	T36.3X6
Trolnitrate (phosphate)	T46.3X1	T46.3X2	T46.3X3	T46.3X4	T46.3X5	T46.3X6
Tromantadine	T37.5X1	T37.5X2	T37.5X3	T37.5X4	T37.5X5	T37.5X6
Trometamol	T50.2X1	T50.2X2	T50.2X3	T50.2X4	T50.2X5	T50.2X6
Tromethamine	T50.2X1	T50.2X2	T50.2X3	T50.2X4	T50.2X5	T50.2X6
Tronothane	T41.3X1	T41.3X2	T41.3X3	T41.3X4	T41.3X5	T41.3X6
Tropacine	T44.3X1	T44.3X2	T44.3X3	T44.3X4	T44.3X5	T44.3X6
Tropatepine	T44.3X1	T44.3X2	T44.3X3	T44.3X4	T44.3X5	T44.3X6
Tropicamide	T44.3X1	T44.3X2	T44.3X3	T44.3X4	T44.3X5	T44.3X6
Trospium chloride	T44.3X1	T44.3X2	T44.3X3	T44.3X4	T44.3X5	T44.3X6
Troxerutin	T46.991	T46.992	T46.993	T46.994	T46.995	T46.996
Troxidone	T42.2X1	T42.2X2	T42.2X3	T42.2X4	T42.2X5	T42.2X6
Tryparsamide	T37.3X1	T37.3X2	T37.3X3	T37.3X4	T37.3X5	T37.3X6
Trypsin	T45.3X1	T45.3X2	T45.3X3	T45.3X4	T45.3X5	T45.3X6
Tryptizol	T43.011	T43.012	T43.013	T43.014	T43.015	T43.016
TSH	T38.811	T38.812	T38.813	T38.814	T38.815	T38.816
Tuaminoheptane	T48.5X1	T48.5X2	T48.5X3	T48.5X4	T48.5X5	T48.5X6
Tuberculin, purified protein derivative (PPD)	T50.8X1	T50.8X2	T50.8X3	T50.8X4	T50.8X5	T50.8X6
Tubocurare	T48.1X1	T48.1X2	T48.1X3	T48.1X4	T48.1X5	T48.1X6
Tubocurarine (chloride)	T48.1X1	T48.1X2	T48.1X3	T48.1X4	T48.1X5	T48.1X6
Tulobuterol	T48.6X1	T48.6X2	T48.6X3	T48.6X4	T48.6X5	T48.6X6
Turpentine (spirits of)	T52.8X1	T52.8X2	T52.8X3	T52.8X4	—	—
vapor	T52.8X1	T52.8X2	T52.8X3	T52.8X4	—	—
Tybamate	T43.591	T43.592	T43.593	T43.594	T43.595	T43.596
Tyloxapol	T48.4X1	T48.4X2	T48.4X3	T48.4X4	T48.4X5	T48.4X6
Tymazoline	T48.5X1	T48.5X2	T48.5X3	T48.5X4	T48.5X5	T48.5X6
Typhoid-paratyphoid vaccine	T50.A91	T50.A92	T50.A93	T50.A94	T50.A95	T50.A96
Typhus vaccine	T50.A91	T50.A92	T50.A93	T50.A94	T50.A95	T50.A96
Tyropanoate	T50.8X1	T50.8X2	T50.8X3	T50.8X4	T50.8X5	T50.8X6
Tyrothricin	T49.6X1	T49.6X2	T49.6X3	T49.6X4	T49.6X5	T49.6X6
ENT agent	T49.6X1	T49.6X2	T49.6X3	T49.6X4	T49.6X5	T49.6X6
ophthalmic preparation	T49.5X1	T49.5X2	T49.5X3	T49.5X4	T49.5X5	T49.5X6

Additional Character May Be Required — Refer to the Tabular List for Character Selection   ▽ Subterms under main terms may continue to next column or page

Table of Drugs and Chemicals

Substance	Poisoning, Accidental (unintentional)	Poisoning, Intentional Self-harm	Poisoning, Assault	Poisoning, Undetermined	Adverse Effect	Underdosing
Ufenamate	T39.391	T39.392	T39.393	T39.394	T39.395	T39.396
Ultraviolet light protectant	T49.3X1	T49.3X2	T49.3X3	T49.3X4	T49.3X5	T49.3X6
Undecenoic acid	T49.0X1	T49.0X2	T49.0X3	T49.0X4	T49.0X5	T49.0X6
Undecoylium	T49.0X1	T49.0X2	T49.0X3	T49.0X4	T49.0X5	T49.0X6
Undecylenic acid (derivatives)	T49.0X1	T49.0X2	T49.0X3	T49.0X4	T49.0X5	T49.0X6
Unna's boot	T49.3X1	T49.3X2	T49.3X3	T49.3X4	T49.3X5	T49.3X6
Unsaturated fatty acid	T46.6X1	T46.6X2	T46.6X3	T46.6X4	T46.6X5	T46.6X6
Uracil mustard	T45.1X1	T45.1X2	T45.1X3	T45.1X4	T45.1X5	T45.1X6
Uramustine	T45.1X1	T45.1X2	T45.1X3	T45.1X4	T45.1X5	T45.1X6
Urapidil	T46.5X1	T46.5X2	T46.5X3	T46.5X4	T46.5X5	T46.5X6
Urari	T48.1X1	T48.1X2	T48.1X3	T48.1X4	T48.1X5	T48.1X6
Urate oxidase	T50.4X1	T50.4X2	T50.4X3	T50.4X4	T50.4X5	T50.4X6
Urea	T47.3X1	T47.3X2	T47.3X3	T47.3X4	T47.3X5	T47.3X6
peroxide	T49.0X1	T49.0X2	T49.0X3	T49.0X4	T49.0X5	T49.0X6
stibamine	T37.4X1	T37.4X2	T37.4X3	T37.4X4	T37.4X5	T37.4X6
topical	T49.8X1	T49.8X2	T49.8X3	T49.8X4	T49.8X5	T49.8X6
Urethane	T45.1X1	T45.1X2	T45.1X3	T45.1X4	T45.1X5	T45.1X6
Urginea (maritima) (scilla) — see Squill						
Uric acid metabolism drug NEC	T50.4X1	T50.4X2	T50.4X3	T50.4X4	T50.4X5	T50.4X6
Uricosuric agent	T50.4X1	T50.4X2	T50.4X3	T50.4X4	T50.4X5	T50.4X6
Urinary anti-infective	T37.8X1	T37.8X2	T37.8X3	T37.8X4	T37.8X5	T37.8X6
Urofollitropin		T38.812	T38.813	T38.814	T38.815	T38.816
Urokinase	T45.611	T45.612	T45.613	T45.614	T45.615	T45.616
Urokon	T50.8X1	T50.8X2	T50.8X3	T50.8X4	T50.8X5	T50.8X6
Ursodeoxycholic acid	T50.991	T50.992	T50.993	T50.994	T50.995	T50.996
Ursodiol	T50.991	T50.992	T50.993	T50.994	T50.995	T50.996
Urtica	T62.2X1	T62.2X2	T62.2X3	T62.2X4	—	—
Utility gas — see Gas, utility						
Vaccine NEC	T50.Z91	T50.Z92	T50.Z93	T50.Z94	T50.Z95	T50.Z96
antineoplastic	T50.Z91	T50.Z92	T50.Z93	T50.Z94	T50.Z95	T50.Z96
bacterial NEC	T50.A91	T50.A92	T50.A93	T50.A94	T50.A95	T50.A96
with						
other bacterial component	T50.A21	T50.A22	T50.A23	T50.A24	T50.A25	T50.A26
pertussis component	T50.A11	T50.A12	T50.A13	T50.A14	T50.A15	T50.A16
viral-rickettsial component	T50.A21	T50.A22	T50.A23	T50.A24	T50.A25	T50.A26
mixed NEC	T50.A21	T50.A22	T50.A23	T50.A24	T50.A25	T50.A26
BCG	T50.A91	T50.A92	T50.A93	T50.A94	T50.A95	T50.A96
cholera	T50.A91	T50.A92	T50.A93	T50.A94	T50.A95	T50.A96
diphtheria	T50.A91	T50.A92	T50.A93	T50.A94	T50.A95	T50.A96
with tetanus	T50.A21	T50.A22	T50.A23	T50.A24	T50.A25	T50.A26
and pertussis	T50.A11	T50.A12	T50.A13	T50.A14	T50.A15	T50.A16
influenza	T50.B91	T50.B92	T50.B93	T50.B94	T50.B95	T50.B96
measles	T50.B91	T50.B92	T50.B93	T50.B94	T50.B95	T50.B96
with mumps and rubella	T50.B91	T50.B92	T50.B93	T50.B94	T50.B95	T50.B96
meningococcal	T50.A91	T50.A92	T50.A93	T50.A94	T50.A95	T50.A96
mumps	T50.B91	T50.B92	T50.B93	T50.B94	T50.B95	T50.B96
paratyphoid	T50.A91	T50.A92	T50.A93	T50.A94	T50.A95	T50.A96
pertussis	T50.A11	T50.A12	T50.A13	T50.A14	T50.A15	T50.A16
with diphtheria	T50.A11	T50.A12	T50.A13	T50.A14	T50.A15	T50.A16
and tetanus	T50.A11	T50.A12	T50.A13	T50.A14	T50.A15	T50.A16
with other component	T50.A11	T50.A12	T50.A13	T50.A14	T50.A15	T50.A16
plague	T50.A91	T50.A92	T50.A93	T50.A94	T50.A95	T50.A96
poliomyelitis	T50.B91	T50.B92	T50.B93	T50.B94	T50.B95	T50.B96
poliovirus	T50.B91	T50.B92	T50.B93	T50.B94	T50.B95	T50.B96
rabies	T50.B91	T50.B92	T50.B93	T50.B94	T50.B95	T50.B96
respiratory syncytial virus	T50.B91	T50.B92	T50.B93	T50.B94	T50.B95	T50.B96
rickettsial NEC	T50.A91	T50.A92	T50.A93	T50.A94	T50.A95	T50.A96
with bacterial component	T50.A21	T50.A22	T50.A23	T50.A24	T50.A25	T50.A26
Rocky Mountain spotted fever	T50.A91	T50.A92	T50.A93	T50.A94	T50.A95	T50.A96
rubella	T50.B91	T50.B92	T50.B93	T50.B94	T50.B95	T50.B96
sabin oral	T50.B91	T50.B92	T50.B93	T50.B94	T50.B95	T50.B96
smallpox	T50.B11	T50.B12	T50.B13	T50.B14	T50.B15	T50.B16
TAB	T50.A91	T50.A92	T50.A93	T50.A94	T50.A95	T50.A96
tetanus	T50.A91	T50.A92	T50.A93	T50.A94	T50.A95	T50.A96
typhoid	T50.A91	T50.A92	T50.A93	T50.A94	T50.A95	T50.A96
typhus	T50.A91	T50.A92	T50.A93	T50.A94	T50.A95	T50.A96
viral NEC	T50.B91	T50.B92	T50.B93	T50.B94	T50.B95	T50.B96
yellow fever	T50.B91	T50.B92	T50.B93	T50.B94	T50.B95	T50.B96
Vaccinia immune globulin	T50.Z11	T50.Z12	T50.Z13	T50.Z14	T50.Z15	T50.Z16
Vaginal contraceptives	T49.8X1	T49.8X2	T49.8X3	T49.8X4	T49.8X5	T49.8X6
Valerian						
root	T42.6X1	T42.6X2	T42.6X3	T42.6X4	T42.6X5	T42.6X6
tincture	T42.6X1	T42.6X2	T42.6X3	T42.6X4	T42.6X5	T42.6X6
Valethamate bromide	T44.3X1	T44.3X2	T44.3X3	T44.3X4	T44.3X5	T44.3X6
Valisone	T49.0X1	T49.0X2	T49.0X3	T49.0X4	T49.0X5	T49.0X6
Valium	T42.4X1	T42.4X2	T42.4X3	T42.4X4	T42.4X5	T42.4X6
Valmid	T42.6X1	T42.6X2	T42.6X3	T42.6X4	T42.6X5	T42.6X6
Valnoctamide	T42.6X1	T42.6X2	T42.6X3	T42.6X4	T42.6X5	T42.6X6
Valproate (sodium)	T42.6X1	T42.6X2	T42.6X3	T42.6X4	T42.6X5	T42.6X6
Valproic acid	T42.6X1	T42.6X2	T42.6X3	T42.6X4	T42.6X5	T42.6X6
Valpromide	T42.6X1	T42.6X2	T42.6X3	T42.6X4	T42.6X5	T42.6X6
Vanadium	T56.891	T56.892	T56.893	T56.894	—	—
Vancomycin	T36.8X1	T36.8X2	T36.8X3	T36.8X4	T36.8X5	T36.8X6
Vapor — see also Gas	T59.91	T59.92	T59.93	T59.94	—	—
kiln (carbon monoxide)	T58.8X1	T58.8X2	T58.8X3	T58.8X4	—	—
lead — see lead						
specified source NEC	T59.891	T59.892	T59.893	T59.894	—	—
Vardenafil	T46.7X1	T46.7X2	T46.7X3	T46.7X4	T46.7X5	T46.7X6
Varicose reduction drug	T46.8X1	T46.8X2	T46.8X3	T46.8X4	T46.8X5	T46.8X6
Varnish	T65.4X1	T65.4X2	T65.4X3	T65.4X4	—	—
cleaner	T52.91	T52.92	T52.93	T52.94	—	—
Vaseline	T49.3X1	T49.3X2	T49.3X3	T49.3X4	T49.3X5	T49.3X6
Vasodilan	T46.7X1	T46.7X2	T46.7X3	T46.7X4	T46.7X5	T46.7X6
Vasodilator						
coronary NEC	T46.3X1	T46.3X2	T46.3X3	T46.3X4	T46.3X5	T46.3X6
peripheral NEC	T46.7X1	T46.7X2	T46.7X3	T46.7X4	T46.7X5	T46.7X6
Vasopressin	T38.891	T38.892	T38.893	T38.894	T38.895	T38.896
Vasopressor drugs	T38.891	T38.892	T38.893	T38.894	T38.895	T38.896
Vecuronium bromide	T48.1X1	T48.1X2	T48.1X3	T48.1X4	T48.1X5	T48.1X6
Vegetable extract, astringent	T49.2X1	T49.2X2	T49.2X3	T49.2X4	T49.2X5	T49.2X6
Venlafaxine	T43.211	T43.212	T43.213	T43.214	T43.215	T43.216
Venom, venomous (bite) (sting)	T63.91	T63.92	T63.93	T63.94	—	—
amphibian NEC	T63.831	T63.832	T63.833	T63.834	—	—
animal NEC	T63.891	T63.892	T63.893	T63.894	—	—
ant	T63.421	T63.422	T63.423	T63.424	—	—
arthropod NEC	T63.481	T63.482	T63.483	T63.484	—	—
bee	T63.441	T63.442	T63.443	T63.444	—	—
centipede	T63.411	T63.412	T63.413	T63.414	—	—
fish	T63.591	T63.592	T63.593	T63.594	—	—
frog	T63.811	T63.812	T63.813	T63.814	—	—
hornet	T63.451	T63.452	T63.453	T63.454	—	—
insect NEC	T63.481	T63.482	T63.483	T63.484	—	—
lizard	T63.121	T63.122	T63.123	T63.124	—	—
marine						
animals	T63.691	T63.692	T63.693	T63.694	—	—
bluebottle	T63.611	T63.612	T63.613	T63.614	—	—
jellyfish NEC	T63.621	T63.622	T63.623	T63.624	—	—
Portugese Man-o-war	T63.611	T63.612	T63.613	T63.614	—	—
sea anemone	T63.631	T63.632	T63.633	T63.634	—	—
specified NEC	T63.691	T63.692	T63.693	T63.694	—	—
fish	T63.591	T63.592	T63.593	T63.594	—	—
plants	T63.711	T63.712	T63.713	T63.714	—	—
sting ray	T63.511	T63.512	T63.513	T63.514	—	—
millipede (tropical)	T63.411	T63.412	T63.413	T63.414	—	—
plant NEC	T63.791	T63.792	T63.793	T63.794	—	—
marine	T63.711	T63.712	T63.713	T63.714	—	—
reptile	T63.191	T63.192	T63.193	T63.194	—	—
gila monster	T63.111	T63.112	T63.113	T63.114	—	—
lizard NEC	T63.121	T63.122	T63.123	T63.124	—	—
scorpion	T63.2X1	T63.2X2	T63.2X3	T63.2X4	—	—
snake	T63.001	T63.002	T63.003	T63.004	—	—
African NEC	T63.081	T63.082	T63.083	T63.084	—	—
American (North) (South) NEC	T63.061	T63.062	T63.063	T63.064	—	—
Asian	T63.081	T63.082	T63.083	T63.084	—	—
Australian	T63.071	T63.072	T63.073	T63.074	—	—
cobra	T63.041	T63.042	T63.043	T63.044	—	—
coral snake	T63.021	T63.022	T63.023	T63.024	—	—
rattlesnake	T63.011	T63.012	T63.013	T63.014	—	—
specified NEC	T63.091	T63.092	T63.093	T63.094	—	—
taipan	T63.031	T63.032	T63.033	T63.034	—	—
specified NEC	T63.891	T63.892	T63.893	T63.894	—	—
spider	T63.301	T63.302	T63.303	T63.304	—	—
black widow	T63.311	T63.312	T63.313	T63.314	—	—
brown recluse	T63.331	T63.332	T63.333	T63.334	—	—
specified NEC	T63.391	T63.392	T63.393	T63.394	—	—
tarantula	T63.321	T63.322	T63.323	T63.324	—	—
sting ray	T63.511	T63.512	T63.513	T63.514	—	—
toad	T63.821	T63.822	T63.823	T63.824	—	—
wasp	T63.461	T63.462	T63.463	T63.464	—	—
Venous sclerosing drug NEC	T46.8X1	T46.8X2	T46.8X3	T46.8X4	T46.8X5	T46.8X6
Ventolin — see Albuterol						
Veramon	T42.3X1	T42.3X2	T42.3X3	T42.3X4	T42.3X5	T42.3X6
Verapamil	T46.1X1	T46.1X2	T46.1X3	T46.1X4	T46.1X5	T46.1X6
Veratrine	T46.5X1	T46.5X2	T46.5X3	T46.5X4	T46.5X5	T46.5X6

Ufenamate — Veratrine

Table of Drugs and Chemicals

Veratrum — Zinc

Substance	Poisoning, Accidental (unintentional)	Poisoning, Intentional Self-harm	Poisoning, Assault	Poisoning, Undetermined	Adverse Effect	Under-dosing
Veratrum						
album	T62.2X1	T62.2X2	T62.2X3	T62.2X4	—	—
alkaloids	T46.5X1	T46.5X2	T46.5X3	T46.5X4	T46.5X5	T46.5X6
viride	T62.2X1	T62.2X2	T62.2X3	T62.2X4	—	—
Verdigris	T60.3X1	T60.3X2	T60.3X3	T60.3X4	—	—
Veronal	T42.3X1	T42.3X2	T42.3X3	T42.3X4	T42.3X5	T42.3X6
Veroxil	T37.4X1	T37.4X2	T37.4X3	T37.4X4	T37.4X5	T37.4X6
Versenate	T50.6X1	T50.6X2	T50.6X3	T50.6X4	T50.6X5	T50.6X6
Versidyne	T39.8X1	T39.8X2	T39.8X3	T39.8X4	T39.8X5	T39.8X6
Vetrabutine	T48.0X1	T48.0X2	T48.0X3	T48.0X4	T48.0X5	T48.0X6
Vidarabine	T37.5X1	T37.5X2	T37.5X3	T37.5X4	T37.5X5	T37.5X6
Vienna						
green	T57.0X1	T57.0X2	T57.0X3	T57.0X4	—	—
insecticide	T60.2X1	T60.2X2	T60.2X3	T60.2X4	—	—
red	T57.0X1	T57.0X2	T57.0X3	T57.0X4	—	—
pharmaceutical dye	T50.991	T50.992	T50.993	T50.994	T50.995	T50.996
Vigabatrin	T42.6X1	T42.6X2	T42.6X3	T42.6X4	T42.6X5	T42.6X6
Viloxazine	T43.291	T43.292	T43.293	T43.294	T43.295	T43.296
Viminol	T39.8X1	T39.8X2	T39.8X3	T39.8X4	T39.8X5	T39.8X6
Vinbarbital, vinbarbitone	T42.3X1	T42.3X2	T42.3X3	T42.3X4	T42.3X5	T42.3X6
Vinblastine	T45.1X1	T45.1X2	T45.1X3	T45.1X4	T45.1X5	T45.1X6
Vinburnine	T46.7X1	T46.7X2	T46.7X3	T46.7X4	T46.7X5	T46.7X6
Vincamine	T45.1X1	T45.1X2	T45.1X3	T45.1X4	T45.1X5	T45.1X6
Vincristine	T45.1X1	T45.1X2	T45.1X3	T45.1X4	T45.1X5	T45.1X6
Vindesine	T45.1X1	T45.1X2	T45.1X3	T45.1X4	T45.1X5	T45.1X6
Vinesthene, vinethene	T41.0X1	T41.0X2	T41.0X3	T41.0X4	T41.0X5	T41.0X6
Vinorelbine tartrate	T45.1X1	T45.1X2	T45.1X3	T45.1X4	T45.1X5	T45.1X6
Vinpocetine	T46.7X1	T46.7X2	T46.7X3	T46.7X4	T46.7X5	T46.7X6
Vinyl						
acetate	T65.891	T65.892	T65.893	T65.894	—	—
bital	T42.3X1	T42.3X2	T42.3X3	T42.3X4	T42.3X5	T42.3X6
bromide	T65.891	T65.892	T65.893	T65.894	—	—
chloride	T59.891	T59.892	T59.893	T59.894	—	—
ether	T41.0X1	T41.0X2	T41.0X3	T41.0X4	T41.0X5	T41.0X6
Vinylbital	T42.3X1	T42.3X2	T42.3X3	T42.3X4	T42.3X5	T42.3X6
Vinylidene chloride	T65.891	T65.892	T65.893	T65.894	—	—
Vioform	T37.8X1	T37.8X2	T37.8X3	T37.8X4	T37.8X5	T37.8X6
topical	T49.0X1	T49.0X2	T49.0X3	T49.0X4	T49.0X5	T49.0X6
Viomycin	T36.8X1	T36.8X2	T36.8X3	T36.8X4	T36.8X5	T36.8X6
Viosterol	T45.2X1	T45.2X2	T45.2X3	T45.2X4	T45.2X5	T45.2X6
Viper (venom)	T63.091	T63.092	T63.093	T63.094	—	—
Viprynium	T37.4X1	T37.4X2	T37.4X3	T37.4X4	T37.4X5	T37.4X6
Viquidil	T46.7X1	T46.7X2	T46.7X3	T46.7X4	T46.7X5	T46.7X6
Viral vaccine NEC	T50.B91	T50.B92	T50.B93	T50.B94	T50.B95	T50.B96
Virginiamycin	T36.8X1	T36.8X2	T36.8X3	T36.8X4	T36.8X5	T36.8X6
Virugon	T37.5X1	T37.5X2	T37.5X3	T37.5X4	T37.5X5	T37.5X6
Viscous agent	T50.901	T50.902	T50.903	T50.904	T50.905	T50.906
Visine	T49.5X1	T49.5X2	T49.5X3	T49.5X4	T49.5X5	T49.5X6
Visnadine	T46.3X1	T46.3X2	T46.3X3	T46.3X4	T46.3X5	T46.3X6
Vitamin NEC	T45.2X1	T45.2X2	T45.2X3	T45.2X4	T45.2X5	T45.2X6
A	T45.2X1	T45.2X2	T45.2X3	T45.2X4	T45.2X5	T45.2X6
B1	T45.2X1	T45.2X2	T45.2X3	T45.2X4	T45.2X5	T45.2X6
B2	T45.2X1	T45.2X2	T45.2X3	T45.2X4	T45.2X5	T45.2X6
B6	T45.2X1	T45.2X2	T45.2X3	T45.2X4	T45.2X5	T45.2X6
B12	T45.2X1	T45.2X2	T45.2X3	T45.2X4	T45.2X5	T45.2X6
B15	T45.2X1	T45.2X2	T45.2X3	T45.2X4	T45.2X5	T45.2X6
B NEC	T45.2X1	T45.2X2	T45.2X3	T45.2X4	T45.2X5	T45.2X6
nicotinic acid	T46.7X1	T46.7X2	T46.7X3	T46.7X4	T46.7X5	T46.7X6
C	T45.2X1	T45.2X2	T45.2X3	T45.2X4	T45.2X5	T45.2X6
D	T45.2X1	T45.2X2	T45.2X3	T45.2X4	T45.2X5	T45.2X6
D2	T45.2X1	T45.2X2	T45.2X3	T45.2X4	T45.2X5	T45.2X6
D3	T45.2X1	T45.2X2	T45.2X3	T45.2X4	T45.2X5	T45.2X6
E	T45.2X1	T45.2X2	T45.2X3	T45.2X4	T45.2X5	T45.2X6
E acetate	T45.2X1	T45.2X2	T45.2X3	T45.2X4	T45.2X5	T45.2X6
hematopoietic	T45.8X1	T45.8X2	T45.8X3	T45.8X4	T45.8X5	T45.8X6
K1	T45.7X1	T45.7X2	T45.7X3	T45.7X4	T45.7X5	T45.7X6
K2	T45.7X1	T45.7X2	T45.7X3	T45.7X4	T45.7X5	T45.7X6
K NEC	T45.7X1	T45.7X2	T45.7X3	T45.7X4	T45.7X5	T45.7X6
PP	T45.2X1	T45.2X2	T45.2X3	T45.2X4	T45.2X5	T45.2X6
ulceroprotectant	T47.1X1	T47.1X2	T47.1X3	T47.1X4	T47.1X5	T47.1X6
Vleminckx's solution	T49.4X1	T49.4X2	T49.4X3	T49.4X4	T49.4X5	T49.4X6
Voltaren — see Diclofenac						
sodium						
Warfarin	T45.511	T45.512	T45.513	T45.514	T45.515	T45.516
rodenticide	T60.4X1-	T60.4X2-	T60.4X3-	T60.4X4-	—	—
sodium	T45.511	T45.512	T45.513	T45.514	T45.515	T45.516
Wasp (sting)	T63.461	T63.462	T63.463	T63.464	—	—
Water						
balance drug	T50.3X1	T50.3X2	T50.3X3	T50.3X4	T50.3X5	T50.3X6
distilled	T50.3X1	T50.3X2	T50.3X3	T50.3X4	T50.3X5	T50.3X6
gas — see Gas, water						

Substance	Poisoning, Accidental (unintentional)	Poisoning, Intentional Self-harm	Poisoning, Assault	Poisoning, Undetermined	Adverse Effect	Under-dosing
Water — continued						
gas — see Gas, water — continued						
incomplete combustion of — see Carbon, monoxide, fuel, utility						
hemlock	T62.2X1	T62.2X2	T62.2X3	T62.2X4	—	—
moccasin (venom)	T63.061	T63.062	T63.063	T63.064	—	—
purified	T50.3X1	T50.3X2	T50.3X3	T50.3X4	T50.3X5	T50.3X6
Wax (paraffin) (petroleum)	T52.0X1	T52.0X2	T52.0X3	T52.0X4	—	—
automobile	T65.891	T65.892	T65.893	T65.894	—	—
floor	T52.0X1	T52.0X2	T52.0X3	T52.0X4	—	—
Weed killers NEC	T60.3X1	T60.3X2	T60.3X3	T60.3X4	—	—
Welldorm	T42.6X1	T42.6X2	T42.6X3	T42.6X4	T42.6X5	T42.6X6
White						
arsenic	T57.0X1	T57.0X2	T57.0X3	T57.0X4	—	—
hellebore	T62.2X1	T62.2X2	T62.2X3	T62.2X4	—	—
lotion (keratolytic)	T49.4X1	T49.4X2	T49.4X3	T49.4X4	T49.4X5	T49.4X6
spirit	T52.0X1	T52.0X2	T52.0X3	T52.0X4	—	—
Whitewash	T65.891	T65.892	T65.893	T65.894	—	—
Whole blood (human)	T45.8X1	T45.8X2	T45.8X3	T45.8X4	T45.8X5	T45.8X6
Wild						
black cherry	T62.2X1	T62.2X2	T62.2X3	T62.2X4	—	—
poisonous plants NEC	T62.2X1	T62.2X2	T62.2X3	T62.2X4	—	—
Window cleaning fluid	T65.891	T65.892	T65.893	T65.894	—	—
Wintergreen (oil)	T49.3X1	T49.3X2	T49.3X3	T49.3X4	T49.3X5	T49.3X6
Wisterine	T62.2X1	T62.2X2	T62.2X3	T62.2X4	—	—
Witch hazel	T49.2X1	T49.2X2	T49.2X3	T49.2X4	T49.2X5	T49.2X6
Wood alcohol or spirit	T51.1X1	T51.1X2	T51.1X3	T51.1X4	—	—
Wool fat (hydrous)	T49.3X1	T49.3X2	T49.3X3	T49.3X4	T49.3X5	T49.3X6
Woorali	T48.1X1	T48.1X2	T48.1X3	T48.1X4	T48.1X5	T48.1X6
Wormseed, American	T37.4X1	T37.4X2	T37.4X3	T37.4X4	T37.4X5	T37.4X6
Xamoterol	T44.5X1	T44.5X2	T44.5X3	T44.5X4	T44.5X5	T44.5X6
Xanthine diuretics	T50.2X1	T50.2X2	T50.2X3	T50.2X4	T50.2X5	T50.2X6
Xanthinol nicotinate	T46.7X1	T46.7X2	T46.7X3	T46.7X4	T46.7X5	T46.7X6
Xanthotoxin	T49.3X1	T49.3X2	T49.3X3	T49.3X4	T49.3X5	T49.3X6
Xantinol nicotinate	T46.7X1	T46.7X2	T46.7X3	T46.7X4	T46.7X5	T46.7X6
Xantocillin	T36.0X1	T36.0X2	T36.0X3	T36.0X4	T36.0X5	T36.0X6
Xenon (127Xe) (133Xe)	T50.8X1	T50.8X2	T50.8X3	T50.8X4	T50.8X5	T50.8X6
Xenysalate	T49.4X1	T49.4X2	T49.4X3	T49.4X4	T49.4X5	T49.4X6
Xibornol	T37.8X1	T37.8X2	T37.8X3	T37.8X4	T37.8X5	T37.8X6
Xigris	T45.511	T45.512	T45.513	T45.514	T45.515	T45.516
Xipamide	T50.2X1	T50.2X2	T50.2X3	T50.2X4	T50.2X5	T50.2X6
Xylene (vapor)	T52.2X1	T52.2X2	T52.2X3	T52.2X4	—	—
Xylocaine (infiltration) (topical)	T41.3X1	T41.3X2	T41.3X3	T41.3X4	T41.3X5	T41.3X6
nerve block (peripheral) (plexus)	T41.3X1	T41.3X2	T41.3X3	T41.3X4	T41.3X5	T41.3X6
spinal	T41.3X1	T41.3X2	T41.3X3	T41.3X4	T41.3X5	T41.3X6
Xylol (vapor)	T52.2X1	T52.2X2	T52.2X3	T52.2X4	—	—
Xylometazoline	T48.5X1	T48.5X2	T48.5X3	T48.5X4	T48.5X5	T48.5X6
Yeast	T45.2X1	T45.2X2	T45.2X3	T45.2X4	T45.2X5	T45.2X6
dried	T45.2X1	T45.2X2	T45.2X3	T45.2X4	T45.2X5	T45.2X6
Yellow						
fever vaccine	T50.B91	T50.B92	T50.B93	T50.B94	T50.B95	T50.B96
jasmine	T62.2X1	T62.2X2	T62.2X3	T62.2X4	—	—
phenolphthalein	T47.2X1	T47.2X2	T47.2X3	T47.2X4	T47.2X5	T47.2X6
Yew	T62.2X1	T62.2X2	T62.2X3	T62.2X4	—	—
Yohimbic acid	T40.991	T40.992	T40.993	T40.994	T40.995	T40.996
Zactane	T39.8X1	T39.8X2	T39.8X3	T39.8X4	T39.8X5	T39.8X6
Zalcitabine	T37.5X1	T37.5X2	T37.5X3	T37.5X4	T37.5X5	T37.5X6
Zaroxolyn	T50.2X1	T50.2X2	T50.2X3	T50.2X4	T50.2X5	T50.2X6
Zephiran (topical)	T49.0X1	T49.0X2	T49.0X3	T49.0X4	T49.0X5	T49.0X6
ophthalmic preparation	T49.5X1	T49.5X2	T49.5X3	T49.5X4	T49.5X5	T49.5X6
Zeranol	T38.7X1	T38.7X2	T38.7X3	T38.7X4	T38.7X5	T38.7X6
Zerone	T51.1X1	T51.1X2	T51.1X3	T51.1X4	—	—
Zidovudine	T37.5X1	T37.5X2	T37.5X3	T37.5X4	T37.5X5	T37.5X6
Zimeldine	T43.221	T43.222	T43.223	T43.224	T43.225	T43.226
Zinc (compounds) (fumes) (vapor)	T56.5X1	T56.5X2	T56.5X3	T56.5X4	—	—
NEC	T49.0X1	T49.0X2	T49.0X3	T49.0X4	T49.0X5	T49.0X6
anti-infectives	T49.0X1	T49.0X2	T49.0X3	T49.0X4	T49.0X5	T49.0X6
antivaricose	T46.8X1	T46.8X2	T46.8X3	T46.8X4	T46.8X5	T46.8X6
bacitracin	T49.0X1	T49.0X2	T49.0X3	T49.0X4	T49.0X5	T49.0X6
chloride (mouthwash)	T49.6X1	T49.6X2	T49.6X3	T49.6X4	T49.6X5	T49.6X6
chromate	T56.5X1	T56.5X2	T56.5X3	T56.5X4	—	—
gelatin	T49.3X1	T49.3X2	T49.3X3	T49.3X4	T49.3X5	T49.3X6
oxide	T49.3X1	T49.3X2	T49.3X3	T49.3X4	T49.3X5	T49.3X6
plaster	T49.3X1	T49.3X2	T49.3X3	T49.3X4	T49.3X5	T49.3X6
peroxide	T49.0X1	T49.0X2	T49.0X3	T49.0X4	T49.0X5	T49.0X6
pesticides	T56.5X1	T56.5X2	T56.5X3	T56.5X4	—	—
phosphide	T60.4X1	T60.4X2	T60.4X3	T60.4X4	—	—
pyrithionate	T49.4X1	T49.4X2	T49.4X3	T49.4X4	T49.4X5	T49.4X6
stearate	T49.3X1	T49.3X2	T49.3X3	T49.3X4	T49.3X5	T49.3X6

Additional Character May Be Required — Refer to the Tabular List for Character Selection   ▽ Subterms under main terms may continue to next column or page

Substance	Poisoning, Accidental (unintentional)	Poisoning, Intentional Self-harm	Poisoning, Assault	Poisoning, Undetermined	Adverse Effect	Under-dosing
Zinc (compounds) (fumes) (vapor) **NEC** — *continued*						
sulfate	T49.5X1	T49.5X2	T49.5X3	T49.5X4	T49.5X5	T49.5X6
ENT agent	T49.6X1	T49.6X2	T49.6X3	T49.6X4	T49.6X5	T49.6X6
ophthalmic solution	T49.5X1	T49.5X2	T49.5X3	T49.5X4	T49.5X5	T49.5X6
topical NEC	T49.0X1	T49.0X2	T49.0X3	T49.0X4	T49.0X5	T49.0X6
undecylenate	T49.0X1	T49.0X2	T49.0X3	T49.0X4	T49.0X5	T49.0X6
Zineb	T60.0X1	T60.0X2	T60.0X3	T60.0X4	—	—
Zinostatin	T45.1X1	T45.1X2	T45.1X3	T45.1X4	T45.1X5	T45.1X6
Zipeprol	T48.3X1	T48.3X2	T48.3X3	T48.3X4	T48.3X5	T48.3X6
Zofenopril	T46.4X1	T46.4X2	T46.4X3	T46.4X4	T46.4X5	T46.4X6
Zolpidem	T42.6X1	T42.6X2	T42.6X3	T42.6X4	T42.6X5	T42.6X6
Zomepirac	T39.391	T39.392	T39.393	T39.394	T39.395	T39.396
Zopiclone	T42.6X1	T42.6X2	T42.6X3	T42.6X4	T42.6X5	T42.6X6
Zorubicin	T45.1X1	T45.1X2	T45.1X3	T45.1X4	T45.1X5	T45.1X6
Zotepine	T43.591	T43.592	T43.593	T43.594	T43.595	T43.596
Zovant	T45.511	T45.512	T45.513	T45.514	T45.515	T45.516
Zoxazolamine	T42.8X1	T42.8X2	T42.8X3	T42.8X4	T42.8X5	T42.8X6
Zuclopenthixol	T43.4X1	T43.4X2	T43.4X3	T43.4X4	T43.4X5	T43.4X6
Zygadenus (venenosus)	T62.2X1	T62.2X2	T62.2X3	T62.2X4	—	—
Zyprexa	T43.591	T43.592	T43.593	T43.594	T43.595	T43.596

External Causes Index

Abandonment — Accident

A

Abandonment (causing exposure to weather conditions)
    (with intent to injure or kill) NEC X58 ☑
Abuse (adult) (child) (mental) (physical) (sexual) X58 ☑
Accident (to) X58 ☑
    aircraft (in transit) (powered) — *see also* Accident,
        transport, aircraft
        due to, caused by cataclysm — *see* Forces of nature,
            by type
    animal-drawn vehicle — *see* Accident, transport, ani-
        mal-drawn vehicle occupant
    animal-rider — *see* Accident, transport, animal-rider
    automobile — *see* Accident, transport, car occupant
    bare foot water skier V94.4 ☑
    boat, boating — *see also* Accident, watercraft
        striking swimmer
            powered V94.11 ☑
            unpowered V94.12 ☑
    bus — *see* Accident, transport, bus occupant
    cable car, not on rails V98.0 ☑
        on rails — *see* Accident, transport, streetcar occu-
            pant
    car — *see* Accident, transport, car occupant
    caused by, due to
        animal NEC W64 ☑
        chain hoist W24.0 ☑
        cold (excessive) — *see* Exposure, cold
        corrosive liquid, substance — *see* Table of Drugs
            and Chemicals
        cutting or piercing instrument — *see* Contact, with,
            by type of instrument
        drive belt W24.0 ☑
        electric
            current — *see* Exposure, electric current
            motor — *see also* Contact, with, by type of ma-
                chine W31.3 ☑
            current (of) W86.8 ☑
        environmental factor NEC X58 ☑
        explosive material — *see* Explosion
        fire, flames — *see* Exposure, fire
        firearm missile — *see* Discharge, firearm by type
        heat (excessive) — *see* Heat
        hot — *see* Contact, with, hot
        ignition — *see* Ignition
        lifting device W24.0 ☑
        lightning — *see* subcategory T75.0 ☑
            causing fire — *see* Exposure, fire
        machine, machinery — *see* Contact, with, by type
            of machine
        natural factor NEC X58 ☑
        pulley (block) W24.0 ☑
        radiation — *see* Radiation
        steam X13.1 ☑
            inhalation X13.0 ☑
            pipe X16 ☑
        thunderbolt — *see* subcategory T75.0 ☑
            causing fire — *see* Exposure, fire
        transmission device W24.1 ☑
    coach — *see* Accident, transport, bus occupant
    coal car — *see* Accident, transport, industrial vehicle
        occupant
    diving — *see also* Fall, into, water
        with
            drowning or submersion — *see* Drowning
    forklift — *see* Accident, transport, industrial vehicle
        occupant
    heavy transport vehicle NOS — *see* Accident, transport,
        truck occupant
    ice yacht V98.2 ☑
    in
        medical, surgical procedure
            as, or due to misadventure — *see* Misadventure
            causing an abnormal reaction or later complica-
                tion without mention of misadventure —
                see also Complication of or following, by
                type of procedure Y84.9
    land yacht V98.1 ☑
    late effect of — *see* W00-X58 with 7th character S
    logging car — *see* Accident, transport, industrial vehicle
        occupant
    machine, machinery — *see also* Contact, with, by type
        of machine
        on board watercraft V93.69 ☑
            explosion — *see* Explosion, in, watercraft

Accident — *continued*
    machine, machinery — *see also* Contact, with, by type
        of machine — *continued*
        on board watercraft — *continued*
            fire — *see* Burn, on board watercraft
            powered craft V93.63 ☑
                ferry boat V93.61 ☑
                fishing boat V93.62 ☑
                jetskis V93.63 ☑
                liner V93.61 ☑
                merchant ship V93.60 ☑
                passenger ship V93.61 ☑
                sailboat V93.64 ☑
    mine tram — *see* Accident, transport, industrial vehicle
        occupant
    mobility scooter (motorized) — *see* Accident, transport,
        pedestrian, conveyance, specified type NEC
    motor scooter — *see* Accident, transport, motorcyclist
    motor vehicle NOS (traffic) — *see also* Accident, trans-
        port V89.2 ☑
        nontraffic V89.0 ☑
        three-wheeled NOS — *see* Accident, transport,
            three-wheeled motor vehicle occupant
    motorcycle NOS — *see* Accident, transport, motorcyclist
    nonmotor vehicle NOS (nontraffic) — *see also* Accident,
        transport V89.1 ☑
        traffic NOS V89.3 ☑
    nontraffic (victim's mode of transport NOS) V88.9 ☑
        collision (between) V88.7 ☑
            bus and truck V88.5 ☑
            car and:
                bus V88.3 ☑
                pickup V88.2 ☑
                three-wheeled motor vehicle V88.0 ☑
                train V88.6 ☑
                truck V88.4 ☑
                two-wheeled motor vehicle V88.0 ☑
                van V88.2 ☑
            specified vehicle NEC and:
                three-wheeled motor vehicle V88.1 ☑
                two-wheeled motor vehicle V88.1 ☑
        known mode of transport — *see* Accident, transport,
            by type of vehicle
        noncollision V88.8 ☑
    on board watercraft V93.89 ☑
        powered craft V93.83 ☑
            ferry boat V93.81 ☑
            fishing boat V93.82 ☑
            jetskis V93.83 ☑
            liner V93.81 ☑
            merchant ship V93.80 ☑
            passenger ship V93.81 ☑
        unpowered craft V93.88 ☑
            canoe V93.85 ☑
            inflatable V93.86 ☑
                in tow
                    recreational V94.31 ☑
                    specified NEC V94.32 ☑
            kayak V93.85 ☑
            sailboat V93.84 ☑
            surf-board V93.88 ☑
            water skis V93.87 ☑
            windsurfer V93.88 ☑
    parachutist V97.29 ☑
        entangled in object V97.21 ☑
        injured on landing V97.22 ☑
    pedal cycle — *see* Accident, transport, pedal cyclist
    pedestrian (on foot)
        with
            another pedestrian W51 ☑
                on pedestrian conveyance NEC V00.09 ☑
                with fall W03 ☑
                    due to ice or snow W00.0 ☑
            roller skater (in-line) V00.01 ☑
            skate boarder V00.02 ☑
            transport vehicle — *see* Accident, transport
        on pedestrian conveyance — *see* Accident, trans-
            port, pedestrian, conveyance
    pick-up truck or van — *see* Accident, transport, pickup
        truck occupant
    quarry truck — *see* Accident, transport, industrial vehi-
        cle occupant
    railway vehicle (any) (in motion) — *see* Accident,
        transport, railway vehicle occupant
        due to cataclysm — *see* Forces of nature, by type

Accident — *continued*
    scooter (non-motorized) — *see* Accident, transport,
        pedestrian, conveyance, scooter
    sequelae of — *see* categories W00-X58 with 7th char-
        acter S
    skateboard — *see* Accident, transport, pedestrian,
        conveyance, skateboard
    ski(ing) — *see* Accident, transport, pedestrian, con-
        veyance
        lift V98.3 ☑
    specified cause NEC X58 ☑
    streetcar — *see* Accident, transport, streetcar occupant
    traffic (victim's mode of transport NOS) V87.9 ☑
        collision (between) V87.7 ☑
            bus and truck V87.5 ☑
            car and:
                bus V87.3 ☑
                pickup V87.2 ☑
                three-wheeled motor vehicle V87.0 ☑
                train V87.6 ☑
                truck V87.4 ☑
                two-wheeled motor vehicle V87.0 ☑
                van V87.2 ☑
            specified vehicle NEC V86.39 ☑
                and
                    three-wheeled motor vehicle V87.1 ☑
                    two-wheeled motor vehicle V87.1 ☑
                driver V86.09 ☑
                passenger V86.19 ☑
                person on outside V86.29 ☑
                while boarding or alighting V86.49 ☑
        known mode of transport — *see* Accident, transport,
            by type of vehicle
        noncollision V87.8 ☑
    transport (involving injury to) V99 ☑
        18 wheeler — *see* Accident, transport, truck occu-
            pant
        agricultural vehicle occupant (nontraffic) V84.9 ☑
            driver V84.5 ☑
            hanger-on V84.7 ☑
            passenger V84.6 ☑
            traffic V84.3 ☑
                driver V84.0 ☑
                hanger-on V84.2 ☑
                passenger V84.1 ☑
            while boarding or alighting V84.4 ☑
        aircraft NEC V97.89 ☑
            military NEC V97.818 ☑
                civilian injured by V97.811 ☑
                with civilian aircraft V97.810 ☑
            occupant injured (in)
                nonpowered craft accident V96.9 ☑
                    balloon V96.00 ☑
                        collision V96.03 ☑
                        crash V96.01 ☑
                        explosion V96.05 ☑
                        fire V96.04 ☑
                        forced landing V96.02 ☑
                        specified type NEC V96.09 ☑
                  glider V96.20 ☑
                    collision V96.23 ☑
                    crash V96.21 ☑
                    explosion V96.25 ☑
                    fire V96.24 ☑
                    forced landing V96.22 ☑
                    specified type NEC V96.29 ☑
                hang glider V96.10 ☑
                    collision V96.13 ☑
                    crash V96.11 ☑
                    explosion V96.15 ☑
                    fire V96.14 ☑
                    forced landing V96.12 ☑
                    specified type NEC V96.19 ☑
                specified craft NEC V96.8 ☑
             powered craft accident V95.9 ☑
                fixed wing NEC
                    commercial V95.30 ☑
                        collision V95.33 ☑
                        crash V95.31 ☑
                        explosion V95.35 ☑
                        fire V95.34 ☑
                        forced landing V95.32 ☑
                        specified type NEC V95.39 ☑
                  private V95.20 ☑
                    collision V95.23 ☑
                    crash V95.21 ☑

Accident — continued
  transport — continued
    aircraft — continued
      occupant injured — continued
        powered craft accident — continued
          fixed wing — continued
            private — continued
              explosion V95.25 ☑
              fire V95.24 ☑
              forced landing V95.22 ☑
              specified type NEC V95.29 ☑
          glider V95.10 ☑
            collision V95.13 ☑
            crash V95.11 ☑
            explosion V95.15 ☑
            fire V95.14 ☑
            forced landing V95.12 ☑
            specified type NEC V95.19 ☑
          helicopter V95.00 ☑
            collision V95.03 ☑
            crash V95.01 ☑
            explosion V95.05 ☑
            fire V95.04 ☑
            forced landing V95.02 ☑
            specified type NEC V95.09 ☑
          spacecraft V95.40 ☑
            collision V95.43 ☑
            crash V95.41 ☑
            explosion V95.45 ☑
            fire V95.44 ☑
            forced landing V95.42 ☑
            specified type NEC V95.49 ☑
          specified craft NEC V95.8 ☑
          ultralight V95.10 ☑
            collision V95.13 ☑
            crash V95.11 ☑
            explosion V95.15 ☑
            fire V95.14 ☑
            forced landing V95.12 ☑
            specified type NEC V95.19 ☑
        specified accident NEC V97.0 ☑
        while boarding or alighting V97.1 ☑
      person (injured by)
        falling from, in or on aircraft V97.0 ☑
        machinery on aircraft V97.89 ☑
        on ground with aircraft involvement V97.39 ☑
        rotating propeller V97.32 ☑
        struck by object falling from aircraft V97.31 ☑
        sucked into aircraft jet V97.33 ☑
        while boarding or alighting aircraft V97.1 ☑
    airport (battery-powered) passenger vehicle — see Accident, transport, industrial vehicle occupant
    all-terrain vehicle occupant (nontraffic) V86.95 ☑
      driver V86.55 ☑
      dune buggy — see Accident, transport, dune buggy occupant
      hanger-on V86.75 ☑
      passenger V86.65 ☑
      snowmobile — see Accident, transport, snowmobile occupant
      specified type NEC V86.99 ☑
        driver V86.59 ☑
        passenger V86.69 ☑
        person on outside V86.79 ☑
      traffic V86.35 ☑
        driver V86.05 ☑
        hanger-on V86.25 ☑
        passenger V86.15 ☑
      while boarding or alighting V86.45 ☑
    ambulance occupant (traffic) V86.31 ☑
      driver V86.01 ☑
      hanger-on V86.21 ☑
      nontraffic V86.91 ☑
        driver V86.51 ☑
        hanger-on V86.71 ☑
        passenger V86.61 ☑
      passenger V86.11 ☑
      while boarding or alighting V86.41 ☑
    animal-drawn vehicle occupant (in) V80.929 ☑
      collision (with)
        animal V80.12 ☑
          being ridden V80.711 ☑
        animal-drawn vehicle V80.721 ☑
        bus V80.42 ☑

Accident — continued
  transport — continued
    animal-drawn vehicle occupant — continued
      collision — continued
        car V80.42 ☑
        fixed or stationary object V80.82 ☑
        military vehicle V80.920 ☑
        nonmotor vehicle V80.791 ☑
        pedal cycle V80.22 ☑
        pedestrian V80.12 ☑
        pickup V80.42 ☑
        railway train or vehicle V80.62 ☑
        specified motor vehicle NEC V80.52 ☑
        streetcar V80.731 ☑
        truck V80.42 ☑
        two- or three-wheeled motor vehicle V80.32 ☑
        van V80.42 ☑
      noncollision V80.02 ☑
      specified circumstance NEC V80.928 ☑
    animal-rider V80.919 ☑
      collision (with)
        animal V80.11 ☑
          being ridden V80.710 ☑
        animal-drawn vehicle V80.720 ☑
        bus V80.41 ☑
        car V80.41 ☑
        fixed or stationary object V80.81 ☑
        military vehicle V80.910 ☑
        nonmotor vehicle V80.790 ☑
        pedal cycle V80.21 ☑
        pedestrian V80.11 ☑
        pickup V80.41 ☑
        railway train or vehicle V80.61 ☑
        specified motor vehicle NEC V80.51 ☑
        streetcar V80.730 ☑
        truck V80.41 ☑
        two- or three-wheeled motor vehicle V80.31 ☑
        van V80.41 ☑
      noncollision V80.018 ☑
        specified as horse rider V80.010 ☑
      specified circumstance NEC V80.918 ☑
    armored car — see Accident, transport, truck occupant
    battery-powered truck (baggage) (mail) — see Accident, transport, industrial vehicle occupant
    bus occupant V79.9 ☑
      collision (with)
        animal (traffic) V70.9 ☑
          being ridden (traffic) V76.9 ☑
            nontraffic V76.3 ☑
            while boarding or alighting V76.4 ☑
          nontraffic V70.3 ☑
          while boarding or alighting V70.4 ☑
        animal-drawn vehicle (traffic) V76.9 ☑
          nontraffic V76.3 ☑
          while boarding or alighting V76.4 ☑
        bus (traffic) V74.9 ☑
          nontraffic V74.3 ☑
          while boarding or alighting V74.4 ☑
        car (traffic) V73.9 ☑
          nontraffic V73.3 ☑
          while boarding or alighting V73.4 ☑
        motor vehicle NOS (traffic) V79.60 ☑
          nontraffic V79.20 ☑
          specified type NEC (traffic) V79.69 ☑
            nontraffic V79.29 ☑
        pedal cycle (traffic) V71.9 ☑
          nontraffic V71.3 ☑
          while boarding or alighting V71.4 ☑
        pickup truck (traffic) V73.9 ☑
          nontraffic V73.3 ☑
          while boarding or alighting V73.4 ☑
        railway vehicle (traffic) V75.9 ☑
          nontraffic V75.3 ☑
          while boarding or alighting V75.4 ☑
        specified vehicle NEC (traffic) V76.9 ☑
          nontraffic V76.3 ☑
          while boarding or alighting V76.4 ☑
        stationary object (traffic) V77.9 ☑
          nontraffic V77.3 ☑
          while boarding or alighting V77.4 ☑
        streetcar (traffic) V76.9 ☑
          nontraffic V76.3 ☑
          while boarding or alighting V76.4 ☑

Accident — continued
  transport — continued
    bus occupant — continued
      collision — continued
        three wheeled motor vehicle (traffic) V72.9 ☑
          nontraffic V72.3 ☑
          while boarding or alighting V72.4 ☑
        truck (traffic) V74.9 ☑
          nontraffic V74.3 ☑
          while boarding or alighting V74.4 ☑
        two wheeled motor vehicle (traffic) V72.9 ☑
          nontraffic V72.3 ☑
          while boarding or alighting V72.4 ☑
        van (traffic) V73.9 ☑
          nontraffic V73.3 ☑
          while boarding or alighting V73.4 ☑
      driver
        collision (with)
          animal (traffic) V70.5 ☑
            being ridden (traffic) V76.5 ☑
              nontraffic V76.0 ☑
            nontraffic V70.0 ☑
          animal-drawn vehicle (traffic) V76.5 ☑
            nontraffic V76.0 ☑
          bus (traffic) V74.5 ☑
            nontraffic V74.0 ☑
          car (traffic) V73.5 ☑
            nontraffic V73.0 ☑
          motor vehicle NOS (traffic) V79.40 ☑
            nontraffic V79.00 ☑
            specified type NEC (traffic) V79.49 ☑
              nontraffic V79.09 ☑
          pedal cycle (traffic) V71.5 ☑
            nontraffic V71.0 ☑
          pickup truck (traffic) V73.5 ☑
            nontraffic V73.0 ☑
          railway vehicle (traffic) V75.5 ☑
            nontraffic V75.0 ☑
          specified vehicle NEC (traffic) V76.5 ☑
            nontraffic V76.0 ☑
          stationary object (traffic) V77.5 ☑
            nontraffic V77.0 ☑
          streetcar (traffic) V76.5 ☑
            nontraffic V76.0 ☑
          three wheeled motor vehicle (traffic) V72.5 ☑
            nontraffic V72.0 ☑
          truck (traffic) V74.5 ☑
            nontraffic V74.0 ☑
          two wheeled motor vehicle (traffic) V72.5 ☑
            nontraffic V72.0 ☑
          van (traffic) V73.5 ☑
            nontraffic V73.0 ☑
        noncollision accident (traffic) V78.5 ☑
          nontraffic V78.0 ☑
      hanger-on
        collision (with)
          animal (traffic) V70.7 ☑
            being ridden (traffic) V76.7 ☑
              nontraffic V76.2 ☑
            nontraffic V70.2 ☑
          animal-drawn vehicle (traffic) V76.7 ☑
            nontraffic V76.2 ☑
          bus (traffic) V74.7 ☑
            nontraffic V74.2 ☑
          car (traffic) V73.7 ☑
            nontraffic V73.2 ☑
          pedal cycle (traffic) V71.7 ☑
            nontraffic V71.2 ☑
          pickup truck (traffic) V73.7 ☑
            nontraffic V73.2 ☑
          railway vehicle (traffic) V75.7 ☑
            nontraffic V75.2 ☑
          specified vehicle NEC (traffic) V76.7 ☑
            nontraffic V76.2 ☑
          stationary object (traffic) V77.7 ☑
            nontraffic V77.2 ☑
          streetcar (traffic) V76.7 ☑
            nontraffic V76.2 ☑
          three wheeled motor vehicle (traffic) V72.7 ☑
            nontraffic V72.2 ☑
          truck (traffic) V74.7 ☑
            nontraffic V74.2 ☑

Accident — *continued*
  transport — *continued*
    bus occupant — *continued*
      hanger-on — *continued*
        collision — *continued*
          two wheeled motor vehicle (traffic) V72.7 ☑
            nontraffic V72.2 ☑
          van (traffic) V73.7 ☑
            nontraffic V73.2 ☑
        noncollision accident (traffic) V78.7 ☑
          nontraffic V78.2 ☑
      noncollision accident (traffic) V78.9 ☑
        nontraffic V78.3 ☑
        while boarding or alighting V78.4 ☑
      nontraffic V79.3 ☑
      passenger
        collision (with)
          animal (traffic) V70.6 ☑
            being ridden (traffic) V76.6 ☑
              nontraffic V76.1 ☑
            nontraffic V70.1 ☑
          animal-drawn vehicle (traffic) V76.6 ☑
            nontraffic V76.1 ☑
          bus (traffic) V74.6 ☑
            nontraffic V74.1 ☑
          car (traffic) V73.6 ☑
            nontraffic V73.1 ☑
          motor vehicle NOS (traffic) V79.50 ☑
            nontraffic V79.10 ☑
            specified type NEC (traffic) V79.59 ☑
              nontraffic V79.19 ☑
          pedal cycle (traffic) V71.6 ☑
            nontraffic V71.1 ☑
          pickup truck (traffic) V73.6 ☑
            nontraffic V73.1 ☑
          railway vehicle (traffic) V75.6 ☑
            nontraffic V75.1 ☑
          specified vehicle NEC (traffic) V76.6 ☑
            nontraffic V76.1 ☑
          stationary object (traffic) V77.6 ☑
            nontraffic V77.1 ☑
          streetcar (traffic) V76.6 ☑
            nontraffic V76.1 ☑
          three wheeled motor vehicle (traffic) V72.6 ☑
            nontraffic V72.1 ☑
          truck (traffic) V74.6 ☑
            nontraffic V74.1 ☑
          two wheeled motor vehicle (traffic) V72.6 ☑
            nontraffic V72.1 ☑
          van (traffic) V73.6 ☑
            nontraffic V73.1 ☑
        noncollision accident (traffic) V78.6 ☑
          nontraffic V78.1 ☑
      specified type NEC V79.88 ☑
      military vehicle V79.81 ☑
    cable car, not on rails V98.0 ☑
      on rails — *see* Accident, transport, streetcar occupant
    car occupant V49.9 ☑
      ambulance occupant — *see* Accident, transport, ambulance occupant
      collision (with)
        animal (traffic) V40.9 ☑
          being ridden (traffic) V46.9 ☑
            nontraffic V46.3 ☑
            while boarding or alighting V46.4 ☑
          nontraffic V40.3 ☑
          while boarding or alighting V40.4 ☑
        animal-drawn vehicle (traffic) V46.9 ☑
          nontraffic V46.3 ☑
          while boarding or alighting V46.4 ☑
        bus (traffic) V44.9 ☑
          nontraffic V44.3 ☑
          while boarding or alighting V44.4 ☑
        car (traffic) V43.92 ☑
          nontraffic V43.32 ☑
          while boarding or alighting V43.42 ☑
        motor vehicle NOS (traffic) V49.60 ☑
          nontraffic V49.20 ☑
          specified type NEC (traffic) V49.69 ☑
            nontraffic V49.29 ☑
        pedal cycle (traffic) V41.9 ☑
          nontraffic V41.3 ☑

Accident — *continued*
  transport — *continued*
    car occupant — *continued*
      collision — *continued*
        pedal cycle — *continued*
          while boarding or alighting V41.4 ☑
        pickup truck (traffic) V43.93 ☑
          nontraffic V43.33 ☑
          while boarding or alighting V43.43 ☑
        railway vehicle (traffic) V45.9 ☑
          nontraffic V45.3 ☑
          while boarding or alighting V45.4 ☑
        specified vehicle NEC (traffic) V46.9 ☑
          nontraffic V46.3 ☑
          while boarding or alighting V46.4 ☑
        sport utility vehicle (traffic) V43.91 ☑
          nontraffic V43.31 ☑
          while boarding or alighting V43.41 ☑
        stationary object (traffic) V47.9 ☑
          nontraffic V47.3 ☑
          while boarding or alighting V47.4 ☑
        streetcar (traffic) V46.9 ☑
          nontraffic V46.3 ☑
          while boarding or alighting V46.4 ☑
        three wheeled motor vehicle (traffic) V42.9 ☑
          nontraffic V42.3 ☑
          while boarding or alighting V42.4 ☑
        truck (traffic) V44.9 ☑
          nontraffic V44.3 ☑
          while boarding or alighting V44.4 ☑
        two wheeled motor vehicle (traffic) V42.9 ☑
          nontraffic V42.3 ☑
          while boarding or alighting V42.4 ☑
        van (traffic) V43.94 ☑
          nontraffic V43.34 ☑
          while boarding or alighting V43.44 ☑
      driver
        collision (with)
          animal (traffic) V40.5 ☑
            being ridden (traffic) V46.5 ☑
              nontraffic V46.0 ☑
            nontraffic V40.0 ☑
          animal-drawn vehicle (traffic) V46.5 ☑
            nontraffic V46.0 ☑
          bus (traffic) V44.5 ☑
            nontraffic V44.0 ☑
          car (traffic) V43.52 ☑
            nontraffic V43.02 ☑
          motor vehicle NOS (traffic) V49.40 ☑
            nontraffic V49.00 ☑
            specified type NEC (traffic) V49.49 ☑
              nontraffic V49.09 ☑
          pedal cycle (traffic) V41.5 ☑
            nontraffic V41.0 ☑
          pickup truck (traffic) V43.53 ☑
            nontraffic V43.03 ☑
          railway vehicle (traffic) V45.5 ☑
            nontraffic V45.0 ☑
          specified vehicle NEC (traffic) V46.5 ☑
            nontraffic V46.0 ☑
          sport utility vehicle (traffic) V43.51 ☑
            nontraffic V43.01 ☑
          stationary object (traffic) V47.5 ☑
            nontraffic V47.0 ☑
          streetcar (traffic) V46.5 ☑
            nontraffic V46.0 ☑
          three wheeled motor vehicle (traffic) V42.5 ☑
            nontraffic V42.0 ☑
          truck (traffic) V44.5 ☑
            nontraffic V44.0 ☑
          two wheeled motor vehicle (traffic) V42.5 ☑
            nontraffic V42.0 ☑
          van (traffic) V43.54 ☑
            nontraffic V43.04 ☑
        noncollision accident (traffic) V48.5 ☑
          nontraffic V48.0 ☑
      hanger-on
        collision (with)
          animal (traffic) V40.7 ☑
            being ridden (traffic) V46.7 ☑
              nontraffic V46.2 ☑
            nontraffic V40.2 ☑
          animal-drawn vehicle (traffic) V46.7 ☑
            nontraffic V46.2 ☑

Accident — *continued*
  transport — *continued*
    car occupant — *continued*
      hanger-on — *continued*
        collision — *continued*
          bus (traffic) V44.7 ☑
            nontraffic V44.2 ☑
          car (traffic) V43.72 ☑
            nontraffic V43.22 ☑
          pedal cycle (traffic) V41.7 ☑
            nontraffic V41.2 ☑
          pickup truck (traffic) V43.73 ☑
            nontraffic V43.23 ☑
          railway vehicle (traffic) V45.7 ☑
            nontraffic V45.2 ☑
          specified vehicle NEC (traffic) V46.7 ☑
            nontraffic V46.2 ☑
          sport utility vehicle (traffic) V43.71 ☑
            nontraffic V43.21 ☑
          stationary object (traffic) V47.7 ☑
            nontraffic V47.2 ☑
          streetcar (traffic) V46.7 ☑
            nontraffic V46.2 ☑
          three wheeled motor vehicle (traffic) V42.7 ☑
            nontraffic V42.2 ☑
          truck (traffic) V44.7 ☑
            nontraffic V44.2 ☑
          two wheeled motor vehicle (traffic) V42.7 ☑
            nontraffic V42.2 ☑
          van (traffic) V43.74 ☑
            nontraffic V43.24 ☑
        noncollision accident (traffic) V48.7 ☑
          nontraffic V48.2 ☑
      noncollision accident (traffic) V48.9 ☑
        nontraffic V48.3 ☑
        while boarding or alighting V48.4 ☑
      nontraffic V49.3 ☑
      passenger
        collision (with)
          animal (traffic) V40.6 ☑
            being ridden (traffic) V46.6 ☑
              nontraffic V46.1 ☑
            nontraffic V40.1 ☑
          animal-drawn vehicle (traffic) V46.6 ☑
            nontraffic V46.1 ☑
          bus (traffic) V44.6 ☑
            nontraffic V44.1 ☑
          car (traffic) V43.62 ☑
            nontraffic V43.12 ☑
          motor vehicle NOS (traffic) V49.50 ☑
            nontraffic V49.10 ☑
            specified type NEC (traffic) V49.59 ☑
              nontraffic V49.19 ☑
          pedal cycle (traffic) V41.6 ☑
            nontraffic V41.1 ☑
          pickup truck (traffic) V43.63 ☑
            nontraffic V43.13 ☑
          railway vehicle (traffic) V45.6 ☑
            nontraffic V45.1 ☑
          specified vehicle NEC (traffic) V46.6 ☑
            nontraffic V46.1 ☑
          sport utility vehicle (traffic) V43.61 ☑
            nontraffic V43.11 ☑
          stationary object (traffic) V47.6 ☑
            nontraffic V47.1 ☑
          streetcar (traffic) V46.6 ☑
            nontraffic V46.1 ☑
          three wheeled motor vehicle (traffic) V42.6 ☑
            nontraffic V42.1 ☑
          truck (traffic) V44.6 ☑
            nontraffic V44.1 ☑
          two wheeled motor vehicle (traffic) V42.6 ☑
            nontraffic V42.1 ☑
          van (traffic) V43.64 ☑
            nontraffic V43.14 ☑
        noncollision accident (traffic) V48.6 ☑
          nontraffic V48.1 ☑
      specified type NEC V49.88 ☑
      military vehicle V49.81 ☑
    coal car — *see* Accident, transport, industrial vehicle occupant
    construction vehicle occupant (nontraffic) V85.9 ☑

☑ Additional Character Required — Refer to the Tabular List for Character Selection   ▽ Subterms under main terms may continue to next column or page

Accident — *continued*
  transport — *continued*
    construction vehicle occupant — *continued*
      driver V85.5 ☑
      hanger-on V85.7 ☑
      passenger V85.6 ☑
      traffic V85.3 ☑
        driver V85.0 ☑
        hanger-on V85.2 ☑
        passenger V85.1 ☑
      while boarding or alighting V85.4 ☑
    dirt bike rider (nontraffic) V86.96 ☑
      driver V86.56 ☑
      hanger-on V86.76 ☑
      passenger V86.66 ☑
      traffic V86.36 ☑
        driver V86.06 ☑
        hanger-on V86.26 ☑
        passenger V86.16 ☑
      while boarding or alighting V86.46 ☑
    due to cataclysm — *see* Forces of nature, by type
    dune buggy occupant (nontraffic) V86.93 ☑
      driver V86.53 ☑
      hanger-on V86.73 ☑
      passenger V86.63 ☑
      traffic V86.33 ☑
        driver V86.03 ☑
        hanger-on V86.23 ☑
        passenger V86.13 ☑
      while boarding or alighting V86.43 ☑
    forklift — *see* Accident, transport, industrial vehicle occupant
    go cart — *see* Accident, transport, all-terrain vehicle occupant
    golf cart — *see* Accident, transport, all-terrain vehicle occupant
    heavy transport vehicle occupant — *see* Accident, transport, truck occupant
    ice yacht V98.2 ☑
    industrial vehicle occupant (nontraffic) V83.9 ☑
      driver V83.5 ☑
      hanger-on V83.7 ☑
      passenger V83.6 ☑
      traffic V83.3 ☑
        driver V83.0 ☑
        hanger-on V83.2 ☑
        passenger V83.1 ☑
      while boarding or alighting V83.4 ☑
    interurban electric car — *see* Accident, transport, streetcar
    land yacht V98.1 ☑
    logging car — *see* Accident, transport, industrial vehicle occupant
    military vehicle occupant (traffic) V86.34 ☑
      driver V86.04 ☑
      hanger-on V86.24 ☑
      nontraffic V86.94 ☑
        driver V86.54 ☑
        hanger-on V86.74 ☑
        passenger V86.64 ☑
      passenger V86.14 ☑
      while boarding or alighting V86.44 ☑
    mine tram — *see* Accident, transport, industrial vehicle occupant
    motor vehicle NEC occupant (traffic) V89.2 ☑
    motorcoach — *see* Accident, transport, bus occupant
    motor/cross bike rider — *see also* Accident, transport, dirt bike rider V86.96 ☑
    motorcyclist V29.9 ☑
      collision (with)
        animal (traffic) V20.9 ☑
          being ridden (traffic) V26.9 ☑
            nontraffic V26.2 ☑
            while boarding or alighting V26.3 ☑
          nontraffic V20.2 ☑
          while boarding or alighting V20.3 ☑
        animal-drawn vehicle (traffic) V26.9 ☑
          nontraffic V26.2 ☑
          while boarding or alighting V26.3 ☑
        bus (traffic) V24.9 ☑
          nontraffic V24.2 ☑
          while boarding or alighting V24.3 ☑
        car (traffic) V23.9 ☑
          nontraffic V23.2 ☑
          while boarding or alighting V23.3 ☑

Accident — *continued*
  transport — *continued*
    motorcyclist — *continued*
      collision — *continued*
        motor vehicle NOS (traffic) V29.60 ☑
          nontraffic V29.20 ☑
          specified type NEC (traffic) V29.69 ☑
            nontraffic V29.29 ☑
        pedal cycle (traffic) V21.9 ☑
          nontraffic V21.2 ☑
          while boarding or alighting V21.3 ☑
        pickup truck (traffic) V23.9 ☑
          nontraffic V23.2 ☑
          while boarding or alighting V23.3 ☑
        railway vehicle (traffic) V25.9 ☑
          nontraffic V25.2 ☑
          while boarding or alighting V25.3 ☑
        specified vehicle NEC (traffic) V26.9 ☑
          nontraffic V26.2 ☑
          while boarding or alighting V26.3 ☑
        stationary object (traffic) V27.9 ☑
          nontraffic V27.2 ☑
          while boarding or alighting V27.3 ☑
        streetcar (traffic) V26.9 ☑
          nontraffic V26.2 ☑
          while boarding or alighting V26.3 ☑
        three wheeled motor vehicle (traffic) V22.9 ☑
          nontraffic V22.2 ☑
          while boarding or alighting V22.3 ☑
        truck (traffic) V24.9 ☑
          nontraffic V24.2 ☑
          while boarding or alighting V24.3 ☑
        two wheeled motor vehicle (traffic) V22.9 ☑
          nontraffic V22.2 ☑
          while boarding or alighting V22.3 ☑
        van (traffic) V23.9 ☑
          nontraffic V23.2 ☑
          while boarding or alighting V23.3 ☑
      driver
        collision (with)
          animal (traffic) V20.4 ☑
            being ridden (traffic) V26.4 ☑
              nontraffic V26.0 ☑
            nontraffic V20.0 ☑
          animal-drawn vehicle (traffic) V26.4 ☑
            nontraffic V26.0 ☑
          bus (traffic) V24.4 ☑
            nontraffic V24.0 ☑
          car (traffic) V23.4 ☑
            nontraffic V23.0 ☑
          motor vehicle NOS (traffic) V29.40 ☑
            nontraffic V29.00 ☑
            specified type NEC (traffic) V29.49 ☑
              nontraffic V29.09 ☑
          pedal cycle (traffic) V21.4 ☑
            nontraffic V21.0 ☑
          pickup truck (traffic) V23.4 ☑
            nontraffic V23.0 ☑
          railway vehicle (traffic) V25.4 ☑
            nontraffic V25.0 ☑
          specified vehicle NEC (traffic) V26.4 ☑
            nontraffic V26.0 ☑
          stationary object (traffic) V27.4 ☑
            nontraffic V27.0 ☑
          streetcar (traffic) V26.4 ☑
            nontraffic V26.0 ☑
          three wheeled motor vehicle (traffic) V22.4 ☑
            nontraffic V22.0 ☑
          truck (traffic) V24.4 ☑
            nontraffic V24.0 ☑
          two wheeled motor vehicle (traffic) V22.4 ☑
            nontraffic V22.0 ☑
          van (traffic) V23.4 ☑
            nontraffic V23.0 ☑
        noncollision accident (traffic) V28.4 ☑
          nontraffic V28.0 ☑
      noncollision accident (traffic) V28.9 ☑
        nontraffic V28.2 ☑
        while boarding or alighting V28.3 ☑
      nontraffic V29.3 ☑
      passenger
        collision (with)
          animal (traffic) V20.5 ☑
            being ridden (traffic) V26.5 ☑

Accident — *continued*
  transport — *continued*
    motorcyclist — *continued*
      passenger — *continued*
        collision — *continued*
          animal — *continued*
            being ridden — *continued*
              nontraffic V26.1 ☑
            nontraffic V20.1 ☑
          animal-drawn vehicle (traffic) V26.5 ☑
            nontraffic V26.1 ☑
          bus (traffic) V24.5 ☑
            nontraffic V24.1 ☑
          car (traffic) V23.5 ☑
            nontraffic V23.1 ☑
          motor vehicle NOS (traffic) V29.50 ☑
            nontraffic V29.10 ☑
            specified type NEC (traffic) V29.59 ☑
              nontraffic V29.19 ☑
          pedal cycle (traffic) V21.5 ☑
            nontraffic V21.1 ☑
          pickup truck (traffic) V23.5 ☑
            nontraffic V23.1 ☑
          railway vehicle (traffic) V25.5 ☑
            nontraffic V25.1 ☑
          specified vehicle NEC (traffic) V26.5 ☑
            nontraffic V26.1 ☑
          stationary object (traffic) V27.5 ☑
            nontraffic V27.1 ☑
          streetcar (traffic) V26.5 ☑
            nontraffic V26.1 ☑
          three wheeled motor vehicle (traffic) V22.5 ☑
            nontraffic V22.1 ☑
          truck (traffic) V24.5 ☑
            nontraffic V24.1 ☑
          two wheeled motor vehicle (traffic) V22.5 ☑
            nontraffic V22.1 ☑
          van (traffic) V23.5 ☑
            nontraffic V23.1 ☑
        noncollision accident (traffic) V28.5 ☑
          nontraffic V28.1 ☑
    specified type NEC V29.88 ☑
    military vehicle V29.81 ☑
    occupant (of)
      aircraft (powered) V95.9 ☑
        fixed wing
          commercial — *see* Accident, transport, aircraft, occupant, powered, fixed wing, commercial
          private — *see* Accident, transport, aircraft, occupant, powered, fixed wing, private
        nonpowered V96.9 ☑
        specified NEC V95.8 ☑
      airport battery-powered vehicle — *see* Accident, transport, industrial vehicle occupant
      all-terrain vehicle (ATV) — *see* Accident, transport, all-terrain vehicle occupant
      animal-drawn vehicle — *see* Accident, transport, animal-drawn vehicle occupant
      automobile — *see* Accident, transport, car occupant
      balloon V96.00 ☑
      battery-powered vehicle — *see* Accident, transport, industrial vehicle occupant
      bicycle — *see* Accident, transport, pedal cyclist
        motorized — *see* Accident, transport, motorcycle rider
      boat NEC — *see* Accident, watercraft
      bulldozer — *see* Accident, transport, construction vehicle occupant
      bus — *see* Accident, transport, bus occupant
      cable car (on rails) — *see also* Accident, transport, streetcar occupant
        not on rails V98.0 ☑
      car — *see also* Accident, transport, car occupant
        cable (on rails) — *see also* Accident, transport, streetcar occupant
        not on rails V98.0 ☑
      coach — *see* Accident, transport, bus occupant
      coal-car — *see* Accident, transport, industrial vehicle occupant
      digger — *see* Accident, transport, construction vehicle occupant

Accident — *continued*
  transport — *continued*
    occupant — *continued*
      dump truck — *see* Accident, transport, construction vehicle occupant
      earth-leveler — *see* Accident, transport, construction vehicle occupant
      farm machinery (self-propelled) — *see* Accident, transport, agricultural vehicle occupant
      forklift — *see* Accident, transport, industrial vehicle occupant
      glider (unpowered) V96.20 ☑
        hang V96.10 ☑
        powered (microlight) (ultralight) — *see* Accident, transport, aircraft, occupant, powered, glider
      glider (unpowered) NEC V96.20 ☑
      hang-glider V96.10 ☑
      harvester — *see* Accident, transport, agricultural vehicle occupant
      heavy (transport) vehicle — *see* Accident, transport, truck occupant
      helicopter — *see* Accident, transport, aircraft, occupant, helicopter
      ice-yacht V98.2 ☑
      kite (carrying person) V96.8 ☑
      land-yacht V98.1 ☑
      logging car — *see* Accident, transport, industrial vehicle occupant
      mechanical shovel — *see* Accident, transport, construction vehicle occupant
      microlight — *see* Accident, transport, aircraft, occupant, powered, glider
      minibus — *see* Accident, transport, pickup truck occupant
      minivan — *see* Accident, transport, pickup truck occupant
      moped — *see* Accident, transport, motorcycle
      motor scooter — *see* Accident, transport, motorcycle
      motorcycle (with sidecar) — *see* Accident, transport, motorcycle
      off-road motor-vehicle — *see also* Accident, transport, all-terrain vehicle occupant V86.99 ☑
      pedal cycle — *see also* Accident, transport, pedal cyclist
      pick-up (truck) — *see* Accident, transport, pickup truck occupant
      railway (train) (vehicle) (subterranean) (elevated) — *see* Accident, transport, railway vehicle occupant
      rickshaw — *see* Accident, transport, pedal cycle
        motorized — *see* Accident, transport, three-wheeled motor vehicle
        pedal driven — *see* Accident, transport, pedal cyclist
      road-roller — *see* Accident, transport, construction vehicle occupant
      ship NOS V94.9 ☑
      ski-lift (chair) (gondola) V98.3 ☑
      snowmobile — *see* Accident, transport, snowmobile occupant
      spacecraft, spaceship — *see* Accident, transport, aircraft, occupant, spacecraft
      sport utility vehicle — *see* Accident, transport, pickup truck occupant
      streetcar (interurban) (operating on public street or highway) — *see* Accident, transport, streetcar occupant
      SUV — *see* Accident, transport, pickup truck occupant
      téléférique V98.0 ☑
      three-wheeled vehicle (motorized) — *see also* Accident, transport, three-wheeled motor vehicle occupant
        nonmotorized — *see* Accident, transport, pedal cycle
      tractor (farm) (and trailer) — *see* Accident, transport, agricultural vehicle occupant
      train — *see* Accident, transport, railway vehicle occupant
      tram — *see* Accident, transport, streetcar occupant
        in mine or quarry — *see* Accident, transport, industrial vehicle occupant
      tricycle — *see* Accident, transport, pedal cycle

Accident — *continued*
  transport — *continued*
    occupant — *continued*
      tricycle — *see* Accident, transport, pedal cycle — *continued*
        motorized — *see* Accident, transport, three-wheeled motor vehicle
      trolley — *see* Accident, transport, streetcar occupant
        in mine or quarry — *see* Accident, transport, industrial vehicle occupant
        tub, in mine or quarry — *see* Accident, transport, industrial vehicle occupant
      ultralight — *see* Accident, transport, aircraft, occupant, powered, glider
      van — *see* Accident, transport, van occupant
      vehicle NEC V89.9 ☑
        heavy transport — *see* Accident, transport, truck occupant
        motor (traffic) NEC V89.2 ☑
        nontraffic NEC V89.0 ☑
      watercraft NOS V94.9 ☑
        causing drowning — *see* Drowning, resulting from accident to boat
    off-road motor-vehicle — *see also* Accident, transport, all-terrain vehicle occupant V86.99 ☑
    parachutist V97.29 ☑
      after accident to aircraft — *see* Accident, transport, aircraft
      entangled in object V97.21 ☑
      injured on landing V97.22 ☑
    pedal cyclist V19.9 ☑
      collision (with)
        animal (traffic) V10.9 ☑
          being ridden (traffic) V16.9 ☑
            nontraffic V16.2 ☑
            while boarding or alighting V16.3 ☑
          nontraffic V10.2 ☑
          while boarding or alighting V10.3 ☑
        animal-drawn vehicle (traffic) V16.9 ☑
          nontraffic V16.2 ☑
          while boarding or alighting V16.3 ☑
        bus (traffic) V14.9 ☑
          nontraffic V14.2 ☑
          while boarding or alighting V14.3 ☑
        car (traffic) V13.9 ☑
          nontraffic V13.2 ☑
          while boarding or alighting V13.3 ☑
        motor vehicle NOS (traffic) V19.60 ☑
          nontraffic V19.20 ☑
          specified type NEC (traffic) V19.69 ☑
            nontraffic V19.29 ☑
        pedal cycle (traffic) V11.9 ☑
          nontraffic V11.2 ☑
          while boarding or alighting V11.3 ☑
        pickup truck (traffic) V13.9 ☑
          nontraffic V13.2 ☑
          while boarding or alighting V13.3 ☑
        railway vehicle (traffic) V15.9 ☑
          nontraffic V15.2 ☑
          while boarding or alighting V15.3 ☑
        specified vehicle NEC (traffic) V16.9 ☑
          nontraffic V16.2 ☑
          while boarding or alighting V16.3 ☑
        stationary object (traffic) V17.9 ☑
          nontraffic V17.2 ☑
          while boarding or alighting V17.3 ☑
        streetcar (traffic) V16.9 ☑
          nontraffic V16.2 ☑
          while boarding or alighting V16.3 ☑
        three wheeled motor vehicle (traffic) V12.9 ☑
          nontraffic V12.2 ☑
          while boarding or alighting V12.3 ☑
        truck (traffic) V14.9 ☑
          nontraffic V14.2 ☑
          while boarding or alighting V14.3 ☑
        two wheeled motor vehicle (traffic) V12.9 ☑
          nontraffic V12.2 ☑
          while boarding or alighting V12.3 ☑
        van (traffic) V13.9 ☑
          nontraffic V13.2 ☑
          while boarding or alighting V13.3 ☑
      driver
        collision (with)
          animal (traffic) V10.4 ☑
            being ridden (traffic) V16.4 ☑

Accident — *continued*
  transport — *continued*
    pedal cyclist — *continued*
      driver — *continued*
        collision — *continued*
          animal — *continued*
            being ridden — *continued*
              nontraffic V16.0 ☑
            nontraffic V10.0 ☑
          animal-drawn vehicle (traffic) V16.4 ☑
            nontraffic V16.0 ☑
          bus (traffic) V14.4 ☑
            nontraffic V14.0 ☑
          car (traffic) V13.4 ☑
            nontraffic V13.0 ☑
          motor vehicle NOS (traffic) V19.40 ☑
            nontraffic V19.00 ☑
            specified type NEC (traffic) V19.49 ☑
              nontraffic V19.09 ☑
          pedal cycle (traffic) V11.4 ☑
            nontraffic V11.0 ☑
          pickup truck (traffic) V13.4 ☑
            nontraffic V13.0 ☑
          railway vehicle (traffic) V15.4 ☑
            nontraffic V15.0 ☑
          specified vehicle NEC (traffic) V16.4 ☑
            nontraffic V16.0 ☑
          stationary object (traffic) V17.4 ☑
            nontraffic V17.0 ☑
          streetcar (traffic) V16.4 ☑
            nontraffic V16.0 ☑
          three wheeled motor vehicle (traffic) V12.4 ☑
            nontraffic V12.0 ☑
          truck (traffic) V14.4 ☑
            nontraffic V14.0 ☑
          two wheeled motor vehicle (traffic) V12.4 ☑
            nontraffic V12.0 ☑
          van (traffic) V13.4 ☑
            nontraffic V13.0 ☑
        noncollision accident (traffic) V18.4 ☑
          nontraffic V18.0 ☑
      noncollision accident (traffic) V18.9 ☑
        nontraffic V18.2 ☑
        while boarding or alighting V18.3 ☑
      nontraffic V19.3 ☑
      passenger
        collision (with)
          animal (traffic) V10.5 ☑
            being ridden (traffic) V16.5 ☑
              nontraffic V16.1 ☑
            nontraffic V10.1 ☑
          animal-drawn vehicle (traffic) V16.5 ☑
            nontraffic V16.1 ☑
          bus (traffic) V14.5 ☑
            nontraffic V14.1 ☑
          car (traffic) V13.5 ☑
            nontraffic V13.1 ☑
          motor vehicle NOS (traffic) V19.50 ☑
            nontraffic V19.10 ☑
            specified type NEC (traffic) V19.59 ☑
              nontraffic V19.19 ☑
          pedal cycle (traffic) V11.5 ☑
            nontraffic V11.1 ☑
          pickup truck (traffic) V13.5 ☑
            nontraffic V13.1 ☑
          railway vehicle (traffic) V15.5 ☑
            nontraffic V15.1 ☑
          specified vehicle NEC (traffic) V16.5 ☑
            nontraffic V16.1 ☑
          stationary object (traffic) V17.5 ☑
            nontraffic V17.1 ☑
          streetcar (traffic) V16.5 ☑
            nontraffic V16.1 ☑
          three wheeled motor vehicle (traffic) V12.5 ☑
            nontraffic V12.1 ☑
          truck (traffic) V14.5 ☑
            nontraffic V14.1 ☑
          two wheeled motor vehicle (traffic) V12.5 ☑
            nontraffic V12.1 ☑
          van (traffic) V13.5 ☑
            nontraffic V13.1 ☑
        noncollision accident (traffic) V18.5 ☑

402

☑ Additional Character Required — Refer to the Tabular List for Character Selection   ▽ Subterms under main terms may continue to next column or page

Accident — *continued*
  transport — *continued*
    pedal cyclist — *continued*
      passenger — *continued*
        noncollision accident — *continued*
          nontraffic V18.1 ☑
        specified type NEC V19.88 ☑
        military vehicle V19.81 ☑
    pedestrian
      conveyance (occupant) V09.9 ☑
        baby stroller V00.828 ☑
          collision (with) V09.9 ☑
            animal being ridden or animal drawn
                vehicle V06.99 ☑
              nontraffic V06.09 ☑
              traffic V06.19 ☑
            bus or heavy transport V04.99 ☑
              nontraffic V04.09 ☑
              traffic V04.19 ☑
            car V03.99 ☑
              nontraffic V03.09 ☑
              traffic V03.19 ☑
            pedal cycle V01.99 ☑
              nontraffic V01.09 ☑
              traffic V01.19 ☑
            pick-up truck or van V03.99 ☑
              nontraffic V03.09 ☑
              traffic V03.19 ☑
            railway (train) (vehicle) V05.99 ☑
              nontraffic V05.09 ☑
              traffic V05.19 ☑
            stationary object V00.822 ☑
            streetcar V06.99 ☑
              nontraffic V06.09 ☑
              traffic V06.19 ☑
            two- or three-wheeled motor vehicle
                V02.99 ☑
              nontraffic V02.09 ☑
              traffic V02.19 ☑
            vehicle V09.9 ☑
              animal-drawn V06.99 ☑
                nontraffic V06.09 ☑
                traffic V06.19 ☑
              motor
                nontraffic V09.00 ☑
                traffic V09.20 ☑
          fall V00.821 ☑
          nontraffic V09.1 ☑
            involving motor vehicle NEC V09.00 ☑
          traffic V09.3 ☑
            involving motor vehicle NEC V09.20 ☑
        flat-bottomed NEC V00.388 ☑
          collision (with) V09.9 ☑
            animal being ridden or animal drawn
                vehicle V06.99 ☑
              nontraffic V06.09 ☑
              traffic V06.19 ☑
            bus or heavy transport V04.99 ☑
              nontraffic V04.09 ☑
              traffic V04.19 ☑
            car V03.99 ☑
              nontraffic V03.09 ☑
              traffic V03.19 ☑
            pedal cycle V01.99 ☑
              nontraffic V01.09 ☑
              traffic V01.19 ☑
            pick-up truck or van V03.99 ☑
              nontraffic V03.09 ☑
              traffic V03.19 ☑
            railway (train) (vehicle) V05.99 ☑
              nontraffic V05.09 ☑
              traffic V05.19 ☑
            stationary object V00.382 ☑
            streetcar V06.99 ☑
              nontraffic V06.09 ☑
              traffic V06.19 ☑
            two- or three-wheeled motor vehicle
                V02.99 ☑
              nontraffic V02.09 ☑
              traffic V02.19 ☑
            vehicle V09.9 ☑
              animal-drawn V06.99 ☑
                nontraffic V06.09 ☑
                traffic V06.19 ☑
              motor
                nontraffic V09.00 ☑

Accident — *continued*
  transport — *continued*
    pedestrian — *continued*
      conveyance — *continued*
        flat-bottomed — *continued*
          collision — *continued*
            vehicle — *continued*
              motor — *continued*
                traffic V09.20 ☑
          fall V00.381 ☑
          nontraffic V09.1 ☑
            involving motor vehicle NEC V09.00 ☑
          snow
            board — *see* Accident, transport,
                pedestrian, conveyance, snow
                board
            ski — *see* Accident, transport, pedes-
                trian, conveyance, skis (snow)
          traffic V09.3 ☑
            involving motor vehicle NEC V09.20 ☑
        gliding type NEC V00.288 ☑
          collision (with) V09.9 ☑
            animal being ridden or animal drawn
                vehicle V06.99 ☑
              nontraffic V06.09 ☑
              traffic V06.19 ☑
            bus or heavy transport V04.99 ☑
              nontraffic V04.09 ☑
              traffic V04.19 ☑
            car V03.99 ☑
              nontraffic V03.09 ☑
              traffic V03.19 ☑
            pedal cycle V01.99 ☑
              nontraffic V01.09 ☑
              traffic V01.19 ☑
            pick-up truck or van V03.99 ☑
              nontraffic V03.09 ☑
              traffic V03.19 ☑
            railway (train) (vehicle) V05.99 ☑
              nontraffic V05.09 ☑
              traffic V05.19 ☑
            stationary object V00.282 ☑
            streetcar V06.99 ☑
              nontraffic V06.09 ☑
              traffic V02.19 ☑
            two- or three-wheeled motor vehicle
                V02.99 ☑
              nontraffic V02.09 ☑
              traffic V02.19 ☑
            vehicle V09.9 ☑
              animal-drawn V06.99 ☑
                nontraffic V06.09 ☑
                traffic V06.19 ☑
              motor
                nontraffic V09.00 ☑
                traffic V09.20 ☑
          fall V00.281 ☑
        heelies — *see* Accident, transport,
            pedestrian, conveyance, heelies
        ice skate — *see* Accident, transport,
            pedestrian, conveyance, ice skate
        nontraffic V09.1 ☑
          involving motor vehicle NEC V09.00 ☑
        sled — *see* Accident, transport, pedestri-
            an, conveyance, sled
        traffic V09.3 ☑
          involving motor vehicle NEC V09.20 ☑
        wheelies — *see* Accident, transport,
            pedestrian, conveyance, heelies
      heelies V00.158 ☑
        colliding with stationary object
            V00.152 ☑
        fall V00.151 ☑
      ice skates V00.218 ☑
        collision (with) V09.9 ☑
          animal being ridden or animal drawn
              vehicle V06.99 ☑
            nontraffic V06.09 ☑
            traffic V06.19 ☑
          bus or heavy transport V04.99 ☑
            nontraffic V04.09 ☑
            traffic V04.19 ☑
          car V03.99 ☑
            nontraffic V03.09 ☑
            traffic V03.19 ☑
          pedal cycle V01.99 ☑

Accident — *continued*
  transport — *continued*
    pedestrian — *continued*
      conveyance — *continued*
        ice skates — *continued*
          collision — *continued*
            pedal cycle — *continued*
              nontraffic V01.09 ☑
              traffic V01.19 ☑
            pick-up truck or van V03.99 ☑
              nontraffic V03.09 ☑
              traffic V03.19 ☑
            railway (train) (vehicle) V05.99 ☑
              nontraffic V05.09 ☑
              traffic V05.19 ☑
            stationary object V00.212 ☑
            streetcar V06.99 ☑
              nontraffic V06.09 ☑
              traffic V06.19 ☑
            two- or three-wheeled motor vehicle
                V02.99 ☑
              nontraffic V02.09 ☑
              traffic V02.19 ☑
            vehicle V09.9 ☑
              animal-drawn V06.99 ☑
                nontraffic V06.09 ☑
                traffic V06.19 ☑
              motor
                nontraffic V09.00 ☑
                traffic V09.20 ☑
          fall V00.211 ☑
          nontraffic V09.1 ☑
            involving motor vehicle NEC V09.00 ☑
          traffic V09.3 ☑
            involving motor vehicle NEC V09.20 ☑
        motorized mobility scooter V00.838 ☑
          collision with stationary object
              V00.832 ☑
          fall from V00.831 ☑
        nontraffic V09.1 ☑
          involving motor vehicle V09.00 ☑
            military V09.01 ☑
            specified type NEC V09.09 ☑
        roller skates (non in-line) V00.128 ☑
          collision (with) V09.9 ☑
            animal being ridden or animal drawn
                vehicle V06.91 ☑
              nontraffic V06.01 ☑
              traffic V06.11 ☑
            bus or heavy transport V04.91 ☑
              nontraffic V04.01 ☑
              traffic V04.11 ☑
            car V03.91 ☑
              nontraffic V03.01 ☑
              traffic V03.11 ☑
            pedal cycle V01.91 ☑
              nontraffic V01.01 ☑
              traffic V01.11 ☑
            pick-up truck or van V03.91 ☑
              nontraffic V03.01 ☑
              traffic V03.11 ☑
            railway (train) (vehicle) V05.91 ☑
              nontraffic V05.01 ☑
              traffic V05.11 ☑
            stationary object V00.122 ☑
            streetcar V06.91 ☑
              nontraffic V06.01 ☑
              traffic V06.11 ☑
            two- or three-wheeled motor vehicle
                V02.91 ☑
              nontraffic V02.01 ☑
              traffic V02.11 ☑
            vehicle V09.9 ☑
              animal-drawn V06.91 ☑
                nontraffic V06.01 ☑
                traffic V06.11 ☑
              motor
                nontraffic V09.00 ☑
                traffic V09.20 ☑
          fall V00.121 ☑
          in-line V00.118 ☑
            collision — *see also* Accident, trans-
                port, pedestrian, conveyance
                occupant, roller skates, collision
                with stationary object V00.112 ☑
            fall V00.111 ☑

Accident — *continued*
  transport — *continued*
    pedestrian — *continued*
      conveyance — *continued*
        roller skates — *continued*
          nontraffic V09.1 ☑
            involving motor vehicle NEC V09.00 ☑
          traffic V09.3 ☑
            involving motor vehicle NEC V09.20 ☑
        rolling shoes V00.158 ☑
          colliding with stationary object V00.152 ☑
          fall V00.151 ☑
        rolling type NEC V00.188 ☑
          collision (with) V09.9 ☑
            animal being ridden or animal drawn vehicle V06.99 ☑
              nontraffic V06.09 ☑
              traffic V06.19 ☑
            bus or heavy transport V04.99 ☑
              nontraffic V04.09 ☑
              traffic V04.19 ☑
            car V03.99 ☑
              nontraffic V03.09 ☑
              traffic V03.19 ☑
            pedal cycle V01.99 ☑
              nontraffic V01.09 ☑
              traffic V01.19 ☑
            pick-up truck or van V03.99 ☑
              nontraffic V03.09 ☑
              traffic V03.19 ☑
            railway (train) (vehicle) V05.99 ☑
              nontraffic V05.09 ☑
              traffic V05.19 ☑
            stationary object V00.182 ☑
            streetcar V06.99 ☑
              nontraffic V06.09 ☑
              traffic V06.19 ☑
            two- or three-wheeled motor vehicle V02.99 ☑
              nontraffic V02.09 ☑
              traffic V02.19 ☑
            vehicle V09.9 ☑
              animal-drawn V06.99 ☑
                nontraffic V06.09 ☑
                traffic V06.19 ☑
              motor
                nontraffic V09.00 ☑
                traffic V09.20 ☑
          fall V00.181 ☑
        in-line roller skate — *see* Accident, transport, pedestrian, conveyance, roller skate, in-line
        nontraffic V09.1 ☑
          involving motor vehicle NEC V09.00 ☑
        roller skate — *see* Accident, transport, pedestrian, conveyance, roller skate
        scooter (non-motorized) — *see* Accident, transport, pedestrian, conveyance, scooter
        skateboard — *see* Accident, transport, pedestrian, conveyance, skate-board
        traffic V09.3 ☑
          involving motor vehicle NEC V09.20 ☑
        scooter (non-motorized) V00.148 ☑
          collision (with) V09.9 ☑
            animal being ridden or animal drawn vehicle V06.99 ☑
              nontraffic V06.09 ☑
              traffic V06.19 ☑
            bus or heavy transport V04.99 ☑
              nontraffic V04.09 ☑
              traffic V04.19 ☑
            car V03.99 ☑
              nontraffic V03.09 ☑
              traffic V03.19 ☑
            pedal cycle V01.99 ☑
              nontraffic V01.09 ☑
              traffic V01.19 ☑
            pick-up truck or van V03.99 ☑
              nontraffic V03.09 ☑
              traffic V03.19 ☑
            railway (train) (vehicle) V05.99 ☑
              nontraffic V05.09 ☑

Accident — *continued*
  transport — *continued*
    pedestrian — *continued*
      conveyance — *continued*
        scooter — *continued*
          collision — *continued*
            railway — *continued*
              traffic V05.19 ☑
            stationary object V00.142 ☑
            streetcar V06.99 ☑
              nontraffic V06.09 ☑
              traffic V06.19 ☑
            two- or three-wheeled motor vehicle V02.99 ☑
              nontraffic V02.09 ☑
              traffic V02.19 ☑
            vehicle V09.9 ☑
              animal-drawn V06.99 ☑
                nontraffic V06.09 ☑
                traffic V06.19 ☑
              motor
                nontraffic V09.00 ☑
                traffic V09.20 ☑
          fall V00.141 ☑
          nontraffic V09.1 ☑
            involving motor vehicle NEC V09.00 ☑
          traffic V09.3 ☑
            involving motor vehicle NEC V09.20 ☑
        skate board V00.138 ☑
          collision (with) V09.9 ☑
            animal being ridden or animal drawn vehicle V06.92 ☑
              nontraffic V06.02 ☑
              traffic V06.12 ☑
            bus or heavy transport V04.92 ☑
              nontraffic V04.02 ☑
              traffic V04.12 ☑
            car V03.92 ☑
              nontraffic V03.02 ☑
              traffic V03.12 ☑
            pedal cycle V01.92 ☑
              nontraffic V01.02 ☑
              traffic V01.12 ☑
            pick-up truck or van V03.92 ☑
              nontraffic V03.02 ☑
              traffic V03.12 ☑
            railway (train) (vehicle) V05.92 ☑
              nontraffic V05.02 ☑
              traffic V05.12 ☑
            stationary object V00.132 ☑
            streetcar V06.92 ☑
              nontraffic V06.02 ☑
              traffic V06.12 ☑
            two- or three-wheeled motor vehicle V02.92 ☑
              nontraffic V02.02 ☑
              traffic V02.12 ☑
            vehicle V09.9 ☑
              animal-drawn V06.92 ☑
                nontraffic V06.02 ☑
                traffic V06.12 ☑
              motor
                nontraffic V09.00 ☑
                traffic V09.20 ☑
          fall V00.131 ☑
          nontraffic V09.1 ☑
            involving motor vehicle NEC V09.00 ☑
          traffic V09.3 ☑
            involving motor vehicle NEC V09.20 ☑
        skis (snow) V00.328 ☑
          collision (with) V09.9 ☑
            animal being ridden or animal drawn vehicle V06.99 ☑
              nontraffic V06.09 ☑
              traffic V06.19 ☑
            bus or heavy transport V04.99 ☑
              nontraffic V04.09 ☑
              traffic V04.19 ☑
            car V03.99 ☑
              nontraffic V03.09 ☑
              traffic V03.19 ☑
            pedal cycle V01.99 ☑
              nontraffic V01.09 ☑
              traffic V01.19 ☑
            pick-up truck or van V03.99 ☑
              nontraffic V03.09 ☑

Accident — *continued*
  transport — *continued*
    pedestrian — *continued*
      conveyance — *continued*
        skis — *continued*
          collision — *continued*
            pick-up truck or van — *continued*
              traffic V03.19 ☑
            railway (train) (vehicle) V05.99 ☑
              nontraffic V05.09 ☑
              traffic V05.19 ☑
            stationary object V00.322 ☑
            streetcar V06.99 ☑
              nontraffic V06.09 ☑
              traffic V06.19 ☑
            two- or three-wheeled motor vehicle V02.99 ☑
              nontraffic V02.09 ☑
              traffic V02.19 ☑
            vehicle V09.9 ☑
              animal-drawn V06.99 ☑
                nontraffic V06.09 ☑
                traffic V06.19 ☑
              motor
                nontraffic V09.00 ☑
                traffic V09.20 ☑
          fall V00.321 ☑
          nontraffic V09.1 ☑
            involving motor vehicle NEC V09.00 ☑
          traffic V09.3 ☑
            involving motor vehicle NEC V09.20 ☑
        sled V00.228 ☑
          collision (with) V09.9 ☑
            animal being ridden or animal drawn vehicle V06.99 ☑
              nontraffic V06.09 ☑
              traffic V06.19 ☑
            bus or heavy transport V04.99 ☑
              nontraffic V04.09 ☑
              traffic V04.19 ☑
            car V03.99 ☑
              nontraffic V03.09 ☑
              traffic V03.19 ☑
            pedal cycle V01.99 ☑
              nontraffic V01.09 ☑
              traffic V01.19 ☑
            pick-up truck or van V03.99 ☑
              nontraffic V03.09 ☑
              traffic V03.19 ☑
            railway (train) (vehicle) V05.99 ☑
              nontraffic V05.09 ☑
              traffic V05.19 ☑
            stationary object V00.222 ☑
            streetcar V06.99 ☑
              nontraffic V06.09 ☑
              traffic V06.19 ☑
            two- or three-wheeled motor vehicle V02.99 ☑
              nontraffic V02.09 ☑
              traffic V02.19 ☑
            vehicle V09.9 ☑
              animal-drawn V06.99 ☑
                nontraffic V06.09 ☑
                traffic V06.19 ☑
              motor
                nontraffic V09.00 ☑
                traffic V09.20 ☑
          fall V00.221 ☑
          nontraffic V09.1 ☑
            involving motor vehicle NEC V09.00 ☑
          traffic V09.3 ☑
            involving motor vehicle NEC V09.20 ☑
        snow board V00.318 ☑
          collision (with) V09.9 ☑
            animal being ridden or animal drawn vehicle V06.99 ☑
              nontraffic V06.09 ☑
              traffic V06.19 ☑
            bus or heavy transport V04.99 ☑
              nontraffic V04.09 ☑
              traffic V04.19 ☑
            car V03.99 ☑
              nontraffic V03.09 ☑
              traffic V03.19 ☑
            pedal cycle V01.99 ☑
              nontraffic V01.09 ☑

☑ Additional Character Required — Refer to the Tabular List for Character Selection   ▽ Subterms under main terms may continue to next column or page

Accident — *continued*
 transport — *continued*
  pedestrian — *continued*
   conveyance — *continued*
    snow board — *continued*
     collision — *continued*
      pedal cycle — *continued*
       traffic V01.19 ☑
      pick-up truck or van V03.99 ☑
       nontraffic V03.09 ☑
       traffic V03.19 ☑
      railway (train) (vehicle) V05.99 ☑
       nontraffic V05.09 ☑
       traffic V05.19 ☑
      stationary object V00.312 ☑
      streetcar V06.99 ☑
       nontraffic V06.09 ☑
       traffic V06.19 ☑
      two- or three-wheeled motor vehicle V02.99 ☑
       nontraffic V02.09 ☑
       traffic V02.19 ☑
      vehicle V09.9 ☑
       animal-drawn V06.99 ☑
        nontraffic V06.09 ☑
        traffic V06.19 ☑
       motor
        nontraffic V09.00 ☑
        traffic V09.20 ☑
     fall V00.311 ☑
     nontraffic V09.1 ☑
      involving motor vehicle NEC V09.00 ☑
     traffic V09.3 ☑
      involving motor vehicle NEC V09.20 ☑
    specified type NEC V00.898 ☑
     collision (with) V09.9 ☑
      animal being ridden or animal drawn vehicle V06.99 ☑
       nontraffic V06.09 ☑
       traffic V06.19 ☑
      bus or heavy transport V04.99 ☑
       nontraffic V04.09 ☑
       traffic V04.19 ☑
      car V03.99 ☑
       nontraffic V03.09 ☑
       traffic V03.19 ☑
      pedal cycle V01.99 ☑
       nontraffic V01.09 ☑
       traffic V01.19 ☑
      pick-up truck or van V03.99 ☑
       nontraffic V03.09 ☑
       traffic V03.19 ☑
      railway (train) (vehicle) V05.99 ☑
       nontraffic V05.09 ☑
       traffic V05.19 ☑
      stationary object V00.892 ☑
      streetcar V06.99 ☑
       nontraffic V06.09 ☑
       traffic V06.19 ☑
      two- or three-wheeled motor vehicle V02.99 ☑
       nontraffic V02.09 ☑
       traffic V02.19 ☑
      vehicle V09.9 ☑
       animal-drawn V06.99 ☑
        nontraffic V06.09 ☑
        traffic V06.19 ☑
       motor
        nontraffic V09.00 ☑
        traffic V09.20 ☑
     fall V00.891 ☑
     nontraffic V09.1 ☑
      involving motor vehicle NEC V09.00 ☑
     traffic V09.3 ☑
      involving motor vehicle NEC V09.20 ☑
    traffic V09.3 ☑
     involving motor vehicle V09.20 ☑
      military V09.21 ☑
     specified type NEC V09.29 ☑
    wheelchair (powered) V00.818 ☑
     collision (with) V09.9 ☑
      animal being ridden or animal drawn vehicle V06.99 ☑
       nontraffic V06.09 ☑
       traffic V06.19 ☑
      bus or heavy transport V04.99 ☑

Accident — *continued*
 transport — *continued*
  pedestrian — *continued*
   conveyance — *continued*
    wheelchair — *continued*
     collision — *continued*
      bus or heavy transport — *continued*
       nontraffic V04.09 ☑
       traffic V04.19 ☑
      car V03.99 ☑
       nontraffic V03.09 ☑
       traffic V03.19 ☑
      pedal cycle V01.99 ☑
       nontraffic V01.09 ☑
       traffic V01.19 ☑
      pick-up truck or van V03.99 ☑
       nontraffic V03.09 ☑
       traffic V03.19 ☑
      railway (train) (vehicle) V05.99 ☑
       nontraffic V05.09 ☑
       traffic V05.19 ☑
      stationary object V00.812 ☑
      streetcar V06.99 ☑
       nontraffic V06.09 ☑
       traffic V06.19 ☑
      two- or three-wheeled motor vehicle V02.99 ☑
       nontraffic V02.09 ☑
       traffic V02.19 ☑
      vehicle V09.9 ☑
       animal-drawn V06.99 ☑
        nontraffic V06.09 ☑
        traffic V06.19 ☑
       motor
        nontraffic V09.00 ☑
        traffic V09.20 ☑
     fall V00.811 ☑
     nontraffic V09.1 ☑
      involving motor vehicle NEC V09.00 ☑
     traffic V09.3 ☑
      involving motor vehicle NEC V09.20 ☑
    wheeled shoe V00.158 ☑
     colliding with stationary object V00.152 ☑
     fall V00.151 ☑
  on foot — *see also* Accident, pedestrian
   collision (with)
    animal being ridden or animal drawn vehicle V06.90 ☑
     nontraffic V06.00 ☑
     traffic V06.10 ☑
    bus or heavy transport V04.90 ☑
     nontraffic V04.00 ☑
     traffic V04.10 ☑
    car V03.90 ☑
     nontraffic V03.00 ☑
     traffic V03.10 ☑
    pedal cycle V01.90 ☑
     nontraffic V01.00 ☑
     traffic V01.10 ☑
    pick-up truck or van V03.90 ☑
     nontraffic V03.00 ☑
     traffic V03.10 ☑
    railway (train) (vehicle) V05.90 ☑
     nontraffic V05.00 ☑
     traffic V05.10 ☑
    streetcar V06.90 ☑
     nontraffic V06.00 ☑
     traffic V06.10 ☑
    two- or three-wheeled motor vehicle V02.90 ☑
     nontraffic V02.00 ☑
     traffic V02.10 ☑
    vehicle V09.9 ☑
     animal-drawn V06.90 ☑
      nontraffic V06.00 ☑
      traffic V06.10 ☑
     motor
   nontraffic V09.1 ☑
    involving motor vehicle V09.00 ☑
     military V09.01 ☑
    specified type NEC V09.09 ☑
   traffic V09.3 ☑
    involving motor vehicle V09.20 ☑
     military V09.21 ☑

Accident — *continued*
 transport — *continued*
  pedestrian — *continued*
   on foot — *see also* Accident, pedestrian — con-
    tinued
    traffic — *continued*
     involving motor vehicle — *continued*
      specified type NEC V09.29 ☑
  person NEC (unknown way or transportation) V99 ☑
   collision (between)
    bus (with)
     heavy transport vehicle (traffic) V87.5 ☑
      nontraffic V88.5 ☑
    car (with)
     bus (traffic) V87.3 ☑
      nontraffic V88.3 ☑
     heavy transport vehicle (traffic) V87.4 ☑
      nontraffic V88.4 ☑
     nontraffic V88.5 ☑
     pick-up truck or van (traffic) V87.2 ☑
      nontraffic V88.2 ☑
     train or railway vehicle (traffic) V87.6 ☑
      nontraffic V88.6 ☑
     two-or three-wheeled motor vehicle (traffic) V87.0 ☑
      nontraffic V88.0 ☑
     motor vehicle (traffic) NEC V87.7 ☑
      nontraffic V88.7 ☑
     two-or three-wheeled vehicle (with) (traffic)
      motor vehicle NEC V87.1 ☑
      nontraffic V88.1 ☑
    nonmotor vehicle (collision) (noncollision) (traf-
     fic) V87.9 ☑
    nontraffic V88.9 ☑
  pickup truck occupant V59.9 ☑
   collision (with)
    animal (traffic) V50.9 ☑
     being ridden (traffic) V56.9 ☑
      nontraffic V56.3 ☑
      while boarding or alighting V56.4 ☑
     nontraffic V50.3 ☑
     while boarding or alighting V50.4 ☑
    animal-drawn vehicle (traffic) V56.9 ☑
     nontraffic V56.3 ☑
     while boarding or alighting V56.4 ☑
    bus (traffic) V54.9 ☑
     nontraffic V54.3 ☑
     while boarding or alighting V54.4 ☑
    car (traffic) V53.9 ☑
     nontraffic V53.3 ☑
     while boarding or alighting V53.4 ☑
    motor vehicle NOS (traffic) V59.60 ☑
     nontraffic V59.20 ☑
     specified type NEC (traffic) V59.69 ☑
      nontraffic V59.29 ☑
    pedal cycle (traffic) V51.9 ☑
     nontraffic V51.3 ☑
     while boarding or alighting V51.4 ☑
    pickup truck (traffic) V53.9 ☑
     nontraffic V53.3 ☑
     while boarding or alighting V53.4 ☑
    railway vehicle (traffic) V55.9 ☑
     nontraffic V55.3 ☑
     while boarding or alighting V55.4 ☑
    specified vehicle NEC (traffic) V56.9 ☑
     nontraffic V56.3 ☑
     while boarding or alighting V56.4 ☑
    stationary object (traffic) V57.9 ☑
     nontraffic V57.3 ☑
     while boarding or alighting V57.4 ☑
    streetcar (traffic) V56.9 ☑
     nontraffic V56.3 ☑
     while boarding or alighting V56.4 ☑
    three wheeled motor vehicle (traffic) V52.9 ☑
     nontraffic V52.3 ☑
     while boarding or alighting V52.4 ☑
    truck (traffic) V54.9 ☑
     nontraffic V54.3 ☑
     while boarding or alighting V54.4 ☑
    two wheeled motor vehicle (traffic) V52.9 ☑
     nontraffic V52.3 ☑
     while boarding or alighting V52.4 ☑
    van (traffic) V53.9 ☑
     nontraffic V53.3 ☑
     while boarding or alighting V53.4 ☑

▽ Subterms under main terms may continue to next column or page ☑ Additional Character Required — Refer to the Tabular List for Character Selection 405

Accident — Accident

Accident — *continued*
  transport — *continued*
    pickup truck occupant — *continued*
      driver
        collision (with)
          animal (traffic) V50.5 ☑
            being ridden (traffic) V56.5 ☑
              nontraffic V56.0 ☑
            nontraffic V50.0 ☑
          animal-drawn vehicle (traffic) V56.5 ☑
            nontraffic V56.0 ☑
          bus (traffic) V54.5 ☑
            nontraffic V54.0 ☑
          car (traffic) V53.5 ☑
            nontraffic V53.0 ☑
          motor vehicle NOS (traffic) V59.40 ☑
            nontraffic V59.00 ☑
            specified type NEC (traffic) V59.49 ☑
              nontraffic V59.09 ☑
          pedal cycle (traffic) V51.5 ☑
            nontraffic V51.0 ☑
          pickup truck (traffic) V53.5 ☑
            nontraffic V53.0 ☑
          railway vehicle (traffic) V55.5 ☑
            nontraffic V55.0 ☑
          specified vehicle NEC (traffic) V56.5 ☑
            nontraffic V56.0 ☑
          stationary object (traffic) V57.5 ☑
            nontraffic V57.0 ☑
          streetcar (traffic) V56.5 ☑
            nontraffic V56.0 ☑
          three wheeled motor vehicle (traffic) V52.5 ☑
            nontraffic V52.0 ☑
          truck (traffic) V54.5 ☑
            nontraffic V54.0 ☑
          two wheeled motor vehicle (traffic) V52.5 ☑
            nontraffic V52.0 ☑
          van (traffic) V53.5 ☑
            nontraffic V53.0 ☑
        noncollision accident (traffic) V58.5 ☑
          nontraffic V58.0 ☑
      hanger-on
        collision (with)
          animal (traffic) V50.7 ☑
            being ridden (traffic) V56.7 ☑
              nontraffic V56.2 ☑
            nontraffic V50.2 ☑
          animal-drawn vehicle (traffic) V56.7 ☑
            nontraffic V56.2 ☑
          bus (traffic) V54.7 ☑
            nontraffic V54.2 ☑
          car (traffic) V53.7 ☑
            nontraffic V53.2 ☑
          pedal cycle (traffic) V51.7 ☑
            nontraffic V51.2 ☑
          pickup truck (traffic) V53.7 ☑
            nontraffic V53.2 ☑
          railway vehicle (traffic) V55.7 ☑
            nontraffic V55.2 ☑
          specified vehicle NEC (traffic) V56.7 ☑
            nontraffic V56.2 ☑
          stationary object (traffic) V57.7 ☑
            nontraffic V57.2 ☑
          streetcar (traffic) V56.7 ☑
            nontraffic V56.2 ☑
          three wheeled motor vehicle (traffic) V52.7 ☑
            nontraffic V52.2 ☑
          truck (traffic) V54.7 ☑
            nontraffic V54.2 ☑
          two wheeled motor vehicle (traffic) V52.7 ☑
            nontraffic V52.2 ☑
          van (traffic) V53.7 ☑
            nontraffic V53.2 ☑
        noncollision accident (traffic) V58.7 ☑
          nontraffic V58.2 ☑
      noncollision accident (traffic) V58.9 ☑
        nontraffic V58.3 ☑
        while boarding or alighting V58.4 ☑
      nontraffic V59.3 ☑
      passenger
        collision (with)
          animal (traffic) V50.6 ☑

Accident — *continued*
  transport — *continued*
    pickup truck occupant — *continued*
      passenger — *continued*
        collision — *continued*
          animal — *continued*
            being ridden (traffic) V56.6 ☑
              nontraffic V56.1 ☑
            nontraffic V50.1 ☑
          animal-drawn vehicle (traffic) V56.6 ☑
            nontraffic V56.1 ☑
          bus (traffic) V54.6 ☑
            nontraffic V54.1 ☑
          car (traffic) V53.6 ☑
            nontraffic V53.1 ☑
          motor vehicle NOS (traffic) V59.50 ☑
            nontraffic V59.10 ☑
            specified type NEC (traffic) V59.59 ☑
              nontraffic V59.19 ☑
          pedal cycle (traffic) V51.6 ☑
            nontraffic V51.1 ☑
          pickup truck (traffic) V53.6 ☑
            nontraffic V53.1 ☑
          railway vehicle (traffic) V55.6 ☑
            nontraffic V55.1 ☑
          specified vehicle NEC (traffic) V56.6 ☑
            nontraffic V56.1 ☑
          stationary object (traffic) V57.6 ☑
            nontraffic V57.1 ☑
          streetcar (traffic) V56.6 ☑
            nontraffic V56.1 ☑
          three wheeled motor vehicle (traffic) V52.6 ☑
            nontraffic V52.1 ☑
          truck (traffic) V54.6 ☑
            nontraffic V54.1 ☑
          two wheeled motor vehicle (traffic) V52.6 ☑
            nontraffic V52.1 ☑
          van (traffic) V53.6 ☑
            nontraffic V53.1 ☑
        noncollision accident (traffic) V58.6 ☑
          nontraffic V58.1 ☑
      specified type NEC V59.88 ☑
      military vehicle V59.81 ☑
    quarry truck — *see* Accident, transport, industrial vehicle occupant
    race car — *see* Accident, transport, motor vehicle NEC occupant
    railway vehicle occupant V81.9 ☑
      collision (with) V81.3 ☑
        motor vehicle (non-military) (traffic) V81.1 ☑
          military V81.83 ☑
          nontraffic V81.0 ☑
        rolling stock V81.2 ☑
        specified object NEC V81.3 ☑
      during derailment V81.7 ☑
        with antecedent collision — *see* Accident, transport, railway vehicle occupant, collision
      explosion V81.81 ☑
      fall (in railway vehicle) V81.5 ☑
        during derailment V81.7 ☑
          with antecedent collision — *see* Accident, transport, railway vehicle occupant, collision
        from railway vehicle V81.6 ☑
          during derailment V81.7 ☑
            with antecedent collision — *see* Accident, transport, railway vehicle occupant, collision
          while boarding or alighting V81.4 ☑
      fire V81.81 ☑
      object falling onto train V81.82 ☑
      specified type NEC V81.89 ☑
      while boarding or alighting V81.4 ☑
    ski lift V98.3 ☑
    snowmobile occupant (nontraffic) V86.92 ☑
      driver V86.52 ☑
      hanger-on V86.72 ☑
      passenger V86.62 ☑
      traffic V86.32 ☑
        driver V86.02 ☑
        hanger-on V86.22 ☑
        passenger V86.12 ☑
      while boarding or alighting V86.42 ☑

Accident — *continued*
  transport — *continued*
    specified NEC V98.8 ☑
    sport utility vehicle occupant — *see also* Accident, transport, pickup truck occupant
    streetcar occupant V82.9 ☑
      collision (with) V82.3 ☑
        motor vehicle (traffic) V82.1 ☑
          nontraffic V82.0 ☑
        rolling stock V82.2 ☑
      during derailment V82.7 ☑
        with antecedent collision — *see* Accident, transport, streetcar occupant, collision
      fall (in streetcar) V82.5 ☑
        during derailment V82.7 ☑
          with antecedent collision — *see* Accident, transport, streetcar occupant, collision
        from streetcar V82.6 ☑
          during derailment V82.7 ☑
            with antecedent collision — *see* Accident, transport, streetcar occupant, collision
          while boarding or alighting V82.4 ☑
        while boarding or alighting V82.4 ☑
      specified type NEC V82.8 ☑
      while boarding or alighting V82.4 ☑
    three-wheeled motor vehicle occupant V39.9 ☑
      collision (with)
        animal (traffic) V30.9 ☑
          being ridden (traffic) V36.9 ☑
            nontraffic V36.3 ☑
            while boarding or alighting V36.4 ☑
          nontraffic V30.3 ☑
          while boarding or alighting V30.4 ☑
        animal-drawn vehicle (traffic) V36.9 ☑
          nontraffic V36.3 ☑
          while boarding or alighting V36.4 ☑
        bus (traffic) V34.9 ☑
          nontraffic V34.3 ☑
          while boarding or alighting V34.4 ☑
        car (traffic) V33.9 ☑
          nontraffic V33.3 ☑
          while boarding or alighting V33.4 ☑
        motor vehicle NOS (traffic) V39.60 ☑
          nontraffic V39.20 ☑
          specified type NEC (traffic) V39.69 ☑
            nontraffic V39.29 ☑
        pedal cycle (traffic) V31.9 ☑
          nontraffic V31.3 ☑
          while boarding or alighting V31.4 ☑
        pickup truck (traffic) V33.9 ☑
          nontraffic V33.3 ☑
          while boarding or alighting V33.4 ☑
        railway vehicle (traffic) V35.9 ☑
          nontraffic V35.3 ☑
          while boarding or alighting V35.4 ☑
        specified vehicle NEC (traffic) V36.9 ☑
          nontraffic V36.3 ☑
          while boarding or alighting V36.4 ☑
        stationary object (traffic) V37.9 ☑
          nontraffic V37.3 ☑
          while boarding or alighting V37.4 ☑
        streetcar (traffic) V36.9 ☑
          nontraffic V36.3 ☑
          while boarding or alighting V36.4 ☑
        three wheeled motor vehicle (traffic) V32.9 ☑
          nontraffic V32.3 ☑
          while boarding or alighting V32.4 ☑
        truck (traffic) V34.9 ☑
          nontraffic V34.3 ☑
          while boarding or alighting V34.4 ☑
        two wheeled motor vehicle (traffic) V32.9 ☑
          nontraffic V32.3 ☑
          while boarding or alighting V32.4 ☑
        van (traffic) V33.9 ☑
          nontraffic V33.3 ☑
          while boarding or alighting V33.4 ☑
      driver
        collision (with)
          animal (traffic) V30.5 ☑
            being ridden (traffic) V36.5 ☑
              nontraffic V36.0 ☑
            nontraffic V30.0 ☑
          animal-drawn vehicle (traffic) V36.5 ☑
            nontraffic V36.0 ☑

Accident — *continued*
  transport — *continued*
    three-wheeled motor vehicle occupant — *continued*
      driver — *continued*
        collision — *continued*
          bus (traffic) V34.5 ☑
            nontraffic V34.0 ☑
          car (traffic) V33.5 ☑
            nontraffic V33.0 ☑
          motor vehicle NOS (traffic) V39.40 ☑
            nontraffic V39.00 ☑
            specified type NEC (traffic) V39.49 ☑
              nontraffic V39.09 ☑
          pedal cycle (traffic) V31.5 ☑
            nontraffic V31.0 ☑
          pickup truck (traffic) V33.5 ☑
            nontraffic V33.0 ☑
          railway vehicle (traffic) V35.5 ☑
            nontraffic V35.0 ☑
          specified vehicle NEC (traffic) V36.5 ☑
            nontraffic V36.0 ☑
          stationary object (traffic) V37.5 ☑
            nontraffic V37.0 ☑
          streetcar (traffic) V36.5 ☑
            nontraffic V36.0 ☑
          three wheeled motor vehicle (traffic) V32.5 ☑
            nontraffic V32.0 ☑
          truck (traffic) V34.5 ☑
            nontraffic V34.0 ☑
          two wheeled motor vehicle (traffic) V32.5 ☑
            nontraffic V32.0 ☑
          van (traffic) V33.5 ☑
            nontraffic V33.0 ☑
          noncollision accident (traffic) V38.5 ☑
            nontraffic V38.0 ☑
      hanger-on
        collision (with)
          animal (traffic) V30.7 ☑
            being ridden (traffic) V36.7 ☑
              nontraffic V36.2 ☑
            nontraffic V30.2 ☑
          animal-drawn vehicle (traffic) V36.7 ☑
            nontraffic V36.2 ☑
          bus (traffic) V34.7 ☑
            nontraffic V34.2 ☑
          car (traffic) V33.7 ☑
            nontraffic V33.2 ☑
          pedal cycle (traffic) V31.7 ☑
            nontraffic V31.2 ☑
          pickup truck (traffic) V33.7 ☑
            nontraffic V33.2 ☑
          railway vehicle (traffic) V35.7 ☑
            nontraffic V35.2 ☑
          specified vehicle NEC (traffic) V36.7 ☑
            nontraffic V36.2 ☑
          stationary object (traffic) V37.7 ☑
            nontraffic V37.2 ☑
          streetcar (traffic) V36.7 ☑
            nontraffic V36.2 ☑
          three wheeled motor vehicle (traffic) V32.7 ☑
            nontraffic V32.2 ☑
          truck (traffic) V34.7 ☑
            nontraffic V34.2 ☑
          two wheeled motor vehicle (traffic) V32.7 ☑
            nontraffic V32.2 ☑
          van (traffic) V33.7 ☑
            nontraffic V33.2 ☑
          noncollision accident (traffic) V38.7 ☑
            nontraffic V38.2 ☑
        noncollision accident (traffic) V38.9 ☑
          nontraffic V38.3 ☑
          while boarding or alighting V38.4 ☑
        nontraffic V39.3 ☑
      passenger
        collision (with)
          animal (traffic) V30.6 ☑
            being ridden (traffic) V36.6 ☑
              nontraffic V36.1 ☑
            nontraffic V30.1 ☑
          animal-drawn vehicle (traffic) V36.6 ☑
            nontraffic V36.1 ☑

Accident — *continued*
  transport — *continued*
    three-wheeled motor vehicle occupant — *continued*
      passenger — *continued*
        collision — *continued*
          bus (traffic) V34.6 ☑
            nontraffic V34.1 ☑
          car (traffic) V33.6 ☑
            nontraffic V33.1 ☑
          motor vehicle NOS (traffic) V39.50 ☑
            nontraffic V39.10 ☑
            specified type NEC (traffic) V39.59 ☑
              nontraffic V39.19 ☑
          pedal cycle (traffic) V31.6 ☑
            nontraffic V31.1 ☑
          pickup truck (traffic) V33.6 ☑
            nontraffic V33.1 ☑
          railway vehicle (traffic) V35.6 ☑
            nontraffic V35.1 ☑
          specified vehicle NEC (traffic) V36.6 ☑
            nontraffic V36.1 ☑
          stationary object (traffic) V37.6 ☑
            nontraffic V37.1 ☑
          streetcar (traffic) V36.6 ☑
            nontraffic V36.1 ☑
          three wheeled motor vehicle (traffic) V32.6 ☑
            nontraffic V32.1 ☑
          truck (traffic) V34.6 ☑
            nontraffic V34.1 ☑
          two wheeled motor vehicle (traffic) V32.6 ☑
            nontraffic V32.1 ☑
          van (traffic) V33.6 ☑
            nontraffic V33.1 ☑
          noncollision accident (traffic) V38.6 ☑
            nontraffic V38.1 ☑
      specified type NEC V39.89 ☑
      military vehicle V39.81 ☑
    tractor (farm) (and trailer) — *see* Accident, transport, agricultural vehicle occupant
    tram — *see* Accident, transport, streetcar
      in mine or quarry — *see* Accident, transport, industrial vehicle occupant
    trolley — *see* Accident, transport, streetcar
      in mine or quarry — *see* Accident, transport, industrial vehicle occupant
    truck (heavy) occupant V69.9 ☑
      collision (with)
        animal (traffic) V60.9 ☑
          being ridden (traffic) V66.9 ☑
            nontraffic V66.3 ☑
            while boarding or alighting V66.4 ☑
          nontraffic V60.3 ☑
          while boarding or alighting V60.4 ☑
        animal-drawn vehicle (traffic) V66.9 ☑
          nontraffic V66.3 ☑
          while boarding or alighting V66.4 ☑
        bus (traffic) V64.9 ☑
          nontraffic V64.3 ☑
          while boarding or alighting V64.4 ☑
        car (traffic) V63.9 ☑
          nontraffic V63.3 ☑
          while boarding or alighting V63.4 ☑
        motor vehicle NOS (traffic) V69.60 ☑
          nontraffic V69.20 ☑
          specified type NEC (traffic) V69.69 ☑
            nontraffic V69.29 ☑
        pedal cycle (traffic) V61.9 ☑
          nontraffic V61.3 ☑
          while boarding or alighting V61.4 ☑
        pickup truck (traffic) V63.9 ☑
          nontraffic V63.3 ☑
          while boarding or alighting V63.4 ☑
        railway vehicle (traffic) V65.9 ☑
          nontraffic V65.3 ☑
          while boarding or alighting V65.4 ☑
        specified vehicle NEC (traffic) V66.9 ☑
          nontraffic V66.3 ☑
          while boarding or alighting V66.4 ☑
        stationary object (traffic) V67.9 ☑
          nontraffic V67.3 ☑
          while boarding or alighting V67.4 ☑
        streetcar (traffic) V66.9 ☑
          nontraffic V66.3 ☑

Accident — *continued*
  transport — *continued*
    truck occupant — *continued*
      collision — *continued*
        streetcar — *continued*
          while boarding or alighting V66.4 ☑
        three wheeled motor vehicle (traffic) V62.9 ☑
          nontraffic V62.3 ☑
          while boarding or alighting V62.4 ☑
        truck (traffic) V64.9 ☑
          nontraffic V64.3 ☑
          while boarding or alighting V64.4 ☑
        two wheeled motor vehicle (traffic) V62.9 ☑
          nontraffic V62.3 ☑
          while boarding or alighting V62.4 ☑
        van (traffic) V63.9 ☑
          nontraffic V63.3 ☑
          while boarding or alighting V63.4 ☑
      driver
        collision (with)
          animal (traffic) V60.5 ☑
            being ridden (traffic) V66.5 ☑
              nontraffic V66.0 ☑
            nontraffic V60.0 ☑
          animal-drawn vehicle (traffic) V66.5 ☑
            nontraffic V66.0 ☑
          bus (traffic) V64.5 ☑
            nontraffic V64.0 ☑
          car (traffic) V63.5 ☑
            nontraffic V63.0 ☑
          motor vehicle NOS (traffic) V69.40 ☑
            nontraffic V69.00 ☑
            specified type NEC (traffic) V69.49 ☑
              nontraffic V69.09 ☑
          pedal cycle (traffic) V61.5 ☑
            nontraffic V61.0 ☑
          pickup truck (traffic) V63.5 ☑
            nontraffic V63.0 ☑
          railway vehicle (traffic) V65.5 ☑
            nontraffic V65.0 ☑
          specified vehicle NEC (traffic) V66.5 ☑
            nontraffic V66.0 ☑
          stationary object (traffic) V67.5 ☑
            nontraffic V67.0 ☑
          streetcar (traffic) V66.5 ☑
            nontraffic V66.0 ☑
          three wheeled motor vehicle (traffic) V62.5 ☑
            nontraffic V62.0 ☑
          truck (traffic) V64.5 ☑
            nontraffic V64.0 ☑
          two wheeled motor vehicle (traffic) V62.5 ☑
            nontraffic V62.0 ☑
          van (traffic) V63.5 ☑
            nontraffic V63.0 ☑
          noncollision accident (traffic) V68.5 ☑
            nontraffic V68.0 ☑
      dump — *see* Accident, transport, construction vehicle occupant
      hanger-on
        collision (with)
          animal (traffic) V60.7 ☑
            being ridden (traffic) V66.7 ☑
              nontraffic V66.2 ☑
            nontraffic V60.2 ☑
          animal-drawn vehicle (traffic) V66.7 ☑
            nontraffic V66.2 ☑
          bus (traffic) V64.7 ☑
            nontraffic V64.2 ☑
          car (traffic) V63.7 ☑
            nontraffic V63.2 ☑
          pedal cycle (traffic) V61.7 ☑
            nontraffic V61.2 ☑
          pickup truck (traffic) V63.7 ☑
            nontraffic V63.2 ☑
          railway vehicle (traffic) V65.7 ☑
            nontraffic V65.2 ☑
          specified vehicle NEC (traffic) V66.7 ☑
            nontraffic V66.2 ☑
          stationary object (traffic) V67.7 ☑
            nontraffic V67.2 ☑
          streetcar (traffic) V66.7 ☑
            nontraffic V66.2 ☑
          three wheeled motor vehicle (traffic) V62.7 ☑

▽ Subterms under main terms may continue to next column or page   ☑ Additional Character Required — Refer to the Tabular List for Character Selection   407

Accident — Accident

Accident — *continued*
  transport — *continued*
    truck occupant — *continued*
      hanger-on — *continued*
        collision — *continued*
          three wheeled motor vehicle — *continued*
            nontraffic V62.2 ☑
          truck (traffic) V64.7 ☑
            nontraffic V64.2 ☑
          two wheeled motor vehicle (traffic) V62.7 ☑
            nontraffic V62.2 ☑
          van (traffic) V63.7 ☑
            nontraffic V63.2 ☑
        noncollision accident (traffic) V68.7 ☑
          nontraffic V68.2 ☑
      noncollision accident (traffic) V68.9 ☑
        nontraffic V68.3 ☑
      while boarding or alighting V68.4 ☑
      nontraffic V69.3 ☑
      passenger
        collision (with)
          animal (traffic) V60.6 ☑
            being ridden (traffic) V66.6 ☑
              nontraffic V66.1- ☑
            nontraffic V60.1 ☑
          animal-drawn vehicle (traffic) V66.6 ☑
            nontraffic V66.1 ☑
          bus (traffic) V64.6 ☑
            nontraffic V64.1 ☑
          car (traffic) V63.6 ☑
            nontraffic V63.1 ☑
          motor vehicle NOS (traffic) V69.50 ☑
            nontraffic V69.10 ☑
            specified type NEC (traffic) V69.59 ☑
              nontraffic V69.19 ☑
          pedal cycle (traffic) V61.6 ☑
            nontraffic V61.1 ☑
          pickup truck (traffic) V63.6 ☑
            nontraffic V63.1 ☑
          railway vehicle (traffic) V65.6 ☑
            nontraffic V65.1 ☑
          specified vehicle NEC (traffic) V66.6 ☑
            nontraffic V66.1 ☑
          stationary object (traffic) V67.6 ☑
            nontraffic V67.1 ☑
          streetcar (traffic) V66.6 ☑
            nontraffic V66.1 ☑
          three wheeled motor vehicle (traffic) V62.6 ☑
            nontraffic V62.1 ☑
          truck (traffic) V64.6 ☑
            nontraffic V64.1 ☑
          two wheeled motor vehicle (traffic) V62.6 ☑
            nontraffic V62.1 ☑
          van (traffic) V63.6 ☑
            nontraffic V63.1 ☑
        noncollision accident (traffic) V68.6 ☑
          nontraffic V68.1 ☑
      pickup — *see* Accident, transport, pickup truck occupant
      specified type NEC V69.88 ☑
      military vehicle V69.81 ☑
    van occupant V59.9 ☑
      collision (with)
        animal (traffic) V50.9 ☑
          being ridden (traffic) V56.9 ☑
            nontraffic V56.3 ☑
            while boarding or alighting V56.4 ☑
          nontraffic V50.3 ☑
          while boarding or alighting V50.4 ☑
        animal-drawn vehicle (traffic) V56.9 ☑
          nontraffic V56.3 ☑
          while boarding or alighting V56.4 ☑
        bus (traffic) V54.9 ☑
          nontraffic V54.3 ☑
          while boarding or alighting V54.4 ☑
        car (traffic) V53.9 ☑
          nontraffic V53.3 ☑
          while boarding or alighting V53.4 ☑
        motor vehicle NOS (traffic) V59.60 ☑
          nontraffic V59.20 ☑
          specified type NEC (traffic) V59.69 ☑
            nontraffic V59.29 ☑

Accident — *continued*
  transport — *continued*
    van occupant — *continued*
      collision — *continued*
        pedal cycle (traffic) V51.9 ☑
          nontraffic V51.3 ☑
          while boarding or alighting V51.4 ☑
        pickup truck (traffic) V53.9 ☑
          nontraffic V53.3 ☑
          while boarding or alighting V53.4 ☑
        railway vehicle (traffic) V55.9 ☑
          nontraffic V55.3 ☑
          while boarding or alighting V55.4 ☑
        specified vehicle NEC (traffic) V56.9 ☑
          nontraffic V56.3 ☑
          while boarding or alighting V56.4 ☑
        stationary object (traffic) V57.9 ☑
          nontraffic V57.3 ☑
          while boarding or alighting V57.4 ☑
        streetcar (traffic) V56.9 ☑
          nontraffic V56.3 ☑
          while boarding or alighting V56.4 ☑
        three wheeled motor vehicle (traffic) V52.9 ☑
          nontraffic V52.3 ☑
          while boarding or alighting V52.4 ☑
        truck (traffic) V54.9 ☑
          nontraffic V54.3 ☑
          while boarding or alighting V54.4 ☑
        two wheeled motor vehicle (traffic) V52.9 ☑
          nontraffic V52.3 ☑
          while boarding or alighting V52.4 ☑
        van (traffic) V53.9 ☑
          nontraffic V53.3 ☑
          while boarding or alighting V53.4 ☑
      driver
        collision (with)
          animal (traffic) V50.5 ☑
            being ridden (traffic) V56.5 ☑
              nontraffic V56.0 ☑
            nontraffic V50.0 ☑
          animal-drawn vehicle (traffic) V56.5 ☑
            nontraffic V56.0 ☑
          bus (traffic) V54.5 ☑
            nontraffic V54.0 ☑
          car (traffic) V53.5 ☑
            nontraffic V53.0 ☑
          motor vehicle NOS (traffic) V59.40 ☑
            nontraffic V59.00 ☑
            specified type NEC (traffic) V59.49 ☑
              nontraffic V59.09 ☑
          pedal cycle (traffic) V51.5 ☑
            nontraffic V51.0 ☑
          pickup truck (traffic) V53.5 ☑
            nontraffic V53.0 ☑
          railway vehicle (traffic) V55.5 ☑
            nontraffic V55.0 ☑
          specified vehicle NEC (traffic) V56.5 ☑
            nontraffic V56.0 ☑
          stationary object (traffic) V57.5 ☑
            nontraffic V57.0 ☑
          streetcar (traffic) V56.5 ☑
            nontraffic V56.0 ☑
          three wheeled motor vehicle (traffic) V52.5 ☑
            nontraffic V52.0 ☑
          truck (traffic) V54.5 ☑
            nontraffic V54.0 ☑
          two wheeled motor vehicle (traffic) V52.5 ☑
            nontraffic V52.0 ☑
          van (traffic) V53.5 ☑
            nontraffic V53.0 ☑
        noncollision accident (traffic) V58.5 ☑
          nontraffic V58.0 ☑
      hanger-on
        collision (with)
          animal (traffic) V50.7 ☑
            being ridden (traffic) V56.7 ☑
              nontraffic V56.2 ☑
            nontraffic V50.2 ☑
          animal-drawn vehicle (traffic) V56.7 ☑
            nontraffic V56.2 ☑
          bus (traffic) V54.7 ☑
            nontraffic V54.2 ☑
          car (traffic) V53.7 ☑
            nontraffic V53.2 ☑

Accident — *continued*
  transport — *continued*
    van occupant — *continued*
      hanger-on — *continued*
        collision — *continued*
          pedal cycle (traffic) V51.7 ☑
            nontraffic V51.2 ☑
          pickup truck (traffic) V53.7 ☑
            nontraffic V53.2 ☑
          railway vehicle (traffic) V55.7 ☑
            nontraffic V55.2 ☑
          specified vehicle NEC (traffic) V56.7 ☑
            nontraffic V56.2 ☑
          stationary object (traffic) V57.7 ☑
            nontraffic V57.2 ☑
          streetcar (traffic) V56.7 ☑
            nontraffic V56.2 ☑
          three wheeled motor vehicle (traffic) V52.7 ☑
            nontraffic V52.2 ☑
          truck (traffic) V54.7 ☑
            nontraffic V54.2 ☑
          two wheeled motor vehicle (traffic) V52.7 ☑
            nontraffic V52.2 ☑
          van (traffic) V53.7 ☑
            nontraffic V53.2 ☑
        noncollision accident (traffic) V58.7 ☑
          nontraffic V58.2 ☑
      noncollision accident (traffic) V58.9 ☑
        nontraffic V58.3 ☑
      while boarding or alighting V58.4 ☑
      nontraffic V59.3 ☑
      passenger
        collision (with)
          animal (traffic) V50.6 ☑
            being ridden (traffic) V56.6 ☑
              nontraffic V56.1 ☑
            nontraffic V50.1 ☑
          animal-drawn vehicle (traffic) V56.6 ☑
            nontraffic V56.1 ☑
          bus (traffic) V54.6 ☑
            nontraffic V54.1 ☑
          car (traffic) V53.6 ☑
            nontraffic V53.1 ☑
          motor vehicle NOS (traffic) V59.50 ☑
            nontraffic V59.10 ☑
            specified type NEC (traffic) V59.59 ☑
              nontraffic V59.19 ☑
          pedal cycle (traffic) V51.6 ☑
            nontraffic V51.1 ☑
          pickup truck (traffic) V53.6 ☑
            nontraffic V53.1 ☑
          railway vehicle (traffic) V55.6 ☑
            nontraffic V55.1 ☑
          specified vehicle NEC (traffic) V56.6 ☑
            nontraffic V56.1 ☑
          stationary object (traffic) V57.6 ☑
            nontraffic V57.1 ☑
          streetcar (traffic) V56.6 ☑
            nontraffic V56.1 ☑
          three wheeled motor vehicle (traffic) V52.6 ☑
            nontraffic V52.1 ☑
          truck (traffic) V54.6 ☑
            nontraffic V54.1 ☑
          two wheeled motor vehicle (traffic) V52.6 ☑
            nontraffic V52.1 ☑
          van (traffic) V53.6 ☑
            nontraffic V53.1 ☑
        noncollision accident (traffic) V58.6 ☑
          nontraffic V58.1 ☑
      specified type NEC V59.88 ☑
      military vehicle V59.81 ☑
    watercraft occupant — *see* Accident, watercraft
  vehicle NEC V89.9 ☑
    animal-drawn NEC — *see* Accident, transport, animal-drawn vehicle occupant
    special
      agricultural — *see* Accident, transport, agricultural vehicle occupant
      construction — *see* Accident, transport, construction vehicle occupant
      industrial — *see* Accident, transport, industrial vehicle occupant

☑ Additional Character Required — Refer to the Tabular List for Character Selection   ▽ Subterms under main terms may continue to next column or page

Accident — *continued*
  vehicle — *continued*
    three-wheeled NEC (motorized) — *see* Accident, transport, three-wheeled motor vehicle occupant
    watercraft V94.9 ☑
      causing
        drowning — *see* Drowning, due to, accident to, watercraft
        injury NEC V91.89 ☑
          crushed between craft and object V91.19 ☑
            powered craft V91.13 ☑
              ferry boat V91.11 ☑
              fishing boat V91.12 ☑
              jetskis V91.13 ☑
              liner V91.11 ☑
              merchant ship V91.10 ☑
              passenger ship V91.11 ☑
            unpowered craft V91.18 ☑
              canoe V91.15 ☑
              inflatable V91.16 ☑
              kayak V91.15 ☑
              sailboat V91.14 ☑
              surf-board V91.18 ☑
              windsurfer V91.18 ☑
          fall on board V91.29 ☑
            powered craft V91.23 ☑
              ferry boat V91.21 ☑
              fishing boat V91.22 ☑
              jetskis V91.23 ☑
              liner V91.21 ☑
              merchant ship V91.20 ☑
              passenger ship V91.21 ☑
            unpowered craft
              canoe V91.25 ☑
              inflatable V91.26 ☑
              kayak V91.25 ☑
              sailboat V91.24 ☑
          fire on board causing burn V91.09 ☑
            powered craft V91.03 ☑
              ferry boat V91.01 ☑
              fishing boat V91.02 ☑
              jetskis V91.03 ☑
              liner V91.01 ☑
              merchant ship V91.00 ☑
              passenger ship V91.01 ☑
            unpowered craft V91.08 ☑
              canoe V91.05 ☑
              inflatable V91.06 ☑
              kayak V91.05 ☑
              sailboat V91.04 ☑
              surf-board V91.08 ☑
              water skis V91.07 ☑
              windsurfer V91.08 ☑
          hit by falling object V91.39 ☑
            powered craft V91.33 ☑
              ferry boat V91.31 ☑
              fishing boat V91.32 ☑
              jetskis V91.33 ☑
              liner V91.31 ☑
              merchant ship V91.30 ☑
              passenger ship V91.31 ☑
            unpowered craft V91.38 ☑
              canoe V91.35 ☑
              inflatable V91.36 ☑
              kayak V91.35 ☑
              sailboat V91.34 ☑
              surf-board V91.38 ☑
              water skis V91.37 ☑
              windsurfer V91.38 ☑
          specified type NEC V91.89 ☑
            powered craft V91.83 ☑
              ferry boat V91.81 ☑
              fishing boat V91.82 ☑
              jetskis V91.83 ☑
              liner V91.81 ☑
              merchant ship V91.80 ☑
              passenger ship V91.81 ☑
            unpowered craft V91.88 ☑
              canoe V91.85 ☑
              inflatable V91.86 ☑
              kayak V91.85 ☑
              sailboat V91.84 ☑
              surf-board V91.88 ☑
              water skis V91.87 ☑
              windsurfer V91.88 ☑

Accident — *continued*
  watercraft — *continued*
    due to, caused by cataclysm — *see* Forces of nature, by type
    military NEC V94.818 ☑
      civilian in water injured by V94.811 ☑
      with civilian watercraft V94.810 ☑
    nonpowered, struck by
      nonpowered vessel V94.22 ☑
      powered vessel V94.21 ☑
    specified type NEC V94.89 ☑
    striking swimmer
      powered V94.11 ☑
      unpowered V94.12 ☑
Acid throwing (assault) Y08.89 ☑
Activity (involving) (of victim at time of event) Y93.9
  aerobic and step exercise (class) Y93.A3 (*following* Y93.7)
  alpine skiing Y93.23
  animal care NEC Y93.K9 (*following* Y93.7)
  arts and handcrafts NEC Y93.D9 (*following* Y93.7)
  athletics played as a team or group NEC Y93.69
  athletics played individually NEC Y93.59
  athletics NEC Y93.79
  baking Y93.G3 (*following* Y93.7)
  ballet Y93.41
  barbells Y93.B3 (*following* Y93.7)
  BASE (Building, Antenna, Span, Earth) jumping Y93.33
  baseball Y93.64
  basketball Y93.67
  bathing (personal) Y93.E1 (*following* Y93.7)
  beach volleyball Y93.68
  bike riding Y93.55
  blackout game Y93.85
  boogie boarding Y93.18
  bowling Y93.54
  boxing Y93.71
  brass instrument playing Y93.J4 (*following* Y93.7)
  building construction Y93.H3 (*following* Y93.7)
  bungee jumping Y93.34
  calisthenics Y93.A2 (*following* Y93.7)
  canoeing (in calm and turbulent water) Y93.16
  capture the flag Y93.6A
  cardiorespiratory exercise NEC Y93.A9 (*following* Y93.7)
  caregiving (providing) NEC Y93.F9 (*following* Y93.7)
    bathing Y93.F1 (*following* Y93.7)
    lifting Y93.F2 (*following* Y93.7)
  cellular
    communication device Y93.C2 (*following* Y93.7)
    telephone Y93.C2 (*following* Y93.7)
  challenge course Y93.A5 (*following* Y93.7)
  cheerleading Y93.45
  choking game Y93.85
  circuit training Y93.A4 (*following* Y93.7)
  cleaning
    floor Y93.E5 (*following* Y93.7)
  climbing NEC Y93.39
    mountain Y93.31
    rock Y93.31
    wall Y93.31
  clothing care and maintenance NEC Y93.E9 (*following* Y93.7)
  combatives Y93.75
  computer
    keyboarding Y93.C1 (*following* Y93.7)
    technology NEC Y93.C9 (*following* Y93.7)
  confidence course Y93.A5 (*following* Y93.7)
  construction (building) Y93.H3 (*following* Y93.7)
  cooking and baking Y93.G3 (*following* Y93.7)
  cool down exercises Y93.A2 (*following* Y93.7)
  cricket Y93.69
  crocheting Y93.D1 (*following* Y93.7)
  cross country skiing Y93.24
  dancing (all types) Y93.41
  digging
    dirt Y93.H1 (*following* Y93.7)
  dirt digging Y93.H1 (*following* Y93.7)
  dishwashing Y93.G1 (*following* Y93.7)
  diving (platform) (springboard) Y93.12
    underwater Y93.15
  dodge ball Y93.6A
  downhill skiing Y93.23
  drum playing Y93.J2 (*following* Y93.7)
  dumbbells Y93.B3 (*following* Y93.7)
  electronic
    devices NEC Y93.C9 (*following* Y93.7)
      hand held interactive Y93.C2 (*following* Y93.7)

Activity — *continued*
  electronic — *continued*
    game playing (using) (with)
      interactive device Y93.C2 (*following* Y93.7)
      keyboard or other stationary device Y93.C1 (*following* Y93.7)
  elliptical machine Y93.A1 (*following* Y93.7)
  exercise(s)
    machines ((primarily) for)
      cardiorespiratory conditioning Y93.A1 (*following* Y93.7)
      muscle strengthening Y93.B1 (*following* Y93.7)
    muscle strengthening (non-machine) NEC Y93.B9 (*following* Y93.7)
  external motion NEC Y93.I9 (*following* Y93.7)
    rollercoaster Y93.I1 (*following* Y93.7)
  fainting game Y93.85
  field hockey Y93.65
  figure skating (pairs) (singles) Y93.21
  flag football Y93.62
  floor mopping and cleaning Y93.E5 (*following* Y93.7)
  food preparation and clean up Y93.G1 (*following* Y93.7)
  football (American) NOS Y93.61
    flag Y93.62
    tackle Y93.61
    touch Y93.62
  four square Y93.6A
  free weights Y93.B3 (*following* Y93.7)
  frisbee (ultimate) Y93.74
  furniture
    building Y93.D3 (*following* Y93.7)
    finishing Y93.D3 (*following* Y93.7)
    repair Y93.D3 (*following* Y93.7)
  game playing (electronic)
    using interactive device Y93.C2 (*following* Y93.7)
    using keyboard or other stationary device Y93.C1 (*following* Y93.7)
  gardening Y93.H2 (*following* Y93.7)
  golf Y93.53
  grass drills Y93.A6 (*following* Y93.7)
  grilling and smoking food Y93.G2 (*following* Y93.7)
  grooming and shearing an animal Y93.K3 (*following* Y93.7)
  guerilla drills Y93.A6 (*following* Y93.7)
  gymnastics (rhythmic) Y93.43
  hand held interactive electronic device Y93.C2 (*following* Y93.7)
  handball Y93.73
  handcrafts NEC Y93.D9 (*following* Y93.7)
  hang gliding Y93.35
  hiking (on level or elevated terrain) Y93.01
  hockey (ice) Y93.22
    field Y93.65
  horseback riding Y93.52
  household (interior) maintenance NEC Y93.E9 (*following* Y93.7)
  ice NEC Y93.29
    dancing Y93.21
    hockey Y93.22
    skating Y93.21
  inline roller skating Y93.51
  ironing Y93.E4 (*following* Y93.7)
  judo Y93.75
  jumping jacks Y93.A2 (*following* Y93.7)
  jumping rope Y93.56
  jumping (off) NEC Y93.39
    BASE (Building, Antenna, Span, Earth) Y93.33
    bungee Y93.34
    jacks Y93.A2 (*following* Y93.7)
    rope Y93.56
  karate Y93.75
  kayaking (in calm and turbulent water) Y93.16
  keyboarding (computer) Y93.C1 (*following* Y93.7)
  kickball Y93.6A
  knitting Y93.D1 (*following* Y93.7)
  lacrosse Y93.65
  land maintenance NEC Y93.H9 (*following* Y93.7)
  landscaping Y93.H2 (*following* Y93.7)
  laundry Y93.E2 (*following* Y93.7)
  machines (exercise)
    primarily for cardiorespiratory conditioning Y93.A1 (*following* Y93.7)
    primarily for muscle strengthening Y93.B1 (*following* Y93.7)
  maintenance
    exterior building NEC Y93.H9 (*following* Y93.7)
    household (interior) NEC Y93.E9 (*following* Y93.7)
    land Y93.H9 (*following* Y93.7)
    property Y93.H9 (*following* Y93.7)

Activity — continued

marching (on level or elevated terrain) Y93.01
martial arts Y93.75
microwave oven Y93.G3 (following Y93.7)
milking an animal Y93.K2 (following Y93.7)
mopping (floor) Y93.E5 (following Y93.7)
mountain climbing Y93.31
muscle strengthening
    exercises (non-machine) NEC Y93.B9 (following Y93.7)
    machines Y93.B1 (following Y93.7)
musical keyboard (electronic) playing Y93.J1 (following Y93.7)
nordic skiing Y93.24
obstacle course Y93.A5 (following Y93.7)
oven (microwave) Y93.G3 (following Y93.7)
packing up and unpacking in moving to a new residence Y93.E6 (following Y93.7)
parasailing Y93.19
pass out game Y93.85
percussion instrument playing NEC Y93.J2 (following Y93.7)
personal
    bathing and showering Y93.E1 (following Y93.7)
    hygiene NEC Y93.E8 (following Y93.7)
    showering Y93.E1 (following Y93.7)
physical games generally associated with school recess, summer camp and children Y93.6A
physical training NEC Y93.A9 (following Y93.7)
piano playing Y93.J1 (following Y93.7)
pilates Y93.B4 (following Y93.7)
platform diving Y93.12
playing musical instrument
    brass instrument Y93.J4 (following Y93.7)
    drum Y93.J2 (following Y93.7)
    musical keyboard (electronic) Y93.J1 (following Y93.7)
    percussion instrument NEC Y93.J2 (following Y93.7)
    piano Y93.J1 (following Y93.7)
    string instrument Y93.J3 (following Y93.7)
    winds instrument Y93.J4 (following Y93.7)
property maintenance
    exterior NEC Y93.H9 (following Y93.7)
    interior NEC Y93.E9 (following Y93.7)
pruning (garden and lawn) Y93.H2 (following Y93.7)
pull-ups Y93.B2 (following Y93.7)
push-ups Y93.B2 (following Y93.7)
racquetball Y93.73
rafting (in calm and turbulent water) Y93.16
raking (leaves) Y93.H1 (following Y93.7)
rappelling Y93.32
refereeing a sports activity Y93.81
residential relocation Y93.E6 (following Y93.7)
rhythmic gymnastics Y93.43
rhythmic movement NEC Y93.49
riding
    horseback Y93.52
    rollercoaster Y93.I1 (following Y93.7)
rock climbing Y93.31
roller skating (inline) Y93.51
rollercoaster riding Y93.I1 (following Y93.7)
rough housing and horseplay Y93.83
rowing (in calm and turbulent water) Y93.16
rugby Y93.63
running Y93.02
SCUBA diving Y93.15
sewing Y93.D2 (following Y93.7)
shoveling Y93.H1 (following Y93.7)
    dirt Y93.H1 (following Y93.7)
    snow Y93.H1 (following Y93.7)
showering (personal) Y93.E1 (following Y93.7)
sit-ups Y93.B2 (following Y93.7)
skateboarding Y93.51
skating (ice) Y93.21
    roller Y93.51
skiing (alpine) (downhill) Y93.23
    cross country Y93.24
    nordic Y93.24
    water Y93.17
sledding (snow) Y93.23
sleeping (sleep) Y93.84
smoking and grilling food Y93.G2 (following Y93.7)
snorkeling Y93.15
snow NEC Y93.29
    boarding Y93.23
    shoveling Y93.H1 (following Y93.7)
    sledding Y93.23
    tubing Y93.23
soccer Y93.66

Activity — continued

softball Y93.64
specified NEC Y93.89
spectator at an event Y93.82
sports NEC Y93.79
    sports played as a team or group NEC Y93.69
    sports played individually NEC Y93.59
springboard diving Y93.12
squash Y93.73
stationary bike Y93.A1 (following Y93.7)
step (stepping) exercise (class) Y93.A3 (following Y93.7)
stepper machine Y93.A1 (following Y93.7)
stove Y93.G3 (following Y93.7)
string instrument playing Y93.J3 (following Y93.7)
surfing Y93.18
    wind Y93.18
swimming Y93.11
tackle football Y93.61
tap dancing Y93.41
tennis Y93.73
tobogganing Y93.23
touch football Y93.62
track and field events (non-running) Y93.57
    running Y93.02
trampoline Y93.44
treadmill Y93.A1 (following Y93.7)
trimming shrubs Y93.H2 (following Y93.7)
tubing (in calm and turbulent water) Y93.16
    snow Y93.23
ultimate frisbee Y93.74
underwater diving Y93.15
unpacking in moving to a new residence Y93.E6 (following Y93.7)
use of stove, oven and microwave oven Y93.G3 (following Y93.7)
vacuuming Y93.E3 (following Y93.7)
volleyball (beach) (court) Y93.68
wake boarding Y93.17
walking (on level or elevated terrain) Y93.01
    an animal Y93.K1 (following Y93.7)
walking an animal Y93.K1 (following Y93.7)
wall climbing Y93.31
warm up and cool down exercises Y93.A2 (following Y93.7)
water NEC Y93.19
    aerobics Y93.14
    craft NEC Y93.19
    exercise Y93.14
    polo Y93.13
    skiing Y93.17
    sliding Y93.18
    survival training and testing Y93.19
weeding (garden and lawn) Y93.H2 (following Y93.7)
wind instrument playing Y93.J4 (following Y93.7)
windsurfing Y93.18
wrestling Y93.72
yoga Y93.42

Adverse effect of drugs — see Table of Drugs and Chemicals

Aerosinusitis — see Air, pressure

After-effect, late — see Sequelae

Air
blast in war operations — see War operations, air blast
pressure
    change, rapid
        during
            ascent W94.29 ☑
                while (in) (surfacing from)
                    aircraft W94.23 ☑
                    deep water diving W94.21 ☑
                    underground W94.22 ☑
            descent W94.39 ☑
                in
                    aircraft W94.31 ☑
                    water W94.32 ☑
    high, prolonged W94.0 ☑
    low, prolonged W94.12 ☑
        due to residence or long visit at high altitude W94.11 ☑

Alpine sickness W94.11 ☑

Altitude sickness W94.11 ☑

Anaphylactic shock, anaphylaxis — see Table of Drugs and Chemicals

Andes disease W94.11 ☑

Arachnidism, arachnoidism X58 ☑

Arson (with intent to injure or kill) X97 ☑

Asphyxia, asphyxiation

by
    food (bone) (seed) — see categories T17 and T18 ☑
    gas — see also Table of Drugs and Chemicals
        legal
            execution — see Legal, intervention, gas
            intervention — see Legal, intervention, gas
from
    fire — see also Exposure, fire
        in war operations — see War operations, fire
    ignition — see Ignition
    vomitus T17.81 ☑
in war operations — see War operations, restriction of airway

Aspiration

food (any type) (into respiratory tract) (with asphyxia, obstruction respiratory tract, suffocation) — see categories T17 and T18 ☑
foreign body — see Foreign body, aspiration
vomitus (with asphyxia, obstruction respiratory tract, suffocation) T17.81 ☑

Assassination (attempt) — see Assault

Assault (homicidal) (by) (in) Y09

arson X97 ☑
bite (of human being) Y04.1 ☑
bodily force Y04.8 ☑
    bite Y04.1 ☑
    bumping into Y04.2 ☑
    sexual — see subcategories T74.0, T76.0 ☑
    unarmed fight Y04.0 ☑
bomb X96.9 ☑
    antipersonnel X96.0 ☑
    fertilizer X96.3 ☑
    gasoline X96.1 ☑
    letter X96.2 ☑
    petrol X96.1 ☑
    pipe X96.3 ☑
    specified NEC X96.8 ☑
brawl (hand) (fists) (foot) (unarmed) Y04.0 ☑
burning, burns (by fire) NEC X97 ☑
    acid Y08.89 ☑
    caustic, corrosive substance Y08.89 ☑
    chemical from swallowing caustic, corrosive substance — see Table of Drugs and Chemicals
    cigarette(s) X97 ☑
    hot object X98.9 ☑
        fluid NEC X98.2 ☑
        household appliance X98.3 ☑
        specified NEC X98.8 ☑
        steam X98.0 ☑
        tap water X98.1 ☑
        vapors X98.0 ☑
    scalding — see Assault, burning
    steam X98.0 ☑
    vitriol Y08.89 ☑
caustic, corrosive substance (gas) Y08.89 ☑
crashing of
    aircraft Y08.81 ☑
    motor vehicle Y03.8 ☑
        pushed in front of Y02.0 ☑
        run over Y03.0 ☑
        specified NEC Y03.8 ☑
cutting or piercing instrument X99.9 ☑
    dagger X99.2 ☑
    glass X99.0 ☑
    knife X99.1 ☑
    specified NEC X99.8 ☑
    sword X99.2 ☑
dagger X99.2 ☑
drowning (in) X92.9 ☑
    bathtub X92.0 ☑
    natural water X92.3 ☑
    specified NEC X92.8 ☑
    swimming pool X92.1 ☑
        following fall X92.2 ☑
dynamite X96.8 ☑
explosive(s) (material) X96.9 ☑
fight (hand) (fists) (foot) (unarmed) Y04.0 ☑
    with weapon — see Assault, by type of weapon
fire X97 ☑
firearm X95.9 ☑
    airgun X95.01 ☑
    handgun X93 ☑
    hunting rifle X94.1 ☑
    larger X94.9 ☑
        specified NEC X94.8 ☑

410 | ☑ Additional Character Required — Refer to the Tabular List for Character Selection | ▽ Subterms under main terms may continue to next column or page

Activity — Assault

Assault — *continued*
  firearm — *continued*
    machine gun X94.2 ☑
    shotgun X94.0 ☑
    specified NEC X95.8 ☑
  from high place Y01 ☑
  gunshot (wound) NEC — *see* Assault, firearm, by type
  incendiary device X97 ☑
  injury Y09
    to child due to criminal abortion attempt NEC
      Y08.89 ☑
  knife X99.1 ☑
  late effect of — *see* categories X92-Y08 with 7th character S
  placing before moving object NEC Y02.8 ☑
    motor vehicle Y02.0 ☑
  poisoning — *see* categories T36-T65 with 7th character S
  puncture, any part of body — *see* Assault, cutting or piercing instrument
  pushing
    before moving object NEC Y02.8 ☑
      motor vehicle Y02.0 ☑
      subway train Y02.1 ☑
      train Y02.1 ☑
    from high place Y01 ☑
  rape T74.2- ☑
  scalding — *see* Assault, burning
  sequelae of — *see* categories X92-Y08 with 7th character S
  sexual (by bodily force) T74.2- ☑
  shooting — *see* Assault, firearm
  specified means NEC Y08.89 ☑
  stab, any part of body — *see* Assault, cutting or piercing instrument
  steam X98.0 ☑
  striking against
    other person Y04.2 ☑
    sports equipment Y08.09 ☑
      baseball bat Y08.02 ☑
      hockey stick Y08.01 ☑
  struck by
    sports equipment Y08.09 ☑
      baseball bat Y08.02 ☑
      hockey stick Y08.01 ☑
  submersion — *see* Assault, drowning
  violence Y09
  weapon Y09
    blunt Y00 ☑
    cutting or piercing — *see* Assault, cutting or piercing instrument
    firearm — *see* Assault, firearm
  wound Y09
    cutting — *see* Assault, cutting or piercing instrument
    gunshot — *see* Assault, firearm
    knife X99.1 ☑
    piercing — *see* Assault, cutting or piercing instrument
    puncture — *see* Assault, cutting or piercing instrument
    stab — *see* Assault, cutting or piercing instrument
Attack by mammals NEC W55.89 ☑
Avalanche — *see* Landslide
Aviator's disease — *see* Air, pressure

B

Barotitis, barodontalgia, barosinusitis, barotrauma
  (otitic) (sinus) — *see* Air, pressure
Battered (baby) (child) (person) (syndrome) X58 ☑
Bayonet wound W26.1 ☑
  in
    legal intervention — *see* Legal, intervention, sharp object, bayonet
    war operations — *see* War operations, combat
  stated as undetermined whether accidental or intentional Y28.8 ☑
  suicide (attempt) X78.2 ☑
Bean in nose — *see* categories T17 and T18 ☑
Bed set on fire NEC — *see* Exposure, fire, uncontrolled, building, bed
Beheading (by guillotine)
  homicide X99.9 ☑
  legal execution — *see* Legal, intervention
Bending, injury in (prolonged) (static) X50.1 ☑

Bends — *see* Air, pressure, change
Bite, bitten by
  alligator W58.01 ☑
  arthropod (nonvenomous) NEC W57 ☑
  bull W55.21 ☑
  cat W55.01 ☑
  cow W55.21 ☑
  crocodile W58.11 ☑
  dog W54.0 ☑
  goat W55.31 ☑
  hoof stock NEC W55.31 ☑
  horse W55.11 ☑
  human being (accidentally) W50.3 ☑
    with intent to injure or kill Y04.1 ☑
    as, or caused by, a crowd or human stampede (with fall) W52 ☑
    assault Y04.1 ☑
    homicide (attempt) Y04.1 ☑
    in
      fight Y04.1 ☑
  insect (nonvenomous) W57 ☑
  lizard (nonvenomous) W59.01 ☑
  mammal NEC W55.81 ☑
    marine W56.31 ☑
  marine animal (nonvenomous) W56.81 ☑
  millipede W57 ☑
  moray eel W56.51 ☑
  mouse W53.01 ☑
  person(s) (accidentally) W50.3 ☑
    with intent to injure or kill Y04.1 ☑
    as, or caused by, a crowd or human stampede (with fall) W52 ☑
    assault Y04.1 ☑
    homicide (attempt) Y04.1 ☑
    in
      fight Y04.1 ☑
  pig W55.41 ☑
  raccoon W55.51 ☑
  rat W53.11 ☑
  reptile W59.81 ☑
    lizard W59.01 ☑
    snake W59.11 ☑
    turtle W59.21 ☑
      terrestrial W59.81 ☑
  rodent W53.81 ☑
    mouse W53.01 ☑
    rat W53.11 ☑
    specified NEC W53.81 ☑
    squirrel W53.21 ☑
  shark W56.41 ☑
  sheep W55.31 ☑
  snake (nonvenomous) W59.11 ☑
  spider (nonvenomous) W57 ☑
  squirrel W53.21 ☑
Blast (air) in war operations — *see* War operations, blast
Blizzard X37.2 ☑
Blood alcohol level Y90.9
  less than 20mg/100ml Y90.0
  presence in blood, level not specified Y90.9
  20-39mg/100ml Y90.1
  40-59mg/100ml Y90.2
  60-79mg/100ml Y90.3
  80-99mg/100ml Y90.4
  100-119mg/100ml Y90.5
  120-199mg/100ml Y90.6
  200-239mg/100ml Y90.7
Blow X58 ☑
  by law-enforcing agent, police (on duty) — *see* Legal, intervention, manhandling
  blunt object — *see* Legal, intervention, blunt object
Blowing up — *see* Explosion
Brawl (hand) (fists) (foot) Y04.0 ☑
Breakage (accidental) (part of)
  ladder (causing fall) W11 ☑
  scaffolding (causing fall) W12 ☑
Broken
  glass, contact with — *see* Contact, with, glass
  power line (causing electric shock) W85 ☑
Bumping against, into (accidentally)
  object NEC W22.8 ☑
    caused by crowd or human stampede (with fall) W52 ☑
    sports equipment W21.9 ☑
    with fall — *see* Fall, due to, bumping against, object
  person(s) W51 ☑
    with fall W03 ☑

Bumping against, into — *continued*
  person(s) — *continued*
    with fall — *continued*
      due to ice or snow W00.0 ☑
    assault Y04.2 ☑
    caused by, a crowd or human stampede (with fall) W52 ☑
    homicide (attempt) Y04.2 ☑
  sports equipment W21.9 ☑
Burn, burned, burning (accidental) (by) (from) (on)
  acid NEC — *see* Table of Drugs and Chemicals
  bed linen — *see* Exposure, fire, uncontrolled, in building, bed
  blowtorch X08.8 ☑
    with ignition of clothing NEC X06.2 ☑
      nightwear X05 ☑
  bonfire, campfire (controlled) — *see also* Exposure, fire, controlled, not in building)
    uncontrolled — *see* Exposure, fire, uncontrolled, not in building
  candle X08.8 ☑
    with ignition of clothing NEC X06.2 ☑
      nightwear X05 ☑
  caustic liquid, substance (external) (internal) NEC — *see* Table of Drugs and Chemicals
  chemical (external) (internal) — *see also* Table of Drugs and Chemicals
    in war operations — *see* War operations. fire
  cigar(s) or cigarette(s) X08.8 ☑
    with ignition of clothing NEC X06.2 ☑
      nightwear X05 ☑
  clothes, clothing NEC (from controlled fire) X06.2 ☑
    with conflagration — *see* Exposure, fire, uncontrolled, building
      not in building or structure — *see* Exposure, fire, uncontrolled, not in building
  cooker (hot) X15.8 ☑
    stated as undetermined whether accidental or intentional Y27.3 ☑
    suicide (attempt) X77.3 ☑
  electric blanket X16 ☑
  engine (hot) X17 ☑
  fire, flames — *see* Exposure, fire
  flare, Very pistol — *see* Discharge, firearm NEC
  heat
    from appliance (electrical) (household) X15.8 ☑
      cooker X15.8 ☑
      hotplate X15.2 ☑
      kettle X15.8 ☑
      light bulb X15.8 ☑
      saucepan X15.3 ☑
      skillet X15.3 ☑
      stated as undetermined whether accidental or intentional Y27.3 ☑
      stove X15.0 ☑
      suicide (attempt) X77.3 ☑
      toaster X15.1 ☑
    in local application or packing during medical or surgical procedure Y63.5
  heating
    appliance, radiator or pipe X16 ☑
  homicide (attempt) — *see* Assault, burning
  hot
    air X14.1 ☑
    cooker X15.8 ☑
    drink X10.0 ☑
    engine X17 ☑
    fat X10.2 ☑
    fluid NEC X12 ☑
    food X10.1 ☑
    gases X14.1 ☑
    heating appliance X16 ☑
    household appliance NEC X15.8 ☑
    kettle X15.8 ☑
    liquid NEC X12 ☑
    machinery X17 ☑
    metal (molten) (liquid) NEC X18 ☑
    object (not producing fire or flames) NEC X19 ☑
    oil (cooking) X10.2 ☑
    pipe(s) X16 ☑
    radiator X16 ☑
    saucepan (glass) (metal) X15.3 ☑
    stove (kitchen) X15.0 ☑
    substance NEC X19 ☑
      caustic or corrosive NEC — *see* Table of Drugs and Chemicals

Burn, burned, burning — *continued*
hot — *continued*
    toaster X15.1 ☑
    tool X17 ☑
    vapor X13.1 ☑
    water (tap) — *see* Contact, with, hot, tap water
hotplate X15.2 ☑
    suicide (attempt) X77.3 ☑
ignition — *see* Ignition
in war operations — *see* War operations, fire
inflicted by other person X97 ☑
    by hot objects, hot vapor, and steam — *see* Assault, burning, hot object
    internal, from swallowed caustic, corrosive liquid, substance — *see* Table of Drugs and Chemicals
iron (hot) X15.8 ☑
    stated as undetermined whether accidental or intentional Y27.3 ☑
    suicide (attempt) X77.3 ☑
kettle (hot) X15.8 ☑
    stated as undetermined whether accidental or intentional Y27.3 ☑
    suicide (attempt) X77.3 ☑
lamp (flame) X08.8 ☑
    with ignition of clothing NEC X06.2 ☑
        nightwear X05 ☑
lighter (cigar) (cigarette) X08.8 ☑
    with ignition of clothing NEC X06.2 ☑
        nightwear X05 ☑
lightning — *see* subcategory T75.0 ☑
    causing fire — *see* Exposure, fire
liquid (boiling) (hot) NEC X12 ☑
    stated as undetermined whether accidental or intentional Y27.2 ☑
    suicide (attempt) X77.2 ☑
local application of externally applied substance in medical or surgical care Y63.5
machinery (hot) X17 ☑
matches X08.8 ☑
    with ignition of clothing NEC X06.2 ☑
        nightwear X05 ☑
mattress — *see* Exposure, fire, uncontrolled, building, bed
medicament, externally applied Y63.5
metal (hot) (liquid) (molten) NEC X18 ☑
nightwear (nightclothes, nightdress, gown, pajamas, robe) X05 ☑
object (hot) NEC X19 ☑
on board watercraft
    due to
        accident to watercraft V91.09 ☑
            powered craft V91.03 ☑
                ferry boat V91.01 ☑
                fishing boat V91.02 ☑
                jetskis V91.03 ☑
                liner V91.01 ☑
                merchant ship V91.00 ☑
                passenger ship V91.01 ☑
            unpowered craft V91.08 ☑
                canoe V91.05 ☑
                inflatable V91.06 ☑
                kayak V91.05 ☑
                sailboat V91.04 ☑
                surf-board V91.08 ☑
                water skis V91.07 ☑
                windsurfer V91.08 ☑
        fire on board V93.09 ☑
            ferry boat V93.01 ☑
            fishing boat V93.02 ☑
            jetskis V93.03 ☑
            liner V93.01 ☑
            merchant ship V93.00 ☑
            passenger ship V93.01 ☑
            powered craft NEC V93.03 ☑
            sailboat V93.04 ☑
        specified heat source NEC on board V93.19 ☑
            ferry boat V93.11 ☑
            fishing boat V93.12 ☑
            jetskis V93.13 ☑
            liner V93.11 ☑
            merchant ship V93.10 ☑
            passenger ship V93.11 ☑
            powered craft NEC V93.13 ☑
            sailboat V93.14 ☑
pipe (hot) X16 ☑
    smoking X08.8 ☑

Burn, burned, burning — *continued*
pipe — *continued*
    smoking — *continued*
        with ignition of clothing NEC X06.2 ☑
            nightwear X05 ☑
powder — *see* Powder burn
radiator (hot) X16 ☑
saucepan (hot) (glass) (metal) X15.3 ☑
    stated as undetermined whether accidental or intentional Y27.3 ☑
    suicide (attempt) X77.3 ☑
self-inflicted X76 ☑
    stated as undetermined whether accidental or intentional Y26 ☑
stated as undetermined whether accidental or intentional Y27.0 ☑
steam X13.1 ☑
    pipe X16 ☑
    stated as undetermined whether accidental or intentional Y27.8 ☑
    stated as undetermined whether accidental or intentional Y27.0 ☑
    suicide (attempt) X77.0 ☑
stove (hot) (kitchen) X15.0 ☑
    stated as undetermined whether accidental or intentional Y27.3 ☑
    suicide (attempt) X77.3 ☑
substance (hot) NEC X19 ☑
    boiling X12 ☑
        stated as undetermined whether accidental or intentional Y27.2 ☑
        suicide (attempt) X77.2 ☑
    molten (metal) X18 ☑
suicide (attempt) NEC X76 ☑
    hot
        household appliance X77.3 ☑
        object X77.9 ☑
therapeutic misadventure
    heat in local application or packing during medical or surgical procedure Y63.5
    overdose of radiation Y63.2
toaster (hot) X15.1 ☑
    stated as undetermined whether accidental or intentional Y27.3 ☑
    suicide (attempt) X77.3 ☑
tool (hot) X17 ☑
torch, welding X08.8 ☑
    with ignition of clothing NEC X06.2 ☑
        nightwear X05 ☑
trash fire (controlled) — *see* Exposure, fire, controlled, not in building
    uncontrolled — *see* Exposure, fire, uncontrolled, not in building
vapor (hot) X13.1 ☑
    stated as undetermined whether accidental or intentional Y27.0 ☑
    suicide (attempt) X77.0 ☑
Very pistol — *see* Discharge, firearm NEC
Butted by animal W55.82 ☑
    bull W55.22 ☑
    cow W55.22 ☑
    goat W55.32 ☑
    horse W55.12 ☑
    pig W55.42 ☑
    sheep W55.32 ☑

C

Caisson disease — *see* Air, pressure, change
Campfire (exposure to) (controlled) — *see also* Exposure, fire, controlled, not in building
    uncontrolled — *see* Exposure, fire, uncontrolled, not in building
Capital punishment (any means) — *see* Legal, intervention
Car sickness T75.3 ☑
Casualty (not due to war) NEC X58 ☑
    war — *see* War operations
Cat
    bite W55.01 ☑
    scratch W55.03 ☑
Cataclysm, cataclysmic (any injury) NEC — *see* Forces of nature
Catching fire — *see* Exposure, fire

Caught
between
    folding object W23.0 ☑
    objects (moving) (stationary and moving) W23.0 ☑
        and machinery — *see* Contact, with, by type of machine
        stationary W23.1 ☑
    sliding door and door frame W23.0 ☑
by, in
    machinery (moving parts of) — *see* Contact, with, by type of machine
    washing-machine wringer W23.0 ☑
under packing crate (due to losing grip) W23.1 ☑
Cave-in caused by cataclysmic earth surface movement or eruption — *see* Landslide
Change(s) in air pressure — *see* Air, pressure, change
Choked, choking (on) (any object except food or vomitus)
    food (bone) (seed) — *see* categories T17 and T18 ☑
    vomitus T17.81- ☑
Civil insurrection — *see* War operations
Cloudburst (any injury) X37.8 ☑
Cold, exposure to (accidental) (excessive) (extreme) (natural) (place) NEC — *see* Exposure, cold
Collapse
building W20.1 ☑
    burning (uncontrolled fire) X00.2 ☑
dam or man-made structure (causing earth movement) X36.0 ☑
machinery — *see* Contact, with, by type of machine
structure W20.1 ☑
    burning (uncontrolled fire) X00.2 ☑
Collision (accidental) NEC — *see also* Accident, transport V89.9 ☑
pedestrian W51 ☑
    with fall W03 ☑
        due to ice or snow W00.0 ☑
        involving pedestrian conveyance — *see* Accident, transport, pedestrian, conveyance
    and
        crowd or human stampede (with fall) W52 ☑
        object W22.8 ☑
            with fall — *see* Fall, due to, bumping against, object
person(s) — *see* Collision, pedestrian
transport vehicle NEC V89.9 ☑
    and
        avalanche, fallen or not moving — *see* Accident, transport
            falling or moving — *see* Landslide
        landslide, fallen or not moving — *see* Accident, transport
            falling or moving — *see* Landslide
    due to cataclysm — *see* Forces of nature, by type
    intentional, purposeful suicide (attempt) — *see* Suicide, collision
Combustion, spontaneous — *see* Ignition
Complication (delayed) **of or following** (medical or surgical procedure) Y84.9
with misadventure — *see* Misadventure
amputation of limb(s) Y83.5
anastomosis (arteriovenous) (blood vessel) (gastrojejunal) (tendon) (natural or artificial material) Y83.2
aspiration (of fluid) Y84.4
    tissue Y84.8
biopsy Y84.8
blood
    sampling Y84.7
    transfusion
        procedure Y84.8
bypass Y83.2
catheterization (urinary) Y84.6
    cardiac Y84.0
colostomy Y83.3
cystostomy Y83.3
dialysis (kidney) Y84.1
drug — *see* Table of Drugs and Chemicals
due to misadventure — *see* Misadventure
duodenostomy Y83.3
electroshock therapy Y84.3
external stoma, creation of Y83.3
formation of external stoma Y83.3
gastrostomy Y83.3
graft Y83.2
hypothermia (medically-induced) Y84.8

Complication (delayed) **of or following** — *continued*

  implant, implantation (of)
    artificial
      internal device (cardiac pacemaker) (electrodes in brain) (heart valve prosthesis) (orthopedic) Y83.1
      material or tissue (for anastomosis or bypass) Y83.2
        with creation of external stoma Y83.3
      natural tissues (for anastomosis or bypass) Y83.2
        with creation of external stoma Y83.3
  infusion Y84.8
    procedure Y84.8
  injection — *see* Table of Drugs and Chemicals
    procedure Y84.8
  insertion of gastric or duodenal sound Y84.5
  insulin-shock therapy Y84.3
  paracentesis (abdominal) (thoracic) (aspirative) Y84.4
  procedures other than surgical operation — *see* Complication of or following, by type of procedure
  radiological procedure or therapy Y84.2
  removal of organ (partial) (total) NEC Y83.6
  sampling
    blood Y84.7
    fluid NEC Y84.4
    tissue Y84.8
  shock therapy Y84.3
  surgical operation NEC — *see also* Complication of or following, by type of operation Y83.9
    reconstructive NEC Y83.4
      with
        anastomosis, bypass or graft Y83.2
        formation of external stoma Y83.3
    specified NEC Y83.8
  transfusion — *see also* Table of Drugs and Chemicals
    procedure Y84.8
  transplant, transplantation (heart) (kidney) (liver) (whole organ, any) Y83.0
    partial organ Y83.4
  ureterostomy Y83.3
  vaccination — *see also* Table of Drugs and Chemicals
    procedure Y84.8

Compression
  divers' squeeze — *see* Air, pressure, change
  trachea by
    food (lodged in esophagus) — *see* categories T17 and T18 ☑
    vomitus (lodged in esophagus) T17.81- ☑

Conflagration — *see* Exposure, fire, uncontrolled

Constriction (external)
  hair W49.01 ☑
  jewelry W49.04 ☑
  ring W49.04 ☑
  rubber band W49.03 ☑
  specified item NEC W49.09 ☑
  string W49.02 ☑
  thread W49.02 ☑

Contact (accidental)
  with
    abrasive wheel (metalworking) W31.1 ☑
    alligator W58.09 ☑
      bite W58.01 ☑
      crushing W58.03 ☑
      strike W58.02 ☑
    amphibian W62.9 ☑
      frog W62.0 ☑
      toad W62.1 ☑
    animal (nonvenomous) NEC W64 ☑
      marine W56.89 ☑
        bite W56.81 ☑
        dolphin — *see* Contact, with, dolphin
        fish NEC — *see* Contact, with, fish
        mammal — *see* Contact, with, mammal, marine
        orca — *see* Contact, with, orca
        sea lion — *see* Contact, with, sea lion
        shark — *see* Contact, with, shark
        strike W56.82 ☑
    animate mechanical force NEC W64 ☑
    arrow W21.89 ☑
      not thrown, projected or falling W45.8 ☑
    arthropods (nonvenomous) W57 ☑
    axe W27.0 ☑
    band-saw (industrial) W31.2 ☑
    bayonet — *see* Bayonet wound
    bee(s) X58 ☑

Contact — *continued*
  with — *continued*
    bench-saw (industrial) W31.2 ☑
    bird W61.99 ☑
      bite W61.91 ☑
      chicken — *see* Contact, with, chicken
      duck — *see* Contact, with, duck
      goose — *see* Contact, with, goose
      macaw — *see* Contact, with, macaw
      parrot — *see* Contact, with, parrot
      psittacine — *see* Contact, with, psittacine
      strike W61.92 ☑
      turkey — *see* Contact, with, turkey
    blender W29.0 ☑
    boiling water X12 ☑
      stated as undetermined whether accidental or intentional Y27.2 ☑
      suicide (attempt) X77.2 ☑
    bore, earth-drilling or mining (land) (seabed) W31.0 ☑
    buffalo — *see* Contact, with, hoof stock NEC
    bull W55.29 ☑
      bite W55.21 ☑
      gored W55.22 ☑
      strike W55.22 ☑
    bumper cars W31.81 ☑
    camel — *see* Contact, with, hoof stock NEC
    can
      lid W26.8 ☑
      opener W27.4 ☑
        powered W29.0 ☑
    cat W55.09 ☑
      bite W55.01 ☑
      scratch W55.03 ☑
    caterpillar (venomous) X58 ☑
    centipede (venomous) X58 ☑
    chain
      hoist W24.0 ☑
        agricultural operations W30.89 ☑
      saw W29.3 ☑
    chicken W61.39 ☑
      peck W61.33 ☑
      strike W61.32 ☑
    chisel W27.0 ☑
    circular saw W31.2 ☑
    cobra X58 ☑
    combine (harvester) W30.0 ☑
    conveyer belt W24.1 ☑
    cooker (hot) X15.8 ☑
      stated as undetermined whether accidental or intentional Y27.3 ☑
      suicide (attempt) X77.3 ☑
    coral X58 ☑
    cotton gin W31.82 ☑
    cow W55.29 ☑
      bite W55.21 ☑
      strike W55.22 ☑
    crane W24.0 ☑
      agricultural operations W30.89 ☑
    crocodile W58.19 ☑
      bite W58.11 ☑
      crushing W58.13 ☑
      strike W58.12 ☑
    dagger W26.1 ☑
      stated as undetermined whether accidental or intentional Y28.2 ☑
      suicide (attempt) X78.2 ☑
    dairy equipment W31.82 ☑
    dart W21.89 ☑
      not thrown, projected or falling W45.8 ☑
    deer — *see* Contact, with, hoof stock NEC
    derrick W24.0 ☑
      agricultural operations W30.89 ☑
        hay W30.2 ☑
    dog W54.8 ☑
      bite W54.0 ☑
      strike W54.1 ☑
    dolphin W56.09 ☑
      bite W56.01 ☑
      strike W56.02 ☑
    donkey — *see* Contact, with, hoof stock NEC
    drill (powered) W29.8 ☑
      earth (land) (seabed) W31.0 ☑
      nonpowered W27.8 ☑
    drive belt W24.0 ☑
      agricultural operations W30.89 ☑

Contact — *continued*
  with — *continued*
    dry ice — *see* Exposure, cold, man-made
    dryer (clothes) (powered) (spin) W29.2 ☑
    duck W61.69 ☑
      bite W61.61 ☑
      strike W61.62 ☑
    earth (-)
      drilling machine (industrial) W31.0 ☑
      scraping machine in stationary use W31.83 ☑
    edge of stiff paper W26.2 ☑
    electric
      beater W29.0 ☑
      blanket X16 ☑
      fan W29.2 ☑
        commercial W31.82 ☑
      knife W29.1 ☑
      mixer W29.0 ☑
    elevator (building) W24.0 ☑
      agricultural operations W30.89 ☑
        grain W30.3 ☑
    engine(s), hot NEC X17 ☑
    excavating machine W31.0 ☑
    farm machine W30.9 ☑
    feces — *see* Contact, with, by type of animal
    fer de lance X58 ☑
    fish W56.59 ☑
      bite W56.51 ☑
      shark — *see* Contact, with, shark
      strike W56.52 ☑
    flying horses W31.81 ☑
    forging (metalworking) machine W31.1 ☑
    fork W27.4 ☑
    forklift (truck) W24.0 ☑
      agricultural operations W30.89 ☑
    frog W62.0 ☑
    garden
      cultivator (powered) W29.3 ☑
        riding W30.89 ☑
      fork W27.1 ☑
    gas turbine W31.3 ☑
    Gila monster X58 ☑
    giraffe — *see* Contact, with, hoof stock NEC
    glass (sharp) (broken) W25 ☑
      assault X99.0 ☑
      due to fall — *see* Fall, by type
      stated as undetermined whether accidental or intentional Y28.0 ☑
      suicide (attempt) X78.0 ☑
      with subsequent fall W18.02 ☑
    goat W55.39 ☑
      bite W55.31 ☑
      strike W55.32 ☑
    goose W61.59 ☑
      bite W61.51 ☑
      strike W61.52 ☑
    hand
      saw W27.0 ☑
      tool (not powered) NEC W27.8 ☑
        powered W29.8 ☑
    harvester W30.0 ☑
    hay-derrick W30.2 ☑
    heating
      appliance (hot) X16 ☑
      pad (electric) X16 ☑
    heat NEC X19 ☑
      from appliance (electrical) (household) — *see* Contact, with, hot, household appliance
      heating appliance X16 ☑
    hedge-trimmer (powered) W29.3 ☑
    hoe W27.1 ☑
    hoist (chain) (shaft) NEC W24.0 ☑
      agricultural W30.89 ☑
    hoof stock NEC W55.39 ☑
      bite W55.31 ☑
      strike W55.32 ☑
    hornet(s) X58 ☑
    horse W55.19 ☑
      bite W55.11 ☑
      strike W55.12 ☑
    hot
      air X14.1 ☑
        inhalation X14.0 ☑
      cooker X15.8 ☑
      drinks X10.0 ☑
      engine X17 ☑

Contact — *continued*
    with — *continued*
        hot — *continued*
            fats X10.2 ☑
            fluids NEC X12 ☑
                assault X98.2 ☑
                suicide (attempt) X77.2 ☑
                undetermined whether accidental or intentional Y27.2 ☑
            food X10.1 ☑
            gases X14.1 ☑
                inhalation X14.0 ☑
            heating appliance X16 ☑
            household appliance X15.8 ☑
                assault X98.3 ☑
                cooker X15.8 ☑
                hotplate X15.2 ☑
                kettle X15.8 ☑
                light bulb X15.8 ☑
                object NEC X19 ☑
                    assault X98.8 ☑
                    stated as undetermined whether accidental or intentional Y27.9 ☑
                    suicide (attempt) X77.8 ☑
                saucepan X15.3 ☑
                skillet X15.3 ☑
                stated as undetermined whether accidental or intentional Y27.3 ☑
                stove X15.0 ☑
                suicide (attempt) X77.3 ☑
                toaster X15.1 ☑
            kettle X15.8 ☑
            light bulb X15.8 ☑
            liquid NEC — *see also* Burn X12 ☑
                drinks X10.0 ☑
                stated as undetermined whether accidental or intentional Y27.2 ☑
                suicide (attempt) X77.2 ☑
                tap water X11.8 ☑
                    stated as undetermined whether accidental or intentional Y27.1 ☑
                    suicide (attempt) X77.1 ☑
            machinery X17 ☑
            metal (molten) (liquid) NEC X18 ☑
            object (not producing fire or flames) NEC X19 ☑
            oil (cooking) X10.2 ☑
            pipe X16 ☑
            plate X15.2 ☑
            radiator X16 ☑
            saucepan (glass) (metal) X15.3 ☑
            skillet X15.3 ☑
            stove (kitchen) X15.0 ☑
            substance NEC X19 ☑
            tap-water X11.8 ☑
                assault X98.1 ☑
                heated on stove X12 ☑
                    stated as undetermined whether accidental or intentional Y27.2 ☑
                    suicide (attempt) X77.2 ☑
                in bathtub X11.0 ☑
                running X11.1 ☑
                    stated as undetermined whether accidental or intentional Y27.1 ☑
                    suicide (attempt) X77.1 ☑
            toaster X15.1 ☑
            tool X17 ☑
            vapors X13.1 ☑
                inhalation X13.0 ☑
            water (tap) X11.8 ☑
                boiling X12 ☑
                    stated as undetermined whether accidental or intentional Y27.2 ☑
                    suicide (attempt) X77.2 ☑
                heated on stove X12 ☑
                    stated as undetermined whether accidental or intentional Y27.2 ☑
                    suicide (attempt) X77.2 ☑
                in bathtub X11.0 ☑
                running X11.1 ☑
                    stated as undetermined whether accidental or intentional Y27.1 ☑
                    suicide (attempt) X77.1 ☑
            hotplate X15.2 ☑
            ice-pick W27.4 ☑
            insect (nonvenomous) NEC W57 ☑
            kettle (hot) X15.8 ☑

Contact — *continued*
    with — *continued*
        knife W26.0 ☑
            assault X99.1 ☑
            electric W29.1 ☑
            stated as undetermined whether accidental or intentional Y28.1 ☑
            suicide (attempt) X78.1 ☑
        lathe (metalworking) W31.1 ☑
            turnings W45.8 ☑
            woodworking W31.2 ☑
        lawnmower (powered) (ridden) W28 ☑
            causing electrocution W86.8 ☑
            suicide (attempt) X83.1 ☑
            unpowered W27.1 ☑
        lift, lifting (devices) W24.0 ☑
            agricultural operations W30.89 ☑
            shaft W24.0 ☑
        liquefied gas — *see* Exposure, cold, man-made
        liquid air, hydrogen, nitrogen — *see* Exposure, cold, man-made
        lizard (nonvenomous) W59.09 ☑
            bite W59.01 ☑
            strike W59.02 ☑
        llama — *see* Contact, with, hoof stock NEC
        macaw W61.19 ☑
            bite W61.11 ☑
            strike W61.12 ☑
        machine, machinery W31.9 ☑
            abrasive wheel W31.1 ☑
            agricultural including animal-powered W30.9 ☑
                combine harvester W30.0 ☑
                grain storage elevator W30.3 ☑
                hay derrick W30.2 ☑
                power take-off device W30.1 ☑
                reaper W30.0 ☑
                specified NEC W30.89 ☑
                thresher W30.0 ☑
                transport vehicle, stationary W30.81 ☑
            band saw W31.2 ☑
            bench saw W31.2 ☑
            circular saw W31.2 ☑
            commercial NEC W31.82 ☑
            drilling, metal (industrial) W31.1 ☑
            earth-drilling W31.0 ☑
            earthmoving or scraping W31.89 ☑
            excavating W31.89 ☑
            forging machine W31.1 ☑
            gas turbine W31.3 ☑
            hot X17 ☑
            internal combustion engine W31.3 ☑
            land drill W31.0 ☑
            lathe W31.1 ☑
            lifting (devices) W24.0 ☑
            metal drill W31.1 ☑
            metalworking (industrial) W31.1 ☑
            milling, metal W31.1 ☑
            mining W31.0 ☑
            molding W31.2 ☑
            overhead plane W31.2 ☑
            power press, metal W31.1 ☑
            prime mover W31.3 ☑
            printing W31.89 ☑
            radial saw W31.2 ☑
            recreational W31.81 ☑
            roller-coaster W31.81 ☑
            rolling mill, metal W31.1 ☑
            sander W31.2 ☑
            seabed drill W31.0 ☑
            shaft
                hoist W31.0 ☑
                lift W31.0 ☑
            specified NEC W31.89 ☑
            spinning W31.89 ☑
            steam engine W31.3 ☑
            transmission W24.1 ☑
            undercutter W31.0 ☑
            water driven turbine W31.3 ☑
            weaving W31.89 ☑
            woodworking or forming (industrial) W31.2 ☑
        mammal (feces) (urine) W55.89 ☑
            bull — *see* Contact, with, bull
            cat — *see* Contact, with, cat
            cow — *see* Contact, with, cow
            goat — *see* Contact, with, goat
            hoof stock — *see* Contact, with, hoof stock

Contact — *continued*
    with — *continued*
        mammal — *continued*
            horse — *see* Contact, with, horse
            marine W56.39 ☑
                dolphin — *see* Contact, with, dolphin
                orca — *see* Contact, with, orca
                sea lion — *see* Contact, with, sea lion
                specified NEC W56.39 ☑
                    bite W56.31 ☑
                    strike W56.32 ☑
            pig — *see* Contact, with, pig
            raccoon — *see* Contact, with, raccoon
            rodent — *see* Contact, with, rodent
            sheep — *see* Contact, with, sheep
            specified NEC W55.89 ☑
                bite W55.81 ☑
                strike W55.82 ☑
        marine
            animal W56.89 ☑
                bite W56.81 ☑
                dolphin — *see* Contact, with, dolphin
                fish NEC — *see* Contact, with, fish
                mammal — *see* Contact, with, mammal, marine
                orca — *see* Contact, with, orca
                sea lion — *see* Contact, with, sea lion
                shark — *see* Contact, with, shark
                strike W56.82 ☑
        meat
            grinder (domestic) W29.0 ☑
                industrial W31.82 ☑
                nonpowered W27.4 ☑
            slicer (domestic) W29.0 ☑
                industrial W31.82 ☑
        merry go round W31.81 ☑
        metal, hot (liquid) (molten) NEC X18 ☑
        millipede W57 ☑
        nail W45.0 ☑
            gun W29.4 ☑
        needle (sewing) W27.3 ☑
            hypodermic W46.0 ☑
                contaminated W46.1 ☑
        object (blunt) NEC
            hot NEC X19 ☑
            legal intervention — *see* Legal, intervention, blunt object
            sharp NEC W45.8 ☑
                inflicted by other person NEC W45.8 ☑
                    stated as
                        intentional homicide (attempt) — *see* Assault, cutting or piercing instrument
                legal intervention — *see* Legal, intervention, sharp object
                self-inflicted X78.9 ☑
        orca W56.29 ☑
            bite W56.21 ☑
            strike W56.22 ☑
        overhead plane W31.2 ☑
        paper (as sharp object) W26.2 ☑
        paper-cutter W27.5 ☑
        parrot W61.09 ☑
            bite W61.01 ☑
            strike W61.02 ☑
        pig W55.49 ☑
            bite W55.41 ☑
            strike W55.42 ☑
        pipe, hot X16 ☑
        pitchfork W27.1 ☑
        plane (metal) (wood) W27.0 ☑
            overhead W31.2 ☑
        plant thorns, spines, sharp leaves or other mechanisms W60 ☑
        powered
            garden cultivator W29.3 ☑
            household appliance, implement, or machine W29.8 ☑
            saw (industrial) W31.2 ☑
                hand W29.8 ☑
        printing machine W31.89 ☑
        psittacine bird W61.29 ☑
            bite W61.21 ☑
            macaw — *see* Contact, with, macaw
            parrot — *see* Contact, with, parrot
            strike W61.22 ☑

Contact — *continued*
  with — *continued*
    pulley (block) (transmission) W24.0 ☑
      agricultural operations W30.89 ☑
    raccoon W55.59 ☑
      bite W55.51 ☑
      strike W55.52 ☑
    radial-saw (industrial) W31.2 ☑
    radiator (hot) X16 ☑
    rake W27.1 ☑
    rattlesnake X58 ☑
    reaper W30.0 ☑
    reptile W59.89 ☑
      lizard — *see* Contact, with, lizard
      snake — *see* Contact, with, snake
      specified NEC W59.89 ☑
        bite W59.81 ☑
        crushing W59.83 ☑
        strike W59.82 ☑
      turtle — *see* Contact, with, turtle
    rivet gun (powered) W29.4 ☑
    road scraper — *see* Accident, transport, construction
      vehicle
    rodent (feces) (urine) W53.89 ☑
      bite W53.81 ☑
      mouse W53.09 ☑
        bite W53.01 ☑
      rat W53.19 ☑
        bite W53.11 ☑
      specified NEC W53.89 ☑
        bite W53.81 ☑
      squirrel W53.29 ☑
        bite W53.21 ☑
    roller coaster W31.81 ☑
    rope NEC W24.0 ☑
      agricultural operations W30.89 ☑
    saliva — *see* Contact, with, by type of animal
    sander W29.8 ☑
      industrial W31.2 ☑
    saucepan (hot) (glass) (metal) X15.3 ☑
    saw W27.0 ☑
      band (industrial) W31.2 ☑
      bench (industrial) W31.2 ☑
      chain W29.3 ☑
      hand W27.0 ☑
    sawing machine, metal W31.1 ☑
    scissors W27.2 ☑
    scorpion X58 ☑
    screwdriver W27.0 ☑
      powered W29.8 ☑
    sea
      anemone, cucumber or urchin (spine) X58 ☑
      lion W56.19 ☑
        bite W56.11 ☑
        strike W56.12 ☑
    serpent — *see* Contact, with, snake, by type
    sewing-machine (electric) (powered) W29.2 ☑
      not powered W27.8 ☑
    shaft (hoist) (lift) (transmission) NEC W24.0 ☑
      agricultural W30.89 ☑
    shark W56.49 ☑
      bite W56.41 ☑
      strike W56.42 ☑
    sharp object(s) W26.9 ☑
      specified NEC W26.8 ☑
    shears (hand) W27.2 ☑
      powered (industrial) W31.1 ☑
        domestic W29.2 ☑
    sheep W55.39 ☑
      bite W55.31 ☑
      strike W55.32 ☑
    shovel W27.8 ☑
      steam — *see* Accident, transport, construction
        vehicle
    snake (nonvenomous) W59.19 ☑
      bite W59.11 ☑
      crushing W59.13 ☑
      strike W59.12 ☑
    spade W27.1 ☑
    spider (venomous) X58 ☑
    spin-drier W29.2 ☑
    spinning machine W31.89 ☑
    splinter W45.8 ☑
    sports equipment W21.9 ☑
    staple gun (powered) W29.8 ☑
    steam X13.1 ☑

Contact — *continued*
  with — *continued*
    steam — *continued*
      engine W31.3 ☑
      inhalation X13.0 ☑
      pipe X16 ☑
      shovel W31.89 ☑
    stove (hot) (kitchen) X15.0 ☑
    substance, hot NEC X19 ☑
      molten (metal) X18 ☑
    sword W26.1 ☑
      assault X99.2 ☑
      stated as undetermined whether accidental or
        intentional Y28.2 ☑
      suicide (attempt) X78.2 ☑
    tarantula X58 ☑
    thresher W30.0 ☑
    tin can lid W26.8 ☑
    toad W62.1 ☑
    toaster (hot) X15.1 ☑
    tool W27.8 ☑
      hand (not powered) W27.8 ☑
        auger W27.0 ☑
        axe W27.0 ☑
        can opener W27.4 ☑
        chisel W27.0 ☑
        fork W27.4 ☑
        garden W27.1 ☑
        handsaw W27.0 ☑
        hoe W27.1 ☑
        ice-pick W27.4 ☑
        kitchen utensil W27.4 ☑
        manual
          lawn mower W27.1 ☑
          sewing machine W27.8 ☑
        meat grinder W27.4 ☑
        needle (sewing) W27.3 ☑
          hypodermic W46.0 ☑
            contaminated W46.1 ☑
        paper cutter W27.5 ☑
        pitchfork W27.1 ☑
        rake W27.1 ☑
        scissors W27.2 ☑
        screwdriver W27.0 ☑
        specified NEC W27.8 ☑
        workbench W27.0 ☑
      hot X17 ☑
      powered W29.8 ☑
        blender W29.0 ☑
          commercial W31.82 ☑
        can opener W29.0 ☑
          commercial W31.82 ☑
        chainsaw W29.3 ☑
        clothes dryer W29.2 ☑
          commercial W31.82 ☑
        dishwasher W29.2 ☑
          commercial W31.82 ☑
        edger W29.3 ☑
        electric fan W29.2 ☑
          commercial W31.82 ☑
        electric knife W29.1 ☑
        food processor W29.0 ☑
          commercial W31.82 ☑
        garbage disposal W29.0 ☑
          commercial W31.82 ☑
        garden tool W29.3 ☑
        hedge trimmer W29.3 ☑
        ice maker W29.0 ☑
          commercial W31.82 ☑
        kitchen appliance W29.0 ☑
          commercial W31.82 ☑
        lawn mower W28 ☑
        meat grinder W29.0 ☑
          commercial W31.82 ☑
        mixer W29.0 ☑
          commercial W31.82 ☑
        rototiller W29.3 ☑
        sewing machine W29.2 ☑
          commercial W31.82 ☑
        washing machine W29.2 ☑
          commercial W31.82 ☑
    transmission device (belt, cable, chain, gear, pinion,
      shaft) W24.1 ☑
      agricultural operations W30.89 ☑
    turbine (gas) (water-driven) W31.3 ☑
    turkey W61.49 ☑

Contact — *continued*
  with — *continued*
    turkey — *continued*
      peck W61.43 ☑
      strike W61.42 ☑
    turtle (nonvenomous) W59.29 ☑
      bite W59.21 ☑
      strike W59.22 ☑
      terrestrial W59.89 ☑
        bite W59.81 ☑
        crushing W59.83 ☑
        strike W59.82 ☑
    under-cutter W31.0 ☑
    urine — *see* Contact, with, by type of animal
    vehicle
      agricultural use (transport) — *see* Accident,
        transport, agricultural vehicle
        not on public highway W30.81 ☑
      industrial use (transport) — *see* Accident, trans-
        port, industrial vehicle
        not on public highway W31.83 ☑
      off-road use (transport) — *see* Accident, trans-
        port, all-terrain or off-road vehicle
        not on public highway W31.83 ☑
      special construction use (transport) — *see* Acci-
        dent, transport, construction vehicle
        not on public highway W31.83 ☑
    venomous
      animal X58 ☑
      arthropods X58 ☑
      lizard X58 ☑
      marine animal NEC X58 ☑
      marine plant NEC X58 ☑
      millipedes (tropical) X58 ☑
      plant(s) X58 ☑
      snake X58 ☑
      spider X58 ☑
      viper X58 ☑
    washing-machine (powered) W29.2 ☑
    wasp X58 ☑
    weaving-machine W31.89 ☑
    winch W24.0 ☑
      agricultural operations W30.89 ☑
    wire NEC W24.0 ☑
      agricultural operations W30.89 ☑
    wood slivers W45.8 ☑
    yellow jacket X58 ☑
    zebra — *see* Contact, with, hoof stock NEC
  pressure X50.9 ☑
  stress X50.9 ☑
Coup de soleil X32 ☑
Crash
  aircraft (in transit) (powered) V95.9 ☑
    balloon V96.01 ☑
    fixed wing NEC (private) V95.21 ☑
      commercial V95.31 ☑
    glider V96.21 ☑
      hang V96.11 ☑
      powered V95.11 ☑
    helicopter V95.01 ☑
    in war operations — *see* War operations, destruction
      of aircraft
    microlight V95.11 ☑
    nonpowered V96.9 ☑
      specified NEC V96.8 ☑
    powered NEC V95.8 ☑
    stated as
      homicide (attempt) Y08.81 ☑
      suicide (attempt) X83.0 ☑
    ultralight V95.11 ☑
  spacecraft V95.41 ☑
  transport vehicle NEC — *see also* Accident, transport
    V89.9 ☑
    homicide (attempt) Y03.8 ☑
    motor NEC (traffic) V89.2 ☑
      homicide (attempt) Y03.8 ☑
      suicide (attempt) — *see* Suicide, collision
Cruelty (mental) (physical) (sexual) X58 ☑
Crushed (accidentally) X58 ☑
  between objects (moving) (stationary and moving)
    W23.0 ☑
    stationary W23.1 ☑
  by
    alligator W58.03 ☑
    avalanche NEC — *see* Landslide
    cave-in W20.0 ☑

Crushed — continued
 by — continued
  cave-in — continued
   caused by cataclysmic earth surface movement
    — see Landslide
  crocodile W58.13 ☑
  crowd or human stampede W52 ☑
  falling
   aircraft V97.39 ☑
    in war operations — see War operations, destruction of aircraft
   earth, material W20.0 ☑
    caused by cataclysmic earth surface movement — see Landslide
   object NEC W20.8 ☑
  landslide NEC — see Landslide
  lizard (nonvenomous) W59.09 ☑
  machinery — see Contact, with, by type of machine
  reptile NEC W59.89 ☑
  snake (nonvenomous) W59.13 ☑
 in
  machinery — see Contact, with, by type of machine
Cut, cutting (any part of body) (accidental) — see also
  Contact, with, by object or machine
 during medical or surgical treatment as misadventure
  — see Index to Diseases and Injuries, Complications
 homicide (attempt) — see Assault, cutting or piercing
  instrument
 inflicted by other person — see Assault, cutting or
  piercing instrument
 legal
  execution — see Legal, intervention
  intervention — see Legal, intervention, sharp object
 machine NEC — see also Contact, with, by type of machine W31.9 ☑
 self-inflicted — see Suicide, cutting or piercing instrument
 suicide (attempt) — see Suicide, cutting or piercing
  instrument
Cyclone (any injury) X37.1 ☑

D

Decapitation (accidental circumstances) NEC X58 ☑
 homicide X99.9 ☑
 legal execution — see Legal, intervention
Dehydration from lack of water X58 ☑
Deprivation X58 ☑
Derailment (accidental)
 railway (rolling stock) (train) (vehicle) (without antecedent collision) V81.7 ☑
  with antecedent collision — see Accident, transport,
   railway vehicle occupant
 streetcar (without antecedent collision) V82.7 ☑
  with antecedent collision — see Accident, transport,
   streetcar occupant
Descent
 parachute (voluntary) (without accident to aircraft)
  V97.29 ☑
  due to accident to aircraft — see Accident, transport,
   aircraft
Desertion X58 ☑
Destitution X58 ☑
Disability, late effect or sequela of injury — see Sequelae
Discharge (accidental)
 airgun W34.010 ☑
  assault X95.01 ☑
  homicide (attempt) X95.01 ☑
  stated as undetermined whether accidental or intentional Y24.0 ☑
  suicide (attempt) X74.01 ☑
 BB gun — see Discharge, airgun
 firearm (accidental) W34.00 ☑
  assault X95.9 ☑
  handgun (pistol) (revolver) W32.0 ☑
   assault X93 ☑
   homicide (attempt) X93 ☑
   legal intervention — see Legal, intervention,
    firearm, handgun
   stated as undetermined whether accidental or
    intentional Y22 ☑
   suicide (attempt) X72 ☑
  homicide (attempt) X95.9 ☑
  hunting rifle W33.02 ☑

Discharge — continued
 firearm — continued
  hunting rifle — continued
   assault X94.1 ☑
   homicide (attempt) X94.1 ☑
   legal intervention
    injuring
     bystander Y35.032 ☑
     law enforcement personnel Y35.031 ☑
     suspect Y35.033 ☑
     unspecified person Y35.039 ☑
   stated as undetermined whether accidental or
    intentional Y23.1 ☑
   suicide (attempt) X73.1 ☑
  larger W33.00 ☑
   assault X94.9 ☑
   homicide (attempt) X94.9 ☑
   hunting rifle — see Discharge, firearm, hunting
    rifle
   legal intervention — see Legal, intervention,
    firearm by type of firearm
   machine gun — see Discharge, firearm, machine
    gun
   shotgun — see Discharge, firearm, shotgun
   specified NEC W33.09 ☑
    assault X94.8 ☑
    homicide (attempt) X94.8 ☑
    legal intervention
     injuring
      bystander Y35.092 ☑
      law enforcement personnel
       Y35.091 ☑
      suspect Y35.093 ☑
      unspecified person Y35.099 ☑
    stated as undetermined whether accidental
     or intentional Y23.8 ☑
    suicide (attempt) X73.8 ☑
   stated as undetermined whether accidental or
    intentional Y23.9 ☑
   suicide (attempt) X73.9 ☑
  legal intervention
   injuring
    bystander Y35.002 ☑
    law enforcement personnel Y35.001 ☑
    suspect Y35.03 ☑
    unspecified person Y35.009 ☑
   using rubber bullet
    injuring
     bystander Y35.042 ☑
     law enforcement personnel Y35.041 ☑
     suspect Y35.043 ☑
     unspecified person Y35.049 ☑
  machine gun W33.03 ☑
   assault X94.2 ☑
   homicide (attempt) X94.2 ☑
   legal intervention — see Legal, intervention,
    firearm, machine gun
   stated as undetermined whether accidental or
    intentional Y23.3 ☑
   suicide (attempt) X73.2 ☑
  pellet gun — see Discharge, airgun
  shotgun W33.01 ☑
   assault X94.0 ☑
   homicide (attempt) X94.0 ☑
   legal intervention — see Legal, intervention,
    firearm, specified NEC
   stated as undetermined whether accidental or
    intentional Y23.0 ☑
   suicide (attempt) X73.0 ☑
  specified NEC W34.09 ☑
   assault X95.8 ☑
   homicide (attempt) X95.8 ☑
   legal intervention — see Legal, intervention,
    firearm, specified NEC
   stated as undetermined whether accidental or
    intentional Y24.8 ☑
   suicide (attempt) X74.8 ☑
  stated as undetermined whether accidental or intentional Y24.9 ☑
  suicide (attempt) X74.9 ☑
 Very pistol W34.09 ☑
  assault X95.8 ☑
  homicide (attempt) X95.8 ☑
  stated as undetermined whether accidental or
   intentional Y24.8 ☑
  suicide (attempt) X74.8 ☑

Discharge — continued
 firework(s) W39 ☑
  stated as undetermined whether accidental or intentional Y25 ☑
 gas-operated gun NEC W34.018 ☑
  airgun — see Discharge, airgun
  assault X95.09 ☑
  homicide (attempt) X95.09 ☑
  paintball gun — see Discharge, paintball gun
  stated as undetermined whether accidental or intentional Y24.8 ☑
  suicide (attempt) X74.09 ☑
 gun NEC — see also Discharge, firearm NEC
  air — see Discharge, airgun
  BB — see Discharge, airgun
  for single hand use — see Discharge, firearm,
   handgun
  hand — see Discharge, firearm, handgun
  machine — see Discharge, firearm, machine gun
  other specified — see Discharge, firearm NEC
  paintball — see Discharge, paintball gun
  pellet — see Discharge, airgun
 handgun — see Discharge, firearm, handgun
 machine gun — see Discharge, firearm, machine gun
 paintball gun W34.011 ☑
  assault X95.02 ☑
  homicide (attempt) X95.02 ☑
  stated as undetermined whether accidental or intentional Y24.8 ☑
  suicide (attempt) X74.02 ☑
 pistol — see Discharge, firearm, handgun
  flare — see Discharge, firearm, Very pistol
  pellet — see Discharge, airgun
  Very — see Discharge, firearm, Very pistol
 revolver — see Discharge, firearm, handgun
 rifle (hunting) — see Discharge, firearm, hunting rifle
 shotgun — see Discharge, firearm, shotgun
 spring-operated gun NEC W34.018 ☑
  assault X95.09 ☑
  homicide (attempt) X95.09 ☑
  stated as undetermined whether accidental or intentional Y24.8 ☑
  suicide (attempt) X74.09 ☑
Disease
 Andes W94.11 ☑
 aviator's — see Air, pressure
 range W94.11 ☑
Diver's disease, palsy, paralysis, squeeze — see Air,
  pressure
Diving (into water) — see Accident, diving
Dog bite W54.0 ☑
Dragged by transport vehicle NEC — see also Accident,
  transport V09.9 ☑
Drinking poison (accidental) — see Table of Drugs and
  Chemicals
Dropped (accidentally) **while being carried or supported by other person** W04 ☑
Drowning (accidental) W74 ☑
 assault X92.9 ☑
 due to
  accident (to)
   machinery — see Contact, with, by type of machine
   watercraft V90.89 ☑
    burning V90.29 ☑
     powered V90.23 ☑
      fishing boat V90.22 ☑
      jetskis V90.23 ☑
      merchant ship V90.20 ☑
      passenger ship V90.21 ☑
     unpowered V90.28 ☑
      canoe V90.25 ☑
      inflatable V90.26 ☑
      kayak V90.25 ☑
      sailboat V90.24 ☑
      water skis V90.27 ☑
    crushed V90.39 ☑
     powered V90.33 ☑
      fishing boat V90.32 ☑
      jetskis V90.33 ☑
      merchant ship V90.30 ☑
      passenger ship V90.31 ☑
     unpowered V90.38 ☑
      canoe V90.35 ☑
      inflatable V90.36 ☑
      kayak V90.35 ☑

Drowning — *continued*
  due to — *continued*
    accident — *continued*
      watercraft — *continued*
        crushed — *continued*
          unpowered — *continued*
            sailboat V90.34 ☑
            water skis V90.37 ☑
        overturning V90.09 ☑
          powered V90.03 ☑
            fishing boat V90.02 ☑
            jetskis V90.03 ☑
            merchant ship V90.00 ☑
            passenger ship V90.01 ☑
          unpowered V90.08 ☑
            canoe V90.05 ☑
            inflatable V90.06 ☑
            kayak V90.05 ☑
            sailboat V90.04 ☑
        sinking V90.19 ☑
          powered V90.13 ☑
            fishing boat V90.12 ☑
            jetskis V90.13 ☑
            merchant ship V90.10 ☑
            passenger ship V90.11 ☑
          unpowered V90.18 ☑
            canoe V90.15 ☑
            inflatable V90.16 ☑
            kayak V90.15 ☑
            sailboat V90.14 ☑
        specified type NEC V90.89 ☑
          powered V90.83 ☑
            fishing boat V90.82 ☑
            jetskis V90.83 ☑
            merchant ship V90.80 ☑
            passenger ship V90.81 ☑
          unpowered V90.88 ☑
            canoe V90.85 ☑
            inflatable V90.86 ☑
            kayak V90.85 ☑
            sailboat V90.84 ☑
            water skis V90.87 ☑
    avalanche — *see* Landslide
    cataclysmic
      earth surface movement NEC — *see* Forces of
        nature, earth movement
      storm — *see* Forces of nature, cataclysmic storm
    cloudburst X37.8 ☑
    cyclone X37.1 ☑
    fall overboard (from) V92.09 ☑
      powered craft V92.03 ☑
        ferry boat V92.01 ☑
        fishing boat V92.02 ☑
        jetskis V92.03 ☑
        liner V92.01 ☑
        merchant ship V92.00 ☑
        passenger ship V92.01 ☑
      resulting from
        accident to watercraft — *see* Drowning, due
          to, accident to, watercraft
        being washed overboard (from) V92.29 ☑
          powered craft V92.23 ☑
            ferry boat V92.21 ☑
            fishing boat V92.22 ☑
            jetskis V92.23 ☑
            liner V92.21 ☑
            merchant ship V92.20 ☑
            passenger ship V92.21 ☑
          unpowered craft V92.28 ☑
            canoe V92.25 ☑
            inflatable V92.26 ☑
            kayak V92.25 ☑
            sailboat V92.24 ☑
            surf-board V92.28 ☑
            water skis V92.27 ☑
            windsurfer V92.28 ☑
        motion of watercraft V92.19 ☑
          powered craft V92.13 ☑
            ferry boat V92.11 ☑
            fishing boat V92.12 ☑
            jetskis V92.13 ☑
            liner V92.11 ☑
            merchant ship V92.10 ☑
            passenger ship V92.11 ☑
          unpowered craft
            canoe V92.15 ☑

Drowning — *continued*
  due to — *continued*
    fall overboard — *continued*
      resulting from — *continued*
        motion of watercraft — *continued*
          unpowered craft — *continued*
            inflatable V92.16 ☑
            kayak V92.15 ☑
            sailboat V92.14 ☑
        unpowered craft V92.08 ☑
          canoe V92.05 ☑
          inflatable V92.06 ☑
          kayak V92.05 ☑
          sailboat V92.04 ☑
          surf-board V92.08 ☑
          water skis V92.07 ☑
          windsurfer V92.08 ☑
    hurricane X37.0 ☑
    jumping into water from watercraft (involved in
      accident) — *see also* Drowning, due to, acci-
      dent to, watercraft
      without accident to or on watercraft W16.711 ☑
    tidal wave NEC — *see* Forces of nature, tidal wave
    torrential rain X37.8 ☑
  following
    fall
      into
        bathtub W16.211 ☑
        bucket W16.221 ☑
        fountain — *see* Drowning, following, fall, into,
          water, specified NEC
        quarry — *see* Drowning, following, fall, into,
          water, specified NEC
        reservoir — *see* Drowning, following, fall, into,
          water, specified NEC
        swimming-pool W16.011 ☑
          stated as undetermined whether acciden-
            tal or intentional Y21.3 ☑
          striking
            bottom W16.021 ☑
            wall W16.031 ☑
          suicide (attempt) X71.2 ☑
        water NOS W16.41 ☑
          natural (lake) (open sea) (river) (stream)
            (pond) W16.111 ☑
            striking
              bottom W16.121 ☑
              side W16.131 ☑
          specified NEC W16.311 ☑
            striking
              bottom W16.321 ☑
              wall W16.331 ☑
      overboard NEC — *see* Drowning, due to, fall
        overboard
    jump or dive
      from boat W16.711 ☑
        striking bottom W16.721 ☑
      into
        fountain — *see* Drowning, following, jump
          or dive, into, water, specified NEC
        quarry — *see* Drowning, following, jump or
          dive, into, water, specified NEC
        reservoir — *see* Drowning, following, jump
          or dive, into, water, specified NEC
        swimming-pool W16.511 ☑
          striking
            bottom W16.521 ☑
            wall W16.531 ☑
          suicide (attempt) X71.2 ☑
        water NOS W16.91 ☑
          natural (lake) (open sea) (river) (stream)
            (pond) W16.611 ☑
          specified NEC W16.811 ☑
            bottom W16.821 ☑
            striking
              bottom W16.821 ☑
              wall W16.831 ☑
           striking
            bottom W16.821 ☑
            wall W16.831 ☑
            striking bottom W16.621 ☑
    homicide (attempt) X92.9 ☑
  in
    bathtub (accidental) W65 ☑
      assault X92.0 ☑
      following fall W16.211 ☑

Drowning — *continued*
  in — *continued*
    bathtub — *continued*
      following fall — *continued*
        stated as undetermined whether accidental
          or intentional Y21.1 ☑
      stated as undetermined whether accidental or
        intentional Y21.0 ☑
      suicide (attempt) X71.0 ☑
    lake — *see* Drowning, in, natural water
    natural water (lake) (open sea) (river) (stream)
      (pond) W69 ☑
      assault X92.3 ☑
      following
        dive or jump W16.611 ☑
          striking bottom W16.621 ☑
        fall W16.111 ☑
          striking
            bottom W16.121 ☑
            side W16.131 ☑
      stated as undetermined whether accidental or
        intentional Y21.4 ☑
      suicide (attempt) X71.3 ☑
    quarry — *see* Drowning, in, specified place NEC
    quenching tank — *see* Drowning, in, specified place
      NEC
    reservoir — *see* Drowning, in, specified place NEC
    river — *see* Drowning, in, natural water
    sea — *see* Drowning, in, natural water
    specified place NEC W73 ☑
      assault X92.8 ☑
      following
        dive or jump W16.811 ☑
          striking
            bottom W16.821 ☑
            wall W16.831 ☑
        fall W16.311 ☑
          striking
            bottom W16.321 ☑
            wall W16.331 ☑
      stated as undetermined whether accidental or
        intentional Y21.8 ☑
      suicide (attempt) X71.8 ☑
    stream — *see* Drowning, in, natural water
    swimming-pool W67 ☑
      assault X92.1 ☑
      following fall X92.2 ☑
      following
        dive or jump W16.511 ☑
          striking
            bottom W16.521 ☑
            wall W16.531 ☑
        fall W16.011 ☑
          striking
            bottom W16.021 ☑
            wall W16.031 ☑
      stated as undetermined whether accidental or
        intentional Y21.2 ☑
        following fall Y21.3 ☑
      suicide (attempt) X71.1 ☑
        following fall X71.2 ☑
    war operations — *see* War operations, restriction
      of airway
  resulting from accident to watercraft — *see* Drowning,
    due to, accident, watercraft
  self-inflicted X71.9 ☑
  stated as undetermined whether accidental or inten-
    tional Y21.9 ☑
  suicide (attempt) X71.9 ☑

E

Earth falling (on) W20.0 ☑
  caused by cataclysmic earth surface movement or
    eruption — *see* Landslide
Earth (surface) **movement NEC** — *see* Forces of nature,
  earth movement
Earthquake (any injury) X34 ☑
Effect(s) (adverse) **of**
  air pressure (any) — *see* Air, pressure
  cold, excessive (exposure to) — *see* Exposure, cold
  heat (excessive) — *see* Heat
  hot place (weather) — *see* Heat
  insolation X30 ☑
  late — *see* Sequelae
  motion — *see* Motion

Effect(s) (adverse) **of** — *continued*
  nuclear explosion or weapon in war operations — *see*
      War operations, nuclear weapon
  radiation — *see* Radiation
  travel — *see* Travel
Electric shock (accidental) (by) (in) — *see* Exposure,
      electric current
Electrocution (accidental) — *see* Exposure, electric cur-
      rent
Endotracheal tube wrongly placed during anesthetic
      procedure
Entanglement
  in
      bed linen, causing suffocation T71 ☑
      wheel of pedal cycle V19.88 ☑
Entry of foreign body or material — *see* Foreign body
Environmental pollution related condition — *see*
      category Z57
Execution, legal (any method) — *see* Legal, intervention
Exhaustion
  cold — *see* Exposure, cold
  due to excessive exertion — *see also* Overexertion
      X50.9 ☑
  heat — *see* Heat
Explosion (accidental) (of) (with secondary fire) W40.9 ☑
  acetylene W40.1 ☑
  aerosol can W36.1 ☑
  air tank (compressed) (in machinery) W36.2 ☑
  aircraft (in transit) (powered) NEC V95.9 ☑
      balloon V96.05 ☑
      fixed wing NEC (private) V95.25 ☑
          commercial V95.35 ☑
      glider V96.25 ☑
      hang V96.15 ☑
      powered V95.15 ☑
      helicopter V95.05 ☑
      in war operations — *see* War operations, destruction
          of aircraft
      microlight V95.15 ☑
      nonpowered V96.9 ☑
          specified NEC V96.8 ☑
      powered NEC V95.8 ☑
      stated as
          homicide (attempt) Y03.8 ☑
          suicide (attempt) X83.0 ☑
      ultralight V95.15 ☑
  anesthetic gas in operating room W40.1 ☑
  antipersonnel bomb W40.8 ☑
      assault X96.0 ☑
      homicide (attempt) X96.0 ☑
      suicide (attempt) X75 ☑
  assault X96.9 ☑
  bicycle tire W37.0 ☑
  blasting (cap) (materials) W40.0 ☑
  boiler (machinery), not on transport vehicle W35 ☑
      on watercraft — *see* Explosion, in, watercraft
  butane W40.1 ☑
  caused by other person X96.9 ☑
  coal gas W40.1 ☑
  detonator W40.0 ☑
  dump (munitions) W40.8 ☑
  dynamite W40.0 ☑
      in
          assault X96.8 ☑
          homicide (attempt) X96.8 ☑
          legal intervention
              injuring
                  bystander Y35.112 ☑
                  law enforcement personnel Y35.111 ☑
                  suspect Y35.113 ☑
                  unspecified person Y35.119 ☑
          suicide (attempt) X75 ☑
  explosive (material) W40.9 ☑
      gas W40.1 ☑
      in blasting operation W40.0 ☑
      specified NEC W40.8 ☑
          in
              assault X96.8 ☑
              homicide (attempt) X96.8 ☑
              legal intervention
                  injuring
                      bystander Y35.192 ☑
                      law enforcement personnel
                          Y35.191 ☑
                      suspect Y35.193 ☑
                      unspecified person Y35.199 ☑

Explosion — *continued*
  explosive — *continued*
      specified — *continued*
          in — *continued*
              suicide (attempt) X75 ☑
  factory (munitions) W40.8 ☑
  fertilizer bomb W40.8 ☑
      assault X96.3 ☑
      homicide (attempt) X96.3 ☑
      suicide (attempt) X75 ☑
  firearm (parts) NEC W34.19 ☑
      airgun W34.110 ☑
      BB gun W34.110 ☑
      gas, air or spring-operated gun NEC W34.118 ☑
      hangun W32.1 ☑
      hunting rifle W33.12 ☑
      larger firearm W33.10 ☑
          specified NEC W33.19 ☑
      machine gun W33.13 ☑
      paintball gun W34.111 ☑
      pellet gun W34.110 ☑
      shotgun W33.11 ☑
      Very pistol [flare] W34.19 ☑
  fire-damp W40.1 ☑
  fireworks W39 ☑
  gas (coal) (explosive) W40.1 ☑
      cylinder W36.9 ☑
          aerosol can W36.1 ☑
          air tank W36.2 ☑
          pressurized W36.3 ☑
          specified NEC W36.8 ☑
  gasoline (fumes) (tank) not in moving motor vehicle
      W40.1 ☑
      bomb W40.8 ☑
          assault X96.1 ☑
          homicide (attempt) X96.1 ☑
          suicide (attempt) X75 ☑
      in motor vehicle — *see* Accident, transport, by type
          of vehicle
  grain store W40.8 ☑
  grenade W40.8 ☑
      in
          assault X96.8 ☑
          homicide (attempt) X96.8 ☑
          legal intervention
              injuring
                  bystander Y35.192 ☑
                  law enforcement personnel Y35.191 ☑
                  suspect Y35.193 ☑
                  unspecified person Y35.199 ☑
          suicide (attempt) X75 ☑
  handgun (parts) — *see* Explosion, firearm, hangun
      (parts)
  homicide (attempt) X96.9 ☑
      antipersonnel bomb — *see* Explosion, antipersonnel
          bomb
      fertilizer bomb — *see* Explosion, fertilizer bomb
      gasoline bomb — *see* Explosion, gasoline bomb
      letter bomb — *see* Explosion, letter bomb
      pipe bomb — *see* Explosion, pipe bomb
      specified NEC X96.8 ☑
  hose, pressurized W37.8 ☑
  hot water heater, tank (in machinery) W35 ☑
      on watercraft — *see* Explosion, in, watercraft
  in, on
      dump W40.8 ☑
      factory W40.8 ☑
      mine (of explosive gases) NEC W40.1 ☑
      watercraft V93.59 ☑
          powered craft V93.53 ☑
              ferry boat V93.51 ☑
              fishing boat V93.52 ☑
              jetskis V93.53 ☑
              liner V93.51 ☑
              merchant ship V93.50 ☑
              passenger ship V93.51 ☑
              sailboat V93.54 ☑
  letter bomb W40.8 ☑
      assault X96.2 ☑
      homicide (attempt) X96.2 ☑
      suicide (attempt) X75 ☑
  machinery — *see also* Contact, with, by type of ma-
      chine
      on board watercraft — *see* Explosion, in, watercraft
      pressure vessel — *see* Explosion, by type of vessel
  methane W40.1 ☑

Explosion — *continued*
  mine W40.1 ☑
  missile NEC W40.8 ☑
  mortar bomb W40.8 ☑
      in
          assault X96.8 ☑
          homicide (attempt) X96.8 ☑
          legal intervention
              injuring
                  bystander Y35.192 ☑
                  law enforcement personnel Y35.191 ☑
                  suspect Y35.193 ☑
                  unspecified person Y35.199 ☑
          suicide (attempt) X75 ☑
  munitions (dump) (factory) W40.8 ☑
  pipe, pressurized W37.8 ☑
      bomb W40.8 ☑
          assault X96.4 ☑
          homicide (attempt) X96.4 ☑
          suicide (attempt) X75 ☑
  pressure, pressurized
      cooker W38 ☑
      gas tank (in machinery) W36.3 ☑
      hose W37.8 ☑
      pipe W37.8 ☑
      specified device NEC W38 ☑
      tire W37.8 ☑
          bicycle W37.0 ☑
      vessel (in machinery) W38 ☑
  propane W40.1 ☑
  self-inflicted X75 ☑
  shell (artillery) NEC W40.8 ☑
      during war operations — *see* War operations, explo-
          sion
      in
          legal intervention
              injuring
                  bystander Y35.122 ☑
                  law enforcement personnel Y35.121 ☑
                  suspect Y35.123 ☑
                  unspecified person Y35.129 ☑
      war — *see* War operations, explosion
  spacecraft V95.45 ☑
  stated as undetermined whether accidental or inten-
      tional Y25 ☑
  steam or water lines (in machinery) W37.8 ☑
  stove W40.9 ☑
  suicide (attempt) X75 ☑
  tire, pressurized W37.8 ☑
      bicycle W37.0 ☑
  undetermined whether accidental or intentional Y25 ☑
  vehicle tire NEC W37.8 ☑
      bicycle W37.0 ☑
  war operations — *see* War operations, explosion
Exposure (to) X58 ☑
  air pressure change — *see* Air, pressure
  cold (accidental) (excessive) (extreme) (natural) (place)
      X31 ☑
      assault Y08.89 ☑
      due to
          man-made conditions W93.8 ☑
              dry ice (contact) W93.01 ☑
                  inhalation W93.02 ☑
              liquid air (contact) (hydrogen) (nitrogen)
                  W93.11 ☑
                  inhalation W93.12 ☑
              refrigeration unit (deep freeze) W93.2 ☑
          suicide (attempt) X83.2 ☑
          weather (conditions) X31 ☑
      homicide (attempt) Y08.89 ☑
      self-inflicted X83.2 ☑
  due to abandonment or neglect X58 ☑
  electric current W86.8 ☑
      appliance (faulty) W86.8 ☑
          domestic W86.0 ☑
      caused by other person Y08.89 ☑
      conductor (faulty) W86.1 ☑
      control apparatus (faulty) W86.1 ☑
      electric power generating plant, distribution station
          W86.1 ☑
      electroshock gun — *see* Exposure, electric current,
          taser
      high-voltage cable W85 ☑
      homicide (attempt) Y08.89 ☑
      legal execution — *see* Legal, intervention, specified
          means NEC

☑ Additional Character Required — Refer to the Tabular List for Character Selection   Subterms under main terms may continue to next column or page

Exposure — *continued*
  electric current — *continued*
    lightning — *see subcategory* T75.0 ☑
    live rail W86.8 ☑
    misadventure in medical or surgical procedure in
      electroshock therapy Y63.4
    motor (electric) (faulty) W86.8 ☑
      domestic W86.0 ☑
    self-inflicted X83.1 ☑
    specified NEC W86.8 ☑
      domestic W86.0 ☑
    stun gun — *see* Exposure, electric current, taser
    suicide (attempt) X83.1 ☑
    taser W86.8 ☑
      assault Y08.89 ☑
      legal intervention — *see category* Y35 ☑
      self-harm (intentional) X83.8 ☑
      undetermined intent Y33 ☑
    third rail W86.8 ☑
    transformer (faulty) W86.1 ☑
    transmission lines W85 ☑
  environmental tobacco smoke X58 ☑
  excessive
    cold — *see* Exposure, cold
    heat (natural) NEC X30 ☑
      man-made W92 ☑
  factor(s) NOS X58 ☑
    environmental NEC X58 ☑
    man-made NEC W99 ☑
    natural NEC — *see* Forces of nature
    specified NEC X58 ☑
  fire, flames (accidental) X08.8 ☑
    assault X97 ☑
    campfire — *see* Exposure, fire, controlled, not in
      building
    controlled (in)
      with ignition (of) clothing — *see also* Ignition,
        clothes X06.2 ☑
        nightwear X05 ☑
      bonfire — *see* Exposure, fire, controlled, not in
        building
      brazier (in building or structure) — *see also* Ex-
        posure, fire, controlled, building
        not in building or structure — *see* Exposure,
          fire, controlled, not in building
      building or structure X02.0 ☑
        with
          fall from building X02.3 ☑
          from building X02.5 ☑
          injury due to building collapse X02.2 ☑
          smoke inhalation X02.1 ☑
        hit by object from building X02.4 ☑
        specified mode of injury NEC X02.8 ☑
      fireplace, furnace or stove — *see* Exposure, fire,
        controlled, building
      not in building or structure X03.0 ☑
        with
          fall X03.3 ☑
          smoke inhalation X03.1 ☑
        hit by object X03.4 ☑
        specified mode of injury NEC X03.8 ☑
      trash — *see* Exposure, fire, controlled, not in
        building
    fireplace — *see* Exposure, fire, controlled, building
    fittings or furniture (in building or structure) (uncon-
      trolled) — *see* Exposure, fire, uncontrolled,
      building
    forest (uncontrolled) — *see* Exposure, fire, uncon-
      trolled, not in building
    grass (uncontrolled) — *see* Exposure, fire, uncon-
      trolled, not in building
    hay (uncontrolled) — *see* Exposure, fire, uncon-
      trolled, not in building
    homicide (attempt) X97 ☑
    ignition of highly flammable material X04 ☑
    in, of, on, starting in
      machinery — *see* Contact, with, by type of ma-
        chine
      motor vehicle (in motion) — *see also* Accident,
        transport, occupant by type of vehicle
        V87.8 ☑
        with collision — *see* Collision
      railway rolling stock, train, vehicle V81.81 ☑
        with collision — *see* Accident, transport, rail-
          way vehicle occupant
      street car (in motion) V82.8 ☑

Exposure — *continued*
  fire, flames — *continued*
    in, of, on, starting in — *continued*
      street car — *continued*
        with collision — *see* Accident, transport,
          streetcar occupant
      transport vehicle NEC — *see also* Accident,
        transport
        with collision — *see* Collision
      war operations — *see also* War operations, fire
        from nuclear explosion — *see* War operations,
          nuclear weapons
      watercraft (in transit) (not in transit) V91.09 ☑
        localized — *see* Burn, on board watercraft,
          due to, fire on board
        powered craft V91.03 ☑
          ferry boat V91.01 ☑
          fishing boat V91.02 ☑
          jet skis V91.03 ☑
          liner V91.01 ☑
          merchant ship V91.00 ☑
          passenger ship V91.01 ☑
        unpowered craft V91.08 ☑
          canoe V91.05 ☑
          inflatable V91.06 ☑
          kayak V91.05 ☑
          sailboat V91.04 ☑
          surf-board V91.08 ☑
          waterskis V91.07 ☑
          windsurfer V91.08 ☑
    lumber (uncontrolled) — *see* Exposure, fire, uncon-
      trolled, not in building
    mine (uncontrolled) — *see* Exposure, fire, uncon-
      trolled, not in building
    prairie (uncontrolled) — *see* Exposure, fire, uncon-
      trolled, not in building
    resulting from
      explosion — *see* Explosion
      lightning X08.8 ☑
    self-inflicted X76 ☑
    specified NEC X08.8 ☑
    started by other person X97 ☑
    stated as undetermined whether accidental or inten-
      tional Y26 ☑
    stove — *see* Exposure, fire, controlled, building
    suicide (attempt) X76 ☑
    tunnel (uncontrolled) — *see* Exposure, fire, uncon-
      trolled, not in building
    uncontrolled
      in building or structure X00.0 ☑
        with
          fall from building X00.3 ☑
          injury due to building collapse X00.2 ☑
          jump from building X00.5 ☑
          smoke inhalation X00.1 ☑
        bed X08.00 ☑
          due to
            cigarette X08.01 ☑
            specified material NEC X08.09 ☑
        furniture NEC X08.20 ☑
          due to
            cigarette X08.21 ☑
            specified material NEC X08.29 ☑
        hit by object from building X00.4 ☑
        sofa X08.10 ☑
          due to
            cigarette X08.11 ☑
            specified material NEC X08.19 ☑
        specified mode of injury NEC X00.8 ☑
      not in building or structure (any) X01.0 ☑
        with
          fall X01.3 ☑
          smoke inhalation X01.1 ☑
        hit by object X01.4 ☑
        specified mode of injury NEC X01.8 ☑
    undetermined whether accidental or intentional
      Y26 ☑
  forces of nature NEC — *see* Forces of nature
  G-forces (abnormal) W49.9 ☑
  gravitational forces (abnormal) W49.9 ☑
  heat (natural) NEC — *see* Heat
  high-pressure jet (hydraulic) (pneumatic) W49.9 ☑
  hydraulic jet W49.9 ☑
  inanimate mechanical force W49.9 ☑
  jet, high-pressure (hydraulic) (pneumatic) W49.9 ☑
  lightning — *see subcategory* T75.0 ☑

Exposure — *continued*
  lightning — *see subcategory* — *continued*
    causing fire — *see* Exposure, fire
  mechanical forces NEC W49.9 ☑
    animate NEC W64 ☑
    inanimate NEC W49.9 ☑
  noise W42.9 ☑
    supersonic W42.0 ☑
  noxious substance — *see* Table of Drugs and Chemicals
  pneumatic jet W49.9 ☑
  prolonged in deep-freeze unit or refrigerator W93.2 ☑
  radiation — *see* Radiation
  smoke — *see also* Exposure, fire
    tobacco, second hand Z77.22
  specified factors NEC X58 ☑
  sunlight X32 ☑
    man-made (sun lamp) W89.8 ☑
      tanning bed W89.1 ☑
  supersonic waves W42.0 ☑
  transmission line(s), electric W85 ☑
  vibration W49.9 ☑
  waves
    infrasound W49.9 ☑
    sound W42.9 ☑
    supersonic W42.0 ☑
  weather NEC — *see* Forces of nature
External cause status Y99.9
  child assisting in compensated work for family Y99.8
  civilian activity done for financial or other compensa-
    tion Y99.0
  civilian activity done for income or pay Y99.0
  family member assisting in compensated work for
    other family member Y99.8
  hobby not done for income Y99.8
  leisure activity Y99.8
  military activity Y99.1
  off-duty activity of military personnel Y99.8
  recreation or sport not for income or while a student
    Y99.8
  specified NEC Y99.8
  student activity Y99.8
  volunteer activity Y99.2

F

Factors, supplemental
  alcohol
    blood level
      less than 20mg/100ml Y90.0
      presence in blood, level not specified Y90.9
      20-39mg/100ml Y90.1
      40-59mg/100ml Y90.2
      60-79mg/100ml Y90.3
      80-99mg/100ml Y90.4
      100-119mg/100ml Y90.5
      120-199mg/100ml Y90.6
      200-239mg/100ml Y90.7
      240mg/100ml or more Y90.8
    presence in blood, but level not specified Y90.9
  environmental-pollution-related condition- *see* Z57 ☑
  nosocomial condition Y95
  work-related condition Y99.0
Failure
  in suture or ligature during surgical procedure Y65.2
  mechanical, of instrument or apparatus (any) (during
    any medical or surgical procedure) Y65.8
  sterile precautions (during medical and surgical care)
    — *see* Misadventure, failure, sterile precautions,
    by type of procedure
  to
    introduce tube or instrument Y65.4
      endotracheal tube during anesthesia Y65.3
    make curve (transport vehicle) NEC — *see* Accident,
      transport
    remove tube or instrument Y65.4
Fall, falling (accidental) W19 ☑
  building W20.1 ☑
    burning (uncontrolled fire) X00.3 ☑
  down
    embankment W17.81 ☑
    escalator W10.0 ☑
    hill W17.81 ☑
    ladder W11 ☑
    ramp W10.2 ☑
    stairs, steps W10.9 ☑

Fall, falling — *continued*
  due to
    bumping against
      object W18.00 ☑
        sharp glass W18.02 ☑
        specified NEC W18.09 ☑
        sports equipment W18.01 ☑
      person W03 ☑
        due to ice or snow W00.0 ☑
        on pedestrian conveyance — *see* Accident, transport, pedestrian, conveyance
    collision with another person W03 ☑
      due to ice or snow W00.0 ☑
      involving pedestrian conveyance — *see* Accident, transport, pedestrian, conveyance
    grocery cart tipping over W17.82 ☑
    ice or snow W00.9 ☑
      from one level to another W00.2 ☑
      on stairs or steps W00.1 ☑
      involving pedestrian conveyance — *see* Accident, transport, pedestrian, conveyance
      on same level W00.0 ☑
    slipping (on moving sidewalk) W01.0 ☑
      with subsequent striking against object W01.10 ☑
        furniture W01.190 ☑
        sharp object W01.119 ☑
          glass W01.110 ☑
          power tool or machine W01.111 ☑
          specified NEC W01.118 ☑
        specified NEC W01.198 ☑
    striking against
      object W18.00 ☑
        sharp glass W18.02 ☑
        specified NEC W18.09 ☑
        sports equipment W18.01 ☑
      person W03 ☑
        due to ice or snow W00.0 ☑
        on pedestrian conveyance — *see* Accident, transport, pedestrian, conveyance
  earth (with asphyxia or suffocation (by pressure)) — *see* Earth, falling
  from, off, out of
    aircraft NEC (with accident to aircraft NEC) W97.0 ☑
      while boarding or alighting V97.1 ☑
    balcony W13.0 ☑
    bed W06 ☑
    boat, ship, watercraft NEC (with drowning or submersion) — *see* Drowning, due to, fall overboard
      with hitting bottom or object V94.0 ☑
    bridge W13.1 ☑
    building W13.9 ☑
      burning (uncontrolled fire) X00.3 ☑
    cavity W17.2 ☑
    chair W07 ☑
    cherry picker W17.89 ☑
    cliff W15 ☑
    dock W17.4 ☑
    embankment W17.81 ☑
    escalator W10.0 ☑
    flagpole W13.8 ☑
    furniture NEC W08 ☑
    grocery cart W17.82 ☑
    haystack W17.89 ☑
    high place NEC W17.89 ☑
      stated as undetermined whether accidental or intentional Y30 ☑
    hole W17.2 ☑
    incline W10.2 ☑
    ladder W11 ☑
    lifting device W17.89 ☑
    machine, machinery — *see also* Contact, with, by type of machine
      not in operation W17.89 ☑
    manhole W17.1 ☑
    mobile elevated work platform [MEWP] W17.89 ☑
    motorized mobility scooter W05.2 ☑
    one level to another NEC W17.89 ☑
      intentional, purposeful, suicide (attempt) X80 ☑
      stated as undetermined whether accidental or intentional Y30 ☑
    pit W17.2 ☑
    playground equipment W09.8 ☑
      jungle gym W09.2 ☑
      slide W09.0 ☑

Fall, falling — *continued*
  from, off, out of — *continued*
    playground equipment — *continued*
      swing W09.1 ☑
    quarry W17.89 ☑
    railing W13.9 ☑
    ramp W10.2 ☑
    roof W13.2 ☑
    scaffolding W12 ☑
    scooter (nonmotorized) W05.1 ☑
      motorized mobility W05.2 ☑
    sky lift W17.89 ☑
    stairs, steps W10.9 ☑
      curb W10.1 ☑
      due to ice or snow W00.1 ☑
      escalator W10.0 ☑
      incline W10.2 ☑
      ramp W10.2 ☑
      sidewalk curb W10.1 ☑
      specified NEC W10.8 ☑
    stepladder W11 ☑
    storm drain W17.1 ☑
    streetcar NEC V82.6 ☑
      while boarding or alighting V82.4 ☑
      with antecedent collision — *see* Accident, transport, streetcar occupant
    structure NEC W13.8 ☑
      burning (uncontrolled fire) X00.3 ☑
    table W08 ☑
    toilet W18.11 ☑
      with subsequent striking against object W18.12 ☑
    train NEC V81.6 ☑
      during derailment (without antecedent collision) V81.7 ☑
      with antecedent collision — *see* Accident, transport, railway vehicle occupant
      while boarding or alighting V81.4 ☑
    transport vehicle after collision — *see* Accident, transport, by type of vehicle, collision
    tree W14 ☑
    vehicle (in motion) NEC — *see also* Accident, transport V89.9 ☑
      motor NEC — *see also* Accident, transport, occupant, by type of vehicle V87.8 ☑
      stationary W17.89 ☑
        while boarding or alighting — *see* Accident, transport, by type of vehicle, while boarding or alighting
    viaduct W13.8 ☑
    wall W13.8 ☑
    watercraft — *see also* Drowning, due to, fall overboard
      with hitting bottom or object V94.0 ☑
    well W17.0 ☑
    wheelchair, non-moving W05.0 ☑
      powered — *see* Accident, transport, pedestrian, conveyance occupant, specified type NEC
    window W13.4 ☑
  in, on
    aircraft NEC V97.0 ☑
      while boarding or alighting V97.1 ☑
      with accident to aircraft V97.0 ☑
    bathtub (empty) W18.2 ☑
      filled W16.212 ☑
        causing drowning W16.211 ☑
    escalator W10.0 ☑
    incline W10.2 ☑
    ladder W11 ☑
    machine, machinery — *see* Contact, with, by type of machine
    object, edged, pointed or sharp (with cut) — *see* Fall, by type
    playground equipment W09.8 ☑
      jungle gym W09.2 ☑
      slide W09.0 ☑
      swing W09.1 ☑
    ramp W10.2 ☑
    scaffolding W12 ☑
    shower W18.2 ☑
      causing drowning W16.211 ☑
    staircase, stairs, steps W10.9 ☑
      curb W10.1 ☑
      due to ice or snow W00.1 ☑
      escalator W10.0 ☑
      incline W10.2 ☑

Fall, falling — *continued*
  in, on — *continued*
    staircase, stairs, steps — *continued*
      specified NEC W10.8 ☑
    streetcar (without antecedent collision) V82.5 ☑
      with antecedent collision — *see* Accident, transport, streetcar occupant
      while boarding or alighting V82.4 ☑
    train (without antecedent collision) V81.5 ☑
      with antecedent collision — *see* Accident, transport, railway vehicle occupant
      during derailment (without antecedent collision) V81.7 ☑
        with antecedent collision — *see* Accident, transport, railway vehicle occupant
      while boarding or alighting V81.4 ☑
    transport vehicle after collision — *see* Accident, transport, by type of vehicle, collision
    watercraft V93.39 ☑
      due to
        accident to craft V91.29 ☑
          powered craft V91.23 ☑
            ferry boat V91.21 ☑
            fishing boat V91.22 ☑
            jetskis V91.23 ☑
            liner V91.21 ☑
            merchant ship V91.20 ☑
            passenger ship V91.21 ☑
          unpowered craft
            canoe V91.25 ☑
            inflatable V91.26 ☑
            kayak V91.25 ☑
            sailboat V91.24 ☑
        powered craft V93.33 ☑
          ferry boat V93.31 ☑
          fishing boat V93.32 ☑
          jetskis V93.33 ☑
          liner V93.31 ☑
          merchant ship V93.30 ☑
          passenger ship V93.31 ☑
        unpowered craft V93.38 ☑
          canoe V93.35 ☑
          inflatable V93.36 ☑
          kayak V93.35 ☑
          sailboat V93.34 ☑
          surf-board V93.38 ☑
          windsurfer V93.38 ☑
  into
    cavity W17.2 ☑
    dock W17.4 ☑
    fire — *see* Exposure, fire, by type
    haystack W17.89 ☑
    hole W17.2 ☑
    lake — *see* Fall, into, water
    manhole W17.1 ☑
    moving part of machinery — *see* Contact, with, by type of machine
    ocean — *see* Fall, into, water
    opening in surface NEC W17.89 ☑
    pit W17.2 ☑
    pond — *see* Fall, into, water
    quarry W17.89 ☑
    river — *see* Fall, into, water
    shaft W17.89 ☑
    storm drain W17.1 ☑
    stream — *see* Fall, into, water
    swimming pool — *see also* Fall, into, water, in, swimming pool
      empty W17.3 ☑
    tank W17.89 ☑
    water W16.42 ☑
      causing drowning W16.41 ☑
      from watercraft — *see* Drowning, due to, fall overboard
      hitting diving board W21.4 ☑
      in
        bathtub W16.212 ☑
          causing drowning W16.211 ☑
        bucket W16.222 ☑
          causing drowning W16.221 ☑
        natural body of water W16.112 ☑
          causing drowning W16.111 ☑
          striking
            bottom W16.122 ☑
              causing drowning W16.121 ☑
            side W16.132 ☑

☑ **Additional Character Required** — Refer to the Tabular List for Character Selection   ▽ **Subterms under main terms may continue to next column or page**

Fall, falling — *continued*
  into — *continued*
    water — *continued*
      in — *continued*
        natural body of water — *continued*
          striking — *continued*
            side — *continued*
              causing drowning W16.131 ☑
        specified water NEC W16.312 ☑
          causing drowning W16.311 ☑
          striking
            bottom W16.322 ☑
              causing drowning W16.321 ☑
            wall W16.332 ☑
              causing drowning W16.331 ☑
      swimming pool W16.012 ☑
        causing drowning W16.011 ☑
        striking
          bottom W16.022 ☑
            causing drowning W16.031 ☑
          wall W16.032 ☑
            causing drowning W16.021 ☑
      utility bucket W16.222 ☑
        causing drowning W16.221 ☑
    well W17.0 ☑
  involving
    bed W06 ☑
    chair W07 ☑
    furniture NEC W08 ☑
    glass — *see* Fall, by type
    playground equipment W09.8 ☑
      jungle gym W09.2 ☑
      slide W09.0 ☑
      swing W09.1 ☑
    roller blades — *see* Accident, transport, pedestrian,
      conveyance
    skateboard(s) — *see* Accident, transport, pedestrian,
      conveyance
    skates (ice) (in line) (roller) — *see* Accident, trans-
      port, pedestrian, conveyance
    skis — *see* Accident, transport, pedestrian, con-
      veyance
    table W08 ☑
    wheelchair, non-moving W05.0 ☑
      powered — *see* Accident, transport, pedestrian,
        conveyance, specified type NEC
  object — *see* Struck by, object, falling
  off
    toilet W18.11 ☑
      with subsequent striking against object
        W18.12 ☑
  on same level W18.30 ☑
    due to
      specified NEC W18.39 ☑
      stepping on an object W18.31 ☑
  out of
    bed W06 ☑
    building NEC W13.8 ☑
    chair W07 ☑
    furniture NEC W08 ☑
    wheelchair, non-moving W05.0 ☑
      powered — *see* Accident, transport, pedestrian,
        conveyance, specified type NEC
    window W13.4 ☑
  over
    animal W01.0 ☑
    cliff W15 ☑
    embankment W17.81 ☑
    small object W01.0 ☑
  rock W20.8 ☑
  same level W18.30 ☑
    from
      being crushed, pushed, or stepped on by a crowd
        or human stampede W52 ☑
      collision, pushing, shoving, by or with other
        person W03 ☑
      slipping, stumbling, tripping W01.0 ☑
    involving ice or snow W00.0 ☑
      involving skates (ice) (roller), skateboard, skis —
        see Accident, transport, pedestrian, con-
        veyance
  snowslide (avalanche) — *see* Landslide
  stone W20.8 ☑
  structure W20.1 ☑
    burning (uncontrolled fire) X00.3 ☑

Fall, falling — *continued*
  through
    bridge W13.1 ☑
    floor W13.3 ☑
    roof W13.2 ☑
    wall W13.8 ☑
    window W13.4 ☑
  timber W20.8 ☑
  tree (caused by lightning) W20.8 ☑
  while being carried or supported by other person(s)
    W04 ☑
Fallen on by
  animal (not being ridden) NEC W55.89 ☑
Felo-de-se — *see* Suicide
Fight (hand) (fists) (foot) — *see* Assault, fight
Fire (accidental) — *see* Exposure, fire
Firearm discharge — *see* Discharge, firearm
**Fireball effects from nuclear explosion in war oper-
  ations** — *see* War operations, nuclear weapons
Fireworks (explosion) W39 ☑
Flash burns from explosion — *see* Explosion
Flood (any injury) (caused by) X38 ☑
  collapse of man-made structure causing earth move-
    ment X36.0 ☑
  tidal wave — *see* Forces of nature, tidal wave
Food (any type) in
  air passages (with asphyxia, obstruction, or suffocation)
    — *see* categories T17 and T18 ☑
  alimentary tract causing asphyxia (due to compression
    of trachea) — *see* categories T17 and T18 ☑
Forces of nature X39.8 ☑
  avalanche X36.1 ☑
    causing transport accident — *see* Accident, trans-
      port, by type of vehicle
  blizzard X37.2 ☑
  cataclysmic storm X37.9 ☑
    with flood X38 ☑
    blizzard X37.2 ☑
    cloudburst X37.8 ☑
    cyclone X37.1 ☑
    dust storm X37.3 ☑
    hurricane X37.0 ☑
    specified storm NEC X37.8 ☑
    storm surge X37.0 ☑
    tornado X37.1 ☑
    twister X37.1 ☑
    typhoon X37.0 ☑
  cloudburst X37.8 ☑
  cold (natural) X31 ☑
  cyclone X37.1 ☑
  dam collapse causing earth movement X36.0 ☑
  dust storm X37.3 ☑
  earth movement X36.1 ☑
    caused by dam or structure collapse X36.0 ☑
    earthquake X34 ☑
  earthquake X34 ☑
  flood (caused by) X38 ☑
    dam collapse X36.0 ☑
    tidal wave — *see* Forces of nature, tidal wave
  heat (natural) X30 ☑
  hurricane X37.0 ☑
  landslide X36.1 ☑
    causing transport accident — *see* Accident, trans-
      port, by type of vehicle
  lightning — *see* subcategory T75.0 ☑
    causing fire — *see* Exposure, fire
  mudslide X36.1 ☑
    causing transport accident — *see* Accident, trans-
      port, by type of vehicle
  radiation (natural) X39.08 ☑
    radon X39.01 ☑
  radon X39.01 ☑
  specified force NEC X39.8 ☑
  storm surge X37.0 ☑
  structure collapse causing earth movement X36.0 ☑
  sunlight X32 ☑
  tidal wave X37.41 ☑
    due to
      earthquake X37.41 ☑
      landslide X37.43 ☑
      storm X37.42 ☑
      volcanic eruption X37.41 ☑
  tornado X37.1 ☑
  tsunami X37.41 ☑
  twister X37.1 ☑
  typhoon X37.0 ☑

Forces of nature — *continued*
  volcanic eruption X35 ☑
Foreign body
  aspiration — *see* Index to Diseases and Injuries, Foreign
    body, respiratory tract
  embedded in skin W45 ☑
  entering through skin W45.8 ☑
    can lid W26.8 ☑
    nail W45.0 ☑
    paper W26.2 ☑
    specified NEC W45.8 ☑
    splinter W45.8 ☑
Forest fire (exposure to) — *see* Exposure, fire, uncontrolled, not in building
Found injured X58 ☑
  from exposure (to) — *see* Exposure
  on
    highway, road(way), street V89.9 ☑
    railway right of way V81.9 ☑
Fracture (circumstances unknown or unspecified) X58 ☑
  due to specified cause NEC X58 ☑
Freezing — *see* Exposure, cold
Frostbite X31 ☑
  due to man-made conditions — *see* Exposure, cold,
    man-made
Frozen — *see* Exposure, cold

G

Gored by bull W55.22 ☑
Gunshot wound W34.00 ☑

H

Hailstones, injured by X39.8 ☑
Hanged herself or himself — *see* Hanging, self-inflicted
Hanging (accidental) — *see also* category T71 ☑
  legal execution — *see* Legal, intervention, specified
    means NEC
Heat (effects of) (excessive) X30 ☑
  due to
    man-made conditions W92 ☑
      on board watercraft V93.29 ☑
        fishing boat V93.22 ☑
        merchant ship V93.20 ☑
        passenger ship V93.21 ☑
        sailboat V93.24 ☑
        specified powered craft NEC V93.23 ☑
    weather (conditions) X30 ☑
  from
    electric heating apparatus causing burning X16 ☑
    nuclear explosion in war operations — *see* War op-
      erations, nuclear weapons
  inappropriate in local application or packing in medical
    or surgical procedure Y63.5
Hemorrhage
  delayed following medical or surgical treatment with-
    out mention of misadventure — *see* Index to
    Diseases and Injuries, Complication(s)
  during medical or surgical treatment as misadventure
    — *see* Index to Diseases and Injuries, Complica-
    tion(s)
High
  altitude (effects) — *see* Air, pressure, low
  level of radioactivity, effects — *see* Radiation
  pressure (effects) — *see* Air, pressure, high
  temperature, effects — *see* Heat
Hit, hitting (accidental) by — *see* Struck by
Hitting against — *see* Striking against
Homicide (attempt) (justifiable) — *see* Assault
Hot
  place, effects — *see also* Heat
  weather, effects X30 ☑
House fire (uncontrolled) — *see* Exposure, fire, uncon-
  trolled, building
Humidity, causing problem X39.8 ☑
Hunger X58 ☑
Hurricane (any injury) X37.0 ☑
Hypobarism, hypobaropathy — *see* Air, pressure, low

I

Ictus
  caloris — *see also* Heat
  solaris X30 ☑
Ignition (accidental) — *see also* Exposure, fire X08.8 ☑

Ignition — *continued*
  anesthetic gas in operating room W40.1 ☑
  apparel X06.2 ☑
    from highly flammable material X04 ☑
    nightwear X05 ☑
  bed linen (sheets) (spreads) (pillows) (mattress) — *see* Exposure, fire, uncontrolled, building, bed
  benzine X04 ☑
  clothes, clothing NEC (from controlled fire) X06.2 ☑
    from
      highly flammable material X04 ☑
  ether X04 ☑
    in operating room W40.1 ☑
  explosive material — *see* Explosion
  gasoline X04 ☑
  jewelry (plastic) (any) X06.0 ☑
  kerosene X04 ☑
  material
    explosive — *see* Explosion
    highly flammable with secondary explosion X04 ☑
  nightwear X05 ☑
  paraffin X04 ☑
  petrol X04 ☑
Immersion (accidental) — *see also* Drowning
  hand or foot due to cold (excessive) X31 ☑
Implantation of quills of porcupine W55.89 ☑
Inanition (from) (hunger) X58 ☑
  thirst X58 ☑
Inappropriate operation performed
  correct operation on wrong side or body part (wrong side) (wrong site) Y65.53
  operation intended for another patient done on wrong patient Y65.52
  wrong operation performed on correct patient Y65.51
Inattention after, at birth (homicidal intent) (infanticidal intent) X58 ☑
Incident, adverse
  device
    anesthesiology Y70.8
      accessory Y70.2
      diagnostic Y70.0
      miscellaneous Y70.8
      monitoring Y70.0
      prosthetic Y70.2
      rehabilitative Y70.1
      surgical Y70.3
      therapeutic Y70.1
    cardiovascular Y71.8
      accessory Y71.2
      diagnostic Y71.0
      miscellaneous Y71.8
      monitoring Y71.0
      prosthetic Y71.2
      rehabilitative Y71.1
      surgical Y71.3
      therapeutic Y71.1
    gastroenterology Y73.8
      accessory Y73.2
      diagnostic Y73.0
      miscellaneous Y73.8
      monitoring Y73.0
      prosthetic Y73.2
      rehabilitative Y73.1
      surgical Y73.3
      therapeutic Y73.1
    general
      hospital Y74.8
        accessory Y74.2
        diagnostic Y74.0
        miscellaneous Y74.8
        monitoring Y74.0
        prosthetic Y74.2
        rehabilitative Y74.1
        surgical Y74.3
        therapeutic Y74.1
      surgical Y81.8
        accessory Y81.2
        diagnostic Y81.0
        miscellaneous Y81.8
        monitoring Y81.0
        prosthetic Y81.2
        rehabilitative Y81.1
        surgical Y81.3
        therapeutic Y81.1
    gynecological Y76.8
      accessory Y76.2
      diagnostic Y76.0
      miscellaneous Y76.8

Incident, adverse — *continued*
  device — *continued*
    gynecological — *continued*
      monitoring Y76.0
      prosthetic Y76.2
      rehabilitative Y76.1
      surgical Y76.3
      therapeutic Y76.1
    medical Y82.9
      specified type NEC Y82.8
    neurological Y75.8
      accessory Y75.2
      diagnostic Y75.0
      miscellaneous Y75.8
      monitoring Y75.0
      prosthetic Y75.2
      rehabilitative Y75.1
      surgical Y75.3
      therapeutic Y75.1
    obstetrical Y76.8
      accessory Y76.2
      diagnostic Y76.0
      miscellaneous Y76.8
      monitoring Y76.0
      prosthetic Y76.2
      rehabilitative Y76.1
      surgical Y76.3
      therapeutic Y76.1
    ophthalmic Y77.8
      accessory Y77.2
      diagnostic Y77.0
      miscellaneous Y77.8
      monitoring Y77.0
      prosthetic Y77.2
      rehabilitative Y77.1
      surgical Y77.3
      therapeutic Y77.1
    orthopedic Y79.8
      accessory Y79.2
      diagnostic Y79.0
      miscellaneous Y79.8
      monitoring Y79.2
      prosthetic Y79.2
      rehabilitative Y79.1
      surgical Y79.3
      therapeutic Y79.1
    otorhinolaryngological Y72.8
      accessory Y72.2
      diagnostic Y72.0
      miscellaneous Y72.8
      monitoring Y72.0
      prosthetic Y72.2
      rehabilitative Y72.1
      surgical Y72.3
      therapeutic Y72.1
    personal use Y74.8
      accessory Y74.2
      diagnostic Y74.0
      miscellaneous Y74.8
      monitoring Y74.0
      prosthetic Y74.2
      rehabilitative Y74.1
      surgical Y74.3
      therapeutic Y74.1
    physical medicine Y80.8
      accessory Y80.2
      diagnostic Y80.0
      miscellaneous Y80.8
      monitoring Y80.0
      prosthetic Y80.2
      rehabilitative Y80.1
      surgical Y80.3
      therapeutic Y80.1
    plastic surgical Y81.8
      accessory Y81.2
      diagnostic Y81.0
      miscellaneous Y81.8
      monitoring Y81.0
      prosthetic Y81.2
      rehabilitative Y81.1
      surgical Y81.3
      therapeutic Y81.1
    radiological Y78.8
      accessory Y78.2
      diagnostic Y78.0
      miscellaneous Y78.8
      monitoring Y78.0
      prosthetic Y78.2
      rehabilitative Y78.1

Incident, adverse — *continued*
  device — *continued*
    radiological — *continued*
      surgical Y78.3
      therapeutic Y78.1
    urology Y73.8
      accessory Y73.2
      diagnostic Y73.0
      miscellaneous Y73.8
      monitoring Y73.0
      prosthetic Y73.2
      rehabilitative Y73.1
      surgical Y73.3
      therapeutic Y73.1
Incineration (accidental) — *see* Exposure, fire
Infanticide — *see* Assault
Infrasound waves (causing injury) W49.9 ☑
Ingestion
  foreign body (causing injury) (with obstruction) — *see* Foreign body, alimentary canal
  poisonous
    plant(s) X58 ☑
    substance NEC — *see* Table of Drugs and Chemicals
Inhalation
  excessively cold substance, man-made — *see* Exposure, cold, man-made
  food (any type) (into respiratory tract) (with asphyxia, obstruction respiratory tract, suffocation) — *see* categories T17 and T18 ☑
  foreign body — *see* Foreign body, aspiration
  gastric contents (with asphyxia, obstruction respiratory passage, suffocation) T17.81- ☑
  hot air or gases X14.0 ☑
  liquid air, hydrogen, nitrogen W93.12 ☑
    suicide (attempt) X83.2 ☑
  steam X13.0 ☑
    assault X98.0 ☑
    stated as undetermined whether accidental or intentional Y27.0 ☑
    suicide (attempt) X77.0 ☑
  toxic gas — *see* Table of Drugs and Chemicals
  vomitus (with asphyxia, obstruction respiratory passage, suffocation) T17.81- ☑
Injury, injured (accidental(ly)) NOS X58 ☑
  by, caused by, from
    assault — *see* Assault
    law-enforcing agent, police, in course of legal intervention — *see* Legal intervention
    suicide (attempt) X83.8 ☑
  due to, in
    civil insurrection — *see* War operations
    fight — *see also* Assault, fight Y04.0 ☑
    war operations — *see* War operations
  homicide — *see also* Assault Y09
  inflicted (by)
    in course of arrest (attempted), suppression of disturbance, maintenance of order, by law-enforcing agents — *see* Legal intervention
    other person
      stated as
        accidental X58 ☑
        intentional, homicide (attempt) — *see* Assault
        undetermined whether accidental or intentional Y33 ☑
  purposely (inflicted) by other person(s) — *see* Assault
  self-inflicted X83.8 ☑
    stated as accidental X58 ☑
  specified cause NEC X58 ☑
  undetermined whether accidental or intentional Y33 ☑
Insolation, effects X30 ☑
Insufficient nourishment X58 ☑
Interruption of respiration (by)
  food (lodged in esophagus) — *see* categories T17 and T18 ☑
  vomitus (lodged in esophagus) T17.81- ☑
Intervention, legal — *see* Legal intervention
Intoxication
  drug — *see* Table of Drugs and Chemicals
  poison — *see* Table of Drugs and Chemicals

J

Jammed (accidentally)
  between objects (moving) (stationary and moving) W23.0 ☑
    stationary W23.1 ☑

Jumped, jumping
before moving object NEC X81.8 ☑
motor vehicle X81.0 ☑
subway train X81.1 ☑
train X81.1 ☑
undetermined whether accidental or intentional
Y31 ☑
from
boat (into water) voluntarily, without accident (to
or on boat) W16.712 ☑
striking bottom W16.722 ☑
causing drowning W16.721 ☑
with
accident to or on boat — see Accident, watercraft
drowning or submersion W16.711 ☑
suicide (attempt) X71.3 ☑
building — see also Jumped, from, high place
W13.9 ☑
burning (uncontrolled fire) X00.5 ☑
high place NEC W17.89 ☑
suicide (attempt) X80 ☑
undetermined whether accidental or intentional
Y30 ☑
structure — see also Jumped, from, high place
W13.9 ☑
burning (uncontrolled fire) X00.5 ☑
into water W16.92 ☑
causing drowning W16.91 ☑
from, off watercraft — see Jumped, from, boat
in
natural body W16.612 ☑
causing drowning W16.611 ☑
striking bottom W16.622 ☑
causing drowning W16.621 ☑
specified place NEC W16.812 ☑
causing drowning W16.811 ☑
striking
bottom W16.822 ☑
causing drowning W16.821 ☑
wall W16.832 ☑
causing drowning W16.831 ☑
swimming pool W16.512 ☑
causing drowning W16.511 ☑
striking
bottom W16.522 ☑
causing drowning W16.521 ☑
wall W16.532 ☑
causing drowning W16.531 ☑
suicide (attempt) X71.3 ☑

K

Kicked by
animal NEC W55.82 ☑
person(s) (accidentally) W50.1 ☑
with intent to injure or kill Y04.0 ☑
as, or caused by, a crowd or human stampede (with
fall) W52 ☑
assault Y04.0 ☑
homicide (attempt) Y04.0 ☑
in
fight Y04.0 ☑
legal intervention
injuring
bystander Y35.812 ☑
law enforcement personnel Y35.811 ☑
suspect Y35.813 ☑
unspecified person Y35.819 ☑
Kicking
against
object W22.8 ☑
sports equipment W21.9 ☑
stationary W22.09 ☑
sports equipment W21.89 ☑
person — see Striking against, person
sports equipment W21.9 ☑
carpet stretcher with knee X50.3 ☑
Killed, killing (accidentally) NOS — see also Injury X58 ☑
in
action — see War operations
brawl, fight (hand) (fists) (foot) Y04.0 ☑
by weapon — see also Assault
cutting, piercing — see Assault, cutting or
piercing instrument

Killed, killing — continued
in — continued
brawl, fight — continued
by weapon — see also Assault — continued
firearm — see Discharge, firearm, by type,
homicide
self
stated as
accident NOS X58 ☑
suicide — see Suicide
undetermined whether accidental or intentional
Y33 ☑
Kneeling (prolonged (static) X50.1 ☑
Knocked down (accidentally) (by) NOS X58 ☑
animal (not being ridden) NEC — see also Struck by,
by type of animal
crowd or human stampede W52 ☑
person W51 ☑
in brawl, fight Y04.0 ☑
transport vehicle NEC — see also Accident, transport
V09.9 ☑

L

Laceration NEC — see Injury
Lack of
care (helpless person) (infant) (newborn) X58 ☑
food except as result of abandonment or neglect
X58 ☑
due to abandonment or neglect X58 ☑
water except as result of transport accident X58 ☑
due to transport accident — see Accident, transport,
by type
helpless person, infant, newborn X58 ☑
Landslide (falling on transport vehicle) X36.1 ☑
caused by collapse of man-made structure X36.0 ☑
Late effect — see Sequelae
Legal
execution (any method) — see Legal, intervention
intervention (by)
baton — see Legal, intervention, blunt object, baton
bayonet — see Legal, intervention, sharp object,
bayonet
blow — see Legal, intervention, manhandling
blunt object
baton
injuring
bystander Y35.312 ☑
law enforcement personnel Y35.311 ☑
suspect Y35.313 ☑
unspecified person Y35.319 ☑
injuring
bystander Y35.302 ☑
law enforcement personnel Y35.301 ☑
suspect Y35.303 ☑
unspecified person Y35.309 ☑
specified NEC
injuring
bystander Y35.392 ☑
law enforcement personnel Y35.391 ☑
suspect Y35.393 ☑
unspecified person Y35.399 ☑
stave
injuring
bystander Y35.392 ☑
law enforcement personnel Y35.391 ☑
suspect Y35.393 ☑
unspecified person Y35.399 ☑
bomb — see Legal, intervention, explosive
conducted energy device
injuring
bystander Y35.832 ☑
law enforcement personnel Y35.831 ☑
suspect Y35.833 ☑
unspecified person Y35.839 ☑
cutting or piercing instrument — see Legal, intervention, sharp object
dynamite — see Legal, intervention, explosive, dynamite
electroshock device (taser)
injuring
bystander Y35.832 ☑
law enforcement personnel Y35.831 ☑
suspect Y35.833 ☑
unspecified person Y35.839 ☑

Legal — continued
intervention — continued
explosive(s)
dynamite
injuring
bystander Y35.112 ☑
law enforcement personnel Y35.111 ☑
suspect Y35.113 ☑
unspecified person Y35.119 ☑
grenade
injuring
bystander Y35.192 ☑
law enforcement personnel Y35.191 ☑
suspect Y35.193 ☑
unspecified person Y35.199 ☑
injuring
bystander Y35.102 ☑
law enforcement personnel Y35.101 ☑
suspect Y35.103 ☑
unspecified person Y35.109 ☑
mortar bomb
injuring
bystander Y35.192 ☑
law enforcement personnel Y35.191 ☑
suspect Y35.193 ☑
unspecified person Y35.199 ☑
shell
injuring
bystander Y35.122 ☑
law enforcement personnel Y35.121 ☑
suspect Y35.123 ☑
unspecified person Y35.129 ☑
specified NEC
injuring
bystander Y35.192 ☑
law enforcement personnel Y35.191 ☑
suspect Y35.193 ☑
unspecified person Y35.199 ☑
firearm(s) (discharge)
handgun
injuring
bystander Y35.022 ☑
law enforcement personnel Y35.021 ☑
suspect Y35.023 ☑
unspecified person Y35.029 ☑
injuring
bystander Y35.002 ☑
law enforcement personnel Y35.001 ☑
suspect Y35.003 ☑
unspecified person Y35.009 ☑
machine gun
injuring
bystander Y35.012 ☑
law enforcement personnel Y35.011 ☑
suspect Y35.013 ☑
unspecified person Y35.019 ☑
rifle pellet
injuring
bystander Y35.032 ☑
law enforcement personnel Y35.031 ☑
suspect Y35.033 ☑
unspecified person Y35.039 ☑
rubber bullet
injuring
bystander Y35.042 ☑
law enforcement personnel Y35.041 ☑
suspect Y35.043 ☑
unspecified person Y35.049 ☑
shotgun — see Legal, intervention, firearm,
specified NEC
specified NEC
injuring
bystander Y35.092 ☑
law enforcement personnel Y35.091 ☑
suspect Y35.093 ☑
unspecified person Y35.099 ☑
gas (asphyxiation) (poisoning)
injuring
bystander Y35.202 ☑
law enforcement personnel Y35.201 ☑
suspect Y35.203 ☑
unspecified person Y35.209 ☑
specified NEC
injuring
bystander Y35.292 ☑
law enforcement personnel Y35.291 ☑
suspect Y35.293 ☑

Legal — continued
  intervention — continued
    gas — continued
      specified — continued
        injuring — continued
          unspecified person Y35.299 ☑
      tear gas
        injuring
          bystander Y35.212 ☑
          law enforcement personnel Y35.211 ☑
          suspect Y35.213 ☑
          unspecified person Y35.219 ☑
    grenade — see Legal, intervention, explosive, grenade
    injuring
      bystander Y35.92 ☑
      law enforcement personnel Y35.91 ☑
      suspect Y35.93 ☑
      unspecified person Y35.99 ☑
    late effect (of) — see with 7th character S Y35 ☑
    manhandling
      injuring
        bystander Y35.812 ☑
        law enforcement personnel Y35.811 ☑
        suspect Y35.813 ☑
        unspecified person Y35.819 ☑
    sequelae (of) — see with 7th character S Y35
    sharp objects
      bayonet
        injuring
          bystander Y35.412 ☑
          law enforcement personnel Y35.411 ☑
          suspect Y35.413 ☑
          unspecified person Y35.419 ☑
      injuring
        bystander Y35.402 ☑
        law enforcement personnel Y35.401 ☑
        suspect Y35.403 ☑
        unspecified person Y35.409 ☑
      specified NEC
        injuring
          bystander Y35.492 ☑
          law enforcement personnel Y35.491 ☑
          suspect Y35.493 ☑
          unspecified person Y35.499 ☑
    specified means NEC
      injuring
        bystander Y35.892 ☑
        law enforcement personnel Y35.891 ☑
        suspect Y35.893 ☑
    stabbing — see Legal, intervention, sharp object
    stave — see Legal, intervention, blunt object, stave
    stun gun
      injuring
        bystander Y35.832 ☑
        law enforcement personnel Y35.831 ☑
        suspect Y35.833 ☑
        unspecified person Y35.839 ☑
    taser
      injuring
        bystander Y35.832 ☑
        law enforcement personnel Y35.831 ☑
        suspect Y35.833 ☑
        unspecified person Y35.839 ☑
    tear gas — see Legal, intervention, gas, tear gas
    truncheon — see Legal, intervention, blunt object, stave

Lifting — see also Overexertion
  heavy objects X50.0 ☑
  weights X50.0 ☑
Lightning (shock) (stroke) (struck by) — see subcategory T75.0 ☑
  causing fire — see Exposure, fire
Loss of control (transport vehicle) NEC — see Accident, transport
Lost at sea NOS — see Drowning, due to, fall overboard
Low
  pressure (effects) — see Air, pressure, low
  temperature (effects) — see Exposure, cold
Lying before train, vehicle or other moving object X81.8 ☑
  subway train X81.1 ☑
  train X81.1 ☑
  undetermined whether accidental or intentional Y31 ☑
Lynching — see Assault

M

Malfunction (mechanism or component) (of)
  firearm W34.10 ☑
    airgun W34.110 ☑
    BB gun W34.110 ☑
    gas, air or spring-operated gun NEC W34.118 ☑
    handgun W32.1 ☑
    hunting rifle W33.12 ☑
    larger firearm W33.10 ☑
      specified NEC W33.19 ☑
    machine gun W33.13 ☑
    paintball gun W34.111 ☑
    pellet gun W34.110 ☑
    shotgun W33.11 ☑
    specified NEC W34.19 ☑
    Very pistol [flare] W34.19 ☑
  handgun — see Malfunction, firearm, handgun
Maltreatment — see Perpetrator
Mangled (accidentally) NOS X58 ☑
Manhandling (in brawl, fight) Y04.0 ☑
  legal intervention — see Legal, intervention, manhandling
Manslaughter (nonaccidental) — see Assault
Mauled by animal NEC W55.89 ☑
Medical procedure, complication of (delayed or as an abnormal reaction without mention of misadventure) — see Complication of or following, by specified type of procedure
  due to or as a result of misadventure — see Misadventure
Melting (due to fire) — see also Exposure, fire
  apparel NEC X06.3 ☑
  clothes, clothing NEC X06.3 ☑
    nightwear X05 ☑
  fittings or furniture (burning building) (uncontrolled fire) X00.8 ☑
  nightwear X05 ☑
  plastic jewelry X06.1 ☑
Mental cruelty X58 ☑
Military operations (injuries to military and civilians occuring during peacetime on military property and during routine military exercises and operations) (by) (from) (involving) Y37.90- ☑
  air blast Y37.20- ☑
  aircraft
    destruction — see Military operations, destruction of aircraft
    airway restriction — see Military operations, restriction of airways
    asphyxiation — see Military operations, restriction of airways
  biological weapons Y37.6X- ☑
  blast Y37.20- ☑
  blast fragments Y37.20- ☑
  blast wave Y37.20- ☑
  blast wind Y37.20- ☑
  bomb Y37.20- ☑
    dirty Y37.50- ☑
    gasoline Y37.31- ☑
    incendiary Y37.31- ☑
    petrol Y37.31- ☑
  bullet Y37.43- ☑
    incendiary Y37.32- ☑
    rubber Y37.41- ☑
  chemical weapons Y37.7X- ☑
  combat
    hand to hand (unarmed) combat Y37.44- ☑
    using blunt or piercing object Y37.45- ☑
  conflagration — see Military operations, fire
  conventional warfare NEC Y37.49- ☑
  depth-charge Y37.01- ☑
  destruction of aircraft Y37.10- ☑
    due to
      air to air missile Y37.11- ☑
      collision with other aircraft Y37.12- ☑
      detonation (accidental) of onboard munitions and explosives Y37.14- ☑
      enemy fire or explosives Y37.11- ☑
      explosive placed on aircraft Y37.11- ☑
      onboard fire Y37.13- ☑
      rocket propelled grenade [RPG] Y37.11- ☑
      small arms fire Y37.11- ☑
      surface to air missile Y37.11- ☑
    specified NEC Y37.19- ☑

Military operations — continued
  detonation (accidental) of
    onboard marine weapons Y37.05- ☑
    own munitions or munitions launch device Y37.24- ☑
  dirty bomb Y37.50- ☑
  explosion (of) Y37.20- ☑
    aerial bomb Y37.21- ☑
    bomb NOS — see also Military operations, bomb(s) Y37.20- ☑
    fragments Y37.20- ☑
    grenade Y37.29- ☑
    guided missile Y37.22- ☑
    improvised explosive device [IED] (person-borne) (roadside) (vehicle-borne) Y37.23- ☑
    land mine Y37.29- ☑
    marine mine (at sea) (in harbor) Y37.02- ☑
    marine weapon Y37.00- ☑
      specified NEC Y37.09- ☑
    own munitions or munitions launch device (accidental) Y37.24- ☑
    sea-based artillery shell Y37.03- ☑
    specified NEC Y37.29- ☑
    torpedo Y37.04- ☑
  fire Y37.30- ☑
    specified NEC Y37.39- ☑
  firearms
    discharge Y37.43- ☑
    pellets Y37.42- ☑
  flamethrower Y37.33- ☑
  fragments (from) (of)
    improvised explosive device [IED] (person-borne) (roadside) (vehicle-borne) Y37.26- ☑
    munitions Y37.25- ☑
    specified NEC Y37.29- ☑
    weapons Y37.27- ☑
  friendly fire Y37.92- ☑
  hand to hand (unarmed) combat Y37.44- ☑
  hot substances — see Military operations, fire
  incendiary bullet Y37.32- ☑
  nuclear weapon (effects of) Y37.50- ☑
    acute radiation exposure Y37.54- ☑
    blast pressure Y37.51- ☑
    direct blast Y37.51- ☑
    direct heat Y37.53- ☑
    fallout exposure Y37.54- ☑
    fireball Y37.53- ☑
    indirect blast (struck or crushed by blast debris) (being thrown by blast) Y37.52- ☑
    ionizing radiation (immediate exposure) Y37.54- ☑
    nuclear radiation Y37.54- ☑
    radiation
      ionizing (immediate exposure) Y37.54- ☑
      nuclear Y37.54- ☑
      thermal Y37.53- ☑
    secondary effects Y37.54- ☑
    specified NEC Y37.59- ☑
    thermal radiation Y37.53- ☑
  restriction of air (airway)
    intentional Y37.46- ☑
    unintentional Y37.47- ☑
  rubber bullets Y37.41- ☑
  shrapnel NOS Y37.29- ☑
  suffocation — see Military operations, restriction of airways
  unconventional warfare NEC Y37.7X- ☑
  underwater blast NOS Y37.00- ☑
  warfare
    conventional NEC Y37.49- ☑
    unconventional NEC Y37.7X- ☑
  weapon of mass destruction [WMD] Y37.91- ☑
  weapons
    biological weapons Y37.6X- ☑
    chemical Y37.7X- ☑
    nuclear (effects of) Y37.50- ☑
      acute radiation exposure Y37.54- ☑
      blast pressure Y37.51- ☑
      direct blast Y37.51- ☑
      direct heat Y37.53- ☑
      fallout exposure Y37.54- ☑
      fireball Y37.53- ☑
      radiation
        ionizing (immediate exposure) Y37.54- ☑
        nuclear Y37.54- ☑
        thermal Y37.53- ☑
      secondary effects Y37.54- ☑

424

☑ **Additional Character Required** — Refer to the Tabular List for Character Selection   ▽ Subterms under main terms may continue to next column or page

Military operations — *continued*
  weapons — *continued*
    nuclear — *continued*
      specified NEC Y37.59- ☑
    of mass destruction [WMD] Y37.91- ☑
Misadventure(s) **to patient**(s) **during surgical or medical care** Y69
  contaminated medical or biological substance (blood, drug, fluid) Y64.9
    administered (by) NEC Y64.9
      immunization Y64.1
      infusion Y64.0
      injection Y64.1
      specified means NEC Y64.8
      transfusion Y64.0
      vaccination Y64.1
  excessive amount of blood or other fluid during transfusion or infusion Y63.0
  failure
    in dosage Y63.9
      electroshock therapy Y63.4
      inappropriate temperature (too hot or too cold) in local application and packing Y63.5
      infusion
        excessive amount of fluid Y63.0
        incorrect dilution of fluid Y63.1
      insulin-shock therapy Y63.4
      nonadministration of necessary drug or biological substance Y63.6
      overdose — *see* Table of Drugs and Chemicals
        radiation, in therapy Y63.2
      radiation
        overdose Y63.2
      specified procedure NEC Y63.8
      transfusion
        excessive amount of blood Y63.0
  mechanical, of instrument or apparatus (any) (during any procedure) Y65.8
  sterile precautions (during procedure) Y62.9
    aspiration of fluid or tissue (by puncture or catheterization, except heart) Y62.6
    biopsy (except needle aspiration) Y62.8
      needle (aspirating) Y62.6
    blood sampling Y62.6
    catheterization Y62.6
      heart Y62.5
    dialysis (kidney) Y62.2
    endoscopic examination Y62.4
    enema Y62.8
    immunization Y62.3
    infusion Y62.1
    injection Y62.3
    needle biopsy Y62.6
    paracentesis (abdominal) (thoracic) Y62.6
    perfusion Y62.2
    puncture (lumbar) Y62.6
    removal of catheter or packing Y62.8
    specified procedure NEC Y62.8
    surgical operation Y62.0
    transfusion Y62.1
    vaccination Y62.3
  suture or ligature during surgical procedure Y65.2
  to introduce or to remove tube or instrument — *see* Failure, to
  hemorrhage — *see* Index to Diseases and Injuries, Complication(s)
  inadvertent exposure of patient to radiation Y63.3
  inappropriate
    operation performed — *see* Inappropriate operation performed
    temperature (too hot or too cold) in local application or packing Y63.5
  infusion — *see also* Misadventure, by type, infusion Y69
    excessive amount of fluid Y63.0
    incorrect dilution of fluid Y63.1
    wrong fluid Y65.1
  mismatched blood in transfusion Y65.0
  nonadministration of necessary drug or biological substance Y63.6
  overdose — *see* Table of Drugs and Chemicals
    radiation (in therapy) Y63.2
  perforation — *see* Index to Diseases and Injuries, Complication(s)
  performance of inappropriate operation — *see* Inappropriate operation performed
  puncture — *see* Index to Diseases and Injuries, Complication(s)

Misadventure(s) **to patient**(s) **during surgical or medical care** — *continued*
  specified type NEC Y65.8
    failure
      suture or ligature during surgical operation Y65.2
      to introduce or to remove tube or instrument — *see* Failure, to
    infusion of wrong fluid Y65.1
    performance of inappropriate operation — *see* Inappropriate operation performed
    transfusion of mismatched blood Y65.0
    wrong
      fluid in infusion Y65.1
      placement of endotracheal tube during anesthetic procedure Y65.3
  transfusion — *see* Misadventure, by type, transfusion
    excessive amount of blood Y63.0
    mismatched blood Y65.0
  wrong
    drug given in error — *see* Table of Drugs and Chemicals
    fluid in infusion Y65.1
    placement of endotracheal tube during anesthetic procedure Y65.3
Mismatched blood in transfusion Y65.0
Motion sickness T75.3 ☑
Mountain sickness W94.11 ☑
Mudslide (of cataclysmic nature) — *see* Landslide
Murder (attempt) — *see* Assault

N

Nail
  contact with W45.0 ☑
    gun W29.4 ☑
  embedded in skin W45.0 ☑
Neglect (criminal) (homicidal intent) X58 ☑
Noise (causing injury) (pollution) W42.9 ☑
  supersonic W42.0 ☑
Nonadministration (of)
  drug or biological substance (necessary) Y63.6
  surgical and medical care Y66
Nosocomial condition Y95

O

Object
  falling
    from, in, on, hitting
      machinery — *see* Contact, with, by type of machine
    set in motion by
      accidental explosion or rupture of pressure vessel W38 ☑
      firearm — *see* Discharge, firearm, by type
      machine(ry) — *see* Contact, with, by type of machine
Overdose (drug) — *see* Table of Drugs and Chemicals
  radiation Y63.2
Overexertion X50.9 ☑
  from
    prolonged static or awkward postures X50.1 ☑
    repetitive movements X50.3 ☑
    specified strenuous movements or postures NEC X50.9 ☑
    strenuous movement or load X50.0 ☑
Overexposure (accidental) (to)
  cold — *see also* Exposure, cold X31 ☑
    due to man-made conditions — *see* Exposure, cold, man-made
  heat — *see also* Heat X30 ☑
  radiation — *see* Radiation
  radioactivity W88.0 ☑
  sun (sunburn) X32 ☑
  weather NEC — *see* Forces of nature
  wind NEC — *see* Forces of nature
Overheated — *see* Heat
Overturning (accidental)
  machinery — *see* Contact, with, by type of machine
  transport vehicle NEC — *see also* Accident, transport V89.9 ☑
  watercraft (causing drowning, submersion) — *see also* Drowning, due to, accident to, watercraft, overturning
    causing injury except drowning or submersion — *see* Accident, watercraft, causing, injury NEC

P

Parachute descent (voluntary) (without accident to aircraft) V97.29 ☑
  due to accident to aircraft — *see* Accident, transport, aircraft
Pecked by bird W61.99 ☑
Perforation during medical or surgical treatment as misadventure — *see* Index to Diseases and Injuries, Complication(s)
Perpetrator, perpetration, of assault, maltreatment and neglect (by) Y07.9
  boyfriend Y07.03
  brother Y07.410
    stepbrother Y07.435
  coach Y07.53
  cousin
    female Y07.491
    male Y07.490
  daycare provider Y07.519
    at-home
      adult care Y07.512
      childcare Y07.510
    care center
      adult care Y07.513
      childcare Y07.511
  family member NEC Y07.499
  father Y07.11
    adoptive Y07.13
    foster Y07.420
    stepfather Y07.430
  foster father Y07.420
  foster mother Y07.421
  girl friend Y07.04
  healthcare provider Y07.529
    mental health Y07.521
    specified NEC Y07.528
  husband Y07.01
  instructor Y07.53
  mother Y07.12
    adoptive Y07.14
    foster Y07.421
    stepmother Y07.433
  multiple perpetrators Y07.6
  nonfamily member Y07.50
    specified NEC Y07.59
  nurse Y07.528
  occupational therapist Y07.528
  partner of parent
    female Y07.434
    male Y07.432
  physical therapist Y07.528
  sister Y07.411
  speech therapist Y07.528
  stepbrother Y07.435
  stepfather Y07.430
  stepmother Y07.433
  stepsister Y07.436
  teacher Y07.53
  wife Y07.02
Piercing — *see* Contact, with, by type of object or machine
Pinched
  between objects (moving) (stationary and moving) W23.0 ☑
  stationary W23.1 ☑
Pinned under machine(ry) — *see* Contact, with, by type of machine
Place of occurrence Y92.9
  abandoned house Y92.89
  airplane Y92.813
  airport Y92.520
  ambulatory health services establishment NEC Y92.538
  ambulatory surgery center Y92.530
  amusement park Y92.831
  apartment (co-op) — *see* Place of occurrence, residence, apartment
  assembly hall Y92.29
  bank Y92.510
  barn Y92.71
  baseball field Y92.320
  basketball court Y92.310
  beach Y92.832
  boarding house — *see* Place of occurrence, residence, boarding house
  boat Y92.814
  bowling alley Y92.39

ⓦ **Subterms under main terms may continue to next column or page**   ☑ **Additional Character Required — Refer to the Tabular List for Character Selection**   **425**

Military operations — Place of occurrence

Place of occurrence — *continued*
bridge Y92.89
building under construction Y92.61
bus Y92.811
    station Y92.521
cafe Y92.511
campsite Y92.833
campus — *see* Place of occurrence, school
canal Y92.89
car Y92.810
casino Y92.59
children's home — *see* Place of occurrence, residence, institutional, orphanage
church Y92.22
cinema Y92.26
clubhouse Y92.29
coal pit Y92.64
college (community) Y92.214
condominium — *see* Place of occurrence, residence, apartment
construction area — *see* Place of occurrence, industrial and construction area
convalescent home — *see* Place of occurrence, residence, institutional, nursing home
court-house Y92.240
cricket ground Y92.328
cultural building Y92.258
    art gallery Y92.250
    museum Y92.251
    music hall Y92.252
    opera house Y92.253
    specified NEC Y92.258
    theater Y92.254
dancehall Y92.252
day nursery Y92.210
dentist office Y92.531
derelict house Y92.89
desert Y92.820
dockyard Y92.62
dock NOS Y92.89
doctor's office Y92.531
dormitory — *see* Place of occurrence, residence, institutional, school dormitory
dry dock Y92.62
factory (building) (premises) Y92.63
farm (land under cultivation) (outbuildings) Y92.79
    barn Y92.71
    chicken coop Y92.72
    field Y92.73
    hen house Y92.72
    house — *see* Place of occurrence, residence, house
    orchard Y92.74
    specified NEC Y92.79
football field Y92.321
forest Y92.821
freeway Y92.411
gallery Y92.250
garage (commercial) Y92.59
    boarding house Y92.044
    military base Y92.135
    mobile home Y92.025
    nursing home Y92.124
    orphanage Y92.114
    private house Y92.015
    reform school Y92.155
gas station Y92.524
gasworks Y92.69
golf course Y92.39
gravel pit Y92.64
grocery Y92.512
gymnasium Y92.39
handball court Y92.318
harbor Y92.89
harness racing course Y92.39
healthcare provider office Y92.531
highway (interstate) Y92.411
hill Y92.828
hockey rink Y92.330
home — *see* Place of occurrence, residence
hospice — *see* Place of occurrence, residence, institutional, nursing home
hospital Y92.239
    cafeteria Y92.233
    corridor Y92.232
    operating room Y92.234
    patient
        bathroom Y92.231
        room Y92.230

Place of occurrence — *continued*
hospital — *continued*
    specified NEC Y92.238
hotel Y92.59
house — *see also* Place of occurrence, residence
    abandoned Y92.89
    under construction Y92.61
industrial and construction area (yard) Y92.69
    building under construction Y92.61
    dock Y92.62
    dry dock Y92.62
    factory Y92.63
    gasworks Y92.69
    mine Y92.64
    oil rig Y92.65
    pit Y92.64
    power station Y92.69
    shipyard Y92.62
    specified NEC Y92.69
    tunnel under construction Y92.69
    workshop Y92.69
kindergarten Y92.211
lacrosse field Y92.328
lake Y92.828
library Y92.241
mall Y92.59
market Y92.512
marsh Y92.828
military
    base — *see* Place of occurrence, residence, institutional, military base
    training ground Y92.84
mine Y92.64
mosque Y92.22
motel Y92.59
motorway (interstate) Y92.411
mountain Y92.828
movie-house Y92.26
museum Y92.251
music-hall Y92.252
not applicable Y92.9
nuclear power station Y92.69
nursing home — *see* Place of occurrence, residence, institutional, nursing home
office building Y92.59
offshore installation Y92.65
oil rig Y92.65
old people's home — *see* Place of occurrence, residence, institutional, specified NEC
opera-house Y92.253
orphanage — *see* Place of occurrence, residence, institutional, orphanage
outpatient surgery center Y92.530
park (public) Y92.830
    amusement Y92.831
parking garage Y92.89
    lot Y92.481
pavement Y92.480
physician office Y92.531
polo field Y92.328
pond Y92.828
post office Y92.242
power station Y92.69
prairie Y92.828
prison — *see* Place of occurrence, residence, institutional, prison
public
    administration building Y92.248
        city hall Y92.243
        courthouse Y92.240
        library Y92.241
        post office Y92.242
        specified NEC Y92.248
    building NEC Y92.29
    hall Y92.29
    place NOS Y92.89
race course Y92.39
radio station Y92.59
railway line (bridge) Y92.85
ranch (outbuildings) — *see* Place of occurrence, farm
recreation area Y92.838
    amusement park Y92.831
    beach Y92.832
    campsite Y92.833
    park (public) Y92.830
    seashore Y92.832
    specified NEC Y92.838

Place of occurrence — *continued*
reform school - — *see* Place of occurrence, residence, institutional, reform school
religious institution Y92.22
residence (non-institutional) (private) Y92.009
    apartment Y92.039
        bathroom Y92.031
        bedroom Y92.032
        kitchen Y92.030
        specified NEC Y92.038
    bathroom Y92.002
    bedroom Y92.003
    boarding house Y92.049
        bathroom Y92.041
        bedroom Y92.042
        driveway Y92.043
        garage Y92.044
        garden Y92.046
        kitchen Y92.040
        specified NEC Y92.048
        swimming pool Y92.045
        yard Y92.046
    dining room Y92.001
    garden Y92.007
    home Y92.009
    house, single family Y92.019
        bathroom Y92.012
        bedroom Y92.013
        dining room Y92.011
        driveway Y92.014
        garage Y92.015
        garden Y92.017
        kitchen Y92.010
        specified NEC Y92.018
        swimming pool Y92.016
        yard Y92.017
    institutional Y92.10
        children's home — *see* Place of occurrence, residence, institutional, orphanage
        hospice — *see* Place of occurrence, residence, institutional, nursing home
        military base Y92.139
            barracks Y92.133
            garage Y92.135
            garden Y92.137
            kitchen Y92.130
            mess hall Y92.131
            specified NEC Y92.138
            swimming pool Y92.136
            yard Y92.137
        nursing home Y92.129
            bathroom Y92.121
            bedroom Y92.122
            driveway Y92.123
            garage Y92.124
            garden Y92.126
            kitchen Y92.120
            specified NEC Y92.128
            swimming pool Y92.125
            yard Y92.126
        orphanage Y92.119
            bathroom Y92.111
            bedroom Y92.112
            driveway Y92.113
            garage Y92.114
            garden Y92.116
            kitchen Y92.110
            specified NEC Y92.118
            swimming pool Y92.115
            yard Y92.116
        prison Y92.149
            bathroom Y92.142
            cell Y92.143
            courtyard Y92.147
            dining room Y92.141
            kitchen Y92.140
            specified NEC Y92.148
            swimming pool Y92.146
        reform school Y92.159
            bathroom Y92.152
            bedroom Y92.153
            dining room Y92.151
            driveway Y92.154
            garage Y92.155
            garden Y92.157
            kitchen Y92.150
            specified NEC Y92.158
            swimming pool Y92.156
            yard Y92.157

☑ **Additional Character Required** — Refer to the Tabular List for Character Selection   ▽ **Subterms under main terms may continue to next column or page**

Place of occurrence — *continued*
  residence — *continued*
    institutional — *continued*
      school dormitory Y92.169
        bathroom Y92.162
        bedroom Y92.163
        dining room Y92.161
        kitchen Y92.160
        specified NEC Y92.168
      specified NEC Y92.199
        bathroom Y92.192
        bedroom Y92.193
        dining room Y92.191
        driveway Y92.194
        garage Y92.195
        garden Y92.197
        kitchen Y92.190
        specified NEC Y92.198
        swimming pool Y92.196
        yard Y92.197
    kitchen Y92.000
    mobile home Y92.029
      bathroom Y92.022
      bedroom Y92.023
      dining room Y92.021
      driveway Y92.024
      garage Y92.025
      garden Y92.027
      kitchen Y92.020
      specified NEC Y92.028
      swimming pool Y92.026
      yard Y92.027
    specified place in residence NEC Y92.008
    specified residence type NEC Y92.099
      bathroom Y92.091
      bedroom Y92.092
      driveway Y92.093
      garage Y92.094
      garden Y92.096
      kitchen Y92.090
      specified NEC Y92.098
      swimming pool Y92.095
      yard Y92.096
  restaurant Y92.511
  riding school Y92.39
  river Y92.828
  road Y92.410
  rodeo ring Y92.39
  rugby field Y92.328
  same day surgery center Y92.530
  sand pit Y92.64
  school (private) (public) (state) Y92.219
    college Y92.214
    daycare center Y92.210
    elementary school Y92.211
    high school Y92.213
    kindergarten Y92.211
    middle school Y92.212
    specified NEC Y92.218
    trace school Y92.215
    university Y92.214
    vocational school Y92.215
  sea (shore) Y92.832
  senior citizen center Y92.29
  service area
    airport Y92.520
    bus station Y92.521
    gas station Y92.524
    highway rest stop Y92.523
    railway station Y92.522
  shipyard Y92.62
  shop (commercial) Y92.513
  sidewalk Y92.480
  silo Y92.79
  skating rink (roller) Y92.331
    ice Y92.330
  slaughter house Y92.86
  soccer field Y92.322
  specified place NEC Y92.89
  sports area Y92.39
    athletic
      court Y92.318
        basketball Y92.310
        specified NEC Y92.318
        squash Y92.311
        tennis Y92.312
      field Y92.328
        baseball Y92.320
        cricket ground Y92.328

Place of occurrence — *continued*
  sports area — *continued*
    athletic — *continued*
      field — *continued*
        football Y92.321
        hockey Y92.328
        soccer Y92.322
        specified NEC Y92.328
    golf course Y92.39
    gymnasium Y92.39
    riding school Y92.39
    skating rink (roller) Y92.331
      ice Y92.330
    stadium Y92.39
    swimming pool Y92.34
  squash court Y92.311
  stadium Y92.39
  steeplechasing course Y92.39
  store Y92.512
  stream Y92.828
  street and highway Y92.410
    bike path Y92.482
    freeway Y92.411
    highway ramp Y92.415
    interstate highway Y92.411
    local residential or business street Y92.414
    motorway Y92.411
    parking lot Y92.481
    parkway Y92.412
    sidewalk Y92.480
    specified NEC Y92.488
    state road Y92.413
  subway car Y92.816
  supermarket Y92.512
  swamp Y92.828
  swimming pool (public) Y92.34
    private (at) Y92.095
      boarding house Y92.045
      military base Y92.136
      mobile home Y92.026
      nursing home Y92.125
      orphanage Y92.115
      prison Y92.146
      reform school Y92.156
      single family residence Y92.016
  synagogue Y92.22
  television station Y92.59
  tennis court Y92.312
  theater Y92.254
  trade area Y92.59
    bank Y92.510
    cafe Y92.511
    casino Y92.59
    garage Y92.59
    hotel Y92.59
    market Y92.512
    office building Y92.59
    radio station Y92.59
    restaurant Y92.511
    shop Y92.513
    shopping mall Y92.59
    store Y92.512
    supermarket Y92.512
    television station Y92.59
    warehouse Y92.59
  trailer park, residential — *see* Place of occurrence, residence, mobile home
  trailer site NOS Y92.89
  train Y92.815
    station Y92.522
  truck Y92.812
  tunnel under construction Y92.69
  university Y92.214
  urgent (health) care center Y92.532
  vehicle (transport) Y92.818
    airplane Y92.813
    boat Y92.814
    bus Y92.811
    car Y92.810
    specified NEC Y92.818
    subway car Y92.816
    train Y92.815
    truck Y92.812
  warehouse Y92.59
  water reservoir Y92.89
  wilderness area Y92.828
    desert Y92.820
    forest Y92.821
    marsh Y92.828

Place of occurrence — *continued*
  wilderness area — *continued*
    mountain Y92.828
    prairie Y92.828
    specified NEC Y92.828
    swamp Y92.828
  workshop Y92.69
  yard, private Y92.096
    boarding house Y92.046
    mobile home Y92.027
    single family house Y92.017
  youth center Y92.29
  zoo (zoological garden) Y92.834
Plumbism — *see* Table of Drugs and Chemicals, lead
Poisoning (accidental) (by) — *see also* Table of Drugs and Chemicals
  by plant, thorns, spines, sharp leaves or other mechanisms NEC X58 ☑
  carbon monoxide
    generated by
      motor vehicle — *see* Accident, transport
      watercraft (in transit) (not in transit) V93.89 ☑
        ferry boat V93.81 ☑
        fishing boat V93.82 ☑
        jet skis V93.83 ☑
        liner V93.81 ☑
        merchant ship V93.80 ☑
        passenger ship V93.81 ☑
        powered craft NEC V93.83 ☑
  caused by injection of poisons into skin by plant thorns, spines, sharp leaves X58 ☑
  marine or sea plants (venomous) X58 ☑
  execution — *see* Legal, intervention, gas
  intervention
    by gas — *see* Legal, intervention, gas
    other specified means — *see* Legal, intervention, specified means NEC
  exhaust gas
    generated by
      motor vehicle — *see* Accident, transport
      watercraft (in transit) (not in transit) V93.89 ☑
        ferry boat V93.81 ☑
        fishing boat V93.82 ☑
        jet skis V93.83 ☑
        liner V93.81 ☑
        merchant ship V93.80 ☑
        passenger ship V93.81 ☑
        powered craft NEC V93.83 ☑
  fumes or smoke due to
    explosion — *see also* Explosion W40.9 ☑
    fire — *see* Exposure, fire
    ignition — *see* Ignition
  gas
    in legal intervention — *see* Legal, intervention, gas
    legal execution — *see* Legal, intervention, gas
  in war operations — *see* War operations
  legal
Powder burn (by) (from)
  airgun W34.110 ☑
  BB gun W34.110 ☑
  firearm NEC W34.19 ☑
  gas, air or spring-operated gun NEC W34.118 ☑
  handgun W32.1 ☑
  hunting rifle W33.12 ☑
  larger firearm W33.10 ☑
    specified NEC W33.19 ☑
  machine gun W33.13 ☑
  paintball gun W34.111 ☑
  pellet gun W34.110 ☑
  shotgun W33.11 ☑
  Very pistol [flare] W34.19 ☑
Premature cessation (of) **surgical and medical care** Y66
Privation (food) (water) X58 ☑
Procedure (operation)
  correct, on wrong side or body part (wrong side) (wrong site) Y65.53
  intended for another patient done on wrong patient Y65.52
  performed on patient not scheduled for surgery Y65.52
  performed on wrong patient Y65.52
  wrong, performed on correct patient Y65.51
Prolonged
  sitting in transport vehicle — *see* Travel, by type of vehicle

Prolonged — *continued*
  stay in
    high altitude as cause of anoxia, barodontalgia,
      barotitis or hypoxia W94.11
    weightless environment X52 ✓
Pulling, excessive — *see also* Overexertion X50.9- ✓
Puncture, puncturing — *see also* Contact, with, by type
  of object or machine
  by
    plant thorns, spines, sharp leaves or other mecha-
      nisms NEC W60 ✓
    during medical or surgical treatment as misadventure
      — *see* Index to Diseases and Injuries, Complica-
      tion(s)
Pushed, pushing (accidental) (injury in)
  by other person(s) (accidental) W51 ✓
    as, or caused by, a crowd or human stampede (with
      fall) W52 ✓
    before moving object NEC Y02.8 ✓
      motor vehicle Y02.0 ✓
      subway train Y02.1 ✓
      train Y02.1 ✓
    from
      high place NEC
        in accidental circumstances W17.89 ✓
        stated as
          intentional, homicide (attempt) Y01 ✓
          undetermined whether accidental or in-
            tentional Y30 ✓
      transport vehicle NEC — *see also* Accident,
        transport V89.9 ✓
        stated as
          intentional, homicide (attempt) Y08.89 ✓
    with fall W03 ✓
      due to ice or snow W00.0 ✓
  overexertion X50.9 ✓

R

Radiation (exposure to)
  arc lamps W89.0 ✓
  atomic power plant (malfunction) NEC W88.1 ✓
  complication of or abnormal reaction to medical radio-
    therapy Y84.2
  electromagnetic, ionizing W88.0 ✓
  gamma rays W88.1 ✓
  in
    war operations (from or following nuclear explosion)
      — *see* War operations
  inadvertent exposure of patient (receiving test or
    therapy) Y63.3
  infrared (heaters and lamps) W90.1 ✓
    excessive heat from W92 ✓
  ionized, ionizing (particles, artificially accelerated)
    radioisotopes W88.1 ✓
    specified NEC W88.8 ✓
    x-rays W88.0 ✓
  isotopes, radioactive — *see* Radiation, radioactive iso-
    topes
  laser(s) W90.2 ✓
    in war operations — *see* War operations
    misadventure in medical care Y63.2
  light sources (man-made visible and ultraviolet)
    W89.9 ✓
    natural X32 ✓
    specified NEC W89.8 ✓
    tanning bed W89.1 ✓
    welding light W89.0 ✓
  man-made visible light W89.9 ✓
    specified NEC W89.8 ✓
    tanning bed W89.1 ✓
    welding light W89.0 ✓
  microwave W90.8 ✓
  misadventure in medical or surgical procedure Y63.2
  natural NEC X39.08 ✓
    radon X39.01 ✓
  overdose (in medical or surgical procedure) Y63.2
  radar W90.0 ✓
  radioactive isotopes (any) W88.1 ✓
    atomic power plant malfunction W88.1 ✓
    misadventure in medical or surgical treatment Y63.2
  radiofrequency W90.0 ✓
  radium NEC W88.1 ✓
  sun X32 ✓
  ultraviolet (light) (man-made) W89.9 ✓
    natural X32 ✓

Radiation — *continued*
  ultraviolet — *continued*
    specified NEC W89.8 ✓
    tanning bed W89.1 ✓
    welding light W89.0 ✓
  welding arc, torch, or light W89.0 ✓
    excessive heat from W92 ✓
  x-rays (hard) (soft) W88.0 ✓
Range disease W94.11
Rape (attempted) T74.2- ✓
Rat bite W53.11
Reaching (prolonged) (static) X50.1 ✓
Reaction, abnormal to medical procedure — *see also*
  Complication of or following, by type of procedure
  Y84.9
  biologicals — *see* Table of Drugs and Chemicals
  drugs — *see* Table of Drugs and Chemicals
  vaccine — *see* Table of Drugs and Chemicals
  with misadventure — *see* Misadventure
Recoil
  airgun W34.110 ✓
  BB gun W34.110 ✓
  firearm NEC W34.19 ✓
  gas, air or spring-operated gun NEC W34.118 ✓
  handgun W32.1 ✓
  hunting rifle W33.12 ✓
  larger firearm W33.10 ✓
    specified NEC W33.19 ✓
  machine gun W33.13 ✓
  paintball gun W34.111 ✓
  pellet W34.110 ✓
  shotgun W33.11 ✓
  Very pistol [flare] W34.19 ✓
Reduction in
  atmospheric pressure — *see* Air, pressure, change
Rock falling on or hitting (accidentally) (person)
  W20.8 ✓
  in cave-in W20.0 ✓
Run over (accidentally) (by)
  animal (not being ridden) NEC W55.89 ✓
  machinery — *see* Contact, with, by specified type of
    machine
  transport vehicle NEC — *see also* Accident, transport
    V09.9 ✓
    intentional homicide (attempt) Y03.0 ✓
    motor NEC V09.20 ✓
      intentional homicide (attempt) Y03.0 ✓
Running
  before moving object X81.8 ✓
    motor vehicle X81.0 ✓
Running off, away
  animal (being ridden) — *see also* Accident, transport
    V80.918 ✓
    not being ridden W55.89 ✓
  animal-drawn vehicle NEC — *see also* Accident, trans-
    port V80.928 ✓
  highway, road(way), street
    transport vehicle NEC — *see also* Accident, transport
      V89.9 ✓
Rupture pressurized devices — *see* Explosion, by type
  of device

S

Saturnism — *see* Table of Drugs and Chemicals, lead
Scald, scalding (accidental) (by) (from) (in) X19 ✓
  air (hot) X14.1 ✓
  gases (hot) X14.1 ✓
  homicide (attempt) — *see* Assault, burning, hot object
  inflicted by other person
    stated as intentional, homicide (attempt) — *see*
      Assault, burning, hot object
  liquid (boiling) (hot) NEC X12 ✓
    stated as undetermined whether accidental or inten-
      tional Y27.2 ✓
    suicide (attempt) X77.2 ✓
  local application of externally applied substance in
    medical or surgical care Y63.5
  metal (molten) (liquid) (hot) NEC X18 ✓
  self-inflicted X77.9 ✓
  stated as undetermined whether accidental or inten-
    tional Y27.8 ✓
  steam X13.1 ✓
    assault X98.0 ✓
    stated as undetermined whether accidental or inten-
      tional Y27.0 ✓

Scald, scalding — *continued*
  steam — *continued*
    suicide (attempt) X77.0 ✓
  suicide (attempt) X77.9 ✓
  vapor (hot) X13.1 ✓
    assault X98.0 ✓
    stated as undetermined whether accidental or inten-
      tional Y27.0 ✓
    suicide (attempt) X77.0 ✓
Scratched by
  cat W55.03 ✓
  person(s) (accidentally) W50.4 ✓
    with intent to injure or kill Y04.0 ✓
    as, or caused by, a crowd or human stampede (with
      fall) W52 ✓
    assault Y04.0 ✓
    homicide (attempt) Y04.0 ✓
    in
      fight Y04.0 ✓
      legal intervention
        injuring
          bystander Y35.892 ✓
          law enforcement personnel Y35.891 ✓
          suspect Y35.893 ✓
Seasickness T75.3 ✓
Self-harm NEC — *see also* External cause by type, undetermined whether accidental or intentional
  intentional — *see* Suicide
  poisoning NEC — *see* Table of Drugs and Chemicals,
    poisoning, accidental
Self-inflicted (injury) **NEC** — *see also* External cause by
  type, undetermined whether accidental or intentional
  intentional — *see* Suicide
  poisoning NEC — *see* Table of Drugs and Chemicals,
    poisoning, accidental
Sequelae (of)
  accident NEC — *see* W00-X58 with 7th character S
  assault (homicidal) (any means) — *see* X92-Y08 with
    7th character S
  homicide, attempt (any means) — *see* X92-Y08 with
    7th character S
  injury undetermined whether accidentally or purposely
    inflicted — *see* Y21-Y33 with 7th character S
  intentional self-harm (classifiable to X71-X83) — *see*
    X71-X83 with 7th character S
  legal intervention — *see* with 7th character S Y35
  motor vehicle accident — *see* V00-V99 with 7th char-
    acter S
  suicide, attempt (any means) — *see* X71-X83 with 7th
    character S
  transport accident — *see* V00-V99 with 7th character
    S
  war operations — *see* War operations
Shock
  electric — *see* Exposure, electric current
  from electric appliance (any) (faulty) W86.8 ✓
    domestic W86.0 ✓
    suicide (attempt) X83.1 ✓
Shooting, shot (accidental(ly)) — *see also* Discharge,
  firearm, by type
  herself or himself — *see* Discharge, firearm by type,
    self-inflicted
  homicide (attempt) — *see* Discharge, firearm by type,
    homicide
  in war operations — *see* War operations
  inflicted by other person — *see* Discharge, firearm by
    type, homicide
    accidental — *see* Discharge, firearm, by type of
      firearm
  legal
    execution — *see* Legal, intervention, firearm
    intervention — *see* Legal, intervention, firearm
  self-inflicted — *see* Discharge, firearm by type, suicide
    accidental — *see* Discharge, firearm, by type of
      firearm
  suicide (attempt) — *see* Discharge, firearm by type,
    suicide
Shoving (accidentally) **by other person** — *see* Pushed,
  by other person
Sickness
  alpine W94.11 ✓
  motion — *see* Motion
  mountain W94.11 ✓
Sinking (accidental)
  watercraft (causing drowning, submersion) — *see also*
    Drowning, due to, accident to, watercraft, sinking

428

☑ **Additional Character Required** — Refer to the Tabular List for Character Selection   ▽ **Subterms under main terms may continue to next column or page**

Prolonged — Sinking

Sinking — *continued*
watercraft — *see also* Drowning, due to, accident to, watercraft, sinking — *continued*
causing injury except drowning or submersion — *see* Accident, watercraft, causing, injury NEC
Siriasis X32 ☑
Sitting (prolonged) (static) X50.1 ☑
Slashed wrists — *see* Cut, self-inflicted
Slipping (accidental) (on same level) (with fall) W01.0 ☑
on
ice W00.0 ☑
with skates — *see* Accident, transport, pedestrian, conveyance
mud W01.0 ☑
oil W01.0 ☑
snow W00.0 ☑
with skis — *see* Accident, transport, pedestrian, conveyance
surface (slippery) (wet) NEC W01.0 ☑
without fall W18.40 ☑
due to
specified NEC W18.49 ☑
stepping from one level to another W18.43 ☑
stepping into hole or opening W18.42 ☑
stepping on object W18.41 ☑
Sliver, wood, contact with W45.8 ☑
Smoldering (due to fire) — *see* Exposure, fire
Sodomy (attempted) **by force** T74.2 ☑
Sound waves (causing injury) W42.9 ☑
supersonic W42.0 ☑
Splinter, contact with W45.8 ☑
Stab, stabbing — *see* Cut
Standing (prolonged) (static) X50.1 ☑
Starvation X58 ☑
Status of external cause Y99.9
child assisting in compensated work for family Y99.8
civilian activity done for financial or other compensation Y99.0
civilian activity done for income or pay Y99.0
family member assisting in compensated work for other family member Y99.8
hobby not done for income Y99.8
leisure activity Y99.8
military activity Y99.1
off-duty activity of military personnel Y99.8
recreation or sport not for income or while a student Y99.8
specified NEC Y99.8
student activity Y99.8
volunteer activity Y99.2
Stepped on
by
animal (not being ridden) NEC W55.89 ☑
crowd or human stampede W52 ☑
person W50.0 ☑
Stepping on
object W22.8 ☑
sports equipment W21.9 ☑
stationary W22.09 ☑
sports equipment W21.89 ☑
with fall W18.31 ☑
person W51 ☑
by crowd or human stampede W52 ☑
sports equipment W21.9 ☑
Sting
arthropod, nonvenomous W57 ☑
insect, nonvenomous W57 ☑
Storm (cataclysmic) — *see* Forces of nature, cataclysmic storm
Straining, excessive — *see also* Overexertion X50.9 ☑
Strangling — *see* Strangulation
Strangulation (accidental) T71 ☑
Strenuous movements — *see also* Overexertion X50.9 ☑
Striking against
airbag (automobile) W22.10 ☑
driver side W22.11 ☑
front passenger side W22.12 ☑
specified NEC W22.19 ☑
bottom when
diving or jumping into water (in) W16.822 ☑
causing drowning W16.821 ☑
from boat W16.722 ☑
causing drowning W16.721 ☑
natural body W16.622 ☑
causing drowning W16.821 ☑

Striking against — *continued*
bottom when — *continued*
diving or jumping into water — *continued*
swimming pool W16.522 ☑
causing drowning W16.521 ☑
falling into water (in) W16.322 ☑
causing drowning W16.321 ☑
fountain — *see* Striking against, bottom when, falling into water, specified NEC
natural body W16.122 ☑
causing drowning W16.121 ☑
reservoir — *see* Striking against, bottom when, falling into water, specified NEC
specified NEC W16.322 ☑
causing drowning W16.321 ☑
swimming pool W16.022 ☑
causing drowning W16.021 ☑
diving board (swimming-pool) W21.4 ☑
object W22.8 ☑
caused by crowd or human stampede (with fall) W52 ☑
furniture W22.03 ☑
lamppost W22.02 ☑
sports equipment W21.9 ☑
stationary W22.09 ☑
sports equipment W21.89 ☑
wall W22.01 ☑
with
drowning or submersion — *see* Drowning
fall — *see* Fall, due to, bumping against, object
person(s) W51 ☑
as, or caused by, a crowd or human stampede (with fall) W52 ☑
assault Y04.2 ☑
homicide (attempt) Y04.2 ☑
with fall W03 ☑
due to ice or snow W00.0 ☑
sports equipment W21.9 ☑
wall (when) W22.01 ☑
diving or jumping into water (in) W16.832 ☑
causing drowning W16.831 ☑
swimming pool W16.532 ☑
causing drowning W16.531 ☑
falling into water (in) W16.332 ☑
causing drowning W16.331 ☑
fountain — *see* Striking against, wall when, falling into water, specified NEC
natural body W16.132 ☑
causing drowning W16.131 ☑
reservoir — *see* Striking against, wall when, falling into water, specified NEC
specified NEC W16.332 ☑
causing drowning W16.331 ☑
swimming pool W16.032 ☑
causing drowning W16.031 ☑
swimming pool (when) W22.042 ☑
causing drowning W22.041 ☑
diving or jumping into water W16.532 ☑
causing drowning W16.531 ☑
falling into water W16.032 ☑
causing drowning W16.031 ☑
Struck (accidentally) **by**
airbag (automobile) W22.10 ☑
driver side W22.11 ☑
front passenger side W22.12 ☑
specified NEC W22.19 ☑
alligator W58.02 ☑
animal (not being ridden) NEC W55.89 ☑
avalanche — *see* Landslide
ball (hit) (thrown) W21.00 ☑
assault Y08.09 ☑
baseball W21.03 ☑
basketball W21.05 ☑
football W21.01 ☑
golf ball W21.04 ☑
soccer W21.02 ☑
softball W21.07 ☑
specified NEC W21.09 ☑
volleyball W21.06 ☑
bat or racquet
baseball bat W21.11 ☑
assault Y08.02 ☑
golf club W21.13 ☑
assault Y08.09 ☑
specified NEC W21.19 ☑
assault Y08.09 ☑

Struck (accidentally) **by** — *continued*
bat or racquet — *continued*
tennis racquet W21.12 ☑
assault Y08.09 ☑
bullet — *see also* Discharge, firearm by type
in war operations — *see* War operations
crocodile W58.12 ☑
dog W54.1 ☑
flare, Very pistol — *see* Discharge, firearm NEC
hailstones X39.8 ☑
hockey (ice)
field
puck W21.221 ☑
stick W21.211 ☑
puck W21.220 ☑
stick W21.210 ☑
assault Y08.01 ☑
landslide — *see* Landslide
law-enforcement agent (on duty) — *see* Legal, intervention, manhandling
with blunt object — *see* Legal, intervention, blunt object
lightning T75.0 ☑
causing fire — *see* Exposure, fire
machine — *see* Contact, with, by type of machine
mammal NEC W55.89 ☑
marine W56.32 ☑
marine animal W56.82 ☑
missile
firearm — *see* Discharge, firearm by type
in war operations — *see* War operations, missile
object W22.8 ☑
blunt W22.8 ☑
assault Y00 ☑
suicide (attempt) X79 ☑
undetermined whether accidental or intentional Y29 ☑
falling W20.8 ☑
from, in, on
building W20.1 ☑
burning (uncontrolled fire) X00.4 ☑
cataclysmic
earth surface movement NEC — *see* Landslide
storm — *see* Forces of nature, cataclysmic storm
cave-in W20.0 ☑
earthquake X34 ☑
machine (in operation) — *see* Contact, with, by type of machine
structure W20.1 ☑
burning X00.4 ☑
transport vehicle (in motion) — *see* Accident, transport, by type of vehicle
watercraft V93.49 ☑
due to
accident to craft V91.39 ☑
powered craft V91.33 ☑
ferry boat V91.31 ☑
fishing boat V91.32 ☑
jetskis V91.33 ☑
liner V91.31 ☑
merchant ship V91.30 ☑
passenger ship V91.31 ☑
unpowered craft V91.38 ☑
canoe V91.35 ☑
inflatable V91.36 ☑
kayak V91.35 ☑
sailboat V91.34 ☑
surf-board V91.38 ☑
windsurfer V91.38 ☑
powered craft V93.43 ☑
ferry boat V93.41 ☑
fishing boat V93.42 ☑
jetskis V93.43 ☑
liner V93.41 ☑
merchant ship V93.40 ☑
passenger ship V93.41 ☑
unpowered craft V93.48 ☑
sailboat V93.44 ☑
surf-board V93.48 ☑
windsurfer V93.48 ☑
moving NEC W20.8 ☑
projected W20.8 ☑
assault Y00 ☑
in sports W21.9 ☑

Struck (accidentally) **by** — *continued*
  object — *continued*
    projected — *continued*
      in sports — *continued*
        assault Y08.09 ☑
        ball W21.00 ☑
          baseball W21.03 ☑
          basketball W21.05 ☑
          football W21.01 ☑
          golf ball W21.04 ☑
          soccer W21.02 ☑
          softball W21.07 ☑
          specified NEC W21.09 ☑
          volleyball W21.06 ☑
        bat or racquet
          baseball bat W21.11 ☑
            assault Y08.02 ☑
          golf club W21.13 ☑
            assault Y08.09 ☑
          specified NEC W21.19 ☑
            assault Y08.09 ☑
          tennis racquet W21.12 ☑
            assault Y08.09 ☑
        hockey (ice)
          field
            puck W21.221 ☑
            stick W21.211 ☑
          puck W21.220 ☑
          stick W21.210 ☑
            assault Y08.01 ☑
        specified NEC W21.89 ☑
    set in motion by explosion — *see* Explosion
    thrown W20.8 ☑
      assault Y00 ☑
      in sports W21.9 ☑
        assault Y08.09 ☑
        ball W21.00 ☑
          baseball W21.03 ☑
          basketball W21.05 ☑
          football W21.01 ☑
          golf ball W21.04 ☑
          soccer W21.02 ☑
          soft ball W21.07 ☑
          specified NEC W21.09 ☑
          volleyball W21.06 ☑
        bat or racquet
          baseball bat W21.11 ☑
            assault Y08.02 ☑
          golf club W21.13 ☑
            assault Y08.09 ☑
          specified NEC W21.19 ☑
            assault Y08.09 ☑
          tennis racquet W21.12 ☑
            assault Y08.09 ☑
        hockey (ice)
          field
            puck W21.221 ☑
            stick W21.211 ☑
          puck W21.220 ☑
          stick W21.210 ☑
            assault Y08.01 ☑
        specified NEC W21.89 ☑
  other person(s) W50.0 ☑
    with
      blunt object W22.8 ☑
        intentional, homicide (attempt) Y00 ☑
        sports equipment W21.9 ☑
        undetermined whether accidental or intentional Y29 ☑
      fall W03 ☑
        due to ice or snow W00.0 ☑
    as, or caused by, a crowd or human stampede (with fall) W52 ☑
      assault Y04.2 ☑
    homicide (attempt) Y04.2 ☑
    in legal intervention
      injuring
        bystander Y35.812 ☑
        law enforcement personnel Y35.811 ☑
        suspect Y35.813 ☑
        unspecified person Y35.819 ☑
    sports equipment W21.9 ☑
  police (on duty) — *see* Legal, intervention, manhandling
    with blunt object — *see* Legal, intervention, blunt object

Struck (accidentally) **by** — *continued*
  sports equipment W21.9 ☑
    assault Y08.09 ☑
    ball W21.00 ☑
      baseball W21.03 ☑
      basketball W21.05 ☑
      football W21.01 ☑
      golf ball W21.04 ☑
      soccer W21.02 ☑
      soft ball W21.07 ☑
      specified NEC W21.09 ☑
      volleyball W21.06 ☑
    bat or racquet
      baseball bat W21.11 ☑
        assault Y08.02 ☑
      golf club W21.13 ☑
        assault Y08.09 ☑
      specified NEC W21.19 ☑
      tennis racquet W21.12 ☑
        assault Y08.09 ☑
    cleats (shoe) W21.31 ☑
    foot wear NEC W21.39 ☑
    football helmet W21.81 ☑
    hockey (ice)
      field
        puck W21.221 ☑
        stick W21.211 ☑
      puck W21.220 ☑
      stick W21.210 ☑
        assault Y08.01 ☑
    skate blades W21.32 ☑
    specified NEC W21.89 ☑
      assault Y08.09 ☑
  thunderbolt — *see* subcategory T75.0 ☑
    causing fire — *see* Exposure, fire
  transport vehicle NEC — *see also* Accident, transport V09.9 ☑
    intentional, homicide (attempt) Y03.0 ☑
    motor NEC — *see also* Accident, transport V09.20 ☑
      homicide Y03.0 ☑
  vehicle (transport) NEC — *see* Accident, transport, by type of vehicle
    stationary (falling from jack, hydraulic lift, ramp) W20.8 ☑

Stumbling
  over
    animal NEC W01.0 ☑
      with fall W18.09 ☑
    carpet, rug or (small) object W22.8 ☑
      with fall W18.09 ☑
    person W51 ☑
      with fall W03 ☑
        due to ice or snow W00.0 ☑
  without fall W18.40 ☑
    due to
      specified NEC W18.49 ☑
      stepping from one level to another W18.43 ☑
      stepping into hole or opening W18.42 ☑
      stepping on object W18.41 ☑
Submersion (accidental) — *see* Drowning
Suffocation (accidental) (by external means) (by pressure) (mechanical) — *see also* category T71 ☑
  due to, by
    avalanche — *see* Landslide
    explosion — *see* Explosion
    fire — *see* Exposure, fire
    food, any type (aspiration) (ingestion) (inhalation) — *see* categories T17 and T18 ☑
    ignition — *see* Ignition
    landslide — *see* Landslide
    machine(ry) — *see* Contact, with, by type of machine
    vomitus (aspiration) (inhalation) T17.81- ☑
  in
    burning building X00.8 ☑
Suicide, suicidal (attempted) (by) X83.8 ☑
  blunt object X79 ☑
  burning, burns X76 ☑
    hot object X77.9 ☑
      fluid NEC X77.2 ☑
      household appliance X77.3 ☑
      specified NEC X77.8 ☑
      steam X77.0 ☑
      tap water X77.1 ☑
      vapors X77.0 ☑
  caustic substance — *see* Table of Drugs and Chemicals

Suicide, suicidal — *continued*
  cold, extreme X83.2 ☑
  collision of motor vehicle with
    motor vehicle X82.0 ☑
    specified NEC X82.8 ☑
    train X82.1 ☑
    tree X82.2 ☑
  crashing of aircraft X83.0 ☑
  cut (any part of body) X78.9 ☑
  cutting or piercing instrument X78.9 ☑
    dagger X78.2 ☑
    glass X78.0 ☑
    knife X78.1 ☑
    specified NEC X78.8 ☑
    sword X78.2 ☑
  drowning (in) X71.9 ☑
    bathtub X71.0 ☑
    natural water X71.3 ☑
    specified NEC X71.8 ☑
    swimming pool X71.1 ☑
      following fall X71.2 ☑
  electrocution X83.1 ☑
  explosive(s) (material) X75 ☑
  fire, flames X76 ☑
  firearm X74.9 ☑
    airgun X74.01 ☑
    handgun X72 ☑
    hunting rifle X73.1 ☑
    larger X73.9 ☑
      specified NEC X73.8 ☑
    machine gun X73.2 ☑
    shotgun X73.0 ☑
    specified NEC X74.8 ☑
  hanging X83.8 ☑
  hot object — *see* Suicide, burning, hot object
  jumping
    before moving object X81.8 ☑
      motor vehicle X81.0 ☑
      subway train X81.1 ☑
      train X81.1 ☑
    from high place X80 ☑
  late effect of attempt — *see* X71-X83 with 7th character S
  lying before moving object, train, vehicle X81.8 ☑
  poisoning — *see* Table of Drugs and Chemicals
  puncture (any part of body) — *see* Suicide, cutting or piercing instrument
  scald — *see* Suicide, burning, hot object
  sequelae of attempt — *see* X71-X83 with 7th character S
  sharp object (any) — *see* Suicide, cutting or piercing instrument
  shooting — *see* Suicide, firearm
  specified means NEC X83.8 ☑
  stab (any part of body) — *see* Suicide, cutting or piercing instrument
  steam, hot vapors X77.0 ☑
  strangulation X83.8 ☑
  submersion — *see* Suicide, drowning
  suffocation X83.8 ☑
  wound NEC X83.8 ☑
Sunstroke X32 ☑
Supersonic waves (causing injury) W42.0 ☑
Surgical procedure, complication of (delayed or as an abnormal reaction without mention of misadventure) — *see also* Complication of or following, by type of procedure
  due to or as a result of misadventure — *see* Misadventure
Swallowed, swallowing
  foreign body — *see* Foreign body, alimentary canal
  poison — *see* Table of Drugs and Chemicals
  substance
    caustic or corrosive — *see* Table of Drugs and Chemicals
    poisonous — *see* Table of Drugs and Chemicals

T

Tackle in sport W03 ☑
Terrorism (involving) Y38.80 ☑
  biological weapons Y38.6X- ☑
  chemical weapons Y38.7X- ☑
  conflagration Y38.3X- ☑
  drowning and submersion Y38.89- ☑
  explosion Y38.2X- ☑

☑ Additional Character Required — Refer to the Tabular List for Character Selection   ▽ Subterms under main terms may continue to next column or page

Terrorism — *continued*
  explosion — *continued*
    destruction of aircraft Y38.1X- ☑
      marine weapons Y38.0X- ☑
    fire Y38.3X- ☑
    firearms Y38.4X- ☑
    hot substances Y38.3X- ☑
    lasers Y38.89- ☑
    nuclear weapons Y38.5X- ☑
    piercing or stabbing instruments Y38.89- ☑
    secondary effects Y38.9X- ☑
    specified method NEC Y38.89- ☑
    suicide bomber Y38.81- ☑
Thirst X58 ☑
Threat to breathing
  aspiration — *see* Aspiration
  due to cave-in, falling earth or substance NEC T71 ☑
Thrown (accidentally)
  against part (any) of or object in transport vehicle (in
      motion) NEC — *see also* Accident, transport
  from
    high place, homicide (attempt) Y01 ☑
    machinery — *see* Contact, with, by type of machine
    transport vehicle NEC — *see also* Accident, transport
        V89.9 ☑
  off — *see* Thrown, from
Thunderbolt — *see* subcategory T75.0 ☑
  causing fire — *see* Exposure, fire
Tidal wave (any injury) **NEC** — *see* Forces of nature, tidal
    wave
Took
  overdose (drug) — *see* Table of Drugs and Chemicals
  poison — *see* Table of Drugs and Chemicals
Tornado (any injury) X37.1 ☑
Torrential rain (any injury) X37.8 ☑
Torture X58 ☑
Trampled by animal NEC W55.89 ☑
Trapped (accidentally)
  between objects (moving) (stationary and moving) —
      see Caught
  by part (any) of
    motorcycle V29.88 ☑
    pedal cycle V19.88 ☑
    transport vehicle NEC — *see also* Accident, transport
        V89.9 ☑
Travel (effects) (sickness) T75.3 ☑
Tree falling on or hitting (accidentally) (person)
    W20.8 ☑
Tripping
  over
    animal W01.0 ☑
      with fall W01.0 ☑
    carpet, rug or (small) object W22.8 ☑
      with fall W18.09 ☑
    person W51 ☑
      with fall W03 ☑
        due to ice or snow W00.0 ☑
    without fall W18.40 ☑
      due to
        specified NEC W18.49 ☑
        stepping from one level to another W18.43 ☑
        stepping into hole or opening W18.42 ☑
        stepping on object W18.41 ☑
Twisted by person(s) (accidentally) W50.2 ☑
  with intent to injure or kill Y04.0 ☑
  as, or caused by, a crowd or human stampede (with
      fall) W52 ☑
  assault Y04.0 ☑
  homicide (attempt) Y04.0 ☑
  in
    fight Y04.0 ☑
    legal intervention — *see* Legal, intervention, man-
        handling
Twisting (prolonged) (static) X50.1- ☑

U

**Underdosing of necessary drugs, medicaments or
    biological substances** Y63.6
Undetermined intent (contact) (exposure)
  automobile collision Y32 ☑
  blunt object Y29 ☑
  drowning (submersion) (in) Y21.9 ☑
    bathtub Y21.0 ☑
      after fall Y21.1 ☑

Undetermined intent — *continued*
  drowning — *continued*
    natural water (lake) (ocean) (pond) (river) (stream)
        Y21.4 ☑
    specified place NEC Y21.8 ☑
    swimming pool Y21.2 ☑
      after fall Y21.3 ☑
  explosive material Y25 ☑
  fall, jump or push from high place Y30 ☑
  falling, lying or running before moving object Y31 ☑
  fire Y26 ☑
  firearm discharge Y24.9 ☑
    airgun (BB) (pellet) Y24.0 ☑
    handgun (pistol) (revolver) Y22 ☑
    hunting rifle Y23.1 ☑
    larger Y23.9 ☑
      hunting rifle Y23.1 ☑
      machine gun Y23.3 ☑
      military Y23.2 ☑
      shotgun Y23.0 ☑
      specified type NEC Y23.8 ☑
    machine gun Y23.3 ☑
    military Y23.2 ☑
    shotgun Y23.0 ☑
    specified type NEC Y24.8 ☑
    Very pistol Y24.8 ☑
  hot object Y27.9 ☑
    fluid NEC Y27.2 ☑
    household appliance Y27.3 ☑
    specified object NEC Y27.8 ☑
    steam Y27.0 ☑
    tap water Y27.1 ☑
    vapor Y27.0 ☑
  jump, fall or push from high place Y30 ☑
  lying, falling or running before moving object Y31 ☑
  motor vehicle crash Y32 ☑
  push, fall or jump from high place Y30 ☑
  running, falling or lying before moving object Y31 ☑
  sharp object Y28.9 ☑
    dagger Y28.2 ☑
    glass Y28.0 ☑
    knife Y28.1 ☑
    specified object NEC Y28.8 ☑
    sword Y28.2 ☑
  smoke Y26 ☑
  specified event NEC Y33 ☑
Use of hand as hammer X50.3 ☑

V

Vibration (causing injury) W49.9 ☑
Victim (of)
  avalanche — *see* Landslide
  earth movements NEC — *see* Forces of nature, earth
      movement
  earthquake X34 ☑
  flood — *see* Flood
  landslide — *see* Landslide
  lightning — *see* subcategory T75.0 ☑
    causing fire — *see* Exposure, fire
  storm (cataclysmic) NEC — *see* Forces of nature, cata-
      clysmic storm
  volcanic eruption X35 ☑
Volcanic eruption (any injury) X35 ☑
Vomitus, gastric contents in air passages (with asphyx-
    ia, obstruction or suffocation) T17.81- ☑

W

Walked into stationary object (any) W22.09 ☑
  furniture W22.03 ☑
  lamppost W22.02 ☑
  wall W22.01 ☑
War operations (injuries to military personnel and civil-
    ians during war, civil insurrection and peacekeeping
    missions) (by) (from) (involving) Y36.90 ☑
  after cessation of hostilities Y36.89- ☑
    explosion (of)
      bomb placed during war operations Y36.82- ☑
      mine placed during war operations Y36.81- ☑
    specified NEC Y36.88- ☑
  air blast Y36.20- ☑
  aircraft
    destruction — *see* War operations, destruction of
        aircraft

War operations — *continued*
  airway restriction — *see* War operations, restriction of
      airways
  asphyxiation — *see* War operations, restriction of air-
      ways
  biological weapons Y36.6X- ☑
  blast Y36.20- ☑
  blast fragments Y36.20- ☑
  blast wave Y36.20- ☑
  blast wind Y36.20- ☑
  bomb Y36.20- ☑
    dirty Y36.50- ☑
    gasoline Y36.31- ☑
    incendiary Y36.31- ☑
    petrol Y36.31- ☑
  bullet Y36.43- ☑
    incendiary Y36.32- ☑
    rubber Y36.41- ☑
  chemical weapons Y36.7X- ☑
  combat
    hand to hand (unarmed) combat Y36.44- ☑
    using blunt or piercing object Y36.45- ☑
  conflagration — *see* War operations, fire
  conventional warfare NEC Y36.49- ☑
  depth charge Y36.01 ☑
  destruction of aircraft Y36.10- ☑
    due to
      air to air missile Y36.11- ☑
      collision with other aircraft Y36.12- ☑
      detonation (accidental) of onboard munitions
          and explosives Y36.14- ☑
      enemy fire or explosives Y36.11- ☑
      explosive placed on aircraft Y36.11- ☑
      onboard fire Y36.13- ☑
      rocket propelled grenade [RPG] Y36.11- ☑
      small arms fire Y36.11- ☑
      surface to air missile Y36.11- ☑
    specified NEC Y36.19- ☑
  detonation (accidental) of
    onboard marine weapons Y36.05- ☑
    own munitions or munitions launch device
        Y36.24- ☑
  dirty bomb Y36.50- ☑
  explosion (of) Y36.20- ☑
    aerial bomb Y36.21- ☑
    after cessation of hostilities
      bomb placed during war operations Y36.82- ☑
      mine placed during war operations Y36.81- ☑
    bomb NOS — *see also* War operations, bomb(s)
        Y36.20- ☑
    fragments Y36.20- ☑
    grenade Y36.29- ☑
    guided missile Y36.22- ☑
    improvised explosive device [IED] (person-borne)
        (roadside) (vehicle-borne) Y36.23- ☑
    land mine Y36.29- ☑
    marine mine (at sea) (in harbor) Y36.02- ☑
    marine weapon Y36.00- ☑
      specified NEC Y36.09- ☑
    own munitions or munitions launch device (acciden-
        tal) Y36.24- ☑
    sea-based artillery shell Y36.03- ☑
    specified NEC Y36.29- ☑
    torpedo Y36.04- ☑
  fire Y36.30- ☑
    specified NEC Y36.39- ☑
  firearms
    discharge Y36.43- ☑
    pellets Y36.42- ☑
  flamethrower Y36.33- ☑
  fragments (from) (of)
    improvised explosive device [IED] (person-borne)
        (roadside) (vehicle-borne) Y36.26- ☑
    munitions Y36.25- ☑
    specified NEC Y36.29- ☑
    weapons Y36.27- ☑
  friendly fire Y36.92 ☑
  hand to hand (unarmed) combat Y36.44- ☑
  hot substances — *see* War operations, fire
  incendiary bullet Y36.32- ☑
  nuclear weapon (effects of) Y36.50- ☑
    acute radiation exposure Y36.54- ☑
    blast pressure Y36.51- ☑
    direct blast Y36.51- ☑
    direct heat Y36.53- ☑
    fallout exposure Y36.54- ☑

War operations — *continued*
nuclear weapon — *continued*
  fireball Y36.53- ☑
  indirect blast (struck or crushed by blast debris)
    (being thrown by blast) Y36.52- ☑
  ionizing radiation (immediate exposure) Y36.54- ☑
  nuclear radiation Y36.54- ☑
  radiation
    ionizing (immediate exposure) Y36.54- ☑
    nuclear Y36.54- ☑
    thermal Y36.53- ☑
  secondary effects Y36.54- ☑
  specified NEC Y36.59- ☑
  thermal radiation Y36.53- ☑
restriction of air (airway)
  intentional Y36.46- ☑
  unintentional Y36.47- ☑
rubber bullets Y36.41- ☑
shrapnel NOS Y36.29- ☑
suffocation — *see* War operations, restriction of airways
unconventional warfare NEC Y36.7X- ☑
underwater blast NOS Y36.00- ☑

War operations — *continued*
warfare
  conventional NEC Y36.49- ☑
  unconventional NEC Y36.7X- ☑
weapon of mass destruction [WMD] Y36.91 ☑
weapons
  biological weapons Y36.6X- ☑
  chemical Y36.7X- ☑
  nuclear (effects of) Y36.50- ☑
    acute radiation exposure Y36.54- ☑
    blast pressure Y36.51- ☑
    direct blast Y36.51- ☑
    direct heat Y36.53- ☑
    fallout exposure Y36.54- ☑
    fireball Y36.53- ☑
    radiation
      ionizing (immediate exposure) Y36.54- ☑
      nuclear Y36.54- ☑
      thermal Y36.53- ☑
    secondary effects Y36.54- ☑
    specified NEC Y36.59- ☑

War operations — *continued*
weapons — *continued*
  of mass destruction [WMD] Y36.91 ☑
Washed
away by flood — *see* Flood
off road by storm (transport vehicle) — *see* Forces of
  nature, cataclysmic storm
Weather exposure NEC — *see* Forces of nature
Weightlessness (causing injury) (effects of) (in spacecraft,
  real or simulated) X52 ☑
Work related condition Y99.0
Wound (accidental) NEC — *see also* Injury X58 ☑
battle — *see also* War operations Y36.90 ☑
gunshot — *see* Discharge, firearm by type
Wreck transport vehicle NEC — *see also* Accident,
  transport V89.9 ☑
Wrong
device implanted into correct surgical site Y65.51
fluid in infusion Y65.1
patient, procedure performed on Y65.52
procedure (operation) on correct patient Y65.51

ICD-10-CM Tabular List of Diseases and Injuries

Chapter 1. Certain Infectious and Parasitic Diseases (A00–B99)

Chapter-specific Guidelines with Coding Examples

The chapter-specific guidelines from the ICD-10-CM Official Guidelines for Coding and Reporting have been provided below. Along with these guidelines are coding examples, contained in the shaded boxes, that have been developed to help illustrate the coding and/or sequencing guidance found in these guidelines.

a. Human immunodeficiency virus (HIV) infections

1) Code only confirmed cases

Code only confirmed cases of HIV infection/illness. This is an exception to the hospital inpatient guideline Section II, H.

In this context, "confirmation" does not require documentation of positive serology or culture for HIV; the provider's diagnostic statement that the patient is HIV positive, or has an HIV-related illness is sufficient.

> Patient admitted with anemia with possible HIV infection
>
> **D64.9**   **Anemia, unspecified**
>
> *Explanation:* Only the anemia is coded in this scenario because it has not been confirmed that an HIV infection is present. This is an exception to the guideline Section II, H for hospital inpatient coding.

2) Selection and sequencing of HIV codes

(a) Patient admitted for HIV-related condition

If a patient is admitted for an HIV-related condition, the principal diagnosis should be B20, Human immunodeficiency virus [HIV] disease followed by additional diagnosis codes for all reported HIV-related conditions.

> HIV with PCP
>
> **B20**   **Human immunodeficiency virus [HIV] disease**
>
> **B59**   **Pneumocystosis**
>
> *Explanation:* Pneumonia due to *Pneumocystis carinii* is an HIV related condition, so the HIV diagnosis code is reported first, followed by the code for the pneumonia.

(b) Patient with HIV disease admitted for unrelated condition

If a patient with HIV disease is admitted for an unrelated condition (such as a traumatic injury), the code for the unrelated condition (e.g., the nature of injury code) should be the principal diagnosis. Other diagnoses would be B20 followed by additional diagnosis codes for all reported HIV-related conditions.

> Unstable angina, native coronary artery atherosclerosis, HIV
>
> **I25.110**   **Atherosclerotic heart disease of native coronary artery with unstable angina pectoris**
>
> **B20**   **Human immunodeficiency virus [HIV] disease**
>
> *Explanation:* The arteriosclerotic coronary artery disease and the unstable angina are not related to HIV, so those conditions are reported first using a combination code, and HIV is reported secondarily.

(c) Whether the patient is newly diagnosed

Whether the patient is newly diagnosed or has had previous admissions/encounters for HIV conditions is irrelevant to the sequencing decision.

> Newly diagnosed multiple cutaneous Kaposi's sarcoma lesions in previously diagnosed HIV disease
>
> **B20**   **Human immunodeficiency virus [HIV] disease**
>
> **C46.0**   **Kaposi's sarcoma of skin**
>
> *Explanation:* Even though the HIV was diagnosed on a previous encounter, it is still sequenced first when coded with an HIV related condition. Kaposi's sarcoma is an HIV-related condition.

(d) Asymptomatic human immunodeficiency virus

Z21, Asymptomatic human immunodeficiency virus [HIV] infection status, is to be applied when the patient without any documentation of symptoms is listed as being "HIV positive," "known HIV," "HIV test positive," or similar terminology. Do not use this code if the term "AIDS" is used or if the patient is treated for any HIV-related illness or is described as having any condition(s) resulting from his/her HIV positive status; use B20 in these cases.

> Patient admitted with acute appendicitis. Status positive HIV test on Atripla, with no prior symptoms
>
> **K35.80**   **Unspecified acute appendicitis**
>
> **Z21**   **Asymptomatic human immunodeficiency virus [HIV] infection status**
>
> *Explanation:* Code Z21 is sequenced second since documentation indicates that the patient has had a positive HIV test but has been asymptomatic. Being on medication for HIV is not an indication that code B20 is used instead of Z21. Unless there has been documentation that the patient has had current or prior symptoms or HIV-related complications, code B20 is not used. The appendicitis is not an AIDS-related complication and is sequenced first.

(e) Patients with inconclusive HIV serology

Patients with inconclusive HIV serology, but no definitive diagnosis or manifestations of the illness, may be assigned code R75, Inconclusive laboratory evidence of human immunodeficiency virus [HIV].

(f) Previously diagnosed HIV-related illness

Patients with any known prior diagnosis of an HIV-related illness should be coded to B20. Once a patient has developed an HIV-related illness, the patient should always be assigned code B20 on every subsequent admission/encounter. Patients previously diagnosed with any HIV illness (B20) should never be assigned to R75 or Z21, Asymptomatic human immunodeficiency virus [HIV] infection status.

(g) HIV infection in pregnancy, childbirth and the puerperium

During pregnancy, childbirth or the puerperium, a patient admitted (or presenting for a health care encounter) because of an HIV-related illness should receive a principal diagnosis code of O98.7-, Human immunodeficiency [HIV] disease complicating pregnancy, childbirth and the puerperium, followed by B20 and the code(s) for the HIV-related illness(es). Codes from Chapter 15 always take sequencing priority.

Patients with asymptomatic HIV infection status admitted (or presenting for a health care encounter) during pregnancy, childbirth, or the puerperium should receive codes of O98.7- and Z21.

(h) Encounters for testing for HIV

If a patient is being seen to determine his/her HIV status, use code Z11.4, Encounter for screening for human immunodeficiency virus [HIV]. Use additional codes for any associated high risk behavior.

If a patient with signs or symptoms is being seen for HIV testing, code the signs and symptoms. An additional counseling code Z71.7, Human immunodeficiency virus [HIV] counseling, may be used if counseling is provided during the encounter for the test.

When a patient returns to be informed of his/her HIV test results and the test result is negative, use code Z71.7, Human immunodeficiency virus [HIV] counseling.

If the results are positive, see previous guidelines and assign codes as appropriate.

b. Infectious agents as the cause of diseases classified to other chapters

Certain infections are classified in chapters other than Chapter 1 and no organism is identified as part of the infection code. In these instances, it is necessary to use an additional code from Chapter 1 to identify the organism. A code from category B95, Streptococcus, Staphylococcus, and Enterococcus as the cause of diseases classified to other chapters, B96, Other bacterial agents as the cause of diseases classified to other chapters, or B97, Viral agents as the cause of diseases classified to other chapters, is to be used as an additional code to identify the organism. An instructional note will be found at the infection code advising that an additional organism code is required.

E. coli UTI

N39.Ø	Urinary tract infection, site not specified
B96.2Ø	Unspecified Escherichia coli [E.coli] as the cause of diseases classified elsewhere

Explanation: An instructional note under the code for the urinary tract infection indicates to code also the specific organism.

c. Infections resistant to antibiotics

Many bacterial infections are resistant to current antibiotics. It is necessary to identify all infections documented as antibiotic resistant. Assign a code from category Z16, Resistance to antimicrobial drugs, following the infection code only if the infection code does not identify drug resistance.

d. Sepsis, severe sepsis, and septic shock

1) Coding of sepsis and severe sepsis

(a) Sepsis

For a diagnosis of sepsis, assign the appropriate code for the underlying systemic infection. If the type of infection or causal organism is not further specified, assign code A41.9, Sepsis, unspecified organism.

A code from subcategory R65.2, Severe sepsis, should not be assigned unless severe sepsis or an associated acute organ dysfunction is documented.

(i) Negative or inconclusive blood cultures and sepsis

Negative or inconclusive blood cultures do not preclude a diagnosis of sepsis in patients with clinical evidence of the condition; however, the provider should be queried.

(ii) Urosepsis

The term urosepsis is a nonspecific term. It is not to be considered synonymous with sepsis. It has no default code in the Alphabetic Index. Should a provider use this term, he/she must be queried for clarification.

(iii) Sepsis with organ dysfunction

If a patient has sepsis and associated acute organ dysfunction or multiple organ dysfunction (MOD), follow the instructions for coding severe sepsis.

(iv) Acute organ dysfunction that is not clearly associated with the sepsis

If a patient has sepsis and an acute organ dysfunction, but the medical record documentation indicates that the acute organ dysfunction is related to a medical condition other than the sepsis, do not assign a code from subcategory R65.2, Severe sepsis. An acute organ dysfunction must be associated with the sepsis in order to assign the severe sepsis code. If the documentation is not clear as to whether an acute organ dysfunction is related to the sepsis or another medical condition, query the provider.

Sepsis and acute respiratory failure due to COPD exacerbation

A41.9	Sepsis, unspecified organism
J44.1	Chronic obstructive pulmonary disease with (acute) exacerbation
J96.ØØ	Acute respiratory failure, unspecified whether with hypoxia or hypercapnia

Explanation: Although acute organ dysfunction is present in the form of acute respiratory failure, severe sepsis (R65.2) is not coded in this example, as the acute respiratory failure is attributed to the COPD exacerbation rather than the sepsis. Sequencing of these codes would be determined by the circumstances of the admission.

(b) Severe sepsis

The coding of severe sepsis requires a minimum of 2 codes: first a code for the underlying systemic infection, followed by a code from subcategory R65.2, Severe sepsis. If the causal organism is not documented, assign code A41.9, Sepsis, unspecified organism, for the infection. Additional code(s) for the associated acute organ dysfunction are also required.

Due to the complex nature of severe sepsis, some cases may require querying the provider prior to assignment of the codes.

2) Septic shock

(a) Septic shock generally refers to circulatory failure associated with severe sepsis, and therefore, it represents a type of acute organ dysfunction.

For cases of septic shock, the code for the systemic infection should be sequenced first, followed by code R65.21, Severe sepsis with septic shock or code T81.12, Postprocedural septic shock. Any additional codes for the other acute organ dysfunctions should also be assigned. As noted in the sequencing instructions in the Tabular List, the code for septic shock cannot be assigned as a principal diagnosis.

Sepsis with septic shock

A41.9	Sepsis, unspecified organism
R65.21	Severe sepsis with septic shock

Explanation: Documentation of septic shock automatically implies severe sepsis as it is a form of acute organ dysfunction. Septic shock is not coded as the principal diagnosis; it is always preceded by the code for the systemic infection.

3) Sequencing of severe sepsis

If severe sepsis is present on admission, and meets the definition of principal diagnosis, the underlying systemic infection should be assigned as principal diagnosis followed by the appropriate code from subcategory R65.2 as required by the sequencing rules in the Tabular List. A code from subcategory R65.2 can never be assigned as a principal diagnosis. When severe sepsis develops during an encounter (it was not present on admission), the underlying systemic infection and the appropriate code from subcategory R65.2 should be assigned as secondary diagnoses. Severe sepsis may be present on admission, but the diagnosis may not be confirmed until sometime after admission. If the documentation is not clear whether severe sepsis was present on admission, the provider should be queried.

4) Sepsis *or* severe sepsis with a localized infection

If the reason for admission is sepsis or severe sepsis and a localized infection, such as pneumonia or cellulitis, a code(s) for the underlying systemic infection should be assigned first and the code for the localized infection should be assigned as a secondary diagnosis. If the patient has severe sepsis, a code from subcategory R65.2 should also be assigned as a secondary diagnosis. If the patient is admitted with a localized infection, such as pneumonia, and sepsis/severe sepsis doesn't develop until after admission, the localized infection should be assigned first, followed by the appropriate sepsis/severe sepsis codes.

Patient presents with acute renal failure due to severe sepsis from *Pseudomonas* pneumonia

A41.52	Sepsis due to Pseudomonas
J15.1	Pneumonia due to Pseudomonas
R65.2Ø	Severe sepsis without septic shock
N17.9	Acute kidney failure, unspecified

Explanation: If all conditions are present on admission, the systemic infection (sepsis) is sequenced first followed by the codes for the localized infection (pneumonia), severe sepsis and any organ dysfunction. If only the pneumonia was present on admission with the sepsis and resulting renal failure developing later in the admission, then the pneumonia would be sequenced first.

5) Sepsis due to a postprocedural infection

(a) Documentation of causal relationship

As with all postprocedural complications, code assignment is based on the provider's documentation of the relationship between the infection and the procedure.

(b) Sepsis due to a postprocedural infection

For infections following a procedure, a code from T81.4Ø, to T81.43 Infection following a procedure, or a code from O86.ØØ to O86.Ø3, Infection of obstetric surgical wound, that identifies the site of the infection should be coded first, if known. Assign an additional code for sepsis following a procedure (T81.44) or sepsis following an obstetrical procedure (O86.Ø4). Use an additional code to identify the infectious agent. If the patient has severe sepsis, the appropriate code from subcategory R65.2 should also be assigned with the additional code(s) for any acute organ dysfunction.

For infections following infusion, transfusion, therapeutic injection, or immunization, a code from subcategory T80.2, Infections following infusion, transfusion, and therapeutic injection, or code T88.Ø-, Infection following immunization, should be coded first, followed by the code for the specific infection. If the patient has severe sepsis, the appropriate code from subcategory R65.2 should also be assigned, with the additional codes(s) for any acute organ dysfunction.

(c) Postprocedural infection and postprocedural septic shock

If a postprocedural infection has resulted in postprocedural septic shock, assign the codes indicated above for sepsis due to a postprocedural infection, followed by code T81.12-, Postprocedural septic shock. Do not assign code R65.21, Severe sepsis with septic shock. Additional code(s) should be assigned for any acute organ dysfunction.

Septic shock following abdominal procedure with intramuscular abscess	
T81.42XA	**Infection following a procedure, deep incisional surgical site, initial encounter**
T81.44XA	**Sepsis following a procedure, initial encounter**
A41.9	**Sepsis, unspecified organism**
T81.12XA	**Postprocedural septic shock, initial encounter**

Explanation: The first code reported identifies the site of the postprocedural infection with intramuscular abscess coded to "deep incisional surgical site." If sepsis occurred as a result of the postprocedural infection, code T81.44- should be coded as a secondary diagnosis, followed by a code for the specific type of sepsis. Postprocedural septic shock is captured by code T81.12- and not with code R65.21. If any other acute organ dysfunction was documented as associated with the postprocedural sepsis, additional codes could be assigned to represent those conditions.

6) Sepsis and severe sepsis associated with a noninfectious process (condition)

In some cases a noninfectious process (condition), such as trauma, may lead to an infection which can result in sepsis or severe sepsis. If sepsis or severe sepsis is documented as associated with a noninfectious condition, such as a burn or serious injury, and this condition meets the definition for principal diagnosis, the code for the noninfectious condition should be sequenced first, followed by the code for the resulting infection. If severe sepsis is present, a code from subcategory R65.2 should also be assigned with any associated organ dysfunction(s) codes. It is not necessary to assign a code from subcategory R65.1, Systemic inflammatory response syndrome (SIRS) of non-infectious origin, for these cases.

If the infection meets the definition of principal diagnosis, it should be sequenced before the non-infectious condition. When both the associated non-infectious condition and the infection meet the definition of principal diagnosis, either may be assigned as principal diagnosis.

Only one code from category R65, Symptoms and signs specifically associated with systemic inflammation and infection, should be assigned. Therefore, when a non-infectious condition leads to an infection resulting in severe sepsis, assign the appropriate code from subcategory R65.2, Severe sepsis. Do not additionally assign a code from subcategory R65.1, Systemic inflammatory response syndrome (SIRS) of non-infectious origin.

See Section I.C.18. SIRS due to non-infectious process

Patient admitted with multiple third-degree burns of right upper arm develops severe MSSA sepsis with septic shock, three days into admission	
T22.391A	**Burn of third degree of multiple sites of right shoulder and upper arm limb, except wrist and hand, initial encounter**
A41.01	**Sepsis due to Methicillin susceptible Staphylococcus aureus**
R65.21	**Severe sepsis with septic shock**

Explanation: Severe sepsis is coded rather than SIRS from R65 because it is documented as a severe systemic infectious response with septic shock to a noninfectious condition. The code for the systemic infection is not used as the principal diagnosis because it was not present on admission. The patient was admitted for the burn injury.

7) Sepsis and septic shock complicating abortion, pregnancy, childbirth, and the puerperium

See Section I.C.15. Sepsis and septic shock complicating abortion, pregnancy, childbirth and the puerperium

8) Newborn sepsis

See Section I.C.16. f. Bacterial sepsis of Newborn

e. Methicillin resistant Staphylococcus aureus (MRSA) conditions

1) Selection and sequencing of MRSA codes

(a) Combination codes for MRSA infection

When a patient is diagnosed with an infection that is due to methicillin resistant *Staphylococcus aureus* (MRSA), and that infection has a combination code that includes the causal organism (e.g., sepsis, pneumonia) assign the appropriate combination code for the condition (e.g., code A41.02, Sepsis due to Methicillin resistant Staphylococcus aureus or code J15.212, Pneumonia due to Methicillin resistant Staphylococcus aureus). Do not assign code B95.62, Methicillin resistant Staphylococcus aureus infection as the cause of diseases classified elsewhere, as an additional code, because the combination code includes the type of infection and the MRSA organism. Do not assign a code from subcategory Z16.11, Resistance to penicillins, as an additional diagnosis.

See Section C.1. for instructions on coding and sequencing of sepsis and severe sepsis.

(b) Other codes for MRSA infection

When there is documentation of a current infection (e.g., wound infection, stitch abscess, urinary tract infection) due to MRSA, and that infection does not have a combination code that includes the causal organism, assign the appropriate code to identify the condition along with code B95.62, Methicillin resistant Staphylococcus aureus infection as the cause of diseases classified elsewhere for the MRSA infection. Do not assign a code from subcategory Z16.11, Resistance to penicillins.

(c) Methicillin susceptible Staphylococcus aureus (MSSA) and MRSA colonization

The condition or state of being colonized or carrying MSSA or MRSA is called colonization or carriage, while an individual person is described as being colonized or being a carrier. Colonization means that MSSA or MSRA is present on or in the body without necessarily causing illness. A positive MRSA colonization test might be documented by the provider as "MRSA screen positive" or "MRSA nasal swab positive".

Assign code Z22.322, Carrier or suspected carrier of Methicillin resistant Staphylococcus aureus, for patients documented as having MRSA colonization. Assign code Z22.321, Carrier or suspected carrier of Methicillin susceptible Staphylococcus aureus, for patients documented as having MSSA colonization. Colonization is not necessarily indicative of a disease process or as the cause of a specific condition the patient may have unless documented as such by the provider.

(d) MRSA colonization and infection

If a patient is documented as having both MRSA colonization and infection during a hospital admission, code Z22.322, Carrier or suspected carrier of Methicillin resistant Staphylococcus aureus, and a code for the MRSA infection may both be assigned.

f. Zika virus infections

1) Code only confirmed cases

Code only a confirmed diagnosis of Zika virus (A92.5, Zika virus disease) as documented by the provider. This is an exception to the hospital inpatient guideline Section II, H. In this context, "confirmation" does not require documentation of the type of test performed; the **provider's** diagnostic statement that the condition is confirmed is sufficient. This code should be assigned regardless of the stated mode of transmission.

If the provider documents "suspected", "possible" or "probable" Zika, do not assign code A92.5. Assign a code(s) explaining the reason for encounter (such as fever, rash, or joint pain) or Z20.821, Contact with and (suspected) exposure to Zika virus.

A 45-year-old female recently returned from a Caribbean vacation complaining of fever, headache, joint and muscle aches and is admitted for suspected influenza. Infectious Disease consult diagnoses Zika virus. Patient discharged with Zika virus disease and instructions for hydration, rest, acetaminophen, and follow-up with Infectious Disease.	
A92.5	**Zika virus disease**

Explanation: Although only a confirmed diagnosis should be coded, when a provider documents a diagnosis of Zika virus, code A92.5 Zika virus disease, is reported whether or not there is any indication of the type of tests performed. If the patient is pregnant, code first a code from category O98.5- Other viral diseases complicating pregnancy, childbirth and the puerperium, followed by code (A92.5) for the confirmed Zika virus. See also guideline 1.C.15.a.1.

Chapter 1. Certain Infectious and Parasitic Diseases (A00-B99)

INCLUDES diseases generally recognized as communicable or transmissible
Use additional code to identify resistance to antimicrobial drugs (Z16.-)

EXCLUDES 1 certain localized infections — see body system-related chapters

EXCLUDES 2 carrier or suspected carrier of infectious disease (Z22.-)
infectious and parasitic diseases complicating pregnancy, childbirth and the puerperium (O98.-)
infectious and parasitic diseases specific to the perinatal period (P35-P39)
influenza and other acute respiratory infections (J00-J22)

This chapter contains the following blocks:

A00-A09   Intestinal infectious diseases
A15-A19   Tuberculosis
A20-A28   Certain zoonotic bacterial diseases
A30-A49   Other bacterial diseases
A50-A64   Infections with a predominantly sexual mode of transmission
A65-A69   Other spirochetal diseases
A70-A74   Other diseases caused by chlamydiae
A75-A79   Rickettsioses
A80-A89   Viral and prion infections of the central nervous system
A90-A99   Arthropod-borne viral fevers and viral hemorrhagic fevers
B00-B09   Viral infections characterized by skin and mucous membrane lesions
B10   Other human herpesviruses
B15-B19   Viral hepatitis
B20   Human immunodeficiency virus [HIV] disease
B25-B34   Other viral diseases
B35-B49   Mycoses
B50-B64   Protozoal diseases
B65-B83   Helminthiases
B85-B89   Pediculosis, acariasis and other infestations
B90-B94   Sequelae of infectious and parasitic diseases
B95-B97   Bacterial and viral infectious agents
B99   Other infectious diseases

Intestinal infectious diseases (A00-A09)

✓4ᵗʰ A00 Cholera

DEF: Acute infection of the bowel due to vibrio cholerae that presents with profuse diarrhea, cramps, and vomiting, resulting in severe dehydration, electrolyte imbalance, and death. It is spread through ingestion of food or water contaminated with feces of infected persons.
CC Excl: For CC codes in category A00: PDX collection 2

A00.0   Cholera due to Vibrio cholerae 01, biovar cholerae   CC
Classical cholera

A00.1   Cholera due to Vibrio cholerae 01, biovar eltor   CC
Cholera eltor

A00.9   Cholera, unspecified   CC

✓4ᵗʰ A01 Typhoid and paratyphoid fevers

DEF: Typhoid fever: Acute generalized illness caused by *Salmonella typhi*. Clinical features include fever, headache, abdominal pain, cough, toxemia, leukopenia, abnormal pulse, rose spots on the skin, bacteremia, hyperplasia of intestinal lymph nodes, mesenteric lymphadenopathy, and Peyer's patches in the intestines.
DEF: Paratyphoid fever: Prolonged febrile illness, caused by *Salmonella* serotypes other than *S. typhi*, especially *S. enterica* serotypes paratyphi A, B, and C.
CC Excl: For CC codes in category A01: PDX collection 3

✓5ᵗʰ A01.0 Typhoid fever
Infection due to Salmonella typhi

A01.00   Typhoid fever, unspecified   CC

A01.01   Typhoid meningitis   CC

A01.02   Typhoid fever with heart involvement   CC
Typhoid endocarditis
Typhoid myocarditis

A01.03   Typhoid pneumonia   CC HCC

A01.04   Typhoid arthritis   CC HCC

A01.05   Typhoid osteomyelitis   CC HCC

A01.09   Typhoid fever with other complications   CC

A01.1   Paratyphoid fever A   CC

A01.2   Paratyphoid fever B   CC

A01.3   Paratyphoid fever C   CC

A01.4   Paratyphoid fever, unspecified   CC
Infection due to Salmonella paratyphi NOS

✓4ᵗʰ A02 Other salmonella infections

INCLUDES infection or foodborne intoxication due to any Salmonella species other than S. typhi and S. paratyphi

A02.0   Salmonella enteritis   CC
Salmonellosis
TIP: Dehydration (E86.0) is a complication of salmonella enteritis and may be reported separately.
CC Excl: PDX collection 4

A02.1   Salmonella sepsis   HIV MCC HCC
CC Excl: PDX collection 5

✓5ᵗʰ A02.2 Localized salmonella infections

A02.20   Localized salmonella infection, unspecified   HIV

A02.21   Salmonella meningitis   HIV MCC
CC Excl: PDX collection 6

A02.22   Salmonella pneumonia   HIV MCC HCC
CC Excl: PDX collection 7

A02.23   Salmonella arthritis   HIV CC HCC
CC Excl: PDX collection 8

A02.24   Salmonella osteomyelitis   HIV CC HCC
CC Excl: PDX collection 9

A02.25   Salmonella pyelonephritis   HIV CC
Salmonella tubulo-interstitial nephropathy
CC Excl: PDX collection 10

A02.29   Salmonella with other localized infection   HIV CC
CC Excl: PDX collection 10

A02.8   Other specified salmonella infections   HIV CC
CC Excl: PDX collection 11

A02.9   Salmonella infection, unspecified   HIV CC
CC Excl: PDX collection 12

✓4ᵗʰ A03 Shigellosis

DEF: Infection caused by the genus the *Shigella*, of the family *Enterobacteriaceae* that is known to cause an acute dysenteric infection of the bowel with fever, drowsiness, anorexia, nausea, vomiting, bloody diarrhea, abdominal cramps, and distention.

A03.0   Shigellosis due to Shigella dysenteriae   CC
Group A shigellosis [Shiga-Kruse dysentery]
CC Excl: PDX collection 13

A03.1   Shigellosis due to Shigella flexneri
Group B shigellosis

A03.2   Shigellosis due to Shigella boydii
Group C shigellosis

A03.3   Shigellosis due to Shigella sonnei
Group D shigellosis

A03.8   Other shigellosis

A03.9   Shigellosis, unspecified
Bacillary dysentery NOS

✓4ᵗʰ A04 Other bacterial intestinal infections

EXCLUDES 1 bacterial foodborne intoxications, NEC (A05.-)
tuberculous enteritis (A18.32)

DEF: Escherichia coli: Gram negative, anaerobic of the family *Enterobacteriaceae* found in the large intestine of warm-blooded animals, generally as a nonpathologic entity aiding in digestion. They become pathogenic when an opportunity to grow somewhere outside this relationship presents itself, such as ingestion of fecal contaminated food or water.
CC Excl: For CC codes in category A04, unless otherwise noted:
For codes A04.0-A04.4: PDX collection 14
For codes A04.5-A04.8: PDX collection 15

A04.0   Enteropathogenic Escherichia coli infection   CC

A04.1   Enterotoxigenic Escherichia coli infection   CC

A04.2   Enteroinvasive Escherichia coli infection   CC

A04.3   Enterohemorrhagic Escherichia coli infection   CC
DEF: *E. coli* infection penetrating the intestinal mucosa, producing microscopic ulceration and bleeding.

A04.4   Other intestinal Escherichia coli infections   CC
Escherichia coli enteritis NOS

A04.5   Campylobacter enteritis   CC
TIP: For Guillain-Barre syndrome occurring as a sequela of *Campylobacter enteritis*, assign code G61.0 as the first-listed diagnosis followed by B94.8 for the sequelae.

A04.6   Enteritis due to Yersinia enterocolitica   CC
EXCLUDES 1 extraintestinal yersiniosis (A28.2)

✓5ᵗʰ **A04.7 Enterocolitis due to Clostridium difficile**

Foodborne intoxication by Clostridium difficile
Pseudomembraneous colitis
AHA: 2017,4Q,4

     A04.71 Enterocolitis due to Clostridium   CC
              difficile, recurrent

     A04.72 Enterocolitis due to Clostridium   CC
              difficile, not specified as recurrent

A04.8 Other specified bacterial intestinal infections   CC

A04.9 Bacterial intestinal infection, unspecified   CC

Bacterial enteritis NOS
CC Excl: PDX collection 16

✓4ᵗʰ **A05 Other bacterial foodborne intoxications, not elsewhere classified**

   EXCLUDES 1   *Clostridium difficile foodborne intoxication and infection (A04.7-)*
              Escherichia coli infection (A04.0-A04.4)
              listeriosis (A32.-)
              salmonella foodborne intoxication and infection (A02.-)
              toxic effect of noxious foodstuffs (T61-T62)

   CC Excl: For CC codes in category A05, unless ortherwise noted: PDX collection 17

   A05.0 Foodborne staphylococcal intoxication   CC

     TIP: Assign code A04.8 to report a staphylococcal infection when it is caused by the ingestion of contaminated food but not caused by *S. aureus* toxins.

   A05.1 Botulism food poisoning   CC

     Botulism NOS
     Classical foodborne intoxication due to Clostridium botulinum
     EXCLUDES 1   *infant botulism (A48.51)*
              wound botulism (A48.52)
     DEF: Muscle-paralyzing neurotoxic disease caused by ingesting pre-formed toxin from the bacterium *Clostridium botulinum*. It causes vomiting and diarrhea, vision problems, slurred speech, difficulty swallowing, paralysis, and death.
     CC Excl: PDX collection 18

   A05.2 Foodborne Clostridium perfringens   CC
        [Clostridium welchii] intoxication

     Enteritis necroticans
     Pig-bel
     CC Excl: PDX collection 19

   A05.3 Foodborne Vibrio parahaemolyticus   CC
        intoxication

   A05.4 Foodborne Bacillus cereus intoxication   CC

   A05.5 Foodborne Vibrio vulnificus intoxication   CC

   A05.8 Other specified bacterial foodborne   CC
        intoxications

   A05.9 Bacterial foodborne intoxication, unspecified

✓4ᵗʰ **A06 Amebiasis**

   INCLUDES   infection due to Entamoeba histolytica
   EXCLUDES 1   *other protozoal intestinal diseases (A07.-)*
   EXCLUDES 2   *acanthamebiasis (B60.1-)*
              Naegleriasis (B60.2)

   DEF: Infection with a single cell protozoan known as the amoeba. Transmission occurs through ingestion of feces, contaminated food or water, use of human feces as fertilizer, or person-to-person contact.

   A06.0 Acute amebic dysentery   CC

     Acute amebiasis
     Intestinal amebiasis NOS
     CC Excl: PDX collection 20

   A06.1 Chronic intestinal amebiasis   CC
     CC Excl: PDX collection 20

   A06.2 Amebic nondysenteric colitis   CC
     CC Excl: PDX collection 21

   A06.3 Ameboma of intestine   CC
     Ameboma NOS
     CC Excl: PDX collection 22

   A06.4 Amebic liver abscess   MCC
     Hepatic amebiasis
     CC Excl: PDX collection 23

   A06.5 Amebic lung abscess   MCC HCC
     Amebic abscess of lung (and liver)
     CC Excl: PDX collection 24

A06.6 Amebic brain abscess   MCC

Amebic abscess of brain (and liver) (and lung)
CC Excl: PDX collection 25

A06.7 Cutaneous amebiasis

✓5ᵗʰ **A06.8 Amebic infection of other sites**

   CC Excl: For CC codes in subcategory A06.8: PDX collection 22

   A06.81 Amebic cystitis   CC

   A06.82 Other amebic genitourinary   CC
         infections

     Amebic balanitis
     Amebic vesiculitis
     Amebic vulvovaginitis

   A06.89 Other amebic infections   CC
     Amebic appendicitis
     Amebic splenic abscess

A06.9 Amebiasis, unspecified

✓4ᵗʰ **A07 Other protozoal intestinal diseases**

   DEF: Protozoa: Group comprised of the simplest, single celled organisms, ranging in size from micro to macroscopic. They can live alone or in colonies, and do not show any differentiation in tissues. Most are motile and can live free in nature, but some are parasitic, causing disease in the variety of hosts they inhabit.

   CC Excl: For CC codes in category A07, unless otherwise noted: PDX collection 26

   A07.0 Balantidiasis
     Balantidial dysentery

   A07.1 Giardiasis [lambliasis]   CC
     DEF: Infection caused by the flagellate protozoan *Giardia lamblia* causing gastrointestinal problems such as vomiting, chronic diarrhea, and weight loss. The most common parasite in the US, this is usually transmitted by ingesting contaminated water while in the cyst state and latches onto the wall of the small intestine.

   A07.2 Cryptosporidiosis   CC HCC
     DEF: Microscopic parasite found in water and one of the most common causes of waterborne gastrointestinal infectious disease in the United States. It is usually transmitted by ingesting contaminated drinking water or recreational water and causes profuse watery diarrhea, flatulence, abdominal pain, and cramping.

   A07.3 Isosporiasis   HIV CC
     Infection due to Isospora belli and Isospora hominis
     Intestinal coccidiosis
     Isosporosis

   A07.4 Cyclosporiasis   CC
     CC Excl: PDX collection 27

   A07.8 Other specified protozoal intestinal diseases   CC
     Intestinal microsporidiosis
     Intestinal trichomoniasis
     Sarcocystosis
     Sarcosporidiosis

   A07.9 Protozoal intestinal disease, unspecified   CC
     Flagellate diarrhea
     Protozoal colitis
     Protozoal diarrhea
     Protozoal dysentery

✓4ᵗʰ **A08 Viral and other specified intestinal infections**

   EXCLUDES 1   *influenza with involvement of gastrointestinal tract (J09.X3, J10.2, J11.2)*

   CC Excl: For CC codes in category A08: PDX collection 28

   A08.0 Rotaviral enteritis   CC

✓5ᵗʰ **A08.1 Acute gastroenteropathy due to Norwalk agent and other small round viruses**

   A08.11 Acute gastroenteropathy due to   CC
         Norwalk agent
     Acute gastroenteropathy due to Norovirus
     Acute gastroenteropathy due to Norwalk-like agent

   A08.19 Acute gastroenteropathy due to   CC
         other small round viruses
     Acute gastroenteropathy due to small round virus [SRV] NOS

   A08.2 Adenoviral enteritis   CC

✓5ᵗʰ **A08.3 Other viral enteritis**

   A08.31 Calicivirus enteritis   CC

   A08.32 Astrovirus enteritis   CC

✓ Additional Character Required   ✓x7ᵗʰ Placeholder   Unacceptable PDx   Questionable PDx   Manifestation   Unspecified Dx   H1-H14 HAC   HCC CMS-HCC Dx   HIV HIV Dx

ICD-10-CM 2020   437

Chapter 1. Certain Infectious and Parasitic Diseases

A08.39 Other viral enteritis   `CC`
Coxsackie virus enteritis
Echovirus enteritis
Enterovirus enteritis NEC
Torovirus enteritis

A08.4 Viral intestinal infection, unspecified
Viral enteritis NOS
Viral gastroenteritis NOS
Viral gastroenteropathy NOS
AHA: 2016,3Q,12

A08.8 Other specified intestinal infections

A09 Infectious gastroenteritis and colitis, unspecified
Infectious colitis NOS
Infectious enteritis NOS
Infectious gastroenteritis NOS
> *EXCLUDES 1*   colitis NOS (K52.9)
> diarrhea NOS (R19.7)
> enteritis NOS (K52.9)
> gastroenteritis NOS (K52.9)
> noninfective gastroenteritis and colitis, unspecified (K52.9)

DEF: Colitis: Inflammation of mucous membranes of the colon.
DEF: Enteritis: Inflammation of mucous membranes of the small intestine.
DEF: Gastroenteritis: Inflammation of mucous membranes of the stomach and intestines.

Tuberculosis (A15-A19)

INCLUDES   infections due to Mycobacterium tuberculosis and Mycobacterium bovis
EXCLUDES 1   congenital tuberculosis (P37.0)
> nonspecific reaction to test for tuberculosis without active tuberculosis (R76.1-)
> pneumoconiosis associated with tuberculosis, any type in A15 (J65)
> positive PPD (R76.11)
> positive tuberculin skin test without active tuberculosis (R76.11)
> sequelae of tuberculosis (B90.-)
> silicotuberculosis (J65)

DEF: Bacterial infection that typically spreads by inhalation of an airborne agent that usually attacks the lungs, but may also affect other organs.

✓4ᵗʰ A15 Respiratory tuberculosis
> **CC Excl:** For CC codes in category A15, unless otherwise noted: PDX collection 29

A15.0 Tuberculosis of lung   `HIV` `CC`
Tuberculous bronchiectasis
Tuberculous fibrosis of lung
Tuberculous pneumonia
Tuberculous pneumothorax

Tuberculosis of Lung

Granulomas from Mycobacterium tuberculosis

A15.4 Tuberculosis of intrathoracic lymph nodes   `HIV` `CC`
Tuberculosis of hilar lymph nodes
Tuberculosis of mediastinal lymph nodes
Tuberculosis of tracheobronchial lymph nodes
> *EXCLUDES 1*   tuberculosis specified as primary (A15.7)

A15.5 Tuberculosis of larynx, trachea and bronchus   `HIV` `CC`
Tuberculosis of bronchus
Tuberculosis of glottis
Tuberculosis of larynx
Tuberculosis of trachea

A15.6 Tuberculous pleurisy   `HIV` `CC`
Tuberculosis of pleura Tuberculous empyema
> *EXCLUDES 1*   primary respiratory tuberculosis (A15.7)

A15.7 Primary respiratory tuberculosis   `HIV` `CC`
> **CC Excl:** PDX collection 30

A15.8 Other respiratory tuberculosis   `HIV` `CC`
Mediastinal tuberculosis
Nasopharyngeal tuberculosis
Tuberculosis of nose
Tuberculosis of sinus [any nasal]
> **CC Excl:** PDX collection 31

A15.9 Respiratory tuberculosis unspecified   `HIV` `CC`
> **CC Excl:** PDX collection 31

✓4ᵗʰ A17 Tuberculosis of nervous system

A17.0 Tuberculous meningitis   `HIV` `MCC`
Tuberculosis of meninges (cerebral)(spinal)
Tuberculous leptomeningitis
> *EXCLUDES 1*   tuberculous meningoencephalitis (A17.82)
> **CC Excl:** PDX collection 32

A17.1 Meningeal tuberculoma   `HIV` `MCC`
Tuberculoma of meninges (cerebral) (spinal)
> *EXCLUDES 2*   tuberculoma of brain and spinal cord (A17.81)
> **CC Excl:** PDX collection 32

✓5ᵗʰ A17.8 Other tuberculosis of nervous system

A17.81 Tuberculoma of brain and spinal cord   `HIV` `MCC`
Tuberculous abscess of brain and spinal cord
> **CC Excl:** PDX collection 33

A17.82 Tuberculous meningoencephalitis   `HIV` `MCC`
Tuberculous myelitis
> **CC Excl:** PDX collection 33

A17.83 Tuberculous neuritis   `HIV` `MCC`
Tuberculous mononeuropathy
> **CC Excl:** No Excl

A17.89 Other tuberculosis of nervous system   `HIV` `MCC`
Tuberculous polyneuropathy
> **CC Excl:** PDX collection 34

A17.9 Tuberculosis of nervous system, unspecified   `HIV` `CC`
> **CC Excl:** PDX collection 35

✓4ᵗʰ A18 Tuberculosis of other organs

✓5ᵗʰ A18.0 Tuberculosis of bones and joints

A18.01 Tuberculosis of spine   `HIV` `CC`
Pott's disease or curvature of spine
Tuberculous arthritis
Tuberculous osteomyelitis of spine
Tuberculous spondylitis
> **CC Excl:** PDX collection 36

A18.02 Tuberculous arthritis of other joints   `HIV` `CC`
Tuberculosis of hip (joint)
Tuberculosis of knee (joint)
> **CC Excl:** PDX collection 37

A18.03 Tuberculosis of other bones   `HIV` `CC`
Tuberculous mastoiditis
Tuberculous osteomyelitis
> **CC Excl:** PDX collection 38

A18.09 Other musculoskeletal tuberculosis   `HIV` `CC`
Tuberculous myositis
Tuberculous synovitis
Tuberculous tenosynovitis
> **CC Excl:** PDX collection 39

✓5ᵗʰ A18.1 Tuberculosis of genitourinary system

A18.10 Tuberculosis of genitourinary system, unspecified   `HIV` `CC`
> **CC Excl:** PDX collection 40

A18.11 Tuberculosis of kidney and ureter   `HIV` `CC`
> **CC Excl:** PDX collection 41

A18.12 Tuberculosis of bladder   `HIV` `CC`
     CC Excl: PDX collection 41

A18.13 Tuberculosis of other urinary organs   `HIV` `CC`
     Tuberculous urethritis
     CC Excl: PDX collection 41

A18.14 Tuberculosis of prostate   `HIV` `CC` `A` `♂`
     CC Excl: PDX collection 42

A18.15 Tuberculosis of other male genital organs   `HIV` `CC` `♂`
     CC Excl: PDX collection 42

A18.16 Tuberculosis of cervix   `HIV` `CC` `♀`
     CC Excl: PDX collection 43

A18.17 Tuberculous female pelvic inflammatory disease   `HIV` `CC` `♀`
     Tuberculous endometritis
     Tuberculous oophoritis and salpingitis
     CC Excl: PDX collection 43

A18.18 Tuberculosis of other female genital organs   `HIV` `CC` `♀`
     Tuberculous ulceration of vulva
     CC Excl: PDX collection 43

A18.2 Tuberculous peripheral lymphadenopathy   `HIV` `CC`
     Tuberculous adenitis
     EXCLUDES 2   *tuberculosis of bronchial and mediastinal lymph nodes (A15.4)*
         tuberculosis of mesenteric and retroperitoneal lymph nodes (A18.39)
         tuberculous tracheobronchial adenopathy (A15.4)
     CC Excl: PDX collection 44

√5ᵗʰ **A18.3 Tuberculosis of intestines, peritoneum and mesenteric glands**
     CC Excl: For CC/MCC codes in subcategory A18.3: PDX collection 45

A18.31 Tuberculous peritonitis   `HIV` `MCC`
     Tuberculous ascites
     DEF: Tuberculous inflammation of the membrane lining the abdomen.

A18.32 Tuberculous enteritis   `HIV` `CC`
     Tuberculosis of anus and rectum
     Tuberculosis of intestine (large) (small)

A18.39 Retroperitoneal tuberculosis   `HIV` `CC`
     Tuberculosis of mesenteric glands
     Tuberculosis of retroperitoneal (lymph glands)

A18.4 Tuberculosis of skin and subcutaneous tissue   `HIV` `CC`
     Erythema induratum, tuberculous
     Lupus excedens
     Lupus vulgaris NOS
     Lupus vulgaris of eyelid
     Scrofuloderma
     Tuberculosis of external ear
     EXCLUDES 2   *lupus erythematosus (L93.-)*
         lupus NOS (M32.9)
         ▶*systemic lupus erythematosus*◀ *(M32.-)*
     CC Excl: PDX collection 30

√5ᵗʰ **A18.5 Tuberculosis of eye**
     EXCLUDES 2   *lupus vulgaris of eyelid (A18.4)*
     CC Excl: For CC codes in subcategory A18.5: PDX collection 46

A18.50 Tuberculosis of eye, unspecified   `HIV` `CC`

A18.51 Tuberculous episcleritis   `HIV` `CC`

A18.52 Tuberculous keratitis   `HIV` `CC`
     Tuberculous interstitial keratitis
     Tuberculous keratoconjunctivitis (interstitial) (phlyctenular)

A18.53 Tuberculous chorioretinitis   `HIV` `CC`

A18.54 Tuberculous iridocyclitis   `HIV` `CC`

A18.59 Other tuberculosis of eye   `HIV` `CC`
     Tuberculous conjunctivitis

A18.6 Tuberculosis of (inner) (middle) ear   `HIV` `CC`
     Tuberculous otitis media
     EXCLUDES 2   *tuberculosis of external ear (A18.4)*
         tuberculous mastoiditis (A18.03)
     CC Excl: PDX collection 47

A18.7 Tuberculosis of adrenal glands   `HIV` `CC`
     Tuberculous Addison's disease
     CC Excl: PDX collection 48

√5ᵗʰ **A18.8 Tuberculosis of other** specified organs

A18.81 Tuberculosis of thyroid gland   `HIV` `CC`
     CC Excl: PDX collection 49

A18.82 Tuberculosis of other endocrine glands   `HIV` `CC`
     Tuberculosis of pituitary gland
     Tuberculosis of thymus gland
     CC Excl: PDX collection 35

A18.83 Tuberculosis of digestive tract organs, **not elsewhere classified**   `HIV` `CC`
     EXCLUDES 1   *tuberculosis of intestine (A18.32)*
     CC Excl: PDX collection 45

A18.84 Tuberculosis of heart   `HIV` `CC`
     Tuberculous cardiomyopathy
     Tuberculous endocarditis
     Tuberculous myocarditis
     Tuberculous pericarditis
     CC Excl: PDX collection 35

A18.85 Tuberculosis of spleen   `HIV` `CC`
     CC Excl: PDX collection 50

A18.89 Tuberculosis of other sites   `HIV` `CC`
     Tuberculosis of muscle
     Tuberculous cerebral arteritis
     CC Excl: PDX collection 35

√4ᵗʰ **A19 Miliary tuberculosis**
     `INCLUDES`   disseminated tuberculosis
         generalized tuberculosis
         tuberculous polyserositis
     CC Excl: For MCC codes in category A19: PDX collection 51

A19.0 Acute miliary tuberculosis of a single specified site   `HIV` `MCC`

A19.1 Acute miliary tuberculosis of multiple sites   `HIV` `MCC`

A19.2 Acute miliary tuberculosis, unspecified   `HIV` `MCC`

A19.8 Other miliary tuberculosis   `HIV` `MCC`

A19.9 Miliary tuberculosis, unspecified   `HIV` `MCC`

Certain zoonotic bacterial diseases (A20-A28)

√4ᵗʰ **A20 Plague**
     `INCLUDES`   infection due to Yersinia pestis

A20.0 Bubonic plague   `MCC`
     CC Excl: PDX collection 52

A20.1 Cellulocutaneous plague   `MCC`
     CC Excl: PDX collection 52

A20.2 Pneumonic plague   `MCC` `HCC`
     CC Excl: PDX collection 53

A20.3 Plague meningitis   `MCC`
     CC Excl: PDX collection 54

A20.7 Septicemic plague   `MCC` `HCC`
     CC Excl: PDX collection 55

A20.8 Other forms of plague   `MCC`
     Abortive plague
     Asymptomatic plague
     Pestis minor
     CC Excl: PDX collection 54

A20.9 Plague, unspecified   `MCC`
     CC Excl: PDX collection 56

√4ᵗʰ **A21 Tularemia**
     `INCLUDES`   deer-fly fever
         infection due to Francisella tularensis
         rabbit fever
     DEF: Febrile disease transmitted to humans by the bites of deer flies, fleas, and ticks, by inhaling aerosolized *F. tularensis*, or by ingesting contaminated food or water. Patients quickly develop fever, chills, weakness, headache, backache, and malaise.

A21.0 Ulceroglandular tularemia   `CC`
     CC Excl: PDX collection 57

A21.1 Oculoglandular tularemia   `CC`
     Ophthalmic tularemia
     CC Excl: PDX collection 58

✔ Additional Character Required   √x7ᵗʰ Placeholder   Unacceptable PDx   Questionable PDx   Manifestation   Unspecified Dx   `H1`-`H4` HAC   `HCC` CMS-HCC Dx   `HIV` HIV Dx

ICD-10-CM 2020   **439**

A21.2 Pulmonary tularemia `CC` `HCC`
CC Excl: PDX collection 59

A21.3 Gastrointestinal tularemia `CC`
Abdominal tularemia
CC Excl: PDX collection 60

A21.7 Generalized tularemia `CC`
CC Excl: PDX collection 61

A21.8 Other forms of tularemia `CC`
CC Excl: PDX collection 61

A21.9 Tularemia, unspecified `CC`
CC Excl: PDX collection 61

✓4ᵗʰ A22 Anthrax
`INCLUDES` infection due to Bacillus anthracis

A22.0 Cutaneous anthrax `CC`
Malignant carbuncle
Malignant pustule
CC Excl: PDX collection 62

A22.1 Pulmonary anthrax `MCC` `HCC`
Inhalation anthrax
Ragpicker's disease
Woolsorter's disease
CC Excl: PDX collection 63

A22.2 Gastrointestinal anthrax `CC`
CC Excl: PDX collection 64

A22.7 Anthrax sepsis `MCC` `HCC`
CC Excl: PDX collection 5

A22.8 Other forms of anthrax `CC`
Anthrax meningitis
CC Excl: PDX collection 65

A22.9 Anthrax, unspecified `CC`
CC Excl: PDX collection 66

✓4ᵗʰ A23 Brucellosis
`INCLUDES` Malta fever
Mediterranean fever
undulant fever

A23.0 Brucellosis due to Brucella melitensis
A23.1 Brucellosis due to Brucella abortus
A23.2 Brucellosis due to Brucella suis
A23.3 Brucellosis due to Brucella canis
A23.8 Other brucellosis `CC`
CC Excl: PDX collection 67
A23.9 Brucellosis, unspecified `CC`
CC Excl: PDX collection 67

✓4ᵗʰ A24 Glanders and melioidosis
CC Excl: For CC codes in category A24, unless otherwise noted: PDX collection 69

A24.0 Glanders `CC`
Infection due to Pseudomonas mallei
Malleus
CC Excl: PDX collection 68

A24.1 Acute and fulminating melioidosis `CC`
Melioidosis pneumonia
Melioidosis sepsis

A24.2 Subacute and chronic melioidosis `CC`
A24.3 Other melioidosis `CC`
A24.9 Melioidosis, unspecified `CC`
Infection due to Pseudomonas pseudomallei NOS
Whitmore's disease

✓4ᵗʰ A25 Rat-bite fevers
CC Excl: For CC codes in category A25: PDX collection 70

A25.0 Spirillosis `CC`
Sodoku

A25.1 Streptobacillosis `CC`
Epidemic arthritic erythema
Haverhill fever
Streptobacillary rat-bite fever

A25.9 Rat-bite fever, unspecified `CC`

✓4ᵗʰ A26 Erysipeloid
DEF: Acute cutaneous infection typically caused by trauma to the skin. Presenting as cellulitis, it may become systemic affecting other organs. It is gram positive bacillus and mainly acquired by those who routinely handle meat.

A26.0 Cutaneous erysipeloid
Erythema migrans

A26.7 Erysipelothrix sepsis `MCC` `HCC`
CC Excl: PDX collection 71

A26.8 Other forms of erysipeloid
A26.9 Erysipeloid, unspecified

✓4ᵗʰ A27 Leptospirosis
CC Excl: For CC codes in category A27: PDX collection 72

A27.0 Leptospirosis icterohemorrhagica `CC`
Leptospiral or spirochetal jaundice (hemorrhagic)
Weil's disease

✓5ᵗʰ A27.8 Other forms of leptospirosis
A27.81 Aseptic meningitis in leptospirosis `MCC`
CC Excl: PDX collection 73
A27.89 Other forms of leptospirosis `CC`
A27.9 Leptospirosis, unspecified `CC`

✓4ᵗʰ A28 Other zoonotic bacterial diseases, not elsewhere classified
CC Excl: For CC codes in category A28, unless otherwise noted: PDX collection 74

A28.0 Pasteurellosis `CC`
A28.1 Cat-scratch disease `CC`
Cat-scratch fever
CC Excl: PDX collection 75
A28.2 Extraintestinal yersiniosis `CC`
`EXCLUDES 1` enteritis due to Yersinia enterocolitica (A04.6)
plague (A20.-)
A28.8 Other specified zoonotic bacterial diseases, not elsewhere classified `CC`
A28.9 Zoonotic bacterial disease, unspecified `CC`

Other bacterial diseases (A30-A49)

AHA: 2016,3Q,8-14

✓4ᵗʰ A30 Leprosy [Hansen's disease]
`INCLUDES` infection due to Mycobacterium leprae
`EXCLUDES 1` sequelae of leprosy (B92)

A30.0 Indeterminate leprosy `CC`
I leprosy
CC Excl: PDX collection 76

A30.1 Tuberculoid leprosy `CC`
TT leprosy
CC Excl: PDX collection 77

A30.2 Borderline tuberculoid leprosy `CC`
BT leprosy
CC Excl: PDX collection 78

A30.3 Borderline leprosy `CC`
BB leprosy
CC Excl: PDX collection 78

A30.4 Borderline lepromatous leprosy `CC`
BL leprosy
CC Excl: PDX collection 78

A30.5 Lepromatous leprosy `CC`
LL leprosy
CC Excl: PDX collection 79

A30.8 Other forms of leprosy `CC`
CC Excl: PDX collection 80

A30.9 Leprosy, unspecified `CC`
CC Excl: PDX collection 81

Chapter 1. Certain Infectious and Parasitic Diseases

✓4ᵗʰ **A31 Infection due to other mycobacteria**

    EXCLUDES 2   leprosy (A30.-)

                 tuberculosis (A15-A19)

    CC Excl: For CC codes in category A31, unless otherwise noted: PDX collection 83

    A31.0 Pulmonary mycobacterial infection   `CC` `HCC`

         Infection due to Mycobacterium avium

         Infection due to Mycobacterium intracellulare [Battey bacillus]

         Infection due to Mycobacterium kansasii

         CC Excl: PDX collection 82

    A31.1 Cutaneous mycobacterial infection   `CC`

         Buruli ulcer

         Infection due to Mycobacterium marinum

         Infection due to Mycobacterium ulcerans

    A31.2 Disseminated mycobacterium avium-intracellulare complex (DMAC)   `HIV` `CC` `HCC`

         MAC sepsis

    A31.8 Other mycobacterial infections   `HIV` `CC`

    A31.9 Mycobacterial infection, unspecified   `HIV` `CC`

         Atypical mycobacterial infection NOS

         Mycobacteriosis NOS

✓4ᵗʰ **A32 Listeriosis**

    INCLUDES   listerial foodborne infection

    EXCLUDES 1   neonatal (disseminated) listeriosis (P37.2)

    CC Excl: For CC codes in category A32: PDX collection 74

    A32.0 Cutaneous listeriosis   `CC`

✓5ᵗʰ   **A32.1 Listerial meningitis and meningoencephalitis**

         A32.11 Listerial meningitis   `CC`

         A32.12 Listerial meningoencephalitis   `CC`

    A32.7 Listerial sepsis   `MCC` `HCC`

         CC Excl: PDX collection 71

✓5ᵗʰ   **A32.8 Other forms of listeriosis**

         A32.81 Oculoglandular listeriosis   `CC`

         A32.82 Listerial endocarditis   `CC`

         A32.89 Other forms of listeriosis   `CC`

                 Listerial cerebral arteritis

    A32.9 Listeriosis, unspecified   `CC`

A33 Tetanus neonatorum   `MCC` `N`

    CC Excl: PDX collection 84

A34 Obstetrical tetanus   `CC` `M` ♀

    CC Excl: PDX collection 85

A35 Other tetanus   `MCC`

     Tetanus NOS

    EXCLUDES 1   obstetrical tetanus (A34)

                 tetanus neonatorum (A33)

    DEF: Tetanus: Acute, often fatal, infectious disease caused by the anaerobic, spore-forming bacillus *Clostridium tetani*. The bacillus enters the body through a contaminated wound, burns, surgical wounds, or cutaneous ulcers. Symptoms include lockjaw, spasms, seizures, and paralysis.

    CC Excl: PDX collection 86

✓4ᵗʰ **A36 Diphtheria**

    CC Excl: For CC codes in category A36, unless otherwise noted: PDX collection 87

    A36.0 Pharyngeal diphtheria   `CC`

         Diphtheritic membranous angina

         Tonsillar diphtheria

    A36.1 Nasopharyngeal diphtheria   `CC`

    A36.2 Laryngeal diphtheria   `CC`

         Diphtheritic laryngotracheitis

    A36.3 Cutaneous diphtheria   `CC`

         EXCLUDES 2   erythrasma (L08.1)

✓5ᵗʰ   **A36.8 Other diphtheria**

         A36.81 Diphtheritic cardiomyopathy   `CC` `HCC`

                 Diphtheritic myocarditis

                 CC Excl: PDX collection 88

         A36.82 Diphtheritic radiculomyelitis   `CC`

         A36.83 Diphtheritic polyneuritis   `CC`

         A36.84 Diphtheritic tubulo-interstitial nephropathy   `CC`

         A36.85 Diphtheritic cystitis   `CC`

         A36.86 Diphtheritic conjunctivitis   `CC`

         A36.89 Other diphtheritic complications   `CC`

                 Diphtheritic peritonitis

    A36.9 Diphtheria, unspecified   `CC`

✓4ᵗʰ **A37 Whooping cough**

    DEF: Acute, highly contagious respiratory tract infection caused by *Bordetella pertussis* and *B. bronchiseptica*. Whooping cough is known by its characteristic paroxysmal cough.

    CC Excl: For codes in category A37:

    For MCC codes: PDX collection 90

    For CC codes: PDX collection 89

✓5ᵗʰ   **A37.0 Whooping cough due to Bordetella pertussis**

         A37.00 Whooping cough due to Bordetella pertussis without pneumonia   `CC`

         A37.01 Whooping cough due to Bordetella pertussis with pneumonia   `MCC`

✓5ᵗʰ   **A37.1 Whooping cough due to Bordetella parapertussis**

         A37.10 Whooping cough due to Bordetella parapertussis without pneumonia   `CC`

         A37.11 Whooping cough due to Bordetella parapertussis with pneumonia   `MCC`

✓5ᵗʰ   **A37.8 Whooping cough due to other Bordetella species**

         A37.80 Whooping cough due to other Bordetella species without pneumonia   `CC`

         A37.81 Whooping cough due to other Bordetella species with pneumonia   `MCC`

✓5ᵗʰ   **A37.9 Whooping cough, unspecified species**

         A37.90 Whooping cough, unspecified species without pneumonia   `CC`

         A37.91 Whooping cough, unspecified species with pneumonia   `MCC`

✓4ᵗʰ **A38 Scarlet fever**

    INCLUDES   scarlatina

    EXCLUDES 2   streptococcal sore throat (J02.0)

    DEF: Acute contagious disease caused by Group A bacteria, the same bacterium that causes strep throat. Individuals with strep throat can develop scarlet fever particularly if the infection is not treated with antibiotics. It is characterized by a red blush to the skin of the chest and abdomen and swelling of the nose, throat, and mouth.

    CC Excl: For CC codes in category A38: PDX collection 91

    A38.0 Scarlet fever with otitis media   `CC`

    A38.1 Scarlet fever with myocarditis   `CC`

    A38.8 Scarlet fever with other complications   `CC`

    A38.9 Scarlet fever, uncomplicated   `CC`

         Scarlet fever, NOS

✓4ᵗʰ **A39 Meningococcal infection**

    DEF: Condition caused by *Neisseria meningitidis*, a bacteria that may invade the spinal cord, brain, heart, joints, optic nerve, or bloodstream.

    A39.0 Meningococcal meningitis   `MCC`

         CC Excl: PDX collection 92

    A39.1 Waterhouse-Friderichsen syndrome   `MCC` `HCC`

         Meningococcal hemorrhagic adrenalitis

         Meningococcic adrenal syndrome

         CC Excl: PDX collection 93

    A39.2 Acute meningococcemia   `MCC` `HCC`

         CC Excl: PDX collection 94

    A39.3 Chronic meningococcemia   `MCC` `HCC`

         CC Excl: PDX collection 94

    A39.4 Meningococcemia, unspecified   `MCC` `HCC`

         CC Excl: PDX collection 94

✓5ᵗʰ   **A39.5 Meningococcal heart disease**

         A39.50 Meningococcal carditis, unspecified   `MCC`

                 CC Excl: PDX collection 95

         A39.51 Meningococcal endocarditis   `MCC`

                 CC Excl: PDX collection 96

         A39.52 Meningococcal myocarditis   `MCC`

                 CC Excl: PDX collection 97

         A39.53 Meningococcal pericarditis   `MCC`

                 CC Excl: PDX collection 98

☑ Additional Character Required   ✓x7ᵗʰ Placeholder   Unacceptable PDx   Questionable PDx   Manifestation   Unspecified Dx   `H1`-`H14` HAC   `HCC` CMS-HCC Dx   `HIV` HIV Dx

ICD-10-CM 2020   441

✓5ᵗʰ A39.8   Other meningococcal infections

     A39.81   Meningococcal encephalitis `MCC`

         CC Excl: PDX collection 99

     A39.82   Meningococcal retrobulbar neuritis `CC`

         CC Excl: PDX collection 100

     A39.83   Meningococcal arthritis `CC` `HCC`

         CC Excl: PDX collection 101

     A39.84   Postmeningococcal arthritis `CC` `HCC`

         CC Excl: PDX collection 101

     A39.89   Other meningococcal infections `CC`

         Meningococcal conjunctivitis

         CC Excl: PDX collection 102

A39.9   Meningococcal infection, unspecified `CC`

     Meningococcal disease NOS

     CC Excl: PDX collection 102

✓4ᵗʰ A40   Streptococcal sepsis

     Code first:

     postprocedural streptococcal sepsis (T81.4-)

     streptococcal sepsis during labor (O75.3)

     streptococcal sepsis following abortion or ectopic or molar pregnancy (O03-O07, O08.0)

     streptococcal sepsis following immunization (T88.0)

     streptococcal sepsis following infusion, transfusion or therapeutic injection (T80.2-)

     EXCLUDES 1   *neonatal (P36.0-P36.1)*

         puerperal sepsis (O85)

         sepsis due to Streptococcus, group D (A41.81)

     AHA: 2018,4Q,89; 2018,1Q,16; 2016,1Q,32

     CC Excl: For MCC codes in category A40, unless otherwise noted: PDX collection 71

     A40.0   Sepsis due to streptococcus, group A `MCC` `HCC`

     A40.1   Sepsis due to streptococcus, group B `MCC` `HCC`

         AHA: 2019,1Q,14

     A40.3   Sepsis due to Streptococcus pneumoniae `MCC` `HCC`

         Pneumococcal sepsis

         CC Excl: No Excl

     A40.8   Other streptococcal sepsis `MCC` `HCC`

     A40.9   Streptococcal sepsis, unspecified `HIV` `MCC` `HCC`

✓4ᵗʰ A41   Other sepsis

     Code first:

     postprocedural sepsis (T81.4-)

     sepsis during labor (O75.3)

     sepsis following abortion, ectopic or molar pregnancy (O03-O07, O08.0)

     sepsis following immunization (T88.0)

     sepsis following infusion, transfusion or therapeutic injection (T80.2-)

     EXCLUDES 1   *bacteremia NOS (R78.81)*

         neonatal (P36.-)

         puerperal sepsis (O85)

         streptococcal sepsis (A40.-)

     EXCLUDES 2   *sepsis (due to) (in) actinomycotic (A42.7)*

         sepsis (due to) (in) anthrax (A22.7)

         sepsis (due to) (in) candidal (B37.7)

         sepsis (due to) (in) Erysipelothrix (A26.7)

         sepsis (due to) (in) extraintestinal yersiniosis (A28.2)

         sepsis (due to) (in) gonococcal (A54.86)

         sepsis (due to) (in) herpesviral (B00.7)

         sepsis (due to) (in) listerial (A32.7)

         sepsis (due to) (in) melioidosis (A24.1)

         sepsis (due to) (in) meningococcal (A39.2-A39.4)

         sepsis (due to) (in) plague (A20.7)

         sepsis (due to) (in) tularemia (A21.7)

         toxic shock syndrome (A48.3)

     AHA: 2018,4Q,18; 2018,1Q,16; 2016,1Q,32; 2014,2Q,13

     CC Excl: For MCC codes in category A41: PDX collection 71

     ✓5ᵗʰ A41.0   Sepsis due to Staphylococcus aureus

         A41.01   Sepsis due to Methicillin susceptible Staphylococcus aureus `HIV` `MCC` `HCC`

             MSSA sepsis

             Staphylococcus aureus sepsis NOS

         A41.02   Sepsis due to Methicillin resistant Staphylococcus aureus `HIV` `MCC` `HCC`

     A41.1   Sepsis due to other specified staphylococcus `HIV` `MCC` `HCC`

         Coagulase negative staphylococcus sepsis

     A41.2   Sepsis due to unspecified staphylococcus `HIV` `MCC` `HCC`

     A41.3   Sepsis due to Hemophilus influenzae `HIV` `MCC` `HCC`

     A41.4   Sepsis due to anaerobes `HIV` `MCC` `HCC`

         EXCLUDES 1   *gas gangrene (A48.0)*

     ✓5ᵗʰ A41.5   Sepsis due to other Gram-negative organisms

         A41.50   Gram-negative sepsis, unspecified `HIV` `MCC` `HCC`

             Gram-negative sepsis NOS

         A41.51   Sepsis due to Escherichia coli [E. coli] `HIV` `MCC` `HCC`

         A41.52   Sepsis due to Pseudomonas `HIV` `MCC` `HCC`

             Pseudomonas aeroginosa

         A41.53   Sepsis due to Serratia `HIV` `MCC` `HCC`

         A41.59   Other Gram-negative sepsis `HIV` `MCC` `HCC`

     ✓5ᵗʰ A41.8   Other specified sepsis

         A41.81   Sepsis due to Enterococcus `HIV` `MCC` `HCC`

             TIP: *E. faecium,* is a species of *Enterococcus* that is highly resistant to multiple antibiotics. Assign a code from category Z16 when resistance to antimicrobial drugs is documented.

         A41.89   Other specified sepsis `HIV` `MCC` `HCC`

             AHA: 2017,1Q,51; 2016,3Q,8-14

             TIP: Viral sepsis is coded here; assign an additional code to identify the specific viral agent or illness.

     A41.9   Sepsis, unspecified organism `HIV` `MCC` `HCC`

         Septicemia NOS

✓4ᵗʰ A42   Actinomycosis

     EXCLUDES 1   *actinomycetoma (B47.1)*

     A42.0   Pulmonary actinomycosis `HIV` `CC` `HCC`

         CC Excl: PDX collection 103

     A42.1   Abdominal actinomycosis `HIV` `CC`

         CC Excl: PDX collection 104

     A42.2   Cervicofacial actinomycosis `HIV` `CC`

         CC Excl: PDX collection 105

     A42.7   Actinomycotic sepsis `HIV` `MCC` `HCC`

         CC Excl: PDX collection 71

     ✓5ᵗʰ A42.8   Other forms of actinomycosis

         CC Excl: For CC codes in subcategory A42.8: PDX collection 106

         A42.81   Actinomycotic meningitis `HIV` `CC`

         A42.82   Actinomycotic encephalitis `HIV` `CC`

         A42.89   Other forms of actinomycosis `HIV` `CC`

     A42.9   Actinomycosis, unspecified `HIV` `CC`

         CC Excl: PDX collection 106

✓4ᵗʰ A43   Nocardiosis

     DEF: Rare bacterial infection occurring most often in those with weakened immune systems. Can be acquired in soil, decaying plants, or standing water. It typically begins in the lungs and has a tendency to spread to other body systems.

     A43.0   Pulmonary nocardiosis `HIV` `CC` `HCC`

         CC Excl: PDX collection 103

     A43.1   Cutaneous nocardiosis `HIV` `CC`

         CC Excl: PDX collection 107

     A43.8   Other forms of nocardiosis `HIV` `CC`

         CC Excl: PDX collection 106

     A43.9   Nocardiosis, unspecified `HIV` `CC`

         CC Excl: PDX collection 106

✓4ᵗʰ A44   Bartonellosis

     CC Excl: For CC codes in category A44: PDX collection 108

     A44.0   Systemic bartonellosis `CC`

         Oroya fever

     A44.1   Cutaneous and mucocutaneous bartonellosis `CC`

         Verruga peruana

     A44.8   Other forms of bartonellosis `CC`

     A44.9   Bartonellosis, unspecified `CC`

A46   Erysipelas

     EXCLUDES 1   *postpartum or puerperal erysipelas (O86.89)*

     DEF: Skin infection affecting the upper dermis and superficial dermal lymphatics. Lesion edges are well-demarcated with distinct raised borders. It is often caused by group A *Streptococci.*

N Newborn: 0   P Pediatric: 0-17   M Maternity: 9-64   A Adult: 15-124   MCC Major Complication/Comorbidity   CC Complication/Comorbidity   SW Severe Wound Dx

442   ICD-10-CM 2020

Chapter 1. Certain Infectious and Parasitic Diseases

✓4ᵗʰ A48 Other bacterial diseases, not elsewhere classified

> EXCLUDES 1   *actinomycetoma (B47.1)*

A48.0 Gas gangrene   MCC HCC
> Clostridial cellulitis
> Clostridial myonecrosis
> **AHA:** 2017,4Q,102
> **CC Excl:** PDX collection 109

A48.1 Legionnaires' disease   HIV MCC HCC
> **DEF:** Severe and often fatal infection by *Legionella pneumophila*. Symptoms include high fever, gastrointestinal pain, headache, myalgia, dry cough, and pneumonia and it is usually transmitted through airborne water droplets via air conditioning systems or hot tubs.
> **CC Excl:** PDX collection 110

A48.2 Nonpneumonic Legionnaires' disease [Pontiac fever]

A48.3 Toxic shock syndrome   MCC HCC
> Use additional code to identify the organism (B95, B96)
> EXCLUDES 1   *endotoxic shock NOS (R57.8)*
>   *sepsis NOS (A41.9)*
> **DEF:** Bacteria producing an endotoxin, such as *Staphylococci*, flood the body with the toxins producing a high fever, vomiting and diarrhea, decreasing blood pressure, a skin rash, and shock.
> **Synonym(s):** *TSS.*
> **CC Excl:** PDX collection 111

A48.4 Brazilian purpuric fever
> Systemic Hemophilus aegyptius infection

✓5ᵗʰ A48.5 Other specified botulism
> Non-foodborne intoxication due to toxins of Clostridium botulinum [C. botulinum]
> EXCLUDES 1   *food poisoning due to toxins of Clostridium botulinum (A05.1)*

A48.51 Infant botulism   CC P
> **CC Excl:** PDX collection 18

A48.52 Wound botulism   CC
> Non-foodborne botulism NOS
> Use additional code for associated wound
> **CC Excl:** PDX collection 18

A48.8 Other specified bacterial diseases

✓4ᵗʰ A49 Bacterial infection of unspecified site

> EXCLUDES 1   *bacterial agents as the cause of diseases classified elsewhere (B95-B96)*
>   *chlamydial infection NOS (A74.9)*
>   *meningococcal infection NOS (A39.9)*
>   *rickettsial infection NOS (A79.9)*
>   *spirochetal infection NOS (A69.9)*

✓5ᵗʰ A49.0 Staphylococcal infection, unspecified site

A49.01 Methicillin susceptible Staphylococcus aureus infection, unspecified site
> Methicillin susceptible Staphylococcus aureus (MSSA) infection
> Staphylococcus aureus infection NOS

A49.02 Methicillin resistant Staphylococcus aureus infection, unspecified site
> Methicillin resistant Staphylococcus aureus (MRSA) infection

A49.1 Streptococcal infection, unspecified site
A49.2 Hemophilus influenzae infection, unspecified site
A49.3 Mycoplasma infection, unspecified site
A49.8 Other bacterial infections of unspecified site
A49.9 Bacterial infection, unspecified
> EXCLUDES 1   *bacteremia NOS (R78.81)*

Infections with a predominantly sexual mode of transmission (A50-A64)

> EXCLUDES 1   *human immunodeficiency virus [HIV] disease (B20)*
>   *nonspecific and nongonococcal urethritis (N34.1)*
>   *Reiter's disease (M02.3-)*

✓4ᵗʰ A50 Congenital syphilis

> **CC Excl: For CC/MCC codes in category A50, unless otherwise noted:** PDX collection 112

✓5ᵗʰ A50.0 Early congenital syphilis, symptomatic
> Any congenital syphilitic condition specified as early or manifest less than two years after birth.

A50.01 Early congenital syphilitic oculopathy   CC

A50.02 Early congenital syphilitic osteochondropathy   CC

A50.03 Early congenital syphilitic pharyngitis   CC
> Early congenital syphilitic laryngitis

A50.04 Early congenital syphilitic pneumonia   CC

A50.05 Early congenital syphilitic rhinitis   CC

A50.06 Early cutaneous congenital syphilis   CC

A50.07 Early mucocutaneous congenital syphilis   CC

A50.08 Early visceral congenital syphilis   CC

A50.09 Other early congenital syphilis, symptomatic

A50.1 Early congenital syphilis, latent
> Congenital syphilis without clinical manifestations, with positive serological reaction and negative spinal fluid test, less than two years after birth.

A50.2 Early congenital syphilis, unspecified   CC
> Congenital syphilis NOS less than two years after birth.
> **CC Excl:** PDX collection 113

✓5ᵗʰ A50.3 Late congenital syphilitic oculopathy
> EXCLUDES 1   *Hutchinson's triad (A50.53)*

A50.30 Late congenital syphilitic oculopathy, unspecified   CC

A50.31 Late congenital syphilitic interstitial keratitis   CC

A50.32 Late congenital syphilitic chorioretinitis   CC

A50.39 Other late congenital syphilitic oculopathy   CC

✓5ᵗʰ A50.4 Late congenital neurosyphilis [juvenile neurosyphilis]
> Use additional code to identify any associated mental disorder
> EXCLUDES 1   *Hutchinson's triad (A50.53)*

A50.40 Late congenital neurosyphilis, unspecified   CC
> Juvenile neurosyphilis NOS
> **CC Excl:** PDX collection 114

A50.41 Late congenital syphilitic meningitis   MCC
> **CC Excl:** PDX collection 115

A50.42 Late congenital syphilitic encephalitis   MCC
> **CC Excl:** PDX collection 114

A50.43 Late congenital syphilitic polyneuropathy   CC
> **CC Excl:** PDX collection 114

A50.44 Late congenital syphilitic optic nerve atrophy   CC

A50.45 Juvenile general paresis   CC
> Dementia paralytica juvenilis
> Juvenile tabetoparetic neurosyphilis
> **CC Excl:** PDX collection 114

A50.49 Other late congenital neurosyphilis   CC
> Juvenile tabes dorsalis
> **CC Excl:** PDX collection 114

✓5ᵗʰ A50.5 Other late congenital syphilis, symptomatic
> Any congenital syphilitic condition specified as late or manifest two years or more after birth.

A50.51 Clutton's joints   CC

A50.52 Hutchinson's teeth   CC

A50.53 Hutchinson's triad   CC

A50.54 Late congenital cardiovascular syphilis   CC

A50.55 Late congenital syphilitic arthropathy   CC HCC

A50.56 Late congenital syphilitic osteochondropathy   CC

A50.57 Syphilitic saddle nose   CC

A50.59 Other late congenital syphilis, symptomatic   CC

A50.6 Late congenital syphilis, latent
> Congenital syphilis without clinical manifestations, with positive serological reaction and negative spinal fluid test, two years or more after birth.

A50.7 Late congenital syphilis, unspecified
> Congenital syphilis NOS two years or more after birth.

A50.9 Congenital syphilis, unspecified

✓ Additional Character Required   ✓x7ᵗʰ Placeholder   Unacceptable PDx   Questionable PDx   Manifestation   Unspecified Dx   H1-H14 HAC   HCC CMS-HCC Dx   HIV HIV Dx

ICD-10-CM 2020   443

Chapter 1. Certain Infectious and Parasitic Diseases

A51–A53.0

√4ᵗʰ **A51 Early syphilis**

DEF: Syphilis: Sexually transmitted disease caused by the treponema pallidum spirochete. Syphilis usually exhibits cutaneous manifestations and may exist for years without symptoms.

A51.0 Primary genital syphilis
Syphilitic chancre NOS

A51.1 Primary anal syphilis

A51.2 Primary syphilis of other sites

√5ᵗʰ **A51.3 Secondary syphilis of skin and mucous membranes**

DEF: Transitory or chronic cutaneous eruptions that present within two to 10 weeks following an initial syphilis infection that may include nontender lymphadenopathy along with alopecia and condylomata lata.

A51.31 Condyloma latum   CC
CC Excl: PDX collection 112

A51.32 Syphilitic alopecia   CC
CC Excl: PDX collection 116

A51.39 Other secondary syphilis of skin   CC
Syphilitic leukoderma
Syphilitic mucous patch
EXCLUDES 1   late syphilitic leukoderma (A52.79)
CC Excl: PDX collection 112

√5ᵗʰ **A51.4 Other secondary syphilis**

A51.41 Secondary syphilitic meningitis   MCC
CC Excl: PDX collection 117

A51.42 Secondary syphilitic female pelvic   CC ♀
disease
CC Excl: PDX collection 113

A51.43 Secondary syphilitic oculopathy   CC
Secondary syphilitic chorioretinitis
Secondary syphilitic iridocyclitis, iritis
Secondary syphilitic uveitis
CC Excl: PDX collection 112

A51.44 Secondary syphilitic nephritis   CC
CC Excl: PDX collection 113

A51.45 Secondary syphilitic hepatitis   CC
CC Excl: PDX collection 118

A51.46 Secondary syphilitic osteopathy   CC
CC Excl: PDX collection 119

A51.49 Other secondary syphilitic   CC
conditions
Secondary syphilitic lymphadenopathy
Secondary syphilitic myositis
CC Excl: No Excl

A51.5 Early syphilis, latent
Syphilis (acquired) without clinical manifestations, with positive serological reaction and negative spinal fluid test, less than two years after infection.

A51.9 Early syphilis, unspecified

√4ᵗʰ **A52 Late syphilis**

√5ᵗʰ **A52.0 Cardiovascular and cerebrovascular syphilis**
CC Excl: For CC codes in subcategory A52.0: PDX collection 114

A52.00 Cardiovascular syphilis, unspecified   CC

A52.01 Syphilitic aneurysm of aorta   CC

A52.02 Syphilitic aortitis   CC

A52.03 Syphilitic endocarditis   CC
Syphilitic aortic valve incompetence or stenosis
Syphilitic mitral valve stenosis
Syphilitic pulmonary valve regurgitation

A52.04 Syphilitic cerebral arteritis   CC

A52.05 Other cerebrovascular syphilis   CC
Syphilitic cerebral aneurysm (ruptured)
(non-ruptured)
Syphilitic cerebral thrombosis

A52.06 Other syphilitic heart involvement   CC
Syphilitic coronary artery disease
Syphilitic myocarditis
Syphilitic pericarditis

A52.09 Other cardiovascular syphilis   CC

√5ᵗʰ **A52.1 Symptomatic neurosyphilis**
CC Excl: For CC/MCC codes in subcategory A52.1, unless otherwise noted: PDX collection 114

A52.10 Symptomatic neurosyphilis,   CC
unspecified

A52.11 Tabes dorsalis   CC
Locomotor ataxia (progressive)
Tabetic neurosyphilis

A52.12 Other cerebrospinal syphilis   CC

A52.13 Late syphilitic meningitis   MCC
CC Excl: PDX collection 115

A52.14 Late syphilitic encephalitis   MCC

A52.15 Late syphilitic neuropathy   CC
Late syphilitic acoustic neuritis
Late syphilitic optic (nerve) atrophy
Late syphilitic polyneuropathy
Late syphilitic retrobulbar neuritis

A52.16 Charcôt's arthropathy (tabetic)   CC
DEF: Progressive neurologic arthropathy in which chronic degeneration of joints in the weight-bearing areas with peripheral hypertrophy occurs as a complication of a neuropathy disorder. Supporting structures relax from a loss of sensation resulting in chronic joint instability.

A52.17 General paresis   CC
Dementia paralytica

A52.19 Other symptomatic neurosyphilis   CC
Syphilitic parkinsonism

A52.2 Asymptomatic neurosyphilis   CC
CC Excl: PDX collection 114

A52.3 Neurosyphilis, unspecified   CC
Gumma (syphilitic)
Syphilis (late)
Syphiloma
CC Excl: PDX collection 114

√5ᵗʰ **A52.7 Other symptomatic late syphilis**
CC Excl: For CC codes in subcategory A52.7, unless otherwise noted: PDX collection 116

A52.71 Late syphilitic oculopathy   CC
Late syphilitic chorioretinitis
Late syphilitic episcleritis
CC Excl: PDX collection 120

A52.72 Syphilis of lung and bronchus   CC

A52.73 Symptomatic late syphilis of other   CC
respiratory organs

A52.74 Syphilis of liver and other viscera   CC
Late syphilitic peritonitis

A52.75 Syphilis of kidney and ureter   CC
Syphilitic glomerular disease

A52.76 Other genitourinary symptomatic   CC
late syphilis
Late syphilitic female pelvic inflammatory disease

A52.77 Syphilis of bone and joint   CC

A52.78 Syphilis of other musculoskeletal   CC
tissue
Late syphilitic bursitis
Syphilis [stage unspecified] of bursa
Syphilis [stage unspecified] of muscle
Syphilis [stage unspecified] of synovium
Syphilis [stage unspecified] of tendon

A52.79 Other symptomatic late syphilis   CC
Late syphilitic leukoderma
Syphilis of adrenal gland
Syphilis of pituitary gland
Syphilis of thyroid gland
Syphilitic splenomegaly
EXCLUDES 1   syphilitic leukoderma (secondary) (A51.39)

A52.8 Late syphilis, latent
Syphilis (acquired) without clinical manifestations, with positive serological reaction and negative spinal fluid test, two years or more after infection.

A52.9 Late syphilis, unspecified

√4ᵗʰ **A53 Other and unspecified syphilis**

A53.0 Latent syphilis, unspecified as early or late
Latent syphilis NOS
Positive serological reaction for syphilis

N Newborn: 0   P Pediatric: 0-17   M Maternity: 9-64   A Adult: 15-124   MCC Major Complication/Comorbidity   CC Complication/Comorbidity   SW Severe Wound Dx

444   ICD-10-CM 2020

A53.9 **Syphilis, unspecified**
Infection due to Treponema pallidum NOS
Syphilis (acquired) NOS
EXCLUDES 1   *syphilis NOS under two years of age (A50.2)*

✓4ᵗʰ **A54** **Gonococcal infection**
DEF: Sexually transmitted bacterial infection caused by *Neisseria gonorrhoeae.* Women are often asymptomatic, while men tend to develop urinary symptoms quickly.

✓5ᵗʰ **A54.0** **Gonococcal infection of** lower genitourinary tract without periurethral or accessory gland abscess
EXCLUDES 1   *gonococcal infection with genitourinary gland abscess (A54.1)*
gonococcal infection with periurethral abscess (A54.1)
CC Excl: For CC codes in subcategory A54.0: PDX collection 121

A54.00 **Gonococcal infection of lower genitourinary tract, unspecified**   CC

A54.01 **Gonococcal** cystitis and urethritis, unspecified   CC

A54.02 **Gonococcal** vulvovaginitis, unspecified   CC ♀

A54.03 **Gonococcal** cervicitis, unspecified   CC ♀

A54.09 **Other gonococcal infection of lower genitourinary tract**   CC

A54.1 **Gonococcal infection of** lower genitourinary tract with periurethral and accessory gland abscess   CC
Gonococcal Bartholin's gland abscess
CC Excl: PDX collection 121

✓5ᵗʰ **A54.2** **Gonococcal pelviperitonitis and other gonococcal genitourinary infection**
CC Excl: For CC codes in subcategory A54.2: PDX collection 121

A54.21 **Gonococcal infection of** kidney and ureter   CC

A54.22 **Gonococcal** prostatitis   CC ♂

A54.23 **Gonococcal infection of other** male genital organs   CC ♂
Gonococcal epididymitis
Gonococcal orchitis

A54.24 **Gonococcal** female pelvic inflammatory disease   CC ♀
Gonococcal pelviperitonitis
EXCLUDES 1   *gonococcal peritonitis (A54.85)*

A54.29 **Other gonococcal genitourinary infections**   CC

✓5ᵗʰ **A54.3** **Gonococcal infection of** eye
CC Excl: For CC codes in subcategory A54.3: PDX collection 116

A54.30 **Gonococcal infection of eye, unspecified**   CC

A54.31 **Gonococcal** conjunctivitis   CC
Ophthalmia neonatorum due to gonococcus

A54.32 **Gonococcal** iridocyclitis   CC

A54.33 **Gonococcal** keratitis   CC

A54.39 **Other gonococcal eye infection**   CC
Gonococcal endophthalmia

✓5ᵗʰ **A54.4** **Gonococcal infection of** musculoskeletal system
CC Excl: For CC codes in subcategory A54.4: PDX collection 122

A54.40 **Gonococcal infection of musculoskeletal system, unspecified**   CC HCC

A54.41 **Gonococcal** spondylopathy   CC HCC

A54.42 **Gonococcal** arthritis   CC HCC
EXCLUDES 2   *gonococcal infection of spine (A54.41)*

A54.43 **Gonococcal** osteomyelitis   CC HCC
EXCLUDES 2   *gonococcal infection of spine (A54.41)*

A54.49 **Gonococcal infection of other** musculoskeletal tissue   CC HCC
Gonococcal bursitis
Gonococcal myositis
Gonococcal synovitis
Gonococcal tenosynovitis

A54.5 **Gonococcal** pharyngitis

A54.6 **Gonococcal infection of** anus and rectum

✓5ᵗʰ **A54.8** **Other gonococcal infections**

A54.81 **Gonococcal** meningitis   MCC
CC Excl: PDX collection 117

A54.82 **Gonococcal** brain abscess   CC
CC Excl: PDX collection 123

A54.83 **Gonococcal** heart infection   CC
Gonococcal endocarditis
Gonococcal myocarditis
Gonococcal pericarditis
CC Excl: PDX collection 124

A54.84 **Gonococcal** pneumonia   CC HCC
CC Excl: PDX collection 123

A54.85 **Gonococcal** peritonitis   CC HCC
EXCLUDES 1   *gonococcal pelviperitonitis (A54.24)*
CC Excl: PDX collection 125

A54.86 **Gonococcal** sepsis   MCC HCC
CC Excl: PDX collection 71

A54.89 **Other gonococcal infections**   CC
Gonococcal keratoderma
Gonococcal lymphadenitis
CC Excl: PDX collection 123

A54.9 **Gonococcal infection, unspecified**   CC
CC Excl: PDX collection 123

A55 **Chlamydial lymphogranuloma (venereum)**
Climatic or tropical bubo
Durand-Nicolas-Favre disease
Esthiomene
Lymphogranuloma inguinale

✓4ᵗʰ **A56** **Other sexually transmitted chlamydial diseases**
INCLUDES   sexually transmitted diseases due to Chlamydia trachomatis
EXCLUDES 1   *neonatal chlamydial conjunctivitis (P39.1)*
neonatal chlamydial pneumonia (P23.1)
EXCLUDES 2   *chlamydial lymphogranuloma (A55)*
conditions classified to A74.-
DEF: Chlamydia trachomatis: Bacterium that causes a common venereal disease. Symptoms of chlamydia are usually mild or absent, however, serious complications may cause irreversible damage, including cystitis, pelvic inflammatory disease, and infertility in women and discharge from the penis, prostatitis, and infertility in men. Genital chlamydial infection can cause arthritis, skin lesions, and inflammation of the eye and urethra.
Synonym(s): Reiter's syndrome.

✓5ᵗʰ **A56.0** **Chlamydial infection of** lower genitourinary tract

A56.00 **Chlamydial infection of lower genitourinary tract, unspecified**

A56.01 **Chlamydial** cystitis and urethritis

A56.02 **Chlamydial** vulvovaginitis   ♀

A56.09 **Other chlamydial infection of lower genitourinary tract**
Chlamydial cervicitis

✓5ᵗʰ **A56.1** **Chlamydial infection of** pelviperitoneum and other genitourinary organs

A56.11 **Chlamydial** female pelvic inflammatory disease   ♀

A56.19 **Other chlamydial genitourinary infection**
Chlamydial epididymitis
Chlamydial orchitis

A56.2 **Chlamydial infection of genitourinary tract, unspecified**

A56.3 **Chlamydial infection of** anus and rectum

A56.4 **Chlamydial infection of** pharynx

A56.8 **Sexually transmitted chlamydial infection of other sites**

A57 **Chancroid**
Ulcus molle
DEF: Localized infection by *Haemophilus ducreyi,* causing genital ulcers and infecting the inguinal lymph nodes.

A58 **Granuloma inguinale**
Donovanosis

✓4ᵗʰ **A59 Trichomoniasis**

> EXCLUDES 2   *intestinal trichomoniasis (A07.8)*
>
> **DEF:** Infection with the parasitic, flagellated protozoa of the genus *Trichomonas*. This protozoon is found in the intestinal and genitourinary tracts of humans and in the mouth around tartar, cavities, and areas of periodontal disease.

  ✓5ᵗʰ **A59.0 Urogenital trichomoniasis**

    A59.00 Urogenital trichomoniasis, unspecified
      Fluor (vaginalis) due to Trichomonas
      Leukorrhea (vaginalis) due to Trichomonas

    A59.01 Trichomonal vulvovaginitis ♀

    A59.02 Trichomonal prostatitis ♂

    A59.03 Trichomonal cystitis and urethritis

    A59.09 Other urogenital trichomoniasis
      Trichomonas cervicitis

  A59.8 Trichomoniasis of other sites

  A59.9 Trichomoniasis, unspecified

✓4ᵗʰ **A60 Anogenital herpesviral [herpes simplex] infections**

  ✓5ᵗʰ **A60.0 Herpesviral infection of genitalia and urogenital tract**

    A60.00 Herpesviral infection of urogenital system, unspecified HIV

    A60.01 Herpesviral infection of penis HIV ♂

    A60.02 Herpesviral infection of other male genital organs ♂

    A60.03 Herpesviral cervicitis ♀

    A60.04 Herpesviral vulvovaginitis HIV ♀
      Herpesviral [herpes simplex] ulceration
      Herpesviral [herpes simplex] vaginitis
      Herpesviral [herpes simplex] vulvitis

    A60.09 Herpesviral infection of other urogenital tract HIV

  A60.1 Herpesviral infection of perianal skin and rectum HIV

  A60.9 Anogenital herpesviral infection, unspecified HIV

✓4ᵗʰ **A63 Other predominantly sexually transmitted diseases, not elsewhere classified**

> EXCLUDES 2   *molluscum contagiosum (B08.1)*
>   *papilloma of cervix (D26.0)*

  A63.0 Anogenital (venereal) warts
    Anogenital warts due to (human) papillomavirus [HPV]
    Condyloma acuminatum

  A63.8 Other specified predominantly sexually transmitted diseases

A64 Unspecified sexually transmitted disease

Other spirochetal diseases (A65-A69)

> EXCLUDES 2   *leptospirosis (A27.-)*
>   *syphilis (A50-A53)*

CC Excl: For CC codes in categories A65-A69, unless otherwise noted: PDX collection 108

A65 Nonvenereal syphilis
  Bejel
  Endemic syphilis
  Njovera

✓4ᵗʰ **A66 Yaws**

> INCLUDES   bouba
>   frambesia (tropica)
>   pian

  A66.0 Initial lesions of yaws
    Chancre of yaws
    Frambesia, initial or primary
    Initial frambesial ulcer
    Mother yaw

  A66.1 Multiple papillomata and wet crab yaws
    Frambesioma
    Pianoma
    Plantar or palmar papilloma of yaws

  A66.2 Other early skin lesions of yaws
    Cutaneous yaws, less than five years after infection
    Early yaws (cutaneous) (macular) (maculopapular) (micropapular) (papular)
    Frambeside of early yaws

  A66.3 Hyperkeratosis of yaws
    Ghoul hand
    Hyperkeratosis, palmar or plantar (early) (late) due to yaws
    Worm-eaten soles

  A66.4 Gummata and ulcers of yaws
    Gummatous frambeside
    Nodular late yaws (ulcerated)

  A66.5 Gangosa
    Rhinopharyngitis mutilans

  A66.6 Bone and joint lesions of yaws HCC
    Yaws ganglion
    Yaws goundou
    Yaws gumma, bone
    Yaws gummatous osteitis or periostitis
    Yaws hydrarthrosis
    Yaws osteitis
    Yaws periostitis (hypertrophic)

  A66.7 Other manifestations of yaws
    Juxta-articular nodules of yaws
    Mucosal yaws

  A66.8 Latent yaws
    Yaws without clinical manifestations, with positive serology

  A66.9 Yaws, unspecified

✓4ᵗʰ **A67 Pinta [carate]**

  A67.0 Primary lesions of pinta
    Chancre (primary) of pinta
    Papule (primary) of pinta

  A67.1 Intermediate lesions of pinta
    Erythematous plaques of pinta
    Hyperchromic lesions of pinta
    Hyperkeratosis of pinta
    Pintids

  A67.2 Late lesions of pinta
    Achromic skin lesions of pinta
    Cicatricial skin lesions of pinta
    Dyschromic skin lesions of pinta

  A67.3 Mixed lesions of pinta
    Achromic with hyperchromic skin lesions of pinta [carate]

  A67.9 Pinta, unspecified

✓4ᵗʰ **A68 Relapsing fevers**

> INCLUDES   recurrent fever
> EXCLUDES 2   *Lyme disease (A69.2-)*

  A68.0 Louse-borne relapsing fever CC
    Relapsing fever due to Borrelia recurrentis

  A68.1 Tick-borne relapsing fever CC
    Relapsing fever due to any Borrelia species other than Borrelia recurrentis

  A68.9 Relapsing fever, unspecified CC

✓4ᵗʰ **A69 Other spirochetal infections**

  A69.0 Necrotizing ulcerative stomatitis
    Cancrum oris
    Fusospirochetal gangrene
    Noma
    Stomatitis gangrenosa

  A69.1 Other Vincent's infections CC
    Fusospirochetal pharyngitis
    Necrotizing ulcerative (acute) gingivitis
    Necrotizing ulcerative (acute) gingivostomatitis
    Spirochetal stomatitis
    Trench mouth
    Vincent's angina
    Vincent's gingivitis
    CC Excl: PDX collection 126

  ✓5ᵗʰ **A69.2 Lyme disease**
    Erythema chronicum migrans due to Borrelia burgdorferi
    DEF: Recurrent multisystem disorder through tick bites that begins with lesions of erythema chronicum migrans and is followed by arthritis of the large joints, myalgia, malaise, and neurological and cardiac manifestations.

    A69.20 Lyme disease, unspecified

    A69.21 Meningitis due to Lyme disease CC

N Newborn: 0   P Pediatric: 0-17   M Maternity: 9-64   A Adult: 15-124   MCC Major Complication/Comorbidity   CC Complication/Comorbidity   SW Severe Wound Dx

446   ICD-10-CM 2020

A69.22 Other neurologic disorders in Lyme disease `CC`
Cranial neuritis
Meningoencephalitis
Polyneuropathy

A69.23 Arthritis due to Lyme disease `CC` `HCC`

A69.29 Other conditions associated with Lyme disease `CC`
Myopericarditis due to Lyme disease
AHA: 2016,3Q,12

A69.8 Other specified spirochetal infections

A69.9 Spirochetal infection, unspecified

Other diseases caused by chlamydiae (A70-A74)

EXCLUDES 1   sexually transmitted chlamydial diseases (A55-A56)

A70 Chlamydia psittaci infections
Ornithosis
Parrot fever
Psittacosis
CC Excl: PDX collection 127

√4ᵗʰ **A71 Trachoma**

EXCLUDES 1   sequelae of trachoma (B94.0)

A71.0 Initial stage of trachoma
Trachoma dubium

A71.1 Active stage of trachoma
Granular conjunctivitis (trachomatous)
Trachomatous follicular conjunctivitis
Trachomatous pannus

A71.9 Trachoma, unspecified

√4ᵗʰ **A74 Other diseases caused by chlamydiae**

EXCLUDES 1   neonatal chlamydial conjunctivitis (P39.1)
neonatal chlamydial pneumonia (P23.1)
Reiter's disease (M02.3-)
sexually transmitted chlamydial diseases (A55-A56)

EXCLUDES 2   chlamydial pneumonia (J16.0)

A74.0 Chlamydial conjunctivitis
Paratrachoma

√5ᵗʰ **A74.8 Other chlamydial diseases**

A74.81 Chlamydial peritonitis

A74.89 Other chlamydial diseases

A74.9 Chlamydial infection, unspecified
Chlamydiosis NOS

Rickettsioses (A75-A79)

DEF: Rickettsia: Condition caused by bacteria that live in lice/ticks transmitted to humans through bites.
CC Excl: For CC codes in categories A75-A79, unless otherwise noted: PDX collection 108

√4ᵗʰ **A75 Typhus fever**

EXCLUDES 1   rickettsiosis due to Ehrlichia sennetsu (A79.81)

A75.0 Epidemic louse-borne typhus fever due to Rickettsia prowazekii `CC`
Classical typhus (fever)
Epidemic (louse-borne) typhus

A75.1 Recrudescent typhus [Brill's disease] `CC`
Brill-Zinsser disease

A75.2 Typhus fever due to Rickettsia typhi `CC`
Murine (flea-borne) typhus

A75.3 Typhus fever due to Rickettsia tsutsugamushi `CC`
Scrub (mite-borne) typhus
Tsutsugamushi fever

A75.9 Typhus fever, unspecified `CC`
Typhus (fever) NOS
CC Excl: PDX collection 128

√4ᵗʰ **A77 Spotted fever [tick-borne rickettsioses]**

A77.0 Spotted fever due to Rickettsia rickettsii `CC`
Rocky Mountain spotted fever
Sao Paulo fever

A77.1 Spotted fever due to Rickettsia conorii `CC`
African tick typhus
Boutonneuse fever
India tick typhus
Kenya tick typhus
Marseilles fever
Mediterranean tick fever

A77.2 Spotted fever due to Rickettsia siberica `CC`
North Asian tick fever
Siberian tick typhus

A77.3 Spotted fever due to Rickettsia australis `CC`
Queensland tick typhus

√5ᵗʰ **A77.4 Ehrlichiosis**

EXCLUDES 1   Rickettsiosis due to Ehrlichia sennetsu (A79.81)

A77.40 Ehrlichiosis, unspecified `CC`

A77.41 Ehrlichiosis chafeensis [E. chafeensis] `CC`

A77.49 Other ehrlichiosis `CC`

A77.8 Other spotted fevers `CC`

A77.9 Spotted fever, unspecified `CC`
Tick-borne typhus NOS

A78 Q fever `CC`
Infection due to Coxiella burnetii
Nine Mile fever
Quadrilateral fever

√4ᵗʰ **A79 Other rickettsioses**

A79.0 Trench fever `CC`
Quintan fever
Wolhynian fever

A79.1 Rickettsialpox due to Rickettsia akari `CC`
Kew Garden fever
Vesicular rickettsiosis
CC Excl: PDX collection 114

√5ᵗʰ **A79.8 Other specified rickettsioses**

A79.81 Rickettsiosis due to Ehrlichia sennetsu `CC`
CC Excl: PDX collection 114

A79.89 Other specified rickettsioses `CC`
CC Excl: PDX collection 114

A79.9 Rickettsiosis, unspecified `CC`
Rickettsial infection NOS
CC Excl: PDX collection 114

Viral and prion infections of the central nervous system (A80-A89)

EXCLUDES 1   postpolio syndrome (G14)
sequelae of poliomyelitis (B91)
sequelae of viral encephalitis (B94.1)

√4ᵗʰ **A80 Acute poliomyelitis**

CC Excl: For MCC codes in category A80: PDX collection 130

A80.0 Acute paralytic poliomyelitis, vaccine-associated `MCC`

A80.1 Acute paralytic poliomyelitis, wild virus, imported `MCC`

A80.2 Acute paralytic poliomyelitis, wild virus, indigenous `MCC`

√5ᵗʰ **A80.3 Acute paralytic poliomyelitis, other and unspecified**

A80.30 Acute paralytic poliomyelitis, unspecified `MCC`

A80.39 Other acute paralytic poliomyelitis `MCC`

A80.4 Acute nonparalytic poliomyelitis

A80.9 Acute poliomyelitis, unspecified

☑ Additional Character Required   √x7ᵗʰ Placeholder   <u>Unacceptable PDx</u>   Questionable PDx   Manifestation   <u>Unspecified Dx</u>   `H1`-`H14` HAC   `HCC` CMS-HCC Dx   `HIV` HIV Dx

ICD-10-CM 2020   **447**

Chapter 1. Certain Infectious and Parasitic Diseases

☑4ᵗʰ **A81 Atypical virus infections of central nervous system**

    INCLUDES   diseases of the central nervous system caused by prions

    Use additional code to identify:

      dementia with behavioral disturbance (F02.81)

      dementia without behavioral disturbance (F02.80)

☑5ᵗʰ **A81.0 Creutzfeldt-Jakob disease**

    DEF: Communicable, rare spongiform encephalopathy occurring later in life with progressive destruction of the pyramidal and extrapyramidal systems eventually leading to death. Progressive dementia, wasting of muscles, tremor, and other symptoms are present.

    CC Excl: For CC codes in subcategory A81.0: PDX collection 131

    A81.00 Creutzfeldt-Jakob disease, unspecified   `CC` `HCC`

      Jakob-Creutzfeldt disease, unspecified

    A81.01 Variant Creutzfeldt-Jakob disease   `CC` `HCC`

      vCJD

    A81.09 Other Creutzfeldt-Jakob disease   `CC` `HCC`

      CJD

      Familial Creutzfeldt-Jakob disease

      Iatrogenic Creutzfeldt-Jakob disease

      Sporadic Creutzfeldt-Jakob disease

      Subacute spongiform encephalopathy (with dementia)

A81.1 Subacute sclerosing panencephalitis   `CC` `HCC`

    Dawson's inclusion body encephalitis

    Van Bogaert's sclerosing leukoencephalopathy

    CC Excl: PDX collection 132

A81.2 Progressive multifocal leukoencephalopathy   `HIV` `CC` `HCC`

    Multifocal leukoencephalopathy NOS

    CC Excl: PDX collection 133

☑5ᵗʰ **A81.8 Other atypical virus infections of central nervous system**

    CC Excl: For CC codes in subcategory A81.8, unless otherwise noted: PDX collection 135

    A81.81 Kuru   `CC` `HCC`

      CC Excl: PDX collection 134

    A81.82 Gerstmann-Sträussler-Scheinker syndrome   `HIV` `CC` `HCC`

      GSS syndrome

    A81.83 Fatal familial insomnia   `HIV` `CC` `HCC`

      FFI

    A81.89 Other atypical virus infections of central nervous system   `HIV` `CC` `HCC`

A81.9 Atypical virus infection of central nervous system, unspecified   `HIV` `CC` `HCC`

    Prion diseases of the central nervous system NOS

    CC Excl: PDX collection 134

☑4ᵗʰ **A82 Rabies**

    CC Excl: For CC codes in category A82: PDX collection 136

A82.0 Sylvatic rabies   `CC`

A82.1 Urban rabies   `CC`

A82.9 Rabies, unspecified   `CC`

☑4ᵗʰ **A83 Mosquito-borne viral encephalitis**

    INCLUDES   mosquito-borne viral meningoencephalitis

    EXCLUDES 2   Venezuelan equine encephalitis (A92.2)

      West Nile fever (A92.3-)

      West Nile virus (A92.3-)

    CC Excl: For MCC codes in category A83: PDX collection 137

A83.0 Japanese encephalitis   `MCC`

A83.1 Western equine encephalitis   `MCC`

A83.2 Eastern equine encephalitis   `MCC`

A83.3 St Louis encephalitis   `MCC`

A83.4 Australian encephalitis   `MCC`

    Kunjin virus disease

A83.5 California encephalitis   `MCC`

    California meningoencephalitis

    La Crosse encephalitis

A83.6 Rocio virus disease   `MCC`

A83.8 Other mosquito-borne viral encephalitis   `MCC`

A83.9 Mosquito-borne viral encephalitis, unspecified   `MCC`

☑4ᵗʰ **A84 Tick-borne viral encephalitis**

    INCLUDES   tick-borne viral meningoencephalitis

    CC Excl: For MCC codes in category A84: PDX collection 137

A84.0 Far Eastern tick-borne encephalitis [Russian spring-summer encephalitis]   `MCC`

A84.1 Central European tick-borne encephalitis   `MCC`

A84.8 Other tick-borne viral encephalitis   `MCC`

    Louping ill

    Powassan virus disease

A84.9 Tick-borne viral encephalitis, unspecified   `MCC`

☑4ᵗʰ **A85 Other viral encephalitis, not elsewhere classified**

    INCLUDES   specified viral encephalomyelitis NEC

      specified viral meningoencephalitis NEC

    EXCLUDES 1   benign myalgic encephalomyelitis (G93.3)

      encephalitis due to cytomegalovirus (B25.8)

      encephalitis due to herpesvirus NEC (B10.0-)

      encephalitis due to herpesvirus [herpes simplex] (B00.4)

      encephalitis due to measles virus (B05.0)

      encephalitis due to mumps virus (B26.2)

      encephalitis due to poliomyelitis virus (A80.-)

      encephalitis due to zoster (B02.0)

      lymphocytic choriomeningitis (A87.2)

    CC Excl: For CC codes in category A85: PDX collection 138

A85.0 Enteroviral encephalitis   `HIV` `CC`

    Enteroviral encephalomyelitis

A85.1 Adenoviral encephalitis   `HIV` `CC`

    Adenoviral meningoencephalitis

A85.2 Arthropod-borne viral encephalitis, unspecified   `MCC`

    EXCLUDES 1   West nile virus with encephalitis (A92.31)

    CC Excl: PDX collection 137

A85.8 Other specified viral encephalitis   `HIV` `CC`

    Encephalitis lethargica

    Von Economo-Cruchet disease

A86 Unspecified viral encephalitis   `HIV` `CC`

    Viral encephalomyelitis NOS

    Viral meningoencephalitis NOS

    CC Excl: PDX collection 139

☑4ᵗʰ **A87 Viral meningitis**

    EXCLUDES 1   meningitis due to herpesvirus [herpes simplex] (B00.3)

      meningitis due to measles virus (B05.1)

      meningitis due to mumps virus (B26.1)

      meningitis due to poliomyelitis virus (A80.-)

      meningitis due to zoster (B02.1)

    DEF: Meningitis: Inflammation of the meningeal layers of the brain and spine.

    CC Excl: For CC codes in category A87, unless otherwise noted: PDX collection 140

A87.0 Enteroviral meningitis   `CC`

    Coxsackievirus meningitis

    Echovirus meningitis

A87.1 Adenoviral meningitis   `CC`

A87.2 Lymphocytic choriomeningitis   `CC`

    Lymphocytic meningoencephalitis

    CC Excl: PDX collection 141

A87.8 Other viral meningitis   `CC`

A87.9 Viral meningitis, unspecified   `CC`

☑4ᵗʰ **A88 Other viral infections of central nervous system, not elsewhere classified**

    EXCLUDES 1   viral encephalitis NOS (A86)

      viral meningitis NOS (A87.9)

A88.0 Enteroviral exanthematous fever [Boston exanthem]   `CC`

    CC Excl: PDX collection 137

A88.1 Epidemic vertigo

A88.8 Other specified viral infections of central nervous system   `HIV` `CC`

    CC Excl: PDX collection 138

A89 Unspecified viral infection of central nervous system   `HIV` `CC`

    CC Excl: PDX collection 139

`N` Newborn: 0   `P` Pediatric: 0-17   `M` Maternity: 9-64   `A` Adult: 15-124   `MCC` Major Complication/Comorbidity   `CC` Complication/Comorbidity   `SW` Severe Wound Dx

Arthropod-borne viral fevers and viral hemorrhagic fevers (A90-A99)

A90 Dengue fever [classical dengue] `CC`

>>**EXCLUDES 1**   *dengue hemorrhagic fever (A91)*
>>**AHA:** 2016,3Q,13
>>**CC Excl:** PDX collection 142

A91 Dengue hemorrhagic fever `CC`

>>**CC Excl:** PDX collection 143

✓4ᵗʰ **A92 Other mosquito-borne viral fevers**

>>**EXCLUDES 1**   *Ross River disease (B33.1)*
>>**CC Excl: For codes in category A92:**
>>**For MCC codes:** PDX collection 145
>>**For CC codes, unless otherwise noted:** PDX collection 144

>**A92.0 Chikungunya virus disease** `CC`
>>Chikungunya (hemorrhagic) fever
>>**CC Excl:** PDX collection 143

>**A92.1 O'nyong-nyong fever** `CC`

>**A92.2 Venezuelan equine fever** `CC`
>>Venezuelan equine encephalitis
>>Venezuelan equine encephalomyelitis virus disease

>✓5ᵗʰ **A92.3 West Nile virus infection**
>>West Nile fever
>>**AHA:** 2016,3Q,12

>>**A92.30 West Nile virus infection, unspecified** `MCC`
>>>West Nile fever NOS
>>>West Nile fever without complications
>>>West Nile virus NOS

>>**A92.31 West Nile virus infection with encephalitis** `MCC`
>>>West Nile encephalitis
>>>West Nile encephalomyelitis

>>**A92.32 West Nile virus infection with other neurologic manifestation** `MCC`
>>>Use additional code to specify the neurologic manifestation

>>**A92.39 West Nile virus infection with other complications** `MCC`
>>>Use additional code to specify the other conditions

>**A92.4 Rift Valley fever** `CC`

>**A92.5 Zika virus disease** `CC`
>>Zika virus fever
>>Zika virus infection
>>Zika NOS
>>**EXCLUDES 1**   *congenital Zika virus disease (P35.4)*
>>**AHA:** 2016,4Q,4-7
>>**DEF:** Virus transmitted via a bite from an infected Aedes species mosquito. Common symptoms of the virus include fever, rash, joint pain, and conjunctivitis; they are usually mild in nature and may last from several days to a week. Most people who have the Zika virus do not require medical attention; however, in pregnant women, the Zika virus can cause a serious birth defect called microcephaly, as well as other severe fetal brain defects.

>**A92.8 Other specified mosquito-borne viral fevers** `CC`

>**A92.9 Mosquito-borne viral fever, unspecified** `CC`
>>**CC Excl:** PDX collection 143

✓4ᵗʰ **A93 Other arthropod-borne viral fevers, not elsewhere classified**
>>**CC Excl: For CC codes in category A93, unless otherwise noted:** PDX collection 143

>**A93.0 Oropouche virus disease** `CC`
>>Oropouche fever
>>**CC Excl:** PDX collection 144

>**A93.1 Sandfly fever** `CC`
>>Pappataci fever
>>Phlebotomus fever

>**A93.2 Colorado tick fever** `CC`

>**A93.8 Other specified arthropod-borne viral fevers** `CC`
>>Piry virus disease
>>Vesicular stomatitis virus disease [Indiana fever]

A94 Unspecified arthropod-borne viral fever `CC`
>>Arboviral fever NOS
>>Arbovirus infection NOS
>>**CC Excl:** PDX collection 143

✓4ᵗʰ **A95 Yellow fever**
>>**CC Excl: For CC codes in category A95:** PDX collection 146

>**A95.0 Sylvatic yellow fever** `CC`
>>Jungle yellow fever

>**A95.1 Urban yellow fever** `CC`

>**A95.9 Yellow fever, unspecified** `CC`

✓4ᵗʰ **A96 Arenaviral hemorrhagic fever**
>>**CC Excl: For CC codes in category A96:** PDX collection 147

>**A96.0 Junin hemorrhagic fever** `CC`
>>Argentinian hemorrhagic fever

>**A96.1 Machupo hemorrhagic fever** `CC`
>>Bolivian hemorrhagic fever

>**A96.2 Lassa fever**

>**A96.8 Other arenaviral hemorrhagic fevers** `CC`

>**A96.9 Arenaviral hemorrhagic fever, unspecified** `CC`

✓4ᵗʰ **A98 Other viral hemorrhagic fevers, not elsewhere classified**
>>**EXCLUDES 1**   *chikungunya hemorrhagic fever (A92.0)*
>>>>>>>>> *dengue hemorrhagic fever (A91)*
>>**CC Excl: For CC codes in category A98, unless otherwise noted:** PDX collection 143

>**A98.0 Crimean-Congo hemorrhagic fever** `CC`
>>Central Asian hemorrhagic fever

>**A98.1 Omsk hemorrhagic fever** `CC`

>**A98.2 Kyasanur Forest disease** `CC`

>**A98.3 Marburg virus disease**

>**A98.4 Ebola virus disease**

>**A98.5 Hemorrhagic fever with renal syndrome** `CC`
>>Epidemic hemorrhagic fever
>>Korean hemorrhagic fever
>>Russian hemorrhagic fever
>>Hantaan virus disease
>>Hantavirus disease with renal manifestations
>>Nephropathia epidemica
>>Songo fever
>>**EXCLUDES 1**   *hantavirus (cardio)-pulmonary syndrome (B33.4)*
>>**CC Excl:** PDX collection 148

>**A98.8 Other specified viral hemorrhagic fevers** `CC`

A99 Unspecified viral hemorrhagic fever `CC`
>>**CC Excl:** PDX collection 143

Viral infections characterized by skin and mucous membrane lesions (B00-B09)

✓4ᵗʰ **B00 Herpesviral [herpes simplex] infections**
>>**EXCLUDES 1**   *congenital herpesviral infections (P35.2)*
>>**EXCLUDES 2**   *anogenital herpesviral infection (A60.-)*
>>>>>>>>> *gammaherpesviral mononucleosis (B27.0-)*
>>>>>>>>> *herpangina (B08.5)*

>**B00.0 Eczema herpeticum** `HIV`
>>Kaposi's varicelliform eruption

>**B00.1 Herpesviral vesicular dermatitis** `HIV`
>>Herpes simplex facialis
>>Herpes simplex labialis
>>Herpes simplex otitis externa
>>Vesicular dermatitis of ear
>>Vesicular dermatitis of lip

>**B00.2 Herpesviral gingivostomatitis and pharyngotonsillitis** `HIV` `CC`
>>Herpesviral pharyngitis
>>**CC Excl:** PDX collection 149

>**B00.3 Herpesviral meningitis** `HIV` `MCC`
>>**CC Excl:** PDX collection 150

Chapter 1. Certain Infectious and Parasitic Diseases

B00.4 Herpesviral encephalitis `HIV` `MCC`

Herpesviral meningoencephalitis
Simian B disease

> **EXCLUDES 1** *herpesviral encephalitis due to herpesvirus 6 and 7 (B10.01, B10.09)*
> *non-simplex herpesviral encephalitis (B10.0-)*

CC Excl: PDX collection 151

✓5th **B00.5 Herpesviral ocular disease**

CC Excl: For CC codes in subcategory B00.5: PDX collection 152

    B00.50 Herpesviral ocular disease, unspecified `HIV` `CC`

    B00.51 Herpesviral iridocyclitis `HIV` `CC`

Herpesviral iritis
Herpesviral uveitis, anterior

    B00.52 Herpesviral keratitis `HIV` `CC`

Herpesviral keratoconjunctivitis

    B00.53 Herpesviral conjunctivitis `HIV` `CC`

    B00.59 Other herpesviral disease of eye `HIV` `CC`

Herpesviral dermatitis of eyelid

B00.7 Disseminated herpesviral disease `HIV` `MCC` `HCC`

Herpesviral sepsis
CC Excl: PDX collection 153

✓5th **B00.8 Other forms of herpesviral infections**

    B00.81 Herpesviral hepatitis `HIV` `CC`

CC Excl: PDX collection 154

    B00.82 Herpes simplex myelitis `MCC` `HCC`

CC Excl: PDX collection 155

    B00.89 Other herpesviral infection `HIV` `CC`

Herpesviral whitlow
CC Excl: PDX collection 156

B00.9 Herpesviral infection, unspecified `HIV`

Herpes simplex infection NOS

✓4th **B01 Varicella [chickenpox]**

CC Excl: For CC codes in category B01: PDX collection 157

B01.0 Varicella meningitis `CC`

✓6th **B01.1 Varicella encephalitis, myelitis and encephalomyelitis**

Postchickenpox encephalitis, myelitis and encephalomyelitis

    B01.11 Varicella encephalitis and encephalomyelitis `MCC`

Postchickenpox encephalitis and encephalomyelitis
CC Excl: PDX collection 158

    B01.12 Varicella myelitis `MCC` `HCC`

Postchickenpox myelitis
CC Excl: PDX collection 159

B01.2 Varicella pneumonia `MCC`

CC Excl: PDX collection 160

✓5th **B01.8 Varicella with other complications**

    B01.81 Varicella keratitis `CC`

    B01.89 Other varicella complications `CC`

B01.9 Varicella without complication `CC`

Varicella NOS

✓4th **B02 Zoster [herpes zoster]**

> **INCLUDES** shingles
> zona

B02.0 Zoster encephalitis `HIV` `CC`

Zoster meningoencephalitis
CC Excl: PDX collection 161

B02.1 Zoster meningitis `HIV` `MCC`

AHA: 2019,1Q,18
CC Excl: PDX collection 162

✓5th **B02.2 Zoster with other nervous system involvement**

CC Excl: For CC codes in subcategory B02.2: PDX collection 161

    B02.21 Postherpetic geniculate ganglionitis `HIV` `CC`

    B02.22 Postherpetic trigeminal neuralgia `HIV` `CC`

    B02.23 Postherpetic polyneuropathy `HIV` `CC`

    B02.24 Postherpetic myelitis `MCC` `HCC`

Herpes zoster myelitis
CC Excl: PDX collection 163

    B02.29 Other postherpetic nervous system involvement `HIV` `CC`

Postherpetic radiculopathy

✓5th **B02.3 Zoster ocular disease**

CC Excl: For CC codes in subcategory B02.3: PDX collection 164

    B02.30 Zoster ocular disease, unspecified `HIV` `CC`

    B02.31 Zoster conjunctivitis `HIV` `CC`

    B02.32 Zoster iridocyclitis `HIV` `CC`

    B02.33 Zoster keratitis `HIV` `CC`

Herpes zoster keratoconjunctivitis

    B02.34 Zoster scleritis `HIV` `CC`

    B02.39 Other herpes zoster eye disease `HIV` `CC`

Zoster blepharitis

B02.7 Disseminated zoster `HIV` `CC`

CC Excl: PDX collection 165

B02.8 Zoster with other complications `HIV` `CC`

Herpes zoster otitis externa
CC Excl: PDX collection 165

B02.9 Zoster without complications `HIV`

Zoster NOS

B03 Smallpox `CC`

> **NOTE** In 1980 the 33rd World Health Assembly declared that smallpox had been eradicated.
> The classification is maintained for surveillance purposes.

CC Excl: PDX collection 166

B04 Monkeypox `CC`

CC Excl: PDX collection 167

✓4th **B05 Measles**

> **INCLUDES** morbilli
> **EXCLUDES 1** *subacute sclerosing panencephalitis (A81.1)*

B05.0 Measles complicated by encephalitis `MCC`

Postmeasles encephalitis
CC Excl: PDX collection 168

B05.1 Measles complicated by meningitis `CC`

Postmeasles meningitis
CC Excl: PDX collection 169

B05.2 Measles complicated by pneumonia `MCC`

Postmeasles pneumonia
CC Excl: PDX collection 170

B05.3 Measles complicated by otitis media

Postmeasles otitis media

B05.4 Measles with intestinal complications `CC`

CC Excl: PDX collection 169

✓5th **B05.8 Measles with other complications**

    B05.81 Measles keratitis and keratoconjunctivitis `CC`

CC Excl: PDX collection 171

    B05.89 Other measles complications `CC`

CC Excl: PDX collection 169

B05.9 Measles without complication

Measles NOS

✓4th **B06 Rubella [German measles]**

> **EXCLUDES 1** *congenital rubella (P35.0)*

DEF: Highly contagious virus in which the symptoms are mild and short-lived in most people. Rubella during pregnancy, however, can result in abortion, stillbirth, or congenital defects.

CC Excl: For CC/MCC codes in category B06, unless otherwise noted: PDX collection 172

✓5th **B06.0 Rubella with neurological complications**

    B06.00 Rubella with neurological complication, unspecified `CC`

    B06.01 Rubella encephalitis `MCC`

Rubella meningoencephalitis

    B06.02 Rubella meningitis `CC`

    B06.09 Other neurological complications of rubella `CC`

✓5th **B06.8 Rubella with other complications**

    B06.81 Rubella pneumonia `CC`

    B06.82 Rubella arthritis `CC` `HCC`

CC Excl: PDX collection 173

    B06.89 Other rubella complications `CC`

`N` Newborn: 0   `P` Pediatric: 0-17   `M` Maternity: 9-64   `A` Adult: 15-124   `MCC` Major Complication/Comorbidity   `CC` Complication/Comorbidity   `SW` Severe Wound Dx

450   ICD-10-CM 2020

B06.9   **Rubella without complication**
Rubella NOS

✓4th **B07**   **Viral warts**

    INCLUDES   verruca simplex
                  verruca vulgaris
                  viral warts due to human papillomavirus
    EXCLUDES 2   anogenital (venereal) warts (A63.0)
                  papilloma of bladder (D41.4)
                  papilloma of cervix (D26.0)
                  papilloma larynx (D14.1)

B07.0   **Plantar wart**
Verruca plantaris

B07.8   **Other viral warts**
Common wart
Flat wart
Verruca plana

B07.9   **Viral wart, unspecified**

✓4th **B08**   **Other viral infections characterized by skin and mucous membrane lesions, not elsewhere classified**
    EXCLUDES 1   vesicular stomatitis virus disease (A93.8)

✓5th   **B08.0**   **Other orthopoxvirus infections**
      EXCLUDES 2   monkeypox (B04)

✓6th   **B08.01**   **Cowpox and vaccinia not from vaccine**

       B08.010   **Cowpox**
             DEF: Disease contracted by milking infected cows. The vesicles usually appear on the fingers, hands, and adjacent areas and usually disappear without scarring. Other symptoms include local edema, lymphangitis, and regional lymphadenitis with or without fever.

       B08.011   **Vaccinia not from vaccine**
           EXCLUDES 1   vaccinia (from vaccination) (generalized) (T88.1)

    B08.02   **Orf virus disease**
Contagious pustular dermatitis
Ecthyma contagiosum

    B08.03   **Pseudocowpox [milker's node]**

    B08.04   **Paravaccinia, unspecified**

    B08.09   **Other orthopoxvirus infections**
Orthopoxvirus infection NOS

  B08.1   **Molluscum contagiosum**
       DEF: Benign poxvirus infection causing small bumps on the skin or conjunctiva and is transmitted by close contact.

✓5th   **B08.2**   **Exanthema subitum [sixth disease]**
Roseola infantum

    B08.20   **Exanthema subitum [sixth disease], unspecified**   P
Roseola infantum, unspecified

    B08.21   **Exanthema subitum [sixth disease] due to human herpesvirus 6**   P
Roseola infantum due to human herpesvirus 6

    B08.22   **Exanthema subitum [sixth disease] due to human herpesvirus 7**   P
Roseola infantum due to human herpesvirus 7

  B08.3   **Erythema infectiosum [fifth disease]**   CC
       DEF: Infection with human parvovirus B19, mainly occurring in children. Symptoms include a low-grade fever, malaise, or a "cold" a few days before the appearance of a mild rash illness that presents as a "slapped-cheek" rash on the face and a lacy red rash on the trunk and limbs.
       CC Excl: PDX collection 174

  B08.4   **Enteroviral vesicular stomatitis with exanthem**
Hand, foot and mouth disease

  B08.5   **Enteroviral vesicular pharyngitis**
Herpangina
       DEF: Acute infectious Coxsackie virus infection causing throat lesions, fever, and vomiting that generally affects children in the summer.

✓5th   **B08.6**   **Parapoxvirus infections**

    B08.60   **Parapoxvirus infection, unspecified**

    B08.61   **Bovine stomatitis**

    B08.62   **Sealpox**

    B08.69   **Other parapoxvirus infections**

✓5th   **B08.7**   **Yatapoxvirus infections**

    B08.70   **Yatapoxvirus infection, unspecified**

    B08.71   **Tanapox virus disease**   CC
       CC Excl: PDX collection 167

    B08.72   **Yaba pox virus disease**
Yaba monkey tumor disease

    B08.79   **Other yatapoxvirus infections**

  B08.8   **Other specified viral infections characterized by skin and mucous membrane lesions**
Enteroviral lymphonodular pharyngitis
Foot-and-mouth disease
Poxvirus NEC

B09   **Unspecified viral infection characterized by skin and mucous membrane lesions**
Viral enanthema NOS
Viral exanthema NOS

Other human herpesviruses (B10)

✓4th **B10**   **Other human herpesviruses**
    EXCLUDES 2   cytomegalovirus (B25.9)
                  Epstein-Barr virus (B27.0-)
                  herpes NOS (B00.9)
                  herpes simplex (B00.-)
                  herpes zoster (B02.-)
                  human herpesvirus NOS (B00.-)
                  human herpesvirus 1 and 2 (B00.-)
                  human herpesvirus 3 (B01.-, B02.0-)
                  human herpesvirus 4 (B27.0-)
                  human herpesvirus 5 (B25.-)
                  varicella (B01.-)
                  zoster (B02.-)

✓5th   **B10.0**   **Other human herpesvirus encephalitis**
      EXCLUDES 2   herpes encephalitis NOS (B00.4)
                    herpes simplex encephalitis (B00.4)
                    human herpesvirus encephalitis (B00.4)
                    simian B herpes virus encephalitis (B00.4)

    B10.01   **Human herpesvirus 6 encephalitis**   HIV MCC
       CC Excl: PDX collection 151

    B10.09   **Other human herpesvirus encephalitis**   HIV MCC
Human herpesvirus 7 encephalitis
       CC Excl: PDX collection 151

✓5th   **B10.8**   **Other human herpesvirus infection**

    B10.81   **Human herpesvirus 6 infection**

    B10.82   **Human herpesvirus 7 infection**

    B10.89   **Other human herpesvirus infection**
Human herpesvirus 8 infection
Kaposi's sarcoma-associated herpesvirus infection

Viral hepatitis (B15-B19)

    EXCLUDES 1   sequelae of viral hepatitis (B94.2)
    EXCLUDES 2   cytomegaloviral hepatitis (B25.1)
                  herpesviral [herpes simplex] hepatitis (B00.81)
DEF: Hepatitis A: HAV infection that is self-limiting with flulike symptoms. Transmission is fecal-oral.
DEF: Hepatitis B: HBV infection that can be chronic and systemic. Transmission is bodily fluids.
DEF: Hepatitis C: HCV infection that can be chronic and systemic. Transmission is blood transfusion and unidentified agents.
DEF: Hepatitis D (delta): HDV that occurs only in the presence of hepatitis B virus. Transmission is contaminated blood in contact with mucous membranes.
DEF: Hepatitis E: HEV is an epidemic form. Transmission is fecal-oral, most often from contaminated water.
CC Excl: For CC/MCC codes in categories B15-B19: PDX collection 175

✓4th **B15**   **Acute hepatitis A**

  B15.0   **Hepatitis A with hepatic coma**   MCC

  B15.9   **Hepatitis A without hepatic coma**   CC
Hepatitis A (acute)(viral) NOS

✓4th **B16**   **Acute hepatitis B**
    AHA: 2016,3Q,13

  B16.0   **Acute hepatitis B with delta-agent with hepatic coma**   MCC

  B16.1   **Acute hepatitis B with delta-agent without hepatic coma**   CC

  B16.2   **Acute hepatitis B without delta-agent with hepatic coma**   MCC

☑ Additional Character Required   ✓x7th Placeholder   Unacceptable PDx   Questionable PDx   Manifestation   Unspecified Dx   H1-H4 HAC   HCC CMS-HCC Dx   HIV HIV Dx

ICD-10-CM 2020   451

B16.9   **Acute hepatitis B** without delta-agent and without hepatic coma   `CC`
     Hepatitis B (acute) (viral) NOS

✓4ᵗʰ **B17**   **Other** acute **viral hepatitis**

     B17.0   **Acute** delta-(super) infection **of hepatitis B carrier**   `CC`

     ✓5ᵗʰ **B17.1**   **Acute** hepatitis C

         B17.10   **Acute hepatitis C** without hepatic coma   `CC`
             Acute hepatitis C NOS

         B17.11   **Acute hepatitis C** with hepatic coma   `MCC`

     B17.2   **Acute** hepatitis E   `CC`

     B17.8   **Other specified acute viral hepatitis**   `CC`
         Hepatitis non-A non-B (acute) (viral) NEC

     B17.9   **Acute viral hepatitis, unspecified**   `CC`
         Acute hepatitis NOS
         Acute infectious hepatitis NOS

✓4ᵗʰ **B18**   **Chronic** viral hepatitis

     INCLUDES   carrier of viral hepatitis
     AHA: 2017,1Q,41

     B18.0   **Chronic viral hepatitis B** with delta-agent   `CC` `HCC`

     B18.1   **Chronic viral hepatitis B** without delta-agent   `CC` `HCC`
         Carrier of viral hepatitis B
         Chronic (viral) hepatitis B

     B18.2   **Chronic viral** hepatitis C   `HCC`
         Carrier of viral hepatitis C
         AHA: 2018,1Q,4

     B18.8   **Other chronic viral hepatitis**   `CC` `HCC`
         Carrier of other viral hepatitis

     B18.9   **Chronic viral hepatitis, unspecified**   `CC` `HCC`
         Carrier of unspecified viral hepatitis

✓4ᵗʰ **B19**   **Unspecified viral hepatitis**

     B19.0   **Unspecified viral hepatitis** with hepatic coma   `MCC`

     ✓5ᵗʰ **B19.1**   **Unspecified viral** hepatitis B

         B19.10   **Unspecified viral hepatitis B** without hepatic coma   `CC`
             Unspecified viral hepatitis B NOS

         B19.11   **Unspecified viral hepatitis B** with hepatic coma   `MCC`

     ✓5ᵗʰ **B19.2**   **Unspecified viral** hepatitis C

         B19.20   **Unspecified viral hepatitis C** without hepatic coma
             Viral hepatitis C NOS

         B19.21   **Unspecified viral hepatitis C** with hepatic coma   `MCC`

     B19.9   **Unspecified viral hepatitis** without hepatic coma   `CC`
         Viral hepatitis NOS

Human immunodeficiency virus [HIV] disease (B20)

B20   **Human immunodeficiency virus [HIV] disease**   `CC` `HCC`

     INCLUDES   acquired immune deficiency syndrome [AIDS]
         AIDS-related complex [ARC]
         HIV infection, symptomatic
     Code first Human immunodeficiency virus [HIV] disease complicating pregnancy, childbirth and the puerperium, if applicable (O98.7-)
     Use additional code(s) to identify all manifestations of HIV infection
     EXCLUDES 1   asymptomatic human immunodeficiency virus [HIV] infection status (Z21)
         exposure to HIV virus (Z20.6)
         inconclusive serologic evidence of HIV (R75)
     AHA: 2019,1Q,8-11
     CC Excl: PDX collection 176

Other viral diseases (B25-B34)

✓4ᵗʰ **B25**   **Cytomegaloviral disease**

     EXCLUDES 1   congenital cytomegalovirus infection (P35.1)
         cytomegaloviral mononucleosis (B27.1-)

     B25.0   **Cytomegaloviral** pneumonitis   `MCC` `HCC`
         CC Excl: PDX collection 110

     B25.1   **Cytomegaloviral** hepatitis   `CC` `HCC`
         CC Excl: No Excl

     B25.2   **Cytomegaloviral** pancreatitis   `MCC` `HCC`
         CC Excl: PDX collection 177

     B25.8   **Other cytomegaloviral diseases**   `HIV` `CC` `HCC`
         Cytomegaloviral encephalitis
         CC Excl: PDX collection 178

     B25.9   **Cytomegaloviral disease, unspecified**   `HIV` `CC` `HCC`
         CC Excl: PDX collection 178

✓4ᵗʰ **B26**   **Mumps**

     INCLUDES   epidemic parotitis
         infectious parotitis

     B26.0   **Mumps** orchitis   `CC` ♂
         CC Excl: PDX collection 179

     B26.1   **Mumps** meningitis   `MCC`
         CC Excl: PDX collection 180

     B26.2   **Mumps** encephalitis   `MCC`
         CC Excl: PDX collection 181

     B26.3   **Mumps** pancreatitis   `CC`
         CC Excl: PDX collection 182

     ✓5ᵗʰ **B26.8**   **Mumps with other complications**
         CC Excl: For CC codes in subcategory B26.8, unless otherwise noted: PDX collection 184

         B26.81   **Mumps** hepatitis   `CC`
             CC Excl: PDX collection 183

         B26.82   **Mumps** myocarditis   `CC`

         B26.83   **Mumps** nephritis   `CC`

         B26.84   **Mumps** polyneuropathy   `CC`
             CC Excl: PDX collection 185

         B26.85   **Mumps** arthritis   `CC` `HCC`

         B26.89   **Other mumps complications**   `CC`

     B26.9   **Mumps without complication**
         Mumps NOS
         Mumps parotitis NOS

✓4ᵗʰ **B27**   **Infectious mononucleosis**

     INCLUDES   glandular fever
         monocytic angina
         Pfeiffer's disease

     ✓5ᵗʰ **B27.0**   **Gammaherpesviral** mononucleosis
         Mononucleosis due to Epstein-Barr virus

         B27.00   **Gammaherpesviral mononucleosis** without complication

         B27.01   **Gammaherpesviral mononucleosis** with polyneuropathy

         B27.02   **Gammaherpesviral mononucleosis** with meningitis

         B27.09   **Gammaherpesviral mononucleosis** with other complications
             Hepatomegaly in gammaherpesviral mononucleosis

     ✓5ᵗʰ **B27.1**   **Cytomegaloviral** mononucleosis

         B27.10   **Cytomegaloviral mononucleosis** without complications

         B27.11   **Cytomegaloviral mononucleosis** with polyneuropathy

         B27.12   **Cytomegaloviral mononucleosis** with meningitis

         B27.19   **Cytomegaloviral mononucleosis** with other complication
             Hepatomegaly in cytomegaloviral mononucleosis

     ✓5ᵗʰ **B27.8**   **Other infectious mononucleosis**

         B27.80   **Other infectious mononucleosis** without complication

         B27.81   **Other infectious mononucleosis** with polyneuropathy

         B27.82   **Other infectious mononucleosis** with meningitis

         B27.89   **Other infectious mononucleosis** with other complication
             Hepatomegaly in other infectious mononucleosis

     ✓5ᵗʰ **B27.9**   **Infectious mononucleosis, unspecified**

         B27.90   **Infectious mononucleosis, unspecified** without complication

         B27.91   **Infectious mononucleosis, unspecified** with polyneuropathy

         B27.92   **Infectious mononucleosis, unspecified** with meningitis

N Newborn: 0   P Pediatric: 0-17   M Maternity: 9-64   A Adult: 15-124   MCC Major Complication/Comorbidity   CC Complication/Comorbidity   SW Severe Wound Dx

452   ICD-10-CM 2020

B27.99   **Infectious mononucleosis, unspecified with other complication**
Hepatomegaly in unspecified infectious mononucleosis

☑4ᵗʰ **B30**   **Viral conjunctivitis**
     EXCLUDES 1   *herpesviral [herpes simplex] ocular disease (B00.5)*
                ocular zoster (B02.3)

Viral Conjunctivitis

Normal conjunctiva

Inflamed conjunctiva

B30.0   **Keratoconjunctivitis due to adenovirus**
Epidemic keratoconjunctivitis
Shipyard eye

B30.1   **Conjunctivitis due to adenovirus**
Acute adenoviral follicular conjunctivitis
Swimming-pool conjunctivitis

B30.2   **Viral pharyngoconjunctivitis**

B30.3   **Acute epidemic hemorrhagic conjunctivitis (enteroviral)**
Conjunctivitis due to coxsackievirus 24
Conjunctivitis due to enterovirus 70
Hemorrhagic conjunctivitis (acute)(epidemic)

B30.8   **Other viral conjunctivitis**
Newcastle conjunctivitis

B30.9   **Viral conjunctivitis, unspecified**

☑4ᵗʰ **B33**   **Other viral diseases, not elsewhere classified**

B33.0   **Epidemic myalgia**
Bornholm disease

B33.1   **Ross River disease**   CC
Epidemic polyarthritis and exanthema
Ross River fever
CC Excl: PDX collection 144

☑5ᵗʰ **B33.2**   **Viral carditis**
Coxsackie (virus) carditis

     B33.20   **Viral carditis, unspecified**   CC
          CC Excl: PDX collection 186

     B33.21   **Viral endocarditis**   CC
          CC Excl: PDX collection 187

     B33.22   **Viral myocarditis**   CC
          CC Excl: PDX collection 186

     B33.23   **Viral pericarditis**   CC
          CC Excl: PDX collection 188

     B33.24   **Viral cardiomyopathy**   HCC

B33.3   **Retrovirus infections, not elsewhere classified**
Retrovirus infection NOS

B33.4   **Hantavirus (cardio)-pulmonary syndrome [HPS] [HCPS]**   CC
Hantavirus disease with pulmonary manifestations
Sin nombre virus disease
Use additional code to identify any associated acute kidney failure (N17.9)
     EXCLUDES 1   *hantavirus disease with renal manifestations (A98.5)*
                hemorrhagic fever with renal manifestations (A98.5)
CC Excl: PDX collection 189

B33.8   **Other specified viral diseases**
     EXCLUDES 1   *anogenital human papillomavirus infection (A63.0)*
                viral warts due to human papillomavirus infection (B07)

☑4ᵗʰ **B34**   **Viral infection of unspecified site**
     EXCLUDES 1   *anogenital human papillomavirus infection (A63.0)*
                cytomegaloviral disease NOS (B25.9)
                herpesvirus [herpes simplex] infection NOS (B00.9)
                retrovirus infection NOS (B33.3)
                viral agents as the cause of diseases classified elsewhere (B97.-)
                viral warts due to human papillomavirus infection (B07)

B34.0   **Adenovirus infection, unspecified**

B34.1   **Enterovirus infection, unspecified**
Coxsackievirus infection NOS
Echovirus infection NOS

B34.2   **Coronavirus infection, unspecified**
     EXCLUDES 1   *pneumonia due to SARS-associated coronavirus (J12.81)*

B34.3   **Parvovirus infection, unspecified**   CC
     CC Excl: PDX collection 174

B34.4   **Papovavirus infection, unspecified**

B34.8   **Other viral infections of unspecified site**

B34.9   **Viral infection, unspecified**
Viremia NOS
AHA: 2016,3Q,10

Mycoses (B35-B49)

EXCLUDES 2   *hypersensitivity pneumonitis due to organic dust (J67.-)*
                mycosis fungoides (C84.0-)

☑4ᵗʰ **B35**   **Dermatophytosis**
     INCLUDES   favus
                infections due to species of Epidermophyton, Micro-sporum and Trichophyton
                tinea, any type except those in B36.-
DEF: Contagious superficial fungal infection of the skin that invades and grows in dead keratin.

B35.0   **Tinea barbae and tinea capitis**
Beard ringworm
Kerion
Scalp ringworm
Sycosis, mycotic

B35.1   **Tinea unguium**
Dermatophytic onychia
Dermatophytosis of nail
Onychomycosis
Ringworm of nails

B35.2   **Tinea manuum**
Dermatophytosis of hand
Hand ringworm

B35.3   **Tinea pedis**
Athlete's foot
Dermatophytosis of foot
Foot ringworm

B35.4   **Tinea corporis**
Ringworm of the body

B35.5   **Tinea imbricata**
Tokelau

B35.6   **Tinea cruris**
Dhobi itch
Groin ringworm
Jock itch

B35.8   **Other dermatophytoses**
Disseminated dermatophytosis
Granulomatous dermatophytosis

B35.9   **Dermatophytosis, unspecified**
Ringworm NOS

☑4ᵗʰ **B36**   **Other superficial mycoses**

B36.0   **Pityriasis versicolor**
Tinea flava
Tinea versicolor

B36.1 Tinea nigra
Keratomycosis nigricans palmaris
Microsporosis nigra
Pityriasis nigra

B36.2 White piedra
Tinea blanca

B36.3 Black piedra

B36.8 Other specified superficial mycoses

B36.9 Superficial mycosis, unspecified

√4ᵗʰ B37 Candidiasis

INCLUDES   candidosis
moniliasis

EXCLUDES 1   neonatal candidiasis (P37.5)

DEF: Candida: Genus of yeast-like fungi that are commonly found in the mouth, skin, intestinal tract, and vagina. It may cause a white, cheesy discharge.

B37.Ø Candidal stomatitis   HIV CC
Oral thrush
CC Excl: PDX collection 190

B37.1 Pulmonary candidiasis   HIV MCC HCC
Candidal bronchitis
Candidal pneumonia
CC Excl: PDX collection 190

B37.2 Candidiasis of skin and nail   HIV
Candidal onychia
Candidal paronychia
EXCLUDES 2   diaper dermatitis (L22)

B37.3 Candidiasis of vulva and vagina   ♀
Candidal vulvovaginitis
Monilial vulvovaginitis
Vaginal thrush

√5ᵗʰ B37.4 Candidiasis of other urogenital sites

B37.41 Candidal cystitis and urethritis   CC H6
CC Excl: PDX collection 191

B37.42 Candidal balanitis   ♂

B37.49 Other urogenital candidiasis   CC H6
Candidal pyelonephritis
CC Excl: PDX collection 191

B37.5 Candidal meningitis   HIV MCC
CC Excl: PDX collection 192

B37.6 Candidal endocarditis   HIV MCC
CC Excl: PDX collection 190

B37.7 Candidal sepsis   MCC HCC
Disseminated candidiasis
Systemic candidiasis
AHA: 2014,4Q,46
TIP: This code is assigned when sepsis is documented as due to any *Candida* type. If non-*Candida albicans* is documented, code B48.8 Other specified mycoses, is assigned.
CC Excl: PDX collection 193

√5ᵗʰ B37.8 Candidiasis of other sites
CC Excl: For CC codes in subcategory B37.8, unless otherwise noted: PDX collection 190

B37.81 Candidal esophagitis   HIV MCC HCC

B37.82 Candidal enteritis   HIV MCC
Candidal proctitis

B37.83 Candidal cheilitis   HIV CC

B37.84 Candidal otitis externa   HIV CC

B37.89 Other sites of candidiasis   HIV CC
Candidal osteomyelitis
CC Excl: PDX collection 194

B37.9 Candidiasis, unspecified   HIV
Thrush NOS

√4ᵗʰ B38 Coccidioidomycosis

B38.Ø Acute pulmonary coccidioidomycosis   HIV CC HCC
CC Excl: PDX collection 195

B38.1 Chronic pulmonary coccidioidomycosis   HIV CC HCC
CC Excl: PDX collection 196

B38.2 Pulmonary coccidioidomycosis, unspecified   HIV CC HCC
CC Excl: PDX collection 196

B38.3 Cutaneous coccidioidomycosis   HIV CC
CC Excl: PDX collection 197

B38.4 Coccidioidomycosis meningitis   HIV MCC
DEF: *Coccidioides immitis* infection of the lining of the brain and/or spinal cord.
CC Excl: PDX collection 198

B38.7 Disseminated coccidioidomycosis   HIV CC
Generalized coccidioidomycosis
CC Excl: PDX collection 199

√5ᵗʰ B38.8 Other forms of coccidioidomycosis

B38.81 Prostatic coccidioidomycosis   HIV CC ♂
CC Excl: PDX collection 197

B38.89 Other forms of coccidioidomycosis   HIV CC
CC Excl: PDX collection 199

B38.9 Coccidioidomycosis, unspecified   HIV CC
CC Excl: PDX collection 199

√4ᵗʰ B39 Histoplasmosis
Code first associated AIDS (B2Ø)
Use additional code for any associated manifestations, such as:
endocarditis (I39)
meningitis (GØ2)
pericarditis (I32)
retinitis (H32)
DEF: Type of lung infection caused by breathing in fungal spores often found in the droppings of bats and birds or soil contaminated by their droppings.
CC Excl: For MCC codes in category B39: PDX collection 200

Histoplasmosis

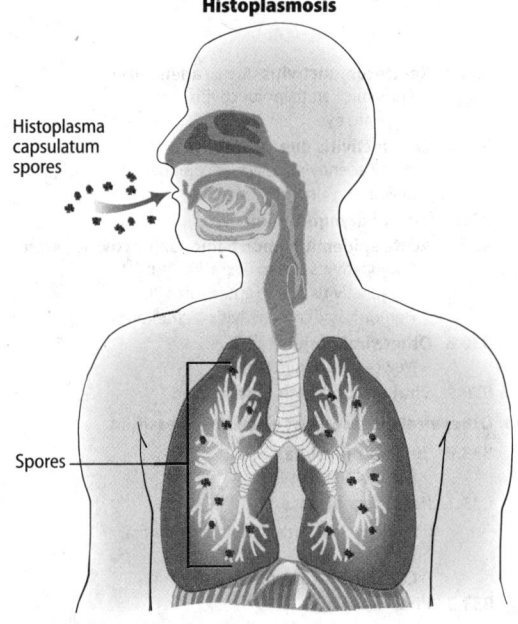

Histoplasma capsulatum spores

Spores

B39.Ø Acute pulmonary histoplasmosis capsulati   HIV MCC HCC

B39.1 Chronic pulmonary histoplasmosis capsulati   HIV MCC HCC

B39.2 Pulmonary histoplasmosis capsulati, unspecified   HIV MCC HCC

B39.3 Disseminated histoplasmosis capsulati   HIV CC
Generalized histoplasmosis capsulati
CC Excl: PDX collection 201

B39.4 Histoplasmosis capsulati, unspecified   HIV
American histoplasmosis

B39.5 Histoplasmosis duboisii   HIV
African histoplasmosis

B39.9 Histoplasmosis, unspecified   HIV

√4ᵗʰ B40 Blastomycosis
EXCLUDES 1   Brazilian blastomycosis (B41.-)
keloidal blastomycosis (B48.Ø)
CC Excl: For CC codes in category B40: PDX collection 202

B40.Ø Acute pulmonary blastomycosis   CC HCC

B40.1 Chronic pulmonary blastomycosis   CC HCC

B40.2 Pulmonary blastomycosis, unspecified   CC HCC

B40.3 Cutaneous blastomycosis   CC

B40.7   **Disseminated blastomycosis**   `CC`
    Generalized blastomycosis

✓5th **B40.8**   **Other forms of blastomycosis**

    B40.81   **Blastomycotic meningoencephalitis**   `CC`
      Meningomyelitis due to blastomycosis

    B40.89   **Other forms of blastomycosis**   `CC`

B40.9   **Blastomycosis, unspecified**   `CC`

✓4th **B41**   **Paracoccidioidomycosis**

    INCLUDES   Brazilian blastomycosis
           Lutz' disease

    CC Excl: For CC codes in category B41: PDX collection 203

B41.0   **Pulmonary paracoccidioidomycosis**   `CC` `HCC`

B41.7   **Disseminated paracoccidioidomycosis**   `CC`
    Generalized paracoccidioidomycosis

B41.8   **Other forms of paracoccidioidomycosis**   `CC`

B41.9   **Paracoccidioidomycosis, unspecified**   `CC`

✓4th **B42**   **Sporotrichosis**

B42.0   **Pulmonary sporotrichosis**

B42.1   **Lymphocutaneous sporotrichosis**

B42.7   **Disseminated sporotrichosis**
    Generalized sporotrichosis

✓5th **B42.8**   **Other forms of sporotrichosis**

    B42.81   **Cerebral sporotrichosis**
      Meningitis due to sporotrichosis

    B42.82   **Sporotrichosis arthritis**   `HCC`

    B42.89   **Other forms of sporotrichosis**

B42.9   **Sporotrichosis, unspecified**

✓4th **B43**   **Chromomycosis and pheomycotic abscess**

B43.0   **Cutaneous chromomycosis**
    Dermatitis verrucosa

B43.1   **Pheomycotic brain abscess**
    Cerebral chromomycosis

B43.2   **Subcutaneous pheomycotic abscess and cyst**

B43.8   **Other forms of chromomycosis**

B43.9   **Chromomycosis, unspecified**

✓4th **B44**   **Aspergillosis**

    INCLUDES   aspergilloma

    CC Excl: For CC codes in category B44, unless otherwise noted: PDX collection 204

B44.0   **Invasive pulmonary aspergillosis**   `MCC` `HCC`
    CC Excl: PDX collection 110

B44.1   **Other pulmonary aspergillosis**   `CC` `HCC`

B44.2   **Tonsillar aspergillosis**   `CC` `HCC`

B44.7   **Disseminated aspergillosis**   `CC` `HCC`
    Generalized aspergillosis

✓5th **B44.8**   **Other forms of aspergillosis**

    B44.81   **Allergic bronchopulmonary aspergillosis**   `CC` `HCC`
      CC Excl: PDX collection 205

    B44.89   **Other forms of aspergillosis**   `CC` `HCC`

B44.9   **Aspergillosis, unspecified**   `CC` `HCC`

✓4th **B45**   **Cryptococcosis**

    CC Excl: For CC codes in category B45: PDX collection 206

B45.0   **Pulmonary cryptococcosis**   `HIV` `CC` `HCC`

B45.1   **Cerebral cryptococcosis**   `MCC` `HCC`
    Cryptococcal meningitis
    Cryptococcosis meningocerebralis
    CC Excl: PDX collection 207

B45.2   **Cutaneous cryptococcosis**   `HIV` `CC` `HCC`

B45.3   **Osseous cryptococcosis**   `HIV` `CC` `HCC`

B45.7   **Disseminated cryptococcosis**   `HIV` `CC` `HCC`
    Generalized cryptococcosis

B45.8   **Other forms of cryptococcosis**   `HIV` `CC` `HCC`

B45.9   **Cryptococcosis, unspecified**   `HIV` `CC` `HCC`

✓4th **B46**   **Zygomycosis**

    CC Excl: For MCC codes in category B46: PDX collection 208

B46.0   **Pulmonary mucormycosis**   `MCC` `HCC`

B46.1   **Rhinocerebral mucormycosis**   `MCC` `HCC`

B46.2   **Gastrointestinal mucormycosis**   `MCC` `HCC`

B46.3   **Cutaneous mucormycosis**   `MCC` `HCC`
    Subcutaneous mucormycosis

B46.4   **Disseminated mucormycosis**   `MCC` `HCC`
    Generalized mucormycosis

B46.5   **Mucormycosis, unspecified**   `MCC` `HCC`

B46.8   **Other zygomycoses**   `MCC` `HCC`
    Entomophthoromycosis

B46.9   **Zygomycosis, unspecified**   `MCC` `HCC`
    Phycomycosis NOS

✓4th **B47**   **Mycetoma**

B47.0   **Eumycetoma**   `CC`
    Madura foot, mycotic
    Maduromycosis
    CC Excl: PDX collection 209

B47.1   **Actinomycetoma**   `HIV` `CC`
    CC Excl: PDX collection 106

B47.9   **Mycetoma, unspecified**   `HIV` `CC`
    Madura foot NOS
    CC Excl: PDX collection 210

✓4th **B48**   **Other mycoses, not elsewhere classified**

B48.0   **Lobomycosis**
    Keloidal blastomycosis
    Lobo's disease

B48.1   **Rhinosporidiosis**

B48.2   **Allescheriasis**   `CC`
    Infection due to Pseudallescheria boydii
    EXCLUDES 1   eumycetoma (B47.0)
    CC Excl: PDX collection 211

B48.3   **Geotrichosis**   `CC`
    Geotrichum stomatitis
    CC Excl: PDX collection 212

B48.4   **Penicillosis**   `CC` `HCC`
    CC Excl: PDX collection 204

B48.8   **Other specified mycoses**   `HIV` `CC` `HCC`
    Adiaspiromycosis
    Infection of tissue and organs by Alternaria
    Infection of tissue and organs by Drechslera
    Infection of tissue and organs by Fusarium
    Infection of tissue and organs by saprophytic fungi NEC
    AHA: 2014,4Q,46; 2014,2Q,13
    TIP: This code is assigned when sepsis is documented as due to non-*Candida albicans*. If sepsis is due to any *Candida* type, code B37.7 Candidal sepsis, is assigned.
    CC Excl: PDX collection 213

B49   **Unspecified mycosis**   `CC`
    Fungemia NOS
    CC Excl: PDX collection 212

Protozoal diseases (B50-B64)

    EXCLUDES 1   amebiasis (A06.-)
          other protozoal intestinal diseases (A07.-)

✓4th **B50**   **Plasmodium falciparum malaria**

    INCLUDES   mixed infections of Plasmodium falciparum with any other Plasmodium species

    CC Excl: For CC/MCC codes in category B50: PDX collection 214

B50.0   **Plasmodium falciparum malaria with cerebral complications**   `CC`
    Cerebral malaria NOS

B50.8   **Other severe and complicated Plasmodium falciparum malaria**   `CC`
    Severe or complicated Plasmodium falciparum malaria NOS

B50.9   **Plasmodium falciparum malaria, unspecified**   `MCC`

✓4th **B51**   **Plasmodium vivax malaria**

    INCLUDES   mixed infections of Plasmodium vivax with other Plasmodium species, except Plasmodium falciparum

    EXCLUDES 1   *Plasmodium vivax with Plasmodium falciparum (B50.-)*

B51.0   **Plasmodium vivax malaria with rupture of spleen**   `CC`
    CC Excl: PDX collection 214

✓ Additional Character Required   ✓x7th Placeholder   Unacceptable PDx   Questionable PDx   Manifestation   Unspecified Dx   H1-H14 HAC   HCC CMS-HCC Dx   HIV HIV Dx

B51.8 Plasmodium vivax malaria with other **complications** `CC`
     CC Excl: PDX collection 214

B51.9 Plasmodium vivax malaria without **complication** `CC`
     Plasmodium vivax malaria NOS
     CC Excl: PDX collection 215

✓4ᵗʰ **B52 Plasmodium** malariae **malaria**
     INCLUDES   mixed infections of Plasmodium malariae with other Plasmodium species, except Plasmodium falciparum and Plasmodium vivax
     EXCLUDES 1   *Plasmodium falciparum (B50.-)*
             Plasmodium vivax (B51.-)

B52.0 Plasmodium malariae malaria with nephropathy `CC`
     CC Excl: PDX collection 216

B52.8 Plasmodium malariae malaria with other **complications** `CC`
     CC Excl: PDX collection 214

B52.9 Plasmodium malariae malaria without **complication** `CC`
     Plasmodium malariae malaria NOS
     CC Excl: PDX collection 214

✓4ᵗʰ **B53 Other specified malaria**
     CC Excl: For CC codes in subcategory B53: PDX collection 214

B53.0 Plasmodium ovale malaria `CC`
     EXCLUDES 1   *Plasmodium ovale with Plasmodium falciparum (B50.-)*
             Plasmodium ovale with Plasmodium malariae (B52.-)
             Plasmodium ovale with Plasmodium vivax (B51.-)

B53.1 Malaria due to simian plasmodia `CC`
     EXCLUDES 1   *malaria due to simian plasmodia with Plasmodium falciparum (B50.-)*
             malaria due to simian plasmodia with Plasmodium malariae (B52.-)
             malaria due to simian plasmodia with Plasmodium ovale (B53.0)
             malaria due to simian plasmodia with Plasmodium vivax (B51.-)

B53.8 Other malaria, not elsewhere classified `CC`

B54 Unspecified malaria `CC`
     CC Excl: PDX collection 217

✓4ᵗʰ **B55 Leishmaniasis**
     CC Excl: For CC codes in category B55: PDX collection 218

B55.0 Visceral leishmaniasis `CC`
     Kala-azar
     Post-kala-azar dermal leishmaniasis

B55.1 Cutaneous leishmaniasis `CC`

B55.2 Mucocutaneous leishmaniasis `CC`

B55.9 Leishmaniasis, unspecified `CC`

✓4ᵗʰ **B56 African trypanosomiasis**
     CC Excl: For CC codes in category B56: PDX collection 218

B56.0 Gambiense trypanosomiasis `CC`
     Infection due to Trypanosoma brucei gambiense
     West African sleeping sickness

B56.1 Rhodesiense trypanosomiasis `CC`
     East African sleeping sickness
     Infection due to Trypanosoma brucei rhodesiense

B56.9 African trypanosomiasis, unspecified `CC`
     Sleeping sickness NOS

✓4ᵗʰ **B57 Chagas' disease**
     INCLUDES   American trypanosomiasis
                  infection due to Trypanosoma cruzi
     CC Excl: For CC codes in category B57, unless otherwise noted: PDX collection 218

B57.0 Acute Chagas' disease with heart involvement `CC`
     Acute Chagas' disease with myocarditis
     CC Excl: PDX collection 219

B57.1 Acute Chagas' disease without **heart involvement** `CC`
     Acute Chagas' disease NOS

B57.2 Chagas' disease (chronic) with heart involvement `CC`
     American trypanosomiasis NOS
     Chagas' disease (chronic) NOS
     Chagas' disease (chronic) with myocarditis
     Trypanosomiasis NOS
     CC Excl: PDX collection 219

✓5ᵗʰ **B57.3 Chagas' disease (chronic) with digestive system involvement**

B57.30 Chagas' disease with digestive system involvement, unspecified `CC`

B57.31 Megaesophagus in Chagas' disease `CC`

B57.32 Megacolon in Chagas' disease `CC`

B57.39 Other digestive system involvement in Chagas' disease `CC`

✓5ᵗʰ **B57.4 Chagas' disease (chronic) with nervous system involvement**

B57.40 Chagas' disease with nervous system involvement, unspecified `CC`

B57.41 Meningitis in Chagas' disease `CC`

B57.42 Meningoencephalitis in Chagas' disease `CC`

B57.49 Other nervous system involvement in Chagas' disease `CC`

B57.5 Chagas' disease (chronic) with other organ involvement `CC`

✓4ᵗʰ **B58 Toxoplasmosis**
     INCLUDES   infection due to Toxoplasma gondii
     EXCLUDES 1   *congenital toxoplasmosis (P37.1)*

✓5ᵗʰ **B58.0 Toxoplasma oculopathy**

B58.00 Toxoplasma oculopathy, unspecified `HIV` `CC`
     CC Excl: PDX collection 220

B58.01 Toxoplasma chorioretinitis `HIV` `CC`
     CC Excl: PDX collection 221

B58.09 Other toxoplasma oculopathy `HIV` `CC`
     Toxoplasma uveitis
     CC Excl: PDX collection 222

B58.1 Toxoplasma hepatitis `HIV` `CC`
     CC Excl: PDX collection 223

B58.2 Toxoplasma meningoencephalitis `HIV` `MCC` `HCC`
     CC Excl: PDX collection 224

B58.3 Pulmonary toxoplasmosis `HIV` `MCC` `HCC`
     CC Excl: PDX collection 225

✓5ᵗʰ **B58.8 Toxoplasmosis with other organ involvement**
     CC Excl: For CC codes in subcategory B58.8: PDX collection 220

B58.81 Toxoplasma myocarditis `HIV` `MCC`
     CC Excl: PDX collection 226

B58.82 Toxoplasma myositis `HIV` `CC`

B58.83 Toxoplasma tubulo-interstitial nephropathy `HIV` `CC`
     Toxoplasma pyelonephritis

B58.89 Toxoplasmosis with other organ involvement `HIV` `CC`

B58.9 Toxoplasmosis, unspecified `HIV` `CC`
     CC Excl: PDX collection 227

B59 Pneumocystosis `HIV` `MCC` `HCC`
     Pneumonia due to Pneumocystis carinii
     Pneumonia due to Pneumocystis jiroveci
     CC Excl: PDX collection 228

✓4ᵗʰ **B60 Other protozoal diseases, not elsewhere classified**
     EXCLUDES 1   *cryptosporidiosis (A07.2)*
             intestinal microsporidiosis (A07.8)
             isosporiasis (A07.3)
     CC Excl: For CC codes in category B60, unless otherwise noted: PDX collection 229

B60.0 Babesiosis `CC`
     Piroplasmosis
     CC Excl: PDX collection 218

✓5ᵗʰ **B60.1 Acanthamebiasis**

B60.10 Acanthamebiasis, unspecified `CC`

B60.11 Meningoencephalitis due to Acanthamoeba (culbertsoni)

B60.12 Conjunctivitis due to Acanthamoeba

B60.13 Keratoconjunctivitis due to Acanthamoeba

B60.19 Other acanthamebic disease `CC`

N Newborn: 0   P Pediatric: 0-17   M Maternity: 9-64   A Adult: 15-124   `MCC` Major Complication/Comorbidity   `CC` Complication/Comorbidity   `SW` Severe Wound Dx

456   ICD-10-CM 2020

B60.2 **Naegleriasis** `CC`
Primary amebic meningoencephalitis

B60.8 **Other specified protozoal diseases** `HIV`
Microsporidiosis

B64 Unspecified protozoal disease

Helminthiases (B65-B83)

✓4ᵗʰ **B65 Schistosomiasis [bilharziasis]**
  INCLUDES   snail fever
  CC Excl: For CC codes in category B65: PDX collection 230

B65.0 **Schistosomiasis due to Schistosoma haematobium [urinary schistosomiasis]** `CC`

B65.1 **Schistosomiasis due to Schistosoma mansoni [intestinal schistosomiasis]** `CC`

B65.2 **Schistosomiasis due to Schistosoma japonicum** `CC`
Asiatic schistosomiasis

B65.3 **Cercarial dermatitis** `CC`
Swimmer's itch

B65.8 **Other schistosomiasis** `CC`
Infection due to Schistosoma intercalatum
Infection due to Schistosoma mattheei
Infection due to Schistosoma mekongi

B65.9 **Schistosomiasis, unspecified** `CC`

✓4ᵗʰ **B66 Other fluke infections**
  CC Excl: For CC codes in category B66: PDX collection 231

B66.0 **Opisthorchiasis** `CC`
Infection due to cat liver fluke
Infection due to Opisthorchis (felineus)(viverrini)

B66.1 **Clonorchiasis** `CC`
Chinese liver fluke disease
Infection due to Clonorchis sinensis
Oriental liver fluke disease

B66.2 **Dicroceliasis** `CC`
Infection due to Dicrocoelium dendriticum
Lancet fluke infection

B66.3 **Fascioliasis** `CC`
Infection due to Fasciola gigantica
Infection due to Fasciola hepatica
Infection due to Fasciola indica
Sheep liver fluke disease

B66.4 **Paragonimiasis** `CC` `HCC`
Infection due to Paragonimus species
Lung fluke disease
Pulmonary distomiasis

B66.5 **Fasciolopsiasis** `CC`
Infection due to Fasciolopsis buski
Intestinal distomiasis

B66.8 **Other specified fluke infections** `CC`
Echinostomiasis
Heterophyiasis
Metagonimiasis
Nanophyetiasis
Watsoniasis

B66.9 **Fluke infection, unspecified**

✓4ᵗʰ **B67 Echinococcosis**
  INCLUDES   hydatidosis

B67.0 **Echinococcus granulosus infection of liver** `CC`
  CC Excl: PDX collection 232

B67.1 **Echinococcus granulosus infection of lung** `CC` `HCC`
  CC Excl: PDX collection 233

B67.2 **Echinococcus granulosus infection of bone** `CC`
  CC Excl: PDX collection 234

✓5ᵗʰ B67.3 **Echinococcus granulosus infection, other and multiple sites**

B67.31 **Echinococcus granulosus infection, thyroid gland** `CC`
  CC Excl: PDX collection 235

B67.32 **Echinococcus granulosus infection, multiple sites** `CC`
  CC Excl: PDX collection 234

B67.39 **Echinococcus granulosus infection, other sites** `CC`
  CC Excl: PDX collection 234

B67.4 **Echinococcus granulosus infection, unspecified** `CC`
Dog tapeworm (infection)
  CC Excl: PDX collection 236

B67.5 **Echinococcus multilocularis infection of liver** `CC`
  CC Excl: PDX collection 237

✓5ᵗʰ B67.6 **Echinococcus multilocularis infection, other and multiple sites**

B67.61 **Echinococcus multilocularis infection, multiple sites** `CC`
  CC Excl: PDX collection 238

B67.69 **Echinococcus multilocularis infection, other sites** `CC`
  CC Excl: PDX collection 238

B67.7 **Echinococcus multilocularis infection, unspecified** `CC`
  CC Excl: PDX collection 239

B67.8 **Echinococcosis, unspecified, of liver** `CC`
  CC Excl: PDX collection 240

✓5ᵗʰ B67.9 **Echinococcosis, other and unspecified**

B67.90 **Echinococcosis, unspecified** `CC`
Echinococcosis NOS
  CC Excl: PDX collection 240

B67.99 **Other echinococcosis** `CC`
  CC Excl: PDX collection 240

✓4ᵗʰ **B68 Taeniasis**
  EXCLUDES 1   cysticercosis (B69.-)

B68.0 **Taenia solium taeniasis** `CC`
Pork tapeworm (infection)
  CC Excl: PDX collection 241

B68.1 **Taenia saginata taeniasis** `CC`
Beef tapeworm (infection)
Infection due to adult tapeworm Taenia saginata
  CC Excl: PDX collection 242

B68.9 **Taeniasis, unspecified** `CC`
  CC Excl: PDX collection 242

✓4ᵗʰ **B69 Cysticercosis**
  INCLUDES   cysticerciasis infection due to larval form of Taenia solium
  DEF: Condition that is developed when larvae or eggs of the tapeworm *Taenia solium* are ingested, most commonly in fecally contaminated water or undercooked pork.
  CC Excl: For CC codes in category B69: PDX collection 242

B69.0 **Cysticercosis of central nervous system** `CC`

B69.1 **Cysticercosis of eye** `CC`

✓5ᵗʰ B69.8 **Cysticercosis of other sites**

B69.81 **Myositis in cysticercosis** `CC`

B69.89 **Cysticercosis of other sites** `CC`

B69.9 **Cysticercosis, unspecified** `CC`

✓4ᵗʰ **B70 Diphyllobothriasis and sparganosis**

B70.0 **Diphyllobothriasis** `CC`
Diphyllobothrium (adult) (latum) (pacificum) infection
Fish tapeworm (infection)
  EXCLUDES 2   larval diphyllobothriasis (B70.1)
  CC Excl: PDX collection 242

B70.1 **Sparganosis** `CC`
Infection due to Sparganum (mansoni) (proliferum)
Infection due to Spirometra larva
Larval diphyllobothriasis
Spirometrosis
  CC Excl: PDX collection 242

✓4ᵗʰ **B71 Other cestode infections**
  CC Excl: For CC codes in category B71: PDX collection 242

B71.0 **Hymenolepiasis** `CC`
Dwarf tapeworm infection
Rat tapeworm (infection)

B71.1 **Dipylidiasis** `CC`

B71.8 **Other specified cestode infections** `CC`
Coenurosis

✔ Additional Character Required   ✓x7ᵗʰ Placeholder   Unacceptable PDx   Questionable PDx   Manifestation   Unspecified Dx   H1-H14 HAC   HCC CMS-HCC Dx   HIV HIV Dx

ICD-10-CM 2020   457

Chapter 1. Certain Infectious and Parasitic Diseases

B71.9 Cestode infection, unspecified
Tapeworm (infection) NOS

B72 Dracunculiasis [CC]
INCLUDES guinea worm infection
infection due to Dracunculus medinensis
CC Excl: PDX collection 243

✓4ᵗʰ B73 Onchocerciasis
INCLUDES onchocerca volvulus infection
onchocercosis
river blindness
CC Excl: For CC codes in category B73: PDX collection 243

✓5ᵗʰ B73.0 Onchocerciasis with eye disease
B73.00 Onchocerciasis with eye involvement, unspecified [CC]
B73.01 Onchocerciasis with endophthalmitis [CC]
B73.02 Onchocerciasis with glaucoma [CC]
B73.09 Onchocerciasis with other eye involvement [CC]
Infestation of eyelid due to onchocerciasis

B73.1 Onchocerciasis without eye disease [CC]

✓4ᵗʰ B74 Filariasis
EXCLUDES 2 onchocerciasis (B73)
tropical (pulmonary) eosinophilia NOS (J82)
CC Excl: For CC codes in category B74: PDX collection 243

B74.0 Filariasis due to Wuchereria bancrofti [CC]
Bancroftian elephantiasis
Bancroftian filariasis
B74.1 Filariasis due to Brugia malayi [CC]
B74.2 Filariasis due to Brugia timori [CC]
B74.3 Loiasis [CC]
Calabar swelling
Eyeworm disease of Africa
Loa loa infection
B74.4 Mansonelliasis [CC]
Infection due to Mansonella ozzardi
Infection due to Mansonella perstans
Infection due to Mansonella streptocerca
B74.8 Other filariases [CC]
Dirofilariasis
B74.9 Filariasis, unspecified [CC]

B75 Trichinellosis [CC]
INCLUDES infection due to Trichinella species
trichiniasis
DEF: Infection by *Trichinella spiralis*, the smallest of the parasitic nematodes, that is transmitted by eating undercooked pork or bear meat.
Synonym(s): *Trichinosis.*
CC Excl: PDX collection 244

✓4ᵗʰ B76 Hookworm diseases
INCLUDES uncinariasis
CC Excl: For CC codes in category B76: PDX collection 245

B76.0 Ancylostomiasis [CC]
Infection due to Ancylostoma species
B76.1 Necatoriasis [CC]
Infection due to Necator americanus
B76.8 Other hookworm diseases [CC]
B76.9 Hookworm disease, unspecified [CC]
Cutaneous larva migrans NOS

✓4ᵗʰ B77 Ascariasis
INCLUDES ascaridiasis
roundworm infection
CC Excl: For CC codes in category B77: PDX collection 246

B77.0 Ascariasis with intestinal complications [CC]
✓5ᵗʰ B77.8 Ascariasis with other complications
B77.81 Ascariasis pneumonia [MCC]
CC Excl: PDX collection 247
B77.89 Ascariasis with other complications [CC]
B77.9 Ascariasis, unspecified [CC]

✓4ᵗʰ B78 Strongyloidiasis
EXCLUDES 1 trichostrongyliasis (B81.2)
CC Excl: For CC codes in category B78: PDX collection 246
B78.0 Intestinal strongyloidiasis [HIV][CC]
B78.1 Cutaneous strongyloidiasis
B78.7 Disseminated strongyloidiasis [HIV][CC]
B78.9 Strongyloidiasis, unspecified [HIV][CC]

B79 Trichuriasis [CC]
INCLUDES trichocephaliasis
whipworm (disease)(infection)
CC Excl: PDX collection 246

B80 Enterobiasis [CC]
INCLUDES oxyuriasis
pinworm infection
threadworm infection
CC Excl: PDX collection 246

✓4ᵗʰ B81 Other intestinal helminthiases, not elsewhere classified
EXCLUDES 1 angiostrongyliasis due to:
angiostrongylus cantonensis (B83.2)
parastrongylus cantonensis (B83.2)

B81.0 Anisakiasis [CC]
Infection due to Anisakis larva
CC Excl: PDX collection 246
B81.1 Intestinal capillariasis [CC]
Capillariasis NOS
Infection due to Capillaria philippinensis
EXCLUDES 2 hepatic capillariasis (B83.8)
CC Excl: PDX collection 246
B81.2 Trichostrongyliasis [CC]
CC Excl: PDX collection 246
B81.3 Intestinal angiostrongyliasis [CC]
Angiostrongyliasis due to:
angiostrongylus costaricensis
parastrongylus costaricensis
CC Excl: PDX collection 248
B81.4 Mixed intestinal helminthiases [CC]
Infection due to intestinal helminths classified to more than one of the categories B65.0-B81.3 and B81.8
Mixed helminthiasis NOS
CC Excl: PDX collection 248
B81.8 Other specified intestinal helminthiases [CC]
Infection due to Oesophagostomum species [esophagostomiasis]
Infection due to Ternidens diminutus [ternidensiasis]
CC Excl: PDX collection 248

✓4ᵗʰ B82 Unspecified intestinal parasitism
B82.0 Intestinal helminthiasis, unspecified [CC]
CC Excl: PDX collection 248
B82.9 Intestinal parasitism, unspecified

✓4ᵗʰ B83 Other helminthiases
EXCLUDES 1 capillariasis NOS (B81.1)
EXCLUDES 2 intestinal capillariasis (B81.1)
B83.0 Visceral larva migrans
Toxocariasis
B83.1 Gnathostomiasis
Wandering swelling
B83.2 Angiostrongyliasis due to Parastrongylus cantonensis
Eosinophilic meningoencephalitis due to Parastrongylus cantonensis
EXCLUDES 2 intestinal angiostrongyliasis (B81.3)
B83.3 Syngamiasis
Syngamosis
B83.4 Internal hirudiniasis
EXCLUDES 2 external hirudiniasis (B88.3)
B83.8 Other specified helminthiases
Acanthocephaliasis
Gongylonemiasis
Hepatic capillariasis
Metastrongyliasis
Thelaziasis

B83.9   **Helminthiasis, unspecified**
Worms NOS
EXCLUDES 1   *intestinal helminthiasis NOS (B82.0)*

Pediculosis, acariasis and other infestations (B85-B89)

✓4ᵗʰ **B85**   **Pediculosis and phthiriasis**

B85.0   **Pediculosis due to Pediculus humanus capitis**
Head-louse infestation

B85.1   **Pediculosis due to Pediculus humanus corporis**
Body-louse infestation

B85.2   **Pediculosis, unspecified**

B85.3   **Phthiriasis**
Infestation by crab-louse
Infestation by Phthirus pubis

B85.4   **Mixed pediculosis and phthiriasis**
Infestation classifiable to more than one of the categories B85.0-B85.3

B86   **Scabies**
Sarcoptic itch
DEF: Mite infestation that is caused by *Sarcoptes scabiei*. Scabies causes intense itching and sometimes secondary infection.

✓4ᵗʰ **B87**   **Myiasis**
INCLUDES   infestation by larva of flies

B87.0   **Cutaneous myiasis**
Creeping myiasis

B87.1   **Wound myiasis**
Traumatic myiasis

B87.2   **Ocular myiasis**

B87.3   **Nasopharyngeal myiasis**
Laryngeal myiasis

B87.4   **Aural myiasis**

✓5ᵗʰ **B87.8**   **Myiasis of other sites**

     B87.81   **Genitourinary myiasis**

     B87.82   **Intestinal myiasis**

     B87.89   **Myiasis of other sites**

B87.9   **Myiasis, unspecified**

✓4ᵗʰ **B88**   **Other infestations**

B88.0   **Other acariasis**
Acarine dermatitis
Dermatitis due to Demodex species
Dermatitis due to Dermanyssus gallinae
Dermatitis due to Liponyssoides sanguineus
Trombiculosis
EXCLUDES 2   *scabies (B86)*

B88.1   **Tungiasis [sandflea infestation]**

B88.2   **Other arthropod infestations**
Scarabiasis

B88.3   **External hirudiniasis**
Leech infestation NOS
EXCLUDES 2   *internal hirudiniasis (B83.4)*

B88.8   **Other specified infestations**
Ichthyoparasitism due to Vandellia cirrhosa
Linguatulosis
Porocephaliasis

B88.9   **Infestation, unspecified**
Infestation (skin) NOS
Infestation by mites NOS
Skin parasites NOS

B89   **Unspecified parasitic disease**

Sequelae of infectious and parasitic diseases (B90-B94)

NOTE   Categories B90-B94 are to be used to indicate conditions in categories A00-B89 as the cause of sequelae, which are themselves classified elsewhere. The "sequelae" include conditions specified as such; they also include residuals of diseases classifiable to the above categories if there is evidence that the disease itself is no longer present. Codes from these categories are not to be used for chronic infections. Code chronic current infections to active infectious disease as appropriate.

Code first condition resulting from (sequela) the infectious or parasitic disease

✓4ᵗʰ **B90**   **Sequelae of tuberculosis**

B90.0   **Sequelae of central nervous system tuberculosis**

B90.1   **Sequelae of genitourinary tuberculosis**

B90.2   **Sequelae of tuberculosis of bones and joints**

B90.8   **Sequelae of tuberculosis of other organs**
EXCLUDES 2   *sequelae of respiratory tuberculosis (B90.9)*

B90.9   **Sequelae of respiratory and unspecified tuberculosis**
Sequelae of tuberculosis NOS

B91   **Sequelae of poliomyelitis**
EXCLUDES 1   *postpolio syndrome (G14)*

B92   **Sequelae of leprosy**

✓4ᵗʰ **B94**   **Sequelae of other and unspecified infectious and parasitic diseases**

B94.0   **Sequelae of trachoma**

B94.1   **Sequelae of viral encephalitis**

B94.2   **Sequelae of viral hepatitis**

B94.8   **Sequelae of other specified infectious and parasitic diseases**
AHA: 2017,4Q,109

B94.9   **Sequelae of unspecified infectious and parasitic disease**

Bacterial and viral infectious agents (B95-B97)

NOTE   These categories are provided for use as supplementary or additional codes to identify the infectious agent(s) in diseases classified elsewhere.

AHA: 2018,4Q,34; 2018,1Q,16

✓4ᵗʰ **B95**   **Streptococcus, Staphylococcus, and Enterococcus as the cause of diseases classified elsewhere**

B95.0   **Streptococcus, group A, as the cause of diseases classified elsewhere**

B95.1   **Streptococcus, group B, as the cause of diseases classified elsewhere**
AHA: 2019,2Q,8-10

B95.2   **Enterococcus as the cause of diseases classified elsewhere**

B95.3   **Streptococcus pneumoniae as the cause of diseases classified elsewhere**

B95.4   **Other streptococcus as the cause of diseases classified elsewhere**

B95.5   **Unspecified streptococcus as the cause of diseases classified elsewhere**

✓5ᵗʰ **B95.6**   **Staphylococcus aureus as the cause of diseases classified elsewhere**

     B95.61   **Methicillin susceptible Staphylococcus aureus infection as the cause of diseases classified elsewhere**
Methicillin susceptible Staphylococcus aureus (MSSA) infection as the cause of diseases classified elsewhere
Staphylococcus aureus infection NOS as the cause of diseases classified elsewhere

     B95.62   **Methicillin resistant Staphylococcus aureus infection as the cause of diseases classified elsewhere**
Methicillin resistant staphylococcus aureus (MRSA) infection as the cause of diseases classified elsewhere
AHA: 2016,1Q,12

B95.7   **Other staphylococcus as the cause of diseases classified elsewhere**

B95.8   **Unspecified staphylococcus as the cause of diseases classified elsewhere**

✓4ᵗʰ **B96**   **Other bacterial agents as the cause of diseases classified elsewhere**

B96.0   **Mycoplasma pneumoniae [M. pneumoniae] as the cause of diseases classified elsewhere**
Pleuro-pneumonia-like-organism [PPLO]

B96.1   **Klebsiella pneumoniae [K. pneumoniae] as the cause of diseases classified elsewhere**

✓5ᵗʰ **B96.2**   **Escherichia coli [E. coli] as the cause of diseases classified elsewhere**

     B96.20   **Unspecified Escherichia coli [E. coli] as the cause of diseases classified elsewhere**
Escherichia coli [E. coli] NOS

☑ Additional Character Required   ✓7ᵗʰ Placeholder   Unacceptable PDx   Questionable PDx   Manifestation   Unspecified Dx   H1 H14 HAC   HCC CMS HCC Dx   HIV HIV Dx

ICD-10-CM 2020   459

Chapter 1. Certain Infectious and Parasitic Diseases

B83.9–B96.20

Chapter 1. Certain Infectious and Parasitic Diseases

B96.21–B99.9

▲ **B96.21 Shiga toxin-producing Escherichia coli [E. coli] [STEC] O157 as the cause of diseases classified elsewhere**
     E. coli O157:H- (nonmotile) with confirmation of Shiga toxin
     E. coli O157 with confirmation of Shiga toxin when H antigen is unknown, or is not H7
     O157:H7 Escherichia coli [E.coli] with or without confirmation of Shiga toxin-production
     Shiga toxin-producing Escherichia coli [E.coli] O157:H7 with or without confirmation of Shiga toxin-production
     STEC O157:H7 with or without confirmation of Shiga toxin-production

▲ **B96.22 Other specified Shiga toxin-producing Escherichia coli [E. coli] [STEC] as the cause of diseases classified elsewhere**
     Non-O157 Shiga toxin-producing Escherichia coli [E.coli]
     Non-O157 Shiga toxin-producing Escherichia coli [E.coli] with known O group

▲ **B96.23 Unspecified Shiga toxin-producing Escherichia coli [E. coli] [STEC] as the cause of diseases classified elsewhere**
     Shiga toxin-producing Escherichia coli [E. coli] with unspecified O group
     STEC NOS

B96.29 Other Escherichia coli [E. coli] as the cause of diseases classified elsewhere
     Non-Shiga toxin-producing E. coli

B96.3 Hemophilus influenzae [H. influenzae] as the cause of diseases classified elsewhere

B96.4 Proteus (mirabilis) (morganii) as the cause of diseases classified elsewhere

B96.5 Pseudomonas (aeruginosa) (mallei) (pseudomallei) as the cause of diseases classified elsewhere
     AHA: 2015,1Q,18

B96.6 Bacteroides fragilis [B. fragilis] as the cause of diseases classified elsewhere

B96.7 Clostridium perfringens [C. perfringens] as the cause of diseases classified elsewhere

√5ᵗʰ **B96.8 Other specified bacterial agents as the cause of diseases classified elsewhere**

     B96.81 Helicobacter pylori [H. pylori] as the cause of diseases classified elsewhere

     B96.82 Vibrio vulnificus as the cause of diseases classified elsewhere

     B96.89 Other specified bacterial agents as the cause of diseases classified elsewhere

√4ᵗʰ **B97 Viral agents as the cause of diseases classified elsewhere**
     AHA: 2016,3Q,8-10,14

B97.0 Adenovirus as the cause of diseases classified elsewhere

√5ᵗʰ **B97.1 Enterovirus as the cause of diseases classified elsewhere**

     B97.10 Unspecified enterovirus as the cause of diseases classified elsewhere

     B97.11 Coxsackievirus as the cause of diseases classified elsewhere

     B97.12 Echovirus as the cause of diseases classified elsewhere

     B97.19 Other enterovirus as the cause of diseases classified elsewhere

√5ᵗʰ **B97.2 Coronavirus as the cause of diseases classified elsewhere**

     B97.21 SARS-associated coronavirus as the cause of diseases classified elsewhere   **cc**
         EXCLUDES 1   pneumonia due to SARS-associated coronavirus (J12.81)
         CC Excl: PDX collection 249

     B97.29 Other coronavirus as the cause of diseases classified elsewhere

√5ᵗʰ **B97.3 Retrovirus as the cause of diseases classified elsewhere**
         EXCLUDES 1   human immunodeficiency virus [HIV] disease (B20)

     B97.30 Unspecified retrovirus as the cause of diseases classified elsewhere

     B97.31 Lentivirus as the cause of diseases classified elsewhere

     B97.32 Oncovirus as the cause of diseases classified elsewhere

     B97.33 Human T-cell lymphotrophic virus, type I [HTLV-I] as the cause of diseases classified elsewhere   **cc**
         CC Excl: PDX collection 250

     B97.34 Human T-cell lymphotrophic virus, type II [HTLV-II] as the cause of diseases classified elsewhere   **cc**
         CC Excl: PDX collection 251

     B97.35 Human immunodeficiency virus, type 2 [HIV 2] as the cause of diseases classified elsewhere   **cc** **HCC**
         CC Excl: PDX collection 252

     B97.39 Other retrovirus as the cause of diseases classified elsewhere

B97.4 Respiratory syncytial virus as the cause of diseases classified elsewhere
     ▶RSV as the cause of diseases classified elsewhere◀
     ▶Code first related disorders, such as:◀
         ▶otitis media (H65.-)◀
         ▶upper respiratory infection (J06.9)◀
         EXCLUDES 2   ▶acute bronchiolitis due to respiratory syncytial virus (RSV) (J21.0)◀
                 ▶acute bronchitis due to respiratory syncytial virus (RSV) (J20.5)◀
                 ▶respiratory syncytial virus (RSV) pneumonia (J12.1)◀

B97.5 Reovirus as the cause of diseases classified elsewhere

B97.6 Parvovirus as the cause of diseases classified elsewhere

B97.7 Papillomavirus as the cause of diseases classified elsewhere

√5ᵗʰ **B97.8 Other viral agents as the cause of diseases classified elsewhere**

     B97.81 Human metapneumovirus as the cause of diseases classified elsewhere

     B97.89 Other viral agents as the cause of diseases classified elsewhere

Other infectious diseases (B99)

√4ᵗʰ **B99 Other and unspecified infectious diseases**

     B99.8 Other infectious disease   **HIV**

     B99.9 Unspecified infectious disease

N Newborn: 0   **P** Pediatric: 0-17   **M** Maternity: 9-64   **A** Adult: 15-124   **MCC** Major Complication/Comorbidity   **CC** Complication/Comorbidity   **SW** Severe Wound Dx

460
     ICD-10-CM 2020

Chapter 2. Neoplasms (C00–D49)

Chapter-specific Guidelines with Coding Examples

The chapter-specific guidelines from the ICD-10-CM Official Guidelines for Coding and Reporting have been provided below. Along with these guidelines are coding examples, contained in the shaded boxes, that have been developed to help illustrate the coding and/or sequencing guidance found in these guidelines.

General guidelines

Chapter 2 of the ICD-10-CM contains the codes for most benign and all malignant neoplasms. Certain benign neoplasms, such as prostatic adenomas, may be found in the specific body system chapters. To properly code a neoplasm it is necessary to determine from the record if the neoplasm is benign, in-situ, malignant, or of uncertain histologic behavior. If malignant, any secondary (metastatic) sites should also be determined.

Primary malignant neoplasms overlapping site boundaries

A primary malignant neoplasm that overlaps two or more contiguous (next to each other) sites should be classified to the subcategory/code .8 ('overlapping lesion'), unless the combination is specifically indexed elsewhere. For multiple neoplasms of the same site that are not contiguous such as tumors in different quadrants of the same breast, codes for each site should be assigned.

> A 73-year-old white female with a large rapidly growing malignant tumor in the left breast extending from the upper outer quadrant into the axillary tail
>
> **C50.812**   **Malignant neoplasm of overlapping sites of left female breast**
>
> *Explanation*: Because this is a single large tumor that overlaps two contiguous sites, a single code for overlapping sites is assigned.

> A 52-year old white female with two distinct lesions of the right breast, one (0.5 cm) in the upper outer quadrant and a second (1.5 cm) in the lower outer quadrant; path report indicates both lesions are malignant
>
> **C50.411**   **Malignant neoplasm of upper-outer quadrant of right female breast**
>
> **C50.511**   **Malignant neoplasm of lower-outer quadrant of right female breast**
>
> *Explanation*: This patient has two distinct malignant lesions of right breast in adjacent quadrants. Because the lesions are not contiguous, two codes are reported.

Malignant neoplasm of ectopic tissue

Malignant neoplasms of ectopic tissue are to be coded to the site of origin mentioned, e.g., ectopic pancreatic malignant neoplasms involving the stomach are coded to malignant neoplasm of pancreas, unspecified (C25.9).

The neoplasm table in the Alphabetic Index should be referenced first. However, if the histological term is documented, that term should be referenced first, rather than going immediately to the Neoplasm Table, in order to determine which column in the Neoplasm Table is appropriate. For example, if the documentation indicates "adenoma," refer to the term in the Alphabetic Index to review the entries under this term and the instructional note to "see also neoplasm, by site, benign." The table provides the proper code based on the type of neoplasm and the site. It is important to select the proper column in the table that corresponds to the type of neoplasm. The Tabular List should then be referenced to verify that the correct code has been selected from the table and that a more specific site code does not exist.

See Section I.C.21. Factors influencing health status and contact with health services, Status, for information regarding Z15.0, codes for genetic susceptibility to cancer.

a. Treatment directed at the malignancy

If the treatment is directed at the malignancy, designate the malignancy as the principal diagnosis.

The only exception to this guideline is if a patient admission/encounter is solely for the administration of chemotherapy, immunotherapy or external beam radiation therapy, assign the appropriate Z51.-- code as the first-listed or principal diagnosis, and the diagnosis or problem for which the service is being performed as a secondary diagnosis.

b. Treatment of secondary site

When a patient is admitted because of a primary neoplasm with metastasis and treatment is directed toward the secondary site only, the secondary neoplasm is designated as the principal diagnosis even though the primary malignancy is still present.

> Patient with primary prostate cancer with metastasis to lungs admitted for wedge resection of mass in right lung
>
> **C78.01**   **Secondary malignant neoplasm of right lung**
>
> **C61**   **Malignant neoplasm of prostate**
>
> *Explanation*: Since the admission is for treatment of the lung metastasis, the secondary lung metastasis is sequenced before the primary prostate cancer.

c. Coding and sequencing of complications

Coding and sequencing of complications associated with the malignancies or with the therapy thereof are subject to the following guidelines:

1) Anemia associated with malignancy

When admission/encounter is for management of an anemia associated with the malignancy, and the treatment is only for anemia, the appropriate code for the malignancy is sequenced as the principal or first-listed diagnosis followed by the appropriate code for the anemia (such as code D63.0, Anemia in neoplastic disease).

> Patient is admitted for treatment of anemia in advanced colon cancer
>
> **C18.9**   **Malignant neoplasm of colon, unspecified**
>
> **D63.0**   **Anemia in neoplastic disease**
>
> *Explanation*: Even though the admission was solely to treat the anemia, this guideline indicates that the code for the malignancy is sequenced first.

2) Anemia associated with chemotherapy, immunotherapy and radiation therapy

When the admission/encounter is for management of an anemia associated with an adverse effect of the administration of chemotherapy or immunotherapy and the only treatment is for the anemia, the anemia code is sequenced first followed by the appropriate codes for the neoplasm and the adverse effect (T45.1X5, Adverse effect of antineoplastic and immunosuppressive drugs).

> A 56-year-old Hispanic male with grade II follicular lymphoma involving multiple lymph node sites referred for blood transfusion to treat anemia due to chemotherapy
>
> **D64.81**   **Anemia due to antineoplastic chemotherapy**
>
> **C82.18**   **Follicular lymphoma grade II, lymph nodes of multiple sites**
>
> **T45.1X5A**   **Adverse effect of antineoplastic and immunosuppressive drugs, initial encounter**
>
> *Explanation*: The code for the anemia is sequenced first followed by the code for the malignant neoplasm and lastly the code for the adverse effect.

When the admission/encounter is for management of an anemia associated with an adverse effect of radiotherapy, the anemia code should be sequenced first, followed by the appropriate neoplasm code and code Y84.2, Radiological procedure and radiotherapy as the cause of abnormal reaction of the patient, or of later complication, without mention of misadventure at the time of the procedure.

A 55-year-old male with a large malignant rectal tumor has been receiving external radiation therapy to shrink the tumor prior to planned surgery. He is admitted today for a blood transfusion to treat anemia related to radiation therapy.

D64.89   **Other specified anemias**

C20   **Malignant neoplasm of rectum**

Y84.2   **Radiological procedure and radiotherapy as the cause of abnormal reaction of the patient, or of later complication, without mention of misadventure at the time of the procedure**

Explanation: The code for the anemia is sequenced first, followed by the code for the malignancy, and lastly the code for the abnormal reaction due to radiotherapy.

3) Management of dehydration due to the malignancy

When the admission/encounter is for management of dehydration due to the malignancy and only the dehydration is being treated (intravenous rehydration), the dehydration is sequenced first, followed by the code(s) for the malignancy.

4) Treatment of a complication resulting from a surgical procedure

When the admission/encounter is for treatment of a complication resulting from a surgical procedure, designate the complication as the principal or first-listed diagnosis if treatment is directed at resolving the complication.

d. Primary malignancy previously excised

When a primary malignancy has been previously excised or eradicated from its site and there is no further treatment directed to that site and there is no evidence of any existing primary malignancy at that site, a code from category Z85, Personal history of malignant neoplasm, should be used to indicate the former site of the malignancy. Any mention of extension, invasion, or metastasis to another site is coded as a secondary malignant neoplasm to that site. The secondary site may be the principal or first-listed **diagnosis** with the Z85 code used as a secondary code.

History of breast cancer, left radical mastectomy 18 months ago with no current treatment; bronchoscopy with lung biopsy shows metastatic disease in the right lung

C78.01   **Secondary malignant neoplasm of right lung**

Z85.3   **Personal history of malignant neoplasm of breast**

Explanation: The patient has undergone a diagnostic procedure that revealed metastatic breast cancer in the right lung. The code for the secondary (metastatic) site is sequenced first followed by a personal history code to identify the former site of the primary malignancy.

e. Admissions/encounters involving chemotherapy, immunotherapy and radiation therapy

1) Episode of care involves surgical removal of neoplasm

When an episode of care involves the surgical removal of a neoplasm, primary or secondary site, followed by adjunct chemotherapy or radiation treatment during the same episode of care, the code for the neoplasm should be assigned as principal or first-listed diagnosis.

2) Patient admission/encounter solely for administration of chemotherapy, immunotherapy and radiation therapy

If a patient admission/encounter is solely for the administration of chemotherapy, immunotherapy or external beam radiation therapy assign code Z51.0, Encounter for antineoplastic radiation therapy, or Z51.11, Encounter for antineoplastic chemotherapy, or Z51.12, Encounter for antineoplastic immunotherapy as the first-listed or principal diagnosis. If a patient receives more than one of these therapies during the same admission more than one of these codes may be assigned, in any sequence.

The malignancy for which the therapy is being administered should be assigned as a secondary diagnosis.

If a patient admission/encounter is for the insertion or implantation of radioactive elements (e.g., brachytherapy) the appropriate code for the malignancy is sequenced as the principal or first-listed diagnosis. Code Z51.0 should not be assigned.

3) Patient admitted for radiation therapy, chemotherapy or immunotherapy and develops complications

When a patient is admitted for the purpose of external beam radiotherapy, immunotherapy or chemotherapy and develops complications such as uncontrolled nausea and vomiting or dehydration, the principal or first-listed diagnosis is Z51.0, Encounter for antineoplastic radiation therapy, or Z51.11, Encounter for antineoplastic chemotherapy, or Z51.12, Encounter for antineoplastic immunotherapy followed by any codes for the complications.

When a patient is admitted for the purpose of insertion or implantation of radioactive elements (e.g., brachytherapy) and develops complications such as uncontrolled nausea and vomiting or dehydration, the principal or first-listed diagnosis is the appropriate code for the malignancy followed by any codes for the complications.

A patient with prostate cancer was admitted for brachytherapy seed implantation and consequently developed urinary retention.

C61   **Malignant neoplasm of prostate**

R33.9   **Retention of urine, unspecified**

Explanation: A code for the malignancy should be listed as the principal diagnosis when insertion of a radioactive element is the reason for admission, even when a complication related to that radioactive element occurs. Codes describing the complications should be listed as secondary codes.

f. Admission/encounter to determine extent of malignancy

When the reason for admission/encounter is to determine the extent of the malignancy, or for a procedure such as paracentesis or thoracentesis, the primary malignancy or appropriate metastatic site is designated as the principal or first-listed diagnosis, even though chemotherapy or radiotherapy is administered.

Patient with left lung cancer with malignant pleural effusion admitted for paracentesis and initiation/administration of chemotherapy

C34.92   **Malignant neoplasm of unspecified part of left bronchus or lung**

J91.0   **Malignant pleural effusion**

Z51.11   **Encounter for antineoplastic chemotherapy**

Explanation: The lung cancer is sequenced before the chemotherapy in this instance because the paracentesis for the malignant effusion is also being performed. An instructional note under the malignant effusion instructs that the lung cancer be sequenced first.

g. Symptoms, signs, and abnormal findings listed in Chapter 18 associated with neoplasms

Symptoms, signs, and ill-defined conditions listed in Chapter 18 characteristic of, or associated with, an existing primary or secondary site malignancy cannot be used to replace the malignancy as principal or first-listed diagnosis, regardless of the number of admissions or encounters for treatment and care of the neoplasm.

See Section I.C.21. Factors influencing health status and contact with health services, Encounter for prophylactic organ removal.

h. Admission/encounter for pain control/management

See Section I.C.6. for information on coding admission/encounter for pain control/management.

i. Malignancy in two or more noncontiguous sites

A patient may have more than one malignant tumor in the same organ. These tumors may represent different primaries or metastatic disease, depending on the site. Should the documentation be unclear, the provider should be queried as to the status of each tumor so that the correct codes can be assigned.

j. Disseminated malignant neoplasm, unspecified

Code C80.0, Disseminated malignant neoplasm, unspecified, is for use only in those cases where the patient has advanced metastatic disease and no known primary or secondary sites are specified. It should not be used in place of assigning codes for the primary site and all known secondary sites.

Patient who has had no medical care for many years is seen today and diagnosed with carcinomatosis

C80.0   **Disseminated malignant neoplasm, unspecified**

Explanation: Carcinomatosis NOS is an "includes" note under this code. Should seldom be used but is available for use in cases such as this.

k. Malignant neoplasm without specification of site

Code C80.1, Malignant (primary) neoplasm, unspecified, equates to Cancer, unspecified. This code should only be used when no determination can be made as to the primary site of a malignancy. This code should rarely be used in the inpatient setting.

l. Sequencing of neoplasm codes

1) Encounter for treatment of primary malignancy

If the reason for the encounter is for treatment of a primary malignancy, assign the malignancy as the principal/first-listed diagnosis. The primary site is to be sequenced first, followed by any metastatic sites.

2) Encounter for treatment of secondary malignancy

When an encounter is for a primary malignancy with metastasis and treatment is directed toward the metastatic (secondary) site(s) only, the metastatic site(s) is designated as the principal/first-listed diagnosis. The primary malignancy is coded as an additional code.

> Patient has primary colon cancer with metastasis to rib and is evaluated for possible excision of portion of rib bone
>
> **C79.51 Secondary malignant neoplasm of bone**
>
> **C18.9 Malignant neoplasm of colon, unspecified**
>
> *Explanation*: The treatment for this encounter is focused on the metastasis to the rib bone rather than the primary colon cancer, thus indicating that the bone metastasis is sequenced as the first-listed code.

3) Malignant neoplasm in a pregnant patient

When a pregnant woman has a malignant neoplasm, a code from subcategory O9A.1-, Malignant neoplasm complicating pregnancy, childbirth, and the puerperium, should be sequenced first, followed by the appropriate code from Chapter 2 to indicate the type of neoplasm.

> A 30-year-old pregnant female in second trimester evaluated for thyroid malignancy
>
> **O9A.112 Malignant neoplasm complicating pregnancy, second trimester**
>
> **C73 Malignant neoplasm of thyroid gland**
>
> *Explanation*: Codes from chapter 15 describing complications of pregnancy are sequenced as first-listed codes, further specified by codes from other chapters such as neoplastic, unless the pregnancy is documented as incidental to the condition. See also guideline 1.C.15.a.1.

4) Encounter for complication associated with a neoplasm

When an encounter is for management of a complication associated with a neoplasm, such as dehydration, and the treatment is only for the complication, the complication is coded first, followed by the appropriate code(s) for the neoplasm.

The exception to this guideline is anemia. When the admission/encounter is for management of an anemia associated with the malignancy, and the treatment is only for anemia, the appropriate code for the malignancy is sequenced as the principal or first-listed diagnosis followed by code D63.0, Anemia in neoplastic disease.

> Patient with pancreatic cancer is seen for initiation of TPN for cancer-related moderate protein-calorie malnutrition
>
> **E44.0 Moderate protein-calorie malnutrition**
>
> **C25.9 Malignant neoplasm of pancreas, unspecified**
>
> *Explanation*: The encounter is to initiate treatment for malnutrition, a common complication of many types of neoplasms, and is sequenced first.

5) Complication from surgical procedure for treatment of a neoplasm

When an encounter is for treatment of a complication resulting from a surgical procedure performed for the treatment of the neoplasm, designate the complication as the principal/first-listed diagnosis. See **the** guideline regarding the coding of a current malignancy versus personal history to determine if the code for the neoplasm should also be assigned.

6) Pathologic fracture due to a neoplasm

When an encounter is for a pathological fracture due to a neoplasm, and the focus of treatment is the fracture, a code from subcategory M84.5, Pathological fracture in neoplastic disease, should be sequenced first, followed by the code for the neoplasm.

If the focus of treatment is the neoplasm with an associated pathological fracture, the neoplasm code should be sequenced first, followed by a code from M84.5 for the pathological fracture.

m. Current malignancy versus personal history of malignancy

When a primary malignancy has been excised but further treatment, such as an additional surgery for the malignancy, radiation therapy or chemotherapy is directed to that site, the primary malignancy code should be used until treatment is completed.

> Female patient with ongoing chemotherapy after right mastectomy for breast cancer
>
> **C50.911 Malignant neoplasm of unspecified site of right female breast**
>
> **Z90.11 Acquired absence of right breast and nipple**
>
> *Explanation*: Even though the breast has been removed, the breast cancer is still being treated with chemotherapy and therefore is still coded as a current condition rather than personal history.

When a primary malignancy has been previously excised or eradicated from its site, there is no further treatment (of the malignancy) directed to that site, and there is no evidence of any existing primary malignancy at that site, a code from category Z85, Personal history of malignant neoplasm, should be used to indicate the former site of the malignancy.

Subcategories Z85.0 – Z85.7 should only be assigned for the former site of a primary malignancy, not the site of a secondary malignancy. Codes from subcategory Z85.8-, may be assigned for the former site(s) of either a primary or secondary malignancy included in this subcategory.

See Section I.C.21. Factors influencing health status and contact with health services, History (of)

n. Leukemia, multiple myeloma, and malignant plasma cell neoplasms in remission versus personal history

The categories for leukemia, and category C90, Multiple myeloma and malignant plasma cell neoplasms, have codes indicating whether or not the leukemia has achieved remission. There are also codes Z85.6, Personal history of leukemia, and Z85.79, Personal history of other malignant neoplasms of lymphoid, hematopoietic and related tissues. If the documentation is unclear as to whether the leukemia has achieved remission, the provider should be queried.

See Section I.C.21. Factors influencing health status and contact with health services, History (of)

o. Aftercare following surgery for neoplasm

See Section I.C.21. Factors influencing health status and contact with health services, Aftercare

p. Follow-up care for completed treatment of a malignancy

See Section I.C.21. Factors influencing health status and contact with health services, Follow-up

q. Prophylactic organ removal for prevention of malignancy

See Section I.C. 21, Factors influencing health status and contact with health services, Prophylactic organ removal

r. Malignant neoplasm associated with transplanted organ

A malignant neoplasm of a transplanted organ should be coded as a transplant complication. Assign first the appropriate code from category T86.-, Complications of transplanted organs and tissue, followed by code C80.2, Malignant neoplasm associated with transplanted organ. Use an additional code for the specific malignancy.

Chapter 2. Neoplasms

Chapter 2. Neoplasms (C00-D49)

NOTE

Functional activity

All neoplasms are classified in this chapter, whether they are functionally active or not. An additional code from Chapter 4 may be used, to identify functional activity associated with any neoplasm.

Morphology [Histology]

Chapter 2 classifies neoplasms primarily by site (topography), with broad groupings for behavior, malignant, in situ, benign, etc. The Table of Neoplasms should be used to identify the correct topography code. In a few cases, such as for malignant melanoma and certain neuroendocrine tumors, the morphology (histologic type) is included in the category and codes.

Primary malignant neoplasms overlapping site boundaries

A primary malignant neoplasm that overlaps two or more contiguous (next to each other) sites should be classified to the subcategory/code .8 ("overlapping lesion"), unless the combination is specifically indexed elsewhere. For multiple neoplasms of the same site that are not contiguous, such as tumors in different quadrants of the same breast, codes for each site should be assigned.

Malignant neoplasm of ectopic tissue

Malignant neoplasms of ectopic tissue are to be coded to the site mentioned, e.g., ectopic pancreatic malignant neoplasms are coded to pancreas, unspecified (C25.9).

AHA: 2017,4Q,103; 2017,1Q,4,5-6,8

This chapter contains the following blocks:

C00-C14   Malignant neoplasms of lip, oral cavity and pharynx
C15-C26   Malignant neoplasms of digestive organs
C30-C39   Malignant neoplasms of respiratory and intrathoracic organs
C40-C41   Malignant neoplasms of bone and articular cartilage
C43-C44   Melanoma and other malignant neoplasms of skin
C45-C49   Malignant neoplasms of mesothelial and soft tissue
C50   Malignant neoplasms of breast
C51-C58   Malignant neoplasms of female genital organs
C60-C63   Malignant neoplasms of male genital organs
C64-C68   Malignant neoplasms of urinary tract
C69-C72   Malignant neoplasms of eye, brain and other parts of central nervous system
C73-C75   Malignant neoplasms of thyroid and other endocrine glands
C7A   Malignant neuroendocrine tumors
C7B   Secondary neuroendocrine tumors
C76-C80   Malignant neoplasms of ill-defined, other secondary and unspecified sites
C81-C96   Malignant neoplasms of lymphoid, hematopoietic and related tissue
D00-D09   In situ neoplasms
D10-D36   Benign neoplasms, except benign neuroendocrine tumors
D3A   Benign neuroendocrine tumors
D37-D48   Neoplasms of uncertain behavior, polycythemia vera and myelodysplastic syndromes
D49   Neoplasms of unspecified behavior

MALIGNANT NEOPLASMS(C00-C96)

Malignant neoplasms, stated or presumed to be primary (of specified sites), and certain specified histologies, except neuroendocrine, and of lymphoid, hematopoietic and related tissue (C00-C75)

Malignant neoplasms of lip, oral cavity and pharynx (C00-C14)

☑4ᵗʰ **C00 Malignant neoplasm of lip**

Use additional code to identify:
   alcohol abuse and dependence (F10.-)
   history of tobacco dependence (Z87.891)
   tobacco dependence (F17.-)
   tobacco use (Z72.0)
   EXCLUDES 1   malignant melanoma of lip (C43.0)
         Merkel cell carcinoma of lip (C4A.0)
         other and unspecified malignant neoplasm of skin of lip (C44.0-)

   C00.0 Malignant neoplasm of external upper lip
     Malignant neoplasm of lipstick area of upper lip
     Malignant neoplasm of upper lip NOS
     Malignant neoplasm of vermilion border of upper lip

   C00.1 Malignant neoplasm of external lower lip
     Malignant neoplasm of lower lip NOS
     Malignant neoplasm of lipstick area of lower lip
     Malignant neoplasm of vermilion border of lower lip

   C00.2 Malignant neoplasm of external lip, unspecified
     Malignant neoplasm of vermilion border of lip NOS

   C00.3 Malignant neoplasm of upper lip, inner aspect
     Malignant neoplasm of buccal aspect of upper lip
     Malignant neoplasm of frenulum of upper lip
     Malignant neoplasm of mucosa of upper lip
     Malignant neoplasm of oral aspect of upper lip

   C00.4 Malignant neoplasm of lower lip, inner aspect
     Malignant neoplasm of buccal aspect of lower lip
     Malignant neoplasm of frenulum of lower lip
     Malignant neoplasm of mucosa of lower lip
     Malignant neoplasm of oral aspect of lower lip

   C00.5 Malignant neoplasm of lip, unspecified, inner aspect
     Malignant neoplasm of buccal aspect of lip, unspecified
     Malignant neoplasm of frenulum of lip, unspecified
     Malignant neoplasm of mucosa of lip, unspecified
     Malignant neoplasm of oral aspect of lip, unspecified

   C00.6 Malignant neoplasm of commissure of lip, unspecified

   C00.8 Malignant neoplasm of overlapping sites of lip

   C00.9 Malignant neoplasm of lip, unspecified

C01 Malignant neoplasm of base of tongue   HCC

   Malignant neoplasm of dorsal surface of base of tongue
   Malignant neoplasm of fixed part of tongue NOS
   Malignant neoplasm of posterior third of tongue
   Use additional code to identify:
     alcohol abuse and dependence (F10.-)
     history of tobacco dependence (Z87.891)
     tobacco dependence (F17.-)
     tobacco use (Z72.0)

Malignant Neoplasm of Tongue

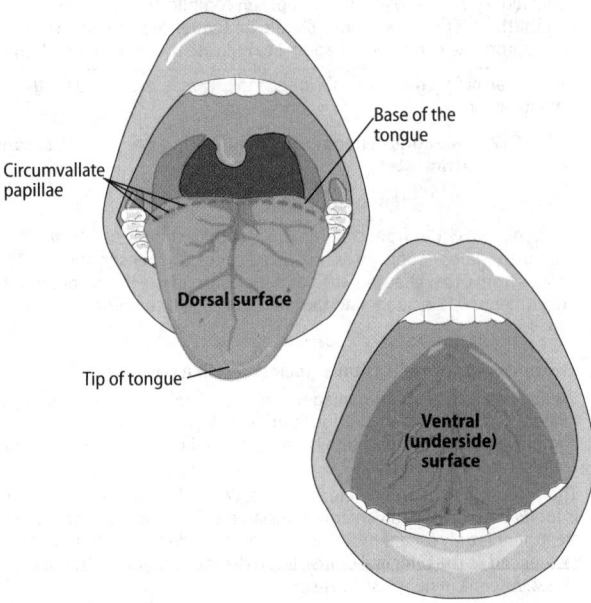

Base of the tongue

Circumvallate papillae

Dorsal surface

Tip of tongue

Ventral (underside) surface

☑4ᵗʰ **C02 Malignant neoplasm of other and unspecified parts of tongue**

   Use additional code to identify:
     alcohol abuse and dependence (F10.-)
     history of tobacco dependence (Z87.891)
     tobacco dependence (F17.-)
     tobacco use (Z72.0)

   C02.0 Malignant neoplasm of dorsal surface of tongue   HCC
     Malignant neoplasm of anterior two-thirds of tongue, dorsal surface
     EXCLUDES 2   malignant neoplasm of dorsal surface of base of tongue (C01)

   C02.1 Malignant neoplasm of border of tongue   HCC
     Malignant neoplasm of tip of tongue

   C02.2 Malignant neoplasm of ventral surface of tongue   HCC
     Malignant neoplasm of anterior two-thirds of tongue, ventral surface
     Malignant neoplasm of frenulum linguae

N Newborn: 0   P Pediatric: 0-17   M Maternity: 9-64   A Adult: 15-124   MCC Major Complication/Comorbidity   CC Complication/Comorbidity   SW Severe Wound Dx

464   ICD-10-CM 2020

C02.3 **Malignant neoplasm of anterior two-thirds of tongue, part unspecified** `HCC`
    Malignant neoplasm of middle third of tongue NOS
    Malignant neoplasm of mobile part of tongue NOS

C02.4 **Malignant neoplasm of lingual tonsil** `HCC`
    EXCLUDES 2   *malignant neoplasm of tonsil NOS (C09.9)*

C02.8 **Malignant neoplasm of overlapping sites of tongue** `HCC`
    Malignant neoplasm of two or more contiguous sites of tongue

C02.9 **Malignant neoplasm of tongue, unspecified** `HCC`

✓4ᵗʰ C03 **Malignant neoplasm of gum**
    INCLUDES   malignant neoplasm of alveolar (ridge) mucosa
              malignant neoplasm of gingiva
    Use additional code to identify:
      alcohol abuse and dependence (F10.-)
      history of tobacco dependence (Z87.891)
      tobacco dependence (F17.-)
      tobacco use (Z72.0)
    EXCLUDES 2   *malignant odontogenic neoplasms (C41.0-C41.1)*

C03.0 **Malignant neoplasm of upper gum** `HCC`

C03.1 **Malignant neoplasm of lower gum** `HCC`

C03.9 **Malignant neoplasm of gum, unspecified** `HCC`

✓4ᵗʰ C04 **Malignant neoplasm of floor of mouth**
    Use additional code to identify:
      alcohol abuse and dependence (F10.-)
      history of tobacco dependence (Z87.891)
      tobacco dependence (F17.-)
      tobacco use (Z72.0)

C04.0 **Malignant neoplasm of anterior floor of mouth** `HCC`
    Malignant neoplasm of anterior to the premolar-canine junction

C04.1 **Malignant neoplasm of lateral floor of mouth** `HCC`

C04.8 **Malignant neoplasm of overlapping sites of floor of mouth** `HCC`

C04.9 **Malignant neoplasm of floor of mouth, unspecified** `HCC`

✓4ᵗʰ C05 **Malignant neoplasm of palate**
    Use additional code to identify:
      alcohol abuse and dependence (F10.-)
      history of tobacco dependence (Z87.891)
      tobacco dependence (F17.-)
      tobacco use (Z72.0)
    EXCLUDES 1   *Kaposi's sarcoma of palate (C46.2)*

C05.0 **Malignant neoplasm of hard palate** `HCC`

C05.1 **Malignant neoplasm of soft palate** `HCC`
    EXCLUDES 2   *malignant neoplasm of nasopharyngeal surface of soft palate (C11.3)*

C05.2 **Malignant neoplasm of uvula** `HCC`

C05.8 **Malignant neoplasm of overlapping sites of palate** `HCC`

C05.9 **Malignant neoplasm of palate, unspecified** `HCC`
    Malignant neoplasm of roof of mouth

✓4ᵗʰ C06 **Malignant neoplasm of other and unspecified parts of mouth**
    Use additional code to identify:
      alcohol abuse and dependence (F10.-)
      history of tobacco dependence (Z87.891)
      tobacco dependence (F17.-)
      tobacco use (Z72.0)

C06.0 **Malignant neoplasm of cheek mucosa** `HCC`
    Malignant neoplasm of buccal mucosa NOS
    Malignant neoplasm of internal cheek

C06.1 **Malignant neoplasm of vestibule of mouth** `HCC`
    Malignant neoplasm of buccal sulcus (upper) (lower)
    Malignant neoplasm of labial sulcus (upper) (lower)

C06.2 **Malignant neoplasm of retromolar area** `HCC`

✓6ᵗʰ C06.8 **Malignant neoplasm of overlapping sites of other and unspecified parts of mouth**

C06.80 **Malignant neoplasm of overlapping sites of unspecified parts of mouth** `HCC`

C06.89 **Malignant neoplasm of overlapping sites of other parts of mouth** `HCC`
    "book leaf" neoplasm [ventral surface of tongue and floor of mouth]

C06.9 **Malignant neoplasm of mouth, unspecified** `HCC`
    Malignant neoplasm of minor salivary gland, unspecified site
    Malignant neoplasm of oral cavity NOS

C07 **Malignant neoplasm of parotid gland** `HCC`
    Use additional code to identify:
      alcohol abuse and dependence (F10.-)
      exposure to environmental tobacco smoke (Z77.22)
      exposure to tobacco smoke in the perinatal period (P96.81)
      history of tobacco dependence (Z87.891)
      occupational exposure to environmental tobacco smoke (Z57.31)
      tobacco dependence (F17.-)
      tobacco use (Z72.0)

✓4ᵗʰ C08 **Malignant neoplasm of other and unspecified major salivary glands**
    INCLUDES   malignant neoplasm of salivary ducts
    Use additional code to identify:
      alcohol abuse and dependence (F10.-)
      exposure to environmental tobacco smoke (Z77.22)
      exposure to tobacco smoke in the perinatal period (P96.81)
      history of tobacco dependence (Z87.891)
      occupational exposure to environmental tobacco smoke (Z57.31)
      tobacco dependence (F17.-)
      tobacco use (Z72.0)
    EXCLUDES 1   *malignant neoplasms of specified minor salivary glands which are classified according to their anatomical location*
    EXCLUDES 2   *malignant neoplasms of minor salivary glands NOS (C06.9)*
                  malignant neoplasm of parotid gland (C07)

C08.0 **Malignant neoplasm of submandibular gland** `HCC`
    Malignant neoplasm of submaxillary gland

C08.1 **Malignant neoplasm of sublingual gland** `HCC`

C08.9 **Malignant neoplasm of major salivary gland, unspecified** `HCC`
    Malignant neoplasm of salivary gland (major) NOS

✓4ᵗʰ C09 **Malignant neoplasm of tonsil**
    Use additional code to identify:
      alcohol abuse and dependence (F10.-)
      exposure to environmental tobacco smoke (Z77.22)
      exposure to tobacco smoke in the perinatal period (P96.81)
      history of tobacco dependence (Z87.891)
      occupational exposure to environmental tobacco smoke (Z57.31)
      tobacco dependence (F17.-)
      tobacco use (Z72.0)
    EXCLUDES 2   *malignant neoplasm of lingual tonsil (C02.4)*
                  malignant neoplasm of pharyngeal tonsil (C11.1)

C09.0 **Malignant neoplasm of tonsillar fossa** `HCC`

C09.1 **Malignant neoplasm of tonsillar pillar (anterior) (posterior)** `HCC`

C09.8 **Malignant neoplasm of overlapping sites of tonsil** `HCC`

C09.9 **Malignant neoplasm of tonsil, unspecified** `HCC`
    Malignant neoplasm of tonsil NOS
    Malignant neoplasm of faucial tonsils
    Malignant neoplasm of palatine tonsils

✓4ᵗʰ C10 **Malignant neoplasm of oropharynx**
    Use additional code to identify:
      alcohol abuse and dependence (F10.-)
      exposure to environmental tobacco smoke (Z77.22)
      exposure to tobacco smoke in the perinatal period (P96.81)
      history of tobacco dependence (Z87.891)
      occupational exposure to environmental tobacco smoke (Z57.31)
      tobacco dependence (F17.-)
      tobacco use (Z72.0)
    EXCLUDES 2   *malignant neoplasm of tonsil (C09.-)*
    DEF: Oropharynx: Middle portion of pharynx (throat); communicates with the oral cavity, nasopharynx and laryngopharynx.

C10.0 **Malignant neoplasm of vallecula** `HCC`

C10.1 **Malignant neoplasm of anterior surface of epiglottis** `HCC`
    Malignant neoplasm of epiglottis, free border [margin]
    Malignant neoplasm of glossoepiglottic fold(s)
    EXCLUDES 2   *malignant neoplasm of epiglottis (suprahyoid portion) NOS (C32.1)*

C10.2 **Malignant neoplasm of lateral wall of oropharynx** `HCC`

C10.3 **Malignant neoplasm of posterior wall of oropharynx** `HCC`

✓ Additional Character Required   ✓7ᵗʰ Placeholder   Unacceptable PDx   Questionable PDx   Manifestation   Unspecified Dx   H1-H14 HAC   HCC CMS-HCC Dx   HIV HIV Dx

Chapter 2. Neoplasms

C10.4   **Malignant neoplasm of** branchial cleft   `HCC`

     Malignant neoplasm of branchial cyst [site of neoplasm]

C10.8   **Malignant neoplasm of** overlapping sites of oropharynx   `HCC`

     Malignant neoplasm of junctional region of oropharynx

C10.9   **Malignant neoplasm of oropharynx, unspecified**   `HCC`

√4ᵗʰ **C11**   **Malignant neoplasm of** nasopharynx

     Use additional code to identify:
        exposure to environmental tobacco smoke (Z77.22)
        exposure to tobacco smoke in the perinatal period (P96.81)
        history of tobacco dependence (Z87.891)
        occupational exposure to environmental tobacco smoke (Z57.31)
        tobacco dependence (F17.-)
        tobacco use (Z72.0)
     DEF: Nasopharynx: Upper portion of pharynx (throat); communicates with the nasal cavities, oropharynx and tympanic cavities.

C11.0   **Malignant neoplasm of** superior wall of nasopharynx   `HCC`

     Malignant neoplasm of roof of nasopharynx

C11.1   **Malignant neoplasm of** posterior wall of nasopharynx   `HCC`

     Malignant neoplasm of adenoid
     Malignant neoplasm of pharyngeal tonsil

C11.2   **Malignant neoplasm of** lateral wall of nasopharynx   `HCC`

     Malignant neoplasm of fossa of Rosenmüller
     Malignant neoplasm of opening of auditory tube
     Malignant neoplasm of pharyngeal recess

C11.3   **Malignant neoplasm of** anterior wall of nasopharynx   `HCC`

     Malignant neoplasm of floor of nasopharynx
     Malignant neoplasm of nasopharyngeal (anterior) (posterior) surface of soft palate
     Malignant neoplasm of posterior margin of nasal choana
     Malignant neoplasm of posterior margin of nasal septum

C11.8   **Malignant neoplasm of** overlapping sites of nasopharynx   `HCC`

C11.9   **Malignant neoplasm of nasopharynx, unspecified**   `HCC`

     Malignant neoplasm of nasopharyngeal wall NOS

C12   **Malignant neoplasm of** pyriform sinus   `HCC`

     Malignant neoplasm of pyriform fossa
     Use additional code to identify:
        exposure to environmental tobacco smoke (Z77.22)
        exposure to tobacco smoke in the perinatal period (P96.81)
        history of tobacco dependence (Z87.891)
        occupational exposure to environmental tobacco smoke (Z57.31)
        tobacco dependence (F17.-)
        tobacco use (Z72.0)

√4ᵗʰ **C13**   **Malignant neoplasm of** hypopharynx

     Use additional code to identify:
        exposure to environmental tobacco smoke (Z77.22)
        exposure to tobacco smoke in the perinatal period (P96.81)
        history of tobacco dependence (Z87.891)
        occupational exposure to environmental tobacco smoke (Z57.31)
        tobacco dependence (F17.-)
        tobacco use (Z72.0)
     EXCLUDES 2   *malignant neoplasm of pyriform sinus (C12)*
     DEF: Hypopharynx: Lower portion of pharynx (throat); communicates with the oropharynx and the esophagus. **Synonyms:** *laryngopharynx.*

C13.0   **Malignant neoplasm of** postcricoid region   `HCC`

C13.1   **Malignant neoplasm of** aryepiglottic fold, hypopharyngeal aspect   `HCC`

     Malignant neoplasm of aryepiglottic fold, marginal zone
     Malignant neoplasm of aryepiglottic fold NOS
     Malignant neoplasm of interarytenoid fold, marginal zone
     Malignant neoplasm of interarytenoid fold NOS
     EXCLUDES 2   *malignant neoplasm of aryepiglottic fold or interarytenoid fold, laryngeal aspect (C32.1)*

C13.2   **Malignant neoplasm of** posterior wall of hypopharynx   `HCC`

C13.8   **Malignant neoplasm of** overlapping sites of hypopharynx   `HCC`

C13.9   **Malignant neoplasm of hypopharynx, unspecified**   `HCC`

     Malignant neoplasm of hypopharyngeal wall NOS

√4ᵗʰ **C14**   **Malignant neoplasm of** other and ill-defined sites in the lip, oral cavity and pharynx

     Use additional code to identify:
        alcohol abuse and dependence (F10.-)
        exposure to environmental tobacco smoke (Z77.22)
        exposure to tobacco smoke in the perinatal period (P96.81)
        history of tobacco dependence (Z87.891)
        occupational exposure to environmental tobacco smoke (Z57.31)
        tobacco dependence (F17.-)
        tobacco use (Z72.0)
     EXCLUDES 1   *malignant neoplasm of oral cavity NOS (C06.9)*

C14.0   **Malignant neoplasm of pharynx, unspecified**   `HCC`

C14.2   **Malignant neoplasm of** Waldeyer's ring   `HCC`

     DEF: Waldeyer's ring: Ring of lymphoid tissue that is made up of the two palatine tonsils, the pharyngeal tonsil (adenoid), and the lingual tonsil. It functions as the defense against infection and assists with the development of the immune system.

C14.8   **Malignant neoplasm of** overlapping sites of lip, oral cavity and pharynx   `HCC`

     Primary malignant neoplasm of two or more contiguous sites of lip, oral cavity and pharynx
     EXCLUDES 1   *"book leaf" neoplasm [ventral surface of tongue and floor of mouth] (C06.89)*

Malignant neoplasms of digestive organs (C15-C26)

     EXCLUDES 1   *Kaposi's sarcoma of gastrointestinal sites (C46.4)*
     EXCLUDES 2   *gastrointestinal stromal tumors (C49.A-)*

√4ᵗʰ **C15**   **Malignant neoplasm of** esophagus

     Use additional code to identify:
        alcohol abuse and dependence (F10.-)

C15.3   **Malignant neoplasm of** upper third of esophagus   `HCC`

C15.4   **Malignant neoplasm of** middle third of esophagus   `HCC`

C15.5   **Malignant neoplasm of** lower third of esophagus   `HCC`

     EXCLUDES 1   *malignant neoplasm of cardio-esophageal junction (C16.0)*

C15.8   **Malignant neoplasm of** overlapping sites of esophagus   `HCC`

C15.9   **Malignant neoplasm of esophagus, unspecified**   `HCC`

√4ᵗʰ **C16**   **Malignant neoplasm of** stomach

     Use additional code to identify:
        alcohol abuse and dependence (F10.-)
     EXCLUDES 2   *malignant carcinoid tumor of the stomach (C7A.092)*

C16.0   **Malignant neoplasm of** cardia   `HCC`

     Malignant neoplasm of cardiac orifice
     Malignant neoplasm of cardio-esophageal junction
     Malignant neoplasm of esophagus and stomach
     Malignant neoplasm of gastro-esophageal junction

C16.1   **Malignant neoplasm of** fundus of stomach   `HCC`

C16.2   **Malignant neoplasm of** body of stomach   `HCC`

C16.3   **Malignant neoplasm of** pyloric antrum   `HCC`

     Malignant neoplasm of gastric antrum

C16.4   **Malignant neoplasm of** pylorus   `HCC`

     Malignant neoplasm of prepylorus
     Malignant neoplasm of pyloric canal

C16.5   **Malignant neoplasm of** lesser curvature of stomach, unspecified   `HCC`

     Malignant neoplasm of lesser curvature of stomach, not classifiable to C16.1-C16.4

C16.6   **Malignant neoplasm of** greater curvature of stomach, unspecified   `HCC`

     Malignant neoplasm of greater curvature of stomach, not classifiable to C16.0-C16.4

C16.8   **Malignant neoplasm of** overlapping sites of stomach   `HCC`

C16.9   **Malignant neoplasm of stomach, unspecified**   `HCC`

     Gastric cancer NOS

√4ᵗʰ **C17**   **Malignant neoplasm of** small intestine

     EXCLUDES 1   *malignant carcinoid tumors of the small intestine (C7A.01)*
     AHA: 2016,1Q,19

C17.0   **Malignant neoplasm of** duodenum   `HCC`

C17.1   **Malignant neoplasm of** jejunum   `HCC`

C17.2   Malignant neoplasm of ileum   `HCC`
> *EXCLUDES 1*   *malignant neoplasm of ileocecal valve (C18.Ø)*

C17.3   Meckel's diverticulum, malignant   `HCC`
> *EXCLUDES 1*   *Meckel's diverticulum, congenital (Q43.Ø)*
> **DEF:** Congenital, abnormal remnant of embryonic digestive system development that leaves a sacculation or outpouching from the wall of the small intestine near the terminal part of the ileum made of acid-secreting tissue as in the stomach.

C17.8   Malignant neoplasm of overlapping sites of small intestine   `HCC`

C17.9   Malignant neoplasm of small intestine, unspecified   `HCC`

✓4ᵗʰ **C18**   Malignant neoplasm of colon
> *EXCLUDES 1*   *malignant carcinoid tumors of the colon (C7A.Ø2-)*

Colon

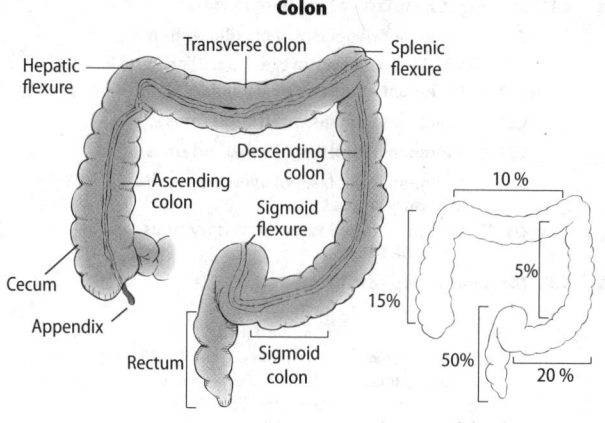

Anatomical distribution of large bowel cancers

C18.Ø   Malignant neoplasm of cecum   `HCC`
> Malignant neoplasm of ileocecal valve

C18.1   Malignant neoplasm of appendix   `HCC`

C18.2   Malignant neoplasm of ascending colon   `HCC`

C18.3   Malignant neoplasm of hepatic flexure   `HCC`

C18.4   Malignant neoplasm of transverse colon   `HCC`

C18.5   Malignant neoplasm of splenic flexure   `HCC`

C18.6   Malignant neoplasm of descending colon   `HCC`

C18.7   Malignant neoplasm of sigmoid colon   `HCC`
> Malignant neoplasm of sigmoid (flexure)
> *EXCLUDES 1*   *malignant neoplasm of rectosigmoid junction (C19)*

C18.8   Malignant neoplasm of overlapping sites of colon   `HCC`

C18.9   Malignant neoplasm of colon, unspecified   `HCC`
> Malignant neoplasm of large intestine NOS

C19   Malignant neoplasm of rectosigmoid junction   `HCC`
> Malignant neoplasm of colon with rectum
> Malignant neoplasm of rectosigmoid (colon)
> *EXCLUDES 1*   *malignant carcinoid tumors of the colon (C7A.Ø2-)*

C2Ø   Malignant neoplasm of rectum   `HCC`
> Malignant neoplasm of rectal ampulla
> *EXCLUDES 1*   *malignant carcinoid tumor of the rectum (C7A.Ø26)*

✓4ᵗʰ **C21**   Malignant neoplasm of anus and anal canal
> *EXCLUDES 2*   *malignant carcinoid tumors of the colon (C7A.Ø2-)*
> *malignant melanoma of anal margin (C43.51)*
> *malignant melanoma of anal skin (C43.51)*
> *malignant melanoma of perianal skin (C43.51)*
> *other and unspecified malignant neoplasm of anal margin (C44.5ØØ, C44.51Ø, C44.52Ø, C44.59Ø)*
> *other and unspecified malignant neoplasm of anal skin (C44.5ØØ, C44.51Ø, C44.52Ø, C44.59Ø)*
> *other and unspecified malignant neoplasm of perianal skin (C44.5ØØ, C44.51Ø, C44.52Ø, C44.59Ø)*

C21.Ø   Malignant neoplasm of anus, unspecified   `HCC`

C21.1   Malignant neoplasm of anal canal   `HCC`
> Malignant neoplasm of anal sphincter

C21.2   Malignant neoplasm of cloacogenic zone   `HCC`

C21.8   Malignant neoplasm of overlapping sites of rectum, anus and anal canal   `HCC`
> Malignant neoplasm of anorectal junction
> Malignant neoplasm of anorectum
> Primary malignant neoplasm of two or more contiguous sites of rectum, anus and anal canal

✓4ᵗʰ **C22**   Malignant neoplasm of liver and intrahepatic bile ducts
> Use additional code to identify:
> alcohol abuse and dependence (F1Ø.-)
> hepatitis B (B16.-, B18.Ø-B18.1)
> hepatitis C (B17.1-, B18.2)
> *EXCLUDES 1*   *malignant neoplasm of biliary tract NOS (C24.9)*
> *secondary malignant neoplasm of liver and intrahepatic bile duct (C78.7)*

C22.Ø   Liver cell carcinoma   `HCC`
> Hepatocellular carcinoma
> Hepatoma
> **AHA:** 2016,1Q,18

C22.1   Intrahepatic bile duct carcinoma   `HCC`
> Cholangiocarcinoma
> *EXCLUDES 1*   *malignant neoplasm of hepatic duct (C24.Ø)*

C22.2   Hepatoblastoma   `HCC`

C22.3   Angiosarcoma of liver   `HCC`
> Kupffer cell sarcoma

C22.4   Other sarcomas of liver   `HCC`

C22.7   Other specified carcinomas of liver   `HCC`

C22.8   Malignant neoplasm of liver, primary, unspecified as to type   `HCC`

C22.9   Malignant neoplasm of liver, not specified as primary or secondary   `HCC`

C23   Malignant neoplasm of gallbladder   `HCC`

✓4ᵗʰ **C24**   Malignant neoplasm of other and unspecified parts of biliary tract
> *EXCLUDES 1*   *malignant neoplasm of intrahepatic bile duct (C22.1)*

C24.Ø   Malignant neoplasm of extrahepatic bile duct   `HCC`
> Malignant neoplasm of biliary duct or passage NOS
> Malignant neoplasm of common bile duct
> Malignant neoplasm of cystic duct
> Malignant neoplasm of hepatic duct

C24.1   Malignant neoplasm of ampulla of Vater   `HCC`
> **DEF:** Malignant neoplasm in the area of dilation at the juncture of the common bile and pancreatic ducts near the opening into the lumen of the duodenum.

C24.8   Malignant neoplasm of overlapping sites of biliary tract   `HCC`
> Malignant neoplasm involving both intrahepatic and extrahepatic bile ducts
> Primary malignant neoplasm of two or more contiguous sites of biliary tract

C24.9   Malignant neoplasm of biliary tract, unspecified   `HCC`

☑ Additional Character Required   ✓x7ᵗʰ Placeholder   Unacceptable PDx   Questionable PDx   Manifestation   Unspecified Dx   H1–H14 HAC   `HCC` CMS-HCC Dx   HIV HIV Dx

ICD-10-CM 2020   467

Chapter 2. Neoplasms

✓4ᵗʰ **C25 Malignant neoplasm of pancreas**

Code also exocrine pancreatic insufficiency (K86.81)
Use additional code to identify:
   alcohol abuse and dependence (F10.-)

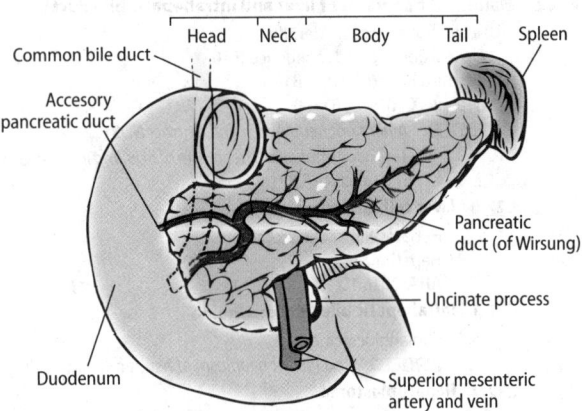

Pancreas

Common bile duct
Accesory pancreatic duct
Head   Neck   Body   Tail   Spleen
Duodenum
Pancreatic duct (of Wirsung)
Uncinate process
Superior mesenteric artery and vein

C25.0 Malignant neoplasm of head of pancreas   HCC

C25.1 Malignant neoplasm of body of pancreas   HCC

C25.2 Malignant neoplasm of tail of pancreas   HCC

C25.3 Malignant neoplasm of pancreatic duct   HCC

C25.4 Malignant neoplasm of endocrine pancreas   HCC
   Malignant neoplasm of islets of Langerhans
   Use additional code to identify any functional activity

C25.7 Malignant neoplasm of other parts of pancreas   HCC
   Malignant neoplasm of neck of pancreas

C25.8 Malignant neoplasm of overlapping sites of pancreas   HCC

C25.9 Malignant neoplasm of pancreas, unspecified   HCC

✓4ᵗʰ **C26 Malignant neoplasm of other and ill-defined digestive organs**

   EXCLUDES 1   malignant neoplasm of peritoneum and retroperitoneum (C48.-)

C26.0 Malignant neoplasm of intestinal tract, part unspecified   HCC
   Malignant neoplasm of intestine NOS

C26.1 Malignant neoplasm of spleen   HCC
   EXCLUDES 1   Hodgkin lymphoma (C81.-)
           non-Hodgkin lymphoma (C82-C85)

C26.9 Malignant neoplasm of ill-defined sites within the digestive system   HCC
   Malignant neoplasm of alimentary canal or tract NOS
   Malignant neoplasm of gastrointestinal tract NOS
   EXCLUDES 1   malignant neoplasm of abdominal NOS (C76.2)
           malignant neoplasm of intra-abdominal NOS (C76.2)

Malignant neoplasms of respiratory and intrathoracic organs (C30-C39)

INCLUDES   malignant neoplasm of middle ear
EXCLUDES 1   mesothelioma (C45.-)

✓4ᵗʰ **C30 Malignant neoplasm of nasal cavity and middle ear**

C30.0 Malignant neoplasm of nasal cavity   HCC
   Malignant neoplasm of cartilage of nose
   Malignant neoplasm of nasal concha
   Malignant neoplasm of internal nose
   Malignant neoplasm of septum of nose
   Malignant neoplasm of vestibule of nose
   EXCLUDES 1   malignant neoplasm of nasal bone (C41.0)
           malignant neoplasm of nose NOS (C76.0)
           malignant neoplasm of olfactory bulb (C72.2-)
           malignant neoplasm of posterior margin of nasal septum and choana (C11.3)
           malignant melanoma of skin of nose (C43.31)
           malignant neoplasm of turbinates (C41.0)
           other and unspecified malignant neoplasm of skin of nose (C44.301, C44.311, C44.321, C44.391)

C30.1 Malignant neoplasm of middle ear   HCC
   Malignant neoplasm of antrum tympanicum
   Malignant neoplasm of auditory tube
   Malignant neoplasm of eustachian tube
   Malignant neoplasm of inner ear
   Malignant neoplasm of mastoid air cells
   Malignant neoplasm of tympanic cavity
   EXCLUDES 1   malignant neoplasm of auricular canal (external) (C43.2-,C44.2-)
           malignant neoplasm of bone of ear (meatus) (C41.0)
           malignant neoplasm of cartilage of ear (C49.0)
           malignant melanoma of skin of (external) ear (C43.2-)
           other and unspecified malignant neoplasm of skin of (external) ear (C44.2-)

✓4ᵗʰ **C31 Malignant neoplasm of accessory sinuses**

C31.0 Malignant neoplasm of maxillary sinus   HCC
   Malignant neoplasm of antrum (Highmore) (maxillary)

C31.1 Malignant neoplasm of ethmoidal sinus   HCC

C31.2 Malignant neoplasm of frontal sinus   HCC

C31.3 Malignant neoplasm of sphenoid sinus   HCC

C31.8 Malignant neoplasm of overlapping sites of accessory sinuses   HCC

C31.9 Malignant neoplasm of accessory sinus, unspecified   HCC

✓4ᵗʰ **C32 Malignant neoplasm of larynx**

Use additional code to identify:
   alcohol abuse and dependence (F10.-)
   exposure to environmental tobacco smoke (Z77.22)
   exposure to tobacco smoke in the perinatal period (P96.81)
   history of tobacco dependence (Z87.891)
   occupational exposure to environmental tobacco smoke (Z57.31)
   tobacco dependence (F17.-)
   tobacco use (Z72.0)

C32.0 Malignant neoplasm of glottis   HCC
   Malignant neoplasm of intrinsic larynx
   Malignant neoplasm of laryngeal commissure (anterior)(posterior)
   Malignant neoplasm of vocal cord (true) NOS

C32.1 Malignant neoplasm of supraglottis   HCC
   Malignant neoplasm of aryepiglottic fold or interarytenoid fold, laryngeal aspect
   Malignant neoplasm of epiglottis (suprahyoid portion) NOS
   Malignant neoplasm of extrinsic larynx
   Malignant neoplasm of false vocal cord
   Malignant neoplasm of posterior (laryngeal) surface of epiglottis
   Malignant neoplasm of ventricular bands
   EXCLUDES 2   malignant neoplasm of anterior surface of epiglottis (C10.1)
           malignant neoplasm of aryepiglottic fold or interarytenoid fold, hypopharyngeal aspect (C13.1)
           malignant neoplasm of aryepiglottic fold or interarytenoid fold, marginal zone (C13.1)
           malignant neoplasm of aryepiglottic fold or interarytenoid fold NOS (C13.1)

C32.2 Malignant neoplasm of subglottis   HCC

C32.3 Malignant neoplasm of laryngeal cartilage   HCC

C32.8 Malignant neoplasm of overlapping sites of larynx   HCC

C32.9 Malignant neoplasm of larynx, unspecified   HCC

C33 Malignant neoplasm of trachea   HCC

Use additional code to identify:
   exposure to environmental tobacco smoke (Z77.22)
   exposure to tobacco smoke in the perinatal period (P96.81)
   history of tobacco dependence (Z87.891)
   occupational exposure to environmental tobacco smoke (Z57.31)
   tobacco dependence (F17.-)
   tobacco use (Z72.0)

N Newborn: 0   P Pediatric: 0-17   M Maternity: 9-64   A Adult: 15-124   MCC Major Complication/Comorbidity   CC Complication/Comorbidity   SW Severe Wound Dx

468   ICD-10-CM 2020

√4ᵗʰ **C34 Malignant neoplasm of** bronchus and lung

Use additional code to identify:
exposure to environmental tobacco smoke (Z77.22)
exposure to tobacco smoke in the perinatal period (P96.81)
history of tobacco dependence (Z87.891)
occupational exposure to environmental tobacco smoke (Z57.31)
tobacco dependence (F17.-)
tobacco use (Z72.0)

   EXCLUDES 1   Kaposi's sarcoma of lung (C46.5-)
        malignant carcinoid tumor of the bronchus and lung (C7A.090)

AHA: 2019,1Q,16

TIP: When documented, assign code I31.3 for associated malignant pericardial effusion. If the sole reason for admission is to treat the effusion with no treatment of the lung malignancy rendered, code I31.3 may be sequenced first.

√5ᵗʰ **C34.0 Malignant neoplasm of** main bronchus

Malignant neoplasm of carina
Malignant neoplasm of hilus (of lung)

   C34.00 Malignant neoplasm of unspecified main bronchus   HCC

   C34.01 Malignant neoplasm of right **main bronchus**   HCC

   C34.02 Malignant neoplasm of left **main bronchus**   HCC

√5ᵗʰ **C34.1 Malignant neoplasm of** upper lobe, **bronchus or lung**

   C34.10 Malignant neoplasm of upper lobe, unspecified bronchus or lung   HCC

   C34.11 Malignant neoplasm of upper lobe, right **bronchus or lung**   HCC

   C34.12 Malignant neoplasm of upper lobe, left **bronchus or lung**   HCC

C34.2 Malignant neoplasm of middle lobe, **bronchus or lung**   HCC

√5ᵗʰ **C34.3 Malignant neoplasm of** lower lobe, **bronchus or lung**

   C34.30 Malignant neoplasm of lower lobe, unspecified bronchus or lung   HCC

   C34.31 Malignant neoplasm of lower lobe, right **bronchus or lung**   HCC

   C34.32 Malignant neoplasm of lower lobe, left **bronchus or lung**   HCC

√5ᵗʰ **C34.8 Malignant neoplasm of** overlapping sites **of bronchus and lung**

   C34.80 Malignant neoplasm of overlapping sites of unspecified bronchus and lung   HCC

   C34.81 Malignant neoplasm of overlapping sites of right **bronchus and lung**   HCC

   C34.82 Malignant neoplasm of overlapping sites of left **bronchus and lung**   HCC

√5ᵗʰ **C34.9 Malignant neoplasm of unspecified part of bronchus or lung**

   C34.90 Malignant neoplasm of unspecified part of unspecified bronchus or lung   HCC

     Lung cancer NOS

   C34.91 Malignant neoplasm of unspecified part of right **bronchus or lung**   HCC

   C34.92 Malignant neoplasm of unspecified part of left **bronchus or lung**   HCC

C37 Malignant neoplasm of thymus   HCC

   EXCLUDES 1   malignant carcinoid tumor of the thymus (C7A.091)

√4ᵗʰ **C38 Malignant neoplasm of** heart, mediastinum and pleura

   EXCLUDES 1   mesothelioma (C45.-)

C38.0 Malignant neoplasm of heart   HCC

   Malignant neoplasm of pericardium

   EXCLUDES 1   malignant neoplasm of great vessels (C49.3)

C38.1 Malignant neoplasm of anterior mediastinum   HCC

C38.2 Malignant neoplasm of posterior mediastinum   HCC

C38.3 Malignant neoplasm of mediastinum, **part unspecified**   HCC

C38.4 Malignant neoplasm of pleura   HCC

C38.8 Malignant neoplasm of overlapping sites **of heart, mediastinum and pleura**   HCC

√4ᵗʰ **C39 Malignant neoplasm of other and ill-defined sites in the respiratory system and intrathoracic organs**

Use additional code to identify:
exposure to environmental tobacco smoke (Z77.22)
exposure to tobacco smoke in the perinatal period (P96.81)
history of tobacco dependence (Z87.891)
occupational exposure to environmental tobacco smoke (Z57.31)
tobacco dependence (F17.-)
tobacco use (Z72.0)

   EXCLUDES 1   intrathoracic malignant neoplasm NOS (C76.1)
        thoracic malignant neoplasm NOS (C76.1)

C39.0 Malignant neoplasm of upper **respiratory tract, part unspecified**   HCC

C39.9 Malignant neoplasm of lower **respiratory tract, part unspecified**   HCC

   Malignant neoplasm of respiratory tract NOS

Malignant neoplasms of bone and articular cartilage (C40-C41)

   INCLUDES   malignant neoplasm of cartilage (articular) (joint)
        malignant neoplasm of periosteum

   EXCLUDES 1   malignant neoplasm of bone marrow NOS (C96.9)
        malignant neoplasm of synovia (C49.-)

√4ᵗʰ **C40 Malignant neoplasm of** bone and articular cartilage of limbs

Use additional code to identify major osseous defect, if applicable (M89.7-)

√5ᵗʰ **C40.0 Malignant neoplasm of** scapula and long bones of upper limb

   C40.00 Malignant neoplasm of scapula and long bones of unspecified upper limb   HCC

   C40.01 Malignant neoplasm of scapula and long bones of right **upper limb**   HCC

   C40.02 Malignant neoplasm of scapula and long bones of left **upper limb**   HCC

√5ᵗʰ **C40.1 Malignant neoplasm of** short bones of upper limb

   C40.10 Malignant neoplasm of short bones of unspecified upper limb   HCC

   C40.11 Malignant neoplasm of short bones of right **upper limb**   HCC

   C40.12 Malignant neoplasm of short bones of left **upper limb**   HCC

√5ᵗʰ **C40.2 Malignant neoplasm of** long bones of lower limb

   C40.20 Malignant neoplasm of long bones of unspecified lower limb   HCC

   C40.21 Malignant neoplasm of long bones of right **lower limb**   HCC

   C40.22 Malignant neoplasm of long bones of left **lower limb**   HCC

√5ᵗʰ **C40.3 Malignant neoplasm of** short bones of lower limb

   C40.30 Malignant neoplasm of short bones of unspecified lower limb   HCC

   C40.31 Malignant neoplasm of short bones of right **lower limb**   HCC

   C40.32 Malignant neoplasm of short bones of left **lower limb**   HCC

√5ᵗʰ **C40.8 Malignant neoplasm of** overlapping sites **of bone and articular cartilage of limb**

   C40.80 Malignant neoplasm of overlapping sites of bone and articular cartilage of unspecified limb   HCC

   C40.81 Malignant neoplasm of overlapping sites of bone and articular cartilage of right **limb**   CC HCC

     CC Excl: PDX collection 293

   C40.82 Malignant neoplasm of overlapping sites of bone and articular cartilage of left **limb**   HCC

√5ᵗʰ **C40.9 Malignant neoplasm of unspecified bones and articular cartilage of limb**

   C40.90 Malignant neoplasm of unspecified bones and articular cartilage of unspecified limb   HCC

   C40.91 Malignant neoplasm of unspecified bones and articular cartilage of right **limb**   HCC

   C40.92 Malignant neoplasm of unspecified bones and articular cartilage of left **limb**   HCC

✓ Additional Character Required   ✓x7ᵗʰ Placeholder   Unacceptable PDx   Questionable PDx   Manifestation   Unspecified Dx   H1-H14 HAC   HCC CMS-HCC Dx   HIV HIV Dx

ICD-10-CM 2020   469

✓4ᵗʰ C41 Malignant neoplasm of bone and articular cartilage of other and unspecified sites

> EXCLUDES 1   malignant neoplasm of bones of limbs (C40.-)
> malignant neoplasm of cartilage of ear (C49.0)
> malignant neoplasm of cartilage of eyelid (C49.0)
> malignant neoplasm of cartilage of larynx (C32.3)
> malignant neoplasm of cartilage of limbs (C40.-)
> malignant neoplasm of cartilage of nose (C30.0)

C41.0 Malignant neoplasm of bones of skull and face   HCC

> Malignant neoplasm of maxilla (superior)
> Malignant neoplasm of orbital bone
> > EXCLUDES 2   carcinoma, any type except intraosseous or odontogenic of:
> > maxillary sinus (C31.0)
> > upper jaw (C03.0)
> > malignant neoplasm of jaw bone (lower) (C41.1)

C41.1 Malignant neoplasm of mandible   HCC

> Malignant neoplasm of inferior maxilla
> Malignant neoplasm of lower jaw bone
> > EXCLUDES 2   carcinoma, any type except intraosseous or odontogenic of:
> > jaw NOS (C03.9)
> > lower (C03.1)
> > malignant neoplasm of upper jaw bone (C41.0)

C41.2 Malignant neoplasm of vertebral column   HCC

> EXCLUDES 1   malignant neoplasm of sacrum and coccyx (C41.4)

C41.3 Malignant neoplasm of ribs, sternum and clavicle   HCC

C41.4 Malignant neoplasm of pelvic bones, sacrum and coccyx   HCC

C41.9 Malignant neoplasm of bone and articular cartilage, unspecified   HCC

Melanoma and other malignant neoplasms of skin (C43-C44)

✓4ᵗʰ C43 Malignant melanoma of skin

> EXCLUDES 1   melanoma in situ (D03.-)
> EXCLUDES 2   malignant melanoma of skin of genital organs (C51-C52, C60.-, C63.-)
> Merkel cell carcinoma (C4A.-)
> sites other than skin - code to malignant neoplasm of the site

C43.0 Malignant melanoma of lip   HCC

> EXCLUDES 1   malignant neoplasm of vermilion border of lip (C00.0-C00.2)

✓6ᵗʰ C43.1 Malignant melanoma of eyelid, including canthus

> AHA: 2018,4Q,4

> **C43.10 Malignant melanoma of unspecified eyelid, including canthus**   HCC

> **✓6ᵗʰ C43.11 Malignant melanoma of right eyelid, including canthus**

> > **C43.111 Malignant melanoma of right upper eyelid, including canthus**   HCC

> > **C43.112 Malignant melanoma of right lower eyelid, including canthus**   HCC

> **✓6ᵗʰ C43.12 Malignant melanoma of left eyelid, including canthus**

> > **C43.121 Malignant melanoma of left upper eyelid, including canthus**   HCC

> > **C43.122 Malignant melanoma of left lower eyelid, including canthus**   HCC

✓5ᵗʰ C43.2 Malignant melanoma of ear and external auricular canal

> **C43.20 Malignant melanoma of unspecified ear and external auricular canal**   HCC

> **C43.21 Malignant melanoma of right ear and external auricular canal**   HCC

> **C43.22 Malignant melanoma of left ear and external auricular canal**   HCC

✓5ᵗʰ C43.3 Malignant melanoma of other and unspecified parts of face

> **C43.30 Malignant melanoma of unspecified part of face**   HCC

> **C43.31 Malignant melanoma of nose**   HCC

> **C43.39 Malignant melanoma of other parts of face**   HCC

C43.4 Malignant melanoma of scalp and neck   HCC

✓5ᵗʰ C43.5 Malignant melanoma of trunk

> EXCLUDES 2   malignant neoplasm of anus NOS (C21.0)
> malignant neoplasm of scrotum (C63.2)

> **C43.51 Malignant melanoma of anal skin**   HCC

> > Malignant melanoma of anal margin
> > Malignant melanoma of perianal skin

> **C43.52 Malignant melanoma of skin of breast**   HCC

> **C43.59 Malignant melanoma of other part of trunk**   HCC

✓5ᵗʰ C43.6 Malignant melanoma of upper limb, including shoulder

> **C43.60 Malignant melanoma of unspecified upper limb, including shoulder**   HCC

> **C43.61 Malignant melanoma of right upper limb, including shoulder**   HCC

> **C43.62 Malignant melanoma of left upper limb, including shoulder**   HCC

✓5ᵗʰ C43.7 Malignant melanoma of lower limb, including hip

> **C43.70 Malignant melanoma of unspecified lower limb, including hip**   HCC

> **C43.71 Malignant melanoma of right lower limb, including hip**   HCC

> **C43.72 Malignant melanoma of left lower limb, including hip**   HCC

C43.8 Malignant melanoma of overlapping sites of skin   HCC

C43.9 Malignant melanoma of skin, unspecified   HCC

> Malignant melanoma of unspecified site of skin
> Melanoma (malignant) NOS

✓4ᵗʰ C4A Merkel cell carcinoma

> DEF: Malignant cutaneous cancer predominantly found in elderly patients with sun exposure that usually presents as a flesh-colored or bluish-red lump typically seen on the neck, head, and face.

C4A.0 Merkel cell carcinoma of lip   HCC

> EXCLUDES 1   malignant neoplasm of vermilion border of lip (C00.0-C00.2)

✓5ᵗʰ C4A.1 Merkel cell carcinoma of eyelid, including canthus

> AHA: 2018,4Q,4

> **C4A.10 Merkel cell carcinoma of unspecified eyelid, including canthus**   HCC

> **✓6ᵗʰ C4A.11 Merkel cell carcinoma of right eyelid, including canthus**

> > **C4A.111 Merkel cell carcinoma of right upper eyelid, including canthus**   HCC

> > **C4A.112 Merkel cell carcinoma of right lower eyelid, including canthus**   HCC

> **✓6ᵗʰ C4A.12 Merkel cell carcinoma of left eyelid, including canthus**

> > **C4A.121 Merkel cell carcinoma of left upper eyelid, including canthus**   HCC

> > **C4A.122 Merkel cell carcinoma of left lower eyelid, including canthus**   HCC

✓5ᵗʰ C4A.2 Merkel cell carcinoma of ear and external auricular canal

> **C4A.20 Merkel cell carcinoma of unspecified ear and external auricular canal**   HCC

> **C4A.21 Merkel cell carcinoma of right ear and external auricular canal**   HCC

> **C4A.22 Merkel cell carcinoma of left ear and external auricular canal**   HCC

✓5ᵗʰ C4A.3 Merkel cell carcinoma of other and unspecified parts of face

> **C4A.30 Merkel cell carcinoma of unspecified part of face**   HCC

> **C4A.31 Merkel cell carcinoma of nose**   HCC

> **C4A.39 Merkel cell carcinoma of other parts of face**   HCC

C4A.4 Merkel cell carcinoma of scalp and neck   HCC

✓5ᵗʰ C4A.5 Merkel cell carcinoma of trunk

> EXCLUDES 2   malignant neoplasm of anus NOS (C21.0)
> malignant neoplasm of scrotum (C63.2)

> **C4A.51 Merkel cell carcinoma of anal skin**   HCC

> > Merkel cell carcinoma of anal margin
> > Merkel cell carcinoma of perianal skin

> **C4A.52 Merkel cell carcinoma of skin of breast**   HCC

> **C4A.59 Merkel cell carcinoma of other part of trunk**   HCC

N Newborn: 0   P Pediatric: 0-17   M Maternity: 9-64   A Adult: 15-124   MCC Major Complication/Comorbidity   CC Complication/Comorbidity   SW Severe Wound Dx

470   ICD–10-CM 2020

√5ᵗʰ **C4A.6 Merkel cell carcinoma** of upper limb, including shoulder

    C4A.60 Merkel cell carcinoma of unspecified upper limb, including shoulder `HCC`

    C4A.61 Merkel cell carcinoma of right **upper limb, including shoulder** `HCC`

    C4A.62 Merkel cell carcinoma of left **upper limb, including shoulder** `HCC`

√5ᵗʰ **C4A.7 Merkel cell carcinoma of** lower limb, including hip

    C4A.70 Merkel cell carcinoma of unspecified lower limb, including hip `HCC`

    C4A.71 Merkel cell carcinoma of right **lower limb, including hip** `HCC`

    C4A.72 Merkel cell carcinoma of left **lower limb, including hip** `HCC`

C4A.8 Merkel cell carcinoma of overlapping sites `HCC`

C4A.9 Merkel cell carcinoma, unspecified `HCC`

    Merkel cell carcinoma of unspecified site

    Merkel cell carcinoma NOS

√4ᵗʰ **C44 Other and unspecified malignant neoplasm** of skin

    `INCLUDES`   malignant neoplasm of sebaceous glands

                   malignant neoplasm of sweat glands

    `EXCLUDES 1`   *Kaposi's sarcoma of skin (C46.0)*

                   malignant melanoma of skin (C43.-)

                   malignant neoplasm of skin of genital organs (C51-C52, C60.-, C63.2)

                   Merkel cell carcinoma (C4A.-)

DEF: Basal cell carcinoma: Abnormal growth of skin cells that arises from the deepest layer of the epidermis and may present as an open sore, red patches, pink growth, or scar. Typically caused by sun exposure, it is one of the most common forms of skin cancer.

DEF: Squamous cell carcinoma: Uncontrolled growth of abnormal skin cells that arises from the outer layers of the skin (epidermis) and may present as an open sore. It is characterized by a firm, red nodule, elevated growth with a central depression, or a flat sore with a scaly crust.

√5ᵗʰ **C44.0 Other and unspecified malignant neoplasm of skin of lip**

    `EXCLUDES 1`   *malignant neoplasm of lip (C00.-)*

    C44.00 Unspecified malignant neoplasm of skin of lip

    C44.01 Basal cell carcinoma of skin of lip

    C44.02 Squamous cell carcinoma of skin of lip

    C44.09 Other specified malignant neoplasm of skin of lip

√5ᵗʰ **C44.1 Other and unspecified malignant neoplasm of skin of** eyelid, including canthus

    `EXCLUDES 1`   *connective tissue of eyelid (C49.0)*

    AHA: 2018,4Q,4

√6ᵗʰ **C44.10 Unspecified malignant neoplasm of skin of eyelid, including canthus**

    C44.101 Unspecified malignant neoplasm of skin of unspecified eyelid, including canthus

√7ᵗʰ **C44.102 Unspecified malignant neoplasm of skin of right eyelid, including canthus**

    C44.1021 Unspecified malignant neoplasm of skin of right upper **eyelid, including canthus**

    C44.1022 Unspecified malignant neoplasm of skin of right lower **eyelid, including canthus**

√7ᵗʰ **C44.109 Unspecified malignant neoplasm of skin of** left **eyelid, including canthus**

    C44.1091 Unspecified malignant neoplasm of skin of left upper **eyelid, including canthus**

    C44.1092 Unspecified malignant neoplasm of skin of left lower **eyelid, including canthus**

√6ᵗʰ **C44.11 Basal cell carcinoma of skin of eyelid, including canthus**

    C44.111 Basal cell carcinoma of skin of unspecified eyelid, including canthus

√7ᵗʰ **C44.112 Basal cell carcinoma of skin of** right **eyelid, including canthus**

    C44.1121 Basal cell carcinoma of skin of right upper **eyelid, including canthus**

    C44.1122 Basal cell carcinoma of skin of right lower **eyelid, including canthus**

√7ᵗʰ **C44.119 Basal cell carcinoma of skin of** left **eyelid, including canthus**

    C44.1191 Basal cell carcinoma of skin of left upper **eyelid, including canthus**

    C44.1192 Basal cell carcinoma of skin of left lower **eyelid, including canthus**

√6ᵗʰ **C44.12 Squamous cell carcinoma of skin of eyelid, including canthus**

    C44.121 Squamous cell carcinoma of skin of unspecified eyelid, including canthus

√7ᵗʰ **C44.122 Squamous cell carcinoma of skin of** right **eyelid, including canthus**

    C44.1221 Squamous cell carcinoma of skin of right upper **eyelid, including canthus**

    C44.1222 Squamous cell carcinoma of skin of right lower **eyelid, including canthus**

√7ᵗʰ **C44.129 Squamous cell carcinoma of skin of** left **eyelid, including canthus**

    C44.1291 Squamous cell carcinoma of skin of left upper **eyelid, including canthus**

    C44.1292 Squamous cell carcinoma of skin of left lower **eyelid, including canthus**

√6ᵗʰ **C44.13 Sebaceous cell carcinoma of skin of eyelid, including canthus**

    C44.131 Sebaceous cell carcinoma of skin of unspecified eyelid, including canthus

√7ᵗʰ **C44.132 Sebaceous cell carcinoma of skin of** right **eyelid, including canthus**

    C44.1321 Sebaceous cell carcinoma of skin of right upper **eyelid, including canthus**

    C44.1322 Sebaceous cell carcinoma of skin of right lower **eyelid, including canthus**

√7ᵗʰ **C44.139 Sebaceous cell carcinoma of skin of** left **eyelid, including canthus**

    C44.1391 Sebaceous cell carcinoma of skin of left upper **eyelid, including canthus**

    C44.1392 Sebaceous cell carcinoma of skin of left lower **eyelid, including canthus**

√6ᵗʰ **C44.19 Other specified malignant neoplasm of skin of eyelid, including canthus**

    C44.191 Other specified malignant neoplasm of skin of unspecified eyelid, including canthus

√7ᵗʰ **C44.192 Other specified malignant neoplasm of skin of** right **eyelid, including canthus**

    C44.1921 Other specified malignant neoplasm of skin of right upper **eyelid, including canthus**

    C44.1922 Other specified malignant neoplasm of skin of right lower **eyelid, including canthus**

√7ᵗʰ **C44.199 Other specified malignant neoplasm of skin of** left **eyelid, including canthus**

    C44.1991 Other specified malignant neoplasm of skin of left upper **eyelid, including canthus**

    C44.1992 Other specified malignant neoplasm of skin of left lower **eyelid, including canthus**

√5ᵗʰ **C44.2 Other and unspecified malignant neoplasm of skin of** ear and external auricular canal

    `EXCLUDES 1`   *connective tissue of ear (C49.0)*

√6ᵗʰ **C44.20 Unspecified malignant neoplasm of skin of ear and external auricular canal**

    C44.201 Unspecified malignant neoplasm of skin of unspecified ear and external auricular canal

    C44.202 Unspecified malignant neoplasm of skin of right **ear and external auricular canal**

    C44.209 Unspecified malignant neoplasm of skin of left **ear and external auricular canal**

√6ᵗʰ **C44.21 Basal cell carcinoma of skin of ear and external auricular canal**

    C44.211 Basal cell carcinoma of skin of unspecified ear and external auricular canal

☑ Additional Character Required   √x7ᵗʰ Placeholder   Unacceptable PDx   Questionable PDx   Manifestation   Unspecified Dx   H1-H14 HAC   HCC CMS-HCC Dx   HIV HIV Dx

ICD-10-CM 2020   471

C4A.6–C44.211

C44.212 Basal cell carcinoma of skin of right ear and external auricular canal

C44.219 Basal cell carcinoma of skin of left ear and external auricular canal

√6th **C44.22** Squamous cell carcinoma of skin of ear and external auricular canal

C44.221 Squamous cell carcinoma of skin of unspecified ear and external auricular canal

C44.222 Squamous cell carcinoma of skin of right ear and external auricular canal

C44.229 Squamous cell carcinoma of skin of left ear and external auricular canal

√6th **C44.29** Other specified malignant neoplasm of skin of ear and external auricular canal

C44.291 Other specified malignant neoplasm of skin of unspecified ear and external auricular canal

C44.292 Other specified malignant neoplasm of skin of right ear and external auricular canal

C44.299 Other specified malignant neoplasm of skin of left ear and external auricular canal

√5th **C44.3** Other and unspecified malignant neoplasm of skin of other and unspecified parts of face

√6th **C44.30** Unspecified malignant neoplasm of skin of other and unspecified parts of face

C44.300 Unspecified malignant neoplasm of skin of unspecified part of face

C44.301 Unspecified malignant neoplasm of skin of nose

C44.309 Unspecified malignant neoplasm of skin of other parts of face

√6th **C44.31** Basal cell carcinoma of skin of other and unspecified parts of face

C44.310 Basal cell carcinoma of skin of unspecified parts of face

C44.311 Basal cell carcinoma of skin of nose

C44.319 Basal cell carcinoma of skin of other parts of face

√6th **C44.32** Squamous cell carcinoma of skin of other and unspecified parts of face

C44.320 Squamous cell carcinoma of skin of unspecified parts of face

C44.321 Squamous cell carcinoma of skin of nose

C44.329 Squamous cell carcinoma of skin of other parts of face

√6th **C44.39** Other specified malignant neoplasm of skin of other and unspecified parts of face

C44.390 Other specified malignant neoplasm of skin of unspecified parts of face

C44.391 Other specified malignant neoplasm of skin of nose

C44.399 Other specified malignant neoplasm of skin of other parts of face

√5th **C44.4** Other and unspecified malignant neoplasm of skin of scalp and neck

C44.40 Unspecified malignant neoplasm of skin of scalp and neck

C44.41 Basal cell carcinoma of skin of scalp and neck

C44.42 Squamous cell carcinoma of skin of scalp and neck

C44.49 Other specified malignant neoplasm of skin of scalp and neck

√5th **C44.5** Other and unspecified malignant neoplasm of skin of trunk

EXCLUDES 1   anus NOS (C21.0)

scrotum (C63.2)

√6th **C44.50** Unspecified malignant neoplasm of skin of trunk

C44.500 Unspecified malignant neoplasm of anal skin

Unspecified malignant neoplasm of anal margin

Unspecified malignant neoplasm of perianal skin

C44.501 Unspecified malignant neoplasm of skin of breast

C44.509 Unspecified malignant neoplasm of skin of other part of trunk

√6th **C44.51** Basal cell carcinoma of skin of trunk

C44.510 Basal cell carcinoma of anal skin

Basal cell carcinoma of anal margin

Basal cell carcinoma of perianal skin

C44.511 Basal cell carcinoma of skin of breast

C44.519 Basal cell carcinoma of skin of other part of trunk

√6th **C44.52** Squamous cell carcinoma of skin of trunk

C44.520 Squamous cell carcinoma of anal skin

Squamous cell carcinoma of anal margin

Squamous cell carcinoma of perianal skin

C44.521 Squamous cell carcinoma of skin of breast

C44.529 Squamous cell carcinoma of skin of other part of trunk

√6th **C44.59** Other specified malignant neoplasm of skin of trunk

C44.590 Other specified malignant neoplasm of anal skin

Other specified malignant neoplasm of anal margin

Other specified malignant neoplasm of perianal skin

C44.591 Other specified malignant neoplasm of skin of breast

C44.599 Other specified malignant neoplasm of skin of other part of trunk

√5th **C44.6** Other and unspecified malignant neoplasm of skin of upper limb, including shoulder

√6th **C44.60** Unspecified malignant neoplasm of skin of upper limb, including shoulder

C44.601 Unspecified malignant neoplasm of skin of unspecified upper limb, including shoulder

C44.602 Unspecified malignant neoplasm of skin of right upper limb, including shoulder.

C44.609 Unspecified malignant neoplasm of skin of left upper limb, including shoulder

√6th **C44.61** Basal cell carcinoma of skin of upper limb, including shoulder

C44.611 Basal cell carcinoma of skin of unspecified upper limb, including shoulder

C44.612 Basal cell carcinoma of skin of right upper limb, including shoulder

C44.619 Basal cell carcinoma of skin of left upper limb, including shoulder

√6th **C44.62** Squamous cell carcinoma of skin of upper limb, including shoulder

C44.621 Squamous cell carcinoma of skin of unspecified upper limb, including shoulder

C44.622 Squamous cell carcinoma of skin of right upper limb, including shoulder

C44.629 Squamous cell carcinoma of skin of left upper limb, including shoulder

√6th **C44.69** Other specified malignant neoplasm of skin of upper limb, including shoulder

C44.691 Other specified malignant neoplasm of skin of unspecified upper limb, including shoulder

C44.692 Other specified malignant neoplasm of skin of right upper limb, including shoulder

C44.699 Other specified malignant neoplasm of skin of left upper limb, including shoulder

√5th **C44.7** Other and unspecified malignant neoplasm of skin of lower limb, including hip

√6th **C44.70** Unspecified malignant neoplasm of skin of lower limb, including hip

C44.701 Unspecified malignant neoplasm of skin of unspecified lower limb, including hip

C44.702 Unspecified malignant neoplasm of skin of right lower limb, including hip

C44.709 Unspecified malignant neoplasm of skin of left lower limb, including hip

√6th **C44.71** Basal cell carcinoma of skin of lower limb, including hip

C44.711 Basal cell carcinoma of skin of unspecified lower limb, including hip

C44.712 Basal cell carcinoma of skin of right lower limb, including hip

C44.719 Basal cell carcinoma of skin of left lower limb, including hip

N Newborn: 0   P Pediatric: 0-17   M Maternity: 9-64   A Adult: 15-124   MCC Major Complication/Comorbidity   CC Complication/Comorbidity   SW Severe Wound Dx

472   ICD-10-CM 2020

✓6ᵗʰ **C44.72 Squamous cell carcinoma** of skin of lower limb, including hip

C44.721 Squamous cell carcinoma of skin of unspecified lower limb, including hip

C44.722 Squamous cell carcinoma of skin of right lower limb, including hip

C44.729 Squamous cell carcinoma of skin of left lower limb, including hip

✓6ᵗʰ **C44.79 Other specified malignant neoplasm of skin of lower** limb, including hip

C44.791 Other specified malignant neoplasm of skin of unspecified lower limb, including hip

C44.792 Other specified malignant neoplasm of skin of right lower limb, including hip

C44.799 Other specified malignant neoplasm of skin of left lower limb, including hip

✓5ᵗʰ **C44.8 Other and unspecified malignant neoplasm of** overlapping sites of skin

C44.80 Unspecified malignant neoplasm of overlapping sites of skin

C44.81 Basal cell carcinoma of overlapping sites of skin

C44.82 Squamous cell carcinoma of overlapping sites of skin

C44.89 Other specified malignant neoplasm of overlapping sites of skin

✓5ᵗʰ **C44.9 Other and unspecified malignant neoplasm of skin,** unspecified

C44.90 Unspecified malignant neoplasm of skin, unspecified

Malignant neoplasm of unspecified site of skin

C44.91 Basal cell carcinoma of skin, unspecified

C44.92 Squamous cell carcinoma of skin, unspecified

C44.99 Other specified malignant neoplasm of skin, unspecified

Malignant neoplasms of mesothelial and soft tissue (C45-C49)

✓4ᵗʰ **C45 Mesothelioma**

DEF: Rare type of cancer that forms in the thin layer of protective tissue that covers the majority of internal organs (mesothelium).

C45.0 Mesothelioma of pleura   HCC

EXCLUDES 1   *other malignant neoplasm of pleura (C38.4)*

AHA: 2017,2Q,11

TIP: For pleural mesothelioma that has metastasized to the chest wall, assign this code for the primary site along with C79.89 for metastatic cancer in the chest wall.

C45.1 Mesothelioma of peritoneum   HCC

Mesothelioma of cul-de-sac
Mesothelioma of mesentery
Mesothelioma of mesocolon
Mesothelioma of omentum
Mesothelioma of peritoneum (parietal) (pelvic)

EXCLUDES 1   *other malignant neoplasm of soft tissue of peritoneum (C48.-)*

C45.2 Mesothelioma of pericardium   HCC

EXCLUDES 1   *other malignant neoplasm of pericardium (C38.0)*

C45.7 Mesothelioma of other sites   HCC

C45.9 Mesothelioma, unspecified   HCC

✓4ᵗʰ **C46 Kaposi's sarcoma**

Code first any human immunodeficiency virus [HIV] disease (B20)
DEF: Malignant neoplasm that causes patches of abnormal tissue to grow under the skin, in the lining of the mouth, nose, and throat, in lymph nodes, or in other visceral organs. Kaposi's sarcoma is caused by human herpesvirus8 (HHV8).

C46.0 Kaposi's sarcoma of skin   HIV HCC

C46.1 Kaposi's sarcoma of soft tissue   HIV HCC

Kaposi's sarcoma of blood vessel
Kaposi's sarcoma of connective tissue
Kaposi's sarcoma of fascia
Kaposi's sarcoma of ligament
Kaposi's sarcoma of lymphatic(s) NEC
Kaposi's sarcoma of muscle

EXCLUDES 2   *Kaposi's sarcoma of lymph glands and nodes (C46.3)*

C46.2 Kaposi's sarcoma of palate   HIV HCC

C46.3 Kaposi's sarcoma of lymph nodes   HIV HCC

C46.4 Kaposi's sarcoma of gastrointestinal sites   HIV HCC

✓5ᵗʰ **C46.5 Kaposi's sarcoma of** lung

AHA: 2019,1Q,16
TIP: When associated malignant pericardial effusion is documented, assign code I31.3. If the sole reason for admission is to treat the effusion with no treatment of the lung malignancy rendered, code I31.3 may be sequenced first.

C46.50 Kaposi's sarcoma of unspecified lung   HIV HCC

C46.51 Kaposi's sarcoma of right lung   HIV HCC

C46.52 Kaposi's sarcoma of left lung   HIV HCC

C46.7 Kaposi's sarcoma of other sites   HIV HCC

C46.9 Kaposi's sarcoma, unspecified   HIV HCC

Kaposi's sarcoma of unspecified site

✓4ᵗʰ **C47 Malignant neoplasm of peripheral nerves and autonomic nervous** system

INCLUDES   malignant neoplasm of sympathetic and parasympathetic nerves and ganglia

EXCLUDES 1   *Kaposi's sarcoma of soft tissue (C46.1)*

C47.0 Malignant neoplasm of peripheral nerves of head, face and neck   HCC

EXCLUDES 1   *malignant neoplasm of peripheral nerves of orbit (C69.6-)*

✓6ᵗʰ **C47.1 Malignant neoplasm of peripheral nerves of** upper limb, including shoulder

C47.10 Malignant neoplasm of peripheral nerves of unspecified upper limb, including shoulder   HCC

C47.11 Malignant neoplasm of peripheral nerves of right upper limb, including shoulder   HCC

C47.12 Malignant neoplasm of peripheral nerves of left upper limb, including shoulder   HCC

✓5ᵗʰ **C47.2 Malignant neoplasm of peripheral nerves of** lower limb, including hip

C47.20 Malignant neoplasm of peripheral nerves of unspecified lower limb, including hip   HCC

C47.21 Malignant neoplasm of peripheral nerves of right lower limb, including hip   HCC

C47.22 Malignant neoplasm of peripheral nerves of left lower limb, including hip   HCC

C47.3 Malignant neoplasm of peripheral nerves of thorax   HCC

C47.4 Malignant neoplasm of peripheral nerves of abdomen   HCC

C47.5 Malignant neoplasm of peripheral nerves of pelvis   HCC

C47.6 Malignant neoplasm of peripheral nerves of trunk, unspecified   HCC

Malignant neoplasm of peripheral nerves of unspecified part of trunk

C47.8 Malignant neoplasm of overlapping sites of peripheral nerves and autonomic nervous system   HCC

C47.9 Malignant neoplasm of peripheral nerves and autonomic nervous system, unspecified   HCC

Malignant neoplasm of unspecified site of peripheral nerves and autonomic nervous system

✓4ᵗʰ **C48 Malignant neoplasm of** retroperitoneum and peritoneum

EXCLUDES 1   *Kaposi's sarcoma of connective tissue (C46.1)*
                mesothelioma (C45.-)

C48.0 Malignant neoplasm of retroperitoneum   HCC

C48.1 Malignant neoplasm of specified parts of peritoneum   HCC

Malignant neoplasm of cul-de-sac
Malignant neoplasm of mesentery
Malignant neoplasm of mesocolon
Malignant neoplasm of omentum
Malignant neoplasm of parietal peritoneum
Malignant neoplasm of pelvic peritoneum

C48.2 Malignant neoplasm of peritoneum, unspecified   HCC

C48.8 Malignant neoplasm of overlapping sites of retroperitoneum and peritoneum   HCC

Chapter 2. Neoplasms

C49–C50.112

✓4th **C49 Malignant neoplasm of other connective and soft tissue**

     INCLUDES   malignant neoplasm of blood vessel
               malignant neoplasm of bursa
               malignant neoplasm of cartilage
               malignant neoplasm of fascia
               malignant neoplasm of fat
               malignant neoplasm of ligament, except uterine
               malignant neoplasm of lymphatic vessel
               malignant neoplasm of muscle
               malignant neoplasm of synovia
               malignant neoplasm of tendon (sheath)

     EXCLUDES 1   *malignant neoplasm of cartilage (of):*
               articular (C40-C41)
               larynx (C32.3)
               nose (C30.0)
             malignant neoplasm of connective tissue of breast (C50.-)

     EXCLUDES 2   *Kaposi's sarcoma of soft tissue (C46.1)*
             malignant neoplasm of heart (C38.0)
             malignant neoplasm of peripheral nerves and autonomic nervous system (C47.-)
             malignant neoplasm of peritoneum (C48.2)
             malignant neoplasm of retroperitoneum (C48.0)
             malignant neoplasm of uterine ligament (C57.3)
             mesothelioma (C45.-)

C49.0 Malignant neoplasm of connective and soft tissue of head, face and neck   HCC
     Malignant neoplasm of connective tissue of ear
     Malignant neoplasm of connective tissue of eyelid
       EXCLUDES 1   *connective tissue of orbit (C69.6-)*

✓5th **C49.1 Malignant neoplasm of connective and soft tissue of upper limb, including shoulder**

     C49.10 Malignant neoplasm of connective and soft tissue of unspecified upper limb, including shoulder   HCC

     C49.11 Malignant neoplasm of connective and soft tissue of right upper limb, including shoulder   HCC

     C49.12 Malignant neoplasm of connective and soft tissue of left upper limb, including shoulder   HCC

✓5th **C49.2 Malignant neoplasm of connective and soft tissue of lower limb, including hip**

     C49.20 Malignant neoplasm of connective and soft tissue of unspecified lower limb, including hip   HCC

     C49.21 Malignant neoplasm of connective and soft tissue of right lower limb, including hip   HCC

     C49.22 Malignant neoplasm of connective and soft tissue of left lower limb, including hip   HCC

C49.3 Malignant neoplasm of connective and soft tissue of thorax   HCC
     Malignant neoplasm of axilla
     Malignant neoplasm of diaphraqm
     Malignant neoplasm of great vessels
       EXCLUDES 1   *malignant neoplasm of breast (C50.-)*
             malignant neoplasm of heart (C38.0)
             malignant neoplasm of mediastinum (C38.1-C38.3)
             malignant neoplasm of thymus (C37)
     AHA: 2015,3Q,19

C49.4 Malignant neoplasm of connective and soft tissue of abdomen   HCC
     Malignant neoplasm of abdominal wall
     Malignant neoplasm of hypochondrium

C49.5 Malignant neoplasm of connective and soft tissue of pelvis   HCC
     Malignant neoplasm of buttock
     Malignant neoplasm of groin
     Malignant neoplasm of perineum

C49.6 Malignant neoplasm of connective and soft tissue of trunk, unspecified   HCC
     Malignant neoplasm of back NOS

C49.8 Malignant neoplasm of overlapping sites of connective and soft tissue   HCC
     Primary malignant neoplasm of two or more contiguous sites of connective and soft tissue

C49.9 Malignant neoplasm of connective and soft tissue, unspecified   HCC

✓5th **C49.A Gastrointestinal stromal tumor**
     AHA: 2016,4Q,8
     DEF: Uncommon malignant tumor found in the GI tract that originates from interstitial cells of the autonomic nervous system. Most occur in the stomach or small intestine but can originate anywhere in the GI tract.

     C49.A0 Gastrointestinal stromal tumor, unspecified site   HCC

     C49.A1 Gastrointestinal stromal tumor of esophagus   HCC

     C49.A2 Gastrointestinal stromal tumor of stomach   HCC

     C49.A3 Gastrointestinal stromal tumor of small intestine   HCC

     C49.A4 Gastrointestinal stromal tumor of large intestine   HCC

     C49.A5 Gastrointestinal stromal tumor of rectum   HCC

     C49.A9 Gastrointestinal stromal tumor of other sites   HCC

Malignant neoplasms of breast (C50)

✓4th **C50 Malignant neoplasm of breast**

     INCLUDES   connective tissue of breast
               Paget's disease of breast
               Paget's disease of nipple
     Use additional code to identify estrogen receptor status (Z17.0, Z17.1)
     EXCLUDES 1   *skin of breast (C44.501, C44.511, C44.521, C44.591)*
     AHA: 2017,4Q,19

Female Breast

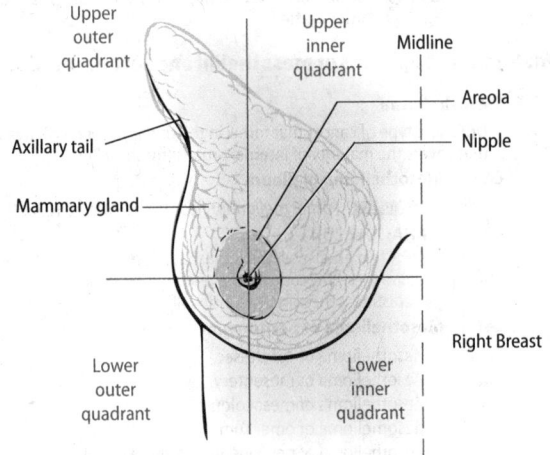

Upper outer quadrant
Upper inner quadrant
Midline
Areola
Nipple
Axillary tail
Mammary gland
Lower outer quadrant
Lower inner quadrant
Right Breast

✓5th **C50.0 Malignant neoplasm of nipple and areola**

     ✓6th **C50.01 Malignant neoplasm of nipple and areola, female**

         C50.011 Malignant neoplasm of nipple and areola, right female breast   HCC ♀

         C50.012 Malignant neoplasm of nipple and areola, left female breast   HCC ♀

         C50.019 Malignant neoplasm of nipple and areola, unspecified female breast   HCC ♀

     ✓6th **C50.02 Malignant neoplasm of nipple and areola, male**

         C50.021 Malignant neoplasm of nipple and areola, right male breast   HCC ♂

         C50.022 Malignant neoplasm of nipple and areola, left male breast   HCC ♂

         C50.029 Malignant neoplasm of nipple and areola, unspecified male breast   HCC ♂

✓5th **C50.1 Malignant neoplasm of central portion of breast**

     ✓6th **C50.11 Malignant neoplasm of central portion of breast, female**

         C50.111 Malignant neoplasm of central portion of right female breast   HCC ♀

         C50.112 Malignant neoplasm of central portion of left female breast   HCC ♀

N Newborn: 0   P Pediatric: 0-17   M Maternity: 9-64   A Adult: 15-124   MCC Major Complication/Comorbidity   CC Complication/Comorbidity   SW Severe Wound Dx

474   ICD-10-CM 2020

C50.119 Malignant neoplasm of central portion of unspecified female breast ☐ HCC ♀

✓6ᵗʰ **C50.12** Malignant neoplasm of central portion of breast, male

    C50.121 Malignant neoplasm of central portion of right male breast ☐ HCC ♂

    C50.122 Malignant neoplasm of central portion of left male breast ☐ HCC ♂

    C50.129 Malignant neoplasm of central portion of unspecified male breast ☐ HCC ♂

✓5ᵗʰ **C50.2** Malignant neoplasm of upper-inner quadrant of breast

  ✓6ᵗʰ **C50.21** Malignant neoplasm of upper-inner quadrant of breast, female

    C50.211 Malignant neoplasm of upper-inner quadrant of right female breast ☐ HCC ♀

    C50.212 Malignant neoplasm of upper-inner quadrant of left female breast ☐ HCC ♀

    C50.219 Malignant neoplasm of upper-inner quadrant of unspecified female breast ☐ HCC ♀

  ✓6ᵗʰ **C50.22** Malignant neoplasm of upper-inner quadrant of breast, male

    C50.221 Malignant neoplasm of upper-inner quadrant of right male breast ☐ HCC ♂

    C50.222 Malignant neoplasm of upper-inner quadrant of left male breast ☐ HCC ♂

    C50.229 Malignant neoplasm of upper-inner quadrant of unspecified male breast ☐ HCC ♂

✓5ᵗʰ **C50.3** Malignant neoplasm of lower-inner quadrant of breast

  ✓6ᵗʰ **C50.31** Malignant neoplasm of lower-inner quadrant of breast, female

    C50.311 Malignant neoplasm of lower-inner quadrant of right female breast ☐ HCC ♀

    C50.312 Malignant neoplasm of lower-inner quadrant of left female breast ☐ HCC ♀

    C50.319 Malignant neoplasm of lower-inner quadrant of unspecified female breast ☐ HCC ♀

  ✓6ᵗʰ **C50.32** Malignant neoplasm of lower-inner quadrant of breast, male

    C50.321 Malignant neoplasm of lower-inner quadrant of right male breast ☐ HCC ♂

    C50.322 Malignant neoplasm of lower-inner quadrant of left male breast ☐ HCC ♂

    C50.329 Malignant neoplasm of lower-inner quadrant of unspecified male breast ☐ HCC ♂

✓5ᵗʰ **C50.4** Malignant neoplasm of upper-outer quadrant of breast

  ✓6ᵗʰ **C50.41** Malignant neoplasm of upper-outer quadrant of breast, female

    C50.411 Malignant neoplasm of upper-outer quadrant of right female breast ☐ HCC ♀

    C50.412 Malignant neoplasm of upper-outer quadrant of left female breast ☐ HCC ♀

    C50.419 Malignant neoplasm of upper-outer quadrant of unspecified female breast ☐ HCC ♀

  ✓6ᵗʰ **C50.42** Malignant neoplasm of upper-outer quadrant of breast, male

    C50.421 Malignant neoplasm of upper-outer quadrant of right male breast ☐ HCC ♂

    C50.422 Malignant neoplasm of upper-outer quadrant of left male breast ☐ HCC ♂

    C50.429 Malignant neoplasm of upper-outer quadrant of unspecified male breast ☐ HCC ♂

✓5ᵗʰ **C50.5** Malignant neoplasm of lower-outer quadrant of breast

  ✓6ᵗʰ **C50.51** Malignant neoplasm of lower-outer quadrant of breast, female

    C50.511 Malignant neoplasm of lower-outer quadrant of right female breast ☐ HCC ♀

    C50.512 Malignant neoplasm of lower-outer quadrant of left female breast ☐ HCC ♀

    C50.519 Malignant neoplasm of lower-outer quadrant of unspecified female breast ☐ HCC ♀

  ✓6ᵗʰ **C50.52** Malignant neoplasm of lower-outer quadrant of breast, male

    C50.521 Malignant neoplasm of lower-outer quadrant of right male breast ☐ HCC ♂

    C50.522 Malignant neoplasm of lower-outer quadrant of left male breast ☐ HCC ♂

    C50.529 Malignant neoplasm of lower-outer quadrant of unspecified male breast ☐ HCC ♂

✓5ᵗʰ **C50.6** Malignant neoplasm of axillary tail of breast

  ✓6ᵗʰ **C50.61** Malignant neoplasm of axillary tail of breast, female

    C50.611 Malignant neoplasm of axillary tail of right female breast ☐ HCC ♀

    C50.612 Malignant neoplasm of axillary tail of left female breast ☐ HCC ♀

    C50.619 Malignant neoplasm of axillary tail of unspecified female breast ☐ HCC ♀

  ✓6ᵗʰ **C50.62** Malignant neoplasm of axillary tail of breast, male

    C50.621 Malignant neoplasm of axillary tail of right male breast ☐ HCC ♂

    C50.622 Malignant neoplasm of axillary tail of left male breast ☐ HCC ♂

    C50.629 Malignant neoplasm of axillary tail of unspecified male breast ☐ HCC ♂

✓5ᵗʰ **C50.8** Malignant neoplasm of overlapping sites of breast

  ✓6ᵗʰ **C50.81** Malignant neoplasm of overlapping sites of breast, female

    C50.811 Malignant neoplasm of overlapping sites of right female breast ☐ HCC ♀

    C50.812 Malignant neoplasm of overlapping sites of left female breast ☐ HCC ♀

    C50.819 Malignant neoplasm of overlapping sites of unspecified female breast ☐ HCC ♀

  ✓6ᵗʰ **C50.82** Malignant neoplasm of overlapping sites of breast, male

    C50.821 Malignant neoplasm of overlapping sites of right male breast ☐ HCC ♂

    C50.822 Malignant neoplasm of overlapping sites of left male breast ☐ HCC ♂

    C50.829 Malignant neoplasm of overlapping sites of unspecified male breast ☐ HCC ♂

✓5ᵗʰ **C50.9** Malignant neoplasm of breast of unspecified site

  ✓6ᵗʰ **C50.91** Malignant neoplasm of breast of unspecified site, female

    C50.911 Malignant neoplasm of unspecified site of right female breast ☐ HCC ♀

    C50.912 Malignant neoplasm of unspecified site of left female breast ☐ HCC ♀

    C50.919 Malignant neoplasm of unspecified site of unspecified female breast ☐ HCC ♀

  ✓6ᵗʰ **C50.92** Malignant neoplasm of breast of unspecified site, male

    C50.921 Malignant neoplasm of unspecified site of right male breast ☐ HCC ♂

    C50.922 Malignant neoplasm of unspecified site of left male breast ☐ HCC ♂

Chapter 2. Neoplasms

C50.929 Malignant neoplasm of unspecified site of unspecified male breast `HCC` ♂

Malignant neoplasms of female genital organs (C51-C58)

INCLUDES   malignant neoplasm of skin of female genital organs

✓4ᵗʰ **C51 Malignant neoplasm of vulva**

EXCLUDES 1   carcinoma in situ of vulva (D07.1)

C51.0 Malignant neoplasm of labium majus `HCC` ♀
Malignant neoplasm of Bartholin's [greater vestibular] gland

C51.1 Malignant neoplasm of labium minus `HCC` ♀

C51.2 Malignant neoplasm of clitoris `HCC` ♀

C51.8 Malignant neoplasm of overlapping sites of vulva `HCC` ♀

C51.9 Malignant neoplasm of vulva, unspecified `HCC` ♀
Malignant neoplasm of external female genitalia NOS
Malignant neoplasm of pudendum

C52 Malignant neoplasm of vagina `HCC` ♀

EXCLUDES 1   carcinoma in situ of vagina (D07.2)

✓4ᵗʰ **C53 Malignant neoplasm of cervix uteri**

EXCLUDES 1   carcinoma in situ of cervix uteri (D06.-)

AHA: 2017,4Q,103

C53.0 Malignant neoplasm of endocervix `HCC` ♀

C53.1 Malignant neoplasm of exocervix `HCC` ♀

C53.8 Malignant neoplasm of overlapping sites of cervix uteri `HCC` ♀

C53.9 Malignant neoplasm of cervix uteri, unspecified `HCC` ♀

✓4ᵗʰ **C54 Malignant neoplasm of corpus uteri**

C54.0 Malignant neoplasm of isthmus uteri `HCC` ♀
Malignant neoplasm of lower uterine segment

C54.1 Malignant neoplasm of endometrium `HCC` ♀

C54.2 Malignant neoplasm of myometrium `HCC` ♀

C54.3 Malignant neoplasm of fundus uteri `HCC` ♀

C54.8 Malignant neoplasm of overlapping sites of corpus uteri `HCC` ♀

C54.9 Malignant neoplasm of corpus uteri, unspecified `HCC` ♀

C55 Malignant neoplasm of uterus, part unspecified `HCC` ♀

✓4ᵗʰ **C56 Malignant neoplasm of ovary**

Use additional code to identify any functional activity

C56.1 Malignant neoplasm of right ovary `HCC` ♀

C56.2 Malignant neoplasm of left ovary `HCC` ♀

C56.9 Malignant neoplasm of unspecified ovary `HCC` ♀

✓4ᵗʰ **C57 Malignant neoplasm of other and unspecified female genital organs**

✓5ᵗʰ **C57.0 Malignant neoplasm of fallopian tube**
Malignant neoplasm of oviduct
Malignant neoplasm of uterine tube

C57.00 Malignant neoplasm of unspecified fallopian tube `HCC` ♀

C57.01 Malignant neoplasm of right fallopian tube `HCC` ♀

C57.02 Malignant neoplasm of left fallopian tube `HCC` ♀

✓5ᵗʰ **C57.1 Malignant neoplasm of broad ligament**

C57.10 Malignant neoplasm of unspecified broad ligament `HCC` ♀

C57.11 Malignant neoplasm of right broad ligament `HCC` ♀

C57.12 Malignant neoplasm of left broad ligament `HCC` ♀

✓5ᵗʰ **C57.2 Malignant neoplasm of round ligament**

C57.20 Malignant neoplasm of unspecified round ligament `HCC` ♀

C57.21 Malignant neoplasm of right round ligament `HCC` ♀

C57.22 Malignant neoplasm of left round ligament `HCC` ♀

C57.3 Malignant neoplasm of parametrium `HCC` ♀
Malignant neoplasm of uterine ligament NOS

C57.4 Malignant neoplasm of uterine adnexa, unspecified `HCC` ♀

C57.7 Malignant neoplasm of other specified female genital organs `HCC` ♀
Malignant neoplasm of wolffian body or duct

C57.8 Malignant neoplasm of overlapping sites of female genital organs `HCC` ♀
Primary malignant neoplasm of two or more contiguous sites of the female genital organs whose point of origin cannot be determined
Primary tubo-ovarian malignant neoplasm whose point of origin cannot be determined
Primary utero-ovarian malignant neoplasm whose point of origin cannot be determined

C57.9 Malignant neoplasm of female genital organ, unspecified `HCC` ♀
Malignant neoplasm of female genitourinary tract NOS

C58 Malignant neoplasm of placenta `HCC` `M` ♀

INCLUDES   choriocarcinoma NOS
choriocarcinoma NOS
chorionepithelioma NOS

EXCLUDES 1   chorioadenoma (destruens) (D39.2)
hydatidiform mole NOS (O01.9)
invasive hydatidiform mole (D39.2)
male choriocarcinoma NOS (C62.9-)
malignant hydatidiform mole (D39.2)

Malignant neoplasms of male genital organs (C60-C63)

INCLUDES   malignant neoplasm of skin of male genital organs

✓4ᵗʰ **C60 Malignant neoplasm of penis**

C60.0 Malignant neoplasm of prepuce `HCC` ♂
Malignant neoplasm of foreskin

C60.1 Malignant neoplasm of glans penis `HCC` ♂

C60.2 Malignant neoplasm of body of penis `HCC` ♂
Malignant neoplasm of corpus cavernosum

C60.8 Malignant neoplasm of overlapping sites of penis `HCC` ♂

C60.9 Malignant neoplasm of penis, unspecified `HCC` ♂
Malignant neoplasm of skin of penis NOS

C61 Malignant neoplasm of prostate `HCC` ♂
Use additional code to identify:
hormone sensitivity status (Z19.1-Z19.2)
rising PSA following treatment for malignant neoplasm of prostate (R97.21)

EXCLUDES 1   malignant neoplasm of seminal vesicle (C63.7)

AHA: 2017,1Q,17

✓4ᵗʰ **C62 Malignant neoplasm of testis**
Use additional code to identify any functional activity

✓5ᵗʰ **C62.0 Malignant neoplasm of undescended testis**
Malignant neoplasm of ectopic testis
Malignant neoplasm of retained testis

C62.00 Malignant neoplasm of unspecified undescended testis `HCC` ♂

C62.01 Malignant neoplasm of undescended right testis `HCC` ♂

C62.02 Malignant neoplasm of undescended left testis `HCC` ♂

✓5ᵗʰ **C62.1 Malignant neoplasm of descended testis**
Malignant neoplasm of scrotal testis

C62.10 Malignant neoplasm of unspecified descended testis `HCC` ♂

C62.11 Malignant neoplasm of descended right testis `HCC` ♂

C62.12 Malignant neoplasm of descended left testis `HCC` ♂

✓5ᵗʰ **C62.9 Malignant neoplasm of testis, unspecified whether descended or undescended**

C62.90 Malignant neoplasm of unspecified testis, unspecified whether descended or undescended `HCC` ♂
Malignant neoplasm of testis NOS

C62.91 Malignant neoplasm of right testis, unspecified whether descended or undescended `HCC` ♂

C62.92 Malignant neoplasm of left testis, unspecified whether descended or undescended `HCC` ♂

✓4th **C63** **Malignant neoplasm of** other and unspecified male genital organs

  ✓5th **C63.0** **Malignant neoplasm of** epididymis

    C63.00 **Malignant neoplasm of unspecified epididymis**   HCC ♂

    C63.01 **Malignant neoplasm of** right **epididymis**   HCC ♂

    C63.02 **Malignant neoplasm of** left **epididymis**   HCC ♂

  ✓5th **C63.1** **Malignant neoplasm of** spermatic cord

    C63.10 **Malignant neoplasm of unspecified spermatic cord**   HCC ♂

    C63.11 **Malignant neoplasm of** right **spermatic cord**

    C63.12 **Malignant neoplasm of** left **spermatic cord**

  C63.2 **Malignant neoplasm of** scrotum   HCC ♂
    Malignant neoplasm of skin of scrotum

  C63.7 **Malignant neoplasm of other specified male genital organs**   HCC ♂
    Malignant neoplasm of seminal vesicle
    Malignant neoplasm of tunica vaginalis

  C63.8 **Malignant neoplasm of** overlapping sites **of male genital organs**   HCC ♂
    Primary malignant neoplasm of two or more contiguous sites of male genital organs whose point of origin cannot be determined

  C63.9 **Malignant neoplasm of male genital organ, unspecified**   HCC ♂
    Malignant neoplasm of male genitourinary tract NOS

Malignant neoplasms of urinary tract (C64-C68)

✓4th **C64** **Malignant neoplasm of** kidney, except renal pelvis

  EXCLUDES 1   malignant carcinoid tumor of the kidney (C7A.093)
    malignant neoplasm of renal calyces (C65.-)
    malignant neoplasm of renal pelvis (C65.-)

  C64.1 **Malignant neoplasm of** right **kidney, except renal pelvis**   HCC

  C64.2 **Malignant neoplasm of** left **kidney, except renal pelvis**   HCC

  C64.9 **Malignant neoplasm of unspecified kidney, except renal pelvis**   HCC

✓4th **C65** **Malignant neoplasm of** renal pelvis

  INCLUDES   malignant neoplasm of pelviureteric junction
    malignant neoplasm of renal calyces

  C65.1 **Malignant neoplasm of** right **renal pelvis**   HCC

  C65.2 **Malignant neoplasm of** left **renal pelvis**   HCC

  C65.9 **Malignant neoplasm of unspecified renal pelvis**   HCC

✓4th **C66** **Malignant neoplasm of** ureter

  EXCLUDES 1   malignant neoplasm of ureteric orifice of bladder (C67.6)

  C66.1 **Malignant neoplasm of** right **ureter**   HCC

  C66.2 **Malignant neoplasm of** left **ureter**   HCC

  C66.9 **Malignant neoplasm of unspecified ureter**   HCC

✓4th **C67** **Malignant neoplasm of** bladder

  C67.0 **Malignant neoplasm of** trigone **of bladder**   HCC

  C67.1 **Malignant neoplasm of** dome **of bladder**   HCC

  C67.2 **Malignant neoplasm of** lateral wall **of bladder**   HCC

  C67.3 **Malignant neoplasm of** anterior wall **of bladder**   HCC

  C67.4 **Malignant neoplasm of** posterior wall **of bladder**   HCC

  C67.5 **Malignant neoplasm of** bladder neck   HCC
    Malignant neoplasm of internal urethral orifice

  C67.6 **Malignant neoplasm of** ureteric orifice   HCC

  C67.7 **Malignant neoplasm of** urachus   HCC

  C67.8 **Malignant neoplasm of** overlapping sites **of bladder**   HCC

  C67.9 **Malignant neoplasm of bladder, unspecified**   HCC
    AHA: 2016,1Q,19

✓4th **C68** **Malignant neoplasm of other and unspecified** urinary organs

  EXCLUDES 1   malignant neoplasm of female genitourinary tract NOS (C57.9)
    malignant neoplasm of male genitourinary tract NOS (C63.9)

  AHA: 2016,1Q,14

  C68.0 **Malignant neoplasm of** urethra   HCC

    EXCLUDES 1   malignant neoplasm of urethral orifice of bladder (C67.5)

  C68.1 **Malignant neoplasm of** paraurethral glands   CC HCC
    CC Excl: PDX collection 312

  C68.8 **Malignant neoplasm of** overlapping sites **of urinary organs**   HCC
    Primary malignant neoplasm of two or more contiguous sites of urinary organs whose point of origin cannot be determined

  C68.9 **Malignant neoplasm of urinary organ, unspecified**   HCC
    Malignant neoplasm of urinary system NOS

Malignant neoplasms of eye, brain and other parts of central nervous system (C69-C72)

✓4th **C69** **Malignant neoplasm of** eye and adnexa

  EXCLUDES 1   malignant neoplasm of connective tissue of eyelid (C49.0)
    malignant neoplasm of eyelid (skin) (C43.1-, C44.1-)
    malignant neoplasm of optic nerve (C72.3-)

  ✓5th **C69.0** **Malignant neoplasm of** conjunctiva

    C69.00 **Malignant neoplasm of unspecified conjunctiva**   HCC

    C69.01 **Malignant neoplasm of** right **conjunctiva**   HCC

    C69.02 **Malignant neoplasm of** left **conjunctiva**   HCC

  ✓5th **C69.1** **Malignant neoplasm of** cornea

    C69.10 **Malignant neoplasm of unspecified cornea**   HCC

    C69.11 **Malignant neoplasm of** right **cornea**   HCC

    C69.12 **Malignant neoplasm of** left **cornea**   HCC

  ✓5th **C69.2** **Malignant neoplasm of** retina

    EXCLUDES 1   dark area on retina (D49.81)
      neoplasm of unspecified behavior of retina and choroid (D49.81)
      retinal freckle (D49.81)

    C69.20 **Malignant neoplasm of unspecified retina**   HCC

    C69.21 **Malignant neoplasm of** right **retina**   HCC

    C69.22 **Malignant neoplasm of** left **retina**   HCC

  ✓5th **C69.3** **Malignant neoplasm of** choroid

    C69.30 **Malignant neoplasm of unspecified choroid**   HCC

    C69.31 **Malignant neoplasm of** right **choroid**   HCC

    C69.32 **Malignant neoplasm of** left **choroid**   HCC

  ✓5th **C69.4** **Malignant neoplasm of** ciliary body

    C69.40 **Malignant neoplasm of unspecified ciliary body**   HCC

    C69.41 **Malignant neoplasm of** right **ciliary body**   HCC

    C69.42 **Malignant neoplasm of** left **ciliary body**   HCC

  ✓5th **C69.5** **Malignant neoplasm of** lacrimal gland and duct
    Malignant neoplasm of lacrimal sac
    Malignant neoplasm of nasolacrimal duct

    C69.50 **Malignant neoplasm of unspecified lacrimal gland and duct**   HCC

    C69.51 **Malignant neoplasm of** right **lacrimal gland and duct**   HCC

    C69.52 **Malignant neoplasm of** left **lacrimal gland and duct**   HCC

  ✓5th **C69.6** **Malignant neoplasm of** orbit
    Malignant neoplasm of connective tissue of orbit
    Malignant neoplasm of extraocular muscle
    Malignant neoplasm of peripheral nerves of orbit
    Malignant neoplasm of retrobulbar tissue
    Malignant neoplasm of retro-ocular tissue
    EXCLUDES 1   malignant neoplasm of orbital bone (C41.0)

    C69.60 **Malignant neoplasm of unspecified orbit**   HCC

    C69.61 **Malignant neoplasm of** right **orbit**   HCC

    C69.62 **Malignant neoplasm of** left **orbit**   HCC

✔ Additional Character Required   ✓x7th Placeholder   Unacceptable PDx   Questionable PDx   Manifestation   Unspecified Dx   H1-H14 HAC   HCC CMS-HCC Dx   HIV HIV Dx

ICD-10-CM 2020   477

✓5ᵗʰ **C69.8** **Malignant neoplasm of** overlapping sites **of eye and adnexa**

    C69.80 **Malignant neoplasm of overlapping sites of** unspecified **eye and adnexa** `HCC`

    C69.81 **Malignant neoplasm of overlapping sites of** right **eye and adnexa** `HCC`

    C69.82 **Malignant neoplasm of overlapping sites of** left **eye and adnexa** `HCC`

✓5ᵗʰ **C69.9** **Malignant neoplasm of unspecified site of eye**

    Malignant neoplasm of eyeball

    C69.90 **Malignant neoplasm of unspecified site of** unspecified **eye** `HCC`

    C69.91 **Malignant neoplasm of unspecified site of** right **eye** `HCC`

    C69.92 **Malignant neoplasm of unspecified site of** left **eye** `HCC`

✓4ᵗʰ **C70** **Malignant neoplasm of** meninges

    C70.0 **Malignant neoplasm of** cerebral **meninges** `HCC`

    C70.1 **Malignant neoplasm of** spinal **meninges** `HCC`

    C70.9 **Malignant neoplasm of meninges, unspecified** `HCC`

✓4ᵗʰ **C71** **Malignant neoplasm of** brain

    EXCLUDES 1 *malignant neoplasm of cranial nerves (C72.2-C72.5)*
        retrobulbar malignant neoplasm (C69.6-)

Lobes of the Brain

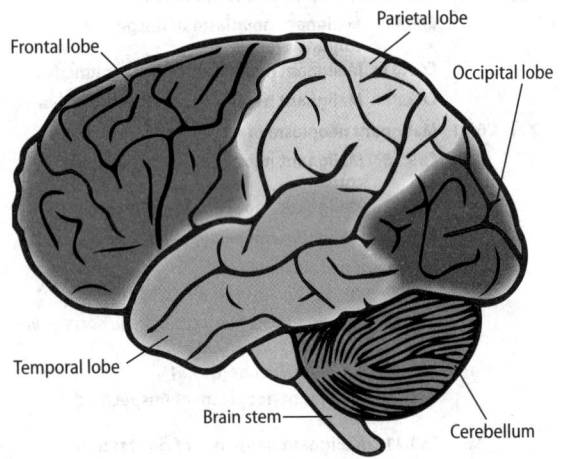

    C71.0 **Malignant neoplasm of** cerebrum, except lobes **and ventricles** `HCC`

        Malignant neoplasm of supratentorial NOS

    C71.1 **Malignant neoplasm of** frontal **lobe** `HCC`

    C71.2 **Malignant neoplasm of** temporal **lobe** `HCC`

    C71.3 **Malignant neoplasm of** parietal **lobe** `HCC`

    C71.4 **Malignant neoplasm of** occipital **lobe** `HCC`

    C71.5 **Malignant neoplasm of** cerebral **ventricle** `HCC`

        EXCLUDES 1 *malignant neoplasm of fourth cerebral ventricle (C71.7)*

    C71.6 **Malignant neoplasm of** cerebellum `HCC`

    C71.7 **Malignant neoplasm of** brain stem `HCC`

        Malignant neoplasm of fourth cerebral ventricle

        Infratentorial malignant neoplasm NOS

    C71.8 **Malignant neoplasm of** overlapping sites **of brain** `HCC`

    C71.9 **Malignant neoplasm of brain, unspecified** `HCC`

        AHA: 2014,3Q,3

✓4ᵗʰ **C72** **Malignant neoplasm of** spinal cord, cranial nerves **and other parts of** central nervous system

    EXCLUDES 1 *malignant neoplasm of meninges (C70.-)*
        malignant neoplasm of peripheral nerves and autonomic nervous system (C47.-)

    C72.0 **Malignant neoplasm of** spinal cord `HCC`

    C72.1 **Malignant neoplasm of** cauda equina `HCC`

✓5ᵗʰ   **C72.2** **Malignant neoplasm of** olfactory nerve

        Malignant neoplasm of olfactory bulb

    C72.20 **Malignant neoplasm of unspecified olfactory nerve** `HCC`

    C72.21 **Malignant neoplasm of** right olfactory nerve `HCC`

    C72.22 **Malignant neoplasm of** left olfactory nerve `HCC`

✓5ᵗʰ **C72.3** **Malignant neoplasm of** optic nerve

    C72.30 **Malignant neoplasm of unspecified optic nerve** `HCC`

    C72.31 **Malignant neoplasm of** right optic nerve `HCC`

    C72.32 **Malignant neoplasm of** left optic nerve `HCC`

✓5ᵗʰ **C72.4** **Malignant neoplasm of** acoustic nerve

    C72.40 **Malignant neoplasm of unspecified acoustic nerve** `HCC`

    C72.41 **Malignant neoplasm of** right acoustic nerve `HCC`

    C72.42 **Malignant neoplasm of** left acoustic nerve `HCC`

✓5ᵗʰ **C72.5** **Malignant neoplasm of other and unspecified** cranial nerves

    C72.50 **Malignant neoplasm of unspecified cranial nerve** `HCC`

        Malignant neoplasm of cranial nerve NOS

    C72.59 **Malignant neoplasm of other cranial nerves** `HCC`

    C72.9 **Malignant neoplasm of central nervous system, unspecified** `HCC`

        Malignant neoplasm of unspecified site of central nervous system

        Malignant neoplasm of nervous system NOS

Malignant neoplasms of thyroid and other endocrine glands (C73-C75)

C73 **Malignant neoplasm of** thyroid gland `HCC`

    Use additional code to identify any functional activity

✓4ᵗʰ **C74** **Malignant neoplasm of** adrenal gland

    TIP: If an adrenal gland tumor is described as functional (producing too much of a hormone), additional codes should be assigned to report the functional activity.

✓5ᵗʰ   **C74.0** **Malignant neoplasm of** cortex of adrenal gland

    C74.00 **Malignant neoplasm of cortex of unspecified adrenal gland** `HCC`

    C74.01 **Malignant neoplasm of cortex of** right **adrenal gland** `HCC`

    C74.02 **Malignant neoplasm of cortex of** left **adrenal gland** `HCC`

✓5ᵗʰ   **C74.1** **Malignant neoplasm of** medulla of adrenal gland

    C74.10 **Malignant neoplasm of medulla of unspecified adrenal gland** `HCC`

    C74.11 **Malignant neoplasm of medulla of** right **adrenal gland** `HCC`

    C74.12 **Malignant neoplasm of medulla of** left **adrenal gland** `HCC`

✓5ᵗʰ   **C74.9** **Malignant neoplasm of unspecified part of adrenal gland**

    C74.90 **Malignant neoplasm of unspecified part of unspecified adrenal gland** `HCC`

    C74.91 **Malignant neoplasm of unspecified part of** right **adrenal gland** `HCC`

    C74.92 **Malignant neoplasm of unspecified part of** left **adrenal gland** `HCC`

✓4ᵗʰ **C75** **Malignant neoplasm of other** endocrine glands and related structures

    EXCLUDES 1 *malignant carcinoid tumors (C7A.0-)*
        malignant neoplasm of adrenal gland (C74.-)
        malignant neoplasm of endocrine pancreas (C25.4)
        malignant neoplasm of islets of Langerhans (C25.4)
        malignant neoplasm of ovary (C56.-)
        malignant neoplasm of testis (C62.-)
        malignant neoplasm of thymus (C37)
        malignant neoplasm of thyroid gland (C73)
        malignant neuroendocrine tumors (C7A.-)

    C75.0 **Malignant neoplasm of** parathyroid **gland** `HCC`

    C75.1 **Malignant neoplasm of** pituitary **gland** `HCC`

    C75.2 **Malignant neoplasm of** craniopharyngeal duct `HCC`

    C75.3 **Malignant neoplasm of** pineal **gland** `HCC`

    C75.4 **Malignant neoplasm of** carotid body `HCC`

    C75.5 **Malignant neoplasm of** aortic body **and other** paraganglia `HCC`

C75.8 Malignant neoplasm with pluriglandular involvement, unspecified `HCC`

C75.9 Malignant neoplasm of endocrine gland, unspecified `HCC`

Malignant neuroendocrine tumors (C7A)

✓4ᵗʰ **C7A** Malignant neuroendocrine tumors

Code also any associated multiple endocrine neoplasia [MEN] syndromes (E31.2-)

Use additional code to identify any associated endocrine syndrome, such as:

carcinoid syndrome (E34.0)

EXCLUDES 2   malignant pancreatic islet cell tumors (C25.4)
Merkel cell carcinoma (C4A.-)

DEF: Tumors comprised of cells that are capable of producing hormonal syndromes in which the normal hormonal balance required to support body system functions is adversely affected.

✓5ᵗʰ **C7A.0** Malignant carcinoid tumors

DEF: Specific type of slow-growing benign or malignant neuroendocrine tumors. Carcinoid tumors occur most commonly in the hormone producing cells of the gastrointestinal tracts and can also occur in the pancreas, testes, ovaries, or lungs.

C7A.00 Malignant carcinoid tumor of unspecified site `HCC`

✓6ᵗʰ **C7A.01** Malignant carcinoid tumors of the small intestine

C7A.010 Malignant carcinoid tumor of the duodenum `HCC`

C7A.011 Malignant carcinoid tumor of the jejunum `HCC`

C7A.012 Malignant carcinoid tumor of the ileum `HCC`

C7A.019 Malignant carcinoid tumor of the small intestine, unspecified portion `HCC`

✓6ᵗʰ **C7A.02** Malignant carcinoid tumors of the appendix, large intestine, and rectum

C7A.020 Malignant carcinoid tumor of the appendix `HCC`

C7A.021 Malignant carcinoid tumor of the cecum `HCC`

C7A.022 Malignant carcinoid tumor of the ascending colon `HCC`

C7A.023 Malignant carcinoid tumor of the transverse colon `HCC`

C7A.024 Malignant carcinoid tumor of the descending colon `HCC`

C7A.025 Malignant carcinoid tumor of the sigmoid colon `HCC`

C7A.026 Malignant carcinoid tumor of the rectum `HCC`

C7A.029 Malignant carcinoid tumor of the large intestine, unspecified portion `HCC`

Malignant carcinoid tumor of the colon NOS

✓6ᵗʰ **C7A.09** Malignant carcinoid tumors of other sites

C7A.090 Malignant carcinoid tumor of the bronchus and lung `HCC`

AHA: 2019,1Q,16

TIP: When associated malignant pericardial effusion is documented, assign code I31.3. If the sole reason for admission is to treat the effusion with no treatment of the lung malignancy rendered, code I31.3 may be sequenced first.

C7A.091 Malignant carcinoid tumor of the thymus `HCC`

C7A.092 Malignant carcinoid tumor of the stomach `HCC`

C7A.093 Malignant carcinoid tumor of the kidney `HCC`

C7A.094 Malignant carcinoid tumor of the foregut, unspecified `HCC`

C7A.095 Malignant carcinoid tumor of the midgut, unspecified `HCC`

C7A.096 Malignant carcinoid tumor of the hindgut, unspecified `HCC`

C7A.098 Malignant carcinoid tumors of other sites `HCC`

C7A.1 Malignant poorly differentiated neuroendocrine tumors `HCC`

Malignant poorly differentiated neuroendocrine tumor NOS

High grade neuroendocrine carcinoma, any site

Malignant poorly differentiated neuroendocrine carcinoma, any site

C7A.8 Other malignant neuroendocrine tumors `HCC`

Secondary neuroendocrine tumors (C7B)

✓4ᵗʰ **C7B** Secondary neuroendocrine tumors

Use additional code to identify any functional activity

✓5ᵗʰ **C7B.0** Secondary carcinoid tumors

C7B.00 Secondary carcinoid tumors, unspecified site `HCC`

C7B.01 Secondary carcinoid tumors of distant lymph nodes `HCC`

C7B.02 Secondary carcinoid tumors of liver `HCC`

C7B.03 Secondary carcinoid tumors of bone `HCC`

C7B.04 Secondary carcinoid tumors of peritoneum `HCC`

Mesentery metastasis of carcinoid tumor

C7B.09 Secondary carcinoid tumors of other sites `HCC`

C7B.1 Secondary Merkel cell carcinoma `HCC`

Merkel cell carcinoma nodal presentation

Merkel cell carcinoma visceral metastatic presentation

C7B.8 Other secondary neuroendocrine tumors `HCC`

Malignant neoplasms of ill-defined, other secondary and unspecified sites (C76-C80)

✓4ᵗʰ **C76** Malignant neoplasm of other and ill-defined sites

EXCLUDES 1   malignant neoplasm of female genitourinary tract NOS (C57.9)

malignant neoplasm of male genitourinary tract NOS (C63.9)

malignant neoplasm of lymphoid, hematopoietic and related tissue (C81-C96)

malignant neoplasm of skin (C44.-)

malignant neoplasm of unspecified site NOS (C80.1)

C76.0 Malignant neoplasm of head, face and neck `HCC`

Malignant neoplasm of cheek NOS

Malignant neoplasm of nose NOS

C76.1 Malignant neoplasm of thorax `HCC`

Intrathoracic malignant neoplasm NOS

Malignant neoplasm of axilla NOS

Thoracic malignant neoplasm NOS

C76.2 Malignant neoplasm of abdomen `HCC`

C76.3 Malignant neoplasm of pelvis `HCC`

Malignant neoplasm of groin NOS

Malignant neoplasm of sites overlapping systems within the pelvis

Rectovaginal (septum) malignant neoplasm

Rectovesical (septum) malignant neoplasm

✓5ᵗʰ **C76.4** Malignant neoplasm of upper limb

C76.40 Malignant neoplasm of unspecified upper limb `HCC`

C76.41 Malignant neoplasm of right upper limb `HCC`

C76.42 Malignant neoplasm of left upper limb `HCC`

✓5ᵗʰ **C76.5** Malignant neoplasm of lower limb

C76.50 Malignant neoplasm of unspecified lower limb `HCC`

C76.51 Malignant neoplasm of right lower limb `HCC`

C76.52 Malignant neoplasm of left lower limb `HCC`

C76.8 Malignant neoplasm of other specified ill-defined sites `HCC`

Malignant neoplasm of overlapping ill-defined sites

Chapter 2. Neoplasms

C77–C80.2

✓4ᵗʰ **C77 Secondary and unspecified malignant neoplasm of lymph nodes**

EXCLUDES 1   *malignant neoplasm of lymph nodes, specified as primary (C81-C86, C88, C96.-)*
mesentary metastasis of carcinoid tumor (C7B.04)
secondary carcinoid tumors of distant lymph nodes (C7B.01)

C77.0 Secondary and unspecified malignant neoplasm of lymph nodes of head, face and neck HCC
Secondary and unspecified malignant neoplasm of supraclavicular lymph nodes

C77.1 Secondary and unspecified malignant neoplasm of intrathoracic lymph nodes HCC

C77.2 Secondary and unspecified malignant neoplasm of intra-abdominal lymph nodes HCC

C77.3 Secondary and unspecified malignant neoplasm of axilla and upper limb lymph nodes HCC
Secondary and unspecified malignant neoplasm of pectoral lymph nodes

C77.4 Secondary and unspecified malignant neoplasm of inguinal and lower limb lymph nodes HCC

C77.5 Secondary and unspecified malignant neoplasm of intrapelvic lymph nodes HCC

C77.8 Secondary and unspecified malignant neoplasm of lymph nodes of multiple regions HCC

C77.9 Secondary and unspecified malignant neoplasm of lymph node, unspecified HCC

✓4ᵗʰ **C78 Secondary malignant neoplasm of respiratory and digestive organs**

EXCLUDES 1   *secondary carcinoid tumors of liver (C7B.02)*
secondary carcinoid tumors of peritoneum (C7B.04)

EXCLUDES 2   *lymph node metastases (C77.0)*

✓5ᵗʰ **C78.0 Secondary malignant neoplasm of lung**

AHA: 2019,1Q,16

C78.00 Secondary malignant neoplasm of unspecified lung HCC

C78.01 Secondary malignant neoplasm of right lung HCC

C78.02 Secondary malignant neoplasm of left lung HCC

C78.1 Secondary malignant neoplasm of mediastinum HCC

C78.2 Secondary malignant neoplasm of pleura HCC

✓5ᵗʰ **C78.3 Secondary malignant neoplasm of other and unspecified respiratory organs**

C78.30 Secondary malignant neoplasm of unspecified respiratory organ HCC

C78.39 Secondary malignant neoplasm of other respiratory organs HCC

C78.4 Secondary malignant neoplasm of small intestine HCC

C78.5 Secondary malignant neoplasm of large intestine and rectum HCC

C78.6 Secondary malignant neoplasm of retroperitoneum and peritoneum HCC

AHA: 2017,2Q,12

C78.7 Secondary malignant neoplasm of liver and intrahepatic bile duct HCC

✓5ᵗʰ **C78.8 Secondary malignant neoplasm of other and unspecified digestive organs**

C78.80 Secondary malignant neoplasm of unspecified digestive organ HCC

C78.89 Secondary malignant neoplasm of other digestive organs HCC
Code also exocrine pancreatic insufficiency (K86.81)

✓4ᵗʰ **C79 Secondary malignant neoplasm of other and unspecified sites**

EXCLUDES 1   *secondary carcinoid tumors (C7B.-)*
secondary neuroendocrine tumors (C7B.-)

✓5ᵗʰ **C79.0 Secondary malignant neoplasm of kidney and renal pelvis**

C79.00 Secondary malignant neoplasm of unspecified kidney and renal pelvis HCC

C79.01 Secondary malignant neoplasm of right kidney and renal pelvis HCC

C79.02 Secondary malignant neoplasm of left kidney and renal pelvis HCC

✓5ᵗʰ **C79.1 Secondary malignant neoplasm of bladder and other and unspecified urinary organs**

C79.10 Secondary malignant neoplasm of unspecified urinary organs HCC

C79.11 Secondary malignant neoplasm of bladder HCC

EXCLUDES 2   *lymph node metastases (C77.0)*

C79.19 Secondary malignant neoplasm of other urinary organs HCC

C79.2 Secondary malignant neoplasm of skin HCC

EXCLUDES 1   *secondary Merkel cell carcinoma (C7B.1)*

✓5ᵗʰ **C79.3 Secondary malignant neoplasm of brain and cerebral meninges**

C79.31 Secondary malignant neoplasm of brain HCC

C79.32 Secondary malignant neoplasm of cerebral meninges HCC

✓5ᵗʰ **C79.4 Secondary malignant neoplasm of other and unspecified parts of nervous system**

C79.40 Secondary malignant neoplasm of unspecified part of nervous system HCC

C79.49 Secondary malignant neoplasm of other parts of nervous system HCC

✓5ᵗʰ **C79.5 Secondary malignant neoplasm of bone and bone marrow**

EXCLUDES 1   *secondary carcinoid tumors of bone (C7B.03)*

C79.51 Secondary malignant neoplasm of bone HCC
TIP: Do not assign in addition to a code from subcategory C90.0 when multiple myeloma is described as metastatic to the bone; bone involvement is integral to multiple myeloma.

C79.52 Secondary malignant neoplasm of bone marrow HCC

✓5ᵗʰ **C79.6 Secondary malignant neoplasm of ovary**

C79.60 Secondary malignant neoplasm of unspecified ovary HCC ♀

C79.61 Secondary malignant neoplasm of right ovary HCC ♀

C79.62 Secondary malignant neoplasm of left ovary HCC ♀

✓5ᵗʰ **C79.7 Secondary malignant neoplasm of adrenal gland**

C79.70 Secondary malignant neoplasm of unspecified adrenal gland HCC

C79.71 Secondary malignant neoplasm of right adrenal gland HCC

C79.72 Secondary malignant neoplasm of left adrenal gland HCC

✓5ᵗʰ **C79.8 Secondary malignant neoplasm of other specified sites**

C79.81 Secondary malignant neoplasm of breast HCC

C79.82 Secondary malignant neoplasm of genital organs HCC

C79.89 Secondary malignant neoplasm of other specified sites HCC

AHA: 2017,2Q,11

C79.9 Secondary malignant neoplasm of unspecified site HCC
Metastatic cancer NOS
Metastatic disease NOS

EXCLUDES 1   *carcinomatosis NOS (C80.0)*
generalized cancer NOS (C80.0)
malignant (primary) neoplasm of unspecified site (C80.1)

✓4ᵗʰ **C80 Malignant neoplasm without specification of site**

EXCLUDES 1   *malignant carcinoid tumor of unspecified site (C7A.00)*
malignant neoplasm of specified multiple sites — code to each site

C80.0 Disseminated malignant neoplasm, unspecified HCC
Carcinomatosis NOS
Generalized cancer, unspecified site (primary) (secondary)
Generalized malignancy, unspecified site (primary) (secondary)

C80.1 Malignant (primary) neoplasm, unspecified HCC
Cancer NOS
Cancer unspecified site (primary)
Carcinoma unspecified site (primary)
Malignancy unspecified site (primary)

EXCLUDES 1   *secondary malignant neoplasm of unspecified site (C79.9)*

C80.2 Malignant neoplasm associated with transplanted organ HCC
Code first complication of transplanted organ (T86.-)
Use additional code to identify the specific malignancy

N Newborn: 0   P Pediatric: 0-17   M Maternity: 9-64   A Adult: 15-124   MCC Major Complication/Comorbidity   CC Complication/Comorbidity   SW Severe Wound Dx

480   ICD-10-CM 2020

Malignant neoplasms of lymphoid, hematopoietic and related tissue (C81-C96)

EXCLUDES 2   *Kaposi's sarcoma of lymph nodes (C46.3)*
secondary and unspecified neoplasm of lymph nodes (C77.-)
secondary neoplasm of bone marrow (C79.52)
secondary neoplasm of spleen (C78.89)

✓4th C81 Hodgkin lymphoma

EXCLUDES 1   *personal history of Hodgkin lymphoma (Z85.71)*

DEF: Malignant disorder of lymphoid cells characterized by the presence of progressively swollen lymph nodes and spleen that may also involve the liver. A diagnosis of Hodgkin's lymphoma can be confirmed by the presence of Reed-Sternberg cells. *Synonym(s):* Hodgkin disease.

✓5th C81.0 Nodular lymphocyte predominant Hodgkin lymphoma

- C81.00 Nodular lymphocyte predominant Hodgkin lymphoma, unspecified site   HCC
- C81.01 Nodular lymphocyte predominant Hodgkin lymphoma, lymph nodes of head, face, and neck   HCC
- C81.02 Nodular lymphocyte predominant Hodgkin lymphoma, intrathoracic lymph nodes   HCC
- C81.03 Nodular lymphocyte predominant Hodgkin lymphoma, intra-abdominal lymph nodes   HCC
- C81.04 Nodular lymphocyte predominant Hodgkin lymphoma, lymph nodes of axilla and upper limb   HCC
- C81.05 Nodular lymphocyte predominant Hodgkin lymphoma, lymph nodes of inguinal region and lower limb   HCC
- C81.06 Nodular lymphocyte predominant Hodgkin lymphoma, intrapelvic lymph nodes   HCC
- C81.07 Nodular lymphocyte predominant Hodgkin lymphoma, spleen   HCC
- C81.08 Nodular lymphocyte predominant Hodgkin lymphoma, lymph nodes of multiple sites   HCC
- C81.09 Nodular lymphocyte predominant Hodgkin lymphoma, extranodal and solid organ sites   HCC

✓5th C81.1 Nodular sclerosis Hodgkin lymphoma

Nodular sclerosis classical Hodgkin lymphoma

- C81.10 Nodular sclerosis Hodgkin lymphoma, unspecified site   HCC
- C81.11 Nodular sclerosis Hodgkin lymphoma, lymph nodes of head, face, and neck   HCC
- C81.12 Nodular sclerosis Hodgkin lymphoma, intrathoracic lymph nodes   HCC
- C81.13 Nodular sclerosis Hodgkin lymphoma, intra-abdominal lymph nodes   HCC
- C81.14 Nodular sclerosis Hodgkin lymphoma, lymph nodes of axilla and upper limb   HCC
- C81.15 Nodular sclerosis Hodgkin lymphoma, lymph nodes of inguinal region and lower limb   HCC
- C81.16 Nodular sclerosis Hodgkin lymphoma, intrapelvic lymph nodes   HCC
- C81.17 Nodular sclerosis Hodgkin lymphoma, spleen   HCC
- C81.18 Nodular sclerosis Hodgkin lymphoma, lymph nodes of multiple sites   HCC
- C81.19 Nodular sclerosis Hodgkin lymphoma, extranodal and solid organ sites   HCC

✓5th C81.2 Mixed cellularity Hodgkin lymphoma

Mixed cellularity classical Hodgkin lymphoma

- C81.20 Mixed cellularity Hodgkin lymphoma, unspecified site   HCC
- C81.21 Mixed cellularity Hodgkin lymphoma, lymph nodes of head, face, and neck   HCC
- C81.22 Mixed cellularity Hodgkin lymphoma, intrathoracic lymph nodes   HCC
- C81.23 Mixed cellularity Hodgkin lymphoma, intra-abdominal lymph nodes   HCC
- C81.24 Mixed cellularity Hodgkin lymphoma, lymph nodes of axilla and upper limb   HCC
- C81.25 Mixed cellularity Hodgkin lymphoma, lymph nodes of inguinal region and lower limb   HCC
- C81.26 Mixed cellularity Hodgkin lymphoma, intrapelvic lymph nodes   HCC
- C81.27 Mixed cellularity Hodgkin lymphoma, spleen   HCC
- C81.28 Mixed cellularity Hodgkin lymphoma, lymph nodes of multiple sites   HCC
- C81.29 Mixed cellularity Hodgkin lymphoma, extranodal and solid organ sites   HCC

✓5th C81.3 Lymphocyte depleted Hodgkin lymphoma

Lymphocyte depleted classical Hodgkin lymphoma

- C81.30 Lymphocyte depleted Hodgkin lymphoma, unspecified site   HCC
- C81.31 Lymphocyte depleted Hodgkin lymphoma, lymph nodes of head, face, and neck   HCC
- C81.32 Lymphocyte depleted Hodgkin lymphoma, intrathoracic lymph nodes   HCC
- C81.33 Lymphocyte depleted Hodgkin lymphoma, intra-abdominal lymph nodes   HCC
- C81.34 Lymphocyte depleted Hodgkin lymphoma, lymph nodes of axilla and upper limb   HCC
- C81.35 Lymphocyte depleted Hodgkin lymphoma, lymph nodes of inguinal region and lower limb   HCC
- C81.36 Lymphocyte depleted Hodgkin lymphoma, intrapelvic lymph nodes   HCC
- C81.37 Lymphocyte depleted Hodgkin lymphoma, spleen   HCC
- C81.38 Lymphocyte depleted Hodgkin lymphoma, lymph nodes of multiple sites   HCC
- C81.39 Lymphocyte depleted Hodgkin lymphoma, extranodal and solid organ sites   HCC

✓5th C81.4 Lymphocyte-rich Hodgkin lymphoma

Lymphocyte-rich classical Hodgkin lymphoma

EXCLUDES 1   *nodular lymphocyte predominant Hodgkin lymphoma (C81.0-)*

- C81.40 Lymphocyte-rich Hodgkin lymphoma, unspecified site   HCC
- C81.41 Lymphocyte-rich Hodgkin lymphoma, lymph nodes of head, face, and neck   HCC
- C81.42 Lymphocyte-rich Hodgkin lymphoma, intrathoracic lymph nodes   HCC
- C81.43 Lymphocyte-rich Hodgkin lymphoma, intra-abdominal lymph nodes   HCC
- C81.44 Lymphocyte-rich Hodgkin lymphoma, lymph nodes of axilla and upper limb   HCC
- C81.45 Lymphocyte-rich Hodgkin lymphoma, lymph nodes of inguinal region and lower limb   HCC
- C81.46 Lymphocyte-rich Hodgkin lymphoma, intrapelvic lymph nodes   HCC
- C81.47 Lymphocyte-rich Hodgkin lymphoma, spleen   HCC
- C81.48 Lymphocyte-rich Hodgkin lymphoma, lymph nodes of multiple sites   HCC
- C81.49 Lymphocyte-rich Hodgkin lymphoma, extranodal and solid organ sites   HCC

✓5th C81.7 Other Hodgkin lymphoma

Classical Hodgkin lymphoma NOS
Other classical Hodgkin lymphoma

- C81.70 Other Hodgkin lymphoma, unspecified site   HCC
- C81.71 Other Hodgkin lymphoma, lymph nodes of head, face, and neck   HCC
- C81.72 Other Hodgkin lymphoma, intrathoracic lymph nodes   HCC
- C81.73 Other Hodgkin lymphoma, intra-abdominal lymph nodes   HCC
- C81.74 Other Hodgkin lymphoma, lymph nodes of axilla and upper limb   HCC
- C81.75 Other Hodgkin lymphoma, lymph nodes of inguinal region and lower limb   HCC
- C81.76 Other Hodgkin lymphoma, intrapelvic lymph nodes   HCC
- C81.77 Other Hodgkin lymphoma, spleen   HCC
- C81.78 Other Hodgkin lymphoma, lymph nodes of multiple sites   HCC

✔ Additional Character Required   ✓x7th Placeholder   Unacceptable PDx   Questionable PDx   Manifestation   Unspecified Dx   H1-H14 HAC   HCC CMS-HCC Dx   HIV HIV Dx
ICD-10-CM 2020   481

C81–C81.78

C81.79 Other Hodgkin lymphoma, extranodal and solid organ sites `HCC`

✓5ᵗʰ **C81.9** Hodgkin lymphoma, unspecified

C81.90 Hodgkin lymphoma, unspecified, unspecified site `HCC`

C81.91 Hodgkin lymphoma, unspecified, lymph nodes of head, face, and neck `HCC`

C81.92 Hodgkin lymphoma, unspecified, intrathoracic lymph nodes `HCC`

C81.93 Hodgkin lymphoma, unspecified, intra-abdominal lymph nodes `HCC`

C81.94 Hodgkin lymphoma, unspecified, lymph nodes of axilla and upper limb `HCC`

C81.95 Hodgkin lymphoma, unspecified, lymph nodes of inguinal region and lower limb `HCC`

C81.96 Hodgkin lymphoma, unspecified, intrapelvic lymph nodes `HCC`

C81.97 Hodgkin lymphoma, unspecified, spleen `HCC`

C81.98 Hodgkin lymphoma, unspecified, lymph nodes of multiple sites `HCC`

C81.99 Hodgkin lymphoma, unspecified, extranodal and solid organ sites `HCC`

✓4ᵗʰ **C82** Follicular lymphoma

INCLUDES follicular lymphoma with or without diffuse areas

EXCLUDES 1 *mature T/NK-cell lymphomas (C84.-)*
personal history of non-Hodgkin lymphoma (Z85.72)

DEF: Most common subgroup of non-Hodgkin lymphomas (NHL), accounting for 20 to 30 percent of all NHLs. NHL is a B-cell lymphoma that is slow growing and characterized by the circular pattern of malignant cell growth with the cells clustered into identifiable nodules or follicles.

✓5ᵗʰ **C82.0** Follicular lymphoma grade I

C82.00 Follicular lymphoma grade I, unspecified site `HCC`

C82.01 Follicular lymphoma grade I, lymph nodes of head, face, and neck `HCC`

C82.02 Follicular lymphoma grade I, intrathoracic lymph nodes `HCC`

C82.03 Follicular lymphoma grade I, intra-abdominal lymph nodes `HCC`

C82.04 Follicular lymphoma grade I, lymph nodes of axilla and upper limb `HCC`

C82.05 Follicular lymphoma grade I, lymph nodes of inguinal region and lower limb `HCC`

C82.06 Follicular lymphoma grade I, intrapelvic lymph nodes `HCC`

C82.07 Follicular lymphoma grade I, spleen `HCC`

C82.08 Follicular lymphoma grade I, lymph nodes of multiple sites `HCC`

C82.09 Follicular lymphoma grade I, extranodal and solid organ sites `HCC`

✓5ᵗʰ **C82.1** Follicular lymphoma grade II

C82.10 Follicular lymphoma grade II, unspecified site `HCC`

C82.11 Follicular lymphoma grade II, lymph nodes of head, face, and neck `HCC`

C82.12 Follicular lymphoma grade II, intrathoracic lymph nodes `HCC`

C82.13 Follicular lymphoma grade II, intra-abdominal lymph nodes `HCC`

C82.14 Follicular lymphoma grade II, lymph nodes of axilla and upper limb `HCC`

C82.15 Follicular lymphoma grade II, lymph nodes of inguinal region and lower limb `HCC`

C82.16 Follicular lymphoma grade II, intrapelvic lymph nodes `HCC`

C82.17 Follicular lymphoma grade II, spleen `CC` `HCC`

    CC Excl: PDX collection 424

C82.18 Follicular lymphoma grade II, lymph nodes of multiple sites `HCC`

C82.19 Follicular lymphoma grade II, extranodal and solid organ sites `HCC`

✓5ᵗʰ **C82.2** Follicular lymphoma grade III, unspecified

C82.20 Follicular lymphoma grade III, unspecified, unspecified site `HCC`

C82.21 Follicular lymphoma grade III, unspecified, lymph nodes of head, face, and neck `HCC`

C82.22 Follicular lymphoma grade III, unspecified, intrathoracic lymph nodes `HCC`

C82.23 Follicular lymphoma grade III, unspecified, intra-abdominal lymph nodes `HCC`

C82.24 Follicular lymphoma grade III, unspecified, lymph nodes of axilla and upper limb `HCC`

C82.25 Follicular lymphoma grade III, unspecified, lymph nodes of inguinal region and lower limb `HCC`

C82.26 Follicular lymphoma grade III, unspecified, intrapelvic lymph nodes `HCC`

C82.27 Follicular lymphoma grade III, unspecified, spleen `HCC`

C82.28 Follicular lymphoma grade III, unspecified, lymph nodes of multiple sites `HCC`

C82.29 Follicular lymphoma grade III, unspecified, extranodal and solid organ sites `HCC`

✓5ᵗʰ **C82.3** Follicular lymphoma grade IIIa

C82.30 Follicular lymphoma grade IIIa, unspecified site `HCC`

C82.31 Follicular lymphoma grade IIIa, lymph nodes of head, face, and neck `HCC`

C82.32 Follicular lymphoma grade IIIa, intrathoracic lymph nodes `HCC`

C82.33 Follicular lymphoma grade IIIa, intra-abdominal lymph nodes `HCC`

C82.34 Follicular lymphoma grade IIIa, lymph nodes of axilla and upper limb `HCC`

C82.35 Follicular lymphoma grade IIIa, lymph nodes of inguinal region and lower limb `HCC`

C82.36 Follicular lymphoma grade IIIa, intrapelvic lymph nodes `HCC`

C82.37 Follicular lymphoma grade IIIa, spleen `HCC`

C82.38 Follicular lymphoma grade IIIa, lymph nodes of multiple sites `HCC`

C82.39 Follicular lymphoma grade IIIa, extranodal and solid organ sites `HCC`

✓5ᵗʰ **C82.4** Follicular lymphoma grade IIIb

C82.40 Follicular lymphoma grade IIIb, unspecified site `HCC`

C82.41 Follicular lymphoma grade IIIb, lymph nodes of head, face, and neck `HCC`

C82.42 Follicular lymphoma grade IIIb, intrathoracic lymph nodes `HCC`

C82.43 Follicular lymphoma grade IIIb, intra-abdominal lymph nodes `HCC`

C82.44 Follicular lymphoma grade IIIb, lymph nodes of axilla and upper limb `HCC`

C82.45 Follicular lymphoma grade IIIb, lymph nodes of inguinal region and lower limb `HCC`

C82.46 Follicular lymphoma grade IIIb, intrapelvic lymph nodes `HCC`

C82.47 Follicular lymphoma grade IIIb, spleen `HCC`

C82.48 Follicular lymphoma grade IIIb, lymph nodes of multiple sites `HCC`

C82.49 Follicular lymphoma grade IIIb, extranodal and solid organ sites `HCC`

✓5ᵗʰ **C82.5** Diffuse follicle center lymphoma

C82.50 Diffuse follicle center lymphoma, unspecified site `HIV` `HCC`

C82.51 Diffuse follicle center lymphoma, lymph nodes of head, face, and neck `HIV` `HCC`

C82.52 Diffuse follicle center lymphoma, intrathoracic lymph nodes `HIV` `HCC`

C82.53 Diffuse follicle center lymphoma, intra-abdominal lymph nodes `HIV` `HCC`

C82.54 Diffuse follicle center lymphoma, lymph nodes of axilla and upper limb `HIV` `HCC`

C82.55 Diffuse follicle center lymphoma, lymph nodes of inguinal region and lower limb `HIV` `HCC`

C82.56 Diffuse follicle center lymphoma, intrapelvic lymph nodes `HIV` `HCC`

C82.57 Diffuse follicle center lymphoma, spleen `HIV` `HCC`

C82.58 Diffuse follicle center lymphoma, lymph nodes of multiple sites `HIV` `HCC`

C82.59 Diffuse follicle center lymphoma, extranodal and solid organ sites `HIV` `HCC`

√5ᵗʰ **C82.6** Cutaneous follicle center lymphoma

    C82.60 Cutaneous follicle center lymphoma, unspecified site `HCC`

    C82.61 Cutaneous follicle center lymphoma, lymph nodes of head, face, and neck `HCC`

    C82.62 Cutaneous follicle center lymphoma, intrathoracic lymph nodes `HCC`

    C82.63 Cutaneous follicle center lymphoma, intra-abdominal lymph nodes `HCC`

    C82.64 Cutaneous follicle center lymphoma, lymph nodes of axilla and upper limb `HCC`

    C82.65 Cutaneous follicle center lymphoma, lymph nodes of inguinal region and lower limb `HCC`

    C82.66 Cutaneous follicle center lymphoma, intrapelvic lymph nodes `HCC`

    C82.67 Cutaneous follicle center lymphoma, spleen `HCC`

    C82.68 Cutaneous follicle center lymphoma, lymph nodes of multiple sites `HCC`

    C82.69 Cutaneous follicle center lymphoma, extranodal and solid organ sites `HCC`

√5ᵗʰ **C82.8** Other types of follicular lymphoma

    C82.80 Other types of follicular lymphoma, unspecified site `HCC`

    C82.81 Other types of follicular lymphoma, lymph nodes of head, face, and neck `HCC`

    C82.82 Other types of follicular lymphoma, intrathoracic lymph nodes `HCC`

    C82.83 Other types of follicular lymphoma, intra-abdominal lymph nodes `HCC`

    C82.84 Other types of follicular lymphoma, lymph nodes of axilla and upper limb `HCC`

    C82.85 Other types of follicular lymphoma, lymph nodes of inguinal region and lower limb `HCC`

    C82.86 Other types of follicular lymphoma, intrapelvic lymph nodes `HCC`

    C82.87 Other types of follicular lymphoma, spleen `HCC`

    C82.88 Other types of follicular lymphoma, lymph nodes of multiple sites `HCC`

    C82.89 Other types of follicular lymphoma, extranodal and solid organ sites `HCC`

√5ᵗʰ **C82.9** Follicular lymphoma, unspecified

    C82.90 Follicular lymphoma, unspecified, unspecified site `HCC`

    C82.91 Follicular lymphoma, unspecified, lymph nodes of head, face, and neck `HCC`

    C82.92 Follicular lymphoma, unspecified, intrathoracic lymph nodes `HCC`

    C82.93 Follicular lymphoma, unspecified, intra-abdominal lymph nodes `HCC`

    C82.94 Follicular lymphoma, unspecified, lymph nodes of axilla and upper limb `HCC`

    C82.95 Follicular lymphoma, unspecified, lymph nodes of inguinal region and lower limb `HCC`

    C82.96 Follicular lymphoma, unspecified, intrapelvic lymph nodes `HCC`

    C82.97 Follicular lymphoma, unspecified, spleen `HCC`

    C82.98 Follicular lymphoma, unspecified, lymph nodes of multiple sites `HCC`

    C82.99 Follicular lymphoma, unspecified, extranodal and solid organ sites `HCC`

√4ᵗʰ **C83** Non-follicular lymphoma

    EXCLUDES 1   personal history of non-Hodgkin lymphoma (Z85.72)

√5ᵗʰ **C83.0** Small cell B-cell lymphoma

    Lymphoplasmacytic lymphoma

    Nodal marginal zone lymphoma

    Non-leukemic variant of B-CLL

    Splenic marginal zone lymphoma

    EXCLUDES 1   chronic lymphocytic leukemia (C91.1)

                    mature T/NK-cell lymphomas (C84.-)

                    Waldenström macroglobulinemia (C88.0)

    DEF: Nonfollicular lymphoma that is rare, slow growing, and usually found in the older population.

    C83.00 Small cell B-cell lymphoma, unspecified site `HIV` `CC` `HCC`

        CC Excl: PDX collection 435

    C83.01 Small cell B-cell lymphoma, lymph nodes of head, face, and neck `HIV` `CC` `HCC`

        CC Excl: PDX collection 436

    C83.02 Small cell B-cell lymphoma, intrathoracic lymph nodes `HIV` `HCC`

    C83.03 Small cell B-cell lymphoma, intra-abdominal lymph nodes `HIV` `HCC`

    C83.04 Small cell B-cell lymphoma, lymph nodes of axilla and upper limb `HIV` `HCC`

    C83.05 Small cell B-cell lymphoma, lymph nodes of inguinal region and lower limb `HIV` `HCC`

    C83.06 Small cell B-cell lymphoma, intrapelvic lymph nodes `HIV` `HCC`

    C83.07 Small cell B-cell lymphoma, spleen `HIV` `HCC`

    C83.08 Small cell B-cell lymphoma, lymph nodes of multiple sites `HIV` `HCC`

    C83.09 Small cell B-cell lymphoma, extranodal and solid organ sites `HIV` `HCC`

√5ᵗʰ **C83.1** Mantle cell lymphoma

    Centrocytic lymphoma

    Malignant lymphomatous polyposis

    DEF: Rare form of B-cell non-Hodgkin lymphoma named for the location of the tumor cell production, the mantle zone of the lymph nodes.

    C83.10 Mantle cell lymphoma, unspecified site `HIV` `HCC`

    C83.11 Mantle cell lymphoma, lymph nodes of head, face, and neck `HIV` `HCC`

    C83.12 Mantle cell lymphoma, intrathoracic lymph nodes `HIV` `HCC`

    C83.13 Mantle cell lymphoma, intra-abdominal lymph nodes `HIV` `HCC`

    C83.14 Mantle cell lymphoma, lymph nodes of axilla and upper limb `HIV` `HCC`

    C83.15 Mantle cell lymphoma, lymph nodes of inguinal region and lower limb `HIV` `HCC`

    C83.16 Mantle cell lymphoma, intrapelvic lymph nodes `HIV` `HCC`

    C83.17 Mantle cell lymphoma, spleen `HIV` `HCC`

    C83.18 Mantle cell lymphoma, lymph nodes of multiple sites `HIV` `HCC`

    C83.19 Mantle cell lymphoma, extranodal and solid organ sites `HIV` `HCC`

√5ᵗʰ **C83.3** Diffuse large B-cell lymphoma

    Anaplastic diffuse large B-cell lymphoma

    CD30-positive diffuse large B-cell lymphoma

    Centroblastic diffuse large B-cell lymphoma

    Diffuse large B-cell lymphoma, subtype not specified

    Immunoblastic diffuse large B-cell lymphoma

    Plasmablastic diffuse large B-cell lymphoma

    T-cell rich diffuse large B-cell lymphoma

    EXCLUDES 1   *mediastinal (thymic) large B-cell lymphoma (C85.2-)*

                  mature T/NK-cell lymphomas (C84.-)

    DEF: Nonfollicular lymphoma that is one of the more common types of lymphoma. This cancer is fast growing and affects any age but is found mostly in the older population.

    C83.30 Diffuse large B-cell lymphoma, unspecified site `HIV` `HCC`

    C83.31 Diffuse large B-cell lymphoma, lymph nodes of head, face, and neck `HIV` `HCC`

    C83.32 Diffuse large B-cell lymphoma, intrathoracic lymph nodes `HIV` `HCC`

    C83.33 Diffuse large B-cell lymphoma, intra-abdominal lymph nodes `HIV` `HCC`

    C83.34 Diffuse large B-cell lymphoma, lymph nodes of axilla and upper limb `HIV` `HCC`

    C83.35 Diffuse large B-cell lymphoma, lymph nodes of inguinal region and lower limb `HIV` `HCC`

    C83.36 Diffuse large B-cell lymphoma, intrapelvic lymph nodes `HIV` `HCC`

    C83.37 Diffuse large B-cell lymphoma, spleen `HIV` `HCC`

    C83.38 Diffuse large B-cell lymphoma, lymph nodes of multiple sites `HIV` `HCC`

    C83.39 Diffuse large B-cell lymphoma, extranodal and solid organ sites `HIV` `HCC`

✔ Additional Character Required   √x7ᵗʰ Placeholder   <u>Unacceptable PDx</u>   Questionable PDx   Manifestation   <u>Unspecified Dx</u>   H1-H14 HAC   `HCC` CMS-HCC Dx   `HIV` HIV Dx

ICD-10-CM 2020   483

Chapter 2. Neoplasms

C83.5–C84.19

✓5ᵗʰ C83.5 Lymphoblastic (diffuse) lymphoma

B-precursor lymphoma
Lymphoblastic B-cell lymphoma
Lymphoblastic lymphoma NOS
Lymphoblastic T-cell lymphoma
T-precursor lymphoma

DEF: Type of non-Hodgkin lymphoma considered lymphoma or leukemia—the determination is made based on the amount of bone marrow involvement. The cells are small to medium immature T-cells that often originate in the thymus where many of the T-cells are made.

C83.50 Lymphoblastic (diffuse) lymphoma, unspecified site `HCC`

C83.51 Lymphoblastic (diffuse) lymphoma, lymph nodes of head, face, and neck `HCC`

C83.52 Lymphoblastic (diffuse) lymphoma, intrathoracic lymph nodes `HCC`

C83.53 Lymphoblastic (diffuse) lymphoma, intra-abdominal lymph nodes `HCC`

C83.54 Lymphoblastic (diffuse) lymphoma, lymph nodes of axilla and upper limb `HCC`

C83.55 Lymphoblastic (diffuse) lymphoma, lymph nodes of inguinal region and lower limb `HCC`

C83.56 Lymphoblastic (diffuse) lymphoma, intrapelvic lymph nodes `HCC`

C83.57 Lymphoblastic (diffuse) lymphoma, spleen `HCC`

C83.58 Lymphoblastic (diffuse) lymphoma, lymph nodes of multiple sites `HCC`

C83.59 Lymphoblastic (diffuse) lymphoma, extranodal and solid organ sites `HCC`

✓5ᵗʰ C83.7 Burkitt lymphoma

Atypical Burkitt lymphoma
Burkitt-like lymphoma

EXCLUDES 1   mature B-cell leukemia Burkitt type (C91.A-)

DEF: Malignancy of the lymphatic system, most often seen as a large bone-deteriorating lesion within the jaw or as an abdominal mass. It is a form of non-Hodgkin's lymphoma and is recognized as the fastest growing human tumor.

C83.70 Burkitt lymphoma, unspecified site `HIV` `HCC`

C83.71 Burkitt lymphoma, lymph nodes of head, face, and neck `HIV` `HCC`

C83.72 Burkitt lymphoma, intrathoracic lymph nodes `HIV` `HCC`

C83.73 Burkitt lymphoma, intra-abdominal lymph nodes `HIV` `HCC`

C83.74 Burkitt lymphoma, lymph nodes of axilla and upper limb `HIV` `HCC`

C83.75 Burkitt lymphoma, lymph nodes of inguinal region and lower limb `HIV` `HCC`

C83.76 Burkitt lymphoma, intrapelvic lymph nodes `HIV` `HCC`

C83.77 Burkitt lymphoma, spleen `HIV` `HCC`

C83.78 Burkitt lymphoma, lymph nodes of multiple sites `HIV` `HCC`

C83.79 Burkitt lymphoma, extranodal and solid organ sites `HIV` `HCC`

✓5ᵗʰ C83.8 Other non-follicular lymphoma

Intravascular large B-cell lymphoma
Lymphoid granulomatosis
Primary effusion B-cell lymphoma

EXCLUDES 1   mediastinal (thymic) large B-cell lymphoma (C85.2-)
          T-cell rich B-cell lymphoma (C83.3-)

C83.80 Other non-follicular lymphoma, unspecified site `HIV` `HCC`

C83.81 Other non-follicular lymphoma, lymph nodes of head, face, and neck `HIV` `HCC`

C83.82 Other non-follicular lymphoma, intrathoracic lymph nodes `HIV` `HCC`

C83.83 Other non-follicular lymphoma, intra-abdominal lymph nodes `HIV` `HCC`

C83.84 Other non-follicular lymphoma, lymph nodes of axilla and upper limb `HIV` `HCC`

C83.85 Other non-follicular lymphoma, lymph nodes of inguinal region and lower limb `HIV` `HCC`

C83.86 Other non-follicular lymphoma, intrapelvic lymph nodes `HIV` `HCC`

C83.87 Other non-follicular lymphoma, spleen `HIV` `HCC`

C83.88 Other non-follicular lymphoma, lymph nodes of multiple sites `HIV` `HCC`

C83.89 Other non-follicular lymphoma, extranodal and solid organ sites `HIV` `HCC`

✓5ᵗʰ C83.9 Non-follicular (diffuse) lymphoma, unspecified

C83.90 Non-follicular (diffuse) lymphoma, unspecified, unspecified site `HIV` `HCC`

C83.91 Non-follicular (diffuse) lymphoma, unspecified, lymph nodes of head, face, and neck `HIV` `HCC`

C83.92 Non-follicular (diffuse) lymphoma, unspecified, intrathoracic lymph nodes `HIV` `HCC`

C83.93 Non-follicular (diffuse) lymphoma, unspecified, intra-abdominal lymph nodes `HIV` `HCC`

C83.94 Non-follicular (diffuse) lymphoma, unspecified, lymph nodes of axilla and upper limb `HIV` `HCC`

C83.95 Non-follicular (diffuse) lymphoma, unspecified, lymph nodes of inguinal region and lower limb `HIV` `HCC`

C83.96 Non-follicular (diffuse) lymphoma, unspecified, intrapelvic lymph nodes `HIV` `HCC`

C83.97 Non-follicular (diffuse) lymphoma, unspecified, spleen `HIV` `HCC`

C83.98 Non-follicular (diffuse) lymphoma, unspecified, lymph nodes of multiple sites `HIV` `HCC`

C83.99 Non-follicular (diffuse) lymphoma, unspecified, extranodal and solid organ sites `HIV` `HCC`

✓4ᵗʰ C84 Mature T/NK-cell lymphomas

EXCLUDES 1   personal history of non-Hodgkin lymphoma (Z85.72)

✓5ᵗʰ C84.0 Mycosis fungoides

EXCLUDES 1   peripheral T-cell lymphoma, not classified (C84.4-)

DEF: Most common form of cutaneous T-cell lymphoma. A type of non-Hodgkin lymphoma in which white blood cells become cancerous and affect the skin and sometimes internal organs.

Synonym(s): Alibert-Bazin syndrome.

C84.00 Mycosis fungoides, unspecified site `HCC`

C84.01 Mycosis fungoides, lymph nodes of head, face, and neck `HCC`

C84.02 Mycosis fungoides, intrathoracic lymph nodes `HCC`

C84.03 Mycosis fungoides, intra-abdominal lymph nodes `HCC`

C84.04 Mycosis fungoides, lymph nodes of axilla and upper limb `HCC`

C84.05 Mycosis fungoides, lymph nodes of inguinal region and lower limb `HCC`

C84.06 Mycosis fungoides, intrapelvic lymph nodes `HCC`

C84.07 Mycosis fungoides, spleen `HCC`

C84.08 Mycosis fungoides, lymph nodes of multiple sites `HCC`

C84.09 Mycosis fungoides, extranodal and solid organ sites `HCC`

✓5ᵗʰ C84.1 Sézary disease

DEF: Extension of mycosis fungoides that affects the blood and all of the skin, appearing as sunburn, rather than patches. It spreads to the lymph nodes and is often linked to a weakened immune system.

C84.10 Sézary disease, unspecified site `HCC`

C84.11 Sézary disease, lymph nodes of head, face, and neck `HCC`

C84.12 Sézary disease, intrathoracic lymph nodes `HCC`

C84.13 Sézary disease, intra-abdominal lymph nodes `HCC`

C84.14 Sézary disease, lymph nodes of axilla and upper limb `HCC`

C84.15 Sézary disease, lymph nodes of inguinal region and lower limb `HCC`

C84.16 Sézary disease, intrapelvic lymph nodes `HCC`

C84.17 Sézary disease, spleen `HCC`

C84.18 Sézary disease, lymph nodes of multiple sites `HCC`

C84.19 Sézary disease, extranodal and solid organ sites `HCC`

✓5ᵗʰ C84.4 Peripheral T-cell lymphoma, not classified

Lennert's lymphoma
Lymphoepithelioid lymphoma
Mature T-cell lymphoma, not elsewhere classified

C84.40 Peripheral T-cell lymphoma, not classified, unspecified site `HIV` `HCC`

C84.41 Peripheral T-cell lymphoma, not classified, lymph nodes of head, face, and neck `HIV` `HCC`

C84.42 Peripheral T-cell lymphoma, not classified, intrathoracic lymph nodes `HIV` `HCC`

C84.43 Peripheral T-cell lymphoma, not classified, intra-abdominal lymph nodes `HIV` `HCC`

C84.44 Peripheral T-cell lymphoma, not classified, lymph nodes of axilla and upper limb `HIV` `HCC`

C84.45 Peripheral T-cell lymphoma, not classified, lymph nodes of inguinal region and lower limb `HIV` `HCC`

C84.46 Peripheral T-cell lymphoma, not classified, intrapelvic lymph nodes `HIV` `HCC`

C84.47 Peripheral T-cell lymphoma, not classified, spleen `HIV` `HCC`

C84.48 Peripheral T-cell lymphoma, not classified, lymph nodes of multiple sites `HIV` `HCC`

C84.49 Peripheral T-cell lymphoma, not classified, extranodal and solid organ sites `HIV` `HCC`

✓5ᵗʰ C84.6 Anaplastic large cell lymphoma, ALK-positive

Anaplastic large cell lymphoma, CD30-positive

C84.60 Anaplastic large cell lymphoma, ALK-positive, unspecified site `HIV` `HCC`

C84.61 Anaplastic large cell lymphoma, ALK-positive, lymph nodes of head, face, and neck `HIV` `HCC`

C84.62 Anaplastic large cell lymphoma, ALK-positive, intrathoracic lymph nodes `HIV` `HCC`

C84.63 Anaplastic large cell lymphoma, ALK-positive, intra-abdominal lymph nodes `HIV` `HCC`

C84.64 Anaplastic large cell lymphoma, ALK-positive, lymph nodes of axilla and upper limb `HIV` `HCC`

C84.65 Anaplastic large cell lymphoma, ALK-positive, lymph nodes of inguinal region and lower limb `HIV` `HCC`

C84.66 Anaplastic large cell lymphoma, ALK-positive, intrapelvic lymph nodes `HIV` `HCC`

C84.67 Anaplastic large cell lymphoma, ALK-positive, spleen `HIV` `HCC`

C84.68 Anaplastic large cell lymphoma, ALK-positive, lymph nodes of multiple sites `HIV` `HCC`

C84.69 Anaplastic large cell lymphoma, ALK-positive, extranodal and solid organ sites `HIV` `HCC`

✓5ᵗʰ C84.7 Anaplastic large cell lymphoma, ALK-negative

EXCLUDES 1   *primary cutaneous CD30-positive T-cell proliferations (C86.6-)*

C84.70 Anaplastic large cell lymphoma, ALK-negative, unspecified site `HIV` `HCC`

C84.71 Anaplastic large cell lymphoma, ALK-negative, lymph nodes of head, face, and neck `HIV` `HCC`

C84.72 Anaplastic large cell lymphoma, ALK-negative, intrathoracic lymph nodes `HIV` `HCC`

C84.73 Anaplastic large cell lymphoma, ALK-negative, intra-abdominal lymph nodes `HIV` `HCC`

C84.74 Anaplastic large cell lymphoma, ALK-negative, lymph nodes of axilla and upper limb `HIV` `HCC`

C84.75 Anaplastic large cell lymphoma, ALK-negative, lymph nodes of inguinal region and lower limb `HIV` `HCC`

C84.76 Anaplastic large cell lymphoma, ALK-negative, intrapelvic lymph nodes `HIV` `HCC`

C84.77 Anaplastic large cell lymphoma, ALK-negative, spleen `HIV` `HCC`

C84.78 Anaplastic large cell lymphoma, ALK-negative, lymph nodes of multiple sites `HIV` `HCC`

C84.79 Anaplastic large cell lymphoma, ALK-negative, extranodal and solid organ sites `HIV` `HCC`

✓5ᵗʰ C84.A Cutaneous T-cell lymphoma, unspecified

C84.A0 Cutaneous T-cell lymphoma, unspecified, unspecified site `HIV` `HCC`

C84.A1 Cutaneous T-cell lymphoma, unspecified, lymph nodes of head, face, and neck `HIV` `HCC`

C84.A2 Cutaneous T-cell lymphoma, unspecified, intrathoracic lymph nodes `HIV` `HCC`

C84.A3 Cutaneous T-cell lymphoma, unspecified, intra-abdominal lymph nodes `HIV` `HCC`

C84.A4 Cutaneous T-cell lymphoma, unspecified, lymph nodes of axilla and upper limb `HIV` `HCC`

C84.A5 Cutaneous T-cell lymphoma, unspecified, lymph nodes of inguinal region and lower limb `HIV` `HCC`

C84.A6 Cutaneous T-cell lymphoma, unspecified, intrapelvic lymph nodes `HIV` `HCC`

C84.A7 Cutaneous T-cell lymphoma, unspecified, spleen `HIV` `HCC`

C84.A8 Cutaneous T-cell lymphoma, unspecified, lymph nodes of multiple sites `HIV` `HCC`

C84.A9 Cutaneous T-cell lymphoma, unspecified, extranodal and solid organ sites `HIV` `HCC`

✓5ᵗʰ C84.Z Other mature T/NK-cell lymphomas

NOTE   If T-cell lineage or involvement is mentioned in conjunction with a specific lymphoma, code to the more specific description.

EXCLUDES 1   *angioimmunoblastic T-cell lymphoma (C86.5)*
blastic NK-cell lymphoma (C86.4)
enteropathy-type T-cell lymphoma (C86.2)
extranodal NK-cell lymphoma, nasal type (C86.0)
hepatosplenic T-cell lymphoma (C86.1)
primary cutaneous CD30-positive T-cell proliferations (C86.6)
subcutaneous panniculitis-like T-cell lymphoma (C86.3)
T-cell leukemia (C91.1-)

C84.Z0 Other mature T/NK-cell lymphomas, unspecified site `HIV` `HCC`

C84.Z1 Other mature T/NK-cell lymphomas, lymph nodes of head, face, and neck `HIV` `HCC`

C84.Z2 Other mature T/NK-cell lymphomas, intrathoracic lymph nodes `HIV` `HCC`

C84.Z3 Other mature T/NK-cell lymphomas, intra-abdominal lymph nodes `HIV` `HCC`

C84.Z4 Other mature T/NK-cell lymphomas, lymph nodes of axilla and upper limb `HIV` `HCC`

C84.Z5 Other mature T/NK-cell lymphomas, lymph nodes of inguinal region and lower limb `HIV` `HCC`

C84.Z6 Other mature T/NK-cell lymphomas, intrapelvic lymph nodes `HIV` `HCC`

C84.Z7 Other mature T/NK-cell lymphomas, spleen `HIV` `HCC`

C84.Z8 Other mature T/NK-cell lymphomas, lymph nodes of multiple sites `HIV` `HCC`

C84.Z9 Other mature T/NK-cell lymphomas, extranodal and solid organ sites `HIV` `HCC`

✓5ᵗʰ C84.9 Mature T/NK-cell lymphomas, unspecified

NK/T cell lymphoma NOS

EXCLUDES 1   *mature T-cell lymphoma, not elsewhere classified (C84.4-)*

C84.90 Mature T/NK-cell lymphomas, unspecified, unspecified site `HIV` `HCC`

C84.91 Mature T/NK-cell lymphomas, unspecified, lymph nodes of head, face, and neck `HIV` `HCC`

C84.92 Mature T/NK-cell lymphomas, unspecified, intrathoracic lymph nodes `HIV` `HCC`

C84.93 Mature T/NK-cell lymphomas, unspecified, intra-abdominal lymph nodes `HIV` `HCC`

C84.94 Mature T/NK-cell lymphomas, unspecified, lymph nodes of axilla and upper limb `HIV` `HCC`

C84.95 Mature T/NK-cell lymphomas, unspecified, lymph nodes of inguinal region and lower limb `HIV` `HCC`

C84.96 **Mature T/NK-cell lymphomas, unspecified, intrapelvic lymph nodes** `HIV` `HCC`

C84.97 **Mature T/NK-cell lymphomas, unspecified, spleen** `HIV` `HCC`

C84.98 **Mature T/NK-cell lymphomas, unspecified, lymph nodes of multiple sites** `HIV` `HCC`

C84.99 **Mature T/NK-cell lymphomas, unspecified, extranodal and solid organ sites** `HIV` `HCC`

√4ᵗʰ **C85 Other specified and unspecified types of non-Hodgkin lymphoma**

EXCLUDES 1   *other specified types of T/NK-cell lymphoma (C86.-)*
personal history of non-Hodgkin lymphoma (Z85.72)

√5ᵗʰ **C85.1 Unspecified B-cell lymphoma**

NOTE   If B-cell lineage or involvement is mentioned in conjunction with a specific lymphoma, code to the more specific description.

C85.10 **Unspecified B-cell lymphoma, unspecified site** `HIV` `HCC`

C85.11 **Unspecified B-cell lymphoma, lymph nodes of head, face, and neck** `HIV` `HCC`

C85.12 **Unspecified B-cell lymphoma, intrathoracic lymph nodes** `HIV` `HCC`

C85.13 **Unspecified B-cell lymphoma, intra-abdominal lymph nodes** `HIV` `HCC`

C85.14 **Unspecified B-cell lymphoma, lymph nodes of axilla and upper limb** `HIV` `HCC`

C85.15 **Unspecified B-cell lymphoma, lymph nodes of inguinal region and lower limb** `HIV` `HCC`

C85.16 **Unspecified B-cell lymphoma, intrapelvic lymph nodes** `HIV` `HCC`

C85.17 **Unspecified B-cell lymphoma, spleen** `HIV` `HCC`

C85.18 **Unspecified B-cell lymphoma, lymph nodes of multiple sites** `HIV` `HCC`

C85.19 **Unspecified B-cell lymphoma, extranodal and solid organ sites** `HIV` `HCC`

√5ᵗʰ **C85.2 Mediastinal (thymic) large B-cell lymphoma**

C85.20 **Mediastinal (thymic) large B-cell lymphoma, unspecified site** `HIV` `HCC`

C85.21 **Mediastinal (thymic) large B-cell lymphoma, lymph nodes of head, face, and neck** `HIV` `HCC`

C85.22 **Mediastinal (thymic) large B-cell lymphoma, intrathoracic lymph nodes** `HIV` `HCC`

C85.23 **Mediastinal (thymic) large B-cell lymphoma, intra-abdominal lymph nodes** `HIV` `HCC`

C85.24 **Mediastinal (thymic) large B-cell lymphoma, lymph nodes of axilla and upper limb** `HIV` `HCC`

C85.25 **Mediastinal (thymic) large B-cell lymphoma, lymph nodes of inguinal region and lower limb** `HIV` `HCC`

C85.26 **Mediastinal (thymic) large B-cell lymphoma, intrapelvic lymph nodes** `HIV` `HCC`

C85.27 **Mediastinal (thymic) large B-cell lymphoma, spleen** `HIV` `HCC`

C85.28 **Mediastinal (thymic) large B-cell lymphoma, lymph nodes of multiple sites** `HIV` `HCC`

C85.29 **Mediastinal (thymic) large B-cell lymphoma, extranodal and solid organ sites** `HIV` `HCC`

√5ᵗʰ **C85.8 Other specified types of non-Hodgkin lymphoma**

C85.80 **Other specified types of non-Hodgkin lymphoma, unspecified site** `HIV` `HCC`

C85.81 **Other specified types of non-Hodgkin lymphoma, lymph nodes of head, face, and neck** `HIV` `HCC`

C85.82 **Other specified types of non-Hodgkin lymphoma, intrathoracic lymph nodes** `HIV` `HCC`

C85.83 **Other specified types of non-Hodgkin lymphoma, intra-abdominal lymph nodes** `HIV` `HCC`

C85.84 **Other specified types of non-Hodgkin lymphoma, lymph nodes of axilla and upper limb** `HIV` `HCC`

C85.85 **Other specified types of non-Hodgkin lymphoma, lymph nodes of inguinal region and lower limb** `HIV` `HCC`

C85.86 **Other specified types of non-Hodgkin lymphoma, intrapelvic lymph nodes** `HIV` `HCC`

C85.87 **Other specified types of non-Hodgkin lymphoma, spleen** `HIV` `HCC`

C85.88 **Other specified types of non-Hodgkin lymphoma, lymph nodes of multiple sites** `HIV` `HCC`

C85.89 **Other specified types of non-Hodgkin lymphoma, extranodal and solid organ sites** `HIV` `HCC`

√5ᵗʰ **C85.9 Non-Hodgkin lymphoma, unspecified**

Lymphoma NOS
Malignant lymphoma NOS
Non-Hodgkin lymphoma NOS

C85.90 **Non-Hodgkin lymphoma, unspecified, unspecified site** `HIV` `HCC`

C85.91 **Non-Hodgkin lymphoma, unspecified, lymph nodes of head, face, and neck** `HIV` `HCC`

C85.92 **Non-Hodgkin lymphoma, unspecified, intrathoracic lymph nodes** `HIV` `HCC`

C85.93 **Non-Hodgkin lymphoma, unspecified, intra-abdominal lymph nodes** `HIV` `HCC`

C85.94 **Non-Hodgkin lymphoma, unspecified, lymph nodes of axilla and upper limb** `HIV` `HCC`

C85.95 **Non-Hodgkin lymphoma, unspecified, lymph nodes of inguinal region and lower limb** `HIV` `HCC`

C85.96 **Non-Hodgkin lymphoma, unspecified, intrapelvic lymph nodes** `HIV` `HCC`

C85.97 **Non-Hodgkin lymphoma, unspecified, spleen** `HIV` `HCC`

C85.98 **Non-Hodgkin lymphoma, unspecified, lymph nodes of multiple sites** `HIV` `HCC`

C85.99 **Non-Hodgkin lymphoma, unspecified, extranodal and solid organ sites** `HIV` `HCC`

√4ᵗʰ **C86 Other specified types of T/NK-cell lymphoma**

EXCLUDES 1   *anaplastic large cell lymphoma, ALK negative (C84.7-)*
anaplastic large cell lymphoma, ALK positive (C84.6-)
mature T/NK-cell lymphomas (C84.-)
other specified types of non-Hodgkin lymphoma (C85.8-)

C86.0 **Extranodal NK/T-cell lymphoma, nasal type** `HIV` `HCC`

C86.1 **Hepatosplenic T-cell lymphoma** `HIV` `HCC`

Alpha-beta and gamma delta types

C86.2 **Enteropathy-type (intestinal) T-cell lymphoma** `HIV` `HCC`

Enteropathy associated T-cell lymphoma

C86.3 **Subcutaneous panniculitis-like T-cell lymphoma** `HIV` `HCC`

C86.4 **Blastic NK-cell lymphoma** `HIV` `HCC`

Blastic plasmacytoid dendritic cell neoplasm (BPDCN)

C86.5 **Angioimmunoblastic T-cell lymphoma** `HIV` `HCC`

Angioimmunoblastic lymphadenopathy with dysproteinemia (AILD)

C86.6 **Primary cutaneous CD30-positive T-cell proliferations** `HIV` `HCC`

Lymphomatoid papulosis
Primary cutaneous anaplastic large cell lymphoma
Primary cutaneous CD30-positive large T-cell lymphoma

√4ᵗʰ **C88 Malignant immunoproliferative diseases and certain other B-cell lymphomas**

EXCLUDES 1   *B-cell lymphoma, unspecified (C85.1-)*
personal history of other malignant neoplasms of lymphoid, hematopoietic and related tissues (Z85.79)

C88.0 **Waldenström macroglobulinemia** `HCC`

Lymphoplasmacytic lymphoma with IgM-production
Macroglobulinemia (idiopathic) (primary)

EXCLUDES 1   *small cell B-cell lymphoma (C83.0)*

C88.2 **Heavy chain disease** `HCC`

Franklin disease
Gamma heavy chain disease
Mu heavy chain disease

C88.3 **Immunoproliferative small intestinal disease** `HCC`

Alpha heavy chain disease
Mediterranean lymphoma

C88.4 **Extranodal marginal zone B-cell lymphoma of mucosa-associated lymphoid tissue [MALT-lymphoma]** `HIV` `HCC`

Lymphoma of skin-associated lymphoid tissue [SALT-lymphoma]

Lymphoma of bronchial-associated lymphoid tissue [BALT-lymphoma]

EXCLUDES 1   *high malignant (diffuse large B-cell) lymphoma (C83.3-)*

C88.8 **Other malignant immunoproliferative diseases** `HCC`

C88.9 **Malignant immunoproliferative disease, unspecified** `HCC`

Immunoproliferative disease NOS

✓4ᵗʰ **C90** **Multiple myeloma and malignant plasma cell neoplasms**

EXCLUDES 1   *personal history of other malignant neoplasms of lymphoid, hematopoietic and related tissues (Z85.79)*

AHA: 2019,2Q,30

✓5ᵗʰ **C90.0** **Multiple myeloma**

Kahler's disease

Medullary plasmacytoma

Myelomatosis

Plasma cell myeloma

EXCLUDES 1   *solitary myeloma (C90.3-)*

          solitary plasmactyoma (C90.3-)

TIP: Do not assign an additional code for bone metastasis (C79.51) when multiple myeloma is described as metastatic to the bone; bone involvement is integral to this disease process.

C90.00 **Multiple myeloma not having achieved remission** `HCC`

Multiple myeloma with failed remission

Multiple myeloma NOS

C90.01 **Multiple myeloma in remission** `HCC`

C90.02 **Multiple myeloma in relapse** `HCC`

✓5ᵗʰ **C90.1** **Plasma cell leukemia**

Plasmacytic leukemia

AHA: 2019,2Q,30

C90.10 **Plasma cell leukemia not having achieved remission** `HCC`

Plasma cell leukemia with failed remission

Plasma cell leukemia NOS

C90.11 **Plasma cell leukemia in remission** `HCC`

C90.12 **Plasma cell leukemia in relapse** `HCC`

✓5ᵗʰ **C90.2** **Extramedullary plasmacytoma**

C90.20 **Extramedullary plasmacytoma not having achieved remission** `HCC`

Extramedullary plasmacytoma with failed remission

Extramedullary plasmacytoma NOS

C90.21 **Extramedullary plasmacytoma in remission** `HCC`

C90.22 **Extramedullary plasmacytoma in relapse** `HCC`

✓5ᵗʰ **C90.3** **Solitary plasmacytoma**

Localized malignant plasma cell tumor NOS

Plasmacytoma NOS

Solitary myeloma

C90.30 **Solitary plasmacytoma not having achieved remission** `HCC`

Solitary plasmacytoma with failed remission

Solitary plasmacytoma NOS

C90.31 **Solitary plasmacytoma in remission** `HCC`

C90.32 **Solitary plasmacytoma in relapse** `HCC`

✓4ᵗʰ **C91** **Lymphoid leukemia**

EXCLUDES 1   *personal history of leukemia (Z85.6)*

DEF: Malignant proliferation of immature lymphocytes (white blood cells that make up lymphoid tissue), called lymphoblasts, that originate in the bone marrow. Can be acute (ALL) or chronic (CLL).

✓5ᵗʰ **C91.0** **Acute lymphoblastic leukemia [ALL]**

NOTE   ▶Codes in subcategory C91.0- should only be used for T-cell and B-cell precursor leukemia◀

C91.00 **Acute lymphoblastic leukemia not having achieved remission** `HCC`

Acute lymphoblastic leukemia with failed remission

Acute lymphoblastic leukemia NOS

C91.01 **Acute lymphoblastic leukemia, in remission** `HCC`

C91.02 **Acute lymphoblastic leukemia, in relapse** `HCC`

✓5ᵗʰ **C91.1** **Chronic lymphocytic leukemia of B-cell type**

Lymphoplasmacytic leukemia

Richter syndrome

EXCLUDES 1   *lymphoplasmacytic lymphoma (C83.0-)*

C91.10 **Chronic lymphocytic leukemia of B-cell type not having achieved remission** `HCC`

Chronic lymphocytic leukemia of B-cell type with failed remission

Chronic lymphocytic leukemia of B-cell type NOS

C91.11 **Chronic lymphocytic leukemia of B-cell type in remission** `HCC`

C91.12 **Chronic lymphocytic leukemia of B-cell type in relapse** `HCC`

✓5ᵗʰ **C91.3** **Prolymphocytic leukemia of B-cell type**

C91.30 **Prolymphocytic leukemia of B-cell type not having achieved remission** `HCC`

Prolymphocytic leukemia of B-cell type with failed remission

Prolymphocytic leukemia of B-cell type NOS

C91.31 **Prolymphocytic leukemia of B-cell type, in remission** `HCC`

C91.32 **Prolymphocytic leukemia of B-cell type, in relapse** `HCC`

✓5ᵗʰ **C91.4** **Hairy cell leukemia**

Leukemic reticuloendotheliosis

DEF: Rare type of leukemia that is slow growing and often also considered a type of lymphoma. The small B-cell lymphocytes appear with "hairy" projections under a microscope and are found mostly in the bone marrow, spleen, and blood.

C91.40 **Hairy cell leukemia not having achieved remission** `HCC`

Hairy cell leukemia with failed remission

Hairy cell leukemia NOS

C91.41 **Hairy cell leukemia, in remission** `HCC`

C91.42 **Hairy cell leukemia, in relapse** `HCC`

✓5ᵗʰ **C91.5** **Adult T-cell lymphoma/leukemia (HTLV-1-associated)**

Acute variant of adult T-cell lymphoma/leukemia (HTLV-1-associated)

Chronic variant of adult T-cell lymphoma/leukemia (HTLV-1-associated)

Lymphomatoid variant of adult T-cell lymphoma/leukemia (HTLV-1-associated)

Smouldering variant of adult T-cell lymphoma/leukemia (HTLV-1-associated)

C91.50 **Adult T-cell lymphoma/leukemia (HTLV-1-associated) not having achieved remission** `HCC` `A`

Adult T-cell lymphoma/leukemia (HTLV-1-associated) with failed remission

Adult T-cell lymphoma/leukemia (HTLV-1-associated) NOS

C91.51 **Adult T-cell lymphoma/leukemia (HTLV-1-associated), in remission** `HCC` `A`

C91.52 **Adult T-cell lymphoma/leukemia (HTLV-1-associated), in relapse** `HCC` `A`

✓5ᵗʰ **C91.6** **Prolymphocytic leukemia of T-cell type**

C91.60 **Prolymphocytic leukemia of T-cell type not having achieved remission** `HCC`

Prolymphocytic leukemia of T-cell type with failed remission

Prolymphocytic leukemia of T-cell type NOS

C91.61 **Prolymphocytic leukemia of T-cell type, in remission** `HCC`

C91.62 **Prolymphocytic leukemia of T-cell type, in relapse** `HCC`

✓5ᵗʰ **C91.A** **Mature B-cell leukemia Burkitt-type**

EXCLUDES 1   *Burkitt lymphoma (C83.7-)*

C91.A0 **Mature B-cell leukemia Burkitt-type not having achieved remission** `HCC`

Mature B-cell leukemia Burkitt-type with failed remission

Mature B-cell leukemia Burkitt-type NOS

C91.A1 **Mature B-cell leukemia Burkitt-type, in remission** `HCC`

C91.A2 **Mature B-cell leukemia Burkitt-type, in relapse** `HCC`

✔ Additional Character Required   ✓x7ᵗʰ Placeholder   Unacceptable PDx   Questionable PDx   Manifestation   Unspecified Dx   `H1`-`H14` HAC   `HCC` CMS-HCC Dx   `HIV` HIV Dx

ICD-10-CM 2020   487

√5ᵗʰ **C91.Z** **Other lymphoid leukemia**

T-cell large granular lymphocytic leukemia (associated with rheumatoid arthritis)

C91.ZØ **Other lymphoid leukemia not having achieved remission** `HCC`

Other lymphoid leukemia with failed remission
Other lymphoid leukemia NOS

C91.Z1 **Other lymphoid leukemia, in remission** `HCC`

C91.Z2 **Other lymphoid leukemia, in relapse** `HCC`

√5ᵗʰ **C91.9** **Lymphoid leukemia, unspecified**

C91.9Ø **Lymphoid leukemia, unspecified not having achieved remission** `HCC`

Lymphoid leukemia with failed remission
Lymphoid leukemia NOS

C91.91 **Lymphoid leukemia, unspecified, in remission** `HCC`

C91.92 **Lymphoid leukemia, unspecified, in relapse** `HCC`

√4ᵗʰ **C92** **Myeloid leukemia**

INCLUDES granulocytic leukemia
myelogenous leukemia

EXCLUDES 1 *personal history of leukemia (Z85.6)*

AHA: 2019,1Q,16

DEF: Cancer that develops in immature myelocytes called myeloblasts. These are the cells that become white blood cells (except lymphocytes), red blood cells, or platelet making cells. Can be acute (AML) or chronic (CML).

TIP: Pancytopenia, although common in some types of myeloid leukemia's, is not always inherent. When it is documented, code D61.818 can be assigned in addition to a code from this category.

√5ᵗʰ **C92.Ø** **Acute myeloblastic leukemia**

Acute myeloblastic leukemia, minimal differentiation
Acute myeloblastic leukemia (with maturation)
Acute myeloblastic leukemia 1/ETO
Acute myeloblastic leukemia MØ
Acute myeloblastic leukemia M1
Acute myeloblastic leukemia M2
Acute myeloblastic leukemia with t(8;21)
Acute myeloblastic leukemia (without a FAB classification) NOS
Refractory anemia with excess blasts in transformation [RAEBT]

EXCLUDES 1 *acute exacerbation of chronic myeloid leukemia (C92.1Ø)*
refractory anemia with excess of blasts not in transformation (D46.2-)

AHA: 2018,4Q,87

C92.ØØ **Acute myeloblastic leukemia, not having achieved remission** `HCC`

Acute myeloblastic leukemia with failed remission
Acute myeloblastic leukemia NOS

C92.Ø1 **Acute myeloblastic leukemia, in remission** `HCC`

C92.Ø2 **Acute myeloblastic leukemia, in relapse** `HCC`

√5ᵗʰ **C92.1** **Chronic myeloid leukemia, BCR/ABL-positive**

Chronic myelogenous leukemia, Philadelphia chromosome (Ph1) positive
Chronic myelogenous leukemia, t(9;22) (q34;q11)
Chronic myelogenous leukemia with crisis of blast cells

EXCLUDES 1 *atypical chronic myeloid leukemia BCR/ABL-negative (C92.2-)*
chronic myelomonocytic leukemia (C93.1-)
chronic myeloproliferative disease (D47.1)

C92.1Ø **Chronic myeloid leukemia, BCR/ABL-positive, not having achieved remission** `HCC`

Chronic myeloid leukemia, BCR/ABL-positive with failed remission
Chronic myeloid leukemia, BCR/ABL-positive NOS

C92.11 **Chronic myeloid leukemia, BCR/ABL-positive, in remission** `HCC`

C92.12 **Chronic myeloid leukemia, BCR/ABL-positive, in relapse** `HCC`

√5ᵗʰ **C92.2** **Atypical chronic myeloid leukemia, BCR/ABL-negative**

C92.2Ø **Atypical chronic myeloid leukemia, BCR/ABL-negative, not having achieved remission** `HCC`

Atypical chronic myeloid leukemia, BCR/ABL-negative with failed remission
Atypical chronic myeloid leukemia, BCR/ABL-negative NOS

C92.21 **Atypical chronic myeloid leukemia, BCR/ABL-negative, in remission** `HCC`

C92.22 **Atypical chronic myeloid leukemia, BCR/ABL-negative, in relapse** `HCC`

√5ᵗʰ **C92.3** **Myeloid sarcoma**

A malignant tumor of immature myeloid cells
Chloroma
Granulocytic sarcoma

C92.3Ø **Myeloid sarcoma, not having achieved remission** `HCC`

Myeloid sarcoma with failed remission
Myeloid sarcoma NOS

C92.31 **Myeloid sarcoma, in remission** `HCC`

C92.32 **Myeloid sarcoma, in relapse** `HCC`

√5ᵗʰ **C92.4** **Acute promyelocytic leukemia**

AML M3
AML Me with t(15;17) and variants

C92.4Ø **Acute promyelocytic leukemia, not having achieved remission** `HCC`

Acute promyelocytic leukemia with failed remission
Acute promyelocytic leukemia NOS

C92.41 **Acute promyelocytic leukemia, in remission** `HCC`

C92.42 **Acute promyelocytic leukemia, in relapse** `HCC`

√5ᵗʰ **C92.5** **Acute myelomonocytic leukemia**

AML M4
AML M4 Eo with inv(16) or t(16;16)

C92.5Ø **Acute myelomonocytic leukemia, not having achieved remission** `HCC`

Acute myelomonocytic leukemia with failed remission
Acute myelomonocytic leukemia NOS

C92.51 **Acute myelomonocytic leukemia, in remission** `HCC`

C92.52 **Acute myelomonocytic leukemia, in relapse** `HCC`

√5ᵗʰ **C92.6** **Acute myeloid leukemia with 11q23-abnormality**

Acute myeloid leukemia with variation of MLL-gene

C92.6Ø **Acute myeloid leukemia with 11q23-abnormality not having achieved remission** `HCC`

Acute myeloid leukemia with 11q23-abnormality with failed remission
Acute myeloid leukemia with 11q23-abnormality NOS

C92.61 **Acute myeloid leukemia with 11q23-abnormality in remission** `HCC`

C92.62 **Acute myeloid leukemia with 11q23-abnormality in relapse** `HCC`

√5ᵗʰ **C92.A** **Acute myeloid leukemia with multilineage dysplasia**

Acute myeloid leukemia with dysplasia of remaining hematopoesis and/or myelodysplastic disease in its history

C92.AØ **Acute myeloid leukemia with multilineage dysplasia, not having achieved remission** `HCC`

Acute myeloid leukemia with multilineage dysplasia with failed remission
Acute myeloid leukemia with multilineage dysplasia NOS

C92.A1 **Acute myeloid leukemia with multilineage dysplasia, in remission** `HCC`

C92.A2 **Acute myeloid leukemia with multilineage dysplasia, in relapse** `HCC`

√5ᵗʰ **C92.Z** **Other myeloid leukemia**

C92.ZØ **Other myeloid leukemia not having achieved remission** `HCC`

Myeloid leukemia NEC with failed remission
Myeloid leukemia NEC

C92.Z1 **Other myeloid leukemia, in remission** `HCC`

C92.Z2 **Other myeloid leukemia, in relapse** `HCC`

☑5ᵗʰ **C92.9   Myeloid leukemia, unspecified**

    C92.90   Myeloid leukemia, unspecified, not HCC
      having achieved remission
        Myeloid leukemia, unspecified with failed remission
        Myeloid leukemia, unspecified NOS

    C92.91   Myeloid leukemia, unspecified in HCC
      remission

    C92.92   Myeloid leukemia, unspecified in relapse HCC

☑4ᵗʰ **C93   Monocytic leukemia**

    INCLUDES monocytoid leukemia
    EXCLUDES 1 *personal history of leukemia (Z85.6)*

☑5ᵗʰ **C93.0   Acute monoblastic/monocytic leukemia**

    AML M5
    AML M5a
    AML M5b

    C93.00   Acute monoblastic/monocytic leukemia, HCC
      not having achieved remission
        Acute monoblastic/monocytic leukemia with failed
          remission
        Acute monoblastic/monocytic leukemia NOS

    C93.01   Acute monoblastic/monocytic leukemia, HCC
      in remission

    C93.02   Acute monoblastic/monocytic leukemia, HCC
      in relapse

☑5ᵗʰ **C93.1   Chronic myelomonocytic leukemia**

    Chronic monocytic leukemia
    CMML-1
    CMML-2
    CMML with eosinophilia

    C93.10   Chronic myelomonocytic leukemia not HCC
      having achieved remission
        Chronic myelomonocytic leukemia with failed
          remission
        Chronic myelomonocytic leukemia NOS

    C93.11   Chronic myelomonocytic leukemia, in HCC
      remission

    C93.12   Chronic myelomonocytic leukemia, in HCC
      relapse

☑5ᵗʰ **C93.3   Juvenile myelomonocytic leukemia**

    C93.30   Juvenile myelomonocytic leukemia, not HCC P
      having achieved remission
        Juvenile myelomonocytic leukemia with failed
          remission
        Juvenile myelomonocytic leukemia NOS

    C93.31   Juvenile myelomonocytic leukemia, in HCC P
      remission

    C93.32   Juvenile myelomonocytic leukemia, in HCC P
      relapse

☑5ᵗʰ **C93.Z   Other monocytic leukemia**

    C93.Z0   Other monocytic leukemia, not having HCC
      achieved remission
        Other monocytic leukemia NOS

    C93.Z1   Other monocytic leukemia, in remission HCC

    C93.Z2   Other monocytic leukemia, in relapse HCC

☑5ᵗʰ **C93.9   Monocytic leukemia, unspecified**

    C93.90   Monocytic leukemia, unspecified, not HCC
      having achieved remission
        Monocytic leukemia, unspecified with failed remission
        Monocytic leukemia, unspecified NOS

    C93.91   Monocytic leukemia, unspecified in HCC
      remission

    C93.92   Monocytic leukemia, unspecified in HCC
      relapse

☑4ᵗʰ **C94   Other leukemias of specified cell type**

    EXCLUDES 1 *leukemic reticuloendotheliosis (C91.4-)*
      myelodysplastic syndromes (D46.-)
      personal history of leukemia (Z85.6)
      plasma cell leukemia (C90.1-)

☑5ᵗʰ **C94.0   Acute erythroid leukemia**

    Acute myeloid leukemia M6(a)(b)
    Erythroleukemia
    DEF: Erythroleukemia: Malignant blood dyscrasia (a
    myeloproliferative disorder).

    C94.00   Acute erythroid leukemia, not having HCC
      achieved remission
        Acute erythroid leukemia with failed remission
        Acute erythroid leukemia NOS

    C94.01   Acute erythroid leukemia, in remission HCC

    C94.02   Acute erythroid leukemia, in relapse HCC

☑5ᵗʰ **C94.2   Acute megakaryoblastic leukemia**

    Acute myeloid leukemia M7
    Acute megakaryocytic leukemia

    C94.20   Acute megakaryoblastic leukemia not HCC
      having achieved remission
        Acute megakaryoblastic leukemia with failed
          remission
        Acute megakaryoblastic leukemia NOS

    C94.21   Acute megakaryoblastic leukemia, in HCC
      remission

    C94.22   Acute megakaryoblastic leukemia, in HCC
      relapse

☑5ᵗʰ **C94.3   Mast cell leukemia**

    AHA: 2017,4Q,5

    C94.30   Mast cell leukemia not having achieved HCC
      remission
        Mast cell leukemia with failed remission
        Mast cell leukemia NOS

    C94.31   Mast cell leukemia, in remission HCC

    C94.32   Mast cell leukemia, in relapse HCC

☑5ᵗʰ **C94.4   Acute panmyelosis with myelofibrosis**

    Acute myelofibrosis
    EXCLUDES 1 *myelofibrosis NOS (D75.81)*
      secondary myelofibrosis NOS (D75.81)

    C94.40   Acute panmyelosis with myelofibrosis HCC
      not having achieved remission
        Acute myelofibrosis NOS
        Acute panmyelosis with myelofibrosis with failed
          remission
        Acute panmyelosis NOS

    C94.41   Acute panmyelosis with myelofibrosis, HCC
      in remission

    C94.42   Acute panmyelosis with myelofibrosis, HCC
      in relapse

    C94.6   Myelodysplastic disease, not classified HCC

      Myeloproliferative disease, not classified

☑5ᵗʰ **C94.8   Other specified leukemias**

    Aggressive NK-cell leukemia
    Acute basophilic leukemia

    C94.80   Other specified leukemias not having HCC
      achieved remission
        Other specified leukemia with failed remission
        Other specified leukemias NOS

    C94.81   Other specified leukemias, in remission HCC

    C94.82   Other specified leukemias, in relapse HCC

☑ Additional Character Required   ✓ₓ7ᵗʰ Placeholder   Unacceptable PDx   Questionable PDx   Manifestation   Unspecified Dx   H1-H14 HAC   HCC CMS-HCC Dx   HIV HIV Dx

Chapter 2. Neoplasms

C95–D01.49

✓4ᵗʰ **C95 Leukemia of unspecified** cell type

> EXCLUDES 1   *personal history of leukemia (Z85.6)*

✓5ᵗʰ **C95.0 Acute** leukemia of unspecified cell type

> Acute bilineal leukemia
> Acute mixed lineage leukemia
> Biphenotypic acute leukemia
> Stem cell leukemia of unclear lineage
>
> EXCLUDES 1   *acute exacerbation of unspecified chronic leukemia (C95.10)*

> **C95.00 Acute leukemia of unspecified cell type** not having achieved remission
> > Acute leukemia of unspecified cell type with failed remission
> > Acute leukemia NOS   HCC

> **C95.01 Acute leukemia of unspecified cell type,** in remission   HCC

> **C95.02 Acute leukemia of unspecified cell type,** in relapse   HCC

✓5ᵗʰ **C95.1 Chronic** leukemia of unspecified cell type

> **C95.10 Chronic leukemia of unspecified cell type** not having achieved remission   HCC
> > Chronic leukemia of unspecified cell type with failed remission
> > Chronic leukemia NOS

> **C95.11 Chronic leukemia of unspecified cell type,** in remission   HCC

> **C95.12 Chronic leukemia of unspecified cell type,** in relapse   HCC

✓5ᵗʰ **C95.9 Leukemia, unspecified**

> **C95.90 Leukemia, unspecified** not having achieved remission   HCC
> > Leukemia, unspecified with failed remission
> > Leukemia NOS

> **C95.91 Leukemia, unspecified, in remission**   HCC

> **C95.92 Leukemia, unspecified, in relapse**   HCC

✓4ᵗʰ **C96 Other and unspecified malignant neoplasms of lymphoid, hematopoietic and related tissue**

> EXCLUDES 1   *personal history of other malignant neoplasms of lymphoid, hematopoietic and related tissues (Z85.79)*

> **C96.0 Multifocal and multisystemic (disseminated) Langerhans-cell histiocytosis**   HCC
> > Histiocytosis X, multisystemic
> > Letterer-Siwe disease
> >
> > EXCLUDES 1   *adult pulmonary Langerhans cell histiocytosis (J84.82)*
> > *multifocal and unisystemic Langerhans-cell histiocytosis (C96.5)*
> > *unifocal Langerhans-cell histiocytosis (C96.6)*

✓5ᵗʰ **C96.2 Malignant mast cell neoplasm**

> EXCLUDES 1   *indolent mastocytosis (D47.02)*
> *mast cell leukemia (C94.30)*
> *mastocytosis (congenital) (cutaneous) (Q82.2)*

> **AHA:** 2017,4Q,5

> **DEF:** Mast cell: Type of white blood cell found in the loose connective tissue of blood vessels and bronchioles responsible for acute hypersensitivity reactions, including anaphylactic shock. The IgE receptors on these cells bind with allergens causing cell degranulation and diffuse, widespread histamine release that results in airway constriction and vasodilation with decreased systemic blood pressure.

> **C96.20 Malignant mast cell neoplasm, unspecified**   HCC

> **C96.21 Aggressive systemic mastocytosis**   HCC

> **C96.22 Mast cell sarcoma**   HCC

> **C96.29 Other malignant mast cell neoplasm**   HCC

> **C96.4 Sarcoma of dendritic cells (accessory cells)**   HCC
> > Follicular dendritic cell sarcoma
> > Interdigitating dendritic cell sarcoma
> > Langerhans cell sarcoma

> **C96.5 Multifocal and unisystemic Langerhans-cell histiocytosis**   HCC
> > Hand-Schüller-Christian disease
> > Histiocytosis X, multifocal
> >
> > EXCLUDES 1   *multifocal and multisystemic (disseminated) Langerhans-cell histiocytosis (C96.0)*
> > *unifocal Langerhans-cell histiocytosis (C96.6)*

> **C96.6 Unifocal Langerhans-cell histiocytosis**   HCC
> > Eosinophilic granuloma
> > Histiocytosis X, unifocal
> > Histiocytosis X NOS
> > Langerhans-cell histiocytosis NOS
> >
> > EXCLUDES 1   *multifocal and multisysemic (disseminated) Langerhans-cell histiocytosis (C96.0)*
> > *multifocal and unisystemic Langerhans-cell histiocytosis (C96.5)*

> **C96.A Histiocytic sarcoma**   HCC
> > Malignant histiocytosis

> **C96.Z Other specified malignant neoplasms of lymphoid, hematopoietic and related tissue**   HCC

> **C96.9 Malignant neoplasm of lymphoid, hematopoietic and related tissue, unspecified**   HCC

In situ neoplasms (D00-D09)

> INCLUDES   Bowen's disease
> erythroplasia
> grade III intraepithelial neoplasia
> Queyrat's erythroplasia

✓4ᵗʰ **D00 Carcinoma in situ of** oral cavity, esophagus and stomach

> EXCLUDES 1   *melanoma in situ (D03.-)*

✓5ᵗʰ **D00.0 Carcinoma in situ of** lip, oral cavity and pharynx

> Use additional code to identify:
> exposure to environmental tobacco smoke (Z77.22)
> exposure to tobacco smoke in the perinatal period (P96.81)
> history of tobacco dependence (Z87.891)
> occupational exposure to environmental tobacco smoke (Z57.31)
> tobacco dependence (F17.-)
> tobacco use (Z72.0)
>
> EXCLUDES 1   *carcinoma in situ of aryepiglottic fold or interarytenoid fold, laryngeal aspect (D02.0)*
> *carcinoma in situ of epiglottis NOS (D02.0)*
> *carcinoma in situ of epiglottis suprahyoid portion (D02.0)*
> *carcinoma in situ of skin of lip (D03.0, D04.0)*

> **D00.00 Carcinoma in situ of oral cavity, unspecified site**

> **D00.01 Carcinoma in situ of** labial mucosa and vermilion border

> **D00.02 Carcinoma in situ of** buccal mucosa

> **D00.03 Carcinoma in situ of** gingiva and edentulous alveolar ridge

> **D00.04 Carcinoma in situ of** soft palate

> **D00.05 Carcinoma in situ of** hard palate

> **D00.06 Carcinoma in situ of** floor of mouth

> **D00.07 Carcinoma in situ of** tongue

> **D00.08 Carcinoma in situ of** pharynx
> > Carcinoma in situ of aryepiglottic fold NOS
> > Carcinoma in situ of hypopharyngeal aspect of aryepiglottic fold
> > Carcinoma in situ of marginal zone of aryepiglottic fold

> **D00.1 Carcinoma in situ of** esophagus

> **D00.2 Carcinoma in situ of** stomach

✓4ᵗʰ **D01 Carcinoma in situ of other and unspecified** digestive organs

> EXCLUDES 1   *melanoma in situ (D03.-)*

> **D01.0 Carcinoma in situ of** colon
> > EXCLUDES 1   *carcinoma in situ of rectosigmoid junction (D01.1)*

> **D01.1 Carcinoma in situ of** rectosigmoid junction

> **D01.2 Carcinoma in situ of** rectum

> **D01.3 Carcinoma in situ of** anus and anal canal
> > Anal intraepithelial neoplasia III [AIN III]
> > Severe dysplasia of anus
> >
> > EXCLUDES 1   *anal intraepithelial neoplasia I and II [AIN I and AIN II] (K62.82)*
> > *carcinoma in situ of anal margin (D04.5)*
> > *carcinoma in situ of anal skin (D04.5)*
> > *carcinoma in situ of perianal skin (D04.5)*

✓5ᵗʰ **D01.4 Carcinoma in situ of other and unspecified parts of** intestine

> EXCLUDES 1   *carcinoma in situ of ampulla of Vater (D01.5)*

> **D01.40 Carcinoma in situ of unspecified part of intestine**

> **D01.49 Carcinoma in situ of other parts of intestine**

N Newborn: 0   P Pediatric: 0-17   M Maternity: 9-64   A Adult: 15-124   MCC Major Complication/Comorbidity   CC Complication/Comorbidity   SW Severe Wound Dx

490   ICD-10-CM 2020

D01.5 Carcinoma in situ of liver, gallbladder and bile ducts
     Carcinoma in situ of ampulla of Vater

D01.7 Carcinoma in situ of other specified digestive organs
     Carcinoma in situ of pancreas

D01.9 Carcinoma in situ of digestive organ, unspecified

✓4ᵗʰ **D02** Carcinoma in situ of middle ear and respiratory system
     Use additional code to identify:
     exposure to environmental tobacco smoke (Z77.22)
     exposure to tobacco smoke in the perinatal period (P96.81)
     history of tobacco dependence (Z87.891)
     occupational exposure to environmental tobacco smoke (Z57.31)
     tobacco dependence (F17.-)
     tobacco use (Z72.0)
     EXCLUDES 1   *melanoma in situ (D03.-)*

D02.0 Carcinoma in situ of larynx
     Carcinoma in situ of aryepiglottic fold or interarytenoid fold, laryngeal aspect
     Carcinoma in situ of epiglottis (suprahyoid portion)
     EXCLUDES 1   *carcinoma in situ of aryepiglottic fold or interarytenoid fold NOS (D00.08)*
         carcinoma in situ of hypopharyngeal aspect (D00.08)
         carcinoma in situ of marginal zone (D00.08)

D02.1 Carcinoma in situ of trachea

✓5ᵗʰ **D02.2** Carcinoma in situ of bronchus and lung

     D02.20 Carcinoma in situ of unspecified bronchus and lung
     D02.21 Carcinoma in situ of right bronchus and lung
     D02.22 Carcinoma in situ of left bronchus and lung

D02.3 Carcinoma in situ of other parts of respiratory system
     Carcinoma in situ of accessory sinuses
     Carcinoma in situ of middle ear
     Carcinoma in situ of nasal cavities
     EXCLUDES 1   *carcinoma in situ of ear (external) (skin) (D04.2-)*
         carcinoma in situ of nose NOS (D09.8)
         carcinoma in situ of skin of nose (D04.3)

D02.4 Carcinoma in situ of respiratory system, unspecified

✓4ᵗʰ **D03** Melanoma in situ

D03.0 Melanoma in situ of lip   HCC

✓5ᵗʰ **D03.1** Melanoma in situ of eyelid, including canthus

     AHA: 2018,4Q,4

     D03.10 Melanoma in situ of unspecified eyelid, including canthus   HCC

     ✓6ᵗʰ **D03.11** Melanoma in situ of right eyelid, including canthus

         D03.111 Melanoma in situ of right upper eyelid, including canthus

         D03.112 Melanoma in situ of right lower eyelid, including canthus   HCC

     ✓6ᵗʰ **D03.12** Melanoma in situ of left eyelid, including canthus

         D03.121 Melanoma in situ of left upper eyelid, including canthus   HCC

         D03.122 Melanoma in situ of left lower eyelid, including canthus   HCC

✓5ᵗʰ **D03.2** Melanoma in situ of ear and external auricular canal

     D03.20 Melanoma in situ of unspecified ear and external auricular canal   HCC

     D03.21 Melanoma in situ of right ear and external auricular canal   HCC

     D03.22 Melanoma in situ of left ear and external auricular canal   HCC

✓5ᵗʰ **D03.3** Melanoma in situ of other and unspecified parts of face

     D03.30 Melanoma in situ of unspecified part of face   HCC

     D03.39 Melanoma in situ of other parts of face   HCC

D03.4 Melanoma in situ of scalp and neck   HCC

✓5ᵗʰ **D03.5** Melanoma in situ of trunk

     D03.51 Melanoma in situ of anal skin   HCC
         Melanoma in situ of anal margin
         Melanoma in situ of perianal skin

     D03.52 Melanoma in situ of breast (skin) (soft tissue)   HCC

     D03.59 Melanoma in situ of other part of trunk   HCC

✓5ᵗʰ **D03.6** Melanoma in situ of upper limb, including shoulder

     D03.60 Melanoma in situ of unspecified upper limb, including shoulder   HCC

     D03.61 Melanoma in situ of right upper limb, including shoulder   HCC

     D03.62 Melanoma in situ of left upper limb, including shoulder   HCC

✓5ᵗʰ **D03.7** Melanoma in situ of lower limb, including hip

     D03.70 Melanoma in situ of unspecified lower limb, including hip   HCC

     D03.71 Melanoma in situ of right lower limb, including hip   HCC

     D03.72 Melanoma in situ of left lower limb, including hip   HCC

D03.8 Melanoma in situ of other sites   HCC
     Melanoma in situ of scrotum
     EXCLUDES 1   *carcinoma in situ of scrotum (D07.61)*

D03.9 Melanoma in situ, unspecified   HCC

✓4ᵗʰ **D04** Carcinoma in situ of skin
     EXCLUDES 1   *erythroplasia of Queyrat (penis) NOS (D07.4)*
         melanoma in situ (D03.-)

D04.0 Carcinoma in situ of skin of lip
     EXCLUDES 1   *carcinoma in situ of vermilion border of lip (D00.01)*
     EXCLUDES 2   ▶*carcinoma in situ of vermilion border of lip (D00.01)*◀

✓5ᵗʰ **D04.1** Carcinoma in situ of skin of eyelid, including canthus

     AHA: 2018,4Q,4

     D04.10 Carcinoma in situ of skin of unspecified eyelid, including canthus

     ✓6ᵗʰ **D04.11** Carcinoma in situ of skin of right eyelid, including canthus

         D04.111 Carcinoma in situ of skin of right upper eyelid, including canthus

         D04.112 Carcinoma in situ of skin of right lower eyelid, including canthus

     ✓6ᵗʰ **D04.12** Carcinoma in situ of skin of left eyelid, including canthus

         D04.121 Carcinoma in situ of skin of left upper eyelid, including canthus

         D04.122 Carcinoma in situ of skin of left lower eyelid, including canthus

✓5ᵗʰ **D04.2** Carcinoma in situ of skin of ear and external auricular canal

     D04.20 Carcinoma in situ of skin of unspecified ear and external auricular canal

     D04.21 Carcinoma in situ of skin of right ear and external auricular canal

     D04.22 Carcinoma in situ of skin of left ear and external auricular canal

✓5ᵗʰ **D04.3** Carcinoma in situ of skin of other and unspecified parts of face

     D04.30 Carcinoma in situ of skin of unspecified part of face

     D04.39 Carcinoma in situ of skin of other parts of face

D04.4 Carcinoma in situ of skin of scalp and neck

D04.5 Carcinoma in situ of skin of trunk
     Carcinoma in situ of anal margin
     Carcinoma in situ of anal skin
     Carcinoma in situ of perianal skin
     Carcinoma in situ of skin of breast
     EXCLUDES 1   *carcinoma in situ of anus NOS (D01.3)*
         carcinoma in situ of scrotum (D07.61)
         carcinoma in situ of skin of genital organs (D07.-)

✓5ᵗʰ **D04.6** Carcinoma in situ of skin of upper limb, including shoulder

     D04.60 Carcinoma in situ of skin of unspecified upper limb, including shoulder

     D04.61 Carcinoma in situ of skin of right upper limb, including shoulder

     D04.62 Carcinoma in situ of skin of left upper limb, including shoulder

✓5ᵗʰ **D04.7** Carcinoma in situ of skin of lower limb, including hip

     D04.70 Carcinoma in situ of skin of unspecified lower limb, including hip

     D04.71 Carcinoma in situ of skin of right lower limb, including hip

     D04.72 Carcinoma in situ of skin of left lower limb, including hip

D04.8 Carcinoma in situ of skin of other sites

D04.9 Carcinoma in situ of skin, unspecified

✔ Additional Character Required   ✓ x 7ᵗʰ Placeholder   Unacceptable PDx   Questionable PDx   Manifestation   Unspecified Dx   H1 -H14 HAC   HCC CMS-HCC Dx   HIV HIV Dx

ICD-10-CM 2020   491

Chapter 2. Neoplasms

D05–D11.9

√4ᵗʰ **D05 Carcinoma in situ of** breast

> EXCLUDES 1   *carcinoma in situ of skin of breast (D04.5)*
> *melanoma in situ of breast (skin) (D03.5)*
> *Paget's disease of breast or nipple (C50.-)*

√5ᵗʰ **D05.0 Lobular carcinoma in situ of breast**

> **D05.00 Lobular carcinoma in situ of unspecified breast**
> **D05.01 Lobular carcinoma in situ of** right **breast**
> **D05.02 Lobular carcinoma in situ of** left **breast**

√5ᵗʰ **D05.1 Intraductal carcinoma in situ of breast**

> **D05.10 Intraductal carcinoma in situ of unspecified breast**
> **D05.11 Intraductal carcinoma in situ of** right **breast**
> **D05.12 Intraductal carcinoma in situ of** left **breast**

√5ᵗʰ **D05.8 Other specified type of carcinoma in situ of breast**

> **D05.80 Other specified type of carcinoma in situ of unspecified breast**
> **D05.81 Other specified type of carcinoma in situ of** right **breast**
> **D05.82 Other specified type of carcinoma in situ of** left **breast**

√5ᵗʰ **D05.9 Unspecified type of carcinoma in situ of breast**

> **D05.90 Unspecified type of carcinoma in situ of unspecified breast**
> **D05.91 Unspecified type of carcinoma in situ of** right **breast**
> **D05.92 Unspecified type of carcinoma in situ of** left **breast**

√4ᵗʰ **D06 Carcinoma in situ of** cervix uteri

> INCLUDES   cervical adenocarcinoma in situ
> cervical intraepithelial glandular neoplasia
> cervical intraepithelial neoplasia III [CIN III]
> severe dysplasia of cervix uteri
>
> EXCLUDES 1   *cervical intraepithelial neoplasia II [CIN II] (N87.1)*
> *cytologic evidence of malignancy of cervix without histologic confirmation (R87.614)*
> *high grade squamous intraepithelial lesion (HGSIL) of cervix (R87.613)*
> *melanoma in situ of cervix (D03.5)*
> *moderate cervical dysplasia (N87.1)*

D06.0 Carcinoma in situ of endocervix ♀
D06.1 Carcinoma in situ of exocervix ♀
D06.7 Carcinoma in situ of other parts of cervix ♀
D06.9 Carcinoma in situ of cervix, unspecified ♀

√4ᵗʰ **D07 Carcinoma in situ of other and unspecified** genital organs

> EXCLUDES 1   *melanoma in situ of trunk (D03.5)*

D07.0 Carcinoma in situ of endometrium ♀
D07.1 Carcinoma in situ of vulva ♀
> Severe dysplasia of vulva
> Vulvar intraepithelial neoplasia III [VIN III]
> EXCLUDES 1   *moderate dysplasia of vulva (N90.1)*
> *vulvar intraepithelial neoplasia II [VIN II] (N90.1)*

D07.2 Carcinoma in situ of vagina ♀
> Severe dysplasia of vagina
> Vaginal intraepithelial neoplasia III [VAIN III]
> EXCLUDES 1   *moderate dysplasia of vagina (N89.1)*
> *vaginal intraepithelial neoplasia II [VIN II] (N89.1)*

√5ᵗʰ **D07.3 Carcinoma in situ of other and unspecified** female genital organs

> **D07.30 Carcinoma in situ of unspecified female genital organs** ♀
> **D07.39 Carcinoma in situ of other female genital organs** ♀

D07.4 Carcinoma in situ of penis ♂
> Erythroplasia of Queyrat NOS
D07.5 Carcinoma in situ of prostate ♂
> Prostatic intraepithelial neoplasia III [PIN III]
> Severe dysplasia of prostate
> EXCLUDES 1   *dysplasia (mild) (moderate) of prostate (N42.3-)*
> *prostatic intraepithelial neoplasia II [PIN II] (N42.3-)*

√5ᵗʰ **D07.6 Carcinoma in situ of other and unspecified** male genital organs

> **D07.60 Carcinoma in situ of unspecified male genital organs** ♂
> **D07.61 Carcinoma in situ of** scrotum ♂
> **D07.69 Carcinoma in situ of other male genital organs** ♂

√4ᵗʰ **D09 Carcinoma in situ of other and unspecified** sites

> EXCLUDES 1   *melanoma in situ (D03.-)*

D09.0 Carcinoma in situ of bladder
√5ᵗʰ **D09.1 Carcinoma in situ of other and unspecified** urinary organs

> **D09.10 Carcinoma in situ of unspecified urinary organ**
> **D09.19 Carcinoma in situ of other urinary organs**

√5ᵗʰ **D09.2 Carcinoma in situ of** eye

> EXCLUDES 1   *carcinoma in situ of skin of eyelid (D04.1-)*
>
> **D09.20 Carcinoma in situ of unspecified eye**
> **D09.21 Carcinoma in situ of** right **eye**
> **D09.22 Carcinoma in situ of** left **eye**

D09.3 Carcinoma in situ of thyroid **and other** endocrine glands
> EXCLUDES 1   *carcinoma in situ of endocrine pancreas (D01.7)*
> *carcinoma in situ of ovary (D07.39)*
> *carcinoma in situ of testis (D07.69)*

D09.8 Carcinoma in situ of other specified sites
D09.9 Carcinoma in situ, unspecified

Benign neoplasms, except benign neuroendocrine tumors (D10-D36)

√4ᵗʰ **D10 Benign neoplasm of** mouth and pharynx

D10.0 Benign neoplasm of lip
> Benign neoplasm of lip (frenulum) (inner aspect) (mucosa) (vermilion border)
> EXCLUDES 1   *benign neoplasm of skin of lip (D22.0, D23.0)*

D10.1 Benign neoplasm of tongue
> Benign neoplasm of lingual tonsil

D10.2 Benign neoplasm of floor **of mouth**

√5ᵗʰ **D10.3 Benign neoplasm of other and unspecified parts of mouth**

> **D10.30 Benign neoplasm of unspecified part of mouth**
> **D10.39 Benign neoplasm of other parts of mouth**
> Benign neoplasm of minor salivary gland NOS
> EXCLUDES 1   *benign odontogenic neoplasms (D16.4-D16.5)*
> *benign neoplasm of mucosa of lip (D10.0)*
> *benign neoplasm of nasopharyngeal surface of soft palate (D10.6)*

D10.4 Benign neoplasm of tonsil
> Benign neoplasm of tonsil (faucial) (palatine)
> EXCLUDES 1   *benign neoplasm of lingual tonsil (D10.1)*
> *benign neoplasm of pharyngeal tonsil (D10.6)*
> *benign neoplasm of tonsillar fossa (D10.5)*
> *benign neoplasm of tonsillar pillars (D10.5)*

D10.5 Benign neoplasm of other parts of oropharynx
> Benign neoplasm of epiglottis, anterior aspect
> Benign neoplasm of tonsillar fossa
> Benign neoplasm of tonsillar pillars
> Benign neoplasm of vallecula
> EXCLUDES 1   *benign neoplasm of epiglottis NOS (D14.1)*
> *benign neoplasm of epiglottis, suprahyoid portion (D14.1)*
> **DEF:** Oropharynx: Middle portion of pharynx (throat); communicates with the oral cavity, nasopharynx and laryngopharynx.

D10.6 Benign neoplasm of nasopharynx
> Benign neoplasm of pharyngeal tonsil
> Benign neoplasm of posterior margin of septum and choanae
> **DEF:** Nasopharynx: Upper portion of pharynx (throat); communicates with the nasal cavities, oropharynx and tympanic cavities.

D10.7 Benign neoplasm of hypopharynx
> **DEF:** Hypopharynx: Lower portion of pharynx (throat); communicates with the oropharynx and the esophagus.
> *Synonyms:* laryngopharynx.

D10.9 Benign neoplasm of pharynx, unspecified

√4ᵗʰ **D11 Benign neoplasm of** major salivary glands

> EXCLUDES 1   *benign neoplasms of specified minor salivary glands which are classified according to their anatomical location*
> *benign neoplasms of minor salivary glands NOS (D10.39)*

D11.0 Benign neoplasm of parotid gland
D11.7 Benign neoplasm of other major salivary glands
> Benign neoplasm of sublingual salivary gland
> Benign neoplasm of submandibular salivary gland
D11.9 Benign neoplasm of major salivary gland, unspecified

✓4th D12 Benign neoplasm of colon, rectum, anus and anal canal
> *EXCLUDES 1* benign carcinoid tumors of the large intestine, and rectum (D3A.02-)
> ▶polyp of colon NOS (K63.5)◀

AHA: 2018,2Q,14; 2017,1Q,15; 2015,2Q,14

TIP: Code K63.5 Polyp of colon, is assigned when documentation states hyperplastic colon polyps, regardless of the site in the colon. Slow-growing, hyperplastic polyps are not precancerous and are classified differently from benign or adenomatous polyps.

D12.0 Benign neoplasm of cecum
Benign neoplasm of ileocecal valve

D12.1 Benign neoplasm of appendix
> *EXCLUDES 1* benign carcinoid tumor of the appendix (D3A.020)

D12.2 Benign neoplasm of ascending colon

D12.3 Benign neoplasm of transverse colon
Benign neoplasm of hepatic flexure
Benign neoplasm of splenic flexure
AHA: 2017,1Q,16

D12.4 Benign neoplasm of descending colon

D12.5 Benign neoplasm of sigmoid colon

D12.6 Benign neoplasm of colon, unspecified
Adenomatosis of colon
Benign neoplasm of large intestine NOS
Polyposis (hereditary) of colon
> *EXCLUDES 1* inflammatory polyp of colon (K51.4-)
> polyp of colon NOS (K63.5)

D12.7 Benign neoplasm of rectosigmoid junction

D12.8 Benign neoplasm of rectum
> *EXCLUDES 1* benign carcinoid tumor of the rectum (D3A.026)
AHA: 2018,1Q,6

D12.9 Benign neoplasm of anus and anal canal
Benign neoplasm of anus NOS
> *EXCLUDES 1* benign neoplasm of anal margin (D22.5, D23.5)
> benign neoplasm of anal skin (D22.5, D23.5)
> benign neoplasm of perianal skin (D22.5, D23.5)

✓4th D13 Benign neoplasm of other and ill-defined parts of digestive system
> *EXCLUDES 1* benign stromal tumors of digestive system (D21.4)

D13.0 Benign neoplasm of esophagus

D13.1 Benign neoplasm of stomach
> *EXCLUDES 1* benign carcinoid tumor of the stomach (D3A.092)

D13.2 Benign neoplasm of duodenum
> *EXCLUDES 1* benign carcinoid tumor of the duodenum (D3A.010)

✓5th D13.3 Benign neoplasm of other and unspecified parts of small intestine
> *EXCLUDES 1* benign carcinoid tumors of the small intestine (D3A.01-)
> benign neoplasm of ileocecal valve (D12.0)

  D13.30 Benign neoplasm of unspecified part of small intestine

  D13.39 Benign neoplasm of other parts of small intestine

D13.4 Benign neoplasm of liver
Benign neoplasm of intrahepatic bile ducts

D13.5 Benign neoplasm of extrahepatic bile ducts

D13.6 Benign neoplasm of pancreas
> *EXCLUDES 1* benign neoplasm of endocrine pancreas (D13.7)

D13.7 Benign neoplasm of endocrine pancreas
Benign neoplasm of islets of Langerhans
Islet cell tumor
Use additional code to identify any functional activity

D13.9 Benign neoplasm of ill-defined sites within the digestive system
Benign neoplasm of digestive system NOS
Benign neoplasm of intestine NOS
Benign neoplasm of spleen

✓4th D14 Benign neoplasm of middle ear and respiratory system

D14.0 Benign neoplasm of middle ear, nasal cavity and accessory sinuses
Benign neoplasm of cartilage of nose
> *EXCLUDES 1* benign neoplasm of auricular canal (external) (D22.2-, D23.2-)
> benign neoplasm of bone of ear (D16.4)
> benign neoplasm of bone of nose (D16.4)
> benign neoplasm of cartilage of ear (D21.0)
> benign neoplasm of ear (external)(skin) (D22.2-, D23.2-)
> benign neoplasm of nose NOS (D36.7)
> benign neoplasm of skin of nose (D22.39, D23.39)
> benign neoplasm of olfactory bulb (D33.3)
> benign neoplasm of posterior margin of septum and choanae (D10.6)
> polyp of accessory sinus (J33.8)
> polyp of ear (middle) (H74.4)
> polyp of nasal (cavity) (J33.-)

D14.1 Benign neoplasm of larynx
Adenomatous polyp of larynx
Benign neoplasm of epiglottis (suprahyoid portion)
> *EXCLUDES 1* benign neoplasm of epiglottis, anterior aspect (D10.5)
> polyp (nonadenomatous) of vocal cord or larynx (J38.1)

D14.2 Benign neoplasm of trachea

✓5th D14.3 Benign neoplasm of bronchus and lung
> *EXCLUDES 1* benign carcinoid tumor of the bronchus and lung (D3A.090)

  D14.30 Benign neoplasm of unspecified bronchus and lung
  D14.31 Benign neoplasm of right bronchus and lung
  D14.32 Benign neoplasm of left bronchus and lung

D14.4 Benign neoplasm of respiratory system, unspecified

✓4th D15 Benign neoplasm of other and unspecified intrathoracic organs
> *EXCLUDES 1* benign neoplasm of mesothelial tissue (D19.-)

D15.0 Benign neoplasm of thymus
> *EXCLUDES 1* benign carcinoid tumor of the thymus (D3A.091)

D15.1 Benign neoplasm of heart
> *EXCLUDES 1* benign neoplasm of great vessels (D21.3)

D15.2 Benign neoplasm of mediastinum

D15.7 Benign neoplasm of other specified intrathoracic organs

D15.9 Benign neoplasm of intrathoracic organ, unspecified

✓4th D16 Benign neoplasm of bone and articular cartilage
> *EXCLUDES 1* benign neoplasm of connective tissue of ear (D21.0)
> benign neoplasm of connective tissue of eyelid (D21.0)
> benign neoplasm of connective tissue of larynx (D14.1)
> benign neoplasm of connective tissue of nose (D14.0)
> benign neoplasm of synovia (D21.-)

✓5th D16.0 Benign neoplasm of scapula and long bones of upper limb
  D16.00 Benign neoplasm of scapula and long bones of unspecified upper limb
  D16.01 Benign neoplasm of scapula and long bones of right upper limb
  D16.02 Benign neoplasm of scapula and long bones of left upper limb

✓5th D16.1 Benign neoplasm of short bones of upper limb
  D16.10 Benign neoplasm of short bones of unspecified upper limb
  D16.11 Benign neoplasm of short bones of right upper limb
  D16.12 Benign neoplasm of short bones of left upper limb

✓5th D16.2 Benign neoplasm of long bones of lower limb
  D16.20 Benign neoplasm of long bones of unspecified lower limb
  D16.21 Benign neoplasm of long bones of right lower limb
  D16.22 Benign neoplasm of long bones of left lower limb

✓5th D16.3 Benign neoplasm of short bones of lower limb
  D16.30 Benign neoplasm of short bones of unspecified lower limb
  D16.31 Benign neoplasm of short bones of right lower limb
  D16.32 Benign neoplasm of short bones of left lower limb

Chapter 2. Neoplasms *(left margin)*

D16.4   **Benign neoplasm of bones of** skull and face
Benign neoplasm of maxilla (superior)
Benign neoplasm of orbital bone
Keratocyst of maxilla
Keratocystic odontogenic tumor of maxilla
    EXCLUDES 2   *benign neoplasm of lower jaw bone (D16.5)*

D16.5   **Benign neoplasm of** lower jaw bone
Keratocyst of mandible
Keratocystic odontogenic tumor of mandible

D16.6   **Benign neoplasm of** vertebral column
    EXCLUDES 1   *benign neoplasm of sacrum and coccyx (D16.8)*

D16.7   **Benign neoplasm of** ribs, sternum and clavicle

D16.8   **Benign neoplasm of** pelvic bones, sacrum and coccyx

D16.9   **Benign neoplasm of bone and articular cartilage, unspecified**

✓4th **D17**   **Benign** lipomatous **neoplasm**

D17.0   **Benign lipomatous neoplasm of** skin and subcutaneous tissue **of head, face and neck**

D17.1   **Benign lipomatous neoplasm of** skin and subcutaneous tissue **of trunk**

✓5th **D17.2**   **Benign lipomatous neoplasm of** skin and subcutaneous tissue **of limb**

    D17.20   **Benign lipomatous neoplasm of skin and subcutaneous tissue of unspecified limb**

    D17.21   **Benign lipomatous neoplasm of skin and subcutaneous tissue of** right arm

    D17.22   **Benign lipomatous neoplasm of skin and subcutaneous tissue of** left arm

    D17.23   **Benign lipomatous neoplasm of skin and subcutaneous tissue of** right leg

    D17.24   **Benign lipomatous neoplasm of skin and subcutaneous tissue of** left leg

✓5th **D17.3**   **Benign lipomatous neoplasm of** skin and subcutaneous tissue **of other and unspecified sites**

    D17.30   **Benign lipomatous neoplasm of skin and subcutaneous tissue of unspecified sites**

    D17.39   **Benign lipomatous neoplasm of skin and subcutaneous tissue of other sites**

D17.4   **Benign lipomatous neoplasm of** intrathoracic organs

D17.5   **Benign lipomatous neoplasm of** intra-abdominal organs
    EXCLUDES 1   *benign lipomatous neoplasm of peritoneum and retroperitoneum (D17.79)*

D17.6   **Benign lipomatous neoplasm of** spermatic cord   ♂

✓5th **D17.7**   **Benign lipomatous neoplasm of other sites**

    D17.71   **Benign lipomatous neoplasm of** kidney

    D17.72   **Benign lipomatous neoplasm of other** genitourinary organ

    D17.79   **Benign lipomatous neoplasm of other sites**
Benign lipomatous neoplasm of peritoneum
Benign lipomatous neoplasm of retroperitoneum

D17.9   **Benign lipomatous neoplasm, unspecified**
Lipoma NOS

✓4th **D18**   **Hemangioma and lymphangioma, any site**
    EXCLUDES 1   *benign neoplasm of glomus jugulare (D35.6)*
blue or pigmented nevus (D22.-)
nevus NOS (D22.-)
vascular nevus (Q82.5)

✓5th **D18.0**   **Hemangioma**
Angioma NOS
Cavernous nevus
DEF: Common benign tumor usually occurring in infancy that is composed of newly formed blood vessels due to malformation of the angioblastic tissue.

    D18.00   **Hemangioma unspecified site**

    D18.01   **Hemangioma of** skin and subcutaneous tissue

    D18.02   **Hemangioma of** intracranial structures   HCC

    D18.03   **Hemangioma of** intra-abdominal structures

    D18.09   **Hemangioma of other sites**

D18.1   **Lymphangioma, any site**
AHA: 2018,3Q,31; 2018,2Q,13

✓4th **D19**   **Benign neoplasm of** mesothelial tissue

D19.0   **Benign neoplasm of mesothelial tissue of** pleura

D19.1   **Benign neoplasm of mesothelial tissue of** peritoneum

D19.7   **Benign neoplasm of mesothelial tissue of other sites**

D19.9   **Benign neoplasm of mesothelial tissue, unspecified**
Benign mesothelioma NOS

✓4th **D20**   **Benign neoplasm of soft tissue of** retroperitoneum and peritoneum
    EXCLUDES 1   *benign lipomatous neoplasm of peritoneum and retroperitoneum (D17.79)*
benign neoplasm of mesothelial tissue (D19.-)

D20.0   **Benign neoplasm of soft tissue of** retroperitoneum

D20.1   **Benign neoplasm of soft tissue of** peritoneum

✓4th **D21**   **Other benign neoplasms of** connective and other soft tissue
    INCLUDES   benign neoplasm of blood vessel
benign neoplasm of bursa
benign neoplasm of cartilage
benign neoplasm of fascia
benign neoplasm of fat
benign neoplasm of ligament, except uterine
benign neoplasm of lymphatic channel
benign neoplasm of muscle
benign neoplasm of synovia
benign neoplasm of tendon (sheath)
benign stromal tumors
    EXCLUDES 1   *benign neoplasm of articular cartilage (D16.-)*
benign neoplasm of cartilage of larynx (D14.1)
benign neoplasm of cartilage of nose (D14.0)
benign neoplasm of connective tissue of breast (D24.-)
benign neoplasm of peripheral nerves and autonomic nervous system (D36.1-)
benign neoplasm of peritoneum (D20.1)
benign neoplasm of retroperitoneum (D20.0)
benign neoplasm of uterine ligament, any (D28.2)
benign neoplasm of vascular tissue (D18.-)
hemangioma (D18.0-)
lipomatous neoplasm (D17.-)
lymphangioma (D18.1)
uterine leiomyoma (D25.-)

D21.0   **Benign neoplasm of connective and other soft tissue of** head, face and neck
Benign neoplasm of connective tissue of ear
Benign neoplasm of connective tissue of eyelid
    EXCLUDES 1   *benign neoplasm of connective tissue of orbit (D31.6-)*

✓5th **D21.1**   **Benign neoplasm of connective and other soft tissue of** upper limb, including shoulder

    D21.10   **Benign neoplasm of connective and other soft tissue of unspecified upper limb, including shoulder**

    D21.11   **Benign neoplasm of connective and other soft tissue of** right upper limb, including shoulder

    D21.12   **Benign neoplasm of connective and other soft tissue of** left upper limb, including shoulder

✓5th **D21.2**   **Benign neoplasm of connective and other soft tissue of** lower limb, including hip

    D21.20   **Benign neoplasm of connective and other soft tissue of unspecified lower limb, including hip**

    D21.21   **Benign neoplasm of connective and other soft tissue of** right lower limb, including hip

    D21.22   **Benign neoplasm of connective and other soft tissue of** left lower limb, including hip

D21.3   **Benign neoplasm of connective and other soft tissue of** thorax
Benign neoplasm of axilla
Benign neoplasm of diaphragm
Benign neoplasm of great vessels
    EXCLUDES 1   *benign neoplasm of heart (D15.1)*
benign neoplasm of mediastinum (D15.2)
benign neoplasm of thymus (D15.0)

D21.4   **Benign neoplasm of connective and other soft tissue of** abdomen
Benign stromal tumors of abdomen

D21.5   **Benign neoplasm of connective and other soft tissue of** pelvis
    EXCLUDES 1   *benign neoplasm of any uterine ligament (D28.2)*
uterine leiomyoma (D25.-)

D21.6   **Benign neoplasm of connective and other soft tissue of** trunk, unspecified
▶Benign neoplasm of connective and other soft tissue back NOS◀

D21.9   **Benign neoplasm of connective and other soft tissue, unspecified**

✓4ᵗʰ **D22 Melanocytic nevi**

INCLUDES   atypical nevus
             blue hairy pigmented nevus
             nevus NOS

D22.0 Melanocytic nevi of lip

✓5ᵗʰ **D22.1 Melanocytic nevi of eyelid, including canthus**

     AHA: 2018,4Q,4

     D22.10 Melanocytic nevi of unspecified eyelid, including canthus

     ✓6ᵗʰ **D22.11 Melanocytic nevi of right eyelid, including canthus**

         D22.111 Melanocytic nevi of right upper eyelid, including canthus

         D22.112 Melanocytic nevi of right lower eyelid, including canthus

     ✓6ᵗʰ **D22.12 Melanocytic nevi of left eyelid, including canthus**

         D22.121 Melanocytic nevi of left upper eyelid, including canthus

         D22.122 Melanocytic nevi of left lower eyelid, including canthus

✓5ᵗʰ **D22.2 Melanocytic nevi of ear and external auricular canal**

     D22.20 Melanocytic nevi of unspecified ear and external auricular canal

     D22.21 Melanocytic nevi of right ear and external auricular canal

     D22.22 Melanocytic nevi of left ear and external auricular canal

✓5ᵗʰ **D22.3 Melanocytic nevi of other and unspecified parts of face**

     D22.30 Melanocytic nevi of unspecified part of face

     D22.39 Melanocytic nevi of other parts of face

D22.4 Melanocytic nevi of scalp and neck

D22.5 Melanocytic nevi of trunk

     Melanocytic nevi of anal margin
     Melanocytic nevi of anal skin
     Melanocytic nevi of perianal skin
     Melanocytic nevi of skin of breast

✓5ᵗʰ **D22.6 Melanocytic nevi of upper limb, including shoulder**

     D22.60 Melanocytic nevi of unspecified upper limb, including shoulder

     D22.61 Melanocytic nevi of right upper limb, including shoulder

     D22.62 Melanocytic nevi of left upper limb, including shoulder

✓5ᵗʰ **D22.7 Melanocytic nevi of lower limb, including hip**

     D22.70 Melanocytic nevi of unspecified lower limb, including hip

     D22.71 Melanocytic nevi of right lower limb, including hip

     D22.72 Melanocytic nevi of left lower limb, including hip

D22.9 Melanocytic nevi, unspecified

✓4ᵗʰ **D23 Other benign neoplasms of skin**

INCLUDES   benign neoplasm of hair follicles
             benign neoplasm of sebaceous glands
             benign neoplasm of sweat glands

EXCLUDES 1   benign lipomatous neoplasms of skin (D17.0-D17.3)
             ~~melanocytic nevi (D22.-)~~

EXCLUDES 2   ▶melanocytic nevi (D22.-)◀

D23.0 Other benign neoplasm of skin of lip

     EXCLUDES 1   benign neoplasm of vermilion border of lip (D10.0)

✓5ᵗʰ **D23.1 Other benign neoplasm of skin of eyelid, including canthus**

     AHA: 2018,4Q,4

     D23.10 Other benign neoplasm of skin of unspecified eyelid, including canthus

     ✓6ᵗʰ **D23.11 Other benign neoplasm of skin of right eyelid, including canthus**

         D23.111 Other benign neoplasm of skin of right upper eyelid, including canthus

         D23.112 Other benign neoplasm of skin of right lower eyelid, including canthus

     ✓6ᵗʰ **D23.12 Other benign neoplasm of skin of left eyelid, including canthus**

         D23.121 Other benign neoplasm of skin of left upper eyelid, including canthus

         D23.122 Other benign neoplasm of skin of left lower eyelid, including canthus

✓5ᵗʰ **D23.2 Other benign neoplasm of skin of ear and external auricular canal**

     D23.20 Other benign neoplasm of skin of unspecified ear and external auricular canal

     D23.21 Other benign neoplasm of skin of right ear and external auricular canal

     D23.22 Other benign neoplasm of skin of left ear and external auricular canal

✓5ᵗʰ **D23.3 Other benign neoplasm of skin of other and unspecified parts of face**

     D23.30 Other benign neoplasm of skin of unspecified part of face

     D23.39 Other benign neoplasm of skin of other parts of face

D23.4 Other benign neoplasm of skin of scalp and neck

D23.5 Other benign neoplasm of skin of trunk

     Other benign neoplasm of anal margin
     Other benign neoplasm of anal skin
     Other benign neoplasm of perianal skin
     Other benign neoplasm of skin of breast

     EXCLUDES 1   benign neoplasm of anus NOS (D12.9)

✓5ᵗʰ **D23.6 Other benign neoplasm of skin of upper limb, including shoulder**

     D23.60 Other benign neoplasm of skin of unspecified upper limb, including shoulder

     D23.61 Other benign neoplasm of skin of right upper limb, including shoulder

     D23.62 Other benign neoplasm of skin of left upper limb, including shoulder

✓5ᵗʰ **D23.7 Other benign neoplasm of skin of lower limb, including hip**

     D23.70 Other benign neoplasm of skin of unspecified lower limb, including hip

     D23.71 Other benign neoplasm of skin of right lower limb, including hip

     D23.72 Other benign neoplasm of skin of left lower limb, including hip

D23.9 Other benign neoplasm of skin, unspecified

✓4ᵗʰ **D24 Benign neoplasm of breast**

INCLUDES   benign neoplasm of connective tissue of breast
             benign neoplasm of soft parts of breast
             fibroadenoma of breast

EXCLUDES 2   adenofibrosis of breast (N60.2)
             benign cyst of breast (N60.-)
             benign mammary dysplasia (N60.-)
             benign neoplasm of skin of breast (D22.5, D23.5)
             fibrocystic disease of breast (N60.-)

D24.1 Benign neoplasm of right breast

D24.2 Benign neoplasm of left breast

D24.9 Benign neoplasm of unspecified breast

✓4ᵗʰ **D25 Leiomyoma of uterus**

INCLUDES   uterine fibroid
             uterine fibromyoma
             uterine myoma

Uterine Leiomyomas (Fibroids)

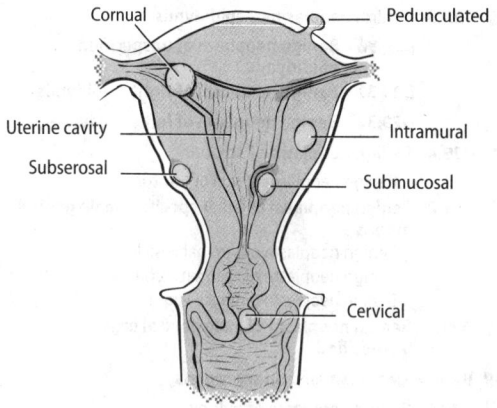

D25.0 Submucous leiomyoma of uterus ♀

D25.1 Intramural leiomyoma of uterus ♀

     Interstitial leiomyoma of uterus

Chapter 2. Neoplasms

D25.2   **Subserosal** leiomyoma of uterus   ♀
      Subperitoneal leiomyoma of uterus

D25.9   **Leiomyoma of uterus, unspecified**   ♀

☑4ᵗʰ **D26**   **Other benign neoplasms of uterus**

D26.0   **Other benign neoplasm of cervix uteri**   ♀

D26.1   **Other benign neoplasm of corpus uteri**   ♀

D26.7   **Other benign neoplasm of other parts of uterus**   ♀

D26.9   **Other benign neoplasm of uterus, unspecified**   ♀

☑4ᵗʰ **D27**   **Benign neoplasm of ovary**
      Use additional code to identify any functional activity
      EXCLUDES 2   *corpus albicans cyst (N83.2-)*
         corpus luteum cyst (N83.1-)
         endometrial cyst (N80.1)
         follicular (atretic) cyst (N83.0-)
         graafian follicle cyst (N83.0-)
         ovarian cyst NEC (N83.2-)
         ovarian retention cyst (N83.2-)

D27.0   **Benign neoplasm of right ovary**   ♀

D27.1   **Benign neoplasm of left ovary**   ♀

D27.9   **Benign neoplasm of unspecified ovary**   ♀

☑4ᵗʰ **D28**   **Benign neoplasm of other and unspecified female genital organs**
      INCLUDES   adenomatous polyp
         benign neoplasm of skin of female genital organs
         benign teratoma
      EXCLUDES 1   *epoophoron cyst (Q50.5)*
         fimbrial cyst (Q50.4)
         Gartner's duct cyst (Q52.4)
         parovarian cyst (Q50.5)

D28.0   **Benign neoplasm of vulva**   ♀

D28.1   **Benign neoplasm of vagina**   ♀

D28.2   **Benign neoplasm of uterine tubes and ligaments**   ♀
      Benign neoplasm of fallopian tube
      Benign neoplasm of uterine ligament (broad) (round)

D28.7   **Benign neoplasm of other specified female genital organs**   ♀

D28.9   **Benign neoplasm of female genital organ, unspecified**   ♀

☑4ᵗʰ **D29**   **Benign neoplasm of male genital organs**
      INCLUDES   benign neoplasm of skin of male genital organs

D29.0   **Benign neoplasm of penis**   ♂

D29.1   **Benign neoplasm of prostate**   ♂
      EXCLUDES 1   *enlarged prostate (N40.-)*

☑5ᵗʰ D29.2   **Benign neoplasm of testis**
      Use additional code to identify any functional activity

    D29.20   **Benign neoplasm of unspecified testis**   ♂

    D29.21   **Benign neoplasm of right testis**   ♂

    D29.22   **Benign neoplasm of left testis**   ♂

☑5ᵗʰ D29.3   **Benign neoplasm of epididymis**

    D29.30   **Benign neoplasm of unspecified epididymis**   ♂

    D29.31   **Benign neoplasm of right epididymis**   ♂

    D29.32   **Benign neoplasm of left epididymis**   ♂

D29.4   **Benign neoplasm of scrotum**   ♂
      Benign neoplasm of skin of scrotum

D29.8   **Benign neoplasm of other specified male genital organs**   ♂
      Benign neoplasm of seminal vesicle
      Benign neoplasm of spermatic cord
      Benign neoplasm of tunica vaginalis

D29.9   **Benign neoplasm of male genital organ, unspecified**   ♂

☑4ᵗʰ **D30**   **Benign neoplasm of urinary organs**

☑5ᵗʰ D30.0   **Benign neoplasm of kidney**
      EXCLUDES 1   *benign carcinoid tumor of the kidney (D3A.093)*
         benign neoplasm of renal calyces (D30.1-)
         benign neoplasm of renal pelvis (D30.1-)

    D30.00   **Benign neoplasm of unspecified kidney**

    D30.01   **Benign neoplasm of right kidney**

    D30.02   **Benign neoplasm of left kidney**

☑5ᵗʰ D30.1   **Benign neoplasm of renal pelvis**

    D30.10   **Benign neoplasm of unspecified renal pelvis**

    D30.11   **Benign neoplasm of right renal pelvis**

    D30.12   **Benign neoplasm of left renal pelvis**

☑5ᵗʰ D30.2   **Benign neoplasm of ureter**
      EXCLUDES 1   *benign neoplasm of ureteric orifice of bladder (D30.3)*

    D30.20   **Benign neoplasm of unspecified ureter**

    D30.21   **Benign neoplasm of right ureter**

    D30.22   **Benign neoplasm of left ureter**

D30.3   **Benign neoplasm of bladder**
      Benign neoplasm of ureteric orifice of bladder
      Benign neoplasm of urethral orifice of bladder

D30.4   **Benign neoplasm of urethra**
      EXCLUDES 1   *benign neoplasm of urethral orifice of bladder (D30.3)*

D30.8   **Benign neoplasm of other specified urinary organs**
      Benign neoplasm of paraurethral glands

D30.9   **Benign neoplasm of urinary organ, unspecified**
      Benign neoplasm of urinary system NOS

☑4ᵗʰ **D31**   **Benign neoplasm of eye and adnexa**
      EXCLUDES 1   *benign neoplasm of connective tissue of eyelid (D21.0)*
         benign neoplasm of optic nerve (D33.3)
         benign neoplasm of skin of eyelid (D22.1-, D23.1-)

☑5ᵗʰ D31.0   **Benign neoplasm of conjunctiva**

    D31.00   **Benign neoplasm of unspecified conjunctiva**

    D31.01   **Benign neoplasm of right conjunctiva**

    D31.02   **Benign neoplasm of left conjunctiva**

☑5ᵗʰ D31.1   **Benign neoplasm of cornea**

    D31.10   **Benign neoplasm of unspecified cornea**

    D31.11   **Benign neoplasm of right cornea**

    D31.12   **Benign neoplasm of left cornea**

☑5ᵗʰ D31.2   **Benign neoplasm of retina**
      EXCLUDES 1   *dark area on retina (D49.81)*
         hemangioma of retina (D49.81)
         neoplasm of unspecified behavior of retina and choroid (D49.81)
         retinal freckle (D49.81)

    D31.20   **Benign neoplasm of unspecified retina**

    D31.21   **Benign neoplasm of right retina**

    D31.22   **Benign neoplasm of left retina**

☑5ᵗʰ D31.3   **Benign neoplasm of choroid**

    D31.30   **Benign neoplasm of unspecified choroid**

    D31.31   **Benign neoplasm of right choroid**

    D31.32   **Benign neoplasm of left choroid**

☑5ᵗʰ D31.4   **Benign neoplasm of ciliary body**

    D31.40   **Benign neoplasm of unspecified ciliary body**

    D31.41   **Benign neoplasm of right ciliary body**

    D31.42   **Benign neoplasm of left ciliary body**

☑5ᵗʰ D31.5   **Benign neoplasm of lacrimal gland and duct**
      Benign neoplasm of lacrimal sac
      Benign neoplasm of nasolacrimal duct

    D31.50   **Benign neoplasm of unspecified lacrimal gland and duct**

    D31.51   **Benign neoplasm of right lacrimal gland and duct**

    D31.52   **Benign neoplasm of left lacrimal gland and duct**

☑5ᵗʰ D31.6   **Benign neoplasm of unspecified site of orbit**
      Benign neoplasm of connective tissue of orbit
      Benign neoplasm of extraocular muscle
      Benign neoplasm of peripheral nerves of orbit
      Benign neoplasm of retrobulbar tissue
      Benign neoplasm of retro-ocular tissue
      EXCLUDES 1   *benign neoplasm of orbital bone (D16.4)*

    D31.60   **Benign neoplasm of unspecified site of unspecified orbit**

    D31.61   **Benign neoplasm of unspecified site of right orbit**

    D31.62   **Benign neoplasm of unspecified site of left orbit**

☑5ᵗʰ D31.9   **Benign neoplasm of unspecified part of eye**
      Benign neoplasm of eyeball

    D31.90   **Benign neoplasm of unspecified part of unspecified eye**

    D31.91   **Benign neoplasm of unspecified part of right eye**

    D31.92   **Benign neoplasm of unspecified part of left eye**

☑4ᵗʰ **D32**   **Benign neoplasm of meninges**

D32.0   **Benign neoplasm of cerebral meninges**   HCC

N Newborn: 0   P Pediatric: 0-17   M Maternity: 9-64   A Adult: 15-124   MCC Major Complication/Comorbidity   CC Complication/Comorbidity   SW Severe Wound Dx

496   ICD-10-CM 2020

D32.1   **Benign neoplasm of spinal meninges**   HCC

D32.9   **Benign neoplasm of meninges, unspecified**   HCC

     Meningioma NOS

✓4ᵗʰ **D33**   **Benign neoplasm of brain and other parts of central nervous system**

     EXCLUDES 1   angioma (D18.0-)

           benign neoplasm of meninges (D32.-)

           benign neoplasm of peripheral nerves and autonomic nervous system (D36.1-)

           hemangioma (D18.0-)

           neurofibromatosis (Q85.0-)

           retro-ocular benign neoplasm (D31.6-)

D33.0   **Benign neoplasm of brain, supratentorial**   HCC

     Benign neoplasm of cerebral ventricle

     Benign neoplasm of cerebrum

     Benign neoplasm of frontal lobe

     Benign neoplasm of occipital lobe

     Benign neoplasm of parietal lobe

     Benign neoplasm of temporal lobe

     EXCLUDES 1   benign neoplasm of fourth ventricle (D33.1)

D33.1   **Benign neoplasm of brain, infratentorial**   HCC

     Benign neoplasm of brain stem

     Benign neoplasm of cerebellum

     Benign neoplasm of fourth ventricle

D33.2   **Benign neoplasm of brain, unspecified**   HCC

D33.3   **Benign neoplasm of cranial nerves**   HCC

     Benign neoplasm of olfactory bulb

D33.4   **Benign neoplasm of spinal cord**   HCC

D33.7   **Benign neoplasm of other specified parts of central nervous system**   HCC

D33.9   **Benign neoplasm of central nervous system, unspecified**   HCC

     Benign neoplasm of nervous system (central) NOS

D34   **Benign neoplasm of thyroid gland**

     Use additional code to identify any functional activity

✓4ᵗʰ **D35**   **Benign neoplasm of other and unspecified endocrine glands**

     Use additional code to identify any functional activity

     EXCLUDES 1   benign neoplasm of endocrine pancreas (D13.7)

           benign neoplasm of ovary (D27.-)

           benign neoplasm of testis (D29.2.-)

           benign neoplasm of thymus (D15.0)

✓5ᵗʰ D35.0   **Benign neoplasm of adrenal gland**

     D35.00   **Benign neoplasm of unspecified adrenal gland**

     D35.01   **Benign neoplasm of right adrenal gland**

     D35.02   **Benign neoplasm of left adrenal gland**

D35.1   **Benign neoplasm of parathyroid gland**

D35.2   **Benign neoplasm of pituitary gland**   HCC

     AHA: 2014,3Q,22

D35.3   **Benign neoplasm of craniopharyngeal duct**   HCC

D35.4   **Benign neoplasm of pineal gland**   HCC

D35.5   **Benign neoplasm of carotid body**

D35.6   **Benign neoplasm of aortic body and other paraganglia**

     Benign tumor of glomus jugulare

D35.7   **Benign neoplasm of other specified endocrine glands**

D35.9   **Benign neoplasm of endocrine gland, unspecified**

     Benign neoplasm of unspecified endocrine gland

✓4ᵗʰ **D36**   **Benign neoplasm of other and unspecified sites**

D36.0   **Benign neoplasm of lymph nodes**

     EXCLUDES 1   lymphangioma (D18.1)

✓5ᵗʰ D36.1   **Benign neoplasm of peripheral nerves and autonomic nervous system**

     EXCLUDES 1   benign neoplasm of peripheral nerves of orbit (D31.6-)

           neurofibromatosis (Q85.0-)

     D36.10   **Benign neoplasm of peripheral nerves and autonomic nervous system, unspecified**

     D36.11   **Benign neoplasm of peripheral nerves and autonomic nervous system of face, head, and neck**

     D36.12   **Benign neoplasm of peripheral nerves and autonomic nervous system, upper limb, including shoulder**

     D36.13   **Benign neoplasm of peripheral nerves and autonomic nervous system of lower limb, including hip**

     D36.14   **Benign neoplasm of peripheral nerves and autonomic nervous system of thorax**

     D36.15   **Benign neoplasm of peripheral nerves and autonomic nervous system of abdomen**

     D36.16   **Benign neoplasm of peripheral nerves and autonomic nervous system of pelvis**

     D36.17   **Benign neoplasm of peripheral nerves and autonomic nervous system of trunk, unspecified**

D36.7   **Benign neoplasm of other specified sites**

     ▶Benign neoplasm of back NOS◄

     Benign neoplasm of nose NOS

D36.9   **Benign neoplasm, unspecified site**

Benign neuroendocrine tumors (D3A)

✓4ᵗʰ **D3A**   **Benign neuroendocrine tumors**

     Code also any associated multiple endocrine neoplasia [MEN] syndromes (E31.2-)

     Use additional code to identify any associated endocrine syndrome, such as:

     carcinoid syndrome (E34.0)

     EXCLUDES 2   benign pancreatic islet cell tumors (D13.7)

✓5ᵗʰ D3A.0   **Benign carcinoid tumors**

     D3A.00   **Benign carcinoid tumor of unspecified site**

           Carcinoid tumor NOS

     ✓6ᵗʰ D3A.01   **Benign carcinoid tumors of the small intestine**

         D3A.010   **Benign carcinoid tumor of the duodenum**

         D3A.011   **Benign carcinoid tumor of the jejunum**

         D3A.012   **Benign carcinoid tumor of the ileum**

         D3A.019   **Benign carcinoid tumor of the small intestine, unspecified portion**

     ✓6ᵗʰ D3A.02   **Benign carcinoid tumors of the appendix, large intestine, and rectum**

         D3A.020   **Benign carcinoid tumor of the appendix**

         D3A.021   **Benign carcinoid tumor of the cecum**

         D3A.022   **Benign carcinoid tumor of the ascending colon**

         D3A.023   **Benign carcinoid tumor of the transverse colon**

         D3A.024   **Benign carcinoid tumor of the descending colon**

         D3A.025   **Benign carcinoid tumor of the sigmoid colon**

         D3A.026   **Benign carcinoid tumor of the rectum**

         D3A.029   **Benign carcinoid tumor of the large intestine, unspecified portion**

           Benign carcinoid tumor of the colon NOS

     ✓6ᵗʰ D3A.09   **Benign carcinoid tumors of other sites**

         D3A.090   **Benign carcinoid tumor of the bronchus and lung**

         D3A.091   **Benign carcinoid tumor of the thymus**

         D3A.092   **Benign carcinoid tumor of the stomach**

         D3A.093   **Benign carcinoid tumor of the kidney**

         D3A.094   **Benign carcinoid tumor of the foregut, unspecified**

         D3A.095   **Benign carcinoid tumor of the midgut, unspecified**

         D3A.096   **Benign carcinoid tumor of the hindgut, unspecified**

         D3A.098   **Benign carcinoid tumors of other sites**

D3A.8   **Other benign neuroendocrine tumors**

     Neuroendocrine tumor NOS

✔ Additional Character Required   ✓x7ᵗʰ Placeholder   Unacceptable PDx   Questionable PDx   Manifestation   Unspecified Dx   H1-H1d HAC   HCC CMS-HCC Dx   HIV HIV Dx

ICD-10-CM 2020   **497**

Chapter 2. Neoplasms (side margin)
D37–D41.1Ø (side margin)

Neoplasms of uncertain behavior, polycythemia vera and myelodysplastic syndromes (D37-D48)

NOTE Categories D37-D44, and D48 classify by site neoplasms of uncertain behavior, i.e., histologic confirmation whether the neoplasm is malignant or benign cannot be made.

EXCLUDES 1 neoplasms of unspecified behavior (D49.-)

√4ᵗʰ **D37 Neoplasm of uncertain behavior of** oral cavity and digestive organs

EXCLUDES 1 stromal tumors of uncertain behavior of digestive system (D48.1)

√5ᵗʰ **D37.Ø Neoplasm of uncertain behavior of** lip, oral cavity and pharynx

EXCLUDES 1 neoplasm of uncertain behavior of aryepiglottic fold or interarytenoid fold, laryngeal aspect (D38.Ø)
neoplasm of uncertain behavior of epiglottis NOS (D38.Ø)
neoplasm of uncertain behavior of skin of lip (D48.5)
neoplasm of uncertain behavior of suprahyoid portion of epiglottis (D38.Ø)

D37.Ø1 Neoplasm of uncertain behavior of lip
Neoplasm of uncertain behavior of vermilion border of lip

D37.Ø2 Neoplasm of uncertain behavior of tongue

√6ᵗʰ **D37.Ø3 Neoplasm of uncertain behavior of the** major salivary glands

D37.Ø3Ø Neoplasm of uncertain behavior of the parotid salivary glands

D37.Ø31 Neoplasm of uncertain behavior of the sublingual salivary glands

D37.Ø32 Neoplasm of uncertain behavior of the submandibular salivary glands

D37.Ø39 Neoplasm of uncertain behavior of the major salivary glands, unspecified

D37.Ø4 Neoplasm of uncertain behavior of the minor salivary glands
Neoplasm of uncertain behavior of submucosal salivary glands of lip
Neoplasm of uncertain behavior of submucosal salivary glands of cheek
Neoplasm of uncertain behavior of submucosal salivary glands of hard palate
Neoplasm of uncertain behavior of submucosal salivary glands of soft palate

D37.Ø5 Neoplasm of uncertain behavior of pharynx
Neoplasm of uncertain behavior of aryepiglottic fold of pharynx NOS
Neoplasm of uncertain behavior of hypopharyngeal aspect of aryepiglottic fold of pharynx
Neoplasm of uncertain behavior of marginal zone of aryepiglottic fold of pharynx

D37.Ø9 Neoplasm of uncertain behavior of other specified sites of the oral cavity

D37.1 Neoplasm of uncertain behavior of stomach

D37.2 Neoplasm of uncertain behavior of small intestine

D37.3 Neoplasm of uncertain behavior of appendix

D37.4 Neoplasm of uncertain behavior of colon

D37.5 Neoplasm of uncertain behavior of rectum
Neoplasm of uncertain behavior of rectosigmoid junction

D37.6 Neoplasm of uncertain behavior of liver, gallbladder and bile ducts
Neoplasm of uncertain behavior of ampulla of Vater

D37.8 Neoplasm of uncertain behavior of other specified digestive organs
Neoplasm of uncertain behavior of anal canal
Neoplasm of uncertain behavior of anal sphincter
Neoplasm of uncertain behavior of anus NOS
Neoplasm of uncertain behavior of esophagus
Neoplasm of uncertain behavior of intestine NOS
Neoplasm of uncertain behavior of pancreas

EXCLUDES 1 neoplasm of uncertain behavior of anal margin (D48.5)
neoplasm of uncertain behavior of anal skin (D48.5)
neoplasm of uncertain behavior of perianal skin (D48.5)

D37.9 Neoplasm of uncertain behavior of digestive organ, unspecified

√4ᵗʰ **D38 Neoplasm of uncertain behavior of** middle ear and respiratory and intrathoracic organs

EXCLUDES 1 neoplasm of uncertain behavior of heart (D48.7)

D38.Ø Neoplasm of uncertain behavior of larynx
Neoplasm of uncertain behavior of aryepiglottic fold or interarytenoid fold, laryngeal aspect
Neoplasm of uncertain behavior of epiglottis (suprahyoid portion)

EXCLUDES 1 neoplasm of uncertain behavior of aryepiglottic fold or interarytenoid fold NOS (D37.Ø5)
neoplasm of uncertain behavior of hypopharyngeal aspect of aryepiglottic fold (D37.Ø5)
neoplasm of uncertain behavior of marginal zone of aryepiglottic fold (D37.Ø5)

D38.1 Neoplasm of uncertain behavior of trachea, bronchus and lung

D38.2 Neoplasm of uncertain behavior of pleura

D38.3 Neoplasm of uncertain behavior of mediastinum

D38.4 Neoplasm of uncertain behavior of thymus

D38.5 Neoplasm of uncertain behavior of other respiratory organs
Neoplasm of uncertain behavior of accessory sinuses
Neoplasm of uncertain behavior of cartilage of nose
Neoplasm of uncertain behavior of middle ear
Neoplasm of uncertain behavior of nasal cavities

EXCLUDES 1 neoplasm of uncertain behavior of ear (external) (skin) (D48.5)
neoplasm of uncertain behavior of nose NOS (D48.7)
neoplasm of uncertain behavior of skin of nose (D48.5)

D38.6 Neoplasm of uncertain behavior of respiratory organ, unspecified

√4ᵗʰ **D39 Neoplasm of uncertain behavior of** female genital organs

D39.Ø Neoplasm of uncertain behavior of uterus ♀

√5ᵗʰ **D39.1 Neoplasm of uncertain behavior of** ovary
Use additional code to identify any functional activity

D39.1Ø Neoplasm of uncertain behavior of unspecified ovary ♀

D39.11 Neoplasm of uncertain behavior of right ovary ♀

D39.12 Neoplasm of uncertain behavior of left ovary ♀

D39.2 Neoplasm of uncertain behavior of placenta Ⓜ ♀
Chorioadenoma destruens
Invasive hydatidiform mole
Malignant hydatidiform mole

EXCLUDES 1 hydatidiform mole NOS (OØ1.9)

D39.8 Neoplasm of uncertain behavior of other specified female genital organs ♀
Neoplasm of uncertain behavior of skin of female genital organs

D39.9 Neoplasm of uncertain behavior of female genital organ, unspecified ♀

√4ᵗʰ **D4Ø Neoplasm of uncertain behavior of** male genital organs

D4Ø.Ø Neoplasm of uncertain behavior of prostate ♂

√5ᵗʰ **D4Ø.1 Neoplasm of uncertain behavior of** testis

D4Ø.1Ø Neoplasm of uncertain behavior of unspecified testis ♂

D4Ø.11 Neoplasm of uncertain behavior of right testis ♂

D4Ø.12 Neoplasm of uncertain behavior of left testis ♂

D4Ø.8 Neoplasm of uncertain behavior of other specified male genital organs ♂
Neoplasm of uncertain behavior of skin of male genital organs

D4Ø.9 Neoplasm of uncertain behavior of male genital organ, unspecified ♂

√4ᵗʰ **D41 Neoplasm of uncertain behavior of** urinary organs

√5ᵗʰ **D41.Ø Neoplasm of uncertain behavior of** kidney

EXCLUDES 1 neoplasm of uncertain behavior of renal pelvis (D41.1-)

D41.ØØ Neoplasm of uncertain behavior of unspecified kidney

D41.Ø1 Neoplasm of uncertain behavior of right kidney

D41.Ø2 Neoplasm of uncertain behavior of left kidney

√5ᵗʰ **D41.1 Neoplasm of uncertain behavior of** renal pelvis

D41.1Ø Neoplasm of uncertain behavior of unspecified renal pelvis

D41.11　Neoplasm of uncertain behavior of right renal pelvis
D41.12　Neoplasm of uncertain behavior of left renal pelvis
√5ᵗʰ **D41.2**　**Neoplasm of uncertain behavior of** ureter
    D41.2Ø　**Neoplasm of uncertain behavior of unspecified ureter**
    D41.21　Neoplasm of uncertain behavior of right ureter
    D41.22　Neoplasm of uncertain behavior of left ureter
D41.3　Neoplasm of uncertain behavior of urethra
D41.4　Neoplasm of uncertain behavior of bladder
D41.8　Neoplasm of uncertain behavior of other specified urinary organs
D41.9　Neoplasm of uncertain behavior of unspecified urinary organ

√4ᵗʰ **D42**　**Neoplasm of uncertain behavior of** meninges
    D42.Ø　**Neoplasm of uncertain behavior of** cerebral meninges　HCC
    D42.1　**Neoplasm of uncertain behavior of** spinal meninges　HCC
    D42.9　**Neoplasm of uncertain behavior of meninges, unspecified**　HCC

√4ᵗʰ **D43**　**Neoplasm of uncertain behavior of** brain and central nervous system
    EXCLUDES 1　*neoplasm of uncertain behavior of peripheral nerves and autonomic nervous system (D48.2)*
    D43.Ø　**Neoplasm of uncertain behavior of** brain, supratentorial　HCC
        Neoplasm of uncertain behavior of cerebral ventricle
        Neoplasm of uncertain behavior of cerebrum
        Neoplasm of uncertain behavior of frontal lobe
        Neoplasm of uncertain behavior of occipital lobe
        Neoplasm of uncertain behavior of parietal lobe
        Neoplasm of uncertain behavior of temporal lobe
        EXCLUDES 1　*neoplasm of uncertain behavior of fourth ventricle (D43.1)*
    D43.1　**Neoplasm of uncertain behavior of** brain, infratentorial　HCC
        Neoplasm of uncertain behavior of brain stem
        Neoplasm of uncertain behavior of cerebellum
        Neoplasm of uncertain behavior of fourth ventricle
    D43.2　**Neoplasm of uncertain behavior of** brain, unspecified　HCC
    D43.3　**Neoplasm of uncertain behavior of** cranial nerves　HCC
    D43.4　**Neoplasm of uncertain behavior of** spinal cord　HCC
    D43.8　**Neoplasm of uncertain behavior of other** specified parts of central nervous system　HCC
    D43.9　**Neoplasm of uncertain behavior of central nervous system, unspecified**　HCC
        Neoplasm of uncertain behavior of nervous system (central) NOS

√4ᵗʰ **D44**　**Neoplasm of uncertain behavior of** endocrine glands
    EXCLUDES 1　*multiple endocrine adenomatosis (E31.2-)*
        multiple endocrine neoplasia (E31.2-)
        neoplasm of uncertain behavior of endocrine pancreas (D37.8)
        neoplasm of uncertain behavior of ovary (D39.1-)
        neoplasm of uncertain behavior of testis (D40.1-)
        neoplasm of uncertain behavior of thymus (D38.4)
    D44.Ø　**Neoplasm of uncertain behavior of** thyroid gland
√5ᵗʰ **D44.1**　**Neoplasm of uncertain behavior of** adrenal gland
        Use additional code to identify any functional activity
        D44.1Ø　**Neoplasm of uncertain behavior of unspecified adrenal gland**
        D44.11　**Neoplasm of uncertain behavior of** right **adrenal gland**
        D44.12　**Neoplasm of uncertain behavior of** left **adrenal gland**
    D44.2　**Neoplasm of uncertain behavior of** parathyroid gland
    D44.3　**Neoplasm of uncertain behavior of** pituitary gland　HCC
        Use additional code to identify any functional activity
    D44.4　**Neoplasm of uncertain behavior of craniopharyngeal duct**　HCC
    D44.5　**Neoplasm of uncertain behavior of** pineal gland　HCC
    D44.6　**Neoplasm of uncertain behavior of** carotid body　HCC
    D44.7　**Neoplasm of uncertain behavior of** aortic body and other paraganglia　HCC
        AHA: 2016,4Q,26
    D44.9　**Neoplasm of uncertain behavior of unspecified endocrine gland**

D45　**Polycythemia vera**　HCC
    EXCLUDES 1　*familial polycythemia (D75.Ø)*
        secondary polycythemia (D75.1)
    DEF: Abnormal proliferation of all bone marrow elements, increased red cell mass, and total blood volume. The etiology is unknown, but it is frequently associated with splenomegaly, leukocytosis, and thrombocythemia.

√4ᵗʰ **D46**　**Myelodysplastic syndromes**
    Use additional code for adverse effect, if applicable, to identify drug (T36-T5Ø with fifth or sixth character 5)
    EXCLUDES 2　*drug-induced aplastic anemia (D61.1)*
    D46.Ø　**Refractory anemia** without ring sideroblasts, **so stated**　HCC
        Refractory anemia without sideroblasts, without excess of blasts
    D46.1　**Refractory anemia** with ring sideroblasts　HCC
        RARS
√5ᵗʰ **D46.2**　**Refractory anemia** with excess of blasts [RAEB]
        D46.2Ø　**Refractory anemia with excess of blasts, unspecified**　HCC
            RAEB NOS
        D46.21　**Refractory anemia with excess of** blasts 1　HCC
            RAEB 1
        D46.22　**Refractory anemia with excess of** blasts 2　HCC
            RAEB 2
    D46.A　**Refractory** cytopenia with multilineage dysplasia　HCC
    D46.B　**Refractory** cytopenia with multilineage dysplasia and ring sideroblasts　HCC
        RCMD RS
    D46.C　**Myelodysplastic syndrome** with isolated del(5q) chromosomal abnormality　HCC
        Myelodysplastic syndrome with 5q deletion
        5q minus syndrome NOS
    D46.4　**Refractory anemia, unspecified**　HCC
    D46.Z　**Other myelodysplastic syndromes**　HCC
        EXCLUDES 1　*chronic myelomonocytic leukemia (C93.1-)*
    D46.9　**Myelodysplastic syndrome, unspecified**　HCC
        Myelodysplasia NOS

√4ᵗʰ **D47**　**Other neoplasms of uncertain behavior of** lymphoid, hematopoietic and related tissue
√5ᵗʰ **D47.Ø**　**Mast cell neoplasms of uncertain behavior**
        EXCLUDES 1　*congenital cutaneous mastocytosis (Q82.2)*
            histiocytic neoplasms of uncertain behavior (D47.Z9)
            malignant mast cell neoplasm (C96.2-)
        AHA: 2017,4Q,5
        D47.Ø1　Cutaneous **mastocytosis**
            Diffuse cutaneous mastocytosis
            Maculopapular cutaneous mastocytosis
            Solitary mastocytoma
            Telangiectasia macularis eruptiva perstans
            Urticaria pigmentosa
            EXCLUDES 1　*congenital (diffuse) (maculopapular) cutaneous mastocytosis (Q82.2)*
                congenital urticaria pigmentosa (Q82.2)
                extracutaneous mastocytoma (D47.Ø9)

D47.02 Systemic mastocytosis
Indolent systemic mastocytosis
Isolated bone marrow mastocytosis
Smoldering systemic mastocytosis
Systemic mastocytosis, with an associated
hematological non-mast cell lineage disease
(SM-AHNMD)
Code also, if applicable, any associated hematological
non-mast cell lineage disease, such as:
acute myeloid leukemia (C92.6-, C92.A-)
chronic myelomonocytic leukemia (C93.1-)
essential thrombocytosis (D47.3)
hypereosinophilic syndrome (D72.1)
myelodysplastic syndrome (D46.9)
myeloproliferative syndrome (D47.1)
non-Hodgkin lymphoma (C82-C85)
plasma cell myeloma (C90.0-)
polycythemia vera (D45)
EXCLUDES 1 *aggressive systemic mastocytosis (C96.21)*
mast cell leukemia (C94.3-)

D47.09 Other mast cell neoplasms of uncertain behavior
Extracutaneous mastocytoma
Mast cell tumor NOS
Mastocytoma NOS
Mastocytosis NOS

D47.1 Chronic myeloproliferative disease `HCC`
Chronic neutrophilic leukemia
Myeloproliferative disease, unspecified
EXCLUDES 1 *atypical chronic myeloid leukemia BCR/ABL-negative (C92.2-)*
chronic myeloid leukemia BCR/ABL-positive (C92.1-)
myelofibrosis NOS (D75.81)
myelophthisic anemia (D61.82)
myelophthisis (D61.82)
secondary myelofibrosis NOS (D75.81)

D47.2 Monoclonal gammopathy
Monoclonal gammopathy of undetermined significance [MGUS]

D47.3 Essential (hemorrhagic) thrombocythemia `HCC`
Essential thrombocytosis
Idiopathic hemorrhagic thrombocythemia
DEF: Chronic myeloproliferative neoplasm involving production of excess blood platelets that may result in abnormal clotting or hemorrhaging.

D47.4 Osteomyelofibrosis `HCC`
Chronic idiopathic myelofibrosis
Myelofibrosis (idiopathic) (with myeloid metaplasia)
Myelosclerosis (megakaryocytic) with myeloid metaplasia
Secondary myelofibrosis in myeloproliferative disease
EXCLUDES 1 *acute myelofibrosis (C94.4-)*

✓5ᵗʰ **D47.Z Other specified neoplasms of uncertain behavior of lymphoid, hematopoietic and related tissue**
AHA: 2016,4Q,8

D47.Z1 Post-transplant lymphoproliferative disorder (PTLD) `HCC`
Code first complications of transplanted organs and tissue (T86.-)
DEF: Excessive proliferation of B-cell lymphocytes following Epstein-Barr virus infection in organ transplant patients. It may progress to non-Hodgkin lymphoma.

D47.Z2 Castleman disease `HCC`
Code also if applicable human herpesvirus 8 infection (B10.89)
EXCLUDES 2 *Kaposi's sarcoma (C46-)*
DEF: Rare disease of the lymph nodes and lymphoid tissues that closely mimics lymphoma.

D47.Z9 Other specified neoplasms of uncertain `HCC`
behavior of lymphoid, hematopoietic and related tissue
Histiocytic tumors of uncertain behavior

D47.9 Neoplasm of uncertain behavior of lymphoid, `HCC`
hematopoietic and related tissue, unspecified
Lymphoproliferative disease NOS

✓4ᵗʰ **D48 Neoplasm of uncertain behavior of other and unspecified sites**
EXCLUDES 1 *neurofibromatosis (nonmalignant) (Q85.0-)*

D48.0 Neoplasm of uncertain behavior of bone and articular cartilage
EXCLUDES 1 *neoplasm of uncertain behavior of cartilage of ear (D48.1)*
neoplasm of uncertain behavior of cartilage of larynx (D38.0)
neoplasm of uncertain behavior of cartilage of nose (D38.5)
neoplasm of uncertain behavior of connective tissue of eyelid (D48.1)
neoplasm of uncertain behavior of synovia (D48.1)

D48.1 Neoplasm of uncertain behavior of connective and other soft tissue
Neoplasm of uncertain behavior of connective tissue of ear
Neoplasm of uncertain behavior of connective tissue of eyelid
Stromal tumors of uncertain behavior of digestive system
EXCLUDES 1 *neoplasm of uncertain behavior of articular cartilage (D48.0)*
neoplasm of uncertain behavior of cartilage of larynx (D38.0)
neoplasm of uncertain behavior of cartilage of nose (D38.5)
neoplasm of uncertain behavior of connective tissue of breast (D48.6-)

D48.2 Neoplasm of uncertain behavior of peripheral nerves and autonomic nervous system
EXCLUDES 1 *neoplasm of uncertain behavior of peripheral nerves of orbit (D48.7)*

D48.3 Neoplasm of uncertain behavior of retroperitoneum

D48.4 Neoplasm of uncertain behavior of peritoneum

D48.5 Neoplasm of uncertain behavior of skin
Neoplasm of uncertain behavior of anal margin
Neoplasm of uncertain behavior of anal skin
Neoplasm of uncertain behavior of perianal skin
Neoplasm of uncertain behavior of skin of breast
EXCLUDES 1 *neoplasm of uncertain behavior of anus NOS (D37.8)*
neoplasm of uncertain behavior of skin of genital organs (D39.8, D40.8)
neoplasm of uncertain behavior of vermilion border of lip (D37.0)

✓5ᵗʰ **D48.6 Neoplasm of uncertain behavior of breast**
Neoplasm of uncertain behavior of connective tissue of breast
Cystosarcoma phyllodes
EXCLUDES 1 *neoplasm of uncertain behavior of skin of breast (D48.5)*

D48.60 Neoplasm of uncertain behavior of unspecified breast
D48.61 Neoplasm of uncertain behavior of right breast
D48.62 Neoplasm of uncertain behavior of left breast

D48.7 Neoplasm of uncertain behavior of other specified sites
Neoplasm of uncertain behavior of eye
Neoplasm of uncertain behavior of heart
Neoplasm of uncertain behavior of peripheral nerves of orbit
EXCLUDES 1 *neoplasm of uncertain behavior of connective tissue (D48.1)*
neoplasm of uncertain behavior of skin of eyelid (D48.5)

D48.9 Neoplasm of uncertain behavior, unspecified

Neoplasms of unspecified behavior (D49)

✓4th D49   Neoplasms of unspecified behavior

NOTE   Category D49 classifies by site neoplasms of unspecified morphology and behavior. The term "mass", unless otherwise stated, is not to be regarded as a neoplastic growth.

INCLUDES   "growth" NOS
neoplasm NOS
new growth NOS
tumor NOS

EXCLUDES 1   neoplasms of uncertain behavior (D37-D44, D48)

D49.0   Neoplasm of unspecified behavior of digestive system

EXCLUDES 1   neoplasm of unspecified behavior of margin of anus (D49.2)
neoplasm of unspecified behavior of perianal skin (D49.2)
neoplasm of unspecified behavior of skin of anus (D49.2)

D49.1   Neoplasm of unspecified behavior of respiratory system

D49.2   Neoplasm of unspecified behavior of bone, soft tissue, and skin

EXCLUDES 1   neoplasm of unspecified behavior of anal canal (D49.0)
neoplasm of unspecified behavior of anus NOS (D49.0)
neoplasm of unspecified behavior of bone marrow (D49.89)
neoplasm of unspecified behavior of cartilage of larynx (D49.1)
neoplasm of unspecified behavior of cartilage of nose (D49.1)
neoplasm of unspecified behavior of connective tissue of breast (D49.3)
neoplasm of unspecified behavior of skin of genital organs (D49.59)
neoplasm of unspecified behavior of vermilion border of lip (D49.0)

D49.3   Neoplasm of unspecified behavior of breast

EXCLUDES 1   neoplasm of unspecified behavior of skin of breast (D49.2)

D49.4   Neoplasm of unspecified behavior of bladder

✓5th D49.5   Neoplasm of unspecified behavior of other genitourinary organs

AHA: 2016,4Q,9

✓6th D49.51   Neoplasm of unspecified behavior of kidney

D49.511   Neoplasm of unspecified behavior of right kidney

D49.512   Neoplasm of unspecified behavior of left kidney

D49.519   Neoplasm of unspecified behavior of unspecified kidney

D49.59   Neoplasm of unspecified behavior of other genitourinary organ

D49.6   Neoplasm of unspecified behavior of brain   **HCC**

EXCLUDES 1   neoplasm of unspecified behavior of cerebral meninges (D49.7)
neoplasm of unspecified behavior of cranial nerves (D49.7)

D49.7   Neoplasm of unspecified behavior of endocrine glands and other parts of nervous system

EXCLUDES 1   neoplasm of unspecified behavior of peripheral, sympathetic, and parasympathetic nerves and ganglia (D49.2)

✓5th D49.8   Neoplasm of unspecified behavior of other specified sites

EXCLUDES 1   neoplasm of unspecified behavior of eyelid (skin) (D49.2)
neoplasm of unspecified behavior of eyelid cartilage (D49.2)
neoplasm of unspecified behavior of great vessels (D49.2)
neoplasm of unspecified behavior of optic nerve (D49.7)

D49.81   Neoplasm of unspecified behavior of retina and choroid
Dark area on retina
Retinal freckle

D49.89   Neoplasm of unspecified behavior of other specified sites

D49.9   Neoplasm of unspecified behavior of unspecified site

✔ Additional Character Required   ✓x7th Placeholder   Unacceptable PDx   Questionable PDx   Manifestation   Unspecified Dx   H1-H14 HAC   HCC CMS-HCC Dx   HIV HIV Dx
ICD-10-CM 2020   501

D49–D49.9

Chapter 3. Diseases of the Blood and Blood-forming Organs and Certain Disorders Involving the Immune Mechanism (D5Ø–D89)

Chapter-specific Guidelines with Coding Examples
Reserved for future guideline expansion

Chapter 3. Diseases of the Blood and Blood-forming Organs

Chapter 3. Diseases of the Blood and Blood-forming Organs and Certain Disorders Involving the Immune Mechanism (D50-D89)

EXCLUDES 2   autoimmune disease (systemic) NOS (M35.9)
certain conditions originating in the perinatal period (P00-P96)
complications of pregnancy, childbirth and the puerperium (O00-O9A)
congenital malformations, deformations and chromosomal abnormalities (Q00-Q99)
endocrine, nutritional and metabolic diseases (E00-E88)
human immunodeficiency virus [HIV] disease (B20)
injury, poisoning and certain other consequences of external causes (S00-T88)
neoplasms (C00-D49)
symptoms, signs and abnormal clinical and laboratory findings, not elsewhere classified (R00-R94)

This chapter contains the following blocks:

D50-D53   Nutritional anemias
D55-D59   Hemolytic anemias
D60-D64   Aplastic and other anemias and other bone marrow failure syndromes
D65-D69   Coagulation defects, purpura and other hemorrhagic conditions
D70-D77   Other disorders of blood and blood-forming organs
D78   Intraoperative and postprocedural complications of the spleen
D80-D89   Certain disorders involving the immune mechanism

Nutritional anemias (D50-D53)

DEF: Nutritional anemia: The result of inadequate intake or absorption of a vitamin or mineral that impacts the production of red blood cells or causes them to develop abnormally affecting the size and shape.

TIP: Documentation must identify a link between anemia and the nutritional deficiency; low levels of a particular nutrient may occur concurrently with anemia but not cause the anemia.

✓4ᵗʰ D50   Iron deficiency anemia

INCLUDES   asiderotic anemia
hypochromic anemia

D50.0   Iron deficiency anemia secondary to blood loss (chronic)
Posthemorrhagic anemia (chronic)
EXCLUDES 1   acute posthemorrhagic anemia (D62)
congenital anemia from fetal blood loss (P61.3)

D50.1   Sideropenic dysphagia
Kelly-Paterson syndrome
Plummer-Vinson syndrome

D50.8   Other iron deficiency anemias
Iron deficiency anemia due to inadequate dietary iron intake

D50.9   Iron deficiency anemia, unspecified

✓4ᵗʰ D51   Vitamin B12 deficiency anemia

EXCLUDES 1   vitamin B12 deficiency (E53.8)

D51.0   Vitamin B12 deficiency anemia due to intrinsic factor deficiency
Addison anemia
Biermer anemia
Pernicious (congenital) anemia
Congenital intrinsic factor deficiency
DEF: Chronic progressive anemia due to vitamin B12 malabsorption, caused by lack of secretion of intrinsic factor, which is produced by the gastric mucosa of the stomach.

D51.1   Vitamin B12 deficiency anemia due to selective vitamin B12 malabsorption with proteinuria
Imerslund (Gräsbeck) syndrome
Megaloblastic hereditary anemia

D51.2   Transcobalamin II deficiency

D51.3   Other dietary vitamin B12 deficiency anemia
Vegan anemia

D51.8   Other vitamin B12 deficiency anemias

D51.9   Vitamin B12 deficiency anemia, unspecified

✓4ᵗʰ D52   Folate deficiency anemia

EXCLUDES 1   folate deficiency without anemia (E53.8)

DEF: Deficiency in a B complex vitamin needed for the production of healthy red blood cells. Lack of folate, or folic acid, and other absorption conditions can cause anemia resulting in large, misshapen red blood cells called megaloblasts.

D52.0   Dietary folate deficiency anemia
Nutritional megaloblastic anemia
DEF: Result of a poor diet with inadequate intake of folate, which is needed to produce healthy red blood cells.

D52.1   Drug-induced folate deficiency anemia
Use additional code for adverse effect, if applicable, to identify drug (T36-T50 with fifth or sixth character 5)

D52.8   Other folate deficiency anemias

D52.9   Folate deficiency anemia, unspecified
Folic acid deficiency anemia NOS

✓4ᵗʰ D53   Other nutritional anemias

INCLUDES   megaloblastic anemia unresponsive to vitamin B12 or folate therapy

D53.0   Protein deficiency anemia
Amino-acid deficiency anemia
Orotaciduric anemia
EXCLUDES 1   Lesch-Nyhan syndrome (E79.1)

D53.1   Other megaloblastic anemias, not elsewhere classified
Megaloblastic anemia NOS
EXCLUDES 1   Di Guglielmo's disease (C94.0)

D53.2   Scorbutic anemia
EXCLUDES 1   scurvy (E54)

D53.8   Other specified nutritional anemias
Anemia associated with deficiency of copper
Anemia associated with deficiency of molybdenum
Anemia associated with deficiency of zinc
EXCLUDES 1   nutritional deficiencies without anemia, such as:
copper deficiency NOS (E61.0)
molybdenum deficiency NOS (E61.5)
zinc deficiency NOS (E60)

D53.9   Nutritional anemia, unspecified
Simple chronic anemia
EXCLUDES 1   anemia NOS (D64.9)
AHA: 2018,4Q,88

Hemolytic anemias (D55-D59)

✓4ᵗʰ D55   Anemia due to enzyme disorders

EXCLUDES 1   drug-induced enzyme deficiency anemia (D59.2)

D55.0   Anemia due to glucose-6-phosphate dehydrogenase [G6PD] deficiency   HCC
Favism
G6PD deficiency anemia
EXCLUDES 1   ▶glucose-6-phosphate dehydrogenase (G6PD) deficiency without anemia (D75.A)◀

D55.1   Anemia due to other disorders of glutathione metabolism   HCC
Anemia (due to) enzyme deficiencies, except G6PD, related to the hexose monophosphate [HMP] shunt pathway
Anemia (due to) hemolytic nonspherocytic (hereditary), type I

D55.2   Anemia due to disorders of glycolytic enzymes   HCC
Hemolytic nonspherocytic (hereditary) anemia, type II
Hexokinase deficiency anemia
Pyruvate kinase [PK] deficiency anemia
Triose-phosphate isomerase deficiency anemia
EXCLUDES 1   disorders of glycolysis not associated with anemia (E74.8)

D55.3   Anemia due to disorders of nucleotide metabolism   HCC

D55.8   Other anemias due to enzyme disorders   HCC

D55.9   Anemia due to enzyme disorder, unspecified   HCC

✔4ᵗʰ **D56 Thalassemia**

> EXCLUDES 1   *sickle-cell thalassemia (D57.4-)*

> **DEF:** Group of inherited disorders of hemoglobin metabolism causing mild to severe anemia. It is usually found in people of Mediterranean, African, Chinese, or Asian descent.

Thalassemia

Misshapen RBC

Misshapen RBC

Healthy RBC

D56.0 Alpha thalassemia   HCC

   Alpha thalassemia major
   Hemoglobin H Constant Spring
   Hemoglobin H disease
   Hydrops fetalis due to alpha thalassemia
   Severe alpha thalassemia
   Triple gene defect alpha thalassemia
   Use additional code, if applicable, for hydrops fetalis due to alpha thalassemia (P56.99)

> EXCLUDES 1   *alpha thalassemia trait or minor (D56.3)*
> *asymptomatic alpha thalassemia (D56.3)*
> *hydrops fetalis due to isoimmunization (P56.0)*
> *hydrops fetalis not due to immune hemolysis (P83.2)*

> **DEF:** HBA1 and HBA2 genetic variant of chromosome 16 prevalent among those of African and Southeast Asian descent. Alpha thalassemia is associated with a wide spectrum of anemic presentation and includes hemoglobin H disease subtypes.

D56.1 Beta thalassemia   HCC

   Beta thalassemia major
   Cooley's anemia
   Homozygous beta thalassemia
   Severe beta thalassemia
   Thalassemia intermedia
   Thalassemia major

> EXCLUDES 1   *beta thalassemia minor (D56.3)*
> *beta thalassemia trait (D56.3)*
> *delta-beta thalassemia (D56.2)*
> *hemoglobin E-beta thalassemia (D56.5)*
> *sickle-cell beta thalassemia (D57.4-)*

D56.2 Delta-beta thalassemia   HCC

   Homozygous delta-beta thalassemia

> EXCLUDES 1   *delta-beta thalassemia minor (D56.3)*
> *delta-beta thalassemia trait (D56.3)*

D56.3 Thalassemia minor

   Alpha thalassemia minor
   Alpha thalassemia silent carrier
   Alpha thalassemia trait
   Beta thalassemia minor
   Beta thalassemia trait
   Delta-beta thalassemia minor
   Delta-beta thalassemia trait
   Thalassemia trait NOS

> EXCLUDES 1   *alpha thalassemia (D56.0)*
> *beta thalassemia (D56.1)*
> *delta-beta thalassemia (D56.2)*
> *hemoglobin E-beta thalassemia (D56.5)*
> *sickle-cell trait (D57.3)*

> **DEF:** Solitary abnormal gene that identifies a carrier of the disease, yet with an absence of symptoms or a clinically mild anemic presentation.

D56.4 Hereditary persistence of fetal hemoglobin [HPFH]   HCC

D56.5 Hemoglobin E-beta thalassemia   HCC

> EXCLUDES 1   *beta thalassemia (D56.1)*
> *beta thalassemia minor (D56.3)*
> *beta thalassemia trait (D56.3)*
> *delta-beta thalassemia (D56.2)*
> *delta-beta thalassemia trait (D56.3)*
> *hemoglobin E disease (D58.2)*
> *other hemoglobinopathies (D58.2)*
> *sickle-cell beta thalassemia (D57.4-)*

D56.8 Other thalassemias   HCC

   Dominant thalassemia
   Hemoglobin C thalassemia
   Mixed thalassemia
   Thalassemia with other hemoglobinopathy

> EXCLUDES 1   *hemoglobin C disease (D58.2)*
> *hemoglobin E disease (D58.2)*
> *other hemoglobinopathies (D58.2)*
> *sickle-cell anemia (D57.-)*
> *sickle-cell thalassemia (D57.4)*

D56.9 Thalassemia, unspecified

   Mediterranean anemia (with other hemoglobinopathy)

✔4ᵗʰ **D57 Sickle-cell disorders**

   Use additional code for any associated fever (R50.81)

> EXCLUDES 1   *other hemoglobinopathies (D58.-)*

> **DEF:** Severe, chronic inherited diseases caused by a genetic variation in hemoglobin protein of the red blood cell. The gene mutation causes the red blood cell to become hard, sticky, and crescent or sickle shaped making it harder for red blood cells to travel through the bloodstream disrupting blood flow and decreasing oxygen transport to tissues.

Sickle cell

Sickle cells

Normal RBCs

✔5ᵗʰ **D57.0 Hb-SS disease with crisis**

   Sickle-cell disease NOS with crisis
   Hb-SS disease with vasoocclusive pain

   D57.00 Hb-SS disease with crisis, unspecified   HCC

   D57.01 Hb-SS disease with acute chest syndrome   HCC

   D57.02 Hb-SS disease with splenic sequestration   HCC

✔ Additional Character Required   ✔x7ᵗʰ Placeholder   Unacceptable PDx   Questionable PDx   Manifestation   Unspecified Dx   H1-H14 HAC   HCC CMS-HCC Dx   HIV HIV Dx

ICD-10-CM 2020

505

D56–D57.02

Chapter 3. Diseases of the Blood and Blood-forming Organs

D57.1 Sickle-cell disease without crisis   `HCC`
Hb-SS disease without crisis
Sickle-cell anemia NOS
Sickle-cell disease NOS
Sickle-cell disorder NOS

✓5ᵗʰ **D57.2 Sickle-cell/Hb-C disease**
Hb-SC disease
Hb-S/Hb-C disease

    D57.20 Sickle-cell/Hb-C disease without crisis   `HCC`

    ✓6ᵗʰ **D57.21 Sickle-cell/Hb-C disease with crisis**

        D57.211 Sickle-cell/Hb-C disease with acute chest syndrome   `HCC`

        D57.212 Sickle-cell/Hb-C disease with splenic sequestration   `MCC` `HCC`
          CC Excl: PDX collection 496

        D57.219 Sickle-cell/Hb-C disease with crisis, unspecified   `HCC`
          Sickle-cell/Hb-C disease with crisis NOS

D57.3 Sickle-cell trait   `HCC`
Hb-S trait
Heterozygous hemoglobin S
DEF: Heterozygous genetic makeup characterized by one gene for normal hemoglobin and one for sickle-cell hemoglobin. The clinical disease is rarely present.

✓5ᵗʰ **D57.4 Sickle-cell thalassemia**
Sickle-cell beta thalassemia
Thalassemia Hb-S disease

    D57.40 Sickle-cell thalassemia without crisis   `HCC`
      Microdrepanocytosis
      Sickle-cell thalassemia NOS

    ✓6ᵗʰ **D57.41 Sickle-cell thalassemia with crisis**
      Sickle-cell thalassemia with vasoocclusive pain

        D57.411 Sickle-cell thalassemia with acute chest syndrome   `HCC`

        D57.412 Sickle-cell thalassemia with splenic sequestration   `MCC` `HCC`
          CC Excl: PDX collection 496

        D57.419 Sickle-cell thalassemia with crisis, unspecified   `HCC`
          Sickle-cell thalassemia with crisis NOS

✓5ᵗʰ **D57.8 Other sickle-cell disorders**
Hb-SD disease
Hb-SE disease

    D57.80 Other sickle-cell disorders without crisis   `HCC`

    ✓6ᵗʰ **D57.81 Other sickle-cell disorders with crisis**

        D57.811 Other sickle-cell disorders with acute chest syndrome   `HCC`

        D57.812 Other sickle-cell disorders with splenic sequestration   `HCC`

        D57.819 Other sickle-cell disorders with crisis, unspecified   `HCC`
          Other sickle-cell disorders with crisis NOS

✓4ᵗʰ **D58 Other hereditary hemolytic anemias**
    `EXCLUDES 1`   hemolytic anemia of the newborn (P55.-)

    D58.0 Hereditary spherocytosis   `HCC`
      Acholuric (familial) jaundice
      Congenital (spherocytic) hemolytic icterus
      Minkowski-Chauffard syndrome
      DEF: Inherited condition caused by mutations to genes responsible for the production of proteins that form the membranes of red blood cells. The shape and flexibility of the red blood cell membrane is altered diminishing the cells ability to traverse the spleen, therefore becoming trapped and destroyed before the red blood cell has reached maturity.

    D58.1 Hereditary elliptocytosis   `HCC`
      Elliptocytosis (congenital)
      Ovalocytosis (congenital) (hereditary)

D58.2 Other hemoglobinopathies   `HCC`
Abnormal hemoglobin NOS
Congenital Heinz body anemia
Hb-C disease
Hb-D disease
Hb-E disease
Hemoglobinopathy NOS
Unstable hemoglobin hemolytic disease
    `EXCLUDES 1`   familial polycythemia (D75.0)
          Hb-M disease (D74.0)
          hemoglobin E-beta thalassemia (D56.5)
          hereditary persistence of fetal hemoglobin [HPFH] (D56.4)
          high-altitude polycythemia (D75.1)
          methemoglobinemia (D74.-)
          other hemoglobinopathies with thalassemia (D56.8)

D58.8 Other specified hereditary hemolytic anemias   `HCC`
Stomatocytosis

D58.9 Hereditary hemolytic anemia, unspecified   `HCC`

✓4ᵗʰ **D59 Acquired hemolytic anemia**
DEF: Non-hereditary anemia characterized by premature destruction of red blood cells caused by infectious organisms, poisons, and physical agents.
CC Excl: For CC/MCC codes in category D59: PDX collection 496

    D59.0 Drug-induced autoimmune hemolytic anemia   `HCC`
      Use additional code for adverse effect, if applicable, to identify drug (T36-T50 with fifth or sixth character 5)

    D59.1 Other autoimmune hemolytic anemias   `HCC`
      Autoimmune hemolytic disease (cold type) (warm type)
      Chronic cold hemagglutinin disease
      Cold agglutinin disease
      Cold agglutinin hemoglobinuria
      Cold type (secondary) (symptomatic) hemolytic anemia
      Warm type (secondary) (symptomatic) hemolytic anemia
      `EXCLUDES 1`   Evans syndrome (D69.41)
          hemolytic disease of newborn (P55.-)
          paroxysmal cold hemoglobinuria (D59.6)

    D59.2 Drug-induced nonautoimmune hemolytic anemia   `HCC`
      Drug-induced enzyme deficiency anemia
      Use additional code for adverse effect, if applicable, to identify drug (T36-T50 with fifth or sixth character 5)

    D59.3 Hemolytic-uremic syndrome   `MCC` `HCC`
      Use additional code to identify associated:
        E. coli infection (B96.2-)
        Pneumococcal pneumonia (J13)
        Shigella dysenteriae (A03.9)
      DEF: Condition typically precipitated by infection causing low platelets and destruction of red blood cells resulting in hemolytic anemia. This cell damage and blockage of renal capillaries lead to kidney failure. Mainly affects children.

    D59.4 Other nonautoimmune hemolytic anemias   `CC` `HCC`
      Mechanical hemolytic anemia
      Microangiopathic hemolytic anemia
      Toxic hemolytic anemia

    D59.5 Paroxysmal nocturnal hemoglobinuria [Marchiafava-Micheli]   `HCC`
      `EXCLUDES 1`   hemoglobinuria NOS (R82.3)

    D59.6 Hemoglobinuria due to hemolysis from other external causes   `HCC`
      Hemoglobinuria from exertion
      March hemoglobinuria
      Paroxysmal cold hemoglobinuria
      Use additional code (Chapter 20) to identify external cause
      `EXCLUDES 1`   hemoglobinuria NOS (R82.3)

    D59.8 Other acquired hemolytic anemias   `HCC`

    D59.9 Acquired hemolytic anemia, unspecified   `CC` `HCC`
      Idiopathic hemolytic anemia, chronic

`N` Newborn: 0   `P` Pediatric: 0-17   `M` Maternity: 9-64   `A` Adult: 15-124   `MCC` Major Complication/Comorbidity   `CC` Complication/Comorbidity   `SW` Severe Wound Dx

506   ICD-10-CM 2020

Aplastic and other anemias and other bone marrow failure syndromes (D60-D64)

✓4ᵗʰ D60 Acquired pure red cell aplasia [erythroblastopenia]

> **INCLUDES**   red cell aplasia (acquired) (adult) (with thymoma)
>
> **EXCLUDES 1**   congenital red cell aplasia (D61.01)
>
> **DEF:** Bone marrow failure characterized by underproduction of red blood cells while white blood cell and platelet production remains normal.
>
> **CC Excl: For MCC codes in category D60:** PDX collection 496

    D60.0 Chronic acquired pure red cell aplasia   MCC HCC

    D60.1 Transient acquired pure red cell aplasia   MCC HCC

    D60.8 Other acquired pure red cell aplasias   MCC HCC

    D60.9 Acquired pure red cell aplasia, unspecified   MCC HCC

✓4ᵗʰ D61 Other aplastic anemias and other bone marrow failure syndromes

> **EXCLUDES 1**   neutropenia (D70.-)
>
> **AHA:** 2014,4Q,22
>
> **DEF:** Aplastic anemia: Bone marrow failure characterized by underproduction of red bloods cells, white blood cells and platelets.
>
> **CC Excl: For CC/MCC codes in category D61, unless otherwise noted:** PDX collection 496

    ✓5ᵗʰ D61.0 Constitutional aplastic anemia

       D61.01 Constitutional (pure) red blood cell aplasia   CC HCC

          Blackfan-Diamond syndrome

          Congenital (pure) red cell aplasia

          Familial hypoplastic anemia

          Primary (pure) red cell aplasia

          Red cell (pure) aplasia of infants

          EXCLUDES 1   acquired red cell aplasia (D60.9)

          CC Excl: PDX collection 498

       D61.09 Other constitutional aplastic anemia   CC HCC

          Fanconi's anemia

          Pancytopenia with malformations

          CC Excl: PDX collection 499

    D61.1 Drug-induced aplastic anemia   MCC HCC

       Use additional code for adverse effect, if applicable, to identify drug (T36-T50 with fifth or sixth character 5)

    D61.2 Aplastic anemia due to other external agents   MCC HCC

       Code first, if applicable, toxic effects of substances chiefly nonmedicinal as to source (T51-T65)

    D61.3 Idiopathic aplastic anemia   MCC HCC

    ✓5ᵗʰ D61.8 Other specified aplastic anemias and other bone marrow failure syndromes

       CC Excl: For CC codes in subcategory D61.8: PDX collection 500

       ✓6ᵗʰ D61.81 Pancytopenia

          EXCLUDES 1   pancytopenia (due to) (with) aplastic anemia (D61.9)

            pancytopenia (due to) (with) bone marrow infiltration (D61.82)

            pancytopenia (due to) (with) congenital (pure) red cell aplasia (D61.01)

            pancytopenia (due to) (with) hairy cell leukemia (C91.4-)

            pancytopenia (due to) (with) human immunodeficiency virus disease (B20)

            pancytopenia (due to) (with) leukoerythroblastic anemia (D61.82)

            pancytopenia (due to) (with) myeloproliferative disease (D47.1)

          EXCLUDES 2   pancytopenia (due to) (with) myelodysplastic syndromes (D46.-)

          DEF: Shortage of all three blood cells: white, red, and platelets.

          D61.810 Antineoplastic chemotherapy induced pancytopenia   CC HCC

            EXCLUDES 2   aplastic anemia due to antineoplastic chemotherapy (D61.1)

          D61.811 Other drug-induced pancytopenia   CC HCC

            EXCLUDES 2   aplastic anemia due to drugs (D61.1)

          D61.818 Other pancytopenia   CC HCC

            AHA: 2019,1Q,16

            TIP: Assign this code in addition to myeloid leukemia codes (C92.-) when pancytopenia is documented. Although common in some types of myeloid leukemia, pancytopenia is not always inherent.

       D61.82 Myelophthisis   CC HCC

          Leukoerythroblastic anemia

          Myelophthisic anemia

          Panmyelophthisis

          Code also the underlying disorder, such as:

            malignant neoplasm of breast (C50.-)

            tuberculosis (A15.-)

          EXCLUDES 1   idiopathic myelofibrosis (D47.1)

            myelofibrosis NOS (D75.81)

            myelofibrosis with myeloid metaplasia (D47.4)

            primary myelofibrosis (D47.1)

            secondary myelofibrosis (D75.81)

          DEF: Condition that occurs when normal hematopoietic tissue in the bone marrow is replaced with abnormal tissue, such as fibrous tissue or tumors. Most commonly seen during the advanced stages of cancer.

       D61.89 Other specified aplastic anemias and other bone marrow failure syndromes   MCC HCC

          CC Excl: PDX collection 496

    D61.9 Aplastic anemia, unspecified   HCC

       Hypoplastic anemia NOS

       Medullary hypoplasia

D62 Acute posthemorrhagic anemia

> **EXCLUDES 1**   anemia due to chronic blood loss (D50.0)
>
>   blood loss anemia NOS (D50.0)
>
>   congenital anemia from fetal blood loss (P61.3)

✓4ᵗʰ D63 Anemia in chronic diseases classified elsewhere

    D63.0 Anemia in neoplastic disease

       Code first neoplasm (C00-D49)

       EXCLUDES 1   aplastic anemia due to antineoplastic chemotherapy (D61.1)

       EXCLUDES 2   anemia due to antineoplastic chemotherapy (D64.81)

    D63.1 Anemia in chronic kidney disease

       Erythropoietin resistant anemia (EPO resistant anemia)

       Code first underlying chronic kidney disease (CKD) (N18.-)

    D63.8 Anemia in other chronic diseases classified elsewhere

       Code first underlying disease, such as:

       diphyllobothriasis (B70.0)

       hookworm disease (B76.0-B76.9)

       hypothyroidism (E00.0-E03.9)

       malaria (B50.0-B54)

       symptomatic late syphilis (A52.79)

       tuberculosis (A18.89)

✓4ᵗʰ D64 Other anemias

> **EXCLUDES 1**   refractory anemia (D46.-)
>
>   refractory anemia with excess blasts in transformation [RAEB T] (C92.0-)
>
> **DEF:** Sideroblastic anemia: Hereditary or secondary disorder in which the red blood cells cannot effectively use iron, a nutrient needed to make hemoglobin. Although the iron can enter the red blood cell it is not assimilated into the hemoglobin molecule and builds up ringed sideroblasts around the cell nucleus.

    D64.0 Hereditary sideroblastic anemia   HCC

       Sex-linked hypochromic sideroblastic anemia

    D64.1 Secondary sideroblastic anemia due to disease   HCC

       Code first underlying disease

    D64.2 Secondary sideroblastic anemia due to drugs and toxins   HCC

       Code first poisoning due to drug or toxin, if applicable (T36-T65 with fifth or sixth character 1-4 or 6)

       Use additional code for adverse effect, if applicable, to identify drug (T36-T50 with fifth or sixth character 5)

    D64.3 Other sideroblastic anemias   HCC

       Sideroblastic anemia NOS

       Pyridoxine-responsive sideroblastic anemia NEC

✓ Additional Character Required   ✓x7ᵗʰ Placeholder   <u>Unacceptable PDx</u>   Questionable PDx   Manifestation   Unspecified Dx   H1-H14 HAC   HCC CMS-HCC Dx   HIV HIV Dx

ICD-10-CM 2020   507

D64.4 Congenital dyserythropoietic anemia
Dyshematopoietic anemia (congenital)
> EXCLUDES 1   *Blackfan-Diamond syndrome (D61.01)*
> *Di Guglielmo's disease (C94.0)*

✓5ᵗʰ D64.8 Other specified anemias

D64.81 Anemia due to antineoplastic chemotherapy
Antineoplastic chemotherapy induced anemia
> EXCLUDES 1   *aplastic anemia due to antineoplastic chemotherapy (D61.1)*
> EXCLUDES 2   *anemia in neoplastic disease (D63.0)*

AHA: 2014,4Q,22
DEF: Reversible adverse effect of chemotherapy, causing inhibition of bone marrow production. A decrease in red blood cell production prevents adequate oxygenation of the tissues and organs causing fatigue, shortness of breath (SOB), and exacerbation of other medical conditions.

D64.89 Other specified anemias
Infantile pseudoleukemia

D64.9 Anemia, unspecified
AHA: 2018,4Q,88; 2017,1Q,7

Coagulation defects, purpura and other hemorrhagic conditions (D65-D69)

D65 Disseminated intravascular coagulation [defibrination syndrome]   MCC   HCC
Afibrinogenemia, acquired
Consumption coagulopathy
Diffuse or disseminated intravascular coagulation [DIC]
Fibrinolytic hemorrhage, acquired
Fibrinolytic purpura
Purpura fulminans
> EXCLUDES 1   *disseminated intravascular coagulation (complicating):*
> *abortion or ectopic or molar pregnancy (O00-O07, O08.1)*
> *in newborn (P60)*
> *pregnancy, childbirth and the puerperium (O45.0, O46.0, O67.0, O72.3)*

CC Excl: PDX collection 502

Coagulation

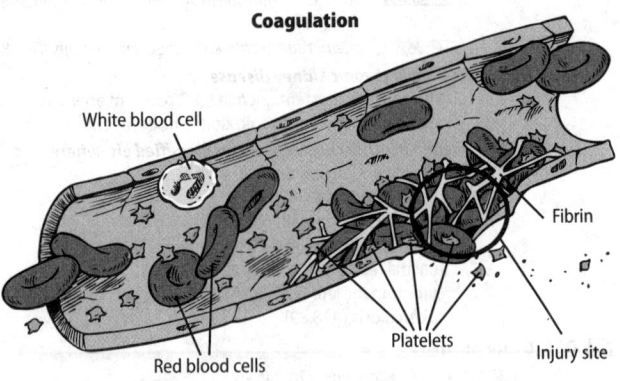
White blood cell
Fibrin
Platelets
Red blood cells
Injury site

D66 Hereditary factor VIII deficiency   MCC   HCC
Classical hemophilia
Deficiency factor VIII (with functional defect)
Hemophilia A
Hemophilia NOS
> EXCLUDES 1   *factor VIII deficiency with vascular defect (D68.0)*

DEF: Hereditary, sex-linked lack of antihemophilic globulin (AHG) (factor VIII) that causes abnormal coagulation characterized by increased bleeding; large bruises of skin; bleeding in the mouth, nose, and gastrointestinal tract; and hemorrhages into joints, resulting in swelling and impaired function.
CC Excl: PDX collection 502

D67 Hereditary factor IX deficiency   MCC   HCC
Christmas disease
Factor IX deficiency (with functional defect)
Hemophilia B
Plasma thromboplastin component [PTC] deficiency
CC Excl: PDX collection 502

✓4ᵗʰ D68 Other coagulation defects
> EXCLUDES 1   *abnormal coagulation profile (R79.1)*
> *coagulation defects complicating abortion or ectopic or molar pregnancy (O00-O07, O08.1)*
> *coagulation defects complicating pregnancy, childbirth and the puerperium (O45.0, O46.0, O67.0, O72.3)*

AHA: 2016,1Q,14
CC Excl: For CC codes in category D68, unless otherwise noted: PDX collection 502

D68.0 Von Willebrand's disease   CC   HCC
Angiohemophilia
Factor VIII deficiency with vascular defect
Vascular hemophilia
> EXCLUDES 1   *capillary fragility (hereditary) (D69.8)*
> *factor VIII deficiency NOS (D66)*
> *factor VIII deficiency with functional defect (D66)*

DEF: Congenital, abnormal blood coagulation caused by deficient blood factor VII. Symptoms include excess or prolonged bleeding.

D68.1 Hereditary factor XI deficiency   CC   HCC
Hemophilia C
Plasma thromboplastin antecedent [PTA] deficiency
Rosenthal's disease

D68.2 Hereditary deficiency of other clotting factors   CC   HCC
AC globulin deficiency
Congenital afibrinogenemia
Deficiency of factor I [fibrinogen]
Deficiency of factor II [prothrombin]
Deficiency of factor V [labile]
Deficiency of factor VII [stable]
Deficiency of factor X [Stuart-Prower]
Deficiency of factor XII [Hageman]
Deficiency of factor XIII [fibrin stabilizing]
Dysfibrinogenemia (congenital)
Hypoproconvertinemia
Owren's disease
Proaccelerin deficiency

✓5ᵗʰ D68.3 Hemorrhagic disorder due to circulating anticoagulants

✓6ᵗʰ D68.31 Hemorrhagic disorder due to intrinsic circulating anticoagulants, antibodies, or inhibitors

D68.311 Acquired hemophilia   CC   HCC
Autoimmune hemophilia
Autoimmune inhibitors to clotting factors
Secondary hemophilia
CC Excl: PDX collection 503

D68.312 Antiphospholipid antibody with hemorrhagic disorder   CC   HCC
Lupus anticoagulant (LAC) with hemorrhagic disorder
Systemic lupus erythematosus [SLE] inhibitor with hemorrhagic disorder
> EXCLUDES 1   *antiphospholipid antibody, finding without diagnosis (R76.0)*
> *antiphospholipid antibody syndrome (D68.61)*
> *antiphospholipid antibody with hypercoagulable state (D68.61)*
> *lupus anticoagulant (LAC) finding without diagnosis (R76.0)*
> *lupus anticoagulant (LAC) with hypercoagulable state (D68.62)*
> *systemic lupus erythematosus [SLE] inhibitor finding without diagnosis (R76.0)*
> *systemic lupus erythematosus [SLE] inhibitor with hypercoagulable state (D68.62)*

CC Excl: PDX collection 504

N Newborn: 0   P Pediatric: 0-17   M Maternity: 9-64   A Adult: 15-124   MCC Major Complication/Comorbidity   CC Complication/Comorbidity   SW Severe Wound Dx

508   ICD-10-CM 2020

D68.318   Other hemorrhagic disorder due to intrinsic circulating anticoagulants, antibodies, or inhibitors   `CC` `HCC`

Antithromboplastinemia

Antithromboplastinogenemia

Hemorrhagic disorder due to intrinsic increase in antithrombin

Hemorrhagic disorder due to intrinsic increase in anti-VIIIa

Hemorrhagic disorder due to intrinsic increase in anti-IXa

Hemorrhagic disorder due to intrinsic increase in anti-XIa

CC Excl: PDX collection 503

D68.32   Hemorrhagic disorder due to extrinsic circulating anticoagulants   `CC` `HCC`

Drug-induced hemorrhagic disorder

Hemorrhagic disorder due to increase in anti-IIa

Hemorrhagic disorder due to increase in anti-Xa

Hyperheparinemia

Use additional code for adverse effect, if applicable, to identify drug (T45.515, T45.525)

AHA: 2016,1Q,14-15

TIP: Do not assign to identify routine therapeutic anticoagulation effects; assign only for documented adverse effects.

D68.4   Acquired coagulation factor deficiency   `CC` `HCC`

Deficiency of coagulation factor due to liver disease

Deficiency of coagulation factor due to vitamin K deficiency

EXCLUDES 1   *vitamin K deficiency of newborn (P53)*

✓5ᵗʰ **D68.5   Primary thrombophilia**

Primary hypercoagulable states

EXCLUDES 1   *antiphospholipid syndrome (D68.61)*

lupus anticoagulant (D68.62)

secondary activated protein C resistance (D68.69)

secondary antiphospholipid antibody syndrome (D68.69)

secondary lupus anticoagulant with hypercoagulable state (D68.69)

secondary systemic lupus erythematosus [SLE] inhibitor with hypercoagulable state (D68.69)

systemic lupus erythematosus [SLE] inhibitor finding without diagnosis (R76.0)

systemic lupus erythematosus [SLE] inhibitor with hemorrhagic disorder (D68.312)

thrombotic thrombocytopenic purpura (M31.1)

DEF: Thrombophilia: Increased tendency of the blood to clot, which can lead to thrombus or embolus formation.

D68.51   Activated protein C resistance   `HCC`

Factor V Leiden mutation

D68.52   Prothrombin gene mutation   `HCC`

D68.59   Other primary thrombophilia   `HCC`

Antithrombin III deficiency

Hypercoagulable state NOS

Primary hypercoagulable state NEC

Primary thrombophilia NEC

Protein C deficiency

Protein S deficiency

Thrombophilia NOS

✓5ᵗʰ **D68.6   Other thrombophilia**

Other hypercoagulable states

EXCLUDES 1   *diffuse or disseminated intravascular coagulation [DIC] (D65)*

heparin induced thrombocytopenia (HIT) (D75.82)

hyperhomocysteinemia (E72.11)

D68.61   Antiphospholipid syndrome   `HCC`

Anticardiolipin syndrome

Antiphospholipid antibody syndrome

EXCLUDES 1   *anti-phospholipid antibody, finding without diagnosis (R76.0)*

anti-phospholipid antibody with hemorrhagic disorder (D68.312)

lupus anticoagulant syndrome (D68.62)

D68.62   Lupus anticoagulant syndrome   `HCC`

Lupus anticoagulant

Presence of systemic lupus erythematosus [SLE] inhibitor

EXCLUDES 1   *anticardiolipin syndrome (D68.61)*

antiphospholipid syndrome (D68.61)

lupus anticoagulant (LAC) finding without diagnosis (R76.0)

lupus anticoagulant (LAC) with hemorrhagic disorder (D68.312)

D68.69   Other thrombophilia   `HCC`

Hypercoagulable states NEC

Secondary hypercoagulable state NOS

D68.8   Other specified coagulation defects   `CC` `HCC`

EXCLUDES 1   *hemorrhagic disease of newborn (P53)*

D68.9   Coagulation defect, unspecified   `CC` `HCC`

✓4ᵗʰ **D69   Purpura and other hemorrhagic conditions**

EXCLUDES 1   *benign hypergammaglobulinemic purpura (D89.0)*

cryoglobulinemic purpura (D89.1)

essential (hemorrhagic) thrombocythemia (D47.3)

hemorrhagic thrombocythemia (D47.3)

purpura fulminans (D65)

thrombotic thrombocytopenic purpura (M31.1)

Waldenström hypergammaglobulinemic purpura (D89.0)

CC Excl: For CC codes in category D69: PDX collection 502

D69.0   Allergic purpura   `CC` `HCC`

Allergic vasculitis

Nonthrombocytopenic hemorrhagic purpura

Nonthrombocytopenic idiopathic purpura

Purpura anaphylactoid

Purpura Henoch(-Schönlein)

Purpura rheumatica

Vascular purpura

EXCLUDES 1   *thrombocytopenic hemorrhagic purpura (D69.3)*

DEF: Any hemorrhagic condition, thrombocytic or nonthrombocytopenic in origin, caused by a presumed allergic reaction.

D69.1   Qualitative platelet defects   `CC` `HCC`

Bernard-Soulier [giant platelet] syndrome

Glanzmann's disease

Grey platelet syndrome

Thromboasthenia (hemorrhagic) (hereditary)

Thrombocytopathy

EXCLUDES 1   *von Willebrand's disease (D68.0)*

D69.2   Other nonthrombocytopenic purpura   `HCC`

Purpura NOS

Purpura simplex

Senile purpura

D69.3   Immune thrombocytopenic purpura   `CC` `HCC`

Hemorrhagic (thrombocytopenic) purpura

Idiopathic thrombocytopenic purpura

Tidal platelet dysgenesis

DEF: Tidal platelet dysgenesis: Fluctuation of platelet counts from normal to very low within periods of 20 to 40 days and may involve autoimmune platelet destruction.

✓5ᵗʰ **D69.4   Other primary thrombocytopenia**

EXCLUDES 1   *transient neonatal thrombocytopenia (P61.0)*

Wiskott-Aldrich syndrome (D82.0)

D69.41   Evans syndrome   `CC` `HCC`

D69.42   Congenital and hereditary thrombocytopenia purpura   `CC` `HCC`

Congenital thrombocytopenia

Hereditary thrombocytopenia

Code first congenital or hereditary disorder, such as: thrombocytopenia with absent radius (TAR syndrome) (Q87.2)

D69.49   Other primary thrombocytopenia   `HCC`

Megakaryocytic hypoplasia

Primary thrombocytopenia NOS

☑ Additional Character Required   ✓x7ᵗʰ Placeholder   Unacceptable PDx   Questionable PDx   Manifestation   Unspecified Dx   H1-H14 HAC   HCC CMS-HCC Dx   HIV HIV Dx

ICD-10-CM 2020

509

Chapter 3. Diseases of the Blood and Blood-forming Organs

✓5ᵗʰ **D69.5 Secondary thrombocytopenia**

EXCLUDES 1   *heparin induced thrombocytopenia (HIT) (D75.82)*

transient thrombocytopenia of newborn (P61.0)

D69.51 Posttransfusion purpura

Posttransfusion purpura from whole blood (fresh) or blood products

PTP

D69.59 Other secondary thrombocytopenia

AHA: 2014,4Q,22

D69.6 Thrombocytopenia, unspecified   HCC

D69.8 Other specified hemorrhagic conditions   HCC

Capillary fragility (hereditary)

Vascular pseudohemophilia

D69.9 Hemorrhagic condition, unspecified   HCC

Other disorders of blood and blood-forming organs (D70-D77)

✓4ᵗʰ **D70 Neutropenia**

INCLUDES   agranulocytosis

decreased absolute neurophile count (ANC)

Use additional code for any associated:

fever (R50.81)

mucositis (J34.81, K12.3-, K92.81, N76.81)

EXCLUDES 1   *neutropenic splenomegaly (D73.81)*

transient neonatal neutropenia (P61.5)

DEF: Abnormally low number of neutrophils. Neutrophils are phagocytic, meaning they surround and consume harmful pathogens, primarily bacteria. When neutrophil counts decrease the risk of infection increases.

D70.0 Congenital agranulocytosis   CC   HCC

Congenital neutropenia

Infantile genetic agranulocytosis

Kostmann's disease

D70.1 Agranulocytosis secondary to cancer chemotherapy   CC   HCC

Code also underlying neoplasm

Use additional code for adverse effect, if applicable, to identify drug (T45.1X5)

AHA: 2014,4Q,22

D70.2 Other drug-induced agranulocytosis   CC   HCC

Use additional code for adverse effect, if applicable, to identify drug (T36-T50 with fifth or sixth character 5)

D70.3 Neutropenia due to infection   CC   HCC

D70.4 Cyclic neutropenia   CC   HCC

Cyclic hematopoiesis

Periodic neutropenia

D70.8 Other neutropenia   CC   HCC

D70.9 Neutropenia, unspecified   CC   HCC

D71 Functional disorders of polymorphonuclear neutrophils   CC   HCC

Cell membrane receptor complex [CR3] defect

Chronic (childhood) granulomatous disease

Congenital dysphagocytosis

Progressive septic granulomatosis

✓4ᵗʰ **D72 Other disorders of white blood cells**

EXCLUDES 1   *basophilia (D72.824)*

immunity disorders (D80-D89)

neutropenia (D70)

preleukemia (syndrome) (D46.9)

D72.0 Genetic anomalies of leukocytes   HCC

Alder (granulation) (granulocyte) anomaly

Alder syndrome

Hereditary leukocytic hypersegmentation

Hereditary leukocytic hyposegmentation

Hereditary leukomelanopathy

May-Hegglin (granulation) (granulocyte) anomaly

May-Hegglin syndrome

Pelger-Huët (granulation) (granulocyte) anomaly

Pelger-Huët syndrome

EXCLUDES 1   *Chédiak (-Steinbrinck)-Higashi syndrome (E70.330)*

D72.1 Eosinophilia

Allergic eosinophilia

Hereditary eosinophilia

EXCLUDES 1   *Löffler's syndrome (J82)*

pulmonary eosinophilia (J82)

✓5ᵗʰ **D72.8 Other specified disorders of white blood cells**

EXCLUDES 1   *leukemia (C91-C95)*

✓6ᵗʰ **D72.81 Decreased white blood cell count**

EXCLUDES 1   *neutropenia (D70.-)*

D72.810 Lymphocytopenia

Decreased lymphocytes

D72.818 Other decreased white blood cell count

Basophilic leukopenia

Eosinophilic leukopenia

Monocytopenia

Other decreased leukocytes

Plasmacytopenia

D72.819 Decreased white blood cell count, unspecified

Decreased leukocytes, unspecified

Leukocytopenia, unspecified

Leukopenia

EXCLUDES 1   *malignant leukopenia (D70.9)*

✓6ᵗʰ **D72.82 Elevated white blood cell count**

EXCLUDES 1   *eosinophilia (D72.1)*

D72.820 Lymphocytosis (symptomatic)

Elevated lymphocytes

D72.821 Monocytosis (symptomatic)

EXCLUDES 1   *infectious mononucleosis (B27.-)*

D72.822 Plasmacytosis

D72.823 Leukemoid reaction

Basophilic leukemoid reaction

Leukemoid reaction NOS

Lymphocytic leukemoid reaction

Monocytic leukemoid reaction

Myelocytic leukemoid reaction

Neutrophilic leukemoid reaction

D72.824 Basophilia

DEF: Increase in the basophils of the blood, a type of white blood cell, often seen in conjunction with neoplastic disorders.

D72.825 Bandemia

Bandemia without diagnosis of specific infection

EXCLUDES 1   *confirmed infection — code to infection*

leukemia (C91.-, C92.-, C93.-, C94.-, C95.-)

DEF: Increase in early neutrophil cells, called band cells that may indicate infection.

D72.828 Other elevated white blood cell count

D72.829 Elevated white blood cell count, unspecified

Elevated leukocytes, unspecified

Leukocytosis, unspecified

D72.89 Other specified disorders of white blood cells

Abnormality of white blood cells NEC

D72.9 Disorder of white blood cells, unspecified

Abnormal leukocyte differential NOS

✓4ᵗʰ **D73 Diseases of spleen**

D73.0 Hyposplenism

Atrophy of spleen

EXCLUDES 1   *asplenia (congenital) (Q89.01)*

postsurgical absence of spleen (Z90.81)

D73.1 Hypersplenism

EXCLUDES 1   *neutropenic splenomegaly (D73.81)*

primary splenic neutropenia (D73.81)

splenitis, splenomegaly in late syphilis (A52.79)

splenitis, splenomegaly in tuberculosis (A18.85)

splenomegaly NOS (R16.1)

splenomegaly congenital (Q89.0)

D73.2 Chronic congestive splenomegaly

D73.3 Abscess of spleen

D73.4 Cyst of spleen

N Newborn: 0   P Pediatric: 0-17   M Maternity: 9-64   A Adult: 15-124   MCC Major Complication/Comorbidity   CC Complication/Comorbidity   SW Severe Wound Dx

510   ICD-10-CM 2020

D73.5 Infarction of spleen
Splenic rupture, nontraumatic
Torsion of spleen
> EXCLUDES 1   *rupture of spleen due to Plasmodium vivax malaria (B51.0)*
> *traumatic rupture of spleen (S36.03-)*

✓5ᵗʰ **D73.8 Other diseases of spleen**

D73.81 Neutropenic splenomegaly
Werner-Schultz disease

D73.89 Other diseases of spleen
Fibrosis of spleen NOS
Perisplenitis
Splenitis NOS

D73.9 Disease of spleen, unspecified

✓4ᵗʰ **D74 Methemoglobinemia**

> **CC Excl: For CC codes in category D74:** PDX collection 506

D74.0 Congenital methemoglobinemia   CC
Congenital NADH-methemoglobin reductase deficiency
Hemoglobin-M [Hb-M] disease
Methemoglobinemia, hereditary

D74.8 Other methemoglobinemias   CC
Acquired methemoglobinemia (with sulfhemoglobinemia)
Toxic methemoglobinemia

D74.9 Methemoglobinemia, unspecified   CC

✓4ᵗʰ **D75 Other and unspecified diseases of blood and blood-forming organs**
> EXCLUDES 2   *acute lymphadenitis (L04.-)*
> *chronic lymphadenitis (I88.1)*
> *enlarged lymph nodes (R59.-)*
> *hypergammaglobulinemia NOS (D89.2)*
> *lymphadenitis NOS (I88.9)*
> *mesenteric lymphadenitis (acute) (chronic) (I88.0)*

D75.0 Familial erythrocytosis
Benign polycythemia
Familial polycythemia
> EXCLUDES 1   *hereditary ovalocytosis (D58.1)*

D75.1 Secondary polycythemia
Acquired polycythemia
Emotional polycythemia
Erythrocytosis NOS
Hypoxemic polycythemia
Nephrogenous polycythemia
Polycythemia due to erythropoietin
Polycythemia due to fall in plasma volume
Polycythemia due to high altitude
Polycythemia due to stress
Polycythemia NOS
Relative polycythemia
> EXCLUDES 1   *polycythemia neonatorum (P61.1)*
> *polycythemia vera (D45)*

DEF: Elevated number of red blood cells in circulating blood as a result of reduced oxygen supply to the tissues.

✓5ᵗʰ **D75.8 Other specified diseases of blood and blood-forming organs**

D75.81 Myelofibrosis   CC HCC
Myelofibrosis NOS
Secondary myelofibrosis NOS
Code first the underlying disorder, such as:
   malignant neoplasm of breast (C50.-)
Use additional code, if applicable, for associated therapy-related myelodysplastic syndrome (D46.-)
Use additional code for adverse effect, if applicable, to identify drug (T45.1X5)
> EXCLUDES 1   *acute myelofibrosis (C94.4-)*
> *idiopathic myelofibrosis (D47.1)*
> *leukoerythroblastic anemia (D61.82)*
> *myelofibrosis with myeloid metaplasia (D47.4)*
> *myelophthisic anemia (D61.82)*
> *myelophthisis (D61.82)*
> *primary myelofibrosis (D47.1)*

> **CC Excl:** PDX collection 488

D75.82 Heparin induced thrombocytopenia (HIT)   CC HCC
DEF: Immune-mediated reaction to heparin therapy causing an abrupt fall in platelet count and serious complications such as pulmonary embolism, stroke, AMI, or DVT.

D75.89 Other specified diseases of blood and blood-forming organs

D75.9 Disease of blood and blood-forming organs, unspecified

D75.A Glucose-6-phosphate dehydrogenase (G6PD) deficiency without anemia
> EXCLUDES 1   *glucose-6-phosphate dehydrogenase (G6PD) deficiency with anemia (D55.0)*

✓4ᵗʰ **D76 Other specified diseases with participation of lymphoreticular and reticulohistiocytic tissue**
> EXCLUDES 1   *(Abt-) Letterer-Siwe disease (C96.0)*
> *eosinophilic granuloma (C96.6)*
> *Hand-Schüller-Christian disease (C96.5)*
> *histiocytic medullary reticulosis (C96.9)*
> *histiocytic sarcoma (C96.A)*
> *histiocytosis X, multifocal (C96.5)*
> *histiocytosis X, unifocal (C96.6)*
> *Langerhans-cell histiocytosis, multifocal (C96.5)*
> *Langerhans-cell histiocytosis NOS (C96.6)*
> *Langerhans-cell histiocytosis, unifocal (C96.6)*
> *leukemic reticuloendotheliosis (C91.4-)*
> *lipomelanotic reticulosis (I89.8)*
> *malignant histiocytosis (C96.A)*
> *malignant reticulosis (C86.0)*
> *nonlipid reticuloendotheliosis (C96.0)*

> **CC Excl: For CC codes in category D76:** PDX collection 507

D76.1 Hemophagocytic lymphohistiocytosis   CC HCC
Familial hemophagocytic reticulosis
Histiocytoses of mononuclear phagocytes

D76.2 Hemophagocytic syndrome, infection-associated   CC HCC
Use additional code to identify infectious agent or disease

D76.3 Other histiocytosis syndromes   CC HCC
Reticulohistiocytoma (giant-cell)
Sinus histiocytosis with massive lymphadenopathy
Xanthogranuloma

D77 Other disorders of blood and blood-forming organs in diseases classified elsewhere
Code first underlying disease, such as:
   amyloidosis (E85.-)
   congenital early syphilis (A50.0)
   echinococcosis (B67.0-B67.9)
   malaria (B50.0-B54)
   schistosomiasis [bilharziasis] (B65.0-B65.9)
   vitamin C deficiency (E54)
> EXCLUDES 1   *rupture of spleen due to Plasmodium vivax malaria (B51.0)*
> *splenitis, splenomegaly in late syphilis (A52.79)*
> *splenitis, splenomegaly in tuberculosis (A18.85)*

Intraoperative and postprocedural complications of the spleen (D78)

> **CC Excl: For CC codes in category D78, unless otherwise noted:** PDX collection 508

✓4ᵗʰ **D78 Intraoperative and postprocedural complications of the spleen**
AHA: 2016,4Q,9-10

✓5ᵗʰ **D78.0 Intraoperative hemorrhage and hematoma of the spleen complicating a procedure**
> EXCLUDES 1   *intraoperative hemorrhage and hematoma of the spleen due to accidental puncture or laceration during a procedure (D78.1-)*

D78.01 Intraoperative hemorrhage and hematoma of the spleen complicating a procedure on the spleen   CC

D78.02 Intraoperative hemorrhage and hematoma of the spleen complicating other procedure   CC

✓ Additional Character Required   ✓x7ᵗʰ Placeholder   Unacceptable PDx   Questionable PDx   Manifestation   Unspecified Dx   H1–H14 HAC   HCC CMS-HCC Dx   HIV HIV Dx

ICD-10-CM 2020   511

Chapter 3. Diseases of the Blood and Blood-forming Organs

D78.1–D82.4

√5ᵗʰ **D78.1** Accidental puncture and laceration of the spleen during a procedure

     D78.11 Accidental puncture and laceration of the spleen during a procedure on the spleen   cc
         CC Excl: PDX collection 509

     D78.12 Accidental puncture and laceration of the spleen during other procedure   cc
         CC Excl: PDX collection 509

√5ᵗʰ **D78.2** Postprocedural hemorrhage of the spleen following a procedure

     D78.21 Postprocedural hemorrhage of the spleen following a procedure on the spleen   cc

     D78.22 Postprocedural hemorrhage of the spleen following other procedure   cc

√5ᵗʰ **D78.3** Postprocedural hematoma and seroma of the spleen following a procedure

     D78.31 Postprocedural hematoma of the spleen following a procedure on the spleen   cc

     D78.32 Postprocedural hematoma of the spleen following other procedure   cc

     D78.33 Postprocedural seroma of the spleen following a procedure on the spleen   cc

     D78.34 Postprocedural seroma of the spleen following other procedure   cc

√5ᵗʰ **D78.8** Other intraoperative and postprocedural complications of the spleen
     Use additional code, if applicable, to further specify disorder

     D78.81 Other intraoperative complications of the spleen   cc
         CC Excl: PDX collection 510

     D78.89 Other postprocedural complications of the spleen   cc
         CC Excl: PDX collection 510

Certain disorders involving the immune mechanism (D80-D89)

INCLUDES   defects in the complement system
     immunodeficiency disorders, except human immunodeficiency virus [HIV] disease
     sarcoidosis

EXCLUDES 1   autoimmune disease (systemic) NOS (M35.9)
     functional disorders of polymorphonuclear neutrophils (D71)
     human immunodeficiency virus [HIV] disease (B20)

CC Excl: For CC codes in categories D80-D89 unless otherwise noted: PDX collection 511

√4ᵗʰ **D80** Immunodeficiency with predominantly antibody defects

     D80.0 Hereditary hypogammaglobulinemia   cc hcc
         Autosomal recessive agammaglobulinemia (Swiss type)
         X-linked agammaglobulinemia [Bruton] (with growth hormone deficiency)

     D80.1 Nonfamilial hypogammaglobulinemia   cc hcc
         Agammaglobulinemia with immunoglobulin-bearing B-lymphocytes
         Common variable agammaglobulinemia [CVAgamma]
         Hypogammaglobulinemia NOS
         CC Excl: PDX collection 512

     D80.2 Selective deficiency of immunoglobulin A [IgA]   cc hcc
         CC Excl: PDX collection 512

     D80.3 Selective deficiency of immunoglobulin G [IgG] subclasses   cc hcc

     D80.4 Selective deficiency of immunoglobulin M [IgM]   cc hcc

     D80.5 Immunodeficiency with increased immunoglobulin M [IgM]   cc hcc

     D80.6 Antibody deficiency with near-normal immunoglobulins or with hyperimmunoglobulinemia   cc hcc

     D80.7 Transient hypogammaglobulinemia of infancy   cc hcc

     D80.8 Other immunodeficiencies with predominantly antibody defects   cc hcc
         Kappa light chain deficiency

     D80.9 Immunodeficiency with predominantly antibody defects, unspecified   cc hcc

√4ᵗʰ **D81** Combined immunodeficiencies

EXCLUDES 1   autosomal recessive agammaglobulinemia (Swiss type) (D80.0)

     D81.0 Severe combined immunodeficiency [SCID] with reticular dysgenesis   cc hcc

     D81.1 Severe combined immunodeficiency [SCID] with low T- and B-cell numbers   cc hcc

     D81.2 Severe combined immunodeficiency [SCID] with low or normal B-cell numbers   cc hcc

▲ √5ᵗʰ **D81.3** Adenosine deaminase [ADA] deficiency

     ● **D81.30** Adenosine deaminase deficiency, unspecified   cc
         ADA deficiency NOS

     D81.31 Severe combined immunodeficiency due to adenosine deaminase deficiency   cc
         ADA deficiency with SCID
         Adenosine deaminase [ADA] deficiency with severe combined immunodeficiency

     ● **D81.32** Adenosine deaminase 2 deficiency   cc
         ADA2 deficiency
         Adenosine deaminase deficiency type 2
         Code also, if applicable, any associated manifestations, such as:
           polyarteritis nodosa (M30.0)
           stroke (I63.-)

     ● **D81.39** Other adenosine deaminase deficiency   cc
         Adenosine deaminase [ADA] deficiency type 1, NOS
         Adenosine deaminase [ADA] deficiency type 1, without SCID
         Adenosine deaminase [ADA] deficiency type 1, without severe combined immunodeficiency
         Partial ADA deficiency (type 1)
         Partial adenosine deaminase deficiency (type 1)

     D81.4 Nezelof's syndrome   cc hcc

     D81.5 Purine nucleoside phosphorylase [PNP] deficiency   cc hcc
         CC Excl: PDX collection 513

     D81.6 Major histocompatibility complex class I deficiency   cc hcc
         Bare lymphocyte syndrome

     D81.7 Major histocompatibility complex class II deficiency   cc hcc

√5ᵗʰ **D81.8** Other combined immunodeficiencies

     √6ᵗʰ **D81.81** Biotin-dependent carboxylase deficiency
         Multiple carboxylase deficiency
         EXCLUDES 1   biotin-dependent carboxylase deficiency due to dietary deficiency of biotin (E53.8)

         D81.810 Biotinidase deficiency

         D81.818 Other biotin-dependent carboxylase deficiency
           Holocarboxylase synthetase deficiency
           Other multiple carboxylase deficiency

         D81.819 Biotin-dependent carboxylase deficiency, unspecified
           Multiple carboxylase deficiency, unspecified

     D81.89 Other combined immunodeficiencies   cc hcc

     D81.9 Combined immunodeficiency, unspecified   cc hcc
         Severe combined immunodeficiency disorder [SCID] NOS

√4ᵗʰ **D82** Immunodeficiency associated with other major defects

EXCLUDES 1   ataxia telangiectasia [Louis-Bar] (G11.3)

     D82.0 Wiskott-Aldrich syndrome   cc hcc
         Immunodeficiency with thrombocytopenia and eczema

     D82.1 Di George's syndrome   cc hcc
         Pharyngeal pouch syndrome
         Thymic alymphoplasia
         Thymic aplasia or hypoplasia with immunodeficiency

     D82.2 Immunodeficiency with short-limbed stature   hcc

     D82.3 Immunodeficiency following hereditary defective response to Epstein-Barr virus   hcc
         X-linked lymphoproliferative disease

     D82.4 Hyperimmunoglobulin E [IgE] syndrome   hcc

N Newborn: 0   P Pediatric: 0-17   M Maternity: 9-64   A Adult: 15-124   MCC Major Complication/Comorbidity   CC Complication/Comorbidity   SW Severe Wound Dx

512   ICD-10-CM 2020

D82.8　Immunodeficiency associated with other specified major defects　`HCC`

D82.9　Immunodeficiency associated with major defect, unspecified　`HCC`

`√4ᵗʰ` **D83**　**Common variable immunodeficiency**

D83.0　Common variable immunodeficiency with predominant abnormalities of B-cell numbers and function　`CC` `HCC`

D83.1　Common variable immunodeficiency with predominant immunoregulatory T-cell disorders　`CC` `HCC`

D83.2　Common variable immunodeficiency with autoantibodies to B- or T-cells　`CC` `HCC`

D83.8　Other common variable immunodeficiencies　`CC` `HCC`

D83.9　Common variable immunodeficiency, unspecified　`CC` `HCC`

`√4ᵗʰ` **D84**　**Other immunodeficiencies**

D84.0　Lymphocyte function antigen-1 [LFA-1] defect　`HCC`

D84.1　Defects in the complement system　`HCC`
　　　　C1 esterase inhibitor [C1-INH] deficiency

D84.8　Other specified immunodeficiencies　`CC` `HCC`

D84.9　Immunodeficiency, unspecified　`CC` `HCC`

`√4ᵗʰ` **D86**　**Sarcoidosis**

DEF: Clustering of immune cells resulting in granuloma formation. Often affects the lungs and lymphatic system but can occur in other body sites.

D86.0　Sarcoidosis of lung　`HCC`

D86.1　Sarcoidosis of lymph nodes

D86.2　Sarcoidosis of lung with sarcoidosis of lymph nodes　`HCC`

D86.3　Sarcoidosis of skin

`√5ᵗʰ` **D86.8**　Sarcoidosis of other sites

D86.81　Sarcoid meningitis

D86.82　Multiple cranial nerve palsies in sarcoidosis　`HCC`

D86.83　Sarcoid iridocyclitis

D86.84　Sarcoid pyelonephritis
　　　　Tubulo-interstitial nephropathy in sarcoidosis

D86.85　Sarcoid myocarditis

D86.86　Sarcoid arthropathy
　　　　Polyarthritis in sarcoidosis

D86.87　Sarcoid myositis

D86.89　Sarcoidosis of other sites
　　　　Hepatic granuloma
　　　　Uveoparotid fever [Heerfordt]

D86.9　Sarcoidosis, unspecified

`√4ᵗʰ` **D89**　**Other disorders involving the immune mechanism, not elsewhere classified**

`EXCLUDES 1`　hyperglobulinemia NOS (R77.1)
　　　　monoclonal gammopathy (of undetermined significance) (D47.2)

`EXCLUDES 2`　transplant failure and rejection (T86.-)

D89.0　Polyclonal hypergammaglobulinemia
　　　　Benign hypergammaglobulinemic purpura
　　　　Polyclonal gammopathy NOS

D89.1　Cryoglobulinemia　`HCC`
　　　　Cryoglobulinemic purpura
　　　　Cryoglobulinemic vasculitis
　　　　Essential cryoglobulinemia
　　　　Idiopathic cryoglobulinemia
　　　　Mixed cryoglobulinemia
　　　　Primary cryoglobulinemia
　　　　Secondary cryoglobulinemia

D89.2　Hypergammaglobulinemia, unspecified

D89.3　Immune reconstitution syndrome　`HCC`
　　　　Immune reconstitution inflammatory syndrome [IRIS]
　　　　Use additional code for adverse effect, if applicable, to identify drug (T36-T50 with fifth or sixth character 5)

`√5ᵗʰ` **D89.4**　**Mast cell activation syndrome and related disorders**

`EXCLUDES 1`　aggressive systemic mastocytosis (C96.21)
　　　　congenital cutaneous mastocytosis (Q82.2)
　　　　(non-congenital) cutaneous mastocytosis (D47.01)
　　　　(indolent) systemic mastocytosis (D47.02)
　　　　malignant mast cell neoplasm (C96.2-)
　　　　malignant mastocytoma (C96.29)
　　　　mast cell leukemia (C94.3-)
　　　　mast cell sarcoma (C96.22)
　　　　mastocytoma NOS (D47.09)
　　　　other mast cell neoplasms of uncertain behavior (D47.09)
　　　　systemic mastocytosis associated with a clonal hematologic non-mast cell lineage disease (SM-AHNMD) (D47.02)

AHA: 2016,4Q,11

D89.40　Mast cell activation, unspecified　`HCC`
　　　　Mast cell activation disorder, unspecified
　　　　Mast cell activation syndrome, NOS

D89.41　Monoclonal mast cell activation syndrome　`HCC`

D89.42　Idiopathic mast cell activation syndrome　`HCC`

D89.43　Secondary mast cell activation　`HCC`
　　　　Secondary mast cell activation syndrome
　　　　Code also underlying etiology, if known

D89.49　Other mast cell activation disorder　`HCC`
　　　　Other mast cell activation syndrome

`√5ᵗʰ` **D89.8**　Other specified disorders involving the immune mechanism, not elsewhere classified

`√6ᵗʰ` **D89.81**　Graft-versus-host disease
　　　　Code first underlying cause, such as:
　　　　　complications of transplanted organs and tissue (T86.-)
　　　　　complications of blood transfusion (T80.89)
　　　　Use additional code to identify associated manifestations, such as:
　　　　　desquamative dermatitis (L30.8)
　　　　　diarrhea (R19.7)
　　　　　elevated bilirubin (R17)
　　　　　hair loss (L65.9)
　　　　CC Excl: For CC codes in subcategory D89.81: PDX collection 514

D89.810　Acute graft-versus-host disease　`CC` `HCC`

D89.811　Chronic graft-versus-host disease　`CC` `HCC`

D89.812　Acute on chronic graft-versus-host disease　`CC` `HCC`

D89.813　Graft-versus-host disease, unspecified　`CC` `HCC`

D89.82　Autoimmune lymphoproliferative syndrome [ALPS]　`HCC`
　　　　DEF: Rare genetic alteration of the Fas protein that impairs normal cellular apoptosis (normal cell death), causing abnormal accumulation of lymphocytes in the lymph glands, liver, and spleen. Symptoms include neutropenia, anemia, and thrombocytopenia.

D89.89　Other specified disorders involving the immune mechanism, not elsewhere classified　`HCC`
　　　　`EXCLUDES 1`　human immunodeficiency virus disease (B20)
　　　　AHA: 2017,4Q,109

D89.9　Disorder involving the immune mechanism, unspecified　`HCC`
　　　　Immune disease NOS
　　　　AHA: 2015,3Q,22

☑ Additional Character Required　　`√x7ᵗʰ` Placeholder　　Unacceptable PDx　　Questionable PDx　　Manifestation　　Unspecified Dx　　`H1`-`H14` HAC　　`HCC` CMS-HCC Dx　　`HIV` HIV Dx

ICD-10-CM 2020　　**513**

Chapter 4. Endocrine, Nutritional and Metabolic Diseases (E00–E89)

Chapter-specific Guidelines with Coding Examples

The chapter-specific guidelines from the ICD-10-CM Official Guidelines for Coding and Reporting have been provided below. Along with these guidelines are coding examples, contained in the shaded boxes, that have been developed to help illustrate the coding and/or sequencing guidance found in these guidelines.

a. Diabetes mellitus

The diabetes mellitus codes are combination codes that include the type of diabetes mellitus, the body system affected, and the complications affecting that body system. As many codes within a particular category as are necessary to describe all of the complications of the disease may be used. They should be sequenced based on the reason for a particular encounter. Assign as many codes from categories E08–E13 as needed to identify all of the associated conditions that the patient has.

> Patient is seen for poorly controlled diabetes, type 2, with diabetic polyneuropathy and diabetic retinopathy with macular edema
>
> **E11.65**   **Type 2 diabetes mellitus with hyperglycemia**
>
> **E11.311**   **Type 2 diabetes mellitus with unspecified diabetic retinopathy with macular edema**
>
> **E11.42**   **Type 2 diabetes mellitus with diabetic polyneuropathy**
>
> *Explanation*: Use as many codes to describe the diabetic complications as needed. Many are combination codes that describe more than one condition. Code first the reason for the encounter. "Poorly controlled" is described as "with hyperglycemia." Diabetes documented as "uncontrolled" is not assumed to be hyperglycemic but can be classified to either hyperglycemia or hypoglycemia. If documentation is not clear, the provider must be queried so that the appropriate code can be reported.

1) Type of diabetes

The age of a patient is not the sole determining factor, though most type 1 diabetics develop the condition before reaching puberty. For this reason type 1 diabetes mellitus is also referred to as juvenile diabetes.

> A 45-year-old patient is diagnosed with type 1 diabetes
>
> **E10.9**   **Type 1 diabetes mellitus without complications**
>
> *Explanation*: Although most type 1 diabetics are diagnosed in childhood or adolescence, it can also begin in adults.

2) Type of diabetes mellitus not documented

If the type of diabetes mellitus is not documented in the medical record the default is E11.-, Type 2 diabetes mellitus.

> H & P lists diabetes and hypertension on patient problem list
>
> **E11.9**   **Type 2 diabetes mellitus without complications**
>
> **I10**   **Essential (primary) hypertension**
>
> *Explanation*: Since the type of diabetes was not documented and no complications were noted, the default code is E11.9.

3) Diabetes mellitus and the use of insulin and oral hypoglycemics

If the documentation in a medical record does not indicate the type of diabetes but does indicate that the patient uses insulin, code E11-, Type 2 diabetes mellitus, should be assigned. An additional code should be assigned from category Z79 to identify the long-term (current) use of insulin or oral hypoglycemic drugs. If the patient is treated with both oral medications and insulin, only the code for long-term (current) use of insulin should be assigned. Code Z79.4 should not be assigned if insulin is given temporarily to bring a type 2 patient's blood sugar under control during an encounter.

> Diabetic patient on daily metformin is admitted in ketoacidosis; insulin given to stabilize blood sugars and discontinued at discharge
>
> **E11.10**   **Type 2 diabetes mellitus with ketoacidosis without coma**
>
> **Z79.84**   **Long term (current) use of oral hypoglycemic drugs**
>
> *Explanation*: Type 2 is the default for diabetes when not further specified in the documentation. Although insulin was given to the patient during the encounter, it was discontinued at discharge, indicating that the patient does not regularly use insulin. Applying code Z79.4 to represent long-term use of insulin would be inappropriate.

4) Diabetes mellitus in pregnancy and gestational diabetes

See Section I.C.15. Diabetes mellitus in pregnancy.

See Section I.C.15. Gestational (pregnancy induced) diabetes

5) Complications due to insulin pump malfunction

(a) Underdose of insulin due to insulin pump failure

An underdose of insulin due to an insulin pump failure should be assigned to a code from subcategory T85.6, Mechanical complication of other specified internal and external prosthetic devices, implants and grafts, that specifies the type of pump malfunction, as the principal or first-listed code, followed by code T38.3X6-, Underdosing of insulin and oral hypoglycemic [antidiabetic] drugs. Additional codes for the type of diabetes mellitus and any associated complications due to the underdosing should also be assigned.

> A 24-year-old type 1 diabetic male treated in ED for hyperglycemia; insulin pump found to be malfunctioning and underdosing
>
> **T85.614A**   **Breakdown (mechanical) of insulin pump, initial encounter**
>
> **T38.3X6A**   **Underdosing of insulin and oral hypoglycemic [antidiabetic] drugs, initial encounter**
>
> **E10.65**   **Type 1 diabetes mellitus with hyperglycemia**
>
> *Explanation*: The complication code for the mechanical breakdown of the pump is sequenced first, followed by the underdosing code and type of diabetes with complication. Code all other diabetic complication codes necessary to describe the patient's condition.

(b) Overdose of insulin due to insulin pump failure

The principal or first-listed code for an encounter due to an insulin pump malfunction resulting in an overdose of insulin, should also be T85.6-, Mechanical complication of other specified internal and external prosthetic devices, implants and grafts, followed by code T38.3X1-, Poisoning by insulin and oral hypoglycemic [antidiabetic] drugs, accidental (unintentional).

> A 24-year-old type 1 diabetic male found down with diabetic coma, brought into ED and treated for hypoglycemia; insulin pump found to be malfunctioning and overdosing
>
> **T85.614A**   **Breakdown (mechanical) of insulin pump, initial encounter**
>
> **T38.3X1A**   **Poisoning by insulin and oral hypoglycemic [antidiabetic] drugs, accidental (unintentional), initial encounter**
>
> **E10.641**   **Type 1 diabetes mellitus with hypoglycemia with coma**
>
> *Explanation*: The complication code for the mechanical breakdown of the pump is sequenced first, followed by the poisoning code and type of diabetes with complication. All the characters in the combination code must be used to form a valid code and to fully describe the type of diabetes, the hypoglycemia, and the coma.

6) Secondary diabetes mellitus

Codes under categories E08, Diabetes mellitus due to underlying condition, E09, Drug or chemical induced diabetes mellitus, and E13, Other specified diabetes mellitus, identify complications/manifestations associated with secondary diabetes mellitus. Secondary diabetes is always caused by another condition or event (e.g., cystic fibrosis, malignant neoplasm of pancreas, pancreatectomy, adverse effect of drug, or poisoning).

(a) Secondary diabetes mellitus and the use of insulin or oral hypoglycemic drugs

For patients with secondary diabetes mellitus who routinely use insulin or oral hypoglycemic drugs, an additional code from category Z79 should be assigned to identify the long-term (current) use of insulin or oral hypoglycemic drugs. If the patient is treated with both oral medications and insulin, only the code for long-term (current) use of insulin should be assigned. Code Z79.4 should not be assigned if insulin is given temporarily to bring a secondary diabetic patient's blood sugar under control during an encounter.

> The patient, maintained on metformin and insulin, was admitted for treatment of diabetic gangrene. The patient developed diabetes secondary to Nelson's syndrome.
>
> **E24.1**   Nelson's syndrome
>
> **E08.52**   Diabetes mellitus due to underlying condition with diabetic peripheral angiopathy with gangrene
>
> **Z79.4**   Long term (current) use of insulin
>
> *Explanation*: When diabetes is caused by an underlying condition, the underlying condition should always be sequenced before any codes representing the diabetes. Patients with secondary diabetes may be maintained on both insulin and an oral hypoglycemic. Report only the code for the long-term use of insulin when both oral hypoglycemic and insulin are prescribed.

(b) Assigning and sequencing secondary diabetes codes and its causes

The sequencing of the secondary diabetes codes in relationship to codes for the cause of the diabetes is based on the Tabular List instructions for categories E08, E09 and E13.

(i) Secondary diabetes mellitus due to pancreatectomy

For postpancreatectomy diabetes mellitus (lack of insulin due to the surgical removal of all or part of the pancreas), assign code E89.1, Postprocedural hypoinsulinemia. Assign a code from category E13 and a code from subcategory Z90.41, Acquired absence of pancreas, as additional codes.

> Patient with newly diagnosed diabetes after surgical removal of part of pancreas is discharged with referral for consult to initiate insulin.
>
> **E89.1**   Postprocedural hypoinsulinemia
>
> **E13.9**   Other specified diabetes mellitus without complications
>
> **Z90.411**   Acquired partial absence of pancreas
>
> *Explanation*: Sequence the postprocedural complication of the hypoinsulinemia due to the partial removal of the pancreas as the first-listed code, followed by the other specified diabetes (NEC) with or without complications and the partial or total acquired absence of the pancreas. Code Z79.4 Long term (current) use of insulin, is not added because the insulin has not yet been started.

(ii) Secondary diabetes due to drugs

Secondary diabetes may be caused by an adverse effect of correctly administered medications, poisoning or sequela of poisoning.

See section I.C.19.e for coding of adverse effects and poisoning, and section I.C.20 for external cause code reporting.

> Initial encounter for corticosteroid-induced diabetes mellitus
>
> **E09.9**   Drug or chemical induced diabetes mellitus without complications
>
> **T38.0X5A**   Adverse effect of glucocorticoids and synthetic analogues, initial encounter
>
> *Explanation*: If the diabetes is caused by an adverse effect of a drug, the diabetic condition is coded first. If it occurs from a poisoning or overdose, the poisoning code causing the diabetes is sequenced first.

Chapter 4. Endocrine, Nutritional and Metabolic Diseases (E00-E89)

NOTE All neoplasms, whether functionally active or not, are classified in Chapter 2. Appropriate codes in this chapter (i.e. E05.8, E07.0, E16-E31, E34.-) may be used as additional codes to indicate either functional activity by neoplasms and ectopic endocrine tissue or hyperfunction and hypofunction of endocrine glands associated with neoplasms and other conditions classified elsewhere.

EXCLUDES 1 transitory endocrine and metabolic disorders specific to newborn (P70-P74)

AHA: 2018,2Q,6

This chapter contains the following blocks:

E00-E07	Disorders of thyroid gland
E08-E13	Diabetes mellitus
E15-E16	Other disorders of glucose regulation and pancreatic internal secretion
E20-E35	Disorders of other endocrine glands
E36	Intraoperative complications of endocrine system
E40-E46	Malnutrition
E50-E64	Other nutritional deficiencies
E65-E68	Overweight, obesity and other hyperalimentation
E70-E88	Metabolic disorders
E89	Postprocedural endocrine and metabolic complications and disorders, not elsewhere classified

Disorders of thyroid gland (E00-E07)

✓4ᵗʰ E00 Congenital iodine-deficiency syndrome

Use additional code (F70-F79) to identify associated intellectual disabilities

EXCLUDES 1 subclinical iodine-deficiency hypothyroidism (E02)

E00.0 Congenital iodine-deficiency syndrome, neurological type
Endemic cretinism, neurological type

E00.1 Congenital iodine-deficiency syndrome, myxedematous type
Endemic hypothyroid cretinism
Endemic cretinism, myxedematous type

E00.2 Congenital iodine-deficiency syndrome, mixed type
Endemic cretinism, mixed type

E00.9 Congenital iodine-deficiency syndrome, unspecified
Congenital iodine-deficiency hypothyroidism NOS
Endemic cretinism NOS

✓4ᵗʰ E01 Iodine-deficiency related thyroid disorders and allied conditions

EXCLUDES 1 congenital iodine-deficiency syndrome (E00.-)
subclinical iodine-deficiency hypothyroidism (E02)

E01.0 Iodine-deficiency related diffuse (endemic) goiter

E01.1 Iodine-deficiency related multinodular (endemic) goiter
Iodine-deficiency related nodular goiter

E01.2 Iodine-deficiency related (endemic) goiter, unspecified
Endemic goiter NOS

E01.8 Other iodine-deficiency related thyroid disorders and allied conditions
Acquired iodine-deficiency hypothyroidism NOS

E02 Subclinical iodine-deficiency hypothyroidism

✓4ᵗʰ E03 Other hypothyroidism

EXCLUDES 1 iodine-deficiency related hypothyroidism (E00-E02)
postprocedural hypothyroidism (E89.0)

DEF: Hypothyroidism: Underproduction of thyroid hormone.

E03.0 Congenital hypothyroidism with diffuse goiter
Congenital parenchymatous goiter (nontoxic)
Congenital goiter (nontoxic) NOS

EXCLUDES 1 transitory congenital goiter with normal function (P72.0)

E03.1 Congenital hypothyroidism without goiter
Aplasia of thyroid (with myxedema)
Congenital atrophy of thyroid
Congenital hypothyroidism NOS

E03.2 Hypothyroidism due to medicaments and other exogenous substances
Code first poisoning due to drug or toxin, if applicable (T36-T65 with fifth or sixth character 1-4 or 6)
Use additional code for adverse effect, if applicable, to identify drug (T36-T50 with fifth or sixth character 5)

E03.3 Postinfectious hypothyroidism

E03.4 Atrophy of thyroid (acquired)
EXCLUDES 1 congenital atrophy of thyroid (E03.1)

E03.5 Myxedema coma MCC HCC
CC Excl: PDX collection 515

E03.8 Other specified hypothyroidism

E03.9 Hypothyroidism, unspecified
Myxedema NOS

✓4ᵗʰ E04 Other nontoxic goiter

EXCLUDES 1 congenital goiter (NOS) (diffuse) (parenchymatous) (E03.0)
iodine-deficiency related goiter (E00-E02)

E04.0 Nontoxic diffuse goiter
Diffuse (colloid) nontoxic goiter
Simple nontoxic goiter

E04.1 Nontoxic single thyroid nodule
Colloid nodule (cystic) (thyroid)
Nontoxic uninodular goiter
Thyroid (cystic) nodule NOS
DEF: Enlarged thyroid, commonly due to decreased thyroid production, with a single nodule. No clinical hypothyroidism.

E04.2 Nontoxic multinodular goiter
Cystic goiter NOS
Multinodular (cystic) goiter NOS
DEF: Enlarged thyroid, commonly due to decreased thyroid production with multiple nodules. No clinical hypothyroidism.

E04.8 Other specified nontoxic goiter

E04.9 Nontoxic goiter, unspecified
Goiter NOS
Nodular goiter (nontoxic) NOS

✓4ᵗʰ E05 Thyrotoxicosis [hyperthyroidism]

EXCLUDES 1 chronic thyroiditis with transient thyrotoxicosis (E06.2)
neonatal thyrotoxicosis (P72.1)

DEF: Excessive quantities of hormones from the thyroid gland caused by overproduction or loss of storage ability.
CC Excl: For MCC codes in category E05: PDX collection 516

✓5ᵗʰ E05.0 Thyrotoxicosis with diffuse goiter
Exophthalmic or toxic goiter NOS
Graves' disease
Toxic diffuse goiter
DEF: Diffuse thyroid enlargement accompanied by hyperthyroidism, bulging eyes, and dermopathy.

E05.00 Thyrotoxicosis with diffuse goiter without thyrotoxic crisis or storm

E05.01 Thyrotoxicosis with diffuse goiter with thyrotoxic crisis or storm MCC

Goiter

Pyramidal lobe
Thyroid cartilage
Healthy thyroid
Goiter (hyperfunctioning thyroid)

✓5ᵗʰ E05.1 Thyrotoxicosis with toxic single thyroid nodule
Thyrotoxicosis with toxic uninodular goiter
DEF: Symptomatic hyperthyroidism with a single nodule on the enlarged thyroid gland. Onset of symptoms can be abrupt and include extreme nervousness, insomnia, weight loss, tremors, and psychosis or coma.

E05.10 Thyrotoxicosis with toxic single thyroid nodule without thyrotoxic crisis or storm

E05.11 Thyrotoxicosis with toxic single thyroid nodule with thyrotoxic crisis or storm MCC

✓5ᵗʰ E05.2 Thyrotoxicosis with toxic multinodular goiter
Toxic nodular goiter NOS

E05.20 Thyrotoxicosis with toxic multinodular goiter without thyrotoxic crisis or storm

E05.21 Thyrotoxicosis with toxic multinodular goiter with thyrotoxic crisis or storm MCC

√5ᵗʰ **E05.3 Thyrotoxicosis** from ectopic thyroid tissue

E05.30 Thyrotoxicosis from ectopic thyroid tissue without thyrotoxic crisis or storm

E05.31 Thyrotoxicosis from ectopic thyroid tissue with thyrotoxic crisis or storm `MCC`

√5ᵗʰ **E05.4 Thyrotoxicosis factitia**

E05.40 Thyrotoxicosis factitia without thyrotoxic crisis or storm

E05.41 Thyrotoxicosis factitia with thyrotoxic crisis or storm `MCC`

√5ᵗʰ **E05.8 Other thyrotoxicosis**

Overproduction of thyroid-stimulating hormone

E05.80 Other thyrotoxicosis without thyrotoxic crisis or storm

E05.81 Other thyrotoxicosis with thyrotoxic crisis or storm `MCC`

√5ᵗʰ **E05.9 Thyrotoxicosis, unspecified**

Hyperthyroidism NOS

E05.90 Thyrotoxicosis, unspecified without thyrotoxic crisis or storm

E05.91 Thyrotoxicosis, unspecified with thyrotoxic crisis or storm `MCC`

√4ᵗʰ **E06 Thyroiditis**

`EXCLUDES 1` *postpartum thyroiditis (O90.5)*

DEF: Inflammation of the thyroid gland.

E06.0 Acute thyroiditis `CC`

Abscess of thyroid
Pyogenic thyroiditis
Suppurative thyroiditis
Use additional code (B95-B97) to identify infectious agent
CC Excl: PDX collection 517

E06.1 Subacute thyroiditis

de Quervain thyroiditis
Giant-cell thyroiditis
Granulomatous thyroiditis
Nonsuppurative thyroiditis
Viral thyroiditis

`EXCLUDES 1` *autoimmune thyroiditis (E06.3)*

E06.2 Chronic thyroiditis with transient thyrotoxicosis

`EXCLUDES 1` *autoimmune thyroiditis (E06.3)*

E06.3 Autoimmune thyroiditis

Hashimoto's thyroiditis
Hashitoxicosis (transient)
Lymphadenoid goiter
Lymphocytic thyroiditis
Struma lymphomatosa

E06.4 Drug-induced thyroiditis

Use additional code for adverse effect, if applicable, to identify drug (T36-T50 with fifth or sixth character 5)

E06.5 Other chronic thyroiditis

Chronic fibrous thyroiditis
Chronic thyroiditis NOS
Ligneous thyroiditis
Riedel thyroiditis

E06.9 Thyroiditis, unspecified

√4ᵗʰ **E07 Other disorders of thyroid**

E07.0 Hypersecretion of calcitonin

C-cell hyperplasia of thyroid
Hypersecretion of thyrocalcitonin

E07.1 Dyshormogenetic goiter

Familial dyshormogenetic goiter
Pendred's syndrome

`EXCLUDES 1` *transitory congenital goiter with normal function (P72.0)*

√5ᵗʰ **E07.8 Other specified disorders of thyroid**

E07.81 Sick-euthyroid syndrome `CC`

Euthyroid sick-syndrome
DEF: Thyroid dysfunction caused by abnormal levels of thyroid hormones T3 and/or T4. This syndrome is often associated with starvation or critical illness.

E07.89 Other specified disorders of thyroid

Abnormality of thyroid-binding globulin
Hemorrhage of thyroid
Infarction of thyroid

E07.9 Disorder of thyroid, unspecified

Diabetes mellitus (E08-E13)

AHA: 2018,4Q,88; 2018,3Q,3-4; 2018,2Q,6; 2017,4Q,6; 2017,1Q,42; 2016,4Q,11-13; 2016,2Q,36; 2016,1Q,11-13

√4ᵗʰ **E08 Diabetes mellitus** due to underlying condition

Code first the underlying condition, such as:
congenital rubella (P35.0)
Cushing's syndrome (E24.-)
cystic fibrosis (E84.-)
malignant neoplasm (C00-C96)
malnutrition (E40-E46)
pancreatitis and other diseases of the pancreas (K85-K86.-)
Use additional code to identify control using:
insulin (Z79.4)
oral antidiabetic drugs (Z79.84)
oral hypoglycemic drugs (Z79.84)

`EXCLUDES 1` *drug or chemical induced diabetes mellitus (E09.-)*
gestational diabetes (O24.4-)
neonatal diabetes mellitus (P70.2)
postpancreatectomy diabetes mellitus (E13.-)
postprocedural diabetes mellitus (E13.-)
secondary diabetes mellitus NEC (E13.-)
type 1 diabetes mellitus (E10.-)
type 2 diabetes mellitus (E11.-)

AHA: 2013,4Q,114; 2013,3Q,20

CC Excl: For MCC codes in category E08: PDX collection 518

√5ᵗʰ **E08.0 Diabetes mellitus due to underlying condition with hyperosmolarity**

DEF: Diabetic hyperosmolarity: Extremely high levels of glucose in the blood without ketones.

E08.00 Diabetes mellitus due to underlying condition with hyperosmolarity without nonketotic hyperglycemic-hyperosmolar coma (NKHHC) `MCC` `H9` `HCC`

E08.01 Diabetes mellitus due to underlying condition with hyperosmolarity with coma `MCC` `H9` `HCC`

√5ᵗʰ **E08.1 Diabetes mellitus due to underlying condition with ketoacidosis**

DEF: Diabetic ketoacidosis: Potentially life-threatening complication due to a shortage of insulin in which the body switches to burning fatty acids and producing acidic ketone bodies.

E08.10 Diabetes mellitus due to underlying condition with ketoacidosis without coma `MCC` `H9` `HCC`

E08.11 Diabetes mellitus due to underlying condition with ketoacidosis with coma `MCC` `HCC`

√5ᵗʰ **E08.2 Diabetes mellitus due to underlying condition with kidney complications**

E08.21 Diabetes mellitus due to underlying condition with diabetic nephropathy `HCC`

Diabetes mellitus due to underlying condition with intercapillary glomerulosclerosis
Diabetes mellitus due to underlying condition with intracapillary glomerulonephrosis
Diabetes mellitus due to underlying condition with Kimmelstiel-Wilson disease

E08.22 Diabetes mellitus due to underlying condition with diabetic chronic kidney disease `HCC`

Use additional code to identify stage of chronic kidney disease (N18.1-N18.6)

E08.29 Diabetes mellitus due to underlying condition with other diabetic kidney complication `HCC`

Renal tubular degeneration in diabetes mellitus due to underlying condition

Ⓝ Newborn: 0   Ⓟ Pediatric: 0-17   Ⓜ Maternity: 9-64   Ⓐ Adult: 15-124   `MCC` Major Complication/Comorbidity   `CC` Complication/Comorbidity   `SW` Severe Wound Dx

518   ICD-10-CM 2020

√5ᵗʰ **E08.3 Diabetes mellitus due to underlying condition with ophthalmic complications**

One of the following 7th characters is to be assigned to codes in subcategories E08.32, E08.33, E08.34, E08.35, and E08.37 to designate laterality of the disease:
1   right eye
2   left eye
3   bilateral
9   unspecified eye

√6ᵗʰ **E08.31 Diabetes mellitus due to underlying condition with unspecified diabetic** retinopathy

DEF: Diabetic retinopathy: Diabetic complication from damage to the retinal vessels resulting in vision problems that can progress to blindness.

E08.311 Diabetes mellitus due to underlying condition with unspecified diabetic retinopathy with macular edema   HCC

E08.319 Diabetes mellitus due to underlying condition with unspecified diabetic retinopathy without macular edema   HCC

√6ᵗʰ **E08.32 Diabetes mellitus due to underlying condition with** mild nonproliferative **diabetic** retinopathy

Diabetes mellitus due to underlying condition with nonproliferative diabetic retinopathy NOS

√7ᵗʰ *E08.321 Diabetes mellitus due to underlying condition with mild nonproliferative diabetic retinopathy with macular edema*   HCC

√7ᵗʰ *E08.329 Diabetes mellitus due to underlying condition with mild nonproliferative diabetic retinopathy without macular edema*   HCC

√6ᵗʰ **E08.33 Diabetes mellitus due to underlying condition with** moderate nonproliferative diabetic retinopathy

√7ᵗʰ *E08.331 Diabetes mellitus due to underlying condition with moderate nonproliferative diabetic retinopathy with macular edema*   HCC

√7ᵗʰ *E08.339 Diabetes mellitus due to underlying condition with moderate nonproliferative diabetic retinopathy without macular edema*   HCC

√6ᵗʰ **E08.34 Diabetes mellitus due to underlying condition with** severe nonproliferative diabetic retinopathy

√7ᵗʰ *E08.341 Diabetes mellitus due to underlying condition with severe nonproliferative diabetic retinopathy with macular edema*   HCC

√7ᵗʰ *E08.349 Diabetes mellitus due to underlying condition with severe nonproliferative diabetic retinopathy without macular edema*   HCC

√6ᵗʰ **E08.35 Diabetes mellitus due to underlying condition with** proliferative diabetic retinopathy

√7ᵗʰ *E08.351 Diabetes mellitus due to underlying condition with proliferative diabetic retinopathy with macular edema*   HCC

√7ᵗʰ *E08.352 Diabetes mellitus due to underlying condition with proliferative diabetic retinopathy with traction retinal detachment involving the macula*   HCC

√7ᵗʰ *E08.353 Diabetes mellitus due to underlying condition with proliferative diabetic retinopathy with traction retinal detachment not involving the macula*   HCC

√7ᵗʰ *E08.354 Diabetes mellitus due to underlying condition with proliferative diabetic retinopathy with combined traction retinal detachment and rhegmatogenous retinal detachment*   HCC

√7ᵗʰ *E08.355 Diabetes mellitus due to underlying condition with stable proliferative diabetic retinopathy*   HCC

√7ᵗʰ *E08.359 Diabetes mellitus due to underlying condition with proliferative diabetic retinopathy without macular edema*   HCC

E08.36 Diabetes mellitus due to underlying condition with diabetic cataract   HCC

AHA: 2019,2Q,30-31; 2016,4Q,142

√x7ᵗʰ **E08.37 Diabetes mellitus due to underlying condition with diabetic** macular edema, resolved following treatment   HCC

E08.39 Diabetes mellitus due to underlying condition with other diabetic ophthalmic complication   HCC

Use additional code to identify manifestation, such as:
diabetic glaucoma (H40-H42)

√5ᵗʰ **E08.4 Diabetes mellitus due to underlying condition with** neurological complications

E08.40 Diabetes mellitus due to underlying condition with diabetic neuropathy, *unspecified*   HCC

E08.41 Diabetes mellitus due to underlying condition with diabetic mononeuropathy   HCC

E08.42 Diabetes mellitus due to underlying condition with diabetic polyneuropathy   HCC

Diabetes mellitus due to underlying condition with diabetic neuralgia

E08.43 Diabetes mellitus due to underlying condition with diabetic autonomic (poly)neuropathy   HCC

Diabetes mellitus due to underlying condition with diabetic gastroparesis

AHA: 2013,4Q,114

E08.44 Diabetes mellitus due to underlying condition with diabetic amyotrophy   HCC

E08.49 Diabetes mellitus due to underlying condition with other diabetic neurological complication   HCC

√5ᵗʰ **E08.5 Diabetes mellitus due to underlying condition with** circulatory complications

E08.51 Diabetes mellitus due to underlying condition with diabetic peripheral angiopathy without gangrene   HCC

AHA: 2018,2Q,7

E08.52 Diabetes mellitus due to underlying condition with diabetic peripheral angiopathy with gangrene   CC HCC

Diabetes mellitus due to underlying condition with diabetic gangrene

AHA: 2018,2Q,7; 2017,4Q,102

CC Excl: PDX collection 519

E08.59 Diabetes mellitus due to underlying condition with other circulatory complications   HCC

☑ Additional Character Required   √x7ᵗʰ Placeholder   Unacceptable PDx   Questionable PDx   Manifestation   Unspecified Dx   H1-H14 HAC   HCC CMS-HCC Dx   HIV HIV Dx

ICD-10-CM 2020

519

Chapter 4. Endocrine, Nutritional and Metabolic Diseases

E08.6–E09.311

✓5ᵗʰ **E08.6 Diabetes mellitus due to underlying condition with other specified complications**

✓6ᵗʰ **E08.61 Diabetes mellitus due to underlying condition with diabetic arthropathy**

E08.610 Diabetes mellitus due to underlying condition with diabetic neuropathic arthropathy HCC

Diabetes mellitus due to underlying condition with Charcôt's joints

DEF: Charcot's joint: Progressive neurologic arthropathy in which chronic degeneration of joints in the weight-bearing areas with peripheral hypertrophy occurs as a complication of a neuropathy disorder. Supporting structures relax from a loss of sensation resulting in chronic joint instability.

E08.618 Diabetes mellitus due to underlying condition with other diabetic arthropathy HCC

AHA: 2018,2Q,6

✓6ᵗʰ **E08.62 Diabetes mellitus due to underlying condition with skin complications**

E08.620 Diabetes mellitus due to underlying condition with diabetic dermatitis HCC

Diabetes mellitus due to underlying condition with diabetic necrobiosis lipoidica

E08.621 Diabetes mellitus due to underlying condition with foot ulcer HCC

Use additional code to identify site of ulcer (L97.4-, L97.5-)

E08.622 Diabetes mellitus due to underlying condition with other skin ulcer HCC

Use additional code to identify site of ulcer (L97.1-L97.9, L98.41-L98.49)

AHA: 2017,4Q,17

E08.628 Diabetes mellitus due to underlying condition with other skin complications HCC

AHA: 2017,4Q,100-101

✓6ᵗʰ **E08.63 Diabetes mellitus due to underlying condition with oral complications**

E08.630 Diabetes mellitus due to underlying condition with periodontal disease HCC

E08.638 Diabetes mellitus due to underlying condition with other oral complications HCC

✓6ᵗʰ **E08.64 Diabetes mellitus due to underlying condition with hypoglycemia**

E08.641 Diabetes mellitus due to underlying condition with hypoglycemia with coma MCC HCC

E08.649 Diabetes mellitus due to underlying condition with hypoglycemia without coma HCC

AHA: 2016,3Q,42; 2015,3Q,21

E08.65 Diabetes mellitus due to underlying condition with hyperglycemia HCC

E08.69 Diabetes mellitus due to underlying condition with other specified complication HCC

Use additional code to identify complication

AHA: 2016,4Q,141; 2016,1Q,13

E08.8 Diabetes mellitus due to underlying condition with unspecified complications HCC

E08.9 Diabetes mellitus due to underlying condition without complications HCC

✓4ᵗʰ **E09 Drug or chemical induced diabetes mellitus**

Code first poisoning due to drug or toxin, if applicable (T36-T65 with fifth or sixth character 1-4 or 6)

Use additional code for adverse effect, if applicable, to identify drug (T36-T50 with fifth or sixth character 5)

Use additional code to identify control using:

insulin (Z79.4)

oral antidiabetic drugs (Z79.84)

oral hypoglycemic drugs (Z79.84)

EXCLUDES 1 diabetes mellitus due to underlying condition (E08.-)

gestational diabetes (O24.4-)

neonatal diabetes mellitus (P70.2)

postpancreatectomy diabetes mellitus (E13.-)

postprocedural diabetes mellitus (E13.-)

secondary diabetes mellitus NEC (E13.-)

type 1 diabetes mellitus (E10.-)

type 2 diabetes mellitus (E11.-)

AHA: 2013,4Q,114; 2013,3Q,20

CC Excl: For MCC codes in category E09: PDX collection 518

✓5ᵗʰ **E09.0 Drug or chemical induced diabetes mellitus with hyperosmolarity**

DEF: Diabetic hyperosmolarity: Extremely high levels of glucose in the blood without ketones.

E09.00 Drug or chemical induced diabetes mellitus with hyperosmolarity without nonketotic hyperglycemic-hyperosmolar coma (NKHHC) MCC H9 HCC

E09.01 Drug or chemical induced diabetes mellitus with hyperosmolarity with coma MCC H9 HCC

✓5ᵗʰ **E09.1 Drug or chemical induced diabetes mellitus with ketoacidosis**

DEF: Diabetic ketoacidosis: Potentially life-threatening complication due to a shortage of insulin in which the body switches to burning fatty acids and producing acidic ketone bodies.

E09.10 Drug or chemical induced diabetes mellitus with ketoacidosis without coma MCC H9 HCC

E09.11 Drug or chemical induced diabetes mellitus with ketoacidosis with coma MCC HCC

✓5ᵗʰ **E09.2 Drug or chemical induced diabetes mellitus with kidney complications**

E09.21 Drug or chemical induced diabetes mellitus with diabetic nephropathy HCC

Drug or chemical induced diabetes mellitus with intercapillary glomerulosclerosis

Drug or chemical induced diabetes mellitus with intracapillary glomerulonephrosis

Drug or chemical induced diabetes mellitus with Kimmelstiel-Wilson disease

E09.22 Drug or chemical induced diabetes mellitus with diabetic chronic kidney disease HCC

Use additional code to identify stage of chronic kidney disease (N18.1-N18.6)

E09.29 Drug or chemical induced diabetes mellitus with other diabetic kidney complication HCC

Drug or chemical induced diabetes mellitus with renal tubular degeneration

✓5ᵗʰ **E09.3 Drug or chemical induced diabetes mellitus with ophthalmic complications**

One of the following 7th characters is to be assigned to codes in subcategories E09.32, E09.33, E09.34, E09.35, and E09.37 to designate laterality of the disease:

1   right eye

2   left eye

3   bilateral

9   unspecified eye

✓6ᵗʰ **E09.31 Drug or chemical induced diabetes mellitus with unspecified diabetic retinopathy**

DEF: Diabetic retinopathy: Diabetic complication from damage to the retinal vessels resulting in vision problems that can progress to blindness.

E09.311 Drug or chemical induced diabetes mellitus with unspecified diabetic retinopathy with macular edema HCC

N Newborn: 0   P Pediatric: 0-17   M Maternity: 9-64   A Adult: 15-124   MCC Major Complication/Comorbidity   CC Complication/Comorbidity   SW Severe Wound Dx

520   ICD-10-CM 2020

E09.319 Drug or chemical induced diabetes mellitus with unspecified diabetic retinopathy without macular edema   HCC

√6ᵗʰ **E09.32** Drug or chemical induced diabetes mellitus with mild nonproliferative diabetic retinopathy
Drug or chemical induced diabetes mellitus with nonproliferative diabetic retinopathy NOS

√7ᵗʰ **E09.321** Drug or chemical induced diabetes mellitus with mild nonproliferative diabetic retinopathy with macular edema   HCC

√7ᵗʰ **E09.329** Drug or chemical induced diabetes mellitus with mild nonproliferative diabetic retinopathy without macular edema   HCC

√6ᵗʰ **E09.33** Drug or chemical induced diabetes mellitus with moderate nonproliferative diabetic retinopathy

√7ᵗʰ **E09.331** Drug or chemical induced diabetes mellitus with moderate nonproliferative diabetic retinopathy with macular edema   HCC

√7ᵗʰ **E09.339** Drug or chemical induced diabetes mellitus with moderate nonproliferative diabetic retinopathy without macular edema   HCC

√6ᵗʰ **E09.34** Drug or chemical induced diabetes mellitus with severe nonproliferative diabetic retinopathy

√7ᵗʰ **E09.341** Drug or chemical induced diabetes mellitus with severe nonproliferative diabetic retinopathy with macular edema   HCC

√7ᵗʰ **E09.349** Drug or chemical induced diabetes mellitus with severe nonproliferative diabetic retinopathy without macular edema   HCC

√6ᵗʰ **E09.35** Drug or chemical induced diabetes mellitus with proliferative diabetic retinopathy

√7ᵗʰ **E09.351** Drug or chemical induced diabetes mellitus with proliferative diabetic retinopathy with macular edema   HCC

√7ᵗʰ **E09.352** Drug or chemical induced diabetes mellitus with proliferative diabetic retinopathy with traction retinal detachment involving the macula   HCC

√7ᵗʰ **E09.353** Drug or chemical induced diabetes mellitus with proliferative diabetic retinopathy with traction retinal detachment not involving the macula   HCC

√7ᵗʰ **E09.354** Drug or chemical induced diabetes mellitus with proliferative diabetic retinopathy with combined traction retinal detachment and rhegmatogenous retinal detachment   HCC

√7ᵗʰ **E09.355** Drug or chemical induced diabetes mellitus with stable proliferative diabetic retinopathy   HCC

√7ᵗʰ **E09.359** Drug or chemical induced diabetes mellitus with proliferative diabetic retinopathy without macular edema   HCC

E09.36 Drug or chemical induced diabetes mellitus with diabetic cataract   HCC
AHA: 2019,2Q,30-31; 2016,4Q,142

√x7ᵗʰ **E09.37** Drug or chemical induced diabetes mellitus with diabetic macular edema, resolved following treatment   HCC

E09.39 Drug or chemical induced diabetes mellitus with other diabetic ophthalmic complication   HCC
Use additional code to identify manifestation, such as:
diabetic glaucoma (H40-H42)

√5ᵗʰ **E09.4** Drug or chemical induced diabetes mellitus with neurological complications

E09.40 Drug or chemical induced diabetes mellitus with neurological complications with diabetic neuropathy, unspecified   HCC

E09.41 Drug or chemical induced diabetes mellitus with neurological complications with diabetic mononeuropathy   HCC

E09.42 Drug or chemical induced diabetes mellitus with neurological complications with diabetic polyneuropathy   HCC
Drug or chemical induced diabetes mellitus with diabetic neuralgia

E09.43 Drug or chemical induced diabetes mellitus with neurological complications with diabetic autonomic (poly)neuropathy   HCC
Drug or chemical induced diabetes mellitus with diabetic gastroparesis
AHA: 2013,4Q,114

E09.44 Drug or chemical induced diabetes mellitus with neurological complications with diabetic amyotrophy   HCC

E09.49 Drug or chemical induced diabetes mellitus with neurological complications with other diabetic neurological complication   HCC

√5ᵗʰ **E09.5** Drug or chemical induced diabetes mellitus with circulatory complications

E09.51 Drug or chemical induced diabetes mellitus with diabetic peripheral angiopathy without gangrene   HCC
AHA: 2018,2Q,7

E09.52 Drug or chemical induced diabetes mellitus with diabetic peripheral angiopathy with gangrene   CC   HCC
Drug or chemical induced diabetes mellitus with diabetic gangrene
AHA: 2018,2Q,7; 2017,4Q,102
CC Excl: PDX collection 519

E09.59 Drug or chemical induced diabetes mellitus with other circulatory complications   HCC

√5ᵗʰ **E09.6** Drug or chemical induced diabetes mellitus with other specified complications

√6ᵗʰ **E09.61** Drug or chemical induced diabetes mellitus with diabetic arthropathy

E09.610 Drug or chemical induced diabetes mellitus with diabetic neuropathic arthropathy   HCC
Drug or chemical induced diabetes mellitus with Charcôt's joints
DEF: Charcot's joint: Progressive neurologic arthropathy in which chronic degeneration of joints in the weight-bearing areas with peripheral hypertrophy occurs as a complication of a neuropathy disorder. Supporting structures relax from a loss of sensation resulting in chronic joint instability.

E09.618 Drug or chemical induced diabetes mellitus with other diabetic arthropathy   HCC
AHA: 2018,2Q,6

✓6ᵗʰ **E09.62 Drug or chemical induced diabetes mellitus with skin complications**

    E09.620 Drug or chemical induced diabetes mellitus with diabetic dermatitis HCC
       Drug or chemical induced diabetes mellitus with diabetic necrobiosis lipoidica

    E09.621 Drug or chemical induced diabetes mellitus with foot ulcer HCC
       Use additional code to identify site of ulcer (L97.4-, L97.5-)

    E09.622 Drug or chemical induced diabetes mellitus with other skin ulcer HCC
       Use additional code to identify site of ulcer (L97.1-L97.9, L98.41-L98.49)
       AHA: 2017,4Q,17

    E09.628 Drug or chemical induced diabetes mellitus with other skin complications HCC
       AHA: 2017,4Q,100-101

✓6ᵗʰ **E09.63 Drug or chemical induced diabetes mellitus with oral complications**

    E09.630 Drug or chemical induced diabetes mellitus with periodontal disease HCC

    E09.638 Drug or chemical induced diabetes mellitus with other oral complications HCC

✓6ᵗʰ **E09.64 Drug or chemical induced diabetes mellitus with hypoglycemia**

    E09.641 Drug or chemical induced diabetes mellitus with hypoglycemia with coma MCC HCC

    E09.649 Drug or chemical induced diabetes mellitus with hypoglycemia without coma HCC
       AHA: 2016,3Q,42; 2015,3Q,21

E09.65 Drug or chemical induced diabetes mellitus with hyperglycemia CC HCC

E09.69 Drug or chemical induced diabetes mellitus with other specified complication CC HCC
    Use additional code to identify complication
    AHA: 2016,4Q,141; 2016,1Q,13

E09.8 Drug or chemical induced diabetes mellitus with unspecified complications CC HCC

E09.9 Drug or chemical induced diabetes mellitus without complications CC HCC

✓4ᵗʰ **E10 Type 1 diabetes mellitus**

INCLUDES   brittle diabetes (mellitus)
    diabetes (mellitus) due to autoimmune process
    diabetes (mellitus) due to immune mediated pancreatic islet beta-cell destruction
    idiopathic diabetes (mellitus)
    juvenile onset diabetes (mellitus)
    ketosis-prone diabetes (mellitus)

EXCLUDES 1   *diabetes mellitus due to underlying condition (E08.-)*
    drug or chemical induced diabetes mellitus (E09.-)
    gestational diabetes (O24.4-)
    hyperglycemia NOS (R73.9)
    neonatal diabetes mellitus (P70.2)
    postpancreatectomy diabetes mellitus (E13.-)
    postprocedural diabetes mellitus (E13.-)
    secondary diabetes mellitus NEC (E13.-)
    type 2 diabetes mellitus (E11.-)

AHA: 2013,4Q,114; 2013,3Q,20
CC Excl: For MCC codes in category E10: PDX collection 520

✓5ᵗʰ **E10.1 Type 1 diabetes mellitus with ketoacidosis**
    AHA: 2013,3Q,20
    DEF: Diabetic ketoacidosis: Potentially life-threatening complication due to a shortage of insulin in which the body switches to burning fatty acids and producing acidic ketone bodies.

    E10.10 Type 1 diabetes mellitus with ketoacidosis without coma MCC H9 HCC

E10.11 Type 1 diabetes mellitus with ketoacidosis with coma MCC HCC

✓5ᵗʰ **E10.2 Type 1 diabetes mellitus with kidney complications**

    E10.21 Type 1 diabetes mellitus with diabetic nephropathy HCC
       Type 1 diabetes mellitus with intercapillary glomerulosclerosis
       Type 1 diabetes mellitus with intracapillary glomerulonephrosis
       Type 1 diabetes mellitus with Kimmelstiel-Wilson disease

    E10.22 Type 1 diabetes mellitus with diabetic chronic kidney disease HCC
       Use additional code to identify stage of chronic kidney disease (N18.1-N18.6)

    E10.29 Type 1 diabetes mellitus with other diabetic kidney complication HCC
       Type 1 diabetes mellitus with renal tubular degeneration
       AHA: 2016,1Q,13

✓5ᵗʰ **E10.3 Type 1 diabetes mellitus with ophthalmic complications**

> One of the following 7th characters is to be assigned to codes in subcategories E10.32, E10.33, E10.34, E10.35, and E10.37 to designate laterality of the disease:
> 1   right eye
> 2   left eye
> 3   bilateral
> 9   unspecified eye

✓6ᵗʰ **E10.31 Type 1 diabetes mellitus with unspecified diabetic retinopathy**
    DEF: Diabetic retinopathy: Diabetic complication from damage to the retinal vessels resulting in vision problems that can progress to blindness.

    E10.311 Type 1 diabetes mellitus with unspecified diabetic retinopathy with macular edema HCC

    E10.319 Type 1 diabetes mellitus with unspecified diabetic retinopathy without macular edema HCC

✓6ᵗʰ **E10.32 Type 1 diabetes mellitus with mild nonproliferative diabetic retinopathy**
    Type 1 diabetes mellitus with nonproliferative diabetic retinopathy NOS

    ✓7ᵗʰ **E10.321 Type 1 diabetes mellitus with mild nonproliferative diabetic retinopathy with macular edema** HCC

    ✓7ᵗʰ **E10.329 Type 1 diabetes mellitus with mild nonproliferative diabetic retinopathy without macular edema** HCC

✓6ᵗʰ **E10.33 Type 1 diabetes mellitus with moderate nonproliferative diabetic retinopathy**

    ✓7ᵗʰ **E10.331 Type 1 diabetes mellitus with moderate nonproliferative diabetic retinopathy with macular edema** HCC

    ✓7ᵗʰ **E10.339 Type 1 diabetes mellitus with moderate nonproliferative diabetic retinopathy without macular edema** HCC

✓6ᵗʰ **E10.34 Type 1 diabetes mellitus with severe nonproliferative diabetic retinopathy**

    ✓7ᵗʰ **E10.341 Type 1 diabetes mellitus with severe nonproliferative diabetic retinopathy with macular edema** HCC

    ✓7ᵗʰ **E10.349 Type 1 diabetes mellitus with severe nonproliferative diabetic retinopathy without macular edema** HCC

✓6ᵗʰ **E10.35** **Type 1 diabetes mellitus with proliferative diabetic retinopathy**

✓7ᵗʰ **E10.351** **Type 1 diabetes mellitus with proliferative diabetic retinopathy with macular edema**　HCC

✓7ᵗʰ **E10.352** **Type 1 diabetes mellitus with proliferative diabetic retinopathy with traction retinal detachment involving the macula**　HCC

✓7ᵗʰ **E10.353** **Type 1 diabetes mellitus with proliferative diabetic retinopathy with traction retinal detachment not involving the macula**　HCC

✓7ᵗʰ **E10.354** **Type 1 diabetes mellitus with proliferative diabetic retinopathy with combined traction retinal detachment and rhegmatogenous retinal detachment**　HCC

✓7ᵗʰ **E10.355** **Type 1 diabetes mellitus with stable proliferative diabetic retinopathy**　HCC

✓7ᵗʰ **E10.359** **Type 1 diabetes mellitus with proliferative diabetic retinopathy without macular edema**　HCC

E10.36 **Type 1 diabetes mellitus with diabetic cataract**　HCC
AHA: 2019,2Q,30-31; 2016,4Q,142

✓x 7ᵗʰ **E10.37** **Type 1 diabetes mellitus with diabetic macular edema, resolved following treatment**　HCC

E10.39 **Type 1 diabetes mellitus with other diabetic ophthalmic complication**　HCC
Use additional code to identify manifestation, such as:
diabetic glaucoma (H40-H42)

✓5ᵗʰ **E10.4** **Type 1 diabetes mellitus with neurological complications**

E10.40 **Type 1 diabetes mellitus with diabetic neuropathy, unspecified**　HCC

E10.41 **Type 1 diabetes mellitus with diabetic mononeuropathy**　HCC

E10.42 **Type 1 diabetes mellitus with diabetic polyneuropathy**　HCC
Type 1 diabetes mellitus with diabetic neuralgia

E10.43 **Type 1 diabetes mellitus with diabetic autonomic (poly)neuropathy**　HCC
Type 1 diabetes mellitus with diabetic gastroparesis
AHA: 2013,4Q,114

E10.44 **Type 1 diabetes mellitus with diabetic amyotrophy**　HCC

E10.49 **Type 1 diabetes mellitus with other diabetic neurological complication**　HCC

✓5ᵗʰ **E10.5** **Type 1 diabetes mellitus with circulatory complications**

E10.51 **Type 1 diabetes mellitus with diabetic peripheral angiopathy without gangrene**　HCC
AHA: 2018,2Q,7

E10.52 **Type 1 diabetes mellitus with diabetic peripheral angiopathy with gangrene**　CC　HCC
Type 1 diabetes mellitus with diabetic gangrene
AHA: 2018,2Q,7; 2017,4Q,102
CC Excl: PDX collection 519

E10.59 **Type 1 diabetes mellitus with other circulatory complications**　HCC

✓5ᵗʰ **E10.6** **Type 1 diabetes mellitus with other specified complications**

✓6ᵗʰ **E10.61** **Type 1 diabetes mellitus with diabetic arthropathy**

E10.610 **Type 1 diabetes mellitus with diabetic neuropathic arthropathy**　HCC
Type 1 diabetes mellitus with Charcôt's joints
DEF: Charcot's joint: Progressive neurologic arthropathy in which chronic degeneration of joints in the weight-bearing areas with peripheral hypertrophy occurs as a complication of a neuropathy disorder. Supporting structures relax from a loss of sensation resulting in chronic joint instability.

E10.618 **Type 1 diabetes mellitus with other diabetic arthropathy**　HCC
AHA: 2018,2Q,6

✓6ᵗʰ **E10.62** **Type 1 diabetes mellitus with skin complications**

E10.620 **Type 1 diabetes mellitus with diabetic dermatitis**　HCC
Type 1 diabetes mellitus with diabetic necrobiosis lipoidica

E10.621 **Type 1 diabetes mellitus with foot ulcer**　HCC
Use additional code to identify site of ulcer (L97.4-, L97.5-)

E10.622 **Type 1 diabetes mellitus with other skin ulcer**　HCC
Use additional code to identify site of ulcer (L97.1-L97.9, L98.41-L98.49)
AHA: 2017,4Q,17

E10.628 **Type 1 diabetes mellitus with other skin complications**　HCC
AHA: 2017,4Q,100-101

✓6ᵗʰ **E10.63** **Type 1 diabetes mellitus with oral complications**

E10.630 **Type 1 diabetes mellitus with periodontal disease**　HCC

E10.638 **Type 1 diabetes mellitus with other oral complications**　HCC

✓6ᵗʰ **E10.64** **Type 1 diabetes mellitus with hypoglycemia**

E10.641 **Type 1 diabetes mellitus with hypoglycemia with coma**　MCC　HCC

E10.649 **Type 1 diabetes mellitus with hypoglycemia without coma**　HCC
AHA: 2016,3Q,42; 2016,1Q,13; 2015,3Q,21

E10.65 **Type 1 diabetes mellitus with hyperglycemia**　HCC
AHA: 2013,3Q,20

E10.69 **Type 1 diabetes mellitus with other specified complication**　HCC
Use additional code to identify complication
AHA: 2016,4Q,141; 2016,1Q,13

E10.8 **Type 1 diabetes mellitus with unspecified complications**　HCC

E10.9 **Type 1 diabetes mellitus without complications**　HCC

✓4th **E11 Type 2 diabetes mellitus**

INCLUDES   diabetes (mellitus) due to insulin secretory defect

diabetes NOS

insulin resistant diabetes (mellitus)

Use additional code to identify control using:

insulin (Z79.4)

oral antidiabetic drugs (Z79.84)

oral hypoglycemic drugs (Z79.84)

EXCLUDES 1   *diabetes mellitus due to underlying condition (E08.-)*

drug or chemical induced diabetes mellitus (E09.-)

gestational diabetes (O24.4-)

neonatal diabetes mellitus (P70.2)

postpancreatectomy diabetes mellitus (E13.-)

postprocedural diabetes mellitus (E13.-)

secondary diabetes mellitus NEC (E13.-)

type 1 diabetes mellitus (E10.-)

AHA: 2016,2Q,10; 2013,4Q,114; 2013,3Q,20; 2013,1Q,26

CC Excl: For MCC codes in category E11: PDX collection 518

✓5th **E11.0 Type 2 diabetes mellitus with hyperosmolarity**

DEF: Diabetic hyperosmolarity: Extremely high levels of glucose in the blood without ketones.

E11.00 Type 2 diabetes mellitus with hyperosmolarity without nonketotic hyperglycemic-hyperosmolar coma (NKHHC)   H9   HCC

E11.01 Type 2 diabetes mellitus with hyperosmolarity with coma   MCC   H9   HCC

✓5th **E11.1 Type 2 diabetes mellitus with ketoacidosis**

DEF: Diabetic ketoacidosis: Potentially life-threatening complication due to a shortage of insulin in which the body switches to burning fatty acids and producing acidic ketone bodies.

E11.10 Type 2 diabetes mellitus with ketoacidosis without coma   MCC   HCC

E11.11 Type 2 diabetes mellitus with ketoacidosis with coma   MCC   HCC

✓5th **E11.2 Type 2 diabetes mellitus with kidney complications**

E11.21 Type 2 diabetes mellitus with diabetic nephropathy   HCC

Type 2 diabetes mellitus with intercapillary glomerulosclerosis

Type 2 diabetes mellitus with intracapillary glomerulonephrosis

Type 2 diabetes mellitus with Kimmelstiel-Wilson disease

E11.22 Type 2 diabetes mellitus with diabetic chronic kidney disease   HCC

Use additional code to identify stage of chronic kidney disease (N18.1-N18.6)

AHA: 2016,1Q,12

E11.29 Type 2 diabetes mellitus with other diabetic kidney complication   HCC

Type 2 diabetes mellitus with renal tubular degeneration

✓5th **E11.3 Type 2 diabetes mellitus with ophthalmic complications**

One of the following 7th characters is to be assigned to codes in subcategories E11.32, E11.33, E11.34, E11.35, and E11.37 to designate laterality of the disease:

1   right eye

2   left eye

3   bilateral

9   unspecified eye

✓6th **E11.31 Type 2 diabetes mellitus with unspecified diabetic retinopathy**

DEF: Diabetic retinopathy: Diabetic complication from damage to the retinal vessels resulting in vision problems that can progress to blindness.

E11.311 Type 2 diabetes mellitus with unspecified diabetic retinopathy with macular edema   HCC

E11.319 Type 2 diabetes mellitus with unspecified diabetic retinopathy without macular edema   HCC

✓6th **E11.32 Type 2 diabetes mellitus with mild nonproliferative diabetic retinopathy**

Type 2 diabetes mellitus with nonproliferative diabetic retinopathy NOS

✓7th **E11.321 Type 2 diabetes mellitus with mild nonproliferative diabetic retinopathy with macular edema**   HCC

✓7th **E11.329 Type 2 diabetes mellitus with mild nonproliferative diabetic retinopathy without macular edema**   HCC

✓6th **E11.33 Type 2 diabetes mellitus with moderate nonproliferative diabetic retinopathy**

✓7th **E11.331 Type 2 diabetes mellitus with moderate nonproliferative diabetic retinopathy with macular edema**   HCC

✓7th **E11.339 Type 2 diabetes mellitus with moderate nonproliferative diabetic retinopathy without macular edema**   HCC

✓6th **E11.34 Type 2 diabetes mellitus with severe nonproliferative diabetic retinopathy**

✓7th **E11.341 Type 2 diabetes mellitus with severe nonproliferative diabetic retinopathy with macular edema**   HCC

✓7th **E11.349 Type 2 diabetes mellitus with severe nonproliferative diabetic retinopathy without macular edema**   HCC

✓6th **E11.35 Type 2 diabetes mellitus with proliferative diabetic retinopathy**

✓7th **E11.351 Type 2 diabetes mellitus with proliferative diabetic retinopathy with macular edema**   HCC

✓7th **E11.352 Type 2 diabetes mellitus with proliferative diabetic retinopathy with traction retinal detachment involving the macula**   HCC

✓7th **E11.353 Type 2 diabetes mellitus with proliferative diabetic retinopathy with traction retinal detachment not involving the macula**   HCC

✓7th **E11.354 Type 2 diabetes mellitus with proliferative diabetic retinopathy with combined traction retinal detachment and rhegmatogenous retinal detachment**   HCC

✓7th **E11.355 Type 2 diabetes mellitus with stable proliferative diabetic retinopathy**   HCC

✓7th **E11.359 Type 2 diabetes mellitus with proliferative diabetic retinopathy without macular edema**   HCC

E11.36 Type 2 diabetes mellitus with diabetic cataract   HCC

AHA: 2019,2Q,30-31; 2016,4Q,142

✓x7th **E11.37 Type 2 diabetes mellitus with diabetic macular edema, resolved following treatment**   HCC

E11.39 Type 2 diabetes mellitus with other diabetic ophthalmic complication   HCC

Use additional code to identify manifestation, such as:

diabetic glaucoma (H40-H42)

✓5th **E11.4 Type 2 diabetes mellitus with neurological complications**

E11.40 Type 2 diabetes mellitus with diabetic neuropathy, unspecified   HCC

AHA: 2013,4Q,129

E11.41 Type 2 diabetes mellitus with diabetic mononeuropathy   HCC

N Newborn: 0   P Pediatric: 0-17   M Maternity: 9-64   A Adult: 15-124   MCC Major Complication/Comorbidity   CC Complication/Comorbidity   SW Severe Wound Dx

524   ICD-10-CM 2020

E11.42   **Type 2 diabetes mellitus with diabetic polyneuropathy**   `HCC`
Type 2 diabetes mellitus with diabetic neuralgia
AHA: 2016,1Q,12

E11.43   **Type 2 diabetes mellitus with diabetic autonomic (poly)neuropathy**   `HCC`
Type 2 diabetes mellitus with diabetic gastroparesis
AHA: 2013,4Q,114

E11.44   **Type 2 diabetes mellitus with diabetic amyotrophy**   `HCC`

E11.49   **Type 2 diabetes mellitus with other diabetic neurological complication**   `HCC`

√5th **E11.5**   **Type 2 diabetes mellitus with circulatory complications**

E11.51   **Type 2 diabetes mellitus with diabetic peripheral angiopathy without gangrene**   `HCC`
AHA: 2018,2Q,7

E11.52   **Type 2 diabetes mellitus with diabetic peripheral angiopathy with gangrene**   `CC` `HCC`
Type 2 diabetes mellitus with diabetic gangrene
AHA: 2018,2Q,7; 2017,4Q,102
CC Excl: PDX collection 519

E11.59   **Type 2 diabetes mellitus with other circulatory complications**   `HCC`

√5th **E11.6**   **Type 2 diabetes mellitus with other specified complications**

√6th **E11.61**   **Type 2 diabetes mellitus with diabetic arthropathy**

E11.610   **Type 2 diabetes mellitus with diabetic neuropathic arthropathy**   `HCC`
Type 2 diabetes mellitus with Charcôt's joints
DEF: Charcot's joint: Progressive neurologic arthropathy in which chronic degeneration of joints in the weight-bearing areas with peripheral hypertrophy occurs as a complication of a neuropathy disorder. Supporting structures relax from a loss of sensation resulting in chronic joint instability.

E11.618   **Type 2 diabetes mellitus with other diabetic arthropathy**   `HCC`
AHA: 2018,2Q,6

√6th **E11.62**   **Type 2 diabetes mellitus with skin complications**

E11.620   **Type 2 diabetes mellitus with diabetic dermatitis**   `HCC`
Type 2 diabetes mellitus with diabetic necrobiosis lipoidica

E11.621   **Type 2 diabetes mellitus with foot ulcer**   `HCC`
Use additional code to identify site of ulcer (L97.4-, L97.5-)
AHA: 2016,1Q,12

E11.622   **Type 2 diabetes mellitus with other skin ulcer**   `HCC`
Use additional code to identify site of ulcer (L97.1-L97.9, L98.41-L98.49)
AHA: 2017,4Q,17

E11.628   **Type 2 diabetes mellitus with other skin complications**   `HCC`
AHA: 2017,4Q,100-101

√6th **E11.63**   **Type 2 diabetes mellitus with oral complications**

E11.630   **Type 2 diabetes mellitus with periodontal disease**   `HCC`

E11.638   **Type 2 diabetes mellitus with other oral complications**   `HCC`

√6th **E11.64**   **Type 2 diabetes mellitus with hypoglycemia**

E11.641   **Type 2 diabetes mellitus with hypoglycemia with coma**   `MCC` `HCC`

E11.649   **Type 2 diabetes mellitus with hypoglycemia without coma**   `HCC`
AHA: 2016,3Q,42; 2015,3Q,21

E11.65   **Type 2 diabetes mellitus with hyperglycemia**   `HCC`
AHA: 2013,3Q,20

E11.69   **Type 2 diabetes mellitus with other specified complication**   `HCC`
Use additional code to identify complication
AHA: 2016,4Q,141; 2016,1Q,13

E11.8   **Type 2 diabetes mellitus with unspecified complications**   `HCC`

E11.9   **Type 2 diabetes mellitus without complications**   `HCC`

√4th **E13**   **Other specified diabetes mellitus**

`INCLUDES`   diabetes mellitus due to genetic defects of beta-cell function
diabetes mellitus due to genetic defects in insulin action
postpancreatectomy diabetes mellitus
postprocedural diabetes mellitus
secondary diabetes mellitus NEC
Use additional code to identify control using:
insulin (Z79.4)
oral antidiabetic drugs (Z79.84)
oral hypoglycemic drugs (Z79.84)

`EXCLUDES 1`   *diabetes (mellitus) due to autoimmune process (E10.-)*
diabetes (mellitus) due to immune mediated pancreatic islet beta-cell destruction (E10.-)
diabetes mellitus due to underlying condition (E08.-)
drug or chemical induced diabetes mellitus (E09.-)
gestational diabetes (O24.4-)
neonatal diabetes mellitus (P70.2)
type 1 diabetes mellitus (E10.-)

AHA: 2018,3Q,4; 2016,1Q,11-13; 2013,4Q,114; 2013,3Q,20
TIP: Use this category when the diabetes is documented as diabetes type 1.5. Synonymous terms used in the documentation may also include combined diabetes type 1 and type 2, latent autoimmune diabetes of adults (LADA), slow-progressing type 1 diabetes, or double diabetes.
TIP: When postprocedural or postpancreatectomy hypoinsulinemia (E89.1) is documented with postprocedural or postpancreatectomy diabetes mellitus (E13.-), code E89.1 should be sequenced first.
CC Excl: For MCC codes in category E13: PDX collection 518

√5th **E13.0**   **Other specified diabetes mellitus with hyperosmolarity**
DEF: Diabetic hyperosmolarity: Extremely high levels of glucose in the blood without ketones.

E13.00   **Other specified diabetes mellitus with hyperosmolarity without nonketotic hyperglycemic-hyperosmolar coma (NKHHC)**   `MCC` `H9` `HCC`
`EXCLUDES 2`   *type 2 diabetes mellitus (E11.-)*

E13.01   **Other specified diabetes mellitus with hyperosmolarity with coma**   `MCC` `H9` `HCC`

√5th **E13.1**   **Other specified diabetes mellitus with ketoacidosis**
AHA: 2016,2Q,10; 2013,1Q,26
DEF: Diabetic ketoacidosis: Potentially life-threatening complication due to a shortage of insulin in which the body switches to burning fatty acids and producing acidic ketone bodies.

E13.10   **Other specified diabetes mellitus with ketoacidosis without coma**   `MCC` `H9` `HCC`

E13.11   **Other specified diabetes mellitus with ketoacidosis with coma**   `MCC` `HCC`

√5th **E13.2**   **Other specified diabetes mellitus with kidney complications**

E13.21   **Other specified diabetes mellitus with diabetic nephropathy**   `HCC`
Other specified diabetes mellitus with intercapillary glomerulosclerosis
Other specified diabetes mellitus with intracapillary glomerulonephrosis
Other specified diabetes mellitus with Kimmelstiel-Wilson disease

E13.22   **Other specified diabetes mellitus with diabetic chronic kidney disease**   `HCC`
Use additional code to identify stage of chronic kidney disease (N18.1-N18.6)

E13.29   **Other specified diabetes mellitus with other diabetic kidney complication**   `HCC`
Other specified diabetes mellitus with renal tubular degeneration

✓5ᵗʰ E13.3 Other specified diabetes mellitus with ophthalmic complications

One of the following 7th characters is to be assigned to codes in subcategories E13.32, E13.33, E13.34, E13.35, and E13.37 to designate laterality of the disease:
1   right eye
2   left eye
3   bilateral
9   unspecified eye

✓6ᵗʰ E13.31 Other specified diabetes mellitus with unspecified diabetic retinopathy

DEF: Diabetic retinopathy: Diabetic complication from damage to the retinal vessels resulting in vision problems that can progress to blindness.

E13.311 Other specified diabetes mellitus with unspecified diabetic retinopathy with macular edema HCC

E13.319 Other specified diabetes mellitus with unspecified diabetic retinopathy without macular edema HCC

✓6ᵗʰ E13.32 Other specified diabetes mellitus with mild nonproliferative diabetic retinopathy

Other specified diabetes mellitus with nonproliferative diabetic retinopathy NOS

✓7ᵗʰ E13.321 Other specified diabetes mellitus with mild nonproliferative diabetic retinopathy with macular edema HCC

✓7ᵗʰ E13.329 Other specified diabetes mellitus with mild nonproliferative diabetic retinopathy without macular edema HCC

✓6ᵗʰ E13.33 Other specified diabetes mellitus with moderate nonproliferative diabetic retinopathy

✓7ᵗʰ E13.331 Other specified diabetes mellitus with moderate nonproliferative diabetic retinopathy with macular edema HCC

✓7ᵗʰ E13.339 Other specified diabetes mellitus with moderate nonproliferative diabetic retinopathy without macular edema HCC

✓6ᵗʰ E13.34 Other specified diabetes mellitus with severe nonproliferative diabetic retinopathy

✓7ᵗʰ E13.341 Other specified diabetes mellitus with severe nonproliferative diabetic retinopathy with macular edema HCC

✓7ᵗʰ E13.349 Other specified diabetes mellitus with severe nonproliferative diabetic retinopathy without macular edema HCC

✓6ᵗʰ E13.35 Other specified diabetes mellitus with proliferative diabetic retinopathy

✓7ᵗʰ E13.351 Other specified diabetes mellitus with proliferative diabetic retinopathy with macular edema HCC

✓7ᵗʰ E13.352 Other specified diabetes mellitus with proliferative diabetic retinopathy with traction retinal detachment involving the macula HCC

✓7ᵗʰ E13.353 Other specified diabetes mellitus with proliferative diabetic retinopathy with traction retinal detachment not involving the macula HCC

✓7ᵗʰ E13.354 Other specified diabetes mellitus with proliferative diabetic retinopathy with combined traction retinal detachment and rhegmatogenous retinal detachment HCC

✓7ᵗʰ E13.355 Other specified diabetes mellitus with stable proliferative diabetic retinopathy HCC

✓7ᵗʰ E13.359 Other specified diabetes mellitus with proliferative diabetic retinopathy without macular edema HCC

E13.36 Other specified diabetes mellitus with diabetic cataract HCC

AHA: 2019,2Q,30-31; 2016,4Q,142

✓x7ᵗʰ E13.37 Other specified diabetes mellitus with diabetic macular edema, resolved following treatment HCC

E13.39 Other specified diabetes mellitus with other diabetic ophthalmic complication HCC

Use additional code to identify manifestation, such as:

diabetic glaucoma (H40-H42)

✓5ᵗʰ E13.4 Other specified diabetes mellitus with neurological complications

E13.40 Other specified diabetes mellitus with diabetic neuropathy, unspecified HCC

E13.41 Other specified diabetes mellitus with diabetic mononeuropathy HCC

E13.42 Other specified diabetes mellitus with diabetic polyneuropathy HCC

Other specified diabetes mellitus with diabetic neuralgia

E13.43 Other specified diabetes mellitus with diabetic autonomic (poly)neuropathy HCC

Other specified diabetes mellitus with diabetic gastroparesis

AHA: 2013,4Q,114

E13.44 Other specified diabetes mellitus with diabetic amyotrophy HCC

E13.49 Other specified diabetes mellitus with other diabetic neurological complication HCC

✓5ᵗʰ E13.5 Other specified diabetes mellitus with circulatory complications

E13.51 Other specified diabetes mellitus with diabetic peripheral angiopathy without gangrene HCC

AHA: 2018,2Q,7

E13.52 Other specified diabetes mellitus with diabetic peripheral angiopathy with gangrene CC HCC

Other specified diabetes mellitus with diabetic gangrene

AHA: 2018,2Q,7; 2017,4Q,102
CC Excl: PDX collection 519

E13.59 Other specified diabetes mellitus with other circulatory complications HCC

✓5ᵗʰ E13.6 Other specified diabetes mellitus with other specified complications

✓6ᵗʰ E13.61 Other specified diabetes mellitus with diabetic arthropathy

E13.610 Other specified diabetes mellitus with diabetic neuropathic arthropathy HCC

Other specified diabetes mellitus with Charcôt's joints

DEF: Charcôt's joint: Progressive neurologic arthropathy in which chronic degeneration of joints in the weight-bearing areas with peripheral hypertrophy occurs as a complication of a neuropathy disorder. Supporting structures relax from a loss of sensation resulting in chronic joint instability.

E13.618 Other specified diabetes mellitus with other diabetic arthropathy HCC

AHA: 2018,2Q,6

N Newborn: 0   P Pediatric: 0-17   M Maternity: 9-64   A Adult: 15-124   MCC Major Complication/Comorbidity   CC Complication/Comorbidity   SW Severe Wound Dx

E13.3–E13.618

526   ICD-10-CM 2020

√6ᵗʰ **E13.62 Other specified diabetes mellitus with skin complications**

    E13.620 Other specified diabetes mellitus with diabetic dermatitis `HCC`

        Other specified diabetes mellitus with diabetic necrobiosis lipoidica

    E13.621 Other specified diabetes mellitus with foot ulcer `HCC`

        Use additional code to identify site of ulcer (L97.4-, L97.5-)

    E13.622 Other specified diabetes mellitus with other skin ulcer `HCC`

        Use additional code to identify site of ulcer (L97.1-L97.9, L98.41-L98.49)

        AHA: 2017,4Q,17

    E13.628 Other specified diabetes mellitus with other skin complications `HCC`

        AHA: 2017,4Q,100-101

√6ᵗʰ **E13.63 Other specified diabetes mellitus with oral complications**

    E13.630 Other specified diabetes mellitus with periodontal disease `HCC`

    E13.638 Other specified diabetes mellitus with other oral complications `HCC`

√6ᵗʰ **E13.64 Other specified diabetes mellitus with hypoglycemia**

    E13.641 Other specified diabetes mellitus with hypoglycemia with coma `MCC` `HCC`

    E13.649 Other specified diabetes mellitus with hypoglycemia without coma `HCC`

        AHA: 2016,3Q,42; 2015,3Q,21

  E13.65 Other specified diabetes mellitus with hyperglycemia `HCC`

  E13.69 Other specified diabetes mellitus with other specified complication `HCC`

    Use additional code to identify complication

    AHA: 2016,4Q,141; 2016,1Q,13

E13.8 Other specified diabetes mellitus with unspecified complications `HCC`

E13.9 Other specified diabetes mellitus without complications `HCC`

Other disorders of glucose regulation and pancreatic internal secretion (E15-E16)

E15 Nondiabetic hypoglycemic coma `CC` `H9` `HCC`

  INCLUDES   drug-induced insulin coma in nondiabetic

    hyperinsulinism with hypoglycemic coma

    hypoglycemic coma NOS

  CC Excl: PDX collection 520

√4ᵗʰ **E16 Other disorders of pancreatic internal secretion**

  E16.0 Drug-induced hypoglycemia without coma

    Use additional code for adverse effect, if applicable, to identify drug (T36-T50 with fifth or sixth character 5)

    EXCLUDES 1   *diabetes with hypoglycemia without coma (E09.649)*

  E16.1 Other hypoglycemia

    Functional hyperinsulinism

    Functional nonhyperinsulinemic hypoglycemia

    Hyperinsulinism NOS

    Hyperplasia of pancreatic islet beta cells NOS

    EXCLUDES 1   *diabetes with hypoglycemia (E08.649, E10.649, E11.649, E13.649)*

        hypoglycemia in infant of diabetic mother (P70.1)

        neonatal hypoglycemia (P70.4)

  E16.2 Hypoglycemia, unspecified

    EXCLUDES 1   *diabetes with hypoglycemia (E08.649, E10.649, E11.649, E13.649)*

    AHA: 2016,3Q,42

    TIP: Assign for nondiabetic hypoglycemic encephalopathy not further clarified in the documentation.

  E16.3 Increased secretion of glucagon

    Hyperplasia of pancreatic endocrine cells with glucagon excess

  E16.4 Increased secretion of gastrin

    Hypergastrinemia

    Hyperplasia of pancreatic endocrine cells with gastrin excess

    Zollinger-Ellison syndrome

  E16.8 Other specified disorders of pancreatic internal secretion

    Increased secretion from endocrine pancreas of growth hormone-releasing hormone

    Increased secretion from endocrine pancreas of pancreatic polypeptide

    Increased secretion from endocrine pancreas of somatostatin

    Increased secretion from endocrine pancreas of vasoactive-intestinal polypeptide

  E16.9 Disorder of pancreatic internal secretion, unspecified

    Islet-cell hyperplasia NOS

    Pancreatic endocrine cell hyperplasia NOS

Disorders of other endocrine glands (E20-E35)

  EXCLUDES 1   *galactorrhea (N64.3)*

    gynecomastia (N62)

√4ᵗʰ **E20 Hypoparathyroidism**

  EXCLUDES 1   *Di George's syndrome (D82.1)*

    postprocedural hypoparathyroidism (E89.2)

    tetany NOS (R29.0)

    transitory neonatal hypoparathyroidism (P71.4)

  E20.0 Idiopathic hypoparathyroidism `HCC`

    DEF: Abnormally low secretion of parathyroid hormones, with unknown cause, which causes decreased calcium and increased phosphorus in the blood, resulting in muscle cramps, tetany, tingling, or burning in the lips, fingers, and toes, and cataracts.

  E20.1 Pseudohypoparathyroidism

  E20.8 Other hypoparathyroidism `HCC`

  E20.9 Hypoparathyroidism, unspecified `HCC`

    Parathyroid tetany

√4ᵗʰ **E21 Hyperparathyroidism and other disorders of parathyroid gland**

  EXCLUDES 1   *adult osteomalacia (M83.-)*

    ectopic hyperparathyroidism (E34.2)

    familial hypocalciuric hypercalcemia (E83.52)

    hungry bone syndrome (E83.81)

    infantile and juvenile osteomalacia (E55.0)

  E21.0 Primary hyperparathyroidism `HCC`

    Hyperplasia of parathyroid

    Osteitis fibrosa cystica generalisata [von Recklinghausen's disease of bone]

    DEF: Parathyroid dysfunction commonly caused by hyperplasia of two or more glands. Symptoms include hypercalcemia and increased parathyroid hormone levels.

  E21.1 Secondary hyperparathyroidism, not elsewhere classified `HCC`

    EXCLUDES 1   *secondary hyperparathyroidism of renal origin (N25.81)*

  E21.2 Other hyperparathyroidism `HCC`

    Tertiary hyperparathyroidism

    EXCLUDES 1   *familial hypocalciuric hypercalcemia (E83.52)*

  E21.3 Hyperparathyroidism, unspecified `HCC`

  E21.4 Other specified disorders of parathyroid gland `HCC`

  E21.5 Disorder of parathyroid gland, unspecified `HCC`

☑ Additional Character Required   √x7ᵗʰ Placeholder   Unacceptable PDx   Questionable PDx   Manifestation   Unspecified Dx   H1-H14 HAC   HCC CMS-HCC Dx   HIV HIV Dx

ICD-10-CM 2020

527

Chapter 4. Endocrine, Nutritional and Metabolic Diseases

E22–E27.1

✓4ᵗʰ E22 Hyperfunction of pituitary gland

EXCLUDES 1
- Cushing's syndrome (E24.-)
- Nelson's syndrome (E24.1)
- overproduction of ACTH not associated with Cushing's disease (E27.0)
- overproduction of pituitary ACTH (E24.0)
- overproduction of thyroid-stimulating hormone (E05.8-)

CC Excl: For CC codes in category E22, unless otherwise noted: PDX collection 521

E22.0 Acromegaly and pituitary gigantism   HCC
Overproduction of growth hormone

EXCLUDES 1
- constitutional gigantism (E34.4)
- constitutional tall stature (E34.4)
- increased secretion from endocrine pancreas of growth hormone-releasing hormone (E16.8)

DEF: Acromegaly: Chronic condition caused by overproduction of the pituitary growth hormone resulting in enlarged skeletal parts and facial features.

E22.1 Hyperprolactinemia   CC HCC
Use additional code for adverse effect, if applicable, to identify drug (T36-T50 with fifth or sixth character 5)

E22.2 Syndrome of inappropriate secretion of antidiuretic hormone   CC HCC
CC Excl: PDX collection 522

E22.8 Other hyperfunction of pituitary gland   CC HCC
Central precocious puberty

E22.9 Hyperfunction of pituitary gland, unspecified   CC HCC

✓4ᵗʰ E23 Hypofunction and other disorders of the pituitary gland

INCLUDES the listed conditions whether the disorder is in the pituitary or the hypothalamus

EXCLUDES 1 postprocedural hypopituitarism (E89.3)

E23.0 Hypopituitarism   HCC
Fertile eunuch syndrome
Hypogonadotropic hypogonadism
Idiopathic growth hormone deficiency
Isolated deficiency of gonadotropin
Isolated deficiency of growth hormone
Isolated deficiency of pituitary hormone
Kallmann's syndrome
Lorain-Levi short stature
Necrosis of pituitary gland (postpartum)
Panhypopituitarism
Pituitary cachexia
Pituitary insufficiency NOS
Pituitary short stature
Sheehan's syndrome
Simmonds' disease

E23.1 Drug-induced hypopituitarism   HCC
Use additional code for adverse effect, if applicable, to identify drug (T36-T50 with fifth or sixth character 5)

E23.2 Diabetes insipidus   CC HCC
EXCLUDES 1 nephrogenic diabetes insipidus (N25.1)
CC Excl: PDX collection 524

E23.3 Hypothalamic dysfunction, not elsewhere classified   HCC
EXCLUDES 1
- Prader-Willi syndrome ▶(Q87.11)◀
- Russell-Silver syndrome ▶(Q87.19)◀

E23.6 Other disorders of pituitary gland   HCC
Abscess of pituitary
Adiposogenital dystrophy

E23.7 Disorder of pituitary gland, unspecified   HCC

✓4ᵗʰ E24 Cushing's syndrome
EXCLUDES 1 congenital adrenal hyperplasia (E25.0)
DEF: Abdominal striae, acne, hypertension, decreased carbohydrate tolerance, moon face, obesity, protein catabolism, and psychiatric disturbances resulting from increased adrenocortical secretion of cortisol caused by ACTH-dependent adrenocortical hyperplasia or tumor, or by steroid effects.
CC Excl: For CC codes in category E24: PDX collection 525

E24.0 Pituitary-dependent Cushing's disease   CC HCC
Overproduction of pituitary ACTH
Pituitary-dependent hypercorticalism

E24.1 Nelson's syndrome   HCC

E24.2 Drug-induced Cushing's syndrome   CC HCC
Use additional code for adverse effect, if applicable, to identify drug (T36-T50 with fifth or sixth character 5)

E24.3 Ectopic ACTH syndrome   CC HCC

E24.4 Alcohol-induced pseudo-Cushing's syndrome   CC HCC

E24.8 Other Cushing's syndrome   CC HCC

E24.9 Cushing's syndrome, unspecified   CC HCC

✓4ᵗʰ E25 Adrenogenital disorders

INCLUDES
- adrenogenital syndromes, virilizing or feminizing, whether acquired or due to adrenal hyperplasia
- consequent on inborn enzyme defects in hormone synthesis
- female adrenal pseudohermaphroditism
- female heterosexual precocious pseudopuberty
- male isosexual precocious pseudopuberty
- male macrogenitosomia praecox
- male sexual precocity with adrenal hyperplasia
- male virilization (female)

EXCLUDES 1
- indeterminate sex and pseudohermaphroditism (Q56)
- chromosomal abnormalities (Q90-Q99)

E25.0 Congenital adrenogenital disorders associated with enzyme deficiency   HCC
Congenital adrenal hyperplasia
21-Hydroxylase deficiency
Salt-losing congenital adrenal hyperplasia

E25.8 Other adrenogenital disorders   HCC
Idiopathic adrenogenital disorder
Use additional code for adverse effect, if applicable, to identify drug (T36-T50 with fifth or sixth character 5)

E25.9 Adrenogenital disorder, unspecified   HCC
Adrenogenital syndrome NOS

✓4ᵗʰ E26 Hyperaldosteronism

✓5ᵗʰ E26.0 Primary hyperaldosteronism

E26.01 Conn's syndrome   HCC
Code also adrenal adenoma (D35.0-)

E26.02 Glucocorticoid-remediable aldosteronism   HCC
Familial aldosteronism type I
DEF: Rare autosomal dominant familial form of primary aldosteronism in which the secretion of aldosterone is under the influence of adrenocorticotrophic hormone (ACTH) rather than the renin-angiotensin mechanism. Moderate hypersecretion of aldosterone and suppressed plasma renin activity that are rapidly reversed by administration of glucosteroids. Symptoms include hypertension and mild hypokalemia.

E26.09 Other primary hyperaldosteronism   HCC
Primary aldosteronism due to adrenal hyperplasia (bilateral)

E26.1 Secondary hyperaldosteronism   HCC

✓5ᵗʰ E26.8 Other hyperaldosteronism

E26.81 Bartter's syndrome   HCC

E26.89 Other hyperaldosteronism   HCC

E26.9 Hyperaldosteronism, unspecified   HCC
Aldosteronism NOS
Hyperaldosteronism NOS

✓4ᵗʰ E27 Other disorders of adrenal gland
CC Excl: For CC codes in category E27: PDX collection 526

E27.0 Other adrenocortical overactivity   CC HCC
Overproduction of ACTH, not associated with Cushing's disease
Premature adrenarche
EXCLUDES 1 Cushing's syndrome (E24.-)

E27.1 Primary adrenocortical insufficiency   CC HCC
Addison's disease
Autoimmune adrenalitis
EXCLUDES 1
- Addison only phenotype adrenoleukodystrophy (E71.528)
- amyloidosis (E85.-)
- tuberculous Addison's disease (A18.7)
- Waterhouse-Friderichsen syndrome (A39.1)

N Newborn: 0   P Pediatric: 0-17   M Maternity: 9-64   A Adult: 15-124   MCC Major Complication/Comorbidity   CC Complication/Comorbidity   SW Severe Wound Dx

528   ICD-10-CM 2020

E27.2 Addisonian crisis `CC` `HCC`
Adrenal crisis
Adrenocortical crisis
DEF: Life-threatening condition that occurs when there is not enough cortisol excreted from the adrenal glands. This condition may be due to injury to the adrenal glands or to the pituitary gland, which controls adrenal hormone secretion, or when a patient stops hydrocortisone treatment too quickly or too early.

E27.3 Drug-induced adrenocortical insufficiency `CC` `HCC`
Use additional code for adverse effect, if applicable, to identify drug (T36-T50 with fifth or sixth character 5)

√5ᵗʰ E27.4 Other and unspecified adrenocortical insufficiency
EXCLUDES 1   adrenoleukodystrophy [Addison-Schilder] (E71.528)
Waterhouse-Friderichsen syndrome (A39.1)

    E27.40 Unspecified adrenocortical insufficiency `CC` `HCC`
Adrenocortical insufficiency NOS
Hypoaldosteronism

    E27.49 Other adrenocortical insufficiency `CC` `HCC`
Adrenal hemorrhage
Adrenal infarction

E27.5 Adrenomedullary hyperfunction `CC` `HCC`
Adrenomedullary hyperplasia
Catecholamine hypersecretion

E27.8 Other specified disorders of adrenal gland `HCC`
Abnormality of cortisol-binding globulin

E27.9 Disorder of adrenal gland, unspecified `HCC`

√4ᵗʰ E28 Ovarian dysfunction
EXCLUDES 1   isolated gonadotropin deficiency (E23.0)
postprocedural ovarian failure (E89.4-)

E28.0 Estrogen excess ♀
Use additional code for adverse effect, if applicable, to identify drug (T36-T50 with fifth or sixth character 5)

E28.1 Androgen excess ♀
Hypersecretion of ovarian androgens
Use additional code for adverse effect, if applicable, to identify drug (T36-T50 with fifth or sixth character 5)

E28.2 Polycystic ovarian syndrome ♀
Sclerocystic ovary syndrome
Stein-Leventhal syndrome
DEF: Common hormonal disorder among women of reproductive age that involves enlarged ovaries with numerous small cysts located along the outer ovarian edge.

√5ᵗʰ E28.3 Primary ovarian failure
EXCLUDES 1   pure gonadal dysgenesis (Q99.1)
Turner's syndrome (Q96.-)

    √6ᵗʰ E28.31 Premature menopause

      E28.310 Symptomatic premature menopause `A` ♀
Symptoms such as flushing, sleeplessness, headache, lack of concentration, associated with premature menopause

      E28.319 Asymptomatic premature menopause `A` ♀
Premature menopause NOS

    E28.39 Other primary ovarian failure ♀
Decreased estrogen
Resistant ovary syndrome

E28.8 Other ovarian dysfunction ♀
Ovarian hyperfunction NOS
EXCLUDES 1   postprocedural ovarian failure (E89.4-)

E28.9 Ovarian dysfunction, unspecified ♀

√4ᵗʰ E29 Testicular dysfunction
EXCLUDES 1   androgen insensitivity syndrome (E34.5-)
azoospermia or oligospermia NOS (N46.0-N46.1)
isolated gonadotropin deficiency (E23.0)
Klinefelter's syndrome (Q98.0-Q98.1, Q98.4)

E29.0 Testicular hyperfunction ♂
Hypersecretion of testicular hormones

E29.1 Testicular hypofunction ♂
Defective biosynthesis of testicular androgen NOS
5-delta-Reductase deficiency (with male pseudohermaphroditism)
Testicular hypogonadism NOS
Use additional code for adverse effect, if applicable, to identify drug (T36-T50 with fifth or sixth character 5)
EXCLUDES 1   postprocedural testicular hypofunction (E89.5)

E29.8 Other testicular dysfunction ♂

E29.9 Testicular dysfunction, unspecified ♂

√4ᵗʰ E30 Disorders of puberty, not elsewhere classified

E30.0 Delayed puberty
Constitutional delay of puberty
Delayed sexual development

E30.1 Precocious puberty `P`
Precocious menstruation
EXCLUDES 1   Albright (-McCune) (-Sternberg) syndrome (Q78.1)
central precocious puberty (E22.8)
congenital adrenal hyperplasia (E25.0)
female heterosexual precocious pseudopuberty (E25.-)
male isosexual precocious pseudopuberty (E25.-)

E30.8 Other disorders of puberty `P`
Premature thelarche

E30.9 Disorder of puberty, unspecified

√4ᵗʰ E31 Polyglandular dysfunction
EXCLUDES 1   ataxia telangiectasia [Louis-Bar] (G11.3)
dystrophia myotonica [Steinert] (G71.11)
pseudohypoparathyroidism (E20.1)

E31.0 Autoimmune polyglandular failure `HCC`
Schmidt's syndrome

E31.1 Polyglandular hyperfunction `HCC`
EXCLUDES 1   multiple endocrine adenomatosis (E31.2-)
multiple endocrine neoplasia (E31.2-)

√5ᵗʰ E31.2 Multiple endocrine neoplasia [MEN] syndromes
Multiple endocrine adenomatosis
Code also any associated malignancies and other conditions associated with the syndromes
DEF: Group of conditions in which several endocrine glands grow excessively (such as in adenomatous hyperplasia) and/or develop benign or malignant tumors. Tumors and hyperplasia associated with MEN often produce excess hormones, which impede normal physiology. There is no comprehensive cure known for MEN syndrome. Treatment is directed at the hyperplasia or tumors in each individual gland. Tumors are usually surgically removed and oral medications or hormonal injections are used to correct hormone imbalances.

    E31.20 Multiple endocrine neoplasia [MEN] syndrome, unspecified `HCC`
Multiple endocrine adenomatosis NOS
Multiple endocrine neoplasia [MEN] syndrome NOS

    E31.21 Multiple endocrine neoplasia [MEN] type I `HCC`
Wermer's syndrome

    E31.22 Multiple endocrine neoplasia [MEN] type IIA `HCC`
Sipple's syndrome

    E31.23 Multiple endocrine neoplasia [MEN] type IIB `HCC`

E31.8 Other polyglandular dysfunction `HCC`

E31.9 Polyglandular dysfunction, unspecified `HCC`

√4ᵗʰ E32 Diseases of thymus
EXCLUDES 1   aplasia or hypoplasia of thymus with immunodeficiency (D82.1)
myasthenia gravis (G70.0)

E32.0 Persistent hyperplasia of thymus `HCC`
Hypertrophy of thymus

E32.1 Abscess of thymus `CC` `HCC`
CC Excl: PDX collection 527

E32.8 Other diseases of thymus `HCC`
EXCLUDES 1   aplasia or hypoplasia with immunodeficiency (D82.1)
thymoma (D15.0)

E32.9 Disease of thymus, unspecified `HCC`

✔ Additional Character Required   Placeholder   Unacceptable PDx   Questionable PDx   Manifestation   Unspecified Dx   HAC   CMS-HCC Dx   HIV Dx

✓4ᵗʰ E34 Other endocrine disorders

EXCLUDES 1   *pseudohypoparathyroidism (E20.1)*

E34.0 Carcinoid syndrome   CC HCC

> NOTE   May be used as an additional code to identify functional activity associated with a carcinoid tumor.
>
> **CC Excl:** PDX collection 528

E34.1 Other hypersecretion of intestinal hormones

E34.2 Ectopic hormone secretion, not elsewhere classified

EXCLUDES 1   *ectopic ACTH syndrome (E24.3)*

E34.3 Short stature due to endocrine disorder
Constitutional short stature
Laron-type short stature

EXCLUDES 1   *achondroplastic short stature (Q77.4)*
hypochondroplastic short stature (Q77.4)
nutritional short stature (E45)
pituitary short stature (E23.0)
progeria (E34.8)
renal short stature (N25.0)
Russell-Silver syndrome ▶(Q87.19)◀
short-limbed stature with immunodeficiency (D82.2)
short stature in specific dysmorphic syndromes — code to syndrome — see Alphabetical Index
short stature NOS (R62.52)

E34.4 Constitutional tall stature   HCC
Constitutional gigantism

✓5ᵗʰ E34.5 Androgen insensitivity syndrome

> **DEF:** X-linked recessive condition in which individuals that are chromosomally male fail to develop normal male external genitalia due to an abnormality on the X chromosome that prohibits the body, completely or in part, from recognizing the androgens produced. *Synonym(s): AIS*

E34.50 Androgen insensitivity syndrome, unspecified
Androgen insensitivity NOS

E34.51 Complete androgen insensitivity syndrome
Complete androgen insensitivity
de Quervain syndrome
Goldberg-Maxwell syndrome

E34.52 Partial androgen insensitivity syndrome
Partial androgen insensitivity
Reifenstein syndrome

E34.8 Other specified endocrine disorders
Pineal gland dysfunction
Progeria

EXCLUDES 2   *pseudohypoparathyroidism (E20.1)*

E34.9 Endocrine disorder, unspecified
Endocrine disturbance NOS
Hormone disturbance NOS

E35 *Disorders of endocrine glands in diseases classified elsewhere*
Code first underlying disease, such as:
late congenital syphilis of thymus gland [Dubois disease] (A50.5)
Use additional code, if applicable, to identify:
sequelae of tuberculosis of other organs (B90.8)

EXCLUDES 1   *Echinococcus granulosus infection of thyroid gland (B67.3)*
meningococcal hemorrhagic adrenalitis (A39.1)
syphilis of endocrine gland (A52.79)
tuberculosis of adrenal gland, except calcification (A18.7)
tuberculosis of endocrine gland NEC (A18.82)
tuberculosis of thyroid gland (A18.81)
Waterhouse-Friderichsen syndrome (A39.1)

Intraoperative complications of endocrine system (E36)

✓4ᵗʰ E36 Intraoperative complications of endocrine system

EXCLUDES 2   *postprocedural endocrine and metabolic complications and disorders, not elsewhere classified (E89.-)*

✓5ᵗʰ E36.0 Intraoperative hemorrhage and hematoma of an endocrine system organ or structure complicating a procedure

EXCLUDES 1   *intraoperative hemorrhage and hematoma of an endocrine system organ or structure due to accidental puncture or laceration during a procedure (E36.1-)*

E36.01 Intraoperative hemorrhage and hematoma of an endocrine system organ or structure complicating an endocrine system procedure   CC
CC Excl: PDX collection 529

E36.02 Intraoperative hemorrhage and hematoma of an endocrine system organ or structure complicating other procedure   CC
CC Excl: PDX collection 529

✓5ᵗʰ E36.1 Accidental puncture and laceration of an endocrine system organ or structure during a procedure

E36.11 Accidental puncture and laceration of an endocrine system organ or structure during an endocrine system procedure   CC
CC Excl: PDX collection 509

E36.12 Accidental puncture and laceration of an endocrine system organ or structure during other procedure   CC
CC Excl: PDX collection 509

E36.8 Other intraoperative complications of endocrine system
Use additional code, if applicable, to further specify disorder

Malnutrition (E40-E46)

EXCLUDES 1   *intestinal malabsorption (K90.-)*
sequelae of protein-calorie malnutrition (E64.0)
EXCLUDES 2   *nutritional anemias (D50-D53)*
starvation (T73.0)
AHA: 2017,4Q,108; 2017,3Q,25
TIP: Assign additional code for BMI from category Z68, when documented. BMI can be based on documentation from clinicians who are not the patient's provider.
CC Excl: For CC/MCC codes in categories E40-E46: PDX collection 530

E40 Kwashiorkor   MCC HCC
Severe malnutrition with nutritional edema with dyspigmentation of skin and hair

EXCLUDES 1   *marasmic kwashiorkor (E42)*

E41 Nutritional marasmus   MCC HCC
Severe malnutrition with marasmus

EXCLUDES 1   *marasmic kwashiorkor (E42)*
AHA: 2017,3Q,24
DEF: Protein-calorie malabsorption or malnutrition in children characterized by tissue wasting, dehydration, and subcutaneous fat depletion. It may occur with infectious disease.

E42 Marasmic kwashiorkor   CC HCC
Intermediate form severe protein-calorie malnutrition
Severe protein-calorie malnutrition with signs of both kwashiorkor and marasmus

E43 Unspecified severe protein-calorie malnutrition   CC HCC
Starvation edema
AHA: 2017,4Q,108

✓4ᵗʰ E44 Protein-calorie malnutrition of moderate and mild degree

E44.0 Moderate protein-calorie malnutrition   MCC HCC

E44.1 Mild protein-calorie malnutrition   CC HCC

E45 Retarded development following protein-calorie malnutrition   CC HCC
Nutritional short stature
Nutritional stunting
Physical retardation due to malnutrition

E46 **Unspecified protein-calorie malnutrition**   `CC` `HCC`

Malnutrition NOS

Protein-calorie imbalance NOS

> *EXCLUDES 1*   *nutritional deficiency NOS (E63.9)*

AHA: 2018,4Q,82

Other nutritional deficiencies (E50-E64)

> *EXCLUDES 2*   *nutritional anemias (D50-D53)*

CC Excl: For CC codes in categories E50-E64, unless otherwise noted: PDX collection 531

✓4ᵗʰ **E50** **Vitamin A deficiency**

> *EXCLUDES 1*   *sequelae of vitamin A deficiency (E64.1)*

E50.0 **Vitamin A deficiency with conjunctival xerosis**

E50.1 **Vitamin A deficiency with Bitot's spot and conjunctival xerosis**

Bitot's spot in the young child

DEF: Vitamin A deficiency with conjunctival dryness and superficial spots of keratinized epithelium.

E50.2 **Vitamin A deficiency with corneal xerosis**

E50.3 **Vitamin A deficiency with corneal ulceration and xerosis**

E50.4 **Vitamin A deficiency with keratomalacia**

DEF: Vitamin A deficiency creating corneal dryness that progresses to corneal insensitivity, softness, and necrosis. It is usually bilateral.

E50.5 **Vitamin A deficiency with night blindness**

E50.6 **Vitamin A deficiency with xerophthalmic scars of cornea**

E50.7 **Other ocular manifestations of vitamin A deficiency**

Xerophthalmia NOS

E50.8 **Other manifestations of vitamin A deficiency**

Follicular keratosis

Xeroderma

E50.9 **Vitamin A deficiency, unspecified**

Hypovitaminosis A NOS

✓4ᵗʰ **E51** **Thiamine deficiency**

> *EXCLUDES 1*   *sequelae of thiamine deficiency (E64.8)*

✓5ᵗʰ **E51.1** **Beriberi**

E51.11 **Dry beriberi**   `CC`

Beriberi NOS

Beriberi with polyneuropathy

E51.12 **Wet beriberi**   `CC`

Beriberi with cardiovascular manifestations

Cardiovascular beriberi

Shoshin disease

E51.2 **Wernicke's encephalopathy**   `MCC`

DEF: Deficiency of vitamin B1 resulting in a triad of acute mental confusion, ataxia, and ophthalmoplegia. The vast majority of affected patients are alcoholics.

E51.8 **Other manifestations of thiamine deficiency**   `CC`

E51.9 **Thiamine deficiency, unspecified**   `CC`

E52 **Niacin deficiency [pellagra]**

Niacin (-tryptophan) deficiency

Nicotinamide deficiency

Pellagra (alcoholic)

> *EXCLUDES 1*   *sequelae of niacin deficiency (E64.8)*

✓4ᵗʰ **E53** **Deficiency of other B group vitamins**

> *EXCLUDES 1*   *sequelae of vitamin B deficiency (E64.8)*

E53.0 **Riboflavin deficiency**   `CC`

Ariboflavinosis

Vitamin B2 deficiency

E53.1 **Pyridoxine deficiency**

Vitamin B6 deficiency

> *EXCLUDES 1*   *pyridoxine-responsive sideroblastic anemia (D64.3)*

E53.8 **Deficiency of other specified B group vitamins**

Biotin deficiency

Cyanocobalamin deficiency

Folate deficiency

Folic acid deficiency

Pantothenic acid deficiency

Vitamin B12 deficiency

> *EXCLUDES 1*   *folate deficiency anemia (D52.-)*
> *vitamin B12 deficiency anemia (D51.-)*

E53.9 **Vitamin B deficiency, unspecified**

E54 **Ascorbic acid deficiency**

Deficiency of vitamin C

Scurvy

> *EXCLUDES 1*   *scorbutic anemia (D53.2)*
> *sequelae of vitamin C deficiency (E64.2)*

DEF: Vitamin C deficiency causing swollen gums, myalgia, weight loss, and weakness.

✓4ᵗʰ **E55** **Vitamin D deficiency**

> *EXCLUDES 1*   *adult osteomalacia (M83.-)*
> *osteoporosis (M80.-)*
> *sequelae of rickets (E64.3)*

E55.0 **Rickets, active**   `CC`

Infantile osteomalacia

Juvenile osteomalacia

> *EXCLUDES 1*   *celiac rickets (K90.0)*
> *Crohn's rickets (K50.-)*
> *hereditary vitamin D-dependent rickets (E83.32)*
> *inactive rickets (E64.3)*
> *renal rickets (N25.0)*
> *sequelae of rickets (E64.3)*
> *vitamin D-resistant rickets (E83.31)*

DEF: Rickets: Softening or weakening of the bones due to a lack of vitamin D, calcium, and phosphate.

CC Excl: PDX collection 532

E55.9 **Vitamin D deficiency, unspecified**

Avitaminosis D

✓4ᵗʰ **E56** **Other vitamin deficiencies**

> *EXCLUDES 1*   *sequelae of other vitamin deficiencies (E64.8)*

E56.0 **Deficiency of vitamin E**

E56.1 **Deficiency of vitamin K**

> *EXCLUDES 1*   *deficiency of coagulation factor due to vitamin K deficiency (D68.4)*
> *vitamin K deficiency of newborn (P53)*

E56.8 **Deficiency of other vitamins**

E56.9 **Vitamin deficiency, unspecified**

E58 **Dietary calcium deficiency**

> *EXCLUDES 1*   *disorders of calcium metabolism (E83.5-)*
> *sequelae of calcium deficiency (E64.8)*

E59 **Dietary selenium deficiency**

Keshan disease

> *EXCLUDES 1*   *sequelae of selenium deficiency (E64.8)*

E60 **Dietary zinc deficiency**

✓4ᵗʰ **E61** **Deficiency of other nutrient elements**

Use additional code for adverse effect, if applicable, to identify drug (T36-T50 with fifth or sixth character 5)

> *EXCLUDES 1*   *disorders of mineral metabolism (E83.-)*
> *iodine deficiency related thyroid disorders (E00-E02)*
> *sequelae of malnutrition and other nutritional deficiencies (E64.-)*

E61.0 **Copper deficiency**

E61.1 **Iron deficiency**

> *EXCLUDES 1*   *iron deficiency anemia (D50.-)*

E61.2 **Magnesium deficiency**

E61.3 **Manganese deficiency**

E61.4 **Chromium deficiency**

E61.5 **Molybdenum deficiency**

E61.6 **Vanadium deficiency**

E61.7 **Deficiency of multiple nutrient elements**

E61.8 **Deficiency of other specified nutrient elements**

E61.9 **Deficiency of nutrient element, unspecified**

✓4ᵗʰ **E63** **Other nutritional deficiencies**

> *EXCLUDES 1*   *dehydration (E86.0)*
> *failure to thrive, adult (R62.7)*
> *failure to thrive, child (R62.51)*
> *feeding problems in newborn (P92.-)*
> *sequelae of malnutrition and other nutritional deficiencies (E64.-)*

E63.0 **Essential fatty acid [EFA] deficiency**

E63.1 **Imbalance of constituents of food intake**

E63.8 **Other specified nutritional deficiencies**

E63.9 **Nutritional deficiency, unspecified**

☑ Additional Character Required   ✓x7ᵗʰ Placeholder   Unacceptable PDx   Questionable PDx   Manifestation   Unspecified Dx   `H1`-`H14` HAC   `HCC` CMS-HCC Dx   `HIV` HIV Dx

ICD-10-CM 2020   531

Chapter 4. Endocrine, Nutritional and Metabolic Diseases

✓4ᵗʰ E64 Sequelae of malnutrition and other nutritional deficiencies

> **NOTE**   This category is to be used to indicate conditions in categories E43, E44, E46, E50-E63 as the cause of sequelae, which are themselves classified elsewhere. The 'sequelae' include conditions specified as such; they also include the late effects of diseases classifiable to the above categories if the disease itself is no longer present

Code first condition resulting from (sequela) of malnutrition and other nutritional deficiencies

E64.0 Sequelae of protein-calorie malnutrition
> *EXCLUDES 2*   retarded development following protein-calorie malnutrition (E45)
> **CC Excl:** PDX collection 530

E64.1 Sequelae of vitamin A deficiency

E64.2 Sequelae of vitamin C deficiency

E64.3 Sequelae of rickets

E64.8 Sequelae of other nutritional deficiencies

E64.9 Sequelae of unspecified nutritional deficiency

Overweight, obesity and other hyperalimentation (E65-E68)

E65 Localized adiposity
Fat pad

✓4ᵗʰ E66 Overweight and obesity

Code first obesity complicating pregnancy, childbirth and the puerperium, if applicable (O99.21-)
Use additional code to identify body mass index (BMI), if known (Z68.-)
> *EXCLUDES 1*   adiposogenital dystrophy (E23.6)
> lipomatosis NOS (E88.2)
> lipomatosis dolorosa [Dercum] (E88.2)
> Prader-Willi syndrome ▶(Q87.11)◄

AHA: 2018,4Q,77,79-80
TIP: Do not assign a BMI code (Z68.-) when a pregnant patient is documented as being overweight or obese. Only a code from subcategory O99.21- and a code from this category should be assigned.

✓5ᵗʰ E66.0 Obesity due to excess calories
    E66.01 Morbid (severe) obesity due to excess calories   H11 HCC
> *EXCLUDES 1*   morbid (severe) obesity with alveolar hypoventilation (E66.2)

    E66.09 Other obesity due to excess calories

E66.1 Drug-induced obesity
> Use additional code for adverse effect, if applicable, to identify drug (T36-T50 with fifth or sixth character 5)

E66.2 Morbid (severe) obesity with alveolar hypoventilation   CC HCC
> Obesity hypoventilation syndrome (OHS)
> Pickwickian syndrome
> **CC Excl:** PDX collection 533

E66.3 Overweight
> **AHA:** 2018,4Q,78

E66.8 Other obesity

E66.9 Obesity, unspecified
> Obesity NOS

✓4ᵗʰ E67 Other hyperalimentation
> *EXCLUDES 1*   hyperalimentation NOS (R63.2)
> sequelae of hyperalimentation (E68)

E67.0 Hypervitaminosis A

E67.1 Hypercarotenemia
> **DEF:** Elevated blood carotene level as a result of excessive carotenoid ingestion or an inability to convert carotenoids to vitamin A. Characteristics often include yellow discoloration of the skin, which may follow overeating of carotenoid-rich foods such as carrots, sweet potatoes, or squash.

E67.2 Megavitamin-B6 syndrome

E67.3 Hypervitaminosis D

E67.8 Other specified hyperalimentation

E68 Sequelae of hyperalimentation
Code first condition resulting from (sequela) of hyperalimentation

Metabolic disorders (E70-E88)

> *EXCLUDES 1*   androgen insensitivity syndrome (E34.5-)
> congenital adrenal hyperplasia (E25.0)
> Ehlers-Danlos syndrome ▶(Q79.6-)◄
> hemolytic anemias attributable to enzyme disorders (D55.-)
> Marfan's syndrome (Q87.4)
> 5-alpha-reductase deficiency (E29.1)

AHA: 2018,2Q,6

✓4ᵗʰ E70 Disorders of aromatic amino-acid metabolism
CC Excl: For CC codes in category E70: PDX collection 534

E70.0 Classical phenylketonuria   CC HCC

E70.1 Other hyperphenylalaninemias   CC HCC

✓5ᵗʰ E70.2 Disorders of tyrosine metabolism
> *EXCLUDES 1*   transitory tyrosinemia of newborn (P74.5)

    E70.20 Disorder of tyrosine metabolism, unspecified   CC HCC

    E70.21 Tyrosinemia   CC HCC
> Hypertyrosinemia

    E70.29 Other disorders of tyrosine metabolism   CC HCC
> Alkaptonuria
> Ochronosis

✓5ᵗʰ E70.3 Albinism
> **DEF:** Absence of pigment in skin, hair, and eyes. This genetic condition is often accompanied by astigmatism, photophobia, and nystagmus.

    E70.30 Albinism, unspecified   CC HCC

    ✓6ᵗʰ E70.31 Ocular albinism
        E70.310 X-linked ocular albinism   CC HCC
        E70.311 Autosomal recessive ocular albinism   CC HCC
        E70.318 Other ocular albinism   CC HCC
        E70.319 Ocular albinism, unspecified   CC HCC

    ✓6ᵗʰ E70.32 Oculocutaneous albinism
> *EXCLUDES 1*   Chediak-Higashi syndrome (E70.330)
> Hermansky-Pudlak syndrome (E70.331)

        E70.320 Tyrosinase negative oculocutaneous albinism   CC HCC
> Albinism I
> Oculocutaneous albinism ty-neg

        E70.321 Tyrosinase positive oculocutaneous albinism   CC HCC
> Albinism II
> Oculocutaneous albinism ty-pos

        E70.328 Other oculocutaneous albinism   CC HCC
> Cross syndrome

        E70.329 Oculocutaneous albinism, unspecified   CC HCC

    ✓6ᵗʰ E70.33 Albinism with hematologic abnormality
        E70.330 Chediak-Higashi syndrome   CC HCC
        E70.331 Hermansky-Pudlak syndrome   CC HCC
        E70.338 Other albinism with hematologic abnormality   CC HCC
        E70.339 Albinism with hematologic abnormality, unspecified   CC HCC

    E70.39 Other specified albinism   CC HCC
> Piebaldism

✓5ᵗʰ E70.4 Disorders of histidine metabolism
    E70.40 Disorders of histidine metabolism, unspecified   CC HCC
    E70.41 Histidinemia   CC HCC
    E70.49 Other disorders of histidine metabolism   CC HCC

E70.5 Disorders of tryptophan metabolism   CC HCC

E70.8 Other disorders of aromatic amino-acid metabolism   CC HCC

E70.9 Disorder of aromatic amino-acid metabolism, unspecified   CC HCC

N Newborn: 0   P Pediatric: 0-17   M Maternity: 9-64   A Adult: 15-124   MCC Major Complication/Comorbidity   CC Complication/Comorbidity   SW Severe Wound Dx

532   ICD-10-CM 2020

☑4ᵗʰ **E71 Disorders of branched-chain amino-acid metabolism and fatty-acid metabolism**

   E71.0 Maple-syrup-urine disease `CC` `HCC`
      CC Excl: PDX collection 534

☑5ᵗʰ **E71.1 Other disorders of branched-chain amino-acid metabolism**
      CC Excl: For CC codes in subcategory E71.1: PDX collection 534

    ☑6ᵗʰ **E71.11 Branched-chain organic acidurias**
      E71.110 Isovaleric acidemia `CC` `HCC`
      E71.111 3-methylglutaconic aciduria `CC` `HCC`
      E71.118 Other branched-chain organic acidurias `CC` `HCC`

    ☑6ᵗʰ **E71.12 Disorders of propionate metabolism**
      E71.120 Methylmalonic acidemia `CC` `HCC`
      E71.121 Propionic acidemia `CC` `HCC`
      E71.128 Other disorders of propionate metabolism `CC` `HCC`

    E71.19 Other disorders of branched-chain amino-acid metabolism `CC` `HCC`
      Hyperleucine-isoleucinemia
      Hypervalinemia

   E71.2 Disorder of branched-chain amino-acid metabolism, unspecified `CC` `HCC`
      CC Excl: PDX collection 534

☑5ᵗʰ **E71.3 Disorders of fatty-acid metabolism**
    EXCLUDES 1 peroxisomal disorders (E71.5)
       Refsum's disease (G60.1)
       Schilder's disease (G37.0)
    EXCLUDES 2 carnitine deficiency due to inborn error of metabolism (E71.42)
    CC Excl: For CC codes in subcategory E71.3, unless otherwise noted: PDX collection 535

    E71.30 Disorder of fatty-acid metabolism, unspecified

    ☑6ᵗʰ **E71.31 Disorders of fatty-acid oxidation**
      E71.310 Long chain/very long chain acyl CoA dehydrogenase deficiency `CC` `HCC`
        LCAD
        VLCAD
      E71.311 Medium chain acyl CoA dehydrogenase deficiency `CC` `HCC`
        MCAD
      E71.312 Short chain acyl CoA dehydrogenase deficiency `CC` `HCC`
        SCAD
      E71.313 Glutaric aciduria type II `CC` `HCC`
        Glutaric aciduria type II A
        Glutaric aciduria type II B
        Glutaric aciduria type II C
        EXCLUDES 1 glutaric aciduria (type 1) NOS (E72.3)
      E71.314 Muscle carnitine palmitoyltransferase deficiency `CC` `HCC`
      E71.318 Other disorders of fatty-acid oxidation `CC` `HCC`

    E71.32 Disorders of ketone metabolism `CC` `HCC`

    E71.39 Other disorders of fatty-acid metabolism `CC` `HCC`
      CC Excl: PDX collection 492

☑5ᵗʰ **E71.4 Disorders of carnitine metabolism**
    EXCLUDES 1 muscle carnitine palmitoyltransferase deficiency (E71.314)

    E71.40 Disorder of carnitine metabolism, unspecified `HCC`

    E71.41 Primary carnitine deficiency `HCC`

    E71.42 Carnitine deficiency due to inborn errors of metabolism `HCC`
      Code also associated inborn error or metabolism

    E71.43 Iatrogenic carnitine deficiency `HCC`
      Carnitine deficiency due to hemodialysis
      Carnitine deficiency due to Valproic acid therapy

    ☑6ᵗʰ **E71.44 Other secondary carnitine deficiency**
      E71.440 Ruvalcaba-Myhre-Smith syndrome `HCC`
      E71.448 Other secondary carnitine deficiency `HCC`

☑5ᵗʰ **E71.5 Peroxisomal disorders**
    EXCLUDES 1 Schilder's disease (G37.0)
    CC Excl: For CC codes in subcategory E71.5: PDX collection 536

    E71.50 Peroxisomal disorder, unspecified `CC` `HCC`

    ☑6ᵗʰ **E71.51 Disorders of peroxisome biogenesis**
      Group 1 peroxisomal disorders
      EXCLUDES 1 Refsum's disease (G60.1)
      E71.510 Zellweger syndrome `CC` `HCC`
      E71.511 Neonatal adrenoleukodystrophy `CC` `HCC`
        EXCLUDES 1 X-linked adrenoleukodystrophy (E71.42-)
      E71.518 Other disorders of peroxisome biogenesis `CC` `HCC`

    ☑6ᵗʰ **E71.52 X-linked adrenoleukodystrophy**
      E71.520 Childhood cerebral X-linked adrenoleukodystrophy `CC` `HCC`
      E71.521 Adolescent X-linked adrenoleukodystrophy `CC` `HCC`
      E71.522 Adrenomyeloneuropathy `CC` `HCC`
      E71.528 Other X-linked adrenoleukodystrophy `CC` `HCC`
        Addison only phenotype adrenoleukodystrophy
        Addison-Schilder adrenoleukodystrophy
      E71.529 X-linked adrenoleukodystrophy, unspecified type `CC` `HCC`

    E71.53 Other group 2 peroxisomal disorders `CC` `HCC`

    ☑6ᵗʰ **E71.54 Other peroxisomal disorders**
      E71.540 Rhizomelic chondrodysplasia punctata `CC` `HCC`
        EXCLUDES 1 chondrodysplasia punctata NOS (Q77.3)
      E71.541 Zellweger-like syndrome `CC` `HCC`
      E71.542 Other group 3 peroxisomal disorders `CC` `HCC`
      E71.548 Other peroxisomal disorders `CC` `HCC`

☑4ᵗʰ **E72 Other disorders of amino-acid metabolism**
   EXCLUDES 1 disorders of:
      aromatic amino-acid metabolism (E70.-)
      branched-chain amino-acid metabolism (E71.0-E71.2)
      fatty-acid metabolism (E71.3)
      purine and pyrimidine metabolism (E79.-)
      gout (M1A.-, M10.-)
   CC Excl: For CC codes in category E72, unless otherwise noted: PDX collection 534

☑5ᵗʰ **E72.0 Disorders of amino-acid transport**
    EXCLUDES 1 disorders of tryptophan metabolism (E70.5)

    E72.00 Disorders of amino-acid transport, unspecified `CC` `HCC`

    E72.01 Cystinuria `CC` `HCC`

    E72.02 Hartnup's disease `CC` `HCC`

    E72.03 Lowe's syndrome `CC` `HCC`
      Use additional code for associated glaucoma (H42)
      CC Excl: No Excl

    E72.04 Cystinosis `CC` `HCC`
      Fanconi (-de Toni) (-Debré) syndrome with cystinosis
      EXCLUDES 1 Fanconi (-de Toni) (-Debré) syndrome without cystinosis (E72.09)

    E72.09 Other disorders of amino-acid transport `CC` `HCC`
      Fanconi (-de Toni) (-Debré) syndrome, unspecified

☑5ᵗʰ **E72.1 Disorders of sulfur-bearing amino-acid metabolism**
    EXCLUDES 1 cystinosis (E72.04)
      cystinuria (E72.01)
      transcobalamin II deficiency (D51.2)

    E72.10 Disorders of sulfur-bearing amino-acid metabolism, unspecified `CC` `HCC`

    E72.11 Homocystinuria `CC` `HCC`
      Cystathionine synthase deficiency

Chapter 4. Endocrine, Nutritional and Metabolic Diseases

E72.12–E74.9

E72.12   **Methylenetetrahydrofolate reductase deficiency**   CC HCC

E72.19   **Other disorders of sulfur-bearing amino-acid metabolism**   CC HCC
Cystathioninuria
Methioninemia
Sulfite oxidase deficiency

√5th **E72.2**   **Disorders of urea cycle metabolism**
    EXCLUDES 1   *disorders of ornithine metabolism (E72.4)*

    E72.20   **Disorder of urea cycle metabolism, unspecified**   CC HCC
      Hyperammonemia
      EXCLUDES 1   *hyperammonemia- hyperornithinemia-homocitrullinemia syndrome E72.4*
             transient hyperammonemia of newborn (P74.6)

    E72.21   **Argininemia**   CC HCC

    E72.22   **Arginosuccinic aciduria**   CC HCC

    E72.23   **Citrullinemia**   CC HCC

    E72.29   **Other disorders of urea cycle metabolism**   CC HCC

E72.3   **Disorders of lysine and hydroxylysine metabolism**   CC HCC
Glutaric aciduria NOS
Glutaric aciduria (type I)
Hydroxylysinemia
Hyperlysinemia
    EXCLUDES 1   *glutaric aciduria type II (E71.313)*
             Refsum's disease (G60.1)
             Zellweger syndrome (E71.510)

E72.4   **Disorders of ornithine metabolism**   CC HCC
Hyperammonemia-Hyperornithinemia-Homocitrullinemia syndrome
Ornithinemia (types I, II)
Ornithine transcarbamylase deficiency
    EXCLUDES 1   *hereditary choroidal dystrophy (H31.2-)*

√5th **E72.5**   **Disorders of glycine metabolism**

    E72.50   **Disorder of glycine metabolism, unspecified**   CC HCC

    E72.51   **Non-ketotic hyperglycinemia**   CC HCC

    E72.52   **Trimethylaminuria**   CC HCC

    E72.53   **Primary hyperoxaluria**   CC HCC
      Oxalosis
      Oxaluria
      AHA: 2018,4Q,29

    E72.59   **Other disorders of glycine metabolism**   CC HCC
      D-glycericacidemia
      Hyperhydroxyprolinemia
      Hyperprolinemia (types I, II)
      Sarcosinemia

√5th **E72.8**   **Other specified disorders of amino-acid metabolism**
    AHA: 2018,4Q,5

    E72.81   **Disorders of gamma aminobutyric acid metabolism**   CC HCC
      4-hydroxybutyric aciduria
      Disorders of GABA metabolism
      GABA metabolic defect
      GABA transaminase deficiency
      GABA-T deficiency
      Gamma-hydroxybutyric aciduria
      SSADHD
      Succinic semialdehyde dehydrogenase deficiency

    E72.89   **Other specified disorders of amino-acid metabolism**   CC HCC
      Disorders of beta-amino-acid metabolism
      Disorders of gamma-glutamyl cycle

E72.9   **Disorder of amino-acid metabolism, unspecified**   CC HCC

√4th **E73**   **Lactose intolerance**
    DEF: Inability to break down sugar in dairy products due to a deficiency in the enzyme lactase.

E73.0   **Congenital lactase deficiency**

E73.1   **Secondary lactase deficiency**

E73.8   **Other lactose intolerance**

E73.9   **Lactose intolerance, unspecified**

√4th **E74**   **Other disorders of carbohydrate metabolism**
    EXCLUDES 1   *diabetes mellitus (E08-E13)*
             hypoglycemia NOS (E16.2)
             increased secretion of glucagon (E16.3)
             mucopolysaccharidosis (E76.0-E76.3)
    CC Excl: For CC codes in category E74: PDX collection 534

√5th **E74.0**   **Glycogen storage disease**

    E74.00   **Glycogen storage disease, unspecified**   CC HCC

    E74.01   **von Gierke disease**   CC HCC
      Type I glycogen storage disease

    E74.02   **Pompe disease**   CC HCC
      Cardiac glycogenosis
      Type II glycogen storage disease

    E74.03   **Cori disease**   CC HCC
      Forbes disease
      Type III glycogen storage disease

    E74.04   **McArdle disease**   CC HCC
      Type V glycogen storage disease

    E74.09   **Other glycogen storage disease**   CC HCC
      Andersen disease
      Hers disease
      Tauri disease
      Glycogen storage disease, types 0, IV, VI-XI
      Liver phosphorylase deficiency
      Muscle phosphofructokinase deficiency

√5th **E74.1**   **Disorders of fructose metabolism**
    EXCLUDES 1   *muscle phosphofructokinase deficiency (E74.09)*

    E74.10   **Disorder of fructose metabolism, unspecified**

    E74.11   **Essential fructosuria**
      Fructokinase deficiency

    E74.12   **Hereditary fructose intolerance**
      Fructosemia

    E74.19   **Other disorders of fructose metabolism**
      Fructose-1, 6-diphosphatase deficiency

√5th **E74.2**   **Disorders of galactose metabolism**

    E74.20   **Disorders of galactose metabolism, unspecified**   CC HCC

    E74.21   **Galactosemia**   CC HCC
      DEF: Any of three genetic disorders caused by a defective galactose metabolism. Symptoms include failure to thrive in infancy, jaundice, liver and spleen damage, cataracts, and mental retardation.

    E74.29   **Other disorders of galactose metabolism**   CC HCC
      Galactokinase deficiency

√5th **E74.3**   **Other disorders of intestinal carbohydrate absorption**
    EXCLUDES 2   *lactose intolerance (E73.-)*

    E74.31   **Sucrase-isomaltase deficiency**

    E74.39   **Other disorders of intestinal carbohydrate absorption**
      Disorder of intestinal carbohydrate absorption NOS
      Glucose-galactose malabsorption
      Sucrase deficiency

E74.4   **Disorders of pyruvate metabolism and gluconeogenesis**   CC HCC
Deficiency of phosphoenolpyruvate carboxykinase
Deficiency of pyruvate carboxylase
Deficiency of pyruvate dehydrogenase
    EXCLUDES 1   *disorders of pyruvate metabolism and gluconeogenesis with anemia (D55.-)*
             Leigh's syndrome (G31.82)

E74.8   **Other specified disorders of carbohydrate metabolism**   CC HCC
Essential pentosuria
Renal glycosuria

E74.9   **Disorder of carbohydrate metabolism, unspecified**   HCC

N Newborn: 0   P Pediatric: 0-17   M Maternity: 9-64   A Adult: 15-124   MCC Major Complication/Comorbidity   CC Complication/Comorbidity   SW Severe Wound Dx

534   ICD-10-CM 2020

√4ᵗʰ **E75** **Disorders of** sphingolipid **metabolism and other** lipid storage **disorders**

> **EXCLUDES 1**   *mucolipidosis, types I-III (E77.0-E77.1)*
>   *Refsum's disease (G60.1)*

CC Excl: For CC codes in category E75, unless otherwise noted: PDX collection 537

√5ᵗʰ   **E75.0**   **GM2 gangliosidosis**

     E75.00   **GM2 gangliosidosis, unspecified**   `CC` `HCC`

     E75.01   **Sandhoff disease**   `CC` `HCC`

     E75.02   **Tay-Sachs disease**   `CC` `HCC`

> **DEF:** Genetic mutation of the HEXA gene that inhibits the breakdown of a toxic substance called ganglioside. The accumulation of ganglioside results in destruction of the neurons in the brain and spinal cord.

Tay-Sachs Disease

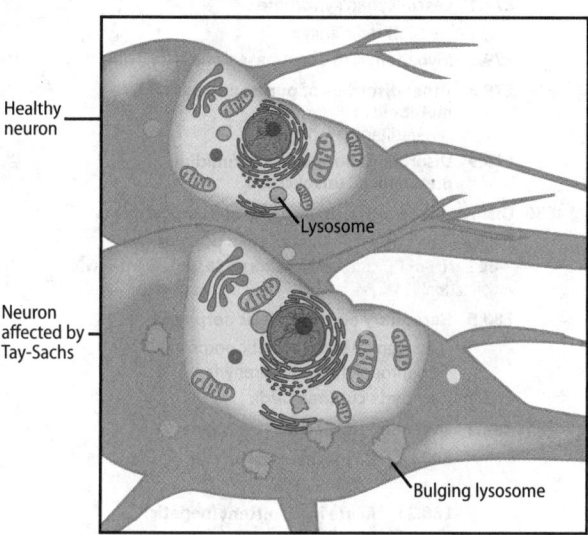

Healthy neuron

Lysosome

Neuron affected by Tay-Sachs

Bulging lysosome

     E75.09   **Other GM2 gangliosidosis**   `CC` `HCC`

        Adult GM2 gangliosidosis
        Juvenile GM2 gangliosidosis

√5ᵗʰ   **E75.1**   **Other and unspecified gangliosidosis**

     E75.10   **Unspecified gangliosidosis**   `CC` `HCC`

        Gangliosidosis NOS

     E75.11   **Mucolipidosis IV**   `CC` `HCC`

     E75.19   **Other gangliosidosis**   `CC` `HCC`

        GM1 gangliosidosis
        GM3 gangliosidosis

√5ᵗʰ   **E75.2**   **Other sphingolipidosis**

> **EXCLUDES 1**   *adrenoleukodystrophy [Addison-Schilder] (E71.528)*

CC Excl: For CC codes in subcategory E75.2: PDX collection 538

     E75.21   **Fabry (-Anderson) disease**   `HCC`

     E75.22   **Gaucher disease**   `HCC`

     E75.23   **Krabbe disease**   `CC` `HCC`

√6ᵗʰ   **E75.24**   **Niemann-Pick disease**

     E75.240   **Niemann-Pick disease type A**   `HCC`

     E75.241   **Niemann-Pick disease type B**   `HCC`

     E75.242   **Niemann-Pick disease type C**   `HCC`

     E75.243   **Niemann-Pick disease type D**   `HCC`

     E75.248   **Other Niemann-Pick disease**   `HCC`

     E75.249   **Niemann-Pick disease, unspecified**   `HCC`

     E75.25   **Metachromatic leukodystrophy**   `CC` `HCC`

     E75.26   **Sulfatase deficiency**   `CC` `HCC`

        Multiple sulfatase deficiency (MSD)
        AHA: 2018,4Q,5-6

     E75.29   **Other sphingolipidosis**   `CC` `HCC`

        Farber's syndrome
        Sulfatide lipidosis

   E75.3   **Sphingolipidosis, unspecified**   `HCC`

   E75.4   **Neuronal ceroid lipofuscinosis**   `CC` `HCC`

        Batten disease
        Bielschowsky-Jansky disease
        Kufs disease
        Spielmeyer-Vogt disease

   E75.5   **Other lipid storage disorders**

        Cerebrotendinous cholesterosis [van Bogaert-Scherer-Epstein]
        Wolman's disease

   E75.6   **Lipid storage disorder, unspecified**

√4ᵗʰ **E76** **Disorders of** glycosaminoglycan **metabolism**

CC Excl: For CC codes in category E76: PDX collection 539

√5ᵗʰ   **E76.0**   **Mucopolysaccharidosis, type I**

     E76.01   **Hurler's syndrome**   `CC` `HCC`

     E76.02   **Hurler-Scheie syndrome**   `CC` `HCC`

     E76.03   **Scheie's syndrome**   `CC` `HCC`

   E76.1   **Mucopolysaccharidosis, type II**   `CC` `HCC`

        Hunter's syndrome

√5ᵗʰ   **E76.2**   **Other mucopolysaccharidoses**

√6ᵗʰ   **E76.21**   **Morquio mucopolysaccharidoses**

     E76.210   **Morquio A mucopolysaccharidoses**   `CC` `HCC`

        Classic Morquio syndrome
        Morquio syndrome A
        Mucopolysaccharidosis, type IVA

     E76.211   **Morquio B mucopolysaccharidoses**   `CC` `HCC`

        Morquio-like mucopolysaccharidoses
        Morquio-like syndrome
        Morquio syndrome B
        Mucopolysaccharidosis, type IVB

     E76.219   **Morquio mucopolysaccharidoses, unspecified**   `CC` `HCC`

        Morquio syndrome
        Mucopolysaccharidosis, type IV

     E76.22   **Sanfilippo mucopolysaccharidoses**   `CC` `HCC`

        Mucopolysaccharidosis, type III (A) (B) (C) (D)
        Sanfilippo A syndrome
        Sanfilippo B syndrome
        Sanfilippo C syndrome
        Sanfilippo D syndrome

     E76.29   **Other mucopolysaccharidoses**   `CC` `HCC`

        beta-Glucuronidase deficiency
        Maroteaux-Lamy (mild) (severe) syndrome
        Mucopolysaccharidosis, types VI, VII

   E76.3   **Mucopolysaccharidosis, unspecified**   `CC` `HCC`

   E76.8   **Other disorders of glucosaminoglycan metabolism**   `CC` `HCC`

   E76.9   **Glucosaminoglycan metabolism disorder, unspecified**   `CC` `HCC`

√4ᵗʰ **E77** **Disorders of** glycoprotein **metabolism**

   E77.0   **Defects in post-translational modification of lysosomal enzymes**   `HCC`

        Mucolipidosis II [I-cell disease]
        Mucolipidosis III [pseudo-Hurler polydystrophy]

   E77.1   **Defects in glycoprotein degradation**   `HCC`

        Aspartylglucosaminuria
        Fucosidosis
        Mannosidosis
        Sialidosis [mucolipidosis I]

   E77.8   **Other disorders of glycoprotein metabolism**   `HCC`

   E77.9   **Disorder of glycoprotein metabolism, unspecified**   `HCC`

✓ Additional Character Required   √x7ᵗʰ Placeholder   Unacceptable PDx   Questionable PDx   Manifestation   Unspecified Dx   `H1`-`H14` HAC   `HCC` CMS-HCC Dx   `HIV` HIV Dx

ICD-10-CM 2020   535

Chapter 4. Endocrine, Nutritional and Metabolic Diseases   E75–E77.9

✓4ᵗʰ **E78** **Disorders of** lipoprotein metabolism and other lipidemias

    EXCLUDES 1   sphingolipidosis (E75.0-E75.3)

✓5ᵗʰ **E78.0** **Pure hypercholesterolemia**

    AHA: 2016,4Q,13-14

    E78.00 **Pure hypercholesterolemia, unspecified**

         Fredrickson's hyperlipoproteinemia, type IIa

         Hyperbetalipoproteinemia

         Low-density-lipoprotein-type [LDL] hyperlipoproteinemia

         (Pure) hypercholesterolemia NOS

    E78.01 **Familial hypercholesterolemia**

E78.1 **Pure hyperglyceridemia**

     Elevated fasting triglycerides

     Endogenous hyperglyceridemia

     Fredrickson's hyperlipoproteinemia, type IV

     Hyperlipidemia, group B

     Hyperprebetalipoproteinemia

     Very-low-density-lipoprotein-type [VLDL] hyperlipoproteinemia

E78.2 **Mixed hyperlipidemia**

     Broad- or floating-betalipoproteinemia

     Combined hyperlipidemia NOS

     Elevated cholesterol with elevated triglycerides NEC

     Fredrickson's hyperlipoproteinemia, type IIb or III

     Hyperbetalipoproteinemia with prebetalipoproteinemia

     Hypercholesteremia with endogenous hyperglyceridemia

     Hyperlipidemia, group C

     Tubo-eruptive xanthoma

     Xanthoma tuberosum

    EXCLUDES 1   cerebrotendinous cholesterosis [van Bogaert-Scherer-Epstein] (E75.5)

         familial combined hyperlipidemia (E78.49)

E78.3 **Hyperchylomicronemia**

     Chylomicron retention disease

     Fredrickson's hyperlipoproteinemia, type I or V

     Hyperlipidemia, group D

     Mixed hyperglyceridemia

✓5ᵗʰ **E78.4** **Other hyperlipidemia**

    AHA: 2018,4Q,6

    E78.41 **Elevated Lipoprotein(a)**

         Elevated Lp(a)

    E78.49 **Other hyperlipidemia**

         Familial combined hyperlipidemia

E78.5 **Hyperlipidemia, unspecified**

E78.6 **Lipoprotein deficiency**

     Abetalipoproteinemia

     Depressed HDL cholesterol

     High-density lipoprotein deficiency

     Hypoalphalipoproteinemia

     Hypobetalipoproteinemia (familial)

     Lecithin cholesterol acyltransferase deficiency

     Tangier disease

✓5ᵗʰ **E78.7** **Disorders of** bile acid and cholesterol metabolism

    EXCLUDES 1   Niemann-Pick disease type C (E75.242)

    E78.70 **Disorder of bile acid and cholesterol metabolism, unspecified**

    E78.71 **Barth syndrome**   CC

        CC Excl: PDX collection 540

    E78.72 **Smith-Lemli-Opitz syndrome**   CC

        CC Excl: PDX collection 540

    E78.79 **Other disorders of bile acid and cholesterol metabolism**

✓5ᵗʰ **E78.8** **Other disorders of lipoprotein metabolism**

    E78.81 **Lipoid dermatoarthritis**

    E78.89 **Other lipoprotein metabolism disorders**

E78.9 **Disorder of lipoprotein metabolism, unspecified**

✓4ᵗʰ **E79** **Disorders of** purine and pyrimidine metabolism

    EXCLUDES 1   Ataxia-telangiectasia ▶(Q87.19)◄

         Bloom's syndrome (Q82.8)

         Cockayne's syndrome ▶(Q87.19)◄

         calculus of kidney (N20.0)

         combined immunodeficiency disorders (D81.-)

         Fanconi's anemia (D61.09)

         gout (M1A.-, M10.-)

         orotaciduric anemia (D53.0)

         progeria (E34.8)

         Werner's syndrome (E34.8)

         xeroderma pigmentosum (Q82.1)

    CC Excl: For CC codes in category E79: PDX collection 513

E79.0 **Hyperuricemia without signs of inflammatory arthritis and tophaceous disease**

     Asymptomatic hyperuricemia

E79.1 **Lesch-Nyhan syndrome**   CC   HCC

     HGPRT deficiency

E79.2 **Myoadenylate deaminase deficiency**   CC   HCC

E79.8 **Other disorders of purine and pyrimidine metabolism**   CC   HCC

     Hereditary xanthinuria

E79.9 **Disorder of purine and pyrimidine metabolism, unspecified**   CC   HCC

✓4ᵗʰ **E80** **Disorders of** porphyrin and bilirubin metabolism

    INCLUDES   defects of catalase and peroxidase

    CC Excl: For CC codes in category E80, unless otherwise noted: PDX collection 513

E80.0 **Hereditary erythropoietic porphyria**   CC   HCC

     Congenital erythropoietic porphyria

     Erythropoietic protoporphyria

E80.1 **Porphyria cutanea tarda**   CC   HCC

✓5ᵗʰ **E80.2** **Other and unspecified porphyria**

    E80.20 **Unspecified porphyria**   CC   HCC

         Porphyria NOS

    E80.21 **Acute intermittent (hepatic) porphyria**   CC   HCC

    E80.29 **Other porphyria**   CC   HCC

         Hereditary coproporphyria

E80.3 **Defects of catalase and peroxidase**   CC   HCC

     Acatalasia [Takahara]

    CC Excl: PDX collection 492

E80.4 **Gilbert syndrome**

E80.5 **Crigler-Najjar syndrome**

E80.6 **Other disorders of bilirubin metabolism**

     Dubin-Johnson syndrome

     Rotor's syndrome

E80.7 **Disorder of bilirubin metabolism, unspecified**

✓4ᵗʰ **E83** **Disorders of** mineral metabolism

    EXCLUDES 1   dietary mineral deficiency (E58-E61)

         parathyroid disorders (E20-E21)

         vitamin D deficiency (E55.-)

✓5ᵗʰ **E83.0** **Disorders of** copper metabolism

    E83.00 **Disorder of copper metabolism, unspecified**

    E83.01 **Wilson's disease**

         Code also associated Kayser Fleischer ring (H18.04-)

    E83.09 **Other disorders of copper metabolism**

         Menkes' (kinky hair) (steely hair) disease

✓5ᵗʰ **E83.1** **Disorders of** iron metabolism

    EXCLUDES 1   iron deficiency anemia (D50.-)

         sideroblastic anemia (D64.0-D64.3)

    E83.10 **Disorder of iron metabolism, unspecified**

    ✓6ᵗʰ **E83.11** **Hemochromatosis**

        EXCLUDES 1   GALD (P78.84)

             gestational alloimmune liver disease (P78.84)

             neonatal hemochromatosis (P78.84)

        E83.110 **Hereditary hemochromatosis**   HCC

             Bronzed diabetes

             Pigmentary cirrhosis (of liver)

             Primary (hereditary) hemochromatosis

N Newborn: 0   P Pediatric: 0-17   M Maternity: 9-64   A Adult: 15-124   MCC Major Complication/Comorbidity   CC Complication/Comorbidity   SW Severe Wound Dx

536   ICD-10-CM 2020

E83.111 **Hemochromatosis** due to repeated red blood cell transfusions `CC`

Iron overload due to repeated red blood cell transfusions

Transfusion (red blood cell) associated hemochromatosis

E83.118 **Other hemochromatosis**

E83.119 **Hemochromatosis, unspecified**

E83.19 **Other disorders of iron metabolism**

Use additional code, if applicable, for idiopathic pulmonary hemosiderosis (J84.03)

E83.2 **Disorders of zinc metabolism**

Acrodermatitis enteropathica

✓5ᵗʰ E83.3 **Disorders of phosphorus metabolism and phosphatases**

EXCLUDES 1   *adult osteomalacia (M83.-)*
              osteoporosis (M80.-)

E83.30 **Disorder of phosphorus metabolism, unspecified**

E83.31 **Familial hypophosphatemia**

Vitamin D-resistant osteomalacia

Vitamin D-resistant rickets

EXCLUDES 1   *vitamin D-deficiency rickets (E55.0)*

E83.32 **Hereditary vitamin D-dependent rickets (type 1) (type 2)**

25-hydroxyvitamin D 1-alpha-hydroxylase deficiency

Pseudovitamin D deficiency

Vitamin D receptor defect

E83.39 **Other disorders of phosphorus metabolism** `CC`

Acid phosphatase deficiency

Hypophosphatasia

✓5ᵗʰ E83.4 **Disorders of magnesium metabolism**

E83.40 **Disorders of magnesium metabolism, unspecified**

E83.41 **Hypermagnesemia**

AHA: 2016,4Q,54

E83.42 **Hypomagnesemia**

E83.49 **Other disorders of magnesium metabolism**

✓5ᵗʰ E83.5 **Disorders of calcium metabolism**

EXCLUDES 1   *chondrocalcinosis (M11.1-M11.2)*
              hungry bone syndrome (E83.81)
              hyperparathyroidism (E21.0-E21.3)

E83.50 **Unspecified disorder of calcium metabolism**

E83.51 **Hypocalcemia** `CC`

E83.52 **Hypercalcemia**

Familial hypocalciuric hypercalcemia

E83.59 **Other disorders of calcium metabolism**

✓5ᵗʰ E83.8 **Other disorders of mineral metabolism**

E83.81 **Hungry bone syndrome**

E83.89 **Other disorders of mineral metabolism**

E83.9 **Disorder of mineral metabolism, unspecified**

✓4ᵗʰ E84 **Cystic fibrosis**

INCLUDES   mucoviscidosis

Code also exocrine pancreatic insufficiency (K86.81)

DEF: Genetic disorder affecting the respiratory, digestive, and reproductive systems in infants to young adults by disturbing exocrine gland function and causing chronic pulmonary disease with excess mucus production and pancreatic deficiency.

CC Excl: For CC/MC codes in category E84: PDX collection 541

E84.0 **Cystic fibrosis with pulmonary manifestations** `MCC` `HCC`

Use additional code to identify any infectious organism present, such as:

Pseudomonas (B96.5)

✓5ᵗʰ E84.1 **Cystic fibrosis with intestinal manifestations**

E84.11 **Meconium ileus in cystic fibrosis** `MCC` `HCC` `N`

EXCLUDES 1   *meconium ileus not due to cystic fibrosis (P76.0)*

E84.19 **Cystic fibrosis with other intestinal manifestations** `CC` `HCC`

Distal intestinal obstruction syndrome

E84.8 **Cystic fibrosis with other manifestations** `CC` `HCC`

E84.9 **Cystic fibrosis, unspecified** `CC` `HCC`

✓4ᵗʰ E85 **Amyloidosis**

EXCLUDES 2   *Alzheimer's disease (G30.0-)*

DEF: Conditions of diverse etiologies characterized by the accumulation of insoluble fibrillar proteins (amyloid) in various organs and tissues of the body, compromising vital functions.

CC Excl: For CC codes in category E85: PDX collection 542

E85.0 **Non-neuropathic heredofamilial amyloidosis** `CC` `HCC`

Hereditary amyloid nephropathy

Code also associated disorders, such as:

autoinflammatory syndromes (M04.-)

EXCLUDES 2   *transthyretin-related (ATTR) familial amyloid cardiomyopathy (E85.4)*

E85.1 **Neuropathic heredofamilial amyloidosis** `CC` `HCC`

Amyloid polyneuropathy (Portuguese)

Transthyretin-related (ATTR) familial amyloid polyneuropathy

AHA: 2012,4Q,99

E85.2 **Heredofamilial amyloidosis, unspecified** `CC` `HCC`

E85.3 **Secondary systemic amyloidosis** `CC` `HCC`

Hemodialysis-associated amyloidosis

E85.4 **Organ-limited amyloidosis** `CC` `HCC`

Localized amyloidosis

Transthyretin-related (ATTR) familial amyloid cardiomyopathy

✓5ᵗʰ E85.8 **Other amyloidosis**

AHA: 2017,4Q,7

E85.81 **Light chain (AL) amyloidosis** `CC` `HCC`

E85.82 **Wild-type transthyretin-related (ATTR) amyloidosis** `CC` `HCC`

Senile systemic amyloidosis (SSA)

E85.89 **Other amyloidosis** `CC` `HCC`

E85.9 **Amyloidosis, unspecified** `CC` `HCC`

✓4ᵗʰ E86 **Volume depletion**

Use additional code(s) for any associated disorders of electrolyte and acid-base balance (E87.-)

EXCLUDES 1   *dehydration of newborn (P74.1)*
              hypovolemic shock NOS (R57.1)
              postprocedural hypovolemic shock (T81.19)
              traumatic hypovolemic shock (T79.4)

AHA: 2019,2Q,7; 2018,2Q,6

E86.0 **Dehydration**

AHA: 2019,2Q,7; 2019,1Q,12; 2014,1Q,7

TIP: Can be assigned in addition to hypernatremia (E87.0) or hyponatremia (E87.1), when documented.

E86.1 **Hypovolemia**

Depletion of volume of plasma

E86.9 **Volume depletion, unspecified**

DEF: Depletion of total body water (dehydration) and/or contraction of total intravascular plasma (hypovolemia).

✓4ᵗʰ E87 **Other disorders of fluid, electrolyte and acid-base balance**

EXCLUDES 1   *diabetes insipidus (E23.2)*
              electrolyte imbalance associated with hyperemesis gravidarum (O21.1)
              electrolyte imbalance following ectopic or molar pregnancy (O08.5)
              familial periodic paralysis (G72.3)

AHA: 2018,2Q,6

CC Excl: For CC codes in category E87: PDX collection 543

E87.0 **Hyperosmolality and hypernatremia** `CC`

Sodium [Na] excess

Sodium [Na] overload

AHA: 2014,1Q,7

TIP: Assign an additional code for dehydration (E86.0), when documented.

E87.1 **Hypo-osmolality and hyponatremia** `CC`

Sodium [Na] deficiency

EXCLUDES 1   *syndrome of inappropriate secretion of antidiuretic hormone (E22.2)*

AHA: 2014,1Q,7

TIP: Assign an additional code for dehydration (E86.0), when documented.

✔ Additional Character Required   ✓x7ᵗʰ Placeholder   Unacceptable PDx   Questionable PDx   Manifestation   Unspecified Dx   `H1`-`H14` HAC   `HCC` CMS-HCC Dx   `HIV` HIV Dx

ICD-10-CM 2020   537

Chapter 4. Endocrine, Nutritional and Metabolic Diseases

E87.2–E89.3

E87.2 Acidosis `CC`
    Acidosis NOS
    Lactic acidosis
    Metabolic acidosis
    Respiratory acidosis
    EXCLUDES 1   *diabetic acidosis — see categories E08-E10, E13 with ketoacidosis*
    DEF: Reduction of alkaline in the blood and tissues caused by an increase in acid and decrease in bicarbonate.

E87.3 Alkalosis `CC`
    Alkalosis NOS
    Metabolic alkalosis
    Respiratory alkalosis

E87.4 Mixed disorder of acid-base balance `CC`

E87.5 Hyperkalemia
    Potassium [K] excess
    Potassium [K] overload

E87.6 Hypokalemia
    Potassium [K] deficiency

√5th E87.7 Fluid overload
    EXCLUDES 1   *edema NOS (R60.9)*
                 fluid retention (R60.9)

    E87.70 Fluid overload, unspecified
    E87.71 Transfusion associated circulatory overload
        Fluid overload due to transfusion (blood) (blood components)
        TACO
    E87.79 Other fluid overload

E87.8 Other disorders of electrolyte and fluid balance, not elsewhere classified
    Electrolyte imbalance NOS
    Hyperchloremia
    Hypochloremia

√4th E88 Other and unspecified metabolic disorders
    Use additional codes for associated conditions
    EXCLUDES 1   *histiocytosis X (chronic) (C96.6)*

√5th E88.0 Disorders of plasma-protein metabolism, not elsewhere classified
    EXCLUDES 1   *disorder of lipoprotein metabolism (E78.-)*
                 monoclonal gammopathy (of undetermined significance) (D47.2)
                 polyclonal hypergammaglobulinemia (D89.0)
                 Waldenström macroglobulinemia (C88.0)

    E88.01 Alpha-1-antitrypsin deficiency `HCC`
        AAT deficiency

    E88.02 Plasminogen deficiency `CC`
        Dysplasminogenemia
        Hypoplasminogenemia
        Type 1 plasminogen deficiency
        Type 2 plasminogen deficiency
        Code also, if applicable, ligneous conjunctivitis (H10.51)
        Use additional code for associated findings, such as:
            hydrocephalus (G91.4)
            ligneous conjunctivitis (H10.51)
            otitis media (H67.-)
            respiratory disorder related to plasminogen deficiency (J99)
        AHA: 2018,4Q,6-7
        CC Excl: PDX collection 2034

    E88.09 Other disorders of plasma-protein metabolism, not elsewhere classified
        Bisalbuminemia

E88.1 Lipodystrophy, not elsewhere classified
    Lipodystrophy NOS
    EXCLUDES 1   *Whipple's disease (K90.81)*

E88.2 Lipomatosis, not elsewhere classified
    Lipomatosis NOS
    Lipomatosis (Check) dolorosa [Dercum]

E88.3 Tumor lysis syndrome `MCC`
    Tumor lysis syndrome (spontaneous)
    Tumor lysis syndrome following antineoplastic drug chemotherapy
    Use additional code for adverse effect, if applicable, to identify drug (T45.1X5)
    AHA: 2019,2Q,24
    DEF: Potentially fatal metabolic complication of tumor necrosis caused by spontaneous or treatment-related accumulation of byproducts from dying cancer cells. Symptoms include hyperkalemia, hyperphosphatemia, hypocalcemia, hyperuricemia, and hyperuricosuria.
    CC Excl: PDX collection 544

√5th E88.4 Mitochondrial metabolism disorders
    EXCLUDES 1   *disorders of pyruvate metabolism (E74.4)*
                 Kearns-Sayre syndrome (H49.81)
                 Leber's disease (H47.22)
                 Leigh's encephalopathy (G31.82)
                 mitochondrial myopathy, NEC (G71.3)
                 Reye's syndrome (G93.7)
    CC Excl: For CC codes in subcategory E88.4: PDX collection 545

    E88.40 Mitochondrial metabolism disorder, unspecified `CC` `HCC`
    E88.41 MELAS syndrome `CC` `HCC`
        Mitochondrial myopathy, encephalopathy, lactic acidosis and stroke-like episodes
    E88.42 MERRF syndrome `CC` `HCC`
        Myoclonic epilepsy associated with ragged-red fibers
        Code also progressive myoclonic epilepsy (G40.3-)
    E88.49 Other mitochondrial metabolism disorders `CC` `HCC`

√5th E88.8 Other specified metabolic disorders
    E88.81 Metabolic syndrome
        Dysmetabolic syndrome X
        Use additional codes for associated manifestations, such as:
            obesity (E66.-)
        DEF: Group of health risks that increase the likelihood of developing heart disease, stroke, and diabetes. These risks include certain parameters for blood pressure, cholesterol, and glucose levels.
    E88.89 Other specified metabolic disorders `HCC`
        Launois-Bensaude adenolipomatosis
        EXCLUDES 1   *adult pulmonary Langerhans cell histiocytosis (J84.82)*

E88.9 Metabolic disorder, unspecified

Postprocedural endocrine and metabolic complications and disorders, not elsewhere classified (E89)

CC Excl: For CC codes in category E89, unless otherwise noted: PDX collection 546

√4th E89 Postprocedural endocrine and metabolic complications and disorders, not elsewhere classified
    EXCLUDES 2   *intraoperative complications of endocrine system organ or structure (E36.0-, E36.1-, E36.8)*

E89.0 Postprocedural hypothyroidism
    Postirradiation hypothyroidism
    Postsurgical hypothyroidism

E89.1 Postprocedural hypoinsulinemia `CC`
    Postpancreatectomy hyperglycemia
    Postsurgical hypoinsulinemia
    Use additional code, if applicable, to identify:
        acquired absence of pancreas (Z90.41-)
        diabetes mellitus (postpancreatectomy) (postprocedural) (E13.-)
        insulin use (Z79.4)
    EXCLUDES 1   *transient postprocedural hyperglycemia (R73.9)*
                 transient postprocedural hypoglycemia (E16.2)
    CC Excl: PDX collection 520

E89.2 Postprocedural hypoparathyroidism `HCC`
    Parathyroprival tetany

E89.3 Postprocedural hypopituitarism `HCC`
    Postirradiation hypopituitarism

N Newborn: 0   P Pediatric: 0-17   M Maternity: 9-64   A Adult: 15-124   **MCC** Major Complication/Comorbidity   **CC** Complication/Comorbidity   **SW** Severe Wound Dx

538

ICD-10-CM 2020

√5ᵗʰ E89.4 Postprocedural ovarian failure

    E89.40 Asymptomatic postprocedural ♀
        ovarian failure
        Postprocedural ovarian failure NOS

    E89.41 Symptomatic postprocedural ♀
        ovarian failure
        Symptoms such as flushing, sleeplessness, headache, lack of concentration, associated with postprocedural menopause

E89.5 Postprocedural testicular hypofunction ♂

E89.6 Postprocedural adrenocortical (-medullary) `CC` `HCC`
    hypofunction
    CC Excl: PDX collection 526

√5ᵗʰ E89.8 Other postprocedural endocrine and metabolic complications and disorders
    AHA: 2016,4Q,9-10

    √6ᵗʰ E89.81 Postprocedural hemorrhage of an endocrine system organ or structure following a procedure

        E89.810 Postprocedural `CC`
            hemorrhage of an endocrine system organ or structure following an endocrine system procedure

        E89.811 Postprocedural `CC`
            hemorrhage of an endocrine system organ or structure following other procedure

    √6ᵗʰ E89.82 Postprocedural hematoma and seroma of an endocrine system organ or structure

        E89.820 Postprocedural hematoma `CC`
            of an endocrine system organ or structure following an endocrine system procedure

        E89.821 Postprocedural hematoma `CC`
            of an endocrine system organ or structure following other procedure

        E89.822 Postprocedural seroma of `CC`
            an endocrine system organ or structure following an endocrine system procedure

        E89.823 Postprocedural seroma of `CC`
            an endocrine system organ or structure following other procedure

    E89.89 Other postprocedural endocrine and `CC`
        metabolic complications and disorders
        Use additional code, if applicable, to further specify disorder

Chapter 5. Mental, Behavioral and Neurodevelopmental Disorders (F01–F99)

Chapter-specific Guidelines with Coding Examples

The chapter-specific guidelines from the ICD-10-CM Official Guidelines for Coding and Reporting have been provided below. Along with these guidelines are coding examples, contained in the shaded boxes, that have been developed to help illustrate the coding and/or sequencing guidance found in these guidelines.

a. Pain disorders related to psychological factors

Assign code F45.41, for pain that is exclusively related to psychological disorders. As indicated by the Excludes 1 note under category G89, a code from category G89 should not be assigned with code F45.41.

> Perceived abdominal pain determined to be persistent somatoform pain disorder
>
> **F45.41**   **Pain disorder exclusively related to psychological factors**
>
> *Explanation*: This pain was diagnosed as being exclusively psychological; therefore, no code from category G89 is added.

Code F45.42, Pain disorders with related psychological factors, should be used with a code from category G89, Pain, not elsewhere classified, if there is documentation of a psychological component for a patient with acute or chronic pain.

See Section I.C.6. Pain

b. Mental and behavioral disorders due to psychoactive substance use

1) In remission

Selection of codes for "in remission" for categories F10-F19, Mental and behavioral disorders due to psychoactive substance use (categories F10-F19 with -11, -.21) requires the provider's clinical judgment. The appropriate codes for "in remission" are assigned only on the basis of provider documentation (as defined in the Official Guidelines for Coding and Reporting), unless otherwise instructed by the classification.

Mild substance use disorders in early or sustained remission are classified to the appropriate codes for substance abuse in remission, and moderate or severe substance use disorders in early or sustained remission are classified to the appropriate codes for substance dependence in remission.

> Insomnia in patient with history of methamphetamine abuse; lab results indicate no current drug use
>
> **G47.00**   **Insomnia, unspecified**
>
> **F15.10**   **Other stimulant abuse, uncomplicated**
>
> *Explanation*: Insomnia is a common side-effect of stimulant use, such as methamphetamines. Although lab tests do not indicate that the patient is currently using methamphetamines, there is no specific documentation stating that the stimulant abuse is in remission. "History of" abuse does not equate to "in remission" in this instance.

2) Psychoactive substance use, abuse and dependence

When the provider documentation refers to use, abuse and dependence of the same substance (e.g. alcohol, opioid, cannabis, etc.), only one code should be assigned to identify the pattern of use based on the following hierarchy:

- If both use and abuse are documented, assign only the code for abuse
- If both abuse and dependence are documented, assign only the code for dependence
- If use, abuse and dependence are all documented, assign only the code for dependence
- If both use and dependence are documented, assign only the code for dependence.

> History and physical notes cannabis dependence; progress note says cannabis abuse
>
> **F12.20**   **Cannabis dependence, uncomplicated**
>
> *Explanation*: In the hierarchy, the dependence code is used if both abuse and dependence are documented.

> Discharge summary says cocaine abuse; progress notes list cocaine use
>
> **F14.10**   **Cocaine abuse, uncomplicated**
>
> *Explanation*: In the hierarchy, the abuse code is used if both abuse and use are documented.

3) Psychoactive substance use, unspecified

As with all other unspecified diagnoses, the codes for unspecified psychoactive substance use disorders (F10.9-, F11.9-, F12.9-, F13.9-, F14.9-, F15.9-, F16.9-, F18.9-, F19.9-) should only be assigned based on provider documentation and when they meet the definition of a reportable diagnosis (see Section III, Reporting Additional Diagnoses). These codes are to be used only when the psychoactive substance use is associated with a physical, mental or behavioral disorder, and such a relationship is documented by the provider.

c. Factitious disorder

Factitious disorder imposed on self or Munchausen's syndrome is a disorder in which a person falsely reports or causes his or her own physical or psychological signs or symptoms. For patients with documented factitious disorder on self or Munchausen's syndrome, assign the appropriate code from subcategory F68.1-, Factitious disorder imposed on self.

Munchausen's syndrome by proxy (MSBP) is a disorder in which a caregiver (perpetrator) falsely reports or causes an illness or injury in another person (victim) under his or her care, such as a child, an elderly adult, or a person who has a disability. The condition is also referred to as "factitious disorder imposed on another" or "factitious disorder by proxy." The perpetrator, not the victim, receives this diagnosis. Assign code F68.A, Factitious disorder imposed on another, to the perpetrator's record. For the victim of a patient suffering from MSBP, assign the appropriate code from categories T74, Adult and child abuse, neglect and other maltreatment, confirmed, or T76, Adult and child abuse, neglect and other maltreatment, suspected.

See Section I.C.19.f. Adult and child abuse, neglect and other maltreatment

Chapter 5. Mental, Behavioral and Neurodevelopmental Disorders (F01-F99)

INCLUDES   disorders of psychological development

EXCLUDES 2   *symptoms, signs and abnormal clinical laboratory findings, not elsewhere classified (R00-R99)*

This chapter contains the following blocks:

F01-F09   Mental disorders due to known physiological conditions
F10-F19   Mental and behavioral disorders due to psychoactive substance use
F20-F29   Schizophrenia, schizotypal, delusional, and other non-mood psychotic disorders
F30-F39   Mood [affective] disorders
F40-F48   Anxiety, dissociative, stress-related, somatoform and other nonpsychotic mental disorders
F50-F59   Behavioral syndromes associated with physiological disturbances and physical factors
F60-F69   Disorders of adult personality and behavior
F70-F79   Intellectual disabilities
F80-F89   Pervasive and specific developmental disorders
F90-F98   Behavioral and emotional disorders with onset usually occurring in childhood and adolescence
F99   Unspecified mental disorder

Mental disorders due to known physiological conditions (F01-F09)

NOTE   This block comprises a range of mental disorders grouped together on the basis of their having in common a demonstrable etiology in cerebral disease, brain injury, or other insult leading to cerebral dysfunction. The dysfunction may be primary, as in diseases, injuries, and insults that affect the brain directly and selectively; or secondary, as in systemic diseases and disorders that attack the brain only as one of the multiple organs or systems of the body that are involved.

√4ᵗʰ **F01   Vascular dementia**

Vascular dementia as a result of infarction of the brain due to vascular disease, including hypertensive cerebrovascular disease.

INCLUDES   arteriosclerotic dementia

Code first the underlying physiological condition or sequelae of cerebrovascular disease.

√5ᵗʰ **F01.5   Vascular dementia**

F01.50   Vascular dementia without behavioral disturbance   HCC A

Major neurocognitive disorder without behavioral disturbance

F01.51   Vascular dementia with behavioral disturbance   CC HCC A

Major neurocognitive disorder due to vascular disease, with behavioral disturbance
Major neurocognitive disorder with aggressive behavior
Major neurocognitive disorder with combative behavior
Major neurocognitive disorder with violent behavior
Vascular dementia with aggressive behavior
Vascular dementia with combative behavior
Vascular dementia with violent behavior
Use additional code, if applicable, to identify wandering in vascular dementia (Z91.83)

CC Excl: PDX collection 547

√4ᵗʰ **F02   Dementia in other diseases classified elsewhere**

INCLUDES   major neurocognitive disorder in other diseases classified elsewhere

Code first the underlying physiological condition, such as:
Alzheimer's (G30.-)
cerebral lipidosis (E75.4)
Creutzfeldt-Jakob disease (A81.0-)
dementia with Lewy bodies (G31.83)
dementia with Parkinsonism (G31.83)
epilepsy and recurrent seizures (G40.-)
frontotemporal dementia (G31.09)
hepatolenticular degeneration (E83.0)
human immunodeficiency virus [HIV] disease (B20)
Huntington's disease (G10)
hypercalcemia (E83.52)
hypothyroidism, acquired (E00-E03.-)
intoxications (T36-T65)
Jakob-Creutzfeldt disease (A81.0-)
multiple sclerosis (G35)
neurosyphilis (A52.17)
niacin deficiency [pellagra] (E52)
Parkinson's disease (G20)
Pick's disease (G31.01)
polyarteritis nodosa (M30.0)
prion disease (A81.9)
systemic lupus erythematosus (M32.-)
traumatic brain injury (S06.-)
trypanosomiasis (B56.-, B57.-)
vitamin B deficiency (E53.8)

EXCLUDES 2   *dementia in alcohol and psychoactive substance disorders (F10-F19, with .17, .27, .97)*
vascular dementia (F01.5-)

√5ᵗʰ **F02.8   Dementia in other diseases classified elsewhere**

AHA: 2017,2Q,7; 2016,4Q,141; 2016,2Q,6

TIP: A code from this subcategory should always be assigned with a code from category G30 when Alzheimer's disease is documented, even in the absence of documented dementia.

F02.80   *Dementia in other diseases classified elsewhere without behavioral disturbance*   HCC

Dementia in other diseases classified elsewhere NOS
Major neurocognitive disorder in other diseases classified elsewhere

F02.81   *Dementia in other diseases classified elsewhere with behavioral disturbance*   CC HCC

Dementia in other diseases classified elsewhere with aggressive behavior
Dementia in other diseases classified elsewhere with combative behavior
Dementia in other diseases classified elsewhere with violent behavior
Major neurocognitive disorder in other diseases classified elsewhere with aggressive behavior
Major neurocognitive disorder in other diseases classified elsewhere with combative behavior
Major neurocognitive disorder in other diseases classified elsewhere with violent behavior
Use additional code, if applicable, to identify wandering in dementia in conditions classified elsewhere (Z91.83)

CC Excl: PDX collection 548

N Newborn: 0   P Pediatric: 0-17   M Maternity: 9-64   A Adult: 15-124   MCC Major Complication/Comorbidity   CC Complication/Comorbidity   SW Severe Wound Dx

542   ICD-10-CM 2020

✓4ᵗʰ **F03 Unspecified dementia**
Presenile dementia NOS
Presenile psychosis NOS
Primary degenerative dementia NOS
Senile dementia NOS
Senile dementia depressed or paranoid type
Senile psychosis NOS
EXCLUDES 1 *senility NOS (R41.81)*
EXCLUDES 2 *mild memory disturbance due to known physiological condition (F06.8)*
senile dementia with delirium or acute confusional state (F05)

✓5ᵗʰ **F03.9 Unspecified dementia**

F03.90 Unspecified dementia without behavioral disturbance HIV HCC A
Dementia NOS
AHA: 2012,4Q,92

F03.91 Unspecified dementia with behavioral disturbance CC HCC A
Unspecified dementia with aggressive behavior
Unspecified dementia with combative behavior
Unspecified dementia with violent behavior
Use additional code, if applicable, to identify wandering in unspecified dementia (Z91.83)
CC Excl: PDX collection 548

F04 Amnestic disorder due to known physiological condition HCC
Korsakov's psychosis or syndrome, nonalcoholic
Code first the underlying physiological condition
EXCLUDES 1 *amnesia NOS (R41.3)*
anterograde amnesia (R41.1)
dissociative amnesia (F44.0)
retrograde amnesia (R41.2)
EXCLUDES 2 *alcohol-induced or unspecified Korsakov's syndrome (F10.26, F10.96)*
Korsakov's syndrome induced by other psychoactive substances (F13.26, F13.96, F19.16, F19.26, F19.96)

F05 Delirium due to known physiological condition CC
Acute or subacute brain syndrome
Acute or subacute confusional state (nonalcoholic)
Acute or subacute infective psychosis
Acute or subacute organic reaction
Acute or subacute psycho-organic syndrome
Delirium of mixed etiology
Delirium superimposed on dementia
Sundowning
Code first the underlying physiological condition
EXCLUDES 1 *delirium NOS (R41.0)*
EXCLUDES 2 *delirium tremens alcohol-induced or unspecified (F10.231, F10.921)*
AHA: 2019,2Q,34
CC Excl: PDX collection 549

✓4ᵗʰ **F06 Other mental disorders due to known physiological condition**
INCLUDES mental disorders due to endocrine disorder
mental disorders due to exogenous hormone
mental disorders due to exogenous toxic substance
mental disorders due to primary cerebral disease
mental disorders due to somatic illness
mental disorders due to systemic disease affecting the brain
Code first the underlying physiological condition
EXCLUDES 1 *unspecified dementia (F03)*
EXCLUDES 2 *delirium due to known physiological condition (F05)*
dementia as classified in F01-F02
other mental disorders associated with alcohol and other psychoactive substances (F10-F19)

F06.0 Psychotic disorder with hallucinations due to known physiological condition CC
Organic hallucinatory state (nonalcoholic)
EXCLUDES 2 *hallucinations and perceptual disturbance induced by alcohol and other psychoactive substances (F10-F19 with .151, .251, .951)*
schizophrenia (F20.-)
CC Excl: PDX collection 550

F06.1 Catatonic disorder due to known physiological condition
Catatonia associated with another mental disorder
Catatonia NOS
EXCLUDES 1 *catatonic stupor (R40.1)*
stupor NOS (R40.1)
EXCLUDES 2 *catatonic schizophrenia (F20.2)*
dissociative stupor (F44.2)
DEF: Catatonic: Abnormal neuropsychiatric state characterized by stupor, immobility or purposeless movements, or unresponsiveness in a person who otherwise appears awake.

F06.2 Psychotic disorder with delusions due to known physiological condition CC
Paranoid and paranoid-hallucinatory organic states
Schizophrenia-like psychosis in epilepsy
EXCLUDES 2 *alcohol and drug-induced psychotic disorder (F10-F19 with .150, .250, .950)*
brief psychotic disorder (F23)
delusional disorder (F22)
schizophrenia (F20.-)
CC Excl: PDX collection 550

✓5ᵗʰ **F06.3 Mood disorder due to known physiological condition**
EXCLUDES 2 *mood disorders due to alcohol and other psychoactive substances (F10-F19 with .14, .24, .94)*
mood disorders, not due to known physiological condition or unspecified (F30-F39)

F06.30 Mood disorder due to known physiological condition, unspecified CC

F06.31 Mood disorder due to known physiological condition with depressive features CC
Depressive disorder due to known physiological condition, with depressive features

F06.32 Mood disorder due to known physiological condition with major depressive-like episode
Depressive disorder due to known physiological condition, with major depressive-like episode

F06.33 Mood disorder due to known physiological condition with manic features
Bipolar and related disorder due to a known physiological condition, with manic features
Bipolar and related disorder due to known physiological condition, with manic- or hypomanic-like episodes

F06.34 Mood disorder due to known physiological condition with mixed features
Bipolar and related disorder due to known physiological condition, with mixed features
Depressive disorder due to known physiological condition, with mixed features

F06.4 Anxiety disorder due to known physiological condition CC
EXCLUDES 2 *anxiety disorders due to alcohol and other psychoactive substances (F10-F19 with .180, .280, .980)*
anxiety disorders, not due to known physiological condition or unspecified (F40.-, F41.-)

F06.8 Other specified mental disorders due to known physiological condition HIV
Epileptic psychosis NOS
Obsessive-compulsive and related disorder due to a known physiological condition
Organic dissociative disorder
Organic emotionally labile [asthenic] disorder

Chapter 5. Mental, Behavioral and Neurodevelopmental Disorders

F07–F10.239

✓4ᵗʰ **F07 Personality and behavioral disorders due to known physiological condition**

Code first the underlying physiological condition

F07.0 **Personality** change due to known physiological condition

Frontal lobe syndrome

Limbic epilepsy personality syndrome

Lobotomy syndrome

Organic personality disorder

Organic pseudopsychopathic personality

Organic pseudoretarded personality

Postleucotomy syndrome

Code first underlying physiological condition

EXCLUDES 1   *mild cognitive impairment (G31.84)*

postconcussional syndrome (F07.81)

postencephalitic syndrome (F07.89)

signs and symptoms involving emotional state (R45.-)

EXCLUDES 2   *specific personality disorder (F60.-)*

✓5ᵗʰ **F07.8 Other personality and behavioral disorders due to known physiological condition**

F07.81 **Postconcussional syndrome**   CC

Postcontusional syndrome (encephalopathy)

Post-traumatic brain syndrome, nonpsychotic

Use additional code to identify associated

post-traumatic headache, if applicable (G44.3-)

EXCLUDES 1   *current concussion (brain) (S06.0-)*

postencephalitic syndrome (F07.89)

DEF: Concussion symptoms that persist for weeks or months after a head injury. These symptoms may include headache, giddiness, fatigue, insomnia, mood fluctuation, and a subjective feeling of impaired intellectual function with extreme reaction to normal stressors.

F07.89 **Other personality and behavioral disorders due to known physiological condition**

Postencephalitic syndrome

Right hemispheric organic affective disorder

F07.9 **Unspecified personality and behavioral disorder due to known physiological condition**   HIV

Organic psychosyndrome

F09 Unspecified mental disorder due to known physiological condition   HIV CC

Mental disorder NOS due to known physiological condition

Organic brain syndrome NOS

Organic mental disorder NOS

Organic psychosis NOS

Symptomatic psychosis NOS

Code first the underlying physiological condition

EXCLUDES 1   *psychosis NOS (F29)*

Mental and behavioral disorders due to psychoactive substance use (F10-F19)

AHA: 2018,4Q,69-70; 2017,4Q,8; 2017,2Q,27

CC Excl: For CC codes in categories F10-F19, unless otherwise noted: PDX collection 550

✓4ᵗʰ **F10** **Alcohol** related disorders

Use additional code for blood alcohol level, if applicable (Y90.-)

✓5ᵗʰ **F10.1 Alcohol** abuse

EXCLUDES 1   *alcohol dependence (F10.2-)*

alcohol use, unspecified (F10.9-)

AHA: 2018,1Q,16; 2015,2Q,15

TIP: Alcohol withdrawal is classified to dependence only (F10.23-); there is no combination code for alcohol abuse with withdrawal. When alcohol abuse and alcohol withdrawal are documented for the same encounter, query the provider for clarification.

TIP: Assign when documentation indicates alcohol withdrawal without dependence; do not assign an additional code for withdrawal.

F10.10 **Alcohol abuse, uncomplicated**

Alcohol use disorder, mild

F10.11 **Alcohol abuse, in remission**

Alcohol use disorder, mild, in early remission

Alcohol use disorder, mild, in sustained remission

✓6ᵗʰ **F10.12 Alcohol abuse with intoxication**

F10.120 **Alcohol abuse with intoxication, uncomplicated**   HCC

F10.121 **Alcohol abuse with intoxication delirium**   CC HCC

F10.129 **Alcohol abuse with intoxication, unspecified**   HCC

F10.14 **Alcohol abuse with alcohol-induced mood disorder**   CC HCC

Alcohol use disorder, mild, with alcohol-induced bipolar or related disorder

Alcohol use disorder, mild, with alcohol-induced depressive disorder

✓6ᵗʰ **F10.15** **Alcohol abuse with alcohol-induced psychotic disorder**

F10.150 **Alcohol abuse with alcohol-induced psychotic disorder with delusions**   HCC

F10.151 **Alcohol abuse with alcohol-induced psychotic disorder with hallucinations**   CC HCC

DEF: Psychosis lasting less than six months with slight or no clouding of consciousness in which auditory hallucinations predominate.

F10.159 **Alcohol abuse with alcohol-induced psychotic disorder, unspecified**   CC HCC

✓6ᵗʰ **F10.18** **Alcohol abuse with other alcohol-induced disorders**

F10.180 **Alcohol abuse with alcohol-induced anxiety disorder**   CC HCC

F10.181 **Alcohol abuse with alcohol-induced sexual dysfunction**   CC HCC

F10.182 **Alcohol abuse with alcohol-induced sleep disorder**   HCC

F10.188 **Alcohol abuse with other alcohol-induced disorder**   CC HCC

F10.19 **Alcohol abuse with unspecified alcohol-induced disorder**   HCC

✓5ᵗʰ **F10.2 Alcohol** dependence

EXCLUDES 1   *alcohol abuse (F10.1-)*

alcohol use, unspecified (F10.9-)

EXCLUDES 2   *toxic effect of alcohol (T51.0-)*

F10.20 **Alcohol dependence, uncomplicated**   HCC

Alcohol use disorder, moderate

Alcohol use disorder, severe

F10.21 **Alcohol dependence, in remission**   HCC

Alcohol use disorder, moderate, in early remission

Alcohol use disorder, moderate, in sustained remission

Alcohol use disorder, severe, in early remission

Alcohol use disorder, severe, in sustained remission

✓6ᵗʰ **F10.22** **Alcohol dependence with intoxication**

Acute drunkenness (in alcoholism)

EXCLUDES 2   *alcohol dependence with withdrawal (F10.23-)*

F10.220 **Alcohol dependence with intoxication, uncomplicated**   HCC

F10.221 **Alcohol dependence with intoxication delirium**   CC HCC

F10.229 **Alcohol dependence with intoxication, unspecified**   HCC

✓6ᵗʰ **F10.23** **Alcohol dependence with withdrawal**

EXCLUDES 2   *alcohol dependence with intoxication (F10.22-)*

AHA: 2018,1Q,16; 2015,2Q,15

TIP: Do not assign a code from this subcategory when documentation indicates alcohol withdrawal without dependence.

F10.230 **Alcohol dependence with withdrawal, uncomplicated**   CC HCC

F10.231 **Alcohol dependence with withdrawal delirium**   CC HCC

F10.232 **Alcohol dependence with withdrawal with perceptual disturbance**   CC HCC

F10.239 **Alcohol dependence with withdrawal, unspecified**   CC HCC

N Newborn: 0   P Pediatric: 0-17   M Maternity: 9-64   A Adult: 15-124   MCC Major Complication/Comorbidity   CC Complication/Comorbidity   SW Severe Wound Dx

544   ICD-10-CM 2020

F10.24 **Alcohol dependence with alcohol-induced mood disorder** `CC` `HCC`

Alcohol use disorder, moderate, with alcohol-induced bipolar or related disorder

Alcohol use disorder, moderate, with alcohol-induced depressive disorder

Alcohol use disorder, severe, with alcohol-induced bipolar or related disorder

Alcohol use disorder, severe, with alcohol-induced depressive disorder

√6ᵗʰ **F10.25** **Alcohol dependence with alcohol-induced psychotic disorder**

     F10.250 **Alcohol dependence with alcohol-induced psychotic disorder with delusions** `HCC`

     F10.251 **Alcohol dependence with alcohol-induced psychotic disorder with hallucinations** `CC` `HCC`

     F10.259 **Alcohol dependence with alcohol-induced psychotic disorder, unspecified** `CC` `HCC`

F10.26 **Alcohol dependence with alcohol-induced persisting amnestic disorder** `HCC`

Alcohol use disorder, moderate, with alcohol-induced major neurocognitive disorder, amnestic-confabulatory type

Alcohol use disorder, severe, with alcohol-induced major neurocognitive disorder, amnestic-confabulatory type

DEF: Prominent and lasting reduced memory span and disordered time appreciation and confabulation that occurs in alcoholics as sequel to acute alcoholic psychosis.

F10.27 **Alcohol dependence with alcohol-induced persisting dementia** `CC` `HCC`

Alcohol use disorder, moderate, with alcohol-induced major neurocognitive disorder, nonamnestic-confabulatory type

Alcohol use disorder, severe, with alcohol-induced major neurocognitive disorder, nonamnestic-confabulatory type

√6ᵗʰ **F10.28** **Alcohol dependence with other alcohol-induced disorders**

     F10.280 **Alcohol dependence with alcohol-induced anxiety disorder** `CC` `HCC`

     F10.281 **Alcohol dependence with alcohol-induced sexual dysfunction** `CC` `HCC`

     F10.282 **Alcohol dependence with alcohol-induced sleep disorder** `HCC`

     F10.288 **Alcohol dependence with other alcohol-induced disorder** `CC` `HCC`

         Alcohol use disorder, moderate, with alcohol-induced mild neurocognitive disorder

         Alcohol use disorder, severe, with alcohol-induced mild neurocognitive disorder

F10.29 **Alcohol dependence with unspecified alcohol-induced disorder** `CC` `HCC`

√5ᵗʰ **F10.9** **Alcohol use, unspecified**

     EXCLUDES 1   *alcohol abuse (F10.1-)*

                alcohol dependence (F10.2-)

     AHA: 2018, 2Q, 10-11

     TIP: Assign a substance use code only when the provider documents a relationship between the use and an associated physical, mental, or behavioral disorder. As with all diagnoses, substance use codes must meet the definition of a reportable diagnosis.

√6ᵗʰ **F10.92** **Alcohol use, unspecified with intoxication**

     F10.920 **Alcohol use, unspecified with intoxication, uncomplicated** `HCC`

         AHA: 2018, 2Q, 10-11

     F10.921 **Alcohol use, unspecified with intoxication delirium** `CC` `HCC`

     F10.929 **Alcohol use, unspecified with intoxication, unspecified** `HCC`

F10.94 **Alcohol use, unspecified with alcohol-induced mood disorder** `CC` `HCC`

Alcohol induced bipolar or related disorder, without use disorder

Alcohol induced depressive disorder, without use disorder

√6ᵗʰ **F10.95** **Alcohol use, unspecified with alcohol-induced psychotic disorder**

     F10.950 **Alcohol use, unspecified with alcohol-induced psychotic disorder with delusions** `HCC`

     F10.951 **Alcohol use, unspecified with alcohol-induced psychotic disorder with hallucinations** `CC` `HCC`

     F10.959 **Alcohol use, unspecified with alcohol-induced psychotic disorder, unspecified** `CC` `HCC`

         Alcohol-induced psychotic disorder without use disorder

F10.96 **Alcohol use, unspecified with alcohol-induced persisting amnestic disorder** `HCC`

Alcohol-induced major neurocognitive disorder, amnestic-confabulatory type, without use disorder

F10.97 **Alcohol use, unspecified with alcohol-induced persisting dementia** `HCC`

Alcohol-induced major neurocognitive disorder, nonamnestic-confabulatory type, without use disorder

√6ᵗʰ **F10.98** **Alcohol use, unspecified with other alcohol-induced disorders**

     F10.980 **Alcohol use, unspecified with alcohol-induced anxiety disorder** `CC` `HCC`

         Alcohol induced anxiety disorder, without use disorder

     F10.981 **Alcohol use, unspecified with alcohol-induced sexual dysfunction** `CC` `HCC`

         Alcohol induced sexual dysfunction, without use disorder

     F10.982 **Alcohol use, unspecified with alcohol-induced sleep disorder** `HCC`

         Alcohol induced sleep disorder, without use disorder

     F10.988 **Alcohol use, unspecified with other alcohol-induced disorder** `CC` `HCC`

         Alcohol induced mild neurocognitive disorder, without use disorder

F10.99 **Alcohol use, unspecified with unspecified alcohol-induced disorder** `HCC`

√4ᵗʰ **F11** **Opioid related disorders**

√5ᵗʰ **F11.1** **Opioid abuse**

     EXCLUDES 1   *opioid dependence (F11.2-)*

                opioid use, unspecified (F11.9-)

     F11.10 **Opioid abuse, uncomplicated** `HCC`

         Opioid use disorder, mild

     F11.11 **Opioid abuse, in remission** `HCC`

         Opioid use disorder, mild, in early remission

         Opioid use disorder, mild, in sustained remission

√6ᵗʰ **F11.12** **Opioid abuse with intoxication**

     F11.120 **Opioid abuse with intoxication, uncomplicated** `HCC`

     F11.121 **Opioid abuse with intoxication delirium** `CC` `HCC`

     F11.122 **Opioid abuse with intoxication with perceptual disturbance** `HCC`

     F11.129 **Opioid abuse with intoxication, unspecified** `HCC`

✅ Additional Character Required   √x7ᵗʰ Placeholder   Unacceptable PDx   Questionable PDx   Manifestation   Unspecified Dx   `H1`-`H14` HAC   `HCC` CMS-HCC Dx   `HIV` HIV Dx

ICD-10-CM 2020   545

F11.14 Opioid abuse with opioid-induced mood disorder   `HCC`

Opioid use disorder, mild, with opioid-induced depressive disorder

✓6th **F11.15** Opioid abuse with opioid-induced psychotic disorder

     F11.150 Opioid abuse with opioid-induced psychotic disorder with delusions   `CC` `HCC`

     F11.151 Opioid abuse with opioid-induced psychotic disorder with hallucinations   `CC` `HCC`

     F11.159 Opioid abuse with opioid-induced psychotic disorder, unspecified   `HCC`

✓6th **F11.18** Opioid abuse with other opioid-induced disorder

     F11.181 Opioid abuse with opioid-induced sexual dysfunction   `HCC`

     F11.182 Opioid abuse with opioid-induced sleep disorder   `HCC`

     F11.188 Opioid abuse with other opioid-induced disorder   `HCC`

F11.19 Opioid abuse with unspecified opioid-induced disorder   `HCC`

✓5th **F11.2** Opioid dependence

   EXCLUDES 1   opioid abuse (F11.1-)
               opioid use, unspecified (F11.9-)
   EXCLUDES 2   opioid poisoning (T40.0-T40.2-)

F11.20 Opioid dependence, uncomplicated   `CC` `HCC`

Opioid use disorder, moderate
Opioid use disorder, severe
CC Excl: No Excl

F11.21 Opioid dependence, in remission   `HCC`

Opioid use disorder, moderate, in early remission
Opioid use disorder, moderate, in sustained remission
Opioid use disorder, severe, in early remission
Opioid use disorder, severe, in sustained remission

✓6th **F11.22** Opioid dependence with intoxication

   EXCLUDES 1   opioid dependence with withdrawal (F11.23)

     F11.220 Opioid dependence with intoxication, uncomplicated   `HCC`

     F11.221 Opioid dependence with intoxication delirium   `CC` `HCC`

     F11.222 Opioid dependence with intoxication with perceptual disturbance   `CC` `HCC`
           CC Excl: No Excl

     F11.229 Opioid dependence with intoxication, unspecified   `HCC`

F11.23 Opioid dependence with withdrawal   `CC` `HCC`

   EXCLUDES 1   opioid dependence with intoxication (F11.22-)

F11.24 Opioid dependence with opioid-induced mood disorder   `HCC`

Opioid use disorder, moderate, with opioid induced depressive disorder

✓6th **F11.25** Opioid dependence with opioid-induced psychotic disorder

     F11.250 Opioid dependence with opioid-induced psychotic disorder with delusions   `CC` `HCC`

     F11.251 Opioid dependence with opioid-induced psychotic disorder with hallucinations   `CC` `HCC`

     F11.259 Opioid dependence with opioid-induced psychotic disorder, unspecified   `CC` `HCC`
           CC Excl: No Excl

✓6th **F11.28** Opioid dependence with other opioid-induced disorder

     F11.281 Opioid dependence with opioid-induced sexual dysfunction   `CC` `HCC`
           CC Excl: No Excl

     F11.282 Opioid dependence with opioid-induced sleep disorder   `CC` `HCC`
           CC Excl: No Excl

     F11.288 Opioid dependence with other opioid-induced disorder   `CC` `HCC`
           CC Excl: No Excl

F11.29 Opioid dependence with unspecified opioid-induced disorder   `HCC`

✓5th **F11.9** Opioid use, unspecified

   EXCLUDES 1   opioid abuse (F11.1-)
               opioid dependence (F11.2-)

TIP: Assign a substance use code only when the provider documents a relationship between the use and an associated physical, mental, or behavioral disorder. As with all diagnoses, substance use codes must meet the definition of a reportable diagnosis.

F11.90 Opioid use, unspecified, uncomplicated
       AHA: 2018,2Q,10-11

✓6th **F11.92** Opioid use, unspecified with intoxication

   EXCLUDES 1   opioid use, unspecified with withdrawal (F11.93)

     F11.920 Opioid use, unspecified with intoxication, uncomplicated   `HCC`

     F11.921 Opioid use, unspecified with intoxication delirium   `CC` `HCC`
           Opioid-induced delirium

     F11.922 Opioid use, unspecified with intoxication with perceptual disturbance   `HCC`

     F11.929 Opioid use, unspecified with intoxication, unspecified   `HCC`

F11.93 Opioid use, unspecified with withdrawal   `CC` `HCC`

   EXCLUDES 1   opioid use, unspecified with intoxication (F11.92-)

F11.94 Opioid use, unspecified with opioid-induced mood disorder   `HCC`

Opioid induced depressive disorder, without use disorder

✓6th **F11.95** Opioid use, unspecified with opioid-induced psychotic disorder

     F11.950 Opioid use, unspecified with opioid-induced psychotic disorder with delusions   `CC` `HCC`

     F11.951 Opioid use, unspecified with opioid-induced psychotic disorder with hallucinations   `CC` `HCC`

     F11.959 Opioid use, unspecified with opioid-induced psychotic disorder, unspecified   `HCC`

✓6th **F11.98** Opioid use, unspecified with other specified opioid-induced disorder

     F11.981 Opioid use, unspecified with opioid-induced sexual dysfunction   `HCC`
           Opioid induced sexual dysfunction, without use disorder

     F11.982 Opioid use, unspecified with opioid-induced sleep disorder   `HCC`
           Opioid induced sleep disorder, without use disorder

     F11.988 Opioid use, unspecified with other opioid-induced disorder   `HCC`
           Opioid induced anxiety disorder, without use disorder

F11.99 Opioid use, unspecified with unspecified opioid-induced disorder   `HCC`

`N` Newborn: 0   `P` Pediatric: 0-17   `M` Maternity: 9-64   `A` Adult: 15-124   `MCC` Major Complication/Comorbidity   `CC` Complication/Comorbidity   `SW` Severe Wound Dx

546   ICD-10-CM 2020

√4ᵗʰ **F12** Cannabis **related disorders**

     INCLUDES   marijuana

√5ᵗʰ **F12.1** **Cannabis** abuse

     EXCLUDES 1   *cannabis dependence (F12.2-)*
              cannabis use, unspecified (F12.9-)

     F12.10 **Cannabis abuse,** uncomplicated
           Cannabis use disorder, mild

     F12.11 **Cannabis abuse,** in remission
           Cannabis use disorder, mild, in early remission
           Cannabis use disorder, mild, in sustained remission

√6ᵗʰ **F12.12** **Cannabis abuse with** intoxication

         F12.120 **Cannabis abuse with**   HCC
                   intoxication,
                   uncomplicated

         F12.121 **Cannabis abuse with**   CC HCC
                   intoxication delirium

         F12.122 **Cannabis abuse with**   HCC
                   intoxication with
                   perceptual disturbance

         F12.129 **Cannabis abuse with**   HCC
                   intoxication, unspecified

√6ᵗʰ **F12.15** **Cannabis abuse with** psychotic disorder

         F12.150 **Cannabis abuse with**   CC HCC
                   psychotic disorder with
                   delusions

         F12.151 **Cannabis abuse with**   CC HCC
                   psychotic disorder with
                   hallucinations

         F12.159 **Cannabis abuse with**   HCC
                   psychotic disorder, unspecified

√6ᵗʰ **F12.18** **Cannabis abuse with other cannabis-induced disorder**

         F12.180 **Cannabis abuse with**   HCC
                   cannabis-induced anxiety
                   disorder

         F12.188 **Cannabis abuse with other**   HCC
                   cannabis-induced disorder
                   Cannabis use disorder, mild, with
                       cannabis-induced sleep disorder

     F12.19 **Cannabis abuse with unspecified**   HCC
           cannabis-induced disorder

√5ᵗʰ **F12.2** **Cannabis** dependence

     EXCLUDES 1   *cannabis abuse (F12.1-)*
              cannabis use, unspecified (F12.9-)
     EXCLUDES 2   *cannabis poisoning (T40.7-)*

     F12.20 **Cannabis dependence,**   HCC
           uncomplicated
           Cannabis use disorder, moderate
           Cannabis use disorder, severe

     F12.21 **Cannabis dependence,** in remission   HCC
           Cannabis use disorder, moderate, in early remission
           Cannabis use disorder, moderate, in sustained
              remission
           Cannabis use disorder, severe, in early remission
           Cannabis use disorder, severe, in sustained remission

√6ᵗʰ **F12.22** **Cannabis dependence with** intoxication

         F12.220 **Cannabis dependence**   HCC
                   with intoxication,
                   uncomplicated

         F12.221 **Cannabis dependence**   CC HCC
                   with intoxication delirium

         F12.222 **Cannabis dependence**   HCC
                   with intoxication with
                   perceptual disturbance

         F12.229 **Cannabis dependence**   HCC
                   with intoxication, unspecified

     F12.23 **Cannabis dependence with**   HCC
           withdrawal
           AHA: 2018,4Q,7

√6ᵗʰ **F12.25** **Cannabis dependence with** psychotic disorder

         F12.250 **Cannabis dependence**   CC HCC
                   with psychotic disorder
                   with delusions

         F12.251 **Cannabis dependence**   CC HCC
                   with psychotic disorder
                   with hallucinations

         F12.259 **Cannabis dependence**   HCC
                   with psychotic disorder, unspecified

√6ᵗʰ **F12.28** **Cannabis dependence with other cannabis-induced disorder**

         F12.280 **Cannabis dependence**   HCC
                   with cannabis-induced
                   anxiety disorder

         F12.288 **Cannabis dependence**   HCC
                   with other
                   cannabis-induced disorder
                   Cannabis use disorder, moderate, with
                       cannabis-induced sleep disorder
                   Cannabis use disorder, severe, with
                       cannabis-induced sleep disorder

     F12.29 **Cannabis dependence with**   HCC
           unspecified cannabis-induced
           disorder

√5ᵗʰ **F12.9** **Cannabis use, unspecified**

     EXCLUDES 1   *cannabis abuse (F12.1-)*
              cannabis dependence (F12.2-)

     TIP: Assign a substance use code only when the provider documents a relationship between the use and an associated physical, mental, or behavioral disorder. As with all diagnoses, substance use codes must meet the definition of a reportable diagnosis.

     F12.90 **Cannabis use, unspecified,** uncomplicated
           AHA: 2018,2Q,10-11

√6ᵗʰ **F12.92** **Cannabis use, unspecified with** intoxication

         F12.920 **Cannabis use, unspecified**   HCC
                   with intoxication,
                   uncomplicated

         F12.921 **Cannabis use, unspecified**   CC HCC
                   with intoxication delirium

         F12.922 **Cannabis use, unspecified**   HCC
                   with intoxication with
                   perceptual disturbance

         F12.929 **Cannabis use, unspecified**   HCC
                   with intoxication, unspecified

     F12.93 **Cannabis use, unspecified with**   HCC
           withdrawal
           AHA: 2018,4Q,7

√6ᵗʰ **F12.95** **Cannabis use, unspecified with** psychotic disorder

         F12.950 **Cannabis use, unspecified**   CC HCC
                   with psychotic disorder
                   with delusions

         F12.951 **Cannabis use, unspecified**   CC HCC
                   with psychotic disorder
                   with hallucinations

         F12.959 **Cannabis use, unspecified**   HCC
                   with psychotic disorder, unspecified
                   Cannabis induced psychotic disorder,
                       without use disorder

√6ᵗʰ **F12.98** **Cannabis use, unspecified with other cannabis-induced disorder**

         F12.980 **Cannabis use, unspecified**   HCC
                   with anxiety disorder
                   Cannabis induced anxiety disorder,
                       without use disorder

         F12.988 **Cannabis use, unspecified**   HCC
                   with other
                   cannabis-induced disorder
                   Cannabis induced sleep disorder, without
                       use disorder

     F12.99 **Cannabis use, unspecified with**   HCC
           unspecified cannabis-induced disorder

√4ᵗʰ **F13** **Sedative, hypnotic, or anxiolytic related disorders**

√5ᵗʰ **F13.1** **Sedative, hypnotic or anxiolytic-related** abuse

     EXCLUDES 1   *sedative, hypnotic or anxiolytic-related dependence (F13.2-)*
              sedative, hypnotic, or anxiolytic use, unspecified (F13.9-)

     F13.10 **Sedative, hypnotic or anxiolytic**   HCC
           abuse, uncomplicated
           Sedative, hypnotic, or anxiolytic use disorder, mild

☑ Additional Character Required   √x7ᵗʰ Placeholder   Unacceptable PDx   Questionable PDx   Manifestation   Unspecified Dx   H1-H14 HAC   HCC CMS-HCC Dx   HIV HIV Dx

ICD-10-CM 2020   547

F13.11 Sedative, hypnotic or anxiolytic abuse, in remission HCC
Sedative, hypnotic or anxiolytic use disorder, mild, in early remission
Sedative, hypnotic or anxiolytic use disorder, mild, in sustained remission

✓6ᵗʰ **F13.12 Sedative, hypnotic or anxiolytic abuse with intoxication**

F13.120 Sedative, hypnotic or anxiolytic abuse with intoxication, uncomplicated HCC

F13.121 Sedative, hypnotic or anxiolytic abuse with intoxication delirium CC HCC

F13.129 Sedative, hypnotic or anxiolytic abuse with intoxication, unspecified HCC

F13.14 Sedative, hypnotic or anxiolytic abuse with sedative, hypnotic or anxiolytic-induced mood disorder HCC
Sedative, hypnotic, or anxiolytic use disorder, mild, with sedative, hypnotic, or anxiolytic-induced bipolar or related disorder
Sedative, hypnotic, or anxiolytic use disorder, mild, with sedative, hypnotic, or anxiolytic-induced depressive disorder

✓6ᵗʰ **F13.15 Sedative, hypnotic or anxiolytic abuse with sedative, hypnotic or anxiolytic-induced psychotic disorder**

F13.150 Sedative, hypnotic or anxiolytic abuse with sedative, hypnotic or anxiolytic-induced psychotic disorder with delusions CC HCC

F13.151 Sedative, hypnotic or anxiolytic abuse with sedative, hypnotic or anxiolytic-induced psychotic disorder with hallucinations CC HCC

F13.159 Sedative, hypnotic or anxiolytic abuse with sedative, hypnotic or anxiolytic-induced psychotic disorder, unspecified HCC

✓6ᵗʰ **F13.18 Sedative, hypnotic or anxiolytic abuse with other sedative, hypnotic or anxiolytic-induced disorders**

F13.180 Sedative, hypnotic or anxiolytic abuse with sedative, hypnotic or anxiolytic-induced anxiety disorder HCC

F13.181 Sedative, hypnotic or anxiolytic abuse with sedative, hypnotic or anxiolytic-induced sexual dysfunction HCC

F13.182 Sedative, hypnotic or anxiolytic abuse with sedative, hypnotic or anxiolytic-induced sleep disorder HCC

F13.188 Sedative, hypnotic or anxiolytic abuse with other sedative, hypnotic or anxiolytic-induced disorder HCC

F13.19 Sedative, hypnotic or anxiolytic abuse with unspecified sedative, hypnotic or anxiolytic-induced disorder HCC

✓5ᵗʰ **F13.2 Sedative, hypnotic or anxiolytic-related dependence**
EXCLUDES 1 sedative, hypnotic or anxiolytic-related abuse (F13.1-)
sedative, hypnotic, or anxiolytic use, unspecified (F13.9-)
EXCLUDES 2 sedative, hypnotic, or anxiolytic poisoning (T42.-)

F13.20 Sedative, hypnotic or anxiolytic dependence, uncomplicated CC HCC
CC Excl: No Excl

F13.21 Sedative, hypnotic or anxiolytic dependence, in remission HCC
Sedative, hypnotic or anxiolytic use disorder, moderate, in early remission
Sedative, hypnotic or anxiolytic use disorder, moderate, in sustained remission
Sedative, hypnotic or anxiolytic use disorder, severe, in early remission
Sedative, hypnotic or anxiolytic use disorder, severe, in sustained remission

✓6ᵗʰ **F13.22 Sedative, hypnotic or anxiolytic dependence with intoxication**
EXCLUDES 1 sedative, hypnotic or anxiolytic dependence with withdrawal (F13.23-)

F13.220 Sedative, hypnotic or anxiolytic dependence with intoxication, uncomplicated HCC

F13.221 Sedative, hypnotic or anxiolytic dependence with intoxication delirium CC HCC

F13.229 Sedative, hypnotic or anxiolytic dependence with intoxication, unspecified HCC

✓6ᵗʰ **F13.23 Sedative, hypnotic or anxiolytic dependence with withdrawal**
Sedative, hypnotic, or anxiolytic use disorder, moderate
Sedative, hypnotic, or anxiolytic use disorder, severe
EXCLUDES 1 sedative, hypnotic or anxiolytic dependence with intoxication (F13.22-)

F13.230 Sedative, hypnotic or anxiolytic dependence with withdrawal, uncomplicated CC HCC

F13.231 Sedative, hypnotic or anxiolytic dependence with withdrawal delirium CC HCC

F13.232 Sedative, hypnotic or anxiolytic dependence with withdrawal with perceptual disturbance CC HCC
Sedative, hypnotic, or anxiolytic withdrawal with perceptual disturbances

F13.239 Sedative, hypnotic or anxiolytic dependence with withdrawal, unspecified CC HCC
Sedative, hypnotic, or anxiolytic withdrawal without perceptual disturbances

F13.24 Sedative, hypnotic or anxiolytic dependence with sedative, hypnotic or anxiolytic-induced mood disorder HCC
Sedative, hypnotic, or anxiolytic use disorder, moderate, with sedative, hypnotic, or anxiolytic-induced bipolar or related disorder
Sedative, hypnotic, or anxiolytic use disorder, moderate, with sedative, hypnotic, or anxiolytic-induced depressive disorder
Sedative, hypnotic, or anxiolytic use disorder, severe, with sedative, hypnotic, or anxiolytic-induced bipolar or related disorder
Sedative, hypnotic, or anxiolytic use disorder, severe, with sedative, hypnotic, or anxiolytic-induced depressive disorder

✓6ᵗʰ **F13.25 Sedative, hypnotic or anxiolytic dependence with sedative, hypnotic or anxiolytic-induced psychotic disorder**

F13.250 Sedative, hypnotic or anxiolytic dependence with sedative, hypnotic or anxiolytic-induced psychotic disorder with delusions CC HCC

F13.251 Sedative, hypnotic or anxiolytic dependence with sedative, hypnotic or anxiolytic-induced psychotic disorder with hallucinations `CC` `HCC`

F13.259 Sedative, hypnotic or anxiolytic dependence with sedative, hypnotic or anxiolytic-induced psychotic disorder, unspecified `CC` `HCC`
CC Excl: No Excl

F13.26 Sedative, hypnotic or anxiolytic dependence with sedative, hypnotic or anxiolytic-induced persisting amnestic disorder `CC` `HCC`
CC Excl: No Excl

F13.27 Sedative, hypnotic or anxiolytic dependence with sedative, hypnotic or anxiolytic-induced persisting dementia `CC` `HCC`
Sedative, hypnotic, or anxiolytic use disorder, moderate, with sedative, hypnotic, or anxiolytic induced major neurocognitive disorder
Sedative, hypnotic, or anxiolytic use disorder, severe, with sedative, hypnotic, or anxiolytic-induced major neurocognitive disorder

✓6th **F13.28** Sedative, hypnotic or anxiolytic dependence with other sedative, hypnotic or anxiolytic-induced disorders

F13.280 Sedative, hypnotic or anxiolytic dependence with sedative, hypnotic or anxiolytic-induced anxiety disorder `CC` `HCC`
CC Excl: No Excl

F13.281 Sedative, hypnotic or anxiolytic dependence with sedative, hypnotic or anxiolytic-induced sexual dysfunction `CC` `HCC`
CC Excl: No Excl

F13.282 Sedative, hypnotic or anxiolytic dependence with sedative, hypnotic or anxiolytic-induced sleep disorder `CC` `HCC`
CC Excl: No Excl

F13.288 Sedative, hypnotic or anxiolytic dependence with other sedative, hypnotic or anxiolytic-induced disorder `CC` `HCC`
Sedative, hypnotic, or anxiolytic use disorder, moderate, with sedative, hypnotic, or anxiolytic-induced mild neurocognitive disorder
Sedative, hypnotic, or anxiolytic use disorder, severe, with sedative, hypnotic, or anxiolytic-induced mild neurocognitive disorder
CC Excl: No Excl

F13.29 Sedative, hypnotic or anxiolytic dependence with unspecified sedative, hypnotic or anxiolytic-induced disorder `HCC`

✓5th **F13.9** Sedative, hypnotic or anxiolytic-related use, unspecified
EXCLUDES 1   sedative, hypnotic or anxiolytic-related abuse (F13.1-)
sedative, hypnotic or anxiolytic-related dependence (F13.2-)
TIP: Assign a substance use code only when the provider documents a relationship between the use and an associated physical, mental, or behavioral disorder. As with all diagnoses, substance use codes must meet the definition of a reportable diagnosis.

F13.90 Sedative, hypnotic, or anxiolytic use, unspecified, uncomplicated
AHA: 2018,2Q,10-11

✓6th **F13.92** Sedative, hypnotic or anxiolytic use, unspecified with intoxication
EXCLUDES 1   sedative, hypnotic or anxiolytic use, unspecified with withdrawal (F13.93-)

F13.920 Sedative, hypnotic or anxiolytic use, unspecified with intoxication, uncomplicated `HCC`

F13.921 Sedative, hypnotic or anxiolytic use, unspecified with intoxication delirium `CC` `HCC`
Sedative, hypnotic, or anxiolytic-induced delirium

F13.929 Sedative, hypnotic or anxiolytic use, unspecified with intoxication, unspecified `HCC`

✓6th **F13.93** Sedative, hypnotic or anxiolytic use, unspecified with withdrawal
EXCLUDES 1   sedative, hypnotic or anxiolytic use, unspecified with intoxication (F13.92-)

F13.930 Sedative, hypnotic or anxiolytic use, unspecified with withdrawal, uncomplicated `CC` `HCC`

F13.931 Sedative, hypnotic or anxiolytic use, unspecified with withdrawal delirium `CC` `HCC`

F13.932 Sedative, hypnotic or anxiolytic use, unspecified with withdrawal with perceptual disturbances `CC` `HCC`

F13.939 Sedative, hypnotic or anxiolytic use, unspecified with withdrawal, unspecified `CC` `HCC`

F13.94 Sedative, hypnotic or anxiolytic use, unspecified with sedative, hypnotic or anxiolytic-induced mood disorder `HCC`
Sedative, hypnotic, or anxiolytic-induced bipolar or related disorder, without use disorder
Sedative, hypnotic, or anxiolytic-induced depressive disorder, without use disorder

✓6th **F13.95** Sedative, hypnotic or anxiolytic use, unspecified with sedative, hypnotic or anxiolytic-induced psychotic disorder

F13.950 Sedative, hypnotic or anxiolytic use, unspecified with sedative, hypnotic or anxiolytic-induced psychotic disorder with delusions `CC` `HCC`

F13.951 Sedative, hypnotic or anxiolytic use, unspecified with sedative, hypnotic or anxiolytic-induced psychotic disorder with hallucinations `CC` `HCC`

F13.959 Sedative, hypnotic or anxiolytic use, unspecified with sedative, hypnotic or anxiolytic-induced psychotic disorder, unspecified `HCC`
Sedative, hypnotic, or anxiolytic-induced psychotic disorder, without use disorder

F13.96 Sedative, hypnotic or anxiolytic use, unspecified with sedative, hypnotic or anxiolytic-induced persisting amnestic disorder `HCC`

F13.97 Sedative, hypnotic or anxiolytic use, unspecified with sedative, hypnotic or anxiolytic-induced persisting dementia `CC` `HCC`
Sedative, hypnotic, or anxiolytic-induced major neurocognitive disorder, without use disorder

✓6ᵗʰ F13.98 Sedative, hypnotic or anxiolytic use, unspecified with other sedative, hypnotic or anxiolytic-induced disorders

    F13.980 Sedative, hypnotic or anxiolytic use, unspecified with sedative, hypnotic or anxiolytic-induced anxiety disorder   HCC

       Sedative, hypnotic, or anxiolytic-induced anxiety disorder, without use disorder

    F13.981 Sedative, hypnotic or anxiolytic use, unspecified with sedative, hypnotic or anxiolytic-induced sexual dysfunction   HCC

       Sedative, hypnotic, or anxiolytic-induced sexual dysfunction disorder, without use disorder

    F13.982 Sedative, hypnotic or anxiolytic use, unspecified with sedative, hypnotic or anxiolytic-induced sleep disorder   HCC

       Sedative, hypnotic, or anxiolytic-induced sleep disorder, without use disorder

    F13.988 Sedative, hypnotic or anxiolytic use, unspecified with other sedative, hypnotic or anxiolytic-induced disorder   HCC

       Sedative, hypnotic, or anxiolytic-induced mild neurocognitive disorder

F13.99 Sedative, hypnotic or anxiolytic use, unspecified with unspecified sedative, hypnotic or anxiolytic-induced disorder   HCC

✓4ᵗʰ F14 Cocaine related disorders

    EXCLUDES 2   other stimulant-related disorders (F15.-)

✓5ᵗʰ F14.1 Cocaine abuse

    EXCLUDES 1   cocaine dependence (F14.2-)
              cocaine use, unspecified (F14.9-)

    F14.10 Cocaine abuse, uncomplicated   HCC

       Cocaine use disorder, mild

    F14.11 Cocaine abuse, in remission   HCC

       Cocaine use disorder, mild, in early remission
       Cocaine use disorder, mild, in sustained remission

  ✓6ᵗʰ F14.12 Cocaine abuse with intoxication

    F14.120 Cocaine abuse with intoxication, uncomplicated   HCC

    F14.121 Cocaine abuse with intoxication with delirium   CC HCC

    F14.122 Cocaine abuse with intoxication with perceptual disturbance   HCC

    F14.129 Cocaine abuse with intoxication, unspecified   HCC

    F14.14 Cocaine abuse with cocaine-induced mood disorder   HCC

       Cocaine use disorder, mild, with cocaine-induced bipolar or related disorder
       Cocaine use disorder, mild, with cocaine-induced depressive disorder

  ✓6ᵗʰ F14.15 Cocaine abuse with cocaine-induced psychotic disorder

    F14.150 Cocaine abuse with cocaine-induced psychotic disorder with delusions   CC HCC

    F14.151 Cocaine abuse with cocaine-induced psychotic disorder with hallucinations   CC HCC

    F14.159 Cocaine abuse with cocaine-induced psychotic disorder, unspecified   HCC

  ✓6ᵗʰ F14.18 Cocaine abuse with other cocaine-induced disorder

    F14.180 Cocaine abuse with cocaine-induced anxiety disorder   HCC

    F14.181 Cocaine abuse with cocaine-induced sexual dysfunction   HCC

    F14.182 Cocaine abuse with cocaine-induced sleep disorder   HCC

    F14.188 Cocaine abuse with other cocaine-induced disorder   HCC

       Cocaine use disorder, mild, with cocaine-induced obsessive compulsive or related disorder

F14.19 Cocaine abuse with unspecified cocaine-induced disorder   HCC

✓5ᵗʰ F14.2 Cocaine dependence

    EXCLUDES 1   cocaine abuse (F14.1-)
              cocaine use, unspecified (F14.9-)

    EXCLUDES 2   cocaine poisoning (T40.5-)

    F14.20 Cocaine dependence, uncomplicated   HCC

       Cocaine use disorder, moderate
       Cocaine use disorder, severe

    F14.21 Cocaine dependence, in remission   HCC

       Cocaine use disorder, moderate, in early remission
       Cocaine use disorder, moderate, in sustained remission
       Cocaine use disorder, severe, in early remission
       Cocaine use disorder, severe, in sustained remission

  ✓6ᵗʰ F14.22 Cocaine dependence with intoxication

    EXCLUDES 1   cocaine dependence with withdrawal (F14.23)

    F14.220 Cocaine dependence with intoxication, uncomplicated   HCC

    F14.221 Cocaine dependence with intoxication delirium   CC HCC

    F14.222 Cocaine dependence with intoxication with perceptual disturbance   CC HCC
       CC Excl: No Excl

    F14.229 Cocaine dependence with intoxication, unspecified   CC HCC
       CC Excl: No Excl

    F14.23 Cocaine dependence with withdrawal   CC HCC

    EXCLUDES 1   cocaine dependence with intoxication (F14.22-)

    F14.24 Cocaine dependence with cocaine-induced mood disorder   HCC

       Cocaine use disorder, moderate, with cocaine-induced bipolar or related disorder
       Cocaine use disorder, moderate, with cocaine-induced depressive disorder
       Cocaine use disorder, severe, with cocaine-induced bipolar or related disorder
       Cocaine use disorder, severe, with cocaine-induced depressive disorder

  ✓6ᵗʰ F14.25 Cocaine dependence with cocaine-induced psychotic disorder

    F14.250 Cocaine dependence with cocaine-induced psychotic disorder with delusions   CC HCC

    F14.251 Cocaine dependence with cocaine-induced psychotic disorder with hallucinations   CC HCC

    F14.259 Cocaine dependence with cocaine-induced psychotic disorder, unspecified   CC HCC
       CC Excl: No Excl

  ✓6ᵗʰ F14.28 Cocaine dependence with other cocaine-induced disorder

    F14.280 Cocaine dependence with cocaine-induced anxiety disorder   CC HCC
       CC Excl: No Excl

    F14.281 Cocaine dependence with cocaine-induced sexual dysfunction   CC HCC
       CC Excl: No Excl

N Newborn: 0   P Pediatric: 0-17   M Maternity: 9-64   A Adult: 15-124   MCC Major Complication/Comorbidity   CC Complication/Comorbidity   SW Severe Wound Dx

550   ICD-10-CM 2020

F14.282 Cocaine dependence with cocaine-induced sleep **disorder** `CC` `HCC`
CC Excl: No Excl

F14.288 Cocaine dependence with other cocaine-induced disorder `CC` `HCC`
Cocaine use disorder, moderate, with cocaine-induced obsessive compulsive or related disorder
Cocaine use disorder, severe, with cocaine-induced obsessive compulsive or related disorder
CC Excl: No Excl

F14.29 Cocaine dependence with unspecified cocaine-induced disorder `HCC`

√5ᵗʰ **F14.9 Cocaine use, unspecified**
EXCLUDES 1   *cocaine abuse (F14.1-)*
       cocaine dependence (F14.2-)
TIP: Assign a substance use code only when the provider documents a relationship between the use and an associated physical, mental, or behavioral disorder. As with all diagnoses, substance use codes must meet the definition of a reportable diagnosis.

F14.90 Cocaine use, unspecified, uncomplicated
AHA: 2018,2Q,10-11

√6ᵗʰ **F14.92 Cocaine use, unspecified with** intoxication

F14.920 Cocaine use, unspecified with intoxication, uncomplicated `HCC`

F14.921 Cocaine use, unspecified with intoxication delirium `CC` `HCC`

F14.922 Cocaine use, unspecified with intoxication with perceptual disturbance `HCC`

F14.929 Cocaine use, unspecified with intoxication, unspecified `HCC`

F14.94 Cocaine use, unspecified with cocaine-induced mood disorder `HCC`
Cocaine induced bipolar or related disorder, without use disorder
Cocaine induced depressive disorder, without use disorder

√6ᵗʰ **F14.95 Cocaine use, unspecified with cocaine-induced** psychotic disorder

F14.950 Cocaine use, unspecified with cocaine-induced psychotic disorder with delusions `CC` `HCC`

F14.951 Cocaine use, unspecified with cocaine-induced psychotic disorder with hallucinations `CC` `HCC`

F14.959 Cocaine use, unspecified with cocaine-induced psychotic disorder, unspecified `HCC`
Cocaine induced psychotic disorder, without use disorder

√6ᵗʰ **F14.98 Cocaine use, unspecified with other specified cocaine-induced disorder**

F14.980 Cocaine use, unspecified with cocaine-induced anxiety disorder `HCC`
Cocaine induced anxiety disorder, without use disorder

F14.981 Cocaine use, unspecified with cocaine-induced sexual dysfunction `HCC`
Cocaine induced sexual dysfunction, without use disorder

F14.982 Cocaine use, unspecified with cocaine-induced sleep disorder `HCC`
Cocaine induced sleep disorder, without use disorder

F14.988 Cocaine use, unspecified with other cocaine-induced disorder `HCC`
Cocaine induced obsessive compulsive or related disorder

F14.99 Cocaine use, unspecified with unspecified cocaine-induced disorder `HCC`

√4ᵗʰ **F15 Other** stimulant **related disorders**
INCLUDES   amphetamine-related disorders
       caffeine
EXCLUDES 2   *cocaine-related disorders (F14.-)*

√5ᵗʰ **F15.1 Other stimulant** abuse
EXCLUDES 1   *other stimulant dependence (F15.2-)*
       other stimulant use, unspecified (F15.9-)

F15.10 Other stimulant abuse, uncomplicated `HCC`
Amphetamine type substance use disorder, mild
Other or unspecified stimulant use disorder, mild

F15.11 Other stimulant abuse, in remission `HCC`
Amphetamine type substance use disorder, mild, in early remission
Amphetamine type substance use disorder, mild, in sustained remission
Other or unspecified stimulant use disorder, mild, in early remission
Other or unspecified stimulant use disorder, mild, in sustained remission

√6ᵗʰ **F15.12 Other stimulant abuse with** intoxication

F15.120 Other stimulant abuse with intoxication, uncomplicated `HCC`

F15.121 Other stimulant abuse with intoxication delirium `CC` `HCC`

F15.122 Other stimulant abuse with intoxication with perceptual disturbance `HCC`
Amphetamine or other stimulant use disorder, mild, with amphetamine or other stimulant intoxication, with perceptual disturbances

F15.129 Other stimulant abuse with intoxication, unspecified `HCC`
Amphetamine or other stimulant use disorder, mild, with amphetamine or other stimulant intoxication, without perceptual disturbances

F15.14 Other stimulant abuse with stimulant-induced mood disorder `HCC`
Amphetamine or other stimulant use disorder, mild, with amphetamine or other stimulant induced bipolar or related disorder
Amphetamine or other stimulant use disorder, mild, with amphetamine or other stimulant induced depressive disorder

√6ᵗʰ **F15.15 Other stimulant abuse with stimulant-induced** psychotic disorder

F15.150 Other stimulant abuse with stimulant-induced psychotic disorder with delusions `CC` `HCC`

F15.151 Other stimulant abuse with stimulant-induced psychotic disorder with hallucinations `CC` `HCC`

F15.159 Other stimulant abuse with stimulant-induced psychotic disorder, unspecified `HCC`

√6ᵗʰ **F15.18 Other stimulant abuse with other stimulant-induced disorder**

F15.180 Other stimulant abuse with stimulant-induced anxiety disorder `HCC`

F15.181 Other stimulant abuse with stimulant-induced sexual dysfunction `HCC`

Chapter 5. Mental, Behavioral and Neurodevelopmental Disorders

F15.182   Other stimulant abuse with stimulant-induced sleep disorder   `HCC`

F15.188   Other stimulant abuse with other stimulant-induced disorder   `HCC`
> Amphetamine or other stimulant use disorder, mild, with amphetamine or other stimulant induced obsessive-compulsive or related disorder

F15.19   Other stimulant abuse with unspecified stimulant-induced disorder   `HCC`

✓5ᵗʰ **F15.2**   Other stimulant **dependence**
> EXCLUDES 1   *other stimulant abuse (F15.1-)*
>   *other stimulant use, unspecified (F15.9-)*

F15.20   Other stimulant dependence, uncomplicated   `CC` `HCC`
> Amphetamine type substance use disorder, moderate
> Amphetamine type substance use disorder, severe
> Other or unspecified stimulant use disorder, moderate
> Other or unspecified stimulant use disorder, severe
> **CC Excl:** No Excl

F15.21   Other stimulant dependence, in remission   `HCC`
> Amphetamine type substance use disorder, moderate, in early remission
> Amphetamine type substance use disorder, moderate, in sustained remission
> Amphetamine type substance use disorder, severe, in early remission
> Amphetamine type substance use disorder, severe, in sustained remission
> Other or unspecified stimulant use disorder, moderate, in early remission
> Other or unspecified stimulant use disorder, moderate, in sustained remission
> Other or unspecified stimulant use disorder, severe, in early remission
> Other or unspecified stimulant use disorder, severe, in sustained remission

✓6ᵗʰ **F15.22**   Other stimulant dependence with **intoxication**
> EXCLUDES 1   *other stimulant dependence with withdrawal (F15.23)*

F15.220   Other stimulant dependence with intoxication, uncomplicated   `HCC`

F15.221   Other stimulant dependence with intoxication delirium   `CC` `HCC`

F15.222   Other stimulant dependence with intoxication with perceptual disturbance   `CC` `HCC`
> Amphetamine or other stimulant use disorder, moderate, with amphetamine or other stimulant intoxication, with perceptual disturbances
> Amphetamine or other stimulant use disorder, severe, with amphetamine or other stimulant intoxication, with perceptual disturbances
> **CC Excl:** No Excl

F15.229   Other stimulant dependence with intoxication, unspecified   `HCC`
> Amphetamine or other stimulant use disorder, moderate, with amphetamine or other stimulant intoxication, without perceptual disturbances
> Amphetamine or other stimulant use disorder, severe, with amphetamine or other stimulant intoxication, without perceptual disturbances

F15.23   Other stimulant dependence with withdrawal   `CC` `HCC`
> Amphetamine or other stimulant withdrawal
> EXCLUDES 1   *other stimulant dependence with intoxication (F15.22)*

F15.24   Other stimulant dependence with stimulant-induced mood disorder   `HCC`
> Amphetamine or other stimulant use disorder, moderate, with amphetamine or other stimulant-induced bipolar or related disorder
> Amphetamine or other stimulant use disorder, moderate, with amphetamine or other stimulant induced depressive disorder
> Amphetamine or other stimulant use disorder, severe, with amphetamine or other stimulant-induced bipolar or related disorder
> Amphetamine or other stimulant use disorder, severe, with amphetamine or other stimulant-induced depressive disorder

✓6ᵗʰ **F15.25**   Other stimulant dependence with stimulant-induced **psychotic disorder**

F15.250   Other stimulant dependence with stimulant-induced psychotic disorder with delusions   `CC` `HCC`

F15.251   Other stimulant dependence with stimulant-induced psychotic disorder with hallucinations   `CC` `HCC`

F15.259   Other stimulant dependence with stimulant-induced psychotic disorder, unspecified   `CC` `HCC`
> **CC Excl:** No Excl

✓6ᵗʰ **F15.28**   Other stimulant dependence with other stimulant-induced disorder

F15.280   Other stimulant dependence with stimulant-induced anxiety disorder   `CC` `HCC`
> **CC Excl:** No Excl

F15.281   Other stimulant dependence with stimulant-induced sexual dysfunction   `CC` `HCC`
> **CC Excl:** No Excl

F15.282   Other stimulant dependence with stimulant-induced sleep disorder   `CC` `HCC`
> **CC Excl:** No Excl

F15.288   Other stimulant dependence with other stimulant-induced disorder   `CC` `HCC`
> Amphetamine or other stimulant use disorder, moderate, with amphetamine or other stimulant induced obsessive compulsive or related disorder
> Amphetamine or other stimulant use disorder, severe, with amphetamine or other stimulant induced obsessive compulsive or related disorder
> **CC Excl:** No Excl

F15.29   Other stimulant dependence with unspecified stimulant-induced disorder   `HCC`

✓5ᵗʰ **F15.9**   Other stimulant **use, unspecified**
> EXCLUDES 1   *other stimulant abuse (F15.1-)*
>   *other stimulant dependence (F15.2-)*
> **TIP:** Assign a substance use code only when the provider documents a relationship between the use and an associated physical, mental, or behavioral disorder. As with all diagnoses, substance use codes must meet the definition of a reportable diagnosis.

F15.90   Other stimulant use, unspecified, uncomplicated
> **AHA:** 2018,2Q,10-11

N Newborn: 0   P Pediatric: 0-17   M Maternity: 9-64   A Adult: 15-124   `MCC` Major Complication/Comorbidity   `CC` Complication/Comorbidity   `SW` Severe Wound Dx

552   ICD-10-CM 2020

✓6ᵗʰ **F15.92** **Other stimulant use, unspecified with** intoxication

> EXCLUDES 1   other stimulant use, unspecified with withdrawal (F15.93)

F15.920 **Other stimulant use, unspecified with intoxication, uncomplicated**   HCC

F15.921 **Other stimulant use, unspecified with intoxication** delirium   CC HCC

> Amphetamine or other stimulant-induced delirium

F15.922 **Other stimulant use, unspecified with intoxication with** perceptual disturbance   HCC

F15.929 **Other stimulant use, unspecified with intoxication, unspecified**   HCC

> Caffeine intoxication

F15.93 **Other stimulant use, unspecified with** withdrawal   CC HCC

> Caffeine withdrawal

> EXCLUDES 1   other stimulant use, unspecified with intoxication (F15.92-)

F15.94 **Other stimulant use, unspecified with stimulant-induced** mood disorder   HCC

> Amphetamine or other stimulant-induced bipolar or related disorder, without use disorder
> Amphetamine or other stimulant-induced depressive disorder, without use disorder

✓6ᵗʰ **F15.95** **Other stimulant use, unspecified with stimulant-induced** psychotic disorder

F15.950 **Other stimulant use, unspecified with stimulant-induced psychotic disorder with** delusions   CC HCC

F15.951 **Other stimulant use, unspecified with stimulant-induced psychotic disorder with** hallucinations   CC HCC

F15.959 **Other stimulant use, unspecified with stimulant-induced psychotic disorder, unspecified**   HCC

> Amphetamine or other stimulant-induced psychotic disorder, without use disorder

✓6ᵗʰ **F15.98** **Other stimulant use, unspecified with other stimulant-induced disorder**

F15.980 **Other stimulant use, unspecified with stimulant-induced** anxiety disorder   HCC

> Amphetamine or other stimulant-induced anxiety disorder, without use disorder
> Caffeine induced anxiety disorder, without use disorder

F15.981 **Other stimulant use, unspecified with stimulant-induced** sexual dysfunction   HCC

> Amphetamine or other stimulant-induced sexual dysfunction, without use disorder

F15.982 **Other stimulant use, unspecified with stimulant-induced** sleep disorder   HCC

> Amphetamine or other stimulant-induced sleep disorder, without use disorder
> Caffeine induced sleep disorder, without use disorder

F15.988 **Other stimulant use, unspecified with other stimulant-induced disorder**   HCC

> Amphetamine or other stimulant-induced obsessive compulsive or related disorder, without use disorder

F15.99 **Other stimulant use, unspecified with unspecified stimulant-induced disorder**   HCC

✓4ᵗʰ **F16** **Hallucinogen** related disorders

> INCLUDES   ecstasy
>   PCP
>   phencyclidine

> AHA: 2018,4Q,31

✓5ᵗʰ **F16.1** **Hallucinogen** abuse

> EXCLUDES 1   hallucinogen dependence (F16.2-)
>   hallucinogen use, unspecified (F16.9-)

F16.10 **Hallucinogen abuse,** uncomplicated   HCC

> Other hallucinogen use disorder, mild
> Phencyclidine use disorder, mild

F16.11 **Hallucinogen abuse,** in remission   HCC

> Other hallucinogen use disorder, mild, in early remission
> Other hallucinogen use disorder, mild, in sustained remission
> Phencyclidine use disorder, mild, in early remission
> Phencyclidine use disorder, mild, in sustained remission

✓6ᵗʰ **F16.12** **Hallucinogen abuse with** intoxication

F16.120 **Hallucinogen abuse with intoxication,** uncomplicated   HCC

F16.121 **Hallucinogen abuse with intoxication with** delirium   CC HCC

F16.122 **Hallucinogen abuse with intoxication with** perceptual disturbance   HCC

F16.129 **Hallucinogen abuse with intoxication, unspecified**   HCC

F16.14 **Hallucinogen abuse with hallucinogen-induced** mood disorder   HCC

> Other hallucinogen use disorder, mild, with other hallucinogen induced bipolar or related disorder
> Other hallucinogen use disorder, mild, with other hallucinogen induced depressive disorder
> Phencyclidine use disorder, mild, with phencyclidine induced bipolar or related disorder
> Phencyclidine use disorder, mild, with phencyclidine induced depressive disorder

✓6ᵗʰ **F16.15** **Hallucinogen abuse with hallucinogen-induced** psychotic disorder

F16.150 **Hallucinogen abuse with hallucinogen-induced psychotic disorder with** delusions   CC HCC

F16.151 **Hallucinogen abuse with hallucinogen-induced psychotic disorder with** hallucinations   CC HCC

F16.159 **Hallucinogen abuse with hallucinogen-induced psychotic disorder, unspecified**   HCC

✓6ᵗʰ **F16.18** **Hallucinogen abuse with other hallucinogen-induced disorder**

F16.180 **Hallucinogen abuse with hallucinogen-induced** anxiety disorder   HCC

F16.183 **Hallucinogen abuse with** hallucinogen persisting perception disorder (flashbacks)   HCC

F16.188 **Hallucinogen abuse with other hallucinogen-induced disorder**   HCC

F16.19 **Hallucinogen abuse with unspecified hallucinogen-induced disorder**   HCC

✓ Additional Character Required   ✓x7ᵗʰ Placeholder   Unacceptable PDx   Questionable PDx   Manifestation   Unspecified Dx   H1 - H14 HAC   HCC CMS-HCC Dx   HIV HIV Dx

ICD-10-CM 2020   553

Chapter 5. Mental, Behavioral and Neurodevelopmental Disorders

✓5ᵗʰ **F16.2**   **Hallucinogen** dependence

     EXCLUDES 1   *hallucinogen abuse (F16.1-)*

                hallucinogen use, unspecified (F16.9-)

     F16.20   **Hallucinogen dependence,**   CC HCC
              uncomplicated

              Other hallucinogen use disorder, moderate

              Other hallucinogen use disorder, severe

              Phencyclidine use disorder, moderate

              Phencyclidine use disorder, severe

              CC Excl: No Excl

     F16.21   **Hallucinogen dependence, in**   HCC
              remission

              Other hallucinogen use disorder, moderate, in early remission

              Other hallucinogen use disorder, moderate, in sustained remission

              Other hallucinogen use disorder, severe, in early remission

              Other hallucinogen use disorder, severe, in sustained remission

              Phencyclidine use disorder, moderate, in early remission

              Phencyclidine use disorder, moderate, in sustained remission

              Phencyclidine use disorder, severe, in early remission

              Phencyclidine use disorder, severe, in sustained remission

✓6ᵗʰ   **F16.22**   **Hallucinogen dependence with** intoxication

     F16.220   **Hallucinogen dependence**   HCC
               with intoxication,
               uncomplicated

     F16.221   **Hallucinogen dependence**   CC HCC
               with intoxication with
               delirium

     F16.229   **Hallucinogen dependence**   HCC
               with intoxication,
               unspecified

     F16.24   **Hallucinogen dependence with**   HCC
              hallucinogen-induced mood
              disorder

              Other hallucinogen use disorder, moderate, with other hallucinogen induced bipolar or related disorder

              Other hallucinogen use disorder, moderate, with other hallucinogen induced depressive disorder

              Other hallucinogen use disorder, severe, with other hallucinogen-induced bipolar or related disorder

              Other hallucinogen use disorder, severe, with other hallucinogen-induced depressive disorder

              Phencyclidine use disorder, moderate, with phencyclidine induced bipolar or related disorder

              Phencyclidine use disorder, moderate, with phencyclidine induced depressive disorder

              Phencyclidine use disorder, severe, with phencyclidine induced bipolar or related disorder

              Phencyclidine use disorder, severe, with phencyclidine-induced depressive disorder

✓6ᵗʰ   **F16.25**   **Hallucinogen dependence with**
            hallucinogen-induced psychotic disorder

     F16.250   **Hallucinogen dependence**   CC HCC
               with
               hallucinogen-induced
               psychotic disorder with
               delusions

     F16.251   **Hallucinogen dependence**   CC HCC
               with
               hallucinogen-induced
               psychotic disorder with
               hallucinations

     F16.259   **Hallucinogen dependence**   CC HCC
               with
               hallucinogen-induced
               psychotic disorder,
               unspecified
                CC Excl: No Excl

✓6ᵗʰ   **F16.28**   **Hallucinogen dependence with** other
            hallucinogen-induced disorder

     F16.280   **Hallucinogen dependence**   CC HCC
               with
               hallucinogen-induced
               anxiety disorder
               CC Excl: No Excl

     F16.283   **Hallucinogen dependence**   CC HCC
               with hallucinogen
               persisting perception
               disorder (flashbacks)
               CC Excl: No Excl

     F16.288   **Hallucinogen dependence**   CC HCC
               with other
               hallucinogen-induced
               disorder
               CC Excl: No Excl

     F16.29   **Hallucinogen dependence with**   HCC
              unspecified hallucinogen-induced
              disorder

✓5ᵗʰ **F16.9**   **Hallucinogen** use, **unspecified**

     EXCLUDES 1   *hallucinogen abuse (F16.1-)*

                hallucinogen dependence (F16.2-)

     TIP: Assign a substance use code only when the provider documents a relationship between the use and an associated physical, mental, or behavioral disorder. As with all diagnoses, substance use codes must meet the definition of a reportable diagnosis.

     F16.90   **Hallucinogen use, unspecified,** uncomplicated
              AHA: 2018,2Q,10-11

✓6ᵗʰ   **F16.92**   **Hallucinogen use, unspecified with** intoxication

     F16.920   **Hallucinogen use,**   HCC
               unspecified with
               intoxication,
               uncomplicated

     F16.921   **Hallucinogen use,**   CC HCC
               unspecified with
               intoxication with delirium
                Other hallucinogen intoxication delirium

     F16.929   **Hallucinogen use,**   HCC
               unspecified with
               intoxication, unspecified

     F16.94   **Hallucinogen use, unspecified with**   HCC
              hallucinogen-induced mood
              disorder

              Other hallucinogen induced bipolar or related disorder, without use disorder

              Other hallucinogen induced depressive disorder, without use disorder

              Phencyclidine induced bipolar or related disorder, without use disorder

              Phencyclidine induced depressive disorder, without use disorder

✓6ᵗʰ   **F16.95**   **Hallucinogen use, unspecified with**
            hallucinogen-induced psychotic disorder

     F16.950   **Hallucinogen use,**   CC HCC
               unspecified with
               hallucinogen-induced
               psychotic disorder with
               delusions

     F16.951   **Hallucinogen use,**   CC HCC
               unspecified with
               hallucinogen-induced
               psychotic disorder with
               hallucinations

     F16.959   **Hallucinogen use,**   HCC
               unspecified with
               hallucinogen-induced
               psychotic disorder,
               unspecified

                Other hallucinogen induced psychotic disorder, without use disorder

                Phencyclidine induced psychotic disorder, without use disorder

Ⓝ Newborn: 0   Ⓟ Pediatric: 0-17   Ⓜ Maternity: 9-64   Ⓐ Adult: 15-124   MCC Major Complication/Comorbidity   CC Complication/Comorbidity   SW Severe Wound Dx

554   **ICD-10-CM 2020**

☑6ᵗʰ **F16.98** **Hallucinogen use, unspecified with other specified hallucinogen-induced disorder**

F16.980 **Hallucinogen use, unspecified with hallucinogen-induced anxiety disorder** `HCC`

Other hallucinogen-induced anxiety disorder, without use disorder

Phencyclidine induced anxiety disorder, without use disorder

F16.983 **Hallucinogen use, unspecified with hallucinogen persisting perception disorder (flashbacks)** `HCC`

F16.988 **Hallucinogen use, unspecified with other hallucinogen-induced disorder** `HCC`

F16.99 **Hallucinogen use, unspecified with unspecified hallucinogen-induced disorder** `HCC`

☑4ᵗʰ **F17** **Nicotine dependence**

`EXCLUDES 1` *history of tobacco dependence (Z87.891)*
tobacco use NOS (Z72.0)

`EXCLUDES 2` *tobacco use (smoking) during pregnancy, childbirth and the puerperium (O99.33-)*
toxic effect of nicotine (T65.2-)

AHA: 2013,4Q,108-109

☑5ᵗʰ **F17.2** **Nicotine dependence**

☑6ᵗʰ **F17.20** **Nicotine dependence, unspecified**

F17.200 **Nicotine dependence, unspecified, uncomplicated**

Tobacco use disorder, mild

Tobacco use disorder, moderate

Tobacco use disorder, severe

AHA: 2016,1Q,36

TIP: Assign when provider documentation indicates "smoker" without further specification.

F17.201 **Nicotine dependence, unspecified, in remission**

Tobacco use disorder, mild, in early remission

Tobacco use disorder, mild, in sustained remission

Tobacco use disorder, moderate, in early remission

Tobacco use disorder, moderate, in sustained remission

Tobacco use disorder, severe, in early remission

Tobacco use disorder, severe, in sustained remission

F17.203 **Nicotine dependence unspecified, with withdrawal** `CC`

Tobacco withdrawal

F17.208 **Nicotine dependence, unspecified, with other nicotine-induced disorders**

F17.209 **Nicotine dependence, unspecified, with unspecified nicotine-induced disorders**

☑6ᵗʰ **F17.21** **Nicotine dependence, cigarettes**

F17.210 **Nicotine dependence, cigarettes, uncomplicated**

AHA: 2017,2Q,28-29

F17.211 **Nicotine dependence, cigarettes, in remission**

Tobacco use disorder, cigarettes, mild, in early remission

Tobacco use disorder, cigarettes, mild, in sustained remission

Tobacco use disorder, cigarettes, moderate, in early remission

Tobacco use disorder, cigarettes, moderate, in sustained remission

Tobacco use disorder, cigarettes, severe, in early remission

Tobacco use disorder, cigarettes, severe, in sustained remission

F17.213 **Nicotine dependence, cigarettes, with withdrawal** `CC`

F17.218 **Nicotine dependence, cigarettes, with other nicotine-induced disorders**

F17.219 **Nicotine dependence, cigarettes, with unspecified nicotine-induced disorders**

☑6ᵗʰ **F17.22** **Nicotine dependence, chewing tobacco**

F17.220 **Nicotine dependence, chewing tobacco, uncomplicated**

F17.221 **Nicotine dependence, chewing tobacco, in remission**

Tobacco use disorder, chewing tobacco, mild, in early remission

Tobacco use disorder, chewing tobacco, mild, in sustained remission

Tobacco use disorder, chewing tobacco, moderate, in early remission

Tobacco use disorder, chewing tobacco, moderate, in sustained remission

Tobacco use disorder, chewing tobacco, severe, in early remission

Tobacco use disorder, chewing tobacco, severe, in sustained remission

F17.223 **Nicotine dependence, chewing tobacco, with withdrawal** `CC`

F17.228 **Nicotine dependence, chewing tobacco, with other nicotine-induced disorders**

F17.229 **Nicotine dependence, chewing tobacco, with unspecified nicotine-induced disorders**

☑6ᵗʰ **F17.29** **Nicotine dependence, other tobacco product**

F17.290 **Nicotine dependence, other tobacco product, uncomplicated**

AHA: 2017,2Q,28-29

F17.291 **Nicotine dependence, other tobacco product, in remission**

Tobacco use disorder, other tobacco product, mild, in early remission

Tobacco use disorder, other tobacco product, mild, in sustained remission

Tobacco use disorder, other tobacco product, moderate, in early remission

Tobacco use disorder, other tobacco product, moderate, in sustained remission

Tobacco use disorder, other tobacco product, severe, in early remission

Tobacco use disorder, other tobacco product, severe, in sustained remission

F17.293 **Nicotine dependence, other tobacco product, with withdrawal** `CC`

F17.298 **Nicotine dependence, other tobacco product, with other nicotine-induced disorders**

F17.299 **Nicotine dependence, other tobacco product, with unspecified nicotine-induced disorders**

☑ Additional Character Required   ☑x7ᵗʰ Placeholder   Unacceptable PDx   Questionable PDx   Manifestation   Unspecified Dx   H1 -H14 HAC   HCC CMS-HCC Dx   HIV HIV Dx

ICD-10-CM 2020

555

Chapter 5. Mental, Behavioral and Neurodevelopmental Disorders

✓4ᵗʰ F18 Inhalant related disorders

INCLUDES   volatile solvents

✓5ᵗʰ F18.1 Inhalant abuse

EXCLUDES 1   *inhalant dependence (F18.2-)*
inhalant use, unspecified (F18.9-)

F18.10 Inhalant abuse, uncomplicated HCC
    Inhalant use disorder, mild

F18.11 Inhalant abuse, in remission HCC
    Inhalant use disorder, mild, in early remission
    Inhalant use disorder, mild, in sustained remission

✓6ᵗʰ F18.12 Inhalant abuse with intoxication

F18.120 Inhalant abuse with intoxication, uncomplicated HCC

F18.121 Inhalant abuse with intoxication delirium CC HCC

F18.129 Inhalant abuse with intoxication, unspecified HCC

F18.14 Inhalant abuse with inhalant-induced mood disorder HCC
    Inhalant use disorder, mild, with inhalant induced depressive disorder

✓6ᵗʰ F18.15 Inhalant abuse with inhalant-induced psychotic disorder

F18.150 Inhalant abuse with inhalant-induced psychotic disorder with delusions CC HCC

F18.151 Inhalant abuse with inhalant-induced psychotic disorder with hallucinations CC HCC

F18.159 Inhalant abuse with inhalant-induced psychotic disorder, unspecified HCC

F18.17 Inhalant abuse with inhalant-induced dementia CC HCC
    Inhalant use disorder, mild, with inhalant induced major neurocognitive disorder

✓6ᵗʰ F18.18 Inhalant abuse with other inhalant-induced disorders

F18.180 Inhalant abuse with inhalant-induced anxiety disorder HCC

F18.188 Inhalant abuse with other inhalant-induced disorder HCC
    Inhalant use disorder, mild, with inhalant induced mild neurocognitive disorder

F18.19 Inhalant abuse with unspecified inhalant-induced disorder HCC

✓5ᵗʰ F18.2 Inhalant dependence

EXCLUDES 1   *inhalant abuse (F18.1-)*
inhalant use, unspecified (F18.9-)

F18.20 Inhalant dependence, uncomplicated CC HCC
    Inhalant use disorder, moderate
    Inhalant use disorder, severe
    CC Excl: No Excl

F18.21 Inhalant dependence, in remission HCC
    Inhalant use disorder, moderate, in early remission
    Inhalant use disorder, moderate, in sustained remission
    Inhalant use disorder, severe, in early remission
    Inhalant use disorder, severe, in sustained remission

✓6ᵗʰ F18.22 Inhalant dependence with intoxication

F18.220 Inhalant dependence with intoxication, uncomplicated HCC

F18.221 Inhalant dependence with intoxication delirium CC HCC

F18.229 Inhalant dependence with intoxication, unspecified HCC

F18.24 Inhalant dependence with inhalant-induced mood disorder HCC
    Inhalant use disorder, moderate, with inhalant induced depressive disorder
    Inhalant use disorder, severe, with inhalant induced depressive disorder

✓6ᵗʰ F18.25 Inhalant dependence with inhalant-induced psychotic disorder

F18.250 Inhalant dependence with inhalant-induced psychotic disorder with delusions CC HCC

F18.251 Inhalant dependence with inhalant-induced psychotic disorder with hallucinations CC HCC

F18.259 Inhalant dependence with inhalant-induced psychotic disorder, unspecified CC HCC
    CC Excl: No Excl

F18.27 Inhalant dependence with inhalant-induced dementia CC HCC
    Inhalant use disorder, moderate, with inhalant induced major neurocognitive disorder
    Inhalant use disorder, severe, with inhalant induced major neurocognitive disorder

✓6ᵗʰ F18.28 Inhalant dependence with other inhalant-induced disorders

F18.280 Inhalant dependence with inhalant-induced anxiety disorder CC HCC
    CC Excl: No Excl

F18.288 Inhalant dependence with other inhalant-induced disorder CC HCC
    Inhalant use disorder, moderate, with inhalant-induced mild neurocognitive disorder
    Inhalant use disorder, severe, with inhalant-induced mild neurocognitive disorder
    CC Excl: No Excl

F18.29 Inhalant dependence with unspecified inhalant-induced disorder HCC

✓5ᵗʰ F18.9 Inhalant use, unspecified

EXCLUDES 1   *inhalant abuse (F18.1-)*
inhalant dependence (F18.2-)

F18.90 Inhalant use, unspecified, uncomplicated
    AHA: 2018,2Q,10-11

✓6ᵗʰ F18.92 Inhalant use, unspecified with intoxication

F18.920 Inhalant use, unspecified with intoxication, uncomplicated HCC

F18.921 Inhalant use, unspecified with intoxication with delirium CC HCC

F18.929 Inhalant use, unspecified with intoxication, unspecified HCC

F18.94 Inhalant use, unspecified with inhalant-induced mood disorder HCC
    Inhalant induced depressive disorder

✓6ᵗʰ F18.95 Inhalant use, unspecified with inhalant-induced psychotic disorder

F18.950 Inhalant use, unspecified with inhalant-induced psychotic disorder with delusions CC HCC

F18.951 Inhalant use, unspecified with inhalant-induced psychotic disorder with hallucinations CC HCC

F18.959 Inhalant use, unspecified with inhalant-induced psychotic disorder, unspecified HCC

N Newborn: 0   P Pediatric: 0-17   M Maternity: 9-64   A Adult: 15-124   MCC Major Complication/Comorbidity   CC Complication/Comorbidity   SW Severe Wound Dx

556   ICD-10-CM 2020

F18.97 **Inhalant use, unspecified with inhalant-induced** persisting dementia   `CC` `HCC`
  Inhalant-induced major neurocognitive disorder

✓6th **F18.98** **Inhalant use, unspecified with other inhalant-induced disorders**
  F18.980 **Inhalant use, unspecified with inhalant-induced** anxiety disorder   `HCC`
  F18.988 **Inhalant use, unspecified with other inhalant-induced disorder**   `HCC`
    Inhalant-induced mild neurocognitive disorder

F18.99 **Inhalant use, unspecified with unspecified inhalant-induced disorder**   `HCC`

✓4th **F19** **Other** psychoactive **substance related disorders**
  INCLUDES polysubstance drug use (indiscriminate drug use)

✓5th **F19.1** **Other psychoactive substance** abuse
  EXCLUDES 1 other psychoactive substance dependence (F19.2-)
    other psychoactive substance use, unspecified (F19.9-)

  F19.10 **Other psychoactive substance abuse,** uncomplicated   `HCC`
    Other (or unknown) substance use disorder, mild

  F19.11 **Other psychoactive substance abuse,** in remission   `HCC`
    Other (or unknown) substance use disorder, mild, in early remission
    Other (or unknown) substance use disorder, mild, in sustained remission

✓6th **F19.12** **Other psychoactive substance abuse with** intoxication
  F19.120 **Other psychoactive substance abuse with intoxication,** uncomplicated   `HCC`
  F19.121 **Other psychoactive substance abuse with intoxication** delirium   `CC` `HCC`
  F19.122 **Other psychoactive substance abuse with intoxication with** perceptual disturbances   `HCC`
  F19.129 **Other psychoactive substance abuse with intoxication,** unspecified   `HCC`

  F19.14 **Other psychoactive substance abuse with psychoactive substance-induced** mood disorder   `HCC`
    Other (or unknown) substance use disorder, mild, with other (or unknown) substance-induced bipolar or related disorder
    Other (or unknown) substance use disorder, mild, with other (or unknown) substance-induced depressive disorder

✓6th **F19.15** **Other psychoactive substance abuse with psychoactive substance-induced** psychotic disorder
  F19.150 **Other psychoactive substance abuse with psychoactive substance-induced psychotic disorder with** delusions   `CC` `HCC`
  F19.151 **Other psychoactive substance abuse with psychoactive substance-induced psychotic disorder with** hallucinations   `CC` `HCC`
  F19.159 **Other psychoactive substance abuse with psychoactive substance-induced psychotic disorder,** unspecified   `HCC`

  F19.16 **Other psychoactive substance abuse with psychoactive substance-induced** persisting amnestic disorder

F19.17 **Other psychoactive substance abuse with psychoactive substance-induced** persisting dementia   `CC` `HCC`
  Other (or unknown) substance use disorder, mild, with other (or unknown) substance-induced major neurocognitive disorder

✓6th **F19.18** **Other psychoactive substance abuse with other psychoactive substance-induced disorders**
  F19.180 **Other psychoactive substance abuse with psychoactive substance-induced** anxiety disorder   `HCC`
  F19.181 **Other psychoactive substance abuse with psychoactive substance-induced** sexual dysfunction   `HCC`
  F19.182 **Other psychoactive substance abuse with psychoactive substance-induced** sleep disorder   `HCC`
  F19.188 **Other psychoactive substance abuse with other psychoactive substance-induced disorder**   `HCC`
    Other (or unknown) substance use disorder, mild, with other (or unknown) substance induced mild neurocognitive disorder
    Other (or unknown) substance use disorder, mild, with other (or unknown) substance induced obsessive-compulsive or related disorder

F19.19 **Other psychoactive substance abuse with unspecified psychoactive substance-induced disorder**   `HCC`

✓5th **F19.2** **Other psychoactive substance** dependence
  EXCLUDES 1 other psychoactive substance abuse (F19.1-)
    other psychoactive substance use, unspecified (F19.9-)

  F19.20 **Other psychoactive substance dependence,** uncomplicated   `CC` `HCC`
    Other (or unknown) substance use disorder, moderate
    Other (or unknown) substance use disorder, severe
    CC Excl: No Excl

  F19.21 **Other psychoactive substance dependence,** in remission   `HCC`
    Other (or unknown) substance use disorder, moderate, in early remission
    Other (or unknown) substance use disorder, moderate, in sustained remission
    Other (or unknown) substance use disorder, severe, in early remission
    Other (or unknown) substance use disorder, severe, in sustained remission

✓6th **F19.22** **Other psychoactive substance dependence with** intoxication
  EXCLUDES 1 other psychoactive substance dependence with withdrawal (F19.23-)
  F19.220 **Other psychoactive substance dependence with intoxication,** uncomplicated   `HCC`
  F19.221 **Other psychoactive substance dependence with intoxication** delirium   `CC` `HCC`
  F19.222 **Other psychoactive substance dependence with intoxication with** perceptual disturbance   `CC` `HCC`
    CC Excl: No Excl
  F19.229 **Other psychoactive substance dependence with intoxication,** unspecified   `HCC`

✓6th **F19.23 Other psychoactive substance dependence with withdrawal**

>*EXCLUDES 1*   other psychoactive substance dependence with intoxication (F19.22-)

   F19.230 Other psychoactive substance dependence with withdrawal, uncomplicated CC HCC

   F19.231 Other psychoactive substance dependence with withdrawal delirium CC HCC

   F19.232 Other psychoactive substance dependence with withdrawal with perceptual disturbance CC HCC

   F19.239 Other psychoactive substance dependence with withdrawal, unspecified CC HCC

F19.24 Other psychoactive substance dependence with psychoactive substance-induced mood disorder HCC

   Other (or unknown) substance use disorder, moderate, with other (or unknown) substance induced bipolar or related disorder

   Other (or unknown) substance use disorder, moderate, with other (or unknown) substance induced depressive disorder

   Other (or unknown) substance use disorder, severe, with other (or unknown) substance induced bipolar or related disorder

   Other (or unknown) substance use disorder, severe, with other (or unknown) substance induced depressive disorder

✓6th **F19.25 Other psychoactive substance dependence with psychoactive substance-induced psychotic disorder**

   F19.250 Other psychoactive substance dependence with psychoactive substance-induced psychotic disorder with delusions CC HCC

   F19.251 Other psychoactive substance dependence with psychoactive substance-induced psychotic disorder with hallucinations CC HCC

   F19.259 Other psychoactive substance dependence with psychoactive substance-induced psychotic disorder, unspecified CC HCC
     CC Excl: No Excl

F19.26 Other psychoactive substance dependence with psychoactive substance-induced persisting amnestic disorder CC HCC
     CC Excl: No Excl

F19.27 Other psychoactive substance dependence with psychoactive substance-induced persisting dementia CC HCC

   Other (or unknown) substance use disorder, moderate, with other (or unknown) substance induced major neurocognitive disorder

   Other (or unknown) substance use disorder, severe, with other (or unknown) substance induced major neurocognitive disorder

✓6th **F19.28 Other psychoactive substance dependence with other psychoactive substance-induced disorders**

   F19.280 Other psychoactive substance dependence with psychoactive substance-induced anxiety disorder CC HCC
     CC Excl: No Excl

   F19.281 Other psychoactive substance dependence with psychoactive substance-induced sexual dysfunction CC HCC
     CC Excl: No Excl

   F19.282 Other psychoactive substance dependence with psychoactive substance-induced sleep disorder CC HCC
     CC Excl: No Excl

   F19.288 Other psychoactive substance dependence with other psychoactive substance-induced disorder CC HCC

     Other (or unknown) substance use disorder, moderate, with other (or unknown) substance induced mild neurocognitive disorder

     Other (or unknown) substance use disorder, severe, with other (or unknown) substance induced mild neurocognitive disorder

     Other (or unknown) substance use disorder, moderate, with other (or unknown) substance induced obsessive compulsive or related disorder

     Other (or unknown) substance use disorder, severe, with other (or unknown) substance induced obsessive-compulsive or related disorder

     CC Excl: No Excl

F19.29 Other psychoactive substance dependence with unspecified psychoactive substance-induced disorder HCC

✓5th **F19.9 Other psychoactive substance use, unspecified**

>*EXCLUDES 1*   other psychoactive substance abuse (F19.1-)
>other psychoactive substance dependence (F19.2-)

F19.90 Other psychoactive substance use, unspecified, uncomplicated
     AHA: 2018,2Q,10-11

✓6th **F19.92 Other psychoactive substance use, unspecified with intoxication**

>*EXCLUDES 1*   other psychoactive substance use, unspecified with withdrawal (F19.93)

   F19.920 Other psychoactive substance use, unspecified with intoxication, uncomplicated HCC

   F19.921 Other psychoactive substance use, unspecified with intoxication with delirium CC HCC

     Other (or unknown) substance-induced delirium

   F19.922 Other psychoactive substance use, unspecified with intoxication with perceptual disturbance HCC

   F19.929 Other psychoactive substance use, unspecified with intoxication, unspecified HCC

✓6th **F19.93 Other psychoactive substance use, unspecified with withdrawal**

>*EXCLUDES 1*   other psychoactive substance use, unspecified with intoxication (F19.92-)

   F19.930 Other psychoactive substance use, unspecified with withdrawal, uncomplicated CC HCC

   F19.931 Other psychoactive substance use, unspecified with withdrawal delirium CC HCC

N Newborn: 0   P Pediatric: 0-17   M Maternity: 9-64   A Adult: 15-124   MCC Major Complication/Comorbidity   CC Complication/Comorbidity   SW Severe Wound Dx

558   ICD-10-CM 2020

F19.932 Other psychoactive substance use, unspecified with withdrawal with perceptual disturbance   `CC` `HCC`

F19.939 Other psychoactive substance use, unspecified with withdrawal, unspecified   `CC` `HCC`

F19.94 Other psychoactive substance use, unspecified with psychoactive substance-induced mood disorder   `HCC`

Other (or unknown) substance-induced bipolar or related disorder, without use disorder

Other (or unknown) substance-induced depressive disorder, without use disorder

√6ᵗʰ **F19.95** Other psychoactive substance use, unspecified with psychoactive substance-induced psychotic disorder

F19.950 Other psychoactive substance use, unspecified with psychoactive substance-induced psychotic disorder with delusions   `CC` `HCC`

F19.951 Other psychoactive substance use, unspecified with psychoactive substance-induced psychotic disorder with hallucinations   `CC` `HCC`

F19.959 Other psychoactive substance use, unspecified with psychoactive substance-induced psychotic disorder, unspecified   `HCC`

Other or unknown substance-induced psychotic disorder, without use disorder

F19.96 Other psychoactive substance use, unspecified with psychoactive substance-induced persisting amnestic disorder   `HCC`

F19.97 Other psychoactive substance use, unspecified with psychoactive substance-induced persisting dementia   `CC` `HCC`

Other (or unknown) substance-induced major neurocognitive disorder, without use disorder

√6ᵗʰ **F19.98** Other psychoactive substance use, unspecified with other psychoactive substance-induced disorders

F19.980 Other psychoactive substance use, unspecified with psychoactive substance-induced anxiety disorder   `HCC`

Other (or unknown) substance-induced anxiety disorder, without use disorder

F19.981 Other psychoactive substance use, unspecified with psychoactive substance-induced sexual dysfunction   `HCC`

Other (or unknown) substance-induced sexual dysfunction, without use disorder

F19.982 Other psychoactive substance use, unspecified with psychoactive substance-induced sleep disorder   `HCC`

Other (or unknown) substance-induced sleep disorder, without use disorder

F19.988 Other psychoactive substance use, unspecified with other psychoactive substance-induced disorder   `HCC`

Other (or unknown) substance-induced mild neurocognitive disorder, without use disorder

Other (or unknown) substance-induced obsessive-compulsive or related disorder, without use disorder

F19.99 Other psychoactive substance use, unspecified with unspecified psychoactive substance-induced disorder   `HCC`

Schizophrenia, schizotypal, delusional, and other non-mood psychotic disorders (F20-F29)

√4ᵗʰ **F20 Schizophrenia**

EXCLUDES 1
  brief psychotic disorder (F23)
  cyclic schizophrenia (F25.0)
  mood [affective] disorders with psychotic symptoms (F30.2, F31.2, F31.5, F31.64, F32.3, F33.3)
  schizoaffective disorder (F25.-)
  schizophrenic reaction NOS (F23)

EXCLUDES 2
  schizophrenic reaction in:
    alcoholism (F10.15-, F10.25-, F10.95-)
    brain disease (F06.2)
    epilepsy (F06.2)
    psychoactive drug use (F11-F19 with .15. .25, .95)
    schizotypal disorder (F21)

DEF: Group of disorders with disturbances in thought (delusions, hallucinations), mood (blunted, flattened, inappropriate affect), and sense of self. Schizophrenia also includes bizarre, purposeless behavior, repetitious activity, or inactivity.

CC Excl: For CC codes in category F20: PDX collection 551

F20.0 Paranoid schizophrenia   `CC` `HCC`

Paraphrenic schizophrenia

EXCLUDES 1   *involutional paranoid state (F22)*
          paranoia (F22)

DEF: Preoccupied with delusional suspicions and auditory hallucinations related to a single theme. This type of schizophrenia is usually hostile, grandiose, threatening, persecutory, and occasionally hypochondriacal.

F20.1 Disorganized schizophrenia   `CC` `HCC`

Hebephrenic schizophrenia
Hebephrenia

F20.2 Catatonic schizophrenia   `CC` `HCC`

Schizophrenic catalepsy
Schizophrenic catatonia
Schizophrenic flexibilitas cerea

EXCLUDES 1   *catatonic stupor (R40.1)*

DEF: Extreme changes in motor activity. One extreme is a decreased response or reaction to the environment and the other is spontaneous activity.

F20.3 Undifferentiated schizophrenia   `HCC`

Atypical schizophrenia

EXCLUDES 1   *acute schizophrenia-like psychotic disorder (F23)*
EXCLUDES 2   *post-schizophrenic depression (F32.89)*

F20.5 Residual schizophrenia   `CC` `HCC`

Restzustand (schizophrenic)
Schizophrenic residual state

√5ᵗʰ **F20.8 Other schizophrenia**

F20.81 Schizophreniform disorder   `CC` `HCC`

Schizophreniform psychosis NOS

F20.89 Other schizophrenia   `CC` `HCC`

Cenesthopathic schizophrenia
Simple schizophrenia

F20.9 Schizophrenia, unspecified   `HCC`

AHA: 2019,2Q,32

F21 Schizotypal disorder   `HCC`

Borderline schizophrenia
Latent schizophrenia
Latent schizophrenic reaction
Prepsychotic schizophrenia
Prodromal schizophrenia
Pseudoneurotic schizophrenia
Pseudopsychopathic schizophrenia
Schizotypal personality disorder

EXCLUDES 2   *Asperger's syndrome (F84.5)*
          schizoid personality disorder (F60.1)

DEF: Disorder characterized by various oddities of thinking, perception, communication, and behavior that may be manifested as magical thinking, ideas of reference, paranoid ideation, recurrent illusions and derealization (depersonalization), or social isolation.

☑ Additional Character Required   √x7ᵗʰ Placeholder   Unacceptable PDx   Questionable PDx   Manifestation   Unspecified Dx   H1 - H14 HAC   HCC CMS-HCC Dx   HIV HIV Dx

ICD-10-CM 2020   **559**

F22　Delusional disorders　`CC` `HCC`
　　　Delusional dysmorphophobia
　　　Involutional paranoid state
　　　Paranoia
　　　Paranoia querulans
　　　Paranoid psychosis
　　　Paranoid state
　　　Paraphrenia (late)
　　　Sensitiver Beziehungswahn
　　　`EXCLUDES 1`　*mood [affective] disorders with psychotic symptoms (F30.2,*
　　　　　　　　F31.2, F31.5, F31.64, F32.3, F33.3)
　　　　　　　　paranoid schizophrenia (F20.0)
　　　`EXCLUDES 2`　*paranoid personality disorder (F60.0)*
　　　　　　　　paranoid psychosis, psychogenic (F23)
　　　　　　　　paranoid reaction (F23)

F23　Brief psychotic disorder　`CC` `HCC`
　　　Paranoid reaction
　　　Psychogenic paranoid psychosis
　　　`EXCLUDES 2`　*mood [affective] disorders with psychotic symptoms (F30.2,*
　　　　　　　　F31.2, F31.5, F31.64, F32.3, F33.3)
　　　AHA: 2019,2Q,32
　　　CC Excl: No Excl

F24　Shared psychotic disorder　`HCC`
　　　Folie à deux
　　　Induced paranoid disorder
　　　Induced psychotic disorder

✓4ᵗʰ　**F25　Schizoaffective disorders**
　　　`EXCLUDES 1`　*mood [affective] disorders with psychotic symptoms (F30.2,*
　　　　　　　　F31.2, F31.5, F31.64, F32.3, F33.3)
　　　　　　　　schizophrenia (F20.-)
　　　F25.0　Schizoaffective disorder, bipolar type　`HCC`
　　　　　Cyclic schizophrenia
　　　　　Schizoaffective disorder, manic type
　　　　　Schizoaffective disorder, mixed type
　　　　　Schizoaffective psychosis, bipolar type
　　　F25.1　Schizoaffective disorder, depressive type　`HCC`
　　　　　Schizoaffective psychosis, depressive type
　　　F25.8　Other schizoaffective disorders　`HCC`
　　　F25.9　Schizoaffective disorder, unspecified　`HCC`
　　　　　Schizoaffective psychosis NOS

F28　Other psychotic disorder not due to a substance or `HIV` `CC` `HCC`
　　　known physiological condition
　　　Chronic hallucinatory psychosis
　　　Other specified schizophrenia spectrum and other psychotic disorder

F29　Unspecified psychosis not due to a substance or `HIV` `CC` `HCC`
　　　known physiological condition
　　　Psychosis NOS
　　　Unspecified schizophrenia spectrum and other psychotic disorder
　　　`EXCLUDES 1`　*mental disorder NOS (F99)*
　　　　　　　　unspecified mental disorder due to known physiological
　　　　　　　　condition (F09)

Mood [affective] disorders (F30-F39)

✓4ᵗʰ　**F30　Manic episode**
　　　`INCLUDES`　bipolar disorder, single manic episode
　　　　　　　mixed affective episode
　　　`EXCLUDES 1`　*bipolar disorder (F31.-)*
　　　　　　　major depressive disorder, recurrent (F33.-)
　　　　　　　major depressive disorder, single episode (F32.-)
　　　DEF: Mania: Characterized by abnormal states of elation or excitement
　　　out of keeping with the individual's circumstances and varying from
　　　enhanced liveliness (hypomania) to violent, almost uncontrollable,
　　　excitement. Aggression and anger, flight of ideas, distractibility, impaired
　　　judgment, and grandiose ideas are common.
　　　CC Excl: For CC codes in category F30, unless otherwise noted: PDX
　　　collection 551

　　✓5ᵗʰ　**F30.1　Manic episode without psychotic symptoms**
　　　　　F30.10　Manic episode without psychotic　`CC` `HCC`
　　　　　　　　　symptoms, unspecified
　　　　　F30.11　Manic episode without psychotic　`CC` `HCC`
　　　　　　　　　symptoms, mild
　　　　　F30.12　Manic episode without psychotic　`CC` `HCC`
　　　　　　　　　symptoms, moderate

　　　　　F30.13　Manic episode, severe, without　`CC` `HCC`
　　　　　　　　　psychotic symptoms
　　　　　　　　　CC Excl: PDX collection 552
　　　F30.2　Manic episode, severe with psychotic　`CC` `HCC`
　　　　　symptoms
　　　　　Manic stupor
　　　　　Mania with mood-congruent psychotic symptoms
　　　　　Mania with mood-incongruent psychotic symptoms
　　　F30.3　Manic episode in partial remission　`HCC`
　　　F30.4　Manic episode in full remission　`HCC`
　　　F30.8　Other manic episodes　`HCC`
　　　　　Hypomania
　　　F30.9　Manic episode, unspecified　`CC` `HCC`
　　　　　Mania NOS

✓4ᵗʰ　**F31　Bipolar disorder**
　　　`INCLUDES`　bipolar I disorder
　　　　　　　bipolar type I disorder
　　　　　　　manic-depressive illness
　　　　　　　manic-depressive psychosis
　　　　　　　manic-depressive reaction
　　　`EXCLUDES 1`　*bipolar disorder, single manic episode (F30.-)*
　　　　　　　major depressive disorder, recurrent (F33.-)
　　　　　　　major depressive disorder, single episode (F32.-)
　　　`EXCLUDES 2`　*cyclothymia (F34.0)*
　　　CC Excl: For CC codes in category F31, unless otherwise noted: PDX
　　　collection 551

　　　F31.0　Bipolar disorder, current episode hypomanic　`CC` `HCC`
　　✓5ᵗʰ　**F31.1　Bipolar disorder, current episode manic without psychotic**
　　　　　features
　　　　　F31.10　Bipolar disorder, current episode　`CC` `HCC`
　　　　　　　　　manic without psychotic features,
　　　　　　　　　unspecified
　　　　　F31.11　Bipolar disorder, current episode　`CC` `HCC`
　　　　　　　　　manic without psychotic features,
　　　　　　　　　mild
　　　　　F31.12　Bipolar disorder, current episode　`CC` `HCC`
　　　　　　　　　manic without psychotic features,
　　　　　　　　　moderate
　　　　　F31.13　Bipolar disorder, current episode　`CC` `HCC`
　　　　　　　　　manic without psychotic features,
　　　　　　　　　severe
　　　　　　　　　CC Excl: PDX collection 553
　　　F31.2　Bipolar disorder, current episode manic　`CC` `HCC`
　　　　　severe with psychotic features
　　　　　Bipolar disorder, current episode manic with mood-congruent
　　　　　　　psychotic symptoms
　　　　　Bipolar disorder, current episode manic with mood-incongruent
　　　　　　　psychotic symptoms
　　　　　Bipolar I disorder, current or most recent episode manic with
　　　　　　　psychotic features
　　✓5ᵗʰ　**F31.3　Bipolar disorder, current episode depressed, mild or**
　　　　　moderate severity
　　　　　F31.30　Bipolar disorder, current episode　`CC` `HCC`
　　　　　　　　　depressed, mild or moderate
　　　　　　　　　severity, unspecified
　　　　　F31.31　Bipolar disorder, current episode　`CC` `HCC`
　　　　　　　　　depressed, mild
　　　　　F31.32　Bipolar disorder, current episode　`CC` `HCC`
　　　　　　　　　depressed, moderate
　　　F31.4　Bipolar disorder, current episode depressed,　`CC` `HCC`
　　　　　severe, without psychotic features
　　　　　CC Excl: PDX collection 554
　　　F31.5　Bipolar disorder, current episode depressed,　`CC` `HCC`
　　　　　severe, with psychotic features
　　　　　Bipolar disorder, current episode depressed with
　　　　　　　mood-congruent psychotic symptoms
　　　　　Bipolar disorder, current episode depressed with
　　　　　　　mood-incongruent psychotic symptoms
　　　　　Bipolar I disorder, current or most recent episode depressed,
　　　　　　　with psychotic features
　　✓5ᵗʰ　**F31.6　Bipolar disorder, current episode mixed**
　　　　　F31.60　Bipolar disorder, current episode　`CC` `HCC`
　　　　　　　　　mixed, unspecified
　　　　　F31.61　Bipolar disorder, current episode　`CC` `HCC`
　　　　　　　　　mixed, mild
　　　　　F31.62　Bipolar disorder, current episode　`CC` `HCC`
　　　　　　　　　mixed, moderate

F31.63 **Bipolar disorder, current episode mixed, severe, without psychotic features** CC HCC
      CC Excl: PDX collection 554

F31.64 **Bipolar disorder, current episode mixed, severe, with psychotic features** CC HCC
      Bipolar disorder, current episode mixed with mood-congruent psychotic symptoms
      Bipolar disorder, current episode mixed with mood-incongruent psychotic symptoms

✓5ᵗʰ **F31.7** **Bipolar disorder, currently in remission**

F31.70 **Bipolar disorder, currently in remission, most recent episode unspecified** HCC

F31.71 **Bipolar disorder, in partial remission, most recent episode hypomanic** HCC

F31.72 **Bipolar disorder, in full remission, most recent episode hypomanic** HCC

F31.73 **Bipolar disorder, in partial remission, most recent episode manic** HCC

F31.74 **Bipolar disorder, in full remission, most recent episode manic** HCC

F31.75 **Bipolar disorder, in partial remission, most recent episode depressed** HCC

F31.76 **Bipolar disorder, in full remission, most recent episode depressed** HCC

F31.77 **Bipolar disorder, in partial remission, most recent episode mixed** HCC

F31.78 **Bipolar disorder, in full remission, most recent episode mixed** HCC

✓5ᵗʰ **F31.8** **Other bipolar disorders**

F31.81 **Bipolar II disorder** HCC
      Bipolar disorder, type 2

F31.89 **Other bipolar disorder** HCC
      Recurrent manic episodes NOS

F31.9 **Bipolar disorder, unspecified** HCC
      Manic depression

✓4ᵗʰ **F32** **Major depressive disorder, single episode**

  INCLUDES single episode of agitated depression
            single episode of depressive reaction
            single episode of major depression
            single episode of psychogenic depression
            single episode of reactive depression
            single episode of vital depression

  EXCLUDES 1 bipolar disorder (F31.-)
             manic episode (F30.-)
             recurrent depressive disorder (F33.-)
  EXCLUDES 2 adjustment disorder (F43.2)

  DEF: Mood disorder that produces depression that may exhibit as sadness, low self-esteem, or guilt feelings. Other manifestations may be withdrawal from friends and family and interrupted sleep.
  CC Excl: For CC codes in category F32: PDX collection 555

F32.0 **Major depressive disorder, single episode, mild** HCC

F32.1 **Major depressive disorder, single episode, moderate** CC HCC

F32.2 **Major depressive disorder, single episode, severe without psychotic features** CC HCC

F32.3 **Major depressive disorder, single episode, severe with psychotic features** CC HCC
      Single episode of major depression with mood-congruent psychotic symptoms
      Single episode of major depression with mood-incongruent psychotic symptoms
      Single episode of major depression with psychotic symptoms
      Single episode of psychogenic depressive psychosis
      Single episode of psychotic depression
      Single episode of reactive depressive psychosis

F32.4 **Major depressive disorder, single episode, in partial remission** HCC

F32.5 **Major depressive disorder, single episode, in full remission** HCC

✓5ᵗʰ **F32.8** **Other depressive episodes**
      AHA: 2016,4Q,14

F32.81 **Premenstrual dysphoric disorder** ♀
      EXCLUDES 1 premenstrual tension syndrome (N94.3)
      DEF: Severe manifestation of premenstrual syndrome (PMS) that can be disabling and destructive to day-to-day activities. It can exacerbate pre-existing emotional disorders, like depression and anxiety, and cause feelings of loss of control, fatigue, and irritability.

F32.89 **Other specified depressive episodes**
      Atypical depression
      Post-schizophrenic depression
      Single episode of 'masked' depression NOS

F32.9 **Major depressive disorder, single episode, unspecified**
      Depression NOS
      Depressive disorder NOS
      Major depression NOS
      AHA: 2013,4Q,107

✓4ᵗʰ **F33** **Major depressive disorder, recurrent**

  INCLUDES recurrent episodes of depressive reaction
            recurrent episodes of endogenous depression
            recurrent episodes of major depression
            recurrent episodes of psychogenic depression
            recurrent episodes of reactive depression
            recurrent episodes of seasonal depressive disorder
            recurrent episodes of vital depression

  EXCLUDES 1 bipolar disorder (F31.-)
             manic episode (F30.-)

  DEF: Mood disorder that produces depression that may exhibit as sadness, low self-esteem, or guilt feelings. Other manifestations may be withdrawal from friends and family and interrupted sleep.
  CC Excl: For CC codes in category F33, unless otherwise noted: PDX collection 555

F33.0 **Major depressive disorder, recurrent, mild** HCC

F33.1 **Major depressive disorder, recurrent, moderate** CC HCC

F33.2 **Major depressive disorder, recurrent, severe without psychotic features** CC HCC

F33.3 **Major depressive disorder, recurrent, severe with psychotic symptoms** CC HCC
      Endogenous depression with psychotic symptoms
      Major depressive disorder, recurrent, with psychotic features
      Recurrent severe episodes of major depression with mood-congruent psychotic symptoms
      Recurrent severe episodes of major depression with mood-incongruent psychotic symptoms
      Recurrent severe episodes of major depression with psychotic symptoms
      Recurrent severe episodes of psychogenic depressive psychosis
      Recurrent severe episodes of psychotic depression
      Recurrent severe episodes of reactive depressive psychosis
      CC Excl: PDX collection 551

✓5ᵗʰ **F33.4** **Major depressive disorder, recurrent, in remission**

F33.40 **Major depressive disorder, recurrent, in remission, unspecified** CC HCC

F33.41 **Major depressive disorder, recurrent, in partial remission** HCC

F33.42 **Major depressive disorder, recurrent, in full remission** HCC

F33.8 **Other recurrent depressive disorders** CC HCC
      Recurrent brief depressive episodes
      CC Excl: PDX collection 551

F33.9 **Major depressive disorder, recurrent, unspecified** CC HCC
      Monopolar depression NOS

✓4ᵗʰ **F34** **Persistent mood [affective] disorders**

F34.0 **Cyclothymic disorder**
      Affective personality disorder
      Cycloid personality
      Cyclothymia
      Cyclothymic personality
      DEF: Mood disorder characterized by fast and repeated alterations between hypomanic and depressed moods.

F34.1 **Dysthymic disorder**
Depressive neurosis
Depressive personality disorder
Dysthymia
Neurotic depression
Persistent anxiety depression
Persistent depressive disorder
EXCLUDES 2 *anxiety depression (mild or not persistent) (F41.8)*
DEF: Depression without psychosis. It is a less severe but persistent depression and is considered a mild to moderate chronic form of depression.

✓5th F34.8 **Other persistent mood [affective] disorders**
AHA: 2016,4Q,14

F34.81 **Disruptive mood dysregulation disorder** CC HCC
CC Excl: PDX collection 551

F34.89 **Other specified persistent mood disorders** CC HCC
CC Excl: PDX collection 551

F34.9 **Persistent mood [affective] disorder, unspecified** CC HCC
CC Excl: PDX collection 551

F39 **Unspecified mood [affective] disorder** HCC
Affective psychosis NOS

Anxiety, dissociative, stress-related, somatoform and other nonpsychotic mental disorders (F40-F48)

✓4th F40 **Phobic anxiety disorders**
DEF: Phobia: Broad-range anxiety with abnormally intense dread of certain objects or specific situations that would not normally have that effect.

✓5th F40.0 **Agoraphobia**
DEF: Profound anxiety or fear of leaving familiar settings like home, or being in unfamiliar locations or with strangers or crowds. Agoraphobia may or may not be preceded by recurrent panic attacks.

F40.00 **Agoraphobia, unspecified**
F40.01 **Agoraphobia with panic disorder**
Panic disorder with agoraphobia
EXCLUDES 1 *panic disorder without agoraphobia (F41.0)*

F40.02 **Agoraphobia without panic disorder**

✓5th F40.1 **Social phobias**
Anthropophobia
Social anxiety disorder
Social anxiety disorder of childhood
Social neurosis

F40.10 **Social phobia, unspecified**
F40.11 **Social phobia, generalized**

✓5th F40.2 **Specific (isolated) phobias**
EXCLUDES 2 *dysmorphophobia (nondelusional) (F45.22)*
nosophobia (F45.22)

✓6th F40.21 **Animal type phobia**
F40.210 **Arachnophobia**
Fear of spiders
F40.218 **Other animal type phobia**

✓6th F40.22 **Natural environment type phobia**
F40.220 **Fear of thunderstorms**
F40.228 **Other natural environment type phobia**

✓6th F40.23 **Blood, injection, injury type phobia**
F40.230 **Fear of blood**
F40.231 **Fear of injections and transfusions**
F40.232 **Fear of other medical care**
F40.233 **Fear of injury**

✓6th F40.24 **Situational type phobia**
F40.240 **Claustrophobia**
F40.241 **Acrophobia**
F40.242 **Fear of bridges**
F40.243 **Fear of flying**
F40.248 **Other situational type phobia**

✓6th F40.29 **Other specified phobia**
F40.290 **Androphobia**
Fear of men
F40.291 **Gynephobia**
Fear of women
F40.298 **Other specified phobia**

F40.8 **Other phobic anxiety disorders**
Phobic anxiety disorder of childhood
F40.9 **Phobic anxiety disorder, unspecified**
Phobia NOS
Phobic state NOS

✓4th F41 **Other anxiety disorders**
EXCLUDES 2 *anxiety in:*
acute stress reaction (F43.0)
neurasthenia (F48.8)
psychophysiologic disorders (F45.-)
transient adjustment reaction (F43.2)
separation anxiety (F93.0)

F41.0 **Panic disorder [episodic paroxysmal anxiety]**
Panic attack
Panic state
EXCLUDES 1 *panic disorder with agoraphobia (F40.01)*
DEF: Neurotic disorder characterized by recurrent panic or anxiety, apprehension, fear, or terror. Symptoms include shortness of breath, palpitations, dizziness, and shakiness; fear of dying may persist.

F41.1 **Generalized anxiety disorder**
Anxiety neurosis
Anxiety reaction
Anxiety state
Overanxious disorder
EXCLUDES 2 *neurasthenia (F48.8)*

F41.3 **Other mixed anxiety disorders**
F41.8 **Other specified anxiety disorders**
Anxiety depression (mild or not persistent)
Anxiety hysteria
Mixed anxiety and depressive disorder
F41.9 **Anxiety disorder, unspecified**
Anxiety NOS

✓4th F42 **Obsessive-compulsive disorder**
EXCLUDES 2 *obsessive-compulsive personality (disorder) (F60.5)*
obsessive-compulsive symptoms occurring in depression (F32-F33)
obsessive-compulsive symptoms occurring in schizophrenia (F20.-)
AHA: 2016,4Q,14-15

F42.2 **Mixed obsessional thoughts and acts**
F42.3 **Hoarding disorder**
F42.4 **Excoriation (skin-picking) disorder**
EXCLUDES 1 *factitial dermatitis (L98.1)*
other specified behavioral and emotional disorders with onset usually occurring in early childhood and adolescence (F98.8)

F42.8 **Other obsessive-compulsive disorder**
Anancastic neurosis
Obsessive-compulsive neurosis
F42.9 **Obsessive-compulsive disorder, unspecified**

✓4th F43 **Reaction to severe stress, and adjustment disorders**
F43.0 **Acute stress reaction**
Acute crisis reaction
Acute reaction to stress
Combat and operational stress reaction
Combat fatigue
Crisis state
Psychic shock

✓5th F43.1 **Post-traumatic stress disorder (PTSD)**
Traumatic neurosis
DEF: Preoccupation with traumatic events beyond normal experience (i.e., rape, personal assault, etc.) that may also include recurring flashbacks of the trauma. Symptoms include difficulty remembering, sleeping, or concentrating, and guilt feelings for surviving.

F43.10 **Post-traumatic stress disorder, unspecified**
F43.11 **Post-traumatic stress disorder, acute**
F43.12 **Post-traumatic stress disorder, chronic**

✓5th F43.2 **Adjustment disorders**
Culture shock
Grief reaction
Hospitalism in children
EXCLUDES 2 *separation anxiety disorder of childhood (F93.0)*

F43.20 **Adjustment disorder, unspecified**

F43.21 Adjustment disorder with depressed mood
   AHA: 2014,1Q,25
F43.22 Adjustment disorder with anxiety
F43.23 Adjustment disorder with mixed anxiety and depressed mood
F43.24 Adjustment disorder with disturbance of conduct
F43.25 Adjustment disorder with mixed disturbance of emotions and conduct
F43.29 Adjustment disorder with other symptoms
F43.8 Other reactions to severe stress
   Other specified trauma and stressor-related disorder
F43.9 Reaction to severe stress, unspecified
   Trauma and stressor-related disorder, NOS

✓4ᵗʰ **F44 Dissociative and conversion disorders**
   INCLUDES conversion hysteria
            conversion reaction
            hysteria
            hysterical psychosis
   EXCLUDES 2 malingering [conscious simulation] (Z76.5)

F44.0 Dissociative amnesia HCC
   EXCLUDES 1 amnesia NOS (R41.3)
              anterograde amnesia (R41.1)
              dissociative amnesia with dissociative fugue (F44.1)
              retrograde amnesia (R41.2)
   EXCLUDES 2 alcohol-or other psychoactive substance-induced amnestic disorder (F10, F13, F19 with .26, .96)
              amnestic disorder due to known physiological condition (F04)
              postictal amnesia in epilepsy (G40.-)

F44.1 Dissociative fugue HCC
   Dissociative amnesia with dissociative fugue
   EXCLUDES 2 postictal fugue in epilepsy (G40.-)
   DEF: Dissociative hysteria identified by memory loss and flight from familiar surroundings to a completely separate environment. Episodes may last hours or days. Conscious activity is not associated with perception of surroundings and there is no later memory of the episode.

F44.2 Dissociative stupor
   EXCLUDES 1 catatonic stupor (R40.1)
              stupor NOS (R40.1)
   EXCLUDES 2 catatonic disorder due to known physiological condition (F06.1)
              depressive stupor (F32, F33)
              manic stupor (F30, F31)

F44.4 Conversion disorder with motor symptom or deficit
   Conversion disorder with abnormal movement
   Conversion disorder with speech symptoms
   Conversion disorder with swallowing symptoms
   Conversion disorder with weakness/paralysis
   Dissociative motor disorders
   Psychogenic aphonia
   Psychogenic dysphonia

F44.5 Conversion disorder with seizures or convulsions
   Conversion disorder with attacks or seizures
   Dissociative convulsions
   AHA: 2019,1Q,19

F44.6 Conversion disorder with sensory symptom or deficit
   Conversion disorder with anesthesia or sensory loss
   Conversion disorder with special sensory symptoms
   Dissociative anesthesia and sensory loss
   Psychogenic deafness

F44.7 Conversion disorder with mixed symptom presentation
✓5ᵗʰ **F44.8 Other dissociative and conversion disorders**
   F44.81 Dissociative identity disorder HCC
      Multiple personality disorder
   F44.89 Other dissociative and conversion disorders
      Ganser's syndrome
      Psychogenic confusion
      Psychogenic twilight state
      Trance and possession disorders
F44.9 Dissociative and conversion disorder, unspecified
   Dissociative disorder NOS

✓4ᵗʰ **F45 Somatoform disorders**
   EXCLUDES 2 dissociative and conversion disorders (F44.-)
              factitious disorders (F68.1-, F68.A)
              hair-plucking (F63.3)
              lalling (F80.0)
              lisping (F80.0)
              malingering [conscious simulation] (Z76.5)
              nail-biting (F98.8)
              psychological or behavioral factors associated with disorders or diseases classified elsewhere (F54)
              sexual dysfunction, not due to a substance or known physiological condition (F52.-)
              thumb-sucking (F98.8)
              tic disorders (in childhood and adolescence) (F95.-)
              Tourette's syndrome (F95.2)
              trichotillomania (F63.3)
   DEF: Types of disorders causing inconsistent physical symptoms that cannot be explained.

F45.0 Somatization disorder
   Briquet's disorder
   Multiple psychosomatic disorder
F45.1 Undifferentiated somatoform disorder
   Somatic symptom disorder
   Undifferentiated psychosomatic disorder
✓5ᵗʰ **F45.2 Hypochondriacal disorders**
   EXCLUDES 2 delusional dysmorphophobia (F22)
              fixed delusions about bodily functions or shape (F22)

   F45.20 Hypochondriacal disorder, unspecified
   F45.21 Hypochondriasis
      Hypochondriacal neurosis
      Illness anxiety disorder
   F45.22 Body dysmorphic disorder
      Dysmorphophobia (nondelusional)
      Nosophobia
   F45.29 Other hypochondriacal disorders
✓5ᵗʰ **F45.4 Pain disorders related to psychological factors**
   EXCLUDES 1 pain NOS (R52)
   F45.41 Pain disorder exclusively related to psychological factors
      Somatoform pain disorder (persistent)
   F45.42 Pain disorder with related psychological factors
      Code also associated acute or chronic pain (G89.-)
F45.8 Other somatoform disorders
   Psychogenic dysmenorrhea
   Psychogenic dysphagia, including 'globus hystericus'
   Psychogenic pruritus
   Psychogenic torticollis
   Somatoform autonomic dysfunction
   Teeth grinding
   EXCLUDES 1 sleep related teeth grinding (G47.63)
F45.9 Somatoform disorder, unspecified
   Psychosomatic disorder NOS

✓4ᵗʰ **F48 Other nonpsychotic mental disorders**
   F48.1 Depersonalization-derealization syndrome HCC
   F48.2 Pseudobulbar affect
      Involuntary emotional expression disorder
      Code first underlying cause, if known, such as:
         amyotrophic lateral sclerosis (G12.21)
         multiple sclerosis (G35)
         sequelae of cerebrovascular disease (I69.-)
         sequelae of traumatic intracranial injury (S06.-)
   F48.8 Other specified nonpsychotic mental disorders
      Dhat syndrome
      Neurasthenia
      Occupational neurosis, including writer's cramp
      Psychasthenia
      Psychasthenic neurosis
      Psychogenic syncope
   F48.9 Nonpsychotic mental disorder, unspecified
      Neurosis NOS

Chapter 5. Mental, Behavioral and Neurodevelopmental Disorders

Behavioral syndromes associated with physiological disturbances and physical factors (F50-F59)

✓4ᵗʰ F50 Eating disorders

EXCLUDES 1   anorexia NOS (R63.0)
     feeding difficulties (R63.3)
     feeding problems of newborn (P92.-)
     polyphagia (R63.2)

EXCLUDES 2   feeding disorder in infancy or childhood (F98.2-)

AHA: 2018,4Q,82

TIP: Assign additional code for BMI from category Z68, when documented. BMI can be based on documentation from clinicians who are not the patient's provider.

CC Excl: For CC codes in category F50, unless otherwise noted: PDX collection 556

✓5ᵗʰ F50.0 Anorexia nervosa

EXCLUDES 1   loss of appetite (R63.0)
     psychogenic loss of appetite (F50.89)

DEF: Psychological eating disorder characterized by an intense fear of gaining weight and an unrealistic perception of body image that perpetuates the feeling of being fat or having too much fat. Avoidance of food and restrictive or unhealthy eating are common.

F50.00   **Anorexia nervosa, unspecified**   CC

F50.01   **Anorexia nervosa, restricting type**   CC

F50.02   **Anorexia nervosa, binge eating/purging type**   CC
     EXCLUDES 1   bulimia nervosa (F50.2)

F50.2 Bulimia nervosa   CC

Bulimia NOS
Hyperorexia nervosa

EXCLUDES 1   anorexia nervosa, binge eating/purging type (F50.02)

DEF: Episodic pattern of overeating (binge eating) followed by purging or extreme exercise accompanied by an awareness of the abnormal eating pattern with a fear of not being able to stop eating.

CC Excl: PDX collection 557

✓5ᵗʰ F50.8 Other eating disorders

EXCLUDES 2   pica of infancy and childhood (F98.3)

AHA: 2017,4Q,9; 2016,4Q,15-16

F50.81   **Binge eating disorder**

F50.82   **Avoidant/restrictive food intake disorder**

F50.89   **Other specified eating disorder**
     Pica in adults
     Psychogenic loss of appetite

F50.9 Eating disorder, unspecified

Atypical anorexia nervosa
Atypical bulimia nervosa
Feeding or eating disorder, unspecified
Other specified feeding disorder

✓4ᵗʰ F51 Sleep disorders not due to a substance or known physiological condition

EXCLUDES 2   organic sleep disorders (G47.-)

✓5ᵗʰ F51.0 Insomnia not due to a substance or known physiological condition

EXCLUDES 2   alcohol related insomnia (F10.182, F10.282, F10.982)
     drug-related insomnia (F11.182, F11.282, F11.982, F13.182, F13.282, F13.982, F14.182, F14.282, F14.982, F15.182, F15.282, F15.982, F19.182, F19.282, F19.982)
     insomnia NOS (G47.0-)
     insomnia due to known physiological condition (G47.0-)
     organic insomnia (G47.0-)
     sleep deprivation (Z72.820)

F51.01   **Primary insomnia**
     Idiopathic insomnia

F51.02   **Adjustment insomnia**

F51.03   **Paradoxical insomnia**

F51.04   **Psychophysiologic insomnia**

F51.05   **Insomnia due to other mental disorder**
     Code also associated mental disorder

F51.09   **Other insomnia not due to a substance or known physiological condition**

✓5ᵗʰ F51.1 Hypersomnia not due to a substance or known physiological condition

EXCLUDES 2   alcohol related hypersomnia (F10.182, F10.282, F10.982)
     drug-related hypersomnia (F11.182, F11.282, F11.982, F13.182, F13.282, F13.982, F14.182, F14.282, F14.982, F15.182, F15.282, F15.982, F19.182, F19.282, F19.982)
     hypersomnia NOS (G47.10)
     hypersomnia due to known physiological condition (G47.10)
     idiopathic hypersomnia (G47.11, G47.12)
     narcolepsy (G47.4-)

F51.11   **Primary hypersomnia**

F51.12   **Insufficient sleep syndrome**
     EXCLUDES 1   sleep deprivation (Z72.820)

F51.13   **Hypersomnia due to other mental disorder**
     Code also associated mental disorder

F51.19   **Other hypersomnia not due to a substance or known physiological condition**

F51.3 Sleepwalking [somnambulism]

Non-rapid eye movement sleep arousal disorders, sleepwalking type

F51.4 Sleep terrors [night terrors]

Non-rapid eye movement sleep arousal disorders, sleep terror type

F51.5 Nightmare disorder

Dream anxiety disorder

F51.8 Other sleep disorders not due to a substance or known physiological condition

F51.9 Sleep disorder not due to a substance or known physiological condition, unspecified

Emotional sleep disorder NOS

✓4ᵗʰ F52 Sexual dysfunction not due to a substance or known physiological condition

EXCLUDES 2   Dhat syndrome (F48.8)

F52.0 Hypoactive sexual desire disorder

Lack or loss of sexual desire
Male hypoactive sexual desire disorder
Sexual anhedonia

EXCLUDES 1   decreased libido (R68.82)

F52.1 Sexual aversion disorder

Sexual aversion and lack of sexual enjoyment

✓5ᵗʰ F52.2 Sexual arousal disorders

Failure of genital response

F52.21   **Male erectile disorder**   ♂
     Erectile disorder
     Psychogenic impotence
     EXCLUDES 1   impotence of organic origin (N52.-)
         impotence NOS (N52.-)

F52.22   **Female sexual arousal disorder**   ♀
     Female sexual interest/arousal disorder

✓5ᵗʰ F52.3 Orgasmic disorder

Inhibited orgasm
Psychogenic anorgasmy

F52.31   **Female orgasmic disorder**   ♀

F52.32   **Male orgasmic disorder**   ♂
     Delayed ejaculation

F52.4 Premature ejaculation   ♂

F52.5 Vaginismus not due to a substance or known physiological condition   ♀

Psychogenic vaginismus

EXCLUDES 2   vaginismus (due to a known physiological condition) (N94.2)

DEF: Psychogenic response resulting in painful contractions of the vaginal canal muscles. This condition can be severe enough to prevent sexual intercourse.

F52.6 Dyspareunia not due to a substance or known physiological condition

Genito-pelvic pain penetration disorder
Psychogenic dyspareunia

EXCLUDES 2   dyspareunia (due to a known physiological condition) (N94.1-)

N Newborn: 0   **P** Pediatric: 0-17   **M** Maternity: 9-64   **A** Adult: 15-124   **MCC** Major Complication/Comorbidity   **CC** Complication/Comorbidity   **SW** Severe Wound Dx

564   ICD-10-CM 2020

F52.8 Other sexual dysfunction not due to a substance or known physiological condition

Excessive sexual drive

Nymphomania

Satyriasis

F52.9 Unspecified sexual dysfunction not due to a substance or known physiological condition

Sexual dysfunction NOS

✓4ᵗʰ **F53 Mental and behavioral disorders associated with the puerperium, not elsewhere classified**

EXCLUDES 1   *mood disorders with psychotic features (F30.2, F31.2, F31.5, F31.64, F32.3, F33.3)*

postpartum dysphoria (O90.6)

psychosis in schizophrenia, schizotypal, delusional, and other psychotic disorders (F20-F29)

AHA: 2018,4Q,8

F53.0 Postpartum depression   M ♀

Postnatal depression, NOS

Postpartum depression, NOS

F53.1 Puerperal psychosis   HCC M ♀

Postpartum psychosis

Puerperal psychosis, NOS

F54 *Psychological and behavioral factors associated with disorders or diseases classified elsewhere*

Psychological factors affecting physical conditions

Code first the associated physical disorder, such as:

asthma (J45.-)

dermatitis (L23-L25)

gastric ulcer (K25.-)

mucous colitis (K58.-)

ulcerative colitis (K51.-)

urticaria (L50.-)

EXCLUDES 2   *tension-type headache (G44.2)*

✓4ᵗʰ **F55 Abuse of non-psychoactive substances**

EXCLUDES 2   *abuse of psychoactive substances (F10-F19)*

F55.0 Abuse of antacids

F55.1 Abuse of herbal or folk remedies

F55.2 Abuse of laxatives

F55.3 Abuse of steroids or hormones

F55.4 Abuse of vitamins

F55.8 Abuse of other non-psychoactive substances

F59 Unspecified behavioral syndromes associated with physiological disturbances and physical factors

Psychogenic physiological dysfunction NOS

Disorders of adult personality and behavior (F60-F69)

✓4ᵗʰ **F60 Specific personality disorders**

F60.0 Paranoid personality disorder   HCC

Expansive paranoid personality (disorder)

Fanatic personality (disorder)

Paranoid personality (disorder)

Querulant personality (disorder)

Sensitive paranoid personality (disorder)

EXCLUDES 2   *paranoia (F22)*

paranoia querulans (F22)

paranoid psychosis (F22)

paranoid schizophrenia (F20.0)

paranoid state (F22)

F60.1 Schizoid personality disorder   HCC

EXCLUDES 2   *Asperger's syndrome (F84.5)*

delusional disorder (F22)

schizoid disorder of childhood (F84.5)

schizophrenia (F20.-)

schizotypal disorder (F21)

F60.2 Antisocial personality disorder   HCC

Amoral personality (disorder)

Asocial personality (disorder)

Dissocial personality disorder

Psychopathic personality (disorder)

Sociopathic personality (disorder)

EXCLUDES 1   *conduct disorders (F91.-)*

EXCLUDES 2   *borderline personality disorder (F60.3)*

F60.3 Borderline personality disorder   HCC

Aggressive personality (disorder)

Emotionally unstable personality disorder

Explosive personality (disorder)

EXCLUDES 2   *antisocial personality disorder (F60.2)*

F60.4 Histrionic personality disorder   HCC

Hysterical personality (disorder)

Psychoinfantile personality (disorder)

F60.5 Obsessive-compulsive personality disorder   HCC

Anankastic personality (disorder)

Compulsive personality (disorder)

Obsessional personality (disorder)

EXCLUDES 2   *obsessive-compulsive disorder (F42-)*

F60.6 Avoidant personality disorder   HCC

Anxious personality disorder

F60.7 Dependent personality disorder   HCC

Asthenic personality (disorder)

Inadequate personality (disorder)

Passive personality (disorder)

DEF: Lack of self-confidence, fear of abandonment, and an obsessive need to be taken care of.

✓5ᵗʰ **F60.8 Other specific personality disorders**

F60.81 Narcissistic personality disorder   HCC

F60.89 Other specific personality disorders   HCC

Eccentric personality disorder

"Haltlose" type personality disorder

Immature personality disorder

Passive-aggressive personality disorder

Psychoneurotic personality disorder

Self-defeating personality disorder

F60.9 Personality disorder, unspecified   HCC

Character disorder NOS

Character neurosis NOS

Pathological personality NOS

✓4ᵗʰ **F63 Impulse disorders**

EXCLUDES 2   *habitual excessive use of alcohol or psychoactive substances (F10-F19)*

impulse disorders involving sexual behavior (F65.-)

F63.0 Pathological gambling

Compulsive gambling

Gambling disorder

EXCLUDES 1   *gambling and betting NOS (Z72.6)*

EXCLUDES 2   *excessive gambling by manic patients (F30, F31)*

gambling in antisocial personality disorder (F60.2)

F63.1 Pyromania

Pathological fire-setting

EXCLUDES 2   *fire-setting (by) (in):*

adult with antisocial personality disorder (F60.2)

alcohol or psychoactive substance intoxication (F10-F19)

conduct disorders (F91.-)

mental disorders due to known physiological condition (F01-F09)

schizophrenia (F20.-)

F63.2 Kleptomania

Pathological stealing

EXCLUDES 1   *shoplifting as the reason for observation for suspected mental disorder (Z03.8)*

EXCLUDES 2   *depressive disorder with stealing (F31-F33)*

stealing due to underlying mental condition - code to mental condition

stealing in mental disorders due to known physiological condition (F01-F09)

F63.3 Trichotillomania

Hair plucking

EXCLUDES 2   *other stereotyped movement disorder (F98.4)*

✓5ᵗʰ **F63.8 Other impulse disorders**

F63.81 Intermittent explosive disorder

F63.89 Other impulse disorders   CC

F63.9 Impulse disorder, unspecified   CC

Impulse control disorder NOS

✓ Additional Character Required   ✓x7ᵗʰ Placeholder   Unacceptable PDx   Questionable PDx   Manifestation   Unspecified Dx   H1-H10 HAC   HCC CMS-HCC Dx   HIV HIV Dx

ICD-10-CM 2020   565

✓4ᵗʰ **F64 Gender identity disorders**

    AHA: 2016,4Q,16

   F64.0 Transsexualism

     Gender identity disorder in adolescence and adulthood

     Gender dysphoria in adolescents and adults

   F64.1 Dual role transvestism

     Use additional code to identify sex reassignment status (Z87.890)

     EXCLUDES 1   *gender identity disorder in childhood (F64.2)*

     EXCLUDES 2   *fetishistic transvestism (F65.1)*

   F64.2 Gender identity disorder of childhood   P

     Gender dysphoria in children

     EXCLUDES 1   *gender identity disorder in adolescence and adulthood (F64.0)*

     EXCLUDES 2   *sexual maturation disorder (F66)*

   F64.8 Other gender identity disorders

     Other specified gender dysphoria

   F64.9 Gender identity disorder, unspecified

     Gender dysphoria, unspecified

     Gender-role disorder NOS

✓4ᵗʰ **F65 Paraphilias**

   F65.0 Fetishism

     Fetishistic disorder

   F65.1 Transvestic fetishism

     Fetishistic transvestism

     Transvestic disorder

   F65.2 Exhibitionism

     Exhibitionistic disorder

   F65.3 Voyeurism

     Voyeuristic disorder

   F65.4 Pedophilia

     Pedophilic disorder

✓5ᵗʰ **F65.5 Sadomasochism**

     F65.50 Sadomasochism, unspecified

     F65.51 Sexual masochism

      Sexual masochism disorder

     F65.52 Sexual sadism

      Sexual sadism disorder

✓5ᵗʰ **F65.8 Other paraphilias**

     F65.81 Frotteurism

      Frotteuristic disorder

     F65.89 Other paraphilias

      Necrophilia

      Other specified paraphilic disorder

   F65.9 Paraphilia, unspecified

     Paraphilic disorder, unspecified

     Sexual deviation NOS

F66 Other sexual disorders

     Sexual maturation disorder

     Sexual relationship disorder

✓4ᵗʰ **F68 Other disorders of adult personality and behavior**

    AHA: 2018,4Q,9,65

    CC Excl: For CC codes in category F68: PDX collection 551

✓5ᵗʰ **F68.1 Factitious disorder imposed on self**

     Compensation neurosis

     Elaboration of physical symptoms for psychological reasons

     Hospital hopper syndrome

     Münchausen's syndrome

     Peregrinating patient

     EXCLUDES 2   *factitial dermatitis (L98.1)*

      person feigning illness (with obvious motivation) (Z76.5)

     F68.10 Factitious disorder imposed on self, unspecified   CC

     F68.11 Factitious disorder imposed on self, with predominantly psychological signs and symptoms

     F68.12 Factitious disorder imposed on self, with predominantly physical signs and symptoms   CC

     F68.13 Factitious disorder imposed on self, with combined psychological and physical signs and symptoms

   F68.A Factitious disorder imposed on another   CC

     Factitious disorder by proxy

     Münchausen's by proxy

   F68.8 Other specified disorders of adult personality and behavior

F69 Unspecified disorder of adult personality and behavior   A

Intellectual disabilities (F70-F79)

Code first any associated physical or developmental disorders

EXCLUDES 1   *borderline intellectual functioning, IQ above 70 to 84 (R41.83)*

F70 Mild intellectual disabilities

     IQ level 50-55 to approximately 70

     Mild mental subnormality

F71 Moderate intellectual disabilities

     IQ level 35-40 to 50-55

     Moderate mental subnormality

F72 Severe intellectual disabilities

     IQ 20-25 to 35-40

     Severe mental subnormality

F73 Profound intellectual disabilities

     IQ level below 20-25

     Profound mental subnormality

F78 Other intellectual disabilities

F79 Unspecified intellectual disabilities

     Mental deficiency NOS

     Mental subnormality NOS

Pervasive and specific developmental disorders (F80-F89)

✓4ᵗʰ **F80 Specific developmental disorders of speech and language**

   F80.0 Phonological disorder

     Dyslalia

     Functional speech articulation disorder

     Lalling

     Lisping

     Phonological developmental disorder

     Speech articulation developmental disorder

     Speech-sound disorder

     EXCLUDES 1   *speech articulation impairment due to aphasia NOS (R47.01)*

      speech articulation impairment due to apraxia (R48.2)

     EXCLUDES 2   *speech articulation impairment due to hearing loss (F80.4)*

      speech articulation impairment due to intellectual disabilities (F70-F79)

      speech articulation impairment with expressive language developmental disorder (F80.1)

      speech articulation impairment with mixed receptive expressive language developmental disorder (F80.2)

   F80.1 Expressive language disorder

     Developmental dysphasia or aphasia, expressive type

     EXCLUDES 1   *mixed receptive-expressive language disorder (F80.2)*

      dysphasia and aphasia NOS (R47.-)

     EXCLUDES 2   *acquired aphasia with epilepsy [Landau-Kleffner] (G40.80-)*

      selective mutism (F94.0)

      intellectual disabilities (F70-F79)

      pervasive developmental disorders (F84.-)

   F80.2 Mixed receptive-expressive language disorder

     Developmental dysphasia or aphasia, receptive type

     Developmental Wernicke's aphasia

     EXCLUDES 1   *central auditory processing disorder (H93.25)*

      dysphasia or aphasia NOS (R47.-)

      expressive language disorder (F80.1)

      expressive type dysphasia or aphasia (F80.1)

      word deafness (H93.25)

     EXCLUDES 2   *acquired aphasia with epilepsy [Landau-Kleffner] (G40.80-)*

      pervasive developmental disorders (F84.-)

      selective mutism (F94.0)

      intellectual disabilities (F70-F79)

   F80.4 Speech and language development delay due to hearing loss

     Code also type of hearing loss (H90.-, H91.-)

N Newborn: 0   P Pediatric: 0-17   M Maternity: 9-64   A Adult: 15-124   MCC Major Complication/Comorbidity   CC Complication/Comorbidity   SW Severe Wound Dx

566   ICD-10-CM 2020

F80.8 Other developmental disorders of speech and language
AHA: 2017,1Q,27

F80.81 Childhood onset fluency disorder
Cluttering NOS
Stuttering NOS
EXCLUDES 1 adult onset fluency disorder (F98.5)
fluency disorder in conditions classified elsewhere (R47.82)
fluency disorder (stuttering) following cerebrovascular disease (I69. with final characters -23)

F80.82 Social pragmatic communication disorder
EXCLUDES 1 Asperger's syndrome (F84.5)
autistic disorder (F84.0)
AHA: 2016,4Q,16

F80.89 Other developmental disorders of speech and language

F80.9 Developmental disorder of speech and language, unspecified
Communication disorder NOS
Language disorder NOS

F81 Specific developmental disorders of scholastic skills

F81.0 Specific reading disorder
"Backward reading"
Developmental dyslexia
Specific learning disorder, with impairment in reading
Specific reading retardation
EXCLUDES 1 alexia NOS (R48.0)
dyslexia NOS (R48.0)
DEF: Serious impairment of reading skills unexplained in relation to general intelligence and teaching processes.

F81.2 Mathematics disorder
Developmental acalculia
Developmental arithmetical disorder
Developmental Gerstmann's syndrome
Specific learning disorder, with impairment in mathematics
EXCLUDES 1 acalculia NOS (R48.8)
EXCLUDES 2 arithmetical difficulties associated with a reading disorder (F81.0)
arithmetical difficulties associated with a spelling disorder (F81.81)
arithmetical difficulties due to inadequate teaching (Z55.8)

F81.8 Other developmental disorders of scholastic skills

F81.81 Disorder of written expression
Specific learning disorder, with impairment in written expression
Specific spelling disorder

F81.89 Other developmental disorders of scholastic skills

F81.9 Developmental disorder of scholastic skills, unspecified
Knowledge acquisition disability NOS
Learning disability NOS
Learning disorder NOS

F82 Specific developmental disorder of motor function
Clumsy child syndrome
Developmental coordination disorder
Developmental dyspraxia
EXCLUDES 1 abnormalities of gait and mobility (R26.-)
lack of coordination (R27.-)
EXCLUDES 2 lack of coordination secondary to intellectual disabilities (F70-F79)

F84 Pervasive developmental disorders
Use additional code to identify any associated medical condition and intellectual disabilities.

F84.0 Autistic disorder
Autism spectrum disorder
Infantile autism
Infantile psychosis
Kanner's syndrome
EXCLUDES 1 Asperger's syndrome (F84.5)
AHA: 2017,1Q,27

F84.2 Rett's syndrome
EXCLUDES 1 Asperger's syndrome (F84.5)
autistic disorder (F84.0)
other childhood disintegrative disorder (F84.3)

F84.3 Other childhood disintegrative disorder CC P
Dementia infantilis
Disintegrative psychosis
Heller's syndrome
Symbiotic psychosis
Use additional code to identify any associated neurological condition
EXCLUDES 1 Asperger's syndrome (F84.5)
autistic disorder (F84.0)
Rett's syndrome (F84.2)
CC Excl: PDX collection 551

F84.5 Asperger's syndrome
Asperger's disorder
Autistic psychopathy
Schizoid disorder of childhood
DEF: High-functioning form of autism. Children with this syndrome usually develop speech on schedule, are generally very intelligent, and communicate well, but have considerable social shortcomings. Synonym(s): AS.

F84.8 Other pervasive developmental disorders
Overactive disorder associated with intellectual disabilities and stereotyped movements

F84.9 Pervasive developmental disorder, unspecified
Atypical autism

F88 Other disorders of psychological development
Developmental agnosia
Global developmental delay
Other specified neurodevelopmental disorder

F89 Unspecified disorder of psychological development
Developmental disorder NOS
Neurodevelopmental disorder NOS

Behavioral and emotional disorders with onset usually occurring in childhood and adolescence (F90-F98)

NOTE Codes within categories F90-F98 may be used regardless of the age of a patient. These disorders generally have onset within the childhood or adolescent years, but may continue throughout life or not be diagnosed until adulthood

F90 Attention-deficit hyperactivity disorders
INCLUDES attention deficit disorder with hyperactivity
attention deficit syndrome with hyperactivity
EXCLUDES 2 anxiety disorders (F40.-, F41.-)
mood [affective] disorders (F30-F39)
pervasive developmental disorders (F84.-)
schizophrenia (F20.-)

F90.0 Attention-deficit hyperactivity disorder, predominantly inattentive type
Attention-deficit/hyperactivity disorder, predominantly inattentive presentation

F90.1 Attention-deficit hyperactivity disorder, predominantly hyperactive type
Attention-deficit/hyperactivity disorder, predominantly hyperactive impulsive presentation

F90.2 Attention-deficit hyperactivity disorder, combined type
Attention-deficit/hyperactivity disorder, combined presentation

F90.8 Attention-deficit hyperactivity disorder, other type

F90.9 Attention-deficit hyperactivity disorder, unspecified type
Attention-deficit hyperactivity disorder of childhood or adolescence NOS
Attention-deficit hyperactivity disorder NOS

F91 Conduct disorders
EXCLUDES 1 antisocial behavior (Z72.81-)
antisocial personality disorder (F60.2)
EXCLUDES 2 conduct problems associated with attention-deficit hyperactivity disorder (F90.-)
mood [affective] disorders (F30-F39)
pervasive developmental disorders (F84.-)
schizophrenia (F20.-)

F91.0 Conduct disorder confined to family context

F91.1 Conduct disorder, childhood-onset type
Unsocialized conduct disorder
Conduct disorder, solitary aggressive type
Unsocialized aggressive disorder

Chapter 5. Mental, Behavioral and Neurodevelopmental Disorders

F91.2   **Conduct disorder, adolescent-onset type**
     Socialized conduct disorder
     Conduct disorder, group type

F91.3   **Oppositional defiant disorder**

F91.8   **Other conduct disorders**
     Other specified conduct disorder
     Other specified disruptive disorder

F91.9   **Conduct disorder, unspecified**
     Behavioral disorder NOS
     Conduct disorder NOS
     Disruptive behavior disorder NOS
     Disruptive disorder NOS

✓4ᵗʰ **F93**   **Emotional disorders with onset specific to childhood**

F93.0   **Separation anxiety disorder of childhood**
     EXCLUDES 2   mood [affective] disorders (F30-F39)
         nonpsychotic mental disorders (F40-F48)
         phobic anxiety disorder of childhood (F40.8)
         social phobia (F40.1)

F93.8   **Other childhood emotional disorders**
     Identity disorder
     EXCLUDES 2   gender identity disorder of childhood (F64.2)

F93.9   **Childhood emotional disorder, unspecified**

✓4ᵗʰ **F94**   **Disorders of social functioning with onset specific to childhood and adolescence**

F94.0   **Selective mutism**
     Elective mutism
     EXCLUDES 2   pervasive developmental disorders (F84.-)
         schizophrenia (F20.-)
         specific developmental disorders of speech and language (F80.-)
         transient mutism as part of separation anxiety in young children (F93.0)

F94.1   **Reactive attachment disorder of childhood**
     Use additional code to identify any associated failure to thrive or growth retardation
     EXCLUDES 1   disinhibited attachment disorder of childhood (F94.2)
         normal variation in pattern of selective attachment
     EXCLUDES 2   Asperger's syndrome (F84.5)
         maltreatment syndromes (T74.-)
         sexual or physical abuse in childhood, resulting in psychosocial problems (Z62.81-)

F94.2   **Disinhibited attachment disorder of childhood**
     Affectionless psychopathy
     Institutional syndrome
     EXCLUDES 1   reactive attachment disorder of childhood (F94.1)
     EXCLUDES 2   Asperger's syndrome (F84.5)
         attention-deficit hyperactivity disorders (F90.-)
         hospitalism in children (F43.2-)

F94.8   **Other childhood disorders of social functioning**

F94.9   **Childhood disorder of social functioning, unspecified**

✓4ᵗʰ **F95**   **Tic disorder**

F95.0   **Transient tic disorder**
     Provisional tic disorder

F95.1   **Chronic motor or vocal tic disorder**

F95.2   **Tourette's disorder**
     Combined vocal and multiple motor tic disorder [de la Tourette]
     Tourette's syndrome

F95.8   **Other tic disorders**

F95.9   **Tic disorder, unspecified**
     Tic NOS

✓4ᵗʰ **F98**   **Other behavioral and emotional disorders with onset usually occurring in childhood and adolescence**
     EXCLUDES 2   breath-holding spells (R06.89)
         gender identity disorder of childhood (F64.2)
         Kleine-Levin syndrome (G47.13)
         obsessive-compulsive disorder (F42-)
         sleep disorders not due to a substance or known physiological condition (F51.-)

F98.0   **Enuresis not due to a substance or known physiological condition**
     Enuresis (primary) (secondary) of nonorganic origin
     Functional enuresis
     Psychogenic enuresis
     Urinary incontinence of nonorganic origin
     EXCLUDES 1   enuresis NOS (R32)

F98.1   **Encopresis not due to a substance or known physiological condition**
     Functional encopresis
     Incontinence of feces of nonorganic origin
     Psychogenic encopresis
     Use additional code to identify the cause of any coexisting constipation
     EXCLUDES 1   encopresis NOS (R15.-)

✓5ᵗʰ **F98.2**   **Other feeding disorders of infancy and childhood**
     EXCLUDES 1   feeding difficulties (R63.3)
     EXCLUDES 2   anorexia nervosa and other eating disorders (F50.-)
         feeding problems of newborn (P92.-)
         pica of infancy or childhood (F98.3)

F98.21   **Rumination disorder of infancy**

F98.29   **Other feeding disorders of infancy and early childhood**

F98.3   **Pica of infancy and childhood**

F98.4   **Stereotyped movement disorders**
     Stereotype/habit disorder
     EXCLUDES 1   abnormal involuntary movements (R25.-)
     EXCLUDES 2   compulsions in obsessive-compulsive disorder (F42-)
         hair plucking (F63.3)
         movement disorders of organic origin (G20-G25)
         nail-biting (F98.8)
         nose-picking (F98.8)
         stereotypies that are part of a broader psychiatric condition (F01-F95)
         thumb-sucking (F98.8)
         tic disorders (F95.-)
         trichotillomania (F63.3)

F98.5   **Adult onset fluency disorder**
     EXCLUDES 1   childhood onset fluency disorder (F80.81)
         dysphasia (R47.02)
         fluency disorder in conditions classified elsewhere (R47.82)
         fluency disorder (stuttering) following cerebrovascular disease (I69. with final characters -23)
         tic disorders (F95.-)

F98.8   **Other specified behavioral and emotional disorders with onset usually occurring in childhood and adolescence**
     Excessive masturbation
     Nail-biting
     Nose-picking
     Thumb-sucking

F98.9   **Unspecified behavioral and emotional disorders with onset usually occurring in childhood and adolescence**

Unspecified mental disorder (F99)

F99   **Mental disorder, not otherwise specified**
     Mental illness NOS
     EXCLUDES 1   unspecified mental disorder due to known physiological condition (F09)

🅝 Newborn: 0   🅟 Pediatric: 0-17   🅜 Maternity: 9-64   🅐 Adult: 15-124   MCC Major Complication/Comorbidity   CC Complication/Comorbidity   SW Severe Wound Dx

568   ICD-10-CM 2020

Chapter 6. Diseases of the Nervous System (G00-G99)

Chapter-specific Guidelines with Coding Examples

The chapter-specific guidelines from the ICD-10-CM Official Guidelines for Coding and Reporting have been provided below. Along with these guidelines are coding examples, contained in the shaded boxes, that have been developed to help illustrate the coding and/or sequencing guidance found in these guidelines.

a. Dominant/nondominant side

Codes from category G81, Hemiplegia and hemiparesis, and subcategories G83.1, Monoplegia of lower limb, G83.2, Monoplegia of upper limb, and G83.3, Monoplegia, unspecified, identify whether the dominant or nondominant side is affected. Should the affected side be documented, but not specified as dominant or nondominant, and the classification system does not indicate a default, code selection is as follows:

- For ambidextrous patients, the default should be dominant.
- If the left side is affected, the default is non-dominant.
- If the right side is affected, the default is dominant.

> Hemiplegia affecting left side of ambidextrous patient
>
> **G81.92   Hemiplegia, unspecified affecting left dominant side**
>
> *Explanation*: Documentation states that the left side is affected and dominant is used for ambidextrous persons.

> Right spastic hemiplegia, unknown whether patient is right- or left-handed
>
> **G81.11   Spastic hemiplegia affecting right dominant side**
>
> *Explanation*: Since it is unknown whether the patient is right- or left-handed, if the right side is affected, the default is dominant.

b. Pain—category G89

1) General coding information

Codes in category G89, Pain, not elsewhere classified, may be used in conjunction with codes from other categories and chapters to provide more detail about acute or chronic pain and neoplasm-related pain, unless otherwise indicated below.

If the pain is not specified as acute or chronic, post-thoracotomy, postprocedural, or neoplasm-related, do not assign codes from category G89.

A code from category G89 should not be assigned if the underlying (definitive) diagnosis is known, unless the reason for the encounter is pain control/ management and not management of the underlying condition.

When an admission or encounter is for a procedure aimed at treating the underlying condition (e.g., spinal fusion, kyphoplasty), a code for the underlying condition (e.g., vertebral fracture, spinal stenosis) should be assigned as the principal diagnosis. No code from category G89 should be assigned.

> Elderly patient with back pain is admitted for kyphoplasty for age-related osteopathic compression fracture at vertebra T3
>
> **M80.08XA   Age-related osteoporosis with current pathological fracture, vertebra(e), initial encounter for fracture**
>
> *Explanation*: No code is assigned for the pain as it is inherent in the underlying condition being treated.

(a) Category G89 codes as principal or first-listed diagnosis

Category G89 codes are acceptable as principal diagnosis or the first-listed code:

- When pain control or pain management is the reason for the admission/encounter (e.g., a patient with displaced intervertebral disc, nerve impingement and severe back pain presents for injection of steroid into the spinal canal). The underlying cause of the pain should be reported as an additional diagnosis, if known.

- When a patient is admitted for the insertion of a neurostimulator for pain control, assign the appropriate pain code as the principal or first-listed diagnosis. When an admission or encounter is for a procedure aimed at treating the underlying condition and a neurostimulator is inserted for pain control during the same admission/encounter, a code for the underlying condition should be assigned as the principal diagnosis and the appropriate pain code should be assigned as a secondary diagnosis.

> Patient with chronic pain from lumbar spondylosis with radiculopathy not relieved by surgery is admitted for insertion of neurostimulator.
>
> **G89.29   Other chronic pain**
>
> **M47.26   Other spondylosis with radiculopathy, lumbar region**
>
> *Explanation*: Since the patient is admitted specifically for a neurostimulator implantation for pain management and not to treat the underlying spondylosis, the chronic pain code is sequenced first, followed by the underlying condition. Neither code M54.16 nor M54.5 is necessary because M47.26 describes the radiculopathy and the site.

(b) Use of category G89 codes in conjunction with site specific pain codes

(i) Assigning category G89 and site-specific pain codes

Codes from category G89 may be used in conjunction with codes that identify the site of pain (including codes from chapter 18) if the category G89 code provides additional information. For example, if the code describes the site of the pain, but does not fully describe whether the pain is acute or chronic, then both codes should be assigned.

> During hospital stay, patient is seen by orthopaedics to evaluate chronic left shoulder pain.
>
> **M25.512   Pain in left shoulder**
>
> **G89.29   Other chronic pain**
>
> *Explanation*: No underlying condition has been determined yet so the pain would be the reason for the visit. The M25 pain code in this instance does not fully describe the condition as it does not represent that the pain is chronic. The G89 chronic pain code is assigned to provide specificity.

(ii) Sequencing of category G89 codes with site-specific pain codes

The sequencing of category G89 codes with site-specific pain codes (including chapter 18 codes), is dependent on the circumstances of the encounter/admission as follows:

- If the encounter is for pain control or pain management, assign the code from category G89 followed by the code identifying the specific site of pain (e.g., encounter for pain management for acute neck pain from trauma is assigned code G89.11, Acute pain due to trauma, followed by code M54.2, Cervicalgia, to identify the site of pain).

> Management of acute, traumatic right knee pain
>
> **G89.11   Acute pain due to trauma**
>
> **M25.561   Pain in right knee**
>
> *Explanation*: The reason for the encounter is to manage or control the pain, not to treat or evaluate an underlying condition. The G89 pain code is assigned as the principal diagnosis but in this instance does not fully describe the condition as it does not include the site and laterality. The M25 pain code is added to provide this information.

Chapter 6. Diseases of the Nervous System

- If the encounter is for any other reason except pain control or pain management, and a related definitive diagnosis has not been established (confirmed) by the provider, assign the code for the specific site of pain first, followed by the appropriate code from category G89.

Tests are performed to investigate the source of the patient's chronic epigastric abdominal pain

R10.13	**Epigastric pain**
G89.29	**Other chronic pain**

Explanation: In this instance the patient's epigastric pain is not being treated; rather the source of the pain is being investigated. A code from chapter 18 for epigastric pain is sequenced before the additional specificity of the G89 code for the chronic pain.

2) Pain due to devices, implants and grafts
See Section I.C.19. Pain due to medical devices

3) Postoperative pain
The provider's documentation should be used to guide the coding of postoperative pain, as well as *Section III. Reporting Additional Diagnoses* and *Section IV. Diagnostic Coding and Reporting in the Outpatient Setting.*

The default for post-thoracotomy and other postoperative pain not specified as acute or chronic is the code for the acute form.

Routine or expected postoperative pain immediately after surgery should not be coded.

Pain pump dose is increased for the patient's unexpected, extreme pain post-thoracotomy

G89.12	**Acute post-thoracotomy pain**

Explanation: When acute or chronic is not documented, default to acute. The use of "unexpected, extreme" and the increase of medication dosage indicate that the pain was more than routine or expected.

(a) Postoperative pain not associated with specific postoperative complication

Postoperative pain not associated with a specific postoperative complication is assigned to the appropriate postoperative pain code in category G89.

(b) Postoperative pain associated with specific postoperative complication

Postoperative pain associated with a specific postoperative complication (such as painful wire sutures) is assigned to the appropriate code(s) found in Chapter 19, Injury, poisoning, and certain other consequences of external causes. If appropriate, use additional code(s) from category G89 to identify acute or chronic pain (G89.18 or G89.28).

4) Chronic pain
Chronic pain is classified to subcategory G89.2. There is no time frame defining when pain becomes chronic pain. The provider's documentation should be used to guide use of these codes.

5) Neoplasm related pain
Code G89.3 is assigned to pain documented as being related, associated or due to cancer, primary or secondary malignancy, or tumor. This code is assigned regardless of whether the pain is acute or chronic.

This code may be assigned as the principal or first-listed code when the stated reason for the admission/encounter is documented as pain control/pain management. The underlying neoplasm should be reported as an additional diagnosis.

Pain medication adjustment for chronic pain from bone metastasis

G89.3	**Neoplasm related pain (acute)(chronic)**
C79.51	**Secondary malignant neoplasm of bone**

Explanation: Since the encounter was for pain medication management, the pain, rather than the neoplasm, was the reason for the encounter and is sequenced first. This "neoplasm-related pain" code includes both acute and chronic pain.

When the reason for the admission/encounter is management of the neoplasm and the pain associated with the neoplasm is also documented, code G89.3 may be assigned as an additional diagnosis. It is not necessary to assign an additional code for the site of the pain.

See Section I.C.2 for instructions on the sequencing of neoplasms for all other stated reasons for the admission/encounter (except for pain control/pain management).

Patient with lung cancer presents with acute hip pain and is evaluated and found to have iliac bone metastasis

C79.51	**Secondary malignant neoplasm of bone**
C34.90	**Malignant neoplasm of unspecified part of unspecified bronchus or lung**
G89.3	**Neoplasm related pain (acute)(chronic)**

Explanation: The reason for the encounter was the evaluation and diagnosis of the bone metastasis, whose code would be assigned as first-listed, followed by codes for the primary neoplasm and the pain due to the iliac bone metastasis.

6) Chronic pain syndrome
Central pain syndrome (G89.0) and chronic pain syndrome (G89.4) are different than the term "chronic pain," and therefore codes should only be used when the provider has specifically documented this condition.

See Section I.C.5. Pain disorders related to psychological factors

Chapter 6. Diseases of the Nervous System (G00-G99)

EXCLUDES 2   certain conditions originating in the perinatal period (P04-P96)
certain infectious and parasitic diseases (A00-B99)
complications of pregnancy, childbirth and the puerperium (O00-O9A)
congenital malformations, deformations, and chromosomal abnormalities (Q00-Q99)
endocrine, nutritional and metabolic diseases (E00-E88)
injury, poisoning and certain other consequences of external causes (S00-T88)
neoplasms (C00-D49)
symptoms, signs and abnormal clinical and laboratory findings, not elsewhere classified (R00-R94)

This chapter contains the following blocks:

G00-G09   Inflammatory diseases of the central nervous system
G10-G14   Systemic atrophies primarily affecting the central nervous system
G20-G26   Extrapyramidal and movement disorders
G30-G32   Other degenerative diseases of the nervous system
G35-G37   Demyelinating diseases of the central nervous system
G40-G47   Episodic and paroxysmal disorders
G50-G59   Nerve, nerve root and plexus disorders
G60-G65   Polyneuropathies and other disorders of the peripheral nervous system
G70-G73   Diseases of myoneural junction and muscle
G80-G83   Cerebral palsy and other paralytic syndromes
G89-G99   Other disorders of the nervous system

Inflammatory diseases of the central nervous system (G00-G09)

✓4th G00   Bacterial meningitis, not elsewhere classified

INCLUDES   bacterial arachnoiditis
bacterial leptomeningitis
bacterial meningitis
bacterial pachymeningitis

EXCLUDES 1   bacterial meningoencephalitis (G04.2)
bacterial meningomyelitis (G04.2)

DEF: Inflammation of meningeal layers of the brain and spinal cord due to a bacterial infection.

CC Excl: For MCC codes in category G00: PDX collection 207

G00.0   Hemophilus meningitis   MCC
Meningitis due to Hemophilus influenzae

G00.1   Pneumococcal meningitis   MCC
Meningtitis due to Streptococcal pneumoniae

G00.2   Streptococcal meningitis   MCC
Use additional code to further identify organism (B95.0-B95.5)

G00.3   Staphylococcal meningitis   MCC
Use additional code to further identify organism (B95.61-B95.8)

G00.8   Other bacterial meningitis   MCC
Meningitis due to Escherichia coli
Meningitis due to Friedländer's bacillus
Meningitis due to Klebsiella
Use additional code to further identify organism (B96.-)

G00.9   Bacterial meningitis, unspecified   MCC
Meningitis due to gram-negative bacteria, unspecified
Purulent meningitis NOS
Pyogenic meningitis NOS
Suppurative meningitis NOS

G01   Meningitis in bacterial diseases classified elsewhere   MCC
Code first underlying disease

EXCLUDES 1   meningitis (in):
gonococcal (A54.81)
leptospirosis (A27.81)
listeriosis (A32.11)
Lyme disease (A69.21)
meningococcal (A39.0)
neurosyphilis (A52.13)
tuberculosis (A17.0)
meningoencephalitis and meningomyelitis in bacterial diseases classified elsewhere (G05)

CC Excl: PDX collection 207

G02   Meningitis in other infectious and parasitic diseases classified elsewhere   MCC
Code first underlying disease, such as:
African trypanosomiasis (B56.-)
poliovirus infection (A80.-)

EXCLUDES 1   candidal meningitis (B37.5)
coccidioidomycosis meningitis (B38.4)
cryptococcal meningitis (B45.1)
herpesviral [herpes simplex] meningitis (B00.3)
infectious mononucleosis complicated by meningitis (B27.- with fourth character 2)
measles complicated by meningitis (B05.1)
meningoencephalitis and meningomyelitis in other infectious and parasitic diseases classified elsewhere (G05)
mumps meningitis (B26.1)
rubella meningitis (B06.02)
varicella [chickenpox] meningitis (B01.0)
zoster meningitis (B02.1)

CC Excl: PDX collection 559

✓4th G03   Meningitis due to other and unspecified causes

INCLUDES   arachnoiditis NOS
leptomeningitis NOS
meningitis NOS
pachymeningitis NOS

EXCLUDES 1   meningoencephalitis (G04.-)
meningomyelitis (G04.-)

CC Excl: For CC/MCC codes in category G03, unless otherwise noted: PDX collection 207

G03.0   Nonpyogenic meningitis   MCC
Aseptic meningitis
Nonbacterial meningitis
DEF: Type of meningitis where no bacterial, viral, or other infectious source exists that explains the meningitis symptomology.

G03.1   Chronic meningitis   CC

G03.2   Benign recurrent meningitis [Mollaret]   CC
DEF: Aseptic or noninfectious inflammation of the meninges with the presence of Mollaret cells in the spinal fluid. The patient experiences recurrent bouts of inflammation, lasting anywhere from two to five days.
CC Excl: PDX collection 140

G03.8   Meningitis due to other specified causes   MCC

G03.9   Meningitis, unspecified   MCC
Arachnoiditis (spinal) NOS

✓4th G04   Encephalitis, myelitis and encephalomyelitis

INCLUDES   acute ascending myelitis
meningoencephalitis
meningomyelitis

EXCLUDES 1   encephalopathy NOS (G93.40)

EXCLUDES 2   acute transverse myelitis (G37.3-)
alcoholic encephalopathy (G31.2)
benign myalgic encephalomyelitis (G93.3)
multiple sclerosis (G35)
subacute necrotizing myelitis (G37.4)
toxic encephalitis (G92)
toxic encephalopathy (G92)

DEF: Encephalitis: Inflammation of the brain, often caused by viral or bacterial infection.
DEF: Encephalomyelitis: Inflammatory disease, often viral in nature, that affects the brain and spinal cord.
DEF: Myelitis: Inflammation of the spinal cord.
CC Excl: For CC/MCC codes in category G04, unless otherwise noted: PDX collection 560

✓5th G04.0   Acute disseminated encephalitis and encephalomyelitis (ADEM)

EXCLUDES 1   acute necrotizing hemorrhagic encephalopathy (G04.3-)
other noninfectious acute disseminated encephalomyelitis (noninfectious ADEM) (G04.81)

G04.00   Acute disseminated encephalitis and encephalomyelitis, unspecified   MCC

G04.01 Postinfectious acute disseminated encephalitis and encephalomyelitis (postinfectious ADEM) `MCC`
> *EXCLUDES 1*   post chickenpox encephalitis (B01.1)
> post measles encephalitis (B05.0)
> post measles myelitis (B05.1)

G04.02 Postimmunization acute disseminated encephalitis, myelitis and encephalomyelitis `MCC`
Encephalitis, post immunization
Encephalomyelitis, post immunization
Use additional code to identify the vaccine (T50.A-, T50.B-, T50.Z-)
CC Excl: No Excl

G04.1 Tropical spastic paraplegia `CC` `HCC`
CC Excl: PDX collection 561

G04.2 Bacterial meningoencephalitis and meningomyelitis, not elsewhere classified `MCC`
CC Excl: PDX collection 207

✓5ᵗʰ **G04.3 Acute necrotizing hemorrhagic encephalopathy**
> *EXCLUDES 1*   acute disseminated encephalitis and encephalomyelitis (G04.0-)

    G04.30 Acute necrotizing hemorrhagic encephalopathy, unspecified `MCC`
    CC Excl: No Excl

    G04.31 Postinfectious acute necrotizing hemorrhagic encephalopathy `MCC`

    G04.32 Postimmunization acute necrotizing hemorrhagic encephalopathy `MCC`
    Use additional code to identify the vaccine (T50.A-, T50.B-, T50.Z-)
    CC Excl: No Excl

    G04.39 Other acute necrotizing hemorrhagic encephalopathy `MCC`
    Code also underlying etiology, if applicable
    CC Excl: No Excl

✓5ᵗʰ **G04.8 Other encephalitis, myelitis and encephalomyelitis**
Code also any associated seizure (G40.-, R56.9)

    G04.81 Other encephalitis and encephalomyelitis `HIV` `MCC`
    Noninfectious acute disseminated encephalomyelitis (noninfectious ADEM)

    G04.89 Other myelitis `HIV` `MCC` `HCC`

✓5ᵗʰ **G04.9 Encephalitis, myelitis and encephalomyelitis, unspecified**

    G04.90 Encephalitis and encephalomyelitis, unspecified `HIV` `MCC`
    Ventriculitis (cerebral) NOS
    CC Excl: PDX collection 562

    G04.91 Myelitis, unspecified `HIV` `MCC` `HCC`
    CC Excl: PDX collection 562

✓4ᵗʰ **G05 Encephalitis, myelitis and encephalomyelitis in diseases classified elsewhere**
Code first underlying disease, such as:
human immunodeficiency virus [HIV] disease (B20)
poliovirus (A80.-)
suppurative otitis media (H66.01-H66.4)
trichinellosis (B75)
> *EXCLUDES 1*   adenoviral encephalitis, myelitis and encephalomyelitis (A85.1)
> congenital toxoplasmosis encephalitis, myelitis and encephalomyelitis (P37.1)
> cytomegaloviral encephalitis, myelitis and encephalomyelitis (B25.8)
> encephalitis, myelitis and encephalomyelitis (in) measles (B05.0)
> encephalitis, myelitis and encephalomyelitis (in) systemic lupus erythematosus (M32.19)
> enteroviral encephalitis, myelitis and encephalomyelitis (A85.0)
> eosinophilic meningoencephalitis (B83.2)
> herpesviral [herpes simplex] encephalitis, myelitis and encephalomyelitis (B00.4)
> listerial encephalitis, myelitis and encephalomyelitis (A32.12)
> meningococcal encephalitis, myelitis and encephalomyelitis (A39.81)
> mumps encephalitis, myelitis and encephalomyelitis (B26.2)
> postchickenpox encephalitis, myelitis and encephalomyelitis (B01.1-)
> rubella encephalitis, myelitis and encephalomyelitis (B06.01)
> toxoplasmosis encephalitis, myelitis and encephalomyelitis (B58.2)
> zoster encephalitis, myelitis and encephalomyelitis (B02.0)

G05.3 Encephalitis and encephalomyelitis in diseases classified elsewhere `MCC`
Meningoencephalitis in diseases classified elsewhere
CC Excl: PDX collection 560

G05.4 Myelitis in diseases classified elsewhere `MCC` `HCC`
Meningomyelitis in diseases classified elsewhere
CC Excl: PDX collection 560

✓4ᵗʰ **G06 Intracranial and intraspinal abscess and granuloma**
Use additional code (B95-B97) to identify infectious agent
DEF: Abscess: Circumscribed collection of pus resulting from bacteria, frequently associated with swelling and other signs of inflammation.
DEF: Granuloma: Abnormal, dense collections or cells forming a mass or nodule of chronically inflamed tissue with granulations that is usually associated with an infective process.

G06.0 Intracranial abscess and granuloma `MCC`
Brain [any part] abscess (embolic)
Cerebellar abscess (embolic)
Cerebral abscess (embolic)
Intracranial epidural abscess or granuloma
Intracranial extradural abscess or granuloma
Intracranial subdural abscess or granuloma
Otogenic abscess (embolic)
> *EXCLUDES 1*   tuberculous intracranial abscess and granuloma (A17.81)

CC Excl: PDX collection 563

G06.1 Intraspinal abscess and granuloma `MCC`
Abscess (embolic) of spinal cord [any part]
Intraspinal epidural abscess or granuloma
Intraspinal extradural abscess or granuloma
Intraspinal subdural abscess or granuloma
> *EXCLUDES 1*   tuberculous intraspinal abscess and granuloma (A17.81)

CC Excl: PDX collection 564

G06.2 Extradural and subdural abscess, unspecified `MCC`
CC Excl: PDX collection 565

N Newborn: 0   P Pediatric: 0-17   M Maternity: 9-64   A Adult: 15-124   `MCC` Major Complication/Comorbidity   `CC` Complication/Comorbidity   `SW` Severe Wound Dx

572   ICD-10-CM 2020

G07 Intracranial and intraspinal abscess and granuloma in diseases classified elsewhere MCC

Code first underlying disease, such as:
schistosomiasis granuloma of brain (B65.-)

EXCLUDES 1   abscess of brain:
amebic (A06.6)
chromomycotic (B43.1)
gonococcal (A54.82)
tuberculous (A17.81)
tuberculoma of meninges (A17.1)

CC Excl: PDX collection 565

G08 Intracranial and intraspinal phlebitis and thrombophlebitis MCC

Septic embolism of intracranial or intraspinal venous sinuses and veins
Septic endophlebitis of intracranial or intraspinal venous sinuses and veins
Septic phlebitis of intracranial or intraspinal venous sinuses and veins
Septic thrombophlebitis of intracranial or intraspinal venous sinuses and veins
Septic thrombosis of intracranial or intraspinal venous sinuses and veins

EXCLUDES 1   intracranial phlebitis and thrombophlebitis complicating:
abortion, ectopic or molar pregnancy (O00–O07, O08.7)
pregnancy, childbirth and the puerperium (O22.5, O87.3)
nonpyogenic intracranial phlebitis and thrombophlebitis (I67.6)

EXCLUDES 2   intracranial phlebitis and thrombophlebitis complicating nonpyogenic intraspinal phlebitis and thrombophlebitis (G95.1)

DEF: Inflammation and formation of a blood clot in a vein within the brain or spine, or their linings.
CC Excl: PDX collection 565

G09 Sequelae of inflammatory diseases of central nervous system

NOTE   Category G09 is to be used to indicate conditions whose primary classification is to G00–G08 as the cause of sequelae, themselves classifiable elsewhere. The "sequelae" include conditions specified as residuals.

Code first condition resulting from (sequela) of inflammatory diseases of central nervous system

Systemic atrophies primarily affecting the central nervous system (G10-G14)

G10 Huntington's disease HCC

Huntington's chorea
Huntington's dementia
Code also dementia in other diseases classified elsewhere without behavioral disturbance (F02.80)

DEF: Genetic disease caused by degeneration of nerve cells in the brain, characterized by chronic progressive mental deterioration. Dementia and death occur within 15 to 20 years of onset.

G11 Hereditary ataxia

EXCLUDES 2   cerebral palsy (G80.-)
hereditary and idiopathic neuropathy (G60.-)
metabolic disorders (E70-E88)

DEF: Ataxia: Defect in muscular control or coordination due to a central nervous system disorder, particularly when voluntary muscular movements are attempted.

G11.0 Congenital nonprogressive ataxia HCC

G11.1 Early-onset cerebellar ataxia HCC

Early-onset cerebellar ataxia with essential tremor
Early-onset cerebellar ataxia with myoclonus [Hunt's ataxia]
Early-onset cerebellar ataxia with retained tendon reflexes
Friedreich's ataxia (autosomal recessive)
X-linked recessive spinocerebellar ataxia

G11.2 Late-onset cerebellar ataxia HCC A

G11.3 Cerebellar ataxia with defective DNA repair HCC

Ataxia telangiectasia [Louis-Bar]

EXCLUDES 2   Cockayne's syndrome ▶(Q87.19)◀
other disorders of purine and pyrimidine metabolism (E79.-)
xeroderma pigmentosum (Q82.1)

G11.4 Hereditary spastic paraplegia HCC

G11.8 Other hereditary ataxias HCC

G11.9 Hereditary ataxia, unspecified HCC

Hereditary cerebellar ataxia NOS
Hereditary cerebellar degeneration
Hereditary cerebellar disease
Hereditary cerebellar syndrome

G12 Spinal muscular atrophy and related syndromes

G12.0 Infantile spinal muscular atrophy, type I [Werdnig-Hoffman] HCC

G12.1 Other inherited spinal muscular atrophy HCC

Adult form spinal muscular atrophy
Childhood form, type II spinal muscular atrophy
Distal spinal muscular atrophy
Juvenile form, type III spinal muscular atrophy [Kugelberg-Welander]
Progressive bulbar palsy of childhood [Fazio-Londe]
Scapuloperoneal form spinal muscular atrophy

G12.2 Motor neuron disease

AHA: 2017,4Q,9-10
For CC codes in subcategory G12.2: PDX collection 570

G12.20 Motor neuron disease, unspecified HCC
G12.21 Amyotrophic lateral sclerosis HCC A
G12.22 Progressive bulbar palsy HCC
G12.23 Primary lateral sclerosis CC HCC
G12.24 Familial motor neuron disease CC HCC
G12.25 Progressive spinal muscle atrophy CC HCC
G12.29 Other motor neuron disease HCC

G12.8 Other spinal muscular atrophies and related syndromes HCC

G12.9 Spinal muscular atrophy, unspecified HCC

G13 Systemic atrophies primarily affecting central nervous system in diseases classified elsewhere

G13.0 Paraneoplastic neuromyopathy and neuropathy HCC

Carcinomatous neuromyopathy
Sensorial paraneoplastic neuropathy [Denny Brown]
Code first underlying neoplasm (C00-D49)

G13.1 Other systemic atrophy primarily affecting central nervous system in neoplastic disease HCC

Paraneoplastic limbic encephalopathy
Code first underlying neoplasm (C00-D49)

G13.2 Systemic atrophy primarily affecting the central nervous system in myxedema HCC

Code first underlying disease, such as:
hypothyroidism (E03.-)
myxedematous congenital iodine deficiency (E00.1)

G13.8 Systemic atrophy primarily affecting central nervous system in other diseases classified elsewhere HCC

Code first underlying disease

G14 Postpolio syndrome

INCLUDES   postpolio myelitic syndrome
EXCLUDES 1   sequelae of poliomyelitis (B91)

Extrapyramidal and movement disorders (G20-G26)

G20 Parkinson's disease HCC

Hemiparkinsonism
Idiopathic Parkinsonism or Parkinson's disease
Paralysis agitans
Parkinsonism or Parkinson's disease NOS
Primary Parkinsonism or Parkinson's disease

EXCLUDES 1   dementia with Parkinsonism (G31.83)

AHA: 2017,2Q,7; 2016,2Q,6
TIP: Repeated falls (R29.6) are not integral to Parkinson's disease and can be separately coded.

✓4th **G21 Secondary parkinsonism**

     EXCLUDES 1   *dementia with Parkinsonism (G31.83)*
                  Huntington's disease (G10)
                  Shy-Drager syndrome (G90.3)
                  syphilitic Parkinsonism (A52.19)

     CC Excl: For CC/MCC codes in category G21, unless otherwise noted: PDX collection 572

     G21.0 Malignant neuroleptic syndrome `MCC`

         Use additional code for adverse effect, if applicable, to identify drug (T43.3X5, T43.4X5, T43.505, T43.595)

         EXCLUDES 1   *neuroleptic induced parkinsonism (G21.11)*

         CC Excl: PDX collection 571

     ✓5th **G21.1 Other drug-induced secondary parkinsonism**

         G21.11 Neuroleptic induced parkinsonism `CC` `HCC`

                 Use additional code for adverse effect, if applicable, to identify drug (T43.3X5, T43.4X5, T43.505, T43.595)

                 EXCLUDES 1   *malignant neuroleptic syndrome (G21.0)*

         G21.19 Other drug induced secondary parkinsonism `CC` `HCC`

                 Other medication-induced parkinsonism

                 Use additional code for adverse effect, if applicable, to identify drug (T36-T50 with fifth or sixth character 5)

     G21.2 Secondary parkinsonism due to other external agents `CC` `HCC`

         Code first (T51-T65) to identify external agent

     G21.3 Postencephalitic parkinsonism `CC` `HCC`

     G21.4 Vascular parkinsonism `HCC`

     G21.8 Other secondary parkinsonism `CC` `HCC`

     G21.9 Secondary parkinsonism, unspecified `CC` `HCC`

✓4th **G23 Other degenerative diseases of basal ganglia**

     EXCLUDES 2   *multi-system degeneration of the autonomic nervous system (G90.3)*

     CC Excl: For CC codes in category G23: PDX collection 573

     G23.0 Hallervorden-Spatz disease `CC` `HCC`

         Pigmentary pallidal degeneration

     G23.1 Progressive supranuclear ophthalmoplegia [Steele-Richardson-Olszewski] `HCC`

         Progressive supranuclear palsy

     G23.2 Striatonigral degeneration `HCC`

     G23.8 Other specified degenerative diseases of basal ganglia `CC` `HCC`

         Calcification of basal ganglia

     G23.9 Degenerative disease of basal ganglia, unspecified `CC` `HCC`

✓4th **G24 Dystonia**

     INCLUDES   dyskinesia

     EXCLUDES 2   *athetoid cerebral palsy (G80.3)*

     DEF: Disorder of abnormal muscle tone, excessive or inadequate. Involuntary movements and prolonged muscle contractions result in tremors, abnormalities in posture, and twisting body motions that affect an isolated area or the whole body.

     CC Excl: For CC codes in category G24: PDX collection 574

     ✓5th **G24.0 Drug induced dystonia**

         Use additional code for adverse effect, if applicable, to identify drug (T36-T50 with fifth or sixth character 5)

         G24.01 Drug induced subacute dyskinesia `CC`

                 Drug induced blepharospasm
                 Drug induced orofacial dyskinesia
                 Neuroleptic induced tardive dyskinesia
                 Tardive dyskinesia

         G24.02 Drug induced acute dystonia `CC`

                 Acute dystonic reaction to drugs
                 Neuroleptic induced acute dystonia

         G24.09 Other drug induced dystonia `CC`

     G24.1 Genetic torsion dystonia

         Dystonia deformans progressiva
         Dystonia musculorum deformans
         Familial torsion dystonia
         Idiopathic familial dystonia
         Idiopathic (torsion) dystonia NOS
         (Schwalbe-) Ziehen-Oppenheim disease

     G24.2 Idiopathic nonfamilial dystonia `CC`

     G24.3 Spasmodic torticollis

         EXCLUDES 1   *congenital torticollis (Q68.0)*
                 hysterical torticollis (F44.4)
                 ocular torticollis (R29.891)
                 psychogenic torticollis (F45.8)
                 torticollis NOS (M43.6)
                 traumatic recurrent torticollis (S13.4)

         DEF: Twisted, unnatural position of the neck due to contracted cervical muscles that pull the head to one side or cause involuntary shaking of the head.

     G24.4 Idiopathic orofacial dystonia

         Orofacial dyskinesia

         EXCLUDES 1   *drug induced orofacial dyskinesia (G24.01)*

     G24.5 Blepharospasm

         EXCLUDES 1   *drug induced blepharospasm (G24.01)*

         DEF: Involuntary contraction of the orbicularis oculi muscle, resulting in the eyelids being completely closed.

     G24.8 Other dystonia

         Acquired torsion dystonia NOS

     G24.9 Dystonia, unspecified

         Dyskinesia NOS

✓4th **G25 Other extrapyramidal and movement disorders**

     EXCLUDES 2   *sleep related movement disorders (G47.6-)*

     G25.0 Essential tremor

         Familial tremor

         EXCLUDES 1   *tremor NOS (R25.1)*

     G25.1 Drug-induced tremor

         Use additional code for adverse effect, if applicable, to identify drug (T36-T50 with fifth or sixth character 5)

     G25.2 Other specified forms of tremor

         Intention tremor

     G25.3 Myoclonus

         Drug-induced myoclonus
         Palatal myoclonus

         Use additional code for adverse effect, if applicable, to identify drug (T36-T50 with fifth or sixth character 5)

         EXCLUDES 1   *facial myokymia (G51.4)*
                 myoclonic epilepsy (G40.-)

         DEF: Spasmodic, brief, involuntary muscle contractions that can be due to an undetermined etiology, drug-induced, or caused by a disease process.

     G25.4 Drug-induced chorea

         Use additional code for adverse effect, if applicable, to identify drug (T36-T50 with fifth or sixth character 5)

     G25.5 Other chorea

         Chorea NOS

         EXCLUDES 1   *chorea NOS with heart involvement (I02.0)*
                 Huntington's chorea (G10)
                 rheumatic chorea (I02.-)
                 Sydenham's chorea (I02.-)

     ✓5th **G25.6 Drug induced tics and other tics of organic origin**

         G25.61 Drug induced tics

                 Use additional code for adverse effect, if applicable, to identify drug (T36-T50 with fifth or sixth character 5)

         G25.69 Other tics of organic origin

                 EXCLUDES 1   *habit spasm (F95.9)*
                         tic NOS (F95.9)
                         Tourette's syndrome (F95.2)

     ✓5th **G25.7 Other and unspecified drug induced movement disorders**

         Use additional code for adverse effect, if applicable, to identify drug (T36-T50 with fifth or sixth character 5)

         G25.70 Drug induced movement disorder, unspecified

         G25.71 Drug induced akathisia

                 Drug induced acathisia
                 Neuroleptic induced acute akathisia
                 Tardive akathisia

         G25.79 Other drug induced movement disorders

     ✓5th **G25.8 Other specified extrapyramidal and movement disorders**

         G25.81 Restless legs syndrome

                 DEF: Neurological disorder of unknown etiology creating an irresistible urge to move the legs, which may temporarily relieve the symptoms. This syndrome is accompanied by motor restlessness and sensations of pain, burning, prickling, or tingling.

N Newborn: 0   P Pediatric: 0-17   M Maternity: 9-64   A Adult: 15-124   MCC Major Complication/Comorbidity   CC Complication/Comorbidity   SW Severe Wound Dx

574   ICD-10-CM 2020

G25.82   **Stiff-man syndrome**   `CC`
          CC Excl: PDX collection 575
G25.83   **Benign shuddering attacks**
G25.89   **Other specified extrapyramidal and movement disorders**
G25.9   **Extrapyramidal and movement disorder, unspecified**   `CC`
          CC Excl: PDX collection 575

G26   *Extrapyramidal and movement disorders in diseases classified elsewhere*
      Code first underlying disease

Other degenerative diseases of the nervous system (G30-G32)

✓4ᵗʰ **G30**   **Alzheimer's disease**
      INCLUDES   Alzheimer's dementia senile and presenile forms
      Use additional code to identify:
         delirium, if applicable (F05)
         dementia with behavioral disturbance (F02.81)
         dementia without behavioral disturbance (F02.80)
      EXCLUDES 1   senile degeneration of brain NEC (G31.1)
                    senile dementia NOS (F03)
                    senility NOS (R41.81)
      AHA: 2017,1Q,43
      TIP: A code from subcategory F02.8 should always be assigned with a code from this category, even in the absence of documented dementia.
      TIP: Functional quadriplegia (R53.2) is not integral to Alzheimer's disease and can be coded in addition to codes from category G30.
      G30.0   **Alzheimer's disease with early onset**   `HCC`
      G30.1   **Alzheimer's disease with late onset**   `HCC` `A`
      G30.8   **Other Alzheimer's disease**   `HCC`
      G30.9   **Alzheimer's disease, unspecified**   `HCC`
                AHA: 2016,2Q,6; 2012,4Q,95

✓4ᵗʰ **G31**   **Other degenerative diseases of nervous system, not elsewhere classified**
      ▶For codes G31.0–G31.83, G31.85–G31.9, use additional code to identify:◀
         dementia with behavioral disturbance (F02.81)
         dementia without behavioral disturbance (F02.80)
      EXCLUDES 2   Reye's syndrome (G93.7)
      ✓5ᵗʰ **G31.0**   **Frontotemporal dementia**
            G31.01   **Pick's disease**   `HCC`
                      Primary progressive aphasia
                      Progressive isolated aphasia
                      DEF: Progressive frontotemporal dementia with asymmetrical atrophy of the frontal and temporal regions of the cerebral cortex and abnormal rounded brain cells called Pick cells with the presence of abnormal staining of protein (called tau). Symptoms include prominent apathy, behavioral changes such as disinhibition and restlessness, echolalia, impairment of language, memory, and intellect, increased carelessness, poor personal hygiene, and decreased attention span.
            G31.09   **Other frontotemporal dementia**   `HCC`
                      Frontal dementia
      G31.1   **Senile degeneration of brain, not elsewhere classified**   `HCC`
                EXCLUDES 1   Alzheimer's disease (G30.-)
                              senility NOS (R41.81)
      G31.2   **Degeneration of nervous system due to alcohol**   `CC` `HCC`
                Alcoholic cerebellar ataxia
                Alcoholic cerebellar degeneration
                Alcoholic cerebral degeneration
                Alcoholic encephalopathy
                Dysfunction of the autonomic nervous system due to alcohol
                Code also associated alcoholism (F10.-)
      ✓5ᵗʰ **G31.8**   **Other specified degenerative diseases of nervous system**
            G31.81   **Alpers disease**   `CC` `HCC`
                      Grey-matter degeneration
                      CC Excl: PDX collection 537
            G31.82   **Leigh's disease**   `CC` `HCC`
                      Subacute necrotizing encephalopathy
                      CC Excl: PDX collection 537

G31.83   **Dementia with Lewy bodies**   `HCC`
          Dementia with Parkinsonism
          Lewy body dementia
          Lewy body disease
          AHA: 2017,2Q,7; 2016,4Q,141
          DEF: Cerebral dementia with neurophysiologic changes, increased hippocampal volume, hypoperfusion in the occipital lobes, beta amyloid deposits with neurofibrillary tangles, and atrophy of the cortex and brainstem. Hallmark neuropsychological characteristics include fluctuating cognition with pronounced variation in attention and alertness, recurrent hallucinations, and Parkinsonism.
G31.84   **Mild cognitive impairment, so stated**
          Mild neurocognitive disorder
          EXCLUDES 1   age related cognitive decline (R41.81)
                        altered mental status (R41.82)
                        cerebral degeneration (G31.9)
                        change in mental status (R41.82)
                        cognitive deficits following (sequelae of) cerebral hemorrhage or infarction (I69.01-, I69.11-, I69.21-, I69.31-, I69.81-, I69.91-)
                        cognitive impairment due to intracranial or head injury (S06.-)
                        dementia (F01.-, F02.-, F03)
                        mild memory disturbance (F06.8)
                        neurologic neglect syndrome (R41.4)
                        personality change, nonpsychotic (F68.8)
G31.85   **Corticobasal degeneration**   `HCC`
G31.89   **Other specified degenerative diseases of nervous system**   `HCC`
G31.9   **Degenerative disease of nervous system, unspecified**   `HCC`

✓4ᵗʰ **G32**   **Other degenerative disorders of nervous system in diseases classified elsewhere**
      G32.0   *Subacute combined degeneration of spinal cord in diseases classified elsewhere*   `CC` `HCC`
                Dana-Putnam syndrome
                Sclerosis of spinal cord (combined) (dorsolateral) (posterolateral)
                Code first underlying disease, such as:
                   anemia (D51.9)
                   dietary (D51.3)
                   pernicious (D51.0)
                   vitamin B12 deficiency (E53.8)
                EXCLUDES 1   syphilitic combined degeneration of spinal cord (A52.11)
                CC Excl: PDX collection 576
      ✓5ᵗʰ **G32.8**   **Other specified degenerative disorders of nervous system in diseases classified elsewhere**
            Code first underlying disease, such as:
               amyloidosis cerebral degeneration (E85.-)
               cerebral degeneration (due to) hypothyroidism (E00.0-E03.9)
               cerebral degeneration (due to) neoplasm (C00-D49)
               cerebral degeneration (due to) vitamin B deficiency, except thiamine (E52-E53.-)
            EXCLUDES 1   superior hemorrhagic polioencephalitis [Wernicke's encephalopathy] (E51.2)
            G32.81   *Cerebellar ataxia in diseases classified elsewhere*   `CC` `HCC`
                      Code first underlying disease, such as:
                         celiac disease (with gluten ataxia) (K90.0)
                         cerebellar ataxia (in) neoplastic disease (paraneoplastic cerebellar degeneration) (C00-D49)
                         non-celiac gluten ataxia (M35.9)
                      EXCLUDES 1   systemic atrophy primarily affecting the central nervous system in alcoholic cerebellar ataxia (G31.2)
                                    systemic atrophy primarily affecting the central nervous system in myxedema (G13.2)
                      CC Excl: PDX collection 567
            G32.89   *Other specified degenerative disorders of nervous system in diseases classified elsewhere*
                      Degenerative encephalopathy in diseases classified elsewhere

Chapter 6. Diseases of the Nervous System

Demyelinating diseases of the central nervous system (G35-G37)

CC Excl: For CC codes in categories G35-G37, unless otherwise noted: PDX collection 578

G35   Multiple sclerosis   `HCC`

     Disseminated multiple sclerosis
     Generalized multiple sclerosis
     Multiple sclerosis NOS
     Multiple sclerosis of brain stem
     Multiple sclerosis of cord

`√4ᵗʰ` **G36   Other acute disseminated demyelination**

     EXCLUDES 1   postinfectious encephalitis and encephalomyelitis NOS (G04.01)

     DEF: Demyelination: Abnormal loss of myelin, the protective white matter that insulates nerve endings and facilitates neuroreception and neurotransmission. When this substance is damaged, the nerve is short-circuited, resulting in impaired or loss of function.

     G36.0   Neuromyelitis optica [Devic]   `CC` `HCC`

         Demyelination in optic neuritis
         EXCLUDES 1   optic neuritis NOS (H46)
         CC Excl: PDX collection 577

     G36.1   Acute and subacute hemorrhagic leukoencephalitis [Hurst]   `CC` `HCC`

     G36.8   Other specified acute disseminated demyelination   `CC` `HCC`

     G36.9   Acute disseminated demyelination, unspecified   `HIV` `CC` `HCC`

`√4ᵗʰ` **G37   Other demyelinating diseases of central nervous system**

     G37.0   Diffuse sclerosis of central nervous system   `CC` `HCC`

         Periaxial encephalitis
         Schilder's disease
         EXCLUDES 1   X linked adrenoleukodystrophy (E71.52-)
         CC Excl: PDX collection 579

     G37.1   Central demyelination of corpus callosum   `CC` `HCC`

     G37.2   Central pontine myelinolysis   `CC` `HCC`

     G37.3   Acute transverse myelitis in demyelinating disease of central nervous system   `CC` `HCC`

         Acute transverse myelitis NOS
         Acute transverse myelopathy
         EXCLUDES 1   multiple sclerosis (G35)
                   neuromyelitis optica [Devic] (G36.0)
         CC Excl: PDX collection 580

     G37.4   Subacute necrotizing myelitis of central nervous system   `HIV` `MCC` `HCC`

         CC Excl: PDX collection 562

     G37.5   Concentric sclerosis [Balo] of central nervous system   `CC` `HCC`

         CC Excl: PDX collection 579

     G37.8   Other specified demyelinating diseases of central nervous system   `CC` `HCC`

     G37.9   Demyelinating disease of central nervous system, unspecified   `HIV` `CC` `HCC`

Episodic and paroxysmal disorders (G40-G47)

`√4ᵗʰ` **G40   Epilepsy and recurrent seizures**

     NOTE   The following terms are to be considered equivalent to intractable: pharmacoresistant (pharmacologically resistant), treatment resistant, refractory (medically) and poorly controlled

     EXCLUDES 1   conversion disorder with seizures (F44.5)
                   convulsions NOS (R56.9)
                   post traumatic seizures (R56.1)
                   seizure (convulsive) NOS (R56.9)
                   seizure of newborn (P90)

     EXCLUDES 2   hippocampal sclerosis (G93.81)
                   mesial temporal sclerosis (G93.81)
                   temporal sclerosis (G93.81)
                   Todd's paralysis (G83.84)

     CC Excl: For codes in category G40:
     For MCC codes: PDX collection 583
     For CC codes, unless otherwise noted: PDX collection 582

`√5ᵗʰ` **G40.0   Localization-related (focal) (partial) idiopathic epilepsy and epileptic syndromes with seizures of localized onset**

         Benign childhood epilepsy with centrotemporal EEG spikes
         Childhood epilepsy with occipital EEG paroxysms
         EXCLUDES 1   adult onset localization-related epilepsy (G40.1-, G40.2-)

`√6ᵗʰ`   **G40.00   Localization-related (focal) (partial) idiopathic epilepsy and epileptic syndromes with seizures of localized onset, not intractable**

         Localization-related (focal) (partial) idiopathic epilepsy and epileptic syndromes with seizures of localized onset without intractability

         G40.001   Localization-related (focal) (partial) idiopathic epilepsy and epileptic syndromes with seizures of localized onset, not intractable, with status epilepticus   `CC` `HCC`

                 CC Excl: PDX collection 581

         G40.009   Localization-related (focal) (partial) idiopathic epilepsy and epileptic syndromes with seizures of localized onset, not intractable, without status epilepticus   `CC` `HCC`

                 Localization-related (focal) (partial) idiopathic epilepsy and epileptic syndromes with seizures of localized onset NOS
                 CC Excl: PDX collection 581

`√6ᵗʰ`   **G40.01   Localization-related (focal) (partial) idiopathic epilepsy and epileptic syndromes with seizures of localized onset, intractable**

         G40.011   Localization-related (focal) (partial) idiopathic epilepsy and epileptic syndromes with seizures of localized onset, intractable, with status epilepticus   `CC` `HCC`

         G40.019   Localization-related (focal) (partial) idiopathic epilepsy and epileptic syndromes with seizures of localized onset, intractable, without status epilepticus   `CC` `HCC`

`N` Newborn: 0   `P` Pediatric: 0-17   `M` Maternity: 9-64   `A` Adult: 15-124   `MCC` Major Complication/Comorbidity   `CC` Complication/Comorbidity   `SW` Severe Wound Dx

576   ICD-10-CM 2020

✓5ᵗʰ **G40.1** **Localization-related (focal) (partial) symptomatic epilepsy and epileptic syndromes with** simple partial seizures

Attacks without alteration of consciousness

Epilepsia partialis continua [Kozhevnikof]

Simple partial seizures developing into secondarily generalized seizures

✓6ᵗʰ **G40.10** **Localization-related (focal) (partial) symptomatic epilepsy and epileptic syndromes with simple partial seizures,** not intractable

Localization-related (focal) (partial) symptomatic epilepsy and epileptic syndromes with simple partial seizures without intractability

G40.101 **Localization-related (focal) (partial) symptomatic epilepsy and epileptic syndromes with simple partial seizures, not intractable, with status epilepticus**   CC HCC

CC Excl: PDX collection 581

G40.109 **Localization-related (focal) (partial) symptomatic epilepsy and epileptic syndromes with simple partial seizures, not intractable, without status epilepticus**   CC HCC

Localization-related (focal) (partial) symptomatic epilepsy and epileptic syndromes with simple partial seizures NOS

CC Excl: PDX collection 581

✓6ᵗʰ **G40.11** **Localization-related (focal) (partial) symptomatic epilepsy and epileptic syndromes with simple partial seizures,** intractable

G40.111 **Localization-related (focal) (partial) symptomatic epilepsy and epileptic syndromes with simple partial seizures, intractable, with status epilepticus**   CC HCC

G40.119 **Localization-related (focal) (partial) symptomatic epilepsy and epileptic syndromes with simple partial seizures, intractable,** without status epilepticus   CC HCC

✓5ᵗʰ **G40.2** **Localization-related (focal) (partial) symptomatic epilepsy and epileptic syndromes with** complex partial seizures

Attacks with alteration of consciousness, often with automatisms

Complex partial seizures developing into secondarily generalized seizures

✓6ᵗʰ **G40.20** **Localization-related (focal) (partial) symptomatic epilepsy and epileptic syndromes with complex partial seizures,** not intractable

Localization-related (focal) (partial) symptomatic epilepsy and epileptic syndromes with complex partial seizures without intractability

G40.201 **Localization-related (focal) (partial) symptomatic epilepsy and epileptic syndromes with complex partial seizures, not intractable, with status epilepticus**   CC HCC

CC Excl: PDX collection 581

G40.209 **Localization-related (focal) (partial) symptomatic epilepsy and epileptic syndromes with complex partial seizures, not intractable,** without status epilepticus   CC HCC

Localization-related (focal) (partial) symptomatic epilepsy and epileptic syndromes with complex partial seizures NOS

CC Excl: PDX collection 581

✓6ᵗʰ **G40.21** **Localization-related (focal) (partial) symptomatic epilepsy and epileptic syndromes with complex partial seizures,** intractable

G40.211 **Localization-related (focal) (partial) symptomatic epilepsy and epileptic syndromes with complex partial seizures, intractable, with status epilepticus**   CC HCC

G40.219 **Localization-related (focal) (partial) symptomatic epilepsy and epileptic syndromes with complex partial seizures, intractable,** without status epilepticus   CC HCC

✓5ᵗʰ **G40.3** **Generalized** idiopathic epilepsy and epileptic syndromes

Code also MERRF syndrome, if applicable (E88.42)

✓6ᵗʰ **G40.30** **Generalized idiopathic epilepsy and epileptic syndromes,** not intractable

Generalized idiopathic epilepsy and epileptic syndromes without intractability

G40.301 **Generalized idiopathic epilepsy and epileptic syndromes, not intractable, with status epilepticus**   MCC HCC

G40.309 **Generalized idiopathic epilepsy and epileptic syndromes, not intractable,** without status epilepticus   HCC

Generalized idiopathic epilepsy and epileptic syndromes NOS

✓6ᵗʰ **G40.31** **Generalized idiopathic epilepsy and epileptic syndromes,** intractable

G40.311 **Generalized idiopathic epilepsy and epileptic syndromes, intractable,** with status epilepticus   MCC HCC

G40.319 **Generalized idiopathic epilepsy and epileptic syndromes, intractable,** without status epilepticus   MCC HCC

✓5ᵗʰ **G40.A** **Absence** epileptic syndrome

Childhood absence epilepsy [pyknolepsy]

Juvenile absence epilepsy

Absence epileptic syndrome, NOS

✓6ᵗʰ **G40.A0** **Absence epileptic syndrome,** not intractable

G40.A01 **Absence epileptic syndrome, not intractable, with status epilepticus**   HCC

G40.A09 **Absence epileptic syndrome, not intractable,** without status epilepticus   HCC

✓6ᵗʰ **G40.A1** **Absence epileptic syndrome,** intractable

G40.A11 **Absence epileptic syndrome, intractable,** with status epilepticus   CC HCC

G40.A19 **Absence epileptic syndrome, intractable,** without status epilepticus   CC HCC

✓5ᵗʰ **G40.B** **Juvenile** myoclonic epilepsy [impulsive petit mal]

✓6ᵗʰ **G40.B0** **Juvenile myoclonic epilepsy,** not intractable

G40.B01 **Juvenile myoclonic epilepsy, not intractable,** with status epilepticus   CC HCC

G40.B09 **Juvenile myoclonic epilepsy, not intractable,** without status epilepticus   CC HCC

✓6ᵗʰ **G40.B1** **Juvenile myoclonic epilepsy,** intractable

G40.B11 **Juvenile myoclonic epilepsy, intractable,** with status epilepticus   CC HCC

G40.B19 **Juvenile myoclonic epilepsy, intractable,** without status epilepticus   CC HCC

√5ᵗʰ G40.4 Other generalized epilepsy and epileptic syndromes
Epilepsy with grand mal seizures on awakening
Epilepsy with myoclonic absences
Epilepsy with myoclonic-astatic seizures
Grand mal seizure NOS
Nonspecific atonic epileptic seizures
Nonspecific clonic epileptic seizures
Nonspecific myoclonic epileptic seizures
Nonspecific tonic epileptic seizures
Nonspecific tonic-clonic epileptic seizures
Symptomatic early myoclonic encephalopathy

√6ᵗʰ G40.40 Other generalized epilepsy and epileptic syndromes, not intractable
Other generalized epilepsy and epileptic syndromes without intractability
Other generalized epilepsy and epileptic syndromes NOS

    G40.401 Other generalized epilepsy and epileptic syndromes, not intractable, with status epilepticus HCC

    G40.409 Other generalized epilepsy and epileptic syndromes, not intractable, without status epilepticus HCC

√6ᵗʰ G40.41 Other generalized epilepsy and epileptic syndromes, intractable

    G40.411 Other generalized epilepsy and epileptic syndromes, intractable, with status epilepticus CC HCC

    G40.419 Other generalized epilepsy and epileptic syndromes, intractable, without status epilepticus CC HCC

√5ᵗʰ G40.5 Epileptic seizures related to external causes
Epileptic seizures related to alcohol
Epileptic seizures related to drugs
Epileptic seizures related to hormonal changes
Epileptic seizures related to sleep deprivation
Epileptic seizures related to stress
Code also, if applicable, associated epilepsy and recurrent seizures (G40.-)
Use additional code for adverse effect, if applicable, to identify drug (T36-T50 with fifth or sixth character 5)

√6ᵗʰ G40.50 Epileptic seizures related to external causes, not intractable

    G40.501 Epileptic seizures related to external causes, not intractable, with status epilepticus CC HCC

    G40.509 Epileptic seizures related to external causes, not intractable, without status epilepticus CC HCC
Epileptic seizures related to external causes, NOS

√5ᵗʰ G40.8 Other epilepsy and recurrent seizures
Epilepsies and epileptic syndromes undetermined as to whether they are focal or generalized
Landau-Kleffner syndrome

√6ᵗʰ G40.80 Other epilepsy

    G40.801 Other epilepsy, not intractable, with status epilepticus CC HCC
Other epilepsy without intractability with status epilepticus

    G40.802 Other epilepsy, not intractable, without status epilepticus CC HCC
Other epilepsy NOS
Other epilepsy without intractability without status epilepticus

    G40.803 Other epilepsy, intractable, with status epilepticus CC HCC

    G40.804 Other epilepsy, intractable, without status epilepticus CC HCC

√6ᵗʰ G40.81 Lennox-Gastaut syndrome
DEF: Severe form of epilepsy with usual onset in early childhood. Seizures are frequent and difficult to treat, causing falls and intellectual impairment.

    G40.811 Lennox-Gastaut syndrome, not intractable, with status epilepticus CC HCC

    G40.812 Lennox-Gastaut syndrome, not intractable, without status epilepticus CC HCC

    G40.813 Lennox-Gastaut syndrome, intractable, with status epilepticus CC HCC

    G40.814 Lennox-Gastaut syndrome, intractable, without status epilepticus CC HCC

√6ᵗʰ G40.82 Epileptic spasms
Infantile spasms
Salaam attacks
West's syndrome

    G40.821 Epileptic spasms, not intractable, with status epilepticus CC HCC
CC Excl: PDX collection 581

    G40.822 Epileptic spasms, not intractable, without status epilepticus CC HCC
CC Excl: PDX collection 581

    G40.823 Epileptic spasms, intractable, with status epilepticus CC HCC

    G40.824 Epileptic spasms, intractable, without status epilepticus CC HCC

    G40.89 Other seizures CC HCC
EXCLUDES 1 post traumatic seizures (R56.1)
recurrent seizures NOS (G40.909)
seizure NOS (R56.9)

√5ᵗʰ G40.9 Epilepsy, unspecified
AHA: 2019,1Q,19

√6ᵗʰ G40.90 Epilepsy, unspecified, not intractable
Epilepsy, unspecified, without intractability

    G40.901 Epilepsy, unspecified, not intractable, with status epilepticus HCC

    G40.909 Epilepsy, unspecified, not intractable, without status epilepticus HCC
Epilepsy NOS
Epileptic convulsions NOS
Epileptic fits NOS
Epileptic seizures NOS
Recurrent seizures NOS
Seizure disorder NOS

√6ᵗʰ G40.91 Epilepsy, unspecified, intractable
Intractable seizure disorder NOS

    G40.911 Epilepsy, unspecified, intractable, with status epilepticus CC HCC

    G40.919 Epilepsy, unspecified, intractable, without status epilepticus CC HCC

√4ᵗʰ **G43** **Migraine**

> **NOTE** The following terms are to be considered equivalent to intractable: pharmacoresistant (pharmacologically resistant), treatment resistant, refractory (medically) and poorly controlled

> Use additional code for adverse effect, if applicable, to identify drug (T36-T50 with fifth or sixth character 5)
>
> *EXCLUDES 1*   *headache NOS (R51)*
>   *lower half migraine (G44.00)*
> *EXCLUDES 2*   *headache syndromes (G44.-)*
>
> **DEF:** Headaches that occur periodically on one or both sides of the head that may be associated with nausea and vomiting, sensitivity to light and sound, dizziness, distorted vision, and cognitive disturbances.

√5ᵗʰ **G43.0** **Migraine** without aura

> Common migraine
> *EXCLUDES 1*   *chronic migraine without aura (G43.7-)*

> √6ᵗʰ **G43.00** **Migraine without aura,** not intractable
> > Migraine without aura without mention of refractory migraine
> >
> > **G43.001** **Migraine without aura, not intractable, with status migrainosus**
> > **G43.009** **Migraine without aura, not intractable, without status migrainosus**
> > > Migraine without aura NOS

> √6ᵗʰ **G43.01** **Migraine without aura,** intractable
> > Migraine without aura with refractory migraine
> >
> > **G43.011** **Migraine without aura, intractable, with status migrainosus**
> > **G43.019** **Migraine without aura, intractable, without status migrainosus**

√5ᵗʰ **G43.1** **Migraine** with aura

> Basilar migraine
> Classical migraine
> Migraine equivalents
> Migraine preceded or accompanied by transient focal neurological phenomena
> Migraine triggered seizures
> Migraine with acute-onset aura
> Migraine with aura without headache (migraine equivalents)
> Migraine with prolonged aura
> Migraine with typical aura
> Retinal migraine
> Code also any associated seizure (G40.-, R56.9)
> *EXCLUDES 1*   *persistent migraine aura (G43.5-, G43.6-)*

> √6ᵗʰ **G43.10** **Migraine with aura,** not intractable
> > Migraine with aura without mention of refractory migraine
> >
> > **G43.101** **Migraine with aura, not intractable, with status migrainosus**
> > **G43.109** **Migraine with aura, not intractable, without status migrainosus**
> > > Migraine with aura NOS

> √6ᵗʰ **G43.11** **Migraine with aura,** intractable
> > Migraine with aura with refractory migraine
> >
> > **G43.111** **Migraine with aura, intractable, with status migrainosus**
> > **G43.119** **Migraine with aura, intractable, without status migrainosus**

√5ᵗʰ **G43.4** Hemiplegic **migraine**

> Familial migraine
> Sporadic migraine

> √6ᵗʰ **G43.40** **Hemiplegic migraine,** not intractable
> > Hemiplegic migraine without refractory migraine
> >
> > **G43.401** **Hemiplegic migraine, not intractable, with status migrainosus**
> > **G43.409** **Hemiplegic migraine, not intractable, without status migrainosus**
> > > Hemiplegic migraine NOS

> √6ᵗʰ **G43.41** **Hemiplegic migraine,** intractable
> > Hemiplegic migraine with refractory migraine
> >
> > **G43.411** **Hemiplegic migraine, intractable, with status migrainosus**
> > **G43.419** **Hemiplegic migraine, intractable, without status migrainosus**

√5ᵗʰ **G43.5** Persistent **migraine** aura without cerebral infarction

> √6ᵗʰ **G43.50** **Persistent migraine aura without cerebral infarction,** not intractable
> > Persistent migraine aura without cerebral infarction, without refractory migraine
> >
> > **G43.501** **Persistent migraine aura without cerebral infarction, not intractable,** with status migrainosus
> > **G43.509** **Persistent migraine aura without cerebral infarction, not intractable,** without status migrainosus
> > > Persistent migraine aura NOS

> √6ᵗʰ **G43.51** **Persistent migraine aura without cerebral infarction,** intractable
> > Persistent migraine aura without cerebral infarction, with refractory migraine
> >
> > **G43.511** **Persistent migraine aura without cerebral infarction, intractable,** with status migrainosus
> > **G43.519** **Persistent migraine aura without cerebral infarction, intractable,** without status migrainosus

√5ᵗʰ **G43.6** Persistent **migraine** aura with cerebral infarction

> Code also the type of cerebral infarction (I63.-)
> **CC Excl:** For CC codes in subcategory G43.6, unless otherwise noted: PDX collection 584

> √6ᵗʰ **G43.60** **Persistent migraine aura with cerebral infarction,** not intractable
> > Persistent migraine aura with cerebral infarction, without refractory migraine
> >
> > **G43.601** **Persistent migraine aura with cerebral infarction, not intractable, with status migrainosus** `CC`
> > **G43.609** **Persistent migraine aura with cerebral infarction, not intractable, without status migrainosus** `CC`
> > > **CC Excl:** PDX collection 585

> √6ᵗʰ **G43.61** **Persistent migraine aura with cerebral infarction,** intractable
> > Persistent migraine aura with cerebral infarction, with refractory migraine
> >
> > **G43.611** **Persistent migraine aura with cerebral infarction, intractable, with status migrainosus** `CC`
> > **G43.619** **Persistent migraine aura with cerebral infarction, intractable, without status migrainosus** `CC`

√5ᵗʰ **G43.7** Chronic **migraine** without aura

> Transformed migraine
> *EXCLUDES 1*   *migraine without aura (G43.0-)*

> √6ᵗʰ **G43.70** **Chronic migraine without aura,** not intractable
> > Chronic migraine without aura, without refractory migraine
> >
> > **G43.701** **Chronic migraine without aura, not intractable,** with status migrainosus
> > **G43.709** **Chronic migraine without aura, not intractable,** without status migrainosus
> > > Chronic migraine without aura NOS

> √6ᵗʰ **G43.71** **Chronic migraine without aura,** intractable
> > Chronic migraine without aura, with refractory migraine
> >
> > **G43.711** **Chronic migraine without aura, intractable,** with status migrainosus
> > **G43.719** **Chronic migraine without aura, intractable,** without status migrainosus

√5ᵗʰ **G43.A** Cyclical vomiting

> *EXCLUDES 1*   ▶*cyclical vomiting syndrome unrelated to migraine (R11.15)*◀

> ▲ **G43.A0** **Cyclical vomiting, in migraine,** not intractable
> > Cyclical vomiting, without refractory migraine
>
> ▲ **G43.A1** **Cyclical vomiting, in migraine,** intractable
> > Cyclical vomiting, with refractory migraine

☑ Additional Character Required   √x7ᵗʰ Placeholder   Unacceptable PDx   Questionable PDx   Manifestation   Unspecified Dx   H1-H10 HAC   HCC CMS-HCC Dx   HIV HIV Dx

✓5ᵗʰ **G43.B** Ophthalmoplegic **migraine**

G43.B0 **Ophthalmoplegic migraine,** not intractable
Ophthalmoplegic migraine, without refractory migraine

G43.B1 **Ophthalmoplegic migraine,** intractable
Ophthalmoplegic migraine, with refractory migraine

✓5ᵗʰ **G43.C** Periodic headache **syndromes in child or adult**

G43.C0 **Periodic headache syndromes in child or adult,** not intractable
Periodic headache syndromes in child or adult, without refractory migraine

G43.C1 **Periodic headache syndromes in child or adult,** intractable
Periodic headache syndromes in child or adult, with refractory migraine

✓5ᵗʰ **G43.D** Abdominal **migraine**

G43.D0 **Abdominal migraine,** not intractable
Abdominal migraine, without refractory migraine

G43.D1 **Abdominal migraine,** intractable
Abdominal migraine, with refractory migraine

✓5ᵗʰ **G43.8** **Other migraine**

✓6ᵗʰ **G43.80** **Other migraine,** not intractable
Other migraine, without refractory migraine

G43.801 **Other migraine, not intractable,** with status migrainosus

G43.809 **Other migraine, not intractable,** without status migrainosus

✓6ᵗʰ **G43.81** **Other migraine,** intractable
Other migraine, with refractory migraine

G43.811 **Other migraine, intractable,** with status migrainosus

G43.819 **Other migraine, intractable,** without status migrainosus

✓6ᵗʰ **G43.82** Menstrual **migraine,** not intractable

Menstrual headache, not intractable
Menstrual migraine, without refractory migraine
Menstrually related migraine, not intractable
Pre-menstrual headache, not intractable
Pre-menstrual migraine, not intractable
Pure menstrual migraine, not intractable
Code also associated premenstrual tension syndrome (N94.3)

G43.821 **Menstrual migraine, not intractable,** with status migrainosus ♀

G43.829 **Menstrual migraine, not intractable,** without status migrainosus ♀
Menstrual migraine NOS

✓6ᵗʰ **G43.83** Menstrual **migraine,** intractable

Menstrual headache, intractable
Menstrual migraine, with refractory migraine
Menstrually related migraine, intractable
Pre-menstrual headache, intractable
Pre-menstrual migraine, intractable
Pure menstrual migraine, intractable
Code also associated premenstrual tension syndrome (N94.3)

G43.831 **Menstrual migraine, intractable,** with status migrainosus ♀

G43.839 **Menstrual migraine, intractable,** without status migrainosus ♀

✓5ᵗʰ **G43.9** **Migraine, unspecified**

✓6ᵗʰ **G43.90** **Migraine, unspecified,** not intractable
Migraine, unspecified, without refractory migraine

G43.901 **Migraine, unspecified, not intractable, with status migrainosus**
Status migrainosus NOS

G43.909 **Migraine, unspecified, not intractable,** without status migrainosus
Migraine NOS

✓6ᵗʰ **G43.91** **Migraine, unspecified,** intractable
Migraine, unspecified, with refractory migraine

G43.911 **Migraine, unspecified, intractable, with** status migrainosus

G43.919 **Migraine, unspecified, intractable,** without status migrainosus

✓4ᵗʰ **G44** Other headache **syndromes**

EXCLUDES 1   *headache NOS (R51)*

EXCLUDES 2   *atypical facial pain (G50.1)*
headache due to lumbar puncture (G97.1)
migraines (G43.-)
trigeminal neuralgia (G50.0)

✓5ᵗʰ **G44.0** Cluster headaches **and other trigeminal autonomic cephalgias (TAC)**
DEF: Cluster headache: Characteristic grouping or clustering of headaches that can last for a number of weeks or months and then completely disappear for months or years. They are typically not associated with gastrointestinal upset or light sensitivity as experienced in migraines.

✓6ᵗʰ **G44.00** **Cluster headache syndrome, unspecified**
Ciliary neuralgia
Cluster headache NOS
Histamine cephalgia
Lower half migraine
Migrainous neuralgia

G44.001 **Cluster headache syndrome, unspecified, intractable**

G44.009 **Cluster headache syndrome, unspecified,** not intractable
Cluster headache syndrome NOS

✓6ᵗʰ **G44.01** Episodic **cluster headache**

G44.011 **Episodic cluster headache,** intractable

G44.019 **Episodic cluster headache,** not intractable
Episodic cluster headache NOS

✓6ᵗʰ **G44.02** Chronic **cluster headache**

G44.021 **Chronic cluster headache,** intractable

G44.029 **Chronic cluster headache,** not intractable
Chronic cluster headache NOS

✓6ᵗʰ **G44.03** Episodic paroxysmal hemicrania
Paroxysmal hemicrania NOS

G44.031 **Episodic paroxysmal hemicrania,** intractable

G44.039 **Episodic paroxysmal hemicrania,** not intractable
Episodic paroxysmal hemicrania NOS

✓6ᵗʰ **G44.04** Chronic **paroxysmal hemicrania**

G44.041 **Chronic paroxysmal hemicrania,** intractable

G44.049 **Chronic paroxysmal hemicrania,** not intractable
Chronic paroxysmal hemicrania NOS

✓6ᵗʰ **G44.05** Short lasting unilateral neuralgiform headache with conjunctival injection and tearing (SUNCT)

G44.051 **Short lasting unilateral neuralgiform headache with conjunctival injection and tearing (SUNCT),** intractable

G44.059 **Short lasting unilateral neuralgiform headache with conjunctival injection and tearing (SUNCT),** not intractable
Short lasting unilateral neuralgiform headache with conjunctival injection and tearing (SUNCT) NOS

✓6ᵗʰ **G44.09** Other trigeminal autonomic cephalgias **(TAC)**

G44.091 **Other trigeminal autonomic cephalgias (TAC),** intractable

G44.099 **Other trigeminal autonomic cephalgias (TAC),** not intractable

G44.1 Vascular **headache, not elsewhere classified**

EXCLUDES 2   *cluster headache (G44.0)*
complicated headache syndromes (G44.5-)
drug-induced headache (G44.4-)
migraine (G43.-)
other specified headache syndromes (G44.8-)
post-traumatic headache (G44.3-)
tension-type headache (G44.2-)

✓5ᵗʰ **G44.2** Tension-type **headache**

✓6ᵗʰ **G44.20** **Tension-type headache, unspecified**

G44.201 **Tension-type headache, unspecified,** intractable

N Newborn: 0   P Pediatric: 0-17   M Maternity: 9-64   A Adult: 15-124   MCC Major Complication/Comorbidity   CC Complication/Comorbidity   SW Severe Wound Dx

580   ICD-10-CM 2020

G44.209 Tension-type headache, unspecified, not intractable

Tension headache NOS

✓6ᵗʰ **G44.21** Episodic tension-type headache

G44.211 Episodic tension-type headache, intractable

G44.219 Episodic tension-type headache, not intractable

Episodic tension-type headache NOS

✓6ᵗʰ **G44.22** Chronic tension-type headache

G44.221 Chronic tension-type headache, intractable

G44.229 Chronic tension-type headache, not intractable

Chronic tension-type headache NOS

✓5ᵗʰ **G44.3** Post-traumatic headache

✓6ᵗʰ **G44.30** Post-traumatic headache, unspecified

G44.301 Post-traumatic headache, unspecified, intractable

G44.309 Post-traumatic headache, unspecified, not intractable

Post-traumatic headache NOS

✓6ᵗʰ **G44.31** Acute post-traumatic headache

G44.311 Acute post-traumatic headache, intractable

G44.319 Acute post-traumatic headache, not intractable

Acute post-traumatic headache NOS

✓6ᵗʰ **G44.32** Chronic post-traumatic headache

G44.321 Chronic post-traumatic headache, intractable

G44.329 Chronic post-traumatic headache, not intractable

Chronic post-traumatic headache NOS

✓5ᵗʰ **G44.4** Drug-induced headache, not elsewhere classified

Medication overuse headache

Use additional code for adverse effect, if applicable, to identify drug (T36-T50 with fifth or sixth character 5)

G44.40 Drug-induced headache, not elsewhere classified, not intractable

G44.41 Drug-induced headache, not elsewhere classified, intractable

✓5ᵗʰ **G44.5** Complicated headache syndromes

G44.51 Hemicrania continua

DEF: Persistent primary headache of unknown causation occurring on one side of the face and head. May last for more than three months, with daily and continuous pain of moderate intensity with severe exacerbations.

G44.52 New daily persistent headache (NDPH)

G44.53 Primary thunderclap headache

G44.59 Other complicated headache syndrome

✓5ᵗʰ **G44.8** Other specified headache syndromes

G44.81 Hypnic headache

G44.82 Headache associated with sexual activity

Orgasmic headache

Preorgasmic headache

G44.83 Primary cough headache

G44.84 Primary exertional headache

G44.85 Primary stabbing headache

G44.89 Other headache syndrome

✓4ᵗʰ **G45** Transient cerebral ischemic attacks and related syndromes

EXCLUDES 1   neonatal cerebral ischemia (P91.0)

transient retinal artery occlusion (H34.0-)

AHA: 2018,2Q,9

DEF: Transient cerebral ischemic attack: Intermittent or brief cerebral dysfunction from lack of oxygenation with no persistent neurological deficits associated with occlusive vascular disease. TIA may denote an impending cerebrovascular accident.

G45.0 Vertebro-basilar artery syndrome

G45.1 Carotid artery syndrome (hemispheric)

G45.2 Multiple and bilateral precerebral artery syndromes

G45.3 Amaurosis fugax

G45.4 Transient global amnesia

EXCLUDES 1   amnesia NOS (R41.3)

G45.8 Other transient cerebral ischemic attacks and related syndromes   CC

CC Excl: PDX collection 586

G45.9 Transient cerebral ischemic attack, unspecified   CC

Spasm of cerebral artery

TIA

Transient cerebral ischemia NOS

CC Excl: PDX collection 586

✓4ᵗʰ **G46** Vascular syndromes of brain in cerebrovascular diseases

Code first underlying cerebrovascular disease (I60-I69)

CC Excl: For CC codes in category G46: PDX collection 586

G46.0 Middle cerebral artery syndrome   CC

G46.1 Anterior cerebral artery syndrome   CC

G46.2 Posterior cerebral artery syndrome   CC

G46.3 Brain stem stroke syndrome

Benedikt syndrome

Claude syndrome

Foville syndrome

Millard-Gubler syndrome

Wallenberg syndrome

Weber syndrome

G46.4 Cerebellar stroke syndrome

G46.5 Pure motor lacunar syndrome

G46.6 Pure sensory lacunar syndrome

G46.7 Other lacunar syndromes

G46.8 Other vascular syndromes of brain in cerebrovascular diseases

✓4ᵗʰ **G47** Sleep disorders

EXCLUDES 2   nightmares (F51.5)

nonorganic sleep disorders (F51.-)

sleep terrors (F51.4)

sleepwalking (F51.3)

✓5ᵗʰ **G47.0** Insomnia

EXCLUDES 2   alcohol related insomnia (F10.182, F10.282, F10.982)

drug-related insomnia (F11.182, F11.282, F11.982, F13.182, F13.282, F13.982, F14.182, F14.282, F14.982, F15.182, F15.282, F15.982, F19.182, F19.282, F19.982)

idiopathic insomnia (F51.01)

insomnia due to a mental disorder (F51.05)

insomnia not due to a substance or known physiological condition (F51.0-)

nonorganic insomnia (F51.0-)

primary insomnia (F51.01)

sleep apnea (G47.3-)

G47.00 Insomnia, unspecified

Insomnia NOS

G47.01 Insomnia due to medical condition

Code also associated medical condition

G47.09 Other insomnia

✓5ᵗʰ **G47.1** Hypersomnia

EXCLUDES 2   alcohol-related hypersomnia (F10.182, F10.282, F10.982)

drug-related hypersomnia (F11.182, F11.282, F11.982, F13.182, F13.282, F13.982, F14.182, F14.282, F14.982, F15.182, F15.282, F15.982, F19.182, F19.282, F19.982)

hypersomnia due to a mental disorder (F51.13)

hypersomnia not due to a substance or known physiological condition (F51.1-)

primary hypersomnia (F51.11)

sleep apnea (G47.3-)

G47.10 Hypersomnia, unspecified

Hypersomnia NOS

G47.11 Idiopathic hypersomnia with long sleep time

Idiopathic hypersomnia NOS

G47.12 Idiopathic hypersomnia without long sleep time

G47.13 Recurrent hypersomnia

Kleine-Levin syndrome

Menstrual related hypersomnia

G47.14 Hypersomnia due to medical condition

Code also associated medical condition

G47.19 Other hypersomnia

✓ Additional Character Required   ✓x7ᵗʰ Placeholder   Unacceptable PDx   Questionable PDx   Manifestation   Unspecified Dx   H1-H14 HAC   HCC CMS-HCC Dx   HIV HIV Dx

ICD-10-CM 2020

581

Chapter 6. Diseases of the Nervous System

☑5ᵗʰ G47.2 Circadian rhythm sleep disorders
Disorders of the sleep wake schedule
Inversion of nyctohemeral rhythm
Inversion of sleep rhythm
DEF: Circadian rhythm: Daily cycle (24-hour period) of physical, mental and behavioral changes. It is largely influenced by environmental ques, such as changes in light or temperature. *Synonyms: sleep/wake cycle.*

G47.20 Circadian rhythm sleep disorder, unspecified type
Sleep wake schedule disorder NOS

G47.21 Circadian rhythm sleep disorder, delayed sleep phase type
Delayed sleep phase syndrome

G47.22 Circadian rhythm sleep disorder, advanced sleep phase type

G47.23 Circadian rhythm sleep disorder, irregular sleep wake type
Irregular sleep-wake pattern

G47.24 Circadian rhythm sleep disorder, free running type
Circadian rhythm sleep disorder, non-24-hour sleep-wake type

G47.25 Circadian rhythm sleep disorder, jet lag type

G47.26 Circadian rhythm sleep disorder, shift work type

G47.27 *Circadian rhythm sleep disorder in conditions classified elsewhere*
Code first underlying condition

G47.29 Other circadian rhythm sleep disorder

☑5ᵗʰ G47.3 Sleep apnea
Code also any associated underlying condition
EXCLUDES 1   apnea NOS (R06.81)
     Cheyne-Stokes breathing (R06.3)
     pickwickian syndrome (E66.2)
     sleep apnea of newborn (P28.3)

G47.30 Sleep apnea, unspecified
Sleep apnea NOS

G47.31 Primary central sleep apnea
Idiopathic central sleep apnea

G47.32 High altitude periodic breathing

G47.33 Obstructive sleep apnea (adult) (pediatric)
Obstructive sleep apnea hypopnea
EXCLUDES 1   obstructive sleep apnea of newborn (P28.3)

G47.34 Idiopathic sleep related nonobstructive alveolar hypoventilation
Sleep related hypoxia

G47.35 Congenital central alveolar hypoventilation syndrome

G47.36 *Sleep related hypoventilation in conditions classified elsewhere*
Sleep related hypoxemia in conditions classified elsewhere
Code first underlying condition

G47.37 *Central sleep apnea in conditions classified elsewhere*
Code first underlying condition

G47.39 Other sleep apnea

☑5ᵗʰ G47.4 Narcolepsy and cataplexy

☑6ᵗʰ G47.41 Narcolepsy
     G47.411 Narcolepsy with cataplexy
     G47.419 Narcolepsy without cataplexy
         Narcolepsy NOS

☑6ᵗʰ G47.42 Narcolepsy in conditions classified elsewhere
Code first underlying condition
     G47.421 *Narcolepsy in conditions classified elsewhere with cataplexy*
     G47.429 *Narcolepsy in conditions classified elsewhere without cataplexy*

☑5ᵗʰ G47.5 Parasomnia
EXCLUDES 1   alcohol induced parasomnia (F10.182, F10.282, F10.982)
     drug induced parasomnia (F11.182, F11.282, F11.982, F13.182, F13.282, F13.982, F14.182, F14.282, F14.982, F15.182, F15.282, F15.982, F19.182, F19.282, F19.982)
     parasomnia not due to a substance or known physiological condition (F51.8)

G47.50 Parasomnia, unspecified
Parasomnia NOS

G47.51 Confusional arousals

G47.52 REM sleep behavior disorder
G47.53 Recurrent isolated sleep paralysis
G47.54 *Parasomnia in conditions classified elsewhere*
Code first underlying condition
G47.59 Other parasomnia

☑5ᵗʰ G47.6 Sleep related movement disorders
EXCLUDES 2   restless legs syndrome (G25.81)
G47.61 Periodic limb movement disorder
G47.62 Sleep related leg cramps
G47.63 Sleep related bruxism
EXCLUDES 1   psychogenic bruxism (F45.8)
G47.69 Other sleep related movement disorders

G47.8 Other sleep disorders
Other specified sleep-wake disorder

G47.9 Sleep disorder, unspecified
Sleep disorder NOS
Unspecified sleep-wake disorder

Nerve, nerve root and plexus disorders (G50-G59)

EXCLUDES 1   current traumatic nerve, nerve root and plexus disorders — see Injury, nerve by body region
     neuralgia NOS (M79.2)
     neuritis NOS (M79.2)
     peripheral neuritis in pregnancy (O26.82-)
     radiculitis NOS (M54.1-)

☑4ᵗʰ G50 Disorders of trigeminal nerve
INCLUDES   disorders of 5th cranial nerve

Trigeminal and Facial Nerve Branches

G50.0 Trigeminal neuralgia
Syndrome of paroxysmal facial pain
Tic douloureux

G50.1 Atypical facial pain
G50.8 Other disorders of trigeminal nerve
G50.9 Disorder of trigeminal nerve, unspecified

☑4ᵗʰ G51 Facial nerve disorders
INCLUDES   disorders of 7th cranial nerve

G51.0 Bell's palsy
Facial palsy

G51.1 Geniculate ganglionitis
EXCLUDES 1   postherpetic geniculate ganglionitis (B02.21)

G51.2 Melkersson's syndrome
Melkersson-Rosenthal syndrome

☑5ᵗʰ G51.3 Clonic hemifacial spasm
AHA: 2018,4Q,10
G51.31 Clonic hemifacial spasm, right
G51.32 Clonic hemifacial spasm, left
G51.33 Clonic hemifacial spasm, bilateral
G51.39 Clonic hemifacial spasm, unspecified

G51.4 Facial myokymia
G51.8 Other disorders of facial nerve
G51.9 Disorder of facial nerve, unspecified

☑4ᵗʰ **G52 Disorders of other cranial nerves**

    EXCLUDES 2   *disorders of acoustic [8th] nerve (H93.3)*
                    disorders of optic [2nd] nerve (H46, H47.0)
                    paralytic strabismus due to nerve palsy (H49.0-H49.2)

    G52.0 Disorders of olfactory nerve
        Disorders of 1st cranial nerve

    G52.1 Disorders of glossopharyngeal nerve
        Disorder of 9th cranial nerve
        Glossopharyngeal neuralgia

    G52.2 Disorders of vagus nerve
        Disorders of pneumogastric [10th] nerve

    G52.3 Disorders of hypoglossal nerve
        Disorders of 12th cranial nerve

    G52.7 Disorders of multiple cranial nerves
        Polyneuritis cranialis

    G52.8 Disorders of other specified cranial nerves

    G52.9 Cranial nerve disorder, unspecified

G53 Cranial nerve disorders in diseases classified elsewhere
    Code first underlying disease, such as:
      neoplasm (C00-D49)

    EXCLUDES 1   *multiple cranial nerve palsy in sarcoidosis (D86.82)*
                    multiple cranial nerve palsy in syphilis (A52.15)
                    postherpetic geniculate ganglionitis (B02.21)
                    postherpetic trigeminal neuralgia (B02.22)

☑4ᵗʰ **G54 Nerve root and plexus disorders**

    EXCLUDES 1   *current traumatic nerve root and plexus disorders — see nerve injury by body region*
                    intervertebral disc disorders (M50-M51)
                    neuralgia or neuritis NOS (M79.2)
                    neuritis or radiculitis brachial NOS (M54.13)
                    neuritis or radiculitis lumbar NOS (M54.16)
                    neuritis or radiculitis lumbosacral NOS (M54.17)
                    neuritis or radiculitis thoracic NOS (M54.14)
                    radiculitis NOS (M54.10)
                    radiculopathy NOS (M54.10)
                    spondylosis (M47.-)

    G54.0 Brachial plexus disorders
        Thoracic outlet syndrome
        DEF: Acquired disorder affecting the spinal nerves that send signals to the shoulder, arm, and hand, causing corresponding motor and sensory dysfunction. This disorder is characterized by regional paresthesia, pain, muscle weakness, and in severe cases paralysis.

    G54.1 Lumbosacral plexus disorders

    G54.2 Cervical root disorders, not elsewhere classified

    G54.3 Thoracic root disorders, not elsewhere classified

    G54.4 Lumbosacral root disorders, not elsewhere classified

    G54.5 Neuralgic amyotrophy
        Parsonage-Aldren-Turner syndrome
        Shoulder-girdle neuritis
        EXCLUDES 1 *neuralgic amyotrophy in diabetes mellitus (E08-E13 with .44)*

    G54.6 Phantom limb syndrome with pain   HCC

    G54.7 Phantom limb syndrome without pain   HCC
        Phantom limb syndrome NOS

    G54.8 Other nerve root and plexus disorders

    G54.9 Nerve root and plexus disorder, unspecified

G55 Nerve root and plexus compressions in diseases classified elsewhere
    Code first underlying disease, such as:
      neoplasm (C00-D49)

    EXCLUDES 1   *nerve root compression (due to) (in) ankylosing spondylitis (M45.-)*
                    nerve root compression (due to) (in) dorsopathies (M53.-, M54.-)
                    nerve root compression (due to) (in) intervertebral disc disorders (M50.1.-, M51.1.-)
                    nerve root compression (due to) (in) spondylopathies (M46.-, M48.-)
                    nerve root compression (due to) (in) spondylosis (M47.0-M47.2-)

☑4ᵗʰ **G56 Mononeuropathies of upper limb**

    EXCLUDES 1   *current traumatic nerve disorder — see nerve injury by body region*

    AHA: 2016,4Q,17-18

Nerves of Upper Limb

Radial

Deep branch of radial
Ulnar
Superficial branch of radial
Median

  ☑5ᵗʰ **G56.0 Carpal tunnel syndrome**
        DEF: Swelling and inflammation in the tendons or bursa surrounding the median nerve caused by repetitive activity. The resulting compression on the nerve causes pain, numbness, and tingling especially to the palm, index, middle finger, and thumb.

        G56.00 Carpal tunnel syndrome, unspecified upper limb
        G56.01 Carpal tunnel syndrome, right upper limb
        G56.02 Carpal tunnel syndrome, left upper limb
        G56.03 Carpal tunnel syndrome, bilateral upper limbs

  ☑5ᵗʰ **G56.1 Other lesions of median nerve**
        G56.10 Other lesions of median nerve, unspecified upper limb
        G56.11 Other lesions of median nerve, right upper limb
        G56.12 Other lesions of median nerve, left upper limb
        G56.13 Other lesions of median nerve, bilateral upper limbs

  ☑5ᵗʰ **G56.2 Lesion of ulnar nerve**
        Tardy ulnar nerve palsy
        G56.20 Lesion of ulnar nerve, unspecified upper limb
        G56.21 Lesion of ulnar nerve, right upper limb
        G56.22 Lesion of ulnar nerve, left upper limb
        G56.23 Lesion of ulnar nerve, bilateral upper limbs

  ☑5ᵗʰ **G56.3 Lesion of radial nerve**
        G56.30 Lesion of radial nerve, unspecified upper limb
        G56.31 Lesion of radial nerve, right upper limb
        G56.32 Lesion of radial nerve, left upper limb
        G56.33 Lesion of radial nerve, bilateral upper limbs

  ☑5ᵗʰ **G56.4 Causalgia of upper limb**
        Complex regional pain syndrome II of upper limb
        EXCLUDES 1 *complex regional pain syndrome I of lower limb (G90.52-)*
                    complex regional pain syndrome I of upper limb (G90.51-)
                    complex regional pain syndrome II of lower limb (G57.7-)
                    reflex sympathetic dystrophy of lower limb (G90.52-)
                    reflex sympathetic dystrophy of upper limb (G90.51-)
        G56.40 Causalgia of unspecified upper limb
        G56.41 Causalgia of right upper limb
        G56.42 Causalgia of left upper limb
        G56.43 Causalgia of bilateral upper limbs

  ☑5ᵗʰ **G56.8 Other specified mononeuropathies of upper limb**
        Interdigital neuroma of upper limb
        G56.80 Other specified mononeuropathies of unspecified upper limb

Chapter 6. Diseases of the Nervous System

G56.81   Other specified mononeuropathies of right upper limb

G56.82   Other specified mononeuropathies of left upper limb

G56.83   Other specified mononeuropathies of bilateral upper limbs

√5th **G56.9**   **Unspecified mononeuropathy of upper limb**

     G56.90   Unspecified mononeuropathy of unspecified upper limb

     G56.91   Unspecified mononeuropathy of right upper limb

     G56.92   Unspecified mononeuropathy of left upper limb

     G56.93   Unspecified mononeuropathy of bilateral upper limbs

√4th **G57**   **Mononeuropathies of lower limb**

     EXCLUDES 1   current traumatic nerve disorder — see nerve injury by body region

     AHA: 2016,4Q,17-18

Nerves of Lower Limb

Obturator nerve

Sciatic nerve

Femoral nerve

Saphenous nerve

Common fibular (peroneal) nerve

Deep fibular (peroneal) nerve

Tibial nerve

Superficial fibular (peroneal) nerve

√5th **G57.0**   **Lesion of sciatic nerve**

     EXCLUDES 1   sciatica NOS (M54.3-)

     EXCLUDES 2   sciatica attributed to intervertebral disc disorder (M51.1.-)

     G57.00   Lesion of sciatic nerve, unspecified lower limb

     G57.01   Lesion of sciatic nerve, right lower limb

     G57.02   Lesion of sciatic nerve, left lower limb

     G57.03   Lesion of sciatic nerve, bilateral lower limbs

√5th **G57.1**   **Meralgia paresthetica**

     Lateral cutaneous nerve of thigh syndrome

     G57.10   Meralgia paresthetica, unspecified lower limb

     G57.11   Meralgia paresthetica, right lower limb

     G57.12   Meralgia paresthetica, left lower limb

     G57.13   Meralgia paresthetica, bilateral lower limbs

√5th **G57.2**   **Lesion of femoral nerve**

     G57.20   Lesion of femoral nerve, unspecified lower limb

     G57.21   Lesion of femoral nerve, right lower limb

     G57.22   Lesion of femoral nerve, left lower limb

     G57.23   Lesion of femoral nerve, bilateral lower limbs

√5th **G57.3**   **Lesion of lateral popliteal nerve**

     Peroneal nerve palsy

     G57.30   Lesion of lateral popliteal nerve, unspecified lower limb

     G57.31   Lesion of lateral popliteal nerve, right lower limb

     G57.32   Lesion of lateral popliteal nerve, left lower limb

     G57.33   Lesion of lateral popliteal nerve, bilateral lower limbs

√5th **G57.4**   **Lesion of medial popliteal nerve**

     G57.40   Lesion of medial popliteal nerve, unspecified lower limb

     G57.41   Lesion of medial popliteal nerve, right lower limb

     G57.42   Lesion of medial popliteal nerve, left lower limb

     G57.43   Lesion of medial popliteal nerve, bilateral lower limbs

√5th **G57.5**   **Tarsal tunnel syndrome**

     G57.50   Tarsal tunnel syndrome, unspecified lower limb

     G57.51   Tarsal tunnel syndrome, right lower limb

     G57.52   Tarsal tunnel syndrome, left lower limb

     G57.53   Tarsal tunnel syndrome, bilateral lower limbs

√5th **G57.6**   **Lesion of plantar nerve**

     Morton's metatarsalgia

     G57.60   Lesion of plantar nerve, unspecified lower limb

     G57.61   Lesion of plantar nerve, right lower limb

     G57.62   Lesion of plantar nerve, left lower limb

     G57.63   Lesion of plantar nerve, bilateral lower limbs

√5th **G57.7**   **Causalgia of lower limb**

     Complex regional pain syndrome II of lower limb

     EXCLUDES 1   complex regional pain syndrome I of lower limb (G90.52-)

                      complex regional pain syndrome I of upper limb (G90.51-)

                      complex regional pain syndrome II of upper limb (G56.4-)

                      reflex sympathetic dystrophy of lower limb (G90.52-)

                      reflex sympathetic dystrophy of upper limb (G90.51-)

     G57.70   Causalgia of unspecified lower limb

     G57.71   Causalgia of right lower limb

     G57.72   Causalgia of left lower limb

     G57.73   Causalgia of bilateral lower limbs

√5th **G57.8**   **Other specified mononeuropathies of lower limb**

     Interdigital neuroma of lower limb

     G57.80   Other specified mononeuropathies of unspecified lower limb

     G57.81   Other specified mononeuropathies of right lower limb

     G57.82   Other specified mononeuropathies of left lower limb

     G57.83   Other specified mononeuropathies of bilateral lower limbs

√5th **G57.9**   **Unspecified mononeuropathy of lower limb**

     G57.90   Unspecified mononeuropathy of unspecified lower limb

     G57.91   Unspecified mononeuropathy of right lower limb

     G57.92   Unspecified mononeuropathy of left lower limb

     G57.93   Unspecified mononeuropathy of bilateral lower limbs

√4th **G58**   **Other mononeuropathies**

     G58.0   Intercostal neuropathy

     G58.7   Mononeuritis multiplex

     G58.8   Other specified mononeuropathies

     G58.9   Mononeuropathy, unspecified

G59   ***Mononeuropathy in diseases classified elsewhere***

     Code first underlying disease

     EXCLUDES 1   diabetic mononeuropathy (E08-E13 with .41)

                      syphilitic nerve paralysis (A52.19)

                      syphilitic neuritis (A52.15)

                      tuberculous mononeuropathy (A17.83)

N Newborn: 0   P Pediatric: 0-17   M Maternity: 9-64   A Adult: 15-124   MCC Major Complication/Comorbidity   CC Complication/Comorbidity   SW Severe Wound Dx

584   ICD-10-CM 2020

Polyneuropathies and other disorders of the peripheral nervous system (G60-G65)

EXCLUDES 1   neuralgia NOS (M79.2)
neuritis NOS (M79.2)
peripheral neuritis in pregnancy (O26.82-)
radiculitis NOS (M54.10)

✔4ᵗʰ G60 Hereditary and idiopathic neuropathy

G60.0 Hereditary motor and sensory neuropathy
Charcôt-Marie-Tooth disease
Déjérine-Sottas disease
Hereditary motor and sensory neuropathy, types I-IV
Hypertrophic neuropathy of infancy
Peroneal muscular atrophy (axonal type) (hypertrophic type)
Roussy-Levy syndrome

G60.1 Refsum's disease   CC
Infantile Refsum disease
DEF: Genetic disorder of the lipid metabolism characterized by retinitis pigmentosa, degenerative nerve disease, ataxia, and dry, rough, scaly skin.
CC Excl: PDX collection 588

G60.2 Neuropathy in association with hereditary ataxia

G60.3 Idiopathic progressive neuropathy

G60.8 Other hereditary and idiopathic neuropathies
Dominantly inherited sensory neuropathy
Morvan's disease
Nelaton's syndrome
Recessively inherited sensory neuropathy

G60.9 Hereditary and idiopathic neuropathy, unspecified

✔4ᵗʰ G61 Inflammatory polyneuropathy

G61.0 Guillain-Barre syndrome   CC   HCC
Acute (post-)infective polyneuritis
Miller Fisher syndrome
AHA: 2014,2Q,4
DEF: Autoimmune disorder due to an immune response to foreign antigens with paraplegia of limbs, flaccid paralysis, ophthalmoplegia, ataxia, and areflexia. In most cases, this disorder is triggered by a mild viral infection, surgery, or following an immunization.
TIP: Guillain-Barre syndrome can occur as a sequela of *Campylobacter enteritis.* Assign code B94.8 for the sequelae as an additional diagnosis.
CC Excl: PDX collection 92

G61.1 Serum neuropathy   HCC
Use additional code for adverse effect, if applicable, to identify serum (T50.-)

✔5ᵗʰ G61.8 Other inflammatory polyneuropathies

G61.81 Chronic inflammatory demyelinating polyneuritis   CC   HCC
CC Excl: PDX collection 589

G61.82 Multifocal motor neuropathy   HCC
MMN
AHA: 2016,4Q,18

G61.89 Other inflammatory polyneuropathies   HCC

G61.9 Inflammatory polyneuropathy, unspecified   HCC

✔4ᵗʰ G62 Other and unspecified polyneuropathies

G62.0 Drug-induced polyneuropathy   HCC
Use additional code for adverse effect, if applicable, to identify drug (T36-T50 with fifth or sixth character 5)

G62.1 Alcoholic polyneuropathy   HCC

G62.2 Polyneuropathy due to other toxic agents   HCC
Code first (T51-T65) to identify toxic agent

✔5ᵗʰ G62.8 Other specified polyneuropathies

G62.81 Critical illness polyneuropathy   CC   HCC
Acute motor neuropathy
CC Excl: PDX collection 590

G62.82 Radiation-induced polyneuropathy   HCC
Use additional external cause code (W88-W90, X39.0-) to identify cause

G62.89 Other specified polyneuropathies
AHA: 2016,2Q,11

G62.9 Polyneuropathy, unspecified
Neuropathy NOS

G63 Polyneuropathy in diseases classified elsewhere   HCC
Code first underlying disease, such as:
amyloidosis (E85.-)
endocrine disease, except diabetes (E00-E07, E15-E16, E20-E34)
metabolic diseases (E70-E88)
neoplasm (C00-D49)
nutritional deficiency (E40-E64)

EXCLUDES 1   polyneuropathy (in):
diabetes mellitus (E08-E13 with .42)
diphtheria (A36.83)
infectious mononucleosis (B27.0-B27.9 with 1)
Lyme disease (A69.22)
mumps (B26.84)
postherpetic (B02.23)
rheumatoid arthritis ▶(M05.5-)◀
scleroderma (M34.83)
systemic lupus erythematosus (M32.19)

AHA: 2012,4Q,99

G64 Other disorders of peripheral nervous system
Disorder of peripheral nervous system NOS

✔4ᵗʰ G65 Sequelae of inflammatory and toxic polyneuropathies
Code first condition resulting from (sequela) of inflammatory and toxic polyneuropathies

G65.0 Sequelae of Guillain-Barré syndrome   HCC

G65.1 Sequelae of other inflammatory polyneuropathy   HCC

G65.2 Sequelae of toxic polyneuropathy   HCC

Diseases of myoneural junction and muscle (G70-G73)

✔4ᵗʰ G70 Myasthenia gravis and other myoneural disorders
EXCLUDES 1   botulism (A05.1, A48.51-A48.52)
transient neonatal myasthenia gravis (P94.0)
CC Excl: For CC/MCC codes in category G70: PDX collection 591

✔5ᵗʰ G70.0 Myasthenia gravis
DEF: Autoimmune neuromuscular disorder caused by antibodies to the acetylcholine receptors at the neuromuscular junction, interfering with proper binding of the neurotransmitter from the neuron to the target muscle, causing muscle weakness, fatigue, and exhaustion, without pain or atrophy.

G70.00 Myasthenia gravis without (acute) exacerbation   HCC
Myasthenia gravis NOS

G70.01 Myasthenia gravis with (acute) exacerbation   MCC   HCC
Myasthenia gravis in crisis

G70.1 Toxic myoneural disorders   HCC
Code first (T51-T65) to identify toxic agent

G70.2 Congenital and developmental myasthenia   HCC

✔5ᵗʰ G70.8 Other specified myoneural disorders

G70.80 Lambert-Eaton syndrome, unspecified   CC   HCC
Lambert-Eaton syndrome NOS

G70.81 Lambert-Eaton syndrome in disease classified elsewhere   CC   HCC
Code first underlying disease
EXCLUDES 1   Lambert-Eaton syndrome in neoplastic disease (G73.1)

G70.89 Other specified myoneural disorders   HCC

G70.9 Myoneural disorder, unspecified   HCC

✔4ᵗʰ G71 Primary disorders of muscles
EXCLUDES 2   arthrogryposis multiplex congenita (Q74.3)
metabolic disorders (E70-E88)
myositis (M60.-)

✔5ᵗʰ G71.0 Muscular dystrophy
AHA: 2018,4Q,11-12

G71.00 Muscular dystrophy, unspecified   HCC

G71.01 Duchenne or Becker muscular dystrophy   HCC
Autosomal recessive, childhood type, muscular dystrophy resembling Duchenne or Becker muscular dystrophy
Benign [Becker] muscular dystrophy
Severe [Duchenne] muscular dystrophy

✔ Additional Character Required   ✔x7ᵗʰ Placeholder   Unacceptable PDx   Questionable PDx   Manifestation   Unspecified Dx   H1-H1x HAC   HCC CMS-HCC Dx   HIV HIV Dx

ICD-10-CM 2020   585

Chapter 6. Diseases of the Nervous System

G71.Ø2   Facioscapulohumeral muscular dystrophy   `HCC`
   Scapulohumeral muscular dystrophy

G71.Ø9   Other specified muscular dystrophies   `HCC`
   Benign scapuloperoneal muscular dystrophy with early contractures [Emery-Dreifuss]
   Congenital muscular dystrophy NOS
   Congenital muscular dystrophy with specific morphological abnormalities of the muscle fiber
   Distal muscular dystrophy
   Limb-girdle muscular dystrophy
   Ocular muscular dystrophy
   Oculopharyngeal muscular dystrophy
   Scapuloperoneal muscular dystrophy

√5ᵗʰ **G71.1   Myotonic disorders**

G71.11   Myotonic muscular dystrophy   `HCC`
   Dystrophia myotonica [Steinert]
   Myotonia atrophica
   Myotonic dystrophy
   Proximal myotonic myopathy (PROMM)
   Steinert disease

G71.12   Myotonia congenita
   Acetazolamide responsive myotonia congenita
   Dominant myotonia congenita [Thomsen disease]
   Myotonia levior
   Recessive myotonia congenita [Becker disease]

G71.13   Myotonic chondrodystrophy
   Chondrodystrophic myotonia
   Congenital myotonic chondrodystrophy
   Schwartz-Jampel disease

G71.14   Drug induced myotonia
   Use additional code for adverse effect, if applicable, to identify drug (T36-T5Ø with fifth or sixth character 5)

G71.19   Other specified myotonic disorders
   Myotonia fluctuans
   Myotonia permanens
   Neuromyotonia [Isaacs]
   Paramyotonia congenita (of von Eulenburg)
   Pseudomyotonia
   Symptomatic myotonia

G71.2   Congenital myopathies   `CC` `HCC`
   Central core disease
   Fiber-type disproportion
   Minicore disease
   Multicore disease
   Myotubular (centronuclear) myopathy
   Nemaline myopathy
   EXCLUDES 1   arthrogryposis multiplex congenita (Q74.3)
   CC Excl: PDX collection 592

G71.3   Mitochondrial myopathy, not elsewhere classified
   EXCLUDES 1   *Kearns-Sayre syndrome (H49.81)*
     Leber's disease (H47.21)
     Leigh's encephalopathy (G31.82)
     mitochondrial metabolism disorders (E88.4.-)
     Reye's syndrome (G93.7)

G71.8   Other primary disorders of muscles

G71.9   Primary disorder of muscle, unspecified
   Hereditary myopathy NOS

√4ᵗʰ **G72   Other and unspecified myopathies**
   EXCLUDES 1   *arthrogryposis multiplex congenita (Q74.3)*
     dermatopolymyositis (M33.-)
     ischemic infarction of muscle (M62.2-)
     myositis (M6Ø.-)
     polymyositis (M33.2.-)
   CC Excl: For CC codes in category G72, unless otherwise noted: PDX collection 593

G72.Ø   Drug-induced myopathy   `CC`
   Use additional code for adverse effect, if applicable, to identify drug (T36-T5Ø with fifth or sixth character 5)

G72.1   Alcoholic myopathy   `CC`
   Use additional code to identify alcoholism (F1Ø.-)

G72.2   Myopathy due to other toxic agents   `CC`
   Code first (T51-T65) to identify toxic agent

G72.3   Periodic paralysis
   Familial periodic paralysis
   Hyperkalemic periodic paralysis (familial)
   Hypokalemic periodic paralysis (familial)
   Myotonic periodic paralysis (familial)
   Normokalemic paralysis (familial)
   Potassium sensitive periodic paralysis
   EXCLUDES 1   *paramyotonia congenita (of von Eulenburg) (G71.19)*

√5ᵗʰ **G72.4   Inflammatory and immune myopathies, not elsewhere classified**

G72.41   Inclusion body myositis [IBM]

G72.49   Other inflammatory and immune myopathies, not elsewhere classified
   Inflammatory myopathy NOS

√5ᵗʰ **G72.8   Other specified myopathies**

G72.81   Critical illness myopathy   `CC`
   Acute necrotizing myopathy
   Acute quadriplegic myopathy
   Intensive care (ICU) myopathy
   Myopathy of critical illness
   CC Excl: PDX collection 594

G72.89   Other specified myopathies

G72.9   Myopathy, unspecified

√4ᵗʰ **G73   Disorders of myoneural junction and muscle in diseases classified elsewhere**

G73.1   *Lambert-Eaton syndrome in neoplastic disease*   `CC` `HCC`
   Code first underlying neoplasm (CØØ-D49)
   EXCLUDES 1   *Lambert-Eaton syndrome not associated with neoplasm (G7Ø.8Ø-G7Ø.81)*
   CC Excl: PDX collection 591

G73.3   *Myasthenic syndromes in other diseases classified elsewhere*   `CC` `HCC`
   Code first underlying disease, such as:
   neoplasm (CØØ-D49)
   thyrotoxicosis (EØ5.-)
   CC Excl: PDX collection 591

G73.7   *Myopathy in diseases classified elsewhere*
   Code first underlying disease, such as:
   hyperparathyroidism (E21.Ø, E21.3)
   hypoparathyroidism (E2Ø.-)
   glycogen storage disease (E74.Ø)
   lipid storage disorders (E75.-)
   EXCLUDES 1   *myopathy in:*
     rheumatoid arthritis (MØ5.32)
     sarcoidosis (D86.87)
     scleroderma (M34.82)
     sicca syndrome [Sjögren] (M35.Ø3)
     systemic lupus erythematosus (M32.19)

Cerebral palsy and other paralytic syndromes (G8Ø-G83)

√4ᵗʰ **G8Ø   Cerebral palsy**
   EXCLUDES 1   *hereditary spastic paraplegia (G11.4)*

G8Ø.Ø   Spastic quadriplegic cerebral palsy   `CC` `HCC`
   Congenital spastic paralysis (cerebral)

G8Ø.1   Spastic diplegic cerebral palsy   `HCC`
   Spastic cerebral palsy NOS

G8Ø.2   Spastic hemiplegic cerebral palsy   `HCC`

G8Ø.3   Athetoid cerebral palsy   `HCC`
   Double athetosis (syndrome)
   Dyskinetic cerebral palsy
   Dystonic cerebral palsy
   Vogt disease

G8Ø.4   Ataxic cerebral palsy   `HCC`

G8Ø.8   Other cerebral palsy   `HCC`
   Mixed cerebral palsy syndromes

G8Ø.9   Cerebral palsy, unspecified   `HCC`
   Cerebral palsy NOS

N Newborn: 0   P Pediatric: 0-17   M Maternity: 9-64   A Adult: 15-124   MCC Major Complication/Comorbidity   CC Complication/Comorbidity   SW Severe Wound Dx

586   ICD-10-CM 2020

✓4ᵗʰ **G81 Hemiplegia and hemiparesis**

> **NOTE** This category is to be used only when hemiplegia (complete)(incomplete) is reported without further specification, or is stated to be old or longstanding but of unspecified cause. The category is also for use in multiple coding to identify these types of hemiplegia resulting from any cause.

> **EXCLUDES 1** congenital cerebral palsy (G80.-)
> hemiplegia and hemiparesis due to sequela of cerebrovascular disease (I69.05-, I69.15-, I69.25-, I69.35-, I69.85-, I69.95-)

> **AHA:** 2015,1Q,25

> **TIP:** If the documentation specifies the affected side but not whether it is the dominant or nondominant side, the default is as follows: for ambidextrous patients, the default is dominant; when the left side is affected, the default is nondominant; and when the right side is affected, the default is dominant.

> **CC Excl: For CC codes in category G81:** PDX collection 561

✓5ᵗʰ **G81.0 Flaccid hemiplegia**

G81.00	Flaccid hemiplegia affecting unspecified side	CC HCC
G81.01	Flaccid hemiplegia affecting right dominant side	CC HCC
G81.02	Flaccid hemiplegia affecting left dominant side	CC HCC
G81.03	Flaccid hemiplegia affecting right nondominant side	CC HCC
G81.04	Flaccid hemiplegia affecting left nondominant side	CC HCC

✓5ᵗʰ **G81.1 Spastic hemiplegia**

G81.10	Spastic hemiplegia affecting unspecified side	CC HCC
G81.11	Spastic hemiplegia affecting right dominant side	CC HCC
G81.12	Spastic hemiplegia affecting left dominant side	CC HCC
G81.13	Spastic hemiplegia affecting right nondominant side	CC HCC
G81.14	Spastic hemiplegia affecting left nondominant side	CC HCC

✓5ᵗʰ **G81.9 Hemiplegia, unspecified**

> **AHA:** 2014,1Q,23

G81.90	Hemiplegia, unspecified affecting unspecified side	CC HCC
G81.91	Hemiplegia, unspecified affecting right dominant side	CC HCC
G81.92	Hemiplegia, unspecified affecting left dominant side	CC HCC
G81.93	Hemiplegia, unspecified affecting right nondominant side	CC HCC
G81.94	Hemiplegia, unspecified affecting left nondominant side	CC HCC

✓4ᵗʰ **G82 Paraplegia (paraparesis) and quadriplegia (quadriparesis)**

> **NOTE** This category is to be used only when the listed conditions are reported without further specification, or are stated to be old or longstanding but of unspecified cause. The category is also for use in multiple coding to identify these conditions resulting from any cause

> **EXCLUDES 1** congenital cerebral palsy (G80.-)
> functional quadriplegia (R53.2)
> hysterical paralysis (F44.4)

✓5ᵗʰ **G82.2 Paraplegia**

> Paralysis of both lower limbs NOS
> Paraparesis (lower) NOS
> Paraplegia (lower) NOS
> **AHA:** 2017,3Q,3
> **CC Excl: For CC codes in subcategory G82.2:** PDX collection 561

G82.20	Paraplegia, unspecified	CC HCC
G82.21	Paraplegia, complete	CC HCC
G82.22	Paraplegia, incomplete	CC HCC

✓5ᵗʰ **G82.5 Quadriplegia**

> **CC Excl: For MCC codes in subcategory G82.5:** PDX collection 595

G82.50	Quadriplegia, unspecified	MCC HCC
G82.51	Quadriplegia, C1-C4 complete	MCC HCC
G82.52	Quadriplegia, C1-C4 incomplete	MCC HCC

| G82.53 | Quadriplegia, C5-C7 complete | MCC HCC |
| G82.54 | Quadriplegia, C5-C7 incomplete | MCC HCC |

✓4ᵗʰ **G83 Other paralytic syndromes**

> **NOTE** This category is to be used only when the listed conditions are reported without further specification, or are stated to be old or longstanding but of unspecified cause. The category is also for use in multiple coding to identify these conditions resulting from any cause.

> **INCLUDES** paralysis (complete) (incomplete), except as in G80-G82

G83.0 Diplegia of upper limbs   CC HCC

> Diplegia (upper)
> Paralysis of both upper limbs
> **CC Excl:** PDX collection 599

✓5ᵗʰ **G83.1 Monoplegia of lower limb**

> Paralysis of lower limb

> **EXCLUDES 1** monoplegia of lower limbs due to sequela of cerebrovascular disease (I69.04-, I69.14-, I69.24-, I69.34-, I69.84-, I69.94-)

> **TIP:** If the documentation specifies the affected side but not whether it is the dominant or nondominant side, the default is as follows: for ambidextrous patients, the default is dominant; when the left side is affected, the default is nondominant; and when the right side is affected, the default is dominant.

G83.10	Monoplegia of lower limb affecting unspecified side	HCC
G83.11	Monoplegia of lower limb affecting right dominant side	HCC
G83.12	Monoplegia of lower limb affecting left dominant side	HCC
G83.13	Monoplegia of lower limb affecting right nondominant side	HCC
G83.14	Monoplegia of lower limb affecting left nondominant side	HCC

✓5ᵗʰ **G83.2 Monoplegia of upper limb**

> Paralysis of upper limb

> **EXCLUDES 1** monoplegia of upper limbs due to sequela of cerebrovascular disease (I69.03-, I69.13-, I69.23-, I69.33-, I69.83-, I69.93-)

> **TIP:** If the documentation specifies the affected side but not whether it is the dominant or nondominant side, the default is as follows: for ambidextrous patients, the default is dominant; when the left side is affected, the default is nondominant; and when the right side is affected, the default is dominant.

G83.20	Monoplegia of upper limb affecting unspecified side	HCC
G83.21	Monoplegia of upper limb affecting right dominant side	HCC
G83.22	Monoplegia of upper limb affecting left dominant side	HCC
G83.23	Monoplegia of upper limb affecting right nondominant side	HCC
G83.24	Monoplegia of upper limb affecting left nondominant side	HCC

✓5ᵗʰ **G83.3 Monoplegia, unspecified**

> **TIP:** If the documentation specifies the affected side but not whether it is the dominant or nondominant side, the default is as follows: for ambidextrous patients, the default is dominant; when the left side is affected, the default is nondominant; and when the right side is affected, the default is dominant.

G83.30	Monoplegia, unspecified affecting unspecified side	HCC
G83.31	Monoplegia, unspecified affecting right dominant side	HCC
G83.32	Monoplegia, unspecified affecting left dominant side	HCC
G83.33	Monoplegia, unspecified affecting right nondominant side	HCC
G83.34	Monoplegia, unspecified affecting left nondominant side	HCC

✔ Additional Character Required   ✓x7ᵗʰ Placeholder   Unacceptable PDx   Questionable PDx   Manifestation   Unspecified Dx   H1-H14 HAC   HCC CMS-HCC Dx   HIV HIV Dx

ICD-10-CM 2020   587

G83.4　Cauda equina syndrome `CC` `HCC`
Neurogenic bladder due to cauda equina syndrome
> *EXCLUDES 1*　cord bladder NOS (G95.89)
> neurogenic bladder NOS (N31.9)

DEF: Compression of the spinal nerve roots presenting with pain and tingling radiating down the buttocks, back of the thigh and calf, and into the foot in a sciatic manner with aching in the bladder, perineum, and sacrum. Loss of bowel and bladder control may also occur.
CC Excl: PDX collection 600

G83.5　Locked-in state `MCC` `HCC`
CC Excl: PDX collection 601

✓5ᵗʰ **G83.8　Other specified paralytic syndromes**
> *EXCLUDES 1*　paralytic syndromes due to current spinal cord injury — code to spinal cord injury (S14, S24, S34)

　　G83.81　Brown-Séquard syndrome `HCC`
　　G83.82　Anterior cord syndrome `HCC`
　　G83.83　Posterior cord syndrome `HCC`
　　G83.84　Todd's paralysis (postepileptic) `HCC`
　　G83.89　Other specified paralytic syndromes `HCC`
G83.9　Paralytic syndrome, unspecified `HCC`

Other disorders of the nervous system (G89-G99)

✓4ᵗʰ **G89　Pain, not elsewhere classified**
Code also related psychological factors associated with pain (F45.42)
> *EXCLUDES 1*　generalized pain NOS (R52)
> pain disorders exclusively related to psychological factors (F45.41)
> pain NOS (R52)
> *EXCLUDES 2*　atypical face pain (G50.1)
> headache syndromes (G44.-)
> localized pain, unspecified type — code to pain by site, such as:
> > abdomen pain (R10.-)
> > back pain (M54.9)
> > breast pain (N64.4)
> > chest pain (R07.1-R07.9)
> > ear pain (H92.0-)
> > eye pain (H57.1)
> > headache (R51)
> > joint pain (M25.5-)
> > limb pain (M79.6-)
> > lumbar region pain (M54.5)
> > painful urination (R30.9)
> > pelvic and perineal pain (R10.2)
> > renal colic (N23)
> > shoulder pain (M25.51-)
> > spine pain (M54.-)
> > throat pain (R07.0)
> > tongue pain (K14.6)
> > tooth pain (K08.8)
> migraines (G43.-)
> myalgia (M79.1-)
> pain from prosthetic devices, implants, and grafts (T82.84, T83.84, T84.84, T85.84-)
> phantom limb syndrome with pain (G54.6)
> vulvar vestibulitis (N94.810)
> vulvodynia (N94.81-)

　　G89.0　Central pain syndrome
　　Déjérine-Roussy syndrome
　　Myelopathic pain syndrome
　　Thalamic pain syndrome (hyperesthetic)

✓5ᵗʰ **G89.1　Acute pain, not elsewhere classified**
　　G89.11　Acute pain due to trauma
　　G89.12　Acute post-thoracotomy pain
　　　　Post-thoracotomy pain NOS
　　G89.18　Other acute postprocedural pain
　　　　Postoperative pain NOS
　　　　Postprocedural pain NOS

✓5ᵗʰ **G89.2　Chronic pain, not elsewhere classified**
> *EXCLUDES 1*　causalgia, lower limb (G57.7-)
> causalgia, upper limb (G56.4-)
> central pain syndrome (G89.0)
> chronic pain syndrome (G89.4)
> complex regional pain syndrome II, lower limb (G57.7-)
> complex regional pain syndrome II, upper limb (G56.4-)
> neoplasm related chronic pain (G89.3)
> reflex sympathetic dystrophy (G90.5-)

　　G89.21　Chronic pain due to trauma
　　G89.22　Chronic post-thoracotomy pain
　　G89.28　Other chronic postprocedural pain
　　　　Other chronic postoperative pain
　　G89.29　Other chronic pain
G89.3　Neoplasm related pain (acute) (chronic)
　　Cancer associated pain
　　Pain due to malignancy (primary) (secondary)
　　Tumor associated pain
G89.4　Chronic pain syndrome
　　Chronic pain associated with significant psychosocial dysfunction

✓4ᵗʰ **G90　Disorders of autonomic nervous system**
> *EXCLUDES 1*　dysfunction of the autonomic nervous system due to alcohol (G31.2)

✓5ᵗʰ **G90.0　Idiopathic peripheral autonomic neuropathy**
　　G90.01　Carotid sinus syncope
　　　　Carotid sinus syndrome
　　　　DEF: Vagal activation caused by pressure on the carotid sinus baroreceptors. Sympathetic nerve impulses may cause sinus arrest or AV block.
　　G90.09　Other idiopathic peripheral autonomic neuropathy
　　　　Idiopathic peripheral autonomic neuropathy NOS
G90.1　Familial dysautonomia [Riley-Day] `CC` `HCC`
G90.2　Horner's syndrome
　　Bernard(-Horner) syndrome
　　Cervical sympathetic dystrophy or paralysis
G90.3　Multi-system degeneration of the autonomic nervous system `CC` `HCC`
　　Neurogenic orthostatic hypotension [Shy-Drager]
> *EXCLUDES 1*　orthostatic hypotension NOS (I95.1)

　　CC Excl: PDX collection 573
G90.4　Autonomic dysreflexia
　　Use additional code to identify the cause, such as:
　　　fecal impaction (K56.41)
　　　pressure ulcer (pressure area) (L89.-)
　　　urinary tract infection (N39.0)

✓5ᵗʰ **G90.5　Complex regional pain syndrome I (CRPS I)**
　　Reflex sympathetic dystrophy
> *EXCLUDES 1*　causalgia of lower limb (G57.7-)
> causalgia of upper limb (G56.4-)
> complex regional pain syndrome II of lower limb (G57.7-)
> complex regional pain syndrome II of upper limb (G56.4-)

　　CC Excl: For CC codes in subcategory G90.5, unless otherwise noted: PDX collection 603

　　G90.50　Complex regional pain syndrome I, unspecified `CC`
　　　　CC Excl: PDX collection 602

✓6ᵗʰ **G90.51　Complex regional pain syndrome I of upper limb**
　　　　G90.511　Complex regional pain syndrome I of right upper limb `CC`
　　　　G90.512　Complex regional pain syndrome I of left upper limb `CC`
　　　　G90.513　Complex regional pain syndrome I of upper limb, bilateral `CC`
　　　　G90.519　Complex regional pain syndrome I of unspecified upper limb `CC`

`N` Newborn: 0　　`P` Pediatric: 0-17　　`M` Maternity: 9-64　　`A` Adult: 15-124　　`MCC` Major Complication/Comorbidity　　`CC` Complication/Comorbidity　　`SW` Severe Wound Dx

✓6ᵗʰ **G90.52** **Complex regional pain syndrome I of** lower limb

     G90.521 **Complex regional pain syndrome I of** right **lower limb** `CC`

     G90.522 **Complex regional pain syndrome I of** left **lower limb** `CC`

     G90.523 **Complex regional pain syndrome I of lower limb,** bilateral `CC`

     G90.529 **Complex regional pain syndrome I of unspecified lower limb** `CC`

   G90.59 **Complex regional pain syndrome I of other specified site** `CC`

G90.8 **Other disorders of autonomic nervous system**

G90.9 **Disorder of the autonomic nervous system, unspecified**

✓4ᵗʰ **G91** **Hydrocephalus**

   `INCLUDES` acquired hydrocephalus

   `EXCLUDES 1` *Arnold-Chiari syndrome with hydrocephalus (Q07.-)*
        congenital hydrocephalus (Q03.-)
        spina bifida with hydrocephalus (Q05.-)

   DEF: Abnormal buildup of cerebrospinal fluid in the brain causing dilation of the ventricles.

   CC Excl: For CC codes in category G91, unless otherwise noted: PDX collection 605

Hydrocephalus (Acquired)

Normal ventricles   Hydrocephalic ventricles

G91.0 **Communicating hydrocephalus** `CC` `HCC`

   Secondary normal pressure hydrocephalus
   CC Excl: PDX collection 604

G91.1 **Obstructive hydrocephalus** `CC` `HCC`

   DEF: Obstruction of the cerebrospinal fluid passage from the brain into the spinal canal characterized by headaches, drowsiness, poor coordination, urinary incontinence, nausea, vomiting, and papilledema.

G91.2 **(Idiopathic) normal pressure hydrocephalus** `CC` `HCC`

   Normal pressure hydrocephalus NOS
   CC Excl: PDX collection 604

G91.3 **Post-traumatic hydrocephalus, unspecified** `CC` `HCC`

G91.4 *Hydrocephalus in diseases classified elsewhere* `HCC`

   Code first underlying condition, such as:
     congenital syphilis (A50.4-)
     neoplasm (C00-D49)
     plasminogen deficiency (E88.02)
     `EXCLUDES 1` *hydrocephalus due to congenital toxoplasmosis (P37.1)*
   AHA: 2014,3Q,3

G91.8 **Other hydrocephalus** `CC` `HCC`

G91.9 **Hydrocephalus, unspecified** `CC` `HCC`

G92 **Toxic encephalopathy** `MCC`

   Toxic encephalitis
   Toxic metabolic encephalopathy
   Code first, if applicable, drug induced (T36-T50)
   Code first (T51-T65) to identify toxic agent
   AHA: 2017,1Q,39-40
   DEF: Brain tissue degeneration due to a toxic substance.
   CC Excl: PDX collection 606

✓4ᵗʰ **G93** **Other disorders of brain**

G93.0 **Cerebral cysts**

   Arachnoid cyst
   Porencephalic cyst, acquired
   `EXCLUDES 1` *acquired periventricular cysts of newborn (P91.1)*
     congenital cerebral cysts (Q04.6)

G93.1 **Anoxic brain damage, not elsewhere classified** `CC` `HCC`

   `EXCLUDES 1` *cerebral anoxia due to anesthesia during labor and delivery (O74.3)*
     cerebral anoxia due to anesthesia during the puerperium (O89.2)
     neonatal anoxia (P84)

   DEF: Brain injury not resulting from birth trauma that is due to lack of oxygen. Brain cells, when deprived of oxygen; begin to expire after 4 minutes.
   CC Excl: PDX collection 607

G93.2 **Benign intracranial hypertension**

   `EXCLUDES 1` *hypertensive encephalopathy (I67.4)*

G93.3 **Postviral fatigue syndrome**

   Benign myalgic encephalomyelitis
   `EXCLUDES 1` *chronic fatigue syndrome NOS (R53.82)*

✓5ᵗʰ **G93.4** **Other and unspecified encephalopathy**

   `EXCLUDES 1` *alcoholic encephalopathy (G31.2)*
     encephalopathy in diseases classified elsewhere (G94)
     hypertensive encephalopathy (I67.4)
     toxic (metabolic) encephalopathy (G92)

   G93.40 **Encephalopathy, unspecified** `HIV` `CC`

     AHA: 2017,2Q,8
     CC Excl: PDX collection 608

   G93.41 **Metabolic encephalopathy** `HIV` `MCC`

     Septic encephalopathy
     AHA: 2017,2Q,8; 2016,3Q,42; 2015,3Q,21
     TIP: Assign separately when documented with diabetic hypoglycemia (E08.649, E09.649, E10.649, E11.649, E13.649).
     CC Excl: PDX collection 609

   G93.49 **Other encephalopathy** `HIV` `CC`

     Encephalopathy NEC
     AHA: 2018,4Q,16; 2018,2Q,22,24; 2017,2Q,9
     CC Excl: PDX collection 610

G93.5 **Compression of brain** `CC` `HCC`

   Arnold-Chiari type 1 compression of brain
   Compression of brain (stem)
   Herniation of brain (stem)
   `EXCLUDES 1` *diffuse traumatic compression of brain (S06.2-)*
     focal traumatic compression of brain (S06.3-)

G93.6 **Cerebral edema** `MCC` `HCC`

   `EXCLUDES 1` *cerebral edema due to birth injury (P11.0)*
     traumatic cerebral edema (S06.1-)
   CC Excl: PDX collection 612

G93.7 **Reye's syndrome** `MCC` `HCC` `P`

   Code first poisoning due to salicylates, if applicable (T39.0-, with sixth character 1-4)
   Use additional code for adverse effect due to salicylates, if applicable (T39.0-, with sixth character 5)
   DEF: Rare childhood illness often developed after a viral upper respiratory infection. Symptoms include vomiting, elevated serum transaminase, brain swelling, disturbances of consciousness, seizures, and changes in liver and other viscera and it can be fatal.
   CC Excl: PDX collection 613

✓5ᵗʰ **G93.8** **Other specified disorders of brain**

   G93.81 **Temporal sclerosis**

     Hippocampal sclerosis
     Mesial temporal sclerosis

   G93.82 **Brain death** `CC`

G93.89   **Other specified disorders of brain**
Postradiation encephalopathy

G93.9   **Disorder of brain, unspecified**   HIV

G94   Other disorders of brain in diseases classified elsewhere
Code first underlying disease
EXCLUDES 1   *encephalopathy in congenital syphilis (A50.49)*
     encephalopathy in influenza (J09.X9, J10.81, J11.81)
     encephalopathy in syphilis (A52.19)
     hydrocephalus in diseases classified elsewhere (G91.4)
AHA: 2018,2Q,22; 2017,2Q,8-9

✓4th G95   Other and unspecified diseases of spinal cord
EXCLUDES 2   *myelitis (G04.-)*

G95.0   **Syringomyelia and syringobulbia**   CC HCC
CC Excl: PDX collection 614

✓5th **G95.1**   **Vascular myelopathies**
EXCLUDES 2   *intraspinal phlebitis and thrombophlebitis, except*
     non-pyogenic (G08)

G95.11   **Acute infarction of spinal cord**   MCC HCC
(embolic) (nonembolic)
Anoxia of spinal cord
Arterial thrombosis of spinal cord
CC Excl: PDX collection 603

G95.19   **Other vascular myelopathies**   CC HCC
Edema of spinal cord
Hematomyelia
Nonpyogenic intraspinal phlebitis and
     thrombophlebitis
Subacute necrotic myelopathy

✓5th **G95.2**   **Other and unspecified cord compression**

G95.20   **Unspecified cord compression**   HIV CC HCC
CC Excl: PDX collection 615

G95.29   **Other cord compression**   HIV CC HCC
CC Excl: PDX collection 615

✓5th **G95.8**   **Other specified diseases of spinal cord**
EXCLUDES 1   *neurogenic bladder NOS (N31.9)*
     neurogenic bladder due to cauda equina syndrome
       (G83.4)
     neuromuscular dysfunction of bladder without spinal
       cord lesion (N31.-)

G95.81   **Conus medullaris syndrome**   CC HCC
CC Excl: PDX collection 603

G95.89   **Other specified diseases of spinal**   CC HCC
cord
Cord bladder NOS
Drug-induced myelopathy
Radiation-induced myelopathy
EXCLUDES 1   *myelopathy NOS (G95.9)*
CC Excl: PDX collection 603

G95.9   **Disease of spinal cord, unspecified**   HIV CC HCC
Myelopathy NOS
CC Excl: PDX collection 615

✓4th G96   Other disorders of central nervous system
G96.0   **Cerebrospinal fluid leak**   CC
EXCLUDES 1   *cerebrospinal fluid leak from spinal puncture (G97.0)*
AHA: 2018,2Q,13
DEF: Cerebrospinal fluid discharging from the nose or the ear
caused by a fracture of the frontal bone with tearing of dura mater
and arachnoid. It is characterized by watery drainage usually from
only one side of the nose or one ear, headache, vision changes,
and hearing loss.
CC Excl: PDX collection 616

✓5th **G96.1**   **Disorders of meninges, not elsewhere classified**

G96.11   **Dural tear**   CC
EXCLUDES 1   *accidental puncture or laceration of dura*
     during a procedure (G97.41)
AHA: 2014,4Q,24
CC Excl: PDX collection 509

G96.12   **Meningeal adhesions (cerebral) (spinal)**

G96.19   **Other disorders of meninges, not elsewhere**
classified

G96.8   **Other specified disorders of central nervous system**

G96.9   **Disorder of central nervous system,**   HIV
unspecified

✓4th G97   Intraoperative and postprocedural complications and disorders of nervous system, not elsewhere classified
EXCLUDES 2   *intraoperative and postprocedural cerebrovascular infarction*
     (I97.81-, I97.82-)
AHA: 2016,4Q,9-10

G97.0   **Cerebrospinal fluid leak from spinal puncture**   CC
CC Excl: PDX collection 617

Spinal Puncture

Spinal cord
Epidural space
Subarachnoid space
Vertebra
Spinal needle

Lumbar area

G97.1   **Other reaction to spinal and lumbar puncture**
Headache due to lumbar puncture

G97.2   **Intracranial hypotension following ventricular**   CC
shunting
CC Excl: PDX collection 617

✓5th **G97.3**   **Intraoperative hemorrhage and hematoma of a nervous**
system organ or structure complicating a procedure
EXCLUDES 1   *intraoperative hemorrhage and hematoma of a*
     nervous system organ or structure due to
     accidental puncture and laceration during a
     procedure (G97.4-)

G97.31   **Intraoperative hemorrhage and**   CC
hematoma of a nervous system
organ or structure complicating a
nervous system procedure
CC Excl: PDX collection 618

G97.32   **Intraoperative hemorrhage and**   CC
hematoma of a nervous system
organ or structure complicating
other procedure
CC Excl: PDX collection 618

✓5th **G97.4**   **Accidental puncture and laceration of a nervous system**
organ or structure during a procedure
CC Excl: For CC codes in subcategory G97.4: PDX collection 509

G97.41   **Accidental puncture or laceration of**   CC
dura during a procedure
Incidental (inadvertent) durotomy
AHA: 2014,4Q,24

G97.48   **Accidental puncture and laceration**   CC
of other nervous system organ or
structure during a nervous system
procedure

G97.49   **Accidental puncture and laceration**   CC
of other nervous system organ or
structure during other procedure

✓5th **G97.5**   **Postprocedural hemorrhage of a nervous system organ or**
structure following a procedure

G97.51   **Postprocedural hemorrhage of a**   CC
nervous system organ or structure
following a nervous system
procedure
CC Excl: PDX collection 619

G97.52   **Postprocedural hemorrhage of a**   CC
nervous system organ or structure
following other procedure
CC Excl: PDX collection 619

✓5ᵗʰ **G97.6** Postprocedural hematoma and seroma **of a nervous system organ or structure following a procedure**
>> **CC Excl: For CC codes in subcategory G97.6:** PDX collection 619

> **G97.61** **Postprocedural** hematoma **of a nervous system organ or structure following a** nervous system procedure   `CC`

> **G97.62** **Postprocedural** hematoma **of a nervous system organ or structure following** other procedure   `CC`

> **G97.63** **Postprocedural** seroma **of a nervous system organ or structure following a** nervous system procedure   `CC`

> **G97.64** **Postprocedural** seroma **of a nervous system organ or structure following** other procedure   `CC`

✓5ᵗʰ **G97.8** **Other intraoperative and postprocedural complications and disorders of nervous system**
> Use additional code to further specify disorder

> **G97.81** **Other intraoperative complications of nervous system**   `CC`
>> **CC Excl:** PDX collection 617

> **G97.82** **Other postprocedural complications and disorders of nervous system**   `CC`
>> **CC Excl:** PDX collection 617

✓4ᵗʰ **G98** **Other disorders of nervous system not elsewhere classified**
> [INCLUDES]   nervous system disorder NOS

> **G98.0** **Neurogenic arthritis, not elsewhere classified**
> Nonsyphilitic neurogenic arthropathy NEC
> Nonsyphilitic neurogenic spondylopathy NEC
>> [EXCLUDES 1]   *spondylopathy (in):*
>>> *syringomyelia and syringobulbia (G95.0)*
>>> *tabes dorsalis (A52.11)*

> **G98.8** **Other disorders of nervous system**   `HIV`
> Nervous system disorder NOS

✓4ᵗʰ **G99** **Other disorders of nervous system in diseases classified elsewhere**

> **G99.0** *Autonomic neuropathy in diseases classified*   `CC` *elsewhere*
> Code first underlying disease, such as:
> amyloidosis (E85.-)
> gout (M1A.-, M10.-)
> hyperthyroidism (E05.-)
>> [EXCLUDES 1]   *diabetic autonomic neuropathy (E08-E13 with .43)*
> **CC Excl:** PDX collection 620

> **G99.2** *Myelopathy in diseases classified elsewhere*   `CC` `HCC`
> Code first underlying disease, such as:
> neoplasm (C00-D49)
>> [EXCLUDES 1]   *myelopathy in:*
>>> *intervertebral disease (M50.0-, M51.0-)*
>>> *spondylosis (M47.0-, M47.1-)*
> **AHA:** 2018,3Q,18-19
> **TIP:** Use this code in addition to a spondylolisthesis code (M43.1-) or a spinal stenosis code (M48.0-) when either of these disorders is documented as the cause of the myelopathy.
> **CC Excl:** PDX collection 603

> **G99.8** *Other specified disorders of nervous system in diseases classified elsewhere*
> Code first underlying disorder, such as:
> amyloidosis (E85.-)
> avitaminosis (E56.9)
>> [EXCLUDES 1]   *nervous system involvement in:*
>>> *cysticercosis (B69.0)*
>>> *rubella (B06.0-)*
>>> *syphilis (A52.1-)*

Chapter 7. Diseases of the Eye and Adnexa (H00–H59)

Chapter-specific Guidelines with Coding Examples

The chapter-specific guidelines from the ICD-10-CM Official Guidelines for Coding and Reporting have been provided below. Along with these guidelines are coding examples, contained in the shaded boxes, that have been developed to help illustrate the coding and/or sequencing guidance found in these guidelines.

a. Glaucoma

1) Assigning glaucoma codes

Assign as many codes from category H40, Glaucoma, as needed to identify the type of glaucoma, the affected eye, and the glaucoma stage.

2) Bilateral glaucoma with same type and stage

When a patient has bilateral glaucoma and both eyes are documented as being the same type and stage, and there is a code for bilateral glaucoma, report only the code for the type of glaucoma, bilateral, with the seventh character for the stage.

> Bilateral severe stage pigmentary glaucoma
>
> **H40.1333   Pigmentary glaucoma, bilateral, severe stage**
>
> *Explanation*: In this scenario, the patient has the same type and stage of glaucoma in both eyes. As this type of glaucoma has a code for bilateral, assign only the code for the bilateral glaucoma with the seventh character for the stage.

When a patient has bilateral glaucoma and both eyes are documented as being the same type and stage, and the classification does not provide a code for bilateral glaucoma (i.e. subcategories H40.10 and H40.20) report only one code for the type of glaucoma with the appropriate seventh character for the stage.

> Bilateral open-angle glaucoma; not specified as to type and stage indeterminate in both eyes
>
> **H40.10X4   Unspecified open-angle glaucoma, indeterminate stage**
>
> *Explanation*: In this scenario, the patient has glaucoma of the same type and stage of both eyes, but there is no code specifically for bilateral glaucoma. Only one code is assigned with the appropriate seventh character for the stage.

3) Bilateral glaucoma stage with different types or stages

When a patient has bilateral glaucoma and each eye is documented as having a different type or stage, and the classification distinguishes laterality, assign the appropriate code for each eye rather than the code for bilateral glaucoma.

When a patient has bilateral glaucoma and each eye is documented as having a different type, and the classification does not distinguish laterality (i.e. subcategories H40.10 and H40.20), assign one code for each type of glaucoma with the appropriate seventh character for the stage.

> Documentation relates mild, unspecified primary angle-closure glaucoma of the left eye with mild unspecified open-angle glaucoma of the right eye
>
> **H40.20X1   Unspecified primary angle-closure glaucoma, mild stage**
>
> **H40.10X1   Unspecified open-angle glaucoma, mild stage**
>
> *Explanation*: In this scenario the patient has a different type of glaucoma in each eye and the classification does not distinguish laterality. A code for each type of glaucoma is assigned, each with the appropriate seventh character for the stage.

When a patient has bilateral glaucoma and each eye is documented as having the same type, but different stage, and the classification does not distinguish laterality (i.e. subcategories H40.10 and H40.20), assign a code for the type of glaucoma for each eye with the seventh character for the specific glaucoma stage documented for each eye.

> Bilateral open-angle glaucoma, not specified as to type; the right eye is documented to be in mild stage and the left eye as being in moderate stage
>
> **H40.10X1   Unspecified open-angle glaucoma, mild stage**
>
> **H40.10X2   Unspecified open-angle glaucoma, moderate stage**
>
> *Explanation*: In this scenario the patient has the same type of glaucoma in each eye but each eye is at a different stage, and the classification does not distinguish laterality at this subcategory level. Two codes are assigned; both codes represent the same type of glaucoma but each has a different seventh character identifying the appropriate stage for each eye.

4) Patient admitted with glaucoma and stage evolves during the admission

If a patient is admitted with glaucoma and the stage progresses during the admission, assign the code for highest stage documented.

> Patient admitted with mild low-tension glaucoma of the right eye, which progresses to moderate stage during the patient's stay
>
> **H40.1212   Low-tension glaucoma, right eye, moderate stage**
>
> *Explanation*: When the glaucoma stage progresses during an admission, assign only the code for the highest stage documented.

5) Indeterminate stage glaucoma

Assignment of the seventh character "4" for "indeterminate stage" should be based on the clinical documentation. The seventh character "4" is used for glaucomas whose stage cannot be clinically determined. This seventh character should not be confused with the seventh character "0", unspecified, which should be assigned when there is no documentation regarding the stage of the glaucoma.

b. Blindness

If "blindness" or "low vision" of both eyes is documented but the visual impairment category is not documented, assign code H54.3, Unqualified visual loss, both eyes. If "blindness" or "low vision" in one eye is documented but the visual impairment category is not documented, assign a code from H54.6-, Unqualified visual loss, one eye. If "blindness" or "visual loss" is documented without any information about whether one or both eyes are affected, assign code H54.7, Unspecified visual loss.

> Blindness in 89-year-old male
>
> **H54.7   Unspecified visual loss**
>
> *Explanation*: Blindness is stated, but there is no mention of whether one or both eyes are affected or the severity of this visual impairment.

Chapter 7. Diseases of the Eye and Adnexa

Chapter 7. Diseases of the Eye and Adnexa (H00–H59)

NOTE   Use an external cause code following the code for the eye condition, if applicable, to identify the cause of the eye condition

EXCLUDES 2   *certain conditions originating in the perinatal period (P04-P96)*
certain infectious and parasitic diseases (A00-B99)
complications of pregnancy, childbirth and the puerperium (O00-O9A)
congenital malformations, deformations, and chromosomal abnormalities (Q00-Q99)
diabetes mellitus related eye conditions (E09.3-, E10.3-, E11.3-, E13.3-)
endocrine, nutritional and metabolic diseases (E00-E88)
injury (trauma) of eye and orbit (S05.-)
injury, poisoning and certain other consequences of external causes (S00-T88)
neoplasms (C00-D49)
symptoms, signs and abnormal clinical and laboratory findings, not elsewhere classified (R00-R94)
syphilis related eye disorders (A50.01, A50.3-, A51.43, A52.71)

This chapter contains the following blocks:

H00-H05	Disorders of eyelid, lacrimal system and orbit
H10-H11	Disorders of conjunctiva
H15-H22	Disorders of sclera, cornea, iris and ciliary body
H25-H28	Disorders of lens
H30-H36	Disorders of choroid and retina
H40-H42	Glaucoma
H43-H44	Disorders of vitreous body and globe
H46-H47	Disorders of optic nerve and visual pathways
H49-H52	Disorders of ocular muscles, binocular movement, accommodation and refraction
H53-H54	Visual disturbances and blindness
H55-H57	Other disorders of eye and adnexa
H59	Intraoperative and postprocedural complications and disorders of eye and adnexa, not elsewhere classified

Disorders of eyelid, lacrimal system and orbit (H00-H05)

EXCLUDES 2   *open wound of eyelid (S01.1-)*
superficial injury of eyelid (S00.1-, S00.2-)

√4ᵗʰ **H00 Hordeolum and chalazion**

√5ᵗʰ   **H00.0 Hordeolum (externum) (internum) of eyelid**

DEF: Acute localized infection of the gland of Zeis (external hordeolum) or Molt or of the meibomian glands (internal hordeolum) of the orbit.

√6ᵗʰ   **H00.01 Hordeolum externum**

Hordeolum NOS
Stye

   H00.011 Hordeolum externum right upper **eyelid**
   H00.012 Hordeolum externum right lower **eyelid**
   H00.013 Hordeolum externum right eye, unspecified eyelid
   H00.014 Hordeolum externum left upper **eyelid**
   H00.015 Hordeolum externum left lower **eyelid**
   H00.016 Hordeolum externum left eye, unspecified eyelid
   H00.019 Hordeolum externum unspecified eye, unspecified eyelid

√6ᵗʰ   **H00.02 Hordeolum internum**

Infection of meibomian gland

   H00.021 Hordeolum internum right upper **eyelid**
   H00.022 Hordeolum internum right lower **eyelid**
   H00.023 Hordeolum internum right eye, unspecified eyelid
   H00.024 Hordeolum internum left upper **eyelid**
   H00.025 Hordeolum internum left lower **eyelid**
   H00.026 Hordeolum internum left eye, unspecified eyelid
   H00.029 Hordeolum internum unspecified eye, unspecified eyelid

√6ᵗʰ   **H00.03 Abscess of eyelid**

Furuncle of eyelid

   H00.031 Abscess of right upper **eyelid**
   H00.032 Abscess of right lower **eyelid**
   H00.033 Abscess of eyelid right eye, unspecified eyelid
   H00.034 Abscess of left upper **eyelid**
   H00.035 Abscess of left lower **eyelid**
   H00.036 Abscess of eyelid left eye, unspecified eyelid
   H00.039 Abscess of eyelid unspecified eye, unspecified eyelid

√5ᵗʰ **H00.1 Chalazion**

Meibomian (gland) cyst

EXCLUDES 2   *infected meibomian gland (H00.02-)*

DEF: Noninfectious, obstructive mass in the oil gland of the eyelid that results in a small chronic lump or inflammation.

   H00.11 Chalazion right upper **eyelid**
   H00.12 Chalazion right lower **eyelid**
   H00.13 Chalazion right eye, unspecified eyelid
   H00.14 Chalazion left upper **eyelid**
   H00.15 Chalazion left lower **eyelid**
   H00.16 Chalazion left eye, unspecified eyelid
   H00.19 Chalazion unspecified eye, unspecified eyelid

√4ᵗʰ **H01 Other inflammation of eyelid**

√5ᵗʰ   **H01.0 Blepharitis**

EXCLUDES 1   *blepharoconjunctivitis (H10.5-)*

√6ᵗʰ   **H01.00 Unspecified blepharitis**

AHA: 2018,4Q,13

   H01.001 Unspecified blepharitis right upper **eyelid**
   H01.002 Unspecified blepharitis right lower **eyelid**
   H01.003 Unspecified blepharitis right eye, unspecified eyelid
   H01.004 Unspecified blepharitis left upper **eyelid**
   H01.005 Unspecified blepharitis left lower **eyelid**
   H01.006 Unspecified blepharitis left eye, unspecified eyelid
   H01.009 Unspecified blepharitis unspecified eye, unspecified eyelid
   H01.00A Unspecified blepharitis right eye, upper and lower eyelids
   H01.00B Unspecified blepharitis left eye, upper and lower eyelids

√6ᵗʰ   **H01.01 Ulcerative blepharitis**

AHA: 2018,4Q,13

   H01.011 Ulcerative blepharitis right upper **eyelid**
   H01.012 Ulcerative blepharitis right lower **eyelid**
   H01.013 Ulcerative blepharitis right eye, unspecified eyelid
   H01.014 Ulcerative blepharitis left upper **eyelid**
   H01.015 Ulcerative blepharitis left lower **eyelid**
   H01.016 Ulcerative blepharitis left eye, unspecified eyelid
   H01.019 Ulcerative blepharitis unspecified eye, unspecified eyelid
   H01.01A Ulcerative blepharitis right eye, upper and lower eyelids
   H01.01B Ulcerative blepharitis left eye, upper and lower eyelids

√6ᵗʰ   **H01.02 Squamous blepharitis**

AHA: 2018,4Q,13

   H01.021 Squamous blepharitis right upper **eyelid**
   H01.022 Squamous blepharitis right lower **eyelid**
   H01.023 Squamous blepharitis right eye, unspecified eyelid
   H01.024 Squamous blepharitis left upper **eyelid**
   H01.025 Squamous blepharitis left lower **eyelid**
   H01.026 Squamous blepharitis left eye, unspecified eyelid
   H01.029 Squamous blepharitis unspecified eye, unspecified eyelid
   H01.02A Squamous blepharitis right eye, upper and lower eyelids
   H01.02B Squamous blepharitis left eye, upper and lower eyelids

√5ᵗʰ   **H01.1 Noninfectious dermatoses of eyelid**

√6ᵗʰ   **H01.11 Allergic dermatitis of eyelid**

Contact dermatitis of eyelid

   H01.111 Allergic dermatitis of right upper **eyelid**
   H01.112 Allergic dermatitis of right lower **eyelid**
   H01.113 Allergic dermatitis of right eye, unspecified eyelid
   H01.114 Allergic dermatitis of left upper **eyelid**
   H01.115 Allergic dermatitis of left lower **eyelid**
   H01.116 Allergic dermatitis of left eye, unspecified eyelid
   H01.119 Allergic dermatitis of unspecified eye, unspecified eyelid

N Newborn: 0   P Pediatric: 0-17   M Maternity: 9-64   A Adult: 15-124   **MCC** Major Complication/Comorbidity   **CC** Complication/Comorbidity   **SW** Severe Wound Dx

594   ICD-10-CM 2020

√6ᵗʰ **H01.12 Discoid lupus erythematosus of eyelid**
- H01.121 Discoid lupus erythematosus of right upper eyelid
- H01.122 Discoid lupus erythematosus of right lower eyelid
- H01.123 Discoid lupus erythematosus of right eye, unspecified eyelid
- H01.124 Discoid lupus erythematosus of left upper eyelid
- H01.125 Discoid lupus erythematosus of left lower eyelid
- H01.126 Discoid lupus erythematosus of left eye, unspecified eyelid
- H01.129 Discoid lupus erythematosus of unspecified eye, unspecified eyelid

√6ᵗʰ **H01.13 Eczematous dermatitis of eyelid**
- H01.131 Eczematous dermatitis of right upper eyelid
- H01.132 Eczematous dermatitis of right lower eyelid
- H01.133 Eczematous dermatitis of right eye, unspecified eyelid
- H01.134 Eczematous dermatitis of left upper eyelid
- H01.135 Eczematous dermatitis of left lower eyelid
- H01.136 Eczematous dermatitis of left eye, unspecified eyelid
- H01.139 Eczematous dermatitis of unspecified eye, unspecified eyelid

√6ᵗʰ **H01.14 Xeroderma of eyelid**
- H01.141 Xeroderma of right upper eyelid
- H01.142 Xeroderma of right lower eyelid
- H01.143 Xeroderma of right eye, unspecified eyelid
- H01.144 Xeroderma of left upper eyelid
- H01.145 Xeroderma of left lower eyelid
- H01.146 Xeroderma of left eye, unspecified eyelid
- H01.149 Xeroderma of unspecified eye, unspecified eyelid

H01.8 Other specified inflammations of eyelid

H01.9 Unspecified inflammation of eyelid
Inflammation of eyelid NOS

√4ᵗʰ **H02 Other disorders of eyelid**
EXCLUDES 1 congenital malformations of eyelid (Q10.0-Q10.3)

Entropion and Ectropion

Normal eyelid | Entropion | Ectropion

√5ᵗʰ **H02.0 Entropion and trichiasis of eyelid**
DEF: Entropion: Inversion of the eyelid, turning the edge in toward the eyeball and causing irritation from contact of the lashes with the surface of the eye.
DEF: Trichiasis: Condition wherein the eyelid is in a normal position but lashes are ingrown or misdirected in their growth so that they irritate the tissues of the eye.

√6ᵗʰ **H02.00 Unspecified entropion of eyelid**
- H02.001 Unspecified entropion of right upper eyelid
- H02.002 Unspecified entropion of right lower eyelid
- H02.003 Unspecified entropion of right eye, unspecified eyelid
- H02.004 Unspecified entropion of left upper eyelid
- H02.005 Unspecified entropion of left lower eyelid
- H02.006 Unspecified entropion of left eye, unspecified eyelid
- H02.009 Unspecified entropion of unspecified eye, unspecified eyelid

√6ᵗʰ **H02.01 Cicatricial entropion of eyelid**
- H02.011 Cicatricial entropion of right upper eyelid
- H02.012 Cicatricial entropion of right lower eyelid
- H02.013 Cicatricial entropion of right eye, unspecified eyelid
- H02.014 Cicatricial entropion of left upper eyelid
- H02.015 Cicatricial entropion of left lower eyelid
- H02.016 Cicatricial entropion of left eye, unspecified eyelid
- H02.019 Cicatricial entropion of unspecified eye, unspecified eyelid

√6ᵗʰ **H02.02 Mechanical entropion of eyelid**
- H02.021 Mechanical entropion of right upper eyelid
- H02.022 Mechanical entropion of right lower eyelid
- H02.023 Mechanical entropion of right eye, unspecified eyelid
- H02.024 Mechanical entropion of left upper eyelid
- H02.025 Mechanical entropion of left lower eyelid
- H02.026 Mechanical entropion of left eye, unspecified eyelid
- H02.029 Mechanical entropion of unspecified eye, unspecified eyelid

√6ᵗʰ **H02.03 Senile entropion of eyelid**
- H02.031 Senile entropion of right upper eyelid Ⓐ
- H02.032 Senile entropion of right lower eyelid Ⓐ
- H02.033 Senile entropion of right eye, unspecified eyelid Ⓐ
- H02.034 Senile entropion of left upper eyelid Ⓐ
- H02.035 Senile entropion of left lower eyelid Ⓐ
- H02.036 Senile entropion of left eye, unspecified eyelid Ⓐ
- H02.039 Senile entropion of unspecified eye, unspecified eyelid Ⓐ

√6ᵗʰ **H02.04 Spastic entropion of eyelid**
- H02.041 Spastic entropion of right upper eyelid
- H02.042 Spastic entropion of right lower eyelid
- H02.043 Spastic entropion of right eye, unspecified eyelid
- H02.044 Spastic entropion of left upper eyelid
- H02.045 Spastic entropion of left lower eyelid
- H02.046 Spastic entropion of left eye, unspecified eyelid
- H02.049 Spastic entropion of unspecified eye, unspecified eyelid

√6ᵗʰ **H02.05 Trichiasis without entropion**
- H02.051 Trichiasis without entropion right upper eyelid
- H02.052 Trichiasis without entropion right lower eyelid
- H02.053 Trichiasis without entropion right eye, unspecified eyelid
- H02.054 Trichiasis without entropion left upper eyelid
- H02.055 Trichiasis without entropion left lower eyelid
- H02.056 Trichiasis without entropion left eye, unspecified eyelid
- H02.059 Trichiasis without entropion unspecified eye, unspecified eyelid

√5ᵗʰ **H02.1 Ectropion of eyelid**
DEF: Drooping of the lower eyelid away from the eye or outward turning or eversion of the edge of the eyelid, exposing the palpebral conjunctiva and causing irritation.

√6ᵗʰ **H02.10 Unspecified ectropion of eyelid**
- H02.101 Unspecified ectropion of right upper eyelid
- H02.102 Unspecified ectropion of right lower eyelid
- H02.103 Unspecified ectropion of right eye, unspecified eyelid
- H02.104 Unspecified ectropion of left upper eyelid
- H02.105 Unspecified ectropion of left lower eyelid

Chapter 7. Diseases of the Eye and Adnexa

H02.106 Unspecified ectropion of left eye, unspecified eyelid
H02.109 Unspecified ectropion of unspecified eye, unspecified eyelid

✓6ᵗʰ **H02.11 Cicatricial ectropion of eyelid**
H02.111 Cicatricial ectropion of right upper eyelid
H02.112 Cicatricial ectropion of right lower eyelid
H02.113 Cicatricial ectropion of right eye, unspecified eyelid
H02.114 Cicatricial ectropion of left upper eyelid
H02.115 Cicatricial ectropion of left lower eyelid
H02.116 Cicatricial ectropion of left eye, unspecified eyelid
H02.119 Cicatricial ectropion of unspecified eye, unspecified eyelid

✓6ᵗʰ **H02.12 Mechanical ectropion of eyelid**
H02.121 Mechanical ectropion of right upper eyelid
H02.122 Mechanical ectropion of right lower eyelid
H02.123 Mechanical ectropion of right eye, unspecified eyelid
H02.124 Mechanical ectropion of left upper eyelid
H02.125 Mechanical ectropion of left lower eyelid
H02.126 Mechanical ectropion of left eye, unspecified eyelid
H02.129 Mechanical ectropion of unspecified eye, unspecified eyelid

✓6ᵗʰ **H02.13 Senile ectropion of eyelid**
H02.131 Senile ectropion of right upper eyelid   Ⓐ
H02.132 Senile ectropion of right lower eyelid   Ⓐ
H02.133 Senile ectropion of right eye, unspecified eyelid   Ⓐ
H02.134 Senile ectropion of left upper eyelid   Ⓐ
H02.135 Senile ectropion of left lower eyelid   Ⓐ
H02.136 Senile ectropion of left eye, unspecified eyelid   Ⓐ
H02.139 Senile ectropion of unspecified eye, unspecified eyelid   Ⓐ

✓6ᵗʰ **H02.14 Spastic ectropion of eyelid**
H02.141 Spastic ectropion of right upper eyelid
H02.142 Spastic ectropion of right lower eyelid
H02.143 Spastic ectropion of right eye, unspecified eyelid
H02.144 Spastic ectropion of left upper eyelid
H02.145 Spastic ectropion of left lower eyelid
H02.146 Spastic ectropion of left eye, unspecified eyelid
H02.149 Spastic ectropion of unspecified eye, unspecified eyelid

✓6ᵗʰ **H02.15 Paralytic ectropion of eyelid**
AHA: 2018,4Q,13
H02.151 Paralytic ectropion of right upper eyelid
H02.152 Paralytic ectropion of right lower eyelid
H02.153 Paralytic ectropion of right eye, unspecified eyelid
H02.154 Paralytic ectropion of left upper eyelid
H02.155 Paralytic ectropion of left lower eyelid
H02.156 Paralytic ectropion of left eye, unspecified eyelid
H02.159 Paralytic ectropion of unspecified eye, unspecified eyelid

✓5ᵗʰ **H02.2 Lagophthalmos**
AHA: 2018,4Q,14
DEF: Condition of the eye that prevents it from closing completely.

✓6ᵗʰ **H02.20 Unspecified lagophthalmos**
H02.201 Unspecified lagophthalmos right upper eyelid
H02.202 Unspecified lagophthalmos right lower eyelid
H02.203 Unspecified lagophthalmos right eye, unspecified eyelid
H02.204 Unspecified lagophthalmos left upper eyelid
H02.205 Unspecified lagophthalmos left lower eyelid
H02.206 Unspecified lagophthalmos left eye, unspecified eyelid
H02.209 Unspecified lagophthalmos unspecified eye, unspecified eyelid
H02.20A Unspecified lagophthalmos right eye, upper and lower eyelids
H02.20B Unspecified lagophthalmos left eye, upper and lower eyelids
H02.20C Unspecified lagophthalmos, bilateral, upper and lower eyelids

✓6ᵗʰ **H02.21 Cicatricial lagophthalmos**
H02.211 Cicatricial lagophthalmos right upper eyelid
H02.212 Cicatricial lagophthalmos right lower eyelid
H02.213 Cicatricial lagophthalmos right eye, unspecified eyelid
H02.214 Cicatricial lagophthalmos left upper eyelid
H02.215 Cicatricial lagophthalmos left lower eyelid
H02.216 Cicatricial lagophthalmos left eye, unspecified eyelid
H02.219 Cicatricial lagophthalmos unspecified eye, unspecified eyelid
H02.21A Cicatricial lagophthalmos right eye, upper and lower eyelids
H02.21B Cicatricial lagophthalmos left eye, upper and lower eyelids
H02.21C Cicatricial lagophthalmos, bilateral, upper and lower eyelids

✓6ᵗʰ **H02.22 Mechanical lagophthalmos**
H02.221 Mechanical lagophthalmos right upper eyelid
H02.222 Mechanical lagophthalmos right lower eyelid
H02.223 Mechanical lagophthalmos right eye, unspecified eyelid
H02.224 Mechanical lagophthalmos left upper eyelid
H02.225 Mechanical lagophthalmos left lower eyelid
H02.226 Mechanical lagophthalmos left eye, unspecified eyelid
H02.229 Mechanical lagophthalmos unspecified eye, unspecified eyelid
H02.22A Mechanical lagophthalmos right eye, upper and lower eyelids
H02.22B Mechanical lagophthalmos left eye, upper and lower eyelids
H02.22C Mechanical lagophthalmos, bilateral, upper and lower eyelids

✓6ᵗʰ **H02.23 Paralytic lagophthalmos**
H02.231 Paralytic lagophthalmos right upper eyelid
H02.232 Paralytic lagophthalmos right lower eyelid
H02.233 Paralytic lagophthalmos right eye, unspecified eyelid
H02.234 Paralytic lagophthalmos left upper eyelid
H02.235 Paralytic lagophthalmos left lower eyelid
H02.236 Paralytic lagophthalmos left eye, unspecified eyelid
H02.239 Paralytic lagophthalmos unspecified eye, unspecified eyelid
H02.23A Paralytic lagophthalmos right eye, upper and lower eyelids
H02.23B Paralytic lagophthalmos left eye, upper and lower eyelids
H02.23C Paralytic lagophthalmos, bilateral, upper and lower eyelids

✓5ᵗʰ **H02.3 Blepharochalasis**
Pseudoptosis
DEF: Loss of elasticity and relaxation of skin of the eyelid, thickened or indurated skin on the eyelid associated with recurrent episodes of edema, and intracellular atrophy.
H02.30 Blepharochalasis unspecified eye, unspecified eyelid
H02.31 Blepharochalasis right upper eyelid
H02.32 Blepharochalasis right lower eyelid
H02.33 Blepharochalasis right eye, unspecified eyelid
H02.34 Blepharochalasis left upper eyelid

H02.35   **Blepharochalasis** left lower eyelid

H02.36   **Blepharochalasis** left eye, unspecified eyelid

√6ᵗʰ **H02.4**   **Ptosis of eyelid**

    √6ᵗʰ **H02.40**   **Unspecified ptosis of eyelid**

         H02.401   **Unspecified ptosis of** right **eyelid**

         H02.402   **Unspecified ptosis of** left **eyelid**

         H02.403   **Unspecified ptosis of** bilateral **eyelids**

         H02.409   **Unspecified ptosis of** unspecified **eyelid**

    √6ᵗʰ **H02.41**   **Mechanical ptosis of eyelid**

         H02.411   **Mechanical ptosis of** right **eyelid**

         H02.412   **Mechanical ptosis of** left **eyelid**

         H02.413   **Mechanical ptosis of** bilateral **eyelids**

         H02.419   **Mechanical ptosis of** unspecified **eyelid**

    √6ᵗʰ **H02.42**   **Myogenic ptosis of eyelid**

         H02.421   **Myogenic ptosis of** right **eyelid**

         H02.422   **Myogenic ptosis of** left **eyelid**

         H02.423   **Myogenic ptosis of** bilateral **eyelids**

         H02.429   **Myogenic ptosis of** unspecified **eyelid**

    √6ᵗʰ **H02.43**   **Paralytic ptosis of eyelid**

         Neurogenic ptosis of eyelid

         H02.431   **Paralytic ptosis of** right **eyelid**

         H02.432   **Paralytic ptosis of** left **eyelid**

         H02.433   **Paralytic ptosis of** bilateral **eyelids**

         H02.439   **Paralytic ptosis unspecified eyelid**

√5ᵗʰ **H02.5**   **Other disorders affecting eyelid function**

     EXCLUDES 2   *blepharospasm (G24.5)*

           organic tic (G25.69)

           psychogenic tic (F95.-)

    √6ᵗʰ **H02.51**   **Abnormal innervation syndrome**

         H02.511   **Abnormal innervation syndrome** right upper **eyelid**

         H02.512   **Abnormal innervation syndrome** right lower **eyelid**

         H02.513   **Abnormal innervation syndrome** right eye, unspecified **eyelid**

         H02.514   **Abnormal innervation syndrome** left upper **eyelid**

         H02.515   **Abnormal innervation syndrome** left lower **eyelid**

         H02.516   **Abnormal innervation syndrome** left eye, unspecified **eyelid**

         H02.519   **Abnormal innervation syndrome** unspecified eye, unspecified **eyelid**

    √6ᵗʰ **H02.52**   **Blepharophimosis**

         Ankyloblepharon

         H02.521   **Blepharophimosis** right upper **eyelid**

         H02.522   **Blepharophimosis** right lower **eyelid**

         H02.523   **Blepharophimosis** right eye, unspecified **eyelid**

         H02.524   **Blepharophimosis** left upper **eyelid**

         H02.525   **Blepharophimosis** left lower **eyelid**

         H02.526   **Blepharophimosis** left eye, unspecified **eyelid**

         H02.529   **Blepharophimosis unspecified eye, unspecified lid**

    √6ᵗʰ **H02.53**   **Eyelid retraction**

         Eyelid lag

         H02.531   **Eyelid retraction** right upper **eyelid**

         H02.532   **Eyelid retraction** right lower **eyelid**

         H02.533   **Eyelid retraction** right eye, unspecified **eyelid**

         H02.534   **Eyelid retraction** left upper **eyelid**

         H02.535   **Eyelid retraction** left lower **eyelid**

         H02.536   **Eyelid retraction** left eye, unspecified **eyelid**

         H02.539   **Eyelid retraction unspecified eye, unspecified lid**

     H02.59   **Other disorders affecting eyelid function**

         Deficient blink reflex

         Sensory disorders

√5ᵗʰ **H02.6**   **Xanthelasma of eyelid**

     DEF: Condition in which there are small yellow tumors that occur on the eyelid, usually appearing near the nose.

     H02.60   **Xanthelasma of** unspecified eye, unspecified eyelid

     H02.61   **Xanthelasma of** right upper **eyelid**

     H02.62   **Xanthelasma of** right lower **eyelid**

     H02.63   **Xanthelasma of** right eye, unspecified eyelid

     H02.64   **Xanthelasma of** left upper **eyelid**

H02.65   **Xanthelasma of** left lower **eyelid**

H02.66   **Xanthelasma of** left eye, unspecified eyelid

√5ᵗʰ **H02.7**   **Other and unspecified degenerative disorders of eyelid and periocular area**

     H02.70   **Unspecified degenerative disorders of eyelid and periocular area**

    √6ᵗʰ **H02.71**   **Chloasma of eyelid and periocular area**

         Dyspigmentation of eyelid

         Hyperpigmentation of eyelid

         H02.711   **Chloasma of** right upper **eyelid and periocular area**

         H02.712   **Chloasma of** right lower **eyelid and periocular area**

         H02.713   **Chloasma of** right eye, unspecified eyelid **and periocular area**

         H02.714   **Chloasma of** left upper **eyelid and periocular area**

         H02.715   **Chloasma of** left lower **eyelid and periocular area**

         H02.716   **Chloasma of** left eye, unspecified eyelid **and periocular area**

         H02.719   **Chloasma of unspecified eye, unspecified eyelid and periocular area**

    √6ᵗʰ **H02.72**   **Madarosis of eyelid and periocular area**

         Hypotrichosis of eyelid

         H02.721   **Madarosis of** right upper **eyelid and periocular area**

         H02.722   **Madarosis of** right lower **eyelid and periocular area**

         H02.723   **Madarosis of** right eye, unspecified eyelid **and periocular area**

         H02.724   **Madarosis of** left upper **eyelid and periocular area**

         H02.725   **Madarosis of** left lower **eyelid and periocular area**

         H02.726   **Madarosis of** left eye, unspecified eyelid **and periocular area**

         H02.729   **Madarosis of unspecified eye, unspecified eyelid and periocular area**

    √6ᵗʰ **H02.73**   **Vitiligo of eyelid and periocular area**

         Hypopigmentation of eyelid

         H02.731   **Vitiligo of** right upper **eyelid and periocular area**

         H02.732   **Vitiligo of** right lower **eyelid and periocular area**

         H02.733   **Vitiligo of** right eye, unspecified eyelid **and periocular area**

         H02.734   **Vitiligo of** left upper **eyelid and periocular area**

         H02.735   **Vitiligo of** left lower **eyelid and periocular area**

         H02.736   **Vitiligo of** left eye, unspecified eyelid **and periocular area**

         H02.739   **Vitiligo of unspecified eye, unspecified eyelid and periocular area**

     H02.79   **Other degenerative disorders of eyelid and periocular area**

√5ᵗʰ **H02.8**   **Other specified disorders of eyelid**

    √6ᵗʰ **H02.81**   **Retained foreign body in eyelid**

         Use additional code to identify the type of retained foreign body (Z18.-)

         EXCLUDES 1   *laceration of eyelid with foreign body (S01.12-)*

            retained intraocular foreign body (H44.6-, H44.7-)

            superficial foreign body of eyelid and periocular area (S00.25-)

         H02.811   **Retained foreign body in** right upper **eyelid**

         H02.812   **Retained foreign body in** right lower **eyelid**

         H02.813   **Retained foreign body in** right eye, unspecified eyelid

         H02.814   **Retained foreign body in** left upper **eyelid**

         H02.815   **Retained foreign body in** left lower **eyelid**

         H02.816   **Retained foreign body in** left eye, unspecified eyelid

         H02.819   **Retained foreign body in unspecified eye, unspecified eyelid**

☑ Additional Character Required   √x7ᵗʰ Placeholder   Unacceptable PDx   Questionable PDx   Manifestation   Unspecified Dx   H1–H14 HAC   HCC CMS-HCC Dx   HIV HIV Dx

ICD-10-CM 2020   597

Chapter 7. Diseases of the Eye and Adnexa

H02.82–H04.149

√6ᵗʰ **H02.82 Cysts** of eyelid
> Sebaceous cyst of eyelid
> **H02.821 Cysts** of right upper **eyelid**
> **H02.822 Cysts** of right lower **eyelid**
> **H02.823 Cysts** of right eye, unspecified **eyelid**
> **H02.824 Cysts** of left upper **eyelid**
> **H02.825 Cysts** of left lower **eyelid**
> **H02.826 Cysts** of left eye, unspecified **eyelid**
> **H02.829 Cysts** of unspecified eye, unspecified eyelid

√6ᵗʰ **H02.83 Dermatochalasis** of eyelid
> **DEF:** Acquired form of connective tissue disorder associated with decreased elastic tissue and abnormal elastin formation, resulting in loss of elasticity of the skin of the eyelid. It is generally associated with aging.
> **H02.831 Dermatochalasis** of right upper **eyelid**
> **H02.832 Dermatochalasis** of right lower **eyelid**
> **H02.833 Dermatochalasis** of right eye, unspecified eyelid
> **H02.834 Dermatochalasis** of left upper **eyelid**
> **H02.835 Dermatochalasis** of left lower **eyelid**
> **H02.836 Dermatochalasis** of left eye, unspecified eyelid
> **H02.839 Dermatochalasis** of unspecified eye, unspecified eyelid

√6ᵗʰ **H02.84 Edema** of eyelid
> Hyperemia of eyelid
> **H02.841 Edema** of right upper **eyelid**
> **H02.842 Edema** of right lower **eyelid**
> **H02.843 Edema** of right eye, unspecified eyelid
> **H02.844 Edema** of left upper **eyelid**
> **H02.845 Edema** of left lower **eyelid**
> **H02.846 Edema** of left eye, unspecified eyelid
> **H02.849 Edema** of unspecified eye, unspecified eyelid

√6ᵗʰ **H02.85 Elephantiasis** of eyelid
> **H02.851 Elephantiasis** of right upper **eyelid**
> **H02.852 Elephantiasis** of right lower **eyelid**
> **H02.853 Elephantiasis** of right eye, unspecified eyelid
> **H02.854 Elephantiasis** of left upper **eyelid**
> **H02.855 Elephantiasis** of left lower **eyelid**
> **H02.856 Elephantiasis** of left eye, unspecified eyelid
> **H02.859 Elephantiasis** of unspecified eye, unspecified eyelid

√6ᵗʰ **H02.86 Hypertrichosis** of eyelid
> **H02.861 Hypertrichosis** of right upper **eyelid**
> **H02.862 Hypertrichosis** of right lower **eyelid**
> **H02.863 Hypertrichosis** of right eye, unspecified eyelid
> **H02.864 Hypertrichosis** of left upper **eyelid**
> **H02.865 Hypertrichosis** of left lower **eyelid**
> **H02.866 Hypertrichosis** of left eye, unspecified eyelid
> **H02.869 Hypertrichosis** of unspecified eye, unspecified eyelid

√6ᵗʰ **H02.87 Vascular anomalies** of eyelid
> **H02.871 Vascular anomalies** of right upper **eyelid**
> **H02.872 Vascular anomalies** of right lower **eyelid**
> **H02.873 Vascular anomalies** of right eye, unspecified eyelid
> **H02.874 Vascular anomalies** of left upper **eyelid**
> **H02.875 Vascular anomalies** of left lower **eyelid**
> **H02.876 Vascular anomalies** of left eye, unspecified eyelid
> **H02.879 Vascular anomalies** of unspecified eye, unspecified eyelid

√6ᵗʰ **H02.88 Meibomian gland dysfunction** of eyelid
> **AHA:** 2018,4Q,14-15
> **H02.881 Meibomian gland dysfunction** right upper eyelid
> **H02.882 Meibomian gland dysfunction** right lower eyelid
> **H02.883 Meibomian gland dysfunction** of right eye, unspecified eyelid
> **H02.884 Meibomian gland dysfunction** left upper eyelid
> **H02.885 Meibomian gland dysfunction** left lower eyelid

H02.886 Meibomian gland dysfunction of left eye, unspecified eyelid
H02.889 Meibomian gland dysfunction of unspecified eye, unspecified eyelid
H02.88A Meibomian gland dysfunction right eye, upper and lower **eyelids**
H02.88B Meibomian gland dysfunction left eye, upper and lower **eyelids**

H02.89 Other specified disorders of eyelid
> Hemorrhage of eyelid

H02.9 Unspecified disorder of eyelid
> Disorder of eyelid NOS

√4ᵗʰ **H04 Disorders of lacrimal system**
> **EXCLUDES 1**   *congenital malformations of lacrimal system (Q10.4-Q10.6)*

√5ᵗʰ **H04.0 Dacryoadenitis**
> **DEF:** Inflammation of the lacrimal gland.

√6ᵗʰ **H04.00 Unspecified dacryoadenitis**
> **H04.001 Unspecified dacryoadenitis,** right **lacrimal gland**
> **H04.002 Unspecified dacryoadenitis,** left **lacrimal gland**
> **H04.003 Unspecified dacryoadenitis,** bilateral **lacrimal glands**
> **H04.009 Unspecified dacryoadenitis, unspecified lacrimal gland**

√6ᵗʰ **H04.01 Acute dacryoadenitis**
> **H04.011 Acute dacryoadenitis,** right **lacrimal gland**
> **H04.012 Acute dacryoadenitis,** left **lacrimal gland**
> **H04.013 Acute dacryoadenitis,** bilateral **lacrimal glands**
> **H04.019 Acute dacryoadenitis, unspecified lacrimal gland**

√6ᵗʰ **H04.02 Chronic dacryoadenitis**
> **H04.021 Chronic dacryoadenitis,** right **lacrimal gland**
> **H04.022 Chronic dacryoadenitis,** left **lacrimal gland**
> **H04.023 Chronic dacryoadenitis,** bilateral **lacrimal gland**
> **H04.029 Chronic dacryoadenitis, unspecified lacrimal gland**

√6ᵗʰ **H04.03 Chronic enlargement of lacrimal gland**
> **H04.031 Chronic enlargement of** right **lacrimal gland**
> **H04.032 Chronic enlargement of** left **lacrimal gland**
> **H04.033 Chronic enlargement of** bilateral **lacrimal glands**
> **H04.039 Chronic enlargement of unspecified lacrimal gland**

√5ᵗʰ **H04.1 Other disorders of lacrimal gland**

√6ᵗʰ **H04.11 Dacryops**
> **H04.111 Dacryops of** right **lacrimal gland**
> **H04.112 Dacryops of** left **lacrimal gland**
> **H04.113 Dacryops of** bilateral **lacrimal glands**
> **H04.119 Dacryops of unspecified lacrimal gland**

√6ᵗʰ **H04.12 Dry eye syndrome**
> Tear film insufficiency, NOS
> **H04.121 Dry eye syndrome of** right **lacrimal gland**
> **H04.122 Dry eye syndrome of** left **lacrimal gland**
> **H04.123 Dry eye syndrome of** bilateral **lacrimal glands**
> **H04.129 Dry eye syndrome of unspecified lacrimal gland**

√6ᵗʰ **H04.13 Lacrimal cyst**
> Lacrimal cystic degeneration
> **H04.131 Lacrimal cyst,** right **lacrimal gland**
> **H04.132 Lacrimal cyst,** left **lacrimal gland**
> **H04.133 Lacrimal cyst,** bilateral **lacrimal glands**
> **H04.139 Lacrimal cyst, unspecified lacrimal gland**

√6ᵗʰ **H04.14 Primary lacrimal gland atrophy**
> **H04.141 Primary lacrimal gland atrophy,** right **lacrimal gland**
> **H04.142 Primary lacrimal gland atrophy,** left **lacrimal gland**
> **H04.143 Primary lacrimal gland atrophy,** bilateral **lacrimal glands**
> **H04.149 Primary lacrimal gland atrophy, unspecified lacrimal gland**

N Newborn: 0   P Pediatric: 0-17   M Maternity: 9-64   A Adult: 15-124   MCC Major Complication/Comorbidity   CC Complication/Comorbidity   SW Severe Wound Dx

598   ICD-10-CM 2020

✓6ᵗʰ **H04.15** Secondary lacrimal gland atrophy

    H04.151 Secondary lacrimal gland atrophy, right lacrimal gland

    H04.152 Secondary lacrimal gland atrophy, left lacrimal gland

    H04.153 Secondary lacrimal gland atrophy, bilateral lacrimal glands

    H04.159 Secondary lacrimal gland atrophy, unspecified lacrimal gland

✓6ᵗʰ **H04.16** Lacrimal gland dislocation

    H04.161 Lacrimal gland dislocation, right lacrimal gland

    H04.162 Lacrimal gland dislocation, left lacrimal gland

    H04.163 Lacrimal gland dislocation, bilateral lacrimal glands

    H04.169 Lacrimal gland dislocation, unspecified lacrimal gland

  H04.19 Other specified disorders of lacrimal gland

✓5ᵗʰ **H04.2** Epiphora

    DEF: Excessive tearing or overflow of tears down the cheeks often due to a stricture in the lacrimal passages but can be caused by other conditions.

✓6ᵗʰ **H04.20** Unspecified epiphora

    H04.201 Unspecified epiphora, right side

    H04.202 Unspecified epiphora, left side

    H04.203 Unspecified epiphora, bilateral

    H04.209 Unspecified epiphora, unspecified side

✓6ᵗʰ **H04.21** Epiphora due to excess lacrimation

    H04.211 Epiphora due to excess lacrimation, right lacrimal gland

    H04.212 Epiphora due to excess lacrimation, left lacrimal gland

    H04.213 Epiphora due to excess lacrimation, bilateral lacrimal glands

    H04.219 Epiphora due to excess lacrimation, unspecified lacrimal gland

✓6ᵗʰ **H04.22** Epiphora due to insufficient drainage

    H04.221 Epiphora due to insufficient drainage, right side

    H04.222 Epiphora due to insufficient drainage, left side

    H04.223 Epiphora due to insufficient drainage, bilateral

    H04.229 Epiphora due to insufficient drainage, unspecified side

✓5ᵗʰ **H04.3** Acute and unspecified inflammation of lacrimal passages

    EXCLUDES 1   neonatal dacryocystitis (P39.1)

✓6ᵗʰ **H04.30** Unspecified dacryocystitis

    H04.301 Unspecified dacryocystitis of right lacrimal passage

    H04.302 Unspecified dacryocystitis of left lacrimal passage

    H04.303 Unspecified dacryocystitis of bilateral lacrimal passages

    H04.309 Unspecified dacryocystitis of unspecified lacrimal passage

✓6ᵗʰ **H04.31** Phlegmonous dacryocystitis

    H04.311 Phlegmonous dacryocystitis of right lacrimal passage

    H04.312 Phlegmonous dacryocystitis of left lacrimal passage

    H04.313 Phlegmonous dacryocystitis of bilateral lacrimal passages

    H04.319 Phlegmonous dacryocystitis of unspecified lacrimal passage

✓6ᵗʰ **H04.32** Acute dacryocystitis

    Acute dacryopericystitis

    H04.321 Acute dacryocystitis of right lacrimal passage

    H04.322 Acute dacryocystitis of left lacrimal passage

    H04.323 Acute dacryocystitis of bilateral lacrimal passages

    H04.329 Acute dacryocystitis of unspecified lacrimal passage

✓6ᵗʰ **H04.33** Acute lacrimal canaliculitis

    H04.331 Acute lacrimal canaliculitis of right lacrimal passage

    H04.332 Acute lacrimal canaliculitis of left lacrimal passage

    H04.333 Acute lacrimal canaliculitis of bilateral lacrimal passages

    H04.339 Acute lacrimal canaliculitis of unspecified lacrimal passage

✓5ᵗʰ **H04.4** Chronic inflammation of lacrimal passages

✓6ᵗʰ **H04.41** Chronic dacryocystitis

    H04.411 Chronic dacryocystitis of right lacrimal passage

    H04.412 Chronic dacryocystitis of left lacrimal passage

    H04.413 Chronic dacryocystitis of bilateral lacrimal passages

    H04.419 Chronic dacryocystitis of unspecified lacrimal passage

✓6ᵗʰ **H04.42** Chronic lacrimal canaliculitis

    H04.421 Chronic lacrimal canaliculitis of right lacrimal passage

    H04.422 Chronic lacrimal canaliculitis of left lacrimal passage

    H04.423 Chronic lacrimal canaliculitis of bilateral lacrimal passages

    H04.429 Chronic lacrimal canaliculitis of unspecified lacrimal passage

✓6ᵗʰ **H04.43** Chronic lacrimal mucocele

    H04.431 Chronic lacrimal mucocele of right lacrimal passage

    H04.432 Chronic lacrimal mucocele of left lacrimal passage

    H04.433 Chronic lacrimal mucocele of bilateral lacrimal passages

    H04.439 Chronic lacrimal mucocele of unspecified lacrimal passage

✓5ᵗʰ **H04.5** Stenosis and insufficiency of lacrimal passages

✓6ᵗʰ **H04.51** Dacryolith

    H04.511 Dacryolith of right lacrimal passage

    H04.512 Dacryolith of left lacrimal passage

    H04.513 Dacryolith of bilateral lacrimal passages

    H04.519 Dacryolith of unspecified lacrimal passage

✓6ᵗʰ **H04.52** Eversion of lacrimal punctum

    H04.521 Eversion of right lacrimal punctum

    H04.522 Eversion of left lacrimal punctum

    H04.523 Eversion of bilateral lacrimal punctum

    H04.529 Eversion of unspecified lacrimal punctum

✓6ᵗʰ **H04.53** Neonatal obstruction of nasolacrimal duct

    EXCLUDES 1   congenital stenosis and stricture of lacrimal duct (Q10.5)

    H04.531 Neonatal obstruction of right nasolacrimal duct   N

    H04.532 Neonatal obstruction of left nasolacrimal duct   N

    H04.533 Neonatal obstruction of bilateral nasolacrimal duct   N

    H04.539 Neonatal obstruction of unspecified nasolacrimal duct   N

✓6ᵗʰ **H04.54** Stenosis of lacrimal canaliculi

    H04.541 Stenosis of right lacrimal canaliculi

    H04.542 Stenosis of left lacrimal canaliculi

    H04.543 Stenosis of bilateral lacrimal canaliculi

    H04.549 Stenosis of unspecified lacrimal canaliculi

✓6ᵗʰ **H04.55** Acquired stenosis of nasolacrimal duct

    H04.551 Acquired stenosis of right nasolacrimal duct

    H04.552 Acquired stenosis of left nasolacrimal duct

    H04.553 Acquired stenosis of bilateral nasolacrimal duct

    H04.559 Acquired stenosis of unspecified nasolacrimal duct

✓6ᵗʰ **H04.56** Stenosis of lacrimal punctum

    H04.561 Stenosis of right lacrimal punctum

    H04.562 Stenosis of left lacrimal punctum

    H04.563 Stenosis of bilateral lacrimal punctum

    H04.569 Stenosis of unspecified lacrimal punctum

✓6ᵗʰ **H04.57** Stenosis of lacrimal sac

    H04.571 Stenosis of right lacrimal sac

Additional Character Required   ✓x7ᵗʰ Placeholder   Unacceptable PDx   Questionable PDx   Manifestation   Unspecified Dx   H1-H1⁴ HAC   HCC CMS-HCC Dx   HIV HIV Dx

ICD-10-CM 2020

599

H04.572 Stenosis of left lacrimal sac
H04.573 Stenosis of bilateral lacrimal sac
H04.579 Stenosis of unspecified lacrimal sac

✓6ᵗʰ **H04.6 Other changes of lacrimal passages**
  ✓6ᵗʰ **H04.61 Lacrimal fistula**
      H04.611 Lacrimal fistula right lacrimal passage SW
      H04.612 Lacrimal fistula left lacrimal passage SW
      H04.613 Lacrimal fistula bilateral lacrimal passages SW
      H04.619 Lacrimal fistula unspecified lacrimal passage SW
    H04.69 Other changes of lacrimal passages
✓5ᵗʰ **H04.8 Other disorders of lacrimal system**
  ✓6ᵗʰ **H04.81 Granuloma of lacrimal passages**
      H04.811 Granuloma of right lacrimal passage
      H04.812 Granuloma of left lacrimal passage
      H04.813 Granuloma of bilateral lacrimal passages
      H04.819 Granuloma of unspecified lacrimal passage
    H04.89 Other disorders of lacrimal system
  H04.9 Disorder of lacrimal system, unspecified

✓4ᵗʰ **H05 Disorders of orbit**
    EXCLUDES 1 congenital malformation of orbit (Q10.7)
  ✓5ᵗʰ **H05.0 Acute inflammation of orbit**
      H05.00 Unspecified acute inflammation of orbit
    ✓6ᵗʰ **H05.01 Cellulitis of orbit**
        Abscess of orbit
        CC Excl: For CC codes in subcategory H05.01: PDX collection 621
        H05.011 Cellulitis of right orbit CC
        H05.012 Cellulitis of left orbit CC
        H05.013 Cellulitis of bilateral orbits CC
        H05.019 Cellulitis of unspecified orbit CC
    ✓6ᵗʰ **H05.02 Osteomyelitis of orbit**
        CC Excl: For CC codes in subcategory H05.02: PDX collection 622
        H05.021 Osteomyelitis of right orbit CC
        H05.022 Osteomyelitis of left orbit CC
        H05.023 Osteomyelitis of bilateral orbits CC
        H05.029 Osteomyelitis of unspecified orbit CC
    ✓6ᵗʰ **H05.03 Periostitis of orbit**
        CC Excl: For CC codes in subcategory H05.03: PDX collection 623
        H05.031 Periostitis of right orbit CC
        H05.032 Periostitis of left orbit CC
        H05.033 Periostitis of bilateral orbits CC
        H05.039 Periostitis of unspecified orbit CC
    ✓6ᵗʰ **H05.04 Tenonitis of orbit**
        H05.041 Tenonitis of right orbit
        H05.042 Tenonitis of left orbit
        H05.043 Tenonitis of bilateral orbits
        H05.049 Tenonitis of unspecified orbit
  ✓5ᵗʰ **H05.1 Chronic inflammatory disorders of orbit**
      H05.10 Unspecified chronic inflammatory disorders of orbit
    ✓6ᵗʰ **H05.11 Granuloma of orbit**
        Pseudotumor (inflammatory) of orbit
        H05.111 Granuloma of right orbit
        H05.112 Granuloma of left orbit
        H05.113 Granuloma of bilateral orbits
        H05.119 Granuloma of unspecified orbit
    ✓6ᵗʰ **H05.12 Orbital myositis**
        H05.121 Orbital myositis, right orbit
        H05.122 Orbital myositis, left orbit
        H05.123 Orbital myositis, bilateral
        H05.129 Orbital myositis, unspecified orbit

  ✓5ᵗʰ **H05.2 Exophthalmic conditions**
      H05.20 Unspecified exophthalmos
    ✓6ᵗʰ **H05.21 Displacement (lateral) of globe**
        H05.211 Displacement (lateral) of globe, right eye
        H05.212 Displacement (lateral) of globe, left eye
        H05.213 Displacement (lateral) of globe, bilateral
        H05.219 Displacement (lateral) of globe, unspecified eye
    ✓6ᵗʰ **H05.22 Edema of orbit**
        Orbital congestion
        H05.221 Edema of right orbit
        H05.222 Edema of left orbit
        H05.223 Edema of bilateral orbit
        H05.229 Edema of unspecified orbit
    ✓6ᵗʰ **H05.23 Hemorrhage of orbit**
        H05.231 Hemorrhage of right orbit
        H05.232 Hemorrhage of left orbit
        H05.233 Hemorrhage of bilateral orbit
        H05.239 Hemorrhage of unspecified orbit
    ✓6ᵗʰ **H05.24 Constant exophthalmos**
        H05.241 Constant exophthalmos, right eye
        H05.242 Constant exophthalmos, left eye
        H05.243 Constant exophthalmos, bilateral
        H05.249 Constant exophthalmos, unspecified eye
    ✓6ᵗʰ **H05.25 Intermittent exophthalmos**
        H05.251 Intermittent exophthalmos, right eye
        H05.252 Intermittent exophthalmos, left eye
        H05.253 Intermittent exophthalmos, bilateral
        H05.259 Intermittent exophthalmos, unspecified eye
    ✓6ᵗʰ **H05.26 Pulsating exophthalmos**
        H05.261 Pulsating exophthalmos, right eye
        H05.262 Pulsating exophthalmos, left eye
        H05.263 Pulsating exophthalmos, bilateral
        H05.269 Pulsating exophthalmos, unspecified eye
  ✓5ᵗʰ **H05.3 Deformity of orbit**
      EXCLUDES 1 congenital deformity of orbit (Q10.7)
                      hypertelorism (Q75.2)
      H05.30 Unspecified deformity of orbit
    ✓6ᵗʰ **H05.31 Atrophy of orbit**
        H05.311 Atrophy of right orbit
        H05.312 Atrophy of left orbit
        H05.313 Atrophy of bilateral orbit
        H05.319 Atrophy of unspecified orbit
    ✓6ᵗʰ **H05.32 Deformity of orbit due to bone disease**
        Code also associated bone disease
        H05.321 Deformity of right orbit due to bone disease
        H05.322 Deformity of left orbit due to bone disease
        H05.323 Deformity of bilateral orbits due to bone disease
        H05.329 Deformity of unspecified orbit due to bone disease
    ✓6ᵗʰ **H05.33 Deformity of orbit due to trauma or surgery**
        H05.331 Deformity of right orbit due to trauma or surgery
        H05.332 Deformity of left orbit due to trauma or surgery
        H05.333 Deformity of bilateral orbits due to trauma or surgery
        H05.339 Deformity of unspecified orbit due to trauma or surgery
    ✓6ᵗʰ **H05.34 Enlargement of orbit**
        H05.341 Enlargement of right orbit
        H05.342 Enlargement of left orbit
        H05.343 Enlargement of bilateral orbits
        H05.349 Enlargement of unspecified orbit
    ✓6ᵗʰ **H05.35 Exostosis of orbit**
        H05.351 Exostosis of right orbit
        H05.352 Exostosis of left orbit
        H05.353 Exostosis of bilateral orbits
        H05.359 Exostosis of unspecified orbit
  ✓5ᵗʰ **H05.4 Enophthalmos**
    ✓6ᵗʰ **H05.40 Unspecified enophthalmos**
        H05.401 Unspecified enophthalmos, right eye

N Newborn: 0   P Pediatric: 0-17   M Maternity: 9-64   A Adult: 15-124   **MCC** Major Complication/Comorbidity   **CC** Complication/Comorbidity   **SW** Severe Wound Dx

✓6ᵗʰ **H05.402** Unspecified enophthalmos, **left** eye

✓6ᵗʰ **H05.403** Unspecified enophthalmos, **bilateral**

H05.409 Unspecified enophthalmos, **unspecified** eye

✓6ᵗʰ **H05.41** **Enophthalmos** due to atrophy of orbital tissue

H05.411 **Enophthalmos due to atrophy of orbital tissue, right** eye

H05.412 **Enophthalmos due to atrophy of orbital tissue, left** eye

H05.413 **Enophthalmos due to atrophy of orbital tissue, bilateral**

H05.419 **Enophthalmos due to atrophy of orbital tissue, unspecified** eye

✓6ᵗʰ **H05.42** **Enophthalmos** due to trauma or surgery

H05.421 **Enophthalmos due to trauma or surgery, right** eye

H05.422 **Enophthalmos due to trauma or surgery, left** eye

H05.423 **Enophthalmos due to trauma or surgery, bilateral**

H05.429 **Enophthalmos due to trauma or surgery, unspecified** eye

✓5ᵗʰ **H05.5** **Retained (old) foreign body following penetrating wound of orbit**

Retrobulbar foreign body

Use additional code to identify the type of retained foreign body (Z18.-)

EXCLUDES 1   *current penetrating wound of orbit (S05.4-)*

EXCLUDES 2   *retained foreign body of eyelid (H02.81-)*

         retained intraocular foreign body (H44.6-, H44.7-)

H05.50 **Retained (old) foreign body following penetrating wound of unspecified orbit**

H05.51 **Retained (old) foreign body following penetrating wound of right orbit**

H05.52 **Retained (old) foreign body following penetrating wound of left orbit**

H05.53 **Retained (old) foreign body following penetrating wound of bilateral orbits**

✓5ᵗʰ **H05.8** **Other disorders of orbit**

✓6ᵗʰ **H05.81** **Cyst of orbit**

Encephalocele of orbit

H05.811 **Cyst of right orbit**

H05.812 **Cyst of left orbit**

H05.813 **Cyst of bilateral orbits**

H05.819 **Cyst of unspecified orbit**

✓6ᵗʰ **H05.82** **Myopathy of extraocular muscles**

H05.821 **Myopathy of extraocular muscles, right orbit**

H05.822 **Myopathy of extraocular muscles, left orbit**

H05.823 **Myopathy of extraocular muscles, bilateral**

H05.829 **Myopathy of extraocular muscles, unspecified orbit**

H05.89 **Other disorders of orbit**

H05.9 **Unspecified disorder of orbit**

Disorders of conjunctiva (H10-H11)

✓4ᵗʰ **H10** **Conjunctivitis**

EXCLUDES 1   *keratoconjunctivitis (H16.2-)*

✓5ᵗʰ **H10.0** **Mucopurulent conjunctivitis**

✓6ᵗʰ **H10.01** **Acute follicular conjunctivitis**

H10.011 **Acute follicular conjunctivitis, right** eye

H10.012 **Acute follicular conjunctivitis, left** eye

H10.013 **Acute follicular conjunctivitis, bilateral**

H10.019 **Acute follicular conjunctivitis, unspecified** eye

✓6ᵗʰ **H10.02** **Other mucopurulent conjunctivitis**

H10.021 **Other mucopurulent conjunctivitis, right** eye

H10.022 **Other mucopurulent conjunctivitis, left** eye

H10.023 **Other mucopurulent conjunctivitis, bilateral**

H10.029 **Other mucopurulent conjunctivitis, unspecified** eye

✓5ᵗʰ **H10.1** **Acute atopic** conjunctivitis

Acute papillary conjunctivitis

H10.10 **Acute atopic conjunctivitis, unspecified** eye

H10.11 **Acute atopic conjunctivitis, right** eye

H10.12 **Acute atopic conjunctivitis, left** eye

H10.13 **Acute atopic conjunctivitis, bilateral**

✓5ᵗʰ **H10.2** **Other** acute conjunctivitis

✓6ᵗʰ **H10.21** **Acute toxic** conjunctivitis

Acute chemical conjunctivitis

Code first (T51-T65) to identify chemical and intent

EXCLUDES 1   *burn and corrosion of eye and adnexa (T26.-)*

H10.211 **Acute toxic conjunctivitis, right** eye

H10.212 **Acute toxic conjunctivitis, left** eye

H10.213 **Acute toxic conjunctivitis, bilateral**

H10.219 **Acute toxic conjunctivitis, unspecified** eye

✓6ᵗʰ **H10.22** **Pseudomembranous** conjunctivitis

H10.221 **Pseudomembranous conjunctivitis, right** eye

H10.222 **Pseudomembranous conjunctivitis, left** eye

H10.223 **Pseudomembranous conjunctivitis, bilateral**

H10.229 **Pseudomembranous conjunctivitis, unspecified** eye

✓6ᵗʰ **H10.23** **Serous** conjunctivitis, except viral

EXCLUDES 1   *viral conjunctivitis (B30.-)*

H10.231 **Serous conjunctivitis, except viral, right** eye

H10.232 **Serous conjunctivitis, except viral, left** eye

H10.233 **Serous conjunctivitis, except viral, bilateral**

H10.239 **Serous conjunctivitis, except viral, unspecified** eye

✓5ᵗʰ **H10.3** **Unspecified** acute conjunctivitis

EXCLUDES 1   *ophthalmia neonatorum NOS (P39.1)*

H10.30 **Unspecified acute conjunctivitis, unspecified** eye

H10.31 **Unspecified acute conjunctivitis, right** eye

H10.32 **Unspecified acute conjunctivitis, left** eye

H10.33 **Unspecified acute conjunctivitis, bilateral**

✓5ᵗʰ **H10.4** **Chronic** conjunctivitis

✓6ᵗʰ **H10.40** **Unspecified chronic conjunctivitis**

H10.401 **Unspecified chronic conjunctivitis, right** eye

H10.402 **Unspecified chronic conjunctivitis, left** eye

H10.403 **Unspecified chronic conjunctivitis, bilateral**

H10.409 **Unspecified chronic conjunctivitis, unspecified** eye

✓6ᵗʰ **H10.41** **Chronic** giant papillary **conjunctivitis**

H10.411 **Chronic giant papillary conjunctivitis, right** eye

H10.412 **Chronic giant papillary conjunctivitis, left** eye

H10.413 **Chronic giant papillary conjunctivitis, bilateral**

H10.419 **Chronic giant papillary conjunctivitis, unspecified** eye

✓6ᵗʰ **H10.42** **Simple** chronic conjunctivitis

H10.421 **Simple chronic conjunctivitis, right** eye

H10.422 **Simple chronic conjunctivitis, left** eye

H10.423 **Simple chronic conjunctivitis, bilateral**

H10.429 **Simple chronic conjunctivitis, unspecified** eye

✓6ᵗʰ **H10.43** **Chronic** follicular **conjunctivitis**

H10.431 **Chronic follicular conjunctivitis, right** eye

H10.432 **Chronic follicular conjunctivitis, left** eye

H10.433 **Chronic follicular conjunctivitis, bilateral**

H10.439 **Chronic follicular conjunctivitis, unspecified** eye

H10.44 **Vernal** conjunctivitis

EXCLUDES 1   *vernal keratoconjunctivitis with limbar and corneal involvement (H16.26-)*

H10.45 **Other chronic** allergic **conjunctivitis**

✓ Additional Character Required   ✓x7ᵗʰ Placeholder   Unacceptable PDx   Questionable PDx   Manifestation   Unspecified Dx   H1-H14 HAC   HCC CMS-HCC Dx   HIV HIV Dx

✓5ᵗʰ **H10.5 Blepharoconjunctivitis**

  ✓6ᵗʰ **H10.50 Unspecified blepharoconjunctivitis**

    H10.501 Unspecified blepharoconjunctivitis, right eye

    H10.502 Unspecified blepharoconjunctivitis, left eye

    H10.503 Unspecified blepharoconjunctivitis, bilateral

    H10.509 Unspecified blepharoconjunctivitis, unspecified eye

  ✓6ᵗʰ **H10.51 Ligneous conjunctivitis**

    Code also underlying condition if known, such as: plasminogen deficiency (E88.02)

    H10.511 Ligneous conjunctivitis, right eye

    H10.512 Ligneous conjunctivitis, left eye

    H10.513 Ligneous conjunctivitis, bilateral

    H10.519 Ligneous conjunctivitis, unspecified eye

  ✓6ᵗʰ **H10.52 Angular blepharoconjunctivitis**

    H10.521 Angular blepharoconjunctivitis, right eye

    H10.522 Angular blepharoconjunctivitis, left eye

    H10.523 Angular blepharoconjunctivitis, bilateral

    H10.529 Angular blepharoconjunctivitis, unspecified eye

  ✓6ᵗʰ **H10.53 Contact blepharoconjunctivitis**

    H10.531 Contact blepharoconjunctivitis, right eye

    H10.532 Contact blepharoconjunctivitis, left eye

    H10.533 Contact blepharoconjunctivitis, bilateral

    H10.539 Contact blepharoconjunctivitis, unspecified eye

✓5ᵗʰ **H10.8 Other conjunctivitis**

  ✓6ᵗʰ **H10.81 Pingueculitis**

    EXCLUDES 1 *pinguecula (H11.15-)*

    H10.811 Pingueculitis, right eye

    H10.812 Pingueculitis, left eye

    H10.813 Pingueculitis, bilateral

    H10.819 Pingueculitis, unspecified eye

  ✓6ᵗʰ **H10.82 Rosacea conjunctivitis**

    Code first underlying rosacea dermatitis (L71.-)

    AHA: 2018,4Q,15

    H10.821 Rosacea conjunctivitis, right eye

    H10.822 Rosacea conjunctivitis, left eye

    H10.823 Rosacea conjunctivitis, bilateral

    H10.829 Rosacea conjunctivitis, unspecified eye

  H10.89 Other conjunctivitis

  H10.9 Unspecified conjunctivitis

✓4ᵗʰ **H11 Other disorders of conjunctiva**

  EXCLUDES 1 *keratoconjunctivitis (H16.2-)*

✓5ᵗʰ **H11.0 Pterygium of eye**

  EXCLUDES 1 *pseudopterygium (H11.81-)*

  DEF: Benign, wedge-shaped, conjunctival thickening that advances from the inner corner of the eye toward the cornea.

Pterygium

Pterygium

  ✓6ᵗʰ **H11.00 Unspecified pterygium of eye**

    H11.001 Unspecified pterygium of right eye

    H11.002 Unspecified pterygium of left eye

    H11.003 Unspecified pterygium of eye, bilateral

    H11.009 Unspecified pterygium of unspecified eye

  ✓6ᵗʰ **H11.01 Amyloid pterygium**

    H11.011 Amyloid pterygium of right eye

    H11.012 Amyloid pterygium of left eye

    H11.013 Amyloid pterygium of eye, bilateral

    H11.019 Amyloid pterygium of unspecified eye

  ✓6ᵗʰ **H11.02 Central pterygium of eye**

    H11.021 Central pterygium of right eye

    H11.022 Central pterygium of left eye

    H11.023 Central pterygium of eye, bilateral

    H11.029 Central pterygium of unspecified eye

  ✓6ᵗʰ **H11.03 Double pterygium of eye**

    H11.031 Double pterygium of right eye

    H11.032 Double pterygium of left eye

    H11.033 Double pterygium of eye, bilateral

    H11.039 Double pterygium of unspecified eye

  ✓6ᵗʰ **H11.04 Peripheral pterygium of eye, stationary**

    H11.041 Peripheral pterygium, stationary, right eye

    H11.042 Peripheral pterygium, stationary, left eye

    H11.043 Peripheral pterygium, stationary, bilateral

    H11.049 Peripheral pterygium, stationary, unspecified eye

  ✓6ᵗʰ **H11.05 Peripheral pterygium of eye, progressive**

    H11.051 Peripheral pterygium, progressive, right eye

    H11.052 Peripheral pterygium, progressive, left eye

    H11.053 Peripheral pterygium, progressive, bilateral

    H11.059 Peripheral pterygium, progressive, unspecified eye

  ✓6ᵗʰ **H11.06 Recurrent pterygium of eye**

    H11.061 Recurrent pterygium of right eye

    H11.062 Recurrent pterygium of left eye

    H11.063 Recurrent pterygium of eye, bilateral

    H11.069 Recurrent pterygium of unspecified eye

✓5ᵗʰ **H11.1 Conjunctival degenerations and deposits**

  EXCLUDES 2 *pseudopterygium (H11.81)*

  H11.10 Unspecified conjunctival degenerations

  ✓6ᵗʰ **H11.11 Conjunctival deposits**

    H11.111 Conjunctival deposits, right eye

    H11.112 Conjunctival deposits, left eye

    H11.113 Conjunctival deposits, bilateral

    H11.119 Conjunctival deposits, unspecified eye

  ✓6ᵗʰ **H11.12 Conjunctival concretions**

    H11.121 Conjunctival concretions, right eye

    H11.122 Conjunctival concretions, left eye

    H11.123 Conjunctival concretions, bilateral

    H11.129 Conjunctival concretions, unspecified eye

  ✓6ᵗʰ **H11.13 Conjunctival pigmentations**

    Conjunctival argyrosis [argyria]

    H11.131 Conjunctival pigmentations, right eye

    H11.132 Conjunctival pigmentations, left eye

    H11.133 Conjunctival pigmentations, bilateral

    H11.139 Conjunctival pigmentations, unspecified eye

  ✓6ᵗʰ **H11.14 Conjunctival xerosis, unspecified**

    EXCLUDES 1 *xerosis of conjunctiva due to vitamin A deficiency (E50.0, E50.1)*

    DEF: Abnormal dryness of the conjunctiva due to lack of insufficient tears or conjunctival secretions.

    H11.141 Conjunctival xerosis, unspecified, right eye

    H11.142 Conjunctival xerosis, unspecified, left eye

    H11.143 Conjunctival xerosis, unspecified, bilateral

    H11.149 Conjunctival xerosis, unspecified, unspecified eye

N Newborn: 0   P Pediatric: 0-17   M Maternity: 9-64   A Adult: 15-124   MCC Major Complication/Comorbidity   CC Complication/Comorbidity   SW Severe Wound Dx

602   ICD-10-CM 2020

✓6ᵗʰ **H11.15** Pinguecula

EXCLUDES 1   pingueculitis (H10.81-)

DEF: Proliferation on the conjunctiva near the sclerocorneal junction, usually of the side of the nose and usually in older patients.

Pinguecula

Pinguecula

H11.151   Pinguecula, right eye
H11.152   Pinguecula, left eye
H11.153   Pinguecula, bilateral
H11.159   Pinguecula, unspecified eye

✓5ᵗʰ **H11.2** Conjunctival scars

✓6ᵗʰ   **H11.21** Conjunctival adhesions and strands (localized)

H11.211   Conjunctival adhesions and strands (localized), right eye
H11.212   Conjunctival adhesions and strands (localized), left eye
H11.213   Conjunctival adhesions and strands (localized), bilateral
H11.219   Conjunctival adhesions and strands (localized), unspecified eye

✓6ᵗʰ   **H11.22** Conjunctival granuloma

H11.221   Conjunctival granuloma, right eye
H11.222   Conjunctival granuloma, left eye
H11.223   Conjunctival granuloma, bilateral
H11.229   Conjunctival granuloma, unspecified

✓6ᵗʰ   **H11.23** Symblepharon

H11.231   Symblepharon, right eye
H11.232   Symblepharon, left eye
H11.233   Symblepharon, bilateral
H11.239   Symblepharon, unspecified eye

✓6ᵗʰ   **H11.24** Scarring of conjunctiva

H11.241   Scarring of conjunctiva, right eye
H11.242   Scarring of conjunctiva, left eye
H11.243   Scarring of conjunctiva, bilateral
H11.249   Scarring of conjunctiva, unspecified eye

✓5ᵗʰ **H11.3** Conjunctival hemorrhage

Subconjunctival hemorrhage

H11.30   Conjunctival hemorrhage, unspecified eye
H11.31   Conjunctival hemorrhage, right eye
H11.32   Conjunctival hemorrhage, left eye
H11.33   Conjunctival hemorrhage, bilateral

✓5ᵗʰ **H11.4** Other conjunctival vascular disorders and cysts

✓6ᵗʰ   **H11.41** Vascular abnormalities of conjunctiva

Conjunctival aneurysm

H11.411   Vascular abnormalities of conjunctiva, right eye
H11.412   Vascular abnormalities of conjunctiva, left eye
H11.413   Vascular abnormalities of conjunctiva, bilateral
H11.419   Vascular abnormalities of conjunctiva, unspecified eye

✓6ᵗʰ   **H11.42** Conjunctival edema

H11.421   Conjunctival edema, right eye
H11.422   Conjunctival edema, left eye
H11.423   Conjunctival edema, bilateral
H11.429   Conjunctival edema, unspecified eye

✓6ᵗʰ   **H11.43** Conjunctival hyperemia

H11.431   Conjunctival hyperemia, right eye

H11.432   Conjunctival hyperemia, left eye
H11.433   Conjunctival hyperemia, bilateral
H11.439   Conjunctival hyperemia, unspecified eye

✓6ᵗʰ   **H11.44** Conjunctival cysts

H11.441   Conjunctival cysts, right eye
H11.442   Conjunctival cysts, left eye
H11.443   Conjunctival cysts, bilateral
H11.449   Conjunctival cysts, unspecified eye

✓5ᵗʰ **H11.8** Other specified disorders of conjunctiva

✓6ᵗʰ   **H11.81** Pseudopterygium of conjunctiva

H11.811   Pseudopterygium of conjunctiva, right eye
H11.812   Pseudopterygium of conjunctiva, left eye
H11.813   Pseudopterygium of conjunctiva, bilateral
H11.819   Pseudopterygium of conjunctiva, unspecified eye

✓6ᵗʰ   **H11.82** Conjunctivochalasis

H11.821   Conjunctivochalasis, right eye
H11.822   Conjunctivochalasis, left eye
H11.823   Conjunctivochalasis, bilateral
H11.829   Conjunctivochalasis, unspecified eye

H11.89   Other specified disorders of conjunctiva

H11.9 Unspecified disorder of conjunctiva

Disorders of sclera, cornea, iris and ciliary body (H15-H22)

✓4ᵗʰ **H15** Disorders of sclera

✓5ᵗʰ **H15.0** Scleritis

✓6ᵗʰ   **H15.00** Unspecified scleritis

H15.001   Unspecified scleritis, right eye
H15.002   Unspecified scleritis, left eye
H15.003   Unspecified scleritis, bilateral
H15.009   Unspecified scleritis, unspecified eye

✓6ᵗʰ   **H15.01** Anterior scleritis

H15.011   Anterior scleritis, right eye
H15.012   Anterior scleritis, left eye
H15.013   Anterior scleritis, bilateral
H15.019   Anterior scleritis, unspecified eye

✓6ᵗʰ   **H15.02** Brawny scleritis

H15.021   Brawny scleritis, right eye
H15.022   Brawny scleritis, left eye
H15.023   Brawny scleritis, bilateral
H15.029   Brawny scleritis, unspecified eye

✓6ᵗʰ   **H15.03** Posterior scleritis

Sclerotenonitis

H15.031   Posterior scleritis, right eye
H15.032   Posterior scleritis, left eye
H15.033   Posterior scleritis, bilateral
H15.039   Posterior scleritis, unspecified eye

✓6ᵗʰ   **H15.04** Scleritis with corneal involvement

H15.041   Scleritis with corneal involvement, right eye
H15.042   Scleritis with corneal involvement, left eye
H15.043   Scleritis with corneal involvement, bilateral
H15.049   Scleritis with corneal involvement, unspecified eye

✓6ᵗʰ   **H15.05** Scleromalacia perforans

H15.051   Scleromalacia perforans, right eye
H15.052   Scleromalacia perforans, left eye
H15.053   Scleromalacia perforans, bilateral
H15.059   Scleromalacia perforans, unspecified eye

✓6ᵗʰ   **H15.09** Other scleritis

Scleral abscess

H15.091   Other scleritis, right eye
H15.092   Other scleritis, left eye
H15.093   Other scleritis, bilateral
H15.099   Other scleritis, unspecified eye

✓5ᵗʰ **H15.1** Episcleritis

✓6ᵗʰ   **H15.10** Unspecified episcleritis

H15.101   Unspecified episcleritis, right eye
H15.102   Unspecified episcleritis, left eye
H15.103   Unspecified episcleritis, bilateral
H15.109   Unspecified episcleritis, unspecified eye

☑ Additional Character Required   ✓x7ᵗʰ Placeholder   Unacceptable PDx   Questionable PDx   Manifestation   Unspecified Dx   H1-H14 HAC   HCC CMS-HCC Dx   HIV HIV Dx

ICD-10-CM 2020

603

✓6ᵗʰ **H15.11** Episcleritis periodica fugax
- **H15.111** Episcleritis periodica fugax, right eye
- **H15.112** Episcleritis periodica fugax, left eye
- **H15.113** Episcleritis periodica fugax, bilateral
- **H15.119** Episcleritis periodica fugax, unspecified eye

✓6ᵗʰ **H15.12** Nodular episcleritis
- **H15.121** Nodular episcleritis, right eye
- **H15.122** Nodular episcleritis, left eye
- **H15.123** Nodular episcleritis, bilateral
- **H15.129** Nodular episcleritis, unspecified eye

✓5ᵗʰ **H15.8** Other disorders of sclera
> EXCLUDES 2   blue sclera (Q13.5)
>   degenerative myopia (H44.2-)

✓6ᵗʰ **H15.81** Equatorial staphyloma
- **H15.811** Equatorial staphyloma, right eye
- **H15.812** Equatorial staphyloma, left eye
- **H15.813** Equatorial staphyloma, bilateral
- **H15.819** Equatorial staphyloma, unspecified eye

✓6ᵗʰ **H15.82** Localized anterior staphyloma
- **H15.821** Localized anterior staphyloma, right eye
- **H15.822** Localized anterior staphyloma, left eye
- **H15.823** Localized anterior staphyloma, bilateral
- **H15.829** Localized anterior staphyloma, unspecified eye

✓6ᵗʰ **H15.83** Staphyloma posticum
- **H15.831** Staphyloma posticum, right eye
- **H15.832** Staphyloma posticum, left eye
- **H15.833** Staphyloma posticum, bilateral
- **H15.839** Staphyloma posticum, unspecified eye

✓6ᵗʰ **H15.84** Scleral ectasia
- **H15.841** Scleral ectasia, right eye
- **H15.842** Scleral ectasia, left eye
- **H15.843** Scleral ectasia, bilateral
- **H15.849** Scleral ectasia, unspecified eye

✓6ᵗʰ **H15.85** Ring staphyloma
- **H15.851** Ring staphyloma, right eye
- **H15.852** Ring staphyloma, left eye
- **H15.853** Ring staphyloma, bilateral
- **H15.859** Ring staphyloma, unspecified eye

H15.89 Other disorders of sclera

H15.9 Unspecified disorder of sclera

✓4ᵗʰ **H16 Keratitis**
> **DEF:** Condition in which the cornea becomes inflamed and irritated.

✓5ᵗʰ **H16.0** Corneal ulcer

✓6ᵗʰ **H16.00** Unspecified corneal ulcer
- **H16.001** Unspecified corneal ulcer, right eye
- **H16.002** Unspecified corneal ulcer, left eye
- **H16.003** Unspecified corneal ulcer, bilateral
- **H16.009** Unspecified corneal ulcer, unspecified eye

✓6ᵗʰ **H16.01** Central corneal ulcer
- **H16.011** Central corneal ulcer, right eye
- **H16.012** Central corneal ulcer, left eye
- **H16.013** Central corneal ulcer, bilateral
- **H16.019** Central corneal ulcer, unspecified eye

✓6ᵗʰ **H16.02** Ring corneal ulcer
- **H16.021** Ring corneal ulcer, right eye
- **H16.022** Ring corneal ulcer, left eye
- **H16.023** Ring corneal ulcer, bilateral
- **H16.029** Ring corneal ulcer, unspecified eye

✓6ᵗʰ **H16.03** Corneal ulcer with hypopyon
- **H16.031** Corneal ulcer with hypopyon, right eye
- **H16.032** Corneal ulcer with hypopyon, left eye
- **H16.033** Corneal ulcer with hypopyon, bilateral
- **H16.039** Corneal ulcer with hypopyon, unspecified eye

✓6ᵗʰ **H16.04** Marginal corneal ulcer
- **H16.041** Marginal corneal ulcer, right eye
- **H16.042** Marginal corneal ulcer, left eye
- **H16.043** Marginal corneal ulcer, bilateral
- **H16.049** Marginal corneal ulcer, unspecified eye

✓6ᵗʰ **H16.05** Mooren's corneal ulcer
- **H16.051** Mooren's corneal ulcer, right eye
- **H16.052** Mooren's corneal ulcer, left eye

H16.053 Mooren's corneal ulcer, bilateral
H16.059 Mooren's corneal ulcer, unspecified eye

✓6ᵗʰ **H16.06** Mycotic corneal ulcer
- **H16.061** Mycotic corneal ulcer, right eye
- **H16.062** Mycotic corneal ulcer, left eye
- **H16.063** Mycotic corneal ulcer, bilateral
- **H16.069** Mycotic corneal ulcer, unspecified eye

✓6ᵗʰ **H16.07** Perforated corneal ulcer
- **H16.071** Perforated corneal ulcer, right eye
- **H16.072** Perforated corneal ulcer, left eye
- **H16.073** Perforated corneal ulcer, bilateral
- **H16.079** Perforated corneal ulcer, unspecified eye

✓5ᵗʰ **H16.1** Other and unspecified superficial keratitis without conjunctivitis

✓6ᵗʰ **H16.10** Unspecified superficial keratitis
- **H16.101** Unspecified superficial keratitis, right eye
- **H16.102** Unspecified superficial keratitis, left eye
- **H16.103** Unspecified superficial keratitis, bilateral
- **H16.109** Unspecified superficial keratitis, unspecified eye

✓6ᵗʰ **H16.11** Macular keratitis
> Areolar keratitis
> Nummular keratitis
> Stellate keratitis
> Striate keratitis
- **H16.111** Macular keratitis, right eye
- **H16.112** Macular keratitis, left eye
- **H16.113** Macular keratitis, bilateral
- **H16.119** Macular keratitis, unspecified eye

✓6ᵗʰ **H16.12** Filamentary keratitis
- **H16.121** Filamentary keratitis, right eye
- **H16.122** Filamentary keratitis, left eye
- **H16.123** Filamentary keratitis, bilateral
- **H16.129** Filamentary keratitis, unspecified eye

✓6ᵗʰ **H16.13** Photokeratitis
> Snow blindness
> Welders keratitis
- **H16.131** Photokeratitis, right eye
- **H16.132** Photokeratitis, left eye
- **H16.133** Photokeratitis, bilateral
- **H16.139** Photokeratitis, unspecified eye

✓6ᵗʰ **H16.14** Punctate keratitis
- **H16.141** Punctate keratitis, right eye
- **H16.142** Punctate keratitis, left eye
- **H16.143** Punctate keratitis, bilateral
- **H16.149** Punctate keratitis, unspecified eye

✓5ᵗʰ **H16.2** Keratoconjunctivitis

✓6ᵗʰ **H16.20** Unspecified keratoconjunctivitis
> Superficial keratitis with conjunctivitis NOS
- **H16.201** Unspecified keratoconjunctivitis, right eye
- **H16.202** Unspecified keratoconjunctivitis, left eye
- **H16.203** Unspecified keratoconjunctivitis, bilateral
- **H16.209** Unspecified keratoconjunctivitis, unspecified eye

✓6ᵗʰ **H16.21** Exposure keratoconjunctivitis
- **H16.211** Exposure keratoconjunctivitis, right eye
- **H16.212** Exposure keratoconjunctivitis, left eye
- **H16.213** Exposure keratoconjunctivitis, bilateral
- **H16.219** Exposure keratoconjunctivitis, unspecified eye

✓6ᵗʰ **H16.22** Keratoconjunctivitis sicca, not specified as Sjögren's
> EXCLUDES 1   Sjögren's syndrome (M35.01)
- **H16.221** Keratoconjunctivitis sicca, not specified as Sjögren's, right eye
- **H16.222** Keratoconjunctivitis sicca, not specified as Sjögren's, left eye
- **H16.223** Keratoconjunctivitis sicca, not specified as Sjögren's, bilateral
- **H16.229** Keratoconjunctivitis sicca, not specified as Sjögren's, unspecified eye

✓6ᵗʰ **H16.23** Neurotrophic keratoconjunctivitis
- **H16.231** Neurotrophic keratoconjunctivitis, right eye
- **H16.232** Neurotrophic keratoconjunctivitis, left eye

ⓃNewborn: 0   ⓅPediatric: 0-17   ⓂMaternity: 9-64   ⒶAdult: 15-124   ᴹᶜᶜMajor Complication/Comorbidity   ᶜᶜComplication/Comorbidity   ˢʷSevere Wound Dx

604   ICD-10-CM 2020

H16.233 Neurotrophic keratoconjunctivitis, bilateral

H16.239 Neurotrophic keratoconjunctivitis, unspecified eye

√6th **H16.24** Ophthalmia nodosa

H16.241 Ophthalmia nodosa, right eye

H16.242 Ophthalmia nodosa, left eye

H16.243 Ophthalmia nodosa, bilateral

H16.249 Ophthalmia nodosa, unspecified eye

√6th **H16.25** Phlyctenular keratoconjunctivitis

H16.251 Phlyctenular keratoconjunctivitis, right eye

H16.252 Phlyctenular keratoconjunctivitis, left eye

H16.253 Phlyctenular keratoconjunctivitis, bilateral

H16.259 Phlyctenular keratoconjunctivitis, unspecified eye

√6th **H16.26** Vernal keratoconjunctivitis, with limbar and corneal involvement

> EXCLUDES 1   *vernal conjunctivitis without limbar and corneal involvement (H10.44)*

H16.261 Vernal keratoconjunctivitis, with limbar and corneal involvement, right eye

H16.262 Vernal keratoconjunctivitis, with limbar and corneal involvement, left eye

H16.263 Vernal keratoconjunctivitis, with limbar and corneal involvement, bilateral

H16.269 Vernal keratoconjunctivitis, with limbar and corneal involvement, unspecified eye

√6th **H16.29** Other keratoconjunctivitis

H16.291 Other keratoconjunctivitis, right eye

H16.292 Other keratoconjunctivitis, left eye

H16.293 Other keratoconjunctivitis, bilateral

H16.299 Other keratoconjunctivitis, unspecified eye

√5th **H16.3** Interstitial and deep keratitis

√6th **H16.30** Unspecified interstitial keratitis

H16.301 Unspecified interstitial keratitis, right eye

H16.302 Unspecified interstitial keratitis, left eye

H16.303 Unspecified interstitial keratitis, bilateral

H16.309 Unspecified interstitial keratitis, unspecified eye

√6th **H16.31** Corneal abscess

H16.311 Corneal abscess, right eye

H16.312 Corneal abscess, left eye

H16.313 Corneal abscess, bilateral

H16.319 Corneal abscess, unspecified eye

√6th **H16.32** Diffuse interstitial keratitis

> Cogan's syndrome

H16.321 Diffuse interstitial keratitis, right eye

H16.322 Diffuse interstitial keratitis, left eye

H16.323 Diffuse interstitial keratitis, bilateral

H16.329 Diffuse interstitial keratitis, unspecified eye

√6th **H16.33** Sclerosing keratitis

H16.331 Sclerosing keratitis, right eye

H16.332 Sclerosing keratitis, left eye

H16.333 Sclerosing keratitis, bilateral

H16.339 Sclerosing keratitis, unspecified eye

√6th **H16.39** Other interstitial and deep keratitis

H16.391 Other interstitial and deep keratitis, right eye

H16.392 Other interstitial and deep keratitis, left eye

H16.393 Other interstitial and deep keratitis, bilateral

H16.399 Other interstitial and deep keratitis, unspecified eye

√5th **H16.4** Corneal neovascularization

√6th **H16.40** Unspecified corneal neovascularization

H16.401 Unspecified corneal neovascularization, right eye

H16.402 Unspecified corneal neovascularization, left eye

H16.403 Unspecified corneal neovascularization, bilateral

H16.409 Unspecified corneal neovascularization, unspecified eye

√6th **H16.41** Ghost vessels (corneal)

H16.411 Ghost vessels (corneal), right eye

H16.412 Ghost vessels (corneal), left eye

H16.413 Ghost vessels (corneal), bilateral

H16.419 Ghost vessels (corneal), unspecified eye

√6th **H16.42** Pannus (corneal)

H16.421 Pannus (corneal), right eye

H16.422 Pannus (corneal), left eye

H16.423 Pannus (corneal), bilateral

H16.429 Pannus (corneal), unspecified eye

√6th **H16.43** Localized vascularization of cornea

H16.431 Localized vascularization of cornea, right eye

H16.432 Localized vascularization of cornea, left eye

H16.433 Localized vascularization of cornea, bilateral

H16.439 Localized vascularization of cornea, unspecified eye

√6th **H16.44** Deep vascularization of cornea

H16.441 Deep vascularization of cornea, right eye

H16.442 Deep vascularization of cornea, left eye

H16.443 Deep vascularization of cornea, bilateral

H16.449 Deep vascularization of cornea, unspecified eye

H16.8 Other keratitis

H16.9 Unspecified keratitis

√4th **H17** Corneal scars and opacities

√5th **H17.0** Adherent leukoma

H17.00 Adherent leukoma, unspecified eye

H17.01 Adherent leukoma, right eye

H17.02 Adherent leukoma, left eye

H17.03 Adherent leukoma, bilateral

√5th **H17.1** Central corneal opacity

H17.10 Central corneal opacity, unspecified eye

H17.11 Central corneal opacity, right eye

H17.12 Central corneal opacity, left eye

H17.13 Central corneal opacity, bilateral

√5th **H17.8** Other corneal scars and opacities

√6th **H17.81** Minor opacity of cornea

> Corneal nebula

H17.811 Minor opacity of cornea, right eye

H17.812 Minor opacity of cornea, left eye

H17.813 Minor opacity of cornea, bilateral

H17.819 Minor opacity of cornea, unspecified eye

√6th **H17.82** Peripheral opacity of cornea

H17.821 Peripheral opacity of cornea, right eye

H17.822 Peripheral opacity of cornea, left eye

H17.823 Peripheral opacity of cornea, bilateral

H17.829 Peripheral opacity of cornea, unspecified eye

H17.89 Other corneal scars and opacities

H17.9 Unspecified corneal scar and opacity

√4th **H18** Other disorders of cornea

√5th **H18.0** Corneal pigmentations and deposits

√6th **H18.00** Unspecified corneal deposit

H18.001 Unspecified corneal deposit, right eye

H18.002 Unspecified corneal deposit, left eye

H18.003 Unspecified corneal deposit, bilateral

H18.009 Unspecified corneal deposit, unspecified eye

√6th **H18.01** Anterior corneal pigmentations

> Staehli's line

H18.011 Anterior corneal pigmentations, right eye

H18.012 Anterior corneal pigmentations, left eye

H18.013 Anterior corneal pigmentations, bilateral

H18.019 Anterior corneal pigmentations, unspecified eye

√6th **H18.02** Argentous corneal deposits

H18.021 Argentous corneal deposits, right eye

H18.022 Argentous corneal deposits, left eye

H18.023 Argentous corneal deposits, bilateral

H18.029 Argentous corneal deposits, unspecified eye

☑ Additional Character Required   √x7th Placeholder   Unacceptable PDx   Questionable PDx   Manifestation   Unspecified Dx   H1-H14 HAC   HCC CMS-HCC Dx   HIV HIV Dx

ICD-10-CM 2020

605

✓6th **H18.03** Corneal deposits in metabolic disorders
     Code also associated metabolic disorder
- **H18.031** Corneal deposits in metabolic disorders, right eye
- **H18.032** Corneal deposits in metabolic disorders, left eye
- **H18.033** Corneal deposits in metabolic disorders, bilateral
- **H18.039** Corneal deposits in metabolic disorders, unspecified eye

✓6th **H18.04** Kayser-Fleischer ring
     Code also associated Wilson's disease (E83.01)
- **H18.041** Kayser-Fleischer ring, right eye
- **H18.042** Kayser-Fleischer ring, left eye
- **H18.043** Kayser-Fleischer ring, bilateral
- **H18.049** Kayser-Fleischer ring, unspecified eye

✓6th **H18.05** Posterior corneal pigmentations
     Krukenberg's spindle
- **H18.051** Posterior corneal pigmentations, right eye
- **H18.052** Posterior corneal pigmentations, left eye
- **H18.053** Posterior corneal pigmentations, bilateral
- **H18.059** Posterior corneal pigmentations, unspecified eye

✓6th **H18.06** Stromal corneal pigmentations
     Hematocornea
- **H18.061** Stromal corneal pigmentations, right eye
- **H18.062** Stromal corneal pigmentations, left eye
- **H18.063** Stromal corneal pigmentations, bilateral
- **H18.069** Stromal corneal pigmentations, unspecified eye

✓5th **H18.1** Bullous keratopathy
     DEF: Corneal swelling due to a damaged corneal endothelium. Bullous keratopathy is characterized by recurring, rupturing epithelial blisters causing glaucoma, iridocyclitis, and Fuchs dystrophy.
- **H18.10** Bullous keratopathy, unspecified eye
- **H18.11** Bullous keratopathy, right eye
- **H18.12** Bullous keratopathy, left eye
- **H18.13** Bullous keratopathy, bilateral

✓5th **H18.2** Other and unspecified corneal edema
- **H18.20** Unspecified corneal edema

✓6th **H18.21** Corneal edema secondary to contact lens
     EXCLUDES 2   other corneal disorders due to contact lens (H18.82-)
- **H18.211** Corneal edema secondary to contact lens, right eye
- **H18.212** Corneal edema secondary to contact lens, left eye
- **H18.213** Corneal edema secondary to contact lens, bilateral
- **H18.219** Corneal edema secondary to contact lens, unspecified eye

✓6th **H18.22** Idiopathic corneal edema
- **H18.221** Idiopathic corneal edema, right eye
- **H18.222** Idiopathic corneal edema, left eye
- **H18.223** Idiopathic corneal edema, bilateral
- **H18.229** Idiopathic corneal edema, unspecified eye

✓6th **H18.23** Secondary corneal edema
- **H18.231** Secondary corneal edema, right eye
- **H18.232** Secondary corneal edema, left eye
- **H18.233** Secondary corneal edema, bilateral
- **H18.239** Secondary corneal edema, unspecified eye

✓5th **H18.3** Changes of corneal membranes
- **H18.30** Unspecified corneal membrane change

✓6th **H18.31** Folds and rupture in Bowman's membrane
- **H18.311** Folds and rupture in Bowman's membrane, right eye
- **H18.312** Folds and rupture in Bowman's membrane, left eye
- **H18.313** Folds and rupture in Bowman's membrane, bilateral
- **H18.319** Folds and rupture in Bowman's membrane, unspecified eye

✓6th **H18.32** Folds in Descemet's membrane
- **H18.321** Folds in Descemet's membrane, right eye
- **H18.322** Folds in Descemet's membrane, left eye
- **H18.323** Folds in Descemet's membrane, bilateral
- **H18.329** Folds in Descemet's membrane, unspecified eye

✓6th **H18.33** Rupture in Descemet's membrane
- **H18.331** Rupture in Descemet's membrane, right eye
- **H18.332** Rupture in Descemet's membrane, left eye
- **H18.333** Rupture in Descemet's membrane, bilateral
- **H18.339** Rupture in Descemet's membrane, unspecified eye

✓5th **H18.4** Corneal degeneration
     EXCLUDES 1   Mooren's ulcer (H16.0-)
                 recurrent erosion of cornea (H18.83-)
- **H18.40** Unspecified corneal degeneration

✓6th **H18.41** Arcus senilis
     Senile corneal changes
- **H18.411** Arcus senilis, right eye
- **H18.412** Arcus senilis, left eye
- **H18.413** Arcus senilis, bilateral
- **H18.419** Arcus senilis, unspecified eye

✓6th **H18.42** Band keratopathy
- **H18.421** Band keratopathy, right eye
- **H18.422** Band keratopathy, left eye
- **H18.423** Band keratopathy, bilateral
- **H18.429** Band keratopathy, unspecified eye

H18.43 Other calcerous corneal degeneration

✓6th **H18.44** Keratomalacia
     EXCLUDES 1   keratomalacia due to vitamin A deficiency (E50.4)
- **H18.441** Keratomalacia, right eye
- **H18.442** Keratomalacia, left eye
- **H18.443** Keratomalacia, bilateral
- **H18.449** Keratomalacia, unspecified eye

✓6th **H18.45** Nodular corneal degeneration
- **H18.451** Nodular corneal degeneration, right eye
- **H18.452** Nodular corneal degeneration, left eye
- **H18.453** Nodular corneal degeneration, bilateral
- **H18.459** Nodular corneal degeneration, unspecified eye

✓6th **H18.46** Peripheral corneal degeneration
- **H18.461** Peripheral corneal degeneration, right eye
- **H18.462** Peripheral corneal degeneration, left eye
- **H18.463** Peripheral corneal degeneration, bilateral
- **H18.469** Peripheral corneal degeneration, unspecified eye

H18.49 Other corneal degeneration

✓5th **H18.5** Hereditary corneal dystrophies
- **H18.50** Unspecified hereditary corneal dystrophies
- **H18.51** Endothelial corneal dystrophy
     Fuchs' dystrophy
- **H18.52** Epithelial (juvenile) corneal dystrophy
- **H18.53** Granular corneal dystrophy
- **H18.54** Lattice corneal dystrophy
- **H18.55** Macular corneal dystrophy
- **H18.59** Other hereditary corneal dystrophies

✓5th **H18.6** Keratoconus

✓6th **H18.60** Keratoconus, unspecified
- **H18.601** Keratoconus, unspecified, right eye
- **H18.602** Keratoconus, unspecified, left eye
- **H18.603** Keratoconus, unspecified, bilateral
- **H18.609** Keratoconus, unspecified, unspecified eye

✓6th **H18.61** Keratoconus, stable
- **H18.611** Keratoconus, stable, right eye
- **H18.612** Keratoconus, stable, left eye
- **H18.613** Keratoconus, stable, bilateral
- **H18.619** Keratoconus, stable, unspecified eye

✓6th **H18.62** Keratoconus, unstable
     Acute hydrops
- **H18.621** Keratoconus, unstable, right eye
- **H18.622** Keratoconus, unstable, left eye
- **H18.623** Keratoconus, unstable, bilateral

N Newborn: 0   P Pediatric: 0-17   M Maternity: 9-64   A Adult: 15-124   MCC Major Complication/Comorbidity   CC Complication/Comorbidity   SW Severe Wound Dx

606   ICD-10-CM 2020

     H18.629 Keratoconus, unstable, unspecified eye

✓5ᵗʰ **H18.7** Other and unspecified corneal deformities

     EXCLUDES 1   *congenital malformations of cornea (Q13.3-Q13.4)*

     H18.70 Unspecified corneal deformity

✓6ᵗʰ **H18.71** Corneal ectasia

     H18.711 Corneal ectasia, right eye
     H18.712 Corneal ectasia, left eye
     H18.713 Corneal ectasia, bilateral
     H18.719 Corneal ectasia, unspecified eye

✓6ᵗʰ **H18.72** Corneal staphyloma

     H18.721 Corneal staphyloma, right eye
     H18.722 Corneal staphyloma, left eye
     H18.723 Corneal staphyloma, bilateral
     H18.729 Corneal staphyloma, unspecified eye

✓6ᵗʰ **H18.73** Descemetocele

     H18.731 Descemetocele, right eye
     H18.732 Descemetocele, left eye
     H18.733 Descemetocele, bilateral
     H18.739 Descemetocele, unspecified eye

✓6ᵗʰ **H18.79** Other corneal deformities

     H18.791 Other corneal deformities, right eye
     H18.792 Other corneal deformities, left eye
     H18.793 Other corneal deformities, bilateral
     H18.799 Other corneal deformities, unspecified eye

✓5ᵗʰ **H18.8** Other specified disorders of cornea

✓6ᵗʰ **H18.81** Anesthesia and hypoesthesia of cornea

     H18.811 Anesthesia and hypoesthesia of cornea, right eye
     H18.812 Anesthesia and hypoesthesia of cornea, left eye
     H18.813 Anesthesia and hypoesthesia of cornea, bilateral
     H18.819 Anesthesia and hypoesthesia of cornea, unspecified eye

✓6ᵗʰ **H18.82** Corneal disorder due to contact lens

     EXCLUDES 2   *corneal edema due to contact lens (H18.21-)*

     H18.821 Corneal disorder due to contact lens, right eye
     H18.822 Corneal disorder due to contact lens, left eye
     H18.823 Corneal disorder due to contact lens, bilateral
     H18.829 Corneal disorder due to contact lens, unspecified eye

✓6ᵗʰ **H18.83** Recurrent erosion of cornea

     H18.831 Recurrent erosion of cornea, right eye
     H18.832 Recurrent erosion of cornea, left eye
     H18.833 Recurrent erosion of cornea, bilateral
     H18.839 Recurrent erosion of cornea, unspecified eye

✓6ᵗʰ **H18.89** Other specified disorders of cornea

     H18.891 Other specified disorders of cornea, right eye
     H18.892 Other specified disorders of cornea, left eye
     H18.893 Other specified disorders of cornea, bilateral
     H18.899 Other specified disorders of cornea, unspecified eye

H18.9 Unspecified disorder of cornea

✓4ᵗʰ **H20** Iridocyclitis

CC Excl: For CC codes in category H20: PDX collection 624

✓5ᵗʰ **H20.0** Acute and subacute iridocyclitis

     Acute anterior uveitis
     Acute cyclitis
     Acute iritis
     Subacute anterior uveitis
     Subacute cyclitis
     Subacute iritis

     EXCLUDES 1   *iridocyclitis, iritis, uveitis (due to) (in) diabetes mellitus (E08-E13 with .39)*
     iridocyclitis, iritis, uveitis (due to) (in) diphtheria (A36.89)
     iridocyclitis, iritis, uveitis (due to) (in) gonococcal (A54.32)
     iridocyclitis, iritis, uveitis (due to) (in) herpes (simplex) (B00.51)
     iridocyclitis, iritis, uveitis (due to) (in) herpes zoster (B02.32)
     iridocyclitis, iritis, uveitis (due to) (in) late congenital syphilis (A50.39)
     iridocyclitis, iritis, uveitis (due to) (in) late syphilis (A52.71)
     iridocyclitis, iritis, uveitis (due to) (in) sarcoidosis (D86.83)
     iridocyclitis, iritis, uveitis (due to) (in) syphilis (A51.43)
     iridocyclitis, iritis, uveitis (due to) (in) toxoplasmosis (B58.09)
     iridocyclitis, iritis, uveitis (due to) (in) tuberculosis (A18.54)

     H20.00 Unspecified acute and subacute iridocyclitis   CC

✓6ᵗʰ **H20.01** Primary iridocyclitis

     H20.011 Primary iridocyclitis, right eye   CC
     H20.012 Primary iridocyclitis, left eye   CC
     H20.013 Primary iridocyclitis, bilateral   CC
     H20.019 Primary iridocyclitis, unspecified eye   CC

✓6ᵗʰ **H20.02** Recurrent acute iridocyclitis

     H20.021 Recurrent acute iridocyclitis, right eye   CC
     H20.022 Recurrent acute iridocyclitis, left eye   CC
     H20.023 Recurrent acute iridocyclitis, bilateral   CC
     H20.029 Recurrent acute iridocyclitis, unspecified eye   CC

✓6ᵗʰ **H20.03** Secondary infectious iridocyclitis

     H20.031 Secondary infectious iridocyclitis, right eye   CC
     H20.032 Secondary infectious iridocyclitis, left eye   CC
     H20.033 Secondary infectious iridocyclitis, bilateral   CC
     H20.039 Secondary infectious iridocyclitis, unspecified eye   CC

✓6ᵗʰ **H20.04** Secondary noninfectious iridocyclitis

     H20.041 Secondary noninfectious iridocyclitis, right eye
     H20.042 Secondary noninfectious iridocyclitis, left eye
     H20.043 Secondary noninfectious iridocyclitis, bilateral
     H20.049 Secondary noninfectious iridocyclitis, unspecified eye

✓6ᵗʰ **H20.05** Hypopyon

     H20.051 Hypopyon, right eye
     H20.052 Hypopyon, left eye
     H20.053 Hypopyon, bilateral
     H20.059 Hypopyon, unspecified eye

☑ Additional Character Required   ✓x7ᵗʰ Placeholder   Unacceptable PDx   Questionable PDx   Manifestation   Unspecified Dx   H1-H14 HAC   HCC CMS-HCC Dx   HIV HIV Dx

ICD-10-CM 2020

607

Chapter 7. Diseases of the Eye and Adnexa *(side margin)*

√5ᵗʰ **H20.1 Chronic iridocyclitis**
Use additional code for any associated cataract (H26.21-)
EXCLUDES 2   *posterior cyclitis (H30.2-)*

   H20.10 Chronic iridocyclitis, unspecified eye
   H20.11 Chronic iridocyclitis, right eye
   H20.12 Chronic iridocyclitis, left eye
   H20.13 Chronic iridocyclitis, bilateral

√5ᵗʰ **H20.2 Lens-induced iridocyclitis**

   H20.20 Lens-induced iridocyclitis, unspecified eye
   H20.21 Lens-induced iridocyclitis, right eye
   H20.22 Lens-induced iridocyclitis, left eye
   H20.23 Lens-induced iridocyclitis, bilateral

√5ᵗʰ **H20.8 Other iridocyclitis**
EXCLUDES 2   *glaucomatocyclitis crises (H40.4-)*
       posterior cyclitis (H30.2-)
       sympathetic uveitis (H44.13-)

√6ᵗʰ **H20.81 Fuchs' heterochromic cyclitis**
   H20.811 Fuchs' heterochromic cyclitis, right eye
   H20.812 Fuchs' heterochromic cyclitis, left eye
   H20.813 Fuchs' heterochromic cyclitis, bilateral
   H20.819 Fuchs' heterochromic cyclitis, unspecified eye

√6ᵗʰ **H20.82 Vogt-Koyanagi syndrome**
   H20.821 Vogt-Koyanagi syndrome, right eye
   H20.822 Vogt-Koyanagi syndrome, left eye
   H20.823 Vogt-Koyanagi syndrome, bilateral
   H20.829 Vogt-Koyanagi syndrome, unspecified eye

H20.9 Unspecified iridocyclitis   CC
Uveitis NOS

√4ᵗʰ **H21 Other disorders of iris and ciliary body**
EXCLUDES 2   *sympathetic uveitis (H44.1-)*

√5ᵗʰ **H21.0 Hyphema**
EXCLUDES 1   *traumatic hyphema (S05.1-)*

Hyphema

Iris
Cornea
Hyphema

   H21.00 Hyphema, unspecified eye
   H21.01 Hyphema, right eye
   H21.02 Hyphema, left eye
   H21.03 Hyphema, bilateral

√5ᵗʰ **H21.1 Other vascular disorders of iris and ciliary body**
Neovascularization of iris or ciliary body
Rubeosis iridis
Rubeosis of iris

√6ᵗʰ **H21.1X Other vascular disorders of iris and ciliary body**
   H21.1X1 Other vascular disorders of iris and ciliary body, right eye
   H21.1X2 Other vascular disorders of iris and ciliary body, left eye
   H21.1X3 Other vascular disorders of iris and ciliary body, bilateral
   H21.1X9 Other vascular disorders of iris and ciliary body, unspecified eye

√5ᵗʰ **H21.2 Degeneration of iris and ciliary body**

√6ᵗʰ **H21.21 Degeneration of chamber angle**
   H21.211 Degeneration of chamber angle, right eye
   H21.212 Degeneration of chamber angle, left eye
   H21.213 Degeneration of chamber angle, bilateral
   H21.219 Degeneration of chamber angle, unspecified eye

√6ᵗʰ **H21.22 Degeneration of ciliary body**
   H21.221 Degeneration of ciliary body, right eye
   H21.222 Degeneration of ciliary body, left eye
   H21.223 Degeneration of ciliary body, bilateral
   H21.229 Degeneration of ciliary body, unspecified eye

√6ᵗʰ **H21.23 Degeneration of iris (pigmentary)**
Translucency of iris
   H21.231 Degeneration of iris (pigmentary), right eye
   H21.232 Degeneration of iris (pigmentary), left eye
   H21.233 Degeneration of iris (pigmentary), bilateral
   H21.239 Degeneration of iris (pigmentary), unspecified eye

√6ᵗʰ **H21.24 Degeneration of pupillary margin**
   H21.241 Degeneration of pupillary margin, right eye
   H21.242 Degeneration of pupillary margin, left eye
   H21.243 Degeneration of pupillary margin, bilateral
   H21.249 Degeneration of pupillary margin, unspecified eye

√6ᵗʰ **H21.25 Iridoschisis**
   H21.251 Iridoschisis, right eye
   H21.252 Iridoschisis, left eye
   H21.253 Iridoschisis, bilateral
   H21.259 Iridoschisis, unspecified eye

√6ᵗʰ **H21.26 Iris atrophy (essential) (progressive)**
   H21.261 Iris atrophy (essential) (progressive), right eye
   H21.262 Iris atrophy (essential) (progressive), left eye
   H21.263 Iris atrophy (essential) (progressive), bilateral
   H21.269 Iris atrophy (essential) (progressive), unspecified eye

√6ᵗʰ **H21.27 Miotic pupillary cyst**
   H21.271 Miotic pupillary cyst, right eye
   H21.272 Miotic pupillary cyst, left eye
   H21.273 Miotic pupillary cyst, bilateral
   H21.279 Miotic pupillary cyst, unspecified eye

H21.29 Other iris atrophy

√5ᵗʰ **H21.3 Cyst of iris, ciliary body and anterior chamber**
EXCLUDES 2   *miotic pupillary cyst (H21.27-)*

√6ᵗʰ **H21.30 Idiopathic cysts of iris, ciliary body or anterior chamber**
Cyst of iris, ciliary body or anterior chamber NOS
   H21.301 Idiopathic cysts of iris, ciliary body or anterior chamber, right eye
   H21.302 Idiopathic cysts of iris, ciliary body or anterior chamber, left eye
   H21.303 Idiopathic cysts of iris, ciliary body or anterior chamber, bilateral
   H21.309 Idiopathic cysts of iris, ciliary body or anterior chamber, unspecified eye

√6ᵗʰ **H21.31 Exudative cysts of iris or anterior chamber**
   H21.311 Exudative cysts of iris or anterior chamber, right eye
   H21.312 Exudative cysts of iris or anterior chamber, left eye
   H21.313 Exudative cysts of iris or anterior chamber, bilateral
   H21.319 Exudative cysts of iris or anterior chamber, unspecified eye

√6ᵗʰ **H21.32 Implantation cysts of iris, ciliary body or anterior chamber**
   H21.321 Implantation cysts of iris, ciliary body or anterior chamber, right eye
   H21.322 Implantation cysts of iris, ciliary body or anterior chamber, left eye
   H21.323 Implantation cysts of iris, ciliary body or anterior chamber, bilateral
   H21.329 Implantation cysts of iris, ciliary body or anterior chamber, unspecified eye

N Newborn: 0   P Pediatric: 0-17   M Maternity: 9-64   A Adult: 15-124   MCC Major Complication/Comorbidity   CC Complication/Comorbidity   SW Severe Wound Dx

608   ICD-10-CM 2020

√6th **H21.33 Parasitic cyst of iris, ciliary body or anterior chamber**

CC Excl: For CC codes in subcategory H21.33: PDX collection 625

H21.331 Parasitic cyst of iris, ciliary body or anterior chamber, **right eye** `CC`

H21.332 Parasitic cyst of iris, ciliary body or anterior chamber, **left eye** `CC`

H21.333 Parasitic cyst of iris, ciliary body or anterior chamber, **bilateral** `CC`

H21.339 Parasitic cyst of iris, ciliary body or anterior chamber, **unspecified eye** `CC`

√6th **H21.34 Primary cyst of pars plana**

H21.341 Primary cyst of pars plana, **right eye**
H21.342 Primary cyst of pars plana, **left eye**
H21.343 Primary cyst of pars plana, **bilateral**
H21.349 Primary cyst of pars plana, **unspecified eye**

√6th **H21.35 Exudative cyst of pars plana**

DEF: Protein, fatty-filled bullous elevation of the nonpigmented outermost ciliary epithelium of pars plana, due to fluid leak from blood vessels.

H21.351 Exudative cyst of pars plana, **right eye**
H21.352 Exudative cyst of pars plana, **left eye**
H21.353 Exudative cyst of pars plana, **bilateral**
H21.359 Exudative cyst of pars plana, **unspecified eye**

√5th **H21.4 Pupillary membranes**

Iris bombé
Pupillary occlusion
Pupillary seclusion

EXCLUDES 1   congenital pupillary membranes (Q13.8)

H21.40 Pupillary membranes, **unspecified eye**
H21.41 Pupillary membranes, **right eye**
H21.42 Pupillary membranes, **left eye**
H21.43 Pupillary membranes, **bilateral**

√5th **H21.5 Other and unspecified adhesions and disruptions of iris and ciliary body**

EXCLUDES 1   corectopia (Q13.2)

√6th **H21.50 Unspecified adhesions of iris**

Synechia (iris) NOS

H21.501 Unspecified adhesions of iris, **right eye**
H21.502 Unspecified adhesions of iris, **left eye**
H21.503 Unspecified adhesions of iris, **bilateral**
H21.509 Unspecified adhesions of iris and ciliary body, **unspecified eye**

√6th **H21.51 Anterior synechiae (iris)**

H21.511 Anterior synechiae (iris), **right eye**
H21.512 Anterior synechiae (iris), **left eye**
H21.513 Anterior synechiae (iris), **bilateral**
H21.519 Anterior synechiae (iris), **unspecified eye**

√6th **H21.52 Goniosynechiae**

H21.521 Goniosynechiae, **right eye**
H21.522 Goniosynechiae, **left eye**
H21.523 Goniosynechiae, **bilateral**
H21.529 Goniosynechiae, **unspecified eye**

√6th **H21.53 Iridodialysis**

H21.531 Iridodialysis, **right eye**
H21.532 Iridodialysis, **left eye**
H21.533 Iridodialysis, **bilateral**
H21.539 Iridodialysis, **unspecified eye**

√6th **H21.54 Posterior synechiae (iris)**

H21.541 Posterior synechiae (iris), **right eye**
H21.542 Posterior synechiae (iris), **left eye**
H21.543 Posterior synechiae (iris), **bilateral**
H21.549 Posterior synechiae (iris), **unspecified eye**

√6th **H21.55 Recession of chamber angle**

H21.551 Recession of chamber angle, **right eye**
H21.552 Recession of chamber angle, **left eye**
H21.553 Recession of chamber angle, **bilateral**
H21.559 Recession of chamber angle, **unspecified eye**

√6th **H21.56 Pupillary abnormalities**

Deformed pupil
Ectopic pupil
Rupture of sphincter, pupil

EXCLUDES 1   congenital deformity of pupil (Q13.2-)

H21.561 Pupillary abnormality, **right eye**
H21.562 Pupillary abnormality, **left eye**
H21.563 Pupillary abnormality, **bilateral**
H21.569 Pupillary abnormality, **unspecified eye**

√5th **H21.8 Other specified disorders of iris and ciliary body**

H21.81 Floppy iris syndrome

Intraoperative floppy iris syndrome (IFIS)
Use additional code for adverse effect, if applicable, to identify drug (T36-T50 with fifth or sixth character 5)

H21.82 Plateau iris syndrome (post-iridectomy) (postprocedural)

H21.89 Other specified disorders of iris and ciliary body

H21.9 Unspecified disorder of iris and ciliary body

H22 Disorders of iris and ciliary body in diseases classified elsewhere

Code first underlying disease, such as:
gout (M1A.-, M10.-)
leprosy (A30.-)
parasitic disease (B89)

Disorders of lens (H25-H28)

√4th **H25 Age-related cataract**

Senile cataract

EXCLUDES 2   capsular glaucoma with pseudoexfoliation of lens (H40.1-)

Cataracts

Normal lens

Clouded lens

Lens affected by cataracts

√5th **H25.0 Age-related incipient cataract**

√6th **H25.01 Cortical age-related cataract**

H25.011 Cortical age-related cataract, **right eye** `A`
H25.012 Cortical age-related cataract, **left eye** `A`
H25.013 Cortical age-related cataract, **bilateral** `A`
H25.019 Cortical age-related cataract, **unspecified eye** `A`

√6th **H25.03 Anterior subcapsular polar age-related cataract**

H25.031 Anterior subcapsular polar age-related cataract, **right eye** `A`
H25.032 Anterior subcapsular polar age-related cataract, **left eye** `A`
H25.033 Anterior subcapsular polar age-related cataract, **bilateral** `A`
H25.039 Anterior subcapsular polar age-related cataract, **unspecified eye** `A`

✓6ᵗʰ H25.04 Posterior subcapsular polar age-related cataract

H25.041 Posterior subcapsular polar age-related cataract, right eye Ⓐ

H25.042 Posterior subcapsular polar age-related cataract, left eye Ⓐ

H25.043 Posterior subcapsular polar age-related cataract, bilateral Ⓐ

H25.049 Posterior subcapsular polar age-related cataract, unspecified eye Ⓐ

✓6ᵗʰ H25.09 Other age-related incipient cataract

Coronary age-related cataract
Punctate age-related cataract
Water clefts

H25.091 Other age-related incipient cataract, right eye Ⓐ

H25.092 Other age-related incipient cataract, left eye Ⓐ

H25.093 Other age-related incipient cataract, bilateral Ⓐ

H25.099 Other age-related incipient cataract, unspecified eye Ⓐ

✓5ᵗʰ H25.1 Age-related nuclear cataract

Cataracta brunescens
Nuclear sclerosis cataract
AHA: 2019,2Q,31; 2016,1Q,32

H25.10 Age-related nuclear cataract, unspecified eye Ⓐ

H25.11 Age-related nuclear cataract, right eye Ⓐ

H25.12 Age-related nuclear cataract, left eye Ⓐ

H25.13 Age-related nuclear cataract, bilateral Ⓐ

✓5ᵗʰ H25.2 Age-related cataract, morgagnian type

Age-related hypermature cataract

H25.20 Age-related cataract, morgagnian type, unspecified eye Ⓐ

H25.21 Age-related cataract, morgagnian type, right eye Ⓐ

H25.22 Age-related cataract, morgagnian type, left eye Ⓐ

H25.23 Age-related cataract, morgagnian type, bilateral Ⓐ

✓5ᵗʰ H25.8 Other age-related cataract

✓6ᵗʰ H25.81 Combined forms of age-related cataract

AHA: 2019,2Q,30

H25.811 Combined forms of age-related cataract, right eye Ⓐ

H25.812 Combined forms of age-related cataract, left eye Ⓐ

H25.813 Combined forms of age-related cataract, bilateral Ⓐ

H25.819 Combined forms of age-related cataract, unspecified eye Ⓐ

H25.89 Other age-related cataract Ⓐ

H25.9 Unspecified age-related cataract Ⓐ

✓4ᵗʰ H26 Other cataract

EXCLUDES 1 congenital cataract (Q12.0)

✓5ᵗʰ H26.0 Infantile and juvenile cataract

✓6ᵗʰ H26.00 Unspecified infantile and juvenile cataract

H26.001 Unspecified infantile and juvenile cataract, right eye Ⓟ

H26.002 Unspecified infantile and juvenile cataract, left eye Ⓟ

H26.003 Unspecified infantile and juvenile cataract, bilateral Ⓟ

H26.009 Unspecified infantile and juvenile cataract, unspecified eye Ⓟ

✓6ᵗʰ H26.01 Infantile and juvenile cortical, lamellar, or zonular cataract

H26.011 Infantile and juvenile cortical, lamellar, or zonular cataract, right eye Ⓟ

H26.012 Infantile and juvenile cortical, lamellar, or zonular cataract, left eye Ⓟ

H26.013 Infantile and juvenile cortical, lamellar, or zonular cataract, bilateral Ⓟ

H26.019 Infantile and juvenile cortical, lamellar, or zonular cataract, unspecified eye Ⓟ

✓6ᵗʰ H26.03 Infantile and juvenile nuclear cataract

H26.031 Infantile and juvenile nuclear cataract, right eye Ⓟ

H26.032 Infantile and juvenile nuclear cataract, left eye Ⓟ

H26.033 Infantile and juvenile nuclear cataract, bilateral Ⓟ

H26.039 Infantile and juvenile nuclear cataract, unspecified eye Ⓟ

✓6ᵗʰ H26.04 Anterior subcapsular polar infantile and juvenile cataract

H26.041 Anterior subcapsular polar infantile and juvenile cataract, right eye Ⓟ

H26.042 Anterior subcapsular polar infantile and juvenile cataract, left eye Ⓟ

H26.043 Anterior subcapsular polar infantile and juvenile cataract, bilateral Ⓟ

H26.049 Anterior subcapsular polar infantile and juvenile cataract, unspecified eye Ⓟ

✓6ᵗʰ H26.05 Posterior subcapsular polar infantile and juvenile cataract

H26.051 Posterior subcapsular polar infantile and juvenile cataract, right eye Ⓟ

H26.052 Posterior subcapsular polar infantile and juvenile cataract, left eye Ⓟ

H26.053 Posterior subcapsular polar infantile and juvenile cataract, bilateral Ⓟ

H26.059 Posterior subcapsular polar infantile and juvenile cataract, unspecified eye Ⓟ

✓6ᵗʰ H26.06 Combined forms of infantile and juvenile cataract

H26.061 Combined forms of infantile and juvenile cataract, right eye Ⓟ

H26.062 Combined forms of infantile and juvenile cataract, left eye Ⓟ

H26.063 Combined forms of infantile and juvenile cataract, bilateral Ⓟ

H26.069 Combined forms of infantile and juvenile cataract, unspecified eye Ⓟ

H26.09 Other infantile and juvenile cataract Ⓟ

✓5ᵗʰ H26.1 Traumatic cataract

Use additional code (Chapter 20) to identify external cause

✓6ᵗʰ H26.10 Unspecified traumatic cataract

H26.101 Unspecified traumatic cataract, right eye
H26.102 Unspecified traumatic cataract, left eye
H26.103 Unspecified traumatic cataract, bilateral
H26.109 Unspecified traumatic cataract, unspecified eye

✓6ᵗʰ H26.11 Localized traumatic opacities

H26.111 Localized traumatic opacities, right eye
H26.112 Localized traumatic opacities, left eye
H26.113 Localized traumatic opacities, bilateral
H26.119 Localized traumatic opacities, unspecified eye

√6ᵗʰ **H26.12** Partially resolved traumatic cataract

     H26.121 Partially resolved traumatic cataract, right eye

     H26.122 Partially resolved traumatic cataract, left eye

     H26.123 Partially resolved traumatic cataract, bilateral

     H26.129 Partially resolved traumatic cataract, unspecified eye

√6ᵗʰ **H26.13** Total traumatic cataract

     H26.131 Total traumatic cataract, right eye

     H26.132 Total traumatic cataract, left eye

     H26.133 Total traumatic cataract, bilateral

     H26.139 Total traumatic cataract, unspecified eye

√5ᵗʰ **H26.2** Complicated cataract

     H26.20 Unspecified complicated cataract

         Cataracta complicata NOS

√6ᵗʰ   **H26.21** Cataract with neovascularization

     Code also associated condition, such as:

         chronic iridocyclitis (H20.1-)

     H26.211 Cataract with neovascularization, right eye

     H26.212 Cataract with neovascularization, left eye

     H26.213 Cataract with neovascularization, bilateral

     H26.219 Cataract with neovascularization, unspecified eye

√6ᵗʰ   **H26.22** Cataract secondary to ocular disorders (degenerative) (inflammatory)

     Code also associated ocular disorder

     H26.221 Cataract secondary to ocular disorders (degenerative) (inflammatory), right eye

     H26.222 Cataract secondary to ocular disorders (degenerative) (inflammatory), left eye

     H26.223 Cataract secondary to ocular disorders (degenerative) (inflammatory), bilateral

     H26.229 Cataract secondary to ocular disorders (degenerative) (inflammatory), unspecified eye

√6ᵗʰ   **H26.23** Glaucomatous flecks (subcapsular)

     Code first underlying glaucoma (H40-H42)

     H26.231 Glaucomatous flecks (subcapsular), right eye

     H26.232 Glaucomatous flecks (subcapsular), left eye

     H26.233 Glaucomatous flecks (subcapsular), bilateral

     H26.239 Glaucomatous flecks (subcapsular), unspecified eye

√5ᵗʰ **H26.3** Drug-induced cataract

     Toxic cataract

     Use additional code for adverse effect, if applicable, to identify drug (T36-T50 with fifth or sixth character 5)

     H26.30 Drug-induced cataract, unspecified eye

     H26.31 Drug-induced cataract, right eye

     H26.32 Drug-induced cataract, left eye

     H26.33 Drug-induced cataract, bilateral

√5ᵗʰ **H26.4** Secondary cataract

     H26.40 Unspecified secondary cataract

√6ᵗʰ   **H26.41** Soemmering's ring

     H26.411 Soemmering's ring, right eye

     H26.412 Soemmering's ring, left eye

     H26.413 Soemmering's ring, bilateral

     H26.419 Soemmering's ring, unspecified eye

√6ᵗʰ   **H26.49** Other secondary cataract

     AHA: 2018,2Q,14

     H26.491 Other secondary cataract, right eye

     H26.492 Other secondary cataract, left eye

     H26.493 Other secondary cataract, bilateral

     H26.499 Other secondary cataract, unspecified eye

H26.8 Other specified cataract

H26.9 Unspecified cataract

√4ᵗʰ **H27** Other disorders of lens

     EXCLUDES 1   congenital lens malformations (Q12.-)

         mechanical complications of intraocular lens implant (T85.2)

         pseudophakia (Z96.1)

√5ᵗʰ **H27.0** Aphakia

     Acquired absence of lens

     Acquired aphakia

     Aphakia due to trauma

     EXCLUDES 1   cataract extraction status (Z98.4-)

         congenital absence of lens (Q12.3)

         congenital aphakia (Q12.3)

     H27.00 Aphakia, unspecified eye

     H27.01 Aphakia, right eye

     H27.02 Aphakia, left eye

     H27.03 Aphakia, bilateral

√5ᵗʰ **H27.1** Dislocation of lens

     H27.10 Unspecified dislocation of lens

√6ᵗʰ   **H27.11** Subluxation of lens

     H27.111 Subluxation of lens, right eye

     H27.112 Subluxation of lens, left eye

     H27.113 Subluxation of lens, bilateral

     H27.119 Subluxation of lens, unspecified eye

√6ᵗʰ   **H27.12** Anterior dislocation of lens

     H27.121 Anterior dislocation of lens, right eye

     H27.122 Anterior dislocation of lens, left eye

     H27.123 Anterior dislocation of lens, bilateral

     H27.129 Anterior dislocation of lens, unspecified eye

√6ᵗʰ   **H27.13** Posterior dislocation of lens

     H27.131 Posterior dislocation of lens, right eye

     H27.132 Posterior dislocation of lens, left eye

     H27.133 Posterior dislocation of lens, bilateral

     H27.139 Posterior dislocation of lens, unspecified eye

H27.8 Other specified disorders of lens

H27.9 Unspecified disorder of lens

H28 *Cataract in diseases classified elsewhere*

     Code first underlying disease, such as:

         hypoparathyroidism (E20.-)

         myotonia (G71.1-)

         myxedema (E03.-)

         protein-calorie malnutrition (E40-E46)

     EXCLUDES 1   cataract in diabetes mellitus (E08.36, E09.36, E10.36, E11.36, E13.36)

Disorders of choroid and retina (H30-H36)

√4ᵗʰ **H30** Chorioretinal inflammation

     CC Excl: For CC codes in category H30: PDX collection 626

√5ᵗʰ **H30.0** Focal chorioretinal inflammation

     Focal chorioretinitis

     Focal choroiditis

     Focal retinitis

     Focal retinochoroiditis

√6ᵗʰ   **H30.00** Unspecified focal chorioretinal inflammation

     Focal chorioretinitis NOS

     Focal choroiditis NOS

     Focal retinitis NOS

     Focal retinochoroiditis NOS

     H30.001 Unspecified focal chorioretinal inflammation, right eye

     H30.002 Unspecified focal chorioretinal inflammation, left eye

     H30.003 Unspecified focal chorioretinal inflammation, bilateral

     H30.009 Unspecified focal chorioretinal inflammation, unspecified eye

√6ᵗʰ   **H30.01** Focal chorioretinal inflammation, juxtapapillary

     H30.011 Focal chorioretinal inflammation, juxtapapillary, right eye

     H30.012 Focal chorioretinal inflammation, juxtapapillary, left eye

     H30.013 Focal chorioretinal inflammation, juxtapapillary, bilateral

     H30.019 Focal chorioretinal inflammation, juxtapapillary, unspecified eye

✔ Additional Character Required   √x7ᵗʰ Placeholder   Unacceptable PDx   Questionable PDx   Manifestation   Unspecified Dx   H1-H16 HAC   HCC CMS-HCC Dx   HIV HIV Dx

ICD-10-CM 2020   611

√6ᵗʰ **H30.02 Focal chorioretinal inflammation of** posterior pole

     H30.021 Focal chorioretinal inflammation of posterior pole, right **eye**

     H30.022 Focal chorioretinal inflammation of posterior pole, left **eye**

     H30.023 Focal chorioretinal inflammation of posterior pole, bilateral

     H30.029 Focal chorioretinal inflammation of posterior pole, unspecified eye

√6ᵗʰ **H30.03 Focal chorioretinal inflammation,** peripheral

     H30.031 Focal chorioretinal inflammation, peripheral, right **eye**

     H30.032 Focal chorioretinal inflammation, peripheral, left **eye**

     H30.033 Focal chorioretinal inflammation, peripheral, bilateral

     H30.039 Focal chorioretinal inflammation, peripheral, unspecified eye

√6ᵗʰ **H30.04 Focal chorioretinal inflammation,** macular or paramacular

     H30.041 Focal chorioretinal inflammation, macular or paramacular, right **eye**

     H30.042 Focal chorioretinal inflammation, macular or paramacular, left **eye**

     H30.043 Focal chorioretinal inflammation, macular or paramacular, bilateral

     H30.049 Focal chorioretinal inflammation, macular or paramacular, unspecified eye

√5ᵗʰ **H30.1** Disseminated **chorioretinal inflammation**

   Disseminated chorioretinitis
   Disseminated choroiditis
   Disseminated retinitis
   Disseminated retinochoroiditis
   EXCLUDES 2   exudative retinopathy (H35.02-)

√6ᵗʰ **H30.10 Unspecified disseminated chorioretinal inflammation**

   Disseminated chorioretinitis NOS
   Disseminated choroiditis NOS
   Disseminated retinitis NOS
   Disseminated retinochoroiditis NOS

     H30.101 Unspecified disseminated chorioretinal inflammation, right **eye**   CC

     H30.102 Unspecified disseminated chorioretinal inflammation, left **eye**   CC

     H30.103 Unspecified disseminated chorioretinal inflammation, bilateral   CC

     H30.109 Unspecified disseminated chorioretinal inflammation, unspecified eye   CC

√6ᵗʰ **H30.11 Disseminated chorioretinal inflammation of** posterior pole

     H30.111 Disseminated chorioretinal inflammation of posterior pole, right **eye**   CC

     H30.112 Disseminated chorioretinal inflammation of posterior pole, left **eye**   CC

     H30.113 Disseminated chorioretinal inflammation of posterior pole, bilateral   CC

     H30.119 Disseminated chorioretinal inflammation of posterior pole, unspecified eye   CC

√6ᵗʰ **H30.12 Disseminated chorioretinal inflammation,** peripheral

     H30.121 Disseminated chorioretinal inflammation, peripheral right **eye**   CC

     H30.122 Disseminated chorioretinal inflammation, peripheral, left **eye**   CC

     H30.123 Disseminated chorioretinal inflammation, peripheral, bilateral   CC

     H30.129 Disseminated chorioretinal inflammation, peripheral, unspecified eye   CC

√6ᵗʰ **H30.13 Disseminated chorioretinal inflammation,** generalized

     H30.131 Disseminated chorioretinal inflammation, generalized, right **eye**   CC

     H30.132 Disseminated chorioretinal inflammation, generalized, left **eye**   CC

     H30.133 Disseminated chorioretinal inflammation, generalized, bilateral   CC

     H30.139 Disseminated chorioretinal inflammation, generalized, unspecified eye   CC

√6ᵗʰ **H30.14** Acute posterior multifocal placoid pigment epitheliopathy

     H30.141 Acute posterior multifocal placoid pigment epitheliopathy, right **eye**   CC

     H30.142 Acute posterior multifocal placoid pigment epitheliopathy, left **eye**   CC

     H30.143 Acute posterior multifocal placoid pigment epitheliopathy, bilateral   CC

     H30.149 Acute posterior multifocal placoid pigment epitheliopathy, unspecified eye   CC

√5ᵗʰ **H30.2 Posterior cyclitis**

   Pars planitis

     H30.20 Posterior cyclitis, unspecified eye

     H30.21 Posterior cyclitis, right **eye**

     H30.22 Posterior cyclitis, left **eye**

     H30.23 Posterior cyclitis, bilateral

√5ᵗʰ **H30.8 Other chorioretinal inflammations**

√6ᵗʰ **H30.81 Harada's disease**

     H30.811 Harada's disease, right **eye**

     H30.812 Harada's disease, left **eye**

     H30.813 Harada's disease, bilateral

     H30.819 Harada's disease, unspecified eye

√6ᵗʰ **H30.89 Other chorioretinal inflammations**

     H30.891 Other chorioretinal inflammations, right **eye**   CC

     H30.892 Other chorioretinal inflammations, left **eye**   CC

     H30.893 Other chorioretinal inflammations, bilateral   CC

     H30.899 Other chorioretinal inflammations, unspecified eye   CC

√5ᵗʰ **H30.9 Unspecified chorioretinal inflammation**

   Chorioretinitis NOS
   Choroiditis NOS
   Neuroretinitis NOS
   Retinitis NOS
   Retinochoroiditis NOS

     H30.90 Unspecified chorioretinal inflammation, unspecified eye   CC

     H30.91 Unspecified chorioretinal inflammation, right **eye**   CC

     H30.92 Unspecified chorioretinal inflammation, left **eye**   CC

     H30.93 Unspecified chorioretinal inflammation, bilateral   CC

Chapter 7. Diseases of the Eye and Adnexa

☑4ᵗʰ **H31 Other disorders of choroid**

     CC Excl: For CC codes in category H31: PDX collection 627

☑5ᵗʰ **H31.0 Chorioretinal scars**

     EXCLUDES 2   *postsurgical chorioretinal scars (H59.81-)*

     ☑6ᵗʰ **H31.00 Unspecified chorioretinal scars**

         H31.001 Unspecified chorioretinal scars, right eye

         H31.002 Unspecified chorioretinal scars, left eye

         H31.003 Unspecified chorioretinal scars, bilateral

         H31.009 Unspecified chorioretinal scars, unspecified eye

     ☑6ᵗʰ **H31.01 Macula scars of posterior pole (postinflammatory) (post-traumatic)**

         EXCLUDES 1   *postprocedural chorioretinal scar (H59.81-)*

         H31.011 Macula scars of posterior pole (postinflammatory) (post-traumatic), right eye

         H31.012 Macula scars of posterior pole (postinflammatory) (post-traumatic), left eye

         H31.013 Macula scars of posterior pole (postinflammatory) (post-traumatic), bilateral

         H31.019 Macula scars of posterior pole (postinflammatory) (post-traumatic), unspecified eye

     ☑6ᵗʰ **H31.02 Solar retinopathy**

         H31.021 Solar retinopathy, right eye

         H31.022 Solar retinopathy, left eye

         H31.023 Solar retinopathy, bilateral

         H31.029 Solar retinopathy, unspecified eye

     ☑6ᵗʰ **H31.09 Other chorioretinal scars**

         H31.091 Other chorioretinal scars, right eye

         H31.092 Other chorioretinal scars, left eye

         H31.093 Other chorioretinal scars, bilateral

         H31.099 Other chorioretinal scars, unspecified eye

☑5ᵗʰ **H31.1 Choroidal degeneration**

     EXCLUDES 2   *angioid streaks of macula (H35.33)*

     ☑6ᵗʰ **H31.10 Unspecified choroidal degeneration**

         Choroidal sclerosis NOS

         H31.101 Choroidal degeneration, unspecified, right eye

         H31.102 Choroidal degeneration, unspecified, left eye

         H31.103 Choroidal degeneration, unspecified, bilateral

         H31.109 Choroidal degeneration, unspecified, unspecified eye

     ☑6ᵗʰ **H31.11 Age-related choroidal atrophy**

         H31.111 Age-related choroidal atrophy, right eye   A

         H31.112 Age-related choroidal atrophy, left eye   A

         H31.113 Age-related choroidal atrophy, bilateral   A

         H31.119 Age-related choroidal atrophy, unspecified eye   A

     ☑6ᵗʰ **H31.12 Diffuse secondary atrophy of choroid**

         H31.121 Diffuse secondary atrophy of choroid, right eye

         H31.122 Diffuse secondary atrophy of choroid, left eye

         H31.123 Diffuse secondary atrophy of choroid, bilateral

         H31.129 Diffuse secondary atrophy of choroid, unspecified eye

☑5ᵗʰ **H31.2 Hereditary choroidal dystrophy**

     EXCLUDES 2   *hyperornithinemia (E72.4)*

                       ornithinemia (E72.4)

     H31.20 Hereditary choroidal dystrophy, unspecified

     H31.21 Choroideremia

     H31.22 Choroidal dystrophy (central areolar) (generalized) (peripapillary)

     H31.23 Gyrate atrophy, choroid

     H31.29 Other hereditary choroidal dystrophy

☑5ᵗʰ **H31.3 Choroidal hemorrhage and rupture**

     ☑6ᵗʰ **H31.30 Unspecified choroidal hemorrhage**

         H31.301 Unspecified choroidal hemorrhage, right eye

         H31.302 Unspecified choroidal hemorrhage, left eye

         H31.303 Unspecified choroidal hemorrhage, bilateral

         H31.309 Unspecified choroidal hemorrhage, unspecified eye

     ☑6ᵗʰ **H31.31 Expulsive choroidal hemorrhage**

         H31.311 Expulsive choroidal hemorrhage, right eye

         H31.312 Expulsive choroidal hemorrhage, left eye

         H31.313 Expulsive choroidal hemorrhage, bilateral

         H31.319 Expulsive choroidal hemorrhage, unspecified eye

     ☑6ᵗʰ **H31.32 Choroidal rupture**

         H31.321 Choroidal rupture, right eye   CC

         H31.322 Choroidal rupture, left eye   CC

         H31.323 Choroidal rupture, bilateral   CC

         H31.329 Choroidal rupture, unspecified eye   CC

☑5ᵗʰ **H31.4 Choroidal detachment**

     ☑6ᵗʰ **H31.40 Unspecified choroidal detachment**

         H31.401 Unspecified choroidal detachment, right eye   CC

         H31.402 Unspecified choroidal detachment, left eye   CC

         H31.403 Unspecified choroidal detachment, bilateral   CC

         H31.409 Unspecified choroidal detachment, unspecified eye   CC

     ☑6ᵗʰ **H31.41 Hemorrhagic choroidal detachment**

         H31.411 Hemorrhagic choroidal detachment, right eye   CC

         H31.412 Hemorrhagic choroidal detachment, left eye   CC

         H31.413 Hemorrhagic choroidal detachment, bilateral   CC

         H31.419 Hemorrhagic choroidal detachment, unspecified eye   CC

     ☑6ᵗʰ **H31.42 Serous choroidal detachment**

         H31.421 Serous choroidal detachment, right eye   CC

         H31.422 Serous choroidal detachment, left eye   CC

         H31.423 Serous choroidal detachment, bilateral   CC

         H31.429 Serous choroidal detachment, unspecified eye   CC

     H31.8 Other specified disorders of choroid

     H31.9 Unspecified disorder of choroid

H32 Chorioretinal disorders in diseases classified elsewhere

     Code first underlying disease, such as:

     congenital toxoplasmosis (P37.1)

     histoplasmosis (B39.-)

     leprosy (A30.-)

     EXCLUDES 1   *chorioretinitis (in):*

            toxoplasmosis (acquired) (B58.01)

            tuberculosis (A18.53)

Chapter 7. Diseases of the Eye and Adnexa

H31-H32

☑ Additional Character Required   ☑7ᵗʰ Placeholder   Unacceptable PDx   Questionable PDx   Manifestation   Unspecified Dx   H1-H14 HAC   HCC CMS-HCC Dx   HIV HIV Dx

ICD-10-CM 2020

613

✓4ᵗʰ H33 Retinal detachments and breaks

    EXCLUDES 1   *detachment of retinal pigment epithelium (H35.72-, H35.73-)*

CC Excl: For CC codes in category H33, unless otherwise noted: PDX collection 628

Retinal Detachment

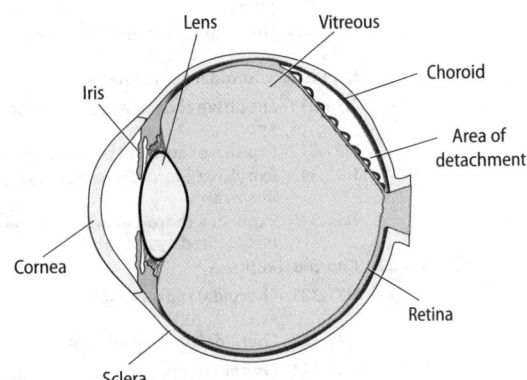

✓5ᵗʰ H33.0 Retinal detachment with retinal break

    Rhegmatogenous retinal detachment

    EXCLUDES 1   *serous retinal detachment (without retinal break) (H33.2-)*

  ✓6ᵗʰ H33.00 Unspecified retinal detachment with retinal break

    H33.001 Unspecified retinal detachment with retinal break, **right** eye

    H33.002 Unspecified retinal detachment with retinal break, **left** eye

    H33.003 Unspecified retinal detachment with retinal break, **bilateral**

    H33.009 Unspecified retinal detachment with retinal break, **unspecified eye**

  ✓6ᵗʰ H33.01 Retinal detachment with single break

    H33.011 Retinal detachment with single break, **right** eye

    H33.012 Retinal detachment with single break, **left** eye

    H33.013 Retinal detachment with single break, **bilateral**

    H33.019 Retinal detachment with single break, **unspecified eye**

  ✓6ᵗʰ H33.02 Retinal detachment with multiple breaks

    H33.021 Retinal detachment with multiple breaks, **right** eye

    H33.022 Retinal detachment with multiple breaks, **left** eye

    H33.023 Retinal detachment with multiple breaks, **bilateral**

    H33.029 Retinal detachment with multiple breaks, **unspecified eye**

  ✓6ᵗʰ H33.03 Retinal detachment with giant retinal tear

    H33.031 Retinal detachment with giant retinal tear, **right eye**

    H33.032 Retinal detachment with giant retinal tear, **left eye**

    H33.033 Retinal detachment with giant retinal tear, **bilateral**

    H33.039 Retinal detachment with giant retinal tear, **unspecified eye**

  ✓6ᵗʰ H33.04 Retinal detachment with retinal dialysis

    H33.041 Retinal detachment with retinal dialysis, **right eye**

    H33.042 Retinal detachment with retinal dialysis, **left eye**

    H33.043 Retinal detachment with retinal dialysis, **bilateral**

    H33.049 Retinal detachment with retinal dialysis, **unspecified eye**

  ✓6ᵗʰ H33.05 Total retinal detachment

    H33.051 Total retinal detachment, **right eye**

    H33.052 Total retinal detachment, **left eye**

    H33.053 Total retinal detachment, **bilateral**

    H33.059 Total retinal detachment, **unspecified eye**

✓5ᵗʰ H33.1 Retinoschisis and retinal cysts

    EXCLUDES 1   *congenital retinoschisis (Q14.1)*

                     microcystoid degeneration of retina (H35.42-)

  ✓6ᵗʰ H33.10 Unspecified retinoschisis

    H33.101 Unspecified retinoschisis, **right eye**

    H33.102 Unspecified retinoschisis, **left eye**

    H33.103 Unspecified retinoschisis, **bilateral**

    H33.109 Unspecified retinoschisis, **unspecified eye**

  ✓6ᵗʰ H33.11 Cyst of ora serrata

    H33.111 Cyst of ora serrata, **right eye**

    H33.112 Cyst of ora serrata, **left eye**

    H33.113 Cyst of ora serrata, **bilateral**

    H33.119 Cyst of ora serrata, **unspecified eye**

  ✓6ᵗʰ H33.12 Parasitic cyst of retina

    CC Excl: For CC codes in subcategory H33.12: PDX collection 625

    H33.121 Parasitic cyst of retina, **right eye**   `CC`

    H33.122 Parasitic cyst of retina, **left eye**   `CC`

    H33.123 Parasitic cyst of retina, **bilateral**   `CC`

    H33.129 Parasitic cyst of retina, **unspecified eye**   `CC`

  ✓6ᵗʰ H33.19 Other retinoschisis and retinal cysts

    Pseudocyst of retina

    H33.191 Other retinoschisis and retinal cysts, **right eye**

    H33.192 Other retinoschisis and retinal cysts, **left eye**

    H33.193 Other retinoschisis and retinal cysts, **bilateral**

    H33.199 Other retinoschisis and retinal cysts, **unspecified eye**

✓5ᵗʰ H33.2 Serous retinal detachment

    Retinal detachment NOS

    Retinal detachment without retinal break

    EXCLUDES 1   *central serous chorioretinopathy (H35.71-)*

    H33.20 Serous retinal detachment, **unspecified eye**   `CC`

    H33.21 Serous retinal detachment, **right eye**   `CC`

    H33.22 Serous retinal detachment, **left eye**   `CC`

    H33.23 Serous retinal detachment, **bilateral**   `CC`

✓5ᵗʰ H33.3 Retinal breaks without detachment

    EXCLUDES 1   *chorioretinal scars after surgery for detachment (H59.81-)*

                     peripheral retinal degeneration without break (H35.4-)

  ✓6ᵗʰ H33.30 Unspecified retinal break

    H33.301 Unspecified retinal break, **right eye**

    H33.302 Unspecified retinal break, **left eye**

    H33.303 Unspecified retinal break, **bilateral**

    H33.309 Unspecified retinal break, **unspecified eye**

  ✓6ᵗʰ H33.31 Horseshoe tear of retina without detachment

    Operculum of retina without detachment

    H33.311 Horseshoe tear of retina without detachment, **right eye**

    H33.312 Horseshoe tear of retina without detachment, **left eye**

    H33.313 Horseshoe tear of retina without detachment, **bilateral**

    H33.319 Horseshoe tear of retina without detachment, **unspecified eye**

  ✓6ᵗʰ H33.32 Round hole of retina without detachment

    H33.321 Round hole, **right eye**

    H33.322 Round hole, **left eye**

    H33.323 Round hole, **bilateral**

    H33.329 Round hole, **unspecified eye**

  ✓6ᵗʰ H33.33 Multiple defects of retina without detachment

    H33.331 Multiple defects of retina without detachment, **right eye**

    H33.332 Multiple defects of retina without detachment, **left eye**

    H33.333 Multiple defects of retina without detachment, **bilateral**

N Newborn: 0   **P** Pediatric: 0-17   **M** Maternity: 9-64   **A** Adult: 15-124   **MCC** Major Complication/Comorbidity   **CC** Complication/Comorbidity   **SW** Severe Wound Dx

614   ICD-10-CM 2020

       H33.339   **Multiple defects of retina without detachment, unspecified eye**

✓5ᵗʰ **H33.4**   **Traction detachment of retina**

     Proliferative vitreo-retinopathy with retinal detachment

     H33.40   **Traction detachment of retina, unspecified eye**   `cc`

     H33.41   **Traction detachment of retina, right eye**   `cc`

     H33.42   **Traction detachment of retina, left eye**   `cc`

     H33.43   **Traction detachment of retina, bilateral**   `cc`

   H33.8   **Other retinal detachments**   `cc`

✓4ᵗʰ **H34**   **Retinal vascular occlusions**

     EXCLUDES 1   *amaurosis fugax (G45.3)*

     CC Excl: For CC codes in category H34: PDX collection 587

✓5ᵗʰ **H34.0**   **Transient retinal artery occlusion**

     H34.00   **Transient retinal artery occlusion, unspecified eye**   `cc`

     H34.01   **Transient retinal artery occlusion, right eye**   `cc`

     H34.02   **Transient retinal artery occlusion, left eye**   `cc`

     H34.03   **Transient retinal artery occlusion, bilateral**   `cc`

✓5ᵗʰ **H34.1**   **Central retinal artery occlusion**

     H34.10   **Central retinal artery occlusion, unspecified eye**   `cc`

     H34.11   **Central retinal artery occlusion, right eye**   `cc`

     H34.12   **Central retinal artery occlusion, left eye**   `cc`

     H34.13   **Central retinal artery occlusion, bilateral**   `cc`

✓5ᵗʰ **H34.2**   **Other retinal artery occlusions**

   ✓6ᵗʰ **H34.21**   **Partial retinal artery occlusion**

     Hollenhorst's plaque

     Retinal microembolism

     H34.211   **Partial retinal artery occlusion, right eye**   `cc`

     H34.212   **Partial retinal artery occlusion, left eye**   `cc`

     H34.213   **Partial retinal artery occlusion, bilateral**   `cc`

     H34.219   **Partial retinal artery occlusion, unspecified eye**   `cc`

   ✓6ᵗʰ **H34.23**   **Retinal artery branch occlusion**

     H34.231   **Retinal artery branch occlusion, right eye**   `cc`

     H34.232   **Retinal artery branch occlusion, left eye**   `cc`

     H34.233   **Retinal artery branch occlusion, bilateral**   `cc`

     H34.239   **Retinal artery branch occlusion, unspecified eye**   `cc`

✓5ᵗʰ **H34.8**   **Other retinal vascular occlusions**

     AHA: 2016,4Q,19

   ✓6ᵗʰ **H34.81**   **Central retinal vein occlusion**

     One of the following 7th characters is to be assigned to codes in subcategory H34.81 to designate the severity of the occlusion:
     0   with macular edema
     1   with retinal neovascularization
     2   stable
       old central retinal vein occlusion

     ✓7ᵗʰ **H34.811**   **Central retinal vein occlusion, right eye**   `cc`

     ✓7ᵗʰ **H34.812**   **Central retinal vein occlusion, left eye**   `cc`

     ✓7ᵗʰ **H34.813**   **Central retinal vein occlusion, bilateral**   `cc`

     ✓7ᵗʰ **H34.819**   **Central retinal vein occlusion, unspecified eye**   `cc`

   ✓6ᵗʰ **H34.82**   **Venous engorgement**

     Incipient retinal vein occlusion

     Partial retinal vein occlusion

     H34.821   **Venous engorgement, right eye**

     H34.822   **Venous engorgement, left eye**

     H34.823   **Venous engorgement, bilateral**

     H34.829   **Venous engorgement, unspecified eye**

   ✓6ᵗʰ **H34.83**   **Tributary (branch) retinal vein occlusion**

     One of the following 7th characters is to be assigned to codes in subcategory H34.83 to designate the severity of the occlusion:
     0   with macular edema
     1   with retinal neovascularization
     2   stable
       old tributary (branch) retinal vein occlusion

     ✓7ᵗʰ **H34.831**   **Tributary (branch) retinal vein occlusion, right eye**

     ✓7ᵗʰ **H34.832**   **Tributary (branch) retinal vein occlusion, left eye**

     ✓7ᵗʰ **H34.833**   **Tributary (branch) retinal vein occlusion, bilateral**

     ✓7ᵗʰ **H34.839**   **Tributary (branch) retinal vein occlusion, unspecified eye**

   H34.9   **Unspecified retinal vascular occlusion**

✓4ᵗʰ **H35**   **Other retinal disorders**

     EXCLUDES 2   *diabetic retinal disorders (E08.311-E08.359, E09.311-E09.359, E10.311-E10.359, E11.311-E11.359, E13.311-E13.359)*

✓5ᵗʰ **H35.0**   **Background retinopathy and retinal vascular changes**

     Code also any associated hypertension (I10.-)

     H35.00   **Unspecified background retinopathy**

   ✓6ᵗʰ **H35.01**   **Changes in retinal vascular appearance**

     Retinal vascular sheathing

     H35.011   **Changes in retinal vascular appearance, right eye**

     H35.012   **Changes in retinal vascular appearance, left eye**

     H35.013   **Changes in retinal vascular appearance, bilateral**

     H35.019   **Changes in retinal vascular appearance, unspecified eye**

   ✓6ᵗʰ **H35.02**   **Exudative retinopathy**

     Coats retinopathy

     H35.021   **Exudative retinopathy, right eye**

     H35.022   **Exudative retinopathy, left eye**

     H35.023   **Exudative retinopathy, bilateral**

     H35.029   **Exudative retinopathy, unspecified eye**

   ✓6ᵗʰ **H35.03**   **Hypertensive retinopathy**

     H35.031   **Hypertensive retinopathy, right eye**

     H35.032   **Hypertensive retinopathy, left eye**

     H35.033   **Hypertensive retinopathy, bilateral**

     H35.039   **Hypertensive retinopathy, unspecified eye**

   ✓6ᵗʰ **H35.04**   **Retinal micro-aneurysms, unspecified**

     H35.041   **Retinal micro-aneurysms, unspecified, right eye**

     H35.042   **Retinal micro-aneurysms, unspecified, left eye**

     H35.043   **Retinal micro-aneurysms, unspecified, bilateral**

     H35.049   **Retinal micro-aneurysms, unspecified, unspecified eye**

   ✓6ᵗʰ **H35.05**   **Retinal neovascularization, unspecified**

     H35.051   **Retinal neovascularization, unspecified, right eye**

     H35.052   **Retinal neovascularization, unspecified, left eye**

     H35.053   **Retinal neovascularization, unspecified, bilateral**

     H35.059   **Retinal neovascularization, unspecified, unspecified eye**

   ✓6ᵗʰ **H35.06**   **Retinal vasculitis**

     Eales disease

     Retinal perivasculitis

     DEF: Sight-threatening intraocular inflammation of the retinal blood vessels that causes minimal, partial, or even complete blindness.

     H35.061   **Retinal vasculitis, right eye**

     H35.062   **Retinal vasculitis, left eye**

     H35.063   **Retinal vasculitis, bilateral**

     H35.069   **Retinal vasculitis, unspecified eye**

   ✓6ᵗʰ **H35.07**   **Retinal telangiectasis**

     H35.071   **Retinal telangiectasis, right eye**

     H35.072   **Retinal telangiectasis, left eye**

✓ Additional Character Required   ✓x7ᵗʰ Placeholder   Unacceptable PDx   Questionable PDx   Manifestation   Unspecified Dx   H1-H14 HAC   HCC CMS-HCC Dx   HIV HIV Dx

ICD-10-CM 2020

615

H33.339–H35.072

Chapter 7. Diseases of the Eye and Adnexa

        H35.Ø73 **Retinal telangiectasis,** bilateral
        H35.Ø79 **Retinal telangiectasis,** unspecified eye
    H35.Ø9 **Other intraretinal microvascular abnormalities**
        Retinal varices

✓5ᵗʰ **H35.1** **Retinopathy of prematurity**

  ✓6ᵗʰ **H35.1Ø** **Retinopathy of prematurity, unspecified**
        Retinopathy of prematurity NOS
        H35.1Ø1 **Retinopathy of prematurity, unspecified,** right **eye**
        H35.1Ø2 **Retinopathy of prematurity, unspecified,** left **eye**
        H35.1Ø3 **Retinopathy of prematurity, unspecified,** bilateral
        H35.1Ø9 **Retinopathy of prematurity, unspecified, unspecified eye**

  ✓6ᵗʰ **H35.11** **Retinopathy of prematurity, stage Ø**
        H35.111 **Retinopathy of prematurity, stage Ø,** right **eye**
        H35.112 **Retinopathy of prematurity, stage Ø,** left **eye**
        H35.113 **Retinopathy of prematurity, stage Ø,** bilateral
        H35.119 **Retinopathy of prematurity, stage Ø, unspecified eye**

  ✓6ᵗʰ **H35.12** **Retinopathy of prematurity, stage 1**
        H35.121 **Retinopathy of prematurity, stage 1,** right **eye**
        H35.122 **Retinopathy of prematurity, stage 1,** left **eye**
        H35.123 **Retinopathy of prematurity, stage 1,** bilateral
        H35.129 **Retinopathy of prematurity, stage 1, unspecified eye**

  ✓6ᵗʰ **H35.13** **Retinopathy of prematurity, stage 2**
        H35.131 **Retinopathy of prematurity, stage 2,** right **eye**
        H35.132 **Retinopathy of prematurity, stage 2,** left **eye**
        H35.133 **Retinopathy of prematurity, stage 2,** bilateral
        H35.139 **Retinopathy of prematurity, stage 2, unspecified eye**

  ✓6ᵗʰ **H35.14** **Retinopathy of prematurity, stage 3**
        H35.141 **Retinopathy of prematurity, stage 3,** right **eye**
        H35.142 **Retinopathy of prematurity, stage 3,** left **eye**
        H35.143 **Retinopathy of prematurity, stage 3,** bilateral
        H35.149 **Retinopathy of prematurity, stage 3, unspecified eye**

  ✓6ᵗʰ **H35.15** **Retinopathy of prematurity, stage 4**
        H35.151 **Retinopathy of prematurity, stage 4,** right **eye**
        H35.152 **Retinopathy of prematurity, stage 4,** left **eye**
        H35.153 **Retinopathy of prematurity, stage 4,** bilateral
        H35.159 **Retinopathy of prematurity, stage 4, unspecified eye**

  ✓6ᵗʰ **H35.16** **Retinopathy of prematurity, stage 5**
        H35.161 **Retinopathy of prematurity, stage 5,** right **eye**
        H35.162 **Retinopathy of prematurity, stage 5,** left **eye**
        H35.163 **Retinopathy of prematurity, stage 5,** bilateral
        H35.169 **Retinopathy of prematurity, stage 5, unspecified eye**

  ✓6ᵗʰ **H35.17** **Retrolental fibroplasia**
        H35.171 **Retrolental fibroplasia,** right **eye**
        H35.172 **Retrolental fibroplasia,** left **eye**
        H35.173 **Retrolental fibroplasia,** bilateral
        H35.179 **Retrolental fibroplasia, unspecified eye**

✓5ᵗʰ **H35.2** **Other non-diabetic proliferative retinopathy**
    Proliferative vitreo-retinopathy
      EXCLUDES 1   *proliferative vitreo-retinopathy with retinal detachment (H33.4-)*
  H35.2Ø **Other non-diabetic proliferative retinopathy, unspecified eye**

H35.21 **Other non-diabetic proliferative retinopathy,** right **eye**
H35.22 **Other non-diabetic proliferative retinopathy,** left **eye**
H35.23 **Other non-diabetic proliferative retinopathy,** bilateral

✓6ᵗʰ **H35.3** **Degeneration of macula and posterior pole**

  H35.3Ø **Unspecified macular degeneration**   🅰
    Age-related macular degeneration

  ✓6ᵗʰ **H35.31** **Nonexudative age-related macular degeneration**
    Atrophic age-related macular degeneration
    Dry age-related macular degeneration
    AHA: 2016,4Q,20-21

> One of the following 7th characters is to be assigned to each code in subcategory H35.31 to designate the stage of the disease:
> Ø   stage unspecified
> 1   early dry stage
> 2   intermediate dry stage
> 3   advanced atrophic without subfoveal involvement
>   advanced dry stage
> 4   advanced atrophic with subfoveal involvement

    ✓7ᵗʰ **H35.311** **Nonexudative age-related macular degeneration,** right **eye** 🅰
    ✓7ᵗʰ **H35.312** **Nonexudative age-related macular degeneration,** left **eye** 🅰
    ✓7ᵗʰ **H35.313** **Nonexudative age-related macular degeneration,** bilateral 🅰
    ✓7ᵗʰ **H35.319** **Nonexudative age-related macular degeneration, unspecified eye** 🅰

  ✓6ᵗʰ **H35.32** **Exudative age-related macular degeneration**
    Wet age-related macular degeneration
    AHA: 2016,4Q,20-21

> One of the following 7th characters is to be assigned to each code in subcategory H35.32 to designate the stage of the disease:
> Ø   stage unspecified
> 1   with active choroidal neovascularization
> 2   with inactive choroidal neovascularization
>   with involuted or regressed neovascularization
> 3   with inactive scar

    ✓7ᵗʰ **H35.321** **Exudative age-related macular degeneration,** right **eye** MCC 🅰
    ✓7ᵗʰ **H35.322** **Exudative age-related macular degeneration,** left **eye** MCC 🅰
    ✓7ᵗʰ **H35.323** **Exudative age-related macular degeneration,** bilateral MCC 🅰
    ✓7ᵗʰ **H35.329** **Exudative age-related macular degeneration, unspecified eye** MCC 🅰

  H35.33 **Angioid streaks of macula**
    DEF: Degeneration of the choroid; characterized by broad, irregular, dark brown streaks radiating from optic disc; occurs with pseudoxanthoma elasticum or Paget's disease.

  ✓6ᵗʰ **H35.34** **Macular cyst, hole, or pseudohole**
    H35.341 **Macular cyst, hole, or pseudohole,** right **eye**
    H35.342 **Macular cyst, hole, or pseudohole,** left **eye**
    H35.343 **Macular cyst, hole, or pseudohole,** bilateral
    H35.349 **Macular cyst, hole, or pseudohole, unspecified eye**

  ✓6ᵗʰ **H35.35** **Cystoid macular degeneration**
    EXCLUDES 1   *cystoid macular edema following cataract surgery (H59.Ø3-)*
    H35.351 **Cystoid macular degeneration,** right **eye**
    H35.352 **Cystoid macular degeneration,** left **eye**
    H35.353 **Cystoid macular degeneration,** bilateral

🅽 Newborn: 0   🅿 Pediatric: 0-17   🅼 Maternity: 9-64   🅰 Adult: 15-124   MCC Major Complication/Comorbidity   CC Complication/Comorbidity   SW Severe Wound Dx

616   ICD-10-CM 2020

H35.359 Cystoid macular degeneration, unspecified eye

✓6ᵗʰ **H35.36** Drusen (degenerative) of macula

　AHA: 2017,1Q,51; 2016,4Q,21

　H35.361 Drusen (degenerative) of macula, right eye

　H35.362 Drusen (degenerative) of macula, left eye

　H35.363 Drusen (degenerative) of macula, bilateral

　H35.369 Drusen (degenerative) of macula, unspecified eye

✓6ᵗʰ **H35.37** Puckering of macula

　H35.371 Puckering of macula, right eye

　H35.372 Puckering of macula, left eye

　H35.373 Puckering of macula, bilateral

　H35.379 Puckering of macula, unspecified eye

✓6ᵗʰ **H35.38** Toxic maculopathy

　Code first poisoning due to drug or toxin, if applicable (T36-T65 with fifth or sixth character 1-4 or 6)

　Use additional code for adverse effect, if applicable, to identify drug (T36-T50 with fifth or sixth character 5)

　H35.381 Toxic maculopathy, right eye

　H35.382 Toxic maculopathy, left eye

　H35.383 Toxic maculopathy, bilateral

　H35.389 Toxic maculopathy, unspecified eye

✓5ᵗʰ **H35.4** Peripheral retinal degeneration

　EXCLUDES 1　hereditary retinal degeneration (dystrophy) (H35.5-)

　　peripheral retinal degeneration with retinal break (H33.3-)

　H35.40 Unspecified peripheral retinal degeneration

✓6ᵗʰ **H35.41** Lattice degeneration of retina

　Palisade degeneration of retina

　DEF: Degeneration of the retina, often bilateral, that is usually benign. It is characterized by lines intersecting at irregular intervals in the peripheral retina. Retinal thinning and retinal holes may occur.

　H35.411 Lattice degeneration of retina, right eye

　H35.412 Lattice degeneration of retina, left eye

　H35.413 Lattice degeneration of retina, bilateral

　H35.419 Lattice degeneration of retina, unspecified eye

✓6ᵗʰ **H35.42** Microcystoid degeneration of retina

　H35.421 Microcystoid degeneration of retina, right eye

　H35.422 Microcystoid degeneration of retina, left eye

　H35.423 Microcystoid degeneration of retina, bilateral

　H35.429 Microcystoid degeneration of retina, unspecified eye

✓6ᵗʰ **H35.43** Paving stone degeneration of retina

　H35.431 Paving stone degeneration of retina, right eye

　H35.432 Paving stone degeneration of retina, left eye

　H35.433 Paving stone degeneration of retina, bilateral

　H35.439 Paving stone degeneration of retina, unspecified eye

✓6ᵗʰ **H35.44** Age-related reticular degeneration of retina

　H35.441 Age-related reticular degeneration of retina, right eye　Ａ

　H35.442 Age-related reticular degeneration of retina, left eye　Ａ

　H35.443 Age-related reticular degeneration of retina, bilateral　Ａ

　H35.449 Age-related reticular degeneration of retina, unspecified eye　Ａ

✓6ᵗʰ **H35.45** Secondary pigmentary degeneration

　H35.451 Secondary pigmentary degeneration, right eye

　H35.452 Secondary pigmentary degeneration, left eye

　H35.453 Secondary pigmentary degeneration, bilateral

H35.459 Secondary pigmentary degeneration, unspecified eye

✓6ᵗʰ **H35.46** Secondary vitreoretinal degeneration

　H35.461 Secondary vitreoretinal degeneration, right eye

　H35.462 Secondary vitreoretinal degeneration, left eye

　H35.463 Secondary vitreoretinal degeneration, bilateral

　H35.469 Secondary vitreoretinal degeneration, unspecified eye

✓5ᵗʰ **H35.5** Hereditary retinal dystrophy

　EXCLUDES 1　dystrophies primarily involving Bruch's membrane (H31.1-)

　H35.50 Unspecified hereditary retinal dystrophy

　H35.51 Vitreoretinal dystrophy

　H35.52 Pigmentary retinal dystrophy

　　Albipunctate retinal dystrophy

　　Retinitis pigmentosa

　　Tapetoretinal dystrophy

　H35.53 Other dystrophies primarily involving the sensory retina

　　Stargardt's disease

　H35.54 Dystrophies primarily involving the retinal pigment epithelium

　　Vitelliform retinal dystrophy

✓5ᵗʰ **H35.6** Retinal hemorrhage

　H35.60 Retinal hemorrhage, unspecified eye

　H35.61 Retinal hemorrhage, right eye

　H35.62 Retinal hemorrhage, left eye

　H35.63 Retinal hemorrhage, bilateral

✓5ᵗʰ **H35.7** Separation of retinal layers

　EXCLUDES 1　retinal detachment (serous) (H33.2-)

　　rhegmatogenous retinal detachment (H33.0-)

　CC Excl: For CC codes in subcategory H35.7: PDX collection 628

　H35.70 Unspecified separation of retinal layers　CC

✓6ᵗʰ **H35.71** Central serous chorioretinopathy

　H35.711 Central serous chorioretinopathy, right eye

　H35.712 Central serous chorioretinopathy, left eye

　H35.713 Central serous chorioretinopathy, bilateral

　H35.719 Central serous chorioretinopathy, unspecified eye

✓6ᵗʰ **H35.72** Serous detachment of retinal pigment epithelium

　H35.721 Serous detachment of retinal pigment epithelium, right eye　CC

　H35.722 Serous detachment of retinal pigment epithelium, left eye　CC

　H35.723 Serous detachment of retinal pigment epithelium, bilateral　CC

　H35.729 Serous detachment of retinal pigment epithelium, unspecified eye　CC

✓6ᵗʰ **H35.73** Hemorrhagic detachment of retinal pigment epithelium

　H35.731 Hemorrhagic detachment of retinal pigment epithelium, right eye　CC

　H35.732 Hemorrhagic detachment of retinal pigment epithelium, left eye　CC

　H35.733 Hemorrhagic detachment of retinal pigment epithelium, bilateral　CC

　H35.739 Hemorrhagic detachment of retinal pigment epithelium, unspecified eye　CC

✓5ᵗʰ **H35.8** Other specified retinal disorders

　EXCLUDES 2　retinal hemorrhage (H35.6-)

　H35.81 Retinal edema

　　Retinal cotton wool spots

✔ Additional Character Required　✓x7ᵗʰ Placeholder　Unacceptable PDx　Questionable PDx　Manifestation　Unspecified Dx　H1-H4 HAC　HCC CMS-HCC Dx　HIV HIV Dx

ICD-10-CM 2020　　　　617

H35.82   **Retinal ischemia**   `CC`
    CC Excl: PDX collection 629

H35.89   **Other specified retinal disorders**

H35.9   **Unspecified retinal disorder**

H36   ***Retinal disorders in diseases classified elsewhere***
    Code first underlying disease, such as:
      lipid storage disorders (E75.-)
      sickle-cell disorders (D57.-)
    EXCLUDES 1   *arteriosclerotic retinopathy (H35.0-)*
           diabetic retinopathy (E08.3-, E09.3-, E10.3-, E11.3-, E13.3-)

Glaucoma (H40-H42)

✔4ᵗʰ **H40**   **Glaucoma**
    EXCLUDES 1   *absolute glaucoma (H44.51-)*
           congenital glaucoma (Q15.0)
           traumatic glaucoma due to birth injury (P15.3)

Open Angle/Angle Closure Glaucoma

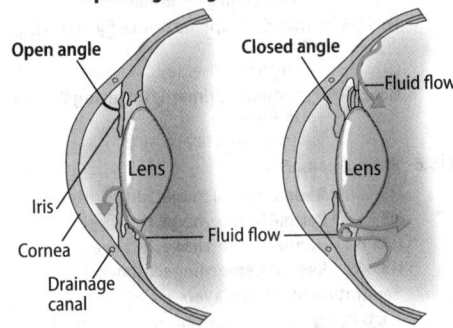

Open angle   Closed angle   Fluid flow   Lens   Iris   Fluid flow   Cornea   Drainage canal

✔5ᵗʰ **H40.0**   **Glaucoma suspect**

   ✔6ᵗʰ **H40.00**   **Preglaucoma, unspecified**
      H40.001   Preglaucoma, unspecified, **right eye**
      H40.002   Preglaucoma, unspecified, **left eye**
      H40.003   Preglaucoma, unspecified, **bilateral**
      H40.009   Preglaucoma, unspecified, **unspecified eye**

   ✔6ᵗʰ **H40.01**   **Open angle with borderline findings, low risk**
      Open angle, low risk
      H40.011   Open angle with borderline findings, low risk, **right eye**
      H40.012   Open angle with borderline findings, low risk, **left eye**
      H40.013   Open angle with borderline findings, low risk, **bilateral**
      H40.019   Open angle with borderline findings, low risk, **unspecified eye**

   ✔6ᵗʰ **H40.02**   **Open angle with borderline findings, high risk**
      Open angle, high risk
      H40.021   Open angle with borderline findings, high risk, **right eye**
      H40.022   Open angle with borderline findings, high risk, **left eye**
      H40.023   Open angle with borderline findings, high risk, **bilateral**
      H40.029   Open angle with borderline findings, high risk, **unspecified eye**

   ✔6ᵗʰ **H40.03**   **Anatomical narrow angle**
      Primary angle closure suspect
      H40.031   Anatomical narrow angle, **right eye**
      H40.032   Anatomical narrow angle, **left eye**
      H40.033   Anatomical narrow angle, **bilateral**
      H40.039   Anatomical narrow angle, **unspecified eye**

   ✔6ᵗʰ **H40.04**   **Steroid responder**
      H40.041   Steroid responder, **right eye**
      H40.042   Steroid responder, **left eye**
      H40.043   Steroid responder, **bilateral**
      H40.049   Steroid responder, **unspecified eye**

   ✔6ᵗʰ **H40.05**   **Ocular hypertension**
      H40.051   Ocular hypertension, **right eye**
      H40.052   Ocular hypertension, **left eye**
      H40.053   Ocular hypertension, **bilateral**
      H40.059   Ocular hypertension, **unspecified eye**

   ✔6ᵗʰ **H40.06**   **Primary angle closure without glaucoma damage**
      H40.061   Primary angle closure without glaucoma damage, **right eye**
      H40.062   Primary angle closure without glaucoma damage, **left eye**
      H40.063   Primary angle closure without glaucoma damage, **bilateral**
      H40.069   Primary angle closure without glaucoma damage, **unspecified eye**

✔5ᵗʰ **H40.1**   **Open-angle glaucoma**

> One of the following 7th characters is to be assigned to each code in subcategories H40.10, H40.11, H40.12, H40.13, and H40.14 to designate the stage of glaucoma.
> 0   stage unspecified
> 1   mild stage
> 2   moderate stage
> 3   severe stage
> 4   indeterminate stage

   ✔x7ᵗʰ **H40.10**   **Unspecified open-angle glaucoma**
      TIP: Only one code from this subcategory should be assigned when both left and right eyes are the same stage.

   ✔6ᵗʰ **H40.11**   **Primary open-angle glaucoma**
      Chronic simple glaucoma
      AHA: 2016,4Q,22
    ✔7ᵗʰ **H40.111**   Primary open-angle glaucoma, **right eye**
    ✔7ᵗʰ **H40.112**   Primary open-angle glaucoma, **left eye**
    ✔7ᵗʰ **H40.113**   Primary open-angle glaucoma, **bilateral**
    ✔7ᵗʰ **H40.119**   Primary open-angle glaucoma, **unspecified eye**

   ✔6ᵗʰ **H40.12**   **Low-tension glaucoma**
    ✔7ᵗʰ **H40.121**   Low-tension glaucoma, **right eye**
    ✔7ᵗʰ **H40.122**   Low-tension glaucoma, **left eye**
    ✔7ᵗʰ **H40.123**   Low-tension glaucoma, **bilateral**
    ✔7ᵗʰ **H40.129**   Low-tension glaucoma, **unspecified eye**

   ✔6ᵗʰ **H40.13**   **Pigmentary glaucoma**
    ✔7ᵗʰ **H40.131**   Pigmentary glaucoma, **right eye**
    ✔7ᵗʰ **H40.132**   Pigmentary glaucoma, **left eye**
    ✔7ᵗʰ **H40.133**   Pigmentary glaucoma, **bilateral**
    ✔7ᵗʰ **H40.139**   Pigmentary glaucoma, **unspecified eye**

   ✔6ᵗʰ **H40.14**   **Capsular glaucoma with pseudoexfoliation of lens**
    ✔7ᵗʰ **H40.141**   Capsular glaucoma with pseudoexfoliation of lens, **right eye**
    ✔7ᵗʰ **H40.142**   Capsular glaucoma with pseudoexfoliation of lens, **left eye**
    ✔7ᵗʰ **H40.143**   Capsular glaucoma with pseudoexfoliation of lens, **bilateral**
    ✔7ᵗʰ **H40.149**   Capsular glaucoma with pseudoexfoliation of lens, **unspecified eye**

   ✔6ᵗʰ **H40.15**   **Residual stage of open-angle glaucoma**
      H40.151   Residual stage of open-angle glaucoma, **right eye**
      H40.152   Residual stage of open-angle glaucoma, **left eye**
      H40.153   Residual stage of open-angle glaucoma, **bilateral**
      H40.159   Residual stage of open-angle glaucoma, **unspecified eye**

✔5ᵗʰ **H40.2**   **Primary angle-closure glaucoma**
    EXCLUDES 1   *aqueous misdirection (H40.83-)*
           malignant glaucoma (H40.83-)

> One of the following 7th characters is to be assigned to code H40.20 and H40.22- to designate the stage of glaucoma.
> 0   stage unspecified
> 1   mild stage
> 2   moderate stage
> 3   severe stage
> 4   indeterminate stage

   ✔x7ᵗʰ **H40.20**   **Unspecified primary angle-closure glaucoma**
      TIP: Only one code from this subcategory should be assigned when both left and right eyes are the same stage.

N Newborn: 0   **P** Pediatric: 0-17   **M** Maternity: 9-64   **A** Adult: 15-124   **MCC** Major Complication/Comorbidity   **CC** Complication/Comorbidity   **SW** Severe Wound Dx

618   ICD-10-CM 2020

√6th **H40.21 Acute angle-closure glaucoma**

Acute angle-closure glaucoma attack
Acute angle-closure glaucoma crisis
CC Excl: For CC codes in subcategory H40.21: PDX collection 630

     H40.211 Acute angle-closure glaucoma, right eye `CC`

     H40.212 Acute angle-closure glaucoma, left eye `CC`

     H40.213 Acute angle-closure glaucoma, bilateral `CC`

     H40.219 Acute angle-closure glaucoma, unspecified eye `CC`

√6th **H40.22 Chronic angle-closure glaucoma**

Chronic primary angle closure glaucoma

√7th   **H40.221 Chronic angle-closure glaucoma, right eye**

√7th   **H40.222 Chronic angle-closure glaucoma, left eye**

√7th   **H40.223 Chronic angle-closure glaucoma, bilateral**

√7th   **H40.229 Chronic angle-closure glaucoma, unspecified eye**

√6th **H40.23 Intermittent angle-closure glaucoma**

     H40.231 Intermittent angle-closure glaucoma, right eye

     H40.232 Intermittent angle-closure glaucoma, left eye

     H40.233 Intermittent angle-closure glaucoma, bilateral

     H40.239 Intermittent angle-closure glaucoma, unspecified eye

√6th **H40.24 Residual stage of angle-closure glaucoma**

     H40.241 Residual stage of angle-closure glaucoma, right eye

     H40.242 Residual stage of angle-closure glaucoma, left eye

     H40.243 Residual stage of angle-closure glaucoma, bilateral

     H40.249 Residual stage of angle-closure glaucoma, unspecified eye

√5th **H40.3 Glaucoma secondary to eye trauma**

Code also underlying condition

One of the following 7th characters is to be assigned to each code in subcategory H40.3- to designate the stage of glaucoma.
Ø   stage unspecified
1   mild stage
2   moderate stage
3   severe stage
4   indeterminate stage

√x7th **H40.30 Glaucoma secondary to eye trauma, unspecified eye**

√x7th **H40.31 Glaucoma secondary to eye trauma, right eye**

√x7th **H40.32 Glaucoma secondary to eye trauma, left eye**

√x7th **H40.33 Glaucoma secondary to eye trauma, bilateral**

√5th **H40.4 Glaucoma secondary to eye inflammation**

Code also underlying condition

One of the following 7th characters is to be assigned to each code in subcategory H40.4- to designate the stage of glaucoma.
Ø   stage unspecified
1   mild stage
2   moderate stage
3   severe stage
4   indeterminate stage

√x7th **H40.40 Glaucoma secondary to eye inflammation, unspecified eye**

√x7th **H40.41 Glaucoma secondary to eye inflammation, right eye**

√x7th **H40.42 Glaucoma secondary to eye inflammation, left eye**

√x7th **H40.43 Glaucoma secondary to eye inflammation, bilateral**

√5th **H40.5 Glaucoma secondary to other eye disorders**

Code also underlying eye disorder

One of the following 7th characters is to be assigned to each code in subcategory H40.5- to designate the stage of glaucoma.
Ø   stage unspecified
1   mild stage
2   moderate stage
3   severe stage
4   indeterminate stage

√x7th **H40.50 Glaucoma secondary to other eye disorders, unspecified eye**

√x7th **H40.51 Glaucoma secondary to other eye disorders, right eye**

√x7th **H40.52 Glaucoma secondary to other eye disorders, left eye**

√x7th **H40.53 Glaucoma secondary to other eye disorders, bilateral**

√5th **H40.6 Glaucoma secondary to drugs**

Use additional code for adverse effect, if applicable, to identify drug (T36-T50 with fifth or sixth character 5)

One of the following 7th characters is to be assigned to each code in subcategory H40.6- to designate the stage of glaucoma
Ø   stage unspecified
1   mild stage
2   moderate stage
3   severe stage
4   indeterminate stage

√x7th **H40.60 Glaucoma secondary to drugs, unspecified eye**

√x7th **H40.61 Glaucoma secondary to drugs, right eye**

√x7th **H40.62 Glaucoma secondary to drugs, left eye**

√x7th **H40.63 Glaucoma secondary to drugs, bilateral**

√5th **H40.8 Other glaucoma**

√6th **H40.81 Glaucoma with increased episcleral venous pressure**

     H40.811 Glaucoma with increased episcleral venous pressure, right eye

     H40.812 Glaucoma with increased episcleral venous pressure, left eye

     H40.813 Glaucoma with increased episcleral venous pressure, bilateral

     H40.819 Glaucoma with increased episcleral venous pressure, unspecified eye

√6th **H40.82 Hypersecretion glaucoma**

     H40.821 Hypersecretion glaucoma, right eye

     H40.822 Hypersecretion glaucoma, left eye

     H40.823 Hypersecretion glaucoma, bilateral

     H40.829 Hypersecretion glaucoma, unspecified eye

√6th **H40.83 Aqueous misdirection**

Malignant glaucoma

     H40.831 Aqueous misdirection, right eye

     H40.832 Aqueous misdirection, left eye

     H40.833 Aqueous misdirection, bilateral

     H40.839 Aqueous misdirection, unspecified eye

     H40.89 Other specified glaucoma

H40.9 Unspecified glaucoma

H42 Glaucoma in diseases classified elsewhere

Code first underlying condition, such as:
amyloidosis (E85.-)
aniridia (Q13.1)
glaucoma (in) diabetes mellitus (E08.39, E09.39, E10.39, E11.39, E13.39)
Lowe's syndrome (E72.03)
Reiger's anomaly (Q13.81)
specified metabolic disorder (E70-E88)
EXCLUDES 1   glaucoma (in) onchocerciasis (B73.02)
             glaucoma (in) syphilis (A52.71)
             glaucoma (in) tuberculous (A18.59)

Disorders of vitreous body and globe (H43-H44)

✓4ᵗʰ H43 Disorders of vitreous body

✓5ᵗʰ H43.Ø Vitreous prolapse
- *EXCLUDES 1*   traumatic vitreous prolapse (SØ5.2-)
  vitreous syndrome following cataract surgery (H59.Ø-)
- **H43.ØØ** Vitreous prolapse, unspecified eye
- H43.Ø1 Vitreous prolapse, right eye
- H43.Ø2 Vitreous prolapse, left eye
- H43.Ø3 Vitreous prolapse, bilateral

✓5ᵗʰ H43.1 Vitreous hemorrhage
- **H43.10** Vitreous hemorrhage, unspecified eye   `HCC`
- H43.11 Vitreous hemorrhage, right eye   `HCC`
- H43.12 Vitreous hemorrhage, left eye   `HCC`
- H43.13 Vitreous hemorrhage, bilateral   `HCC`

✓5ᵗʰ H43.2 Crystalline deposits in vitreous body
- **H43.20** Crystalline deposits in vitreous body, unspecified eye
- H43.21 Crystalline deposits in vitreous body, right eye
- H43.22 Crystalline deposits in vitreous body, left eye
- H43.23 Crystalline deposits in vitreous body, bilateral

✓5ᵗʰ H43.3 Other vitreous opacities
- **✓6ᵗʰ H43.31 Vitreous membranes and strands**
  - H43.311 Vitreous membranes and strands, right eye
  - H43.312 Vitreous membranes and strands, left eye
  - H43.313 Vitreous membranes and strands, bilateral
  - **H43.319** Vitreous membranes and strands, unspecified eye
- **✓6ᵗʰ H43.39 Other vitreous opacities**
  - Vitreous floaters
  - H43.391 Other vitreous opacities, right eye
  - H43.392 Other vitreous opacities, left eye
  - H43.393 Other vitreous opacities, bilateral
  - **H43.399** Other vitreous opacities, unspecified eye

✓5ᵗʰ H43.8 Other disorders of vitreous body
- *EXCLUDES 1*   proliferative vitreo-retinopathy with retinal detachment (H33.4-)
- *EXCLUDES 2*   vitreous abscess (H44.Ø2-)
- **✓6ᵗʰ H43.81 Vitreous degeneration**
  - Vitreous detachment
  - H43.811 Vitreous degeneration, right eye
  - H43.812 Vitreous degeneration, left eye
  - H43.813 Vitreous degeneration, bilateral
  - **H43.819** Vitreous degeneration, unspecified eye
- **✓6ᵗʰ H43.82 Vitreomacular adhesion**
  - Vitreomacular traction
  - H43.821 Vitreomacular adhesion, right eye   `A`
  - H43.822 Vitreomacular adhesion, left eye   `A`
  - H43.823 Vitreomacular adhesion, bilateral   `A`
  - **H43.829** Vitreomacular adhesion, unspecified eye   `A`
- H43.89 Other disorders of vitreous body
- **H43.9 Unspecified disorder of vitreous body**

✓4ᵗʰ H44 Disorders of globe
- **INCLUDES** disorders affecting multiple structures of eye
- CC Excl: For CC codes in cateogry H44, unless otherwise noted: PDX collection 625

✓5ᵗʰ H44.Ø Purulent endophthalmitis
- Use additional code to identify organism
- *EXCLUDES 1*   bleb associated endophthalmitis (H59.4-)
- **✓6ᵗʰ H44.ØØ Unspecified purulent endophthalmitis**
  - H44.ØØ1 Unspecified purulent endophthalmitis, right eye   `CC`
  - H44.ØØ2 Unspecified purulent endophthalmitis, left eye   `CC`
  - H44.ØØ3 Unspecified purulent endophthalmitis, bilateral   `CC`
  - H44.ØØ9 Unspecified purulent endophthalmitis, unspecified eye   `CC`
- **✓6ᵗʰ H44.Ø1 Panophthalmitis (acute)**
  - H44.Ø11 Panophthalmitis (acute), right eye   `CC`
  - H44.Ø12 Panophthalmitis (acute), left eye   `CC`
  - H44.Ø13 Panophthalmitis (acute), bilateral   `CC`
  - **H44.Ø19** Panophthalmitis (acute), unspecified eye   `CC`
- **✓6ᵗʰ H44.Ø2 Vitreous abscess (chronic)**
  - CC Excl: For CC codes in subcategory H44.Ø2: PDX collection 631
  - H44.Ø21 Vitreous abscess (chronic), right eye   `CC`
  - H44.Ø22 Vitreous abscess (chronic), left eye   `CC`
  - H44.Ø23 Vitreous abscess (chronic), bilateral   `CC`
  - **H44.Ø29** Vitreous abscess (chronic), unspecified eye   `CC`

✓5ᵗʰ H44.1 Other endophthalmitis
- *EXCLUDES 1*   bleb associated endophthalmitis (H59.4-)
- *EXCLUDES 2*   ophthalmia nodosa (H16.2-)
- **✓6ᵗʰ H44.11 Panuveitis**
  - **DEF:** Inflammation of all layers of the uvea of the eye, including the choroid, iris, and ciliary body. It also typically involves the lens, retina, optic nerve, and vitreous and causes reduced vision or blindness.
  - CC Excl: For CC codes in subcategory H44.11: PDX collection 632
  - H44.111 Panuveitis, right eye   `CC`
  - H44.112 Panuveitis, left eye   `CC`
  - H44.113 Panuveitis, bilateral   `CC`
  - **H44.119** Panuveitis, unspecified eye   `CC`
- **✓6ᵗʰ H44.12 Parasitic endophthalmitis, unspecified**
  - **H44.121** Parasitic endophthalmitis, unspecified, right eye   `CC`
  - **H44.122** Parasitic endophthalmitis, unspecified, left eye   `CC`
  - **H44.123** Parasitic endophthalmitis, unspecified, bilateral   `CC`
  - **H44.129** Parasitic endophthalmitis, unspecified, unspecified eye   `CC`
- **✓6ᵗʰ H44.13 Sympathetic uveitis**
  - CC Excl: For CC codes in subcategory H44.13: PDX collection 632
  - H44.131 Sympathetic uveitis, right eye   `CC`
  - H44.132 Sympathetic uveitis, left eye   `CC`
  - H44.133 Sympathetic uveitis, bilateral   `CC`
  - **H44.139** Sympathetic uveitis, unspecified eye   `CC`
- H44.19 Other endophthalmitis   `CC`

✓5ᵗʰ H44.2 Degenerative myopia
- Malignant myopia
- **AHA:** 2017,4Q,10-11
- **H44.20** Degenerative myopia, unspecified eye
- H44.21 Degenerative myopia, right eye
- H44.22 Degenerative myopia, left eye
- H44.23 Degenerative myopia, bilateral
- **✓6ᵗʰ H44.2A Degenerative myopia with choroidal neovascularization**
  - Use additional code for any associated choroid disorders (H31.-)
  - H44.2A1 Degenerative myopia with choroidal neovascularization, right eye
  - H44.2A2 Degenerative myopia with choroidal neovascularization, left eye
  - H44.2A3 Degenerative myopia with choroidal neovascularization, bilateral eye
  - **H44.2A9** Degenerative myopia with choroidal neovascularization, unspecified eye

---

`N` Newborn: 0   `P` Pediatric: 0-17   `M` Maternity: 9-64   `A` Adult: 15-124   `MCC` Major Complication/Comorbidity   `CC` Complication/Comorbidity   `SW` Severe Wound Dx

✓6ᵗʰ **H44.2B Degenerative myopia** with macular hole

    H44.2B1 Degenerative myopia with macular hole, right eye

    H44.2B2 Degenerative myopia with macular hole, left eye

    H44.2B3 Degenerative myopia with macular hole, bilateral eye

    H44.2B9 Degenerative myopia with macular hole, unspecified eye

✓6ᵗʰ **H44.2C Degenerative myopia** with retinal detachment

    Use additional code to identify the retinal detachment (H33.-)

    H44.2C1 Degenerative myopia with retinal detachment, right eye

    H44.2C2 Degenerative myopia with retinal detachment, left eye

    H44.2C3 Degenerative myopia with retinal detachment, bilateral eye

    H44.2C9 Degenerative myopia with retinal detachment, unspecified eye

✓6ᵗʰ **H44.2D Degenerative myopia** with foveoschisis

    H44.2D1 Degenerative myopia with foveoschisis, right eye

    H44.2D2 Degenerative myopia with foveoschisis, left eye

    H44.2D3 Degenerative myopia with foveoschisis, bilateral eye

    H44.2D9 Degenerative myopia with foveoschisis, unspecified eye

✓6ᵗʰ **H44.2E Degenerative myopia with other maculopathy**

    H44.2E1 Degenerative myopia with other maculopathy, right eye

    H44.2E2 Degenerative myopia with other maculopathy, left eye

    H44.2E3 Degenerative myopia with other maculopathy, bilateral eye

    H44.2E9 Degenerative myopia with other maculopathy, unspecified eye

✓5ᵗʰ **H44.3 Other and unspecified degenerative disorders of globe**

    H44.30 Unspecified degenerative disorder of globe

✓6ᵗʰ **H44.31 Chalcosis**

    H44.311 Chalcosis, right eye

    H44.312 Chalcosis, left eye

    H44.313 Chalcosis, bilateral

    H44.319 Chalcosis, unspecified eye

✓6ᵗʰ **H44.32 Siderosis of eye**

    DEF: Iron pigment deposits within tissue of the eyeball caused by high iron content of the blood. Symptoms include cataracts, rust-colored anterior subcapsular deposits, iris heterochromia, pupillary mydriasis, and depressed electroretinogram amplitudes.

    H44.321 Siderosis of eye, right eye

    H44.322 Siderosis of eye, left eye

    H44.323 Siderosis of eye, bilateral

    H44.329 Siderosis of eye, unspecified eye

✓6ᵗʰ **H44.39 Other degenerative disorders of globe**

    H44.391 Other degenerative disorders of globe, right eye

    H44.392 Other degenerative disorders of globe, left eye

    H44.393 Other degenerative disorders of globe, bilateral

    H44.399 Other degenerative disorders of globe, unspecified eye

✓5ᵗʰ **H44.4 Hypotony of eye**

    H44.40 Unspecified hypotony of eye

✓6ᵗʰ **H44.41 Flat anterior chamber hypotony of eye**

    H44.411 Flat anterior chamber hypotony of right eye

    H44.412 Flat anterior chamber hypotony of left eye

    H44.413 Flat anterior chamber hypotony of eye, bilateral

    H44.419 Flat anterior chamber hypotony of unspecified eye

✓6ᵗʰ **H44.42 Hypotony of eye due to** ocular fistula

    H44.421 Hypotony of right eye due to ocular fistula

    H44.422 Hypotony of left eye due to ocular fistula

    H44.423 Hypotony of eye due to ocular fistula, bilateral

    H44.429 Hypotony of unspecified eye due to ocular fistula

✓6ᵗʰ **H44.43 Hypotony of eye due to other ocular disorders**

    H44.431 Hypotony of eye due to other ocular disorders, right eye

    H44.432 Hypotony of eye due to other ocular disorders, left eye

    H44.433 Hypotony of eye due to other ocular disorders, bilateral

    H44.439 Hypotony of eye due to other ocular disorders, unspecified eye

✓6ᵗʰ **H44.44 Primary hypotony of eye**

    H44.441 Primary hypotony of right eye

    H44.442 Primary hypotony of left eye

    H44.443 Primary hypotony of eye, bilateral

    H44.449 Primary hypotony of unspecified eye

✓5ᵗʰ **H44.5 Degenerated conditions of globe**

    H44.50 Unspecified degenerated conditions of globe

✓6ᵗʰ **H44.51 Absolute glaucoma**

    H44.511 Absolute glaucoma, right eye

    H44.512 Absolute glaucoma, left eye

    H44.513 Absolute glaucoma, bilateral

    H44.519 Absolute glaucoma, unspecified eye

✓6ᵗʰ **H44.52 Atrophy of globe**

    Phthisis bulbi

    H44.521 Atrophy of globe, right eye

    H44.522 Atrophy of globe, left eye

    H44.523 Atrophy of globe, bilateral

    H44.529 Atrophy of globe, unspecified eye

✓6ᵗʰ **H44.53 Leucocoria**

    H44.531 Leucocoria, right eye

    H44.532 Leucocoria, left eye

    H44.533 Leucocoria, bilateral

    H44.539 Leucocoria, unspecified eye

✓5ᵗʰ **H44.6 Retained (old) intraocular foreign body,** magnetic

    Use additional code to identify magnetic foreign body (Z18.11)

    EXCLUDES 1   *current intraocular foreign body (S05.-)*

    EXCLUDES 2   *retained foreign body in eyelid (H02.81-)*

    retained (old) foreign body following penetrating wound of orbit (H05.5-)

    retained (old) intraocular foreign body, nonmagnetic (H44.7-)

✓6ᵗʰ **H44.60 Unspecified retained (old) intraocular foreign body, magnetic**

    H44.601 Unspecified retained (old) intraocular foreign body, magnetic, right eye

    H44.602 Unspecified retained (old) intraocular foreign body, magnetic, left eye

    H44.603 Unspecified retained (old) intraocular foreign body, magnetic, bilateral

    H44.609 Unspecified retained (old) intraocular foreign body, magnetic, unspecified eye

✓6ᵗʰ **H44.61 Retained (old) magnetic foreign body in** anterior chamber

    H44.611 Retained (old) magnetic foreign body in anterior chamber, right eye

    H44.612 Retained (old) magnetic foreign body in anterior chamber, left eye

    H44.613 Retained (old) magnetic foreign body in anterior chamber, bilateral

    H44.619 Retained (old) magnetic foreign body in anterior chamber, unspecified eye

✓6ᵗʰ **H44.62 Retained (old) magnetic foreign body in** iris or ciliary body

    H44.621 Retained (old) magnetic foreign body in iris or ciliary body, right eye

    H44.622 Retained (old) magnetic foreign body in iris or ciliary body, left eye

    H44.623 Retained (old) magnetic foreign body in iris or ciliary body, bilateral

    H44.629 Retained (old) magnetic foreign body in iris or ciliary body, unspecified eye

✓6ᵗʰ **H44.63 Retained (old) magnetic foreign body in** lens

    H44.631 Retained (old) magnetic foreign body in lens, right eye

    H44.632 Retained (old) magnetic foreign body in lens, left eye

✓ Additional Character Required   ✓x7ᵗʰ Placeholder   Unacceptable PDx   Questionable PDx   Manifestation   Unspecified Dx   H1-H4 HAC   HCC CMS-HCC Dx   HIV HIV Dx

ICD-10-CM 2020

621

H44.2B–H44.632

H44.633 Retained (old) magnetic foreign body in lens, bilateral

H44.639 Retained (old) magnetic foreign body in lens, unspecified eye

√6ᵗʰ **H44.64** Retained (old) magnetic foreign body in posterior wall of globe

H44.641 Retained (old) magnetic foreign body in posterior wall of globe, right eye

H44.642 Retained (old) magnetic foreign body in posterior wall of globe, left eye

H44.643 Retained (old) magnetic foreign body in posterior wall of globe, bilateral

H44.649 Retained (old) magnetic foreign body in posterior wall of globe, unspecified eye

√6ᵗʰ **H44.65** Retained (old) magnetic foreign body in vitreous body

H44.651 Retained (old) magnetic foreign body in vitreous body, right eye

H44.652 Retained (old) magnetic foreign body in vitreous body, left eye

H44.653 Retained (old) magnetic foreign body in vitreous body, bilateral

H44.659 Retained (old) magnetic foreign body in vitreous body, unspecified eye

√6ᵗʰ **H44.69** Retained (old) intraocular foreign body, magnetic, in other or multiple sites

H44.691 Retained (old) intraocular foreign body, magnetic, in other or multiple sites, right eye

H44.692 Retained (old) intraocular foreign body, magnetic, in other or multiple sites, left eye

H44.693 Retained (old) intraocular foreign body, magnetic, in other or multiple sites, bilateral

H44.699 Retained (old) intraocular foreign body, magnetic, in other or multiple sites, unspecified eye

√5ᵗʰ **H44.7** Retained (old) intraocular foreign body, nonmagnetic

Use additional code to identify nonmagnetic foreign body (Z18.Ø1-Z18.1Ø, Z18.12, Z18.2-Z18.9)

EXCLUDES 1   *current intraocular foreign body (SØ5.-)*

EXCLUDES 2   *retained foreign body in eyelid (HØ2.81-)*

retained (old) foreign body following penetrating wound of orbit (HØ5.5-)

retained (old) intraocular foreign body, magnetic (H44.6-)

√6ᵗʰ **H44.7Ø** Unspecified retained (old) intraocular foreign body, nonmagnetic

H44.7Ø1 Unspecified retained (old) intraocular foreign body, nonmagnetic, right eye

H44.7Ø2 Unspecified retained (old) intraocular foreign body, nonmagnetic, left eye

H44.7Ø3 Unspecified retained (old) intraocular foreign body, nonmagnetic, bilateral

H44.7Ø9 Unspecified retained (old) intraocular foreign body, nonmagnetic, unspecified eye

Retained (old) intraocular foreign body NOS

√6ᵗʰ **H44.71** Retained (nonmagnetic) (old) foreign body in anterior chamber

H44.711 Retained (nonmagnetic) (old) foreign body in anterior chamber, right eye

H44.712 Retained (nonmagnetic) (old) foreign body in anterior chamber, left eye

H44.713 Retained (nonmagnetic) (old) foreign body in anterior chamber, bilateral

H44.719 Retained (nonmagnetic) (old) foreign body in anterior chamber, unspecified eye

√6ᵗʰ **H44.72** Retained (nonmagnetic) (old) foreign body in iris or ciliary body

H44.721 Retained (nonmagnetic) (old) foreign body in iris or ciliary body, right eye

H44.722 Retained (nonmagnetic) (old) foreign body in iris or ciliary body, left eye

H44.723 Retained (nonmagnetic) (old) foreign body in iris or ciliary body, bilateral

H44.729 Retained (nonmagnetic) (old) foreign body in iris or ciliary body, unspecified eye

√6ᵗʰ **H44.73** Retained (nonmagnetic) (old) foreign body in lens

H44.731 Retained (nonmagnetic) (old) foreign body in lens, right eye

H44.732 Retained (nonmagnetic) (old) foreign body in lens, left eye

H44.733 Retained (nonmagnetic) (old) foreign body in lens, bilateral

H44.739 Retained (nonmagnetic) (old) foreign body in lens, unspecified eye

√6ᵗʰ **H44.74** Retained (nonmagnetic) (old) foreign body in posterior wall of globe

H44.741 Retained (nonmagnetic) (old) foreign body in posterior wall of globe, right eye

H44.742 Retained (nonmagnetic) (old) foreign body in posterior wall of globe, left eye

H44.743 Retained (nonmagnetic) (old) foreign body in posterior wall of globe, bilateral

H44.749 Retained (nonmagnetic) (old) foreign body in posterior wall of globe, unspecified eye

√6ᵗʰ **H44.75** Retained (nonmagnetic) (old) foreign body in vitreous body

H44.751 Retained (nonmagnetic) (old) foreign body in vitreous body, right eye

H44.752 Retained (nonmagnetic) (old) foreign body in vitreous body, left eye

H44.753 Retained (nonmagnetic) (old) foreign body in vitreous body, bilateral

H44.759 Retained (nonmagnetic) (old) foreign body in vitreous body, unspecified eye

√6ᵗʰ **H44.79** Retained (old) intraocular foreign body, nonmagnetic, in other or multiple sites

H44.791 Retained (old) intraocular foreign body, nonmagnetic, in other or multiple sites, right eye

H44.792 Retained (old) intraocular foreign body, nonmagnetic, in other or multiple sites, left eye

H44.793 Retained (old) intraocular foreign body, nonmagnetic, in other or multiple sites, bilateral

H44.799 Retained (old) intraocular foreign body, nonmagnetic, in other or multiple sites, unspecified eye

√5ᵗʰ **H44.8** Other disorders of globe

√6ᵗʰ **H44.81** Hemophthalmos

DEF: Pool of blood within the eyeball, not from a current injury.

H44.811 Hemophthalmos, right eye

H44.812 Hemophthalmos, left eye

H44.813 Hemophthalmos, bilateral

H44.819 Hemophthalmos, unspecified eye

√6ᵗʰ **H44.82** Luxation of globe

H44.821 Luxation of globe, right eye

H44.822 Luxation of globe, left eye

H44.823 Luxation of globe, bilateral

H44.829 Luxation of globe, unspecified eye

H44.89 Other disorders of globe

H44.9 Unspecified disorder of globe

Disorders of optic nerve and visual pathways (H46-H47)

√4ᵗʰ **H46** Optic neuritis

EXCLUDES 2   *ischemic optic neuropathy (H47.Ø1-)*

neuromyelitis optica [Devic] (G36.Ø)

CC Excl: For CC codes in category H46: PDX collection 633

√5ᵗʰ **H46.Ø** Optic papillitis

H46.ØØ Optic papillitis, unspecified eye   CC

H46.Ø1 Optic papillitis, right eye   CC

H46.Ø2 Optic papillitis, left eye   CC

H46.Ø3 Optic papillitis, bilateral   CC

√5ᵗʰ **H46.1** Retrobulbar neuritis

Retrobulbar neuritis NOS

EXCLUDES 1   *syphilitic retrobulbar neuritis (A52.15)*

H46.1Ø Retrobulbar neuritis, unspecified eye   CC

H46.11 Retrobulbar neuritis, right eye   CC

H46.12 Retrobulbar neuritis, left eye   CC

N Newborn: 0   P Pediatric: 0-17   M Maternity: 9-64   A Adult: 15-124   MCC Major Complication/Comorbidity   CC Complication/Comorbidity   SW Severe Wound Dx

622   ICD-10-CM 2020

H46.13   **Retrobulbar neuritis,** bilateral   `CC`

H46.2   **Nutritional** optic neuropathy

H46.3   **Toxic** optic neuropathy
     Code first (T51-T65) to identify cause

H46.8   **Other optic neuritis**   `CC`

H46.9   **Unspecified optic neuritis**   `CC`

✓4ᵗʰ **H47**   **Other disorders of optic [2nd] nerve and visual pathways**

   ✓5ᵗʰ **H47.0**   **Disorders of optic nerve, not elsewhere classified**

     ✓6ᵗʰ **H47.01**   **Ischemic** optic neuropathy

       H47.011   **Ischemic optic neuropathy, right** eye
       H47.012   **Ischemic optic neuropathy, left** eye
       H47.013   **Ischemic optic neuropathy, bilateral**
       H47.019   **Ischemic optic neuropathy, unspecified eye**

     ✓6ᵗʰ **H47.02**   **Hemorrhage** in optic nerve sheath

       H47.021   **Hemorrhage in optic nerve sheath, right eye**
       H47.022   **Hemorrhage in optic nerve sheath, left eye**
       H47.023   **Hemorrhage in optic nerve sheath, bilateral**
       H47.029   **Hemorrhage in optic nerve sheath, unspecified eye**

     ✓6ᵗʰ **H47.03**   **Optic nerve** hypoplasia

       H47.031   **Optic nerve hypoplasia, right** eye
       H47.032   **Optic nerve hypoplasia, left** eye
       H47.033   **Optic nerve hypoplasia, bilateral**
       H47.039   **Optic nerve hypoplasia, unspecified eye**

     ✓6ᵗʰ **H47.09**   **Other disorders of optic nerve, not elsewhere classified**
       Compression of optic nerve
       H47.091   **Other disorders of optic nerve, not elsewhere classified, right** eye
       H47.092   **Other disorders of optic nerve, not elsewhere classified, left** eye
       H47.093   **Other disorders of optic nerve, not elsewhere classified, bilateral**
       H47.099   **Other disorders of optic nerve, not elsewhere classified, unspecified eye**

   ✓5ᵗʰ **H47.1**   **Papilledema**
     DEF: Swelling of the optic papilla, the raised area connected to the optic disk made up of nerves that enter the eyeball. It may be caused by increased intracranial pressure, decreased ocular pressure, or a retinal disorder.

     H47.10   **Unspecified papilledema**   `CC`
       CC Excl: PDX collection 634

     H47.11   **Papilledema associated with increased intracranial pressure**   `CC`
       CC Excl: PDX collection 634

     H47.12   **Papilledema associated with** decreased ocular pressure

     H47.13   **Papilledema associated with** retinal disorder

     ✓6ᵗʰ **H47.14**   **Foster-Kennedy syndrome**
       H47.141   **Foster-Kennedy syndrome, right** eye
       H47.142   **Foster-Kennedy syndrome, left** eye
       H47.143   **Foster-Kennedy syndrome, bilateral**
       H47.149   **Foster-Kennedy syndrome, unspecified eye**

   ✓5ᵗʰ **H47.2**   **Optic atrophy**

     H47.20   **Unspecified optic atrophy**

     ✓6ᵗʰ **H47.21**   **Primary** optic atrophy
       H47.211   **Primary optic atrophy, right** eye
       H47.212   **Primary optic atrophy, left** eye
       H47.213   **Primary optic atrophy, bilateral**
       H47.219   **Primary optic atrophy, unspecified eye**

     H47.22   **Hereditary** optic atrophy
       Leber's optic atrophy

     ✓6ᵗʰ **H47.23**   **Glaucomatous** optic atrophy
       H47.231   **Glaucomatous optic atrophy, right** eye
       H47.232   **Glaucomatous optic atrophy, left** eye
       H47.233   **Glaucomatous optic atrophy, bilateral**
       H47.239   **Glaucomatous optic atrophy, unspecified eye**

     ✓6ᵗʰ **H47.29**   **Other optic atrophy**
       Temporal pallor of optic disc
       H47.291   **Other optic atrophy, right** eye
       H47.292   **Other optic atrophy, left** eye

       H47.293   **Other optic atrophy, bilateral**
       H47.299   **Other optic atrophy, unspecified eye**

   ✓5ᵗʰ **H47.3**   **Other disorders of optic disc**

     ✓6ᵗʰ **H47.31**   **Coloboma** of optic disc
       H47.311   **Coloboma of optic disc, right** eye
       H47.312   **Coloboma of optic disc, left** eye
       H47.313   **Coloboma of optic disc, bilateral**
       H47.319   **Coloboma of optic disc, unspecified eye**

     ✓6ᵗʰ **H47.32**   **Drusen** of optic disc
       H47.321   **Drusen of optic disc, right** eye
       H47.322   **Drusen of optic disc, left** eye
       H47.323   **Drusen of optic disc, bilateral**
       H47.329   **Drusen of optic disc, unspecified eye**

     ✓6ᵗʰ **H47.33**   **Pseudopapilledema** of optic disc
       H47.331   **Pseudopapilledema of optic disc, right** eye
       H47.332   **Pseudopapilledema of optic disc, left** eye
       H47.333   **Pseudopapilledema of optic disc, bilateral**
       H47.339   **Pseudopapilledema of optic disc, unspecified eye**

     ✓6ᵗʰ **H47.39**   **Other disorders of optic disc**
       H47.391   **Other disorders of optic disc, right** eye
       H47.392   **Other disorders of optic disc, left** eye
       H47.393   **Other disorders of optic disc, bilateral**
       H47.399   **Other disorders of optic disc, unspecified eye**

   ✓5ᵗʰ **H47.4**   **Disorders of optic chiasm**
     Code also underlying condition
     CC Excl: For CC codes in subcategory H47.4: PDX collection 635

     H47.41   **Disorders of optic chiasm in (due to)** inflammatory disorders   `CC`

     H47.42   **Disorders of optic chiasm in (due to)** neoplasm   `CC`

     H47.43   **Disorders of optic chiasm in (due to)** vascular disorders   `CC`

     H47.49   **Disorders of optic chiasm in (due to) other disorders**   `CC`

   ✓5ᵗʰ **H47.5**   **Disorders of other visual pathways**
     Disorders of optic tracts, geniculate nuclei and optic radiations
     Code also underlying condition
     CC Excl: For CC codes in subcategory H47.5: PDX collection 635

     ✓6ᵗʰ **H47.51**   **Disorders of visual pathways in (due to)** inflammatory disorders
       H47.511   **Disorders of visual pathways in (due to) inflammatory disorders, right** side   `CC`
       H47.512   **Disorders of visual pathways in (due to) inflammatory disorders, left** side   `CC`
       H47.519   **Disorders of visual pathways in (due to) inflammatory disorders, unspecified side**   `CC`

     ✓6ᵗʰ **H47.52**   **Disorders of visual pathways in (due to)** neoplasm
       H47.521   **Disorders of visual pathways in (due to) neoplasm, right** side   `CC`
       H47.522   **Disorders of visual pathways in (due to) neoplasm, left** side   `CC`
       H47.529   **Disorders of visual pathways in (due to) neoplasm, unspecified side**   `CC`

     ✓6ᵗʰ **H47.53**   **Disorders of visual pathways in (due to)** vascular disorders
       H47.531   **Disorders of visual pathways in (due to) vascular disorders, right** side   `CC`
       H47.532   **Disorders of visual pathways in (due to) vascular disorders, left** side   `CC`

☑ Additional Character Required   ✓x7ᵗʰ Placeholder   **Unacceptable PDx**   Questionable PDx   Manifestation   Unspecified Dx   **HI-HI5** HAC   **HCC** CMS-HCC Dx   **HIV** HIV Dx

ICD-10-CM 2020

623

H47.539 **Disorders of visual pathways in (due to) vascular disorders, unspecified side** `CC`

✓5th **H47.6** **Disorders of visual cortex**

Code also underlying condition

EXCLUDES 1   injury to visual cortex ▶S04.04-◀

CC Excl: For CC codes in subcategory H47.6: PDX collection 636

✓6th **H47.61** **Cortical blindness**

H47.611 **Cortical blindness, right side of brain**
H47.612 **Cortical blindness, left side of brain**
H47.619 **Cortical blindness, unspecified side of brain**

✓6th **H47.62** **Disorders of visual cortex in (due to) inflammatory disorders**

H47.621 **Disorders of visual cortex in (due to) inflammatory disorders, right side of brain** `CC`

H47.622 **Disorders of visual cortex in (due to) inflammatory disorders, left side of brain** `CC`

H47.629 **Disorders of visual cortex in (due to) inflammatory disorders, unspecified side of brain** `CC`

✓6th **H47.63** **Disorders of visual cortex in (due to) neoplasm**

H47.631 **Disorders of visual cortex in (due to) neoplasm, right side of brain** `CC`

H47.632 **Disorders of visual cortex in (due to) neoplasm, left side of brain** `CC`

H47.639 **Disorders of visual cortex in (due to) neoplasm, unspecified side of brain** `CC`

✓6th **H47.64** **Disorders of visual cortex in (due to) vascular disorders**

H47.641 **Disorders of visual cortex in (due to) vascular disorders, right side of brain** `CC`

H47.642 **Disorders of visual cortex in (due to) vascular disorders, left side of brain** `CC`

H47.649 **Disorders of visual cortex in (due to) vascular disorders, unspecified side of brain** `CC`

H47.9 **Unspecified disorder of visual pathways**

Disorders of ocular muscles, binocular movement, accommodation and refraction (H49-H52)

EXCLUDES 2   nystagmus and other irregular eye movements (H55)

✓4th **H49** **Paralytic strabismus**

EXCLUDES 2   internal ophthalmoplegia (H52.51-)
internuclear ophthalmoplegia (H51.2-)
progressive supranuclear ophthalmoplegia (G23.1)

DEF: Strabismus: Misalignment of the eyes with the inability to move and focus in the same direction due to conditions affecting the muscles controlling them.

✓5th **H49.0** **Third [oculomotor] nerve palsy**

H49.00 **Third [oculomotor] nerve palsy, unspecified eye**
H49.01 **Third [oculomotor] nerve palsy, right eye**
H49.02 **Third [oculomotor] nerve palsy, left eye**
H49.03 **Third [oculomotor] nerve palsy, bilateral**

✓5th **H49.1** **Fourth [trochlear] nerve palsy**

H49.10 **Fourth [trochlear] nerve palsy, unspecified eye**
H49.11 **Fourth [trochlear] nerve palsy, right eye**
H49.12 **Fourth [trochlear] nerve palsy, left eye**
H49.13 **Fourth [trochlear] nerve palsy, bilateral**

✓5th **H49.2** **Sixth [abducent] nerve palsy**

H49.20 **Sixth [abducent] nerve palsy, unspecified eye**
H49.21 **Sixth [abducent] nerve palsy, right eye**
H49.22 **Sixth [abducent] nerve palsy, left eye**
H49.23 **Sixth [abducent] nerve palsy, bilateral**

✓5th **H49.3** **Total (external) ophthalmoplegia**

H49.30 **Total (external) ophthalmoplegia, unspecified eye**

H49.31 **Total (external) ophthalmoplegia, right eye**
H49.32 **Total (external) ophthalmoplegia, left eye**
H49.33 **Total (external) ophthalmoplegia, bilateral**

✓5th **H49.4** **Progressive external ophthalmoplegia**

EXCLUDES 1   Kearns-Sayre syndrome (H49.81-)

H49.40 **Progressive external ophthalmoplegia, unspecified eye**

H49.41 **Progressive external ophthalmoplegia, right eye**
H49.42 **Progressive external ophthalmoplegia, left eye**
H49.43 **Progressive external ophthalmoplegia, bilateral**

✓5th **H49.8** **Other paralytic strabismus**

✓6th **H49.81** **Kearns-Sayre syndrome**

Progressive external ophthalmoplegia with pigmentary retinopathy
Use additional code for other manifestation, such as:
heart block (I45.9)

CC Excl: For CC codes in subcategory H49.81: PDX collection 545

H49.811 **Kearns-Sayre syndrome, right eye** `CC` `HCC`

H49.812 **Kearns-Sayre syndrome, left eye** `CC` `HCC`

H49.813 **Kearns-Sayre syndrome, bilateral** `CC` `HCC`

H49.819 **Kearns-Sayre syndrome, unspecified eye** `CC` `HCC`

✓6th **H49.88** **Other paralytic strabismus**

External ophthalmoplegia NOS

H49.881 **Other paralytic strabismus, right eye**
H49.882 **Other paralytic strabismus, left eye**
H49.883 **Other paralytic strabismus, bilateral**
H49.889 **Other paralytic strabismus, unspecified eye**

H49.9 **Unspecified paralytic strabismus**

✓4th **H50** **Other strabismus**

DEF: Strabismus: Misalignment of the eyes with the inability to move and focus in the same direction due to conditions affecting the muscles controlling them.

✓5th **H50.0** **Esotropia**

Convergent concomitant strabismus

EXCLUDES 1   intermittent esotropia (H50.31-, H50.32)

H50.00 **Unspecified esotropia**

✓6th **H50.01** **Monocular esotropia**

H50.011 **Monocular esotropia, right eye**
H50.012 **Monocular esotropia, left eye**

✓6th **H50.02** **Monocular esotropia with A pattern**

H50.021 **Monocular esotropia with A pattern, right eye**
H50.022 **Monocular esotropia with A pattern, left eye**

✓6th **H50.03** **Monocular esotropia with V pattern**

H50.031 **Monocular esotropia with V pattern, right eye**
H50.032 **Monocular esotropia with V pattern, left eye**

✓6th **H50.04** **Monocular esotropia with other noncomitancies**

H50.041 **Monocular esotropia with other noncomitancies, right eye**
H50.042 **Monocular esotropia with other noncomitancies, left eye**

H50.05 **Alternating esotropia**
H50.06 **Alternating esotropia with A pattern**
H50.07 **Alternating esotropia with V pattern**

H50.08   Alternating esotropia with other noncomitancies

Eye Muscle Diseases

R.   L.
Monocular (one eye only) esotropia (inward)

Monocular exotropia (outward)

Monocular hypertropia (upward)

√5ᵗʰ **H50.1   Exotropia**

Divergent concomitant strabismus

EXCLUDES 1   *intermittent exotropia (H50.33-, H50.34)*

H50.10   **Unspecified exotropia**

√6ᵗʰ H50.11   Monocular exotropia

H50.111 **Monocular exotropia, right eye**
H50.112 **Monocular exotropia, left eye**

√6ᵗʰ H50.12   Monocular exotropia with A pattern

H50.121 **Monocular exotropia with A pattern, right eye**
H50.122 **Monocular exotropia with A pattern, left eye**

√6ᵗʰ H50.13   Monocular exotropia with V pattern

H50.131 **Monocular exotropia with V pattern, right eye**
H50.132 **Monocular exotropia with V pattern, left eye**

√6ᵗʰ H50.14   Monocular exotropia with other noncomitancies

H50.141 **Monocular exotropia with other noncomitancies, right eye**
H50.142 **Monocular exotropia with other noncomitancies, left eye**

H50.15   Alternating exotropia
H50.16   Alternating exotropia with A pattern
H50.17   Alternating exotropia with V pattern
H50.18   Alternating exotropia with other noncomitancies

√5ᵗʰ **H50.2   Vertical strabismus**

Hypertropia

H50.21   Vertical strabismus, right eye
H50.22   Vertical strabismus, left eye

√5ᵗʰ **H50.3   Intermittent heterotropia**

H50.30   **Unspecified intermittent heterotropia**

√6ᵗʰ H50.31   Intermittent monocular esotropia

H50.311 **Intermittent monocular esotropia, right eye**
H50.312 **Intermittent monocular esotropia, left eye**

H50.32   Intermittent alternating esotropia

√6ᵗʰ H50.33   Intermittent monocular exotropia

H50.331 **Intermittent monocular exotropia, right eye**
H50.332 **Intermittent monocular exotropia, left eye**

H50.34   Intermittent alternating exotropia

√5ᵗʰ **H50.4   Other and unspecified heterotropia**

H50.40   **Unspecified heterotropia**

√6ᵗʰ H50.41   Cyclotropia

H50.411 **Cyclotropia, right eye**
H50.412 **Cyclotropia, left eye**

H50.42   Monofixation syndrome

H50.43   Accommodative component in esotropia

√5ᵗʰ H50.5   Heterophoria

H50.50   **Unspecified heterophoria**
H50.51   Esophoria
H50.52   Exophoria
H50.53   Vertical heterophoria
H50.54   Cyclophoria
H50.55   Alternating heterophoria

√5ᵗʰ H50.6   Mechanical strabismus

H50.60   **Mechanical strabismus, unspecified**

√6ᵗʰ H50.61   Brown's sheath syndrome

H50.611 Brown's sheath syndrome, right eye
H50.612 Brown's sheath syndrome, left eye

H50.69   Other mechanical strabismus

Strabismus due to adhesions
Traumatic limitation of duction of eye muscle

√5ᵗʰ H50.8   Other specified strabismus

√6ᵗʰ H50.81   Duane's syndrome

H50.811 Duane's syndrome, right eye
H50.812 Duane's syndrome, left eye

H50.89   Other specified strabismus

H50.9   **Unspecified strabismus**

√4ᵗʰ **H51   Other disorders of binocular movement**

H51.0   Palsy (spasm) of conjugate gaze

√5ᵗʰ H51.1   Convergence insufficiency and excess

H51.11   Convergence insufficiency
H51.12   Convergence excess

√5ᵗʰ H51.2   Internuclear ophthalmoplegia

H51.20   **Internuclear ophthalmoplegia, unspecified eye**
H51.21   Internuclear ophthalmoplegia, right eye
H51.22   Internuclear ophthalmoplegia, left eye
H51.23   Internuclear ophthalmoplegia, bilateral

H51.8   Other specified disorders of binocular movement
H51.9   **Unspecified disorder of binocular movement**

√4ᵗʰ **H52   Disorders of refraction and accommodation**

√5ᵗʰ H52.0   Hypermetropia

H52.00   **Hypermetropia, unspecified eye**
H52.01   Hypermetropia, right eye
H52.02   Hypermetropia, left eye
H52.03   Hypermetropia, bilateral

√5ᵗʰ H52.1   Myopia

EXCLUDES 1   *degenerative myopia (H44.2-)*

H52.10   **Myopia, unspecified eye**
H52.11   Myopia, right eye
H52.12   Myopia, left eye
H52.13   Myopia, bilateral

√5ᵗʰ H52.2   Astigmatism

√6ᵗʰ H52.20   **Unspecified astigmatism**

H52.201 **Unspecified astigmatism, right eye**
H52.202 **Unspecified astigmatism, left eye**
H52.203 **Unspecified astigmatism, bilateral**
H52.209 **Unspecified astigmatism, unspecified eye**

√6ᵗʰ H52.21   Irregular astigmatism

H52.211 Irregular astigmatism, right eye
H52.212 Irregular astigmatism, left eye
H52.213 Irregular astigmatism, bilateral
H52.219 **Irregular astigmatism, unspecified eye**

√6ᵗʰ H52.22   Regular astigmatism

H52.221 Regular astigmatism, right eye
H52.222 Regular astigmatism, left eye
H52.223 Regular astigmatism, bilateral
H52.229 **Regular astigmatism, unspecified eye**

√5ᵗʰ H52.3   Anisometropia and aniseikonia

H52.31   Anisometropia
H52.32   Aniseikonia

H52.4   Presbyopia

√5ᵗʰ H52.5   Disorders of accommodation

√6ᵗʰ H52.51   Internal ophthalmoplegia (complete) (total)

H52.511 Internal ophthalmoplegia (complete) (total), right eye
H52.512 Internal ophthalmoplegia (complete) (total), left eye

Chapter 7. Diseases of the Eye and Adnexa

H52.513 Internal ophthalmoplegia (complete) (total), **bilateral**

H52.519 Internal ophthalmoplegia (complete) (total), unspecified eye

√6ᵗʰ **H52.52** **Paresis of accommodation**

H52.521 Paresis of accommodation, **right** eye
H52.522 Paresis of accommodation, **left** eye
H52.523 Paresis of accommodation, **bilateral**
H52.529 Paresis of accommodation, unspecified eye

√6ᵗʰ **H52.53** **Spasm of accommodation**

H52.531 Spasm of accommodation, **right** eye
H52.532 Spasm of accommodation, **left** eye
H52.533 Spasm of accommodation, **bilateral**
H52.539 Spasm of accommodation, unspecified eye

H52.6 Other disorders of refraction
H52.7 Unspecified disorder of refraction

Visual disturbances and blindness (H53-H54)

√4ᵗʰ **H53** **Visual disturbances**

√5ᵗʰ **H53.0** **Amblyopia ex anopsia**

> **EXCLUDES 1**   amblyopia due to vitamin A deficiency (E50.5)

√6ᵗʰ **H53.00** **Unspecified amblyopia**

H53.001 Unspecified amblyopia, **right** eye
H53.002 Unspecified amblyopia, **left** eye
H53.003 Unspecified amblyopia, **bilateral**
H53.009 Unspecified amblyopia, unspecified eye

√6ᵗʰ **H53.01** **Deprivation amblyopia**

H53.011 Deprivation amblyopia, **right** eye
H53.012 Deprivation amblyopia, **left** eye
H53.013 Deprivation amblyopia, **bilateral**
H53.019 Deprivation amblyopia, unspecified eye

√6ᵗʰ **H53.02** **Refractive amblyopia**

H53.021 Refractive amblyopia, **right** eye
H53.022 Refractive amblyopia, **left** eye
H53.023 Refractive amblyopia, **bilateral**
H53.029 Refractive amblyopia, unspecified eye

√6ᵗʰ **H53.03** **Strabismic amblyopia**

> **EXCLUDES 1**   strabismus (H50.-)

H53.031 Strabismic amblyopia, **right** eye
H53.032 Strabismic amblyopia, **left** eye
H53.033 Strabismic amblyopia, **bilateral**
H53.039 Strabismic amblyopia, unspecified eye

√6ᵗʰ **H53.04** **Amblyopia suspect**

> **AHA:** 2016,4Q,22-23

H53.041 Amblyopia suspect, **right** eye
H53.042 Amblyopia suspect, **left** eye
H53.043 Amblyopia suspect, **bilateral**
H53.049 Amblyopia suspect, unspecified eye

√5ᵗʰ **H53.1** **Subjective visual disturbances**

> **EXCLUDES 1**   subjective visual disturbances due to vitamin A deficiency (E50.5)
>   visual hallucinations (R44.1)

> **CC Excl: CC codes in subcategory H53.1:** PDX collection 637

H53.10 Unspecified subjective visual disturbances
H53.11 Day blindness
> Hemeralopia

√6ᵗʰ **H53.12** **Transient visual loss**

> Scintillating scotoma
> **EXCLUDES 1**   amaurosis fugax (G45.3-)
>   transient retinal artery occlusion (H34.0-)

H53.121 Transient visual loss, **right** eye   CC
H53.122 Transient visual loss, **left** eye   CC
H53.123 Transient visual loss, **bilateral**   CC
H53.129 Transient visual loss, unspecified eye   CC

√6ᵗʰ **H53.13** **Sudden visual loss**

H53.131 Sudden visual loss, **right** eye   CC
H53.132 Sudden visual loss, **left** eye   CC
H53.133 Sudden visual loss, **bilateral**   CC
H53.139 Sudden visual loss, unspecified eye   CC

√6ᵗʰ **H53.14** **Visual discomfort**

> Asthenopia
> Photophobia

H53.141 Visual discomfort, **right** eye
H53.142 Visual discomfort, **left** eye
H53.143 Visual discomfort, **bilateral**
H53.149 Visual discomfort, unspecified

H53.15 Visual **distortions** of shape and size
> Metamorphopsia
H53.16 **Psychophysical** visual disturbances
H53.19 Other subjective visual disturbances
> Visual halos

H53.2 **Diplopia**
> Double vision

√5ᵗʰ **H53.3** **Other and unspecified disorders of binocular vision**

H53.30 Unspecified disorder of binocular vision
H53.31 Abnormal retinal correspondence
H53.32 Fusion with defective stereopsis
H53.33 Simultaneous visual perception without fusion
H53.34 Suppression of binocular vision

√5ᵗʰ **H53.4** **Visual field defects**

H53.40 Unspecified visual field defects

√6ᵗʰ **H53.41** **Scotoma involving central area**

> Central scotoma

H53.411 Scotoma involving central area, **right** eye
H53.412 Scotoma involving central area, **left** eye
H53.413 Scotoma involving central area, **bilateral**
H53.419 Scotoma involving central area, unspecified eye

√6ᵗʰ **H53.42** **Scotoma of blind spot area**

> Enlarged blind spot

H53.421 Scotoma of blind spot area, **right** eye
H53.422 Scotoma of blind spot area, **left** eye
H53.423 Scotoma of blind spot area, **bilateral**
H53.429 Scotoma of blind spot area, unspecified eye

√6ᵗʰ **H53.43** **Sector or arcuate defects**

> Arcuate scotoma
> Bjerrum scotoma

H53.431 Sector or arcuate defects, **right** eye
H53.432 Sector or arcuate defects, **left** eye
H53.433 Sector or arcuate defects, **bilateral**
H53.439 Sector or arcuate defects, unspecified eye

√6ᵗʰ **H53.45** **Other localized visual field defect**

> Peripheral visual field defect
> Ring scotoma NOS
> Scotoma NOS

H53.451 Other localized visual field defect, **right** eye
H53.452 Other localized visual field defect, **left** eye
H53.453 Other localized visual field defect, **bilateral**
H53.459 Other localized visual field defect, unspecified eye

√6ᵗʰ **H53.46** **Homonymous bilateral field defects**

> Homonymous hemianopia
> Homonymous hemianopsia
> Quadrant anopia
> Quadrant anopsia

H53.461 Homonymous bilateral field defects, **right** side
H53.462 Homonymous bilateral field defects, **left** side
H53.469 Homonymous bilateral field defects, unspecified side
> Homonymous bilateral field defects NOS

H53.47 **Heteronymous** bilateral field defects
> Heteronymous hemianop(s)ia

√6ᵗʰ **H53.48** **Generalized contraction** of visual field

H53.481 Generalized contraction of visual field, **right** eye
H53.482 Generalized contraction of visual field, **left** eye

N Newborn: 0   P Pediatric: 0-17   M Maternity: 9-64   A Adult: 15-124   MCC Major Complication/Comorbidity   CC Complication/Comorbidity   SW Severe Wound Dx

626   ICD-10-CM 2020

H53.483 Generalized contraction of visual field, bilateral

H53.489 Generalized contraction of visual field, unspecified eye

☑5ᵗʰ **H53.5 Color vision deficiencies**

Color blindness

EXCLUDES 2 *day blindness (H53.11)*

H53.50 Unspecified color vision deficiencies

Color blindness NOS

H53.51 Achromatopsia

DEF: Nonprogressive genetic visual disorder characterized by complete color blindness, decreased vision, and light sensitivity.

H53.52 Acquired color vision deficiency

H53.53 Deuteranomaly

Deuteranopia

DEF: Male-only genetic disorder causing difficulty in distinguishing green and red; no shortened spectrum.

H53.54 Protanomaly

Protanopia

H53.55 Tritanomaly

Tritanopia

H53.59 Other color vision deficiencies

☑5ᵗʰ **H53.6 Night blindness**

EXCLUDES 1 *night blindness due to vitamin A deficiency (E50.5)*

H53.60 Unspecified night blindness

H53.61 Abnormal dark adaptation curve

H53.62 Acquired night blindness

H53.63 Congenital night blindness

H53.69 Other night blindness

☑5ᵗʰ **H53.7 Vision sensitivity deficiencies**

H53.71 Glare sensitivity

H53.72 Impaired contrast sensitivity

H53.8 Other visual disturbances

H53.9 Unspecified visual disturbance

☑4ᵗʰ **H54 Blindness and low vision**

NOTE For definition of visual impairment categories see table below

Code first any associated underlying cause of the blindness

EXCLUDES 1 *amaurosis fugax (G45.3)*

AHA: 2017,4Q,11-12

☑5ᵗʰ **H54.0 Blindness, both eyes**

Visual impairment categories 3, 4, 5 in both eyes.

☑6ᵗʰ **H54.0X Blindness, both eyes, different category levels**

☑7ᵗʰ **H54.0X3 Blindness right eye, category 3**

H54.0X33 Blindness right eye category 3, blindness left eye category 3

H54.0X34 Blindness right eye category 3, blindness left eye category 4

H54.0X35 Blindness right eye category 3, blindness left eye category 5

☑7ᵗʰ **H54.0X4 Blindness right eye, category 4**

H54.0X43 Blindness right eye category 4, blindness left eye category 3

H54.0X44 Blindness right eye category 4, blindness left eye category 4

H54.0X45 Blindness right eye category 4, blindness left eye category 5

☑7ᵗʰ **H54.0X5 Blindness right eye, category 5**

H54.0X53 Blindness right eye category 5, blindness left eye category 3

H54.0X54 Blindness right eye category 5, blindness left eye category 4

H54.0X55 Blindness right eye category 5, blindness left eye category 5

☑5ᵗʰ **H54.1 Blindness, one eye, low vision other eye**

Visual impairment categories 3, 4, 5 in one eye, with categories 1 or 2 in the other eye.

H54.10 Blindness, one eye, low vision other eye, unspecified eyes

☑6ᵗʰ **H54.11 Blindness, right eye, low vision left eye**

☑7ᵗʰ **H54.113 Blindness right eye category 3, low vision left eye**

H54.1131 Blindness right eye category 3, low vision left eye category 1

H54.1132 Blindness right eye category 3, low vision left eye category 2

☑7ᵗʰ **H54.114 Blindness right eye category 4, low vision left eye**

H54.1141 Blindness right eye category 4, low vision left eye category 1

H54.1142 Blindness right eye category 4, low vision left eye category 2

☑7ᵗʰ **H54.115 Blindness right eye category 5, low vision left eye**

H54.1151 Blindness right eye category 5, low vision left eye category 1

H54.1152 Blindness right eye category 5, low vision left eye category 2

☑6ᵗʰ **H54.12 Blindness, left eye, low vision right eye**

☑7ᵗʰ **H54.121 Low vision right eye category 1, blindness left eye**

H54.1213 Low vision right eye category 1, blindness left eye category 3

H54.1214 Low vision right eye category 1, blindness left eye category 4

H54.1215 Low vision right eye category 1, blindness left eye category 5

☑7ᵗʰ **H54.122 Low vision right eye category 2, blindness left eye**

H54.1223 Low vision right eye category 2, blindness left eye category 3

H54.1224 Low vision right eye category 2, blindness left eye category 4

H54.1225 Low vision right eye category 2, blindness left eye category 5

☑5ᵗʰ **H54.2 Low vision, both eyes**

Visual impairment categories 1 or 2 in both eyes.

☑6ᵗʰ **H54.2X Low vision, both eyes, different category levels**

☑7ᵗʰ **H54.2X1 Low vision, right eye, category 1**

H54.2X11 Low vision right eye category 1, low vision left eye category 1

H54.2X12 Low vision right eye category 1, low vision left eye category 2

☑7ᵗʰ **H54.2X2 Low vision, right eye, category 2**

H54.2X21 Low vision right eye category 2, low vision left eye category 1

H54.2X22 Low vision right eye category 2, low vision left eye category 2

H54.3 Unqualified visual loss, both eyes

Visual impairment category 9 in both eyes.

TIP: Assign only when both eyes are documented as affected by blindness or low vision but the visual impairment category is not documented.

☑5ᵗʰ **H54.4 Blindness, one eye**

Visual impairment categories 3, 4, 5 in one eye [normal vision in other eye]

H54.40 Blindness, one eye, unspecified eye

☑6ᵗʰ **H54.41 Blindness, right eye, normal vision left eye**

☑7ᵗʰ **H54.413 Blindness, right eye, category 3**

H54.413A Blindness right eye category 3, normal vision left eye

☑7ᵗʰ **H54.414 Blindness, right eye, category 4**

H54.414A Blindness right eye category 4, normal vision left eye

☑7ᵗʰ **H54.415 Blindness, right eye, category 5**

H54.415A Blindness right eye category 5, normal vision left eye

☑6ᵗʰ **H54.42 Blindness, left eye, normal vision right eye**

☑7ᵗʰ **H54.42A Blindness, left eye, category 3-5**

H54.42A3 Blindness left eye category 3, normal vision right eye

H54.42A4 Blindness left eye category 4, normal vision right eye

H54.42A5 Blindness left eye category 5, normal vision right eye

☑ Additional Character Required   ☑x7ᵗʰ Placeholder   Unacceptable PDx   Questionable PDx   Manifestation   Unspecified Dx   H1–H14 HAC   HCC CMS-HCC Dx   HIV HIV Dx

ICD-10-CM 2020

627

☑5ᵗʰ **H54.5 Low vision, one eye**
Visual impairment categories 1 or 2 in one eye [normal vision in other eye].

    H54.50 Low vision, one eye, unspecified eye

    ☑6ᵗʰ **H54.51 Low vision, right eye, normal vision left eye**

      ☑7ᵗʰ **H54.511 Low vision, right eye, category 1-2**

        H54.511A Low vision right eye category 1, normal vision left eye

        H54.512A Low vision right eye category 2, normal vision left eye

    ☑7ᵗʰ **H54.52 Low vision, left eye, normal vision right eye**

      ☑7ᵗʰ **H54.52A Low vision, left eye, category 1-2**

        H54.52A1 Low vision left eye category 1, normal vision right eye

        H54.52A2 Low vision left eye category 2, normal vision right eye

☑5ᵗʰ **H54.6 Unqualified visual loss, one eye**
Visual impairment category 9 in one eye [normal vision in other eye].

   TIP: Assign a code from this category only when one eye is documented as affected by blindness or low vision but the visual impairment category is not documented.

    H54.60 Unqualified visual loss, one eye, unspecified

    H54.61 Unqualified visual loss, right eye, normal vision left eye

    H54.62 Unqualified visual loss, left eye, normal vision right eye

H54.7 Unspecified visual loss
Visual impairment category 9 NOS

   TIP: Assign only when documentation specifies blindness, visual loss, or low vision but not whether one or both eyes are affected or the visual impairment category.

H54.8 Legal blindness, as defined in USA
Blindness NOS according to USA definition

   EXCLUDES 1 *legal blindness with specification of impairment level (H54.0-H54.7)*

   NOTE The table below gives a classification of severity of visual impairment recommended by a WHO Study Group on the Prevention of Blindness, Geneva, 6-10 November 1972.

The term "low vision" in category H54 comprises categories 1 and 2 of the table, the term "blindness" categories 3, 4 and 5, and the term "unqualified visual loss" category 9.

If the extent of the visual field is taken into account, patients with a field no greater than 10 but greater than 5 around central fixation should be placed in category 3 and patients with a field no greater than 5 around central fixation should be placed in category 4, even if the central acuity is not impaired.

Category of visual impairment	Visual acuity with best possible correction	
	Maximum less than:	Minimum equal to or better than:
1	6/18 3/10 (0.3) 20/70	6/60 1/10 (0.1) 20/200
2	6/60 1/10 (0.1) 20/200	3/60 1/20 (0.05) 20/400
3	3/60 1/200 (0.05) 20/400	1/60 (finger counting at one meter) 1/50 (0.02) 5/300 (20/1200)
4	1/60 (finger counting at one meter) 1/50 (0.02) 5/300	Light perception
5	No light perception	
9	Undetermined or unspecified	

Other disorders of eye and adnexa (H55-H57)

☑4ᵗʰ **H55 Nystagmus and other irregular eye movements**

   ☑5ᵗʰ **H55.0 Nystagmus**

    DEF: Rapid, rhythmic, involuntary movements of the eyeball in vertical, horizontal, rotational, or mixed directions.

    H55.00 Unspecified nystagmus

    H55.01 Congenital nystagmus

    H55.02 Latent nystagmus

    H55.03 Visual deprivation nystagmus

    H55.04 Dissociated nystagmus

    H55.09 Other forms of nystagmus

   ☑5ᵗʰ **H55.8 Other irregular eye movements**

    H55.81 Saccadic eye movements

    H55.89 Other irregular eye movements

☑4ᵗʰ **H57 Other disorders of eye and adnexa**

   ☑5ᵗʰ **H57.0 Anomalies of pupillary function**

    H57.00 Unspecified anomaly of pupillary function

    H57.01 Argyll Robertson pupil, atypical

     EXCLUDES 1 *syphilitic Argyll Robertson pupil (A52.19)*

    H57.02 Anisocoria

    H57.03 Miosis

    H57.04 Mydriasis

   ☑6ᵗʰ **H57.05 Tonic pupil**

    H57.051 Tonic pupil, right eye

    H57.052 Tonic pupil, left eye

    H57.053 Tonic pupil, bilateral

    H57.059 Tonic pupil, unspecified eye

    H57.09 Other anomalies of pupillary function

   ☑5ᵗʰ **H57.1 Ocular pain**

    H57.10 Ocular pain, unspecified eye

    H57.11 Ocular pain, right eye

    H57.12 Ocular pain, left eye

    H57.13 Ocular pain, bilateral

   ☑5ᵗʰ **H57.8 Other specified disorders of eye and adnexa**

    AHA: 2018,4Q,15-16

   ☑6ᵗʰ **H57.81 Brow ptosis**

    H57.811 Brow ptosis, right

    H57.812 Brow ptosis, left

    H57.813 Brow ptosis, bilateral

    H57.819 Brow ptosis, unspecified

    H57.89 Other specified disorders of eye and adnexa

   H57.9 Unspecified disorder of eye and adnexa

Intraoperative and postprocedural complications and disorders of eye and adnexa, not elsewhere classified (H59)

☑4ᵗʰ **H59 Intraoperative and postprocedural complications and disorders of eye and adnexa, not elsewhere classified**

   EXCLUDES 1 *mechanical complication of intraocular lens (T85.2)*
mechanical complication of other ocular prosthetic devices, implants and grafts (T85.3)
pseudophakia (Z96.1)
secondary cataracts (H26.4-)

   ☑5ᵗʰ **H59.0 Disorders of the eye following cataract surgery**

    CC Excl: For CC codes in subcategory H59.0: PDX collection 638

   ☑6ᵗʰ **H59.01 Keratopathy (bullous aphakic) following cataract surgery**
Vitreal corneal syndrome
Vitreous (touch) syndrome

    H59.011 Keratopathy (bullous aphakic) following cataract surgery, right eye `CC`

    H59.012 Keratopathy (bullous aphakic) following cataract surgery, left eye `CC`

    H59.013 Keratopathy (bullous aphakic) following cataract surgery, bilateral `CC`

    H59.019 Keratopathy (bullous aphakic) following cataract surgery, unspecified eye `CC`

Ⓝ Newborn: 0   Ⓟ Pediatric: 0-17   Ⓜ Maternity: 9-64   Ⓐ Adult: 15-124   **MCC** Major Complication/Comorbidity   **CC** Complication/Comorbidity   **SW** Severe Wound Dx

628   ICD-10-CM 2020

✓6th **H59.02** Cataract (lens) fragments in eye following cataract surgery

H59.021 Cataract (lens) fragments in eye following cataract surgery, right eye

H59.022 Cataract (lens) fragments in eye following cataract surgery, left eye

H59.023 Cataract (lens) fragments in eye following cataract surgery, bilateral

H59.029 Cataract (lens) fragments in eye following cataract surgery, unspecified eye

✓6th **H59.03** Cystoid macular edema following cataract surgery

H59.031 Cystoid macular edema following cataract surgery, right eye CC

H59.032 Cystoid macular edema following cataract surgery, left eye CC

H59.033 Cystoid macular edema following cataract surgery, bilateral CC

H59.039 Cystoid macular edema following cataract surgery, unspecified eye CC

✓6th **H59.09** Other disorders of the eye following cataract surgery

H59.091 Other disorders of the right eye following cataract surgery CC

H59.092 Other disorders of the left eye following cataract surgery CC

H59.093 Other disorders of the eye following cataract surgery, bilateral CC

H59.099 Other disorders of unspecified eye following cataract surgery CC

✓5th **H59.1** Intraoperative hemorrhage and hematoma of eye and adnexa complicating a procedure

EXCLUDES 1 intraoperative hemorrhage and hematoma of eye and adnexa due to accidental puncture or laceration during a procedure (H59.2-)

CC Excl: For CC codes in subcategory H59.1: PDX collection 639

✓6th **H59.11** Intraoperative hemorrhage and hematoma of eye and adnexa complicating an ophthalmic procedure

H59.111 Intraoperative hemorrhage and hematoma of right eye and adnexa complicating an ophthalmic procedure CC

H59.112 Intraoperative hemorrhage and hematoma of left eye and adnexa complicating an ophthalmic procedure CC

H59.113 Intraoperative hemorrhage and hematoma of eye and adnexa complicating an ophthalmic procedure, bilateral CC

H59.119 Intraoperative hemorrhage and hematoma of unspecified eye and adnexa complicating an ophthalmic procedure CC

✓6th **H59.12** Intraoperative hemorrhage and hematoma of eye and adnexa complicating other procedure

H59.121 Intraoperative hemorrhage and hematoma of right eye and adnexa complicating other procedure CC

H59.122 Intraoperative hemorrhage and hematoma of left eye and adnexa complicating other procedure CC

H59.123 Intraoperative hemorrhage and hematoma of eye and adnexa complicating other procedure, bilateral CC

H59.129 Intraoperative hemorrhage and hematoma of unspecified eye and adnexa complicating other procedure CC

✓5th **H59.2** Accidental puncture and laceration of eye and adnexa during a procedure

CC Excl: For CC codes in subcategory H59.2: PDX collection 509

✓6th **H59.21** Accidental puncture and laceration of eye and adnexa during an ophthalmic procedure

H59.211 Accidental puncture and laceration of right eye and adnexa during an ophthalmic procedure CC

H59.212 Accidental puncture and laceration of left eye and adnexa during an ophthalmic procedure CC

H59.213 Accidental puncture and laceration of eye and adnexa during an ophthalmic procedure, bilateral CC

H59.219 Accidental puncture and laceration of unspecified eye and adnexa during an ophthalmic procedure CC

✓6th **H59.22** Accidental puncture and laceration of eye and adnexa during other procedure

H59.221 Accidental puncture and laceration of right eye and adnexa during other procedure CC

H59.222 Accidental puncture and laceration of left eye and adnexa during other procedure CC

H59.223 Accidental puncture and laceration of eye and adnexa during other procedure, bilateral CC

H59.229 Accidental puncture and laceration of unspecified eye and adnexa during other procedure CC

✓5th **H59.3** Postprocedural hemorrhage, hematoma, and seroma of eye and adnexa following a procedure

AHA: 2016,4Q,9-10

CC Excl: For CC codes in subcategory H59.3: PDX collection 639

✓6th **H59.31** Postprocedural hemorrhage of eye and adnexa following an ophthalmic procedure

H59.311 Postprocedural hemorrhage of right eye and adnexa following an ophthalmic procedure CC

H59.312 Postprocedural hemorrhage of left eye and adnexa following an ophthalmic procedure CC

H59.313 Postprocedural hemorrhage of eye and adnexa following an ophthalmic procedure, bilateral CC

H59.319 Postprocedural hemorrhage of unspecified eye and adnexa following an ophthalmic procedure CC

✓6th **H59.32** Postprocedural hemorrhage of eye and adnexa following other procedure

H59.321 Postprocedural hemorrhage of right eye and adnexa following other procedure CC

H59.322 Postprocedural hemorrhage of left eye and adnexa following other procedure CC

✔ Additional Character Required   ✓x7th Placeholder   Unacceptable PDx   Questionable PDx   Manifestation   Unspecified Dx   H1 - H14 HAC   HCC CMS-HCC Dx   HIV HIV Dx

ICD-10-CM 2020   629

Chapter 7. Diseases of the Eye and Adnexa

H59.323–H59.89

    H59.323 **Postprocedural hemorrhage of eye and adnexa following other procedure, bilateral** `CC`

    H59.329 **Postprocedural hemorrhage of unspecified eye and adnexa following other procedure** `CC`

✓6ᵗʰ **H59.33 Postprocedural hematoma of eye and adnexa following an ophthalmic procedure**

    H59.331 **Postprocedural hematoma of right eye and adnexa following an ophthalmic procedure** `CC`

    H59.332 **Postprocedural hematoma of left eye and adnexa following an ophthalmic procedure** `CC`

    H59.333 **Postprocedural hematoma of eye and adnexa following an ophthalmic procedure, bilateral** `CC`

    H59.339 **Postprocedural hematoma of unspecified eye and adnexa following an ophthalmic procedure** `CC`

✓6ᵗʰ **H59.34 Postprocedural hematoma of eye and adnexa following other procedure**

    H59.341 **Postprocedural hematoma of right eye and adnexa following other procedure** `CC`

    H59.342 **Postprocedural hematoma of left eye and adnexa following other procedure** `CC`

    H59.343 **Postprocedural hematoma of eye and adnexa following other procedure, bilateral** `CC`

    H59.349 **Postprocedural hematoma of unspecified eye and adnexa following other procedure** `CC`

✓6ᵗʰ **H59.35 Postprocedural seroma of eye and adnexa following an ophthalmic procedure**

    H59.351 **Postprocedural seroma of right eye and adnexa following an ophthalmic procedure** `CC`

    H59.352 **Postprocedural seroma of left eye and adnexa following an ophthalmic procedure** `CC`

    H59.353 **Postprocedural seroma of eye and adnexa following an ophthalmic procedure, bilateral** `CC`

    H59.359 **Postprocedural seroma of unspecified eye and adnexa following an ophthalmic procedure** `CC`

✓6ᵗʰ **H59.36 Postprocedural seroma of eye and adnexa following other procedure**

    H59.361 **Postprocedural seroma of right eye and adnexa following other procedure** `CC`

    H59.362 **Postprocedural seroma of left eye and adnexa following other procedure** `CC`

    H59.363 **Postprocedural seroma of eye and adnexa following other procedure, bilateral** `CC`

    H59.369 **Postprocedural seroma of unspecified eye and adnexa following other procedure** `CC`

✓5ᵗʰ **H59.4 Inflammation (infection) of postprocedural bleb**

    Postprocedural blebitis

    EXCLUDES 1   *filtering (vitreous) bleb after glaucoma surgery status (Z98.83)*

    H59.40 **Inflammation (infection) of postprocedural bleb, unspecified**

    H59.41 **Inflammation (infection) of postprocedural bleb, stage 1**

    H59.42 **Inflammation (infection) of postprocedural bleb, stage 2**

    H59.43 **Inflammation (infection) of postprocedural bleb, stage 3**

    Bleb endophthalmitis

✓5ᵗʰ **H59.8 Other intraoperative and postprocedural complications and disorders of eye and adnexa, not elsewhere classified**

    CC Excl: For CC codes in subcategory H59.8: PDX collection 638

✓6ᵗʰ **H59.81 Chorioretinal scars after surgery for detachment**

    H59.811 **Chorioretinal scars after surgery for detachment, right eye** `CC`

    H59.812 **Chorioretinal scars after surgery for detachment, left eye** `CC`

    H59.813 **Chorioretinal scars after surgery for detachment, bilateral** `CC`

    H59.819 **Chorioretinal scars after surgery for detachment, unspecified eye** `CC`

    H59.88 **Other intraoperative complications of eye and adnexa, not elsewhere classified** `CC`

    H59.89 **Other postprocedural complications and disorders of eye and adnexa, not elsewhere classified** `CC`

N Newborn: 0   P Pediatric: 0-17   M Maternity: 9-64   A Adult: 15-124   MCC Major Complication/Comorbidity   CC Complication/Comorbidity   SW Severe Wound Dx

630   ICD-10-CM 2020

Chapter 8. Diseases of the Ear and Mastoid Process (H60–H95)

Chapter-specific Guidelines with Coding Examples
Reserved for future guideline expansion.

Chapter 8. Diseases of the Ear and Mastoid Process (H60-H95)

NOTE   Use an external cause code following the code for the ear condition, if applicable, to identify the cause of the ear condition

EXCLUDES 2   *certain conditions originating in the perinatal period (P04-P96)*
certain infectious and parasitic diseases (A00-B99)
complications of pregnancy, childbirth and the puerperium (O00-O9A)
congenital malformations, deformations and chromosomal abnormalities (Q00-Q99)
endocrine, nutritional and metabolic diseases (E00-E88)
injury, poisoning and certain other consequences of external causes (S00-T88)
neoplasms (C00-D49)
symptoms, signs and abnormal clinical and laboratory findings, not elsewhere classified (R00-R94)

This chapter contains the following blocks:
H60-H62   Diseases of external ear
H65-H75   Diseases of middle ear and mastoid
H80-H83   Diseases of inner ear
H90-H94   Other disorders of ear
H95   Intraoperative and postprocedural complications and disorders of ear and mastoid process, not elsewhere classified

Diseases of external ear (H60-H62)

✓4ᵗʰ H60 Otitis externa

TIP: When the specific infectious agent is identified, a code from Chapter 1 is assigned instead of a code from this category.

✓5ᵗʰ H60.0 Abscess of external ear
    Boil of external ear
    Carbuncle of auricle or external auditory canal
    Furuncle of external ear
    H60.00 Abscess of external ear, unspecified ear
    H60.01 Abscess of right external ear
    H60.02 Abscess of left external ear
    H60.03 Abscess of external ear, bilateral

✓5ᵗʰ H60.1 Cellulitis of external ear
    Cellulitis of auricle
    Cellulitis of external auditory canal
    H60.10 Cellulitis of external ear, unspecified ear
    H60.11 Cellulitis of right external ear
    H60.12 Cellulitis of left external ear
    H60.13 Cellulitis of external ear, bilateral

✓5ᵗʰ H60.2 Malignant otitis externa
    CC Excl: For CC codes in subcategory H60.2: PDX collection 640
    H60.20 Malignant otitis externa, unspecified ear   **CC**
    H60.21 Malignant otitis externa, right ear   **CC**
    H60.22 Malignant otitis externa, left ear   **CC**
    H60.23 Malignant otitis externa, bilateral   **CC**

✓5ᵗʰ H60.3 Other infective otitis externa

    ✓6ᵗʰ H60.31 Diffuse otitis externa
       H60.311 Diffuse otitis externa, right ear
       H60.312 Diffuse otitis externa, left ear
       H60.313 Diffuse otitis externa, bilateral
       H60.319 Diffuse otitis externa, unspecified ear

    ✓6ᵗʰ H60.32 Hemorrhagic otitis externa
       H60.321 Hemorrhagic otitis externa, right ear
       H60.322 Hemorrhagic otitis externa, left ear
       H60.323 Hemorrhagic otitis externa, bilateral
       H60.329 Hemorrhagic otitis externa, unspecified ear

    ✓6ᵗʰ H60.33 Swimmer's ear
       DEF: Commonly occurs when water gets trapped in the ear after swimming.
       H60.331 Swimmer's ear, right ear
       H60.332 Swimmer's ear, left ear
       H60.333 Swimmer's ear, bilateral
       H60.339 Swimmer's ear, unspecified ear

    ✓6ᵗʰ H60.39 Other infective otitis externa
       H60.391 Other infective otitis externa, right ear
       H60.392 Other infective otitis externa, left ear
       H60.393 Other infective otitis externa, bilateral
       H60.399 Other infective otitis externa, unspecified ear

✓5ᵗʰ H60.4 Cholesteatoma of external ear
    Keratosis obturans of external ear (canal)
    EXCLUDES 2   *cholesteatoma of middle ear (H71.-)*
       recurrent cholesteatoma of postmastoidectomy cavity (H95.0-)
    DEF: Cholesteatoma: Noncancerous cyst-like mass of cell debris, including cholesterol and epithelial cells resulting from trauma, repeated or improperly healed infections, and congenital enclosure of epidermal cells.
    H60.40 Cholesteatoma of external ear, unspecified ear
    H60.41 Cholesteatoma of right external ear
    H60.42 Cholesteatoma of left external ear
    H60.43 Cholesteatoma of external ear, bilateral

✓5ᵗʰ H60.5 Acute noninfective otitis externa

    ✓6ᵗʰ H60.50 Unspecified acute noninfective otitis externa
       Acute otitis externa NOS
       H60.501 Unspecified acute noninfective otitis externa, right ear
       H60.502 Unspecified acute noninfective otitis externa, left ear
       H60.503 Unspecified acute noninfective otitis externa, bilateral
       H60.509 Unspecified acute noninfective otitis externa, unspecified ear

    ✓6ᵗʰ H60.51 Acute actinic otitis externa
       H60.511 Acute actinic otitis externa, right ear
       H60.512 Acute actinic otitis externa, left ear
       H60.513 Acute actinic otitis externa, bilateral
       H60.519 Acute actinic otitis externa, unspecified ear

    ✓6ᵗʰ H60.52 Acute chemical otitis externa
       H60.521 Acute chemical otitis externa, right ear
       H60.522 Acute chemical otitis externa, left ear
       H60.523 Acute chemical otitis externa, bilateral
       H60.529 Acute chemical otitis externa, unspecified ear

    ✓6ᵗʰ H60.53 Acute contact otitis externa
       H60.531 Acute contact otitis externa, right ear
       H60.532 Acute contact otitis externa, left ear
       H60.533 Acute contact otitis externa, bilateral
       H60.539 Acute contact otitis externa, unspecified ear

    ✓6ᵗʰ H60.54 Acute eczematoid otitis externa
       H60.541 Acute eczematoid otitis externa, right ear
       H60.542 Acute eczematoid otitis externa, left ear
       H60.543 Acute eczematoid otitis externa, bilateral
       H60.549 Acute eczematoid otitis externa, unspecified ear

    ✓6ᵗʰ H60.55 Acute reactive otitis externa
       H60.551 Acute reactive otitis externa, right ear
       H60.552 Acute reactive otitis externa, left ear
       H60.553 Acute reactive otitis externa, bilateral
       H60.559 Acute reactive otitis externa, unspecified ear

    ✓6ᵗʰ H60.59 Other noninfective acute otitis externa
       H60.591 Other noninfective acute otitis externa, right ear
       H60.592 Other noninfective acute otitis externa, left ear
       H60.593 Other noninfective acute otitis externa, bilateral
       H60.599 Other noninfective acute otitis externa, unspecified ear

✓5ᵗʰ H60.6 Unspecified chronic otitis externa
    H60.60 Unspecified chronic otitis externa, unspecified ear
    H60.61 Unspecified chronic otitis externa, right ear
    H60.62 Unspecified chronic otitis externa, left ear
    H60.63 Unspecified chronic otitis externa, bilateral

✓5ᵗʰ H60.8 Other otitis externa
    ✓6ᵗʰ H60.8X Other otitis externa
       H60.8X1 Other otitis externa, right ear
       H60.8X2 Other otitis externa, left ear
       H60.8X3 Other otitis externa, bilateral
       H60.8X9 Other otitis externa, unspecified ear

✓5ᵗʰ H60.9 Unspecified otitis externa
    H60.90 Unspecified otitis externa, unspecified ear
    H60.91 Unspecified otitis externa, right ear

N Newborn: 0   **P** Pediatric: 0-17   **M** Maternity: 9-64   **A** Adult: 15-124   **MCC** Major Complication/Comorbidity   **CC** Complication/Comorbidity   **SW** Severe Wound Dx

632   ICD-10-CM 2020

| H60.92 | Unspecified otitis externa, left ear |
| H60.93 | Unspecified otitis externa, bilateral |

✓4ᵗʰ **H61** **Other disorders of external ear**

✓5ᵗʰ **H61.0** **Chondritis and perichondritis of external ear**

Chondrodermatitis nodularis chronica helicis
Perichondritis of auricle
Perichondritis of pinna

✓6ᵗʰ **H61.00** **Unspecified perichondritis of external ear**

H61.001	Unspecified perichondritis of right external ear
H61.002	Unspecified perichondritis of left external ear
H61.003	Unspecified perichondritis of external ear, bilateral
H61.009	Unspecified perichondritis of external ear, unspecified ear

✓6ᵗʰ **H61.01** **Acute perichondritis of external ear**

H61.011	Acute perichondritis of right external ear
H61.012	Acute perichondritis of left external ear
H61.013	Acute perichondritis of external ear, bilateral
H61.019	Acute perichondritis of external ear, unspecified ear

✓6ᵗʰ **H61.02** **Chronic perichondritis of external ear**

H61.021	Chronic perichondritis of right external ear
H61.022	Chronic perichondritis of left external ear
H61.023	Chronic perichondritis of external ear, bilateral
H61.029	Chronic perichondritis of external ear, unspecified ear

✓6ᵗʰ **H61.03** **Chondritis of external ear**

Chondritis of auricle
Chondritis of pinna
AHA: 2015,1Q,18
DEF: Infection that has progressed into the cartilage and presents as indurated and edematous skin over the pinna. Vascular compromise occurs with tissue necrosis and deformity.

H61.031	Chondritis of right external ear
H61.032	Chondritis of left external ear
H61.033	Chondritis of external ear, bilateral
H61.039	Chondritis of external ear, unspecified ear

✓5ᵗʰ **H61.1** **Noninfective disorders of pinna**

EXCLUDES 2   *cauliflower ear (M95.1-)*
              gouty tophi of ear (M1A.-)

✓6ᵗʰ **H61.10** **Unspecified noninfective disorders of pinna**

Disorder of pinna NOS

H61.101	Unspecified noninfective disorders of pinna, right ear
H61.102	Unspecified noninfective disorders of pinna, left ear
H61.103	Unspecified noninfective disorders of pinna, bilateral
H61.109	Unspecified noninfective disorders of pinna, unspecified ear

✓6ᵗʰ **H61.11** **Acquired deformity of pinna**

Acquired deformity of auricle
EXCLUDES 2   *cauliflower ear (M95.1-)*

H61.111	Acquired deformity of pinna, right ear
H61.112	Acquired deformity of pinna, left ear
H61.113	Acquired deformity of pinna, bilateral
H61.119	Acquired deformity of pinna, unspecified ear

✓6ᵗʰ **H61.12** **Hematoma of pinna**

Hematoma of auricle

H61.121	Hematoma of pinna, right ear
H61.122	Hematoma of pinna, left ear
H61.123	Hematoma of pinna, bilateral
H61.129	Hematoma of pinna, unspecified ear

✓6ᵗʰ **H61.19** **Other noninfective disorders of pinna**

H61.191	Noninfective disorders of pinna, right ear
H61.192	Noninfective disorders of pinna, left ear
H61.193	Noninfective disorders of pinna, bilateral
H61.199	Noninfective disorders of pinna, unspecified ear

✓5ᵗʰ **H61.2** **Impacted cerumen**

Wax in ear

H61.20	Impacted cerumen, unspecified ear
H61.21	Impacted cerumen, right ear
H61.22	Impacted cerumen, left ear
H61.23	Impacted cerumen, bilateral

✓5ᵗʰ **H61.3** **Acquired stenosis of external ear canal**

Collapse of external ear canal
EXCLUDES 1   *postprocedural stenosis of external ear canal (H95.81-)*

✓6ᵗʰ **H61.30** **Acquired stenosis of external ear canal, unspecified**

H61.301	Acquired stenosis of right external ear canal, unspecified
H61.302	Acquired stenosis of left external ear canal, unspecified
H61.303	Acquired stenosis of external ear canal, unspecified, bilateral
H61.309	Acquired stenosis of external ear canal, unspecified, unspecified ear

✓6ᵗʰ **H61.31** **Acquired stenosis of external ear canal secondary to trauma**

H61.311	Acquired stenosis of right external ear canal secondary to trauma
H61.312	Acquired stenosis of left external ear canal secondary to trauma
H61.313	Acquired stenosis of external ear canal secondary to trauma, bilateral
H61.319	Acquired stenosis of external ear canal secondary to trauma, unspecified ear

✓6ᵗʰ **H61.32** **Acquired stenosis of external ear canal secondary to inflammation and infection**

DEF: Narrowing of the external ear canal due to chronic inflammation or infection.

H61.321	Acquired stenosis of right external ear canal secondary to inflammation and infection
H61.322	Acquired stenosis of left external ear canal secondary to inflammation and infection
H61.323	Acquired stenosis of external ear canal secondary to inflammation and infection, bilateral
H61.329	Acquired stenosis of external ear canal secondary to inflammation and infection, unspecified ear

✓6ᵗʰ **H61.39** **Other acquired stenosis of external ear canal**

H61.391	Other acquired stenosis of right external ear canal
H61.392	Other acquired stenosis of left external ear canal
H61.393	Other acquired stenosis of external ear canal, bilateral
H61.399	Other acquired stenosis of external ear canal, unspecified ear

✓5ᵗʰ **H61.8** **Other specified disorders of external ear**

✓6ᵗʰ **H61.81** **Exostosis of external canal**

H61.811	Exostosis of right external canal
H61.812	Exostosis of left external canal
H61.813	Exostosis of external canal, bilateral
H61.819	Exostosis of external canal, unspecified ear

✓6ᵗʰ **H61.89** **Other specified disorders of external ear**

H61.891	Other specified disorders of right external ear
H61.892	Other specified disorders of left external ear
H61.893	Other specified disorders of external ear, bilateral
H61.899	Other specified disorders of external ear, unspecified ear

✓5ᵗʰ **H61.9** **Disorder of external ear, unspecified**

H61.90	Disorder of external ear, unspecified, unspecified ear
H61.91	Disorder of right external ear, unspecified
H61.92	Disorder of left external ear, unspecified
H61.93	Disorder of external ear, unspecified, bilateral

☑ Additional Character Required   ✓x7ᵗʰ Placeholder   Unacceptable PDx   Questionable PDx   Manifestation   Unspecified Dx   H1-H14 HAC   HCC CMS-HCC Dx   HIV HIV Dx

ICD-10-CM 2020   633

☑4ᵗʰ **H62 Disorders of external ear in diseases classified elsewhere**

  ☑5ᵗʰ **H62.4 Otitis externa in other diseases classified elsewhere**

    Code first underlying disease, such as:
      erysipelas (A46)
      impetigo (L01.0)

    EXCLUDES 1   *otitis externa (in):*
        candidiasis (B37.84)
        herpes viral [herpes simplex] (B00.1)
        herpes zoster (B02.8)

    H62.40   *Otitis externa in other diseases classified elsewhere, unspecified ear*

    H62.41   *Otitis externa in other diseases classified elsewhere, right ear*

    H62.42   *Otitis externa in other diseases classified elsewhere, left ear*

    H62.43   *Otitis externa in other diseases classified elsewhere, bilateral*

  ☑5ᵗʰ **H62.8 Other disorders of external ear in diseases classified elsewhere**

    Code first underlying disease, such as:
      gout (M1A.-, M10.-)

    ☑6ᵗʰ **H62.8X Other disorders of external ear in diseases classified elsewhere**

      H62.8X1   *Other disorders of right external ear in diseases classified elsewhere*

      H62.8X2   *Other disorders of left external ear in diseases classified elsewhere*

      H62.8X3   *Other disorders of external ear in diseases classified elsewhere, bilateral*

      H62.8X9   *Other disorders of external ear in diseases classified elsewhere, unspecified ear*

Diseases of middle ear and mastoid (H65-H75)

☑4ᵗʰ **H65 Nonsuppurative otitis media**

  INCLUDES   nonsuppurative otitis media with myringitis

  Use additional code for any associated perforated tympanic membrane (H72.-)

  ▶Use additional code, if applicable, to identify:◀
    exposure to environmental tobacco smoke (Z77.22)
    exposure to tobacco smoke in the perinatal period (P96.81)
    history of tobacco dependence (Z87.891)
    ▶infectious agent (B95-B97)◀
    occupational exposure to environmental tobacco smoke (Z57.31)
    tobacco dependence (F17.-)
    tobacco use (Z72.0)

  ☑5ᵗʰ **H65.0 Acute serous otitis media**

    Acute and subacute secretory otitis

    H65.00   **Acute serous otitis media, unspecified ear**

    H65.01   **Acute serous otitis media, right ear**

    H65.02   **Acute serous otitis media, left ear**

    H65.03   **Acute serous otitis media, bilateral**

    H65.04   **Acute serous otitis media, recurrent, right ear**

    H65.05   **Acute serous otitis media, recurrent, left ear**

    H65.06   **Acute serous otitis media, recurrent, bilateral**

    H65.07   **Acute serous otitis media, recurrent, unspecified ear**

  ☑5ᵗʰ **H65.1 Other acute nonsuppurative otitis media**

    EXCLUDES 1   *otitic barotrauma (T70.0)*
        otitis media (acute) NOS (H66.9)

    ☑6ᵗʰ **H65.11 Acute and subacute allergic otitis media (mucoid) (sanguinous) (serous)**

      H65.111   **Acute and subacute allergic otitis media (mucoid) (sanguinous) (serous), right ear**

      H65.112   **Acute and subacute allergic otitis media (mucoid) (sanguinous) (serous), left ear**

      H65.113   **Acute and subacute allergic otitis media (mucoid) (sanguinous) (serous), bilateral**

      H65.114   **Acute and subacute allergic otitis media (mucoid) (sanguinous) (serous), recurrent, right ear**

      H65.115   **Acute and subacute allergic otitis media (mucoid) (sanguinous) (serous), recurrent, left ear**

      H65.116   **Acute and subacute allergic otitis media (mucoid) (sanguinous) (serous), recurrent, bilateral**

      H65.117   **Acute and subacute allergic otitis media (mucoid) (sanguinous) (serous), recurrent, unspecified ear**

      H65.119   **Acute and subacute allergic otitis media (mucoid) (sanguinous) (serous), unspecified ear**

    ☑6ᵗʰ **H65.19 Other acute nonsuppurative otitis media**

      Acute and subacute mucoid otitis media
      Acute and subacute nonsuppurative otitis media NOS
      Acute and subacute sanguinous otitis media
      Acute and subacute seromucinous otitis media

      H65.191   **Other acute nonsuppurative otitis media, right ear**

      H65.192   **Other acute nonsuppurative otitis media, left ear**

      H65.193   **Other acute nonsuppurative otitis media, bilateral**

      H65.194   **Other acute nonsuppurative otitis media, recurrent, right ear**

      H65.195   **Other acute nonsuppurative otitis media, recurrent, left ear**

      H65.196   **Other acute nonsuppurative otitis media, recurrent, bilateral**

      H65.197   **Other acute nonsuppurative otitis media recurrent, unspecified ear**

      H65.199   **Other acute nonsuppurative otitis media, unspecified ear**

  ☑5ᵗʰ **H65.2 Chronic serous otitis media**

    Chronic tubotympanal catarrh

    H65.20   **Chronic serous otitis media, unspecified ear**

    H65.21   **Chronic serous otitis media, right ear**

    H65.22   **Chronic serous otitis media, left ear**

    H65.23   **Chronic serous otitis media, bilateral**

  ☑5ᵗʰ **H65.3 Chronic mucoid otitis media**

    Chronic mucinous otitis media
    Chronic secretory otitis media
    Chronic transudative otitis media
    Glue ear

    EXCLUDES 1   *adhesive middle ear disease (H74.1)*

    H65.30   **Chronic mucoid otitis media, unspecified ear**

    H65.31   **Chronic mucoid otitis media, right ear**

    H65.32   **Chronic mucoid otitis media, left ear**

    H65.33   **Chronic mucoid otitis media, bilateral**

  ☑5ᵗʰ **H65.4 Other chronic nonsuppurative otitis media**

    ☑6ᵗʰ **H65.41 Chronic allergic otitis media**

      H65.411   **Chronic allergic otitis media, right ear**

      H65.412   **Chronic allergic otitis media, left ear**

      H65.413   **Chronic allergic otitis media, bilateral**

      H65.419   **Chronic allergic otitis media, unspecified ear**

    ☑6ᵗʰ **H65.49 Other chronic nonsuppurative otitis media**

      Chronic exudative otitis media
      Chronic nonsuppurative otitis media NOS
      Chronic otitis media with effusion (nonpurulent)
      Chronic seromucinous otitis media

      H65.491   **Other chronic nonsuppurative otitis media, right ear**

      H65.492   **Other chronic nonsuppurative otitis media, left ear**

      H65.493   **Other chronic nonsuppurative otitis media, bilateral**

      H65.499   **Other chronic nonsuppurative otitis media, unspecified ear**

  ☑5ᵗʰ **H65.9 Unspecified nonsuppurative otitis media**

    Allergic otitis media NOS
    Catarrhal otitis media NOS
    Exudative otitis media NOS
    Mucoid otitis media NOS
    Otitis media with effusion (nonpurulent) NOS
    Secretory otitis media NOS
    Seromucinous otitis media NOS
    Serous otitis media NOS
    Transudative otitis media NOS

    H65.90   **Unspecified nonsuppurative otitis media, unspecified ear**

    H65.91   **Unspecified nonsuppurative otitis media, right ear**

    H65.92   **Unspecified nonsuppurative otitis media, left ear**

    H65.93   **Unspecified nonsuppurative otitis media, bilateral**

N Newborn: 0   P Pediatric: 0-17   M Maternity: 9-64   A Adult: 15-124   MCC Major Complication/Comorbidity   CC Complication/Comorbidity   SW Severe Wound Dx

634   ICD-10-CM 2020

√4ᵗʰ **H66** **Suppurative and unspecified otitis media**

> INCLUDES   suppurative and unspecified otitis media with myringitis
> Use additional code to identify:
> exposure to environmental tobacco smoke (Z77.22)
> exposure to tobacco smoke in the perinatal period (P96.81)
> history of tobacco dependence (Z87.891)
> occupational exposure to environmental tobacco smoke (Z57.31)
> tobacco dependence (F17.-)
> tobacco use (Z72.0)
> **AHA:** 2016,1Q,34

√5ᵗʰ **H66.0** **Acute suppurative otitis media**

> √6ᵗʰ **H66.00** **Acute suppurative otitis media** without spontaneous rupture of ear drum
>
> > **H66.001** **Acute suppurative otitis media without spontaneous rupture of ear drum,** right ear
> >
> > **H66.002** **Acute suppurative otitis media without spontaneous rupture of ear drum,** left ear
> >
> > **H66.003** **Acute suppurative otitis media without spontaneous rupture of ear drum,** bilateral
> >
> > **H66.004** **Acute suppurative otitis media without spontaneous rupture of ear drum,** recurrent, right ear
> >
> > **H66.005** **Acute suppurative otitis media without spontaneous rupture of ear drum,** recurrent, left ear
> >
> > **H66.006** **Acute suppurative otitis media without spontaneous rupture of ear drum,** recurrent, bilateral
> >
> > **H66.007** **Acute suppurative otitis media without spontaneous rupture of ear drum,** recurrent, unspecified ear
> >
> > **H66.009** **Acute suppurative otitis media without spontaneous rupture of ear drum,** unspecified ear
>
> √6ᵗʰ **H66.01** **Acute suppurative otitis media** with spontaneous rupture of ear drum
>
> > **DEF:** Sudden, severe inflammation of the middle ear, causing pressure that perforates the ear drum tissue.
> >
> > **H66.011** **Acute suppurative otitis media with spontaneous rupture of ear drum,** right ear
> >
> > **H66.012** **Acute suppurative otitis media with spontaneous rupture of ear drum,** left ear
> >
> > **H66.013** **Acute suppurative otitis media with spontaneous rupture of ear drum,** bilateral
> >
> > **H66.014** **Acute suppurative otitis media with spontaneous rupture of ear drum,** recurrent, right ear
> >
> > **H66.015** **Acute suppurative otitis media with spontaneous rupture of ear drum,** recurrent, left ear
> >
> > **H66.016** **Acute suppurative otitis media with spontaneous rupture of ear drum,** recurrent, bilateral
> >
> > **H66.017** **Acute suppurative otitis media with spontaneous rupture of ear drum,** recurrent, unspecified ear
> >
> > **H66.019** **Acute suppurative otitis media with spontaneous rupture of ear drum,** unspecified ear

√5ᵗʰ **H66.1** **Chronic tubotympanic suppurative otitis media**

> Benign chronic suppurative otitis media
> Chronic tubotympanic disease
> Use additional code for any associated perforated tympanic membrane (H72.-)
>
> **H66.10** **Chronic tubotympanic suppurative otitis media, unspecified**
>
> **H66.11** **Chronic tubotympanic suppurative otitis media, right ear**
>
> **H66.12** **Chronic tubotympanic suppurative otitis media, left ear**
>
> **H66.13** **Chronic tubotympanic suppurative otitis media, bilateral**

√5ᵗʰ **H66.2** **Chronic atticoantral suppurative otitis media**

> Chronic atticoantral disease
> Use additional code for any associated perforated tympanic membrane (H72.-)
>
> **H66.20** **Chronic atticoantral suppurative otitis media, unspecified ear**

H66.21 **Chronic atticoantral suppurative otitis media,** right ear

H66.22 **Chronic atticoantral suppurative otitis media,** left ear

H66.23 **Chronic atticoantral suppurative otitis media,** bilateral

√5ᵗʰ **H66.3** **Other chronic suppurative otitis media**

> Chronic suppurative otitis media NOS
> Use additional code for any associated perforated tympanic membrane (H72.-)
>
> > EXCLUDES 1   tuberculous otitis media (A18.6)
>
> √6ᵗʰ **H66.3X** **Other chronic suppurative otitis media**
>
> > **H66.3X1** **Other chronic suppurative otitis media,** right ear
> >
> > **H66.3X2** **Other chronic suppurative otitis media,** left ear
> >
> > **H66.3X3** **Other chronic suppurative otitis media,** bilateral
> >
> > **H66.3X9** **Other chronic suppurative otitis media,** unspecified ear

√5ᵗʰ **H66.4** **Suppurative otitis media, unspecified**

> Purulent otitis media NOS
> Use additional code for any associated perforated tympanic membrane (H72.-)
>
> **H66.40** **Suppurative otitis media, unspecified, unspecified ear**
>
> **H66.41** **Suppurative otitis media, unspecified,** right ear
>
> **H66.42** **Suppurative otitis media, unspecified,** left ear
>
> **H66.43** **Suppurative otitis media, unspecified,** bilateral

√5ᵗʰ **H66.9** **Otitis media, unspecified**

> Otitis media NOS
> Acute otitis media NOS
> Chronic otitis media NOS
> Use additional code for any associated perforated tympanic membrane (H72.-)
>
> **H66.90** **Otitis media, unspecified, unspecified ear**
>
> **H66.91** **Otitis media, unspecified,** right ear
>
> **H66.92** **Otitis media, unspecified,** left ear
>
> **H66.93** **Otitis media, unspecified,** bilateral

√4ᵗʰ **H67** **Otitis media in diseases classified elsewhere**

> Code first underlying disease, such as:
> plasminogen deficiency (E88.02)
> viral disease NEC (B00-B34)
> Use additional code for any associated perforated tympanic membrane (H72.-)
>
> > EXCLUDES 1   otitis media in:
> > influenza (J09.X9, J10.83, J11.83)
> > measles (B05.3)
> > scarlet fever (A38.0)
> > tuberculosis (A18.6)
>
> *H67.1* *Otitis media in diseases classified elsewhere,* right ear
>
> *H67.2* *Otitis media in diseases classified elsewhere,* left ear
>
> *H67.3* *Otitis media in diseases classified elsewhere,* bilateral
>
> *H67.9* *Otitis media in diseases classified elsewhere, unspecified ear*

√4ᵗʰ **H68** **Eustachian salpingitis and obstruction**

> **DEF:** Eustachian tube: Internal channel between the tympanic cavity and the nasopharynx that equalizes internal pressure to the outside pressure and drains mucous production from the middle ear.

√5ᵗʰ **H68.0** **Eustachian salpingitis**

> √6ᵗʰ **H68.00** **Unspecified Eustachian salpingitis**
>
> > **H68.001** **Unspecified Eustachian salpingitis,** right ear
> >
> > **H68.002** **Unspecified Eustachian salpingitis,** left ear
> >
> > **H68.003** **Unspecified Eustachian salpingitis,** bilateral
> >
> > **H68.009** **Unspecified Eustachian salpingitis, unspecified ear**
>
> √6ᵗʰ **H68.01** **Acute Eustachian salpingitis**
>
> > **H68.011** **Acute Eustachian salpingitis,** right ear
> >
> > **H68.012** **Acute Eustachian salpingitis,** left ear
> >
> > **H68.013** **Acute Eustachian salpingitis,** bilateral
> >
> > **H68.019** **Acute Eustachian salpingitis, unspecified ear**
>
> √6ᵗʰ **H68.02** **Chronic Eustachian salpingitis**
>
> > **H68.021** **Chronic Eustachian salpingitis,** right ear
> >
> > **H68.022** **Chronic Eustachian salpingitis,** left ear

☑ Additional Character Required   √x 7ᵗʰ Placeholder   Unacceptable PDx   Questionable PDx   Manifestation   Unspecified Dx   H1-H14 HAC   HCC CMS-HCC Dx   HIV HIV Dx

ICD-10-CM 2020   635

          H68.023   Chronic Eustachian salpingitis, **bilateral**

          H68.029   Chronic Eustachian salpingitis, **unspecified ear**

✓5ᵗʰ **H68.1**   **Obstruction** of Eustachian tube

     Stenosis of Eustachian tube

     Stricture of Eustachian tube

     ✓6ᵗʰ **H68.10**   **Unspecified obstruction** of Eustachian tube

          H68.101   Unspecified obstruction of Eustachian tube, **right ear**

          H68.102   Unspecified obstruction of Eustachian tube, **left ear**

          H68.103   Unspecified obstruction of Eustachian tube, **bilateral**

          H68.109   Unspecified obstruction of Eustachian tube, **unspecified ear**

     ✓6ᵗʰ **H68.11**   **Osseous obstruction** of Eustachian tube

          H68.111   Osseous obstruction of Eustachian tube, **right ear**

          H68.112   Osseous obstruction of Eustachian tube, **left ear**

          H68.113   Osseous obstruction of Eustachian tube, **bilateral**

          H68.119   Osseous obstruction of Eustachian tube, **unspecified ear**

     ✓6ᵗʰ **H68.12**   **Intrinsic cartilagenous obstruction** of Eustachian tube

          H68.121   Intrinsic cartilagenous obstruction of Eustachian tube, **right ear**

          H68.122   Intrinsic cartilagenous obstruction of Eustachian tube, **left ear**

          H68.123   Intrinsic cartilagenous obstruction of Eustachian tube, **bilateral**

          H68.129   Intrinsic cartilagenous obstruction of Eustachian tube, **unspecified ear**

     ✓6ᵗʰ **H68.13**   **Extrinsic cartilagenous obstruction** of Eustachian tube

           Compression of Eustachian tube

          H68.131   Extrinsic cartilagenous obstruction of Eustachian tube, **right ear**

          H68.132   Extrinsic cartilagenous obstruction of Eustachian tube, **left ear**

          H68.133   Extrinsic cartilagenous obstruction of Eustachian tube, **bilateral**

          H68.139   Extrinsic cartilagenous obstruction of Eustachian tube, **unspecified ear**

✓4ᵗʰ **H69**   **Other and unspecified disorders of Eustachian tube**

     DEF: Eustachian tube: Internal channel between the tympanic cavity and the nasopharynx that equalizes internal pressure to the outside pressure and drains mucous production from the middle ear.

     ✓5ᵗʰ **H69.0**   **Patulous Eustachian tube**

        H69.00   Patulous Eustachian tube, **unspecified ear**

        H69.01   Patulous Eustachian tube, **right ear**

        H69.02   Patulous Eustachian tube, **left ear**

        H69.03   Patulous Eustachian tube, **bilateral**

     ✓5ᵗʰ **H69.8**   **Other specified disorders of Eustachian tube**

        H69.80   Other specified disorders of Eustachian tube, **unspecified ear**

        H69.81   Other specified disorders of Eustachian tube, **right ear**

        H69.82   Other specified disorders of Eustachian tube, **left ear**

        H69.83   Other specified disorders of Eustachian tube, **bilateral**

     ✓5ᵗʰ **H69.9**   **Unspecified Eustachian tube disorder**

        H69.90   Unspecified Eustachian tube disorder, **unspecified ear**

        H69.91   Unspecified Eustachian tube disorder, **right ear**

        H69.92   Unspecified Eustachian tube disorder, **left ear**

        H69.93   Unspecified Eustachian tube disorder, **bilateral**

✓4ᵗʰ **H70**   **Mastoiditis and related conditions**

     ✓5ᵗʰ **H70.0**   **Acute mastoiditis**

         Abscess of mastoid

         Empyema of mastoid

         CC Excl: For CC codes in subcategory H70.0: PDX collection 641

         ✓6ᵗʰ **H70.00**   **Acute mastoiditis** without complications

          H70.001   Acute mastoiditis without complications, **right ear**   CC

          H70.002   Acute mastoiditis without complications, **left ear**   CC

          H70.003   Acute mastoiditis without complications, **bilateral**   CC

          H70.009   Acute mastoiditis without complications, unspecified ear   CC

         ✓6ᵗʰ **H70.01**   **Subperiosteal abscess** of mastoid

          H70.011   Subperiosteal abscess of mastoid, **right ear**   CC

          H70.012   Subperiosteal abscess of mastoid, **left ear**   CC

          H70.013   Subperiosteal abscess of mastoid, **bilateral**   CC

          H70.019   Subperiosteal abscess of mastoid, **unspecified ear**   CC

         ✓6ᵗʰ **H70.09**   **Acute mastoiditis with other complications**

          H70.091   Acute mastoiditis with other complications, **right ear**   CC

          H70.092   Acute mastoiditis with other complications, **left ear**   CC

          H70.093   Acute mastoiditis with other complications, **bilateral**   CC

          H70.099   Acute mastoiditis with other complications, unspecified ear   CC

     ✓5ᵗʰ **H70.1**   **Chronic mastoiditis**

         Caries of mastoid

         Fistula of mastoid

         EXCLUDES 1   *tuberculous mastoiditis (A18.03)*

        H70.10   Chronic mastoiditis, **unspecified ear**

        H70.11   Chronic mastoiditis, **right ear**

        H70.12   Chronic mastoiditis, **left ear**

        H70.13   Chronic mastoiditis, **bilateral**

     ✓5ᵗʰ **H70.2**   **Petrositis**

         Inflammation of petrous bone

         ✓6ᵗʰ **H70.20**   **Unspecified petrositis**

          H70.201   Unspecified petrositis, **right ear**

          H70.202   Unspecified petrositis, **left ear**

          H70.203   Unspecified petrositis, **bilateral**

          H70.209   Unspecified petrositis, **unspecified ear**

         ✓6ᵗʰ **H70.21**   **Acute petrositis**

           DEF: Sudden, severe inflammation of the petrous temporal bone behind the ear, associated with a middle ear infection.

          H70.211   Acute petrositis, **right ear**

          H70.212   Acute petrositis, **left ear**

          H70.213   Acute petrositis, **bilateral**

          H70.219   Acute petrositis, **unspecified ear**

         ✓6ᵗʰ **H70.22**   **Chronic petrositis**

          H70.221   Chronic petrositis, **right ear**

          H70.222   Chronic petrositis, **left ear**

          H70.223   Chronic petrositis, **bilateral**

          H70.229   Chronic petrositis, **unspecified ear**

     ✓5ᵗʰ **H70.8**   **Other mastoiditis and related conditions**

         EXCLUDES 1   *preauricular sinus and cyst (Q18.1)*

                     sinus, fistula, and cyst of branchial cleft (Q18.0)

         ✓6ᵗʰ **H70.81**   **Postauricular fistula**

          H70.811   Postauricular fistula, **right ear**   SW

          H70.812   Postauricular fistula, **left ear**   SW

          H70.813   Postauricular fistula, **bilateral**   SW

          H70.819   Postauricular fistula, **unspecified ear**   SW

         ✓6ᵗʰ **H70.89**   **Other mastoiditis and related conditions**

          H70.891   Other mastoiditis and related conditions, **right ear**

          H70.892   Other mastoiditis and related conditions, **left ear**

          H70.893   Other mastoiditis and related conditions, **bilateral**

          H70.899   Other mastoiditis and related conditions, **unspecified ear**

N Newborn: 0   P Pediatric: 0-17   M Maternity: 9-64   A Adult: 15-124   MCC Major Complication/Comorbidity   CC Complication/Comorbidity   SW Severe Wound Dx

636   ICD-10-CM 2020

✓5ᵗʰ **H70.9**   **Unspecified mastoiditis**

     H70.90   **Unspecified mastoiditis, unspecified ear**

     H70.91   **Unspecified mastoiditis, right ear**

     H70.92   **Unspecified mastoiditis, left ear**

     H70.93   **Unspecified mastoiditis, bilateral**

✓4ᵗʰ **H71**   **Cholesteatoma of middle ear**

     EXCLUDES 2   *cholesteatoma of external ear (H60.4-)*

                   recurrent cholesteatoma of postmastoidectomy cavity (H95.0-)

     DEF: Cholesteatoma: Noncancerous cyst-like mass of cell debris, including cholesterol and epithelial cells resulting from trauma, repeated or improperly healed infections, and congenital enclosure of epidermal cells.

Cholesteatoma of Middle Ear

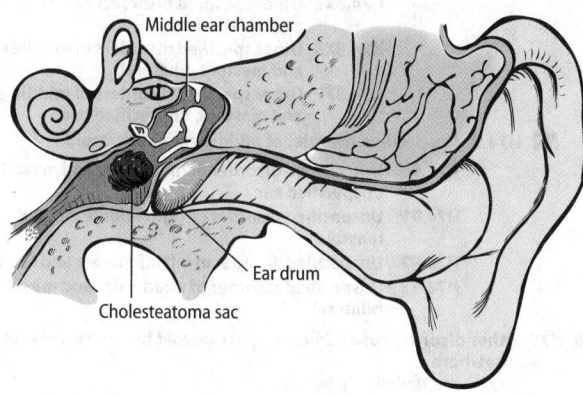

✓5ᵗʰ **H71.0**   **Cholesteatoma of attic**

     H71.00   **Cholesteatoma of attic, unspecified ear**

     H71.01   **Cholesteatoma of attic, right ear**

     H71.02   **Cholesteatoma of attic, left ear**

     H71.03   **Cholesteatoma of attic, bilateral**

✓5ᵗʰ **H71.1**   **Cholesteatoma of tympanum**

     H71.10   **Cholesteatoma of tympanum, unspecified ear**

     H71.11   **Cholesteatoma of tympanum, right ear**

     H71.12   **Cholesteatoma of tympanum, left ear**

     H71.13   **Cholesteatoma of tympanum, bilateral**

✓5ᵗʰ **H71.2**   **Cholesteatoma of mastoid**

     H71.20   **Cholesteatoma of mastoid, unspecified ear**

     H71.21   **Cholesteatoma of mastoid, right ear**

     H71.22   **Cholesteatoma of mastoid, left ear**

     H71.23   **Cholesteatoma of mastoid, bilateral**

✓5ᵗʰ **H71.3**   **Diffuse cholesteatosis**

     H71.30   **Diffuse cholesteatosis, unspecified ear**

     H71.31   **Diffuse cholesteatosis, right ear**

     H71.32   **Diffuse cholesteatosis, left ear**

     H71.33   **Diffuse cholesteatosis, bilateral**

✓5ᵗʰ **H71.9**   **Unspecified cholesteatoma**

     H71.90   **Unspecified cholesteatoma, unspecified ear**

     H71.91   **Unspecified cholesteatoma, right ear**

     H71.92   **Unspecified cholesteatoma, left ear**

     H71.93   **Unspecified cholesteatoma, bilateral**

✓4ᵗʰ **H72**   **Perforation of tympanic membrane**

     INCLUDES   persistent post-traumatic perforation of ear drum

                postinflammatory perforation of ear drum

     Code first any associated otitis media (H65.-, H66.1-, H66.2-, H66.3-, H66.4-, H66.9-, H67.-)

     EXCLUDES 1   *acute suppurative otitis media with rupture of the tympanic membrane (H66.01-)*

                   traumatic rupture of ear drum (S09.2-)

✓5ᵗʰ **H72.0**   **Central perforation of tympanic membrane**

     H72.00   **Central perforation of tympanic membrane, unspecified ear**

     H72.01   **Central perforation of tympanic membrane, right ear**

     H72.02   **Central perforation of tympanic membrane, left ear**

     H72.03   **Central perforation of tympanic membrane, bilateral**

✓5ᵗʰ **H72.1**   **Attic perforation of tympanic membrane**

     Perforation of pars flaccida

     H72.10   **Attic perforation of tympanic membrane, unspecified ear**

     H72.11   **Attic perforation of tympanic membrane, right ear**

     H72.12   **Attic perforation of tympanic membrane, left ear**

     H72.13   **Attic perforation of tympanic membrane, bilateral**

✓5ᵗʰ **H72.2**   **Other marginal perforations of tympanic membrane**

     ✓6ᵗʰ **H72.2X**   **Other marginal perforations of tympanic membrane**

         H72.2X1   **Other marginal perforations of tympanic membrane, right ear**

         H72.2X2   **Other marginal perforations of tympanic membrane, left ear**

         H72.2X3   **Other marginal perforations of tympanic membrane, bilateral**

         H72.2X9   **Other marginal perforations of tympanic membrane, unspecified ear**

✓5ᵗʰ **H72.8**   **Other perforations of tympanic membrane**

     ✓6ᵗʰ **H72.81**   **Multiple perforations of tympanic membrane**

         H72.811   **Multiple perforations of tympanic membrane, right ear**

         H72.812   **Multiple perforations of tympanic membrane, left ear**

         H72.813   **Multiple perforations of tympanic membrane, bilateral**

         H72.819   **Multiple perforations of tympanic membrane, unspecified ear**

     ✓6ᵗʰ **H72.82**   **Total perforations of tympanic membrane**

         H72.821   **Total perforations of tympanic membrane, right ear**

         H72.822   **Total perforations of tympanic membrane, left ear**

         H72.823   **Total perforations of tympanic membrane, bilateral**

         H72.829   **Total perforations of tympanic membrane, unspecified ear**

✓5ᵗʰ **H72.9**   **Unspecified perforation of tympanic membrane**

     H72.90   **Unspecified perforation of tympanic membrane, unspecified ear**

     H72.91   **Unspecified perforation of tympanic membrane, right ear**

     H72.92   **Unspecified perforation of tympanic membrane, left ear**

     H72.93   **Unspecified perforation of tympanic membrane, bilateral**

✓4ᵗʰ **H73**   **Other disorders of tympanic membrane**

     ✓5ᵗʰ **H73.0**   **Acute myringitis**

         EXCLUDES 1   *acute myringitis with otitis media (H65, H66)*

         ✓6ᵗʰ **H73.00**   **Unspecified acute myringitis**

             Acute tympanitis NOS

             H73.001   **Acute myringitis, right ear**

             H73.002   **Acute myringitis, left ear**

             H73.003   **Acute myringitis, bilateral**

             H73.009   **Acute myringitis, unspecified ear**

         ✓6ᵗʰ **H73.01**   **Bullous myringitis**

             DEF: Bacterial or viral otitis media that is characterized by the appearance of serous or hemorrhagic blebs on the ear drum and sudden onset of severe pain in ear.

             H73.011   **Bullous myringitis, right ear**

             H73.012   **Bullous myringitis, left ear**

             H73.013   **Bullous myringitis, bilateral**

             H73.019   **Bullous myringitis, unspecified ear**

         ✓6ᵗʰ **H73.09**   **Other acute myringitis**

             H73.091   **Other acute myringitis, right ear**

             H73.092   **Other acute myringitis, left ear**

             H73.093   **Other acute myringitis, bilateral**

             H73.099   **Other acute myringitis, unspecified ear**

     ✓5ᵗʰ **H73.1**   **Chronic myringitis**

         Chronic tympanitis

         EXCLUDES 1   *chronic myringitis with otitis media (H65, H66)*

         H73.10   **Chronic myringitis, unspecified ear**

         H73.11   **Chronic myringitis, right ear**

         H73.12   **Chronic myringitis, left ear**

         H73.13   **Chronic myringitis, bilateral**

     ✓5ᵗʰ **H73.2**   **Unspecified myringitis**

         H73.20   **Unspecified myringitis, unspecified ear**

         H73.21   **Unspecified myringitis, right ear**

✓ Additional Character Required   ✓x7ᵗʰ Placeholder   Unacceptable PDx   Questionable PDx   Manifestation   Unspecified Dx   H1 – H14 HAC   HCC CMS-HCC Dx   HIV HIV Dx

ICD-10-CM 2020   **637**

Chapter 8. Diseases of the Ear and Mastoid Process

H73.22   Unspecified myringitis, left ear

H73.23   Unspecified myringitis, bilateral

☑5ᵗʰ **H73.8**   Other specified disorders of tympanic membrane

    ☑6ᵗʰ **H73.81**   Atrophic flaccid tympanic membrane

       H73.811   Atrophic flaccid tympanic membrane, right ear

       H73.812   Atrophic flaccid tympanic membrane, left ear

       H73.813   Atrophic flaccid tympanic membrane, bilateral

       H73.819   Atrophic flaccid tympanic membrane, unspecified ear

    ☑6ᵗʰ **H73.82**   Atrophic nonflaccid tympanic membrane

       H73.821   Atrophic nonflaccid tympanic membrane, right ear

       H73.822   Atrophic nonflaccid tympanic membrane, left ear

       H73.823   Atrophic nonflaccid tympanic membrane, bilateral

       H73.829   Atrophic nonflaccid tympanic membrane, unspecified ear

    ☑6ᵗʰ **H73.89**   Other specified disorders of tympanic membrane

       H73.891   Other specified disorders of tympanic membrane, right ear

       H73.892   Other specified disorders of tympanic membrane, left ear

       H73.893   Other specified disorders of tympanic membrane, bilateral

       H73.899   Other specified disorders of tympanic membrane, unspecified ear

☑5ᵗʰ **H73.9**   Unspecified disorder of tympanic membrane

    H73.90   Unspecified disorder of tympanic membrane, unspecified ear

    H73.91   Unspecified disorder of tympanic membrane, right ear

    H73.92   Unspecified disorder of tympanic membrane, left ear

    H73.93   Unspecified disorder of tympanic membrane, bilateral

☑4ᵗʰ **H74**   Other disorders of middle ear mastoid

    EXCLUDES 2   mastoiditis (H70.-)

☑5ᵗʰ **H74.0**   Tympanosclerosis

    DEF: Calcification of tissue in the ear drum, middle ear bones, and middle ear canal.

    H74.01   Tympanosclerosis, right ear

    H74.02   Tympanosclerosis, left ear

    H74.03   Tympanosclerosis, bilateral

    H74.09   Tympanosclerosis, unspecified ear

☑5ᵗʰ **H74.1**   Adhesive middle ear disease

    Adhesive otitis

    EXCLUDES 1   glue ear (H65.3-)

    H74.11   Adhesive right middle ear disease

    H74.12   Adhesive left middle ear disease

    H74.13   Adhesive middle ear disease, bilateral

    H74.19   Adhesive middle ear disease, unspecified ear

☑5ᵗʰ **H74.2**   Discontinuity and dislocation of ear ossicles

    H74.20   Discontinuity and dislocation of ear ossicles, unspecified ear

    H74.21   Discontinuity and dislocation of right ear ossicles

    H74.22   Discontinuity and dislocation of left ear ossicles

    H74.23   Discontinuity and dislocation of ear ossicles, bilateral

☑5ᵗʰ **H74.3**   Other acquired abnormalities of ear ossicles

    ☑6ᵗʰ **H74.31**   Ankylosis of ear ossicles

       H74.311   Ankylosis of ear ossicles, right ear

       H74.312   Ankylosis of ear ossicles, left ear

       H74.313   Ankylosis of ear ossicles, bilateral

       H74.319   Ankylosis of ear ossicles, unspecified ear

    ☑6ᵗʰ **H74.32**   Partial loss of ear ossicles

       H74.321   Partial loss of ear ossicles, right ear

       H74.322   Partial loss of ear ossicles, left ear

       H74.323   Partial loss of ear ossicles, bilateral

       H74.329   Partial loss of ear ossicles, unspecified ear

    ☑6ᵗʰ **H74.39**   Other acquired abnormalities of ear ossicles

       H74.391   Other acquired abnormalities of right ear ossicles

H74.392   Other acquired abnormalities of left ear ossicles

H74.393   Other acquired abnormalities of ear ossicles, bilateral

H74.399   Other acquired abnormalities of ear ossicles, unspecified ear

☑5ᵗʰ **H74.4**   Polyp of middle ear

    H74.40   Polyp of middle ear, unspecified ear

    H74.41   Polyp of right middle ear

    H74.42   Polyp of left middle ear

    H74.43   Polyp of middle ear, bilateral

☑5ᵗʰ **H74.8**   Other specified disorders of middle ear and mastoid

    ☑6ᵗʰ **H74.8X**   Other specified disorders of middle ear and mastoid

       H74.8X1   Other specified disorders of right middle ear and mastoid

       H74.8X2   Other specified disorders of left middle ear and mastoid

       H74.8X3   Other specified disorders of middle ear and mastoid, bilateral

       H74.8X9   Other specified disorders of middle ear and mastoid, unspecified ear

☑5ᵗʰ **H74.9**   Unspecified disorder of middle ear and mastoid

    H74.90   Unspecified disorder of middle ear and mastoid, unspecified ear

    H74.91   Unspecified disorder of right middle ear and mastoid

    H74.92   Unspecified disorder of left middle ear and mastoid

    H74.93   Unspecified disorder of middle ear and mastoid, bilateral

☑4ᵗʰ **H75**   Other disorders of middle ear and mastoid in diseases classified elsewhere

    Code first underlying disease

☑5ᵗʰ **H75.0**   Mastoiditis in infectious and parasitic diseases classified elsewhere

    EXCLUDES 1   mastoiditis (in):

       syphilis (A52.77)

       tuberculosis (A18.03)

    H75.00   *Mastoiditis in infectious and parasitic diseases classified elsewhere, unspecified ear*

    H75.01   *Mastoiditis in infectious and parasitic diseases classified elsewhere, right ear*

    H75.02   *Mastoiditis in infectious and parasitic diseases classified elsewhere, left ear*

    H75.03   *Mastoiditis in infectious and parasitic diseases classified elsewhere, bilateral*

☑5ᵗʰ **H75.8**   Other specified disorders of middle ear and mastoid in diseases classified elsewhere

    H75.80   *Other specified disorders of middle ear and mastoid in diseases classified elsewhere, unspecified ear*

    H75.81   *Other specified disorders of right middle ear and mastoid in diseases classified elsewhere*

    H75.82   *Other specified disorders of left middle ear and mastoid in diseases classified elsewhere*

    H75.83   *Other specified disorders of middle ear and mastoid in diseases classified elsewhere, bilateral*

Diseases of inner ear (H80-H83)

☑4ᵗʰ **H80**   Otosclerosis

    INCLUDES   otospongiosis

☑5ᵗʰ **H80.0**   Otosclerosis involving oval window, nonobliterative

    H80.00   Otosclerosis involving oval window, nonobliterative, unspecified ear

    H80.01   Otosclerosis involving oval window, nonobliterative, right ear

    H80.02   Otosclerosis involving oval window, nonobliterative, left ear

    H80.03   Otosclerosis involving oval window, nonobliterative, bilateral

☑5ᵗʰ **H80.1**   Otosclerosis involving oval window, obliterative

    H80.10   Otosclerosis involving oval window, obliterative, unspecified ear

    H80.11   Otosclerosis involving oval window, obliterative, right ear

    H80.12   Otosclerosis involving oval window, obliterative, left ear

    H80.13   Otosclerosis involving oval window, obliterative, bilateral

✓5ᵗʰ **H80.2　Cochlear otosclerosis**

　　Otosclerosis involving otic capsule
　　Otosclerosis involving round window

　　H80.20　Cochlear otosclerosis, unspecified ear
　　H80.21　Cochlear otosclerosis, right ear
　　H80.22　Cochlear otosclerosis, left ear
　　H80.23　Cochlear otosclerosis, bilateral

✓5ᵗʰ **H80.8　Other otosclerosis**

　　H80.80　Other otosclerosis, unspecified ear
　　H80.81　Other otosclerosis, right ear
　　H80.82　Other otosclerosis, left ear
　　H80.83　Other otosclerosis, bilateral

✓5ᵗʰ **H80.9　Unspecified otosclerosis**

　　H80.90　Unspecified otosclerosis, unspecified ear
　　H80.91　Unspecified otosclerosis, right ear
　　H80.92　Unspecified otosclerosis, left ear
　　H80.93　Unspecified otosclerosis, bilateral

✓4ᵗʰ **H81　Disorders of vestibular function**

　　EXCLUDES 1　epidemic vertigo (A88.1)
　　　　　　　　vertigo NOS (R42)

✓5ᵗʰ **H81.0　Ménière's disease**

　　Labyrinthine hydrops
　　Ménière's syndrome or vertigo
　　DEF: Distended membranous labyrinth of the middle ear from fluctuating pressure of fluid (hydrops) that causes vertigo, tinnitus, pressure, and hearing loss that may last on and off for several hours. Episodes may occur in clusters or may subside for weeks, months, or even years.

　　H81.01　Ménière's disease, right ear
　　H81.02　Ménière's disease, left ear
　　H81.03　Ménière's disease, bilateral
　　H81.09　Ménière's disease, unspecified ear

✓5ᵗʰ **H81.1　Benign paroxysmal vertigo**

　　H81.10　Benign paroxysmal vertigo, unspecified ear
　　H81.11　Benign paroxysmal vertigo, right ear
　　H81.12　Benign paroxysmal vertigo, left ear
　　H81.13　Benign paroxysmal vertigo, bilateral

✓5ᵗʰ **H81.2　Vestibular neuronitis**

　　DEF: Transient benign vertigo caused by inflammation of the vestibular nerve. It is characterized by response to caloric stimulation on one side and nystagmus with rhythmic movement of the eyes. Normal auditory function is present.

　　H81.20　Vestibular neuronitis, unspecified ear
　　H81.21　Vestibular neuronitis, right ear
　　H81.22　Vestibular neuronitis, left ear
　　H81.23　Vestibular neuronitis, bilateral

✓5ᵗʰ **H81.3　Other peripheral vertigo**

　　✓6ᵗʰ **H81.31　Aural vertigo**

　　　　H81.311　Aural vertigo, right ear
　　　　H81.312　Aural vertigo, left ear
　　　　H81.313　Aural vertigo, bilateral
　　　　H81.319　Aural vertigo, unspecified ear

　　✓6ᵗʰ **H81.39　Other peripheral vertigo**

　　　　Lermoyez' syndrome
　　　　Otogenic vertigo
　　　　Peripheral vertigo NOS

　　　　H81.391　Other peripheral vertigo, right ear
　　　　H81.392　Other peripheral vertigo, left ear
　　　　H81.393　Other peripheral vertigo, bilateral
　　　　H81.399　Other peripheral vertigo, unspecified ear

▲　**H81.4　Vertigo of central origin**

　　Central positional nystagmus
　　H81.41　~~Vertigo of central origin, right ear~~
　　H81.42　~~Vertigo of central origin, left ear~~
　　H81.43　~~Vertigo of central origin, bilateral~~
　　H81.49　~~Vertigo of central origin, unspecified ear~~

✓5ᵗʰ **H81.8　Other disorders of vestibular function**

　　✓6ᵗʰ **H81.8X　Other disorders of vestibular function**

　　　　H81.8X1　Other disorders of vestibular function, right ear
　　　　H81.8X2　Other disorders of vestibular function, left ear
　　　　H81.8X3　Other disorders of vestibular function, bilateral
　　　　H81.8X9　Other disorders of vestibular function, unspecified ear

✓5ᵗʰ **H81.9　Unspecified disorder of vestibular function**

　　Vertiginous syndrome NOS

　　H81.90　Unspecified disorder of vestibular function, unspecified ear
　　H81.91　Unspecified disorder of vestibular function, right ear
　　H81.92　Unspecified disorder of vestibular function, left ear
　　H81.93　Unspecified disorder of vestibular function, bilateral

✓4ᵗʰ **H82　Vertiginous syndromes in diseases classified elsewhere**

　　Code first underlying disease
　　EXCLUDES 1　epidemic vertigo (A88.1)

　　H82.1　Vertiginous syndromes in diseases classified elsewhere, right ear
　　H82.2　Vertiginous syndromes in diseases classified elsewhere, left ear
　　H82.3　Vertiginous syndromes in diseases classified elsewhere, bilateral
　　H82.9　Vertiginous syndromes in diseases classified elsewhere, unspecified ear

✓4ᵗʰ **H83　Other diseases of inner ear**

　　✓5ᵗʰ **H83.0　Labyrinthitis**

　　　　DEF: Inflammation of the inner ear, or labyrinth, characterized by pus, vertigo, dizziness, nausea, and hearing loss.

　　　　H83.01　Labyrinthitis, right ear
　　　　H83.02　Labyrinthitis, left ear
　　　　H83.03　Labyrinthitis, bilateral
　　　　H83.09　Labyrinthitis, unspecified ear

　　✓5ᵗʰ **H83.1　Labyrinthine fistula**

　　　　H83.11　Labyrinthine fistula, right ear
　　　　H83.12　Labyrinthine fistula, left ear　　SW
　　　　H83.13　Labyrinthine fistula, bilateral　　SW
　　　　H83.19　Labyrinthine fistula, unspecified ear　　SW

　　✓5ᵗʰ **H83.2　Labyrinthine dysfunction**

　　　　Labyrinthine hypersensitivity
　　　　Labyrinthine hypofunction
　　　　Labyrinthine loss of function
　　　　DEF: Decreased function of the labyrinth sensors.

　　　　✓6ᵗʰ **H83.2X　Labyrinthine dysfunction**

　　　　　　H83.2X1　Labyrinthine dysfunction, right ear
　　　　　　H83.2X2　Labyrinthine dysfunction, left ear
　　　　　　H83.2X3　Labyrinthine dysfunction, bilateral
　　　　　　H83.2X9　Labyrinthine dysfunction, unspecified ear

　　✓5ᵗʰ **H83.3　Noise effects on inner ear**

　　　　Acoustic trauma of inner ear
　　　　Noise-induced hearing loss of inner ear

　　　　✓6ᵗʰ **H83.3X　Noise effects on inner ear**

　　　　　　H83.3X1　Noise effects on right inner ear
　　　　　　H83.3X2　Noise effects on left inner ear
　　　　　　H83.3X3　Noise effects on inner ear, bilateral
　　　　　　H83.3X9　Noise effects on inner ear, unspecified ear

　　✓5ᵗʰ **H83.8　Other specified diseases of inner ear**

　　　　✓6ᵗʰ **H83.8X　Other specified diseases of inner ear**

　　　　　　H83.8X1　Other specified diseases of right inner ear
　　　　　　H83.8X2　Other specified diseases of left inner ear
　　　　　　H83.8X3　Other specified diseases of inner ear, bilateral
　　　　　　H83.8X9　Other specified diseases of inner ear, unspecified ear

　　✓5ᵗʰ **H83.9　Unspecified disease of inner ear**

　　　　H83.90　Unspecified disease of inner ear, unspecified ear
　　　　H83.91　Unspecified disease of right inner ear
　　　　H83.92　Unspecified disease of left inner ear
　　　　H83.93　Unspecified disease of inner ear, bilateral

✅ Additional Character Required　　✓x7ᵗʰ Placeholder　　Unacceptable PDx　　Questionable PDx　　Manifestation　　Unspecified Dx　　H1-H14 HAC　　HCC CMS-HCC Dx　　HIV HIV Dx

Other disorders of ear (H90-H94)

✓4ᵗʰ H90 Conductive and sensorineural hearing loss

EXCLUDES 1 *deaf nonspeaking NEC (H91.3)*
deafness NOS (H91.9-)
hearing loss NOS (H91.9-)
noise-induced hearing loss (H83.3-)
ototoxic hearing loss (H91.0-)
sudden (idiopathic) hearing loss (H91.2-)

AHA: 2015,2Q,7

DEF: Conductive hearing loss: Hearing Loss due to the inability of sound waves to move from the outer (external ear) to the inner ear.

DEF: Sensorineural hearing loss: Hearing loss that occurs from damage to the hair cells of the inner ear or problems with the nerve pathways from the inner ear to the brain.

H90.0 Conductive hearing loss, **bilateral**

✓5ᵗʰ H90.1 Conductive hearing loss, **unilateral** with unrestricted hearing on the contralateral side

    H90.11 Conductive hearing loss, unilateral, **right** ear, with unrestricted hearing on the contralateral side

    H90.12 Conductive hearing loss, unilateral, **left** ear, with unrestricted hearing on the contralateral side

H90.2 Conductive hearing loss, unspecified
    Conductive deafness NOS

H90.3 Sensorineural hearing loss, **bilateral**

✓5ᵗʰ H90.4 Sensorineural hearing loss, **unilateral** with unrestricted hearing on the contralateral side

    H90.41 Sensorineural hearing loss, unilateral, **right** ear, with unrestricted hearing on the contralateral side

    H90.42 Sensorineural hearing loss, unilateral, **left** ear, with unrestricted hearing on the contralateral side

H90.5 Unspecified sensorineural hearing loss
    Central hearing loss NOS
    Congenital deafness NOS
    Neural hearing loss NOS
    Perceptive hearing loss NOS
    Sensorineural deafness NOS
    Sensory hearing loss NOS

    EXCLUDES 1 *abnormal auditory perception (H93.2-)*
    psychogenic deafness (F44.6)

H90.6 Mixed conductive and sensorineural hearing loss, bilateral
    AHA: 2015,2Q,7

✓5ᵗʰ H90.7 Mixed conductive and sensorineural hearing loss, unilateral with unrestricted hearing on the contralateral side

    H90.71 Mixed conductive and sensorineural hearing loss, unilateral, **right** ear, with unrestricted hearing on the contralateral side

    H90.72 Mixed conductive and sensorineural hearing loss, unilateral, **left** ear, with unrestricted hearing on the contralateral side

H90.8 Mixed conductive and sensorineural hearing loss, unspecified

✓5ᵗʰ H90.A Conductive and sensorineural hearing loss with restricted hearing on the contralateral side
    AHA: 2016,4Q,23-25

    ✓6ᵗʰ H90.A1 Conductive hearing loss, unilateral, with restricted hearing on the contralateral side

        H90.A11 Conductive hearing loss, unilateral, **right** ear with restricted hearing on the contralateral side

        H90.A12 Conductive hearing loss, unilateral, **left** ear with restricted hearing on the contralateral side

    ✓6ᵗʰ H90.A2 Sensorineural hearing loss, unilateral, with restricted hearing on the contralateral side

        H90.A21 Sensorineural hearing loss, unilateral, **right** ear, with restricted hearing on the contralateral side

        H90.A22 Sensorineural hearing loss, unilateral, **left** ear, with restricted hearing on the contralateral side

    ✓6ᵗʰ H90.A3 Mixed conductive and sensorineural hearing loss, unilateral with restricted hearing on the contralateral side

        H90.A31 Mixed conductive and sensorineural hearing loss, unilateral, **right** ear with restricted hearing on the contralateral side

        H90.A32 Mixed conductive and sensorineural hearing, unilateral, **left** ear with restricted hearing on the contralateral side

✓4ᵗʰ H91 Other and unspecified hearing loss

EXCLUDES 1 *abnormal auditory perception (H93.2-)*
hearing loss as classified in H90.-
impacted cerumen (H61.2-)
noise-induced hearing loss (H83.3-)
psychogenic deafness (F44.6)
transient ischemic deafness (H93.01-)

✓5ᵗʰ H91.0 Ototoxic hearing loss

    Code first poisoning due to drug or toxin, if applicable (T36-T65 with fifth or sixth character 1-4 or 6)

    Use additional code for adverse effect, if applicable, to identify drug (T36-T50 with fifth or sixth character 5)

    H91.01 Ototoxic hearing loss, **right** ear

    H91.02 Ototoxic hearing loss, **left** ear

    H91.03 Ototoxic hearing loss, **bilateral**

    H91.09 Ototoxic hearing loss, unspecified ear

✓5ᵗʰ H91.1 Presbycusis
    Presbyacusia

    H91.10 Presbycusis, unspecified ear

    H91.11 Presbycusis, right ear

    H91.12 Presbycusis, left ear

    H91.13 Presbycusis, bilateral

✓5ᵗʰ H91.2 Sudden idiopathic hearing loss
    Sudden hearing loss NOS

    H91.20 Sudden idiopathic hearing loss, unspecified ear

    H91.21 Sudden idiopathic hearing loss, right ear

    H91.22 Sudden idiopathic hearing loss, left ear

    H91.23 Sudden idiopathic hearing loss, bilateral

H91.3 Deaf nonspeaking, not elsewhere classified

✓5ᵗʰ H91.8 Other specified hearing loss

    ✓6ᵗʰ H91.8X Other specified hearing loss

        H91.8X1 Other specified hearing loss, right ear

        H91.8X2 Other specified hearing loss, left ear

        H91.8X3 Other specified hearing loss, bilateral

        H91.8X9 Other specified hearing loss, unspecified ear

✓5ᵗʰ H91.9 Unspecified hearing loss
    Deafness NOS
    High frequency deafness
    Low frequency deafness

    H91.90 Unspecified hearing loss, unspecified ear

    H91.91 Unspecified hearing loss, right ear

    H91.92 Unspecified hearing loss, left ear

    H91.93 Unspecified hearing loss, bilateral

✓4ᵗʰ H92 Otalgia and effusion of ear

✓5ᵗʰ H92.0 Otalgia

    H92.01 Otalgia, right ear

    H92.02 Otalgia, left ear

    H92.03 Otalgia, bilateral

    H92.09 Otalgia, unspecified ear

✓5ᵗʰ H92.1 Otorrhea

    EXCLUDES 1 *leakage of cerebrospinal fluid through ear (G96.0)*

    H92.10 Otorrhea, unspecified ear

    H92.11 Otorrhea, right ear

    H92.12 Otorrhea, left ear

    H92.13 Otorrhea, bilateral

✓5ᵗʰ H92.2 Otorrhagia

    EXCLUDES 1 *traumatic otorrhagia — code to injury*

    H92.20 Otorrhagia, unspecified ear

    H92.21 Otorrhagia, right ear

    H92.22 Otorrhagia, left ear

    H92.23 Otorrhagia, bilateral

✓4ᵗʰ H93 Other disorders of ear, not elsewhere classified

✓5ᵗʰ H93.0 Degenerative and vascular disorders of ear

    EXCLUDES 1 *presbycusis (H91.1)*

    ✓6ᵗʰ H93.01 Transient ischemic deafness

        H93.011 Transient ischemic deafness, right ear

        H93.012 Transient ischemic deafness, left ear

        H93.013 Transient ischemic deafness, bilateral

        H93.019 Transient ischemic deafness, unspecified ear

N Newborn: 0   **P** Pediatric: 0-17   **M** Maternity: 9-64   **A** Adult: 15-124   **MCC** Major Complication/Comorbidity   **CC** Complication/Comorbidity   **SW** Severe Wound Dx

640   ICD-10-CM 2020

√6ᵗʰ **H93.09 Unspecified degenerative and vascular disorders of ear**

     H93.091 Unspecified degenerative and vascular disorders of right ear

     H93.092 Unspecified degenerative and vascular disorders of left ear

     H93.093 Unspecified degenerative and vascular disorders of ear, bilateral

     H93.099 Unspecified degenerative and vascular disorders of unspecified ear

√5ᵗʰ **H93.1 Tinnitus**

     H93.11 Tinnitus, right ear

     H93.12 Tinnitus, left ear

     H93.13 Tinnitus, bilateral

     H93.19 Tinnitus, unspecified ear

√5ᵗʰ **H93.A Pulsatile tinnitus**

     AHA: 2016,4Q,25-26

     H93.A1 Pulsatile tinnitus, right ear

     H93.A2 Pulsatile tinnitus, left ear

     H93.A3 Pulsatile tinnitus, bilateral

     H93.A9 Pulsatile tinnitus, unspecified ear

√5ᵗʰ **H93.2 Other abnormal auditory perceptions**

     EXCLUDES 2   *auditory hallucinations (R44.0)*

     √6ᵗʰ **H93.21 Auditory recruitment**

       H93.211 Auditory recruitment, right ear

       H93.212 Auditory recruitment, left ear

       H93.213 Auditory recruitment, bilateral

       H93.219 Auditory recruitment, unspecified ear

     √6ᵗʰ **H93.22 Diplacusis**

       H93.221 Diplacusis, right ear

       H93.222 Diplacusis, left ear

       H93.223 Diplacusis, bilateral

       H93.229 Diplacusis, unspecified ear

     √6ᵗʰ **H93.23 Hyperacusis**

       DEF: Exceptionally acute sense of hearing caused by such conditions as Bell's palsy. This term may also refer to painful sensitivity to sounds.

       H93.231 Hyperacusis, right ear

       H93.232 Hyperacusis, left ear

       H93.233 Hyperacusis, bilateral

       H93.239 Hyperacusis, unspecified ear

     √6ᵗʰ **H93.24 Temporary auditory threshold shift**

       H93.241 Temporary auditory threshold shift, right ear

       H93.242 Temporary auditory threshold shift, left ear

       H93.243 Temporary auditory threshold shift, bilateral

       H93.249 Temporary auditory threshold shift, unspecified ear

     H93.25 Central auditory processing disorder

       Congenital auditory imperception

       Word deafness

       EXCLUDES 1   *mixed receptive-expressive language disorder (F80.2)*

     √6ᵗʰ **H93.29 Other abnormal auditory perceptions**

       H93.291 Other abnormal auditory perceptions, right ear

       H93.292 Other abnormal auditory perceptions, left ear

       H93.293 Other abnormal auditory perceptions, bilateral

       H93.299 Other abnormal auditory perceptions, unspecified ear

√5ᵗʰ **H93.3 Disorders of acoustic nerve**

     Disorder of 8th cranial nerve

     EXCLUDES 1   *acoustic neuroma (D33.3)*

           syphilitic acoustic neuritis (A52.15)

     √6ᵗʰ **H93.3X Disorders of acoustic nerve**

       H93.3X1 Disorders of right acoustic nerve

       H93.3X2 Disorders of left acoustic nerve

       H93.3X3 Disorders of bilateral acoustic nerves

       H93.3X9 Disorders of unspecified acoustic nerve

√5ᵗʰ **H93.8 Other specified disorders of ear**

     √6ᵗʰ **H93.8X Other specified disorders of ear**

       H93.8X1 Other specified disorders of right ear

       H93.8X2 Other specified disorders of left ear

       H93.8X3 Other specified disorders of ear, bilateral

       H93.8X9 Other specified disorders of ear, unspecified ear

√5ᵗʰ **H93.9 Unspecified disorder of ear**

     H93.90 Unspecified disorder of ear, unspecified ear

     H93.91 Unspecified disorder of right ear

     H93.92 Unspecified disorder of left ear

     H93.93 Unspecified disorder of ear, bilateral

√4ᵗʰ **H94 Other disorders of ear in diseases classified elsewhere**

     √5ᵗʰ **H94.0 Acoustic neuritis in infectious and parasitic diseases classified elsewhere**

       Code first underlying disease, such as:

         parasitic disease (B65-B89)

       EXCLUDES 1   *acoustic neuritis (in):*

           herpes zoster (B02.29)

           syphilis (A52.15)

       H94.00 Acoustic neuritis in infectious and parasitic diseases classified elsewhere, unspecified ear

       H94.01 Acoustic neuritis in infectious and parasitic diseases classified elsewhere, right ear

       H94.02 Acoustic neuritis in infectious and parasitic diseases classified elsewhere, left ear

       H94.03 Acoustic neuritis in infectious and parasitic diseases classified elsewhere, bilateral

     √5ᵗʰ **H94.8 Other specified disorders of ear in diseases classified elsewhere**

       Code first underlying disease, such as:

         congenital syphilis (A50.0)

       EXCLUDES 1   *aural myiasis (B87.4)*

           syphilitic labyrinthitis (A52.79)

       H94.80 Other specified disorders of ear in diseases classified elsewhere, unspecified ear

       H94.81 Other specified disorders of right ear in diseases classified elsewhere

       H94.82 Other specified disorders of left ear in diseases classified elsewhere

       H94.83 Other specified disorders of ear in diseases classified elsewhere, bilateral

Intraoperative and postprocedural complications and disorders of ear and mastoid process, not elsewhere classified (H95)

CC Excl: For CC codes in category H95, unless otherwise noted: PDX collection 642

√4ᵗʰ **H95 Intraoperative and postprocedural complications and disorders of ear and mastoid process, not elsewhere classified**

     AHA: 2016,4Q,9-10

     √5ᵗʰ **H95.0 Recurrent cholesteatoma of postmastoidectomy cavity**

       H95.00 Recurrent cholesteatoma of postmastoidectomy cavity, unspecified ear

       H95.01 Recurrent cholesteatoma of postmastoidectomy cavity, right ear

       H95.02 Recurrent cholesteatoma of postmastoidectomy cavity, left ear

       H95.03 Recurrent cholesteatoma of postmastoidectomy cavity, bilateral ears

     √5ᵗʰ **H95.1 Other disorders of ear and mastoid process following mastoidectomy**

     √6ᵗʰ **H95.11 Chronic inflammation of postmastoidectomy cavity**

       H95.111 Chronic inflammation of postmastoidectomy cavity, right ear

       H95.112 Chronic inflammation of postmastoidectomy cavity, left ear

       H95.113 Chronic inflammation of postmastoidectomy cavity, bilateral ears

       H95.119 Chronic inflammation of postmastoidectomy cavity, unspecified ear

     √6ᵗʰ **H95.12 Granulation of postmastoidectomy cavity**

       H95.121 Granulation of postmastoidectomy cavity, right ear

       H95.122 Granulation of postmastoidectomy cavity, left ear

       H95.123 Granulation of postmastoidectomy cavity, bilateral ears

       H95.129 Granulation of postmastoidectomy cavity, unspecified ear

☑ Additional Character Required   √x7ᵗʰ Placeholder   Unacceptable PDx   Questionable PDx   Manifestation   Unspecified Dx   H1-H14 HAC   HCC CMS-HCC Dx   HIV HIV Dx

ICD-10-CM 2020

641

✓6ᵗʰ **H95.13 Mucosal cyst of postmastoidectomy cavity**

     H95.131 Mucosal cyst of postmastoidectomy cavity, **right** ear

     H95.132 Mucosal cyst of postmastoidectomy cavity, **left** ear

     H95.133 Mucosal cyst of postmastoidectomy cavity, **bilateral** ears

     H95.139 Mucosal cyst of postmastoidectomy cavity, unspecified ear

✓6ᵗʰ **H95.19 Other disorders following mastoidectomy**

     H95.191 Other disorders following mastoidectomy, **right** ear

     H95.192 Other disorders following mastoidectomy, **left** ear

     H95.193 Other disorders following mastoidectomy, **bilateral** ears

     H95.199 Other disorders following mastoidectomy, unspecified ear

✓5ᵗʰ **H95.2 Intraoperative hemorrhage and hematoma of ear and mastoid process complicating a procedure**

     EXCLUDES 1   intraoperative hemorrhage and hematoma of ear and mastoid process due to accidental puncture or laceration during a procedure (H95.3-)

     H95.21 Intraoperative hemorrhage and hematoma of ear and mastoid process complicating a procedure on the ear and mastoid process   `CC`

     H95.22 Intraoperative hemorrhage and hematoma of ear and mastoid process complicating other procedure   `CC`

✓5ᵗʰ **H95.3 Accidental puncture and laceration of ear and mastoid process during a procedure**

     H95.31 Accidental puncture and laceration of the ear and mastoid process during a procedure on the ear and mastoid process   `CC`

        CC Excl: PDX collection 509

     H95.32 Accidental puncture and laceration of the ear and mastoid process during other procedure   `CC`

        CC Excl: PDX collection 509

✓5ᵗʰ **H95.4 Postprocedural hemorrhage of ear and mastoid process following a procedure**

     H95.41 Postprocedural hemorrhage of ear and mastoid process following a procedure on the ear and mastoid process   `CC`

     H95.42 Postprocedural hemorrhage of ear and mastoid process following other procedure   `CC`

✓5ᵗʰ **H95.5 Postprocedural hematoma and seroma of ear and mastoid process following a procedure**

     H95.51 Postprocedural hematoma of ear and mastoid process following a procedure on the ear and mastoid process   `CC`

     H95.52 Postprocedural hematoma of ear and mastoid process following other procedure   `CC`

     H95.53 Postprocedural seroma of ear and mastoid process following a procedure on the ear and mastoid process   `CC`

     H95.54 Postprocedural seroma of ear and mastoid process following other procedure   `CC`

✓5ᵗʰ **H95.8 Other intraoperative and postprocedural complications and disorders of the ear and mastoid process, not elsewhere classified**

     EXCLUDES 2   postprocedural complications and disorders following mastoidectomy (H95.0-, H95.1-)

     For CC codes in subcategory H95.8: PDX collection 643

     ✓6ᵗʰ **H95.81 Postprocedural stenosis of external ear canal**

        H95.811 Postprocedural stenosis of right external ear canal   `CC`

        H95.812 Postprocedural stenosis of left external ear canal   `CC`

        H95.813 Postprocedural stenosis of external ear canal, bilateral   `CC`

        H95.819 Postprocedural stenosis of unspecified external ear canal   `CC`

     H95.88 Other intraoperative complications and disorders of the ear and mastoid process, not elsewhere classified   `CC`

        Use additional code, if applicable, to further specify disorder

     H95.89 Other postprocedural complications and disorders of the ear and mastoid process, not elsewhere classified   `CC`

        Use additional code, if applicable, to further specify disorder

N Newborn: 0   **P** Pediatric: 0-17   **M** Maternity: 9-64   **A** Adult: 15-124   **MCC** Major Complication/Comorbidity   **CC** Complication/Comorbidity   **SW** Severe Wound Dx

642   ICD-10-CM 2020

Chapter 9. Diseases of the Circulatory System (I00–I99)

Chapter-specific Guidelines with Coding Examples

The chapter-specific guidelines from the ICD-10-CM Official Guidelines for Coding and Reporting have been provided below. Along with these guidelines are coding examples, contained in the shaded boxes, that have been developed to help illustrate the coding and/or sequencing guidance found in these guidelines.

a. Hypertension

The classification presumes a causal relationship between hypertension and heart involvement and between hypertension and kidney involvement, as the two conditions are linked by the term "with" in the Alphabetic Index. These conditions should be coded as related even in the absence of provider documentation explicitly linking them, unless the documentation clearly states the conditions are unrelated.

For hypertension and conditions not specifically linked by relational terms such as "with," "associated with" or "due to" in the classification, provider documentation must link the conditions in order to code them as related.

1) Hypertension with heart disease

Hypertension with heart conditions classified to I50.- or I51.4-I51.7, I51.89, I51.9, are assigned to a code from category I11, Hypertensive heart disease. Use additional code(s) from category I50, Heart failure, to identify the type(s) of heart failure in those patients with heart failure.

The same heart conditions (I50.-, I51.4-I51.7, I51.89, I51.9) with hypertension are coded separately if the provider has documented they are unrelated to the hypertension. Sequence according to the circumstances of the admission/encounter.

> Patient is admitted in left heart failure. Patient also has a history of hypertension managed by medication.
>
> **I11.0**   **Hypertensive heart disease with heart failure**
>
> **I50.1**   **Left ventricular failure, unspecified**
>
> *Explanation*: Without a diagnostic statement to the contrary, hypertension and heart failure have an assumed causal relationship, and a combination code should be used. An additional code to identify the type of heart failure (I50.-) should also be provided.

2) Hypertensive chronic kidney disease

Assign codes from category I12, Hypertensive chronic kidney disease, when both hypertension and a condition classifiable to category N18, Chronic kidney disease (CKD), are present. CKD should not be coded as hypertensive if the provider indicates the CKD is not related to the hypertension.

The appropriate code from category N18 should be used as a secondary code with a code from category I12 to identify the stage of chronic kidney disease.

See Section I.C.14. Chronic kidney disease.

If a patient has hypertensive chronic kidney disease and acute renal failure, an additional code for the acute renal failure is required.

> Patient is admitted with stage IV chronic kidney disease (CKD) due to polycystic kidney disease. Patient also is on lisinopril for hypertension.
>
> **N18.4**   **Chronic kidney disease, stage 4 (severe)**
>
> **Q61.3**   **Polycystic kidney, unspecified**
>
> **I10**   **Essential (primary) hypertension**
>
> *Explanation*: A combination code describing a relationship between hypertension and CKD is not used because the physician documentation identifies the polycystic kidney disease as the cause for the CKD.

3) Hypertensive heart and chronic kidney disease

Assign codes from combination category I13, Hypertensive heart and chronic kidney disease, when there is hypertension with both heart and kidney involvement. If heart failure is present, assign an additional code from category I50 to identify the type of heart failure.

The appropriate code from category N18, Chronic kidney disease, should be used as a secondary code with a code from category I13 to identify the stage of chronic kidney disease.

See Section I.C.14. Chronic kidney disease.

The codes in category I13, Hypertensive heart and chronic kidney disease, are combination codes that include hypertension, heart disease and chronic kidney disease. The Includes note at I13 specifies that the conditions included at I11 and I12 are included together in I13. If a patient has hypertension, heart disease and chronic kidney disease, then a code

from I13 should be used, not individual codes for hypertension, heart disease and chronic kidney disease, or codes from I11 or I12.

For patients with both acute renal failure and chronic kidney disease, an additional code for acute renal failure is required.

> Hypertensive heart and kidney disease with congestive heart failure and stage 2 chronic kidney disease
>
> **I13.0**   **Hypertensive heart and chronic kidney disease with heart failure and stage 1 through stage 4 chronic kidney disease, or unspecified chronic kidney disease**
>
> **I50.9**   **Heart failure, unspecified**
>
> **N18.2**   **Chronic kidney disease, stage 2 (mild)**
>
> *Explanation*: Combination codes in category I13 are used to report conditions classifiable to *both* categories I11 and I12. Do not report conditions classifiable to I11 and I12 separately. Use additional codes to report type of heart failure and stage of CKD.

4) Hypertensive cerebrovascular disease

For hypertensive cerebrovascular disease, first assign the appropriate code from categories I60-I69, followed by the appropriate hypertension code.

> Rupture of cerebral aneurysm caused by malignant hypertension
>
> **I60.7**   **Nontraumatic subarachnoid hemorrhage from unspecified intracranial artery**
>
> **I10**   **Essential (primary) hypertension**
>
> *Explanation*: Hypertensive cerebrovascular disease requires two codes: the appropriate I60–I69 code followed by the appropriate hypertension code.

5) Hypertensive retinopathy

Subcategory H35.0, Background retinopathy and retinal vascular changes, should be used with a code from category I10 – I15, Hypertensive disease to include the systemic hypertension. The sequencing is based on the reason for the encounter.

6) Hypertension, secondary

Secondary hypertension is due to an underlying condition. Two codes are required: one to identify the underlying etiology and one from category I15 to identify the hypertension. Sequencing of codes is determined by the reason for admission/encounter.

> Renovascular hypertension due to renal artery atherosclerosis
>
> **I15.0**   **Renovascular hypertension**
>
> **I70.1**   **Atherosclerosis of renal artery**
>
> *Explanation*: Secondary hypertension requires two codes: a code to identify the etiology and the appropriate I15 code.

7) Hypertension, transient

Assign code R03.0, Elevated blood pressure reading without diagnosis of hypertension, unless patient has an established diagnosis of hypertension. Assign code O13.-, Gestational [pregnancy-induced] hypertension without significant proteinuria, or O14.-, Pre-eclampsia, for transient hypertension of pregnancy.

8) Hypertension, controlled

This diagnostic statement usually refers to an existing state of hypertension under control by therapy. Assign the appropriate code from categories I10-I15, Hypertensive diseases.

9) Hypertension, uncontrolled

Uncontrolled hypertension may refer to untreated hypertension or hypertension not responding to current therapeutic regimen. In either case, assign the appropriate code from categories I10-I15, Hypertensive diseases.

10) Hypertensive crisis

Assign a code from category I16, Hypertensive crisis, for documented hypertensive urgency, hypertensive emergency or unspecified hypertensive crisis. Code also any identified hypertensive disease (I10-I15). The sequencing is based on the reason for the encounter.

11) Pulmonary hypertension

Pulmonary hypertension is classified to category I27, Other pulmonary heart diseases. For secondary pulmonary hypertension (I27.1, I27.2-), code also any associated conditions or adverse effects of drugs or toxins.

The sequencing is based on the reason for the encounter, except for adverse effects of drugs (See Section I.C.19.e.).

b. Atherosclerotic coronary artery disease and angina

ICD-10-CM has combination codes for atherosclerotic heart disease with angina pectoris. The subcategories for these codes are I25.11, Atherosclerotic heart disease of native coronary artery with angina pectoris and I25.7, Atherosclerosis of coronary artery bypass graft(s) and coronary artery of transplanted heart with angina pectoris.

When using one of these combination codes it is not necessary to use an additional code for angina pectoris. A causal relationship can be assumed in a patient with both atherosclerosis and angina pectoris, unless the documentation indicates the angina is due to something other than the atherosclerosis.

If a patient with coronary artery disease is admitted due to an acute myocardial infarction (AMI), the AMI should be sequenced before the coronary artery disease.

See Section I.C.9. Acute myocardial infarction (AMI)

c. Intraoperative and postprocedural cerebrovascular accident

Medical record documentation should clearly specify the cause- and- effect relationship between the medical intervention and the cerebrovascular accident in order to assign a code for intraoperative or postprocedural cerebrovascular accident.

Proper code assignment depends on whether it was an infarction or hemorrhage and whether it occurred intraoperatively or postoperatively. If it was a cerebral hemorrhage, code assignment depends on the type of procedure performed.

Embolic cerebral infarction of the right middle cerebral artery that occurred during hip replacement surgery. The surgeon documented as due to the surgery.

I97.811	**Intraoperative cerebrovascular infarction during other surgery**
I63.411	**Cerebral infarction due to embolism of right middle cerebral artery**

Explanation: Code assignment for intraoperative or postprocedural cerebrovascular accident is based on the provider's documentation of a cause-and-effect relationship between the condition and the procedure. Proper code assignment also depends on whether the cerebrovascular accident was an infarction or hemorrhage, occurred intraoperatively or postoperatively, and the type of procedure performed.

---

d. Sequelae of cerebrovascular disease

1) Category I69, Sequelae of cerebrovascular disease

Category I69 is used to indicate conditions classifiable to categories I60-I67 as the causes of sequela (neurologic deficits), themselves classified elsewhere. These "late effects" include neurologic deficits that persist after initial onset of conditions classifiable to categories I60-I67. The neurologic deficits caused by cerebrovascular disease may be present from the onset or may arise at any time after the onset of the condition classifiable to categories I60-I67.

Codes from category I69, Sequelae of cerebrovascular disease, that specify hemiplegia, hemiparesis and monoplegia identify whether the dominant or nondominant side is affected. Should the affected side be documented, but not specified as dominant or nondominant, and the classification system does not indicate a default, code selection is as follows:

- For ambidextrous patients, the default should be dominant.
- If the left side is affected, the default is non-dominant.
- If the right side is affected, the default is dominant.

2) Codes from category I69 with codes from I60–I67

Codes from category I69 may be assigned on a health care record with codes from I60-I67, if the patient has a current cerebrovascular disease and deficits from an old cerebrovascular disease.

3) Codes from category I69 and personal history of transient ischemic attack (TIA) and cerebral infarction (Z86.73)

Codes from category I69 should not be assigned if the patient does not have neurologic deficits.

See Section I.C.21. 4. History (of) for use of personal history codes

e. Acute myocardial infarction (AMI)

1) Type 1 ST elevation myocardial infarction (STEMI) and non ST elevation myocardial infarction (NSTEMI)

The ICD-10-CM codes for type 1 acute myocardial infarction (AMI) identify the site, such as anterolateral wall or true posterior wall. Subcategories I21.0-I21.2 and code I21.3 are used for type 1 ST elevation myocardial infarction (STEMI). Code I21.4, Non-ST elevation (NSTEMI) myocardial infarction, is used for type 1 non ST elevation myocardial infarction (NSTEMI) and nontransmural MIs.

If a type 1 NSTEMI evolves to STEMI, assign the STEMI code. If a type 1 STEMI converts to NSTEMI due to thrombolytic therapy, it is still coded as STEMI.

For encounters occurring while the myocardial infarction is equal to, or less than, four weeks old, including transfers to another acute setting or a postacute setting, and the myocardial infarction meets the definition for "other diagnoses" (see Section III, Reporting Additional Diagnoses), codes from category I21 may continue to be reported. For encounters after the 4 week time frame and the patient is still receiving care related to the myocardial infarction, the appropriate aftercare code should be assigned, rather than a code from category I21. For old or healed myocardial infarctions not requiring further care, code I25.2, Old myocardial infarction, may be assigned.

2) Acute myocardial infarction, unspecified

Code I21.9, Acute myocardial infarction, unspecified, is the default for unspecified acute myocardial infarction or unspecified type. If only type 1 STEMI or transmural MI without the site is documented, assign code I21.3, ST elevation (STEMI) myocardial infarction of unspecified site.

3) AMI documented as nontransmural or subendocardial but site provided

If an AMI is documented as nontransmural or subendocardial, but the site is provided, it is still coded as a subendocardial AMI.

See Section I.C.21.3 for information on coding status post administration of tPA in a different facility within the last 24 hours.

4) Subsequent acute myocardial infarction

A code from category I22, Subsequent ST elevation (STEMI) and non-ST elevation (NSTEMI) myocardial infarction, is to be used when a patient who has suffered a type 1 or unspecified AMI has a new AMI within the 4 week time frame of the initial AMI. A code from category I22 must be used in conjunction with a code from category I21. The sequencing of the I22 and I21 codes depends on the circumstances of the encounter.

Do not assign code I22 for subsequent myocardial infarctions other than type 1 or unspecified. For subsequent type 2 AMI assign only code I21.A1. For subsequent type 4 or type 5 AMI, assign only code I21.A9.

If a subsequent myocardial infarction of one type occurs within 4 weeks of a myocardial infarction of a different type, assign the appropriate codes from category I21 to identify each type. Do not assign a code from I22. Codes from category I22 should only be assigned if both the initial and subsequent myocardial infarctions are type 1 or unspecified.

5) Other types of myocardial infarction

The ICD-10-CM provides codes for different types of myocardial infarction. Type 1 myocardial infarctions are assigned to codes I21.0-I21.4.

Type 2 myocardial infarction (myocardial infarction due to demand ischemia or secondary to ischemic **im**balance) is assigned to code I21.A1, Myocardial infarction type 2 with the underlying cause **coded first**. Do not assign code I24.8, Other forms of acute ischemic heart disease, for the demand ischemia. **If** a type 2 AMI is described as NSTEMI or STEMI, only assign code I21.A1. Codes I21.01-I21.4 should only be assigned for type 1 AMIs.

Acute myocardial infarctions type 3, 4a, 4b, 4c and 5 are assigned to code I21.A9, Other myocardial infarction type.

The "Code also" and "Code first" notes should be followed related to complications, and for coding of postprocedural myocardial infarctions during or following cardiac surgery.

Myocardial infarction involving the left circumflex artery occurring during PTCA with stent insertion to treat coronary artery disease

I25.10	**Atherosclerotic heart disease of native coronary artery without angina pectoris**
I97.790	**Other intraoperative cardiac functional disturbances during cardiac surgery**
I21.A9	**Other myocardial infarction type**

Explanation: A myocardial infarction occurring during a revascularization procedure is not considered a type 1 myocardial infarction (MI) and should not be coded to a type 1 MI code (I21.0-, I21.1-, I21.2-, I21.3) even when the specific site of the MI is documented. According to the code first instruction at I21.A9, the complication code (I97.790) should be sequenced before code I21.A9.

Chapter 9. Diseases of the Circulatory System (I00-I99)

EXCLUDES 2   certain conditions originating in the perinatal period (P04-P96)
certain infectious and parasitic diseases (A00-B99)
complications of pregnancy, childbirth and the puerperium (O00-O9A)
congenital malformations, deformations, and chromosomal abnormalities (Q00-Q99)
endocrine, nutritional and metabolic diseases (E00-E88)
injury, poisoning and certain other consequences of external causes (S00-T88)
neoplasms (C00-D49)
symptoms, signs and abnormal clinical and laboratory findings, not elsewhere classified (R00-R94)
systemic connective tissue disorders (M30-M36)
transient cerebral ischemic attacks and related syndromes (G45.-)

This chapter contains the following blocks:

I00-I02   Acute rheumatic fever
I05-I09   Chronic rheumatic heart diseases
I10-I16   Hypertensive diseases
I20-I25   Ischemic heart diseases
I26-I28   Pulmonary heart disease and diseases of pulmonary circulation
I30-I52   Other forms of heart disease
I60-I69   Cerebrovascular diseases
I70-I79   Diseases of arteries, arterioles and capillaries
I80-I89   Diseases of veins, lymphatic vessels and lymph nodes, not elsewhere classified
I95-I99   Other and unspecified disorders of the circulatory system

Acute rheumatic fever (I00-I02)

DEF: Inflammatory disease that can follow a throat infection by group A streptococci. Complications can involve the joints (arthritis), subcutaneous tissue (nodules), skin (erythema marginatum), heart (carditis), or brain (chorea).

I00   Rheumatic fever without heart involvement

     INCLUDES   arthritis, rheumatic, acute or subacute
     EXCLUDES 1   rheumatic fever with heart involvement (I01.0-I01.9)

✓4ᵗʰ   I01   Rheumatic fever with heart involvement

     EXCLUDES 1   chronic diseases of rheumatic origin (I05-I09) unless rheumatic fever is also present or there is evidence of reactivation or activity of the rheumatic process

     I01.0   Acute rheumatic pericarditis   **CC**

         Any condition in I00 with pericarditis
         Rheumatic pericarditis (acute)
         EXCLUDES 1   acute pericarditis not specified as rheumatic (I30.-)
         CC Excl: PDX collection 188

     I01.1   Acute rheumatic endocarditis   **CC**

         Any condition in I00 with endocarditis or valvulitis
         Acute rheumatic valvulitis
         CC Excl: PDX collection 644

     I01.2   Acute rheumatic myocarditis   **CC**

         Any condition in I00 with myocarditis
         CC Excl: PDX collection 186

     I01.8   Other acute rheumatic heart disease   **CC**

         Any condition in I00 with other or multiple types of heart involvement
         Acute rheumatic pancarditis
         CC Excl: PDX collection 645

     I01.9   Acute rheumatic heart disease, unspecified   **CC**

         Any condition in I00 with unspecified type of heart involvement
         Rheumatic carditis, acute
         Rheumatic heart disease, active or acute
         CC Excl: PDX collection 646

✓4ᵗʰ   I02   Rheumatic chorea

     INCLUDES   Sydenham's chorea
     EXCLUDES 1   chorea NOS (G25.5)
                  Huntington's chorea (G10)

     I02.0   Rheumatic chorea with heart involvement   **CC**

         Chorea NOS with heart involvement
         Rheumatic chorea with heart involvement of any type classifiable under I01.-
         CC Excl: PDX collection 645

     I02.9   Rheumatic chorea without heart involvement   **CC**

         Rheumatic chorea NOS
         CC Excl: PDX collection 646

Chronic rheumatic heart diseases (I05-I09)

✓4ᵗʰ   I05   Rheumatic mitral valve diseases

     INCLUDES   conditions classifiable to both I05.0 and I05.2-I05.9, whether specified as rheumatic or not
     EXCLUDES 1   mitral valve disease specified as nonrheumatic (I34.-)
                  mitral valve disease with aortic and/or tricuspid valve involvement (I08.-)

     I05.0   Rheumatic mitral stenosis

         Mitral (valve) obstruction (rheumatic)
         DEF: Narrowing of the mitral valve between the left atrium and left ventricle due to rheumatic fever. Symptoms include shortness of breath during or after exercise, fatigue, palpitations, chest discomfort, and swelling of feet or legs.

     I05.1   Rheumatic mitral insufficiency

         Rheumatic mitral incompetence
         Rheumatic mitral regurgitation
         EXCLUDES 1   mitral insufficiency not specified as rheumatic (I34.0)

     I05.2   Rheumatic mitral stenosis with insufficiency

         Rheumatic mitral stenosis with incompetence or regurgitation

     I05.8   Other rheumatic mitral valve diseases

         Rheumatic mitral (valve) failure

     I05.9   Rheumatic mitral valve disease, unspecified

         Rheumatic mitral (valve) disorder (chronic) NOS

✓4ᵗʰ   I06   Rheumatic aortic valve diseases

     EXCLUDES 1   aortic valve disease not specified as rheumatic (I35.-)
                  aortic valve disease with mitral and/or tricuspid valve involvement (I08.-)

     I06.0   Rheumatic aortic stenosis

         Rheumatic aortic (valve) obstruction

     I06.1   Rheumatic aortic insufficiency

         Rheumatic aortic incompetence
         Rheumatic aortic regurgitation

     I06.2   Rheumatic aortic stenosis with insufficiency

         Rheumatic aortic stenosis with incompetence or regurgitation

     I06.8   Other rheumatic aortic valve diseases

     I06.9   Rheumatic aortic valve disease, unspecified

         Rheumatic aortic (valve) disease NOS

✓4ᵗʰ   I07   Rheumatic tricuspid valve diseases

     INCLUDES   rheumatic tricuspid valve diseases specified as rheumatic or unspecified
     EXCLUDES 1   tricuspid valve disease specified as nonrheumatic (I36.-)
                  tricuspid valve disease with aortic and/or mitral valve involvement (I08.-)

     I07.0   Rheumatic tricuspid stenosis

         Tricuspid (valve) stenosis (rheumatic)

     I07.1   Rheumatic tricuspid insufficiency

         Tricuspid (valve) insufficiency (rheumatic)

     I07.2   Rheumatic tricuspid stenosis and insufficiency

     I07.8   Other rheumatic tricuspid valve diseases

     I07.9   Rheumatic tricuspid valve disease, unspecified

         Rheumatic tricuspid valve disorder NOS

✓4ᵗʰ   I08   Multiple valve diseases

     INCLUDES   multiple valve diseases specified as rheumatic or unspecified
     EXCLUDES 1   endocarditis, valve unspecified (I38)
                  multiple valve disease specified a nonrheumatic (I34.-, I35.-, I36.-, I37.-, I38.-, Q22.-, Q23.-, Q24.8-)
                  rheumatic valve disease NOS (I09.1)

     I08.0   Rheumatic disorders of both mitral and aortic valves

         Involvement of both mitral and aortic valves specified as rheumatic or unspecified
         AHA: 2019,2Q,5

     I08.1   Rheumatic disorders of both mitral and tricuspid valves

     I08.2   Rheumatic disorders of both aortic and tricuspid valves

     I08.3   Combined rheumatic disorders of mitral, aortic and tricuspid valves

     I08.8   Other rheumatic multiple valve diseases

     I08.9   Rheumatic multiple valve disease, unspecified

✓4ᵗʰ   I09   Other rheumatic heart diseases

     I09.0   Rheumatic myocarditis   **CC**

         EXCLUDES 1   myocarditis not specified as rheumatic (I51.4)
         CC Excl: PDX collection 647

✓ Additional Character Required   ✓x7ᵗʰ Placeholder   <u>Unacceptable PDx</u>   Questionable PDx   Manifestation   <u>Unspecified Dx</u>   H1-H19 HAC   HCC CMS-HCC Dx   HIV HIV Dx

ICD-10-CM 2020   645

Chapter 9. Diseases of the Circulatory System

I09.1   **Rheumatic diseases of endocardium, valve unspecified**
Rheumatic endocarditis (chronic)
Rheumatic valvulitis (chronic)
EXCLUDES 1   *endocarditis, valve unspecified (I38)*

I09.2   **Chronic rheumatic pericarditis**   CC
Adherent pericardium, rheumatic
Chronic rheumatic mediastinopericarditis
Chronic rheumatic myopericarditis
EXCLUDES 1   *chronic pericarditis not specified as rheumatic (I31.-)*
CC Excl: PDX collection 188

✓5th **I09.8**   **Other specified rheumatic heart diseases**

    I09.81   **Rheumatic heart failure**   CC HCC
Use additional code to identify type of heart failure (I50.-)
DEF: Decreased cardiac output, edema, and hypertension due to rheumatic heart disease.
CC Excl: PDX collection 648

    I09.89   **Other specified rheumatic heart diseases**
Rheumatic disease of pulmonary valve

I09.9   **Rheumatic heart disease, unspecified**
Rheumatic carditis
EXCLUDES 1   *rheumatoid carditis (M05.31)*

Hypertensive diseases (I10-I16)

Use additional code to identify:
exposure to environmental tobacco smoke (Z77.22)
history of tobacco dependence (Z87.891)
occupational exposure to environmental tobacco smoke (Z57.31)
tobacco dependence (F17.-)
tobacco use (Z72.0)
EXCLUDES 1   *neonatal hypertension (P29.2)*
primary pulmonary hypertension (I27.0)
EXCLUDES 2   *hypertensive disease complicating pregnancy, childbirth and the puerperium (O10-O11, O13-O16)*

I10   **Essential (primary) hypertension**
INCLUDES   high blood pressure
hypertension (arterial) (benign) (essential) (malignant) (primary) (systemic)
EXCLUDES 1   *hypertensive disease complicating pregnancy, childbirth and the puerperium (O10-O11, O13-O16)*
EXCLUDES 2   *essential (primary) hypertension involving vessels of brain (I60-I69)*
essential (primary) hypertension involving vessels of eye (H35.0-)
AHA: 2018,2Q,9; 2016,4Q,27

✓4th **I11**   **Hypertensive heart disease**
INCLUDES   any condition in I50.-, I51.4-I51.9 due to hypertension
AHA: 2018,2Q,9
TIP: Do not assign a code from this category when provider documentation indicates the heart disease is attributable to another cause.

    I11.0   **Hypertensive heart disease with heart failure**   HCC
Hypertensive heart failure
Use additional code to identify type of heart failure (I50.-)
AHA: 2017,1Q,47

    I11.9   **Hypertensive heart disease without heart failure**
Hypertensive heart disease NOS

✓4th **I12**   **Hypertensive chronic kidney disease**
INCLUDES   any condition in N18 and N26 — due to hypertension
arteriosclerosis of kidney
arteriosclerotic nephritis (chronic) (interstitial)
hypertensive nephropathy
nephrosclerosis
EXCLUDES 1   *hypertension due to kidney disease (I15.0, I15.1)*
renovascular hypertension (I15.0)
secondary hypertension (I15.-)
EXCLUDES 2   *acute kidney failure (N17.-)*
AHA: 2018,4Q,88; 2016,3Q,22
TIP: Do not assign a code from this category when provider documentation indicates the chronic kidney disease (CKD) is attributable to another cause.

    I12.0   **Hypertensive chronic kidney disease with stage 5**   CC HCC
chronic kidney disease or end stage renal disease
Use additional code to identify the stage of chronic kidney disease (N18.5, N18.6)
CC Excl: PDX collection 649

I12.9   **Hypertensive chronic kidney disease with stage 1 through stage 4 chronic kidney disease, or unspecified chronic kidney disease**
Hypertensive chronic kidney disease NOS
Hypertensive renal disease NOS
Use additional code to identify the stage of chronic kidney disease (N18.1-N18.4, N18.9)

✓4th **I13**   **Hypertensive heart and chronic kidney disease**
INCLUDES   any condition in I11.- with any condition in I12.-
cardiorenal disease
cardiovascular renal disease
TIP: Do not assign a code from this category when provider documentation indicates the heart and/or chronic kidney disease is attributable to another cause.
CC Excl: For CC codes in category I13: PDX collection 650

    I13.0   **Hypertensive heart and chronic kidney disease**   CC HCC
with heart failure and stage 1 through stage 4 chronic kidney disease, or unspecified chronic kidney disease
Use additional code to identify type of heart failure (I50.-)
Use additional code to identify stage of chronic kidney disease (N18.1-N18.4, N18.9)

✓5th **I13.1**   **Hypertensive heart and chronic kidney disease without heart failure**

    I13.10   **Hypertensive heart and chronic kidney disease without heart failure, with stage 1 through stage 4 chronic kidney disease, or unspecified chronic kidney disease**
Hypertensive heart disease and hypertensive chronic kidney disease NOS
Use additional code to identify the stage of chronic kidney disease (N18.1-N18.4, N18.9)

    I13.11   **Hypertensive heart and chronic kidney disease without heart failure, with stage 5 chronic kidney disease, or end stage renal disease**   CC HCC
Use additional code to identify the stage of chronic kidney disease (N18.5, N18.6)

    I13.2   **Hypertensive heart and chronic kidney disease with heart failure and with stage 5 chronic kidney disease, or end stage renal disease**   CC HCC
Use additional code to identify type of heart failure (I50.-)
Use additional code to identify the stage of chronic kidney disease (N18.5, N18.6)

✓4th **I15**   **Secondary hypertension**
Code also underlying condition
EXCLUDES 1   *postprocedural hypertension (I97.3)*
EXCLUDES 2   *secondary hypertension involving vessels of brain (I60-I69)*
secondary hypertension involving vessels of eye (H35.0-)

    I15.0   **Renovascular hypertension**
    I15.1   **Hypertension secondary to other renal disorders**
AHA: 2016,3Q,22
    I15.2   **Hypertension secondary to endocrine disorders**
    I15.8   **Other secondary hypertension**
    I15.9   **Secondary hypertension, unspecified**

✓4th **I16**   **Hypertensive crisis**
Code also any identified hypertensive disease (I10-I15)
AHA: 2016,4Q,26-28
    I16.0   **Hypertensive urgency**
    I16.1   **Hypertensive emergency**   CC
CC Excl: No Excl
    I16.9   **Hypertensive crisis, unspecified**   CC
CC Excl: No Excl

Ischemic heart diseases (I20-I25)

Use additional code to identify presence of hypertension (I10-I16)

√4ᵗʰ I20 Angina pectoris

Use additional code to identify:
exposure to environmental tobacco smoke (Z77.22)
history of tobacco dependence (Z87.891)
occupational exposure to environmental tobacco smoke (Z57.31)
tobacco dependence (F17.-)
tobacco use (Z72.0)

EXCLUDES 1   *angina pectoris with atherosclerotic heart disease of native coronary arteries (I25.1-)*
atherosclerosis of coronary artery bypass graft(s) and coronary artery of transplanted heart with angina pectoris (I25.7-)
postinfarction angina (I23.7)

DEF: Chest pain due to reduced blood flow resulting in a lack of oxygen to the heart muscles.

I20.0   Unstable angina   CC   HCC

Accelerated angina
Crescendo angina
De novo effort angina
Intermediate coronary syndrome
Preinfarction syndrome
Worsening effort angina
DEF: Condition representing an intermediate stage between angina of effort and acute myocardial infarction.
CC Excl: PDX collection 651

I20.1   Angina pectoris with documented spasm   CC   HCC

Angiospastic angina
Prinzmetal angina
Spasm-induced angina
Variant angina
CC Excl: PDX collection 652

I20.8   Other forms of angina pectoris   HCC

Angina equivalent
Angina of effort
Coronary slow flow syndrome
Stable angina
Stenocardia
Use additional code(s) for symptoms associated with angina equivalent

I20.9   Angina pectoris, unspecified   HCC

Angina NOS
Anginal syndrome
Cardiac angina
Ischemic chest pain

√4ᵗʰ I21 Acute myocardial infarction

INCLUDES   cardiac infarction
coronary (artery) embolism
coronary (artery) occlusion
coronary (artery) rupture
coronary (artery) thrombosis
infarction of heart, myocardium, or ventricle
myocardial infarction specified as acute or with a stated duration of 4 weeks (28 days) or less from onset

Use additional code, if applicable, to identify:
exposure to environmental tobacco smoke (Z77.22)
history of tobacco dependence (Z87.891)
occupational exposure to environmental tobacco smoke (Z57.31)
status post administration of tPA (rtPA) in a different facility within the last 24 hours prior to admission to current facility (Z92.82)
tobacco dependence (F17.-)
tobacco use (Z72.0)

EXCLUDES 2   *old myocardial infarction (I25.2)*
postmyocardial infarction syndrome (I24.1)
subsequent type 1 myocardial infarction (I22.-)

AHA: 2019,2Q,5; 2018,4Q,68; 2018,3Q,5; 2017,4Q,12-14; 2017,1Q,44-45; 2016,4Q,140; 2015,2Q,16; 2013,1Q,25; 2012,4Q,96,102-103

TIP: When chronic total occlusion and myocardial infarction are documented as being in different vessels, assign code I25.82 Chronic total occlusion of coronary artery, in addition to the myocardial infarction code.

CC Excl: For MCC codes in category I21: PDX collection 653

√5ᵗʰ I21.0   ST elevation (STEMI) myocardial infarction of anterior wall

Type 1 ST elevation myocardial infarction of anterior wall
DEF: ST elevation myocardial infarction: Complete obstruction of one or more coronary arteries causing decreased blood flow (ischemia) and necrosis of myocardial muscle cells.

I21.01   ST elevation (STEMI) myocardial infarction involving left main coronary artery   CC   HCC

I21.02   ST elevation (STEMI) myocardial infarction involving left anterior descending coronary artery   CC   HCC

ST elevation (STEMI) myocardial infarction involving diagonal coronary artery
AHA: 2013,1Q,25

I21.09   ST elevation (STEMI) myocardial infarction involving other coronary artery of anterior wall   CC   HCC

Acute transmural myocardial infarction of anterior wall
Anteroapical transmural (Q wave) infarction (acute)
Anterolateral transmural (Q wave) infarction (acute)
Anteroseptal transmural (Q wave) infarction (acute)
Transmural (Q wave) infarction (acute) (of) anterior (wall) NOS
AHA: 2012,4Q,102-103

√5ᵗʰ I21.1   ST elevation (STEMI) myocardial infarction of inferior wall

Type 1 ST elevation myocardial infarction of inferior wall
DEF: ST elevation myocardial infarction: Complete obstruction of one or more coronary arteries causing decreased blood flow (ischemia) and necrosis of myocardial muscle cells.

I21.11   ST elevation (STEMI) myocardial infarction involving right coronary artery   CC   HCC

Inferoposterior transmural (Q wave) infarction (acute)

I21.19   ST elevation (STEMI) myocardial infarction involving other coronary artery of inferior wall   CC   HCC

Acute transmural myocardial infarction of inferior wall
Inferolateral transmural (Q wave) infarction (acute)
Transmural (Q wave) infarction (acute) (of) diaphragmatic wall
Transmural (Q wave) infarction (acute) (of) inferior (wall) NOS

EXCLUDES 2   *ST elevation (STEMI) myocardial infarction involving left circumflex coronary artery (I21.21)*

AHA: 2012,4Q,96

✓5ᵗʰ I21.2   ST elevation (STEMI) myocardial infarction of other sites

Type 1 ST elevation myocardial infarction of other sites

DEF: ST elevation myocardial infarction: Complete obstruction of one or more coronary arteries causing decreased blood flow (ischemia) and necrosis of myocardial muscle cells.

I21.21   ST elevation (STEMI) myocardial   `CC` `HCC`
infarction involving left circumflex coronary artery

ST elevation (STEMI) myocardial infarction involving oblique marginal coronary artery

I21.29   ST elevation (STEMI) myocardial   `CC` `HCC`
infarction involving other sites

Acute transmural myocardial infarction of other sites

Apical-lateral transmural (Q wave) infarction (acute)

Basal-lateral transmural (Q wave) infarction (acute)

High lateral transmural (Q wave) infarction (acute)

Lateral (wall) NOS transmural (Q wave) infarction (acute)

Posterior (true) transmural (Q wave) infarction (acute)

Posterobasal transmural (Q wave) infarction (acute)

Posterolateral transmural (Q wave) infarction (acute)

Posteroseptal transmural (Q wave) infarction (acute)

Septal transmural (Q wave) infarction (acute) NOS

I21.3   ST elevation (STEMI) myocardial infarction of   `CC` `HCC`
unspecified site

Acute transmural myocardial infarction of unspecified site

Transmural (Q wave) myocardial infarction NOS

Type 1 ST elevation myocardial infarction of unspecified site

DEF: ST elevation myocardial infarction: Complete obstruction of one or more coronary arteries causing decreased blood flow (ischemia) and necrosis of myocardial muscle cells.

I21.4   Non-ST elevation (NSTEMI) myocardial infarction   `MCC` `HCC`

Acute subendocardial myocardial infarction

Non-Q wave myocardial infarction NOS

Nontransmural myocardial infarction NOS

Type 1 non-ST elevation myocardial infarction

AHA: 2019,2Q,33; 2017,1Q,44-45

DEF: Partial obstruction of one or more coronary arteries that causes decreased blood flow (ischemia) and may cause partial thickness necrosis of myocardial muscle cells.

I21.9   Acute myocardial infarction, unspecified   `MCC` `HCC`

Myocardial infarction (acute) NOS

✓5ᵗʰ I21.A   Other type of myocardial infarction

AHA: 2019,2Q,5

I21.A1   Myocardial infarction type 2   `MCC` `HCC`

Myocardial infarction due to demand ischemia

Myocardial infarction secondary to ischemic imbalance

▶Code first the underlying cause, such as:◀

▶anemia (D50.0-D64.9)◀

▶chronic obstructive pulmonary disease (J44.-)◀

▶paroxysmal tachycardia (I47.0-I47.9)◀

▶shock (R57.0-R57.9)◀

~~Code also the underlying cause, if known and applicable, such as:~~

~~anemia (D50.0-D64.9)~~

~~chronic obstructive pulmonary disease (J44.-)~~

~~heart failure (I50.-)~~

~~paroxysmal tachycardia (I47.0-I47.9)~~

~~renal failure (N17.0-N19)~~

~~shock (R57.0-R57.9)~~

AHA: 2017,4Q,13-14

DEF: Often referred to as due to demand ischemia, myocardial infarction (MI) type 2 refers to an MI due to ischemia and necrosis resulting from an oxygen imbalance to the heart. This mismatch between oxygen decreased supply and increased demand is caused by conditions other than coronary artery disease such as vasospasm, embolism, anemia, hypertension, hypotension, or arrhythmias.

I21.A9   Other myocardial infarction type   `MCC` `HCC`

Myocardial infarction associated with revascularization procedure

Myocardial infarction type 3

Myocardial infarction type 4a

Myocardial infarction type 4b

Myocardial infarction type 4c

Myocardial infarction type 5

Code first, if applicable, postprocedural myocardial infarction following cardiac surgery (I97.190), or postprocedural myocardial infarction during cardiac surgery (I97.790)

Code also complication, if known and applicable, such as:

(acute) stent occlusion (T82.897-)

(acute) stent stenosis ▶(T82.855-)◀

(acute) stent thrombosis (T82.867-)

cardiac arrest due to underlying cardiac condition (I46.2)

complication of percutaneous coronary intervention (PCI) (I97.89)

occlusion of coronary artery bypass graft (T82.218-)

AHA: 2019,2Q,33

✓4ᵗʰ I22   Subsequent ST elevation (STEMI) and non-ST elevation (NSTEMI) myocardial infarction

`INCLUDES`   acute myocardial infarction occurring within four weeks (28 days) of a previous acute myocardial infarction, regardless of site

cardiac infarction

coronary (artery) embolism

coronary (artery) occlusion

coronary (artery) rupture

coronary (artery) thrombosis

infarction of heart, myocardium, or ventricle

recurrent myocardial infarction

reinfarction of myocardium

rupture of heart, myocardium, or ventricle

subsequent type 1 myocardial infarction

Use additional code, if applicable, to identify:

exposure to environmental tobacco smoke (Z77.22)

history of tobacco dependence (Z87.891)

occupational exposure to environmental tobacco smoke (Z57.31)

status post administration of tPA (rtPA) in a different facility within the last 24 hours prior to admission to current facility (Z92.82)

tobacco dependence (F17.-)

tobacco use (Z72.0)

`EXCLUDES 1`   subsequent myocardial infarction, type 2 (I21.A1)

subsequent myocardial infarction of other type (type 3) (type 4) (type 5) (I21.A9)

AHA: 2018,4Q,68; 2018,3Q,5; 2017,4Q,12-13; 2017,2Q,11; 2013,1Q,25; 2012,4Q,97,102-103

DEF: Non-ST elevation myocardial infarction: Partial obstruction of one or more coronary arteries that causes decreased blood flow (ischemia) and may cause partial thickness necrosis of myocardial muscle cells.

DEF: ST elevation myocardial infarction: Complete obstruction of one or more coronary arteries causing decreased blood flow (ischemia) and necrosis of myocardial muscle cells.

TIP: When chronic total occlusion and myocardial infarction are documented as being in different vessels, assign code I25.82 Chronic total occlusion of coronary artery, in addition to the myocardial infarction code.

I22.0   Subsequent ST elevation (STEMI) myocardial   `CC` `HCC`
infarction of anterior wall

Subsequent acute transmural myocardial infarction of anterior wall

Subsequent transmural (Q wave) infarction (acute)(of) anterior (wall) NOS

Subsequent anteroapical transmural (Q wave) infarction (acute)

Subsequent anterolateral transmural (Q wave) infarction (acute)

Subsequent anteroseptal transmural (Q wave) infarction (acute)

`N` Newborn: 0   `P` Pediatric: 0-17   `M` Maternity: 9-64   `A` Adult: 15-124   `MCC` Major Complication/Comorbidity   `CC` Complication/Comorbidity   `SW` Severe Wound Dx

648   ICD-10-CM 2020

I22.1 Subsequent ST elevation (STEMI) myocardial infarction of inferior wall `CC` `HCC`

Subsequent acute transmural myocardial infarction of inferior wall

Subsequent transmural (Q wave) infarction (acute)(of) diaphragmatic wall

Subsequent transmural (Q wave) infarction (acute)(of) inferior (wall) NOS

Subsequent inferolateral transmural (Q wave) infarction (acute)

Subsequent inferoposterior transmural (Q wave) infarction (acute)

AHA: 2012,4Q,102

I22.2 Subsequent non-ST elevation (NSTEMI) myocardial infarction `CC` `HCC`

Subsequent acute subendocardial myocardial infarction

Subsequent non-Q wave myocardial infarction NOS

Subsequent nontransmural myocardial infarction NOS

I22.8 Subsequent ST elevation (STEMI) myocardial infarction of other sites `CC` `HCC`

Subsequent acute transmural myocardial infarction of other sites

Subsequent apical-lateral transmural (Q wave) myocardial infarction (acute)

Subsequent basal-lateral transmural (Q wave) myocardial infarction (acute)

Subsequent high lateral transmural (Q wave) myocardial infarction (acute)

Subsequent transmural (Q wave) myocardial infarction (acute)(of) lateral (wall) NOS

Subsequent posterior (true) transmural (Q wave) myocardial infarction (acute)

Subsequent posterobasal transmural (Q wave) myocardial infarction (acute)

Subsequent posterolateral transmural (Q wave) myocardial infarction (acute)

Subsequent posteroseptal transmural (Q wave) myocardial infarction (acute)

Subsequent septal NOS transmural (Q wave) myocardial infarction (acute)

I22.9 Subsequent ST elevation (STEMI) myocardial infarction of unspecified site `CC` `HCC`

Subsequent acute myocardial infarction of unspecified site

Subsequent myocardial infarction (acute) NOS

✓4ᵗʰ I23 Certain current complications following ST elevation (STEMI) and non-ST elevation (NSTEMI) myocardial infarction (within the 28 day period)

AHA: 2017,2Q,11

DEF: ST elevation myocardial infarction: Complete obstruction of one or more coronary arteries causing decreased blood flow (ischemia) and necrosis of myocardial muscle cells.

DEF: Non-ST elevation myocardial infarction: Partial obstruction of one or more coronary arteries that causes decreased blood flow (ischemia) and may cause partial thickness necrosis of myocardial muscle cells.

CC Excl: For CC codes in category I23: PDX collection 654

I23.0 Hemopericardium as current complication following acute myocardial infarction `CC` `HCC` `A`

EXCLUDES 1   hemopericardium not specified as current complication following acute myocardial infarction (I31.2)

I23.1 Atrial septal defect as current complication following acute myocardial infarction `CC` `HCC` `A`

EXCLUDES 1   acquired atrial septal defect not specified as current complication following acute myocardial infarction (I51.0)

I23.2 Ventricular septal defect as current complication following acute myocardial infarction `CC` `HCC` `A`

EXCLUDES 1   acquired ventricular septal defect not specified as current complication following acute myocardial infarction (I51.0)

I23.3 Rupture of cardiac wall without hemopericardium as current complication following acute myocardial infarction `CC` `HCC` `A`

I23.4 Rupture of chordae tendineae as current complication following acute myocardial infarction `MCC` `HCC`

EXCLUDES 1   rupture of chordae tendineae not specified as current complication following acute myocardial infarction (I51.1)

CC Excl: PDX collection 655

I23.5 Rupture of papillary muscle as current complication following acute myocardial infarction `MCC` `HCC`

EXCLUDES 1   rupture of papillary muscle not specified as current complication following acute myocardial infarction (I51.2)

CC Excl: PDX collection 656

I23.6 Thrombosis of atrium, auricular appendage, and ventricle as current complications following acute myocardial infarction `CC` `HCC` `A`

EXCLUDES 1   thrombosis of atrium, auricular appendage, and ventricle not specified as current complication following acute myocardial infarction (I51.3)

I23.7 Postinfarction angina `CC` `HCC` `A`

AHA: 2015,2Q,16

TIP: When postinfarction angina occurs with atherosclerotic coronary artery disease, code both I23.7 and I25.118 for atherosclerotic disease with other forms of angina pectoris.

I23.8 Other current complications following acute myocardial infarction `CC` `HCC` `A`

✓4ᵗʰ I24 Other acute ischemic heart diseases

EXCLUDES 1   angina pectoris (I20.-)

transient myocardial ischemia in newborn (P29.4)

CC Excl: For CC codes in category I24, unless otherwise noted: PDX collection 657

I24.0 Acute coronary thrombosis not resulting in myocardial infarction `CC` `HCC`

Acute coronary (artery) (vein) embolism not resulting in myocardial infarction

Acute coronary (artery) (vein) occlusion not resulting in myocardial infarction

Acute coronary (artery) (vein) thromboembolism not resulting in myocardial infarction

EXCLUDES 1   atherosclerotic heart disease (I25.1-)

AHA: 2013,1Q,24

I24.1 Dressler's syndrome `CC` `HCC`

Postmyocardial infarction syndrome

EXCLUDES 1   postinfarction angina (I23.7)

DEF: Fever, leukocytosis, chest pain, evidence of pericarditis, pleurisy, and pneumonia occurring days or weeks after a myocardial infarction.

CC Excl: PDX collection 658

I24.8 Other forms of acute ischemic heart disease `CC` `HCC`

EXCLUDES 1   myocardial infarction due to demand ischemia (I21.A1)

AHA: 2017,4Q,13

I24.9 Acute ischemic heart disease, unspecified `CC` `HCC`

EXCLUDES 1   ischemic heart disease (chronic) NOS (I25.9)

✓4ᵗʰ **I25 Chronic ischemic heart disease**
Use additional code to identify:
chronic total occlusion of coronary artery (I25.82)
exposure to environmental tobacco smoke (Z77.22)
history of tobacco dependence (Z87.891)
occupational exposure to environmental tobacco smoke (Z57.31)
tobacco dependence (F17.-)
tobacco use (Z72.0)

✓5ᵗʰ **I25.1 Atherosclerotic heart disease of native coronary artery**
Atherosclerotic cardiovascular disease
Coronary (artery) atheroma
Coronary (artery) atherosclerosis
Coronary (artery) disease
Coronary (artery) sclerosis
Use additional code, if applicable, to identify:
coronary atherosclerosis due to calcified coronary lesion (I25.84)
coronary atherosclerosis due to lipid rich plaque (I25.83)
EXCLUDES 2   *atheroembolism (I75.-)*
atherosclerosis of coronary artery bypass graft(s) and transplanted heart (I25.7-)

Atheromas

Atheromas (fatty tissue and/or plaque)   Lumen

I25.10 Atherosclerotic heart disease of native coronary artery without angina pectoris   🅰
Atherosclerotic heart disease NOS
AHA: 2015,2Q,16; 2012,4Q,92

✓6ᵗʰ **I25.11 Atherosclerotic heart disease of native coronary artery with angina pectoris**

I25.110 Atherosclerotic heart disease of native coronary artery with unstable angina pectoris   CC HCC 🅰
EXCLUDES 1   *unstable angina without atherosclerotic heart disease (I20.0)*
CC Excl: PDX collection 651

I25.111 Atherosclerotic heart disease of native coronary artery with angina pectoris with documented spasm   HCC 🅰
EXCLUDES 1   *angina pectoris with documented spasm without atherosclerotic heart disease (I20.1)*

I25.118 Atherosclerotic heart disease of native coronary artery with other forms of angina pectoris   HCC 🅰
EXCLUDES 1   *other forms of angina pectoris without atherosclerotic heart disease (I20.8)*

AHA: 2015,2Q,16
TIP: When postinfarction angina occurs with atherosclerotic coronary artery disease, code both I23.7 and I25.118 for atherosclerotic disease with other forms of angina pectoris.

I25.119 Atherosclerotic heart disease of native coronary artery with unspecified angina pectoris   HCC 🅰
Atherosclerotic heart disease with angina NOS
Atherosclerotic heart disease with ischemic chest pain
EXCLUDES 1   *unspecified angina pectoris without atherosclerotic heart disease (I20.9)*

I25.2 Old myocardial infarction
Healed myocardial infarction
Past myocardial infarction diagnosed by ECG or other investigation, but currently presenting no symptoms

I25.3 Aneurysm of heart   CC
Mural aneurysm
Ventricular aneurysm
CC Excl: PDX collection 659

✓5ᵗʰ **I25.4 Coronary artery aneurysm and dissection**

I25.41 Coronary artery aneurysm
Coronary arteriovenous fistula, acquired
EXCLUDES 1   *congenital coronary (artery) aneurysm (Q24.5)*

I25.42 Coronary artery dissection   MCC
DEF: Tear in the intimal arterial wall of a coronary artery resulting in the sudden intrusion of blood within the layers of the wall.
CC Excl: PDX collection 660

I25.5 Ischemic cardiomyopathy
EXCLUDES 2   *coronary atherosclerosis (I25.1-, I25.7-)*

I25.6 Silent myocardial ischemia

✓5ᵗʰ **I25.7 Atherosclerosis of coronary artery bypass graft(s) and coronary artery of transplanted heart with angina pectoris**
Use additional code, if applicable, to identify:
coronary atherosclerosis due to calcified coronary lesion (I25.84)
coronary atherosclerosis due to lipid rich plaque (I25.83)
EXCLUDES 1   *atherosclerosis of bypass graft(s) of transplanted heart without angina pectoris (I25.812)*
atherosclerosis of coronary artery bypass graft(s) without angina pectoris (I25.810)
atherosclerosis of native coronary artery of transplanted heart without angina pectoris (I25.811)

✓6ᵗʰ **I25.70 Atherosclerosis of coronary artery bypass graft(s), unspecified, with angina pectoris**

I25.700 Atherosclerosis of coronary artery bypass graft(s), unspecified, with unstable angina pectoris   CC HCC 🅰
EXCLUDES 1   *unstable angina pectoris without atherosclerosis of coronary artery bypass graft (I20.0)*
CC Excl: PDX collection 651

I25.701 Atherosclerosis of coronary artery bypass graft(s), unspecified, with angina pectoris with documented spasm   HCC 🅰
EXCLUDES 1   *angina pectoris with documented spasm without atherosclerosis of coronary artery bypass graft (I20.1)*

I25.708 Atherosclerosis of coronary artery bypass graft(s), unspecified, with other forms of angina pectoris   HCC 🅰
EXCLUDES 1   *other forms of angina pectoris without atherosclerosis of coronary artery bypass graft (I20.8)*

I25.709 Atherosclerosis of coronary artery bypass graft(s), unspecified, with unspecified angina pectoris   HCC 🅰
EXCLUDES 1   *unspecified angina pectoris without atherosclerosis of coronary artery bypass graft (I20.9)*

✓6ᵗʰ **I25.71** **Atherosclerosis of** autologous vein **coronary artery bypass graft(s) with angina pectoris**
CC Excl: For CC codes in subcategory I25.71, unless otherwise noted: PDX collection 662

I25.710 **Atherosclerosis of autologous** CC HCC A **vein coronary artery bypass graft(s) with** unstable **angina pectoris**
EXCLUDES 1   unstable angina without atherosclerosis of autologous vein coronary artery bypass graft(s) (I20.0)
EXCLUDES 2   embolism or thrombus of coronary artery bypass graft(s) (T82.8-)
CC Excl: PDX collection 661

I25.711 **Atherosclerosis of autologous** CC HCC A **vein coronary artery bypass graft(s) with angina pectoris with** documented spasm
EXCLUDES 1   angina pectoris with documented spasm without atherosclerosis of autologous vein coronary artery bypass graft(s) (I20.1)

I25.718 **Atherosclerosis of autologous** CC HCC A **vein coronary artery bypass graft(s) with other forms of angina pectoris**
EXCLUDES 1   other forms of angina pectoris without atherosclerosis of autologous vein coronary artery bypass graft(s) (I20.8)

I25.719 **Atherosclerosis of autologous** CC HCC A **vein coronary artery bypass graft(s) with unspecified angina pectoris**
EXCLUDES 1   unspecified angina pectoris without atherosclerosis of autologous vein coronary artery bypass graft(s) (I20.9)

✓6ᵗʰ **I25.72** **Atherosclerosis of** autologous artery **coronary artery bypass graft(s) with angina pectoris**
Atherosclerosis of internal mammary artery graft with angina pectoris
CC Excl: For CC codes in subcategories I25.72, unless otherwise noted: PDX collection 662

I25.720 **Atherosclerosis of autologous** CC HCC A **artery coronary artery bypass graft(s) with** unstable **angina pectoris**
EXCLUDES 1   unstable angina without atherosclerosis of autologous artery coronary artery bypass graft(s) (I20.0)
CC Excl: PDX collection 661

I25.721 **Atherosclerosis of autologous** CC HCC A **artery coronary artery bypass graft(s) with angina pectoris with** documented spasm
EXCLUDES 1   angina pectoris with documented spasm without atherosclerosis of autologous artery coronary artery bypass graft(s) (I20.1)

I25.728 **Atherosclerosis of autologous** CC HCC A **artery coronary artery bypass graft(s) with other forms of angina pectoris**
EXCLUDES 1   other forms of angina pectoris without atherosclerosis of autologous artery coronary artery bypass graft(s) (I20.8)

I25.729 **Atherosclerosis of autologous** CC HCC A **artery coronary artery bypass graft(s) with unspecified angina pectoris**
EXCLUDES 1   unspecified angina pectoris without atherosclerosis of autologous artery coronary artery bypass graft(s) (I20.9)

✓6ᵗʰ **I25.73** **Atherosclerosis of** nonautologous biological **coronary artery bypass graft(s) with angina pectoris**
CC Excl: For CC codes in subcategories I25.73, unless otherwise noted: PDX collection 662

I25.730 **Atherosclerosis of** CC HCC A **nonautologous biological coronary artery bypass graft(s) with** unstable **angina pectoris**
EXCLUDES 1   unstable angina without atherosclerosis of nonautologous biological coronary artery bypass graft(s) (I20.0)
CC Excl: PDX collection 661

I25.731 **Atherosclerosis of** CC HCC A **nonautologous biological coronary artery bypass graft(s) with angina pectoris with** documented spasm
EXCLUDES 1   angina pectoris with documented spasm without atherosclerosis of nonautologous biological coronary artery bypass graft(s) (I20.1)

I25.738 **Atherosclerosis of** CC HCC A **nonautologous biological coronary artery bypass graft(s) with other forms of angina pectoris**
EXCLUDES 1   other forms of angina pectoris without atherosclerosis of nonautologous biological coronary artery bypass graft(s) (I20.8)

I25.739 **Atherosclerosis of** CC HCC A **nonautologous biological coronary artery bypass graft(s) with unspecified angina pectoris**
EXCLUDES 1   unspecified angina pectoris without atherosclerosis of nonautologous biological coronary artery bypass graft(s) (I20.9)

✓6ᵗʰ **I25.75** **Atherosclerosis of** native **coronary artery of** transplanted heart **with angina pectoris**
EXCLUDES 1   atherosclerosis of native coronary artery of transplanted heart without angina pectoris (I25.811)
CC Excl: For CC codes in subcategory I25.75, unless otherwise noted: PDX collection 664

I25.750 **Atherosclerosis of native** CC HCC **coronary artery of transplanted heart with** unstable **angina**
CC Excl: PDX collection 663

I25.751 **Atherosclerosis of native** CC HCC **coronary artery of transplanted heart with angina pectoris with** documented spasm

I25.758 **Atherosclerosis of native** CC HCC **coronary artery of transplanted heart with other forms of angina pectoris**

I25.759 **Atherosclerosis of native** CC HCC **coronary artery of transplanted heart with unspecified angina pectoris**

✓6ᵗʰ I25.76 Atherosclerosis of bypass graft of coronary artery of transplanted heart with angina pectoris

> EXCLUDES 1   atherosclerosis of bypass graft of coronary artery of transplanted heart without angina pectoris (I25.812)

> **CC Excl: For CC codes in subcategory I25.76, unless otherwise noted:** PDX collection 666

I25.760 Atherosclerosis of bypass graft CC HCC A **of coronary artery of transplanted heart with unstable angina**
> **CC Excl:** PDX collection 665

I25.761 Atherosclerosis of bypass graft CC HCC A **of coronary artery of transplanted heart with angina pectoris with documented spasm**

I25.768 Atherosclerosis of bypass graft CC HCC A **of coronary artery of transplanted heart with other forms of angina pectoris**

I25.769 Atherosclerosis of bypass graft CC HCC A **of coronary artery of transplanted heart with unspecified angina pectoris**

✓6ᵗʰ I25.79 Atherosclerosis of other coronary artery bypass graft(s) with angina pectoris

> **CC Excl: For CC codes in subcategory I25.79, unless otherwise noted:** No Excl

I25.790 Atherosclerosis of other CC HCC A **coronary artery bypass graft(s) with unstable angina pectoris**
> EXCLUDES 1   unstable angina without atherosclerosis of other coronary artery bypass graft(s) (I20.0)

> **CC Excl:** PDX collection 651

I25.791 Atherosclerosis of other CC HCC A **coronary artery bypass graft(s) with angina pectoris with documented spasm**
> EXCLUDES 1   angina pectoris with documented spasm without atherosclerosis of other coronary artery bypass graft(s) (I20.1)

I25.798 Atherosclerosis of other CC HCC A **coronary artery bypass graft(s) with other forms of angina pectoris**
> EXCLUDES 1   other forms of angina pectoris without atherosclerosis of other coronary artery bypass graft(s) (I20.8)

I25.799 Atherosclerosis of other CC HCC A **coronary artery bypass graft(s) with unspecified angina pectoris**
> EXCLUDES 1   unspecified angina pectoris without atherosclerosis of other coronary artery bypass graft(s) (I20.9)

✓5ᵗʰ I25.8 Other forms of chronic ischemic heart disease

✓6ᵗʰ I25.81 Atherosclerosis of other coronary vessels without angina pectoris
> Use additional code, if applicable, to identify:
> coronary atherosclerosis due to calcified coronary lesion (I25.84)
> coronary atherosclerosis due to lipid rich plaque (I25.83)

> EXCLUDES 1   ~~atherosclerotic heart disease of native coronary artery without angina pectoris (I25.10)~~

> EXCLUDES 2   ▶atherosclerotic heart disease of native coronary artery without angina pectoris (I25.10)◀

I25.810 Atherosclerosis of coronary CC A **artery bypass graft(s) without angina pectoris**
> Atherosclerosis of coronary artery bypass graft NOS
> EXCLUDES 1   atherosclerosis of coronary bypass graft(s) with angina pectoris (I25.70-I25.73-, I25.79-)

> **CC Excl:** No Excl

I25.811 Atherosclerosis of native CC **coronary artery of transplanted heart without angina pectoris**
> Atherosclerosis of native coronary artery of transplanted heart NOS
> EXCLUDES 1   atherosclerosis of native coronary artery of transplanted heart with angina pectoris (I25.75-)

> **CC Excl:** PDX collection 664

I25.812 Atherosclerosis of bypass graft CC A **of coronary artery of transplanted heart without angina pectoris**
> Atherosclerosis of bypass graft of transplanted heart NOS
> EXCLUDES 1   atherosclerosis of bypass graft of transplanted heart with angina pectoris (I25.76)

> **CC Excl:** PDX collection 666

I25.82 Chronic total occlusion of coronary artery
> Complete occlusion of coronary artery
> Total occlusion of coronary artery
> Code first coronary atherosclerosis (I25.1-, I25.7-, I25.81-)
> EXCLUDES 1   acute coronary occlusion with myocardial infarction (I21.0-I21.9, I22.-)
> acute coronary occlusion without myocardial infarction (I24.0)

> **AHA:** 2018,3Q,5
> **DEF:** Complete blockage of the coronary artery due to plaque accumulation over an extended period of time, resulting in substantial reduction of blood flow. Symptoms include angina or chest pain.
> **TIP:** Report this code in addition to a code from category I21 or I22 when the chronic total occlusion and the myocardial infarction are documented as being in different vessels.

I25.83 Coronary atherosclerosis due to lipid rich plaque A
> Code first coronary atherosclerosis (I25.1-, I25.7-, I25.81-)

I25.84 Coronary atherosclerosis due to calcified coronary lesion
> Coronary atherosclerosis due to severely calcified coronary lesion
> Code first coronary atherosclerosis (I25.1-, I25.7-, I25.81-)

I25.89 Other forms of chronic ischemic heart disease

I25.9 Chronic ischemic heart disease, unspecified
> Ischemic heart disease (chronic) NOS

N Newborn: 0   P Pediatric: 0-17   M Maternity: 9-64   A Adult: 15-124   MCC Major Complication/Comorbidity   CC Complication/Comorbidity   SW Severe Wound Dx

652   ICD-10-CM 2020

Pulmonary heart disease and diseases of pulmonary circulation (I26-I28)

✓4th I26　Pulmonary embolism

INCLUDES　pulmonary (acute)(artery)(vein) infarction
pulmonary (acute) (artery)(vein) thromboembolism
pulmonary (acute)(artery)(vein) thrombosis

EXCLUDES 2　*chronic pulmonary embolism (I27.82)*
personal history of pulmonary embolism (Z86.711)
pulmonary embolism complicating abortion, ectopic or molar pregnancy (O00-O07, O08.2)
pulmonary embolism complicating pregnancy, childbirth and the puerperium (O88.-)
pulmonary embolism due to trauma (T79.0, T79.1)
pulmonary embolism due to complications of surgical and medical care (T80.0, T81.7-, T82.8-)
septic (non-pulmonary) arterial embolism (I76)

✓5th I26.0　Pulmonary embolism with acute cor pulmonale

DEF: Cor pulmonale: Heart-lung disease appearing in identifiable forms as chronic or acute. The chronic form of this heart-lung disease is marked by dilation, hypertrophy and failure of the right ventricle due to a disease that has affected the function of the lungs, excluding congenital or left heart diseases and is also called chronic cardiopulmonary disease. The acute form is an overload of the right ventricle from a rapid onset of pulmonary hypertension, usually arising from a pulmonary embolism.

CC Excl: For MCC codes in subcategory I26.0: PDX collection 667

I26.01　Septic pulmonary embolism with acute cor pulmonale MCC HCC
Code first underlying infection

I26.02　Saddle embolus of pulmonary artery with acute cor pulmonale MCC H10 HCC

I26.09　Other pulmonary embolism with acute cor pulmonale MCC H10 HCC
Acute cor pulmonale NOS
AHA: 2014,4Q,21

✓5th I26.9　Pulmonary embolism without acute cor pulmonale

I26.90　Septic pulmonary embolism without acute cor pulmonale MCC HCC
Code first underlying infection
CC Excl: PDX collection 668

I26.92　Saddle embolus of pulmonary artery without acute cor pulmonale MCC H10 HCC
CC Excl: PDX collection 669

● **I26.93　Single subsegmental pulmonary embolism without acute cor pulmonale** MCC
Subsegmental pulmonary embolism NOS

● **I26.94　Multiple subsegmental pulmonary emboli without acute cor pulmonale** MCC

I26.99　Other pulmonary embolism without acute cor pulmonale MCC H10 HCC
Acute pulmonary embolism NOS
Pulmonary embolism NOS
AHA: 2019,2Q,22
CC Excl: PDX collection 670

✓4th I27　Other pulmonary heart diseases

I27.0　Primary pulmonary hypertension CC HCC
Heritable pulmonary arterial hypertension
Idiopathic pulmonary arterial hypertension
Primary group 1 pulmonary hypertension
Primary pulmonary arterial hypertension

EXCLUDES 1　*persistent pulmonary hypertension of newborn (P29.30)*
pulmonary hypertension NOS (I27.20)
secondary pulmonary arterial hypertension (I27.21)
secondary pulmonary hypertension (I27.29)

DEF: Condition that occurs when pressure within the pulmonary artery is elevated and vascular resistance is observed in the lungs.
CC Excl: PDX collection 671

I27.1　Kyphoscoliotic heart disease CC HCC
CC Excl: PDX collection 533

✓5th I27.2　Other secondary pulmonary hypertension
Code also associated underlying condition
EXCLUDES 1　*Eisenmenger's syndrome (I27.83)*
AHA: 2017,4Q,14-15; 2014,4Q,21
DEF: Condition that occurs when pressure within the pulmonary artery is elevated and vascular resistance is observed in the lungs.

I27.20　Pulmonary hypertension, unspecified HCC
Pulmonary hypertension NOS

I27.21　Secondary pulmonary arterial hypertension HCC
(Associated) (drug-induced) (toxin-induced) pulmonary arterial hypertension NOS
(Associated) (drug-induced) (toxin-induced) (secondary) group 1 pulmonary hypertension
Code also associated conditions if applicable, or adverse effects of drugs or toxins, such as:
adverse effect of appetite depressants (T50.5X5)
congenital heart disease (Q20-Q28)
human immunodeficiency virus [HIV] disease (B20)
polymyositis (M33.2-)
portal hypertension (K76.6)
rheumatoid arthritis (M05.-)
schistosomiasis (B65.-)
Sjögren syndrome (M35.0-)
systemic sclerosis (M34.-)

I27.22　Pulmonary hypertension due to left heart disease HCC
Group 2 pulmonary hypertension
Code also associated left heart disease, if known, such as:
multiple valve disease (I08.-)
rheumatic aortic valve diseases (I06.-)
rheumatic mitral valve diseases (I05.-)

I27.23　Pulmonary hypertension due to lung diseases and hypoxia HCC
Group 3 pulmonary hypertension
Code also associated lung disease, if known, such as:
bronchiectasis (J47.-)
cystic fibrosis with pulmonary manifestations (E84.0)
interstitial lung disease (J84.-)
pleural effusion (J90)
sleep apnea (G47.3-)

I27.24　Chronic thromboembolic pulmonary hypertension HCC
Group 4 pulmonary hypertension
Code also associated pulmonary embolism, if applicable (I26.-, I27.82)

I27.29　Other secondary pulmonary hypertension HCC
Group 5 pulmonary hypertension
Pulmonary hypertension with unclear multifactorial mechanisms
Pulmonary hypertension due to hematologic disorders
Pulmonary hypertension due to metabolic disorders
Pulmonary hypertension due to other systemic disorders
Code also other associated disorders, if known, such as:
chronic myeloid leukemia (C92.10- C92.22)
essential thrombocythemia (D47.3)
Gaucher disease (E75.22)
hypertensive chronic kidney disease with end stage renal disease (I12.0, I13.11, I13.2)
hyperthyroidism (E05.-)
hypothyroidism (E00-E03)
polycythemia vera (D45)
sarcoidosis (D86.-)
AHA: 2016,2Q,8

Chapter 9. Diseases of the Circulatory System

✓5ᵗʰ **I27.8 Other specified pulmonary heart diseases**

I27.81 Cor pulmonale (chronic) CC HCC

Cor pulmonale NOS

EXCLUDES 1 *acute cor pulmonale (I26.0-)*

AHA: 2014,4Q,21

DEF: Heart-lung disease appearing in identifiable forms as chronic or acute. The chronic form of this heart-lung disease is marked by dilation, hypertrophy and failure of the right ventricle due to a disease that has affected the function of the lungs, excluding congenital or left heart diseases and is also called chronic cardiopulmonary disease. The acute form is an overload of the right ventricle from a rapid onset of pulmonary hypertension, usually arising from a pulmonary embolism.

I27.82 Chronic pulmonary embolism CC HCC

Use additional code, if applicable, for associated long-term (current) use of anticoagulants (Z79.01)

EXCLUDES 1 *personal history of pulmonary embolism (Z86.711)*

DEF: Long-standing condition commonly associated with pulmonary hypertension in which small blood clots travel to the lungs repeatedly over many weeks, months, or years, requiring continuation of established anticoagulant or thrombolytic therapy.

CC Excl: PDX collection 669

I27.83 Eisenmenger's syndrome HCC

Eisenmenger's complex

(Irreversible) Eisenmenger's disease

Pulmonary hypertension with right to left shunt related to congenital heart disease

Code also underlying heart defect, if known, such as:

atrial septal defect (Q21.1)
Eisenmenger's defect (Q21.8)
patent ductus arteriosus (Q25.0)
ventricular septal defect (Q21.0)

DEF: Pulmonary hypertension with congenital communication between two circulations resulting in a right to left shunt. This causes reduced oxygen saturation in the arterial blood, leading to cyanosis and organ damage. Once it develops, this life-threating condition is irreversible.

I27.89 Other specified pulmonary heart diseases HCC

I27.9 Pulmonary heart disease, unspecified HCC

Chronic cardiopulmonary disease

✓4ᵗʰ **I28 Other diseases of pulmonary vessels**

I28.0 Arteriovenous fistula of pulmonary vessels CC HCC

EXCLUDES 1 *congenital arteriovenous fistula (Q25.72)*

CC Excl: PDX collection 672

I28.1 Aneurysm of pulmonary artery CC HCC

EXCLUDES 1 *congenital aneurysm (Q25.79)*
congenital arteriovenous aneurysm (Q25.72)

CC Excl: PDX collection 672

I28.8 Other diseases of pulmonary vessels HCC

Pulmonary arteritis
Pulmonary endarteritis
Rupture of pulmonary vessels
Stenosis of pulmonary vessels
Stricture of pulmonary vessels

I28.9 Disease of pulmonary vessels, unspecified HCC

Other forms of heart disease (I30-I52)

✓4ᵗʰ **I30 Acute pericarditis**

INCLUDES acute mediastinopericarditis
acute myopericarditis
acute pericardial effusion
acute pleuropericarditis
acute pneumopericarditis

EXCLUDES 1 *Dressler's syndrome (I24.1)*
rheumatic pericarditis (acute) (I01.0)
viral pericarditis due to Coxsakie virus (B33.23)

DEF: Pericarditis: Inflammation affecting the pericardium, the fibroserous membrane that surrounds the heart.

CC Excl: For CC codes in category I30: PDX collection 673

I30.0 Acute nonspecific idiopathic pericarditis CC

I30.1 Infective pericarditis CC

Pneumococcal pericarditis
Pneumopyopericardium
Purulent pericarditis
Pyopericarditis
Pyopericardium
Pyopneumopericardium
Staphylococcal pericarditis
Streptococcal pericarditis
Suppurative pericarditis
Viral pericarditis

Use additional code (B95-B97) to identify infectious agent

I30.8 Other forms of acute pericarditis CC

I30.9 Acute pericarditis, unspecified CC

✓4ᵗʰ **I31 Other diseases of pericardium**

EXCLUDES 1 *diseases of pericardium specified as rheumatic (I09.2)*
postcardiotomy syndrome (I97.0)
traumatic injury to pericardium (S26.-)

I31.0 Chronic adhesive pericarditis CC

Accretio cordis
Adherent pericardium
Adhesive mediastinopericarditis

CC Excl: PDX collection 674

I31.1 Chronic constrictive pericarditis CC

Concretio cordis
Pericardial calcification

CC Excl: PDX collection 674

I31.2 Hemopericardium, not elsewhere classified CC

EXCLUDES 1 *hemopericardium as current complication following acute myocardial infarction (I23.0)*

DEF: Presence of blood in the pericardial sac (pericardium). It can lead to potentially fatal cardiac tamponade if enough blood enters the pericardial cavity.

CC Excl: PDX collection 674

I31.3 Pericardial effusion (noninflammatory) CC

Chylopericardium

EXCLUDES 1 *acute pericardial effusion (I30.9)*

AHA: 2019,1Q,16

TIP: Assign this code for documented malignant pericardial effusion. If the sole reason for admission is to treat the effusion with no treatment rendered for the associated malignancy, this code may be sequenced first.

CC Excl: PDX collection 188

I31.4 Cardiac tamponade CC

Code first underlying cause

DEF: Life-threatening condition in which fluid or blood accumulates in the space between the muscle of the heart (myocardium) and the outer sac that covers the heart (pericardium), resulting in compression of the heart.

CC Excl: PDX collection 188

Cardiac Tamponade

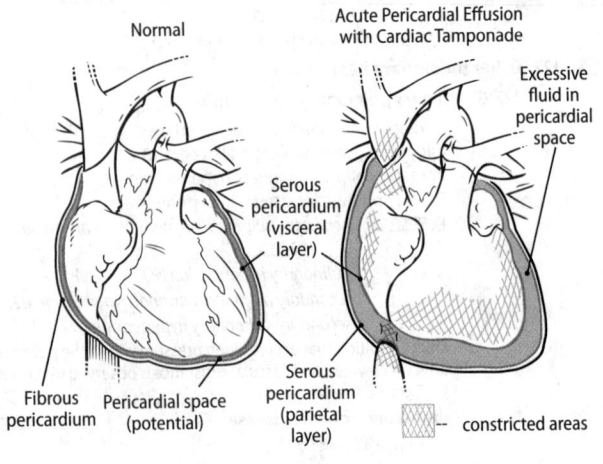

I31.8   **Other specified diseases of pericardium**   `CC`
     Epicardial plaques
     Focal pericardial adhesions
     CC Excl: PDX collection 188

I31.9   **Disease of pericardium, unspecified**   `CC`
     Pericarditis (chronic) NOS
     CC Excl: PDX collection 188

I32   *Pericarditis in diseases classified elsewhere*   `CC`
     Code first underlying disease
     EXCLUDES 1   *pericarditis (in):*
         coxsackie (virus) (B33.23)
         gonococcal (A54.83)
         meningococcal (A39.53)
         rheumatoid (arthritis) (M05.31)
         syphilitic (A52.06)
         systemic lupus erythematosus (M32.12)
         tuberculosis (A18.84)
     DEF: Pericarditis: Inflammation affecting the pericardium, the fibroserous membrane that surrounds the heart.
     CC Excl: PDX collection 673

✓4ᵗʰ   **I33**   **Acute and subacute endocarditis**
     EXCLUDES 1   *acute rheumatic endocarditis (I01.1)*
         endocarditis NOS (I38)
     DEF: Endocarditis: Inflammatory disease of the interior lining of the heart chamber and heart valves.

   I33.0   **Acute and subacute infective endocarditis**   `HIV` `MCC`
     Bacterial endocarditis (acute) (subacute)
     Infective endocarditis (acute) (subacute) NOS
     Endocarditis lenta (acute) (subacute)
     Malignant endocarditis (acute) (subacute)
     Purulent endocarditis (acute) (subacute)
     Septic endocarditis (acute) (subacute)
     Ulcerative endocarditis (acute) (subacute)
     Vegetative endocarditis (acute) (subacute)
     Use additional code (B95-B97) to identify infectious agent
     CC Excl: PDX collection 675

   I33.9   **Acute and subacute endocarditis, unspecified**   `HIV` `MCC`
     Acute endocarditis NOS
     Acute myoendocarditis NOS
     Acute periendocarditis NOS
     Subacute endocarditis NOS
     Subacute myoendocarditis NOS
     Subacute periendocarditis NOS
     CC Excl: PDX collection 675

✓4ᵗʰ   **I34**   **Nonrheumatic mitral valve disorders**
     EXCLUDES 1   *mitral valve disease (I05.9)*
         mitral valve failure (I05.8)
         mitral valve stenosis (I05.0)
         mitral valve disorder of unspecified cause with diseases of aortic and/or tricuspid valve(s) (I08.-)
         mitral valve disorder of unspecified cause with mitral stenosis or obstruction (I05.0)
         mitral valve disorder specified as congenital (Q23.2, Q23.9)
         mitral valve disorder specified as rheumatic (I05.-)

   I34.0   **Nonrheumatic mitral (valve) insufficiency**
     Nonrheumatic mitral (valve) incompetence NOS
     Nonrheumatic mitral (valve) regurgitation NOS

   I34.1   **Nonrheumatic mitral (valve) prolapse**
     Floppy nonrheumatic mitral valve syndrome
     EXCLUDES 1   *Marfan's syndrome (Q87.4-)*

   I34.2   **Nonrheumatic mitral (valve) stenosis**
   I34.8   **Other nonrheumatic mitral valve disorders**
   I34.9   **Nonrheumatic mitral valve disorder, unspecified**

✓4ᵗʰ   **I35**   **Nonrheumatic aortic valve disorders**
     EXCLUDES 1   *aortic valve disorder of unspecified cause but with diseases of mitral and/or tricuspid valve(s) (I08.-)*
         aortic valve disorder specified as congenital (Q23.0, Q23.1)
         aortic valve disorder specified as rheumatic (I06.-)
         hypertrophic subaortic stenosis (I42.1)

   I35.0   **Nonrheumatic aortic (valve) stenosis**
   I35.1   **Nonrheumatic aortic (valve) insufficiency**
     Nonrheumatic aortic (valve) incompetence NOS
     Nonrheumatic aortic (valve) regurgitation NOS

   I35.2   **Nonrheumatic aortic (valve) stenosis with insufficiency**
   I35.8   **Other nonrheumatic aortic valve disorders**

   I35.9   **Nonrheumatic aortic valve disorder, unspecified**

✓4ᵗʰ   **I36**   **Nonrheumatic tricuspid valve disorders**
     EXCLUDES 1   *tricuspid valve disorders of unspecified cause (I07.-)*
         tricuspid valve disorders specified as congenital (Q22.4, Q22.8, Q22.9)
         tricuspid valve disorders specified as rheumatic (I07.-)
         tricuspid valve disorders with aortic and/or mitral valve involvement (I08.-)

   I36.0   **Nonrheumatic tricuspid (valve) stenosis**
   I36.1   **Nonrheumatic tricuspid (valve) insufficiency**
     Nonrheumatic tricuspid (valve) incompetence
     Nonrheumatic tricuspid (valve) regurgitation

   I36.2   **Nonrheumatic tricuspid (valve) stenosis with insufficiency**
   I36.8   **Other nonrheumatic tricuspid valve disorders**
   I36.9   **Nonrheumatic tricuspid valve disorder, unspecified**

✓4ᵗʰ   **I37**   **Nonrheumatic pulmonary valve disorders**
     EXCLUDES 1   *pulmonary valve disorder specified as congenital (Q22.1, Q22.2, Q22.3)*
         pulmonary valve disorder specified as rheumatic (I09.89)

   I37.0   **Nonrheumatic pulmonary valve stenosis**
   I37.1   **Nonrheumatic pulmonary valve insufficiency**
     Nonrheumatic pulmonary valve incompetence
     Nonrheumatic pulmonary valve regurgitation

   I37.2   **Nonrheumatic pulmonary valve stenosis with insufficiency**
   I37.8   **Other nonrheumatic pulmonary valve disorders**
   I37.9   **Nonrheumatic pulmonary valve disorder, unspecified**

I38   **Endocarditis, valve unspecified**   `CC`
     INCLUDES   endocarditis (chronic) NOS
         valvular incompetence NOS
         valvular insufficiency NOS
         valvular regurgitation NOS
         valvular stenosis NOS
         valvulitis (chronic) NOS
     EXCLUDES 1   *congenital insufficiency of cardiac valve NOS (Q24.8)*
         congenital stenosis of cardiac valve NOS (Q24.8)
         endocardial fibroelastosis (I42.4)
         endocarditis specified as rheumatic (I09.1)
     DEF: Endocarditis: Inflammatory disease of the interior lining of the heart chamber and heart valves.
     CC Excl: PDX collection 676

I39   *Endocarditis and heart valve disorders in diseases classified elsewhere*   `CC`
     Code first underlying disease, such as:
     Q fever (A78)
     EXCLUDES 1   *endocardial involvement in:*
         candidiasis (B37.6)
         gonococcal infection (A54.83)
         Libman-Sacks disease (M32.11)
         listerosis (A32.82)
         meningococcal infection (A39.51)
         rheumatoid arthritis (M05.31)
         syphilis (A52.03)
         tuberculosis (A18.84)
         typhoid fever (A01.02)
     DEF: Endocarditis: Inflammatory disease of the interior lining of the heart chamber and heart valves.
     CC Excl: PDX collection 676

✓4ᵗʰ   **I40**   **Acute myocarditis**
     INCLUDES   subacute myocarditis
     EXCLUDES 1   *acute rheumatic myocarditis (I01.2)*
     DEF: Myocarditis: Inflammation of the middle layer of the heart, which is composed of muscle tissue.
     CC Excl: For MCC codes in category I40: PDX collection 677

   I40.0   **Infective myocarditis**   `HIV` `MCC`
     Septic myocarditis
     Use additional code (B95-B97) to identify infectious agent

   I40.1   **Isolated myocarditis**   `HIV` `MCC`
     Fiedler's myocarditis
     Giant cell myocarditis
     Idiopathic myocarditis

   I40.8   **Other acute myocarditis**   `HIV` `MCC`
   I40.9   **Acute myocarditis, unspecified**   `HIV` `MCC`

☑ Additional Character Required   ✓x7ᵗʰ Placeholder   Unacceptable PDx   Questionable PDx   Manifestation   Unspecified Dx   **H1**-**H14** HAC   `HCC` CMS-HCC Dx   `HIV` HIV Dx

ICD-10-CM 2020   **655**

I41 Myocarditis in diseases classified elsewhere `MCC`

Code first underlying disease, such as:
  typhus (A75.0-A75.9)

EXCLUDES 1 myocarditis (in):
    Chagas' disease (chronic) (B57.2)
    acute (B57.0)
    coxsackie (virus) infection (B33.22)
    diphtheritic (A36.81)
    gonococcal (A54.83)
    influenzal (J09.X9, J10.82, J11.82)
    meningococcal (A39.52)
    mumps (B26.82)
    rheumatoid arthritis (M05.31)
    sarcoid (D86.85)
    syphilis (A52.06)
    toxoplasmosis (B58.81)
    tuberculous (A18.84)

DEF: Myocarditis: Inflammation of the middle layer of the heart, which is composed of muscle tissue.
CC Excl: PDX collection 677

✓4th I42 Cardiomyopathy

INCLUDES myocardiopathy

Code first pre-existing cardiomyopathy complicating pregnancy and puerperium (O99.4)

EXCLUDES 2 *ischemic cardiomyopathy (I25.5)*
    peripartum cardiomyopathy (O90.3)
    ventricular hypertrophy (I51.7)

CC Excl: For CC codes in category I42: PDX collection 678

I42.0 Dilated cardiomyopathy `CC` `HCC`
  Congestive cardiomyopathy

I42.1 Obstructive hypertrophic cardiomyopathy `HCC`
  Hypertrophic subaortic stenosis (idiopathic)
  DEF: Cardiomyopathy marked by left ventricle hypertrophy and an enlarged septum that result in obstructed blood flow, arrhythmias, mitral regurgitation, and sudden cardiac death.
  TIP: When this condition is described as inherited, assign code Q24.8.

I42.2 Other hypertrophic cardiomyopathy `HCC`
  Nonobstructive hypertrophic cardiomyopathy

I42.3 Endomyocardial (eosinophilic) disease `HCC`
  Endomyocardial (tropical) fibrosis
  Löffler's endocarditis

I42.4 Endocardial fibroelastosis `HCC`
  Congenital cardiomyopathy
  Elastomyofibrosis

I42.5 Other restrictive cardiomyopathy `HCC`
  Constrictive cardiomyopathy NOS

I42.6 Alcoholic cardiomyopathy `CC` `HCC`
  Code also presence of alcoholism (F10.-)

I42.7 Cardiomyopathy due to drug and external agent `CC` `HCC`
  Code first poisoning due to drug or toxin, if applicable (T36-T65 with fifth or sixth character 1-4 or 6)
  Use additional code for adverse effect, if applicable, to identify drug (T36-T50 with fifth or sixth character 5)

I42.8 Other cardiomyopathies `CC` `HCC`

I42.9 Cardiomyopathy, unspecified `CC` `HCC`
  Cardiomyopathy (primary) (secondary) NOS

I43 Cardiomyopathy in diseases classified elsewhere `CC` `HCC`

Code first underlying disease, such as:
  amyloidosis (E85.-)
  glycogen storage disease (E74.0)
  gout (M10.0-)
  thyrotoxicosis (E05.0-E05.9-)

EXCLUDES 1 cardiomyopathy (in):
    coxsackie (virus) (B33.24)
    diphtheria (A36.81)
    sarcoidosis (D86.85)
    tuberculosis (A18.84)

CC Excl: PDX collection 678

✓4th I44 Atrioventricular and left bundle-branch block

I44.0 Atrioventricular block, first degree

I44.1 Atrioventricular block, second degree
  Atrioventricular block, type I and II
  Möbitz block, type I and II
  Second degree block, type I and II
  Wenckebach's block

I44.2 Atrioventricular block, complete `CC` `HCC`
  Complete heart block NOS
  Third degree block
  AHA: 2019,2Q,4
  CC Excl: PDX collection 679

✓5th I44.3 Other and unspecified atrioventricular block
  Atrioventricular block NOS

  I44.30 Unspecified atrioventricular block
  I44.39 Other atrioventricular block

I44.4 Left anterior fascicular block

I44.5 Left posterior fascicular block

✓5th I44.6 Other and unspecified fascicular block

  I44.60 Unspecified fascicular block
    Left bundle-branch hemiblock NOS

  I44.69 Other fascicular block

I44.7 Left bundle-branch block, unspecified

Conduction Disorders

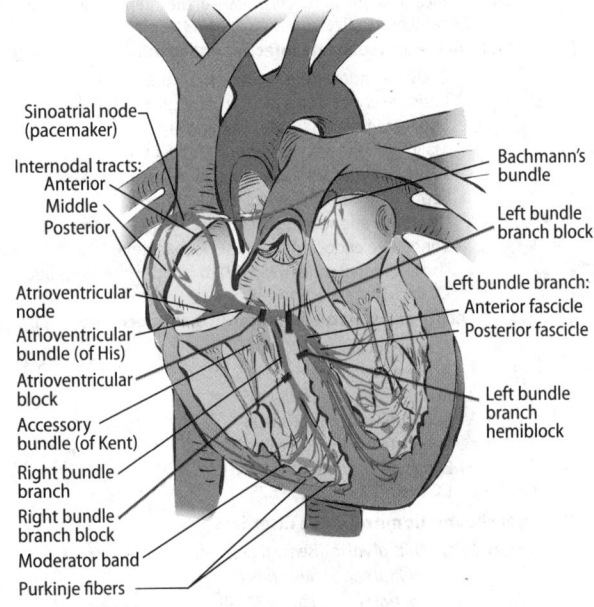

Sinoatrial node (pacemaker)
Internodal tracts:
  Anterior
  Middle
  Posterior
Atrioventricular node
Atrioventricular bundle (of His)
Atrioventricular block
Accessory bundle (of Kent)
Right bundle branch
Right bundle branch block
Moderator band
Purkinje fibers
Bachmann's bundle
Left bundle branch block
Left bundle branch:
  Anterior fascicle
  Posterior fascicle
Left bundle branch hemiblock

✓4th I45 Other conduction disorders

CC Excl: For CC codes in category I45: PDX collection 679

I45.0 Right fascicular block

✓5th I45.1 Other and unspecified right bundle-branch block

  I45.10 Unspecified right bundle-branch block
    Right bundle-branch block NOS

  I45.19 Other right bundle-branch block

I45.2 Bifascicular block `CC`

I45.3 Trifascicular block `CC`

I45.4 Nonspecific intraventricular block
  Bundle-branch block NOS

I45.5 Other specified heart block
  Sinoatrial block
  Sinoauricular block
  EXCLUDES 1 *heart block NOS (I45.9)*

I45.6 Pre-excitation syndrome
  Accelerated atrioventricular conduction
  Accessory atrioventricular conduction
  Anomalous atrioventricular excitation
  Lown-Ganong-Levine syndrome
  Pre-excitation atrioventricular conduction
  Wolff-Parkinson-White syndrome

`N` Newborn: 0   `P` Pediatric: 0-17   `M` Maternity: 9-64   `A` Adult: 15-124   `MCC` Major Complication/Comorbidity   `CC` Complication/Comorbidity   `SW` Severe Wound Dx

656   ICD-10-CM 2020

✓5ᵗʰ **I45.8**   **Other specified conduction disorders**

I45.81   **Long QT syndrome**
DEF: Condition characterized by recurrent syncope, malignant arrhythmias, and sudden death. This syndrome has a characteristic prolonged Q-T interval on an electrocardiogram.

I45.89   **Other specified conduction disorders**
Atrioventricular [AV] dissociation
Interference dissociation
Isorhythmic dissociation
Nonparoxysmal AV nodal tachycardia
AHA: 2013,2Q,31

I45.9   **Conduction disorder, unspecified**
Heart block NOS
Stokes-Adams syndrome

✓4ᵗʰ **I46**   **Cardiac arrest**
     EXCLUDES 1   *cardiogenic shock (R57.0)*
AHA: 2019,2Q,4-5

I46.2   **Cardiac arrest due to underlying cardiac condition**   HCC
Code first underlying cardiac condition

I46.8   **Cardiac arrest due to other underlying condition**   HCC
Code first underlying condition

I46.9   **Cardiac arrest, cause unspecified**   HCC

✓4ᵗʰ **I47**   **Paroxysmal tachycardia**
Code first tachycardia complicating:
    abortion or ectopic or molar pregnancy (O00-O07, O08.8)
    obstetric surgery and procedures (O75.4)
     EXCLUDES 1   *tachycardia NOS (R00.0)*
                sinoauricular tachycardia NOS (R00.0)
                sinus [sinusal] tachycardia NOS (R00.0)
CC Excl: For CC codes in category I47: PDX collection 679

I47.0   **Re-entry ventricular arrhythmia**   CC HCC

I47.1   **Supraventricular tachycardia**   CC HCC
Atrial (paroxysmal) tachycardia
Atrioventricular [AV] (paroxysmal) tachycardia
Atrioventricular re-entrant (nodal) tachycardia [AVNRT] [AVRT]
Junctional (paroxysmal) tachycardia
Nodal (paroxysmal) tachycardia

I47.2   **Ventricular tachycardia**   CC HCC
AHA: 2013,3Q,23

I47.9   **Paroxysmal tachycardia, unspecified**   HCC
Bouveret (-Hoffman) syndrome

✓4ᵗʰ **I48**   **Atrial fibrillation and flutter**
CC Excl: For CC codes in category I48: PDX collection 679

I48.0   **Paroxysmal atrial fibrillation**   HCC
AHA: 2018,3Q,6

▲ ✓5ᵗʰ **I48.1**   **Persistent atrial fibrillation**
     EXCLUDES 1   ▶*permanent atrial fibrillation (I48.21)*◀
AHA: 2019,2Q,3; 2018,3Q,6

● **I48.11**   **Longstanding persistent atrial fibrillation**   CC

● **I48.19**   **Other persistent atrial fibrillation**   CC
Chronic persistent atrial fibrillation
Persistent atrial fibrillation, NOS

▲ ✓5ᵗʰ **I48.2**   **Chronic atrial fibrillation**
~~Permanent atrial fibrillation~~
AHA: 2019,2Q,3; 2018,3Q,6

● **I48.20**   **Chronic atrial fibrillation, unspecified**   CC
     EXCLUDES 1   *chronic persistent atrial fibrillation (I48.19)*

● **I48.21**   **Permanent atrial fibrillation**   CC

I48.3   **Typical atrial flutter**   CC HCC
Type I atrial flutter

I48.4   **Atypical atrial flutter**   CC HCC
Type II atrial flutter

✓5ᵗʰ **I48.9**   **Unspecified atrial fibrillation and atrial flutter**

I48.91   **Unspecified atrial fibrillation**   HCC

I48.92   **Unspecified atrial flutter**   CC HCC

✓4ᵗʰ **I49**   **Other cardiac arrhythmias**
Code first cardiac arrhythmia complicating:
    abortion or ectopic or molar pregnancy (O00-O07, O08.8)
    obstetric surgery and procedures (O75.4)
     EXCLUDES 1   *neonatal dysrhythmia (P29.1-)*
                sinoatrial bradycardia (R00.1)
                sinus bradycardia (R00.1)
                vagal bradycardia (R00.1)
     EXCLUDES 2   *bradycardia NOS (R00.1)*
CC Excl: For CC codes in category I49: PDX collection 679

✓5ᵗʰ **I49.0**   **Ventricular fibrillation and flutter**

I49.01   **Ventricular fibrillation**   CC HCC

I49.02   **Ventricular flutter**   CC HCC

I49.1   **Atrial premature depolarization**
Atrial premature beats

I49.2   **Junctional premature depolarization**   CC HCC

I49.3   **Ventricular premature depolarization**

✓5ᵗʰ **I49.4**   **Other and unspecified premature depolarization**

I49.40   **Unspecified premature depolarization**
Premature beats NOS

I49.49   **Other premature depolarization**
Ectopic beats
Extrasystoles
Extrasystolic arrhythmias
Premature contractions

I49.5   **Sick sinus syndrome**   HCC
Tachycardia-bradycardia syndrome
AHA: 2019,1Q,33
TIP: The presence of a pacemaker controls but does not cure sick sinus syndrome and therefore is considered a reportable chronic condition. When a pacemaker is evaluated by a provider, this code and code Z95.0 Presence of cardiac pacemaker, should be reported, even in the absence of any notable changes or management.

I49.8   **Other specified cardiac arrhythmias**
Brugada syndrome
Coronary sinus rhythm disorder
Ectopic rhythm disorder
Nodal rhythm disorder

I49.9   **Cardiac arrhythmia, unspecified**
Arrhythmia (cardiac) NOS

✓4ᵗʰ **I50**   **Heart failure**
Code first:
    heart failure complicating abortion or ectopic or molar pregnancy (O00-O07, O08.8)
    heart failure due to hypertension (I11.0)
    heart failure due to hypertension with chronic kidney disease (I13.-)
    heart failure following surgery (I97.13-)
    obstetric surgery and procedures (O75.4)
    rheumatic heart failure (I09.81)
     EXCLUDES 1   *neonatal cardiac failure (P29.0)*
     EXCLUDES 2   *cardiac arrest (I46.-)*
AHA: 2018,4Q,67; 2018,2Q,9; 2017,1Q,47; 2014,1Q,25; 2013,2Q,33
CC Excl: For CC/MCC codes in category I50, unless otherwise noted: PDX collection 682

I50.1   **Left ventricular failure, unspecified**   CC HCC
Cardiac asthma
Edema of lung with heart disease NOS
Edema of lung with heart failure
Left heart failure
Pulmonary edema with heart disease NOS
Pulmonary edema with heart failure
     EXCLUDES 1   *edema of lung without heart disease or heart failure (J81.-)*
                pulmonary edema without heart disease or failure (J81.-)
CC Excl: PDX collection 681

✔ Additional Character Required   ✔x7ᵗʰ Placeholder   Unacceptable PDx   Questionable PDx   Manifestation   Unspecified Dx   H1 - H14 HAC   HCC CMS-HCC Dx   HIV HIV Dx

ICD-10-CM 2020   **657**

√5ᵗʰ **I50.2 Systolic (congestive) heart failure**

Heart failure with reduced ejection fraction [HFrEF]
Systolic left ventricular heart failure
Code also end stage heart failure, if applicable (I50.84)

> EXCLUDES 1   combined systolic (congestive) and diastolic (congestive) heart failure (I50.4-)

AHA: 2017,1Q,46; 2016,1Q,10

I50.20 Unspecified systolic (congestive) heart failure `CC` `HCC`

I50.21 Acute systolic (congestive) heart failure `MCC` `HCC`
> CC Excl: PDX collection 2025

I50.22 Chronic systolic (congestive) heart failure `HCC`

I50.23 Acute on chronic systolic (congestive) heart failure `MCC` `HCC`

√5ᵗʰ **I50.3 Diastolic (congestive) heart failure**

Diastolic left ventricular heart failure
Heart failure with normal ejection fraction
Heart failure with preserved ejection fraction [HFpEF]
Code also end stage heart failure, if applicable (I50.84)

> EXCLUDES 1   combined systolic (congestive) and diastolic (congestive) heart failure (I50.4-)

AHA: 2017,1Q,46; 2016,1Q,10

I50.30 Unspecified diastolic (congestive) heart failure `CC` `HCC`

I50.31 Acute diastolic (congestive) heart failure `MCC` `HCC`
> CC Excl: PDX collection 2025

I50.32 Chronic diastolic (congestive) heart failure `HCC`

I50.33 Acute on chronic diastolic (congestive) heart failure `MCC` `HCC`

√5ᵗʰ **I50.4 Combined systolic (congestive) and diastolic (congestive) heart failure**

Combined systolic and diastolic left ventricular heart failure
Heart failure with reduced ejection fraction and diastolic dysfunction
Code also end stage heart failure, if applicable (I50.84)

AHA: 2017,1Q,46; 2016,1Q,10

I50.40 Unspecified combined systolic (congestive) and diastolic (congestive) heart failure `CC` `HCC`

I50.41 Acute combined systolic (congestive) and diastolic (congestive) heart failure `MCC` `HCC`

I50.42 Chronic combined systolic (congestive) and diastolic (congestive) heart failure `HCC`

I50.43 Acute on chronic combined systolic (congestive) and diastolic (congestive) heart failure `MCC` `HCC`

√5ᵗʰ **I50.8 Other heart failure**

AHA: 2017,4Q,15-16

√6ᵗʰ **I50.81 Right heart failure**

Right ventricular failure

I50.810 Right heart failure, unspecified `HCC`

Right heart failure without mention of left heart failure
Right ventricular failure NOS

I50.811 Acute right heart failure `HCC`

Acute isolated right heart failure
Acute (isolated) right ventricular failure

I50.812 Chronic right heart failure `HCC`

Chronic isolated right heart failure
Chronic (isolated) right ventricular failure

I50.813 Acute on chronic right heart failure `HCC`

Acute on chronic isolated right heart failure
Acute on chronic (isolated) right ventricular failure
Acute decompensation of chronic (isolated) right ventricular failure
Acute exacerbation of chronic (isolated) right ventricular failure

I50.814 Right heart failure due to left heart failure `HCC`

Right ventricular failure secondary to left ventricular failure
Code also the type of left ventricular failure, if known (I50.2-I50.43)

> EXCLUDES 1   right heart failure with but not due to left heart failure (I50.82)

I50.82 Biventricular heart failure `HCC`

Code also the type of left ventricular failure as systolic, diastolic, or combined, if known (I50.2-I50.43)

I50.83 High output heart failure `HCC`

> DEF: Occurs when the high demand for blood exceeds the capacity of a normally functioning heart to meet the demand.

I50.84 End stage heart failure `HCC`

Stage D heart failure
Code also the type of heart failure as systolic, diastolic, or combined, if known (I50.2-I50.43)

I50.89 Other heart failure `HCC`

I50.9 Heart failure, unspecified `HCC`

Cardiac, heart or myocardial failure NOS
Congestive heart disease
Congestive heart failure NOS

> EXCLUDES 2   ▶fluid overload unrelated to congestive heart failure◀ (E87.70)

AHA: 2017,4Q,15-16; 2017,1Q,45-46; 2014,4Q,21; 2012,4Q,92

√4ᵗʰ **I51 Complications and ill-defined descriptions of heart disease**

> EXCLUDES 1   any condition in I51.4-I51.9 due to hypertension (I11.-)
> any condition in I51.4-I51.9 due to hypertension and chronic kidney disease (I13.-)
> heart disease specified as rheumatic (I00-I09)

I51.0 Cardiac septal defect, acquired `CC` `A`

Acquired septal atrial defect (old)
Acquired septal auricular defect (old)
Acquired septal ventricular defect (old)

> EXCLUDES 1   cardiac septal defect as current complication following acute myocardial infarction (I23.1, I23.2)

> DEF: Abnormal communication between opposite heart chambers due to a defect of the septum. It is not present at birth.

CC Excl: PDX collection 654

I51.1 Rupture of chordae tendineae, not elsewhere classified `CC` `HCC`

> EXCLUDES 1   rupture of chordae tendineae as current complication following acute myocardial infarction (I23.4)

I51.2 Rupture of papillary muscle, not elsewhere classified `CC` `HCC`

> EXCLUDES 1   rupture of papillary muscle as current complication following acute myocardial infarction (I23.5)

I51.3 Intracardiac thrombosis, not elsewhere classified `CC`

Apical thrombosis (old)
Atrial thrombosis (old)
Auricular thrombosis (old)
Mural thrombosis (old)
Ventricular thrombosis (old)

> EXCLUDES 1   intracardiac thrombosis as current complication following acute myocardial infarction (I23.6)

AHA: 2013,1Q,24

I51.4 Myocarditis, unspecified `HCC`

Chronic (interstitial) myocarditis
Myocardial fibrosis
Myocarditis NOS

> EXCLUDES 1   acute or subacute myocarditis (I40.-)

AHA: 2018,4Q,67; 2018,2Q,9

I51.5 Myocardial degeneration `HCC`

Fatty degeneration of heart or myocardium
Myocardial disease
Senile degeneration of heart or myocardium

AHA: 2018,4Q,67; 2018,2Q,9

Ⓝ Newborn: 0   Ⓟ Pediatric: 0-17   Ⓜ Maternity: 9-64   Ⓐ Adult: 15-124   `MCC` Major Complication/Comorbidity   `CC` Complication/Comorbidity   `SW` Severe Wound Dx

658   ICD-10-CM 2020

I51.7 Cardiomegaly
Cardiac dilatation
Cardiac hypertrophy
Ventricular dilatation
AHA: 2018,4Q,67; 2018,2Q,9

√5ᵗʰ **I51.8 Other ill-defined heart diseases**
AHA: 2018,2Q,9

I51.81 Takotsubo syndrome   `CC`
Reversible left ventricular dysfunction following
sudden emotional stress
Stress induced cardiomyopathy
Takotsubo cardiomyopathy
Transient left ventricular apical ballooning syndrome
DEF: Complex of symptoms mimicking myocardial
infarct in absence of heart disease, with the majority
of cases occurring in postmenopausal women. Heart
muscles are temporarily weakened, and a sudden,
massive surge of adrenalin stuns the heart, greatly
reducing the ability to pump blood.
CC Excl: PDX collection 683

I51.89 Other ill-defined heart diseases
Carditis (acute)(chronic)
Pancarditis (acute)(chronic)
AHA: 2019,2Q,5; 2018,4Q,67

I51.9 Heart disease, unspecified
AHA: 2018,4Q,67; 2018,2Q,9

I52 Other heart disorders in diseases classified elsewhere
Code first underlying disease, such as:
congenital syphilis (A50.5)
mucopolysaccharidosis (E76.3)
schistosomiasis (B65.0-B65.9)
EXCLUDES 1   heart disease (in):
gonococcal infection (A54.83)
meningococcal infection (A39.50)
rheumatoid arthritis (M05.31)
syphilis (A52.06)

Cerebrovascular diseases (I60-I69)

Use additional code to identify presence of:
alcohol abuse and dependence (F10.-)
exposure to environmental tobacco smoke (Z77.22)
history of tobacco dependence (Z87.891)
hypertension (I10-I16)
occupational exposure to environmental tobacco smoke (Z57.31)
tobacco dependence (F17.-)
tobacco use (Z72.0)
EXCLUDES 1   traumatic intracranial hemorrhage (S06.-)
AHA: 2014,3Q,5; 2012,4Q,91-92

√4ᵗʰ **I60 Nontraumatic subarachnoid hemorrhage**
EXCLUDES 1   syphilitic ruptured cerebral aneurysm (A52.05)
EXCLUDES 2   sequelae of subarachnoid hemorrhage (I69.0-)
CC Excl: For MCC codes in category I60: PDX collection 684

√5ᵗʰ **I60.0 Nontraumatic subarachnoid hemorrhage from carotid siphon and bifurcation**

I60.00 Nontraumatic subarachnoid hemorrhage `MCC` `HCC`
from unspecified carotid siphon and bifurcation

I60.01 Nontraumatic subarachnoid hemorrhage `MCC` `HCC`
from right carotid siphon and bifurcation

I60.02 Nontraumatic subarachnoid hemorrhage `MCC` `HCC`
from left carotid siphon and bifurcation

√5ᵗʰ **I60.1 Nontraumatic subarachnoid hemorrhage from middle cerebral artery**

I60.10 Nontraumatic subarachnoid hemorrhage `MCC` `HCC`
from unspecified middle cerebral artery

I60.11 Nontraumatic subarachnoid hemorrhage `MCC` `HCC`
from right middle cerebral artery

I60.12 Nontraumatic subarachnoid hemorrhage `MCC` `HCC`
from left middle cerebral artery

I60.2 Nontraumatic subarachnoid hemorrhage from `MCC` `HCC`
anterior communicating artery

√5ᵗʰ **I60.3 Nontraumatic subarachnoid hemorrhage from posterior communicating artery**

I60.30 Nontraumatic subarachnoid hemorrhage `MCC` `HCC`
from unspecified posterior communicating artery

I60.31 Nontraumatic subarachnoid hemorrhage `MCC` `HCC`
from right posterior communicating artery

I60.32 Nontraumatic subarachnoid hemorrhage `MCC` `HCC`
from left posterior communicating artery

I60.4 Nontraumatic subarachnoid hemorrhage from `MCC` `HCC`
basilar artery

√5ᵗʰ **I60.5 Nontraumatic subarachnoid hemorrhage from vertebral artery**

I60.50 Nontraumatic subarachnoid hemorrhage `MCC` `HCC`
from unspecified vertebral artery

I60.51 Nontraumatic subarachnoid hemorrhage `MCC` `HCC`
from right vertebral artery

I60.52 Nontraumatic subarachnoid hemorrhage `MCC` `HCC`
from left vertebral artery

I60.6 Nontraumatic subarachnoid hemorrhage from `MCC` `HCC`
other intracranial arteries

I60.7 Nontraumatic subarachnoid hemorrhage from `MCC` `HCC`
unspecified intracranial artery
Ruptured (congenital) berry aneurysm
Ruptured (congenital) cerebral aneurysm
Subarachnoid hemorrhage (nontraumatic) from cerebral artery
NOS
Subarachnoid hemorrhage (nontraumatic) from communicating
artery NOS
EXCLUDES 1   berry aneurysm, nonruptured (I67.1)

I60.8 Other nontraumatic subarachnoid hemorrhage `MCC` `HCC`
Meningeal hemorrhage
Rupture of cerebral arteriovenous malformation

I60.9 Nontraumatic subarachnoid hemorrhage, `MCC` `HCC`
unspecified

√4ᵗʰ **I61 Nontraumatic intracerebral hemorrhage**
EXCLUDES 2   sequelae of intracerebral hemorrhage (I69.1-)
AHA: 2017,2Q,9-10
CC Excl: For MCC codes in category I61: PDX collection 684

I61.0 Nontraumatic intracerebral hemorrhage in `MCC` `HCC`
hemisphere, subcortical
Deep intracerebral hemorrhage (nontraumatic)
AHA: 2016,4Q,27

I61.1 Nontraumatic intracerebral hemorrhage in `MCC` `HCC`
hemisphere, cortical
Cerebral lobe hemorrhage (nontraumatic)
Superficial intracerebral hemorrhage (nontraumatic)

I61.2 Nontraumatic intracerebral hemorrhage in `MCC` `HCC`
hemisphere, unspecified

I61.3 Nontraumatic intracerebral hemorrhage in brain `MCC` `HCC`
stem

I61.4 Nontraumatic intracerebral hemorrhage in `MCC` `HCC`
cerebellum

I61.5 Nontraumatic intracerebral hemorrhage, `MCC` `HCC`
intraventricular

I61.6 Nontraumatic intracerebral hemorrhage, multiple `MCC` `HCC`
localized

I61.8 Other nontraumatic intracerebral hemorrhage `MCC` `HCC`

I61.9 Nontraumatic intracerebral hemorrhage, `MCC` `HCC`
unspecified

√4ᵗʰ **I62 Other and unspecified nontraumatic intracranial hemorrhage**
EXCLUDES 2   sequelae of intracranial hemorrhage (I69.2)
CC Excl: For CC/MCC codes in category I62: PDX collection 684

√5ᵗʰ **I62.0 Nontraumatic subdural hemorrhage**

I62.00 Nontraumatic subdural hemorrhage, `MCC` `HCC`
unspecified

I62.01 Nontraumatic acute subdural `MCC` `HCC`
hemorrhage

I62.02 Nontraumatic subacute subdural `MCC` `HCC`
hemorrhage

I62.03 Nontraumatic chronic subdural `CC` `HCC`
hemorrhage

I62.1 Nontraumatic extradural hemorrhage `MCC` `HCC`
Nontraumatic epidural hemorrhage

I62.9 Nontraumatic intracranial hemorrhage, `CC` `HCC`
unspecified

√4ᵗʰ **I63 Cerebral infarction**

INCLUDES   occlusion and stenosis of cerebral and precerebral arteries, resulting in cerebral infarction

Use additional code, if applicable, to identify status post administration of tPA (rtPA) in a different facility within the last 24 hours prior to admission to current facility (Z92.82)

Use additional code, if known, to indicate National Institutes of Health Stroke Scale (NIHSS) score (R29.7-)

EXCLUDES 2   *sequelae of cerebral infarction (I69.3-)*

AHA: 2017,2Q,9-10; 2016,4Q,28,61-62; 2014,1Q,23

TIP: Weakness on one side of the body documented as secondary to stroke is synonymous with hemiparesis/hemiplegia (G81.-). Weakness of one limb documented as secondary to stroke is synonymous with monoplegia (G83.1-, G83.2-, G83.3-).

√5ᵗʰ **I63.0 Cerebral infarction due to thrombosis of precerebral arteries**

     I63.00 Cerebral infarction due to thrombosis of unspecified precerebral artery MCC HCC
       CC Excl: PDX collection 685

     √6ᵗʰ **I63.01 Cerebral infarction due to thrombosis of vertebral artery**
       CC Excl: For MCC codes in subcategory I63.01: PDX collection 686

       I63.011 Cerebral infarction due to thrombosis of right vertebral artery MCC HCC

       I63.012 Cerebral infarction due to thrombosis of left vertebral artery MCC HCC

       I63.013 Cerebral infarction due to thrombosis of bilateral vertebral arteries MCC HCC

       I63.019 Cerebral infarction due to thrombosis of unspecified vertebral artery MCC HCC

     I63.02 Cerebral infarction due to thrombosis of basilar artery MCC HCC
       CC Excl: PDX collection 685

     √6ᵗʰ **I63.03 Cerebral infarction due to thrombosis of carotid artery**
       CC Excl: For MCC codes in subcategory I63.03: PDX collection 687

       I63.031 Cerebral infarction due to thrombosis of right carotid artery MCC HCC

       I63.032 Cerebral infarction due to thrombosis of left carotid artery MCC HCC

       I63.033 Cerebral infarction due to thrombosis of bilateral carotid arteries MCC HCC

       I63.039 Cerebral infarction due to thrombosis of unspecified carotid artery MCC HCC

     I63.09 Cerebral infarction due to thrombosis of other precerebral artery MCC HCC
       CC Excl: PDX collection 685

√5ᵗʰ **I63.1 Cerebral infarction due to embolism of precerebral arteries**

     I63.10 Cerebral infarction due to embolism of unspecified precerebral artery MCC HCC
       CC Excl: PDX collection 685

     √6ᵗʰ **I63.11 Cerebral infarction due to embolism of vertebral artery**
       CC Excl: For MCC codes in subcategory I63.13: PDX collection 686

       I63.111 Cerebral infarction due to embolism of right vertebral artery MCC HCC

       I63.112 Cerebral infarction due to embolism of left vertebral artery MCC HCC

       I63.113 Cerebral infarction due to embolism of bilateral vertebral arteries MCC HCC

       I63.119 Cerebral infarction due to embolism of unspecified vertebral artery MCC HCC

     I63.12 Cerebral infarction due to embolism of basilar artery MCC HCC
       CC Excl: PDX collection 685

     √6ᵗʰ **I63.13 Cerebral infarction due to embolism of carotid artery**
       CC Excl: For MCC codes in subcategory I63.13: PDX collection 687

       I63.131 Cerebral infarction due to embolism of right carotid artery MCC HCC

       I63.132 Cerebral infarction due to embolism of left carotid artery MCC HCC

       I63.133 Cerebral infarction due to embolism of bilateral carotid arteries MCC HCC

       I63.139 Cerebral infarction due to embolism of unspecified carotid artery MCC HCC

     I63.19 Cerebral infarction due to embolism of other precerebral artery MCC HCC
       CC Excl: PDX collection 685

√5ᵗʰ **I63.2 Cerebral infarction due to unspecified occlusion or stenosis of precerebral arteries**

     I63.20 Cerebral infarction due to unspecified occlusion or stenosis of unspecified precerebral arteries MCC HCC
       CC Excl: PDX collection 685

     √6ᵗʰ **I63.21 Cerebral infarction due to unspecified occlusion or stenosis of vertebral arteries**
       CC Excl: For MCC codes in subcategory I63.21: PDX collection 686

       I63.211 Cerebral infarction due to unspecified occlusion or stenosis of right vertebral artery MCC HCC

       I63.212 Cerebral infarction due to unspecified occlusion or stenosis of left vertebral artery MCC HCC

       I63.213 Cerebral infarction due to unspecified occlusion or stenosis of bilateral vertebral arteries MCC HCC

       I63.219 Cerebral infarction due to unspecified occlusion or stenosis of unspecified vertebral artery MCC HCC

     I63.22 Cerebral infarction due to unspecified occlusion or stenosis of basilar artery MCC HCC
       CC Excl: PDX collection 685

     √6ᵗʰ **I63.23 Cerebral infarction due to unspecified occlusion or stenosis of carotid arteries**
       CC Excl: For MCC codes in subcategory I63.23: PDX collection 687

       I63.231 Cerebral infarction due to unspecified occlusion or stenosis of right carotid arteries MCC HCC

       I63.232 Cerebral infarction due to unspecified occlusion or stenosis of left carotid arteries MCC HCC

       I63.233 Cerebral infarction due to unspecified occlusion or stenosis of bilateral carotid arteries MCC HCC

       I63.239 Cerebral infarction due to unspecified occlusion or stenosis of unspecified carotid artery MCC HCC

     I63.29 Cerebral infarction due to unspecified occlusion or stenosis of other precerebral arteries MCC HCC
       CC Excl: PDX collection 685

√5ᵗʰ **I63.3 Cerebral infarction due to thrombosis of cerebral arteries**
     CC Excl: For MCC codes in subcategory I63.3: PDX collection 688

     I63.30 Cerebral infarction due to thrombosis of unspecified cerebral artery MCC HCC

     √6ᵗʰ **I63.31 Cerebral infarction due to thrombosis of middle cerebral artery**

       I63.311 Cerebral infarction due to thrombosis of right middle cerebral artery MCC HCC

       I63.312 Cerebral infarction due to thrombosis of left middle cerebral artery MCC HCC

N Newborn: 0   P Pediatric: 0-17   M Maternity: 9-64   A Adult: 15-124   MCC Major Complication/Comorbidity   CC Complication/Comorbidity   SW Severe Wound Dx

660   ICD-10-CM 2020

I63.313   **Cerebral infarction due to thrombosis of** bilateral **middle cerebral arteries**   MCC HCC

I63.319   **Cerebral infarction due to thrombosis of unspecified middle cerebral artery**   MCC HCC

✓6ᵗʰ   **I63.32**   **Cerebral infarction due to thrombosis of** anterior **cerebral artery**

    I63.321   **Cerebral infarction due to thrombosis of** right **anterior cerebral artery**   MCC HCC

    I63.322   **Cerebral infarction due to thrombosis of** left **anterior cerebral artery**   MCC HCC

    I63.323   **Cerebral infarction due to thrombosis of** bilateral **anterior cerebral arteries**   MCC HCC

    I63.329   **Cerebral infarction due to thrombosis of unspecified anterior cerebral artery**   MCC HCC

✓6ᵗʰ   **I63.33**   **Cerebral infarction due to thrombosis of** posterior **cerebral artery**

    I63.331   **Cerebral infarction due to thrombosis of** right **posterior cerebral artery**   MCC HCC

    I63.332   **Cerebral infarction due to thrombosis of** left **posterior cerebral artery**   MCC HCC

    I63.333   **Cerebral infarction due to thrombosis of** bilateral **posterior cerebral arteries**   MCC HCC

    I63.339   **Cerebral infarction due to thrombosis of unspecified posterior cerebral artery**   MCC HCC

✓6ᵗʰ   **I63.34**   **Cerebral infarction due to thrombosis of** cerebellar **artery**

    I63.341   **Cerebral infarction due to thrombosis of** right **cerebellar artery**   MCC HCC

    I63.342   **Cerebral infarction due to thrombosis of** left **cerebellar artery**   MCC HCC

    I63.343   **Cerebral infarction due to thrombosis of** bilateral **cerebellar arteries**   MCC HCC

    I63.349   **Cerebral infarction due to thrombosis of unspecified cerebellar artery**   MCC HCC

  I63.39   **Cerebral infarction due to thrombosis of other cerebral artery**   MCC HCC

✓5ᵗʰ   **I63.4**   **Cerebral infarction due to** embolism of cerebral **arteries**

    CC Excl: For MCC codes in subcategory I63.4: PDX collection 688

  I63.40   **Cerebral infarction due to embolism of unspecified cerebral artery**   MCC HCC

✓6ᵗʰ   **I63.41**   **Cerebral infarction due to embolism of** middle **cerebral artery**

    I63.411   **Cerebral infarction due to embolism of** right **middle cerebral artery**   MCC HCC

    I63.412   **Cerebral infarction due to embolism of** left **middle cerebral artery**   MCC HCC

    I63.413   **Cerebral infarction due to embolism of** bilateral **middle cerebral arteries**   MCC HCC

    I63.419   **Cerebral infarction due to embolism of unspecified middle cerebral artery**   MCC HCC

✓6ᵗʰ   **I63.42**   **Cerebral infarction due to embolism of** anterior **cerebral artery**

    I63.421   **Cerebral infarction due to embolism of** right **anterior cerebral artery**   MCC HCC

    I63.422   **Cerebral infarction due to embolism of** left **anterior cerebral artery**   MCC HCC

    I63.423   **Cerebral infarction due to embolism of** bilateral **anterior cerebral arteries**   MCC HCC

    I63.429   **Cerebral infarction due to embolism of unspecified anterior cerebral artery**   MCC HCC

✓6ᵗʰ   **I63.43**   **Cerebral infarction due to embolism of** posterior **cerebral artery**

    I63.431   **Cerebral infarction due to embolism of** right **posterior cerebral artery**   MCC HCC

    I63.432   **Cerebral infarction due to embolism of** left **posterior cerebral artery**   MCC HCC

    I63.433   **Cerebral infarction due to embolism of** bilateral **posterior cerebral arteries**   MCC HCC

    I63.439   **Cerebral infarction due to embolism of unspecified posterior cerebral artery**   MCC HCC

✓6ᵗʰ   **I63.44**   **Cerebral infarction due to embolism of** cerebellar **artery**

    I63.441   **Cerebral infarction due to embolism of** right **cerebellar artery**   MCC HCC

    I63.442   **Cerebral infarction due to embolism of** left **cerebellar artery**   MCC HCC

    I63.443   **Cerebral infarction due to embolism of** bilateral **cerebellar arteries**   MCC HCC

    I63.449   **Cerebral infarction due to embolism of unspecified cerebellar artery**   MCC HCC

  I63.49   **Cerebral infarction due to embolism of other cerebral artery**   MCC HCC

✓5ᵗʰ   **I63.5**   **Cerebral infarction due to unspecified** occlusion or stenosis of cerebral **arteries**

    CC Excl: For MCC codes in subcategory I63.5: PDX collection 688

  I63.50   **Cerebral infarction due to unspecified occlusion or stenosis of unspecified cerebral artery**   MCC HCC

✓6ᵗʰ   **I63.51**   **Cerebral infarction due to unspecified occlusion or stenosis of** middle **cerebral artery**

    I63.511   **Cerebral infarction due to unspecified occlusion or stenosis of** right **middle cerebral artery**   MCC HCC

    I63.512   **Cerebral infarction due to unspecified occlusion or stenosis of** left **middle cerebral artery**   MCC HCC

    I63.513   **Cerebral infarction due to unspecified occlusion or stenosis of** bilateral **middle cerebral arteries**   MCC HCC

    I63.519   **Cerebral infarction due to unspecified occlusion or stenosis of unspecified middle cerebral artery**   MCC HCC

✓6ᵗʰ   **I63.52**   **Cerebral infarction due to unspecified occlusion or stenosis of** anterior **cerebral artery**

    I63.521   **Cerebral infarction due to unspecified occlusion or stenosis of** right **anterior cerebral artery**   MCC HCC

    I63.522   **Cerebral infarction due to unspecified occlusion or stenosis of** left **anterior cerebral artery**   MCC HCC

    I63.523   **Cerebral infarction due to unspecified occlusion or stenosis of** bilateral **anterior cerebral arteries**   MCC HCC

    I63.529   **Cerebral infarction due to unspecified occlusion or stenosis of unspecified anterior cerebral artery**   MCC HCC

✓6ᵗʰ   **I63.53**   **Cerebral infarction due to unspecified occlusion or stenosis of** posterior **cerebral artery**

    I63.531   **Cerebral infarction due to unspecified occlusion or stenosis of** right **posterior cerebral artery**   MCC HCC

    I63.532   **Cerebral infarction due to unspecified occlusion or stenosis of** left **posterior cerebral artery**   MCC HCC

✔ Additional Character Required   ✓x7ᵗʰ Placeholder   Unacceptable PDx   Questionable PDx   Manifestation   Unspecified Dx   H1 - H14 HAC   HCC CMS-HCC Dx   HIV HIV Dx

I63.533 Cerebral infarction due to unspecified occlusion or stenosis of bilateral posterior cerebral arteries `MCC` `HCC`

I63.539 Cerebral infarction due to unspecified occlusion or stenosis of unspecified posterior cerebral artery `MCC` `HCC`

√6ᵗʰ **I63.54** Cerebral infarction due to unspecified occlusion or stenosis of cerebellar artery

I63.541 Cerebral infarction due to unspecified occlusion or stenosis of right cerebellar artery `MCC` `HCC`

I63.542 Cerebral infarction due to unspecified occlusion or stenosis of left cerebellar artery `MCC` `HCC`

I63.543 Cerebral infarction due to unspecified occlusion or stenosis of bilateral cerebellar arteries `MCC` `HCC`

I63.549 Cerebral infarction due to unspecified occlusion or stenosis of unspecified cerebellar artery `MCC` `HCC`

I63.59 Cerebral infarction due to unspecified occlusion or stenosis of other cerebral artery `MCC` `HCC`

I63.6 Cerebral infarction due to cerebral venous thrombosis, nonpyogenic `MCC` `HCC`
CC Excl: PDX collection 688

√5ᵗʰ **I63.8** Other cerebral infarction
AHA: 2018,4Q,16

I63.81 Other cerebral infarction due to occlusion or stenosis of small artery `MCC` `HCC`
Lacunar infarction
CC Excl: PDX collection 688

I63.89 Other cerebral infarction `MCC` `HCC`
CC Excl: PDX collection 688

I63.9 Cerebral infarction, unspecified `MCC` `HCC`
Stroke NOS
EXCLUDES 2   transient cerebral ischemic attacks and related syndromes (G45.-)
AHA: 2015,1Q,25
TIP: When provider documentation does not identify the location of an infarction, imaging reports can be used to pinpoint the location and lead to a more specific infarction code.
CC Excl: PDX collection 688

√4ᵗʰ **I65 Occlusion and stenosis of precerebral arteries, not resulting in cerebral infarction**
INCLUDES   embolism of precerebral artery
narrowing of precerebral artery
obstruction (complete) (partial) of precerebral artery
thrombosis of precerebral artery
EXCLUDES 1   insufficiency, NOS, of precerebral artery (G45.-)
insufficiency of precerebral arteries causing cerebral infarction (I63.Ø-I63.2)
AHA: 2018,2Q,9

√5ᵗʰ **I65.Ø** Occlusion and stenosis of vertebral artery
I65.Ø1 Occlusion and stenosis of right vertebral artery
I65.Ø2 Occlusion and stenosis of left vertebral artery
I65.Ø3 Occlusion and stenosis of bilateral vertebral arteries `CC`
I65.Ø9 Occlusion and stenosis of unspecified vertebral artery

I65.1 Occlusion and stenosis of basilar artery

√5ᵗʰ **I65.2** Occlusion and stenosis of carotid artery
I65.21 Occlusion and stenosis of right carotid artery
I65.22 Occlusion and stenosis of left carotid artery
I65.23 Occlusion and stenosis of bilateral carotid arteries
I65.29 Occlusion and stenosis of unspecified carotid artery

I65.8 Occlusion and stenosis of other precerebral arteries
I65.9 Occlusion and stenosis of unspecified precerebral artery
Occlusion and stenosis of precerebral artery NOS

√4ᵗʰ **I66 Occlusion and stenosis of cerebral arteries, not resulting in cerebral infarction**
INCLUDES   embolism of cerebral artery
narrowing of cerebral artery
obstruction (complete) (partial) of cerebral artery
thrombosis of cerebral artery
EXCLUDES 1   occlusion and stenosis of cerebral artery causing cerebral infarction (I63.3-I63.5)

√5ᵗʰ **I66.Ø** Occlusion and stenosis of middle cerebral artery
I66.Ø1 Occlusion and stenosis of right middle cerebral artery
I66.Ø2 Occlusion and stenosis of left middle cerebral artery
I66.Ø3 Occlusion and stenosis of bilateral middle cerebral arteries
I66.Ø9 Occlusion and stenosis of unspecified middle cerebral artery

√5ᵗʰ **I66.1** Occlusion and stenosis of anterior cerebral artery
I66.11 Occlusion and stenosis of right anterior cerebral artery
I66.12 Occlusion and stenosis of left anterior cerebral artery
I66.13 Occlusion and stenosis of bilateral anterior cerebral arteries
I66.19 Occlusion and stenosis of unspecified anterior cerebral artery

√5ᵗʰ **I66.2** Occlusion and stenosis of posterior cerebral artery
I66.21 Occlusion and stenosis of right posterior cerebral artery
I66.22 Occlusion and stenosis of left posterior cerebral artery
I66.23 Occlusion and stenosis of bilateral posterior cerebral arteries
I66.29 Occlusion and stenosis of unspecified posterior cerebral artery

I66.3 Occlusion and stenosis of cerebellar arteries
I66.8 Occlusion and stenosis of other cerebral arteries
Occlusion and stenosis of perforating arteries
I66.9 Occlusion and stenosis of unspecified cerebral artery

√4ᵗʰ **I67 Other cerebrovascular diseases**
EXCLUDES 2   sequelae of the listed conditions (I69.8)
I67.Ø Dissection of cerebral arteries, nonruptured `MCC` `HCC`
EXCLUDES 1   ruptured cerebral arteries (I6Ø.7)
CC Excl: PDX collection 689

N Newborn: 0   P Pediatric: 0-17   M Maternity: 9-64   A Adult: 15-124   `MCC` Major Complication/Comorbidity   `CC` Complication/Comorbidity   `SW` Severe Wound Dx

662   ICD-10-CM 2020

I67.1 Cerebral aneurysm, nonruptured
Cerebral aneurysm NOS
Cerebral arteriovenous fistula, acquired
Internal carotid artery aneurysm, intracranial portion
Internal carotid artery aneurysm, NOS
> **EXCLUDES 1**   congenital cerebral aneurysm, nonruptured (Q28.-)
> ruptured cerebral aneurysm (I60.7)

Berry Aneurysm

Berry aneurysms form at the site of a weakness in an arterial wall, often at a junction

Berry aneurysm

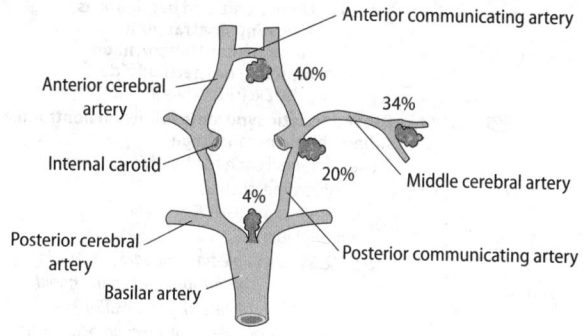

Anterior communicating artery
Anterior cerebral artery
Internal carotid
Posterior cerebral artery
Basilar artery
Posterior communicating artery
Middle cerebral artery
40%
34%
20%
4%

Common sites of berry aneurysms in the circle of Willis arteries

I67.2 Cerebral atherosclerosis   [A]
Atheroma of cerebral and precerebral arteries

I67.3 Progressive vascular leukoencephalopathy   [HIV] [CC] [HCC]
Binswanger's disease
CC Excl: PDX collection 133

I67.4 Hypertensive encephalopathy   [CC]
> **EXCLUDES 2**   insufficiency, NOS, of precerebral arteries (G45.2)

CC Excl: PDX collection 690

I67.5 Moyamoya disease   [CC]
DEF: Cerebrovascular ischemia. Vessels occlude and rupture, causing tiny hemorrhages at the base of brain. It affects predominantly Japanese people.
CC Excl: PDX collection 691

I67.6 Nonpyogenic thrombosis of intracranial venous system   [CC]
Nonpyogenic thrombosis of cerebral vein
Nonpyogenic thrombosis of intracranial venous sinus
> **EXCLUDES 1**   nonpyogenic thrombosis of intracranial venous system causing infarction (I63.6)

CC Excl: PDX collection 692

I67.7 Cerebral arteritis, not elsewhere classified   [CC]
Granulomatous angiitis of the nervous system
> **EXCLUDES 1**   allergic granulomatous angiitis (M30.1)

CC Excl: PDX collection 693

✓5ᵗʰ I67.8 Other specified cerebrovascular diseases
CC Excl: For CC codes in subcategory I67.8, unless otherwise noted: PDX collection 694

I67.81 Acute cerebrovascular insufficiency   [CC]
Acute cerebrovascular insufficiency unspecified as to location or reversibility

I67.82 Cerebral ischemia   [CC]
Chronic cerebral ischemia

I67.83 Posterior reversible encephalopathy syndrome   [HIV] [MCC]
PRES
CC Excl: PDX collection 610

✓6ᵗʰ I67.84 Cerebral vasospasm and vasoconstriction

I67.841 Reversible cerebrovascular vasoconstriction syndrome   [CC]
Call-Fleming syndrome
Code first underlying condition, if applicable, such as eclampsia (O15.00-O15.9)
CC Excl: PDX collection 586

I67.848 Other cerebrovascular vasospasm and vasoconstriction   [CC]
CC Excl: PDX collection 586

✓6ᵗʰ I67.85 Hereditary cerebrovascular diseases
AHA: 2018,4Q,17

I67.850 Cerebral autosomal dominant arteriopathy with subcortical infarcts and leukoencephalopathy   [CC]
CADASIL
Code also any associated diagnoses, such as:
epilepsy (G40.-)
stroke (I63.-)
vascular dementia (F01.-)

I67.858 Other hereditary cerebrovascular disease   [CC]

I67.89 Other cerebrovascular disease

I67.9 Cerebrovascular disease, unspecified

✓4ᵗʰ I68 Cerebrovascular disorders in diseases classified elsewhere

I68.0 Cerebral amyloid angiopathy
Code first underlying amyloidosis (E85.-)

I68.2 Cerebral arteritis in other diseases classified elsewhere   [CC]
Code first underlying disease
> **EXCLUDES 1**   cerebral arteritis (in):
> listerosis (A32.89)
> syphilis (A52.04)
> systemic lupus erythematosus (M32.19)
> tuberculosis (A18.89)

CC Excl: PDX collection 693

I68.8 Other cerebrovascular disorders in diseases classified elsewhere
Code first underlying disease
> **EXCLUDES 1**   syphilitic cerebral aneurysm (A52.05)

✓4ᵗʰ I69 Sequelae of cerebrovascular disease

NOTE   Category I69 is to be used to indicate conditions in I60-I67 as the cause of sequelae. The "sequelae" include conditions specified as such or as residuals which may occur at any time after the onset of the causal condition

> **EXCLUDES 1**   personal history of cerebral infarction without residual deficit (Z86.73)
> personal history of prolonged reversible ischemic neurologic deficit (PRIND) (Z86.73)
> personal history of reversible ischemic neurolocgial deficit (RIND) (Z86.73)
> sequelae of traumatic intracranial injury (S06.-)

AHA: 2017,1Q,47; 2016,4Q,28; 2015,1Q,25; 2012,4Q,106
TIP: Weakness on one side of the body (unilateral weakness) documented as secondary to old cerebrovascular disease is synonymous with hemiparesis/hemiplegia. Weakness of one limb documented as secondary to old cerebrovascular disease is synonymous with monoplegia.
TIP: For codes describing hemiplegia, hemiparesis, and monoplegia; if the documentation identifies the affected side but not whether it is the dominant or nondominant side, the default is as follows: for ambidextrous patients, the default is dominant; when the left side is affected, the default is nondominant; and when the right side is affected, the default is dominant.

✓5ᵗʰ I69.0 Sequelae of nontraumatic subarachnoid hemorrhage

I69.00 Unspecified sequelae of nontraumatic subarachnoid hemorrhage

✓6ᵗʰ I69.01 Cognitive deficits following nontraumatic subarachnoid hemorrhage

I69.010 Attention and concentration deficit following nontraumatic subarachnoid hemorrhage

I69.011 Memory deficit following nontraumatic subarachnoid hemorrhage

Chapter 9. Diseases of the Circulatory System

I69.012 Visuospatial deficit and spatial neglect following nontraumatic subarachnoid hemorrhage

I69.013 Psychomotor deficit following nontraumatic subarachnoid hemorrhage

I69.014 Frontal lobe and executive function deficit following nontraumatic subarachnoid hemorrhage

I69.015 Cognitive social or emotional deficit following nontraumatic subarachnoid hemorrhage

I69.018 Other symptoms and signs involving cognitive functions following nontraumatic subarachnoid hemorrhage

I69.019 Unspecified symptoms and signs involving cognitive functions following nontraumatic subarachnoid hemorrhage

✓6th I69.02 Speech and language deficits following nontraumatic subarachnoid hemorrhage

I69.020 Aphasia following nontraumatic subarachnoid hemorrhage

I69.021 Dysphasia following nontraumatic subarachnoid hemorrhage

I69.022 Dysarthria following nontraumatic subarachnoid hemorrhage

I69.023 Fluency disorder following nontraumatic subarachnoid hemorrhage

Stuttering following nontraumatic subarachnoid hemorrhage

I69.028 Other speech and language deficits following nontraumatic subarachnoid hemorrhage

✓6th I69.03 Monoplegia of upper limb following nontraumatic subarachnoid hemorrhage

AHA: 2017,1Q,47

I69.031 Monoplegia of upper limb following nontraumatic subarachnoid hemorrhage affecting right dominant side   HCC

I69.032 Monoplegia of upper limb following nontraumatic subarachnoid hemorrhage affecting left dominant side   HCC

I69.033 Monoplegia of upper limb following nontraumatic subarachnoid hemorrhage affecting right non-dominant side   HCC

I69.034 Monoplegia of upper limb following nontraumatic subarachnoid hemorrhage affecting left non-dominant side   HCC

I69.039 Monoplegia of upper limb following nontraumatic subarachnoid hemorrhage affecting unspecified side   HCC

✓6th I69.04 Monoplegia of lower limb following nontraumatic subarachnoid hemorrhage

AHA: 2017,1Q,47

I69.041 Monoplegia of lower limb following nontraumatic subarachnoid hemorrhage affecting right dominant side   HCC

I69.042 Monoplegia of lower limb following nontraumatic subarachnoid hemorrhage affecting left dominant side   HCC

I69.043 Monoplegia of lower limb following nontraumatic subarachnoid hemorrhage affecting right non-dominant side   HCC

I69.044 Monoplegia of lower limb following nontraumatic subarachnoid hemorrhage affecting left non-dominant side   HCC

I69.049 Monoplegia of lower limb following nontraumatic subarachnoid hemorrhage affecting unspecified side   HCC

✓6th I69.05 Hemiplegia and hemiparesis following nontraumatic subarachnoid hemorrhage

AHA: 2015,1Q,25

I69.051 Hemiplegia and hemiparesis following nontraumatic subarachnoid hemorrhage affecting right dominant side   CC HCC

CC Excl: PDX collection 695

I69.052 Hemiplegia and hemiparesis following nontraumatic subarachnoid hemorrhage affecting left dominant side   CC HCC

CC Excl: PDX collection 695

I69.053 Hemiplegia and hemiparesis following nontraumatic subarachnoid hemorrhage affecting right non-dominant side   CC HCC

CC Excl: PDX collection 696

I69.054 Hemiplegia and hemiparesis following nontraumatic subarachnoid hemorrhage affecting left non-dominant side   CC HCC

CC Excl: PDX collection 696

I69.059 Hemiplegia and hemiparesis following nontraumatic subarachnoid hemorrhage affecting unspecified side   CC HCC

CC Excl: PDX collection 697

✓6th I69.06 Other paralytic syndrome following nontraumatic subarachnoid hemorrhage

Use additional code to identify type of paralytic syndrome, such as:
locked-in state (G83.5)
quadriplegia (G82.5-)

EXCLUDES 1 hemiplegia/hemiparesis following nontraumatic subarachnoid hemorrhage (I69.05-)
monoplegia of lower limb following nontraumatic subarachnoid hemorrhage (I69.04-)
monoplegia of upper limb following nontraumatic subarachnoid hemorrhage (I69.03-)

I69.061 Other paralytic syndrome following nontraumatic subarachnoid hemorrhage affecting right dominant side   HCC

I69.062 Other paralytic syndrome following nontraumatic subarachnoid hemorrhage affecting left dominant side   HCC

I69.063 Other paralytic syndrome following nontraumatic subarachnoid hemorrhage affecting right non-dominant side   HCC

I69.064 Other paralytic syndrome following nontraumatic subarachnoid hemorrhage affecting left non-dominant side   HCC

I69.065 Other paralytic syndrome following nontraumatic subarachnoid hemorrhage, bilateral   HCC

I69.069 Other paralytic syndrome following nontraumatic subarachnoid hemorrhage affecting unspecified side   HCC

✓6th I69.09 Other sequelae of nontraumatic subarachnoid hemorrhage

I69.090 Apraxia following nontraumatic subarachnoid hemorrhage

I69.091 Dysphagia following nontraumatic subarachnoid hemorrhage

Use additional code to identify the type of dysphagia, if known (R13.1-)

I69.092 Facial weakness following nontraumatic subarachnoid hemorrhage

Facial droop following nontraumatic subarachnoid hemorrhage

N Newborn: 0   P Pediatric: 0-17   M Maternity: 9-64   A Adult: 15-124   MCC Major Complication/Comorbidity   CC Complication/Comorbidity   SW Severe Wound Dx

664   ICD-10-CM 2020

I69.093   **Ataxia following nontraumatic subarachnoid hemorrhage**

I69.098   **Other sequelae following nontraumatic subarachnoid hemorrhage**

Alterations of sensation following nontraumatic subarachnoid hemorrhage

Disturbance of vision following nontraumatic subarachnoid hemorrhage

Use additional code to identify the sequelae

√5th   I69.1   Sequelae of nontraumatic intracerebral hemorrhage

    I69.10   Unspecified sequelae of nontraumatic intracerebral hemorrhage

    √6th   I69.11   Cognitive deficits following nontraumatic intracerebral hemorrhage

I69.110   **Attention and concentration deficit following nontraumatic intracerebral hemorrhage**

I69.111   **Memory deficit following nontraumatic intracerebral hemorrhage**

I69.112   **Visuospatial deficit and spatial neglect following nontraumatic intracerebral hemorrhage**

I69.113   **Psychomotor deficit following nontraumatic intracerebral hemorrhage**

I69.114   **Frontal lobe and executive function deficit following nontraumatic intracerebral hemorrhage**

I69.115   **Cognitive social or emotional deficit following nontraumatic intracerebral hemorrhage**

I69.118   **Other symptoms and signs involving cognitive functions following nontraumatic intracerebral hemorrhage**

I69.119   **Unspecified symptoms and signs involving cognitive functions following nontraumatic intracerebral hemorrhage**

    √6th   I69.12   Speech and language deficits following nontraumatic intracerebral hemorrhage

I69.120   **Aphasia following nontraumatic intracerebral hemorrhage**

I69.121   **Dysphasia following nontraumatic intracerebral hemorrhage**

I69.122   **Dysarthria following nontraumatic intracerebral hemorrhage**

I69.123   **Fluency disorder following nontraumatic intracerebral hemorrhage**

Stuttering following nontraumatic intracerebral hemorrhage

I69.128   **Other speech and language deficits following nontraumatic intracerebral hemorrhage**

    √6th   I69.13   Monoplegia of upper limb following nontraumatic intracerebral hemorrhage

AHA: 2017,1Q,47

I69.131   **Monoplegia of upper limb following nontraumatic intracerebral hemorrhage affecting right dominant side**   HCC

I69.132   **Monoplegia of upper limb following nontraumatic intracerebral hemorrhage affecting left dominant side**   HCC

I69.133   **Monoplegia of upper limb following nontraumatic intracerebral hemorrhage affecting right non-dominant side**   HCC

I69.134   **Monoplegia of upper limb following nontraumatic intracerebral hemorrhage affecting left non-dominant side**   HCC

I69.139   **Monoplegia of upper limb following nontraumatic intracerebral hemorrhage affecting unspecified side**   HCC

√6th   I69.14   Monoplegia of lower limb following nontraumatic intracerebral hemorrhage

AHA: 2017,1Q,47

I69.141   **Monoplegia of lower limb following nontraumatic intracerebral hemorrhage affecting right dominant side**   HCC

I69.142   **Monoplegia of lower limb following nontraumatic intracerebral hemorrhage affecting left dominant side**   HCC

I69.143   **Monoplegia of lower limb following nontraumatic intracerebral hemorrhage affecting right non-dominant side**   HCC

I69.144   **Monoplegia of lower limb following nontraumatic intracerebral hemorrhage affecting left non-dominant side**   HCC

I69.149   **Monoplegia of lower limb following nontraumatic intracerebral hemorrhage affecting unspecified side**   HCC

√6th   I69.15   Hemiplegia and hemiparesis following nontraumatic intracerebral hemorrhage

AHA: 2015,1Q,25

I69.151   **Hemiplegia and hemiparesis following nontraumatic intracerebral hemorrhage affecting right dominant side**   CC HCC

     CC Excl: PDX collection 695

I69.152   **Hemiplegia and hemiparesis following nontraumatic intracerebral hemorrhage affecting left dominant side**   CC HCC

     CC Excl: PDX collection 695

I69.153   **Hemiplegia and hemiparesis following nontraumatic intracerebral hemorrhage affecting right non-dominant side**   CC HCC

     CC Excl: PDX collection 696

I69.154   **Hemiplegia and hemiparesis following nontraumatic intracerebral hemorrhage affecting left non-dominant side**   CC HCC

     CC Excl: PDX collection 696

I69.159   **Hemiplegia and hemiparesis following nontraumatic intracerebral hemorrhage affecting unspecified side**   CC HCC

     CC Excl: PDX collection 697

√6th   I69.16   Other paralytic syndrome following nontraumatic intracerebral hemorrhage

Use additional code to identify type of paralytic syndrome, such as:

locked-in state (G83.5)

quadriplegia (G82.5-)

EXCLUDES 1   hemiplegia/hemiparesis following nontraumatic intracerebral hemorrhage (I69.15-)

monoplegia of lower limb following nontraumatic intracerebral hemorrhage (I69.14-)

monoplegia of upper limb following nontraumatic intracerebral hemorrhage (I69.13-)

I69.161   **Other paralytic syndrome following nontraumatic intracerebral hemorrhage affecting right dominant side**   HCC

I69.162   **Other paralytic syndrome following nontraumatic intracerebral hemorrhage affecting left dominant side**   HCC

I69.163   **Other paralytic syndrome following nontraumatic intracerebral hemorrhage affecting right non-dominant side**   HCC

☑ Additional Character Required   √x7th Placeholder   Unacceptable PDx   Questionable PDx   Manifestation   Unspecified Dx   H1-H4 HAC   HCC CMS-HCC Dx   HIV HIV Dx

ICD-10-CM 2020

665

    I69.164   Other paralytic syndrome following nontraumatic intracerebral hemorrhage affecting left non-dominant side   `HCC`

    I69.165   Other paralytic syndrome following nontraumatic intracerebral hemorrhage, bilateral   `HCC`

    I69.169   Other paralytic syndrome following nontraumatic intracerebral hemorrhage affecting unspecified side   `HCC`

✓6th   **I69.19**   Other sequelae of nontraumatic intracerebral hemorrhage

    I69.190   Apraxia following nontraumatic intracerebral hemorrhage

    I69.191   Dysphagia following nontraumatic intracerebral hemorrhage
         Use additional code to identify the type of dysphagia, if known (R13.1-)

    I69.192   Facial weakness following nontraumatic intracerebral hemorrhage
         Facial droop following nontraumatic intracerebral hemorrhage

    I69.193   Ataxia following nontraumatic intracerebral hemorrhage

    I69.198   Other sequelae of nontraumatic intracerebral hemorrhage
         Alteration of sensations following nontraumatic intracerebral hemorrhage
         Disturbance of vision following nontraumatic intracerebral hemorrhage
         Use additional code to identify the sequelae

✓5th   **I69.2**   Sequelae of other nontraumatic intracranial hemorrhage

    I69.20   Unspecified sequelae of other nontraumatic intracranial hemorrhage

✓6th   **!I69.21**   Cognitive deficits following other nontraumatic intracranial hemorrhage

    I69.210   Attention and concentration deficit following other nontraumatic intracranial hemorrhage

    I69.211   Memory deficit following other nontraumatic intracranial hemorrhage

    I69.212   Visuospatial deficit and spatial neglect following other nontraumatic intracranial hemorrhage

    I69.213   Psychomotor deficit following other nontraumatic intracranial hemorrhage

    I69.214   Frontal lobe and executive function deficit following other nontraumatic intracranial hemorrhage

    I69.215   Cognitive social or emotional deficit following other nontraumatic intracranial hemorrhage

    I69.218   Other symptoms and signs involving cognitive functions following other nontraumatic intracranial hemorrhage

    I69.219   Unspecified symptoms and signs involving cognitive functions following other nontraumatic intracranial hemorrhage

✓6th   **I69.22**   Speech and language deficits following other nontraumatic intracranial hemorrhage

    I69.220   Aphasia following other nontraumatic intracranial hemorrhage

    I69.221   Dysphasia following other nontraumatic intracranial hemorrhage

    I69.222   Dysarthria following other nontraumatic intracranial hemorrhage

    I69.223   Fluency disorder following other nontraumatic intracranial hemorrhage
         Stuttering following other nontraumatic intracranial hemorrhage

    I69.228   Other speech and language deficits following other nontraumatic intracranial hemorrhage

✓6th   **I69.23**   Monoplegia of upper limb following other nontraumatic intracranial hemorrhage
     AHA: 2017,1Q,47

    I69.231   Monoplegia of upper limb following other nontraumatic intracranial hemorrhage affecting right dominant side   `HCC`

    I69.232   Monoplegia of upper limb following other nontraumatic intracranial hemorrhage affecting left dominant side   `HCC`

    I69.233   Monoplegia of upper limb following other nontraumatic intracranial hemorrhage affecting right non-dominant side   `HCC`

    I69.234   Monoplegia of upper limb following other nontraumatic intracranial hemorrhage affecting left non-dominant side   `HCC`

    I69.239   Monoplegia of upper limb following other nontraumatic intracranial hemorrhage affecting unspecified side   `HCC`

✓6th   **I69.24**   Monoplegia of lower limb following other nontraumatic intracranial hemorrhage
     AHA: 2017,1Q,47

    I69.241   Monoplegia of lower limb following other nontraumatic intracranial hemorrhage affecting right dominant side   `HCC`

    I69.242   Monoplegia of lower limb following other nontraumatic intracranial hemorrhage affecting left dominant side   `HCC`

    I69.243   Monoplegia of lower limb following other nontraumatic intracranial hemorrhage affecting right non-dominant side   `HCC`

    I69.244   Monoplegia of lower limb following other nontraumatic intracranial hemorrhage affecting left non-dominant side   `HCC`

    I69.249   Monoplegia of lower limb following other nontraumatic intracranial hemorrhage affecting unspecified side   `HCC`

✓6th   **I69.25**   Hemiplegia and hemiparesis following other nontraumatic intracranial hemorrhage
     AHA: 2015,1Q,25

    I69.251   Hemiplegia and hemiparesis following other nontraumatic intracranial hemorrhage affecting right dominant side   `CC` `HCC`
         CC Excl: PDX collection 695

    I69.252   Hemiplegia and hemiparesis following other nontraumatic intracranial hemorrhage affecting left dominant side   `CC` `HCC`
         CC Excl: PDX collection 695

    I69.253   Hemiplegia and hemiparesis following other nontraumatic intracranial hemorrhage affecting right non-dominant side   `CC` `HCC`
         CC Excl: PDX collection 696

    I69.254   Hemiplegia and hemiparesis following other nontraumatic intracranial hemorrhage affecting left non-dominant side   `CC` `HCC`
         CC Excl: PDX collection 696

    I69.259   Hemiplegia and hemiparesis following other nontraumatic intracranial hemorrhage affecting unspecified side   `CC` `HCC`
         CC Excl: PDX collection 697

N Newborn: 0   P Pediatric: 0-17   M Maternity: 9-64   A Adult: 15-124   MCC Major Complication/Comorbidity   CC Complication/Comorbidity   SW Severe Wound Dx

666   ICD-10-CM 2020

✓6ᵗʰ **I69.26** **Other paralytic syndrome following other nontraumatic intracranial hemorrhage**

Use additional code to identify type of paralytic syndrome, such as:

locked-in state (G83.5)

quadriplegia (G82.5-)

> **EXCLUDES 1**   *hemiplegia/hemiparesis following other nontraumatic intracranial hemorrhage (I69.25-)*
> *monoplegia of lower limb following other nontraumatic intracranial hemorrhage (I69.24-)*
> *monoplegia of upper limb following other nontraumatic intracranial hemorrhage (I69.23-)*

  I69.261 **Other paralytic syndrome following other nontraumatic intracranial hemorrhage affecting right dominant side**   `HCC`

  I69.262 **Other paralytic syndrome following other nontraumatic intracranial hemorrhage affecting left dominant side**   `HCC`

  I69.263 **Other paralytic syndrome following other nontraumatic intracranial hemorrhage affecting right non-dominant side**   `HCC`

  I69.264 **Other paralytic syndrome following other nontraumatic intracranial hemorrhage affecting left non-dominant side**   `HCC`

  I69.265 **Other paralytic syndrome following other nontraumatic intracranial hemorrhage, bilateral**   `HCC`

  I69.269 **Other paralytic syndrome following other nontraumatic intracranial hemorrhage affecting unspecified side**   `HCC`

✓6ᵗʰ **I69.29** **Other sequelae of other nontraumatic intracranial hemorrhage**

  I69.290 **Apraxia following other nontraumatic intracranial hemorrhage**

  I69.291 **Dysphagia following other nontraumatic intracranial hemorrhage**

Use additional code to identify the type of dysphagia, if known (R13.1-)

  I69.292 **Facial weakness following other nontraumatic intracranial hemorrhage**

Facial droop following other nontraumatic intracranial hemorrhage

  I69.293 **Ataxia following other nontraumatic intracranial hemorrhage**

  I69.298 **Other sequelae of other nontraumatic intracranial hemorrhage**

Alteration of sensation following other nontraumatic intracranial hemorrhage

Disturbance of vision following other nontraumatic intracranial hemorrhage

Use additional code to identify the sequelae

✓5ᵗʰ **I69.3** **Sequelae of cerebral infarction**

Sequelae of stroke NOS

AHA: 2013,4Q,127-128; 2012,4Q,92,94

  I69.30 **Unspecified sequelae of cerebral infarction**

✓6ᵗʰ **I69.31** **Cognitive deficits following cerebral infarction**

  I69.310 **Attention and concentration deficit following cerebral infarction**

  I69.311 **Memory deficit following cerebral infarction**

  I69.312 **Visuospatial deficit and spatial neglect following cerebral infarction**

  I69.313 **Psychomotor deficit following cerebral infarction**

  I69.314 **Frontal lobe and executive function deficit following cerebral infarction**

  I69.315 **Cognitive social or emotional deficit following cerebral infarction**

  I69.318 **Other symptoms and signs involving cognitive functions following cerebral infarction**

  I69.319 **Unspecified symptoms and signs involving cognitive functions following cerebral infarction**

✓6ᵗʰ **I69.32** **Speech and language deficits following cerebral infarction**

  I69.320 **Aphasia following cerebral infarction**

  I69.321 **Dysphasia following cerebral infarction**

    AHA: 2012,4Q,91

  I69.322 **Dysarthria following cerebral infarction**

> **EXCLUDES 2**   *transient ischemic attack (TIA) (G45.9)*

  I69.323 **Fluency disorder following cerebral infarction**

Stuttering following cerebral infarction

  I69.328 **Other speech and language deficits following cerebral infarction**

✓6ᵗʰ **I69.33** **Monoplegia of upper limb following cerebral infarction**

AHA: 2017,1Q,47

  I69.331 **Monoplegia of upper limb following cerebral infarction affecting right dominant side**   `HCC`

  I69.332 **Monoplegia of upper limb following cerebral infarction affecting left dominant side**   `HCC`

  I69.333 **Monoplegia of upper limb following cerebral infarction affecting right non-dominant side**   `HCC`

  I69.334 **Monoplegia of upper limb following cerebral infarction affecting left non-dominant side**   `HCC`

  I69.339 **Monoplegia of upper limb following cerebral infarction affecting unspecified side**   `HCC`

✓6ᵗʰ **I69.34** **Monoplegia of lower limb following cerebral infarction**

AHA: 2017,1Q,47

  I69.341 **Monoplegia of lower limb following cerebral infarction affecting right dominant side**   `HCC`

  I69.342 **Monoplegia of lower limb following cerebral infarction affecting left dominant side**   `HCC`

  I69.343 **Monoplegia of lower limb following cerebral infarction affecting right non-dominant side**   `HCC`

  I69.344 **Monoplegia of lower limb following cerebral infarction affecting left non-dominant side**   `HCC`

  I69.349 **Monoplegia of lower limb following cerebral infarction affecting unspecified side**   `HCC`

✓6ᵗʰ **I69.35** **Hemiplegia and hemiparesis following cerebral infarction**

AHA: 2015,1Q,25

  I69.351 **Hemiplegia and hemiparesis following cerebral infarction affecting right dominant side**   `CC` `HCC`

> **EXCLUDES 2**   *transient ischemic attack (TIA) (G45.9)*

    CC Excl: PDX collection 695

  I69.352 **Hemiplegia and hemiparesis following cerebral infarction affecting left dominant side**   `CC` `HCC`

    CC Excl: PDX collection 695

  I69.353 **Hemiplegia and hemiparesis following cerebral infarction affecting right non-dominant side**   `CC` `HCC`

    CC Excl: PDX collection 696

  I69.354 **Hemiplegia and hemiparesis following cerebral infarction affecting left non-dominant side**   `CC` `HCC`

    AHA: 2012,4Q,91

    CC Excl: PDX collection 696

✔ Additional Character Required   ✓x7ᵗʰ Placeholder   Unacceptable PDx   Questionable PDx   Manifestation   Unspecified Dx   H1 - H14 HAC   HCC CMS-HCC Dx   HIV HIV Dx

ICD-10-CM 2020

667

Chapter 9. Diseases of the Circulatory System

I69.359 **Hemiplegia and hemiparesis following cerebral infarction affecting unspecified side** `CC` `HCC`
CC Excl: PDX collection 697

√6ᵗʰ I69.36 **Other paralytic syndrome following cerebral infarction**
Use additional code to identify type of paralytic syndrome, such as:
locked-in state (G83.5)
quadriplegia (G82.5-)
EXCLUDES 1   *hemiplegia/hemiparesis following cerebral infarction (I69.35-)*
monoplegia of lower limb following cerebral infarction (I69.34-)
monoplegia of upper limb following cerebral infarction (I69.33-)

I69.361 **Other paralytic syndrome following cerebral infarction affecting right dominant side** `HCC`

I69.362 **Other paralytic syndrome following cerebral infarction affecting left dominant side** `HCC`

I69.363 **Other paralytic syndrome following cerebral infarction affecting right non-dominant side** `HCC`

I69.364 **Other paralytic syndrome following cerebral infarction affecting left non-dominant side** `HCC`

I69.365 **Other paralytic syndrome following cerebral infarction, bilateral** `HCC`

I69.369 **Other paralytic syndrome following cerebral infarction affecting unspecified side** `HCC`

√6ᵗʰ I69.39 **Other sequelae of cerebral infarction**

I69.390 **Apraxia following cerebral infarction**

I69.391 **Dysphagia following cerebral infarction**
Use additional code to identify the type of dysphagia, if known (R13.1-)

I69.392 **Facial weakness following cerebral infarction**
Facial droop following cerebral infarction

I69.393 **Ataxia following cerebral infarction**

I69.398 **Other sequelae of cerebral infarction**
Alteration of sensation following cerebral infarction
Disturbance of vision following cerebral infarction
Use additional code to identify the sequelae

√6ᵗʰ I69.8 **Sequelae of other cerebrovascular diseases**
EXCLUDES 1   *sequelae of traumatic intracranial injury (S06.-)*

I69.80 **Unspecified sequelae of other cerebrovascular disease**

√6ᵗʰ I69.81 **Cognitive deficits following other cerebrovascular disease**

I69.810 **Attention and concentration deficit following other cerebrovascular disease**

I69.811 **Memory deficit following other cerebrovascular disease**

I69.812 **Visuospatial deficit and spatial neglect following other cerebrovascular disease**

I69.813 **Psychomotor deficit following other cerebrovascular disease**

I69.814 **Frontal lobe and executive function deficit following other cerebrovascular disease**

I69.815 **Cognitive social or emotional deficit following other cerebrovascular disease**

I69.818 **Other symptoms and signs involving cognitive functions following other cerebrovascular disease**

I69.819 **Unspecified symptoms and signs involving cognitive functions following other cerebrovascular disease**

√6ᵗʰ I69.82 **Speech and language deficits following other cerebrovascular disease**

I69.820 **Aphasia following other cerebrovascular disease**

I69.821 **Dysphasia following other cerebrovascular disease**

I69.822 **Dysarthria following other cerebrovascular disease**

I69.823 **Fluency disorder following other cerebrovascular disease**
Stuttering following other cerebrovascular disease

I69.828 **Other speech and language deficits following other cerebrovascular disease**

√6ᵗʰ I69.83 **Monoplegia of upper limb following other cerebrovascular disease**
AHA: 2017,1Q,47

I69.831 **Monoplegia of upper limb following other cerebrovascular disease affecting right dominant side** `HCC`

I69.832 **Monoplegia of upper limb following other cerebrovascular disease affecting left dominant side** `HCC`

I69.833 **Monoplegia of upper limb following other cerebrovascular disease affecting right non-dominant side** `HCC`

I69.834 **Monoplegia of upper limb following other cerebrovascular disease affecting left non-dominant side** `HCC`

I69.839 **Monoplegia of upper limb following other cerebrovascular disease affecting unspecified side** `HCC`

√6ᵗʰ I69.84 **Monoplegia of lower limb following other cerebrovascular disease**
AHA: 2017,1Q,47

I69.841 **Monoplegia of lower limb following other cerebrovascular disease affecting right dominant side** `HCC`

I69.842 **Monoplegia of lower limb following other cerebrovascular disease affecting left dominant side** `HCC`

I69.843 **Monoplegia of lower limb following other cerebrovascular disease affecting right non-dominant side** `HCC`

I69.844 **Monoplegia of lower limb following other cerebrovascular disease affecting left non-dominant side** `HCC`

I69.849 **Monoplegia of lower limb following other cerebrovascular disease affecting unspecified side** `HCC`

√6ᵗʰ I69.85 **Hemiplegia and hemiparesis following other cerebrovascular disease**
AHA: 2015,1Q,25

I69.851 **Hemiplegia and hemiparesis following other cerebrovascular disease affecting right dominant side** `CC` `HCC`
CC Excl: PDX collection 695

I69.852 **Hemiplegia and hemiparesis following other cerebrovascular disease affecting left dominant side** `CC` `HCC`
CC Excl: PDX collection 695

I69.853 **Hemiplegia and hemiparesis following other cerebrovascular disease affecting right non-dominant side** `CC` `HCC`
CC Excl: PDX collection 696

I69.854   **Hemiplegia and hemiparesis following other cerebrovascular disease affecting left non-dominant side** `CC` `HCC`
> CC Excl: PDX collection 696

I69.859   **Hemiplegia and hemiparesis following other cerebrovascular disease affecting unspecified side** `CC` `HCC`
> CC Excl: PDX collection 697

√6ᵗʰ   **I69.86**   **Other paralytic syndrome following other cerebrovascular disease**
> Use additional code to identify type of paralytic syndrome, such as:
> locked-in state (G83.5)
> quadriplegia (G82.5-)
>
> *EXCLUDES 1*   *hemiplegia/hemiparesis following other cerebrovascular disease (I69.85-)*
> *monoplegia of lower limb following other cerebrovascular disease (I69.84-)*
> *monoplegia of upper limb following other cerebrovascular disease (I69.83-)*

I69.861   **Other paralytic syndrome following other cerebrovascular disease affecting right dominant side** `HCC`

I69.862   **Other paralytic syndrome following other cerebrovascular disease affecting left dominant side** `HCC`

I69.863   **Other paralytic syndrome following other cerebrovascular disease affecting right non-dominant side** `HCC`

I69.864   **Other paralytic syndrome following other cerebrovascular disease affecting left non-dominant side** `HCC`

I69.865   **Other paralytic syndrome following other cerebrovascular disease, bilateral** `HCC`

I69.869   **Other paralytic syndrome following other cerebrovascular disease affecting unspecified side** `HCC`

√6ᵗʰ   **I69.89**   **Other sequelae of other cerebrovascular disease**

I69.890   **Apraxia following other cerebrovascular disease**

I69.891   **Dysphagia following other cerebrovascular disease**
> Use additional code to identify the type of dysphagia, if known (R13.1-)

I69.892   **Facial weakness following other cerebrovascular disease**
> Facial droop following other cerebrovascular disease

I69.893   **Ataxia following other cerebrovascular disease**

I69.898   **Other sequelae of other cerebrovascular disease**
> Alteration of sensation following other cerebrovascular disease
> Disturbance of vision following other cerebrovascular disease
> Use additional code to identify the sequelae

√5ᵗʰ   **I69.9**   **Sequelae of unspecified cerebrovascular diseases**
> *EXCLUDES 1*   *sequelae of stroke (I69.3)*
> *sequelae of traumatic intracranial injury (S06.-)*

I69.90   **Unspecified sequelae of unspecified cerebrovascular disease**

√6ᵗʰ   **I69.91**   **Cognitive deficits following unspecified cerebrovascular disease**

I69.910   **Attention and concentration deficit following unspecified cerebrovascular disease**

I69.911   **Memory deficit following unspecified cerebrovascular disease**

I69.912   **Visuospatial deficit and spatial neglect following unspecified cerebrovascular disease**

I69.913   **Psychomotor deficit following unspecified cerebrovascular disease**

I69.914   **Frontal lobe and executive function deficit following unspecified cerebrovascular disease**

I69.915   **Cognitive social or emotional deficit following unspecified cerebrovascular disease**

I69.918   **Other symptoms and signs involving cognitive functions following unspecified cerebrovascular disease**

I69.919   **Unspecified symptoms and signs involving cognitive functions following unspecified cerebrovascular disease**

√6ᵗʰ   **I69.92**   **Speech and language deficits following unspecified cerebrovascular disease**

I69.920   **Aphasia following unspecified cerebrovascular disease**

I69.921   **Dysphasia following unspecified cerebrovascular disease**

I69.922   **Dysarthria following unspecified cerebrovascular disease**

I69.923   **Fluency disorder following unspecified cerebrovascular disease**
> Stuttering following unspecified cerebrovascular disease

I69.928   **Other speech and language deficits following unspecified cerebrovascular disease**

√6ᵗʰ   **I69.93**   **Monoplegia of upper limb following unspecified cerebrovascular disease**
> AHA: 2017,1Q,47

I69.931   **Monoplegia of upper limb following unspecified cerebrovascular disease affecting right dominant side** `HCC`

I69.932   **Monoplegia of upper limb following unspecified cerebrovascular disease affecting left dominant side** `HCC`

I69.933   **Monoplegia of upper limb following unspecified cerebrovascular disease affecting right non-dominant side** `HCC`

I69.934   **Monoplegia of upper limb following unspecified cerebrovascular disease affecting left non-dominant side** `HCC`

I69.939   **Monoplegia of upper limb following unspecified cerebrovascular disease affecting unspecified side** `HCC`

√6ᵗʰ   **I69.94**   **Monoplegia of lower limb following unspecified cerebrovascular disease**
> AHA: 2017,1Q,47

I69.941   **Monoplegia of lower limb following unspecified cerebrovascular disease affecting right dominant side** `HCC`

I69.942   **Monoplegia of lower limb following unspecified cerebrovascular disease affecting left dominant side** `HCC`

I69.943   **Monoplegia of lower limb following unspecified cerebrovascular disease affecting right non-dominant side** `HCC`

I69.944   **Monoplegia of lower limb following unspecified cerebrovascular disease affecting left non-dominant side** `HCC`

I69.949   **Monoplegia of lower limb following unspecified cerebrovascular disease affecting unspecified side** `HCC`

✔ Additional Character Required
ICD-10-CM 2020
   √x7ᵗʰ Placeholder   Unacceptable PDx   Questionable PDx   Manifestation   Unspecified Dx   H1-H14 HAC   HCC CMS-HCC Dx   HIV HIV Dx

669

√6ᵗʰ **I69.95** Hemiplegia and hemiparesis following unspecified cerebrovascular disease
AHA: 2015,1Q,25

     I69.951 Hemiplegia and hemiparesis following unspecified cerebrovascular disease affecting right dominant side   CC   HCC
        CC Excl: PDX collection 695

     I69.952 Hemiplegia and hemiparesis following unspecified cerebrovascular disease affecting left dominant side   CC   HCC
        CC Excl: PDX collection 695

     I69.953 Hemiplegia and hemiparesis following unspecified cerebrovascular disease affecting right non-dominant side   CC   HCC
        CC Excl: PDX collection 696

     I69.954 Hemiplegia and hemiparesis following unspecified cerebrovascular disease affecting left non-dominant side   CC   HCC
        CC Excl: PDX collection 696

     I69.959 Hemiplegia and hemiparesis following unspecified cerebrovascular disease affecting unspecified side   CC   HCC
        CC Excl: PDX collection 697

√6ᵗʰ **I69.96** Other paralytic syndrome following unspecified cerebrovascular disease
Use additional code to identify type of paralytic syndrome, such as:
locked-in state (G83.5)
quadriplegia (G82.5-)

        EXCLUDES 1   *hemiplegia/hemiparesis following unspecified cerebrovascular disease (I69.95-)*
monoplegia of lower limb following unspecified cerebrovascular disease (I69.94-)
monoplegia of upper limb following unspecified cerebrovascular disease (I69.93-)

     I69.961 Other paralytic syndrome following unspecified cerebrovascular disease affecting right dominant side   HCC

     I69.962 Other paralytic syndrome following unspecified cerebrovascular disease affecting left dominant side   HCC

     I69.963 Other paralytic syndrome following unspecified cerebrovascular disease affecting right non-dominant side   HCC

     I69.964 Other paralytic syndrome following unspecified cerebrovascular disease affecting left non-dominant side   HCC

     I69.965 Other paralytic syndrome following unspecified cerebrovascular disease, bilateral   HCC

     I69.969 Other paralytic syndrome following unspecified cerebrovascular disease affecting unspecified side   HCC

√6ᵗʰ **I69.99** Other sequelae of unspecified cerebrovascular disease

     I69.990 Apraxia following unspecified cerebrovascular disease

     I69.991 Dysphagia following unspecified cerebrovascular disease
        Use additional code to identify the type of dysphagia, if known (R13.1-)

     I69.992 Facial weakness following unspecified cerebrovascular disease
        Facial droop following unspecified cerebrovascular disease

     I69.993 Ataxia following unspecified cerebrovascular disease

     I69.998 Other sequelae following unspecified cerebrovascular disease
        Alteration in sensation following unspecified cerebrovascular disease
        Disturbance of vision following unspecified cerebrovascular disease
        Use additional code to identify the sequelae

Diseases of arteries, arterioles and capillaries (I70-I79)

√4ᵗʰ **I70** **Atherosclerosis**

     INCLUDES   arterial degeneration
arteriolosclerosis
arteriosclerosis
arteriosclerotic vascular disease
arteriovascular degeneration
atheroma
endarteritis deformans or obliterans
senile arteritis
senile endarteritis
vascular degeneration

Use additional code to identify:
exposure to environmental tobacco smoke (Z77.22)
history of tobacco dependence (Z87.891)
occupational exposure to environmental tobacco smoke (Z57.31)
tobacco dependence (F17.-)
tobacco use (Z72.0)

     EXCLUDES 2   *arteriosclerotic cardiovascular disease (I25.1-)*
arteriosclerotic heart disease (I25.1-)
atheroembolism (I75.-)
cerebral atherosclerosis (I67.2)
coronary atherosclerosis (I25.1-)
mesenteric atherosclerosis (K55.1)
precerebral atherosclerosis (I67.2)
primary pulmonary atherosclerosis (I27.0)

I70.0 **Atherosclerosis of aorta**   HCC   A

I70.1 **Atherosclerosis of renal artery**   HCC   A
     Goldblatt's kidney
     EXCLUDES 2   *atherosclerosis of renal arterioles (I12.-)*

√5ᵗʰ **I70.2** **Atherosclerosis of native arteries of the extremities**
Mönckeberg's (medial) sclerosis
Use additional code, if applicable, to identify chronic total occlusion of artery of extremity (I70.92)
     EXCLUDES 2   *atherosclerosis of bypass graft of extremities (I70.30-I70.79)*
AHA: 2018,3Q,4; 2018,2Q,7

√6ᵗʰ **I70.20** **Unspecified atherosclerosis of native arteries of extremities**

     I70.201 Unspecified atherosclerosis of native arteries of extremities, right leg   HCC   A

     I70.202 Unspecified atherosclerosis of native arteries of extremities, left leg   HCC   A

     I70.203 Unspecified atherosclerosis of native arteries of extremities, bilateral legs   HCC   A

     I70.208 Unspecified atherosclerosis of native arteries of extremities, other extremity   HCC   A

     I70.209 Unspecified atherosclerosis of native arteries of extremities, unspecified extremity   HCC   A

√6ᵗʰ **I70.21** **Atherosclerosis of native arteries of extremities with intermittent claudication**

     I70.211 Atherosclerosis of native arteries of extremities with intermittent claudication, right leg   HCC   A

     I70.212 Atherosclerosis of native arteries of extremities with intermittent claudication, left leg   HCC   A

     I70.213 Atherosclerosis of native arteries of extremities with intermittent claudication, bilateral legs   HCC   A

I70.218   **Atherosclerosis of native arteries of extremities with intermittent claudication, other extremity**   HCC A

I70.219   **Atherosclerosis of native arteries of extremities with intermittent claudication, unspecified extremity**   HCC A

✓6th I70.22   **Atherosclerosis of native arteries of extremities with rest pain**

    INCLUDES   any condition classifiable to I70.21-

I70.221   **Atherosclerosis of native arteries of extremities with rest pain, right leg**   HCC A

I70.222   **Atherosclerosis of native arteries of extremities with rest pain, left leg**   HCC A

I70.223   **Atherosclerosis of native arteries of extremities with rest pain, bilateral legs**   HCC A

I70.228   **Atherosclerosis of native arteries of extremities with rest pain, other extremity**   HCC A

I70.229   **Atherosclerosis of native arteries of extremities with rest pain, unspecified extremity**   HCC A

✓6th I70.23   **Atherosclerosis of native arteries of right leg with ulceration**

    INCLUDES   any condition classifiable to I70.211 and I70.221

    Use additional code to identify severity of ulcer (L97.-)

I70.231   **Atherosclerosis of native arteries of right leg with ulceration of thigh**   HCC A

I70.232   **Atherosclerosis of native arteries of right leg with ulceration of calf**   HCC A

I70.233   **Atherosclerosis of native arteries of right leg with ulceration of ankle**   HCC A

I70.234   **Atherosclerosis of native arteries of right leg with ulceration of heel and midfoot**   HCC A

     Atherosclerosis of native arteries of right leg with ulceration of plantar surface of midfoot

I70.235   **Atherosclerosis of native arteries of right leg with ulceration of other part of foot**   HCC A

     Atherosclerosis of native arteries of right leg extremities with ulceration of toe

I70.238   **Atherosclerosis of native arteries of right leg with ulceration of other part of lower leg**   HCC A

I70.239   **Atherosclerosis of native arteries of right leg with ulceration of unspecified site**   HCC A

✓6th I70.24   **Atherosclerosis of native arteries of left leg with ulceration**

    INCLUDES   any condition classifiable to I70.212 and I70.222

    Use additional code to identify severity of ulcer (L97.-)

I70.241   **Atherosclerosis of native arteries of left leg with ulceration of thigh**   HCC A

I70.242   **Atherosclerosis of native arteries of left leg with ulceration of calf**   HCC A

I70.243   **Atherosclerosis of native arteries of left leg with ulceration of ankle**   HCC A

I70.244   **Atherosclerosis of native arteries of left leg with ulceration of heel and midfoot**   HCC A

     Atherosclerosis of native arteries of left leg with ulceration of plantar surface of midfoot

I70.245   **Atherosclerosis of native arteries of left leg with ulceration of other part of foot**   HCC A

     Atherosclerosis of native arteries of left leg extremities with ulceration of toe

I70.248   **Atherosclerosis of native arteries of left leg with ulceration of other part of lower leg**   HCC A

I70.249   **Atherosclerosis of native arteries of left leg with ulceration of unspecified site**   HCC A

I70.25   **Atherosclerosis of native arteries of other extremities with ulceration**   HCC A

    INCLUDES   any condition classifiable to I70.218 and I70.228

    Use additional code to identify the severity of the ulcer (L98.49-)

✓6th I70.26   **Atherosclerosis of native arteries of extremities with gangrene**

    INCLUDES   any condition classifiable to I70.21-, I70.22-, I70.23-, I70.24-, and I70.25-

    Use additional code to identify the severity of any ulcer (L97.-, L98.49-), if applicable

    CC Excl: For CC codes in subcategory I70.26: PDX collection 519

I70.261   **Atherosclerosis of native arteries of extremities with gangrene, right leg**   CC HCC A

I70.262   **Atherosclerosis of native arteries of extremities with gangrene, left leg**   CC HCC A

I70.263   **Atherosclerosis of native arteries of extremities with gangrene, bilateral legs**   CC HCC A

I70.268   **Atherosclerosis of native arteries of extremities with gangrene, other extremity**   CC HCC A

I70.269   **Atherosclerosis of native arteries of extremities with gangrene, unspecified extremity**   CC HCC A

✓6th I70.29   **Other atherosclerosis of native arteries of extremities**

I70.291   **Other atherosclerosis of native arteries of extremities, right leg**   HCC A

I70.292   **Other atherosclerosis of native arteries of extremities, left leg**   HCC A

I70.293   **Other atherosclerosis of native arteries of extremities, bilateral legs**   HCC A

I70.298   **Other atherosclerosis of native arteries of extremities, other extremity**   HCC A

I70.299   **Other atherosclerosis of native arteries of extremities, unspecified extremity**   HCC A

✓6th I70.3   **Atherosclerosis of unspecified type of bypass graft(s) of the extremities**

    Use additional code, if applicable, to identify chronic total occlusion of artery of extremity (I70.92)

    EXCLUDES 1   embolism or thrombus of bypass graft(s) of extremities (T82.8-)

✓6th I70.30   **Unspecified atherosclerosis of unspecified type of bypass graft(s) of the extremities**

I70.301   **Unspecified atherosclerosis of unspecified type of bypass graft(s) of the extremities, right leg**   HCC A

I70.302   **Unspecified atherosclerosis of unspecified type of bypass graft(s) of the extremities, left leg**   HCC A

I70.303   **Unspecified atherosclerosis of unspecified type of bypass graft(s) of the extremities, bilateral legs**   HCC A

I70.308   **Unspecified atherosclerosis of unspecified type of bypass graft(s) of the extremities, other extremity**   HCC A

✓ Additional Character Required   ✓x7th Placeholder   Unacceptable PDx   Questionable PDx   Manifestation   Unspecified Dx   H1 - H14 HAC   HCC CMS-HCC Dx   HIV HIV Dx

ICD-10-CM 2020   671

I70.309 Unspecified atherosclerosis of unspecified type of bypass graft(s) of the extremities, unspecified extremity `HCC` `A`

✓6ᵗʰ **I70.31** Atherosclerosis of unspecified type of bypass graft(s) of the extremities with intermittent claudication

  I70.311 Atherosclerosis of unspecified type of bypass graft(s) of the extremities with intermittent claudication, right leg `HCC` `A`

  I70.312 Atherosclerosis of unspecified type of bypass graft(s) of the extremities with intermittent claudication, left leg `HCC` `A`

  I70.313 Atherosclerosis of unspecified type of bypass graft(s) of the extremities with intermittent claudication, bilateral legs `HCC` `A`

  I70.318 Atherosclerosis of unspecified type of bypass graft(s) of the extremities with intermittent claudication, other extremity `HCC` `A`

  I70.319 Atherosclerosis of unspecified type of bypass graft(s) of the extremities with intermittent claudication, unspecified extremity `HCC` `A`

✓6ᵗʰ **I70.32** Atherosclerosis of unspecified type of bypass graft(s) of the extremities with rest pain
  [INCLUDES] any condition classifiable to I70.31-

  I70.321 Atherosclerosis of unspecified type of bypass graft(s) of the extremities with rest pain, right leg `HCC` `A`

  I70.322 Atherosclerosis of unspecified type of bypass graft(s) of the extremities with rest pain, left leg `HCC` `A`

  I70.323 Atherosclerosis of unspecified type of bypass graft(s) of the extremities with rest pain, bilateral legs `HCC` `A`

  I70.328 Atherosclerosis of unspecified type of bypass graft(s) of the extremities with rest pain, other extremity `HCC` `A`

  I70.329 Atherosclerosis of unspecified type of bypass graft(s) of the extremities with rest pain, unspecified extremity `HCC` `A`

✓6ᵗʰ **I70.33** Atherosclerosis of unspecified type of bypass graft(s) of the right leg with ulceration
  [INCLUDES] any condition classifiable to I70.311 and I70.321
  Use additional code to identify severity of ulcer (L97.-)
  CC Excl: For CC codes in subcategory I70.33: PDX collection 698

  I70.331 Atherosclerosis of unspecified type of bypass graft(s) of the right leg with ulceration of thigh `CC` `HCC` `A`

  I70.332 Atherosclerosis of unspecified type of bypass graft(s) of the right leg with ulceration of calf `CC` `HCC` `A`

  I70.333 Atherosclerosis of unspecified type of bypass graft(s) of the right leg with ulceration of ankle `CC` `HCC` `A`

  I70.334 Atherosclerosis of unspecified type of bypass graft(s) of the right leg with ulceration of heel and midfoot `CC` `HCC` `A`
    Atherosclerosis of unspecified type of bypass graft(s) of right leg with ulceration of plantar surface of midfoot

I70.335 Atherosclerosis of unspecified type of bypass graft(s) of the right leg with ulceration of other part of foot `HCC` `A`
  Atherosclerosis of unspecified type of bypass graft(s) of the right leg with ulceration of toe

I70.338 Atherosclerosis of unspecified type of bypass graft(s) of the right leg with ulceration of other part of lower leg `CC` `HCC` `A`

I70.339 Atherosclerosis of unspecified type of bypass graft(s) of the right leg with ulceration of unspecified site `CC` `HCC` `A`

✓6ᵗʰ **I70.34** Atherosclerosis of unspecified type of bypass graft(s) of the left leg with ulceration
  [INCLUDES] any condition classifiable to I70.312 and I70.322
  Use additional code to identify severity of ulcer (L97.-)
  CC Excl: For CC codes in subcategory I70.34: PDX collection 698

  I70.341 Atherosclerosis of unspecified type of bypass graft(s) of the left leg with ulceration of thigh `CC` `HCC` `A`

  I70.342 Atherosclerosis of unspecified type of bypass graft(s) of the left leg with ulceration of calf `CC` `HCC` `A`

  I70.343 Atherosclerosis of unspecified type of bypass graft(s) of the left leg with ulceration of ankle `CC` `HCC` `A`

  I70.344 Atherosclerosis of unspecified type of bypass graft(s) of the left leg with ulceration of heel and midfoot `CC` `HCC` `A`
    Atherosclerosis of unspecified type of bypass graft(s) of left leg with ulceration of plantar surface of midfoot

  I70.345 Atherosclerosis of unspecified type of bypass graft(s) of the left leg with ulceration of other part of foot `HCC` `A`
    Atherosclerosis of unspecified type of bypass graft(s) of the left leg with ulceration of toe

  I70.348 Atherosclerosis of unspecified type of bypass graft(s) of the left leg with ulceration of other part of lower leg `CC` `HCC` `A`

  I70.349 Atherosclerosis of unspecified type of bypass graft(s) of the left leg with ulceration of unspecified site `CC` `HCC` `A`

I70.35 Atherosclerosis of unspecified type of bypass graft(s) of other extremity with ulceration `HCC` `A`
  [INCLUDES] any condition classifiable to I70.318 and I70.328
  Use additional code to identify severity of ulcer (L98.49-)

✓6ᵗʰ **I70.36** Atherosclerosis of unspecified type of bypass graft(s) of the extremities with gangrene
  [INCLUDES] any condition classifiable to I70.31-, I70.32-, I70.33-, I70.34-, I70.35
  Use additional code to identify the severity of any ulcer (L97.-, L98.49-), if applicable
  CC Excl: For CC codes in subcategory I70.36: PDX collection 519

  I70.361 Atherosclerosis of unspecified type of bypass graft(s) of the extremities with gangrene, right leg `CC` `HCC` `A`

  I70.362 Atherosclerosis of unspecified type of bypass graft(s) of the extremities with gangrene, left leg `CC` `HCC` `A`

  I70.363 Atherosclerosis of unspecified type of bypass graft(s) of the extremities with gangrene, bilateral legs `CC` `HCC` `A`

N Newborn: 0   P Pediatric: 0-17   M Maternity: 9-64   A Adult: 15-124   MCC Major Complication/Comorbidity   CC Complication/Comorbidity   SW Severe Wound Dx

672   ICD-10-CM 2020

I70.368   Atherosclerosis of unspecified `CC` `HCC` `A` type of bypass graft(s) of the extremities with gangrene, other extremity

I70.369   Atherosclerosis of unspecified `CC` `HCC` `A` type of bypass graft(s) of the extremities with gangrene, unspecified extremity

√6ᵗʰ I70.39   Other atherosclerosis of unspecified type of bypass graft(s) of the extremities

I70.391   Other atherosclerosis of `HCC` `A` unspecified type of bypass graft(s) of the extremities, right leg

I70.392   Other atherosclerosis of `HCC` `A` unspecified type of bypass graft(s) of the extremities, left leg

I70.393   Other atherosclerosis of `HCC` `A` unspecified type of bypass graft(s) of the extremities, bilateral legs

I70.398   Other atherosclerosis of `HCC` `A` unspecified type of bypass graft(s) of the extremities, other extremity

I70.399   Other atherosclerosis of `HCC` `A` unspecified type of bypass graft(s) of the extremities, unspecified extremity

√6ᵗʰ I70.4   **Atherosclerosis of autologous vein bypass graft(s) of the extremities**

Use additional code, if applicable, to identify chronic total occlusion of artery of extremity (I70.92)

√6ᵗʰ I70.40   Unspecified atherosclerosis of autologous vein bypass graft(s) of the extremities

I70.401   Unspecified atherosclerosis of `HCC` `A` autologous vein bypass graft(s) of the extremities, right leg

I70.402   Unspecified atherosclerosis of `HCC` `A` autologous vein bypass graft(s) of the extremities, left leg

I70.403   Unspecified atherosclerosis of `HCC` `A` autologous vein bypass graft(s) of the extremities, bilateral legs

I70.408   Unspecified atherosclerosis of `HCC` `A` autologous vein bypass graft(s) of the extremities, other extremity

I70.409   Unspecified atherosclerosis of `HCC` `A` autologous vein bypass graft(s) of the extremities, unspecified extremity

√6ᵗʰ I70.41   Atherosclerosis of autologous vein bypass graft(s) of the extremities with intermittent claudication

I70.411   Atherosclerosis of autologous `HCC` `A` vein bypass graft(s) of the extremities with intermittent claudication, right leg

I70.412   Atherosclerosis of autologous `HCC` `A` vein bypass graft(s) of the extremities with intermittent claudication, left leg

I70.413   Atherosclerosis of autologous `HCC` `A` vein bypass graft(s) of the extremities with intermittent claudication, bilateral legs

I70.418   Atherosclerosis of autologous `HCC` `A` vein bypass graft(s) of the extremities with intermittent claudication, other extremity

I70.419   Atherosclerosis of autologous `HCC` `A` vein bypass graft(s) of the extremities with intermittent claudication, unspecified extremity

√6ᵗʰ I70.42   Atherosclerosis of autologous vein bypass graft(s) of the extremities with rest pain

INCLUDES   any condition classifiable to I70.41-

I70.421   Atherosclerosis of autologous `HCC` `A` vein bypass graft(s) of the extremities with rest pain, right leg

I70.422   Atherosclerosis of autologous `HCC` `A` vein bypass graft(s) of the extremities with rest pain, left leg

I70.423   Atherosclerosis of autologous `HCC` `A` vein bypass graft(s) of the extremities with rest pain, bilateral legs

I70.428   Atherosclerosis of autologous `HCC` `A` vein bypass graft(s) of the extremities with rest pain, other extremity

I70.429   Atherosclerosis of autologous `HCC` `A` vein bypass graft(s) of the extremities with rest pain, unspecified extremity

√6ᵗʰ I70.43   Atherosclerosis of autologous vein bypass graft(s) of the right leg with ulceration

INCLUDES   any condition classifiable to I70.411 and I70.421

Use additional code to identify severity of ulcer (L97.-)

CC Excl: For CC codes in subcategory I70.43: PDX collection 698

I70.431   Atherosclerosis of autologous `CC` `HCC` `A` vein bypass graft(s) of the right leg with ulceration of thigh

I70.432   Atherosclerosis of autologous `CC` `HCC` `A` vein bypass graft(s) of the right leg with ulceration of calf

I70.433   Atherosclerosis of autologous `CC` `HCC` `A` vein bypass graft(s) of the right leg with ulceration of ankle

I70.434   Atherosclerosis of autologous `CC` `HCC` `A` vein bypass graft(s) of the right leg with ulceration of heel and midfoot

Atherosclerosis of autologous vein bypass graft(s) of right leg with ulceration of plantar surface of midfoot

I70.435   Atherosclerosis of autologous `HCC` `A` vein bypass graft(s) of the right leg with ulceration of other part of foot

Atherosclerosis of autologous vein bypass graft(s) of right leg with ulceration of toe

I70.438   Atherosclerosis of autologous `CC` `HCC` `A` vein bypass graft(s) of the right leg with ulceration of other part of lower leg

I70.439   Atherosclerosis of autologous `CC` `HCC` `A` vein bypass graft(s) of the right leg with ulceration of unspecified site

√6ᵗʰ I70.44   Atherosclerosis of autologous vein bypass graft(s) of the left leg with ulceration

INCLUDES   any condition classifiable to I70.412 and I70.422

Use additional code to identify severity of ulcer (L97.-)

CC Excl: For CC codes in subcategory I70.44: PDX collection 698

I70.441   Atherosclerosis of autologous `CC` `HCC` `A` vein bypass graft(s) of the left leg with ulceration of thigh

I70.442   Atherosclerosis of autologous `CC` `HCC` `A` vein bypass graft(s) of the left leg with ulceration of calf

I70.443   Atherosclerosis of autologous `CC` `HCC` `A` vein bypass graft(s) of the left leg with ulceration of ankle

✔ Additional Character Required   √x7ᵗʰ Placeholder   Unacceptable PDx   Questionable PDx   Manifestation   Unspecified Dx   H1 - H14 HAC   HCC CMS-HCC Dx   HIV HIV Dx

ICD-10-CM 2020

673

I70.368–I70.443

I70.444 **Atherosclerosis of autologous** CC HCC A
vein bypass graft(s) of the left
leg with ulceration of heel and
midfoot
> Atherosclerosis of autologous vein bypass graft(s) of left leg with ulceration of plantar surface of midfoot

I70.445 **Atherosclerosis of autologous** HCC A
vein bypass graft(s) of the left
leg with ulceration of other
part of foot
> Atherosclerosis of autologous vein bypass graft(s) of left leg with ulceration of toe

I70.448 **Atherosclerosis of autologous** CC HCC A
vein bypass graft(s) of the left
leg with ulceration of other
part of lower leg

I70.449 **Atherosclerosis of autologous** CC HCC A
vein bypass graft(s) of the left
leg with ulceration of
unspecified site

I70.45 **Atherosclerosis of autologous vein** HCC A
bypass graft(s) of other extremity with
ulceration
> INCLUDES   any condition classifiable to I70.418, I70.428, and I70.438
>
> Use additional code to identify severity of ulcer (L98.49)

✓6ᵗʰ **I70.46** **Atherosclerosis of autologous vein bypass graft(s)**
of the extremities with gangrene
> INCLUDES   any condition classifiable to I70.41-, I70.42-, and I70.43-, I70.44-, I70.45
>
> Use additional code to identify the severity of any ulcer (L97.-, L98.49-), if applicable
>
> CC Excl: For CC codes in subcategory I70.46: PDX collection 519

I70.461 **Atherosclerosis of autologous** CC HCC A
vein bypass graft(s) of the
extremities with gangrene,
right leg

I70.462 **Atherosclerosis of autologous** CC HCC A
vein bypass graft(s) of the
extremities with gangrene, left
leg

I70.463 **Atherosclerosis of autologous** CC HCC A
vein bypass graft(s) of the
extremities with gangrene,
bilateral legs

I70.468 **Atherosclerosis of autologous** CC HCC A
vein bypass graft(s) of the
extremities with gangrene,
other extremity

I70.469 **Atherosclerosis of autologous** CC HCC A
vein bypass graft(s) of the
extremities with gangrene,
unspecified extremity

✓6ᵗʰ **I70.49** **Other atherosclerosis of autologous vein bypass**
graft(s) of the extremities

I70.491 **Other atherosclerosis of** HCC A
autologous vein bypass
graft(s) of the extremities,
right leg

I70.492 **Other atherosclerosis of** HCC A
autologous vein bypass
graft(s) of the extremities, left
leg

I70.493 **Other atherosclerosis of** HCC A
autologous vein bypass
graft(s) of the extremities,
bilateral legs

I70.498 **Other atherosclerosis of** HCC A
autologous vein bypass
graft(s) of the extremities,
other extremity

I70.499 **Other atherosclerosis of** HCC A
autologous vein bypass
graft(s) of the extremities,
unspecified extremity

✓5ᵗʰ **I70.5** **Atherosclerosis of** nonautologous biological bypass graft(s)
of the extremities
> Use additional code, if applicable, to identify chronic total occlusion of artery of extremity (I70.92)

✓6ᵗʰ **I70.50** **Unspecified atherosclerosis of nonautologous**
biological bypass graft(s) of the extremities

I70.501 **Unspecified atherosclerosis of** HCC A
nonautologous biological
bypass graft(s) of the
extremities, right leg

I70.502 **Unspecified atherosclerosis of** HCC A
nonautologous biological
bypass graft(s) of the
extremities, left leg

I70.503 **Unspecified atherosclerosis of** HCC A
nonautologous biological
bypass graft(s) of the
extremities, bilateral legs

I70.508 **Unspecified atherosclerosis of** HCC A
nonautologous biological
bypass graft(s) of the
extremities, other extremity

I70.509 **Unspecified atherosclerosis of** HCC A
nonautologous biological
bypass graft(s) of the
extremities, unspecified
extremity

✓6ᵗʰ **I70.51** **Atherosclerosis of nonautologous biological bypass**
graft(s) of the extremities intermittent claudication

I70.511 **Atherosclerosis of** HCC A
nonautologous biological
bypass graft(s) of the
extremities with intermittent
claudication, right leg

I70.512 **Atherosclerosis of** HCC A
nonautologous biological
bypass graft(s) of the
extremities with intermittent
claudication, left leg

I70.513 **Atherosclerosis of** HCC A
nonautologous biological
bypass graft(s) of the
extremities with intermittent
claudication, bilateral legs

I70.518 **Atherosclerosis of** HCC A
nonautologous biological
bypass graft(s) of the
extremities with intermittent
claudication, other extremity

I70.519 **Atherosclerosis of** HCC A
nonautologous biological
bypass graft(s) of the
extremities with intermittent
claudication, unspecified
extremity

✓6ᵗʰ **I70.52** **Atherosclerosis of nonautologous biological bypass**
graft(s) of the extremities with rest pain
> INCLUDES   any condition classifiable to I70.51-

I70.521 **Atherosclerosis of** HCC A
nonautologous biological
bypass graft(s) of the
extremities with rest pain,
right leg

I70.522 **Atherosclerosis of** HCC A
nonautologous biological
bypass graft(s) of the
extremities with rest pain, left
leg

I70.523 **Atherosclerosis of** HCC A
nonautologous biological
bypass graft(s) of the
extremities with rest pain,
bilateral legs

I70.528 **Atherosclerosis of** HCC A
nonautologous biological
bypass graft(s) of the
extremities with rest pain,
other extremity

I70.529 **Atherosclerosis of** HCC A
nonautologous biological
bypass graft(s) of the
extremities with rest pain,
unspecified extremity

✓6ᵗʰ **I70.53** **Atherosclerosis of nonautologous biological bypass graft(s) of the right leg with ulceration**

[INCLUDES] any condition classifiable to I70.511 and I70.521

Use additional code to identify severity of ulcer (L97.-)

CC Excl: For CC codes in subcategory I70.53: PDX collection 698

I70.531 **Atherosclerosis of nonautologous biological bypass graft(s) of the right leg with ulceration of thigh** `CC` `HCC` `A`

I70.532 **Atherosclerosis of nonautologous biological bypass graft(s) of the right leg with ulceration of calf** `CC` `HCC` `A`

I70.533 **Atherosclerosis of nonautologous biological bypass graft(s) of the right leg with ulceration of ankle** `CC` `HCC` `A`

I70.534 **Atherosclerosis of nonautologous biological bypass graft(s) of the right leg with ulceration of heel and midfoot** `CC` `HCC` `A`

Atherosclerosis of nonautologous biological bypass graft(s) of right leg with ulceration of plantar surface of midfoot

I70.535 **Atherosclerosis of nonautologous biological bypass graft(s) of the right leg with ulceration of other part of foot** `HCC` `A`

Atherosclerosis of nonautologous biological bypass graft(s) of the right leg with ulceration of toe

I70.538 **Atherosclerosis of nonautologous biological bypass graft(s) of the right leg with ulceration of other part of lower leg** `CC` `HCC` `A`

I70.539 **Atherosclerosis of nonautologous biological bypass graft(s) of the right leg with ulceration of unspecified site** `CC` `HCC` `A`

✓6ᵗʰ **I70.54** **Atherosclerosis of nonautologous biological bypass graft(s) of the left leg with ulceration**

[INCLUDES] any condition classifiable to I70.512 and I70.522

Use additional code to identify severity of ulcer (L97.-)

CC Excl: For CC codes in subcategory I70.54: PDX collection 698

I70.541 **Atherosclerosis of nonautologous biological bypass graft(s) of the left leg with ulceration of thigh** `CC` `HCC` `A`

I70.542 **Atherosclerosis of nonautologous biological bypass graft(s) of the left leg with ulceration of calf** `CC` `HCC` `A`

I70.543 **Atherosclerosis of nonautologous biological bypass graft(s) of the left leg with ulceration of ankle** `CC` `HCC` `A`

I70.544 **Atherosclerosis of nonautologous biological bypass graft(s) of the left leg with ulceration of heel and midfoot** `CC` `HCC` `A`

Atherosclerosis of nonautologous biological bypass graft(s) of left leg with ulceration of plantar surface of midfoot

I70.545 **Atherosclerosis of nonautologous biological bypass graft(s) of the left leg with ulceration of other part of foot** `HCC` `A`

Atherosclerosis of nonautologous biological bypass graft(s) of the left leg with ulceration of toe

I70.548 **Atherosclerosis of nonautologous biological bypass graft(s) of the left leg with ulceration of other part of lower leg** `CC` `HCC` `A`

I70.549 **Atherosclerosis of nonautologous biological bypass graft(s) of the left leg with ulceration of unspecified site** `CC` `HCC` `A`

I70.55 **Atherosclerosis of nonautologous biological bypass graft(s) of other extremity with ulceration** `HCC` `A`

[INCLUDES] any condition classifiable to I70.518, I70.528, and I70.538

Use additional code to identify severity of ulcer (L98.49)

✓6ᵗʰ **I70.56** **Atherosclerosis of nonautologous biological bypass graft(s) of the extremities with gangrene**

[INCLUDES] any condition classifiable to I70.51-, I70.52-, and I70.53-, I70.54-, I70.55

Use additional code to identify the severity of any ulcer (L97.-, L98.49-), if applicable

CC Excl: For CC codes in subcategory I70.56: PDX collection 519

I70.561 **Atherosclerosis of nonautologous biological bypass graft(s) of the extremities with gangrene, right leg** `CC` `HCC` `A`

I70.562 **Atherosclerosis of nonautologous biological bypass graft(s) of the extremities with gangrene, left leg** `CC` `HCC` `A`

I70.563 **Atherosclerosis of nonautologous biological bypass graft(s) of the extremities with gangrene, bilateral legs** `CC` `HCC` `A`

I70.568 **Atherosclerosis of nonautologous biological bypass graft(s) of the extremities with gangrene, other extremity** `CC` `HCC` `A`

I70.569 **Atherosclerosis of nonautologous biological bypass graft(s) of the extremities with gangrene, unspecified extremity** `CC` `HCC` `A`

✓6ᵗʰ **I70.59** **Other atherosclerosis of nonautologous biological bypass graft(s) of the extremities**

I70.591 **Other atherosclerosis of nonautologous biological bypass graft(s) of the extremities, right leg** `HCC` `A`

I70.592 **Other atherosclerosis of nonautologous biological bypass graft(s) of the extremities, left leg** `HCC` `A`

I70.593 **Other atherosclerosis of nonautologous biological bypass graft(s) of the extremities, bilateral legs** `HCC` `A`

I70.598 **Other atherosclerosis of nonautologous biological bypass graft(s) of the extremities, other extremity** `HCC` `A`

I70.599 **Other atherosclerosis of nonautologous biological bypass graft(s) of the extremities, unspecified extremity** `HCC` `A`

✓6ᵗʰ **I70.6** **Atherosclerosis of nonbiological bypass graft(s) of the extremities**

Use additional code, if applicable, to identify chronic total occlusion of artery of extremity (I70.92)

✓6ᵗʰ **I70.60** **Unspecified atherosclerosis of nonbiological bypass graft(s) of the extremities**

I70.601 **Unspecified atherosclerosis of nonbiological bypass graft(s) of the extremities, right leg** `HCC` `A`

I70.602 **Unspecified atherosclerosis of nonbiological bypass graft(s) of the extremities, left leg** `HCC` `A`

☑ Additional Character Required　✓ˣ⁷ᵗʰ Placeholder　Unacceptable PDx　Questionable PDx　Manifestation　Unspecified Dx　`H1`-`H14` HAC　`HCC` CMS-HCC Dx　`HIV` HIV Dx

I70.603 Unspecified atherosclerosis of `HCC` `A`
nonbiological bypass graft(s)
of the extremities, bilateral
legs

I70.608 Unspecified atherosclerosis of `HCC` `A`
nonbiological bypass graft(s)
of the extremities, other
extremity

I70.609 Unspecified atherosclerosis of `HCC` `A`
nonbiological bypass graft(s)
of the extremities, unspecified
extremity

√6ᵗʰ **I70.61** Atherosclerosis of nonbiological bypass graft(s) of
the extremities with intermittent claudication

I70.611 Atherosclerosis of `HCC` `A`
nonbiological bypass graft(s)
of the extremities with
intermittent claudication, right
leg

I70.612 Atherosclerosis of `HCC` `A`
nonbiological bypass graft(s)
of the extremities with
intermittent claudication, left
leg

I70.613 Atherosclerosis of `HCC` `A`
nonbiological bypass graft(s)
of the extremities with
intermittent claudication,
bilateral legs

I70.618 Atherosclerosis of `HCC` `A`
nonbiological bypass graft(s)
of the extremities with
intermittent claudication,
other extremity

I70.619 Atherosclerosis of `HCC` `A`
nonbiological bypass graft(s)
of the extremities with
intermittent claudication,
unspecified extremity

√6ᵗʰ **I70.62** Atherosclerosis of nonbiological bypass graft(s) of
the extremities with rest pain

INCLUDES   any condition classifiable to I70.61-

I70.621 Atherosclerosis of `HCC` `A`
nonbiological bypass graft(s)
of the extremities with rest
pain, right leg

I70.622 Atherosclerosis of `HCC` `A`
nonbiological bypass graft(s)
of the extremities with rest
pain, left leg

I70.623 Atherosclerosis of `HCC` `A`
nonbiological bypass graft(s)
of the extremities with rest
pain, bilateral legs

I70.628 Atherosclerosis of `HCC` `A`
nonbiological bypass graft(s)
of the extremities with rest
pain, other extremity

I70.629 Atherosclerosis of `HCC` `A`
nonbiological bypass graft(s)
of the extremities with rest
pain, unspecified extremity

√6ᵗʰ **I70.63** Atherosclerosis of nonbiological bypass graft(s) of
the right leg with ulceration

INCLUDES   any condition classifiable to I70.611 and
I70.621

Use additional code to identify severity of ulcer (L97.-)

CC Excl: For CC codes in subcategory I70.63: PDX
collection 698

I70.631 Atherosclerosis of `CC` `HCC` `A`
nonbiological bypass graft(s)
of the right leg with ulceration
of thigh

I70.632 Atherosclerosis of `CC` `HCC` `A`
nonbiological bypass graft(s)
of the right leg with ulceration
of calf

I70.633 Atherosclerosis of `CC` `HCC` `A`
nonbiological bypass graft(s)
of the right leg with ulceration
of ankle

I70.634 Atherosclerosis of `CC` `HCC` `A`
nonbiological bypass graft(s)
of the right leg with ulceration
of heel and midfoot

Atherosclerosis of nonbiological bypass
graft(s) of right leg with ulceration of
plantar surface of midfoot

I70.635 Atherosclerosis of `HCC` `A`
nonbiological bypass graft(s)
of the right leg with ulceration
of other part of foot

Atherosclerosis of nonbiological bypass
graft(s) of the right leg with ulceration
of toe

I70.638 Atherosclerosis of `CC` `HCC` `A`
nonbiological bypass graft(s)
of the right leg with ulceration
of other part of lower leg

I70.639 Atherosclerosis of `CC` `HCC` `A`
nonbiological bypass graft(s)
of the right leg with ulceration
of unspecified site

√6ᵗʰ **I70.64** Atherosclerosis of nonbiological bypass graft(s) of
the left leg with ulceration

INCLUDES   any condition classifiable to I70.612 and
I70.622

Use additional code to identify severity of ulcer (L97.-)

CC Excl: For CC codes in subcategory I70.64: PDX
collection 698

I70.641 Atherosclerosis of `CC` `HCC` `A`
nonbiological bypass graft(s)
of the left leg with ulceration
of thigh

I70.642 Atherosclerosis of `CC` `HCC` `A`
nonbiological bypass graft(s)
of the left leg with ulceration
of calf

I70.643 Atherosclerosis of `CC` `HCC` `A`
nonbiological bypass graft(s)
of the left leg with ulceration
of ankle

I70.644 Atherosclerosis of `CC` `HCC` `A`
nonbiological bypass graft(s)
of the left leg with ulceration
of heel and midfoot

Atherosclerosis of nonbiological bypass
graft(s) of left leg with ulceration of
plantar surface of midfoot

I70.645 Atherosclerosis of `HCC` `A`
nonbiological bypass graft(s)
of the left leg with ulceration
of other part of foot

Atherosclerosis of nonbiological bypass
graft(s) of the left leg with ulceration
of toe

I70.648 Atherosclerosis of `CC` `HCC` `A`
nonbiological bypass graft(s)
of the left leg with ulceration
of other part of lower leg

I70.649 Atherosclerosis of `CC` `HCC` `A`
nonbiological bypass graft(s)
of the left leg with ulceration
of unspecified site

I70.65 Atherosclerosis of nonbiological bypass `HCC` `A`
graft(s) of other extremity with
ulceration

INCLUDES   any condition classifiable to I70.618 and
I70.628

Use additional code to identify severity of ulcer
(L98.49)

√6ᵗʰ **I70.66** Atherosclerosis of nonbiological bypass graft(s) of
the extremities with gangrene

INCLUDES   any condition classifiable to I70.61-,
I70.62-, I70.63-, I70.64-, I70.65

Use additional code to identify the severity of any
ulcer (L97.-, L98.49-), if applicable

CC Excl: For CC codes in subcategory I70.66: PDX
collection 519

I70.661 Atherosclerosis of `CC` `HCC` `A`
nonbiological bypass graft(s)
of the extremities with
gangrene, right leg

`N` Newborn: 0   `P` Pediatric: 0-17   `M` Maternity: 9-64   `A` Adult: 15-124   `MCC` Major Complication/Comorbidity   `CC` Complication/Comorbidity   `SW` Severe Wound Dx

676   ICD-10-CM 2020

I70.662 Atherosclerosis of nonbiological bypass graft(s) of the extremities with gangrene, left leg   CC HCC A

I70.663 Atherosclerosis of nonbiological bypass graft(s) of the extremities with gangrene, bilateral legs   CC HCC A

I70.668 Atherosclerosis of nonbiological bypass graft(s) of the extremities with gangrene, other extremity   CC HCC A

I70.669 Atherosclerosis of nonbiological bypass graft(s) of the extremities with gangrene, unspecified extremity   CC HCC A

√6th **I70.69** Other atherosclerosis of nonbiological bypass graft(s) of the extremities

I70.691 Other atherosclerosis of nonbiological bypass graft(s) of the extremities, right leg   HCC A

I70.692 Other atherosclerosis of nonbiological bypass graft(s) of the extremities, left leg   HCC A

I70.693 Other atherosclerosis of nonbiological bypass graft(s) of the extremities, bilateral legs   HCC A

I70.698 Other atherosclerosis of nonbiological bypass graft(s) of the extremities, other extremity   HCC A

I70.699 Other atherosclerosis of nonbiological bypass graft(s) of the extremities, unspecified extremity   HCC A

√5th **I70.7** Atherosclerosis of other type of bypass graft(s) of the extremities

Use additional code, if applicable, to identify chronic total occlusion of artery of extremity (I70.92)

√6th **I70.70** Unspecified atherosclerosis of other type of bypass graft(s) of the extremities

I70.701 Unspecified atherosclerosis of other type of bypass graft(s) of the extremities, right leg   HCC A

I70.702 Unspecified atherosclerosis of other type of bypass graft(s) of the extremities, left leg   HCC A

I70.703 Unspecified atherosclerosis of other type of bypass graft(s) of the extremities, bilateral legs   HCC A

I70.708 Unspecified atherosclerosis of other type of bypass graft(s) of the extremities, other extremity   HCC A

I70.709 Unspecified atherosclerosis of other type of bypass graft(s) of the extremities, unspecified extremity   HCC A

√6th **I70.71** Atherosclerosis of other type of bypass graft(s) of the extremities with intermittent claudication

I70.711 Atherosclerosis of other type of bypass graft(s) of the extremities with intermittent claudication, right leg   HCC A

I70.712 Atherosclerosis of other type of bypass graft(s) of the extremities with intermittent claudication, left leg   HCC A

I70.713 Atherosclerosis of other type of bypass graft(s) of the extremities with intermittent claudication, bilateral legs   HCC A

I70.718 Atherosclerosis of other type of bypass graft(s) of the extremities with intermittent claudication, other extremity   HCC A

I70.719 Atherosclerosis of other type of bypass graft(s) of the extremities with intermittent claudication, unspecified extremity   HCC A

√6th **I70.72** Atherosclerosis of other type of bypass graft(s) of the extremities with rest pain

INCLUDES   any condition classifiable to I70.71-

I70.721 Atherosclerosis of other type of bypass graft(s) of the extremities with rest pain, right leg   HCC A

I70.722 Atherosclerosis of other type of bypass graft(s) of the extremities with rest pain, left leg   HCC A

I70.723 Atherosclerosis of other type of bypass graft(s) of the extremities with rest pain, bilateral legs   HCC A

I70.728 Atherosclerosis of other type of bypass graft(s) of the extremities with rest pain, other extremity   HCC A

I70.729 Atherosclerosis of other type of bypass graft(s) of the extremities with rest pain, unspecified extremity   HCC A

√6th **I70.73** Atherosclerosis of other type of bypass graft(s) of the right leg with ulceration

INCLUDES   any condition classifiable to I70.711 and I70.721

Use additional code to identify severity of ulcer (L97.-)

CC Excl: For CC codes in subcategory I70.73: PDX collection 698

I70.731 Atherosclerosis of other type of bypass graft(s) of the right leg with ulceration of thigh   CC HCC A

I70.732 Atherosclerosis of other type of bypass graft(s) of the right leg with ulceration of calf   CC HCC A

I70.733 Atherosclerosis of other type of bypass graft(s) of the right leg with ulceration of ankle   CC HCC A

I70.734 Atherosclerosis of other type of bypass graft(s) of the right leg with ulceration of heel and midfoot   CC HCC A

Atherosclerosis of other type of bypass graft(s) of right leg with ulceration of plantar surface of midfoot

I70.735 Atherosclerosis of other type of bypass graft(s) of the right leg with ulceration of other part of foot   HCC A

Atherosclerosis of other type of bypass graft(s) of right leg with ulceration of toe

I70.738 Atherosclerosis of other type of bypass graft(s) of the right leg with ulceration of other part of lower leg   CC HCC A

I70.739 Atherosclerosis of other type of bypass graft(s) of the right leg with ulceration of unspecified site   CC HCC A

√6th **I70.74** Atherosclerosis of other type of bypass graft(s) of the left leg with ulceration

INCLUDES   any condition classifiable to I70.712 and I70.722

Use additional code to identify severity of ulcer (L97.-)

CC Excl: For CC codes in subcategory I70.74: PDX collection 698

I70.741 Atherosclerosis of other type of bypass graft(s) of the left leg with ulceration of thigh   CC HCC A

I70.742 Atherosclerosis of other type of bypass graft(s) of the left leg with ulceration of calf   CC HCC A

I70.743 Atherosclerosis of other type of bypass graft(s) of the left leg with ulceration of ankle   CC HCC A

✔ Additional Character Required   √x7th Placeholder   Unacceptable PDx   Questionable PDx   Manifestation   Unspecified Dx   H1-H14 HAC   HCC CMS-HCC Dx   HIV HIV Dx

ICD-10-CM 2020   **677**

I70.744 **Atherosclerosis of other type** `CC` `HCC` `A`
of bypass graft(s) of the left leg
with ulceration of heel and
midfoot

    Atherosclerosis of other type of bypass
graft(s) of left leg with ulceration of
plantar surface of midfoot

I70.745 **Atherosclerosis of other type** `HCC` `A`
of bypass graft(s) of the left leg
with ulceration of other part of
foot

    Atherosclerosis of other type of bypass
graft(s) of left leg with ulceration of
toe

I70.748 **Atherosclerosis of other type** `CC` `HCC` `A`
of bypass graft(s) of the left leg
with ulceration of other part of
lower leg

I70.749 **Atherosclerosis of other type** `CC` `HCC` `A`
of bypass graft(s) of the left leg
with ulceration of unspecified
site

I70.75 **Atherosclerosis of other type of bypass** `HCC` `A`
graft(s) of other extremity with
ulceration

   INCLUDES   any condition classifiable to I70.718 and
I70.728

   Use additional code to identify severity of ulcer
(L98.49)

√6ᵗʰ **I70.76** **Atherosclerosis of other type of bypass graft(s) of**
the extremities with gangrene

   INCLUDES   any condition classifiable to I70.71-,
I70.72-, I70.73-, I70.74-, I70.75

   Use additional code to identify the severity of any
ulcer (L97.-, L98.49-), if applicable

CC Excl: For CC codes in subcategory I70.76: PDX
collection 519

I70.761 **Atherosclerosis of other type** `CC` `HCC` `A`
of bypass graft(s) of the
extremities with gangrene,
right leg

I70.762 **Atherosclerosis of other type** `CC` `HCC` `A`
of bypass graft(s) of the
extremities with gangrene, left
leg

I70.763 **Atherosclerosis of other type** `CC` `HCC` `A`
of bypass graft(s) of the
extremities with gangrene,
bilateral legs

I70.768 **Atherosclerosis of other type** `CC` `HCC` `A`
of bypass graft(s) of the
extremities with gangrene,
other extremity

I70.769 **Atherosclerosis of other type** `CC` `HCC` `A`
of bypass graft(s) of the
extremities with gangrene,
unspecified extremity

√6ᵗʰ **I70.79** **Other atherosclerosis of other type of bypass**
graft(s) of the extremities

I70.791 **Other atherosclerosis of other** `HCC` `A`
type of bypass graft(s) of the
extremities, right leg

I70.792 **Other atherosclerosis of other** `HCC` `A`
type of bypass graft(s) of the
extremities, left leg

I70.793 **Other atherosclerosis of other** `HCC` `A`
type of bypass graft(s) of the
extremities, bilateral legs

I70.798 **Other atherosclerosis of other** `HCC` `A`
type of bypass graft(s) of the
extremities, other extremity

I70.799 **Other atherosclerosis of other** `HCC` `A`
type of bypass graft(s) of the
extremities, unspecified
extremity

I70.8 **Atherosclerosis of other arteries** `A`

    TIP: Arteriosclerosis of the iliac arteries is coded here.

√5ᵗʰ **I70.9** **Other and unspecified atherosclerosis**

I70.90 **Unspecified atherosclerosis** `A`

I70.91 **Generalized atherosclerosis** `A`

I70.92 **Chronic total occlusion** of artery of the `CC` `HCC` `A`
extremities

    Complete occlusion of artery of the extremities

    Total occlusion of artery of the extremities

    Code first atherosclerosis of arteries of the extremities
(I70.2-, I70.3-, I70.4-, I70.5-, I70.6-, I70.7-)

    CC Excl: PDX collection 699

√4ᵗʰ **I71** **Aortic aneurysm and dissection**

   EXCLUDES 1   aortic ectasia (I77.81-)

       syphilitic aortic aneurysm (A52.01)

       traumatic aortic aneurysm (S25.09, S35.09)

CC Excl: For MCC codes in category I71: PDX collection 700

√5ᵗʰ **I71.0** **Dissection of aorta**

I71.00 **Dissection of unspecified site of aorta** `CC` `HCC`

I71.01 **Dissection of** thoracic **aorta** `MCC` `HCC`

I71.02 **Dissection of** abdominal **aorta** `MCC` `HCC`

I71.03 **Dissection of** thoracoabdominal **aorta** `MCC` `HCC`

I71.1 **Thoracic aortic aneurysm, ruptured** `MCC` `HCC`

I71.2 **Thoracic aortic aneurysm, without rupture** `HCC`

I71.3 **Abdominal aortic aneurysm, ruptured** `MCC` `HCC`

I71.4 **Abdominal aortic aneurysm, without rupture** `HCC`

I71.5 **Thoracoabdominal aortic aneurysm, ruptured** `MCC` `HCC`

I71.6 **Thoracoabdominal aortic aneurysm, without** `HCC`
rupture

I71.8 **Aortic aneurysm of unspecified site, ruptured** `MCC` `HCC`

    Rupture of aorta NOS

I71.9 **Aortic aneurysm of unspecified site, without** `HCC`
rupture

    Aneurysm of aorta

    Dilatation of aorta

    Hyaline necrosis of aorta

√4ᵗʰ **I72** **Other aneurysm**

   INCLUDES   aneurysm (cirsoid) (false) (ruptured)

   EXCLUDES 2   acquired aneurysm (I77.0)

       aneurysm (of) aorta (I71.-)

       aneurysm (of) arteriovenous NOS (Q27.3-)

       carotid artery dissection (I77.71)

       cerebral (nonruptured) aneurysm (I67.1)

       coronary aneurysm (I25.4)

       coronary artery dissection (I25.42)

       dissection of artery NEC (I77.79)

       dissection of precerebral artery, congenital (nonruptured)
(Q28.1)

       heart aneurysm (I25.3)

       iliac artery dissection (I77.72)

       precerebral artery, congential (nonruptured) (Q28.1)

       pulmonary artery aneurysm (I28.1)

       renal artery dissection (I77.73)

       retinal aneurysm (H35.0)

       ruptured cerebral aneurysm (I60.7)

       varicose aneurysm (I77.0)

       vertebral artery dissection (I77.74)

AHA: 2016,4Q,28-29

I72.0 **Aneurysm of** carotid **artery** `HCC`

    Aneurysm of common carotid artery

    Aneurysm of external carotid artery

    Aneurysm of internal carotid artery, extracranial portion

   EXCLUDES 1   aneurysm of internal carotid artery, intracranial
portion (I67.1)

       aneurysm of internal carotid artery NOS (I67.1)

I72.1 **Aneurysm of artery of** upper extremity `HCC`

I72.2 **Aneurysm of** renal **artery** `HCC`

I72.3 **Aneurysm of** iliac **artery** `HCC`

I72.4 **Aneurysm of artery of** lower extremity `HCC`

    AHA: 2019,2Q,21

N Newborn: 0   P Pediatric: 0-17   M Maternity: 9-64   A Adult: 15-124   MCC Major Complication/Comorbidity   CC Complication/Comorbidity   SW Severe Wound Dx

678   ICD-10-CM 2020

I72.5 Aneurysm of other precerebral arteries `HCC`
Aneurysm of basilar artery (trunk)
EXCLUDES 2   *aneurysm of carotid artery (I72.0)*
aneurysm of vertebral artery (I72.6)
dissection of carotid artery (I77.71)
dissection of other precerebral arteries (I77.75)
dissection of vertebral artery (I77.74)

I72.6 Aneurysm of vertebral artery `HCC`
EXCLUDES 2   *dissection of vertebral artery (I77.74)*

I72.8 Aneurysm of other specified arteries `HCC`

I72.9 Aneurysm of unspecified site `HCC`

Aneurysm

Layers of muscular and elastic tissue — Outer layer
Inner layer — Aneurysm

√4ᵗʰ I73 Other peripheral vascular diseases
EXCLUDES 2   *chilblains (T69.1)*
frostbite (T33-T34)
immersion hand or foot (T69.0-)
spasm of cerebral artery (G45.9)
AHA: 2018,4Q,87

√5ᵗʰ I73.0 Raynaud's syndrome
Raynaud's disease
Raynaud's phenomenon (secondary)
DEF: Constriction of the arteries of the digits caused by cold or by nerve or arterial damage and can be prompted by stress or emotion. Blood cannot reach the skin and soft tissues and the skin turns white with blue mottling.

I73.00 Raynaud's syndrome without gangrene
I73.01 Raynaud's syndrome with gangrene `CC` `HCC`
CC Excl: PDX collection 519

I73.1 Thromboangiitis obliterans [Buerger's disease] `HCC`
DEF: Inflammatory disease of the extremity blood vessels, mainly the lower blood vessels. This disease is associated with heavy tobacco use. The arteries are more affected than veins. It occurs primarily in young men and leads to tissue ischemia and gangrene.

√5ᵗʰ I73.8 Other specified peripheral vascular diseases
EXCLUDES 1   *diabetic (peripheral) angiopathy (E08-E13 with .51-.52)*
I73.81 Erythromelalgia `HCC`
I73.89 Other specified peripheral vascular diseases `HCC`
Acrocyanosis
Erythrocyanosis
Simple acroparesthesia [Schultze's type]
Vasomotor acroparesthesia [Nothnagel's type]

I73.9 Peripheral vascular disease, unspecified `HCC`
Intermittent claudication
Peripheral angiopathy NOS
Spasm of artery
EXCLUDES 1   *atherosclerosis of the extremities (I70.2-I70.7-)*
AHA: 2018,2Q,7

√4ᵗʰ I74 Arterial embolism and thrombosis
INCLUDES embolic infarction
embolic occlusion
thrombotic infarction
thrombotic occlusion
Code first:
embolism and thrombosis complicating abortion or ectopic or molar pregnancy (O00-O07, O08.2)
embolism and thrombosis complicating pregnancy, childbirth and the puerperium (O88.-)
EXCLUDES 2   *atheroembolism (I75.-)*
basilar embolism and thrombosis (I63.0-I63.2, I65.1)
carotid embolism and thrombosis (I63.0-I63.2, I65.2)
cerebral embolism and thrombosis (I63.3-I63.5, I66.-)
coronary embolism and thrombosis (I21-I25)
mesenteric embolism and thrombosis (K55.0-)
ophthalmic embolism and thrombosis (H34.-)
precerebral embolism and thrombosis NOS (I63.0-I63.2, I65.9)
pulmonary embolism and thrombosis (I26.-)
renal embolism and thrombosis (N28.0)
retinal embolism and thrombosis (H34.-)
septic embolism and thrombosis (I76)
vertebral embolism and thrombosis (I63.0-I63.2, I65.0)

√5ᵗʰ I74.0 Embolism and thrombosis of abdominal aorta
I74.01 Saddle embolus of abdominal aorta `MCC` `HCC`
CC Excl: PDX collection 669
I74.09 Other arterial embolism and thrombosis of abdominal aorta `CC` `HCC`
Aortic bifurcation syndrome
Aortoiliac obstruction
Leriche's syndrome
CC Excl: PDX collection 669

√5ᵗʰ I74.1 Embolism and thrombosis of other and unspecified parts of aorta
I74.10 Embolism and thrombosis of unspecified parts of aorta `CC` `HCC`
CC Excl: PDX collection 669
I74.11 Embolism and thrombosis of thoracic aorta `CC` `HCC`
CC Excl: PDX collection 701
I74.19 Embolism and thrombosis of other parts of aorta `CC` `HCC`
CC Excl: PDX collection 669

I74.2 Embolism and thrombosis of arteries of the upper extremities `CC` `HCC`
CC Excl: PDX collection 702
I74.3 Embolism and thrombosis of arteries of the lower extremities `CC` `HCC`
CC Excl: PDX collection 703
I74.4 Embolism and thrombosis of arteries of extremities, unspecified `CC` `HCC`
Peripheral arterial embolism NOS
CC Excl: PDX collection 703
I74.5 Embolism and thrombosis of iliac artery `CC` `HCC`
CC Excl: PDX collection 704
I74.8 Embolism and thrombosis of other arteries `CC` `HCC`
CC Excl: PDX collection 705
I74.9 Embolism and thrombosis of unspecified artery `CC` `HCC`
CC Excl: PDX collection 705

√4ᵗʰ I75 Atheroembolism
INCLUDES atherothrombotic microembolism
cholesterol embolism
√5ᵗʰ I75.0 Atheroembolism of extremities
√6ᵗʰ I75.01 Atheroembolism of upper extremity
CC Excl: For CC codes in subcategory I75.01: PDX collection 706
I75.011 Atheroembolism of right upper extremity `CC` `HCC`
I75.012 Atheroembolism of left upper extremity `CC` `HCC`
I75.013 Atheroembolism of bilateral upper extremities `CC` `HCC`
I75.019 Atheroembolism of unspecified upper extremity `CC` `HCC`

√6ᵗʰ **I75.02** **Atheroembolism of** lower **extremity**

CC Excl: For CC codes in subcategory I75.02: PDX collection 707

     I75.021 **Atheroembolism of** right **lower extremity** CC HCC

     I75.022 **Atheroembolism of** left **lower extremity** CC HCC

     I75.023 **Atheroembolism of** bilateral **lower extremities** CC HCC

     I75.029 **Atheroembolism of unspecified lower extremity** CC HCC

√5ᵗʰ **I75.8** **Atheroembolism of other sites**

     I75.81 **Atheroembolism of** kidney CC HCC

      Use additional code for any associated acute kidney failure and chronic kidney disease (N17.-, N18.-)

      CC Excl: PDX collection 708

     I75.89 **Atheroembolism of other site** CC HCC

      CC Excl: PDX collection 709

I76 **Septic arterial embolism** CC HCC

Code first underlying infection, such as:
   infective endocarditis (I33.0)
   lung abscess (J85.-)
Use additional code to identify the site of the embolism (I74.-)

EXCLUDES 2   septic pulmonary embolism (I26.01, I26.90)

CC Excl: PDX collection 705

√4ᵗʰ **I77** **Other disorders of arteries and arterioles**

EXCLUDES 2   collagen (vascular) diseases (M30-M36)
     hypersensitivity angiitis (M31.0)
     pulmonary artery (I28.-)

I77.0 **Arteriovenous fistula, acquired** HCC

Aneurysmal varix
Arteriovenous aneurysm, acquired

EXCLUDES 1   arteriovenous aneurysm NOS (Q27.3-)
     presence of arteriovenous shunt (fistula) for dialysis (Z99.2)
     traumatic — see injury of blood vessel by body region

EXCLUDES 2   cerebral (I67.1)
     coronary (I25.4)

DEF: Communication between an artery and vein caused by trauma or invasive procedures.

I77.1 **Stricture of artery** HCC

Narrowing of artery

I77.2 **Rupture of artery** CC HCC

Erosion of artery
Fistula of artery
Ulcer of artery

EXCLUDES 1   traumatic rupture of artery — see injury of blood vessel by body region

CC Excl: PDX collection 710

I77.3 **Arterial fibromuscular dysplasia** HCC

Fibromuscular hyperplasia (of) carotid artery
Fibromuscular hyperplasia (of) renal artery

I77.4 **Celiac artery compression syndrome** CC HCC

CC Excl: PDX collection 711

I77.5 **Necrosis of artery** CC HCC

CC Excl: PDX collection 712

I77.6 **Arteritis, unspecified** HCC

Aortitis NOS
Endarteritis NOS

EXCLUDES 1   arteritis or endarteritis:
     aortic arch (M31.4)
     cerebral NEC (I67.7)
     coronary (I25.89)
     deformans (I70.-)
     giant cell (M31.5, M31.6)
     obliterans (I70.-)
     senile (I70.-)

√6ᵗʰ **I77.7** **Other arterial dissection**

EXCLUDES 2   dissection of aorta (I71.0-)
     dissection of coronary artery (I25.42)

AHA: 2016,4Q,28-29

CC Excl: For MCC codes in subcategory I77.7: PDX collection 689

     I77.70 **Dissection of unspecified artery** MCC HCC

     I77.71 **Dissection of** carotid **artery** MCC HCC

     I77.72 **Dissection of** iliac **artery** MCC HCC

     I77.73 **Dissection of** renal **artery** MCC HCC

     I77.74 **Dissection of** vertebral **artery** MCC HCC

      EXCLUDES 2   aneurysm of vertebral artery (I72.6)

     I77.75 **Dissection of other precerebral arteries** MCC HCC

      Dissection of basilar artery (trunk)

      EXCLUDES 2   aneurysm of carotid artery (I72.0)
       aneurysm of other precerebral arteries (I72.5)
       aneurysm of vertebral artery (I72.6)
       dissection of carotid artery (I77.71)
       dissection of vertebral artery (I77.74)

     I77.76 **Dissection of artery of** upper extremity MCC HCC

     I77.77 **Dissection of artery of** lower extremity MCC HCC

     I77.79 **Dissection of other specified artery** MCC HCC

√5ᵗʰ **I77.8** **Other specified disorders of arteries and arterioles**

   √6ᵗʰ **I77.81** **Aortic ectasia**

     Ectasis aorta

     EXCLUDES 1   aortic aneurysm and dissection (I71.0-)

     I77.810 Thoracic **aortic ectasia** HCC

     I77.811 Abdominal **aortic ectasia** HCC

     I77.812 Thoracoabdominal **aortic ectasia** HCC

     I77.819 **Aortic ectasia, unspecified site** HCC

   I77.89 **Other specified disorders of arteries and arterioles** HCC

I77.9 **Disorder of arteries and arterioles, unspecified** HCC

AHA: 2018,2Q,7

√4ᵗʰ **I78** **Diseases of capillaries**

I78.0 **Hereditary hemorrhagic telangiectasia** HCC

Rendu-Osler-Weber disease

I78.1 **Nevus, non-neoplastic**

Araneus nevus
Senile nevus
Spider nevus
Stellar nevus

EXCLUDES 1   nevus NOS (D22.-)
     vascular NOS (Q82.5)

EXCLUDES 2   blue nevus (D22.-)
     flammeus nevus (Q82.5)
     hairy nevus (D22.-)
     melanocytic nevus (D22.-)
     pigmented nevus (D22.-)
     portwine nevus (Q82.5)
     sanguineous nevus (Q82.5)
     strawberry nevus (Q82.5)
     verrucous nevus (Q82.5)

AHA: 2019,1Q,21

I78.8 **Other diseases of capillaries**

I78.9 **Disease of capillaries, unspecified**

√4ᵗʰ **I79** **Disorders of arteries, arterioles and capillaries in diseases classified elsewhere**

I79.0 **Aneurysm of aorta in diseases classified elsewhere** HCC

Code first underlying disease

EXCLUDES 1   syphilitic aneurysm (A52.01)

I79.1 **Aortitis in diseases classified elsewhere** HCC

Code first underlying disease

EXCLUDES 1   syphilitic aortitis (A52.02)

I79.8 **Other disorders of arteries, arterioles and capillaries in diseases classified elsewhere** HCC

Code first underlying disease, such as:
   amyloidosis (E85.-)

EXCLUDES 1   diabetic (peripheral) angiopathy (E08-E13 with .51-.52)
     syphilitic endarteritis (A52.09)
     tuberculous endarteritis (A18.89)

N Newborn: 0   P Pediatric: 0-17   M Maternity: 9-64   A Adult: 15-124   MCC Major Complication/Comorbidity   CC Complication/Comorbidity   SW Severe Wound Dx

680   ICD-10-CM 2020

Diseases of veins, lymphatic vessels and lymph nodes, not elsewhere classified (I80-I89)

✓4ᵗʰ **I80 Phlebitis and thrombophlebitis**

INCLUDES   endophlebitis
     inflammation, vein
     periphlebitis
     suppurative phlebitis

Code first:
     phlebitis and thrombophlebitis complicating abortion, ectopic or molar pregnancy (O00-O07, O08.7)
     phlebitis and thrombophlebitis complicating pregnancy, childbirth and the puerperium (O22.-, O87.-)

EXCLUDES 1   *venous embolism and thrombosis of lower extremities (I82.4-, I82.5-, I82.81-)*

CC Excl: For CC codes in category I80: PDX collection 713

✓5ᵗʰ **I80.0 Phlebitis and thrombophlebitis of** superficial vessels of lower extremities
     Phlebitis and thrombophlebitis of femoropopliteal vein

I80.00 Phlebitis and thrombophlebitis of superficial vessels of unspecified lower extremity

I80.01 Phlebitis and thrombophlebitis of superficial vessels of right **lower extremity**

I80.02 Phlebitis and thrombophlebitis of superficial vessels of left **lower extremity**

I80.03 Phlebitis and thrombophlebitis of superficial vessels of lower extremities, bilateral

✓5ᵗʰ **I80.1 Phlebitis and thrombophlebitis of** femoral vein
     ▶Phlebitis and thrombophlebitis of common femoral vein◀
     ▶Phlebitis and thrombophlebitis of deep femoral vein◀

I80.10 Phlebitis and thrombophlebitis of unspecified femoral vein CC HCC

I80.11 Phlebitis and thrombophlebitis of right **femoral vein** CC HCC

I80.12 Phlebitis and thrombophlebitis of left **femoral vein** CC HCC

I80.13 Phlebitis and thrombophlebitis of femoral vein, bilateral CC HCC

✓5ᵗʰ **I80.2 Phlebitis and thrombophlebitis of other and unspecified** deep vessels of lower extremities

✓6ᵗʰ **I80.20 Phlebitis and thrombophlebitis of unspecified deep vessels of lower extremities**

I80.201 Phlebitis and thrombophlebitis of unspecified deep vessels of right **lower extremity** CC HCC

I80.202 Phlebitis and thrombophlebitis of unspecified deep vessels of left **lower extremity** CC HCC

I80.203 Phlebitis and thrombophlebitis of unspecified deep vessels of lower extremities, bilateral CC HCC

I80.209 Phlebitis and thrombophlebitis of unspecified deep vessels of unspecified lower extremity CC HCC

✓6ᵗʰ **I80.21 Phlebitis and thrombophlebitis of** iliac vein
     ▶Phlebitis and thrombophlebitis of common iliac vein◀
     ▶Phlebitis and thrombophlebitis of external iliac vein◀
     ▶Phlebitis and thrombophlebitis of internal iliac vein◀

I80.211 Phlebitis and thrombophlebitis of right **iliac vein** CC HCC

I80.212 Phlebitis and thrombophlebitis of left **iliac vein** CC HCC

I80.213 Phlebitis and thrombophlebitis of iliac vein, bilateral CC HCC

I80.219 Phlebitis and thrombophlebitis of unspecified iliac vein CC HCC

✓6ᵗʰ **I80.22 Phlebitis and thrombophlebitis of** popliteal vein

I80.221 Phlebitis and thrombophlebitis of right **popliteal vein** CC HCC

I80.222 Phlebitis and thrombophlebitis of left **popliteal vein** CC HCC

I80.223 Phlebitis and thrombophlebitis of popliteal vein, bilateral CC HCC

I80.229 Phlebitis and thrombophlebitis of unspecified popliteal vein CC HCC

✓6ᵗʰ **I80.23 Phlebitis and thrombophlebitis of** tibial vein
     ▶Phlebitis and thrombophlebitis of anterior tibial vein◀
     ▶Phlebitis and thrombophlebitis of posterior tibial vein◀

I80.231 Phlebitis and thrombophlebitis of right **tibial vein** CC HCC

I80.232 Phlebitis and thrombophlebitis of left **tibial vein** CC HCC

I80.233 Phlebitis and thrombophlebitis of tibial vein, bilateral CC HCC

I80.239 Phlebitis and thrombophlebitis of unspecified tibial vein CC HCC

✓6ᵗʰ **I80.24 Phlebitis and thrombophlebitis of** peroneal vein

I80.241 Phlebitis and thrombophlebitis of right **peroneal vein** CC

I80.242 Phlebitis and thrombophlebitis of left **peroneal vein**

I80.243 Phlebitis and thrombophlebitis of peroneal vein, bilateral

I80.249 Phlebitis and thrombophlebitis of unspecified peroneal vein CC

✓6ᵗʰ **I80.25 Phlebitis and thrombophlebitis of** calf muscular vein
     Phlebitis and thrombophlebitis of calf muscular vein, NOS
     Phlebitis and thrombophlebitis of gastrocnemial vein
     Phlebitis and thrombophlebitis of soleal vein

I80.251 Phlebitis and thrombophlebitis of right **calf muscular vein**

I80.252 Phlebitis and thrombophlebitis of left **calf muscular vein**

I80.253 Phlebitis and thrombophlebitis of calf muscular vein, bilateral

I80.259 Phlebitis and thrombophlebitis of unspecified calf muscular vein

✓6ᵗʰ **I80.29 Phlebitis and thrombophlebitis of other deep vessels of lower extremities**

I80.291 Phlebitis and thrombophlebitis of other deep vessels of right **lower extremity** CC HCC

I80.292 Phlebitis and thrombophlebitis of other deep vessels of left **lower extremity** CC HCC

I80.293 Phlebitis and thrombophlebitis of other deep vessels of lower extremity, bilateral CC HCC

I80.299 Phlebitis and thrombophlebitis of other deep vessels of unspecified lower extremity CC HCC

I80.3 Phlebitis and thrombophlebitis of lower extremities, unspecified

I80.8 Phlebitis and thrombophlebitis of other sites

I80.9 Phlebitis and thrombophlebitis of unspecified site

I81 Portal vein thrombosis MCC

Portal (vein) obstruction

EXCLUDES 2   *hepatic vein thrombosis (I82.0)*
            phlebitis of portal vein (K75.1)

CC Excl: PDX collection 714

☑ Additional Character Required   ✓x7ᵗʰ Placeholder   Unacceptable PDx   Questionable PDx   Manifestation   Unspecified Dx   H1-H14 HAC   HCC CMS-HCC Dx   HIV HIV Dx

ICD-10-CM 2020   681

Chapter 9. Diseases of the Circulatory System

✓4th **I82 Other venous embolism and thrombosis**

Code first venous embolism and thrombosis complicating:
abortion, ectopic or molar pregnancy (O00-O07, O08.7)
pregnancy, childbirth and the puerperium (O22.-, O87.-)

EXCLUDES 2   venous embolism and thrombosis (of):
cerebral (I63.6, I67.6)
coronary (I21-I25)
intracranial and intraspinal, septic or NOS (G08)
intracranial, nonpyogenic (I67.6)
intraspinal, nonpyogenic (G95.1)
mesenteric (K55.0-)
portal (I81)
pulmonary (I26.-)

CC Excl: For CC codes in category I82, unless otherwise noted: PDX collection 717

I82.0   Budd-Chiari syndrome   MCC HCC

Hepatic vein thrombosis
DEF: Thrombosis or other obstruction of the hepatic veins. Symptoms include an enlarged liver, extensive collateral vessels, intractable ascites, and severe portal hypertension.
CC Excl: PDX collection 715

I82.1   Thrombophlebitis migrans   CC

CC Excl: PDX collection 716

✓5th **I82.2   Embolism and thrombosis of vena cava and other thoracic veins**

✓6th **I82.21   Embolism and thrombosis of superior vena cava**

I82.210   Acute embolism and thrombosis of superior vena cava   CC HCC

Embolism and thrombosis of superior vena cava NOS

I82.211   Chronic embolism and thrombosis of superior vena cava   CC HCC

✓6th **I82.22   Embolism and thrombosis of inferior vena cava**

I82.220   Acute embolism and thrombosis of inferior vena cava   MCC HCC

Embolism and thrombosis of inferior vena cava NOS
CC Excl: PDX collection 718

I82.221   Chronic embolism and thrombosis of inferior vena cava   MCC HCC

CC Excl: PDX collection 718

✓6th **I82.29   Embolism and thrombosis of other thoracic veins**

Embolism and thrombosis of brachiocephalic (innominate) vein

I82.290   Acute embolism and thrombosis of other thoracic veins   CC HCC

I82.291   Chronic embolism and thrombosis of other thoracic veins   CC HCC

I82.3   Embolism and thrombosis of renal vein   CC MCC

CC Excl: PDX collection 719

✓5th **I82.4   Acute embolism and thrombosis of deep veins of lower extremity**

✓6th **I82.40   Acute embolism and thrombosis of unspecified deep veins of lower extremity**

Deep vein thrombosis NOS
DVT NOS

EXCLUDES 1   acute embolism and thrombosis of unspecified deep veins of distal lower extremity (I82.4Z-)
acute embolism and thrombosis of unspecified deep veins of proximal lower extremity (I82.4Y-)

I82.401   Acute embolism and thrombosis of unspecified deep veins of right lower extremity   CC H10 HCC

I82.402   Acute embolism and thrombosis of unspecified deep veins of left lower extremity   CC H10 HCC

I82.403   Acute embolism and thrombosis of unspecified deep veins of lower extremity, bilateral   CC H10 HCC

I82.409   Acute embolism and thrombosis of unspecified deep veins of unspecified lower extremity   CC H10 HCC

✓6th **I82.41   Acute embolism and thrombosis of femoral vein**

▶Acute embolism and thrombosis of common femoral vein◀
▶Acute embolism and thrombosis of deep femoral vein◀

I82.411   Acute embolism and thrombosis of right femoral vein   CC H10 HCC

I82.412   Acute embolism and thrombosis of left femoral vein   CC H10 HCC

I82.413   Acute embolism and thrombosis of femoral vein, bilateral   CC H10 HCC

I82.419   Acute embolism and thrombosis of unspecified femoral vein   CC H10 HCC

✓6th **I82.42   Acute embolism and thrombosis of iliac vein**

▶Acute embolism and thrombosis of common iliac vein◀
▶Acute embolism and thrombosis of external iliac vein◀
▶Acute embolism and thrombosis of internal iliac vein◀

I82.421   Acute embolism and thrombosis of right iliac vein   CC H10 HCC

I82.422   Acute embolism and thrombosis of left iliac vein   CC H10 HCC

I82.423   Acute embolism and thrombosis of iliac vein, bilateral   CC H10 HCC

I82.429   Acute embolism and thrombosis of unspecified iliac vein   CC H10 HCC

✓6th **I82.43   Acute embolism and thrombosis of popliteal vein**

I82.431   Acute embolism and thrombosis of right popliteal vein   CC H10 HCC

I82.432   Acute embolism and thrombosis of left popliteal vein   CC H10 HCC

I82.433   Acute embolism and thrombosis of popliteal vein, bilateral   CC H10 HCC

I82.439   Acute embolism and thrombosis of unspecified popliteal vein   CC H10 HCC

✓6th **I82.44   Acute embolism and thrombosis of tibial vein**

▶Acute embolism and thrombosis of anterior tibial vein◀
▶Acute embolism and thrombosis of posterior tibial vein◀

I82.441   Acute embolism and thrombosis of right tibial vein   CC H10 HCC

I82.442   Acute embolism and thrombosis of left tibial vein   CC H10 HCC

I82.443   Acute embolism and thrombosis of tibial vein, bilateral   CC H10 HCC

I82.449   Acute embolism and thrombosis of unspecified tibial vein   CC H10 HCC

✓6th **I82.45   Acute embolism and thrombosis of peroneal vein**

I82.451   Acute embolism and thrombosis of right peroneal vein   CC

I82.452   Acute embolism and thrombosis of left peroneal vein   CC

I82.453   Acute embolism and thrombosis of peroneal vein, bilateral   CC

I82.459   Acute embolism and thrombosis of unspecified peroneal vein   CC

N Newborn: 0   P Pediatric: 0-17   M Maternity: 9-64   A Adult: 15-124   MCC Major Complication/Comorbidity   CC Complication/Comorbidity   SW Severe Wound Dx

682   ICD-10-CM 2020

● √6ᵗʰ **I82.46**   **Acute embolism and thrombosis of** calf muscular vein
     Acute embolism and thrombosis of calf muscular vein, NOS
     Acute embolism and thrombosis of gastrocnemial vein
     Acute embolism and thrombosis of soleal vein

●   **I82.461**   **Acute embolism and thrombosis of** right **calf muscular vein**

●   **I82.462**   **Acute embolism and thrombosis of** left **calf muscular vein**

●   **I82.463**   **Acute embolism and thrombosis of calf muscular vein,** bilateral

●   **I82.469**   **Acute embolism and thrombosis of unspecified calf muscular vein**

√6ᵗʰ **I82.49**   **Acute embolism and thrombosis of other specified deep vein of lower extremity**

   I82.491   **Acute embolism and thrombosis of other specified deep vein of** right **lower extremity**   CC H10 HCC

   I82.492   **Acute embolism and thrombosis of other specified deep vein of** left **lower extremity**   CC H10 HCC

   I82.493   **Acute embolism and thrombosis of other specified deep vein of lower extremity,** bilateral   CC H10 HCC

   I82.499   **Acute embolism and thrombosis of other specified deep vein of unspecified lower extremity**   CC H10 HCC

√6ᵗʰ **I82.4Y**   **Acute embolism and thrombosis of unspecified deep veins of** proximal **lower extremity**
     Acute embolism and thrombosis of deep vein of thigh NOS
     Acute embolism and thrombosis of deep vein of upper leg NOS

   I82.4Y1   **Acute embolism and thrombosis of unspecified deep veins of** right **proximal lower extremity**   CC H10 HCC

   I82.4Y2   **Acute embolism and thrombosis of unspecified deep veins of** left **proximal lower extremity**   CC H10 HCC

   I82.4Y3   **Acute embolism and thrombosis of unspecified deep veins of proximal lower extremity,** bilateral   CC H10 HCC

   I82.4Y9   **Acute embolism and thrombosis of unspecified deep veins of unspecified proximal lower extremity**   CC H10 HCC

√6ᵗʰ **I82.4Z**   **Acute embolism and thrombosis of unspecified deep veins of** distal **lower extremity**
     Acute embolism and thrombosis of deep vein of calf NOS
     Acute embolism and thrombosis of deep vein of lower leg NOS

   I82.4Z1   **Acute embolism and thrombosis of unspecified deep veins of** right **distal lower extremity**   CC H10 HCC

   I82.4Z2   **Acute embolism and thrombosis of unspecified deep veins of** left **distal lower extremity**   CC H10 HCC

   I82.4Z3   **Acute embolism and thrombosis of unspecified deep veins of distal lower extremity,** bilateral   CC H10 HCC

   I82.4Z9   **Acute embolism and thrombosis of unspecified deep veins of unspecified distal lower extremity**   CC H10 HCC

√5ᵗʰ **I82.5**   Chronic **embolism and thrombosis of** deep veins of lower extremity
     Use additional code, if applicable, for associated long-term (current) use of anticoagulants (Z79.01)
     EXCLUDES 1   *personal history of venous embolism and thrombosis (Z86.718)*

√6ᵗʰ **I82.50**   **Chronic embolism and thrombosis of unspecified deep veins of lower extremity**
     EXCLUDES 1   *chronic embolism and thrombosis of unspecified deep veins of distal lower extremity (I82.5Z-)*
     chronic embolism and thrombosis of unspecified deep veins of proximal lower extremity (I82.5Y-)

   I82.501   **Chronic embolism and thrombosis of unspecified deep veins of** right **lower extremity**   CC HCC

   I82.502   **Chronic embolism and thrombosis of unspecified deep veins of** left **lower extremity**   CC HCC

   I82.503   **Chronic embolism and thrombosis of unspecified deep veins of lower extremity,** bilateral   CC HCC

   I82.509   **Chronic embolism and thrombosis of unspecified deep veins of unspecified lower extremity**   CC HCC

√6ᵗʰ **I82.51**   **Chronic embolism and thrombosis of** femoral vein
     ▶Chronic embolism and thrombosis of common femoral vein◀
     ▶Chronic embolism and thrombosis of deep femoral vein◀

   I82.511   **Chronic embolism and thrombosis of** right **femoral vein**   CC HCC

   I82.512   **Chronic embolism and thrombosis of** left **femoral vein**   CC HCC

   I82.513   **Chronic embolism and thrombosis of femoral vein,** bilateral   CC HCC

   I82.519   **Chronic embolism and thrombosis of unspecified femoral vein**   CC HCC

√6ᵗʰ **I82.52**   **Chronic embolism and thrombosis of** iliac vein
     ▶Chronic embolism and thrombosis of common iliac vein◀
     ▶Chronic embolism and thrombosis of external iliac vein◀
     ▶Chronic embolism and thrombosis of internal iliac vein◀

   I82.521   **Chronic embolism and thrombosis of** right **iliac vein**   CC HCC

   I82.522   **Chronic embolism and thrombosis of** left **iliac vein**   CC HCC

   I82.523   **Chronic embolism and thrombosis of iliac vein,** bilateral   CC HCC

   I82.529   **Chronic embolism and thrombosis of unspecified iliac vein**   CC HCC

√6ᵗʰ **I82.53**   **Chronic embolism and thrombosis of** popliteal vein

   I82.531   **Chronic embolism and thrombosis of** right **popliteal vein**   CC HCC

   I82.532   **Chronic embolism and thrombosis of** left **popliteal vein**   CC HCC

   I82.533   **Chronic embolism and thrombosis of popliteal vein,** bilateral   CC HCC

   I82.539   **Chronic embolism and thrombosis of unspecified popliteal vein**   CC HCC

✔ Additional Character Required   √x7ᵗʰ Placeholder   Unacceptable PDx   Questionable PDx   Manifestation   Unspecified Dx   H1-H14 HAC   HCC CMS-HCC Dx   HIV HIV Dx

ICD-10-CM 2020   683

Chapter 9. Diseases of the Circulatory System

I82.54–I82.701

√6ᵗʰ **I82.54** **Chronic embolism and thrombosis of** tibial vein
> ▶Chronic embolism and thrombosis of anterior tibial vein◀
> ▶Chronic embolism and thrombosis of posterior tibial vein◀

I82.541 Chronic embolism and thrombosis of right tibial vein `CC` `HCC`

I82.542 Chronic embolism and thrombosis of left tibial vein `CC` `HCC`

I82.543 Chronic embolism and thrombosis of tibial vein, bilateral

I82.549 Chronic embolism and thrombosis of unspecified tibial vein `CC` `HCC`

√6ᵗʰ **I82.55** **Chronic embolism and thrombosis of** peroneal vein

I82.551 Chronic embolism and thrombosis of right peroneal vein `CC`

I82.552 Chronic embolism and thrombosis of left peroneal vein `CC`

I82.553 Chronic embolism and thrombosis of peroneal vein, bilateral `CC`

I82.559 Chronic embolism and thrombosis of unspecified peroneal vein `CC`

√6ᵗʰ **I82.56** **Chronic embolism and thrombosis of** calf muscular vein
> Chronic embolism and thrombosis of calf muscular vein NOS
> Chronic embolism and thrombosis of gastrocnemial vein
> Chronic embolism and thrombosis of soleal vein

I82.561 Chronic embolism and thrombosis of right calf muscular vein

I82.562 Chronic embolism and thrombosis of left calf muscular vein

I82.563 Chronic embolism and thrombosis of calf muscular vein, bilateral

I82.569 Chronic embolism and thrombosis of unspecified calf muscular vein

√6ᵗʰ **I82.59** **Chronic embolism and thrombosis of other specified deep vein of lower extremity**

I82.591 Chronic embolism and thrombosis of other specified deep vein of right lower extremity `CC` `HCC`

I82.592 Chronic embolism and thrombosis of other specified deep vein of left lower extremity `CC` `HCC`

I82.593 Chronic embolism and thrombosis of other specified deep vein of lower extremity, bilateral `CC` `HCC`

I82.599 Chronic embolism and thrombosis of other specified deep vein of unspecified lower extremity `CC` `HCC`

√6ᵗʰ **I82.5Y** **Chronic embolism and thrombosis of unspecified deep veins of** proximal **lower extremity**
> Chronic embolism and thrombosis of deep veins of thigh NOS
> Chronic embolism and thrombosis of deep veins of upper leg NOS

I82.5Y1 Chronic embolism and thrombosis of unspecified deep veins of right proximal lower extremity `CC` `HCC`

I82.5Y2 Chronic embolism and thrombosis of unspecified deep veins of left proximal lower extremity `CC` `HCC`

I82.5Y3 Chronic embolism and thrombosis of unspecified deep veins of proximal lower extremity, bilateral `CC` `HCC`

I82.5Y9 Chronic embolism and thrombosis of unspecified deep veins of unspecified proximal lower extremity `CC` `HCC`

√6ᵗʰ **I82.5Z** **Chronic embolism and thrombosis of unspecified deep veins of** distal **lower extremity**
> Chronic embolism and thrombosis of deep veins of calf NOS
> Chronic embolism and thrombosis of deep veins of lower leg NOS

I82.5Z1 Chronic embolism and thrombosis of unspecified deep veins of right distal lower extremity `CC` `HCC`

I82.5Z2 Chronic embolism and thrombosis of unspecified deep veins of left distal lower extremity `CC` `HCC`

I82.5Z3 Chronic embolism and thrombosis of unspecified deep veins of distal lower extremity, bilateral `CC` `HCC`

I82.5Z9 Chronic embolism and thrombosis of unspecified deep veins of unspecified distal lower extremity `CC` `HCC`

√5ᵗʰ **I82.6** Acute embolism and thrombosis of veins of upper extremity

√6ᵗʰ **I82.60** **Acute embolism and thrombosis of unspecified veins of upper extremity**

I82.601 Acute embolism and thrombosis of unspecified veins of right upper extremity `CC`

I82.602 Acute embolism and thrombosis of unspecified veins of left upper extremity `CC`

I82.603 Acute embolism and thrombosis of unspecified veins of upper extremity, bilateral `CC`

I82.609 Acute embolism and thrombosis of unspecified veins of unspecified upper extremity `CC`

√6ᵗʰ **I82.61** **Acute embolism and thrombosis of** superficial veins **of upper extremity**
> Acute embolism and thrombosis of antecubital vein
> Acute embolism and thrombosis of basilic vein
> Acute embolism and thrombosis of cephalic vein

I82.611 Acute embolism and thrombosis of superficial veins of right upper extremity `CC`

I82.612 Acute embolism and thrombosis of superficial veins of left upper extremity `CC`

I82.613 Acute embolism and thrombosis of superficial veins of upper extremity, bilateral `CC`

I82.619 Acute embolism and thrombosis of superficial veins of unspecified upper extremity `CC`

√6ᵗʰ **I82.62** **Acute embolism and thrombosis of** deep veins **of upper extremity**
> Acute embolism and thrombosis of brachial vein
> Acute embolism and thrombosis of radial vein
> Acute embolism and thrombosis of ulnar vein

I82.621 Acute embolism and thrombosis of deep veins of right upper extremity `CC` `HCC`

I82.622 Acute embolism and thrombosis of deep veins of left upper extremity `CC` `HCC`

I82.623 Acute embolism and thrombosis of deep veins of upper extremity, bilateral `CC` `HCC`

I82.629 Acute embolism and thrombosis of deep veins of unspecified upper extremity `CC` `HCC`

√5ᵗʰ **I82.7** Chronic embolism and thrombosis of veins of upper extremity
> Use additional code, if applicable, for associated long-term (current) use of anticoagulants (Z79.01)
> **EXCLUDES 1**   *personal history of venous embolism and thrombosis (Z86.718)*

√6ᵗʰ **I82.70** **Chronic embolism and thrombosis of unspecified veins of upper extremity**

I82.701 Chronic embolism and thrombosis of unspecified veins of right upper extremity `CC`

Ⓝ Newborn: 0   Ⓟ Pediatric: 0-17   Ⓜ Maternity: 9-64   Ⓐ Adult: 15-124   `MCC` Major Complication/Comorbidity   `CC` Complication/Comorbidity   `SW` Severe Wound Dx

684   ICD-10-CM 2020

I82.702 Chronic embolism and thrombosis of unspecified veins of left upper extremity `CC`

I82.703 Chronic embolism and thrombosis of unspecified veins of upper extremity, bilateral `CC`

I82.709 Chronic embolism and thrombosis of unspecified veins of unspecified upper extremity `CC`

✓6th **I82.71** Chronic embolism and thrombosis of superficial veins of upper extremity
Chronic embolism and thrombosis of antecubital vein
Chronic embolism and thrombosis of basilic vein
Chronic embolism and thrombosis of cephalic vein

I82.711 Chronic embolism and thrombosis of superficial veins of right upper extremity `CC`

I82.712 Chronic embolism and thrombosis of superficial veins of left upper extremity `CC`

I82.713 Chronic embolism and thrombosis of superficial veins of upper extremity, bilateral `CC`

I82.719 Chronic embolism and thrombosis of superficial veins of unspecified upper extremity `CC`

✓6th **I82.72** Chronic embolism and thrombosis of deep veins of upper extremity
Chronic embolism and thrombosis of brachial vein
Chronic embolism and thrombosis of radial vein
Chronic embolism and thrombosis of ulnar vein

I82.721 Chronic embolism and thrombosis of deep veins of right upper extremity `CC` `HCC`

I82.722 Chronic embolism and thrombosis of deep veins of left upper extremity `CC` `HCC`

I82.723 Chronic embolism and thrombosis of deep veins of upper extremity, bilateral `CC` `HCC`

I82.729 Chronic embolism and thrombosis of deep veins of unspecified upper extremity `CC` `HCC`

✓5th **I82.A** Embolism and thrombosis of axillary vein

✓6th **I82.A1** Acute embolism and thrombosis of axillary vein

I82.A11 Acute embolism and thrombosis of right axillary vein `CC` `HCC`

I82.A12 Acute embolism and thrombosis of left axillary vein `CC` `HCC`

I82.A13 Acute embolism and thrombosis of axillary vein, bilateral `CC` `HCC`

I82.A19 Acute embolism and thrombosis of unspecified axillary vein `CC` `HCC`

✓6th **I82.A2** Chronic embolism and thrombosis of axillary vein

I82.A21 Chronic embolism and thrombosis of right axillary vein `CC` `HCC`

I82.A22 Chronic embolism and thrombosis of left axillary vein `CC` `HCC`

I82.A23 Chronic embolism and thrombosis of axillary vein, bilateral `CC` `HCC`

I82.A29 Chronic embolism and thrombosis of unspecified axillary vein `CC` `HCC`

✓5th **I82.B** Embolism and thrombosis of subclavian vein

✓6th **I82.B1** Acute embolism and thrombosis of subclavian vein

I82.B11 Acute embolism and thrombosis of right subclavian vein `CC` `HCC`

I82.B12 Acute embolism and thrombosis of left subclavian vein `CC` `HCC`

I82.B13 Acute embolism and thrombosis of subclavian vein, bilateral `CC` `HCC`

I82.B19 Acute embolism and thrombosis of unspecified subclavian vein `CC` `HCC`

✓6th **I82.B2** Chronic embolism and thrombosis of subclavian vein

I82.B21 Chronic embolism and thrombosis of right subclavian vein `CC` `HCC`

I82.B22 Chronic embolism and thrombosis of left subclavian vein `CC` `HCC`

I82.B23 Chronic embolism and thrombosis of subclavian vein, bilateral `CC` `HCC`

I82.B29 Chronic embolism and thrombosis of unspecified subclavian vein `CC` `HCC`

✓5th **I82.C** Embolism and thrombosis of internal jugular vein

✓6th **I82.C1** Acute embolism and thrombosis of internal jugular vein

I82.C11 Acute embolism and thrombosis of right internal jugular vein `CC` `HCC`

I82.C12 Acute embolism and thrombosis of left internal jugular vein `CC` `HCC`

I82.C13 Acute embolism and thrombosis of internal jugular vein, bilateral `CC` `HCC`

I82.C19 Acute embolism and thrombosis of unspecified internal jugular vein `CC` `HCC`

✓6th **I82.C2** Chronic embolism and thrombosis of internal jugular vein

I82.C21 Chronic embolism and thrombosis of right internal jugular vein `CC` `HCC`

I82.C22 Chronic embolism and thrombosis of left internal jugular vein `CC` `HCC`

I82.C23 Chronic embolism and thrombosis of internal jugular vein, bilateral `CC` `HCC`

I82.C29 Chronic embolism and thrombosis of unspecified internal jugular vein `CC` `HCC`

✓5th **I82.8** Embolism and thrombosis of other specified veins
Use additional code, if applicable, for associated long-term (current) use of anticoagulants (Z79.01)

✓6th **I82.81** Embolism and thrombosis of superficial veins of lower extremities
Embolism and thrombosis of saphenous vein (greater) (lesser)

I82.811 Embolism and thrombosis of superficial veins of right lower extremity `CC`

I82.812 Embolism and thrombosis of superficial veins of left lower extremity `CC`

I82.813 Embolism and thrombosis of superficial veins of lower extremities, bilateral `CC`

I82.819 Embolism and thrombosis of superficial veins of unspecified lower extremity `CC`

✓6th **I82.89** Embolism and thrombosis of other specified veins

I82.890 Acute embolism and thrombosis of other specified veins `CC`

I82.891 Chronic embolism and thrombosis of other specified veins `CC`

✓5th **I82.9** Embolism and thrombosis of unspecified vein

I82.90 Acute embolism and thrombosis of unspecified vein `CC`
Embolism of vein NOS
Thrombosis (vein) NOS

I82.91 Chronic embolism and thrombosis of unspecified vein `CC`

Chapter 9. Diseases of the Circulatory System

√4th **I83 Varicose veins of lower extremities**

> EXCLUDES 1   *varicose veins complicating pregnancy (O22.0-)*
> *varicose veins complicating the puerperium (O87.4)*

√5th **I83.0 Varicose veins of lower extremities with** ulcer

> Use additional code to identify severity of ulcer (L97.-)

√6th **I83.00 Varicose veins of unspecified lower extremity with ulcer**

I83.001 Varicose veins of unspecified lower extremity with ulcer of thigh HCC A

I83.002 Varicose veins of unspecified lower extremity with ulcer of calf HCC A

I83.003 Varicose veins of unspecified lower extremity with ulcer of ankle HCC A

I83.004 Varicose veins of unspecified lower extremity with ulcer of heel and midfoot HCC A
> Varicose veins of unspecified lower extremity with ulcer of plantar surface of midfoot

I83.005 Varicose veins of unspecified lower extremity with ulcer other part of foot HCC A
> Varicose veins of unspecified lower extremity with ulcer of toe

I83.008 Varicose veins of unspecified lower extremity with ulcer other part of lower leg HCC A

I83.009 Varicose veins of unspecified lower extremity with ulcer of unspecified site HCC A

√6th **I83.01 Varicose veins of** right **lower extremity with ulcer**

I83.011 Varicose veins of right lower extremity with ulcer of thigh HCC A

I83.012 Varicose veins of right lower extremity with ulcer of calf HCC A

I83.013 Varicose veins of right lower extremity with ulcer of ankle HCC A

I83.014 Varicose veins of right lower extremity with ulcer of heel and midfoot HCC A
> Varicose veins of right lower extremity with ulcer of plantar surface of midfoot

I83.015 Varicose veins of right lower extremity with ulcer other part of foot HCC A
> Varicose veins of right lower extremity with ulcer of toe

I83.018 Varicose veins of right lower extremity with ulcer other part of lower leg HCC A

I83.019 Varicose veins of right lower extremity with ulcer of unspecified site HCC A

√6th **I83.02 Varicose veins of** left **lower extremity with ulcer**

I83.021 Varicose veins of left lower extremity with ulcer of thigh HCC A

I83.022 Varicose veins of left lower extremity with ulcer of calf HCC A

I83.023 Varicose veins of left lower extremity with ulcer of ankle HCC A

I83.024 Varicose veins of left lower extremity with ulcer of heel and midfoot HCC A
> Varicose veins of left lower extremity with ulcer of plantar surface of midfoot

I83.025 Varicose veins of left lower extremity with ulcer other part of foot HCC A
> Varicose veins of left lower extremity with ulcer of toe

I83.028 Varicose veins of left lower extremity with ulcer other part of lower leg HCC A

I83.029 Varicose veins of left lower extremity with ulcer of unspecified site HCC A

√5th **I83.1 Varicose veins of lower extremities with** inflammation

I83.10 Varicose veins of unspecified lower extremity with inflammation A

I83.11 Varicose veins of right **lower extremity with inflammation** A

I83.12 Varicose veins of left **lower extremity with inflammation** A

√5th **I83.2 Varicose veins of lower extremities with both** ulcer and inflammation

> Use additional code to identify severity of ulcer (L97.-)
> **CC Excl: For CC codes in subcategory I83.2:** PDX collection 720

√6th **I83.20 Varicose veins of** unspecified **lower extremity with both ulcer and inflammation**

I83.201 Varicose veins of unspecified lower extremity with both ulcer of thigh and inflammation CC HCC A

I83.202 Varicose veins of unspecified lower extremity with both ulcer of calf and inflammation CC HCC A

I83.203 Varicose veins of unspecified lower extremity with both ulcer of ankle and inflammation CC HCC A

I83.204 Varicose veins of unspecified lower extremity with both ulcer of heel and midfoot and inflammation CC HCC A
> Varicose veins of unspecified lower extremity with both ulcer of plantar surface of midfoot and inflammation

I83.205 Varicose veins of unspecified lower extremity with both ulcer of other part of foot and inflammation CC HCC A
> Varicose veins of unspecified lower extremity with both ulcer of toe and inflammation

I83.208 Varicose veins of unspecified lower extremity with both ulcer of other part of lower extremity and inflammation CC HCC A

I83.209 Varicose veins of unspecified lower extremity with both ulcer of unspecified site and inflammation CC HCC A

√6th **I83.21 Varicose veins of** right **lower extremity with both ulcer and inflammation**

I83.211 Varicose veins of right lower extremity with both ulcer of thigh and inflammation CC HCC A

I83.212 Varicose veins of right lower extremity with both ulcer of calf and inflammation CC HCC A

I83.213 Varicose veins of right lower extremity with both ulcer of ankle and inflammation CC HCC A

I83.214 Varicose veins of right lower extremity with both ulcer of heel and midfoot and inflammation CC HCC A
> Varicose veins of right lower extremity with both ulcer of plantar surface of midfoot and inflammation

I83.215 Varicose veins of right lower extremity with both ulcer other part of foot and inflammation CC HCC A
> Varicose veins of right lower extremity with both ulcer of toe and inflammation

I83.218 Varicose veins of right lower extremity with both ulcer of other part of lower extremity and inflammation CC HCC A

I83.219 Varicose veins of right lower extremity with both ulcer of unspecified site and inflammation CC HCC A

√6th **I83.22 Varicose veins of** left **lower extremity with both ulcer and inflammation**

I83.221 Varicose veins of left lower extremity with both ulcer of thigh and inflammation CC HCC A

I83.222 Varicose veins of left lower extremity with both ulcer of calf and inflammation CC HCC A

N Newborn: 0   P Pediatric: 0-17   M Maternity: 9-64   A Adult: 15-124   MCC Major Complication/Comorbidity   CC Complication/Comorbidity   SW Severe Wound Dx

686   ICD-10-CM 2020

I83.223   **Varicose veins of left lower extremity with both ulcer of ankle and inflammation** `CC` `HCC` `A`

I83.224   **Varicose veins of left lower extremity with both ulcer of heel and midfoot and inflammation** `CC` `HCC` `A`

> Varicose veins of left lower extremity with both ulcer of plantar surface of midfoot and inflammation

I83.225   **Varicose veins of left lower extremity with both ulcer other part of foot and inflammation** `CC` `HCC` `A`

> Varicose veins of left lower extremity with both ulcer of toe and inflammation

I83.228   **Varicose veins of left lower extremity with both ulcer of other part of lower extremity and inflammation** `CC` `HCC` `A`

I83.229   **Varicose veins of left lower extremity with both ulcer of unspecified site and inflammation** `CC` `HCC` `A`

√5ᵗʰ **I83.8   Varicose veins of lower extremities with other complications**

√6ᵗʰ **I83.81   Varicose veins of lower extremities with pain**

I83.811   **Varicose veins of right lower extremity with pain** `A`

I83.812   **Varicose veins of left lower extremity with pain** `A`

I83.813   **Varicose veins of bilateral lower extremities with pain** `A`

I83.819   **Varicose veins of unspecified lower extremity with pain** `A`

√6ᵗʰ **I83.89   Varicose veins of lower extremities with other complications**

> Varicose veins of lower extremities with edema
> Varicose veins of lower extremities with swelling

I83.891   **Varicose veins of right lower extremity with other complications** `A`

I83.892   **Varicose veins of left lower extremity with other complications** `A`

I83.893   **Varicose veins of bilateral lower extremities with other complications** `A`

I83.899   **Varicose veins of unspecified lower extremity with other complications** `A`

√5ᵗʰ **I83.9   Asymptomatic varicose veins of lower extremities**

> Phlebectasia of lower extremities
> Varicose veins of lower extremities
> Varix of lower extremities

I83.90   **Asymptomatic varicose veins of unspecified lower extremity** `A`

> Varicose veins NOS

I83.91   **Asymptomatic varicose veins of right lower extremity** `A`

I83.92   **Asymptomatic varicose veins of left lower extremity** `A`

I83.93   **Asymptomatic varicose veins of bilateral lower extremities** `A`

√4ᵗʰ **I85   Esophageal varices**

> Use additional code to identify:
> alcohol abuse and dependence (F10.-)

√5ᵗʰ **I85.0   Esophageal varices**

> Idiopathic esophageal varices
> Primary esophageal varices

I85.00   **Esophageal varices without bleeding** `CC` `HCC`

> Esophageal varices NOS
> **CC Excl:** PDX collection 721

I85.01   **Esophageal varices with bleeding** `MCC` `HCC`

> **CC Excl:** PDX collection 722

√5ᵗʰ **I85.1   Secondary esophageal varices**

> Esophageal varices secondary to alcoholic liver disease
> Esophageal varices secondary to cirrhosis of liver
> Esophageal varices secondary to schistosomiasis
> Esophageal varices secondary to toxic liver disease
> Code first underlying disease

I85.10   **Secondary esophageal varices without bleeding** `CC` `HCC`

> **CC Excl:** PDX collection 723

I85.11   **Secondary esophageal varices with bleeding** `MCC` `HCC`

> **CC Excl:** PDX collection 724

√4ᵗʰ **I86   Varicose veins of other sites**

> `EXCLUDES 1`   *varicose veins of unspecified site (I83.9-)*
> `EXCLUDES 2`   *retinal varices (H35.0-)*

I86.0   Sublingual varices

> **DEF:** Distended, tortuous veins beneath the tongue.

I86.1   Scrotal varices ♂

> Varicocele

I86.2   Pelvic varices

I86.3   Vulval varices ♀

> `EXCLUDES 1`   *vulval varices complicating childbirth and the puerperium (O87.8)*
> *vulval varices complicating pregnancy (O22.1-)*

I86.4   Gastric varices

I86.8   Varicose veins of other specified sites `A`

> Varicose ulcer of nasal septum

√4ᵗʰ **I87   Other disorders of veins**

√5ᵗʰ **I87.0   Postthrombotic syndrome**

> Chronic venous hypertension due to deep vein thrombosis
> Postphlebitic syndrome
> `EXCLUDES 1`   *chronic venous hypertension without deep vein thrombosis (I87.3-)*
> **CC Excl: For CC codes in subcategory I87.0:** PDX collection 725

√6ᵗʰ **I87.00   Postthrombotic syndrome without complications**

> Asymptomatic postthrombotic syndrome

I87.001   **Postthrombotic syndrome without complications of right lower extremity**

I87.002   **Postthrombotic syndrome without complications of left lower extremity**

I87.003   **Postthrombotic syndrome without complications of bilateral lower extremity**

I87.009   **Postthrombotic syndrome without complications of unspecified extremity**

> Postthrombotic syndrome NOS

√6ᵗʰ **I87.01   Postthrombotic syndrome with ulcer**

> Use additional code to specify site and severity of ulcer (L97.-)

I87.011   **Postthrombotic syndrome with ulcer of right lower extremity** `CC` `HCC`

I87.012   **Postthrombotic syndrome with ulcer of left lower extremity** `CC` `HCC`

I87.013   **Postthrombotic syndrome with ulcer of bilateral lower extremity** `CC` `HCC`

I87.019   **Postthrombotic syndrome with ulcer of unspecified lower extremity** `CC` `HCC`

√6ᵗʰ **I87.02   Postthrombotic syndrome with inflammation**

I87.021   **Postthrombotic syndrome with inflammation of right lower extremity**

I87.022   **Postthrombotic syndrome with inflammation of left lower extremity**

I87.023   **Postthrombotic syndrome with inflammation of bilateral lower extremity**

I87.029   **Postthrombotic syndrome with inflammation of unspecified lower extremity**

√6ᵗʰ **I87.03   Postthrombotic syndrome with ulcer and inflammation**

> Use additional code to specify site and severity of ulcer (L97.-)

I87.031   **Postthrombotic syndrome with ulcer and inflammation of right lower extremity** `CC` `HCC`

I87.032   **Postthrombotic syndrome with ulcer and inflammation of left lower extremity** `CC` `HCC`

✔ Additional Character Required   √x7ᵗʰ Placeholder   <u>Unacceptable PDx</u>   Questionable PDx   Manifestation   <u>Unspecified Dx</u>   H1 - H14 HAC   `HCC` CMS-HCC Dx   `HIV` HIV Dx

ICD-10-CM 2020   687

           I87.033 Postthrombotic syndrome with ulcer and inflammation of **bilateral lower** extremity `CC` `HCC`

           I87.039 Postthrombotic syndrome with ulcer and inflammation of unspecified lower extremity `CC` `HCC`

     ✓6th **I87.09** Postthrombotic syndrome with other complications

           I87.091 Postthrombotic syndrome with other complications of **right lower** extremity

           I87.092 Postthrombotic syndrome with other complications of **left lower** extremity

           I87.093 Postthrombotic syndrome with other complications of **bilateral lower** extremity

           I87.099 Postthrombotic syndrome with other complications of unspecified lower extremity

I87.1   **Compression of vein** `CC`

     Stricture of vein

     Vena cava syndrome (inferior) (superior)

     EXCLUDES 2   *compression of pulmonary vein (I28.8)*

     CC Excl: PDX collection 726

I87.2   **Venous insufficiency (chronic) (peripheral)**

     Stasis dermatitis

     EXCLUDES 1   *stasis dermatitis with varicose veins of lower extremities (I83.1-, I83.2-)*

     DEF: Insufficient drainage of venous blood in any part of the body that results in edema or dermatosis.

✓5th **I87.3**   **Chronic venous hypertension (idiopathic)**

     Stasis edema

     EXCLUDES 1   *chronic venous hypertension due to deep vein thrombosis (I87.0-)*

                varicose veins of lower extremities (I83.-)

     CC Excl: For CC codes in subcategory I87.3: PDX collection 727

     ✓6th **I87.30**   **Chronic venous hypertension (idiopathic) without complications**

         Asymptomatic chronic venous hypertension (idiopathic)

           I87.301 Chronic venous hypertension (idiopathic) without complications of **right lower** extremity

           I87.302 Chronic venous hypertension (idiopathic) without complications of **left lower** extremity

           I87.303 Chronic venous hypertension (idiopathic) without complications of **bilateral lower** extremity

           I87.309 Chronic venous hypertension (idiopathic) without complications of unspecified lower extremity

                Chronic venous hypertension NOS

     ✓6th **I87.31**   Chronic venous hypertension (idiopathic) with **ulcer**

         Use additional code to specify site and severity of ulcer (L97.-)

           I87.311 Chronic venous hypertension (idiopathic) with ulcer of **right lower** extremity `CC` `HCC`

           I87.312 Chronic venous hypertension (idiopathic) with ulcer of **left lower** extremity `CC` `HCC`

           I87.313 Chronic venous hypertension (idiopathic) with ulcer of **bilateral lower** extremity `CC` `HCC`

           I87.319 Chronic venous hypertension (idiopathic) with ulcer of unspecified lower extremity `CC` `HCC`

     ✓6th **I87.32**   Chronic venous hypertension (idiopathic) with **inflammation**

           I87.321 Chronic venous hypertension (idiopathic) with inflammation of **right lower** extremity

           I87.322 Chronic venous hypertension (idiopathic) with inflammation of **left lower** extremity

           I87.323 Chronic venous hypertension (idiopathic) with inflammation of **bilateral lower** extremity

           I87.329 Chronic venous hypertension (idiopathic) with inflammation of unspecified lower extremity

     ✓6th **I87.33**   Chronic venous hypertension (idiopathic) with **ulcer and inflammation**

         Use additional code to specify site and severity of ulcer (L97.-)

           I87.331 Chronic venous hypertension (idiopathic) with ulcer and inflammation of **right lower** extremity `CC` `HCC`

           I87.332 Chronic venous hypertension (idiopathic) with ulcer and inflammation of **left lower** extremity `CC` `HCC`

           I87.333 Chronic venous hypertension (idiopathic) with ulcer and inflammation of **bilateral lower** extremity `CC` `HCC`

           I87.339 Chronic venous hypertension (idiopathic) with ulcer and inflammation of unspecified lower extremity `CC` `HCC`

     ✓6th **I87.39**   Chronic venous hypertension (idiopathic) with other complications

           I87.391 Chronic venous hypertension (idiopathic) with other complications of **right lower** extremity

           I87.392 Chronic venous hypertension (idiopathic) with other complications of **left lower** extremity

           I87.393 Chronic venous hypertension (idiopathic) with other complications of **bilateral lower** extremity

           I87.399 Chronic venous hypertension (idiopathic) with other complications of unspecified lower extremity

I87.8   **Other specified disorders of veins**

     Phlebosclerosis

     Venofibrosis

I87.9   **Disorder of vein, unspecified**

✓4th **I88**   **Nonspecific lymphadenitis**

     EXCLUDES 1   *acute lymphadenitis, except mesenteric (L04.-)*

                enlarged lymph nodes NOS (R59.-)

                human immunodeficiency virus [HIV] disease resulting in generalized lymphadenopathy (B20)

I88.0   **Nonspecific mesenteric lymphadenitis**

     Mesenteric lymphadenitis (acute)(chronic)

I88.1   **Chronic lymphadenitis, except mesenteric**

     Adenitis

     Lymphadenitis

I88.8   **Other nonspecific lymphadenitis**

I88.9   **Nonspecific lymphadenitis, unspecified**

     Lymphadenitis NOS

✓4th **I89**   **Other noninfective disorders of lymphatic vessels and lymph nodes**

     EXCLUDES 1   *chylocele, tunica vaginalis (nonfilarial) NOS (N50.89)*

                enlarged lymph nodes NOS (R59.-)

                filarial chylocele (B74.-)

                hereditary lymphedema (Q82.0)

I89.0   **Lymphedema, not elsewhere classified**

     Elephantiasis (nonfilarial) NOS

     Lymphangiectasis

     Obliteration, lymphatic vessel

     Praecox lymphedema

     Secondary lymphedema

     EXCLUDES 1   *postmastectomy lymphedema (I97.2)*

I89.1   **Lymphangitis**

     Chronic lymphangitis

     Lymphangitis NOS

     Subacute lymphangitis

     EXCLUDES 1   *acute lymphangitis (L03.-)*

I89.8   **Other specified noninfective disorders of lymphatic vessels and lymph nodes**

     Chylocele (nonfilarial)

     Chylous ascites

     Chylous cyst

     Lipomelanotic reticulosis

     Lymph node or vessel fistula

     Lymph node or vessel infarction

     Lymph node or vessel rupture

N Newborn: 0   P Pediatric: 0-17   M Maternity: 9-64   A Adult: 15-124   MCC Major Complication/Comorbidity   CC Complication/Comorbidity   SW Severe Wound Dx

688   ICD-10-CM 2020

I89.9   **Noninfective disorder of lymphatic vessels and lymph nodes, unspecified**
Disease of lymphatic vessels NOS

Other and unspecified disorders of the circulatory system (I95-I99)

✓4ᵗʰ **I95 Hypotension**

> EXCLUDES 1   *cardiovascular collapse (R57.9) (~R57.9)*
> *maternal hypotension syndrome (O26.5-)*
> *nonspecific low blood pressure reading NOS (R03.1)*

I95.0   **Idiopathic hypotension**

I95.1   **Orthostatic hypotension**
Hypotension, postural
> EXCLUDES 1   *neurogenic orthostatic hypotension [Shy-Drager] (G90.3)*
> *orthostatic hypotension due to drugs (I95.2)*

I95.2   **Hypotension due to drugs**
Orthostatic hypotension due to drugs
Use additional code for adverse effect, if applicable, to identify drug (T36-T50 with fifth or sixth character 5)

I95.3   **Hypotension of hemodialysis**
Intra-dialytic hypotension

✓5ᵗʰ **I95.8**   **Other hypotension**

I95.81   **Postprocedural hypotension**

I95.89   **Other hypotension**
Chronic hypotension

I95.9   **Hypotension, unspecified**

I96 Gangrene, not elsewhere classified   CC HCC
Gangrenous cellulitis
> EXCLUDES 1   *gangrene in atherosclerosis of native arteries of the extremities (I70.26)*
> *gangrene in hernia (K40.1, K40.4, K41.1, K41.4, K42.1, K43.1-, K44.1, K45.1, K46.1)*
> *gangrene in other peripheral vascular diseases (I73.-)*
> *gangrene of certain specified sites — see Alphabetical Index*
> *gas gangrene (A48.0)*
> *pyoderma gangrenosum (L88)*
> EXCLUDES 2   *gangrene in diabetes mellitus (E08-E13 with .52)*
AHA: 2018,4Q,87; 2018,3Q,3; 2017,3Q,6; 2013,2Q,34
CC Excl: PDX collection 519

✓4ᵗʰ **I97 Intraoperative and postprocedural complications and disorders of circulatory system, not elsewhere classified**
> EXCLUDES 2   *postprocedural shock (T81.1-)*
AHA: 2019,2Q,21

I97.0   **Postcardiotomy syndrome**

✓5ᵗʰ **I97.1**   **Other postprocedural cardiac functional disturbances**
> EXCLUDES 2   *acute pulmonary insufficiency following thoracic surgery (J95.1)*
> *intraoperative cardiac functional disturbances (I97.7-)*
CC Excl: For CC codes in subcategory I97.1: PDX collection 728

✓6ᵗʰ **I97.11**   **Postprocedural cardiac insufficiency**

I97.110   **Postprocedural cardiac insufficiency following cardiac surgery**   CC

I97.111   **Postprocedural cardiac insufficiency following other surgery**   CC

✓6ᵗʰ **I97.12**   **Postprocedural cardiac arrest**

I97.120   **Postprocedural cardiac arrest following cardiac surgery**   CC

I97.121   **Postprocedural cardiac arrest following other surgery**   CC

✓6ᵗʰ **I97.13**   **Postprocedural heart failure**
Use additional code to identify the heart failure (I50.-)

I97.130   **Postprocedural heart failure following cardiac surgery**   CC

I97.131   **Postprocedural heart failure following other surgery**   CC

✓6ᵗʰ **I97.19**   **Other postprocedural cardiac functional disturbances**
Use additional code, if applicable, to further specify disorder

I97.190   **Other postprocedural cardiac functional disturbances following cardiac surgery**   CC
Use additional code, if applicable, for type 4 or type 5 myocardial infarction, to further specify disorder
AHA: 2019,2Q,33

I97.191   **Other postprocedural cardiac functional disturbances following other surgery**   CC

I97.2   **Postmastectomy lymphedema syndrome**   A
Elephantiasis due to mastectomy
Obliteration of lymphatic vessels

I97.3   **Postprocedural hypertension**

✓5ᵗʰ **I97.4**   **Intraoperative hemorrhage and hematoma of a circulatory system organ or structure complicating a procedure**
> EXCLUDES 1   *intraoperative hemorrhage and hematoma of a circulatory system organ or structure due to accidental puncture and laceration during a procedure (I97.5-)*
> EXCLUDES 2   *intraoperative cerebrovascular hemorrhage complicating a procedure (G97.3-)*
CC Excl: For CC codes in subcategory I97.4: PDX collection 729

✓6ᵗʰ **I97.41**   **Intraoperative hemorrhage and hematoma of a circulatory system organ or structure complicating a circulatory system procedure**

I97.410   **Intraoperative hemorrhage and hematoma of a circulatory system organ or structure complicating a cardiac catheterization**   CC

I97.411   **Intraoperative hemorrhage and hematoma of a circulatory system organ or structure complicating a cardiac bypass**   CC

I97.418   **Intraoperative hemorrhage and hematoma of a circulatory system organ or structure complicating other circulatory system procedure**   CC

I97.42   **Intraoperative hemorrhage and hematoma of a circulatory system organ or structure complicating other procedure**   CC

✓5ᵗʰ **I97.5**   **Accidental puncture and laceration of a circulatory system organ or structure during a procedure**
> EXCLUDES 2   *accidental puncture and laceration of brain during a procedure (G97.4-)*

I97.51   **Accidental puncture and laceration of a circulatory system organ or structure during a circulatory system procedure**   CC
AHA: 2019,2Q,24
CC Excl: PDX collection 509

I97.52   **Accidental puncture and laceration of a circulatory system organ or structure during other procedure**   CC
CC Excl: PDX collection 509

✓5ᵗʰ **I97.6**   **Postprocedural hemorrhage, hematoma and seroma of a circulatory system organ or structure following a procedure**
> EXCLUDES 2   *postprocedural cerebrovascular hemorrhage complicating a procedure (G97.5-)*
AHA: 2016,4Q,9-10
CC Excl: For CC codes in subcategory I97.6: PDX collection 729

✓6ᵗʰ **I97.61**   **Postprocedural hemorrhage of a circulatory system organ or structure following a circulatory system procedure**

I97.610   **Postprocedural hemorrhage of a circulatory system organ or structure following a cardiac catheterization**   CC

I97.611   **Postprocedural hemorrhage of a circulatory system organ or structure following cardiac bypass**   CC

I97.618   **Postprocedural hemorrhage of a circulatory system organ or structure following other circulatory system procedure**   CC

Chapter 9. Diseases of the Circulatory System

I97.62–I99.9

√6ᵗʰ **I97.62 Postprocedural hemorrhage, hematoma and seroma** of a circulatory system organ or structure following other procedure

    I97.620 Postprocedural hemorrhage of a circulatory system organ or structure following other procedure   `CC`

    I97.621 Postprocedural hematoma of a circulatory system organ or structure following other procedure   `CC`

    I97.622 Postprocedural seroma of a circulatory system organ or structure following other procedure   `CC`

√6ᵗʰ **I97.63 Postprocedural hematoma** of a circulatory system organ or structure following a circulatory system procedure

    I97.630 Postprocedural hematoma of a circulatory system organ or structure following a cardiac catheterization   `CC`

    I97.631 Postprocedural hematoma of a circulatory system organ or structure following cardiac bypass   `CC`

    I97.638 Postprocedural hematoma of a circulatory system organ or structure following other circulatory system procedure   `CC`

√6ᵗʰ **I97.64 Postprocedural seroma** of a circulatory system organ or structure following a circulatory system procedure

    I97.640 Postprocedural seroma of a circulatory system organ or structure following a cardiac catheterization   `CC`

    I97.641 Postprocedural seroma of a circulatory system organ or structure following cardiac bypass   `CC`

    I97.648 Postprocedural seroma of a circulatory system organ or structure following other circulatory system procedure   `CC`

√5ᵗʰ **I97.7 Intraoperative cardiac functional disturbances**

    EXCLUDES 2   *acute pulmonary insufficiency following thoracic surgery (J95.1)*

         postprocedural cardiac functional disturbances (I97.1-)

    CC Excl: For CC codes in subcategory I97.7: PDX collection 728

√6ᵗʰ **I97.71 Intraoperative cardiac arrest**

    I97.710 Intraoperative cardiac arrest during cardiac surgery   `CC`

    I97.711 Intraoperative cardiac arrest during other surgery   `CC`

√6ᵗʰ **I97.79 Other intraoperative cardiac functional disturbances**

    Use additional code, if applicable, to further specify disorder

    I97.790 Other intraoperative cardiac functional disturbances during cardiac surgery   `CC`

    I97.791 Other intraoperative cardiac functional disturbances during other surgery   `CC`

√5ᵗʰ **I97.8 Other intraoperative and postprocedural complications and disorders of the circulatory system, not elsewhere classified**

    Use additional code, if applicable, to further specify disorder

    CC Excl: For CC codes in subcatgory I97.8, unless otherwise noted: PDX collection 617

√6ᵗʰ **I97.81 Intraoperative cerebrovascular infarction**

    I97.810 Intraoperative cerebrovascular infarction during cardiac surgery   `CC` `HCC`

    I97.811 Intraoperative cerebrovascular infarction during other surgery   `CC` `HCC`

√6ᵗʰ **I97.82 Postprocedural cerebrovascular infarction**

    I97.820 Postprocedural cerebrovascular infarction following cardiac surgery   `CC` `HCC`

    I97.821 Postprocedural cerebrovascular infarction following other surgery   `CC` `HCC`

    I97.88 Other intraoperative complications of the circulatory system, not elsewhere classified   `CC`

      CC Excl: PDX collection 728

    I97.89 Other postprocedural complications and disorders of the circulatory system, not elsewhere classified   `CC`

      AHA: 2019,2Q,33

      CC Excl: PDX collection 728

√4ᵗʰ **I99 Other and unspecified disorders of circulatory system**

    I99.8 Other disorder of circulatory system

    I99.9 Unspecified disorder of circulatory system

N Newborn: 0   P Pediatric: 0-17   M Maternity: 9-64   A Adult: 15-124   MCC Major Complication/Comorbidity   CC Complication/Comorbidity   SW Severe Wound Dx

690   ICD-10-CM 2020

Chapter 10. Diseases of the Respiratory System (J00–J99)

Chapter-specific Guidelines with Coding Examples

The chapter-specific guidelines from the ICD-10-CM Official Guidelines for Coding and Reporting have been provided below. Along with these guidelines are coding examples, contained in the shaded boxes, that have been developed to help illustrate the coding and/or sequencing guidance found in these guidelines.

a. Chronic obstructive pulmonary disease [COPD] and asthma

1) Acute exacerbation of chronic obstructive bronchitis and asthma

The codes in categories J44 and J45 distinguish between uncomplicated cases and those in acute exacerbation. An acute exacerbation is a worsening or a decompensation of a chronic condition. An acute exacerbation is not equivalent to an infection superimposed on a chronic condition, though an exacerbation may be triggered by an infection.

Vancomycin IV was started to treat a patient with acute pneumonia due to *Streptococcus pneumoniae*. Patient also with acute exacerbation of COPD continued on home meds.

J13   **Pneumonia due to Streptococcus pneumoniae**

J44.0   **Chronic obstructive pulmonary disease with (acute) lower respiratory infection**

J44.1   **Chronic obstructive pulmonary disease with (acute) exacerbation**

Explanation: ICD-10-CM uses combination codes to create organism-specific classifications for acute pneumonia. Category J44 codes include combination codes with severity components, which differentiate between COPD with acute lower respiratory infection (acute pneumonia), COPD with acute exacerbation, and COPD without mention of a complication (unspecified).

An acute exacerbation is a worsening or a decompensation of a chronic condition. An acute exacerbation is not equivalent to an infection superimposed on a chronic condition, though an exacerbation may be triggered by an infection, as in this example. Treatment of the pneumonia necessitated the inpatient admission. Instructional notes at J44.0 say to "code also to identify the infection," which informs the coder that another code must be assigned if applicable. Sequencing of the pneumonia and COPD exacerbation are governed by the Section II, "Selection of Principal Diagnosis," guidelines. In this case it was the pneumonia that was "chiefly responsible for occasioning the admission" with the IV vancomycin treatment.

Exacerbation of moderate persistent asthma with status asthmaticus

J45.42   **Moderate persistent asthma with status asthmaticus**

Explanation: Category J45 Asthma includes severity-specific subcategories and fifth-character codes to distinguish between uncomplicated cases, those in acute exacerbation, and those with status asthmaticus.

---

b. Acute respiratory failure

1) Acute respiratory failure as principal diagnosis

A code from subcategory J96.0, Acute respiratory failure, or subcategory J96.2, Acute and chronic respiratory failure, may be assigned as a principal diagnosis when it is the condition established after study to be chiefly responsible for occasioning the admission to the hospital, and the selection is supported by the Alphabetic Index and Tabular List. However, chapter-specific coding guidelines (such as obstetrics, poisoning, HIV, newborn) that provide sequencing direction take precedence.

Acute hypoxic respiratory failure due to COPD exacerbation

J96.01   **Acute respiratory failure with hypoxia**

J44.1   **Chronic obstructive pulmonary disease with (acute) exacerbation**

Explanation: Category J96 classifies respiratory failure with combination codes that designate the severity and the presence of hypoxia and hypercapnia. Code J96.01 is sequenced as the first-listed diagnosis, as the reason for the admission. Respiratory failure may be assigned as a principal diagnosis when it is the condition established after study to be chiefly responsible for occasioning the admission to the hospital and the selection is supported by the Alphabetic Index and Tabular List.

---

2) Acute respiratory failure as secondary diagnosis

Respiratory failure may be listed as a secondary diagnosis if it occurs after admission, or if it is present on admission, but does not meet the definition of principal diagnosis.

Acute respiratory failure due to accidental oxycodone overdose

T40.2X1A   **Poisoning by other opioids, accidental (unintentional), initial encounter**

J96.00   **Acute respiratory failure, unspecified whether with hypoxia or hypercapnia**

Explanation: Respiratory failure may be assigned as a principal diagnosis when it is the condition established after study to be chiefly responsible for occasioning the admission to the hospital, and the selection is supported by the Alphabetic Index and Tabular List. However, chapter-specific coding guidelines, such as poisoning, that provide sequencing direction take precedence. When coding a poisoning or reaction to the improper use of a medication (e.g. overdose, wrong substance given or taken in error, wrong route of administration), first assign the appropriate code from categories T36–T50. Use additional code(s) for all manifestations of the poisoning. In this instance, the respiratory failure is a manifestation of the poisoning and is sequenced as a secondary diagnosis.

Acute pneumococcal pneumonia with subsequent development of acute respiratory failure

J13   **Pneumonia due to Streptococcus pneumoniae**

J96.00   **Acute respiratory failure, unspecified whether with hypoxia or hypercapnia**

Explanation: Acute respiratory failure may be listed as a secondary diagnosis if it occurs after admission, or if it is present on admission but does not meet the definition of principal diagnosis.

---

3) Sequencing of acute respiratory failure and another acute condition

When a patient is admitted with respiratory failure and another acute condition, (e.g., myocardial infarction, cerebrovascular accident, aspiration pneumonia), the principal diagnosis will not be the same in every situation. This applies whether the other acute condition is a respiratory or nonrespiratory condition. Selection of the principal diagnosis will be dependent on the circumstances of admission. If both the respiratory failure and the other acute condition are equally responsible for occasioning the admission to the hospital, and there are no chapter-specific sequencing rules, the guideline regarding two or more diagnoses that equally meet the definition for principal diagnosis (*Section II, C.*) may be applied in these situations.

If the documentation is not clear as to whether acute respiratory failure and another condition are equally responsible for occasioning the admission, query the provider for clarification.

Acute pneumococcal pneumonia and acute respiratory failure, both present on admission

J96.00   **Acute respiratory failure, unspecified whether with hypoxia or hypercapnia**

J13   **Pneumonia due to Streptococcus pneumoniae**

Explanation: When a patient is admitted with respiratory failure and another acute condition, such as a bacterial pneumonia, the principal diagnosis is not the same in every situation. This applies whether the other acute condition is a respiratory or nonrespiratory condition. The principal diagnosis depends on the circumstances of admission.

---

c. Influenza due to certain identified influenza viruses

Code only confirmed cases of influenza due to certain identified influenza viruses (category J09), and due to other identified influenza virus (category J10). This is an exception to the hospital inpatient guideline Section II, H. (Uncertain Diagnosis).

In this context, "confirmation" does not require documentation of positive laboratory testing specific for avian or other novel influenza A or other identified influenza virus. However, coding should be based on the provider's diagnostic statement that the patient has avian influenza, or other novel influenza A, for category J09, or has another particular identified strain of influenza, such as H1N1 or H3N2, but not identified as novel or variant, for category J10.

If the provider records "suspected" or "possible" or "probable" avian influenza, or novel influenza, or other identified influenza, then the appropriate influenza code from category J11, Influenza due to unidentified influenza virus, should be assigned. A code from category J09, Influenza due to certain identified influenza viruses, should not be assigned nor should a code from category J10, Influenza due to other identified influenza virus.

Influenza due to avian influenza virus with pneumonia

J09.X1   Influenza due to identified novel influenza A virus with pneumonia

Explanation: Codes in category J09 Influenza due to certain identified influenza viruses should be assigned only for confirmed cases. "Confirmation" does not require positive laboratory testing of a specific influenza virus but does need to be based on the provider's diagnostic statement, which should not include terms such as "possible," "probable," or "suspected."

d. Ventilator associated pneumonia

1) Documentation of ventilator associated pneumonia

As with all procedural or postprocedural complications, code assignment is based on the provider's documentation of the relationship between the condition and the procedure.

Code J95.851, Ventilator associated pneumonia, should be assigned only when the provider has documented ventilator associated pneumonia (VAP). An additional code to identify the organism (e.g., Pseudomonas aeruginosa, code B96.5) should also be assigned. Do not assign an additional code from categories J12-J18 to identify the type of pneumonia.

Code J95.851 should not be assigned for cases where the patient has pneumonia and is on a mechanical ventilator and the provider has not specifically stated that the pneumonia is ventilator-associated pneumonia. If the documentation is unclear as to whether the patient has a pneumonia that is a complication attributable to the mechanical ventilator, query the provider.

2) Ventilator associated pneumonia develops after admission

A patient may be admitted with one type of pneumonia (e.g., code J13, Pneumonia due to Streptococcus pneumonia) and subsequently develop VAP. In this instance, the principal diagnosis would be the appropriate code from categories J12-J18 for the pneumonia diagnosed at the time of admission. Code J95.851, Ventilator associated pneumonia, would be assigned as an additional diagnosis when the provider has also documented the presence of ventilator associated pneumonia.

Patient with pneumonia due to *Klebsiella pneumoniae* develops superimposed MRSA ventilator-associated pneumonia

J15.0   Pneumonia due to Klebsiella pneumoniae

J95.851   Ventilator associated pneumonia

B95.62   Methicillin resistant Staphylococcus aureus infection as the cause of diseases classified elsewhere

Explanation: Code assignment for ventilator-associated pneumonia is based on the provider's documentation of the relationship between the condition and the procedure and is reported only when the provider has documented ventilator-associated pneumonia (VAP).

A patient may be admitted with one type of pneumonia and subsequently develop VAP. In this example, the principal diagnosis code describes the pneumonia diagnosed at the time of admission, with code J95.851 Ventilator associated pneumonia, assigned as secondary.

Chapter 10. Diseases of the Respiratory System
(J00-J99)

NOTE   When a respiratory condition is described as occurring in more than one site and is not specifically indexed, it should be classified to the lower anatomic site (e.g., tracheobronchitis to bronchitis in J40).

Use additional code, where applicable, to identify:
    exposure to environmental tobacco smoke (Z77.22)
    exposure to tobacco smoke in the perinatal period (P96.81)
    history of tobacco dependence (Z87.891)
    occupational exposure to environmental tobacco smoke (Z57.31)
    tobacco dependence (F17.-)
    tobacco use (Z72.0)

EXCLUDES 2   *certain conditions originating in the perinatal period (P04-P96)*
    certain infectious and parasitic diseases (A00-B99)
    complications of pregnancy, childbirth and the puerperium (O00-O9A)
    congenital malformations, deformations and chromosomal abnormalities (Q00-Q99)
    endocrine, nutritional and metabolic diseases (E00-E88)
    injury, poisoning and certain other consequences of external causes (S00-T88)
    neoplasms (C00-D49)
    smoke inhalation (T59.81-)
    symptoms, signs and abnormal clinical and laboratory findings, not elsewhere classified (R00-R94)

This chapter contains the following blocks:

J00-J06	Acute upper respiratory infections
J09-J18	Influenza and pneumonia
J20-J22	Other acute lower respiratory infections
J30-J39	Other diseases of upper respiratory tract
J40-J47	Chronic lower respiratory diseases
J60-J70	Lung diseases due to external agents
J80-J84	Other respiratory diseases principally affecting the interstitium
J85-J86	Suppurative and necrotic conditions of the lower respiratory tract
J90-J94	Other diseases of the pleura
J95	Intraoperative and postprocedural complications and disorders of respiratory system, not elsewhere classified
J96-J99	Other diseases of the respiratory system

Acute upper respiratory infections (J00-J06)

EXCLUDES 1   *chronic obstructive pulmonary disease with acute lower respiratory infection (J44.0)*
    influenza virus with other respiratory manifestations (J09.X2, J10.1, J11.1)

J00   Acute nasopharyngitis [common cold]
    Acute rhinitis
    Coryza (acute)
    Infective nasopharyngitis NOS
    Infective rhinitis
    Nasal catarrh, acute
    Nasopharyngitis NOS

    EXCLUDES 1   *acute pharyngitis (J02.-)*
        acute sore throat NOS (J02.9)
        pharyngitis NOS (J02.9)
        rhinitis NOS (J31.0)
        sore throat NOS (J02.9)

    EXCLUDES 2   *allergic rhinitis (J30.1-J30.9)*
        chronic pharyngitis (J31.2)
        chronic rhinitis (J31.0)
        chronic sore throat (J31.2)
        nasopharyngitis, chronic (J31.1)
        vasomotor rhinitis (J30.0)

    DEF: Acute inflammation of the mucous membranes that extends from the nares to the pharynx. It is characterized by nasal obstruction, sneezing, runny nose, and sore throat.

J01   Acute sinusitis
    INCLUDES   acute abscess of sinus
        acute empyema of sinus
        acute infection of sinus
        acute inflammation of sinus
        acute suppuration of sinus
    Use additional code (B95-B97) to identify infectious agent
    EXCLUDES 1   *sinusitis NOS (J32.9)*
    EXCLUDES 2   *chronic sinusitis (J32.0-J32.8)*

    J01.0   Acute maxillary sinusitis
        Acute antritis
        J01.00   Acute maxillary sinusitis, unspecified
        J01.01   Acute recurrent maxillary sinusitis

    J01.1   Acute frontal sinusitis
        J01.10   Acute frontal sinusitis, unspecified
        J01.11   Acute recurrent frontal sinusitis

    J01.2   Acute ethmoidal sinusitis
        J01.20   Acute ethmoidal sinusitis, unspecified
        J01.21   Acute recurrent ethmoidal sinusitis

    J01.3   Acute sphenoidal sinusitis
        J01.30   Acute sphenoidal sinusitis, unspecified
        J01.31   Acute recurrent sphenoidal sinusitis

    J01.4   Acute pansinusitis
        J01.40   Acute pansinusitis, unspecified
        J01.41   Acute recurrent pansinusitis

    J01.8   Other acute sinusitis
        J01.80   Other acute sinusitis
             Acute sinusitis involving more than one sinus but not pansinusitis
        J01.81   Other acute recurrent sinusitis
             Acute recurrent sinusitis involving more than one sinus but not pansinusitis

    J01.9   Acute sinusitis, unspecified
        J01.90   Acute sinusitis, unspecified
        J01.91   Acute recurrent sinusitis, unspecified

J02   Acute pharyngitis
    INCLUDES   acute sore throat
    EXCLUDES 1   *acute laryngopharyngitis (J06.0)*
        peritonsillar abscess (J36)
        pharyngeal abscess (J39.1)
        retropharyngeal abscess (J39.0)
    EXCLUDES 2   *chronic pharyngitis (J31.2)*

    J02.0   Streptococcal pharyngitis
        Septic pharyngitis
        Streptococcal sore throat
        EXCLUDES 2   *scarlet fever (A38.-)*

    J02.8   Acute pharyngitis due to other specified organisms
        Use additional code (B95-B97) to identify infectious agent
        EXCLUDES 1   *acute pharyngitis due to coxsackie virus (B08.5)*
             acute pharyngitis due to gonococcus (A54.5)
             acute pharyngitis due to herpes [simplex] virus (B00.2)
             acute pharyngitis due to infectious mononucleosis (B27.-)
             enteroviral vesicular pharyngitis (B08.5)

    J02.9   Acute pharyngitis, unspecified
        Gangrenous pharyngitis (acute)
        Infective pharyngitis (acute) NOS
        Pharyngitis (acute) NOS
        Sore throat (acute) NOS
        Suppurative pharyngitis (acute)
        Ulcerative pharyngitis (acute)

J03   Acute tonsillitis
    EXCLUDES 1   *acute sore throat (J02.-)*
        hypertrophy of tonsils (J35.1)
        peritonsillar abscess (J36)
        sore throat NOS (J02.9)
        streptococcal sore throat (J02.0)
    EXCLUDES 2   *chronic tonsillitis (J35.0)*

    J03.0   Streptococcal tonsillitis
        J03.00   Acute streptococcal tonsillitis, unspecified
        J03.01   Acute recurrent streptococcal tonsillitis

    J03.8   Acute tonsillitis due to other specified organisms
        Use additional code (B95-B97) to identify infectious agent
        EXCLUDES 1   *diphtheritic tonsillitis (A36.0)*
             herpesviral pharyngotonsillitis (B00.2)
             streptococcal tonsillitis (J03.0)
             tuberculous tonsillitis (A15.8)
             Vincent's tonsillitis (A69.1)
        J03.80   Acute tonsillitis due to other specified organisms
        J03.81   Acute recurrent tonsillitis due to other specified organisms

Chapter 10. Diseases of the Respiratory System

J03.9–J10.00

✓5ᵗʰ **J03.9** **Acute tonsillitis, unspecified**
Follicular tonsillitis (acute)
Gangrenous tonsillitis (acute)
Infective tonsillitis (acute)
Tonsillitis (acute) NOS
Ulcerative tonsillitis (acute)

     J03.90 **Acute tonsillitis, unspecified**
     J03.91 **Acute recurrent tonsillitis, unspecified**

✓4ᵗʰ **J04** **Acute laryngitis and tracheitis**
Use additional code (B95-B97) to identify infectious agent
     EXCLUDES 1   *acute obstructive laryngitis [croup] and epiglottitis (J05.-)*
     EXCLUDES 2   *laryngismus (stridulus) (J38.5)*

   J04.0 **Acute laryngitis**
Edematous laryngitis (acute)
Laryngitis (acute) NOS
Subglottic laryngitis (acute)
Suppurative laryngitis (acute)
Ulcerative laryngitis (acute)
     EXCLUDES 1   *acute obstructive laryngitis (J05.0)*
     EXCLUDES 2   *chronic laryngitis (J37.0)*

✓5ᵗʰ **J04.1** **Acute tracheitis**
Acute viral tracheitis
Catarrhal tracheitis (acute)
Tracheitis (acute) NOS
     EXCLUDES 2   *chronic tracheitis (J42)*

     J04.10 **Acute tracheitis without obstruction**
     J04.11 **Acute tracheitis with obstruction**   MCC
       CC Excl: PDX collection 730

   J04.2 **Acute laryngotracheitis**
Laryngotracheitis NOS
Tracheitis (acute) with laryngitis (acute)
     EXCLUDES 1   *acute obstructive laryngotracheitis (J05.0)*
     EXCLUDES 2   *chronic laryngotracheitis (J37.1)*

✓5ᵗʰ **J04.3** **Supraglottitis, unspecified**

     J04.30 **Supraglottitis, unspecified, without obstruction**
     J04.31 **Supraglottitis, unspecified, with obstruction**   MCC
       CC Excl: PDX collection 731

✓4ᵗʰ **J05** **Acute obstructive laryngitis [croup] and epiglottitis**
Use additional code (B95-B97) to identify infectious agent

   J05.0 **Acute obstructive laryngitis [croup]**
Obstructive laryngitis (acute) NOS
Obstructive laryngotracheitis NOS
DEF: Acute laryngeal obstruction due to allergies, foreign bodies, or in the majority of cases a viral infection. Symptoms include a harsh, barking cough, hoarseness, and a persistent, high-pitched respiratory sound (stridor).

✓5ᵗʰ **J05.1** **Acute epiglottitis**
     EXCLUDES 2   *epiglottitis, chronic (J37.0)*

     J05.10 **Acute epiglottitis without obstruction**   CC
Epiglottitis NOS
       CC Excl: PDX collection 732
     J05.11 **Acute epiglottitis with obstruction**   MCC
       CC Excl: PDX collection 730

✓4ᵗʰ **J06** **Acute upper respiratory infections of multiple and unspecified sites**
     EXCLUDES 1   *acute respiratory infection NOS (J22)*
                streptococcal pharyngitis (J02.0)

   J06.0 **Acute laryngopharyngitis**
   J06.9 **Acute upper respiratory infection, unspecified**
Upper respiratory disease, acute
Upper respiratory infection NOS
▶Use additional code (B95-B97) to identify infectious agent, if known, such as:◀
▶respiratory syncytial virus (RSV) (B97.4)◀

Influenza and pneumonia (J09-J18)

   EXCLUDES 2   *allergic or eosinophilic pneumonia (J82)*
               aspiration pneumonia NOS (J69.0)
               meconium pneumonia (P24.01)
               neonatal aspiration pneumonia (P24.-)
               pneumonia due to solids and liquids (J69.-)
               congenital pneumonia (P23.9)
               lipid pneumonia (J69.1)
               rheumatic pneumonia (I00)
               ventilator associated pneumonia (J95.851)

AHA: 2017,4Q,96
TIP: Documentation of lobar pneumonia or multilobar pneumonia should be coded to J18.1 when the specific organism causing the pneumonia is not identified. When the organism is documented, lobar pneumonia or multilobar pneumonia should be coded using categories J12-J16, depending on the organism that is present.
TIP: Hemoptysis (R04.2) is not customarily associated with pneumonia and may be reported separately.
CC Excl: For MCC codes in categories J09-J18, unless otherwise noted: PDX collection 110

✓4ᵗʰ **J09** **Influenza due to certain identified influenza viruses**
     EXCLUDES 1   *influenza A/H1N1 (J10.-)*
               influenza due to other identified influenza virus (J10.-)
               influenza due to unidentified influenza virus (J11.-)
               seasonal influenza due to other identified influenza virus (J10.-)
               seasonal influenza due to unidentified influenza virus (J11.-)

✓5ᵗʰ **J09.X** **Influenza due to identified novel influenza A virus**
Avian influenza
Bird influenza
Influenza A/H5N1
Influenza of other animal origin, not bird or swine
Swine influenza virus (viruses that normally cause infections in pigs)
AHA: 2016,3Q,10

   J09.X1 **Influenza due to identified novel influenza A virus with pneumonia**   HIV   MCC
Code also, if applicable, associated:
lung abscess (J85.1)
other specified type of pneumonia

   J09.X2 **Influenza due to identified novel influenza A virus with other respiratory manifestations**
Influenza due to identified novel influenza A virus NOS
Influenza due to identified novel influenza A virus with laryngitis
Influenza due to identified novel influenza A virus with pharyngitis
Influenza due to identified novel influenza A virus with upper respiratory symptoms
Use additional code, if applicable, for associated:
pleural effusion (J91.8)
sinusitis (J01.-)

   J09.X3 **Influenza due to identified novel influenza A virus with gastrointestinal manifestations**
Influenza due to identified novel influenza A virus gastroenteritis
     EXCLUDES 1   *'intestinal flu' [viral gastroenteritis] (A08.-)*

   J09.X9 **Influenza due to identified novel influenza A virus with other manifestations**
Influenza due to identified novel influenza A virus with encephalopathy
Influenza due to identified novel influenza A virus with myocarditis
Influenza due to identified novel influenza A virus with otitis media
Use additional code to identify manifestation

✓4ᵗʰ **J10** **Influenza due to other identified influenza virus**
     EXCLUDES 1   *influenza due to avian influenza virus (J09.X-)*
               influenza due to swine flu (J09.X-)
               influenza due to unidentifed influenza virus (J11.-)

✓5ᵗʰ **J10.0** **Influenza due to other identified influenza virus with pneumonia**
Code also associated lung abscess, if applicable (J85.1)

   J10.00 **Influenza due to other identified influenza virus with unspecified type of pneumonia**   MCC

N Newborn: 0   P Pediatric: 0-17   M Maternity: 9-64   A Adult: 15-124   MCC Major Complication/Comorbidity   CC Complication/Comorbidity   SW Severe Wound Dx

694   ICD-10-CM 2020

J10.01 Influenza due to other identified influenza virus with the same other identified influenza virus pneumonia MCC

J10.08 Influenza due to other identified influenza virus with other specified pneumonia HIV MCC
Code also other specified type of pneumonia
CC Excl: PDX collection 733

J10.1 Influenza due to other identified influenza virus with other respiratory manifestations CC
Influenza due to other identified influenza virus NOS
Influenza due to other identified influenza virus with laryngitis
Influenza due to other identified influenza virus with pharyngitis
Influenza due to other identified influenza virus with upper respiratory symptoms
Use additional code for associated pleural effusion, if applicable (J91.8)
Use additional code for associated sinusitis, if applicable (J01.-)
AHA: 2016,3Q,10-11

J10.2 Influenza due to other identified influenza virus with gastrointestinal manifestations
Influenza due to other identified influenza virus gastroenteritis
EXCLUDES 1 "intestinal flu" [viral gastroenteritis] (A08.-)

√5th **J10.8 Influenza due to other identified influenza virus with other manifestations**

J10.81 Influenza due to other identified influenza virus with encephalopathy

J10.82 Influenza due to other identified influenza virus with myocarditis

J10.83 Influenza due to other identified influenza virus with otitis media
Use additional code for any associated perforated tympanic membrane (H72.-)

J10.89 Influenza due to other identified influenza virus with other manifestations
Use additional codes to identify the manifestations

√4th **J11 Influenza due to unidentified influenza virus**

√5th **J11.0 Influenza due to unidentified influenza virus with pneumonia**
Code also associated lung abscess, if applicable (J85.1)
AHA: 2016,3Q,11

J11.00 Influenza due to unidentified influenza virus with unspecified type of pneumonia MCC
Influenza with pneumonia NOS

J11.08 Influenza due to unidentified influenza virus with specified pneumonia MCC
Code also other specified type of pneumonia

J11.1 Influenza due to unidentified influenza virus with other respiratory manifestations
Influenza NOS
Influenzal laryngitis NOS
Influenzal pharyngitis NOS
Influenza with upper respiratory symptoms NOS
Use additional code for associated pleural effusion, if applicable (J91.8)
Use additional code for associated sinusitis, if applicable (J01.-)

J11.2 Influenza due to unidentified influenza virus with gastrointestinal manifestations
Influenza gastroenteritis NOS
EXCLUDES 1 "intestinal flu" [viral gastroenteritis] (A08.-)

√5th **J11.8 Influenza due to unidentified influenza virus with other manifestations**

J11.81 Influenza due to unidentified influenza virus with encephalopathy
Influenzal encephalopathy NOS

J11.82 Influenza due to unidentified influenza virus with myocarditis
Influenzal myocarditis NOS

J11.83 Influenza due to unidentified influenza virus with otitis media
Influenzal otitis media NOS
Use additional code for any associated perforated tympanic membrane (H72.-)

J11.89 Influenza due to unidentified influenza virus with other manifestations
Use additional codes to identify the manifestations

√4th **J12 Viral pneumonia, not elsewhere classified**
INCLUDES bronchopneumonia due to viruses other than influenza viruses
Code first associated influenza, if applicable (J09.X1, J10.0-, J11.0-)
Code also associated abscess, if applicable (J85.1)
EXCLUDES 1 aspiration pneumonia due to anesthesia during labor and delivery (O74.0)
aspiration pneumonia due to anesthesia during pregnancy (O29)
aspiration pneumonia due to anesthesia during puerperium (O89.0)
aspiration pneumonia due to solids and liquids (J69.-)
aspiration pneumonia NOS (J69.0)
congenital pneumonia (P23.0)
congenital rubella pneumonitis (P35.0)
interstitial pneumonia NOS (J84.9)
lipid pneumonia (J69.1)
neonatal aspiration pneumonia (P24.-)
AHA: 2019,1Q,35; 2018,3Q,24; 2016,3Q,15; 2013,4Q,118
CC Excl: For MCC codes in category J12, unless otherwise noted: PDX collection 734

J12.0 Adenoviral pneumonia MCC

J12.1 Respiratory syncytial virus pneumonia MCC
▶RSV pneumonia◀

J12.2 Parainfluenza virus pneumonia MCC

J12.3 Human metapneumovirus pneumonia HIV MCC

√5th **J12.8 Other viral pneumonia**

J12.81 Pneumonia due to SARS-associated coronavirus HIV MCC
Severe acute respiratory syndrome NOS
DEF: Severe adult respiratory syndrome caused by the coronavirus, specified as inflammation of the lungs with consolidation.
CC Excl: PDX collection 735

J12.89 Other viral pneumonia HIV MCC

J12.9 Viral pneumonia, unspecified HIV MCC

J13 Pneumonia due to Streptococcus pneumoniae HIV MCC HCC
Bronchopneumonia due to S. pneumoniae
Code first associated influenza, if applicable (J09.X1, J10.0-, J11.0-)
Code also associated abscess, if applicable (J85.1)
EXCLUDES 1 congenital pneumonia due to S. pneumoniae (P23.6)
lobar pneumonia, unspecified organism (J18.1)
pneumonia due to other streptococci (J15.3-J15.4)
AHA: 2019,1Q,35; 2018,3Q,24; 2016,3Q,15; 2013,4Q,118

J14 Pneumonia due to Hemophilus influenzae HIV MCC HCC
Bronchopneumonia due to H. influenzae
Code first associated influenza, if applicable (J09.X1, J10.0-, J11.0-)
Code also associated abscess, if applicable (J85.1)
EXCLUDES 1 congenital pneumonia due to H. influenzae (P23.6)
AHA: 2019,1Q,35; 2018,3Q,24; 2016,3Q,15; 2013,4Q,118

√4th **J15 Bacterial pneumonia, not elsewhere classified**
INCLUDES Bronchopneumonia due to bacteria other than S. pneumoniae and H. influenzae
Code first associated influenza, if applicable (J09.X1, J10.0-, -J11.0-)
Code also associated abscess, if applicable (J85.1)
EXCLUDES 1 chlamydial pneumonia (J16.0)
congenital pneumonia (P23.-)
Legionnaires' disease (A48.1)
spirochetal pneumonia (A69.8)
AHA: 2019,1Q,35; 2018,3Q,24; 2016,3Q,15; 2013,4Q,118

J15.0 Pneumonia due to Klebsiella pneumoniae HIV MCC HCC

J15.1 Pneumonia due to Pseudomonas HIV MCC HCC

√5th **J15.2 Pneumonia due to staphylococcus**

J15.20 Pneumonia due to staphylococcus, unspecified HIV MCC HCC

√6th **J15.21 Pneumonia due to Staphylococcus aureus**

J15.211 Pneumonia due to methicillin susceptible Staphylococcus aureus HIV MCC HCC
MSSA pneumonia
Pneumonia due to Staphylococcus aureus NOS

Chapter 10. Diseases of the Respiratory System

J15.212   **Pneumonia due to methicillin resistant Staphylococcus aureus**   `HIV` `MCC` `HCC`

J15.29   **Pneumonia due to other staphylococcus**   `HIV` `MCC` `HCC`

J15.3   **Pneumonia due to streptococcus, group B**   `HIV` `MCC` `HCC`

J15.4   **Pneumonia due to other streptococci**   `HIV` `MCC` `HCC`

     `EXCLUDES 1`   *pneumonia due to streptococcus, group B (J15.3)*
              pneumonia due to Streptococcus pneumoniae (J13)

J15.5   **Pneumonia due to Escherichia coli**   `HIV` `MCC` `HCC`

J15.6   **Pneumonia due to other Gram-negative bacteria**

     Pneumonia due to other aerobic Gram-negative bacteria
     Pneumonia due to Serratia marcescens

J15.7   **Pneumonia due to Mycoplasma pneumoniae**   `MCC`

J15.8   **Pneumonia due to other specified bacteria**   `HIV` `MCC` `HCC`

J15.9   **Unspecified bacterial pneumonia**   `HIV` `MCC`

     Pneumonia due to gram-positive bacteria

`√4th` **J16**   **Pneumonia due to other infectious organisms, not elsewhere classified**

     Code first associated influenza, if applicable (J09.X1, J10.0-, J11.0-)
     Code also associated abscess, if applicable (J85.1)

     `EXCLUDES 1`   *congenital pneumonia (P23.-)*
              ornithosis (A70)
              pneumocystosis (B59)
              pneumonia NOS (J18.9)

     AHA: 2019,1Q,35; 2018,3Q,24; 2016,3Q,15; 2013,4Q,118

J16.0   **Chlamydial pneumonia**   `MCC`

J16.8   **Pneumonia due to other specified infectious organisms**   `MCC`

J17   *Pneumonia in diseases classified elsewhere*   `MCC`

     Code first underlying disease, such as:
       Q fever (A78)
       rheumatic fever (I00)
       schistosomiasis (B65.0-B65.9)

     `EXCLUDES 1`   *candidial pneumonia (B37.1)*
              chlamydial pneumonia (J16.0)
              gonorrheal pneumonia (A54.84)
              histoplasmosis pneumonia (B39.0-B39.2)
              measles pneumonia (B05.2)
              nocardiosis pneumonia (A43.0)
              pneumocystosis (B59)
              pneumonia due to Pneumocystis carinii (B59)
              pneumonia due to Pneumocystis jiroveci (B59)
              pneumonia in actinomycosis (A42.0)
              pneumonia in anthrax (A22.1)
              pneumonia in ascariasis (B77.81)
              pneumonia in aspergillosis (B44.0-B44.1)
              pneumonia in coccidioidomycosis (B38.0-B38.2)
              pneumonia in cytomegalovirus disease (B25.0)
              pneumonia in toxoplasmosis (B58.3)
              rubella pneumonia (B06.81)
              salmonella pneumonia (A02.22)
              spirochetal infection NEC with pneumonia (A69.8)
              tularemia pneumonia (A21.2)
              typhoid fever with pneumonia (A01.03)
              varicella pneumonia (B01.2)
              whooping cough with pneumonia (A37 with fifth character 1)

     AHA: 2019,1Q,35; 2016,3Q,15; 2013,4Q,118

`√4th` **J18**   **Pneumonia, unspecified organism**

     Code first associated influenza, if applicable (J09.X1, J10.0-, J11.0-)

     `EXCLUDES 1`   *abscess of lung with pneumonia (J85.1)*
              aspiration pneumonia due to anesthesia during labor and delivery (O74.0)
              aspiration pneumonia due to anesthesia during pregnancy (O29)
              aspiration pneumonia due to anesthesia during puerperium (O89.0)
              aspiration pneumonia due to solids and liquids (J69.-)
              aspiration pneumonia NOS (J69.0)
              congenital pneumonia (P23.0)
              drug-induced interstitial lung disorder (J70.2-J70.4)
              interstitial pneumonia NOS (J84.9)
              lipid pneumonia (J69.1)
              neonatal aspiration pneumonia (P24.-)
              pneumonitis due to external agents (J67-J70)
              pneumonitis due to fumes and vapors (J68.0)
              usual interstitial pneumonia (J84.17)

     AHA: 2019,1Q,35; 2016,3Q,15; 2013,4Q,118

J18.0   **Bronchopneumonia, unspecified organism**   `MCC`

     `EXCLUDES 1`   *hypostatic bronchopneumonia (J18.2)*
              lipid pneumonia (J69.1)
     `EXCLUDES 2`   *acute bronchiolitis (J21.-)*
              chronic bronchiolitis (J44.9)

J18.1   **Lobar pneumonia, unspecified organism**   `HIV` `MCC` `HCC`

     AHA: 2018,3Q,24

     TIP: Use this code for documented lobar pneumonia or multilobar pneumonia when the causal organism is not identified. If the causal organism is identified, codes from categories J12-J16 should be used, depending on the organism that is present.

J18.2   **Hypostatic pneumonia, unspecified organism**   `CC`

     Hypostatic bronchopneumonia
     Passive pneumonia
     CC Excl: PDX collection 736

J18.8   **Other pneumonia, unspecified organism**   `HIV` `MCC`

J18.9   **Pneumonia, unspecified organism**   `HIV` `MCC`

     AHA: 2019,2Q,28; 2014,3Q,4; 2013,4Q,119; 2012,4Q,94

Other acute lower respiratory infections (J20-J22)

     `EXCLUDES 2`   *chronic obstructive pulmonary disease with acute lower respiratory infection (J44.0)*

`√4th` **J20**   **Acute bronchitis**

     `INCLUDES`   acute and subacute bronchitis (with) bronchospasm
              acute and subacute bronchitis (with) tracheitis
              acute and subacute bronchitis (with) tracheobronchitis, acute
              acute and subacute fibrinous bronchitis
              acute and subacute membranous bronchitis
              acute and subacute purulent bronchitis
              acute and subacute septic bronchitis

     `EXCLUDES 1`   *bronchitis NOS (J40)*
              tracheobronchitis NOS (J40)

     `EXCLUDES 2`   *acute bronchitis with bronchiectasis (J47.0)*
              acute bronchitis with chronic obstructive asthma (J44.0)
              acute bronchitis with chronic obstructive pulmonary disease (J44.0)
              allergic bronchitis NOS (J45.909-)
              bronchitis due to chemicals, fumes and vapors (J68.0)
              chronic bronchitis NOS (J42)
              chronic mucopurulent bronchitis (J41.1)
              chronic obstructive bronchitis (J44.-)
              chronic obstructive tracheobronchitis (J44.-)
              chronic simple bronchitis (J41.0)
              chronic tracheobronchitis (J42)

     AHA: 2019,1Q,35; 2016,3Q,10,16

     DEF: Acute inflammation of the main branches of the bronchial tree due to infectious or irritant agents. Symptoms include cough with a varied production of sputum, fever, substernal soreness, and lung rales. Bronchitis usually lasts three to 10 days.

J20.0   **Acute bronchitis due to Mycoplasma pneumoniae**

J20.1   **Acute bronchitis due to Hemophilus influenzae**

J20.2   **Acute bronchitis due to streptococcus**

J20.3   **Acute bronchitis due to coxsackievirus**

J20.4   **Acute bronchitis due to parainfluenza virus**

`N` Newborn: 0   `P` Pediatric: 0-17   `M` Maternity: 9-64   `A` Adult: 15-124   `MCC` Major Complication/Comorbidity   `CC` Complication/Comorbidity   `SW` Severe Wound Dx

696   ICD-10-CM 2020

J20.5   **Acute bronchitis due to** respiratory syncytial virus
► Acute bronchitis due to RSV ◄

J20.6   **Acute bronchitis due to** rhinovirus

J20.7   **Acute bronchitis due to** echovirus

J20.8   **Acute bronchitis due to other specified organisms**

J20.9   **Acute bronchitis, unspecified**

✓4ᵗʰ **J21**   **Acute bronchiolitis**

> INCLUDES   acute bronchiolitis with bronchospasm
>
> EXCLUDES 2   *respiratory bronchiolitis interstitial lung disease (J84.115)*
>
> CC Excl: For CC codes in category J21, unless otherwise noted: PDX collection 738

J21.0   **Acute bronchiolitis due to** respiratory syncytial virus   CC
► Acute bronchiolitis due to RSV ◄
CC Excl: PDX collection 737

J21.1   **Acute bronchiolitis due to** human metapneumovirus   CC

J21.8   **Acute bronchiolitis due to other specified organisms**   CC

J21.9   **Acute bronchiolitis, unspecified**   CC
Bronchiolitis (acute)
> EXCLUDES 1   *chronic bronchiolitis (J44.-)*

J22   **Unspecified acute lower respiratory infection**
Acute (lower) respiratory (tract) infection NOS
> EXCLUDES 1   *upper respiratory infection (acute) (J06.9)*

Other diseases of upper respiratory tract (J30-J39)

✓4ᵗʰ **J30**   **Vasomotor and allergic rhinitis**

> INCLUDES   spasmodic rhinorrhea
>
> EXCLUDES 1   *allergic rhinitis with asthma (bronchial) (J45.909)*
> *rhinitis NOS (J31.0)*

J30.0   **Vasomotor** rhinitis
DEF: Noninfectious and nonallergic type of rhinitis for which the cause is often unknown. Symptoms often mimic those of allergic rhinitis with a diagnosis of vasomotor rhinitis typically made after ruling out allergens as the cause.

J30.1   **Allergic** rhinitis **due to** pollen
Allergy NOS due to pollen
Hay fever
Pollinosis

J30.2   **Other** seasonal allergic **rhinitis**

J30.5   **Allergic rhinitis** due to food

✓5ᵗʰ **J30.8**   **Other allergic rhinitis**

J30.81   **Allergic rhinitis due to** animal **(cat) (dog)** hair and dander

J30.89   **Other allergic rhinitis**
Perennial allergic rhinitis

J30.9   **Allergic rhinitis, unspecified**

✓4ᵗʰ **J31**   **Chronic rhinitis, nasopharyngitis and pharyngitis**

Use additional code to identify:
exposure to environmental tobacco smoke (Z77.22)
exposure to tobacco smoke in the perinatal period (P96.81)
history of tobacco dependence (Z87.891)
occupational exposure to environmental tobacco smoke (Z57.31)
tobacco dependence (F17.-)
tobacco use (Z72.0)

J31.0   **Chronic rhinitis**
Atrophic rhinitis (chronic)
Granulomatous rhinitis (chronic)
Hypertrophic rhinitis (chronic)
Obstructive rhinitis (chronic)
Ozena
Purulent rhinitis (chronic)
Rhinitis (chronic) NOS
Ulcerative rhinitis (chronic)
> EXCLUDES 1   *allergic rhinitis (J30.1-J30.9)*
> *vasomotor rhinitis (J30.0)*

DEF: Persistent inflammation of the mucous membranes of the nose, characterized by a postnasal drip.

J31.1   **Chronic nasopharyngitis**
> EXCLUDES 2   *acute nasopharyngitis (J00)*

DEF: Persistent inflammation of the mucous membranes extending from the nares to the pharynx. It is characterized by constant irritation in the nasopharynx and postnasal drip.

J31.2   **Chronic pharyngitis**
Atrophic pharyngitis (chronic)
Chronic sore throat
Granular pharyngitis (chronic)
Hypertrophic pharyngitis (chronic)
> EXCLUDES 2   *acute pharyngitis (J02.9)*

✓4ᵗʰ **J32**   **Chronic sinusitis**

> INCLUDES   sinus abscess
> sinus empyema
> sinus infection
> sinus suppuration

Use additional code to identify:
exposure to environmental tobacco smoke (Z77.22)
exposure to tobacco smoke in the perinatal period (P96.81)
history of tobacco dependence (Z87.891)
infectious agent (B95-B97)
occupational exposure to environmental tobacco smoke (Z57.31)
tobacco dependence (F17.-)
tobacco use (Z72.0)
> EXCLUDES 2   *acute sinusitis (J01.-)*

J32.0   **Chronic** maxillary **sinusitis**
Antritis (chronic)
Maxillary sinusitis NOS

J32.1   **Chronic** frontal **sinusitis**
Frontal sinusitis NOS

J32.2   **Chronic** ethmoidal **sinusitis**
Ethmoidal sinusitis NOS
> EXCLUDES 1   *Woakes' ethmoiditis (J33.1)*

J32.3   **Chronic** sphenoidal **sinusitis**
Sphenoidal sinusitis NOS

J32.4   **Chronic** pansinusitis
Pansinusitis NOS

J32.8   **Other chronic sinusitis**
Sinusitis (chronic) involving more than one sinus but not pansinusitis

J32.9   **Chronic sinusitis, unspecified**
Sinusitis (chronic) NOS

✓4ᵗʰ **J33**   **Nasal polyp**

Use additional code to identify:
exposure to environmental tobacco smoke (Z77.22)
exposure to tobacco smoke in the perinatal period (P96.81)
history of tobacco dependence (Z87.891)
occupational exposure to environmental tobacco smoke (Z57.31)
tobacco dependence (F17.-)
tobacco use (Z72.0)
> EXCLUDES 1   *adenomatous polyps (D14.0)*

J33.0   **Polyp of nasal cavity**
Choanal polyp
Nasopharyngeal polyp

J33.1   **Polypoid sinus degeneration**
Woakes' syndrome or ethmoiditis

J33.8   **Other polyp of sinus**
Accessory polyp of sinus
Ethmoidal polyp of sinus
Maxillary polyp of sinus
Sphenoidal polyp of sinus

J33.9   **Nasal polyp, unspecified**

✓4ᵗʰ **J34**   **Other and unspecified disorders of nose and nasal sinuses**
> EXCLUDES 2   *varicose ulcer of nasal septum (I86.8)*

J34.0   **Abscess, furuncle and carbuncle of nose**
Cellulitis of nose
Necrosis of nose
Ulceration of nose

J34.1   **Cyst and mucocele of nose and nasal sinus**

J34.2   **Deviated nasal septum**
Deflection or deviation of septum (nasal) (acquired)
> EXCLUDES 1   *congenital deviated nasal septum (Q67.4)*

DEF: Condition in which the nasal septum, a thin wall composed of cartilage and bone that separates the two nostrils, is crooked or displaced from the midline.

J34.3   **Hypertrophy of nasal turbinates**
DEF: Overgrowth of bones within the nasal turbinate, which are ridges of bone and soft tissue that project from the sidewalls of the nasal passages. Hypertrophy can cause obstruction of the nasal passages.

✓ Additional Character Required   ✓x7ᵗʰ Placeholder   Unacceptable PDx   Questionable PDx   Manifestation   Unspecified Dx   H1-H14 HAC   HCC CMS-HCC Dx   HIV HIV Dx

ICD-10-CM 2020   697

J20.5–J34.3

Chapter 10. Diseases of the Respiratory System

J34.8-J39.1

√5ᵗʰ **J34.8 Other specified disorders of nose and nasal sinuses**

    J34.81 Nasal mucositis (ulcerative)

      Code also type of associated therapy, such as:
        antineoplastic and immunosuppressive drugs
        (T45.1X-)
        radiological procedure and radiotherapy (Y84.2)
      EXCLUDES 2   *gastrointestinal mucositis (ulcerative)*
           (K92.81)
           mucositis (ulcerative) of vagina and vulva
           (N76.81)
           oral mucositis (ulcerative) (K12.3-)

    J34.89 Other specified disorders of nose and nasal sinuses
      Perforation of nasal septum NOS
      Rhinolith

  J34.9 Unspecified disorder of nose and nasal sinuses

√4ᵗʰ **J35 Chronic diseases of tonsils and adenoids**

  Use additional code to identify:
    exposure to environmental tobacco smoke (Z77.22)
    exposure to tobacco smoke in the perinatal period (P96.81)
    history of tobacco dependence (Z87.891)
    occupational exposure to environmental tobacco smoke (Z57.31)
    tobacco dependence (F17.-)
    tobacco use (Z72.0)

√5ᵗʰ **J35.0 Chronic tonsillitis and adenoiditis**
    EXCLUDES 2   *acute tonsillitis (J03.-)*

    J35.01 Chronic tonsillitis
    J35.02 Chronic adenoiditis
    J35.03 Chronic tonsillitis and adenoiditis

  J35.1 Hypertrophy of tonsils
    Enlargement of tonsils
    EXCLUDES 1   *hypertrophy of tonsils with tonsillitis (J35.0-)*

  J35.2 Hypertrophy of adenoids
    Enlargement of adenoids
    EXCLUDES 1   *hypertrophy of adenoids with adenoiditis (J35.0-)*

  J35.3 Hypertrophy of tonsils with hypertrophy of adenoids
    EXCLUDES 1   *hypertrophy of tonsils and adenoids with tonsillitis*
           and adenoiditis (J35.03)

  J35.8 Other chronic diseases of tonsils and adenoids
    Adenoid vegetations
    Amygdalolith
    Calculus, tonsil
    Cicatrix of tonsil (and adenoid)
    Tonsillar tag
    Ulcer of tonsil

  J35.9 Chronic disease of tonsils and adenoids, unspecified
    Disease (chronic) of tonsils and adenoids NOS

J36 Peritonsillar abscess   **CC**

  INCLUDES   abscess of tonsil
        peritonsillar cellulitis
        quinsy

  Use additional code (B95-B97) to identify infectious agent
  EXCLUDES 1   *acute tonsillitis (J03.-)*
        chronic tonsillitis (J35.0)
        retropharyngeal abscess (J39.0)
        tonsillitis NOS (J03.9-)

  CC Excl: PDX collection 739

√4ᵗʰ **J37 Chronic laryngitis and laryngotracheitis**

  Use additional code to identify:
    exposure to environmental tobacco smoke (Z77.22)
    exposure to tobacco smoke in the perinatal period (P96.81)
    history of tobacco dependence (Z87.891)
    infectious agent (B95-B97)
    occupational exposure to environmental tobacco smoke (Z57.31)
    tobacco dependence (F17.-)
    tobacco use (Z72.0)

  J37.0 Chronic laryngitis
    Catarrhal laryngitis
    Hypertrophic laryngitis
    Sicca laryngitis
    EXCLUDES 2   *acute laryngitis (J04.0)*
        obstructive (acute) laryngitis (J05.0)

  J37.1 Chronic laryngotracheitis
    Laryngitis, chronic, with tracheitis (chronic)
    Tracheitis, chronic, with laryngitis
    EXCLUDES 1   *chronic tracheitis (J42)*
    EXCLUDES 2   *acute laryngotracheitis (J04.2)*
        acute tracheitis (J04.1)

√4ᵗʰ **J38 Diseases of vocal cords and larynx, not elsewhere classified**

  Use additional code to identify:
    exposure to environmental tobacco smoke (Z77.22)
    exposure to tobacco smoke in the perinatal period (P96.81)
    history of tobacco dependence (Z87.891)
    occupational exposure to environmental tobacco smoke (Z57.31)
    tobacco dependence (F17.-)
    tobacco use (Z72.0)
  EXCLUDES 1   *congenital laryngeal stridor (P28.89)*
        obstructive laryngitis (acute) (J05.0)
        postprocedural subglottic stenosis (J95.5)
        stridor (R06.1)
        ulcerative laryngitis (J04.0)

√5ᵗʰ **J38.0 Paralysis of vocal cords and larynx**
    Laryngoplegia
    Paralysis of glottis

    J38.00 Paralysis of vocal cords and larynx, unspecified
    J38.01 Paralysis of vocal cords and larynx, unilateral
    J38.02 Paralysis of vocal cords and larynx, bilateral

  J38.1 Polyp of vocal cord and larynx
    EXCLUDES 1   *adenomatous polyps (D14.1)*

  J38.2 Nodules of vocal cords
    Chorditis (fibrinous)(nodosa)(tuberosa)
    Singer's nodes
    Teacher's nodes

  J38.3 Other diseases of vocal cords
    Abscess of vocal cords
    Cellulitis of vocal cords
    Granuloma of vocal cords
    Leukokeratosis of vocal cords
    Leukoplakia of vocal cords

  J38.4 Edema of larynx
    Edema (of) glottis
    Subglottic edema
    Supraglottic edema
    EXCLUDES 1   *acute obstructive laryngitis [croup] (J05.0)*
        edematous laryngitis (J04.0)

  J38.5 Laryngeal spasm
    Laryngismus (stridulus)

  J38.6 Stenosis of larynx

  J38.7 Other diseases of larynx
    Abscess of larynx
    Cellulitis of larynx
    Disease of larynx NOS
    Necrosis of larynx
    Pachyderma of larynx
    Perichondritis of larynx
    Ulcer of larynx

√4ᵗʰ **J39 Other diseases of upper respiratory tract**
  EXCLUDES 1   *acute respiratory infection NOS (J22)*
        acute upper respiratory infection (J06.9)
        upper respiratory inflammation due to chemicals, gases,
          fumes or vapors (J68.2)

  J39.0 Retropharyngeal and parapharyngeal abscess   **CC**
    Peripharyngeal abscess
    EXCLUDES 1   *peritonsillar abscess (J36)*
    DEF: Purulent infection behind the pharynx and the front of the
    precerebral fascia, characterized by neck stiffness, cervical
    lymphadenopathy, sore throat, fever, and stridor.
    CC Excl: PDX collection 740

  J39.1 Other abscess of pharynx   **CC**
    Cellulitis of pharynx
    Nasopharyngeal abscess
    CC Excl: PDX collection 740

N Newborn: 0   P Pediatric: 0-17   M Maternity: 9-64   A Adult: 15-124   MCC Major Complication/Comorbidity   CC Complication/Comorbidity   SW Severe Wound Dx

698   ICD-10-CM 2020

J39.2 **Other diseases of pharynx**
Cyst of pharynx
Edema of pharynx
> EXCLUDES 2 *chronic pharyngitis (J31.2)*
> *ulcerative pharyngitis (J02.9)*

J39.3 **Upper respiratory tract hypersensitivity reaction, site unspecified**
> EXCLUDES 1 *hypersensitivity reaction of upper respiratory tract, such as:*
> *extrinsic allergic alveolitis (J67.9)*
> *pneumoconiosis (J60-J67.9)*

J39.8 **Other specified diseases of upper respiratory tract**
J39.9 **Disease of upper respiratory tract, unspecified**

Chronic lower respiratory diseases (J40-J47)

> EXCLUDES 1 *bronchitis due to chemicals, gases, fumes and vapors (J68.0)*
> EXCLUDES 2 *cystic fibrosis (E84.-)*

J40 **Bronchitis, not specified as acute or chronic**
Bronchitis NOS
Bronchitis with tracheitis NOS
Catarrhal bronchitis
Tracheobronchitis NOS
Use additional code to identify:
exposure to environmental tobacco smoke (Z77.22)
exposure to tobacco smoke in the perinatal period (P96.81)
history of tobacco dependence (Z87.891)
occupational exposure to environmental tobacco smoke (Z57.31)
tobacco dependence (F17.-)
tobacco use (Z72.0)
> EXCLUDES 1 *acute bronchitis (J20.-)*
> *allergic bronchitis NOS (J45.909-)*
> *asthmatic bronchitis NOS (J45.9-)*
> *bronchitis due to chemicals, gases, fumes and vapors (J68.0)*

√4ᵗʰ **J41** **Simple and mucopurulent chronic bronchitis**
Use additional code to identify:
exposure to environmental tobacco smoke (Z77.22)
exposure to tobacco smoke in the perinatal period (P96.81)
history of tobacco dependence (Z87.891)
occupational exposure to environmental tobacco smoke (Z57.31)
tobacco dependence (F17.-)
tobacco use (Z72.0)
> EXCLUDES 1 *chronic bronchitis NOS (J42)*
> *chronic obstructive bronchitis (J44.-)*

J41.0 **Simple chronic bronchitis** `HCC`
J41.1 **Mucopurulent chronic bronchitis** `HCC`
J41.8 **Mixed simple and mucopurulent chronic bronchitis** `HCC`

J42 **Unspecified chronic bronchitis** `HCC`
Chronic bronchitis NOS
Chronic tracheitis
Chronic tracheobronchitis
Use additional code to identify:
exposure to environmental tobacco smoke (Z77.22)
exposure to tobacco smoke in the perinatal period (P96.81)
history of tobacco dependence (Z87.891)
occupational exposure to environmental tobacco smoke (Z57.31)
tobacco dependence (F17.-)
tobacco use (Z72.0)
> EXCLUDES 1 *chronic asthmatic bronchitis (J44.-)*
> *chronic bronchitis with airways obstruction (J44.-)*
> *chronic emphysematous bronchitis (J44.-)*
> *chronic obstructive pulmonary disease NOS (J44.9)*
> *simple and mucopurulent chronic bronchitis (J41.-)*

√4ᵗʰ **J43** **Emphysema**
Use additional code to identify:
exposure to environmental tobacco smoke (Z77.22)
history of tobacco dependence (Z87.891)
occupational exposure to environmental tobacco smoke (Z57.31)
tobacco dependence (F17.-)
tobacco use (Z72.0)
> EXCLUDES 1 *compensatory emphysema (J98.3)*
> *emphysema due to inhalation of chemicals, gases, fumes or vapors (J68.4)*
> *emphysema with chronic (obstructive) bronchitis (J44.-)*
> *emphysematous (obstructive) bronchitis (J44.-)*
> *interstitial emphysema (J98.2)*
> *mediastinal emphysema (J98.2)*
> *neonatal interstitial emphysema (P25.0)*
> *surgical (subcutaneous) emphysema (T81.82)*
> *traumatic subcutaneous emphysema (T79.7)*

DEF: Pathological condition in which there is destructive enlargement of the air sacs in the lungs resulting in damage and lack of elasticity to the alveolar walls, commonly seen in long-term smokers.

Emphysema

Healthy alveoli
Patent bronchiole
Well-vascularized
Dilated alveoli
Excess mucus

Alveoli w/ Emphysema
Collapsed bronchiole
Enlarged alveoli
Broken/fewer capillaries
Alveolar membranes break down

J43.0 **Unilateral pulmonary emphysema [MacLeod's syndrome]** `HCC`
Swyer-James syndrome
Unilateral emphysema
Unilateral hyperlucent lung
Unilateral pulmonary artery functional hypoplasia
Unilateral transparency of lung

J43.1 **Panlobular emphysema** `HCC`
Panacinar emphysema

J43.2 **Centrilobular emphysema** `HCC`

J43.8 **Other emphysema** `HCC`

J43.9 **Emphysema, unspecified** `HCC`
Bullous emphysema (lung)(pulmonary)
Emphysema (lung)(pulmonary) NOS
Emphysematous bleb
Vesicular emphysema (lung)(pulmonary)
AHA: 2019,1Q,34-36; 2017,4Q,97-98

✓4th J44 Other chronic obstructive pulmonary disease

INCLUDES   asthma with chronic obstructive pulmonary disease
chronic asthmatic (obstructive) bronchitis
chronic bronchitis with airways obstruction
chronic bronchitis with emphysema
chronic emphysematous bronchitis
chronic obstructive asthma
chronic obstructive bronchitis
chronic obstructive tracheobronchitis

Code also type of asthma, if applicable (J45.-)
Use additional code to identify:
  exposure to environmental tobacco smoke (Z77.22)
  history of tobacco dependence (Z87.891)
  occupational exposure to environmental tobacco smoke (Z57.31)
  tobacco dependence (F17.-)
  tobacco use (Z72.Ø)

EXCLUDES 1   *bronchiectasis (J47.-)*
chronic bronchitis NOS (J42)
chronic simple and mucopurulent bronchitis (J41.-)
chronic tracheitis (J42)
chronic tracheobronchitis (J42)
emphysema without chronic bronchitis (J43.-)

AHA: 2019,1Q,34-36; 2017,4Q,97-98; 2017,1Q,25-26; 2016,3Q,15-16; 2013,4Q,109

▲ **J44.Ø** **Chronic obstructive pulmonary disease with**   **CC** **HCC**
    (acute) lower respiratory infection
      Code also to identify the infection
      AHA: 2019,1Q,35; 2017,4Q,96; 2017,1Q,24-25
      TIP: Do not assign when only aspiration pneumonia is present. Aspiration pneumonis is not classified as a respiratory infection.

J44.1 **Chronic obstructive pulmonary disease with**   **CC** **HCC**
    (acute) exacerbation
    Decompensated COPD
    Decompensated COPD with (acute) exacerbation
      EXCLUDES 2   *chronic obstructive pulmonary disease [COPD] with acute bronchitis (J44.Ø)*
           lung diseases due to external agents (J6Ø-J7Ø)
      AHA: 2019,1Q,34; 2017,4Q,96; 2017,1Q,26; 2016,1Q,36
      TIP: Exacerbation of COPD should not be assumed based upon worsening of a concomitant respiratory disease or when COPD is described as end-stage.
      CC Excl: PDX collection 741

J44.9 **Chronic obstructive pulmonary disease,**   **HCC**
    unspecified
    Chronic obstructive airway disease NOS
    Chronic obstructive lung disease NOS
      EXCLUDES 2   *lung diseases due to external agents (J6Ø-J7Ø)*
      AHA: 2019,1Q,36; 2017,4Q,96-97; 2016,1Q,36; 2014,4Q,21; 2013,4Q,109

✓4th J45 Asthma

INCLUDES   allergic (predominantly) asthma
allergic bronchitis NOS
allergic rhinitis with asthma
atopic asthma
extrinsic allergic asthma
hay fever with asthma
idiosyncratic asthma
intrinsic nonallergic asthma
nonallergic asthma

Use additional code to identify:
  exposure to environmental tobacco smoke (Z77.22)
  exposure to tobacco smoke in the perinatal period (P96.81)
  history of tobacco dependence (Z87.891)
  occupational exposure to environmental tobacco smoke (Z57.31)
  tobacco dependence (F17.-)
  tobacco use (Z72.Ø)

EXCLUDES 1   *detergent asthma (J69.8)*
eosinophilic asthma (J82)
miner's asthma (J6Ø)
wheezing NOS (RØ6.2)
wood asthma (J67.8)

EXCLUDES 2   *asthma with chronic obstructive pulmonary disease (J44.9)*
chronic asthmatic (obstructive) bronchitis (J44.9)
chronic obstructive asthma (J44.9)

AHA: 2019,1Q,36; 2017,1Q,25-26; 2012,4Q,99
DEF: Status asthmaticus: Severe, intractable episode of asthma that is unresponsive to normal therapeutic measures.
CC Excl: For CC codes in category J45: PDX collection 742

Asthma

Respiratory bronchiole — Smooth muscle fibers — Contraction of smooth muscle fibers — Mucus lining bronchial tubes — Alveoli — Extra mucus secretion in inflamed bronchial tubes — Air trapped within alveoli — Normal alveoli — Asthmatic alveoli

✓5th **J45.2** **Mild intermittent asthma**

    J45.2Ø **Mild intermittent asthma, uncomplicated**
        Mild intermittent asthma NOS

    J45.21 **Mild intermittent asthma with**   **CC**
        (acute) exacerbation

    J45.22 **Mild intermittent asthma with status**   **CC**
        asthmaticus

✓5th **J45.3** **Mild persistent asthma**

    J45.3Ø **Mild persistent asthma, uncomplicated**
        Mild persistent asthma NOS

    J45.31 **Mild persistent asthma with (acute)**   **CC**
        exacerbation
          AHA: 2016,1Q,35

    J45.32 **Mild persistent asthma with status**   **CC**
        asthmaticus

✓5th **J45.4** **Moderate persistent asthma**

    J45.4Ø **Moderate persistent asthma, uncomplicated**
        Moderate persistent asthma NOS

    J45.41 **Moderate persistent asthma with**   **CC**
        (acute) exacerbation
          AHA: 2017,1Q,26

    J45.42 **Moderate persistent asthma with**   **CC**
        status asthmaticus

N Newborn: 0   **P** Pediatric: 0-17   **M** Maternity: 9-64   **A** Adult: 15-124   **MCC** Major Complication/Comorbidity   **CC** Complication/Comorbidity   **SW** Severe Wound Dx

700   ICD-10-CM 2020

√5ᵗʰ **J45.5** Severe persistent **asthma**

  J45.50 **Severe persistent asthma,** uncomplicated
    Severe persistent asthma NOS

  J45.51 **Severe persistent asthma with (acute)** exacerbation   `MCC`

  J45.52 **Severe persistent asthma with** status **asthmaticus**   `CC`

√5ᵗʰ **J45.9** **Other and unspecified asthma**

  √6ᵗʰ **J45.90** **Unspecified asthma**
    Asthmatic bronchitis NOS
    Childhood asthma NOS
    Late onset asthma
    AHA: 2017,4Q,96; 2017,1Q,25

    J45.901 **Unspecified asthma with (acute)** exacerbation   `CC`

    J45.902 **Unspecified asthma with** status asthmaticus   `CC`

    J45.909 **Unspecified asthma,** uncomplicated
      Asthma NOS
      EXCLUDES 2   *lung diseases due to external agents (J60-J70)*
      AHA: 2017,1Q,25

  √6ᵗʰ **J45.99** **Other asthma**

    J45.990 **Exercise induced bronchospasm**

    J45.991 **Cough variant** asthma

    J45.998 **Other asthma**

√4ᵗʰ **J47** **Bronchiectasis**

  INCLUDES   bronchiolectasis
  Use additional code to identify:
    exposure to environmental tobacco smoke (Z77.22)
    exposure to tobacco smoke in the perinatal period (P96.81)
    history of tobacco dependence (Z87.891)
    occupational exposure to environmental tobacco smoke (Z57.31)
    tobacco dependence (F17.-)
    tobacco use (Z72.0)
  EXCLUDES 1   *congenital bronchiectasis (Q33.4)*
      tuberculous bronchiectasis (current disease) (A15.0)
  DEF: Dilation of the bronchi with mucus production and persistent cough due to infection or chronic conditions that causes diminished lung capacity and frequent infections of the lung.

  J47.0 **Bronchiectasis with** acute lower respiratory **infection**   `CC` `HCC`
    Bronchiectasis with acute bronchitis
    Use additional code to identify the infection
    CC Excl: PDX collection 743

  J47.1 **Bronchiectasis with (acute)** exacerbation   `CC` `HCC`
    CC Excl: PDX collection 743

  J47.9 **Bronchiectasis,** uncomplicated   `HCC`
    Bronchiectasis NOS

Lung diseases due to external agents (J60-J70)

EXCLUDES 2   *asthma (J45.-)*
    malignant neoplasm of bronchus and lung (C34.-)
DEF: Pneumoconiosis: Condition caused by inhaling inorganic dust particles, typically associated with occupations that require regular exposure to mineral dusts. A form of interstitial lung disease that contributes to the inflammation of the air sacs, causing the lung tissue to harden.
CC Excl: For CC/MCC codes in categories J60-J70: PDX collection 110

J60 **Coalworker's** pneumoconiosis   `HCC` `A`
  Anthracosilicosis
  Anthracosis
  Black lung disease
  Coalworker's lung
  EXCLUDES 1   *coalworker pneumoconiosis with tuberculosis, any type in A15 (J65)*

J61 **Pneumoconiosis due to** asbestos and other mineral **fibers**   `HCC` `A`
  Asbestosis
  EXCLUDES 1   *pleural plaque with asbestosis (J92.0)*
      pneumoconiosis with tuberculosis, any type in A15 (J65)

√4ᵗʰ **J62** **Pneumoconiosis due to** dust containing silica
  INCLUDES   silicotic fibrosis (massive) of lung
  EXCLUDES 1   *pneumoconiosis with tuberculosis, any type in A15 (J65)*
  J62.0 **Pneumoconiosis due to** talc dust   `HCC`

  J62.8 **Pneumoconiosis due to** other dust containing silica   `HCC`
    Silicosis NOS

√4ᵗʰ **J63** **Pneumoconiosis due to other** inorganic dusts
  EXCLUDES 1   *pneumoconiosis with tuberculosis, any type in A15 (J65)*

  J63.0 **Aluminosis (of lung)**   `HCC`

  J63.1 **Bauxite fibrosis (of lung)**   `HCC`

  J63.2 **Berylliosis**   `HCC`

  J63.3 **Graphite fibrosis (of lung)**   `HCC`

  J63.4 **Siderosis**   `HCC`

  J63.5 **Stannosis**   `HCC`

  J63.6 **Pneumoconiosis due to other specified inorganic dusts**   `HCC`

J64 **Unspecified pneumoconiosis**   `HCC`
  EXCLUDES 1   *pneumonoconiosis with tuberculosis, any type in A15 (J65)*

J65 **Pneumoconiosis** associated with tuberculosis   `HCC`
  Any condition in J60-J64 with tuberculosis, any type in A15
  Silicotuberculosis

√4ᵗʰ **J66** **Airway disease due to specific** organic dust
  EXCLUDES 2   *allergic alveolitis (J67.-)*
      asbestosis (J61)
      bagassosis (J67.1)
      farmer's lung (J67.0)
      hypersensitivity pneumonitis due to organic dust (J67.-)
      reactive airways dysfunction syndrome (J68.3)

  J66.0 **Byssinosis**   `HCC`
    Airway disease due to cotton dust

  J66.1 **Flax-dressers' disease**   `HCC`

  J66.2 **Cannabinosis**   `HCC`

  J66.8 **Airway disease due to other specific organic dusts**   `HCC`

√4ᵗʰ **J67** **Hypersensitivity pneumonitis due to organic dust**
  INCLUDES   allergic alveolitis and pneumonitis due to inhaled organic dust and particles of fungal, actinomycetic or other origin
  EXCLUDES 1   *pneumonitis due to inhalation of chemicals, gases, fumes or vapors (J68.0)*

  J67.0 **Farmer's lung**   `HCC`
    Harvester's lung
    Haymaker's lung
    Moldy hay disease

  J67.1 **Bagassosis**   `HCC`
    Bagasse disease
    Bagasse pneumonitis

  J67.2 **Bird fancier's lung**   `HCC`
    Budgerigar fancier's disease or lung
    Pigeon fancier's disease or lung

  J67.3 **Suberosis**   `HCC`
    Corkhandler's disease or lung
    Corkworker's disease or lung

  J67.4 **Maltworker's lung**   `HCC`
    Alveolitis due to Aspergillus clavatus

  J67.5 **Mushroom-worker's lung**   `HCC`

  J67.6 **Maple-bark-stripper's lung**   `HCC`
    Alveolitis due to Cryptostroma corticale
    Cryptostromosis

  J67.7 **Air conditioner and humidifier lung**   `CC` `HCC`
    Allergic alveolitis due to fungal, thermophilic actinomycetes and other organisms growing in ventilation [air conditioning] systems

  J67.8 **Hypersensitivity pneumonitis due to other organic dusts**   `CC` `HCC`
    Cheese-washer's lung
    Coffee-worker's lung
    Fish-meal worker's lung
    Furrier's lung
    Sequoiosis

☑ Additional Character Required   √x7ᵗʰ Placeholder   Unacceptable PDx   Questionable PDx   Manifestation   Unspecified Dx   H1-H14 HAC   HCC CMS-HCC Dx   HIV HIV Dx

ICD-10-CM 2020

701

J67.9 **Hypersensitivity pneumonitis due to** `CC` `HCC`
unspecified organic dust
Allergic alveolitis (extrinsic) NOS
Hypersensitivity pneumonitis NOS

✓4ᵗʰ **J68** **Respiratory conditions due to inhalation of chemicals, gases, fumes and vapors**
Code first (T51-T65) to identify cause
Use additional code to identify associated respiratory conditions, such as:
acute respiratory failure (J96.0-)

J68.0 **Bronchitis and pneumonitis due to chemicals,** `CC` `HCC`
gases, fumes and vapors
Chemical bronchitis (acute)
AHA: 2019,2Q,31

J68.1 **Pulmonary edema due to chemicals, gases,** `MCC` `HCC`
fumes and vapors
Chemical pulmonary edema (acute) (chronic)
EXCLUDES 1   *pulmonary edema (acute) (chronic) NOS (J81.-)*

J68.2 **Upper respiratory inflammation due to** `HCC`
**chemicals, gases, fumes and vapors, not
elsewhere classified**

J68.3 **Other acute and subacute respiratory** `HCC`
**conditions due to chemicals, gases, fumes and
vapors**
Reactive airways dysfunction syndrome

J68.4 **Chronic respiratory conditions due to** `HCC`
chemicals, gases, fumes and vapors
Emphysema (diffuse) (chronic) due to inhalation of chemicals, gases, fumes and vapors
Obliterative bronchiolitis (chronic) (subacute) due to inhalation of chemicals, gases, fumes and vapors
Pulmonary fibrosis (chronic) due to inhalation of chemicals, gases, fumes and vapors
EXCLUDES 1   *chronic pulmonary edema due to chemicals, gases, fumes and vapors (J68.1)*

J68.8 **Other respiratory conditions due to chemicals,** `HCC`
gases, fumes and vapors

J68.9 **Unspecified respiratory condition due to** `HCC`
chemicals, gases, fumes and vapors

✓4ᵗʰ **J69** **Pneumonitis due to solids and liquids**
EXCLUDES 1   *neonatal aspiration syndromes (P24.-)*
postprocedural pneumonitis (J95.4)
AHA: 2017,1Q,24
DEF: Pneumonitis: Noninfectious inflammation of the walls of the alveoli in the lung tissue due to inhalation of food, vomit, oils, essences, or other solids or liquids.

J69.0 **Pneumonitis due to inhalation of food and** `MCC` `HCC`
vomit
Aspiration pneumonia NOS
Aspiration pneumonia (due to) food (regurgitated)
Aspiration pneumonia (due to) gastric secretions
Aspiration pneumonia (due to) milk
Aspiration pneumonia (due to) vomit
Code also any associated foreign body in respiratory tract (T17.-)
EXCLUDES 1   *chemical pneumonitis due to anesthesia (J95.4)*
obstetric aspiration pneumonitis (O74.0)
AHA: 2019,2Q,6,31

J69.1 **Pneumonitis due to inhalation of oils and** `MCC` `HCC`
essences
Exogenous lipoid pneumonia
Lipid pneumonia NOS
Code first (T51-T65) to identify substance
EXCLUDES 1   *endogenous lipoid pneumonia (J84.89)*

J69.8 **Pneumonitis due to inhalation of other solids** `MCC` `HCC`
and liquids
Pneumonitis due to aspiration of blood
Pneumonitis due to aspiration of detergent
Code first (T51-T65) to identify substance

✓4ᵗʰ **J70** **Respiratory conditions due to other external agents**

J70.0 **Acute pulmonary manifestations due to** `CC` `HCC`
radiation
Radiation pneumonitis
Use additional code (W88-W90, X39.0-) to identify the external cause

J70.1 **Chronic and other pulmonary manifestations** `CC` `HCC`
due to radiation
Fibrosis of lung following radiation
Use additional code (W88-W90, X39.0-) to identify the external cause

J70.2 **Acute drug-induced interstitial lung disorders** `HCC`
Use additional code for adverse effect, if applicable, to identify drug (T36-T50 with fifth or sixth character 5)
EXCLUDES 1   *interstitial pneumonia NOS (J84.9)*
lymphoid interstitial pneumonia (J84.2)
AHA: 2019,2Q,28

J70.3 **Chronic drug-induced interstitial lung** `HCC`
disorders
Use additional code for adverse effect, if applicable, to identify drug (T36-T50 with fifth or sixth character 5)
EXCLUDES 1   *interstitial pneumonia NOS (J84.9)*
lymphoid interstitial pneumonia (J84.2)

J70.4 **Drug-induced interstitial lung disorders,** `HCC`
unspecified
Use additional code for adverse effect, if applicable, to identify drug (T36-T50 with fifth or sixth character 5)
EXCLUDES 1   *interstitial pneumonia NOS (J84.9)*
lymphoid interstitial pneumonia (J84.2)
AHA: 2019,2Q,28

J70.5 **Respiratory conditions due to smoke** `HCC`
inhalation
Smoke inhalation NOS
EXCLUDES 1   *smoke inhalation due to chemicals, gases, fumes and vapors (J68.9)*
AHA: 2013,4Q,121

J70.8 **Respiratory conditions due to other specified** `HCC`
external agents
Code first (T51-T65) to identify the external agent

J70.9 **Respiratory conditions due to unspecified** `HCC`
external agent
Code first (T51-T65) to identify the external agent

Other respiratory diseases principally affecting the interstitium (J80-J84)

J80 **Acute respiratory distress syndrome** `MCC` `HCC`
Acute respiratory distress syndrome in adult or child
Adult hyaline membrane disease
EXCLUDES 1   *respiratory distress syndrome in newborn (perinatal) (P22.0)*
AHA: 2017,1Q,26
DEF: Lung inflammation or injury resulting in a build-up of fluid in the air sacs, preventing the passage of oxygen from the air into the bloodstream.
CC Excl: PDX collection 744

✓4ᵗʰ **J81** **Pulmonary edema**
Use additional code to identify:
exposure to environmental tobacco smoke (Z77.22)
history of tobacco dependence (Z87.891)
occupational exposure to environmental tobacco smoke (Z57.31)
tobacco dependence (F17.-)
tobacco use (Z72.0)
EXCLUDES 1   *chemical (acute) pulmonary edema (J68.1)*
hypostatic pneumonia (J18.2)
passive pneumonia (J18.2)
pulmonary edema due to external agents (J60-J70)
pulmonary edema with heart disease NOS (I50.1)
pulmonary edema with heart failure (I50.1)
DEF: Accumulation of fluid in the air sacs of the lungs, making it difficult to breath.

J81.0 **Acute pulmonary edema** `MCC` `HCC`
Acute edema of lung
CC Excl: PDX collection 745

J81.1 **Chronic pulmonary edema** `CC`
Pulmonary congestion (chronic) (passive)
Pulmonary edema NOS
CC Excl: PDX collection 736

Ⓝ Newborn: 0   Ⓟ Pediatric: 0-17   Ⓜ Maternity: 9-64   Ⓐ Adult: 15-124   `MCC` Major Complication/Comorbidity   `CC` Complication/Comorbidity   `SW` Severe Wound Dx

702   ICD-10-CM 2020

J82 Pulmonary eosinophilia, not elsewhere classified `CC` `HCC`

Allergic pneumonia
Eosinophilic asthma
Eosinophilic pneumonia
Löffler's pneumonia
Tropical (pulmonary) eosinophilia NOS

> **EXCLUDES 1**   *pulmonary eosinophilia due to aspergillosis (B44.-)*
> *pulmonary eosinophilia due to drugs (J70.2-J70.4)*
> *pulmonary eosinophilia due to specified parasitic infection (B50-B83)*
> *pulmonary eosinophilia due to systemic connective tissue disorders (M30-M36)*
> *pulmonary infiltrate NOS (R91.8)*

DEF: Infiltration of eosinophils (white blood cells of the immune system) into the parenchyma of the lungs, resulting in cough, fever, and dyspnea.
CC Excl: PDX collection 746

✓4th **J84 Other interstitial pulmonary diseases**

> **EXCLUDES 1**   *drug-induced interstitial lung disorders (J70.2-J70.4)*
> *interstitial emphysema (J98.2)*
> **EXCLUDES 2**   *lung diseases due to external agents (J60-J70)*

DEF: Interstitial: Within the small spaces or gaps occurring in tissue or organs.
CC Excl: For CC/MCC codes in category J84, unless otherwise noted: PDX collection 747

✓5th **J84.0 Alveolar and parieto-alveolar conditions**

J84.01 Alveolar proteinosis `CC` `HCC`

> **DEF:** Reduced ventilation due to proteinaceous deposits on alveoli. Symptoms include dyspnea, cough, chest pain, weakness, weight loss, and hemoptysis.

J84.02 Pulmonary alveolar microlithiasis `CC` `HCC`

J84.03 *Idiopathic pulmonary hemosiderosis* `CC` `HCC`

> Essential brown induration of lung
> Code first underlying disease, such as:
>   disorders of iron metabolism (E83.1-)
> > **EXCLUDES 1**   *acute idiopathic pulmonary hemorrhage in infants [AIPHI] (R04.81)*
> **DEF:** Fibrosis of the alveolar walls marked by abnormal accumulation of iron as hemosiderin in the lungs. It primarily affects children and symptoms include anemia, fluid in the lungs, and blood in the sputum. Etiology is unknown.

J84.09 Other alveolar and parieto-alveolar conditions `CC` `HCC`

✓5th **J84.1 Other interstitial pulmonary diseases with fibrosis**

> **EXCLUDES 1**   *pulmonary fibrosis (chronic) due to inhalation of chemicals, gases, fumes or vapors (J68.4)*
> *pulmonary fibrosis (chronic) following radiation (J70.1)*

J84.10 Pulmonary fibrosis, unspecified `HCC`

> Capillary fibrosis of lung
> Cirrhosis of lung (chronic) NOS
> Fibrosis of lung (atrophic) (chronic) (confluent) (massive) (perialveolar) (peribronchial) NOS
> Induration of lung (chronic) NOS
> Postinflammatory pulmonary fibrosis

✓6th **J84.11 Idiopathic interstitial pneumonia**

> **EXCLUDES 1**   *lymphoid interstitial pneumonia (J84.2)*
> *pneumocystis pneumonia (B59)*

J84.111 Idiopathic interstitial pneumonia, not otherwise specified `HCC`

J84.112 Idiopathic pulmonary fibrosis `HCC`

> Cryptogenic fibrosing alveolitis
> Idiopathic fibrosing alveolitis

J84.113 Idiopathic non-specific interstitial pneumonitis `HCC`

> > **EXCLUDES 1**   *non-specific interstitial pneumonia NOS, or due to known underlying cause (J84.89)*

J84.114 Acute interstitial pneumonitis `CC` `HCC`

> Hamman-Rich syndrome
> > **EXCLUDES 1**   *pneumocystis pneumonia (B59)*

J84.115 Respiratory bronchiolitis interstitial lung disease `HCC`

J84.116 Cryptogenic organizing pneumonia `CC` `HCC`

> > **EXCLUDES 1**   *organizing pneumonia NOS, or due to known underlying cause (J84.89)*

J84.117 Desquamative interstitial pneumonia `CC` `HCC`

J84.17 *Other interstitial pulmonary diseases with fibrosis in diseases classified elsewhere* `HCC`

> Interstitial pneumonia (nonspecific) (usual) due to collagen vascular disease
> Interstitial pneumonia (nonspecific) (usual) in diseases classified elsewhere
> Organizing pneumonia due to collagen vascular disease
> Organizing pneumonia in diseases classified elsewhere
> Code first underlying disease, such as:
>   progressive systemic sclerosis (M34.0)
>   rheumatoid arthritis (M05.00-M06.9)
>   systemic lupus erythematosis (M32.0-M32.9)

J84.2 Lymphoid interstitial pneumonia `CC` `HCC`

> Lymphoid interstitial pneumonitis

✓5th **J84.8 Other specified interstitial pulmonary diseases**

> **EXCLUDES 1**   *exogenous lipoid pneumonia (J69.1)*
> *unspecified lipoid pneumonia (J69.1)*

J84.81 Lymphangioleiomyomatosis `MCC` `HCC`

> Lymphangiomyomatosis

J84.82 Adult pulmonary Langerhans cell histiocytosis `CC` `HCC` `A`

> Adult PLCH

J84.83 Surfactant mutations of the lung `MCC` `HCC`

> **DEF:** Genetic disorder resulting in insufficient secretion of a complex mixture of phospholipids and proteins that reduce surface tension in the alveoli following the onset of breathing to facilitate lung expansion in the newborn. It is the leading indication for pediatric lung transplantation.
> **CC Excl:** PDX collection 748

✓6th **J84.84 Other interstitial lung diseases of childhood**

> **CC Excl: For MCC codes in subcategory J84.84:** PDX collection 748

J84.841 Neuroendocrine cell hyperplasia of infancy `MCC` `HCC`

J84.842 Pulmonary interstitial glycogenosis `MCC` `HCC`

J84.843 Alveolar capillary dysplasia with vein misalignment `MCC` `HCC`

J84.848 Other interstitial lung diseases of childhood `MCC` `HCC`

J84.89 Other specified interstitial pulmonary diseases `HCC`

> Endogenous lipoid pneumonia
> Interstitial pneumonitis
> Non-specific interstitial pneumonitis NOS
> Organizing pneumonia NOS
> Code first, if applicable:
>   poisoning due to drug or toxin (T51-T65 with fifth or sixth character to indicate intent), for toxic pneumonopathy
>   underlying cause of pneumonopathy, if known
> Use additional code, for adverse effect, to identify drug (T36-T50 with fifth or sixth character 5), if drug-induced
> > **EXCLUDES 1**   *cryptogenic organizing pneumonia (J84.116)*
> > *idiopathic non-specific interstitial pneumonitis (J84.113)*
> > *lymphoid interstitial pneumonia (J84.2)*
> > *lipoid pneumonia, exogenous or unspecified (J69.1)*

AHA: 2019,2Q,28

Chapter 10. Diseases of the Respiratory System

J84.9   Interstitial pulmonary disease, unspecified   `HCC`

Interstitial pneumonia NOS

Suppurative and necrotic conditions of the lower respiratory tract (J85-J86)

`√4ᵗʰ` **J85**   **Abscess of lung and mediastinum**

Use additional code (B95-B97) to identify infectious agent

CC Excl: For MCC codes in category J85, unless otherwise noted: PDX collection 749

J85.Ø   Gangrene and necrosis **of lung**   `MCC` `HCC`

J85.1   Abscess of lung **with pneumonia**   `MCC` `HCC`

Code also the type of pneumonia

J85.2   Abscess of lung **without pneumonia**   `MCC` `HCC`

Abscess of lung NOS

J85.3   **Abscess of mediastinum**   `MCC` `HCC`

CC Excl: PDX collection 750

`√4ᵗʰ` **J86**   **Pyothorax**

Use additional code (B95-B97) to identify infectious agent

`EXCLUDES 1`   *abscess of lung (J85.-)*

pyothorax due to tuberculosis (A15.6)

DEF: Collection of pus in the pleural space that is commonly caused by an infection that spreads from the lung, such as bacterial pneumonia or a lung abscess.

J86.Ø   **Pyothorax with fistula**   `MCC` `HCC` `SW`

Bronchocutaneous fistula

Bronchopleural fistula

Hepatopleural fistula

Mediastinal fistula

Pleural fistula

Thoracic fistula

Any condition classifiable to J86.9 with fistula

DEF: Purulent infection of the respiratory cavity, with communication from a cavity to another structure.

CC Excl: PDX collection 751

J86.9   **Pyothorax without fistula**   `MCC` `HCC`

Abscess of pleura

Abscess of thorax

Empyema (chest) (lung) (pleura)

Fibrinopurulent pleurisy

Purulent pleurisy

Pyopneumothorax

Septic pleurisy

Seropurulent pleurisy

Suppurative pleurisy

CC Excl: PDX collection 751

Other diseases of the pleura (J9Ø-J94)

J9Ø   **Pleural effusion, not elsewhere classified**   `CC`

Encysted pleurisy

Pleural effusion NOS

Pleurisy with effusion (exudative) (serous)

`EXCLUDES 1`   *chylous (pleural) effusion (J94.Ø)*

malignant pleural effusion (J91.Ø))

pleurisy NOS (RØ9.1)

tuberculous pleural effusion (A15.6)

DEF: Collection of lymph and other fluid within the pleural space.

CC Excl: PDX collection 752

`√4ᵗʰ` **J91**   **Pleural effusion in conditions classified elsewhere**

`EXCLUDES 2`   *pleural effusion in heart failure (I5Ø.-)*

pleural effusion in systemic lupus erythematosus (M32.13)

DEF: Collection of lymph and other fluid within the pleural space.

J91.Ø   *Malignant pleural effusion*   `CC`

Code first underlying neoplasm

CC Excl: PDX collection 753

J91.8   *Pleural effusion in other conditions classified elsewhere*   `CC`

Code first underlying disease, such as:

filariasis (B74.Ø-B74.9)

influenza (JØ9.X2, J1Ø.1, J11.1)

AHA: 2015,2Q,15

TIP: Assign this code as a secondary diagnosis to congestive heart failure (I5Ø.-) only if pleural effusion is specifically evaluated or treated.

CC Excl: PDX collection 752

Pleural Effusion

Right lung

Left lung

Pleura

Pleural space

Pleural effusion

`√4ᵗʰ` **J92**   **Pleural plaque**

`INCLUDES`   pleural thickening

DEF: Areas of fibrous thickening that form on the parietal or visceral pleura, the membranes that line the ribs and lungs.

J92.Ø   **Pleural plaque with presence of asbestos**

J92.9   **Pleural plaque without asbestos**

Pleural plaque NOS

`√4ᵗʰ` **J93**   **Pneumothorax and air leak**

`EXCLUDES 1`   *congenital or perinatal pneumothorax (P25.1)*

postprocedural air leak (J95.812)

postprocedural pneumothorax (J95.811)

pyopneumothorax (J86.-)

traumatic pneumothorax (S27.Ø)

tuberculous (current disease) pneumothorax (A15.-)

DEF: Pneumothorax: Lung displacement due to abnormal leakage of air or gas that is trapped in the pleural space formed by the membrane that encloses the lungs and lines the thoracic cavity.

CC Excl: For CC/MCC codes in category J93: PDX collection 754

J93.Ø   **Spontaneous tension pneumothorax**   `MCC`

DEF: Leaking air from the lung into the lining, causing collapse.

`√5ᵗʰ` **J93.1**   **Other spontaneous pneumothorax**

J93.11   **Primary spontaneous pneumothorax**   `CC`

J93.12   **Secondary spontaneous pneumothorax**   `CC`

Code first underlying condition, such as:

catamenial pneumothorax due to endometriosis (N8Ø.8)

cystic fibrosis (E84.-)

eosinophilic pneumonia (J82)

lymphangioleiomyomatosis (J84.81)

malignant neoplasm of bronchus and lung (C34.-)

Marfan's syndrome (Q87.4)

pneumonia due to Pneumocystis carinii (B59)

secondary malignant neoplasm of lung (C78.Ø-)

spontaneous rupture of the esophagus (K22.3)

`√5ᵗʰ` **J93.8**   **Other pneumothorax and air leak**

J93.81   **Chronic pneumothorax**   `CC`

J93.82   **Other air leak**   `CC`

Persistent air leak

`N` Newborn: 0   `P` Pediatric: 0-17   `M` Maternity: 9-64   `A` Adult: 15-124   `MCC` Major Complication/Comorbidity   `CC` Complication/Comorbidity   `SW` Severe Wound Dx

J84.9–J93.82

704   ICD-10-CM 2020

J93.83 **Other pneumothorax** `CC`

Acute pneumothorax
Spontaneous pneumothorax NOS

J93.9 **Pneumothorax, unspecified** `CC`

Pneumothorax NOS

✓4ᵗʰ **J94 Other pleural conditions**

EXCLUDES 1 *pleurisy NOS (R09.1)*
traumatic hemopneumothorax (S27.2)
traumatic hemothorax (S27.1)
tuberculous pleural conditions (current disease) (A15.-)

J94.0 **Chylous effusion** `CC`

Chyliform effusion
DEF: Fluid within the pleural space due to the leaking of lymph contents into the space, usually as a result of thoracic duct damage or injury or mediastinal lymphoma.
CC Excl: PDX collection 752

J94.1 **Fibrothorax**

DEF: Fibrosis within the pleural lining of the lungs commonly seen as a stiff layer surrounding the lung typically attributed to traumatic hemothorax or pleural effusion.

J94.2 **Hemothorax** `CC`

Hemopneumothorax
CC Excl: PDX collection 752

J94.8 **Other specified pleural conditions** `CC`

Hydropneumothorax
Hydrothorax
CC Excl: No Excl

J94.9 **Pleural condition, unspecified**

Intraoperative and postprocedural complications and disorders of respiratory system, not elsewhere classified (J95)

✓4ᵗʰ **J95 Intraoperative and postprocedural complications and disorders of respiratory system, not elsewhere classified**

EXCLUDES 2 *aspiration pneumonia (J69.-)*
emphysema (subcutaneous) resulting from a procedure (T81.82)
hypostatic pneumonia (J18.2)
pulmonary manifestations due to radiation (J70.0-J70.1)

✓5ᵗʰ **J95.0 Tracheostomy complications**

DEF: Tracheostomy: Formation of a tracheal opening on the neck surface with tube insertion to allow for respiration in cases of obstruction or decreased patency. A tracheostomy may be planned or performed on an emergency basis for temporary or long-term use.
CC Excl: For CC codes in subcategory J95.0: PDX collection 755

Tracheostomy

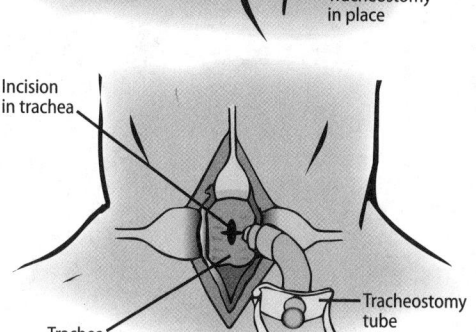

Tracheostomy in place

Incision in trachea

Trachea

Tracheostomy tube

J95.00 **Unspecified tracheostomy complication** `CC` `HCC`

J95.01 **Hemorrhage from tracheostomy stoma** `CC` `HCC`

J95.02 **Infection of tracheostomy stoma** `CC` `HCC`

Use additional code to identify type of infection, such as:
cellulitis of neck (L03.221)
sepsis (A40, A41.-)

J95.03 **Malfunction of tracheostomy stoma** `CC` `HCC`

Mechanical complication of tracheostomy stoma
Obstruction of tracheostomy airway
Tracheal stenosis due to tracheostomy

J95.04 **Tracheo-esophageal fistula following tracheostomy** `CC` `HCC`

J95.09 **Other tracheostomy complication** `CC` `HCC`

J95.1 **Acute pulmonary insufficiency following thoracic surgery** `CC` `HCC`

EXCLUDES 2 *functional disturbances following cardiac surgery (I97.0, I97.1-)*

J95.2 **Acute pulmonary insufficiency following nonthoracic surgery** `MCC` `HCC`

EXCLUDES 2 *functional disturbances following cardiac surgery (I97.0, I97.1-)*

CC Excl: PDX collection 756

J95.3 **Chronic pulmonary insufficiency following surgery** `MCC` `HCC`

EXCLUDES 2 *functional disturbances following cardiac surgery (I97.0, I97.1-)*

CC Excl: PDX collection 756

J95.4 **Chemical pneumonitis due to anesthesia** `CC`

Mendelson's syndrome
Postprocedural aspiration pneumonia
Use additional code for adverse effect, if applicable, to identify drug (T41.- with fifth or sixth character 5)

EXCLUDES 1 *aspiration pneumonitis due to anesthesia complicating labor and delivery (O74.0)*
aspiration pneumonitis due to anesthesia complicating pregnancy (O29)
aspiration pneumonitis due to anesthesia complicating the puerperium (O89.01)

CC Excl: PDX collection 757

J95.5 **Postprocedural subglottic stenosis** `CC`

CC Excl: PDX collection 757

✓5ᵗʰ **J95.6 Intraoperative hemorrhage and hematoma of a respiratory system organ or structure complicating a procedure**

EXCLUDES 1 *intraoperative hemorrhage and hematoma of a respiratory system organ or structure due to accidental puncture and laceration during procedure (J95.7-)*

J95.61 **Intraoperative hemorrhage and hematoma of a respiratory system organ or structure complicating a respiratory system procedure** `CC`
CC Excl: PDX collection 758

J95.62 **Intraoperative hemorrhage and hematoma of a respiratory system organ or structure complicating other procedure** `CC`
CC Excl: PDX collection 758

✓5ᵗʰ **J95.7 Accidental puncture and laceration of a respiratory system organ or structure during a procedure**

EXCLUDES 2 *postprocedural pneumothorax (J95.811)*

J95.71 **Accidental puncture and laceration of a respiratory system organ or structure during a respiratory system procedure** `CC`
CC Excl: PDX collection 509

J95.72 **Accidental puncture and laceration of a respiratory system organ or structure during other procedure** `CC`
CC Excl: PDX collection 509

✓5ᵗʰ **J95.8 Other intraoperative and postprocedural complications and disorders of respiratory system, not elsewhere classified**
AHA: 2016,4Q,9-10

✓6ᵗʰ **J95.81 Postprocedural pneumothorax and air leak**

J95.811 **Postprocedural pneumothorax** `CC` `H14`
CC Excl: PDX collection 754

Chapter 10. Diseases of the Respiratory System

J95.812 Postprocedural air leak `CC`
  CC Excl: PDX collection 754

✓6th **J95.82 Postprocedural respiratory failure**
  EXCLUDES 1   *respiratory failure in other conditions (J96.-)*

  J95.821 Acute postprocedural respiratory failure `CC` `HCC`
    Postprocedural respiratory failure NOS

  J95.822 Acute and chronic postprocedural respiratory failure `MCC` `HCC`
    CC Excl: PDX collection 756

✓6th **J95.83 Postprocedural hemorrhage of a respiratory system organ or structure following a procedure**

  J95.830 Postprocedural hemorrhage of a respiratory system organ or structure following a respiratory system procedure `CC`
    CC Excl: PDX collection 758

  J95.831 Postprocedural hemorrhage of a respiratory system organ or structure following other procedure `CC`
    CC Excl: PDX collection 758

J95.84 Transfusion-related acute lung injury (TRALI) `CC`
  DEF: Relatively rare, but serious, pulmonary complication of blood transfusion, with acute respiratory distress, noncardiogenic pulmonary edema, cyanosis, hypoxemia, hypotension, fever, and chills.
  CC Excl: PDX collection 757

✓6th **J95.85 Complication of respirator [ventilator]**

  J95.850 Mechanical complication of respirator `CC` `HCC`
    EXCLUDES 1   *encounter for respirator [ventilator] dependence during power failure (Z99.12)*
    CC Excl: PDX collection 759

  J95.851 Ventilator associated pneumonia `CC` `HCC`
    Ventilator associated pneumonitis
    Use additional code to identify the organism, if known (B95.-, B96.-, B97.-)
    EXCLUDES 1   *ventilator lung in newborn (P27.8)*
    AHA: 2017,1Q,25
    CC Excl: PDX collection 757

  J95.859 Other complication of respirator [ventilator] `CC` `HCC`
    CC Excl: PDX collection 757

✓6th **J95.86 Postprocedural hematoma and seroma of a respiratory system organ or structure following a procedure**
    CC Excl: For CC codes in subcategory J95.86: PDX collection 758

  J95.860 Postprocedural hematoma of a respiratory system organ or structure following a respiratory system procedure `CC`

  J95.861 Postprocedural hematoma of a respiratory system organ or structure following other procedure `CC`

  J95.862 Postprocedural seroma of a respiratory system organ or structure following a respiratory system procedure `CC`

  J95.863 Postprocedural seroma of a respiratory system organ or structure following other procedure `CC`

J95.88 Other intraoperative complications of respiratory system, not elsewhere classified `CC`
  CC Excl: PDX collection 757

J95.89 Other postprocedural complications and disorders of respiratory system, not elsewhere classified `CC`
  Use additional code to identify disorder, such as:
    aspiration pneumonia (J69.-)
    bacterial or viral pneumonia (J12-J18)
    EXCLUDES 2   *acute pulmonary insufficiency following thoracic surgery (J95.1)*
          postprocedural subglottic stenosis (J95.5)
  CC Excl: PDX collection 757

Other diseases of the respiratory system (J96-J99)

✓4th **J96 Respiratory failure, not elsewhere classified**
  EXCLUDES 1   *acute respiratory distress syndrome (J80)*
    cardiorespiratory failure (R09.2)
    newborn respiratory distress syndrome (P22.0)
    postprocedural respiratory failure (J95.82-)
    respiratory arrest (R09.2)
    respiratory arrest of newborn (P28.81)
    respiratory failure of newborn (P28.5)
  CC Excl: For CC/MCC codes in category J96: PDX collection 744

✓5th **J96.0 Acute respiratory failure**

  J96.00 Acute respiratory failure, unspecified whether with hypoxia or hypercapnia `MCC` `HCC`
    AHA: 2016,3Q,14; 2013,4Q,121

  J96.01 Acute respiratory failure with hypoxia `MCC` `HCC`

  J96.02 Acute respiratory failure with hypercapnia `MCC` `HCC`

✓5th **J96.1 Chronic respiratory failure**

  J96.10 Chronic respiratory failure, unspecified whether with hypoxia or hypercapnia `CC` `HCC`
    AHA: 2016,1Q,38; 2015,1Q,21

  J96.11 Chronic respiratory failure with hypoxia `CC` `HCC`
    AHA: 2013,4Q,129

  J96.12 Chronic respiratory failure with hypercapnia `CC` `HCC`

✓5th **J96.2 Acute and chronic respiratory failure**
    Acute on chronic respiratory failure

  J96.20 Acute and chronic respiratory failure, unspecified whether with hypoxia or hypercapnia `MCC` `HCC`

  J96.21 Acute and chronic respiratory failure with hypoxia `MCC` `HCC`

  J96.22 Acute and chronic respiratory failure with hypercapnia `MCC` `HCC`

✓5th **J96.9 Respiratory failure, unspecified**

  J96.90 Respiratory failure, unspecified, unspecified whether with hypoxia or hypercapnia `MCC` `HCC`

  J96.91 Respiratory failure, unspecified with hypoxia `MCC` `HCC`

  J96.92 Respiratory failure, unspecified with hypercapnia `MCC` `HCC`

✓4ᵗʰ **J98 Other respiratory disorders**

Use additional code to identify:

exposure to environmental tobacco smoke (Z77.22)

exposure to tobacco smoke in the perinatal period (P96.81)

history of tobacco dependence (Z87.891)

occupational exposure to environmental tobacco smoke (Z57.31)

tobacco dependence (F17.-)

tobacco use (Z72.0)

> EXCLUDES 1   *newborn apnea (P28.4)*
> *newborn sleep apnea (P28.3)*
> EXCLUDES 2   *apnea NOS (R06.81)*
> *sleep apnea (G47.3-)*

✓5ᵗʰ **J98.0 Diseases of bronchus, not elsewhere classified**

J98.01 Acute bronchospasm   `CC`

> EXCLUDES 1   *acute bronchiolitis with bronchospasm (J21.-)*
> *acute bronchitis with bronchospasm (J20.-)*
> *asthma (J45.-)*
> *exercise induced bronchospasm (J45.990)*

J98.09 Other diseases of bronchus, not elsewhere classified

Broncholithiasis

Calcification of bronchus

Stenosis of bronchus

Tracheobronchial collapse

Tracheobronchial dyskinesia

Ulcer of bronchus

✓5ᵗʰ **J98.1 Pulmonary collapse**

> EXCLUDES 1   *therapeutic collapse of lung status (Z98.3)*

J98.11 Atelectasis   `CC`

> EXCLUDES 1   *newborn atelectasis*
> *tuberculous atelectasis (current disease) (A15)*

DEF: Collapse of lung tissue affecting part or all of one lung, preventing normal oxygen absorption to healthy tissues.

CC Excl: PDX collection 760

J98.19 Other pulmonary collapse   `CC`

CC Excl: PDX collection 760

J98.2 Interstitial emphysema   `HCC`

Mediastinal emphysema

> EXCLUDES 1   *emphysema NOS (J43.9)*
> *emphysema in newborn (P25.0)*
> *surgical emphysema (subcutaneous) (T81.82)*
> *traumatic subcutaneous emphysema (T79.7)*

J98.3 Compensatory emphysema   `HCC`

DEF: Distention of all or part of the lung caused by disease processes or surgical intervention that decreased volume in another part of the lung, causing an overcompensation reaction. Compensatory emphysema occurs in association with pneumonias, pleural effusions, atelectasis, empyema, and pneumothorax.

J98.4 Other disorders of lung

Calcification of lung

Cystic lung disease (acquired)

Lung disease NOS

Pulmolithiasis

> EXCLUDES 1   *acute interstitial pneumonitis (J84.114)*
> *pulmonary insufficiency following surgery (J95.1-J95.2)*

✓5ᵗʰ **J98.5 Diseases of mediastinum, not elsewhere classified**

> EXCLUDES 2   *abscess of mediastinum (J85.3)*

AHA: 2016,4Q,29

J98.51 Mediastinitis   `MCC` `H8`

Code first underlying condition, if applicable, such as postoperative mediastinitis (T81.-)

CC Excl: No Excl

J98.59 Other diseases of mediastinum, not elsewhere classified   `MCC` `H8`

Fibrosis of mediastinum

Hernia of mediastinum

Retraction of mediastinum

CC Excl: No Excl

J98.6 Disorders of diaphragm

Diaphragmatitis

Paralysis of diaphragm

Relaxation of diaphragm

> EXCLUDES 1   *congenital malformation of diaphragm NEC (Q79.1)*
> *congenital diaphragmatic hernia (Q79.0)*
> EXCLUDES 2   *diaphragmatic hernia (K44.-)*

J98.8 Other specified respiratory disorders

J98.9 Respiratory disorder, unspecified

Respiratory disease (chronic) NOS

J99   ***Respiratory disorders in diseases classified elsewhere***   `HCC`

Code first underlying disease, such as:

amyloidosis (E85.-)

ankylosing spondylitis (M45)

congenital syphilis (A50.5)

cryoglobulinemia (D89.1)

early congenital syphilis (A50.0)

plasminogen deficiency (E88.02)

schistosomiasis (B65.0-B65.9)

> EXCLUDES 1   *respiratory disorders in:*
> *amebiasis (A06.5)*
> *blastomycosis (B40.0-B40.2)*
> *candidiasis (B37.1)*
> *coccidioidomycosis (B38.0-B38.2)*
> *cystic fibrosis with pulmonary manifestations (E84.0)*
> *dermatomyositis (M33.01, M33.11)*
> *histoplasmosis (B39.0-B39.2)*
> *late syphilis (A52.72, A52.73)*
> *polymyositis (M33.21)*
> *sicca syndrome (M35.02)*
> *systemic lupus erythematosus (M32.13)*
> *systemic sclerosis (M34.81)*
> *Wegener's granulomatosis (M31.30-M31.31)*

✓ Additional Character Required   ✓x7ᵗʰ Placeholder   Unacceptable PDx   Questionable PDx   Manifestation   Unspecified Dx   `H1`-`H14` HAC   `HCC` CMS-HCC Dx   `HIV` HIV Dx

ICD-10-CM 2020   707

Chapter 11. Diseases of the Digestive System (KØØ–K95)

Chapter-specific Guidelines with Coding Examples
Reserved for future guideline expansion.

Chapter 11. Diseases of the Digestive System

Chapter 11. Diseases of the Digestive System (K00–K95)

> **EXCLUDES 2**   certain conditions originating in the perinatal period (P04–P96)
> certain infectious and parasitic diseases (A00–B99)
> complications of pregnancy, childbirth and the puerperium (O00–O9A)
> congenital malformations, deformations and chromosomal abnormalities (Q00–Q99)
> endocrine, nutritional and metabolic diseases (E00–E88)
> injury, poisoning and certain other consequences of external causes (S00–T88)
> neoplasms (C00–D49)
> symptoms, signs and abnormal clinical and laboratory findings, not elsewhere classified (R00–R94)

This chapter contains the following blocks:

K00–K14	Diseases of oral cavity and salivary glands
K20–K31	Diseases of esophagus, stomach and duodenum
K35–K38	Diseases of appendix
K40–K46	Hernia
K50–K52	Noninfective enteritis and colitis
K55–K64	Other diseases of intestines
K65–K68	Diseases of peritoneum and retroperitoneum
K70–K77	Diseases of liver
K80–K87	Disorders of gallbladder, biliary tract and pancreas
K90–K95	Other diseases of the digestive system

Diseases of oral cavity and salivary glands (K00–K14)

✓4ᵗʰ K00   Disorders of tooth development and eruption

> **EXCLUDES 2**   embedded and impacted teeth (K01.-)

K00.0   Anodontia
Hypodontia
Oligodontia
> **EXCLUDES 1**   acquired absence of teeth (K08.1-)

DEF: Partial or complete absence of teeth due to a congenital defect involving the tooth bud.

K00.1   Supernumerary teeth
Distomolar
Fourth molar
Mesiodens
Paramolar
Supplementary teeth
> **EXCLUDES 2**   supernumerary roots (K00.2)

K00.2   Abnormalities of size and form of teeth
Concrescence of teeth
Dens evaginatus
Dens in dente
Dens invaginatus
Enamel pearls
Fusion of teeth
Gemination of teeth
Macrodontia
Microdontia
Peg-shaped [conical] teeth
Supernumerary roots
Taurodontism
Tuberculum paramolare
> **EXCLUDES 1**   abnormalities of teeth due to congenital syphilis (A50.5)
> tuberculum Carabelli, which is regarded as a normal variation and should not be coded

K00.3   Mottled teeth
Dental fluorosis
Mottling of enamel
Nonfluoride enamel opacities
> **EXCLUDES 2**   deposits [accretions] on teeth (K03.6)

K00.4   Disturbances in tooth formation
Aplasia and hypoplasia of cementum
Dilaceration of tooth
Enamel hypoplasia (neonatal) (postnatal) (prenatal)
Regional odontodysplasia
Turner's tooth
> **EXCLUDES 1**   Hutchinson's teeth and mulberry molars in congenital syphilis (A50.5)
> **EXCLUDES 2**   mottled teeth (K00.3)

K00.5   Hereditary disturbances in tooth structure, not elsewhere classified
Amelogenesis imperfecta
Dentinogenesis imperfecta
Odontogenesis imperfecta
Dentinal dysplasia
Shell teeth

K00.6   Disturbances in tooth eruption
Dentia praecox
Natal tooth
Neonatal tooth
Premature eruption of tooth
Premature shedding of primary [deciduous] tooth
Prenatal teeth
Retained [persistent] primary tooth
> **EXCLUDES 2**   embedded and impacted teeth (K01.-)

K00.7   Teething syndrome

K00.8   Other disorders of tooth development
Color changes during tooth formation
Intrinsic staining of teeth NOS
> **EXCLUDES 2**   posteruptive color changes (K03.7)

K00.9   Disorder of tooth development, unspecified
Disorder of odontogenesis NOS

✓4ᵗʰ K01   Embedded and impacted teeth
> **EXCLUDES 1**   abnormal position of fully erupted teeth (M26.3-)

K01.0   Embedded teeth

K01.1   Impacted teeth

✓4ᵗʰ K02   Dental caries
> **INCLUDES**   caries of dentine
> dental cavities
> early childhood caries
> pre-eruptive caries
> recurrent caries (dentino enamel junction) (enamel) (to the pulp)
> tooth decay

DEF: Localized section of tooth decay that begins on the tooth surface with destruction of the calcified enamel, allowing bacterial destruction to continue and form cavities and may extend to the dentin and pulp.

Tooth Anatomy

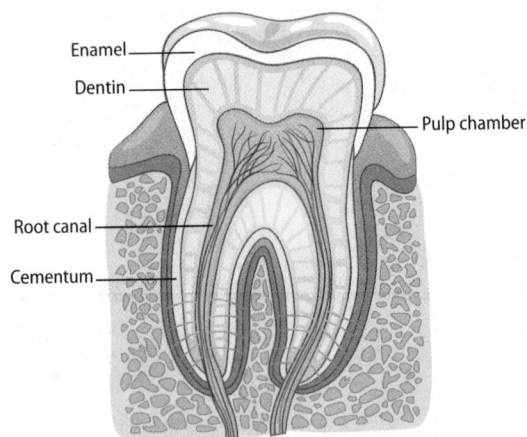

Enamel
Dentin
Pulp chamber
Root canal
Cementum

K02.3   Arrested dental caries
Arrested coronal and root caries

✓5ᵗʰ K02.5   Dental caries on pit and fissure surface
Dental caries on chewing surface of tooth

K02.51   Dental caries on pit and fissure surface limited to enamel
White spot lesions [initial caries] on pit and fissure surface of tooth

K02.52   Dental caries on pit and fissure surface penetrating into dentin
Primary dental caries, cervical origin

K02.53   Dental caries on pit and fissure surface penetrating into pulp

√5ᵗʰ **K02.6 Dental caries on** smooth surface

    K02.61 Dental caries on smooth surface limited to enamel
        White spot lesions [initial caries] on smooth surface of tooth

    K02.62 Dental caries on smooth surface penetrating into dentin

    K02.63 Dental caries on smooth surface penetrating into pulp

    K02.7 Dental root **caries**

    K02.9 Dental caries, unspecified

√4ᵗʰ **K03 Other diseases of hard tissues of teeth**

    EXCLUDES 2   bruxism (F45.8)
            dental caries (K02.-)
            teeth-grinding NOS (F45.8)

    K03.0 Excessive attrition of teeth
        Approximal wear of teeth
        Occlusal wear of teeth
        DEF: Attrition: In dentistry, wearing away or erosion of tooth surface from abrasive food or grinding teeth.

    K03.1 Abrasion of teeth
        Dentifrice abrasion of teeth
        Habitual abrasion of teeth
        Occupational abrasion of teeth
        Ritual abrasion of teeth
        Traditional abrasion of teeth
        Wedge defect NOS

    K03.2 Erosion of teeth
        Erosion of teeth due to diet
        Erosion of teeth due to drugs and medicaments
        Erosion of teeth due to persistent vomiting
        Erosion of teeth NOS
        Idiopathic erosion of teeth
        Occupational erosion of teeth

    K03.3 Pathological resorption of teeth
        Internal granuloma of pulp
        Resorption of teeth (external)

    K03.4 Hypercementosis
        Cementation hyperplasia

    K03.5 Ankylosis of teeth

    K03.6 Deposits [accretions] on teeth
        Betel deposits [accretions] on teeth
        Black deposits [accretions] on teeth
        Extrinsic staining of teeth NOS
        Green deposits [accretions] on teeth
        Materia alba deposits [accretions] on teeth
        Orange deposits [accretions] on teeth
        Staining of teeth NOS
        Subgingival dental calculus
        Supragingival dental calculus
        Tobacco deposits [accretions] on teeth

    K03.7 Posteruptive color changes of dental hard tissues
        EXCLUDES 2   deposits [accretions] on teeth (K03.6)

√5ᵗʰ   **K03.8 Other specified diseases of hard tissues of teeth**

    K03.81 Cracked tooth
        EXCLUDES 1   asymptomatic craze lines in enamel - omit code
                broken or fractured tooth due to trauma (S02.5)

    K03.89 Other specified diseases of hard tissues of teeth

    K03.9 Disease of hard tissues of teeth, unspecified

√4ᵗʰ **K04 Diseases of pulp and periapical tissues**
    AHA: 2016,4Q,29-30

√5ᵗʰ   **K04.0 Pulpitis**
        Acute pulpitis
        Chronic (hyperplastic) (ulcerative) pulpitis

    K04.01 Reversible pulpitis

    K04.02 Irreversible pulpitis   CC
        CC Excl: PDX collection 761

    K04.1 Necrosis of pulp
        Pulpal gangrene

    K04.2 Pulp degeneration
        Denticles
        Pulpal calcifications
        Pulpal stones

    K04.3 Abnormal hard tissue formation in pulp
        Secondary or irregular dentine

    K04.4 Acute apical periodontitis of pulpal origin
        Acute apical periodontitis NOS
        EXCLUDES 1   acute periodontitis (K05.2-)
        DEF: Severe inflammation of the area surrounding the tip of a tooth's root that is often secondary to infection or trauma.

    K04.5 Chronic apical periodontitis
        Apical or periapical granuloma
        Apical periodontitis NOS
        EXCLUDES 1   chronic periodontitis (K05.3-)

    K04.6 Periapical abscess with sinus   SW
        Dental abscess with sinus
        Dentoalveolar abscess with sinus

    K04.7 Periapical abscess without sinus
        Dental abscess without sinus
        Dentoalveolar abscess without sinus

    K04.8 Radicular cyst
        Apical (periodontal) cyst
        Periapical cyst
        Residual radicular cyst
        EXCLUDES 2   lateral periodontal cyst (K09.0)
        DEF: Most common odontogenic cyst in tissue around the tooth apex due to chronic inflammation of dental pulp.

√5ᵗʰ   **K04.9 Other and unspecified diseases of pulp and periapical tissues**

    K04.90 Unspecified diseases of pulp and periapical tissues

    K04.99 Other diseases of pulp and periapical tissues

√4ᵗʰ **K05 Gingivitis and periodontal diseases**
    Use additional code to identify:
        alcohol abuse and dependence (F10.-)
        exposure to environmental tobacco smoke (Z77.22)
        exposure to tobacco smoke in the perinatal period (P96.81)
        history of tobacco dependence (Z87.891)
        occupational exposure to environmental tobacco smoke (Z57.31)
        tobacco dependence (F17.-)
        tobacco use (Z72.0)
    AHA: 2016,4Q,29-30

√5ᵗʰ   **K05.0 Acute gingivitis**
        EXCLUDES 1   acute necrotizing ulcerative gingivitis (A69.1)
                herpesviral [herpes simplex] gingivostomatitis (B00.2)

    K05.00 Acute gingivitis, plaque induced
        Acute gingivitis NOS
        Plaque induced gingival disease

    K05.01 Acute gingivitis, non-plaque induced

√5ᵗʰ   **K05.1 Chronic gingivitis**
        Desquamative gingivitis (chronic)
        Gingivitis (chronic) NOS
        Hyperplastic gingivitis (chronic)
        Pregnancy associated gingivitis
        Simple marginal gingivitis (chronic)
        Ulcerative gingivitis (chronic)
        Code first, if applicable, diseases of the digestive system complicating pregnacy (O99.61-)

    K05.10 Chronic gingivitis, plaque induced
        Chronic gingivitis NOS
        Gingivitis NOS

    K05.11 Chronic gingivitis, non-plaque induced

√5ᵗʰ   **K05.2 Aggressive periodontitis**
        Acute pericoronitis
        EXCLUDES 1   acute apical periodontitis (K04.4)
                periapical abscess (K04.7)
                periapical abscess with sinus (K04.6)

    K05.20 Aggressive periodontitis, unspecified

√6ᵗʰ   **K05.21 Aggressive periodontitis,** localized
        Periodontal abscess

    K05.211 Aggressive periodontitis, localized, slight

    K05.212 Aggressive periodontitis, localized, moderate

    K05.213 Aggressive periodontitis, localized, severe

    K05.219 Aggressive periodontitis, localized, unspecified severity

√6ᵗʰ   **K05.22 Aggressive periodontitis,** generalized

    K05.221 Aggressive periodontitis, generalized, slight

✔ Additional Character Required   √x7ᵗʰ Placeholder   Unacceptable PDx   Questionable PDx   Manifestation   Unspecified Dx   H1-H14 HAC   HCC CMS-HCC Dx   HIV HIV Dx

ICD-10-CM 2020   711

Chapter 11. Diseases of the Digestive System

K05.222 Aggressive periodontitis, generalized, moderate

K05.223 Aggressive periodontitis, generalized, severe

K05.229 Aggressive periodontitis, generalized, unspecified severity

√5th **K05.3 Chronic periodontitis**
Chronic pericoronitis
Complex periodontitis
Periodontitis NOS
Simplex periodontitis
EXCLUDES 1 *chronic apical periodontitis (K04.5)*

K05.30 Chronic periodontitis, unspecified

√6th **K05.31** Chronic periodontitis, localized

K05.311 Chronic periodontitis, localized, slight
K05.312 Chronic periodontitis, localized, moderate
K05.313 Chronic periodontitis, localized, severe
K05.319 Chronic periodontitis, localized, unspecified severity

√6th **K05.32** Chronic periodontitis, generalized

K05.321 Chronic periodontitis, generalized, slight
K05.322 Chronic periodontitis, generalized, moderate
K05.323 Chronic periodontitis, generalized, severe
K05.329 Chronic periodontitis, generalized, unspecified

K05.4 Periodontosis
Juvenile periodontosis

K05.5 Other periodontal diseases
Combined periodontic-endodontic lesion
Narrow gingival width (of periodontal soft tissue)
EXCLUDES 2 *leukoplakia of gingiva (K13.21)*

K05.6 Periodontal disease, unspecified

√4th **K06 Other disorders of gingiva and edentulous alveolar ridge**
EXCLUDES 2 *acute gingivitis (K05.0)*
atrophy of edentulous alveolar ridge (K08.2)
chronic gingivitis (K05.1)
gingivitis NOS (K05.1)
AHA: 2016,4Q,29-30

√5th **K06.0 Gingival recession**
Gingival recession (postinfective) (postprocedural)
AHA: 2017,4Q,16

√6th **K06.01** Gingival recession, localized

K06.010 Localized gingival recession, unspecified
Localized gingival recession, NOS
K06.011 Localized gingival recession, minimal
K06.012 Localized gingival recession, moderate
K06.013 Localized gingival recession, severe

√6th **K06.02** Gingival recession, generalized

K06.020 Generalized gingival recession, unspecified
Generalized gingival recession, NOS
K06.021 Generalized gingival recession, minimal
K06.022 Generalized gingival recession, moderate
K06.023 Generalized gingival recession, severe

K06.1 Gingival enlargement
Gingival fibromatosis

K06.2 Gingival and edentulous alveolar ridge lesions associated with trauma
Irritative hyperplasia of edentulous ridge [denture hyperplasia]
Use additional code (Chapter 20) to identify external cause or denture status (Z97.2)

K06.3 Horizontal alveolar bone loss

K06.8 Other specified disorders of gingiva and edentulous alveolar ridge
Fibrous epulis
Flabby alveolar ridge
Giant cell epulis
Peripheral giant cell granuloma of gingiva
Pyogenic granuloma of gingiva
Vertical ridge deficiency
EXCLUDES 2 *gingival cyst (K09.0)*

K06.9 Disorder of gingiva and edentulous alveolar ridge, unspecified

√4th **K08 Other disorders of teeth and supporting structures**
EXCLUDES 2 *dentofacial anomalies [including malocclusion] (M26.-)*
disorders of jaw (M27.-)
AHA: 2016,4Q,29-30

K08.0 Exfoliation of teeth due to systemic causes
Code also underlying systemic condition

√5th **K08.1 Complete loss of teeth**
Acquired loss of teeth, complete
EXCLUDES 1 *congenital absence of teeth (K00.0)*
exfoliation of teeth due to systemic causes (K08.0)
partial loss of teeth (K08.4-)
DEF: Loss of all teeth as a result of caries, trauma, extraction, periodontal disease, or other specified or unspecified causes.
Synonym(s): complete edentulism

√6th **K08.10** Complete loss of teeth, unspecified cause

K08.101 Complete loss of teeth, unspecified cause, class I
K08.102 Complete loss of teeth, unspecified cause, class II
K08.103 Complete loss of teeth, unspecified cause, class III
K08.104 Complete loss of teeth, unspecified cause, class IV
K08.109 Complete loss of teeth, unspecified cause, unspecified class
Edentulism NOS

√6th **K08.11** Complete loss of teeth due to trauma

K08.111 Complete loss of teeth due to trauma, class I
K08.112 Complete loss of teeth due to trauma, class II
K08.113 Complete loss of teeth due to trauma, class III
K08.114 Complete loss of teeth due to trauma, class IV
K08.119 Complete loss of teeth due to trauma, unspecified class

√6th **K08.12** Complete loss of teeth due to periodontal diseases

K08.121 Complete loss of teeth due to periodontal diseases, class I
K08.122 Complete loss of teeth due to periodontal diseases, class II
K08.123 Complete loss of teeth due to periodontal diseases, class III
K08.124 Complete loss of teeth due to periodontal diseases, class IV
K08.129 Complete loss of teeth due to periodontal diseases, unspecified class

√6th **K08.13** Complete loss of teeth due to caries

K08.131 Complete loss of teeth due to caries, class I
K08.132 Complete loss of teeth due to caries, class II
K08.133 Complete loss of teeth due to caries, class III
K08.134 Complete loss of teeth due to caries, class IV
K08.139 Complete loss of teeth due to caries, unspecified class

√6th **K08.19** Complete loss of teeth due to other specified cause

K08.191 Complete loss of teeth due to other specified cause, class I
K08.192 Complete loss of teeth due to other specified cause, class II
K08.193 Complete loss of teeth due to other specified cause, class III
K08.194 Complete loss of teeth due to other specified cause, class IV
K08.199 Complete loss of teeth due to other specified cause, unspecified class

√5th **K08.2 Atrophy of edentulous alveolar ridge**

K08.20 Unspecified atrophy of edentulous alveolar ridge
Atrophy of the mandible NOS
Atrophy of the maxilla NOS
K08.21 Minimal atrophy of the mandible
Minimal atrophy of the edentulous mandible
K08.22 Moderate atrophy of the mandible
Moderate atrophy of the edentulous mandible

K08.23　Severe **atrophy of the** mandible
　　　　Severe atrophy of the edentulous mandible

K08.24　Minimal **atrophy of** maxilla
　　　　Minimal atrophy of the edentulous maxilla

K08.25　Moderate **atrophy of the** maxilla
　　　　Moderate atrophy of the edentulous maxilla

K08.26　Severe **atrophy of the** maxilla
　　　　Severe atrophy of the edentulous maxilla

K08.3　**Retained dental root**

✓5th K08.4　**Partial loss of teeth**
　　　Acquired loss of teeth, partial
　　　EXCLUDES 1　*complete loss of teeth (K08.1-)*
　　　　　　　　congenital absence of teeth (K00.0)
　　　EXCLUDES 2　*exfoliation of teeth due to systemic causes (K08.0)*

　✓6th K08.40　**Partial loss of teeth, unspecified cause**
　　　K08.401　**Partial loss of teeth, unspecified cause,** class I
　　　K08.402　**Partial loss of teeth, unspecified cause,** class II
　　　K08.403　**Partial loss of teeth, unspecified cause,** class III
　　　K08.404　**Partial loss of teeth, unspecified cause,** class IV
　　　K08.409　**Partial loss of teeth, unspecified cause, unspecified class**
　　　　　　　Tooth extraction status NOS

　✓6th K08.41　**Partial loss of teeth due to** trauma
　　　K08.411　**Partial loss of teeth due to trauma,** class I
　　　K08.412　**Partial loss of teeth due to trauma,** class II
　　　K08.413　**Partial loss of teeth due to trauma,** class III
　　　K08.414　**Partial loss of teeth due to trauma,** class IV
　　　K08.419　**Partial loss of teeth due to trauma, unspecified class**

　✓6th K08.42　**Partial loss of teeth due to** periodontal diseases
　　　K08.421　**Partial loss of teeth due to periodontal diseases,** class I
　　　K08.422　**Partial loss of teeth due to periodontal diseases,** class II
　　　K08.423　**Partial loss of teeth due to periodontal diseases,** class III
　　　K08.424　**Partial loss of teeth due to periodontal diseases,** class IV
　　　K08.429　**Partial loss of teeth due to periodontal diseases, unspecified class**

　✓6th K08.43　**Partial loss of teeth due to** caries
　　　K08.431　**Partial loss of teeth due to caries,** class I
　　　K08.432　**Partial loss of teeth due to caries,** class II
　　　K08.433　**Partial loss of teeth due to caries,** class III
　　　K08.434　**Partial loss of teeth due to caries,** class IV
　　　K08.439　**Partial loss of teeth due to caries, unspecified class**

　✓6th K08.49　**Partial loss of teeth due to other specified cause**
　　　K08.491　**Partial loss of teeth due to other specified cause,** class I
　　　K08.492　**Partial loss of teeth due to other specified cause,** class II
　　　K08.493　**Partial loss of teeth due to other specified cause,** class III
　　　K08.494　**Partial loss of teeth due to other specified cause,** class IV
　　　K08.499　**Partial loss of teeth due to other specified cause, unspecified class**

✓5th K08.5　**Unsatisfactory restoration of tooth**
　　　Defective bridge, crown, filling
　　　Defective dental restoration
　　　EXCLUDES 1　*dental restoration status (Z98.811)*
　　　EXCLUDES 2　*endosseous dental implant failure (M27.6-)*
　　　　　　　　unsatisfactory endodontic treatment (M27.5-)

　K08.50　**Unsatisfactory restoration of tooth, unspecified**
　　　Defective dental restoration NOS

　K08.51　**Open restoration margins of tooth**
　　　Dental restoration failure of marginal integrity
　　　Open margin on tooth restoration
　　　Poor gingival margin to tooth restoration

K08.52　**Unrepairable overhanging of dental restorative materials**
　　　Overhanging of tooth restoration

✓6th K08.53　**Fractured dental restorative material**
　　　EXCLUDES 1　*cracked tooth (K03.81)*
　　　　　　　　traumatic fracture of tooth (S02.5)
　　　K08.530　**Fractured dental restorative material** without loss of material
　　　K08.531　**Fractured dental restorative material** with loss of material
　　　K08.539　**Fractured dental restorative material, unspecified**

K08.54　**Contour of existing restoration of tooth biologically incompatible with oral health**
　　　Dental restoration failure of periodontal anatomical integrity
　　　Unacceptable contours of existing restoration of tooth
　　　Unacceptable morphology of existing restoration of tooth

K08.55　**Allergy to existing dental restorative material**
　　　Use additional code to identify the specific type of allergy

K08.56　**Poor aesthetic of existing restoration of tooth**
　　　Dental restoration aesthetically inadequate or displeasing

K08.59　**Other unsatisfactory restoration of tooth**
　　　Other defective dental restoration

✓5th K08.8　**Other specified disorders of teeth and supporting structures**
　　　K08.81　**Primary occlusal trauma**
　　　K08.82　**Secondary occlusal trauma**
　　　K08.89　**Other specified disorders of teeth and supporting structures**
　　　　　　Enlargement of alveolar ridge NOS
　　　　　　Insufficient anatomic crown height
　　　　　　Insufficient clinical crown length
　　　　　　Irregular alveolar process
　　　　　　Toothache NOS

K08.9　**Disorder of teeth and supporting structures, unspecified**

✓4th **K09　Cysts of oral region, not elsewhere classified**
　　INCLUDES　lesions showing histological features both of aneurysmal cyst and of another fibro-osseous lesion
　　EXCLUDES 2　*cysts of jaw (M27.0-, M27.4-)*
　　　　　　　radicular cyst (K04.8)

K09.0　Developmental odontogenic **cysts**
　　　Dentigerous cyst
　　　Eruption cyst
　　　Follicular cyst
　　　Gingival cyst
　　　Lateral periodontal cyst
　　　Primordial cyst
　　　EXCLUDES 2　*keratocysts (D16.4, D16.5)*
　　　　　　　odontogenic keratocystic tumors (D16.4, D16.5)

K09.1　Developmental (nonodontogenic) **cysts of oral region**
　　　Cyst (of) incisive canal
　　　Cyst (of) palatine of papilla
　　　Globulomaxillary cyst
　　　Median palatal cyst
　　　Nasoalveolar cyst
　　　Nasolabial cyst
　　　Nasopalatine duct cyst

K09.8　**Other cysts of oral region, not elsewhere classified**
　　　Dermoid cyst
　　　Epidermoid cyst
　　　Lymphoepithelial cyst
　　　Epstein's pearl

K09.9　**Cyst of oral region, unspecified**

✓4th **K11　Diseases of salivary glands**
　　Use additional code to identify:
　　alcohol abuse and dependence (F10.-)
　　exposure to environmental tobacco smoke (Z77.22)
　　exposure to tobacco smoke in the perinatal period (P96.81)
　　history of tobacco dependence (Z87.891)
　　occupational exposure to environmental tobacco smoke (Z57.31)
　　tobacco dependence (F17.-)
　　tobacco use (Z72.0)

K11.0　**Atrophy of salivary gland**

☑ Additional Character Required　✓x7th Placeholder　Unacceptable PDx　Questionable PDx　Manifestation　Unspecified Dx　H1-H14 HAC　HCC CMS-HCC Dx　HIV HIV Dx

ICD-10-CM 2020

713

Chapter 11. Diseases of the Digestive System

K11.1   **Hypertrophy of salivary gland**
DEF: Overgrowth of or enlarged salivary gland tissue caused by infection, salivary duct blockage, autoimmune diseases, and benign and malignant tumors.

√5ᵗʰ **K11.2**   **Sialoadenitis**
Parotitis
EXCLUDES 1   epidemic parotitis (B26.-)
mumps (B26.-)
uveoparotid fever [Heerfordt] (D86.89)
DEF: Inflammation of the salivary gland.

    K11.20   **Sialoadenitis, unspecified**
    K11.21   **Acute sialoadenitis**
         EXCLUDES 1   acute recurrent sialoadenitis (K11.22)
    K11.22   **Acute recurrent sialoadenitis**
    K11.23   **Chronic sialoadenitis**

K11.3   **Abscess of salivary gland**

K11.4   **Fistula of salivary gland**   SW
      EXCLUDES 1   congenital fistula of salivary gland (Q38.4)

K11.5   **Sialolithiasis**
Calculus of salivary gland or duct
Stone of salivary gland or duct

K11.6   **Mucocele of salivary gland**
Mucous extravasation cyst of salivary gland
Mucous retention cyst of salivary gland
Ranula

K11.7   **Disturbances of salivary secretion**
Hypoptyalism
Ptyalism
Xerostomia
      EXCLUDES 2   dry mouth NOS (R68.2)

K11.8   **Other diseases of salivary glands**
Benign lymphoepithelial lesion of salivary gland
Mikulicz' disease
Necrotizing sialometaplasia
Sialectasia
Stenosis of salivary duct
Stricture of salivary duct
      EXCLUDES 1   sicca syndrome [Sjögren] (M35.0-)

    K11.9   **Disease of salivary gland, unspecified**
Sialoadenopathy NOS

√4ᵗʰ **K12**   **Stomatitis and related lesions**
Use additional code to identify:
alcohol abuse and dependence (F10.-)
exposure to environmental tobacco smoke (Z77.22)
exposure to tobacco smoke in the perinatal period (P96.81)
history of tobacco dependence (Z87.891)
occupational exposure to environmental tobacco smoke (Z57.31)
tobacco dependence (F17.-)
tobacco use (Z72.0)
      EXCLUDES 1   cancrum oris (A69.0)
cheilitis (K13.0)
gangrenous stomatitis (A69.0)
herpesviral [herpes simplex] gingivostomatitis (B00.2)
noma (A69.0)

    K12.0   **Recurrent oral aphthae**
Aphthous stomatitis (major) (minor)
Bednar's aphthae
Periadenitis mucosa necrotica recurrens
Recurrent aphthous ulcer
Stomatitis herpetiformis
DEF: Disorder of unknown etiology with small oval or round painful ulcers of the mouth marked by a grayish exudate and a red halo effect.

    K12.1   **Other forms of stomatitis**
Stomatitis NOS
Denture stomatitis
Ulcerative stomatitis
Vesicular stomatitis
      EXCLUDES 1   acute necrotizing ulcerative stomatitis (A69.1)
Vincent's stomatitis (A69.1)

    K12.2   **Cellulitis and abscess of mouth**   CC
Cellulitis of mouth (floor)
Submandibular abscess
      EXCLUDES 2   abscess of salivary gland (K11.3)
abscess of tongue (K14.0)
periapical abscess (K04.6-K04.7)
periodontal abscess (K05.21)
peritonsillar abscess (J36)
CC Excl: PDX collection 763

√5ᵗʰ **K12.3**   **Oral mucositis (ulcerative)**
Mucositis (oral) (oropharyneal)
      EXCLUDES 2   gastrointestinal mucositis (ulcerative) (K92.81)
mucositis (ulcerative) of vagina and vulva (N76.81)
nasal mucositis (ulcerative) (J34.81)

    K12.30   **Oral mucositis (ulcerative), unspecified**
    K12.31   **Oral mucositis (ulcerative) due to antineoplastic therapy**
Use additional code for adverse effect, if applicable, to identify antineoplastic and immunosuppressive drugs (T45.1X5)
Use additional code for other antineoplastic therapy, such as:
radiological procedure and radiotherapy (Y84.2)
    K12.32   **Oral mucositis (ulcerative) due to other drugs**
Use additional code for adverse effect, if applicable, to identify drug (T36-T50 with fifth or sixth character 5)
    K12.33   **Oral mucositis (ulcerative) due to radiation**
Use additional external cause code (W88-W90, X39.0-) to identify cause
    K12.39   **Other oral mucositis (ulcerative)**
Viral oral mucositis (ulcerative)

√4ᵗʰ **K13**   **Other diseases of lip and oral mucosa**
INCLUDES   epithelial disturbances of tongue
Use additional code to identify:
alcohol abuse and dependence (F10.-)
exposure to environmental tobacco smoke (Z77.22)
exposure to tobacco smoke in the perinatal period (P96.81)
history of tobacco dependence (Z87.891)
occupational exposure to environmental tobacco smoke (Z57.31)
tobacco dependence (F17.-)
tobacco use (Z72.0)
      EXCLUDES 2   certain disorders of gingiva and edentulous alveolar ridge (K05-K06)
cysts of oral region (K09.-)
diseases of tongue (K14.-)
stomatitis and related lesions (K12.-)

    K13.0   **Diseases of lips**
Abscess of lips
Angular cheilitis
Cellulitis of lips
Cheilitis NOS
Cheilodynia
Cheilosis
Exfoliative cheilitis
Fistula of lips
Glandular cheilitis
Hypertrophy of lips
Perlèche NEC
      EXCLUDES 1   ariboflavinosis (E53.0)
cheilitis due to radiation-related disorders (L55-L59)
congenital fistula of lips (Q38.0)
congenital hypertrophy of lips (Q18.6)
perlèche due to candidiasis (B37.83)
perlèche due to riboflavin deficiency (E53.0)

    K13.1   **Cheek and lip biting**

✓5ᵗʰ **K13.2** **Leukoplakia and other disturbances of oral epithelium, including tongue**

> EXCLUDES 1   *carcinoma in situ of oral epithelium (D00.0-)*
>   *hairy leukoplakia (K13.3)*
>
> **DEF:** Leukoplakia: Thickened white patches or lesions appearing on a mucous membrane, such as oral mucosa or tongue.

     K13.21 **Leukoplakia of oral mucosa, including tongue**
         Leukokeratosis of oral mucosa
         Leukoplakia of gingiva, lips, tongue
>   EXCLUDES 1   *hairy leukoplakia (K13.3)*
>   *leukokeratosis nicotina palati (K13.24)*

     K13.22 **Minimal keratinized residual ridge mucosa**
         Minimal keratinization of alveolar ridge mucosa

     K13.23 **Excessive keratinized residual ridge mucosa**
         Excessive keratinization of alveolar ridge mucosa

     K13.24 **Leukokeratosis nicotina palati**
         Smoker's palate

     K13.29 **Other disturbances of oral epithelium, including tongue**
         Erythroplakia of mouth or tongue
         Focal epithelial hyperplasia of mouth or tongue
         Leukoedema of mouth or tongue
         Other oral epithelium disturbances

K13.3 **Hairy leukoplakia**

K13.4 **Granuloma and granuloma-like lesions of oral mucosa**
     Eosinophilic granuloma
     Granuloma pyogenicum
     Verrucous xanthoma

K13.5 **Oral submucous fibrosis**
     Submucous fibrosis of tongue

K13.6 **Irritative hyperplasia of oral mucosa**
>   EXCLUDES 2   *irritative hyperplasia of edentulous ridge [denture hyperplasia] (K06.2)*

✓5ᵗʰ **K13.7** **Other and unspecified lesions of oral mucosa**

     K13.70 **Unspecified lesions of oral mucosa**
     K13.79 **Other lesions of oral mucosa**
         Focal oral mucinosis

✓4ᵗʰ **K14** **Diseases of tongue**
     Use additional code to identify:
     alcohol abuse and dependence (F10.-)
     exposure to environmental tobacco smoke (Z77.22)
     history of tobacco dependence (Z87.891)
     occupational exposure to environmental tobacco smoke (Z57.31)
     tobacco dependence (F17.-)
     tobacco use (Z72.0)
>   EXCLUDES 2   *erythroplakia (K13.29)*
>   *focal epithelial hyperplasia (K13.29)*
>   *leukedema of tongue (K13.29)*
>   *leukoplakia of tongue (K13.21)*
>   *hairy leukoplakia (K13.3)*
>   *macroglossia (congenital) (Q38.2)*
>   *submucous fibrosis of tongue (K13.5)*

K14.0 **Glossitis**
     Abscess of tongue
     Ulceration (traumatic) of tongue
>   EXCLUDES 1   *atrophic glossitis (K14.4)*
>
> **DEF:** Inflammation and swelling of the tongue that may be associated with infection, adverse drug reactions, smoking, or injury.

K14.1 **Geographic tongue**
     Benign migratory glossitis
     Glossitis areata exfoliativa

K14.2 **Median rhomboid glossitis**

K14.3 **Hypertrophy of tongue papillae**
     Black hairy tongue
     Coated tongue
     Hypertrophy of foliate papillae
     Lingua villosa nigra

K14.4 **Atrophy of tongue papillae**
     Atrophic glossitis

K14.5 **Plicated tongue**
     Fissured tongue
     Furrowed tongue
     Scrotal tongue
>   EXCLUDES 1   *fissured tongue, congenital (Q38.3)*

K14.6 **Glossodynia**
     Glossopyrosis
     Painful tongue

K14.8 **Other diseases of tongue**
     Atrophy of tongue
     Crenated tongue
     Enlargement of tongue
     Glossocele
     Glossoptosis
     Hypertrophy of tongue

K14.9 **Disease of tongue, unspecified**
     Glossopathy NOS

Diseases of esophagus, stomach and duodenum (K20-K31)

> EXCLUDES 2   *hiatus hernia (K44.-)*

✓4ᵗʰ **K20** **Esophagitis**
     Use additional code to identify:
     alcohol abuse and dependence (F10.-)
>   EXCLUDES 1   *erosion of esophagus (K22.1-)*
>   *esophagitis with gastro-esophageal reflux disease (K21.0)*
>   *reflux esophagitis (K21.0)*
>   *ulcerative esophagitis (K22.1-)*
>   EXCLUDES 2   *eosinophilic gastritis or gastroenteritis (K52.81)*

K20.0 **Eosinophilic esophagitis**

K20.8 **Other esophagitis**
     Abscess of esophagus

K20.9 **Esophagitis, unspecified**
     Esophagitis NOS

✓4ᵗʰ **K21** **Gastro-esophageal reflux disease**
>   EXCLUDES 1   *newborn esophageal reflux (P78.83)*

K21.0 **Gastro-esophageal reflux disease with esophagitis**
     Reflux esophagitis

K21.9 **Gastro-esophageal reflux disease without esophagitis**
     Esophageal reflux NOS
     AHA: 2016,1Q,18

✓4ᵗʰ **K22** **Other diseases of esophagus**
>   EXCLUDES 2   *esophageal varices (I85.-)*

K22.0 **Achalasia of cardia**
     Achalasia NOS
     Cardiospasm
>   EXCLUDES 1   *congenital cardiospasm (Q39.5)*
>
> **DEF:** Esophageal motility disorder that is caused by absence of the esophageal peristalsis and impaired relaxation of the lower esophageal sphincter. It is characterized by dysphagia, regurgitation, and heartburn.

✓5ᵗʰ **K22.1** **Ulcer of esophagus**
     Barrett's ulcer
     Erosion of esophagus
     Fungal ulcer of esophagus
     Peptic ulcer of esophagus
     Ulcer of esophagus due to ingestion of chemicals
     Ulcer of esophagus due to ingestion of drugs and medicaments
     Ulcerative esophagitis
     Code first poisoning due to drug or toxin, if applicable (T36-T65 with fifth or sixth character 1-4 or 6)
     Use additional code for adverse effect, if applicable, to identify drug (T36-T50 with fifth or sixth character 5)
>   EXCLUDES 1   *Barrett's esophagus (K22.7-)*
>
> **AHA:** 2018,3Q,22; 2017,3Q,27
>
> **TIP:** Assign a code for "with bleeding" when an esophageal ulcer and bleeding (hematemesis) are documented. The ICD-10-CM classification assumes the two are related without the provider linking the two conditions. Evidence of bleeding during a procedure is not required.
>
> **TIP:** For bleeding ulcers resulting from anticoagulant therapy, code D68.32 Hemorrhagic disorder due to extrinsic circulating anticoagulant, and an adverse-effect code from subcategory T45.5- should also be assigned. Either the bleeding ulcer code or code D68.32 may be sequenced first, depending on the circumstances of admission.

     K22.10 **Ulcer of esophagus without bleeding**   CC
         Ulcer of esophagus NOS
         CC Excl: PDX collection 764

✓ Additional Character Required   ✓x7ᵗʰ Placeholder   Unacceptable PDx   Questionable PDx   Manifestation   Unspecified Dx   H1-H14 HAC   HCC CMS-HCC Dx   HIV HIV Dx

ICD-10-CM 2020

715

K13.2–K22.10

Chapter 11. Diseases of the Digestive System

Chapter 11. Diseases of the Digestive System

K22.11   **Ulcer of esophagus** with bleeding   MCC

> EXCLUDES 2   bleeding esophageal varices (I85.Ø1, I85.11)

CC Excl: PDX collection 765

K22.2   **Esophageal obstruction**

Compression of esophagus
Constriction of esophagus
Stenosis of esophagus
Stricture of esophagus

> EXCLUDES 1   congenital stenosis or stricture of esophagus (Q39.3)

K22.3   **Perforation of esophagus**   MCC

Rupture of esophagus

> EXCLUDES 1   traumatic perforation of (thoracic) esophagus (S27.8-)

CC Excl: PDX collection 766

K22.4   **Dyskinesia of esophagus**

Corkscrew esophagus
Diffuse esophageal spasm
Spasm of esophagus

> EXCLUDES 1   cardiospasm (K22.Ø)

K22.5   **Diverticulum of esophagus, acquired**

Esophageal pouch, acquired

> EXCLUDES 1   diverticulum of esophagus (congenital) (Q39.6)

K22.6   **Gastro-esophageal laceration-hemorrhage syndrome**   MCC

Mallory-Weiss syndrome
CC Excl: PDX collection 767

√5ᵗʰ **K22.7**   **Barrett's esophagus**

Barrett's disease
Barrett's syndrome

> EXCLUDES 1   Barrett's ulcer (K22.1)
>
>   malignant neoplasm of esophagus (C15.-)

DEF: Metaplastic disorder in which specialized columnar epithelial cells replace the normal squamous epithelial cells. Secondary to chronic gastroesophageal reflux damage to the mucosa, this disorder increases the risk of developing adenocarcinoma.

K22.7Ø   **Barrett's esophagus** without dysplasia

Barrett's esophagus NOS

√6ᵗʰ **K22.71**   **Barrett's esophagus** with dysplasia

K22.71Ø   **Barrett's esophagus** with low grade dysplasia

K22.711   **Barrett's esophagus** with high grade dysplasia

K22.719   **Barrett's esophagus** with dysplasia, unspecified

K22.8   **Other specified diseases of esophagus**

Hemorrhage of esophagus NOS

> EXCLUDES 2   esophageal varices (I85.-)
>
>   Paterson-Kelly syndrome (D5Ø.1)

K22.9   **Disease of esophagus, unspecified**

K23   *Disorders of esophagus in diseases classified elsewhere*

Code first underlying disease, such as:
congenital syphilis (A5Ø.5)

> EXCLUDES 1   late syphilis (A52.79)
>
>   megaesophagus due to Chagas' disease (B57.31)
>
>   tuberculosis (A18.83)

√4ᵗʰ **K25**   **Gastric ulcer**

> INCLUDES   erosion (acute) of stomach
>
>   pylorus ulcer (peptic)
>
>   stomach ulcer (peptic)

Use additional code to identify:
alcohol abuse and dependence (F1Ø.-)

> EXCLUDES 1   acute gastritis (K29.Ø-)
>
>   peptic ulcer NOS (K27.-)

AHA: 2017,3Q,27

TIP: Assign a code for "with hemorrhage" when a gastric ulcer and GI bleeding are documented. The ICD-10-CM classification assumes the two are related without the provider linking the two conditions. Evidence of bleeding during a procedure is not required.

TIP: For bleeding ulcers resulting from anticoagulant therapy, code D68.32 Hemorrhagic disorder due to extrinsic circulating anticoagulant, and an adverse-effect code from subcategory T45.5- should also be assigned. Either the bleeding ulcer code or code D68.32 may be sequenced first, depending on the circumstances of admission.

CC Excl: For MCC codes in category K25: PDX collection 765

K25.Ø   **Acute gastric ulcer** with hemorrhage   MCC

K25.1   **Acute gastric ulcer** with perforation   MCC HCC

K25.2   **Acute gastric ulcer** with both hemorrhage and perforation   MCC HCC

K25.3   **Acute gastric ulcer** without hemorrhage or perforation   CC

CC Excl: PDX collection 765

K25.4   **Chronic or unspecified gastric ulcer** with hemorrhage   MCC

K25.5   **Chronic or unspecified gastric ulcer** with perforation   MCC HCC

K25.6   **Chronic or unspecified gastric ulcer** with both hemorrhage and perforation   MCC HCC

K25.7   **Chronic gastric ulcer** without hemorrhage or perforation   CC

K25.9   **Gastric ulcer, unspecified** as acute or chronic, without hemorrhage or perforation   CC

Gastrointestinal Ulcers

K26   **Duodenal ulcer**

> INCLUDES   erosion (acute) of duodenum
>
>   duodenum ulcer (peptic)
>
>   postpyloric ulcer (peptic)

Use additional code to identify:
alcohol abuse and dependence (F1Ø.-)

> EXCLUDES 1   peptic ulcer NOS (K27.-)

AHA: 2017,3Q,27

TIP: Assign a code for "with hemorrhage" when a duodenal ulcer and GI bleeding are documented. The ICD-10-CM classification assumes the two are related without the provider linking the two conditions. Evidence of bleeding during a procedure is not required.

TIP: For bleeding ulcers resulting from anticoagulant therapy, code D68.32 Hemorrhagic disorder due to extrinsic circulating anticoagulant, and an adverse-effect code from subcategory T45.5- should also be assigned. Either the bleeding ulcer code or code D68.32 may be sequenced first, depending on the circumstances of admission.

CC Excl: For MCC codes in category K26: PDX collection 768

K26.Ø   **Acute duodenal ulcer** with hemorrhage   MCC

K26.1   **Acute duodenal ulcer** with perforation   MCC HCC

K26.2   **Acute duodenal ulcer** with both hemorrhage and perforation   MCC HCC

K26.3   **Acute duodenal ulcer** without hemorrhage or perforation   CC

CC Excl: PDX collection 769

K26.4   **Chronic or unspecified duodenal ulcer** with hemorrhage   MCC

AHA: 2016,1Q,14

K26.5   **Chronic or unspecified duodenal ulcer** with perforation   MCC HCC

K26.6   **Chronic or unspecified duodenal ulcer** with both hemorrhage and perforation   MCC HCC

K26.7   **Chronic duodenal ulcer** without hemorrhage or perforation

K26.9   **Duodenal ulcer, unspecified** as acute or chronic, without hemorrhage or perforation

N Newborn: 0   P Pediatric: 0-17   M Maternity: 9-64   A Adult: 15-124   MCC Major Complication/Comorbidity   CC Complication/Comorbidity   SW Severe Wound Dx

716   ICD-10-CM 2020

✔4ᵗʰ K27 Peptic ulcer, site unspecified

INCLUDES   gastroduodenal ulcer NOS
         peptic ulcer NOS

Use additional code to identify:
    alcohol abuse and dependence (F1Ø.-)

EXCLUDES 1   *peptic ulcer of newborn (P78.82)*

AHA: 2017,3Q,27

TIP: Assign a code for "with hemorrhage" when a peptic ulcer and GI bleeding are documented. The ICD-10-CM classification assumes the two are related without the provider linking the two conditions. Evidence of bleeding during a procedure is not required.

TIP: For bleeding ulcers resulting from anticoagulant therapy, code D68.32 Hemorrhagic disorder due to extrinsic circulating anticoagulant, and an adverse-effect code from subcategory T45.5- should also be assigned. Either the bleeding ulcer code or code D68.32 may be sequenced first, depending on the circumstances of admission.

CC Excl: For CC/MCC codes in category K27: PDX collection 768

K27.Ø	Acute **peptic ulcer, site unspecified, with** hemorrhage	MCC
K27.1	Acute **peptic ulcer, site unspecified, with** perforation	MCC HCC
K27.2	Acute **peptic ulcer, site unspecified, with both** hemorrhage and perforation	MCC HCC
K27.3	Acute **peptic ulcer, site unspecified, without** hemorrhage or perforation	CC
K27.4	Chronic **or unspecified peptic ulcer, site unspecified, with hemorrhage**	MCC
K27.5	Chronic **or unspecified peptic ulcer, site unspecified, with perforation**	MCC HCC
K27.6	Chronic **or unspecified peptic ulcer, site unspecified, with both hemorrhage and perforation**	MCC HCC
K27.7	Chronic **peptic ulcer, site unspecified, without hemorrhage or perforation**	
K27.9	Peptic ulcer, site unspecified, unspecified as acute or chronic, without hemorrhage or perforation	

✔4ᵗʰ K28 Gastrojejunal ulcer

INCLUDES   anastomotic ulcer (peptic) or erosion
         gastrocolic ulcer (peptic) or erosion
         gastrointestinal ulcer (peptic) or erosion
         gastrojejunal ulcer (peptic) or erosion
         jejunal ulcer (peptic) or erosion
         marginal ulcer (peptic) or erosion
         stomal ulcer (peptic) or erosion

Use additional code to identify:
    alcohol abuse and dependence (F1Ø.-)

EXCLUDES 1   *primary ulcer of small intestine (K63.3)*

AHA: 2017,3Q,27

TIP: Assign a code for "with hemorrhage" when a gastrojejunal ulcer and GI bleeding are documented. The ICD-10-CM classification assumes the two are related without the provider linking the two conditions. Evidence of bleeding during a procedure is not required.

TIP: For bleeding ulcers resulting from anticoagulant therapy, code D68.32 Hemorrhagic disorder due to extrinsic circulating anticoagulant, and an adverse-effect code from subcategory T45.5- should also be assigned. Either the bleeding ulcer code or code D68.32 may be sequenced first, depending on the circumstances of admission.

CC Excl: For CC/MCC codes in category K28: PDX collection 765

K28.Ø	Acute **gastrojejunal ulcer with hemorrhage**	MCC
K28.1	Acute **gastrojejunal ulcer with perforation**	MCC HCC
K28.2	Acute **gastrojejunal ulcer with both** hemorrhage and perforation	MCC HCC
K28.3	Acute **gastrojejunal ulcer without hemorrhage** or perforation	CC
K28.4	Chronic **or unspecified gastrojejunal ulcer with hemorrhage**	MCC
K28.5	Chronic **or unspecified gastrojejunal ulcer with perforation**	MCC HCC
K28.6	Chronic **or unspecified gastrojejunal ulcer with both hemorrhage and perforation**	MCC HCC
K28.7	Chronic **gastrojejunal ulcer without hemorrhage or perforation**	
K28.9	Gastrojejunal ulcer, unspecified as acute or chronic, without hemorrhage or perforation	

✔4ᵗʰ K29 Gastritis and duodenitis

EXCLUDES 1   *eosinophilic gastritis or gastroenteritis (K52.81)*
         Zollinger-Ellison syndrome (E16.4)

AHA: 2018,3Q,22

TIP: Assign a code for "with bleeding" when gastritis or duodenitis and GI bleeding are documented. The ICD-10-CM classification assumes the two are related without the provider linking the two conditions. Evidence of bleeding during a procedure is not required.

TIP: For bleeding resulting from anticoagulant therapy, code D68.32 Hemorrhagic disorder due to extrinsic circulating anticoagulant, and an adverse-effect code from subcategory T45.5- should also be assigned. Either code K29 or code D68.32 may be sequenced first, depending on the circumstances of admission.

CC Excl: For MCC codes in category K29: PDX collection 770

✔5ᵗʰ K29.Ø Acute gastritis

Use additional code to identify:
    alcohol abuse and dependence (F1Ø.-)

EXCLUDES 1   *erosion (acute) of stomach (K25.-)*

K29.ØØ	Acute gastritis without bleeding	CC
K29.Ø1	Acute gastritis with bleeding	MCC

✔5ᵗʰ K29.2 Alcoholic gastritis

Use additional code to identify:
    alcohol abuse and dependence (F1Ø.-)

K29.2Ø	Alcoholic gastritis without bleeding	
K29.21	Alcoholic gastritis with bleeding	MCC

✔5ᵗʰ K29.3 Chronic superficial gastritis

K29.3Ø	Chronic superficial gastritis without bleeding	
K29.31	Chronic superficial gastritis with bleeding	MCC

✔5ᵗʰ K29.4 Chronic atrophic gastritis

Gastric atrophy

K29.4Ø	Chronic atrophic gastritis without bleeding	
K29.41	Chronic atrophic gastritis with bleeding	MCC

✔5ᵗʰ K29.5 Unspecified chronic gastritis

Chronic antral gastritis
Chronic fundal gastritis

K29.5Ø	Unspecified chronic gastritis without bleeding	
K29.51	Unspecified chronic gastritis with bleeding	MCC

✔5ᵗʰ K29.6 Other gastritis

Giant hypertrophic gastritis
Granulomatous gastritis
Ménétrier's disease

K29.6Ø	Other gastritis without bleeding	
K29.61	Other gastritis with bleeding	MCC

✔5ᵗʰ K29.7 Gastritis, unspecified

K29.7Ø	Gastritis, unspecified, without bleeding	
K29.71	Gastritis, unspecified, with bleeding	MCC

✔5ᵗʰ K29.8 Duodenitis

K29.8Ø	Duodenitis without bleeding	
K29.81	Duodenitis with bleeding	MCC

✔5ᵗʰ K29.9 Gastroduodenitis, unspecified

K29.9Ø	Gastroduodenitis, unspecified, without bleeding	
K29.91	Gastroduodenitis, unspecified, with bleeding	MCC

K3Ø Functional dyspepsia

Indigestion

EXCLUDES 1   *dyspepsia NOS (R1Ø.13)*
         heartburn (R12)
         nervous dyspepsia (F45.8)
         neurotic dyspepsia (F45.8)
         psychogenic dyspepsia (F45.8)

✔4ᵗʰ K31 Other diseases of stomach and duodenum

INCLUDES   functional disorders of stomach

EXCLUDES 2   *diabetic gastroparesis (EØ8.43, EØ9.43, E1Ø.43, E11.43, E13.43)*
         diverticulum of duodenum (K57.ØØ-K57.13)

K31.Ø	Acute dilatation of stomach	CC

Acute distention of stomach

CC Excl: PDX collection 771

✔ Additional Character Required   ✔x7ᵗʰ Placeholder   Unacceptable PDx   Questionable PDx   Manifestation   Unspecified Dx   H1-H14 HAC   HCC CMS-HCC Dx   HIV HIV Dx

ICD-10-CM 2020

717

K31.1 Adult hypertrophic pyloric stenosis `CC` `A`

Pyloric stenosis NOS

EXCLUDES 1 congenital or infantile pyloric stenosis (Q40.0)

CC Excl: PDX collection 772

K31.2 Hourglass stricture and stenosis of stomach

EXCLUDES 1 congenital hourglass stomach (Q40.2)

hourglass contraction of stomach (K31.89)

K31.3 Pylorospasm, not elsewhere classified

EXCLUDES 1 congenital or infantile pylorospasm (Q40.0)

neurotic pylorospasm (F45.8)

psychogenic pylorospasm (F45.8)

K31.4 Gastric diverticulum

EXCLUDES 1 congenital diverticulum of stomach (Q40.2)

K31.5 Obstruction of duodenum `CC`

Constriction of duodenum

Duodenal ileus (chronic)

Stenosis of duodenum

Stricture of duodenum

Volvulus of duodenum

EXCLUDES 1 congenital stenosis of duodenum (Q41.0)

CC Excl: PDX collection 773

K31.6 Fistula of stomach and duodenum `CC` `SW`

Gastrocolic fistula

Gastrojejunocolic fistula

CC Excl: PDX collection 774

K31.7 Polyp of stomach and duodenum `CC`

EXCLUDES 1 adenomatous polyp of stomach (D13.1)

`√5th` **K31.8 Other specified diseases of stomach and duodenum**

`√6th` **K31.81 Angiodysplasia of stomach and duodenum**

TIP: Assign a code for "with bleeding" when angiodysplasia of the stomach or the duodenum and GI bleeding are documented. The ICD-10-CM classification assumes the two are related without the provider linking the two conditions. Evidence of bleeding during a procedure is not required.

K31.811 Angiodysplasia of stomach and duodenum with bleeding `CC`

K31.819 Angiodysplasia of stomach and duodenum without bleeding

Angiodysplasia of stomach and duodenum NOS

K31.82 Dieulafoy lesion (hemorrhagic) of stomach and duodenum `MCC`

EXCLUDES 2 Dieulafoy lesion of intestine (K63.81)

DEF: Abnormally large submucosal artery protruding through a defect in the stomach mucosa or intestines that can cause massive and life-threatening hemorrhaging.

CC Excl: PDX collection 775

K31.83 Achlorhydria

DEF: Absence of hydrochloric acid in gastric secretions due to gastric mucosa atrophy. Achlorhydria is unresponsive to histamines.

K31.84 Gastroparesis

Gastroparalysis

Code first underlying disease, if known, such as:

anorexia nervosa (F50.0-)

diabetes mellitus (E08.43, E09.43, E10.43, E11.43, E13.43)

scleroderma (M34.-)

AHA: 2013,4Q,114

K31.89 Other diseases of stomach and duodenum

AHA: 2017,1Q,28

K31.9 Disease of stomach and duodenum, unspecified

Diseases of appendix (K35-K38)

`√4th` **K35 Acute appendicitis**

AHA: 2018,4Q,17-18

`√5th` **K35.2 Acute appendicitis with generalized peritonitis**

Appendicitis (acute) with generalized (diffuse) peritonitis following rupture or perforation of appendix

K35.20 Acute appendicitis with generalized peritonitis, without abscess

(Acute) appendicitis with generalized peritonitis NOS

K35.21 Acute appendicitis with generalized peritonitis, with abscess

`√5th` **K35.3 Acute appendicitis with localized peritonitis**

K35.30 Acute appendicitis with localized peritonitis, without perforation or gangrene

Acute appendicitis with localized peritonitis NOS

K35.31 Acute appendicitis with localized peritonitis and gangrene, without perforation

K35.32 Acute appendicitis with perforation and localized peritonitis, without abscess

(Acute) appendicitis with perforation NOS

Perforated appendix NOS

Ruptured appendix (with localized peritonitis) NOS

K35.33 Acute appendicitis with perforation and localized peritonitis, with abscess

(Acute) appendicitis with (peritoneal) abscess NOS

Ruptured appendix with localized peritonitis and abscess

`√5th` **K35.8 Other and unspecified acute appendicitis**

CC Excl: For CC codes in subcategory K35.8: PDX collection 776

K35.80 Unspecified acute appendicitis `CC`

Acute appendicitis NOS

Acute appendicitis without (localized) (generalized) peritonitis

`√6th` **K35.89 Other acute appendicitis**

K35.890 Other acute appendicitis without perforation or gangrene `CC`

K35.891 Other acute appendicitis without perforation, with gangrene `CC`

(Acute) appendicitis with gangrene NOS

K36 Other appendicitis

Chronic appendicitis

Recurrent appendicitis

K37 Unspecified appendicitis

EXCLUDES 1 unspecified appendicitis with peritonitis (K35.2-, K35.3-)

`√4th` **K38 Other diseases of appendix**

K38.0 Hyperplasia of appendix

K38.1 Appendicular concretions

Fecalith of appendix

Stercolith of appendix

K38.2 Diverticulum of appendix

K38.3 Fistula of appendix

K38.8 Other specified diseases of appendix

Intussusception of appendix

K38.9 Disease of appendix, unspecified

Hernia (K40-K46)

`NOTE` Hernia with both gangrene and obstruction is classified to hernia with gangrene.

`INCLUDES` acquired hernia

congenital [except diaphragmatic or hiatus] hernia

recurrent hernia

`√4th` **K40 Inguinal hernia**

`INCLUDES` bubonocele

direct inguinal hernia

double inguinal hernia

indirect inguinal hernia

inguinal hernia NOS

oblique inguinal hernia

scrotal hernia

DEF: Within the groin region.

CC Excl: For CC/MCC codes in category K40: PDX collection 777

`√5th` **K40.0 Bilateral inguinal hernia, with obstruction, without gangrene**

Inguinal hernia (bilateral) causing obstruction without gangrene

Incarcerated inguinal hernia (bilateral) without gangrene

Irreducible inguinal hernia (bilateral) without gangrene

Strangulated inguinal hernia (bilateral) without gangrene

K40.00 Bilateral inguinal hernia, with obstruction, without gangrene, not specified as recurrent `CC`

Bilateral inguinal hernia, with obstruction, without gangrene NOS

K40.01 Bilateral inguinal hernia, with obstruction, without gangrene, recurrent `CC`

N Newborn: 0   P Pediatric: 0-17   M Maternity: 9-64   A Adult: 15-124   MCC Major Complication/Comorbidity   CC Complication/Comorbidity   SW Severe Wound Dx

718   ICD-10-CM 2020

✓5ᵗʰ **K40.1** Bilateral **inguinal hernia,** with gangrene

    K40.10 **Bilateral inguinal hernia, with gangrene,** not specified as recurrent   `MCC`
        Bilateral inguinal hernia, with gangrene NOS

    K40.11 **Bilateral inguinal hernia, with gangrene,** recurrent   `MCC`

✓5ᵗʰ **K40.2** Bilateral **inguinal hernia,** without obstruction or gangrene

    K40.20 **Bilateral inguinal hernia, without obstruction or gangrene,** not specified as recurrent
        Bilateral inguinal hernia NOS

    K40.21 **Bilateral inguinal hernia, without obstruction or gangrene,** recurrent

✓5ᵗʰ **K40.3** Unilateral **inguinal hernia,** with obstruction, without gangrene

    Inguinal hernia (unilateral) causing obstruction without gangrene
    Incarcerated inguinal hernia (unilateral) without gangrene
    Irreducible inguinal hernia (unilateral) without gangrene
    Strangulated inguinal hernia (unilateral) without gangrene

    K40.30 **Unilateral inguinal hernia, with obstruction, without gangrene,** not specified as recurrent   `CC`
        Inguinal hernia, with obstruction NOS
        Unilateral inguinal hernia, with obstruction, without gangrene NOS

    K40.31 **Unilateral inguinal hernia, with obstruction, without gangrene,** recurrent   `CC`

✓5ᵗʰ **K40.4** Unilateral **inguinal hernia,** with gangrene

    K40.40 **Unilateral inguinal hernia, with gangrene,** not specified as recurrent   `MCC`
        Inguinal hernia with gangrene NOS
        Unilateral inguinal hernia with gangrene NOS

    K40.41 **Unilateral inguinal hernia, with gangrene,** recurrent   `MCC`

✓5ᵗʰ **K40.9** Unilateral **inguinal hernia,** without obstruction or gangrene

    K40.90 **Unilateral inguinal hernia, without obstruction or gangrene,** not specified as recurrent
        Inguinal hernia NOS
        Unilateral inguinal hernia NOS

    K40.91 **Unilateral inguinal hernia, without obstruction or gangrene,** recurrent

Hernia Sites

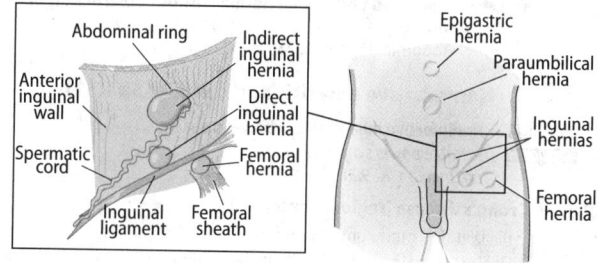

✓4ᵗʰ **K41** Femoral **hernia**

    CC Excl: For codes in category K41:
    For MCC codes: PDX collection 779
    For CC codes: PDX collection 778

✓5ᵗʰ **K41.0** Bilateral **femoral hernia,** with obstruction, without gangrene

    Femoral hernia (bilateral) causing obstruction, without gangrene
    Incarcerated femoral hernia (bilateral), without gangrene
    Irreducible femoral hernia (bilateral), without gangrene
    Strangulated femoral hernia (bilateral), without gangrene

    K41.00 **Bilateral femoral hernia, with obstruction, without gangrene,** not specified as recurrent   `CC`
        Bilateral femoral hernia, with obstruction, without gangrene NOS

    K41.01 **Bilateral femoral hernia, with obstruction, without gangrene,** recurrent   `CC`

✓5ᵗʰ **K41.1** Bilateral **femoral hernia,** with gangrene

    K41.10 **Bilateral femoral hernia, with gangrene,** not specified as recurrent   `MCC`
        Bilateral femoral hernia, with gangrene NOS

    K41.11 **Bilateral femoral hernia, with gangrene,** recurrent   `MCC`

✓5ᵗʰ **K41.2** Bilateral **femoral hernia,** without obstruction or gangrene

    K41.20 **Bilateral femoral hernia, without obstruction or gangrene,** not specified as recurrent
        Bilateral femoral hernia NOS

    K41.21 **Bilateral femoral hernia, without obstruction or gangrene,** recurrent

✓5ᵗʰ **K41.3** Unilateral **femoral hernia,** with obstruction, without gangrene

    Femoral hernia (unilateral) causing obstruction, without gangrene
    Incarcerated femoral hernia (unilateral), without gangrene
    Irreducible femoral hernia (unilateral), without gangrene
    Strangulated femoral hernia (unilateral), without gangrene

    K41.30 **Unilateral femoral hernia, with obstruction, without gangrene,** not specified as recurrent   `CC`
        Femoral hernia, with obstruction NOS
        Unilateral femoral hernia, with obstruction NOS

    K41.31 **Unilateral femoral hernia, with obstruction, without gangrene,** recurrent   `CC`

✓5ᵗʰ **K41.4** Unilateral **femoral hernia,** with gangrene

    K41.40 **Unilateral femoral hernia, with gangrene,** not specified as recurrent   `MCC`
        Femoral hernia, with gangrene NOS
        Unilateral femoral hernia, with gangrene NOS

    K41.41 **Unilateral femoral hernia, with gangrene,** recurrent   `MCC`

✓5ᵗʰ **K41.9** Unilateral **femoral hernia,** without obstruction or gangrene

    K41.90 **Unilateral femoral hernia, without obstruction or gangrene,** not specified as recurrent
        Femoral hernia NOS
        Unilateral femoral hernia NOS

    K41.91 **Unilateral femoral hernia, without obstruction or gangrene,** recurrent

✓4ᵗʰ **K42** Umbilical **hernia**

    `INCLUDES`   paraumbilical hernia
    `EXCLUDES 1`   *omphalocele (Q79.2)*

    K42.0 **Umbilical hernia** with obstruction, without gangrene   `CC`
        Umbilical hernia causing obstruction, without gangrene
        Incarcerated umbilical hernia, without gangrene
        Irreducible umbilical hernia, without gangrene
        Strangulated umbilical hernia, without gangrene
        CC Excl: PDX collection 780

    K42.1 **Umbilical hernia** with gangrene   `MCC`
        Gangrenous umbilical hernia
        CC Excl: PDX collection 781

    K42.9 **Umbilical hernia** without obstruction or gangrene
        Umbilical hernia NOS

✓4ᵗʰ **K43** Ventral **hernia**

    DEF: Condition in which a loop of bowel protrudes through a weakness in the abdominal wall muscles that may occur as a birth defect, past surgical site (incisional), or form at a stomal site (parastomal).
    CC Excl: For codes in category K43:
    For MCC codes: PDX collection 781
    For CC codes: PDX collection 780

    K43.0 **Incisional hernia** with obstruction, without gangrene   `CC`
        Incisional hernia causing obstruction, without gangrene
        Incarcerated incisional hernia, without gangrene
        Irreducible incisional hernia, without gangrene
        Strangulated incisional hernia, without gangrene

    K43.1 **Incisional hernia** with gangrene   `MCC`
        Gangrenous incisional hernia

    K43.2 **Incisional hernia** without obstruction or gangrene
        Incisional hernia NOS

K43.3 Parastomal **hernia** with obstruction, without gangrene   `CC`
    Incarcerated parastomal hernia, without gangrene
    Irreducible parastomal hernia, without gangrene
    Parastomal hernia causing obstruction, without gangrene
    Strangulated parastomal hernia, without gangrene

K43.4 Parastomal **hernia** with gangrene   `MCC`
    Gangrenous parastomal hernia

K43.5 Parastomal **hernia** without obstruction or gangrene
    Parastomal hernia NOS

K43.6 Other and unspecified ventral hernia with obstruction, without gangrene   `CC`
    Epigastric hernia causing obstruction, without gangrene
    Hypogastric hernia causing obstruction, without gangrene
    Incarcerated epigastric hernia without gangrene
    Incarcerated hypogastric hernia without gangrene
    Incarcerated midline hernia without gangrene
    Incarcerated spigelian hernia without gangrene
    Incarcerated subxiphoid hernia without gangrene
    Irreducible epigastric hernia without gangrene
    Irreducible hypogastric hernia without gangrene
    Irreducible midline hernia without gangrene
    Irreducible spigelian hernia without gangrene
    Irreducible subxiphoid hernia without gangrene
    Midline hernia causing obstruction, without gangrene
    Spigelian hernia causing obstruction, without gangrene
    Strangulated epigastric hernia without gangrene
    Strangulated hypogastric hernia without gangrene
    Strangulated midline hernia without gangrene
    Strangulated spigelian hernia without gangrene
    Strangulated subxiphoid hernia without gangrene
    Subxiphoid hernia causing obstruction, without gangrene

K43.7 Other and unspecified ventral hernia with gangrene   `MCC`
    Any condition listed under K43.6 specified as gangrenous

K43.9 Ventral hernia without obstruction or gangrene
    Epigastric hernia
    Ventral hernia NOS

✓4ᵗʰ **K44** Diaphragmatic **hernia**
    INCLUDES   hiatus hernia (esophageal) (sliding)
             paraesophageal hernia
    EXCLUDES 1   *congenital diaphragmatic hernia (Q79.0)*
             congenital hiatus hernia (Q40.1)

DEF: Protrusion of an abdominal organ, usually the stomach, through the esophageal opening within the diaphragm and occurring in two types: the sliding hiatal hernia and the paraesophageal hernia.

Hiatal Hernia

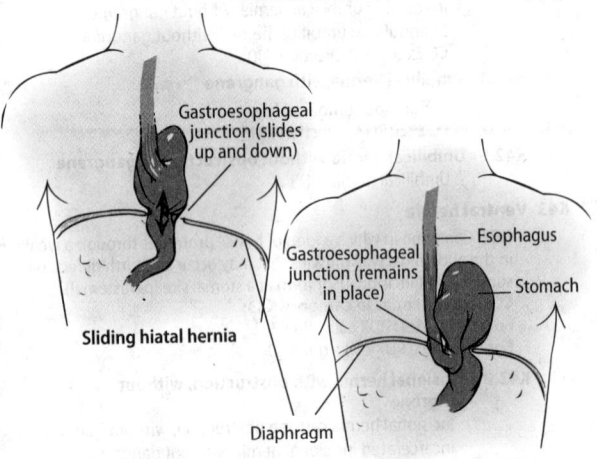

Sliding hiatal hernia

Paraesophageal hiatal hernia

K44.0 Diaphragmatic hernia with obstruction, without gangrene   `CC`
    Diaphragmatic hernia causing obstruction
    Incarcerated diaphragmatic hernia
    Irreducible diaphragmatic hernia
    Strangulated diaphragmatic hernia
    CC Excl: PDX collection 782

K44.1 Diaphragmatic hernia with gangrene   `MCC`
    Gangrenous diaphragmatic hernia
    CC Excl: PDX collection 782

K44.9 Diaphragmatic hernia without obstruction or gangrene
    Diaphragmatic hernia NOS

✓4ᵗʰ **K45** Other abdominal hernia
    INCLUDES   abdominal hernia, specified site NEC
             lumbar hernia
             obturator hernia
             pudendal hernia
             retroperitoneal hernia
             sciatic hernia

K45.0 Other specified abdominal hernia with obstruction, without gangrene   `CC`
    Other specified abdominal hernia causing obstruction
    Other specified incarcerated abdominal hernia
    Other specified irreducible abdominal hernia
    Other specified strangulated abdominal hernia
    CC Excl: PDX collection 783

K45.1 Other specified abdominal hernia with gangrene   `MCC`
    Any condition listed under K45 specified as gangrenous
    CC Excl: PDX collection 784

K45.8 Other specified abdominal hernia without obstruction or gangrene

✓4ᵗʰ **K46** Unspecified abdominal hernia
    INCLUDES   enterocele
             epiplocele
             hernia NOS
             interstitial hernia
             intestinal hernia
             intra-abdominal hernia
    EXCLUDES 1   *vaginal enterocele (N81.5)*

K46.0 Unspecified abdominal hernia with obstruction, without gangrene   `CC`
    Unspecified abdominal hernia causing obstruction
    Unspecified incarcerated abdominal hernia
    Unspecified irreducible abdominal hernia
    Unspecified strangulated abdominal hernia
    CC Excl: PDX collection 783

K46.1 Unspecified abdominal hernia with gangrene   `MCC`
    Any condition listed under K46 specified as gangrenous
    CC Excl: PDX collection 784

K46.9 Unspecified abdominal hernia without obstruction or gangrene
    Abdominal hernia NOS

Noninfective enteritis and colitis (K50-K52)

    INCLUDES   noninfective inflammatory bowel disease
    EXCLUDES 1   *irritable bowel syndrome (K58.-)*
             megacolon (K59.3-)

✓4ᵗʰ **K50** Crohn's disease [regional enteritis]
    INCLUDES   granulomatous enteritis
    Use additional code to identify manifestations, such as:
       pyoderma gangrenosum (L88)
    EXCLUDES 1   *ulcerative colitis (K51.-)*
    AHA: 2012,4Q,104
    DEF: Chronic inflammation of the gastrointestinal tract characterized by chronic granulomatous disease, most commonly affecting the intestines and the terminal ileum.

✓5ᵗʰ **K50.0** Crohn's disease of small intestine
    Crohn's disease [regional enteritis] of duodenum
    Crohn's disease [regional enteritis] of ileum
    Crohn's disease [regional enteritis] of jejunum
    Regional ileitis
    Terminal ileitis
    EXCLUDES 1   *Crohn's disease of both small and large intestine (K50.8-)*

       K50.00 Crohn's disease of small intestine without complications   `HCC`

       ✓6ᵗʰ **K50.01** Crohn's disease of small intestine with complications

           K50.011 Crohn's disease of small intestine with rectal bleeding   `HCC`

K50.012   Crohn's disease of small intestine with intestinal obstruction   `HCC`

K50.013   Crohn's disease of small intestine with fistula   `HCC` `SW`

K50.014   Crohn's disease of small intestine with abscess   `HCC`
     AHA: 2012,4Q,104

K50.018   Crohn's disease of small intestine with other complication   `HCC`

K50.019   Crohn's disease of small intestine with unspecified complications   `HCC`

√5th **K50.1   Crohn's disease of large intestine**

Crohn's disease [regional enteritis] of colon
Crohn's disease [regional enteritis] of large bowel
Crohn's disease [regional enteritis] of rectum
Granulomatous colitis
Regional colitis

   EXCLUDES 1   Crohn's disease of both small and large intestine (K50.8)

K50.10   Crohn's disease of large intestine without complications   `HCC`

√6th K50.11   Crohn's disease of large intestine with complications

K50.111   Crohn's disease of large intestine with rectal bleeding   `HCC`

K50.112   Crohn's disease of large intestine with intestinal obstruction   `HCC`

K50.113   Crohn's disease of large intestine with fistula   `HCC` `SW`

K50.114   Crohn's disease of large intestine with abscess   `HCC`

K50.118   Crohn's disease of large intestine with other complication   `HCC`

K50.119   Crohn's disease of large intestine with unspecified complications   `HCC`

√5th **K50.8   Crohn's disease of both small and large intestine**

K50.80   Crohn's disease of both small and large intestine without complications   `HCC`

√6th K50.81   Crohn's disease of both small and large intestine with complications

K50.811   Crohn's disease of both small and large intestine with rectal bleeding   `HCC`

K50.812   Crohn's disease of both small and large intestine with intestinal obstruction   `HCC`

K50.813   Crohn's disease of both small and large intestine with fistula   `HCC` `SW`

K50.814   Crohn's disease of both small and large intestine with abscess   `HCC`

K50.818   Crohn's disease of both small and large intestine with other complication   `HCC`

K50.819   Crohn's disease of both small and large intestine with unspecified complications   `HCC`

√5th **K50.9   Crohn's disease, unspecified**

K50.90   Crohn's disease, unspecified, without complications   `HCC`
     Crohn's disease NOS
     Regional enteritis NOS

√6th K50.91   Crohn's disease, unspecified, with complications

K50.911   Crohn's disease, unspecified, with rectal bleeding   `HCC`

K50.912   Crohn's disease, unspecified, with intestinal obstruction   `HCC`

K50.913   Crohn's disease, unspecified, with fistula   `HCC` `SW`

K50.914   Crohn's disease, unspecified, with abscess   `HCC`

K50.918   Crohn's disease, unspecified, with other complication   `HCC`

K50.919   Crohn's disease, unspecified, with unspecified complications   `HCC`

√4th **K51   Ulcerative colitis**

Use additional code to identify manifestations, such as:
pyoderma gangrenosum (L88)

   EXCLUDES 1   Crohn's disease [regional enteritis] (K50.-)

√5th **K51.0   Ulcerative (chronic) pancolitis**

Backwash ileitis

K51.00   Ulcerative (chronic) pancolitis without complications   `HCC`
     Ulcerative (chronic) pancolitis NOS

√6th K51.01   Ulcerative (chronic) pancolitis with complications

K51.011   Ulcerative (chronic) pancolitis with rectal bleeding   `HCC`

K51.012   Ulcerative (chronic) pancolitis with intestinal obstruction   `HCC`

K51.013   Ulcerative (chronic) pancolitis with fistula   `HCC` `SW`

K51.014   Ulcerative (chronic) pancolitis with abscess   `HCC`

K51.018   Ulcerative (chronic) pancolitis with other complication   `HCC`

K51.019   Ulcerative (chronic) pancolitis with unspecified complications   `HCC`

√5th **K51.2   Ulcerative (chronic) proctitis**

K51.20   Ulcerative (chronic) proctitis without complications   `HCC`
     Ulcerative (chronic) proctitis NOS

√6th K51.21   Ulcerative (chronic) proctitis with complications

K51.211   Ulcerative (chronic) proctitis with rectal bleeding   `HCC`

K51.212   Ulcerative (chronic) proctitis with intestinal obstruction   `CC` `HCC`
     CC Excl: PDX collection 785

K51.213   Ulcerative (chronic) proctitis with fistula   `HCC` `SW`

K51.214   Ulcerative (chronic) proctitis with abscess   `HCC`

K51.218   Ulcerative (chronic) proctitis with other complication   `HCC`

K51.219   Ulcerative (chronic) proctitis with unspecified complications   `HCC`

√5th **K51.3   Ulcerative (chronic) rectosigmoiditis**

K51.30   Ulcerative (chronic) rectosigmoiditis without complications   `HCC`
     Ulcerative (chronic) rectosigmoiditis NOS

√6th K51.31   Ulcerative (chronic) rectosigmoiditis with complications

K51.311   Ulcerative (chronic) rectosigmoiditis with rectal bleeding   `HCC`

K51.312   Ulcerative (chronic) rectosigmoiditis with intestinal obstruction   `HCC`

K51.313   Ulcerative (chronic) rectosigmoiditis with fistula   `HCC` `SW`

K51.314   Ulcerative (chronic) rectosigmoiditis with abscess   `HCC`

K51.318   Ulcerative (chronic) rectosigmoiditis with other complication   `HCC`

K51.319   Ulcerative (chronic) rectosigmoiditis with unspecified complications   `HCC`

Chapter 11. Diseases of the Digestive System

✓5ᵗʰ **K51.4 Inflammatory polyps of colon**

EXCLUDES 1   *adenomatous polyp of colon (D12.6)*
polyposis of colon (D12.6)
polyps of colon NOS (K63.5)

K51.40 Inflammatory polyps of colon without complications   HCC
Inflammatory polyps of colon NOS

✓6ᵗʰ **K51.41 Inflammatory polyps of colon with complications**

K51.411 Inflammatory polyps of colon with rectal bleeding   HCC

K51.412 Inflammatory polyps of colon with intestinal obstruction   HCC

K51.413 Inflammatory polyps of colon with fistula   CC HCC SW
CC Excl: PDX collection 785

K51.414 Inflammatory polyps of colon with abscess   HCC

K51.418 Inflammatory polyps of colon with other complication   HCC

K51.419 Inflammatory polyps of colon with unspecified complications   HCC

✓5ᵗʰ **K51.5 Left sided colitis**
Left hemicolitis

K51.50 Left sided colitis without complications   HCC
Left sided colitis NOS

✓6ᵗʰ **K51.51 Left sided colitis with complications**

K51.511 Left sided colitis with rectal bleeding   HCC

K51.512 Left sided colitis with intestinal obstruction   HCC

K51.513 Left sided colitis with fistula   HCC SW

K51.514 Left sided colitis with abscess   HCC

K51.518 Left sided colitis with other complication   HCC

K51.519 Left sided colitis with unspecified complications   HCC

✓5ᵗʰ **K51.8 Other ulcerative colitis**
CC Excl: For CC codes in subcategory K51.8: PDX collection 785

K51.80 Other ulcerative colitis without complications   HCC

✓6ᵗʰ **K51.81 Other ulcerative colitis with complications**

K51.811 Other ulcerative colitis with rectal bleeding   CC HCC

K51.812 Other ulcerative colitis with intestinal obstruction   CC HCC

K51.813 Other ulcerative colitis with fistula   CC HCC SW

K51.814 Other ulcerative colitis with abscess   CC HCC

K51.818 Other ulcerative colitis with other complication   CC HCC

K51.819 Other ulcerative colitis with unspecified complications   CC HCC

✓5ᵗʰ **K51.9 Ulcerative colitis, unspecified**
CC Excl: For CC codes in subcategory K51.9: PDX collection 787

K51.90 Ulcerative colitis, unspecified, without complications   HCC

✓6ᵗʰ **K51.91 Ulcerative colitis, unspecified, with complications**

K51.911 Ulcerative colitis, unspecified with rectal bleeding   CC HCC

K51.912 Ulcerative colitis, unspecified with intestinal obstruction   CC HCC

K51.913 Ulcerative colitis, unspecified with fistula   CC HCC SW

K51.914 Ulcerative colitis, unspecified with abscess   CC HCC

K51.918 Ulcerative colitis, unspecified with other complication   CC HCC

K51.919 Ulcerative colitis, unspecified with unspecified complications   CC HCC

✓4ᵗʰ **K52 Other and unspecified noninfective gastroenteritis and colitis**
AHA: 2016,4Q,30-31

K52.0 Gastroenteritis and colitis due to radiation   CC
CC Excl: PDX collection 788

K52.1 Toxic gastroenteritis and colitis   CC
Drug-induced gastroenteritis and colitis
Code first (T51-T65) to identify toxic agent
Use additional code for adverse effect, if applicable, to identify drug (T36-T50 with fifth or sixth character 5)
AHA: 2019,1Q,17
CC Excl: PDX collection 789

✓5ᵗʰ **K52.2 Allergic and dietetic gastroenteritis and colitis**
Food hypersensitivity gastroenteritis or colitis
Use additional code to identify type of food allergy (Z91.01-, Z91.02-)

EXCLUDES 2   *allergic eosinophilic colitis (K52.82)*
allergic eosinophilic esophagitis (K20.0)
allergic eosinophilic gastritis (K52.81)
allergic eosinophilic gastroenteritis (K52.81)
food protein-induced proctocolitis (K52.82)

DEF: True immunoglobulin E (IgE)-mediated allergic reaction of the lining of the stomach, intestines, or colon to food proteins. It causes nausea, vomiting, diarrhea, and abdominal cramping.
TIP: Assign a code for "with hemorrhage" when angiodysplasia and GI bleeding are documented. The ICD-10-CM classification assumes the two are related without the provider linking the two conditions. Evidence of bleeding during a procedure is not required.

K52.21 Food protein-induced enterocolitis syndrome
FPIES
Use additional code for hypovolemic shock, if present (R57.1)

K52.22 Food protein-induced enteropathy

K52.29 Other allergic and dietetic gastroenteritis and colitis
Food hypersensitivity gastroenteritis or colitis
Immediate gastrointestinal hypersensitivity

K52.3 Indeterminate colitis
Colonic inflammatory bowel disease unclassified (IBDU)
EXCLUDES 1   *unspecified colitis (K52.9)*

✓5ᵗʰ **K52.8 Other specified noninfective gastroenteritis and colitis**

K52.81 Eosinophilic gastritis or gastroenteritis
Eosinophilic enteritis
EXCLUDES 2   *eosinophilic esophagitis (K20.0)*
DEF: Disorder involving the accumulation of eosinophil in the lining of the stomach or multiple levels of the gastrointestinal tract, but without a known cause such as connective tissue disease, drug reaction, malignancy, or parasitic infection.

K52.82 Eosinophilic colitis
Allergic proctocolitis
Food-induced eosinophilic proctocolitis
Food protein-induced proctocolitis
Milk protein-induced proctocolitis
DEF: Disorder involving the accumulation of eosinophil in the tissues lining the colon, but without a known cause such as connective tissue disease, drug reaction, malignancy, or parasitic infection. The resultant inflammation may cause extreme abdominal pain, diarrhea, or bloody stool.

✓6ᵗʰ **K52.83 Microscopic colitis**

K52.831 Collagenous colitis
K52.832 Lymphocytic colitis
K52.838 Other microscopic colitis
K52.839 Microscopic colitis, unspecified

K52.89 Other specified noninfective gastroenteritis and colitis
AHA: 2019,1Q,20

N Newborn: 0   P Pediatric: 0-17   M Maternity: 9-64   A Adult: 15-124   MCC Major Complication/Comorbidity   CC Complication/Comorbidity   SW Severe Wound Dx

K52.9 **Noninfective gastroenteritis and colitis, unspecified**
Colitis NOS
Enteritis NOS
Gastroenteritis NOS
Ileitis NOS
Jejunitis NOS
Sigmoiditis NOS

EXCLUDES 1   *diarrhea NOS (R19.7)*
functional diarrhea (K59.1)
infectious gastroenteritis and colitis NOS (A09)
neonatal diarrhea (noninfective) (P78.3)
psychogenic diarrhea (F45.8)

Other diseases of intestines (K55-K64)

☑4ᵗʰ K55 **Vascular disorders of intestine**

EXCLUDES 1   *necrotizing enterocolitis of newborn (P77.-)*

AHA: 2016,4Q,32

CC Excl: For MCC codes in category K55, unless otherwise noted: PDX collection 790

☑5ᵗʰ K55.0 **Acute vascular disorders of intestine**
Infarction of appendices epiploicae
Mesenteric (artery) (vein) embolism
Mesenteric (artery) (vein) infarction
Mesenteric (artery) (vein) thrombosis

☑6ᵗʰ K55.01 **Acute (reversible) ischemia of small intestine**

K55.011 **Focal (segmental) acute (reversible) ischemia of small intestine** MCC HCC

K55.012 **Diffuse acute (reversible) ischemia of small intestine** MCC HCC

K55.019 **Acute (reversible) ischemia of small intestine, extent unspecified** MCC HCC

☑6ᵗʰ K55.02 **Acute infarction of small intestine**
Gangrene of small intestine
Necrosis of small intestine

K55.021 **Focal (segmental) acute infarction of small intestine** MCC HCC

K55.022 **Diffuse acute infarction of small intestine** MCC HCC

K55.029 **Acute infarction of small intestine, extent unspecified** MCC HCC

☑6ᵗʰ K55.03 **Acute (reversible) ischemia of large intestine**
Acute fulminant ischemic colitis
Subacute ischemic colitis

K55.031 **Focal (segmental) acute (reversible) ischemia of large intestine** MCC HCC

K55.032 **Diffuse acute (reversible) ischemia of large intestine** MCC HCC

K55.039 **Acute (reversible) ischemia of large intestine, extent unspecified** MCC HCC

☑6ᵗʰ K55.04 **Acute infarction of large intestine**
Gangrene of large intestine
Necrosis of large intestine

K55.041 **Focal (segmental) acute infarction of large intestine** MCC HCC

K55.042 **Diffuse acute infarction of large intestine** MCC HCC

K55.049 **Acute infarction of large intestine, extent unspecified** MCC HCC

☑6ᵗʰ K55.05 **Acute (reversible) ischemia of intestine, part unspecified**

K55.051 **Focal (segmental) acute (reversible) ischemia of intestine, part unspecified** MCC HCC

K55.052 **Diffuse acute (reversible) ischemia of intestine, part unspecified** MCC HCC

K55.059 **Acute (reversible) ischemia of intestine, part and extent unspecified** MCC HCC

☑6ᵗʰ K55.06 **Acute infarction of intestine, part unspecified**
Acute intestinal infarction
Gangrene of intestine
Necrosis of intestine

K55.061 **Focal (segmental) acute infarction of intestine, part unspecified** MCC HCC

K55.062 **Diffuse acute infarction of intestine, part unspecified** MCC HCC

K55.069 **Acute infarction of intestine, part and extent unspecified** MCC HCC

K55.1 **Chronic vascular disorders of intestine** HCC
Chronic ischemic colitis
Chronic ischemic enteritis
Chronic ischemic enterocolitis
Ischemic stricture of intestine
Mesenteric atherosclerosis
Mesenteric vascular insufficiency

☑5ᵗʰ K55.2 **Angiodysplasia of colon**

AHA: 2018,3Q,21

TIP: Assign a code for "with hemorrhage" when angiodysplasia and GI bleeding are documented. The ICD-10-CM classification assumes the two are related without the provider linking the two conditions. Evidence of bleeding during a procedure is not required.

K55.20 **Angiodysplasia of colon without hemorrhage**

K55.21 **Angiodysplasia of colon with hemorrhage** MCC
DEF: Small vascular abnormalities due to fragile blood vessels in the colon, resulting in blood loss from the gastrointestinal (GI) tract.
CC Excl: PDX collection 770

☑5ᵗʰ K55.3 **Necrotizing enterocolitis**

EXCLUDES 1   *necrotizing enterocolitis of newborn (P77.-)*
EXCLUDES 2   *necrotizing enterocolitis due to Clostridium difficile (A04.7-)*

K55.30 **Necrotizing enterocolitis, unspecified** MCC HCC
Necrotizing enterocolitis, NOS

K55.31 **Stage 1 necrotizing enterocolitis** MCC HCC
Necrotizing enterocolitis without pneumatosis, without perforation

K55.32 **Stage 2 necrotizing enterocolitis** MCC HCC
Necrotizing enterocolitis with pneumatosis, without perforation

K55.33 **Stage 3 necrotizing enterocolitis** MCC HCC
Necrotizing enterocolitis with perforation
Necrotizing enterocolitis with pneumatosis and perforation

K55.8 **Other vascular disorders of intestine** HCC

K55.9 **Vascular disorder of intestine, unspecified** HCC
Ischemic colitis
Ischemic enteritis
Ischemic enterocolitis

☑4ᵗʰ K56 **Paralytic ileus and intestinal obstruction without hernia**

EXCLUDES 1   *congenital stricture or stenosis of intestine (Q41-Q42)*
cystic fibrosis with meconium ileus (E84.11)
ischemic stricture of intestine (K55.1)
meconium ileus NOS (P76.0)
neonatal intestinal obstructions classifiable to P76.-
obstruction of duodenum (K31.5)
postprocedural intestinal obstruction (K91.3-)
stenosis of anus or rectum (K62.4)

CC Excl: For CC codes in category K56: PDX collection 792

K56.0 **Paralytic ileus** CC HCC
Paralysis of bowel
Paralysis of colon
Paralysis of intestine

EXCLUDES 1   *gallstone ileus (K56.3)*
ileus NOS (K56.7)
obstructive ileus NOS (K56.69-)

DEF: Intestinal obstruction due to paralysis of bowel motility or peristalsis.

K56.1 Intussusception   `CC` `HCC`

Intussusception or invagination of bowel
Intussusception or invagination of colon
Intussusception or invagination of intestine
Intussusception or invagination of rectum

EXCLUDES 2   intussusception of appendix (K38.8)

DEF: Intestinal obstruction due to prolapse of a bowel section into an adjacent section. It occurs primarily in children and symptoms include acute abdominal pain, vomiting, and passage of blood and mucus from the rectum.

K56.2 Volvulus   `CC` `HCC`

Strangulation of colon or intestine
Torsion of colon or intestine
Twist of colon or intestine

EXCLUDES 2   volvulus of duodenum (K31.5)

DEF: Twisting, knotting, or entanglement of the bowel on itself that may quickly compromise oxygen supply to the intestinal tissues. A volvulus usually occurs at the sigmoid and ileocecal areas of the intestines.

Volvulus

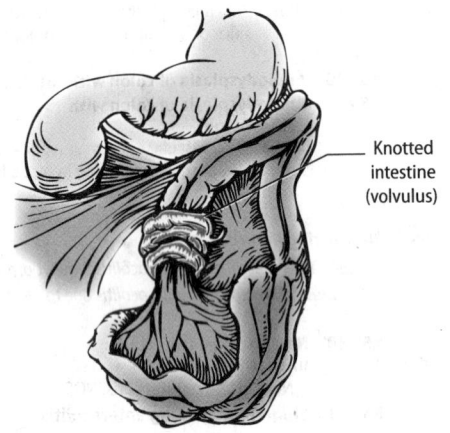

Knotted intestine (volvulus)

K56.3 Gallstone ileus   `CC` `HCC`

Obstruction of intestine by gallstone

✓5ᵗʰ K56.4 Other impaction of intestine

K56.41 Fecal impaction   `CC` `HCC`

EXCLUDES 1   constipation (K59.0-)
incomplete defecation (R15.0)

K56.49 Other impaction of intestine   `CC` `HCC`

✓5ᵗʰ K56.5 Intestinal adhesions [bands] with obstruction (postinfection)

Abdominal hernia due to adhesions with obstruction
Peritoneal adhesions [bands] with intestinal obstruction (postinfection)

AHA: 2017,4Q,16-17

K56.50 Intestinal adhesions [bands], unspecified as to partial versus complete obstruction   `CC` `HCC`

Intestinal adhesions with obstruction NOS

K56.51 Intestinal adhesions [bands], with partial obstruction   `CC` `HCC`

Intestinal adhesions with incomplete obstruction

K56.52 Intestinal adhesions [bands] with complete obstruction   `CC` `HCC`

✓5ᵗʰ K56.6 Other and unspecified intestinal obstruction

AHA: 2017,4Q,16-17; 2017,2Q,12

✓6ᵗʰ K56.60 Unspecified intestinal obstruction

EXCLUDES 1   intestinal obstruction due to specified condition - code to condition

K56.600 Partial intestinal obstruction, unspecified as to cause   `CC` `HCC`

Incomplete intestinal obstruction, NOS

K56.601 Complete intestinal obstruction, unspecified as to cause   `CC` `HCC`

K56.609 Unspecified intestinal obstruction, unspecified as to partial versus complete obstruction   `CC` `HCC`

Intestinal obstruction NOS

✓6ᵗʰ K56.69 Other intestinal obstruction

Enterostenosis NOS
Obstructive ileus NOS
Occlusion of colon or intestine NOS
Stenosis of colon or intestine NOS
Stricture of colon or intestine NOS

EXCLUDES 1   intestinal obstruction due to specified condition - code to condition

K56.690 Other partial intestinal obstruction   `CC` `HCC`

Other incomplete intestinal obstruction

K56.691 Other complete intestinal obstruction   `CC` `HCC`

K56.699 Other intestinal obstruction unspecified as to partial versus complete obstruction   `CC` `HCC`

Other intestinal obstruction, NEC

K56.7 Ileus, unspecified   `CC` `HCC`

EXCLUDES 1   obstructive ileus (K56.69-)

EXCLUDES 2   intestinal obstruction with hernia (K40-K46)

AHA: 2017,1Q,40

✓4ᵗʰ K57 Diverticular disease of intestine

Code also if applicable peritonitis K65.-

EXCLUDES 1   congenital diverticulum of intestine (Q43.8)
Meckel's diverticulum (Q43.0)

EXCLUDES 2   diverticulum of appendix (K38.2)

AHA: 2018,3Q,21

TIP: Assign a code for "with bleeding" when diverticular disease of the intestine and GI bleeding are documented. The ICD-10-CM classification assumes the two are related without the provider linking the two conditions. Evidence of bleeding during a procedure is not required.

CC Excl: For codes in category K57:
For MCC codes: PDX collection 770
For CC codes, unless otherwise noted: PDX collection 794

✓5ᵗʰ K57.0 Diverticulitis of small intestine with perforation and abscess

Diverticulitis of small intestine with peritonitis

EXCLUDES 1   diverticulitis of both small and large intestine with perforation and abscess (K57.4-)

K57.00 Diverticulitis of small intestine with perforation and abscess without bleeding   `CC`

CC Excl: PDX collection 793

K57.01 Diverticulitis of small intestine with perforation and abscess with bleeding   `MCC`

✓5ᵗʰ K57.1 Diverticular disease of small intestine without perforation or abscess

EXCLUDES 1   diverticular disease of both small and large intestine without perforation or abscess (K57.5-)

K57.10 Diverticulosis of small intestine without perforation or abscess without bleeding

Diverticular disease of small intestine NOS

K57.11 Diverticulosis of small intestine without perforation or abscess with bleeding   `MCC`

K57.12 Diverticulitis of small intestine without perforation or abscess without bleeding

K57.13 Diverticulitis of small intestine without perforation or abscess with bleeding   `MCC`

✓5ᵗʰ K57.2 Diverticulitis of large intestine with perforation and abscess

Diverticulitis of colon with peritonitis

EXCLUDES 1   diverticulitis of both small and large intestine with perforation and abscess (K57.4-)

K57.20 Diverticulitis of large intestine with perforation and abscess without bleeding   `CC`

K57.21 Diverticulitis of large intestine with perforation and abscess with bleeding   `MCC`

`N` Newborn: 0   `P` Pediatric: 0-17   `M` Maternity: 9-64   `A` Adult: 15-124   `MCC` Major Complication/Comorbidity   `CC` Complication/Comorbidity   `SW` Severe Wound Dx

724   ICD-10-CM 2020

Chapter 11. Diseases of the Digestive System

√5ᵗʰ **K57.3 Diverticular disease of** large intestine without perforation or abscess

> EXCLUDES 1   *diverticular disease of both small and large intestine without perforation or abscess (K57.5-)*

K57.30 Diverticulosis of large intestine without perforation or abscess without bleeding
> Diverticular disease of colon NOS

K57.31 Diverticulosis of large intestine without perforation or abscess with bleeding   CC

K57.32 Diverticulitis of large intestine without perforation or abscess without bleeding   CC

K57.33 Diverticulitis of large intestine without perforation or abscess with bleeding   CC

√5ᵗʰ **K57.4 Diverticulitis of both** small and large intestine with perforation and abscess
> Diverticulitis of both small and large intestine with peritonitis

K57.40 Diverticulitis of both small and large intestine with perforation and abscess without bleeding   CC

K57.41 Diverticulitis of both small and large intestine with perforation and abscess with bleeding   MCC

√5ᵗʰ **K57.5 Diverticular disease of** both small and large intestine without perforation or abscess

K57.50 Diverticulosis of both small and large intestine without perforation or abscess without bleeding
> Diverticular disease of both small and large intestine NOS

K57.51 Diverticulosis of both small and large intestine without perforation or abscess with bleeding   MCC

K57.52 Diverticulitis of both small and large intestine without perforation or abscess without bleeding   CC

K57.53 Diverticulitis of both small and large intestine without perforation or abscess with bleeding   MCC

√5ᵗʰ **K57.8 Diverticulitis of intestine, part unspecified,** with perforation and abscess
> Diverticulitis of intestine NOS with peritonitis

K57.80 Diverticulitis of intestine, part unspecified, with perforation and abscess without bleeding   CC

K57.81 Diverticulitis of intestine, part unspecified, with perforation and abscess with bleeding   MCC

√5ᵗʰ **K57.9 Diverticular disease of intestine, part unspecified,** without perforation or abscess

K57.90 Diverticulosis of intestine, part unspecified, without perforation or abscess without bleeding
> Diverticular disease of intestine NOS

K57.91 Diverticulosis of intestine, part unspecified, without perforation or abscess with bleeding   MCC

K57.92 Diverticulitis of intestine, part unspecified, without perforation or abscess without bleeding   CC

K57.93 Diverticulitis of intestine, part unspecified, without perforation or abscess with bleeding   MCC

√4ᵗʰ **K58 Irritable bowel syndrome**

> INCLUDES   irritable colon
> spastic colon

AHA: 2016,4Q,32-33

K58.0 Irritable bowel syndrome with diarrhea

K58.1 Irritable bowel syndrome with constipation

K58.2 Mixed irritable bowel syndrome

K58.8 Other irritable bowel syndrome

K58.9 Irritable bowel syndrome without diarrhea
> Irritable bowel syndrome NOS

√4ᵗʰ **K59 Other functional intestinal disorders**

> EXCLUDES 1   *change in bowel habit NOS (R19.4)*
> *intestinal malabsorption (K90.-)*
> *psychogenic intestinal disorders (F45.8)*
> EXCLUDES 2   *functional disorders of stomach (K31.-)*

√5ᵗʰ **K59.0 Constipation**

> ~~Use additional code for adverse effect, if applicable, to identify~~
> ~~drug (T36-T50 with fifth or sixth character 5)~~
> EXCLUDES 1   *fecal impaction (K56.41)*
> *incomplete defecation (R15.0)*

AHA: 2016,4Q,33

K59.00 Constipation, unspecified

K59.01 Slow transit constipation
> **DEF:** Delay in the transit of fecal material through the colon secondary to smooth muscle dysfunction or decreased peristaltic contractions along the colon.

K59.02 Outlet dysfunction constipation

K59.03 Drug induced constipation
> Use additional code for adverse effect, if applicable, to identify drug (T36-T50 with fifth or sixth character 5)

K59.04 Chronic idiopathic constipation
> Functional constipation

K59.09 Other constipation
> Chronic constipation

K59.1 Functional diarrhea
> EXCLUDES 1   *diarrhea NOS (R19.7)*
> *irritable bowel syndrome with diarrhea (K58.0)*

K59.2 Neurogenic bowel, not elsewhere classified   CC
> **DEF:** Disorder of bowel due to a spinal cord lesion due to injury or as a complication of conditions such as multiple sclerosis (MS) or spina bifida. Loss of bowel control is the primary symptom, manifested as constipation or bowel incontinence.
> **CC Excl:** PDX collection 795

√5ᵗʰ **K59.3 Megacolon, not elsewhere classified**
> Dilatation of colon
> Code first, if applicable (T51-T65) to identify toxic agent
> EXCLUDES 1   *congenital megacolon (aganglionic) (Q43.1)*
> *megacolon (due to) (in) Chagas' disease (B57.32)*
> *megacolon (due to) (in) Clostridium difficile (A04.7-)*
> *megacolon (due to) (in) Hirschsprung's disease (Q43.1)*

AHA: 2016,4Q,33-34

K59.31 Toxic megacolon   CC HCC
> **CC Excl:** PDX collection 795

K59.39 Other megacolon   CC
> Megacolon NOS
> **CC Excl:** PDX collection 795

K59.4 Anal spasm
> Proctalgia fugax

K59.8 Other specified functional intestinal disorders
> Atony of colon
> Pseudo-obstruction (acute) (chronic) of intestine

K59.9 Functional intestinal disorder, unspecified

√4ᵗʰ **K60 Fissure and fistula of anal and rectal regions**

> EXCLUDES 1   *fissure and fistula of anal and rectal regions with abscess or cellulitis (K61.-)*
> EXCLUDES 2   *anal sphincter tear (healed) (nontraumatic) (old) (K62.81)*

K60.0 Acute anal fissure

K60.1 Chronic anal fissure

K60.2 Anal fissure, unspecified

K60.3 Anal fistula   SW

K60.4 Rectal fistula   SW
> Fistula of rectum to skin
> EXCLUDES 1   *rectovaginal fistula (N82.3)*
> *vesicorectal fistual (N32.1)*

K60.5 Anorectal fistula   SW

√4ᵗʰ **K61 Abscess of anal and rectal regions**

> INCLUDES   abscess of anal and rectal regions
> cellulitis of anal and rectal regions

K61.0 Anal abscess
> Perianal abscess
> EXCLUDES 2   *intrasphincteric abscess (K61.4)*

☑ Additional Character Required   √x7ᵗʰ Placeholder   Unacceptable PDx   Questionable PDx   Manifestation   Unspecified Dx   H1-H14 HAC   HCC CMS-HCC Dx   HIV HIV Dx

ICD-10-CM 2020   725

Chapter 11. Diseases of the Digestive System

K61.1   **Rectal abscess**
Perirectal abscess
EXCLUDES 1   *ischiorectal abscess (K61.39)*
AHA: 2012,4Q,104

K61.2   **Anorectal abscess**

✓5ᵗʰ **K61.3**   **Ischiorectal abscess**
AHA: 2018,4Q,19

     K61.31   **Horseshoe abscess**

     K61.39   **Other ischiorectal abscess**
Abscess of ischiorectal fossa
Ischiorectal abscess, NOS

K61.4   **Intrasphincteric abscess**
Intersphincteric abscess

K61.5   **Supralevator abscess**
AHA: 2018,4Q,19

✓4ᵗʰ **K62**   **Other diseases of anus and rectum**
INCLUDES   anal canal
EXCLUDES 2   *colostomy and enterostomy malfunction (K94.0-, K94.1-)*
fecal incontinence (R15.-)
hemorrhoids (K64.-)

K62.0   **Anal polyp**

K62.1   **Rectal polyp**
EXCLUDES 1   *adenomatous polyp (D12.8)*
AHA: 2018,1Q,6

K62.2   **Anal prolapse**
Prolapse of anal canal

K62.3   **Rectal prolapse**
Prolapse of rectal mucosa

K62.4   **Stenosis of anus and rectum**
Stricture of anus (sphincter)
AHA: 2019,2Q,13

K62.5   **Hemorrhage of anus and rectum**
EXCLUDES 1   *gastrointestinal bleeding NOS (K92.2)*
melena (K92.1)
neonatal rectal hemorrhage (P54.2)
AHA: 2019,1Q,21

K62.6   **Ulcer of anus and rectum**
Solitary ulcer of anus and rectum
Stercoral ulcer of anus and rectum
EXCLUDES 1   *fissure and fistula of anus and rectum (K60.-)*
ulcerative colitis (K51.-)

K62.7   **Radiation proctitis**
Use additional code to identify the type of radiation (W90.-)
AHA: 2019,1Q,21

✓5ᵗʰ **K62.8**   **Other specified diseases of anus and rectum**
EXCLUDES 2   *ulcerative proctitis (K51.2)*

     K62.81   **Anal sphincter tear (healed) (nontraumatic) (old)**
Tear of anus, nontraumatic
Use additional code for any associated fecal incontinence (R15.-)
EXCLUDES 2   *anal fissure (K60.-)*
anal sphincter tear (healed) (old) complicating delivery (O34.7-)
traumatic tear of anal sphincter (S31.831)

     K62.82   **Dysplasia of anus**
Anal intraepithelial neoplasia I and II (AIN I and II) (histologically confirmed)
Dysplasia of anus NOS
Mild and moderate dysplasia of anus (histologically confirmed)
EXCLUDES 1   *abnormal results from anal cytologic examination without histologic confirmation (R85.61-)*
anal intraepithelial neoplasia III (D01.3)
carcinoma in situ of anus (D01.3)
HGSIL of anus (R85.613)
severe dysplasia of anus (D01.3)

     K62.89   **Other specified diseases of anus and rectum**
Proctitis NOS
Use additional code for any associated fecal incontinence (R15.-)

K62.9   **Disease of anus and rectum, unspecified**

✓4ᵗʰ **K63**   **Other diseases of intestine**

K63.0   **Abscess of intestine**   **CC**
EXCLUDES 1   *abscess of intestine with Crohn's disease (K50.014, K50.114, K50.814, K50.914)*
abscess of intestine with diverticular disease (K57.0, K57.2, K57.4, K57.8)
abscess of intestine with ulcerative colitis (K51.014, K51.214, K51.314, K51.414, K51.514, K51.814, K51.914)
EXCLUDES 2   *abscess of anal and rectal regions (K61.-)*
abscess of appendix (K35.3-)
CC Excl: PDX collection 798

K63.1   **Perforation of intestine (nontraumatic)**   **CC MCC**
Perforation (nontraumatic) of rectum
EXCLUDES 1   *perforation (nontraumatic) of duodenum (K26.-)*
perforation (nontraumatic) of intestine with diverticular disease (K57.0, K57.2, K57.4, K57.8)
EXCLUDES 2   *perforation (nontraumatic) of appendix (K35.2-, K35.3-)*

K63.2   **Fistula of intestine**   **CC SW**
EXCLUDES 1   *fistula of duodenum (K31.6)*
fistula of intestine with Crohn's disease (K50.013, K50.113, K50.813, K50.913)
fistula of intestine with ulcerative colitis (K51.013, K51.213, K51.313, K51.413, K51.513, K51.813, K51.913)
EXCLUDES 2   *fistula of anal and rectal regions (K60.-)*
fistula of appendix (K38.3)
intestinal-genital fistula, female (N82.2-N82.4)
vesicointestinal fistula (N32.1)
AHA: 2017,3Q,4
CC Excl: PDX collection 800

K63.3   **Ulcer of intestine**   **CC**
Primary ulcer of small intestine
EXCLUDES 1   *duodenal ulcer (K26.-)*
gastrointestinal ulcer (K28.-)
gastrojejunal ulcer (K28.-)
jejunal ulcer (K28.-)
peptic ulcer, site unspecified (K27.-)
ulcer of intestine with perforation (K63.1)
ulcer of anus or rectum (K62.6)
ulcerative colitis (K51.-)
CC Excl: PDX collection 801

K63.4   **Enteroptosis**

K63.5   **Polyp of colon**
EXCLUDES 1   *adenomatous polyp of colon ▶(D12.-)◀*
inflammatory polyp of colon (K51.4-)
polyposis of colon (D12.6)
AHA: 2019,1Q,33; 2018,2Q,14; 2017,1Q,15; 2015,2Q,14
TIP: Assign this code when documentation states hyperplastic colon polyp regardless of the site in the colon. Slow-growing, hyperplastic polyps are not precancerous and are classified differently from benign or adenomatous polyps.

✓5ᵗʰ **K63.8**   **Other specified diseases of intestine**

     K63.81   **Dieulafoy lesion of intestine**   **MCC**
EXCLUDES 2   *Dieulafoy lesion of stomach and duodenum (K31.82)*
DEF: Abnormally large submucosal artery protruding through a defect in the stomach mucosa or intestines that can cause massive and life-threatening hemorrhaging.
CC Excl: PDX collection 802

     K63.89   **Other specified diseases of intestine**
AHA: 2013,2Q,31

K63.9   **Disease of intestine, unspecified**

N Newborn: 0   **P** Pediatric: 0-17   **M** Maternity: 9-64   **A** Adult: 15-124   **MCC** Major Complication/Comorbidity   **CC** Complication/Comorbidity   **SW** Severe Wound Dx

726   ICD-10-CM 2020

✓4ᵗʰ K64 Hemorrhoids and perianal venous thrombosis

INCLUDES   piles

EXCLUDES 1   hemorrhoids complicating childbirth and the puerperium (O87.2)

hemorrhoids complicating pregnancy (O22.4)

Hemorrhoids

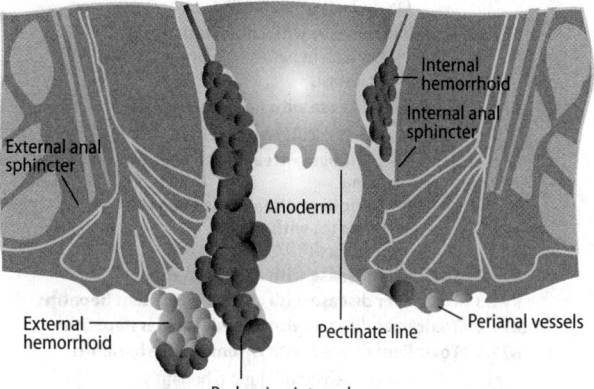

Internal hemorrhoid

Internal anal sphincter

External anal sphincter

Anoderm

External hemorrhoid

Perianal vessels

Pectinate line

Prolapsing internal hemorrhoid

K64.Ø   First degree hemorrhoids
Grade/stage I hemorrhoids
Hemorrhoids (bleeding) without prolapse outside of anal canal

K64.1   Second degree hemorrhoids
Grade/stage II hemorrhoids
Hemorrhoids (bleeding) that prolapse with straining, but retract spontaneously

K64.2   Third degree hemorrhoids
Grade/stage III hemorrhoids
Hemorrhoids (bleeding) that prolapse with straining and require manual replacement back inside anal canal

K64.3   Fourth degree hemorrhoids
Grade/stage IV hemorrhoids
Hemorrhoids (bleeding) with prolapsed tissue that cannot be manually replaced

K64.4   Residual hemorrhoidal skin tags
External hemorrhoids, NOS
Skin tags of anus

K64.5   Perianal venous thrombosis
External hemorrhoids with thrombosis
Perianal hematoma
Thrombosed hemorrhoids NOS

K64.8   Other hemorrhoids
Internal hemorrhoids, without mention of degree
Prolapsed hemorrhoids, degree not specified

K64.9   Unspecified hemorrhoids
Hemorrhoids (bleeding) NOS
Hemorrhoids (bleeding) without mention of degree

Diseases of peritoneum and retroperitoneum (K65-K68)

CC Excl: For CC/MCC codes in categories K65-K68, unless otherwise noted: PDX collection 803

✓4ᵗʰ K65 Peritonitis

Use additional code (B95-B97), to identify infectious agent, if known
Code also if applicable diverticular disease of intestine (K57.-)

EXCLUDES 1   acute appendicitis with generalized peritonitis (K35.2-)

aseptic peritonitis (T81.6)

benign paroxysmal peritonitis (E85.Ø)

chemical peritonitis (T81.6)

gonococcal peritonitis (A54.85)

neonatal peritonitis (P78.Ø-P78.1)

pelvic peritonitis, female (N73.3-N73.5)

periodic familial peritonitis (E85.Ø)

peritonitis due to talc or other foreign substance (T81.6)

peritonitis in chlamydia (A74.81)

peritonitis in diphtheria (A36.89)

peritonitis in syphilis (late) (A52.74)

peritonitis in tuberculosis (A18.31)

peritonitis with or following abortion or ectopic or molar pregnancy (OØØ-OØ7, OØ8.Ø)

peritonitis with or following appendicitis (K35.-)

puerperal peritonitis (O85)

retroperitoneal infections (K68.-)

K65.Ø   Generalized (acute) peritonitis   MCC HCC
Pelvic peritonitis (acute), male
Subphrenic peritonitis (acute)
Suppurative peritonitis (acute)

K65.1   Peritoneal abscess   MCC HCC
Abdominopelvic abscess
Abscess (of) omentum
Abscess (of) peritoneum
Mesenteric abscess
Retrocecal abscess
Subdiaphragmatic abscess
Subhepatic abscess
Subphrenic abscess
AHA: 2019,1Q,15

K65.2   Spontaneous bacterial peritonitis   MCC HCC
EXCLUDES 1   bacterial peritonitis NOS (K65.9)

K65.3   Choleperitonitis   MCC HCC
Peritonitis due to bile
DEF: Inflammation of the peritoneum due to leakage of bile into the peritoneal cavity resulting from rupture of the bile passages or gallbladder.

K65.4   Sclerosing mesenteritis   CC HCC
Fat necrosis of peritoneum
(Idiopathic) sclerosing mesenteric fibrosis
Mesenteric lipodystrophy
Mesenteric panniculitis
Retractile mesenteritis

K65.8   Other peritonitis   MCC HCC
Chronic proliferative peritonitis
Peritonitis due to urine

K65.9   Peritonitis, unspecified   MCC HCC
Bacterial peritonitis NOS
AHA: 2013,2Q,31

✓4ᵗʰ K66 Other disorders of peritoneum

EXCLUDES 2   ascites (R18.-)

peritoneal effusion (chronic) (R18.8)

K66.Ø   Peritoneal adhesions (postprocedural) (postinfection)
Adhesions (of) abdominal (wall)
Adhesions (of) diaphragm
Adhesions (of) intestine
Adhesions (of) male pelvis
Adhesions (of) omentum
Adhesions (of) stomach
Adhesive bands
Mesenteric adhesions
EXCLUDES 1   female pelvic adhesions [bands] (N73.6)

peritoneal adhesions with intestinal obstruction (K56.5-)

☑ Additional Character Required   ✓x7ᵗʰ Placeholder   Unacceptable PDx   Questionable PDx   Manifestation   Unspecified Dx   H1-H14 HAC   HCC CMS-HCC Dx   HIV HIV Dx

ICD-10-CM 2020   727

Chapter 11. Diseases of the Digestive System

K64–K66.Ø

K66.1 Hemoperitoneum `MCC`
> EXCLUDES 1   *traumatic hemoperitoneum (S36.8-)*
> **CC Excl:** PDX collection 804

K66.8 Other specified disorders of peritoneum

K66.9 Disorder of peritoneum, unspecified

K67 *Disorders of peritoneum in infectious diseases classified elsewhere* `MCC` `HCC`
> Code first underlying disease, such as:
> congenital syphilis (A50.0)
> helminthiasis (B65.0-B83.9)
> EXCLUDES 1   *peritonitis in chlamydia (A74.81)*
> *peritonitis in diphtheria (A36.89)*
> *peritonitis in gonococcal (A54.85)*
> *peritonitis in syphilis (late) (A52.74)*
> *peritonitis in tuberculosis (A18.31)*

√4th **K68 Disorders of retroperitoneum**

√5th **K68.1 Retroperitoneal abscess**

K68.11 Postprocedural retroperitoneal abscess `CC` `H11` `H12` `H13`
> EXCLUDES 2   *infection following procedure (T81.4-)*
> **CC Excl:** PDX collection 805

K68.12 Psoas muscle abscess `MCC` `HCC`
> **CC Excl:** PDX collection 806

K68.19 Other retroperitoneal abscess `MCC` `HCC`
> **AHA:** 2019,1Q,15
> **TIP:** This code should be used for a diagnosis of internal presacral abscess. If an intra-abdominal abscess is also present, code K65.1 can also be assigned; sequencing depends on the circumstances of admission.

K68.9 Other disorders of retroperitoneum `MCC`

Diseases of liver (K70-K77)

> EXCLUDES 1   *jaundice NOS (R17)*
> EXCLUDES 2   *hemochromatosis (E83.11-)*
> *Reye's syndrome (G93.7)*
> *viral hepatitis (B15-B19)*
> *Wilson's disease (E83.0)*

√4th **K70 Alcoholic liver disease**
> Use additional code to identify:
> alcohol abuse and dependence (F10.-)

K70.0 Alcoholic fatty liver `A`

√5th **K70.1 Alcoholic hepatitis**

K70.10 Alcoholic hepatitis without ascites `A`

K70.11 Alcoholic hepatitis with ascites `A`

K70.2 Alcoholic fibrosis and sclerosis of liver `A`

√5th **K70.3 Alcoholic cirrhosis of liver**
> Alcoholic cirrhosis NOS

K70.30 Alcoholic cirrhosis of liver without ascites `HCC` `A`

K70.31 Alcoholic cirrhosis of liver with ascites `HCC` `A`
> **AHA:** 2018,1Q,4

√5th **K70.4 Alcoholic hepatic failure**
> Acute alcoholic hepatic failure
> Alcoholic hepatic failure NOS
> Chronic alcoholic hepatic failure
> Subacute alcoholic hepatic failure

K70.40 Alcoholic hepatic failure without coma `HCC` `A`

K70.41 Alcoholic hepatic failure with coma `MCC` `HCC` `A`
> **CC Excl:** PDX collection 807

K70.9 Alcoholic liver disease, unspecified `HCC` `A`

√4th **K71 Toxic liver disease**
> INCLUDES   drug-induced idiosyncratic (unpredictable) liver disease
> drug-induced toxic (predictable) liver disease
> Code first poisoning due to drug or toxin, if applicable (T36-T65 with fifth or sixth character 1-4 or 6)
> Use additional code for adverse effect, if applicable, to identify drug (T36-T50 with fifth or sixth character 5)
> EXCLUDES 2   *alcoholic liver disease (K70.-)*
> *Budd-Chiari syndrome (I82.0)*

K71.0 Toxic liver disease with cholestasis
> Cholestasis with hepatocyte injury
> "Pure" cholestasis

√5th **K71.1 Toxic liver disease with hepatic necrosis**
> Hepatic failure (acute) (chronic) due to drugs

K71.10 Toxic liver disease with hepatic necrosis, without coma

K71.11 Toxic liver disease with hepatic necrosis, with coma `MCC` `HCC`
> **CC Excl:** PDX collection 807

K71.2 Toxic liver disease with acute hepatitis

K71.3 Toxic liver disease with chronic persistent hepatitis

K71.4 Toxic liver disease with chronic lobular hepatitis

√5th **K71.5 Toxic liver disease with chronic active hepatitis**
> Toxic liver disease with lupoid hepatitis

K71.50 Toxic liver disease with chronic active hepatitis without ascites

K71.51 Toxic liver disease with chronic active hepatitis with ascites
> **AHA:** 2018,1Q,4

K71.6 Toxic liver disease with hepatitis, not elsewhere classified

K71.7 Toxic liver disease with fibrosis and cirrhosis of liver

K71.8 Toxic liver disease with other disorders of liver
> Toxic liver disease with focal nodular hyperplasia
> Toxic liver disease with hepatic granulomas
> Toxic liver disease with peliosis hepatis
> Toxic liver disease with veno-occlusive disease of liver

K71.9 Toxic liver disease, unspecified

√4th **K72 Hepatic failure, not elsewhere classified**
> INCLUDES   fulminant hepatitis NEC, with hepatic failure
> hepatic encephalopathy NOS
> liver (cell) necrosis with hepatic failure
> malignant hepatitis NEC, with hepatic failure
> yellow liver atrophy or dystrophy
> EXCLUDES 1   *alcoholic hepatic failure (K70.4)*
> *hepatic failure with toxic liver disease (K71.1-)*
> *icterus of newborn (P55-P59)*
> *postprocedural hepatic failure (K91.82)*
> EXCLUDES 2   *hepatic failure complicating abortion or ectopic or molar pregnancy (O00-O07, O08.8)*
> *hepatic failure complicating pregnancy, childbirth and the puerperium (O26.6-)*
> *viral hepatitis with hepatic coma (B15-B19)*

AHA: 2017,1Q,41

√5th **K72.0 Acute and subacute hepatic failure**
> Acute non-viral hepatitis NOS
> **AHA:** 2015,2Q,17; 2014,2Q,13

K72.00 Acute and subacute hepatic failure without coma `MCC`
> **CC Excl:** PDX collection 808

K72.01 Acute and subacute hepatic failure with coma `MCC` `HCC`
> **CC Excl:** PDX collection 808

√5th **K72.1 Chronic hepatic failure**

K72.10 Chronic hepatic failure without coma `HCC`

K72.11 Chronic hepatic failure with coma `MCC` `HCC`
> **CC Excl:** PDX collection 807

√5th **K72.9 Hepatic failure, unspecified**

K72.90 Hepatic failure, unspecified without coma `HCC`
> **AHA:** 2018,4Q,20; 2016,2Q,35

K72.91 Hepatic failure, unspecified with coma `MCC` `HCC`
> Hepatic coma NOS
> **CC Excl:** PDX collection 807

☑️4ᵗʰ **K73 Chronic hepatitis, not elsewhere classified**

    EXCLUDES 1   *alcoholic hepatitis (chronic) (K70.1-)*

        drug-induced hepatitis (chronic) (K71.-)

        granulomatous hepatitis (chronic) NEC (K75.3)

        reactive, nonspecific hepatitis (chronic) (K75.2)

        viral hepatitis (chronic) (B15-B19)

    K73.0 Chronic persistent hepatitis, not elsewhere classified `HCC`

    K73.1 Chronic lobular hepatitis, not elsewhere classified `HCC`

    K73.2 Chronic active hepatitis, not elsewhere classified `HCC`

    K73.8 Other chronic hepatitis, not elsewhere classified `HCC`

    K73.9 Chronic hepatitis, unspecified `HCC`

☑️4ᵗʰ **K74 Fibrosis and cirrhosis of liver**

    Code also, if applicable, viral hepatitis (acute) (chronic) (B15-B19)

    EXCLUDES 1   *alcoholic cirrhosis (of liver) (K70.3)*

        alcoholic fibrosis of liver (K70.2)

        cardiac sclerosis of liver (K76.1)

        cirrhosis (of liver) with toxic liver disease (K71.7)

        congenital cirrhosis (of liver) (P78.81)

        pigmentary cirrhosis (of liver) (E83.110)

    K74.0 Hepatic fibrosis

    K74.1 Hepatic sclerosis

    K74.2 Hepatic fibrosis with hepatic sclerosis

    K74.3 Primary biliary cirrhosis `HCC`

        Chronic nonsuppurative destructive cholangitis

        Primary biliary cholangitis

        EXCLUDES 2 ▶*primary sclerosing cholangitis*◀ *(K83.01)*

    K74.4 Secondary biliary cirrhosis `HCC`

    K74.5 Biliary cirrhosis, unspecified `HCC`

☑️5ᵗʰ **K74.6 Other and unspecified cirrhosis of liver**

        K74.60 Unspecified cirrhosis of liver `HCC`

            Cirrhosis (of liver) NOS

            AHA: 2018,1Q,4

        K74.69 Other cirrhosis of liver `HCC`

            Cryptogenic cirrhosis (of liver)

            Macronodular cirrhosis (of liver)

            Micronodular cirrhosis (of liver)

            Mixed type cirrhosis (of liver)

            Portal cirrhosis (of liver)

            Postnecrotic cirrhosis (of liver)

☑️4ᵗʰ **K75 Other inflammatory liver diseases**

    EXCLUDES 2   *toxic liver disease (K71.-)*

    K75.0 Abscess of liver `MCC`

        Cholangitic hepatic abscess

        Hematogenic hepatic abscess

        Hepatic abscess NOS

        Lymphogenic hepatic abscess

        Pylephlebitic hepatic abscess

        EXCLUDES 1 *amebic liver abscess (A06.4)*

            cholangitis without liver abscess (K83.09)

            pylephlebitis without liver abscess (K75.1)

        EXCLUDES 2 *acute or subacute hepatitis NOS (B17.9)*

            acute or subacute non-viral hepatitis (K72.0)

            chronic hepatitis NEC (K73.8)

        CC Excl: PDX collection 809

    K75.1 Phlebitis of portal vein `MCC`

        Pylephlebitis

        EXCLUDES 1 *pylephlebitic liver abscess (K75.0)*

        DEF: Inflammation of the portal vein or branches due to diverticulitis, perforated appendicitis, or peritonitis. Symptoms include fever, chills, jaundice, sweating, and abscess in various body parts.

        CC Excl: PDX collection 809

    K75.2 Nonspecific reactive hepatitis

        EXCLUDES 1 *acute or subacute hepatitis (K72.0-)*

            chronic hepatitis NEC (K73.-)

            viral hepatitis (B15-B19)

    K75.3 Granulomatous hepatitis, not elsewhere classified

        EXCLUDES 1 *acute or subacute hepatitis (K72.0-)*

            chronic hepatitis NEC (K73.-)

            viral hepatitis (B15-B19)

    K75.4 Autoimmune hepatitis `HCC`

        Lupoid hepatitis NEC

☑️5ᵗʰ **K75.8 Other specified inflammatory liver diseases**

        K75.81 Nonalcoholic steatohepatitis (NASH)

        K75.89 Other specified inflammatory liver diseases

    K75.9 Inflammatory liver disease, unspecified

        Hepatitis NOS

        EXCLUDES 1 *acute or subacute hepatitis (K72.0-)*

            chronic hepatitis NEC (K73.-)

            viral hepatitis (B15-B19)

    AHA: 2015,2Q,17

☑️4ᵗʰ **K76 Other diseases of liver**

    EXCLUDES 2   *alcoholic liver disease (K70.-)*

        amyloid degeneration of liver (E85.-)

        cystic disease of liver (congenital) (Q44.6)

        hepatic vein thrombosis (I82.0)

        hepatomegaly NOS (R16.0)

        pigmentary cirrhosis (of liver) (E83.110)

        portal vein thrombosis (I81)

        toxic liver disease (K71.-)

    K76.0 Fatty (change of) liver, not elsewhere classified

        Nonalcoholic fatty liver disease (NAFLD)

        EXCLUDES 1 *nonalcoholic steatohepatitis (NASH) (K75.81)*

    K76.1 Chronic passive congestion of liver `CC`

        Cardiac cirrhosis

        Cardiac sclerosis

    K76.2 Central hemorrhagic necrosis of liver `MCC`

        EXCLUDES 1 *liver necrosis with hepatic failure (K72.-)*

        CC Excl: PDX collection 808

    K76.3 Infarction of liver `MCC`

        CC Excl: PDX collection 808

    K76.4 Peliosis hepatis

        Hepatic angiomatosis

    K76.5 Hepatic veno-occlusive disease

        EXCLUDES 1 *Budd-Chiari syndrome (I82.0)*

    K76.6 Portal hypertension `CC` `HCC`

        Use additional code for any associated complications, such as: portal hypertensive gastropathy (K31.89)

        CC Excl: PDX collection 810

    K76.7 Hepatorenal syndrome `MCC` `HCC`

        EXCLUDES 1 *hepatorenal syndrome following labor and delivery (O90.4)*

            postprocedural hepatorenal syndrome (K91.83)

        CC Excl: PDX collection 811

☑️5ᵗʰ **K76.8 Other specified diseases of liver**

        K76.81 Hepatopulmonary syndrome `HCC`

            Code first underlying liver disease, such as:

                alcoholic cirrhosis of liver (K70.3-)

                cirrhosis of liver without mention of alcohol (K74.6-)

        K76.89 Other specified diseases of liver

            Cyst (simple) of liver

            Focal nodular hyperplasia of liver

            Hepatoptosis

    K76.9 Liver disease, unspecified

☑️ Additional Character Required   ✓x7ᵗʰ Placeholder   Unacceptable PDx   Questionable PDx   Manifestation   Unspecified Dx   H1 - H14 HAC   `HCC` CMS-HCC Dx   `HIV` HIV Dx

K77 Liver disorders in diseases classified elsewhere `CC`

Code first underlying disease, such as:
- amyloidosis (E85.-)
- congenital syphilis (A50.0, A50.5)
- congenital toxoplasmosis (P37.1)
- schistosomiasis (B65.0-B65.9)

EXCLUDES 1 alcoholic hepatitis (K70.1-)
alcoholic liver disease (K70.-)
cytomegaloviral hepatitis (B25.1)
herpesviral [herpes simplex] hepatitis (B00.81)
infectious mononucleosis with liver disease (B27.0-B27.9 with .9)
mumps hepatitis (B26.81)
sarcoidosis with liver disease (D86.89)
secondary syphilis with liver disease (A51.45)
syphilis (late) with liver disease (A52.74)
toxoplasmosis (acquired) hepatitis (B58.1)
tuberculosis with liver disease (A18.83)

CC Excl: No Excl

Disorders of gallbladder, biliary tract and pancreas (K80-K87)

✓4ᵗʰ K80 Cholelithiasis

EXCLUDES 1 *retained cholelithiasis following cholecystectomy (K91.86)*
AHA: 2018,4Q,20
DEF: Presence or formation of concretions (calculi or "gallstones") in the gallbladder. The stones contain cholesterol, calcium carbonate, or calcium bilirubinate in pure forms or in various combinations.

Cholelithiasis

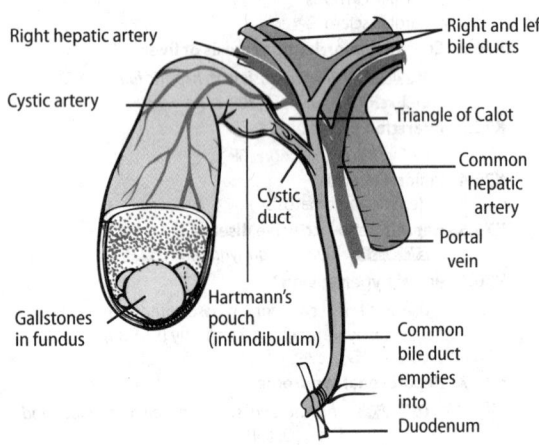

Right hepatic artery — Right and left bile ducts
Cystic artery — Triangle of Calot
Cystic duct — Common hepatic artery
Portal vein
Gallstones in fundus — Hartmann's pouch (infundibulum) — Common bile duct empties into Duodenum

✓5ᵗʰ K80.0 Calculus of gallbladder with acute cholecystitis

Any condition listed in K80.2 with acute cholecystitis
Use additional code if applicable for associated gangrene of gallbladder (K82.A1), or perforation of gallbladder (K82.A2)

K80.00 Calculus of gallbladder with acute cholecystitis without obstruction

K80.01 Calculus of gallbladder with acute cholecystitis with obstruction
CC Excl: PDX collection 813

✓5ᵗʰ K80.1 Calculus of gallbladder with other cholecystitis

Use additional code if applicable for associated gangrene of gallbladder (K82.A1), or perforation of gallbladder (K82.A2)
CC Excl: For CC codes in subcategory K80.1: PDX collection 813

K80.10 Calculus of gallbladder with chronic cholecystitis without obstruction
Cholelithiasis with cholecystitis NOS

K80.11 Calculus of gallbladder with chronic cholecystitis with obstruction `CC`

K80.12 Calculus of gallbladder with acute and chronic cholecystitis without obstruction

K80.13 Calculus of gallbladder with acute and chronic cholecystitis with obstruction `CC`

K80.18 Calculus of gallbladder with other cholecystitis without obstruction

K80.19 Calculus of gallbladder with other cholecystitis with obstruction `CC`

✓5ᵗʰ K80.2 Calculus of gallbladder without cholecystitis

Cholecystolithiasis without cholecystitis
Cholelithiasis (without cholecystitis)
Colic (recurrent) of gallbladder (without cholecystitis)
Gallstone (impacted) of cystic duct (without cholecystitis)
Gallstone (impacted) of gallbladder (without cholecystitis)

K80.20 Calculus of gallbladder without cholecystitis without obstruction

K80.21 Calculus of gallbladder without cholecystitis with obstruction `CC`
CC Excl: PDX collection 813

✓5ᵗʰ K80.3 Calculus of bile duct with cholangitis

Any condition listed in K80.5 with cholangitis
DEF: Cholangitis: Inflammation of the bile ducts.
CC Excl: For CC codes in subcategory K80.3, unless otherwise noted: PDX collection 814

K80.30 Calculus of bile duct with cholangitis, unspecified, without obstruction `CC`

K80.31 Calculus of bile duct with cholangitis, unspecified, with obstruction `CC`
CC Excl: PDX collection 815

K80.32 Calculus of bile duct with acute cholangitis without obstruction `CC`

K80.33 Calculus of bile duct with acute cholangitis with obstruction `CC`
CC Excl: PDX collection 815

K80.34 Calculus of bile duct with chronic cholangitis without obstruction `CC`

K80.35 Calculus of bile duct with chronic cholangitis with obstruction `CC`
CC Excl: PDX collection 815

K80.36 Calculus of bile duct with acute and chronic cholangitis without obstruction `CC`

K80.37 Calculus of bile duct with acute and chronic cholangitis with obstruction `CC`
CC Excl: PDX collection 815

✓5ᵗʰ K80.4 Calculus of bile duct with cholecystitis

Any condition listed in K80.5 with cholecystitis (with cholangitis)
Use additional code if applicable for associated gangrene of gallbladder (K82.A1), or perforation of gallbladder (K82.A2)
AHA: 2019,1Q,17
CC Excl: For CC codes in subcategory K80.4: PDX collection 815

K80.40 Calculus of bile duct with cholecystitis, unspecified, without obstruction `CC`

K80.41 Calculus of bile duct with cholecystitis, unspecified, with obstruction `CC`
AHA: 2019,1Q,17

K80.42 Calculus of bile duct with acute cholecystitis without obstruction `CC`

K80.43 Calculus of bile duct with acute cholecystitis with obstruction `CC`

K80.44 Calculus of bile duct with chronic cholecystitis without obstruction `CC`

K80.45 Calculus of bile duct with chronic cholecystitis with obstruction `CC`

K80.46 Calculus of bile duct with acute and chronic cholecystitis without obstruction `CC`

K80.47 Calculus of bile duct with acute and chronic cholecystitis with obstruction `CC`

✓5ᵗʰ K80.5 Calculus of bile duct without cholangitis or cholecystitis

Choledocholithiasis (without cholangitis or cholecystitis)
Gallstone (impacted) of bile duct NOS (without cholangitis or cholecystitis)
Gallstone (impacted) of common duct (without cholangitis or cholecystitis)
Gallstone (impacted) of hepatic duct (without cholangitis or cholecystitis)
Hepatic cholelithiasis (without cholangitis or cholecystitis)
Hepatic colic (recurrent) (without cholangitis or cholecystitis)
DEF: Cholangitis: Inflammation of the bile ducts.

K80.50 Calculus of bile duct without cholangitis or cholecystitis without obstruction `CC`

K80.51 **Calculus of bile duct without cholangitis or cholecystitis with obstruction** `CC`
CC Excl: PDX collection 815

√5ᵗʰ **K80.6** **Calculus of gallbladder and bile duct with cholecystitis**
Use additional code if applicable for associated gangrene of gallbladder (K82.A1), or perforation of gallbladder (K82.A2)
CC Excl: For CC codes in subcategory K80.6, unless otherwise noted: PDX collection 815

K80.60 **Calculus of gallbladder and bile duct with cholecystitis, unspecified, without obstruction** `CC`

K80.61 **Calculus of gallbladder and bile duct with cholecystitis, unspecified, with obstruction** `CC`

K80.62 **Calculus of gallbladder and bile duct with acute cholecystitis without obstruction** `CC`

K80.63 **Calculus of gallbladder and bile duct with acute cholecystitis with obstruction** `CC`
CC Excl: PDX collection 816

K80.64 **Calculus of gallbladder and bile duct with chronic cholecystitis without obstruction** `CC`

K80.65 **Calculus of gallbladder and bile duct with chronic cholecystitis with obstruction** `CC`

K80.66 **Calculus of gallbladder and bile duct with acute and chronic cholecystitis without obstruction** `CC`
CC Excl: PDX collection 817

K80.67 **Calculus of gallbladder and bile duct with acute and chronic cholecystitis with obstruction** `CC`

√5ᵗʰ **K80.7** **Calculus of gallbladder and bile duct without cholecystitis**

K80.70 **Calculus of gallbladder and bile duct without cholecystitis without obstruction** `CC`

K80.71 **Calculus of gallbladder and bile duct without cholecystitis with obstruction** `CC`
CC Excl: PDX collection 815

√5ᵗʰ **K80.8** **Other cholelithiasis**

K80.80 **Other cholelithiasis without obstruction**

K80.81 **Other cholelithiasis with obstruction** `CC`
CC Excl: PDX collection 815

√4ᵗʰ **K81** **Cholecystitis**
Use additional code if applicable for associated gangrene of gallbladder (K82.A1), or perforation of gallbladder (K82.A2)
EXCLUDES 1 cholecystitis with cholelithiasis (K80.-)
AHA: 2018,4Q,20

K81.0 **Acute cholecystitis** `CC`
Abscess of gallbladder
Angiocholecystitis
Emphysematous (acute) cholecystitis
Empyema of gallbladder
Gangrene of gallbladder
Gangrenous cholecystitis
Suppurative cholecystitis
CC Excl: PDX collection 818

K81.1 **Chronic cholecystitis**

K81.2 **Acute cholecystitis with chronic cholecystitis** `CC`
CC Excl: PDX collection 819

K81.9 **Cholecystitis, unspecified**

√4ᵗʰ **K82** **Other diseases of gallbladder**
EXCLUDES 1 nonvisualization of gallbladder (R93.2)
postcholecystectomy syndrome (K91.5)
CC Excl: For CC codes in category K82: PDX collection 820

K82.0 **Obstruction of gallbladder** `CC`
Occlusion of cystic duct or gallbladder without cholelithiasis
Stenosis of cystic duct or gallbladder without cholelithiasis
Stricture of cystic duct or gallbladder without cholelithiasis
EXCLUDES 1 obstruction of gallbladder with cholelithiasis (K80.-)

K82.1 **Hydrops of gallbladder**
Mucocele of gallbladder

K82.2 **Perforation of gallbladder** `CC`
Rupture of cystic duct or gallbladder
EXCLUDES 1 perforation of gallbladder in cholecystitis (K82.A2)

K82.3 **Fistula of gallbladder** `CC`
Cholecystocolic fistula
Cholecystoduodenal fistula

K82.4 **Cholesterolosis of gallbladder**
Strawberry gallbladder
EXCLUDES 1 cholesterolosis of gallbladder with cholecystitis (K81.-)
cholesterolosis of gallbladder with cholelithiasis (K80.-)

K82.8 **Other specified diseases of gallbladder**
Adhesions of cystic duct or gallbladder
Atrophy of cystic duct or gallbladder
Cyst of cystic duct or gallbladder
Dyskinesia of cystic duct or gallbladder
Hypertrophy of cystic duct or gallbladder
Nonfunctioning of cystic duct or gallbladder
Ulcer of cystic duct or gallbladder

K82.9 **Disease of gallbladder, unspecified**

√5ᵗʰ **K82.A** **Disorders of gallbladder in diseases classified elsewhere**
Code first the type of cholecystitis (K81.-), or cholelithiasis with cholecystitis (K80.00-K80.19, K80.40-K80.47, K80.60-K80.67)
AHA: 2018,4Q,19-20

K82.A1 *Gangrene of gallbladder in cholecystitis*

K82.A2 *Perforation of gallbladder in cholecystitis* `CC`

√4ᵗʰ **K83** **Other diseases of biliary tract**
EXCLUDES 1 postcholecystectomy syndrome (K91.5)
EXCLUDES 2 conditions involving the gallbladder (K81-K82)
conditions involving the cystic duct (K81-K82)

√5ᵗʰ **K83.0** **Cholangitis**
EXCLUDES 1 cholangitic liver abscess (K75.0)
cholangitis with choledocholithiasis (K80.3-, K80.4-)
EXCLUDES 2 chronic nonsuppurative destructive cholangitis (K74.3)
primary biliary cholangitis (K74.3)
primary biliary cirrhosis (K74.3)
AHA: 2018,4Q,20

K83.01 **Primary sclerosing cholangitis** `CC`
CC Excl: PDX collection 814

K83.09 **Other cholangitis** `CC`
Ascending cholangitis
Cholangitis NOS
Primary cholangitis
Recurrent cholangitis
Sclerosing cholangitis
Secondary cholangitis
Stenosing cholangitis
Suppurative cholangitis
CC Excl: PDX collection 814

K83.1 **Obstruction of bile duct** `MCC`
Occlusion of bile duct without cholelithiasis
Stenosis of bile duct without cholelithiasis
Stricture of bile duct without cholelithiasis
EXCLUDES 1 congenital obstruction of bile duct (Q44.3)
obstruction of bile duct with cholelithiasis (K80.-)
AHA: 2016,1Q,18
CC Excl: PDX collection 821

K83.2 **Perforation of bile duct** `MCC`
Rupture of bile duct
CC Excl: PDX collection 822

K83.3 **Fistula of bile duct** `CC`
Choledochoduodenal fistula
AHA: 2019,1Q,17
CC Excl: PDX collection 822

K83.4 **Spasm of sphincter of Oddi**

K83.5 **Biliary cyst**

K83.8 **Other specified diseases of biliary tract**
Adhesions of biliary tract
Atrophy of biliary tract
Hypertrophy of biliary tract
Ulcer of biliary tract

K83.9 **Disease of biliary tract, unspecified**

Chapter 11. Diseases of the Digestive System

K80.51-K83.9

Chapter 11. Diseases of the Digestive System

K85–K91.0

☑4ᵗʰ **K85 Acute pancreatitis**

INCLUDES   acute (recurrent) pancreatitis

     subacute pancreatitis

AHA: 2016,4Q,34

CC Excl: For MCC codes in category K85: PDX collection 177

☑5ᵗʰ **K85.0 Idiopathic acute pancreatitis**

K85.00 Idiopathic acute pancreatitis   MCC
without necrosis or infection

K85.01 Idiopathic acute pancreatitis with   MCC
uninfected necrosis

K85.02 Idiopathic acute pancreatitis with   MCC
infected necrosis

☑5ᵗʰ **K85.1 Biliary acute pancreatitis**

Gallstone pancreatitis

K85.10 Biliary acute pancreatitis without   MCC
necrosis or infection

K85.11 Biliary acute pancreatitis with   MCC
uninfected necrosis

K85.12 Biliary acute pancreatitis with   MCC
infected necrosis

☑5ᵗʰ **K85.2 Alcohol induced acute pancreatitis**

EXCLUDES 2   alcohol induced chronic pancreatitis (K86.0)

K85.20 Alcohol induced acute pancreatitis   MCC
without necrosis or infection

K85.21 Alcohol induced acute pancreatitis   MCC
with uninfected necrosis

K85.22 Alcohol induced acute pancreatitis   MCC
with infected necrosis

☑5ᵗʰ **K85.3 Drug induced acute pancreatitis**

Use additional code for adverse effect, if applicable, to identify drug (T36-T50 with fifth or sixth character 5)

Use additional code to identify drug abuse and dependence (F11.- F17.-)

K85.30 Drug induced acute pancreatitis   MCC
without necrosis or infection

K85.31 Drug induced acute pancreatitis with   MCC
uninfected necrosis

K85.32 Drug induced acute pancreatitis with   MCC
infected necrosis

☑5ᵗʰ **K85.8 Other acute pancreatitis**

K85.80 Other acute pancreatitis without   MCC
necrosis or infection

K85.81 Other acute pancreatitis with   MCC
uninfected necrosis

K85.82 Other acute pancreatitis with   MCC
infected necrosis

☑5ᵗʰ **K85.9 Acute pancreatitis, unspecified**

Pancreatitis NOS

K85.90 Acute pancreatitis without necrosis   MCC
or infection, unspecified

K85.91 Acute pancreatitis with uninfected   MCC
necrosis, unspecified

K85.92 Acute pancreatitis with infected   MCC
necrosis, unspecified

☑4ᵗʰ **K86 Other diseases of pancreas**

EXCLUDES 2   fibrocystic disease of pancreas (E84.-)

     islet cell tumor (of pancreas) (D13.7)

     pancreatic steatorrhea (K90.3)

K86.0 Alcohol-induced chronic pancreatitis   HCC

Use additional code to identify:

     alcohol abuse and dependence (F10.-)

Code also exocrine pancreatic insufficiency (K86.81)

EXCLUDES 2   alcohol induced acute pancreatitis (K85.2-)

K86.1 Other chronic pancreatitis   HCC

Chronic pancreatitis NOS

Infectious chronic pancreatitis

Recurrent chronic pancreatitis

Relapsing chronic pancreatitis

Code also exocrine pancreatic insufficiency (K86.81)

K86.2 Cyst of pancreas

K86.3 Pseudocyst of pancreas

☑5ᵗʰ **K86.8 Other specified diseases of pancreas**

AHA: 2016,4Q,34-35

K86.81 Exocrine pancreatic insufficiency

K86.89 Other specified diseases of pancreas

Aseptic pancreatic necrosis, unrelated to acute pancreatitis

Atrophy of pancreas

Calculus of pancreas

Cirrhosis of pancreas

Fibrosis of pancreas

Pancreatic fat necrosis, unrelated to acute pancreatitis

Pancreatic infantilism

Pancreatic necrosis NOS, unrelated to acute pancreatitis

K86.9 Disease of pancreas, unspecified

K87 Disorders of gallbladder, biliary tract and pancreas in diseases classified elsewhere

Code first underlying disease

EXCLUDES 1   cytomegaloviral pancreatitis (B25.2)

     mumps pancreatitis (B26.3)

     syphilitic gallbladder (A52.74)

     syphilitic pancreas (A52.74)

     tuberculosis of gallbladder (A18.83)

     tuberculosis of pancreas (A18.83)

Other diseases of the digestive system (K90-K95)

☑4ᵗʰ **K90 Intestinal malabsorption**

EXCLUDES 1   intestinal malabsorption following gastrointestinal surgery (K91.2)

AHA: 2017,4Q,108

K90.0 Celiac disease

Celiac disease with steatorrhea

Celiac gluten-sensitive enteropathy

Nontropical sprue

Use additional code for associated disorders including:

     dermatitis herpetiformis (L13.0)

     gluten ataxia (G32.81)

Code also exocrine pancreatic insufficiency (K86.81)

DEF: Malabsorption syndrome due to gluten consumption. Symptoms include fetid, bulky, frothy, oily stools; a distended abdomen; gas; asthenia; electrolyte depletion; and vitamin B, D, and K deficiency.

K90.1 Tropical sprue

Sprue NOS

Tropical steatorrhea

K90.2 Blind loop syndrome, not elsewhere classified

Blind loop syndrome NOS

EXCLUDES 1   congenital blind loop syndrome (Q43.8)

         postsurgical blind loop syndrome (K91.2)

K90.3 Pancreatic steatorrhea

☑5ᵗʰ **K90.4 Other malabsorption due to intolerance**

EXCLUDES 2   celiac gluten-sensitive enteropathy (K90.0)

         lactose intolerance (E73.-)

AHA: 2016,4Q,35-36

K90.41 Non-celiac gluten sensitivity

Gluten sensitivity NOS

Non-celiac gluten sensitive enteropathy

K90.49 Malabsorption due to intolerance, not elsewhere classified

Malabsorption due to intolerance to carbohydrate

Malabsorption due to intolerance to fat

Malabsorption due to intolerance to protein

Malabsorption due to intolerance to starch

☑5ᵗʰ **K90.8 Other intestinal malabsorption**

K90.81 Whipple's disease

K90.89 Other intestinal malabsorption

K90.9 Intestinal malabsorption, unspecified

☑4ᵗʰ **K91 Intraoperative and postprocedural complications and disorders of digestive system, not elsewhere classified**

EXCLUDES 2   complications of artificial opening of digestive system (K94.-)

     complications of bariatric procedures (K95.-)

     gastrojejunal ulcer (K28.-)

     postprocedural (radiation) retroperitoneal abscess (K68.11)

     radiation colitis (K52.0)

     radiation gastroenteritis (K52.0)

     radiation proctitis (K62.7)

AHA: 2016,4Q,9-10

K91.0 Vomiting following gastrointestinal surgery

N Newborn: 0   P Pediatric: 0-17   M Maternity: 9-64   A Adult: 15-124   MCC Major Complication/Comorbidity   CC Complication/Comorbidity   SW Severe Wound Dx

732   ICD-10-CM 2020

K91.1 **Postgastric surgery syndromes**
Dumping syndrome
Postgastrectomy syndrome
Postvagotomy syndrome

K91.2 **Postsurgical malabsorption, not elsewhere classified**
Postsurgical blind loop syndrome
EXCLUDES 1   *malabsorption osteomalacia in adults (M83.2)*
malabsorption osteoporosis, postsurgical (M80.8-, M81.8)

√5ᵗʰ **K91.3** **Postprocedural intestinal obstruction**
AHA: 2017,4Q,16-17; 2017,1Q,40
CC Excl: For CC codes in subcategory K91.3: PDX collection 792

    K91.30 **Postprocedural intestinal**   CC
obstruction, unspecified as to partial versus complete
Postprocedural intestinal obstruction NOS

    K91.31 **Postprocedural partial intestinal**   CC
obstruction
Postprocedural incomplete intestinal obstruction

    K91.32 **Postprocedural complete intestinal**   MCC
obstruction

K91.5 **Postcholecystectomy syndrome**

√5ᵗʰ **K91.6** **Intraoperative hemorrhage and hematoma of a digestive system organ or structure complicating a procedure**
EXCLUDES 1   *intraoperative hemorrhage and hematoma of a digestive system organ or structure due to accidental puncture and laceration during a procedure (K91.7-)*

    K91.61 **Intraoperative hemorrhage and**   CC
hematoma of a digestive system organ or structure complicating a digestive system procedure
CC Excl: PDX collection 829

    K91.62 **Intraoperative hemorrhage and**   CC
hematoma of a digestive system organ or structure complicating other procedure
CC Excl: PDX collection 829

√5ᵗʰ **K91.7** **Accidental puncture and laceration of a digestive system organ or structure during a procedure**

    K91.71 **Accidental puncture and laceration**   CC
of a digestive system organ or structure during a digestive system procedure
CC Excl: PDX collection 509

    K91.72 **Accidental puncture and laceration**   CC
of a digestive system organ or structure during other procedure
AHA: 2019,2Q,23
CC Excl: PDX collection 509

√5ᵗʰ **K91.8** **Other intraoperative and postprocedural complications and disorders of digestive system**
CC Excl: For CC codes in subcategory K91.8, unless otherwise noted: PDX collection 828

    K91.81 **Other intraoperative complications**   CC
of digestive system

    K91.82 **Postprocedural hepatic failure**   CC

    K91.83 **Postprocedural hepatorenal**   CC
syndrome

√6ᵗʰ **K91.84** **Postprocedural hemorrhage of a digestive system organ or structure following a procedure**

      K91.840 **Postprocedural**   CC
hemorrhage of a digestive system organ or structure following a digestive system procedure
AHA: 2016,1Q,15
CC Excl: PDX collection 829

      K91.841 **Postprocedural**   CC
hemorrhage of a digestive system organ or structure following other procedure
CC Excl: PDX collection 829

√6ᵗʰ **K91.85** **Complications of intestinal pouch**

    K91.850 **Pouchitis**   CC   HCC
Inflammation of internal ileoanal pouch
DEF: Inflammatory complication of an existing surgically created ileoanal pouch, resulting in multiple GI complaints, including diarrhea, abdominal pain, rectal bleeding, fecal urgency, or incontinence.

    K91.858 **Other complications of**   CC   HCC
intestinal pouch
AHA: 2019,2Q,13

K91.86 **Retained cholelithiasis following**   CC
cholecystectomy

√6ᵗʰ **K91.87** **Postprocedural hematoma and seroma of a digestive system organ or structure following a procedure**
CC Excl: For CC codes in subcategory K91.87: PDX collection 829

    K91.870 **Postprocedural hematoma**   CC
of a digestive system organ or structure following a digestive system procedure

    K91.871 **Postprocedural hematoma**   CC
of a digestive system organ or structure following other procedure

    K91.872 **Postprocedural seroma of**   CC
a digestive system organ or structure following a digestive system procedure

    K91.873 **Postprocedural seroma of**   CC
a digestive system organ or structure following other procedure

K91.89 **Other postprocedural complications**   CC
and disorders of digestive system
Use additional code, if applicable, to further specify disorder
EXCLUDES 2   *postprocedural retroperitoneal abscess (K68.11)*
AHA: 2017,1Q,40

√4ᵗʰ **K92** **Other diseases of digestive system**
EXCLUDES 1   *neonatal gastrointestinal hemorrhage (P54.0-P54.3)*
CC Excl: For CC codes in category K92, unless otherwise noted: PDX collection 770

K92.0 **Hematemesis**   CC

K92.1 **Melena**   CC
EXCLUDES 1   *occult blood in feces (R19.5)*

K92.2 **Gastrointestinal hemorrhage, unspecified**   CC
Gastric hemorrhage NOS
Intestinal hemorrhage NOS
EXCLUDES 1   *acute hemorrhagic gastritis (K29.01)*
hemorrhage of anus and rectum (K62.5)
angiodysplasia of stomach with hemorrhage (K31.811)
diverticular disease with hemorrhage (K57.-)
gastritis and duodenitis with hemorrhage (K29.-)
peptic ulcer with hemorrhage (K25-K28)

√5ᵗʰ **K92.8** **Other specified diseases of the digestive system**

    K92.81 **Gastrointestinal mucositis**   CC
(ulcerative)
Code also type of associated therapy, such as:
antineoplastic and immunosuppressive drugs (T45.1X-)
radiological procedure and radiotherapy (Y84.2)
EXCLUDES 2   *mucositis (ulcerative) of vagina and vulva (N76.81)*
nasal mucositis (ulcerative) (J34.81)
oral mucositis (ulcerative) (K12.3-)
CC Excl: PDX collection 765

    K92.89 **Other specified diseases of the digestive system**

K92.9 **Disease of digestive system, unspecified**

✓4ᵗʰ **K94** **Complications of artificial openings of the digestive system**

    CC Excl: For CC codes in category K94, unless otherwise noted: PDX collection 830

  ✓5ᵗʰ **K94.0** **Colostomy** complications

      K94.00 **Colostomy complication, unspecified**   HCC

      K94.01 **Colostomy** hemorrhage   CC HCC

      K94.02 **Colostomy** infection   CC HCC

        Use additional code to specify type of infection, such as:
          cellulitis of abdominal wall (L03.311)
          sepsis (A40.-, A41.-)

      K94.03 **Colostomy** malfunction   CC HCC

        Mechanical complication of colostomy
        CC Excl: PDX collection 831

      K94.09 **Other complications of colostomy**   CC HCC

  ✓5ᵗʰ **K94.1** **Enterostomy** complications

      K94.10 **Enterostomy complication, unspecified**   HCC

      K94.11 **Enterostomy** hemorrhage   CC HCC

      K94.12 **Enterostomy** infection   CC HCC

        Use additional code to specify type of infection, such as:
          cellulitis of abdominal wall (L03.311)
          sepsis (A40.-, A41.-)

      K94.13 **Enterostomy** malfunction   CC HCC

        Mechanical complication of enterostomy
        CC Excl: PDX collection 831

      K94.19 **Other complications of enterostomy**   CC HCC

  ✓5ᵗʰ **K94.2** **Gastrostomy** complications

      K94.20 **Gastrostomy complication, unspecified**   HCC

      K94.21 **Gastrostomy** hemorrhage   HCC

      K94.22 **Gastrostomy** infection   CC HCC

        Use additional code to specify type of infection, such as:
          cellulitis of abdominal wall (L03.311)
          sepsis (A40.-, A41.-)
        CC Excl: PDX collection 828

      K94.23 **Gastrostomy** malfunction   CC HCC

        Mechanical complication of gastrostomy
        AHA: 2019,1Q,26
        CC Excl: PDX collection 828

      K94.29 **Other complications of gastrostomy**   HCC

  ✓5ᵗʰ **K94.3** **Esophagostomy** complications

    CC Excl: For CC codes in subcategory K94.3: PDX collection 828

      K94.30 **Esophagostomy complications, unspecified**   CC HCC

      K94.31 **Esophagostomy** hemorrhage   CC HCC

      K94.32 **Esophagostomy** infection   CC HCC

        Use additional code to identify the infection

      K94.33 **Esophagostomy** malfunction   CC HCC

        Mechanical complication of esophagostomy

      K94.39 **Other complications of esophagostomy**   CC HCC

✓4ᵗʰ **K95** **Complications of bariatric procedures**

    CC Excl: For CC codes in category K95: PDX collection 828

  ✓5ᵗʰ **K95.0** **Complications of** gastric band procedure

      K95.01 Infection **due to gastric band procedure**   CC H11

        Use additional code to specify type of infection or organism, such as:
          bacterial and viral infectious agents (B95.-, B96.-)
          cellulitis of abdominal wall (L03.311)
          sepsis (A40.-, A41.-)

      K95.09 **Other complications of gastric band procedure**   CC

        Use additional code, if applicable, to further specify complication

  ✓5ᵗʰ **K95.8** **Complications of other bariatric procedure**

    EXCLUDES 1   *complications of gastric band surgery (K95.0-)*

      K95.81 Infection **due to other bariatric procedure**   CC H11

        Use additional code to specify type of infection or organism, such as:
          bacterial and viral infectious agents (B95.-, B96.-)
          cellulitis of abdominal wall (L03.311)
          sepsis (A40.-, A41.-)

      K95.89 **Other complications of other bariatric procedure**   CC

        Use additional code, if applicable, to further specify complication

N Newborn: 0   P Pediatric: 0-17   M Maternity: 9-64   A Adult: 15-124   MCC Major Complication/Comorbidity   CC Complication/Comorbidity   SW Severe Wound Dx

734   ICD-10-CM 2020

Chapter 12. Diseases of the Skin and Subcutaneous Tissue (L00–L99)

Chapter-specific Guidelines with Coding Examples

The chapter-specific guidelines from the ICD-10-CM Official Guidelines for Coding and Reporting have been provided below. Along with these guidelines are coding examples, contained in the shaded boxes, that have been developed to help illustrate the coding and/or sequencing guidance found in these guidelines.

a. Pressure ulcer stage codes

1) Pressure ulcer stages

Codes **in** category L89, Pressure ulcer, identify the site **and stage** of the pressure ulcer.

The ICD-10-CM classifies pressure ulcer stages based on severity, which is designated by stages 1-4, **deep tissue pressure injury,** unspecified stage, and unstageable.

Assign as many codes from category L89 as needed to identify all the pressure ulcers the patient has, if applicable.

See Section I.B.14 for pressure ulcer stage documentation by clinicians other than patient's provider

---
Nursing notes: Dressings changed daily on stage 4 ulcer on heel and stage 2 ulcer on elbow

Discharge summary: Pressure ulcers on right heel and left elbow

L89.614   Pressure ulcer of right heel, stage 4

L89.022   Pressure ulcer of left elbow, stage 2

Explanation: Right heel and left elbow pressure ulcers were documented by the patient's provider in the discharge summary. Although the stage of these ulcers was not included in the provider's diagnostic statement, it is appropriate to code the stage from documentation from other clinicians involved in the patient's care, such as the nurse's notes, according to section I.B.14. Combination codes from category L89 Pressure ulcer, identify the site of the pressure ulcer as well as the stage. Assign as many codes from category L89 as needed to identify all the pressure ulcers the patient has.

---

2) Unstageable pressure ulcers

Assignment of the code for unstageable pressure ulcer (L89.--0) should be based on the clinical documentation. These codes are used for pressure ulcers whose stage cannot be clinically determined (e.g., the ulcer is covered by eschar or has been treated with a skin or muscle graft). This code should not be confused with the codes for unspecified stage (L89.--9). When there is no documentation regarding the stage of the pressure ulcer, assign the appropriate code for unspecified stage (L89.--9).

Pressure ulcer of the right lower back documented as unstageable due to the presence of thick eschar covering the ulcer

L89.130   Pressure ulcer of right lower back, unstageable

Explanation: Codes for unstageable pressure ulcers are assigned when the stage cannot be clinically determined (e.g., the ulcer is covered by eschar or has been treated with a skin or muscle graft).

---

3) Documented pressure ulcer stage

Assignment of the pressure ulcer stage code should be guided by clinical documentation of the stage or documentation of the terms found in the Alphabetic Index. For clinical terms describing the stage that are not found in the Alphabetic Index, and there is no documentation of the stage, the provider should be queried.

Left heel pressure ulcer with partial thickness skin loss involving the dermis

L89.622   Pressure ulcer of left heel, stage 2

Explanation: Code assignment for the pressure ulcer stage should be guided by either the clinical documentation of the stage or the documentation of terms found in the Alphabetic Index. The clinical documentation describing the left heel pressure ulcer "partial thickness skin loss involving the dermis" matches the ICD-10-CM index parenthetical description for stage 2 "(abrasion, blister, partial thickness skin loss involving epidermis and/or dermis)."

---

4) Patients admitted with pressure ulcers documented as healed

No code is assigned if the documentation states that the pressure ulcer is completely healed **at the time of admission.**

5) Pressure ulcers documented as healing

Pressure ulcers described as healing should be assigned the appropriate pressure ulcer stage code based on the documentation in the medical record. If the documentation does not provide information about the stage of the healing pressure ulcer, assign the appropriate code for unspecified stage.

If the documentation is unclear as to whether the patient has a current (new) pressure ulcer or if the patient is being treated for a healing pressure ulcer, query the provider.

For ulcers that were present on admission but healed at the time of discharge, assign the code for the site and stage of the pressure ulcer at the time of admission.

H & P noted healing stage 2 sacral pressure ulcer. Resolved at time of discharge summary.

L89.152   Pressure ulcer of sacral region, stage 2

Explanation: Although completely healed upon discharge, the pressure ulcer required observation and/or treatment and should be coded based on the site and stage upon admission.

---

6) Patient admitted with pressure ulcer evolving into another stage during the admission

If a patient is admitted to an inpatient hospital with a pressure ulcer at one stage and it progresses to a higher stage, two separate codes should be assigned: one code for the site and stage of the ulcer on admission and a second code for the same ulcer site and the highest stage reported during the stay.

Stage 3 right hip pressure ulcer worsened during admission to a stage 4

L89.213   Pressure ulcer of right hip, stage 3

L89.214   Pressure ulcer of right hip, stage 4

Explanation: A pressure ulcer that progresses from a lower stage to a higher stage is assigned two codes, one for the documented stage upon admission and one for the documented stage at discharge.

---

7) Pressure-induced deep tissue damage

For pressure-induced deep tissue damage or deep tissue pressure injury, assign only the appropriate code for pressure-induced deep tissue damage (L89.--6).

b. Non-pressure chronic ulcers

1) Patients admitted with non-pressure ulcers documented as healed

No code is assigned if the documentation states that the non-pressure ulcer is completely healed **at the time of admission.**

2) Non-pressure ulcers documented as healing

Non-pressure ulcers described as healing should be assigned the appropriate non-pressure ulcer code based on the documentation in the medical record. If the documentation does not provide information about the severity of the healing non-pressure ulcer, assign the appropriate code for unspecified severity.

If the documentation is unclear as to whether the patient has a current (new) non-pressure ulcer or if the patient is being treated for a healing non-pressure ulcer, query the provider.

For ulcers that were present on admission but healed at the time of discharge, assign the code for the site and severity of the non-pressure ulcer at the time of admission.

Admission diagnosis: Chronic ulcer, fat layer exposed, on left ankle

Discharge diagnosis: Resolution of ulcer on the left ankle

L97.322   Non-pressure chronic ulcer of left ankle with fat layer exposed

Explanation: Although the ulcer was documented as resolved (healed) at discharge, a code representing the site and severity of the ulcer upon admission should be appended.

---

3) Patient admitted with non-pressure ulcer that progresses to another severity level during the admission

If a patient is admitted to an inpatient hospital with a non-pressure ulcer at one severity level and it progresses to a higher severity level, two separate codes should be assigned: one code for the site and severity level of the ulcer on admission and a second code for the same ulcer site and the highest severity level reported during the stay.

See Section I.B.14 for pressure ulcer stage documentation by clinicians other than patient's provider

Chapter 12. Diseases of the Skin and Subcutaneous Tissue (L00-L99)

EXCLUDES 2   certain conditions originating in the perinatal period (P04-P96)
certain infectious and parasitic diseases (A00-B99)
complications of pregnancy, childbirth and the puerperium (O00-O9A)
congenital malformations, deformations, and chromosomal abnormalities (Q00-Q99)
endocrine, nutritional and metabolic diseases (E00-E88)
lipomelanotic reticulosis (I89.8)
neoplasms (C00-D49)
symptoms, signs and abnormal clinical and laboratory findings, not elsewhere classified (R00-R94)
systemic connective tissue disorders (M30-M36)
viral warts (B07.-)

This chapter contains the following blocks:
L00-L08   Infections of the skin and subcutaneous tissue
L10-L14   Bullous disorders
L20-L30   Dermatitis and eczema
L40-L45   Papulosquamous disorders
L49-L54   Urticaria and erythema
L55-L59   Radiation-related disorders of the skin and subcutaneous tissue
L60-L75   Disorders of skin appendages
L76   Intraoperative and postprocedural complications of skin and subcutaneous tissue
L80-L99   Other disorders of the skin and subcutaneous tissue

Infections of the skin and subcutaneous tissue (L00-L08)

Use additional code (B95-B97) to identify infectious agent

EXCLUDES 2   hordeolum (H00.0)
infective dermatitis (L30.3)
local infections of skin classified in Chapter 1
lupus panniculitis (L93.2)
panniculitis NOS (M79.3)
panniculitis of neck and back (M54.0-)
perlèche NOS (K13.0)
perlèche due to candidiasis (B37.0)
perlèche due to riboflavin deficiency (E53.0)
pyogenic granuloma (L98.0)
relapsing panniculitis [Weber-Christian] (M35.6)
viral warts (B07.-)
zoster (B02.-)

L00   Staphylococcal scalded skin syndrome
Ritter's disease
Use additional code to identify percentage of skin exfoliation (L49.-)

EXCLUDES 1   bullous impetigo (L01.03)
pemphigus neonatorum (L01.03)
toxic epidermal necrolysis [Lyell] (L51.2)

DEF: Infectious skin disease of children younger than 5 years marked by eruptions ranging from a few localized blisters to widespread, easily ruptured, fine vesicles and bullae affecting almost the entire body. It results in exfoliation of large planes of skin and leaves raw areas.

✓4ᵗʰ L01   Impetigo

EXCLUDES 1   impetigo herpetiformis (L40.1)

DEF: Acute, superficial, highly contagious skin infection commonly occurring in children. Skin lesions usually appear on the face and consist of vesicles and bullae that burst and form yellow crusts.

✓5ᵗʰ **L01.0   Impetigo**
Impetigo contagiosa
Impetigo vulgaris

L01.00   **Impetigo, unspecified**
Impetigo NOS

L01.01   **Non-bullous impetigo**

L01.02   **Bockhart's impetigo**
Impetigo follicularis
Perifolliculitis NOS
Superficial pustular perifolliculitis
DEF: Superficial inflammation of the hair follicles most commonly caused by staph aureus that manifests as rounded, sphere-shaped, pustular eruptions in the areas of the scalp, beard, underarms, extremities, and buttocks.

L01.03   **Bullous impetigo**
Impetigo neonatorum
Pemphigus neonatorum

L01.09   **Other impetigo**
Ulcerative impetigo

L01.1   Impetiginization of other dermatoses

✓4ᵗʰ L02   Cutaneous abscess, furuncle and carbuncle
Use additional code to identify organism (B95-B96)

EXCLUDES 2   abscess of anus and rectal regions (K61.-)
abscess of female genital organs (external) (N76.4)
abscess of male genital organs (external) (N48.2, N49.-)

DEF: Carbuncle: Infection of the skin that arises from a collection of interconnected infected boils or furuncles, usually from hair follicles infected by *Staphylococcus*. This condition can produce pus and form drainage cavities.
DEF: Furuncle: Inflamed, painful abscess, cyst, or nodule on the skin caused by bacteria, often *Staphylococcus*, entering along the hair follicle.

✓5ᵗʰ **L02.0   Cutaneous abscess, furuncle and carbuncle of face**

EXCLUDES 2   abscess of ear, external (H60.0)
abscess of eyelid (H00.0)
abscess of head [any part, except face] (L02.8)
abscess of lacrimal gland (H04.0)
abscess of lacrimal passages (H04.3)
abscess of mouth (K12.2)
abscess of nose (J34.0)
abscess of orbit (H05.0)
submandibular abscess (K12.2)

L02.01   **Cutaneous abscess of face**

L02.02   **Furuncle of face**
Boil of face
Folliculitis of face

L02.03   **Carbuncle of face**

✓5ᵗʰ **L02.1   Cutaneous abscess, furuncle and carbuncle of neck**

L02.11   **Cutaneous abscess of neck**

L02.12   **Furuncle of neck**
Boil of neck
Folliculitis of neck

L02.13   **Carbuncle of neck**

✓5ᵗʰ **L02.2   Cutaneous abscess, furuncle and carbuncle of trunk**

EXCLUDES 1   non-newborn omphalitis (L08.82)
omphalitis of newborn (P38.-)

EXCLUDES 2   abscess of breast (N61.1)
abscess of buttocks (L02.3)
abscess of female external genital organs (N76.4)
abscess of hip (L02.4)
abscess of male external genital organs (N48.2, N49.-)

CC Excl: For CC codes in subcategory L02.2: PDX collection 833

✓6ᵗʰ   L02.21   **Cutaneous abscess of trunk**

L02.211   **Cutaneous abscess of abdominal wall**   **CC**

L02.212   **Cutaneous abscess of back [any part, except buttock]**   **CC**

L02.213   **Cutaneous abscess of chest wall**   **CC**

L02.214   **Cutaneous abscess of groin**   **CC**

L02.215   **Cutaneous abscess of perineum**   **CC**

L02.216   **Cutaneous abscess of umbilicus**   **CC**

L02.219   **Cutaneous abscess of trunk, unspecified**

✓6ᵗʰ   L02.22   **Furuncle of trunk**
Boil of trunk
Folliculitis of trunk

L02.221   **Furuncle of abdominal wall**

L02.222   **Furuncle of back [any part, except buttock]**

L02.223   **Furuncle of chest wall**

L02.224   **Furuncle of groin**

L02.225   **Furuncle of perineum**

L02.226   **Furuncle of umbilicus**

L02.229   **Furuncle of trunk, unspecified**

✓6ᵗʰ   L02.23   **Carbuncle of trunk**

L02.231   **Carbuncle of abdominal wall**

L02.232   **Carbuncle of back [any part, except buttock]**

L02.233   **Carbuncle of chest wall**

L02.234   **Carbuncle of groin**

L02.235   **Carbuncle of perineum**

L02.236   **Carbuncle of umbilicus**

L02.239   **Carbuncle of trunk, unspecified**

Chapter 12. Diseases of the Skin and Subcutaneous Tissue

✓5th **L02.3** **Cutaneous abscess, furuncle and carbuncle of** buttock

     EXCLUDES 1   *pilonidal cyst with abscess (L05.01)*

   L02.31   **Cutaneous abscess** of buttock   CC

       Cutaneous abscess of gluteal region
       CC Excl: PDX collection 834

   L02.32   **Furuncle** of buttock

       Boil of buttock
       Folliculitis of buttock
       Furuncle of gluteal region

   L02.33   **Carbuncle** of buttock

       Carbuncle of gluteal region

✓5th **L02.4** **Cutaneous abscess, furuncle and carbuncle of** limb

     EXCLUDES 2   *cutaneous abscess, furuncle and carbuncle of groin (L02.214, L02.224, L02.234)*

               cutaneous abscess, furuncle and carbuncle of hand (L02.5-)

               cutaneous abscess, furuncle and carbuncle of foot (L02.6-)

     CC Excl: For CC codes in subcategory L02.4: PDX collection 835

   ✓6th **L02.41**   **Cutaneous abscess** of limb

     L02.411   **Cutaneous abscess of** right axilla   CC

     L02.412   **Cutaneous abscess of** left axilla   CC

     L02.413   **Cutaneous abscess of** right upper **limb**

     L02.414   **Cutaneous abscess of** left upper **limb**

     L02.415   **Cutaneous abscess of** right lower **limb**

     L02.416   **Cutaneous abscess of** left lower **limb**

     L02.419   **Cutaneous abscess of limb, unspecified**

   ✓6th **L02.42**   **Furuncle** of limb

       Boil of limb
       Folliculitis of limb

     L02.421   **Furuncle of** right axilla

     L02.422   **Furuncle of** left axilla

     L02.423   **Furuncle of** right upper **limb**

     L02.424   **Furuncle of** left upper **limb**

     L02.425   **Furuncle of** right lower **limb**

     L02.426   **Furuncle of** left lower **limb**

     L02.429   **Furuncle of limb, unspecified**

   ✓6th **L02.43**   **Carbuncle** of limb

     L02.431   **Carbuncle of** right axilla

     L02.432   **Carbuncle of** left axilla

     L02.433   **Carbuncle of** right upper **limb**

     L02.434   **Carbuncle of** left upper **limb**

     L02.435   **Carbuncle of** right lower **limb**

     L02.436   **Carbuncle of** left lower **limb**

     L02.439   **Carbuncle of limb, unspecified**

✓5th **L02.5** **Cutaneous abscess, furuncle and carbuncle of** hand

   ✓6th **L02.51**   **Cutaneous abscess** of hand

     L02.511   **Cutaneous abscess of** right hand

     L02.512   **Cutaneous abscess of** left hand

     L02.519   **Cutaneous abscess of unspecified hand**

   ✓6th **L02.52**   **Furuncle** hand

       Boil of hand
       Folliculitis of hand

     L02.521   **Furuncle** right **hand**

     L02.522   **Furuncle** left **hand**

     L02.529   **Furuncle unspecified hand**

   ✓6th **L02.53**   **Carbuncle** of hand

     L02.531   **Carbuncle of** right hand

     L02.532   **Carbuncle of** left hand

     L02.539   **Carbuncle of unspecified hand**

✓5th **L02.6** **Cutaneous abscess, furuncle and carbuncle of** foot

     CC Excl: For CC codes in subcategory L02.6: PDX collection 838

   ✓6th **L02.61**   **Cutaneous abscess** of foot

     L02.611   **Cutaneous abscess of** right foot   CC

     L02.612   **Cutaneous abscess of** left foot   CC

     L02.619   **Cutaneous abscess of unspecified foot**   CC

   ✓6th **L02.62**   **Furuncle** of foot

       Boil of foot
       Folliculitis of foot

     L02.621   **Furuncle of** right **foot**

     L02.622   **Furuncle of** left **foot**

     L02.629   **Furuncle of unspecified foot**

   ✓6th **L02.63**   **Carbuncle** of foot

     L02.631   **Carbuncle of** right **foot**

     L02.632   **Carbuncle of** left **foot**

     L02.639   **Carbuncle of unspecified foot**

✓5th **L02.8** **Cutaneous abscess, furuncle and carbuncle of other sites**

   ✓6th **L02.81**   **Cutaneous abscess** of other sites

     L02.811   **Cutaneous abscess of** head **[any part, except face]**

     L02.818   **Cutaneous abscess of other sites**

   ✓6th **L02.82**   **Furuncle** of other sites

       Boil of other sites
       Folliculitis of other sites

     L02.821   **Furuncle of** head **[any part, except face]**

     L02.828   **Furuncle of other sites**

   ✓6th **L02.83**   **Carbuncle** of other sites

     L02.831   **Carbuncle of** head **[any part, except face]**

     L02.838   **Carbuncle of other sites**

✓5th **L02.9** **Cutaneous abscess, furuncle and carbuncle, unspecified**

   L02.91   **Cutaneous abscess, unspecified**

   L02.92   **Furuncle, unspecified**

       Boil NOS
       Furunculosis NOS

   L02.93   **Carbuncle, unspecified**

✓4th **L03** **Cellulitis and acute lymphangitis**

     EXCLUDES 2   *cellulitis of anal and rectal region (K61.-)*

               cellulitis of external auditory canal (H60.1)

               cellulitis of eyelid (H00.0)

               cellulitis of female external genital organs (N76.4)

               cellulitis of lacrimal apparatus (H04.3)

               cellulitis of male external genital organs (N48.2, N49.-)

               cellulitis of mouth (K12.2)

               cellulitis of nose (J34.0)

               eosinophilic cellulitis [Wells] (L98.3)

               febrile neutrophilic dermatosis [Sweet] (L98.2)

               lymphangitis (chronic) (subacute) (I89.1)

     AHA: 2017,4Q,100

     DEF: Cellulitis: Infection of the skin and subcutaneous tissues, most often caused by *Staphylococcus* or *Streptococcus* bacteria secondary to a cutaneous lesion. Progression of the inflammation may lead to abscess and tissue death, or even systemic infection-like bacteremia.

     DEF: Lymphangitis: Inflammation of the lymph channels most often caused by *Streptococcus*.

✓5th **L03.0** **Cellulitis and acute lymphangitis of** finger and toe

       Infection of nail
       Onychia
       Paronychia
       Perionychia

   ✓6th **L03.01**   **Cellulitis** of finger

       Felon
       Whitlow

     EXCLUDES 1   *herpetic whitlow (B00.89)*

     DEF: Felon: Superficial bacterial skin infection at the tip of the finger.

     L03.011   **Cellulitis of** right **finger**

     L03.012   **Cellulitis of** left **finger**

     L03.019   **Cellulitis of unspecified finger**

   ✓6th **L03.02**   **Acute lymphangitis** of finger

       Hangnail with lymphangitis of finger

     L03.021   **Acute lymphangitis of** right **finger**

     L03.022   **Acute lymphangitis of** left **finger**

     L03.029   **Acute lymphangitis of unspecified finger**

   ✓6th **L03.03**   **Cellulitis** of toe

     L03.031   **Cellulitis of** right **toe**

     L03.032   **Cellulitis of** left **toe**

     L03.039   **Cellulitis of unspecified toe**

   ✓6th **L03.04**   **Acute lymphangitis** of toe

       Hangnail with lymphangitis of toe

     L03.041   **Acute lymphangitis of** right **toe**

     L03.042   **Acute lymphangitis of** left **toe**

     L03.049   **Acute lymphangitis of unspecified toe**

✓ Additional Character Required   ✓x7th Placeholder   Unacceptable PDx   Questionable PDx   Manifestation   Unspecified Dx   H1-H14 HAC   HCC CMS-HCC Dx   HIV HIV Dx

ICD-10-CM 2020   737

Chapter 12. Diseases of the Skin and Subcutaneous Tissue

✓6ᵗʰ L03.1 Cellulitis and acute lymphangitis of other parts of limb

> CC Excl: For CC codes in subcategory L03.1, unless otherwise noted: PDX collection 835

    ✓6ᵗʰ L03.11 Cellulitis of other parts of limb

> EXCLUDES 2   cellulitis of fingers (L03.01-)
> cellulitis of toes (L03.03-)
> groin (L03.314)

        L03.111 Cellulitis of right axilla   CC

        L03.112 Cellulitis of left axilla   CC

        L03.113 Cellulitis of right upper limb   CC

        L03.114 Cellulitis of left upper limb   CC

        L03.115 Cellulitis of right lower limb   CC

> CC Excl: PDX collection 836

        L03.116 Cellulitis of left lower limb   CC

> CC Excl: PDX collection 836

        L03.119 Cellulitis of unspecified part of limb   CC

> CC Excl: PDX collection 836

    ✓6ᵗʰ L03.12 Acute lymphangitis of other parts of limb

> EXCLUDES 2   acute lymphangitis of fingers (L03.2-)
> acute lymphangitis of groin (L03.324)
> acute lymphangitis of toes (L03.04-)

        L03.121 Acute lymphangitis of right axilla   CC

        L03.122 Acute lymphangitis of left axilla   CC

        L03.123 Acute lymphangitis of right upper limb   CC

        L03.124 Acute lymphangitis of left upper limb   CC

        L03.125 Acute lymphangitis of right lower limb   CC

> CC Excl: PDX collection 836

        L03.126 Acute lymphangitis of left lower limb   CC

> CC Excl: PDX collection 836

        L03.129 Acute lymphangitis of unspecified part of limb   CC

> CC Excl: PDX collection 836

✓5ᵗʰ L03.2 Cellulitis and acute lymphangitis of face and neck

    ✓6ᵗʰ L03.21 Cellulitis and acute lymphangitis of face

        L03.211 Cellulitis of face   CC

> EXCLUDES 2   abscess of orbit (H05.01-)
> cellulitis of ear (H60.1-)
> cellulitis of eyelid (H00.0-)
> cellulitis of head (L03.81)
> cellulitis of lacrimal apparatus (H04.3)
> cellulitis of lip (K13.0)
> cellulitis of mouth (K12.2)
> cellulitis of nose (internal) (J34.0)
> cellulitis of orbit (H05.01-)
> cellulitis of scalp (L03.81)

> AHA: 2013,4Q,123
> CC Excl: PDX collection 840

        L03.212 Acute lymphangitis of face   CC

> CC Excl: No Excl

        L03.213 Periorbital cellulitis   CC

> Preseptal cellulitis
> AHA: 2016,4Q,36
> CC Excl: PDX collection 840

    ✓6ᵗʰ L03.22 Cellulitis and acute lymphangitis of neck

        L03.221 Cellulitis of neck   CC

> CC Excl: PDX collection 832

        L03.222 Acute lymphangitis of neck   CC

> CC Excl: PDX collection 832

✓5ᵗʰ L03.3 Cellulitis and acute lymphangitis of trunk

> CC Excl: For CC codes in subcategory L03.3, unless otherwise noted: PDX collection 833

    ✓6ᵗʰ L03.31 Cellulitis of trunk

> EXCLUDES 2   cellulitis of anal and rectal regions (K61.-)
> cellulitis of breast NOS (N61.0)
> cellulitis of female external genital organs (N76.4)
> cellulitis of male external genital organs (N48.2, N49.-)
> omphalitis of newborn (P38.-)
> puerperal cellulitis of breast (O91.2)

        L03.311 Cellulitis of abdominal wall   CC

> EXCLUDES 2   cellulitis of umbilicus (L03.316)
> cellulitis of groin (L03.314)

        L03.312 Cellulitis of back [any part except buttock]   CC

        L03.313 Cellulitis of chest wall   CC

        L03.314 Cellulitis of groin   CC

        L03.315 Cellulitis of perineum   CC

        L03.316 Cellulitis of umbilicus   CC

        L03.317 Cellulitis of buttock   CC

> CC Excl: PDX collection 834

        L03.319 Cellulitis of trunk, unspecified   CC

    ✓6ᵗʰ L03.32 Acute lymphangitis of trunk

        L03.321 Acute lymphangitis of abdominal wall   CC

        L03.322 Acute lymphangitis of back [any part except buttock]   CC

        L03.323 Acute lymphangitis of chest wall   CC

        L03.324 Acute lymphangitis of groin   CC

        L03.325 Acute lymphangitis of perineum   CC

        L03.326 Acute lymphangitis of umbilicus   CC

        L03.327 Acute lymphangitis of buttock   CC

> CC Excl: PDX collection 834

        L03.329 Acute lymphangitis of trunk, unspecified   CC

✓5ᵗʰ L03.8 Cellulitis and acute lymphangitis of other sites

> CC Excl: For CC codes in subcategory L03.8: PDX collection 839

    ✓6ᵗʰ L03.81 Cellulitis of other sites

        L03.811 Cellulitis of head [any part, except face]   CC

> Cellulitis of scalp
> EXCLUDES 2   cellulitis of face (L03.211)

        L03.818 Cellulitis of other sites   CC

    ✓6ᵗʰ L03.89 Acute lymphangitis of other sites

        L03.891 Acute lymphangitis of head [any part, except face]   CC

        L03.898 Acute lymphangitis of other sites   CC

✓5ᵗʰ L03.9 Cellulitis and acute lymphangitis, unspecified

    L03.90 Cellulitis, unspecified   CC

> CC Excl: PDX collection 839

    L03.91 Acute lymphangitis, unspecified   CC

> EXCLUDES 1   lymphangitis NOS (I89.1)
> CC Excl: PDX collection 839

✓4ᵗʰ L04 Acute lymphadenitis

> INCLUDES   abscess (acute) of lymph nodes, except mesenteric
> acute lymphadenitis, except mesenteric
> EXCLUDES 1   chronic or subacute lymphadenitis, except mesenteric (I88.1)
> enlarged lymph nodes (R59.-)
> human immunodeficiency virus [HIV] disease resulting in generalized lymphadenopathy (B20)
> lymphadenitis NOS (I88.9)
> nonspecific mesenteric lymphadenitis (I88.0)

> DEF: Inflammation or enlargement of the lymph nodes.

    L04.0 Acute lymphadenitis of face, head and neck

N Newborn: 0   P Pediatric: 0-17   M Maternity: 9-64   A Adult: 15-124   MCC Major Complication/Comorbidity   CC Complication/Comorbidity   SW Severe Wound Dx

738   ICD-10-CM 2020

L04.1   **Acute lymphadenitis of** trunk

L04.2   **Acute lymphadenitis of** upper limb
Acute lymphadenitis of axilla
Acute lymphadenitis of shoulder

L04.3   **Acute lymphadenitis of** lower limb
Acute lymphadenitis of hip
EXCLUDES 2   *acute lymphadenitis of groin (L04.1)*

L04.8   **Acute lymphadenitis of other sites**

L04.9   **Acute lymphadenitis, unspecified**

✓4th **L05**   **Pilonidal cyst and sinus**

DEF: Pilonidal cyst: Sac or sinus cavity of trapped epithelial tissues in the sacrococcygeal region, usually associated with ingrown hair.
DEF: Pilonidal sinus: Fistula, tract, or channel that extends from an infected area of ingrown hair to another site within the skin or out to the skin surface.

Pilonidal Cyst

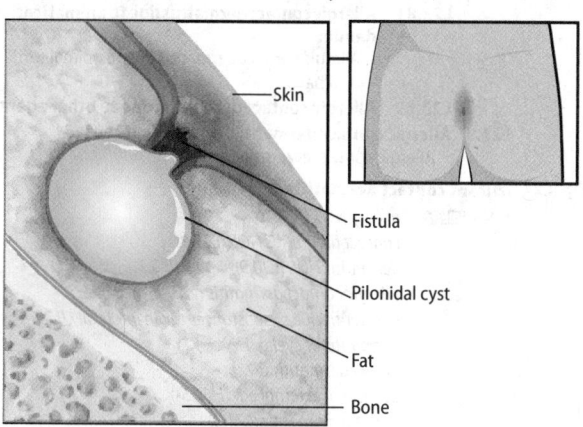

Skin

Fistula

Pilonidal cyst

Fat

Bone

✓5th **L05.0**   **Pilonidal cyst and sinus** with abscess

     L05.01   **Pilonidal** cyst **with abscess**   `CC` `SW`
         Pilonidal abscess
         Pilonidal dimple with abscess
         Postanal dimple with abscess
         EXCLUDES 2   *congenital sacral dimple (Q82.6)*
                  parasacral dimple (Q82.6)
         CC Excl: PDX collection 841

     L05.02   **Pilonidal** sinus **with abscess**   `CC` `SW`
         Coccygeal fistula with abscess
         Coccygeal sinus with abscess
         Pilonidal fistula with abscess
         CC Excl: PDX collection 841

✓5th **L05.9**   **Pilonidal cyst and sinus** without abscess

     L05.91   **Pilonidal** cyst **without abscess**
         Pilonidal dimple
         Postanal dimple
         Pilonidal cyst NOS
         EXCLUDES 2   *congenital sacral dimple (Q82.6)*
                  parasacral dimple (Q82.6)

     L05.92   **Pilonidal** sinus **without abscess**   `SW`
         Coccygeal fistula
         Coccygeal sinus without abscess
         Pilonidal fistula

✓4th **L08**   **Other local infections of skin and subcutaneous tissue**

L08.0   **Pyoderma**
Dermatitis gangrenosa
Purulent dermatitis
Septic dermatitis
Suppurative dermatitis
EXCLUDES 1   *pyoderma gangrenosum (L88)*
            pyoderma vegetans (L08.81)
DEF: Any superficial skin disease commonly characterized by the discharging of pus not attributed to another condition.

L08.1   **Erythrasma**   `HIV` `CC`
DEF: Chronic, superficial skin infection of brown scaly patches, commonly found in skin folds most prevalent in the overweight or diabetic population.
CC Excl: PDX collection 107

✓5th **L08.8**   **Other specified local infections of the skin and subcutaneous tissue**

     L08.81   **Pyoderma vegetans**
         EXCLUDES 1   *pyoderma gangrenosum (L88)*
                  pyoderma NOS (L08.0)

     L08.82   **Omphalitis not of newborn**
         EXCLUDES 1   *omphalitis of newborn (P38.-)*

     L08.89   **Other specified local infections of the skin and subcutaneous tissue**

L08.9   **Local infection of the skin and subcutaneous tissue, unspecified**

Bullous disorders (L10-L14)

EXCLUDES 1   *benign familial pemphigus [Hailey-Hailey] (Q82.8)*
         staphylococcal scalded skin syndrome (L00)
         toxic epidermal necrolysis [Lyell] (L51.2)

CC Excl: For CC codes in categories L10-L14, unless otherwise noted: PDX collection 842

✓4th **L10**   **Pemphigus**

EXCLUDES 1   *pemphigus neonatorum (L01.03)*

L10.0   **Pemphigus** vulgaris   `CC`

L10.1   **Pemphigus** vegetans   `CC`

L10.2   **Pemphigus** foliaceous   `CC`

L10.3   **Brazilian pemphigus [fogo selvagem]**   `CC`

L10.4   **Pemphigus** erythematosus   `CC`
Senear-Usher syndrome

L10.5   **Drug-induced pemphigus**   `CC`
Use additional code for adverse effect, if applicable, to identify drug (T36-T50 with fifth or sixth character 5)

✓5th **L10.8**   **Other pemphigus**

     L10.81   **Paraneoplastic pemphigus**   `CC`

     L10.89   **Other pemphigus**   `CC`

L10.9   **Pemphigus, unspecified**   `CC`

✓4th **L11**   **Other acantholytic disorders**

L11.0   **Acquired keratosis follicularis**
EXCLUDES 1   *keratosis follicularis (congenital) [Darier-White] (Q82.8)*

L11.1   **Transient acantholytic dermatosis [Grover]**

L11.8   **Other specified acantholytic disorders**

L11.9   **Acantholytic disorder, unspecified**

✓4th **L12**   **Pemphigoid**

EXCLUDES 1   *herpes gestationis (O26.4-)*
         impetigo herpetiformis (L40.1)

L12.0   **Bullous pemphigoid**   `CC`

L12.1   **Cicatricial pemphigoid**
Benign mucous membrane pemphigoid
DEF: Chronic autoimmune disease characterized by subepidermal blistering lesions of the mucosa, including the conjunctiva. It is seen predominantly in the elderly and produces adhesions and scarring.

L12.2   **Chronic bullous disease of childhood**   `P`
Juvenile dermatitis herpetiformis

✓5th **L12.3**   **Acquired epidermolysis bullosa**
EXCLUDES 1   *epidermolysis bullosa (congenital) (Q81.-)*
CC Excl: For CC codes in subcategory L12.3: PDX collection 843

     L12.30   **Acquired epidermolysis bullosa, unspecified**   `CC` `HCC`

     L12.31   **Epidermolysis bullosa due to drug**   `CC` `HCC`
         Use additional code for adverse effect, if applicable, to identify drug (T36-T50 with fifth or sixth character 5)

     L12.35   **Other acquired epidermolysis bullosa**   `CC` `HCC`

L12.8   **Other pemphigoid**   `CC`

L12.9   **Pemphigoid, unspecified**   `CC`

☑4ᵗʰ **L13　Other bullous disorders**

L13.0　Dermatitis herpetiformis
Duhring's disease
Hydroa herpetiformis
EXCLUDES 1　*juvenile dermatitis herpetiformis (L12.2)*
senile dermatitis herpetiformis (L12.0)
DEF: Skin disease to which people are genetically predisposed resulting from an immunological response to gluten. Dermatitis herpetiformis is an extremely pruritic eruption of various lesions that frequently heal, leaving hyperpigmentation or hypopigmentation and occasionally scarring. It is usually associated with asymptomatic gluten-sensitive enteropathy.

L13.1　Subcorneal pustular dermatitis
Sneddon-Wilkinson disease

L13.8　Other specified bullous disorders

L13.9　Bullous disorder, unspecified

L14　Bullous disorders in diseases classified elsewhere
Code first underlying disease

Dermatitis and eczema (L20-L30)

NOTE　In this block the terms dermatitis and eczema are used synonymously and interchangeably.

EXCLUDES 2　*chronic (childhood) granulomatous disease (D71)*
dermatitis gangrenosa (L08.0)
dermatitis herpetiformis (L13.0)
dry skin dermatitis (L85.3)
factitial dermatitis (L98.1)
perioral dermatitis (L71.0)
radiation-related disorders of the skin and subcutaneous tissue (L55-L59)
stasis dermatitis (I87.2)

☑4ᵗʰ **L20　Atopic dermatitis**

L20.0　Besnier's prurigo

☑5ᵗʰ **L20.8　Other atopic dermatitis**
EXCLUDES 2　*circumscribed neurodermatitis (L28.0)*

L20.81　Atopic neurodermatitis
Diffuse neurodermatitis

L20.82　Flexural eczema

L20.83　Infantile (acute) (chronic) eczema　Ⓟ

L20.84　Intrinsic (allergic) eczema

L20.89　Other atopic dermatitis

L20.9　Atopic dermatitis, unspecified

☑4ᵗʰ **L21　Seborrheic dermatitis**
EXCLUDES 2　*infective dermatitis (L30.3)*
seborrheic keratosis (L82.-)

L21.0　Seborrhea capitis
Cradle cap
AHA: 2018,1Q,6
TIP: Assign for dandruff in an adult patient.

L21.1　Seborrheic infantile dermatitis　Ⓟ

L21.8　Other seborrheic dermatitis

L21.9　Seborrheic dermatitis, unspecified
Seborrhea NOS

L22　Diaper dermatitis
Diaper erythema
Diaper rash
Psoriasiform diaper rash

☑4ᵗʰ **L23　Allergic contact dermatitis**
EXCLUDES 1　*allergy NOS (T78.40)*
contact dermatitis NOS (L25.9)
dermatitis NOS (L30.9)
EXCLUDES 2　*dermatitis due to substances taken internally (L27.-)*
dermatitis of eyelid (H01.1-)
diaper dermatitis (L22)
eczema of external ear (H60.5-)
irritant contact dermatitis (L24.-)
perioral dermatitis (L71.0)
radiation-related disorders of the skin and subcutaneous tissue (L55-L59)

L23.0　Allergic contact dermatitis due to metals
Allergic contact dermatitis due to chromium
Allergic contact dermatitis due to nickel

L23.1　Allergic contact dermatitis due to adhesives

L23.2　Allergic contact dermatitis due to cosmetics

L23.3　Allergic contact dermatitis due to drugs in contact with skin
Use additional code for adverse effect, if applicable, to identify drug (T36-T50 with fifth or sixth character 5)
EXCLUDES 2　*dermatitis due to ingested drugs and medicaments (L27.0-L27.1)*

L23.4　Allergic contact dermatitis due to dyes

L23.5　Allergic contact dermatitis due to other chemical products
Allergic contact dermatitis due to cement
Allergic contact dermatitis due to insecticide
Allergic contact dermatitis due to plastic
Allergic contact dermatitis due to rubber

L23.6　Allergic contact dermatitis due to food in contact with the skin
EXCLUDES 2　*dermatitis due to ingested food (L27.2)*

L23.7　Allergic contact dermatitis due to plants, except food
EXCLUDES 2　*allergy NOS due to pollen (J30.1)*

☑5ᵗʰ **L23.8　Allergic contact dermatitis due to other agents**

L23.81　Allergic contact dermatitis due to animal (cat) (dog) dander
Allergic contact dermatitis due to animal (cat) (dog) hair

L23.89　Allergic contact dermatitis due to other agents

L23.9　Allergic contact dermatitis, unspecified cause
Allergic contact eczema NOS

☑4ᵗʰ **L24　Irritant contact dermatitis**
EXCLUDES 1　*allergy NOS (T78.40)*
contact dermatitis NOS (L25.9)
dermatitis NOS (L30.9)
EXCLUDES 2　*allergic contact dermatitis (L23.-)*
dermatitis due to substances taken internally (L27.-)
dermatitis of eyelid (H01.1-)
diaper dermatitis (L22)
eczema of external ear (H60.5-)
perioral dermatitis (L71.0)
radiation-related disorders of the skin and subcutaneous tissue (L55-L59)

L24.0　Irritant contact dermatitis due to detergents

L24.1　Irritant contact dermatitis due to oils and greases

L24.2　Irritant contact dermatitis due to solvents
Irritant contact dermatitis due to chlorocompound
Irritant contact dermatitis due to cyclohexane
Irritant contact dermatitis due to ester
Irritant contact dermatitis due to glycol
Irritant contact dermatitis due to hydrocarbon
Irritant contact dermatitis due to ketone

L24.3　Irritant contact dermatitis due to cosmetics

L24.4　Irritant contact dermatitis due to drugs in contact with skin
Use additional code for adverse effect, if applicable, to identify drug (T36-T50 with fifth or sixth character 5)

L24.5　Irritant contact dermatitis due to other chemical products
Irritant contact dermatitis due to cement
Irritant contact dermatitis due to insecticide
Irritant contact dermatitis due to plastic
Irritant contact dermatitis due to rubber

L24.6　Irritant contact dermatitis due to food in contact with skin
EXCLUDES 2　*dermatitis due to ingested food (L27.2)*

L24.7　Irritant contact dermatitis due to plants, except food
EXCLUDES 2　*allergy NOS to pollen (J30.1)*

☑5ᵗʰ **L24.8　Irritant contact dermatitis due to other agents**

L24.81　Irritant contact dermatitis due to metals
Irritant contact dermatitis due to chromium
Irritant contact dermatitis due to nickel

L24.89　Irritant contact dermatitis due to other agents
Irritant contact dermatitis due to dyes

L24.9　Irritant contact dermatitis, unspecified cause
Irritant contact eczema NOS

√4ᵗʰ L25 Unspecified contact dermatitis

EXCLUDES 1   allergic contact dermatitis (L23.-)
              allergy NOS (T78.40)
              dermatitis NOS (L30.9)
              irritant contact dermatitis (L24.-)

EXCLUDES 2   dermatitis due to ingested substances (L27.-)
              dermatitis of eyelid (H01.1-)
              eczema of external ear (H60.5-)
              perioral dermatitis (L71.0)
              radiation-related disorders of the skin and subcutaneous
              tissue (L55-L59)

L25.0 Unspecified contact dermatitis due to cosmetics

L25.1 Unspecified contact dermatitis due to drugs in contact with skin
Use additional code for adverse effect, if applicable, to identify drug (T36-T50 with fifth or sixth character 5)

EXCLUDES 2   dermatitis due to ingested drugs and medicaments (L27.0-L27.1)

L25.2 Unspecified contact dermatitis due to dyes

L25.3 Unspecified contact dermatitis due to other chemical products
Unspecified contact dermatitis due to cement
Unspecified contact dermatitis due to insecticide

L25.4 Unspecified contact dermatitis due to food in contact with skin

EXCLUDES 2   dermatitis due to ingested food (L27.2)

L25.5 Unspecified contact dermatitis due to plants, except food

EXCLUDES 1   nettle rash (L50.9)

EXCLUDES 2   allergy NOS due to pollen (J30.1)

L25.8 Unspecified contact dermatitis due to other agents

L25.9 Unspecified contact dermatitis, unspecified cause
Contact dermatitis (occupational) NOS
Contact eczema (occupational) NOS

L26 Exfoliative dermatitis
Hebra's pityriasis

EXCLUDES 1   Ritter's disease (L00)

√4ᵗʰ L27 Dermatitis due to substances taken internally

EXCLUDES 1   allergy NOS (T78.40)

EXCLUDES 2   adverse food reaction, except dermatitis (T78.0-T78.1)
              contact dermatitis (L23-L25)
              drug photoallergic response (L56.1)
              drug phototoxic response (L56.0)
              urticaria (L50.-)

L27.0 Generalized skin eruption due to drugs and medicaments taken internally   [CC]
Use additional code for adverse effect, if applicable, to identify drug (T36-T50 with fifth or sixth character 5)

L27.1 Localized skin eruption due to drugs and medicaments taken internally   [CC]
Use additional code for adverse effect, if applicable, to identify drug (T36-T50 with fifth or sixth character 5)

L27.2 Dermatitis due to ingested food

EXCLUDES 2   dermatitis due to food in contact with skin (L23.6, L24.6, L25.4)

L27.8 Dermatitis due to other substances taken internally

L27.9 Dermatitis due to unspecified substance taken internally

√4ᵗʰ L28 Lichen simplex chronicus and prurigo

L28.0 Lichen simplex chronicus
Circumscribed neurodermatitis
Lichen NOS

L28.1 Prurigo nodularis

L28.2 Other prurigo
Prurigo NOS
Prurigo Hebra
Prurigo mitis
Urticaria papulosa

√4ᵗʰ L29 Pruritus

EXCLUDES 1   neurotic excoriation (L98.1)
              psychogenic pruritus (F45.8)

L29.0 Pruritus ani

L29.1 Pruritus scroti   ♂

L29.2 Pruritus vulvae   ♀

L29.3 Anogenital pruritus, unspecified

L29.8 Other pruritus

L29.9 Pruritus, unspecified
Itch NOS

√4ᵗʰ L30 Other and unspecified dermatitis

EXCLUDES 2   contact dermatitis (L23-L25)
              dry skin dermatitis (L85.3)
              small plaque parapsoriasis (L41.3)
              stasis dermatitis (I87.2)

L30.0 Nummular dermatitis

L30.1 Dyshidrosis [pompholyx]

L30.2 Cutaneous autosensitization
Candidid [levurid]
Dermatophytid
Eczematid

L30.3 Infective dermatitis
Infectious eczematoid dermatitis

L30.4 Erythema intertrigo

L30.5 Pityriasis alba
AHA: 2018,1Q,6

L30.8 Other specified dermatitis

L30.9 Dermatitis, unspecified
Eczema NOS

Papulosquamous disorders (L40-L45)

√4ᵗʰ L40 Psoriasis

DEF: Chronic autoimmune condition that speeds up skin cell growth, causing excessive immature skin cells to form raised, rounded erythematous lesions covered by dry, silvery scaling patches. Most commonly found on the scalp, elbows, knees, hands, feet, and genitals, it can also affect the joints with stiffness and swelling.

L40.0 Psoriasis vulgaris
Nummular psoriasis
Plaque psoriasis

L40.1 Generalized pustular psoriasis
Impetigo herpetiformis
Von Zumbusch's disease

L40.2 Acrodermatitis continua

L40.3 Pustulosis palmaris et plantaris

L40.4 Guttate psoriasis

√5ᵗʰ L40.5 Arthropathic psoriasis

L40.50 Arthropathic psoriasis, unspecified   [HCC]

L40.51 Distal interphalangeal psoriatic arthropathy   [HCC]

L40.52 Psoriatic arthritis mutilans   [HCC]

L40.53 Psoriatic spondylitis   [HCC]

L40.54 Psoriatic juvenile arthropathy   [HCC]

L40.59 Other psoriatic arthropathy   [HCC]

L40.8 Other psoriasis
Flexural psoriasis

L40.9 Psoriasis, unspecified

√4ᵗʰ L41 Parapsoriasis

EXCLUDES 1   poikiloderma vasculare atrophicans (L94.5)

L41.0 Pityriasis lichenoides et varioliformis acuta
Mucha-Habermann disease

L41.1 Pityriasis lichenoides chronica

L41.3 Small plaque parapsoriasis

L41.4 Large plaque parapsoriasis

L41.5 Retiform parapsoriasis

L41.8 Other parapsoriasis

L41.9 Parapsoriasis, unspecified

L42 Pityriasis rosea

√4ᵗʰ L43 Lichen planus

EXCLUDES 1   lichen planopilaris (L66.1)

L43.0 Hypertrophic lichen planus

L43.1 Bullous lichen planus

L43.2 Lichenoid drug reaction
Use additional code for adverse effect, if applicable, to identify drug (T36-T50 with fifth or sixth character 5)

L43.3 Subacute (active) lichen planus
Lichen planus tropicus

L43.8 Other lichen planus

L43.9 Lichen planus, unspecified

√4ᵗʰ L44 Other papulosquamous disorders

L44.0 Pityriasis rubra pilaris

☑ Additional Character Required   √x7ᵗʰ Placeholder   <u>Unacceptable PDx</u>   Questionable PDx   Manifestation   <u>Unspecified Dx</u>   H1-H14 HAC   HCC CMS-HCC Dx   HIV HIV Dx

ICD-10-CM 2020   741

L44.1 Lichen nitidus
> **DEF:** Chronic, inflammatory, asymptomatic skin disorder, characterized by numerous glistening, flat-topped, discrete, skin-colored micropapules, most often on the penis, lower abdomen, inner thighs, wrists, forearms, breasts, and buttocks.

L44.2 Lichen striatus

L44.3 Lichen ruber moniliformis

L44.4 Infantile papular acrodermatitis [Gianotti-Crosti]   P

L44.8 Other specified papulosquamous disorders

L44.9 Papulosquamous disorder, unspecified

L45 Papulosquamous disorders in diseases classified elsewhere
> Code first underlying disease

Urticaria and erythema (L49-L54)

> EXCLUDES 1   *Lyme disease (A69.2-)*
> *rosacea (L71.-)*

√4th L49 Exfoliation due to erythematous conditions according to extent of body surface involved
> Code first erythematous condition causing exfoliation, such as:
> Ritter's disease (L00)
> ▶(Staphylococcal) scalded skin syndrome◀ (L00)
> Stevens-Johnson syndrome (L51.1)
> Stevens-Johnson syndrome-toxic epidermal necrolysis overlap syndrome (L51.3)
> toxic epidermal necrolysis (L51.2)
> **DEF:** Exfoliation: Falling or sloughing off skin in layers.

L49.0 Exfoliation due to erythematous condition involving less than 10 percent of body surface
> Exfoliation due to erythematous condition NOS

L49.1 Exfoliation due to erythematous condition involving 10-19 percent of body surface

L49.2 Exfoliation due to erythematous condition involving 20-29 percent of body surface

L49.3 Exfoliation due to erythematous condition involving 30-39 percent of body surface   CC
> **CC Excl:** PDX collection 844

L49.4 Exfoliation due to erythematous condition involving 40-49 percent of body surface   CC
> **CC Excl:** PDX collection 845

L49.5 Exfoliation due to erythematous condition involving 50-59 percent of body surface   CC
> **CC Excl:** PDX collection 846

L49.6 Exfoliation due to erythematous condition involving 60-69 percent of body surface   CC
> **CC Excl:** PDX collection 847

L49.7 Exfoliation due to erythematous condition involving 70-79 percent of body surface   CC
> **CC Excl:** PDX collection 848

L49.8 Exfoliation due to erythematous condition involving 80-89 percent of body surface   CC
> **CC Excl:** PDX collection 849

L49.9 Exfoliation due to erythematous condition involving 90 or more percent of body surface   CC
> **CC Excl:** PDX collection 850

√4th L50 Urticaria
> EXCLUDES 1   *allergic contact dermatitis (L23.-)*
> *angioneurotic edema (T78.3)*
> *giant urticaria (T78.3)*
> *hereditary angio-edema (D84.1)*
> *Quincke's edema (T78.3)*
> *serum urticaria (T80.6-)*
> *solar urticaria (L56.3)*
> *urticaria neonatorum (P83.8)*
> *urticaria papulosa (L28.2)*
> *urticaria pigmentosa ▶(D47.01)◀*
> **DEF:** Eruption of itching edema of the skin. **Synonym(s):** hives.

L50.0 Allergic urticaria

L50.1 Idiopathic urticaria

L50.2 Urticaria due to cold and heat
> EXCLUDES 2   *familial cold urticaria (M04.2)*

L50.3 Dermatographic urticaria

L50.4 Vibratory urticaria

L50.5 Cholinergic urticaria

L50.6 Contact urticaria

L50.8 Other urticaria
> Chronic urticaria
> Recurrent periodic urticaria

L50.9 Urticaria, unspecified

√4th L51 Erythema multiforme
> Use additional code for adverse effect, if applicable, to identify drug (T36-T50 with fifth or sixth character 5)
> Use additional code to identify associated manifestations, such as:
> arthropathy associated with dermatological disorders (M14.8-)
> conjunctival edema (H11.42)
> conjunctivitis (H10.22-)
> corneal scars and opacities (H17.-)
> corneal ulcer (H16.0-)
> edema of eyelid (H02.84-)
> inflammation of eyelid (H01.8)
> keratoconjunctivitis sicca (H16.22-)
> mechanical lagophthalmos (H02.22-)
> stomatitis (K12.-)
> symblepharon (H11.23-)
> Use additional code to identify percentage of skin exfoliation (L49.-)
> EXCLUDES 1   *staphylococcal scalded skin syndrome (L00)*
> *Ritter's disease (L00)*
> **DEF:** Acute complex of symptoms with a varied pattern of skin eruptions, such as macular, bullous, popular, nodose, or vesicular lesions on the neck, face, and legs. Erythema (redness of skin and mucous membranes) multiforme (multiple forms) is a hypersensitivity (allergic) reaction that can occur at any age but primarily affects children or young adults.
> **CC Excl:** For CC codes in category L51: PDX collection 843

L51.0 Nonbullous erythema multiforme

L51.1 Stevens-Johnson syndrome   CC HCC

L51.2 Toxic epidermal necrolysis [Lyell]   CC HCC

L51.3 Stevens-Johnson syndrome-toxic epidermal necrolysis overlap syndrome   CC HCC
> SJS-TEN overlap syndrome

L51.8 Other erythema multiforme

L51.9 Erythema multiforme, unspecified
> Erythema iris
> Erythema multiforme major NOS
> Erythema multiforme minor NOS
> Herpes iris

L52 Erythema nodosum
> EXCLUDES 1   *tuberculous erythema nodosum (A18.4)*
> **DEF:** Form of panniculitis (inflammation of the fat layer beneath the skin) most often occurring in women. Commonly seen as a hypersensitivity reaction to infections, drugs, sarcoidosis, and specific enteropathies. The acute stage is associated with fever, malaise, and arthralgia. The lesions are pink to blue in color as tender nodules and are found on the front of the legs below the knees.

√4th L53 Other erythematous conditions
> EXCLUDES 1   *erythema ab igne (L59.0)*
> *erythema due to external agents in contact with skin (L23-L25)*
> *erythema intertrigo (L30.4)*
> **CC Excl:** For CC codes in category L53: PDX collection 851

L53.0 Toxic erythema   CC
> Code first poisoning due to drug or toxin, if applicable (T36-T65 with fifth or sixth character 1-4 or 6)
> Use additional code for adverse effect, if applicable, to identify drug (T36-T50 with fifth or sixth character 5)
> EXCLUDES 1   *neonatal erythema toxicum (P83.1)*

L53.1 Erythema annulare centrifugum   CC

L53.2 Erythema marginatum   CC

L53.3 Other chronic figurate erythema   CC

L53.8 Other specified erythematous conditions

L53.9 Erythematous condition, unspecified
> Erythema NOS
> Erythroderma NOS

L54 Erythema in diseases classified elsewhere
> Code first underlying disease

Radiation-related disorders of the skin and subcutaneous tissue (L55-L59)

√4th L55 Sunburn

L55.0 Sunburn of first degree

L55.1 Sunburn of second degree

N Newborn: 0   P Pediatric: 0-17   M Maternity: 9-64   A Adult: 15-124   MCC Major Complication/Comorbidity   CC Complication/Comorbidity   SW Severe Wound Dx

742   ICD-10-CM 2020

L55.2 **Sunburn of** third degree

L55.9 **Sunburn, unspecified**

✓4ᵗʰ **L56 Other acute skin changes due to ultraviolet radiation**

     Use additional code to identify the source of the ultraviolet radiation (W89, X32)

L56.0 **Drug phototoxic response**

     Use additional code for adverse effect, if applicable, to identify drug (T36-T50 with fifth or sixth character 5)

L56.1 **Drug photoallergic response**

     Use additional code for adverse effect, if applicable, to identify drug (T36-T50 with fifth or sixth character 5)

L56.2 **Photocontact dermatitis [berloque dermatitis]**

L56.3 **Solar urticaria**

L56.4 **Polymorphous light eruption**

L56.5 **Disseminated superficial actinic porokeratosis (DSAP)**

     DEF: Autosomal dominant skin condition occurring in sun-exposed areas of the skin (particularly the arms and legs), characterized by superficial annular, keratotic, brownish-red spots or thickenings with depressed centers and sharp, ridged borders. It may evolve into squamous cell carcinoma.

L56.8 **Other specified acute skin changes due to ultraviolet radiation**

L56.9 **Acute skin change due to ultraviolet radiation, unspecified**

✓4ᵗʰ **L57 Skin changes due to chronic exposure to nonionizing radiation**

     Use additional code to identify the source of the ultraviolet radiation (W89)

L57.0 **Actinic keratosis**

     Keratosis NOS

     Senile keratosis

     Solar keratosis

L57.1 **Actinic reticuloid**

L57.2 **Cutis rhomboidalis nuchae**

L57.3 **Poikiloderma of Civatte**

L57.4 **Cutis laxa senilis**

     Elastosis senilis

L57.5 **Actinic granuloma**

L57.8 **Other skin changes due to chronic exposure to nonionizing radiation**

     Farmer's skin

     Sailor's skin

     Solar dermatitis

L57.9 **Skin changes due to chronic exposure to nonionizing radiation, unspecified**

✓4ᵗʰ **L58 Radiodermatitis**

     Use additional code to identify the source of the radiation (W88, W90)

L58.0 **Acute radiodermatitis**

L58.1 **Chronic radiodermatitis**

L58.9 **Radiodermatitis, unspecified**

✓4ᵗʰ **L59 Other disorders of skin and subcutaneous tissue related to radiation**

L59.0 **Erythema ab igne [dermatitis ab igne]**

L59.8 **Other specified disorders of the skin and subcutaneous tissue related to radiation**

     AHA: 2017,1Q,33

L59.9 **Disorder of the skin and subcutaneous tissue related to radiation, unspecified**

Disorders of skin appendages (L60-L75)

EXCLUDES 1   *congenital malformations of integument (Q84.-)*

✓4ᵗʰ **L60 Nail disorders**

     EXCLUDES 2   *clubbing of nails (R68.3)*

                 onychia and paronychia (L03.0-)

Nail Disorders

Normal

Koilonychia

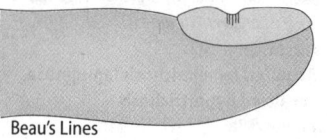

Beau's Lines

L60.0 **Ingrowing nail**

L60.1 **Onycholysis**

L60.2 **Onychogryphosis**

L60.3 **Nail dystrophy**

L60.4 **Beau's lines**

L60.5 **Yellow nail syndrome**

L60.8 **Other nail disorders**

L60.9 **Nail disorder, unspecified**

L62 ***Nail disorders in diseases classified elsewhere***

     Code first underlying disease, such as:

         pachydermoperiostosis (M89.4-)

✓4ᵗʰ **L63 Alopecia areata**

L63.0 **Alopecia (capitis)** totalis

L63.1 **Alopecia** universalis

L63.2 Ophiasis

L63.8 **Other alopecia areata**

L63.9 **Alopecia areata, unspecified**

✓4ᵗʰ **L64 Androgenic alopecia**

     INCLUDES   male-pattern baldness

L64.0 Drug-induced **androgenic alopecia**

     Use additional code for adverse effect, if applicable, to identify drug (T36-T50 with fifth or sixth character 5)

L64.8 **Other androgenic alopecia**

L64.9 **Androgenic alopecia, unspecified**

✓4ᵗʰ **L65 Other nonscarring hair loss**

     Use additional code for adverse effect, if applicable, to identify drug (T36-T50 with fifth or sixth character 5)

     EXCLUDES 1   *trichotillomania (F63.3)*

L65.0 **Telogen effluvium**

     DEF: Form of nonscarring alopecia characterized by shedding of hair from premature telogen development in follicles due to stress, including shock, childbirth, surgery, drugs, or weight loss.

L65.1 **Anagen effluvium**

L65.2 **Alopecia mucinosa**

L65.8 **Other specified nonscarring hair loss**

L65.9 **Nonscarring hair loss, unspecified**

     Alopecia NOS

✓4ᵗʰ **L66 Cicatricial alopecia [scarring hair loss]**

L66.0 **Pseudopelade**

L66.1 **Lichen planopilaris**

     Follicular lichen planus

L66.2 **Folliculitis decalvans**

L66.3 **Perifolliculitis capitis abscedens**

L66.4 **Folliculitis ulerythematosa reticulata**

✓ Additional Character Required   ✓x7ᵗʰ Placeholder   Unacceptable PDx   Questionable PDx   Manifestation   Unspecified Dx   H1-H14 HAC   HCC CMS-HCC Dx   HIV HIV Dx

ICD-10-CM 2020   **743**

Chapter 12. Diseases of the Skin and Subcutaneous Tissue

L66.8 **Other cicatricial alopecia**
  AHA: 2015,1Q,19

L66.9 **Cicatricial alopecia, unspecified**

✓4ᵗʰ L67 **Hair color and hair shaft abnormalities**
  EXCLUDES 1 monilethrix (Q84.1)
    pili annulati (Q84.1)
    telogen effluvium (L65.0)

L67.0 **Trichorrhexis nodosa**

L67.1 **Variations in hair color**
  Canities
  Greyness, hair (premature)
  Heterochromia of hair
  Poliosis circumscripta, acquired
  Poliosis NOS

L67.8 **Other hair color and hair shaft abnormalities**
  Fragilitas crinium

L67.9 **Hair color and hair shaft abnormality, unspecified**

✓4ᵗʰ L68 **Hypertrichosis**
  INCLUDES excess hair
  EXCLUDES 1 congenital hypertrichosis (Q84.2)
    persistent lanugo (Q84.2)

L68.0 **Hirsutism**

L68.1 **Acquired hypertrichosis lanuginosa**

L68.2 **Localized hypertrichosis**

L68.3 **Polytrichia**

L68.8 **Other hypertrichosis**

L68.9 **Hypertrichosis, unspecified**

✓4ᵗʰ L70 **Acne**
  EXCLUDES 2 acne keloid (L73.0)

L70.0 **Acne vulgaris**

L70.1 **Acne conglobata**

L70.2 **Acne varioliformis**
  Acne necrotica miliaris
  DEF: Rare form of acne characterized by development of persistent brown papulopustules followed by scar formation. This type of acne usually presents on the brow and temporoparietal part of the scalp.

L70.3 **Acne tropica**

L70.4 **Infantile acne** P

L70.5 **Acné excoriée**
  Acné excoriée des jeunes filles
  Picker's acne

L70.8 **Other acne**

L70.9 **Acne, unspecified**

✓4ᵗʰ L71 **Rosacea**
  Use additional code for adverse effect, if applicable, to identify drug (T36-T50 with fifth or sixth character 5)

L71.0 **Perioral dermatitis**

L71.1 **Rhinophyma**

L71.8 **Other rosacea**
  AHA: 2018,4Q,15

L71.9 **Rosacea, unspecified**

✓4ᵗʰ L72 **Follicular cysts of skin and subcutaneous tissue**

L72.0 **Epidermal cyst**

✓5ᵗʰ L72.1 **Pilar and trichodermal cyst**

L72.11 **Pilar cyst**

L72.12 **Trichodermal cyst**
  Trichilemmal (proliferating) cyst

L72.2 **Steatocystoma multiplex**

L72.3 **Sebaceous cyst**
  EXCLUDES 2 pilar cyst (L72.11)
    trichilemmal (proliferating) cyst (L72.12)

L72.8 **Other follicular cysts of the skin and subcutaneous tissue**

L72.9 **Follicular cyst of the skin and subcutaneous tissue, unspecified**

✓4ᵗʰ L73 **Other follicular disorders**

L73.0 **Acne keloid**

L73.1 **Pseudofolliculitis barbae**

L73.2 **Hidradenitis suppurativa**

L73.8 **Other specified follicular disorders**
  Sycosis barbae

L73.9 **Follicular disorder, unspecified**

✓4ᵗʰ L74 **Eccrine sweat disorders**
  EXCLUDES 2 generalized hyperhidrosis (R61)
  DEF: Eccrine sweat glands: Glands found in the dermal and hypodermal layer of the skin throughout the body, particularly on the forehead, scalp, axillae, palms, and soles. These glands produce watery and neutral or slightly acidic sweat.

L74.0 **Miliaria rubra**

L74.1 **Miliaria crystallina**

L74.2 **Miliaria profunda**
  Miliaria tropicalis

L74.3 **Miliaria, unspecified**

L74.4 **Anhidrosis**
  Hypohidrosis
  DEF: Inability to sweat normally. When the body can't cool itself through perspiration it can lead to heatstroke, a life-threatening condition.

✓5ᵗʰ L74.5 **Focal hyperhidrosis**

✓6ᵗʰ L74.51 **Primary focal hyperhidrosis**

L74.510 **Primary focal hyperhidrosis, axilla**
L74.511 **Primary focal hyperhidrosis, face**
L74.512 **Primary focal hyperhidrosis, palms**
L74.513 **Primary focal hyperhidrosis, soles**
L74.519 **Primary focal hyperhidrosis, unspecified**

L74.52 **Secondary focal hyperhidrosis**
  Frey's syndrome

L74.8 **Other eccrine sweat disorders**

L74.9 **Eccrine sweat disorder, unspecified**
  Sweat gland disorder NOS

✓4ᵗʰ L75 **Apocrine sweat disorders**
  EXCLUDES 1 dyshidrosis (L30.1)
    hidradenitis suppurativa (L73.2)
  DEF: Apocrine sweat glands: Found in the axilla, areola, and circumanal region, these glands begin to function in puberty and produce viscid milky secretions in response to external stimuli.

L75.0 **Bromhidrosis**

L75.1 **Chromhidrosis**

L75.2 **Apocrine miliaria**
  Fox-Fordyce disease
  DEF: Chronic, usually pruritic disease evidenced by small follicular papular eruptions, especially in the axillary and pubic areas. Apocrine miliaria develops from the closure and rupture of the affected apocrine glands' intraepidermal portion of the ducts.

L75.8 **Other apocrine sweat disorders**

L75.9 **Apocrine sweat disorder, unspecified**

Intraoperative and postprocedural complications of skin and subcutaneous tissue (L76)

✓4ᵗʰ L76 **Intraoperative and postprocedural complications of skin and subcutaneous tissue**
  AHA: 2016,4Q,9-10
  CC Excl: For CC codes in category L76, unless otheerwise noted: PDX collection 852

✓5ᵗʰ L76.0 **Intraoperative hemorrhage and hematoma of skin and subcutaneous tissue complicating a procedure**
  EXCLUDES 1 intraoperative hemorrhage and hematoma of skin and subcutaneous tissue due to accidental puncture and laceration during a procedure (L76.1-)

L76.01 **Intraoperative hemorrhage and hematoma of skin and subcutaneous tissue complicating a dermatologic procedure** CC

L76.02 **Intraoperative hemorrhage and hematoma of skin and subcutaneous tissue complicating other procedure** CC

✓5ᵗʰ L76.1 **Accidental puncture and laceration of skin and subcutaneous tissue during a procedure**

L76.11 **Accidental puncture and laceration of skin and subcutaneous tissue during a dermatologic procedure** CC
  CC Excl: PDX collection 509

L76.12 **Accidental puncture and laceration of skin and subcutaneous tissue during other procedure** CC
  CC Excl: PDX collection 509

N Newborn: 0   P Pediatric: 0-17   M Maternity: 9-64   A Adult: 15-124   MCC Major Complication/Comorbidity   CC Complication/Comorbidity   SW Severe Wound Dx

744

ICD-10-CM 2020

✓5ᵗʰ **L76.2 Postprocedural hemorrhage of skin and subcutaneous tissue following a procedure**
   L76.21 Postprocedural hemorrhage of skin and subcutaneous tissue following a dermatologic procedure `CC`
   L76.22 Postprocedural hemorrhage of skin and subcutaneous tissue following other procedure `CC`

✓5ᵗʰ **L76.3 Postprocedural hematoma and seroma of skin and subcutaneous tissue following a procedure**
   L76.31 Postprocedural hematoma of skin and subcutaneous tissue following a dermatologic procedure `CC`
   L76.32 Postprocedural hematoma of skin and subcutaneous tissue following other procedure `CC`
   L76.33 Postprocedural seroma of skin and subcutaneous tissue following a dermatologic procedure `CC`
   L76.34 Postprocedural seroma of skin and subcutaneous tissue following other procedure `CC`

✓5ᵗʰ **L76.8 Other intraoperative and postprocedural complications of skin and subcutaneous tissue**
Use additional code, if applicable, to further specify disorder
   L76.81 Other intraoperative complications of skin and subcutaneous tissue
   L76.82 Other postprocedural complications of skin and subcutaneous tissue
    AHA: 2017,3Q,6

Other disorders of the skin and subcutaneous tissue (L80-L99)

L80 Vitiligo
EXCLUDES 2   vitiligo of eyelids (H02.73-)
vitiligo of vulva (N90.89)
DEF: Persistent, progressive development of nonpigmented white patches on otherwise normal skin.

✓4ᵗʰ **L81 Other disorders of pigmentation**
EXCLUDES 1   birthmark NOS (Q82.5)
Peutz-Jeghers syndrome (Q85.8)
EXCLUDES 2   nevus — see Alphabetical Index
L81.0 Postinflammatory hyperpigmentation
L81.1 Chloasma
L81.2 Freckles
L81.3 Café au lait spots
L81.4 Other melanin hyperpigmentation
Lentigo
L81.5 Leukoderma, not elsewhere classified
L81.6 Other disorders of diminished melanin formation
L81.7 Pigmented purpuric dermatosis
Angioma serpiginosum
L81.8 Other specified disorders of pigmentation
Iron pigmentation
Tattoo pigmentation
L81.9 Disorder of pigmentation, unspecified

✓4ᵗʰ **L82 Seborrheic keratosis**
INCLUDES   basal cell papilloma
dermatosis papulosa nigra
Leser-Trélat disease
EXCLUDES 2   seborrheic dermatitis (L21.-)
DEF: Common, benign, noninvasive, lightly pigmented, warty growth composed of basaloid cells that usually appear at middle age as soft, easily crumbling plaques on the face, trunk, and extremities.
L82.0 Inflamed seborrheic keratosis
L82.1 Other seborrheic keratosis
Seborrheic keratosis NOS

L83 Acanthosis nigricans
Confluent and reticulated papillomatosis
DEF: Diffuse, velvety hyperplasia of the spinous skin layer of the axilla and other body folds marked by gray, brown, or black pigmentation. In adult form, it is often associated with malignant acanthosis nigricans in a benign, nevoid form relatively generalized.

L84 Corns and callosities
Callus
Clavus

✓4ᵗʰ **L85 Other epidermal thickening**
EXCLUDES 2   hypertrophic disorders of the skin (L91.-)
L85.0 Acquired ichthyosis
EXCLUDES 1   congenital ichthyosis (Q80.-)
L85.1 Acquired keratosis [keratoderma] palmaris et plantaris
EXCLUDES 1   inherited keratosis palmaris et plantaris (Q82.8)
L85.2 Keratosis punctata (palmaris et plantaris)
L85.3 Xerosis cutis
Dry skin dermatitis
L85.8 Other specified epidermal thickening
Cutaneous horn
L85.9 Epidermal thickening, unspecified

L86 Keratoderma in diseases classified elsewhere
Code first underlying disease, such as:
Reiter's disease (M02.3-)
EXCLUDES 1   gonococcal keratoderma (A54.89)
gonococcal keratosis (A54.89)
keratoderma due to vitamin A deficiency (E50.8)
keratosis due to vitamin A deficiency (E50.8)
xeroderma due to vitamin A deficiency (E50.8)

✓4ᵗʰ **L87 Transepidermal elimination disorders**
EXCLUDES 1   granuloma annulare (perforating) (L92.0)
L87.0 Keratosis follicularis et parafollicularis in cutem penetrans
Hyperkeratosis follicularis penetrans
Kyrle disease
L87.1 Reactive perforating collagenosis
L87.2 Elastosis perforans serpiginosa
L87.8 Other transepidermal elimination disorders
L87.9 Transepidermal elimination disorder, unspecified

L88 Pyoderma gangrenosum `CC`
Phagedenic pyoderma
EXCLUDES 1   dermatitis gangrenosa (L08.0)
DEF: Persistent debilitating skin disease characterized by irregular, boggy, blue-red ulcerations, with central healing and undermined edges.
CC Excl: PDX collection 853

✓4ᵗʰ **L89 Pressure ulcer**

INCLUDES
- bed sore
- decubitus ulcer
- plaster ulcer
- pressure area
- pressure sore

Code first any associated gangrene (I96)

EXCLUDES 2
- decubitus (trophic) ulcer of cervix (uteri) (N86)
- diabetic ulcers (E08.621, E08.622, E09.621, E09.622, E10.621, E10.622, E11.621, E11.622, E13.621, E13.622)
- non-pressure chronic ulcer of skin (L97.-)
- skin infections (L00-L08)
- varicose ulcer (I83.0, I83.2)

AHA: 2018,4Q,69; 2018,3Q,3; 2018,2Q,21; 2017,4Q,109; 2017,1Q,49; 2016,4Q,143

TIP: The stage of a diagnosed pressure ulcer can be based on documentation from clinicians who are not the patient's provider.

Four Stages of Pressure Ulcer

Stage 1
Persistent focal edema

Stage 2
Abrasion, blister, partial thickness skin loss involving epidermis and/or dermis

Stage 3
Full thickness skin loss involving damage or necrosis of subcutaneous tissue

Stage 4
Necrosis of soft tissues through to underlying muscle, tendon, or bone

✓5ᵗʰ **L89.0 Pressure ulcer of elbow**

✓6ᵗʰ **L89.00 Pressure ulcer of unspecified elbow**

L89.000 Pressure ulcer of unspecified elbow, unstageable `CC` `HCC` `SW`

L89.001 Pressure ulcer of unspecified elbow, stage 1 `CC`
Healing pressure ulcer of unspecified elbow, stage 1
Pressure pre-ulcer skin changes limited to persistent focal edema, unspecified elbow

L89.002 Pressure ulcer of unspecified elbow, stage 2 `CC` `HCC`
Healing pressure ulcer of unspecified elbow, stage 2
Pressure ulcer with abrasion, blister, partial thickness skin loss involving epidermis and/or dermis, unspecified elbow

L89.003 Pressure ulcer of unspecified elbow, stage 3 `CC` `H4` `HCC` `SW`
Healing pressure ulcer of unspecified elbow, stage 3
Pressure ulcer with full thickness skin loss involving damage or necrosis of subcutaneous tissue, unspecified elbow

L89.004 Pressure ulcer of unspecified elbow, stage 4
Healing pressure ulcer of unspecified elbow, stage 4
Pressure ulcer with necrosis of soft tissues through to underlying muscle, tendon, or bone, unspecified elbow

L89.006 Pressure-induced deep tissue damage of unspecified elbow `CC`

L89.009 Pressure ulcer of unspecified elbow, unspecified stage `CC`
Healing pressure ulcer of elbow NOS
Healing pressure ulcer of unspecified elbow, unspecified stage

✓6ᵗʰ **L89.01 Pressure ulcer of right elbow**

L89.010 Pressure ulcer of right elbow, unstageable `CC` `HCC` `SW`

L89.011 Pressure ulcer of right elbow, stage 1 `CC`
Healing pressure ulcer of right elbow, stage 1
Pressure pre-ulcer skin changes limited to persistent focal edema, right elbow

L89.012 Pressure ulcer of right elbow, stage 2 `CC` `HCC`
Healing pressure ulcer of right elbow, stage 2
Pressure ulcer with abrasion, blister, partial thickness skin loss involving epidermis and/or dermis, right elbow

L89.013 Pressure ulcer of right elbow, stage 3 `CC` `H4` `HCC` `SW`
Healing pressure ulcer of right elbow, stage 3
Pressure ulcer with full thickness skin loss involving damage or necrosis of subcutaneous tissue, right elbow

L89.014 Pressure ulcer of right elbow, stage 4 `CC` `H4` `HCC` `SW`
Healing pressure ulcer of right elbow, stage 4
Pressure ulcer with necrosis of soft tissues through to underlying muscle, tendon, or bone, right elbow

L89.016 Pressure-induced deep tissue damage of right elbow `CC`

L89.019 Pressure ulcer of right elbow, unspecified stage `CC`
Healing pressure right of elbow NOS
Healing pressure ulcer of right elbow, unspecified stage

✓6ᵗʰ **L89.02 Pressure ulcer of left elbow**

L89.020 Pressure ulcer of left elbow, unstageable `CC` `HCC` `SW`

L89.021 Pressure ulcer of left elbow, stage 1 `CC`
Healing pressure ulcer of left elbow, stage 1
Pressure pre-ulcer skin changes limited to persistent focal edema, left elbow

L89.022 Pressure ulcer of left elbow, stage 2 `CC` `HCC`
Healing pressure ulcer of left elbow, stage 2
Pressure ulcer with abrasion, blister, partial thickness skin loss involving epidermis and/or dermis, left elbow

L89.023 Pressure ulcer of left elbow, stage 3 `CC` `H4` `HCC` `SW`
Healing pressure ulcer of left elbow, stage 3
Pressure ulcer with full thickness skin loss involving damage or necrosis of subcutaneous tissue, left elbow

N Newborn: 0   P Pediatric: 0-17   M Maternity: 9-64   A Adult: 15-124   MCC Major Complication/Comorbidity   CC Complication/Comorbidity   SW Severe Wound Dx

746   ICD-10-CM 2020

L89.024 Pressure ulcer of left `CC` `H4` `HCC` `SW`
elbow, stage 4
    Healing pressure ulcer of left elbow, stage 4
    Pressure ulcer with necrosis of soft tissues through to underlying muscle, tendon, or bone, left elbow

L89.026 Pressure-induced deep `CC`
tissue damage **of left**
elbow

L89.029 Pressure ulcer of left `CC`
elbow, unspecified stage
    Healing pressure ulcer of left of elbow NOS
    Healing pressure ulcer of left elbow, unspecified stage

`√5ᵗʰ` **L89.1 Pressure ulcer of** back

  `√6ᵗʰ` **L89.10 Pressure ulcer of unspecified part of back**

L89.100 Pressure ulcer of `CC` `HCC` `SW`
unspecified part of back,
unstageable

L89.101 Pressure ulcer of `CC`
unspecified part of back,
stage 1
    Healing pressure ulcer of unspecified part of back, stage 1
    Pressure pre-ulcer skin changes limited to persistent focal edema, unspecified part of back

L89.102 Pressure ulcer of `CC` `HCC`
unspecified part of back,
stage 2
    Healing pressure ulcer of unspecified part of back, stage 2
    Pressure ulcer with abrasion, blister, partial thickness skin loss involving epidermis and/or dermis, unspecified part of back

L89.103 Pressure ulcer of `CC` `H4` `HCC` `SW`
unspecified part of back,
stage 3
    Healing pressure ulcer of unspecified part of back, stage 3
    Pressure ulcer with full thickness skin loss involving damage or necrosis of subcutaneous tissue, unspecified part of back

L89.104 Pressure ulcer of `CC` `H4` `HCC` `SW`
unspecified part of back,
stage 4
    Healing pressure ulcer of unspecified part of back, stage 4
    Pressure ulcer with necrosis of soft tissues through to underlying muscle, tendon, or bone, unspecified part of back

L89.106 Pressure-induced deep `CC`
tissue damage **of**
unspecified part of back

L89.109 Pressure ulcer of `CC`
unspecified part of back,
unspecified stage
    Healing pressure ulcer of unspecified part of back NOS
    Healing pressure ulcer of unspecified part of back, unspecified stage

  `√6ᵗʰ` **L89.11 Pressure ulcer of** right upper **back**
    Pressure ulcer of right shoulder blade

L89.110 Pressure ulcer of right `CC` `HCC` `SW`
upper back, unstageable

L89.111 Pressure ulcer of right `CC`
upper back, stage 1
    Healing pressure ulcer of right upper back, stage 1
    Pressure pre-ulcer skin changes limited to persistent focal edema, right upper back

L89.112 Pressure ulcer of right `CC` `HCC`
upper back, stage 2
    Healing pressure ulcer of right upper back, stage 2
    Pressure ulcer with abrasion, blister, partial thickness skin loss involving epidermis and/or dermis, right upper back

L89.113 Pressure ulcer of right `CC` `H4` `HCC` `SW`
upper back, stage 3
    Healing pressure ulcer of right upper back, stage 3
    Pressure ulcer with full thickness skin loss involving damage or necrosis of subcutaneous tissue, right upper back

L89.114 Pressure ulcer of right `CC` `H4` `HCC` `SW`
upper back, stage 4
    Healing pressure ulcer of right upper back, stage 4
    Pressure ulcer with necrosis of soft tissues through to underlying muscle, tendon, or bone, right upper back

L89.116 Pressure-induced deep `CC`
tissue damage **of right**
upper back

L89.119 Pressure ulcer of right `CC`
upper back, unspecified
stage
    Healing pressure ulcer of right upper back NOS
    Healing pressure ulcer of right upper back, unspecified stage

  `√6ᵗʰ` **L89.12 Pressure ulcer of** left upper **back**
    Pressure ulcer of left shoulder blade

L89.120 Pressure ulcer of left `CC` `HCC` `SW`
upper back, unstageable

L89.121 Pressure ulcer of left `CC`
upper back, stage 1
    Healing pressure ulcer of left upper back, stage 1
    Pressure pre-ulcer skin changes limited to persistent focal edema, left upper back

L89.122 Pressure ulcer of left `CC` `HCC`
upper back, stage 2
    Healing pressure ulcer of left upper back, stage 2
    Pressure ulcer with abrasion, blister, partial thickness skin loss involving epidermis and/or dermis, left upper back

L89.123 Pressure ulcer of left `CC` `H4` `HCC` `SW`
upper back, stage 3
    Healing pressure ulcer of left upper back, stage 3
    Pressure ulcer with full thickness skin loss involving damage or necrosis of subcutaneous tissue, left upper back

L89.124 Pressure ulcer of left `CC` `H4` `HCC` `SW`
upper back, stage 4
    Healing pressure ulcer of left upper back, stage 4
    Pressure ulcer with necrosis of soft tissues through to underlying muscle, tendon, or bone, left upper back

L89.126 Pressure-induced deep `CC`
tissue damage **of left**
upper back

L89.129 Pressure ulcer of left `CC`
upper back, unspecified
stage
    Healing pressure ulcer of left upper back NOS
    Healing pressure ulcer of left upper back, unspecified stage

  `√6ᵗʰ` **L89.13 Pressure ulcer of** right lower **back**

L89.130 Pressure ulcer of right `CC` `HCC` `SW`
lower back, unstageable

L89.131 Pressure ulcer of right lower back, stage 1 `CC`
>   Healing pressure ulcer of right lower back, stage 1
>   Pressure pre-ulcer skin changes limited to persistent focal edema, right lower back

L89.132 Pressure ulcer of right lower back, stage 2 `CC` `HCC`
>   Healing pressure ulcer of right lower back, stage 2
>   Pressure ulcer with abrasion, blister, partial thickness skin loss involving epidermis and/or dermis, right lower back

L89.133 Pressure ulcer of right lower back, stage 3 `CC` `H4` `HCC` `SW`
>   Healing pressure ulcer of right lower back, stage 3
>   Pressure ulcer with full thickness skin loss involving damage or necrosis of subcutaneous tissue, right lower back

L89.134 Pressure ulcer of right lower back, stage 4 `CC` `H4` `HCC` `SW`
>   Healing pressure ulcer of right lower back, stage 4
>   Pressure ulcer with necrosis of soft tissues through to underlying muscle, tendon, or bone, right lower back

L89.136 Pressure-induced deep tissue damage of right lower back `CC`

L89.139 Pressure ulcer of right lower back, unspecified stage `CC`
>   Healing pressure ulcer of right lower back NOS
>   Healing pressure ulcer of right lower back, unspecified stage

✓6th **L89.14 Pressure ulcer of left lower back**

L89.140 Pressure ulcer of left lower back, unstageable `CC` `HCC` `SW`

L89.141 Pressure ulcer of left lower back, stage 1 `CC`
>   Healing pressure ulcer of left lower back, stage 1
>   Pressure pre-ulcer skin changes limited to persistent focal edema, left lower back

L89.142 Pressure ulcer of left lower back, stage 2 `CC` `HCC`
>   Healing pressure ulcer of left lower back, stage 2
>   Pressure ulcer with abrasion, blister, partial thickness skin loss involving epidermis and/or dermis, left lower back

L89.143 Pressure ulcer of left lower back, stage 3 `CC` `H4` `HCC` `SW`
>   Healing pressure ulcer of left lower back, stage 3
>   Pressure ulcer with full thickness skin loss involving damage or necrosis of subcutaneous tissue, left lower back

L89.144 Pressure ulcer of left lower back, stage 4 `CC` `H4` `HCC` `SW`
>   Healing pressure ulcer of left lower back, stage 4
>   Pressure ulcer with necrosis of soft tissues through to underlying muscle, tendon, or bone, left lower back

L89.146 Pressure-induced deep tissue damage of left lower back `CC`

L89.149 Pressure ulcer of left lower back, unspecified stage `CC`
>   Healing pressure ulcer of left lower back NOS
>   Healing pressure ulcer of left lower back, unspecified stage

✓6th **L89.15 Pressure ulcer of sacral region**
>   Pressure ulcer of coccyx
>   Pressure ulcer of tailbone

L89.150 Pressure ulcer of sacral region, unstageable `CC` `HCC` `SW`

L89.151 Pressure ulcer of sacral region, stage 1 `CC`
>   Healing pressure ulcer of sacral region, stage 1
>   Pressure pre-ulcer skin changes limited to persistent focal edema, sacral region

L89.152 Pressure ulcer of sacral region, stage 2 `CC` `HCC`
>   Healing pressure ulcer of sacral region, stage 2
>   Pressure ulcer with abrasion, blister, partial thickness skin loss involving epidermis and/or dermis, sacral region

L89.153 Pressure ulcer of sacral region, stage 3 `CC` `H4` `HCC` `SW`
>   Healing pressure ulcer of sacral region, stage 3
>   Pressure ulcer with full thickness skin loss involving damage or necrosis of subcutaneous tissue, sacral region

L89.154 Pressure ulcer of sacral region, stage 4 `CC` `H4` `HCC` `SW`
>   Healing pressure ulcer of sacral region, stage 4
>   Pressure ulcer with necrosis of soft tissues through to underlying muscle, tendon, or bone, sacral region

L89.156 Pressure-induced deep tissue damage of sacral region `CC`

L89.159 Pressure ulcer of sacral region, unspecified stage `CC`
>   Healing pressure ulcer of sacral region NOS
>   Healing pressure ulcer of sacral region, unspecified stage

✓5th **L89.2 Pressure ulcer of hip**

✓6th **L89.20 Pressure ulcer of unspecified hip**

L89.200 Pressure ulcer of unspecified hip, unstageable `CC` `HCC` `SW`

L89.201 Pressure ulcer of unspecified hip, stage 1 `CC`
>   Healing pressure ulcer of unspecified hip back, stage 1
>   Pressure pre-ulcer skin changes limited to persistent focal edema, unspecified hip

L89.202 Pressure ulcer of unspecified hip, stage 2 `CC` `HCC`
>   Healing pressure ulcer of unspecified hip, stage 2
>   Pressure ulcer with abrasion, blister, partial thickness skin loss involving epidermis and/or dermis, unspecified hip

L89.203 Pressure ulcer of unspecified hip, stage 3 `CC` `H4` `HCC` `SW`
>   Healing pressure ulcer of unspecified hip, stage 3
>   Pressure ulcer with full thickness skin loss involving damage or necrosis of subcutaneous tissue, unspecified hip

`N` Newborn: 0   `P` Pediatric: 0-17   `M` Maternity: 9-64   `A` Adult: 15-124   `MCC` Major Complication/Comorbidity   `CC` Complication/Comorbidity   `SW` Severe Wound Dx

748   ICD-10-CM 2020

L89.204 Pressure ulcer of `CC` `H4` `HCC` `SW`
unspecified hip, stage 4

   Healing pressure ulcer of unspecified hip,
     stage 4

   Pressure ulcer with necrosis of soft tissues
     through to underlying muscle,
     tendon, or bone, unspecified hip

L89.206 Pressure-induced deep `CC`
tissue damage of
unspecified hip

L89.209 Pressure ulcer of `CC`
unspecified hip,
unspecified stage

   Healing pressure ulcer of unspecified hip
     NOS

   Healing pressure ulcer of unspecified hip,
     unspecified stage

✓6ᵗʰ **L89.21 Pressure ulcer of** right **hip**

L89.210 Pressure ulcer of right hip, `CC` `HCC` `SW`
unstageable

L89.211 Pressure ulcer of right hip, `CC`
stage 1

   Healing pressure ulcer of right hip back,
     stage 1

   Pressure pre-ulcer skin changes limited to
     persistent focal edema, right hip

L89.212 Pressure ulcer of right hip, `CC` `HCC`
stage 2

   Healing pressure ulcer of right hip, stage 2

   Pressure ulcer with abrasion, blister, partial
     thickness skin loss involving
     epidermis and/or dermis, right hip

L89.213 Pressure ulcer of right hip, `CC` `H4` `HCC` `SW`
stage 3

   Healing pressure ulcer of right hip, stage 3

   Pressure ulcer with full thickness skin loss
     involving damage or necrosis of
     subcutaneous tissue, right hip

L89.214 Pressure ulcer of right hip, `CC` `H4` `HCC` `SW`
stage 4

   Healing pressure ulcer of right hip, stage 4

   Pressure ulcer with necrosis of soft tissues
     through to underlying muscle,
     tendon, or bone, right hip

L89.216 Pressure-induced deep `CC`
tissue damage of right hip

L89.219 Pressure ulcer of right hip, `CC`
unspecified stage

   Healing pressure ulcer of right hip NOS

   Healing pressure ulcer of right hip,
     unspecified stage

✓6ᵗʰ **L89.22 Pressure ulcer of** left **hip**

L89.220 Pressure ulcer of left hip, `CC` `HCC` `SW`
unstageable

L89.221 Pressure ulcer of left hip, `CC`
stage 1

   Healing pressure ulcer of left hip back,
     stage 1

   Pressure pre-ulcer skin changes limited to
     persistent focal edema, left hip

L89.222 Pressure ulcer of left hip, `CC` `HCC`
stage 2

   Healing pressure ulcer of left hip, stage 2

   Pressure ulcer with abrasion, blister, partial
     thickness skin loss involving
     epidermis and/or dermis, left hip

L89.223 Pressure ulcer of left hip, `CC` `H4` `HCC` `SW`
stage 3

   Healing pressure ulcer of left hip, stage 3

   Pressure ulcer with full thickness skin loss
     involving damage or necrosis of
     subcutaneous tissue, left hip

L89.224 Pressure ulcer of left hip, `CC` `H4` `HCC` `SW`
stage 4

   Healing pressure ulcer of left hip, stage 4

   Pressure ulcer with necrosis of soft tissues
     through to underlying muscle,
     tendon, or bone, left hip

L89.226 Pressure-induced deep `HCC`
tissue damage of left hip

L89.229 Pressure ulcer of left hip, `CC`
unspecified stage

   Healing pressure ulcer of left hip NOS

   Healing pressure ulcer of left hip,
     unspecified stage

✓5ᵗʰ **L89.3 Pressure ulcer of** buttock

✓6ᵗʰ **L89.30 Pressure ulcer of unspecified buttock**

L89.300 Pressure ulcer of `CC` `HCC` `SW`
unspecified buttock,
unstageable

L89.301 Pressure ulcer of `CC`
unspecified buttock, stage
1

   Healing pressure ulcer of unspecified
     buttock, stage 1

   Pressure pre-ulcer skin changes limited to
     persistent focal edema, unspecified
     buttock

L89.302 Pressure ulcer of `CC` `HCC`
unspecified buttock, stage
2

   Healing pressure ulcer of unspecified
     buttock, stage 2

   Pressure ulcer with abrasion, blister, partial
     thickness skin loss involving
     epidermis and/or dermis, unspecified
     buttock

L89.303 Pressure ulcer of `CC` `H4` `HCC` `SW`
unspecified buttock, stage
3

   Healing pressure ulcer of unspecified
     buttock, stage 3

   Pressure ulcer with full thickness skin loss
     involving damage or necrosis of
     subcutaneous tissue, unspecified
     buttock

L89.304 Pressure ulcer of `CC` `H4` `HCC` `SW`
unspecified buttock, stage
4

   Healing pressure ulcer of unspecified
     buttock, stage 4

   Pressure ulcer with necrosis of soft tissues
     through to underlying muscle,
     tendon, or bone, unspecified buttock

L89.306 Pressure-induced deep `CC`
tissue damage of
unspecified buttock

L89.309 Pressure ulcer of `CC`
unspecified buttock,
unspecified stage

   Healing pressure ulcer of unspecified
     buttock NOS

   Healing pressure ulcer of unspecified
     buttock, unspecified stage

✓6ᵗʰ **L89.31 Pressure ulcer of** right **buttock**

L89.310 Pressure ulcer of right `CC` `HCC` `SW`
buttock, unstageable

L89.311 Pressure ulcer of right `CC`
buttock, stage 1

   Healing pressure ulcer of right buttock,
     stage 1

   Pressure pre-ulcer skin changes limited to
     persistent focal edema, right buttock

L89.312 Pressure ulcer of right `CC` `HCC`
buttock, stage 2

   Healing pressure ulcer of right buttock,
     stage 2

   Pressure ulcer with abrasion, blister, partial
     thickness skin loss involving
     epidermis and/or dermis, right
     buttock

L89.313 Pressure ulcer of right `CC` `H4` `HCC` `SW`
buttock, stage 3

   Healing pressure ulcer of right buttock,
     stage 3

   Pressure ulcer with full thickness skin loss
     involving damage or necrosis of
     subcutaneous tissue, right buttock

L89.314 **Pressure ulcer of right buttock, stage 4** `CC` `H4` `HCC` `SW`
> Healing pressure ulcer of right buttock, stage 4
> Pressure ulcer with necrosis of soft tissues through to underlying muscle, tendon, or bone, right buttock

L89.316 **Pressure-induced deep tissue damage of right buttock** `CC`

L89.319 **Pressure ulcer of right buttock, unspecified stage** `CC`
> Healing pressure ulcer of right buttock NOS
> Healing pressure ulcer of right buttock, unspecified stage

✓6ᵗʰ **L89.32** **Pressure ulcer of left buttock**

L89.320 **Pressure ulcer of left buttock, unstageable** `CC` `HCC` `SW`

L89.321 **Pressure ulcer of left buttock, stage 1** `CC`
> Healing pressure ulcer of left buttock, stage 1
> Pressure pre-ulcer skin changes limited to persistent focal edema, left buttock

L89.322 **Pressure ulcer of left buttock, stage 2** `CC` `HCC`
> Healing pressure ulcer of left buttock, stage 2
> Pressure ulcer with abrasion, blister, partial thickness skin loss involving epidermis and/or dermis, left buttock

L89.323 **Pressure ulcer of left buttock, stage 3** `CC` `H4` `HCC` `SW`
> Healing pressure ulcer of left buttock, stage 3
> Pressure ulcer with full thickness skin loss involving damage or necrosis of subcutaneous tissue, left buttock

L89.324 **Pressure ulcer of left buttock, stage 4** `CC` `H4` `HCC` `SW`
> Healing pressure ulcer of left buttock, stage 4
> Pressure ulcer with necrosis of soft tissues through to underlying muscle, tendon, or bone, left buttock

L89.326 **Pressure-induced deep tissue damage of left buttock** `CC`

L89.329 **Pressure ulcer of left buttock, unspecified stage** `CC`
> Healing pressure ulcer of left buttock NOS
> Healing pressure ulcer of left buttock, unspecified stage

✓5ᵗʰ **L89.4** **Pressure ulcer of contiguous site of back, buttock and hip**

L89.40 **Pressure ulcer of contiguous site of back, buttock and hip, unspecified stage** `CC`
> Healing pressure ulcer of contiguous site of back, buttock and hip NOS
> Healing pressure ulcer of contiguous site of back, buttock and hip, unspecified stage

L89.41 **Pressure ulcer of contiguous site of back, buttock and hip, stage 1** `CC`
> Healing pressure ulcer of contiguous site of back, buttock and hip, stage 1
> Pressure pre-ulcer skin changes limited to persistent focal edema, contiguous site of back, buttock and hip

L89.42 **Pressure ulcer of contiguous site of back, buttock and hip, stage 2** `CC` `HCC`
> Healing pressure ulcer of contiguous site of back, buttock and hip, stage 2
> Pressure ulcer with abrasion, blister, partial thickness skin loss involving epidermis and/or dermis, contiguous site of back, buttock and hip

L89.43 **Pressure ulcer of contiguous site of back, buttock and hip, stage 3** `CC` `H4` `HCC` `SW`
> Healing pressure ulcer of contiguous site of back, buttock and hip, stage 3
> Pressure ulcer with full thickness skin loss involving damage or necrosis of subcutaneous tissue, contiguous site of back, buttock and hip

L89.44 **Pressure ulcer of contiguous site of back, buttock and hip, stage 4** `CC` `H4` `HCC` `SW`
> Healing pressure ulcer of contiguous site of back, buttock and hip, stage 4
> Pressure ulcer with necrosis of soft tissues through to underlying muscle, tendon, or bone, contiguous site of back, buttock and hip

L89.45 **Pressure ulcer of contiguous site of back, buttock and hip, unstageable** `CC` `HCC` `SW`

L89.46 **Pressure-induced deep tissue damage of contiguous site of back, buttock and hip** `CC`

✓5ᵗʰ **L89.5** **Pressure ulcer of ankle**

✓6ᵗʰ **L89.50** **Pressure ulcer of unspecified ankle**

L89.500 **Pressure ulcer of unspecified ankle, unstageable** `CC` `HCC` `SW`

L89.501 **Pressure ulcer of unspecified ankle, stage 1** `CC`
> Healing pressure ulcer of unspecified ankle, stage 1
> Pressure pre-ulcer skin changes limited to persistent focal edema, unspecified ankle

L89.502 **Pressure ulcer of unspecified ankle, stage 2** `CC` `HCC`
> Healing pressure ulcer of unspecified ankle, stage 2
> Pressure ulcer with abrasion, blister, partial thickness skin loss involving epidermis and/or dermis, unspecified ankle

L89.503 **Pressure ulcer of unspecified ankle, stage 3** `CC` `H4` `HCC` `SW`
> Healing pressure ulcer of unspecified ankle, stage 3
> Pressure ulcer with full thickness skin loss involving damage or necrosis of subcutaneous tissue, unspecified ankle

L89.504 **Pressure ulcer of unspecified ankle, stage 4** `CC` `H4` `HCC` `SW`
> Healing pressure ulcer of unspecified ankle, stage 4
> Pressure ulcer with necrosis of soft tissues through to underlying muscle, tendon, or bone, unspecified ankle

L89.506 **Pressure-induced deep tissue damage of unspecified ankle** `CC`

L89.509 **Pressure ulcer of unspecified ankle, unspecified stage** `CC`
> Healing pressure ulcer of unspecified ankle NOS
> Healing pressure ulcer of unspecified ankle, unspecified stage

✓6ᵗʰ **L89.51** **Pressure ulcer of right ankle**

L89.510 **Pressure ulcer of right ankle, unstageable** `CC` `HCC` `SW`

L89.511 **Pressure ulcer of right ankle, stage 1** `CC`
> Healing pressure ulcer of right ankle, stage 1
> Pressure pre-ulcer skin changes limited to persistent focal edema, right ankle

N Newborn: 0   P Pediatric: 0-17   M Maternity: 9-64   A Adult: 15-124   **MCC** Major Complication/Comorbidity   **CC** Complication/Comorbidity   **SW** Severe Wound Dx

ICD-10-CM 2020

750

L89.512   **Pressure ulcer of right ankle,** stage 2   `CC` `HCC`
> Healing pressure ulcer of right ankle, stage 2
> Pressure ulcer with abrasion, blister, partial thickness skin loss involving epidermis and/or dermis, right ankle

L89.513   **Pressure ulcer of right ankle,** stage 3   `CC` `H4` `HCC` `SW`
> Healing pressure ulcer of right ankle, stage 3
> Pressure ulcer with full thickness skin loss involving damage or necrosis of subcutaneous tissue, right ankle

L89.514   **Pressure ulcer of right ankle,** stage 4   `CC` `H4` `HCC` `SW`
> Healing pressure ulcer of right ankle, stage 4
> Pressure ulcer with necrosis of soft tissues through to underlying muscle, tendon, or bone, right ankle

L89.516   **Pressure-induced** deep tissue damage **of right ankle**   `CC`

L89.519   **Pressure ulcer of right ankle, unspecified stage**   `CC`
> Healing pressure ulcer of right ankle NOS
> Healing pressure ulcer of right ankle, unspecified stage

√6ᵗʰ **L89.52**   **Pressure ulcer of** left **ankle**

L89.520   **Pressure ulcer of left ankle,** unstageable   `CC` `HCC` `SW`

L89.521   **Pressure ulcer of left ankle,** stage 1   `CC`
> Healing pressure ulcer of left ankle, stage 1
> Pressure pre-ulcer skin changes limited to persistent focal edema, left ankle

L89.522   **Pressure ulcer of left ankle,** stage 2   `CC` `HCC`
> Healing pressure ulcer of left ankle, stage 2
> Pressure ulcer with abrasion, blister, partial thickness skin loss involving epidermis and/or dermis, left ankle

L89.523   **Pressure ulcer of left ankle,** stage 3   `CC` `H4` `HCC` `SW`
> Healing pressure ulcer of left ankle, stage 3
> Pressure ulcer with full thickness skin loss involving damage or necrosis of subcutaneous tissue, left ankle

L89.524   **Pressure ulcer of left ankle,** stage 4   `CC` `H4` `HCC` `SW`
> Healing pressure ulcer of left ankle, stage 4
> Pressure ulcer with necrosis of soft tissues through to underlying muscle, tendon, or bone, left ankle

L89.526   **Pressure-induced** deep tissue damage **of left ankle**   `CC`

L89.529   **Pressure ulcer of left ankle, unspecified stage**   `CC`
> Healing pressure ulcer of left ankle NOS
> Healing pressure ulcer of left ankle, unspecified stage

√5ᵗʰ **L89.6**   **Pressure ulcer of** heel

√6ᵗʰ **L89.60**   **Pressure ulcer of unspecified heel**

L89.600   **Pressure ulcer of unspecified heel,** unstageable   `CC` `HCC` `SW`

L89.601   **Pressure ulcer of unspecified heel,** stage 1   `CC`
> Healing pressure ulcer of unspecified heel, stage 1
> Pressure pre-ulcer skin changes limited to persistent focal edema, unspecified heel

L89.602   **Pressure ulcer of unspecified heel,** stage 2   `CC` `HCC`
> Healing pressure ulcer of unspecified heel, stage 2
> Pressure ulcer with abrasion, blister, partial thickness skin loss involving epidermis and/or dermis, unspecified heel

L89.603   **Pressure ulcer of unspecified heel,** stage 3   `CC` `H4` `HCC` `SW`
> Healing pressure ulcer of unspecified heel, stage 3
> Pressure ulcer with full thickness skin loss involving damage or necrosis of subcutaneous tissue, unspecified heel

L89.604   **Pressure ulcer of unspecified heel,** stage 4   `CC` `H4` `HCC` `SW`
> Healing pressure ulcer of unspecified heel, stage 4
> Pressure ulcer with necrosis of soft tissues through to underlying muscle, tendon, or bone, unspecified heel

L89.606   **Pressure-induced** deep tissue damage **of unspecified heel**   `CC`

L89.609   **Pressure ulcer of unspecified heel, unspecified stage**   `CC`
> Healing pressure ulcer of unspecified heel NOS
> Healing pressure ulcer of unspecified heel, unspecified stage

√6ᵗʰ **L89.61**   **Pressure ulcer of** right **heel**

L89.610   **Pressure ulcer of right heel,** unstageable   `CC` `HCC` `SW`

L89.611   **Pressure ulcer of right heel,** stage 1   `CC`
> Healing pressure ulcer of right heel, stage 1
> Pressure pre-ulcer skin changes limited to persistent focal edema, right heel

L89.612   **Pressure ulcer of right heel,** stage 2   `CC` `HCC`
> Healing pressure ulcer of right heel, stage 2
> Pressure ulcer with abrasion, blister, partial thickness skin loss involving epidermis and/or dermis, right heel

L89.613   **Pressure ulcer of right heel,** stage 3   `CC` `H4` `HCC` `SW`
> Healing pressure ulcer of right heel, stage 3
> Pressure ulcer with full thickness skin loss involving damage or necrosis of subcutaneous tissue, right heel

L89.614   **Pressure ulcer of right heel,** stage 4   `CC` `H4` `HCC` `SW`
> Healing pressure ulcer of right heel, stage 4
> Pressure ulcer with necrosis of soft tissues through to underlying muscle, tendon, or bone, right heel

L89.616   **Pressure-induced** deep tissue damage **of right heel**   `CC`

L89.619   **Pressure ulcer of right heel, unspecified stage**   `CC`
> Healing pressure ulcer of right heel NOS
> Healing pressure ulcer of right heel, unspecified stage

√6ᵗʰ **L89.62**   **Pressure ulcer of** left **heel**

L89.620   **Pressure ulcer of left heel,** unstageable   `CC` `HCC` `SW`

L89.621   **Pressure ulcer of left heel,** stage 1   `CC`
> Healing pressure ulcer of left heel, stage 1
> Pressure pre-ulcer skin changes limited to persistent focal edema, left heel

✔ Additional Character Required   √x7ᵗʰ Placeholder   Unacceptable PDx   Questionable PDx   Manifestation   Unspecified Dx   H1-H4 HAC   HCC CMS-HCC Dx   HIV HIV Dx

ICD-10-CM 2020   751

Chapter 12. Diseases of the Skin and Subcutaneous Tissue   L89.512–L89.621

Chapter 12. Diseases of the Skin and Subcutaneous Tissue

L89.622   **Pressure ulcer of left heel,** `CC` `HCC`
stage 2
   Healing pressure ulcer of left heel, stage 2
   Pressure ulcer with abrasion, blister, partial
     thickness skin loss involving
     epidermis and/or dermis, left heel

L89.623   **Pressure ulcer of left heel,** `CC` `H4` `HCC` `SW`
stage 3
   Healing pressure ulcer of left heel, stage 3
   Pressure ulcer with full thickness skin loss
     involving damage or necrosis of
     subcutaneous tissue, left heel

L89.624   **Pressure ulcer of left heel,** `CC` `H4` `HCC` `SW`
stage 4
   Healing pressure ulcer of left heel, stage 4
   Pressure ulcer with necrosis of soft tissues
     through to underlying muscle,
     tendon, or bone, left heel

L89.626   **Pressure-induced deep** `CC`
tissue damage of left heel

L89.629   **Pressure ulcer of left heel,** `CC`
unspecified stage
   Healing pressure ulcer of left heel NOS
   Healing pressure ulcer of left heel,
     unspecified stage

✓5ᵗʰ **L89.8**   **Pressure ulcer of other site**

   ✓6ᵗʰ **L89.81**   **Pressure ulcer of head**
     Pressure ulcer of face

L89.810   **Pressure ulcer of head,** `CC` `HCC` `SW`
unstageable

L89.811   **Pressure ulcer of head,** `CC`
stage 1
   Healing pressure ulcer of head, stage 1
   Pressure pre-ulcer skin changes limited to
     persistent focal edema, head

L89.812   **Pressure ulcer of head,** `CC` `HCC`
stage 2
   Healing pressure ulcer of head, stage 2
   Pressure ulcer with abrasion, blister, partial
     thickness skin loss involving
     epidermis and/or dermis, head

L89.813   **Pressure ulcer of head,** `CC` `H4` `HCC` `SW`
stage 3
   Healing pressure ulcer of head, stage 3
   Pressure ulcer with full thickness skin loss
     involving damage or necrosis of
     subcutaneous tissue, head

L89.814   **Pressure ulcer of head,** `CC` `H4` `HCC` `SW`
stage 4
   Healing pressure ulcer of head, stage 4
   Pressure ulcer with necrosis of soft tissues
     through to underlying muscle,
     tendon, or bone, head

L89.816   **Pressure-induced deep** `CC`
tissue damage of head

L89.819   **Pressure ulcer of head,** `CC`
unspecified stage
   Healing pressure ulcer of head NOS
   Healing pressure ulcer of head, unspecified
     stage

   ✓6ᵗʰ **L89.89**   **Pressure ulcer of other site**

L89.890   **Pressure ulcer of other** `CC` `HCC` `SW`
site, unstageable

L89.891   **Pressure ulcer of other** `CC`
site, stage 1
   Healing pressure ulcer of other site, stage 1
   Pressure pre-ulcer skin changes limited to
     persistent focal edema, other site

L89.892   **Pressure ulcer of other** `CC` `HCC`
site, stage 2
   Healing pressure ulcer of other site, stage 2
   Pressure ulcer with abrasion, blister, partial
     thickness skin loss involving
     epidermis and/or dermis, other site

L89.893   **Pressure ulcer of other** `CC` `H4` `HCC` `SW`
site, stage 3
   Healing pressure ulcer of other site, stage 3
   Pressure ulcer with full thickness skin loss
     involving damage or necrosis of
     subcutaneous tissue, other site

L89.894   **Pressure ulcer of other** `CC` `H4` `HCC` `SW`
site, stage 4
   Healing pressure ulcer of other site, stage 4
   Pressure ulcer with necrosis of soft tissues
     through to underlying muscle,
     tendon, or bone, other site

L89.896   **Pressure-induced deep** `CC`
**tissue damage of other
site**

L89.899   **Pressure ulcer of other** `CC`
site, unspecified stage
   Healing pressure ulcer of other site NOS
   Healing pressure ulcer of other site,
     unspecified stage

✓5ᵗʰ **L89.9**   **Pressure ulcer of unspecified site**

L89.90   **Pressure ulcer of unspecified site,** `CC`
unspecified stage
   Healing pressure ulcer of unspecified site NOS
   Healing pressure ulcer of unspecified site, unspecified
     stage

L89.91   **Pressure ulcer of unspecified site,** `CC`
stage 1
   Healing pressure ulcer of unspecified site, stage 1
   Pressure pre-ulcer skin changes limited to persistent
     focal edema, unspecified site

L89.92   **Pressure ulcer of unspecified site,** `CC` `HCC`
stage 2
   Healing pressure ulcer of unspecified site, stage 2
   Pressure ulcer with abrasion, blister, partial thickness
     skin loss involving epidermis and/or dermis,
     unspecified site

L89.93   **Pressure ulcer of unspecified site,** `CC` `H4` `HCC` `SW`
stage 3
   Healing pressure ulcer of unspecified site, stage 3
   Pressure ulcer with full thickness skin loss involving
     damage or necrosis of subcutaneous tissue,
     unspecified site

L89.94   **Pressure ulcer of unspecified site,** `CC` `H4` `HCC` `SW`
stage 4
   Healing pressure ulcer of unspecified site, stage 4
   Pressure ulcer with necrosis of soft tissues through
     to underlying muscle, tendon, or bone,
     unspecified site

L89.95   **Pressure ulcer of unspecified site,** `CC` `HCC` `SW`
unstageable

L89.96   **Pressure-induced deep tissue** `CC`
damage of unspecified site

✓4ᵗʰ **L90**   **Atrophic disorders of skin**

   L90.0   **Lichen sclerosus et atrophicus**
     `EXCLUDES 2`   *lichen sclerosus of external female genital organs*
       (N90.4)
     lichen sclerosus of external male genital organs
       (N48.0)

   L90.1   **Anetoderma of Schweninger-Buzzi**

   L90.2   **Anetoderma of Jadassohn-Pellizzari**

   L90.3   **Atrophoderma of Pasini and Pierini**

   L90.4   **Acrodermatitis chronica atrophicans**

   L90.5   **Scar conditions and fibrosis of skin**
     Adherent scar (skin)
     Cicatrix
     Disfigurement of skin due to scar
     Fibrosis of skin NOS
     Scar NOS
     `EXCLUDES 2`   *hypertrophic scar (L91.0)*
       keloid scar (L91.0)
     AHA: 2016,2Q,5; 2015,1Q,19

   L90.6   **Striae atrophicae**

   L90.8   **Other atrophic disorders of skin**

   L90.9   **Atrophic disorder of skin, unspecified**

☑4ᵗʰ L91 Hypertrophic disorders of skin

L91.0 Hypertrophic scar
Keloid
Keloid scar
EXCLUDES 2   acne keloid (L73.0)
           scar NOS (L90.5)
DEF: Overgrowth of scar tissue due to excess amounts of collagen during connective tissue repair, occurring mainly on the upper trunk and face.

L91.8 Other hypertrophic disorders of the skin
L91.9 Hypertrophic disorder of the skin, unspecified

☑4ᵗʰ L92 Granulomatous disorders of skin and subcutaneous tissue
EXCLUDES 2   actinic granuloma (L57.5)

L92.0 Granuloma annulare
Perforating granuloma annulare
L92.1 Necrobiosis lipoidica, not elsewhere classified
EXCLUDES 1   necrobiosis lipoidica associated with diabetes
           mellitus (E08-E13 with .620)
L92.2 Granuloma faciale [eosinophilic granuloma of skin]
L92.3 Foreign body granuloma of the skin and subcutaneous tissue
Use additional code to identify the type of retained foreign body (Z18.-)
L92.8 Other granulomatous disorders of the skin and subcutaneous tissue
L92.9 Granulomatous disorder of the skin and subcutaneous tissue, unspecified
EXCLUDES 2   umbilical granuloma (P83.81)
AHA: 2017,4Q,21-22

☑4ᵗʰ L93 Lupus erythematosus
Use additional code for adverse effect, if applicable, to identify drug (T36-T50 with fifth or sixth character 5)
EXCLUDES 1   lupus exedens (A18.4)
           lupus vulgaris (A18.4)
           scleroderma (M34.-)
           systemic lupus erythematosus (M32.-)
DEF: Inflammatory, autoimmune skin condition in which the body's autoimmune system attacks healthy tissue of the integumentary system.

L93.0 Discoid lupus erythematosus
Lupus erythematosus NOS
L93.1 Subacute cutaneous lupus erythematosus
L93.2 Other local lupus erythematosus
Lupus erythematosus profundus
Lupus panniculitis

☑4ᵗʰ L94 Other localized connective tissue disorders
EXCLUDES 1   systemic connective tissue disorders (M30-M36)

L94.0 Localized scleroderma [morphea]
Circumscribed scleroderma
L94.1 Linear scleroderma
En coup de sabre lesion
L94.2 Calcinosis cutis
L94.3 Sclerodactyly
L94.4 Gottron's papules
L94.5 Poikiloderma vasculare atrophicans
L94.6 Ainhum
L94.8 Other specified localized connective tissue disorders
L94.9 Localized connective tissue disorder, unspecified

☑4ᵗʰ L95 Vasculitis limited to skin, not elsewhere classified
EXCLUDES 1   angioma serpiginosum (L81.7)
           Henoch(-Schönlein) purpura (D69.0)
           hypersensitivity angiitis (M31.0)
           lupus panniculitis (L93.2)
           panniculitis NOS (M79.3)
           panniculitis of neck and back (M54.0-)
           polyarteritis nodosa (M30.0)
           relapsing panniculitis (M35.6)
           rheumatoid vasculitis (M05.2)
           serum sickness (T80.6-)
           urticaria (L50.-)
           Wegener's granulomatosis (M31.3-)

L95.0 Livedoid vasculitis
Atrophie blanche (en plaque)
L95.1 Erythema elevatum diutinum
L95.8 Other vasculitis limited to the skin
L95.9 Vasculitis limited to the skin, unspecified

☑4ᵗʰ L97 Non-pressure chronic ulcer of lower limb, not elsewhere classified
INCLUDES   chronic ulcer of skin of lower limb NOS
           non-healing ulcer of skin
           non-infected sinus of skin
           trophic ulcer NOS
           tropical ulcer NOS
           ulcer of skin of lower limb NOS
Code first any associated underlying condition, such as:
   any associated gangrene (I96)
   atherosclerosis of the lower extremities (I70.23-, I70.24-, I70.33-, I70.34-, I70.43-, I70.44-, I70.53-, I70.54-, I70.63-, I70.64-, I70.73-, I70.74-)
   chronic venous hypertension (I87.31-, I87.33-)
   diabetic ulcers (E08.621, E08.622, E09.621, E09.622, E10.621, E10.622, E11.621, E11.622, E13.621, E13.622)
   postphlebitic syndrome (I87.01-, I87.03-)
   postthrombotic syndrome (I87.01-, I87.03-)
   varicose ulcer (I83.0-, I83.2-)
EXCLUDES 2   pressure ulcer (pressure area) (L89.-)
           skin infections (L00-L08)
           specific infections classified to A00-B99
AHA: 2018,4Q,69; 2017,4Q,17
TIP: The depth and/or severity of a diagnosed nonpressure ulcer can be determined based on medical record documentation from clinicians who are not the patient's provider.
TIP: Assign a code from this category/subcategory for nonpressure ulcers documented as acute.
CC Excl: For CC codes in category L97: PDX collection 698

☑5ᵗʰ L97.1 Non-pressure chronic ulcer of thigh

☑6ᵗʰ L97.10 Non-pressure chronic ulcer of unspecified thigh

L97.101 Non-pressure chronic ulcer of unspecified thigh limited to breakdown of skin   CC HCC

L97.102 Non-pressure chronic ulcer of unspecified thigh with fat layer exposed   CC HCC SW

L97.103 Non-pressure chronic ulcer of unspecified thigh with necrosis of muscle   CC HCC SW

L97.104 Non-pressure chronic ulcer of unspecified thigh with necrosis of bone   CC HCC SW

L97.105 Non-pressure chronic ulcer of unspecified thigh with muscle involvement without evidence of necrosis   CC HCC

L97.106 Non-pressure chronic ulcer of unspecified thigh with bone involvement without evidence of necrosis   CC HCC

L97.108 Non-pressure chronic ulcer of unspecified thigh with other specified severity   CC HCC

L97.109 Non-pressure chronic ulcer of unspecified thigh with unspecified severity   CC HCC

☑6ᵗʰ L97.11 Non-pressure chronic ulcer of right thigh

L97.111 Non-pressure chronic ulcer of right thigh limited to breakdown of skin   CC HCC

L97.112 Non-pressure chronic ulcer of right thigh with fat layer exposed   CC HCC SW

L97.113 Non-pressure chronic ulcer of right thigh with necrosis of muscle   CC HCC SW

L97.114 Non-pressure chronic ulcer of right thigh with necrosis of bone   CC HCC SW

L97.115 Non-pressure chronic ulcer of right thigh with muscle involvement without evidence of necrosis   CC HCC

L97.116 Non-pressure chronic ulcer of right thigh with bone involvement without evidence of necrosis   CC HCC

L97.118 Non-pressure chronic ulcer of right thigh with other specified severity   CC HCC

L97.119 Non-pressure chronic ulcer of right thigh with unspecified severity `CC` `HCC`

✓6ᵗʰ **L97.12** Non-pressure chronic ulcer of left thigh

L97.121 Non-pressure chronic ulcer of left thigh limited to breakdown of skin `CC` `HCC`

L97.122 Non-pressure chronic ulcer of left thigh with fat layer exposed `CC` `HCC` `SW`

L97.123 Non-pressure chronic ulcer of left thigh with necrosis of muscle `CC` `HCC` `SW`

L97.124 Non-pressure chronic ulcer of left thigh with necrosis of bone `CC` `HCC` `SW`

L97.125 Non-pressure chronic ulcer of left thigh with muscle involvement without evidence of necrosis `CC` `HCC`

L97.126 Non-pressure chronic ulcer of left thigh with bone involvement without evidence of necrosis `CC` `HCC`

L97.128 Non-pressure chronic ulcer of left thigh with other specified severity `CC` `HCC`

L97.129 Non-pressure chronic ulcer of left thigh with unspecified severity `CC` `HCC`

✓5ᵗʰ **L97.2** Non-pressure chronic ulcer of calf

✓6ᵗʰ **L97.20** Non-pressure chronic ulcer of unspecified calf

L97.201 Non-pressure chronic ulcer of unspecified calf limited to breakdown of skin `CC` `HCC`

L97.202 Non-pressure chronic ulcer of unspecified calf with fat layer exposed `CC` `HCC` `SW`

L97.203 Non-pressure chronic ulcer of unspecified calf with necrosis of muscle `CC` `HCC` `SW`

L97.204 Non-pressure chronic ulcer of unspecified calf with necrosis of bone `CC` `HCC` `SW`

L97.205 Non-pressure chronic ulcer of unspecified calf with muscle involvement without evidence of necrosis `CC` `HCC`

L97.206 Non-pressure chronic ulcer of unspecified calf with bone involvement without evidence of necrosis `CC` `HCC`

L97.208 Non-pressure chronic ulcer of unspecified calf with other specified severity `CC` `HCC`

L97.209 Non-pressure chronic ulcer of unspecified calf with unspecified severity `CC` `HCC`

✓6ᵗʰ **L97.21** Non-pressure chronic ulcer of right calf

L97.211 Non-pressure chronic ulcer of right calf limited to breakdown of skin `CC` `HCC`

L97.212 Non-pressure chronic ulcer of right calf with fat layer exposed `CC` `HCC` `SW`

L97.213 Non-pressure chronic ulcer of right calf with necrosis of muscle `CC` `HCC` `SW`

L97.214 Non-pressure chronic ulcer of right calf with necrosis of bone `CC` `HCC` `SW`

L97.215 Non-pressure chronic ulcer of right calf with muscle involvement without evidence of necrosis `CC` `HCC`

L97.216 Non-pressure chronic ulcer of right calf with bone involvement without evidence of necrosis `CC` `HCC`

L97.218 Non-pressure chronic ulcer of right calf with other specified severity `CC` `HCC`

L97.219 Non-pressure chronic ulcer of right calf with unspecified severity `CC` `HCC`

✓6ᵗʰ **L97.22** Non-pressure chronic ulcer of left calf

L97.221 Non-pressure chronic ulcer of left calf limited to breakdown of skin `CC` `HCC`

L97.222 Non-pressure chronic ulcer of left calf with fat layer exposed `CC` `HCC` `SW`

L97.223 Non-pressure chronic ulcer of left calf with necrosis of muscle `CC` `HCC` `SW`

L97.224 Non-pressure chronic ulcer of left calf with necrosis of bone `CC` `HCC` `SW`

L97.225 Non-pressure chronic ulcer of left calf with muscle involvement without evidence of necrosis `CC` `HCC`

L97.226 Non-pressure chronic ulcer of left calf with bone involvement without evidence of necrosis `CC` `HCC`

L97.228 Non-pressure chronic ulcer of left calf with other specified severity `CC` `HCC`

L97.229 Non-pressure chronic ulcer of left calf with unspecified severity `CC` `HCC`

✓5ᵗʰ **L97.3** Non-pressure chronic ulcer of ankle

✓6ᵗʰ **L97.30** Non-pressure chronic ulcer of unspecified ankle

L97.301 Non-pressure chronic ulcer of unspecified ankle limited to breakdown of skin `CC` `HCC`

L97.302 Non-pressure chronic ulcer of unspecified ankle with fat layer exposed `CC` `HCC` `SW`

L97.303 Non-pressure chronic ulcer of unspecified ankle with necrosis of muscle `CC` `HCC` `SW`

L97.304 Non-pressure chronic ulcer of unspecified ankle with necrosis of bone `CC` `HCC` `SW`

L97.305 Non-pressure chronic ulcer of unspecified ankle with muscle involvement without evidence of necrosis `CC` `HCC`

L97.306 Non-pressure chronic ulcer of unspecified ankle with bone involvement without evidence of necrosis `CC` `HCC`

L97.308 Non-pressure chronic ulcer of unspecified ankle with other specified severity `CC` `HCC`

L97.309 Non-pressure chronic ulcer of unspecified ankle with unspecified severity `CC` `HCC`

✓6ᵗʰ **L97.31** Non-pressure chronic ulcer of right ankle

L97.311 Non-pressure chronic ulcer of right ankle limited to breakdown of skin `CC` `HCC`

L97.312 Non-pressure chronic ulcer of right ankle with fat layer exposed `CC` `HCC` `SW`

L97.313 Non-pressure chronic ulcer of right ankle with necrosis of muscle `CC` `HCC` `SW`

L97.314 Non-pressure chronic ulcer of right ankle with necrosis of bone `CC` `HCC` `SW`

L97.315 Non-pressure chronic ulcer of right ankle with muscle involvement without evidence of necrosis `CC` `HCC`

L97.316 Non-pressure chronic ulcer of right ankle with bone involvement without evidence of necrosis `CC` `HCC`

L97.318 Non-pressure chronic ulcer of right ankle with other specified severity `CC` `HCC`

        L97.319 Non-pressure chronic ulcer of right ankle with unspecified severity   `CC` `HCC`

    ✓6th **L97.32** Non-pressure chronic ulcer of left ankle

        L97.321 Non-pressure chronic ulcer of left ankle limited to breakdown of skin   `CC` `HCC`

        L97.322 Non-pressure chronic ulcer of left ankle with fat layer exposed   `CC` `HCC` `SW`

        L97.323 Non-pressure chronic ulcer of left ankle with necrosis of muscle   `CC` `HCC` `SW`

        L97.324 Non-pressure chronic ulcer of left ankle with necrosis of bone   `CC` `HCC` `SW`

        L97.325 Non-pressure chronic ulcer of left ankle with muscle involvement without evidence of necrosis   `CC` `HCC`

        L97.326 Non-pressure chronic ulcer of left ankle with bone involvement without evidence of necrosis   `CC` `HCC`

        L97.328 Non-pressure chronic ulcer of left ankle with other specified severity   `CC` `HCC`

        L97.329 Non-pressure chronic ulcer of left ankle with unspecified severity   `CC` `HCC`

✓5th **L97.4** Non-pressure chronic ulcer of heel and midfoot

    Non-pressure chronic ulcer of plantar surface of midfoot

    ✓6th **L97.40** Non-pressure chronic ulcer of unspecified heel and midfoot

        L97.401 Non-pressure chronic ulcer of unspecified heel and midfoot limited to breakdown of skin   `CC` `HCC`

        L97.402 Non-pressure chronic ulcer of unspecified heel and midfoot with fat layer exposed   `CC` `HCC` `SW`

        L97.403 Non-pressure chronic ulcer of unspecified heel and midfoot with necrosis of muscle   `CC` `HCC` `SW`

        L97.404 Non-pressure chronic ulcer of unspecified heel and midfoot with necrosis of bone   `CC` `HCC` `SW`

        L97.405 Non-pressure chronic ulcer of unspecified heel and midfoot with muscle involvement without evidence of necrosis   `CC` `HCC`

        L97.406 Non-pressure chronic ulcer of unspecified heel and midfoot with bone involvement without evidence of necrosis   `CC` `HCC`

        L97.408 Non-pressure chronic ulcer of unspecified heel and midfoot with other specified severity   `CC` `HCC`

        L97.409 Non-pressure chronic ulcer of unspecified heel and midfoot with unspecified severity   `CC` `HCC`

    ✓6th **L97.41** Non-pressure chronic ulcer of right heel and midfoot

        L97.411 Non-pressure chronic ulcer of right heel and midfoot limited to breakdown of skin   `CC` `HCC`

        L97.412 Non-pressure chronic ulcer of right heel and midfoot with fat layer exposed   `CC` `HCC` `SW`

        L97.413 Non-pressure chronic ulcer of right heel and midfoot with necrosis of muscle   `CC` `HCC` `SW`

        L97.414 Non-pressure chronic ulcer of right heel and midfoot with necrosis of bone   `CC` `HCC` `SW`

        L97.415 Non-pressure chronic ulcer of right heel and midfoot with muscle involvement without evidence of necrosis   `CC` `HCC`

        L97.416 Non-pressure chronic ulcer of right heel and midfoot with bone involvement without evidence of necrosis   `CC` `HCC`

        L97.418 Non-pressure chronic ulcer of right heel and midfoot with other specified severity   `CC` `HCC`

        L97.419 Non-pressure chronic ulcer of right heel and midfoot with unspecified severity   `CC` `HCC`

    ✓6th **L97.42** Non-pressure chronic ulcer of left heel and midfoot

        L97.421 Non-pressure chronic ulcer of left heel and midfoot limited to breakdown of skin   `CC` `HCC`

            AHA: 2016,1Q,12

        L97.422 Non-pressure chronic ulcer of left heel and midfoot with fat layer exposed   `CC` `HCC` `SW`

        L97.423 Non-pressure chronic ulcer of left heel and midfoot with necrosis of muscle   `CC` `HCC` `SW`

        L97.424 Non-pressure chronic ulcer of left heel and midfoot with necrosis of bone   `CC` `HCC` `SW`

        L97.425 Non-pressure chronic ulcer of left heel and midfoot with muscle involvement without evidence of necrosis   `CC` `HCC`

        L97.426 Non-pressure chronic ulcer of left heel and midfoot with bone involvement without evidence of necrosis   `CC` `HCC`

        L97.428 Non-pressure chronic ulcer of left heel and midfoot with other specified severity   `CC` `HCC`

        L97.429 Non-pressure chronic ulcer of left heel and midfoot with unspecified severity   `CC` `HCC`

✓5th **L97.5** Non-pressure chronic ulcer of other part of foot

    Non-pressure chronic ulcer of toe

    ✓6th **L97.50** Non-pressure chronic ulcer of other part of unspecified foot

        L97.501 Non-pressure chronic ulcer of other part of unspecified foot limited to breakdown of skin   `HCC`

        L97.502 Non-pressure chronic ulcer of other part of unspecified foot with fat layer exposed   `HCC` `SW`

        L97.503 Non-pressure chronic ulcer of other part of unspecified foot with necrosis of muscle   `HCC` `SW`

        L97.504 Non-pressure chronic ulcer of other part of unspecified foot with necrosis of bone   `HCC` `SW`

        L97.505 Non-pressure chronic ulcer of other part of unspecified foot with muscle involvement without evidence of necrosis   `CC` `HCC`

        L97.506 Non-pressure chronic ulcer of other part of unspecified foot with bone involvement without evidence of necrosis   `CC` `HCC`

        L97.508 Non-pressure chronic ulcer of other part of unspecified foot with other specified severity   `CC` `HCC`

✓ Additional Character Required ✓x7th Placeholder   Unacceptable PDx   Questionable PDx   Manifestation   Unspecified Dx   H1-H14 HAC   HCC CMS-HCC Dx   HIV HIV Dx

ICD-10-CM 2020

755

L97.509 Non-pressure chronic ulcer of other part of unspecified foot with unspecified severity `HCC`

✓6ᵗʰ **L97.51** Non-pressure chronic ulcer of other part of right foot

L97.511 Non-pressure chronic ulcer of other part of right foot limited to breakdown of skin `HCC`

L97.512 Non-pressure chronic ulcer of other part of right foot with fat layer exposed `HCC` `SW`

L97.513 Non-pressure chronic ulcer of other part of right foot with necrosis of muscle `HCC` `SW`

L97.514 Non-pressure chronic ulcer of other part of right foot with necrosis of bone `HCC` `SW`

L97.515 Non-pressure chronic ulcer of other part of right foot with muscle involvement without evidence of necrosis `CC` `HCC`

L97.516 Non-pressure chronic ulcer of other part of right foot with bone involvement without evidence of necrosis `CC` `HCC`

L97.518 Non-pressure chronic ulcer of other part of right foot with other specified severity `CC` `HCC`

L97.519 Non-pressure chronic ulcer of other part of right foot with unspecified severity `HCC`

✓6ᵗʰ **L97.52** Non-pressure chronic ulcer of other part of left foot

L97.521 Non-pressure chronic ulcer of other part of left foot limited to breakdown of skin `HCC`

L97.522 Non-pressure chronic ulcer of other part of left foot with fat layer exposed `HCC` `SW`

L97.523 Non-pressure chronic ulcer of other part of left foot with necrosis of muscle `HCC` `SW`

L97.524 Non-pressure chronic ulcer of other part of left foot with necrosis of bone `HCC` `SW`

L97.525 Non-pressure chronic ulcer of other part of left foot with muscle involvement without evidence of necrosis `CC` `HCC`

L97.526 Non-pressure chronic ulcer of other part of left foot with bone involvement without evidence of necrosis `CC` `HCC`

L97.528 Non-pressure chronic ulcer of other part of left foot with other specified severity `CC` `HCC`

L97.529 Non-pressure chronic ulcer of other part of left foot with unspecified severity `HCC`

✓5ᵗʰ **L97.8** Non-pressure chronic ulcer of other part of lower leg

✓6ᵗʰ **L97.80** Non-pressure chronic ulcer of other part of unspecified lower leg

L97.801 Non-pressure chronic ulcer of other part of unspecified lower leg limited to breakdown of skin `CC` `HCC`

L97.802 Non-pressure chronic ulcer of other part of unspecified lower leg with fat layer exposed `CC` `HCC` `SW`

L97.803 Non-pressure chronic ulcer of other part of unspecified lower leg with necrosis of muscle `CC` `HCC` `SW`

L97.804 Non-pressure chronic ulcer of other part of unspecified lower leg with necrosis of bone `CC` `HCC` `SW`

L97.805 Non-pressure chronic ulcer of other part of unspecified lower leg with muscle involvement without evidence of necrosis `CC` `HCC`

L97.806 Non-pressure chronic ulcer of other part of unspecified lower leg with bone involvement without evidence of necrosis `CC` `HCC`

L97.808 Non-pressure chronic ulcer of other part of unspecified lower leg with other specified severity `CC` `HCC`

L97.809 Non-pressure chronic ulcer of other part of unspecified lower leg with unspecified severity `CC` `HCC`

✓6ᵗʰ **L97.81** Non-pressure chronic ulcer of other part of right lower leg

L97.811 Non-pressure chronic ulcer of other part of right lower leg limited to breakdown of skin `CC` `HCC`

L97.812 Non-pressure chronic ulcer of other part of right lower leg with fat layer exposed `CC` `HCC` `SW`

L97.813 Non-pressure chronic ulcer of other part of right lower leg with necrosis of muscle `CC` `HCC` `SW`

L97.814 Non-pressure chronic ulcer of other part of right lower leg with necrosis of bone `CC` `HCC` `SW`

L97.815 Non-pressure chronic ulcer of other part of right lower leg with muscle involvement without evidence of necrosis `CC` `HCC`

L97.816 Non-pressure chronic ulcer of other part of right lower leg with bone involvement without evidence of necrosis `CC` `HCC`

L97.818 Non-pressure chronic ulcer of other part of right lower leg with other specified severity `CC` `HCC`

L97.819 Non-pressure chronic ulcer of other part of right lower leg with unspecified severity `CC` `HCC`

✓6ᵗʰ **L97.82** Non-pressure chronic ulcer of other part of left lower leg

L97.821 Non-pressure chronic ulcer of other part of left lower leg limited to breakdown of skin `CC` `HCC`

L97.822 Non-pressure chronic ulcer of other part of left lower leg with fat layer exposed `CC` `HCC` `SW`

L97.823 Non-pressure chronic ulcer of other part of left lower leg with necrosis of muscle `CC` `HCC` `SW`

L97.824 Non-pressure chronic ulcer of other part of left lower leg with necrosis of bone `CC` `HCC` `SW`

L97.825 Non-pressure chronic ulcer of other part of left lower leg with muscle involvement without evidence of necrosis `CC` `HCC`

L97.826 Non-pressure chronic ulcer of other part of left lower leg with bone involvement without evidence of necrosis `CC` `HCC`

L97.828 Non-pressure chronic ulcer of other part of left lower leg with other specified severity `CC` `HCC`

Ⓝ Newborn: 0　　Ⓟ Pediatric: 0-17　　Ⓜ Maternity: 9-64　　Ⓐ Adult: 15-124　　`MCC` Major Complication/Comorbidity　　`CC` Complication/Comorbidity　　`SW` Severe Wound Dx

756　　ICD-10-CM 2020

L97.829   Non-pressure chronic ulcer of other part of left lower leg with unspecified severity   `CC` `HCC`

√5th **L97.9 Non-pressure chronic ulcer of unspecified part of lower leg**

√6th **L97.90   Non-pressure chronic ulcer of unspecified part of unspecified lower leg**

L97.901   Non-pressure chronic ulcer of unspecified part of unspecified lower leg limited to breakdown of skin   `CC` `HCC`

L97.902   Non-pressure chronic ulcer of unspecified part of unspecified lower leg with fat layer exposed   `CC` `HCC` `SW`

L97.903   Non-pressure chronic ulcer of unspecified part of unspecified lower leg with necrosis of muscle   `CC` `HCC` `SW`

L97.904   Non-pressure chronic ulcer of unspecified part of unspecified lower leg with necrosis of bone   `CC` `HCC` `SW`

L97.905   Non-pressure chronic ulcer of unspecified part of unspecified lower leg with muscle involvement without evidence of necrosis   `CC` `HCC`

L97.906   Non-pressure chronic ulcer of unspecified part of unspecified lower leg with bone involvement without evidence of necrosis   `CC` `HCC`

L97.908   Non-pressure chronic ulcer of unspecified part of unspecified lower leg with other specified severity   `CC` `HCC`

L97.909   Non-pressure chronic ulcer of unspecified part of unspecified lower leg with unspecified severity   `CC` `HCC`

√6th **L97.91   Non-pressure chronic ulcer of unspecified part of right lower leg**

L97.911   Non-pressure chronic ulcer of unspecified part of right lower leg limited to breakdown of skin   `CC` `HCC`

L97.912   Non-pressure chronic ulcer of unspecified part of right lower leg with fat layer exposed   `CC` `HCC` `SW`

L97.913   Non-pressure chronic ulcer of unspecified part of right lower leg with necrosis of muscle   `CC` `HCC` `SW`

L97.914   Non-pressure chronic ulcer of unspecified part of right lower leg with necrosis of bone   `CC` `HCC` `SW`

L97.915   Non-pressure chronic ulcer of unspecified part of right lower leg with muscle involvement without evidence of necrosis   `CC` `HCC`

L97.916   Non-pressure chronic ulcer of unspecified part of right lower leg with bone involvement without evidence of necrosis   `CC` `HCC`

L97.918   Non-pressure chronic ulcer of unspecified part of right lower leg with other specified severity   `CC` `HCC`

L97.919   Non-pressure chronic ulcer of unspecified part of right lower leg with unspecified severity   `CC` `HCC`

√6th **L97.92   Non-pressure chronic ulcer of unspecified part of left lower leg**

L97.921   Non-pressure chronic ulcer of unspecified part of left lower leg limited to breakdown of skin   `CC` `HCC` `SW`

L97.922   Non-pressure chronic ulcer of unspecified part of left lower leg with fat layer exposed   `CC` `HCC` `SW`

L97.923   Non-pressure chronic ulcer of unspecified part of left lower leg with necrosis of muscle   `CC` `HCC` `SW`

L97.924   Non-pressure chronic ulcer of unspecified part of left lower leg with necrosis of bone   `CC` `HCC` `SW`

L97.925   Non-pressure chronic ulcer of unspecified part of left lower leg with muscle involvement without evidence of necrosis   `CC` `HCC`

L97.926   Non-pressure chronic ulcer of unspecified part of left lower leg with bone involvement without evidence of necrosis   `CC` `HCC`

L97.928   Non-pressure chronic ulcer of unspecified part of left lower leg with other specified severity   `CC` `HCC`

L97.929   Non-pressure chronic ulcer of unspecified part of left lower leg with unspecified severity   `CC` `HCC`

√4th **L98 Other disorders of skin and subcutaneous tissue, not elsewhere classified**

L98.0 Pyogenic granuloma

EXCLUDES 2   pyogenic granuloma of gingiva (K06.8)

pyogenic granuloma of maxillary alveolar ridge (K04.5)

pyogenic granuloma of oral mucosa (K13.4)

DEF: Solitary polypoid capillary hemangioma often associated with local irritation, trauma, and superimposed inflammation. Located on the skin and gingival or oral mucosa, they bleed easily and may ulcerate and form crusted sores.

L98.1 Factitial dermatitis

Neurotic excoriation

EXCLUDES 1   excoriation (skin-picking) disorder (F42.4)

AHA: 2016,4Q,15

DEF: Self-inflicted skin lesions to satisfy an unconscious psychological or emotional need. Methods used to injure the skin include deep excoriations with a sharp instrument, scarification with a knife, or the application of caustic chemicals and burning, sometimes with a cigarette.

L98.2 Febrile neutrophilic dermatosis [Sweet]

L98.3 Eosinophilic cellulitis [Wells]   `CC`

CC Excl: PDX collection 839

√5th **L98.4 Non-pressure chronic ulcer of skin, not elsewhere classified**

Chronic ulcer of skin NOS

Tropical ulcer NOS

Ulcer of skin NOS

EXCLUDES 2   gangrene (I96)

pressure ulcer (pressure area) (L89.-)

skin infections (L00-L08)

specific infections classified to A00-B99

ulcer of lower limb NEC (L97.-)

varicose ulcer (I83.0-I82.2)

AHA: 2017,4Q,17

TIP: The depth and/or severity of a diagnosed nonpressure ulcer can be determined based on medical record documentation from clinicians who are not the patient's provider.

TIP: Assign a code from this category/subcategory for nonpressure ulcers documented as acute.

CC Excl: For CC codes in subcategory L98.4: PDX collection 698

√6th **L98.41   Non-pressure chronic ulcer of buttock**

L98.411   Non-pressure chronic ulcer of buttock limited to breakdown of skin   `HCC`

L98.412   Non-pressure chronic ulcer of buttock with fat layer exposed   `HCC` `SW`

L98.413   Non-pressure chronic ulcer of buttock with necrosis of muscle   `HCC` `SW`

Chapter 12. Diseases of the Skin and Subcutaneous Tissue

L98.414   **Non-pressure chronic ulcer of buttock** with necrosis of bone   HCC SW

L98.415   **Non-pressure chronic ulcer of buttock** with muscle involvement without evidence of necrosis   CC HCC

L98.416   **Non-pressure chronic ulcer of buttock** with bone involvement without evidence of necrosis   CC HCC

L98.418   **Non-pressure chronic ulcer of buttock** with other specified severity   CC HCC

L98.419   **Non-pressure chronic ulcer of buttock** with unspecified severity   HCC

√6ᵗʰ **L98.42**   **Non-pressure chronic ulcer of** back

L98.421   **Non-pressure chronic ulcer of back** limited to breakdown of skin   HCC

L98.422   **Non-pressure chronic ulcer of back** with fat layer exposed   HCC SW

L98.423   **Non-pressure chronic ulcer of back** with necrosis of muscle   HCC SW

L98.424   **Non-pressure chronic ulcer of back** with necrosis of bone   HCC SW

L98.425   **Non-pressure chronic ulcer of back** with muscle involvement without evidence of necrosis   CC HCC

L98.426   **Non-pressure chronic ulcer of back** with bone involvement without evidence of necrosis   CC HCC

L98.428   **Non-pressure chronic ulcer of back** with other specified severity   CC HCC

L98.429   **Non-pressure chronic ulcer of back** with unspecified severity   HCC

√6ᵗʰ **L98.49**   **Non-pressure chronic ulcer of skin of other sites**

Non-pressure chronic ulcer of skin NOS

L98.491   **Non-pressure chronic ulcer of skin of other sites** limited to breakdown of skin   HCC

L98.492   **Non-pressure chronic ulcer of skin of other sites** with fat layer exposed   HCC SW

L98.493   **Non-pressure chronic ulcer of skin of other sites** with necrosis of muscle   HCC SW

L98.494   **Non-pressure chronic ulcer of skin of other sites** with necrosis of bone   HCC SW

L98.495   **Non-pressure chronic ulcer of skin of other sites** with muscle involvement without evidence of necrosis   CC HCC

L98.496   **Non-pressure chronic ulcer of skin of other sites** with bone involvement without evidence of necrosis   CC HCC

L98.498   **Non-pressure chronic ulcer of skin of other sites** with other specified severity   CC HCC

L98.499   **Non-pressure chronic ulcer of skin of other sites** with unspecified severity   HCC

L98.5   **Mucinosis of the skin**

Focal mucinosis

Lichen myxedematosus

Reticular erythematous mucinosis

EXCLUDES 1   *focal oral mucinosis (K13.79)*

myxedema (E03.9)

L98.6   **Other infiltrative disorders of the skin and subcutaneous tissue**

EXCLUDES 1   *hyalinosis cutis et mucosae (E78.89)*

L98.7   **Excessive and redundant skin and subcutaneous tissue**

Loose or sagging skin, following bariatric surgery weight loss

Loose or sagging skin following dietary weight loss

Loose or sagging skin, NOS

EXCLUDES 2   *acquired excess or redundant skin of eyelid (H02.3-)*

congenital excess or redundant skin of eyelid (Q10.3)

skin changes due to chronic exposure to nonionizing radiation (L57.-)

AHA: 2016,4Q,36

L98.8   **Other specified disorders of the skin and subcutaneous tissue**

AHA: 2013,2Q,32

L98.9   **Disorder of the skin and subcutaneous tissue, unspecified**

L99   ***Other disorders of skin and subcutaneous tissue in diseases classified elsewhere***

Code first underlying disease, such as:

amyloidosis (E85.-)

EXCLUDES 1   *skin disorders in diabetes (E08-E13 with .62)*

skin disorders in gonorrhea (A54.89)

skin disorders in syphilis (A51.31, A52.79)

N Newborn: 0   P Pediatric: 0-17   M Maternity: 9-64   A Adult: 15-124   MCC Major Complication/Comorbidity   CC Complication/Comorbidity   SW Severe Wound Dx

758   ICD-10-CM 2020

Chapter 13. Diseases of the Musculoskeletal System and Connective Tissue (M00–M99)

Chapter-specific Guidelines with Coding Examples

The chapter-specific guidelines from the ICD-10-CM Official Guidelines for Coding and Reporting have been provided below. Along with these guidelines are coding examples, contained in the shaded boxes, that have been developed to help illustrate the coding and/or sequencing guidance found in these guidelines.

a. Site and laterality

Most of the codes within Chapter 13 have site and laterality designations. The site represents the bone, joint or the muscle involved. For some conditions where more than one bone, joint or muscle is usually involved, such as osteoarthritis, there is a "multiple sites" code available. For categories where no multiple site code is provided and more than one bone, joint or muscle is involved, multiple codes should be used to indicate the different sites involved.

> Rheumatoid arthritis of multiple sites without rheumatoid factor
>
> **M06.09**   **Rheumatoid arthritis without rheumatoid factor, multiple sites**
>
> *Explanation:* For some conditions where more than one bone, joint or muscle is usually involved, such as rheumatoid arthritis, there is a "multiple sites" code available.

> Osteomyelitis of the fourth thoracic and second lumbar vertebrae
>
> **M46.24**   **Osteomyelitis of vertebra, thoracic region**
>
> **M46.26**   **Osteomyelitis of vertebra, lumbar region**
>
> *Explanation:* For categories without a multiple site code and more than one bone, joint, or muscle is involved, multiple codes should be used to indicate the different sites involved.

1) Bone versus joint

For certain conditions, the bone may be affected at the upper or lower end, (e.g., avascular necrosis of bone, M87, Osteoporosis, M80, M81). Though the portion of the bone affected may be at the joint, the site designation will be the bone, not the joint.

> Idiopathic avascular necrosis of the femoral head of the left hip joint
>
> **M87.052**   **Idiopathic aseptic necrosis of left femur**
>
> *Explanation:* For certain conditions such as avascular necrosis, the bone may be affected at the joint, but the site designation is the bone, not the joint.

b. Acute traumatic versus chronic or recurrent musculoskeletal conditions

Many musculoskeletal conditions are a result of previous injury or trauma to a site, or are recurrent conditions. Bone, joint or muscle conditions that are the result of a healed injury are usually found in chapter 13. Recurrent bone, joint or muscle conditions are also usually found in chapter 13. Any current, acute injury should be coded to the appropriate injury code from chapter 19. Chronic or recurrent conditions should generally be coded with a code from chapter 13. If it is difficult to determine from the documentation in the record which code is best to describe a condition, query the provider.

> Acute traumatic bucket-handle tear of right medial meniscus
>
> **S83.211A**   **Bucket-handle tear of medial meniscus, current injury, right knee, initial encounter**
>
> *Explanation:* Any current, acute injury is not coded in chapter 13. It should instead be coded to the appropriate injury code from chapter 19.

> Old bucket-handle tear of right medial meniscus
>
> **M23.203**   **Derangement of unspecified medial meniscus due to old tear or injury, right knee**
>
> *Explanation:* Chronic or recurrent conditions should generally be coded with a code from chapter 13.

c. Coding of pathologic fractures

7th character A is for use as long as the patient is receiving active treatment for the fracture. Examples of active treatment are: surgical treatment, emergency department encounter, evaluation and continuing treatment by the same or a different physician. While the patient may be seen by a new or different provider over the course of treatment for a pathological fracture, assignment of the 7th character is based on whether the patient is undergoing active treatment and not whether the provider is seeing the patient for the first time.

> Patient admitted for repair of pathologic fracture of left foot, unknown cause. The surgery will be performed by his orthopedic specialist who he has been seeing for this fracture for the past month.
>
> **M84.475A**   **Pathological fracture, left foot, initial encounter for fracture**
>
> *Explanation:* Seventh character A is for use as long as the patient is receiving active treatment for a pathologic fracture. Examples of active treatment are surgical treatment, emergency department encounter, evaluation, and continuing treatment by the same or a different physician.
>
> The seventh character is based on whether the patient is undergoing active treatment such as surgery, and not whether the provider is seeing the patient for the first time.

7th character D is to be used for encounters after the patient has completed active treatment for the fracture and is receiving routine care for the fracture during the healing or recovery phase. The other 7th characters, listed under each subcategory in the Tabular List, are to be used for subsequent encounters for treatment of problems associated with the healing, such as malunions, nonunions, and sequelae.

Care for complications of surgical treatment for fracture repairs during the healing or recovery phase should be coded with the appropriate complication codes.

See Section I.C.19. Coding of traumatic fractures.

d. Osteoporosis

Osteoporosis is a systemic condition, meaning that all bones of the musculoskeletal system are affected. Therefore, site is not a component of the codes under category M81, Osteoporosis without current pathological fracture. The site codes under category M80, Osteoporosis with current pathological fracture, identify the site of the fracture, not the osteoporosis.

1) Osteoporosis without pathological fracture

Category M81, Osteoporosis without current pathological fracture, is for use for patients with osteoporosis who do not currently have a pathologic fracture due to the osteoporosis, even if they have had a fracture in the past. For patients with a history of osteoporosis fractures, status code Z87.310, Personal history of (healed) osteoporosis fracture, should follow the code from M81.

> Age-related osteoporosis with healed osteoporotic fracture of the lumbar vertebra
>
> **M81.0**   **Age-related osteoporosis without current pathological fracture**
>
> **Z87.310**   **Personal history of (healed) osteoporosis fracture**
>
> *Explanation:* Category M81 is used for patients with osteoporosis who do not currently have a pathologic fracture due to the osteoporosis. To report a previous (healed) fracture, status code Z87.310 Personal history of (healed) osteoporosis fracture, should follow the code from M81.

2) Osteoporosis with current pathological fracture

Category M80, Osteoporosis with current pathological fracture, is for patients who have a current pathologic fracture at the time of an encounter. The codes under M80 identify the site of the fracture. A code from category M80, not a traumatic fracture code, should be used for any patient with known osteoporosis who suffers a fracture, even if the patient had a minor fall or trauma, if that fall or trauma would not usually break a normal, healthy bone.

> Disuse osteoporosis with current fracture of right shoulder sustained lifting a grocery bag, initial encounter
>
> **M80.811A**   **Other osteoporosis with current pathological fracture, right shoulder, initial encounter for fracture**
>
> *Explanation:* A code from category M80, not a traumatic fracture code, should be used for any patient with known osteoporosis who suffers a fracture, even if the patient had a minor fall or trauma, if that fall or trauma would not usually break a normal, healthy bone.

Muscle/Tendon Table

ICD-10-CM categorizes certain muscles and tendons in the upper and lower extremities by their action (e.g., extension, flexion), their anatomical location (e.g., posterior, anterior), and/or whether they are intrinsic or extrinsic to a certain anatomical area. The Muscle/Tendon Table is provided at the beginning of chapters 13 and 19 as a resource to help users when code selection depends on one or more of these characteristics. Please note that this table is not all-inclusive, and proper code assignment should be based on the provider's documentation.

Body Region	Muscle	Extensor Tendon	Flexor Tendon	Other Tendon
Shoulder				
	Deltoid	Posterior deltoid	Anterior deltoid	
	Rotator cuff			
	Infraspinatus			Infraspinatus
	Subscapularis			Subscapularis
	Supraspinatus			Supraspinatus
	Teres minor			Teres minor
	Teres major	Teres major		
Upper arm				
	Anterior muscles			
	Biceps brachii — long head		Biceps brachii — long head	
	Biceps brachii — short head		Biceps brachii — short head	
	Brachialis		Brachialis	
	Coracobrachialis		Coracobrachialis	
	Posterior muscles			
	Triceps brachii	Triceps brachii		
Forearm				
	Anterior muscles			
	Flexors			
	Deep			
	Flexor digitorum profundus		Flexor digitorum profundus	
	Flexor pollicis longus		Flexor pollicis longus	
	Intermediate			
	Flexor digitorum superficialis		Flexor digitorum superficialis	
	Superficial			
	Flexor carpi radialis		Flexor carpi radialis	
	Flexor carpi ulnaris		Flexor carpi ulnaris	
	Palmaris longus		Palmaris longus	
	Pronators			
	Pronator quadratus			Pronator quadratus
	Pronator teres			Pronator teres
	Posterior muscles			
	Extensors			
	Deep			
	Abductor pollicis longus			Abductor pollicis longus
	Extensor indicis	Extensor indicis		
	Extensor pollicis brevis	Extensor pollicis brevis		
	Extensor pollicis longus	Extensor pollicis longus		
	Superficial			
	Brachioradialis			Brachioradialis
	Extensor carpi radialis brevis	Extensor carpi radialis brevis		
	Extensor carpi radialis longus	Extensor carpi radialis longus		
	Extensor carpi ulnaris	Extensor carpi ulnaris		
	Extensor digiti minimi	Extensor digiti minimi		
	Extensor digitorum	Extensor digitorum		
	Anconeus	Anconeus		
	Supinator			Supinator

Body Region	Muscle	Extensor Tendon	Flexor Tendon	Other Tendon
Hand				
Extrinsic — attach to a site in the forearm as well as a site in the hand with action related to hand movement at the wrist				
	Extensor carpi radialis brevis	Extensor carpi radialis brevis		
	Extensor carpi radialis longus	Extensor carpie radialis longus		
	Extensor carpi ulnaris	Extensor carpi ulnaris		
	Flexor carpi radialis		Flexor carpi radialis	
	Flexor carpi ulnaris		Flexor carpi ulnaris	
	Flexor digitorum superficialis		Flexor digitorum superficialis	
	Palmaris longus		Palmaris longus	
Extrinsic — attach to a site in the forearm as well as a site in the hand with action in the hand related to finger movement				
	Adductor pollicis longus			Adductor pollicis longus
	Extensor digiti minimi	Extensor digiti minimi		
	Extensor digitorum	Extensor digitorum		
	Extensor indicis	Extensor indicis		
	Flexor digitorum profundus		Flexor digitorum profundus	
	Flexor digitorum superficialis		Flexor digitorum superficialis	
Extrinsic — attach to a site in the forearm as well as a site in the hand with action in the hand related to thumb movement				
	Extensor pollicis brevis	Extensor pollicis brevis		
	Extensor pollicis longus	Extensor pollicis longus		
	Flexor pollicis longus		Flexor pollicis longus	
Intrinsic — found within the hand only				
	Adductor pollicis			Adductor pollicis
	Dorsal interossei	Dorsal interossei	Dorsal interossei	
	Lumbricals	Lumbricals	Lumbricals	
	Palmaris brevis			Palmaris brevis
	Palmar interossei	Palmar interossei	Palmar interossei	
	Hypothenar muscles			
	Abductor digiti minimi			Abductor digiti minimi
	Flexor digiti minimi brevis		Flexor digiti minimi brevis	
	Oppenens digiti minimi		Oppenens digiti minimi	
	Thenar muscles			
	Abductor pollicis brevis			Abductor pollicis brevis
	Flexor pollicis brevis		Flexor pollicis brevis	
	Oppenens pollicis		Oppenens pollicis	
Thigh				
	Anterior muscles			
	Iliopsoas		Iliopsoas	
	Pectineus		Pectineus	
	Quadriceps	Quadriceps		
	Rectus femoris	Rectus femoris — Extends knee	Rectus femoris — Flexes hip	
	Vastus intermedius	Vastus intermedius		
	Vastus lateralis	Vastus lateralis		
	Vastus medialis	Vastus medialis		
	Sartorius		Sartorius	
	Medial muscles			
	Adductor brevis			Adductor brevis
	Adductor longus			Adductor longus
	Adductor magnus			Adductor magnus
	Gracilis			Gracilis
	Obturator externus			Obturator externus
	Posterior muscles			
	Hamstring	Hamstring — Extends hip	Hamstring — Flexes knee	
	Biceps femoris	Biceps femoris	Biceps femoris	
	Semimembranosus	Semimembranosus	Semimembranosus	
	Semitendinosus	Semitendinosus	Semitendinosus	

Chapter 13. Diseases of the Musculoskeletal System and Connective Tissue

Body Region	Muscle	Extensor Tendon	Flexor Tendon	Other Tendon
Lower leg				
	Anterior muscles			
	Extensor digitorum longus	Extensor digitorum longus		
	Extensor hallucis longus	Extensor hallucis longus		
	Fibularis (peroneus) tertius	Fibularis (peroneus) tertius		
	Tibialis anterior	Tibialis anterior		Tibialis anterior
	Lateral muscles			
	Fibularis (peroneus) brevis		Fibularis (peroneus) brevis	
	Fibularis (peroneus) longus		Fibularis (peroneus) longus	
	Posterior muscles			
	Deep			
	Flexor digitorum longus		Flexor digitorum longus	
	Flexor hallucis longus		Flexor hallucis longus	
	Popliteus		Popliteus	
	Tibialis posterior		Tibialis posterior	
	Superficial			
	Gastrocnemius		Gastrocnemius	
	Plantaris		Plantaris	
	Soleus		Soleus	
				Calcaneal (Achilles)
Ankle/Foot				
Extrinsic — attach to a site in the lower leg as well as a site in the foot with action related to foot movement at the ankle				
	Plantaris		Plantaris	
	Soleus		Soleus	
	Tibialis anterior	Tibialis anterior		
	Tibialis posterior		Tibialis posterior	
Extrinsic — attach to a site in the lower leg as well as a site in the foot with action in the foot related to toe movement				
	Extensor digitorum longus	Extensor digitorum longus		
	Extensor hallicus longus	Extensor hallicus longus		
	Flexor digitorum longus		Flexor digitorum longus	
	Flexor hallucis longus		Flexor hallucis longus	
Intrinsic — found within the ankle/foot only				
	Dorsal muscles			
	Extensor digitorum brevis	Extensor digitorum brevis		
	Extensor hallucis brevis	Extensor hallucis brevis		
	Plantar muscles			
	Abductor digiti minimi		Abductor digiti minimi	
	Abductor hallucis		Abductor hallucis	
	Dorsal interossei	Dorsal interossei	Dorsal interossei	
	Flexor digiti minimi brevis		Flexor digiti minimi brevis	
	Flexor digitorum brevis		Flexor digitorum brevis	
	Flexor hallucis brevis		Flexor hallucis brevis	
	Lumbricals	Lumbricals	Lumbricals	
	Quadratus plantae		Quadratus plantae	
	Plantar interossei	Plantar interossei	Plantar interossei	

Chapter 13. Diseases of the Musculoskeletal System and Connective Tissue (M00-M99)

NOTE Use an external cause code following the code for the musculoskeletal condition, if applicable, to identify the cause of the musculoskeletal condition

EXCLUDES 2 arthropathic psoriasis (L40.5-)
certain conditions originating in the perinatal period (P04-P96)
certain infectious and parasitic diseases (A00-B99)
compartment syndrome (traumatic) (T79.A-)
complications of pregnancy, childbirth and the puerperium (O00-O9A)
congenital malformations, deformations, and chromosomal abnormalities (Q00-Q99)
endocrine, nutritional and metabolic diseases (E00-E88)
injury, poisoning and certain other consequences of external causes (S00-T88)
neoplasms (C00-D49)
symptoms, signs and abnormal clinical and laboratory findings, not elsewhere classified (R00-R94)

This chapter contains the following blocks:
M00-M02 Infectious arthropathies
M04 Autoinflammatory syndromes
M05-M14 Inflammatory polyarthropathies
M15-M19 Osteoarthritis
M20-M25 Other joint disorders
M26-M27 Dentofacial anomalies [including malocclusion] and other disorders of jaw
M30-M36 Systemic connective tissue disorders
M40-M43 Deforming dorsopathies
M45-M49 Spondylopathies
M50-M54 Other dorsopathies
M60-M63 Disorders of muscles
M65-M67 Disorders of synovium and tendon
M70-M79 Other soft tissue disorders
M80-M85 Disorders of bone density and structure
M86-M90 Other osteopathies
M91-M94 Chondropathies
M95 Other disorders of the musculoskeletal system and connective tissue
M96 Intraoperative and postprocedural complications and disorders of musculoskeletal system, not elsewhere classified
M97 Periprosthetic fracture around internal prosthetic joint
M99 Biomechanical lesions, not elsewhere classified

ARTHROPATHIES (M00-M25)

INCLUDES disorders affecting predominantly peripheral (limb) joints

Infectious arthropathies (M00-M02)

NOTE This block comprises arthropathies due to microbiological agents. Distinction is made between the following types of etiological relationship:

a) direct infection of joint, where organisms invade synovial tissue and microbial antigen is present in the joint;

b) indirect infection, which may be of two types: a reactive arthropathy, where microbial infection of the body is established but neither organisms nor antigens can be identified in the joint, and a postinfective arthropathy, where microbial antigen is present but recovery of an organism is inconstant and evidence of local multiplication is lacking.

√4ᵗʰ **M00 Pyogenic arthritis**

DEF: Pyogenic: Relating to or involving pus production, often referred to as suppurative or purulent.

√5ᵗʰ **M00.0 Staphylococcal arthritis and polyarthritis**

Use additional code (B95.61-B95.8) to identify bacterial agent
EXCLUDES 2 infection and inflammatory reaction due to internal joint prosthesis (T84.5-)

M00.00 Staphylococcal arthritis, unspecified joint CC HCC
CC Excl: PDX collection 855

√6ᵗʰ **M00.01 Staphylococcal arthritis, shoulder**
CC Excl: For CC codes in subcategory M00.01: PDX collection 856

M00.011 Staphylococcal arthritis, right shoulder CC HCC

M00.012 Staphylococcal arthritis, left shoulder CC HCC

M00.019 Staphylococcal arthritis, unspecified shoulder CC HCC

√6ᵗʰ **M00.02 Staphylococcal arthritis, elbow**
CC Excl: For CC codes in subcategory M00.02: PDX collection 857

M00.021 Staphylococcal arthritis, right elbow CC HCC

M00.022 Staphylococcal arthritis, left elbow CC HCC

M00.029 Staphylococcal arthritis, unspecified elbow CC HCC

√6ᵗʰ **M00.03 Staphylococcal arthritis, wrist**
Staphylococcal arthritis of carpal bones
CC Excl: For CC codes in subcategory M00.03: PDX collection 858

M00.031 Staphylococcal arthritis, right wrist CC HCC

M00.032 Staphylococcal arthritis, left wrist CC HCC

M00.039 Staphylococcal arthritis, unspecified wrist CC HCC

√6ᵗʰ **M00.04 Staphylococcal arthritis, hand**
Staphylococcal arthritis of metacarpus and phalanges
CC Excl: For CC codes in subcategory M00.04: PDX collection 859

M00.041 Staphylococcal arthritis, right hand CC HCC

M00.042 Staphylococcal arthritis, left hand CC HCC

M00.049 Staphylococcal arthritis, unspecified hand CC HCC

√6ᵗʰ **M00.05 Staphylococcal arthritis, hip**
CC Excl: For CC codes in subcategory M00.05: PDX collection 860

M00.051 Staphylococcal arthritis, right hip CC HCC

M00.052 Staphylococcal arthritis, left hip CC HCC

M00.059 Staphylococcal arthritis, unspecified hip CC HCC

√6ᵗʰ **M00.06 Staphylococcal arthritis, knee**
CC Excl: For CC codes in subcategory M00.06: PDX collection 861

M00.061 Staphylococcal arthritis, right knee CC HCC

M00.062 Staphylococcal arthritis, left knee CC HCC

M00.069 Staphylococcal arthritis, unspecified knee CC HCC

√6ᵗʰ **M00.07 Staphylococcal arthritis, ankle and foot**
Staphylococcal arthritis, tarsus, metatarsus and phalanges
CC Excl: For CC codes in subcategory M00.07: PDX collection 862

M00.071 Staphylococcal arthritis, right ankle and foot CC HCC

M00.072 Staphylococcal arthritis, left ankle and foot CC HCC

M00.079 Staphylococcal arthritis, unspecified ankle and foot CC HCC

M00.08 Staphylococcal arthritis, vertebrae CC HCC
CC Excl: PDX collection 855

M00.09 Staphylococcal polyarthritis CC HCC
CC Excl: PDX collection 855

√5ᵗʰ **M00.1 Pneumococcal arthritis and polyarthritis**

M00.10 Pneumococcal arthritis, unspecified joint CC HCC
CC Excl: PDX collection 855

√6ᵗʰ **M00.11 Pneumococcal arthritis, shoulder**
CC Excl: For CC codes in subcategory M00.11: PDX collection 856

M00.111 Pneumococcal arthritis, right shoulder CC HCC

M00.112 Pneumococcal arthritis, left shoulder CC HCC

M00.119 Pneumococcal arthritis, unspecified shoulder CC HCC

Chapter 13. Diseases of the Musculoskeletal System and Connective Tissue

✓6ᵗʰ **M00.12 Pneumococcal arthritis, elbow**

     CC Excl: For CC codes in subcategory M00.12: PDX collection 857

     M00.121 Pneumococcal arthritis, right elbow   `CC` `HCC`

     M00.122 Pneumococcal arthritis, left elbow   `CC` `HCC`

     M00.129 Pneumococcal arthritis, unspecified elbow   `CC` `HCC`

✓6ᵗʰ **M00.13 Pneumococcal arthritis, wrist**

     Pneumococcal arthritis of carpal bones

     CC Excl: For CC codes in subcategory M00.13: PDX collection 858

     M00.131 Pneumococcal arthritis, right wrist   `CC` `HCC`

     M00.132 Pneumococcal arthritis, left wrist   `CC` `HCC`

     M00.139 Pneumococcal arthritis, unspecified wrist   `CC` `HCC`

✓6ᵗʰ **M00.14 Pneumococcal arthritis, hand**

     Pneumococcal arthritis of metacarpus and phalanges

     CC Excl: For CC codes in subcategory M00.14: PDX collection 859

     M00.141 Pneumococcal arthritis, right hand   `CC` `HCC`

     M00.142 Pneumococcal arthritis, left hand   `CC` `HCC`

     M00.149 Pneumococcal arthritis, unspecified hand   `CC` `HCC`

✓6ᵗʰ **M00.15 Pneumococcal arthritis, hip**

     CC Excl: For CC codes in subcategory M00.15: PDX collection 860

     M00.151 Pneumococcal arthritis, right hip   `CC` `HCC`

     M00.152 Pneumococcal arthritis, left hip   `CC` `HCC`

     M00.159 Pneumococcal arthritis, unspecified hip   `CC` `HCC`

✓6ᵗʰ **M00.16 Pneumococcal arthritis, knee**

     CC Excl: For CC codes in subcategory M00.16: PDX collection 861

     M00.161 Pneumococcal arthritis, right knee   `CC` `HCC`

     M00.162 Pneumococcal arthritis, left knee   `CC` `HCC`

     M00.169 Pneumococcal arthritis, unspecified knee   `CC` `HCC`

✓6ᵗʰ **M00.17 Pneumococcal arthritis, ankle and foot**

     Pneumococcal arthritis, tarsus, metatarsus and phalanges

     CC Excl: For CC codes in subcategory M00.17: PDX collection 862

     M00.171 Pneumococcal arthritis, right ankle and foot   `CC` `HCC`

     M00.172 Pneumococcal arthritis, left ankle and foot   `CC` `HCC`

     M00.179 Pneumococcal arthritis, unspecified ankle and foot   `CC` `HCC`

     M00.18 Pneumococcal arthritis, vertebrae   `CC` `HCC`

     CC Excl: PDX collection 855

     M00.19 Pneumococcal polyarthritis   `CC` `HCC`

     CC Excl: PDX collection 855

✓5ᵗʰ **M00.2 Other streptococcal arthritis and polyarthritis**

     Use additional code (B95.0-B95.2, B95.4-B95.5) to identify bacterial agent

     M00.20 Other streptococcal arthritis, unspecified joint   `CC` `HCC`

     CC Excl: PDX collection 855

✓6ᵗʰ **M00.21 Other streptococcal arthritis, shoulder**

     CC Excl: For CC codes in subcategory M00.21: PDX collection 856

     M00.211 Other streptococcal arthritis, right shoulder   `CC` `HCC`

     M00.212 Other streptococcal arthritis, left shoulder   `CC` `HCC`

     M00.219 Other streptococcal arthritis, unspecified shoulder   `CC` `HCC`

✓6ᵗʰ **M00.22 Other streptococcal arthritis, elbow**

     CC Excl: For CC codes in subcategory M00.22: PDX collection 857

     M00.221 Other streptococcal arthritis, right elbow   `CC` `HCC`

     M00.222 Other streptococcal arthritis, left elbow   `CC` `HCC`

     M00.229 Other streptococcal arthritis, unspecified elbow   `CC` `HCC`

✓6ᵗʰ **M00.23 Other streptococcal arthritis, wrist**

     Other streptococcal arthritis of carpal bones

     CC Excl: For CC codes in subcategory M00.23: PDX collection 858

     M00.231 Other streptococcal arthritis, right wrist   `CC` `HCC`

     M00.232 Other streptococcal arthritis, left wrist   `CC` `HCC`

     M00.239 Other streptococcal arthritis, unspecified wrist   `CC` `HCC`

✓6ᵗʰ **M00.24 Other streptococcal arthritis, hand**

     Other streptococcal arthritis metacarpus and phalanges

     CC Excl: For CC codes in subcategory M00.24: PDX collection 859

     M00.241 Other streptococcal arthritis, right hand   `CC` `HCC`

     M00.242 Other streptococcal arthritis, left hand   `CC` `HCC`

     M00.249 Other streptococcal arthritis, unspecified hand   `CC` `HCC`

✓6ᵗʰ **M00.25 Other streptococcal arthritis, hip**

     CC Excl: For CC codes in subcategory M00.25: PDX collection 860

     M00.251 Other streptococcal arthritis, right hip   `CC` `HCC`

     M00.252 Other streptococcal arthritis, left hip   `CC` `HCC`

     M00.259 Other streptococcal arthritis, unspecified hip   `CC` `HCC`

✓6ᵗʰ **M00.26 Other streptococcal arthritis, knee**

     CC Excl: For CC codes in subcategory M00.26: PDX collection 861

     M00.261 Other streptococcal arthritis, right knee   `CC` `HCC`

     M00.262 Other streptococcal arthritis, left knee   `CC` `HCC`

     M00.269 Other streptococcal arthritis, unspecified knee   `CC` `HCC`

✓6ᵗʰ **M00.27 Other streptococcal arthritis, ankle and foot**

     Other streptococcal arthritis, tarsus, metatarsus and phalanges

     CC Excl: For CC codes in subcategory M00.27: PDX collection 862

     M00.271 Other streptococcal arthritis, right ankle and foot   `CC` `HCC`

     M00.272 Other streptococcal arthritis, left ankle and foot   `CC` `HCC`

     M00.279 Other streptococcal arthritis, unspecified ankle and foot   `CC` `HCC`

     M00.28 Other streptococcal arthritis, vertebrae   `CC` `HCC`

     CC Excl: PDX collection 855

     M00.29 Other streptococcal polyarthritis   `CC` `HCC`

     CC Excl: PDX collection 855

✓5ᵗʰ **M00.8 Arthritis and polyarthritis due to other bacteria**

     Use additional code (B96) to identify bacteria

     M00.80 Arthritis due to other bacteria, unspecified joint   `CC` `HCC`

     CC Excl: PDX collection 855

✓6ᵗʰ **M00.81 Arthritis due to other bacteria, shoulder**

     CC Excl: For CC codes in subcategory M00.81: PDX collection 856

     M00.811 Arthritis due to other bacteria, right shoulder   `CC` `HCC`

N Newborn: 0   P Pediatric: 0-17   M Maternity: 9-64   A Adult: 15-124   **MCC** Major Complication/Comorbidity   **CC** Complication/Comorbidity   **SW** Severe Wound Dx

764   ICD-10-CM 2020

          M00.812 Arthritis due to other bacteria, **left** shoulder `CC` `HCC`

          M00.819 Arthritis due to other bacteria, unspecified shoulder `CC` `HCC`

✓6ᵗʰ **M00.82** Arthritis due to other bacteria, **elbow**

          CC Excl: For CC codes in subcategory M00.82: PDX collection 857

          M00.821 Arthritis due to other bacteria, **right** elbow `CC` `HCC`

          M00.822 Arthritis due to other bacteria, **left** elbow `CC` `HCC`

          M00.829 Arthritis due to other bacteria, unspecified elbow `CC` `HCC`

✓6ᵗʰ **M00.83** Arthritis due to other bacteria, **wrist**

          Arthritis due to other bacteria, carpal bones

          CC Excl: For CC codes in subcategory M00.83: PDX collection 858

          M00.831 Arthritis due to other bacteria, **right** wrist `CC` `HCC`

          M00.832 Arthritis due to other bacteria, **left** wrist `CC` `HCC`

          M00.839 Arthritis due to other bacteria, unspecified wrist `CC` `HCC`

✓6ᵗʰ **M00.84** Arthritis due to other bacteria, **hand**

          Arthritis due to other bacteria, metacarpus and phalanges

          CC Excl: For CC codes in subcategory M00.84: PDX collection 859

          M00.841 Arthritis due to other bacteria, **right** hand `CC` `HCC`

          M00.842 Arthritis due to other bacteria, **left** hand `CC` `HCC`

          M00.849 Arthritis due to other bacteria, unspecified hand `CC` `HCC`

✓6ᵗʰ **M00.85** Arthritis due to other bacteria, **hip**

          CC Excl: For CC codes in subcategory M00.85: PDX collection 860

          M00.851 Arthritis due to other bacteria, **right** hip `CC` `HCC`

          M00.852 Arthritis due to other bacteria, **left** hip `CC` `HCC`

          M00.859 Arthritis due to other bacteria, unspecified hip `CC` `HCC`

✓6ᵗʰ **M00.86** Arthritis due to other bacteria, **knee**

          CC Excl: For CC codes in subcategory M00.86: PDX collection 861

          M00.861 Arthritis due to other bacteria, **right** knee `CC` `HCC`

          M00.862 Arthritis due to other bacteria, **left** knee `CC` `HCC`

          M00.869 Arthritis due to other bacteria, unspecified knee `CC` `HCC`

✓6ᵗʰ **M00.87** Arthritis due to other bacteria, **ankle and foot**

          Arthritis due to other bacteria, tarsus, metatarsus, and phalanges

          CC Excl: For CC codes in subcategory M00.87: PDX collection 862

          M00.871 Arthritis due to other bacteria, **right** ankle and foot `CC` `HCC`

          M00.872 Arthritis due to other bacteria, **left** ankle and foot `CC` `HCC`

          M00.879 Arthritis due to other bacteria, unspecified ankle and foot `CC` `HCC`

    M00.88 Arthritis due to other bacteria, **vertebrae** `CC` `HCC`

          CC Excl: PDX collection 855

    M00.89 **Polyarthritis** due to other bacteria `CC` `HCC`

          CC Excl: PDX collection 855

M00.9 **Pyogenic arthritis, unspecified** `CC` `HCC`

    Infective arthritis NOS

    CC Excl: PDX collection 855

✓4ᵗʰ **M01** **Direct infections of joint in infectious and parasitic diseases classified elsewhere**

    Code first underlying disease, such as:

      leprosy [Hansen's disease] (A30.-)

      mycoses (B35-B49)

      O'nyong-nyong fever (A92.1)

      paratyphoid fever (A01.1-A01.4)

      EXCLUDES 1   arthropathy in Lyme disease (A69.23)

               gonococcal arthritis (A54.42)

               meningococcal arthritis (A39.83)

               mumps arthritis (B26.85)

               postinfective arthropathy (M02.-)

               postmeningococcal arthritis (A39.84)

               reactive arthritis (M02.3)

               rubella arthritis (B06.82)

               sarcoidosis arthritis (D86.86)

               typhoid fever arthritis (A01.04)

               tuberculosis arthritis (A18.01-A18.02)

    CC Excl: For CC codes in category M01, unless otherwise noted: PDX collection 863

✓5ᵗʰ **M01.X** **Direct infection of joint in infectious and parasitic diseases classified elsewhere**

          M01.X0 Direct infection of unspecified joint in infectious and parasitic diseases classified elsewhere `CC` `HCC`

    ✓6ᵗʰ **M01.X1** Direct infection of **shoulder** joint in infectious and parasitic diseases classified elsewhere

          CC Excl: For CC codes in subcategory M01.X1: PDX collection 864

          M01.X11 Direct infection of **right** shoulder in infectious and parasitic diseases classified elsewhere `CC` `HCC`

          M01.X12 Direct infection of **left** shoulder in infectious and parasitic diseases classified elsewhere `CC` `HCC`

          M01.X19 Direct infection of unspecified shoulder in infectious and parasitic diseases classified elsewhere `CC` `HCC`

    ✓6ᵗʰ **M01.X2** Direct infection of **elbow** in infectious and parasitic diseases classified elsewhere

          M01.X21 Direct infection of **right** elbow in infectious and parasitic diseases classified elsewhere `CC` `HCC`

          M01.X22 Direct infection of **left** elbow in infectious and parasitic diseases classified elsewhere `CC` `HCC`

          M01.X29 Direct infection of unspecified elbow in infectious and parasitic diseases classified elsewhere `CC` `HCC`

    ✓6ᵗʰ **M01.X3** Direct infection of **wrist** in infectious and parasitic diseases classified elsewhere

          Direct infection of carpal bones in infectious and parasitic diseases classified elsewhere

          M01.X31 Direct infection of **right** wrist in infectious and parasitic diseases classified elsewhere `CC` `HCC`

          M01.X32 Direct infection of **left** wrist in infectious and parasitic diseases classified elsewhere `CC` `HCC`

          M01.X39 Direct infection of unspecified wrist in infectious and parasitic diseases classified elsewhere `CC` `HCC`

✓6th **M01.X4** Direct infection of hand in infectious and parasitic diseases classified elsewhere

Direct infection of metacarpus and phalanges in infectious and parasitic diseases classified elsewhere

M01.X41 *Direct infection of right hand in infectious and parasitic diseases classified elsewhere* CC HCC

M01.X42 *Direct infection of left hand in infectious and parasitic diseases classified elsewhere* CC HCC

M01.X49 *Direct infection of unspecified hand in infectious and parasitic diseases classified elsewhere* CC HCC

✓6th **M01.X5** Direct infection of hip in infectious and parasitic diseases classified elsewhere

M01.X51 *Direct infection of right hip in infectious and parasitic diseases classified elsewhere* CC HCC

M01.X52 *Direct infection of left hip in infectious and parasitic diseases classified elsewhere* CC HCC

M01.X59 *Direct infection of unspecified hip in infectious and parasitic diseases classified elsewhere* CC HCC

✓6th **M01.X6** Direct infection of knee in infectious and parasitic diseases classified elsewhere

M01.X61 *Direct infection of right knee in infectious and parasitic diseases classified elsewhere* CC HCC

M01.X62 *Direct infection of left knee in infectious and parasitic diseases classified elsewhere* CC HCC

M01.X69 *Direct infection of unspecified knee in infectious and parasitic diseases classified elsewhere* CC HCC

✓6th **M01.X7** Direct infection of ankle and foot in infectious and parasitic diseases classified elsewhere

Direct infection of tarsus, metatarsus and phalanges in infectious and parasitic diseases classified elsewhere

M01.X71 *Direct infection of right ankle and foot in infectious and parasitic diseases classified elsewhere* CC HCC

M01.X72 *Direct infection of left ankle and foot in infectious and parasitic diseases classified elsewhere* CC HCC

M01.X79 *Direct infection of unspecified ankle and foot in infectious and parasitic diseases classified elsewhere* CC HCC

M01.X8 *Direct infection of vertebrae in infectious and parasitic diseases classified elsewhere* CC HCC

M01.X9 *Direct infection of multiple joints in infectious and parasitic diseases classified elsewhere* CC HCC

✓4th **M02** Postinfective and reactive arthropathies

Code first underlying disease, such as:
congenital syphilis [Clutton's joints] (A50.5)
enteritis due to Yersinia enterocolitica (A04.6)
infective endocarditis (I33.0)
viral hepatitis (B15-B19)

EXCLUDES 1 Behçet's disease (M35.2)
direct infections of joint in infectious and parasitic diseases classified elsewhere (M01.-)
mumps arthritis (B26.85)
postmeningococcal arthritis (A39.84)
rheumatic fever (I00)
rubella arthritis (B06.82)
syphilis arthritis (late) (A52.77)
tabetic arthropathy [Charcôt's] (A52.16)

✓5th **M02.0** Arthropathy following intestinal bypass

M02.00 Arthropathy following intestinal bypass, unspecified site

✓6th **M02.01** Arthropathy following intestinal bypass, shoulder

M02.011 Arthropathy following intestinal bypass, right shoulder

M02.012 Arthropathy following intestinal bypass, left shoulder

M02.019 Arthropathy following intestinal bypass, unspecified shoulder

✓6th **M02.02** Arthropathy following intestinal bypass, elbow

M02.021 Arthropathy following intestinal bypass, right elbow

M02.022 Arthropathy following intestinal bypass, left elbow

M02.029 Arthropathy following intestinal bypass, unspecified elbow

✓6th **M02.03** Arthropathy following intestinal bypass, wrist

Arthropathy following intestinal bypass, carpal bones

M02.031 Arthropathy following intestinal bypass, right wrist

M02.032 Arthropathy following intestinal bypass, left wrist

M02.039 Arthropathy following intestinal bypass, unspecified wrist

✓6th **M02.04** Arthropathy following intestinal bypass, hand

Arthropathy following intestinal bypass, metacarpals and phalanges

M02.041 Arthropathy following intestinal bypass, right hand

M02.042 Arthropathy following intestinal bypass, left hand

M02.049 Arthropathy following intestinal bypass, unspecified hand

✓6th **M02.05** Arthropathy following intestinal bypass, hip

M02.051 Arthropathy following intestinal bypass, right hip

M02.052 Arthropathy following intestinal bypass, left hip

M02.059 Arthropathy following intestinal bypass, unspecified hip

✓6th **M02.06** Arthropathy following intestinal bypass, knee

M02.061 Arthropathy following intestinal bypass, right knee

M02.062 Arthropathy following intestinal bypass, left knee

M02.069 Arthropathy following intestinal bypass, unspecified knee

✓6th **M02.07** Arthropathy following intestinal bypass, ankle and foot

Arthropathy following intestinal bypass, tarsus, metatarsus and phalanges

M02.071 Arthropathy following intestinal bypass, right ankle and foot

M02.072 Arthropathy following intestinal bypass, left ankle and foot

M02.079 Arthropathy following intestinal bypass, unspecified ankle and foot

M02.08 Arthropathy following intestinal bypass, vertebrae

M02.09 Arthropathy following intestinal bypass, multiple sites

✓5th **M02.1** Postdysenteric arthropathy

M02.10 Postdysenteric arthropathy, unspecified site HCC

√6ᵗʰ **M02.11 Postdysenteric arthropathy, shoulder**

    M02.111 Postdysenteric arthropathy, **right shoulder** `HCC`

    M02.112 Postdysenteric arthropathy, **left** shoulder `HCC`

    M02.119 Postdysenteric arthropathy, unspecified shoulder `HCC`

√6ᵗʰ **M02.12 Postdysenteric arthropathy, elbow**

    M02.121 Postdysenteric arthropathy, **right** elbow `HCC`

    M02.122 Postdysenteric arthropathy, **left** elbow `HCC`

    M02.129 Postdysenteric arthropathy, unspecified elbow `HCC`

√6ᵗʰ **M02.13 Postdysenteric arthropathy, wrist**

    Postdysenteric arthropathy, carpal bones

    M02.131 Postdysenteric arthropathy, **right** wrist `HCC`

    M02.132 Postdysenteric arthropathy, **left** wrist `HCC`

    M02.139 Postdysenteric arthropathy, unspecified wrist `HCC`

√6ᵗʰ **M02.14 Postdysenteric arthropathy, hand**

    Postdysenteric arthropathy, metacarpus and phalanges

    M02.141 Postdysenteric arthropathy, **right** hand `HCC`

    M02.142 Postdysenteric arthropathy, **left** hand `HCC`

    M02.149 Postdysenteric arthropathy, unspecified hand `HCC`

√6ᵗʰ **M02.15 Postdysenteric arthropathy, hip**

    M02.151 Postdysenteric arthropathy, **right** hip `HCC`

    M02.152 Postdysenteric arthropathy, **left** hip `HCC`

    M02.159 Postdysenteric arthropathy, unspecified hip `HCC`

√6ᵗʰ **M02.16 Postdysenteric arthropathy, knee**

    M02.161 Postdysenteric arthropathy, **right** knee `HCC`

    M02.162 Postdysenteric arthropathy, **left** knee `HCC`

    M02.169 Postdysenteric arthropathy, unspecified knee `HCC`

√6ᵗʰ **M02.17 Postdysenteric arthropathy, ankle and foot**

    Postdysenteric arthropathy, tarsus, metatarsus and phalanges

    M02.171 Postdysenteric arthropathy, **right** ankle and foot `HCC`

    M02.172 Postdysenteric arthropathy, **left** ankle and foot `HCC`

    M02.179 Postdysenteric arthropathy, unspecified ankle and foot `HCC`

  M02.18 Postdysenteric arthropathy, vertebrae `HCC`

  M02.19 Postdysenteric arthropathy, multiple sites `HCC`

√5ᵗʰ **M02.2 Postimmunization arthropathy**

  M02.20 Postimmunization arthropathy, unspecified site

√6ᵗʰ **M02.21 Postimmunization arthropathy, shoulder**

    M02.211 Postimmunization arthropathy, **right** shoulder

    M02.212 Postimmunization arthropathy, **left** shoulder

    M02.219 Postimmunization arthropathy, unspecified shoulder

√6ᵗʰ **M02.22 Postimmunization arthropathy, elbow**

    M02.221 Postimmunization arthropathy, **right** elbow

    M02.222 Postimmunization arthropathy, **left** elbow

    M02.229 Postimmunization arthropathy, unspecified elbow

√6ᵗʰ **M02.23 Postimmunization arthropathy, wrist**

    Postimmunization arthropathy, carpal bones

    M02.231 Postimmunization arthropathy, **right** wrist

    M02.232 Postimmunization arthropathy, **left** wrist

    M02.239 Postimmunization arthropathy, unspecified wrist

√6ᵗʰ **M02.24 Postimmunization arthropathy, hand**

    Postimmunization arthropathy, metacarpus and phalanges

    M02.241 Postimmunization arthropathy, **right** hand

    M02.242 Postimmunization arthropathy, **left** hand

    M02.249 Postimmunization arthropathy, unspecified hand

√6ᵗʰ **M02.25 Postimmunization arthropathy, hip**

    M02.251 Postimmunization arthropathy, **right** hip

    M02.252 Postimmunization arthropathy, **left** hip

    M02.259 Postimmunization arthropathy, unspecified hip

√6ᵗʰ **M02.26 Postimmunization arthropathy, knee**

    M02.261 Postimmunization arthropathy, **right** knee

    M02.262 Postimmunization arthropathy, **left** knee

    M02.269 Postimmunization arthropathy, unspecified knee

√6ᵗʰ **M02.27 Postimmunization arthropathy, ankle and foot**

    Postimmunization arthropathy, tarsus, metatarsus and phalanges

    M02.271 Postimmunization arthropathy, **right** ankle and foot

    M02.272 Postimmunization arthropathy, **left** ankle and foot

    M02.279 Postimmunization arthropathy, unspecified ankle and foot

  M02.28 Postimmunization arthropathy, vertebrae

  M02.29 Postimmunization arthropathy, multiple sites

√5ᵗʰ **M02.3 Reiter's disease**

  Reactive arthritis

  DEF: Arthritis, iridocyclitis, and urethritis, sometimes with diarrhea. While symptoms may recur, arthritis is constant.

  M02.30 Reiter's disease, unspecified site `HCC`

√6ᵗʰ **M02.31 Reiter's disease, shoulder**

    M02.311 Reiter's disease, **right** shoulder `HCC`

    M02.312 Reiter's disease, **left** shoulder `HCC`

    M02.319 Reiter's disease, unspecified shoulder `HCC`

√6ᵗʰ **M02.32 Reiter's disease, elbow**

    M02.321 Reiter's disease, **right** elbow `HCC`

    M02.322 Reiter's disease, **left** elbow `HCC`

    M02.329 Reiter's disease, unspecified elbow `HCC`

√6ᵗʰ **M02.33 Reiter's disease, wrist**

    Reiter's disease, carpal bones

    M02.331 Reiter's disease, **right** wrist `HCC`

    M02.332 Reiter's disease, **left** wrist `HCC`

    M02.339 Reiter's disease, unspecified wrist `HCC`

√6ᵗʰ **M02.34 Reiter's disease, hand**

    Reiter's disease, metacarpus and phalanges

    M02.341 Reiter's disease, **right** hand `HCC`

    M02.342 Reiter's disease, **left** hand `HCC`

    M02.349 Reiter's disease, unspecified hand `HCC`

√6ᵗʰ **M02.35 Reiter's disease, hip**

    M02.351 Reiter's disease, **right** hip `HCC`

    M02.352 Reiter's disease, **left** hip `HCC`

    M02.359 Reiter's disease, unspecified hip `HCC`

√6th **M02.36 Reiter's disease, knee**
> **M02.361 Reiter's disease, right knee** `HCC`
> **M02.362 Reiter's disease, left knee** `HCC`
> **M02.369 Reiter's disease, unspecified knee** `HCC`

√6th **M02.37 Reiter's disease, ankle and foot**
> Reiter's disease, tarsus, metatarsus and phalanges
> **M02.371 Reiter's disease, right ankle and foot** `HCC`
> **M02.372 Reiter's disease, left ankle and foot** `HCC`
> **M02.379 Reiter's disease, unspecified ankle and foot** `HCC`

M02.38 Reiter's disease, vertebrae `HCC`

M02.39 Reiter's disease, multiple sites `HCC`

√5th **M02.8 Other reactive arthropathies**
> **M02.80 Other reactive arthropathies, unspecified site** `HCC`

√6th **M02.81 Other reactive arthropathies, shoulder**
> **M02.811 Other reactive arthropathies, right shoulder** `HCC`
> **M02.812 Other reactive arthropathies, left shoulder** `HCC`
> **M02.819 Other reactive arthropathies, unspecified shoulder** `HCC`

√6th **M02.82 Other reactive arthropathies, elbow**
> **M02.821 Other reactive arthropathies, right elbow** `HCC`
> **M02.822 Other reactive arthropathies, left elbow** `HCC`
> **M02.829 Other reactive arthropathies, unspecified elbow** `HCC`

√6th **M02.83 Other reactive arthropathies, wrist**
> Other reactive arthropathies, carpal bones
> **M02.831 Other reactive arthropathies, right wrist** `HCC`
> **M02.832 Other reactive arthropathies, left wrist** `HCC`
> **M02.839 Other reactive arthropathies, unspecified wrist** `HCC`

√6th **M02.84 Other reactive arthropathies, hand**
> Other reactive arthropathies, metacarpus and phalanges
> **M02.841 Other reactive arthropathies, right hand** `HCC`
> **M02.842 Other reactive arthropathies, left hand** `HCC`
> **M02.849 Other reactive arthropathies, unspecified hand** `HCC`

√6th **M02.85 Other reactive arthropathies, hip**
> **M02.851 Other reactive arthropathies, right hip** `HCC`
> **M02.852 Other reactive arthropathies, left hip** `HCC`
> **M02.859 Other reactive arthropathies, unspecified hip** `HCC`

√6th **M02.86 Other reactive arthropathies, knee**
> **M02.861 Other reactive arthropathies, right knee** `HCC`
> **M02.862 Other reactive arthropathies, left knee** `HCC`
> **M02.869 Other reactive arthropathies, unspecified knee** `HCC`

√6th **M02.87 Other reactive arthropathies, ankle and foot**
> Other reactive arthropathies, tarsus, metatarsus and phalanges
> **M02.871 Other reactive arthropathies, right ankle and foot** `HCC`
> **M02.872 Other reactive arthropathies, left ankle and foot** `HCC`
> **M02.879 Other reactive arthropathies, unspecified ankle and foot** `HCC`

M02.88 Other reactive arthropathies, vertebrae `HCC`

M02.89 Other reactive arthropathies, multiple sites `HCC`

M02.9 Reactive arthropathy, unspecified `HCC`

Autoinflammatory syndromes (M04)

√4th **M04 Autoinflammatory syndromes**
> EXCLUDES 2   Crohn's disease (K50.-)
> AHA: 2016,4Q,37

M04.1 Periodic fever syndromes `HCC`
> Familial Mediterranean fever
> Hyperimmunoglobin D syndrome
> Mevalonate kinase deficiency
> Tumor necrosis factor receptor associated periodic syndrome [TRAPS]

M04.2 Cryopyrin-associated periodic syndromes `HCC`
> Chronic infantile neurological, cutaneous and articular syndrome [CINCA]
> Familial cold autoinflammatory syndrome
> Familial cold urticaria
> Muckle-Wells syndrome
> Neonatal onset multisystemic inflammatory disorder [NOMID]

M04.8 Other autoinflammatory syndromes `HCC`
> Blau syndrome
> Deficiency of interleukin 1 receptor antagonist [DIRA]
> Majeed syndrome
> Periodic fever, aphthous stomatitis, pharyngitis, and adenopathy syndrome [PFAPA]
> Pyogenic arthritis, pyoderma gangrenosum, and acne syndrome [PAPA]

M04.9 Autoinflammatory syndrome, unspecified `HCC`

Inflammatory polyarthropathies (M05-M14)

√4th **M05 Rheumatoid arthritis with rheumatoid factor**
> EXCLUDES 1   rheumatic fever (I00)
>   juvenile rheumatoid arthritis (M08.-)
>   rheumatoid arthritis of spine (M45.-)
> **DEF:** Rheumatoid arthritis: Autoimmune systemic disease that causes chronic inflammation of the joints and other areas of the body, manifested by inflammatory changes in articular structures and synovial membranes, atrophy, and loss in bone density.

√5th **M05.0 Felty's syndrome**
> Rheumatoid arthritis with splenoadenomegaly and leukopenia
> **M05.00 Felty's syndrome, unspecified site** `HCC`

√6th **M05.01 Felty's syndrome, shoulder**
> **M05.011 Felty's syndrome, right shoulder** `HCC`
> **M05.012 Felty's syndrome, left shoulder** `HCC`
> **M05.019 Felty's syndrome, unspecified shoulder** `HCC`

√6th **M05.02 Felty's syndrome, elbow**
> **M05.021 Felty's syndrome, right elbow** `HCC`
> **M05.022 Felty's syndrome, left elbow** `HCC`
> **M05.029 Felty's syndrome, unspecified elbow** `HCC`

√6th **M05.03 Felty's syndrome, wrist**
> Felty's syndrome, carpal bones
> **M05.031 Felty's syndrome, right wrist** `HCC`
> **M05.032 Felty's syndrome, left wrist** `HCC`
> **M05.039 Felty's syndrome, unspecified wrist** `HCC`

√6th **M05.04 Felty's syndrome, hand**
> Felty's syndrome, metacarpus and phalanges
> **M05.041 Felty's syndrome, right hand** `HCC`
> **M05.042 Felty's syndrome, left hand** `HCC`

M05.049 Felty's syndrome, unspecified hand `HCC`

✓6ᵗʰ M05.05 Felty's syndrome, hip

   M05.051 Felty's syndrome, right hip `HCC`

   M05.052 Felty's syndrome, left hip `HCC`

   M05.059 Felty's syndrome, unspecified hip `HCC`

✓6ᵗʰ M05.06 Felty's syndrome, knee

   M05.061 Felty's syndrome, right knee `HCC`

   M05.062 Felty's syndrome, left knee `HCC`

   M05.069 Felty's syndrome, unspecified knee `HCC`

✓6ᵗʰ M05.07 Felty's syndrome, ankle and foot

   Felty's syndrome, tarsus, metatarsus and phalanges

   M05.071 Felty's syndrome, right ankle and foot `HCC`

   M05.072 Felty's syndrome, left ankle and foot `HCC`

   M05.079 Felty's syndrome, unspecified ankle and foot `HCC`

  M05.09 Felty's syndrome, multiple sites `HCC`

✓5ᵗʰ M05.1 Rheumatoid lung disease with rheumatoid arthritis

  DEF: Lung disorders associated with rheumatoid arthritis.

  M05.10 Rheumatoid lung disease with rheumatoid arthritis of unspecified site `HCC`

✓6ᵗʰ M05.11 Rheumatoid lung disease with rheumatoid arthritis of shoulder

   M05.111 Rheumatoid lung disease with rheumatoid arthritis of right shoulder `HCC`

   M05.112 Rheumatoid lung disease with rheumatoid arthritis of left shoulder `HCC`

   M05.119 Rheumatoid lung disease with rheumatoid arthritis of unspecified shoulder `HCC`

✓6ᵗʰ M05.12 Rheumatoid lung disease with rheumatoid arthritis of elbow

   M05.121 Rheumatoid lung disease with rheumatoid arthritis of right elbow `HCC`

   M05.122 Rheumatoid lung disease with rheumatoid arthritis of left elbow `HCC`

   M05.129 Rheumatoid lung disease with rheumatoid arthritis of unspecified elbow `HCC`

✓6ᵗʰ M05.13 Rheumatoid lung disease with rheumatoid arthritis of wrist

   Rheumatoid lung disease with rheumatoid arthritis, carpal bones

   M05.131 Rheumatoid lung disease with rheumatoid arthritis of right wrist `HCC`

   M05.132 Rheumatoid lung disease with rheumatoid arthritis of left wrist `HCC`

   M05.139 Rheumatoid lung disease with rheumatoid arthritis of unspecified wrist `HCC`

✓6ᵗʰ M05.14 Rheumatoid lung disease with rheumatoid arthritis of hand

   Rheumatoid lung disease with rheumatoid arthritis, metacarpus and phalanges

   M05.141 Rheumatoid lung disease with rheumatoid arthritis of right hand `HCC`

   M05.142 Rheumatoid lung disease with rheumatoid arthritis of left hand `HCC`

   M05.149 Rheumatoid lung disease with rheumatoid arthritis of unspecified hand `HCC`

✓6ᵗʰ M05.15 Rheumatoid lung disease with rheumatoid arthritis of hip

   M05.151 Rheumatoid lung disease with rheumatoid arthritis of right hip `HCC`

M05.152 Rheumatoid lung disease with rheumatoid arthritis of left hip `HCC`

M05.159 Rheumatoid lung disease with rheumatoid arthritis of unspecified hip `HCC`

✓6ᵗʰ M05.16 Rheumatoid lung disease with rheumatoid arthritis of knee

   M05.161 Rheumatoid lung disease with rheumatoid arthritis of right knee `HCC`

   M05.162 Rheumatoid lung disease with rheumatoid arthritis of left knee `HCC`

   M05.169 Rheumatoid lung disease with rheumatoid arthritis of unspecified knee `HCC`

✓6ᵗʰ M05.17 Rheumatoid lung disease with rheumatoid arthritis of ankle and foot

   Rheumatoid lung disease with rheumatoid arthritis, tarsus, metatarsus and phalanges

   M05.171 Rheumatoid lung disease with rheumatoid arthritis of right ankle and foot `HCC`

   M05.172 Rheumatoid lung disease with rheumatoid arthritis of left ankle and foot `HCC`

   M05.179 Rheumatoid lung disease with rheumatoid arthritis of unspecified ankle and foot `HCC`

  M05.19 Rheumatoid lung disease with rheumatoid arthritis of multiple sites `HCC`

✓5ᵗʰ M05.2 Rheumatoid vasculitis with rheumatoid arthritis

  M05.20 Rheumatoid vasculitis with rheumatoid arthritis of unspecified site `HCC`

✓6ᵗʰ M05.21 Rheumatoid vasculitis with rheumatoid arthritis of shoulder

   M05.211 Rheumatoid vasculitis with rheumatoid arthritis of right shoulder `HCC`

   M05.212 Rheumatoid vasculitis with rheumatoid arthritis of left shoulder `HCC`

   M05.219 Rheumatoid vasculitis with rheumatoid arthritis of unspecified shoulder `HCC`

✓6ᵗʰ M05.22 Rheumatoid vasculitis with rheumatoid arthritis of elbow

   M05.221 Rheumatoid vasculitis with rheumatoid arthritis of right elbow `HCC`

   M05.222 Rheumatoid vasculitis with rheumatoid arthritis of left elbow `HCC`

   M05.229 Rheumatoid vasculitis with rheumatoid arthritis of unspecified elbow `HCC`

✓6ᵗʰ M05.23 Rheumatoid vasculitis with rheumatoid arthritis of wrist

   Rheumatoid vasculitis with rheumatoid arthritis, carpal bones

   M05.231 Rheumatoid vasculitis with rheumatoid arthritis of right wrist `HCC`

   M05.232 Rheumatoid vasculitis with rheumatoid arthritis of left wrist `HCC`

   M05.239 Rheumatoid vasculitis with rheumatoid arthritis of unspecified wrist `HCC`

✓6ᵗʰ M05.24 Rheumatoid vasculitis with rheumatoid arthritis of hand

   Rheumatoid vasculitis with rheumatoid arthritis, metacarpus and phalanges

   M05.241 Rheumatoid vasculitis with rheumatoid arthritis of right hand `HCC`

   M05.242 Rheumatoid vasculitis with rheumatoid arthritis of left hand `HCC`

☑ Additional Character Required ✓x7ᵗʰ Placeholder Unacceptable PDx Questionable PDx Manifestation Unspecified Dx H1-H14 HAC HCC CMS-HCC Dx HIV HIV Dx

Chapter 13. Diseases of the Musculoskeletal System and Connective Tissue

M05.249–M05.431

M05.249 Rheumatoid vasculitis with rheumatoid arthritis of unspecified hand `HCC`

✓6ᵗʰ M05.25 Rheumatoid vasculitis with rheumatoid arthritis of hip

M05.251 Rheumatoid vasculitis with rheumatoid arthritis of right hip `HCC`

M05.252 Rheumatoid vasculitis with rheumatoid arthritis of left hip `HCC`

M05.259 Rheumatoid vasculitis with rheumatoid arthritis of unspecified hip `HCC`

✓6ᵗʰ M05.26 Rheumatoid vasculitis with rheumatoid arthritis of knee

M05.261 Rheumatoid vasculitis with rheumatoid arthritis of right knee `HCC`

M05.262 Rheumatoid vasculitis with rheumatoid arthritis of left knee `HCC`

M05.269 Rheumatoid vasculitis with rheumatoid arthritis of unspecified knee `HCC`

✓6ᵗʰ M05.27 Rheumatoid vasculitis with rheumatoid arthritis of ankle and foot

Rheumatoid vasculitis with rheumatoid arthritis, tarsus, metatarsus and phalanges

M05.271 Rheumatoid vasculitis with rheumatoid arthritis of right ankle and foot `HCC`

M05.272 Rheumatoid vasculitis with rheumatoid arthritis of left ankle and foot `HCC`

M05.279 Rheumatoid vasculitis with rheumatoid arthritis of unspecified ankle and foot `HCC`

M05.29 Rheumatoid vasculitis with rheumatoid arthritis of multiple sites `HCC`

✓5ᵗʰ M05.3 Rheumatoid heart disease with rheumatoid arthritis

Rheumatoid carditis
Rheumatoid endocarditis
Rheumatoid myocarditis
Rheumatoid pericarditis

M05.30 Rheumatoid heart disease with rheumatoid arthritis of unspecified site `HCC`

✓6ᵗʰ M05.31 Rheumatoid heart disease with rheumatoid arthritis of shoulder

M05.311 Rheumatoid heart disease with rheumatoid arthritis of right shoulder `HCC`

M05.312 Rheumatoid heart disease with rheumatoid arthritis of left shoulder `HCC`

M05.319 Rheumatoid heart disease with rheumatoid arthritis of unspecified shoulder `HCC`

✓6ᵗʰ M05.32 Rheumatoid heart disease with rheumatoid arthritis of elbow

M05.321 Rheumatoid heart disease with rheumatoid arthritis of right elbow `HCC`

M05.322 Rheumatoid heart disease with rheumatoid arthritis of left elbow `HCC`

M05.329 Rheumatoid heart disease with rheumatoid arthritis of unspecified elbow `HCC`

✓6ᵗʰ M05.33 Rheumatoid heart disease with rheumatoid arthritis of wrist

Rheumatoid heart disease with rheumatoid arthritis, carpal bones

M05.331 Rheumatoid heart disease with rheumatoid arthritis of right wrist `HCC`

M05.332 Rheumatoid heart disease with rheumatoid arthritis of left wrist `HCC`

M05.339 Rheumatoid heart disease with rheumatoid arthritis of unspecified wrist `HCC`

✓6ᵗʰ M05.34 Rheumatoid heart disease with rheumatoid arthritis of hand

Rheumatoid heart disease with rheumatoid arthritis, metacarpus and phalanges

M05.341 Rheumatoid heart disease with rheumatoid arthritis of right hand `HCC`

M05.342 Rheumatoid heart disease with rheumatoid arthritis of left hand `HCC`

M05.349 Rheumatoid heart disease with rheumatoid arthritis of unspecified hand `HCC`

✓6ᵗʰ M05.35 Rheumatoid heart disease with rheumatoid arthritis of hip

M05.351 Rheumatoid heart disease with rheumatoid arthritis of right hip `HCC`

M05.352 Rheumatoid heart disease with rheumatoid arthritis of left hip `HCC`

M05.359 Rheumatoid heart disease with rheumatoid arthritis of unspecified hip `HCC`

✓6ᵗʰ M05.36 Rheumatoid heart disease with rheumatoid arthritis of knee

M05.361 Rheumatoid heart disease with rheumatoid arthritis of right knee `HCC`

M05.362 Rheumatoid heart disease with rheumatoid arthritis of left knee `HCC`

M05.369 Rheumatoid heart disease with rheumatoid arthritis of unspecified knee `HCC`

✓6ᵗʰ M05.37 Rheumatoid heart disease with rheumatoid arthritis of ankle and foot

Rheumatoid heart disease with rheumatoid arthritis, tarsus, metatarsus and phalanges

M05.371 Rheumatoid heart disease with rheumatoid arthritis of right ankle and foot `HCC`

M05.372 Rheumatoid heart disease with rheumatoid arthritis of left ankle and foot `HCC`

M05.379 Rheumatoid heart disease with rheumatoid arthritis of unspecified ankle and foot `HCC`

M05.39 Rheumatoid heart disease with rheumatoid arthritis of multiple sites `HCC`

✓5ᵗʰ M05.4 Rheumatoid myopathy with rheumatoid arthritis

M05.40 Rheumatoid myopathy with rheumatoid arthritis of unspecified site `HCC`

✓6ᵗʰ M05.41 Rheumatoid myopathy with rheumatoid arthritis of shoulder

M05.411 Rheumatoid myopathy with rheumatoid arthritis of right shoulder `HCC`

M05.412 Rheumatoid myopathy with rheumatoid arthritis of left shoulder `HCC`

M05.419 Rheumatoid myopathy with rheumatoid arthritis of unspecified shoulder `HCC`

✓6ᵗʰ M05.42 Rheumatoid myopathy with rheumatoid arthritis of elbow

M05.421 Rheumatoid myopathy with rheumatoid arthritis of right elbow `HCC`

M05.422 Rheumatoid myopathy with rheumatoid arthritis of left elbow `HCC`

M05.429 Rheumatoid myopathy with rheumatoid arthritis of unspecified elbow `HCC`

✓6ᵗʰ M05.43 Rheumatoid myopathy with rheumatoid arthritis of wrist

Rheumatoid myopathy with rheumatoid arthritis, carpal bones

M05.431 Rheumatoid myopathy with rheumatoid arthritis of right wrist `HCC`

Ⓝ Newborn: 0   Ⓟ Pediatric: 0-17   Ⓜ Maternity: 9-64   Ⓐ Adult: 15-124   `MCC` Major Complication/Comorbidity   `CC` Complication/Comorbidity   `SW` Severe Wound Dx

770   ICD-10-CM 2020

M05.432 Rheumatoid myopathy with rheumatoid arthritis of **left** wrist `HCC`

M05.439 Rheumatoid myopathy with rheumatoid arthritis of unspecified wrist `HCC`

✓6ᵗʰ **M05.44** Rheumatoid myopathy with rheumatoid arthritis of **hand**
Rheumatoid myopathy with rheumatoid arthritis, metacarpus and phalanges

M05.441 Rheumatoid myopathy with rheumatoid arthritis of **right** hand `HCC`

M05.442 Rheumatoid myopathy with rheumatoid arthritis of **left** hand `HCC`

M05.449 Rheumatoid myopathy with rheumatoid arthritis of unspecified hand `HCC`

✓6ᵗʰ **M05.45** Rheumatoid myopathy with rheumatoid arthritis of **hip**

M05.451 Rheumatoid myopathy with rheumatoid arthritis of **right** hip `HCC`

M05.452 Rheumatoid myopathy with rheumatoid arthritis of **left** hip `HCC`

M05.459 Rheumatoid myopathy with rheumatoid arthritis of unspecified hip `HCC`

✓6ᵗʰ **M05.46** Rheumatoid myopathy with rheumatoid arthritis of **knee**

M05.461 Rheumatoid myopathy with rheumatoid arthritis of **right** knee `HCC`

M05.462 Rheumatoid myopathy with rheumatoid arthritis of **left** knee `HCC`

M05.469 Rheumatoid myopathy with rheumatoid arthritis of unspecified knee `HCC`

✓6ᵗʰ **M05.47** Rheumatoid myopathy with rheumatoid arthritis of **ankle and foot**
Rheumatoid myopathy with rheumatoid arthritis, tarsus, metatarsus and phalanges

M05.471 Rheumatoid myopathy with rheumatoid arthritis of **right** ankle and foot `HCC`

M05.472 Rheumatoid myopathy with rheumatoid arthritis of **left** ankle and foot `HCC`

M05.479 Rheumatoid myopathy with rheumatoid arthritis of unspecified ankle and foot `HCC`

M05.49 Rheumatoid myopathy with rheumatoid arthritis of **multiple sites** `HCC`

✓5ᵗʰ **M05.5** Rheumatoid **polyneuropathy with rheumatoid arthritis**

M05.50 Rheumatoid polyneuropathy with rheumatoid arthritis of unspecified site `HCC`

✓6ᵗʰ **M05.51** Rheumatoid polyneuropathy with rheumatoid arthritis of **shoulder**

M05.511 Rheumatoid polyneuropathy with rheumatoid arthritis of **right** shoulder `HCC`

M05.512 Rheumatoid polyneuropathy with rheumatoid arthritis of **left** shoulder `HCC`

M05.519 Rheumatoid polyneuropathy with rheumatoid arthritis of unspecified shoulder `HCC`

✓6ᵗʰ **M05.52** Rheumatoid polyneuropathy with rheumatoid arthritis of **elbow**

M05.521 Rheumatoid polyneuropathy with rheumatoid arthritis of **right** elbow `HCC`

M05.522 Rheumatoid polyneuropathy with rheumatoid arthritis of **left** elbow `HCC`

M05.529 Rheumatoid polyneuropathy with rheumatoid arthritis of unspecified elbow `HCC`

✓6ᵗʰ **M05.53** Rheumatoid polyneuropathy with rheumatoid arthritis of **wrist**
Rheumatoid polyneuropathy with rheumatoid arthritis, carpal bones

M05.531 Rheumatoid polyneuropathy with rheumatoid arthritis of **right** wrist `HCC`

M05.532 Rheumatoid polyneuropathy with rheumatoid arthritis of **left** wrist `HCC`

M05.539 Rheumatoid polyneuropathy with rheumatoid arthritis of unspecified wrist `HCC`

✓6ᵗʰ **M05.54** Rheumatoid polyneuropathy with rheumatoid arthritis of **hand**
Rheumatoid polyneuropathy with rheumatoid arthritis, metacarpus and phalanges

M05.541 Rheumatoid polyneuropathy with rheumatoid arthritis of **right** hand `HCC`

M05.542 Rheumatoid polyneuropathy with rheumatoid arthritis of **left** hand `HCC`

M05.549 Rheumatoid polyneuropathy with rheumatoid arthritis of unspecified hand `HCC`

✓6ᵗʰ **M05.55** Rheumatoid polyneuropathy with rheumatoid arthritis of **hip**

M05.551 Rheumatoid polyneuropathy with rheumatoid arthritis of **right** hip `HCC`

M05.552 Rheumatoid polyneuropathy with rheumatoid arthritis of **left** hip `HCC`

M05.559 Rheumatoid polyneuropathy with rheumatoid arthritis of unspecified hip `HCC`

✓6ᵗʰ **M05.56** Rheumatoid polyneuropathy with rheumatoid arthritis of **knee**

M05.561 Rheumatoid polyneuropathy with rheumatoid arthritis of **right** knee `HCC`

M05.562 Rheumatoid polyneuropathy with rheumatoid arthritis of **left** knee `HCC`

M05.569 Rheumatoid polyneuropathy with rheumatoid arthritis of unspecified knee `HCC`

✓6ᵗʰ **M05.57** Rheumatoid polyneuropathy with rheumatoid arthritis of **ankle and foot**
Rheumatoid polyneuropathy with rheumatoid arthritis, tarsus, metatarsus and phalanges

M05.571 Rheumatoid polyneuropathy with rheumatoid arthritis of **right** ankle and foot `HCC`

M05.572 Rheumatoid polyneuropathy with rheumatoid arthritis of **left** ankle and foot `HCC`

M05.579 Rheumatoid polyneuropathy with rheumatoid arthritis of unspecified ankle and foot `HCC`

M05.59 Rheumatoid polyneuropathy with rheumatoid arthritis of multiple sites `HCC`

✓5ᵗʰ **M05.6** Rheumatoid arthritis with involvement of other organs and systems

M05.60 Rheumatoid arthritis of unspecified site with involvement of other organs and systems `HCC`

✓6ᵗʰ **M05.61** Rheumatoid arthritis of shoulder with involvement of other organs and systems

    M05.611 Rheumatoid arthritis of right shoulder with involvement of other organs and systems `HCC`

    M05.612 Rheumatoid arthritis of left shoulder with involvement of other organs and systems `HCC`

    M05.619 Rheumatoid arthritis of unspecified shoulder with involvement of other organs and systems `HCC`

✓6ᵗʰ **M05.62** Rheumatoid arthritis of elbow with involvement of other organs and systems

    M05.621 Rheumatoid arthritis of right elbow with involvement of other organs and systems `HCC`

    M05.622 Rheumatoid arthritis of left elbow with involvement of other organs and systems `HCC`

    M05.629 Rheumatoid arthritis of unspecified elbow with involvement of other organs and systems `HCC`

✓6ᵗʰ **M05.63** Rheumatoid arthritis of wrist with involvement of other organs and systems
    Rheumatoid arthritis of carpal bones with involvement of other organs and systems

    M05.631 Rheumatoid arthritis of right wrist with involvement of other organs and systems `HCC`

    M05.632 Rheumatoid arthritis of left wrist with involvement of other organs and systems `HCC`

    M05.639 Rheumatoid arthritis of unspecified wrist with involvement of other organs and systems `HCC`

✓6ᵗʰ **M05.64** Rheumatoid arthritis of hand with involvement of other organs and systems
    Rheumatoid arthritis of metacarpus and phalanges with involvement of other organs and systems

    M05.641 Rheumatoid arthritis of right hand with involvement of other organs and systems `HCC`

    M05.642 Rheumatoid arthritis of left hand with involvement of other organs and systems `HCC`

    M05.649 Rheumatoid arthritis of unspecified hand with involvement of other organs and systems `HCC`

✓6ᵗʰ **M05.65** Rheumatoid arthritis of hip with involvement of other organs and systems

    M05.651 Rheumatoid arthritis of right hip with involvement of other organs and systems `HCC`

    M05.652 Rheumatoid arthritis of left hip with involvement of other organs and systems `HCC`

    M05.659 Rheumatoid arthritis of unspecified hip with involvement of other organs and systems `HCC`

✓6ᵗʰ **M05.66** Rheumatoid arthritis of knee with involvement of other organs and systems

    M05.661 Rheumatoid arthritis of right knee with involvement of other organs and systems `HCC`

    M05.662 Rheumatoid arthritis of left knee with involvement of other organs and systems `HCC`

    M05.669 Rheumatoid arthritis of unspecified knee with involvement of other organs and systems `HCC`

✓6ᵗʰ **M05.67** Rheumatoid arthritis of ankle and foot with involvement of other organs and systems
    Rheumatoid arthritis of tarsus, metatarsus and phalanges with involvement of other organs and systems

    M05.671 Rheumatoid arthritis of right ankle and foot with involvement of other organs and systems `HCC`

    M05.672 Rheumatoid arthritis of left ankle and foot with involvement of other organs and systems `HCC`

    M05.679 Rheumatoid arthritis of unspecified ankle and foot with involvement of other organs and systems `HCC`

M05.69 Rheumatoid arthritis of multiple sites with involvement of other organs and systems `HCC`

✓5ᵗʰ **M05.7** Rheumatoid arthritis with rheumatoid factor without organ or systems involvement

M05.70 Rheumatoid arthritis with rheumatoid factor of unspecified site without organ or systems involvement `HCC`

✓6ᵗʰ **M05.71** Rheumatoid arthritis with rheumatoid factor of shoulder without organ or systems involvement

    M05.711 Rheumatoid arthritis with rheumatoid factor of right shoulder without organ or systems involvement `HCC`

    M05.712 Rheumatoid arthritis with rheumatoid factor of left shoulder without organ or systems involvement `HCC`

    M05.719 Rheumatoid arthritis with rheumatoid factor of unspecified shoulder without organ or systems involvement `HCC`

✓6ᵗʰ **M05.72** Rheumatoid arthritis with rheumatoid factor of elbow without organ or systems involvement

    M05.721 Rheumatoid arthritis with rheumatoid factor of right elbow without organ or systems involvement `HCC`

    M05.722 Rheumatoid arthritis with rheumatoid factor of left elbow without organ or systems involvement `HCC`

    M05.729 Rheumatoid arthritis with rheumatoid factor of unspecified elbow without organ or systems involvement `HCC`

✓6ᵗʰ **M05.73** Rheumatoid arthritis with rheumatoid factor of wrist without organ or systems involvement

    M05.731 Rheumatoid arthritis with rheumatoid factor of right wrist without organ or systems involvement `HCC`

    M05.732 Rheumatoid arthritis with rheumatoid factor of left wrist without organ or systems involvement `HCC`

    M05.739 Rheumatoid arthritis with rheumatoid factor of unspecified wrist without organ or systems involvement `HCC`

N Newborn: 0   P Pediatric: 0-17   M Maternity: 9-64   A Adult: 15-124   `MCC` Major Complication/Comorbidity   `CC` Complication/Comorbidity   `SW` Severe Wound Dx

772   ICD-10-CM 2020

✓6ᵗʰ **M05.74** **Rheumatoid arthritis with rheumatoid factor of hand without organ or systems involvement**

     M05.741 Rheumatoid arthritis with rheumatoid factor of right hand without organ or systems involvement   `HCC`

     M05.742 Rheumatoid arthritis with rheumatoid factor of left hand without organ or systems involvement   `HCC`

     M05.749 Rheumatoid arthritis with rheumatoid factor of unspecified hand without organ or systems involvement   `HCC`

✓6ᵗʰ **M05.75** **Rheumatoid arthritis with rheumatoid factor of hip without organ or systems involvement**

     M05.751 Rheumatoid arthritis with rheumatoid factor of right hip without organ or systems involvement   `HCC`

     M05.752 Rheumatoid arthritis with rheumatoid factor of left hip without organ or systems involvement   `HCC`

     M05.759 Rheumatoid arthritis with rheumatoid factor of unspecified hip without organ or systems involvement   `HCC`

✓6ᵗʰ **M05.76** **Rheumatoid arthritis with rheumatoid factor of knee without organ or systems involvement**

     M05.761 Rheumatoid arthritis with rheumatoid factor of right knee without organ or systems involvement   `HCC`

     M05.762 Rheumatoid arthritis with rheumatoid factor of left knee without organ or systems involvement   `HCC`

     M05.769 Rheumatoid arthritis with rheumatoid factor of unspecified knee without organ or systems involvement   `HCC`

✓6ᵗʰ **M05.77** **Rheumatoid arthritis with rheumatoid factor of ankle and foot without organ or systems involvement**

     M05.771 Rheumatoid arthritis with rheumatoid factor of right ankle and foot without organ or systems involvement   `HCC`

     M05.772 Rheumatoid arthritis with rheumatoid factor of left ankle and foot without organ or systems involvement   `HCC`

     M05.779 Rheumatoid arthritis with rheumatoid factor of unspecified ankle and foot without organ or systems involvement   `HCC`

     M05.79 Rheumatoid arthritis with rheumatoid factor of multiple sites without organ or systems involvement   `HCC`

✓5ᵗʰ **M05.8** **Other rheumatoid arthritis with rheumatoid factor**

     M05.80 Other rheumatoid arthritis with rheumatoid factor of unspecified site   `HCC`

✓6ᵗʰ **M05.81** **Other rheumatoid arthritis with rheumatoid factor of shoulder**

     M05.811 Other rheumatoid arthritis with rheumatoid factor of right shoulder   `HCC`

     M05.812 Other rheumatoid arthritis with rheumatoid factor of left shoulder   `HCC`

     M05.819 Other rheumatoid arthritis with rheumatoid factor of unspecified shoulder   `HCC`

✓6ᵗʰ **M05.82** **Other rheumatoid arthritis with rheumatoid factor of elbow**

     M05.821 Other rheumatoid arthritis with rheumatoid factor of right elbow   `HCC`

     M05.822 Other rheumatoid arthritis with rheumatoid factor of left elbow   `HCC`

     M05.829 Other rheumatoid arthritis with rheumatoid factor of unspecified elbow   `HCC`

✓6ᵗʰ **M05.83** **Other rheumatoid arthritis with rheumatoid factor of wrist**

     M05.831 Other rheumatoid arthritis with rheumatoid factor of right wrist   `HCC`

     M05.832 Other rheumatoid arthritis with rheumatoid factor of left wrist   `HCC`

     M05.839 Other rheumatoid arthritis with rheumatoid factor of unspecified wrist   `HCC`

✓6ᵗʰ **M05.84** **Other rheumatoid arthritis with rheumatoid factor of hand**

     M05.841 Other rheumatoid arthritis with rheumatoid factor of right hand   `HCC`

     M05.842 Other rheumatoid arthritis with rheumatoid factor of left hand   `HCC`

     M05.849 Other rheumatoid arthritis with rheumatoid factor of unspecified hand   `HCC`

✓6ᵗʰ **M05.85** **Other rheumatoid arthritis with rheumatoid factor of hip**

     M05.851 Other rheumatoid arthritis with rheumatoid factor of right hip   `HCC`

     M05.852 Other rheumatoid arthritis with rheumatoid factor of left hip   `HCC`

     M05.859 Other rheumatoid arthritis with rheumatoid factor of unspecified hip   `HCC`

✓6ᵗʰ **M05.86** **Other rheumatoid arthritis with rheumatoid factor of knee**

     M05.861 Other rheumatoid arthritis with rheumatoid factor of right knee   `HCC`

     M05.862 Other rheumatoid arthritis with rheumatoid factor of left knee   `HCC`

     M05.869 Other rheumatoid arthritis with rheumatoid factor of unspecified knee   `HCC`

✓6ᵗʰ **M05.87** **Other rheumatoid arthritis with rheumatoid factor of ankle and foot**

     M05.871 Other rheumatoid arthritis with rheumatoid factor of right ankle and foot   `HCC`

     M05.872 Other rheumatoid arthritis with rheumatoid factor of left ankle and foot   `HCC`

     M05.879 Other rheumatoid arthritis with rheumatoid factor of unspecified ankle and foot   `HCC`

     M05.89 Other rheumatoid arthritis with rheumatoid factor of multiple sites   `HCC`

     M05.9 Rheumatoid arthritis with rheumatoid factor, unspecified   `HCC`

✓4ᵗʰ **M06** **Other rheumatoid arthritis**

     DEF: Rheumatoid arthritis: Autoimmune systemic disease that causes chronic inflammation of the joints and other areas of the body, manifested by inflammatory changes in articular structures and synovial membranes, atrophy, and loss in bone density.

✓5ᵗʰ **M06.0** **Rheumatoid arthritis without rheumatoid factor**

     M06.00 Rheumatoid arthritis without rheumatoid factor, unspecified site   `HCC`

✓6ᵗʰ **M06.01** **Rheumatoid arthritis without rheumatoid factor, shoulder**

     M06.011 Rheumatoid arthritis without rheumatoid factor, right shoulder   `HCC`

✔ Additional Character Required   ✓xʔᵗʰ Placeholder   Unacceptable PDx   Questionable PDx   Manifestation   Unspecified Dx   H1-H14 HAC   HCC CMS-HCC Dx   HIV HIV Dx

ICD-10-CM 2020   773

M06.012 Rheumatoid arthritis without rheumatoid factor, left shoulder `HCC`

M06.019 Rheumatoid arthritis without rheumatoid factor, unspecified shoulder `HCC`

✓6ᵗʰ **M06.02** Rheumatoid arthritis without rheumatoid factor, elbow

   M06.021 Rheumatoid arthritis without rheumatoid factor, right elbow `HCC`

   M06.022 Rheumatoid arthritis without rheumatoid factor, left elbow `HCC`

   M06.029 Rheumatoid arthritis without rheumatoid factor, unspecified elbow `HCC`

✓6ᵗʰ **M06.03** Rheumatoid arthritis without rheumatoid factor, wrist

   M06.031 Rheumatoid arthritis without rheumatoid factor, right wrist `HCC`

   M06.032 Rheumatoid arthritis without rheumatoid factor, left wrist `HCC`

   M06.039 Rheumatoid arthritis without rheumatoid factor, unspecified wrist `HCC`

✓6ᵗʰ **M06.04** Rheumatoid arthritis without rheumatoid factor, hand

   M06.041 Rheumatoid arthritis without rheumatoid factor, right hand `HCC`

   M06.042 Rheumatoid arthritis without rheumatoid factor, left hand `HCC`

   M06.049 Rheumatoid arthritis without rheumatoid factor, unspecified hand `HCC`

✓6ᵗʰ **M06.05** Rheumatoid arthritis without rheumatoid factor, hip

   M06.051 Rheumatoid arthritis without rheumatoid factor, right hip `HCC`

   M06.052 Rheumatoid arthritis without rheumatoid factor, left hip `HCC`

   M06.059 Rheumatoid arthritis without rheumatoid factor, unspecified hip `HCC`

✓6ᵗʰ **M06.06** Rheumatoid arthritis without rheumatoid factor, knee

   M06.061 Rheumatoid arthritis without rheumatoid factor, right knee `HCC`

   M06.062 Rheumatoid arthritis without rheumatoid factor, left knee `HCC`

   M06.069 Rheumatoid arthritis without rheumatoid factor, unspecified knee `HCC`

✓6ᵗʰ **M06.07** Rheumatoid arthritis without rheumatoid factor, ankle and foot

   M06.071 Rheumatoid arthritis without rheumatoid factor, right ankle and foot `HCC`

   M06.072 Rheumatoid arthritis without rheumatoid factor, left ankle and foot `HCC`

   M06.079 Rheumatoid arthritis without rheumatoid factor, unspecified ankle and foot `HCC`

M06.08 Rheumatoid arthritis without rheumatoid factor, vertebrae `HCC`

M06.09 Rheumatoid arthritis without rheumatoid factor, multiple sites `HCC`

M06.1 Adult-onset Still's disease `HCC` `A`

   EXCLUDES 1   Still's disease NOS (M08.2-)

   DEF: Type of systemic arthritis characterized by a transient rash and spiking fevers. This condition may resolve or develop into a chronic condition and may affect internal organs, as well as joints.

   Synonym(s): AOSD

✓5ᵗʰ **M06.2** Rheumatoid bursitis

   M06.20 Rheumatoid bursitis, unspecified site `HCC`

  ✓6ᵗʰ **M06.21** Rheumatoid bursitis, shoulder

     M06.211 Rheumatoid bursitis, right shoulder `HCC`

     M06.212 Rheumatoid bursitis, left shoulder `HCC`

     M06.219 Rheumatoid bursitis, unspecified shoulder `HCC`

  ✓6ᵗʰ **M06.22** Rheumatoid bursitis, elbow

     M06.221 Rheumatoid bursitis, right elbow `HCC`

     M06.222 Rheumatoid bursitis, left elbow `HCC`

     M06.229 Rheumatoid bursitis, unspecified elbow `HCC`

  ✓6ᵗʰ **M06.23** Rheumatoid bursitis, wrist

     M06.231 Rheumatoid bursitis, right wrist `HCC`

     M06.232 Rheumatoid bursitis, left wrist `HCC`

     M06.239 Rheumatoid bursitis, unspecified wrist `HCC`

  ✓6ᵗʰ **M06.24** Rheumatoid bursitis, hand

     M06.241 Rheumatoid bursitis, right hand `HCC`

     M06.242 Rheumatoid bursitis, left hand `HCC`

     M06.249 Rheumatoid bursitis, unspecified hand `HCC`

  ✓6ᵗʰ **M06.25** Rheumatoid bursitis, hip

     M06.251 Rheumatoid bursitis, right hip `HCC`

     M06.252 Rheumatoid bursitis, left hip `HCC`

     M06.259 Rheumatoid bursitis, unspecified hip `HCC`

  ✓6ᵗʰ **M06.26** Rheumatoid bursitis, knee

     M06.261 Rheumatoid bursitis, right knee `HCC`

     M06.262 Rheumatoid bursitis, left knee `HCC`

     M06.269 Rheumatoid bursitis, unspecified knee `HCC`

  ✓6ᵗʰ **M06.27** Rheumatoid bursitis, ankle and foot

     M06.271 Rheumatoid bursitis, right ankle and foot `HCC`

     M06.272 Rheumatoid bursitis, left ankle and foot `HCC`

     M06.279 Rheumatoid bursitis, unspecified ankle and foot `HCC`

   M06.28 Rheumatoid bursitis, vertebrae `HCC`

   M06.29 Rheumatoid bursitis, multiple sites `HCC`

✓5ᵗʰ **M06.3** Rheumatoid nodule

   M06.30 Rheumatoid nodule, unspecified site `HCC`

  ✓6ᵗʰ **M06.31** Rheumatoid nodule, shoulder

     M06.311 Rheumatoid nodule, right shoulder `HCC`

     M06.312 Rheumatoid nodule, left shoulder `HCC`

     M06.319 Rheumatoid nodule, unspecified shoulder `HCC`

  ✓6ᵗʰ **M06.32** Rheumatoid nodule, elbow

     M06.321 Rheumatoid nodule, right elbow `HCC`

     M06.322 Rheumatoid nodule, left elbow `HCC`

     M06.329 Rheumatoid nodule, unspecified elbow `HCC`

  ✓6ᵗʰ **M06.33** Rheumatoid nodule, wrist

     M06.331 Rheumatoid nodule, right wrist `HCC`

N Newborn: 0   P Pediatric: 0-17   M Maternity: 9-64   A Adult: 15-124   MCC Major Complication/Comorbidity   CC Complication/Comorbidity   SW Severe Wound Dx

774   ICD-10-CM 2020

M06.332   Rheumatoid nodule, left wrist   **HCC**

M06.339   Rheumatoid nodule, unspecified wrist

✓6ᵗʰ   M06.34   **Rheumatoid nodule, hand**

M06.341   Rheumatoid nodule, right hand   **HCC**

M06.342   Rheumatoid nodule, left hand   **HCC**

M06.349   Rheumatoid nodule, unspecified hand   **HCC**

✓6ᵗʰ   M06.35   **Rheumatoid nodule, hip**

M06.351   Rheumatoid nodule, right hip   **HCC**

M06.352   Rheumatoid nodule, left hip   **HCC**

M06.359   Rheumatoid nodule, unspecified hip   **HCC**

✓6ᵗʰ   M06.36   **Rheumatoid nodule, knee**

M06.361   Rheumatoid nodule, right knee   **HCC**

M06.362   Rheumatoid nodule, left knee   **HCC**

M06.369   Rheumatoid nodule, unspecified knee   **HCC**

✓6ᵗʰ   M06.37   **Rheumatoid nodule, ankle and foot**

M06.371   Rheumatoid nodule, right ankle and foot   **HCC**

M06.372   Rheumatoid nodule, left ankle and foot   **HCC**

M06.379   Rheumatoid nodule, unspecified ankle and foot   **HCC**

M06.38   **Rheumatoid nodule, vertebrae**   **HCC**

M06.39   **Rheumatoid nodule, multiple sites**   **HCC**

M06.4   **Inflammatory polyarthropathy**   **HCC**

    EXCLUDES 1   polyarthritis NOS (M13.0)

✓5ᵗʰ   M06.8   **Other specified rheumatoid arthritis**

M06.80   Other specified rheumatoid arthritis, unspecified site   **HCC**

✓6ᵗʰ   M06.81   **Other specified rheumatoid arthritis, shoulder**

M06.811   Other specified rheumatoid arthritis, right shoulder   **HCC**

M06.812   Other specified rheumatoid arthritis, left shoulder   **HCC**

M06.819   Other specified rheumatoid arthritis, unspecified shoulder   **HCC**

✓6ᵗʰ   M06.82   **Other specified rheumatoid arthritis, elbow**

M06.821   Other specified rheumatoid arthritis, right elbow   **HCC**

M06.822   Other specified rheumatoid arthritis, left elbow   **HCC**

M06.829   Other specified rheumatoid arthritis, unspecified elbow   **HCC**

✓6ᵗʰ   M06.83   **Other specified rheumatoid arthritis, wrist**

M06.831   Other specified rheumatoid arthritis, right wrist   **HCC**

M06.832   Other specified rheumatoid arthritis, left wrist   **HCC**

M06.839   Other specified rheumatoid arthritis, unspecified wrist   **HCC**

✓6ᵗʰ   M06.84   **Other specified rheumatoid arthritis, hand**

M06.841   Other specified rheumatoid arthritis, right hand   **HCC**

M06.842   Other specified rheumatoid arthritis, left hand   **HCC**

M06.849   Other specified rheumatoid arthritis, unspecified hand   **HCC**

✓6ᵗʰ   M06.85   **Other specified rheumatoid arthritis, hip**

M06.851   Other specified rheumatoid arthritis, right hip   **HCC**

M06.852   Other specified rheumatoid arthritis, left hip   **HCC**

M06.859   Other specified rheumatoid arthritis, unspecified hip   **HCC**

✓6ᵗʰ   M06.86   **Other specified rheumatoid arthritis, knee**

M06.861   Other specified rheumatoid arthritis, right knee   **HCC**

M06.862   Other specified rheumatoid arthritis, left knee   **HCC**

M06.869   Other specified rheumatoid arthritis, unspecified knee   **HCC**

✓6ᵗʰ   M06.87   **Other specified rheumatoid arthritis, ankle and foot**

M06.871   Other specified rheumatoid arthritis, right ankle and foot   **HCC**

M06.872   Other specified rheumatoid arthritis, left ankle and foot   **HCC**

M06.879   Other specified rheumatoid arthritis, unspecified ankle and foot   **HCC**

M06.88   **Other specified rheumatoid arthritis, vertebrae**   **HCC**

M06.89   **Other specified rheumatoid arthritis, multiple sites**   **HCC**

M06.9   **Rheumatoid arthritis, unspecified**   **HCC**

✓4ᵗʰ   **M07   Enteropathic arthropathies**

    Code also associated enteropathy, such as:
      regional enteritis [Crohn's disease] (K50.-)
      ulcerative colitis (K51.-)
    EXCLUDES 1   psoriatic arthropathies (L40.5-)

✓5ᵗʰ   M07.6   **Enteropathic arthropathies**

M07.60   Enteropathic arthropathies, unspecified site

✓6ᵗʰ   M07.61   **Enteropathic arthropathies, shoulder**

M07.611   Enteropathic arthropathies, right shoulder

M07.612   Enteropathic arthropathies, left shoulder

M07.619   Enteropathic arthropathies, unspecified shoulder

✓6ᵗʰ   M07.62   **Enteropathic arthropathies, elbow**

M07.621   Enteropathic arthropathies, right elbow

M07.622   Enteropathic arthropathies, left elbow

M07.629   Enteropathic arthropathies, unspecified elbow

✓6ᵗʰ   M07.63   **Enteropathic arthropathies, wrist**

M07.631   Enteropathic arthropathies, right wrist

M07.632   Enteropathic arthropathies, left wrist

M07.639   Enteropathic arthropathies, unspecified wrist

✓6ᵗʰ   M07.64   **Enteropathic arthropathies, hand**

M07.641   Enteropathic arthropathies, right hand

M07.642   Enteropathic arthropathies, left hand

M07.649   Enteropathic arthropathies, unspecified hand

✓6ᵗʰ   M07.65   **Enteropathic arthropathies, hip**

M07.651   Enteropathic arthropathies, right hip

M07.652   Enteropathic arthropathies, left hip

M07.659   Enteropathic arthropathies, unspecified hip

✓6ᵗʰ   M07.66   **Enteropathic arthropathies, knee**

M07.661   Enteropathic arthropathies, right knee

M07.662   Enteropathic arthropathies, left knee

M07.669   Enteropathic arthropathies, unspecified knee

✓6ᵗʰ   M07.67   **Enteropathic arthropathies, ankle and foot**

M07.671   Enteropathic arthropathies, right ankle and foot

M07.672   Enteropathic arthropathies, left ankle and foot

M07.679   **Enteropathic arthropathies, unspecified ankle and foot**

M07.68   **Enteropathic arthropathies,** vertebrae

M07.69   **Enteropathic arthropathies,** multiple sites

√4ᵗʰ **M08   Juvenile arthritis**

Code also any associated underlying condition, such as:
regional enteritis [Crohn's disease] (K50.-)
ulcerative colitis (K51.-)

EXCLUDES 1   arthropathy in Whipple's disease (M14.8)
Felty's syndrome (M05.0)
juvenile dermatomyositis (M33.0-)
psoriatic juvenile arthropathy (L40.54)

√5ᵗʰ **M08.0   Unspecified juvenile rheumatoid arthritis**

Juvenile rheumatoid arthritis with or without rheumatoid factor

M08.00   **Unspecified juvenile rheumatoid arthritis of unspecified site**   `HCC`

√6ᵗʰ **M08.01   Unspecified juvenile rheumatoid arthritis,** shoulder

M08.011   **Unspecified juvenile rheumatoid arthritis,** right **shoulder**   `HCC`

M08.012   **Unspecified juvenile rheumatoid arthritis,** left **shoulder**   `HCC`

M08.019   **Unspecified juvenile rheumatoid arthritis, unspecified shoulder**   `HCC`

√6ᵗʰ **M08.02   Unspecified juvenile rheumatoid arthritis of** elbow

M08.021   **Unspecified juvenile rheumatoid arthritis,** right **elbow**   `HCC`

M08.022   **Unspecified juvenile rheumatoid arthritis,** left **elbow**   `HCC`

M08.029   **Unspecified juvenile rheumatoid arthritis, unspecified elbow**   `HCC`

√6ᵗʰ **M08.03   Unspecified juvenile rheumatoid arthritis,** wrist

M08.031   **Unspecified juvenile rheumatoid arthritis,** right **wrist**   `HCC`

M08.032   **Unspecified juvenile rheumatoid arthritis,** left **wrist**   `HCC`

M08.039   **Unspecified juvenile rheumatoid arthritis, unspecified wrist**   `HCC`

√6ᵗʰ **M08.04   Unspecified juvenile rheumatoid arthritis,** hand

M08.041   **Unspecified juvenile rheumatoid arthritis,** right **hand**   `HCC`

M08.042   **Unspecified juvenile rheumatoid arthritis,** left **hand**   `HCC`

M08.049   **Unspecified juvenile rheumatoid arthritis, unspecified hand**   `HCC`

√6ᵗʰ **M08.05   Unspecified juvenile rheumatoid arthritis,** hip

M08.051   **Unspecified juvenile rheumatoid arthritis,** right **hip**   `HCC`

M08.052   **Unspecified juvenile rheumatoid arthritis,** left **hip**   `HCC`

M08.059   **Unspecified juvenile rheumatoid arthritis, unspecified hip**   `HCC`

√6ᵗʰ **M08.06   Unspecified juvenile rheumatoid arthritis,** knee

M08.061   **Unspecified juvenile rheumatoid arthritis,** right **knee**   `HCC`

M08.062   **Unspecified juvenile rheumatoid arthritis,** left **knee**   `HCC`

M08.069   **Unspecified juvenile rheumatoid arthritis, unspecified knee**   `HCC`

√6ᵗʰ **M08.07   Unspecified juvenile rheumatoid arthritis,** ankle and foot

M08.071   **Unspecified juvenile rheumatoid arthritis,** right **ankle and foot**   `HCC`

M08.072   **Unspecified juvenile rheumatoid arthritis,** left **ankle and foot**   `HCC`

M08.079   **Unspecified juvenile rheumatoid arthritis, unspecified ankle and foot**   `HCC`

M08.08   **Unspecified juvenile rheumatoid arthritis,** vertebrae   `HCC`

M08.09   **Unspecified juvenile rheumatoid arthritis,** multiple sites   `HCC`

M08.1   Juvenile ankylosing spondylitis   `HCC`

EXCLUDES 1   ankylosing spondylitis in adults (M45.0-)

√5ᵗʰ **M08.2   Juvenile rheumatoid arthritis with systemic onset**

Still's disease NOS

EXCLUDES 1   adult-onset Still's disease (M06.1-)

DEF: Systemic juvenile rheumatoid arthritis characterized by a transient rash and spiking fevers that may affect internal organs, as well as joints.

M08.20   **Juvenile rheumatoid arthritis with systemic onset, unspecified site**   `HCC`

√6ᵗʰ **M08.21   Juvenile rheumatoid arthritis with systemic onset, shoulder**

M08.211   **Juvenile rheumatoid arthritis with systemic onset, right shoulder**   `HCC`

M08.212   **Juvenile rheumatoid arthritis with systemic onset, left shoulder**   `HCC`

M08.219   **Juvenile rheumatoid arthritis with systemic onset, unspecified shoulder**   `HCC`

√6ᵗʰ **M08.22   Juvenile rheumatoid arthritis with systemic onset, elbow**

M08.221   **Juvenile rheumatoid arthritis with systemic onset, right elbow**   `HCC`

M08.222   **Juvenile rheumatoid arthritis with systemic onset, left elbow**   `HCC`

M08.229   **Juvenile rheumatoid arthritis with systemic onset, unspecified elbow**   `HCC`

√6ᵗʰ **M08.23   Juvenile rheumatoid arthritis with systemic onset, wrist**

M08.231   **Juvenile rheumatoid arthritis with systemic onset, right wrist**   `HCC`

M08.232   **Juvenile rheumatoid arthritis with systemic onset, left wrist**   `HCC`

M08.239   **Juvenile rheumatoid arthritis with systemic onset, unspecified wrist**   `HCC`

√6ᵗʰ **M08.24   Juvenile rheumatoid arthritis with systemic onset, hand**

M08.241   **Juvenile rheumatoid arthritis with systemic onset, right hand**   `HCC`

M08.242   **Juvenile rheumatoid arthritis with systemic onset, left hand**   `HCC`

M08.249   **Juvenile rheumatoid arthritis with systemic onset, unspecified hand**   `HCC`

√6ᵗʰ **M08.25   Juvenile rheumatoid arthritis with systemic onset, hip**

M08.251   **Juvenile rheumatoid arthritis with systemic onset, right hip**   `HCC`

M08.252   **Juvenile rheumatoid arthritis with systemic onset, left hip**   `HCC`

M08.259   **Juvenile rheumatoid arthritis with systemic onset, unspecified hip**   `HCC`

√6ᵗʰ **M08.26   Juvenile rheumatoid arthritis with systemic onset, knee**

M08.261   **Juvenile rheumatoid arthritis with systemic onset, right knee**   `HCC`

M08.262   **Juvenile rheumatoid arthritis with systemic onset, left knee**   `HCC`

N Newborn: 0   P Pediatric: 0-17   M Maternity: 9-64   A Adult: 15-124   `MCC` Major Complication/Comorbidity   `CC` Complication/Comorbidity   `SW` Severe Wound Dx

776   ICD-10-CM 2020

M08.269   Juvenile rheumatoid arthritis with systemic onset, unspecified knee   `HCC`

√6ᵗʰ   M08.27   Juvenile rheumatoid arthritis with systemic onset, ankle and foot

    M08.271   Juvenile rheumatoid arthritis with systemic onset, right ankle and foot   `HCC`

    M08.272   Juvenile rheumatoid arthritis with systemic onset, left ankle and foot   `HCC`

    M08.279   Juvenile rheumatoid arthritis with systemic onset, unspecified ankle and foot   `HCC`

M08.28   Juvenile rheumatoid arthritis with systemic onset, vertebrae   `HCC`

M08.29   Juvenile rheumatoid arthritis with systemic onset, multiple sites   `HCC`

M08.3   Juvenile rheumatoid polyarthritis (seronegative)   `HCC`

√5ᵗʰ   M08.4   Pauciarticular juvenile rheumatoid arthritis

    M08.40   Pauciarticular juvenile rheumatoid arthritis, unspecified site   `HCC`

√6ᵗʰ   M08.41   Pauciarticular juvenile rheumatoid arthritis, shoulder

    M08.411   Pauciarticular juvenile rheumatoid arthritis, right shoulder   `HCC`

    M08.412   Pauciarticular juvenile rheumatoid arthritis, left shoulder   `HCC`

    M08.419   Pauciarticular juvenile rheumatoid arthritis, unspecified shoulder   `HCC`

√6ᵗʰ   M08.42   Pauciarticular juvenile rheumatoid arthritis, elbow

    M08.421   Pauciarticular juvenile rheumatoid arthritis, right elbow   `HCC`

    M08.422   Pauciarticular juvenile rheumatoid arthritis, left elbow   `HCC`

    M08.429   Pauciarticular juvenile rheumatoid arthritis, unspecified elbow   `HCC`

√6ᵗʰ   M08.43   Pauciarticular juvenile rheumatoid arthritis, wrist

    M08.431   Pauciarticular juvenile rheumatoid arthritis, right wrist   `HCC`

    M08.432   Pauciarticular juvenile rheumatoid arthritis, left wrist   `HCC`

    M08.439   Pauciarticular juvenile rheumatoid arthritis, unspecified wrist   `HCC`

√6ᵗʰ   M08.44   Pauciarticular juvenile rheumatoid arthritis, hand

    M08.441   Pauciarticular juvenile rheumatoid arthritis, right hand   `HCC`

    M08.442   Pauciarticular juvenile rheumatoid arthritis, left hand   `HCC`

    M08.449   Pauciarticular juvenile rheumatoid arthritis, unspecified hand   `HCC`

√6ᵗʰ   M08.45   Pauciarticular juvenile rheumatoid arthritis, hip

    M08.451   Pauciarticular juvenile rheumatoid arthritis, right hip   `HCC`

    M08.452   Pauciarticular juvenile rheumatoid arthritis, left hip   `HCC`

    M08.459   Pauciarticular juvenile rheumatoid arthritis, unspecified hip   `HCC`

√6ᵗʰ   M08.46   Pauciarticular juvenile rheumatoid arthritis, knee

    M08.461   Pauciarticular juvenile rheumatoid arthritis, right knee   `HCC`

    M08.462   Pauciarticular juvenile rheumatoid arthritis, left knee   `HCC`

M08.469   Pauciarticular juvenile rheumatoid arthritis, unspecified knee   `HCC`

√6ᵗʰ   M08.47   Pauciarticular juvenile rheumatoid arthritis, ankle and foot

    M08.471   Pauciarticular juvenile rheumatoid arthritis, right ankle and foot   `HCC`

    M08.472   Pauciarticular juvenile rheumatoid arthritis, left ankle and foot   `HCC`

    M08.479   Pauciarticular juvenile rheumatoid arthritis, unspecified ankle and foot   `HCC`

M08.48   Pauciarticular juvenile rheumatoid arthritis, vertebrae   `HCC`

√5ᵗʰ   M08.8   Other juvenile arthritis

    M08.80   Other juvenile arthritis, unspecified site   `HCC`

√6ᵗʰ   M08.81   Other juvenile arthritis, shoulder

    M08.811   Other juvenile arthritis, right shoulder   `HCC`

    M08.812   Other juvenile arthritis, left shoulder   `HCC`

    M08.819   Other juvenile arthritis, unspecified shoulder   `HCC`

√6ᵗʰ   M08.82   Other juvenile arthritis, elbow

    M08.821   Other juvenile arthritis, right elbow   `HCC`

    M08.822   Other juvenile arthritis, left elbow   `HCC`

    M08.829   Other juvenile arthritis, unspecified elbow   `HCC`

√6ᵗʰ   M08.83   Other juvenile arthritis, wrist

    M08.831   Other juvenile arthritis, right wrist   `HCC`

    M08.832   Other juvenile arthritis, left wrist   `HCC`

    M08.839   Other juvenile arthritis, unspecified wrist   `HCC`

√6ᵗʰ   M08.84   Other juvenile arthritis, hand

    M08.841   Other juvenile arthritis, right hand   `HCC`

    M08.842   Other juvenile arthritis, left hand   `HCC`

    M08.849   Other juvenile arthritis, unspecified hand   `HCC`

√6ᵗʰ   M08.85   Other juvenile arthritis, hip

    M08.851   Other juvenile arthritis, right hip   `HCC`

    M08.852   Other juvenile arthritis, left hip   `HCC`

    M08.859   Other juvenile arthritis, unspecified hip   `HCC`

√6ᵗʰ   M08.86   Other juvenile arthritis, knee

    M08.861   Other juvenile arthritis, right knee   `HCC`

    M08.862   Other juvenile arthritis, left knee   `HCC`

    M08.869   Other juvenile arthritis, unspecified knee   `HCC`

√6ᵗʰ   M08.87   Other juvenile arthritis, ankle and foot

    M08.871   Other juvenile arthritis, right ankle and foot   `HCC`

    M08.872   Other juvenile arthritis, left ankle and foot   `HCC`

    M08.879   Other juvenile arthritis, unspecified ankle and foot   `HCC`

M08.88   Other juvenile arthritis, other specified site   `HCC`

    Other juvenile arthritis, vertebrae

M08.89   Other juvenile arthritis, multiple sites   `HCC`

√5ᵗʰ   M08.9   Juvenile arthritis, unspecified

    EXCLUDES 1   juvenile rheumatoid arthritis, unspecified (M08.0-)

    M08.90   Juvenile arthritis, unspecified, unspecified site   `HCC`

✔ Additional Character Required   √x7ᵗʰ Placeholder   Unacceptable PDx   Questionable PDx   Manifestation   Unspecified Dx   H1-H14 HAC   HCC CMS-HCC Dx   HIV HIV Dx

ICD-10-CM 2020   777

√6ᵗʰ **M08.91** Juvenile arthritis, unspecified, shoulder

  M08.911 Juvenile arthritis, unspecified, right shoulder `HCC`

  M08.912 Juvenile arthritis, unspecified, left shoulder `HCC`

  M08.919 Juvenile arthritis, unspecified, unspecified shoulder `HCC`

√6ᵗʰ **M08.92** Juvenile arthritis, unspecified, elbow

  M08.921 Juvenile arthritis, unspecified, right elbow `HCC`

  M08.922 Juvenile arthritis, unspecified, left elbow `HCC`

  M08.929 Juvenile arthritis, unspecified, unspecified elbow `HCC`

√6ᵗʰ **M08.93** Juvenile arthritis, unspecified, wrist

  M08.931 Juvenile arthritis, unspecified, right wrist `HCC`

  M08.932 Juvenile arthritis, unspecified, left wrist `HCC`

  M08.939 Juvenile arthritis, unspecified, unspecified wrist `HCC`

√6ᵗʰ **M08.94** Juvenile arthritis, unspecified, hand

  M08.941 Juvenile arthritis, unspecified, right hand `HCC`

  M08.942 Juvenile arthritis, unspecified, left hand `HCC`

  M08.949 Juvenile arthritis, unspecified, unspecified hand `HCC`

√6ᵗʰ **M08.95** Juvenile arthritis, unspecified, hip

  M08.951 Juvenile arthritis, unspecified, right hip `HCC`

  M08.952 Juvenile arthritis, unspecified, left hip `HCC`

  M08.959 Juvenile arthritis, unspecified, unspecified hip `HCC`

√6ᵗʰ **M08.96** Juvenile arthritis, unspecified, knee

  M08.961 Juvenile arthritis, unspecified, right knee `HCC`

  M08.962 Juvenile arthritis, unspecified, left knee `HCC`

  M08.969 Juvenile arthritis, unspecified, unspecified knee `HCC`

√6ᵗʰ **M08.97** Juvenile arthritis, unspecified, ankle and foot

  M08.971 Juvenile arthritis, unspecified, right ankle and foot `HCC`

  M08.972 Juvenile arthritis, unspecified, left ankle and foot `HCC`

  M08.979 Juvenile arthritis, unspecified, unspecified ankle and foot `HCC`

  M08.98 Juvenile arthritis, unspecified, vertebrae `HCC`

  M08.99 Juvenile arthritis, unspecified, multiple sites `HCC`

√4ᵗʰ **M1A** Chronic gout

Use additional code to identify:
autonomic neuropathy in diseases classified elsewhere (G99.0)
calculus of urinary tract in diseases classified elsewhere (N22)
cardiomyopathy in diseases classified elsewhere (I43)
disorders of external ear in diseases classified elsewhere (H61.1-, H62.8-)
disorders of iris and ciliary body in diseases classified elsewhere (H22)
glomerular disorders in diseases classified elsewhere (N08)

`EXCLUDES 1` gout NOS (M10.-)

`EXCLUDES 2` acute gout (M10.-)

The appropriate 7th character is to be added to each code from category M1A.
0   without tophus (tophi)
1   with tophus (tophi)

√5ᵗʰ **M1A.0** Idiopathic chronic gout

Chronic gouty bursitis
Primary chronic gout

√x7ᵗʰ **M1A.00** Idiopathic chronic gout, unspecified site

√6ᵗʰ **M1A.01** Idiopathic chronic gout, shoulder

  √7ᵗʰ **M1A.011** Idiopathic chronic gout, right shoulder

  √7ᵗʰ **M1A.012** Idiopathic chronic gout, left shoulder

  √7ᵗʰ **M1A.019** Idiopathic chronic gout, unspecified shoulder

√6ᵗʰ **M1A.02** Idiopathic chronic gout, elbow

  √7ᵗʰ **M1A.021** Idiopathic chronic gout, right elbow

  √7ᵗʰ **M1A.022** Idiopathic chronic gout, left elbow

  √7ᵗʰ **M1A.029** Idiopathic chronic gout, unspecified elbow

√6ᵗʰ **M1A.03** Idiopathic chronic gout, wrist

  √7ᵗʰ **M1A.031** Idiopathic chronic gout, right wrist

  √7ᵗʰ **M1A.032** Idiopathic chronic gout, left wrist

  √7ᵗʰ **M1A.039** Idiopathic chronic gout, unspecified wrist

√6ᵗʰ **M1A.04** Idiopathic chronic gout, hand

  √7ᵗʰ **M1A.041** Idiopathic chronic gout, right hand

  √7ᵗʰ **M1A.042** Idiopathic chronic gout, left hand

  √7ᵗʰ **M1A.049** Idiopathic chronic gout, unspecified hand

√6ᵗʰ **M1A.05** Idiopathic chronic gout, hip

  √7ᵗʰ **M1A.051** Idiopathic chronic gout, right hip

  √7ᵗʰ **M1A.052** Idiopathic chronic gout, left hip

  √7ᵗʰ **M1A.059** Idiopathic chronic gout, unspecified hip

√6ᵗʰ **M1A.06** Idiopathic chronic gout, knee

  √7ᵗʰ **M1A.061** Idiopathic chronic gout, right knee

  √7ᵗʰ **M1A.062** Idiopathic chronic gout, left knee

  √7ᵗʰ **M1A.069** Idiopathic chronic gout, unspecified knee

√6ᵗʰ **M1A.07** Idiopathic chronic gout, ankle and foot

  √7ᵗʰ **M1A.071** Idiopathic chronic gout, right ankle and foot

  √7ᵗʰ **M1A.072** Idiopathic chronic gout, left ankle and foot

  √7ᵗʰ **M1A.079** Idiopathic chronic gout, unspecified ankle and foot

√x7ᵗʰ **M1A.08** Idiopathic chronic gout, vertebrae

√x7ᵗʰ **M1A.09** Idiopathic chronic gout, multiple sites

√5ᵗʰ **M1A.1** Lead-induced chronic gout

Code first toxic effects of lead and its compounds (T56.0-)

√x7ᵗʰ **M1A.10** Lead-induced chronic gout, unspecified site

√6ᵗʰ **M1A.11** Lead-induced chronic gout, shoulder

  √7ᵗʰ **M1A.111** Lead-induced chronic gout, right shoulder

  √7ᵗʰ **M1A.112** Lead-induced chronic gout, left shoulder

  √7ᵗʰ **M1A.119** Lead-induced chronic gout, unspecified shoulder

√6ᵗʰ **M1A.12** Lead-induced chronic gout, elbow

  √7ᵗʰ **M1A.121** Lead-induced chronic gout, right elbow

  √7ᵗʰ **M1A.122** Lead-induced chronic gout, left elbow

  √7ᵗʰ **M1A.129** Lead-induced chronic gout, unspecified elbow

√6ᵗʰ **M1A.13** Lead-induced chronic gout, wrist

  √7ᵗʰ **M1A.131** Lead-induced chronic gout, right wrist

  √7ᵗʰ **M1A.132** Lead-induced chronic gout, left wrist

M08.91–M1A.132

Ⓝ Newborn: 0   Ⓟ Pediatric: 0-17   Ⓜ Maternity: 9-64   Ⓐ Adult: 15-124   `MCC` Major Complication/Comorbidity   `CC` Complication/Comorbidity   `SW` Severe Wound Dx

778   ICD-10-CM 2020

√7ᵗʰ **M1A.139** Lead-induced chronic gout, unspecified wrist

√6ᵗʰ **M1A.14** Lead-induced chronic gout, hand

   √7ᵗʰ **M1A.141** Lead-induced chronic gout, right hand

   √7ᵗʰ **M1A.142** Lead-induced chronic gout, left hand

   √7ᵗʰ **M1A.149** Lead-induced chronic gout, unspecified hand

√6ᵗʰ **M1A.15** Lead-induced chronic gout, hip

   √7ᵗʰ **M1A.151** Lead-induced chronic gout, right hip

   √7ᵗʰ **M1A.152** Lead-induced chronic gout, left hip

   √7ᵗʰ **M1A.159** Lead-induced chronic gout, unspecified hip

√6ᵗʰ **M1A.16** Lead-induced chronic gout, knee

   √7ᵗʰ **M1A.161** Lead-induced chronic gout, right knee

   √7ᵗʰ **M1A.162** Lead-induced chronic gout, left knee

   √7ᵗʰ **M1A.169** Lead-induced chronic gout, unspecified knee

√6ᵗʰ **M1A.17** Lead-induced chronic gout, ankle and foot

   √7ᵗʰ **M1A.171** Lead-induced chronic gout, right ankle and foot

   √7ᵗʰ **M1A.172** Lead-induced chronic gout, left ankle and foot

   √7ᵗʰ **M1A.179** Lead-induced chronic gout, unspecified ankle and foot

√x7ᵗʰ **M1A.18** Lead-induced chronic gout, vertebrae

√x7ᵗʰ **M1A.19** Lead-induced chronic gout, multiple sites

√5ᵗʰ **M1A.2** Drug-induced chronic gout

    Use additional code for adverse effect, if applicable, to identify drug (T36-T50 with fifth or sixth character 5)

√x7ᵗʰ **M1A.20** Drug-induced chronic gout, unspecified site

√6ᵗʰ **M1A.21** Drug-induced chronic gout, shoulder

   √7ᵗʰ **M1A.211** Drug-induced chronic gout, right shoulder

   √7ᵗʰ **M1A.212** Drug-induced chronic gout, left shoulder

   √7ᵗʰ **M1A.219** Drug-induced chronic gout, unspecified shoulder

√6ᵗʰ **M1A.22** Drug-induced chronic gout, elbow

   √7ᵗʰ **M1A.221** Drug-induced chronic gout, right elbow

   √7ᵗʰ **M1A.222** Drug-induced chronic gout, left elbow

   √7ᵗʰ **M1A.229** Drug-induced chronic gout, unspecified elbow

√6ᵗʰ **M1A.23** Drug-induced chronic gout, wrist

   √7ᵗʰ **M1A.231** Drug-induced chronic gout, right wrist

   √7ᵗʰ **M1A.232** Drug-induced chronic gout, left wrist

   √7ᵗʰ **M1A.239** Drug-induced chronic gout, unspecified wrist

√6ᵗʰ **M1A.24** Drug-induced chronic gout, hand

   √7ᵗʰ **M1A.241** Drug-induced chronic gout, right hand

   √7ᵗʰ **M1A.242** Drug-induced chronic gout, left hand

   √7ᵗʰ **M1A.249** Drug-induced chronic gout, unspecified hand

√6ᵗʰ **M1A.25** Drug-induced chronic gout, hip

   √7ᵗʰ **M1A.251** Drug-induced chronic gout, right hip

   √7ᵗʰ **M1A.252** Drug-induced chronic gout, left hip

   √7ᵗʰ **M1A.259** Drug-induced chronic gout, unspecified hip

√6ᵗʰ **M1A.26** Drug-induced chronic gout, knee

   √7ᵗʰ **M1A.261** Drug-induced chronic gout, right knee

   √7ᵗʰ **M1A.262** Drug-induced chronic gout, left knee

   √7ᵗʰ **M1A.269** Drug-induced chronic gout, unspecified knee

√6ᵗʰ **M1A.27** Drug-induced chronic gout, ankle and foot

   √7ᵗʰ **M1A.271** Drug-induced chronic gout, right ankle and foot

   √7ᵗʰ **M1A.272** Drug-induced chronic gout, left ankle and foot

   √7ᵗʰ **M1A.279** Drug-induced chronic gout, unspecified ankle and foot

√x7ᵗʰ **M1A.28** Drug-induced chronic gout, vertebrae

√x7ᵗʰ **M1A.29** Drug-induced chronic gout, multiple sites

√5ᵗʰ **M1A.3** Chronic gout due to renal impairment

    Code first associated renal disease

√x7ᵗʰ **M1A.30** Chronic gout due to renal impairment, unspecified site

√6ᵗʰ **M1A.31** Chronic gout due to renal impairment, shoulder

   √7ᵗʰ **M1A.311** Chronic gout due to renal impairment, right shoulder

   √7ᵗʰ **M1A.312** Chronic gout due to renal impairment, left shoulder

   √7ᵗʰ **M1A.319** Chronic gout due to renal impairment, unspecified shoulder

√6ᵗʰ **M1A.32** Chronic gout due to renal impairment, elbow

   √7ᵗʰ **M1A.321** Chronic gout due to renal impairment, right elbow

   √7ᵗʰ **M1A.322** Chronic gout due to renal impairment, left elbow

   √7ᵗʰ **M1A.329** Chronic gout due to renal impairment, unspecified elbow

√6ᵗʰ **M1A.33** Chronic gout due to renal impairment, wrist

   √7ᵗʰ **M1A.331** Chronic gout due to renal impairment, right wrist

   √7ᵗʰ **M1A.332** Chronic gout due to renal impairment, left wrist

   √7ᵗʰ **M1A.339** Chronic gout due to renal impairment, unspecified wrist

√6ᵗʰ **M1A.34** Chronic gout due to renal impairment, hand

   √7ᵗʰ **M1A.341** Chronic gout due to renal impairment, right hand

   √7ᵗʰ **M1A.342** Chronic gout due to renal impairment, left hand

   √7ᵗʰ **M1A.349** Chronic gout due to renal impairment, unspecified hand

√6ᵗʰ **M1A.35** Chronic gout due to renal impairment, hip

   √7ᵗʰ **M1A.351** Chronic gout due to renal impairment, right hip

   √7ᵗʰ **M1A.352** Chronic gout due to renal impairment, left hip

   √7ᵗʰ **M1A.359** Chronic gout due to renal impairment, unspecified hip

√6ᵗʰ **M1A.36** Chronic gout due to renal impairment, knee

   √7ᵗʰ **M1A.361** Chronic gout due to renal impairment, right knee

   √7ᵗʰ **M1A.362** Chronic gout due to renal impairment, left knee

   √7ᵗʰ **M1A.369** Chronic gout due to renal impairment, unspecified knee

√6ᵗʰ **M1A.37** Chronic gout due to renal impairment, ankle and foot

   √7ᵗʰ **M1A.371** Chronic gout due to renal impairment, right ankle and foot

   √7ᵗʰ **M1A.372** Chronic gout due to renal impairment, left ankle and foot

   √7ᵗʰ **M1A.379** Chronic gout due to renal impairment, unspecified ankle and foot

√x7ᵗʰ **M1A.38** Chronic gout due to renal impairment, vertebrae

√x7ᵗʰ **M1A.39** Chronic gout due to renal impairment, multiple sites

√5ᵗʰ **M1A.4** Other secondary chronic gout

    Code first associated condition

√x7ᵗʰ **M1A.40** Other secondary chronic gout, unspecified site

√6ᵗʰ **M1A.41** Other secondary chronic gout, shoulder

   √7ᵗʰ **M1A.411** Other secondary chronic gout, right shoulder

   √7ᵗʰ **M1A.412** Other secondary chronic gout, left shoulder

   √7ᵗʰ **M1A.419** Other secondary chronic gout, unspecified shoulder

√6ᵗʰ **M1A.42** Other secondary chronic gout, elbow

   √7ᵗʰ **M1A.421** Other secondary chronic gout, right elbow

   √7ᵗʰ **M1A.422** Other secondary chronic gout, left elbow

   √7ᵗʰ **M1A.429** Other secondary chronic gout, unspecified elbow

√6ᵗʰ **M1A.43** Other secondary chronic gout, wrist

   √7ᵗʰ **M1A.431** Other secondary chronic gout, right wrist

   √7ᵗʰ **M1A.432** Other secondary chronic gout, left wrist

   √7ᵗʰ **M1A.439** Other secondary chronic gout, unspecified wrist

✔ Additional Character Required   √x7ᵗʰ Placeholder   Unacceptable PDx   Questionable PDx   Manifestation   Unspecified Dx   H1-H14 HAC   HCC CMS-HCC Dx   HIV HIV Dx

ICD-10-CM 2020   779

✓6ᵗʰ **M1A.44** Other secondary chronic gout, hand

     ✓7ᵗʰ **M1A.441** Other secondary chronic gout, right **hand**

     ✓7ᵗʰ **M1A.442** Other secondary chronic gout, left **hand**

     ✓7ᵗʰ **M1A.449** Other secondary chronic gout, unspecified **hand**

✓6ᵗʰ **M1A.45** Other secondary chronic gout, hip

     ✓7ᵗʰ **M1A.451** Other secondary chronic gout, right **hip**

     ✓7ᵗʰ **M1A.452** Other secondary chronic gout, left **hip**

     ✓7ᵗʰ **M1A.459** Other secondary chronic gout, unspecified **hip**

✓6ᵗʰ **M1A.46** Other secondary chronic gout, knee

     ✓7ᵗʰ **M1A.461** Other secondary chronic gout, right **knee**

     ✓7ᵗʰ **M1A.462** Other secondary chronic gout, left **knee**

     ✓7ᵗʰ **M1A.469** Other secondary chronic gout, unspecified **knee**

✓6ᵗʰ **M1A.47** Other secondary chronic gout, ankle and foot

     ✓7ᵗʰ **M1A.471** Other secondary chronic gout, right **ankle and foot**

     ✓7ᵗʰ **M1A.472** Other secondary chronic gout, left **ankle and foot**

     ✓7ᵗʰ **M1A.479** Other secondary chronic gout, unspecified **ankle and foot**

✓x7ᵗʰ **M1A.48** Other secondary chronic gout, vertebrae

✓x7ᵗʰ **M1A.49** Other secondary chronic gout, multiple sites

✓x7ᵗʰ **M1A.9** Chronic gout, unspecified

✓4ᵗʰ **M10** **Gout**

Acute gout

Gout attack

Gout flare

Podagra

Use additional code to identify:

     autonomic neuropathy in diseases classified elsewhere (G99.0)

     calculus of urinary tract in diseases classified elsewhere (N22)

     cardiomyopathy in diseases classified elsewhere (I43)

     disorders of external ear in diseases classified elsewhere (H61.1-, H62.8-)

     disorders of iris and ciliary body in diseases classified elsewhere (H22)

     glomerular disorders in diseases classified elsewhere (N08)

EXCLUDES 2   chronic gout (M1A.-)

DEF: Purine and pyrimidine metabolic disorders, manifested by hyperuricemia and recurrent acute inflammatory arthritis. Monosodium urate or monohydrate crystals may be deposited in and around the joints, leading to joint destruction and severe crippling.

✓5ᵗʰ **M10.0** **Idiopathic gout**

Gouty bursitis

Primary gout

     M10.00 Idiopathic gout, unspecified site

✓6ᵗʰ **M10.01** Idiopathic gout, shoulder

     M10.011 Idiopathic gout, right **shoulder**

     M10.012 Idiopathic gout, left **shoulder**

     M10.019 Idiopathic gout, unspecified **shoulder**

✓6ᵗʰ **M10.02** Idiopathic gout, elbow

     M10.021 Idiopathic gout, right **elbow**

     M10.022 Idiopathic gout, left **elbow**

     M10.029 Idiopathic gout, unspecified **elbow**

✓6ᵗʰ **M10.03** Idiopathic gout, wrist

     M10.031 Idiopathic gout, right **wrist**

     M10.032 Idiopathic gout, left **wrist**

     M10.039 Idiopathic gout, unspecified **wrist**

✓6ᵗʰ **M10.04** Idiopathic gout, hand

     M10.041 Idiopathic gout, right **hand**

     M10.042 Idiopathic gout, left **hand**

     M10.049 Idiopathic gout, unspecified **hand**

✓6ᵗʰ **M10.05** Idiopathic gout, hip

     M10.051 Idiopathic gout, right **hip**

     M10.052 Idiopathic gout, left **hip**

     M10.059 Idiopathic gout, unspecified **hip**

✓6ᵗʰ **M10.06** Idiopathic gout, knee

     M10.061 Idiopathic gout, right **knee**

     M10.062 Idiopathic gout, left **knee**

     M10.069 Idiopathic gout, unspecified **knee**

✓6ᵗʰ **M10.07** Idiopathic gout, ankle and foot

     M10.071 Idiopathic gout, right **ankle and foot**

     M10.072 Idiopathic gout, left **ankle and foot**

     M10.079 Idiopathic gout, unspecified ankle and foot

     M10.08 Idiopathic gout, vertebrae

     M10.09 Idiopathic gout, multiple sites

✓5ᵗʰ **M10.1** Lead-induced gout

     Code first toxic effects of lead and its compounds (T56.0-)

     M10.10 Lead-induced gout, unspecified site

✓6ᵗʰ **M10.11** Lead-induced gout, shoulder

     M10.111 Lead-induced gout, right **shoulder**

     M10.112 Lead-induced gout, left **shoulder**

     M10.119 Lead-induced gout, unspecified **shoulder**

✓6ᵗʰ **M10.12** Lead-induced gout, elbow

     M10.121 Lead-induced gout, right **elbow**

     M10.122 Lead-induced gout, left **elbow**

     M10.129 Lead-induced gout, unspecified **elbow**

✓6ᵗʰ **M10.13** Lead-induced gout, wrist

     M10.131 Lead-induced gout, right **wrist**

     M10.132 Lead-induced gout, left **wrist**

     M10.139 Lead-induced gout, unspecified **wrist**

✓6ᵗʰ **M10.14** Lead-induced gout, hand

     M10.141 Lead-induced gout, right **hand**

     M10.142 Lead-induced gout, left **hand**

     M10.149 Lead-induced gout, unspecified **hand**

✓6ᵗʰ **M10.15** Lead-induced gout, hip

     M10.151 Lead-induced gout, right **hip**

     M10.152 Lead-induced gout, left **hip**

     M10.159 Lead-induced gout, unspecified **hip**

✓6ᵗʰ **M10.16** Lead-induced gout, knee

     M10.161 Lead-induced gout, right **knee**

     M10.162 Lead-induced gout, left **knee**

     M10.169 Lead-induced gout, unspecified **knee**

✓6ᵗʰ **M10.17** Lead-induced gout, ankle and foot

     M10.171 Lead-induced gout, right **ankle and foot**

     M10.172 Lead-induced gout, left **ankle and foot**

     M10.179 Lead-induced gout, unspecified ankle and foot

     M10.18 Lead-induced gout, vertebrae

     M10.19 Lead-induced gout, multiple sites

✓5ᵗʰ **M10.2** Drug-induced gout

     Use additional code for adverse effect, if applicable, to identify drug (T36-T50 with fifth or sixth character 5)

     M10.20 Drug-induced gout, unspecified site

✓6ᵗʰ **M10.21** Drug-induced gout, shoulder

     M10.211 Drug-induced gout, right **shoulder**

     M10.212 Drug-induced gout, left **shoulder**

     M10.219 Drug-induced gout, unspecified **shoulder**

✓6ᵗʰ **M10.22** Drug-induced gout, elbow

     M10.221 Drug-induced gout, right **elbow**

     M10.222 Drug-induced gout, left **elbow**

     M10.229 Drug-induced gout, unspecified **elbow**

✓6ᵗʰ **M10.23** Drug-induced gout, wrist

     M10.231 Drug-induced gout, right **wrist**

     M10.232 Drug-induced gout, left **wrist**

     M10.239 Drug-induced gout, unspecified **wrist**

✓6ᵗʰ **M10.24** Drug-induced gout, hand

     M10.241 Drug-induced gout, right **hand**

     M10.242 Drug-induced gout, left **hand**

     M10.249 Drug-induced gout, unspecified **hand**

✓6ᵗʰ **M10.25** Drug-induced gout, hip

     M10.251 Drug-induced gout, right **hip**

     M10.252 Drug-induced gout, left **hip**

     M10.259 Drug-induced gout, unspecified **hip**

✓6ᵗʰ **M10.26** Drug-induced gout, knee

     M10.261 Drug-induced gout, right **knee**

     M10.262 Drug-induced gout, left **knee**

     M10.269 Drug-induced gout, unspecified **knee**

✓6ᵗʰ **M10.27** Drug-induced gout, ankle and foot

     M10.271 Drug-induced gout, right **ankle and foot**

     M10.272 Drug-induced gout, left **ankle and foot**

     M10.279 Drug-induced gout, unspecified ankle and foot

     M10.28 Drug-induced gout, vertebrae

     M10.29 Drug-induced gout, multiple sites

N Newborn: 0   **P** Pediatric: 0-17   **M** Maternity: 9-64   **A** Adult: 15-124   **MCC** Major Complication/Comorbidity   **CC** Complication/Comorbidity   **SW** Severe Wound Dx

780   ICD-10-CM 2020

✓5ᵗʰ **M10.3**   **Gout due to** renal impairment
Code first associated renal disease
- **M10.30**   Gout due to renal impairment, unspecified site
- ✓6ᵗʰ **M10.31**   Gout due to renal impairment, shoulder
  - **M10.311**   Gout due to renal impairment, right shoulder
  - **M10.312**   Gout due to renal impairment, left shoulder
  - **M10.319**   Gout due to renal impairment, unspecified shoulder
- ✓6ᵗʰ **M10.32**   Gout due to renal impairment, elbow
  - **M10.321**   Gout due to renal impairment, right elbow
  - **M10.322**   Gout due to renal impairment, left elbow
  - **M10.329**   Gout due to renal impairment, unspecified elbow
- ✓6ᵗʰ **M10.33**   Gout due to renal impairment, wrist
  - **M10.331**   Gout due to renal impairment, right wrist
  - **M10.332**   Gout due to renal impairment, left wrist
  - **M10.339**   Gout due to renal impairment, unspecified wrist
- ✓6ᵗʰ **M10.34**   Gout due to renal impairment, hand
  - **M10.341**   Gout due to renal impairment, right hand
  - **M10.342**   Gout due to renal impairment, left hand
  - **M10.349**   Gout due to renal impairment, unspecified hand
- ✓6ᵗʰ **M10.35**   Gout due to renal impairment, hip
  - **M10.351**   Gout due to renal impairment, right hip
  - **M10.352**   Gout due to renal impairment, left hip
  - **M10.359**   Gout due to renal impairment, unspecified hip
- ✓6ᵗʰ **M10.36**   Gout due to renal impairment, knee
  - **M10.361**   Gout due to renal impairment, right knee
  - **M10.362**   Gout due to renal impairment, left knee
  - **M10.369**   Gout due to renal impairment, unspecified knee
- ✓6ᵗʰ **M10.37**   Gout due to renal impairment, ankle and foot
  - **M10.371**   Gout due to renal impairment, right ankle and foot
  - **M10.372**   Gout due to renal impairment, left ankle and foot
  - **M10.379**   Gout due to renal impairment, unspecified ankle and foot
- **M10.38**   Gout due to renal impairment, vertebrae
- **M10.39**   Gout due to renal impairment, multiple sites

✓5ᵗʰ **M10.4**   **Other** secondary gout
Code first associated condition
- **M10.40**   Other secondary gout, unspecified site
- ✓6ᵗʰ **M10.41**   Other secondary gout, shoulder
  - **M10.411**   Other secondary gout, right shoulder
  - **M10.412**   Other secondary gout, left shoulder
  - **M10.419**   Other secondary gout, unspecified shoulder
- ✓6ᵗʰ **M10.42**   Other secondary gout, elbow
  - **M10.421**   Other secondary gout, right elbow
  - **M10.422**   Other secondary gout, left elbow
  - **M10.429**   Other secondary gout, unspecified elbow
- ✓6ᵗʰ **M10.43**   Other secondary gout, wrist
  - **M10.431**   Other secondary gout, right wrist
  - **M10.432**   Other secondary gout, left wrist
  - **M10.439**   Other secondary gout, unspecified wrist
- ✓6ᵗʰ **M10.44**   Other secondary gout, hand
  - **M10.441**   Other secondary gout, right hand
  - **M10.442**   Other secondary gout, left hand
  - **M10.449**   Other secondary gout, unspecified hand
- ✓6ᵗʰ **M10.45**   Other secondary gout, hip
  - **M10.451**   Other secondary gout, right hip
  - **M10.452**   Other secondary gout, left hip
  - **M10.459**   Other secondary gout, unspecified hip
- ✓6ᵗʰ **M10.46**   Other secondary gout, knee
  - **M10.461**   Other secondary gout, right knee
  - **M10.462**   Other secondary gout, left knee
  - **M10.469**   Other secondary gout, unspecified knee
- ✓6ᵗʰ **M10.47**   Other secondary gout, ankle and foot
  - **M10.471**   Other secondary gout, right ankle and foot
  - **M10.472**   Other secondary gout, left ankle and foot

- **M10.479**   Other secondary gout, unspecified ankle and foot
- **M10.48**   Other secondary gout, vertebrae
- **M10.49**   Other secondary gout, multiple sites

M10.9   **Gout, unspecified**
Gout NOS

✓4ᵗʰ **M11**   **Other crystal arthropathies**
✓5ᵗʰ **M11.0**   **Hydroxyapatite deposition disease**
> **DEF:** Disease caused by deposits of calcium phosphate crystals in the soft tissues close to the joint (especially tendons) or in the joints. These calcifications can be mono or polyarticular and can cause destruction of the joint involved.

- **M11.00**   Hydroxyapatite deposition disease, unspecified site
- ✓6ᵗʰ **M11.01**   Hydroxyapatite deposition disease, shoulder
  - **M11.011**   Hydroxyapatite deposition disease, right shoulder
  - **M11.012**   Hydroxyapatite deposition disease, left shoulder
  - **M11.019**   Hydroxyapatite deposition disease, unspecified shoulder
- ✓6ᵗʰ **M11.02**   Hydroxyapatite deposition disease, elbow
  - **M11.021**   Hydroxyapatite deposition disease, right elbow
  - **M11.022**   Hydroxyapatite deposition disease, left elbow
  - **M11.029**   Hydroxyapatite deposition disease, unspecified elbow
- ✓6ᵗʰ **M11.03**   Hydroxyapatite deposition disease, wrist
  - **M11.031**   Hydroxyapatite deposition disease, right wrist
  - **M11.032**   Hydroxyapatite deposition disease, left wrist
  - **M11.039**   Hydroxyapatite deposition disease, unspecified wrist
- ✓6ᵗʰ **M11.04**   Hydroxyapatite deposition disease, hand
  - **M11.041**   Hydroxyapatite deposition disease, right hand
  - **M11.042**   Hydroxyapatite deposition disease, left hand
  - **M11.049**   Hydroxyapatite deposition disease, unspecified hand
- ✓6ᵗʰ **M11.05**   Hydroxyapatite deposition disease, hip
  - **M11.051**   Hydroxyapatite deposition disease, right hip
  - **M11.052**   Hydroxyapatite deposition disease, left hip
  - **M11.059**   Hydroxyapatite deposition disease, unspecified hip
- ✓6ᵗʰ **M11.06**   Hydroxyapatite deposition disease, knee
  - **M11.061**   Hydroxyapatite deposition disease, right knee
  - **M11.062**   Hydroxyapatite deposition disease, left knee
  - **M11.069**   Hydroxyapatite deposition disease, unspecified knee
- ✓6ᵗʰ **M11.07**   Hydroxyapatite deposition disease, ankle and foot
  - **M11.071**   Hydroxyapatite deposition disease, right ankle and foot
  - **M11.072**   Hydroxyapatite deposition disease, left ankle and foot
  - **M11.079**   Hydroxyapatite deposition disease, unspecified ankle and foot
- **M11.08**   Hydroxyapatite deposition disease, vertebrae
- **M11.09**   Hydroxyapatite deposition disease, multiple sites

✓5ᵗʰ **M11.1**   **Familial chondrocalcinosis**
- **M11.10**   Familial chondrocalcinosis, unspecified site
- ✓6ᵗʰ **M11.11**   Familial chondrocalcinosis, shoulder
  - **M11.111**   Familial chondrocalcinosis, right shoulder
  - **M11.112**   Familial chondrocalcinosis, left shoulder
  - **M11.119**   Familial chondrocalcinosis, unspecified shoulder
- ✓6ᵗʰ **M11.12**   Familial chondrocalcinosis, elbow
  - **M11.121**   Familial chondrocalcinosis, right elbow
  - **M11.122**   Familial chondrocalcinosis, left elbow
  - **M11.129**   Familial chondrocalcinosis, unspecified elbow
- ✓6ᵗʰ **M11.13**   Familial chondrocalcinosis, wrist
  - **M11.131**   Familial chondrocalcinosis, right wrist

☑ Additional Character Required   ✓x7ᵗʰ Placeholder   **Unacceptable PDx**   Questionable PDx   Manifestation   Unspecified Dx   H1-H14 HAC   HCC CMS-HCC Dx   HIV HIV Dx

ICD-10-CM 2020

781

       M11.132   Familial chondrocalcinosis, left wrist
       M11.139   Familial chondrocalcinosis, unspecified wrist

✓6ᵗʰ   M11.14   Familial chondrocalcinosis, hand
       M11.141   Familial chondrocalcinosis, right hand
       M11.142   Familial chondrocalcinosis, left hand
       M11.149   Familial chondrocalcinosis, unspecified hand

✓6ᵗʰ   M11.15   Familial chondrocalcinosis, hip
       M11.151   Familial chondrocalcinosis, right hip
       M11.152   Familial chondrocalcinosis, left hip
       M11.159   Familial chondrocalcinosis, unspecified hip

✓6ᵗʰ   M11.16   Familial chondrocalcinosis, knee
       M11.161   Familial chondrocalcinosis, right knee
       M11.162   Familial chondrocalcinosis, left knee
       M11.169   Familial chondrocalcinosis, unspecified knee

✓6ᵗʰ   M11.17   Familial chondrocalcinosis, ankle and foot
       M11.171   Familial chondrocalcinosis, right ankle and foot
       M11.172   Familial chondrocalcinosis, left ankle and foot
       M11.179   Familial chondrocalcinosis, unspecified ankle and foot

     M11.18   Familial chondrocalcinosis, vertebrae
     M11.19   Familial chondrocalcinosis, multiple sites

✓5ᵗʰ   M11.2   Other chondrocalcinosis
     Chondrocalcinosis NOS
     AHA: 2018,3Q,20
     TIP: Pseudogout is captured with codes in this subcategory.

     M11.20   Other chondrocalcinosis, unspecified site
✓6ᵗʰ   M11.21   Other chondrocalcinosis, shoulder
       M11.211   Other chondrocalcinosis, right shoulder
       M11.212   Other chondrocalcinosis, left shoulder
       M11.219   Other chondrocalcinosis, unspecified shoulder

✓6ᵗʰ   M11.22   Other chondrocalcinosis, elbow
       M11.221   Other chondrocalcinosis, right elbow
       M11.222   Other chondrocalcinosis, left elbow
       M11.229   Other chondrocalcinosis, unspecified elbow

✓6ᵗʰ   M11.23   Other chondrocalcinosis, wrist
       M11.231   Other chondrocalcinosis, right wrist
       M11.232   Other chondrocalcinosis, left wrist
       M11.239   Other chondrocalcinosis, unspecified wrist

✓6ᵗʰ   M11.24   Other chondrocalcinosis, hand
       M11.241   Other chondrocalcinosis, right hand
       M11.242   Other chondrocalcinosis, left hand
       M11.249   Other chondrocalcinosis, unspecified hand

✓6ᵗʰ   M11.25   Other chondrocalcinosis, hip
       M11.251   Other chondrocalcinosis, right hip
       M11.252   Other chondrocalcinosis, left hip
       M11.259   Other chondrocalcinosis, unspecified hip

✓6ᵗʰ   M11.26   Other chondrocalcinosis, knee
       M11.261   Other chondrocalcinosis, right knee
       M11.262   Other chondrocalcinosis, left knee
       M11.269   Other chondrocalcinosis, unspecified knee

✓6ᵗʰ   M11.27   Other chondrocalcinosis, ankle and foot
       M11.271   Other chondrocalcinosis, right ankle and foot
       M11.272   Other chondrocalcinosis, left ankle and foot
       M11.279   Other chondrocalcinosis, unspecified ankle and foot

     M11.28   Other chondrocalcinosis, vertebrae
     M11.29   Other chondrocalcinosis, multiple sites

✓5ᵗʰ   M11.8   Other specified crystal arthropathies
     M11.80   Other specified crystal arthropathies, unspecified site
✓6ᵗʰ   M11.81   Other specified crystal arthropathies, shoulder
       M11.811   Other specified crystal arthropathies, right shoulder
       M11.812   Other specified crystal arthropathies, left shoulder

       M11.819   Other specified crystal arthropathies, unspecified shoulder
✓6ᵗʰ   M11.82   Other specified crystal arthropathies, elbow
       M11.821   Other specified crystal arthropathies, right elbow
       M11.822   Other specified crystal arthropathies, left elbow
       M11.829   Other specified crystal arthropathies, unspecified elbow

✓6ᵗʰ   M11.83   Other specified crystal arthropathies, wrist
       M11.831   Other specified crystal arthropathies, right wrist
       M11.832   Other specified crystal arthropathies, left wrist
       M11.839   Other specified crystal arthropathies, unspecified wrist

✓6ᵗʰ   M11.84   Other specified crystal arthropathies, hand
       M11.841   Other specified crystal arthropathies, right hand
       M11.842   Other specified crystal arthropathies, left hand
       M11.849   Other specified crystal arthropathies, unspecified hand

✓6ᵗʰ   M11.85   Other specified crystal arthropathies, hip
       M11.851   Other specified crystal arthropathies, right hip
       M11.852   Other specified crystal arthropathies, left hip
       M11.859   Other specified crystal arthropathies, unspecified hip

✓6ᵗʰ   M11.86   Other specified crystal arthropathies, knee
       M11.861   Other specified crystal arthropathies, right knee
       M11.862   Other specified crystal arthropathies, left knee
       M11.869   Other specified crystal arthropathies, unspecified knee

✓6ᵗʰ   M11.87   Other specified crystal arthropathies, ankle and foot
       M11.871   Other specified crystal arthropathies, right ankle and foot
       M11.872   Other specified crystal arthropathies, left ankle and foot
       M11.879   Other specified crystal arthropathies, unspecified ankle and foot

     M11.88   Other specified crystal arthropathies, vertebrae
     M11.89   Other specified crystal arthropathies, multiple sites
     M11.9   Crystal arthropathy, unspecified

✓4ᵗʰ   M12   Other and unspecified arthropathy
     EXCLUDES 1   arthrosis (M15-M19)
           cricoarytenoid arthropathy (J38.7)

✓5ᵗʰ   M12.0   Chronic postrheumatic arthropathy [Jaccoud]
     M12.00   Chronic postrheumatic arthropathy [Jaccoud], unspecified site   HCC
✓6ᵗʰ   M12.01   Chronic postrheumatic arthropathy [Jaccoud], shoulder
       M12.011   Chronic postrheumatic arthropathy [Jaccoud], right shoulder   HCC
       M12.012   Chronic postrheumatic arthropathy [Jaccoud], left shoulder
       M12.019   Chronic postrheumatic arthropathy [Jaccoud], unspecified shoulder   HCC

✓6ᵗʰ   M12.02   Chronic postrheumatic arthropathy [Jaccoud], elbow
       M12.021   Chronic postrheumatic arthropathy [Jaccoud], right elbow   HCC
       M12.022   Chronic postrheumatic arthropathy [Jaccoud], left elbow   HCC
       M12.029   Chronic postrheumatic arthropathy [Jaccoud], unspecified elbow   HCC

✓6ᵗʰ   M12.03   Chronic postrheumatic arthropathy [Jaccoud], wrist
       M12.031   Chronic postrheumatic arthropathy [Jaccoud], right wrist   HCC

         M12.032   Chronic postrheumatic arthropathy [Jaccoud], left wrist   `HCC`

         M12.039   Chronic postrheumatic arthropathy [Jaccoud], unspecified wrist   `HCC`

✓6ᵗʰ   M12.04   Chronic postrheumatic arthropathy [Jaccoud], hand

         M12.041   Chronic postrheumatic arthropathy [Jaccoud], right hand   `HCC`

         M12.042   Chronic postrheumatic arthropathy [Jaccoud], left hand   `HCC`

         M12.049   Chronic postrheumatic arthropathy [Jaccoud], unspecified hand   `HCC`

✓6ᵗʰ   M12.05   Chronic postrheumatic arthropathy [Jaccoud], hip

         M12.051   Chronic postrheumatic arthropathy [Jaccoud], right hip   `HCC`

         M12.052   Chronic postrheumatic arthropathy [Jaccoud], left hip   `HCC`

         M12.059   Chronic postrheumatic arthropathy [Jaccoud], unspecified hip   `HCC`

✓6ᵗʰ   M12.06   Chronic postrheumatic arthropathy [Jaccoud], knee

         M12.061   Chronic postrheumatic arthropathy [Jaccoud], right knee   `HCC`

         M12.062   Chronic postrheumatic arthropathy [Jaccoud], left knee   `HCC`

         M12.069   Chronic postrheumatic arthropathy [Jaccoud], unspecified knee   `HCC`

✓6ᵗʰ   M12.07   Chronic postrheumatic arthropathy [Jaccoud], ankle and foot

         M12.071   Chronic postrheumatic arthropathy [Jaccoud], right ankle and foot   `HCC`

         M12.072   Chronic postrheumatic arthropathy [Jaccoud], left ankle and foot   `HCC`

         M12.079   Chronic postrheumatic arthropathy [Jaccoud], unspecified ankle and foot   `HCC`

     M12.08   Chronic postrheumatic arthropathy [Jaccoud], other specified site   `HCC`

         Chronic postrheumatic arthropathy [Jaccoud], vertebrae

     M12.09   Chronic postrheumatic arthropathy [Jaccoud], multiple sites   `HCC`

✓5ᵗʰ   M12.1   Kaschin-Beck disease

         Osteochondroarthrosis deformans endemica

     M12.10   Kaschin-Beck disease, unspecified site

✓6ᵗʰ   M12.11   Kaschin-Beck disease, shoulder

         M12.111   Kaschin-Beck disease, right shoulder
         M12.112   Kaschin-Beck disease, left shoulder
         M12.119   Kaschin-Beck disease, unspecified shoulder

✓6ᵗʰ   M12.12   Kaschin-Beck disease, elbow

         M12.121   Kaschin-Beck disease, right elbow
         M12.122   Kaschin-Beck disease, left elbow
         M12.129   Kaschin-Beck disease, unspecified elbow

✓6ᵗʰ   M12.13   Kaschin-Beck disease, wrist

         M12.131   Kaschin-Beck disease, right wrist
         M12.132   Kaschin-Beck disease, left wrist
         M12.139   Kaschin-Beck disease, unspecified wrist

✓6ᵗʰ   M12.14   Kaschin-Beck disease, hand

         M12.141   Kaschin-Beck disease, right hand
         M12.142   Kaschin-Beck disease, left hand
         M12.149   Kaschin-Beck disease, unspecified hand

✓6ᵗʰ   M12.15   Kaschin-Beck disease, hip

         M12.151   Kaschin-Beck disease, right hip
         M12.152   Kaschin-Beck disease, left hip
         M12.159   Kaschin-Beck disease, unspecified hip

✓6ᵗʰ   M12.16   Kaschin-Beck disease, knee

         M12.161   Kaschin-Beck disease, right knee
         M12.162   Kaschin-Beck disease, left knee

         M12.169   Kaschin-Beck disease, unspecified knee

✓6ᵗʰ   M12.17   Kaschin-Beck disease, ankle and foot

         M12.171   Kaschin-Beck disease, right ankle and foot
         M12.172   Kaschin-Beck disease, left ankle and foot
         M12.179   Kaschin-Beck disease, unspecified ankle and foot

     M12.18   Kaschin-Beck disease, vertebrae
     M12.19   Kaschin-Beck disease, multiple sites

✓5ᵗʰ   M12.2   Villonodular synovitis (pigmented)

     M12.20   Villonodular synovitis (pigmented), unspecified site

✓6ᵗʰ   M12.21   Villonodular synovitis (pigmented), shoulder

         M12.211   Villonodular synovitis (pigmented), right shoulder
         M12.212   Villonodular synovitis (pigmented), left shoulder
         M12.219   Villonodular synovitis (pigmented), unspecified shoulder

✓6ᵗʰ   M12.22   Villonodular synovitis (pigmented), elbow

         M12.221   Villonodular synovitis (pigmented), right elbow
         M12.222   Villonodular synovitis (pigmented), left elbow
         M12.229   Villonodular synovitis (pigmented), unspecified elbow

✓6ᵗʰ   M12.23   Villonodular synovitis (pigmented), wrist

         M12.231   Villonodular synovitis (pigmented), right wrist
         M12.232   Villonodular synovitis (pigmented), left wrist
         M12.239   Villonodular synovitis (pigmented), unspecified wrist

✓6ᵗʰ   M12.24   Villonodular synovitis (pigmented), hand

         M12.241   Villonodular synovitis (pigmented), right hand
         M12.242   Villonodular synovitis (pigmented), left hand
         M12.249   Villonodular synovitis (pigmented), unspecified hand

✓6ᵗʰ   M12.25   Villonodular synovitis (pigmented), hip

         M12.251   Villonodular synovitis (pigmented), right hip
         M12.252   Villonodular synovitis (pigmented), left hip
         M12.259   Villonodular synovitis (pigmented), unspecified hip

✓6ᵗʰ   M12.26   Villonodular synovitis (pigmented), knee

         M12.261   Villonodular synovitis (pigmented), right knee
         M12.262   Villonodular synovitis (pigmented), left knee
         M12.269   Villonodular synovitis (pigmented), unspecified knee

✓6ᵗʰ   M12.27   Villonodular synovitis (pigmented), ankle and foot

         M12.271   Villonodular synovitis (pigmented), right ankle and foot
         M12.272   Villonodular synovitis (pigmented), left ankle and foot
         M12.279   Villonodular synovitis (pigmented), unspecified ankle and foot

     M12.28   Villonodular synovitis (pigmented), other specified site

         Villonodular synovitis (pigmented), vertebrae

     M12.29   Villonodular synovitis (pigmented), multiple sites

✓5ᵗʰ   M12.3   Palindromic rheumatism

         DEF: Sudden and recurring attacks of moderate to severe joint pain and swelling generally occurring in the hands or feet of unknown etiology. After the attack subsides, the joints appear normal again.

     M12.30   Palindromic rheumatism, unspecified site

✓6ᵗʰ   M12.31   Palindromic rheumatism, shoulder

         M12.311   Palindromic rheumatism, right shoulder
         M12.312   Palindromic rheumatism, left shoulder
         M12.319   Palindromic rheumatism, unspecified shoulder

✓6ᵗʰ   M12.32   Palindromic rheumatism, elbow

         M12.321   Palindromic rheumatism, right elbow
         M12.322   Palindromic rheumatism, left elbow

✔ Additional Character Required   ✓x7ᵗʰ Placeholder   Unacceptable PDx   Questionable PDx   Manifestation   Unspecified Dx   H1-H14 HAC   HCC CMS-HCC Dx   HIV HIV Dx

ICD-10-CM 2020   783

Chapter 13. Diseases of the Musculoskeletal System and Connective Tissue

M12.329 Palindromic rheumatism, unspecified elbow

✓6ᵗʰ M12.33 Palindromic rheumatism, wrist

    M12.331 Palindromic rheumatism, right wrist
    M12.332 Palindromic rheumatism, left wrist
    M12.339 Palindromic rheumatism, unspecified wrist

✓6ᵗʰ M12.34 Palindromic rheumatism, hand

    M12.341 Palindromic rheumatism, right hand
    M12.342 Palindromic rheumatism, left hand
    M12.349 Palindromic rheumatism, unspecified hand

✓6ᵗʰ M12.35 Palindromic rheumatism, hip

    M12.351 Palindromic rheumatism, right hip
    M12.352 Palindromic rheumatism, left hip
    M12.359 Palindromic rheumatism, unspecified hip

✓6ᵗʰ M12.36 Palindromic rheumatism, knee

    M12.361 Palindromic rheumatism, right knee
    M12.362 Palindromic rheumatism, left knee
    M12.369 Palindromic rheumatism, unspecified knee

✓6ᵗʰ M12.37 Palindromic rheumatism, ankle and foot

    M12.371 Palindromic rheumatism, right ankle and foot
    M12.372 Palindromic rheumatism, left ankle and foot
    M12.379 Palindromic rheumatism, unspecified ankle and foot

    M12.38 Palindromic rheumatism, other specified site
        Palindromic rheumatism, vertebrae

    M12.39 Palindromic rheumatism, multiple sites

✓5ᵗʰ M12.4 Intermittent hydrarthrosis

    M12.40 Intermittent hydrarthrosis, unspecified site

✓6ᵗʰ M12.41 Intermittent hydrarthrosis, shoulder

    M12.411 Intermittent hydrarthrosis, right shoulder
    M12.412 Intermittent hydrarthrosis, left shoulder
    M12.419 Intermittent hydrarthrosis, unspecified shoulder

✓6ᵗʰ M12.42 Intermittent hydrarthrosis, elbow

    M12.421 Intermittent hydrarthrosis, right elbow
    M12.422 Intermittent hydrarthrosis, left elbow
    M12.429 Intermittent hydrarthrosis, unspecified elbow

✓6ᵗʰ M12.43 Intermittent hydrarthrosis, wrist

    M12.431 Intermittent hydrarthrosis, right wrist
    M12.432 Intermittent hydrarthrosis, left wrist
    M12.439 Intermittent hydrarthrosis, unspecified wrist

✓6ᵗʰ M12.44 Intermittent hydrarthrosis, hand

    M12.441 Intermittent hydrarthrosis, right hand
    M12.442 Intermittent hydrarthrosis, left hand
    M12.449 Intermittent hydrarthrosis, unspecified hand

✓6ᵗʰ M12.45 Intermittent hydrarthrosis, hip

    M12.451 Intermittent hydrarthrosis, right hip
    M12.452 Intermittent hydrarthrosis, left hip
    M12.459 Intermittent hydrarthrosis, unspecified hip

✓6ᵗʰ M12.46 Intermittent hydrarthrosis, knee

    M12.461 Intermittent hydrarthrosis, right knee
    M12.462 Intermittent hydrarthrosis, left knee
    M12.469 Intermittent hydrarthrosis, unspecified knee

✓6ᵗʰ M12.47 Intermittent hydrarthrosis, ankle and foot

    M12.471 Intermittent hydrarthrosis, right ankle and foot
    M12.472 Intermittent hydrarthrosis, left ankle and foot
    M12.479 Intermittent hydrarthrosis, unspecified ankle and foot

    M12.48 Intermittent hydrarthrosis, other site
    M12.49 Intermittent hydrarthrosis, multiple sites

✓5ᵗʰ M12.5 Traumatic arthropathy

    EXCLUDES 1   *current injury–see Alphabetic Index*
        post-traumatic osteoarthritis of first carpometacarpal joint (M18.2-M18.3)
        post-traumatic osteoarthritis of hip (M16.4-M16.5)
        post-traumatic osteoarthritis of knee (M17.2-M17.3)
        post-traumatic osteoarthritis NOS (M19.1-)
        post-traumatic osteoarthritis of other single joints (M19.1-)

    AHA: 2015,1Q,17

    M12.50 Traumatic arthropathy, unspecified site

✓6ᵗʰ M12.51 Traumatic arthropathy, shoulder

    M12.511 Traumatic arthropathy, right shoulder
    M12.512 Traumatic arthropathy, left shoulder
    M12.519 Traumatic arthropathy, unspecified shoulder

✓6ᵗʰ M12.52 Traumatic arthropathy, elbow

    M12.521 Traumatic arthropathy, right elbow
    M12.522 Traumatic arthropathy, left elbow
    M12.529 Traumatic arthropathy, unspecified elbow

✓6ᵗʰ M12.53 Traumatic arthropathy, wrist

    M12.531 Traumatic arthropathy, right wrist
    M12.532 Traumatic arthropathy, left wrist
    M12.539 Traumatic arthropathy, unspecified wrist

✓6ᵗʰ M12.54 Traumatic arthropathy, hand

    M12.541 Traumatic arthropathy, right hand
    M12.542 Traumatic arthropathy, left hand
    M12.549 Traumatic arthropathy, unspecified hand

✓6ᵗʰ M12.55 Traumatic arthropathy, hip

    M12.551 Traumatic arthropathy, right hip
    M12.552 Traumatic arthropathy, left hip
    M12.559 Traumatic arthropathy, unspecified hip

✓6ᵗʰ M12.56 Traumatic arthropathy, knee

    M12.561 Traumatic arthropathy, right knee
    M12.562 Traumatic arthropathy, left knee
    M12.569 Traumatic arthropathy, unspecified knee

✓6ᵗʰ M12.57 Traumatic arthropathy, ankle and foot

    M12.571 Traumatic arthropathy, right ankle and foot
    M12.572 Traumatic arthropathy, left ankle and foot
    M12.579 Traumatic arthropathy, unspecified ankle and foot

    M12.58 Traumatic arthropathy, other specified site
        Traumatic arthropathy, vertebrae

    M12.59 Traumatic arthropathy, multiple sites

✓5ᵗʰ M12.8 Other specific arthropathies, not elsewhere classified
    Transient arthropathy

    M12.80 Other specific arthropathies, not elsewhere classified, unspecified site

✓6ᵗʰ M12.81 Other specific arthropathies, not elsewhere classified, shoulder

    M12.811 Other specific arthropathies, not elsewhere classified, right shoulder
    M12.812 Other specific arthropathies, not elsewhere classified, left shoulder
    M12.819 Other specific arthropathies, not elsewhere classified, unspecified shoulder

✓6ᵗʰ M12.82 Other specific arthropathies, not elsewhere classified, elbow

    M12.821 Other specific arthropathies, not elsewhere classified, right elbow
    M12.822 Other specific arthropathies, not elsewhere classified, left elbow
    M12.829 Other specific arthropathies, not elsewhere classified, unspecified elbow

✓6ᵗʰ M12.83 Other specific arthropathies, not elsewhere classified, wrist

    M12.831 Other specific arthropathies, not elsewhere classified, right wrist
    M12.832 Other specific arthropathies, not elsewhere classified, left wrist
    M12.839 Other specific arthropathies, not elsewhere classified, unspecified wrist

N Newborn: 0   P Pediatric: 0-17   M Maternity: 9-64   A Adult: 15-124   MCC Major Complication/Comorbidity   CC Complication/Comorbidity   SW Severe Wound Dx

784   ICD-10-CM 2020

√6ᵗʰ **M12.84** Other specific arthropathies, not elsewhere classified, **hand**
- **M12.841** Other specific arthropathies, not elsewhere classified, **right hand**
- **M12.842** Other specific arthropathies, not elsewhere classified, **left hand**
- **M12.849** Other specific arthropathies, not elsewhere classified, unspecified hand

√6ᵗʰ **M12.85** Other specific arthropathies, not elsewhere classified, **hip**
- **M12.851** Other specific arthropathies, not elsewhere classified, **right hip**
- **M12.852** Other specific arthropathies, not elsewhere classified, **left hip**
- **M12.859** Other specific arthropathies, not elsewhere classified, unspecified hip

√6ᵗʰ **M12.86** Other specific arthropathies, not elsewhere classified, **knee**
- **M12.861** Other specific arthropathies, not elsewhere classified, **right knee**
- **M12.862** Other specific arthropathies, not elsewhere classified, **left knee**
- **M12.869** Other specific arthropathies, not elsewhere classified, unspecified knee

√6ᵗʰ **M12.87** Other specific arthropathies, not elsewhere classified, **ankle and foot**
- **M12.871** Other specific arthropathies, not elsewhere classified, **right ankle and foot**
- **M12.872** Other specific arthropathies, not elsewhere classified, **left ankle and foot**
- **M12.879** Other specific arthropathies, not elsewhere classified, unspecified ankle and foot

M12.88 Other specific arthropathies, not elsewhere classified, other specified site

     Other specific arthropathies, not elsewhere classified, vertebrae

M12.89 Other specific arthropathies, not elsewhere classified, **multiple sites**

M12.9 Arthropathy, unspecified

√4ᵗʰ **M13 Other arthritis**

     EXCLUDES 1   arthrosis (M15-M19)
               osteoarthritis (M15-M19)

M13.0 Polyarthritis, unspecified

√5ᵗʰ **M13.1** Monoarthritis, not elsewhere classified

     M13.10 Monoarthritis, not elsewhere classified, unspecified site

√6ᵗʰ **M13.11** Monoarthritis, not elsewhere classified, **shoulder**
- **M13.111** Monoarthritis, not elsewhere classified, **right shoulder**
- **M13.112** Monoarthritis, not elsewhere classified, **left shoulder**
- **M13.119** Monoarthritis, not elsewhere classified, unspecified shoulder

√6ᵗʰ **M13.12** Monoarthritis, not elsewhere classified, **elbow**
- **M13.121** Monoarthritis, not elsewhere classified, **right elbow**
- **M13.122** Monoarthritis, not elsewhere classified, **left elbow**
- **M13.129** Monoarthritis, not elsewhere classified, unspecified elbow

√6ᵗʰ **M13.13** Monoarthritis, not elsewhere classified, **wrist**
- **M13.131** Monoarthritis, not elsewhere classified, **right wrist**
- **M13.132** Monoarthritis, not elsewhere classified, **left wrist**
- **M13.139** Monoarthritis, not elsewhere classified, unspecified wrist

√6ᵗʰ **M13.14** Monoarthritis, not elsewhere classified, **hand**
- **M13.141** Monoarthritis, not elsewhere classified, **right hand**
- **M13.142** Monoarthritis, not elsewhere classified, **left hand**
- **M13.149** Monoarthritis, not elsewhere classified, unspecified hand

√6ᵗʰ **M13.15** Monoarthritis, not elsewhere classified, **hip**
- **M13.151** Monoarthritis, not elsewhere classified, **right hip**
- **M13.152** Monoarthritis, not elsewhere classified, **left hip**
- **M13.159** Monoarthritis, not elsewhere classified, unspecified hip

√6ᵗʰ **M13.16** Monoarthritis, not elsewhere classified, **knee**
- **M13.161** Monoarthritis, not elsewhere classified, **right knee**
- **M13.162** Monoarthritis, not elsewhere classified, **left knee**
- **M13.169** Monoarthritis, not elsewhere classified, unspecified knee

√6ᵗʰ **M13.17** Monoarthritis, not elsewhere classified, **ankle and foot**
- **M13.171** Monoarthritis, not elsewhere classified, **right ankle and foot**
- **M13.172** Monoarthritis, not elsewhere classified, **left ankle and foot**
- **M13.179** Monoarthritis, not elsewhere classified, unspecified ankle and foot

√5ᵗʰ **M13.8 Other specified arthritis**

     Allergic arthritis

     EXCLUDES 1   osteoarthritis (M15-M19)

M13.80 Other specified arthritis, unspecified site

√6ᵗʰ **M13.81** Other specified arthritis, **shoulder**
- **M13.811** Other specified arthritis, **right shoulder**
- **M13.812** Other specified arthritis, **left shoulder**
- **M13.819** Other specified arthritis, unspecified shoulder

√6ᵗʰ **M13.82** Other specified arthritis, **elbow**
- **M13.821** Other specified arthritis, **right elbow**
- **M13.822** Other specified arthritis, **left elbow**
- **M13.829** Other specified arthritis, unspecified elbow

√6ᵗʰ **M13.83** Other specified arthritis, **wrist**
- **M13.831** Other specified arthritis, **right wrist**
- **M13.832** Other specified arthritis, **left wrist**
- **M13.839** Other specified arthritis, unspecified wrist

√6ᵗʰ **M13.84** Other specified arthritis, **hand**
- **M13.841** Other specified arthritis, **right hand**
- **M13.842** Other specified arthritis, **left hand**
- **M13.849** Other specified arthritis, unspecified hand

√6ᵗʰ **M13.85** Other specified arthritis, **hip**
- **M13.851** Other specified arthritis, **right hip**
- **M13.852** Other specified arthritis, **left hip**
- **M13.859** Other specified arthritis, unspecified hip

√6ᵗʰ **M13.86** Other specified arthritis, **knee**
- **M13.861** Other specified arthritis, **right knee**
- **M13.862** Other specified arthritis, **left knee**
- **M13.869** Other specified arthritis, unspecified knee

√6ᵗʰ **M13.87** Other specified arthritis, **ankle and foot**
- **M13.871** Other specified arthritis, **right ankle and foot**
- **M13.872** Other specified arthritis, **left ankle and foot**
- **M13.879** Other specified arthritis, unspecified ankle and foot

M13.88 Other specified arthritis, other site

M13.89 Other specified arthritis, **multiple sites**

☑ Additional Character Required   √x7ᵗʰ Placeholder   Unacceptable PDx   Questionable PDx   Manifestation   Unspecified Dx   H1-H14 HAC   HCC CMS-HCC Dx   HIV HIV Dx

ICD-10-CM 2020

785

Chapter 13. Diseases of the Musculoskeletal System and Connective Tissue

M12.84–M13.89

Chapter 13. Diseases of the Musculoskeletal System and Connective Tissue

☑4ᵗʰ **M14** **Arthropathies in other diseases classified elsewhere**

    EXCLUDES 1   arthropathy in:
         diabetes mellitus (EØ8-E13 with .61-)
         hematological disorders (M36.2-M36.3)
         hypersensitivity reactions (M36.4)
         neoplastic disease (M36.1)
         neurosyphillis (A52.16)
         sarcoidosis (D86.86)
       enteropathic arthropathies (MØ7.-)
       juvenile psoriatic arthropathy (L40.54)
       lipoid dermatoarthritis (E78.81)

☑5ᵗʰ **M14.6** **Charcôt's joint**

     Neuropathic arthropathy
     EXCLUDES 1   Charcôt's joint in diabetes mellitus (EØ8-E13 with .61Ø)
         Charcôt's joint in tabes dorsalis (A52.16)
     DEF: Progressive neurologic arthropathy in which chronic degeneration of joints in the weight-bearing areas with peripheral hypertrophy occurs as a complication of a neuropathy disorder. Supporting structures relax from a loss of sensation resulting in chronic joint instability.

     M14.6Ø Charcôt's joint, unspecified site
     ☑6ᵗʰ **M14.61** Charcôt's joint, shoulder
         M14.611 Charcôt's joint, right shoulder
         M14.612 Charcôt's joint, left shoulder
         M14.619 Charcôt's joint, unspecified shoulder
     ☑6ᵗʰ **M14.62** Charcôt's joint, elbow
         M14.621 Charcôt's joint, right elbow
         M14.622 Charcôt's joint, left elbow
         M14.629 Charcôt's joint, unspecified elbow
     ☑6ᵗʰ **M14.63** Charcôt's joint, wrist
         M14.631 Charcôt's joint, right wrist
         M14.632 Charcôt's joint, left wrist
         M14.639 Charcôt's joint, unspecified wrist
     ☑6ᵗʰ **M14.64** Charcôt's joint, hand
         M14.641 Charcôt's joint, right hand
         M14.642 Charcôt's joint, left hand
         M14.649 Charcôt's joint, unspecified hand
     ☑6ᵗʰ **M14.65** Charcôt's joint, hip
         M14.651 Charcôt's joint, right hip
         M14.652 Charcôt's joint, left hip
         M14.659 Charcôt's joint, unspecified hip
     ☑6ᵗʰ **M14.66** Charcôt's joint, knee
         M14.661 Charcôt's joint, right knee
         M14.662 Charcôt's joint, left knee
         M14.669 Charcôt's joint, unspecified knee
     ☑6ᵗʰ **M14.67** Charcôt's joint, ankle and foot
         M14.671 Charcôt's joint, right ankle and foot
         M14.672 Charcôt's joint, left ankle and foot
         M14.679 Charcôt's joint, unspecified ankle and foot
     M14.68 Charcôt's joint, vertebrae
     M14.69 Charcôt's joint, multiple sites

☑5ᵗʰ **M14.8** **Arthropathies in other specified diseases classified elsewhere**

     Code first underlying disease, such as:
       amyloidosis (E85.-)
       erythema multiforme (L51.-)
       erythema nodosum (L52)
       hemochromatosis (E83.11-)
       hyperparathyroidism (E21.-)
       hypothyroidism (EØØ-EØ3)
       sickle-cell disorders (D57.-)
       thyrotoxicosis [hyperthyroidism] (EØ5.-)
       Whipple's disease (K90.81)

     M14.8Ø *Arthropathies in other specified diseases classified elsewhere, unspecified site*
     ☑6ᵗʰ **M14.81** Arthropathies in other specified diseases classified elsewhere, shoulder
         M14.811 *Arthropathies in other specified diseases classified elsewhere, right shoulder*
         M14.812 *Arthropathies in other specified diseases classified elsewhere, left shoulder*
         M14.819 *Arthropathies in other specified diseases classified elsewhere, unspecified shoulder*

     ☑6ᵗʰ **M14.82** Arthropathies in other specified diseases classified elsewhere, elbow
         M14.821 *Arthropathies in other specified diseases classified elsewhere, right elbow*
         M14.822 *Arthropathies in other specified diseases classified elsewhere, left elbow*
         M14.829 *Arthropathies in other specified diseases classified elsewhere, unspecified elbow*
     ☑6ᵗʰ **M14.83** Arthropathies in other specified diseases classified elsewhere, wrist
         M14.831 *Arthropathies in other specified diseases classified elsewhere, right wrist*
         M14.832 *Arthropathies in other specified diseases classified elsewhere, left wrist*
         M14.839 *Arthropathies in other specified diseases classified elsewhere, unspecified wrist*
     ☑6ᵗʰ **M14.84** Arthropathies in other specified diseases classified elsewhere, hand
         M14.841 *Arthropathies in other specified diseases classified elsewhere, right hand*
         M14.842 *Arthropathies in other specified diseases classified elsewhere, left hand*
         M14.849 *Arthropathies in other specified diseases classified elsewhere, unspecified hand*
     ☑6ᵗʰ **M14.85** Arthropathies in other specified diseases classified elsewhere, hip
         M14.851 *Arthropathies in other specified diseases classified elsewhere, right hip*
         M14.852 *Arthropathies in other specified diseases classified elsewhere, left hip*
         M14.859 *Arthropathies in other specified diseases classified elsewhere, unspecified hip*
     ☑6ᵗʰ **M14.86** Arthropathies in other specified diseases classified elsewhere, knee
         M14.861 *Arthropathies in other specified diseases classified elsewhere, right knee*
         M14.862 *Arthropathies in other specified diseases classified elsewhere, left knee*
         M14.869 *Arthropathies in other specified diseases classified elsewhere, unspecified knee*
     ☑6ᵗʰ **M14.87** Arthropathies in other specified diseases classified elsewhere, ankle and foot
         M14.871 *Arthropathies in other specified diseases classified elsewhere, right ankle and foot*
         M14.872 *Arthropathies in other specified diseases classified elsewhere, left ankle and foot*
         M14.879 *Arthropathies in other specified diseases classified elsewhere, unspecified ankle and foot*
     M14.88 *Arthropathies in other specified diseases classified elsewhere, vertebrae*
     M14.89 *Arthropathies in other specified diseases classified elsewhere, multiple sites*

Osteoarthritis (M15-M19)

EXCLUDES 2   osteoarthritis of spine (M47.-)
TIP: Assign a primary osteoarthritis code when the type of osteoarthritis—primary, secondary, or generalized—is not specified in the documentation. Primary is considered the default.

☑4ᵗʰ **M15** **Polyosteoarthritis**

     INCLUDES   arthritis of multiple sites
     EXCLUDES 1   bilateral involvement of single joint (M16-M19)

     M15.Ø **Primary generalized (osteo)arthritis**
     M15.1 **Heberden's nodes (with arthropathy)**
       Interphalangeal distal osteoarthritis
     M15.2 **Bouchard's nodes (with arthropathy)**
       Juxtaphalangeal distal osteoarthritis
     M15.3 **Secondary multiple arthritis**
       Post-traumatic polyosteoarthritis
     M15.4 **Erosive (osteo)arthritis**
     M15.8 **Other polyosteoarthritis**
     M15.9 **Polyosteoarthritis, unspecified**
       Generalized osteoarthritis NOS

☑4ᵗʰ **M16** **Osteoarthritis of hip**

     AHA: 2016,4Q,146
     M16.Ø **Bilateral primary osteoarthritis of hip**
       AHA: 2018,2Q,15

N Newborn: 0   P Pediatric: 0-17   M Maternity: 9-64   A Adult: 15-124   MCC Major Complication/Comorbidity   CC Complication/Comorbidity   SW Severe Wound Dx

786   ICD-10-CM 2020

☑5ᵗʰ **M16.1** Unilateral primary **osteoarthritis of hip**
> Primary osteoarthritis of hip NOS
> **AHA:** 2018,2Q,15

     M16.10 Unilateral primary osteoarthritis, unspecified hip
     M16.11 Unilateral primary osteoarthritis, right hip
     M16.12 Unilateral primary osteoarthritis, left hip

M16.2 Bilateral **osteoarthritis resulting from hip dysplasia**

☑5ᵗʰ **M16.3** Unilateral **osteoarthritis resulting from hip dysplasia**
> Dysplastic osteoarthritis of hip NOS

     M16.30 Unilateral osteoarthritis resulting from hip dysplasia, unspecified hip
     M16.31 Unilateral osteoarthritis resulting from hip dysplasia, right hip
     M16.32 Unilateral osteoarthritis resulting from hip dysplasia, left hip

M16.4 Bilateral **post-traumatic osteoarthritis of hip**

☑5ᵗʰ **M16.5** Unilateral **post-traumatic osteoarthritis of hip**
> Post-traumatic osteoarthritis of hip NOS

     M16.50 Unilateral post-traumatic osteoarthritis, unspecified hip
     M16.51 Unilateral post-traumatic osteoarthritis, right hip
     M16.52 Unilateral post-traumatic osteoarthritis, left hip

M16.6 Other bilateral secondary osteoarthritis of hip

M16.7 Other unilateral secondary osteoarthritis of hip
> Secondary osteoarthritis of hip NOS

M16.9 Osteoarthritis of hip, unspecified

☑4ᵗʰ **M17** Osteoarthritis of **knee**
> **AHA:** 2016,4Q,146-147

M17.0 Bilateral primary **osteoarthritis of knee**
> **AHA:** 2018,2Q,15

☑5ᵗʰ **M17.1** Unilateral primary **osteoarthritis of knee**
> Primary osteoarthritis of knee NOS
> **AHA:** 2018,2Q,15

     M17.10 Unilateral primary osteoarthritis, unspecified knee
     M17.11 Unilateral primary osteoarthritis, right knee
     M17.12 Unilateral primary osteoarthritis, left knee

M17.2 Bilateral **post-traumatic osteoarthritis of knee**

☑5ᵗʰ **M17.3** Unilateral **post-traumatic osteoarthritis of knee**
> Post-traumatic osteoarthritis of knee NOS

     M17.30 Unilateral post-traumatic osteoarthritis, unspecified knee
     M17.31 Unilateral post-traumatic osteoarthritis, right knee
     M17.32 Unilateral post-traumatic osteoarthritis, left knee

M17.4 Other bilateral secondary **osteoarthritis of knee**

M17.5 Other unilateral secondary **osteoarthritis of knee**
> Secondary osteoarthritis of knee NOS

M17.9 Osteoarthritis of knee, unspecified

☑4ᵗʰ **M18** Osteoarthritis of **first carpometacarpal joint**

M18.0 Bilateral primary **osteoarthritis of first carpometacarpal joints**

☑5ᵗʰ **M18.1** Unilateral primary **osteoarthritis of first carpometacarpal joint**
> Primary osteoarthritis of first carpometacarpal joint NOS

     M18.10 Unilateral primary osteoarthritis of first carpometacarpal joint, unspecified hand
     M18.11 Unilateral primary osteoarthritis of first carpometacarpal joint, right hand
     M18.12 Unilateral primary osteoarthritis of first carpometacarpal joint, left hand

M18.2 Bilateral **post-traumatic osteoarthritis of first carpometacarpal joints**

☑5ᵗʰ **M18.3** Unilateral **post-traumatic osteoarthritis of first carpometacarpal joint**
> Post-traumatic osteoarthritis of first carpometacarpal joint NOS

     M18.30 Unilateral post-traumatic osteoarthritis of first carpometacarpal joint, unspecified hand
     M18.31 Unilateral post-traumatic osteoarthritis of first carpometacarpal joint, right hand
     M18.32 Unilateral post-traumatic osteoarthritis of first carpometacarpal joint, left hand

M18.4 Other bilateral secondary **osteoarthritis of first carpometacarpal joints**

☑5ᵗʰ **M18.5** Other unilateral secondary **osteoarthritis of first carpometacarpal joint**
> Secondary osteoarthritis of first carpometacarpal joint NOS

     M18.50 Other unilateral secondary osteoarthritis of first carpometacarpal joint, unspecified hand

     M18.51 Other unilateral secondary osteoarthritis of first carpometacarpal joint, right hand
     M18.52 Other unilateral secondary osteoarthritis of first carpometacarpal joint, left hand

M18.9 Osteoarthritis of first carpometacarpal joint, unspecified

☑4ᵗʰ **M19** Other and unspecified osteoarthritis
> EXCLUDES 1   *polyarthritis (M15.-)*
> EXCLUDES 2   *arthrosis of spine (M47.-)*
>   *hallux rigidus (M20.2)*
>   *osteoarthritis of spine (M47.-)*

☑5ᵗʰ **M19.0** Primary **osteoarthritis of other joints**
> **AHA:** 2018,2Q,15; 2016,4Q,145

☑6ᵗʰ **M19.01** Primary osteoarthritis, **shoulder**
     M19.011 Primary osteoarthritis, right shoulder
     M19.012 Primary osteoarthritis, left shoulder
     M19.019 Primary osteoarthritis, unspecified shoulder

☑6ᵗʰ **M19.02** Primary osteoarthritis, **elbow**
     M19.021 Primary osteoarthritis, right elbow
     M19.022 Primary osteoarthritis, left elbow
     M19.029 Primary osteoarthritis, unspecified elbow

☑6ᵗʰ **M19.03** Primary osteoarthritis, **wrist**
     M19.031 Primary osteoarthritis, right wrist
     M19.032 Primary osteoarthritis, left wrist
     M19.039 Primary osteoarthritis, unspecified wrist

☑6ᵗʰ **M19.04** Primary osteoarthritis, **hand**
> EXCLUDES 2   *primary osteoarthritis of first carpometacarpal joint (M18.0-, M18.1-)*

     M19.041 Primary osteoarthritis, right hand
     M19.042 Primary osteoarthritis, left hand
     M19.049 Primary osteoarthritis, unspecified hand

☑6ᵗʰ **M19.07** Primary osteoarthritis **ankle and foot**
     M19.071 Primary osteoarthritis, right ankle and foot
     M19.072 Primary osteoarthritis, left ankle and foot
     M19.079 Primary osteoarthritis, unspecified ankle and foot

☑5ᵗʰ **M19.1** Post-traumatic **osteoarthritis of other joints**

☑6ᵗʰ **M19.11** Post-traumatic osteoarthritis, **shoulder**
     M19.111 Post-traumatic osteoarthritis, right shoulder
     M19.112 Post-traumatic osteoarthritis, left shoulder
     M19.119 Post-traumatic osteoarthritis, unspecified shoulder

☑6ᵗʰ **M19.12** Post-traumatic osteoarthritis, **elbow**
     M19.121 Post-traumatic osteoarthritis, right elbow
     M19.122 Post-traumatic osteoarthritis, left elbow
     M19.129 Post-traumatic osteoarthritis, unspecified elbow

☑6ᵗʰ **M19.13** Post-traumatic osteoarthritis, **wrist**
     M19.131 Post-traumatic osteoarthritis, right wrist
     M19.132 Post-traumatic osteoarthritis, left wrist
     M19.139 Post-traumatic osteoarthritis, unspecified wrist

☑6ᵗʰ **M19.14** Post-traumatic osteoarthritis, **hand**
> EXCLUDES 2   *post-traumatic osteoarthritis of first carpometacarpal joint (M18.2-, M18.3-)*

     M19.141 Post-traumatic osteoarthritis, right hand
     M19.142 Post-traumatic osteoarthritis, left hand
     M19.149 Post-traumatic osteoarthritis, unspecified hand

☑6ᵗʰ **M19.17** Post-traumatic osteoarthritis, **ankle and foot**
     M19.171 Post-traumatic osteoarthritis, right ankle and foot
     M19.172 Post-traumatic osteoarthritis, left ankle and foot
     M19.179 Post-traumatic osteoarthritis, unspecified ankle and foot

☑5ᵗʰ **M19.2** Secondary **osteoarthritis of other joints**

☑6ᵗʰ **M19.21** Secondary osteoarthritis, **shoulder**
     M19.211 Secondary osteoarthritis, right shoulder
     M19.212 Secondary osteoarthritis, left shoulder

☑ Additional Character Required   ☑x7ᵗʰ Placeholder   Unacceptable PDx   Questionable PDx   Manifestation   Unspecified Dx   H1-H14 HAC   HCC CMS-HCC Dx   HIV HIV Dx

ICD-10-CM 2020

787

Chapter 13. Diseases of the Musculoskeletal System and Connective Tissue

M16.1–M19.212

M19.219 Secondary osteoarthritis, unspecified shoulder

√6ᵗʰ **M19.22** Secondary osteoarthritis, elbow

M19.221 Secondary osteoarthritis, right elbow
M19.222 Secondary osteoarthritis, left elbow
M19.229 Secondary osteoarthritis, unspecified elbow

√6ᵗʰ **M19.23** Secondary osteoarthritis, wrist

M19.231 Secondary osteoarthritis, right wrist
M19.232 Secondary osteoarthritis, left wrist
M19.239 Secondary osteoarthritis, unspecified wrist

√6ᵗʰ **M19.24** Secondary osteoarthritis, hand

M19.241 Secondary osteoarthritis, right hand
M19.242 Secondary osteoarthritis, left hand
M19.249 Secondary osteoarthritis, unspecified hand

√6ᵗʰ **M19.27** Secondary osteoarthritis, ankle and foot

M19.271 Secondary osteoarthritis, right ankle and foot
M19.272 Secondary osteoarthritis, left ankle and foot
M19.279 Secondary osteoarthritis, unspecified ankle and foot

√5ᵗʰ **M19.9** Osteoarthritis, unspecified site

M19.90 Unspecified osteoarthritis, unspecified site
Arthrosis NOS
Arthritis NOS
Osteoarthritis NOS
AHA: 2016,4Q,147

M19.91 Primary osteoarthritis, unspecified site
Primary osteoarthritis NOS

M19.92 Post-traumatic osteoarthritis, unspecified site
Post-traumatic osteoarthritis NOS

M19.93 Secondary osteoarthritis, unspecified site
Secondary osteoarthritis NOS

Other joint disorders (M20-M25)

EXCLUDES 2   joints of the spine (M40-M54)

√4ᵗʰ **M20** Acquired deformities of fingers and toes

EXCLUDES 1   acquired absence of fingers and toes (Z89.-)
congenital absence of fingers and toes (Q71.3-, Q72.3-)
congenital deformities and malformations of fingers and toes (Q66.-, Q68-Q70, Q74.-)

√5ᵗʰ **M20.0** Deformity of finger(s)

EXCLUDES 1   clubbing of fingers (R68.3)
palmar fascial fibromatosis [Dupuytren] (M72.0)
trigger finger (M65.3)

√6ᵗʰ **M20.00** Unspecified deformity of finger(s)

M20.001 Unspecified deformity of right finger(s)
M20.002 Unspecified deformity of left finger(s)
M20.009 Unspecified deformity of unspecified finger(s)

√6ᵗʰ **M20.01** Mallet finger

M20.011 Mallet finger of right finger(s)
M20.012 Mallet finger of left finger(s)
M20.019 Mallet finger of unspecified finger(s)

√6ᵗʰ **M20.02** Boutonnière deformity

DEF: Deformity of the finger caused by flexion of the proximal interphalangeal joint and hyperextension of the distal joint. The deformity results from rheumatoid arthritis, osteoarthritis, or injury.

M20.021 Boutonnière deformity of right finger(s)
M20.022 Boutonnière deformity of left finger(s)
M20.029 Boutonnière deformity of unspecified finger(s)

√6ᵗʰ **M20.03** Swan-neck deformity

DEF: Flexed distal and hyperextended proximal interphalangeal joint most commonly caused by rheumatoid arthritis.

M20.031 Swan-neck deformity of right finger(s)
M20.032 Swan-neck deformity of left finger(s)
M20.039 Swan-neck deformity of unspecified finger(s)

√6ᵗʰ **M20.09** Other deformity of finger(s)

M20.091 Other deformity of right finger(s)
M20.092 Other deformity of left finger(s)

M20.099 Other deformity of finger(s), unspecified finger(s)

√5ᵗʰ **M20.1** Hallux valgus (acquired)

EXCLUDES 2   bunion (M21.6-)
AHA: 2016,4Q,38
DEF: Deformity in which the great toe deviates toward the other toes and may even be positioned over or under the second toe.

Hallux Valgus

Hallux valgus

Medial eminence of metatarsal bone

Right foot

M20.10 Hallux valgus (acquired), unspecified foot
M20.11 Hallux valgus (acquired), right foot
M20.12 Hallux valgus (acquired), left foot

√5ᵗʰ **M20.2** Hallux rigidus

M20.20 Hallux rigidus, unspecified foot
M20.21 Hallux rigidus, right foot
M20.22 Hallux rigidus, left foot

√5ᵗʰ **M20.3** Hallux varus (acquired)

DEF: Deformity in which the great toe deviates away from the other toes.

M20.30 Hallux varus (acquired), unspecified foot
M20.31 Hallux varus (acquired), right foot
M20.32 Hallux varus (acquired), left foot

√5ᵗʰ **M20.4** Other hammer toe(s) (acquired)

M20.40 Other hammer toe(s) (acquired), unspecified foot
M20.41 Other hammer toe(s) (acquired), right foot
M20.42 Other hammer toe(s) (acquired), left foot

√5ᵗʰ **M20.5** Other deformities of toe(s) (acquired)

√6ᵗʰ **M20.5X** Other deformities of toe(s) (acquired)

M20.5X1 Other deformities of toe(s) (acquired), right foot
M20.5X2 Other deformities of toe(s) (acquired), left foot
M20.5X9 Other deformities of toe(s) (acquired), unspecified foot

√5ᵗʰ **M20.6** Acquired deformities of toe(s), unspecified

M20.60 Acquired deformities of toe(s), unspecified, unspecified foot
M20.61 Acquired deformities of toe(s), unspecified, right foot
M20.62 Acquired deformities of toe(s), unspecified, left foot

√4ᵗʰ **M21** Other acquired deformities of limbs

EXCLUDES 1   acquired absence of limb (Z89.-)
congenital absence of limbs (Q71-Q73)
congenital deformities and malformations of limbs (Q65-Q66, Q68-Q74)

EXCLUDES 2   acquired deformities of fingers or toes (M20.-)
coxa plana (M91.2)

√5ᵗʰ **M21.0** Valgus deformity, not elsewhere classified

EXCLUDES 1   metatarsus valgus (Q66.6)
talipes calcaneovalgus ►(Q66.4-)◄

M21.00 Valgus deformity, not elsewhere classified, unspecified site

---

N Newborn: 0   P Pediatric: 0-17   M Maternity: 9-64   A Adult: 15-124   MCC Major Complication/Comorbidity   CC Complication/Comorbidity   SW Severe Wound Dx

✓6ᵗʰ **M21.02 Valgus deformity, not elsewhere classified, elbow**
     Cubitus valgus
     M21.021 Valgus deformity, not elsewhere classified, right elbow
     M21.022 Valgus deformity, not elsewhere classified, left elbow
     M21.029 Valgus deformity, not elsewhere classified, unspecified elbow

✓6ᵗʰ **M21.05 Valgus deformity, not elsewhere classified, hip**
     M21.051 Valgus deformity, not elsewhere classified, right hip
     M21.052 Valgus deformity, not elsewhere classified, left hip
     M21.059 Valgus deformity, not elsewhere classified, unspecified hip

✓6ᵗʰ **M21.06 Valgus deformity, not elsewhere classified, knee**
     Genu valgum
     Knock knee
     DEF: Genu valga/valgum: Condition in which the thighs slant inward, causing the knees to be angled abnormally close together, leaving the space between the ankles wider than normal.

Genu Valga (knock-knee)

     M21.061 Valgus deformity, not elsewhere classified, right knee
     M21.062 Valgus deformity, not elsewhere classified, left knee
     M21.069 Valgus deformity, not elsewhere classified, unspecified knee

✓6ᵗʰ **M21.07 Valgus deformity, not elsewhere classified, ankle**
     M21.071 Valgus deformity, not elsewhere classified, right ankle
     M21.072 Valgus deformity, not elsewhere classified, left ankle
     M21.079 Valgus deformity, not elsewhere classified, unspecified ankle

✓5ᵗʰ **M21.1 Varus deformity, not elsewhere classified**
     EXCLUDES 1   metatarsus varus ▶(Q66.22-)◀
                   tibia vara (M92.5)

     M21.10 Varus deformity, not elsewhere classified, unspecified site

✓6ᵗʰ **M21.12 Varus deformity, not elsewhere classified, elbow**
     Cubitus varus, elbow
     M21.121 Varus deformity, not elsewhere classified, right elbow
     M21.122 Varus deformity, not elsewhere classified, left elbow
     M21.129 Varus deformity, not elsewhere classified, unspecified elbow

✓6ᵗʰ **M21.15 Varus deformity, not elsewhere classified, hip**
     M21.151 Varus deformity, not elsewhere classified, right hip
     M21.152 Varus deformity, not elsewhere classified, left hip

     M21.159 Varus deformity, not elsewhere classified, unspecified

✓6ᵗʰ **M21.16 Varus deformity, not elsewhere classified, knee**
     Bow leg
     Genu varum
     DEF: Genu varus/varum: Condition in which the thighs and/or legs are bowed in an outward curve with an abnormally increased space between the knees.

Genu Varus (bowleg)

     M21.161 Varus deformity, not elsewhere classified, right knee
     M21.162 Varus deformity, not elsewhere classified, left knee
     M21.169 Varus deformity, not elsewhere classified, unspecified knee

✓6ᵗʰ **M21.17 Varus deformity, not elsewhere classified, ankle**
     M21.171 Varus deformity, not elsewhere classified, right ankle
     M21.172 Varus deformity, not elsewhere classified, left ankle
     M21.179 Varus deformity, not elsewhere classified, unspecified ankle

✓5ᵗʰ **M21.2 Flexion deformity**
     M21.20 Flexion deformity, unspecified site

✓6ᵗʰ **M21.21 Flexion deformity, shoulder**
     M21.211 Flexion deformity, right shoulder
     M21.212 Flexion deformity, left shoulder
     M21.219 Flexion deformity, unspecified shoulder

✓6ᵗʰ **M21.22 Flexion deformity, elbow**
     M21.221 Flexion deformity, right elbow
     M21.222 Flexion deformity, left elbow
     M21.229 Flexion deformity, unspecified elbow

✓6ᵗʰ **M21.23 Flexion deformity, wrist**
     M21.231 Flexion deformity, right wrist
     M21.232 Flexion deformity, left wrist
     M21.239 Flexion deformity, unspecified wrist

✓6ᵗʰ **M21.24 Flexion deformity, finger joints**
     M21.241 Flexion deformity, right finger joints
     M21.242 Flexion deformity, left finger joints
     M21.249 Flexion deformity, unspecified finger joints

✓6ᵗʰ **M21.25 Flexion deformity, hip**
     M21.251 Flexion deformity, right hip
     M21.252 Flexion deformity, left hip
     M21.259 Flexion deformity, unspecified hip

✓6ᵗʰ **M21.26 Flexion deformity, knee**
     M21.261 Flexion deformity, right knee
     M21.262 Flexion deformity, left knee
     M21.269 Flexion deformity, unspecified knee

✓6ᵗʰ **M21.27 Flexion deformity, ankle and toes**
     M21.271 Flexion deformity, right ankle and toes
     M21.272 Flexion deformity, left ankle and toes

           M21.279 Flexion deformity, unspecified ankle and toes

✓5ᵗʰ **M21.3** Wrist or foot drop (acquired)

    ✓6ᵗʰ **M21.33** Wrist drop (acquired)

        M21.331 Wrist drop, right wrist
        M21.332 Wrist drop, left wrist
        M21.339 Wrist drop, unspecified wrist

    ✓6ᵗʰ **M21.37** Foot drop (acquired)

        M21.371 Foot drop, right foot
        M21.372 Foot drop, left foot
        M21.379 Foot drop, unspecified foot

✓5ᵗʰ **M21.4** Flat foot [pes planus] (acquired)

    EXCLUDES 1   congenital pes planus (Q66.5-)

    M21.40 Flat foot [pes planus] (acquired), unspecified foot
    M21.41 Flat foot [pes planus] (acquired), right foot
    M21.42 Flat foot [pes planus] (acquired), left foot

✓5ᵗʰ **M21.5** Acquired clawhand, clubhand, clawfoot and clubfoot

    EXCLUDES 1   clubfoot, not specified as acquired (Q66.89)

    ✓6ᵗʰ **M21.51** Acquired clawhand

        M21.511 Acquired clawhand, right hand
        M21.512 Acquired clawhand, left hand
        M21.519 Acquired clawhand, unspecified hand

    ✓6ᵗʰ **M21.52** Acquired clubhand

        M21.521 Acquired clubhand, right hand
        M21.522 Acquired clubhand, left hand
        M21.529 Acquired clubhand, unspecified hand

    ✓6ᵗʰ **M21.53** Acquired clawfoot

        DEF: High foot arch with hyperextended toes at the metatarsophalangeal joint and flexed toes at the distal joints.
        M21.531 Acquired clawfoot, right foot
        M21.532 Acquired clawfoot, left foot
        M21.539 Acquired clawfoot, unspecified foot

    ✓6ᵗʰ **M21.54** Acquired clubfoot

        DEF: Acquired anomaly of the foot with the heel elevated and rotated outward and the toes pointing inward.
        M21.541 Acquired clubfoot, right foot
        M21.542 Acquired clubfoot, left foot
        M21.549 Acquired clubfoot, unspecified foot

✓5ᵗʰ **M21.6** Other acquired deformities of foot

    EXCLUDES 2   deformities of toe (acquired) (M20.1-M20.6-)

    AHA: 2016,4Q,38

    ✓6ᵗʰ **M21.61** Bunion

        M21.611 Bunion of right foot
        M21.612 Bunion of left foot
        M21.619 Bunion of unspecified foot

    ✓6ᵗʰ **M21.62** Bunionette

        M21.621 Bunionette of right foot
        M21.622 Bunionette of left foot
        M21.629 Bunionette of unspecified foot

    ✓6ᵗʰ **M21.6X** Other acquired deformities of foot

        M21.6X1 Other acquired deformities of right foot
        M21.6X2 Other acquired deformities of left foot
        M21.6X9 Other acquired deformities of unspecified foot

✓5ᵗʰ **M21.7** Unequal limb length (acquired)

    NOTE   The site used should correspond to the shorter limb

    M21.70 Unequal limb length (acquired), unspecified site

    ✓6ᵗʰ **M21.72** Unequal limb length (acquired), humerus

        M21.721 Unequal limb length (acquired), right humerus
        M21.722 Unequal limb length (acquired), left humerus
        M21.729 Unequal limb length (acquired), unspecified humerus

    ✓6ᵗʰ **M21.73** Unequal limb length (acquired), ulna and radius

        M21.731 Unequal limb length (acquired), right ulna
        M21.732 Unequal limb length (acquired), left ulna
        M21.733 Unequal limb length (acquired), right radius
        M21.734 Unequal limb length (acquired), left radius
        M21.739 Unequal limb length (acquired), unspecified ulna and radius

    ✓6ᵗʰ **M21.75** Unequal limb length (acquired), femur

        M21.751 Unequal limb length (acquired), right femur
        M21.752 Unequal limb length (acquired), left femur
        M21.759 Unequal limb length (acquired), unspecified femur

    ✓6ᵗʰ **M21.76** Unequal limb length (acquired), tibia and fibula

        M21.761 Unequal limb length (acquired), right tibia
        M21.762 Unequal limb length (acquired), left tibia
        M21.763 Unequal limb length (acquired), right fibula
        M21.764 Unequal limb length (acquired), left fibula
        M21.769 Unequal limb length (acquired), unspecified tibia and fibula

✓5ᵗʰ **M21.8** Other specified acquired deformities of limbs

    EXCLUDES 2   coxa plana (M91.2)

    M21.80 Other specified acquired deformities of unspecified limb

    ✓6ᵗʰ **M21.82** Other specified acquired deformities of upper arm

        M21.821 Other specified acquired deformities of right upper arm
        M21.822 Other specified acquired deformities of left upper arm
        M21.829 Other specified acquired deformities of unspecified upper arm

    ✓6ᵗʰ **M21.83** Other specified acquired deformities of forearm

        M21.831 Other specified acquired deformities of right forearm
        M21.832 Other specified acquired deformities of left forearm
        M21.839 Other specified acquired deformities of unspecified forearm

    ✓6ᵗʰ **M21.85** Other specified acquired deformities of thigh

        M21.851 Other specified acquired deformities of right thigh
        M21.852 Other specified acquired deformities of left thigh
        M21.859 Other specified acquired deformities of unspecified thigh

    ✓6ᵗʰ **M21.86** Other specified acquired deformities of lower leg

        M21.861 Other specified acquired deformities of right lower leg
        M21.862 Other specified acquired deformities of left lower leg
        M21.869 Other specified acquired deformities of unspecified lower leg

✓5ᵗʰ **M21.9** Unspecified acquired deformity of limb and hand

    M21.90 Unspecified acquired deformity of unspecified limb

    ✓6ᵗʰ **M21.92** Unspecified acquired deformity of upper arm

        M21.921 Unspecified acquired deformity of right upper arm
        M21.922 Unspecified acquired deformity of left upper arm
        M21.929 Unspecified acquired deformity of unspecified upper arm

    ✓6ᵗʰ **M21.93** Unspecified acquired deformity of forearm

        M21.931 Unspecified acquired deformity of right forearm
        M21.932 Unspecified acquired deformity of left forearm
        M21.939 Unspecified acquired deformity of unspecified forearm

    ✓6ᵗʰ **M21.94** Unspecified acquired deformity of hand

        M21.941 Unspecified acquired deformity of hand, right hand
        M21.942 Unspecified acquired deformity of hand, left hand
        M21.949 Unspecified acquired deformity of hand, unspecified hand

    ✓6ᵗʰ **M21.95** Unspecified acquired deformity of thigh

        M21.951 Unspecified acquired deformity of right thigh
        M21.952 Unspecified acquired deformity of left thigh
        M21.959 Unspecified acquired deformity of unspecified thigh

N Newborn: 0   **P** Pediatric: 0-17   **M** Maternity: 9-64   **A** Adult: 15-124   **MCC** Major Complication/Comorbidity   **CC** Complication/Comorbidity   **SW** Severe Wound Dx

790   ICD-10-CM 2020

✓6ᵗʰ **M21.96 Unspecified acquired deformity of** lower leg

    M21.961 Unspecified acquired deformity of right lower leg

    M21.962 Unspecified acquired deformity of left lower leg

    M21.969 Unspecified acquired deformity of unspecified lower leg

✓4ᵗʰ **M22 Disorder of patella**

    EXCLUDES 1   traumatic dislocation of patella (S83.0-)

✓5ᵗʰ **M22.0 Recurrent dislocation of patella**

    M22.00 Recurrent dislocation of patella, unspecified knee

    M22.01 Recurrent dislocation of patella, right **knee**

    M22.02 Recurrent dislocation of patella, left **knee**

✓5ᵗʰ **M22.1 Recurrent subluxation of patella**

    Incomplete dislocation of patella

    M22.10 Recurrent subluxation of patella, unspecified knee

    M22.11 Recurrent subluxation of patella, right **knee**

    M22.12 Recurrent subluxation of patella, left **knee**

✓5ᵗʰ **M22.2 Patellofemoral disorders**

    ✓6ᵗʰ **M22.2X Patellofemoral disorders**

      M22.2X1 Patellofemoral disorders, right **knee**

      M22.2X2 Patellofemoral disorders, left **knee**

      M22.2X9 Patellofemoral disorders, unspecified knee

✓5ᵗʰ **M22.3 Other derangements of patella**

    ✓6ᵗʰ **M22.3X Other derangements of patella**

      M22.3X1 Other derangements of patella, right **knee**

      M22.3X2 Other derangements of patella, left **knee**

      M22.3X9 Other derangements of patella, unspecified knee

✓5ᵗʰ **M22.4 Chondromalacia patellae**

    M22.40 Chondromalacia patellae, unspecified knee

    M22.41 Chondromalacia patellae, right **knee**

    M22.42 Chondromalacia patellae, left **knee**

✓5ᵗʰ **M22.8 Other disorders of patella**

    ✓6ᵗʰ **M22.8X Other disorders of patella**

      M22.8X1 Other disorders of patella, right **knee**

      M22.8X2 Other disorders of patella, left **knee**

      M22.8X9 Other disorders of patella, unspecified knee

✓5ᵗʰ **M22.9 Unspecified disorder of patella**

    M22.90 Unspecified disorder of patella, unspecified knee

    M22.91 Unspecified disorder of patella, right **knee**

    M22.92 Unspecified disorder of patella, left **knee**

✓4ᵗʰ **M23 Internal derangement of knee**

    EXCLUDES 1   ankylosis (M24.66)

       current injury — see injury of knee and lower leg (S80-S89)

       deformity of knee (M21.-)

       osteochondritis dissecans (M93.2)

       recurrent dislocation or subluxation of joints (M24.4)

       recurrent dislocation or subluxation of patella (M22.0-M22.1)

✓5ᵗʰ **M23.0 Cystic meniscus**

    ✓6ᵗʰ **M23.00 Cystic meniscus, unspecified meniscus**

      Cystic meniscus, unspecified lateral meniscus

      Cystic meniscus, unspecified medial meniscus

      M23.000 Cystic meniscus, unspecified lateral **meniscus,** right **knee**

      M23.001 Cystic meniscus, unspecified lateral **meniscus,** left **knee**

      M23.002 Cystic meniscus, unspecified lateral **meniscus, unspecified knee**

      M23.003 Cystic meniscus, unspecified medial **meniscus,** right **knee**

      M23.004 Cystic meniscus, unspecified medial **meniscus,** left **knee**

      M23.005 Cystic meniscus, unspecified medial **meniscus, unspecified knee**

      M23.006 Cystic meniscus, unspecified meniscus, right **knee**

      M23.007 Cystic meniscus, unspecified meniscus, left **knee**

      M23.009 Cystic meniscus, unspecified meniscus, unspecified knee

✓6ᵗʰ **M23.01 Cystic meniscus,** anterior horn of medial **meniscus**

    M23.011 Cystic meniscus, anterior horn of medial meniscus, right **knee**

    M23.012 Cystic meniscus, anterior horn of medial meniscus, left **knee**

    M23.019 Cystic meniscus, anterior horn of medial meniscus, unspecified knee

✓6ᵗʰ **M23.02 Cystic meniscus,** posterior horn of medial **meniscus**

    M23.021 Cystic meniscus, posterior horn of medial meniscus, right **knee**

    M23.022 Cystic meniscus, posterior horn of medial meniscus, left **knee**

    M23.029 Cystic meniscus, posterior horn of medial meniscus, unspecified knee

✓6ᵗʰ **M23.03 Cystic meniscus,** other medial **meniscus**

    M23.031 Cystic meniscus, other medial meniscus, right **knee**

    M23.032 Cystic meniscus, other medial meniscus, left **knee**

    M23.039 Cystic meniscus, other medial meniscus, unspecified knee

✓6ᵗʰ **M23.04 Cystic meniscus,** anterior horn of lateral **meniscus**

    M23.041 Cystic meniscus, anterior horn of lateral meniscus, right **knee**

    M23.042 Cystic meniscus, anterior horn of lateral meniscus, left **knee**

    M23.049 Cystic meniscus, anterior horn of lateral meniscus, unspecified knee

✓6ᵗʰ **M23.05 Cystic meniscus,** posterior horn of lateral **meniscus**

    M23.051 Cystic meniscus, posterior horn of lateral meniscus, right **knee**

    M23.052 Cystic meniscus, posterior horn of lateral meniscus, left **knee**

    M23.059 Cystic meniscus, posterior horn of lateral meniscus, unspecified knee

✓6ᵗʰ **M23.06 Cystic meniscus,** other lateral **meniscus**

    M23.061 Cystic meniscus, other lateral meniscus, right **knee**

    M23.062 Cystic meniscus, other lateral meniscus, left **knee**

    M23.069 Cystic meniscus, other lateral meniscus, unspecified knee

✓5ᵗʰ **M23.2 Derangement of meniscus due to old tear or injury**

    Old bucket-handle tear

    AHA: 2019,2Q,26

Derangement of Meniscus

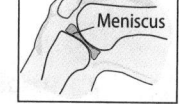

Lateral meniscus · Posterior cruciate ligament · Medial meniscus

Anterior horns · Posterior horns · Patellar ligament · Anterior cruciate ligament

Overhead view of right knee

Bucket handle tear

Radial tear

Meniscus

✓6ᵗʰ **M23.20 Derangement of unspecified meniscus due to old tear or injury**

    Derangement of unspecified lateral meniscus due to old tear or injury

    Derangement of unspecified medial meniscus due to old tear or injury

    M23.200 Derangement of unspecified lateral **meniscus due to old tear or injury,** right **knee**

✔ Additional Character Required   ✓×7ᵗʰ Placeholder   Unacceptable PDx   Questionable PDx   Manifestation   Unspecified Dx   H1-H14 HAC   HCC CMS-HCC Dx   HIV HIV Dx

ICD-10-CM 2020   791

M23.201   Derangement of unspecified lateral meniscus due to old tear or injury, left knee

M23.202   Derangement of unspecified lateral meniscus due to old tear or injury, unspecified knee

M23.203   Derangement of unspecified medial meniscus due to old tear or injury, right knee

M23.204   Derangement of unspecified medial meniscus due to old tear or injury, left knee

M23.205   Derangement of unspecified medial meniscus due to old tear or injury, unspecified knee

M23.206   Derangement of unspecified meniscus due to old tear or injury, right knee

M23.207   Derangement of unspecified meniscus due to old tear or injury, left knee

M23.209   Derangement of unspecified meniscus due to old tear or injury, unspecified knee

√6ᵗʰ M23.21   Derangement of anterior horn of medial meniscus due to old tear or injury

   M23.211   Derangement of anterior horn of medial meniscus due to old tear or injury, right knee

   M23.212   Derangement of anterior horn of medial meniscus due to old tear or injury, left knee

   M23.219   Derangement of anterior horn of medial meniscus due to old tear or injury, unspecified knee

√6ᵗʰ M23.22   Derangement of posterior horn of medial meniscus due to old tear or injury

   M23.221   Derangement of posterior horn of medial meniscus due to old tear or injury, right knee

   M23.222   Derangement of posterior horn of medial meniscus due to old tear or injury, left knee

   M23.229   Derangement of posterior horn of medial meniscus due to old tear or injury, unspecified knee

√6ᵗʰ M23.23   Derangement of other medial meniscus due to old tear or injury

   M23.231   Derangement of other medial meniscus due to old tear or injury, right knee

   M23.232   Derangement of other medial meniscus due to old tear or injury, left knee

   M23.239   Derangement of other medial meniscus due to old tear or injury, unspecified knee

√6ᵗʰ M23.24   Derangement of anterior horn of lateral meniscus due to old tear or injury

   M23.241   Derangement of anterior horn of lateral meniscus due to old tear or injury, right knee

   M23.242   Derangement of anterior horn of lateral meniscus due to old tear or injury, left knee

   M23.249   Derangement of anterior horn of lateral meniscus due to old tear or injury, unspecified knee

√6ᵗʰ M23.25   Derangement of posterior horn of lateral meniscus due to old tear or injury

   M23.251   Derangement of posterior horn of lateral meniscus due to old tear or injury, right knee

   M23.252   Derangement of posterior horn of lateral meniscus due to old tear or injury, left knee

   M23.259   Derangement of posterior horn of lateral meniscus due to old tear or injury, unspecified knee

√6ᵗʰ M23.26   Derangement of other lateral meniscus due to old tear or injury

   M23.261   Derangement of other lateral meniscus due to old tear or injury, right knee

   M23.262   Derangement of other lateral meniscus due to old tear or injury, left knee

   M23.269   Derangement of other lateral meniscus due to old tear or injury, unspecified knee

√5ᵗʰ M23.3   Other meniscus derangements

   Degenerate meniscus
   Detached meniscus
   Retained meniscus

√6ᵗʰ M23.30   Other meniscus derangements, unspecified meniscus

   Other meniscus derangements, unspecified lateral meniscus
   Other meniscus derangements, unspecified medial meniscus

   M23.300   Other meniscus derangements, unspecified lateral meniscus, right knee

   M23.301   Other meniscus derangements, unspecified lateral meniscus, left knee

   M23.302   Other meniscus derangements, unspecified lateral meniscus, unspecified knee

   M23.303   Other meniscus derangements, unspecified medial meniscus, right knee

   M23.304   Other meniscus derangements, unspecified medial meniscus, left knee

   M23.305   Other meniscus derangements, unspecified medial meniscus, unspecified knee

   M23.306   Other meniscus derangements, unspecified meniscus, right knee

   M23.307   Other meniscus derangements, unspecified meniscus, left knee

   M23.309   Other meniscus derangements, unspecified meniscus, unspecified knee

√6ᵗʰ M23.31   Other meniscus derangements, anterior horn of medial meniscus

   M23.311   Other meniscus derangements, anterior horn of medial meniscus, right knee

   M23.312   Other meniscus derangements, anterior horn of medial meniscus, left knee

   M23.319   Other meniscus derangements, anterior horn of medial meniscus, unspecified knee

√6ᵗʰ M23.32   Other meniscus derangements, posterior horn of medial meniscus

   M23.321   Other meniscus derangements, posterior horn of medial meniscus, right knee

   M23.322   Other meniscus derangements, posterior horn of medial meniscus, left knee

   M23.329   Other meniscus derangements, posterior horn of medial meniscus, unspecified knee

√6ᵗʰ M23.33   Other meniscus derangements, other medial meniscus

   M23.331   Other meniscus derangements, other medial meniscus, right knee

   M23.332   Other meniscus derangements, other medial meniscus, left knee

   M23.339   Other meniscus derangements, other medial meniscus, unspecified knee

√6ᵗʰ M23.34   Other meniscus derangements, anterior horn of lateral meniscus

   M23.341   Other meniscus derangements, anterior horn of lateral meniscus, right knee

   M23.342   Other meniscus derangements, anterior horn of lateral meniscus, left knee

   M23.349   Other meniscus derangements, anterior horn of lateral meniscus, unspecified knee

√6ᵗʰ M23.35   Other meniscus derangements, posterior horn of lateral meniscus

   M23.351   Other meniscus derangements, posterior horn of lateral meniscus, right knee

   M23.352   Other meniscus derangements, posterior horn of lateral meniscus, left knee

   M23.359   Other meniscus derangements, posterior horn of lateral meniscus, unspecified knee

√6ᵗʰ M23.36   Other meniscus derangements, other lateral meniscus

   M23.361   Other meniscus derangements, other lateral meniscus, right knee

   M23.362   Other meniscus derangements, other lateral meniscus, left knee

   M23.369   Other meniscus derangements, other lateral meniscus, unspecified knee

N Newborn: 0   P Pediatric: 0-17   M Maternity: 9-64   A Adult: 15-124   MCC Major Complication/Comorbidity   CC Complication/Comorbidity   SW Severe Wound Dx

792   ICD-10-CM 2020

✓5ᵗʰ **M23.4 Loose body in knee**
- **M23.40 Loose body in knee, unspecified knee**
- **M23.41 Loose body in knee, right knee**
- **M23.42 Loose body in knee, left knee**

✓5ᵗʰ **M23.5 Chronic instability of knee**
- **M23.50 Chronic instability of knee, unspecified knee**
- **M23.51 Chronic instability of knee, right knee**
- **M23.52 Chronic instability of knee, left knee**

✓5ᵗʰ **M23.6 Other spontaneous disruption of ligament(s) of knee**
- ✓6ᵗʰ **M23.60 Other spontaneous disruption of unspecified ligament of knee**
  - **M23.601 Other spontaneous disruption of unspecified ligament of right knee**
  - **M23.602 Other spontaneous disruption of unspecified ligament of left knee**
  - **M23.609 Other spontaneous disruption of unspecified ligament of unspecified knee**
- ✓6ᵗʰ **M23.61 Other spontaneous disruption of anterior cruciate ligament of knee**
  - **M23.611 Other spontaneous disruption of anterior cruciate ligament of right knee**
  - **M23.612 Other spontaneous disruption of anterior cruciate ligament of left knee**
  - **M23.619 Other spontaneous disruption of anterior cruciate ligament of unspecified knee**
- ✓6ᵗʰ **M23.62 Other spontaneous disruption of posterior cruciate ligament of knee**
  - **M23.621 Other spontaneous disruption of posterior cruciate ligament of right knee**
  - **M23.622 Other spontaneous disruption of posterior cruciate ligament of left knee**
  - **M23.629 Other spontaneous disruption of posterior cruciate ligament of unspecified knee**
- ✓6ᵗʰ **M23.63 Other spontaneous disruption of medial collateral ligament of knee**
  - **M23.631 Other spontaneous disruption of medial collateral ligament of right knee**
  - **M23.632 Other spontaneous disruption of medial collateral ligament of left knee**
  - **M23.639 Other spontaneous disruption of medial collateral ligament of unspecified knee**
- ✓6ᵗʰ **M23.64 Other spontaneous disruption of lateral collateral ligament of knee**
  - **M23.641 Other spontaneous disruption of lateral collateral ligament of right knee**
  - **M23.642 Other spontaneous disruption of lateral collateral ligament of left knee**
  - **M23.649 Other spontaneous disruption of lateral collateral ligament of unspecified knee**
- ✓6ᵗʰ **M23.67 Other spontaneous disruption of capsular ligament of knee**
  - **M23.671 Other spontaneous disruption of capsular ligament of right knee**
  - **M23.672 Other spontaneous disruption of capsular ligament of left knee**
  - **M23.679 Other spontaneous disruption of capsular ligament of unspecified knee**

✓5ᵗʰ **M23.8 Other internal derangements of knee**
  Laxity of ligament of knee
  Snapping knee
- ✓6ᵗʰ **M23.8X Other internal derangements of knee**
  - **M23.8X1 Other internal derangements of right knee**
  - **M23.8X2 Other internal derangements of left knee**
  - **M23.8X9 Other internal derangements of unspecified knee**

✓5ᵗʰ **M23.9 Unspecified internal derangement of knee**
- **M23.90 Unspecified internal derangement of unspecified knee**
- **M23.91 Unspecified internal derangement of right knee**
- **M23.92 Unspecified internal derangement of left knee**

✓4ᵗʰ **M24 Other specific joint derangements**
- EXCLUDES 1 *current injury — see injury of joint by body region*
- EXCLUDES 2 *ganglion (M67.4)*
  snapping knee (M23.8-)
  temporomandibular joint disorders (M26.6-)

✓5ᵗʰ **M24.0 Loose body in joint**
- EXCLUDES 2 *loose body in knee (M23.4)*
  - **M24.00 Loose body in unspecified joint**
- ✓6ᵗʰ **M24.01 Loose body in shoulder**
  - **M24.011 Loose body in right shoulder**
  - **M24.012 Loose body in left shoulder**
  - **M24.019 Loose body in unspecified shoulder**
- ✓6ᵗʰ **M24.02 Loose body in elbow**
  - **M24.021 Loose body in right elbow**
  - **M24.022 Loose body in left elbow**
  - **M24.029 Loose body in unspecified elbow**
- ✓6ᵗʰ **M24.03 Loose body in wrist**
  - **M24.031 Loose body in right wrist**
  - **M24.032 Loose body in left wrist**
  - **M24.039 Loose body in unspecified wrist**
- ✓6ᵗʰ **M24.04 Loose body in finger joints**
  - **M24.041 Loose body in right finger joint(s)**
  - **M24.042 Loose body in left finger joint(s)**
  - **M24.049 Loose body in unspecified finger joint(s)**
- ✓6ᵗʰ **M24.05 Loose body in hip**
  - **M24.051 Loose body in right hip**
  - **M24.052 Loose body in left hip**
  - **M24.059 Loose body in unspecified hip**
- ✓6ᵗʰ **M24.07 Loose body in ankle and toe joints**
  - **M24.071 Loose body in right ankle**
  - **M24.072 Loose body in left ankle**
  - **M24.073 Loose body in unspecified ankle**
  - **M24.074 Loose body in right toe joint(s)**
  - **M24.075 Loose body in left toe joint(s)**
  - **M24.076 Loose body in unspecified toe joints**
- **M24.08 Loose body, other site**

✓5ᵗʰ **M24.1 Other articular cartilage disorders**
- EXCLUDES 2 *chondrocalcinosis (M11.1, M11.2-)*
  internal derangement of knee (M23.-)
  metastatic calcification (E83.5)
  ochronosis (E70.2)
  - **M24.10 Other articular cartilage disorders, unspecified site**
- ✓6ᵗʰ **M24.11 Other articular cartilage disorders, shoulder**
  - **M24.111 Other articular cartilage disorders, right shoulder**
  - **M24.112 Other articular cartilage disorders, left shoulder**
  - **M24.119 Other articular cartilage disorders, unspecified shoulder**
- ✓6ᵗʰ **M24.12 Other articular cartilage disorders, elbow**
  - **M24.121 Other articular cartilage disorders, right elbow**
  - **M24.122 Other articular cartilage disorders, left elbow**
  - **M24.129 Other articular cartilage disorders, unspecified elbow**
- ✓6ᵗʰ **M24.13 Other articular cartilage disorders, wrist**
  - **M24.131 Other articular cartilage disorders, right wrist**
  - **M24.132 Other articular cartilage disorders, left wrist**
  - **M24.139 Other articular cartilage disorders, unspecified wrist**
- ✓6ᵗʰ **M24.14 Other articular cartilage disorders, hand**
  - **M24.141 Other articular cartilage disorders, right hand**
  - **M24.142 Other articular cartilage disorders, left hand**
  - **M24.149 Other articular cartilage disorders, unspecified hand**
- ✓6ᵗʰ **M24.15 Other articular cartilage disorders, hip**
  - **M24.151 Other articular cartilage disorders, right hip**
  - **M24.152 Other articular cartilage disorders, left hip**
  - **M24.159 Other articular cartilage disorders, unspecified hip**

Chapter 13. Diseases of the Musculoskeletal System and Connective Tissue

√6ᵗʰ **M24.17** Other articular cartilage disorders, ankle and foot

    M24.171 Other articular cartilage disorders, right ankle

    M24.172 Other articular cartilage disorders, left ankle

    M24.173 Other articular cartilage disorders, unspecified ankle

    M24.174 Other articular cartilage disorders, right foot

    M24.175 Other articular cartilage disorders, left foot

    M24.176 Other articular cartilage disorders, unspecified foot

√5ᵗʰ **M24.2** Disorder of ligament

    Instability secondary to old ligament injury

    Ligamentous laxity NOS

    EXCLUDES 1   familial ligamentous laxity (M35.7)

    EXCLUDES 2   internal derangement of knee ▶(M23.5-M23.8X9)◀

    M24.20 Disorder of ligament, unspecified site

√6ᵗʰ **M24.21** Disorder of ligament, shoulder

    M24.211 Disorder of ligament, right shoulder

    M24.212 Disorder of ligament, left shoulder

    M24.219 Disorder of ligament, unspecified shoulder

√6ᵗʰ **M24.22** Disorder of ligament, elbow

    M24.221 Disorder of ligament, right elbow

    M24.222 Disorder of ligament, left elbow

    M24.229 Disorder of ligament, unspecified elbow

√6ᵗʰ **M24.23** Disorder of ligament, wrist

    M24.231 Disorder of ligament, right wrist

    M24.232 Disorder of ligament, left wrist

    M24.239 Disorder of ligament, unspecified wrist

√6ᵗʰ **M24.24** Disorder of ligament, hand

    M24.241 Disorder of ligament, right hand

    M24.242 Disorder of ligament, left hand

    M24.249 Disorder of ligament, unspecified hand

√6ᵗʰ **M24.25** Disorder of ligament, hip

    M24.251 Disorder of ligament, right hip

    M24.252 Disorder of ligament, left hip

    M24.259 Disorder of ligament, unspecified hip

√6ᵗʰ **M24.27** Disorder of ligament, ankle and foot

    M24.271 Disorder of ligament, right ankle

    M24.272 Disorder of ligament, left ankle

    M24.273 Disorder of ligament, unspecified ankle

    M24.274 Disorder of ligament, right foot

    M24.275 Disorder of ligament, left foot

    M24.276 Disorder of ligament, unspecified foot

    M24.28 Disorder of ligament, vertebrae

√5ᵗʰ **M24.3** Pathological dislocation of joint, not elsewhere classified

    EXCLUDES 1   congenital dislocation or displacement of joint — see congenital malformations and deformations of the musculoskeletal system (Q65-Q79)

        current injury — see injury of joints and ligaments by body region

        recurrent dislocation of joint (M24.4-)

    M24.30 Pathological dislocation of unspecified joint, not elsewhere classified

√6ᵗʰ **M24.31** Pathological dislocation of shoulder, not elsewhere classified

    M24.311 Pathological dislocation of right shoulder, not elsewhere classified

    M24.312 Pathological dislocation of left shoulder, not elsewhere classified

    M24.319 Pathological dislocation of unspecified shoulder, not elsewhere classified

√6ᵗʰ **M24.32** Pathological dislocation of elbow, not elsewhere classified

    M24.321 Pathological dislocation of right elbow, not elsewhere classified

    M24.322 Pathological dislocation of left elbow, not elsewhere classified

    M24.329 Pathological dislocation of unspecified elbow, not elsewhere classified

√6ᵗʰ **M24.33** Pathological dislocation of wrist, not elsewhere classified

    M24.331 Pathological dislocation of right wrist, not elsewhere classified

    M24.332 Pathological dislocation of left wrist, not elsewhere classified

    M24.339 Pathological dislocation of unspecified wrist, not elsewhere classified

√6ᵗʰ **M24.34** Pathological dislocation of hand, not elsewhere classified

    M24.341 Pathological dislocation of right hand, not elsewhere classified

    M24.342 Pathological dislocation of left hand, not elsewhere classified

    M24.349 Pathological dislocation of unspecified hand, not elsewhere classified

√6ᵗʰ **M24.35** Pathological dislocation of hip, not elsewhere classified

    M24.351 Pathological dislocation of right hip, not elsewhere classified

    M24.352 Pathological dislocation of left hip, not elsewhere classified

    M24.359 Pathological dislocation of unspecified hip, not elsewhere classified

√6ᵗʰ **M24.36** Pathological dislocation of knee, not elsewhere classified

    M24.361 Pathological dislocation of right knee, not elsewhere classified

    M24.362 Pathological dislocation of left knee, not elsewhere classified

    M24.369 Pathological dislocation of unspecified knee, not elsewhere classified

√6ᵗʰ **M24.37** Pathological dislocation of ankle and foot, not elsewhere classified

    M24.371 Pathological dislocation of right ankle, not elsewhere classified

    M24.372 Pathological dislocation of left ankle, not elsewhere classified

    M24.373 Pathological dislocation of unspecified ankle, not elsewhere classified

    M24.374 Pathological dislocation of right foot, not elsewhere classified

    M24.375 Pathological dislocation of left foot, not elsewhere classified

    M24.376 Pathological dislocation of unspecified foot, not elsewhere classified

√5ᵗʰ **M24.4** Recurrent dislocation of joint

    Recurrent subluxation of joint

    EXCLUDES 2   recurrent dislocation of patella (M22.0-M22.1)

        recurrent vertebral dislocation (M43.3-, M43.4, M43.5-)

    M24.40 Recurrent dislocation, unspecified joint

√6ᵗʰ **M24.41** Recurrent dislocation, shoulder

    M24.411 Recurrent dislocation, right shoulder

    M24.412 Recurrent dislocation, left shoulder

    M24.419 Recurrent dislocation, unspecified shoulder

√6ᵗʰ **M24.42** Recurrent dislocation, elbow

    M24.421 Recurrent dislocation, right elbow

    M24.422 Recurrent dislocation, left elbow

    M24.429 Recurrent dislocation, unspecified elbow

√6ᵗʰ **M24.43** Recurrent dislocation, wrist

    M24.431 Recurrent dislocation, right wrist

    M24.432 Recurrent dislocation, left wrist

    M24.439 Recurrent dislocation, unspecified wrist

√6ᵗʰ **M24.44** Recurrent dislocation, hand and finger(s)

    M24.441 Recurrent dislocation, right hand

    M24.442 Recurrent dislocation, left hand

    M24.443 Recurrent dislocation, unspecified hand

    M24.444 Recurrent dislocation, right finger

    M24.445 Recurrent dislocation, left finger

    M24.446 Recurrent dislocation, unspecified finger

√6ᵗʰ **M24.45** Recurrent dislocation, hip

    M24.451 Recurrent dislocation, right hip

    M24.452 Recurrent dislocation, left hip

    M24.459 Recurrent dislocation, unspecified hip

√6ᵗʰ **M24.46** Recurrent dislocation, knee

    M24.461 Recurrent dislocation, right knee

    M24.462 Recurrent dislocation, left knee

    M24.469 Recurrent dislocation, unspecified knee

√6ᵗʰ **M24.47** Recurrent dislocation, ankle, foot and toes

    M24.471 Recurrent dislocation, right ankle

    M24.472 Recurrent dislocation, left ankle

    M24.473 Recurrent dislocation, unspecified ankle

    M24.474 Recurrent dislocation, right foot

N Newborn: 0   **P** Pediatric: 0-17   **M** Maternity: 9-64   **A** Adult: 15-124   **MCC** Major Complication/Comorbidity   **CC** Complication/Comorbidity   **SW** Severe Wound Dx

794   ICD-10-CM 2020

M24.17–M24.474

M24.475 Recurrent dislocation, left foot
M24.476 Recurrent dislocation, unspecified foot
M24.477 Recurrent dislocation, right toe(s)
M24.478 Recurrent dislocation, left toe(s)
M24.479 Recurrent dislocation, unspecified toe(s)

√5ᵗʰ **M24.5 Contracture of joint**

     EXCLUDES 1   *contracture of muscle without contracture of joint (M62.4-)*
                    contracture of tendon (sheath) without contracture of joint (M62.4-)
                    Dupuytren's contracture (M72.0)
     EXCLUDES 2   *acquired deformities of limbs (M20-M21)*
     AHA: 2016,2Q,6

     M24.50 Contracture, unspecified joint
√6ᵗʰ   **M24.51 Contracture, shoulder**
     M24.511 Contracture, right shoulder
     M24.512 Contracture, left shoulder
     M24.519 Contracture, unspecified shoulder
√6ᵗʰ   **M24.52 Contracture, elbow**
     M24.521 Contracture, right elbow
     M24.522 Contracture, left elbow
     M24.529 Contracture, unspecified elbow
√6ᵗʰ   **M24.53 Contracture, wrist**
     M24.531 Contracture, right wrist
     M24.532 Contracture, left wrist
     M24.539 Contracture, unspecified wrist
√6ᵗʰ   **M24.54 Contracture, hand**
     M24.541 Contracture, right hand
     M24.542 Contracture, left hand
     M24.549 Contracture, unspecified hand
√6ᵗʰ   **M24.55 Contracture, hip**
     M24.551 Contracture, right hip
     M24.552 Contracture, left hip
     M24.559 Contracture, unspecified hip
√6ᵗʰ   **M24.56 Contracture, knee**
     M24.561 Contracture, right knee
     M24.562 Contracture, left knee
     M24.569 Contracture, unspecified knee
√6ᵗʰ   **M24.57 Contracture, ankle and foot**
     M24.571 Contracture, right ankle
     M24.572 Contracture, left ankle
     M24.573 Contracture, unspecified ankle
     M24.574 Contracture, right foot
     M24.575 Contracture, left foot
     M24.576 Contracture, unspecified foot

√5ᵗʰ **M24.6 Ankylosis of joint**

     EXCLUDES 1   *stiffness of joint without ankylosis (M25.6-)*
     EXCLUDES 2   *spine (M43.2-)*
     DEF: Ankylosis: Abnormal union or fusion of bones in a joint, which is normally moveable.

     M24.60 Ankylosis, unspecified joint
√6ᵗʰ   **M24.61 Ankylosis, shoulder**
     M24.611 Ankylosis, right shoulder
     M24.612 Ankylosis, left shoulder
     M24.619 Ankylosis, unspecified shoulder
√6ᵗʰ   **M24.62 Ankylosis, elbow**
     M24.621 Ankylosis, right elbow
     M24.622 Ankylosis, left elbow
     M24.629 Ankylosis, unspecified elbow
√6ᵗʰ   **M24.63 Ankylosis, wrist**
     M24.631 Ankylosis, right wrist
     M24.632 Ankylosis, left wrist
     M24.639 Ankylosis, unspecified wrist
√6ᵗʰ   **M24.64 Ankylosis, hand**
     M24.641 Ankylosis, right hand
     M24.642 Ankylosis, left hand
     M24.649 Ankylosis, unspecified hand
√6ᵗʰ   **M24.65 Ankylosis, hip**
     M24.651 Ankylosis, right hip
     M24.652 Ankylosis, left hip
     M24.659 Ankylosis, unspecified hip
√6ᵗʰ   **M24.66 Ankylosis, knee**
     M24.661 Ankylosis, right knee
     M24.662 Ankylosis, left knee
     M24.669 Ankylosis, unspecified knee

√6ᵗʰ   **M24.67 Ankylosis, ankle and foot**
     M24.671 Ankylosis, right ankle
     M24.672 Ankylosis, left ankle
     M24.673 Ankylosis, unspecified ankle
     M24.674 Ankylosis, right foot
     M24.675 Ankylosis, left foot
     M24.676 Ankylosis, unspecified foot

M24.7 Protrusio acetabuli

     DEF: Intrapelvic protrusion of the acetabulum characterized by the sinking of the floor of the acetabulum, causing the femoral head to protrude. It limits hip movement and is of unknown etiology. **Synonym(s):** *Otto's pelvis.*

√5ᵗʰ **M24.8 Other specific joint derangements, not elsewhere classified**

     EXCLUDES 2   *iliotibial band syndrome (M76.3)*

     M24.80 Other specific joint derangements of unspecified joint, not elsewhere classified
√6ᵗʰ   **M24.81 Other specific joint derangements of shoulder, not elsewhere classified**
     M24.811 Other specific joint derangements of right shoulder, not elsewhere classified
     M24.812 Other specific joint derangements of left shoulder, not elsewhere classified
     M24.819 Other specific joint derangements of unspecified shoulder, not elsewhere classified
√6ᵗʰ   **M24.82 Other specific joint derangements of elbow, not elsewhere classified**
     M24.821 Other specific joint derangements of right elbow, not elsewhere classified
     M24.822 Other specific joint derangements of left elbow, not elsewhere classified
     M24.829 Other specific joint derangements of unspecified elbow, not elsewhere classified
√6ᵗʰ   **M24.83 Other specific joint derangements of wrist, not elsewhere classified**
     M24.831 Other specific joint derangements of right wrist, not elsewhere classified
     M24.832 Other specific joint derangements of left wrist, not elsewhere classified
     M24.839 Other specific joint derangements of unspecified wrist, not elsewhere classified
√6ᵗʰ   **M24.84 Other specific joint derangements of hand, not elsewhere classified**
     M24.841 Other specific joint derangements of right hand, not elsewhere classified
     M24.842 Other specific joint derangements of left hand, not elsewhere classified
     M24.849 Other specific joint derangements of unspecified hand, not elsewhere classified
√6ᵗʰ   **M24.85 Other specific joint derangements of hip, not elsewhere classified**
     Irritable hip
     M24.851 Other specific joint derangements of right hip, not elsewhere classified
     M24.852 Other specific joint derangements of left hip, not elsewhere classified
     M24.859 Other specific joint derangements of unspecified hip, not elsewhere classified
√6ᵗʰ   **M24.87 Other specific joint derangements of ankle and foot, not elsewhere classified**
     M24.871 Other specific joint derangements of right ankle, not elsewhere classified
     M24.872 Other specific joint derangements of left ankle, not elsewhere classified
     M24.873 Other specific joint derangements of unspecified ankle, not elsewhere classified
     M24.874 Other specific joint derangements of right foot, not elsewhere classified
     M24.875 Other specific joint derangements of left foot, not elsewhere classified
     M24.876 Other specific joint derangements of unspecified foot, not elsewhere classified

M24.9 Joint derangement, unspecified

☑ Additional Character Required   √x7ᵗʰ Placeholder   Unacceptable PDx   Questionable PDx   Manifestation   Unspecified Dx   H1-H4 HAC   HCC CMS-HCC Dx   HIV HIV Dx

ICD-10-CM 2020   795

✓4ᵗʰ **M25 Other joint disorder, not elsewhere classified**

     EXCLUDES 2   *abnormality of gait and mobility (R26.-)*
            acquired deformities of limb (M20-M21)
            calcification of bursa (M71.4-)
            calcification of shoulder (joint) (M75.3)
            calcification of tendon (M65.2-)
            difficulty in walking (R26.2)
            temporomandibular joint disorder (M26.6-)

✓5ᵗʰ **M25.0 Hemarthrosis**

     EXCLUDES 1   *current injury — see injury of joint by body region*
            hemophilic arthropathy (M36.2)

     M25.00 Hemarthrosis, unspecified joint   CC
         CC Excl: PDX collection 868

✓6ᵗʰ   **M25.01 Hemarthrosis, shoulder**
         CC Excl: For CC codes in subcategory M25.01: PDX collection 869

         M25.011 Hemarthrosis, right shoulder   CC
         M25.012 Hemarthrosis, left shoulder   CC
         M25.019 Hemarthrosis, unspecified shoulder   CC

✓6ᵗʰ   **M25.02 Hemarthrosis, elbow**
         CC Excl: For CC codes in subcategory M25.02: PDX collection 870

         M25.021 Hemarthrosis, right elbow   CC
         M25.022 Hemarthrosis, left elbow   CC
         M25.029 Hemarthrosis, unspecified elbow   CC

✓6ᵗʰ   **M25.03 Hemarthrosis, wrist**
         CC Excl: For CC codes in subcategory M25.03: PDX collection 871

         M25.031 Hemarthrosis, right wrist   CC
         M25.032 Hemarthrosis, left wrist   CC
         M25.039 Hemarthrosis, unspecified wrist   CC

✓6ᵗʰ   **M25.04 Hemarthrosis, hand**
         CC Excl: For CC codes in subcategory M25.04: PDX collection 872

         M25.041 Hemarthrosis, right hand   CC
         M25.042 Hemarthrosis, left hand   CC
         M25.049 Hemarthrosis, unspecified hand   CC

✓6ᵗʰ   **M25.05 Hemarthrosis, hip**
         CC Excl: For CC codes in subcategory M25.05: PDX collection 868

         M25.051 Hemarthrosis, right hip   CC
         M25.052 Hemarthrosis, left hip   CC
         M25.059 Hemarthrosis, unspecified hip   CC

✓6ᵗʰ   **M25.06 Hemarthrosis, knee**
         CC Excl: For CC codes in subcategory M25.06: PDX collection 873

         M25.061 Hemarthrosis, right knee   CC
         M25.062 Hemarthrosis, left knee   CC
         M25.069 Hemarthrosis, unspecified knee   CC

✓6ᵗʰ   **M25.07 Hemarthrosis, ankle and foot**
         CC Excl: For CC codes in subcategory M25.07: PDX collection 873

         M25.071 Hemarthrosis, right ankle   CC
         M25.072 Hemarthrosis, left ankle   CC
         M25.073 Hemarthrosis, unspecified ankle   CC
         M25.074 Hemarthrosis, right foot   CC
         M25.075 Hemarthrosis, left foot   CC
         M25.076 Hemarthrosis, unspecified foot   CC

     M25.08 Hemarthrosis, other specified site   CC
         Hemarthrosis, vertebrae
         CC Excl: PDX collection 868

✓5ᵗʰ **M25.1 Fistula of joint**

     M25.10 Fistula, unspecified joint   SW

✓6ᵗʰ   **M25.11 Fistula, shoulder**
         M25.111 Fistula, right shoulder   SW
         M25.112 Fistula, left shoulder   SW
         M25.119 Fistula, unspecified shoulder   SW

✓6ᵗʰ   **M25.12 Fistula, elbow**
         M25.121 Fistula, right elbow   SW
         M25.122 Fistula, left elbow   SW
         M25.129 Fistula, unspecified elbow   SW

✓6ᵗʰ   **M25.13 Fistula, wrist**
         M25.131 Fistula, right wrist   SW
         M25.132 Fistula, left wrist   SW
         M25.139 Fistula, unspecified wrist   SW

✓6ᵗʰ   **M25.14 Fistula, hand**
         M25.141 Fistula, right hand   SW
         M25.142 Fistula, left hand   SW
         M25.149 Fistula, unspecified hand   SW

✓6ᵗʰ   **M25.15 Fistula, hip**
         M25.151 Fistula, right hip   SW
         M25.152 Fistula, left hip   SW
         M25.159 Fistula, unspecified hip   SW

✓6ᵗʰ   **M25.16 Fistula, knee**
         M25.161 Fistula, right knee   SW
         M25.162 Fistula, left knee   SW
         M25.169 Fistula, unspecified knee   SW

✓6ᵗʰ   **M25.17 Fistula, ankle and foot**
         M25.171 Fistula, right ankle   SW
         M25.172 Fistula, left ankle   SW
         M25.173 Fistula, unspecified ankle   SW
         M25.174 Fistula, right foot   SW
         M25.175 Fistula, left foot   SW
         M25.176 Fistula, unspecified foot   SW

     M25.18 Fistula, other specified site   SW
         Fistula, vertebrae

✓5ᵗʰ **M25.2 Flail joint**

     DEF: Hinged joint that exhibits an abnormal or excessive degree of range and mobility.

     M25.20 Flail joint, unspecified joint

✓6ᵗʰ   **M25.21 Flail joint, shoulder**
         M25.211 Flail joint, right shoulder
         M25.212 Flail joint, left shoulder
         M25.219 Flail joint, unspecified shoulder

✓6ᵗʰ   **M25.22 Flail joint, elbow**
         M25.221 Flail joint, right elbow
         M25.222 Flail joint, left elbow
         M25.229 Flail joint, unspecified elbow

✓6ᵗʰ   **M25.23 Flail joint, wrist**
         M25.231 Flail joint, right wrist
         M25.232 Flail joint, left wrist
         M25.239 Flail joint, unspecified wrist

✓6ᵗʰ   **M25.24 Flail joint, hand**
         M25.241 Flail joint, right hand
         M25.242 Flail joint, left hand
         M25.249 Flail joint, unspecified hand

✓6ᵗʰ   **M25.25 Flail joint, hip**
         M25.251 Flail joint, right hip
         M25.252 Flail joint, left hip
         M25.259 Flail joint, unspecified hip

✓6ᵗʰ   **M25.26 Flail joint, knee**
         M25.261 Flail joint, right knee
         M25.262 Flail joint, left knee
         M25.269 Flail joint, unspecified knee

✓6ᵗʰ   **M25.27 Flail joint, ankle and foot**
         M25.271 Flail joint, right ankle and foot
         M25.272 Flail joint, left ankle and foot
         M25.279 Flail joint, unspecified ankle and foot

     M25.28 Flail joint, other site

√5th **M25.3　Other instability of joint**

> EXCLUDES 1　instability of joint secondary to old ligament injury (M24.2-)
> instability of joint secondary to removal of joint prosthesis (M96.8-)
> EXCLUDES 2　spinal instabilities (M53.2-)

M25.30　Other instability, unspecified joint

√6th **M25.31　Other instability, shoulder**

M25.311　Other instability, right shoulder
M25.312　Other instability, left shoulder
M25.319　Other instability, unspecified shoulder

√6th **M25.32　Other instability, elbow**

M25.321　Other instability, right elbow
M25.322　Other instability, left elbow
M25.329　Other instability, unspecified elbow

√6th **M25.33　Other instability, wrist**

M25.331　Other instability, right wrist
M25.332　Other instability, left wrist
M25.339　Other instability, unspecified wrist

√6th **M25.34　Other instability, hand**

M25.341　Other instability, right hand
M25.342　Other instability, left hand
M25.349　Other instability, unspecified hand

√6th **M25.35　Other instability, hip**

M25.351　Other instability, right hip
M25.352　Other instability, left hip
M25.359　Other instability, unspecified hip

√6th **M25.36　Other instability, knee**

M25.361　Other instability, right knee
M25.362　Other instability, left knee
M25.369　Other instability, unspecified knee

√6th **M25.37　Other instability, ankle and foot**

M25.371　Other instability, right ankle
M25.372　Other instability, left ankle
M25.373　Other instability, unspecified ankle
M25.374　Other instability, right foot
M25.375　Other instability, left foot
M25.376　Other instability, unspecified foot

√5th **M25.4　Effusion of joint**

> EXCLUDES 1　hydrarthrosis in yaws (A66.6)
> intermittent hydrarthrosis (M12.4-)
> other infective (teno)synovitis (M65.1-)

M25.40　Effusion, unspecified joint

√6th **M25.41　Effusion, shoulder**

M25.411　Effusion, right shoulder
M25.412　Effusion, left shoulder
M25.419　Effusion, unspecified shoulder

√6th **M25.42　Effusion, elbow**

M25.421　Effusion, right elbow
M25.422　Effusion, left elbow
M25.429　Effusion, unspecified elbow

√6th **M25.43　Effusion, wrist**

M25.431　Effusion, right wrist
M25.432　Effusion, left wrist
M25.439　Effusion, unspecified wrist

√6th **M25.44　Effusion, hand**

M25.441　Effusion, right hand
M25.442　Effusion, left hand
M25.449　Effusion, unspecified hand

√6th **M25.45　Effusion, hip**

M25.451　Effusion, right hip
M25.452　Effusion, left hip
M25.459　Effusion, unspecified hip

√6th **M25.46　Effusion, knee**

M25.461　Effusion, right knee
M25.462　Effusion, left knee
M25.469　Effusion, unspecified knee

√6th **M25.47　Effusion, ankle and foot**

M25.471　Effusion, right ankle
M25.472　Effusion, left ankle
M25.473　Effusion, unspecified ankle
M25.474　Effusion, right foot
M25.475　Effusion, left foot
M25.476　Effusion, unspecified foot

M25.48　Effusion, other site

√5th **M25.5　Pain in joint**

> EXCLUDES 2　pain in hand (M79.64-)
> pain in fingers (M79.64-)
> pain in foot (M79.67-)
> pain in limb (M79.6-)
> pain in toes (M79.67-)

M25.50　Pain in unspecified joint

√6th **M25.51　Pain in shoulder**

M25.511　Pain in right shoulder
M25.512　Pain in left shoulder
M25.519　Pain in unspecified shoulder

√6th **M25.52　Pain in elbow**

M25.521　Pain in right elbow
M25.522　Pain in left elbow
M25.529　Pain in unspecified elbow

√6th **M25.53　Pain in wrist**

M25.531　Pain in right wrist
M25.532　Pain in left wrist
M25.539　Pain in unspecified wrist

√6th **M25.54　Pain in joints of hand**

> AHA: 2016,4Q,38

M25.541　Pain in joints of right hand
M25.542　Pain in joints of left hand
M25.549　Pain in joints of unspecified hand
　　　　　Pain in joints of hand NOS

√6th **M25.55　Pain in hip**

M25.551　Pain in right hip
M25.552　Pain in left hip
M25.559　Pain in unspecified hip

√6th **M25.56　Pain in knee**

M25.561　Pain in right knee
M25.562　Pain in left knee
M25.569　Pain in unspecified knee

√6th **M25.57　Pain in ankle and joints of foot**

M25.571　Pain in right ankle and joints of right foot
M25.572　Pain in left ankle and joints of left foot
M25.579　Pain in unspecified ankle and joints of unspecified foot

√5th **M25.6　Stiffness of joint, not elsewhere classified**

> EXCLUDES 1　ankylosis of joint (M24.6-)
> contracture of joint (M24.5-)

M25.60　Stiffness of unspecified joint, not elsewhere classified

√6th **M25.61　Stiffness of shoulder, not elsewhere classified**

M25.611　Stiffness of right shoulder, not elsewhere classified
M25.612　Stiffness of left shoulder, not elsewhere classified
M25.619　Stiffness of unspecified shoulder, not elsewhere classified

√6th **M25.62　Stiffness of elbow, not elsewhere classified**

M25.621　Stiffness of right elbow, not elsewhere classified
M25.622　Stiffness of left elbow, not elsewhere classified
M25.629　Stiffness of unspecified elbow, not elsewhere classified

√6th **M25.63　Stiffness of wrist, not elsewhere classified**

M25.631　Stiffness of right wrist, not elsewhere classified
M25.632　Stiffness of left wrist, not elsewhere classified
M25.639　Stiffness of unspecified wrist, not elsewhere classified

√6th **M25.64　Stiffness of hand, not elsewhere classified**

M25.641　Stiffness of right hand, not elsewhere classified
M25.642　Stiffness of left hand, not elsewhere classified
M25.649　Stiffness of unspecified hand, not elsewhere classified

√6th **M25.65　Stiffness of hip, not elsewhere classified**

M25.651　Stiffness of right hip, not elsewhere classified
M25.652　Stiffness of left hip, not elsewhere classified

☑ Additional Character Required　√x7th Placeholder　Unacceptable PDx　Questionable PDx　Manifestation　Unspecified Dx　H1-H14 HAC　HCC CMS-HCC Dx　HIV HIV Dx

M25.659 Stiffness of unspecified hip, not elsewhere classified

✓6th **M25.66** Stiffness of knee, not elsewhere classified

     M25.661 Stiffness of right knee, not elsewhere classified

     M25.662 Stiffness of left knee, not elsewhere classified

     M25.669 Stiffness of unspecified knee, not elsewhere classified

✓6th **M25.67** Stiffness of ankle and foot, not elsewhere classified

     M25.671 Stiffness of right ankle, not elsewhere classified

     M25.672 Stiffness of left ankle, not elsewhere classified

     M25.673 Stiffness of unspecified ankle, not elsewhere classified

     M25.674 Stiffness of right foot, not elsewhere classified

     M25.675 Stiffness of left foot, not elsewhere classified

     M25.676 Stiffness of unspecified foot, not elsewhere classified

✓5th **M25.7 Osteophyte**

     M25.70 Osteophyte, unspecified joint

✓6th **M25.71** Osteophyte, shoulder

     M25.711 Osteophyte, right shoulder

     M25.712 Osteophyte, left shoulder

     M25.719 Osteophyte, unspecified shoulder

✓6th **M25.72** Osteophyte, elbow

     M25.721 Osteophyte, right elbow

     M25.722 Osteophyte, left elbow

     M25.729 Osteophyte, unspecified elbow

✓6th **M25.73** Osteophyte, wrist

     M25.731 Osteophyte, right wrist

     M25.732 Osteophyte, left wrist

     M25.739 Osteophyte, unspecified wrist

✓6th **M25.74** Osteophyte, hand

     M25.741 Osteophyte, right hand

     M25.742 Osteophyte, left hand

     M25.749 Osteophyte, unspecified hand

✓6th **M25.75** Osteophyte, hip

     M25.751 Osteophyte, right hip

     M25.752 Osteophyte, left hip

     M25.759 Osteophyte, unspecified hip

✓6th **M25.76** Osteophyte, knee

     M25.761 Osteophyte, right knee

     M25.762 Osteophyte, left knee

     M25.769 Osteophyte, unspecified knee

✓6th **M25.77** Osteophyte, ankle and foot

     M25.771 Osteophyte, right ankle

     M25.772 Osteophyte, left ankle

     M25.773 Osteophyte, unspecified ankle

     M25.774 Osteophyte, right foot

     M25.775 Osteophyte, left foot

     M25.776 Osteophyte, unspecified foot

     M25.78 Osteophyte, vertebrae

✓5th **M25.8 Other specified joint disorders**

     M25.80 Other specified joint disorders, unspecified joint

✓6th **M25.81** Other specified joint disorders, shoulder

     M25.811 Other specified joint disorders, right shoulder

     M25.812 Other specified joint disorders, left shoulder

     M25.819 Other specified joint disorders, unspecified shoulder

✓6th **M25.82** Other specified joint disorders, elbow

     M25.821 Other specified joint disorders, right elbow

     M25.822 Other specified joint disorders, left elbow

     M25.829 Other specified joint disorders, unspecified elbow

✓6th **M25.83** Other specified joint disorders, wrist

     M25.831 Other specified joint disorders, right wrist

     M25.832 Other specified joint disorders, left wrist

     M25.839 Other specified joint disorders, unspecified wrist

✓6th **M25.84** Other specified joint disorders, hand

     M25.841 Other specified joint disorders, right hand

     M25.842 Other specified joint disorders, left hand

     M25.849 Other specified joint disorders, unspecified hand

✓6th **M25.85** Other specified joint disorders, hip

     AHA: 2014,4Q,25

     M25.851 Other specified joint disorders, right hip

     M25.852 Other specified joint disorders, left hip

     M25.859 Other specified joint disorders, unspecified hip

✓6th **M25.86** Other specified joint disorders, knee

     M25.861 Other specified joint disorders, right knee

     M25.862 Other specified joint disorders, left knee

     M25.869 Other specified joint disorders, unspecified knee

✓6th **M25.87** Other specified joint disorders, ankle and foot

     M25.871 Other specified joint disorders, right ankle and foot

     M25.872 Other specified joint disorders, left ankle and foot

     M25.879 Other specified joint disorders, unspecified ankle and foot

     M25.9 Joint disorder, unspecified

Dentofacial anomalies [including malocclusion] and other disorders of jaw (M26-M27)

EXCLUDES 1   hemifacial atrophy or hypertrophy (Q67.4)

     unilateral condylar hyperplasia or hypoplasia (M27.8)

✓4th **M26 Dentofacial anomalies [including malocclusion]**

✓5th **M26.0 Major anomalies of jaw size**

     EXCLUDES 1   acromegaly (E22.0)

         Robin's syndrome (Q87.0)

     M26.00 Unspecified anomaly of jaw size

     M26.01 Maxillary hyperplasia

     M26.02 Maxillary hypoplasia

         AHA: 2014,3Q,23

     M26.03 Mandibular hyperplasia

     M26.04 Mandibular hypoplasia

     M26.05 Macrogenia

     M26.06 Microgenia

     M26.07 Excessive tuberosity of jaw

         Entire maxillary tuberosity

     M26.09 Other specified anomalies of jaw size

✓5th **M26.1 Anomalies of jaw-cranial base relationship**

     M26.10 Unspecified anomaly of jaw-cranial base relationship

     M26.11 Maxillary asymmetry

     M26.12 Other jaw asymmetry

     M26.19 Other specified anomalies of jaw-cranial base relationship

✓5th **M26.2 Anomalies of dental arch relationship**

     M26.20 Unspecified anomaly of dental arch relationship

✓6th **M26.21** Malocclusion, Angle's class

     M26.211 Malocclusion, Angle's class I

         Neutro-occlusion

     M26.212 Malocclusion, Angle's class II

         Disto-occlusion Division I

         Disto-occlusion Division II

     M26.213 Malocclusion, Angle's class III

         Mesio-occlusion

     M26.219 Malocclusion, Angle's class, unspecified

✓6th **M26.22** Open occlusal relationship

     M26.220 Open anterior occlusal relationship

         Anterior open bite

     M26.221 Open posterior occlusal relationship

         Posterior open bite

     M26.23 Excessive horizontal overlap

         Excessive horizontal overjet

     M26.24 Reverse articulation

         Crossbite (anterior) (posterior)

     M26.25 Anomalies of interarch distance

N Newborn: 0   **P** Pediatric: 0-17   **M** Maternity: 9-64   **A** Adult: 15-124   **MCC** Major Complication/Comorbidity   **CC** Complication/Comorbidity   **SW** Severe Wound Dx

798   ICD-10-CM 2020

M26.29 Other anomalies of dental arch relationship
Midline deviation of dental arch
Overbite (excessive) deep
Overbite (excessive) horizontal
Overbite (excessive) vertical
Posterior lingual occlusion of mandibular teeth

✓5ᵗʰ **M26.3 Anomalies of tooth position of fully erupted tooth or teeth**
    EXCLUDES 2   *embedded and impacted teeth (K01.-)*

M26.30 Unspecified anomaly of tooth position of fully erupted tooth or teeth
Abnormal spacing of fully erupted tooth or teeth NOS
Displacement of fully erupted tooth or teeth NOS
Transposition of fully erupted tooth or teeth NOS

M26.31 Crowding of fully erupted teeth

M26.32 Excessive spacing of fully erupted teeth
Diastema of fully erupted tooth or teeth NOS

M26.33 Horizontal displacement of fully erupted tooth or teeth
Tipped tooth or teeth
Tipping of fully erupted tooth

M26.34 Vertical displacement of fully erupted tooth or teeth
Extruded tooth
Infraeruption of tooth or teeth
Supraeruption of tooth or teeth

M26.35 Rotation of fully erupted tooth or teeth

M26.36 Insufficient interocclusal distance of fully erupted teeth (ridge)
Lack of adequate intermaxillary vertical dimension of fully erupted teeth

M26.37 Excessive interocclusal distance of fully erupted teeth
Excessive intermaxillary vertical dimension of fully erupted teeth
Loss of occlusal vertical dimension of fully erupted teeth

M26.39 Other anomalies of tooth position of fully erupted tooth or teeth

M26.4 Malocclusion, unspecified

✓5ᵗʰ **M26.5 Dentofacial functional abnormalities**
    EXCLUDES 1   *bruxism (F45.8)*
             teeth-grinding NOS (F45.8)

M26.50 Dentofacial functional abnormalities, unspecified

M26.51 Abnormal jaw closure

M26.52 Limited mandibular range of motion

M26.53 Deviation in opening and closing of the mandible

M26.54 Insufficient anterior guidance
Insufficient anterior occlusal guidance

M26.55 Centric occlusion maximum intercuspation discrepancy
    EXCLUDES 1   *centric occlusion NOS (M26.59)*

M26.56 Non-working side interference
Balancing side interference

M26.57 Lack of posterior occlusal support

M26.59 Other dentofacial functional abnormalities
Centric occlusion (of teeth) NOS
Malocclusion due to abnormal swallowing
Malocclusion due to mouth breathing
Malocclusion due to tongue, lip or finger habits

✓5ᵗʰ **M26.6 Temporomandibular joint disorders**
    EXCLUDES 2   *current temporomandibular joint dislocation (S03.0)*
             current temporomandibular joint sprain (S03.4)
    AHA: 2016,4Q,38-39

Temporomandibular Joint

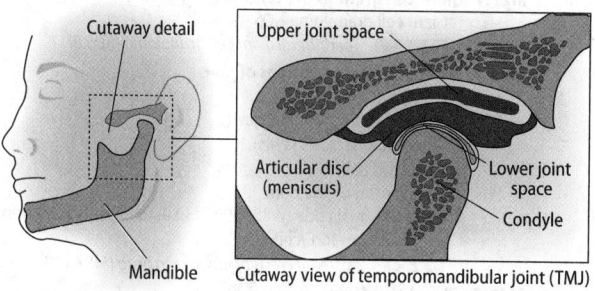

Cutaway detail
Upper joint space
Articular disc (meniscus)
Lower joint space
Condyle
Mandible
Cutaway view of temporomandibular joint (TMJ)

✓6ᵗʰ **M26.60 Temporomandibular joint disorder, unspecified**

M26.601 Right temporomandibular joint disorder, unspecified

M26.602 Left temporomandibular joint disorder, unspecified

M26.603 Bilateral temporomandibular joint disorder, unspecified

M26.609 Unspecified temporomandibular joint disorder, unspecified side
Temporomandibular joint disorder NOS

✓6ᵗʰ **M26.61 Adhesions and ankylosis of temporomandibular joint**

M26.611 Adhesions and ankylosis of right temporomandibular joint

M26.612 Adhesions and ankylosis of left temporomandibular joint

M26.613 Adhesions and ankylosis of bilateral temporomandibular joint

M26.619 Adhesions and ankylosis of temporomandibular joint, unspecified side

✓6ᵗʰ **M26.62 Arthralgia of temporomandibular joint**

M26.621 Arthralgia of right temporomandibular joint

M26.622 Arthralgia of left temporomandibular joint

M26.623 Arthralgia of bilateral temporomandibular joint

M26.629 Arthralgia of temporomandibular joint, unspecified side

✓6ᵗʰ **M26.63 Articular disc disorder of temporomandibular joint**

M26.631 Articular disc disorder of right temporomandibular joint

M26.632 Articular disc disorder of left temporomandibular joint

M26.633 Articular disc disorder of bilateral temporomandibular joint

M26.639 Articular disc disorder of temporomandibular joint, unspecified side

M26.69 Other specified disorders of temporomandibular joint

✓5ᵗʰ **M26.7 Dental alveolar anomalies**

M26.70 Unspecified alveolar anomaly

M26.71 Alveolar maxillary hyperplasia

M26.72 Alveolar mandibular hyperplasia

M26.73 Alveolar maxillary hypoplasia

M26.74 Alveolar mandibular hypoplasia

M26.79 Other specified alveolar anomalies

✓5ᵗʰ **M26.8 Other dentofacial anomalies**

M26.81 Anterior soft tissue impingement
Anterior soft tissue impingement on teeth

M26.82 Posterior soft tissue impingement
Posterior soft tissue impingement on teeth

M26.89 Other dentofacial anomalies

M26.9 Dentofacial anomaly, unspecified

Chapter 13. Diseases of the Musculoskeletal System and Connective Tissue

☑4ᵗʰ M27 Other diseases of jaws

M27.0 Developmental disorders of jaws
Latent bone cyst of jaw
Stafne's cyst
Torus mandibularis
Torus palatinus

M27.1 Giant cell granuloma, central
Giant cell granuloma NOS
EXCLUDES 1   *peripheral giant cell granuloma (K06.8)*

M27.2 Inflammatory conditions of jaws
Osteitis of jaw(s)
Osteomyelitis (neonatal) jaw(s)
Osteoradionecrosis jaw(s)
Periostitis jaw(s)
Sequestrum of jaw bone
Use additional code (W88-W90, X39.0) to identify radiation, if radiation-induced
EXCLUDES 2   *osteonecrosis of jaw due to drug (M87.180)*

M27.3 Alveolitis of jaws
Alveolar osteitis
Dry socket

☑5ᵗʰ M27.4 Other and unspecified cysts of jaw
EXCLUDES 1   *cysts of oral region (K09.-)*
latent bone cyst of jaw (M27.0)
Stafne's cyst (M27.0)

M27.40 Unspecified cyst of jaw
Cyst of jaw NOS

M27.49 Other cysts of jaw
Aneurysmal cyst of jaw
Hemorrhagic cyst of jaw
Traumatic cyst of jaw

☑5ᵗʰ M27.5 Periradicular pathology associated with previous endodontic treatment

M27.51 Perforation of root canal space due to endodontic treatment

M27.52 Endodontic overfill

M27.53 Endodontic underfill

M27.59 Other periradicular pathology associated with previous endodontic treatment

☑5ᵗʰ M27.6 Endosseous dental implant failure

M27.61 Osseointegration failure of dental implant
Hemorrhagic complications of dental implant placement
Iatrogenic osseointegration failure of dental implant
Osseointegration failure of dental implant due to complications of systemic disease
Osseointegration failure of dental implant due to poor bone quality
Pre-integration failure of dental implant NOS
Pre-osseointegration failure of dental implant

M27.62 Post-osseointegration biological failure of dental implant
Failure of dental implant due to lack of attached gingiva
Failure of dental implant due to occlusal trauma (caused by poor prosthetic design)
Failure of dental implant due to parafunctional habits
Failure of dental implant due to periodontal infection (peri-implantitis)
Failure of dental implant due to poor oral hygiene
Iatrogenic post-osseointegration failure of dental implant
Post-osseointegration failure of dental implant due to complications of systemic disease

M27.63 Post-osseointegration mechanical failure of dental implant
Failure of dental prosthesis causing loss of dental implant
Fracture of dental implant
EXCLUDES 2   *cracked tooth (K03.81)*
fractured dental restorative material with loss of material (K08.531)
fractured dental restorative material without loss of material (K08.530)
fractured tooth (S02.5)

M27.69 Other endosseous dental implant failure
Dental implant failure NOS

M27.8 Other specified diseases of jaws
Cherubism
Exostosis
Fibrous dysplasia
Unilateral condylar hyperplasia
Unilateral condylar hypoplasia
EXCLUDES 1   *jaw pain (R68.84)*

M27.9 Disease of jaws, unspecified

Systemic connective tissue disorders (M30-M36)

INCLUDES   autoimmune disease NOS
collagen (vascular) disease NOS
systemic autoimmune disease
systemic collagen (vascular) disease
EXCLUDES 1   *autoimmune disease, single organ or single cell-type-code to relevant condition category*

☑4ᵗʰ M30 Polyarteritis nodosa and related conditions
EXCLUDES 1   *microscopic polyarteritis (M31.7)*
CC Excl: For CC codes in category M30, unless otherwise noted: PDX collection 874

M30.0 Polyarteritis nodosa   `CC` `HCC`

M30.1 Polyarteritis with lung involvement [Churg-Strauss]   `CC` `HCC`
Allergic granulomatous angiitis

M30.2 Juvenile polyarteritis   `CC` `HCC`

M30.3 Mucocutaneous lymph node syndrome [Kawasaki]   `CC` `HCC`
CC Excl: PDX collection 875

M30.8 Other conditions related to polyarteritis nodosa   `CC` `HCC`
Polyangiitis overlap syndrome

☑4ᵗʰ M31 Other necrotizing vasculopathies
CC Excl: For CC/MCC codes in category M31, unless otherwise noted: PDX collection 874

M31.0 Hypersensitivity angiitis   `CC` `HCC`
Goodpasture's syndrome

M31.1 Thrombotic microangiopathy   `MCC` `HCC`
Thrombotic thrombocytopenic purpura

M31.2 Lethal midline granuloma   `CC` `HCC`

☑5ᵗʰ M31.3 Wegener's granulomatosis
Necrotizing respiratory granulomatosis

M31.30 Wegener's granulomatosis without renal involvement   `HCC`
Wegener's granulomatosis NOS

M31.31 Wegener's granulomatosis with renal involvement   `CC` `HCC`

M31.4 Aortic arch syndrome [Takayasu]   `CC` `HCC`

M31.5 Giant cell arteritis with polymyalgia rheumatica   `HCC`

M31.6 Other giant cell arteritis   `HCC`

M31.7 Microscopic polyangiitis   `CC` `HCC`
Microscopic polyarteritis
EXCLUDES 1   *polyarteritis nodosa (M30.0)*

M31.8 Other specified necrotizing vasculopathies   `CC` `HCC`
Hypocomplementemic vasculitis
Septic vasculitis
CC Excl: PDX collection 712

M31.9 Necrotizing vasculopathy, unspecified   `CC` `HCC`
CC Excl: PDX collection 712

☑4ᵗʰ M32 Systemic lupus erythematosus (SLE)
EXCLUDES 1   *lupus erythematosus (discoid) (NOS) (L93.0)*
AHA: 2018,3Q,14
TIP: There is no default code for "lupus NOS." Query the provider for the specific type of lupus in order to assign the appropriate code.

M32.0 Drug-induced systemic lupus erythematosus   `HCC`
Use additional code for adverse effect, if applicable, to identify drug (T36-T50 with fifth or sixth character 5)

☑5ᵗʰ M32.1 Systemic lupus erythematosus with organ or system involvement

M32.10 Systemic lupus erythematosus, organ or system involvement unspecified   `HCC`

Ⓝ Newborn: 0   Ⓟ Pediatric: 0-17   Ⓜ Maternity: 9-64   Ⓐ Adult: 15-124   `MCC` Major Complication/Comorbidity   `CC` Complication/Comorbidity   `SW` Severe Wound Dx

800   ICD-10-CM 2020

M32.11 **Endocarditis** in systemic lupus erythematosus `CC` `HCC`
  Libman-Sacks disease
  CC Excl: PDX collection 676

M32.12 **Pericarditis** in systemic lupus erythematosus `CC` `HCC`
  Lupus pericarditis
  CC Excl: PDX collection 673

M32.13 **Lung involvement** in systemic lupus erythematosus `HCC`
  Pleural effusion due to systemic lupus erythematosus

M32.14 **Glomerular disease** in systemic lupus erythematosus `HCC`
  Lupus renal disease NOS
  AHA: 2013,4Q,125

M32.15 **Tubulo-interstitial nephropathy** in systemic lupus erythematosus `HCC`

M32.19 **Other organ or system involvement** in systemic lupus erythematosus `HCC`

M32.8 Other forms of systemic lupus erythematosus `HCC`

M32.9 Systemic lupus erythematosus, unspecified `HCC`
  SLE NOS
  Systemic lupus erythematosus NOS
  Systemic lupus erythematosus without organ involvement

✓4ᵗʰ **M33** Dermatopolymyositis
  AHA: 2017,4Q,18
  CC Excl: For CC codes in category M33, unless otherwise noted: PDX collection 876

  ✓5ᵗʰ **M33.0** **Juvenile** dermatomyositis

  M33.00 **Juvenile dermatomyositis, organ involvement unspecified** `CC` `HCC`

  M33.01 **Juvenile dermatomyositis with respiratory involvement** `CC` `HCC`

  M33.02 **Juvenile dermatomyositis with myopathy** `CC` `HCC`
    CC Excl: PDX collection 877

  M33.03 **Juvenile dermatomyositis without myopathy** `CC` `HCC`

  M33.09 **Juvenile dermatomyositis with other organ involvement** `CC` `HCC`

  ✓5ᵗʰ **M33.1** Other dermatomyositis
    Adult dermatomyositis

    M33.10 **Other dermatomyositis, organ involvement unspecified** `CC` `HCC`

    M33.11 **Other dermatomyositis with respiratory involvement** `CC` `HCC`

    M33.12 **Other dermatomyositis with myopathy** `CC` `HCC`
      CC Excl: PDX collection 877

    M33.13 **Other dermatomyositis without myopathy** `CC` `HCC`
      Dermatomyositis NOS

    M33.19 **Other dermatomyositis with other organ involvement** `CC` `HCC`

  ✓5ᵗʰ **M33.2** Polymyositis

    M33.20 **Polymyositis, organ involvement unspecified** `CC` `HCC`
      CC Excl: PDX collection 878

    M33.21 **Polymyositis with respiratory involvement** `CC` `HCC`
      CC Excl: PDX collection 878

    M33.22 **Polymyositis with myopathy** `CC` `HCC`
      CC Excl: PDX collection 879

    M33.29 **Polymyositis with other organ involvement** `CC` `HCC`
      CC Excl: PDX collection 878

  ✓5ᵗʰ **M33.9** Dermatopolymyositis, unspecified

    M33.90 **Dermatopolymyositis, unspecified, organ involvement unspecified** `CC` `HCC`

    M33.91 **Dermatopolymyositis, unspecified with respiratory involvement** `CC` `HCC`

    M33.92 **Dermatopolymyositis, unspecified with myopathy** `CC` `HCC`
      CC Excl: PDX collection 877

    M33.93 **Dermatopolymyositis, unspecified without myopathy** `CC` `HCC`

    M33.99 **Dermatopolymyositis, unspecified with other organ involvement** `CC` `HCC`

✓4ᵗʰ **M34** Systemic sclerosis [scleroderma]
  EXCLUDES 1 *circumscribed scleroderma (L94.0)*
    neonatal scleroderma ▶(P83.88)◄

  M34.0 **Progressive** systemic sclerosis `HCC`

  M34.1 **CR(E)ST syndrome** `HCC`
    Combination of calcinosis, Raynaud's phenomenon, esophageal dysfunction, sclerodactyly, telangiectasia

  M34.2 **Systemic sclerosis induced by drug and chemical** `HCC`
    Code first poisoning due to drug or toxin, if applicable (T36-T65 with fifth or sixth character 1-4 or 6)
    Use additional code for adverse effect, if applicable, to identify drug (T36-T50 with fifth or sixth character 5)

  ✓5ᵗʰ **M34.8** Other forms of systemic sclerosis

    M34.81 **Systemic sclerosis with lung involvement** `CC` `HCC`
      CC Excl: No Excl

    M34.82 **Systemic sclerosis with myopathy** `CC` `HCC`
      CC Excl: PDX collection 867

    M34.83 **Systemic sclerosis with polyneuropathy** `HCC`

    M34.89 **Other systemic sclerosis** `HCC`

  M34.9 Systemic sclerosis, unspecified `HCC`

✓4ᵗʰ **M35** Other systemic involvement of connective tissue
  EXCLUDES 1 *reactive perforating collagenosis (L87.1)*

  ✓5ᵗʰ **M35.0** Sicca syndrome [Sjögren]
    DEF: Autoimmune disease associated with keratoconjunctivitis, laryngopharyngitis, rhinitis, dry mouth, enlarged parotid gland, and chronic polyarthritis.

    M35.00 **Sicca syndrome, unspecified** `HCC`

    M35.01 **Sicca syndrome with keratoconjunctivitis** `HCC`

    M35.02 **Sicca syndrome with lung involvement** `HCC`

    M35.03 **Sicca syndrome with myopathy** `CC` `HCC`
      CC Excl: PDX collection 867

    M35.04 **Sicca syndrome with tubulo-interstitial nephropathy** `HCC`
      Renal tubular acidosis in sicca syndrome

    M35.09 **Sicca syndrome with other organ involvement** `HCC`

  M35.1 **Other overlap syndromes** `CC` `HCC`
    Mixed connective tissue disease
    EXCLUDES 1 *polyangiitis overlap syndrome (M30.8)*
    CC Excl: PDX collection 880

  M35.2 **Behçet's disease** `CC` `HCC`
    CC Excl: PDX collection 863

  M35.3 **Polymyalgia rheumatica** `HCC`
    EXCLUDES 1 *polymyalgia rheumatica with giant cell arteritis (M31.5)*

  M35.4 **Diffuse (eosinophilic) fasciitis**

  M35.5 **Multifocal fibrosclerosis** `CC` `HCC`
    CC Excl: PDX collection 880

  M35.6 **Relapsing panniculitis [Weber-Christian]**
    EXCLUDES 1 *lupus panniculitis (L93.2)*
      panniculitis NOS (M79.3-)

  M35.7 **Hypermobility syndrome**
    Familial ligamentous laxity
    EXCLUDES 1 *Ehlers-Danlos syndrome ▶(Q79.6-)◄*
      ligamentous laxity, NOS (M24.2-)

  M35.8 **Other specified systemic involvement of connective tissue** `CC` `HCC`
    CC Excl: PDX collection 880

  M35.9 **Systemic involvement of connective tissue, unspecified** `HCC`
    Autoimmune disease (systemic) NOS
    Collagen (vascular) disease NOS

✓4ᵗʰ **M36** Systemic disorders of connective tissue in diseases classified elsewhere
  EXCLUDES 2 *arthropathies in diseases classified elsewhere (M14.-)*

  M36.0 **Dermato(poly)myositis in neoplastic disease** `CC` `HCC`
    Code first underlying neoplasm (C00-D49)
    CC Excl: PDX collection 876

M36.1 **Arthropathy in neoplastic disease**
Code first underlying neoplasm, such as:
leukemia (C91-C95)
malignant histiocytosis (C96.A)
multiple myeloma (C90.0)

M36.2 **Hemophilic arthropathy**
Hemarthrosis in hemophilic arthropathy
Code first underlying disease, such as:
factor VIII deficiency (D66)
with vascular defect (D68.0)
factor IX deficiency (D67)
hemophilia (classical) (D66)
hemophilia B (D67)
hemophilia C (D68.1)

M36.3 **Arthropathy in other blood disorders**

M36.4 **Arthropathy in hypersensitivity reactions classified elsewhere**
Code first underlying disease, such as:
Henoch (-Schönlein) purpura (D69.0)
serum sickness (T80.6-)

M36.8 **Systemic disorders of connective tissue in other diseases classified elsewhere**   HCC
Code first underlying disease, such as:
alkaptonuria (E70.2)
hypogammaglobulinemia (D80.-)
ochronosis (E70.2)

DORSOPATHIES (M40-M54)

Deforming dorsopathies (M40-M43)

√4ᵗʰ **M40 Kyphosis and lordosis**
   EXCLUDES 1   congenital kyphosis and lordosis (Q76.4)
kyphoscoliosis (M41.-)
postprocedural kyphosis and lordosis (M96.-)

Kyphosis and Lordosis

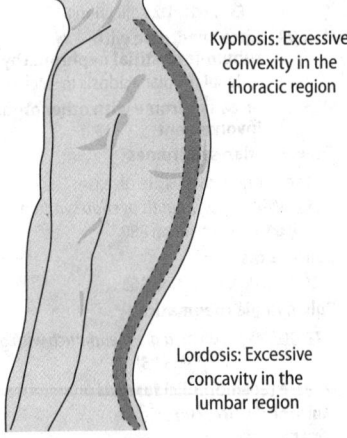

Kyphosis: Excessive convexity in the thoracic region

Lordosis: Excessive concavity in the lumbar region

√5ᵗʰ **M40.0 Postural kyphosis**
   EXCLUDES 1   osteochondrosis of spine (M42.-)
   M40.00 Postural kyphosis, site unspecified
   M40.03 Postural kyphosis, cervicothoracic **region**
   M40.04 Postural kyphosis, thoracic **region**
   M40.05 Postural kyphosis, thoracolumbar **region**

√5ᵗʰ **M40.1 Other secondary kyphosis**
   M40.10 Other secondary kyphosis, site unspecified
   M40.12 Other secondary kyphosis, cervical **region**
   M40.13 Other secondary kyphosis, cervicothoracic **region**
   M40.14 Other secondary kyphosis, thoracic **region**
   M40.15 Other secondary kyphosis, thoracolumbar **region**

√6ᵗʰ **M40.2 Other and unspecified kyphosis**
   √6ᵗʰ **M40.20 Unspecified kyphosis**
     M40.202 Unspecified kyphosis, cervical region
     M40.203 Unspecified kyphosis, cervicothoracic region
     M40.204 Unspecified kyphosis, thoracic **region**
     M40.205 Unspecified kyphosis, thoracolumbar region
     M40.209 Unspecified kyphosis, site unspecified

√6ᵗʰ **M40.29 Other kyphosis**
   M40.292 Other kyphosis, cervical **region**
   M40.293 Other kyphosis, cervicothoracic **region**
   M40.294 Other kyphosis, thoracic **region**
   M40.295 Other kyphosis, thoracolumbar **region**
   M40.299 Other kyphosis, site unspecified

√5ᵗʰ **M40.3 Flatback syndrome**
   M40.30 Flatback syndrome, site unspecified
   M40.35 Flatback syndrome, thoracolumbar **region**
   M40.36 Flatback syndrome, lumbar **region**
   M40.37 Flatback syndrome, lumbosacral **region**

√5ᵗʰ **M40.4 Postural lordosis**
   Acquired lordosis
   M40.40 Postural lordosis, site unspecified
   M40.45 Postural lordosis, thoracolumbar **region**
   M40.46 Postural lordosis, lumbar **region**
   M40.47 Postural lordosis, lumbosacral **region**

√5ᵗʰ **M40.5 Lordosis, unspecified**
   M40.50 Lordosis, unspecified, site unspecified
   M40.55 Lordosis, unspecified, thoracolumbar **region**
   M40.56 Lordosis, unspecified, lumbar **region**
   M40.57 Lordosis, unspecified, lumbosacral **region**

√4ᵗʰ **M41 Scoliosis**
   INCLUDES   kyphoscoliosis
   EXCLUDES 1   congenital scoliosis due to bony malformation (Q76.3)
congenital scoliosis NOS (Q67.5)
kyphoscoliotic heart disease (I27.1)
postprocedural scoliosis (M96.-)
postural congenital scoliosis (Q67.5)

Scoliosis

Lateral curvature of spine

√5ᵗʰ **M41.0 Infantile idiopathic scoliosis**
   AHA: 2014,4Q,26
   M41.00 Infantile idiopathic scoliosis, site unspecified
   M41.02 Infantile idiopathic scoliosis, cervical **region**
   M41.03 Infantile idiopathic scoliosis, cervicothoracic **region**
   M41.04 Infantile idiopathic scoliosis, thoracic **region**
   M41.05 Infantile idiopathic scoliosis, thoracolumbar **region**
   M41.06 Infantile idiopathic scoliosis, lumbar **region**
   M41.07 Infantile idiopathic scoliosis, lumbosacral **region**
   M41.08 Infantile idiopathic scoliosis, sacral and sacrococcygeal **region**

√5ᵗʰ **M41.1 Juvenile and adolescent idiopathic scoliosis**
   √6ᵗʰ **M41.11 Juvenile idiopathic scoliosis**
     AHA: 2014,4Q,28
     M41.112 Juvenile idiopathic scoliosis, cervical **region**
     M41.113 Juvenile idiopathic scoliosis, cervicothoracic **region**
     M41.114 Juvenile idiopathic scoliosis, thoracic **region**
     M41.115 Juvenile idiopathic scoliosis, thoracolumbar **region**

M41.116   Juvenile idiopathic scoliosis, **lumbar region**

M41.117   Juvenile idiopathic scoliosis, **lumbosacral region**

M41.119   Juvenile idiopathic scoliosis, **site unspecified**

✓6ᵗʰ **M41.12**   **Adolescent** scoliosis

M41.122   Adolescent idiopathic scoliosis, **cervical region**

M41.123   Adolescent idiopathic scoliosis, **cervicothoracic region**

M41.124   Adolescent idiopathic scoliosis, **thoracic region**

M41.125   Adolescent idiopathic scoliosis, **thoracolumbar region**

M41.126   Adolescent idiopathic scoliosis, **lumbar region**

M41.127   Adolescent idiopathic scoliosis, **lumbosacral region**

M41.129   Adolescent idiopathic scoliosis, **site unspecified**

✓5ᵗʰ **M41.2**   **Other** idiopathic scoliosis

M41.20   **Other idiopathic scoliosis, site unspecified**

M41.22   Other idiopathic scoliosis, **cervical region**

M41.23   Other idiopathic scoliosis, **cervicothoracic region**

M41.24   Other idiopathic scoliosis, **thoracic region**

M41.25   Other idiopathic scoliosis, **thoracolumbar region**

M41.26   Other idiopathic scoliosis, **lumbar region**

M41.27   Other idiopathic scoliosis, **lumbosacral region**

✓6ᵗʰ **M41.3**   **Thoracogenic** scoliosis

M41.30   **Thoracogenic scoliosis, site unspecified**

M41.34   Thoracogenic scoliosis, **thoracic region**

M41.35   Thoracogenic scoliosis, **thoracolumbar region**

✓5ᵗʰ **M41.4**   **Neuromuscular** scoliosis

Scoliosis secondary to cerebral palsy, Friedreich's ataxia, poliomyelitis and other neuromuscular disorders

Code also underlying condition

AHA: 2014,4Q,27

M41.40   **Neuromuscular scoliosis, site unspecified**

M41.41   Neuromuscular scoliosis, **occipito-atlanto-axial region**

M41.42   Neuromuscular scoliosis, **cervical region**

M41.43   Neuromuscular scoliosis, **cervicothoracic region**

M41.44   Neuromuscular scoliosis, **thoracic region**

M41.45   Neuromuscular scoliosis, **thoracolumbar region**

M41.46   Neuromuscular scoliosis, **lumbar region**

M41.47   Neuromuscular scoliosis, **lumbosacral region**

✓5ᵗʰ **M41.5**   **Other** secondary scoliosis

AHA: 2019,1Q,19

M41.50   **Other secondary scoliosis, site unspecified**

M41.52   Other secondary scoliosis, **cervical region**

M41.53   Other secondary scoliosis, **cervicothoracic region**

M41.54   Other secondary scoliosis, **thoracic region**

M41.55   Other secondary scoliosis, **thoracolumbar region**

M41.56   Other secondary scoliosis, **lumbar region**

M41.57   Other secondary scoliosis, **lumbosacral region**

✓5ᵗʰ **M41.8**   **Other forms of scoliosis**

M41.80   **Other forms of scoliosis, site unspecified**

M41.82   Other forms of scoliosis, **cervical region**

M41.83   Other forms of scoliosis, **cervicothoracic region**

M41.84   Other forms of scoliosis, **thoracic region**

M41.85   Other forms of scoliosis, **thoracolumbar region**

M41.86   Other forms of scoliosis, **lumbar region**

M41.87   Other forms of scoliosis, **lumbosacral region**

M41.9   **Scoliosis, unspecified**

✓4ᵗʰ **M42**   **Spinal osteochondrosis**

✓5ᵗʰ **M42.0**   **Juvenile** osteochondrosis of spine

Calvé's disease

Scheuermann's disease

EXCLUDES 1   *postural kyphosis (M40.0)*

M42.00   **Juvenile osteochondrosis of spine, site unspecified**

M42.01   Juvenile osteochondrosis of spine, **occipito-atlanto-axial region**

M42.02   Juvenile osteochondrosis of spine, **cervical region**

M42.03   Juvenile osteochondrosis of spine, **cervicothoracic region**

M42.04   Juvenile osteochondrosis of spine, **thoracic region**

M42.05   Juvenile osteochondrosis of spine, **thoracolumbar region**

M42.06   Juvenile osteochondrosis of spine, **lumbar region**

M42.07   Juvenile osteochondrosis of spine, **lumbosacral region**

M42.08   Juvenile osteochondrosis of spine, **sacral and sacrococcygeal region**

M42.09   Juvenile osteochondrosis of spine, **multiple sites in spine**

✓5ᵗʰ **M42.1**   **Adult** osteochondrosis of spine

M42.10   **Adult osteochondrosis of spine, site unspecified**   A

M42.11   **Adult osteochondrosis of spine, occipito-atlanto-axial region**   A

M42.12   **Adult osteochondrosis of spine, cervical region**   A

M42.13   **Adult osteochondrosis of spine, cervicothoracic region**   A

M42.14   **Adult osteochondrosis of spine, thoracic region**   A

M42.15   **Adult osteochondrosis of spine, thoracolumbar region**   A

M42.16   **Adult osteochondrosis of spine, lumbar region**   A

M42.17   **Adult osteochondrosis of spine, lumbosacral region**   A

M42.18   **Adult osteochondrosis of** spine, **sacral and sacrococcygeal region**   A

M42.19   **Adult osteochondrosis of spine, multiple sites in spine**   A

M42.9   **Spinal osteochondrosis, unspecified**

✓4ᵗʰ **M43**   **Other deforming dorsopathies**

EXCLUDES 1   *congenital spondylolysis and spondylolisthesis (Q76.2)*

hemivertebra (Q76.3-Q76.4)

Klippel-Feil syndrome (Q76.1)

lumbarization and sacralization (Q76.4)

platyspondylisis (Q76.4)

spina bifida occulta (Q76.0)

spinal curvature in osteoporosis (M80.-)

spinal curvature in Paget's disease of bone [osteitis deformans] (M88.-)

✓6ᵗʰ **M43.0**   **Spondylolysis**

EXCLUDES 1   *congenital spondylolysis (Q76.2)*

spondylolisthesis (M43.1)

M43.00   **Spondylolysis, site unspecified**

M43.01   Spondylolysis, **occipito-atlanto-axial region**

M43.02   Spondylolysis, **cervical region**

M43.03   Spondylolysis, **cervicothoracic region**

M43.04   Spondylolysis, **thoracic region**

M43.05   Spondylolysis, **thoracolumbar region**

M43.06   Spondylolysis, **lumbar region**

M43.07   Spondylolysis, **lumbosacral region**

M43.08   Spondylolysis, **sacral and sacrococcygeal region**

M43.09   Spondylolysis, **multiple sites in spine**

✓6ᵗʰ **M43.1**   **Spondylolisthesis**

EXCLUDES 1   *acute traumatic of lumbosacral region (S33.1)*

acute traumatic of sites other than lumbosacral — code to Fracture, vertebra, by region

congenital spondylolisthesis (Q76.2)

AHA: 2018,3Q,18

TIP: Code also any associated radiculopathy (M54.1-) and/or myelopathy (G99.2).

M43.10   **Spondylolisthesis, site unspecified**

M43.11   Spondylolisthesis, **occipito-atlanto-axial region**

M43.12   Spondylolisthesis, **cervical region**

M43.13   Spondylolisthesis, **cervicothoracic region**

M43.14   Spondylolisthesis, **thoracic region**

M43.15   Spondylolisthesis, **thoracolumbar region**

M43.16   Spondylolisthesis, **lumbar region**

M43.17   Spondylolisthesis, **lumbosacral region**

M43.18   Spondylolisthesis, **sacral and sacrococcygeal region**

M43.19   Spondylolisthesis, **multiple sites in spine**

✓ Additional Character Required   ✓x7ᵗʰ Placeholder   Unacceptable PDx   Questionable PDx   Manifestation   Unspecified Dx   H1-H14 HAC   HCC CMS-HCC Dx   HIV HIV Dx

ICD-10-CM 2020

803

☑5ᵗʰ **M43.2 Fusion of spine**
Ankylosis of spinal joint
 EXCLUDES 1   *ankylosing spondylitis (M45.0-)*
           congenital fusion of spine (Q76.4)
 EXCLUDES 2   *arthrodesis status (Z98.1)*
           pseudoarthrosis after fusion or arthrodesis (M96.0)

     M43.20 Fusion of spine, site unspecified
     M43.21 Fusion of spine, occipito-atlanto-axial region
     M43.22 Fusion of spine, cervical region
     M43.23 Fusion of spine, cervicothoracic region
     M43.24 Fusion of spine, thoracic region
     M43.25 Fusion of spine, thoracolumbar region
     M43.26 Fusion of spine, lumbar region
     M43.27 Fusion of spine, lumbosacral region
     M43.28 Fusion of spine, sacral and sacrococcygeal region

M43.3 Recurrent atlantoaxial dislocation with myelopathy
M43.4 Other recurrent atlantoaxial dislocation
☑5ᵗʰ **M43.5 Other recurrent vertebral dislocation**
 EXCLUDES 1   *biomechanical lesions NEC (M99.-)*

   ☑6ᵗʰ **M43.5X Other recurrent vertebral dislocation**
     M43.5X2 Other recurrent vertebral dislocation, cervical region
     M43.5X3 Other recurrent vertebral dislocation, cervicothoracic region
     M43.5X4 Other recurrent vertebral dislocation, thoracic region
     M43.5X5 Other recurrent vertebral dislocation, thoracolumbar region
     M43.5X6 Other recurrent vertebral dislocation, lumbar region
     M43.5X7 Other recurrent vertebral dislocation, lumbosacral region
     M43.5X8 Other recurrent vertebral dislocation, sacral and sacrococcygeal region
     M43.5X9 Other recurrent vertebral dislocation, site unspecified

M43.6 Torticollis
 EXCLUDES 1   *congenital (sternomastoid) torticollis (Q68.0)*
           current injury — see Injury, of spine, by body region
           ocular torticollis (R29.891)
           psychogenic torticollis (F45.8)
           spasmodic torticollis (G24.3)
           torticollis due to birth injury (P15.2)
 DEF: Twisted, unnatural position of the neck due to contracted cervical muscles that pull the head to one side.

☑5ᵗʰ **M43.8 Other specified deforming dorsopathies**
 EXCLUDES 2   *kyphosis and lordosis (M40.-)*
           scoliosis (M41.-)

   ☑6ᵗʰ **M43.8X Other specified deforming dorsopathies**
     M43.8X1 Other specified deforming dorsopathies, occipito-atlanto-axial region
     M43.8X2 Other specified deforming dorsopathies, cervical region
     M43.8X3 Other specified deforming dorsopathies, cervicothoracic region
     M43.8X4 Other specified deforming dorsopathies, thoracic region
     M43.8X5 Other specified deforming dorsopathies, thoracolumbar region
     M43.8X6 Other specified deforming dorsopathies, lumbar region
     M43.8X7 Other specified deforming dorsopathies, lumbosacral region
     M43.8X8 Other specified deforming dorsopathies, sacral and sacrococcygeal region
     M43.8X9 Other specified deforming dorsopathies, site unspecified

   M43.9 Deforming dorsopathy, unspecified
     Curvature of spine NOS

Spondylopathies (M45-M49)

☑4ᵗʰ **M45 Ankylosing spondylitis**
Rheumatoid arthritis of spine
 EXCLUDES 1   *arthropathy in Reiter's disease (M02.3-)*
           juvenile (ankylosing) spondylitis (M08.1)
 EXCLUDES 2   *Behçet's disease (M35.2)*

   M45.0 Ankylosing spondylitis of multiple sites in spine   `HCC`
   M45.1 Ankylosing spondylitis of occipito-atlanto-axial region   `HCC`
   M45.2 Ankylosing spondylitis of cervical region   `HCC`
   M45.3 Ankylosing spondylitis of cervicothoracic region   `HCC`
   M45.4 Ankylosing spondylitis of thoracic region   `HCC`
   M45.5 Ankylosing spondylitis of thoracolumbar region   `HCC`
   M45.6 Ankylosing spondylitis lumbar region   `HCC`
   M45.7 Ankylosing spondylitis of lumbosacral region   `HCC`
   M45.8 Ankylosing spondylitis sacral and sacrococcygeal region   `HCC`
   M45.9 Ankylosing spondylitis of unspecified sites in spine   `HCC`

☑4ᵗʰ **M46 Other inflammatory spondylopathies**

   ☑5ᵗʰ **M46.0 Spinal enthesopathy**
     Disorder of ligamentous or muscular attachments of spine

     M46.00 Spinal enthesopathy, site unspecified   `HCC`
     M46.01 Spinal enthesopathy, occipito-atlanto-axial region   `HCC`
     M46.02 Spinal enthesopathy, cervical region   `HCC`
     M46.03 Spinal enthesopathy, cervicothoracic region   `HCC`
     M46.04 Spinal enthesopathy, thoracic region   `HCC`
     M46.05 Spinal enthesopathy, thoracolumbar region   `HCC`
     M46.06 Spinal enthesopathy, lumbar region   `HCC`
     M46.07 Spinal enthesopathy, lumbosacral region   `HCC`
     M46.08 Spinal enthesopathy, sacral and sacrococcygeal region   `HCC`
     M46.09 Spinal enthesopathy, multiple sites in spine   `HCC`

   M46.1 Sacroiliitis, not elsewhere classified   `HCC`
     DEF: Inflammation of the sacroiliac joint (situated at the juncture of the sacrum and hip). Symptoms include pain in the buttocks or lower back that can extend down one or both legs.

   ☑5ᵗʰ **M46.2 Osteomyelitis of vertebra**
     CC Excl: For CC codes in subcategory M46.2: PDX collection 881

     M46.20 Osteomyelitis of vertebra, site unspecified   `CC` `HCC`
     M46.21 Osteomyelitis of vertebra, occipito-atlanto-axial region   `CC` `HCC`
     M46.22 Osteomyelitis of vertebra, cervical region   `CC` `HCC`
     M46.23 Osteomyelitis of vertebra, cervicothoracic region   `CC` `HCC`
     M46.24 Osteomyelitis of vertebra, thoracic region   `CC` `HCC`
     M46.25 Osteomyelitis of vertebra, thoracolumbar region   `CC` `HCC`
     M46.26 Osteomyelitis of vertebra, lumbar region   `CC` `HCC`
     M46.27 Osteomyelitis of vertebra, lumbosacral region   `CC` `HCC`
     M46.28 Osteomyelitis of vertebra, sacral and sacrococcygeal region   `CC` `HCC`

   ☑5ᵗʰ **M46.3 Infection of intervertebral disc (pyogenic)**
     Use additional code (B95-B97) to identify infectious agent
     CC Excl: For CC codes in subcategory M46.3: PDX collection 882

     M46.30 Infection of intervertebral disc (pyogenic), site unspecified   `CC` `HCC`

M46.31 **Infection of intervertebral disc (pyogenic),** occipito-atlanto-axial region   `CC` `HCC`

M46.32 **Infection of intervertebral disc (pyogenic),** cervical region   `CC` `HCC`

M46.33 **Infection of intervertebral disc (pyogenic),** cervicothoracic region   `CC` `HCC`

M46.34 **Infection of intervertebral disc (pyogenic),** thoracic region   `CC` `HCC`

M46.35 **Infection of intervertebral disc (pyogenic),** thoracolumbar region   `CC` `HCC`

M46.36 **Infection of intervertebral disc (pyogenic),** lumbar region   `CC` `HCC`

M46.37 **Infection of intervertebral disc (pyogenic),** lumbosacral region   `CC` `HCC`

M46.38 **Infection of intervertebral disc (pyogenic),** sacral and sacrococcygeal region   `CC` `HCC`

M46.39 **Infection of intervertebral disc (pyogenic),** multiple sites in spine   `CC` `HCC`

√5ᵗʰ **M46.4 Discitis, unspecified**

M46.40 **Discitis, unspecified, site unspecified**

M46.41 **Discitis, unspecified,** occipito-atlanto-axial region

M46.42 **Discitis, unspecified,** cervical region

M46.43 **Discitis, unspecified,** cervicothoracic region

M46.44 **Discitis, unspecified,** thoracic region

M46.45 **Discitis, unspecified,** thoracolumbar region

M46.46 **Discitis, unspecified,** lumbar region

M46.47 **Discitis, unspecified,** lumbosacral region

M46.48 **Discitis, unspecified,** sacral and sacrococcygeal region

M46.49 **Discitis, unspecified,** multiple sites in spine

√5ᵗʰ **M46.5 Other infective spondylopathies**

M46.50 **Other infective spondylopathies, site unspecified**   `HCC`

M46.51 **Other infective spondylopathies,** occipito-atlanto-axial region   `HCC`

M46.52 **Other infective spondylopathies,** cervical region   `HCC`

M46.53 **Other infective spondylopathies,** cervicothoracic region   `HCC`

M46.54 **Other infective spondylopathies,** thoracic region   `HCC`

M46.55 **Other infective spondylopathies,** thoracolumbar region   `HCC`

M46.56 **Other infective spondylopathies,** lumbar region   `HCC`

M46.57 **Other infective spondylopathies,** lumbosacral region   `HCC`

M46.58 **Other infective spondylopathies,** sacral and sacrococcygeal region   `HCC`

M46.59 **Other infective spondylopathies,** multiple sites in spine   `HCC`

√5ᵗʰ **M46.8 Other specified inflammatory spondylopathies**

M46.80 **Other specified inflammatory spondylopathies, site unspecified**   `HCC`

M46.81 **Other specified inflammatory spondylopathies,** occipito-atlanto-axial region   `HCC`

M46.82 **Other specified inflammatory spondylopathies,** cervical region   `HCC`

M46.83 **Other specified inflammatory spondylopathies,** cervicothoracic region   `HCC`

M46.84 **Other specified inflammatory spondylopathies,** thoracic region   `HCC`

M46.85 **Other specified inflammatory spondylopathies,** thoracolumbar region   `HCC`

M46.86 **Other specified inflammatory spondylopathies,** lumbar region   `HCC`

M46.87 **Other specified inflammatory spondylopathies,** lumbosacral region   `HCC`

M46.88 **Other specified inflammatory spondylopathies,** sacral and sacrococcygeal region   `HCC`

M46.89 **Other specified inflammatory spondylopathies,** multiple sites in spine   `HCC`

√5ᵗʰ **M46.9 Unspecified inflammatory spondylopathy**

M46.90 **Unspecified inflammatory spondylopathy, site unspecified**   `HCC`

M46.91 **Unspecified inflammatory spondylopathy,** occipito-atlanto-axial region   `HCC`

M46.92 **Unspecified inflammatory spondylopathy,** cervical region   `HCC`

M46.93 **Unspecified inflammatory spondylopathy,** cervicothoracic region   `HCC`

M46.94 **Unspecified inflammatory spondylopathy,** thoracic region   `HCC`

M46.95 **Unspecified inflammatory spondylopathy,** thoracolumbar region   `HCC`

M46.96 **Unspecified inflammatory spondylopathy,** lumbar region   `HCC`

M46.97 **Unspecified inflammatory spondylopathy,** lumbosacral region   `HCC`

M46.98 **Unspecified inflammatory spondylopathy,** sacral and sacrococcygeal region   `HCC`

M46.99 **Unspecified inflammatory spondylopathy,** multiple sites in spine   `HCC`

√4ᵗʰ **M47 Spondylosis**

> `INCLUDES` arthrosis or osteoarthritis of spine
> degeneration of facet joints

> **CC Excl: For CC codes in category M47, unless otherwise noted:** PDX collection 883

√5ᵗʰ **M47.0 Anterior spinal and vertebral artery compression syndromes**

√6ᵗʰ M47.01 **Anterior spinal artery compression syndromes**

M47.011 **Anterior spinal artery compression syndromes, occipito-atlanto-axial region**   `CC`

M47.012 **Anterior spinal artery compression syndromes, cervical region**   `CC`

M47.013 **Anterior spinal artery compression syndromes, cervicothoracic region**   `CC`

M47.014 **Anterior spinal artery compression syndromes, thoracic region**   `CC`

M47.015 **Anterior spinal artery compression syndromes, thoracolumbar region**   `CC`

M47.016 **Anterior spinal artery compression syndromes, lumbar region**   `CC`

M47.019 **Anterior spinal artery compression syndromes, site unspecified**   `CC`

√6ᵗʰ M47.02 **Vertebral artery compression syndromes**

M47.021 **Vertebral artery compression syndromes, occipito-atlanto-axial region**   `CC`

M47.022 **Vertebral artery compression syndromes, cervical region**   `CC`

M47.029 **Vertebral artery compression syndromes, site unspecified**   `CC`

√5ᵗʰ **M47.1 Other spondylosis with myelopathy**

> Spondylogenic compression of spinal cord
> `EXCLUDES 1`   vertebral subluxation ▶(M43.3-M43.5X9)◀

M47.10 **Other spondylosis with myelopathy, site unspecified**   `CC`
> **CC Excl:** PDX collection 884

M47.11 **Other spondylosis with myelopathy,** occipito-atlanto-axial region   `CC`

M47.12 **Other spondylosis with myelopathy,** cervical region   `CC`

M47.13 **Other spondylosis with myelopathy,** cervicothoracic region   `CC`

✔ Additional Character Required   √x7ᵗʰ Placeholder   Unacceptable PDx   Questionable PDx   Manifestation   Unspecified Dx   `H1`-`H14` HAC   `HCC` CMS-HCC Dx   `HIV` HIV Dx

ICD-10-CM 2020

805

Chapter 13. Diseases of the Musculoskeletal System and Connective Tissue

M47.14   Other spondylosis with myelopathy, thoracic region   `CC`
     CC Excl: PDX collection 885

M47.15   Other spondylosis with myelopathy, thoracolumbar region   `CC`
     CC Excl: PDX collection 885

M47.16   Other spondylosis with myelopathy, lumbar region   `CC`
     CC Excl: PDX collection 886

√5ᵗʰ **M47.2**   **Other spondylosis with radiculopathy**

M47.20   Other spondylosis with radiculopathy, site unspecified

M47.21   Other spondylosis with radiculopathy, occipito-atlanto-axial region

M47.22   Other spondylosis with radiculopathy, cervical region

M47.23   Other spondylosis with radiculopathy, cervicothoracic region

M47.24   Other spondylosis with radiculopathy, thoracic region

M47.25   Other spondylosis with radiculopathy, thoracolumbar region

M47.26   Other spondylosis with radiculopathy, lumbar region

M47.27   Other spondylosis with radiculopathy, lumbosacral region

M47.28   Other spondylosis with radiculopathy, sacral and sacrococcygeal region

√5ᵗʰ **M47.8**   **Other spondylosis**

√6ᵗʰ **M47.81**   Spondylosis without myelopathy or radiculopathy
     AHA: 2018,2Q,14

M47.811   Spondylosis without myelopathy or radiculopathy, occipito-atlanto-axial region

M47.812   Spondylosis without myelopathy or radiculopathy, cervical region

M47.813   Spondylosis without myelopathy or radiculopathy, cervicothoracic region

M47.814   Spondylosis without myelopathy or radiculopathy, thoracic region

M47.815   Spondylosis without myelopathy or radiculopathy, thoracolumbar region

M47.816   Spondylosis without myelopathy or radiculopathy, lumbar region

M47.817   Spondylosis without myelopathy or radiculopathy, lumbosacral region

M47.818   Spondylosis without myelopathy or radiculopathy, sacral and sacrococcygeal region

M47.819   Spondylosis without myelopathy or radiculopathy, site unspecified

√6ᵗʰ **M47.89**   Other spondylosis

M47.891   Other spondylosis, occipito-atlanto-axial region

M47.892   Other spondylosis, cervical region

M47.893   Other spondylosis, cervicothoracic region

M47.894   Other spondylosis, thoracic region

M47.895   Other spondylosis, thoracolumbar region

M47.896   Other spondylosis, lumbar region

M47.897   Other spondylosis, lumbosacral region

M47.898   Other spondylosis, sacral and sacrococcygeal region

M47.899   Other spondylosis, site unspecified

M47.9   **Spondylosis, unspecified**

√4ᵗʰ **M48**   **Other spondylopathies**

√5ᵗʰ **M48.0**   **Spinal stenosis**

Caudal stenosis
     AHA: 2018,3Q,18-19
     TIP: Code also any associated radiculopathy (M54.1-) and/or myelopathy (G99.2).

M48.00   Spinal stenosis, site unspecified

M48.01   Spinal stenosis, occipito-atlanto-axial region

M48.02   Spinal stenosis, cervical region

M48.03   Spinal stenosis, cervicothoracic region

M48.04   Spinal stenosis, thoracic region

M48.05   Spinal stenosis, thoracolumbar region

√6ᵗʰ **M48.06**   Spinal stenosis, lumbar region
     AHA: 2018,3Q,19; 2017,4Q,18-19
     DEF: Spinal canal narrowing in the lumbar area with nerve root compression, causing muscle pain, fatigue, and weakness during extension of the lumbar spine. Pain is relieved by sitting or bending.

M48.061   Spinal stenosis, lumbar region without neurogenic claudication
     Spinal stenosis, lumbar region NOS

M48.062   Spinal stenosis, lumbar region with neurogenic claudication

M48.07   Spinal stenosis, lumbosacral region

M48.08   Spinal stenosis, sacral and sacrococcygeal region

√5ᵗʰ **M48.1**   **Ankylosing hyperostosis [Forestier]**

Diffuse idiopathic skeletal hyperostosis [DISH]

M48.10   Ankylosing hyperostosis [Forestier], site unspecified

M48.11   Ankylosing hyperostosis [Forestier], occipito-atlanto-axial region

M48.12   Ankylosing hyperostosis [Forestier], cervical region

M48.13   Ankylosing hyperostosis [Forestier], cervicothoracic region

M48.14   Ankylosing hyperostosis [Forestier], thoracic region

M48.15   Ankylosing hyperostosis [Forestier], thoracolumbar region

M48.16   Ankylosing hyperostosis [Forestier], lumbar region

M48.17   Ankylosing hyperostosis [Forestier], lumbosacral region

M48.18   Ankylosing hyperostosis [Forestier], sacral and sacrococcygeal region

M48.19   Ankylosing hyperostosis [Forestier], multiple sites in spine

√5ᵗʰ **M48.2**   **Kissing spine**

M48.20   Kissing spine, site unspecified

M48.21   Kissing spine, occipito-atlanto-axial region

M48.22   Kissing spine, cervical region

M48.23   Kissing spine, cervicothoracic region

M48.24   Kissing spine, thoracic region

M48.25   Kissing spine, thoracolumbar region

M48.26   Kissing spine, lumbar region

M48.27   Kissing spine, lumbosacral region

√5ᵗʰ **M48.3**   **Traumatic spondylopathy**

CC Excl: For CC codes in subcategory M48.3: PDX collection 887

M48.30   Traumatic spondylopathy, site unspecified   `CC`

M48.31   Traumatic spondylopathy, occipito-atlanto-axial region   `CC`

M48.32   Traumatic spondylopathy, cervical region   `CC`

M48.33   Traumatic spondylopathy, cervicothoracic region   `CC`

M48.34   Traumatic spondylopathy, thoracic region   `CC`

M48.35   Traumatic spondylopathy, thoracolumbar region   `CC`

M48.36   Traumatic spondylopathy, lumbar region   `CC`

M48.37   Traumatic spondylopathy, lumbosacral region   `CC`

M48.38   Traumatic spondylopathy, sacral and sacrococcygeal region   `CC`

N Newborn: 0   P Pediatric: 0-17   M Maternity: 9-64   A Adult: 15-124   MCC Major Complication/Comorbidity   CC Complication/Comorbidity   SW Severe Wound Dx

806   ICD-10-CM 2020

√5ᵗʰ **M48.4 Fatigue fracture of vertebra**

Stress fracture of vertebra

EXCLUDES 1   *pathological fracture NOS (M84.4-)*

pathological fracture of vertebra due to neoplasm (M84.58)

pathological fracture of vertebra due to osteoporosis (M80.-)

pathological fracture of vertebra due to other diagnosis (M84.68)

traumatic fracture of vertebrae (S12.0-S12.3-, S22.0-, S32.0-)

The appropriate 7th character is to be added to each code from subcategory M48.4.
A   initial encounter for fracture
D   subsequent encounter for fracture with routine healing
G   subsequent encounter for fracture with delayed healing
S   sequela of fracture

√x7ᵗʰ **M48.40 Fatigue fracture of vertebra, site unspecified**

√x7ᵗʰ **M48.41 Fatigue fracture of vertebra, occipito-atlanto-axial region**

√x7ᵗʰ **M48.42 Fatigue fracture of vertebra, cervical region**

√x7ᵗʰ **M48.43 Fatigue fracture of vertebra, cervicothoracic region**

√x7ᵗʰ **M48.44 Fatigue fracture of vertebra, thoracic region**

√x7ᵗʰ **M48.45 Fatigue fracture of vertebra, thoracolumbar region**

√x7ᵗʰ **M48.46 Fatigue fracture of vertebra, lumbar region**

√x7ᵗʰ **M48.47 Fatigue fracture of vertebra, lumbosacral region**

√x7ᵗʰ **M48.48 Fatigue fracture of vertebra, sacral and sacrococcygeal region**

√5ᵗʰ **M48.5 Collapsed vertebra, not elsewhere classified**

Collapsed vertebra NOS

Compression fracture of vertebra NOS

Wedging of vertebra NOS

EXCLUDES 1   *current injury — see Injury of spine, by body region*

fatigue fracture of vertebra (M48.4)

pathological fracture NOS (M84.4-)

pathological fracture of vertebra due to neoplasm (M84.58)

pathological fracture of vertebra due to osteoporosis (M80.-)

pathological fracture of vertebra due to other diagnosis (M84.68)

stress fracture of vertebra (M48.4-)

traumatic fracture of vertebra (S12.-, S22.-, S32.-)

The appropriate 7th character is to be added to each code from subcategory M48.5.
A   initial encounter for fracture
D   subsequent encounter for fracture with routine healing
G   subsequent encounter for fracture with delayed healing
S   sequela of fracture

CC Excl: For CC codes in subcategory M48.5: PDX collection 888

6 √x7ᵗʰ **M48.50 Collapsed vertebra, not elsewhere classified, site unspecified**   CC HCC

6 √x7ᵗʰ **M48.51 Collapsed vertebra, not elsewhere classified, occipito-atlanto-axial region**   CC HCC

6 √x7ᵗʰ **M48.52 Collapsed vertebra, not elsewhere classified, cervical region**   CC HCC

6 √x7ᵗʰ **M48.53 Collapsed vertebra, not elsewhere classified, cervicothoracic region**   CC HCC

6 √x7ᵗʰ **M48.54 Collapsed vertebra, not elsewhere classified, thoracic region**   CC HCC

6 √x7ᵗʰ **M48.55 Collapsed vertebra, not elsewhere classified, thoracolumbar region**   CC HCC

6 √x7ᵗʰ **M48.56 Collapsed vertebra, not elsewhere classified, lumbar region**   CC HCC

6 √x7ᵗʰ **M48.57 Collapsed vertebra, not elsewhere classified, lumbosacral region**   CC HCC

6 √x7ᵗʰ **M48.58 Collapsed vertebra, not elsewhere classified, sacral and sacrococcygeal region**   CC HCC

√5ᵗʰ **M48.8 Other specified spondylopathies**

Ossification of posterior longitudinal ligament

√6ᵗʰ **M48.8X Other specified spondylopathies**

M48.8X1 Other specified spondylopathies, occipito-atlanto-axial region   HCC

M48.8X2 Other specified spondylopathies, cervical region   HCC

M48.8X3 Other specified spondylopathies, cervicothoracic region   HCC

M48.8X4 Other specified spondylopathies, thoracic region   HCC

M48.8X5 Other specified spondylopathies, thoracolumbar region   HCC

M48.8X6 Other specified spondylopathies, lumbar region   HCC

M48.8X7 Other specified spondylopathies, lumbosacral region   HCC

M48.8X8 Other specified spondylopathies, sacral and sacrococcygeal region   HCC

M48.8X9 Other specified spondylopathies, site unspecified   HCC

M48.9 Spondylopathy, unspecified

√4ᵗʰ **M49 Spondylopathies in diseases classified elsewhere**

INCLUDES   curvature of spine in diseases classified elsewhere
deformity of spine in diseases classified elsewhere
kyphosis in diseases classified elsewhere
scoliosis in diseases classified elsewhere
spondylopathy in diseases classified elsewhere

Code first underlying disease, such as:
brucellosis (A23.-)
Charcôt-Marie-Tooth disease (G60.0)
enterobacterial infections (A01-A04)
osteitis fibrosa cystica (E21.0)

EXCLUDES 1   *curvature of spine in tuberculosis [Pott's] (A18.01)*

enteropathic arthropathies (M07.-)

gonococcal spondylitis (A54.41)

neuropathic spondylopathy in syringomyelia (G95.0)

neuropathic spondylopathy in tabes dorsalis (A52.11)

neuropathic [tabes dorsalis] spondylitis (A52.11)

nonsyphilitic neuropathic spondylopathy NEC (G98.0)

spondylitis in syphilis (acquired) (A52.77)

tuberculous spondylitis (A18.01)

typhoid fever spondylitis (A01.05)

√5ᵗʰ **M49.8 Spondylopathy in diseases classified elsewhere**

M49.80 Spondylopathy in diseases classified elsewhere, site unspecified   HCC

M49.81 Spondylopathy in diseases classified elsewhere, occipito-atlanto-axial region   HCC

M49.82 Spondylopathy in diseases classified elsewhere, cervical region   HCC

M49.83 Spondylopathy in diseases classified elsewhere, cervicothoracic region   HCC

M49.84 Spondylopathy in diseases classified elsewhere, thoracic region   HCC

M49.85 Spondylopathy in diseases classified elsewhere, thoracolumbar region   HCC

M49.86 Spondylopathy in diseases classified elsewhere, lumbar region   HCC

M49.87 Spondylopathy in diseases classified elsewhere, lumbosacral region   HCC

M49.88 Spondylopathy in diseases classified elsewhere, sacral and sacrococcygeal region   HCC

M49.89 Spondylopathy in diseases classified elsewhere, multiple sites in spine   HCC

✔ Additional Character Required   √x7ᵗʰ Placeholder   Unacceptable PDx   Questionable PDx   Manifestation   Unspecified Dx   H1-H14 HAC   HCC CMS-HCC Dx   HIV HIV Dx

ICD-10-CM 2020

807

Other dorsopathies (M50-M54)

EXCLUDES 1   *current injury — see injury of spine by body region*
discitis NOS (M46.4-)

✓4ᵗʰ **M50 Cervical disc disorders**

NOTE   Code to the most superior level of disorder

INCLUDES   cervicothoracic disc disorders
cervicothoracic disc disorders with cervicalgia

AHA: 2016,4Q,39-40; 2016,1Q,17

✓5ᵗʰ **M50.0 Cervical disc disorder** with myelopathy

AHA: 2018,3Q,19

CC Excl: For CC codes in subcategory M50.0: PDX collection 889

M50.00   Cervical disc disorder with myelopathy, unspecified cervical region   CC

M50.01   Cervical disc disorder with myelopathy, **high cervical** region   CC
C2-C3 disc disorder with myelopathy
C3-C4 disc disorder with myelopathy

✓6ᵗʰ **M50.02**   Cervical disc disorder with myelopathy, mid-cervical region

   M50.020   Cervical disc disorder with myelopathy, mid-cervical region, unspecified level   CC

   M50.021   Cervical disc disorder at **C4-C5 level** with myelopathy   CC
C4-C5 disc disorder with myelopathy

   M50.022   Cervical disc disorder at **C5-C6 level** with myelopathy   CC
C5-C6 disc disorder with myelopathy

   M50.023   Cervical disc disorder at **C6-C7 level** with myelopathy   CC
C6-C7 disc disorder with myelopathy

M50.03   Cervical disc disorder with myelopathy, **cervicothoracic** region   CC
C7-T1 disc disorder with myelopathy

✓5ᵗʰ **M50.1 Cervical disc disorder** with radiculopathy

EXCLUDES 2   *brachial radiculitis NOS (M54.13)*

AHA: 2018,3Q,19

M50.10   Cervical disc disorder with radiculopathy, unspecified cervical region

M50.11   Cervical disc disorder with radiculopathy, **high cervical region**
C2-C3 disc disorder with radiculopathy
C3 radiculopathy due to disc disorder
C3-C4 disc disorder with radiculopathy
C4 radiculopathy due to disc disorder

✓6ᵗʰ **M50.12**   Cervical disc disorder with radiculopathy, mid-cervical region

   M50.120   Mid-cervical disc disorder, unspecified level

   M50.121   Cervical disc disorder at **C4-C5 level** with radiculopathy
C4-C5 disc disorder with radiculopathy
C5 radiculopathy due to disc disorder

   M50.122   Cervical disc disorder at **C5-C6 level** with radiculopathy
C5-C6 disc disorder with radiculopathy
C6 radiculopathy due to disc disorder

   M50.123   Cervical disc disorder at **C6-C7 level** with radiculopathy
C6-C7 disc disorder with radiculopathy
C7 radiculopathy due to disc disorder

M50.13   Cervical disc disorder with radiculopathy, **cervicothoracic** region
C7-T1 disc disorder with radiculopathy
C8 radiculopathy due to disc disorder

✓5ᵗʰ **M50.2 Other cervical disc** displacement

   M50.20   Other cervical disc displacement, unspecified cervical region

M50.21   Other cervical disc displacement, **high cervical** region
Other C2-C3 cervical disc displacement
Other C3-C4 cervical disc displacement

✓6ᵗʰ **M50.22**   Other cervical disc displacement, mid-cervical region

   M50.220   Other cervical disc displacement, mid-cervical region, unspecified level

   M50.221   Other cervical disc displacement at **C4-C5 level**
Other C4-C5 cervical disc displacement

   M50.222   Other cervical disc displacement at **C5-C6 level**
Other C5-C6 cervical disc displacement

   M50.223   Other cervical disc displacement at **C6-C7 level**
Other C6-C7 cervical disc displacement

M50.23   Other cervical disc displacement, **cervicothoracic** region
Other C7-T1 cervical disc displacement

✓5ᵗʰ **M50.3 Other cervical disc** degeneration

   M50.30   Other cervical disc degeneration, unspecified cervical region

M50.31   Other cervical disc degeneration, **high cervical** region
Other C2-C3 cervical disc degeneration
Other C3-C4 cervical disc degeneration

✓6ᵗʰ **M50.32**   Other cervical disc degeneration, mid-cervical region

   M50.320   Other cervical disc degeneration, mid-cervical region, unspecified level

   M50.321   Other cervical disc degeneration at **C4-C5 level**
Other C4-C5 cervical disc degeneration

   M50.322   Other cervical disc degeneration at **C5-C6 level**
Other C5-C6 cervical disc degeneration

   M50.323   Other cervical disc degeneration at **C6-C7 level**
Other C6-C7 cervical disc degeneration

M50.33   Other cervical disc degeneration, **cervicothoracic** region
Other C7-T1 cervical disc degeneration

✓5ᵗʰ **M50.8 Other cervical disc disorders**

   M50.80   Other cervical disc disorders, unspecified cervical region

M50.81   Other cervical disc disorders, **high cervical region**
Other C2-C3 cervical disc disorders
Other C3-C4 cervical disc disorders

✓6ᵗʰ **M50.82**   Other cervical disc disorders, mid-cervical region

   M50.820   Other cervical disc disorders, mid-cervical region, unspecified level

   M50.821   Other cervical disc disorders at **C4-C5 level**
Other C4-C5 cervical disc disorders

   M50.822   Other cervical disc disorders at **C5-C6 level**
Other C5-C6 cervical disc disorders

   M50.823   Other cervical disc disorders at **C6-C7 level**
Other C6-C7 cervical disc disorders

M50.83   Other cervical disc disorders, **cervicothoracic** region
Other C7-T1 cervical disc disorders

✓5ᵗʰ **M50.9 Cervical disc disorder, unspecified**

   M50.90   Cervical disc disorder, unspecified, unspecified cervical region

M50.91   Cervical disc disorder, unspecified, **high cervical** region
C2-C3 cervical disc disorder, unspecified
C3-C4 cervical disc disorder, unspecified

✓6ᵗʰ **M50.92**   Cervical disc disorder, unspecified, mid-cervical region

   M50.920   Unspecified cervical disc disorder, mid-cervical region, unspecified level

   M50.921   Unspecified cervical disc disorder at **C4-C5 level**
Unspecified C4-C5 cervical disc disorder

   M50.922   Unspecified cervical disc disorder at **C5-C6 level**
Unspecified C5-C6 cervical disc disorder

   M50.923   Unspecified cervical disc disorder at **C6-C7 level**
Unspecified C6-C7 cervical disc disorder

Ⓝ Newborn: 0   Ⓟ Pediatric: 0-17   Ⓜ Maternity: 9-64   Ⓐ Adult: 15-124   MCC Major Complication/Comorbidity   CC Complication/Comorbidity   SW Severe Wound Dx

808   ICD-10-CM 2020

M50.93   Cervical disc disorder, unspecified, **cervicothoracic region**
C7-T1 cervical disc disorder, unspecified

√4ᵗʰ **M51**   **Thoracic, thoracolumbar, and lumbosacral intervertebral disc disorders**
     EXCLUDES 2   *cervical and cervicothoracic disc disorders (M50.-)*
                 sacral and sacrococcygeal disorders (M53.3)

√5ᵗʰ **M51.0**   **Thoracic, thoracolumbar and lumbosacral intervertebral disc disorders with myelopathy**
     M51.04   **Intervertebral disc disorders with myelopathy, thoracic region**   CC
            CC Excl: PDX collection 890
     M51.05   **Intervertebral disc disorders with myelopathy, thoracolumbar region**   CC
            CC Excl: PDX collection 890
     M51.06   **Intervertebral disc disorders with myelopathy, lumbar region**   CC
            CC Excl: PDX collection 891

√5ᵗʰ **M51.1**   **Thoracic, thoracolumbar and lumbosacral intervertebral disc disorders with radiculopathy**
     Sciatica due to intervertebral disc disorder
     EXCLUDES 1   *lumbar radiculitis NOS (M54.16)*
                 sciatica NOS (M54.3)
     AHA: 2018,3Q,18
     M51.14   **Intervertebral disc disorders with radiculopathy, thoracic region**
     M51.15   **Intervertebral disc disorders with radiculopathy, thoracolumbar region**
     M51.16   **Intervertebral disc disorders with radiculopathy, lumbar region**
     M51.17   **Intervertebral disc disorders with radiculopathy, lumbosacral region**

√5ᵗʰ **M51.2**   **Other thoracic, thoracolumbar and lumbosacral intervertebral disc displacement**
     Lumbago due to displacement of intervertebral disc

Displacement Intervertebral Disc

Normal Top View   Herniated Top View

Lamina
Nucleus pulposus
Ligamentum flavum
Spinal cord
Spinal nerve
Herniates through annulus
Disc annulus
Nucleus pulposus

     M51.24   **Other intervertebral disc displacement, thoracic region**
     M51.25   **Other intervertebral disc displacement, thoracolumbar region**
     M51.26   **Other intervertebral disc displacement, lumbar region**
     M51.27   **Other intervertebral disc displacement, lumbosacral region**

√5ᵗʰ **M51.3**   **Other thoracic, thoracolumbar and lumbosacral intervertebral disc degeneration**
     AHA: 2018,2Q,15; 2013,3Q,22
     M51.34   **Other intervertebral disc degeneration, thoracic region**
     M51.35   **Other intervertebral disc degeneration, thoracolumbar region**
     M51.36   **Other intervertebral disc degeneration, lumbar region**
     M51.37   **Other intervertebral disc degeneration, lumbosacral region**

√5ᵗʰ **M51.4**   **Schmorl's nodes**
     DEF: Irregular bone defect in the margin of the vertebral body that causes herniation into the end plate of the vertebral body.
     M51.44   **Schmorl's nodes, thoracic region**
     M51.45   **Schmorl's nodes, thoracolumbar region**
     M51.46   **Schmorl's nodes, lumbar region**

     M51.47   **Schmorl's nodes, lumbosacral region**

√5ᵗʰ **M51.8**   **Other thoracic, thoracolumbar and lumbosacral intervertebral disc disorders**
     M51.84   **Other intervertebral disc disorders, thoracic region**
     M51.85   **Other intervertebral disc disorders, thoracolumbar region**
     M51.86   **Other intervertebral disc disorders, lumbar region**
     M51.87   **Other intervertebral disc disorders, lumbosacral region**

M51.9   **Unspecified thoracic, thoracolumbar and lumbosacral intervertebral disc disorder**

√4ᵗʰ **M53**   **Other and unspecified dorsopathies, not elsewhere classified**
     M53.0   **Cervicocranial syndrome**
            Posterior cervical sympathetic syndrome
     M53.1   **Cervicobrachial syndrome**
            EXCLUDES 2   *cervical disc disorder (M50.-)*
                       thoracic outlet syndrome (G54.0)

√5ᵗʰ **M53.2**   **Spinal instabilities**
     √6ᵗʰ **M53.2X**   **Spinal instabilities**
            M53.2X1   **Spinal instabilities, occipito-atlanto-axial region**
            M53.2X2   **Spinal instabilities, cervical region**
            M53.2X3   **Spinal instabilities, cervicothoracic region**
            M53.2X4   **Spinal instabilities, thoracic region**
            M53.2X5   **Spinal instabilities, thoracolumbar region**
            M53.2X6   **Spinal instabilities, lumbar region**
            M53.2X7   **Spinal instabilities, lumbosacral region**
            M53.2X8   **Spinal instabilities, sacral and sacrococcygeal region**
            M53.2X9   **Spinal instabilities, site unspecified**

     M53.3   **Sacrococcygeal disorders, not elsewhere classified**
            Coccygodynia

√5ᵗʰ **M53.8**   **Other specified dorsopathies**
     M53.80   **Other specified dorsopathies, site unspecified**
     M53.81   **Other specified dorsopathies, occipito-atlanto-axial region**
     M53.82   **Other specified dorsopathies, cervical region**
     M53.83   **Other specified dorsopathies, cervicothoracic region**
     M53.84   **Other specified dorsopathies, thoracic region**
     M53.85   **Other specified dorsopathies, thoracolumbar region**
     M53.86   **Other specified dorsopathies, lumbar region**
     M53.87   **Other specified dorsopathies, lumbosacral region**
     M53.88   **Other specified dorsopathies, sacral and sacrococcygeal region**

     M53.9   **Dorsopathy, unspecified**

√4ᵗʰ **M54**   **Dorsalgia**
     EXCLUDES 1   *psychogenic dorsalgia (F45.41)*

√5ᵗʰ **M54.0**   **Panniculitis affecting regions of neck and back**
     EXCLUDES 1   *lupus panniculitis (L93.2)*
                 panniculitis NOS (M79.3)
                 relapsing [Weber-Christian] panniculitis (M35.6)
     M54.00   **Panniculitis affecting regions of neck and back, site unspecified**
     M54.01   **Panniculitis affecting regions of neck and back, occipito-atlanto-axial region**
     M54.02   **Panniculitis affecting regions of neck and back, cervical region**
     M54.03   **Panniculitis affecting regions of neck and back, cervicothoracic region**
     M54.04   **Panniculitis affecting regions of neck and back, thoracic region**
     M54.05   **Panniculitis affecting regions of neck and back, thoracolumbar region**
     M54.06   **Panniculitis affecting regions of neck and back, lumbar region**
     M54.07   **Panniculitis affecting regions of neck and back, lumbosacral region**
     M54.08   **Panniculitis affecting regions of neck and back, sacral and sacrococcygeal region**
     M54.09   **Panniculitis affecting regions, neck and back, multiple sites in spine**

✓5ᵗʰ **M54.1 Radiculopathy**

Brachial neuritis or radiculitis NOS
Lumbar neuritis or radiculitis NOS
Lumbosacral neuritis or radiculitis NOS
Thoracic neuritis or radiculitis NOS
Radiculitis NOS

EXCLUDES 1 *neuralgia and neuritis NOS (M79.2)*
radiculopathy with cervical disc disorder (M50.1)
radiculopathy with lumbar and other intervertebral disc disorder (M51.1-)
radiculopathy with spondylosis (M47.2-)

AHA: 2018,3Q,18

TIP: A code from this subcategory can be used in addition to a spondylolisthesis code (M43.1-) or a spinal stenosis code (M48.0-) when either condition is documented as the cause of the radiculopathy.

M54.10 **Radiculopathy, site unspecified**
M54.11 **Radiculopathy, occipito-atlanto-axial region**
M54.12 **Radiculopathy, cervical region**
M54.13 **Radiculopathy, cervicothoracic region**
M54.14 **Radiculopathy, thoracic region**
M54.15 **Radiculopathy, thoracolumbar region**
M54.16 **Radiculopathy, lumbar region**
M54.17 **Radiculopathy, lumbosacral region**
M54.18 **Radiculopathy, sacral and sacrococcygeal region**

M54.2 Cervicalgia

EXCLUDES 1 *cervicalgia due to intervertebral cervical disc disorder (M50.-)*

✓5ᵗʰ **M54.3 Sciatica**

EXCLUDES 1 *lesion of sciatic nerve (G57.0)*
sciatica due to intervertebral disc disorder (M51.1-)
sciatica with lumbago (M54.4-)

M54.30 **Sciatica, unspecified side**
M54.31 **Sciatica, right side**
M54.32 **Sciatica, left side**

✓5ᵗʰ **M54.4 Lumbago with sciatica**

EXCLUDES 1 *lumbago with sciatica due to intervertebral disc disorder (M51.1-)*

AHA: 2016,2Q,7

M54.40 **Lumbago with sciatica, unspecified side**
M54.41 **Lumbago with sciatica, right side**
M54.42 **Lumbago with sciatica, left side**

M54.5 Low back pain

Loin pain
Lumbago NOS

EXCLUDES 1 *low back strain (S39.012)*
lumbago due to intervertebral disc displacement (M51.2-)
lumbago with sciatica (M54.4-)

M54.6 Pain in thoracic spine

EXCLUDES 1 *pain in thoracic spine due to intervertebral disc disorder (M51.-)*

✓5ᵗʰ **M54.8 Other dorsalgia**

EXCLUDES 1 *dorsalgia in thoracic region (M54.6)*
low back pain (M54.5)

M54.81 **Occipital neuralgia**
M54.89 **Other dorsalgia**

M54.9 **Dorsalgia, unspecified**

Backache NOS
Back pain NOS

SOFT TISSUE DISORDERS (M60-M79)

Disorders of muscles (M60-M63)

EXCLUDES 1 *dermatopolymyositis (M33.-)*
muscular dystrophies and myopathies (G71-G72)
myopathy in amyloidosis (E85.-)
myopathy in polyarteritis nodosa (M30.0)
myopathy in rheumatoid arthritis (M05.32)
myopathy in scleroderma (M34.-)
myopathy in Sjögren's syndrome (M35.03)
myopathy in systemic lupus erythematosus (M32.-)

✓4ᵗʰ **M60 Myositis**

EXCLUDES 2 *inclusion body myositis [IBM] (G72.41)*

✓5ᵗʰ **M60.0 Infective myositis**

Tropical pyomyositis
Use additional code (B95-B97) to identify infectious agent
CC Excl: For CC codes in subcategory M60.0: PDX collection 806

✓6ᵗʰ M60.00 **Infective myositis, unspecified site**

M60.000 **Infective myositis, unspecified right arm** CC
Infective myositis, right upper limb NOS

M60.001 **Infective myositis, unspecified left arm** CC
Infective myositis, left upper limb NOS

M60.002 **Infective myositis, unspecified arm** CC
Infective myositis, upper limb NOS

M60.003 **Infective myositis, unspecified right leg** CC
Infective myositis, right lower limb NOS

M60.004 **Infective myositis, unspecified left leg** CC
Infective myositis, left lower limb NOS

M60.005 **Infective myositis, unspecified leg** CC
Infective myositis, lower limb NOS

M60.009 **Infective myositis, unspecified site** CC

✓6ᵗʰ M60.01 **Infective myositis, shoulder**

M60.011 **Infective myositis, right shoulder** CC
M60.012 **Infective myositis, left shoulder** CC
M60.019 **Infective myositis, unspecified shoulder** CC

✓6ᵗʰ M60.02 **Infective myositis, upper arm**

M60.021 **Infective myositis, right upper arm** CC
M60.022 **Infective myositis, left upper arm** CC
M60.029 **Infective myositis, unspecified upper arm** CC

✓6ᵗʰ M60.03 **Infective myositis, forearm**

M60.031 **Infective myositis, right forearm** CC
M60.032 **Infective myositis, left forearm** CC
M60.039 **Infective myositis, unspecified forearm** CC

✓6ᵗʰ M60.04 **Infective myositis, hand and fingers**

M60.041 **Infective myositis, right hand** CC
M60.042 **Infective myositis, left hand** CC
M60.043 **Infective myositis, unspecified hand** CC
M60.044 **Infective myositis, right finger(s)** CC
M60.045 **Infective myositis, left finger(s)** CC
M60.046 **Infective myositis, unspecified finger(s)** CC

✓6ᵗʰ M60.05 **Infective myositis, thigh**

M60.051 **Infective myositis, right thigh** CC
M60.052 **Infective myositis, left thigh** CC

M60.059 Infective myositis, unspecified thigh `CC`

✓6ᵗʰ M60.06 Infective myositis, lower leg

M60.061 Infective myositis, right lower leg `CC`

M60.062 Infective myositis, left lower leg `CC`

M60.069 Infective myositis, unspecified lower leg `CC`

✓6ᵗʰ M60.07 Infective myositis, ankle, foot and toes

M60.070 Infective myositis, right ankle `CC`

M60.071 Infective myositis, left ankle `CC`

M60.072 Infective myositis, unspecified ankle `CC`

M60.073 Infective myositis, right foot `CC`

M60.074 Infective myositis, left foot `CC`

M60.075 Infective myositis, unspecified foot `CC`

M60.076 Infective myositis, right toe(s) `CC`

M60.077 Infective myositis, left toe(s) `CC`

M60.078 Infective myositis, unspecified toe(s) `CC`

M60.08 Infective myositis, other site `CC`

M60.09 Infective myositis, multiple sites `CC`

✓6ᵗʰ M60.1 Interstitial myositis

M60.10 Interstitial myositis of unspecified site

✓6ᵗʰ M60.11 Interstitial myositis, shoulder

M60.111 Interstitial myositis, right shoulder

M60.112 Interstitial myositis, left shoulder

M60.119 Interstitial myositis, unspecified shoulder

✓6ᵗʰ M60.12 Interstitial myositis, upper arm

M60.121 Interstitial myositis, right upper arm

M60.122 Interstitial myositis, left upper arm

M60.129 Interstitial myositis, unspecified upper arm

✓6ᵗʰ M60.13 Interstitial myositis, forearm

M60.131 Interstitial myositis, right forearm

M60.132 Interstitial myositis, left forearm

M60.139 Interstitial myositis, unspecified forearm

✓6ᵗʰ M60.14 Interstitial myositis, hand

M60.141 Interstitial myositis, right hand

M60.142 Interstitial myositis, left hand

M60.149 Interstitial myositis, unspecified hand

✓6ᵗʰ M60.15 Interstitial myositis, thigh

M60.151 Interstitial myositis, right thigh

M60.152 Interstitial myositis, left thigh

M60.159 Interstitial myositis, unspecified thigh

✓6ᵗʰ M60.16 Interstitial myositis, lower leg

M60.161 Interstitial myositis, right lower leg

M60.162 Interstitial myositis, left lower leg

M60.169 Interstitial myositis, unspecified lower leg

✓6ᵗʰ M60.17 Interstitial myositis, ankle and foot

M60.171 Interstitial myositis, right ankle and foot

M60.172 Interstitial myositis, left ankle and foot

M60.179 Interstitial myositis, unspecified ankle and foot

M60.18 Interstitial myositis, other site

M60.19 Interstitial myositis, multiple sites

✓5ᵗʰ M60.2 Foreign body granuloma of soft tissue, not elsewhere classified

Use additional code to identify the type of retained foreign body (Z18.-)

EXCLUDES 1   foreign body granuloma of skin and subcutaneous tissue (L92.3)

M60.20 Foreign body granuloma of soft tissue, not elsewhere classified, unspecified site

✓6ᵗʰ M60.21 Foreign body granuloma of soft tissue, not elsewhere classified, shoulder

M60.211 Foreign body granuloma of soft tissue, not elsewhere classified, right shoulder

M60.212 Foreign body granuloma of soft tissue, not elsewhere classified, left shoulder

M60.219 Foreign body granuloma of soft tissue, not elsewhere classified, unspecified shoulder

✓6ᵗʰ M60.22 Foreign body granuloma of soft tissue, not elsewhere classified, upper arm

M60.221 Foreign body granuloma of soft tissue, not elsewhere classified, right upper arm

M60.222 Foreign body granuloma of soft tissue, not elsewhere classified, left upper arm

M60.229 Foreign body granuloma of soft tissue, not elsewhere classified, unspecified upper arm

✓6ᵗʰ M60.23 Foreign body granuloma of soft tissue, not elsewhere classified, forearm

M60.231 Foreign body granuloma of soft tissue, not elsewhere classified, right forearm

M60.232 Foreign body granuloma of soft tissue, not elsewhere classified, left forearm

M60.239 Foreign body granuloma of soft tissue, not elsewhere classified, unspecified forearm

✓6ᵗʰ M60.24 Foreign body granuloma of soft tissue, not elsewhere classified, hand

M60.241 Foreign body granuloma of soft tissue, not elsewhere classified, right hand

M60.242 Foreign body granuloma of soft tissue, not elsewhere classified, left hand

M60.249 Foreign body granuloma of soft tissue, not elsewhere classified, unspecified hand

✓6ᵗʰ M60.25 Foreign body granuloma of soft tissue, not elsewhere classified, thigh

M60.251 Foreign body granuloma of soft tissue, not elsewhere classified, right thigh

M60.252 Foreign body granuloma of soft tissue, not elsewhere classified, left thigh

M60.259 Foreign body granuloma of soft tissue, not elsewhere classified, thigh

✓6ᵗʰ M60.26 Foreign body granuloma of soft tissue, not elsewhere classified, lower leg

M60.261 Foreign body granuloma of soft tissue, not elsewhere classified, right lower leg

M60.262 Foreign body granuloma of soft tissue, not elsewhere classified, left lower leg

M60.269 Foreign body granuloma of soft tissue, not elsewhere classified, unspecified lower leg

✓6ᵗʰ M60.27 Foreign body granuloma of soft tissue, not elsewhere classified, ankle and foot

M60.271 Foreign body granuloma of soft tissue, not elsewhere classified, right ankle and foot

M60.272 Foreign body granuloma of soft tissue, not elsewhere classified, left ankle and foot

M60.279 Foreign body granuloma of soft tissue, not elsewhere classified, unspecified ankle and foot

M60.28 Foreign body granuloma of soft tissue, not elsewhere classified, other site

✓5ᵗʰ M60.8 Other myositis

M60.80 Other myositis, unspecified site

✓6ᵗʰ M60.81 Other myositis shoulder

M60.811 Other myositis, right shoulder

M60.812 Other myositis, left shoulder

M60.819 Other myositis, unspecified shoulder

✓6ᵗʰ M60.82 Other myositis, upper arm

M60.821 Other myositis, right upper arm

M60.822 Other myositis, left upper arm

M60.829 Other myositis, unspecified upper arm

✓6ᵗʰ M60.83 Other myositis, forearm

M60.831 Other myositis, right forearm

M60.832 Other myositis, left forearm

M60.839 Other myositis, unspecified forearm

✓6ᵗʰ M60.84 Other myositis, hand

M60.841 Other myositis, right hand

M60.842 Other myositis, left hand

M60.849 Other myositis, unspecified hand

✓6ᵗʰ M60.85 Other myositis, thigh

M60.851 Other myositis, right thigh

✔ Additional Character Required   ✓x7ᵗʰ Placeholder   Unacceptable PDx   Questionable PDx   Manifestation   Unspecified Dx   H1 - H14 HAC   HCC CMS-HCC Dx   HIV HIV Dx

ICD-10-CM 2020

811

M60.852 **Other myositis,** left thigh
M60.859 **Other myositis, unspecified thigh**
✓6ᵗʰ M60.86 **Other myositis,** lower leg
M60.861 **Other myositis,** right lower leg
M60.862 **Other myositis,** left lower leg
M60.869 **Other myositis, unspecified lower leg**
✓6ᵗʰ M60.87 **Other myositis,** ankle and foot
M60.871 **Other myositis,** right ankle and foot
M60.872 **Other myositis,** left ankle and foot
M60.879 **Other myositis, unspecified ankle and foot**
M60.88 **Other myositis, other site**
M60.89 **Other myositis,** multiple sites
M60.9 **Myositis, unspecified**

✓4ᵗʰ **M61 Calcification and ossification of muscle**
✓5ᵗʰ M61.0 **Myositis ossificans** traumatica
M61.00 **Myositis ossificans traumatica, unspecified site**
✓6ᵗʰ M61.01 **Myositis ossificans traumatica,** shoulder
M61.011 **Myositis ossificans traumatica,** right shoulder
M61.012 **Myositis ossificans traumatica,** left shoulder
M61.019 **Myositis ossificans traumatica, unspecified shoulder**
✓6ᵗʰ M61.02 **Myositis ossificans traumatica,** upper arm
M61.021 **Myositis ossificans traumatica,** right upper arm
M61.022 **Myositis ossificans traumatica,** left upper arm
M61.029 **Myositis ossificans traumatica, unspecified upper arm**
✓6ᵗʰ M61.03 **Myositis ossificans traumatica,** forearm
M61.031 **Myositis ossificans traumatica,** right forearm
M61.032 **Myositis ossificans traumatica,** left forearm
M61.039 **Myositis ossificans traumatica, unspecified forearm**
✓6ᵗʰ M61.04 **Myositis ossificans traumatica,** hand
M61.041 **Myositis ossificans traumatica,** right hand
M61.042 **Myositis ossificans traumatica,** left hand
M61.049 **Myositis ossificans traumatica, unspecified hand**
✓6ᵗʰ M61.05 **Myositis ossificans traumatica,** thigh
M61.051 **Myositis ossificans traumatica,** right thigh
M61.052 **Myositis ossificans traumatica,** left thigh
M61.059 **Myositis ossificans traumatica, unspecified thigh**
✓6ᵗʰ M61.06 **Myositis ossificans traumatica,** lower leg
M61.061 **Myositis ossificans traumatica,** right lower leg
M61.062 **Myositis ossificans traumatica,** left lower leg
M61.069 **Myositis ossificans traumatica, unspecified lower leg**
✓6ᵗʰ M61.07 **Myositis ossificans traumatica,** ankle and foot
M61.071 **Myositis ossificans traumatica,** right ankle and foot
M61.072 **Myositis ossificans traumatica,** left ankle and foot
M61.079 **Myositis ossificans traumatica, unspecified ankle and foot**
M61.08 **Myositis ossificans traumatica, other site**
M61.09 **Myositis ossificans traumatica,** multiple sites
✓5ᵗʰ M61.1 **Myositis ossificans** progressiva
Fibrodysplasia ossificans progressiva
M61.10 **Myositis ossificans progressiva, unspecified site**
✓6ᵗʰ M61.11 **Myositis ossificans progressiva,** shoulder
M61.111 **Myositis ossificans progressiva,** right shoulder
M61.112 **Myositis ossificans progressiva,** left shoulder
M61.119 **Myositis ossificans progressiva, unspecified shoulder**
✓6ᵗʰ M61.12 **Myositis ossificans progressiva,** upper arm
M61.121 **Myositis ossificans progressiva,** right upper arm

M61.122 **Myositis ossificans progressiva,** left upper arm
M61.129 **Myositis ossificans progressiva, unspecified arm**
✓6ᵗʰ M61.13 **Myositis ossificans progressiva,** forearm
M61.131 **Myositis ossificans progressiva,** right forearm
M61.132 **Myositis ossificans progressiva,** left forearm
M61.139 **Myositis ossificans progressiva, unspecified forearm**
✓6ᵗʰ M61.14 **Myositis ossificans progressiva,** hand and finger(s)
M61.141 **Myositis ossificans progressiva,** right hand
M61.142 **Myositis ossificans progressiva,** left hand
M61.143 **Myositis ossificans progressiva, unspecified hand**
M61.144 **Myositis ossificans progressiva,** right finger(s)
M61.145 **Myositis ossificans progressiva,** left finger(s)
M61.146 **Myositis ossificans progressiva, unspecified finger(s)**
✓6ᵗʰ M61.15 **Myositis ossificans progressiva,** thigh
M61.151 **Myositis ossificans progressiva,** right thigh
M61.152 **Myositis ossificans progressiva,** left thigh
M61.159 **Myositis ossificans progressiva, unspecified thigh**
✓6ᵗʰ M61.16 **Myositis ossificans progressiva,** lower leg
M61.161 **Myositis ossificans progressiva,** right lower leg
M61.162 **Myositis ossificans progressiva,** left lower leg
M61.169 **Myositis ossificans progressiva, unspecified lower leg**
✓6ᵗʰ M61.17 **Myositis ossificans progressiva,** ankle, foot and toe(s)
M61.171 **Myositis ossificans progressiva,** right ankle
M61.172 **Myositis ossificans progressiva,** left ankle
M61.173 **Myositis ossificans progressiva, unspecified ankle**
M61.174 **Myositis ossificans progressiva,** right foot
M61.175 **Myositis ossificans progressiva,** left foot
M61.176 **Myositis ossificans progressiva, unspecified foot**
M61.177 **Myositis ossificans progressiva,** right toe(s)
M61.178 **Myositis ossificans progressiva,** left toe(s)
M61.179 **Myositis ossificans progressiva, unspecified toe(s)**
M61.18 **Myositis ossificans progressiva, other site**
M61.19 **Myositis ossificans progressiva,** multiple sites
✓5ᵗʰ M61.2 **Paralytic calcification and ossification of muscle**
Myositis ossificans associated with quadriplegia or paraplegia
M61.20 **Paralytic calcification and ossification of muscle, unspecified site**
✓6ᵗʰ M61.21 **Paralytic calcification and ossification of muscle,** shoulder
M61.211 **Paralytic calcification and ossification of muscle,** right shoulder
M61.212 **Paralytic calcification and ossification of muscle,** left shoulder
M61.219 **Paralytic calcification and ossification of muscle, unspecified shoulder**
✓6ᵗʰ M61.22 **Paralytic calcification and ossification of muscle,** upper arm
M61.221 **Paralytic calcification and ossification of muscle,** right upper arm
M61.222 **Paralytic calcification and ossification of muscle,** left upper arm
M61.229 **Paralytic calcification and ossification of muscle, unspecified upper arm**
✓6ᵗʰ M61.23 **Paralytic calcification and ossification of muscle,** forearm
M61.231 **Paralytic calcification and ossification of muscle,** right forearm
M61.232 **Paralytic calcification and ossification of muscle,** left forearm

N Newborn: 0   P Pediatric: 0-17   M Maternity: 9-64   A Adult: 15-124   MCC Major Complication/Comorbidity   CC Complication/Comorbidity   SW Severe Wound Dx

812   ICD-10-CM 2020

M61.239 Paralytic calcification and ossification of muscle, unspecified forearm

✓6ᵗʰ **M61.24** Paralytic calcification and ossification of muscle, hand

M61.241 Paralytic calcification and ossification of muscle, right hand

M61.242 Paralytic calcification and ossification of muscle, left hand

M61.249 Paralytic calcification and ossification of muscle, unspecified hand

✓6ᵗʰ **M61.25** Paralytic calcification and ossification of muscle, thigh

M61.251 Paralytic calcification and ossification of muscle, right thigh

M61.252 Paralytic calcification and ossification of muscle, left thigh

M61.259 Paralytic calcification and ossification of muscle, unspecified thigh

✓6ᵗʰ **M61.26** Paralytic calcification and ossification of muscle, lower leg

M61.261 Paralytic calcification and ossification of muscle, right lower leg

M61.262 Paralytic calcification and ossification of muscle, left lower leg

M61.269 Paralytic calcification and ossification of muscle, unspecified lower leg

✓6ᵗʰ **M61.27** Paralytic calcification and ossification of muscle, ankle and foot

M61.271 Paralytic calcification and ossification of muscle, right ankle and foot

M61.272 Paralytic calcification and ossification of muscle, left ankle and foot

M61.279 Paralytic calcification and ossification of muscle, unspecified ankle and foot

M61.28 Paralytic calcification and ossification of muscle, other site

M61.29 Paralytic calcification and ossification of muscle, multiple sites

✓5ᵗʰ **M61.3** Calcification and ossification of muscles associated with burns

Myositis ossificans associated with burns

M61.30 Calcification and ossification of muscles associated with burns, unspecified site

✓6ᵗʰ **M61.31** Calcification and ossification of muscles associated with burns, shoulder

M61.311 Calcification and ossification of muscles associated with burns, right shoulder

M61.312 Calcification and ossification of muscles associated with burns, left shoulder

M61.319 Calcification and ossification of muscles associated with burns, unspecified shoulder

✓6ᵗʰ **M61.32** Calcification and ossification of muscles associated with burns, upper arm

M61.321 Calcification and ossification of muscles associated with burns, right upper arm

M61.322 Calcification and ossification of muscles associated with burns, left upper arm

M61.329 Calcification and ossification of muscles associated with burns, unspecified upper arm

✓6ᵗʰ **M61.33** Calcification and ossification of muscles associated with burns, forearm

M61.331 Calcification and ossification of muscles associated with burns, right forearm

M61.332 Calcification and ossification of muscles associated with burns, left forearm

M61.339 Calcification and ossification of muscles associated with burns, unspecified forearm

✓6ᵗʰ **M61.34** Calcification and ossification of muscles associated with burns, hand

M61.341 Calcification and ossification of muscles associated with burns, right hand

M61.342 Calcification and ossification of muscles associated with burns, left hand

M61.349 Calcification and ossification of muscles associated with burns, unspecified hand

✓6ᵗʰ **M61.35** Calcification and ossification of muscles associated with burns, thigh

M61.351 Calcification and ossification of muscles associated with burns, right thigh

M61.352 Calcification and ossification of muscles associated with burns, left thigh

M61.359 Calcification and ossification of muscles associated with burns, unspecified thigh

✓6ᵗʰ **M61.36** Calcification and ossification of muscles associated with burns, lower leg

M61.361 Calcification and ossification of muscles associated with burns, right lower leg

M61.362 Calcification and ossification of muscles associated with burns, left lower leg

M61.369 Calcification and ossification of muscles associated with burns, unspecified lower leg

✓6ᵗʰ **M61.37** Calcification and ossification of muscles associated with burns, ankle and foot

M61.371 Calcification and ossification of muscles associated with burns, right ankle and foot

M61.372 Calcification and ossification of muscles associated with burns, left ankle and foot

M61.379 Calcification and ossification of muscles associated with burns, unspecified ankle and foot

M61.38 Calcification and ossification of muscles associated with burns, other site

M61.39 Calcification and ossification of muscles associated with burns, multiple sites

✓5ᵗʰ **M61.4** Other calcification of muscle

> EXCLUDES 1 *calcific tendinitis NOS (M65.2-)*
> *calcific tendinitis of shoulder (M75.3)*

M61.40 Other calcification of muscle, unspecified site

✓6ᵗʰ **M61.41** Other calcification of muscle, shoulder

M61.411 Other calcification of muscle, right shoulder

M61.412 Other calcification of muscle, left shoulder

M61.419 Other calcification of muscle, unspecified shoulder

✓6ᵗʰ **M61.42** Other calcification of muscle, upper arm

M61.421 Other calcification of muscle, right upper arm

M61.422 Other calcification of muscle, left upper arm

M61.429 Other calcification of muscle, unspecified upper arm

✓6ᵗʰ **M61.43** Other calcification of muscle, forearm

M61.431 Other calcification of muscle, right forearm

M61.432 Other calcification of muscle, left forearm

M61.439 Other calcification of muscle, unspecified forearm

✓6ᵗʰ **M61.44** Other calcification of muscle, hand

M61.441 Other calcification of muscle, right hand

M61.442 Other calcification of muscle, left hand

M61.449 Other calcification of muscle, unspecified hand

✓6ᵗʰ **M61.45** Other calcification of muscle, thigh

M61.451 Other calcification of muscle, right thigh

M61.452 Other calcification of muscle, left thigh

M61.459 Other calcification of muscle, unspecified thigh

✓6ᵗʰ **M61.46** Other calcification of muscle, lower leg

M61.461 Other calcification of muscle, right lower leg

M61.462 Other calcification of muscle, left lower leg

M61.469 Other calcification of muscle, unspecified lower leg

✓6ᵗʰ **M61.47** Other calcification of muscle, ankle and foot

M61.471 Other calcification of muscle, right ankle and foot

M61.472 Other calcification of muscle, left ankle and foot

M61.479 Other calcification of muscle, unspecified ankle and foot

M61.48 Other calcification of muscle, other site

M61.49 Other calcification of muscle, multiple sites

✓5ᵗʰ **M61.5** Other ossification of muscle

M61.50 Other ossification of muscle, unspecified site

✓6ᵗʰ M61.51   Other ossification of muscle, shoulder

   M61.511   Other ossification of muscle, right shoulder

   M61.512   Other ossification of muscle, left shoulder

   M61.519   Other ossification of muscle, unspecified shoulder

✓6ᵗʰ M61.52   Other ossification of muscle, upper arm

   M61.521   Other ossification of muscle, right upper arm

   M61.522   Other ossification of muscle, left upper arm

   M61.529   Other ossification of muscle, unspecified upper arm

✓6ᵗʰ M61.53   Other ossification of muscle, forearm

   M61.531   Other ossification of muscle, right forearm

   M61.532   Other ossification of muscle, left forearm

   M61.539   Other ossification of muscle, unspecified forearm

✓6ᵗʰ M61.54   Other ossification of muscle, hand

   M61.541   Other ossification of muscle, right hand

   M61.542   Other ossification of muscle, left hand

   M61.549   Other ossification of muscle, unspecified hand

✓6ᵗʰ M61.55   Other ossification of muscle, thigh

   M61.551   Other ossification of muscle, right thigh

   M61.552   Other ossification of muscle, left thigh

   M61.559   Other ossification of muscle, unspecified thigh

✓6ᵗʰ M61.56   Other ossification of muscle, lower leg

   M61.561   Other ossification of muscle, right lower leg

   M61.562   Other ossification of muscle, left lower leg

   M61.569   Other ossification of muscle, unspecified lower leg

✓6ᵗʰ M61.57   Other ossification of muscle, ankle and foot

   M61.571   Other ossification of muscle, right ankle and foot

   M61.572   Other ossification of muscle, left ankle and foot

   M61.579   Other ossification of muscle, unspecified ankle and foot

  M61.58   Other ossification of muscle, other site

  M61.59   Other ossification of muscle, multiple sites

M61.9   Calcification and ossification of muscle, unspecified

✓4ᵗʰ M62   **Other disorders of muscle**

   EXCLUDES 1   *alcoholic myopathy (G72.1)*
            cramp and spasm (R25.2)
            drug-induced myopathy (G72.0)
            myalgia (M79.1-)
            stiff-man syndrome (G25.82)

   EXCLUDES 2   *nontraumatic hematoma of muscle (M79.81)*

✓5ᵗʰ M62.0   Separation of muscle (nontraumatic)

   Diastasis of muscle

   EXCLUDES 1   *diastasis recti complicating pregnancy, labor and delivery (O71.8)*
            traumatic separation of muscle — see strain of muscle by body region

   M62.00   Separation of muscle (nontraumatic), unspecified site

✓6ᵗʰ M62.01   Separation of muscle (nontraumatic), shoulder

   M62.011   Separation of muscle (nontraumatic), right shoulder

   M62.012   Separation of muscle (nontraumatic), left shoulder

   M62.019   Separation of muscle (nontraumatic), unspecified shoulder

✓6ᵗʰ M62.02   Separation of muscle (nontraumatic), upper arm

   M62.021   Separation of muscle (nontraumatic), right upper arm

   M62.022   Separation of muscle (nontraumatic), left upper arm

   M62.029   Separation of muscle (nontraumatic), unspecified upper arm

✓6ᵗʰ M62.03   Separation of muscle (nontraumatic), forearm

   M62.031   Separation of muscle (nontraumatic), right forearm

   M62.032   Separation of muscle (nontraumatic), left forearm

   M62.039   Separation of muscle (nontraumatic), unspecified forearm

✓6ᵗʰ M62.04   Separation of muscle (nontraumatic), hand

   M62.041   Separation of muscle (nontraumatic), right hand

   M62.042   Separation of muscle (nontraumatic), left hand

   M62.049   Separation of muscle (nontraumatic), unspecified hand

✓6ᵗʰ M62.05   Separation of muscle (nontraumatic), thigh

   M62.051   Separation of muscle (nontraumatic), right thigh

   M62.052   Separation of muscle (nontraumatic), left thigh

   M62.059   Separation of muscle (nontraumatic), unspecified thigh

✓6ᵗʰ M62.06   Separation of muscle (nontraumatic), lower leg

   M62.061   Separation of muscle (nontraumatic), right lower leg

   M62.062   Separation of muscle (nontraumatic), left lower leg

   M62.069   Separation of muscle (nontraumatic), unspecified lower leg

✓6ᵗʰ M62.07   Separation of muscle (nontraumatic), ankle and foot

   M62.071   Separation of muscle (nontraumatic), right ankle and foot

   M62.072   Separation of muscle (nontraumatic), left ankle and foot

   M62.079   Separation of muscle (nontraumatic), unspecified ankle and foot

  M62.08   Separation of muscle (nontraumatic), other site

✓5ᵗʰ M62.1   Other rupture of muscle (nontraumatic)

   EXCLUDES 1   *traumatic rupture of muscle — see strain of muscle by body region*

   EXCLUDES 2   *rupture of tendon (M66.-)*

   M62.10   Other rupture of muscle (nontraumatic), unspecified site

✓6ᵗʰ M62.11   Other rupture of muscle (nontraumatic), shoulder

   M62.111   Other rupture of muscle (nontraumatic), right shoulder

   M62.112   Other rupture of muscle (nontraumatic), left shoulder

   M62.119   Other rupture of muscle (nontraumatic), unspecified shoulder

✓6ᵗʰ M62.12   Other rupture of muscle (nontraumatic), upper arm

   M62.121   Other rupture of muscle (nontraumatic), right upper arm

   M62.122   Other rupture of muscle (nontraumatic), left upper arm

   M62.129   Other rupture of muscle (nontraumatic), unspecified upper arm

✓6ᵗʰ M62.13   Other rupture of muscle (nontraumatic), forearm

   M62.131   Other rupture of muscle (nontraumatic), right forearm

   M62.132   Other rupture of muscle (nontraumatic), left forearm

   M62.139   Other rupture of muscle (nontraumatic), unspecified forearm

✓6ᵗʰ M62.14   Other rupture of muscle (nontraumatic), hand

   M62.141   Other rupture of muscle (nontraumatic), right hand

   M62.142   Other rupture of muscle (nontraumatic), left hand

   M62.149   Other rupture of muscle (nontraumatic), unspecified hand

✓6ᵗʰ M62.15   Other rupture of muscle (nontraumatic), thigh

   M62.151   Other rupture of muscle (nontraumatic), right thigh

   M62.152   Other rupture of muscle (nontraumatic), left thigh

   M62.159   Other rupture of muscle (nontraumatic), unspecified thigh

✓6ᵗʰ M62.16   Other rupture of muscle (nontraumatic), lower leg

   M62.161   Other rupture of muscle (nontraumatic), right lower leg

   M62.162   Other rupture of muscle (nontraumatic), left lower leg

N Newborn: 0   **P** Pediatric: 0-17   **M** Maternity: 9-64   **A** Adult: 15-124   **MCC** Major Complication/Comorbidity   **CC** Complication/Comorbidity   **SW** Severe Wound Dx

814   ICD-10-CM 2020

M62.169 Other rupture of muscle (nontraumatic), unspecified lower leg

√6ᵗʰ **M62.17** Other rupture of muscle (nontraumatic), ankle and foot

    M62.171 Other rupture of muscle (nontraumatic), right ankle and foot

    M62.172 Other rupture of muscle (nontraumatic), left ankle and foot

    M62.179 Other rupture of muscle (nontraumatic), unspecified ankle and foot

  M62.18 Other rupture of muscle (nontraumatic), other site

√5ᵗʰ **M62.2** Nontraumatic ischemic infarction of muscle

    EXCLUDES 1   *compartment syndrome (traumatic) (T79.A-)*

         nontraumatic compartment syndrome (M79.A-)

         rhabdomyolysis (M62.82)

         traumatic ischemia of muscle (T79.6)

         Volkmann's ischemic contracture (T79.6)

  M62.20 Nontraumatic ischemic infarction of muscle, unspecified site

√6ᵗʰ **M62.21** Nontraumatic ischemic infarction of muscle, shoulder

    M62.211 Nontraumatic ischemic infarction of muscle, right shoulder

    M62.212 Nontraumatic ischemic infarction of muscle, left shoulder

    M62.219 Nontraumatic ischemic infarction of muscle, unspecified shoulder

√6ᵗʰ **M62.22** Nontraumatic ischemic infarction of muscle, upper arm

    M62.221 Nontraumatic ischemic infarction of muscle, right upper arm

    M62.222 Nontraumatic ischemic infarction of muscle, left upper arm

    M62.229 Nontraumatic ischemic infarction of muscle, unspecified upper arm

√6ᵗʰ **M62.23** Nontraumatic ischemic infarction of muscle, forearm

    M62.231 Nontraumatic ischemic infarction of muscle, right forearm

    M62.232 Nontraumatic ischemic infarction of muscle, left forearm

    M62.239 Nontraumatic ischemic infarction of muscle, unspecified forearm

√6ᵗʰ **M62.24** Nontraumatic ischemic infarction of muscle, hand

    M62.241 Nontraumatic ischemic infarction of muscle, right hand

    M62.242 Nontraumatic ischemic infarction of muscle, left hand

    M62.249 Nontraumatic ischemic infarction of muscle, unspecified hand

√6ᵗʰ **M62.25** Nontraumatic ischemic infarction of muscle, thigh

    M62.251 Nontraumatic ischemic infarction of muscle, right thigh

    M62.252 Nontraumatic ischemic infarction of muscle, left thigh

    M62.259 Nontraumatic ischemic infarction of muscle, unspecified thigh

√6ᵗʰ **M62.26** Nontraumatic ischemic infarction of muscle, lower leg

    M62.261 Nontraumatic ischemic infarction of muscle, right lower leg

    M62.262 Nontraumatic ischemic infarction of muscle, left lower leg

    M62.269 Nontraumatic ischemic infarction of muscle, unspecified lower leg

√6ᵗʰ **M62.27** Nontraumatic ischemic infarction of muscle, ankle and foot

    M62.271 Nontraumatic ischemic infarction of muscle, right ankle and foot

    M62.272 Nontraumatic ischemic infarction of muscle, left ankle and foot

    M62.279 Nontraumatic ischemic infarction of muscle, unspecified ankle and foot

  M62.28 Nontraumatic ischemic infarction of muscle, other site

  M62.3 Immobility syndrome (paraplegic)   CC

√5ᵗʰ **M62.4** Contracture of muscle

    Contracture of tendon (sheath)

    EXCLUDES 1   *contracture of joint (M24.5-)*

  M62.40 Contracture of muscle, unspecified site

√6ᵗʰ **M62.41** Contracture of muscle, shoulder

    M62.411 Contracture of muscle, right shoulder

    M62.412 Contracture of muscle, left shoulder

    M62.419 Contracture of muscle, unspecified shoulder

√6ᵗʰ **M62.42** Contracture of muscle, upper arm

    M62.421 Contracture of muscle, right upper arm

    M62.422 Contracture of muscle, left upper arm

    M62.429 Contracture of muscle, unspecified upper arm

√6ᵗʰ **M62.43** Contracture of muscle, forearm

    M62.431 Contracture of muscle, right forearm

    M62.432 Contracture of muscle, left forearm

    M62.439 Contracture of muscle, unspecified forearm

√6ᵗʰ **M62.44** Contracture of muscle, hand

    M62.441 Contracture of muscle, right hand

    M62.442 Contracture of muscle, left hand

    M62.449 Contracture of muscle, unspecified hand

√6ᵗʰ **M62.45** Contracture of muscle, thigh

    M62.451 Contracture of muscle, right thigh

    M62.452 Contracture of muscle, left thigh

    M62.459 Contracture of muscle, unspecified thigh

√6ᵗʰ **M62.46** Contracture of muscle, lower leg

    M62.461 Contracture of muscle, right lower leg

    M62.462 Contracture of muscle, left lower leg

    M62.469 Contracture of muscle, unspecified lower leg

√6ᵗʰ **M62.47** Contracture of muscle, ankle and foot

    M62.471 Contracture of muscle, right ankle and foot

    M62.472 Contracture of muscle, left ankle and foot

    M62.479 Contracture of muscle, unspecified ankle and foot

  M62.48 Contracture of muscle, other site

  M62.49 Contracture of muscle, multiple sites

√5ᵗʰ **M62.5** Muscle wasting and atrophy, not elsewhere classified

    Disuse atrophy NEC

    EXCLUDES 1   *neuralgic amyotrophy (G54.5)*

         progressive muscular atrophy (G12.21)

         sarcopenia (M62.84)

    EXCLUDES 2   *pelvic muscle wasting (N81.84)*

  M62.50 Muscle wasting and atrophy, not elsewhere classified, unspecified site

√6ᵗʰ **M62.51** Muscle wasting and atrophy, not elsewhere classified, shoulder

    M62.511 Muscle wasting and atrophy, not elsewhere classified, right shoulder

    M62.512 Muscle wasting and atrophy, not elsewhere classified, left shoulder

    M62.519 Muscle wasting and atrophy, not elsewhere classified, unspecified shoulder

√6ᵗʰ **M62.52** Muscle wasting and atrophy, not elsewhere classified, upper arm

    M62.521 Muscle wasting and atrophy, not elsewhere classified, right upper arm

    M62.522 Muscle wasting and atrophy, not elsewhere classified, left upper arm

    M62.529 Muscle wasting and atrophy, not elsewhere classified, unspecified upper arm

√6ᵗʰ **M62.53** Muscle wasting and atrophy, not elsewhere classified, forearm

    M62.531 Muscle wasting and atrophy, not elsewhere classified, right forearm

    M62.532 Muscle wasting and atrophy, not elsewhere classified, left forearm

    M62.539 Muscle wasting and atrophy, not elsewhere classified, unspecified forearm

√6ᵗʰ **M62.54** Muscle wasting and atrophy, not elsewhere classified, hand

    M62.541 Muscle wasting and atrophy, not elsewhere classified, right hand

    M62.542 Muscle wasting and atrophy, not elsewhere classified, left hand

    M62.549 Muscle wasting and atrophy, not elsewhere classified, unspecified hand

☑ Additional Character Required   √x7ᵗʰ Placeholder   Unacceptable PDx   Questionable PDx   Manifestation   Unspecified Dx   H1-H14 HAC   HCC CMS-HCC Dx   HIV HIV Dx

ICD-10-CM 2020

815

√6th **M62.55** **Muscle wasting and atrophy, not elsewhere classified, thigh**
　　M62.551 Muscle wasting and atrophy, not elsewhere classified, right thigh
　　M62.552 Muscle wasting and atrophy, not elsewhere classified, left thigh
　　M62.559 Muscle wasting and atrophy, not elsewhere classified, unspecified thigh

√6th **M62.56** **Muscle wasting and atrophy, not elsewhere classified, lower leg**
　　M62.561 Muscle wasting and atrophy, not elsewhere classified, right lower leg
　　M62.562 Muscle wasting and atrophy, not elsewhere classified, left lower leg
　　M62.569 Muscle wasting and atrophy, not elsewhere classified, unspecified lower leg

√6th **M62.57** **Muscle wasting and atrophy, not elsewhere classified, ankle and foot**
　　M62.571 Muscle wasting and atrophy, not elsewhere classified, right ankle and foot
　　M62.572 Muscle wasting and atrophy, not elsewhere classified, left ankle and foot
　　M62.579 Muscle wasting and atrophy, not elsewhere classified, unspecified ankle and foot

　　M62.58 **Muscle wasting and atrophy, not elsewhere classified, other site**

　　M62.59 **Muscle wasting and atrophy, not elsewhere classified, multiple sites**

√5th **M62.8** **Other specified disorders of muscle**
　　EXCLUDES 2　nontraumatic hematoma of muscle (M79.81)

　　M62.81 **Muscle weakness (generalized)**
　　　　EXCLUDES 1　muscle weakness in sarcopenia (M62.84)

　　M62.82 **Rhabdomyolysis** CC
　　　　EXCLUDES 1　traumatic rhabdomyolysis (T79.6)
　　　　AHA: 2019,2Q,12
　　　　DEF: Rapid disintegration or destruction of skeletal muscle caused by direct or indirect injury, resulting in the excretion of muscle protein myoglobin into the urine.
　　　　CC Excl: PDX collection 892

√6th **M62.83** **Muscle spasm**
　　M62.830 Muscle spasm of back
　　M62.831 Muscle spasm of calf
　　　　Charley-horse
　　M62.838 Other muscle spasm

　　M62.84 **Sarcopenia**
　　　　Age-related sarcopenia
　　　　Code first underlying disease, if applicable, such as:
　　　　　disorders of myoneural junction and muscle disease in diseases classified elsewhere (G73.-)
　　　　　other and unspecified myopathies (G72.-)
　　　　　primary disorders of muscles (G71.-)
　　　　AHA: 2016,4Q,41

　　M62.89 **Other specified disorders of muscle**
　　　　Muscle (sheath) hernia

M62.9 **Disorder of muscle, unspecified**

√4th **M63** **Disorders of muscle in diseases classified elsewhere**
　　Code first underlying disease, such as:
　　　leprosy (A30.-)
　　　neoplasm (C49.-, C79.89, D21.-, D48.1)
　　　schistosomiasis (B65.-)
　　　trichinellosis (B75)
　　EXCLUDES 1　myopathy in cysticercosis (B69.81)
　　　　myopathy in endocrine diseases (G73.7)
　　　　myopathy in metabolic diseases (G73.7)
　　　　myopathy in sarcoidosis (D86.87)
　　　　myopathy in secondary syphilis (A51.49)
　　　　myopathy in syphilis (late) (A52.78)
　　　　myopathy in toxoplasmosis (B58.82)
　　　　myopathy in tuberculosis (A18.09)

√5th **M63.8** **Disorders of muscle in diseases classified elsewhere**
　　M63.80 *Disorders of muscle in diseases classified elsewhere, unspecified site*
√6th **M63.81** *Disorders of muscle in diseases classified elsewhere, shoulder*
　　M63.811 *Disorders of muscle in diseases classified elsewhere, right shoulder*

　　M63.812 *Disorders of muscle in diseases classified elsewhere, left shoulder*
　　M63.819 *Disorders of muscle in diseases classified elsewhere, unspecified shoulder*
√6th **M63.82** *Disorders of muscle in diseases classified elsewhere, upper arm*
　　M63.821 *Disorders of muscle in diseases classified elsewhere, right upper arm*
　　M63.822 *Disorders of muscle in diseases classified elsewhere, left upper arm*
　　M63.829 *Disorders of muscle in diseases classified elsewhere, unspecified upper arm*
√6th **M63.83** *Disorders of muscle in diseases classified elsewhere, forearm*
　　M63.831 *Disorders of muscle in diseases classified elsewhere, right forearm*
　　M63.832 *Disorders of muscle in diseases classified elsewhere, left forearm*
　　M63.839 *Disorders of muscle in diseases classified elsewhere, unspecified forearm*
√6th **M63.84** *Disorders of muscle in diseases classified elsewhere, hand*
　　M63.841 *Disorders of muscle in diseases classified elsewhere, right hand*
　　M63.842 *Disorders of muscle in diseases classified elsewhere, left hand*
　　M63.849 *Disorders of muscle in diseases classified elsewhere, unspecified hand*
√6th **M63.85** *Disorders of muscle in diseases classified elsewhere, thigh*
　　M63.851 *Disorders of muscle in diseases classified elsewhere, right thigh*
　　M63.852 *Disorders of muscle in diseases classified elsewhere, left thigh*
　　M63.859 *Disorders of muscle in diseases classified elsewhere, unspecified thigh*
√6th **M63.86** *Disorders of muscle in diseases classified elsewhere, lower leg*
　　M63.861 *Disorders of muscle in diseases classified elsewhere, right lower leg*
　　M63.862 *Disorders of muscle in diseases classified elsewhere, left lower leg*
　　M63.869 *Disorders of muscle in diseases classified elsewhere, unspecified lower leg*
√6th **M63.87** *Disorders of muscle in diseases classified elsewhere, ankle and foot*
　　M63.871 *Disorders of muscle in diseases classified elsewhere, right ankle and foot*
　　M63.872 *Disorders of muscle in diseases classified elsewhere, left ankle and foot*
　　M63.879 *Disorders of muscle in diseases classified elsewhere, unspecified ankle and foot*
　　M63.88 *Disorders of muscle in diseases classified elsewhere, other site*
　　M63.89 *Disorders of muscle in diseases classified elsewhere, multiple sites*

Disorders of synovium and tendon (M65-M67)

√4th **M65** **Synovitis and tenosynovitis**
　　EXCLUDES 1　chronic crepitant synovitis of hand and wrist (M70.0-)
　　　　current injury — see injury of ligament or tendon by body region
　　　　soft tissue disorders related to use, overuse and pressure (M70.-)

√5th **M65.0** **Abscess of tendon sheath**
　　Use additional code (B95-B96) to identify bacterial agent.
　　M65.00 Abscess of tendon sheath, unspecified site
√6th **M65.01** Abscess of tendon sheath, shoulder
　　M65.011 Abscess of tendon sheath, right shoulder
　　M65.012 Abscess of tendon sheath, left shoulder
　　M65.019 Abscess of tendon sheath, unspecified shoulder
√6th **M65.02** Abscess of tendon sheath, upper arm
　　M65.021 Abscess of tendon sheath, right upper arm
　　M65.022 Abscess of tendon sheath, left upper arm
　　M65.029 Abscess of tendon sheath, unspecified upper arm
√6th **M65.03** Abscess of tendon sheath, forearm
　　M65.031 Abscess of tendon sheath, right forearm

M65.032   Abscess of tendon sheath, left forearm

M65.039   Abscess of tendon sheath, unspecified forearm

✓6ᵗʰ M65.04   Abscess of tendon sheath, hand

M65.041   Abscess of tendon sheath, right hand

M65.042   Abscess of tendon sheath, left hand

M65.049   Abscess of tendon sheath, unspecified hand

✓6ᵗʰ M65.05   Abscess of tendon sheath, thigh

M65.051   Abscess of tendon sheath, right thigh

M65.052   Abscess of tendon sheath, left thigh

M65.059   Abscess of tendon sheath, unspecified thigh

✓6ᵗʰ M65.06   Abscess of tendon sheath, lower leg

M65.061   Abscess of tendon sheath, right lower leg

M65.062   Abscess of tendon sheath, left lower leg

M65.069   Abscess of tendon sheath, unspecified lower leg

✓6ᵗʰ M65.07   Abscess of tendon sheath, ankle and foot

M65.071   Abscess of tendon sheath, right ankle and foot

M65.072   Abscess of tendon sheath, left ankle and foot

M65.079   Abscess of tendon sheath, unspecified ankle and foot

M65.08   Abscess of tendon sheath, other site

✓5ᵗʰ M65.1   Other infective (teno)synovitis

M65.10   Other infective (teno)synovitis, unspecified site

✓6ᵗʰ M65.11   Other infective (teno)synovitis, shoulder

M65.111   Other infective (teno)synovitis, right shoulder

M65.112   Other infective (teno)synovitis, left shoulder

M65.119   Other infective (teno)synovitis, unspecified shoulder

✓6ᵗʰ M65.12   Other infective (teno)synovitis, elbow

M65.121   Other infective (teno)synovitis, right elbow

M65.122   Other infective (teno)synovitis, left elbow

M65.129   Other infective (teno)synovitis, unspecified elbow

✓6ᵗʰ M65.13   Other infective (teno)synovitis, wrist

M65.131   Other infective (teno)synovitis, right wrist

M65.132   Other infective (teno)synovitis, left wrist

M65.139   Other infective (teno)synovitis, unspecified wrist

✓6ᵗʰ M65.14   Other infective (teno)synovitis, hand

M65.141   Other infective (teno)synovitis, right hand

M65.142   Other infective (teno)synovitis, left hand

M65.149   Other infective (teno)synovitis, unspecified hand

✓6ᵗʰ M65.15   Other infective (teno)synovitis, hip

M65.151   Other infective (teno)synovitis, right hip

M65.152   Other infective (teno)synovitis, left hip

M65.159   Other infective (teno)synovitis, unspecified hip

✓6ᵗʰ M65.16   Other infective (teno)synovitis, knee

M65.161   Other infective (teno)synovitis, right knee

M65.162   Other infective (teno)synovitis, left knee

M65.169   Other infective (teno)synovitis, unspecified knee

✓6ᵗʰ M65.17   Other infective (teno)synovitis, ankle and foot

M65.171   Other infective (teno)synovitis, right ankle and foot

M65.172   Other infective (teno)synovitis, left ankle and foot

M65.179   Other infective (teno)synovitis, unspecified ankle and foot

M65.18   Other infective (teno)synovitis, other site

M65.19   Other infective (teno)synovitis, multiple sites

✓5ᵗʰ M65.2   Calcific tendinitis

> **EXCLUDES 1**   tendinitis as classified in M75-M77
> calcified tendinitis of shoulder (M75.3)

M65.20   Calcific tendinitis, unspecified site

✓6ᵗʰ M65.22   Calcific tendinitis, upper arm

M65.221   Calcific tendinitis, right upper arm

M65.222   Calcific tendinitis, left upper arm

M65.229   Calcific tendinitis, unspecified upper arm

✓6ᵗʰ M65.23   Calcific tendinitis, forearm

M65.231   Calcific tendinitis, right forearm

M65.232   Calcific tendinitis, left forearm

M65.239   Calcific tendinitis, unspecified forearm

✓6ᵗʰ M65.24   Calcific tendinitis, hand

M65.241   Calcific tendinitis, right hand

M65.242   Calcific tendinitis, left hand

M65.249   Calcific tendinitis, unspecified hand

✓6ᵗʰ M65.25   Calcific tendinitis, thigh

M65.251   Calcific tendinitis, right thigh

M65.252   Calcific tendinitis, left thigh

M65.259   Calcific tendinitis, unspecified thigh

✓6ᵗʰ M65.26   Calcific tendinitis, lower leg

M65.261   Calcific tendinitis, right lower leg

M65.262   Calcific tendinitis, left lower leg

M65.269   Calcific tendinitis, unspecified lower leg

✓6ᵗʰ M65.27   Calcific tendinitis, ankle and foot

M65.271   Calcific tendinitis, right ankle and foot

M65.272   Calcific tendinitis, left ankle and foot

M65.279   Calcific tendinitis, unspecified ankle and foot

M65.28   Calcific tendinitis, other site

M65.29   Calcific tendinitis, multiple sites

✓5ᵗʰ M65.3   Trigger finger

Nodular tendinous disease

M65.30   Trigger finger, unspecified finger

✓6ᵗʰ M65.31   Trigger thumb

M65.311   Trigger thumb, right thumb

M65.312   Trigger thumb, left thumb

M65.319   Trigger thumb, unspecified thumb

✓6ᵗʰ M65.32   Trigger finger, index finger

M65.321   Trigger finger, right index finger

M65.322   Trigger finger, left index finger

M65.329   Trigger finger, unspecified index finger

✓6ᵗʰ M65.33   Trigger finger, middle finger

M65.331   Trigger finger, right middle finger

M65.332   Trigger finger, left middle finger

M65.339   Trigger finger, unspecified middle finger

✓6ᵗʰ M65.34   Trigger finger, ring finger

M65.341   Trigger finger, right ring finger

M65.342   Trigger finger, left ring finger

M65.349   Trigger finger, unspecified ring finger

✓6ᵗʰ M65.35   Trigger finger, little finger

M65.351   Trigger finger, right little finger

M65.352   Trigger finger, left little finger

M65.359   Trigger finger, unspecified little finger

M65.4   Radial styloid tenosynovitis [de Quervain]

✓5ᵗʰ M65.8   Other synovitis and tenosynovitis

M65.80   Other synovitis and tenosynovitis, unspecified site

✓6ᵗʰ M65.81   Other synovitis and tenosynovitis, shoulder

M65.811   Other synovitis and tenosynovitis, right shoulder

M65.812   Other synovitis and tenosynovitis, left shoulder

M65.819   Other synovitis and tenosynovitis, unspecified shoulder

✓6ᵗʰ M65.82   Other synovitis and tenosynovitis, upper arm

M65.821   Other synovitis and tenosynovitis, right upper arm

M65.822   Other synovitis and tenosynovitis, left upper arm

M65.829   Other synovitis and tenosynovitis, unspecified upper arm

✓6ᵗʰ M65.83   Other synovitis and tenosynovitis, forearm

M65.831   Other synovitis and tenosynovitis, right forearm

M65.832   Other synovitis and tenosynovitis, left forearm

M65.839   Other synovitis and tenosynovitis, unspecified forearm

✓6ᵗʰ M65.84   Other synovitis and tenosynovitis, hand

M65.841   Other synovitis and tenosynovitis, right hand

M65.842   Other synovitis and tenosynovitis, left hand

M65.849 Other synovitis and tenosynovitis, unspecified hand

√6ᵗʰ **M65.85** Other synovitis and tenosynovitis, thigh

    M65.851 Other synovitis and tenosynovitis, right thigh

    M65.852 Other synovitis and tenosynovitis, left thigh

    M65.859 Other synovitis and tenosynovitis, unspecified thigh

√6ᵗʰ **M65.86** Other synovitis and tenosynovitis, lower leg

    M65.861 Other synovitis and tenosynovitis, right lower leg

    M65.862 Other synovitis and tenosynovitis, left lower leg

    M65.869 Other synovitis and tenosynovitis, unspecified lower leg

√6ᵗʰ **M65.87** Other synovitis and tenosynovitis, ankle and foot

    M65.871 Other synovitis and tenosynovitis, right ankle and foot

    M65.872 Other synovitis and tenosynovitis, left ankle and foot

    M65.879 Other synovitis and tenosynovitis, unspecified ankle and foot

    M65.88 Other synovitis and tenosynovitis, other site

    M65.89 Other synovitis and tenosynovitis, multiple sites

M65.9 Synovitis and tenosynovitis, unspecified

√4ᵗʰ **M66** Spontaneous rupture of synovium and tendon

    INCLUDES   rupture that occurs when a normal force is applied to tissues that are inferred to have less than normal strength

    EXCLUDES 2   rotator cuff syndrome (M75.1-)

    rupture where an abnormal force is applied to normal tissue — see injury of tendon by body region

M66.0 Rupture of popliteal cyst

√5ᵗʰ **M66.1** Rupture of synovium

    Rupture of synovial cyst

    EXCLUDES 2   rupture of popliteal cyst (M66.0)

    M66.10 Rupture of synovium, unspecified joint

√6ᵗʰ **M66.11** Rupture of synovium, shoulder

    M66.111 Rupture of synovium, right shoulder
    M66.112 Rupture of synovium, left shoulder
    M66.119 Rupture of synovium, unspecified shoulder

√6ᵗʰ **M66.12** Rupture of synovium, elbow

    M66.121 Rupture of synovium, right elbow
    M66.122 Rupture of synovium, left elbow
    M66.129 Rupture of synovium, unspecified elbow

√6ᵗʰ **M66.13** Rupture of synovium, wrist

    M66.131 Rupture of synovium, right wrist
    M66.132 Rupture of synovium, left wrist
    M66.139 Rupture of synovium, unspecified wrist

√6ᵗʰ **M66.14** Rupture of synovium, hand and fingers

    M66.141 Rupture of synovium, right hand
    M66.142 Rupture of synovium, left hand
    M66.143 Rupture of synovium, unspecified hand
    M66.144 Rupture of synovium, right finger(s)
    M66.145 Rupture of synovium, left finger(s)
    M66.146 Rupture of synovium, unspecified finger(s)

√6ᵗʰ **M66.15** Rupture of synovium, hip

    M66.151 Rupture of synovium, right hip
    M66.152 Rupture of synovium, left hip
    M66.159 Rupture of synovium, unspecified hip

√6ᵗʰ **M66.17** Rupture of synovium, ankle, foot and toes

    M66.171 Rupture of synovium, right ankle
    M66.172 Rupture of synovium, left ankle
    M66.173 Rupture of synovium, unspecified ankle
    M66.174 Rupture of synovium, right foot
    M66.175 Rupture of synovium, left foot
    M66.176 Rupture of synovium, unspecified foot
    M66.177 Rupture of synovium, right toe(s)
    M66.178 Rupture of synovium, left toe(s)
    M66.179 Rupture of synovium, unspecified toe(s)

    M66.18 Rupture of synovium, other site

√5ᵗʰ **M66.2** Spontaneous rupture of extensor tendons

    TIP: Refer to the Muscle/Tendon table at the beginning of this chapter.

    M66.20 Spontaneous rupture of extensor tendons, unspecified site

√6ᵗʰ **M66.21** Spontaneous rupture of extensor tendons, shoulder

    M66.211 Spontaneous rupture of extensor tendons, right shoulder
    M66.212 Spontaneous rupture of extensor tendons, left shoulder
    M66.219 Spontaneous rupture of extensor tendons, unspecified shoulder

√6ᵗʰ **M66.22** Spontaneous rupture of extensor tendons, upper arm

    M66.221 Spontaneous rupture of extensor tendons, right upper arm
    M66.222 Spontaneous rupture of extensor tendons, left upper arm
    M66.229 Spontaneous rupture of extensor tendons, unspecified upper arm

√6ᵗʰ **M66.23** Spontaneous rupture of extensor tendons, forearm

    M66.231 Spontaneous rupture of extensor tendons, right forearm
    M66.232 Spontaneous rupture of extensor tendons, left forearm
    M66.239 Spontaneous rupture of extensor tendons, unspecified forearm

√6ᵗʰ **M66.24** Spontaneous rupture of extensor tendons, hand

    M66.241 Spontaneous rupture of extensor tendons, right hand
    M66.242 Spontaneous rupture of extensor tendons, left hand
    M66.249 Spontaneous rupture of extensor tendons, unspecified hand

√6ᵗʰ **M66.25** Spontaneous rupture of extensor tendons, thigh

    M66.251 Spontaneous rupture of extensor tendons, right thigh
    M66.252 Spontaneous rupture of extensor tendons, left thigh
    M66.259 Spontaneous rupture of extensor tendons, unspecified thigh

√6ᵗʰ **M66.26** Spontaneous rupture of extensor tendons, lower leg

    M66.261 Spontaneous rupture of extensor tendons, right lower leg
    M66.262 Spontaneous rupture of extensor tendons, left lower leg
    M66.269 Spontaneous rupture of extensor tendons, unspecified lower leg

√6ᵗʰ **M66.27** Spontaneous rupture of extensor tendons, ankle and foot

    M66.271 Spontaneous rupture of extensor tendons, right ankle and foot
    M66.272 Spontaneous rupture of extensor tendons, left ankle and foot
    M66.279 Spontaneous rupture of extensor tendons, unspecified ankle and foot

    M66.28 Spontaneous rupture of extensor tendons, other site

    M66.29 Spontaneous rupture of extensor tendons, multiple sites

√5ᵗʰ **M66.3** Spontaneous rupture of flexor tendons

    TIP: Refer to the Muscle/Tendon table at the beginning of this chapter.

    M66.30 Spontaneous rupture of flexor tendons, unspecified site

√6ᵗʰ **M66.31** Spontaneous rupture of flexor tendons, shoulder

    M66.311 Spontaneous rupture of flexor tendons, right shoulder
    M66.312 Spontaneous rupture of flexor tendons, left shoulder
    M66.319 Spontaneous rupture of flexor tendons, unspecified shoulder

√6ᵗʰ **M66.32** Spontaneous rupture of flexor tendons, upper arm

    M66.321 Spontaneous rupture of flexor tendons, right upper arm
    M66.322 Spontaneous rupture of flexor tendons, left upper arm
    M66.329 Spontaneous rupture of flexor tendons, unspecified upper arm

N Newborn: 0   P Pediatric: 0-17   M Maternity: 9-64   A Adult: 15-124   MCC Major Complication/Comorbidity   CC Complication/Comorbidity   SW Severe Wound Dx

818   ICD-10-CM 2020

☑6ᵗʰ **M66.33** Spontaneous rupture of flexor tendons, forearm

    M66.331 Spontaneous rupture of flexor tendons, right **forearm**

    M66.332 Spontaneous rupture of flexor tendons, left **forearm**

    M66.339 Spontaneous rupture of flexor tendons, unspecified **forearm**

☑6ᵗʰ **M66.34** Spontaneous rupture of flexor tendons, hand

    M66.341 Spontaneous rupture of flexor tendons, right **hand**

    M66.342 Spontaneous rupture of flexor tendons, left **hand**

    M66.349 Spontaneous rupture of flexor tendons, unspecified **hand**

☑6ᵗʰ **M66.35** Spontaneous rupture of flexor tendons, thigh

    M66.351 Spontaneous rupture of flexor tendons, right **thigh**

    M66.352 Spontaneous rupture of flexor tendons, left **thigh**

    M66.359 Spontaneous rupture of flexor tendons, unspecified **thigh**

☑6ᵗʰ **M66.36** Spontaneous rupture of flexor tendons, lower leg

    M66.361 Spontaneous rupture of flexor tendons, right **lower leg**

    M66.362 Spontaneous rupture of flexor tendons, left **lower leg**

    M66.369 Spontaneous rupture of flexor tendons, unspecified **lower leg**

☑6ᵗʰ **M66.37** Spontaneous rupture of flexor tendons, ankle and foot

    M66.371 Spontaneous rupture of flexor tendons, right **ankle and foot**

    M66.372 Spontaneous rupture of flexor tendons, left **ankle and foot**

    M66.379 Spontaneous rupture of flexor tendons, unspecified **ankle and foot**

    M66.38 Spontaneous rupture of flexor tendons, other site

    M66.39 Spontaneous rupture of flexor tendons, multiple sites

☑5ᵗʰ **M66.8** Spontaneous rupture of other tendons

    TIP: Refer to the Muscle/Tendon table at the beginning of this chapter.

    M66.80 Spontaneous rupture of other tendons, unspecified site

☑6ᵗʰ **M66.81** Spontaneous rupture of other tendons, shoulder

    M66.811 Spontaneous rupture of other tendons, right **shoulder**

    M66.812 Spontaneous rupture of other tendons, left **shoulder**

    M66.819 Spontaneous rupture of other tendons, unspecified **shoulder**

☑6ᵗʰ **M66.82** Spontaneous rupture of other tendons, upper arm

    M66.821 Spontaneous rupture of other tendons, right **upper arm**

    M66.822 Spontaneous rupture of other tendons, left **upper arm**

    M66.829 Spontaneous rupture of other tendons, unspecified **upper arm**

☑6ᵗʰ **M66.83** Spontaneous rupture of other tendons, forearm

    M66.831 Spontaneous rupture of other tendons, right **forearm**

    M66.832 Spontaneous rupture of other tendons, left **forearm**

    M66.839 Spontaneous rupture of other tendons, unspecified **forearm**

☑6ᵗʰ **M66.84** Spontaneous rupture of other tendons, hand

    M66.841 Spontaneous rupture of other tendons, right **hand**

    M66.842 Spontaneous rupture of other tendons, left **hand**

    M66.849 Spontaneous rupture of other tendons, unspecified **hand**

☑6ᵗʰ **M66.85** Spontaneous rupture of other tendons, thigh

    M66.851 Spontaneous rupture of other tendons, right **thigh**

    M66.852 Spontaneous rupture of other tendons, left **thigh**

    M66.859 Spontaneous rupture of other tendons, unspecified **thigh**

☑6ᵗʰ **M66.86** Spontaneous rupture of other tendons, lower leg

    M66.861 Spontaneous rupture of other tendons, right **lower leg**

    M66.862 Spontaneous rupture of other tendons, left **lower leg**

    M66.869 Spontaneous rupture of other tendons, unspecified **lower leg**

☑6ᵗʰ **M66.87** Spontaneous rupture of other tendons, ankle and foot

    M66.871 Spontaneous rupture of other tendons, right **ankle and foot**

    M66.872 Spontaneous rupture of other tendons, left **ankle and foot**

    M66.879 Spontaneous rupture of other tendons, unspecified **ankle and foot**

    M66.88 Spontaneous rupture of other tendons, other sites

    M66.89 Spontaneous rupture of other tendons, multiple sites

M66.9 Spontaneous rupture of unspecified tendon

    Rupture at musculotendinous junction, nontraumatic

☑4ᵗʰ **M67** Other disorders of synovium and tendon

    EXCLUDES 1   palmar fascial fibromatosis [Dupuytren] (M72.0)

                tendinitis NOS (M77.9-)

                xanthomatosis localized to tendons (E78.2)

☑5ᵗʰ **M67.0** Short Achilles tendon (acquired)

    M67.00 Short Achilles tendon (acquired), unspecified ankle

    M67.01 Short Achilles tendon (acquired), right ankle

    M67.02 Short Achilles tendon (acquired), left ankle

☑5ᵗʰ **M67.2** Synovial hypertrophy, not elsewhere classified

    EXCLUDES 1   villonodular synovitis (pigmented) (M12.2-)

    M67.20 Synovial hypertrophy, not elsewhere classified, unspecified site

☑6ᵗʰ **M67.21** Synovial hypertrophy, not elsewhere classified, shoulder

    M67.211 Synovial hypertrophy, not elsewhere classified, right **shoulder**

    M67.212 Synovial hypertrophy, not elsewhere classified, left **shoulder**

    M67.219 Synovial hypertrophy, not elsewhere classified, unspecified **shoulder**

☑6ᵗʰ **M67.22** Synovial hypertrophy, not elsewhere classified, upper arm

    M67.221 Synovial hypertrophy, not elsewhere classified, right **upper arm**

    M67.222 Synovial hypertrophy, not elsewhere classified, left **upper arm**

    M67.229 Synovial hypertrophy, not elsewhere classified, unspecified **upper arm**

☑6ᵗʰ **M67.23** Synovial hypertrophy, not elsewhere classified, forearm

    M67.231 Synovial hypertrophy, not elsewhere classified, right **forearm**

    M67.232 Synovial hypertrophy, not elsewhere classified, left **forearm**

    M67.239 Synovial hypertrophy, not elsewhere classified, unspecified **forearm**

☑6ᵗʰ **M67.24** Synovial hypertrophy, not elsewhere classified, hand

    M67.241 Synovial hypertrophy, not elsewhere classified, right **hand**

    M67.242 Synovial hypertrophy, not elsewhere classified, left **hand**

    M67.249 Synovial hypertrophy, not elsewhere classified, unspecified **hand**

☑6ᵗʰ **M67.25** Synovial hypertrophy, not elsewhere classified, thigh

    M67.251 Synovial hypertrophy, not elsewhere classified, right **thigh**

    M67.252 Synovial hypertrophy, not elsewhere classified, left **thigh**

    M67.259 Synovial hypertrophy, not elsewhere classified, unspecified **thigh**

☑6ᵗʰ **M67.26** Synovial hypertrophy, not elsewhere classified, lower leg

    M67.261 Synovial hypertrophy, not elsewhere classified, right **lower leg**

    M67.262 Synovial hypertrophy, not elsewhere classified, left **lower leg**

    M67.269 Synovial hypertrophy, not elsewhere classified, unspecified **lower leg**

☑ Additional Character Required   ☑x7ᵗʰ Placeholder   Unacceptable PDx   Questionable PDx   Manifestation   Unspecified Dx   H1-H14 HAC   HCC CMS-HCC Dx   HIV HIV Dx

ICD-10-CM 2020

819

M67.27 Synovial hypertrophy, not elsewhere classified, ankle and foot
     M67.271 Synovial hypertrophy, not elsewhere classified, right ankle and foot
     M67.272 Synovial hypertrophy, not elsewhere classified, left ankle and foot
     M67.279 Synovial hypertrophy, not elsewhere classified, unspecified ankle and foot
M67.28 Synovial hypertrophy, not elsewhere classified, other site
M67.29 Synovial hypertrophy, not elsewhere classified, multiple sites

M67.3 Transient synovitis
    Toxic synovitis
    EXCLUDES 1   palindromic rheumatism (M12.3-)
    M67.30 Transient synovitis, unspecified site
    M67.31 Transient synovitis, shoulder
     M67.311 Transient synovitis, right shoulder
     M67.312 Transient synovitis, left shoulder
     M67.319 Transient synovitis, unspecified shoulder
    M67.32 Transient synovitis, elbow
     M67.321 Transient synovitis, right elbow
     M67.322 Transient synovitis, left elbow
     M67.329 Transient synovitis, unspecified elbow
    M67.33 Transient synovitis, wrist
     M67.331 Transient synovitis, right wrist
     M67.332 Transient synovitis, left wrist
     M67.339 Transient synovitis, unspecified wrist
    M67.34 Transient synovitis, hand
     M67.341 Transient synovitis, right hand
     M67.342 Transient synovitis, left hand
     M67.349 Transient synovitis, unspecified hand
    M67.35 Transient synovitis, hip
     M67.351 Transient synovitis, right hip
     M67.352 Transient synovitis, left hip
     M67.359 Transient synovitis, unspecified hip
    M67.36 Transient synovitis, knee
     M67.361 Transient synovitis, right knee
     M67.362 Transient synovitis, left knee
     M67.369 Transient synovitis, unspecified knee
    M67.37 Transient synovitis, ankle and foot
     M67.371 Transient synovitis, right ankle and foot
     M67.372 Transient synovitis, left ankle and foot
     M67.379 Transient synovitis, unspecified ankle and foot
    M67.38 Transient synovitis, other site
    M67.39 Transient synovitis, multiple sites

M67.4 Ganglion
    Ganglion of joint or tendon (sheath)
    EXCLUDES 1   ganglion in yaws (A66.6)
    EXCLUDES 2   cyst of bursa (M71.2-M71.3)
           cyst of synovium (M71.2-M71.3)
    DEF: Fluid-filled, benign cyst appearing on a tendon sheath or aponeurosis, frequently connecting to an underlying joint.
    M67.40 Ganglion, unspecified site
    M67.41 Ganglion, shoulder
     M67.411 Ganglion, right shoulder
     M67.412 Ganglion, left shoulder
     M67.419 Ganglion, unspecified shoulder
    M67.42 Ganglion, elbow
     M67.421 Ganglion, right elbow
     M67.422 Ganglion, left elbow
     M67.429 Ganglion, unspecified elbow

M67.43 Ganglion, wrist

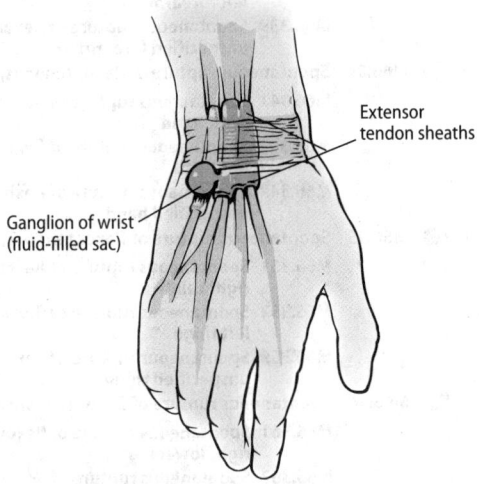

Ganglion of Wrist

Extensor tendon sheaths

Ganglion of wrist (fluid-filled sac)

     M67.431 Ganglion, right wrist
     M67.432 Ganglion, left wrist
     M67.439 Ganglion, unspecified wrist
    M67.44 Ganglion, hand
     M67.441 Ganglion, right hand
     M67.442 Ganglion, left hand
     M67.449 Ganglion, unspecified hand
    M67.45 Ganglion, hip
     M67.451 Ganglion, right hip
     M67.452 Ganglion, left hip
     M67.459 Ganglion, unspecified hip
    M67.46 Ganglion, knee
     M67.461 Ganglion, right knee
     M67.462 Ganglion, left knee
     M67.469 Ganglion, unspecified knee
    M67.47 Ganglion, ankle and foot
     M67.471 Ganglion, right ankle and foot
     M67.472 Ganglion, left ankle and foot
     M67.479 Ganglion, unspecified ankle and foot
    M67.48 Ganglion, other site
    M67.49 Ganglion, multiple sites

M67.5 Plica syndrome
    Plica knee
    M67.50 Plica syndrome, unspecified knee
    M67.51 Plica syndrome, right knee
    M67.52 Plica syndrome, left knee

M67.8 Other specified disorders of synovium and tendon
    M67.80 Other specified disorders of synovium and tendon, unspecified site
    M67.81 Other specified disorders of synovium and tendon, shoulder
     M67.811 Other specified disorders of synovium, right shoulder
     M67.812 Other specified disorders of synovium, left shoulder
     M67.813 Other specified disorders of tendon, right shoulder
     M67.814 Other specified disorders of tendon, left shoulder
     M67.819 Other specified disorders of synovium and tendon, unspecified shoulder
    M67.82 Other specified disorders of synovium and tendon, elbow
     M67.821 Other specified disorders of synovium, right elbow
     M67.822 Other specified disorders of synovium, left elbow
     M67.823 Other specified disorders of tendon, right elbow
     M67.824 Other specified disorders of tendon, left elbow

M67.829 Other specified disorders of synovium and tendon, unspecified elbow
√6ᵗʰ **M67.83** Other specified disorders of synovium and tendon, wrist
   M67.831 Other specified disorders of synovium, right wrist
   M67.832 Other specified disorders of synovium, left wrist
   M67.833 Other specified disorders of tendon, right wrist
   M67.834 Other specified disorders of tendon, left wrist
   M67.839 Other specified disorders of synovium and tendon, unspecified wrist
√6ᵗʰ **M67.84** Other specified disorders of synovium and tendon, hand
   M67.841 Other specified disorders of synovium, right hand
   M67.842 Other specified disorders of synovium, left hand
   M67.843 Other specified disorders of tendon, right hand
   M67.844 Other specified disorders of tendon, left hand
   M67.849 Other specified disorders of synovium and tendon, unspecified hand
√6ᵗʰ **M67.85** Other specified disorders of synovium and tendon, hip
   M67.851 Other specified disorders of synovium, right hip
   M67.852 Other specified disorders of synovium, left hip
   M67.853 Other specified disorders of tendon, right hip
   M67.854 Other specified disorders of tendon, left hip
   M67.859 Other specified disorders of synovium and tendon, unspecified hip
√6ᵗʰ **M67.86** Other specified disorders of synovium and tendon, knee
   M67.861 Other specified disorders of synovium, right knee
   M67.862 Other specified disorders of synovium, left knee
   M67.863 Other specified disorders of tendon, right knee
   M67.864 Other specified disorders of tendon, left knee
   M67.869 Other specified disorders of synovium and tendon, unspecified knee
√6ᵗʰ **M67.87** Other specified disorders of synovium and tendon, ankle and foot
   M67.871 Other specified disorders of synovium, right ankle and foot
   M67.872 Other specified disorders of synovium, left ankle and foot
   M67.873 Other specified disorders of tendon, right ankle and foot
   M67.874 Other specified disorders of tendon, left ankle and foot
   M67.879 Other specified disorders of synovium and tendon, unspecified ankle and foot
M67.88 Other specified disorders of synovium and tendon, other site
M67.89 Other specified disorders of synovium and tendon, multiple sites
√5ᵗʰ **M67.9** Unspecified disorder of synovium and tendon
   M67.90 Unspecified disorder of synovium and tendon, unspecified site
√6ᵗʰ **M67.91** Unspecified disorder of synovium and tendon, shoulder
   M67.911 Unspecified disorder of synovium and tendon, right shoulder
   M67.912 Unspecified disorder of synovium and tendon, left shoulder
   M67.919 Unspecified disorder of synovium and tendon, unspecified shoulder
√6ᵗʰ **M67.92** Unspecified disorder of synovium and tendon, upper arm
   M67.921 Unspecified disorder of synovium and tendon, right upper arm
   M67.922 Unspecified disorder of synovium and tendon, left upper arm

M67.929 Unspecified disorder of synovium and tendon, unspecified upper arm
√6ᵗʰ **M67.93** Unspecified disorder of synovium and tendon, forearm
   M67.931 Unspecified disorder of synovium and tendon, right forearm
   M67.932 Unspecified disorder of synovium and tendon, left forearm
   M67.939 Unspecified disorder of synovium and tendon, unspecified forearm
√6ᵗʰ **M67.94** Unspecified disorder of synovium and tendon, hand
   M67.941 Unspecified disorder of synovium and tendon, right hand
   M67.942 Unspecified disorder of synovium and tendon, left hand
   M67.949 Unspecified disorder of synovium and tendon, unspecified hand
√6ᵗʰ **M67.95** Unspecified disorder of synovium and tendon, thigh
   M67.951 Unspecified disorder of synovium and tendon, right thigh
   M67.952 Unspecified disorder of synovium and tendon, left thigh
   M67.959 Unspecified disorder of synovium and tendon, unspecified thigh
√6ᵗʰ **M67.96** Unspecified disorder of synovium and tendon, lower leg
   M67.961 Unspecified disorder of synovium and tendon, right lower leg
   M67.962 Unspecified disorder of synovium and tendon, left lower leg
   M67.969 Unspecified disorder of synovium and tendon, unspecified lower leg
√6ᵗʰ **M67.97** Unspecified disorder of synovium and tendon, ankle and foot
   M67.971 Unspecified disorder of synovium and tendon, right ankle and foot
   M67.972 Unspecified disorder of synovium and tendon, left ankle and foot
   M67.979 Unspecified disorder of synovium and tendon, unspecified ankle and foot
M67.98 Unspecified disorder of synovium and tendon, other site
M67.99 Unspecified disorder of synovium and tendon, multiple sites

Other soft tissue disorders (M70-M79)

√4ᵗʰ **M70** Soft tissue disorders related to use, overuse and pressure
   INCLUDES soft tissue disorders of occupational origin
   Use additional external cause code to identify activity causing disorder (Y93.-)
   EXCLUDES 1 bursitis NOS (M71.9-)
   EXCLUDES 2 bursitis of shoulder (M75.5)
      enthesopathies (M76-M77)
      pressure ulcer (pressure area) (L89.-)
√5ᵗʰ **M70.0** Crepitant synovitis (acute) (chronic) of hand and wrist
√6ᵗʰ **M70.03** Crepitant synovitis (acute) (chronic), wrist
   M70.031 Crepitant synovitis (acute) (chronic), right wrist
   M70.032 Crepitant synovitis (acute) (chronic), left wrist
   M70.039 Crepitant synovitis (acute) (chronic), unspecified wrist
√6ᵗʰ **M70.04** Crepitant synovitis (acute) (chronic), hand
   M70.041 Crepitant synovitis (acute) (chronic), right hand
   M70.042 Crepitant synovitis (acute) (chronic), left hand
   M70.049 Crepitant synovitis (acute) (chronic), unspecified hand
√5ᵗʰ **M70.1** Bursitis of hand
   M70.10 Bursitis, unspecified hand
   M70.11 Bursitis, right hand
   M70.12 Bursitis, left hand
√5ᵗʰ **M70.2** Olecranon bursitis
   M70.20 Olecranon bursitis, unspecified elbow
   M70.21 Olecranon bursitis, right elbow
   M70.22 Olecranon bursitis, left elbow

√5ᵗʰ **M70.3** **Other bursitis of** elbow
     M70.30 Other bursitis of elbow, unspecified elbow
     M70.31 Other bursitis of elbow, right elbow
     M70.32 Other bursitis of elbow, left elbow

√5ᵗʰ **M70.4** Prepatellar bursitis
     M70.40 Prepatellar bursitis, unspecified knee
     M70.41 Prepatellar bursitis, right knee
     M70.42 Prepatellar bursitis, left knee

Knee Bursae

Suprapatellar bursa — Patella
Femur — Prepatellar bursa
— Infrapatellar bursa
Popliteal bursa — Tibia

√5ᵗʰ **M70.5** **Other bursitis of** knee
     M70.50 Other bursitis of knee, unspecified knee
     M70.51 Other bursitis of knee, right knee
     M70.52 Other bursitis of knee, left knee

√5ᵗʰ **M70.6** Trochanteric **bursitis**
     Trochanteric tendinitis
     M70.60 Trochanteric bursitis, unspecified hip
     M70.61 Trochanteric bursitis, right hip
     M70.62 Trochanteric bursitis, left hip

√5ᵗʰ **M70.7** **Other bursitis of** hip
     Ischial bursitis
     M70.70 Other bursitis of hip, unspecified hip
     M70.71 Other bursitis of hip, right hip
     M70.72 Other bursitis of hip, left hip

√5ᵗʰ **M70.8** **Other soft tissue disorders related to use, overuse and pressure**
     M70.80 Other soft tissue disorders related to use, overuse and pressure of unspecified site

     √6ᵗʰ **M70.81** Other soft tissue disorders related to use, overuse and pressure of shoulder
         M70.811 Other soft tissue disorders related to use, overuse and pressure, right shoulder
         M70.812 Other soft tissue disorders related to use, overuse and pressure, left shoulder
         M70.819 Other soft tissue disorders related to use, overuse and pressure, unspecified shoulder

     √6ᵗʰ **M70.82** Other soft tissue disorders related to use, overuse and pressure of upper arm
         M70.821 Other soft tissue disorders related to use, overuse and pressure, right upper arm
         M70.822 Other soft tissue disorders related to use, overuse and pressure, left upper arm
         M70.829 Other soft tissue disorders related to use, overuse and pressure, unspecified upper arms

     √6ᵗʰ **M70.83** Other soft tissue disorders related to use, overuse and pressure of forearm
         M70.831 Other soft tissue disorders related to use, overuse and pressure, right forearm
         M70.832 Other soft tissue disorders related to use, overuse and pressure, left forearm
         M70.839 Other soft tissue disorders related to use, overuse and pressure, unspecified forearm

√6ᵗʰ **M70.84** Other soft tissue disorders related to use, overuse and pressure of hand
     M70.841 Other soft tissue disorders related to use, overuse and pressure, right hand
     M70.842 Other soft tissue disorders related to use, overuse and pressure, left hand
     M70.849 Other soft tissue disorders related to use, overuse and pressure, unspecified hand

√6ᵗʰ **M70.85** Other soft tissue disorders related to use, overuse and pressure of thigh
     M70.851 Other soft tissue disorders related to use, overuse and pressure, right thigh
     M70.852 Other soft tissue disorders related to use, overuse and pressure, left thigh
     M70.859 Other soft tissue disorders related to use, overuse and pressure, unspecified thigh

√6ᵗʰ **M70.86** Other soft tissue disorders related to use, overuse and pressure lower leg
     M70.861 Other soft tissue disorders related to use, overuse and pressure, right lower leg
     M70.862 Other soft tissue disorders related to use, overuse and pressure, left lower leg
     M70.869 Other soft tissue disorders related to use, overuse and pressure, unspecified leg

√6ᵗʰ **M70.87** Other soft tissue disorders related to use, overuse and pressure of ankle and foot
     M70.871 Other soft tissue disorders related to use, overuse and pressure, right ankle and foot
     M70.872 Other soft tissue disorders related to use, overuse and pressure, left ankle and foot
     M70.879 Other soft tissue disorders related to use, overuse and pressure, unspecified ankle and foot

     M70.88 Other soft tissue disorders related to use, overuse and pressure other site

     M70.89 Other soft tissue disorders related to use, overuse and pressure multiple sites

√5ᵗʰ **M70.9** **Unspecified soft tissue disorder related to use, overuse and pressure**
     M70.90 Unspecified soft tissue disorder related to use, overuse and pressure of unspecified site

     √6ᵗʰ **M70.91** Unspecified soft tissue disorder related to use, overuse and pressure of shoulder
         M70.911 Unspecified soft tissue disorder related to use, overuse and pressure, right shoulder
         M70.912 Unspecified soft tissue disorder related to use, overuse and pressure, left shoulder
         M70.919 Unspecified soft tissue disorder related to use, overuse and pressure, unspecified shoulder

     √6ᵗʰ **M70.92** Unspecified soft tissue disorder related to use, overuse and pressure of upper arm
         M70.921 Unspecified soft tissue disorder related to use, overuse and pressure, right upper arm
         M70.922 Unspecified soft tissue disorder related to use, overuse and pressure, left upper arm
         M70.929 Unspecified soft tissue disorder related to use, overuse and pressure, unspecified upper arm

     √6ᵗʰ **M70.93** Unspecified soft tissue disorder related to use, overuse and pressure of forearm
         M70.931 Unspecified soft tissue disorder related to use, overuse and pressure, right forearm
         M70.932 Unspecified soft tissue disorder related to use, overuse and pressure, left forearm
         M70.939 Unspecified soft tissue disorder related to use, overuse and pressure, unspecified forearm

     √6ᵗʰ **M70.94** Unspecified soft tissue disorder related to use, overuse and pressure of hand
         M70.941 Unspecified soft tissue disorder related to use, overuse and pressure, right hand
         M70.942 Unspecified soft tissue disorder related to use, overuse and pressure, left hand
         M70.949 Unspecified soft tissue disorder related to use, overuse and pressure, unspecified hand

N Newborn: 0   P Pediatric: 0-17   M Maternity: 9-64   A Adult: 15-124   MCC Major Complication/Comorbidity   CC Complication/Comorbidity   SW Severe Wound Dx

822   ICD-10-CM 2020

√6ᵗʰ **M70.95** **Unspecified soft tissue disorder related to use, overuse and pressure of** thigh

    M70.951 Unspecified soft tissue disorder related to use, overuse and pressure, right thigh

    M70.952 Unspecified soft tissue disorder related to use, overuse and pressure, left thigh

    M70.959 Unspecified soft tissue disorder related to use, overuse and pressure, unspecified thigh

√6ᵗʰ **M70.96** **Unspecified soft tissue disorder related to use, overuse and pressure** lower leg

    M70.961 Unspecified soft tissue disorder related to use, overuse and pressure, right lower leg

    M70.962 Unspecified soft tissue disorder related to use, overuse and pressure, left lower leg

    M70.969 Unspecified soft tissue disorder related to use, overuse and pressure, unspecified lower leg

√6ᵗʰ **M70.97** **Unspecified soft tissue disorder related to use, overuse and pressure of** ankle and foot

    M70.971 Unspecified soft tissue disorder related to use, overuse and pressure, right ankle and foot

    M70.972 Unspecified soft tissue disorder related to use, overuse and pressure, left ankle and foot

    M70.979 Unspecified soft tissue disorder related to use, overuse and pressure, unspecified ankle and foot

M70.98 **Unspecified soft tissue disorder related to use, overuse and pressure other**

M70.99 **Unspecified soft tissue disorder related to use, overuse and pressure** multiple sites

√4ᵗʰ **M71** **Other bursopathies**

    EXCLUDES 1   bunion (M20.1)
                  bursitis related to use, overuse or pressure (M70.-)
                  enthesopathies (M76-M77)

√5ᵗʰ **M71.0** **Abscess of bursa**

    Use additional code (B95.-, B96.-) to identify causative organism

    M71.00 **Abscess of bursa, unspecified site**

√6ᵗʰ **M71.01** **Abscess of bursa,** shoulder

    M71.011 Abscess of bursa, right shoulder

    M71.012 Abscess of bursa, left shoulder

    M71.019 Abscess of bursa, unspecified shoulder

√6ᵗʰ **M71.02** **Abscess of bursa,** elbow

    M71.021 Abscess of bursa, right elbow

    M71.022 Abscess of bursa, left elbow

    M71.029 Abscess of bursa, unspecified elbow

√6ᵗʰ **M71.03** **Abscess of bursa,** wrist

    M71.031 Abscess of bursa, right wrist

    M71.032 Abscess of bursa, left wrist

    M71.039 Abscess of bursa, unspecified wrist

√6ᵗʰ **M71.04** **Abscess of bursa,** hand

    M71.041 Abscess of bursa, right hand

    M71.042 Abscess of bursa, left hand

    M71.049 Abscess of bursa, unspecified hand

√6ᵗʰ **M71.05** **Abscess of bursa,** hip

    M71.051 Abscess of bursa, right hip

    M71.052 Abscess of bursa, left hip

    M71.059 Abscess of bursa, unspecified hip

√6ᵗʰ **M71.06** **Abscess of bursa,** knee

    M71.061 Abscess of bursa, right knee

    M71.062 Abscess of bursa, left knee

    M71.069 Abscess of bursa, unspecified knee

√6ᵗʰ **M71.07** **Abscess of bursa,** ankle and foot

    M71.071 Abscess of bursa, right ankle and foot

    M71.072 Abscess of bursa, left ankle and foot

    M71.079 Abscess of bursa, unspecified ankle and foot

M71.08 **Abscess of bursa, other site**

M71.09 **Abscess of bursa,** multiple sites

√5ᵗʰ **M71.1** **Other infective bursitis**

    Use additional code (B95.-, B96.-) to identify causative organism

    M71.10 **Other infective bursitis, unspecified site**

√6ᵗʰ **M71.11** **Other infective bursitis,** shoulder

    M71.111 Other infective bursitis, right shoulder

    M71.112 Other infective bursitis, left shoulder

    M71.119 Other infective bursitis, unspecified shoulder

√6ᵗʰ **M71.12** **Other infective bursitis,** elbow

    M71.121 Other infective bursitis, right elbow

    M71.122 Other infective bursitis, left elbow

    M71.129 Other infective bursitis, unspecified elbow

√6ᵗʰ **M71.13** **Other infective bursitis,** wrist

    M71.131 Other infective bursitis, right wrist

    M71.132 Other infective bursitis, left wrist

    M71.139 Other infective bursitis, unspecified wrist

√6ᵗʰ **M71.14** **Other infective bursitis,** hand

    M71.141 Other infective bursitis, right hand

    M71.142 Other infective bursitis, left hand

    M71.149 Other infective bursitis, unspecified hand

√6ᵗʰ **M71.15** **Other infective bursitis,** hip

    M71.151 Other infective bursitis, right hip

    M71.152 Other infective bursitis, left hip

    M71.159 Other infective bursitis, unspecified hip

√6ᵗʰ **M71.16** **Other infective bursitis,** knee

    M71.161 Other infective bursitis, right knee

    M71.162 Other infective bursitis, left knee

    M71.169 Other infective bursitis, unspecified knee

√6ᵗʰ **M71.17** **Other infective bursitis,** ankle and foot

    M71.171 Other infective bursitis, right ankle and foot

    M71.172 Other infective bursitis, left ankle and foot

    M71.179 Other infective bursitis, unspecified ankle and foot

M71.18 **Other infective bursitis, other site**

M71.19 **Other infective bursitis,** multiple sites

√5ᵗʰ **M71.2** **Synovial cyst of popliteal space [Baker]**

    EXCLUDES 1   synovial cyst of popliteal space with rupture (M66.0)

    DEF: Sac filled with clear synovial fluid in adults, usually secondary to disease inside the joint, located on the back of the knee in the popliteal fossa area. In children, the cyst usually represents a ganglion of one of the tendons in the knee.

Baker's Cyst

Baker's cyst connected to knee joint synovial cavity

    M71.20 **Synovial cyst of popliteal space [Baker], unspecified knee**

    M71.21 **Synovial cyst of popliteal space [Baker],** right knee

    M71.22 **Synovial cyst of popliteal space [Baker],** left knee

√5ᵗʰ **M71.3** **Other bursal cyst**

    Synovial cyst NOS

    EXCLUDES 1   synovial cyst with rupture (M66.1-)

    M71.30 **Other bursal cyst, unspecified site**

√6ᵗʰ **M71.31** **Other bursal cyst,** shoulder

    M71.311 Other bursal cyst, right shoulder

    M71.312 Other bursal cyst, left shoulder

    M71.319 Other bursal cyst, unspecified shoulder

√6ᵗʰ **M71.32** **Other bursal cyst,** elbow

    M71.321 Other bursal cyst, right elbow

☑ Additional Character Required   √x7ᵗʰ Placeholder   Unacceptable PDx   Questionable PDx   Manifestation   Unspecified Dx   H1-H14 HAC   HCC CMS-HCC Dx   HIV HIV Dx

ICD-10-CM 2020   823

M71.322 Other bursal cyst, left elbow
M71.329 Other bursal cyst, unspecified elbow

✓6ᵗʰ M71.33 Other bursal cyst, wrist
M71.331 Other bursal cyst, right wrist
M71.332 Other bursal cyst, left wrist
M71.339 Other bursal cyst, unspecified wrist

✓6ᵗʰ M71.34 Other bursal cyst, hand
M71.341 Other bursal cyst, right hand
M71.342 Other bursal cyst, left hand
M71.349 Other bursal cyst, unspecified hand

✓6ᵗʰ M71.35 Other bursal cyst, hip
M71.351 Other bursal cyst, right hip
M71.352 Other bursal cyst, left hip
M71.359 Other bursal cyst, unspecified hip

✓6ᵗʰ M71.37 Other bursal cyst, ankle and foot
M71.371 Other bursal cyst, right ankle and foot
M71.372 Other bursal cyst, left ankle and foot
M71.379 Other bursal cyst, unspecified ankle and foot

M71.38 Other bursal cyst, other site
M71.39 Other bursal cyst, multiple sites

✓5ᵗʰ M71.4 Calcium deposit in bursa
EXCLUDES 2   calcium deposit in bursa of shoulder (M75.3)

M71.40 Calcium deposit in bursa, unspecified site

✓6ᵗʰ M71.42 Calcium deposit in bursa, elbow
M71.421 Calcium deposit in bursa, right elbow
M71.422 Calcium deposit in bursa, left elbow
M71.429 Calcium deposit in bursa, unspecified elbow

✓6ᵗʰ M71.43 Calcium deposit in bursa, wrist
M71.431 Calcium deposit in bursa, right wrist
M71.432 Calcium deposit in bursa, left wrist
M71.439 Calcium deposit in bursa, unspecified wrist

✓6ᵗʰ M71.44 Calcium deposit in bursa, hand
M71.441 Calcium deposit in bursa, right hand
M71.442 Calcium deposit in bursa, left hand
M71.449 Calcium deposit in bursa, unspecified hand

✓6ᵗʰ M71.45 Calcium deposit in bursa, hip
M71.451 Calcium deposit in bursa, right hip
M71.452 Calcium deposit in bursa, left hip
M71.459 Calcium deposit in bursa, unspecified hip

✓6ᵗʰ M71.46 Calcium deposit in bursa, knee
M71.461 Calcium deposit in bursa, right knee
M71.462 Calcium deposit in bursa, left knee
M71.469 Calcium deposit in bursa, unspecified knee

✓6ᵗʰ M71.47 Calcium deposit in bursa, ankle and foot
M71.471 Calcium deposit in bursa, right ankle and foot
M71.472 Calcium deposit in bursa, left ankle and foot
M71.479 Calcium deposit in bursa, unspecified ankle and foot

M71.48 Calcium deposit in bursa, other site
M71.49 Calcium deposit in bursa, multiple sites

✓5ᵗʰ M71.5 Other bursitis, not elsewhere classified
EXCLUDES 1   bursitis NOS (M71.9-)
EXCLUDES 2   bursitis of shoulder (M75.5)
              bursitis of tibial collateral [Pellegrini-Stieda] (M76.4-)

M71.50 Other bursitis, not elsewhere classified, unspecified site

✓6ᵗʰ M71.52 Other bursitis, not elsewhere classified, elbow
M71.521 Other bursitis, not elsewhere classified, right elbow
M71.522 Other bursitis, not elsewhere classified, left elbow
M71.529 Other bursitis, not elsewhere classified, unspecified elbow

✓6ᵗʰ M71.53 Other bursitis, not elsewhere classified, wrist
M71.531 Other bursitis, not elsewhere classified, right wrist
M71.532 Other bursitis, not elsewhere classified, left wrist
M71.539 Other bursitis, not elsewhere classified, unspecified wrist

✓6ᵗʰ M71.54 Other bursitis, not elsewhere classified, hand
M71.541 Other bursitis, not elsewhere classified, right hand
M71.542 Other bursitis, not elsewhere classified, left hand
M71.549 Other bursitis, not elsewhere classified, unspecified hand

✓6ᵗʰ M71.55 Other bursitis, not elsewhere classified, hip
M71.551 Other bursitis, not elsewhere classified, right hip
M71.552 Other bursitis, not elsewhere classified, left hip
M71.559 Other bursitis, not elsewhere classified, unspecified hip

✓6ᵗʰ M71.56 Other bursitis, not elsewhere classified, knee
M71.561 Other bursitis, not elsewhere classified, right knee
M71.562 Other bursitis, not elsewhere classified, left knee
M71.569 Other bursitis, not elsewhere classified, unspecified knee

✓6ᵗʰ M71.57 Other bursitis, not elsewhere classified, ankle and foot
M71.571 Other bursitis, not elsewhere classified, right ankle and foot
M71.572 Other bursitis, not elsewhere classified, left ankle and foot
M71.579 Other bursitis, not elsewhere classified, unspecified ankle and foot

M71.58 Other bursitis, not elsewhere classified, other site

✓5ᵗʰ M71.8 Other specified bursopathies
M71.80 Other specified bursopathies, unspecified site

✓6ᵗʰ M71.81 Other specified bursopathies, shoulder
M71.811 Other specified bursopathies, right shoulder
M71.812 Other specified bursopathies, left shoulder
M71.819 Other specified bursopathies, unspecified shoulder

✓6ᵗʰ M71.82 Other specified bursopathies, elbow
M71.821 Other specified bursopathies, right elbow
M71.822 Other specified bursopathies, left elbow
M71.829 Other specified bursopathies, unspecified elbow

✓6ᵗʰ M71.83 Other specified bursopathies, wrist
M71.831 Other specified bursopathies, right wrist
M71.832 Other specified bursopathies, left wrist
M71.839 Other specified bursopathies, unspecified wrist

✓6ᵗʰ M71.84 Other specified bursopathies, hand
M71.841 Other specified bursopathies, right hand
M71.842 Other specified bursopathies, left hand
M71.849 Other specified bursopathies, unspecified hand

✓6ᵗʰ M71.85 Other specified bursopathies, hip
M71.851 Other specified bursopathies, right hip
M71.852 Other specified bursopathies, left hip
M71.859 Other specified bursopathies, unspecified hip

✓6ᵗʰ M71.86 Other specified bursopathies, knee
M71.861 Other specified bursopathies, right knee
M71.862 Other specified bursopathies, left knee
M71.869 Other specified bursopathies, unspecified knee

✓6ᵗʰ M71.87 Other specified bursopathies, ankle and foot
M71.871 Other specified bursopathies, right ankle and foot
M71.872 Other specified bursopathies, left ankle and foot
M71.879 Other specified bursopathies, unspecified ankle and foot

M71.88 Other specified bursopathies, other site
M71.89 Other specified bursopathies, multiple sites

M71.9 Bursopathy, unspecified
Bursitis NOS

N Newborn: 0   P Pediatric: 0-17   M Maternity: 9-64   A Adult: 15-124   MCC Major Complication/Comorbidity   CC Complication/Comorbidity   SW Severe Wound Dx

824   ICD-10-CM 2020

✓4ᵗʰ **M72 Fibroblastic disorders**

> EXCLUDES 2   *retroperitoneal fibromatosis (D48.3)*

M72.0 Palmar fascial fibromatosis [Dupuytren]   A

> **DEF:** Dupuytren's contracture: Flexion deformity of a finger, due to shortened, thickened fibrosing of palmar fascia. The cause is unknown, but it is associated with long-standing epilepsy.

M72.1 Knuckle pads

M72.2 Plantar fascial fibromatosis

> Plantar fasciitis
> **DEF:** Rapid-growing and multiplanar nodular swellings and pain in the foot that is not associated with contractures.

M72.4 Pseudosarcomatous fibromatosis

> Nodular fasciitis

M72.6 Necrotizing fasciitis   MCC HCC

> Use additional code (B95.-, B96.-) to identify causative organism
> **CC Excl:** PDX collection 806

M72.8 Other fibroblastic disorders

> Abscess of fascia
> Fasciitis NEC
> Other infective fasciitis
> Use additional code to (B95.-, B96.-) identify causative organism
> > EXCLUDES 1   *diffuse (eosinophilic) fasciitis (M35.4)*
> > *necrotizing fasciitis (M72.6)*
> > *nodular fasciitis (M72.4)*
> > *perirenal fasciitis NOS (N13.5)*
> > *perirenal fasciitis with infection (N13.6)*
> > *plantar fasciitis (M72.2)*

M72.9 Fibroblastic disorder, unspecified

> Fasciitis NOS
> Fibromatosis NOS

✓4ᵗʰ **M75 Shoulder lesions**

> EXCLUDES 2   *shoulder-hand syndrome (M89.0-)*

✓5ᵗʰ **M75.0 Adhesive capsulitis of shoulder**

> Frozen shoulder
> Periarthritis of shoulder
> **AHA:** 2015,2Q,23

> **M75.00 Adhesive capsulitis of unspecified shoulder**
> **M75.01 Adhesive capsulitis of right shoulder**
> **M75.02 Adhesive capsulitis of left shoulder**

✓5ᵗʰ **M75.1 Rotator cuff tear or rupture, not specified as traumatic**

> Rotator cuff syndrome
> Supraspinatus syndrome
> Supraspinatus tear or rupture, not specified as traumatic
> > EXCLUDES 1   *tear of rotator cuff, traumatic (S46.01-)*

> ✓6ᵗʰ **M75.10 Unspecified rotator cuff tear or rupture, not specified as traumatic**
> > **M75.100 Unspecified rotator cuff tear or rupture of unspecified shoulder, not specified as traumatic**
> > **M75.101 Unspecified rotator cuff tear or rupture of right shoulder, not specified as traumatic**
> > **M75.102 Unspecified rotator cuff tear or rupture of left shoulder, not specified as traumatic**

> ✓6ᵗʰ **M75.11 Incomplete rotator cuff tear or rupture not specified as traumatic**
> > **M75.110 Incomplete rotator cuff tear or rupture of unspecified shoulder, not specified as traumatic**
> > **M75.111 Incomplete rotator cuff tear or rupture of right shoulder, not specified as traumatic**
> > **M75.112 Incomplete rotator cuff tear or rupture of left shoulder, not specified as traumatic**

> ✓6ᵗʰ **M75.12 Complete rotator cuff tear or rupture not specified as traumatic**
> > **M75.120 Complete rotator cuff tear or rupture of unspecified shoulder, not specified as traumatic**
> > **M75.121 Complete rotator cuff tear or rupture of right shoulder, not specified as traumatic**   CC
> > **M75.122 Complete rotator cuff tear or rupture of left shoulder, not specified as traumatic**   CC

✓5ᵗʰ **M75.2 Bicipital tendinitis**

> **M75.20 Bicipital tendinitis, unspecified shoulder**
> **M75.21 Bicipital tendinitis, right shoulder**
> **M75.22 Bicipital tendinitis, left shoulder**

✓5ᵗʰ **M75.3 Calcific tendinitis of shoulder**

> Calcified bursa of shoulder

> **M75.30 Calcific tendinitis of unspecified shoulder**
> **M75.31 Calcific tendinitis of right shoulder**
> **M75.32 Calcific tendinitis of left shoulder**

✓5ᵗʰ **M75.4 Impingement syndrome of shoulder**

> **M75.40 Impingement syndrome of unspecified shoulder**
> **M75.41 Impingement syndrome of right shoulder**
> **M75.42 Impingement syndrome of left shoulder**

✓5ᵗʰ **M75.5 Bursitis of shoulder**

> **M75.50 Bursitis of unspecified shoulder**
> **M75.51 Bursitis of right shoulder**
> **M75.52 Bursitis of left shoulder**

✓5ᵗʰ **M75.8 Other shoulder lesions**

> **M75.80 Other shoulder lesions, unspecified shoulder**
> **M75.81 Other shoulder lesions, right shoulder**
> **M75.82 Other shoulder lesions, left shoulder**

✓5ᵗʰ **M75.9 Shoulder lesion, unspecified**

> **M75.90 Shoulder lesion, unspecified, unspecified shoulder**
> **M75.91 Shoulder lesion, unspecified, right shoulder**
> **M75.92 Shoulder lesion, unspecified, left shoulder**

✓4ᵗʰ **M76 Enthesopathies, lower limb, excluding foot**

> EXCLUDES 2   *bursitis due to use, overuse and pressure (M70.-)*
> *enthesopathies of ankle and foot (M77.5-)*

✓5ᵗʰ **M76.0 Gluteal tendinitis**

> **M76.00 Gluteal tendinitis, unspecified hip**
> **M76.01 Gluteal tendinitis, right hip**
> **M76.02 Gluteal tendinitis, left hip**

✓5ᵗʰ **M76.1 Psoas tendinitis**

> **M76.10 Psoas tendinitis, unspecified hip**
> **M76.11 Psoas tendinitis, right hip**
> **M76.12 Psoas tendinitis, left hip**

✓5ᵗʰ **M76.2 Iliac crest spur**

> **M76.20 Iliac crest spur, unspecified hip**
> **M76.21 Iliac crest spur, right hip**
> **M76.22 Iliac crest spur, left hip**

✓5ᵗʰ **M76.3 Iliotibial band syndrome**

> **M76.30 Iliotibial band syndrome, unspecified leg**
> **M76.31 Iliotibial band syndrome, right leg**
> **M76.32 Iliotibial band syndrome, left leg**

✓5ᵗʰ **M76.4 Tibial collateral bursitis [Pellegrini-Stieda]**

> **M76.40 Tibial collateral bursitis [Pellegrini-Stieda], unspecified leg**
> **M76.41 Tibial collateral bursitis [Pellegrini-Stieda], right leg**
> **M76.42 Tibial collateral bursitis [Pellegrini-Stieda], left leg**

✓5ᵗʰ **M76.5 Patellar tendinitis**

> **M76.50 Patellar tendinitis, unspecified knee**
> **M76.51 Patellar tendinitis, right knee**
> **M76.52 Patellar tendinitis, left knee**

✓5ᵗʰ **M76.6 Achilles tendinitis**

> Achilles bursitis
> **M76.60 Achilles tendinitis, unspecified leg**
> **M76.61 Achilles tendinitis, right leg**
> **M76.62 Achilles tendinitis, left leg**

✓5ᵗʰ **M76.7 Peroneal tendinitis**

> **M76.70 Peroneal tendinitis, unspecified leg**
> **M76.71 Peroneal tendinitis, right leg**
> **M76.72 Peroneal tendinitis, left leg**

✓5ᵗʰ **M76.8 Other specified enthesopathies of lower limb, excluding foot**

> ✓6ᵗʰ **M76.81 Anterior tibial syndrome**
> > **M76.811 Anterior tibial syndrome, right leg**
> > **M76.812 Anterior tibial syndrome, left leg**
> > **M76.819 Anterior tibial syndrome, unspecified leg**

> ✓6ᵗʰ **M76.82 Posterior tibial tendinitis**
> > **M76.821 Posterior tibial tendinitis, right leg**
> > **M76.822 Posterior tibial tendinitis, left leg**
> > **M76.829 Posterior tibial tendinitis, unspecified leg**

✅ Additional Character Required   ✓x7ᵗʰ Placeholder   Unacceptable PDx   Questionable PDx   Manifestation   Unspecified Dx   H1-H14 HAC   HCC CMS-HCC Dx   HIV HIV Dx

ICD-10-CM 2020   825

✓6ᵗʰ **M76.89** **Other specified enthesopathies of** lower limb, **excluding foot**
     M76.891 **Other specified enthesopathies of** right **lower limb, excluding foot**
     M76.892 **Other specified enthesopathies of** left **lower limb, excluding foot**
     M76.899 **Other specified enthesopathies of unspecified lower limb, excluding foot**
M76.9 **Unspecified enthesopathy, lower limb, excluding foot**

✓4ᵗʰ **M77** **Other enthesopathies**
     EXCLUDES 1   bursitis NOS (M71.9-)
     EXCLUDES 2   bursitis due to use, overuse and pressure (M70.-)
               osteophyte (M25.7)
               spinal enthesopathy (M46.0-)

✓5ᵗʰ **M77.0** **Medial** epicondylitis
     M77.00 **Medial epicondylitis, unspecified elbow**
     M77.01 **Medial epicondylitis,** right **elbow**
     M77.02 **Medial epicondylitis,** left **elbow**

✓5ᵗʰ **M77.1** **Lateral** epicondylitis
     Tennis elbow
     M77.10 **Lateral epicondylitis, unspecified elbow**
     M77.11 **Lateral epicondylitis,** right **elbow**
     M77.12 **Lateral epicondylitis,** left **elbow**

✓5ᵗʰ **M77.2** **Periarthritis of wrist**
     M77.20 **Periarthritis, unspecified wrist**
     M77.21 **Periarthritis,** right **wrist**
     M77.22 **Periarthritis,** left **wrist**

✓5ᵗʰ **M77.3** **Calcaneal spur**
     DEF: Overgrowth of calcaneus bone on the underside of the heel that causes pain on walking. Calcaneal spur is due to a chronic avulsion injury of the plantar fascia from the calcaneus.
     M77.30 **Calcaneal spur, unspecified foot**
     M77.31 **Calcaneal spur,** right **foot**
     M77.32 **Calcaneal spur,** left **foot**

✓5ᵗʰ **M77.4** **Metatarsalgia**
     EXCLUDES 1   Morton's metatarsalgia (G57.6)
     M77.40 **Metatarsalgia, unspecified foot**
     M77.41 **Metatarsalgia,** right **foot**
     M77.42 **Metatarsalgia,** left **foot**

▲ ✓5ᵗʰ **M77.5** **Other enthesopathy of** foot and ankle
▲   **M77.50** **Other enthesopathy of unspecified foot and ankle**
▲   **M77.51** **Other enthesopathy of** right **foot and ankle**
▲   **M77.52** **Other enthesopathy of** left **foot and ankle**

M77.8 **Other enthesopathies, not elsewhere classified**
M77.9 **Enthesopathy, unspecified**
     Bone spur NOS
     Capsulitis NOS
     Periarthritis NOS
     Tendinitis NOS

✓4ᵗʰ **M79** **Other and unspecified soft tissue disorders, not elsewhere classified**
     EXCLUDES 1   psychogenic rheumatism (F45.8)
               soft tissue pain, psychogenic (F45.41)

M79.0 **Rheumatism, unspecified**
     EXCLUDES 1   fibromyalgia (M79.7)
               palindromic rheumatism (M12.3-)

✓5ᵗʰ **M79.1** **Myalgia**
     Myofascial pain syndrome
     EXCLUDES 1   fibromyalgia (M79.7)
               myositis (M60.-)
     AHA: 2018,4Q,21
     M79.10 **Myalgia, unspecified site**
     M79.11 **Myalgia of** mastication muscle
     M79.12 **Myalgia of** auxiliary muscles, **head and neck**
     M79.18 **Myalgia, other site**

M79.2 **Neuralgia and neuritis, unspecified**
     EXCLUDES 1   brachial radiculitis NOS (M54.1)
               lumbosacral radiculitis NOS (M54.1)
               mononeuropathies (G56-G58)
               radiculitis NOS (M54.1)
               sciatica (M54.3-M54.4)
     TIP: Assign for documented neuropathic pain.

M79.3 **Panniculitis, unspecified**   CC
     EXCLUDES 1   lupus panniculitis (L93.2)
               neck and back panniculitis (M54.0-)
               relapsing [Weber-Christian] panniculitis (M35.6)

M79.4 **Hypertrophy of (infrapatellar) fat pad**
M79.5 **Residual foreign body in soft tissue**
     EXCLUDES 1   foreign body granuloma of skin and subcutaneous tissue (L92.3)
               foreign body granuloma of soft tissue (M60.2-)

✓5ᵗʰ **M79.6** **Pain in limb, hand, foot, fingers and toes**
     EXCLUDES 2   pain in joint (M25.5-)
     ✓6ᵗʰ **M79.60** **Pain in limb, unspecified**
         M79.601 **Pain in** right **arm**
               Pain in right upper limb NOS
         M79.602 **Pain in** left **arm**
               Pain in left upper limb NOS
         M79.603 **Pain in** arm, unspecified
               Pain in upper limb NOS
         M79.604 **Pain in** right **leg**
               Pain in right lower limb NOS
         M79.605 **Pain in** left **leg**
               Pain in left lower limb NOS
         M79.606 **Pain in leg, unspecified**
               Pain in lower limb NOS
         M79.609 **Pain in unspecified limb**
               Pain in limb NOS
     ✓6ᵗʰ **M79.62** **Pain in** upper arm
         Pain in axillary region
         M79.621 **Pain in** right **upper arm**
         M79.622 **Pain in** left **upper arm**
         M79.629 **Pain in unspecified upper arm**
     ✓6ᵗʰ **M79.63** **Pain in** forearm
         M79.631 **Pain in** right **forearm**
         M79.632 **Pain in** left **forearm**
         M79.639 **Pain in unspecified forearm**
     ✓6ᵗʰ **M79.64** **Pain in** hand and fingers
         M79.641 **Pain in** right **hand**
         M79.642 **Pain in** left **hand**
         M79.643 **Pain in unspecified hand**
         M79.644 **Pain in** right **finger(s)**
         M79.645 **Pain in** left **finger(s)**
         M79.646 **Pain in unspecified finger(s)**
     ✓6ᵗʰ **M79.65** **Pain in** thigh
         M79.651 **Pain in** right **thigh**
         M79.652 **Pain in** left **thigh**
         M79.659 **Pain in unspecified thigh**
     ✓6ᵗʰ **M79.66** **Pain in** lower leg
         M79.661 **Pain in** right **lower leg**
         M79.662 **Pain in** left **lower leg**
         M79.669 **Pain in unspecified lower leg**
     ✓6ᵗʰ **M79.67** **Pain in** foot and toes
         M79.671 **Pain in** right **foot**
         M79.672 **Pain in** left **foot**
         M79.673 **Pain in unspecified foot**
         M79.674 **Pain in** right **toe(s)**
         M79.675 **Pain in** left **toe(s)**
         M79.676 **Pain in unspecified toe(s)**

M79.7 **Fibromyalgia**
     Fibromyositis
     Fibrositis
     Myofibrositis

✓5ᵗʰ **M79.A** **Nontraumatic compartment syndrome**
     Code first, if applicable, associated postprocedural complication
     EXCLUDES 1   compartment syndrome NOS (T79.A-)
               fibromyalgia (M79.7)
               nontraumatic ischemic infarction of muscle (M62.2-)
               traumatic compartment syndrome (T79.A-)

     ✓6ᵗʰ **M79.A1** **Nontraumatic compartment syndrome of** upper extremity
         Nontraumatic compartment syndrome of shoulder, arm, forearm, wrist, hand, and fingers
         CC Excl: For CC codes in subcategory M79.A1: PDX collection 893
         M79.A11 **Nontraumatic compartment syndrome of** right **upper extremity**   CC

M79.A12 Nontraumatic compartment syndrome of left upper extremity `CC`

M79.A19 Nontraumatic compartment syndrome of unspecified upper extremity `CC`

√6ᵗʰ **M79.A2 Nontraumatic compartment syndrome of lower extremity**
Nontraumatic compartment syndrome of hip, buttock, thigh, leg, foot, and toes
CC Excl: For CC codes in subcategory M79.A2: PDX collection 894

M79.A21 Nontraumatic compartment syndrome of right lower extremity `CC`

M79.A22 Nontraumatic compartment syndrome of left lower extremity `CC`

M79.A29 Nontraumatic compartment syndrome of unspecified lower extremity `CC`

M79.A3 Nontraumatic compartment syndrome of abdomen `CC`
CC Excl: PDX collection 895

M79.A9 Nontraumatic compartment syndrome of other sites `CC`
CC Excl: PDX collection 896

√5ᵗʰ **M79.8 Other specified soft tissue disorders**

M79.81 Nontraumatic hematoma of soft tissue
Nontraumatic hematoma of muscle
Nontraumatic seroma of muscle and soft tissue

M79.89 Other specified soft tissue disorders
Polyalgia

M79.9 Soft tissue disorder, unspecified

OSTEOPATHIES AND CHONDROPATHIES (M80-M94)

Disorders of bone density and structure (M80-M85)

√4ᵗʰ **M80 Osteoporosis with current pathological fracture**
INCLUDES osteoporosis with current fragility fracture
Use additional code to identify major osseous defect, if applicable (M89.7-)
EXCLUDES 1 collapsed vertebra NOS (M48.5)
pathological fracture NOS (M84.4)
wedging of vertebra NOS (M48.5)
EXCLUDES 2 personal history of (healed) osteoporosis fracture (Z87.310)
AHA: 2018,2Q,12
TIP: The site codes in this category identify the site of the fracture, not the site of the osteoporosis.

The appropriate 7th character is to be added to each code from category M80:
A initial encounter for fracture
D subsequent encounter for fracture with routine healing
G subsequent encounter for fracture with delayed healing
K subsequent encounter for fracture with nonunion
P subsequent encounter for fracture with malunion
S sequela

CC Excl: For codes in category M80:
CC with 7th character A: PDX collection 888
CC with 7th character K or P: PDX collection 897

√5ᵗʰ **M80.0 Age-related osteoporosis with current pathological fracture**
Involutional osteoporosis with current pathological fracture
Osteoporosis NOS with current pathological fracture
Postmenopausal osteoporosis with current pathological fracture
Senile osteoporosis with current pathological fracture

3 √x7ᵗʰ **M80.00 Age-related osteoporosis with current pathological fracture, unspecified site** `CC` `A`

√6ᵗʰ **M80.01 Age-related osteoporosis with current pathological fracture, shoulder**

3 √7ᵗʰ **M80.011 Age-related osteoporosis with current pathological fracture, right shoulder** `CC` `A`

3 √7ᵗʰ **M80.012 Age-related osteoporosis with current pathological fracture, left shoulder** `CC` `A`

3 √7ᵗʰ **M80.019 Age-related osteoporosis with current pathological fracture, unspecified shoulder** `CC` `A`

√6ᵗʰ **M80.02 Age-related osteoporosis with current pathological fracture, humerus**

3 √7ᵗʰ **M80.021 Age-related osteoporosis with current pathological fracture, right humerus** `CC` `A`

3 √7ᵗʰ **M80.022 Age-related osteoporosis with current pathological fracture, left humerus** `CC` `A`

3 √7ᵗʰ **M80.029 Age-related osteoporosis with current pathological fracture, unspecified humerus** `CC` `A`

√6ᵗʰ **M80.03 Age-related osteoporosis with current pathological fracture, forearm**
Age-related osteoporosis with current pathological fracture of wrist

3 √7ᵗʰ **M80.031 Age-related osteoporosis with current pathological fracture, right forearm** `CC` `A`

3 √7ᵗʰ **M80.032 Age-related osteoporosis with current pathological fracture, left forearm** `CC` `A`

3 √7ᵗʰ **M80.039 Age-related osteoporosis with current pathological fracture, unspecified forearm** `CC` `A`

√6ᵗʰ **M80.04 Age-related osteoporosis with current pathological fracture, hand**

3 √7ᵗʰ **M80.041 Age-related osteoporosis with current pathological fracture, right hand** `CC` `A`

3 √7ᵗʰ **M80.042 Age-related osteoporosis with current pathological fracture, left hand** `CC` `A`

3 √7ᵗʰ **M80.049 Age-related osteoporosis with current pathological fracture, unspecified hand** `CC` `A`

√6ᵗʰ **M80.05 Age-related osteoporosis with current pathological fracture, femur**
Age-related osteoporosis with current pathological fracture of hip

3,6 √7ᵗʰ **M80.051 Age-related osteoporosis with current pathological fracture, right femur** `CC` `HCC` `A`

3,6 √7ᵗʰ **M80.052 Age-related osteoporosis with current pathological fracture, left femur** `CC` `HCC` `A`

3,6 √7ᵗʰ **M80.059 Age-related osteoporosis with current pathological fracture, unspecified femur** `CC` `HCC` `A`

√6ᵗʰ **M80.06 Age-related osteoporosis with current pathological fracture, lower leg**

3 √7ᵗʰ **M80.061 Age-related osteoporosis with current pathological fracture, right lower leg** `CC` `A`

3 √7ᵗʰ **M80.062 Age-related osteoporosis with current pathological fracture, left lower leg** `CC` `A`

3 √7ᵗʰ **M80.069 Age-related osteoporosis with current pathological fracture, unspecified lower leg** `CC` `A`

√6ᵗʰ **M80.07 Age-related osteoporosis with current pathological fracture, ankle and foot**

3 √7ᵗʰ **M80.071 Age-related osteoporosis with current pathological fracture, right ankle and foot** `CC` `A`

3 √7ᵗʰ **M80.072 Age-related osteoporosis with current pathological fracture, left ankle and foot** `CC` `A`

3 √7ᵗʰ **M80.079 Age-related osteoporosis with current pathological fracture, unspecified ankle and foot** `CC` `A`

3,6 √x7ᵗʰ **M80.08 Age-related osteoporosis with current pathological fracture, vertebra(e)** `CC` `HCC`

Chapter 13. Diseases of the Musculoskeletal System and Connective Tissue

M80.8–M83.9

☑5ᵗʰ **M80.8** **Other osteoporosis with current pathological fracture**

Drug-induced osteoporosis with current pathological fracture

Idiopathic osteoporosis with current pathological fracture

Osteoporosis of disuse with current pathological fracture

Postoophorectomy osteoporosis with current pathological fracture

Postsurgical malabsorption osteoporosis with current pathological fracture

Post-traumatic osteoporosis with current pathological fracture

Use additional code for adverse effect, if applicable, to identify drug (T36-T50 with fifth or sixth character 5)

3 ☑x7ᵗʰ **M80.80** Other osteoporosis with current pathological fracture, unspecified site   CC

☑6ᵗʰ **M80.81** Other osteoporosis with pathological fracture, shoulder

    3 ☑7ᵗʰ **M80.811** Other osteoporosis with current pathological fracture, right shoulder   CC

    3 ☑7ᵗʰ **M80.812** Other osteoporosis with current pathological fracture, left shoulder   CC

    3 ☑7ᵗʰ **M80.819** Other osteoporosis with current pathological fracture, unspecified shoulder   CC

☑6ᵗʰ **M80.82** Other osteoporosis with current pathological fracture, humerus

    3 ☑7ᵗʰ **M80.821** Other osteoporosis with current pathological fracture, right humerus   CC

    3 ☑7ᵗʰ **M80.822** Other osteoporosis with current pathological fracture, left humerus   CC

    3 ☑7ᵗʰ **M80.829** Other osteoporosis with current pathological fracture, unspecified humerus   CC

☑6ᵗʰ **M80.83** Other osteoporosis with current pathological fracture, forearm

Other osteoporosis with current pathological fracture of wrist

    3 ☑7ᵗʰ **M80.831** Other osteoporosis with current pathological fracture, right forearm   CC

    3 ☑7ᵗʰ **M80.832** Other osteoporosis with current pathological fracture, left forearm   CC

    3 ☑7ᵗʰ **M80.839** Other osteoporosis with current pathological fracture, unspecified forearm   CC

☑6ᵗʰ **M80.84** Other osteoporosis with current pathological fracture, hand

    3 ☑7ᵗʰ **M80.841** Other osteoporosis with current pathological fracture, right hand   CC

    3 ☑7ᵗʰ **M80.842** Other osteoporosis with current pathological fracture, left hand   CC

    3 ☑7ᵗʰ **M80.849** Other osteoporosis with current pathological fracture, unspecified hand   CC

☑6ᵗʰ **M80.85** Other osteoporosis with current pathological fracture, femur

Other osteoporosis with current pathological fracture of hip

    3,6 ☑7ᵗʰ **M80.851** Other osteoporosis with current pathological fracture, right femur   CC HCC

    3,6 ☑7ᵗʰ **M80.852** Other osteoporosis with current pathological fracture, left femur   CC HCC

    3,6 ☑7ᵗʰ **M80.859** Other osteoporosis with current pathological fracture, unspecified femur   CC HCC

☑6ᵗʰ **M80.86** Other osteoporosis with current pathological fracture, lower leg

    3 ☑7ᵗʰ **M80.861** Other osteoporosis with current pathological fracture, right lower leg   CC

    3 ☑7ᵗʰ **M80.862** Other osteoporosis with current pathological fracture, left lower leg   CC

    3 ☑7ᵗʰ **M80.869** Other osteoporosis with current pathological fracture, unspecified lower leg   CC

☑6ᵗʰ **M80.87** Other osteoporosis with current pathological fracture, ankle and foot

    3 ☑7ᵗʰ **M80.871** Other osteoporosis with current pathological fracture, right ankle and foot   CC

    3 ☑7ᵗʰ **M80.872** Other osteoporosis with current pathological fracture, left ankle and foot   CC

    3 ☑7ᵗʰ **M80.879** Other osteoporosis with current pathological fracture, unspecified ankle and foot   CC

3,6 ☑x7ᵗʰ **M80.88** Other osteoporosis with current pathological fracture, vertebra(e)   CC HCC

☑4ᵗʰ **M81** **Osteoporosis without current pathological fracture**

Use additional code to identify:

major osseous defect, if applicable (M89.7-)

personal history of (healed) osteoporosis fracture, if applicable (Z87.310)

   EXCLUDES 1   osteoporosis with current pathological fracture (M80.-)

            Sudeck's atrophy (M89.0)

M81.0 **Age-related osteoporosis without current pathological fracture**   A

Involutional osteoporosis without current pathological fracture

Osteoporosis NOS

Postmenopausal osteoporosis without current pathological fracture

Senile osteoporosis without current pathological fracture

M81.6 **Localized osteoporosis [Lequesne]**

   EXCLUDES 1   Sudeck's atrophy (M89.0)

M81.8 **Other osteoporosis without current pathological fracture**

Drug-induced osteoporosis without current pathological fracture

Idiopathic osteoporosis without current pathological fracture

Osteoporosis of disuse without current pathological fracture

Postoophorectomy osteoporosis without current pathological fracture

Postsurgical malabsorption osteoporosis without current pathological fracture

Post-traumatic osteoporosis without current pathological fracture

Use additional code for adverse effect, if applicable, to identify drug (T36-T50 with fifth or sixth character 5)

☑4ᵗʰ **M83** **Adult osteomalacia**

   EXCLUDES 1   infantile and juvenile osteomalacia (E55.0)

            renal osteodystrophy (N25.0)

            rickets (active) (E55.0)

            rickets (active) sequelae (E64.3)

            vitamin D-resistant osteomalacia (E83.3)

            vitamin D-resistant rickets (active) (E83.3)

M83.0 **Puerperal osteomalacia**   M ♀

M83.1 **Senile osteomalacia**   A

M83.2 **Adult osteomalacia due to malabsorption**   A

Postsurgical malabsorption osteomalacia in adults

M83.3 **Adult osteomalacia due to malnutrition**   A

M83.4 **Aluminum bone disease**

M83.5 **Other drug-induced osteomalacia in adults**   A

Use additional code for adverse effect, if applicable, to identify drug (T36-T50 with fifth or sixth character 5)

M83.8 **Other adult osteomalacia**   A

M83.9 **Adult osteomalacia, unspecified**   A

N Newborn: 0   P Pediatric: 0-17   M Maternity: 9-64   A Adult: 15-124   MCC Major Complication/Comorbidity   CC Complication/Comorbidity   SW Severe Wound Dx

828   ICD-10-CM 2020

✓4ᵗʰ **M84 Disorder of continuity of bone**

       EXCLUDES 2   *traumatic fracture of bone-see fracture, by site*

✓5ᵗʰ **M84.3 Stress fracture**

     Fatigue fracture

     March fracture

     Stress fracture NOS

     Stress reaction

     Use additional external cause code(s) to identify the cause of the stress fracture

       EXCLUDES 1   *pathological fracture due to osteoporosis (M80.-)*

                 pathological fracture NOS (M84.4.-)

                 traumatic fracture (S12.-, S22.-, S32.-, S42.-, S52.-, S62.-, S72.-, S82.-, S92.-)

       EXCLUDES 2   *personal history of (healed) stress (fatigue) fracture (Z87.312)*

                 stress fracture of vertebra (M48.4-)

> The appropriate 7th character is to be added to each code from subcategory M84.3.
> A   initial encounter for fracture
> D   subsequent encounter for fracture with routine healing
> G   subsequent encounter for fracture with delayed healing
> K   subsequent encounter for fracture with nonunion
> P   subsequent encounter for fracture with malunion
> S   sequela

> CC Excl: For codes in subcategory M84.3:
> CC with 7th character K or P: PDX collection 897

⁴ ✓x7ᵗʰ **M84.30 Stress fracture, unspecified site**   CC

✓6ᵗʰ **M84.31 Stress fracture,** shoulder

     ⁴ ✓7ᵗʰ **M84.311 Stress fracture,** right shoulder   CC

     ⁴ ✓7ᵗʰ **M84.312 Stress fracture,** left shoulder

     ⁴ ✓7ᵗʰ **M84.319 Stress fracture, unspecified shoulder**   CC

✓6ᵗʰ **M84.32 Stress fracture,** humerus

     ⁴ ✓7ᵗʰ **M84.321 Stress fracture,** right humerus   CC

     ⁴ ✓7ᵗʰ **M84.322 Stress fracture,** left humerus

     ⁴ ✓7ᵗʰ **M84.329 Stress fracture, unspecified humerus**   CC

✓6ᵗʰ **M84.33 Stress fracture,** ulna and radius

     ⁴ ✓7ᵗʰ **M84.331 Stress fracture,** right ulna   CC

     ⁴ ✓7ᵗʰ **M84.332 Stress fracture,** left ulna

     ⁴ ✓7ᵗʰ **M84.333 Stress fracture,** right radius   CC

     ⁴ ✓7ᵗʰ **M84.334 Stress fracture,** left radius

     ⁴ ✓7ᵗʰ **M84.339 Stress fracture, unspecified ulna and radius**   CC

✓6ᵗʰ **M84.34 Stress fracture,** hand and fingers

     ⁴ ✓7ᵗʰ **M84.341 Stress fracture,** right hand   CC

     ⁴ ✓7ᵗʰ **M84.342 Stress fracture,** left hand

     ⁴ ✓7ᵗʰ **M84.343 Stress fracture, unspecified hand**   CC

     ⁴ ✓7ᵗʰ **M84.344 Stress fracture,** right finger(s)   CC

     ⁴ ✓7ᵗʰ **M84.345 Stress fracture,** left finger(s)

     ⁴ ✓7ᵗʰ **M84.346 Stress fracture, unspecified finger(s)**   CC

✓6ᵗʰ **M84.35 Stress fracture,** pelvis and femur

     Stress fracture, hip

     ⁴ ✓7ᵗʰ **M84.350 Stress fracture,** pelvis   CC

     ⁴ ✓7ᵗʰ **M84.351 Stress fracture,** right femur   CC

     ⁴ ✓7ᵗʰ **M84.352 Stress fracture,** left femur   CC

     ⁴ ✓7ᵗʰ **M84.353 Stress fracture, unspecified femur**   CC

     ⁴ ✓7ᵗʰ **M84.359 Stress fracture, hip, unspecified**   CC

✓6ᵗʰ **M84.36 Stress fracture,** tibia and fibula

     ⁴ ✓7ᵗʰ **M84.361 Stress fracture,** right tibia   CC

     ⁴ ✓7ᵗʰ **M84.362 Stress fracture,** left tibia   CC

     ⁴ ✓7ᵗʰ **M84.363 Stress fracture,** right fibula   CC

     ⁴ ✓7ᵗʰ **M84.364 Stress fracture,** left fibula   CC

     ⁴ ✓7ᵗʰ **M84.369 Stress fracture, unspecified tibia and fibula**   CC

✓6ᵗʰ **M84.37 Stress fracture, ankle, foot and toes**

     ⁴ ✓7ᵗʰ **M84.371 Stress fracture,** right ankle   CC

     ⁴ ✓7ᵗʰ **M84.372 Stress fracture,** left ankle   CC

     ⁴ ✓7ᵗʰ **M84.373 Stress fracture, unspecified ankle**   CC

     ⁴ ✓7ᵗʰ **M84.374 Stress fracture,** right foot   CC

     ⁴ ✓7ᵗʰ **M84.375 Stress fracture,** left foot   CC

     ⁴ ✓7ᵗʰ **M84.376 Stress fracture, unspecified foot**   CC

     ⁴ ✓7ᵗʰ **M84.377 Stress fracture,** right toe(s)   CC

     ⁴ ✓7ᵗʰ **M84.378 Stress fracture,** left toe(s)   CC

     ⁴ ✓7ᵗʰ **M84.379 Stress fracture, unspecified toe(s)**   CC

⁴ ✓x7ᵗʰ **M84.38 Stress fracture, other site**   CC

       EXCLUDES 2   *stress fracture of vertebra (M48.4-)*

✓5ᵗʰ **M84.4 Pathological fracture, not elsewhere classified**

     Chronic fracture

     Pathological fracture NOS

       EXCLUDES 1   *collapsed vertebra NEC (M48.5)*

                 pathological fracture in neoplastic disease (M84.5-)

                 pathological fracture in osteoporosis (M80.-)

                 pathological fracture in other disease (M84.6-)

                 stress fracture (M84.3-)

                 traumatic fracture (S12.-, S22.-, S32.-, S42.-, S52.-, S62.-, S72.-, S82.-, S92.-)

       EXCLUDES 2   *personal history of (healed) pathological fracture (Z87.311)*

> The appropriate 7th character is to be added to each code from subcategory M84.4.
> A   initial encounter for fracture
> D   subsequent encounter for fracture with routine healing
> G   subsequent encounter for fracture with delayed healing
> K   subsequent encounter for fracture with nonunion
> P   subsequent encounter for fracture with malunion
> S   sequela

> CC Excl: For codes in subcategory M84.4:
> CC with 7th character A: PDX collection 888
> CC with 7th character K or P: PDX collection 897

³ ✓x7ᵗʰ **M84.40 Pathological fracture, unspecified site**   CC

✓6ᵗʰ **M84.41 Pathological fracture,** shoulder

     ³ ✓7ᵗʰ **M84.411 Pathological fracture,** right shoulder   CC

     ³ ✓7ᵗʰ **M84.412 Pathological fracture,** left shoulder   CC

     ³ ✓7ᵗʰ **M84.419 Pathological fracture, unspecified shoulder**   CC

✓6ᵗʰ **M84.42 Pathological fracture,** humerus

     ³ ✓7ᵗʰ **M84.421 Pathological fracture,** right humerus   CC

     ³ ✓7ᵗʰ **M84.422 Pathological fracture,** left humerus   CC

     ³ ✓7ᵗʰ **M84.429 Pathological fracture, unspecified humerus**   CC

✓6ᵗʰ **M84.43 Pathological fracture,** ulna and radius

     ³ ✓7ᵗʰ **M84.431 Pathological fracture,** right ulna   CC

     ³ ✓7ᵗʰ **M84.432 Pathological fracture,** left ulna   CC

     ³ ✓7ᵗʰ **M84.433 Pathological fracture,** right radius   CC

     ³ ✓7ᵗʰ **M84.434 Pathological fracture,** left radius   CC

     ³ ✓7ᵗʰ **M84.439 Pathological fracture, unspecified ulna and radius**   CC

✓6ᵗʰ **M84.44 Pathological fracture,** hand and fingers

     ³ ✓7ᵗʰ **M84.441 Pathological fracture,** right hand   CC

     ³ ✓7ᵗʰ **M84.442 Pathological fracture,** left hand   CC

     ³ ✓7ᵗʰ **M84.443 Pathological fracture, unspecified hand**   CC

✓ Additional Character Required   ✓x7ᵗʰ Placeholder   Unacceptable PDx   Questionable PDx   Manifestation   Unspecified Dx   H1-H14 HAC   HCC CMS-HCC Dx   HIV HIV Dx

ICD-10-CM 2020

829

3 √7ᵗʰ **M84.444** Pathological fracture, right finger(s) `CC`

3 √7ᵗʰ **M84.445** Pathological fracture, left finger(s) `CC`

3 √7ᵗʰ **M84.446** Pathological fracture, unspecified finger(s) `CC`

√6ᵗʰ **M84.45** Pathological fracture, femur and pelvis

    AHA: 2016,4Q,43

3,6 √7ᵗʰ **M84.451** Pathological fracture, right femur `CC` `HCC`

3,6 √7ᵗʰ **M84.452** Pathological fracture, left femur `CC` `HCC`

3,6 √7ᵗʰ **M84.453** Pathological fracture, unspecified femur `CC` `HCC`

3 √7ᵗʰ **M84.454** Pathological fracture, pelvis `CC`

3,6 √7ᵗʰ **M84.459** Pathological fracture, hip, unspecified `CC` `HCC`

√6ᵗʰ **M84.46** Pathological fracture, tibia and fibula

3 √7ᵗʰ **M84.461** Pathological fracture, right tibia `CC`

3 √7ᵗʰ **M84.462** Pathological fracture, left tibia `CC`

3 √7ᵗʰ **M84.463** Pathological fracture, right fibula `CC`

3 √7ᵗʰ **M84.464** Pathological fracture, left fibula `CC`

3 √7ᵗʰ **M84.469** Pathological fracture, unspecified tibia and fibula `CC`

√6ᵗʰ **M84.47** Pathological fracture, ankle, foot and toes

3 √7ᵗʰ **M84.471** Pathological fracture, right ankle `CC`

3 √7ᵗʰ **M84.472** Pathological fracture, left ankle `CC`

3 √7ᵗʰ **M84.473** Pathological fracture, unspecified ankle `CC`

3 √7ᵗʰ **M84.474** Pathological fracture, right foot `CC`

3 √7ᵗʰ **M84.475** Pathological fracture, left foot `CC`

3 √7ᵗʰ **M84.476** Pathological fracture, unspecified foot `CC`

3 √7ᵗʰ **M84.477** Pathological fracture, right toe(s) `CC`

3 √7ᵗʰ **M84.478** Pathological fracture, left toe(s) `CC`

3 √7ᵗʰ **M84.479** Pathological fracture, unspecified toe(s) `CC`

3 √x7ᵗʰ **M84.48** Pathological fracture, other site `CC`

√5ᵗʰ **M84.5** Pathological fracture in neoplastic disease

    Code also underlying neoplasm

The appropriate 7th character is to be added to each code from subcategory M84.5.
A   initial encounter for fracture
D   subsequent encounter for fracture with routine healing
G   subsequent encounter for fracture with delayed healing
K   subsequent encounter for fracture with nonunion
P   subsequent encounter for fracture with malunion
S   sequela

CC Excl: For codes in subcategory M84.5:
CC with 7th character A: PDX collection 888
CC with 7th character K or P: PDX collection 897

3 √x7ᵗʰ **M84.50** Pathological fracture in neoplastic disease, unspecified site `CC`

√6ᵗʰ **M84.51** Pathological fracture in neoplastic disease, shoulder

3 √7ᵗʰ **M84.511** Pathological fracture in neoplastic disease, right shoulder `CC`

3 √7ᵗʰ **M84.512** Pathological fracture in neoplastic disease, left shoulder `CC`

3 √7ᵗʰ **M84.519** Pathological fracture in neoplastic disease, unspecified shoulder `CC`

√6ᵗʰ **M84.52** Pathological fracture in neoplastic disease, humerus

3 √7ᵗʰ **M84.521** Pathological fracture in neoplastic disease, right humerus `CC`

3 √7ᵗʰ **M84.522** Pathological fracture in neoplastic disease, left humerus `CC`

3 √7ᵗʰ **M84.529** Pathological fracture in neoplastic disease, unspecified humerus `CC`

√6ᵗʰ **M84.53** Pathological fracture in neoplastic disease, ulna and radius

3 √7ᵗʰ **M84.531** Pathological fracture in neoplastic disease, right ulna `CC`

3 √7ᵗʰ **M84.532** Pathological fracture in neoplastic disease, left ulna `CC`

3 √7ᵗʰ **M84.533** Pathological fracture in neoplastic disease, right radius `CC`

3 √7ᵗʰ **M84.534** Pathological fracture in neoplastic disease, left radius `CC`

3 √7ᵗʰ **M84.539** Pathological fracture in neoplastic disease, unspecified ulna and radius `CC`

√6ᵗʰ **M84.54** Pathological fracture in neoplastic disease, hand

3 √7ᵗʰ **M84.541** Pathological fracture in neoplastic disease, right hand `CC`

3 √7ᵗʰ **M84.542** Pathological fracture in neoplastic disease, left hand `CC`

3 √7ᵗʰ **M84.549** Pathological fracture in neoplastic disease, unspecified hand `CC`

√6ᵗʰ **M84.55** Pathological fracture in neoplastic disease, pelvis and femur

3 √7ᵗʰ **M84.550** Pathological fracture in neoplastic disease, pelvis `CC`

3,6 √7ᵗʰ **M84.551** Pathological fracture in neoplastic disease, right femur `CC` `HCC`

3,6 √7ᵗʰ **M84.552** Pathological fracture in neoplastic disease, left femur `CC` `HCC`

3,6 √7ᵗʰ **M84.553** Pathological fracture in neoplastic disease, unspecified femur `CC` `HCC`

3,6 √7ᵗʰ **M84.559** Pathological fracture in neoplastic disease, hip, unspecified `CC` `HCC`

√6ᵗʰ **M84.56** Pathological fracture in neoplastic disease, tibia and fibula

3 √7ᵗʰ **M84.561** Pathological fracture in neoplastic disease, right tibia `CC`

3 √7ᵗʰ **M84.562** Pathological fracture in neoplastic disease, left tibia `CC`

3 √7ᵗʰ **M84.563** Pathological fracture in neoplastic disease, right fibula `CC`

3 √7ᵗʰ **M84.564** Pathological fracture in neoplastic disease, left fibula `CC`

3 √7ᵗʰ **M84.569** Pathological fracture in neoplastic disease, unspecified tibia and fibula `CC`

√6ᵗʰ **M84.57** Pathological fracture in neoplastic disease, ankle and foot

3 √7ᵗʰ **M84.571** Pathological fracture in neoplastic disease, right ankle `CC`

3 √7ᵗʰ **M84.572** Pathological fracture in neoplastic disease, left ankle `CC`

3 √7ᵗʰ **M84.573** Pathological fracture in neoplastic disease, unspecified ankle `CC`

3 √7ᵗʰ **M84.574** Pathological fracture in neoplastic disease, right foot `CC`

3 √7ᵗʰ **M84.575** Pathological fracture in neoplastic disease, left foot `CC`

N Newborn: 0   P Pediatric: 0-17   M Maternity: 9-64   A Adult: 15-124   `MCC` Major Complication/Comorbidity   `CC` Complication/Comorbidity   `SW` Severe Wound Dx

830   ICD-10-CM 2020

3 ☑7ᵗʰ **M84.576** **Pathological fracture in neoplastic disease, unspecified foot** `CC`

3 ☑x7ᵗʰ **M84.58** **Pathological fracture in neoplastic disease, other specified site** `CC`

           Pathological fracture in neoplastic disease, vertebrae

☑5ᵗʰ **M84.6** **Pathological fracture in other disease**

    Code also underlying condition

    EXCLUDES 1   *pathological fracture in osteoporosis (M80.-)*

> The appropriate 7th character is to be added to each code from subcategory M84.6.
> A   initial encounter for fracture
> D   subsequent encounter for fracture with routine healing
> G   subsequent encounter for fracture with delayed healing
> K   subsequent encounter for fracture with nonunion
> P   subsequent encounter for fracture with malunion
> S   sequela

> **CC Excl: For codes in subcategory M84.6:**
> **CC with 7th character A:** PDX collection 888
> **CC with 7th character K or P:** PDX collection 897

3 ☑x7ᵗʰ **M84.60** **Pathological fracture in other disease, unspecified site** `CC`

☑6ᵗʰ **M84.61** **Pathological fracture in other disease, shoulder**

    3 ☑7ᵗʰ **M84.611** **Pathological fracture in other disease, right shoulder** `CC`

    3 ☑7ᵗʰ **M84.612** **Pathological fracture in other disease, left shoulder** `CC`

    3 ☑7ᵗʰ **M84.619** **Pathological fracture in other disease, unspecified shoulder** `CC`

☑6ᵗʰ **M84.62** **Pathological fracture in other disease, humerus**

    3 ☑7ᵗʰ **M84.621** **Pathological fracture in other disease, right humerus** `CC`

    3 ☑7ᵗʰ **M84.622** **Pathological fracture in other disease, left humerus** `CC`

    3 ☑7ᵗʰ **M84.629** **Pathological fracture in other disease, unspecified humerus** `CC`

☑6ᵗʰ **M84.63** **Pathological fracture in other disease, ulna and radius**

    3 ☑7ᵗʰ **M84.631** **Pathological fracture in other disease, right ulna** `CC`

    3 ☑7ᵗʰ **M84.632** **Pathological fracture in other disease, left ulna** `CC`

    3 ☑7ᵗʰ **M84.633** **Pathological fracture in other disease, right radius** `CC`

    3 ☑7ᵗʰ **M84.634** **Pathological fracture in other disease, left radius** `CC`

    3 ☑7ᵗʰ **M84.639** **Pathological fracture in other disease, unspecified ulna and radius** `CC`

☑6ᵗʰ **M84.64** **Pathological fracture in other disease, hand**

    3 ☑7ᵗʰ **M84.641** **Pathological fracture in other disease, right hand** `CC`

    3 ☑7ᵗʰ **M84.642** **Pathological fracture in other disease, left hand** `CC`

    3 ☑7ᵗʰ **M84.649** **Pathological fracture in other disease, unspecified hand** `CC`

☑6ᵗʰ **M84.65** **Pathological fracture in other disease, pelvis and femur**

    3 ☑7ᵗʰ **M84.650** **Pathological fracture in other disease, pelvis** `CC`

    3,6 ☑7ᵗʰ **M84.651** **Pathological fracture in other disease, right femur** `CC` `HCC`

    3,6 ☑7ᵗʰ **M84.652** **Pathological fracture in other disease, left femur** `CC` `HCC`

    3,6 ☑7ᵗʰ **M84.653** **Pathological fracture in other disease, unspecified femur** `CC` `HCC`

    3,6 ☑7ᵗʰ **M84.659** **Pathological fracture in other disease, hip, unspecified** `CC` `HCC`

☑6ᵗʰ **M84.66** **Pathological fracture in other disease, tibia and fibula**

    3 ☑7ᵗʰ **M84.661** **Pathological fracture in other disease, right tibia** `CC`

3 ☑7ᵗʰ **M84.662** **Pathological fracture in other disease, left tibia** `CC`

3 ☑7ᵗʰ **M84.663** **Pathological fracture in other disease, right fibula** `CC`

3 ☑7ᵗʰ **M84.664** **Pathological fracture in other disease, left fibula** `CC`

3 ☑7ᵗʰ **M84.669** **Pathological fracture in other disease, unspecified tibia and fibula** `CC`

☑6ᵗʰ **M84.67** **Pathological fracture in other disease, ankle and foot**

    3 ☑7ᵗʰ **M84.671** **Pathological fracture in other disease, right ankle** `CC`

    3 ☑7ᵗʰ **M84.672** **Pathological fracture in other disease, left ankle** `CC`

    3 ☑7ᵗʰ **M84.673** **Pathological fracture in other disease, unspecified ankle** `CC`

    3 ☑7ᵗʰ **M84.674** **Pathological fracture in other disease, right foot** `CC`

    3 ☑7ᵗʰ **M84.675** **Pathological fracture in other disease, left foot** `CC`

    3 ☑7ᵗʰ **M84.676** **Pathological fracture in other disease, unspecified foot** `CC`

3 ☑x7ᵗʰ **M84.68** **Pathological fracture in other disease, other site** `CC`

☑6ᵗʰ **M84.7** **Nontraumatic fracture, not elsewhere classified**

  ☑6ᵗʰ **M84.75** **Atypical femoral fracture**

    AHA: 2016,4Q,41-42

> The appropriate 7th character is to be added to each code from M84.75.
> A   initial encounter for fracture
> D   subsequent encounter for fracture with routine healing
> G   subsequent encounter for fracture with delayed healing
> K   subsequent encounter for fracture with nonunion
> P   subsequent encounter for fracture with malunion
> S   sequela

> **CC Excl: For codes in subcategory M84.75:**
> **CC with 7th character A:** PDX collection 888
> **CC with 7th character K or P:** PDX collection 897

    3 ☑7ᵗʰ **M84.750** **Atypical femoral fracture, unspecified** `CC`

    3 ☑7ᵗʰ **M84.751** **Incomplete atypical femoral fracture, right leg** `CC`

    3 ☑7ᵗʰ **M84.752** **Incomplete atypical femoral fracture, left leg** `CC`

    3 ☑7ᵗʰ **M84.753** **Incomplete atypical femoral fracture, unspecified leg** `CC`

    3,6 ☑7ᵗʰ **M84.754** **Complete transverse atypical femoral fracture, right leg** `CC` `HCC`

    3,6 ☑7ᵗʰ **M84.755** **Complete transverse atypical femoral fracture, left leg** `CC` `HCC`

    3,6 ☑7ᵗʰ **M84.756** **Complete transverse atypical femoral fracture, unspecified leg** `CC` `HCC`

    3,6 ☑7ᵗʰ **M84.757** **Complete oblique atypical femoral fracture, right leg** `CC` `HCC`

    3,6 ☑7ᵗʰ **M84.758** **Complete oblique atypical femoral fracture, left leg** `CC` `HCC`

    3,6 ☑7ᵗʰ **M84.759** **Complete oblique atypical femoral fracture, unspecified leg** `CC` `HCC`

☑5ᵗʰ **M84.8** **Other disorders of continuity of bone**

  M84.80 **Other disorders of continuity of bone, unspecified site**

  ☑6ᵗʰ **M84.81** **Other disorders of continuity of bone, shoulder**

    M84.811 **Other disorders of continuity of bone, right shoulder**

    M84.812 **Other disorders of continuity of bone, left shoulder**

    M84.819 **Other disorders of continuity of bone, unspecified shoulder**

☑ Additional Character Required   ☑x7ᵗʰ Placeholder   Unacceptable PDx   Questionable PDx   Manifestation   Unspecified Dx   H1-H14 HAC   HCC CMS-HCC Dx   HIV HIV Dx

ICD-10-CM 2020   831

√6ᵗʰ **M84.82** **Other disorders of continuity of bone,** humerus

    M84.821 **Other disorders of continuity of bone,** right **humerus**

    M84.822 **Other disorders of continuity of bone,** left **humerus**

    M84.829 **Other disorders of continuity of bone, unspecified humerus**

√6ᵗʰ **M84.83** **Other disorders of continuity of bone,** ulna and radius

    M84.831 **Other disorders of continuity of bone,** right **ulna**

    M84.832 **Other disorders of continuity of bone,** left **ulna**

    M84.833 **Other disorders of continuity of bone,** right **radius**

    M84.834 **Other disorders of continuity of bone,** left **radius**

    M84.839 **Other disorders of continuity of bone, unspecified ulna and radius**

√6ᵗʰ **M84.84** **Other disorders of continuity of bone,** hand

    M84.841 **Other disorders of continuity of bone,** right **hand**

    M84.842 **Other disorders of continuity of bone,** left **hand**

    M84.849 **Other disorders of continuity of bone, unspecified hand**

√6ᵗʰ **M84.85** **Other disorders of continuity of bone,** pelvic region and thigh

    M84.851 **Other disorders of continuity of bone,** right **pelvic region and thigh**

    M84.852 **Other disorders of continuity of bone,** left **pelvic region and thigh**

    M84.859 **Other disorders of continuity of bone, unspecified pelvic region and thigh**

√6ᵗʰ **M84.86** **Other disorders of continuity of bone,** tibia and fibula

    M84.861 **Other disorders of continuity of bone,** right **tibia**

    M84.862 **Other disorders of continuity of bone,** left **tibia**

    M84.863 **Other disorders of continuity of bone,** right **fibula**

    M84.864 **Other disorders of continuity of bone,** left **fibula**

    M84.869 **Other disorders of continuity of bone, unspecified tibia and fibula**

√6ᵗʰ **M84.87** **Other disorders of continuity of bone,** ankle and foot

    M84.871 **Other disorders of continuity of bone,** right **ankle and foot**

    M84.872 **Other disorders of continuity of bone,** left **ankle and foot**

    M84.879 **Other disorders of continuity of bone, unspecified ankle and foot**

    M84.88 **Other disorders of continuity of bone, other site**

M84.9 **Disorder of continuity of bone, unspecified**

√4ᵗʰ **M85** **Other disorders of bone density and structure**

    EXCLUDES 1   osteogenesis imperfecta (Q78.0)

         osteopetrosis (Q78.2)

         osteopoikilosis (Q78.8)

         polyostotic fibrous dysplasia (Q78.1)

√5ᵗʰ **M85.0** **Fibrous dysplasia (monostotic)**

    EXCLUDES 2   fibrous dysplasia of jaw (M27.8)

    M85.00 **Fibrous dysplasia (monostotic), unspecified site**

√6ᵗʰ **M85.01** **Fibrous dysplasia (monostotic),** shoulder

    M85.011 **Fibrous dysplasia (monostotic),** right **shoulder**

    M85.012 **Fibrous dysplasia (monostotic),** left **shoulder**

    M85.019 **Fibrous dysplasia (monostotic), unspecified shoulder**

√6ᵗʰ **M85.02** **Fibrous dysplasia (monostotic),** upper arm

    M85.021 **Fibrous dysplasia (monostotic),** right **upper arm**

    M85.022 **Fibrous dysplasia (monostotic),** left **upper arm**

    M85.029 **Fibrous dysplasia (monostotic), unspecified upper arm**

√6ᵗʰ **M85.03** **Fibrous dysplasia (monostotic),** forearm

    M85.031 **Fibrous dysplasia (monostotic),** right **forearm**

    M85.032 **Fibrous dysplasia (monostotic),** left **forearm**

    M85.039 **Fibrous dysplasia (monostotic), unspecified forearm**

√6ᵗʰ **M85.04** **Fibrous dysplasia (monostotic),** hand

    M85.041 **Fibrous dysplasia (monostotic),** right **hand**

    M85.042 **Fibrous dysplasia (monostotic),** left **hand**

    M85.049 **Fibrous dysplasia (monostotic), unspecified hand**

√6ᵗʰ **M85.05** **Fibrous dysplasia (monostotic),** thigh

    M85.051 **Fibrous dysplasia (monostotic),** right **thigh**

    M85.052 **Fibrous dysplasia (monostotic),** left **thigh**

    M85.059 **Fibrous dysplasia (monostotic), unspecified thigh**

√6ᵗʰ **M85.06** **Fibrous dysplasia (monostotic),** lower leg

    M85.061 **Fibrous dysplasia (monostotic),** right **lower leg**

    M85.062 **Fibrous dysplasia (monostotic),** left **lower leg**

    M85.069 **Fibrous dysplasia (monostotic), unspecified lower leg**

√6ᵗʰ **M85.07** **Fibrous dysplasia (monostotic),** ankle and foot

    M85.071 **Fibrous dysplasia (monostotic),** right **ankle and foot**

    M85.072 **Fibrous dysplasia (monostotic),** left **ankle and foot**

    M85.079 **Fibrous dysplasia (monostotic), unspecified ankle and foot**

    M85.08 **Fibrous dysplasia (monostotic), other site**

    M85.09 **Fibrous dysplasia (monostotic),** multiple sites

√5ᵗʰ **M85.1** **Skeletal fluorosis**

    M85.10 **Skeletal fluorosis, unspecified site**

√6ᵗʰ **M85.11** **Skeletal fluorosis,** shoulder

    M85.111 **Skeletal fluorosis,** right **shoulder**

    M85.112 **Skeletal fluorosis,** left **shoulder**

    M85.119 **Skeletal fluorosis, unspecified shoulder**

√6ᵗʰ **M85.12** **Skeletal fluorosis,** upper arm

    M85.121 **Skeletal fluorosis,** right **upper arm**

    M85.122 **Skeletal fluorosis,** left **upper arm**

    M85.129 **Skeletal fluorosis, unspecified upper arm**

√6ᵗʰ **M85.13** **Skeletal fluorosis,** forearm

    M85.131 **Skeletal fluorosis,** right **forearm**

    M85.132 **Skeletal fluorosis,** left **forearm**

    M85.139 **Skeletal fluorosis, unspecified forearm**

√6ᵗʰ **M85.14** **Skeletal fluorosis,** hand

    M85.141 **Skeletal fluorosis,** right **hand**

    M85.142 **Skeletal fluorosis,** left **hand**

    M85.149 **Skeletal fluorosis, unspecified hand**

√6ᵗʰ **M85.15** **Skeletal fluorosis,** thigh

    M85.151 **Skeletal fluorosis,** right **thigh**

    M85.152 **Skeletal fluorosis,** left **thigh**

    M85.159 **Skeletal fluorosis, unspecified thigh**

√6ᵗʰ **M85.16** **Skeletal fluorosis,** lower leg

    M85.161 **Skeletal fluorosis,** right **lower leg**

    M85.162 **Skeletal fluorosis,** left **lower leg**

    M85.169 **Skeletal fluorosis, unspecified lower leg**

√6ᵗʰ **M85.17** **Skeletal fluorosis,** ankle and foot

    M85.171 **Skeletal fluorosis,** right **ankle and foot**

    M85.172 **Skeletal fluorosis,** left **ankle and foot**

    M85.179 **Skeletal fluorosis, unspecified ankle and foot**

    M85.18 **Skeletal fluorosis, other site**

    M85.19 **Skeletal fluorosis,** multiple sites

M85.2 **Hyperostosis of skull**

    DEF: Abnormal bone growth on the inner aspect of the cranial bones.

√5ᵗʰ **M85.3** **Osteitis condensans**

    M85.30 **Osteitis condensans, unspecified site**

√6ᵗʰ **M85.31** **Osteitis condensans,** shoulder

    M85.311 **Osteitis condensans,** right **shoulder**

    M85.312 **Osteitis condensans,** left **shoulder**

N Newborn: 0   P Pediatric: 0-17   M Maternity: 9-64   A Adult: 15-124   MCC Major Complication/Comorbidity   CC Complication/Comorbidity   SW Severe Wound Dx

832   ICD-10-CM 2020

M85.319 Osteitis condensans, unspecified shoulder

✓6ᵗʰ **M85.32 Osteitis condensans, upper arm**

M85.321 Osteitis condensans, right upper arm
M85.322 Osteitis condensans, left upper arm
M85.329 Osteitis condensans, unspecified upper arm

✓6ᵗʰ **M85.33 Osteitis condensans, forearm**

M85.331 Osteitis condensans, right forearm
M85.332 Osteitis condensans, left forearm
M85.339 Osteitis condensans, unspecified forearm

✓6ᵗʰ **M85.34 Osteitis condensans, hand**

M85.341 Osteitis condensans, right hand
M85.342 Osteitis condensans, left hand
M85.349 Osteitis condensans, unspecified hand

✓6ᵗʰ **M85.35 Osteitis condensans, thigh**

M85.351 Osteitis condensans, right thigh
M85.352 Osteitis condensans, left thigh
M85.359 Osteitis condensans, unspecified thigh

✓6ᵗʰ **M85.36 Osteitis condensans, lower leg**

M85.361 Osteitis condensans, right lower leg
M85.362 Osteitis condensans, left lower leg
M85.369 Osteitis condensans, unspecified lower leg

✓6ᵗʰ **M85.37 Osteitis condensans, ankle and foot**

M85.371 Osteitis condensans, right ankle and foot
M85.372 Osteitis condensans, left ankle and foot
M85.379 Osteitis condensans, unspecified ankle and foot

M85.38 Osteitis condensans, other site
M85.39 Osteitis condensans, multiple sites

✓5ᵗʰ **M85.4 Solitary bone cyst**

> EXCLUDES 2   solitary cyst of jaw (M27.4)

M85.40 **Solitary bone cyst, unspecified site**
✓6ᵗʰ **M85.41 Solitary bone cyst, shoulder**

M85.411 Solitary bone cyst, right shoulder
M85.412 Solitary bone cyst, left shoulder
M85.419 Solitary bone cyst, unspecified shoulder

✓6ᵗʰ **M85.42 Solitary bone cyst, humerus**

M85.421 Solitary bone cyst, right humerus
M85.422 Solitary bone cyst, left humerus
M85.429 Solitary bone cyst, unspecified humerus

✓6ᵗʰ **M85.43 Solitary bone cyst, ulna and radius**

M85.431 Solitary bone cyst, right ulna and radius
M85.432 Solitary bone cyst, left ulna and radius
M85.439 Solitary bone cyst, unspecified ulna and radius

✓6ᵗʰ **M85.44 Solitary bone cyst, hand**

M85.441 Solitary bone cyst, right hand
M85.442 Solitary bone cyst, left hand
M85.449 Solitary bone cyst, unspecified hand

✓6ᵗʰ **M85.45 Solitary bone cyst, pelvis**

M85.451 Solitary bone cyst, right pelvis
M85.452 Solitary bone cyst, left pelvis
M85.459 Solitary bone cyst, unspecified pelvis

✓6ᵗʰ **M85.46 Solitary bone cyst, tibia and fibula**

M85.461 Solitary bone cyst, right tibia and fibula
M85.462 Solitary bone cyst, left tibia and fibula
M85.469 Solitary bone cyst, unspecified tibia and fibula

✓6ᵗʰ **M85.47 Solitary bone cyst, ankle and foot**

M85.471 Solitary bone cyst, right ankle and foot
M85.472 Solitary bone cyst, left ankle and foot
M85.479 Solitary bone cyst, unspecified ankle and foot

M85.48 Solitary bone cyst, other site

✓5ᵗʰ **M85.5 Aneurysmal bone cyst**

> EXCLUDES 2   aneurysmal cyst of jaw (M27.4)

DEF: Solitary bone lesion that bulges into the periosteum and is marked by a calcified rim.

M85.50 **Aneurysmal bone cyst, unspecified site**
✓6ᵗʰ **M85.51 Aneurysmal bone cyst, shoulder**

M85.511 Aneurysmal bone cyst, right shoulder
M85.512 Aneurysmal bone cyst, left shoulder
M85.519 Aneurysmal bone cyst, unspecified shoulder

✓6ᵗʰ **M85.52 Aneurysmal bone cyst, upper arm**

M85.521 Aneurysmal bone cyst, right upper arm
M85.522 Aneurysmal bone cyst, left upper arm
M85.529 Aneurysmal bone cyst, unspecified upper arm

✓6ᵗʰ **M85.53 Aneurysmal bone cyst, forearm**

M85.531 Aneurysmal bone cyst, right forearm
M85.532 Aneurysmal bone cyst, left forearm
M85.539 Aneurysmal bone cyst, unspecified forearm

✓6ᵗʰ **M85.54 Aneurysmal bone cyst, hand**

M85.541 Aneurysmal bone cyst, right hand
M85.542 Aneurysmal bone cyst, left hand
M85.549 Aneurysmal bone cyst, unspecified hand

✓6ᵗʰ **M85.55 Aneurysmal bone cyst, thigh**

M85.551 Aneurysmal bone cyst, right thigh
M85.552 Aneurysmal bone cyst, left thigh
M85.559 Aneurysmal bone cyst, unspecified thigh

✓6ᵗʰ **M85.56 Aneurysmal bone cyst, lower leg**

M85.561 Aneurysmal bone cyst, right lower leg
M85.562 Aneurysmal bone cyst, left lower leg
M85.569 Aneurysmal bone cyst, unspecified lower leg

✓6ᵗʰ **M85.57 Aneurysmal bone cyst, ankle and foot**

M85.571 Aneurysmal bone cyst, right ankle and foot
M85.572 Aneurysmal bone cyst, left ankle and foot
M85.579 Aneurysmal bone cyst, unspecified ankle and foot

M85.58 Aneurysmal bone cyst, other site
M85.59 Aneurysmal bone cyst, multiple sites

✓5ᵗʰ **M85.6 Other cyst of bone**

> EXCLUDES 1   cyst of jaw NEC (M27.4)
> osteitis fibrosa cystica generalisata [von Recklinghausen's disease of bone] (E21.0)

M85.60 **Other cyst of bone, unspecified site**
✓6ᵗʰ **M85.61 Other cyst of bone, shoulder**

M85.611 Other cyst of bone, right shoulder
M85.612 Other cyst of bone, left shoulder
M85.619 Other cyst of bone, unspecified shoulder

✓6ᵗʰ **M85.62 Other cyst of bone, upper arm**

M85.621 Other cyst of bone, right upper arm
M85.622 Other cyst of bone, left upper arm
M85.629 Other cyst of bone, unspecified upper arm

✓6ᵗʰ **M85.63 Other cyst of bone, forearm**

M85.631 Other cyst of bone, right forearm
M85.632 Other cyst of bone, left forearm
M85.639 Other cyst of bone, unspecified forearm

✓6ᵗʰ **M85.64 Other cyst of bone, hand**

M85.641 Other cyst of bone, right hand
M85.642 Other cyst of bone, left hand
M85.649 Other cyst of bone, unspecified hand

✓6ᵗʰ **M85.65 Other cyst of bone, thigh**

M85.651 Other cyst of bone, right thigh
M85.652 Other cyst of bone, left thigh
M85.659 Other cyst of bone, unspecified thigh

✓6ᵗʰ **M85.66 Other cyst of bone, lower leg**

M85.661 Other cyst of bone, right lower leg
M85.662 Other cyst of bone, left lower leg
M85.669 Other cyst of bone, unspecified lower leg

✓6ᵗʰ **M85.67 Other cyst of bone, ankle and foot**

M85.671 Other cyst of bone, right ankle and foot
M85.672 Other cyst of bone, left ankle and foot
M85.679 Other cyst of bone, unspecified ankle and foot

M85.68 Other cyst of bone, other site
M85.69 Other cyst of bone, multiple sites

✓5ᵗʰ **M85.8 Other specified disorders of bone density and structure**

Hyperostosis of bones, except skull
Osteosclerosis, acquired

> EXCLUDES 1   diffuse idiopathic skeletal hyperostosis [DISH] (M48.1)
> osteosclerosis congenita (Q77.4)
> osteosclerosis fragilitas (generalista) (Q78.2)
> osteosclerosis myelofibrosis (D75.81)

M85.80 **Other specified disorders of bone density and structure, unspecified site**

☑ Additional Character Required   ✓x7ᵗʰ Placeholder   Unacceptable PDx   Questionable PDx   Manifestation   Unspecified Dx   H1-H1d HAC   HCC CMS-HCC Dx   HIV HIV Dx

ICD-10-CM 2020

833

Chapter 13. Diseases of the Musculoskeletal System and Connective Tissue

✓6th **M85.81** **Other specified disorders of bone density and structure, shoulder**

   M85.811 Other specified disorders of bone density and structure, right shoulder

   M85.812 Other specified disorders of bone density and structure, left shoulder

   M85.819 Other specified disorders of bone density and structure, unspecified shoulder

✓6th **M85.82** **Other specified disorders of bone density and structure, upper arm**

   M85.821 Other specified disorders of bone density and structure, right upper arm

   M85.822 Other specified disorders of bone density and structure, left upper arm

   M85.829 Other specified disorders of bone density and structure, unspecified upper arm

✓6th **M85.83** **Other specified disorders of bone density and structure, forearm**

   M85.831 Other specified disorders of bone density and structure, right forearm

   M85.832 Other specified disorders of bone density and structure, left forearm

   M85.839 Other specified disorders of bone density and structure, unspecified forearm

✓6th **M85.84** **Other specified disorders of bone density and structure, hand**

   M85.841 Other specified disorders of bone density and structure, right hand

   M85.842 Other specified disorders of bone density and structure, left hand

   M85.849 Other specified disorders of bone density and structure, unspecified hand

✓6th **M85.85** **Other specified disorders of bone density and structure, thigh**

   M85.851 Other specified disorders of bone density and structure, right thigh

   M85.852 Other specified disorders of bone density and structure, left thigh

   M85.859 Other specified disorders of bone density and structure, unspecified thigh

✓6th **M85.86** **Other specified disorders of bone density and structure, lower leg**

   M85.861 Other specified disorders of bone density and structure, right lower leg

   M85.862 Other specified disorders of bone density and structure, left lower leg

   M85.869 Other specified disorders of bone density and structure, unspecified lower leg

✓6th **M85.87** **Other specified disorders of bone density and structure, ankle and foot**

   M85.871 Other specified disorders of bone density and structure, right ankle and foot

   M85.872 Other specified disorders of bone density and structure, left ankle and foot

   M85.879 Other specified disorders of bone density and structure, unspecified ankle and foot

   M85.88 Other specified disorders of bone density and structure, other site

   M85.89 Other specified disorders of bone density and structure, multiple sites

M85.9 Disorder of bone density and structure, unspecified

Other osteopathies (M86–M90)

EXCLUDES 1   *postprocedural osteopathies (M96.-)*

✓4th **M86 Osteomyelitis**

Use additional code (B95–B97) to identify infectious agent
Use additional code to identify major osseous defect, if applicable (M89.7-)

   EXCLUDES 1   *osteomyelitis due to:*
     echinococcus (B67.2)
     gonococcus (A54.43)
     salmonella (A02.24)

   EXCLUDES 2   *ostemyelitis of:*
     orbit (H05.0-)
     petrous bone (H70.2-)
     vertebra (M46.2-)

✓5th **M86.0 Acute hematogenous osteomyelitis**

   M86.00 Acute hematogenous osteomyelitis, unspecified site   CC HCC
     CC Excl: PDX collection 898

✓6th **M86.01** **Acute hematogenous osteomyelitis, shoulder**

   CC Excl: For CC codes in subcategory M86.01: PDX collection 899

   M86.011 Acute hematogenous osteomyelitis, right shoulder   CC HCC

   M86.012 Acute hematogenous osteomyelitis, left shoulder   CC HCC

   M86.019 Acute hematogenous osteomyelitis, unspecified shoulder   CC HCC

✓6th **M86.02** **Acute hematogenous osteomyelitis, humerus**

   CC Excl: For CC codes in subcategory M86.02: PDX collection 900

   M86.021 Acute hematogenous osteomyelitis, right humerus   CC HCC

   M86.022 Acute hematogenous osteomyelitis, left humerus   CC HCC

   M86.029 Acute hematogenous osteomyelitis, unspecified humerus   CC HCC

✓6th **M86.03** **Acute hematogenous osteomyelitis, radius and ulna**

   CC Excl: For CC codes in subcategory M86.03: PDX collection 901

   M86.031 Acute hematogenous osteomyelitis, right radius and ulna   CC HCC

   M86.032 Acute hematogenous osteomyelitis, left radius and ulna   CC HCC

   M86.039 Acute hematogenous osteomyelitis, unspecified radius and ulna   CC HCC

✓6th **M86.04** **Acute hematogenous osteomyelitis, hand**

   CC Excl: For CC codes in subcategory M86.04: PDX collection 902

   M86.041 Acute hematogenous osteomyelitis, right hand   CC HCC

   M86.042 Acute hematogenous osteomyelitis, left hand   CC HCC

   M86.049 Acute hematogenous osteomyelitis, unspecified hand   CC HCC

✓6th **M86.05** **Acute hematogenous osteomyelitis, femur**

   CC Excl: For CC codes in subcategory M86.05: PDX collection 903

   M86.051 Acute hematogenous osteomyelitis, right femur   CC HCC

   M86.052 Acute hematogenous osteomyelitis, left femur   CC HCC

   M86.059 Acute hematogenous osteomyelitis, unspecified femur   CC HCC

✓6th **M86.06** **Acute hematogenous osteomyelitis, tibia and fibula**

   CC Excl: For CC codes in subcategory M86.06: PDX collection 904

   M86.061 Acute hematogenous osteomyelitis, right tibia and fibula   CC HCC

   M86.062 Acute hematogenous osteomyelitis, left tibia and fibula   CC HCC

   M86.069 Acute hematogenous osteomyelitis, unspecified tibia and fibula   CC HCC

✓6th **M86.07** **Acute hematogenous osteomyelitis, ankle and foot**

   CC Excl: For CC codes in subcategory M86.07: PDX collection 905

   M86.071 Acute hematogenous osteomyelitis, right ankle and foot   CC HCC

   M86.072 Acute hematogenous osteomyelitis, left ankle and foot   CC HCC

   M86.079 Acute hematogenous osteomyelitis, unspecified ankle and foot   CC HCC

N Newborn: 0   P Pediatric: 0-17   M Maternity: 9-64   A Adult: 15-124   MCC Major Complication/Comorbidity   CC Complication/Comorbidity   SW Severe Wound Dx

834   ICD-10-CM 2020

M85.81–M86.079

M86.08 **Acute hematogenous osteomyelitis, other sites** `CC` `HCC`
    CC Excl: PDX collection 882

M86.09 **Acute hematogenous osteomyelitis, multiple sites** `CC` `HCC`
    CC Excl: PDX collection 898

✓5ᵗʰ M86.1 **Other acute osteomyelitis**

    M86.10 **Other acute osteomyelitis, unspecified site** `CC` `HCC`
        CC Excl: PDX collection 898

    ✓6ᵗʰ M86.11 **Other acute osteomyelitis, shoulder**
        CC Excl: For CC codes in subcategory M86.11: PDX collection 899

        M86.111 **Other acute osteomyelitis, right shoulder** `CC` `HCC`
        M86.112 **Other acute osteomyelitis, left shoulder** `CC` `HCC`
        M86.119 **Other acute osteomyelitis, unspecified shoulder** `CC` `HCC`

    ✓6ᵗʰ M86.12 **Other acute osteomyelitis, humerus**
        CC Excl: For CC codes in subcategory M86.12: PDX collection 900

        M86.121 **Other acute osteomyelitis, right humerus** `CC` `HCC`
        M86.122 **Other acute osteomyelitis, left humerus** `CC` `HCC`
        M86.129 **Other acute osteomyelitis, unspecified humerus** `CC` `HCC`

    ✓6ᵗʰ M86.13 **Other acute osteomyelitis, radius and ulna**
        CC Excl: For CC codes in subcategory M86.13: PDX collection 901

        M86.131 **Other acute osteomyelitis, right radius and ulna** `CC` `HCC`
        M86.132 **Other acute osteomyelitis, left radius and ulna** `CC` `HCC`
        M86.139 **Other acute osteomyelitis, unspecified radius and ulna** `CC` `HCC`

    ✓6ᵗʰ M86.14 **Other acute osteomyelitis, hand**
        CC Excl: For CC codes in subcategory M86.14: PDX collection 902

        M86.141 **Other acute osteomyelitis, right hand** `CC` `HCC`
        M86.142 **Other acute osteomyelitis, left hand** `CC` `HCC`
        M86.149 **Other acute osteomyelitis, unspecified hand** `CC` `HCC`

    ✓6ᵗʰ M86.15 **Other acute osteomyelitis, femur**
        CC Excl: For CC codes in subcategory M86.15: PDX collection 903

        M86.151 **Other acute osteomyelitis, right femur** `CC` `HCC`
        M86.152 **Other acute osteomyelitis, left femur** `CC` `HCC`
        M86.159 **Other acute osteomyelitis, unspecified femur** `CC` `HCC`

    ✓6ᵗʰ M86.16 **Other acute osteomyelitis, tibia and fibula**
        CC Excl: For CC codes in subcategory M86.16: PDX collection 904

        M86.161 **Other acute osteomyelitis, right tibia and fibula** `CC` `HCC`
        M86.162 **Other acute osteomyelitis, left tibia and fibula** `CC` `HCC`
        M86.169 **Other acute osteomyelitis, unspecified tibia and fibula** `CC` `HCC`

    ✓6ᵗʰ M86.17 **Other acute osteomyelitis, ankle and foot**
        CC Excl: For CC codes in subcategory M86.17: PDX collection 905

        M86.171 **Other acute osteomyelitis, right ankle and foot** `CC` `HCC`
        M86.172 **Other acute osteomyelitis, left ankle and foot** `CC` `HCC`
        M86.179 **Other acute osteomyelitis, unspecified ankle and foot** `CC` `HCC`

    M86.18 **Other acute osteomyelitis, other site** `CC` `HCC`
        CC Excl: PDX collection 882

M86.19 **Other acute osteomyelitis, multiple sites** `CC` `HCC`
    CC Excl: PDX collection 898

✓5ᵗʰ M86.2 **Subacute osteomyelitis**

    M86.20 **Subacute osteomyelitis, unspecified site** `CC` `HCC`
        CC Excl: PDX collection 898

    ✓6ᵗʰ M86.21 **Subacute osteomyelitis, shoulder**
        CC Excl: For CC codes in subcategory M86.21: PDX collection 899

        M86.211 **Subacute osteomyelitis, right shoulder** `CC` `HCC`
        M86.212 **Subacute osteomyelitis, left shoulder** `CC` `HCC`
        M86.219 **Subacute osteomyelitis, unspecified shoulder** `CC` `HCC`

    ✓6ᵗʰ M86.22 **Subacute osteomyelitis, humerus**
        CC Excl: For CC codes in subcategory M86.22: PDX collection 900

        M86.221 **Subacute osteomyelitis, right humerus** `CC` `HCC`
        M86.222 **Subacute osteomyelitis, left humerus** `CC` `HCC`
        M86.229 **Subacute osteomyelitis, unspecified humerus** `CC` `HCC`

    ✓6ᵗʰ M86.23 **Subacute osteomyelitis, radius and ulna**
        CC Excl: For CC codes in subcategory M86.23: PDX collection 901

        M86.231 **Subacute osteomyelitis, right radius and ulna** `CC` `HCC`
        M86.232 **Subacute osteomyelitis, left radius and ulna** `CC` `HCC`
        M86.239 **Subacute osteomyelitis, unspecified radius and ulna** `CC` `HCC`

    ✓6ᵗʰ M86.24 **Subacute osteomyelitis, hand**
        CC Excl: For CC codes in subcategory M86.24: PDX collection 902

        M86.241 **Subacute osteomyelitis, right hand** `CC` `HCC`
        M86.242 **Subacute osteomyelitis, left hand** `CC` `HCC`
        M86.249 **Subacute osteomyelitis, unspecified hand** `CC` `HCC`

    ✓6ᵗʰ M86.25 **Subacute osteomyelitis, femur**
        CC Excl: For CC codes in subcategory M86.25: PDX collection 903

        M86.251 **Subacute osteomyelitis, right femur** `CC` `HCC`
        M86.252 **Subacute osteomyelitis, left femur** `CC` `HCC`
        M86.259 **Subacute osteomyelitis, unspecified femur** `CC` `HCC`

    ✓6ᵗʰ M86.26 **Subacute osteomyelitis, tibia and fibula**
        CC Excl: For CC codes in subcategory M86.26: PDX collection 904

        M86.261 **Subacute osteomyelitis, right tibia and fibula** `CC` `HCC`
        M86.262 **Subacute osteomyelitis, left tibia and fibula** `CC` `HCC`
        M86.269 **Subacute osteomyelitis, unspecified tibia and fibula** `CC` `HCC`

    ✓6ᵗʰ M86.27 **Subacute osteomyelitis, ankle and foot**
        CC Excl: For CC codes in subcategory M86.27: PDX collection 905

        M86.271 **Subacute osteomyelitis, right ankle and foot** `CC` `HCC`
        M86.272 **Subacute osteomyelitis, left ankle and foot** `CC` `HCC`
        M86.279 **Subacute osteomyelitis, unspecified ankle and foot** `CC` `HCC`

    M86.28 **Subacute osteomyelitis, other site** `CC` `HCC`
        CC Excl: PDX collection 882

    M86.29 **Subacute osteomyelitis, multiple sites** `CC` `HCC`
        CC Excl: PDX collection 898

✔ Additional Character Required   ✓x7ᵗʰ Placeholder   Unacceptable PDx   Questionable PDx   Manifestation   Unspecified Dx   H1-H14 HAC   HCC CMS-HCC Dx   HIV HIV Dx

ICD-10-CM 2020   835

Chapter 13. Diseases of the Musculoskeletal System and Connective Tissue

M86.08–M86.29

✓5ᵗʰ **M86.3** Chronic multifocal osteomyelitis

CC Excl: For CC codes in subcategory M86.3, unless otherwise noted: PDX collection 881

M86.3Ø Chronic multifocal osteomyelitis, unspecified site `CC` `HCC`

CC Excl: PDX collection 906

✓6ᵗʰ **M86.31** Chronic multifocal osteomyelitis, shoulder

M86.311 Chronic multifocal osteomyelitis, right shoulder `CC` `HCC`

M86.312 Chronic multifocal osteomyelitis, left shoulder `CC` `HCC`

M86.319 Chronic multifocal osteomyelitis, unspecified shoulder `CC` `HCC`

✓6ᵗʰ **M86.32** Chronic multifocal osteomyelitis, humerus

M86.321 Chronic multifocal osteomyelitis, right humerus `CC` `HCC`

M86.322 Chronic multifocal osteomyelitis, left humerus `CC` `HCC`

M86.329 Chronic multifocal osteomyelitis, unspecified humerus `CC` `HCC`

✓6ᵗʰ **M86.33** Chronic multifocal osteomyelitis, radius and ulna

M86.331 Chronic multifocal osteomyelitis, right radius and ulna `CC` `HCC`

M86.332 Chronic multifocal osteomyelitis, left radius and ulna `CC` `HCC`

M86.339 Chronic multifocal osteomyelitis, unspecified radius and ulna `CC` `HCC`

✓6ᵗʰ **M86.34** Chronic multifocal osteomyelitis, hand

M86.341 Chronic multifocal osteomyelitis, right hand `CC` `HCC`

M86.342 Chronic multifocal osteomyelitis, left hand `CC` `HCC`

M86.349 Chronic multifocal osteomyelitis, unspecified hand `CC` `HCC`

✓6ᵗʰ **M86.35** Chronic multifocal osteomyelitis, femur

M86.351 Chronic multifocal osteomyelitis, right femur `CC` `HCC`

M86.352 Chronic multifocal osteomyelitis, left femur `CC` `HCC`

M86.359 Chronic multifocal osteomyelitis, unspecified femur `CC` `HCC`

✓6ᵗʰ **M86.36** Chronic multifocal osteomyelitis, tibia and fibula

M86.361 Chronic multifocal osteomyelitis, right tibia and fibula `CC` `HCC`

M86.362 Chronic multifocal osteomyelitis, left tibia and fibula `CC` `HCC`

M86.369 Chronic multifocal osteomyelitis, unspecified tibia and fibula `CC` `HCC`

✓6ᵗʰ **M86.37** Chronic multifocal osteomyelitis, ankle and foot

M86.371 Chronic multifocal osteomyelitis, right ankle and foot `CC` `HCC`

M86.372 Chronic multifocal osteomyelitis, left ankle and foot `CC` `HCC`

M86.379 Chronic multifocal osteomyelitis, unspecified ankle and foot `CC` `HCC`

M86.38 Chronic multifocal osteomyelitis, other site `CC` `HCC`

M86.39 Chronic multifocal osteomyelitis, multiple sites `CC` `HCC`

✓5ᵗʰ **M86.4** Chronic osteomyelitis with draining sinus

CC Excl: For CC codes in subcategory M86.4, unless otherwise noted: PDX collection 881

M86.4Ø Chronic osteomyelitis with draining sinus, unspecified site `CC` `HCC`

CC Excl: PDX collection 906

✓6ᵗʰ **M86.41** Chronic osteomyelitis with draining sinus, shoulder

M86.411 Chronic osteomyelitis with draining sinus, right shoulder `CC` `HCC`

M86.412 Chronic osteomyelitis with draining sinus, left shoulder `CC` `HCC`

M86.419 Chronic osteomyelitis with draining sinus, unspecified shoulder `CC` `HCC`

✓6ᵗʰ **M86.42** Chronic osteomyelitis with draining sinus, humerus

M86.421 Chronic osteomyelitis with draining sinus, right humerus `CC` `HCC`

M86.422 Chronic osteomyelitis with draining sinus, left humerus `CC` `HCC`

M86.429 Chronic osteomyelitis with draining sinus, unspecified humerus `CC` `HCC`

✓6ᵗʰ **M86.43** Chronic osteomyelitis with draining sinus, radius and ulna

M86.431 Chronic osteomyelitis with draining sinus, right radius and ulna `CC` `HCC`

M86.432 Chronic osteomyelitis with draining sinus, left radius and ulna `CC` `HCC`

M86.439 Chronic osteomyelitis with draining sinus, unspecified radius and ulna `CC` `HCC`

✓6ᵗʰ **M86.44** Chronic osteomyelitis with draining sinus, hand

M86.441 Chronic osteomyelitis with draining sinus, right hand `CC` `HCC`

M86.442 Chronic osteomyelitis with draining sinus, left hand `CC` `HCC`

M86.449 Chronic osteomyelitis with draining sinus, unspecified hand `CC` `HCC`

✓6ᵗʰ **M86.45** Chronic osteomyelitis with draining sinus, femur

M86.451 Chronic osteomyelitis with draining sinus, right femur `CC` `HCC`

M86.452 Chronic osteomyelitis with draining sinus, left femur `CC` `HCC`

M86.459 Chronic osteomyelitis with draining sinus, unspecified femur `CC` `HCC`

✓6ᵗʰ **M86.46** Chronic osteomyelitis with draining sinus, tibia and fibula

M86.461 Chronic osteomyelitis with draining sinus, right tibia and fibula `CC` `HCC`

M86.462 Chronic osteomyelitis with draining sinus, left tibia and fibula `CC` `HCC`

M86.469 Chronic osteomyelitis with draining sinus, unspecified tibia and fibula `CC` `HCC`

✓6ᵗʰ **M86.47** Chronic osteomyelitis with draining sinus, ankle and foot

M86.471 Chronic osteomyelitis with draining sinus, right ankle and foot `CC` `HCC`

M86.472 Chronic osteomyelitis with draining sinus, left ankle and foot `CC` `HCC`

M86.479 Chronic osteomyelitis with draining sinus, unspecified ankle and foot `CC` `HCC`

M86.48 Chronic osteomyelitis with draining sinus, other site `CC` `HCC`

M86.49 Chronic osteomyelitis with draining sinus, multiple sites `CC` `HCC`

N Newborn: 0   P Pediatric: 0-17   M Maternity: 9-64   A Adult: 15-124   `MCC` Major Complication/Comorbidity   `CC` Complication/Comorbidity   `SW` Severe Wound Dx

836   ICD-10-CM 2020

✓6ᵗʰ **M86.5** Other chronic hematogenous **osteomyelitis**

CC Excl: For CC codes in subcategory M86.5, unless otherwise noted: PDX collection 881

  M86.50 Other chronic hematogenous osteomyelitis, unspecified site `CC` `HCC`
    CC Excl: PDX collection 906

✓6ᵗʰ **M86.51** Other chronic hematogenous osteomyelitis, shoulder

    M86.511 Other chronic hematogenous osteomyelitis, right shoulder `CC` `HCC`

    M86.512 Other chronic hematogenous osteomyelitis, left shoulder `CC` `HCC`

    M86.519 Other chronic hematogenous osteomyelitis, unspecified shoulder `CC` `HCC`

✓6ᵗʰ **M86.52** Other chronic hematogenous osteomyelitis, humerus

    M86.521 Other chronic hematogenous osteomyelitis, right humerus `CC` `HCC`

    M86.522 Other chronic hematogenous osteomyelitis, left humerus `CC` `HCC`

    M86.529 Other chronic hematogenous osteomyelitis, unspecified humerus `CC` `HCC`

✓6ᵗʰ **M86.53** Other chronic hematogenous osteomyelitis, radius and ulna

    M86.531 Other chronic hematogenous osteomyelitis, right radius and ulna `CC` `HCC`

    M86.532 Other chronic hematogenous osteomyelitis, left radius and ulna `CC` `HCC`

    M86.539 Other chronic hematogenous osteomyelitis, unspecified radius and ulna `CC` `HCC`

✓6ᵗʰ **M86.54** Other chronic hematogenous osteomyelitis, hand

    M86.541 Other chronic hematogenous osteomyelitis, right hand `CC` `HCC`

    M86.542 Other chronic hematogenous osteomyelitis, left hand `CC` `HCC`

    M86.549 Other chronic hematogenous osteomyelitis, unspecified hand `CC` `HCC`

✓6ᵗʰ **M86.55** Other chronic hematogenous osteomyelitis, femur

    M86.551 Other chronic hematogenous osteomyelitis, right femur `CC` `HCC`

    M86.552 Other chronic hematogenous osteomyelitis, left femur `CC` `HCC`

    M86.559 Other chronic hematogenous osteomyelitis, unspecified femur `CC` `HCC`

✓6ᵗʰ **M86.56** Other chronic hematogenous osteomyelitis, tibia and fibula

    M86.561 Other chronic hematogenous osteomyelitis, right tibia and fibula `CC` `HCC`

    M86.562 Other chronic hematogenous osteomyelitis, left tibia and fibula `CC` `HCC`

    M86.569 Other chronic hematogenous osteomyelitis, unspecified tibia and fibula `CC` `HCC`

✓6ᵗʰ **M86.57** Other chronic hematogenous osteomyelitis, ankle and foot

    M86.571 Other chronic hematogenous osteomyelitis, right ankle and foot `CC` `HCC`

    M86.572 Other chronic hematogenous osteomyelitis, left ankle and foot `CC` `HCC`

    M86.579 Other chronic hematogenous osteomyelitis, unspecified ankle and foot `CC` `HCC`

  M86.58 Other chronic hematogenous osteomyelitis, other site `CC` `HCC`

  M86.59 Other chronic hematogenous osteomyelitis, multiple sites `CC` `HCC`

✓5ᵗʰ **M86.6** Other chronic osteomyelitis

CC Excl: For CC codes in subcategory M86.6, unless otherwise noted: PDX collection 881

  M86.60 Other chronic osteomyelitis, unspecified site `CC` `HCC`
    CC Excl: PDX collection 906

✓6ᵗʰ **M86.61** Other chronic osteomyelitis, shoulder

    M86.611 Other chronic osteomyelitis, right shoulder `CC` `HCC`

    M86.612 Other chronic osteomyelitis, left shoulder `CC` `HCC`

    M86.619 Other chronic osteomyelitis, unspecified shoulder `CC` `HCC`

✓6ᵗʰ **M86.62** Other chronic osteomyelitis, humerus

    M86.621 Other chronic osteomyelitis, right humerus `CC` `HCC`

    M86.622 Other chronic osteomyelitis, left humerus `CC` `HCC`

    M86.629 Other chronic osteomyelitis, unspecified humerus `CC` `HCC`

✓6ᵗʰ **M86.63** Other chronic osteomyelitis, radius and ulna

    M86.631 Other chronic osteomyelitis, right radius and ulna `CC` `HCC`

    M86.632 Other chronic osteomyelitis, left radius and ulna `CC` `HCC`

    M86.639 Other chronic osteomyelitis, unspecified radius and ulna `CC` `HCC`

✓6ᵗʰ **M86.64** Other chronic osteomyelitis, hand

    M86.641 Other chronic osteomyelitis, right hand `CC` `HCC`

    M86.642 Other chronic osteomyelitis, left hand `CC` `HCC`

    M86.649 Other chronic osteomyelitis, unspecified hand `CC` `HCC`

✓6ᵗʰ **M86.65** Other chronic osteomyelitis, thigh

    M86.651 Other chronic osteomyelitis, right thigh `CC` `HCC`

    M86.652 Other chronic osteomyelitis, left thigh `CC` `HCC`

    M86.659 Other chronic osteomyelitis, unspecified thigh `CC` `HCC`

✓6ᵗʰ **M86.66** Other chronic osteomyelitis, tibia and fibula

    M86.661 Other chronic osteomyelitis, right tibia and fibula `CC` `HCC`

    M86.662 Other chronic osteomyelitis, left tibia and fibula `CC` `HCC`

    M86.669 Other chronic osteomyelitis, unspecified tibia and fibula `CC` `HCC`

✔ Additional Character Required   ✓x7ᵗʰ Placeholder   Unacceptable PDx   Questionable PDx   Manifestation   Unspecified Dx   H1 - H14 HAC   HCC CMS-HCC Dx   HIV HIV Dx

ICD-10-CM 2020   837

✓6ᵗʰ **M86.67** **Other chronic osteomyelitis,** ankle and foot

    M86.671 **Other chronic osteomyelitis,** right ankle and foot   CC HCC
       AHA: 2016,1Q,13

    M86.672 **Other chronic osteomyelitis,** left ankle and foot   CC HCC

    M86.679 **Other chronic osteomyelitis, unspecified ankle and foot**   CC HCC

   M86.68 **Other chronic osteomyelitis, other site**   CC HCC

   M86.69 **Other chronic osteomyelitis, multiple sites**   CC HCC

✓5ᵗʰ **M86.8** **Other osteomyelitis**

    Brodie's abscess

    CC Excl: For CC codes in subcategory M86.8, unless otherwise noted: PDX collection 881

✓6ᵗʰ **M86.8X** **Other osteomyelitis**

    M86.8X0 **Other osteomyelitis, multiple sites**   CC HCC

    M86.8X1 **Other osteomyelitis, shoulder**   CC HCC

    M86.8X2 **Other osteomyelitis, upper arm**   CC HCC

    M86.8X3 **Other osteomyelitis, forearm**   CC HCC

    M86.8X4 **Other osteomyelitis,** hand   CC HCC

    M86.8X5 **Other osteomyelitis,** thigh   CC HCC

    M86.8X6 **Other osteomyelitis,** lower leg   CC HCC

    M86.8X7 **Other osteomyelitis,** ankle and foot   CC HCC

    M86.8X8 **Other osteomyelitis, other site**   CC HCC

    M86.8X9 **Other osteomyelitis, unspecified sites**   CC HCC
       CC Excl: PDX collection 906

   M86.9 **Osteomyelitis, unspecified**   CC HCC

    Infection of bone NOS
    Periostitis without osteomyelitis
    CC Excl: PDX collection 906

✓4ᵗʰ **M87** **Osteonecrosis**

    INCLUDES   avascular necrosis of bone

    Use additional code to identify major osseous defect, if applicable (M89.7-)

    EXCLUDES 1   juvenile osteonecrosis (M91-M92)
       osteochondropathies (M90-M93)

    CC Excl: For CC codes in category M87, unless otherwise noted: PDX collection 907

✓5ᵗʰ **M87.0** **Idiopathic aseptic** necrosis of bone

    M87.00 **Idiopathic aseptic necrosis of unspecified bone**   CC HCC

✓6ᵗʰ **M87.01** **Idiopathic aseptic necrosis of** shoulder

    Idiopathic aseptic necrosis of clavicle and scapula

    CC Excl: For CC codes in subcategory M87.01: PDX collection 908

    M87.011 **Idiopathic aseptic necrosis of** right shoulder   CC HCC

    M87.012 **Idiopathic aseptic necrosis of** left shoulder   CC HCC

    M87.019 **Idiopathic aseptic necrosis of unspecified shoulder**   CC HCC

✓6ᵗʰ **M87.02** **Idiopathic aseptic necrosis of** humerus

    CC Excl: For CC codes in subcategory M87.02: PDX collection 908

    M87.021 **Idiopathic aseptic necrosis of** right humerus   CC HCC

    M87.022 **Idiopathic aseptic necrosis of** left humerus   CC HCC

    M87.029 **Idiopathic aseptic necrosis of unspecified humerus**   CC HCC

✓6ᵗʰ **M87.03** **Idiopathic aseptic necrosis of** radius, ulna and carpus

    M87.031 **Idiopathic aseptic necrosis of** right radius   CC HCC

    M87.032 **Idiopathic aseptic necrosis of** left radius   CC HCC

    M87.033 **Idiopathic aseptic necrosis of** unspecified radius   CC HCC

    M87.034 **Idiopathic aseptic necrosis of** right ulna   CC HCC

    M87.035 **Idiopathic aseptic necrosis of** left ulna   CC HCC

    M87.036 **Idiopathic aseptic necrosis of unspecified ulna**   CC HCC

    M87.037 **Idiopathic aseptic necrosis of** right carpus   CC HCC

    M87.038 **Idiopathic aseptic necrosis of** left carpus   CC HCC

    M87.039 **Idiopathic aseptic necrosis of unspecified carpus**   CC HCC

✓6ᵗʰ **M87.04** **Idiopathic aseptic necrosis of** hand and fingers

    Idiopathic aseptic necrosis of metacarpals and phalanges of hands

    M87.041 **Idiopathic aseptic necrosis of** right hand   CC HCC

    M87.042 **Idiopathic aseptic necrosis of** left hand   CC HCC

    M87.043 **Idiopathic aseptic necrosis of unspecified hand**   CC HCC

    M87.044 **Idiopathic aseptic necrosis of** right finger(s)   CC HCC

    M87.045 **Idiopathic aseptic necrosis of** left finger(s)   CC HCC

    M87.046 **Idiopathic aseptic necrosis of unspecified finger(s)**   CC HCC

✓6ᵗʰ **M87.05** **Idiopathic aseptic necrosis of** pelvis and femur

    M87.050 **Idiopathic aseptic necrosis of** pelvis   CC HCC

    M87.051 **Idiopathic aseptic necrosis of** right femur   CC HCC
       CC Excl: PDX collection 909

    M87.052 **Idiopathic aseptic necrosis of** left femur   CC HCC
       CC Excl: PDX collection 909

    M87.059 **Idiopathic aseptic necrosis of unspecified femur**   CC HCC
       CC Excl: PDX collection 909

✓6ᵗʰ **M87.06** **Idiopathic aseptic necrosis of** tibia and fibula

    M87.061 **Idiopathic aseptic necrosis of** right tibia   CC HCC

    M87.062 **Idiopathic aseptic necrosis of** left tibia   CC HCC

    M87.063 **Idiopathic aseptic necrosis of unspecified tibia**   CC HCC

    M87.064 **Idiopathic aseptic necrosis of** right fibula   CC HCC

    M87.065 **Idiopathic aseptic necrosis of** left fibula   CC HCC

    M87.066 **Idiopathic aseptic necrosis of unspecified fibula**   CC HCC

✓6ᵗʰ **M87.07** **Idiopathic aseptic necrosis of** ankle, foot and toes

    Idiopathic aseptic necrosis of metatarsus, tarsus, and phalanges of toes

    M87.071 **Idiopathic aseptic necrosis of** right ankle   CC HCC

    M87.072 **Idiopathic aseptic necrosis of** left ankle   CC HCC

    M87.073 **Idiopathic aseptic necrosis of unspecified ankle**   CC HCC

    M87.074 **Idiopathic aseptic necrosis of** right foot   CC HCC
       CC Excl: PDX collection 910

    M87.075 **Idiopathic aseptic necrosis of** left foot   CC HCC
       CC Excl: PDX collection 910

    M87.076 **Idiopathic aseptic necrosis of unspecified foot**   CC HCC
       CC Excl: PDX collection 910

    M87.077 **Idiopathic aseptic necrosis of** right toe(s)   CC HCC

    M87.078 **Idiopathic aseptic necrosis of** left toe(s)   CC HCC

    M87.079 **Idiopathic aseptic necrosis of unspecified toe(s)**   CC HCC

   M87.08 **Idiopathic aseptic necrosis of bone, other site**   CC HCC

   M87.09 **Idiopathic aseptic necrosis of bone,** multiple sites   CC HCC

N Newborn: 0   P Pediatric: 0-17   M Maternity: 9-64   A Adult: 15-124   MCC Major Complication/Comorbidity   CC Complication/Comorbidity   SW Severe Wound Dx

838   ICD-10-CM 2020

✓5th **M87.1** Osteonecrosis due to drugs
> Use additional code for adverse effect, if applicable, to identify drug (T36-T50 with fifth or sixth character 5)

M87.10 Osteonecrosis due to drugs, unspecified bone   `CC` `HCC`

✓6th **M87.11** Osteonecrosis due to drugs, shoulder

     M87.111 Osteonecrosis due to drugs, right shoulder   `CC` `HCC`

     M87.112 Osteonecrosis due to drugs, left shoulder   `CC` `HCC`

     M87.119 Osteonecrosis due to drugs, unspecified shoulder   `CC` `HCC`

✓6th **M87.12** Osteonecrosis due to drugs, humerus

> **CC Excl: For CC codes in subcategory M87.12:** PDX collection 908

     M87.121 Osteonecrosis due to drugs, right humerus   `CC` `HCC`

     M87.122 Osteonecrosis due to drugs, left humerus   `CC` `HCC`

     M87.129 Osteonecrosis due to drugs, unspecified humerus   `CC` `HCC`

✓6th **M87.13** Osteonecrosis due to drugs of radius, ulna and carpus

     M87.131 Osteonecrosis due to drugs of right radius   `CC` `HCC`

     M87.132 Osteonecrosis due to drugs of left radius   `CC` `HCC`

     M87.133 Osteonecrosis due to drugs of unspecified radius   `CC` `HCC`

     M87.134 Osteonecrosis due to drugs of right ulna   `CC` `HCC`

     M87.135 Osteonecrosis due to drugs of left ulna   `CC` `HCC`

     M87.136 Osteonecrosis due to drugs of unspecified ulna   `CC` `HCC`

     M87.137 Osteonecrosis due to drugs of right carpus   `CC` `HCC`

     M87.138 Osteonecrosis due to drugs of left carpus   `CC` `HCC`

     M87.139 Osteonecrosis due to drugs of unspecified carpus   `CC` `HCC`

✓6th **M87.14** Osteonecrosis due to drugs, hand and fingers

     M87.141 Osteonecrosis due to drugs, right hand   `CC` `HCC`

     M87.142 Osteonecrosis due to drugs, left hand   `CC` `HCC`

     M87.143 Osteonecrosis due to drugs, unspecified hand   `CC` `HCC`

     M87.144 Osteonecrosis due to drugs, right finger(s)   `CC` `HCC`

     M87.145 Osteonecrosis due to drugs, left finger(s)   `CC` `HCC`

     M87.146 Osteonecrosis due to drugs, unspecified finger(s)   `CC` `HCC`

✓6th **M87.15** Osteonecrosis due to drugs, pelvis and femur

> **CC Excl: For CC codes in subcategory M87.15:** PDX collection 909

     M87.150 Osteonecrosis due to drugs, pelvis   `CC` `HCC`

     M87.151 Osteonecrosis due to drugs, right femur   `CC` `HCC`

     M87.152 Osteonecrosis due to drugs, left femur   `CC` `HCC`

     M87.159 Osteonecrosis due to drugs, unspecified femur   `CC` `HCC`

✓6th **M87.16** Osteonecrosis due to drugs, tibia and fibula

     M87.161 Osteonecrosis due to drugs, right tibia   `CC` `HCC`

     M87.162 Osteonecrosis due to drugs, left tibia   `CC` `HCC`

     M87.163 Osteonecrosis due to drugs, unspecified tibia   `CC` `HCC`

     M87.164 Osteonecrosis due to drugs, right fibula   `CC` `HCC`

     M87.165 Osteonecrosis due to drugs, left fibula   `CC` `HCC`

     M87.166 Osteonecrosis due to drugs, unspecified fibula   `CC` `HCC`

✓6th **M87.17** Osteonecrosis due to drugs, ankle, foot and toes

     M87.171 Osteonecrosis due to drugs, right ankle   `CC` `HCC`

     M87.172 Osteonecrosis due to drugs, left ankle   `CC` `HCC`

     M87.173 Osteonecrosis due to drugs, unspecified ankle   `CC` `HCC`

     M87.174 Osteonecrosis due to drugs, right foot   `CC` `HCC`
> **CC Excl:** PDX collection 910

     M87.175 Osteonecrosis due to drugs, left foot   `CC` `HCC`
> **CC Excl:** PDX collection 910

     M87.176 Osteonecrosis due to drugs, unspecified foot   `CC` `HCC`
> **CC Excl:** PDX collection 910

     M87.177 Osteonecrosis due to drugs, right toe(s)   `CC` `HCC`

     M87.178 Osteonecrosis due to drugs, left toe(s)   `CC` `HCC`

     M87.179 Osteonecrosis due to drugs, unspecified toe(s)   `CC` `HCC`

✓6th **M87.18** Osteonecrosis due to drugs, other site

     M87.180 Osteonecrosis due to drugs, jaw   `CC` `HCC`

     M87.188 Osteonecrosis due to drugs, other site   `CC` `HCC`

M87.19 Osteonecrosis due to drugs, multiple sites   `CC` `HCC`

✓5th **M87.2** Osteonecrosis due to previous trauma

M87.20 Osteonecrosis due to previous trauma, unspecified bone   `CC` `HCC`

✓6th **M87.21** Osteonecrosis due to previous trauma, shoulder

     M87.211 Osteonecrosis due to previous trauma, right shoulder   `CC` `HCC`

     M87.212 Osteonecrosis due to previous trauma, left shoulder   `CC` `HCC`

     M87.219 Osteonecrosis due to previous trauma, unspecified shoulder   `CC` `HCC`

✓6th **M87.22** Osteonecrosis due to previous trauma, humerus

> **CC Excl: For CC codes in subcategory M87.22:** PDX collection 908

     M87.221 Osteonecrosis due to previous trauma, right humerus   `CC` `HCC`

     M87.222 Osteonecrosis due to previous trauma, left humerus   `CC` `HCC`

     M87.229 Osteonecrosis due to previous trauma, unspecified humerus   `CC` `HCC`

✓6th **M87.23** Osteonecrosis due to previous trauma of radius, ulna and carpus

     M87.231 Osteonecrosis due to previous trauma of right radius   `CC` `HCC`

     M87.232 Osteonecrosis due to previous trauma of left radius   `CC` `HCC`

     M87.233 Osteonecrosis due to previous trauma of unspecified radius   `CC` `HCC`

     M87.234 Osteonecrosis due to previous trauma of right ulna   `CC` `HCC`

     M87.235 Osteonecrosis due to previous trauma of left ulna   `CC` `HCC`

     M87.236 Osteonecrosis due to previous trauma of unspecified ulna   `CC` `HCC`

     M87.237 Osteonecrosis due to previous trauma of right carpus   `CC` `HCC`

     M87.238 Osteonecrosis due to previous trauma of left carpus   `CC` `HCC`

✔ Additional Character Required   ✓x7th Placeholder   Unacceptable PDx   Questionable PDx   Manifestation   Unspecified Dx   `H1`-`H14` HAC   `HCC` CMS-HCC Dx   `HIV` HIV Dx

ICD-10-CM 2020   **839**

M87.239 Osteonecrosis due to previous trauma of unspecified carpus `CC` `HCC`

✓6ᵗʰ **M87.24** Osteonecrosis due to previous trauma, **hand and fingers**

M87.241 Osteonecrosis due to previous trauma, **right hand** `CC` `HCC`

M87.242 Osteonecrosis due to previous trauma, **left hand** `CC` `HCC`

M87.243 Osteonecrosis due to previous trauma, **unspecified hand** `CC` `HCC`

M87.244 Osteonecrosis due to previous trauma, **right finger(s)** `CC` `HCC`

M87.245 Osteonecrosis due to previous trauma, **left finger(s)** `CC` `HCC`

M87.246 Osteonecrosis due to previous trauma, **unspecified finger(s)** `CC` `HCC`

✓6ᵗʰ **M87.25** Osteonecrosis due to previous trauma, **pelvis and femur**

M87.250 Osteonecrosis due to previous trauma, **pelvis** `CC` `HCC`

M87.251 Osteonecrosis due to previous trauma, **right femur** `CC` `HCC`
　　CC Excl: PDX collection 909

M87.252 Osteonecrosis due to previous trauma, **left femur** `CC` `HCC`
　　CC Excl: PDX collection 909

M87.256 Osteonecrosis due to previous trauma, **unspecified femur** `CC` `HCC`
　　CC Excl: PDX collection 909

✓6ᵗʰ **M87.26** Osteonecrosis due to previous trauma, **tibia and fibula**

M87.261 Osteonecrosis due to previous trauma, **right tibia** `CC` `HCC`

M87.262 Osteonecrosis due to previous trauma, **left tibia** `CC` `HCC`

M87.263 Osteonecrosis due to previous trauma, **unspecified tibia** `CC` `HCC`

M87.264 Osteonecrosis due to previous trauma, **right fibula** `CC` `HCC`

M87.265 Osteonecrosis due to previous trauma, **left fibula** `CC` `HCC`

M87.266 Osteonecrosis due to previous trauma, **unspecified fibula** `CC` `HCC`

✓6ᵗʰ **M87.27** Osteonecrosis due to previous trauma, **ankle, foot and toes**

M87.271 Osteonecrosis due to previous trauma, **right ankle** `CC` `HCC`

M87.272 Osteonecrosis due to previous trauma, **left ankle** `CC` `HCC`

M87.273 Osteonecrosis due to previous trauma, **unspecified ankle** `CC` `HCC`

M87.274 Osteonecrosis due to previous trauma, **right foot** `CC` `HCC`
　　CC Excl: PDX collection 910

M87.275 Osteonecrosis due to previous trauma, **left foot** `CC` `HCC`
　　CC Excl: PDX collection 910

M87.276 Osteonecrosis due to previous trauma, **unspecified foot** `CC` `HCC`
　　CC Excl: PDX collection 910

M87.277 Osteonecrosis due to previous trauma, **right toe(s)** `CC` `HCC`

M87.278 Osteonecrosis due to previous trauma, **left toe(s)** `CC` `HCC`

M87.279 Osteonecrosis due to previous trauma, **unspecified toe(s)** `CC` `HCC`

M87.28 Osteonecrosis due to previous trauma, **other site** `CC` `HCC`

M87.29 Osteonecrosis due to previous trauma, **multiple sites** `CC` `HCC`

✓5ᵗʰ **M87.3** Other **secondary osteonecrosis**

M87.30 Other secondary osteonecrosis, **unspecified bone** `CC` `HCC`

✓6ᵗʰ **M87.31** Other secondary osteonecrosis, **shoulder**

M87.311 Other secondary osteonecrosis, **right shoulder** `CC` `HCC`

M87.312 Other secondary osteonecrosis, **left shoulder** `CC` `HCC`

M87.319 Other secondary osteonecrosis, unspecified **shoulder** `CC` `HCC`

✓6ᵗʰ **M87.32** Other secondary osteonecrosis, **humerus**
　　CC Excl: For CC codes in subcategory M87.32: PDX collection 908

M87.321 Other secondary osteonecrosis, **right humerus** `CC` `HCC`

M87.322 Other secondary osteonecrosis, **left humerus** `CC` `HCC`

M87.329 Other secondary osteonecrosis, unspecified **humerus** `CC` `HCC`

✓6ᵗʰ **M87.33** Other secondary osteonecrosis of **radius, ulna and carpus**

M87.331 Other secondary osteonecrosis of **right radius** `CC` `HCC`

M87.332 Other secondary osteonecrosis of **left radius** `CC` `HCC`

M87.333 Other secondary osteonecrosis of **unspecified radius** `CC` `HCC`

M87.334 Other secondary osteonecrosis of **right ulna** `CC` `HCC`

M87.335 Other secondary osteonecrosis of **left ulna** `CC` `HCC`

M87.336 Other secondary osteonecrosis of **unspecified ulna** `CC` `HCC`

M87.337 Other secondary osteonecrosis of **right carpus** `CC` `HCC`

M87.338 Other secondary osteonecrosis of **left carpus** `CC` `HCC`

M87.339 Other secondary osteonecrosis of **unspecified carpus** `CC` `HCC`

✓6ᵗʰ **M87.34** Other secondary osteonecrosis, **hand and fingers**

M87.341 Other secondary osteonecrosis, **right hand** `CC` `HCC`

M87.342 Other secondary osteonecrosis, **left hand** `CC` `HCC`

M87.343 Other secondary osteonecrosis, unspecified **hand** `CC` `HCC`

M87.344 Other secondary osteonecrosis, **right finger(s)** `CC` `HCC`

M87.345 Other secondary osteonecrosis, **left finger(s)** `CC` `HCC`

M87.346 Other secondary osteonecrosis, unspecified **finger(s)** `CC` `HCC`

✓6ᵗʰ **M87.35** Other secondary osteonecrosis, **pelvis and femur**
　　CC Excl: For CC codes in subcategory M87.35: PDX collection 909

M87.350 Other secondary osteonecrosis, **pelvis** `CC` `HCC`

M87.351 Other secondary osteonecrosis, **right femur** `CC` `HCC`

Ⓝ Newborn: 0　　Ⓟ Pediatric: 0-17　　Ⓜ Maternity: 9-64　　Ⓐ Adult: 15-124　　ᴹᶜᶜ Major Complication/Comorbidity　　`CC` Complication/Comorbidity　　ˢʷ Severe Wound Dx

840　　　　　　　　ICD-10-CM 2020

M87.352 Other secondary osteonecrosis, left femur   `CC` `HCC`

M87.353 Other secondary osteonecrosis, unspecified femur   `CC` `HCC`

√6ᵗʰ **M87.36** Other secondary osteonecrosis, tibia and fibula

M87.361 Other secondary osteonecrosis, right tibia   `CC` `HCC`

M87.362 Other secondary osteonecrosis, left tibia   `CC` `HCC`

M87.363 Other secondary osteonecrosis, unspecified tibia   `CC` `HCC`

M87.364 Other secondary osteonecrosis, right fibula   `CC` `HCC`

M87.365 Other secondary osteonecrosis, left fibula   `CC` `HCC`

M87.366 Other secondary osteonecrosis, unspecified fibula   `CC` `HCC`

√6ᵗʰ **M87.37** Other secondary osteonecrosis, ankle and foot

M87.371 Other secondary osteonecrosis, right ankle   `CC` `HCC`

M87.372 Other secondary osteonecrosis, left ankle   `CC` `HCC`

M87.373 Other secondary osteonecrosis, unspecified ankle   `CC` `HCC`

M87.374 Other secondary osteonecrosis, right foot   `CC` `HCC`
    CC Excl: PDX collection 910

M87.375 Other secondary osteonecrosis, left foot   `CC` `HCC`
    CC Excl: PDX collection 910

M87.376 Other secondary osteonecrosis, unspecified foot   `CC` `HCC`
    CC Excl: PDX collection 910

M87.377 Other secondary osteonecrosis, right toe(s)   `CC` `HCC`

M87.378 Other secondary osteonecrosis, left toe(s)   `CC` `HCC`

M87.379 Other secondary osteonecrosis, unspecified toe(s)   `CC` `HCC`

M87.38 Other secondary osteonecrosis, other site   `CC` `HCC`

M87.39 Other secondary osteonecrosis, multiple sites   `CC` `HCC`

√5ᵗʰ **M87.8** Other osteonecrosis

M87.80 Other osteonecrosis, unspecified bone   `CC` `HCC`

√6ᵗʰ **M87.81** Other osteonecrosis, shoulder

M87.811 Other osteonecrosis, right shoulder   `CC` `HCC`

M87.812 Other osteonecrosis, left shoulder   `CC` `HCC`

M87.819 Other osteonecrosis, unspecified shoulder   `CC` `HCC`

√6ᵗʰ **M87.82** Other osteonecrosis, humerus

    CC Excl: For CC codes in subcategory M87.82: PDX collection 908

M87.821 Other osteonecrosis, right humerus   `CC` `HCC`

M87.822 Other osteonecrosis, left humerus   `CC` `HCC`

M87.829 Other osteonecrosis, unspecified humerus   `CC` `HCC`

√6ᵗʰ **M87.83** Other osteonecrosis of radius, ulna and carpus

M87.831 Other osteonecrosis of right radius   `CC` `HCC`

M87.832 Other osteonecrosis of left radius   `CC` `HCC`

M87.833 Other osteonecrosis of unspecified radius   `CC` `HCC`

M87.834 Other osteonecrosis of right ulna   `CC` `HCC`

M87.835 Other osteonecrosis of left ulna   `CC` `HCC`

M87.836 Other osteonecrosis of unspecified ulna   `CC` `HCC`

M87.837 Other osteonecrosis of right carpus   `CC` `HCC`

M87.838 Other osteonecrosis of left carpus   `CC` `HCC`

M87.839 Other osteonecrosis of unspecified carpus   `CC` `HCC`

√6ᵗʰ **M87.84** Other osteonecrosis, hand and fingers

M87.841 Other osteonecrosis, right hand   `CC` `HCC`

M87.842 Other osteonecrosis, left hand   `CC` `HCC`

M87.843 Other osteonecrosis, unspecified hand   `CC` `HCC`

M87.844 Other osteonecrosis, right finger(s)   `CC` `HCC`

M87.845 Other osteonecrosis, left finger(s)   `CC` `HCC`

M87.849 Other osteonecrosis, unspecified finger(s)   `CC` `HCC`

√6ᵗʰ **M87.85** Other osteonecrosis, pelvis and femur

    CC Excl: For CC codes in subcategory M87.85: PDX collection 909

M87.850 Other osteonecrosis, pelvis   `CC` `HCC`

M87.851 Other osteonecrosis, right femur   `CC` `HCC`

M87.852 Other osteonecrosis, left femur   `CC` `HCC`

M87.859 Other osteonecrosis, unspecified femur   `CC` `HCC`

√6ᵗʰ **M87.86** Other osteonecrosis, tibia and fibula

M87.861 Other osteonecrosis, right tibia   `CC` `HCC`

M87.862 Other osteonecrosis, left tibia   `CC` `HCC`

M87.863 Other osteonecrosis, unspecified tibia   `CC` `HCC`

M87.864 Other osteonecrosis, right fibula   `CC` `HCC`

M87.865 Other osteonecrosis, left fibula   `CC` `HCC`

M87.869 Other osteonecrosis, unspecified fibula   `CC` `HCC`

√6ᵗʰ **M87.87** Other osteonecrosis, ankle, foot and toes

M87.871 Other osteonecrosis, right ankle   `CC` `HCC`

M87.872 Other osteonecrosis, left ankle   `CC` `HCC`

M87.873 Other osteonecrosis, unspecified ankle   `CC` `HCC`

M87.874 Other osteonecrosis, right foot   `CC` `HCC`
    CC Excl: PDX collection 910

M87.875 Other osteonecrosis, left foot   `CC` `HCC`
    CC Excl: PDX collection 910

M87.876 Other osteonecrosis, unspecified foot   `CC` `HCC`
    CC Excl: PDX collection 910

M87.877 Other osteonecrosis, right toe(s)   `CC` `HCC`

M87.878 Other osteonecrosis, left toe(s)   `CC` `HCC`

M87.879 Other osteonecrosis, unspecified toe(s)   `CC` `HCC`

M87.88 Other osteonecrosis, other site   `CC` `HCC`

M87.89 Other osteonecrosis, multiple sites   `CC` `HCC`

M87.9 Osteonecrosis, unspecified   `CC` `HCC`

    Necrosis of bone NOS

√4ᵗʰ **M88** Osteitis deformans [Paget's disease of bone]

    EXCLUDES 1   osteitis deformans in neoplastic disease (M90.6)

    DEF: Bone disease characterized by numerous cycles of bone resorption by the body. Resorption is followed by accelerated repair attempts, causing bone deformities and bowing, with associated fractures and pain.

M88.0 Osteitis deformans of skull

M88.1 Osteitis deformans of vertebrae

√5ᵗʰ **M88.8** Osteitis deformans of other bones

√6ᵗʰ **M88.81** Osteitis deformans of shoulder

M88.811 Osteitis deformans of right shoulder

M88.812 Osteitis deformans of left shoulder

☑ Additional Character Required   √x7ᵗʰ Placeholder   Unacceptable PDx   Questionable PDx   Manifestation   Unspecified Dx   H1-H14 HAC   HCC CMS-HCC Dx   HIV HIV Dx

ICD-10-CM 2020

841

M88.819　Osteitis deformans of unspecified shoulder

✓6ᵗʰ M88.82　Osteitis deformans of upper arm

　M88.821　Osteitis deformans of right upper arm
　M88.822　Osteitis deformans of left upper arm
　M88.829　Osteitis deformans of unspecified upper arm

✓6ᵗʰ M88.83　Osteitis deformans of forearm

　M88.831　Osteitis deformans of right forearm
　M88.832　Osteitis deformans of left forearm
　M88.839　Osteitis deformans of unspecified forearm

✓6ᵗʰ M88.84　Osteitis deformans of hand

　M88.841　Osteitis deformans of right hand
　M88.842　Osteitis deformans of left hand
　M88.849　Osteitis deformans of unspecified hand

✓6ᵗʰ M88.85　Osteitis deformans of thigh

　M88.851　Osteitis deformans of right thigh
　M88.852　Osteitis deformans of left thigh
　M88.859　Osteitis deformans of unspecified thigh

✓6ᵗʰ M88.86　Osteitis deformans of lower leg

　M88.861　Osteitis deformans of right lower leg
　M88.862　Osteitis deformans of left lower leg
　M88.869　Osteitis deformans of unspecified lower leg

✓6ᵗʰ M88.87　Osteitis deformans of ankle and foot

　M88.871　Osteitis deformans of right ankle and foot
　M88.872　Osteitis deformans of left ankle and foot
　M88.879　Osteitis deformans of unspecified ankle and foot

M88.88　Osteitis deformans of other bones
　EXCLUDES 2　osteitis deformans of skull (M88.0)
　　　　　　　osteitis deformans of vertebrae (M88.1)

M88.89　Osteitis deformans of multiple sites

M88.9　Osteitis deformans of unspecified bone

✓4ᵗʰ M89　Other disorders of bone

✓5ᵗʰ M89.0　Algoneurodystrophy
　Shoulder-hand syndrome
　Sudeck's atrophy
　EXCLUDES 1　causalgia, lower limb (G57.7-)
　　　　　　　causalgia, upper limb (G56.4-)
　　　　　　　complex regional pain syndrome II, lower limb (G57.7-)
　　　　　　　complex regional pain syndrome II, upper limb (G56.4-)
　　　　　　　reflex sympathetic dystrophy (G90.5-)

M89.00　Algoneurodystrophy, unspecified site

✓6ᵗʰ M89.01　Algoneurodystrophy, shoulder
　M89.011　Algoneurodystrophy, right shoulder
　M89.012　Algoneurodystrophy, left shoulder
　M89.019　Algoneurodystrophy, unspecified shoulder

✓6ᵗʰ M89.02　Algoneurodystrophy, upper arm
　M89.021　Algoneurodystrophy, right upper arm
　M89.022　Algoneurodystrophy, left upper arm
　M89.029　Algoneurodystrophy, unspecified upper arm

✓6ᵗʰ M89.03　Algoneurodystrophy, forearm
　M89.031　Algoneurodystrophy, right forearm
　M89.032　Algoneurodystrophy, left forearm
　M89.039　Algoneurodystrophy, unspecified forearm

✓6ᵗʰ M89.04　Algoneurodystrophy, hand
　M89.041　Algoneurodystrophy, right hand
　M89.042　Algoneurodystrophy, left hand
　M89.049　Algoneurodystrophy, unspecified hand

✓6ᵗʰ M89.05　Algoneurodystrophy, thigh
　M89.051　Algoneurodystrophy, right thigh
　M89.052　Algoneurodystrophy, left thigh
　M89.059　Algoneurodystrophy, unspecified thigh

✓6ᵗʰ M89.06　Algoneurodystrophy, lower leg
　M89.061　Algoneurodystrophy, right lower leg
　M89.062　Algoneurodystrophy, left lower leg
　M89.069　Algoneurodystrophy, unspecified lower leg

✓6ᵗʰ M89.07　Algoneurodystrophy, ankle and foot
　M89.071　Algoneurodystrophy, right ankle and foot
　M89.072　Algoneurodystrophy, left ankle and foot
　M89.079　Algoneurodystrophy, unspecified ankle and foot

M89.08　Algoneurodystrophy, other site
M89.09　Algoneurodystrophy, multiple sites

✓5ᵗʰ M89.1　Physeal arrest
　Arrest of growth plate
　Epiphyseal arrest
　Growth plate arrest

✓6ᵗʰ M89.12　Physeal arrest, humerus
　M89.121　Complete physeal arrest, right proximal humerus
　M89.122　Complete physeal arrest, left proximal humerus
　M89.123　Partial physeal arrest, right proximal humerus
　M89.124　Partial physeal arrest, left proximal humerus
　M89.125　Complete physeal arrest, right distal humerus
　M89.126　Complete physeal arrest, left distal humerus
　M89.127　Partial physeal arrest, right distal humerus
　M89.128　Partial physeal arrest, left distal humerus
　M89.129　Physeal arrest, humerus, unspecified

✓6ᵗʰ M89.13　Physeal arrest, forearm
　M89.131　Complete physeal arrest, right distal radius
　M89.132　Complete physeal arrest, left distal radius
　M89.133　Partial physeal arrest, right distal radius
　M89.134　Partial physeal arrest, left distal radius
　M89.138　Other physeal arrest of forearm
　M89.139　Physeal arrest, forearm, unspecified

✓6ᵗʰ M89.15　Physeal arrest, femur
　M89.151　Complete physeal arrest, right proximal femur
　M89.152　Complete physeal arrest, left proximal femur
　M89.153　Partial physeal arrest, right proximal femur
　M89.154　Partial physeal arrest, left proximal femur
　M89.155　Complete physeal arrest, right distal femur
　M89.156　Complete physeal arrest, left distal femur
　M89.157　Partial physeal arrest, right distal femur
　M89.158　Partial physeal arrest, left distal femur
　M89.159　Physeal arrest, femur, unspecified

✓6ᵗʰ M89.16　Physeal arrest, lower leg
　M89.160　Complete physeal arrest, right proximal tibia
　M89.161　Complete physeal arrest, left proximal tibia
　M89.162　Partial physeal arrest, right proximal tibia
　M89.163　Partial physeal arrest, left proximal tibia
　M89.164　Complete physeal arrest, right distal tibia
　M89.165　Complete physeal arrest, left distal tibia
　M89.166　Partial physeal arrest, right distal tibia
　M89.167　Partial physeal arrest, left distal tibia
　M89.168　Other physeal arrest of lower leg
　M89.169　Physeal arrest, lower leg, unspecified

M89.18　Physeal arrest, other site

✓5ᵗʰ M89.2　Other disorders of bone development and growth
　M89.20　Other disorders of bone development and growth, unspecified site

✓6ᵗʰ M89.21　Other disorders of bone development and growth, shoulder
　M89.211　Other disorders of bone development and growth, right shoulder
　M89.212　Other disorders of bone development and growth, left shoulder
　M89.219　Other disorders of bone development and growth, unspecified shoulder

✓6ᵗʰ M89.22　Other disorders of bone development and growth, humerus
　M89.221　Other disorders of bone development and growth, right humerus

N Newborn: 0　P Pediatric: 0-17　M Maternity: 9-64　A Adult: 15-124　MCC Major Complication/Comorbidity　CC Complication/Comorbidity　SW Severe Wound Dx

842　　　ICD-10-CM 2020

M89.222 Other disorders of bone development and growth, left humerus

M89.229 Other disorders of bone development and growth, unspecified humerus

✓6ᵗʰ **M89.23** Other disorders of bone development and growth, ulna and radius

M89.231 Other disorders of bone development and growth, right ulna

M89.232 Other disorders of bone development and growth, left ulna

M89.233 Other disorders of bone development and growth, right radius

M89.234 Other disorders of bone development and growth, left radius

M89.239 Other disorders of bone development and growth, unspecified ulna and radius

✓6ᵗʰ **M89.24** Other disorders of bone development and growth, hand

M89.241 Other disorders of bone development and growth, right hand

M89.242 Other disorders of bone development and growth, left hand

M89.249 Other disorders of bone development and growth, unspecified hand

✓6ᵗʰ **M89.25** Other disorders of bone development and growth, femur

M89.251 Other disorders of bone development and growth, right femur

M89.252 Other disorders of bone development and growth, left femur

M89.259 Other disorders of bone development and growth, unspecified femur

✓6ᵗʰ **M89.26** Other disorders of bone development and growth, tibia and fibula

M89.261 Other disorders of bone development and growth, right tibia

M89.262 Other disorders of bone development and growth, left tibia

M89.263 Other disorders of bone development and growth, right fibula

M89.264 Other disorders of bone development and growth, left fibula

M89.269 Other disorders of bone development and growth, unspecified lower leg

✓6ᵗʰ **M89.27** Other disorders of bone development and growth, ankle and foot

M89.271 Other disorders of bone development and growth, right ankle and foot

M89.272 Other disorders of bone development and growth, left ankle and foot

M89.279 Other disorders of bone development and growth, unspecified ankle and foot

M89.28 Other disorders of bone development and growth, other site

M89.29 Other disorders of bone development and growth, multiple sites

✓5ᵗʰ **M89.3** Hypertrophy of bone

M89.30 Hypertrophy of bone, unspecified site

✓6ᵗʰ **M89.31** Hypertrophy of bone, shoulder

M89.311 Hypertrophy of bone, right shoulder

M89.312 Hypertrophy of bone, left shoulder

M89.319 Hypertrophy of bone, unspecified shoulder

✓6ᵗʰ **M89.32** Hypertrophy of bone, humerus

M89.321 Hypertrophy of bone, right humerus

M89.322 Hypertrophy of bone, left humerus

M89.329 Hypertrophy of bone, unspecified humerus

✓6ᵗʰ **M89.33** Hypertrophy of bone, ulna and radius

M89.331 Hypertrophy of bone, right ulna

M89.332 Hypertrophy of bone, left ulna

M89.333 Hypertrophy of bone, right radius

M89.334 Hypertrophy of bone, left radius

M89.339 Hypertrophy of bone, unspecified ulna and radius

✓6ᵗʰ **M89.34** Hypertrophy of bone, hand

M89.341 Hypertrophy of bone, right hand

M89.342 Hypertrophy of bone, left hand

M89.349 Hypertrophy of bone, unspecified hand

✓6ᵗʰ **M89.35** Hypertrophy of bone, femur

M89.351 Hypertrophy of bone, right femur

M89.352 Hypertrophy of bone, left femur

M89.359 Hypertrophy of bone, unspecified femur

✓6ᵗʰ **M89.36** Hypertrophy of bone, tibia and fibula

M89.361 Hypertrophy of bone, right tibia

M89.362 Hypertrophy of bone, left tibia

M89.363 Hypertrophy of bone, right fibula

M89.364 Hypertrophy of bone, left fibula

M89.369 Hypertrophy of bone, unspecified tibia and fibula

✓6ᵗʰ **M89.37** Hypertrophy of bone, ankle and foot

M89.371 Hypertrophy of bone, right ankle and foot

M89.372 Hypertrophy of bone, left ankle and foot

M89.379 Hypertrophy of bone, unspecified ankle and foot

M89.38 Hypertrophy of bone, other site

M89.39 Hypertrophy of bone, multiple sites

✓5ᵗʰ **M89.4** Other hypertrophic osteoarthropathy

Marie-Bamberger disease
Pachydermoperiostosis

M89.40 Other hypertrophic osteoarthropathy, unspecified site

✓6ᵗʰ **M89.41** Other hypertrophic osteoarthropathy, shoulder

M89.411 Other hypertrophic osteoarthropathy, right shoulder

M89.412 Other hypertrophic osteoarthropathy, left shoulder

M89.419 Other hypertrophic osteoarthropathy, unspecified shoulder

✓6ᵗʰ **M89.42** Other hypertrophic osteoarthropathy, upper arm

M89.421 Other hypertrophic osteoarthropathy, right upper arm

M89.422 Other hypertrophic osteoarthropathy, left upper arm

M89.429 Other hypertrophic osteoarthropathy, unspecified upper arm

✓6ᵗʰ **M89.43** Other hypertrophic osteoarthropathy, forearm

M89.431 Other hypertrophic osteoarthropathy, right forearm

M89.432 Other hypertrophic osteoarthropathy, left forearm

M89.439 Other hypertrophic osteoarthropathy, unspecified forearm

✓6ᵗʰ **M89.44** Other hypertrophic osteoarthropathy, hand

M89.441 Other hypertrophic osteoarthropathy, right hand

M89.442 Other hypertrophic osteoarthropathy, left hand

M89.449 Other hypertrophic osteoarthropathy, unspecified hand

✓6ᵗʰ **M89.45** Other hypertrophic osteoarthropathy, thigh

M89.451 Other hypertrophic osteoarthropathy, right thigh

M89.452 Other hypertrophic osteoarthropathy, left thigh

M89.459 Other hypertrophic osteoarthropathy, unspecified thigh

✓6ᵗʰ **M89.46** Other hypertrophic osteoarthropathy, lower leg

M89.461 Other hypertrophic osteoarthropathy, right lower leg

M89.462 Other hypertrophic osteoarthropathy, left lower leg

M89.469 Other hypertrophic osteoarthropathy, unspecified lower leg

✓6ᵗʰ **M89.47** Other hypertrophic osteoarthropathy, ankle and foot

M89.471 Other hypertrophic osteoarthropathy, right ankle and foot

M89.472 Other hypertrophic osteoarthropathy, left ankle and foot

M89.479 Other hypertrophic osteoarthropathy, unspecified ankle and foot

M89.48 Other hypertrophic osteoarthropathy, other site

M89.49 Other hypertrophic osteoarthropathy, multiple sites

√5ᵗʰ **M89.5 Osteolysis**

Use additional code to identify major osseous defect, if applicable (M89.7-)

EXCLUDES 2   periprosthetic osteolysis of internal prosthetic joint (T84.Ø5-)

M89.5Ø Osteolysis, unspecified site

√6ᵗʰ **M89.51 Osteolysis, shoulder**

M89.511 Osteolysis, right shoulder
M89.512 Osteolysis, left shoulder
M89.519 Osteolysis, unspecified shoulder

√6ᵗʰ **M89.52 Osteolysis, upper arm**

M89.521 Osteolysis, right upper arm
M89.522 Osteolysis, left upper arm
M89.529 Osteolysis, unspecified upper arm

√6ᵗʰ **M89.53 Osteolysis, forearm**

M89.531 Osteolysis, right forearm
M89.532 Osteolysis, left forearm
M89.539 Osteolysis, unspecified forearm

√6ᵗʰ **M89.54 Osteolysis, hand**

M89.541 Osteolysis, right hand
M89.542 Osteolysis, left hand
M89.549 Osteolysis, unspecified hand

√6ᵗʰ **M89.55 Osteolysis, thigh**

M89.551 Osteolysis, right thigh
M89.552 Osteolysis, left thigh
M89.559 Osteolysis, unspecified thigh

√6ᵗʰ **M89.56 Osteolysis, lower leg**

M89.561 Osteolysis, right lower leg
M89.562 Osteolysis, left lower leg
M89.569 Osteolysis, unspecified lower leg

√6ᵗʰ **M89.57 Osteolysis, ankle and foot**

M89.571 Osteolysis, right ankle and foot
M89.572 Osteolysis, left ankle and foot
M89.579 Osteolysis, unspecified ankle and foot

M89.58 Osteolysis, other site
M89.59 Osteolysis, multiple sites

√5ᵗʰ **M89.6 Osteopathy after poliomyelitis**

Use additional code (B91) to identify previous poliomyelitis

EXCLUDES 1   postpolio syndrome (G14)

M89.6Ø Osteopathy after poliomyelitis, unspecified site HCC

√6ᵗʰ **M89.61 Osteopathy after poliomyelitis, shoulder**

M89.611 Osteopathy after poliomyelitis, right shoulder HCC
M89.612 Osteopathy after poliomyelitis, left shoulder HCC
M89.619 Osteopathy after poliomyelitis, unspecified shoulder HCC

√6ᵗʰ **M89.62 Osteopathy after poliomyelitis, upper arm**

M89.621 Osteopathy after poliomyelitis, right upper arm HCC
M89.622 Osteopathy after poliomyelitis, left upper arm HCC
M89.629 Osteopathy after poliomyelitis, unspecified upper arm HCC

√6ᵗʰ **M89.63 Osteopathy after poliomyelitis, forearm**

M89.631 Osteopathy after poliomyelitis, right forearm HCC
M89.632 Osteopathy after poliomyelitis, left forearm HCC
M89.639 Osteopathy after poliomyelitis, unspecified forearm HCC

√6ᵗʰ **M89.64 Osteopathy after poliomyelitis, hand**

M89.641 Osteopathy after poliomyelitis, right hand HCC
M89.642 Osteopathy after poliomyelitis, left hand HCC
M89.649 Osteopathy after poliomyelitis, unspecified hand HCC

√6ᵗʰ **M89.65 Osteopathy after poliomyelitis, thigh**

M89.651 Osteopathy after poliomyelitis, right thigh HCC
M89.652 Osteopathy after poliomyelitis, left thigh HCC
M89.659 Osteopathy after poliomyelitis, unspecified thigh HCC

√6ᵗʰ **M89.66 Osteopathy after poliomyelitis, lower leg**

M89.661 Osteopathy after poliomyelitis, right lower leg HCC
M89.662 Osteopathy after poliomyelitis, left lower leg HCC
M89.669 Osteopathy after poliomyelitis, unspecified lower leg HCC

√6ᵗʰ **M89.67 Osteopathy after poliomyelitis, ankle and foot**

M89.671 Osteopathy after poliomyelitis, right ankle and foot HCC
M89.672 Osteopathy after poliomyelitis, left ankle and foot HCC
M89.679 Osteopathy after poliomyelitis, unspecified ankle and foot HCC

M89.68 Osteopathy after poliomyelitis, other site HCC
M89.69 Osteopathy after poliomyelitis, multiple sites HCC

√5ᵗʰ **M89.7 Major osseous defect**

Code first underlying disease, if known, such as:
aseptic necrosis of bone (M87.-)
malignant neoplasm of bone (C4Ø.-)
osteolysis (M89.5)
osteomyelitis (M86.-)
osteonecrosis (M87.-)
osteoporosis (M8Ø.-, M81.-)
periprosthetic osteolysis (T84.Ø5-)

M89.7Ø Major osseous defect, unspecified site

√6ᵗʰ **M89.71 Major osseous defect, shoulder region**

Major osseous defect clavicle or scapula
M89.711 Major osseous defect, right shoulder region
M89.712 Major osseous defect, left shoulder region
M89.719 Major osseous defect, unspecified shoulder region

√6ᵗʰ **M89.72 Major osseous defect, humerus**

M89.721 Major osseous defect, right humerus
M89.722 Major osseous defect, left humerus
M89.729 Major osseous defect, unspecified humerus

√6ᵗʰ **M89.73 Major osseous defect, forearm**

Major osseous defect of radius and ulna
M89.731 Major osseous defect, right forearm
M89.732 Major osseous defect, left forearm
M89.739 Major osseous defect, unspecified forearm

√6ᵗʰ **M89.74 Major osseous defect, hand**

Major osseous defect of carpus, fingers, metacarpus
M89.741 Major osseous defect, right hand
M89.742 Major osseous defect, left hand
M89.749 Major osseous defect, unspecified hand

√6ᵗʰ **M89.75 Major osseous defect, pelvic region and thigh**

Major osseous defect of femur and pelvis
M89.751 Major osseous defect, right pelvic region and thigh
M89.752 Major osseous defect, left pelvic region and thigh
M89.759 Major osseous defect, unspecified pelvic region and thigh

√6ᵗʰ **M89.76 Major osseous defect, lower leg**

Major osseous defect of fibula and tibia
M89.761 Major osseous defect, right lower leg
M89.762 Major osseous defect, left lower leg
M89.769 Major osseous defect, unspecified lower leg

N Newborn: 0   P Pediatric: 0-17   M Maternity: 9-64   A Adult: 15-124   MCC Major Complication/Comorbidity   CC Complication/Comorbidity   SW Severe Wound Dx

844   ICD-10-CM 2020

✓6th **M89.77** Major osseous defect, ankle and foot

Major osseous defect of metatarsus, tarsus, toes

M89.771 Major osseous defect, right ankle and foot

M89.772 Major osseous defect, left ankle and foot

M89.779 Major osseous defect, unspecified ankle and foot

M89.78 Major osseous defect, other site

M89.79 Major osseous defect, multiple sites

✓6th **M89.8** Other specified disorders of bone

Infantile cortical hyperostoses

Post-traumatic subperiosteal ossification

✓6th **M89.8X** Other specified disorders of bone

M89.8X0 Other specified disorders of bone, multiple sites

M89.8X1 Other specified disorders of bone, shoulder

M89.8X2 Other specified disorders of bone, upper arm

M89.8X3 Other specified disorders of bone, forearm

M89.8X4 Other specified disorders of bone, hand

M89.8X5 Other specified disorders of bone, thigh

M89.8X6 Other specified disorders of bone, lower leg

M89.8X7 Other specified disorders of bone, ankle and foot

M89.8X8 Other specified disorders of bone, other site

M89.8X9 Other specified disorders of bone, unspecified site

M89.9 Disorder of bone, unspecified

✓4th **M90** Osteopathies in diseases classified elsewhere

EXCLUDES 1   osteochondritis, osteomyelitis, and osteopathy (in):

cryptococcosis (B45.3)

diabetes mellitus (E08-E13 with .69-)

gonococcal (A54.43)

neurogenic syphilis (A52.11)

renal osteodystrophy (N25.0)

salmonellosis (A02.24)

secondary syphilis (A51.46)

syphilis (late) (A52.77)

✓5th **M90.5** Osteonecrosis in diseases classified elsewhere

Code first underlying disease, such as:

caisson disease (T70.3)

hemoglobinopathy (D50-D64)

CC Excl: For CC codes in subcategory M90.5, unless otherwise noted: PDX collection 907

M90.50 Osteonecrosis in diseases classified elsewhere, unspecified site   CC HCC

✓6th **M90.51** Osteonecrosis in diseases classified elsewhere, shoulder

CC Excl: For CC codes in subcategory M90.51: PDX collection 908

M90.511 Osteonecrosis in diseases classified elsewhere, right shoulder   CC HCC

M90.512 Osteonecrosis in diseases classified elsewhere, left shoulder   CC HCC

M90.519 Osteonecrosis in diseases classified elsewhere, unspecified shoulder   CC HCC

✓6th **M90.52** Osteonecrosis in diseases classified elsewhere, upper arm

M90.521 Osteonecrosis in diseases classified elsewhere, right upper arm   CC HCC

M90.522 Osteonecrosis in diseases classified elsewhere, left upper arm   CC HCC

M90.529 Osteonecrosis in diseases classified elsewhere, unspecified upper arm   CC HCC

✓6th **M90.53** Osteonecrosis in diseases classified elsewhere, forearm

M90.531 Osteonecrosis in diseases classified elsewhere, right forearm   CC HCC

M90.532 Osteonecrosis in diseases classified elsewhere, left forearm   CC HCC

M90.539 Osteonecrosis in diseases classified elsewhere, unspecified forearm   CC HCC

✓6th **M90.54** Osteonecrosis in diseases classified elsewhere, hand

M90.541 Osteonecrosis in diseases classified elsewhere, right hand   CC HCC

M90.542 Osteonecrosis in diseases classified elsewhere, left hand   CC HCC

M90.549 Osteonecrosis in diseases classified elsewhere, unspecified hand   CC HCC

✓6th **M90.55** Osteonecrosis in diseases classified elsewhere, thigh

CC Excl: For CC codes in subcategory M90.55: PDX collection 909

M90.551 Osteonecrosis in diseases classified elsewhere, right thigh   CC HCC

M90.552 Osteonecrosis in diseases classified elsewhere, left thigh   CC HCC

M90.559 Osteonecrosis in diseases classified elsewhere, unspecified thigh   CC HCC

✓6th **M90.56** Osteonecrosis in diseases classified elsewhere, lower leg

M90.561 Osteonecrosis in diseases classified elsewhere, right lower leg   CC HCC

M90.562 Osteonecrosis in diseases classified elsewhere, left lower leg   CC HCC

M90.569 Osteonecrosis in diseases classified elsewhere, unspecified lower leg   CC HCC

✓6th **M90.57** Osteonecrosis in diseases classified elsewhere, ankle and foot

M90.571 Osteonecrosis in diseases classified elsewhere, right ankle and foot   CC HCC

M90.572 Osteonecrosis in diseases classified elsewhere, left ankle and foot   CC HCC

M90.579 Osteonecrosis in diseases classified elsewhere, unspecified ankle and foot   CC HCC

M90.58 Osteonecrosis in diseases classified elsewhere, other site   CC HCC

M90.59 Osteonecrosis in diseases classified elsewhere, multiple sites   CC HCC

✓5th **M90.6** Osteitis deformans in neoplastic diseases

Osteitis deformans in malignant neoplasm of bone

Code first the neoplasm (C40.-, C41.-)

EXCLUDES 1   osteitis deformans [Paget's disease of bone] (M88.-)

M90.60 Osteitis deformans in neoplastic diseases, unspecified site

✓6th **M90.61** Osteitis deformans in neoplastic diseases, shoulder

M90.611 Osteitis deformans in neoplastic diseases, right shoulder

M90.612 Osteitis deformans in neoplastic diseases, left shoulder

M90.619 Osteitis deformans in neoplastic diseases, unspecified shoulder

✓6th **M90.62** Osteitis deformans in neoplastic diseases, upper arm

M90.621 Osteitis deformans in neoplastic diseases, right upper arm

M90.622 Osteitis deformans in neoplastic diseases, left upper arm

M90.629 Osteitis deformans in neoplastic diseases, unspecified upper arm

✓6th **M90.63** Osteitis deformans in neoplastic diseases, forearm

M90.631 Osteitis deformans in neoplastic diseases, right forearm

M90.632 Osteitis deformans in neoplastic diseases, left forearm

M90.639 Osteitis deformans in neoplastic diseases, unspecified forearm

✓ Additional Character Required   ✓x7th Placeholder   Unacceptable PDx   Questionable PDx   Manifestation   Unspecified Dx   H1-H14 HAC   HCC CMS-HCC Dx   HIV HIV Dx

ICD-10-CM 2020

845

Chapter 13. Diseases of the Musculoskeletal System and Connective Tissue

M90.64–M92.10

√6ᵗʰ **M90.64 Osteitis deformans in neoplastic diseases,** hand

    M90.641 Osteitis deformans in neoplastic diseases, right hand

    M90.642 Osteitis deformans in neoplastic diseases, left hand

    M90.649 Osteitis deformans in neoplastic diseases, unspecified hand

√6ᵗʰ **M90.65 Osteitis deformans in neoplastic diseases,** thigh

    M90.651 Osteitis deformans in neoplastic diseases, right thigh

    M90.652 Osteitis deformans in neoplastic diseases, left thigh

    M90.659 Osteitis deformans in neoplastic diseases, unspecified thigh

√6ᵗʰ **M90.66 Osteitis deformans in neoplastic diseases,** lower leg

    M90.661 Osteitis deformans in neoplastic diseases, right lower leg

    M90.662 Osteitis deformans in neoplastic diseases, left lower leg

    M90.669 Osteitis deformans in neoplastic diseases, unspecified lower leg

√6ᵗʰ **M90.67 Osteitis deformans in neoplastic diseases,** ankle and foot

    M90.671 Osteitis deformans in neoplastic diseases, right ankle and foot

    M90.672 Osteitis deformans in neoplastic diseases, left ankle and foot

    M90.679 Osteitis deformans in neoplastic diseases, unspecified ankle and foot

    M90.68 Osteitis deformans in neoplastic diseases, other site

    M90.69 Osteitis deformans in neoplastic diseases, multiple sites

√5ᵗʰ **M90.8 Osteopathy in diseases classified elsewhere**

    Code first underlying disease, such as:
       rickets (E55.0)
       vitamin-D-resistant rickets (E83.3)

    M90.80 Osteopathy in diseases classified elsewhere, unspecified site

√6ᵗʰ **M90.81 Osteopathy in diseases classified elsewhere,** shoulder

    M90.811 Osteopathy in diseases classified elsewhere, right shoulder

    M90.812 Osteopathy in diseases classified elsewhere, left shoulder

    M90.819 Osteopathy in diseases classified elsewhere, unspecified shoulder

√6ᵗʰ **M90.82 Osteopathy in diseases classified elsewhere,** upper arm

    M90.821 Osteopathy in diseases classified elsewhere, right upper arm

    M90.822 Osteopathy in diseases classified elsewhere, left upper arm

    M90.829 Osteopathy in diseases classified elsewhere, unspecified upper arm

√6ᵗʰ **M90.83 Osteopathy in diseases classified elsewhere,** forearm

    M90.831 Osteopathy in diseases classified elsewhere, right forearm

    M90.832 Osteopathy in diseases classified elsewhere, left forearm

    M90.839 Osteopathy in diseases classified elsewhere, unspecified forearm

√6ᵗʰ **M90.84 Osteopathy in diseases classified elsewhere,** hand

    M90.841 Osteopathy in diseases classified elsewhere, right hand

    M90.842 Osteopathy in diseases classified elsewhere, left hand

    M90.849 Osteopathy in diseases classified elsewhere, unspecified hand

√6ᵗʰ **M90.85 Osteopathy in diseases classified elsewhere,** thigh

    M90.851 Osteopathy in diseases classified elsewhere, right thigh

    M90.852 Osteopathy in diseases classified elsewhere, left thigh

    M90.859 Osteopathy in diseases classified elsewhere, unspecified thigh

√6ᵗʰ **M90.86 Osteopathy in diseases classified elsewhere,** lower leg

    M90.861 Osteopathy in diseases classified elsewhere, right lower leg

    M90.862 Osteopathy in diseases classified elsewhere, left lower leg

    M90.869 Osteopathy in diseases classified elsewhere, unspecified lower leg

√6ᵗʰ **M90.87 Osteopathy in diseases classified elsewhere,** ankle and foot

    M90.871 Osteopathy in diseases classified elsewhere, right ankle and foot

    M90.872 Osteopathy in diseases classified elsewhere, left ankle and foot

    M90.879 Osteopathy in diseases classified elsewhere, unspecified ankle and foot

    M90.88 Osteopathy in diseases classified elsewhere, other site

    M90.89 Osteopathy in diseases classified elsewhere, multiple sites

Chondropathies (M91-M94)

EXCLUDES 1   *postprocedural chondropathies (M96.-)*

√4ᵗʰ **M91 Juvenile osteochondrosis of** hip and pelvis

    EXCLUDES 1   *slipped upper femoral epiphysis (nontraumatic) (M93.0)*

M91.0 Juvenile osteochondrosis of pelvis

    Osteochondrosis (juvenile) of acetabulum
    Osteochondrosis (juvenile) of iliac crest [Buchanan]
    Osteochondrosis (juvenile) of ischiopubic synchondrosis [van Neck]
    Osteochondrosis (juvenile) of symphysis pubis [Pierson]

√5ᵗʰ **M91.1 Juvenile osteochondrosis of** head of femur [Legg-Calvé-Perthes]

    M91.10 Juvenile osteochondrosis of head of femur [Legg-Calvé-Perthes], unspecified leg

    M91.11 Juvenile osteochondrosis of head of femur [Legg-Calvé-Perthes], right leg

    M91.12 Juvenile osteochondrosis of head of femur [Legg-Calvé-Perthes], left leg

√5ᵗʰ **M91.2 Coxa plana**

    Hip deformity due to previous juvenile osteochondrosis

    M91.20 Coxa plana, unspecified hip
    M91.21 Coxa plana, right hip
    M91.22 Coxa plana, left hip

√5ᵗʰ **M91.3 Pseudocoxalgia**

    M91.30 Pseudocoxalgia, unspecified hip
    M91.31 Pseudocoxalgia, right hip
    M91.32 Pseudocoxalgia, left hip

√5ᵗʰ **M91.4 Coxa magna**

    M91.40 Coxa magna, unspecified hip
    M91.41 Coxa magna, right hip
    M91.42 Coxa magna, left hip

√5ᵗʰ **M91.8 Other juvenile osteochondrosis of hip and pelvis**

    Juvenile osteochondrosis after reduction of congenital dislocation of hip

    M91.80 Other juvenile osteochondrosis of hip and pelvis, unspecified leg

    M91.81 Other juvenile osteochondrosis of hip and pelvis, right leg

    M91.82 Other juvenile osteochondrosis of hip and pelvis, left leg

√5ᵗʰ **M91.9 Juvenile osteochondrosis of hip and pelvis, unspecified**

    M91.90 Juvenile osteochondrosis of hip and pelvis, unspecified, unspecified leg

    M91.91 Juvenile osteochondrosis of hip and pelvis, unspecified, right leg

    M91.92 Juvenile osteochondrosis of hip and pelvis, unspecified, left leg

√4ᵗʰ **M92 Other juvenile osteochondrosis**

√5ᵗʰ **M92.0 Juvenile osteochondrosis of** humerus

    Osteochondrosis (juvenile) of capitulum of humerus [Panner]
    Osteochondrosis (juvenile) of head of humerus [Haas]

    M92.00 Juvenile osteochondrosis of humerus, unspecified arm

    M92.01 Juvenile osteochondrosis of humerus, right arm

    M92.02 Juvenile osteochondrosis of humerus, left arm

√5ᵗʰ **M92.1 Juvenile osteochondrosis of** radius and ulna

    Osteochondrosis (juvenile) of lower ulna [Burns]
    Osteochondrosis (juvenile) of radial head [Brailsford]

    M92.10 Juvenile osteochondrosis of radius and ulna, unspecified arm

N Newborn: 0   P Pediatric: 0-17   M Maternity: 9-64   A Adult: 15-124   **MCC** Major Complication/Comorbidity   **CC** Complication/Comorbidity   **SW** Severe Wound Dx

    M92.11   **Juvenile osteochondrosis of radius and ulna, right arm**

    M92.12   **Juvenile osteochondrosis of radius and ulna, left arm**

√5th M92.2   **Juvenile osteochondrosis, hand**

   √6th M92.20   **Unspecified juvenile osteochondrosis, hand**

      M92.201   **Unspecified juvenile osteochondrosis, right hand**

      M92.202   **Unspecified juvenile osteochondrosis, left hand**

      M92.209   **Unspecified juvenile osteochondrosis, unspecified hand**

   √6th M92.21   **Osteochondrosis (juvenile) of carpal lunate [Kienböck]**

      M92.211   **Osteochondrosis (juvenile) of carpal lunate [Kienböck], right hand**

      M92.212   **Osteochondrosis (juvenile) of carpal lunate [Kienböck], left hand**

      M92.219   **Osteochondrosis (juvenile) of carpal lunate [Kienböck], unspecified hand**

   √6th M92.22   **Osteochondrosis (juvenile) of metacarpal heads [Mauclaire]**

      M92.221   **Osteochondrosis (juvenile) of metacarpal heads [Mauclaire], right hand**

      M92.222   **Osteochondrosis (juvenile) of metacarpal heads [Mauclaire], left hand**

      M92.229   **Osteochondrosis (juvenile) of metacarpal heads [Mauclaire], unspecified hand**

   √6th M92.29   **Other juvenile osteochondrosis, hand**

      M92.291   **Other juvenile osteochondrosis, right hand**

      M92.292   **Other juvenile osteochondrosis, left hand**

      M92.299   **Other juvenile osteochondrosis, unspecified hand**

√5th M92.3   **Other juvenile osteochondrosis, upper limb**

   M92.30   **Other juvenile osteochondrosis, unspecified upper limb**

   M92.31   **Other juvenile osteochondrosis, right upper limb**

   M92.32   **Other juvenile osteochondrosis, left upper limb**

√5th M92.4   **Juvenile osteochondrosis of patella**

   Osteochondrosis (juvenile) of primary patellar center [Köhler]

   Osteochondrosis (juvenile) of secondary patellar centre [Sinding Larsen]

   M92.40   **Juvenile osteochondrosis of patella, unspecified knee**

   M92.41   **Juvenile osteochondrosis of patella, right knee**

   M92.42   **Juvenile osteochondrosis of patella, left knee**

√5th M92.5   **Juvenile osteochondrosis of tibia and fibula**

   Osteochondrosis (juvenile) of proximal tibia [Blount]

   Osteochondrosis (juvenile) of tibial tubercle [Osgood-Schlatter]

   Tibia vara

   M92.50   **Juvenile osteochondrosis of tibia and fibula, unspecified leg**

   M92.51   **Juvenile osteochondrosis of tibia and fibula, right leg**

   M92.52   **Juvenile osteochondrosis of tibia and fibula, left leg**

√5th M92.6   **Juvenile osteochondrosis of tarsus**

   Osteochondrosis (juvenile) of calcaneum [Sever]

   Osteochondrosis (juvenile) of os tibiale externum [Haglund]

   Osteochondrosis (juvenile) of talus [Diaz]

   Osteochondrosis (juvenile) of tarsal navicular [Köhler]

   M92.60   **Juvenile osteochondrosis of tarsus, unspecified ankle**

   M92.61   **Juvenile osteochondrosis of tarsus, right ankle**

   M92.62   **Juvenile osteochondrosis of tarsus, left ankle**

√5th M92.7   **Juvenile osteochondrosis of metatarsus**

   Osteochondrosis (juvenile) of fifth metatarsus [Iselin]

   Osteochondrosis (juvenile) of second metatarsus [Freiberg]

   M92.70   **Juvenile osteochondrosis of metatarsus, unspecified foot**

   M92.71   **Juvenile osteochondrosis of metatarsus, right foot**

   M92.72   **Juvenile osteochondrosis of metatarsus, left foot**

  M92.8   **Other specified juvenile osteochondrosis**

   Calcaneal apophysitis

   DEF: Calcaneal apophysitis: Inflammation of the calcaneus at the point of Achilles tendon insertion usually occurring in boys ages 8 to 14. Pain, tenderness, and localized swelling are present.

  M92.9   **Juvenile osteochondrosis, unspecified**

   Juvenile apophysitis NOS

   Juvenile epiphysitis NOS

   Juvenile osteochondritis NOS

   Juvenile osteochondrosis NOS

√4th M93   **Other osteochondropathies**

   EXCLUDES 2   *osteochondrosis of spine (M42.-)*

√5th M93.0   **Slipped upper femoral epiphysis (nontraumatic)**

   Use additional code for associated chondrolysis (M94.3)

   √6th M93.00   **Unspecified slipped upper femoral epiphysis (nontraumatic)**

      M93.001   **Unspecified slipped upper femoral epiphysis (nontraumatic), right hip**

      M93.002   **Unspecified slipped upper femoral epiphysis (nontraumatic), left hip**

      M93.003   **Unspecified slipped upper femoral epiphysis (nontraumatic), unspecified hip**

   √6th M93.01   **Acute slipped upper femoral epiphysis (nontraumatic)**

      M93.011   **Acute slipped upper femoral epiphysis (nontraumatic), right hip**

      M93.012   **Acute slipped upper femoral epiphysis (nontraumatic), left hip**

      M93.013   **Acute slipped upper femoral epiphysis (nontraumatic), unspecified hip**

   √6th M93.02   **Chronic slipped upper femoral epiphysis (nontraumatic)**

      M93.021   **Chronic slipped upper femoral epiphysis (nontraumatic), right hip**

      M93.022   **Chronic slipped upper femoral epiphysis (nontraumatic), left hip**

      M93.023   **Chronic slipped upper femoral epiphysis (nontraumatic), unspecified hip**

   √6th M93.03   **Acute on chronic slipped upper femoral epiphysis (nontraumatic)**

      M93.031   **Acute on chronic slipped upper femoral epiphysis (nontraumatic), right hip**

      M93.032   **Acute on chronic slipped upper femoral epiphysis (nontraumatic), left hip**

      M93.033   **Acute on chronic slipped upper femoral epiphysis (nontraumatic), unspecified hip**

  M93.1   **Kienböck's disease of adults**   A

   Adult osteochondrosis of carpal lunates

√5th M93.2   **Osteochondritis dissecans**

   DEF: Avascular necrosis caused by lack of blood flow to the bone and cartilage of a joint causing the bone to die. This can result in splinters or pieces of cartilage breaking off in the joint.

   M93.20   **Osteochondritis dissecans of unspecified site**

   √6th M93.21   **Osteochondritis dissecans of shoulder**

      M93.211   **Osteochondritis dissecans, right shoulder**

      M93.212   **Osteochondritis dissecans, left shoulder**

      M93.219   **Osteochondritis dissecans, unspecified shoulder**

   √6th M93.22   **Osteochondritis dissecans of elbow**

      M93.221   **Osteochondritis dissecans, right elbow**

      M93.222   **Osteochondritis dissecans, left elbow**

      M93.229   **Osteochondritis dissecans, unspecified elbow**

   √6th M93.23   **Osteochondritis dissecans of wrist**

      M93.231   **Osteochondritis dissecans, right wrist**

      M93.232   **Osteochondritis dissecans, left wrist**

      M93.239   **Osteochondritis dissecans, unspecified wrist**

   √6th M93.24   **Osteochondritis dissecans of joints of hand**

      M93.241   **Osteochondritis dissecans, joints of right hand**

      M93.242   **Osteochondritis dissecans, joints of left hand**

      M93.249   **Osteochondritis dissecans, joints of unspecified hand**

   √6th M93.25   **Osteochondritis dissecans of hip**

      M93.251   **Osteochondritis dissecans, right hip**

      M93.252   **Osteochondritis dissecans, left hip**

      M93.259   **Osteochondritis dissecans, unspecified hip**

   √6th M93.26   **Osteochondritis dissecans knee**

      M93.261   **Osteochondritis dissecans, right knee**

      M93.262   **Osteochondritis dissecans, left knee**

☑ Additional Character Required   √x7th Placeholder   Unacceptable PDx   Questionable PDx   Manifestation   Unspecified Dx   H1-H14 HAC   HCC CMS-HCC Dx   HIV HIV Dx

ICD-10-CM 2020   847

M93.269 Osteochondritis dissecans, unspecified knee

✓6ᵗʰ M93.27 Osteochondritis dissecans of ankle and joints of foot

M93.271 Osteochondritis dissecans, right ankle and joints of right foot

M93.272 Osteochondritis dissecans, left ankle and joints of left foot

M93.279 Osteochondritis dissecans, unspecified ankle and joints of foot

M93.28 Osteochondritis dissecans other site

M93.29 Osteochondritis dissecans multiple sites

✓5ᵗʰ M93.8 Other specified osteochondropathies

M93.80 Other specified osteochondropathies of unspecified site

✓6ᵗʰ M93.81 Other specified osteochondropathies of shoulder

M93.811 Other specified osteochondropathies, right shoulder

M93.812 Other specified osteochondropathies, left shoulder

M93.819 Other specified osteochondropathies, unspecified shoulder

✓6ᵗʰ M93.82 Other specified osteochondropathies of upper arm

M93.821 Other specified osteochondropathies, right upper arm

M93.822 Other specified osteochondropathies, left upper arm

M93.829 Other specified osteochondropathies, unspecified upper arm

✓6ᵗʰ M93.83 Other specified osteochondropathies of forearm

M93.831 Other specified osteochondropathies, right forearm

M93.832 Other specified osteochondropathies, left forearm

M93.839 Other specified osteochondropathies, unspecified forearm

✓6ᵗʰ M93.84 Other specified osteochondropathies of hand

M93.841 Other specified osteochondropathies, right hand

M93.842 Other specified osteochondropathies, left hand

M93.849 Other specified osteochondropathies, unspecified hand

✓6ᵗʰ M93.85 Other specified osteochondropathies of thigh

M93.851 Other specified osteochondropathies, right thigh

M93.852 Other specified osteochondropathies, left thigh

M93.859 Other specified osteochondropathies, unspecified thigh

✓6ᵗʰ M93.86 Other specified osteochondropathies lower leg

M93.861 Other specified osteochondropathies, right lower leg

M93.862 Other specified osteochondropathies, left lower leg

M93.869 Other specified osteochondropathies, unspecified lower leg

✓6ᵗʰ M93.87 Other specified osteochondropathies of ankle and foot

M93.871 Other specified osteochondropathies, right ankle and foot

M93.872 Other specified osteochondropathies, left ankle and foot

M93.879 Other specified osteochondropathies, unspecified ankle and foot

M93.88 Other specified osteochondropathies other site

M93.89 Other specified osteochondropathies multiple sites

✓5ᵗʰ M93.9 Osteochondropathy, unspecified

Apophysitis NOS
Epiphysitis NOS
Osteochondritis NOS
Osteochondrosis NOS

M93.90 Osteochondropathy, unspecified of unspecified site

✓6ᵗʰ M93.91 Osteochondropathy, unspecified of shoulder

M93.911 Osteochondropathy, unspecified, right shoulder

M93.912 Osteochondropathy, unspecified, left shoulder

M93.919 Osteochondropathy, unspecified, unspecified shoulder

✓6ᵗʰ M93.92 Osteochondropathy, unspecified of upper arm

M93.921 Osteochondropathy, unspecified, right upper arm

M93.922 Osteochondropathy, unspecified, left upper arm

M93.929 Osteochondropathy, unspecified, unspecified upper arm

✓6ᵗʰ M93.93 Osteochondropathy, unspecified of forearm

M93.931 Osteochondropathy, unspecified, right forearm

M93.932 Osteochondropathy, unspecified, left forearm

M93.939 Osteochondropathy, unspecified, unspecified forearm

✓6ᵗʰ M93.94 Osteochondropathy, unspecified of hand

M93.941 Osteochondropathy, unspecified, right hand

M93.942 Osteochondropathy, unspecified, left hand

M93.949 Osteochondropathy, unspecified, unspecified hand

✓6ᵗʰ M93.95 Osteochondropathy, unspecified of thigh

M93.951 Osteochondropathy, unspecified, right thigh

M93.952 Osteochondropathy, unspecified, left thigh

M93.959 Osteochondropathy, unspecified, unspecified thigh

✓6ᵗʰ M93.96 Osteochondropathy, unspecified lower leg

M93.961 Osteochondropathy, unspecified, right lower leg

M93.962 Osteochondropathy, unspecified, left lower leg

M93.969 Osteochondropathy, unspecified, unspecified lower leg

✓6ᵗʰ M93.97 Osteochondropathy, unspecified of ankle and foot

M93.971 Osteochondropathy, unspecified, right ankle and foot

M93.972 Osteochondropathy, unspecified, left ankle and foot

M93.979 Osteochondropathy, unspecified, unspecified ankle and foot

M93.98 Osteochondropathy, unspecified other site

M93.99 Osteochondropathy, unspecified multiple sites

✓4ᵗʰ M94 Other disorders of cartilage

M94.0 Chondrocostal junction syndrome [Tietze]
Costochondritis

M94.1 Relapsing polychondritis

✓5ᵗʰ M94.2 Chondromalacia

EXCLUDES 1   chondromalacia patellae (M22.4)

M94.20 Chondromalacia, unspecified site

✓6ᵗʰ M94.21 Chondromalacia, shoulder

M94.211 Chondromalacia, right shoulder
M94.212 Chondromalacia, left shoulder
M94.219 Chondromalacia, unspecified shoulder

✓6ᵗʰ M94.22 Chondromalacia, elbow

M94.221 Chondromalacia, right elbow
M94.222 Chondromalacia, left elbow
M94.229 Chondromalacia, unspecified elbow

✓6ᵗʰ M94.23 Chondromalacia, wrist

M94.231 Chondromalacia, right wrist
M94.232 Chondromalacia, left wrist
M94.239 Chondromalacia, unspecified wrist

✓6ᵗʰ M94.24 Chondromalacia, joints of hand

M94.241 Chondromalacia, joints of right hand
M94.242 Chondromalacia, joints of left hand
M94.249 Chondromalacia, joints of unspecified hand

✓6ᵗʰ M94.25 Chondromalacia, hip

M94.251 Chondromalacia, right hip
M94.252 Chondromalacia, left hip
M94.259 Chondromalacia, unspecified hip

✓6ᵗʰ M94.26 Chondromalacia, knee

M94.261 Chondromalacia, right knee
M94.262 Chondromalacia, left knee

Ⓝ Newborn: 0   Ⓟ Pediatric: 0-17   Ⓜ Maternity: 9-64   Ⓐ Adult: 15-124   MCC Major Complication/Comorbidity   CC Complication/Comorbidity   SW Severe Wound Dx

848   ICD-10-CM 2020

✓6ᵗʰ **M94.27 Chondromalacia, ankle and joints of foot**

     M94.269 Chondromalacia, unspecified knee

     M94.271 Chondromalacia, right ankle and joints of right foot

     M94.272 Chondromalacia, left ankle and joints of left foot

     M94.279 Chondromalacia, unspecified ankle and joints of foot

     M94.28 Chondromalacia, other site

     M94.29 Chondromalacia, multiple sites

✓5ᵗʰ **M94.3 Chondrolysis**

     Code first any associated slipped upper femoral epiphysis (nontraumatic) (M93.0-)

     ✓6ᵗʰ **M94.35 Chondrolysis, hip**

         M94.351 Chondrolysis, right hip

         M94.352 Chondrolysis, left hip

         M94.359 Chondrolysis, unspecified hip

✓5ᵗʰ **M94.8 Other specified disorders of cartilage**

     ✓6ᵗʰ **M94.8X Other specified disorders of cartilage**

         M94.8X0 Other specified disorders of cartilage, multiple sites

         M94.8X1 Other specified disorders of cartilage, shoulder

         M94.8X2 Other specified disorders of cartilage, upper arm

         M94.8X3 Other specified disorders of cartilage, forearm

         M94.8X4 Other specified disorders of cartilage, hand

         M94.8X5 Other specified disorders of cartilage, thigh

         M94.8X6 Other specified disorders of cartilage, lower leg

         M94.8X7 Other specified disorders of cartilage, ankle and foot

         M94.8X8 Other specified disorders of cartilage, other site

         M94.8X9 Other specified disorders of cartilage, unspecified sites

     M94.9 Disorder of cartilage, unspecified

Other disorders of the musculoskeletal system and connective tissue (M95)

✓4ᵗʰ **M95 Other acquired deformities of musculoskeletal system and connective tissue**

     EXCLUDES 2   *acquired absence of limbs and organs (Z89-Z90)*

         acquired deformities of limbs (M20-M21)

         congenital malformations and deformations of the musculoskeletal system (Q65-Q79)

         deforming dorsopathies (M40-M43)

         dentofacial anomalies [including malocclusion] (M26.-)

         postprocedural musculoskeletal disorders (M96.-)

     M95.0 Acquired deformity of nose

         EXCLUDES 2   *deviated nasal septum (J34.2)*

✓5ᵗʰ **M95.1 Cauliflower ear**

         EXCLUDES 2   *other acquired deformities of ear (H61.1)*

         DEF: Acquired deformity of the external ear due to injury or subsequent perichondritis.

     M95.10 Cauliflower ear, unspecified ear

     M95.11 Cauliflower ear, right ear

     M95.12 Cauliflower ear, left ear

     M95.2 Other acquired deformity of head

     M95.3 Acquired deformity of neck

     M95.4 Acquired deformity of chest and rib

         AHA: 2014,4Q,26-27

     M95.5 Acquired deformity of pelvis

         EXCLUDES 1   *maternal care for known or suspected disproportion (O33.-)*

     M95.8 Other specified acquired deformities of musculoskeletal system

     M95.9 Acquired deformity of musculoskeletal system, unspecified

Intraoperative and postprocedural complications and disorders of musculoskeletal system, not elsewhere classified (M96)

✓4ᵗʰ **M96 Intraoperative and postprocedural complications and disorders of musculoskeletal system, not elsewhere classified**

     EXCLUDES 2   *arthropathy following intestinal bypass (M02.0-)*

         complications of internal orthopedic prosthetic devices, implants and grafts (T84.-)

         disorders associated with osteoporosis (M80)

         periprosthetic fracture around internal prosthetic joint (M97.-)

         presence of functional implants and other devices (Z96-Z97)

     M96.0 Pseudarthrosis after fusion or arthrodesis   CC

         CC Excl: No Excl

     M96.1 Postlaminectomy syndrome, not elsewhere classified

     M96.2 Postradiation kyphosis

     M96.3 Postlaminectomy kyphosis

     M96.4 Postsurgical lordosis

     M96.5 Postradiation scoliosis

✓5ᵗʰ **M96.6 Fracture of bone following insertion of orthopedic implant, joint prosthesis, or bone plate**

     Intraoperative fracture of bone during insertion of orthopedic implant, joint prosthesis, or bone plate

         EXCLUDES 2   *complication of internal orthopedic devices, implants or grafts (T84.-)*

     CC Excl: For CC codes in subcategory M96.6: PDX collection 911

     ✓6ᵗʰ **M96.62 Fracture of humerus following insertion of orthopedic implant, joint prosthesis, or bone plate**

         M96.621 Fracture of humerus following insertion of orthopedic implant, joint prosthesis, or bone plate, right arm   CC HCC

         M96.622 Fracture of humerus following insertion of orthopedic implant, joint prosthesis, or bone plate, left arm   CC HCC

         M96.629 Fracture of humerus following insertion of orthopedic implant, joint prosthesis, or bone plate, unspecified arm   CC HCC

     ✓6ᵗʰ **M96.63 Fracture of radius or ulna following insertion of orthopedic implant, joint prosthesis, or bone plate**

         M96.631 Fracture of radius or ulna following insertion of orthopedic implant, joint prosthesis, or bone plate, right arm   CC HCC

         M96.632 Fracture of radius or ulna following insertion of orthopedic implant, joint prosthesis, or bone plate, left arm   CC HCC

         M96.639 Fracture of radius or ulna following insertion of orthopedic implant, joint prosthesis, or bone plate, unspecified arm   CC HCC

     M96.65 Fracture of pelvis following insertion of orthopedic implant, joint prosthesis, or bone plate   CC HCC

     ✓6ᵗʰ **M96.66 Fracture of femur following insertion of orthopedic implant, joint prosthesis, or bone plate**

         M96.661 Fracture of femur following insertion of orthopedic implant, joint prosthesis, or bone plate, right leg   CC HCC

         M96.662 Fracture of femur following insertion of orthopedic implant, joint prosthesis, or bone plate, left leg   CC HCC

         M96.669 Fracture of femur following insertion of orthopedic implant, joint prosthesis, or bone plate, unspecified leg   CC HCC

✔ Additional Character Required   ✓x7ᵗʰ Placeholder   Unacceptable PDx   Questionable PDx   Manifestation   Unspecified Dx   H1-H14 HAC   HCC CMS-HCC Dx   HIV HIV Dx

ICD-10-CM 2020

849

√6th **M96.67** **Fracture of** tibia **or** fibula **following insertion of orthopedic implant, joint prosthesis, or bone plate**

M96.671 Fracture of tibia or fibula following insertion of orthopedic implant, joint prosthesis, or bone plate, right leg `CC` `HCC`

M96.672 Fracture of tibia or fibula following insertion of orthopedic implant, joint prosthesis, or bone plate, left leg `CC` `HCC`

M96.679 Fracture of tibia or fibula following insertion of orthopedic implant, joint prosthesis, or bone plate, unspecified leg `CC` `HCC`

M96.69 **Fracture of other bone following insertion of orthopedic implant, joint prosthesis, or bone plate** `CC` `HCC`

√5th **M96.8** **Other intraoperative and postprocedural complications and disorders of musculoskeletal system, not elsewhere classified**

AHA: 2016,4Q,9-10

CC Excl: For CC codes in subcategory M96.8, unless otherwise noted: PDX collection 912

√6th **M96.81** Intraoperative hemorrhage and hematoma **of a** musculoskeletal structure complicating a procedure

EXCLUDES 1 *intraoperative hemorrhage and hematoma of a musculoskeletal structure due to accidental puncture and laceration during a procedure (M96.82-)*

M96.810 Intraoperative hemorrhage and hematoma of a musculoskeletal structure complicating a musculoskeletal system procedure `CC`

M96.811 Intraoperative hemorrhage and hematoma of a musculoskeletal structure complicating other procedure `CC`

√6th **M96.82** Accidental puncture and laceration **of a** musculoskeletal structure during a procedure

M96.820 Accidental puncture and laceration of a musculoskeletal structure during a musculoskeletal system procedure `CC`

CC Excl: PDX collection 509

M96.821 Accidental puncture and laceration of a musculoskeletal structure during other procedure `CC`

CC Excl: PDX collection 509

√6th **M96.83** Postprocedural hemorrhage **of a musculoskeletal structure following a procedure**

M96.830 Postprocedural hemorrhage of a musculoskeletal structure following a musculoskeletal system procedure `CC`

M96.831 Postprocedural hemorrhage of a musculoskeletal structure following other procedure `CC`

√6th **M96.84** Postprocedural hematoma and seroma **of a musculoskeletal structure following a procedure**

M96.840 Postprocedural hematoma of a musculoskeletal structure following a musculoskeletal system procedure `CC`

M96.841 Postprocedural hematoma of a musculoskeletal structure following other procedure `CC`

AHA: 2016,4Q,10

M96.842 Postprocedural seroma of a musculoskeletal structure following a musculoskeletal system procedure `CC`

M96.843 Postprocedural seroma of a musculoskeletal structure following other procedure `CC`

AHA: 2018,3Q,6

M96.89 **Other intraoperative and postprocedural complications and disorders of the musculoskeletal system** `CC`

Instability of joint secondary to removal of joint prosthesis

Use additional code, if applicable, to further specify disorder

CC Excl: PDX collection 643

Periprosthetic fractures around internal prosthetic joint (M97)

√4th **M97** **Periprosthetic fracture around internal prosthetic joint**

EXCLUDES 2 *breakage (fracture) of prosthetic joint (T84.01-)*
fracture of bone following insertion of orthopedic implant, joint prosthesis or bone plate (M96.6-)

AHA: 2016,4Q,42-43

The appropriate 7th character is to be added to each code from category M97.
A initial encounter
D subsequent encounter
S sequela

CC Excl: For CC codes in category M97: PDX collection 911

√5th **M97.0** **Periprosthetic fracture around internal prosthetic hip joint**

AHA: 2018,1Q,21; 2016,4Q,42

√x7th **M97.01** **Periprosthetic fracture around internal prosthetic right hip joint** `CC` `HCC`

√x7th **M97.02** **Periprosthetic fracture around internal prosthetic left hip joint** `CC` `HCC`

√5th **M97.1** **Periprosthetic fracture around internal prosthetic knee joint**

√x7th **M97.11** **Periprosthetic fracture around internal prosthetic right knee joint** `CC`

√x7th **M97.12** **Periprosthetic fracture around internal prosthetic left knee joint** `CC`

√5th **M97.2** **Periprosthetic fracture around internal prosthetic ankle joint**

√x7th **M97.21** **Periprosthetic fracture around internal prosthetic right ankle joint** `CC`

√x7th **M97.22** **Periprosthetic fracture around internal prosthetic left ankle joint** `CC`

√5th **M97.3** **Periprosthetic fracture around internal prosthetic shoulder joint**

√x7th **M97.31** **Periprosthetic fracture around internal prosthetic right shoulder joint** `CC`

√x7th **M97.32** **Periprosthetic fracture around internal prosthetic left shoulder joint** `CC`

√5th **M97.4** **Periprosthetic fracture around internal prosthetic elbow joint**

√x7th **M97.41** **Periprosthetic fracture around internal prosthetic right elbow joint** `CC`

√x7th **M97.42** **Periprosthetic fracture around internal prosthetic left elbow joint** `CC`

√x7th **M97.8** **Periprosthetic fracture around other internal prosthetic joint** `CC`

Periprosthetic fracture around internal prosthetic finger joint
Periprosthetic fracture around internal prosthetic spinal joint
Periprosthetic fracture around internal prosthetic toe joint
Periprosthetic fracture around internal prosthetic wrist joint
Use additional code to identify the joint (Z96.6-)

√x7th **M97.9** **Periprosthetic fracture around unspecified internal prosthetic joint** `CC`

Biomechanical lesions, not elsewhere classified (M99)

✓4ᵗʰ M99 Biomechanical lesions, not elsewhere classified

NOTE This category should not be used if the condition can be classified elsewhere.

DEF: Biomechanical lesion: Term used by osteopathic and chiropractic physicians to describe musculoskeletal conditions treated that are not more appropriately classified elsewhere.

✓5ᵗʰ M99.Ø Segmental and somatic dysfunction

    M99.ØØ Segmental and somatic dysfunction of **head** region

    M99.Ø1 Segmental and somatic dysfunction of **cervical** region

    M99.Ø2 Segmental and somatic dysfunction of **thoracic** region

    M99.Ø3 Segmental and somatic dysfunction of **lumbar** region

    M99.Ø4 Segmental and somatic dysfunction of **sacral** region

    M99.Ø5 Segmental and somatic dysfunction of **pelvic** region

    M99.Ø6 Segmental and somatic dysfunction of **lower extremity**

    M99.Ø7 Segmental and somatic dysfunction of **upper extremity**

    M99.Ø8 Segmental and somatic dysfunction of **rib cage**

    M99.Ø9 Segmental and somatic dysfunction of **abdomen and other** regions

✓5ᵗʰ M99.1 Subluxation complex (vertebral)

    M99.1Ø Subluxation complex (vertebral) of **head** region   **CC** **H5**
         CC Excl: PDX collection 913

    M99.11 Subluxation complex (vertebral) of **cervical** region   **CC** **H5**
         CC Excl: PDX collection 913

    M99.12 Subluxation complex (vertebral) of **thoracic** region

    M99.13 Subluxation complex (vertebral) of **lumbar** region

    M99.14 Subluxation complex (vertebral) of **sacral** region

    M99.15 Subluxation complex (vertebral) of **pelvic** region

    M99.16 Subluxation complex (vertebral) of **lower extremity**

    M99.17 Subluxation complex (vertebral) of **upper extremity**

    M99.18 Subluxation complex (vertebral) of **rib cage**   **CC** **H5**
         CC Excl: PDX collection 914

    M99.19 Subluxation complex (vertebral) of **abdomen and other** regions

✓5ᵗʰ M99.2 Subluxation stenosis of neural canal

    M99.2Ø Subluxation stenosis of neural canal of **head** region

    M99.21 Subluxation stenosis of neural canal of **cervical** region

    M99.22 Subluxation stenosis of neural canal of **thoracic** region

    M99.23 Subluxation stenosis of neural canal of **lumbar** region

    M99.24 Subluxation stenosis of neural canal of **sacral** region

    M99.25 Subluxation stenosis of neural canal of **pelvic** region

    M99.26 Subluxation stenosis of neural canal of **lower extremity**

    M99.27 Subluxation stenosis of neural canal of **upper extremity**

    M99.28 Subluxation stenosis of neural canal of **rib cage**

    M99.29 Subluxation stenosis of neural canal of **abdomen and other** regions

✓5ᵗʰ M99.3 Osseous stenosis of neural canal

    M99.3Ø Osseous stenosis of neural canal of **head** region

    M99.31 Osseous stenosis of neural canal of **cervical** region

    M99.32 Osseous stenosis of neural canal of **thoracic** region

    M99.33 Osseous stenosis of neural canal of **lumbar** region

    M99.34 Osseous stenosis of neural canal of **sacral** region

    M99.35 Osseous stenosis of neural canal of **pelvic** region

    M99.36 Osseous stenosis of neural canal of **lower extremity**

    M99.37 Osseous stenosis of neural canal of **upper extremity**

    M99.38 Osseous stenosis of neural canal of **rib cage**

    M99.39 Osseous stenosis of neural canal of **abdomen and other** regions

✓5ᵗʰ M99.4 Connective tissue stenosis of neural canal

    M99.4Ø Connective tissue stenosis of neural canal of **head** region

    M99.41 Connective tissue stenosis of neural canal of **cervical** region

    M99.42 Connective tissue stenosis of neural canal of **thoracic** region

    M99.43 Connective tissue stenosis of neural canal of **lumbar** region

    M99.44 Connective tissue stenosis of neural canal of **sacral** region

    M99.45 Connective tissue stenosis of neural canal of **pelvic** region

    M99.46 Connective tissue stenosis of neural canal of **lower extremity**

    M99.47 Connective tissue stenosis of neural canal of **upper extremity**

    M99.48 Connective tissue stenosis of neural canal of **rib cage**

    M99.49 Connective tissue stenosis of neural canal of **abdomen and other** regions

✓5ᵗʰ M99.5 Intervertebral disc stenosis of neural canal

    M99.5Ø Intervertebral disc stenosis of neural canal of **head** region

    M99.51 Intervertebral disc stenosis of neural canal of **cervical** region

    M99.52 Intervertebral disc stenosis of neural canal of **thoracic** region

    M99.53 Intervertebral disc stenosis of neural canal of **lumbar** region

    M99.54 Intervertebral disc stenosis of neural canal of **sacral** region

    M99.55 Intervertebral disc stenosis of neural canal of **pelvic** region

    M99.56 Intervertebral disc stenosis of neural canal of **lower extremity**

    M99.57 Intervertebral disc stenosis of neural canal of **upper extremity**

    M99.58 Intervertebral disc stenosis of neural canal of **rib cage**

    M99.59 Intervertebral disc stenosis of neural canal of **abdomen and other** regions

✓5ᵗʰ M99.6 Osseous and subluxation stenosis of intervertebral foramina

    M99.6Ø Osseous and subluxation stenosis of intervertebral foramina of **head** region

    M99.61 Osseous and subluxation stenosis of intervertebral foramina of **cervical** region

    M99.62 Osseous and subluxation stenosis of intervertebral foramina of **thoracic** region

    M99.63 Osseous and subluxation stenosis of intervertebral foramina of **lumbar** region

    M99.64 Osseous and subluxation stenosis of intervertebral foramina of **sacral** region

    M99.65 Osseous and subluxation stenosis of intervertebral foramina of **pelvic** region

    M99.66 Osseous and subluxation stenosis of intervertebral foramina of **lower extremity**

    M99.67 Osseous and subluxation stenosis of intervertebral foramina of **upper extremity**

    M99.68 Osseous and subluxation stenosis of intervertebral foramina of **rib cage**

    M99.69 Osseous and subluxation stenosis of intervertebral foramina of **abdomen and other** regions

✓5ᵗʰ M99.7 Connective tissue and disc stenosis of intervertebral foramina

    M99.7Ø Connective tissue and disc stenosis of intervertebral foramina of **head** region

    M99.71 Connective tissue and disc stenosis of intervertebral foramina of **cervical** region

    M99.72 Connective tissue and disc stenosis of intervertebral foramina of **thoracic** region

    M99.73 Connective tissue and disc stenosis of intervertebral foramina of **lumbar** region

    M99.74 Connective tissue and disc stenosis of intervertebral foramina of **sacral** region

    M99.75 Connective tissue and disc stenosis of intervertebral foramina of **pelvic** region

    M99.76 Connective tissue and disc stenosis of intervertebral foramina of **lower extremity**

    M99.77 Connective tissue and disc stenosis of intervertebral foramina of **upper extremity**

    M99.78 Connective tissue and disc stenosis of intervertebral foramina of **rib cage**

    M99.79 Connective tissue and disc stenosis of intervertebral foramina of **abdomen and other** regions

✓5ᵗʰ M99.8 Other biomechanical lesions

    M99.8Ø Other biomechanical lesions of **head** region

Chapter 13. Diseases of the Musculoskeletal System and Connective Tissue

M99–M99.8Ø

✔ Additional Character Required   **✓x7ᵗʰ** Placeholder   <u>Unacceptable PDx</u>   Questionable PDx   Manifestation   <u>Unspecified Dx</u>   **H1**-**H14** HAC   **HCC** CMS-HCC Dx   **HIV** HIV Dx

ICD-10-CM 2020

851

M99.81   Other biomechanical lesions of cervical region
M99.82   Other biomechanical lesions of thoracic region
M99.83   Other biomechanical lesions of lumbar region
M99.84   Other biomechanical lesions of sacral region
M99.85   Other biomechanical lesions of pelvic region
M99.86   Other biomechanical lesions of lower extremity
M99.87   Other biomechanical lesions of upper extremity
M99.88   Other biomechanical lesions of rib cage
M99.89   Other biomechanical lesions of abdomen and other regions

M99.9   Biomechanical lesion, unspecified

N Newborn: 0   P Pediatric: 0-17   M Maternity: 9-64   A Adult: 15-124   MCC Major Complication/Comorbidity   CC Complication/Comorbidity   SW Severe Wound Dx

852   ICD-10-CM 2020

Chapter 14. Diseases of Genitourinary System (NØØ–N99)

Chapter-specific Guidelines with Coding Examples

The chapter-specific guidelines from the ICD-10-CM Official Guidelines for Coding and Reporting have been provided below. Along with these guidelines are coding examples, contained in the shaded boxes, that have been developed to help illustrate the coding and/or sequencing guidance found in these guidelines.

a. Chronic kidney disease

1) Stages of chronic kidney disease (CKD)

The ICD-10-CM classifies CKD based on severity. The severity of CKD is designated by stages 1-5. Stage 2, code N18.2, equates to mild CKD; stage 3, code N18.3, equates to moderate CKD; and stage 4, code N18.4, equates to severe CKD. Code N18.6, End stage renal disease (ESRD), is assigned when the provider has documented end-stage renal disease (ESRD).

If both a stage of CKD and ESRD are documented, assign code N18.6 only.

Stage 5 chronic kidney disease with ESRD requiring chronic dialysis

N18.6	**End stage renal disease**
Z99.2	**Dependence on renal dialysis**

Explanation: The diagnostic statement indicates the patient has chronic kidney disease, documented both as stage 5 and as ESRD requiring chronic dialysis. Code N18.6 End stage renal disease (ESRD), is assigned when the provider has documented end-stage-renal disease (ESRD). If both a stage of CKD and ESRD are documented, assign code N18.6 only.

---

2) Chronic kidney disease and kidney transplant status

Patients who have undergone kidney transplant may still have some form of chronic kidney disease (CKD) because the kidney transplant may not fully restore kidney function. Therefore, the presence of CKD alone does not constitute a transplant complication. Assign the appropriate N18 code for the patient's stage of CKD and code Z94.Ø, Kidney transplant status. If a transplant complication such as failure or rejection or other transplant complication is documented, see section I.C.19.g for information on coding complications of a kidney transplant. If the documentation is unclear as to whether the patient has a complication of the transplant, query the provider.

Patient with residual chronic kidney disease stage 1 after kidney transplant

N18.1	**Chronic kidney disease, stage 1**
Z94.Ø	**Kidney transplant status**

Explanation: Patients who have undergone kidney transplant may still have some form of chronic kidney disease (CKD) because the kidney transplant may not fully restore kidney function. The presence of CKD alone does not constitute a transplant complication. Assign the appropriate N18 code for the patient's stage of CKD and code Z94.Ø Kidney transplant status.

---

3) Chronic kidney disease with other conditions

Patients with CKD may also suffer from other serious conditions, most commonly diabetes mellitus and hypertension. The sequencing of the CKD code in relationship to codes for other contributing conditions is based on the conventions in the Tabular List.

See I.C.9. Hypertensive chronic kidney disease.

See I.C.19. Chronic kidney disease and kidney transplant complications.

Type 1 diabetic chronic kidney disease, stage 2

E1Ø.22	**Type 1 diabetes mellitus with diabetic chronic kidney disease**
N18.2	**Chronic kidney disease, stage 2 (mild)**

Explanation: Patients with CKD may also suffer from other serious conditions such as diabetes mellitus. The sequencing of the CKD code in relationship to codes for other contributing conditions is based on the conventions in the Tabular List. Diabetic CKD code E1Ø.22 includes an instructional note to "Use additional code to identify stage of chronic kidney disease (N18.1–N18.6)," thus providing sequencing direction.

Chapter 14. Diseases of the Genitourinary System

Chapter 14. Diseases of the Genitourinary System (N00-N99)

EXCLUDES 2   *certain conditions originating in the perinatal period (P04-P96)*
certain infectious and parasitic diseases (A00-B99)
complications of pregnancy, childbirth and the puerperium (O00-O9A)
congenital malformations, deformations and chromosomal abnormalities (Q00-Q99)
endocrine, nutritional and metabolic diseases (E00-E88)
injury, poisoning and certain other consequences of external causes (S00-T88)
neoplasms (C00-D49)
symptoms, signs and abnormal clinical and laboratory findings, not elsewhere classified (R00-R94)

This chapter contains the following blocks:

N00-N08   Glomerular diseases
N10-N16   Renal tubulo-interstitial diseases
N17-N19   Acute kidney failure and chronic kidney disease
N20-N23   Urolithiasis
N25-N29   Other disorders of kidney and ureter
N30-N39   Other diseases of the urinary system
N40-N53   Diseases of male genital organs
N60-N65   Disorders of breast
N70-N77   Inflammatory diseases of female pelvic organs
N80-N98   Noninflammatory disorders of female genital tract
N99   Intraoperative and postprocedural complications and disorders of genitourinary system, not elsewhere classified

Glomerular diseases (N00-N08)

Code also any associated kidney failure (N17-N19).

EXCLUDES 1   *hypertensive chronic kidney disease (I12.-)*

DEF: Glomeruli: Clusters of microscopic blood vessels located within the kidneys containing small pores through which waste products are filtered from the blood and urine is formed.

DEF: Glomerulonephritis: Disease of the kidney with diffuse inflammation of the capillary loops of the glomeruli.

√4ᵗʰ **N00**   **Acute nephritic syndrome**

    INCLUDES   acute glomerular disease
                   acute glomerulonephritis
                   acute nephritis
    EXCLUDES 1   *acute tubulo-interstitial nephritis (N10)*
                      nephritic syndrome NOS (N05.-)

CC Excl: For MCC codes in category N00, unless otherwise noted: PDX collection 915

N00.0   **Acute nephritic syndrome with minor glomerular abnormality**   **MCC**
       Acute nephritic syndrome with minimal change lesion

N00.1   **Acute nephritic syndrome with focal and segmental glomerular lesions**   **MCC**
       Acute nephritic syndrome with focal and segmental hyalinosis
       Acute nephritic syndrome with focal and segmental sclerosis
       Acute nephritic syndrome with focal glomerulonephritis

N00.2   **Acute nephritic syndrome with diffuse membranous glomerulonephritis**   **MCC**

N00.3   **Acute nephritic syndrome with diffuse mesangial proliferative glomerulonephritis**   **MCC**

N00.4   **Acute nephritic syndrome with diffuse endocapillary proliferative glomerulonephritis**   **MCC**

N00.5   **Acute nephritic syndrome with diffuse mesangiocapillary glomerulonephritis**   **MCC**
       Acute nephritic syndrome with membranoproliferative glomerulonephritis, types 1 and 3, or NOS

N00.6   **Acute nephritic syndrome with dense deposit disease**   **MCC**
       Acute nephritic syndrome with membranoproliferative glomerulonephritis, type 2

N00.7   **Acute nephritic syndrome with diffuse crescentic glomerulonephritis**   **MCC**
       Acute nephritic syndrome with extracapillary glomerulonephritis

N00.8   **Acute nephritic syndrome with other morphologic changes**   **MCC**
       Acute nephritic syndrome with proliferative glomerulonephritis NOS
       CC Excl: PDX collection 916

N00.9   **Acute nephritic syndrome with unspecified morphologic changes**   **MCC**

√4ᵗʰ **N01**   **Rapidly progressive nephritic syndrome**

    INCLUDES   rapidly progressive glomerular disease
                   rapidly progressive glomerulonephritis
                   rapidly progressive nephritis
    EXCLUDES 1   *nephritic syndrome NOS (N05.-)*

CC Excl: For MCC codes in category N01: PDX collection 915

N01.0   **Rapidly progressive nephritic syndrome with minor glomerular abnormality**   **MCC**
       Rapidly progressive nephritic syndrome with minimal change lesion

N01.1   **Rapidly progressive nephritic syndrome with focal and segmental glomerular lesions**   **MCC**
       Rapidly progressive nephritic syndrome with focal and segmental hyalinosis
       Rapidly progressive nephritic syndrome with focal and segmental sclerosis
       Rapidly progressive nephritic syndrome with focal glomerulonephritis

N01.2   **Rapidly progressive nephritic syndrome with diffuse membranous glomerulonephritis**   **MCC**

N01.3   **Rapidly progressive nephritic syndrome with diffuse mesangial proliferative glomerulonephritis**   **MCC**

N01.4   **Rapidly progressive nephritic syndrome with diffuse endocapillary proliferative glomerulonephritis**   **MCC**

N01.5   **Rapidly progressive nephritic syndrome with diffuse mesangiocapillary glomerulonephritis**   **MCC**
       Rapidly progressive nephritic syndrome with membranoproliferative glomerulonephritis, types 1 and 3, or NOS

N01.6   **Rapidly progressive nephritic syndrome with dense deposit disease**   **MCC**
       Rapidly progressive nephritic syndrome with membranoproliferative glomerulonephritis, type 2

N01.7   **Rapidly progressive nephritic syndrome with diffuse crescentic glomerulonephritis**   **MCC**
       Rapidly progressive nephritic syndrome with extracapillary glomerulonephritis

N01.8   **Rapidly progressive nephritic syndrome with other morphologic changes**   **MCC**
       Rapidly progressive nephritic syndrome with proliferative glomerulonephritis NOS

N01.9   **Rapidly progressive nephritic syndrome with unspecified morphologic changes**   **MCC**

√4ᵗʰ **N02**   **Recurrent and persistent hematuria**

    EXCLUDES 1   *acute cystitis with hematuria (N30.01)*
                     hematuria NOS (R31.9)
                     hematuria not associated with specified morphologic lesions (R31.-)

CC Excl: For CC codes in category N02, unless otherwise noted: PDX collection 917

N02.0   **Recurrent and persistent hematuria with minor glomerular abnormality**   **CC**
       Recurrent and persistent hematuria with minimal change lesion

N02.1   **Recurrent and persistent hematuria with focal and segmental glomerular lesions**   **CC**
       Recurrent and persistent hematuria with focal and segmental hyalinosis
       Recurrent and persistent hematuria with focal and segmental sclerosis
       Recurrent and persistent hematuria with focal glomerulonephritis

N02.2   **Recurrent and persistent hematuria with diffuse membranous glomerulonephritis**   **CC**

N02.3   **Recurrent and persistent hematuria with diffuse mesangial proliferative glomerulonephritis**   **CC**

N02.4   **Recurrent and persistent hematuria with diffuse endocapillary proliferative glomerulonephritis**   **CC**

N02.5   **Recurrent and persistent hematuria with diffuse mesangiocapillary glomerulonephritis**   **CC**
       Recurrent and persistent hematuria with membranoproliferative glomerulonephritis, types 1 and 3, or NOS

N Newborn: 0   **P** Pediatric: 0-17   **M** Maternity: 9-64   **A** Adult: 15-124   **MCC** Major Complication/Comorbidity   **CC** Complication/Comorbidity   **SW** Severe Wound Dx

854   ICD-10-CM 2020

N02.6 **Recurrent and persistent hematuria with dense deposit disease** `CC`

Recurrent and persistent hematuria with membranoproliferative glomerulonephritis, type 2

N02.7 **Recurrent and persistent hematuria with diffuse crescentic glomerulonephritis** `CC`

Recurrent and persistent hematuria with extracapillary glomerulonephritis

N02.8 **Recurrent and persistent hematuria with other morphologic changes** `CC`

Recurrent and persistent hematuria with proliferative glomerulonephritis NOS

CC Excl: PDX collection 915

N02.9 **Recurrent and persistent hematuria with unspecified morphologic changes** `CC`

AHA: 2017,2Q,5

CC Excl: PDX collection 915

✓4ᵗʰ **N03** **Chronic nephritic syndrome**

INCLUDES   chronic glomerular disease
        chronic glomerulonephritis
        chronic nephritis

EXCLUDES 1   *chronic tubulo-interstitial nephritis (N11.-)*
        diffuse sclerosing glomerulonephritis (N05.8-)
        nephritic syndrome NOS (N05.-)

DEF: Slow, progressive type of nephritis characterized by inflammation of the capillary loops in the glomeruli of the kidney, which leads to renal failure.

CC Excl: For CC codes in category N03: PDX collection 918

N03.0 **Chronic nephritic syndrome with minor glomerular abnormality** `CC`

Chronic nephritic syndrome with minimal change lesion

N03.1 **Chronic nephritic syndrome with focal and segmental glomerular lesions** `CC`

Chronic nephritic syndrome with focal and segmental hyalinosis
Chronic nephritic syndrome with focal and segmental sclerosis
Chronic nephritic syndrome with focal glomerulonephritis

N03.2 **Chronic nephritic syndrome with diffuse membranous glomerulonephritis** `CC`

N03.3 **Chronic nephritic syndrome with diffuse mesangial proliferative glomerulonephritis** `CC`

N03.4 **Chronic nephritic syndrome with diffuse endocapillary proliferative glomerulonephritis** `CC`

N03.5 **Chronic nephritic syndrome with diffuse mesangiocapillary glomerulonephritis** `CC`

Chronic nephritic syndrome with membranoproliferative glomerulonephritis, types 1 and 3, or NOS

N03.6 **Chronic nephritic syndrome with dense deposit disease** `CC`

Chronic nephritic syndrome with membranoproliferative glomerulonephritis, type 2

N03.7 **Chronic nephritic syndrome with diffuse crescentic glomerulonephritis** `CC`

Chronic nephritic syndrome with extracapillary glomerulonephritis

N03.8 **Chronic nephritic syndrome with other morphologic changes** `CC`

Chronic nephritic syndrome with proliferative glomerulonephritis NOS

N03.9 **Chronic nephritic syndrome with unspecified morphologic changes** `CC`

✓4ᵗʰ **N04** **Nephrotic syndrome**

INCLUDES   congenital nephrotic syndrome
        lipoid nephrosis

CC Excl: For CC codes in category N04, unless otherwise noted: PDX collection 917

N04.0 **Nephrotic syndrome with minor glomerular abnormality** `CC`

Nephrotic syndrome with minimal change lesion

N04.1 **Nephrotic syndrome with focal and segmental glomerular lesions** `CC`

Nephrotic syndrome with focal and segmental hyalinosis
Nephrotic syndrome with focal and segmental sclerosis
Nephrotic syndrome with focal glomerulonephritis

N04.2 **Nephrotic syndrome with diffuse membranous glomerulonephritis** `CC`

N04.3 **Nephrotic syndrome with diffuse mesangial proliferative glomerulonephritis** `CC`

N04.4 **Nephrotic syndrome with diffuse endocapillary proliferative glomerulonephritis** `CC`

N04.5 **Nephrotic syndrome with diffuse mesangiocapillary glomerulonephritis** `CC`

Nephrotic syndrome with membranoproliferative glomerulonephritis, types 1 and 3, or NOS

N04.6 **Nephrotic syndrome with dense deposit disease** `CC`

Nephrotic syndrome with membranoproliferative glomerulonephritis, type 2

N04.7 **Nephrotic syndrome with diffuse crescentic glomerulonephritis** `CC`

Nephrotic syndrome with extracapillary glomerulonephritis

CC Excl: PDX collection 915

N04.8 **Nephrotic syndrome with other morphologic changes** `CC`

Nephrotic syndrome with proliferative glomerulonephritis NOS

CC Excl: PDX collection 915

N04.9 **Nephrotic syndrome with unspecified morphologic changes** `CC`

CC Excl: PDX collection 915

✓4ᵗʰ **N05** **Unspecified nephritic syndrome**

INCLUDES   glomerular disease NOS
        glomerulonephritis NOS
        nephritis NOS
        nephropathy NOS and renal disease NOS with morphological lesion specified in .0-.8

EXCLUDES 1   *nephropathy NOS with no stated morphological lesion (N28.9)*
        renal disease NOS with no stated morphological lesion (N28.9)
        tubulo-interstitial nephritis NOS (N12)

CC Excl: For CC codes in category N05: PDX collection 918

N05.0 **Unspecified nephritic syndrome with minor glomerular abnormality**

Unspecified nephritic syndrome with minimal change lesion

N05.1 **Unspecified nephritic syndrome with focal and segmental glomerular lesions**

Unspecified nephritic syndrome with focal and segmental hyalinosis
Unspecified nephritic syndrome with focal and segmental sclerosis
Unspecified nephritic syndrome with focal glomerulonephritis

N05.2 **Unspecified nephritic syndrome with diffuse membranous glomerulonephritis** `CC`

N05.3 **Unspecified nephritic syndrome with diffuse mesangial proliferative glomerulonephritis** `CC`

N05.4 **Unspecified nephritic syndrome with diffuse endocapillary proliferative glomerulonephritis** `CC`

N05.5 **Unspecified nephritic syndrome with diffuse mesangiocapillary glomerulonephritis** `CC`

Unspecified nephritic syndrome with membranoproliferative glomerulonephritis, types 1 and 3, or NOS

N05.6 **Unspecified nephritic syndrome with dense deposit disease**

Unspecified nephritic syndrome with membranoproliferative glomerulonephritis, type 2

N05.7 **Unspecified nephritic syndrome with diffuse crescentic glomerulonephritis**

Unspecified nephritic syndrome with extracapillary glomerulonephritis

N05.8 **Unspecified nephritic syndrome with other morphologic changes**

Unspecified nephritic syndrome with proliferative glomerulonephritis NOS

N05.9 **Unspecified nephritic syndrome with unspecified morphologic changes**

✓4ᵗʰ **N06** **Isolated proteinuria with specified morphological lesion**

EXCLUDES 1   *proteinuria not associated with specific morphologic lesions (R80.0)*

CC Excl: For CC codes in category N06: PDX collection 918

N06.0 **Isolated proteinuria with minor glomerular abnormality**

Isolated proteinuria with minimal change lesion

N06.1 **Isolated proteinuria with focal and segmental glomerular lesions**

Isolated proteinuria with focal and segmental hyalinosis
Isolated proteinuria with focal and segmental sclerosis
Isolated proteinuria with focal glomerulonephritis

N06.2 **Isolated proteinuria with diffuse membranous glomerulonephritis** `CC`

✓ Additional Character Required   ✓x7ᵗʰ Placeholder   Unacceptable PDx   Questionable PDx   Manifestation   Unspecified Dx   H1 - H14 HAC   HCC CMS-HCC Dx   HIV HIV Dx

ICD-10-CM 2020

N02.6–N06.2

855

N06.3 Isolated proteinuria with diffuse mesangial proliferative glomerulonephritis `CC`

N06.4 Isolated proteinuria with diffuse endocapillary proliferative glomerulonephritis `CC`

N06.5 Isolated proteinuria with diffuse mesangiocapillary glomerulonephritis `CC`
Isolated proteinuria with membranoproliferative glomerulonephritis, types 1 and 3, or NOS

N06.6 Isolated proteinuria with dense deposit disease
Isolated proteinuria with membranoproliferative glomerulonephritis, type 2

N06.7 Isolated proteinuria with diffuse crescentic glomerulonephritis
Isolated proteinuria with extracapillary glomerulonephritis

N06.8 Isolated proteinuria with other morphologic lesion
Isolated proteinuria with proliferative glomerulonephritis NOS

N06.9 Isolated proteinuria with unspecified morphologic lesion

✓4ᵗʰ N07 Hereditary nephropathy, not elsewhere classified
EXCLUDES 2 Alport's syndrome (Q87.81-)
hereditary amyloid nephropathy (E85.-)
nail patella syndrome (Q87.2)
non-neuropathic heredofamilial amyloidosis (E85.-)

CC Excl: For CC codes in category N07: PDX collection 918

N07.0 Hereditary nephropathy, not elsewhere classified with minor glomerular abnormality
Hereditary nephropathy, not elsewhere classified with minimal change lesion

N07.1 Hereditary nephropathy, not elsewhere classified with focal and segmental glomerular lesions
Hereditary nephropathy, not elsewhere classified with focal and segmental hyalinosis
Hereditary nephropathy, not elsewhere classified with focal and segmental sclerosis
Hereditary nephropathy, not elsewhere classified with focal glomerulonephritis

N07.2 Hereditary nephropathy, not elsewhere classified with diffuse membranous glomerulonephritis `CC`

N07.3 Hereditary nephropathy, not elsewhere classified with diffuse mesangial proliferative glomerulonephritis `CC`

N07.4 Hereditary nephropathy, not elsewhere classified with diffuse endocapillary proliferative glomerulonephritis `CC`

N07.5 Hereditary nephropathy, not elsewhere classified with diffuse mesangiocapillary glomerulonephritis `CC`
Hereditary nephropathy, not elsewhere classified with membranoproliferative glomerulonephritis, types 1 and 3, or NOS

N07.6 Hereditary nephropathy, not elsewhere classified with dense deposit disease
Hereditary nephropathy, not elsewhere classified with membranoproliferative glomerulonephritis, type 2

N07.7 Hereditary nephropathy, not elsewhere classified with diffuse crescentic glomerulonephritis
Hereditary nephropathy, not elsewhere classified with extracapillary glomerulonephritis

N07.8 Hereditary nephropathy, not elsewhere classified with other morphologic lesions
Hereditary nephropathy, not elsewhere classified with proliferative glomerulonephritis NOS

N07.9 Hereditary nephropathy, not elsewhere classified with unspecified morphologic lesions

N08 *Glomerular disorders in diseases classified elsewhere*
Glomerulonephritis
Nephritis
Nephropathy
Code first underlying disease, such as:
amyloidosis (E85.-)
congenital syphilis (A50.5)
cryoglobulinemia (D89.1)
disseminated intravascular coagulation (D65)
gout (M1A.-, M10.-)
microscopic polyangiitis (M31.7)
multiple myeloma (C90.0-)
sepsis (A40.0-A41.9)
sickle-cell disease (D57.0-D57.8)
EXCLUDES 1 *glomerulonephritis, nephritis and nephropathy (in):*
antiglomerular basement membrane disease (M31.0)
diabetes (E08-E13 with .21)
gonococcal (A54.21)
Goodpasture's syndrome (M31.0)
hemolytic-uremic syndrome (D59.3)
lupus (M32.14)
mumps (B26.83)
syphilis (A52.75)
systemic lupus erythematosus (M32.14)
Wegener's granulomatosis (M31.31)
pyelonephritis in diseases classified elsewhere (N16)
renal tubulo-interstitial disorders classified elsewhere (N16)

Renal tubulo-interstitial diseases (N10-N16)

INCLUDES pyelonephritis
EXCLUDES 1 *pyeloureteritis cystica (N28.85)*

N10 Acute pyelonephritis `H6`
Acute infectious interstitial nephritis
Acute pyelitis
Acute tubulo-interstitial nephritis
Hemoglobin nephrosis
Myoglobin nephrosis
Use additional code (B95-B97), to identify infectious agent

✓4ᵗʰ N11 Chronic tubulo-interstitial nephritis
INCLUDES chronic infectious interstitial nephritis
chronic pyelitis
chronic pyelonephritis
Use additional code (B95-B97), to identify infectious agent

N11.0 Nonobstructive reflux-associated chronic pyelonephritis
Pyelonephritis (chronic) associated with (vesicoureteral) reflux
EXCLUDES 1 *vesicoureteral reflux NOS (N13.70)*

N11.1 Chronic obstructive pyelonephritis `CC`
Pyelonephritis (chronic) associated with anomaly of pelviureteric junction
Pyelonephritis (chronic) associated with anomaly of pyeloureteric junction
Pyelonephritis (chronic) associated with crossing of vessel
Pyelonephritis (chronic) associated with kinking of ureter
Pyelonephritis (chronic) associated with obstruction of ureter
Pyelonephritis (chronic) associated with stricture of pelviureteric junction
Pyelonephritis (chronic) associated with stricture of ureter
EXCLUDES 1 *calculous pyelonephritis (N20.9)*
obstructive uropathy (N13.-)
CC Excl: PDX collection 920

N11.8 Other chronic tubulo-interstitial nephritis `CC`
Nonobstructive chronic pyelonephritis NOS
CC Excl: PDX collection 921

N11.9 Chronic tubulo-interstitial nephritis, unspecified `CC` `H6`
Chronic interstitial nephritis NOS
Chronic pyelitis NOS
Chronic pyelonephritis NOS
CC Excl: PDX collection 922

N Newborn: 0   **P** Pediatric: 0-17   **M** Maternity: 9-64   **A** Adult: 15-124   **MCC** Major Complication/Comorbidity   **CC** Complication/Comorbidity   **SW** Severe Wound Dx

856   ICD-10-CM 2020

N12   Tubulo-interstitial nephritis, not specified as acute or chronic   CC H6
Interstitial nephritis NOS
Pyelitis NOS
Pyelonephritis NOS
EXCLUDES 1   *calculous pyelonephritis (N20.9)*
CC Excl: PDX collection 922

✓4th N13   Obstructive and reflux uropathy
EXCLUDES 2   *calculus of kidney and ureter without hydronephrosis (N20.-)*
congenital obstructive defects of renal pelvis and ureter (Q62.0-Q62.3)
hydronephrosis with ureteropelvic junction obstruction (Q62.11)
obstructive pyelonephritis (N11.1)
DEF: Hydronephrosis: Distension of the kidney caused by an accumulation of urine that cannot flow out due to an obstruction that may be caused by conditions such as kidney stones or vesicoureteral reflux.
CC Excl: For CC codes in category N13, unless otherwise noted: PDX collection 922

N13.0   Hydronephrosis with ureteropelvic junction obstruction   CC
Hydronephrosis due to acquired occlusion of ureteropelvic junction
EXCLUDES 2   *hydronephrosis with ureteropelvic junction obstruction due to calculus (N13.2)*
AHA: 2016,4Q,43

Hydronephrosis/UPJ Obstruction

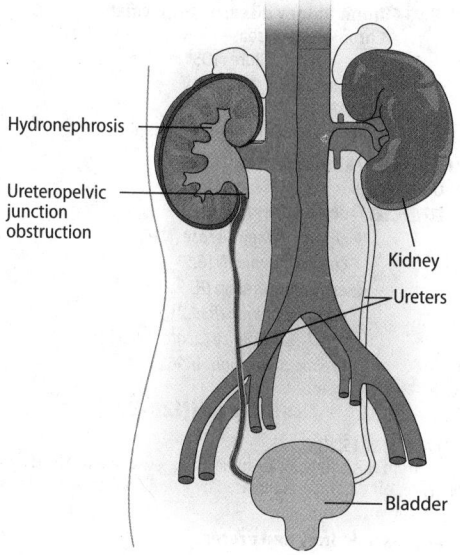

Hydronephrosis
Ureteropelvic junction obstruction
Kidney
Ureters
Bladder

N13.1   Hydronephrosis with ureteral stricture, not elsewhere classified   CC
EXCLUDES 1   *hydronephrosis with ureteral stricture with infection (N13.6)*

N13.2   Hydronephrosis with renal and ureteral calculous obstruction   CC
EXCLUDES 1   *hydronephrosis with renal and ureteral calculous obstruction with infection (N13.6)*

✓5th N13.3   Other and unspecified hydronephrosis
EXCLUDES 1   *hydronephrosis with infection (N13.6)*
N13.30   Unspecified hydronephrosis   CC
N13.39   Other hydronephrosis   CC

N13.4   Hydroureter   CC
EXCLUDES 1   *congenital hydroureter (Q62.3-)*
hydroureter with infection (N13.6)
vesicoureteral-reflux with hydroureter (N13.73-)
DEF: Abnormal enlargement or distension of the ureter with water or urine caused by an obstruction.
CC Excl: PDX collection 923

N13.5   Crossing vessel and stricture of ureter without hydronephrosis
Kinking and stricture of ureter without hydronephrosis
EXCLUDES 1   *crossing vessel and stricture of ureter without hydronephrosis with infection (N13.6)*

N13.6   Pyonephrosis   CC H6
Conditions in N13.0-N13.5 with infection
Obstructive uropathy with infection
Use additional code (B95-B97), to identify infectious agent
AHA: 2018,2Q,21

✓5th N13.7   Vesicoureteral-reflux
EXCLUDES 1   *reflux-associated pyelonephritis (N11.0)*
DEF: Urine passage from the bladder flows backward up into the ureter and kidneys that can lead to bacterial infection and an increase in hydrostatic pressure, causing kidney damage.

Vesicoureteral Reflux

Kidneys
Ureters
Bladder

Normal flow of urine   Urine flowing the wrong way (VUR)

N13.70   Vesicoureteral-reflux, unspecified
Vesicoureteral-reflux NOS
N13.71   Vesicoureteral-reflux without reflux nephropathy
✓6th N13.72   Vesicoureteral-reflux with reflux nephropathy without hydroureter
N13.721   Vesicoureteral-reflux with reflux nephropathy without hydroureter, unilateral
N13.722   Vesicoureteral-reflux with reflux nephropathy without hydroureter, bilateral
N13.729   Vesicoureteral-reflux with reflux nephropathy without hydroureter, unspecified
✓6th N13.73   Vesicoureteral-reflux with reflux nephropathy with hydroureter
N13.731   Vesicoureteral-reflux with reflux nephropathy with hydroureter, unilateral
N13.732   Vesicoureteral-reflux with reflux nephropathy with hydroureter, bilateral
N13.739   Vesicoureteral-reflux with reflux nephropathy with hydroureter, unspecified

N13.8   Other obstructive and reflux uropathy   CC
Urinary tract obstruction due to specified cause
Code first, if applicable, any causal condition, such as:
enlarged prostate (N40.1)
CC Excl: PDX collection 920

N13.9   Obstructive and reflux uropathy, unspecified
Urinary tract obstruction NOS

✓4th N14   Drug- and heavy-metal-induced tubulo-interstitial and tubular conditions
Code first poisoning due to drug or toxin, if applicable (T36-T65 with fifth or sixth character 1-4 or 6)
Use additional code for adverse effect, if applicable, to identify drug (T36-T50 with fifth or sixth character 5)
N14.0   Analgesic nephropathy
N14.1   Nephropathy induced by other drugs, medicaments and biological substances
N14.2   Nephropathy induced by unspecified drug, medicament or biological substance
N14.3   Nephropathy induced by heavy metals
N14.4   Toxic nephropathy, not elsewhere classified

✓4th N15   Other renal tubulo-interstitial diseases
N15.0   Balkan nephropathy
Balkan endemic nephropathy

N15.1 Renal and perinephric abscess   `MCC` `H6`
     CC Excl: PDX collection 919

N15.8 Other specified renal tubulo-interstitial diseases

N15.9 Renal tubulo-interstitial disease, unspecified
     Infection of kidney NOS
     `EXCLUDES 1`   *urinary tract infection NOS (N39.0)*

N16 Renal tubulo-interstitial disorders in diseases classified elsewhere
     Pyelonephritis
     Tubulo-interstitial nephritis
     Code first underlying disease, such as:
       brucellosis (A23.0-A23.9)
       cryoglobulinemia (D89.1)
       glycogen storage disease (E74.0)
       leukemia (C91-C95)
       lymphoma (C81.0-C85.9, C96.0-C96.9)
       multiple myeloma (C90.0-)
       sepsis (A40.0-A41.9)
       Wilson's disease (E83.0)
     `EXCLUDES 1`   *diphtheritic pyelonephritis and tubulo-interstitial nephritis (A36.84)*
         pyelonephritis and tubulo-interstitial nephritis in candidiasis (B37.49)
         pyelonephritis and tubulo-interstitial nephritis in cystinosis (E72.04)
         pyelonephritis and tubulo-interstitial nephritis in salmonella infection (A02.25)
         pyelonephritis and tubulo-interstitial nephritis in sarcoidosis (D86.84)
         pyelonephritis and tubulo-interstitial nephritis in sicca syndrome [Sjogren's] (M35.04)
         pyelonephritis and tubulo-interstitial nephritis in systemic lupus erythematosus (M32.15)
         pyelonephritis and tubulo-interstitial nephritis in toxoplasmosis (B58.83)
         renal tubular degeneration in diabetes (E08-E13 with .29)
         syphilitic pyelonephritis and tubulo-interstitial nephritis (A52.75)

Acute kidney failure and chronic kidney disease (N17-N19)

     `EXCLUDES 2`   *congenital renal failure (P96.0)*
         drug- and heavy-metal-induced tubulo-interstitial and tubular conditions (N14.-)
         extrarenal uremia (R39.2)
         hemolytic-uremic syndrome (D59.3)
         hepatorenal syndrome (K76.7)
         postpartum hepatorenal syndrome (O90.4)
         posttraumatic renal failure (T79.5)
         prerenal uremia (R39.2)
         renal failure complicating abortion or ectopic or molar pregnancy (O00-O07, O08.4)
         renal failure following labor and delivery (O90.4)
         renal failure postprocedural (N99.0)

N17 Acute kidney failure   `4th`
     Code also associated underlying condition
     `EXCLUDES 1`   *posttraumatic renal failure (T79.5)*
     AHA: 2019,2Q,7; 2019,1Q,12; 2013,4Q,124
     CC Excl: For CC/MCC codes in category N17, unless otherwise noted: PDX collection 924

N17.0 Acute kidney failure with tubular necrosis   `MCC` `HCC`
     Acute tubular necrosis
     Renal tubular necrosis
     Tubular necrosis NOS

N17.1 Acute kidney failure with acute cortical necrosis   `MCC` `HCC`
     Acute cortical necrosis
     Cortical necrosis NOS
     Renal cortical necrosis

N17.2 Acute kidney failure with medullary necrosis   `MCC` `HCC`
     Medullary [papillary] necrosis NOS
     Acute medullary [papillary] necrosis
     Renal medullary [papillary] necrosis

N17.8 Other acute kidney failure   `CC` `HCC`
     CC Excl: PDX collection 925

N17.9 Acute kidney failure, unspecified   `CC` `HCC`
     Acute kidney injury (nontraumatic)
     `EXCLUDES 2`   *traumatic kidney injury (S37.0-)*

N18 Chronic kidney disease (CKD)   `4th`
     Code first any associated:
       diabetic chronic kidney disease (E08.22, E09.22, E10.22, E11.22, E13.22)
       hypertensive chronic kidney disease (I12.-, I13.-)
     Use additional code to identify kidney transplant status, if applicable, (Z94.0)
     AHA: 2013,1Q,24

N18.1 Chronic kidney disease, stage 1

N18.2 Chronic kidney disease, stage 2 (mild)

N18.3 Chronic kidney disease, stage 3 (moderate)   `HCC`

N18.4 Chronic kidney disease, stage 4 (severe)   `HCC`

N18.5 Chronic kidney disease, stage 5   `HCC`
     `EXCLUDES 1`   *chronic kidney disease, stage 5 requiring chronic dialysis (N18.6)*
     DEF: End-stage renal disease (ESRD) with a GFR value of 15 ml/min or less not yet requiring chronic dialysis.
     TIP: When both ESRD and CKD 5 are documented, code only for ESRD.

N18.6 End stage renal disease   `CC` `HCC`
     Chronic kidney disease requiring chronic dialysis
     Use additional code to identify dialysis status (Z99.2)
     AHA: 2016,3Q,22; 2016,1Q,12; 2013,4Q,124-125
     TIP: When both ESRD and CKD 5 are documented, code only for ESRD.

N18.9 Chronic kidney disease, unspecified
     Chronic renal disease
     Chronic renal failure NOS
     Chronic renal insufficiency
     Chronic uremia NOS
     Diffuse sclerosing glomerulonephritis NOS

N19 Unspecified kidney failure
     Uremia NOS
     `EXCLUDES 1`   *acute kidney failure (N17.-)*
         chronic kidney disease (N18.-)
         chronic uremia (N18.9)
         extrarenal uremia (R39.2)
         prerenal uremia (R39.2)
         renal insufficiency (acute) (N28.9)
         uremia of newborn (P96.0)

Urolithiasis (N20-N23)

AHA: 2017,1Q,5; 2015,2Q,8
TIP: Codes from this code block can be assigned based on the diagnosis listed in a radiology report when authenticated by a radiologist and available at the time of code assignment.

N20 Calculus of kidney and ureter   `4th`
     Calculous pyelonephritis
     `EXCLUDES 1`   *nephrocalcinosis (E83.5)*
         that with hydronephrosis (N13.2)

N20.0 Calculus of kidney
     Nephrolithiasis NOS
     Renal calculus
     Renal stone
     Staghorn calculus
     Stone in kidney

N20.1 Calculus of ureter   `CC`
     Ureteric stone
     AHA: 2016,3Q,22
     CC Excl: PDX collection 928

N20.2 Calculus of kidney with calculus of ureter   `CC`
     CC Excl: PDX collection 928

N20.9 Urinary calculus, unspecified

N21 Calculus of lower urinary tract   `4th`
     `INCLUDES`   calculus of lower urinary tract with cystitis and urethritis

N21.0 Calculus in bladder
     Calculus in diverticulum of bladder
     Urinary bladder stone
     `EXCLUDES 2`   *staghorn calculus (N20.0)*

N21.1 Calculus in urethra
     `EXCLUDES 2`   *calculus of prostate (N42.0)*

N21.8 Other lower urinary tract calculus

`N` Newborn: 0   `P` Pediatric: 0-17   `M` Maternity: 9-64   `A` Adult: 15-124   `MCC` Major Complication/Comorbidity   `CC` Complication/Comorbidity   `SW` Severe Wound Dx

N21.9   **Calculus of lower urinary tract, unspecified**
> *EXCLUDES 1*   calculus of urinary tract NOS (N20.9)

N22   *Calculus of urinary tract in diseases classified elsewhere*
> Code first underlying disease, such as:
> gout (M1A.-, M10.-)
> schistosomiasis (B65.0-B65.9)

N23   **Unspecified renal colic**

Other disorders of kidney and ureter (N25-N29)

> *EXCLUDES 2*   disorders of kidney and ureter with urolithiasis (N20-N23)

✓4ᵗʰ **N25**   **Disorders resulting from impaired renal tubular function**

     N25.0   **Renal osteodystrophy**
> Azotemic osteodystrophy
> Phosphate-losing tubular disorders
> Renal rickets
> Renal short stature
> *EXCLUDES 2*   metabolic disorders classifiable to E70-E88
> **DEF:** Various bone diseases occurring when kidney function is impaired or fails. Abnormal levels of phosphorous and calcium can lead to osteomalacia, osteoporosis, or osteosclerosis.

     N25.1   **Nephrogenic diabetes insipidus**   `CC` `HCC`
> *EXCLUDES 1*   diabetes insipidus NOS (E23.2)
> **DEF:** Type of diabetes due to the inability of renal tubules to reabsorb water back into the body. It is not responsive to vasopressin (antidiuretic hormone) and it is characterized by excessive thirst and excessive urine production. It may develop into chronic renal insufficiency.
> **CC Excl:** PDX collection 929

✓5ᵗʰ   **N25.8**   **Other disorders resulting from impaired renal tubular function**

     N25.81   **Secondary hyperparathyroidism of renal origin**   `CC` `HCC`
> *EXCLUDES 1*   secondary hyperparathyroidism, non-renal (E21.1)
> *EXCLUDES 2*   metabolic disorders classifiable to E70-E88
> **DEF:** Parathyroid dysfunction caused by chronic renal failure. Phosphate clearance and vitamin D production is impaired resulting in lowered calcium blood levels and an excessive production of parathyroid hormone.
> **CC Excl:** PDX collection 930

     N25.89   **Other disorders resulting from impaired renal tubular function**
> Hypokalemic nephropathy
> Lightwood-Albright syndrome
> Renal tubular acidosis NOS

     N25.9   **Disorder resulting from impaired renal tubular function, unspecified**

✓4ᵗʰ **N26**   **Unspecified contracted kidney**
> *EXCLUDES 1*   contracted kidney due to hypertension (I12.-)
> diffuse sclerosing glomerulonephritis (N05.8.-)
> hypertensive nephrosclerosis (arteriolar) (arteriosclerotic) (I12.-)
> small kidney of unknown cause (N27.-)

     N26.1   **Atrophy of kidney (terminal)**

     N26.2   **Page kidney**

     N26.9   **Renal sclerosis, unspecified**

✓4ᵗʰ **N27**   **Small kidney of unknown cause**
> *INCLUDES*   oligonephronia

     N27.0   **Small kidney, unilateral**

     N27.1   **Small kidney, bilateral**

     N27.9   **Small kidney, unspecified**

✓4ᵗʰ **N28**   **Other disorders of kidney and ureter, not elsewhere classified**

     N28.0   **Ischemia and infarction of kidney**   `CC` `HCC`
> Renal artery embolism
> Renal artery obstruction
> Renal artery occlusion
> Renal artery thrombosis
> Renal infarct
> *EXCLUDES 1*   atherosclerosis of renal artery (extrarenal part) (I70.1)
> congenital stenosis of renal artery (Q27.1)
> Goldblatt's kidney (I70.1)
> **CC Excl:** PDX collection 931

     N28.1   **Cyst of kidney, acquired**
> Cyst (multiple) (solitary) of kidney (acquired)
> *EXCLUDES 1*   cystic kidney disease (congenital) (Q61.-)

✓5ᵗʰ   **N28.8**   **Other specified disorders of kidney and ureter**
> *EXCLUDES 1*   hydroureter (N13.4)
> ureteric stricture with hydronephrosis (N13.1)
> ureteric stricture without hydronephrosis (N13.5)
> **CC Excl:** For CC codes in subcategory N28.8: PDX collection 922

     N28.81   **Hypertrophy of kidney**

     N28.82   **Megaloureter**

     N28.83   **Nephroptosis**

     N28.84   **Pyelitis cystica**   `CC` `H6`

     N28.85   **Pyeloureteritis cystica**   `CC` `H6`

     N28.86   **Ureteritis cystica**   `CC` `H6`

     N28.89   **Other specified disorders of kidney and ureter**

     N28.9   **Disorder of kidney and ureter, unspecified**
> Nephropathy NOS
> Renal disease (acute) NOS
> Renal insufficiency (acute)
> *EXCLUDES 1*   chronic renal insufficiency (N18.9)
> unspecified nephritic syndrome (N05.-)
> **AHA:** 2016,1Q,13

N29   *Other disorders of kidney and ureter in diseases classified elsewhere*
> Code first underlying disease, such as:
> amyloidosis (E85.-)
> nephrocalcinosis (E83.5)
> schistosomiasis (B65.0-B65.9)
> *EXCLUDES 1*   disorders of kidney and ureter in:
>   cystinosis (E72.0)
>   gonorrhea (A54.21)
>   syphilis (A52.75)
>   tuberculosis (A18.11)

Other diseases of the urinary system (N30-N39)

> *EXCLUDES 1*   urinary infection (complicating):
> abortion or ectopic or molar pregnancy (O00-O07, O08.8)
> pregnancy, childbirth and the puerperium (O23.-, O75.3, O86.2-)

✓4ᵗʰ **N30**   **Cystitis**
> Use additional code to identify infectious agent (B95-B97)
> *EXCLUDES 1*   prostatocystitis (N41.3)
> **AHA:** 2017,1Q,6
> **DEF:** Inflammation of the urinary bladder. Symptoms include dysuria, frequency of urination, urgency, and hematuria.
> **CC Excl:** For CC codes in category N30: PDX collection 932

✓6ᵗʰ   **N30.0**   **Acute cystitis**
> *EXCLUDES 1*   irradiation cystitis (N30.4-)
> trigonitis (N30.3-)

     N30.00   **Acute cystitis** without hematuria   `H6`

     N30.01   **Acute cystitis** with hematuria   `H6`

✓5ᵗʰ   **N30.1**   **Interstitial cystitis (chronic)**

     N30.10   **Interstitial cystitis (chronic)** without hematuria

     N30.11   **Interstitial cystitis (chronic)** with hematuria

✓5ᵗʰ   **N30.2**   **Other** chronic cystitis

     N30.20   **Other chronic cystitis** without hematuria

     N30.21   **Other chronic cystitis** with hematuria

✓5ᵗʰ   **N30.3**   **Trigonitis**
> Urethrotrigonitis

     N30.30   **Trigonitis** without hematuria

     N30.31   **Trigonitis** with hematuria

✓5ᵗʰ   **N30.4**   **Irradiation** cystitis

     N30.40   **Irradiation cystitis** without hematuria   `CC`

     N30.41   **Irradiation cystitis** with hematuria   `CC`

✓5ᵗʰ   **N30.8**   **Other cystitis**
> Abscess of bladder

     N30.80   **Other cystitis** without hematuria

     N30.81   **Other cystitis** with hematuria

✓5ᵗʰ   **N30.9**   **Cystitis, unspecified**

     N30.90   **Cystitis, unspecified** without hematuria

     N30.91   **Cystitis, unspecified** with hematuria

✓4ᵗʰ N31 Neuromuscular dysfunction of bladder, not elsewhere classified

Use additional code to identify any associated urinary incontinence (N39.3-N39.4-)

EXCLUDES 1   cord bladder NOS (G95.89)

neurogenic bladder due to cauda equina syndrome (G83.4)

neuromuscular dysfunction due to spinal cord lesion (G95.89)

N31.0 Uninhibited neuropathic bladder, not elsewhere classified

N31.1 Reflex neuropathic bladder, not elsewhere classified

N31.2 Flaccid neuropathic bladder, not elsewhere classified

Atonic (motor) (sensory) neuropathic bladder

Autonomous neuropathic bladder

Nonreflex neuropathic bladder

N31.8 Other neuromuscular dysfunction of bladder

N31.9 Neuromuscular dysfunction of bladder, unspecified

Neurogenic bladder dysfunction NOS

✓4ᵗʰ N32 Other disorders of bladder

EXCLUDES 2   calculus of bladder (N21.0)

cystocele (N81.1-)

hernia or prolapse of bladder, female (N81.1-)

N32.0 Bladder-neck obstruction

Bladder-neck stenosis (acquired)

EXCLUDES 1   congenital bladder-neck obstruction (Q64.3-)

DEF: Bladder outlet and vesicourethral obstruction that occurs as a consequence of benign prostatic hypertrophy or prostatic cancer. It may also occur in either sex due to strictures, radiation, cystoscopy, catheterization, injury, infection, blood clots, bladder cancer, impaction, or other disease that compresses the bladder neck.

N32.1 Vesicointestinal fistula   CC

Vesicorectal fistula

CC Excl: PDX collection 933

N32.2 Vesical fistula, not elsewhere classified   CC

EXCLUDES 1   fistula between bladder and female genital tract (N82.0-N82.1)

CC Excl: PDX collection 933

N32.3 Diverticulum of bladder

EXCLUDES 1   congenital diverticulum of bladder (Q64.6)

diverticulitis of bladder (N30.8-)

✓5ᵗʰ N32.8 Other specified disorders of bladder

N32.81 Overactive bladder

Detrusor muscle hyperactivity

EXCLUDES 1   frequent urination due to specified bladder condition — code to condition

DEF: Sudden involuntary contractions of the muscular wall of the bladder that results in a sudden, strong urge to urinate.

N32.89 Other specified disorders of bladder

Bladder hemorrhage

Bladder hypertrophy

Calcified bladder

Contracted bladder

N32.9 Bladder disorder, unspecified

N33 Bladder disorders in diseases classified elsewhere

Code first underlying disease, such as:

schistosomiasis (B65.0-B65.9)

EXCLUDES 1   bladder disorder in syphilis (A52.76)

bladder disorder in tuberculosis (A18.12)

candidal cystitis (B37.41)

chlamydial cystitis (A56.01)

cystitis in gonorrhea (A54.01)

cystitis in neurogenic bladder (N31.-)

diphtheritic cystitis (A36.85)

neurogenic bladder (N31.-)

syphilitic cystitis (A52.76)

trichomonal cystitis (A59.03)

✓4ᵗʰ N34 Urethritis and urethral syndrome

Use additional code (B95-B97), to identify infectious agent

EXCLUDES 2   Reiter's disease (M02.3-)

urethritis in diseases with a predominantly sexual mode of transmission (A50-A64)

urethrotrigonitis (N30.3-)

AHA: 2017,1Q,6

N34.0 Urethral abscess   CC H6

Abscess (of) Cowper's gland

Abscess (of) Littré's gland

Abscess (of) urethral (gland)

Periurethral abscess

EXCLUDES 1   urethral caruncle (N36.2)

CC Excl: PDX collection 934

N34.1 Nonspecific urethritis

Nongonococcal urethritis

Nonvenereal urethritis

N34.2 Other urethritis

Meatitis, urethral

Postmenopausal urethritis

Ulcer of urethra (meatus)

Urethritis NOS

N34.3 Urethral syndrome, unspecified

✓4ᵗʰ N35 Urethral stricture

EXCLUDES 1   congenital urethral stricture (Q64.3-)

postprocedural urethral stricture (N99.1-)

AHA: 2018,4Q,21-22

✓5ᵗʰ N35.0 Post-traumatic urethral stricture

Urethral stricture due to injury

EXCLUDES 1   postprocedural urethral stricture (N99.1-)

✓6ᵗʰ N35.01 Post-traumatic urethral stricture, male

N35.010 Post-traumatic urethral stricture, male, meatal   ♂

N35.011 Post-traumatic bulbous urethral stricture   ♂

N35.012 Post-traumatic membranous urethral stricture   ♂

N35.013 Post-traumatic anterior urethral stricture   ♂

N35.014 Post-traumatic urethral stricture, male, unspecified   ♂

N35.016 Post-traumatic urethral stricture, male, overlapping sites   ♂

✓6ᵗʰ N35.02 Post-traumatic urethral stricture, female

N35.021 Urethral stricture due to childbirth   ♀

N35.028 Other post-traumatic urethral stricture, female   ♀

✓5ᵗʰ N35.1 Postinfective urethral stricture, not elsewhere classified

EXCLUDES 1   gonococcal urethral stricture (A54.01)

syphilitic urethral stricture (A52.76)

urethral stricture associated with schistosomiasis (B65.-, N29)

✓6ᵗʰ N35.11 Postinfective urethral stricture, not elsewhere classified, male

N35.111 Postinfective urethral stricture, not elsewhere classified, male, meatal   ♂

N35.112 Postinfective bulbous urethral stricture, not elsewhere classified, male   ♂

N35.113 Postinfective membranous urethral stricture, not elsewhere classified, male   ♂

N35.114 Postinfective anterior urethral stricture, not elsewhere classified, male   ♂

N35.116 Postinfective urethral stricture, not elsewhere classified, male, overlapping sites   ♂

N35.119 Postinfective urethral stricture, not elsewhere classified, male, unspecified   ♂

N Newborn: 0   P Pediatric: 0-17   M Maternity: 9-64   A Adult: 15-124   MCC Major Complication/Comorbidity   CC Complication/Comorbidity   SW Severe Wound Dx

860   ICD-10-CM 2020

N35.12   Postinfective urethral stricture, not elsewhere classified, female   ♀

✓5ᵗʰ **N35.8**   **Other urethral stricture**
> EXCLUDES 1   postprocedural urethral stricture (N99.1-)

    ✓6ᵗʰ **N35.81**   **Other urethral stricture, male**
> **N35.811**   Other urethral stricture, male, meatal   ♂
> **N35.812**   Other urethral bulbous stricture, male   ♂
> **N35.813**   Other membranous urethral stricture, male   ♂
> **N35.814**   Other anterior urethral stricture, male   ♂
> **N35.816**   Other urethral stricture, male, overlapping sites   ♂
> **N35.819**   Other urethral stricture, male, unspecified site   ♂

    N35.82   Other urethral stricture, female   ♀

✓5ᵗʰ **N35.9**   **Urethral stricture, unspecified**
    ✓6ᵗʰ **N35.91**   **Urethral stricture, unspecified, male**
> **N35.911**   Unspecified urethral stricture, male, meatal   ♂
> **N35.912**   Unspecified bulbous urethral stricture, male   ♂
> **N35.913**   Unspecified membranous urethral stricture, male   ♂
> **N35.914**   Unspecified anterior urethral stricture, male   ♂
> **N35.916**   Unspecified urethral stricture, male, overlapping sites   ♂
> **N35.919**   Unspecified urethral stricture, male, unspecified site   ♂
>> Pinhole meatus NOS
>> Urethral stricture NOS

    N35.92   Unspecified urethral stricture, female   ♀

▲

✓4ᵗʰ **N36**   **Other disorders of urethra**

N36.0   **Urethral fistula**   CC
> Urethroperineal fistula
> Urethrorectal fistula
> Urinary fistula NOS
> EXCLUDES 1   urethroscrotal fistula (N50.89)
>> urethrovaginal fistula (N82.1)
>> urethrovesicovaginal fistula (N82.1)
> **CC Excl:** PDX collection 935

N36.1   **Urethral diverticulum**
N36.2   **Urethral caruncle**
✓5ᵗʰ **N36.4**   **Urethral functional and muscular disorders**
> Use additional code to identify associated urinary stress incontinence (N39.3)

    N36.41   **Hypermobility of urethra**
    N36.42   **Intrinsic sphincter deficiency (ISD)**
    N36.43   **Combined hypermobility of urethra and intrinsic sphincter deficiency**
    N36.44   **Muscular disorders of urethra**
>> Bladder sphincter dyssynergy

N36.5   **Urethral false passage**
N36.8   **Other specified disorders of urethra**
> EXCLUDES 1   congenital urethrocele (Q64.7)
>> female urethrocele (N81.0)

N36.9   **Urethral disorder, unspecified**

N37   *Urethral disorders in diseases classified elsewhere*
> Code first underlying disease
> EXCLUDES 1   urethritis (in):
>> candidal infection (B37.41)
>> chlamydial (A56.01)
>> gonorrhea (A54.01)
>> syphilis (A52.76)
>> trichomonal infection (A59.03)
>> tuberculosis (A18.13)

✓4ᵗʰ **N39**   **Other disorders of urinary system**
> EXCLUDES 2   hematuria NOS (R31.-)
>> recurrent or persistent hematuria (N02.-)
>> recurrent or persistent hematuria with specified morphological lesion (N02.-)
>> proteinuria NOS (R80.-)

N39.0   **Urinary tract infection, site not specified**   CC H6
> Use additional code (B95-B97), to identify infectious agent
> EXCLUDES 1   candidiasis of urinary tract (B37.4-)
>> neonatal urinary tract infection (P39.3)
>> ▶pyuria (R82.81)◀
>> urinary tract infection of specified site, such as:
>> cystitis (N30.-)
>> urethritis (N34.-)
> **AHA:** 2018,2Q,21,22; 2018,1Q,16; 2017,1Q,6; 2012,4Q,94
> **CC Excl:** PDX collection 936

N39.3   **Stress incontinence (female) (male)**
> Code also any associated overactive bladder (N32.81)
> EXCLUDES 1   mixed incontinence (N39.46)

✓5ᵗʰ **N39.4**   **Other specified urinary incontinence**
> Code also any associated overactive bladder (N32.81)
> EXCLUDES 1   enuresis NOS (R32)
>> functional urinary incontinence (R39.81)
>> urinary incontinence associated with cognitive impairment (R39.81)
>> urinary incontinence NOS (R32)
>> urinary incontinence of nonorganic origin (F98.0)

    N39.41   **Urge incontinence**
> EXCLUDES 1   mixed incontinence (N39.46)

    N39.42   **Incontinence without sensory awareness**
>> Insensible (urinary) incontinence

    N39.43   **Post-void dribbling**
    N39.44   **Nocturnal enuresis**
    N39.45   **Continuous leakage**
    N39.46   **Mixed incontinence**
>> Urge and stress incontinence

    ✓6ᵗʰ **N39.49**   **Other specified urinary incontinence**
>> **AHA:** 2016,4Q,44
>> **N39.490**   **Overflow incontinence**
>> **N39.491**   **Coital incontinence**
>> **N39.492**   **Postural (urinary) incontinence**
>> **N39.498**   **Other specified urinary incontinence**
>>> Reflex incontinence
>>> Total incontinence

N39.8   **Other specified disorders of urinary system**
N39.9   **Disorder of urinary system, unspecified**

Diseases of male genital organs (N40-N53)

✓4ᵗʰ **N40**   **Benign prostatic hyperplasia**
> INCLUDES   adenofibromatous hypertrophy of prostate
>> benign hypertrophy of the prostate
>> benign prostatic hypertrophy
>> BPH
>> enlarged prostate
>> nodular prostate
>> polyp of prostate
> EXCLUDES 1   benign neoplasms of prostate (adenoma, benign) (fibroadenoma) (fibroma) (myoma) (D29.1)
> EXCLUDES 2   malignant neoplasm of prostate (C61)
> **DEF:** Enlargement of the prostate gland due to an abnormal proliferation of fibrostromal tissue in the paraurethral glands. This condition causes impingement of the urethra resulting in obstructed urinary flow.

N40.0   **Benign prostatic hyperplasia without lower urinary tract symptoms**   A ♂
> Enlarged prostate NOS
> Enlarged prostate without LUTS

Chapter 14. Diseases of the Genitourinary System

N40.1 **Benign prostatic hyperplasia with lower urinary tract symptoms**   A ♂

Enlarged prostate with LUTS

Use additional code for associated symptoms, when specified:
incomplete bladder emptying (R39.14)
nocturia (R35.1)
straining on urination (R39.16)
urinary frequency (R35.0)
urinary hesitancy (R39.11)
urinary incontinence (N39.4-)
urinary obstruction (N13.8)
urinary retention (R33.8)
urinary urgency (R39.15)
weak urinary stream (R39.12)
AHA: 2018,4Q,55

N40.2 **Nodular prostate without lower urinary tract symptoms**   A ♂

Nodular prostate without LUTS

N40.3 **Nodular prostate with lower urinary tract symptoms**   A ♂

Use additional code for associated symptoms, when specified:
incomplete bladder emptying (R39.14)
nocturia (R35.1)
straining on urination (R39.16)
urinary frequency (R35.0)
urinary hesitancy (R39.11)
urinary incontinence (N39.4-)
urinary obstruction (N13.8)
urinary retention (R33.8)
urinary urgency (R39.15)
weak urinary stream (R39.12)

✓4ᵗʰ **N41** **Inflammatory diseases of prostate**

Use additional code (B95-B97), to identify infectious agent

N41.0 **Acute prostatitis**   A ♂

N41.1 **Chronic prostatitis**   A ♂

N41.2 **Abscess of prostate**   CC A ♂

CC Excl: PDX collection 937

N41.3 **Prostatocystitis**   A ♂

N41.4 **Granulomatous prostatitis**   A ♂

N41.8 **Other inflammatory diseases of prostate**   A ♂

N41.9 **Inflammatory disease of prostate, unspecified**   A ♂

Prostatitis NOS

✓4ᵗʰ **N42** **Other and unspecified disorders of prostate**

N42.0 **Calculus of prostate**   A ♂

Prostatic stone
DEF: Formation of a small, solid stone often composed of calcium carbonate or calcium phosphate in the prostate gland.

N42.1 **Congestion and hemorrhage of prostate**   A ♂

EXCLUDES 1   enlarged prostate (N40.-)
hematuria (R31.-)
hyperplasia of prostate (N40.-)
inflammatory diseases of prostate (N41.-)

✓5ᵗʰ **N42.3** **Dysplasia of prostate**

AHA: 2016,4Q,44

N42.30 **Unspecified dysplasia of prostate**   ♂

N42.31 **Prostatic intraepithelial neoplasia**   ♂

PIN
Prostatic intraepithelial neoplasia I (PIN I)
Prostatic intraepithelial neoplasia II (PIN II)
EXCLUDES 1   prostatic intraepithelial neoplasia III (PIN III) (D07.5)
DEF: Abnormality of shape and size of the intraepithelial tissues of the prostate. It is a premalignant condition characterized by stalks and absence of a basilar cell layer.

N42.32 **Atypical small acinar proliferation of prostate**   ♂

N42.39 **Other dysplasia of prostate**   ♂

✓5ᵗʰ **N42.8** **Other specified disorders of prostate**

N42.81 **Prostatodynia syndrome**   A ♂

Painful prostate syndrome

N42.82 **Prostatosis syndrome**   A ♂

N42.83 **Cyst of prostate**   A ♂

N42.89 **Other specified disorders of prostate**   A ♂

N42.9 **Disorder of prostate, unspecified**   A ♂

✓4ᵗʰ **N43** **Hydrocele and spermatocele**

INCLUDES   hydrocele of spermatic cord, testis or tunica vaginalis
EXCLUDES 1   congenital hydrocele (P83.5)
DEF: Hydrocele: Serous fluid that collects in the tunica vaginalis of the scrotum along the spermatic cord in males.

N43.0 **Encysted hydrocele**   ♂

N43.1 **Infected hydrocele**   CC ♂

Use additional code (B95-B97), to identify infectious agent
CC Excl: PDX collection 938

N43.2 **Other hydrocele**   ♂

Hydrocele

Testicle
Scrotum

Normal   Noncommunicating hydrocele   Communicating hydrocele   Hydrocele of the cord

N43.3 **Hydrocele, unspecified**   ♂

✓5ᵗʰ **N43.4** **Spermatocele of epididymis**

Spermatic cyst
DEF: Spermatocele: Noncancerous accumulation of fluid and dead sperm cells normally located at the head of the epididymis that exhibits itself as a hard, smooth scrotal mass and do not normally require treatment unless they become enlarged or cause pain.

N43.40 **Spermatocele of epididymis, unspecified**   ♂

N43.41 **Spermatocele of epididymis, single**   ♂

N43.42 **Spermatocele of epididymis, multiple**   ♂

✓4ᵗʰ **N44** **Noninflammatory disorders of testis**

CC Excl: For CC codes in category N44: PDX collection 939

✓5ᵗʰ **N44.0** **Torsion of testis**

N44.00 **Torsion of testis, unspecified**   CC ♂

N44.01 **Extravaginal torsion of spermatic cord**   CC ♂

DEF: Torsion of the spermatic cord just below the tunica vaginalis attachments.

N44.02 **Intravaginal torsion of spermatic cord**   CC ♂

Torsion of spermatic cord NOS

N44.03 **Torsion of appendix testis**   CC ♂

N44.04 **Torsion of appendix epididymis**   CC ♂

N44.1 **Cyst of tunica albuginea testis**   ♂

N44.2 **Benign cyst of testis**   ♂

N44.8 **Other noninflammatory disorders of the testis**   ♂

✓4ᵗʰ **N45** **Orchitis and epididymitis**

Use additional code (B95-B97), to identify infectious agent

N45.1 **Epididymitis**   ♂

N45.2 **Orchitis**   ♂

N45.3 **Epididymo-orchitis**   ♂

N45.4 **Abscess of epididymis or testis**   CC ♂

CC Excl: PDX collection 940

N Newborn: 0   P Pediatric: 0-17   M Maternity: 9-64   A Adult: 15-124   MCC Major Complication/Comorbidity   CC Complication/Comorbidity   SW Severe Wound Dx

N40.1–N45.4

862   ICD-10-CM 2020

✓4ᵗʰ N46 Male infertility

    EXCLUDES 1   vasectomy status (Z98.52)

    ✓5ᵗʰ N46.Ø Azoospermia

        Absolute male infertility

        Male infertility due to germinal (cell) aplasia

        Male infertility due to spermatogenic arrest (complete)

        DEF: Failure of the development of sperm or the absence of sperm in semen.

        N46.Ø1 Organic azoospermia   A ♂

           Azoospermia NOS

        ✓6ᵗʰ N46.Ø2 Azoospermia due to extratesticular causes

           Code also associated cause

           N46.Ø21 Azoospermia due to drug therapy   A ♂

           N46.Ø22 Azoospermia due to infection   A ♂

           N46.Ø23 Azoospermia due to obstruction of efferent ducts   A ♂

           N46.Ø24 Azoospermia due to radiation   A ♂

           N46.Ø25 Azoospermia due to systemic disease   A ♂

           N46.Ø29 Azoospermia due to other extratesticular causes   A ♂

    ✓5ᵗʰ N46.1 Oligospermia

        Male infertility due to germinal cell desquamation

        Male infertility due to hypospermatogenesis

        Male infertility due to incomplete spermatogenic arrest

        DEF: Insufficient production of sperm in semen.

        N46.11 Organic oligospermia   A ♂

           Oligospermia NOS

        ✓6ᵗʰ N46.12 Oligospermia due to extratesticular causes

           Code also associated cause

           N46.121 Oligospermia due to drug therapy   A ♂

           N46.122 Oligospermia due to infection   A ♂

           N46.123 Oligospermia due to obstruction of efferent ducts   A ♂

           N46.124 Oligospermia due to radiation   A ♂

           N46.125 Oligospermia due to systemic disease   A ♂

           N46.129 Oligospermia due to other extratesticular causes   A ♂

    N46.8 Other male infertility   A ♂

    N46.9 Male infertility, unspecified   A ♂

✓4ᵗʰ N47 Disorders of prepuce

    N47.Ø Adherent prepuce, newborn   N ♂

    N47.1 Phimosis   ♂

        DEF: Condition in which the foreskin is contracted and cannot be drawn back behind the glans penis.

    N47.2 Paraphimosis   ♂

    N47.3 Deficient foreskin   ♂

    N47.4 Benign cyst of prepuce   ♂

    N47.5 Adhesions of prepuce and glans penis   ♂

    N47.6 Balanoposthitis   ♂

        Use additional code (B95-B97), to identify infectious agent

        EXCLUDES 1   balanitis (N48.1)

    N47.7 Other inflammatory diseases of prepuce   ♂

        Use additional code (B95-B97), to identify infectious agent

    N47.8 Other disorders of prepuce   ♂

✓4ᵗʰ N48 Other disorders of penis

    N48.Ø Leukoplakia of penis   ♂

        Balanitis xerotica obliterans

        Kraurosis of penis

        Lichen sclerosus of external male genital organs

        EXCLUDES 1   carcinoma in situ of penis (DØ7.4)

    N48.1 Balanitis   ♂

        Use additional code (B95-B97), to identify infectious agent

        EXCLUDES 1   amebic balanitis (AØ6.8)

                 balanitis xerotica obliterans (N48.Ø)

                 candidal balanitis (B37.42)

                 gonococcal balanitis (A54.23)

                 herpesviral [herpes simplex] balanitis (A6Ø.Ø1)

        DEF: Inflammation of the glans penis, most often affecting uncircumcised males.

    ✓5ᵗʰ N48.2 Other inflammatory disorders of penis

        Use additional code (B95-B97), to identify infectious agent

        EXCLUDES 1   balanitis (N48.1)

                 balanitis xerotica obliterans (N48.Ø)

                 balanoposthitis (N47.6)

        N48.21 Abscess of corpus cavernosum and penis   ♂

        N48.22 Cellulitis of corpus cavernosum and penis   ♂

        N48.29 Other inflammatory disorders of penis   ♂

    ✓5ᵗʰ N48.3 Priapism

        Painful erection

        Code first underlying cause

        CC Excl: For CC codes in subcategory N48.3: PDX collection 941

        N48.3Ø Priapism, unspecified   CC ♂

        N48.31 Priapism due to trauma   CC ♂

        N48.32 Priapism due to disease classified elsewhere   CC ♂

        N48.33 Priapism, drug-induced   CC ♂

        N48.39 Other priapism   CC ♂

    N48.5 Ulcer of penis   ♂

    N48.6 Induration penis plastica   ♂

        Peyronie's disease

        Plastic induration of penis

    ✓5ᵗʰ N48.8 Other specified disorders of penis

        N48.81 Thrombosis of superficial vein of penis   ♂

        N48.82 Acquired torsion of penis   ♂

           Acquired torsion of penis NOS

           EXCLUDES 1   congenital torsion of penis (Q55.63)

        N48.83 Acquired buried penis   ♂

           EXCLUDES 1   congenital hidden penis (Q55.64)

        N48.89 Other specified disorders of penis   ♂

    N48.9 Disorder of penis, unspecified   ♂

✓4ᵗʰ N49 Inflammatory disorders of male genital organs, not elsewhere classified

    Use additional code (B95-B97), to identify infectious agent

    EXCLUDES 1   inflammation of penis (N48.1, N48.2-)

              orchitis and epididymitis (N45.-)

    N49.Ø Inflammatory disorders of seminal vesicle   ♂

        Vesiculitis NOS

    N49.1 Inflammatory disorders of spermatic cord, tunica vaginalis and vas deferens   ♂

        Vasitis

    N49.2 Inflammatory disorders of scrotum   ♂

    N49.3 Fournier gangrene   ♂

    N49.8 Inflammatory disorders of other specified male genital organs   ♂

        Inflammation of multiple sites in male genital organs

    N49.9 Inflammatory disorder of unspecified male genital organ   ♂

        Abscess of unspecified male genital organ

        Boil of unspecified male genital organ

        Carbuncle of unspecified male genital organ

        Cellulitis of unspecified male genital organ

✓4ᵗʰ N5Ø Other and unspecified disorders of male genital organs

    EXCLUDES 2   torsion of testis (N44.Ø-)

    N5Ø.Ø Atrophy of testis   ♂

✔ Additional Character Required   ✓x7ᵗʰ Placeholder   Unacceptable PDx   Questionable PDx   Manifestation   Unspecified Dx   H1-H1V HAC   HCC CMS-HCC Dx   HIV HIV Dx

ICD-10-CM 2020

863

Chapter 14. Diseases of the Genitourinary System

N50.1   **Vascular disorders of male genital organs** ♂

Hematocele, NOS, of male genital organs

Hemorrhage of male genital organs

Thrombosis of male genital organs

N50.3   **Cyst of epididymis** ♂

☑5ᵗʰ **N50.8**   **Other specified disorders of male genital organs**

AHA: 2016,4Q,45

☑6ᵗʰ **N50.81**   **Testicular pain**

N50.811   **Right testicular pain** ♂

N50.812   **Left testicular pain** ♂

N50.819   **Testicular pain, unspecified** ♂

N50.82   **Scrotal pain** ♂

N50.89   **Other specified disorders of the male genital organs** ♂

Atrophy of scrotum, seminal vesicle, spermatic cord, tunica vaginalis and vas deferens

Chylocele, tunica vaginalis (nonfilarial) NOS

Edema of scrotum, seminal vesicle, spermatic cord, tunica vaginalis and vas deferens

Hypertrophy of scrotum, seminal vesicle, spermatic cord, tunica vaginalis and vas deferens

Stricture of spermatic cord, tunica vaginalis, and vas deferens

Ulcer of scrotum, seminal vesicle, spermatic cord, testis, tunica vaginalis and vas deferens

Urethroscrotal fistula

N50.9   **Disorder of male genital organs, unspecified** ♂

N51   **Disorders of male genital organs in diseases classified elsewhere** ♂

Code first underlying disease, such as:

filariasis (B74.0-B74.9)

EXCLUDES 1   *amebic balanitis (A06.8)*

candidal balanitis (B37.42)

gonococcal balanitis (A54.23)

gonococcal prostatitis (A54.22)

herpesviral [herpes simplex] balanitis (A60.01)

trichomonal prostatitis (A59.02)

tuberculous prostatitis (A18.14)

☑4ᵗʰ **N52**   **Male erectile dysfunction**

EXCLUDES 1   *psychogenic impotence (F52.21)*

☑5ᵗʰ **N52.0**   **Vasculogenic erectile dysfunction**

N52.01   **Erectile dysfunction due to arterial insufficiency** Ⓐ ♂

N52.02   **Corporo-venous occlusive erectile dysfunction** Ⓐ ♂

N52.03   **Combined arterial insufficiency and corporo-venous occlusive erectile dysfunction** Ⓐ ♂

N52.1   **Erectile dysfunction due to diseases classified elsewhere** Ⓐ ♂

Code first underlying disease

N52.2   **Drug-induced erectile dysfunction** Ⓐ ♂

☑5ᵗʰ **N52.3**   **Postprocedural erectile dysfunction**

AHA: 2016,4Q,45

N52.31   **Erectile dysfunction following radical prostatectomy** Ⓐ ♂

N52.32   **Erectile dysfunction following radical cystectomy** Ⓐ ♂

N52.33   **Erectile dysfunction following urethral surgery** Ⓐ ♂

N52.34   **Erectile dysfunction following simple prostatectomy** Ⓐ ♂

N52.35   **Erectile dysfunction following radiation therapy** Ⓐ ♂

N52.36   **Erectile dysfunction following interstitial seed therapy** Ⓐ ♂

N52.37   **Erectile dysfunction following prostate ablative therapy** Ⓐ ♂

Erectile dysfunction following cryotherapy

Erectile dysfunction following other prostate ablative therapies

Erectile dysfunction following ultrasound ablative therapies

N52.39   **Other and unspecified postprocedural erectile dysfunction** Ⓐ ♂

N52.8   **Other male erectile dysfunction** Ⓐ ♂

N52.9   **Male erectile dysfunction, unspecified** Ⓐ ♂

Impotence NOS

☑4ᵗʰ **N53**   **Other male sexual dysfunction**

EXCLUDES 1   *psychogenic sexual dysfunction (F52.-)*

☑5ᵗʰ **N53.1**   **Ejaculatory dysfunction**

EXCLUDES 1   *premature ejaculation (F52.4)*

N53.11   **Retarded ejaculation** ♂

N53.12   **Painful ejaculation** ♂

N53.13   **Anejaculatory orgasm** ♂

N53.14   **Retrograde ejaculation** ♂

DEF: Form of male sexual dysfunction in which the semen enters the bladder instead of going out through the urethra during ejaculation.

N53.19   **Other ejaculatory dysfunction** ♂

Ejaculatory dysfunction NOS

N53.8   **Other male sexual dysfunction** ♂

N53.9   **Unspecified male sexual dysfunction** ♂

Disorders of breast (N60-N65)

EXCLUDES 1   *disorders of breast associated with childbirth (O91-O92)*

☑4ᵗʰ **N60**   **Benign mammary dysplasia**

INCLUDES   fibrocystic mastopathy

☑5ᵗʰ **N60.0**   **Solitary cyst of breast**

Cyst of breast

N60.01   **Solitary cyst of right breast**

N60.02   **Solitary cyst of left breast**

N60.09   **Solitary cyst of unspecified breast**

☑5ᵗʰ **N60.1**   **Diffuse cystic mastopathy**

Cystic breast

Fibrocystic disease of breast

EXCLUDES 1   *diffuse cystic mastopathy with epithelial proliferation (N60.3-)*

N60.11   **Diffuse cystic mastopathy of right breast** Ⓐ

N60.12   **Diffuse cystic mastopathy of left breast** Ⓐ

N60.19   **Diffuse cystic mastopathy of unspecified breast** Ⓐ

☑5ᵗʰ **N60.2**   **Fibroadenosis of breast**

Adenofibrosis of breast

EXCLUDES 2   *fibroadenoma of breast (D24.-)*

N60.21   **Fibroadenosis of right breast**

N60.22   **Fibroadenosis of left breast**

N60.29   **Fibroadenosis of unspecified breast**

☑5ᵗʰ **N60.3**   **Fibrosclerosis of breast**

Cystic mastopathy with epithelial proliferation

N60.31   **Fibrosclerosis of right breast**

N60.32   **Fibrosclerosis of left breast**

N60.39   **Fibrosclerosis of unspecified breast**

☑5ᵗʰ **N60.4**   **Mammary duct ectasia**

N60.41   **Mammary duct ectasia of right breast**

N60.42   **Mammary duct ectasia of left breast**

N60.49   **Mammary duct ectasia of unspecified breast**

☑5ᵗʰ **N60.8**   **Other benign mammary dysplasias**

N60.81   **Other benign mammary dysplasias of right breast**

N60.82   **Other benign mammary dysplasias of left breast**

N60.89   **Other benign mammary dysplasias of unspecified breast**

☑5ᵗʰ **N60.9**   **Unspecified benign mammary dysplasia**

N60.91   **Unspecified benign mammary dysplasia of right breast**

N60.92   **Unspecified benign mammary dysplasia of left breast**

N60.99   **Unspecified benign mammary dysplasia of unspecified breast**

Ⓝ Newborn: 0   Ⓟ Pediatric: 0-17   Ⓜ Maternity: 9-64   Ⓐ Adult: 15-124   MCC Major Complication/Comorbidity   CC Complication/Comorbidity   SW Severe Wound Dx

N50.1–N60.99

864   ICD-10-CM 2020

Chapter 14. Diseases of the Genitourinary System

☑4ᵗʰ **N61 Inflammatory disorders of breast**

    EXCLUDES 1   *inflammatory carcinoma of breast (C50.9)*

         inflammatory disorder of breast associated with childbirth (O91.-)

         neonatal infective mastitis (P39.0)

         thrombophlebitis of breast [Mondor's disease] (I80.8)

  N61.0 Mastitis without abscess

     Infective mastitis (acute) (nonpuerperal) (subacute)

     Mastitis (acute) (nonpuerperal) (subacute) NOS

     Cellulitis (acute) (nonpuerperal) (subacute) of breast NOS

     Cellulitis (acute) (nonpuerperal) (subacute) of nipple NOS

  N61.1 Abscess of the breast and nipple

     Abscess (acute) (chronic) (nonpuerperal) of areola

     Abscess (acute) (chronic) (nonpuerperal) of breast

     Carbuncle of breast

     Mastitis with abscess

N62 Hypertrophy of breast

  Gynecomastia

  Hypertrophy of breast NOS

  Massive pubertal hypertrophy of breast

    EXCLUDES 1   *breast engorgement of newborn (P83.4)*

         disproportion of reconstructed breast (N65.1)

☑4ᵗʰ **N63 Unspecified lump in breast**

  Nodule(s) NOS in breast

  AHA: 2017,4Q,19

  N63.0 Unspecified lump in unspecified breast

☑5ᵗʰ **N63.1 Unspecified lump in the right breast**

    N63.10 Unspecified lump in the right breast, unspecified quadrant

    N63.11 Unspecified lump in the right breast, upper outer quadrant

    N63.12 Unspecified lump in the right breast, upper inner quadrant

    N63.13 Unspecified lump in the right breast, lower outer quadrant

    N63.14 Unspecified lump in the right breast, lower inner quadrant

    N63.15 Unspecified lump in the right breast, overlapping quadrants

☑5ᵗʰ **N63.2 Unspecified lump in the left breast**

    N63.20 Unspecified lump in the left breast, unspecified quadrant

    N63.21 Unspecified lump in the left breast, upper outer quadrant

    N63.22 Unspecified lump in the left breast, upper inner quadrant

    N63.23 Unspecified lump in the left breast, lower outer quadrant

    N63.24 Unspecified lump in the left breast, lower inner quadrant

    N63.25 Unspecified lump in the left breast, overlapping quadrants

☑5ᵗʰ **N63.3 Unspecified lump in axillary tail**

    N63.31 Unspecified lump in axillary tail of the right breast

    N63.32 Unspecified lump in axillary tail of the left breast

☑5ᵗʰ **N63.4 Unspecified lump in breast, subareolar**

    N63.41 Unspecified lump in right breast, subareolar

    N63.42 Unspecified lump in left breast, subareolar

☑4ᵗʰ **N64 Other disorders of breast**

    EXCLUDES 2   *mechanical complication of breast prosthesis and implant (T85.4-)*

  N64.0 Fissure and fistula of nipple

  N64.1 Fat necrosis of breast

     Fat necrosis (segmental) of breast

     Code first breast necrosis due to breast graft (T85.898)

  N64.2 Atrophy of breast

  N64.3 Galactorrhea not associated with childbirth

  N64.4 Mastodynia

☑5ᵗʰ **N64.5 Other signs and symptoms in breast**

    EXCLUDES 2   *abnormal findings on diagnostic imaging of breast (R92.-)*

    N64.51 Induration of breast

    N64.52 Nipple discharge

       EXCLUDES 1   *abnormal findings in nipple discharge (R89.-)*

    N64.53 Retraction of nipple

    N64.59 Other signs and symptoms in breast

☑5ᵗʰ **N64.8 Other specified disorders of breast**

    N64.81 Ptosis of breast   🅰

       EXCLUDES 1   *ptosis of native breast in relation to reconstructed breast (N65.1)*

    N64.82 Hypoplasia of breast   🅰

     Micromastia

       EXCLUDES 1   *congenital absence of breast (Q83.0)*

           hypoplasia of native breast in relation to reconstructed breast (N65.1)

    N64.89 Other specified disorders of breast

     Galactocele

     Subinvolution of breast (postlactational)

     AHA: 2019,1Q,32; 2018,1Q,3

  N64.9 Disorder of breast, unspecified

☑4ᵗʰ **N65 Deformity and disproportion of reconstructed breast**

  N65.0 Deformity of reconstructed breast   🅰

     Contour irregularity in reconstructed breast

     Excess tissue in reconstructed breast

     Misshapen reconstructed breast

  N65.1 Disproportion of reconstructed breast   🅰

     Breast asymmetry between native breast and reconstructed breast

     Disproportion between native breast and reconstructed breast

Inflammatory diseases of female pelvic organs (N70-N77)

  EXCLUDES 1   *inflammatory diseases of female pelvic organs complicating: abortion or ectopic or molar pregnancy (O00-O07, O08.0)*

         pregnancy, childbirth and the puerperium (O23.-, O75.3, O85, O86.-)

CC Excl: For CC/MCC codes in categories N70-N77, unless otherwise noted: PDX collection 942

☑4ᵗʰ **N70 Salpingitis and oophoritis**

    INCLUDES   abscess (of) fallopian tube

       abscess (of) ovary

       pyosalpinx

       salpingo-oophoritis

       tubo-ovarian abscess

       tubo-ovarian inflammatory disease

    Use additional code (B95-B97), to identify infectious agent

    EXCLUDES 1   *gonococcal infection (A54.24)*

         tuberculous infection (A18.17)

☑5ᵗʰ **N70.0 Acute salpingitis and oophoritis**

    N70.01 Acute salpingitis   CC ♀

    N70.02 Acute oophoritis   CC ♀

    N70.03 Acute salpingitis and oophoritis   CC ♀

☑5ᵗʰ **N70.1 Chronic salpingitis and oophoritis**

     Hydrosalpinx

    N70.11 Chronic salpingitis   ♀

    N70.12 Chronic oophoritis   ♀

    N70.13 Chronic salpingitis and oophoritis   ♀

☑5ᵗʰ **N70.9 Salpingitis and oophoritis, unspecified**

    N70.91 Salpingitis, unspecified   ♀

    N70.92 Oophoritis, unspecified   ♀

    N70.93 Salpingitis and oophoritis, unspecified   ♀

☑4ᵗʰ **N71 Inflammatory disease of uterus, except cervix**

    INCLUDES   endo (myo) metritis

       metritis

       myometritis

       pyometra

       uterine abscess

    Use additional code (B95-B97), to identify infectious agent

    EXCLUDES 1   *hyperplastic endometritis (N85.0-)*

         infection of uterus following delivery (O85, O86.-)

  N71.0 Acute inflammatory disease of uterus   CC ♀

    CC Excl: PDX collection 943

  N71.1 Chronic inflammatory disease of uterus   ♀

  N71.9 Inflammatory disease of uterus, unspecified   ♀

☑ Additional Character Required   ☑x7ᵗʰ Placeholder   Unacceptable PDx   Questionable PDx   Manifestation   Unspecified Dx   H1-H14 HAC   HCC CMS-HCC Dx   HIV HIV Dx

N72 Inflammatory disease of cervix uteri ♀

INCLUDES   cervicitis (with or without erosion or ectropion)
    endocervicitis (with or without erosion or ectropion)
    exocervicitis (with or without erosion or ectropion)

Use additional code (B95-B97), to identify infectious agent

EXCLUDES 1   *erosion and ectropion of cervix without cervicitis (N86)*

✓4ᵗʰ **N73 Other female pelvic inflammatory diseases**

Use additional code (B95-B97), to identify infectious agent

N73.0 Acute parametritis and pelvic cellulitis CC ♀

Abscess of broad ligament
Abscess of parametrium
Pelvic cellulitis, female
DEF: Parametritis: Inflammation of the parametrium.

N73.1 Chronic parametritis and pelvic cellulitis ♀

Any condition in N73.0 specified as chronic
EXCLUDES 1   *tuberculous parametritis and pelvic cellulitis (A18.17)*

N73.2 Unspecified parametritis and pelvic cellulitis ♀

Any condition in N73.0 unspecified whether acute or chronic

N73.3 Female acute pelvic peritonitis MCC ♀

N73.4 Female chronic pelvic peritonitis CC ♀

EXCLUDES 1   *tuberculous pelvic (female) peritonitis (A18.17)*

N73.5 Female pelvic peritonitis, unspecified ♀

N73.6 Female pelvic peritoneal adhesions (postinfective) ♀

EXCLUDES 2   *postprocedural pelvic peritoneal adhesions (N99.4)*
AHA: 2014,1Q,6

N73.8 Other specified female pelvic inflammatory diseases ♀

N73.9 Female pelvic inflammatory disease, unspecified ♀

Female pelvic infection or inflammation NOS

N74 Female pelvic inflammatory disorders in diseases classified elsewhere ♀

Code first underlying disease
EXCLUDES 1   *chlamydial cervicitis (A56.02)*
    chlamydial pelvic inflammatory disease (A56.11)
    gonococcal cervicitis (A54.03)
    gonococcal pelvic inflammatory disease (A54.24)
    herpesviral [herpes simplex] cervicitis (A60.03)
    herpesviral [herpes simplex] pelvic inflammatory disease (A60.09)
    syphilitic cervicitis (A52.76)
    syphilitic pelvic inflammatory disease (A52.76)
    trichomonal cervicitis (A59.09)
    tuberculous cervicitis (A18.16)
    tuberculous pelvic inflammatory disease (A18.17)

✓4ᵗʰ **N75 Diseases of Bartholin's gland**

DEF: Bartholin's gland: Mucous-producing gland found in the vestibular bulbs on either side of the vaginal orifice and connected to the mucosal membrane at the opening by a duct.

N75.0 Cyst of Bartholin's gland ♀

N75.1 Abscess of Bartholin's gland CC ♀

CC Excl: PDX collection 944

N75.8 Other diseases of Bartholin's gland ♀

Bartholinitis

N75.9 Disease of Bartholin's gland, unspecified ♀

✓4ᵗʰ **N76 Other inflammation of vagina and vulva**

Use additional code (B95-B97), to identify infectious agent
EXCLUDES 2   *senile (atrophic) vaginitis (N95.2)*
    vulvar vestibulitis (N94.810)

N76.0 Acute vaginitis ♀

Acute vulvovaginitis
Vaginitis NOS
Vulvovaginitis NOS

N76.1 Subacute and chronic vaginitis ♀

Chronic vulvovaginitis
Subacute vulvovaginitis

N76.2 Acute vulvitis ♀

Vulvitis NOS

N76.3 Subacute and chronic vulvitis ♀

N76.4 Abscess of vulva ♀

Furuncle of vulva

N76.5 Ulceration of vagina ♀

N76.6 Ulceration of vulva ♀

✓5ᵗʰ **N76.8 Other specified inflammation of vagina and vulva**

N76.81 Mucositis (ulcerative) of vagina and vulva CC ♀

Code also type of associated therapy, such as:
    antineoplastic and immunosuppressive drugs (T45.1X-)
    radiological procedure and radiotherapy (Y84.2)
EXCLUDES 2   *gastrointestinal mucositis (ulcerative) (K92.81)*
    nasal mucositis (ulcerative) (J34.81)
    oral mucositis (ulcerative) (K12.3-)
CC Excl: PDX collection 945

N76.89 Other specified inflammation of vagina and vulva ♀

✓4ᵗʰ **N77 Vulvovaginal ulceration and inflammation in diseases classified elsewhere**

N77.0 Ulceration of vulva in diseases classified elsewhere ♀

Code first underlying disease, such as:
    Behçet's disease (M35.2)
EXCLUDES 1   *ulceration of vulva in gonococcal infection (A54.02)*
    ulceration of vulva in herpesviral [herpes simplex] infection (A60.04)
    ulceration of vulva in syphilis (A51.0)
    ulceration of vulva in tuberculosis (A18.18)

N77.1 Vaginitis, vulvitis and vulvovaginitis in diseases classified elsewhere ♀

Code first underlying disease, such as:
    pinworm (B80)
EXCLUDES 1   *candidal vulvovaginitis (B37.3)*
    chlamydial vulvovaginitis (A56.02)
    gonococcal vulvovaginitis (A54.02)
    herpesviral [herpes simplex] vulvovaginitis (A60.04)
    trichomonal vulvovaginitis (A59.01)
    tuberculous vulvovaginitis (A18.18)
    vulvovaginitis in early syphilis (A51.0)
    vulvovaginitis in late syphilis (A52.76)

Noninflammatory disorders of female genital tract (N80-N98)

✓4ᵗʰ **N80 Endometriosis**

DEF: Aberrant uterine mucosal tissue appearing in areas of the pelvic cavity outside of its normal location, lining the uterus, and inflaming surrounding tissues often resulting in infertility or spontaneous abortion.

N80.0 Endometriosis of uterus ♀

Adenomyosis
EXCLUDES 1   *stromal endometriosis (D39.0)*

N80.1 Endometriosis of ovary ♀

N80.2 Endometriosis of fallopian tube ♀

N80.3 Endometriosis of pelvic peritoneum ♀

N80.4 Endometriosis of rectovaginal septum and vagina ♀

N80.5 Endometriosis of intestine ♀

N80.6 Endometriosis in cutaneous scar ♀

N80.8 Other endometriosis ♀

Endometriosis of thorax

N80.9 Endometriosis, unspecified ♀

N Newborn: 0   P Pediatric: 0-17   M Maternity: 9-64   A Adult: 15-124   MCC Major Complication/Comorbidity   CC Complication/Comorbidity   SW Severe Wound Dx

866   ICD-10-CM 2020

☑4ᵗʰ **N81 Female genital prolapse**

> ᴇxᴄʟuᴅᴇꜱ 1 *genital prolapse complicating pregnancy, labor or delivery (O34.5-)*
> *prolapse and hernia of ovary and fallopian tube (N83.4-)*
> *prolapse of vaginal vault after hysterectomy (N99.3)*

Types of Pelvic Organ Prolapse

Urethrocele   **Cystocele**

Rectocele   **Enterocele**

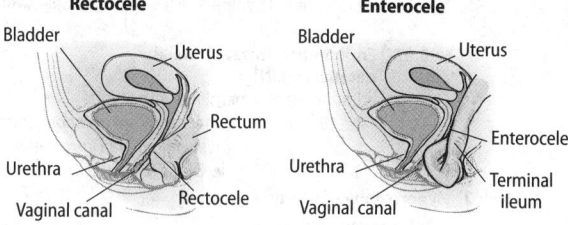

N81.0 Urethrocele   ♀

> ᴇxᴄʟuᴅᴇꜱ 1 *urethrocele with cystocele (N81.1-)*
> *urethrocele with prolapse of uterus (N81.2-N81.4)*

☑5ᵗʰ **N81.1 Cystocele**

Cystocele with urethrocele
Cystourethrocele

> ᴇxᴄʟuᴅᴇꜱ 1 *cystocele with prolapse of uterus (N81.2-N81.4)*

N81.10 Cystocele, unspecified   ♀
Prolapse of (anterior) vaginal wall NOS

N81.11 Cystocele, midline   ♀

N81.12 Cystocele, lateral   ♀
Paravaginal cystocele
DEF: Detachment of the lateral support connections of the vagina at the arcus tendineus fasciae pelvis (ATFP) that results in bladder drop. The bladder herniates into the vagina laterally.

N81.2 Incomplete uterovaginal prolapse   ♀
First degree uterine prolapse
Prolapse of cervix NOS
Second degree uterine prolapse

> ᴇxᴄʟuᴅᴇꜱ 1 *cervical stump prolapse (N81.85)*

N81.3 Complete uterovaginal prolapse   ♀
Procidentia (uteri) NOS
Third degree uterine prolapse

N81.4 Uterovaginal prolapse, unspecified   ♀
Prolapse of uterus NOS

N81.5 Vaginal enterocele   ♀

> ᴇxᴄʟuᴅᴇꜱ 1 *enterocele with prolapse of uterus (N81.2-N81.4)*

N81.6 Rectocele   ♀
Prolapse of posterior vaginal wall
Use additional code for any associated fecal incontinence, if applicable (R15.-)

> ᴇxᴄʟuᴅᴇꜱ 2 *perineocele (N81.81)*
> *rectal prolapse (K62.3)*
> *rectocele with prolapse of uterus (N81.2-N81.4)*

☑5ᵗʰ **N81.8 Other female genital prolapse**

N81.81 Perineocele   ♀

N81.82 Incompetence or weakening of pubocervical tissue   ♀

N81.83 Incompetence or weakening of rectovaginal tissue   ♀

N81.84 Pelvic muscle wasting   ♀
Disuse atrophy of pelvic muscles and anal sphincter

N81.85 Cervical stump prolapse   ♀

N81.89 Other female genital prolapse   ♀
Deficient perineum
Old laceration of muscles of pelvic floor

N81.9 Female genital prolapse, unspecified   ♀

☑4ᵗʰ **N82 Fistulae involving female genital tract**

> ᴇxᴄʟuᴅᴇꜱ 1 *vesicointestinal fistulae (N32.1)*

CC Excl: For CC codes in category N82: PDX collection 946

N82.0 Vesicovaginal fistula   CC SW ♀

N82.1 Other female urinary-genital tract fistulae   CC ♀
Cervicovesical fistula
Ureterovaginal fistula
Urethrovaginal fistula
Uteroureteric fistula
Uterovesical fistula
AHA: 2017,3Q,3

N82.2 Fistula of vagina to small intestine   CC SW ♀

N82.3 Fistula of vagina to large intestine   CC SW ♀
Rectovaginal fistula

N82.4 Other female intestinal-genital tract fistulae   CC SW ♀
Intestinouterine fistula

N82.5 Female genital tract-skin fistulae   CC SW ♀
Uterus to abdominal wall fistula
Vaginoperineal fistula

N82.8 Other female genital tract fistulae   CC ♀

N82.9 Female genital tract fistula, unspecified   CC ♀

☑4ᵗʰ **N83 Noninflammatory disorders of ovary, fallopian tube and broad ligament**

> ᴇxᴄʟuᴅᴇꜱ 2 *hydrosalpinx (N70.1-)*

AHA: 2016,4Q,46

☑5ᵗʰ **N83.0 Follicular cyst of ovary**
Cyst of graafian follicle
Hemorrhagic follicular cyst (of ovary)

N83.00 Follicular cyst of ovary, unspecified side   ♀

N83.01 Follicular cyst of right ovary   ♀

N83.02 Follicular cyst of left ovary   ♀

☑5ᵗʰ **N83.1 Corpus luteum cyst**
Hemorrhagic corpus luteum cyst

N83.10 Corpus luteum cyst of ovary, unspecified side   ♀

N83.11 Corpus luteum cyst of right ovary   ♀

N83.12 Corpus luteum cyst of left ovary   ♀

☑5ᵗʰ **N83.2 Other and unspecified ovarian cysts**

> ᴇxᴄʟuᴅᴇꜱ 1 *developmental ovarian cyst (Q50.1)*
> *neoplastic ovarian cyst (D27.-)*
> *polycystic ovarian syndrome (E28.2)*
> *Stein-Leventhal syndrome (E28.2)*

☑6ᵗʰ **N83.20 Unspecified ovarian cysts**

N83.201 Unspecified ovarian cyst, right side   ♀

N83.202 Unspecified ovarian cyst, left side   ♀

N83.209 Unspecified ovarian cyst, unspecified side   ♀
Ovarian cyst, NOS

☑6ᵗʰ **N83.29 Other ovarian cysts**
Retention cyst of ovary
Simple cyst of ovary

N83.291 Other ovarian cyst, right side   ♀

N83.292 Other ovarian cyst, left side   ♀

N83.299 Other ovarian cyst, unspecified side   ♀

☑5ᵗʰ **N83.3 Acquired atrophy of ovary and fallopian tube**

☑6ᵗʰ **N83.31 Acquired atrophy of ovary**

N83.311 Acquired atrophy of right ovary   ♀

N83.312 Acquired atrophy of left ovary   ♀

N83.319 Acquired atrophy of ovary, unspecified side ♀
Acquired atrophy of ovary, NOS

✓6th **N83.32** Acquired atrophy of fallopian tube
N83.321 Acquired atrophy of right fallopian tube ♀
N83.322 Acquired atrophy of left fallopian tube ♀
N83.329 Acquired atrophy of fallopian tube, unspecified side ♀
Acquired atrophy of fallopian tube, NOS

✓6th **N83.33** Acquired atrophy of ovary and fallopian tube
N83.331 Acquired atrophy of right ovary and fallopian tube ♀
N83.332 Acquired atrophy of left ovary and fallopian tube ♀
N83.339 Acquired atrophy of ovary and fallopian tube, unspecified side ♀
Acquired atrophy of ovary and fallopian tube, NOS

✓5th **N83.4** Prolapse and hernia of ovary and fallopian tube
N83.40 Prolapse and hernia of ovary and fallopian tube, unspecified side ♀
Prolapse and hernia of ovary and fallopian tube, NOS
N83.41 Prolapse and hernia of right ovary and fallopian tube ♀
N83.42 Prolapse and hernia of left ovary and fallopian tube ♀

✓5th **N83.5** Torsion of ovary, ovarian pedicle and fallopian tube
Torsion of accessory tube
CC Excl: For CC codes in subcategory N83.5: PDX collection 947

✓6th **N83.51** Torsion of ovary and ovarian pedicle
N83.511 Torsion of right ovary and ovarian pedicle CC ♀
N83.512 Torsion of left ovary and ovarian pedicle CC ♀
N83.519 Torsion of ovary and ovarian pedicle, unspecified side CC ♀
Torsion of ovary and ovarian pedicle, NOS

✓6th **N83.52** Torsion of fallopian tube
Torsion of hydatid of Morgagni
N83.521 Torsion of right fallopian tube CC ♀
N83.522 Torsion of left fallopian tube CC ♀
N83.529 Torsion of fallopian tube, unspecified side CC ♀
Torsion of fallopian tube, NOS
N83.53 Torsion of ovary, ovarian pedicle and fallopian tube CC ♀

N83.6 Hematosalpinx ♀
EXCLUDES 1 *hematosalpinx (with) (in):*
hematocolpos (N89.7)
hematometra (N85.7)
tubal pregnancy (O00.1-)

N83.7 Hematoma of broad ligament ♀

N83.8 Other noninflammatory disorders of ovary, fallopian tube and broad ligament ♀
Broad ligament laceration syndrome [Allen-Masters]

N83.9 Noninflammatory disorder of ovary, fallopian tube and broad ligament, unspecified ♀

✓4th **N84** Polyp of female genital tract
EXCLUDES 1 *adenomatous polyp (D28.-)*
placental polyp (O90.89)

N84.0 Polyp of corpus uteri ♀
Polyp of endometrium
Polyp of uterus NOS
EXCLUDES 1 *polypoid endometrial hyperplasia (N85.0-)*

N84.1 Polyp of cervix uteri ♀
Mucous polyp of cervix

N84.2 Polyp of vagina ♀

N84.3 Polyp of vulva ♀
Polyp of labia

N84.8 Polyp of other parts of female genital tract ♀

N84.9 Polyp of female genital tract, unspecified ♀

✓4th **N85** Other noninflammatory disorders of uterus, except cervix
EXCLUDES 1 *endometriosis (N80.-)*
inflammatory diseases of uterus (N71.-)
noninflammatory disorders of cervix, except malposition (N86-N88)
polyp of corpus uteri (N84.0)
uterine prolapse (N81.-)

✓5th **N85.0** Endometrial hyperplasia
N85.00 Endometrial hyperplasia, unspecified ♀
Hyperplasia (adenomatous) (cystic) (glandular) of endometrium
Hyperplastic endometritis
N85.01 Benign endometrial hyperplasia ♀
Endometrial hyperplasia (complex) (simple) without atypia
N85.02 Endometrial intraepithelial neoplasia [EIN] ♀
Endometrial hyperplasia with atypia
EXCLUDES 1 *malignant neoplasm of endometrium (with endometrial intraepithelial neoplasia [EIN]) (C54.1)*

N85.2 Hypertrophy of uterus ♀
Bulky or enlarged uterus
EXCLUDES 1 *puerperal hypertrophy of uterus (O90.89)*

N85.3 Subinvolution of uterus ♀
EXCLUDES 1 *puerperal subinvolution of uterus (O90.89)*

N85.4 Malposition of uterus ♀
Anteversion of uterus
Retroflexion of uterus
Retroversion of uterus
EXCLUDES 1 *malposition of uterus complicating pregnancy, labor or delivery (O34.5-, O65.5)*

N85.5 Inversion of uterus ♀
EXCLUDES 1 *current obstetric trauma (O71.2)*
postpartum inversion of uterus (O71.2)
DEF: Abnormality in which the uterus turns inside out.

Inversion of Uterus

Uterus

N85.6 Intrauterine synechiae ♀

N85.7 Hematometra ♀
Hematosalpinx with hematometra
EXCLUDES 1 *hematometra with hematocolpos (N89.7)*
DEF: Accumulation of blood within the uterus.

N85.8 Other specified noninflammatory disorders of uterus ♀
Atrophy of uterus, acquired
Fibrosis of uterus NOS

N85.9 Noninflammatory disorder of uterus, unspecified ♀
Disorder of uterus NOS

N86 Erosion and ectropion of cervix uteri ♀
    Decubitus (trophic) ulcer of cervix
    Eversion of cervix
    EXCLUDES 1   *erosion and ectropion of cervix with cervicitis (N72)*

☑4ᵗʰ **N87 Dysplasia of cervix uteri**
    EXCLUDES 1   *abnormal results from cervical cytologic examination without*
        histologic confirmation (R87.61-)
        carcinoma in situ of cervix uteri (D06.-)
        cervical intraepithelial neoplasia III [CIN III] (D06.-)
        HGSIL of cervix (R87.613)
        severe dysplasia of cervix uteri (D06.-)

N87.0 Mild cervical dysplasia ♀
    Cervical intraepithelial neoplasia I [CIN I]

N87.1 Moderate cervical dysplasia ♀
    Cervical intraepithelial neoplasia II [CIN II]

N87.9 Dysplasia of cervix uteri, unspecified ♀
    Anaplasia of cervix
    Cervical atypism
    Cervical dysplasia NOS

☑4ᵗʰ **N88 Other noninflammatory disorders of cervix uteri**
    EXCLUDES 2   *inflammatory disease of cervix (N72)*
        polyp of cervix (N84.1)

N88.0 Leukoplakia of cervix uteri ♀

N88.1 Old laceration of cervix uteri ♀
    Adhesions of cervix
    EXCLUDES 1   *current obstetric trauma (O71.3)*

N88.2 Stricture and stenosis of cervix uteri ♀
    EXCLUDES 1   *stricture and stenosis of cervix uteri complicating*
        labor (O65.5)

N88.3 Incompetence of cervix uteri ♀
    Investigation and management of (suspected) cervical
    incompetence in a nonpregnant woman
    EXCLUDES 1   *cervical incompetence complicating pregnancy*
        (O34.3-)
    DEF: Inadequate functioning of the cervix marked by abnormal
    widening during pregnancy and causing premature birth or
    miscarriage.

N88.4 Hypertrophic elongation of cervix uteri ♀

N88.8 Other specified noninflammatory disorders ♀
    of cervix uteri
    EXCLUDES 1   *current obstetric trauma (O71.3)*

N88.9 Noninflammatory disorder of cervix uteri, ♀
    unspecified

☑4ᵗʰ **N89 Other noninflammatory disorders of vagina**
    EXCLUDES 1   *abnormal results from vaginal cytologic examination without*
        histologic confirmation (R87.62-)
        carcinoma in situ of vagina (D07.2)
        HGSIL of vagina (R87.623)
        inflammation of vagina (N76.-)
        senile (atrophic) vaginitis (N95.2)
        severe dysplasia of vagina (D07.2)
        trichomonal leukorrhea (A59.00)
        vaginal intraepithelial neoplasia [VAIN], grade III (D07.2)

N89.0 Mild vaginal dysplasia ♀
    Vaginal intraepithelial neoplasia [VAIN], grade I

N89.1 Moderate vaginal dysplasia ♀
    Vaginal intraepithelial neoplasia [VAIN], grade II

N89.3 Dysplasia of vagina, unspecified ♀

N89.4 Leukoplakia of vagina ♀

N89.5 Stricture and atresia of vagina ♀
    Vaginal adhesions
    Vaginal stenosis
    EXCLUDES 1   *congenital atresia or stricture (Q52.4)*
        postprocedural adhesions of vagina (N99.2)

N89.6 Tight hymenal ring ♀
    Rigid hymen
    Tight introitus
    EXCLUDES 1   *imperforate hymen (Q52.3)*

N89.7 Hematocolpos ♀
    Hematocolpos with hematometra or hematosalpinx
    AHA: 2016,4Q,58

N89.8 Other specified noninflammatory disorders ♀
    of vagina
    Leukorrhea NOS
    Old vaginal laceration
    Pessary ulcer of vagina
    EXCLUDES 1   *current obstetric trauma (O70.-, O71.4, O71.7-O71.8)*
        old laceration involving muscles of pelvic floor
        (N81.8)

N89.9 Noninflammatory disorder of vagina, ♀
    unspecified

☑4ᵗʰ **N90 Other noninflammatory disorders of vulva and perineum**
    EXCLUDES 1   *anogenital (venereal) warts (A63.0)*
        carcinoma in situ of vulva (D07.1)
        condyloma acuminatum (A63.0)
        current obstetric trauma (O70.-, O71.7-O71.8)
        inflammation of vulva (N76.-)
        severe dysplasia of vulva (D07.1)
        vulvar intraepithelial neoplasm III [VIN III] (D07.1)

N90.0 Mild vulvar dysplasia ♀
    Vulvar intraepithelial neoplasia [VIN], grade I

N90.1 Moderate vulvar dysplasia ♀
    Vulvar intraepithelial neoplasia [VIN], grade II

N90.3 Dysplasia of vulva, unspecified ♀

N90.4 Leukoplakia of vulva ♀
    Dystrophy of vulva
    Kraurosis of vulva
    Lichen sclerosus of external female genital organs

N90.5 Atrophy of vulva ♀
    Stenosis of vulva

☑6ᵗʰ **N90.6 Hypertrophy of vulva**
    AHA: 2016,4Q,46

N90.60 Unspecified hypertrophy of vulva ♀
    Unspecified hypertrophy of labia

N90.61 Childhood asymmetric labium majus ♀
    enlargement
    CALME

N90.69 Other specified hypertrophy of vulva ♀
    Other specified hypertrophy of labia

N90.7 Vulvar cyst ♀

☑5ᵗʰ **N90.8 Other specified noninflammatory disorders of vulva and**
    perineum

☑6ᵗʰ **N90.81 Female genital mutilation status**
    Female genital cutting status

N90.810 Female genital mutilation ♀
    status, unspecified
    Female genital cutting status, unspecified
    Female genital mutilation status NOS

N90.811 Female genital mutilation ♀
    Type I status
    Clitorectomy status
    Female genital cutting Type I status

N90.812 Female genital mutilation ♀
    Type II status
    Clitorectomy with excision of labia minora
    status
    Female genital cutting Type II status

N90.813 Female genital mutilation ♀
    Type III status
    Female genital cutting Type III status
    Infibulation status

N90.818 Other female genital ♀
    mutilation status
    Female genital cutting Type IV status
    Female genital mutilation Type IV status
    Other female genital cutting status

N90.89 Other specified noninflammatory ♀
    disorders of vulva and perineum
    Adhesions of vulva
    Hypertrophy of clitoris

N90.9 Noninflammatory disorder of vulva and ♀
    perineum, unspecified

☑4ᵗʰ **N91 Absent, scanty and rare menstruation**
    EXCLUDES 1   *ovarian dysfunction (E28.-)*

N91.0 Primary amenorrhea ♀

N91.1 Secondary amenorrhea ♀

☑ Additional Character Required   ✓x7ᵗʰ Placeholder   Unacceptable PDx   Questionable PDx   Manifestation   Unspecified Dx   H1-H14 HAC   HCC CMS-HCC Dx   HIV HIV Dx

N91.2 **Amenorrhea, unspecified** ♀

N91.3 **Primary oligomenorrhea** ♀

N91.4 **Secondary oligomenorrhea** ♀

N91.5 **Oligomenorrhea, unspecified** ♀
> Hypomenorrhea NOS

✓4ᵗʰ **N92** **Excessive, frequent and irregular menstruation**
> EXCLUDES 1   *postmenopausal bleeding (N95.0)*
> *precocious puberty (menstruation) (E30.1)*

N92.0 **Excessive and frequent menstruation with regular cycle** ♀
> Heavy periods NOS
> Menorrhagia NOS
> Polymenorrhea

N92.1 **Excessive and frequent menstruation with irregular cycle** ♀
> Irregular intermenstrual bleeding
> Irregular, shortened intervals between menstrual bleeding
> Menometrorrhagia
> Metrorrhagia

N92.2 **Excessive menstruation at puberty** P ♀
> Excessive bleeding associated with onset of menstrual periods
> Pubertal menorrhagia
> Puberty bleeding

N92.3 **Ovulation bleeding** ♀
> Regular intermenstrual bleeding

N92.4 **Excessive bleeding in the premenopausal period** ♀
> Climacteric menorrhagia or metrorrhagia
> Menopausal menorrhagia or metrorrhagia
> ▶Perimenopausal bleeding◀
> ▶Perimenopausal menorrhagia or metrorrhagia◀
> Preclimacteric menorrhagia or metrorrhagia
> Premenopausal menorrhagia or metrorrhagia

N92.5 **Other specified irregular menstruation** ♀

N92.6 **Irregular menstruation, unspecified** ♀
> Irregular bleeding NOS
> Irregular periods NOS
> EXCLUDES 1   *irregular menstruation with:*
> > *lengthened intervals or scanty bleeding (N91.3-N91.5)*
> > *shortened intervals or excessive bleeding (N92.1)*

✓4ᵗʰ **N93** **Other abnormal uterine and vaginal bleeding**
> EXCLUDES 1   *neonatal vaginal hemorrhage (P54.6)*
> *precocious puberty (menstruation) (E30.1)*
> *pseudomenses (P54.6)*

N93.0 **Postcoital and contact bleeding** ♀

N93.1 **Pre-pubertal vaginal bleeding** ♀
> AHA: 2016,4Q,47

N93.8 **Other specified abnormal uterine and vaginal bleeding** ♀
> Dysfunctional or functional uterine or vaginal bleeding NOS

N93.9 **Abnormal uterine and vaginal bleeding, unspecified** ♀

✓4ᵗʰ **N94** **Pain and other conditions associated with female genital organs and menstrual cycle**

N94.0 **Mittelschmerz** ♀
> DEF: One-sided, lower abdominal pain occurring between menstrual periods that is associated with ovulation.

✓5ᵗʰ **N94.1** **Dyspareunia**
> EXCLUDES 1   *psychogenic dyspareunia (F52.6)*
> AHA: 2016,4Q,47

N94.10 **Unspecified dyspareunia** ♀

N94.11 **Superficial (introital) dyspareunia** ♀

N94.12 **Deep dyspareunia** ♀

N94.19 **Other specified dyspareunia** ♀

N94.2 **Vaginismus** ♀
> EXCLUDES 1   *psychogenic vaginismus (F52.5)*
> DEF: Spontaneous contractions of the muscles surrounding the vagina, causing it to constrict or close.

N94.3 **Premenstrual tension syndrome** ♀
> Code also associated menstrual migraine (G43.82-, G43.83-)
> EXCLUDES 1   *premenstrual dysphoric disorder (F32.81)*

N94.4 **Primary dysmenorrhea** ♀

N94.5 **Secondary dysmenorrhea** ♀

N94.6 **Dysmenorrhea, unspecified** ♀
> EXCLUDES 1   *psychogenic dysmenorrhea (F45.8)*

✓5ᵗʰ **N94.8** **Other specified conditions associated with female genital organs and menstrual cycle**

✓6ᵗʰ **N94.81** **Vulvodynia**

N94.810 **Vulvar vestibulitis** ♀

N94.818 **Other vulvodynia** ♀

N94.819 **Vulvodynia, unspecified** ♀
> Vulvodynia NOS

N94.89 **Other specified conditions associated with female genital organs and menstrual cycle** ♀
> DEF: Hydrocele: Serous fluid that collects in the canal of Nuck in females.

N94.9 **Unspecified condition associated with female genital organs and menstrual cycle** ♀

✓4ᵗʰ **N95** **Menopausal and other perimenopausal disorders**
> Menopausal and other perimenopausal disorders due to naturally occurring (age-related) menopause and perimenopause
> EXCLUDES 1   *excessive bleeding in the premenopausal period (N92.4)*
> *menopausal and perimenopausal disorders due to artificial or premature menopause (E89.4-, E28.31-)*
> *premature menopause (E28.31-)*
> EXCLUDES 2   *postmenopausal osteoporosis (M81.0-)*
> *postmenopausal osteoporosis with current pathological fracture (M80.0-)*
> *postmenopausal urethritis (N34.2)*

N95.0 **Postmenopausal bleeding** ♀

N95.1 **Menopausal and female climacteric states** ♀
> Symptoms such as flushing, sleeplessness, headache, lack of concentration, associated with natural (age-related) menopause
> Use additional code for associated symptoms
> EXCLUDES 1   *asymptomatic menopausal state (Z78.0)*
> > *symptoms associated with artificial menopause (E89.41)*
> > *symptoms associated with premature menopause (E28.310)*

N95.2 **Postmenopausal atrophic vaginitis** ♀
> Senile (atrophic) vaginitis

N95.8 **Other specified menopausal and perimenopausal disorders** ♀

N95.9 **Unspecified menopausal and perimenopausal disorder** ♀

N96 **Recurrent pregnancy loss** ♀
> Investigation or care in a nonpregnant woman with history of recurrent pregnancy loss
> EXCLUDES 1   *recurrent pregnancy loss with current pregnancy (O26.2-)*

✓4ᵗʰ **N97** **Female infertility**
> INCLUDES   inability to achieve a pregnancy
> sterility, female NOS
> EXCLUDES 1   *female infertility associated with:*
> > *hypopituitarism (E23.0)*
> > *Stein-Leventhal syndrome (E28.2)*
> EXCLUDES 2   *incompetence of cervix uteri (N88.3)*
> DEF: Infertility: Inability to conceive for at least one year with regular intercourse.
> DEF: Primary infertility: Infertility occurring in patients who have never conceived.
> DEF: Secondary infertility: Infertility occurring in patients who have previously conceived.

N97.0 **Female infertility associated with anovulation** ♀

N97.1 **Female infertility of tubal origin** ♀
> Female infertility associated with congenital anomaly of tube
> Female infertility due to tubal block
> Female infertility due to tubal occlusion
> Female infertility due to tubal stenosis

N97.2 **Female infertility of** uterine origin   ♀

    Female infertility associated with congenital anomaly of uterus
    Female infertility due to nonimplantation of ovum

N97.8 **Female infertility of other origin**   ♀

N97.9 **Female infertility, unspecified**   ♀

✓4ᵗʰ **N98 Complications associated with artificial fertilization**

    CC Excl: For CC codes in category N98, unless otherwise noted: PDX collection 643

N98.0 **Infection associated with artificial insemination**   CC ♀

    CC Excl: PDX collection 948

N98.1 **Hyperstimulation of ovaries**   CC ♀

    Hyperstimulation of ovaries NOS
    Hyperstimulation of ovaries associated with induced ovulation

N98.2 **Complications of attempted introduction of fertilized ovum following in vitro fertilization**   CC ♀

N98.3 **Complications of attempted introduction of embryo in embryo transfer**   CC ♀

N98.8 **Other complications associated with artificial fertilization**   CC ♀

N98.9 **Complication associated with artificial fertilization, unspecified**   CC ♀

Intraoperative and postprocedural complications and disorders of genitourinary system, not elsewhere classified (N99)

CC Excl: For CC codes in category N99, unless otherwise noted: PDX collection 952

✓4ᵗʰ **N99 Intraoperative and postprocedural complications and disorders of genitourinary system, not elsewhere classified**

    EXCLUDES 2   irradiation cystitis (N30.4-)

       postoophorectomy ostepoorosis with current pathological fracture (M80.8-)

       postoophorectomy osteoporosis without current pathological fracture (M81.8)

N99.0 **Postprocedural (acute) (chronic) kidney failure**

    Use additional code to type of kidney disease

✓5ᵗʰ **N99.1 Postprocedural urethral stricture**

    Postcatheterization urethral stricture

✓6ᵗʰ **N99.11 Postprocedural urethral stricture, male**

    AHA: 2016,4Q,47-48

    N99.110 **Postprocedural urethral stricture, male, meatal**   ♂

    N99.111 **Postprocedural bulbous urethral stricture, male**   ♂

    N99.112 **Postprocedural membranous urethral stricture, male**   ♂

    N99.113 **Postprocedural anterior bulbous urethral stricture, male**   ♂

    N99.114 **Postprocedural urethral stricture, male, unspecified**   ♂

    N99.115 **Postprocedural fossa navicularis urethral stricture**   ♂

    N99.116 **Postprocedural urethral stricture, male, overlapping sites**   ♂

    N99.12 **Postprocedural urethral stricture, female**   ♀

N99.2 **Postprocedural adhesions of vagina**   ♀

N99.3 **Prolapse of vaginal vault after hysterectomy**   ♀

N99.4 **Postprocedural pelvic peritoneal adhesions**

    EXCLUDES 2   pelvic peritoneal adhesions NOS (N73.6)

       postinfective pelvic peritoneal adhesions (N73.6)

✓5ᵗʰ **N99.5 Complications of stoma of urinary tract**

    EXCLUDES 2   mechanical complication of urinary catheter (T83.0-)

    AHA: 2016,4Q,48

✓6ᵗʰ **N99.51 Complication of cystostomy**

    N99.510 **Cystostomy hemorrhage**   CC HCC

       CC Excl: PDX collection 949

    N99.511 **Cystostomy infection**   CC HCC

       CC Excl: PDX collection 950

N99.512 **Cystostomy malfunction**   CC HCC

    CC Excl: PDX collection 951

N99.518 **Other cystostomy complication**   CC HCC

    CC Excl: PDX collection 949

✓6ᵗʰ **N99.52 Complication of incontinent external stoma of urinary tract**

    N99.520 **Hemorrhage of incontinent external stoma of urinary tract**   HCC

    N99.521 **Infection of incontinent external stoma of urinary tract**   HCC

    N99.522 **Malfunction of incontinent external stoma of urinary tract**   HCC

    N99.523 **Herniation of incontinent stoma of urinary tract**   HCC

    N99.524 **Stenosis of incontinent stoma of urinary tract**   HCC

    N99.528 **Other complication of incontinent external stoma of urinary tract**   HCC

✓6ᵗʰ **N99.53 Complication of continent stoma of urinary tract**

    N99.530 **Hemorrhage of continent stoma of urinary tract**   HCC

    N99.531 **Infection of continent stoma of urinary tract**   HCC

    N99.532 **Malfunction of continent stoma of urinary tract**   HCC

    N99.533 **Herniation of continent stoma of urinary tract**   HCC

    N99.534 **Stenosis of continent stoma of urinary tract**   HCC

    N99.538 **Other complication of continent stoma of urinary tract**   HCC

✓5ᵗʰ **N99.6 Intraoperative hemorrhage and hematoma of a genitourinary system organ or structure complicating a procedure**

    EXCLUDES 1   intraoperative hemorrhage and hematoma of a genitourinary system organ or structure due to accidental puncture or laceration during a procedure (N99.7-)

    N99.61 **Intraoperative hemorrhage and hematoma of a genitourinary system organ or structure complicating a genitourinary system procedure**   CC

    N99.62 **Intraoperative hemorrhage and hematoma of a genitourinary system organ or structure complicating other procedure**   CC

✓5ᵗʰ **N99.7 Accidental puncture and laceration of a genitourinary system organ or structure during a procedure**

    N99.71 **Accidental puncture and laceration of a genitourinary system organ or structure during a genitourinary system procedure**   CC

       CC Excl: PDX collection 509

    N99.72 **Accidental puncture and laceration of a genitourinary system organ or structure during other procedure**   CC

       CC Excl: PDX collection 509

✓5ᵗʰ **N99.8 Other intraoperative and postprocedural complications and disorders of genitourinary system**

    AHA: 2016,4Q,9-10

    N99.81 **Other intraoperative complications of genitourinary system**

✓6ᵗʰ **N99.82 Postprocedural hemorrhage of a genitourinary system organ or structure following a procedure**

    N99.820 **Postprocedural hemorrhage of a genitourinary system organ or structure following a genitourinary system procedure**   CC

    N99.821 **Postprocedural hemorrhage of a genitourinary system organ or structure following other procedure**   CC

    N99.83 **Residual ovary syndrome**   ♀

✔ Additional Character Required   ✓x7ᵗʰ Placeholder   Unacceptable PDx   Questionable PDx   Manifestation   Unspecified Dx   H1-H14 HAC   HCC CMS-HCC Dx   HIV HIV Dx

ICD-10-CM 2020   871

Chapter 14. Diseases of the Genitourinary System

✓6ᵗʰ **N99.84** Postprocedural hematoma and seroma of a genitourinary system organ or structure following a procedure

    N99.840 Postprocedural hematoma of a genitourinary system organ or structure following a genitourinary system procedure　[CC]

    N99.841 Postprocedural hematoma of a genitourinary system organ or structure following other procedure　[CC]

    N99.842 Postprocedural seroma of a genitourinary system organ or structure following a genitourinary system procedure　[CC]

    N99.843 Postprocedural seroma of a genitourinary system organ or structure following other procedure　[CC]

● **N99.85** Post endometrial ablation syndrome

  N99.89 Other postprocedural complications and disorders of genitourinary system

[N] Newborn: 0　[P] Pediatric: 0-17　[M] Maternity: 9-64　[A] Adult: 15-124　[MCC] Major Complication/Comorbidity　[CC] Complication/Comorbidity　[SW] Severe Wound Dx

872　　ICD-10-CM 2020

Chapter 15. Pregnancy, Childbirth and the Puerperium (O00–O9A)

Chapter-specific Guidelines with Coding Examples

The chapter-specific guidelines from the ICD-10-CM Official Guidelines for Coding and Reporting have been provided below. Along with these guidelines are coding examples, contained in the shaded boxes, that have been developed to help illustrate the coding and/or sequencing guidance found in these guidelines.

a. General rules for obstetric cases

1) Codes from Chapter 15 and sequencing priority

Obstetric cases require codes from chapter 15, codes in the range O00-O9A, Pregnancy, Childbirth, and the Puerperium. Chapter 15 codes have sequencing priority over codes from other chapters. Additional codes from other chapters may be used in conjunction with chapter 15 codes to further specify conditions. Should the provider document that the pregnancy is incidental to the encounter, then code Z33.1, Pregnant state, incidental, should be used in place of any chapter 15 codes. It is the provider's responsibility to state that the condition being treated is not affecting the pregnancy.

Pregnant patient at 25 weeks' gestation admitted for bladder abscess

O23.12	Infections of bladder in pregnancy, second trimester
N30.80	Other cystitis without hematuria
Z3A.25	25 weeks gestation of pregnancy

Explanation: The documentation does not indicate that the pregnancy is incidental or in any way unaffected by the bladder abscess; therefore, an obstetrics code should be sequenced first. An additional code was provided to identify the specific bladder condition as this information is not called out specifically in the obstetrics code.

---

2) Chapter 15 codes used only on the maternal record

Chapter 15 codes are to be used only on the maternal record, never on the record of the newborn.

3) Final character for trimester

The majority of codes in Chapter 15 have a final character indicating the trimester of pregnancy. The timeframes for the trimesters are indicated at the beginning of the chapter. If trimester is not a component of a code, it is because the condition always occurs in a specific trimester, or the concept of trimester of pregnancy is not applicable. Certain codes have characters for only certain trimesters because the condition does not occur in all trimesters, but it may occur in more than just one.

Assignment of the final character for trimester should be based on the provider's documentation of the trimester (or number of weeks) for the current admission/encounter. This applies to the assignment of trimester for pre-existing conditions as well as those that develop during or are due to the pregnancy. The provider's documentation of the number of weeks may be used to assign the appropriate code identifying the trimester.

Whenever delivery occurs during the current admission, and there is an "in childbirth" option for the obstetric complication being coded, the "in childbirth" code should be assigned.

Pregnant patient at 21 weeks' gestation admitted with excessive vomiting

| O21.2 | Late vomiting of pregnancy |
| Z3A.21 | 21 weeks gestation of pregnancy |

Explanation: Category O21 classifies vomiting in pregnancy. Although code selection is based on whether the vomiting is before or after 20 completed weeks, these codes are not further classified by trimester. If vomiting only in the second trimester was documented, the provider should be queried for the specific week of gestation, as this will affect code selection.

---

4) Selection of trimester for inpatient admissions that encompass more than one trimester

In instances when a patient is admitted to a hospital for complications of pregnancy during one trimester and remains in the hospital into a subsequent trimester, the trimester character for the antepartum complication code should be assigned on the basis of the trimester when the complication developed, not the trimester of the discharge. If the condition developed prior to the current admission/encounter or represents a pre-existing condition, the trimester character for the trimester at the time of the admission/encounter should be assigned.

Patient admitted at 27 6/7 weeks' gestation for hemorrhaging from partial placenta previa; three days after admission at 28 1/7 weeks' gestation, she developed gestational hypertension

O44.32	Partial placenta previa with hemorrhage, second trimester
O13.3	Gestational [pregnancy-induced] hypertension without significant proteinuria, third trimester
Z3A.27	27 weeks gestation of pregnancy

Explanation: The patient presented with hemorrhaging from partial placenta previa while still in her 27th week, which falls within the second trimester. The gestational hypertension did not occur until three days after admission, putting the patient in her 28th week of pregnancy or what is considered to be the third trimester. The weeks of gestation captured by a code from category Z3A should represent only the gestational weeks upon admission.

---

5) Unspecified trimester

Each category that includes codes for trimester has a code for "unspecified trimester." The "unspecified trimester" code should rarely be used, such as when the documentation in the record is insufficient to determine the trimester and it is not possible to obtain clarification.

6) 7th character for fetus identification

Where applicable, a 7th character is to be assigned for certain categories (O31, O32, O33.3 - O33.6, O35, O36, O40, O41, O60.1, O60.2, O64, and O69) to identify the fetus for which the complication code applies.

Assign 7th character "0":

- For single gestations
- When the documentation in the record is insufficient to determine the fetus affected and it is not possible to obtain clarification.
- When it is not possible to clinically determine which fetus is affected.

Maternal patient with twin gestations is seen after ultrasound identifies fetus B to be in breech presentation

| O32.1XX2 | Maternal care for breech presentation, fetus 2 |

Explanation: The documentation indicates that although there are two fetuses, only one fetus is determined to be in breech presentation. Whether fetus 2 or fetus B is used, the coder can assign the seventh character of 2 to identify the second fetus as the one in breech.

---

b. Selection of OB principal or first-listed diagnosis

1) Routine outpatient prenatal visits

For routine outpatient prenatal visits when no complications are present, a code from category Z34, Encounter for supervision of normal pregnancy, should be used as the first-listed diagnosis. These codes should not be used in conjunction with chapter 15 codes.

2) Supervision of high-risk pregnancy

Codes from category O09, Supervision of high-risk pregnancy, are intended for use only during the prenatal period. For complications during the labor or delivery episode as a result of a high-risk pregnancy, assign the applicable complication codes from Chapter 15. If there are no complications during the labor or delivery episode, assign code O80, Encounter for full-term uncomplicated delivery.

For routine prenatal outpatient visits for patients with high-risk pregnancies, a code from category O09, Supervision of high-risk pregnancy, should be used as the first-listed diagnosis. Secondary chapter 15 codes may be used in conjunction with these codes if appropriate.

36-year-old with history of preterm labor admitted in labor with second child at 39 weeks' gestation, delivered healthy baby without complications

O80	Encounter for full-term uncomplicated delivery
Z3A.39	39 weeks gestation of pregnancy
Z37.0	Single live birth

Explanation: Although this patient is over 35 and having her second child (elderly multigravida) and has a history of preterm labor with her first child, no codes from category O09.- should be appended. In the absence of any other complications noted during the encounter, code O80 is the most appropriate code to describe the principal diagnosis.

---

3) Episodes when no delivery occurs

In episodes when no delivery occurs, the principal diagnosis should correspond to the principal complication of the pregnancy which necessitated the encounter. Should more than one complication exist, all of which are treated or monitored, any of the complication codes may be sequenced first.

4) When a delivery occurs

When an obstetric patient is admitted and delivers during that admission, the condition that prompted the admission should be sequenced as the principal diagnosis. If multiple conditions prompted the admission, sequence the one most related to the delivery as the principal diagnosis. A code for any complication of the delivery should be assigned as an additional diagnosis. In cases of cesarean delivery, if the patient was admitted with a condition that resulted in the performance of a cesarean procedure, that condition should be selected as the principal diagnosis. If the reason for the admission was unrelated to the condition resulting in the cesarean delivery, the condition related to the reason for the admission should be selected as the principal diagnosis.

Maternal patient with diet-controlled gestational diabetes was admitted at 38 weeks' gestation in obstructed labor due to footling presentation; cesarean performed for the malpresentation

O64.8XX0	Obstructed labor due to other malposition and malpresentation, not applicable or unspecified
O24.420	Gestational diabetes mellitus in childbirth, diet controlled
Z3A.38	38 weeks gestation of pregnancy
Z37.0	Single live birth

Explanation: The obstructed labor necessitated the cesarean procedure.

At 39 weeks' gestation, a maternal patient presents with hemorrhage with coagulation defect; the next day the patient goes into labor and eventually delivers via cesarean section due to arrested active phase of labor

O46.003	Antepartum hemorrhage with coagulation defect, unspecified, third trimester
O62.1	Secondary uterine inertia
Z3A.39	39 weeks gestation of pregnancy
Z37.0	Single live birth

Explanation: The patient was admitted because of the antepartum hemorrhage with coagulation defect. The arrested active phase, although the reason for the cesarean delivery, did not develop until later into the stay.

5) Outcome of delivery

A code from category Z37, Outcome of delivery, should be included on every maternal record when a delivery has occurred. These codes are not to be used on subsequent records or on the newborn record.

c. Pre-existing conditions versus conditions due to the pregnancy

Certain categories in Chapter 15 distinguish between conditions of the mother that existed prior to pregnancy (pre-existing) and those that are a direct result of pregnancy. When assigning codes from Chapter 15, it is important to assess if a condition was pre-existing prior to pregnancy or developed during or due to the pregnancy in order to assign the correct code.

Categories that do not distinguish between pre-existing and pregnancy-related conditions may be used for either. It is acceptable to use codes specifically for the puerperium with codes complicating pregnancy and childbirth if a condition arises postpartum during the delivery encounter.

d. Pre-existing hypertension in pregnancy

Category O10, Pre-existing hypertension complicating pregnancy, childbirth and the puerperium, includes codes for hypertensive heart and hypertensive chronic kidney disease. When assigning one of the O10 codes that includes hypertensive heart disease or hypertensive chronic kidney disease, it is necessary to add a secondary code from the appropriate hypertension category to specify the type of heart failure or chronic kidney disease.

See Section I.C.9. Hypertension.

e. Fetal conditions affecting the management of the mother

1) Codes from categories O35 and O36

Codes from categories O35, Maternal care for known or suspected fetal abnormality and damage, and O36, Maternal care for other fetal problems, are assigned only when the fetal condition is actually responsible for modifying the management of the mother, i.e., by requiring diagnostic studies, additional observation, special care, or termination of pregnancy. The fact that the fetal condition exists does not justify assigning a code from this series to the mother's record.

A patient is seen in ED for spotting 15 weeks into her pregnancy; the doctors also suspect fetal hydrocephalus.

O26.852	Spotting complicating pregnancy, second trimester
Z3A.15	15 weeks gestation of pregnancy

Explanation: Whether the fetal hydrocephalus was suspected or confirmed, an additional code is not warranted for this condition as the documentation does not indicate that this fetal condition is in any way altering the management of the mother or complicating her pregnancy.

2) In utero surgery

In cases when surgery is performed on the fetus, a diagnosis code from category O35, Maternal care for known or suspected fetal abnormality and damage, should be assigned identifying the fetal condition. Assign the appropriate procedure code for the procedure performed.

No code from Chapter 16, the perinatal codes, should be used on the mother's record to identify fetal conditions. Surgery performed in utero on a fetus is still to be coded as an obstetric encounter.

f. HIV infection in pregnancy, childbirth and the puerperium

During pregnancy, childbirth or the puerperium, a patient admitted because of an HIV-related illness should receive a principal diagnosis from subcategory O98.7-, Human immunodeficiency [HIV] disease complicating pregnancy, childbirth and the puerperium, followed by the code(s) for the HIV-related illness(es).

Patients with asymptomatic HIV infection status admitted during pregnancy, childbirth, or the puerperium should receive codes of O98.7- and Z21, Asymptomatic human immunodeficiency virus [HIV] infection status.

A previously asymptomatic HIV patient who is 13 weeks pregnant is admitted with oral thrush.

O98.711	Human immunodeficiency virus [HIV] disease complicating pregnancy, first trimester
B20	Human immunodeficiency virus [HIV] disease
B37.0	Candidal stomatitis
Z3A.13	13 weeks gestation of pregnancy

Explanation: Because oral thrush is an HIV-related condition, this patient is now considered to have HIV disease. An obstetrics code indicating that HIV is complicating the pregnancy is coded first, followed by B20 for HIV disease as well as a code for the oral thrush.

g. Diabetes mellitus in pregnancy

Diabetes mellitus is a significant complicating factor in pregnancy. Pregnant women who are diabetic should be assigned a code from category O24, Diabetes mellitus in pregnancy, childbirth, and the puerperium, first, followed by the appropriate diabetes code(s) (E08-E13) from Chapter 4.

h. Long term use of insulin and oral hypoglycemics

See section I.C.4.a.3 for information on the long term use of insulin and oral hypoglycemic.

i. Gestational (pregnancy induced) diabetes

Gestational (pregnancy induced) diabetes can occur during the second and third trimester of pregnancy in women who were not diabetic prior to pregnancy. Gestational diabetes can cause complications in the pregnancy similar to those of pre-existing diabetes mellitus. It also puts the woman at greater risk of developing diabetes after the pregnancy. Codes for gestational diabetes are in subcategory O24.4, Gestational diabetes mellitus. No other code from category O24, Diabetes mellitus in pregnancy, childbirth, and the puerperium, should be used with a code from O24.4.

The codes under subcategory O24.4 include diet controlled, insulin controlled, and controlled by oral hypoglycemic drugs. If a patient with gestational diabetes is treated with both diet and insulin, only the code for insulin-controlled is required. If a patient with gestational diabetes is treated with both diet and oral hypoglycemic medications, only the code for "controlled by oral hypoglycemic drugs" is required. Code Z79.4, Long-term (current) use of insulin or code Z79.84, Long-term (current) use of oral hypoglycemic drugs, should not be assigned with codes from subcategory O24.4.

An abnormal glucose tolerance in pregnancy is assigned a code from subcategory O99.81, Abnormal glucose complicating pregnancy, childbirth, and the puerperium.

Patient at 39 weeks term pregnancy with gestational diabetes was admitted in labor and delivered a healthy newborn. Patient is on a diabetic diet with daily metformin.

O24.425   **Gestational diabetes mellitus in childbirth, controlled by oral hypoglycemic drugs**

Z3A.39   **39 weeks gestation of pregnancy**

Z37.0   **Single live birth**

Explanation: When the patient is admitted for delivery and the patient's gestational diabetes is controlled by both diet and oral hypoglycemic medications, only the combination code in subcategory O24.4-Gestational diabetes mellitus, is reported. No code is added for diet controlled diabetes, and no Z code for long-term use of oral hypoglycemics is reported with the O24.4 combination codes.

j. Sepsis and septic shock complicating abortion, pregnancy, childbirth and the puerperium

When assigning a chapter 15 code for sepsis complicating abortion, pregnancy, childbirth, and the puerperium, a code for the specific type of infection should be assigned as an additional diagnosis. If severe sepsis is present, a code from subcategory R65.2, Severe sepsis, and code(s) for associated organ dysfunction(s) should also be assigned as additional diagnoses.

Patient is seen several days after a miscarriage with sepsis; cultures return MSSA

O03.87   **Sepsis following complete or unspecified spontaneous abortion**

B95.61   **Methicillin susceptible Staphylococcus aureus infection as the cause of diseases classified elsewhere**

Explanation: The type of infection that caused this patient to become septic was methicillin susceptible *Staphylococcus aureus* (MSSA), which as a secondary code helps capture all aspects related to this patient's septic condition.

k. Puerperal sepsis

Code O85, Puerperal sepsis, should be assigned with a secondary code to identify the causal organism (e.g., for a bacterial infection, assign a code from category B95-B96, Bacterial infections in conditions classified elsewhere). A code from category A40, Streptococcal sepsis, or A41, Other sepsis, should not be used for puerperal sepsis. If applicable, use additional codes to identify severe sepsis (R65.2-) and any associated acute organ dysfunction.

l. Alcohol, tobacco *and drug* use during pregnancy, childbirth and the puerperium

1) Alcohol use during pregnancy, childbirth and the puerperium

Codes under subcategory O99.31, Alcohol use complicating pregnancy, childbirth, and the puerperium, should be assigned for any pregnancy case when a mother uses alcohol during the pregnancy or postpartum. A secondary code from category F10, Alcohol related disorders, should also be assigned to identify manifestations of the alcohol use.

2) Tobacco use during pregnancy, childbirth and the puerperium

Codes under subcategory O99.33, Smoking (tobacco) complicating pregnancy, childbirth, and the puerperium, should be assigned for any pregnancy case when a mother uses any type of tobacco product during the pregnancy or postpartum. A secondary code from category F17, Nicotine dependence, should also be assigned to identify the type of nicotine dependence.

3) Drug use during pregnancy, childbirth and the puerperium

Codes under subcategory O99.32, Drug use complicating pregnancy, childbirth, and the puerperium, should be assigned for any pregnancy case when a mother uses drugs during the pregnancy or postpartum. This can involve illegal drugs, or inappropriate use or abuse of prescription drugs. Secondary code(s) from categories F11-F16 and F18-F19 should also be assigned to identify manifestations of the drug use.

m. Poisoning, toxic effects, adverse effects and underdosing in a pregnant patient

A code from subcategory O9A.2, Injury, poisoning and certain other consequences of external causes complicating pregnancy, childbirth, and the puerperium, should be sequenced first, followed by the appropriate injury, poisoning, toxic effect, adverse effect or underdosing code, and then the additional code(s) that specifies the condition caused by the poisoning, toxic effect, adverse effect or underdosing.

See Section I.C.19. Adverse effects, poisoning, underdosing and toxic effects.

Patient admitted with accidental carbon monoxide poisoning from a gas heating implement; the patient is 18 weeks' pregnant

O9A.212   **Injury, poisoning and certain other consequences of external causes complicating pregnancy, second trimester**

T58.11XA   **Toxic effect of carbon monoxide from utility gas, accidental (unintentional), initial encounter**

Z3A.18   **18 weeks gestation of pregnancy**

Explanation: Although the carbon monoxide poisoning is the reason the patient was admitted, a code from the obstetrics chapter must be sequenced first. Chapter 15 codes have sequencing priority over codes from other chapters.

n. Normal delivery, code O80

1) Encounter for full term uncomplicated delivery

Code O80 should be assigned when a woman is admitted for a full-term normal delivery and delivers a single, healthy infant without any complications antepartum, during the delivery, or postpartum during the delivery episode. Code O80 is always a principal diagnosis. It is not to be used if any other code from chapter 15 is needed to describe a current complication of the antenatal, delivery, or **postnatal** period. Additional codes from other chapters may be used with code O80 if they are not related to or are in any way complicating the pregnancy.

2) Uncomplicated delivery with resolved antepartum complication

Code O80 may be used if the patient had a complication at some point during the pregnancy, but the complication is not present at the time of the admission for delivery.

Patient presents in labor at 39 weeks' gestation and delivers a healthy newborn; patient had abnormal glucose levels in her first trimester, which have since resolved

O80   **Encounter for full-term uncomplicated delivery**

Z37.0   **Single live birth**

Explanation: The abnormal glucose levels during the first trimester cannot be coded if they are not affecting the patient's current trimester. Without additional complications associated with the pregnancy, fetus, or mother, code O80 is appropriate.

3) Outcome of delivery for O80

Z37.0, Single live birth, is the only outcome of delivery code appropriate for use with O80.

o. The peripartum and postpartum periods

1) Peripartum and postpartum periods

The postpartum period begins immediately after delivery and continues for six weeks following delivery. The peripartum period is defined as the last month of pregnancy to five months postpartum.

2) Peripartum and postpartum complication

A postpartum complication is any complication occurring within the six-week period.

3) Pregnancy-related complications after 6 week period

Chapter 15 codes may also be used to describe pregnancy-related complications after the peripartum or postpartum period if the provider documents that a condition is pregnancy related.

Patient admitted for varicose veins. She had a baby boy three months ago; the varicose veins started to appear one month ago. The doctor attributes the patient's pregnancy as the cause of the varicose veins, which continue to be painful and bother the patient. She is seeking surgical relief.

O87.4   Varicose veins of the lower extremity in the puerperium

Explanation: Although the varicose veins occurred several months after the delivery of the newborn, the doctor attributed the varicose veins to pregnancy and therefore a code from chapter 15 is appropriate.

4) Admission for routine postpartum care following delivery outside hospital

When the mother delivers outside the hospital prior to admission and is admitted for routine postpartum care and no complications are noted, code Z39.0, Encounter for care and examination of mother immediately after delivery, should be assigned as the principal diagnosis.

5) Pregnancy associated cardiomyopathy

Pregnancy associated cardiomyopathy, code O90.3, is unique in that it may be diagnosed in the third trimester of pregnancy but may continue to progress months after delivery. For this reason, it is referred to as peripartum cardiomyopathy. Code O90.3 is only for use when the cardiomyopathy develops as a result of pregnancy in a woman who did not have pre-existing heart disease.

p. Code O94, Sequelae of complication of pregnancy, childbirth, and the puerperium

1) Code O94

Code O94, Sequelae of complication of pregnancy, childbirth, and the puerperium, is for use in those cases when an initial complication of a pregnancy develops a sequelae requiring care or treatment at a future date.

2) After the initial postpartum period

This code may be used at any time after the initial postpartum period.

3) Sequencing of code O94

This code, like all sequela codes, is to be sequenced following the code describing the sequelae of the complication.

q. Termination of pregnancy and spontaneous abortions

1) Abortion with liveborn fetus

When an attempted termination of pregnancy results in a liveborn fetus, assign code Z33.2, Encounter for elective termination of pregnancy and a code from category Z37, Outcome of Delivery.

2) Retained products of conception following an abortion

Subsequent encounters for retained products of conception following a spontaneous abortion or elective termination of pregnancy, without complications are assigned O03.4, Incomplete spontaneous, abortion without complication, or code O07.4, Failed attempted termination of pregnancy without complication. This advice is appropriate even when the patient was discharged previously with a discharge diagnosis of complete abortion. If the patient has a specific complication associated with the spontaneous abortion or elective termination of pregnancy in addition to retained products of conception, assign the appropriate complication code (e.g., O03.-, O04.-, O07.-) instead of code O03.4 or O07.4.

Patient was seen two days ago for complete spontaneous abortion but returns today for urinary tract infection (UTI) with ultrasound showing retained products of conception

O03.38   Urinary tract infection following incomplete spontaneous abortion

Explanation: Although the diagnosis from the patient's previous stay indicated that the patient had a complete abortion, it is now determined that there were actually retained products of conception (POC). An abortion with retained POC is considered incomplete and in this case resulted in the patient developing a UTI.

3) Complications leading to abortion

Codes from Chapter 15 may be used as additional codes to identify any documented complications of the pregnancy in conjunction with codes in categories in O04, O07 and O08.

r. Abuse in a pregnant patient

For suspected or confirmed cases of abuse of a pregnant patient, a code(s) from subcategories O9A.3, Physical abuse complicating pregnancy, childbirth, and the puerperium, O9A.4, Sexual abuse complicating pregnancy, childbirth, and the puerperium, and O9A.5, Psychological abuse complicating pregnancy, childbirth, and the puerperium, should be sequenced first, followed by the appropriate codes (if applicable) to identify any associated current injury due to physical abuse, sexual abuse, and the perpetrator of abuse.

See Section I.C.19. Adult and child abuse, neglect and other maltreatment.

Chapter 15. Pregnancy, Childbirth and the Puerperium (O00-O9A)

> **NOTE** CODES FROM THIS CHAPTER ARE FOR USE ONLY ON MATERNAL RECORDS, NEVER ON NEWBORN RECORDS
>
> Codes from this chapter are for use for conditions related to or aggravated by the pregnancy, childbirth, or by the puerperium (maternal causes or obstetric causes)

> **NOTE** Trimesters are counted from the first day of the last menstrual period. They are defined as follows:
>
> 1st trimester- less than 14 weeks Ø days
>
> 2nd trimester- 14 weeks Ø days to less than 28 weeks Ø days
>
> 3rd trimester- 28 weeks Ø days until delivery

Use additional code from category Z3A, Weeks of gestation, to identify the specific week of the pregnancy, if known.

EXCLUDES 1   *supervision of normal pregnancy (Z34.-)*

EXCLUDES 2   *mental and behavioral disorders associated with the puerperium (F53.-)*
obstetrical tetanus (A34)
postpartum necrosis of pituitary gland (E23.Ø)
puerperal osteomalacia (M83.Ø)

AHA: 2016,1Q,3-5; 2014,3Q,5

This chapter contains the following blocks:

O00-O08 Pregnancy with abortive outcome
O09 Supervision of high risk pregnancy
O10-O16 Edema, proteinuria and hypertensive disorders in pregnancy, childbirth and the puerperium
O20-O29 Other maternal disorders predominantly related to pregnancy
O30-O48 Maternal care related to the fetus and amniotic cavity and possible delivery problems
O60-O77 Complications of labor and delivery
O80-O82 Encounter for delivery
O85-O92 Complications predominantly related to the puerperium
O94-O9A Other obstetric conditions, not elsewhere classified

Pregnancy with abortive outcome (O00-O08)

EXCLUDES 1   *continuing pregnancy in multiple gestation after abortion of one fetus or more (O31.1-, O31.3-)*

TIP: Do not assign a code from category Z3A with codes in this code block.

✔4ᵗʰ O00 Ectopic pregnancy

INCLUDES   ruptured ectopic pregnancy

Use additional code from category O08 to identify any associated complication

AHA: 2016,4Q,48-50; 2014,3Q,17

DEF: Implantation of a fertilized egg outside the uterus, usually in the fallopian tube or abdomen that requires emergency treatment.

CC Excl: For CC codes in category O00: PDX collection 953

Ectopic Pregnancy

Labels: Cornual/interstitial, Isthmic, Ampullar, Infundibular, Tubal (fallopian), Ovarian, Intraligamentous, Abdominal, Intramural/mural, Cervical

✔6ᵗʰ O00.Ø Abdominal pregnancy

EXCLUDES 1   *maternal care for viable fetus in abdominal pregnancy (O36.7-)*

   O00.ØØ Abdominal pregnancy without intrauterine pregnancy   CC M ♀
     Abdominal pregnancy NOS

   O00.Ø1 Abdominal pregnancy with intrauterine pregnancy   CC M ♀

✔5ᵗʰ O00.1 Tubal pregnancy

Fallopian pregnancy
Rupture of (fallopian) tube due to pregnancy
Tubal abortion

AHA: 2017,4Q,20

✔6ᵗʰ O00.10 Tubal pregnancy without intrauterine pregnancy

Tubal pregnancy NOS

   O00.101 Right tubal pregnancy without intrauterine pregnancy   CC M ♀

   O00.102 Left tubal pregnancy without intrauterine pregnancy   CC M ♀

   O00.109 Unspecified tubal pregnancy without intrauterine pregnancy   CC M ♀

✔6ᵗʰ O00.11 Tubal pregnancy with intrauterine pregnancy

   O00.111 Right tubal pregnancy with intrauterine pregnancy   CC M ♀

   O00.112 Left tubal pregnancy with intrauterine pregnancy   CC M ♀

   O00.119 Unspecified tubal pregnancy with intrauterine pregnancy   CC M ♀

✔5ᵗʰ O00.2 Ovarian pregnancy

AHA: 2017,4Q,20

✔6ᵗʰ O00.20 Ovarian pregnancy without intrauterine pregnancy

Ovarian pregnancy NOS

   O00.201 Right ovarian pregnancy without intrauterine pregnancy   CC M ♀

   O00.202 Left ovarian pregnancy without intrauterine pregnancy   CC M ♀

   O00.209 Unspecified ovarian pregnancy without intrauterine pregnancy   CC M ♀

✔6ᵗʰ O00.21 Ovarian pregnancy with intrauterine pregnancy

   O00.211 Right ovarian pregnancy with intrauterine pregnancy   CC M ♀

   O00.212 Left ovarian pregnancy with intrauterine pregnancy   CC M ♀

   O00.219 Unspecified ovarian pregnancy with intrauterine pregnancy   CC M ♀

✔5ᵗʰ O00.8 Other ectopic pregnancy

Cervical pregnancy
Cornual pregnancy
Intraligamentous pregnancy
Mural pregnancy

   O00.80 Other ectopic pregnancy without intrauterine pregnancy   CC M ♀
     Other ectopic pregnancy NOS

   O00.81 Other ectopic pregnancy with intrauterine pregnancy   CC M ♀

✔5ᵗʰ O00.9 Ectopic pregnancy, unspecified

   O00.90 Unspecified ectopic pregnancy without intrauterine pregnancy   CC M ♀
     Ectopic pregnancy NOS

   O00.91 Unspecified ectopic pregnancy with intrauterine pregnancy   CC M ♀

✔4ᵗʰ O01 Hydatidiform mole

Use additional code from category O08 to identify any associated complication

EXCLUDES 1   *chorioadenoma (destruens) (D39.2)*
malignant hydatidiform mole (D39.2)

AHA: 2014,3Q,17

DEF: Abnormal product of pregnancy, marked by a mass of cysts resembling a bunch of grapes due to chorionic villi proliferation and dissolution. It must be surgically removed.

   O01.Ø Classical hydatidiform mole   M ♀
     Complete hydatidiform mole

   O01.1 Incomplete and partial hydatidiform mole   M ♀

   O01.9 Hydatidiform mole, unspecified   M ♀
     Trophoblastic disease NOS
     Vesicular mole NOS

✔ Additional Character Required   ✔x7ᵗʰ Placeholder   Unacceptable PDx   Questionable PDx   Manifestation   Unspecified Dx   H1-H14 HAC   HCC CMS-HCC Dx   HIV HIV Dx

ICD-10-CM 2020   877

Chapter 15. Pregnancy, Childbirth and the Puerperium

☑4ᵗʰ **O02 Other abnormal products of conception**

Use additional code from category O08 to identify any associated complication

> **EXCLUDES 1**   *papyraceous fetus (O31.0-)*

AHA: 2014,3Q,17

O02.0 Blighted ovum and nonhydatidiform mole   M ♀

Carneous mole
Fleshy mole
Intrauterine mole NOS
Molar pregnancy NEC
Pathological ovum

O02.1 Missed abortion   M ♀

Early fetal death, before completion of 20 weeks of gestation, with retention of dead fetus

> **EXCLUDES 1**   *failed induced abortion (O07.-)*
> *fetal death (intrauterine) (late) (O36.4)*
> *missed abortion with blighted ovum (O02.0)*
> *missed abortion with hydatidiform mole (O01.-)*
> *missed abortion with nonhydatidiform (O02.0)*
> *missed abortion with other abnormal products of conception (O02.8-)*
> *missed delivery (O36.4)*
> *stillbirth (P95)*

☑5ᵗʰ **O02.8 Other specified abnormal products of conception**

> **EXCLUDES 1**   *abnormal products of conception with blighted ovum (O02.0)*
> *abnormal products of conception with hydatidiform mole (O01.-)*
> *abnormal products of conception with nonhydatidiform mole (O02.0)*

O02.81 Inappropriate change in quantitative human chorionic gonadotropin (hCG) in early pregnancy   M ♀

Biochemical pregnancy
Chemical pregnancy
Inappropriate level of quantitative human chorionic gonadotropin (hCG) for gestational age in early pregnancy

O02.89 Other abnormal products of conception   M ♀

O02.9 Abnormal product of conception, unspecified   M ♀

☑4ᵗʰ **O03 Spontaneous abortion**

> **NOTE**   Incomplete abortion includes retained products of conception following spontaneous abortion

> **INCLUDES**   miscarriage

CC Excl: For CC/MCC codes in category O03: PDX collection 954

O03.0 Genital tract and pelvic infection following incomplete spontaneous abortion   CC M ♀

Endometritis following incomplete spontaneous abortion
Oophoritis following incomplete spontaneous abortion
Parametritis following incomplete spontaneous abortion
Pelvic peritonitis following incomplete spontaneous abortion
Salpingitis following incomplete spontaneous abortion
Salpingo-oophoritis following incomplete spontaneous abortion

> **EXCLUDES 1**   *sepsis following incomplete spontaneous abortion (O03.37)*
> *urinary tract infection following incomplete spontaneous abortion (O03.38)*

O03.1 Delayed or excessive hemorrhage following incomplete spontaneous abortion   M ♀

Afibrinogenemia following incomplete spontaneous abortion
Defibrination syndrome following incomplete spontaneous abortion
Hemolysis following incomplete spontaneous abortion
Intravascular coagulation following incomplete spontaneous abortion

O03.2 Embolism following incomplete spontaneous abortion   MCC M ♀

Air embolism following incomplete spontaneous abortion
Amniotic fluid embolism following incomplete spontaneous abortion
Blood-clot embolism following incomplete spontaneous abortion
Embolism NOS following incomplete spontaneous abortion
Fat embolism following incomplete spontaneous abortion
Pulmonary embolism following incomplete spontaneous abortion
Pyemic embolism following incomplete spontaneous abortion
Septic or septicopyemic embolism following incomplete spontaneous abortion
Soap embolism following incomplete spontaneous abortion

☑5ᵗʰ **O03.3 Other and unspecified complications following incomplete spontaneous abortion**

O03.30 Unspecified complication following incomplete spontaneous abortion   CC M ♀

O03.31 Shock following incomplete spontaneous abortion   MCC M ♀

Circulatory collapse following incomplete spontaneous abortion
Shock (postprocedural) following incomplete spontaneous abortion

> **EXCLUDES 1**   *shock due to infection following incomplete spontaneous abortion (O03.37)*

O03.32 Renal failure following incomplete spontaneous abortion   MCC M ♀

Kidney failure (acute) following incomplete spontaneous abortion
Oliguria following incomplete spontaneous abortion
Renal shutdown following incomplete spontaneous abortion
Renal tubular necrosis following incomplete spontaneous abortion
Uremia following incomplete spontaneous abortion

O03.33 Metabolic disorder following incomplete spontaneous abortion   CC M ♀

O03.34 Damage to pelvic organs following incomplete spontaneous abortion   CC M ♀

Laceration, perforation, tear or chemical damage of bladder following incomplete spontaneous abortion
Laceration, perforation, tear or chemical damage of bowel following incomplete spontaneous abortion
Laceration, perforation, tear or chemical damage of broad ligament following incomplete spontaneous abortion
Laceration, perforation, tear or chemical damage of cervix following incomplete spontaneous abortion
Laceration, perforation, tear or chemical damage of periurethral tissue following incomplete spontaneous abortion
Laceration, perforation, tear or chemical damage of uterus following incomplete spontaneous abortion
Laceration, perforation, tear or chemical damage of vagina following incomplete spontaneous abortion

O03.35 Other venous complications following incomplete spontaneous abortion   CC M ♀

O03.36 Cardiac arrest following incomplete spontaneous abortion   CC M ♀

O03.37 Sepsis following incomplete spontaneous abortion   CC M ♀

Use additional code to identify infectious agent (B95-B97)
Use additional code to identify severe sepsis, if applicable (R65.2-)

> **EXCLUDES 1**   *septic or septicopyemic embolism following incomplete spontaneous abortion (O03.2)*

N Newborn: 0   P Pediatric: 0-17   M Maternity: 9-64   A Adult: 15-124   MCC Major Complication/Comorbidity   CC Complication/Comorbidity   SW Severe Wound Dx

878   ICD-10-CM 2020

O03.38 **Urinary tract infection** following incomplete **spontaneous abortion**   cc M ♀

Cystitis following incomplete spontaneous abortion

O03.39 **Incomplete spontaneous abortion with other complications**   cc M ♀

O03.4 **Incomplete** spontaneous abortion without complication   M ♀

O03.5 **Genital tract and pelvic infection** following complete or unspecified **spontaneous abortion**   cc M ♀

Endometritis following complete or unspecified spontaneous abortion

Oophoritis following complete or unspecified spontaneous abortion

Parametritis following complete or unspecified spontaneous abortion

Pelvic peritonitis following complete or unspecified spontaneous abortion

Salpingitis following complete or unspecified spontaneous abortion

Salpingo-oophoritis following complete or unspecified spontaneous abortion

> EXCLUDES 1   *sepsis following complete or unspecified spontaneous abortion (O03.87)*
>
> *urinary tract infection following complete or unspecified spontaneous abortion (O03.88)*

O03.6 **Delayed or excessive hemorrhage** following complete or unspecified **spontaneous abortion**   M ♀

Afibrinogenemia following complete or unspecified spontaneous abortion

Defibrination syndrome following complete or unspecified spontaneous abortion

Hemolysis following complete or unspecified spontaneous abortion

Intravascular coagulation following complete or unspecified spontaneous abortion

O03.7 **Embolism** following complete or unspecified **spontaneous abortion**   cc M ♀

Air embolism following complete or unspecified spontaneous abortion

Amniotic fluid embolism following complete or unspecified spontaneous abortion

Blood-clot embolism following complete or unspecified spontaneous abortion

Embolism NOS following complete or unspecified spontaneous abortion

Fat embolism following complete or unspecified spontaneous abortion

Pulmonary embolism following complete or unspecified spontaneous abortion

Pyemic embolism following complete or unspecified spontaneous abortion

Septic or septicopyemic embolism following complete or unspecified spontaneous abortion

Soap embolism following complete or unspecified spontaneous abortion

√5th **O03.8** **Other and unspecified complications following complete or unspecified spontaneous abortion**

O03.80 **Unspecified complication following complete or unspecified spontaneous abortion**   cc M ♀

O03.81 **Shock following complete or unspecified spontaneous abortion**   MCC M ♀

Circulatory collapse following complete or unspecified spontaneous abortion

Shock (postprocedural) following complete or unspecified spontaneous abortion

> EXCLUDES 1   *shock due to infection following complete or unspecified spontaneous abortion (O03.87)*

O03.82 **Renal failure following complete or unspecified spontaneous abortion**   MCC M ♀

Kidney failure (acute) following complete or unspecified spontaneous abortion

Oliguria following complete or unspecified spontaneous abortion

Renal shutdown following complete or unspecified spontaneous abortion

Renal tubular necrosis following complete or unspecified spontaneous abortion

Uremia following complete or unspecified spontaneous abortion

O03.83 **Metabolic disorder following complete or unspecified spontaneous abortion**   cc M ♀

O03.84 **Damage to pelvic organs following complete or unspecified spontaneous abortion**   cc M ♀

Laceration, perforation, tear or chemical damage of bladder following complete or unspecified spontaneous abortion

Laceration, perforation, tear or chemical damage of bowel following complete or unspecified spontaneous abortion

Laceration, perforation, tear or chemical damage of broad ligament following complete or unspecified spontaneous abortion

Laceration, perforation, tear or chemical damage of cervix following complete or unspecified spontaneous abortion

Laceration, perforation, tear or chemical damage of periurethral tissue following complete or unspecified spontaneous abortion

Laceration, perforation, tear or chemical damage of uterus following complete or unspecified spontaneous abortion

Laceration, perforation, tear or chemical damage of vagina following complete or unspecified spontaneous abortion

O03.85 **Other venous complications following complete or unspecified spontaneous abortion**   cc M ♀

O03.86 **Cardiac arrest following complete or unspecified spontaneous abortion**   cc M ♀

O03.87 **Sepsis following complete or unspecified spontaneous abortion**   cc M ♀

Use additional code to identify infectious agent (B95-B97)

Use additional code to identify severe sepsis, if applicable (R65.2-)

> EXCLUDES 1   *septic or septicopyemic embolism following complete or unspecified spontaneous abortion (O03.7)*

O03.88 **Urinary tract infection following complete or unspecified spontaneous abortion**   cc M ♀

Cystitis following complete or unspecified spontaneous abortion

O03.89 **Complete or unspecified spontaneous abortion with other complications**   cc M ♀

O03.9 **Complete or unspecified spontaneous abortion without complication**   M ♀

Miscarriage NOS

Spontaneous abortion NOS

☑4ᵗʰ **O04** Complications **following (induced)** termination of pregnancy

> INCLUDES   complications following (induced) termination of pregnancy
>
> EXCLUDES 1   *encounter for elective termination of pregnancy, uncomplicated (Z33.2)*
>
> *failed attempted termination of pregnancy (O07.-)*
>
> **CC Excl: For CC/MCC codes in category O04, unless otherwise noted:** PDX collection 954

O04.5 **Genital tract and pelvic infection following** CC ♀ **(induced) termination of pregnancy**

Endometritis following (induced) termination of pregnancy
Oophoritis following (induced) termination of pregnancy
Parametritis following (induced) termination of pregnancy
Pelvic peritonitis following (induced) termination of pregnancy
Salpingitis following (induced) termination of pregnancy
Salpingo-oophoritis following (induced) termination of pregnancy

> EXCLUDES 1   *sepsis following (induced) termination of pregnancy (O04.87)*
>
> *urinary tract infection following (induced) termination of pregnancy (O04.88)*

O04.6 **Delayed or excessive hemorrhage following** M ♀ **(induced) termination of pregnancy**

Afibrinogenemia following (induced) termination of pregnancy
Defibrination syndrome following (induced) termination of pregnancy
Hemolysis following (induced) termination of pregnancy
Intravascular coagulation following (induced) termination of pregnancy

O04.7 **Embolism following (induced) termination of** MCC M ♀ **pregnancy**

Air embolism following (induced) termination of pregnancy
Amniotic fluid embolism following (induced) termination of pregnancy
Blood-clot embolism following (induced) termination of pregnancy
Embolism NOS following (induced) termination of pregnancy
Fat embolism following (induced) termination of pregnancy
Pulmonary embolism following (induced) termination of pregnancy
Pyemic embolism following (induced) termination of pregnancy
Septic or septicopyemic embolism following (induced) termination of pregnancy
Soap embolism following (induced) termination of pregnancy

☑5ᵗʰ **O04.8** **(Induced) termination of pregnancy with other and unspecified complications**

O04.80 **(Induced) termination of pregnancy with** CC M ♀ **unspecified complications**

O04.81 **Shock following (induced) termination** MCC M ♀ **of pregnancy**

Circulatory collapse following (induced) termination of pregnancy
Shock (postprocedural) following (induced) termination of pregnancy

> EXCLUDES 1   *shock due to infection following (induced) termination of pregnancy (O04.87)*

O04.82 **Renal failure following (induced)** MCC M ♀ **termination of pregnancy**

Kidney failure (acute) following (induced) termination of pregnancy
Oliguria following (induced) termination of pregnancy
Renal shutdown following (induced) termination of pregnancy
Renal tubular necrosis following (induced) termination of pregnancy
Uremia following (induced) termination of pregnancy

O04.83 **Metabolic disorder following (induced)** CC M ♀ **termination of pregnancy**

O04.84 **Damage to pelvic organs following** CC M ♀ **(induced) termination of pregnancy**

Laceration, perforation, tear or chemical damage of bladder following (induced) termination of pregnancy
Laceration, perforation, tear or chemical damage of bowel following (induced) termination of pregnancy
Laceration, perforation, tear or chemical damage of broad ligament following (induced) termination of pregnancy
Laceration, perforation, tear or chemical damage of cervix following (induced) termination of pregnancy
Laceration, perforation, tear or chemical damage of periurethral tissue following (induced) termination of pregnancy
Laceration, perforation, tear or chemical damage of uterus following (induced) termination of pregnancy
Laceration, perforation, tear or chemical damage of vagina following (induced) termination of pregnancy

O04.85 **Other venous complications following** CC M ♀ **(induced) termination of pregnancy**

O04.86 **Cardiac arrest following (induced)** CC M ♀ **termination of pregnancy**

O04.87 **Sepsis following (induced) termination** CC M ♀ **of pregnancy**

Use additional code to identify infectious agent (B95-B97)
Use additional code to identify severe sepsis, if applicable (R65.2-)

> EXCLUDES 1   *septic or septicopyemic embolism following (induced) termination of pregnancy (O04.7)*
>
> **CC Excl:** PDX collection 955

O04.88 **Urinary tract infection following** CC M ♀ **(induced) termination of pregnancy**

Cystitis following (induced) termination of pregnancy

O04.89 **(Induced) termination of pregnancy with** CC M ♀ **other complications**

☑4ᵗʰ **O07** **Failed attempted termination of pregnancy**

> INCLUDES   failure of attempted induction of termination of pregnancy
>
> incomplete elective abortion
>
> EXCLUDES 1   *incomplete spontaneous abortion (O03.0-)*

O07.0 **Genital tract and pelvic infection following failed** CC M ♀ **attempted termination of pregnancy**

Endometritis following failed attempted termination of pregnancy
Oophoritis following failed attempted termination of pregnancy
Parametritis following failed attempted termination of pregnancy
Pelvic peritonitis following failed attempted termination of pregnancy
Salpingitis following failed attempted termination of pregnancy
Salpingo-oophoritis following failed attempted termination of pregnancy

> EXCLUDES 1   *sepsis following failed attempted termination of pregnancy (O07.37)*
>
> *urinary tract infection following failed attempted termination of pregnancy (O07.38)*
>
> **CC Excl:** PDX collection 956

O07.1 **Delayed or excessive hemorrhage following failed** CC M ♀ **attempted termination of pregnancy**

Afibrinogenemia following failed attempted termination of pregnancy
Defibrination syndrome following failed attempted termination of pregnancy
Hemolysis following failed attempted termination of pregnancy
Intravascular coagulation following failed attempted termination of pregnancy

> **CC Excl:** PDX collection 957

O07.2 Embolism following failed attempted termination of pregnancy `MCC` `M` ♀

  Air embolism following failed attempted termination of pregnancy

  Amniotic fluid embolism following failed attempted termination of pregnancy

  Blood-clot embolism following failed attempted termination of pregnancy

  Embolism NOS following failed attempted termination of pregnancy

  Fat embolism following failed attempted termination of pregnancy

  Pulmonary embolism following failed attempted termination of pregnancy

  Pyemic embolism following failed attempted termination of pregnancy

  Septic or septicopyemic embolism following failed attempted termination of pregnancy

  Soap embolism following failed attempted termination of pregnancy

  CC Excl: PDX collection 958

√5ᵗʰ O07.3 Failed attempted termination of pregnancy with other and unspecified complications

  CC Excl: For CC codes in subcategory O07.3, unless otherwise noted: PDX collection 954

  O07.30 Failed attempted termination of pregnancy with unspecified complications `CC` `M` ♀

  O07.31 Shock following failed attempted termination of pregnancy `MCC` `M` ♀

    Circulatory collapse following failed attempted termination of pregnancy

    Shock (postprocedural) following failed attempted termination of pregnancy

    EXCLUDES 1 *shock due to infection following failed attempted termination of pregnancy (O07.37)*

    CC Excl: PDX collection 959

  O07.32 Renal failure following failed attempted termination of pregnancy `MCC` `M` ♀

    Kidney failure (acute) following failed attempted termination of pregnancy

    Oliguria following failed attempted termination of pregnancy

    Renal shutdown following failed attempted termination of pregnancy

    Renal tubular necrosis following failed attempted termination of pregnancy

    Uremia following failed attempted termination of pregnancy

    CC Excl: PDX collection 960

  O07.33 Metabolic disorder following failed attempted termination of pregnancy `CC` `M` ♀

  O07.34 Damage to pelvic organs following failed attempted termination of pregnancy `CC` `M` ♀

    Laceration, perforation, tear or chemical damage of bladder following failed attempted termination of pregnancy

    Laceration, perforation, tear or chemical damage of bowel following failed attempted termination of pregnancy

    Laceration, perforation, tear or chemical damage of broad ligament following failed attempted termination of pregnancy

    Laceration, perforation, tear or chemical damage of cervix following failed attempted termination of pregnancy

    Laceration, perforation, tear or chemical damage of periurethral tissue following failed attempted termination of pregnancy

    Laceration, perforation, tear or chemical damage of uterus following failed attempted termination of pregnancy

    Laceration, perforation, tear or chemical damage of vagina following failed attempted termination of pregnancy

    CC Excl: PDX collection 961

  O07.35 Other venous complications following failed attempted termination of pregnancy `CC` `M` ♀

O07.36 Cardiac arrest following failed attempted termination of pregnancy `CC` `M` ♀

O07.37 Sepsis following failed attempted termination of pregnancy `CC` `M` ♀

  Use additional code (B95-B97), to identify infectious agent

  Use additional code (R65.2-) to identify severe sepsis, if applicable

  EXCLUDES 1 *septic or septicopyemic embolism following failed attempted termination of pregnancy (O07.2)*

  CC Excl: PDX collection 956

O07.38 Urinary tract infection following failed attempted termination of pregnancy `CC` `M` ♀

  Cystitis following failed attempted termination of pregnancy

O07.39 Failed attempted termination of pregnancy with other complications `CC` `M` ♀

O07.4 Failed attempted termination of pregnancy without complication `M` ♀

√4ᵗʰ O08 Complications following ectopic and molar pregnancy

  This category is for use with categories O00-O02 to identify any associated complications

  CC Excl: For CC/MCC codes in category O08, unless otherwise noted: PDX collection 963

O08.0 Genital tract and pelvic infection following ectopic and molar pregnancy `CC` `M` ♀

  Endometritis following ectopic and molar pregnancy

  Oophoritis following ectopic and molar pregnancy

  Parametritis following ectopic and molar pregnancy

  Pelvic peritonitis following ectopic and molar pregnancy

  Salpingitis following ectopic and molar pregnancy

  Salpingo-oophoritis following ectopic and molar pregnancy

  EXCLUDES 1 *sepsis following ectopic and molar pregnancy (O08.82)*

    urinary tract infection (O08.83)

  CC Excl: PDX collection 85

O08.1 Delayed or excessive hemorrhage following ectopic and molar pregnancy `CC` `M` ♀

  Afibrinogenemia following ectopic and molar pregnancy

  Defibrination syndrome following ectopic and molar pregnancy

  Hemolysis following ectopic and molar pregnancy

  Intravascular coagulation following ectopic and molar pregnancy

  EXCLUDES 1 *delayed or excessive hemorrhage due to incomplete abortion (O03.1)*

  CC Excl: PDX collection 962

O08.2 Embolism following ectopic and molar pregnancy `MCC` `M` ♀

  Air embolism following ectopic and molar pregnancy

  Amniotic fluid embolism following ectopic and molar pregnancy

  Blood-clot embolism following ectopic and molar pregnancy

  Embolism NOS following ectopic and molar pregnancy

  Fat embolism following ectopic and molar pregnancy

  Pulmonary embolism following ectopic and molar pregnancy

  Pyemic embolism following ectopic and molar pregnancy

  Septic or septicopyemic embolism following ectopic and molar pregnancy

  Soap embolism following ectopic and molar pregnancy

O08.3 Shock following ectopic and molar pregnancy `MCC` `M` ♀

  Circulatory collapse following ectopic and molar pregnancy

  Shock (postprocedural) following ectopic and molar pregnancy

  EXCLUDES 1 *shock due to infection following ectopic and molar pregnancy (O08.82)*

O08.4 Renal failure following ectopic and molar pregnancy `MCC` `M` ♀

  Kidney failure (acute) following ectopic and molar pregnancy

  Oliguria following ectopic and molar pregnancy

  Renal shutdown following ectopic and molar pregnancy

  Renal tubular necrosis following ectopic and molar pregnancy

  Uremia following ectopic and molar pregnancy

O08.5 Metabolic disorders following an ectopic and molar pregnancy `CC` `M` ♀

✔ Additional Character Required   √x7ᵗʰ Placeholder   Unacceptable PDx   Questionable PDx   Manifestation   Unspecified Dx   H1-H14 HAC   HCC CMS-HCC Dx   HIV HIV Dx

ICD-10-CM 2020   881

O07.2–O08.5

O08.6 Damage to pelvic organs and tissues **following an ectopic and molar pregnancy** cc M ♀
Laceration, perforation, tear or chemical damage of bladder following an ectopic and molar pregnancy
Laceration, perforation, tear or chemical damage of bowel following an ectopic and molar pregnancy
Laceration, perforation, tear or chemical damage of broad ligament following an ectopic and molar pregnancy
Laceration, perforation, tear or chemical damage of cervix following an ectopic and molar pregnancy
Laceration, perforation, tear or chemical damage of periurethral tissue following an ectopic and molar pregnancy
Laceration, perforation, tear or chemical damage of uterus following an ectopic and molar pregnancy
Laceration, perforation, tear or chemical damage of vagina following an ectopic and molar pregnancy

O08.7 Other venous complications following an ectopic and molar pregnancy cc M ♀

✓5ᵗʰ **O08.8** Other complications following an ectopic and molar pregnancy

O08.81 Cardiac arrest following an ectopic and molar pregnancy cc M ♀

O08.82 Sepsis following ectopic and molar pregnancy cc M ♀
Use additional code (B95-B97), to identify infectious agent
Use additional code (R65.2-) to identify severe sepsis, if applicable
EXCLUDES 1 septic or septicopyemic embolism following ectopic and molar pregnancy (O08.2)
CC Excl: PDX collection 85

O08.83 Urinary tract infection following an ectopic and molar pregnancy cc M ♀
Cystitis following an ectopic and molar pregnancy

O08.89 Other complications following an ectopic and molar pregnancy cc M ♀

O08.9 Unspecified complication following an ectopic and molar pregnancy cc M ♀

Supervision of high risk pregnancy (O09)

✓4ᵗʰ **O09** Supervision of high risk pregnancy
AHA: 2016,4Q,48-50,150

✓5ᵗʰ **O09.0** Supervision of pregnancy with history of infertility
DEF: Infertility: Inability to conceive for at least one year with regular intercourse.

O09.00 Supervision of pregnancy with history of infertility, unspecified trimester M ♀

O09.01 Supervision of pregnancy with history of infertility, first trimester M ♀

O09.02 Supervision of pregnancy with history of infertility, second trimester M ♀

O09.03 Supervision of pregnancy with history of infertility, third trimester M ♀

✓5ᵗʰ **O09.1** Supervision of pregnancy with history of ectopic pregnancy
DEF: Ectopic pregnancy: Implantation of a fertilized egg outside the uterus, usually in the fallopian tube or abdomen that requires emergency treatment.

O09.10 Supervision of pregnancy with history of ectopic pregnancy, unspecified trimester M ♀

O09.11 Supervision of pregnancy with history of ectopic pregnancy, first trimester M ♀

O09.12 Supervision of pregnancy with history of ectopic pregnancy, second trimester M ♀

O09.13 Supervision of pregnancy with history of ectopic pregnancy, third trimester M ♀

✓5ᵗʰ **O09.A** Supervision of pregnancy with history of molar pregnancy
DEF: Molar pregnancy: Trophoblastic neoplasm that mimics pregnancy by proliferating from a pathologic ovum and resulting only in a mass of cysts resembling grapes, 80 percent of which are benign, but require surgical removal.

O09.A0 Supervision of pregnancy with history of molar pregnancy, unspecified trimester M ♀

O09.A1 Supervision of pregnancy with history of molar pregnancy, first trimester M ♀

O09.A2 Supervision of pregnancy with history of molar pregnancy, second trimester M ♀

O09.A3 Supervision of pregnancy with history of molar pregnancy, third trimester M ♀

✓5ᵗʰ **O09.2** Supervision of pregnancy with other poor reproductive or obstetric history
EXCLUDES 2 pregnancy care for patient with history of recurrent pregnancy loss (O26.2-)

✓6ᵗʰ **O09.21** Supervision of pregnancy with history of pre-term labor

O09.211 Supervision of pregnancy with history of pre-term labor, first trimester M ♀

O09.212 Supervision of pregnancy with history of pre-term labor, second trimester M ♀

O09.213 Supervision of pregnancy with history of pre-term labor, third trimester M ♀

O09.219 Supervision of pregnancy with history of pre-term labor, unspecified trimester M ♀

✓6ᵗʰ **O09.29** Supervision of pregnancy with other poor reproductive or obstetric history
Supervision of pregnancy with history of neonatal death
Supervision of pregnancy with history of stillbirth

O09.291 Supervision of pregnancy with other poor reproductive or obstetric history, first trimester M ♀

O09.292 Supervision of pregnancy with other poor reproductive or obstetric history, second trimester M ♀

O09.293 Supervision of pregnancy with other poor reproductive or obstetric history, third trimester M ♀

O09.299 Supervision of pregnancy with other poor reproductive or obstetric history, unspecified trimester M ♀

✓5ᵗʰ **O09.3** Supervision of pregnancy with insufficient antenatal care
Supervision of concealed pregnancy
Supervision of hidden pregnancy

O09.30 Supervision of pregnancy with insufficient antenatal care, unspecified trimester M ♀

O09.31 Supervision of pregnancy with insufficient antenatal care, first trimester M ♀

O09.32 Supervision of pregnancy with insufficient antenatal care, second trimester M ♀

O09.33 Supervision of pregnancy with insufficient antenatal care, third trimester M ♀

✓5ᵗʰ **O09.4** Supervision of pregnancy with grand multiparity

O09.40 Supervision of pregnancy with grand multiparity, unspecified trimester M ♀

O09.41 Supervision of pregnancy with grand multiparity, first trimester M ♀

O09.42 Supervision of pregnancy with grand multiparity, second trimester M ♀

O09.43 Supervision of pregnancy with grand multiparity, third trimester M ♀

✓5ᵗʰ **O09.5** Supervision of elderly primigravida and multigravida
Pregnancy for a female 35 years and older at expected date of delivery

✓6ᵗʰ **O09.51** Supervision of elderly primigravida

O09.511 Supervision of elderly primigravida, first trimester M ♀

O09.512 Supervision of elderly primigravida, second trimester M ♀

O09.513 Supervision of elderly primigravida, third trimester M ♀

O09.519 Supervision of elderly primigravida, unspecified trimester M ♀

✓6ᵗʰ **O09.52** Supervision of elderly multigravida

O09.521 Supervision of elderly multigravida, first trimester M ♀

O09.522 Supervision of elderly multigravida, second trimester M ♀

O09.523 Supervision of elderly multigravida, third trimester M ♀

O09.529 **Supervision of elderly multigravida, unspecified trimester** M ♀

✓5th O09.6 **Supervision of** young primigravida and multigravida

Supervision of pregnancy for a female less than 16 years old at expected date of delivery

✓6th O09.61 **Supervision of** young primigravida

O09.611 **Supervision of young primigravida,** first trimester M ♀

O09.612 **Supervision of young primigravida,** second trimester M ♀

O09.613 **Supervision of young primigravida,** third trimester M ♀

O09.619 **Supervision of young primigravida, unspecified trimester** M ♀

✓6th O09.62 **Supervision of** young multigravida

O09.621 **Supervision of young multigravida,** first trimester M ♀

O09.622 **Supervision of young multigravida,** second trimester M ♀

O09.623 **Supervision of young multigravida,** third trimester M ♀

O09.629 **Supervision of young multigravida, unspecified trimester** M ♀

✓5th O09.7 **Supervision of high risk pregnancy due to** social problems

O09.70 **Supervision of high risk pregnancy due to social problems, unspecified trimester** M ♀

O09.71 **Supervision of high risk pregnancy due to social problems,** first trimester M ♀

O09.72 **Supervision of high risk pregnancy due to social problems,** second trimester M ♀

O09.73 **Supervision of high risk pregnancy due to social problems,** third trimester M ♀

✓5th O09.8 **Supervision of other high risk pregnancies**

✓6th O09.81 **Supervision of pregnancy** resulting from assisted reproductive technology

Supervision of pregnancy resulting from in-vitro fertilization

EXCLUDES 2 gestational carrier status (Z33.3)

O09.811 **Supervision of pregnancy resulting from assisted reproductive technology,** first trimester M ♀

O09.812 **Supervision of pregnancy resulting from assisted reproductive technology,** second trimester M ♀

O09.813 **Supervision of pregnancy resulting from assisted reproductive technology,** third trimester M ♀

O09.819 **Supervision of pregnancy resulting from assisted reproductive technology, unspecified trimester** M ♀

✓6th O09.82 **Supervision of pregnancy with** history of in utero procedure during previous pregnancy

O09.821 **Supervision of pregnancy with history of in utero procedure during previous pregnancy,** first trimester M ♀

O09.822 **Supervision of pregnancy with history of in utero procedure during previous pregnancy,** second trimester M ♀

O09.823 **Supervision of pregnancy with history of in utero procedure during previous pregnancy,** third trimester M ♀

O09.829 **Supervision of pregnancy with history of in utero procedure during previous pregnancy, unspecified trimester** M ♀

EXCLUDES 1 supervision of pregnancy affected by in utero procedure during current pregnancy (O35.7)

✓6th O09.89 **Supervision of other high risk pregnancies**

O09.891 **Supervision of other high risk pregnancies,** first trimester M ♀

O09.892 **Supervision of other high risk pregnancies,** second trimester M ♀

O09.893 **Supervision of other high risk pregnancies,** third trimester M ♀

O09.899 **Supervision of other high risk pregnancies, unspecified trimester** M ♀

✓5th O09.9 **Supervision of high risk pregnancy, unspecified**

O09.90 **Supervision of high risk pregnancy, unspecified, unspecified trimester** M ♀

O09.91 **Supervision of high risk pregnancy, unspecified,** first trimester M ♀

O09.92 **Supervision of high risk pregnancy, unspecified,** second trimester M ♀

O09.93 **Supervision of high risk pregnancy, unspecified,** third trimester M ♀

Edema, proteinuria and hypertensive disorders in pregnancy, childbirth and the puerperium (O10-O16)

AHA: 2016,4Q,50

CC Excl: For CC/MCC codes in categories O10-O16, unless otherwise noted: PDX collection 964

✓4th O10 Pre-existing hypertension complicating pregnancy, childbirth and the puerperium

INCLUDES pre-existing hypertension with pre-existing proteinuria complicating pregnancy, childbirth and the puerperium

EXCLUDES 2 pre-existing hypertension with superimposed pre-eclampsia complicating pregnancy, childbirth and the puerperium (O11.-)

✓5th O10.0 **Pre-existing** essential **hypertension complicating pregnancy, childbirth and the puerperium**

Any condition in I10 specified as a reason for obstetric care during pregnancy, childbirth or the puerperium

✓6th O10.01 **Pre-existing essential hypertension complicating** pregnancy

O10.011 **Pre-existing essential hypertension complicating pregnancy,** first trimester CC M ♀

O10.012 **Pre-existing essential hypertension complicating pregnancy,** second trimester CC M ♀

O10.013 **Pre-existing essential hypertension complicating pregnancy,** third trimester CC M ♀

O10.019 **Pre-existing essential hypertension complicating pregnancy, unspecified trimester** M ♀

O10.02 **Pre-existing essential hypertension complicating** childbirth CC M ♀

O10.03 **Pre-existing essential hypertension complicating the** puerperium M ♀

✓5th O10.1 **Pre-existing hypertensive** heart disease **complicating pregnancy, childbirth and the puerperium**

Any condition in I11 specified as a reason for obstetric care during pregnancy, childbirth or the puerperium

Use additional code from I11 to identify the type of hypertensive heart disease

✓6th O10.11 **Pre-existing hypertensive heart disease complicating** pregnancy

O10.111 **Pre-existing hypertensive heart disease complicating pregnancy,** first trimester M ♀

O10.112 **Pre-existing hypertensive heart disease complicating pregnancy,** second trimester M ♀

O10.113 **Pre-existing hypertensive heart disease complicating pregnancy,** third trimester M ♀

O10.119 **Pre-existing hypertensive heart disease complicating pregnancy, unspecified trimester** M ♀

O10.12 **Pre-existing hypertensive heart disease complicating** childbirth M ♀

O10.13 **Pre-existing hypertensive heart disease complicating the** puerperium M ♀

☑ Additional Character Required   ✓x7th Placeholder   Unacceptable PDx   Questionable PDx   Manifestation   Unspecified Dx   H1-H14 HAC   HCC CMS-HCC Dx   HIV HIV Dx

ICD-10-CM 2020   883

Chapter 15. Pregnancy, Childbirth and the Puerperium

O10.2–O12.25

√5ᵗʰ **O10.2** **Pre-existing hypertensive chronic kidney disease complicating pregnancy, childbirth and the puerperium**
Any condition in I12 specified as a reason for obstetric care during pregnancy, childbirth or the puerperium
Use additional code from I12 to identify the type of hypertensive chronic kidney disease

√6ᵗʰ **O10.21** **Pre-existing hypertensive chronic kidney disease complicating pregnancy**

O10.211 Pre-existing hypertensive chronic kidney disease complicating pregnancy, first trimester   M ♀

O10.212 Pre-existing hypertensive chronic kidney disease complicating pregnancy, second trimester   M ♀

O10.213 Pre-existing hypertensive chronic kidney disease complicating pregnancy, third trimester   M ♀

O10.219 Pre-existing hypertensive chronic kidney disease complicating pregnancy, unspecified trimester   M ♀

O10.22 Pre-existing hypertensive chronic kidney disease complicating childbirth   M ♀

O10.23 Pre-existing hypertensive chronic kidney disease complicating the puerperium   M ♀

√5ᵗʰ **O10.3** **Pre-existing hypertensive heart and chronic kidney disease complicating pregnancy, childbirth and the puerperium**
Any condition in I13 specified as a reason for obstetric care during pregnancy, childbirth or the puerperium
Use additional code from I13 to identify the type of hypertensive heart and chronic kidney disease

√6ᵗʰ **O10.31** **Pre-existing hypertensive heart and chronic kidney disease complicating pregnancy**

O10.311 Pre-existing hypertensive heart and chronic kidney disease complicating pregnancy, first trimester   M ♀

O10.312 Pre-existing hypertensive heart and chronic kidney disease complicating pregnancy, second trimester   M ♀

O10.313 Pre-existing hypertensive heart and chronic kidney disease complicating pregnancy, third trimester   M ♀

O10.319 Pre-existing hypertensive heart and chronic kidney disease complicating pregnancy, unspecified trimester   M ♀

O10.32 Pre-existing hypertensive heart and chronic kidney disease complicating childbirth   M ♀

O10.33 Pre-existing hypertensive heart and chronic kidney disease complicating the puerperium   M ♀

√5ᵗʰ **O10.4** **Pre-existing secondary hypertension complicating pregnancy, childbirth and the puerperium**
Any condition in I15 specified as a reason for obstetric care during pregnancy, childbirth or the puerperium
Use additional code from I15 to identify the type of secondary hypertension

√6ᵗʰ **O10.41** **Pre-existing secondary hypertension complicating pregnancy**

O10.411 Pre-existing secondary hypertension complicating pregnancy, first trimester   CC M ♀

O10.412 Pre-existing secondary hypertension complicating pregnancy, second trimester   CC M ♀

O10.413 Pre-existing secondary hypertension complicating pregnancy, third trimester   CC M ♀

O10.419 Pre-existing secondary hypertension complicating pregnancy, unspecified trimester   M ♀

O10.42 Pre-existing secondary hypertension complicating childbirth   MCC M ♀

O10.43 Pre-existing secondary hypertension complicating the puerperium   CC M ♀

√5ᵗʰ **O10.9** **Unspecified pre-existing hypertension complicating pregnancy, childbirth and the puerperium**

√6ᵗʰ **O10.91** **Unspecified pre-existing hypertension complicating pregnancy**

O10.911 Unspecified pre-existing hypertension complicating pregnancy, first trimester   CC M ♀

O10.912 Unspecified pre-existing hypertension complicating pregnancy, second trimester   CC M ♀

O10.913 Unspecified pre-existing hypertension complicating pregnancy, third trimester   CC M ♀

O10.919 Unspecified pre-existing hypertension complicating pregnancy, unspecified trimester   M ♀

O10.92 Unspecified pre-existing hypertension complicating childbirth   CC M ♀

O10.93 Unspecified pre-existing hypertension complicating the puerperium   M ♀

√4ᵗʰ **O11** **Pre-existing hypertension with pre-eclampsia**

INCLUDES   conditions in O10 complicated by pre-eclampsia
pre-eclampsia superimposed pre-existing in hypertension
Use additional code from O10 to identify the type of hypertension
DEF: Complication of pregnancy manifesting in the development of borderline hypertension, protein in the urine, and unresponsive swelling between the 20th week of pregnancy and the end of the first week following birth in mild to moderate cases. Severe preeclampsia presents with hypertension, associated with marked swelling, proteinuria, abdominal pain, and/or visual changes.

O11.1 Pre-existing hypertension with pre-eclampsia, first trimester   MCC M ♀

O11.2 Pre-existing hypertension with pre-eclampsia, second trimester   MCC M ♀

O11.3 Pre-existing hypertension with pre-eclampsia, third trimester   MCC M ♀

O11.4 Pre-existing hypertension with pre-eclampsia, complicating childbirth   M ♀

O11.5 Pre-existing hypertension with pre-eclampsia, complicating the puerperium   M ♀

O11.9 Pre-existing hypertension with pre-eclampsia, unspecified trimester   M ♀

√4ᵗʰ **O12** **Gestational [pregnancy-induced] edema and proteinuria without hypertension**
CC Excl: For CC codes in category O12: PDX collection 965

√5ᵗʰ **O12.0** **Gestational edema**

O12.00 Gestational edema, unspecified trimester   M ♀

O12.01 Gestational edema, first trimester   M ♀

O12.02 Gestational edema, second trimester   M ♀

O12.03 Gestational edema, third trimester   M ♀

O12.04 Gestational edema, complicating childbirth   M ♀

O12.05 Gestational edema, complicating the puerperium   M ♀

√5ᵗʰ **O12.1** **Gestational proteinuria**

O12.10 Gestational proteinuria, unspecified trimester   M ♀

O12.11 Gestational proteinuria, first trimester   CC M ♀

O12.12 Gestational proteinuria, second trimester   CC M ♀

O12.13 Gestational proteinuria, third trimester   CC M ♀

O12.14 Gestational proteinuria, complicating childbirth   M ♀

O12.15 Gestational proteinuria, complicating the puerperium   M ♀

√5ᵗʰ **O12.2** **Gestational edema with proteinuria**

O12.20 Gestational edema with proteinuria, unspecified trimester   M ♀

O12.21 Gestational edema with proteinuria, first trimester   CC M ♀

O12.22 Gestational edema with proteinuria, second trimester   CC M ♀

O12.23 Gestational edema with proteinuria, third trimester   CC M ♀

O12.24 Gestational edema with proteinuria, complicating childbirth   M ♀

O12.25 Gestational edema with proteinuria, complicating the puerperium   M ♀

✓4ᵗʰ O13   Gestational [pregnancy-induced] hypertension without significant proteinuria

INCLUDES   gestational hypertension NOS
         transient hypertension of pregnancy
AHA: 2016,1Q,5

O13.1   **Gestational [pregnancy-induced] hypertension without significant proteinuria, first trimester**   M ♀

O13.2   **Gestational [pregnancy-induced] hypertension without significant proteinuria, second trimester**   M ♀

O13.3   **Gestational [pregnancy-induced] hypertension without significant proteinuria, third trimester**   M ♀

O13.4   **Gestational [pregnancy-induced] hypertension without significant proteinuria, complicating childbirth**   M ♀

O13.5   **Gestational [pregnancy-induced] hypertension without significant proteinuria, complicating the puerperium**   M ♀

O13.9   **Gestational [pregnancy-induced] hypertension without significant proteinuria, unspecified trimester**   M ♀

✓4ᵗʰ O14   Pre-eclampsia

EXCLUDES 1   pre-existing hypertension with pre-eclampsia (O11)
DEF: Complication of pregnancy manifesting in the development of borderline hypertension, protein in the urine, and unresponsive swelling between the 20th week of pregnancy and the end of the first week following birth in mild to moderate cases. Severe preeclampsia presents with hypertension, associated with marked swelling, proteinuria, abdominal pain, and/or visual changes.

✓5ᵗʰ O14.0   Mild to moderate pre-eclampsia
AHA: 2019,2Q,8

O14.00   **Mild to moderate pre-eclampsia, unspecified trimester**   M ♀

O14.02   **Mild to moderate pre-eclampsia, second trimester**   cc M ♀

O14.03   **Mild to moderate pre-eclampsia, third trimester**   cc M ♀

O14.04   **Mild to moderate pre-eclampsia, complicating childbirth**   M ♀
     AHA: 2019,2Q,8

O14.05   **Mild to moderate pre-eclampsia, complicating the puerperium**   M ♀

✓5ᵗʰ O14.1   Severe pre-eclampsia
EXCLUDES 1   HELLP syndrome (O14.2-)

O14.10   **Severe pre-eclampsia, unspecified trimester**   M ♀

O14.12   **Severe pre-eclampsia, second trimester**   MCC M ♀

O14.13   **Severe pre-eclampsia, third trimester**   MCC M ♀

O14.14   **Severe pre-eclampsia complicating childbirth**   M ♀

O14.15   **Severe pre-eclampsia, complicating the puerperium**   M ♀

✓5ᵗʰ O14.2   HELLP syndrome
Severe pre-eclampsia with hemolysis, elevated liver enzymes and low platelet count (HELLP)

O14.20   **HELLP syndrome (HELLP), unspecified trimester**   M ♀

O14.22   **HELLP syndrome (HELLP), second trimester**   MCC M ♀

O14.23   **HELLP syndrome (HELLP), third trimester**   MCC M ♀

O14.24   **HELLP syndrome, complicating childbirth**   M ♀

O14.25   **HELLP syndrome, complicating the puerperium**   M ♀

✓5ᵗʰ O14.9   Unspecified pre-eclampsia

O14.90   **Unspecified pre-eclampsia, unspecified trimester**   M ♀

O14.92   **Unspecified pre-eclampsia, second trimester**   cc M ♀

O14.93   **Unspecified pre-eclampsia, third trimester**   cc M ♀

O14.94   **Unspecified pre-eclampsia, complicating childbirth**   M ♀

O14.95   **Unspecified pre-eclampsia, complicating the puerperium**   M ♀

✓4ᵗʰ O15   Eclampsia

INCLUDES   convulsions following conditions in O10-O14 and O16
DEF: Tetany and toxemia producing seizure activity or coma in a pregnant patient who most often has presented with prior preeclampsia (i.e., hypertension, albuminuria, and edema).

✓5ᵗʰ O15.0   Eclampsia complicating pregnancy

O15.00   **Eclampsia complicating pregnancy, unspecified trimester**   M ♀

O15.02   **Eclampsia complicating pregnancy, second trimester**   MCC M ♀

O15.03   **Eclampsia complicating pregnancy, third trimester**   MCC M ♀

O15.1   **Eclampsia complicating labor**   MCC M ♀

O15.2   **Eclampsia complicating the puerperium**   MCC M ♀

O15.9   **Eclampsia, unspecified as to time period**   M ♀
     Eclampsia NOS

✓4ᵗʰ O16   Unspecified maternal hypertension

O16.1   **Unspecified maternal hypertension, first trimester**   cc M ♀

O16.2   **Unspecified maternal hypertension, second trimester**   cc M ♀

O16.3   **Unspecified maternal hypertension, third trimester**   cc M ♀

O16.4   **Unspecified maternal hypertension, complicating childbirth**   M ♀

O16.5   **Unspecified maternal hypertension, complicating the puerperium**   M ♀

O16.9   **Unspecified maternal hypertension, unspecified trimester**   M ♀

Other maternal disorders predominantly related to pregnancy (O20-O29)

EXCLUDES 2   maternal care related to the fetus and amniotic cavity and possible delivery problems (O30-O48)
     maternal diseases classifiable elsewhere but complicating pregnancy, labor and delivery, and the puerperium (O98-O99)

✓4ᵗʰ O20   Hemorrhage in early pregnancy

INCLUDES   hemorrhage before completion of 20 weeks gestation
EXCLUDES 1   pregnancy with abortive outcome (O00-O08)

O20.0   **Threatened abortion**   cc M ♀
     Hemorrhage specified as due to threatened abortion
     DEF: Bloody discharge during pregnancy. The cervix may be dilated and pregnancy threatened, but the pregnancy is not terminated.
     CC Excl: PDX collection 966

O20.8   **Other hemorrhage in early pregnancy**   M ♀

O20.9   **Hemorrhage in early pregnancy, unspecified**   cc M ♀
     CC Excl: PDX collection 966

✓4ᵗʰ O21   Excessive vomiting in pregnancy

O21.0   **Mild hyperemesis gravidarum**   M ♀
     Hyperemesis gravidarum, mild or unspecified, starting before the end of the 20th week of gestation

O21.1   **Hyperemesis gravidarum with metabolic disturbance**   M ♀
     Hyperemesis gravidarum, starting before the end of the 20th week of gestation, with metabolic disturbance such as carbohydrate depletion
     Hyperemesis gravidarum, starting before the end of the 20th week of gestation, with metabolic disturbance such as dehydration
     Hyperemesis gravidarum, starting before the end of the 20th week of gestation, with metabolic disturbance such as electrolyte imbalance

O21.2   **Late vomiting of pregnancy**   M ♀
     Excessive vomiting starting after 20 completed weeks of gestation

O21.8   **Other vomiting complicating pregnancy**   M ♀
     Vomiting due to diseases classified elsewhere, complicating pregnancy
     Use additional code, to identify cause

O21.9   **Vomiting of pregnancy, unspecified**   M ♀

Chapter 15. Pregnancy, Childbirth and the Puerperium

O22–O23.33

√4ᵗʰ **O22 Venous complications and hemorrhoids in pregnancy**

> EXCLUDES 1   venous complications of:
> abortion NOS (O03.9)
> ectopic or molar pregnancy (O08.7)
> failed attempted abortion (O07.35)
> induced abortion (O04.85)
> spontaneous abortion (O03.89)
>
> EXCLUDES 2   obstetric pulmonary embolism (O88.-)
> venous complications and hemorrhoids of childbirth and the puerperium (O87.-)

CC Excl: For CC/MCC codes in category O22: PDX collection 967

√5ᵗʰ **O22.0 Varicose veins of lower extremity in pregnancy**

> Varicose veins NOS in pregnancy
> **DEF:** Distended, tortuous veins of the lower extremities associated with pregnancy.

O22.00	Varicose veins of lower extremity in pregnancy, unspecified trimester	Ⓜ ♀
O22.01	Varicose veins of lower extremity in pregnancy, first trimester	Ⓜ ♀
O22.02	Varicose veins of lower extremity in pregnancy, second trimester	Ⓜ ♀
O22.03	Varicose veins of lower extremity in pregnancy, third trimester	Ⓜ ♀

√5ᵗʰ **O22.1 Genital varices in pregnancy**

> Perineal varices in pregnancy
> Vaginal varices in pregnancy
> Vulval varices in pregnancy

O22.10	Genital varices in pregnancy, unspecified trimester	Ⓜ ♀
O22.11	Genital varices in pregnancy, first trimester	Ⓜ ♀
O22.12	Genital varices in pregnancy, second trimester	Ⓜ ♀
O22.13	Genital varices in pregnancy, third trimester	Ⓜ ♀

√5ᵗʰ **O22.2 Superficial thrombophlebitis in pregnancy**

> Phlebitis in pregnancy NOS
> Thrombophlebitis of legs in pregnancy
> Thrombosis in pregnancy NOS
> Use additional code to identify the superficial thrombophlebitis (I80.0-)

O22.20	Superficial thrombophlebitis in pregnancy, unspecified trimester	CC Ⓜ ♀
O22.21	Superficial thrombophlebitis in pregnancy, first trimester	CC Ⓜ ♀
O22.22	Superficial thrombophlebitis in pregnancy, second trimester	CC Ⓜ ♀
O22.23	Superficial thrombophlebitis in pregnancy, third trimester	CC Ⓜ ♀

√5ᵗʰ **O22.3 Deep phlebothrombosis in pregnancy**

> Deep vein thrombosis, antepartum
> Use additional code to identify the deep vein thrombosis (I82.4-, I82.5-, I82.62-, I82.72-)
> Use additional code, if applicable, for associated long-term (current) use of anticoagulants (Z79.01)

O22.30	Deep phlebothrombosis in pregnancy, unspecified trimester	CC Ⓜ ♀
O22.31	Deep phlebothrombosis in pregnancy, first trimester	MCC Ⓜ ♀
O22.32	Deep phlebothrombosis in pregnancy, second trimester	MCC Ⓜ ♀
O22.33	Deep phlebothrombosis in pregnancy, third trimester	MCC Ⓜ ♀

√5ᵗʰ **O22.4 Hemorrhoids in pregnancy**

O22.40	Hemorrhoids in pregnancy, unspecified trimester	CC Ⓜ ♀
O22.41	Hemorrhoids in pregnancy, first trimester	CC Ⓜ ♀
O22.42	Hemorrhoids in pregnancy, second trimester	CC Ⓜ ♀
O22.43	Hemorrhoids in pregnancy, third trimester	CC Ⓜ ♀

√5ᵗʰ **O22.5 Cerebral venous thrombosis in pregnancy**

> Cerebrovenous sinus thrombosis in pregnancy

O22.50	Cerebral venous thrombosis in pregnancy, unspecified trimester	CC Ⓜ ♀
O22.51	Cerebral venous thrombosis in pregnancy, first trimester	CC Ⓜ ♀
O22.52	Cerebral venous thrombosis in pregnancy, second trimester	CC Ⓜ ♀
O22.53	Cerebral venous thrombosis in pregnancy, third trimester	CC Ⓜ ♀

√5ᵗʰ **O22.8 Other venous complications in pregnancy**

√6ᵗʰ **O22.8X Other venous complications in pregnancy**

O22.8X1	Other venous complications in pregnancy, first trimester	CC Ⓜ ♀
O22.8X2	Other venous complications in pregnancy, second trimester	CC Ⓜ ♀
O22.8X3	Other venous complications in pregnancy, third trimester	CC Ⓜ ♀
O22.8X9	Other venous complications in pregnancy, unspecified trimester	CC Ⓜ ♀

√5ᵗʰ **O22.9 Venous complication in pregnancy, unspecified**

> Gestational phlebitis NOS
> Gestational phlebopathy NOS
> Gestational thrombosis NOS

O22.90	Venous complication in pregnancy, unspecified, unspecified trimester	CC Ⓜ ♀
O22.91	Venous complication in pregnancy, unspecified, first trimester	Ⓜ ♀
O22.92	Venous complication in pregnancy, unspecified, second trimester	Ⓜ ♀
O22.93	Venous complication in pregnancy, unspecified, third trimester	Ⓜ ♀

√4ᵗʰ **O23 Infections of genitourinary tract in pregnancy**

> Use additional code to identify organism (B95.-, B96.-)
>
> EXCLUDES 2   gonococcal infections complicating pregnancy, childbirth and the puerperium (O98.2)
> infections with a predominantly sexual mode of transmission NOS complicating pregnancy, childbirth and the puerperium (O98.3)
> syphilis complicating pregnancy, childbirth and the puerperium (O98.1)
> tuberculosis of genitourinary system complicating pregnancy, childbirth and the puerperium (O98.0)
> venereal disease NOS complicating pregnancy, childbirth and the puerperium (O98.3)

AHA: 2018,2Q,20

CC Excl: For CC codes in category O23: PDX collection 968

√5ᵗʰ **O23.0 Infections of kidney in pregnancy**

> Pyelonephritis in pregnancy

O23.00	Infections of kidney in pregnancy, unspecified trimester	Ⓜ ♀
O23.01	Infections of kidney in pregnancy, first trimester	CC Ⓜ ♀
O23.02	Infections of kidney in pregnancy, second trimester	CC Ⓜ ♀
O23.03	Infections of kidney in pregnancy, third trimester	CC Ⓜ ♀

√5ᵗʰ **O23.1 Infections of bladder in pregnancy**

O23.10	Infections of bladder in pregnancy, unspecified trimester	Ⓜ ♀
O23.11	Infections of bladder in pregnancy, first trimester	CC Ⓜ ♀
O23.12	Infections of bladder in pregnancy, second trimester	CC Ⓜ ♀
O23.13	Infections of bladder in pregnancy, third trimester	CC Ⓜ ♀

√5ᵗʰ **O23.2 Infections of urethra in pregnancy**

O23.20	Infections of urethra in pregnancy, unspecified trimester	Ⓜ ♀
O23.21	Infections of urethra in pregnancy, first trimester	CC Ⓜ ♀
O23.22	Infections of urethra in pregnancy, second trimester	CC Ⓜ ♀
O23.23	Infections of urethra in pregnancy, third trimester	CC Ⓜ ♀

√5ᵗʰ **O23.3 Infections of other parts of urinary tract in pregnancy**

O23.30	Infections of other parts of urinary tract in pregnancy, unspecified trimester	Ⓜ ♀
O23.31	Infections of other parts of urinary tract in pregnancy, first trimester	CC Ⓜ ♀
O23.32	Infections of other parts of urinary tract in pregnancy, second trimester	CC Ⓜ ♀
O23.33	Infections of other parts of urinary tract in pregnancy, third trimester	CC Ⓜ ♀

Ⓝ Newborn: 0   Ⓟ Pediatric: 0-17   Ⓜ Maternity: 9-64   Ⓐ Adult: 15-124   MCC Major Complication/Comorbidity   CC Complication/Comorbidity   SW Severe Wound Dx

886   ICD-10-CM 2020

✓5ᵗʰ **O23.4** **Unspecified infection of urinary tract in pregnancy**

    O23.40 **Unspecified infection of urinary tract in pregnancy, unspecified trimester** M ♀

    O23.41 **Unspecified infection of urinary tract in pregnancy, first trimester** cc M ♀

    O23.42 **Unspecified infection of urinary tract in pregnancy, second trimester** cc M ♀

    O23.43 **Unspecified infection of urinary tract in pregnancy, third trimester** cc M ♀

✓5ᵗʰ **O23.5** **Infections of the genital tract in pregnancy**

    ✓6ᵗʰ **O23.51** **Infection of cervix in pregnancy**

        O23.511 **Infections of cervix in pregnancy, first trimester** cc M ♀

        O23.512 **Infections of cervix in pregnancy, second trimester** cc M ♀

        O23.513 **Infections of cervix in pregnancy, third trimester** cc M ♀

        O23.519 **Infections of cervix in pregnancy, unspecified trimester** M ♀

    ✓6ᵗʰ **O23.52** **Salpingo-oophoritis in pregnancy**

        Oophoritis in pregnancy

        Salpingitis in pregnancy

        O23.521 **Salpingo-oophoritis in pregnancy, first trimester** cc M ♀

        O23.522 **Salpingo-oophoritis in pregnancy, second trimester** cc M ♀

        O23.523 **Salpingo-oophoritis in pregnancy, third trimester** cc M ♀

        O23.529 **Salpingo-oophoritis in pregnancy, unspecified trimester** M ♀

    ✓6ᵗʰ **O23.59** **Infection of other part of genital tract in pregnancy**

        O23.591 **Infection of other part of genital tract in pregnancy, first trimester** cc M ♀

        O23.592 **Infection of other part of genital tract in pregnancy, second trimester** cc M ♀

        O23.593 **Infection of other part of genital tract in pregnancy, third trimester** cc M ♀

        O23.599 **Infection of other part of genital tract in pregnancy, unspecified trimester** M ♀

    ✓6ᵗʰ **O23.9** **Unspecified genitourinary tract infection in pregnancy**

        Genitourinary tract infection in pregnancy NOS

    O23.90 **Unspecified genitourinary tract infection in pregnancy, unspecified trimester** M ♀

    O23.91 **Unspecified genitourinary tract infection in pregnancy, first trimester** cc M ♀

    O23.92 **Unspecified genitourinary tract infection in pregnancy, second trimester** cc M ♀

    O23.93 **Unspecified genitourinary tract infection in pregnancy, third trimester** cc M ♀

✓4ᵗʰ **O24** **Diabetes mellitus in pregnancy, childbirth and the puerperium**

    CC Excl: For CC codes in category O24: PDX collection 969

✓5ᵗʰ **O24.0** **Pre-existing type 1 diabetes mellitus, in pregnancy, childbirth and the puerperium**

    Juvenile onset diabetes mellitus, in pregnancy, childbirth and the puerperium

    Ketosis-prone diabetes mellitus in pregnancy, childbirth and the puerperium

    Use additional code from category E10 to further identify any manifestations

    ✓6ᵗʰ **O24.01** **Pre-existing type 1 diabetes mellitus, in pregnancy**

        O24.011 **Pre-existing type 1 diabetes mellitus, in pregnancy, first trimester** cc M ♀

        O24.012 **Pre-existing type 1 diabetes mellitus, in pregnancy, second trimester** cc M ♀

        O24.013 **Pre-existing type 1 diabetes mellitus, in pregnancy, third trimester** cc M ♀

        O24.019 **Pre-existing type 1 diabetes mellitus, in pregnancy, unspecified trimester** cc M ♀

    O24.02 **Pre-existing type 1 diabetes mellitus, in childbirth** cc M ♀

    O24.03 **Pre-existing type 1 diabetes mellitus, in the puerperium** cc M ♀

✓5ᵗʰ **O24.1** **Pre-existing type 2 diabetes mellitus, in pregnancy, childbirth and the puerperium**

    Insulin-resistant diabetes mellitus in pregnancy, childbirth and the puerperium

    Use additional code (for):

        from category E11 to further identify any manifestations

        long-term (current) use of insulin (Z79.4)

    ✓6ᵗʰ **O24.11** **Pre-existing type 2 diabetes mellitus, in pregnancy**

        O24.111 **Pre-existing type 2 diabetes mellitus, in pregnancy, first trimester** cc M ♀

        O24.112 **Pre-existing type 2 diabetes mellitus, in pregnancy, second trimester** cc M ♀

        O24.113 **Pre-existing type 2 diabetes mellitus, in pregnancy, third trimester** cc M ♀

        O24.119 **Pre-existing type 2 diabetes mellitus, in pregnancy, unspecified trimester** cc M ♀

    O24.12 **Pre-existing type 2 diabetes mellitus, in childbirth** cc M ♀

    O24.13 **Pre-existing type 2 diabetes mellitus, in the puerperium** cc M ♀

✓5ᵗʰ **O24.3** **Unspecified pre-existing diabetes mellitus in pregnancy, childbirth and the puerperium**

    Use additional code (for):

        from category E11 to further identify any manifestation

        long-term (current) use of insulin (Z79.4)

    ✓6ᵗʰ **O24.31** **Unspecified pre-existing diabetes mellitus in pregnancy**

        O24.311 **Unspecified pre-existing diabetes mellitus in pregnancy, first trimester** cc M ♀

        O24.312 **Unspecified pre-existing diabetes mellitus in pregnancy, second trimester** cc M ♀

        O24.313 **Unspecified pre-existing diabetes mellitus in pregnancy, third trimester** cc M ♀

        O24.319 **Unspecified pre-existing diabetes mellitus in pregnancy, unspecified trimester** cc M ♀

    O24.32 **Unspecified pre-existing diabetes mellitus in childbirth** cc M ♀

    O24.33 **Unspecified pre-existing diabetes mellitus in the puerperium** cc M ♀

✓5ᵗʰ **O24.4** **Gestational diabetes mellitus**

    Diabetes mellitus arising in pregnancy

    Gestational diabetes mellitus NOS

    AHA: 2016,4Q,50; 2015,4Q,34

    ✓6ᵗʰ **O24.41** **Gestational diabetes mellitus in pregnancy**

        O24.410 **Gestational diabetes mellitus in pregnancy, diet controlled** M ♀

        O24.414 **Gestational diabetes mellitus in pregnancy, insulin controlled** cc M ♀

        O24.415 **Gestational diabetes mellitus in pregnancy, controlled by oral hypoglycemic drugs** cc M ♀

        Gestational diabetes mellitus in pregnancy, controlled by oral antidiabetic drugs

        O24.419 **Gestational diabetes mellitus in pregnancy, unspecified control** M ♀

    ✓6ᵗʰ **O24.42** **Gestational diabetes mellitus in childbirth**

        AHA: 2016,1Q,5

        O24.420 **Gestational diabetes mellitus in childbirth, diet controlled** M ♀

        O24.424 **Gestational diabetes mellitus in childbirth, insulin controlled** cc M ♀

        O24.425 **Gestational diabetes mellitus in childbirth, controlled by oral hypoglycemic drugs** cc M ♀

        Gestational diabetes mellitus in childbirth, controlled by oral antidiabetic drugs

        O24.429 **Gestational diabetes mellitus in childbirth, unspecified control** M ♀

✅ Additional Character Required   ✓x7ᵗʰ Placeholder   Unacceptable PDx   Questionable PDx   Manifestation   Unspecified Dx   H1-H14 HAC   HCC CMS-HCC Dx   HIV HIV Dx

ICD-10-CM 2020   887

Chapter 15. Pregnancy, Childbirth and the Puerperium

✓6ᵗʰ **O24.43 Gestational diabetes mellitus in the** puerperium

    O24.430 Gestational diabetes mellitus in the puerperium, diet controlled   M ♀

    O24.434 Gestational diabetes mellitus in the puerperium, insulin controlled   CC M ♀

    O24.435 Gestational diabetes mellitus in puerperium, controlled by oral hypoglycemic drugs   CC M ♀

        Gestational diabetes mellitus in puerperium, controlled by oral antidiabetic drugs

    O24.439 Gestational diabetes mellitus in the puerperium, unspecified control   M ♀

✓5ᵗʰ **O24.8 Other pre-existing diabetes mellitus in pregnancy, childbirth, and the puerperium**

    Use additional code (for):

        from categories E08, E09 and E13 to further identify any manifestation

        long-term (current) use of insulin (Z79.4)

  ✓6ᵗʰ **O24.81 Other pre-existing diabetes mellitus in** pregnancy

    O24.811 Other pre-existing diabetes mellitus in pregnancy, first trimester   CC M ♀

    O24.812 Other pre-existing diabetes mellitus in pregnancy, second trimester   CC M ♀

    O24.813 Other pre-existing diabetes mellitus in pregnancy, third trimester   CC M ♀

    O24.819 Other pre-existing diabetes mellitus in pregnancy, unspecified trimester   CC M ♀

  O24.82 Other pre-existing diabetes mellitus in childbirth   CC M ♀

  O24.83 Other pre-existing diabetes mellitus in the puerperium   CC M ♀

✓5ᵗʰ **O24.9 Unspecified diabetes mellitus in pregnancy, childbirth and the puerperium**

    Use additional code for long-term (current) use of insulin (Z79.4)

  ✓6ᵗʰ **O24.91 Unspecified diabetes mellitus in** pregnancy

    O24.911 Unspecified diabetes mellitus in pregnancy, first trimester   CC M ♀

    O24.912 Unspecified diabetes mellitus in pregnancy, second trimester   CC M ♀

    O24.913 Unspecified diabetes mellitus in pregnancy, third trimester   CC M ♀

    O24.919 Unspecified diabetes mellitus in pregnancy, unspecified trimester   CC M ♀

  O24.92 Unspecified diabetes mellitus in childbirth   CC M ♀

  O24.93 Unspecified diabetes mellitus in the puerperium   CC M ♀

✓4ᵗʰ **O25 Malnutrition in pregnancy, childbirth and the puerperium**

  ✓5ᵗʰ **O25.1 Malnutrition in** pregnancy

    O25.10 Malnutrition in pregnancy, unspecified trimester   M ♀

    O25.11 Malnutrition in pregnancy, first trimester   M ♀

    O25.12 Malnutrition in pregnancy, second trimester   M ♀

    O25.13 Malnutrition in pregnancy, third trimester   M ♀

  O25.2 Malnutrition in childbirth   M ♀

  O25.3 Malnutrition in the puerperium   M ♀

✓4ᵗʰ **O26 Maternal care for other conditions predominantly related to pregnancy**

  ✓5ᵗʰ **O26.0 Excessive weight gain in pregnancy**

    EXCLUDES 2   gestational edema (O12.0, O12.2)

    O26.00 Excessive weight gain in pregnancy, unspecified trimester   M ♀

    O26.01 Excessive weight gain in pregnancy, first trimester   M ♀

    O26.02 Excessive weight gain in pregnancy, second trimester   M ♀

    O26.03 Excessive weight gain in pregnancy, third trimester   M ♀

✓5ᵗʰ **O26.1 Low weight gain in pregnancy**

  O26.10 Low weight gain in pregnancy, unspecified trimester   M ♀

  O26.11 Low weight gain in pregnancy, first trimester   M ♀

  O26.12 Low weight gain in pregnancy, second trimester   M ♀

  O26.13 Low weight gain in pregnancy, third trimester   M ♀

✓5ᵗʰ **O26.2 Pregnancy care for patient with recurrent pregnancy loss**

  O26.20 Pregnancy care for patient with recurrent pregnancy loss, unspecified trimester   M ♀

  O26.21 Pregnancy care for patient with recurrent pregnancy loss, first trimester   M ♀

  O26.22 Pregnancy care for patient with recurrent pregnancy loss, second trimester   M ♀

  O26.23 Pregnancy care for patient with recurrent pregnancy loss, third trimester   M ♀

✓5ᵗʰ **O26.3 Retained intrauterine contraceptive device in pregnancy**

  O26.30 Retained intrauterine contraceptive device in pregnancy, unspecified trimester   M ♀

  O26.31 Retained intrauterine contraceptive device in pregnancy, first trimester   M ♀

  O26.32 Retained intrauterine contraceptive device in pregnancy, second trimester   M ♀

  O26.33 Retained intrauterine contraceptive device in pregnancy, third trimester   M ♀

✓5ᵗʰ **O26.4 Herpes gestationis**

  DEF: Rare skin disorder of unknown origin that appears on the abdomen in the second and third trimester as intensely itchy blisters that spread to other sites.

  O26.40 Herpes gestationis, unspecified trimester   M ♀

  O26.41 Herpes gestationis, first trimester   M ♀

  O26.42 Herpes gestationis, second trimester   M ♀

  O26.43 Herpes gestationis, third trimester   M ♀

✓5ᵗʰ **O26.5 Maternal hypotension syndrome**

  Supine hypotensive syndrome

  O26.50 Maternal hypotension syndrome, unspecified trimester   M ♀

  O26.51 Maternal hypotension syndrome, first trimester   M ♀

  O26.52 Maternal hypotension syndrome, second trimester   M ♀

  O26.53 Maternal hypotension syndrome, third trimester   M ♀

✓5ᵗʰ **O26.6 Liver and biliary tract disorders in pregnancy, childbirth and the puerperium**

  Use additional code to identify the specific disorder

  EXCLUDES 2   hepatorenal syndrome following labor and delivery (O90.4)

  CC Excl: For CC codes in subcategory O26.6: PDX collection 972

  ✓6ᵗʰ **O26.61 Liver and biliary tract disorders in** pregnancy

    O26.611 Liver and biliary tract disorders in pregnancy, first trimester   CC M ♀

    O26.612 Liver and biliary tract disorders in pregnancy, second trimester   CC M ♀

    O26.613 Liver and biliary tract disorders in pregnancy, third trimester   CC M ♀

    O26.619 Liver and biliary tract disorders in pregnancy, unspecified trimester   M ♀

  O26.62 Liver and biliary tract disorders in childbirth   CC M ♀

  O26.63 Liver and biliary tract disorders in the puerperium   M ♀

✓5ᵗʰ **O26.7 Subluxation of symphysis (pubis) in pregnancy, childbirth and the puerperium**

  EXCLUDES 1   traumatic separation of symphysis (pubis) during childbirth (O71.6)

  ✓6ᵗʰ **O26.71 Subluxation of symphysis (pubis) in** pregnancy

    O26.711 Subluxation of symphysis (pubis) in pregnancy, first trimester   M ♀

    O26.712 Subluxation of symphysis (pubis) in pregnancy, second trimester   M ♀

N Newborn: 0   P Pediatric: 0-17   M Maternity: 9-64   A Adult: 15-124   MCC Major Complication/Comorbidity   CC Complication/Comorbidity   SW Severe Wound Dx

888   ICD-10-CM 2020

O26.713 Subluxation of symphysis (pubis) in pregnancy, third trimester M ♀

O26.719 Subluxation of symphysis (pubis) in pregnancy, unspecified trimester M ♀

O26.72 Subluxation of symphysis (pubis) in childbirth M ♀

O26.73 Subluxation of symphysis (pubis) in the puerperium M ♀

✓5ᵗʰ **O26.8 Other specified pregnancy related conditions**

✓6ᵗʰ **O26.81 Pregnancy related exhaustion and fatigue**

O26.811 Pregnancy related exhaustion and fatigue, first trimester M ♀

O26.812 Pregnancy related exhaustion and fatigue, second trimester M ♀

O26.813 Pregnancy related exhaustion and fatigue, third trimester M ♀

O26.819 Pregnancy related exhaustion and fatigue, unspecified trimester M ♀

✓6ᵗʰ **O26.82 Pregnancy related peripheral neuritis**

O26.821 Pregnancy related peripheral neuritis, first trimester M ♀

O26.822 Pregnancy related peripheral neuritis, second trimester M ♀

O26.823 Pregnancy related peripheral neuritis, third trimester M ♀

O26.829 Pregnancy related peripheral neuritis, unspecified trimester M ♀

✓6ᵗʰ **O26.83 Pregnancy related renal disease**

Use additional code to identify the specific disorder
CC Excl: For CC codes in subcategory O26.83: PDX collection 965

O26.831 Pregnancy related renal disease, first trimester cc M ♀

O26.832 Pregnancy related renal disease, second trimester cc M ♀

O26.833 Pregnancy related renal disease, third trimester cc M ♀

O26.839 Pregnancy related renal disease, unspecified trimester M ♀

✓6ᵗʰ **O26.84 Uterine size-date discrepancy complicating pregnancy**

EXCLUDES 1   *encounter for suspected problem with fetal growth ruled out (Z03.74)*

O26.841 Uterine size-date discrepancy, first trimester M ♀

O26.842 Uterine size-date discrepancy, second trimester M ♀

O26.843 Uterine size-date discrepancy, third trimester M ♀

O26.849 Uterine size-date discrepancy, unspecified trimester M ♀

✓6ᵗʰ **O26.85 Spotting complicating pregnancy**

O26.851 Spotting complicating pregnancy, first trimester M ♀

O26.852 Spotting complicating pregnancy, second trimester M ♀

O26.853 Spotting complicating pregnancy, third trimester M ♀

O26.859 Spotting complicating pregnancy, unspecified trimester M ♀

O26.86 Pruritic urticarial papules and plaques of pregnancy (PUPPP) M ♀
Polymorphic eruption of pregnancy

✓6ᵗʰ **O26.87 Cervical shortening**

EXCLUDES 1   *encounter for suspected cervical shortening ruled out (Z03.75)*
DEF: Cervix that has shortened to less than 25 mm before the 24th week of pregnancy. A shortened cervix is a warning sign for impending premature delivery and is treated by cervical cerclage placement or progesterone.
CC Excl: For CC codes in subcategory O26.87: PDX collection 973

O26.872 Cervical shortening, second trimester cc M ♀

O26.873 Cervical shortening, third trimester cc M ♀

O26.879 Cervical shortening, unspecified trimester cc M ♀

✓6ᵗʰ **O26.89 Other specified pregnancy related conditions**

AHA: 2015,3Q,40

O26.891 Other specified pregnancy related conditions, first trimester M ♀

O26.892 Other specified pregnancy related conditions, second trimester M ♀

O26.893 Other specified pregnancy related conditions, third trimester M ♀

O26.899 Other specified pregnancy related conditions, unspecified trimester M ♀

✓5ᵗʰ **O26.9 Pregnancy related conditions, unspecified**

O26.90 Pregnancy related conditions, unspecified, unspecified trimester M ♀

O26.91 Pregnancy related conditions, unspecified, first trimester M ♀

O26.92 Pregnancy related conditions, unspecified, second trimester M ♀

O26.93 Pregnancy related conditions, unspecified, third trimester M ♀

✓4ᵗʰ **O28 Abnormal findings on antenatal screening of mother**

EXCLUDES 1   *diagnostic findings classified elsewhere — see Alphabetical Index*

O28.0 Abnormal hematological finding on antenatal screening of mother M ♀

O28.1 Abnormal biochemical finding on antenatal screening of mother M ♀

O28.2 Abnormal cytological finding on antenatal screening of mother M ♀

O28.3 Abnormal ultrasonic finding on antenatal screening of mother M ♀

O28.4 Abnormal radiological finding on antenatal screening of mother M ♀

O28.5 Abnormal chromosomal and genetic finding on antenatal screening of mother M ♀

O28.8 Other abnormal findings on antenatal screening of mother M ♀

O28.9 Unspecified abnormal findings on antenatal screening of mother M ♀

✓4ᵗʰ **O29 Complications of anesthesia during pregnancy**

INCLUDES   maternal complications arising from the administration of a general, regional or local anesthetic, analgesic or other sedation during pregnancy
Use additional code, if necessary, to identify the complication
EXCLUDES 2   *complications of anesthesia during labor and delivery (O74.-)*
complications of anesthesia during the puerperium (O89.-)

✓5ᵗʰ **O29.0 Pulmonary complications of anesthesia during pregnancy**

✓6ᵗʰ **O29.01 Aspiration pneumonitis due to anesthesia during pregnancy**
Inhalation of stomach contents or secretions NOS due to anesthesia during pregnancy
Mendelson's syndrome due to anesthesia during pregnancy

O29.011 Aspiration pneumonitis due to anesthesia during pregnancy, first trimester M ♀

O29.012 Aspiration pneumonitis due to anesthesia during pregnancy, second trimester M ♀

O29.013 Aspiration pneumonitis due to anesthesia during pregnancy, third trimester M ♀

O29.019 Aspiration pneumonitis due to anesthesia during pregnancy, unspecified trimester M ♀

✓6ᵗʰ **O29.02 Pressure collapse of lung due to anesthesia during pregnancy**

O29.021 Pressure collapse of lung due to anesthesia during pregnancy, first trimester M ♀

O29.022 Pressure collapse of lung due to anesthesia during pregnancy, second trimester M ♀

☑ Additional Character Required   ✓x7ᵗʰ Placeholder   Unacceptable PDx   Questionable PDx   Manifestation   Unspecified Dx   H1-H14 HAC   HCC CMS-HCC Dx   HIV HIV Dx
ICD-10-CM 2020

889

O29.Ø23   **Pressure collapse of lung due to anesthesia during pregnancy,** third trimester   M♀

O29.Ø29   **Pressure collapse of lung due to anesthesia during pregnancy, unspecified trimester**   M♀

✓6th O29.Ø9   **Other pulmonary complications of anesthesia during pregnancy**

O29.Ø91   **Other pulmonary complications of anesthesia during pregnancy,** first trimester   M♀

O29.Ø92   **Other pulmonary complications of anesthesia during pregnancy,** second trimester   M♀

O29.Ø93   **Other pulmonary complications of anesthesia during pregnancy,** third trimester   M♀

O29.Ø99   **Other pulmonary complications of anesthesia during pregnancy, unspecified trimester**   M♀

✓5th O29.1   **Cardiac complications of anesthesia during pregnancy**

✓6th O29.11   **Cardiac arrest due to anesthesia during pregnancy**

O29.111   **Cardiac arrest due to anesthesia during pregnancy,** first trimester   M♀

O29.112   **Cardiac arrest due to anesthesia during pregnancy,** second trimester   M♀

O29.113   **Cardiac arrest due to anesthesia during pregnancy,** third trimester   M♀

O29.119   **Cardiac arrest due to anesthesia during pregnancy, unspecified trimester**   M♀

✓6th O29.12   **Cardiac failure due to anesthesia during pregnancy**

O29.121   **Cardiac failure due to anesthesia during pregnancy,** first trimester   M♀

O29.122   **Cardiac failure due to anesthesia during pregnancy,** second trimester   M♀

O29.123   **Cardiac failure due to anesthesia during pregnancy,** third trimester   M♀

O29.129   **Cardiac failure due to anesthesia during pregnancy, unspecified trimester**   M♀

✓6th O29.19   **Other cardiac complications of anesthesia during pregnancy**

O29.191   **Other cardiac complications of anesthesia during pregnancy,** first trimester   M♀

O29.192   **Other cardiac complications of anesthesia during pregnancy,** second trimester   M♀

O29.193   **Other cardiac complications of anesthesia during pregnancy,** third trimester   M♀

O29.199   **Other cardiac complications of anesthesia during pregnancy, unspecified trimester**   M♀

✓5th O29.2   **Central nervous system complications of anesthesia during pregnancy**

✓6th O29.21   **Cerebral anoxia due to anesthesia during pregnancy**

O29.211   **Cerebral anoxia due to anesthesia during pregnancy,** first trimester   M♀

O29.212   **Cerebral anoxia due to anesthesia during pregnancy,** second trimester   M♀

O29.213   **Cerebral anoxia due to anesthesia during pregnancy,** third trimester   M♀

O29.219   **Cerebral anoxia due to anesthesia during pregnancy, unspecified trimester**   M♀

✓6th O29.29   **Other central nervous system complications of anesthesia during pregnancy**

O29.291   **Other central nervous system complications of anesthesia during pregnancy,** first trimester   M♀

O29.292   **Other central nervous system complications of anesthesia during pregnancy,** second trimester   M♀

O29.293   **Other central nervous system complications of anesthesia during pregnancy,** third trimester   M♀

O29.299   **Other central nervous system complications of anesthesia during pregnancy, unspecified trimester**   M♀

✓5th O29.3   **Toxic reaction to local anesthesia during pregnancy**

✓6th O29.3X   **Toxic reaction to local anesthesia during pregnancy**

O29.3X1   **Toxic reaction to local anesthesia during pregnancy,** first trimester   M♀

O29.3X2   **Toxic reaction to local anesthesia during pregnancy,** second trimester   M♀

O29.3X3   **Toxic reaction to local anesthesia during pregnancy,** third trimester   M♀

O29.3X9   **Toxic reaction to local anesthesia during pregnancy, unspecified trimester**   M♀

✓5th O29.4   **Spinal and epidural anesthesia induced headache during pregnancy**

O29.4Ø   **Spinal and epidural anesthesia induced headache during pregnancy, unspecified trimester**   M♀

O29.41   **Spinal and epidural anesthesia induced headache during pregnancy,** first trimester   M♀

O29.42   **Spinal and epidural anesthesia induced headache during pregnancy,** second trimester   M♀

O29.43   **Spinal and epidural anesthesia induced headache during pregnancy,** third trimester   M♀

✓5th O29.5   **Other complications of spinal and epidural anesthesia during pregnancy**

✓6th O29.5X   **Other complications of spinal and epidural anesthesia during pregnancy**

O29.5X1   **Other complications of spinal and epidural anesthesia during pregnancy,** first trimester   M♀

O29.5X2   **Other complications of spinal and epidural anesthesia during pregnancy,** second trimester   M♀

O29.5X3   **Other complications of spinal and epidural anesthesia during pregnancy,** third trimester   M♀

O29.5X9   **Other complications of spinal and epidural anesthesia during pregnancy, unspecified trimester**   M♀

✓5th O29.6   **Failed or difficult intubation for anesthesia during pregnancy**

O29.6Ø   **Failed or difficult intubation for anesthesia during pregnancy, unspecified trimester**   M♀

O29.61   **Failed or difficult intubation for anesthesia during pregnancy,** first trimester   M♀

O29.62   **Failed or difficult intubation for anesthesia during pregnancy,** second trimester   M♀

O29.63   **Failed or difficult intubation for anesthesia during pregnancy,** third trimester   M♀

✓5th O29.8   **Other complications of anesthesia during pregnancy**

✓6th O29.8X   **Other complications of anesthesia during pregnancy**

O29.8X1   **Other complications of anesthesia during pregnancy,** first trimester   M♀

N Newborn: 0   P Pediatric: 0-17   M Maternity: 9-64   A Adult: 15-124   MCC Major Complication/Comorbidity   CC Complication/Comorbidity   SW Severe Wound Dx

890   ICD-10-CM 2020

O29.8X2   **Other complications of anesthesia during pregnancy, second trimester**   M ♀

O29.8X3   **Other complications of anesthesia during pregnancy, third trimester**   M ♀

O29.8X9   **Other complications of anesthesia during pregnancy, unspecified trimester**   M ♀

✓5th   O29.9   **Unspecified complication of anesthesia during pregnancy**

O29.90   **Unspecified complication of anesthesia during pregnancy, unspecified trimester**   M ♀

O29.91   **Unspecified complication of anesthesia during pregnancy, first trimester**   M ♀

O29.92   **Unspecified complication of anesthesia during pregnancy, second trimester**   M ♀

O29.93   **Unspecified complication of anesthesia during pregnancy, third trimester**   M ♀

Maternal care related to the fetus and amniotic cavity and possible delivery problems (O30-O48)

✓4th   **O30   Multiple gestation**

Code also any complications specific to multiple gestation

AHA: 2016,4Q,51

CC Excl: For CC codes in category O30: PDX collection 976

✓5th   O30.0   **Twin pregnancy**

✓6th   O30.00   **Twin pregnancy, unspecified number of placenta and unspecified number of amniotic sacs**

O30.001   **Twin pregnancy, unspecified number of placenta and unspecified number of amniotic sacs, first trimester**   M ♀

O30.002   **Twin pregnancy, unspecified number of placenta and unspecified number of amniotic sacs, second trimester**   M ♀

O30.003   **Twin pregnancy, unspecified number of placenta and unspecified number of amniotic sacs, third trimester**   M ♀

O30.009   **Twin pregnancy, unspecified number of placenta and unspecified number of amniotic sacs, unspecified trimester**   M ♀

✓6th   O30.01   **Twin pregnancy, monochorionic/monoamniotic**

Twin pregnancy, one placenta, one amniotic sac

EXCLUDES 1   conjoined twins (O30.02-)

Twin Gestation – Monochorionic/Monoamniotic

O30.011   **Twin pregnancy, monochorionic/monoamniotic, first trimester**   M ♀

O30.012   **Twin pregnancy, monochorionic/monoamniotic, second trimester**   M ♀

O30.013   **Twin pregnancy, monochorionic/monoamniotic, third trimester**   M ♀

O30.019   **Twin pregnancy, monochorionic/monoamniotic, unspecified trimester**   M ♀

✓6th   O30.02   **Conjoined twin pregnancy**

O30.021   **Conjoined twin pregnancy, first trimester**   M ♀

O30.022   **Conjoined twin pregnancy, second trimester**   M ♀

O30.023   **Conjoined twin pregnancy, third trimester**   CC M ♀

O30.029   **Conjoined twin pregnancy, unspecified trimester**   M ♀

✓6th   O30.03   **Twin pregnancy, monochorionic/diamniotic**

Twin pregnancy, one placenta, two amniotic sacs

Twin Gestation – Monochorionic/Diamniotic

1 Chorionic sac
2 Amniotic sacs
2 Fetuses
2 Umbilical cords
1 Placenta

O30.031   **Twin pregnancy, monochorionic/diamniotic, first trimester**   M ♀

O30.032   **Twin pregnancy, monochorionic/diamniotic, second trimester**   M ♀

O30.033   **Twin pregnancy, monochorionic/diamniotic, third trimester**   M ♀

O30.039   **Twin pregnancy, monochorionic/diamniotic, unspecified trimester**   M ♀

✓6th   O30.04   **Twin pregnancy, dichorionic/diamniotic**

Twin pregnancy, two placentae, two amniotic sacs

Twin Gestation – Dichorionic/Diamniotic

2 Chorionic sacs
2 Amniotic sacs
2 Fetuses
2 Umbilical cords
2 Placentas

O30.041   **Twin pregnancy, dichorionic/diamniotic, first trimester**   M ♀

O30.042   **Twin pregnancy, dichorionic/diamniotic, second trimester**   M ♀

O30.043   **Twin pregnancy, dichorionic/diamniotic, third trimester**   M ♀

O30.049   **Twin pregnancy, dichorionic/diamniotic, unspecified trimester**   M ♀

☑ Additional Character Required   ✓x7th Placeholder   Unacceptable PDx   Questionable PDx   Manifestation   Unspecified Dx   H1-H4 HAC   HCC CMS-HCC Dx   HIV HIV Dx

ICD-10-CM 2020   891

Chapter 15. Pregnancy, Childbirth and the Puerperium

✓6th **O30.09** Twin pregnancy, unable to determine number of placenta and number of amniotic sacs

     O30.091 Twin pregnancy, unable to determine number of placenta and number of amniotic sacs, first trimester   Ⓜ ♀

     O30.092 Twin pregnancy, unable to determine number of placenta and number of amniotic sacs, second trimester   Ⓜ ♀

     O30.093 Twin pregnancy, unable to determine number of placenta and number of amniotic sacs, third trimester   Ⓜ ♀

     O30.099 Twin pregnancy, unable to determine number of placenta and number of amniotic sacs, unspecified trimester   Ⓜ ♀

✓5th **O30.1** Triplet pregnancy

   ✓6th **O30.10** Triplet pregnancy, unspecified number of placenta and unspecified number of amniotic sacs
       AHA: 2016,2Q,8

     O30.101 Triplet pregnancy, unspecified number of placenta and unspecified number of amniotic sacs, first trimester   cc Ⓜ ♀

     O30.102 Triplet pregnancy, unspecified number of placenta and unspecified number of amniotic sacs, second trimester   cc Ⓜ ♀

     O30.103 Triplet pregnancy, unspecified number of placenta and unspecified number of amniotic sacs, third trimester   cc Ⓜ ♀

     O30.109 Triplet pregnancy, unspecified number of placenta and unspecified number of amniotic sacs, unspecified trimester   Ⓜ ♀

   ✓6th **O30.11** Triplet pregnancy with two or more monochorionic fetuses

     O30.111 Triplet pregnancy with two or more monochorionic fetuses, first trimester   cc Ⓜ ♀

     O30.112 Triplet pregnancy with two or more monochorionic fetuses, second trimester   cc Ⓜ ♀

     O30.113 Triplet pregnancy with two or more monochorionic fetuses, third trimester   cc Ⓜ ♀

     O30.119 Triplet pregnancy with two or more monochorionic fetuses, unspecified trimester   Ⓜ ♀

   ✓6th **O30.12** Triplet pregnancy with two or more monoamniotic fetuses

     O30.121 Triplet pregnancy with two or more monoamniotic fetuses, first trimester   cc Ⓜ ♀

     O30.122 Triplet pregnancy with two or more monoamniotic fetuses, second trimester   cc Ⓜ ♀

     O30.123 Triplet pregnancy with two or more monoamniotic fetuses, third trimester   cc Ⓜ ♀

     O30.129 Triplet pregnancy with two or more monoamniotic fetuses, unspecified trimester   Ⓜ ♀

   ✓6th **O30.13** Triplet pregnancy, trichorionic/triamniotic
       AHA: 2018,4Q,22

     O30.131 Triplet pregnancy, trichorionic/triamniotic, first trimester   cc Ⓜ ♀

     O30.132 Triplet pregnancy, trichorionic/triamniotic, second trimester   cc Ⓜ ♀

     O30.133 Triplet pregnancy, trichorionic/triamniotic, third trimester   cc Ⓜ ♀

     O30.139 Triplet pregnancy, trichorionic/triamniotic, unspecified trimester   Ⓜ ♀

✓6th **O30.19** Triplet pregnancy, unable to determine number of placenta and number of amniotic sacs

     O30.191 Triplet pregnancy, unable to determine number of placenta and number of amniotic sacs, first trimester   cc Ⓜ ♀

     O30.192 Triplet pregnancy, unable to determine number of placenta and number of amniotic sacs, second trimester   cc Ⓜ ♀

     O30.193 Triplet pregnancy, unable to determine number of placenta and number of amniotic sacs, third trimester   cc Ⓜ ♀

     O30.199 Triplet pregnancy, unable to determine number of placenta and number of amniotic sacs, unspecified trimester   Ⓜ ♀

✓5th **O30.2** Quadruplet pregnancy

   ✓6th **O30.20** Quadruplet pregnancy, unspecified number of placenta and unspecified number of amniotic sacs

     O30.201 Quadruplet pregnancy, unspecified number of placenta and unspecified number of amniotic sacs, first trimester   cc Ⓜ ♀

     O30.202 Quadruplet pregnancy, unspecified number of placenta and unspecified number of amniotic sacs, second trimester   cc Ⓜ ♀

     O30.203 Quadruplet pregnancy, unspecified number of placenta and unspecified number of amniotic sacs, third trimester   cc Ⓜ ♀

     O30.209 Quadruplet pregnancy, unspecified number of placenta and unspecified number of amniotic sacs, unspecified trimester   Ⓜ ♀

   ✓6th **O30.21** Quadruplet pregnancy with two or more monochorionic fetuses

     O30.211 Quadruplet pregnancy with two or more monochorionic fetuses, first trimester   cc Ⓜ ♀

     O30.212 Quadruplet pregnancy with two or more monochorionic fetuses, second trimester   cc Ⓜ ♀

     O30.213 Quadruplet pregnancy with two or more monochorionic fetuses, third trimester   cc Ⓜ ♀

     O30.219 Quadruplet pregnancy with two or more monochorionic fetuses, unspecified trimester   Ⓜ ♀

   ✓6th **O30.22** Quadruplet pregnancy with two or more monoamniotic fetuses

     O30.221 Quadruplet pregnancy with two or more monoamniotic fetuses, first trimester   cc Ⓜ ♀

     O30.222 Quadruplet pregnancy with two or more monoamniotic fetuses, second trimester   cc Ⓜ ♀

     O30.223 Quadruplet pregnancy with two or more monoamniotic fetuses, third trimester   cc Ⓜ ♀

     O30.229 Quadruplet pregnancy with two or more monoamniotic fetuses, unspecified trimester   Ⓜ ♀

   ✓6th **O30.23** Quadruplet pregnancy, quadrachorionic/quadra-amniotic
       AHA: 2018,4Q,22

     O30.231 Quadruplet pregnancy, quadrachorionic/quadra-amniotic, first trimester   cc Ⓜ ♀

     O30.232 Quadruplet pregnancy, quadrachorionic/quadra-amniotic, second trimester   cc Ⓜ ♀

     O30.233 Quadruplet pregnancy, quadrachorionic/quadra-amniotic, third trimester   cc Ⓜ ♀

     O30.239 Quadruplet pregnancy, quadrachorionic/quadra-amniotic, unspecified trimester   Ⓜ ♀

Ⓝ Newborn: 0   Ⓟ Pediatric: 0-17   Ⓜ Maternity: 9-64   Ⓐ Adult: 15-124   MCC Major Complication/Comorbidity   cc Complication/Comorbidity   SW Severe Wound Dx

892   ICD-10-CM 2020

√6ᵗʰ O30.29 **Quadruplet pregnancy,** unable to determine number of placenta and number of amniotic sacs

     O30.291 Quadruplet pregnancy, unable to determine number of placenta and number of amniotic sacs, first trimester   cc M ♀

     O30.292 Quadruplet pregnancy, unable to determine number of placenta and number of amniotic sacs, second trimester   cc M ♀

     O30.293 Quadruplet pregnancy, unable to determine number of placenta and number of amniotic sacs, third trimester   cc M ♀

     O30.299 Quadruplet pregnancy, unable to determine number of placenta and number of amniotic sacs, unspecified trimester   M ♀

√5ᵗʰ O30.8 **Other specified multiple gestation**

     Multiple gestation pregnancy greater then quadruplets

√6ᵗʰ O30.80 **Other specified multiple gestation,** unspecified number of placenta and unspecified number of amniotic sacs

     O30.801 Other specified multiple gestation, unspecified number of placenta and unspecified number of amniotic sacs, first trimester   cc M ♀

     O30.802 Other specified multiple gestation, unspecified number of placenta and unspecified number of amniotic sacs, second trimester   cc M ♀

     O30.803 Other specified multiple gestation, unspecified number of placenta and unspecified number of amniotic sacs, third trimester   cc M ♀

     O30.809 Other specified multiple gestation, unspecified number of placenta and unspecified number of amniotic sacs, unspecified trimester   M ♀

√6ᵗʰ O30.81 **Other specified multiple gestation with** two or more monochorionic fetuses

     O30.811 Other specified multiple gestation with two or more monochorionic fetuses, first trimester   cc M ♀

     O30.812 Other specified multiple gestation with two or more monochorionic fetuses, second trimester   cc M ♀

     O30.813 Other specified multiple gestation with two or more monochorionic fetuses, third trimester   cc M ♀

     O30.819 Other specified multiple gestation with two or more monochorionic fetuses, unspecified trimester   M ♀

√6ᵗʰ O30.82 **Other specified multiple gestation with** two or more monoamniotic fetuses

     O30.821 Other specified multiple gestation with two or more monoamniotic fetuses, first trimester   cc M ♀

     O30.822 Other specified multiple gestation with two or more monoamniotic fetuses, second trimester   cc M ♀

     O30.823 Other specified multiple gestation with two or more monoamniotic fetuses, third trimester   cc M ♀

     O30.829 Other specified multiple gestation with two or more monoamniotic fetuses, unspecified trimester   M ♀

√6ᵗʰ O30.83 **Other specified multiple gestation,** number of chorions and amnions are both equal to the number of fetuses

     Pentachorionic, penta-amniotic pregnancy (quintuplets)

     Hexachorionic, hexa-amniotic pregnancy (sextuplets)

     Heptachorionic, hepta-amniotic pregnancy (septuplets)

     AHA: 2018,4Q,22

     O30.831 Other specified multiple gestation, number of chorions and amnions are both equal to the number of fetuses, first trimester   cc M ♀

     O30.832 Other specified multiple gestation, number of chorions and amnions are both equal to the number of fetuses, second trimester   cc M ♀

     O30.833 Other specified multiple gestation, number of chorions and amnions are both equal to the number of fetuses, third trimester   cc M ♀

     O30.839 Other specified multiple gestation, number of chorions and amnions are both equal to the number of fetuses, unspecified trimester   M ♀

√6ᵗʰ O30.89 **Other specified multiple gestation,** unable to determine number of placenta and number of amniotic sacs

     O30.891 Other specified multiple gestation, unable to determine number of placenta and number of amniotic sacs, first trimester   cc M ♀

     O30.892 Other specified multiple gestation, unable to determine number of placenta and number of amniotic sacs, second trimester   cc M ♀

     O30.893 Other specified multiple gestation, unable to determine number of placenta and number of amniotic sacs, third trimester   cc M ♀

     O30.899 Other specified multiple gestation, unable to determine number of placenta and number of amniotic sacs, unspecified trimester   M ♀

√5ᵗʰ O30.9 **Multiple gestation, unspecified**

     Multiple pregnancy NOS

     O30.90 Multiple gestation, unspecified, unspecified trimester   M ♀

     O30.91 Multiple gestation, unspecified, first trimester   M ♀

     O30.92 Multiple gestation, unspecified, second trimester   M ♀

     O30.93 Multiple gestation, unspecified, third trimester   M ♀

☑ Additional Character Required   √x7ᵗʰ Placeholder   Unacceptable PDx   Questionable PDx   Manifestation   Unspecified Dx   H1-H14 HAC   HCC CMS-HCC Dx   HIV HIV Dx

ICD-10-CM 2020   893

☑4ᵗʰ **O31 Complications specific to multiple gestation**

> EXCLUDES 2   *delayed delivery of second twin, triplet, etc. (O63.2)*
> *malpresentation of one fetus or more (O32.9)*
> *placental transfusion syndromes (O43.0-)*

AHA: 2012,4Q,107

> One of the following 7th characters is to be assigned to each code under category O31. 7th character Ø is for single gestations and multiple gestations where the fetus is unspecified. 7th characters 1 through 9 are for cases of multiple gestations to identify the fetus for which the code applies. The appropriate code from category O3Ø, Multiple gestation, must also be assigned when assigning a code from category O31 that has a 7th character of 1 through 9.
> Ø   not applicable or unspecified
> 1   fetus 1
> 2   fetus 2
> 3   fetus 3
> 4   fetus 4
> 5   fetus 5
> 9   other fetus

☑5ᵗʰ **O31.Ø Papyraceous fetus**

> Fetus compressus
> **DEF:** Fetus that has died, but remains in utero for weeks before delivery, becoming compacted and mummified in appearance, with skin resembling parchment. Occurs most commonly in multigestational pregnancies. *Synonym(s): paper doll fetus.*

   ✓x7ᵗʰ **O31.ØØ Papyraceous fetus, unspecified trimester**   Ⓜ♀

   ✓x7ᵗʰ **O31.Ø1 Papyraceous fetus, first trimester**   Ⓜ♀

   ✓x7ᵗʰ **O31.Ø2 Papyraceous fetus, second trimester**   Ⓜ♀

   ✓x7ᵗʰ **O31.Ø3 Papyraceous fetus, third trimester**   Ⓜ♀

☑5ᵗʰ **O31.1 Continuing pregnancy after spontaneous abortion of one fetus or more**

   ✓x7ᵗʰ **O31.1Ø Continuing pregnancy after spontaneous abortion of one fetus or more, unspecified trimester**   Ⓜ♀

   ✓x7ᵗʰ **O31.11 Continuing pregnancy after spontaneous abortion of one fetus or more, first trimester**   Ⓜ♀

   ✓x7ᵗʰ **O31.12 Continuing pregnancy after spontaneous abortion of one fetus or more, second trimester**   Ⓜ♀

   ✓x7ᵗʰ **O31.13 Continuing pregnancy after spontaneous abortion of one fetus or more, third trimester**   Ⓜ♀

☑5ᵗʰ **O31.2 Continuing pregnancy after intrauterine death of one fetus or more**

   ✓x7ᵗʰ **O31.2Ø Continuing pregnancy after intrauterine death of one fetus or more, unspecified trimester**   Ⓜ♀

   ✓x7ᵗʰ **O31.21 Continuing pregnancy after intrauterine death of one fetus or more, first trimester**   Ⓜ♀

   ✓x7ᵗʰ **O31.22 Continuing pregnancy after intrauterine death of one fetus or more, second trimester**   Ⓜ♀

   ✓x7ᵗʰ **O31.23 Continuing pregnancy after intrauterine death of one fetus or more, third trimester**   Ⓜ♀

☑5ᵗʰ **O31.3 Continuing pregnancy after elective fetal reduction of one fetus or more**

> Continuing pregnancy after selective termination of one fetus or more

   ✓x7ᵗʰ **O31.3Ø Continuing pregnancy after elective fetal reduction of one fetus or more, unspecified trimester**   Ⓜ♀

   ✓x7ᵗʰ **O31.31 Continuing pregnancy after elective fetal reduction of one fetus or more, first trimester**   Ⓜ♀

   ✓x7ᵗʰ **O31.32 Continuing pregnancy after elective fetal reduction of one fetus or more, second trimester**   Ⓜ♀

   ✓x7ᵗʰ **O31.33 Continuing pregnancy after elective fetal reduction of one fetus or more, third trimester**   Ⓜ♀

☑5ᵗʰ **O31.8 Other complications specific to multiple gestation**

   ☑6ᵗʰ **O31.8X Other complications specific to multiple gestation**

> **CC Excl: For CC codes in subcategory O31.8X:** PDX collection 976

     ☑7ᵗʰ **O31.8X1 Other complications specific to multiple gestation, first trimester**   ⒸⒸ Ⓜ♀

     ☑7ᵗʰ **O31.8X2 Other complications specific to multiple gestation, second trimester**   ⒸⒸ Ⓜ♀

     ☑7ᵗʰ **O31.8X3 Other complications specific to multiple gestation, third trimester**   ⒸⒸ Ⓜ♀

     ☑7ᵗʰ **O31.8X9 Other complications specific to multiple gestation, unspecified trimester**   ⒸⒸ Ⓜ♀

☑4ᵗʰ **O32 Maternal care for malpresentation of fetus**

> INCLUDES   the listed conditions as a reason for observation, hospitalization or other obstetric care of the mother, or for cesarean delivery before onset of labor
> EXCLUDES 1   *malpresentation of fetus with obstructed labor (O64.-)*

AHA: 2012,4Q,107

> One of the following 7th characters is to be assigned to each code under category O32. 7th character Ø is for single gestations and multiple gestations where the fetus is unspecified. 7th characters 1 through 9 are for cases of multiple gestations to identify the fetus for which the code applies. The appropriate code from category O3Ø, Multiple gestation, must also be assigned when assigning a code from category O32 that has a 7th character of 1 through 9.
> Ø   not applicable or unspecified
> 1   fetus 1
> 2   fetus 2
> 3   fetus 3
> 4   fetus 4
> 5   fetus 5
> 9   other fetus

✓x7ᵗʰ **O32.Ø Maternal care for unstable lie**   Ⓜ♀

✓x7ᵗʰ **O32.1 Maternal care for breech presentation**   Ⓜ♀

> Maternal care for buttocks presentation
> Maternal care for complete breech
> Maternal care for frank breech
> EXCLUDES 1   *footling presentation (O32.8)*
> *incomplete breech (O32.8)*
> **DEF:** Fetus presentation in a longitudinal lie with the buttocks or feet closest to birth canal that may require external cephalic version or cesarean delivery.

✓x7ᵗʰ **O32.2 Maternal care for transverse and oblique lie**   Ⓜ♀

> Maternal care for oblique presentation
> Maternal care for transverse presentation

✓x7ᵗʰ **O32.3 Maternal care for face, brow and chin presentation**   Ⓜ♀

✓x7ᵗʰ **O32.4 Maternal care for high head at term**   Ⓜ♀

> Maternal care for failure of head to enter pelvic brim

✓x7ᵗʰ **O32.6 Maternal care for compound presentation**   Ⓜ♀

✓x7ᵗʰ **O32.8 Maternal care for other malpresentation of fetus**   Ⓜ♀

> Maternal care for footling presentation
> Maternal care for incomplete breech

✓x7ᵗʰ **O32.9 Maternal care for malpresentation of fetus, unspecified**   Ⓜ♀

Fetal Malpresentation

Breech — Mother's pelvis

Shoulder (arm prolapse)

Face (mentum)

Compound (extremity together with head)

Oblique

Ⓝ Newborn: 0   Ⓟ Pediatric: 0-17   Ⓜ Maternity: 9-64   Ⓐ Adult: 15-124   ᴹᶜᶜ Major Complication/Comorbidity   ⒸⒸ Complication/Comorbidity   ˢʷ Severe Wound Dx

894   ICD-10-CM 2020

✓4th O33 Maternal care for disproportion

INCLUDES the listed conditions as a reason for observation, hospitalization or other obstetric care of the mother, or for cesarean delivery before onset of labor

EXCLUDES 1 disproportion with obstructed labor (O65-O66)

O33.0 Maternal care for disproportion due to deformity of maternal pelvic bones   CC M ♀

Maternal care for disproportion due to pelvic deformity causing disproportion NOS

CC Excl: PDX collection 977

O33.1 Maternal care for disproportion due to generally contracted pelvis   M ♀

Maternal care for disproportion due to contracted pelvis NOS causing disproportion

O33.2 Maternal care for disproportion due to inlet contraction of pelvis   M ♀

Maternal care for disproportion due to inlet contraction (pelvis) causing disproportion

✓x7th O33.3 Maternal care for disproportion due to outlet contraction of pelvis   M ♀

Maternal care for disproportion due to mid-cavity contraction (pelvis)

Maternal care for disproportion due to outlet contraction (pelvis)

One of the following 7th characters is to be assigned to code O33.3. 7th character 0 is for single gestations and multiple gestations where the fetus is unspecified. 7th characters 1 through 9 are for cases of multiple gestations to identify the fetus for which the code applies. The appropriate code from category O30, Multiple gestation, must also be assigned when assigning code O33.3 with a 7th character of 1 through 9.

- 0   not applicable or unspecified
- 1   fetus 1
- 2   fetus 2
- 3   fetus 3
- 4   fetus 4
- 5   fetus 5
- 9   other fetus

✓x7th O33.4 Maternal care for disproportion of mixed maternal and fetal origin   M ♀

One of the following 7th characters is to be assigned to code O33.4. 7th character 0 is for single gestations and multiple gestations where the fetus is unspecified. 7th characters 1 through 9 are for cases of multiple gestations to identify the fetus for which the code applies. The appropriate code from category O30, Multiple gestation, must also be assigned when assigning code O33.4 with a 7th character of 1 through 9.

- 0   not applicable or unspecified
- 1   fetus 1
- 2   fetus 2
- 3   fetus 3
- 4   fetus 4
- 5   fetus 5
- 9   other fetus

✓x7th O33.5 Maternal care for disproportion due to unusually large fetus   M ♀

. Maternal care for disproportion due to disproportion of fetal origin with normally formed fetus

Maternal care for disproportion due to fetal disproportion NOS

One of the following 7th characters is to be assigned to code O33.5. 7th character 0 is for single gestations and multiple gestations where the fetus is unspecified. 7th characters 1 through 9 are for cases of multiple gestations to identify the fetus for which the code applies. The appropriate code from category O30, Multiple gestation, must also be assigned when assigning code O33.5 with a 7th character of 1 through 9.

- 0   not applicable or unspecified
- 1   fetus 1
- 2   fetus 2
- 3   fetus 3
- 4   fetus 4
- 5   fetus 5
- 9   other fetus

✓x7th O33.6 Maternal care for disproportion due to hydrocephalic fetus   M ♀

One of the following 7th characters is to be assigned to code O33.6. 7th character 0 is for single gestations and multiple gestations where the fetus is unspecified. 7th characters 1 through 9 are for cases of multiple gestations to identify the fetus for which the code applies. The appropriate code from category O30, Multiple gestation, must also be assigned when assigning code O33.6 with a 7th character of 1 through 9.

- 0   not applicable or unspecified
- 1   fetus 1
- 2   fetus 2
- 3   fetus 3
- 4   fetus 4
- 5   fetus 5
- 9   other fetus

✓x7th O33.7 Maternal care for disproportion due to other fetal deformities   M ♀

Maternal care for disproportion due to fetal ascites

Maternal care for disproportion due to fetal hydrops

Maternal care for disproportion due to fetal meningomyelocele

Maternal care for disproportion due to fetal sacral teratoma

Maternal care for disproportion due to fetal tumor

EXCLUDES 1 obstructed labor due to other fetal deformities (O66.3)

AHA: 2016,4Q,51

One of the following 7th characters is to be assigned to code O33.7. 7th character 0 is for single gestations and multiple gestations where the fetus is unspecified. 7th characters 1 through 9 are for cases of multiple gestations to identify the fetus for which the code applies. The appropriate code from category O30, Multiple gestation, must also be assigned when assigning code O33.7 with a 7th character of 1 through 9.

- 0   not applicable or unspecified
- 1   fetus 1
- 2   fetus 2
- 3   fetus 3
- 4   fetus 4
- 5   fetus 5
- 9   other fetus

O33.8 Maternal care for disproportion of other origin   M ♀

O33.9 Maternal care for disproportion, unspecified   M ♀

Maternal care for disproportion due to cephalopelvic disproportion NOS

Maternal care for disproportion due to fetopelvic disproportion NOS

✓4th O34 Maternal care for abnormality of pelvic organs

INCLUDES the listed conditions as a reason for hospitalization or other obstetric care of the mother, or for cesarean delivery before onset of labor

Code first any associated obstructed labor (O65.5)

Use additional code for specific condition

✓5th O34.0 Maternal care for congenital malformation of uterus

Maternal care for double uterus

Maternal care for uterus bicornis

O34.00 Maternal care for unspecified congenital malformation of uterus, unspecified trimester   M ♀

O34.01 Maternal care for unspecified congenital malformation of uterus, first trimester   M ♀

O34.02 Maternal care for unspecified congenital malformation of uterus, second trimester   M ♀

O34.03 Maternal care for unspecified congenital malformation of uterus, third trimester   M ♀

✓5th O34.1 Maternal care for benign tumor of corpus uteri

EXCLUDES 2 maternal care for benign tumor of cervix (O34.4-)

maternal care for malignant neoplasm of uterus (O9A.1-)

O34.10 Maternal care for benign tumor of corpus uteri, unspecified trimester   M ♀

O34.11 Maternal care for benign tumor of corpus uteri, first trimester   M ♀

O34.12 Maternal care for benign tumor of corpus uteri, second trimester   M ♀

O34.13 Maternal care for benign tumor of corpus uteri, third trimester   M ♀

☑ Additional Character Required   ✓x7th Placeholder   Unacceptable PDx   Questionable PDx   Manifestation   Unspecified Dx   H1-H14 HAC   HCC CMS-HCC Dx   HIV HIV Dx

ICD-10-CM 2020

895

√5ᵗʰ **O34.2 Maternal care due to** uterine scar from previous surgery

    AHA: 2016,4Q,76

    √6ᵗʰ **O34.21 Maternal care for scar** from previous cesarean delivery

       AHA: 2018,3Q,23; 2016,4Q,51-52

       O34.211 Maternal care for low transverse **scar from previous cesarean delivery**   M ♀

       O34.212 Maternal care for vertical **scar from previous cesarean delivery**   M ♀

         Maternal care for classical scar from previous cesarean delivery

       O34.219 Maternal care for unspecified type scar from previous cesarean delivery   M ♀

    O34.29 Maternal care due to uterine scar from other previous surgery   M ♀

       Maternal care due to uterine scar from other transmural uterine incision

√5ᵗʰ **O34.3 Maternal care for** cervical incompetence

    Maternal care for cerclage with or without cervical incompetence

    Maternal care for Shirodkar suture with or without cervical incompetence

    DEF: Inadequate functioning of the cervix marked by abnormal widening during pregnancy and causing premature birth or miscarriage.

    CC Excl: For MCC codes in subcategory O34.3: PDX collection 973

    O34.30 Maternal care for cervical incompetence, unspecified trimester   M ♀

    O34.31 Maternal care for cervical incompetence, first trimester   MCC M ♀

    O34.32 Maternal care for cervical incompetence, second trimester   MCC M ♀

    O34.33 Maternal care for cervical incompetence, third trimester   MCC M ♀

√5ᵗʰ **O34.4 Maternal care for** other abnormalities of cervix

    O34.40 Maternal care for other abnormalities of cervix, unspecified trimester   M ♀

    O34.41 Maternal care for other abnormalities of cervix, first trimester   M ♀

    O34.42 Maternal care for other abnormalities of cervix, second trimester   M ♀

    O34.43 Maternal care for other abnormalities of cervix, third trimester   M ♀

√5ᵗʰ **O34.5 Maternal care for** other abnormalities of gravid uterus

    √6ᵗʰ **O34.51 Maternal care for** incarceration of gravid uterus

       O34.511 Maternal care for incarceration of gravid uterus, first trimester   M ♀

       O34.512 Maternal care for incarceration of gravid uterus, second trimester   M ♀

       O34.513 Maternal care for incarceration of gravid uterus, third trimester   M ♀

       O34.519 Maternal care for incarceration of gravid uterus, unspecified trimester   M ♀

    √6ᵗʰ **O34.52 Maternal care for** prolapse of gravid uterus

       O34.521 Maternal care for prolapse of gravid uterus, first trimester   M ♀

       O34.522 Maternal care for prolapse of gravid uterus, second trimester   M ♀

       O34.523 Maternal care for prolapse of gravid uterus, third trimester   M ♀

       O34.529 Maternal care for prolapse of gravid uterus, unspecified trimester   M ♀

    √6ᵗʰ **O34.53 Maternal care for** retroversion of gravid uterus

       O34.531 Maternal care for retroversion of gravid uterus, first trimester   M ♀

       O34.532 Maternal care for retroversion of gravid uterus, second trimester   M ♀

       O34.533 Maternal care for retroversion of gravid uterus, third trimester   M ♀

       O34.539 Maternal care for retroversion of gravid uterus, unspecified trimester   M ♀

    √6ᵗʰ **O34.59 Maternal care for other abnormalities of gravid uterus**

       O34.591 Maternal care for other abnormalities of gravid uterus, first trimester   M ♀

       O34.592 Maternal care for other abnormalities of gravid uterus, second trimester   M ♀

       O34.593 Maternal care for other abnormalities of gravid uterus, third trimester   M ♀

       O34.599 Maternal care for other abnormalities of gravid uterus, unspecified trimester   M ♀

√5ᵗʰ **O34.6 Maternal care for** abnormality of vagina

    EXCLUDES 2   maternal care for vaginal varices in pregnancy (O22.1-)

    O34.60 Maternal care for abnormality of vagina, unspecified trimester   M ♀

    O34.61 Maternal care for abnormality of vagina, first trimester   M ♀

    O34.62 Maternal care for abnormality of vagina, second trimester   M ♀

    O34.63 Maternal care for abnormality of vagina, third trimester   M ♀

√5ᵗʰ **O34.7 Maternal care for** abnormality of vulva and perineum

    EXCLUDES 2   maternal care for perineal and vulval varices in pregnancy (O22.1-)

    O34.70 Maternal care for abnormality of vulva and perineum, unspecified trimester   M ♀

    O34.71 Maternal care for abnormality of vulva and perineum, first trimester   M ♀

    O34.72 Maternal care for abnormality of vulva and perineum, second trimester   M ♀

    O34.73 Maternal care for abnormality of vulva and perineum, third trimester   M ♀

√5ᵗʰ **O34.8 Maternal care for** other abnormalities of pelvic organs

    O34.80 Maternal care for other abnormalities of pelvic organs, unspecified trimester   M ♀

    O34.81 Maternal care for other abnormalities of pelvic organs, first trimester   M ♀

    O34.82 Maternal care for other abnormalities of pelvic organs, second trimester   M ♀

    O34.83 Maternal care for other abnormalities of pelvic organs, third trimester   M ♀

√5ᵗʰ **O34.9 Maternal care for abnormality of pelvic organ, unspecified**

    O34.90 Maternal care for abnormality of pelvic organ, unspecified, unspecified trimester   M ♀

    O34.91 Maternal care for abnormality of pelvic organ, unspecified, first trimester   M ♀

    O34.92 Maternal care for abnormality of pelvic organ, unspecified, second trimester   M ♀

    O34.93 Maternal care for abnormality of pelvic organ, unspecified, third trimester   M ♀

N Newborn: 0   P Pediatric: 0-17   M Maternity: 9-64   A Adult: 15-124   MCC Major Complication/Comorbidity   CC Complication/Comorbidity   SW Severe Wound Dx

896   ICD-10-CM 2020

☑4ᵗʰ **O35 Maternal care for known or suspected fetal abnormality and damage**

INCLUDES the listed conditions in the fetus as a reason for hospitalization or other obstetric care to the mother, or for termination of pregnancy

Code also any maternal condition

EXCLUDES 1 encounter for suspected maternal and fetal conditions ruled out (Z03.7-)

One of the following 7th characters is to be assigned to each code under category O35. 7th character 0 is for single gestations and multiple gestations where the fetus is unspecified. 7th characters 1 through 9 are for cases of multiple gestations to identify the fetus for which the code applies. The appropriate code from category O30, Multiple gestation, must also be assigned when assigning a code from category O35 that has a 7th character of 1 through 9.

0 not applicable or unspecified
1 fetus 1
2 fetus 2
3 fetus 3
4 fetus 4
5 fetus 5
9 other fetus

☑x7ᵗʰ **O35.0 Maternal care for (suspected) central nervous system malformation in fetus** M ♀
Maternal care for fetal anencephaly
Maternal care for fetal hydrocephalus
Maternal care for fetal spina bifida
EXCLUDES 2 chromosomal abnormality in fetus (O35.1)

☑x7ᵗʰ **O35.1 Maternal care for (suspected) chromosomal abnormality in fetus** M ♀

☑x7ᵗʰ **O35.2 Maternal care for (suspected) hereditary disease in fetus** M ♀
EXCLUDES 2 chromosomal abnormality in fetus (O35.1)

☑x7ᵗʰ **O35.3 Maternal care for (suspected) damage to fetus from viral disease in mother** M ♀
Maternal care for damage to fetus from maternal cytomegalovirus infection
Maternal care for damage to fetus from maternal rubella

☑x7ᵗʰ **O35.4 Maternal care for (suspected) damage to fetus from alcohol** M ♀

☑x7ᵗʰ **O35.5 Maternal care for (suspected) damage to fetus by drugs** M ♀
Maternal care for damage to fetus from drug addiction

☑x7ᵗʰ **O35.6 Maternal care for (suspected) damage to fetus by radiation** M ♀

☑x7ᵗʰ **O35.7 Maternal care for (suspected) damage to fetus by other medical procedures** M ♀
Maternal care for damage to fetus by amniocentesis
Maternal care for damage to fetus by biopsy procedures
Maternal care for damage to fetus by hematological investigation
Maternal care for damage to fetus by intrauterine contraceptive device
Maternal care for damage to fetus by intrauterine surgery

☑x7ᵗʰ **O35.8 Maternal care for other (suspected) fetal abnormality and damage** M ♀
Maternal care for damage to fetus from maternal listeriosis
Maternal care for damage to fetus from maternal toxoplasmosis

☑x7ᵗʰ **O35.9 Maternal care for (suspected) fetal abnormality and damage, unspecified** M ♀

☑4ᵗʰ **O36 Maternal care for other fetal problems**

INCLUDES the listed conditions in the fetus as a reason for hospitalization or other obstetric care of the mother, or for termination of pregnancy

EXCLUDES 1 encounter for suspected maternal and fetal conditions ruled out (Z03.7-)
placental transfusion syndromes (O43.0-)

EXCLUDES 2 labor and delivery complicated by fetal stress (O77.-)

AHA: 2015,3Q,40

One of the following 7th characters is to be assigned to each code under category O36. 7th character 0 is for single gestations and multiple gestations where the fetus is unspecified. 7th characters 1 through 9 are for cases of multiple gestations to identify the fetus for which the code applies. The appropriate code from category O30, Multiple gestation, must also be assigned when assigning a code from category O36 that has a 7th character of 1 through 9.

0 not applicable or unspecified
1 fetus 1
2 fetus 2
3 fetus 3
4 fetus 4
5 fetus 5
9 other fetus

☑5ᵗʰ **O36.0 Maternal care for rhesus isoimmunization**
Maternal care for Rh incompatibility (with hydrops fetalis)
CC Excl: For CC codes in subcategory O36.0: PDX collection 978

☑6ᵗʰ **O36.01 Maternal care for anti-D [Rh] antibodies**
AHA: 2014,4Q,17

☑7ᵗʰ **O36.011 Maternal care for anti-D [Rh] antibodies, first trimester** cc M ♀

☑7ᵗʰ **O36.012 Maternal care for anti-D [Rh] antibodies, second trimester** cc M ♀

☑7ᵗʰ **O36.013 Maternal care for anti-D [Rh] antibodies, third trimester** cc M ♀

☑7ᵗʰ **O36.019 Maternal care for anti-D [Rh] antibodies, unspecified trimester** M ♀

☑6ᵗʰ **O36.09 Maternal care for other rhesus isoimmunization**

☑7ᵗʰ **O36.091 Maternal care for other rhesus isoimmunization, first trimester** cc M ♀

☑7ᵗʰ **O36.092 Maternal care for other rhesus isoimmunization, second trimester** cc M ♀

☑7ᵗʰ **O36.093 Maternal care for other rhesus isoimmunization, third trimester** cc M ♀

☑7ᵗʰ **O36.099 Maternal care for other rhesus isoimmunization, unspecified trimester** M ♀

☑5ᵗʰ **O36.1 Maternal care for other isoimmunization**
Maternal care for ABO isoimmunization

☑6ᵗʰ **O36.11 Maternal care for Anti-A sensitization**
Maternal care for isoimmunization NOS (with hydrops fetalis)

☑7ᵗʰ **O36.111 Maternal care for Anti-A sensitization, first trimester** M ♀

☑7ᵗʰ **O36.112 Maternal care for Anti-A sensitization, second trimester** M ♀

☑7ᵗʰ **O36.113 Maternal care for Anti-A sensitization, third trimester** M ♀

☑7ᵗʰ **O36.119 Maternal care for Anti-A sensitization, unspecified trimester** M ♀

☑6ᵗʰ **O36.19 Maternal care for other isoimmunization**
Maternal care for Anti-B sensitization

☑7ᵗʰ **O36.191 Maternal care for other isoimmunization, first trimester** cc M ♀

☑7ᵗʰ **O36.192 Maternal care for other isoimmunization, second trimester** M ♀

☑7ᵗʰ **O36.193 Maternal care for other isoimmunization, third trimester** M ♀

☑7ᵗʰ **O36.199 Maternal care for other isoimmunization, unspecified trimester** M ♀

Chapter 15. Pregnancy, Childbirth and the Puerperium

O36.2–O36.93

✓5ᵗʰ **O36.2 Maternal care for hydrops fetalis**

Maternal care for hydrops fetalis NOS

Maternal care for hydrops fetalis not associated with isoimmunization

> **EXCLUDES 1**   *hydrops fetalis associated with ABO isoimmunization (O36.1-)*
>
> *hydrops fetalis associated with rhesus isoimmunization (O36.0-)*

DEF: Hydrops fetalis: Abnormal fluid buildup in at least two of the following fetal organ spaces: the skin (edema), abdomen (ascites), around the heart (pericardia effusion), and around the lung (pleural effusion). Fluid accumulation may also occur in the mother as polyhydramnios and edema of the placenta.

✓x7ᵗʰ **O36.20 Maternal care for hydrops fetalis, unspecified trimester**   M ♀

✓x7ᵗʰ **O36.21 Maternal care for hydrops fetalis, first trimester**   M ♀

✓x7ᵗʰ **O36.22 Maternal care for hydrops fetalis, second trimester**   M ♀

✓x7ᵗʰ **O36.23 Maternal care for hydrops fetalis, third trimester**   M ♀

✓x7ᵗʰ **O36.4 Maternal care for intrauterine death**   CC M ♀

Maternal care for intrauterine fetal death NOS

Maternal care for intrauterine fetal death after completion of 20 weeks of gestation

Maternal care for late fetal death

Maternal care for missed delivery

> **EXCLUDES 1**   *missed abortion (O02.1)*
>
> *stillbirth (P95)*

CC Excl: PDX collection 979

✓5ᵗʰ **O36.5 Maternal care for known or suspected poor fetal growth**

✓6ᵗʰ **O36.51 Maternal care for known or suspected placental insufficiency**

✓7ᵗʰ **O36.511 Maternal care for known or suspected placental insufficiency, first trimester**   M ♀

✓7ᵗʰ **O36.512 Maternal care for known or suspected placental insufficiency, second trimester**   M ♀

✓7ᵗʰ **O36.513 Maternal care for known or suspected placental insufficiency, third trimester**   M ♀

✓7ᵗʰ **O36.519 Maternal care for known or suspected placental insufficiency, unspecified trimester**   M ♀

✓6ᵗʰ **O36.59 Maternal care for other known or suspected poor fetal growth**

Maternal care for known or suspected light-for-dates NOS

Maternal care for known or suspected small-for-dates NOS

✓7ᵗʰ **O36.591 Maternal care for other known or suspected poor fetal growth, first trimester**   M ♀

✓7ᵗʰ **O36.592 Maternal care for other known or suspected poor fetal growth, second trimester**   M ♀

✓7ᵗʰ **O36.593 Maternal care for other known or suspected poor fetal growth, third trimester**   M ♀

✓7ᵗʰ **O36.599 Maternal care for other known or suspected poor fetal growth, unspecified trimester**   M ♀

✓5ᵗʰ **O36.6 Maternal care for excessive fetal growth**

Maternal care for known or suspected large-for-dates

✓x7ᵗʰ **O36.60 Maternal care for excessive fetal growth, unspecified trimester**   M ♀

✓x7ᵗʰ **O36.61 Maternal care for excessive fetal growth, first trimester**   M ♀

✓x7ᵗʰ **O36.62 Maternal care for excessive fetal growth, second trimester**   M ♀

✓x7ᵗʰ **O36.63 Maternal care for excessive fetal growth, third trimester**   M ♀

✓5ᵗʰ **O36.7 Maternal care for viable fetus in abdominal pregnancy**

✓x7ᵗʰ **O36.70 Maternal care for viable fetus in abdominal pregnancy, unspecified trimester**   M ♀

✓x7ᵗʰ **O36.71 Maternal care for viable fetus in abdominal pregnancy, first trimester**   M ♀

✓x7ᵗʰ **O36.72 Maternal care for viable fetus in abdominal pregnancy, second trimester**   M ♀

✓x7ᵗʰ **O36.73 Maternal care for viable fetus in abdominal pregnancy, third trimester**   M ♀

✓5ᵗʰ **O36.8 Maternal care for other specified fetal problems**

✓x7ᵗʰ **O36.80 Pregnancy with inconclusive fetal viability**   M ♀

Encounter to determine fetal viability of pregnancy

AHA: 2019,2Q,29

✓6ᵗʰ **O36.81 Decreased fetal movements**

✓7ᵗʰ **O36.812 Decreased fetal movements, second trimester**   M ♀

✓7ᵗʰ **O36.813 Decreased fetal movements, third trimester**   M ♀

✓7ᵗʰ **O36.819 Decreased fetal movements, unspecified trimester**   M ♀

✓6ᵗʰ **O36.82 Fetal anemia and thrombocytopenia**

✓7ᵗʰ **O36.821 Fetal anemia and thrombocytopenia, first trimester**   M ♀

✓7ᵗʰ **O36.822 Fetal anemia and thrombocytopenia, second trimester**   M ♀

✓7ᵗʰ **O36.823 Fetal anemia and thrombocytopenia, third trimester**   M ♀

✓7ᵗʰ **O36.829 Fetal anemia and thrombocytopenia, unspecified trimester**   M ♀

✓6ᵗʰ **O36.83 Maternal care for abnormalities of the fetal heart rate or rhythm**

► Maternal care for depressed fetal heart rate tones ◄

► Maternal care for fetal bradycardia ◄

► Maternal care for fetal heart rate abnormal variability ◄

► Maternal care for fetal heart rate decelerations ◄

► Maternal care for fetal heart rate irregularity ◄

► Maternal care for fetal tachycardia ◄

► Maternal care for non-reassuring fetal heart rate or rhythm ◄

AHA: 2017,4Q,20

TIP: Assign for documented fetal tachycardia, bradycardia, decelerations, or loss of variability detected during antenatal testing.

✓7ᵗʰ **O36.831 Maternal care for abnormalities of the fetal heart rate or rhythm, first trimester**   M ♀

✓7ᵗʰ **O36.832 Maternal care for abnormalities of the fetal heart rate or rhythm, second trimester**   M ♀

✓7ᵗʰ **O36.833 Maternal care for abnormalities of the fetal heart rate or rhythm, third trimester**   M ♀

✓7ᵗʰ **O36.839 Maternal care for abnormalities of the fetal heart rate or rhythm, unspecified trimester**   M ♀

✓6ᵗʰ **O36.89 Maternal care for other specified fetal problems**

✓7ᵗʰ **O36.891 Maternal care for other specified fetal problems, first trimester**   M ♀

✓7ᵗʰ **O36.892 Maternal care for other specified fetal problems, second trimester**   M ♀

✓7ᵗʰ **O36.893 Maternal care for other specified fetal problems, third trimester**   M ♀

✓7ᵗʰ **O36.899 Maternal care for other specified fetal problems, unspecified trimester**   M ♀

✓5ᵗʰ **O36.9 Maternal care for fetal problem, unspecified**

✓x7ᵗʰ **O36.90 Maternal care for fetal problem, unspecified, unspecified trimester**   M ♀

✓x7ᵗʰ **O36.91 Maternal care for fetal problem, unspecified, first trimester**   M ♀

✓x7ᵗʰ **O36.92 Maternal care for fetal problem, unspecified, second trimester**   M ♀

✓x7ᵗʰ **O36.93 Maternal care for fetal problem, unspecified, third trimester**   M ♀

N Newborn: 0   P Pediatric: 0-17   M Maternity: 9-64   A Adult: 15-124   MCC Major Complication/Comorbidity   CC Complication/Comorbidity   SW Severe Wound Dx

898   ICD-10-CM 2020

✓4th O4Ø Polyhydramnios

INCLUDES hydramnios

EXCLUDES 1 encounter for suspected maternal and fetal conditions ruled out (ZØ3.7-)

AHA: 2016,1Q,4

DEF: Excess amniotic fluid surrounding the fetus, typically defined as a total fluid volume of greater than 24.0 cc.

One of the following 7th characters is to be assigned to each code under category O4Ø. 7th character Ø is for single gestations and multiple gestations where the fetus is unspecified. 7th characters 1 through 9 are for cases of multiple gestations to identify the fetus for which the code applies. The appropriate code from category O3Ø, Multiple gestation, must also be assigned when assigning a code from category O4Ø that has a 7th character of 1 through 9.

Ø not applicable or unspecified
1 fetus 1
2 fetus 2
3 fetus 3
4 fetus 4
5 fetus 5
9 other fetus

✓x7th **O4Ø.1 Polyhydramnios, first trimester** M ♀
✓x7th **O4Ø.2 Polyhydramnios, second trimester** M ♀
✓x7th **O4Ø.3 Polyhydramnios, third trimester** M ♀
✓x7th **O4Ø.9 Polyhydramnios, unspecified trimester** M ♀

✓4th O41 Other disorders of amniotic fluid and membranes

EXCLUDES 1 encounter for suspected maternal and fetal conditions ruled out (ZØ3.7-)

One of the following 7th characters is to be assigned to each code under category O41. 7th character Ø is for single gestations and multiple gestations where the fetus is unspecified. 7th characters 1 through 9 are for cases of multiple gestations to identify the fetus for which the code applies. The appropriate code from category O3Ø, Multiple gestation, must also be assigned when assigning a code from category O41 that has a 7th character of 1 through 9.

Ø not applicable or unspecified
1 fetus 1
2 fetus 2
3 fetus 3
4 fetus 4
5 fetus 5
9 other fetus

✓5th **O41.Ø Oligohydramnios**

Oligohydramnios without rupture of membranes
DEF: Low amniotic fluid, occurring most frequently in the last trimester.
CC Excl: For CC codes in category O41.Ø: PDX collection 982

✓x7th **O41.ØØ Oligohydramnios, unspecified trimester** M ♀
✓x7th **O41.Ø1 Oligohydramnios, first trimester** CC M ♀
✓x7th **O41.Ø2 Oligohydramnios, second trimester** CC M ♀
✓x7th **O41.Ø3 Oligohydramnios, third trimester** CC M ♀

✓5th **O41.1 Infection of amniotic sac and membranes**

CC Excl: For MCC codes in subcategory O41.1: PDX collection 983

✓6th **O41.1Ø Infection of amniotic sac and membranes, unspecified**
✓7th **O41.1Ø1 Infection of amniotic sac and membranes, unspecified, first trimester** MCC M ♀
✓7th **O41.1Ø2 Infection of amniotic sac and membranes, unspecified, second trimester** MCC M ♀
✓7th **O41.1Ø3 Infection of amniotic sac and membranes, unspecified, third trimester** MCC M ♀
✓7th **O41.1Ø9 Infection of amniotic sac and membranes, unspecified, unspecified trimester** M ♀

✓6th **O41.12 Chorioamnionitis**
AHA: 2019,2Q,34
✓7th **O41.121 Chorioamnionitis, first trimester** MCC M ♀
✓7th **O41.122 Chorioamnionitis, second trimester** MCC M ♀
✓7th **O41.123 Chorioamnionitis, third trimester** MCC M ♀

✓7th **O41.129 Chorioamnionitis, unspecified trimester** M ♀

✓6th **O41.14 Placentitis**
✓7th **O41.141 Placentitis, first trimester** MCC M ♀
✓7th **O41.142 Placentitis, second trimester** MCC M ♀
✓7th **O41.143 Placentitis, third trimester** MCC M ♀
✓7th **O41.149 Placentitis, unspecified trimester** M ♀

✓5th **O41.8 Other specified disorders of amniotic fluid and membranes**
✓6th **O41.8X Other specified disorders of amniotic fluid and membranes**
✓7th **O41.8X1 Other specified disorders of amniotic fluid and membranes, first trimester** M ♀
✓7th **O41.8X2 Other specified disorders of amniotic fluid and membranes, second trimester** M ♀
✓7th **O41.8X3 Other specified disorders of amniotic fluid and membranes, third trimester** M ♀
✓7th **O41.8X9 Other specified disorders of amniotic fluid and membranes, unspecified trimester** M ♀

✓5th **O41.9 Disorder of amniotic fluid and membranes, unspecified**
✓x7th **O41.9Ø Disorder of amniotic fluid and membranes, unspecified, unspecified trimester** M ♀
✓x7th **O41.91 Disorder of amniotic fluid and membranes, unspecified, first trimester** M ♀
✓x7th **O41.92 Disorder of amniotic fluid and membranes, unspecified, second trimester** M ♀
✓x7th **O41.93 Disorder of amniotic fluid and membranes, unspecified, third trimester** M ♀

✓4th O42 Premature rupture of membranes
AHA: 2016,1Q,3
✓5th **O42.Ø Premature rupture of membranes, onset of labor within 24 hours of rupture**
O42.ØØ Premature rupture of membranes, onset of labor within 24 hours of rupture, unspecified weeks of gestation M ♀
✓6th **O42.Ø1 Preterm premature rupture of membranes, onset of labor within 24 hours of rupture**
Premature rupture of membranes before 37 completed weeks of gestation
O42.Ø11 Preterm premature rupture of membranes, onset of labor within 24 hours of rupture, first trimester M ♀
O42.Ø12 Preterm premature rupture of membranes, onset of labor within 24 hours of rupture, second trimester M ♀
O42.Ø13 Preterm premature rupture of membranes, onset of labor within 24 hours of rupture, third trimester M ♀
O42.Ø19 Preterm premature rupture of membranes, onset of labor within 24 hours of rupture, unspecified trimester M ♀
O42.Ø2 Full-term premature rupture of membranes, onset of labor within 24 hours of rupture M ♀
Premature rupture of membranes at or after 37 completed weeks of gestation, onset of labor within 24 hours of rupture

✓5th **O42.1 Premature rupture of membranes, onset of labor more than 24 hours following rupture**
AHA: 2016,1Q,5
O42.1Ø Premature rupture of membranes, onset of labor more than 24 hours following rupture, unspecified weeks of gestation M ♀
✓6th **O42.11 Preterm premature rupture of membranes, onset of labor more than 24 hours following rupture**
Premature rupture of membranes before 37 completed weeks of gestation
O42.111 Preterm premature rupture of membranes, onset of labor more than 24 hours following rupture, first trimester M ♀

042.112 Preterm premature rupture of membranes, onset of labor more than 24 hours following rupture, **second trimester** Ⓜ♀

042.113 Preterm premature rupture of membranes, onset of labor more than 24 hours following rupture, **third trimester** Ⓜ♀

042.119 Preterm premature rupture of membranes, onset of labor more than 24 hours following rupture, **unspecified trimester** Ⓜ♀

042.12 **Full-term** premature rupture of membranes, onset of labor more than 24 hours following rupture Ⓜ♀
> Premature rupture of membranes at or after 37 completed weeks of gestation, onset of labor more than 24 hours following rupture

✓5ᵗʰ **042.9** Premature rupture of membranes, unspecified as to length of time between rupture and onset of labor

042.90 Premature rupture of membranes, unspecified as to length of time between rupture and onset of labor, unspecified weeks of gestation Ⓜ♀

✓6ᵗʰ **042.91** **Preterm** premature rupture of membranes, unspecified as to length of time between rupture and onset of labor
> Premature rupture of membranes before 37 completed weeks of gestation

042.911 Preterm premature rupture of membranes, unspecified as to length of time between rupture and onset of labor, **first trimester** Ⓜ♀

042.912 Preterm premature rupture of membranes, unspecified as to length of time between rupture and onset of labor, **second trimester** Ⓜ♀

042.913 Preterm premature rupture of membranes, unspecified as to length of time between rupture and onset of labor, **third trimester** Ⓜ♀

042.919 Preterm premature rupture of membranes, unspecified as to length of time between rupture and onset of labor, **unspecified trimester** Ⓜ♀

042.92 **Full-term** premature rupture of membranes, unspecified as to length of time between rupture and onset of labor Ⓜ♀
> Premature rupture of membranes at or after 37 completed weeks of gestation, unspecified as to length of time between rupture and onset of labor

✓4ᵗʰ **043** **Placental disorders**
> EXCLUDES 2 *maternal care for poor fetal growth due to placental insufficiency (O36.5-)*
> *placenta previa (O44.-)*
> *placental polyp (O90.89)*
> *placentitis (O41.14-)*
> *premature separation of placenta [abruptio placentae] (O45.-)*

✓5ᵗʰ **043.0** **Placental transfusion syndromes**

✓6ᵗʰ **043.01** **Fetomaternal** placental transfusion syndrome
> Maternofetal placental transfusion syndrome

043.011 Fetomaternal placental transfusion syndrome, **first trimester** Ⓜ♀

043.012 Fetomaternal placental transfusion syndrome, **second trimester** Ⓜ♀

043.013 Fetomaternal placental transfusion syndrome, **third trimester** Ⓜ♀

043.019 Fetomaternal placental transfusion syndrome, **unspecified trimester** Ⓜ♀

✓6ᵗʰ **043.02** **Fetus-to-fetus** placental transfusion syndrome
> **DEF:** Condition in which an imbalance in amniotic fluid occurs due to uneven blood flow between twins sharing a placenta.

Twin to Twin Transfusion Syndrome (TTTS)

Healthy twins   Twins with TTTS

043.021 Fetus-to-fetus placental transfusion syndrome, **first trimester** Ⓜ♀

043.022 Fetus-to-fetus placental transfusion syndrome, **second trimester** Ⓜ♀

043.023 Fetus-to-fetus placental transfusion syndrome, **third trimester** Ⓜ♀

043.029 Fetus-to-fetus placental transfusion syndrome, **unspecified trimester** Ⓜ♀

✓5ᵗʰ **043.1** **Malformation of placenta**

✓6ᵗʰ **043.10** **Malformation of placenta, unspecified**
> Abnormal placenta NOS

043.101 Malformation of placenta, unspecified, **first trimester** Ⓜ♀

043.102 Malformation of placenta, unspecified, **second trimester** Ⓜ♀

043.103 Malformation of placenta, unspecified, **third trimester** Ⓜ♀

043.109 Malformation of placenta, unspecified, **unspecified trimester** Ⓜ♀

✓6ᵗʰ **043.11** **Circumvallate** placenta

043.111 Circumvallate placenta, **first trimester** Ⓜ♀

043.112 Circumvallate placenta, **second trimester** Ⓜ♀

043.113 Circumvallate placenta, **third trimester** Ⓜ♀

043.119 Circumvallate placenta, **unspecified trimester** Ⓜ♀

✓6ᵗʰ **043.12** **Velamentous insertion of umbilical cord**

043.121 Velamentous insertion of umbilical cord, **first trimester** Ⓜ♀

043.122 Velamentous insertion of umbilical cord, **second trimester** Ⓜ♀

043.123 Velamentous insertion of umbilical cord, **third trimester** Ⓜ♀

043.129 Velamentous insertion of umbilical cord, **unspecified trimester** Ⓜ♀

✓6ᵗʰ **043.19** **Other malformation of placenta**

043.191 Other malformation of placenta, **first trimester** Ⓜ♀

043.192 Other malformation of placenta, **second trimester** Ⓜ♀

043.193 Other malformation of placenta, **third trimester** Ⓜ♀

043.199 Other malformation of placenta, **unspecified trimester** Ⓜ♀

√5ᵗʰ **O43.2 Morbidly adherent placenta**

Code also associated third stage postpartum hemorrhage, if applicable (O72.0)

    EXCLUDES 1   retained placenta (O73.-)

√6ᵗʰ **O43.21 Placenta** accreta

DEF: Condition where the placenta adheres too deeply to the uterine wall; often associated with placenta previa.

O43.211 Placenta accreta, first trimester   M ♀

O43.212 Placenta accreta, second trimester   M ♀

O43.213 Placenta accreta, third trimester   M ♀

O43.219 Placenta accreta, unspecified trimester   M ♀

√6ᵗʰ **O43.22 Placenta** increta

DEF: Condition where the placenta adheres too deeply to the uterine wall and penetrates the muscle; often associated with placenta previa.

O43.221 Placenta increta, first trimester   M ♀

O43.222 Placenta increta, second trimester   M ♀

O43.223 Placenta increta, third trimester   M ♀

O43.229 Placenta increta, unspecified trimester   M ♀

√6ᵗʰ **O43.23 Placenta** percreta

DEF: Condition where the placenta attaches through the uterine muscle and may invade other organs, resulting in antenatal complications, premature delivery, retention of all or a portion of the placenta, or postpartum bleeding.

O43.231 Placenta percreta, first trimester   M ♀

O43.232 Placenta percreta, second trimester   M ♀

O43.233 Placenta percreta, third trimester   M ♀

O43.239 Placenta percreta, unspecified trimester   M ♀

√5ᵗʰ **O43.8 Other placental disorders**

√6ᵗʰ **O43.81 Placental infarction**

O43.811 Placental infarction, first trimester   M ♀

O43.812 Placental infarction, second trimester   M ♀

O43.813 Placental infarction, third trimester   M ♀

O43.819 Placental infarction, unspecified trimester   M ♀

√6ᵗʰ **O43.89 Other placental disorders**

Placental dysfunction

O43.891 Other placental disorders, first trimester   M ♀

O43.892 Other placental disorders, second trimester   M ♀

O43.893 Other placental disorders, third trimester   M ♀

O43.899 Other placental disorders, unspecified trimester   M ♀

√5ᵗʰ **O43.9 Unspecified placental disorder**

O43.90 Unspecified placental disorder, unspecified trimester   M ♀

O43.91 Unspecified placental disorder, first trimester   M ♀

O43.92 Unspecified placental disorder, second trimester   M ♀

O43.93 Unspecified placental disorder, third trimester   M ♀

√4ᵗʰ **O44 Placenta previa**

AHA: 2016,4Q,52-53

DEF: Placenta implanted in the lower segment of the uterus, which commonly causes hemorrhage in the last trimester of pregnancy.

CC Excl: For CC/MCC codes in category O44: PDX collection 966

√5ᵗʰ **O44.0 Complete placenta previa NOS or** without hemorrhage

Placenta previa NOS

O44.00 Complete placenta previa NOS or without hemorrhage, unspecified trimester   M ♀

O44.01 Complete placenta previa NOS or without hemorrhage, first trimester   CC M ♀

O44.02 Complete placenta previa NOS or without hemorrhage, second trimester   CC M ♀

O44.03 Complete placenta previa NOS or without hemorrhage, third trimester   CC M ♀

√5ᵗʰ **O44.1 Complete** placenta previa with hemorrhage

    EXCLUDES 1   labor and delivery complicated by hemorrhage from vasa previa (O69.4)

O44.10 Complete placenta previa with hemorrhage, unspecified trimester   M ♀

O44.11 Complete placenta previa with hemorrhage, first trimester   MCC M ♀

O44.12 Complete placenta previa with hemorrhage, second trimester   MCC M ♀

O44.13 Complete placenta previa with hemorrhage, third trimester   MCC M ♀

√5ᵗʰ **O44.2 Partial** placenta previa without hemorrhage

Marginal placenta previa, NOS or without hemorrhage

O44.20 Partial placenta previa NOS or without hemorrhage, unspecified trimester   M ♀

O44.21 Partial placenta previa NOS or without hemorrhage, first trimester   CC M ♀

O44.22 Partial placenta previa NOS or without hemorrhage, second trimester   CC M ♀

O44.23 Partial placenta previa NOS or without hemorrhage, third trimester   CC M ♀

√5ᵗʰ **O44.3 Partial** placenta previa with hemorrhage

Marginal placenta previa with hemorrhage

O44.30 Partial placenta previa with hemorrhage, unspecified trimester   M ♀

O44.31 Partial placenta previa with hemorrhage, first trimester   MCC M ♀

O44.32 Partial placenta previa with hemorrhage, second trimester   MCC M ♀

O44.33 Partial placenta previa with hemorrhage, third trimester   MCC M ♀

√5ᵗʰ **O44.4 Low lying** placenta NOS or without hemorrhage

Low implantation of placenta NOS or without hemorrhage

O44.40 Low lying placenta NOS or without hemorrhage, unspecified trimester   M ♀

O44.41 Low lying placenta NOS or without hemorrhage, first trimester   CC M ♀

O44.42 Low lying placenta NOS or without hemorrhage, second trimester   CC M ♀

O44.43 Low lying placenta NOS or without hemorrhage, third trimester   CC M ♀

√5ᵗʰ **O44.5 Low lying** placenta with hemorrhage

Low implantation of placenta with hemorrhage

O44.50 Low lying placenta with hemorrhage, unspecified trimester   M ♀

O44.51 Low lying placenta with hemorrhage, first trimester   MCC M ♀

O44.52 Low lying placenta with hemorrhage, second trimester   MCC M ♀

O44.53 Low lying placenta with hemorrhage, third trimester   MCC M ♀

√4ᵗʰ **O45 Premature separation of placenta [abruptio placentae]**

√5ᵗʰ **O45.0 Premature separation of placenta** with coagulation defect

CC Excl: For MCC codes in subcategory O45.0: PDX collection 985

√6ᵗʰ **O45.00 Premature separation of placenta with coagulation defect, unspecified**

O45.001 Premature separation of placenta with coagulation defect, unspecified, first trimester   MCC M ♀

O45.002 Premature separation of placenta with coagulation defect, unspecified, second trimester   MCC M ♀

O45.003 Premature separation of placenta with coagulation defect, unspecified, third trimester   MCC M ♀

O45.009 Premature separation of placenta with coagulation defect, unspecified, unspecified trimester   M ♀

✓6ᵗʰ **O45.01** Premature separation of placenta with afibrinogenemia

Premature separation of placenta with hypofibrinogenemia

O45.011 Premature separation of placenta with afibrinogenemia, first trimester   MCC M ♀

O45.012 Premature separation of placenta with afibrinogenemia, second trimester   MCC M ♀

O45.013 Premature separation of placenta with afibrinogenemia, third trimester   MCC M ♀

O45.019 Premature separation of placenta with afibrinogenemia, unspecified trimester   M ♀

✓6ᵗʰ **O45.02** Premature separation of placenta with disseminated intravascular coagulation

O45.021 Premature separation of placenta with disseminated intravascular coagulation, first trimester   MCC M ♀

O45.022 Premature separation of placenta with disseminated intravascular coagulation, second trimester   MCC M ♀

O45.023 Premature separation of placenta with disseminated intravascular coagulation, third trimester   MCC M ♀

O45.029 Premature separation of placenta with disseminated intravascular coagulation, unspecified trimester   M ♀

✓6ᵗʰ **O45.09** Premature separation of placenta with other coagulation defect

O45.091 Premature separation of placenta with other coagulation defect, first trimester   MCC M ♀

O45.092 Premature separation of placenta with other coagulation defect, second trimester   MCC M ♀

O45.093 Premature separation of placenta with other coagulation defect, third trimester   MCC M ♀

O45.099 Premature separation of placenta with other coagulation defect, unspecified trimester   M ♀

✓5ᵗʰ **O45.8** Other premature separation of placenta

CC Excl: For MCC codes in subcategory O45.8: PDX collection 986

✓6ᵗʰ **O45.8X** Other premature separation of placenta

O45.8X1 Other premature separation of placenta, first trimester   MCC M ♀

O45.8X2 Other premature separation of placenta, second trimester   MCC M ♀

O45.8X3 Other premature separation of placenta, third trimester   MCC M ♀

O45.8X9 Other premature separation of placenta, unspecified trimester   M ♀

✓5ᵗʰ **O45.9** Premature separation of placenta, unspecified

Abruptio placentae NOS

CC Excl: For MCC codes in subcategory O45.9: PDX collection 986

O45.90 Premature separation of placenta, unspecified, unspecified trimester   M ♀

O45.91 Premature separation of placenta, unspecified, first trimester   MCC M ♀

O45.92 Premature separation of placenta, unspecified, second trimester   MCC M ♀

O45.93 Premature separation of placenta, unspecified, third trimester   MCC M ♀

✓4ᵗʰ **O46** Antepartum hemorrhage, not elsewhere classified

EXCLUDES 1   hemorrhage in early pregnancy (O20.-)
intrapartum hemorrhage NEC (O67.-)
placenta previa (O44.-)
premature separation of placenta [abruptio placentae] (O45.-)

DEF: Uterine hemorrhage prior to delivery that is not related to placenta previa or abruptio placentae.

✓5ᵗʰ **O46.0** Antepartum hemorrhage with coagulation defect

CC Excl: For MCC codes in subcategory O46.0: PDX collection 985

✓6ᵗʰ **O46.00** Antepartum hemorrhage with coagulation defect, unspecified

O46.001 Antepartum hemorrhage with coagulation defect, unspecified, first trimester   MCC M ♀

O46.002 Antepartum hemorrhage with coagulation defect, unspecified, second trimester   MCC M ♀

O46.003 Antepartum hemorrhage with coagulation defect, unspecified, third trimester   MCC M ♀

O46.009 Antepartum hemorrhage with coagulation defect, unspecified, unspecified trimester   M ♀

✓6ᵗʰ **O46.01** Antepartum hemorrhage with afibrinogenemia

Antepartum hemorrhage with hypofibrinogenemia

O46.011 Antepartum hemorrhage with afibrinogenemia, first trimester   MCC M ♀

O46.012 Antepartum hemorrhage with afibrinogenemia, second trimester   MCC M ♀

O46.013 Antepartum hemorrhage with afibrinogenemia, third trimester   MCC M ♀

O46.019 Antepartum hemorrhage with afibrinogenemia, unspecified trimester   M ♀

✓6ᵗʰ **O46.02** Antepartum hemorrhage with disseminated intravascular coagulation

O46.021 Antepartum hemorrhage with disseminated intravascular coagulation, first trimester   MCC M ♀

O46.022 Antepartum hemorrhage with disseminated intravascular coagulation, second trimester   MCC M ♀

O46.023 Antepartum hemorrhage with disseminated intravascular coagulation, third trimester   MCC M ♀

O46.029 Antepartum hemorrhage with disseminated intravascular coagulation, unspecified trimester   M ♀

✓6ᵗʰ **O46.09** Antepartum hemorrhage with other coagulation defect

O46.091 Antepartum hemorrhage with other coagulation defect, first trimester   MCC M ♀

O46.092 Antepartum hemorrhage with other coagulation defect, second trimester   MCC M ♀

O46.093 Antepartum hemorrhage with other coagulation defect, third trimester   MCC M ♀

O46.099 Antepartum hemorrhage with other coagulation defect, unspecified trimester   M ♀

✓5ᵗʰ **O46.8** Other antepartum hemorrhage

✓6ᵗʰ **O46.8X** Other antepartum hemorrhage

O46.8X1 Other antepartum hemorrhage, first trimester   M ♀

O46.8X2 Other antepartum hemorrhage, second trimester   M ♀

O46.8X3 Other antepartum hemorrhage, third trimester   M ♀

O46.8X9 Other antepartum hemorrhage, unspecified trimester   M ♀

✓5ᵗʰ **O46.9** Antepartum hemorrhage, unspecified

O46.90 Antepartum hemorrhage, unspecified, unspecified trimester   M ♀

N Newborn: 0   P Pediatric: 0-17   M Maternity: 9-64   A Adult: 15-124   MCC Major Complication/Comorbidity   CC Complication/Comorbidity   SW Severe Wound Dx

902   ICD-10-CM 2020

O46.91	Antepartum hemorrhage, unspecified, **first trimester**	M ♀

O46.92   Antepartum hemorrhage, unspecified, **second trimester**   M ♀

O46.93   Antepartum hemorrhage, unspecified, **third trimester**   M ♀

✓4ᵗʰ **O47**   **False labor**

    INCLUDES   Braxton Hicks contractions
               threatened labor
    EXCLUDES 1   *preterm labor (O60.-)*
    CC Excl: For CC codes in category O47: PDX collection 987

✓5ᵗʰ **O47.0**   **False labor** before 37 completed weeks of gestation

    O47.00   **False labor before 37 completed weeks of gestation, unspecified trimester**   M ♀

    O47.02   **False labor before 37 completed weeks of gestation, second trimester**   CC M ♀

    O47.03   **False labor before 37 completed weeks of gestation, third trimester**   CC M ♀

O47.1   **False labor** at or after 37 completed weeks of gestation   CC M ♀

O47.9   **False labor, unspecified**   M ♀

✓4ᵗʰ **O48**   **Late pregnancy**

O48.0   **Post-term pregnancy**   M ♀

    Pregnancy over 40 completed weeks to 42 completed weeks gestation

O48.1   **Prolonged pregnancy**   M ♀

    Pregnancy which has advanced beyond 42 completed weeks gestation
    AHA: 2016,1Q,5

Complications of labor and delivery (O60-O77)

✓4ᵗʰ **O60**   **Preterm labor**

    INCLUDES   onset (spontaneous) of labor before 37 completed weeks of gestation
    EXCLUDES 1   *false labor (O47.0-)*
               threatened labor NOS (O47.0-)
    CC Excl: For CC/MCC codes in category O60: PDX collection 987

✓5ᵗʰ **O60.0**   **Preterm labor** without delivery

    O60.00   **Preterm labor without delivery, unspecified trimester**   M ♀

    O60.02   **Preterm labor without delivery, second trimester**   MCC M ♀

    O60.03   **Preterm labor without delivery, third trimester**   MCC M ♀

✓5ᵗʰ **O60.1**   **Preterm labor with preterm delivery**

    AHA: 2016,2Q,10

    One of the following 7th characters is to be assigned to each code under subcategory O60.1. 7th character 0 is for single gestations and multiple gestations where the fetus is unspecified. 7th characters 1 through 9 are for cases of multiple gestations to identify the fetus for which the code applies. The appropriate code from category O30, Multiple gestation, must also be assigned when assigning a code from subcategory O60.1 that has a 7th character of 1 through 9.
     0   not applicable or unspecified
     1   fetus 1
     2   fetus 2
     3   fetus 3
     4   fetus 4
     5   fetus 5
     9   other fetus

    ✓x7ᵗʰ **O60.10**   **Preterm labor with preterm delivery, unspecified trimester**   CC M ♀
                Preterm labor with delivery NOS

    ✓x7ᵗʰ **O60.12**   **Preterm labor second trimester with preterm delivery second trimester**   MCC M ♀

    ✓x7ᵗʰ **O60.13**   **Preterm labor second trimester with preterm delivery third trimester**   MCC M ♀

    ✓x7ᵗʰ **O60.14**   **Preterm labor third trimester with preterm delivery third trimester**   MCC M ♀

✓5ᵗʰ **O60.2**   **Term delivery with preterm labor**

    One of the following 7th characters is to be assigned to each code under subcategory O60.2. 7th character 0 is for single gestations and multiple gestations where the fetus is unspecified. 7th characters 1 through 9 are for cases of multiple gestations to identify the fetus for which the code applies. The appropriate code from category O30, Multiple gestation, must also be assigned when assigning a code from subcategory O60.2 that has a 7th character of 1 through 9.
     0   not applicable or unspecified
     1   fetus 1
     2   fetus 2
     3   fetus 3
     4   fetus 4
     5   fetus 5
     9   other fetus

    ✓x7ᵗʰ **O60.20**   **Term delivery with preterm labor, unspecified trimester**   CC M ♀

    ✓x7ᵗʰ **O60.22**   **Term delivery with preterm labor, second trimester**   MCC M ♀

    ✓x7ᵗʰ **O60.23**   **Term delivery with preterm labor, third trimester**   MCC M ♀

✓4ᵗʰ **O61**   **Failed induction of labor**

O61.0   **Failed medical induction of labor**   M ♀

    Failed induction (of labor) by oxytocin
    Failed induction (of labor) by prostaglandins

O61.1   **Failed instrumental induction of labor**   M ♀

    Failed mechanical induction (of labor)
    Failed surgical induction (of labor)

O61.8   **Other failed induction of labor**   M ♀

O61.9   **Failed induction of labor, unspecified**   M ♀

✓4ᵗʰ **O62**   **Abnormalities of forces of labor**

    DEF: Uterine inertia: Weak or poorly coordinated contractions of the uterus during labor.

O62.0   **Primary inadequate contractions**   M ♀

    Failure of cervical dilatation
    Primary hypotonic uterine dysfunction
    Uterine inertia during latent phase of labor

O62.1   **Secondary uterine inertia**   M ♀

    Arrested active phase of labor
    Secondary hypotonic uterine dysfunction

O62.2   **Other uterine inertia**   M ♀

    Atony of uterus without hemorrhage
    Atony of uterus NOS
    Desultory labor
    Hypotonic uterine dysfunction NOS
    Irregular labor
    Poor contractions
    Slow slope active phase of labor
    Uterine inertia NOS
    EXCLUDES 1   *atony of uterus with hemorrhage (postpartum) (O72.1)*
               postpartum atony of uterus without hemorrhage (O75.89)
    DEF: Uterine atony: Failure of the uterine muscles to contract after the fetus and placenta are delivered.

O62.3   **Precipitate labor**   M ♀

    DEF: Rapid labor with delivery occurring in three hours or less from the onset of contractions.

O62.4   **Hypertonic, incoordinate, and prolonged uterine contractions**   M ♀

    Cervical spasm
    Contraction ring dystocia
    Dyscoordinate labor
    Hour-glass contraction of uterus
    Hypertonic uterine dysfunction
    Incoordinate uterine action
    Tetanic contractions
    Uterine dystocia NOS
    Uterine spasm
    EXCLUDES 1   *dystocia (fetal) (maternal) NOS (O66.9)*

O62.8   **Other abnormalities of forces of labor**   M ♀

O62.9   **Abnormality of forces of labor, unspecified**   M ♀

✓4ᵗʰ **O63 Long labor**

   O63.0 Prolonged first stage (of labor)   Ⓜ ♀

   O63.1 Prolonged second stage (of labor)   Ⓜ ♀

   O63.2 Delayed delivery of second twin, triplet, etc.   Ⓜ ♀

   O63.9 Long labor, unspecified   ⒸⒸ Ⓜ ♀
        Prolonged labor NOS
        CC Excl: PDX collection 988

✓4ᵗʰ **O64 Obstructed labor due to malposition and malpresentation of fetus**

> One of the following 7th characters is to be assigned to each code under category O64. 7th character Ø is for single gestations and multiple gestations where the fetus is unspecified. 7th characters 1 through 9 are for cases of multiple gestations to identify the fetus for which the code applies. The appropriate code from category O30, Multiple gestation, must also be assigned when assigning a code from category O64 that has a 7th character of 1 through 9.
>
> Ø   not applicable or unspecified
> 1   fetus 1
> 2   fetus 2
> 3   fetus 3
> 4   fetus 4
> 5   fetus 5
> 9   other fetus

Fetal Malposition

Breech   Shoulder (arm prolapse)   Mother's pelvis   Compound (extremity together with head)   Face (mentum)   Oblique

✓x7ᵗʰ **O64.0** Obstructed labor due to incomplete rotation of fetal head   Ⓜ ♀
        Deep transverse arrest
        Obstructed labor due to persistent occipitoiliac (position)
        Obstructed labor due to persistent occipitoposterior (position)
        Obstructed labor due to persistent occipitosacral (position)
        Obstructed labor due to persistent occipitotransverse (position)

✓x7ᵗʰ **O64.1** Obstructed labor due to breech presentation   Ⓜ ♀
        Obstructed labor due to buttocks presentation
        Obstructed labor due to complete breech presentation
        Obstructed labor due to frank breech presentation

✓x7ᵗʰ **O64.2** Obstructed labor due to face presentation   Ⓜ ♀
        Obstructed labor due to chin presentation

✓x7ᵗʰ **O64.3** Obstructed labor due to brow presentation   Ⓜ ♀

✓x7ᵗʰ **O64.4** Obstructed labor due to shoulder presentation   Ⓜ ♀
        Prolapsed arm
        EXCLUDES 1   impacted shoulders (O66.0)
                    shoulder dystocia (O66.0)

✓x7ᵗʰ **O64.5** Obstructed labor due to compound presentation   Ⓜ ♀

✓x7ᵗʰ **O64.8** Obstructed labor due to other malposition and malpresentation   Ⓜ ♀
        Obstructed labor due to footling presentation
        Obstructed labor due to incomplete breech presentation

✓x7ᵗʰ **O64.9** Obstructed labor due to malposition and malpresentation, unspecified   Ⓜ ♀

✓4ᵗʰ **O65 Obstructed labor due to maternal pelvic abnormality**

   O65.0 Obstructed labor due to deformed pelvis   Ⓜ ♀

   O65.1 Obstructed labor due to generally contracted pelvis   Ⓜ ♀

   O65.2 Obstructed labor due to pelvic inlet contraction   Ⓜ ♀

   O65.3 Obstructed labor due to pelvic outlet and mid-cavity contraction   Ⓜ ♀

   O65.4 Obstructed labor due to fetopelvic disproportion, unspecified   Ⓜ ♀
        EXCLUDES 1   dystocia due to abnormality of fetus (O66.2-O66.3)

   O65.5 Obstructed labor due to abnormality of maternal pelvic organs   Ⓜ ♀
        Obstructed labor due to conditions listed in O34.-
        Use additional code to identify abnormality of pelvic organs O34.-

   O65.8 Obstructed labor due to other maternal pelvic abnormalities   Ⓜ ♀

   O65.9 Obstructed labor due to maternal pelvic abnormality, unspecified   Ⓜ ♀

✓4ᵗʰ **O66 Other obstructed labor**

   O66.0 Obstructed labor due to shoulder dystocia   Ⓜ ♀
        Impacted shoulders
        DEF: Obstructed labor due to impacted fetal shoulders. It is an emergency condition that may require cesarean section, forceps delivery, vacuum extraction, or symphysiotomy.

   O66.1 Obstructed labor due to locked twins   Ⓜ ♀

   O66.2 Obstructed labor due to unusually large fetus   Ⓜ ♀

   O66.3 Obstructed labor due to other abnormalities of fetus   Ⓜ ♀
        Dystocia due to fetal ascites
        Dystocia due to fetal hydrops
        Dystocia due to fetal meningomyelocele
        Dystocia due to fetal sacral teratoma
        Dystocia due to fetal tumor
        Dystocia due to hydrocephalic fetus
        Use additional code to identify cause of obstruction

✓5ᵗʰ   **O66.4** Failed trial of labor

       O66.40 Failed trial of labor, unspecified   Ⓜ ♀

       O66.41 Failed attempted vaginal birth after previous cesarean delivery   Ⓜ ♀
            Code first rupture of uterus, if applicable (O71.0-, O71.1)

   O66.5 Attempted application of vacuum extractor and forceps   Ⓜ ♀
        Attempted application of vacuum or forceps, with subsequent delivery by forceps or cesarean delivery

   O66.6 Obstructed labor due to other multiple fetuses   Ⓜ ♀

   O66.8 Other specified obstructed labor   Ⓜ ♀
        Use additional code to identify cause of obstruction

   O66.9 Obstructed labor, unspecified   Ⓜ ♀
        Dystocia NOS
        Fetal dystocia NOS
        Maternal dystocia NOS

✓4ᵗʰ **O67 Labor and delivery complicated by intrapartum hemorrhage, not elsewhere classified**
       EXCLUDES 1   antepartum hemorrhage NEC (O46.-)
               placenta previa (O44.-)
               premature separation of placenta [abruptio placentae] (O45.-)
       EXCLUDES 2   postpartum hemorrhage (O72.-)

   O67.0 Intrapartum hemorrhage with coagulation defect   ⓂⒸⒸ Ⓜ ♀
        Intrapartum hemorrhage (excessive) associated with afibrinogenemia
        Intrapartum hemorrhage (excessive) associated with disseminated intravascular coagulation
        Intrapartum hemorrhage (excessive) associated with hyperfibrinolysis
        Intrapartum hemorrhage (excessive) associated with hypofibrinogenemia
        CC Excl: PDX collection 985

   O67.8 Other intrapartum hemorrhage   Ⓜ ♀
        Excessive intrapartum hemorrhage

   O67.9 Intrapartum hemorrhage, unspecified   Ⓜ ♀

Ⓝ Newborn: 0   Ⓟ Pediatric: 0-17   Ⓜ Maternity: 9-64   Ⓐ Adult: 15-124   ⓂⒸⒸ Major Complication/Comorbidity   ⒸⒸ Complication/Comorbidity   ⓈⓌ Severe Wound Dx

904   ICD-10-CM 2020

O68 Labor and delivery complicated by abnormality of fetal acid-base balance cc M ♀

Fetal acidemia complicating labor and delivery
Fetal acidosis complicating labor and delivery
Fetal alkalosis complicating labor and delivery
Fetal metabolic acidemia complicating labor and delivery

EXCLUDES 1 *fetal stress NOS (O77.9)*
labor and delivery complicated by electrocardiographic evidence of fetal stress (O77.8)
labor and delivery complicated by ultrasonic evidence of fetal stress (O77.8)

EXCLUDES 2 *abnormality in fetal heart rate or rhythm (O76)*
labor and delivery complicated by meconium in amniotic fluid (O77.0)

CC Excl: PDX collection 989

✓4ᵗʰ **O69 Labor and delivery complicated by umbilical cord complications**

AHA: 2016,1Q,5

One of the following 7th characters is to be assigned to each code under category O69. 7th character Ø is for single gestations and multiple gestations where the fetus is unspecified. 7th characters 1 through 9 are for cases of multiple gestations to identify the fetus for which the code applies. The appropriate code from category O30, Multiple gestation, must also be assigned when assigning a code from category O69 that has a 7th character of 1 through 9.

Ø   not applicable or unspecified
1   fetus 1
2   fetus 2
3   fetus 3
4   fetus 4
5   fetus 5
9   other fetus

✓x7ᵗʰ **O69.Ø Labor and delivery complicated by prolapse of cord** M ♀

DEF: Abnormal presentation of the fetus marked by a protruding umbilical cord during labor. It can cause fetal death.

✓x7ᵗʰ **O69.1 Labor and delivery complicated by cord around neck, with compression** M ♀

EXCLUDES 1 *labor and delivery complicated by cord around neck, without compression (O69.81)*

✓x7ᵗʰ **O69.2 Labor and delivery complicated by other cord entanglement, with compression** M ♀

Labor and delivery complicated by compression of cord NOS
Labor and delivery complicated by entanglement of cords of twins in monoamniotic sac
Labor and delivery complicated by knot in cord

EXCLUDES 1 *labor and delivery complicated by other cord entanglement, without compression (O69.82)*

✓x7ᵗʰ **O69.3 Labor and delivery complicated by short cord** M ♀

✓x7ᵗʰ **O69.4 Labor and delivery complicated by vasa previa** M ♀

Labor and delivery complicated by hemorrhage from vasa previa

✓x7ᵗʰ **O69.5 Labor and delivery complicated by vascular lesion of cord** M ♀

Labor and delivery complicated by cord bruising
Labor and delivery complicated by cord hematoma
Labor and delivery complicated by thrombosis of umbilical vessels

✓5ᵗʰ **O69.8 Labor and delivery complicated by other cord complications**

✓x7ᵗʰ **O69.81 Labor and delivery complicated by cord around neck, without compression** M ♀

AHA: 2016,1Q,5

✓x7ᵗʰ **O69.82 Labor and delivery complicated by other cord entanglement, without compression** M ♀

✓x7ᵗʰ **O69.89 Labor and delivery complicated by other cord complications** M ♀

✓x7ᵗʰ **O69.9 Labor and delivery complicated by cord complication, unspecified** M ♀

✓4ᵗʰ **O70 Perineal laceration during delivery**

INCLUDES episiotomy extended by laceration
EXCLUDES 1 *obstetric high vaginal laceration alone (O71.4)*
AHA: 2016,2Q,34; 2016,1Q,3-4,5

O70.Ø First degree perineal laceration during delivery M ♀

Perineal laceration, rupture or tear involving fourchette during delivery
Perineal laceration, rupture or tear involving labia during delivery
Perineal laceration, rupture or tear involving skin during delivery
Perineal laceration, rupture or tear involving vagina during delivery
Perineal laceration, rupture or tear involving vulva during delivery
Slight perineal laceration, rupture or tear during delivery

O70.1 Second degree perineal laceration during delivery M ♀

Perineal laceration, rupture or tear during delivery as in O70.0, also involving pelvic floor
Perineal laceration, rupture or tear during delivery as in O70.0, also involving perineal muscles
Perineal laceration, rupture or tear during delivery as in O70.0, also involving vaginal muscles

EXCLUDES 1 *perineal laceration involving anal sphincter (O70.2)*

✓5ᵗʰ **O70.2 Third degree perineal laceration during delivery**

Perineal laceration, rupture or tear during delivery as in O70.1, also involving anal sphincter
Perineal laceration, rupture or tear during delivery as in O70.1, also involving rectovaginal septum
Perineal laceration, rupture or tear during delivery as in O70.1, also involving sphincter NOS

EXCLUDES 1 *anal sphincter tear during delivery without third degree perineal laceration (O70.4)*
perineal laceration involving anal or rectal mucosa (O70.3)

AHA: 2016,4Q,53-54

CC Excl: For CC codes in subcategory O70.2: PDX collection 990

O70.20 Third degree perineal laceration during delivery, unspecified cc M ♀

O70.21 Third degree perineal laceration during delivery, IIIa cc M ♀

Third degree perineal laceration during delivery with less than 50% of external anal sphincter (EAS) thickness torn

O70.22 Third degree perineal laceration during delivery, IIIb cc M ♀

Third degree perineal laceration during delivery with more than 50% external anal sphincter (EAS) thickness torn

O70.23 Third degree perineal laceration during delivery, IIIc cc M ♀

Third degree perineal laceration during delivery with both external anal sphincter (EAS) and internal anal sphincter (IAS) torn

O70.3 Fourth degree perineal laceration during delivery cc M ♀

Perineal laceration, rupture or tear during delivery as in O70.2, also involving anal mucosa
Perineal laceration, rupture or tear during delivery as in O70.2, also involving rectal mucosa

CC Excl: PDX collection 991

O70.4 Anal sphincter tear complicating delivery, not associated with third degree laceration cc M ♀

EXCLUDES 1 *anal sphincter tear with third degree perineal laceration (O70.2)*

CC Excl: PDX collection 992

O70.9 Perineal laceration during delivery, unspecified M ♀

✓4ᵗʰ **O71 Other obstetric trauma**

INCLUDES obstetric damage from instruments

✓5ᵗʰ **O71.Ø Rupture of uterus (spontaneous) before onset of labor**

EXCLUDES 1 *disruption of (current) cesarean delivery wound (O90.0)*
laceration of uterus, NEC (O71.81)

O71.00 Rupture of uterus before onset of labor, unspecified trimester M ♀

✔ Additional Character Required   ✓x7ᵗʰ Placeholder   <u>Unacceptable PDx</u>   Questionable PDx   Manifestation   <u>Unspecified Dx</u>   H1-H14 HAC   HCC CMS-HCC Dx   HIV HIV Dx

ICD-10-CM 2020   905

071.02 Rupture of uterus before onset of labor, second trimester [MCC] [M] ♀
CC Excl: PDX collection 993

071.03 Rupture of uterus before onset of labor, third trimester [MCC] [M] ♀
CC Excl: PDX collection 993

071.1 Rupture of uterus during labor [MCC] [M] ♀
Rupture of uterus not stated as occurring before onset of labor
EXCLUDES 1   *disruption of cesarean delivery wound (O90.0)*
laceration of uterus, NEC (O71.81)
CC Excl: PDX collection 993

071.2 Postpartum inversion of uterus [CC] [M] ♀
CC Excl: PDX collection 994

071.3 Obstetric laceration of cervix [CC] [M] ♀
Annular detachment of cervix
CC Excl: PDX collection 995

071.4 Obstetric high vaginal laceration alone [CC] [M] ♀
Laceration of vaginal wall without perineal laceration
EXCLUDES 1   *obstetric high vaginal laceration with perineal laceration (O70.-)*
AHA: 2016,1Q,5
CC Excl: PDX collection 996

071.5 Other obstetric injury to pelvic organs [CC] [M] ♀
Obstetric injury to bladder
Obstetric injury to urethra
EXCLUDES 2   *obstetric periurethral trauma (O71.82)*
AHA: 2014,4Q,18
CC Excl: PDX collection 993

071.6 Obstetric damage to pelvic joints and ligaments [CC] [M] ♀
Obstetric avulsion of inner symphyseal cartilage
Obstetric damage to coccyx
Obstetric traumatic separation of symphysis (pubis)
CC Excl: PDX collection 997

071.7 Obstetric hematoma of pelvis [CC] [M] ♀
Obstetric hematoma of perineum
Obstetric hematoma of vagina
Obstetric hematoma of vulva
CC Excl: PDX collection 998

√5th **071.8 Other specified obstetric trauma**

071.81   Laceration of uterus, not elsewhere classified [M] ♀

071.82   Other specified trauma to perineum and vulva [M] ♀
Obstetric periurethral trauma
AHA: 2016,1Q,4; 2014,4Q,18

071.89   Other specified obstetric trauma [M] ♀

071.9 Obstetric trauma, unspecified [M] ♀

√4th **072 Postpartum hemorrhage**
INCLUDES   hemorrhage after delivery of fetus or infant

072.0 Third-stage hemorrhage [CC] [M] ♀
Hemorrhage associated with retained, trapped or adherent placenta
Retained placenta NOS
Code also type of adherent placenta (O43.2-)
CC Excl: PDX collection 999

072.1 Other immediate postpartum hemorrhage [CC] [M] ♀
Hemorrhage following delivery of placenta
Postpartum hemorrhage (atonic) NOS
Uterine atony with hemorrhage
EXCLUDES 1   *uterine atony NOS (O62.2)*
uterine atony without hemorrhage (O62.2)
postpartum atony of uterus without hemorrhage (O75.89)
AHA: 2016,1Q,4
DEF: Uterine atony: Failure of the uterine muscles to contract after the fetus and placenta are delivered.
CC Excl: PDX collection 1000

072.2 Delayed and secondary postpartum hemorrhage [CC] [M] ♀
Hemorrhage associated with retained portions of placenta or membranes after the first 24 hours following delivery of placenta
Retained products of conception NOS, following delivery
CC Excl: PDX collection 1001

072.3 Postpartum coagulation defects [M] ♀
Postpartum afibrinogenemia
Postpartum fibrinolysis

√4th **073 Retained placenta and membranes, without hemorrhage**
EXCLUDES 1   *placenta accreta (O43.21-)*
placenta increta (O43.22-)
placenta percreta (O43.23-)
DEF: Postpartum condition resulting from failure to expel placental membrane tissues due to failed contractions of the uterine wall.

073.0 Retained placenta without hemorrhage [M] ♀
Adherent placenta, without hemorrhage
Trapped placenta without hemorrhage

073.1 Retained portions of placenta and membranes, without hemorrhage [M] ♀
Retained products of conception following delivery, without hemorrhage

√4th **074 Complications of anesthesia during labor and delivery**
INCLUDES   maternal complications arising from the administration of a general, regional or local anesthetic, analgesic or other sedation during labor and delivery
Use additional code, if applicable, to identify specific complication

074.0 Aspiration pneumonitis due to anesthesia during labor and delivery [M] ♀
Inhalation of stomach contents or secretions NOS due to anesthesia during labor and delivery
Mendelson's syndrome due to anesthesia during labor and delivery

074.1 Other pulmonary complications of anesthesia during labor and delivery [M] ♀

074.2 Cardiac complications of anesthesia during labor and delivery [M] ♀

074.3 Central nervous system complications of anesthesia during labor and delivery [M] ♀

074.4 Toxic reaction to local anesthesia during labor and delivery [M] ♀

074.5 Spinal and epidural anesthesia-induced headache during labor and delivery [M] ♀

074.6 Other complications of spinal and epidural anesthesia during labor and delivery [M] ♀

074.7 Failed or difficult intubation for anesthesia during labor and delivery [M] ♀

074.8 Other complications of anesthesia during labor and delivery [M] ♀

074.9 Complication of anesthesia during labor and delivery, unspecified [M] ♀

√4th **075 Other complications of labor and delivery, not elsewhere classified**
EXCLUDES 2   *puerperal (postpartum) infection (O86.-)*
puerperal (postpartum) sepsis (O85)

075.0 Maternal distress during labor and delivery [M] ♀

075.1 Shock during or following labor and delivery [MCC] [M] ♀
Obstetric shock following labor and delivery
CC Excl: PDX collection 1002

075.2 Pyrexia during labor, not elsewhere classified [CC] [M] ♀
CC Excl: PDX collection 1003

075.3 Other infection during labor [MCC] [M] ♀
Sepsis during labor
Use additional code (B95-B97), to identify infectious agent
CC Excl: PDX collection 1004

075.4 Other complications of obstetric surgery and procedures [M] ♀
Cardiac arrest following obstetric surgery or procedures
Cardiac failure following obstetric surgery or procedures
Cerebral anoxia following obstetric surgery or procedures
Pulmonary edema following obstetric surgery or procedures
Use additional code to identify specific complication
EXCLUDES 2   *complications of anesthesia during labor and delivery (O74.-)*
disruption of obstetrical (surgical) wound (O90.0-O90.1)
hematoma of obstetrical (surgical) wound (O90.2)
infection of obstetrical (surgical) wound (O86.0-)

075.5 Delayed delivery after artificial rupture of membranes [M] ♀

√5th **075.8 Other specified complications of labor and delivery**

075.81   Maternal exhaustion complicating labor and delivery [M] ♀

O75.82   **Onset (spontaneous) of labor after 37 completed weeks of gestation but before 39 completed weeks gestation, with delivery by (planned) cesarean section**   M ♀

Delivery by (planned) cesarean section occurring after 37 completed weeks of gestation but before 39 completed weeks gestation due to (spontaneous) onset of labor

Code first to specify reason for planned cesarean section such as:

cephalopelvic disproportion (normally formed fetus) (O33.9)

previous cesarean delivery (O34.21)

O75.89   **Other specified complications of labor and delivery**   M ♀

O75.9   **Complication of labor and delivery, unspecified**   M ♀

O76   Abnormality in fetal heart rate and rhythm complicating labor and delivery   CC M ♀

Depressed fetal heart rate tones complicating labor and delivery

Fetal bradycardia complicating labor and delivery

Fetal heart rate decelerations complicating labor and delivery

Fetal heart rate irregularity complicating labor and delivery

Fetal heart rate abnormal variability complicating labor and delivery

Fetal tachycardia complicating labor and delivery

Non-reassuring fetal heart rate or rhythm complicating labor and delivery

EXCLUDES 1   *fetal stress NOS (O77.9)*

labor and delivery complicated by electrocardiographic evidence of fetal stress (O77.8)

labor and delivery complicated by ultrasonic evidence of fetal stress (O77.8)

EXCLUDES 2   *fetal metabolic acidemia (O68)*

other fetal stress (O77.0-O77.1)

AHA: 2013,4Q,118

O77   Other fetal stress complicating labor and delivery

O77.0   **Labor and delivery complicated by meconium in amniotic fluid**   M ♀

AHA: 2013,4Q,117-118

O77.1   **Fetal stress in labor or delivery due to drug administration**   M ♀

O77.8   **Labor and delivery complicated by other evidence of fetal stress**   M ♀

Labor and delivery complicated by electrocardiographic evidence of fetal stress

Labor and delivery complicated by ultrasonic evidence of fetal stress

EXCLUDES 1   *abnormality of fetal acid-base balance (O68)*

abnormality in fetal heart rate or rhythm (O76)

fetal metabolic acidemia (O68)

O77.9   **Labor and delivery complicated by fetal stress, unspecified**   M ♀

EXCLUDES 1   *abnormality of fetal acid-base balance (O68)*

abnormality in fetal heart rate or rhythm (O76)

fetal metabolic acidemia (O68)

Encounter for delivery (O80-O82)

O80   Encounter for full-term uncomplicated delivery   M ♀

NOTE   Delivery requiring minimal or no assistance, with or without episiotomy, without fetal manipulation [e.g., rotation version] or instrumentation [forceps] of a spontaneous, cephalic, vaginal, full-term, single, live-born infant. This code is for use as a single diagnosis code and is not to be used with any other code from chapter 15.

Use additional code to indicate outcome of delivery (Z37.0)

AHA: 2016,4Q,150; 2014,2Q,9

O82   Encounter for cesarean delivery without indication   M ♀

Use additional code to indicate outcome of delivery (Z37.0)

Complications predominantly related to the puerperium (O85-O92)

EXCLUDES 2   *mental and behavioral disorders associated with the puerperium (F53.-)*

obstetrical tetanus (A34)

puerperal osteomalacia (M83.0)

O85   Puerperal sepsis   MCC M ♀

Postpartum sepsis

Puerperal peritonitis

Puerperal pyemia

Use additional code (B95-B97), to identify infectious agent

Use additional code (R65.2-) to identify severe sepsis, if applicable

EXCLUDES 1   *fever of unknown origin following delivery (O86.4)*

genital tract infection following delivery (O86.1-)

obstetric pyemic and septic embolism (O88.3-)

puerperal septic thrombophlebitis (O86.81)

urinary tract infection following delivery (O86.2-)

EXCLUDES 2   *sepsis during labor (O75.3)*

AHA: 2018,4Q,23

CC Excl: PDX collection 1005

O86   Other puerperal infections

Use additional code (B95-B97), to identify infectious agent

EXCLUDES 2   *infection during labor (O75.3)*

obstetrical tetanus (A34)

CC Excl: For codes in category O86:

For MCC codes: PDX collection 1005

For CC codes, unless otherwise noted: PDX collection 968

O86.0   **Infection of obstetric surgical wound**

Infected cesarean delivery wound following delivery

Infected perineal repair following delivery

EXCLUDES 1   *complications of procedures, not elsewhere classified (T81.4-)*

postprocedural fever NOS (R50.82)

postprocedural retroperitoneal abscess (K68.11)

AHA: 2018,4Q,22-23,62

O86.00   **Infection of obstetric surgical wound, unspecified**   M ♀

O86.01   **Infection of obstetric surgical wound, superficial incisional site**   M ♀

Subcutaneous abscess following an obstetrical procedure

Stitch abscess following an obstetrical procedure

O86.02   **Infection of obstetric surgical wound, deep incisional site**   M ♀

Intramuscular abscess following an obstetrical procedure

▶Sub-fascial abscess following an obstetrical procedure◀

O86.03   **Infection of obstetric surgical wound, organ and space site**   M ♀

Intraabdominal abscess following an obstetrical procedure

Subphrenic abscess following an obstetrical procedure

O86.04   **Sepsis following an obstetrical procedure**   MCC M ♀

Use additional code to identify the sepsis

AHA: 2019,2Q,39

O86.09   **Infection of obstetric surgical wound, other surgical site**   M ♀

O86.1   **Other infection of genital tract following delivery**

O86.11   **Cervicitis following delivery**   CC M ♀

O86.12   **Endometritis following delivery**   CC M ♀

CC Excl: PDX collection 1005

O86.13   **Vaginitis following delivery**   CC M ♀

O86.19   **Other infection of genital tract following delivery**   CC M ♀

O86.2   **Urinary tract infection following delivery**

O86.20   **Urinary tract infection following delivery, unspecified**   CC M ♀

Puerperal urinary tract infection NOS

O86.21   **Infection of kidney following delivery**   CC M ♀

O86.22   **Infection of bladder following delivery**   CC M ♀

Infection of urethra following delivery

O86.29   **Other urinary tract infection following delivery**   CC M ♀

✓ Additional Character Required   ✓x7th Placeholder   Unacceptable PDx   Questionable PDx   Manifestation   Unspecified Dx   H1-H4 HAC   HCC CMS-HCC Dx   HIV HIV Dx

ICD-10-CM 2020   907

Chapter 15. Pregnancy, Childbirth and the Puerperium

O86.4 **Pyrexia** of unknown origin following delivery   `CC` M ♀

Puerperal infection NOS following delivery

Puerperal pyrexia NOS following delivery

EXCLUDES 2   *pyrexia during labor (O75.2)*

DEF: Fever of unknown origin experienced by the mother after childbirth.

CC Excl: PDX collection 1006

√5ᵗʰ **O86.8** **Other specified puerperal infections**

O86.81 **Puerperal** septic thrombophlebitis   `MCC` M ♀

O86.89 **Other specified puerperal infections**   `MCC` M ♀

√4ᵗʰ **O87** **Venous complications and hemorrhoids in the puerperium**

INCLUDES   venous complications in labor, delivery and the puerperium

EXCLUDES 2   *obstetric embolism (O88.-)*

puerperal septic thrombophlebitis (O86.81)

venous complications in pregnancy (O22.-)

CC Excl: For CC/MCC codes in category O87: PDX collection 967

O87.0 **Superficial thrombophlebitis in the puerperium**   `CC` M ♀

Puerperal phlebitis NOS

Puerperal thrombosis NOS

O87.1 **Deep phlebothrombosis in the puerperium**   `MCC` M ♀

Deep vein thrombosis, postpartum

Pelvic thrombophlebitis, postpartum

Use additional code to identify the deep vein thrombosis (I82.4-, I82.5-, I82.62-, I82.72-)

Use additional code, if applicable, for associated long-term (current) use of anticoagulants (Z79.01)

O87.2 **Hemorrhoids in the puerperium**   `CC` M ♀

O87.3 **Cerebral venous thrombosis in the puerperium**   `CC` M ♀

Cerebrovenous sinus thrombosis in the puerperium

O87.4 **Varicose veins of lower extremity in the puerperium**   M ♀

O87.8 **Other venous complications in the puerperium**   `CC` M ♀

Genital varices in the puerperium

O87.9 **Venous complication in the puerperium, unspecified**   M ♀

Puerperal phlebopathy NOS

√4ᵗʰ **O88** **Obstetric embolism**

EXCLUDES 1   *embolism complicating abortion NOS (O03.2)*

embolism complicating ectopic or molar pregnancy (O08.2)

embolism complicating failed attempted abortion (O07.2)

embolism complicating induced abortion (O04.7)

embolism complicating spontaneous abortion (O03.2, O03.7)

CC Excl: For CC/MCC codes in category O88: PDX collection 1007

√5ᵗʰ **O88.0** **Obstetric** air embolism

DEF: Sudden blocking of the pulmonary artery or right ventricle with air or nitrogen bubbles.

√6ᵗʰ **O88.01** **Obstetric air embolism in** pregnancy

O88.011 **Air embolism in pregnancy, first trimester**   `MCC` M ♀

O88.012 **Air embolism in pregnancy, second trimester**   `MCC` M ♀

O88.013 **Air embolism in pregnancy, third trimester**   `MCC` M ♀

O88.019 **Air embolism in pregnancy, unspecified trimester**   M ♀

O88.02 **Air embolism in** childbirth   `MCC` M ♀

O88.03 **Air embolism in the** puerperium   `MCC` M ♀

√5ᵗʰ **O88.1** **Amniotic fluid** embolism

Anaphylactoid syndrome in pregnancy

√6ᵗʰ **O88.11** **Amniotic fluid embolism in** pregnancy

O88.111 **Amniotic fluid embolism in pregnancy, first trimester**   `MCC` M ♀

O88.112 **Amniotic fluid embolism in pregnancy, second trimester**   `MCC` M ♀

O88.113 **Amniotic fluid embolism in pregnancy, third trimester**   `MCC` M ♀

O88.119 **Amniotic fluid embolism in pregnancy, unspecified trimester**   M ♀

O88.12 **Amniotic fluid embolism in** childbirth   `MCC` M ♀

O88.13 **Amniotic fluid embolism in the** puerperium   `MCC` M ♀

√5ᵗʰ **O88.2** **Obstetric** thromboembolism

√6ᵗʰ **O88.21** **Thromboembolism in** pregnancy

Obstetric (pulmonary) embolism NOS

O88.211 **Thromboembolism in pregnancy, first trimester**   `MCC` M ♀

O88.212 **Thromboembolism in pregnancy, second trimester**   `MCC` M ♀

O88.213 **Thromboembolism in pregnancy, third trimester**   `MCC` M ♀

O88.219 **Thromboembolism in pregnancy, unspecified trimester**   M ♀

O88.22 **Thromboembolism in** childbirth   `MCC` M ♀

O88.23 **Thromboembolism in the** puerperium   `MCC` M ♀

Puerperal (pulmonary) embolism NOS

√5ᵗʰ **O88.3** **Obstetric** pyemic and septic embolism

√6ᵗʰ **O88.31** **Pyemic and septic embolism in** pregnancy

O88.311 **Pyemic and septic embolism in pregnancy, first trimester**   `MCC` M ♀

O88.312 **Pyemic and septic embolism in pregnancy, second trimester**   `MCC` M ♀

O88.313 **Pyemic and septic embolism in pregnancy, third trimester**   `MCC` M ♀

O88.319 **Pyemic and septic embolism in pregnancy, unspecified trimester**   `CC` M ♀

O88.32 **Pyemic and septic embolism in** childbirth   `MCC` M ♀

O88.33 **Pyemic and septic embolism in the** puerperium   `MCC` M ♀

√5ᵗʰ **O88.8** **Other obstetric embolism**

Obstetric fat embolism

√6ᵗʰ **O88.81** **Other embolism in** pregnancy

O88.811 **Other embolism in pregnancy, first trimester**   `MCC` M ♀

O88.812 **Other embolism in pregnancy, second trimester**   `MCC` M ♀

O88.813 **Other embolism in pregnancy, third trimester**   `MCC` M ♀

O88.819 **Other embolism in pregnancy, unspecified trimester**   M ♀

O88.82 **Other embolism in** childbirth   `MCC` M ♀

O88.83 **Other embolism in the** puerperium   `MCC` M ♀

√4ᵗʰ **O89** **Complications of anesthesia during the puerperium**

INCLUDES   maternal complications arising from the administration of a general, regional or local anesthetic, analgesic or other sedation during the puerperium

Use additional code, if applicable, to identify specific complication

√5ᵗʰ **O89.0** **Pulmonary** complications of anesthesia during the puerperium

O89.01 **Aspiration pneumonitis due to anesthesia during the puerperium**   M ♀

Inhalation of stomach contents or secretions NOS due to anesthesia during the puerperium

Mendelson's syndrome due to anesthesia during the puerperium

O89.09 **Other pulmonary complications of anesthesia during the puerperium**   M ♀

O89.1 **Cardiac complications of anesthesia during the puerperium**   M ♀

O89.2 **Central nervous system complications of anesthesia during the puerperium**   M ♀

O89.3 **Toxic reaction to local anesthesia during the puerperium**   M ♀

O89.4 **Spinal and epidural anesthesia-induced headache during the puerperium**   M ♀

O89.5 **Other complications of spinal and epidural anesthesia during the puerperium**   M ♀

O89.6 **Failed or difficult intubation for anesthesia during the puerperium**   M ♀

O89.8 **Other complications of anesthesia during the puerperium**   M ♀

O89.9 **Complication of anesthesia during the puerperium, unspecified**   M ♀

`N` Newborn: 0   `P` Pediatric: 0-17   `M` Maternity: 9-64   `A` Adult: 15-124   `MCC` Major Complication/Comorbidity   `CC` Complication/Comorbidity   `SW` Severe Wound Dx

908   ICD-10-CM 2020

Chapter 15. Pregnancy, Childbirth and the Puerperium

O86.4–O89.9

✓4ᵗʰ O90 Complications of the puerperium, not elsewhere classified

O90.0 Disruption of cesarean delivery wound M ♀

Dehiscence of cesarean delivery wound

EXCLUDES 1 *rupture of uterus (spontaneous) before onset of labor (O71.0-)*

rupture of uterus during labor (O71.1)

O90.1 Disruption of perineal obstetric wound M ♀

Disruption of wound of episiotomy

Disruption of wound of perineal laceration

Secondary perineal tear

O90.2 Hematoma of obstetric wound M ♀

O90.3 Peripartum cardiomyopathy MCC M ♀

Conditions in I42- arising during pregnancy and the puerperium

EXCLUDES 1 *pre-existing heart disease complicating pregnancy and the puerperium (O99.4-)*

DEF: Any structural or functional abnormality of the ventricular myocardium. It is a noninflammatory disease of obscure or unknown etiology with onset during the postpartum period.

CC Excl: PDX collection 1008

O90.4 Postpartum acute kidney failure MCC M ♀

Hepatorenal syndrome following labor and delivery

CC Excl: PDX collection 1009

O90.5 Postpartum thyroiditis M ♀

O90.6 Postpartum mood disturbance M ♀

Postpartum blues

Postpartum dysphoria

Postpartum sadness

EXCLUDES 1 *postpartum depression (F53.0)*

puerperal psychosis (F53.1)

✓5ᵗʰ O90.8 Other complications of the puerperium, not elsewhere classified

O90.81 Anemia of the puerperium M ♀

Postpartum anemia NOS

EXCLUDES 1 *pre-existing anemia complicating the puerperium (O99.03)*

O90.89 Other complications of the puerperium, not elsewhere classified M ♀

Placental polyp

O90.9 Complication of the puerperium, unspecified M ♀

✓4ᵗʰ O91 Infections of breast associated with pregnancy, the puerperium and lactation

Use additional code to identify infection

✓5ᵗʰ O91.0 Infection of nipple associated with pregnancy, the puerperium and lactation

✓6ᵗʰ O91.01 Infection of nipple associated with pregnancy

Gestational abscess of nipple

O91.011 Infection of nipple associated with pregnancy, first trimester M ♀

O91.012 Infection of nipple associated with pregnancy, second trimester M ♀

O91.013 Infection of nipple associated with pregnancy, third trimester M ♀

O91.019 Infection of nipple associated with pregnancy, unspecified trimester M ♀

O91.02 Infection of nipple associated with the puerperium M ♀

Puerperal abscess of nipple

O91.03 Infection of nipple associated with lactation M ♀

Abscess of nipple associated with lactation

✓5ᵗʰ O91.1 Abscess of breast associated with pregnancy, the puerperium and lactation

✓6ᵗʰ O91.11 Abscess of breast associated with pregnancy

Gestational mammary abscess

Gestational purulent mastitis

Gestational subareolar abscess

O91.111 Abscess of breast associated with pregnancy, first trimester M ♀

O91.112 Abscess of breast associated with pregnancy, second trimester M ♀

O91.113 Abscess of breast associated with pregnancy, third trimester M ♀

O91.119 Abscess of breast associated with pregnancy, unspecified trimester M ♀

O91.12 Abscess of breast associated with the puerperium M ♀

Puerperal mammary abscess

Puerperal purulent mastitis

Puerperal subareolar abscess

O91.13 Abscess of breast associated with lactation M ♀

Mammary abscess associated with lactation

Purulent mastitis associated with lactation

Subareolar abscess associated with lactation

✓5ᵗʰ O91.2 Nonpurulent mastitis associated with pregnancy, the puerperium and lactation

✓6ᵗʰ O91.21 Nonpurulent mastitis associated with pregnancy

Gestational interstitial mastitis

Gestational lymphangitis of breast

Gestational mastitis NOS

Gestational parenchymatous mastitis

O91.211 Nonpurulent mastitis associated with pregnancy, first trimester M ♀

O91.212 Nonpurulent mastitis associated with pregnancy, second trimester M ♀

O91.213 Nonpurulent mastitis associated with pregnancy, third trimester M ♀

O91.219 Nonpurulent mastitis associated with pregnancy, unspecified trimester M ♀

O91.22 Nonpurulent mastitis associated with the puerperium M ♀

Puerperal interstitial mastitis

Puerperal lymphangitis of breast

Puerperal mastitis NOS

Puerperal parenchymatous mastitis

O91.23 Nonpurulent mastitis associated with lactation M ♀

Interstitial mastitis associated with lactation

Lymphangitis of breast associated with lactation

Mastitis NOS associated with lactation

Parenchymatous mastitis associated with lactation

✓4ᵗʰ O92 Other disorders of breast and disorders of lactation associated with pregnancy and the puerperium

✓5ᵗʰ O92.0 Retracted nipple associated with pregnancy, the puerperium, and lactation

✓6ᵗʰ O92.01 Retracted nipple associated with pregnancy

O92.011 Retracted nipple associated with pregnancy, first trimester M ♀

O92.012 Retracted nipple associated with pregnancy, second trimester M ♀

O92.013 Retracted nipple associated with pregnancy, third trimester M ♀

O92.019 Retracted nipple associated with pregnancy, unspecified trimester M ♀

O92.02 Retracted nipple associated with the puerperium M ♀

O92.03 Retracted nipple associated with lactation M ♀

✓5ᵗʰ O92.1 Cracked nipple associated with pregnancy, the puerperium, and lactation

Fissure of nipple, gestational or puerperal

✓6ᵗʰ O92.11 Cracked nipple associated with pregnancy

O92.111 Cracked nipple associated with pregnancy, first trimester M ♀

O92.112 Cracked nipple associated with pregnancy, second trimester M ♀

O92.113 Cracked nipple associated with pregnancy, third trimester M ♀

O92.119 Cracked nipple associated with pregnancy, unspecified trimester M ♀

O92.12 Cracked nipple associated with the puerperium M ♀

O92.13 Cracked nipple associated with lactation M ♀

☑ Additional Character Required   ✓x7ᵗʰ Placeholder   Unacceptable PDx   Questionable PDx   Manifestation   Unspecified Dx   H1-H14 HAC   HCC CMS-HCC Dx   HIV HIV Dx

ICD-10-CM 2020

909

√5ᵗʰ **O92.2 Other and unspecified disorders of breast associated with pregnancy and the puerperium**
- **O92.20 Unspecified disorder of breast associated** M ♀
  with pregnancy and the puerperium
- **O92.29 Other disorders of breast associated with** M ♀
  pregnancy and the puerperium

O92.3 Agalactia M ♀
Primary agalactia
EXCLUDES 1   *elective agalactia (O92.5)*
           secondary agalactia (O92.5)
           therapeutic agalactia (O92.5)
DEF: Absence of milk secretion in a female after delivery.

O92.4 Hypogalactia M ♀

O92.5 Suppressed lactation M ♀
Elective agalactia
Secondary agalactia
Therapeutic agalactia
EXCLUDES 1   *primary agalactia (O92.3)*

O92.6 Galactorrhea M ♀
DEF: Excessive or persistent milk secretion by the breast that may occur in the absence of nursing.

√5ᵗʰ **O92.7 Other and unspecified disorders of lactation**
- **O92.70 Unspecified disorders of lactation** M ♀
- **O92.79 Other disorders of lactation** M ♀
  Puerperal galactocele

Other obstetric conditions, not elsewhere classified (O94-O9A)

O94 Sequelae of complication of pregnancy, childbirth, and M ♀
the puerperium
NOTE   This category is to be used to indicate conditions in O00-O77.-, O85-O94 and O98-O9A.- as the cause of late effects. The sequelae include conditions specified as such, or as late effects, which may occur at any time after the puerperium

Code first condition resulting from (sequela) of complication of pregnancy, childbirth, and the puerperium

√4ᵗʰ **O98 Maternal infectious and parasitic diseases classifiable elsewhere but complicating pregnancy, childbirth and the puerperium**
INCLUDES   the listed conditions when complicating the pregnant state, when aggravated by the pregnancy, or as a reason for obstetric care

Use additional code (Chapter 1), to identify specific infectious or parasitic disease
EXCLUDES 2   *herpes gestationis (O26.4-)*
           infectious carrier state (O99.82-, O99.83-)
           obstetrical tetanus (A34)
           puerperal infection (O86.-)
           puerperal sepsis (O85)
           when the reason for maternal care is that the disease is known or suspected to have affected the fetus (O35-O36)

√5ᵗʰ **O98.0 Tuberculosis complicating pregnancy, childbirth and the puerperium**
Conditions in A15-A19
CC Excl: For CC codes in subcategory O98.0: PDX collection 1011

√6ᵗʰ **O98.01 Tuberculosis complicating pregnancy**
- **O98.011 Tuberculosis complicating** CC M ♀
  pregnancy, first trimester
- **O98.012 Tuberculosis complicating** CC M ♀
  pregnancy, second trimester
- **O98.013 Tuberculosis complicating** CC M ♀
  pregnancy, third trimester
- **O98.019 Tuberculosis complicating** M ♀
  pregnancy, unspecified trimester
- **O98.02 Tuberculosis complicating childbirth** CC M ♀
- **O98.03 Tuberculosis complicating the** CC M ♀
  puerperium

√5ᵗʰ **O98.1 Syphilis complicating pregnancy, childbirth and the puerperium**
Conditions in A50-A53
CC Excl: For CC codes in subcategory O98.1: PDX collection 1012

√6ᵗʰ **O98.11 Syphilis complicating pregnancy**
- **O98.111 Syphilis complicating** CC M ♀
  pregnancy, first trimester
- **O98.112 Syphilis complicating** CC M ♀
  pregnancy, second trimester
- **O98.113 Syphilis complicating** CC M ♀
  pregnancy, third trimester
- **O98.119 Syphilis complicating** M ♀
  pregnancy, unspecified trimester
- **O98.12 Syphilis complicating childbirth** CC M ♀
- **O98.13 Syphilis complicating the puerperium** CC M ♀

√5ᵗʰ **O98.2 Gonorrhea complicating pregnancy, childbirth and the puerperium**
Conditions in A54.-
CC Excl: For CC codes in subcategory O98.2: PDX collection 1012

√6ᵗʰ **O98.21 Gonorrhea complicating pregnancy**
- **O98.211 Gonorrhea complicating** CC M ♀
  pregnancy, first trimester
- **O98.212 Gonorrhea complicating** CC M ♀
  pregnancy, second trimester
- **O98.213 Gonorrhea complicating** CC M ♀
  pregnancy, third trimester
- **O98.219 Gonorrhea complicating** M ♀
  pregnancy, unspecified trimester
- **O98.22 Gonorrhea complicating childbirth** CC M ♀
- **O98.23 Gonorrhea complicating the puerperium** CC M ♀

√5ᵗʰ **O98.3 Other infections with a predominantly sexual mode of transmission complicating pregnancy, childbirth and the puerperium**
Conditions in A55-A64

√6ᵗʰ **O98.31 Other infections with a predominantly sexual mode of transmission complicating pregnancy**
- **O98.311 Other infections with a** M ♀
  predominantly sexual mode of transmission complicating pregnancy, first trimester
- **O98.312 Other infections with a** M ♀
  predominantly sexual mode of transmission complicating pregnancy, second trimester
- **O98.313 Other infections with a** M ♀
  predominantly sexual mode of transmission complicating pregnancy, third trimester
- **O98.319 Other infections with a** M ♀
  predominantly sexual mode of transmission complicating pregnancy, unspecified trimester
- **O98.32 Other infections with a predominantly** M ♀
  sexual mode of transmission complicating childbirth
- **O98.33 Other infections with a predominantly** M ♀
  sexual mode of transmission complicating the puerperium

√5ᵗʰ **O98.4 Viral hepatitis complicating pregnancy, childbirth and the puerperium**
Conditions in B15-B19
CC Excl: For CC codes in subcategory O98.4: PDX collection 1013

√6ᵗʰ **O98.41 Viral hepatitis complicating pregnancy**
- **O98.411 Viral hepatitis complicating** CC M ♀
  pregnancy, first trimester
- **O98.412 Viral hepatitis complicating** CC M ♀
  pregnancy, second trimester
- **O98.413 Viral hepatitis complicating** CC M ♀
  pregnancy, third trimester
- **O98.419 Viral hepatitis complicating** M ♀
  pregnancy, unspecified trimester
- **O98.42 Viral hepatitis complicating childbirth** CC M ♀
- **O98.43 Viral hepatitis complicating the** CC M ♀
  puerperium

N Newborn: 0   P Pediatric: 0-17   M Maternity: 9-64   A Adult: 15-124   MCC Major Complication/Comorbidity   CC Complication/Comorbidity   SW Severe Wound Dx

910   ICD-10-CM 2020

✓5ᵗʰ **O98.5 Other viral diseases complicating pregnancy, childbirth and the puerperium**
     Conditions in A8Ø-BØ9, B25-B34, R87.81-, R87.82-
         EXCLUDES 1   *human immunodeficiency virus [HIV] disease complicating pregnancy, childbirth and the puerperium (O98.7-)*
     CC Excl: For CC codes in subcategory O98.5: PDX collection 1013

     ✓6ᵗʰ **O98.51 Other viral diseases complicating pregnancy**
         O98.511 Other viral diseases complicating pregnancy, first trimester   CC M ♀
         O98.512 Other viral diseases complicating pregnancy, second trimester   CC M ♀
         O98.513 Other viral diseases complicating pregnancy, third trimester   CC M ♀
         O98.519 Other viral diseases complicating pregnancy, unspecified trimester   M ♀
     O98.52 Other viral diseases complicating childbirth   M ♀
     O98.53 Other viral diseases complicating the puerperium   CC M ♀

✓5ᵗʰ **O98.6 Protozoal diseases complicating pregnancy, childbirth and the puerperium**
     Conditions in B5Ø-B64
     CC Excl: For CC codes in subcategory O98.6, unless otherwise noted: PDX collection 1014

     ✓6ᵗʰ **O98.61 Protozoal diseases complicating pregnancy**
         O98.611 Protozoal diseases complicating pregnancy, first trimester   CC M ♀
         O98.612 Protozoal diseases complicating pregnancy, second trimester   CC M ♀
         O98.613 Protozoal diseases complicating pregnancy, third trimester   CC M ♀
         O98.619 Protozoal diseases complicating pregnancy, unspecified trimester   M ♀
     O98.62 Protozoal diseases complicating childbirth   CC M ♀
         CC Excl: PDX collection 1015
     O98.63 Protozoal diseases complicating the puerperium   CC M ♀
         CC Excl: PDX collection 1015

✓5ᵗʰ **O98.7 Human immunodeficiency virus [HIV] disease complicating pregnancy, childbirth and the puerperium**
     Use additional code to identify the type of HIV disease:
     acquired immune deficiency syndrome (AIDS) (B2Ø)
     asymptomatic HIV status (Z21)
     HIV positive NOS (Z21)
     symptomatic HIV disease (B2Ø)
     CC Excl: For CC codes in subcategory O98.7: PDX collection 1013

     ✓6ᵗʰ **O98.71 Human immunodeficiency virus [HIV] disease complicating pregnancy**
         O98.711 Human immunodeficiency virus [HIV] disease complicating pregnancy, first trimester   CC M ♀
         O98.712 Human immunodeficiency virus [HIV] disease complicating pregnancy, second trimester   CC M ♀
         O98.713 Human immunodeficiency virus [HIV] disease complicating pregnancy, third trimester   CC M ♀
         O98.719 Human immunodeficiency virus [HIV] disease complicating pregnancy, unspecified trimester   M ♀
     O98.72 Human immunodeficiency virus [HIV] disease complicating childbirth   CC M ♀
     O98.73 Human immunodeficiency virus [HIV] disease complicating the puerperium   CC M ♀

✓5ᵗʰ **O98.8 Other maternal infectious and parasitic diseases complicating pregnancy, childbirth and the puerperium**
     CC Excl: For CC codes in subcategory O98.8: PDX collection 1013

     ✓6ᵗʰ **O98.81 Other maternal infectious and parasitic diseases complicating pregnancy**
         O98.811 Other maternal infectious and parasitic diseases complicating pregnancy, first trimester   CC M ♀
         O98.812 Other maternal infectious and parasitic diseases complicating pregnancy, second trimester   CC M ♀
         O98.813 Other maternal infectious and parasitic diseases complicating pregnancy, third trimester   CC M ♀
         O98.819 Other maternal infectious and parasitic diseases complicating pregnancy, unspecified trimester   M ♀
     O98.82 Other maternal infectious and parasitic diseases complicating childbirth   CC M ♀
     O98.83 Other maternal infectious and parasitic diseases complicating the puerperium   CC M ♀

✓5ᵗʰ **O98.9 Unspecified maternal infectious and parasitic disease complicating pregnancy, childbirth and the puerperium**
     CC Excl: For CC codes in subcategory O98.9: PDX collection 1013

     ✓6ᵗʰ **O98.91 Unspecified maternal infectious and parasitic disease complicating pregnancy**
         O98.911 Unspecified maternal infectious and parasitic disease complicating pregnancy, first trimester   CC M ♀
         O98.912 Unspecified maternal infectious and parasitic disease complicating pregnancy, second trimester   CC M ♀
         O98.913 Unspecified maternal infectious and parasitic disease complicating pregnancy, third trimester   CC M ♀
         O98.919 Unspecified maternal infectious and parasitic disease complicating pregnancy, unspecified trimester   M ♀
     O98.92 Unspecified maternal infectious and parasitic disease complicating childbirth   CC M ♀
     O98.93 Unspecified maternal infectious and parasitic disease complicating the puerperium   CC M ♀

✓4ᵗʰ **O99 Other maternal diseases classifiable elsewhere but complicating pregnancy, childbirth and the puerperium**
     INCLUDES   conditions which complicate the pregnant state, are aggravated by the pregnancy or are a main reason for obstetric care
     Use additional code to identify specific condition
     EXCLUDES 2   *when the reason for maternal care is that the condition is known or suspected to have affected the fetus (O35-O36)*

     ✓5ᵗʰ **O99.Ø Anemia complicating pregnancy, childbirth and the puerperium**
     Conditions in D5Ø-D64
         EXCLUDES 1   *anemia arising in the puerperium (O9Ø.81)*
                           postpartum anemia NOS (O9Ø.81)

         ✓6ᵗʰ **O99.Ø1 Anemia complicating pregnancy**
         AHA: 2016,1Q,4
         O99.Ø11 Anemia complicating pregnancy, first trimester   M ♀
         O99.Ø12 Anemia complicating pregnancy, second trimester   M ♀
         O99.Ø13 Anemia complicating pregnancy, third trimester   M ♀
         O99.Ø19 Anemia complicating pregnancy, unspecified trimester   M ♀
     O99.Ø2 Anemia complicating childbirth   M ♀
     O99.Ø3 Anemia complicating the puerperium   M ♀
         EXCLUDES 1   *postpartum anemia not pre-existing prior to delivery (O9Ø.81)*

✓ Additional Character Required   ✓x7ᵗʰ Placeholder   Unacceptable PDx   Questionable PDx   Manifestation   Unspecified Dx   H1-H14 HAC   HCC CMS-HCC Dx   HIV HIV Dx

ICD-10-CM 2020   911

✓5ᵗʰ **O99.1 Other diseases of the** blood and blood-forming organs **and certain disorders** involving the immune mechanism **complicating pregnancy, childbirth and the puerperium**
Conditions in D65-D89
EXCLUDES 1　hemorrhage with coagulation defects (O45.-, O46.0-, O67.0, O72.3)

CC Excl: For CC codes in subcategory O99.1, unless otherwise noted: PDX collection 1016

✓6ᵗʰ **O99.11 Other diseases of the blood and blood-forming organs and certain disorders involving the immune mechanism complicating** pregnancy

　O99.111 Other diseases of the blood and blood-forming organs and certain disorders involving the immune mechanism complicating pregnancy, first trimester　cc M ♀

　O99.112 Other diseases of the blood and blood-forming organs and certain disorders involving the immune mechanism complicating pregnancy, second trimester　cc M ♀

　O99.113 Other diseases of the blood and blood-forming organs and certain disorders involving the immune mechanism complicating pregnancy, third trimester　cc M ♀

　O99.119 Other diseases of the blood and blood-forming organs and certain disorders involving the immune mechanism complicating pregnancy, unspecified trimester　cc M ♀
　CC Excl: PDX collection 1017

　O99.12 Other diseases of the blood and blood-forming organs and certain disorders involving the immune mechanism complicating childbirth　cc M ♀

　O99.13 Other diseases of the blood and blood-forming organs and certain disorders involving the immune mechanism complicating the puerperium　cc M ♀

✓5ᵗʰ **O99.2** Endocrine, nutritional and metabolic diseases **complicating pregnancy, childbirth and the puerperium**
Conditions in E00-E88
EXCLUDES 2　diabetes mellitus (O24.-)
　　malnutrition (O25.-)
　　postpartum thyroiditis (O90.5)

✓6ᵗʰ **O99.21 Obesity complicating pregnancy, childbirth, and the puerperium**
Use additional code to identify the type of obesity (E66.-)
AHA: 2018,4Q,80
TIP: Do not assign a BMI code (Z68.-) for obese or overweight patients who are pregnant.

　O99.210 Obesity complicating pregnancy, unspecified trimester　M ♀

　O99.211 Obesity complicating pregnancy, first trimester　M ♀

　O99.212 Obesity complicating pregnancy, second trimester　M ♀

　O99.213 Obesity complicating pregnancy, third trimester　M ♀

　O99.214 Obesity complicating childbirth　M ♀

　O99.215 Obesity complicating the puerperium　M ♀

✓6ᵗʰ **O99.28 Other endocrine, nutritional and metabolic diseases complicating pregnancy, childbirth and the puerperium**

　O99.280 Endocrine, nutritional and metabolic diseases complicating pregnancy, unspecified trimester　M ♀

　O99.281 Endocrine, nutritional and metabolic diseases complicating pregnancy, first trimester　M ♀

　O99.282 Endocrine, nutritional and metabolic diseases complicating pregnancy, second trimester　M ♀

　O99.283 Endocrine, nutritional and metabolic diseases complicating pregnancy, third trimester　M ♀

　O99.284 Endocrine, nutritional and metabolic diseases complicating childbirth　M ♀

　O99.285 Endocrine, nutritional and metabolic diseases complicating the puerperium　M ♀

✓5ᵗʰ **O99.3** Mental disorders **and diseases of the** nervous system **complicating pregnancy, childbirth and the puerperium**
CC Excl: For CC codes in subcategory O99.3, unless otherwise noted: PDX collection 1018

✓6ᵗʰ **O99.31** Alcohol use **complicating pregnancy, childbirth, and the puerperium**
Use additional code(s) from F10 to identify manifestations of the alcohol use

　O99.310 Alcohol use complicating pregnancy, unspecified trimester　M ♀

　O99.311 Alcohol use complicating pregnancy, first trimester　M ♀

　O99.312 Alcohol use complicating pregnancy, second trimester　M ♀

　O99.313 Alcohol use complicating pregnancy, third trimester　M ♀

　O99.314 Alcohol use complicating childbirth　M ♀

　O99.315 Alcohol use complicating the puerperium　M ♀

✓6ᵗʰ **O99.32** Drug use **complicating pregnancy, childbirth, and the puerperium**
Use additional code(s) from F11-F16 and F18-F19 to identify manifestations of the drug use
AHA: 2018,4Q,69-70; 2018,2Q,10
TIP: When drug use is documented during pregnancy, assign first a code from this subcategory followed by an additional code from F11-F16 and F18-F19 identifying the specific drug use even if not documented as associated with a physical, mental, or behavioral disorder. According to chapter 15 guidelines, it is the provider's responsibility to state that the condition being treated is not affecting the pregnancy.

　O99.320 Drug use complicating pregnancy, unspecified trimester　M ♀

　O99.321 Drug use complicating pregnancy, first trimester　cc M ♀

　O99.322 Drug use complicating pregnancy, second trimester　cc M ♀

　O99.323 Drug use complicating pregnancy, third trimester　cc M ♀

　O99.324 Drug use complicating childbirth　cc M ♀

　O99.325 Drug use complicating the puerperium　cc M ♀

✓6ᵗʰ **O99.33** Tobacco use disorder **complicating pregnancy, childbirth, and the puerperium**
Smoking complicating pregnancy, childbirth, and the puerperium
Use additional code from category F17 to identify type of tobacco nicotine dependence

　O99.330 Smoking (tobacco) complicating pregnancy, unspecified trimester　M ♀

　O99.331 Smoking (tobacco) complicating pregnancy, first trimester　M ♀

　O99.332 Smoking (tobacco) complicating pregnancy, second trimester　M ♀

　O99.333 Smoking (tobacco) complicating pregnancy, third trimester　M ♀

　O99.334 Smoking (tobacco) complicating childbirth　M ♀

　O99.335 Smoking (tobacco) complicating the puerperium　M ♀

N Newborn: 0　P Pediatric: 0-17　M Maternity: 9-64　A Adult: 15-124　MCC Major Complication/Comorbidity　CC Complication/Comorbidity　SW Severe Wound Dx

912　ICD-10-CM 2020

√6ᵗʰ **O99.34** **Other mental disorders complicating pregnancy, childbirth, and the puerperium**
▶Conditions in FØ1-FØ9, F2Ø-F99 and F54-F99◀
EXCLUDES 2   *postpartum mood disturbance (O90.6)*
postnatal psychosis (F53.1)
puerperal psychosis (F53.1)

O99.340 **Other mental disorders complicating pregnancy, unspecified trimester**   Ⓜ♀

O99.341 **Other mental disorders complicating pregnancy, first trimester**   Ⓜ♀

O99.342 **Other mental disorders complicating pregnancy, second trimester**   Ⓜ♀

O99.343 **Other mental disorders complicating pregnancy, third trimester**   Ⓜ♀

O99.344 **Other mental disorders complicating childbirth**   Ⓜ♀

O99.345 **Other mental disorders complicating the puerperium**   Ⓜ♀
AHA: 2018,4Q,8

√6ᵗʰ **O99.35** **Diseases of the nervous system complicating pregnancy, childbirth, and the puerperium**
Conditions in GØ0-G99
EXCLUDES 2   *pregnancy related peripheral neuritis (O26.8-)*

O99.350 **Diseases of the nervous system complicating pregnancy, unspecified trimester**   Ⓜ♀

O99.351 **Diseases of the nervous system complicating pregnancy, first trimester**   Ⓜ♀

O99.352 **Diseases of the nervous system complicating pregnancy, second trimester**   Ⓜ♀

O99.353 **Diseases of the nervous system complicating pregnancy, third trimester**   Ⓜ♀

O99.354 **Diseases of the nervous system complicating childbirth**   CC Ⓜ♀
CC Excl: PDX collection 1016

O99.355 **Diseases of the nervous system complicating the puerperium**   CC Ⓜ♀
CC Excl: PDX collection 1016

√5ᵗʰ **O99.4** **Diseases of the circulatory system complicating pregnancy, childbirth and the puerperium**
Conditions in IØ0-I99
EXCLUDES 1   *peripartum cardiomyopathy (O90.3)*
EXCLUDES 2   *hypertensive disorders (O10-O16)*
obstetric embolism (O88.-)
venous complications and cerebrovenous sinus thrombosis in labor, childbirth and the puerperium (O87.-)
venous complications and cerebrovenous sinus thrombosis in pregnancy (O22.-)
AHA: 2016,2Q,8
CC Excl: For CC codes in subcategory O99.4, unless otherwise noted: PDX collection 1019

√6ᵗʰ **O99.41** **Diseases of the circulatory system complicating pregnancy**

O99.411 **Diseases of the circulatory system complicating pregnancy, first trimester**   CC Ⓜ♀

O99.412 **Diseases of the circulatory system complicating pregnancy, second trimester**   CC Ⓜ♀

O99.413 **Diseases of the circulatory system complicating pregnancy, third trimester**   CC Ⓜ♀

O99.419 **Diseases of the circulatory system complicating pregnancy, unspecified trimester**   Ⓜ♀

O99.42 **Diseases of the circulatory system complicating childbirth**   MCC Ⓜ♀
CC Excl: PDX collection 1008

O99.43 **Diseases of the circulatory system complicating the puerperium**   CC Ⓜ♀

√5ᵗʰ **O99.5** **Diseases of the respiratory system complicating pregnancy, childbirth and the puerperium**
Conditions in JØ0-J99

√6ᵗʰ **O99.51** **Diseases of the respiratory system complicating pregnancy**

O99.511 **Diseases of the respiratory system complicating pregnancy, first trimester**   Ⓜ♀

O99.512 **Diseases of the respiratory system complicating pregnancy, second trimester**   Ⓜ♀

O99.513 **Diseases of the respiratory system complicating pregnancy, third trimester**   Ⓜ♀

O99.519 **Diseases of the respiratory system complicating pregnancy, unspecified trimester**   Ⓜ♀

O99.52 **Diseases of the respiratory system complicating childbirth**   Ⓜ♀

O99.53 **Diseases of the respiratory system complicating the puerperium**   Ⓜ♀

√5ᵗʰ **O99.6** **Diseases of the digestive system complicating pregnancy, childbirth and the puerperium**
Conditions in KØ0-K93
EXCLUDES 2   *hemorrhoids in pregnancy (O22.4-)*
liver and biliary tract disorders in pregnancy, childbirth and the puerperium (O26.6-)

√6ᵗʰ **O99.61** **Diseases of the digestive system complicating pregnancy**
AHA: 2016,1Q,4

O99.611 **Diseases of the digestive system complicating pregnancy, first trimester**   Ⓜ♀

O99.612 **Diseases of the digestive system complicating pregnancy, second trimester**   Ⓜ♀

O99.613 **Diseases of the digestive system complicating pregnancy, third trimester**   Ⓜ♀

O99.619 **Diseases of the digestive system complicating pregnancy, unspecified trimester**   Ⓜ♀

O99.62 **Diseases of the digestive system complicating childbirth**   Ⓜ♀

O99.63 **Diseases of the digestive system complicating the puerperium**   Ⓜ♀

√5ᵗʰ **O99.7** **Diseases of the skin and subcutaneous tissue complicating pregnancy, childbirth and the puerperium**
Conditions in LØ0-L99
EXCLUDES 2   *herpes gestationis (O26.4)*
pruritic urticarial papules and plaques of pregnancy (PUPPP) (O26.86)

√6ᵗʰ **O99.71** **Diseases of the skin and subcutaneous tissue complicating pregnancy**

O99.711 **Diseases of the skin and subcutaneous tissue complicating pregnancy, first trimester**   Ⓜ♀

O99.712 **Diseases of the skin and subcutaneous tissue complicating pregnancy, second trimester**   Ⓜ♀

O99.713 **Diseases of the skin and subcutaneous tissue complicating pregnancy, third trimester**   Ⓜ♀

O99.719 **Diseases of the skin and subcutaneous tissue complicating pregnancy, unspecified trimester**   Ⓜ♀

O99.72 **Diseases of the skin and subcutaneous tissue complicating childbirth**   Ⓜ♀

O99.73 **Diseases of the skin and subcutaneous tissue complicating the puerperium**   Ⓜ♀

√5ᵗʰ **O99.8 Other specified diseases and conditions complicating pregnancy, childbirth and the puerperium**
  Conditions in D00-D48, H00-H95, M00-N99, and Q00-Q99
  Use additional code to identify condition
  EXCLUDES 2 *genitourinary infections in pregnancy (O23.-)*
    infection of genitourinary tract following delivery
      ▶*(O86.1-O86.4)*◀
    malignant neoplasm complicating pregnancy, childbirth and the puerperium (O9A.1-)
    maternal care for known or suspected abnormality of maternal pelvic organs (O34.-)
    postpartum acute kidney failure (O90.4)
    traumatic injuries in pregnancy (O9A.2-)
  CC Excl: For CC codes in subcategory O99.8: PDX collection 1013

√6ᵗʰ **O99.81 Abnormal glucose complicating pregnancy, childbirth and the puerperium**
    EXCLUDES 1 *gestational diabetes (O24.4-)*
    O99.810 Abnormal glucose complicating pregnancy Ⓜ♀
    O99.814 Abnormal glucose complicating childbirth Ⓜ♀
    O99.815 Abnormal glucose complicating the puerperium Ⓜ♀

√6ᵗʰ **O99.82 Streptococcus B carrier state complicating pregnancy, childbirth and the puerperium**
    EXCLUDES 1 *carrier of streptococcus group B (GBS) in a nonpregnant woman (Z22.330)*
    DEF: *Streptococcus* group B colonization: Bacteria normally found in the vagina or lower intestine of many healthy adult women that may infect the fetus during childbirth, causing mental or physical handicaps or death. Women who test positive for *streptococcus* Group B during pregnancy are considered a "colonized" status and are treated with IV antibiotics at the time of delivery and may also be treated with oral antibiotics during the pregnancy.
    O99.820 Streptococcus B carrier state complicating pregnancy Ⓜ♀
    O99.824 Streptococcus B carrier state complicating childbirth Ⓜ♀
      AHA: 2019,2Q,8
    O99.825 Streptococcus B carrier state complicating the puerperium Ⓜ♀

√6ᵗʰ **O99.83 Other infection carrier state complicating pregnancy, childbirth and the puerperium**
    Use additional code to identify the carrier state (Z22.-)
    O99.830 Other infection carrier state complicating pregnancy ㏄ Ⓜ♀
    O99.834 Other infection carrier state complicating childbirth ㏄ Ⓜ♀
    O99.835 Other infection carrier state complicating the puerperium ㏄ Ⓜ♀

√6ᵗʰ **O99.84 Bariatric surgery status complicating pregnancy, childbirth and the puerperium**
    Gastric banding status complicating pregnancy, childbirth and the puerperium
    Gastric bypass status for obesity complicating pregnancy, childbirth and the puerperium
    Obesity surgery status complicating pregnancy, childbirth and the puerperium
    O99.840 Bariatric surgery status complicating pregnancy, unspecified trimester Ⓜ♀
    O99.841 Bariatric surgery status complicating pregnancy, first trimester Ⓜ♀
    O99.842 Bariatric surgery status complicating pregnancy, second trimester Ⓜ♀
    O99.843 Bariatric surgery status complicating pregnancy, third trimester Ⓜ♀
    O99.844 Bariatric surgery status complicating childbirth Ⓜ♀
    O99.845 Bariatric surgery status complicating the puerperium Ⓜ♀

  O99.89 Other specified diseases and conditions complicating pregnancy, childbirth and the puerperium Ⓜ♀

√4ᵗʰ **O9A Maternal malignant neoplasms, traumatic injuries and abuse classifiable elsewhere but complicating pregnancy, childbirth and the puerperium**

√5ᵗʰ **O9A.1 Malignant neoplasm complicating pregnancy, childbirth and the puerperium**
  Conditions in C00-C96
  Use additional code to identify neoplasm
  EXCLUDES 2 *maternal care for benign tumor of corpus uteri (O34.1-)*
    maternal care for benign tumor of cervix (O34.4-)
  AHA: 2015,3Q,19

√6ᵗʰ **O9A.11 Malignant neoplasm complicating pregnancy**
    O9A.111 Malignant neoplasm complicating pregnancy, first trimester Ⓜ♀
    O9A.112 Malignant neoplasm complicating pregnancy, second trimester Ⓜ♀
    O9A.113 Malignant neoplasm complicating pregnancy, third trimester Ⓜ♀
    O9A.119 Malignant neoplasm complicating pregnancy, unspecified trimester Ⓜ♀

  O9A.12 Malignant neoplasm complicating childbirth Ⓜ♀

  O9A.13 Malignant neoplasm complicating the puerperium Ⓜ♀

√5ᵗʰ **O9A.2 Injury, poisoning and certain other consequences of external causes complicating pregnancy, childbirth and the puerperium**
  Conditions in S00-T88, except T74 and T76
  Use additional code(s) to identify the injury or poisoning
  EXCLUDES 2 *physical, sexual and psychological abuse complicating pregnancy, childbirth and the puerperium (O9A.3-, O9A.4-, O9A.5-)*

√6ᵗʰ **O9A.21 Injury, poisoning and certain other consequences of external causes complicating pregnancy**
    O9A.211 Injury, poisoning and certain other consequences of external causes complicating pregnancy, first trimester Ⓜ♀
    O9A.212 Injury, poisoning and certain other consequences of external causes complicating pregnancy, second trimester Ⓜ♀
    O9A.213 Injury, poisoning and certain other consequences of external causes complicating pregnancy, third trimester Ⓜ♀
    O9A.219 Injury, poisoning and certain other consequences of external causes complicating pregnancy, unspecified trimester Ⓜ♀

  O9A.22 Injury, poisoning and certain other consequences of external causes complicating childbirth Ⓜ♀

  O9A.23 Injury, poisoning and certain other consequences of external causes complicating the puerperium Ⓜ♀

√5ᵗʰ **O9A.3 Physical abuse complicating pregnancy, childbirth and the puerperium**
  Conditions in T74.11 or T76.11
  Use additional code (if applicable):
    to identify any associated current injury due to physical abuse
    to identify the perpetrator of abuse (Y07.-)
  EXCLUDES 2 *sexual abuse complicating pregnancy, childbirth and the puerperium (O9A.4)*

√6ᵗʰ **O9A.31 Physical abuse complicating pregnancy**
    O9A.311 Physical abuse complicating pregnancy, first trimester Ⓜ♀
    O9A.312 Physical abuse complicating pregnancy, second trimester Ⓜ♀
    O9A.313 Physical abuse complicating pregnancy, third trimester Ⓜ♀
    O9A.319 Physical abuse complicating pregnancy, unspecified trimester Ⓜ♀

  O9A.32 Physical abuse complicating childbirth Ⓜ♀

  O9A.33 Physical abuse complicating the puerperium Ⓜ♀

Ⓝ Newborn: 0   Ⓟ Pediatric: 0-17   Ⓜ Maternity: 9-64   Ⓐ Adult: 15-124   ㎊㏄ Major Complication/Comorbidity   ㏄ Complication/Comorbidity   ㏒ Severe Wound Dx

914   ICD-10-CM 2020

✓5ᵗʰ **O9A.4** Sexual abuse **complicating pregnancy, childbirth and the puerperium**
　　　　Conditions in T74.21 or T76.21
　　　　Use additional code (if applicable):
　　　　　　to identify any associated current injury due to sexual abuse
　　　　　　to identify the perpetrator of abuse (Y07.-)

✓6ᵗʰ **O9A.41** **Sexual abuse complicating** pregnancy

　　　　O9A.411 **Sexual abuse complicating pregnancy,** first trimester　Ⓜ ♀

　　　　O9A.412 **Sexual abuse complicating pregnancy,** second trimester　Ⓜ ♀

　　　　O9A.413 **Sexual abuse complicating pregnancy,** third trimester　Ⓜ ♀

　　　　O9A.419 **Sexual abuse complicating pregnancy, unspecified trimester**　Ⓜ ♀

O9A.42 **Sexual abuse complicating** childbirth　Ⓜ ♀

O9A.43 **Sexual abuse complicating the** puerperium　Ⓜ ♀

✓5ᵗʰ **O9A.5** Psychological abuse **complicating pregnancy, childbirth and the puerperium**
　　　　Conditions in T74.31 or T76.31
　　　　Use additional code to identify the perpetrator of abuse (Y07.-)

✓6ᵗʰ **O9A.51** **Psychological abuse complicating** pregnancy

　　　　O9A.511 **Psychological abuse complicating pregnancy,** first trimester　Ⓜ ♀

　　　　O9A.512 **Psychological abuse complicating pregnancy,** second trimester　Ⓜ ♀

　　　　O9A.513 **Psychological abuse complicating pregnancy,** third trimester　Ⓜ ♀

　　　　O9A.519 **Psychological abuse complicating pregnancy, unspecified trimester**　Ⓜ ♀

O9A.52 **Psychological abuse complicating** childbirth　Ⓜ ♀

O9A.53 **Psychological abuse complicating the** puerperium　Ⓜ ♀

Chapter 16. Certain Conditions Originating in the Perinatal Period (PØØ–P96)

Chapter-specific Guidelines with Coding Examples

The chapter-specific guidelines from the ICD-10-CM Official Guidelines for Coding and Reporting have been provided below. Along with these guidelines are coding examples, contained in the shaded boxes, that have been developed to help illustrate the coding and/or sequencing guidance found in these guidelines.

For coding and reporting purposes the perinatal period is defined as before birth through the 28th day following birth. The following guidelines are provided for reporting purposes

a. General perinatal rules

1) Use of Chapter 16 codes

Codes in this chapter are <u>never</u> for use on the maternal record. Codes from Chapter 15, the obstetric chapter, are never permitted on the newborn record. Chapter 16 codes may be used throughout the life of the patient if the condition is still present.

2) Principal diagnosis for birth record

When coding the birth episode in a newborn record, assign a code from category Z38, Liveborn infants according to place of birth and type of delivery, as the principal diagnosis. A code from category Z38 is assigned only once, to a newborn at the time of birth. If a newborn is transferred to another institution, a code from category Z38 should not be used at the receiving hospital.

A code from category Z38 is used only on the newborn record, not on the mother's record.

> Newborn delivered via vaginal delivery in Rural Hospital A, experienced meconium aspiration resulting in pneumonia. Rural Hospital A is not equipped to handle the extensive respiratory therapy this baby needs and transfers the patient to Metropolis Hospital B, where the pneumonia resolves and the newborn is eventually discharged.
>
> *Rural Hospital A*
>
> **Z38.ØØ   Single liveborn infant, delivered vaginally**
>
> **P24.Ø1   Meconium aspiration with respiratory symptoms**
>
> *Metropolis Hospital B*
>
> **P24.Ø1   Meconium aspiration with respiratory symptoms**
>
> *Explanation:* A code from category Z38 is a one-time use only code. The hospital that actually delivered the newborn, in this case Rural Hospital A, can append a code from category Z38 but for the delivery admission only. Once the patient is transferred or discharged, the Z38 category no longer applies for that patient.
>
> The reason for the transfer to Metropolis Hospital B was for the respiratory symptoms (pneumonia) the newborn was exhibiting secondary to aspirating meconium.

3) Use of codes from other chapters with codes from Chapter 16

Codes from other chapters may be used with codes from chapter 16 if the codes from the other chapters provide more specific detail. Codes for signs and symptoms may be assigned when a definitive diagnosis has not been established. If the reason for the encounter is a perinatal condition, the code from chapter 16 should be sequenced first.

4) Use of Chapter 16 codes after the perinatal period

Should a condition originate in the perinatal period, and continue throughout the life of the patient, the perinatal code should continue to be used regardless of the patient's age.

> A 7-year-old patient with history of birth injury that resulted in Erb's palsy is seen for subscapularis release
>
> **P14.Ø   Erb's paralysis due to birth injury**
>
> *Explanation:* Although in this instance Erb's palsy is specifically related to a birth injury, it has not resolved and continues to be a health concern. A perinatal code is appropriate even though this patient is beyond the perinatal period.

5) Birth process or community acquired conditions

If a newborn has a condition that may be either due to the birth process or community acquired and the documentation does not indicate which it is, the default is due to the birth process and the code from Chapter 16 should be used. If the condition is community-acquired, a code from Chapter 16 should not be assigned.

6) Code all clinically significant conditions

All clinically significant conditions noted on routine newborn examination should be coded. A condition is clinically significant if it requires:

clinical evaluation; or

therapeutic treatment; or

diagnostic procedures; or

extended length of hospital stay; or

increased nursing care and/or monitoring; or

has implications for future health care needs

Note: The perinatal guidelines listed above are the same as the general coding guidelines for "additional diagnoses", except for the final point regarding implications for future health care needs. Codes should be assigned for conditions that have been specified by the provider as having implications for future health care needs.

b. Observation and evaluation of newborns for suspected conditions not found

1) Use of ZØ5 codes

Assign a code from category ZØ5, Observation and evaluation of newborns and infants for suspected conditions ruled out, to identify those instances when a healthy newborn is evaluated for a suspected condition that is determined after study not to be present. Do not use a code from category ZØ5 when the patient has identified signs or symptoms of a suspected problem; in such cases code the sign or symptom.

2) ZØ5 on Other than the birth record

A code from category ZØ5 may also be assigned as a principal or first-listed code for readmissions or encounters when the code from category Z38 code no longer applies. Codes from category ZØ5 are for use only for healthy newborns and infants for which no condition after study is found to be present.

3) ZØ5 on a birth record

A code from category ZØ5 is to be used as a secondary code after the code from category Z38, Liveborn infants according to place of birth and type of delivery.

> Newborn delivered via vaginal delivery; previous ultrasounds showed what appeared to be an abnormality of the right kidney. Kidney function tests were performed and ultrasounds taken and any genitourinary conditions ruled out.
>
> **Z38.ØØ   Single liveborn infant, delivered vaginally**
>
> **ZØ5.6   Observation and evaluation of newborn for suspected genitourinary condition ruled out**
>
> Explanation: The newborn had no signs or symptoms of kidney or other genitourinary condition but was evaluated after delivery due to the abnormal prenatal ultrasound findings. A Z code describing the type and place of birth should be coded first, followed by a ZØ5 category code for the work performed to rule out a suspected genitourinary condition.

c. Coding additional perinatal diagnoses

1) Assigning codes for conditions that require treatment

Assign codes for conditions that require treatment or further investigation, prolong the length of stay, or require resource utilization.

2) Codes for conditions specified as having implications for future health care needs

Assign codes for conditions that have been specified by the provider as having implications for future health care needs.

Note: This guideline should not be used for adult patients.

> An abnormal noise was heard in the left hip of a post-term newborn during a physical examination. The pediatrician would like to follow the patient after discharge as a hip click can be an early sign of hip dysplasia. The newborn was delivered via cesarean at 41 weeks.
>
> **Z38.01   Single liveborn infant, delivered by cesarean**
>
> **P08.21   Post-term newborn**
>
> **R29.4   Clicking hip**
>
> *Explanation:* The abnormal hip noise or click is appended as a secondary diagnosis not only because it is an abnormal finding upon examination, but also due to its potential to be part of a bigger health issue. The hip dysplasia has not yet been diagnosed and does not warrant a code at this time.

d. Prematurity and fetal growth retardation

Providers utilize different criteria in determining prematurity. A code for prematurity should not be assigned unless it is documented. Assignment of codes in categories P05, Disorders of newborn related to slow fetal growth and fetal malnutrition, and P07, Disorders of newborn related to short gestation and low birth weight, not elsewhere classified, should be based on the recorded birth weight and estimated gestational age.

When both birth weight and gestational age are available, two codes from category P07 should be assigned, with the code for birth weight sequenced before the code for gestational age.

e. Low birth weight and immaturity status

Codes from category P07, Disorders of newborn related to short gestation and low birth weight, not elsewhere classified, are for use for a child or adult who was premature or had a low birth weight as a newborn and this is affecting the patient's current health status.

See Section I.C.21. Factors influencing health status and contact with health services, Status.

> A 35-year-old patient, who weighed 659 grams at birth, is seen for heart disease documented as being a consequence of the low birth weight
>
> **I51.9   Heart disease, unspecified**
>
> **P07.02   Extremely low birth weight newborn, 500–749 grams**
>
> *Explanation:* A code from subcategories P07.0- and P07.1- is appropriate, regardless of the age of the patient, as long as the documentation provides a clear link between the patient's current illness and the low birth weight.

f. Bacterial sepsis of newborn

Category P36, Bacterial sepsis of newborn, includes congenital sepsis. If a perinate is documented as having sepsis without documentation of congenital or community acquired, the default is congenital and a code from category P36 should be assigned. If the P36 code includes the causal organism, an additional code from category B95, Streptococcus, Staphylococcus, and Enterococcus as the cause of diseases classified elsewhere, or B96, Other bacterial agents as the cause of diseases classified elsewhere, should not be assigned. If the P36 code does not include the causal organism, assign an additional code from category B96. If applicable, use additional codes to identify severe sepsis (R65.2-) and any associated acute organ dysfunction.

> A full-term infant develops severe sepsis 24 hours after discharge from the hospital and is readmitted; cultures identified *E. coli* as the infective agent
>
> **P36.4   Sepsis of newborn due to Escherichia coli**
>
> **R65.20   Severe sepsis without septic shock**
>
> *Explanation:* Even though this newborn was discharged and could have acquired *E. coli* from his/her external environment, due to the lack of documentation specifying specifically how this pathogen was acquired, the default is to code the *E. coli* sepsis as congenital. A code from chapter 1, "Certain Infectious and Parasitic Diseases," is not required because the perinatal sepsis code identifies both the sepsis and the bacteria causing the sepsis.

g. Stillbirth

Code P95, Stillbirth, is only for use in institutions that maintain separate records for stillbirths. No other code should be used with P95. Code P95 should not be used on the mother's record.

Chapter 16. Certain Conditions Originating in the Perinatal Period (P00-P96)

NOTE   Codes from this chapter are for use on newborn records only, never on maternal records

INCLUDES   conditions that have their origin in the fetal or perinatal period (before birth through the first 28 days after birth) even if morbidity occurs later

EXCLUDES 2   congenital malformations, deformations and chromosomal abnormalities (Q00-Q99)
endocrine, nutritional and metabolic diseases (E00-E88)
injury, poisoning and certain other consequences of external causes (S00-T88)
neoplasms (C00-D49)
tetanus neonatorum (A33)

This chapter contains the following blocks:

P00-P04	Newborn affected by maternal factors and by complications of pregnancy, labor, and delivery
P05-P08	Disorders of newborn related to length of gestation and fetal growth
P09	Abnormal findings on neonatal screening
P10-P15	Birth trauma
P19-P29	Respiratory and cardiovascular disorders specific to the perinatal period
P35-P39	Infections specific to the perinatal period
P50-P61	Hemorrhagic and hematological disorders of newborn
P70-P74	Transitory endocrine and metabolic disorders specific to newborn
P76-P78	Digestive system disorders of newborn
P80-P83	Conditions involving the integument and temperature regulation of newborn
P84	Other problems with newborn
P90-P96	Other disorders originating in the perinatal period

Newborn affected by maternal factors and by complications of pregnancy, labor, and delivery (P00-P04)

NOTE   These codes are for use when the listed maternal conditions are specified as the cause of confirmed morbidity or potential morbidity which have their origin in the perinatal period (before birth through the first 28 days after birth).

AHA: 2016,4Q,54-55

☑4ᵗʰ **P00**   **Newborn affected by maternal conditions that may be unrelated to present pregnancy**

Code first any current condition in newborn

EXCLUDES 2   encounter for observation of newborn for suspected diseases and conditions ruled out (Z05.-)
newborn affected by maternal complications of pregnancy (P01.-)
newborn affected by maternal endocrine and metabolic disorders (P70-P74)
newborn affected by noxious substances transmitted via placenta or breast milk (P04.-)

P00.0   **Newborn affected by maternal hypertensive disorders**
Newborn affected by maternal conditions classifiable to O10-O11, O13-O16

P00.1   **Newborn affected by maternal renal and urinary tract diseases**
Newborn affected by maternal conditions classifiable to N00-N39

P00.2   **Newborn affected by maternal infectious and parasitic diseases**
Newborn affected by maternal infectious disease classifiable to A00-B99, J09 and J10
EXCLUDES 1   maternal genital tract or other localized infections (P00.8)
EXCLUDES 2   infections specific to the perinatal period (P35-P39)
AHA: 2019,2Q,10; 2015,3Q,20

P00.3   **Newborn affected by other maternal circulatory and respiratory diseases**
Newborn affected by maternal conditions classifiable to I00-I99, J00-J99, Q20-Q34 and not included in P00.0, P00.2

P00.4   **Newborn affected by maternal nutritional disorders**
Newborn affected by maternal disorders classifiable to E40-E64
Maternal malnutrition NOS

P00.5   **Newborn affected by maternal injury**
Newborn affected by maternal conditions classifiable to O9A.2-

P00.6   **Newborn affected by surgical procedure on mother**
Newborn affected by amniocentesis
EXCLUDES 1   Cesarean delivery for present delivery (P03.4)
damage to placenta from amniocentesis, Cesarean delivery or surgical induction (P02.1)
previous surgery to uterus or pelvic organs (P03.89)
EXCLUDES 2   newborn affected by complication of (fetal) intrauterine procedure (P96.5)

P00.7   **Newborn affected by other medical procedures on mother, not elsewhere classified**
Newborn affected by radiation to mother
EXCLUDES 1   damage to placenta from amniocentesis, cesarean delivery or surgical induction (P02.1)
newborn affected by other complications of labor and delivery (P03.-)

☑5ᵗʰ **P00.8**   **Newborn affected by other maternal conditions**

P00.81   **Newborn affected by periodontal disease in mother**

P00.89   **Newborn affected by other maternal conditions**
Newborn affected by conditions classifiable to T80-T88
Newborn affected by maternal genital tract or other localized infections
Newborn affected by maternal systemic lupus erythematosus
AHA: 2019,2Q,9

P00.9   **Newborn affected by unspecified maternal condition**

☑4ᵗʰ **P01**   **Newborn affected by maternal complications of pregnancy**
Code first any current condition in newborn
EXCLUDES 2   encounter for observation of newborn for suspected diseases and conditions ruled out (Z05.-)

P01.0   **Newborn affected by incompetent cervix**

P01.1   **Newborn affected by premature rupture of membranes**

P01.2   **Newborn affected by oligohydramnios**
EXCLUDES 1   oligohydramnios due to premature rupture of membranes (P01.1)
DEF: Oligohydramnios: Low amniotic fluid level, resulting in underdeveloped organs in the fetus.

P01.3   **Newborn affected by polyhydramnios**
Newborn affected by hydramnios
DEF: Polyhydramnios: Excess amniotic fluid surrounding the fetus, typically defined as a total fluid volume of greater than 24.0 cc.

P01.4   **Newborn affected by ectopic pregnancy**
Newborn affected by abdominal pregnancy

P01.5   **Newborn affected by multiple pregnancy**
Newborn affected by triplet (pregnancy)
Newborn affected by twin (pregnancy)

P01.6   **Newborn affected by maternal death**

P01.7   **Newborn affected by malpresentation before labor**
Newborn affected by breech presentation before labor
Newborn affected by external version before labor
Newborn affected by face presentation before labor
Newborn affected by transverse lie before labor
Newborn affected by unstable lie before labor

P01.8   **Newborn affected by other maternal complications of pregnancy**

P01.9   **Newborn affected by maternal complication of pregnancy, unspecified**

☑4ᵗʰ **P02**   **Newborn affected by complications of placenta, cord and membranes**
Code first any current condition in newborn
EXCLUDES 2   encounter for observation of newborn for suspected diseases and conditions ruled out (Z05.-)

P02.0   **Newborn affected by placenta previa**
DEF: Placenta developed in the lower segment of the uterus that can cause hemorrhaging leading to preterm delivery.

P02.1   **Newborn affected by other forms of placental separation and hemorrhage**
Newborn affected by abruptio placenta
Newborn affected by accidental hemorrhage
Newborn affected by antepartum hemorrhage
Newborn affected by damage to placenta from amniocentesis, cesarean delivery or surgical induction
Newborn affected by maternal blood loss
Newborn affected by premature separation of placenta

☑5ᵗʰ **P02.2**   **Newborn affected by other and unspecified morphological and functional abnormalities of placenta**

P02.20   **Newborn affected by unspecified morphological and functional abnormalities of placenta**

P02.29 Newborn affected by other morphological and functional abnormalities of placenta
Newborn affected by placental dysfunction
Newborn affected by placental infarction
Newborn affected by placental insufficiency

P02.3 Newborn affected by placental transfusion syndromes
Newborn affected by placental and cord abnormalities resulting in twin-to-twin or other transplacental transfusion

P02.4 Newborn affected by prolapsed cord

P02.5 Newborn affected by other compression of umbilical cord
Newborn affected by umbilical cord (tightly) around neck
Newborn affected by entanglement of umbilical cord
Newborn affected by knot in umbilical cord

✓5ᵗʰ P02.6 Newborn affected by other and unspecified conditions of umbilical cord

　P02.60 Newborn affected by unspecified conditions of umbilical cord

　P02.69 Newborn affected by other conditions of umbilical cord
　　Newborn affected by short umbilical cord
　　Newborn affected by vasa previa
　　EXCLUDES 1 *newborn affected by single umbilical artery (Q27.0)*

✓5ᵗʰ P02.7 Newborn affected by chorioamnionitis
AHA: 2018,4Q,23-24
DEF: Inflammation of the fetal membranes due to maternal infection characterized by fetal tachycardia, respiratory distress, apnea, weak cries, and poor sucking.

　P02.70 Newborn affected by fetal inflammatory response syndrome 　**HCC**
　　Newborn affected by FIRS

　P02.78 Newborn affected by other conditions from chorioamnionitis
　　Newborn affected by amnionitis
　　Newborn affected by membranitis
　　Newborn affected by placentitis

P02.8 Newborn affected by other abnormalities of membranes

P02.9 Newborn affected by abnormality of membranes, unspecified

✓4ᵗʰ P03 Newborn affected by other complications of labor and delivery
Code first any current condition in newborn
EXCLUDES 2 *encounter for observation of newborn for suspected diseases and conditions ruled out (Z05.-)*

P03.0 Newborn affected by breech delivery and extraction

P03.1 Newborn affected by other malpresentation, malposition and disproportion during labor and delivery
Newborn affected by contracted pelvis
Newborn affected by conditions classifiable to O64-O66
Newborn affected by persistent occipitoposterior
Newborn affected by transverse lie

P03.2 Newborn affected by forceps delivery

Forceps Assisted Birth

Forceps extractor

P03.3 Newborn affected by delivery by vacuum extractor [ventouse]

Vacuum Assisted Birth

Vacuum extractor

P03.4 Newborn affected by Cesarean delivery

P03.5 Newborn affected by precipitate delivery
Newborn affected by rapid second stage

P03.6 Newborn affected by abnormal uterine contractions
Newborn affected by conditions classifiable to O62.-, except O62.3
Newborn affected by hypertonic labor
Newborn affected by uterine inertia

✓5ᵗʰ P03.8 Newborn affected by other specified complications of labor and delivery

　✓6ᵗʰ P03.81 Newborn affected by abnormality in fetal (intrauterine) heart rate or rhythm
　　EXCLUDES 1 *neonatal cardiac dysrhythmia (P29.1-)*

　　P03.810 Newborn affected by abnormality in fetal (intrauterine) heart rate or rhythm before the onset of labor

　　P03.811 Newborn affected by abnormality in fetal (intrauterine) heart rate or rhythm during labor

　　P03.819 Newborn affected by abnormality in fetal (intrauterine) heart rate or rhythm, unspecified as to time of onset

　P03.82 Meconium passage during delivery
　　EXCLUDES 1 *meconium aspiration (P24.00, P24.01)*
　　　meconium staining (P96.83)
　　DEF: Fetal intestinal activity that increases in response to a fetomaternal distressed state during delivery. The anal sphincter relaxes and meconium is passed into the amniotic fluid.

　P03.89 Newborn affected by other specified complications of labor and delivery
　　Newborn affected by abnormality of maternal soft tissues
　　Newborn affected by conditions classifiable to O60-O75 and by procedures used in labor and delivery not included in P02.- and P03.0-P03.6
　　Newborn affected by induction of labor

P03.9 Newborn affected by complication of labor and delivery, unspecified

✓4ᵗʰ P04 Newborn affected by noxious substances transmitted via placenta or breast milk
INCLUDES nonteratogenic effects of substances transmitted via placenta
EXCLUDES 2 *congenital malformations (Q00-Q99)*
encounter for observation of newborn for suspected diseases and conditions ruled out (Z05.-)
neonatal jaundice from excessive hemolysis due to drugs or toxins transmitted from mother (P58.4)
newborn in contact with and (suspected) exposures hazardous to health not transmitted via placenta or breast milk (Z77.-)

P04.0 Newborn affected by maternal anesthesia and analgesia in pregnancy, labor and delivery
Newborn affected by reactions and intoxications from maternal opiates and tranquilizers administered for procedures during pregnancy or labor and delivery
EXCLUDES 2 *newborn affected by other maternal medication (P04.1-)*

✓5ᵗʰ **P04.1 Newborn affected by other maternal medication**

Code first withdrawal symptoms from maternal use of drugs of addiction (P96.1)

EXCLUDES 1   dysmorphism due to warfarin (Q86.2)
fetal hydantoin syndrome (Q86.1)

EXCLUDES 2   maternal anesthesia and analgesia in pregnancy, labor and delivery (P04.0)
maternal use of drugs of addiction (P04.4-)

AHA: 2018,4Q,24-25

P04.11 Newborn affected by maternal antineoplastic chemotherapy

P04.12 Newborn affected by maternal cytotoxic drugs

P04.13 Newborn affected by maternal use of anticonvulsants

P04.14 Newborn affected by maternal use of opiates

P04.15 Newborn affected by maternal use of antidepressants

P04.16 Newborn affected by maternal use of amphetamines

P04.17 Newborn affected by maternal use of sedative-hypnotics

P04.1A Newborn affected by maternal use of anxiolytics

P04.18 Newborn affected by other maternal medication

P04.19 Newborn affected by maternal use of unspecified medication

P04.2 Newborn affected by maternal use of tobacco

Newborn affected by exposure in utero to tobacco smoke

EXCLUDES 2   newborn exposure to environmental tobacco smoke (P96.81)

P04.3 Newborn affected by maternal use of alcohol

EXCLUDES 1   fetal alcohol syndrome (Q86.0)

✓5ᵗʰ **P04.4 Newborn affected by maternal use of** drugs of addiction

AHA: 2018,4Q,25

P04.40 Newborn affected by maternal use of unspecified drugs of addiction

P04.41 Newborn affected by maternal use of cocaine

"Crack baby"

P04.42 Newborn affected by maternal use of hallucinogens

EXCLUDES 2   newborn affected by other maternal medication (P04.1-)

P04.49 Newborn affected by maternal use of other drugs of addiction

EXCLUDES 2   newborn affected by maternal anesthesia and analgesia (P04.0)
withdrawal symptoms from maternal use of drugs of addiction (P96.1)

P04.5 Newborn affected by maternal use of nutritional chemical substances

P04.6 Newborn affected by maternal exposure to environmental chemical substances

✓5ᵗʰ **P04.8 Newborn affected by other maternal** noxious substances

AHA: 2018,4Q,25

P04.81 Newborn affected by maternal use of cannabis

P04.89 Newborn affected by other maternal noxious substances

P04.9 Newborn affected by maternal noxious substance, unspecified

Disorders of newborn related to length of gestation and fetal growth (P05-P08)

✓4ᵗʰ **P05 Disorders of newborn related to slow fetal growth and fetal malnutrition**

AHA: 2016,4Q,55-56

✓5ᵗʰ **P05.0 Newborn light for gestational age**

Newborn light-for-dates
Weight below but length above 10th percentile for gestational age

P05.00 Newborn light for gestational age, unspecified weight

P05.01 Newborn light for gestational age, less than 500 grams

P05.02 Newborn light for gestational age, 500-749 grams

P05.03 Newborn light for gestational age, 750-999 grams

P05.04 Newborn light for gestational age, 1000-1249 grams

P05.05 Newborn light for gestational age, 1250-1499 grams

P05.06 Newborn light for gestational age, 1500-1749 grams

P05.07 Newborn light for gestational age, 1750-1999 grams

P05.08 Newborn light for gestational age, 2000-2499 grams

P05.09 Newborn light for gestational age, 2500 grams and over

Newborn light for gestational age, other

✓5ᵗʰ **P05.1 Newborn small for gestational age**

Newborn small-and-light-for-dates
Newborn small-for-dates
Weight and length below 10th percentile for gestational age

P05.10 Newborn small for gestational age, unspecified weight

P05.11 Newborn small for gestational age, less than 500 grams

P05.12 Newborn small for gestational age, 500-749 grams

P05.13 Newborn small for gestational age, 750-999 grams

P05.14 Newborn small for gestational age, 1000-1249 grams

P05.15 Newborn small for gestational age, 1250-1499 grams

P05.16 Newborn small for gestational age, 1500-1749 grams

P05.17 Newborn small for gestational age, 1750-1999 grams

P05.18 Newborn small for gestational age, 2000-2499 grams

P05.19 Newborn small for gestational age, other

Newborn small for gestational age, 2500 grams and over

P05.2 Newborn affected by fetal (intrauterine) malnutrition **not light or small for gestational age**

Infant, not light or small for gestational age, showing signs of fetal malnutrition, such as dry, peeling skin and loss of subcutaneous tissue

EXCLUDES 1   newborn affected by fetal malnutrition with light for gestational age (P05.0-)
newborn affected by fetal malnutrition with small for gestational age (P05.1-)

P05.9 Newborn affected by slow intrauterine growth, unspecified

Newborn affected by fetal growth retardation NOS

✓4ᵗʰ **P07 Disorders of newborn related to short gestation and low birth weight, not elsewhere classified**

NOTE   When both birth weight and gestational age of the newborn are available, both should be coded with birth weight sequenced before gestational age

INCLUDES   the listed conditions, without further specification, as the cause of morbidity or additional care, in newborn

✓5ᵗʰ **P07.0 Extremely low birth weight newborn**

Newborn birth weight 999 g. or less

EXCLUDES 1   low birth weight due to slow fetal growth and fetal malnutrition (P05.-)

P07.00 Extremely low birth weight newborn, unspecified weight

P07.01 Extremely low birth weight newborn, less than 500 grams

P07.02 Extremely low birth weight newborn, 500-749 grams

P07.03 Extremely low birth weight newborn, 750-999 grams

✓5ᵗʰ **P07.1 Other low birth weight newborn**

Newborn birth weight 1000-2499 g.

EXCLUDES 1   low birth weight due to slow fetal growth and fetal malnutrition (P05.-)

P07.10 Other low birth weight newborn, unspecified weight

P07.14 Other low birth weight newborn, 1000-1249 grams

P07.15 Other low birth weight newborn, 1250-1499 grams

P07.16 Other low birth weight newborn, 1500-1749 grams

P07.17 Other low birth weight newborn, 1750-1999 grams

P07.18 Other low birth weight newborn, 2000-2499 grams

✔ Additional Character Required   ✓x7ᵗʰ Placeholder   Unacceptable PDx   Questionable PDx   Manifestation   Unspecified Dx   H1 - H14 HAC   HCC CMS-HCC Dx   HIV HIV Dx

ICD-10-CM 2020   921

Chapter 16. Certain Conditions Originating in the Perinatal Period

P07.2–P11.9

✓5ᵗʰ **P07.2** **Extreme immaturity of newborn**

Less than 28 completed weeks (less than 196 completed days) of gestation.

P07.20 **Extreme immaturity of newborn, unspecified weeks of gestation**

Gestational age less than 28 completed weeks NOS

P07.21 **Extreme immaturity of newborn, gestational age less than 23 completed weeks**

Extreme immaturity of newborn, gestational age less than 23 weeks, 0 days

P07.22 **Extreme immaturity of newborn, gestational age 23 completed weeks**

Extreme immaturity of newborn, gestational age 23 weeks, 0 days through 23 weeks, 6 days

P07.23 **Extreme immaturity of newborn, gestational age 24 completed weeks**

Extreme immaturity of newborn, gestational age 24 weeks, 0 days through 24 weeks, 6 days

P07.24 **Extreme immaturity of newborn, gestational age 25 completed weeks**

Extreme immaturity of newborn, gestational age 25 weeks, 0 days through 25 weeks, 6 days

P07.25 **Extreme immaturity of newborn, gestational age 26 completed weeks**

Extreme immaturity of newborn, gestational age 26 weeks, 0 days through 26 weeks, 6 days

P07.26 **Extreme immaturity of newborn, gestational age 27 completed weeks**

Extreme immaturity of newborn, gestational age 27 weeks, 0 days through 27 weeks, 6 days

✓5ᵗʰ **P07.3** **Preterm [premature] newborn [other]**

28 completed weeks or more but less than 37 completed weeks (196 completed days but less than 259 completed days) of gestation

Prematurity NOS

AHA: 2017,3Q,26

P07.30 **Preterm newborn, unspecified weeks of gestation**

P07.31 **Preterm newborn, gestational age 28 completed weeks**

Preterm newborn, gestational age 28 weeks, 0 days through 28 weeks, 6 days

P07.32 **Preterm newborn, gestational age 29 completed weeks**

Preterm newborn, gestational age 29 weeks, 0 days through 29 weeks, 6 days

P07.33 **Preterm newborn, gestational age 30 completed weeks**

Preterm newborn, gestational age 30 weeks, 0 days through 30 weeks, 6 days

P07.34 **Preterm newborn, gestational age 31 completed weeks**

Preterm newborn, gestational age 31 weeks, 0 days through 31 weeks, 6 days

P07.35 **Preterm newborn, gestational age 32 completed weeks**

Preterm newborn, gestational age 32 weeks, 0 days through 32 weeks, 6 days

P07.36 **Preterm newborn, gestational age 33 completed weeks**

Preterm newborn, gestational age 33 weeks, 0 days through 33 weeks, 6 days

P07.37 **Preterm newborn, gestational age 34 completed weeks**

Preterm newborn, gestational age 34 weeks, 0 days through 34 weeks, 6 days

P07.38 **Preterm newborn, gestational age 35 completed weeks**

Preterm newborn, gestational age 35 weeks, 0 days through 35 weeks, 6 days

P07.39 **Preterm newborn, gestational age 36 completed weeks**

Preterm newborn, gestational age 36 weeks, 0 days through 36 weeks, 6 days

✓4ᵗʰ **P08** **Disorders of newborn related to long gestation and high birth weight**

NOTE   When both birth weight and gestational age of the newborn are available, priority of assignment should be given to birth weight

INCLUDES   the listed conditions, without further specification, as causes of morbidity or additional care, in newborn

P08.0 **Exceptionally large newborn baby**

Usually implies a birth weight of 4500 g. or more

EXCLUDES 1   *syndrome of infant of diabetic mother (P70.1)*

syndrome of infant of mother with gestational diabetes (P70.0)

P08.1 **Other heavy for gestational age newborn**

Other newborn heavy- or large-for-dates regardless of period of gestation

Usually implies a birth weight of 4000 g. to 4499 g.

EXCLUDES 1   *newborn with a birth weight of 4500 or more (P08.0)*

syndrome of infant of diabetic mother (P70.1)

syndrome of infant of mother with gestational diabetes (P70.0).

✓5ᵗʰ **P08.2** **Late newborn, not heavy for gestational age**

AHA: 2014,1Q,14

P08.21 **Post-term newborn**

Newborn with gestation period over 40 completed weeks to 42 completed weeks

P08.22 **Prolonged gestation of newborn**

Newborn with gestation period over 42 completed weeks (294 days or more), not heavy- or large-for-dates.

Postmaturity NOS

Abnormal findings on neonatal screening (P09)

P09 **Abnormal findings on neonatal screening**

Use additional code to identify signs, symptoms and conditions associated with the screening

EXCLUDES 2   *nonspecific serologic evidence of human immunodeficiency virus [HIV] (R75)*

Birth trauma (P10-P15)

CC Excl: For MCC codes in categories P10-P15, unless otherwise noted: PDX collection 1020

✓4ᵗʰ **P10** **Intracranial laceration and hemorrhage due to birth injury**

EXCLUDES 1   *intracranial hemorrhage of newborn NOS (P52.9)*

intracranial hemorrhage of newborn due to anoxia or hypoxia (P52.-)

nontraumatic intracranial hemorrhage of newborn (P52.-)

P10.0 **Subdural hemorrhage due to birth injury**   MCC

Subdural hematoma (localized) due to birth injury

EXCLUDES 1   *subdural hemorrhage accompanying tentorial tear (P10.4)*

P10.1 **Cerebral hemorrhage due to birth injury**   MCC

P10.2 **Intraventricular hemorrhage due to birth injury**   CC

CC Excl: PDX collection 1021

P10.3 **Subarachnoid hemorrhage due to birth injury**   MCC

CC Excl: PDX collection 1022

P10.4 **Tentorial tear due to birth injury**   MCC

P10.8 **Other intracranial lacerations and hemorrhages due to birth injury**   MCC

P10.9 **Unspecified intracranial laceration and hemorrhage due to birth injury**   MCC

✓4ᵗʰ **P11** **Other birth injuries to central nervous system**

P11.0 **Cerebral edema due to birth injury**   MCC

P11.1 **Other specified brain damage due to birth injury**

P11.2 **Unspecified brain damage due to birth injury**   MCC

P11.3 **Birth injury to facial nerve**

Facial palsy due to birth injury

P11.4 **Birth injury to other cranial nerves**

P11.5 **Birth injury to spine and spinal cord**

Fracture of spine due to birth injury

P11.9 **Birth injury to central nervous system, unspecified**   MCC

N Newborn: 0   P Pediatric: 0-17   M Maternity: 9-64   A Adult: 15-124   MCC Major Complication/Comorbidity   CC Complication/Comorbidity   SW Severe Wound Dx

922   ICD-10-CM 2020

✓4ᵗʰ P12 Birth injury to scalp

Birth Injuries to Scalp

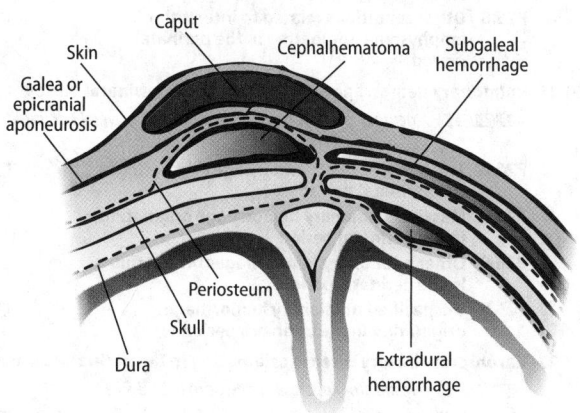

Caput
Skin
Cephalhematoma
Subgaleal hemorrhage
Galea or epicranial aponeurosis
Periosteum
Skull
Dura
Extradural hemorrhage

P12.0 Cephalhematoma due to birth injury
DEF: Condition that occurs in a neonate when blood vessels between the skull and periosteum rupture and blood collects in the subperiosteal space (below the periosteum). It is typically caused by prolonged labor or trauma due to instrument-assisted delivery (e.g., forceps, vacuum extraction), although in rare circumstances, it may indicate a linear skull fracture with intracranial hemorrhage.

P12.1 Chignon (from vacuum extraction) due to birth injury
DEF: Artificial swelling of the scalp that occurs when a collection of interstitial fluid and blood forms in the area of the scalp where the suction cup was applied during a vacuum-assisted delivery.

P12.2 Epicranial subaponeurotic hemorrhage due to birth injury CC
Subgaleal hemorrhage
CC Excl: PDX collection 1023

P12.3 Bruising of scalp due to birth injury

P12.4 Injury of scalp of newborn due to monitoring equipment
Sampling incision of scalp of newborn
Scalp clip (electrode) injury of newborn

✓5ᵗʰ P12.8 Other birth injuries to scalp

P12.81 Caput succedaneum
DEF: Swelling of the scalp as a result of pressure being exerted on the head from the vaginal walls, uterus, or instrumentation used in assisting a delivery (e.g., vacuum).

P12.89 Other birth injuries to scalp

P12.9 Birth injury to scalp, unspecified

✓4ᵗʰ P13 Birth injury to skeleton

EXCLUDES 2   birth injury to spine (P11.5)

P13.0 Fracture of skull due to birth injury

P13.1 Other birth injuries to skull
EXCLUDES 1   cephalhematoma (P12.0)

P13.2 Birth injury to femur

P13.3 Birth injury to other long bones

P13.4 Fracture of clavicle due to birth injury

P13.8 Birth injuries to other parts of skeleton

P13.9 Birth injury to skeleton, unspecified

✓4ᵗʰ P14 Birth injury to peripheral nervous system

P14.0 Erb's paralysis due to birth injury
DEF: Erb's paralysis: Most common type of brachial plexus (peripheral nerve) injury in a neonate that involves nerve damage at the level of C5-C6. Synonym(s): Erb's palsy

P14.1 Klumpke's paralysis due to birth injury

P14.2 Phrenic nerve paralysis due to birth injury

P14.3 Other brachial plexus birth injuries

P14.8 Birth injuries to other parts of peripheral nervous system

P14.9 Birth injury to peripheral nervous system, unspecified

✓4ᵗʰ P15 Other birth injuries

P15.0 Birth injury to liver
Rupture of liver due to birth injury

P15.1 Birth injury to spleen
Rupture of spleen due to birth injury

P15.2 Sternomastoid injury due to birth injury

P15.3 Birth injury to eye
Subconjunctival hemorrhage due to birth injury
Traumatic glaucoma due to birth injury

P15.4 Birth injury to face
Facial congestion due to birth injury

P15.5 Birth injury to external genitalia

P15.6 Subcutaneous fat necrosis due to birth injury

P15.8 Other specified birth injuries
TIP: Use for any injury of newborn from scalpel.

P15.9 Birth injury, unspecified

Respiratory and cardiovascular disorders specific to the perinatal period (P19-P29)

CC Excl: For MCC codes in categories P19-P29, unless otherwise noted: PDX collection 748

✓4ᵗʰ P19 Metabolic acidemia in newborn

INCLUDES   metabolic acidemia in newborn

P19.0 Metabolic acidemia in newborn first noted before onset of labor

P19.1 Metabolic acidemia in newborn first noted during labor

P19.2 Metabolic acidemia noted at birth

P19.9 Metabolic acidemia, unspecified

✓4ᵗʰ P22 Respiratory distress of newborn

EXCLUDES 1   respiratory arrest of newborn (P28.81)
respiratory failure of newborn NOS (P28.5)

AHA: 2019,2Q,29

P22.0 Respiratory distress syndrome of newborn MCC
Cardiorespiratory distress syndrome of newborn
Hyaline membrane disease
Idiopathic respiratory distress syndrome [IRDS or RDS] of newborn
Pulmonary hypoperfusion syndrome
Respiratory distress syndrome, type I
EXCLUDES 2 ▶respiratory arrest of newborn (P28.81)◀
▶respiratory failure of newborn NOS (P28.5)◀
AHA: 2019,2Q,29
DEF: Severe chest contractions upon air intake and expiratory grunting. The infant appears blue due to oxygen deficiency and has a rapid respiratory rate, formerly called hyaline membrane disease.

P22.1 Transient tachypnea of newborn
Idiopathic tachypnea of newborn
Respiratory distress syndrome, type II
Wet lung syndrome
DEF: Rapid, labored breathing of a newborn. It is a short-term problem that begins after birth and lasts about three days.

P22.8 Other respiratory distress of newborn
EXCLUDES 1 ▶respiratory arrest of newborn (P28.81)◀
▶respiratory failure of newborn NOS (P28.5)◀

P22.9 Respiratory distress of newborn, unspecified
EXCLUDES 1 ▶respiratory arrest of newborn (P28.81)◀
▶respiratory failure of newborn NOS (P28.5)◀

✓4ᵗʰ P23 Congenital pneumonia

INCLUDES   infective pneumonia acquired in utero or during birth
EXCLUDES 1   neonatal pneumonia resulting from aspiration (P24.-)

P23.0 Congenital pneumonia due to viral agent MCC
Use additional code (B97) to identify organism
EXCLUDES 1   congenital rubella pneumonitis (P35.0)

P23.1 Congenital pneumonia due to Chlamydia MCC

P23.2 Congenital pneumonia due to staphylococcus MCC

P23.3 Congenital pneumonia due to streptococcus, group B MCC

P23.4 Congenital pneumonia due to Escherichia coli MCC

P23.5 Congenital pneumonia due to Pseudomonas MCC

P23.6 Congenital pneumonia due to other bacterial agents MCC
Congenital pneumonia due to Hemophilus influenzae
Congenital pneumonia due to Klebsiella pneumoniae
Congenital pneumonia due to Mycoplasma
Congenital pneumonia due to Streptococcus, except group B
Use additional code (B95-B96) to identify organism

P23.8 Congenital pneumonia due to other organisms MCC

P23.9 Congenital pneumonia, unspecified MCC

✔ Additional Character Required   ✓x7ᵗʰ Placeholder   Unacceptable PDx   Questionable PDx   Manifestation   Unspecified Dx   H1-H14 HAC   HCC CMS-HCC Dx   HIV HIV Dx

ICD-10-CM 2020   923

Chapter 16. Certain Conditions Originating in the Perinatal Period

P24–P28.81

☑4ᵗʰ **P24 Neonatal aspiration**

[INCLUDES] aspiration in utero and during delivery

☑5ᵗʰ **P24.0 Meconium aspiration**

EXCLUDES 1　meconium passage (without aspiration) during delivery (P03.82)

meconium staining (P96.83)

DEF: Meconium in the trachea or seen on chest x-ray after birth.

P24.00 Meconium aspiration without respiratory symptoms

Meconium aspiration NOS

P24.01 Meconium aspiration with respiratory symptoms　MCC

Meconium aspiration pneumonia

Meconium aspiration pneumonitis

Meconium aspiration syndrome NOS

Use additional code to identify any secondary pulmonary hypertension, if applicable (I27.2-)

DEF: Aspiration of fetal intestinal material during or prior to delivery. If is usually a complication of placental insufficiency, causing pneumonitis and bronchial obstruction (inflammatory reaction of lungs).

☑5ᵗʰ **P24.1 Neonatal aspiration of (clear) amniotic fluid and mucus**

Neonatal aspiration of liquor (amnii)

P24.10 Neonatal aspiration of (clear) amniotic fluid and mucus without respiratory symptoms

Neonatal aspiration of amniotic fluid and mucus NOS

P24.11 Neonatal aspiration of (clear) amniotic fluid and mucus with respiratory symptoms　MCC

Neonatal aspiration of amniotic fluid and mucus with pneumonia

Neonatal aspiration of amniotic fluid and mucus with pneumonitis

Use additional code to identify any secondary pulmonary hypertension, if applicable (I27.2-)

☑5ᵗʰ **P24.2 Neonatal aspiration of blood**

P24.20 Neonatal aspiration of blood without respiratory symptoms

Neonatal aspiration of blood NOS

P24.21 Neonatal aspiration of blood with respiratory symptoms　MCC

Neonatal aspiration of blood with pneumonia

Neonatal aspiration of blood with pneumonitis

Use additional code to identify any secondary pulmonary hypertension, if applicable (I27.2-)

☑5ᵗʰ **P24.3 Neonatal aspiration of milk and regurgitated food**

Neonatal aspiration of stomach contents

P24.30 Neonatal aspiration of milk and regurgitated food without respiratory symptoms

Neonatal aspiration of milk and regurgitated food NOS

P24.31 Neonatal aspiration of milk and regurgitated food with respiratory symptoms　MCC

Neonatal aspiration of milk and regurgitated food with pneumonia

Neonatal aspiration of milk and regurgitated food with pneumonitis

Use additional code to identify any secondary pulmonary hypertension, if applicable (I27.2-)

☑5ᵗʰ **P24.8 Other neonatal aspiration**

P24.80 Other neonatal aspiration without respiratory symptoms

Neonatal aspiration NEC

P24.81 Other neonatal aspiration with respiratory symptoms　MCC

Neonatal aspiration pneumonia NEC

Neonatal aspiration with pneumonitis NEC

Neonatal aspiration with pneumonia NOS

Neonatal aspiration with pneumonitis NOS

Use additional code to identify any secondary pulmonary hypertension, if applicable (I27.2-)

P24.9 Neonatal aspiration, unspecified

☑4ᵗʰ **P25 Interstitial emphysema and related conditions originating in the perinatal period**

P25.0 Interstitial emphysema originating in the perinatal period　MCC

P25.1 Pneumothorax originating in the perinatal period　MCC

P25.2 Pneumomediastinum originating in the perinatal period　MCC

P25.3 Pneumopericardium originating in the perinatal period　MCC

P25.8 Other conditions related to interstitial emphysema originating in the perinatal period　MCC

☑4ᵗʰ **P26 Pulmonary hemorrhage originating in the perinatal period**

EXCLUDES 1　acute idiopathic hemorrhage in infants over 28 days old (R04.81)

P26.0 Tracheobronchial hemorrhage originating in the perinatal period　MCC

P26.1 Massive pulmonary hemorrhage originating in the perinatal period　MCC

P26.8 Other pulmonary hemorrhages originating in the perinatal period　MCC

P26.9 Unspecified pulmonary hemorrhage originating in the perinatal period　MCC

☑4ᵗʰ **P27 Chronic respiratory disease originating in the perinatal period**

EXCLUDES 2　respiratory distress of newborn (P22.0-P22.9)

P27.0 Wilson-Mikity syndrome　MCC

Pulmonary dysmaturity

DEF: Pulmonary insufficiency in newborn babies, especially those with low birth weight. Rapid onset of hypercapnia and cyanosis occur during the first month of life frequently resulting in death.

P27.1 Bronchopulmonary dysplasia originating in the perinatal period　MCC

P27.8 Other chronic respiratory diseases originating in the perinatal period　MCC

Congenital pulmonary fibrosis

Ventilator lung in newborn

P27.9 Unspecified chronic respiratory disease originating in the perinatal period　MCC

☑4ᵗʰ **P28 Other respiratory conditions originating in the perinatal period**

EXCLUDES 1　congenital malformations of the respiratory system (Q30-Q34)

P28.0 Primary atelectasis of newborn　CC

Primary failure to expand terminal respiratory units

Pulmonary hypoplasia associated with short gestation

Pulmonary immaturity NOS

☑5ᵗʰ **P28.1 Other and unspecified atelectasis of newborn**

P28.10 Unspecified atelectasis of newborn　CC

Atelectasis of newborn NOS

P28.11 Resorption atelectasis without respiratory distress syndrome　CC

EXCLUDES 1　resorption atelectasis with respiratory distress syndrome (P22.0)

P28.19 Other atelectasis of newborn　CC

Partial atelectasis of newborn

Secondary atelectasis of newborn

P28.2 Cyanotic attacks of newborn　CC

EXCLUDES 1　apnea of newborn (P28.3-P28.4)

CC Excl: PDX collection 1024

P28.3 Primary sleep apnea of newborn　CC

Central sleep apnea of newborn

Obstructive sleep apnea of newborn

Sleep apnea of newborn NOS

DEF: Unexplained cessation of breathing when a neonate makes no respiratory effort for 20 seconds or longer or when a neonate's breathing cessation is accompanied by cyanosis, bradycardia, or hypotonia.

CC Excl: PDX collection 1025

P28.4 Other apnea of newborn　CC

Apnea of prematurity

Obstructive apnea of newborn

EXCLUDES 1　obstructive sleep apnea of newborn (P28.3)

CC Excl: PDX collection 1026

P28.5 Respiratory failure of newborn　MCC

EXCLUDES 1　respiratory arrest of newborn (P28.81)

respiratory distress of newborn (P22.0-)

AHA: 2019,2Q,29

☑5ᵗʰ **P28.8 Other specified respiratory conditions of newborn**

P28.81 Respiratory arrest of newborn　MCC

CC Excl: PDX collection 1027

N Newborn: 0　　P Pediatric: 0-17　　M Maternity: 9-64　　A Adult: 15-124　　MCC Major Complication/Comorbidity　　CC Complication/Comorbidity　　SW Severe Wound Dx

924　　　　　ICD-10-CM 2020

P28.89   **Other specified respiratory conditions of newborn**
Congenital laryngeal stridor
Sniffles in newborn
Snuffles in newborn
EXCLUDES 1   *early congenital syphilitic rhinitis (A50.05)*

P28.9   **Respiratory condition of newborn, unspecified**
Respiratory depression in newborn

✓4ᵗʰ **P29**   **Cardiovascular disorders originating in the perinatal period**
EXCLUDES 1   *congenital malformations of the circulatory system (Q20–Q28)*

P29.0   **Neonatal cardiac failure**

✓5ᵗʰ **P29.1**   **Neonatal cardiac dysrhythmia**

P29.11   **Neonatal** tachycardia

P29.12   **Neonatal** bradycardia

P29.2   **Neonatal hypertension**

✓5ᵗʰ **P29.3**   **Persistent fetal circulation**
AHA: 2017,4Q,20-21

P29.30   **Pulmonary hypertension of newborn**   `MCC`
Persistent pulmonary hypertension of newborn
DEF: Condition that occurs when pressure within the pulmonary artery is elevated and vascular resistance is observed in the lungs.
CC Excl: PDX collection 1028

P29.38   **Other persistent fetal circulation**   `MCC`
Delayed closure of ductus arteriosus
CC Excl: PDX collection 1028

P29.4   **Transient myocardial ischemia in newborn**

✓5ᵗʰ **P29.8**   **Other cardiovascular disorders originating in the perinatal period**

P29.81   **Cardiac arrest of newborn**   `MCC`
CC Excl: PDX collection 1029

P29.89   **Other cardiovascular disorders originating in the perinatal period**
AHA: 2014,4Q,23

P29.9   **Cardiovascular disorder originating in the perinatal period, unspecified**

Infections specific to the perinatal period (P35-P39)

Infections acquired in utero, during birth via the umbilicus, or during the first 28 days after birth
EXCLUDES 2   *asymptomatic human immunodeficiency virus [HIV] infection status (Z21)*
congenital gonococcal infection (A54.-)
congenital pneumonia (P23.-)
congenital syphilis (A50.-)
human immunodeficiency virus [HIV] disease (B20)
infant botulism (A48.51)
infectious diseases not specific to the perinatal period (A00-B99, J09, J10.-)
intestinal infectious disease (A00-A09)
laboratory evidence of human immunodeficiency virus [HIV] (R75)
tetanus neonatorum (A33)

✓4ᵗʰ **P35**   **Congenital viral diseases**
`INCLUDES`   infections acquired in utero or during birth
CC Excl: For MCC codes in category P35, unless otherwise noted: PDX collection 562

P35.0   **Congenital** rubella **syndrome**   `CC`
Congenital rubella pneumonitis
CC Excl: PDX collection 1030

P35.1   **Congenital** cytomegalovirus **infection**   `MCC`
CC Excl: PDX collection 1030

P35.2   **Congenital** herpesviral [herpes simplex] **infection**   `MCC`

P35.3   **Congenital** viral hepatitis   `MCC`

P35.4   **Congenital** Zika virus **disease**   `MCC`
Use additional code to identify manifestations of congenital Zika virus disease
AHA: 2018,4Q,25-26

P35.8   **Other congenital viral diseases**   `MCC`
Congenital varicella [chickenpox]

P35.9   **Congenital viral disease, unspecified**   `MCC`

✓4ᵗʰ **P36**   **Bacterial sepsis of newborn**
`INCLUDES`   congenital sepsis
Use additional code(s), if applicable, to identify severe sepsis (R65.2-) and associated acute organ dysfunction(s)
CC Excl: For MCC codes in category P36: PDX collection 1031

P36.0   **Sepsis of newborn due to** streptococcus, group B   `MCC` `HCC`

✓5ᵗʰ **P36.1**   **Sepsis of newborn due to other and unspecified** streptococci

P36.10   **Sepsis of newborn due to unspecified streptococci**   `MCC` `HCC`

P36.19   **Sepsis of newborn due to other streptococci**   `MCC` `HCC`

P36.2   **Sepsis of newborn due to** Staphylococcus aureus   `MCC` `HCC`

✓5ᵗʰ **P36.3**   **Sepsis of newborn due to other and unspecified** staphylococci

P36.30   **Sepsis of newborn due to unspecified staphylococci**   `MCC` `HCC`

P36.39   **Sepsis of newborn due to other staphylococci**   `MCC` `HCC`

P36.4   **Sepsis of newborn due to** Escherichia coli   `MCC` `HCC`

P36.5   **Sepsis of newborn due to** anaerobes   `MCC` `HCC`

P36.8   **Other** bacterial sepsis **of newborn**   `MCC` `HCC`
Use additional code from category B96 to identify organism

P36.9   **Bacterial sepsis of newborn, unspecified**   `MCC` `HCC`

✓4ᵗʰ **P37**   **Other congenital infectious and parasitic diseases**
EXCLUDES 2   *congenital syphilis (A50.-)*
infectious neonatal diarrhea (A00-A09)
necrotizing enterocolitis in newborn (P77.-)
noninfectious neonatal diarrhea (P78.3)
ophthalmia neonatorum due to gonococcus (A54.31)
tetanus neonatorum (A33)
CC Excl: For MCC codes in category P37: PDX collection 562

P37.0   **Congenital** tuberculosis   `MCC`

P37.1   **Congenital** toxoplasmosis   `MCC`
Hydrocephalus due to congenital toxoplasmosis

P37.2   **Neonatal (disseminated)** listeriosis   `MCC`

P37.3   **Congenital** falciparum malaria   `MCC`

P37.4   **Other congenital** malaria   `MCC`

P37.5   **Neonatal** candidiasis

P37.8   **Other specified congenital infectious and parasitic diseases**   `MCC`

P37.9   **Congenital infectious or parasitic disease, unspecified**   `MCC`

✓4ᵗʰ **P38**   **Omphalitis of newborn**
EXCLUDES 1   *omphalitis not of newborn (L08.82)*
tetanus omphalitis (A33)
umbilical hemorrhage of newborn (P51.-)
DEF: Omphalitis: Infection and inflammation of the umbilical stump, often due to bacteria that can spread beyond the umbilical stump to the fascia, muscle, or even the umbilical vessels.

P38.1   **Omphalitis** with mild hemorrhage   `CC`
CC Excl: PDX collection 1032

P38.9   **Omphalitis** without hemorrhage   `CC`
Omphalitis of newborn NOS
CC Excl: PDX collection 1032

✓4ᵗʰ **P39**   **Other infections specific to the perinatal period**
Use additional code to identify organism or specific infection
CC Excl: For CC codes in category P39, unless otherwise noted: PDX collection 1033

P39.0   **Neonatal infective** mastitis   `CC`
EXCLUDES 1   *breast engorgement of newborn (P83.4)*
noninfective mastitis of newborn (P83.4)
CC Excl: PDX collection 1032

P39.1   **Neonatal** conjunctivitis and dacryocystitis
Neonatal chlamydial conjunctivitis
Ophthalmia neonatorum NOS
EXCLUDES 1   *gonococcal conjunctivitis (A54.31)*

P39.2   **Intra-amniotic** infection affecting newborn, not elsewhere classified   `CC`

P39.3   **Neonatal** urinary tract infection   `CC`
CC Excl: PDX collection 1034

P39.4   Neonatal skin infection `CC`
> Neonatal pyoderma
> *EXCLUDES 1*   pemphigus neonatorum (L00)
>   staphylococcal scalded skin syndrome (L00)

P39.8   Other specified infections specific to the perinatal period `CC`

P39.9   Infection specific to the perinatal period, unspecified `CC`

Hemorrhagic and hematological disorders of newborn (P50-P61)

EXCLUDES 1   congenital stenosis and stricture of bile ducts (Q44.3)
                       Crigler-Najjar syndrome (E80.5)
                       Dubin-Johnson syndrome (E80.6)
                       Gilbert syndrome (E80.4)
                       hereditary hemolytic anemias (D55-D58)

✓4ᵗʰ **P50   Newborn affected by intrauterine (fetal) blood loss**
> *EXCLUDES 1*   congenital anemia from intrauterine (fetal) blood loss (P61.3)

P50.0   Newborn affected by intrauterine (fetal) blood loss from vasa previa

P50.1   Newborn affected by intrauterine (fetal) blood loss from ruptured cord

P50.2   Newborn affected by intrauterine (fetal) blood loss from placenta

P50.3   Newborn affected by hemorrhage into co-twin

P50.4   Newborn affected by hemorrhage into maternal circulation

P50.5   Newborn affected by intrauterine (fetal) blood loss from cut end of co-twin's cord

P50.8   Newborn affected by other intrauterine (fetal) blood loss

P50.9   Newborn affected by intrauterine (fetal) blood loss, unspecified
> Newborn affected by fetal hemorrhage NOS

✓4ᵗʰ **P51   Umbilical hemorrhage of newborn**
> *EXCLUDES 1*   omphalitis with mild hemorrhage (P38.1)
>   umbilical hemorrhage from cut end of co-twins cord (P50.5)

P51.0   Massive umbilical hemorrhage of newborn

P51.8   Other umbilical hemorrhages of newborn
> Slipped umbilical ligature NOS

P51.9   Umbilical hemorrhage of newborn, unspecified

✓4ᵗʰ **P52   Intracranial nontraumatic hemorrhage of newborn**
> *INCLUDES*   intracranial hemorrhage due to anoxia or hypoxia
> *EXCLUDES 1*   intracranial hemorrhage due to birth injury (P10.-)
>   intracranial hemorrhage due to other injury (S06.-)

> **CC Excl: For codes in category P52:**
> **For MCC codes, unless otherwise noted:** PDX collection 1020
> **For CC codes:** PDX collection 1021

P52.0   Intraventricular (nontraumatic) hemorrhage, grade 1, of newborn `CC`
> Subependymal hemorrhage (without intraventricular extension)
> Bleeding into germinal matrix

P52.1   Intraventricular (nontraumatic) hemorrhage, grade 2, of newborn `CC`
> Subependymal hemorrhage with intraventricular extension
> Bleeding into ventricle

✓5ᵗʰ **P52.2   Intraventricular (nontraumatic) hemorrhage, grade 3 and grade 4, of newborn**

> **P52.21   Intraventricular (nontraumatic) hemorrhage, grade 3, of newborn** `MCC`
> > Subependymal hemorrhage with intraventricular extension with enlargement of ventricle
> > **CC Excl:** PDX collection 1021

> **P52.22   Intraventricular (nontraumatic) hemorrhage, grade 4, of newborn** `MCC`
> > Bleeding into cerebral cortex
> > Subependymal hemorrhage with intracerebral extension
> > **CC Excl:** PDX collection 1021

P52.3   Unspecified intraventricular (nontraumatic) hemorrhage of newborn `CC`

P52.4   Intracerebral (nontraumatic) hemorrhage of newborn `MCC`

P52.5   Subarachnoid (nontraumatic) hemorrhage of newborn `MCC`
> **CC Excl:** PDX collection 1022

P52.6   Cerebellar (nontraumatic) and posterior fossa hemorrhage of newborn `MCC`

P52.8   Other intracranial (nontraumatic) hemorrhages of newborn `MCC`

P52.9   Intracranial (nontraumatic) hemorrhage of newborn, unspecified `MCC`

P53   Hemorrhagic disease of newborn `CC`
> Vitamin K deficiency of newborn
> **CC Excl:** PDX collection 1035

✓4ᵗʰ **P54   Other neonatal hemorrhages**
> *EXCLUDES 1*   newborn affected by (intrauterine) blood loss (P50.-)
>   pulmonary hemorrhage originating in the perinatal period (P26.-)
> **CC Excl: For CC/MCC codes in category P54:** PDX collection 1036

P54.0   Neonatal hematemesis
> *EXCLUDES 1*   neonatal hematemesis due to swallowed maternal blood (P78.2)

P54.1   Neonatal melena `MCC`
> *EXCLUDES 1*   neonatal melena due to swallowed maternal blood (P78.2)

P54.2   Neonatal rectal hemorrhage `MCC`

P54.3   Other neonatal gastrointestinal hemorrhage `MCC`

P54.4   Neonatal adrenal hemorrhage `CC`

P54.5   Neonatal cutaneous hemorrhage
> Neonatal bruising
> Neonatal ecchymoses
> Neonatal petechiae
> Neonatal superficial hematomata
> *EXCLUDES 2*   bruising of scalp due to birth injury (P12.3)
>   cephalhematoma due to birth injury (P12.0)

P54.6   Neonatal vaginal hemorrhage ♀
> Neonatal pseudomenses

P54.8   Other specified neonatal hemorrhages

P54.9   Neonatal hemorrhage, unspecified

✓4ᵗʰ **P55   Hemolytic disease of newborn**

P55.0   Rh isoimmunization of newborn
> **DEF:** Incompatible Rh fetal-maternal blood grouping that prematurely destroys red blood cells. Symptoms include jaundice, asphyxia, pulmonary hypertension, edema, respiratory distress, kernicterus, and coagulopathies. It is detected by a Coombs test.
> **TIP:** A positive Coombs test without documentation of associated Rh isoimmunization should be coded to R79.89 Other specified abnormal findings of blood chemistry.

P55.1   ABO isoimmunization of newborn
> **AHA:** 2015,3Q,20

P55.8   Other hemolytic diseases of newborn
> **AHA:** 2018,3Q,24

P55.9   Hemolytic disease of newborn, unspecified

✓4ᵗʰ **P56   Hydrops fetalis due to hemolytic disease**
> *EXCLUDES 1*   hydrops fetalis NOS (P83.2)
> **CC Excl: For MCC codes in category P56:** PDX collection 1037

P56.0   Hydrops fetalis due to isoimmunization `MCC`

✓5ᵗʰ **P56.9   Hydrops fetalis due to other and unspecified hemolytic disease**

> **P56.90   Hydrops fetalis due to unspecified hemolytic disease** `MCC`

> **P56.99   Hydrops fetalis due to other hemolytic disease** `MCC`

✓4ᵗʰ **P57   Kernicterus**

P57.0   Kernicterus due to isoimmunization `MCC`
> **DEF:** Complication of erythroblastosis fetalis associated with severe neural symptoms, high blood bilirubin levels, and nerve cell destruction. It results in bilirubin-pigmented gray matter of the central nervous system.
> **CC Excl:** PDX collection 1037

P57.8   Other specified kernicterus `MCC`
> *EXCLUDES 1*   Crigler-Najjar syndrome (E80.5)
> **CC Excl:** PDX collection 1038

P57.9   Kernicterus, unspecified `MCC`
> **CC Excl:** PDX collection 1038

✓4ᵗʰ **P58   Neonatal jaundice due to other excessive hemolysis**
> *EXCLUDES 1*   jaundice due to isoimmunization (P55-P57)

P58.0   Neonatal jaundice due to bruising

P58.1   Neonatal jaundice due to bleeding

P58.2   Neonatal jaundice due to infection

P58.3   **Neonatal jaundice due to** polycythemia

☑5ᵗʰ P58.4   **Neonatal jaundice due to** drugs or toxins **transmitted from mother or given to newborn**

> Code first poisoning due to drug or toxin, if applicable (T36-T65 with fifth or sixth character 1-4 or 6)
> Use additional code for adverse effect, if applicable, to identify drug (T36-T50 with fifth or sixth character 5)

    P58.41   **Neonatal jaundice due to drugs or toxins** transmitted from mother

    P58.42   **Neonatal jaundice due to drugs or toxins** given to newborn

P58.5   **Neonatal jaundice due to** swallowed maternal blood

P58.8   **Neonatal jaundice due to other specified excessive hemolysis**

P58.9   **Neonatal jaundice due to excessive hemolysis, unspecified**

☑4ᵗʰ **P59 Neonatal jaundice from other and unspecified causes**

> EXCLUDES 1   *jaundice due to inborn errors of metabolism (E70-E88)*
> *kernicterus (P57.-)*

CC Excl: For MCC codes in category P59: PDX collection 1038

P59.0   **Neonatal jaundice associated with** preterm delivery

> Hyperbilirubinemia of prematurity
> Jaundice due to delayed conjugation associated with preterm delivery

P59.1   **Inspissated bile syndrome**   MCC

> DEF: Biliary obstruction in newborn resulting from obstruction of outflow tract.

☑5ᵗʰ P59.2   **Neonatal jaundice from other and unspecified** hepatocellular damage

> EXCLUDES 1   *congenital viral hepatitis (P35.3)*

    P59.20   **Neonatal jaundice from unspecified hepatocellular damage**   MCC

    P59.29   **Neonatal jaundice from other hepatocellular damage**   MCC

> Neonatal giant cell hepatitis
> Neonatal (idiopathic) hepatitis

P59.3   **Neonatal jaundice from** breast milk inhibitor

P59.8   **Neonatal jaundice from other specified causes**

P59.9   **Neonatal jaundice, unspecified**

> Neonatal physiological jaundice (intense)(prolonged) NOS
> AHA: 2015,3Q,20

P60   **Disseminated intravascular coagulation of newborn**   MCC

> Defibrination syndrome of newborn
> CC Excl: PDX collection 1035

☑4ᵗʰ **P61 Other perinatal hematological disorders**

> EXCLUDES 1   *transient hypogammaglobulinemia of infancy (D80.7)*

P61.0   **Transient neonatal thrombocytopenia**   MCC

> Neonatal thrombocytopenia due to exchange transfusion
> Neonatal thrombocytopenia due to idiopathic maternal thrombocytopenia
> Neonatal thrombocytopenia due to isoimmunization
> DEF: Temporary decrease in blood platelets of a newborn that is secondary to placental insufficiency.
> CC Excl: PDX collection 1035

P61.1   **Polycythemia neonatorum**

> DEF: Abnormal increase of total red blood cells of a newborn that results in hyperviscosity, which slows the flow of blood through small blood vessels.

P61.2   **Anemia of prematurity**   CC

> CC Excl: PDX collection 1039

P61.3   **Congenital anemia from fetal blood loss**   CC

> CC Excl: PDX collection 1039

P61.4   **Other congenital anemias, not elsewhere classified**   CC

> Congenital anemia NOS
> CC Excl: PDX collection 1039

P61.5   **Transient neonatal neutropenia**   MCC

> EXCLUDES 1   *congenital neutropenia (nontransient) (D70.0)*
> DEF: Low blood neutrophil counts of newborn that occurs due to maternal hypertension, sepsis, twin-twin transfusion, alloimmunization, and hemolytic disease.
> CC Excl: PDX collection 1040

P61.6   **Other transient neonatal disorders of coagulation**   CC

> CC Excl: PDX collection 1035

P61.8   **Other specified perinatal hematological disorders**

P61.9   **Perinatal hematological disorder, unspecified**

Transitory endocrine and metabolic disorders specific to newborn (P70-P74)

INCLUDES   transitory endocrine and metabolic disturbances caused by the infant's response to maternal endocrine and metabolic factors, or its adjustment to extrauterine environment

AHA: 2018,2Q,6

☑4ᵗʰ **P70 Transitory disorders of** carbohydrate metabolism **specific to newborn**

P70.0   **Syndrome of infant of mother with** gestational diabetes

> Newborn (with hypoglycemia) affected by maternal gestational diabetes

> EXCLUDES 1   *newborn (with hypoglycemia) affected by maternal (pre-existing) diabetes mellitus (P70.1)*
> *syndrome of infant of a diabetic mother (P70.1)*

P70.1   **Syndrome of infant of a** diabetic mother

> Newborn (with hypoglycemia) affected by maternal (pre-existing) diabetes mellitus

> EXCLUDES 1   *newborn (with hypoglycemia) affected by maternal gestational diabetes (P70.0)*
> *syndrome of infant of mother with gestational diabetes (P70.0)*

P70.2   **Neonatal** diabetes mellitus   CC

> CC Excl: PDX collection 1041

P70.3   **Iatrogenic** neonatal hypoglycemia

P70.4   **Other neonatal hypoglycemia**

> Transitory neonatal hypoglycemia

P70.8   **Other transitory disorders of carbohydrate metabolism of newborn**   CC

> CC Excl: PDX collection 1042

P70.9   **Transitory disorder of carbohydrate metabolism of newborn, unspecified**

☑4ᵗʰ **P71 Transitory neonatal disorders of** calcium and magnesium **metabolism**

CC Excl: For CC codes in category P71: PDX collection 1041

P71.0   **Cow's milk hypocalcemia** in newborn   CC

P71.1   **Other neonatal hypocalcemia**   CC

> EXCLUDES 1   *neonatal hypoparathyroidism (P71.4)*

P71.2   **Neonatal** hypomagnesemia   CC

P71.3   **Neonatal** tetany without calcium or magnesium deficiency   CC

> Neonatal tetany NOS

P71.4   **Transitory neonatal** hypoparathyroidism   CC

P71.8   **Other transitory neonatal disorders of calcium and magnesium metabolism**   CC

> AHA: 2016,4Q,54

P71.9   **Transitory neonatal disorder of calcium and magnesium metabolism, unspecified**   CC

☑4ᵗʰ **P72 Other transitory neonatal** endocrine disorders

> EXCLUDES 1   *congenital hypothyroidism with or without goiter (E03.0-E03.1)*
> *dyshormogenetic goiter (E07.1)*
> *Pendred's syndrome (E07.1)*

CC Excl: For CC codes in category P72, unless otherwise noted: PDX collection 1042

P72.0   **Neonatal goiter, not elsewhere classified**   CC

> Transitory congenital goiter with normal functioning

P72.1   **Transitory** neonatal hyperthyroidism   CC

> Neonatal thyrotoxicosis
> CC Excl: PDX collection 1041

P72.2   **Other transitory neonatal disorders of thyroid function, not elsewhere classified**   CC

> Transitory neonatal hypothyroidism

P72.8   **Other specified transitory neonatal endocrine disorders**   CC

P72.9   **Transitory neonatal endocrine disorder, unspecified**

☑4ᵗʰ **P74 Other transitory neonatal** electrolyte and metabolic **disturbances**

> AHA: 2018,4Q,26-27

CC Excl: For CC codes in category P74: PDX collection 1042

P74.0   **Late metabolic acidosis of newborn**   MCC

> EXCLUDES 1   *(fetal) metabolic acidosis of newborn (P19)*
> CC Excl: PDX collection 1041

P74.1   **Dehydration of newborn**

☑ Additional Character Required   ☑7ᵗʰ Placeholder   Unacceptable PDx   Questionable PDx   Manifestation   Unspecified Dx   H1–H14 HAC   HCC CMS-HCC Dx   HIV HIV Dx

ICD-10-CM 2020   927

Chapter 16. Certain Conditions Originating in the Perinatal Period *(left margin, vertical)*

P74.2–P83.6 *(left margin, vertical)*

✓5ᵗʰ **P74.2 Disturbances of sodium balance of newborn**

P74.21 Hypernatremia of newborn

P74.22 Hyponatremia of newborn

✓5ᵗʰ **P74.3 Disturbances of potassium balance of newborn**

P74.31 Hyperkalemia of newborn

P74.32 Hypokalemia of newborn

✓5ᵗʰ **P74.4 Other transitory electrolyte disturbances of newborn**

P74.41 Alkalosis of newborn CC

Hyperbicarbonatemia

✓6ᵗʰ **P74.42 Disturbances of chlorine balance of newborn**

P74.421 Hyperchloremia of newborn

Hyperchloremic metabolic acidosis

EXCLUDES 2 *late metabolic acidosis of the newborn ▶(P74.0)◀*

P74.422 Hypochloremia of newborn

P74.49 Other transitory electrolyte disturbance of newborn

P74.5 Transitory tyrosinemia of newborn CC

P74.6 Transitory hyperammonemia of newborn CC

P74.8 Other transitory metabolic disturbances of newborn CC

Amino-acid metabolic disorders described as transitory

P74.9 Transitory metabolic disturbance of newborn, unspecified

Digestive system disorders of newborn (P76-P78)

✓4ᵗʰ **P76 Other intestinal obstruction of newborn**

P76.0 Meconium plug syndrome

Meconium ileus NOS

EXCLUDES 1 *meconium ileus in cystic fibrosis (E84.11)*

DEF: Meconium obstruction of a newborn's intestines, resulting from unusually thick or hard meconium.

P76.1 Transitory ileus of newborn CC

EXCLUDES 1 *Hirschsprung's disease (Q43.1)*

CC Excl: PDX collection 1043

P76.2 Intestinal obstruction due to inspissated milk

P76.8 Other specified intestinal obstruction of newborn

EXCLUDES 1 *intestinal obstruction classifiable to K56.-*

P76.9 Intestinal obstruction of newborn, unspecified

✓4ᵗʰ **P77 Necrotizing enterocolitis of newborn**

DEF: Serious intestinal infection and inflammation in preterm infants. Severity is measured by stages and may progress to life-threatening perforation or peritonitis. Resection surgical treatment may be necessary.

CC Excl: For MCC codes in category P77: PDX collection 1044

P77.1 Stage 1 necrotizing enterocolitis in newborn MCC

Necrotizing enterocolitis without pneumatosis, without perforation

DEF: Broad-spectrum symptoms with nonspecific signs, including feeding intolerance, abdominal distention, bradycardia, and metabolic abnormalities.

P77.2 Stage 2 necrotizing enterocolitis in newborn MCC

Necrotizing enterocolitis with pneumatosis, without perforation

DEF: Radiographic confirmation of necrotizing enterocolitis showing intestinal dilatation, fixed loops of bowels, pneumatosis intestinalis, metabolic acidosis, and thrombocytopenia.

P77.3 Stage 3 necrotizing enterocolitis in newborn MCC

Necrotizing enterocolitis with perforation

Necrotizing enterocolitis with pneumatosis and perforation

DEF: Advanced stage in which an infant demonstrates signs of bowel perforation, septic shock, metabolic acidosis, ascites, disseminated intravascular coagulopathy, and neutropenia.

P77.9 Necrotizing enterocolitis in newborn, unspecified MCC

Necrotizing enterocolitis in newborn, NOS

✓4ᵗʰ **P78 Other perinatal digestive system disorders**

EXCLUDES 1 *cystic fibrosis (E84.0-E84.9)*

neonatal gastrointestinal hemorrhages (P54.0-P54.3)

P78.0 Perinatal intestinal perforation MCC

Meconium peritonitis

CC Excl: PDX collection 1044

P78.1 Other neonatal peritonitis

Neonatal peritonitis NOS

P78.2 Neonatal hematemesis and melena due to swallowed maternal blood

P78.3 Noninfective neonatal diarrhea

Neonatal diarrhea NOS

✓5ᵗʰ **P78.8 Other specified perinatal digestive system disorders**

P78.81 Congenital cirrhosis (of liver)

P78.82 Peptic ulcer of newborn

P78.83 Newborn esophageal reflux

Neonatal esophageal reflux

P78.84 Gestational alloimmune liver disease

GALD

Neonatal hemochromatosis

EXCLUDES 1 *hemochromatosis (E83.11-)*

AHA: 2017,4Q,21

DEF: Severe hepatic injury with onset during fetal development with manifestations beginning during fetal life. It is due to maternal antibodies to fetal hepatic cells (hepatocytes) that cross the placenta into the fetal circulation, causing hepatic cell necrosis.

P78.89 Other specified perinatal digestive system disorders

P78.9 Perinatal digestive system disorder, unspecified

Conditions involving the integument and temperature regulation of newborn (P80-P83)

✓4ᵗʰ **P80 Hypothermia of newborn**

DEF: Decrease in newborn body temperature due to their larger ratio of surface area to body weight, thin skin with blood vessels close to the surface, and a limited amount of subcutaneous fat.

P80.0 Cold injury syndrome

Severe and usually chronic hypothermia associated with a pink flushed appearance, edema and neurological and biochemical abnormalities.

EXCLUDES 1 *mild hypothermia of newborn (P80.8)*

P80.8 Other hypothermia of newborn

Mild hypothermia of newborn

P80.9 Hypothermia of newborn, unspecified

✓4ᵗʰ **P81 Other disturbances of temperature regulation of newborn**

P81.0 Environmental hyperthermia of newborn

P81.8 Other specified disturbances of temperature regulation of newborn

P81.9 Disturbance of temperature regulation of newborn, unspecified

Fever of newborn NOS

✓4ᵗʰ **P83 Other conditions of integument specific to newborn**

EXCLUDES 1 *congenital malformations of skin and integument (Q80-Q84)*

hydrops fetalis due to hemolytic disease (P56.-)

neonatal skin infection (P39.4)

staphylococcal scalded skin syndrome (L00)

EXCLUDES 2 *cradle cap (L21.0)*

diaper [napkin] dermatitis (L22)

P83.0 Sclerema neonatorum CC

DEF: Diffuse, rapidly progressing white, waxy, nonpitting hardening of tissue, usually of legs and feet that is life-threatening. It is found in preterm or debilitated infants. Etiology is unknown.

CC Excl: PDX collection 1045

P83.1 Neonatal erythema toxicum

P83.2 Hydrops fetalis not due to hemolytic disease MCC

Hydrops fetalis NOS

DEF: Severe, life-threatening problem of a newborn characterized by severe edema of the entire body. It is unrelated to immune response.

CC Excl: PDX collection 1046

✓5ᵗʰ **P83.3 Other and unspecified edema specific to newborn**

P83.30 Unspecified edema specific to newborn CC

CC Excl: PDX collection 1047

P83.39 Other edema specific to newborn CC

CC Excl: PDX collection 1047

P83.4 Breast engorgement of newborn

Noninfective mastitis of newborn

P83.5 Congenital hydrocele ♂

DEF: Hydrocele: Serous fluid that collects in the tunica vaginalis of the scrotum along the spermatic cord in males.

P83.6 Umbilical polyp of newborn

N Newborn: 0 P Pediatric: 0-17 M Maternity: 9-64 A Adult: 15-124 MCC Major Complication/Comorbidity CC Complication/Comorbidity SW Severe Wound Dx

928 ICD-10-CM 2020

✓5ᵗʰ **P83.8** **Other specified conditions of integument specific to newborn**
　　　AHA: 2017,4Q,21-22

　　P83.81 **Umbilical granuloma**
　　　　EXCLUDES 2　*granulomatous disorder of the skin and subcutaneous tissue, unspecified (L92.9)*

　　P83.88 **Other specified conditions of integument specific to newborn**
　　　　Bronze baby syndrome
　　　　Neonatal scleroderma
　　　　Urticaria neonatorum

P83.9 **Condition of the integument specific to newborn, unspecified**

Other problems with newborn (P84)

P84 **Other problems with newborn**
　　Acidemia of newborn
　　Acidosis of newborn
　　Anoxia of newborn NOS
　　Asphyxia of newborn NOS
　　Hypercapnia of newborn
　　Hypoxemia of newborn
　　Hypoxia of newborn NOS
　　Mixed metabolic and respiratory acidosis of newborn
　　EXCLUDES 1　*intracranial hemorrhage due to anoxia or hypoxia (P52.-)*
　　　　hypoxic ischemic encephalopathy [HIE] (P91.6-)
　　　　late metabolic acidosis of newborn (P74.0)

Other disorders originating in the perinatal period (P90-P96)

P90 **Convulsions of newborn**　　　　MCC
　　EXCLUDES 1　*benign myoclonic epilepsy in infancy (G40.3-)*
　　　　benign neonatal convulsions (familial) (G40.3-)
　　CC Excl: PDX collection 1048

✓4ᵗʰ **P91** **Other disturbances of cerebral status of newborn**
　　CC Excl: For MCC codes in category P91, unless otherwise noted: PDX collection 1049

　　P91.0 **Neonatal cerebral ischemia**　　MCC

　　P91.1 **Acquired periventricular cysts of newborn**　　MCC

　　P91.2 **Neonatal cerebral leukomalacia**　　MCC
　　　　Periventricular leukomalacia
　　　　CC Excl: PDX collection 1022

　　P91.3 **Neonatal cerebral irritability**　　MCC

　　P91.4 **Neonatal cerebral depression**　　MCC

　　P91.5 **Neonatal coma**　　MCC

✓5ᵗʰ **P91.6** **Hypoxic ischemic encephalopathy [HIE]**
　　　　EXCLUDES 1　*neonatal cerebral depression (P91.4)*
　　　　　neonatal cerebral irritability (P91.3)
　　　　　neonatal coma (P91.5)
　　AHA: 2017,4Q,22
　　CC Excl: For CC/MCC codes in subcategory P91.6: PDX collection 1050

　　　P91.60 **Hypoxic ischemic encephalopathy [HIE], unspecified**　　CC

　　　P91.61 **Mild hypoxic ischemic encephalopathy [HIE]**　　CC

　　　P91.62 **Moderate hypoxic ischemic encephalopathy [HIE]**　　CC

　　　P91.63 **Severe hypoxic ischemic encephalopathy [HIE]**　　MCC

✓5ᵗʰ **P91.8** **Other specified disturbances of cerebral status of newborn**
　　AHA: 2017,4Q,22

　　✓6ᵗʰ **P91.81** **Neonatal encephalopathy**
　　　　P91.811 ***Neonatal encephalopathy in diseases classified elsewhere***
　　　　　Code first underlying condition, if known, such as:
　　　　　congenital cirrhosis (of liver) (P78.81)
　　　　　intracranial nontraumatic hemorrhage of newborn (P52.-)
　　　　　kernicterus (P57.-)
　　　　P91.819 **Neonatal encephalopathy, unspecified**

　　　P91.88 **Other specified disturbances of cerebral status of newborn**

P91.9 **Disturbance of cerebral status of newborn, unspecified**

✓4ᵗʰ **P92** **Feeding problems of newborn**
　　EXCLUDES 1　*eating disorders (F50.-)*
　　　　feeding problems in child over 28 days old (R63.3)
　　AHA: 2016,3Q,19
　　TIP: Continue to assign a code from this category for feeding problems in a patient greater than 28 days old when that feeding problem was initially diagnosed between day 0 and day 28. Do not assign code R63.3.

　　✓5ᵗʰ **P92.0** **Vomiting of newborn**
　　　　EXCLUDES 1　*vomiting of child over 28 days old (R11.-)*

　　　P92.01 **Bilious vomiting of newborn**　　MCC
　　　　　EXCLUDES 1　*bilious vomiting in child over 28 days old (R11.14)*
　　　　　CC Excl: PDX collection 1051

　　　P92.09 **Other vomiting of newborn**
　　　　　EXCLUDES 1　*regurgitation of food in newborn (P92.1)*

　　P92.1 **Regurgitation and rumination of newborn**

　　P92.2 **Slow feeding of newborn**

　　P92.3 **Underfeeding of newborn**

　　P92.4 **Overfeeding of newborn**

　　P92.5 **Neonatal difficulty in feeding at breast**
　　　　AHA: 2017,1Q,28

　　P92.6 **Failure to thrive in newborn**
　　　　EXCLUDES 1　*failure to thrive in child over 28 days old (R62.51)*

　　P92.8 **Other feeding problems of newborn**

　　P92.9 **Feeding problem of newborn, unspecified**

✓4ᵗʰ **P93** **Reactions and intoxications due to drugs administered to newborn**
　　INCLUDES　reactions and intoxications due to drugs administered to fetus affecting newborn
　　EXCLUDES 1　*jaundice due to drugs or toxins transmitted from mother or given to newborn (P58.4-)*
　　　　reactions and intoxications from maternal opiates, tranquilizers and other medication (P04.0-P04.1, P04.4-)
　　　　withdrawal symptoms from maternal use of drugs of addiction (P96.1)
　　　　withdrawal symptoms from therapeutic use of drugs in newborn (P96.2)

　　P93.0 **Grey baby syndrome**　　CC
　　　　Grey syndrome from chloramphenicol administration in newborn
　　　　CC Excl: PDX collection 1052

　　P93.8 **Other reactions and intoxications due to drugs administered to newborn**　　CC
　　　　Use additional code for adverse effect, if applicable, to identify drug (T36-T50 with fifth or sixth character 5)
　　　　CC Excl: PDX collection 1052

✓4ᵗʰ **P94** **Disorders of muscle tone of newborn**

　　P94.0 **Transient neonatal myasthenia gravis**　　CC
　　　　EXCLUDES 1　*myasthenia gravis (G70.0)*
　　　　CC Excl: PDX collection 1041

　　P94.1 **Congenital hypertonia**

　　P94.2 **Congenital hypotonia**
　　　　Floppy baby syndrome, unspecified

　　P94.8 **Other disorders of muscle tone of newborn**

　　P94.9 **Disorder of muscle tone of newborn, unspecified**

P95 **Stillbirth**
　　Deadborn fetus NOS
　　Fetal death of unspecified cause
　　Stillbirth NOS
　　EXCLUDES 1　*maternal care for intrauterine death (O36.4)*
　　　　missed abortion (O02.1)
　　　　outcome of delivery, stillbirth (Z37.1, Z37.3, Z37.4, Z37.7)

✓4ᵗʰ **P96** **Other conditions originating in the perinatal period**

　　P96.0 **Congenital renal failure**
　　　　Uremia of newborn

　　P96.1 **Neonatal withdrawal symptoms from maternal use of drugs of addiction**　　CC
　　　　Drug withdrawal syndrome in infant of dependent mother
　　　　Neonatal abstinence syndrome
　　　　EXCLUDES 1　*reactions and intoxications from maternal opiates and tranquilizers administered during labor and delivery (P04.0)*
　　　　AHA: 2018,4Q,24-25
　　　　CC Excl: PDX collection 1052

✓ Additional Character Required　　✓x7ᵗʰ Placeholder　　Unacceptable PDx　　Questionable PDx　　Manifestation　　Unspecified Dx　　H1-H14 HAC　　HCC CMS-HCC Dx　　HIV HIV Dx

ICD-10-CM 2020　　　　929

Chapter 16. Certain Conditions Originating in the Perinatal Period

  P96.2 **Withdrawal symptoms from therapeutic use**   **CC**
     of drugs in newborn
     CC Excl: PDX collection 1052

  P96.3 **Wide cranial sutures of newborn**
     Neonatal craniotabes

  P96.5 **Complication to newborn due to (fetal) intrauterine**
     procedure
     EXCLUDES 2   *newborn affected by amniocentesis (P00.6)*

✓5ᵗʰ **P96.8** **Other specified conditions originating in the perinatal period**

     P96.81 **Exposure to (parental) (environmental) tobacco**
         smoke in the perinatal period
         EXCLUDES 2   *newborn affected by in utero exposure to*
                tobacco (P04.2)
                exposure to environmental tobacco smoke
                    after the perinatal period (Z77.22)

     P96.82 **Delayed separation of umbilical cord**

     P96.83 **Meconium staining**
         EXCLUDES 1   *meconium aspiration (P24.00, P24.01)*
                  meconium passage during delivery
                    (P03.82)

         DEF: Meconium passed in utero causing discoloration
         on the fetal skin and nails or on the umbilicus. This
         staining may be incidental or may be an indicator of
         significant fetal stress that could affect outcomes.

     P96.89 **Other specified conditions originating in the**
         perinatal period
         Use additional code to specify condition

  P96.9 **Condition originating in the perinatal period, unspecified**
     Congenital debility NOS

N Newborn: 0   **P** Pediatric: 0-17   **M** Maternity: 9-64   **A** Adult: 15-124   **MCC** Major Complication/Comorbidity   **CC** Complication/Comorbidity   **SW** Severe Wound Dx

930   **ICD-10-CM 2020**

Chapter 17. Congenital Malformations, Deformations and Chromosomal Abnormalities (Q00–Q99)

Chapter-specific Guidelines with Coding Examples

The chapter-specific guidelines from the ICD-10-CM Official Guidelines for Coding and Reporting have been provided below. Along with these guidelines are coding examples, contained in the shaded boxes, that have been developed to help illustrate the coding and/or sequencing guidance found in these guidelines.

Assign an appropriate code(s) from categories Q00-Q99, Congenital malformations, deformations, and chromosomal abnormalities when a malformation/deformation or chromosomal abnormality is documented. A malformation/deformation/or chromosomal abnormality may be the principal/first-listed diagnosis on a record or a secondary diagnosis.

When a malformation/deformation/or chromosomal abnormality does not have a unique code assignment, assign additional code(s) for any manifestations that may be present.

When the code assignment specifically identifies the malformation/deformation/or chromosomal abnormality, manifestations that are an inherent component of the anomaly should not be coded separately. Additional codes should be assigned for manifestations that are not an inherent component.

8-day-old infant with tetralogy of Fallot and pulmonary stenosis
Q21.3   **Tetralogy of Fallot**
Explanation: Pulmonary stenosis is inherent in the disease process of tetralogy of Fallot. When the code assignment specifically identifies the malformation/deformation/or chromosomal abnormality, manifestations that are inherent components of the anomaly should not be coded separately.

7-month-old infant with Down syndrome and common atrioventricular canal
Q90.9   **Down syndrome, unspecified**
Q21.2   **Atrioventricular septal defect**
Explanation: While a common atrioventricular canal is often associated with patients with Down syndrome, this manifestation is not an inherent component and may be reported separately. When the code assignment specifically identifies the anomaly, manifestations that are inherent components of the condition should not be coded separately. Additional codes should be assigned for manifestations that are not inherent components.

Codes from Chapter 17 may be used throughout the life of the patient. If a congenital malformation or deformity has been corrected, a personal history code should be used to identify the history of the malformation or deformity. Although present at birth, **a** malformation/deformation/or chromosomal abnormality may not be identified until later in life. Whenever the condition is diagnosed by the **provider**, it is appropriate to assign a code from codes Q00-Q99. For the birth admission, the appropriate code from category Z38, Liveborn infants, according to place of birth and type of delivery, should be sequenced as the principal diagnosis, followed by any congenital anomaly codes, Q00- Q99.

Three-year-old with history of corrected ventricular septal defect
Z87.74   **Personal history of (corrected) congenital malformations of heart and circulatory system**
Explanation: If a congenital malformation or deformity has been corrected, a personal history code should be used to identify the history of the malformation or deformity.

Forty-year-old man with headaches diagnosed with congenital arteriovenous malformation of cerebral vessels by brain scan
Q28.2   **Arteriovenous malformation of cerebral vessels**
Explanation: Although present at birth, malformations may not be identified until later in life. Whenever a congenital condition is diagnosed by the physician, it is appropriate to assign a code from the range Q00–Q99.

Newborn with anencephaly delivered vaginally in hospital
Z38.00   **Single liveborn infant, delivered vaginally**
Q00.0   **Anencephaly**
Explanation: For the birth admission, the appropriate code from category Z38 Liveborn infants, according to place of birth and type of delivery, should be sequenced as the principal diagnosis, followed by any congenital anomaly codes, Q00–Q99.

Chapter 17. Congenital Malformations, Deformations and Chromosomal Abnormalities (Q00-Q99)

NOTE Codes from this chapter are not for use on maternal records

EXCLUDES 2 inborn errors of metabolism (E70-E88)

This chapter contains the following blocks:

Q00-Q07 Congenital malformations of the nervous system
Q10-Q18 Congenital malformations of eye, ear, face and neck
Q20-Q28 Congenital malformations of the circulatory system
Q30-Q34 Congenital malformations of the respiratory system
Q35-Q37 Cleft lip and cleft palate
Q38-Q45 Other congenital malformations of the digestive system
Q50-Q56 Congenital malformations of genital organs
Q60-Q64 Congenital malformations of the urinary system
Q65-Q79 Congenital malformations and deformations of the musculoskeletal system
Q80-Q89 Other congenital malformations
Q90-Q99 Chromosomal abnormalities, not elsewhere classified

Congenital malformations of the nervous system (Q00-Q07)

✓4th Q00 Anencephaly and similar malformations

> **CC Excl:** For MCC codes in category Q00, unless otherwise noted: PDX collection 1053

> **Q00.0 Anencephaly**   `MCC` `HCC`
>> Acephaly
>> Acrania
>> Amyelencephaly
>> Hemianencephaly
>> Hemicephaly

> **Q00.1 Craniorachischisis**   `MCC` `HCC`

> **Q00.2 Iniencephaly**   `MCC` `HCC`

✓4th Q01 Encephalocele

> **INCLUDES** Arnold-Chiari syndrome, type III
>> encephalocystocele
>> encephalomyelocele
>> hydroencephalocele
>> hydromeningocele, cranial
>> meningocele, cerebral
>> meningoencephalocele

> **EXCLUDES 1** Meckel-Gruber syndrome (Q61.9)

> **DEF:** Congenital protrusion of brain tissue through a defect in the skull.

> **CC Excl:** For CC codes in category Q01: PDX collection 1054

> **Q01.0 Frontal encephalocele**   `CC` `HCC`

> **Q01.1 Nasofrontal encephalocele**   `CC` `HCC`

> **Q01.2 Occipital encephalocele**   `CC` `HCC`

> **Q01.8 Encephalocele of other sites**   `CC` `HCC`

> **Q01.9 Encephalocele, unspecified**   `CC` `HCC`

Q02 Microcephaly   `HCC`

> **INCLUDES** hydromicrocephaly
>> micrencephalon

> ▶Code first, if applicable, congenital Zika virus disease◀

> ~~Use additional code, if applicable, to identify congenital Zika virus disease~~

> **EXCLUDES 1** Meckel-Gruber syndrome (Q61.9)

> **AHA:** 2018,4Q,26

> **DEF:** Congenital disorder in which the head circumference is more than two standard deviations below the mean for age, sex, race, and gestation and associated with a decreased life expectancy.

✓4th Q03 Congenital hydrocephalus

> **INCLUDES** hydrocephalus in newborn

> **EXCLUDES 1** Arnold-Chiari syndrome, type II (Q07.0-)
>> acquired hydrocephalus (G91.-)
>> hydrocephalus due to congenital toxoplasmosis (P37.1)
>> hydrocephalus with spina bifida (Q05.0-Q05.4)

> **DEF:** Hydrocephalus: Abnormal buildup of cerebrospinal fluid in the brain causing dilation of the ventricles.

Congenital Hydrocephalus

Pressure

Normal ventricles   Hydrocephalic ventricles

> **Q03.0 Malformations of aqueduct of Sylvius**   `HCC`
>> Anomaly of aqueduct of Sylvius
>> Obstruction of aqueduct of Sylvius, congenital
>> Stenosis of aqueduct of Sylvius

> **Q03.1 Atresia of foramina of Magendie and Luschka**   `HCC`
>> Dandy-Walker syndrome

> **Q03.8 Other congenital hydrocephalus**   `HCC`

> **Q03.9 Congenital hydrocephalus, unspecified**   `HCC`

✓4th Q04 Other congenital malformations of brain

> **EXCLUDES 1** cyclopia (Q87.0)
>> macrocephaly (Q75.3)

> **CC Excl:** For codes in category Q04:
> **For MCC codes:** PDX collection 1054
> **For CC codes:** PDX collection 1055

> **Q04.0 Congenital malformations of corpus callosum**   `MCC` `HCC`
>> Agenesis of corpus callosum

> **Q04.1 Arhinencephaly**   `MCC` `HCC`

> **Q04.2 Holoprosencephaly**   `MCC` `HCC`

> **Q04.3 Other reduction deformities of brain**   `MCC` `HCC`
>> Absence of part of brain
>> Agenesis of part of brain
>> Agyria
>> Aplasia of part of brain
>> Hydranencephaly
>> Hypoplasia of part of brain
>> Lissencephaly
>> Microgyria
>> Pachygyria
>> **EXCLUDES 1** congenital malformations of corpus callosum (Q04.0)

> **Q04.4 Septo-optic dysplasia of brain**   `CC` `HCC`

> **Q04.5 Megalencephaly**   `CC` `HCC`

> **Q04.6 Congenital cerebral cysts**   `CC` `HCC`
>> Porencephaly
>> Schizencephaly
>> **EXCLUDES 1** acquired porencephalic cyst (G93.0)

> **Q04.8 Other specified congenital malformations of brain**   `CC` `HCC`
>> Arnold-Chiari syndrome, type IV
>> Macrogyria

> **Q04.9 Congenital malformation of brain, unspecified**   `HCC`
>> Congenital anomaly NOS of brain
>> Congenital deformity NOS of brain
>> Congenital disease or lesion NOS of brain
>> Multiple anomalies NOS of brain, congenital

✓4ᵗʰ Q05 Spina bifida

INCLUDES
hydromeningocele (spinal)
meningocele (spinal)
meningomyelocele
myelocele
myelomeningocele
rachischisis
spina bifida (aperta)(cystica)
syringomyelocele

Use additional code for any associated paraplegia (paraparesis) (G82.2-)

EXCLUDES 1   *Arnold-Chiari syndrome, type II (Q07.0-)*
spina bifida occulta (Q76.0)

DEF: Lack of closure in the vertebral column with protrusion of the spinal cord through the defect, often in the lumbosacral area. This condition can be recognized by the presence of alpha-fetoproteins in the amniotic fluid.

CC Excl: For CC codes in category Q05: PDX collection 1056

Spina Bifida

Spina bifida occulta   Meningocele   Myelomeningocele

Q05.0	**Cervical spina bifida with hydrocephalus**	CC HCC
Q05.1	**Thoracic spina bifida with hydrocephalus**	CC HCC
	Dorsal spina bifida with hydrocephalus	
	Thoracolumbar spina bifida with hydrocephalus	
Q05.2	**Lumbar spina bifida with hydrocephalus**	CC HCC
	Lumbosacral spina bifida with hydrocephalus	
Q05.3	**Sacral spina bifida with hydrocephalus**	CC HCC
Q05.4	**Unspecified spina bifida with hydrocephalus**	CC HCC
Q05.5	**Cervical spina bifida without hydrocephalus**	HCC
Q05.6	**Thoracic spina bifida without hydrocephalus**	HCC
	Dorsal spina bifida NOS	
	Thoracolumbar spina bifida NOS	
Q05.7	**Lumbar spina bifida without hydrocephalus**	HCC
	Lumbosacral spina bifida NOS	
Q05.8	**Sacral spina bifida without hydrocephalus**	HCC
Q05.9	**Spina bifida, unspecified**	HCC

✓4ᵗʰ Q06 Other congenital malformations of spinal cord

Q06.0	**Amyelia**	HCC
Q06.1	**Hypoplasia and dysplasia of spinal cord**	HCC
	Atelomyelia	
	Myelatelia	
	Myelodysplasia of spinal cord	
Q06.2	**Diastematomyelia**	HCC

DEF: Rare congenital anomaly often associated with spina bifida. The spinal cord is separated into longitudinal halves by a bony, cartilaginous or fibrous septum, each half surrounded by a dural sac.

Q06.3	**Other congenital cauda equina malformations**	HCC
Q06.4	**Hydromyelia**	HCC
	Hydrorachis	
Q06.8	**Other specified congenital malformations of spinal cord**	HCC
Q06.9	**Congenital malformation of spinal cord, unspecified**	HCC

Congenital anomaly NOS of spinal cord
Congenital deformity NOS of spinal cord
Congenital disease or lesion NOS of spinal cord

✓4ᵗʰ Q07 Other congenital malformations of nervous system

EXCLUDES 2   *congenital central alveolar hypoventilation syndrome (G47.35)*
familial dysautonomia [Riley-Day] (G90.1)
neurofibromatosis (nonmalignant) (Q85.0-)

CC Excl: For CC codes in category Q07: PDX collection 1056

✓5ᵗʰ Q07.0 Arnold-Chiari syndrome

Arnold-Chiari syndrome, type II

EXCLUDES 1   *Arnold-Chiari syndrome, type III (Q01.-)*
Arnold-Chiari syndrome, type IV (Q04.8)

DEF: Congenital malformation of the brain in which the cerebellum protrudes through the foramen magnum into the spinal canal.

Q07.00	**Arnold-Chiari syndrome without spina bifida or hydrocephalus**	HCC
Q07.01	**Arnold-Chiari syndrome with spina bifida**	HCC
Q07.02	**Arnold-Chiari syndrome with hydrocephalus**	CC HCC
Q07.03	**Arnold-Chiari syndrome with spina bifida and hydrocephalus**	CC HCC
Q07.8	**Other specified congenital malformations of nervous system**	HCC
	Agenesis of nerve	
	Displacement of brachial plexus	
	Jaw-winking syndrome	
	Marcus Gunn's syndrome	
Q07.9	**Congenital malformation of nervous system, unspecified**	HCC

Congenital anomaly NOS of nervous system
Congenital deformity NOS of nervous system
Congenital disease or lesion NOS of nervous system

Congenital malformations of eye, ear, face and neck (Q10-Q18)

EXCLUDES 2   *cleft lip and cleft palate (Q35-Q37)*
congenital malformation of cervical spine (Q05.0, Q05.5, Q67.5, Q76.0-Q76.4)
congenital malformation of larynx (Q31.-)
congenital malformation of lip NEC (Q38.0)
congenital malformation of nose (Q30.-)
congenital malformation of parathyroid gland (Q89.2)
congenital malformation of thyroid gland (Q89.2)

✓4ᵗʰ Q10 Congenital malformations of eyelid, lacrimal apparatus and orbit

EXCLUDES 1   *cryptophthalmos NOS (Q11.2)*
cryptophthalmos syndrome (Q87.0)

Q10.0 Congenital ptosis
DEF: Congenital drooping of the eyelid. Ptosis is mostly idiopathic, but may occur genetically.

Q10.1 Congenital ectropion

Q10.2 Congenital entropion

Q10.3 Other congenital malformations of eyelid
Ablepharon
Blepharophimosis, congenital
Coloboma of eyelid
Congenital absence or agenesis of cilia
Congenital absence or agenesis of eyelid
Congenital accessory eyelid
Congenital accessory eye muscle
Congenital malformation of eyelid NOS

Q10.4 Absence and agenesis of lacrimal apparatus
Congenital absence of punctum lacrimale

Q10.5 Congenital stenosis and stricture of lacrimal duct

Q10.6 Other congenital malformations of lacrimal apparatus
Congenital malformation of lacrimal apparatus NOS

Q10.7 Congenital malformation of orbit

✓4ᵗʰ Q11 Anophthalmos, microphthalmos and macrophthalmos

Q11.0 Cystic eyeball

Q11.1 Other anophthalmos
Anophthalmos NOS
Agenesis of eye
Aplasia of eye

✓ Additional Character Required   ✓x7ᵗʰ Placeholder   Unacceptable PDx   Questionable PDx   Manifestation   Unspecified Dx   H1-H14 HAC   HCC CMS-HCC Dx   HIV HIV Dx

ICD-10-CM 2020   933

Chapter 17. Congenital Malformations, Deformations and Chromosomal Abnormalities

Q11.2 Microphthalmos
Cryptophthalmos NOS
Dysplasia of eye
Hypoplasia of eye
Rudimentary eye
EXCLUDES 1   *cryptophthalmos syndrome (Q87.0)*

Q11.3 Macrophthalmos
EXCLUDES 1   *macrophthalmos in congenital glaucoma (Q15.0)*

✓4ᵗʰ Q12 Congenital lens malformations

Q12.0 Congenital cataract

Q12.1 Congenital displaced lens

Q12.2 Coloboma of lens

Coloboma of Lens

Coloboma

Q12.3 Congenital aphakia

Q12.4 Spherophakia

Q12.8 Other congenital lens malformations
Microphakia

Q12.9 Congenital lens malformation, unspecified

✓4ᵗʰ Q13 Congenital malformations of anterior segment of eye

Q13.0 Coloboma of iris
Coloboma NOS
DEF: Defective or absent section of ocular tissue that may present as mild cupping or a small pit in the ocular disc due to extensive defects in the iris, ciliary body, choroids, and retina.

Q13.1 Absence of iris
Aniridia
Use additional code for associated glaucoma (H42)
DEF: Incompletely formed or absent iris. It affects both eyes and is a dominant trait.

Q13.2 Other congenital malformations of iris
Anisocoria, congenital
Atresia of pupil
Congenital malformation of iris NOS
Corectopia

Q13.3 Congenital corneal opacity

Q13.4 Other congenital corneal malformations
Congenital malformation of cornea NOS
Microcornea
Peter's anomaly

Q13.5 Blue sclera

✓5ᵗʰ Q13.8 Other congenital malformations of anterior segment of eye

Q13.81 Rieger's anomaly
Use additional code for associated glaucoma (H42)

Q13.89 Other congenital malformations of anterior segment of eye

Q13.9 Congenital malformation of anterior segment of eye, unspecified

✓4ᵗʰ Q14 Congenital malformations of posterior segment of eye
EXCLUDES 2   *optic nerve hypoplasia (H47.03-)*

Q14.0 Congenital malformation of vitreous humor
Congenital vitreous opacity

Q14.1 Congenital malformation of retina
Congenital retinal aneurysm

Q14.2 Congenital malformation of optic disc
Coloboma of optic disc

Q14.3 Congenital malformation of choroid

Q14.8 Other congenital malformations of posterior segment of eye
Coloboma of the fundus

Q14.9 Congenital malformation of posterior segment of eye, unspecified

✓4ᵗʰ Q15 Other congenital malformations of eye
EXCLUDES 1   *congenital nystagmus (H55.01)*
ocular albinism (E70.31-)
optic nerve hypoplasia (H47.03-)
retinitis pigmentosa (H35.52)

Q15.0 Congenital glaucoma
Axenfeld's anomaly
Buphthalmos
Glaucoma of childhood
Glaucoma of newborn
Hydrophthalmos
Keratoglobus, congenital, with glaucoma
Macrocornea with glaucoma
Macrophthalmos in congenital glaucoma
Megalocornea with glaucoma

Q15.8 Other specified congenital malformations of eye

Q15.9 Congenital malformation of eye, unspecified
Congenital anomaly of eye
Congenital deformity of eye

✓4ᵗʰ Q16 Congenital malformations of ear causing impairment of hearing
EXCLUDES 1   *congenital deafness (H90.-)*

Q16.0 Congenital absence of (ear) auricle

Q16.1 Congenital absence, atresia and stricture of auditory canal (external)
Congenital atresia or stricture of osseous meatus

Q16.2 Absence of eustachian tube

Q16.3 Congenital malformation of ear ossicles
Congenital fusion of ear ossicles

Q16.4 Other congenital malformations of middle ear
Congenital malformation of middle ear NOS

Q16.5 Congenital malformation of inner ear
Congenital anomaly of membranous labyrinth
Congenital anomaly of organ of Corti

Q16.9 Congenital malformation of ear causing impairment of hearing, unspecified
Congenital absence of ear NOS

✓4ᵗʰ Q17 Other congenital malformations of ear
EXCLUDES 1   *congenital malformations of ear with impairment of hearing (Q16.0-Q16.9)*
preauricular sinus (Q18.1)

Q17.0 Accessory auricle
Accessory tragus
Polyotia
Preauricular appendage or tag
Supernumerary ear
Supernumerary lobule

Q17.1 Macrotia
DEF: Birth defect characterized by abnormal enlargement of the pinna of the ear.

Q17.2 Microtia

Q17.3 Other misshapen ear
Pointed ear

Q17.4 Misplaced ear
Low-set ears
EXCLUDES 1   *cervical auricle (Q18.2)*

Q17.5 Prominent ear
Bat ear

Q17.8 Other specified congenital malformations of ear
Congenital absence of lobe of ear

Q17.9 Congenital malformation of ear, unspecified
Congenital anomaly of ear NOS

✓4ᵗʰ Q18 Other congenital malformations of face and neck
EXCLUDES 1   *cleft lip and cleft palate (Q35-Q37)*
conditions classified to Q67.0-Q67.4
congenital malformations of skull and face bones (Q75.-)
cyclopia (Q87.0)
dentofacial anomalies [including malocclusion] (M26.-)
malformation syndromes affecting facial appearance (Q87.0)
persistent thyroglossal duct (Q89.2)

Q18.0 Sinus, fistula and cyst of branchial cleft
Branchial vestige

Q18.1 Preauricular sinus and cyst   SW
Fistula of auricle, congenital
Cervicoaural fistula

Q18.2 Other branchial cleft malformations
Branchial cleft malformation NOS
Cervical auricle
Otocephaly

Q18.3 Webbing of neck
Pterygium colli
DEF: Congenital malformation characterized by a thick, triangular skinfold that stretches from the lateral side of the neck across the shoulder. It is associated with genetic conditions such as Turner's and Noonan's syndromes.

Q18.4 Macrostomia
DEF: Rare congenital craniofacial bilateral or unilateral anomaly of the mouth due to malformed maxillary and mandibular processes. It results in an abnormally large mouth extending toward the ear.

Q18.5 Microstomia

Q18.6 Macrocheilia
Hypertrophy of lip, congenital

Q18.7 Microcheilia

Q18.8 Other specified congenital malformations of face and neck
Medial cyst of face and neck
Medial fistula of face and neck
Medial sinus of face and neck

Q18.9 Congenital malformation of face and neck, unspecified
Congenital anomaly NOS of face and neck

Congenital malformations of the circulatory system (Q20-Q28)

☑4ᵗʰ Q20 Congenital malformations of cardiac chambers and connections
    EXCLUDES 1   *dextrocardia with situs inversus (Q89.3)*
                     mirror-image atrial arrangement with situs inversus (Q89.3)
    CC Excl: For CC/MCC codes in category Q20: PDX collection 1057

Q20.0 Common arterial trunk   `MCC`
Persistent truncus arteriosus
    EXCLUDES 1   *aortic septal defect (Q21.4)*

Q20.1 Double outlet right ventricle   `MCC`
Taussig-Bing syndrome

Q20.2 Double outlet left ventricle   `MCC`

Q20.3 Discordant ventriculoarterial connection   `MCC`
Dextrotransposition of aorta
Transposition of great vessels (complete)

Q20.4 Double inlet ventricle   `MCC`
Common ventricle
Cor triloculare biatriatum
Single ventricle

Q20.5 Discordant atrioventricular connection   `CC`
Corrected transposition
Levotransposition
Ventricular inversion

Q20.6 Isomerism of atrial appendages
Isomerism of atrial appendages with asplenia or polysplenia

Q20.8 Other congenital malformations of cardiac chambers and connections
Cor binoculare

Q20.9 Congenital malformation of cardiac chambers and connections, unspecified

☑4ᵗʰ Q21 Congenital malformations of cardiac septa
    EXCLUDES 1   *acquired cardiac septal defect (I51.0)*

Q21.0 Ventricular septal defect
Roger's disease

Ventricular Septal Defect

Q21.1 Atrial septal defect
Coronary sinus defect
Patent or persistent foramen ovale
Patent or persistent ostium secundum defect (type II)
Patent or persistent sinus venosus defect

Atrial Septal Defect

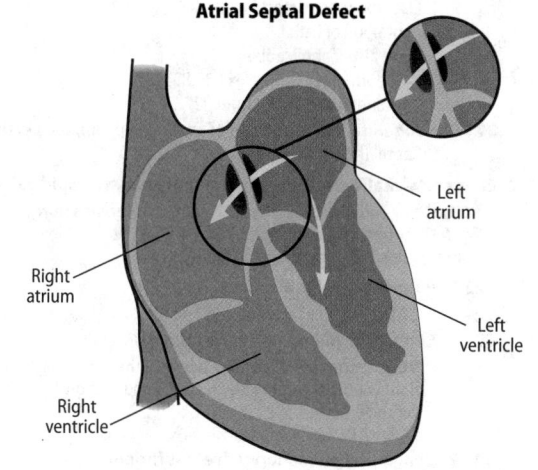

Left atrium
Right atrium
Left ventricle
Right ventricle

Q21.2 Atrioventricular septal defect
Common atrioventricular canal
Endocardial cushion defect
Ostium primum atrial septal defect (type I)

Atrioventricular Septal Defect

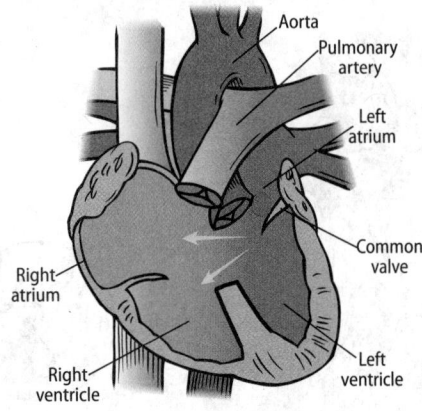

Aorta
Pulmonary artery
Left atrium
Right atrium
Common valve
Right ventricle
Left ventricle

Q21.3 Tetralogy of Fallot `MCC`
Ventricular septal defect with pulmonary stenosis or atresia, dextroposition of aorta and hypertrophy of right ventricle.
AHA: 2014,3Q,16
CC Excl: PDX collection 1057

Q21.4 Aortopulmonary septal defect
Aortic septal defect
Aortopulmonary window

Q21.8 Other congenital malformations of cardiac septa
Eisenmenger's defect
Pentalogy of Fallot
Code also if applicable:
  Eisenmenger's complex (I27.83)
  Eisenmenger's syndrome (I27.83)

Q21.9 Congenital malformation of cardiac septum, unspecified
Septal (heart) defect NOS

✓4ᵗʰ Q22 Congenital malformations of pulmonary and tricuspid valves
CC Excl: For codes in category Q22, unless otherwise noted:
For MCC codes: PDX collection 1061
For CC codes: PDX collection 1060

Q22.0 Pulmonary valve atresia `MCC`
CC Excl: PDX collection 1059

Q22.1 Congenital pulmonary valve stenosis `CC`
DEF: Stenosis of the opening between the pulmonary artery and right ventricle, causing obstructed blood outflow from the right ventricle.
CC Excl: PDX collection 1059

Q22.2 Congenital pulmonary valve insufficiency `CC`
Congenital pulmonary valve regurgitation

Q22.3 Other congenital malformations of pulmonary valve `CC`
Congenital malformation of pulmonary valve NOS
Supernumerary cusps of pulmonary valve

Q22.4 Congenital tricuspid stenosis `MCC`
Congenital tricuspid atresia

Q22.5 Ebstein's anomaly `MCC`
DEF: Malformation of the tricuspid valve characterized by septal and posterior leaflets attaching to the wall of the right ventricle. Ebstein's anomaly causes the right ventricle to fuse with the atrium into a large right atrium and a small ventricle and leads to heart failure and abnormal cardiac rhythm.

Q22.6 Hypoplastic right heart syndrome `MCC`

Q22.8 Other congenital malformations of tricuspid valve `MCC`

Q22.9 Congenital malformation of tricuspid valve, unspecified `MCC`

✓4ᵗʰ Q23 Congenital malformations of aortic and mitral valves

Q23.0 Congenital stenosis of aortic valve
Congenital aortic atresia
Congenital aortic stenosis NOS
EXCLUDES 1 congenital stenosis of aortic valve in hypoplastic left heart syndrome (Q23.4)
congenital subaortic stenosis (Q24.4)
supravalvular aortic stenosis (congenital) (Q25.3)

Q23.1 Congenital insufficiency of aortic valve
Bicuspid aortic valve
Congenital aortic insufficiency

Q23.2 Congenital mitral stenosis
Congenital mitral atresia
DEF: Congenital stenosis of the mitral valve orifice between the left atrium and ventricle, at the supravalvular, valvular, or subvalvular levels, causing obstruction to left ventricular filling.

Q23.3 Congenital mitral insufficiency

Q23.4 Hypoplastic left heart syndrome `MCC`
CC Excl: PDX collection 1061

Q23.8 Other congenital malformations of aortic and mitral valves

Q23.9 Congenital malformation of aortic and mitral valves, unspecified

✓4ᵗʰ Q24 Other congenital malformations of heart
EXCLUDES 1 endocardial fibroelastosis (I42.4)

Q24.0 Dextrocardia `CC`
EXCLUDES 1 dextrocardia with situs inversus (Q89.3)
isomerism of atrial appendages (with asplenia or polysplenia) (Q20.6)
mirror-image atrial arrangement with situs inversus (Q89.3)
DEF: Congenital condition in which the heart is located on the right side of the chest rather than in its normal position on the left.
CC Excl: PDX collection 1062

Q24.1 Levocardia `CC`
CC Excl: PDX collection 1062

Q24.2 Cor triatriatum `MCC`
CC Excl: PDX collection 1063

Q24.3 Pulmonary infundibular stenosis `CC`
Subvalvular pulmonic stenosis
CC Excl: PDX collection 1063

Q24.4 Congenital subaortic stenosis `MCC`
DEF: Congenital heart defect characterized by stenosis of the left ventricular outflow tract due to a fibrous tissue ring or septal hypertrophy below the aortic valve.
CC Excl: PDX collection 1063

Q24.5 Malformation of coronary vessels
Congenital coronary (artery) aneurysm

Q24.6 Congenital heart block `MCC`
CC Excl: PDX collection 1065

Q24.8 Other specified congenital malformations of heart
Congenital diverticulum of left ventricle
Congenital malformation of myocardium
Congenital malformation of pericardium
Malposition of heart
Uhl's disease

Q24.9 Congenital malformation of heart, unspecified
Congenital anomaly of heart
Congenital disease of heart

☑️4ᵗʰ **Q25 Congenital malformations of great arteries**

Q25.0 Patent ductus arteriosus `CC`

Patent ductus Botallo
Persistent ductus arteriosus
DEF: Condition in which the normal channel between the pulmonary artery and the aorta fails to close at birth, causing arterial blood to recirculate in the lungs and inhibiting the blood supply to the aorta. *Synonym(s): PDA.*
CC Excl: PDX collection 1066

Patent Ductus Arteriosus

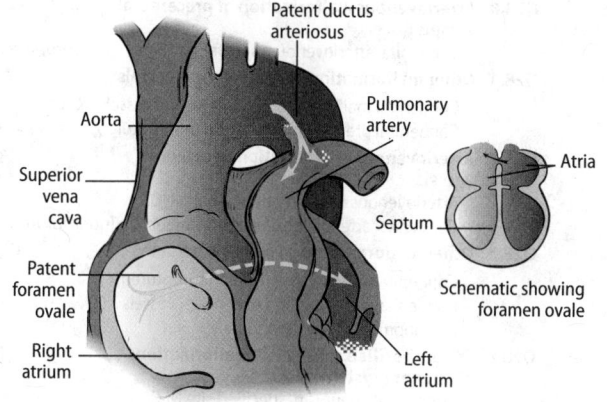

Q25.1 Coarctation of aorta `CC`

Coarctation of aorta (preductal) (postductal)
Stenosis of aorta
AHA: 2016,4Q,56-57
CC Excl: PDX collection 1067

☑️5ᵗʰ **Q25.2 Atresia of aorta**

AHA: 2016,4Q,56-57

Q25.21 Interruption of aortic arch `CC`

Atresia of aortic arch
CC Excl: PDX collection 1068

Q25.29 Other atresia of aorta `CC`

Atresia of aorta
CC Excl: PDX collection 1068

Q25.3 Supravalvular aortic stenosis `CC`

EXCLUDES 1   congenital aortic stenosis NOS (Q23.0)
congenital stenosis of aortic valve (Q23.0)
CC Excl: PDX collection 1068

☑️5ᵗʰ **Q25.4 Other congenital malformations of aorta**

EXCLUDES 1   hypoplasia of aorta in hypoplastic left heart syndrome (Q23.4)
AHA: 2016,4Q,57
CC Excl: For CC codes in subcategory Q25.4: PDX collection 1069

Q25.40 Congenital malformation of aorta unspecified `CC`

Q25.41 Absence and aplasia of aorta `CC`

Q25.42 Hypoplasia of aorta `CC`

Q25.43 Congenital aneurysm of aorta `CC`

Congenital aneurysm of aortic root
Congenital aneurysm of aortic sinus

Q25.44 Congenital dilation of aorta `CC`

Q25.45 Double aortic arch `CC`

Vascular ring of aorta

Aortic Arch Anomalies

Aortic arch — Esophagus — Trachea

Normal aortic arch

Double aortic arch   Right aortic arch

Q25.46 Tortuous aortic arch `CC`

Persistent convolutions of aortic arch

Q25.47 Right aortic arch `CC`

Persistent right aortic arch

Q25.48 Anomalous origin of subclavian artery `CC`

Q25.49 Other congenital malformations of aorta `CC`

Aortic arch
Bovine arch

Q25.5 Atresia of pulmonary artery `MCC`

CC Excl: PDX collection 1070

Q25.6 Stenosis of pulmonary artery `MCC`

Supravalvular pulmonary stenosis
CC Excl: PDX collection 1070

☑️5ᵗʰ **Q25.7 Other congenital malformations of pulmonary artery**

CC Excl: For MCC codes in subcategory Q25.7: PDX collection 1070

Q25.71 Coarctation of pulmonary artery `MCC`

Q25.72 Congenital pulmonary arteriovenous malformation `MCC`

Congenital pulmonary arteriovenous aneurysm

Q25.79 Other congenital malformations of pulmonary artery `MCC`

Aberrant pulmonary artery
Agenesis of pulmonary artery
Congenital aneurysm of pulmonary artery
Congenital anomaly of pulmonary artery
Hypoplasia of pulmonary artery

Q25.8 Other congenital malformations of other great arteries `CC`

CC Excl: PDX collection 1069

Q25.9 Congenital malformation of great arteries, unspecified `CC`

CC Excl: PDX collection 1069

☑️4ᵗʰ **Q26 Congenital malformations of great veins**

Q26.0 Congenital stenosis of vena cava `CC`

Congenital stenosis of vena cava (inferior)(superior)
CC Excl: PDX collection 1071

Q26.1 Persistent left superior vena cava `CC`

CC Excl: PDX collection 1071

Q26.2   Total anomalous pulmonary venous connection   `CC`
Total anomalous pulmonary venous return [TAPVR], subdiaphragmatic
Total anomalous pulmonary venous return [TAPVR], supradiaphragmatic
CC Excl: PDX collection 1072

Q26.3   Partial anomalous pulmonary venous connection   `CC`
Partial anomalous pulmonary venous return
CC Excl: PDX collection 1073

Q26.4   Anomalous pulmonary venous connection, unspecified   `CC`
CC Excl: PDX collection 1073

Q26.5   Anomalous portal venous connection

Q26.6   Portal vein-hepatic artery fistula

Q26.8   Other congenital malformations of great veins   `CC`
Absence of vena cava (inferior) (superior)
Azygos continuation of inferior vena cava
Persistent left posterior cardinal vein
Scimitar syndrome
CC Excl: PDX collection 1071

Q26.9   Congenital malformation of great vein, unspecified   `CC`
Congenital anomaly of vena cava (inferior) (superior) NOS
CC Excl: PDX collection 1074

✓4ᵗʰ **Q27   Other congenital malformations of peripheral vascular system**
EXCLUDES 2   *anomalies of cerebral and precerebral vessels (Q28.0-Q28.3)*
anomalies of coronary vessels (Q24.5)
anomalies of pulmonary artery (Q25.5-Q25.7)
congenital retinal aneurysm (Q14.1)
hemangioma and lymphangioma (D18.-)

Q27.0   Congenital absence and hypoplasia of umbilical artery
Single umbilical artery

Q27.1   Congenital renal artery stenosis

Q27.2   Other congenital malformations of renal artery
Congenital malformation of renal artery NOS
Multiple renal arteries

✓5ᵗʰ **Q27.3   Arteriovenous malformation (peripheral)**
Arteriovenous aneurysm
EXCLUDES 1   *acquired arteriovenous aneurysm (I77.0)*
EXCLUDES 2   *arteriovenous malformation of cerebral vessels (Q28.2)*
arteriovenous malformation of precerebral vessels (Q28.0)
DEF: Arteriovenous malformation: Connecting passage between an artery and a vein.

     Q27.30   Arteriovenous malformation, site unspecified   `CC`
       CC Excl: PDX collection 1075

     Q27.31   Arteriovenous malformation of vessel of upper limb

     Q27.32   Arteriovenous malformation of vessel of lower limb

     Q27.33   Arteriovenous malformation of digestive system vessel
       AHA: 2018,3Q,21

     Q27.34   Arteriovenous malformation of renal vessel

     Q27.39   Arteriovenous malformation, other site

Q27.4   Congenital phlebectasia   `CC`
CC Excl: PDX collection 1075

Q27.8   Other specified congenital malformations of peripheral vascular system
Absence of peripheral vascular system
Atresia of peripheral vascular system
Congenital aneurysm (peripheral)
Congenital stricture, artery
Congenital varix
EXCLUDES 1   *arteriovenous malformation (Q27.3-)*

Q27.9   Congenital malformation of peripheral vascular system, unspecified
Anomaly of artery or vein NOS

✓4ᵗʰ **Q28   Other congenital malformations of circulatory system**
EXCLUDES 1   *congenital aneurysm NOS (Q27.8)*
congenital coronary aneurysm (Q24.5)
ruptured cerebral arteriovenous malformation (I60.8)
ruptured malformation of precerebral vessels (I72.0)
EXCLUDES 2   *congenital peripheral aneurysm (Q27.8)*
congenital pulmonary aneurysm (Q25.79)
congenital retinal aneurysm (Q14.1)
CC Excl: For codes in category Q28:
For MCC codes: PDX collection 1076
For CC codes, unless otherwise noted: PDX collection 1075

Q28.0   Arteriovenous malformation of precerebral vessels   `CC`
Congenital arteriovenous precerebral aneurysm (nonruptured)

Q28.1   Other malformations of precerebral vessels   `CC`
Congenital malformation of precerebral vessels NOS
Congenital precerebral aneurysm (nonruptured)

Q28.2   Arteriovenous malformation of cerebral vessels   `MCC`
Arteriovenous malformation of brain NOS
Congenital arteriovenous cerebral aneurysm (nonruptured)

Q28.3   Other malformations of cerebral vessels   `MCC`
Congenital cerebral aneurysm (nonruptured)
Congenital malformation of cerebral vessels NOS
Developmental venous anomaly

Q28.8   Other specified congenital malformations of circulatory system   `CC`
Congenital aneurysm, specified site NEC
Spinal vessel anomaly

Q28.9   Congenital malformation of circulatory system, unspecified   `CC`
CC Excl: PDX collection 1077

Congenital malformations of the respiratory system (Q30-Q34)

✓4ᵗʰ **Q30   Congenital malformations of nose**
EXCLUDES 1   *congenital deviation of nasal septum (Q67.4)*

Q30.0   Choanal atresia
Atresia of nares (anterior) (posterior)
Congenital stenosis of nares (anterior) (posterior)

Q30.1   Agenesis and underdevelopment of nose
Congenital absent of nose

Q30.2   Fissured, notched and cleft nose

Q30.3   Congenital perforated nasal septum

Q30.8   Other congenital malformations of nose
Accessory nose
Congenital anomaly of nasal sinus wall

Q30.9   Congenital malformation of nose, unspecified

✓4ᵗʰ **Q31   Congenital malformations of larynx**
EXCLUDES 1   *congenital laryngeal stridor NOS (P28.89)*
CC Excl: For CC codes in category Q31: PDX collection 1078

Q31.0   Web of larynx
Glottic web of larynx
Subglottic web of larynx
Web of larynx NOS
DEF: Congenital malformation of the larynx marked by thin, translucent, or thick fibrotic membrane-like structure between the vocal folds. It is characterized by shortness of breath and stridor.

Q31.1   Congenital subglottic stenosis   `CC`

Q31.2   Laryngeal hypoplasia   `CC`

Q31.3   Laryngocele   `CC`

Q31.5   Congenital laryngomalacia   `CC`

Q31.8   Other congenital malformations of larynx   `CC`
Absence of larynx
Agenesis of larynx
Atresia of larynx
Congenital cleft thyroid cartilage
Congenital fissure of epiglottis
Congenital stenosis of larynx NEC
Posterior cleft of cricoid cartilage

Q31.9   Congenital malformation of larynx, unspecified   `CC`

`N` Newborn: 0   `P` Pediatric: 0-17   `M` Maternity: 9-64   `A` Adult: 15-124   `MCC` Major Complication/Comorbidity   `CC` Complication/Comorbidity   `SW` Severe Wound Dx

938   ICD-10-CM 2020

✓4ᵗʰ **Q32** **Congenital malformations of** trachea and bronchus

> EXCLUDES 1   *congenital bronchiectasis (Q33.4)*

CC Excl: For CC codes in category Q32: PDX collection 1078

Q32.0 **Congenital** tracheomalacia   `CC`

Q32.1 **Other congenital malformations of trachea**   `CC`
Atresia of trachea
Congenital anomaly of tracheal cartilage
Congenital dilatation of trachea
Congenital malformation of trachea
Congenital stenosis of trachea
Congenital tracheocele

Q32.2 **Congenital** bronchomalacia   `CC`

Q32.3 **Congenital** stenosis of bronchus   `CC`

Q32.4 **Other congenital malformations of bronchus**   `CC`
Absence of bronchus
Agenesis of bronchus
Atresia of bronchus
Congenital diverticulum of bronchus
Congenital malformation of bronchus NOS

✓4ᵗʰ **Q33** **Congenital malformations of** lung

CC Excl: For MCC codes in category Q33: PDX collection 1079

Q33.0 **Congenital** cystic lung   `CC`
Congenital cystic lung disease
Congenital honeycomb lung
Congenital polycystic lung disease
> EXCLUDES 1   *cystic fibrosis (E84.0)*
> *cystic lung disease, acquired or unspecified (J98.4)*
CC Excl: PDX collection 1079

Q33.1 **Accessory** lobe of lung
Azygos lobe (fissured), lung

Q33.2 **Sequestration** of lung   `MCC`

Q33.3 **Agenesis** of lung   `MCC`
Congenital absence of lung (lobe)

Q33.4 **Congenital** bronchiectasis   `CC`
CC Excl: PDX collection 1080

Q33.5 **Ectopic** tissue in lung

Q33.6 **Congenital** hypoplasia and dysplasia of lung   `MCC`
> EXCLUDES 1   *pulmonary hypoplasia associated with short gestation (P28.0)*

Q33.8 **Other congenital malformations of lung**

Q33.9 **Congenital malformation of lung, unspecified**

✓4ᵗʰ **Q34** **Other congenital malformations of** respiratory system
> EXCLUDES 2   *congenital central alveolar hypoventilation syndrome (G47.35)*

Q34.0 **Anomaly of** pleura

Q34.1 **Congenital cyst of** mediastinum

Q34.8 **Other specified congenital malformations of respiratory system**
Atresia of nasopharynx

Q34.9 **Congenital malformation of respiratory system, unspecified**
Congenital absence of respiratory system
Congenital anomaly of respiratory system NOS

Cleft lip and cleft palate (Q35-Q37)

Use additional code to identify associated malformation of the nose (Q30.2)
> EXCLUDES 1   *Robin's syndrome (Q87.0)*

✓4ᵗʰ **Q35** **Cleft** palate

> INCLUDES   fissure of palate
> palatoschisis
> EXCLUDES 1   *cleft palate with cleft lip (Q37.-)*

DEF: Congenital fissure or defect of the roof of the mouth opening to the nasal cavity due to failure of embryonic cells to fuse completely.

Cleft Palate

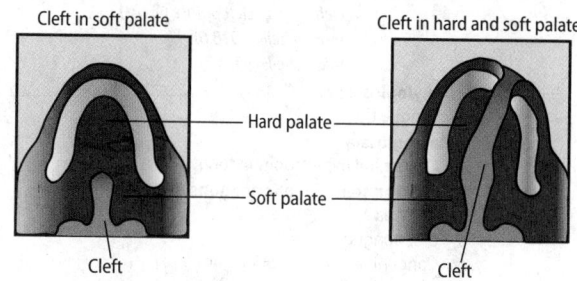

Cleft in soft palate   Cleft in hard and soft palate
Hard palate
Soft palate
Cleft   Cleft

Q35.1 **Cleft** hard palate
Q35.3 **Cleft** soft palate
Q35.5 **Cleft** hard palate with cleft soft palate
Q35.7 **Cleft** uvula
Q35.9 **Cleft palate, unspecified**
Cleft palate NOS

✓4ᵗʰ **Q36** **Cleft** lip

> INCLUDES   cheiloschisis
> congenital fissure of lip
> harelip
> labium leporinum
> EXCLUDES 1   *cleft lip with cleft palate (Q37.-)*

DEF: Congenital fissure or opening in the upper lip due to failure of embryonic cells to fuse completely.

Cleft Lip

Unilateral incomplete   Unilateral complete   Bilateral complete

Q36.0 **Cleft lip,** bilateral
Q36.1 **Cleft lip,** median
Q36.9 **Cleft lip,** unilateral
Cleft lip NOS

✓4ᵗʰ **Q37** **Cleft** palate with cleft lip

> INCLUDES   cheilopalatoschisis

Q37.0 **Cleft** hard palate with bilateral cleft lip
Q37.1 **Cleft** hard palate with unilateral cleft lip
Cleft hard palate with cleft lip NOS
Q37.2 **Cleft** soft palate with bilateral cleft lip
Q37.3 **Cleft** soft palate with unilateral cleft lip
Cleft soft palate with cleft lip NOS
Q37.4 **Cleft** hard and soft palate with bilateral cleft lip
Q37.5 **Cleft** hard and soft palate with unilateral cleft lip
Cleft hard and soft palate with cleft lip NOS
Q37.8 **Unspecified cleft palate with bilateral cleft lip**
Q37.9 **Unspecified cleft palate with unilateral cleft lip**
Cleft palate with cleft lip NOS

Chapter 17. Congenital Malformations, Deformations and Chromosomal Abnormalities

Q38–Q43.0

Other congenital malformations of the digestive system (Q38–Q45)

☑4ᵗʰ Q38 Other congenital malformations of tongue, mouth and pharynx

> **EXCLUDES 1**   dentofacial anomalies (M26.-)
> macrostomia (Q18.4)
> microstomia (Q18.5)

Q38.0 Congenital malformations of lips, not elsewhere classified
Congenital fistula of lip
Congenital malformation of lip NOS
Van der Woude's syndrome
> **EXCLUDES 1**   cleft lip (Q36.-)
> cleft lip with cleft palate (Q37.-)
> macrocheilia (Q18.6)
> microcheilia (Q18.7)

Q38.1 Ankyloglossia
Tongue tie

Q38.2 Macroglossia
Congenital hypertrophy of tongue

Q38.3 Other congenital malformations of tongue
Aglossia
Bifid tongue
Congenital adhesion of tongue
Congenital fissure of tongue
Congenital malformation of tongue NOS
Double tongue
Hypoglossia
Hypoplasia of tongue
Microglossia

Q38.4 Congenital malformations of salivary glands and ducts
Atresia of salivary glands and ducts
Congenital absence of salivary glands and ducts
Congenital accessory salivary glands and ducts
Congenital fistula of salivary gland

Q38.5 Congenital malformations of palate, not elsewhere classified
Congenital absence of uvula
Congenital malformation of palate NOS
Congenital high arched palate
> **EXCLUDES 1**   cleft palate (Q35.-)
> cleft palate with cleft lip (Q37.-)

Q38.6 Other congenital malformations of mouth
Congenital malformation of mouth NOS

Q38.7 Congenital pharyngeal pouch
Congenital diverticulum of pharynx
> **EXCLUDES 1**   pharyngeal pouch syndrome (D82.1)

Q38.8 Other congenital malformations of pharynx
Congenital malformation of pharynx NOS
Imperforate pharynx

☑4ᵗʰ Q39 Congenital malformations of esophagus

> **CC Excl: For codes in category Q39:**
> **For MCC codes:** PDX collection 1081
> **For CC codes:** PDX collection 1082

Q39.0 Atresia of esophagus without fistula   `MCC`
Atresia of esophagus NOS

Q39.1 Atresia of esophagus with tracheo-esophageal fistula   `MCC`
Atresia of esophagus with broncho-esophageal fistula

Q39.2 Congenital tracheo-esophageal fistula without atresia   `MCC`
Congenital tracheo-esophageal fistula NOS

Q39.3 Congenital stenosis and stricture of esophagus   `MCC`

Q39.4 Esophageal web   `CC`

Q39.5 Congenital dilatation of esophagus   `CC`
Congenital cardiospasm

Q39.6 Congenital diverticulum of esophagus   `CC`
Congenital esophageal pouch

Q39.8 Other congenital malformations of esophagus   `CC`
Congenital absence of esophagus
Congenital displacement of esophagus
Congenital duplication of esophagus

Q39.9 Congenital malformation of esophagus, unspecified   `CC`

☑4ᵗʰ Q40 Other congenital malformations of upper alimentary tract

Q40.0 Congenital hypertrophic pyloric stenosis
Congenital or infantile constriction
Congenital or infantile hypertrophy
Congenital or infantile spasm
Congenital or infantile stenosis
Congenital or infantile stricture

Q40.1 Congenital hiatus hernia
Congenital displacement of cardia through esophageal hiatus
> **EXCLUDES 1**   congenital diaphragmatic hernia (Q79.0)

Q40.2 Other specified congenital malformations of stomach
Congenital displacement of stomach
Congenital diverticulum of stomach
Congenital hourglass stomach
Congenital duplication of stomach
Megalogastria
Microgastria

Q40.3 Congenital malformation of stomach, unspecified

Q40.8 Other specified congenital malformations of upper alimentary tract

Q40.9 Congenital malformation of upper alimentary tract, unspecified
Congenital anomaly of upper alimentary tract
Congenital deformity of upper alimentary tract

☑4ᵗʰ Q41 Congenital absence, atresia and stenosis of small intestine

> **INCLUDES**   congenital obstruction, occlusion or stricture of small intestine or intestine NOS

> **EXCLUDES 1**   cystic fibrosis with intestinal manifestation (E84.11)
> meconium ileus NOS (without cystic fibrosis) (P76.0)

> **CC Excl: For CC codes in category Q41:** PDX collection 1083

Q41.0 Congenital absence, atresia and stenosis of duodenum   `CC`

Q41.1 Congenital absence, atresia and stenosis of jejunum   `CC`
Apple peel syndrome
Imperforate jejunum

Q41.2 Congenital absence, atresia and stenosis of ileum   `CC`

Q41.8 Congenital absence, atresia and stenosis of other specified parts of small intestine   `CC`

Q41.9 Congenital absence, atresia and stenosis of small intestine, part unspecified   `CC`
Congenital absence, atresia and stenosis of intestine NOS

☑4ᵗʰ Q42 Congenital absence, atresia and stenosis of large intestine

> **INCLUDES**   congenital obstruction, occlusion and stricture of large intestine

> **CC Excl: For CC codes in category Q42:** PDX collection 1084

Q42.0 Congenital absence, atresia and stenosis of rectum with fistula   `CC`

Q42.1 Congenital absence, atresia and stenosis of rectum without fistula   `CC`
Imperforate rectum

Q42.2 Congenital absence, atresia and stenosis of anus with fistula   `CC`

Q42.3 Congenital absence, atresia and stenosis of anus without fistula   `CC`
Imperforate anus

Q42.8 Congenital absence, atresia and stenosis of other parts of large intestine   `CC`

Q42.9 Congenital absence, atresia and stenosis of large intestine, part unspecified   `CC`

☑4ᵗʰ Q43 Other congenital malformations of intestine

> **CC Excl: For CC codes in category Q43, unless otherwise noted:** PDX collection 1087

Q43.0 Meckel's diverticulum (displaced) (hypertrophic)
Persistent omphalomesenteric duct
Persistent vitelline duct
DEF: Congenital, abnormal remnant of embryonic digestive system development that leaves a sacculation or outpouching from the wall of the small intestine near the terminal part of the ileum made of acid-secreting tissue as in the stomach.

N Newborn: 0   P Pediatric: 0-17   M Maternity: 9-64   A Adult: 15-124   MCC Major Complication/Comorbidity   CC Complication/Comorbidity   SW Severe Wound Dx

940   ICD-10-CM 2020

Q43.1 Hirschsprung's disease   CC

Aganglionosis
Congenital (aganglionic) megacolon
DEF: Congenital enlargement or dilation of the colon, with the absence of nerve cells in a segment of colon distally that causes the inability to defecate.
CC Excl: PDX collection 1085

Q43.2 Other congenital functional disorders of colon   CC

Congenital dilatation of colon
CC Excl: PDX collection 1085

Q43.3 Congenital malformations of intestinal fixation   CC

Congenital omental, anomalous adhesions [bands]
Congenital peritoneal adhesions [bands]
Incomplete rotation of cecum and colon
Insufficient rotation of cecum and colon
Jackson's membrane
Malrotation of colon
Rotation failure of cecum and colon
Universal mesentery
CC Excl: PDX collection 1086

Q43.4 Duplication of intestine   CC

Q43.5 Ectopic anus   CC

Q43.6 Congenital fistula of rectum and anus   CC

EXCLUDES 1   congenital fistula of anus with absence, atresia and stenosis (Q42.2)
congenital fistula of rectum with absence, atresia and stenosis (Q42.0)
congenital rectovaginal fistula (Q52.2)
congenital urethrorectal fistula (Q64.73)
pilonidal fistula or sinus (L05.-)

Q43.7 Persistent cloaca   CC

Cloaca NOS

Q43.8 Other specified congenital malformations of intestine   CC

Congenital blind loop syndrome
Congenital diverticulitis, colon
Congenital diverticulum, intestine
Dolichocolon
Megaloappendix
Megaloduodenum
Microcolon
Transposition of appendix
Transposition of colon
Transposition of intestine
AHA: 2013,2Q,31

Q43.9 Congenital malformation of intestine, unspecified   CC

✓4ᵗʰ **Q44 Congenital malformations of gallbladder, bile ducts and liver**

CC Excl: For codes in category Q44:
For MCC codes: PDX collection 1089
For CC codes, unless otherwise noted: PDX collection 1088

Q44.0 Agenesis, aplasia and hypoplasia of gallbladder   CC

Congenital absence of gallbladder

Q44.1 Other congenital malformations of gallbladder   CC

Congenital malformation of gallbladder NOS
Intrahepatic gallbladder

Q44.2 Atresia of bile ducts   MCC

Q44.3 Congenital stenosis and stricture of bile ducts   MCC

Q44.4 Choledochal cyst   CC

Q44.5 Other congenital malformations of bile ducts   CC

Accessory hepatic duct
Biliary duct duplication
Congenital malformation of bile duct NOS
Cystic duct duplication

Q44.6 Cystic disease of liver   CC

Fibrocystic disease of liver
CC Excl: PDX collection 1090

Q44.7 Other congenital malformations of liver   CC

Accessory liver
Alagille's syndrome
Congenital absence of liver
Congenital hepatomegaly
Congenital malformation of liver NOS

✓4ᵗʰ **Q45 Other congenital malformations of digestive system**

EXCLUDES 2   congenital diaphragmatic hernia (Q79.0)
congenital hiatus hernia (Q40.1)
CC Excl: For CC codes in category Q45: PDX collection 1091

Q45.0 Agenesis, aplasia and hypoplasia of pancreas   CC

Congenital absence of pancreas

Q45.1 Annular pancreas   CC

Q45.2 Congenital pancreatic cyst   CC

Q45.3 Other congenital malformations of pancreas and pancreatic duct   CC

Accessory pancreas
Congenital malformation of pancreas or pancreatic duct NOS
EXCLUDES 1   congenital diabetes mellitus (E10.-)
cystic fibrosis (E84.0-E84.9)
fibrocystic disease of pancreas (E84.-)
neonatal diabetes mellitus (P70.2)

Q45.8 Other specified congenital malformations of digestive system

Absence (complete) (partial) of alimentary tract NOS
Duplication of digestive system
Malposition, congenital of digestive system

Q45.9 Congenital malformation of digestive system, unspecified

Congenital anomaly of digestive system
Congenital deformity of digestive system

Congenital malformations of genital organs (Q50-Q56)

EXCLUDES 1   androgen insensitivity syndrome (E34.5-)
syndromes associated with anomalies in the number and form of chromosomes (Q90-Q99)

✓4ᵗʰ **Q50 Congenital malformations of ovaries, fallopian tubes and broad ligaments**

✓5ᵗʰ **Q50.0 Congenital absence of ovary**

EXCLUDES 1   Turner's syndrome (Q96.-)

Q50.01 Congenital absence of ovary, unilateral   ♀

Q50.02 Congenital absence of ovary, bilateral   ♀

Q50.1 Developmental ovarian cyst   ♀

Q50.2 Congenital torsion of ovary   ♀

✓5ᵗʰ **Q50.3 Other congenital malformations of ovary**

Q50.31 Accessory ovary   ♀

Q50.32 Ovarian streak   ♀

46, XX with streak gonads

Q50.39 Other congenital malformation of ovary   ♀

Congenital malformation of ovary NOS

Q50.4 Embryonic cyst of fallopian tube   ♀

Fimbrial cyst

Q50.5 Embryonic cyst of broad ligament   ♀

Epoophoron cyst
Parovarian cyst

Q50.6 Other congenital malformations of fallopian tube and broad ligament   ♀

Absence of fallopian tube and broad ligament
Accessory fallopian tube and broad ligament
Atresia of fallopian tube and broad ligament
Congenital malformation of fallopian tube or broad ligament NOS

✓4ᵗʰ **Q51 Congenital malformations of uterus and cervix**

Q51.0 Agenesis and aplasia of uterus   ♀

Congenital absence of uterus

✓5ᵗʰ **Q51.1 Doubling of uterus with doubling of cervix and vagina**

Q51.10 Doubling of uterus with doubling of cervix and vagina without obstruction   ♀

Doubling of uterus with doubling of cervix and vagina NOS

Q51.11 Doubling of uterus with doubling of cervix and vagina with obstruction   ♀

✓5ᵗʰ **Q51.2 Other doubling of uterus**
Doubling of uterus NOS
Septate uterus
AHA: 2018,4Q,27

    Q51.20 Other doubling of uterus, unspecified ♀
       Septate uterus, unspecified

    Q51.21 Other complete doubling of uterus ♀
       Complete septate uterus

    Q51.22 Other partial doubling of uterus ♀
       Partial septate uterus

    Q51.28 Other doubling of uterus, other specified ♀
       Septate uterus, other specified

Q51.3 Bicornate uterus ♀
    Bicornate uterus, complete or partial

Q51.4 Unicornate uterus ♀
    Unicornate uterus with or without a separate uterine horn
    Uterus with only one functioning horn

Q51.5 Agenesis and aplasia of cervix ♀
    Congenital absence of cervix

Q51.6 Embryonic cyst of cervix ♀

Q51.7 Congenital fistulae between uterus and digestive and urinary tracts ♀

✓5ᵗʰ **Q51.8 Other congenital malformations of uterus and cervix**

    ✓6ᵗʰ **Q51.81 Other congenital malformations of uterus**

       Q51.810 Arcuate uterus ♀
          Arcuatus uterus

       Q51.811 Hypoplasia of uterus ♀

       Q51.818 Other congenital malformations of uterus ♀
          Müllerian anomaly of uterus NEC

    ✓6ᵗʰ **Q51.82 Other congenital malformations of cervix**

       Q51.820 Cervical duplication ♀

       Q51.821 Hypoplasia of cervix ♀

       Q51.828 Other congenital malformations of cervix ♀

    Q51.9 Congenital malformation of uterus and cervix, unspecified ♀

✓4ᵗʰ **Q52 Other congenital malformations of female genitalia**

    Q52.0 Congenital absence of vagina ♀
       Vaginal agenesis, total or partial

    ✓5ᵗʰ **Q52.1 Doubling of vagina**

       EXCLUDES 1   doubling of vagina with doubling of uterus and cervix (Q51.1-)

       Q52.10 Doubling of vagina, unspecified ♀
          Septate vagina NOS

       Q52.11 Transverse vaginal septum ♀

       ✓6ᵗʰ **Q52.12 Longitudinal vaginal septum**
          AHA: 2016,4Q,58-59

          Q52.120 Longitudinal vaginal septum, nonobstructing ♀

          Q52.121 Longitudinal vaginal septum, obstructing, right side ♀

          Q52.122 Longitudinal vaginal septum, obstructing, left side ♀

          Q52.123 Longitudinal vaginal septum, microperforate, right side ♀

          Q52.124 Longitudinal vaginal septum, microperforate, left side ♀

          Q52.129 Other and unspecified longitudinal vaginal septum ♀

    Q52.2 Congenital rectovaginal fistula ♀
       EXCLUDES 1   cloaca (Q43.7)

    Q52.3 Imperforate hymen ♀
       DEF: Obstructive anomaly of vagina, characterized by complete closure of the membranous fold around the external opening of the vagina, obstructing the vaginal introitus.

Q52.4 Other congenital malformations of vagina ♀
    Canal of Nuck cyst, congenital
    Congenital malformation of vagina NOS
    Embryonic vaginal cyst
    Gartner's duct cyst

Q52.5 Fusion of labia ♀

Q52.6 Congenital malformation of clitoris ♀

✓5ᵗʰ **Q52.7 Other and unspecified congenital malformations of vulva**

    Q52.70 Unspecified congenital malformations of vulva ♀
       Congenital malformation of vulva NOS

    Q52.71 Congenital absence of vulva ♀

    Q52.79 Other congenital malformations of vulva ♀
       Congenital cyst of vulva

Q52.8 Other specified congenital malformations of female genitalia ♀

Q52.9 Congenital malformation of female genitalia, unspecified ♀

✓4ᵗʰ **Q53 Undescended and ectopic testicle**

    ✓5ᵗʰ **Q53.0 Ectopic testis**

       Q53.00 Ectopic testis, unspecified ♂

       Q53.01 Ectopic testis, unilateral ♂

       Q53.02 Ectopic testes, bilateral ♂

    ✓5ᵗʰ **Q53.1 Undescended testicle, unilateral**
       AHA: 2017,4Q,22-23

       Q53.10 Unspecified undescended testicle, unilateral ♂

       ✓6ᵗʰ **Q53.11 Abdominal testis, unilateral**

          Q53.111 Unilateral intraabdominal testis ♂

          Q53.112 Unilateral inguinal testis ♂

       Q53.12 Ectopic perineal testis, unilateral ♂

       Q53.13 Unilateral high scrotal testis ♂

    ✓5ᵗʰ **Q53.2 Undescended testicle, bilateral**
       AHA: 2017,4Q,22-23

       Q53.20 Undescended testicle, unspecified, bilateral ♂

       ✓6ᵗʰ **Q53.21 Abdominal testis, bilateral**

          Q53.211 Bilateral intraabdominal testes ♂

          Q53.212 Bilateral inguinal testes ♂

       Q53.22 Ectopic perineal testis, bilateral ♂

       Q53.23 Bilateral high scrotal testes ♂

    Q53.9 Undescended testicle, unspecified ♂
       Cryptorchism NOS

✓4ᵗʰ **Q54 Hypospadias**

    EXCLUDES 1   epispadias (Q64.0)

    DEF: Abnormal opening of the urethra on the ventral (underside) surface of the penis.

Hypospadias

Balanic (glanular, coronal) hypospadias
Subcoronal hypospadias
Penile hypospadias
Penile raphe
Scrotal hypospadias
Penoscrotal hypospadias
Scrotum
Scrotal raphe
Hypospadias (ventral view)
Perineal hypospadias

    Q54.0 Hypospadias, balanic ♂
       Hypospadias, coronal
       Hypospadias, glandular

    Q54.1 Hypospadias, penile ♂

Ⓝ Newborn: 0   Ⓟ Pediatric: 0-17   Ⓜ Maternity: 9-64   Ⓐ Adult: 15-124   MCC Major Complication/Comorbidity   CC Complication/Comorbidity   SW Severe Wound Dx

942   ICD-10-CM 2020

Q54.2 **Hypospadias,** penoscrotal   ♂

Q54.3 **Hypospadias,** perineal   ♂

Q54.4 Congenital chordee   ♂

     Chordee without hypospadias

Q54.8 **Other hypospadias**   ♂

     Hypospadias with intersex state

Q54.9 **Hypospadias, unspecified**   ♂

√4th **Q55 Other congenital malformations of** male genital organs

     EXCLUDES 1   *congenital hydrocele (P83.5)*

         hypospadias (Q54.-)

Q55.0 **Absence and aplasia of testis**   ♂

     Monorchism

Q55.1 **Hypoplasia of testis and scrotum**   ♂

     Fusion of testes

√5th Q55.2 **Other and unspecified congenital malformations of** testis and scrotum

     Q55.20 **Unspecified congenital**   ♂
         malformations of testis and scrotum

         Congenital malformation of testis or scrotum NOS

     Q55.21 **Polyorchism**   ♂

         DEF: Congenital anomaly in which there are more than two testes.

     Q55.22 **Retractile testis**   ♂

     Q55.23 **Scrotal** transposition   ♂

     Q55.29 **Other congenital malformations of**   ♂
         testis and scrotum

Q55.3 **Atresia of** vas deferens   ♂

     Code first any associated cystic fibrosis (E84.-)

Q55.4 **Other congenital malformations of vas**   ♂
deferens, epididymis, seminal vesicles and prostate

     Absence or aplasia of prostate

     Absence or aplasia of spermatic cord

     Congenital malformation of vas deferens, epididymis, seminal vesicles or prostate NOS

Q55.5 **Congenital** absence and aplasia of penis   ♂

√5th Q55.6 **Other congenital malformations of** penis

     Q55.61 **Curvature** of penis (lateral)   ♂

     Q55.62 **Hypoplasia** of penis   ♂

         Micropenis

     Q55.63 **Congenital torsion** of penis   ♂

         EXCLUDES 1   *acquired torsion of penis (N48.82)*

     Q55.64 **Hidden penis**   ♂

         Buried penis

         Concealed penis

         EXCLUDES 1   *acquired buried penis (N48.83)*

     Q55.69 **Other congenital malformation of**   ♂
         penis

         Congenital malformation of penis NOS

Q55.7 **Congenital** vasocutaneous fistula   ♂

Q55.8 **Other specified congenital malformations of**   ♂
male genital organs

Q55.9 **Congenital malformation of male genital**   ♂
organ, unspecified

     Congenital anomaly of male genital organ

     Congenital deformity of male genital organ

√4th **Q56 Indeterminate sex and pseudohermaphroditism**

     EXCLUDES 1   *46, XX true hermaphrodite (Q99.1)*

         androgen insensitivity syndrome (E34.5-)

         chimera 46, XX/46, XY true hermaphrodite (Q99.0)

         female pseudohermaphroditism with adrenocortical disorder (E25.-)

         pseudohermaphroditism with specified chromosomal anomaly (Q96-Q99)

         pure gonadal dysgenesis (Q99.1)

     DEF: Indeterminate sex: External genitalia that is nondescript, lacking the physical appearance specific to either sex.

     DEF: Pseudohermaphroditism: Presence of gonads of one sex and external genitalia of another sex.

Q56.0 **Hermaphroditism,** not elsewhere classified

     Ovotestis

Q56.1 Male **pseudohermaphroditism, not elsewhere**   ♂
classified

     46, XY with streak gonads

     Male pseudohermaphroditism NOS

Q56.2 Female **pseudohermaphroditism, not**   ♀
elsewhere classified

     Female pseudohermaphroditism NOS

Q56.3 **Pseudohermaphroditism, unspecified**

Q56.4 **Indeterminate sex, unspecified**

     Ambiguous genitalia

Congenital malformations of the urinary system (Q60-Q64)

√4th **Q60 Renal agenesis and other** reduction defects of kidney

     INCLUDES   congenital absence of kidney

         congenital atrophy of kidney

         infantile atrophy of kidney

Q60.0 **Renal** agenesis, unilateral

Q60.1 **Renal** agenesis, bilateral

Q60.2 **Renal agenesis, unspecified**

Q60.3 **Renal** hypoplasia, unilateral

Q60.4 **Renal** hypoplasia, bilateral

Q60.5 **Renal hypoplasia, unspecified**

Q60.6 **Potter's syndrome**

√4th **Q61 Cystic kidney disease**

     EXCLUDES 1   *acquired cyst of kidney (N28.1)*

         Potter's syndrome (Q60.6)

√5th Q61.0 **Congenital renal** cyst

     Q61.00 **Congenital renal cyst, unspecified**

         Cyst of kidney NOS (congenital)

     Q61.01 **Congenital** single **renal cyst**

     Q61.02 **Congenital** multiple **renal cysts**

√5th Q61.1 **Polycystic kidney,** infantile type

     Polycystic kidney, autosomal recessive

     Q61.11 **Cystic dilatation of collecting ducts**

     Q61.19 **Other polycystic kidney, infantile type**

Q61.2 **Polycystic** kidney, adult type

     Polycystic kidney, autosomal dominant

Q61.3 **Polycystic kidney, unspecified**

     AHA: 2016,3Q,22

Q61.4 **Renal** dysplasia

     Multicystic dysplastic kidney

     Multicystic kidney (development)

     Multicystic kidney disease

     Multicystic renal dysplasia

     EXCLUDES 1   *polycystic kidney disease (Q61.11-Q61.3)*

Q61.5 **Medullary cystic kidney**

     Nephronopthisis

     Sponge kidney NOS

     DEF: Sponge kidney: Dilated collecting tubules that are usually asymptomatic. Calcinosis in tubules may cause renal insufficiency.

Q61.8 **Other cystic kidney diseases**   CC

     Fibrocystic kidney

     Fibrocystic renal degeneration or disease

     CC Excl: PDX collection 1095

Q61.9 **Cystic kidney disease, unspecified**   CC

     Meckel-Gruber syndrome

     CC Excl: PDX collection 1093

√4th **Q62 Congenital obstructive defects of** renal pelvis **and congenital malformations of** ureter

     CC Excl: For CC codes in category Q62: PDX collection 1098

Q62.0 **Congenital** hydronephrosis   CC

√5th Q62.1 **Congenital** occlusion of ureter   CC

     Atresia and stenosis of ureter

     Q62.10 **Congenital occlusion of ureter,**   CC
         unspecified

     Q62.11 **Congenital occlusion of**   CC
         ureteropelvic junction

     Q62.12 **Congenital occlusion of**   CC
         ureterovesical orifice

Q62.2 **Congenital** megaureter   CC

     Congenital dilatation of ureter

√5th Q62.3 **Other obstructive defects of renal pelvis and ureter**

     Q62.31 **Congenital** ureterocele, orthotopic   CC

✓ Additional Character Required   √x7th Placeholder   Unacceptable PDx   Questionable PDx   Manifestation   Unspecified Dx   H1-H14 HAC   HCC CMS-HCC Dx   HIV HIV Dx

ICD-10-CM 2020   943

Q62.32 **Cecoureterocele** `CC`

　Ectopic ureterocele

Q62.39 **Other obstructive defects of renal pelvis and ureter** `CC`

　Ureteropelvic junction obstruction NOS

Q62.4 **Agenesis of ureter**

　Congenital absence ureter

Q62.5 **Duplication of ureter**

　Accessory ureter

　Double ureter

✓5ᵗʰ **Q62.6** **Malposition of ureter**

　Q62.60 **Malposition of ureter, unspecified**

　Q62.61 **Deviation of ureter**

　Q62.62 **Displacement of ureter**

　Q62.63 **Anomalous implantation of ureter**

　　Ectopia of ureter

　　Ectopic ureter

　Q62.69 **Other malposition of ureter**

Q62.7 **Congenital vesico-uretero-renal reflux**

Q62.8 **Other congenital malformations of ureter**

　Anomaly of ureter NOS

✓4ᵗʰ **Q63** **Other congenital malformations of kidney**

　EXCLUDES 1　*congenital nephrotic syndrome (N04.-)*

Q63.0 **Accessory kidney**

Q63.1 **Lobulated, fused and horseshoe kidney**

Q63.2 **Ectopic kidney**

　Congenital displaced kidney

　Malrotation of kidney

Q63.3 **Hyperplastic and giant kidney**

　Compensatory hypertrophy of kidney

Q63.8 **Other specified congenital malformations of kidney**

　Congenital renal calculi

Q63.9 **Congenital malformation of kidney, unspecified**

✓4ᵗʰ **Q64** **Other congenital malformations of urinary system**

Q64.0 **Epispadias**

　EXCLUDES 1　*hypospadias (Q54.-)*

Epispadias

Normal external urethral orifice

Glans penis

Foreskin (retracted)

Epispadias

Epispadias (dorsal view)

✓5ᵗʰ **Q64.1** **Exstrophy of urinary bladder**

　CC Excl: For CC codes in subcategory Q64.1: PDX collection 1099

　Q64.10 **Exstrophy of urinary bladder, unspecified** `CC`

　　Ectopia vesicae

　Q64.11 **Supravesical fissure of urinary bladder** `CC`

　Q64.12 **Cloacal exstrophy of urinary bladder** `CC`

　Q64.19 **Other exstrophy of urinary bladder** `CC`

　　Extroversion of bladder

Q64.2 **Congenital posterior urethral valves** `CC`

　CC Excl: PDX collection 1100

✓5ᵗʰ **Q64.3** **Other atresia and stenosis of urethra and bladder neck**

　CC Excl: For CC codes in subcategory Q64.3: PDX collection 1100

　Q64.31 **Congenital bladder neck obstruction** `CC`

　　Congenital obstruction of vesicourethral orifice

　Q64.32 **Congenital stricture of urethra** `CC`

　Q64.33 **Congenital stricture of urinary meatus** `CC`

Q64.39 **Other atresia and stenosis of urethra and bladder neck** `CC`

　Atresia and stenosis of urethra and bladder neck NOS

Q64.4 **Malformation of urachus**

　Cyst of urachus

　Patent urachus

　Prolapse of urachus

Q64.5 **Congenital absence of bladder and urethra**

Q64.6 **Congenital diverticulum of bladder**

✓5ᵗʰ **Q64.7** **Other and unspecified congenital malformations of bladder and urethra**

　EXCLUDES 1　*congenital prolapse of bladder (mucosa) (Q79.4)*

　Q64.70 **Unspecified congenital malformation of bladder and urethra**

　　Malformation of bladder or urethra NOS

　Q64.71 **Congenital prolapse of urethra**

　Q64.72 **Congenital prolapse of urinary meatus**

　Q64.73 **Congenital urethrorectal fistula**

　Q64.74 **Double urethra**

　Q64.75 **Double urinary meatus**

　Q64.79 **Other congenital malformations of bladder and urethra**

Q64.8 **Other specified congenital malformations of urinary system**

Q64.9 **Congenital malformation of urinary system, unspecified**

　Congenital anomaly NOS of urinary system

　Congenital deformity NOS of urinary system

Congenital malformations and deformations of the musculoskeletal system (Q65-Q79)

✓4ᵗʰ **Q65** **Congenital deformities of hip**

　EXCLUDES 1　*clicking hip (R29.4)*

✓5ᵗʰ **Q65.0** **Congenital dislocation of hip, unilateral**

　Q65.00 **Congenital dislocation of unspecified hip, unilateral**

　Q65.01 **Congenital dislocation of right hip, unilateral**

　Q65.02 **Congenital dislocation of left hip, unilateral**

Q65.1 **Congenital dislocation of hip, bilateral**

Q65.2 **Congenital dislocation of hip, unspecified**

✓5ᵗʰ **Q65.3** **Congenital partial dislocation of hip, unilateral**

　Q65.30 **Congenital partial dislocation of unspecified hip, unilateral**

　Q65.31 **Congenital partial dislocation of right hip, unilateral**

　Q65.32 **Congenital partial dislocation of left hip, unilateral**

Q65.4 **Congenital partial dislocation of hip, bilateral**

Q65.5 **Congenital partial dislocation of hip, unspecified**

Q65.6 **Congenital unstable hip**

　Congenital dislocatable hip

✓5ᵗʰ **Q65.8** **Other congenital deformities of hip**

　Q65.81 **Congenital coxa valga**

　Q65.82 **Congenital coxa vara**

　Q65.89 **Other specified congenital deformities of hip**

　　Anteversion of femoral neck

　　Congenital acetabular dysplasia

Q65.9 **Congenital deformity of hip, unspecified**

✓4ᵗʰ **Q66** **Congenital deformities of feet**

　EXCLUDES 1　*reduction defects of feet (Q72.-)*

　　　valgus deformities (acquired) (M21.0-)

　　　varus deformities (acquired) (M21.1-)

▲ ✓5ᵗʰ **Q66.0** **Congenital talipes equinovarus**

　● **Q66.00** **Congenital talipes equinovarus, unspecified foot**

　● **Q66.01** **Congenital talipes equinovarus, right foot**

　● **Q66.02** **Congenital talipes equinovarus, left foot**

▲ ✓5ᵗʰ **Q66.1** **Congenital talipes calcaneovarus**

　● **Q66.10** **Congenital talipes calcaneovarus, unspecified foot**

　● **Q66.11** **Congenital talipes calcaneovarus, right foot**

　● **Q66.12** **Congenital talipes calcaneovarus, left foot**

✓5ᵗʰ **Q66.2** **Congenital metatarsus (primus) varus**

　AHA: 2016,4Q,59

▲ 　✓6ᵗʰ **Q66.21** **Congenital metatarsus primus varus**

　● 　**Q66.211** **Congenital metatarsus primus varus, right foot**

　● 　**Q66.212** **Congenital metatarsus primus varus, left foot**

N Newborn: 0　　P Pediatric: 0-17　　M Maternity: 9-64　　A Adult: 15-124　　MCC Major Complication/Comorbidity　　CC Complication/Comorbidity　　SW Severe Wound Dx

944　　　　　　　　　　　　　　　　　　　　　　　　　　　　　　　　　　ICD-10-CM 2020

Q66.219 Congenital metatarsus primus varus, unspecified foot
▲ ✓6ᵗʰ **Q66.22 Congenital** metatarsus adductus
    Congenital metatarsus varus
● **Q66.221 Congenital metatarsus adductus, right foot**
● **Q66.222 Congenital metatarsus adductus, left foot**
● **Q66.229 Congenital metatarsus adductus, unspecified foot**
▲ ✓5ᵗʰ **Q66.3 Other congenital varus deformities of feet**
    Hallux varus, congenital
● **Q66.30 Other congenital varus deformities of feet, unspecified foot**
● **Q66.31 Other congenital varus deformities of feet, right foot**
● **Q66.32 Other congenital varus deformities of feet, left foot**
▲ ✓5ᵗʰ **Q66.4 Congenital** talipes calcaneovalgus
● **Q66.40 Congenital talipes calcaneovalgus, unspecified foot**
● **Q66.41 Congenital talipes calcaneovalgus, right foot**
● **Q66.42 Congenital talipes calcaneovalgus, left foot**
✓5ᵗʰ **Q66.5 Congenital** pes planus
    Congenital flat foot
    Congenital rigid flat foot
    Congenital spastic (everted) flat foot
    EXCLUDES 1 pes planus, acquired (M21.4)
● **Q66.50 Congenital pes planus, unspecified foot**
● **Q66.51 Congenital pes planus, right foot**
● **Q66.52 Congenital pes planus, left foot**
Q66.6 Other congenital valgus deformities of feet
    Congenital metatarsus valgus
▲ ✓5ᵗʰ **Q66.7 Congenital** pes cavus
● **Q66.70 Congenital pes cavus, unspecified foot**
● **Q66.71 Congenital pes cavus, right foot**
● **Q66.72 Congenital pes cavus, left foot**
✓5ᵗʰ **Q66.8 Other congenital deformities of feet**
● **Q66.80 Congenital vertical talus deformity, unspecified foot**
● **Q66.81 Congenital vertical talus deformity, right foot**
● **Q66.82 Congenital vertical talus deformity, left foot**
● **Q66.89 Other specified congenital deformities of feet**
    Congenital asymmetric talipes
    Congenital clubfoot NOS
    Congenital talipes NOS
    Congenital tarsal coalition
    Hammer toe, congenital
    DEF: Clubfoot: Congenital anomaly of the foot with the heel elevated and rotated outward and the toes pointing inward.
▲ ✓5ᵗʰ **Q66.9 Congenital deformity of feet, unspecified**
● **Q66.90 Congenital deformity of feet, unspecified, unspecified foot**
● **Q66.91 Congenital deformity of feet, unspecified, right foot**
● **Q66.92 Congenital deformity of feet, unspecified, left foot**
✓4ᵗʰ **Q67 Congenital musculoskeletal deformities of** head, face, spine and chest
    EXCLUDES 1 congenital malformation syndromes classified to Q87.-
        Potter's syndrome (Q60.6)
Q67.0 Congenital facial asymmetry
Q67.1 Congenital compression facies
Q67.2 Dolichocephaly
Q67.3 Plagiocephaly
Q67.4 Other congenital deformities of skull, face and jaw
    Congenital depressions in skull
    Congenital hemifacial atrophy or hypertrophy
    Deviation of nasal septum, congenital
    Squashed or bent nose, congenital
    EXCLUDES 1 dentofacial anomalies [including malocclusion] (M26.-)
        syphilitic saddle nose (A50.5)
    DEF: Deviated septum: Condition in which the nasal septum, a thin wall composed of cartilage and bone that separates the two nostrils, is crooked or displaced from the midline.

Q67.5 Congenital deformity of spine cc
    Congenital postural scoliosis
    Congenital scoliosis NOS
    EXCLUDES 1 infantile idiopathic scoliosis (M41.0)
        scoliosis due to congenital bony malformation (Q76.3)
    AHA: 2014,4Q,26
    CC Excl: PDX collection 1101
Q67.6 Pectus excavatum
    Congenital funnel chest
Q67.7 Pectus carinatum
    Congenital pigeon chest
Q67.8 Other congenital deformities of chest cc
    Congenital deformity of chest wall NOS
    CC Excl: PDX collection 1102
✓4ᵗʰ **Q68 Other congenital musculoskeletal deformities**
    EXCLUDES 1 reduction defects of limb(s) (Q71-Q73)
    EXCLUDES 2 congenital myotonic chondrodystrophy (G71.13)
Q68.0 Congenital deformity of sternocleidomastoid muscle
    Congenital contracture of sternocleidomastoid (muscle)
    Congenital (sternomastoid) torticollis
    Sternomastoid tumor (congenital)
Q68.1 Congenital deformity of finger(s) and hand cc
    Congenital clubfinger
    Spade-like hand (congenital)
    CC Excl: PDX collection 1102
Q68.2 Congenital deformity of knee
    Congenital dislocation of knee
    Congenital genu recurvatum
Q68.3 Congenital bowing of femur
    EXCLUDES 1 anteversion of femur (neck) (Q65.89)
Q68.4 Congenital bowing of tibia and fibula
Q68.5 Congenital bowing of long bones of leg, unspecified
Q68.6 Discoid meniscus
Q68.8 Other specified congenital musculoskeletal deformities
    Congenital deformity of clavicle
    Congenital deformity of elbow
    Congenital deformity of forearm
    Congenital deformity of scapula
    Congenital deformity of wrist
    Congenital dislocation of elbow
    Congenital dislocation of shoulder
    Congenital dislocation of wrist
✓4ᵗʰ **Q69 Polydactyly**
Q69.0 Accessory finger(s)
Q69.1 Accessory thumb(s)
Q69.2 Accessory toe(s)
    Accessory hallux
Q69.9 Polydactyly, unspecified
    Supernumerary digit(s) NOS
✓4ᵗʰ **Q70 Syndactyly**
✓5ᵗʰ **Q70.0 Fused fingers**
    Complex syndactyly of fingers with synostosis
● **Q70.00 Fused fingers, unspecified hand**
    Q70.01 Fused fingers, right hand
    Q70.02 Fused fingers, left hand
    Q70.03 Fused fingers, bilateral
✓5ᵗʰ **Q70.1 Webbed fingers**
    Simple syndactyly of fingers without synostosis
● **Q70.10 Webbed fingers, unspecified hand**
    Q70.11 Webbed fingers, right hand
    Q70.12 Webbed fingers, left hand
    Q70.13 Webbed fingers, bilateral
✓5ᵗʰ **Q70.2 Fused toes**
    Complex syndactyly of toes with synostosis
● **Q70.20 Fused toes, unspecified foot**
    Q70.21 Fused toes, right foot
    Q70.22 Fused toes, left foot
    Q70.23 Fused toes, bilateral
✓5ᵗʰ **Q70.3 Webbed toes**
    Simple syndactyly of toes without synostosis
● **Q70.30 Webbed toes, unspecified foot**
    Q70.31 Webbed toes, right foot
    Q70.32 Webbed toes, left foot

Q70.33　**Webbed toes,** bilateral

Q70.4　Polysyndactyly, unspecified

> EXCLUDES 1　*specified syndactyly of hand and feet — code to specified conditions (Q70.0-Q70.3-)*

Q70.9　Syndactyly, unspecified
Symphalangy NOS

✓4th **Q71　Reduction defects of** upper limb

✓5th **Q71.0　Congenital** complete absence **of upper limb**

Q71.00　**Congenital complete absence of unspecified upper limb**

Q71.01　**Congenital complete absence of** right **upper limb**

Q71.02　**Congenital complete absence of** left **upper limb**

Q71.03　**Congenital complete absence of upper limb,** bilateral

✓5th **Q71.1　Congenital** absence of upper arm and forearm with hand present

Q71.10　**Congenital absence of unspecified upper arm and forearm with hand present**

Q71.11　**Congenital absence of** right **upper arm and forearm with hand present**

Q71.12　**Congenital absence of** left **upper arm and forearm with hand present**

Q71.13　**Congenital absence of upper arm and forearm with hand present,** bilateral

✓5th **Q71.2　Congenital** absence of both forearm and hand

Q71.20　**Congenital absence of both forearm and hand, unspecified upper limb**

Q71.21　**Congenital absence of both forearm and hand,** right **upper limb**

Q71.22　**Congenital absence of both forearm and hand,** left **upper limb**

Q71.23　**Congenital absence of both forearm and hand,** bilateral

✓5th **Q71.3　Congenital** absence of hand and finger

Q71.30　**Congenital absence of unspecified hand and finger**

Q71.31　**Congenital absence of** right **hand and finger**

Q71.32　**Congenital absence of** left **hand and finger**

Q71.33　**Congenital absence of hand and finger,** bilateral

✓5th **Q71.4　Longitudinal reduction defect of** radius

Clubhand (congenital)
Radial clubhand

Q71.40　**Longitudinal reduction defect of unspecified radius**

Q71.41　**Longitudinal reduction defect of** right **radius**

Q71.42　**Longitudinal reduction defect of** left **radius**

Q71.43　**Longitudinal reduction defect of radius,** bilateral

✓5th **Q71.5　Longitudinal reduction defect of** ulna

Q71.50　**Longitudinal reduction defect of unspecified ulna**

Q71.51　**Longitudinal reduction defect of** right **ulna**

Q71.52　**Longitudinal reduction defect of** left **ulna**

Q71.53　**Longitudinal reduction defect of ulna,** bilateral

✓5th **Q71.6　Lobster-claw hand**

Q71.60　**Lobster-claw hand, unspecified hand**

Q71.61　**Lobster-claw** right **hand**

Q71.62　**Lobster-claw** left **hand**

Q71.63　**Lobster-claw hand,** bilateral

✓5th **Q71.8　Other reduction defects of** upper limb

✓6th Q71.81　**Congenital** shortening **of upper limb**

Q71.811　**Congenital shortening of** right **upper limb**

Q71.812　**Congenital shortening of** left **upper limb**

Q71.813　**Congenital shortening of upper limb,** bilateral

Q71.819　**Congenital shortening of unspecified upper limb**

✓6th Q71.89　**Other reduction defects of upper limb**

Q71.891　**Other reduction defects of** right **upper limb**

Q71.892　**Other reduction defects of** left **upper limb**

Q71.893　**Other reduction defects of upper limb,** bilateral

Q71.899　**Other reduction defects of unspecified upper limb**

✓5th **Q71.9　Unspecified reduction defect of upper limb**

Q71.90　**Unspecified reduction defect of unspecified upper limb**

Q71.91　**Unspecified reduction defect of** right **upper limb**

Q71.92　**Unspecified reduction defect of** left **upper limb**

Q71.93　**Unspecified reduction defect of upper limb,** bilateral

✓4th **Q72　Reduction defects of** lower limb

✓5th **Q72.0　Congenital** complete absence **of lower limb**

Q72.00　**Congenital complete absence of unspecified lower limb**

Q72.01　**Congenital complete absence of** right **lower limb**

Q72.02　**Congenital complete absence of** left **lower limb**

Q72.03　**Congenital complete absence of lower limb,** bilateral

✓5th **Q72.1　Congenital** absence of thigh and lower leg with foot present

Q72.10　**Congenital absence of unspecified thigh and lower leg with foot present**

Q72.11　**Congenital absence of** right **thigh and lower leg with foot present**

Q72.12　**Congenital absence of** left **thigh and lower leg with foot present**

Q72.13　**Congenital absence of thigh and lower leg with foot present,** bilateral

✓5th **Q72.2　Congenital** absence of both lower leg and foot

Q72.20　**Congenital absence of both lower leg and foot, unspecified lower limb**

Q72.21　**Congenital absence of both lower leg and foot,** right **lower limb**

Q72.22　**Congenital absence of both lower leg and foot,** left **lower limb**

Q72.23　**Congenital absence of both lower leg and foot,** bilateral

✓5th **Q72.3　Congenital** absence of foot and toe(s)

Q72.30　**Congenital absence of unspecified foot and toe(s)**

Q72.31　**Congenital absence of** right **foot and toe(s)**

Q72.32　**Congenital absence of** left **foot and toe(s)**

Q72.33　**Congenital absence of foot and toe(s),** bilateral

✓5th **Q72.4　Longitudinal reduction defect of** femur

Proximal femoral focal deficiency

Q72.40　**Longitudinal reduction defect of unspecified femur**

Q72.41　**Longitudinal reduction defect of** right **femur**

Q72.42　**Longitudinal reduction defect of** left **femur**

Q72.43　**Longitudinal reduction defect of femur,** bilateral

✓5th **Q72.5　Longitudinal reduction defect of** tibia

Q72.50　**Longitudinal reduction defect of unspecified tibia**

Q72.51　**Longitudinal reduction defect of** right **tibia**

Q72.52　**Longitudinal reduction defect of** left **tibia**

Q72.53　**Longitudinal reduction defect of tibia,** bilateral

✓5th **Q72.6　Longitudinal reduction defect of** fibula

Q72.60　**Longitudinal reduction defect of unspecified fibula**

Q72.61　**Longitudinal reduction defect of** right **fibula**

Q72.62　**Longitudinal reduction defect of** left **fibula**

Q72.63　**Longitudinal reduction defect of fibula,** bilateral

✓5th **Q72.7　Split foot**

Q72.70　**Split foot, unspecified lower limb**

Q72.71　**Split foot,** right **lower limb**

Q72.72　**Split foot,** left **lower limb**

Q72.73　**Split foot,** bilateral

✓5th **Q72.8　Other reduction defects of lower limb**

✓6th Q72.81　**Congenital** shortening **of lower limb**

Q72.811　**Congenital shortening of** right **lower limb**

Q72.812　**Congenital shortening of** left **lower limb**

Q72.813　**Congenital shortening of lower limb,** bilateral

Q72.819　**Congenital shortening of unspecified lower limb**

✓6th Q72.89　**Other reduction defects of lower limb**

Q72.891　**Other reduction defects of** right **lower limb**

Q72.892　**Other reduction defects of** left **lower limb**

Q72.893　**Other reduction defects of lower limb,** bilateral

Q72.899　**Other reduction defects of unspecified lower limb**

✓5th **Q72.9　Unspecified reduction defect of lower limb**

Q72.90　**Unspecified reduction defect of unspecified lower limb**

Q72.91　**Unspecified reduction defect of** right **lower limb**

Q72.92　**Unspecified reduction defect of** left **lower limb**

Q72.93　**Unspecified reduction defect of lower limb,** bilateral

☑4ᵗʰ **Q73 Reduction defects of unspecified limb**

Q73.0 Congenital absence of unspecified limb(s)
Amelia NOS

Q73.1 Phocomelia, unspecified limb(s)
Phocomelia NOS

Q73.8 Other reduction defects of unspecified limb(s)
Longitudinal reduction deformity of unspecified limb(s)
Ectromelia of limb NOS
Hemimelia of limb NOS
Reduction defect of limb NOS

☑4ᵗʰ **Q74 Other congenital malformations of limb(s)**

EXCLUDES 1   *polydactyly (Q69.-)*
reduction defect of limb (Q71-Q73)
syndactyly (Q70.-)

Q74.0 Other congenital malformations of upper limb(s), including shoulder girdle
Accessory carpal bones
Cleidocranial dysostosis
Congenital pseudarthrosis of clavicle
Macrodactylia (fingers)
Madelung's deformity
Radioulnar synostosis
Sprengel's deformity
Triphalangeal thumb

Q74.1 Congenital malformation of knee
Congenital absence of patella
Congenital dislocation of patella
Congenital genu valgum
Congenital genu varum
Rudimentary patella
EXCLUDES 1   *congenital dislocation of knee (Q68.2)*
congenital genu recurvatum (Q68.2)
nail patella syndrome (Q87.2)

Q74.2 Other congenital malformations of lower limb(s), including pelvic girdle
Congenital fusion of sacroiliac joint
Congenital malformation of ankle joint
Congenital malformation of sacroiliac joint
EXCLUDES 1   *anteversion of femur (neck) (Q65.89)*

Q74.3 Arthrogryposis multiplex congenita   CC
CC Excl: PDX collection 1102

Q74.8 Other specified congenital malformations of limb(s)

Q74.9 Unspecified congenital malformation of limb(s)
Congenital anomaly of limb(s) NOS

☑4ᵗʰ **Q75 Other congenital malformations of skull and face bones**

EXCLUDES 1   *congenital malformation of face NOS (Q18.-)*
congenital malformation syndromes classified to Q87.-
dentofacial anomalies [including malocclusion] (M26.-)
musculoskeletal deformities of head and face (Q67.0-Q67.4)
skull defects associated with congenital anomalies of brain such as:
anencephaly (Q00.0)
encephalocele (Q01.-)
hydrocephalus (Q03.-)
microcephaly (Q02)

Q75.0 Craniosynostosis
Acrocephaly
Imperfect fusion of skull
Oxycephaly
Trigonocephaly
DEF: Congenital condition in which one or more of the cranial sutures fuse prematurely, creating a deformed or aberrant head shape.

Q75.1 Craniofacial dysostosis
Crouzon's disease

Q75.2 Hypertelorism

Q75.3 Macrocephaly

Q75.4 Mandibulofacial dysostosis
Franceschetti syndrome
Treacher Collins syndrome

Q75.5 Oculomandibular dysostosis

Q75.8 Other specified congenital malformations of skull and face bones
Absence of skull bone, congenital
Congenital deformity of forehead
Platybasia

Q75.9 Congenital malformation of skull and face bones, unspecified
Congenital anomaly of face bones NOS
Congenital anomaly of skull NOS

☑4ᵗʰ **Q76 Congenital malformations of spine and bony thorax**

EXCLUDES 1   *congenital musculoskeletal deformities of spine and chest (Q67.5-Q67.8)*

Q76.0 Spina bifida occulta
EXCLUDES 1   *meningocele (spinal) (Q05.-)*
spina bifida (aperta) (cystica) (Q05.-)

Q76.1 Klippel-Feil syndrome
Cervical fusion syndrome

Q76.2 Congenital spondylolisthesis
Congenital spondylolysis
EXCLUDES 1   *spondylolisthesis (acquired) (M43.1-)*
spondylolysis (acquired) (M43.0-)

Q76.3 Congenital scoliosis due to congenital bony   CC
malformation
Hemivertebra fusion or failure of segmentation with scoliosis
CC Excl: PDX collection 1101

☑5ᵗʰ **Q76.4 Other congenital malformations of spine, not associated with scoliosis**
CC Excl: For CC codes in subcategory Q76.4: PDX collection 1101

☑6ᵗʰ **Q76.41 Congenital kyphosis**

Q76.411 Congenital kyphosis, occipito-atlanto-axial region

Q76.412 Congenital kyphosis, cervical region

Q76.413 Congenital kyphosis, cervicothoracic region

Q76.414 Congenital kyphosis, thoracic region

Q76.415 Congenital kyphosis, thoracolumbar region

Q76.419 Congenital kyphosis, unspecified region

☑6ᵗʰ **Q76.42 Congenital lordosis**

Q76.425 Congenital lordosis, thoracolumbar region   CC

Q76.426 Congenital lordosis, lumbar region   CC

Q76.427 Congenital lordosis, lumbosacral region   CC

Q76.428 Congenital lordosis, sacral and sacrococcygeal region   CC

Q76.429 Congenital lordosis, unspecified region   CC

Q76.49 Other congenital malformations of spine, not associated with scoliosis
Congenital absence of vertebra NOS
Congenital fusion of spine NOS
Congenital malformation of lumbosacral (joint) (region) NOS
Congenital malformation of spine NOS
Hemivertebra NOS
Malformation of spine NOS
Platyspondylisis NOS
Supernumerary vertebra NOS

Q76.5 Cervical rib
Supernumerary rib in cervical region

Q76.6 Other congenital malformations of ribs   CC
Accessory rib
Congenital absence of rib
Congenital fusion of ribs
Congenital malformation of ribs NOS
EXCLUDES 1   *short rib syndrome (Q77.2)*
CC Excl: PDX collection 1103

Q76.7 Congenital malformation of sternum   CC
Congenital absence of sternum
Sternum bifidum
CC Excl: PDX collection 1103

Q76.8 Other congenital malformations of bony thorax   CC
CC Excl: PDX collection 1103

Q76.9 Congenital malformation of bony thorax, unspecified `CC`
   CC Excl: PDX collection 1103

✔4ᵗʰ **Q77 Osteochondrodysplasia with defects of growth of tubular bones and spine**
   EXCLUDES 1   *mucopolysaccharidosis (E76.0-E76.3)*
   EXCLUDES 2   *congenital myotonic chondrodystrophy (G71.13)*

Q77.0 Achondrogenesis
   Hypochondrogenesis

Q77.1 Thanatophoric short stature

Q77.2 Short rib syndrome `CC`
   Asphyxiating thoracic dysplasia [Jeune]
   CC Excl: PDX collection 1103

Q77.3 Chondrodysplasia punctata
   EXCLUDES 1   *Rhizomelic chondrodysplasia punctata (E71.43)*

Q77.4 Achondroplasia
   Hypochondroplasia
   Osteosclerosis congenita

Q77.5 Diastrophic dysplasia

Q77.6 Chondroectodermal dysplasia
   Ellis-van Creveld syndrome

Q77.7 Spondyloepiphyseal dysplasia

Q77.8 Other osteochondrodysplasia with defects of growth of tubular bones and spine

Q77.9 Osteochondrodysplasia with defects of growth of tubular bones and spine, unspecified

✔4ᵗʰ **Q78 Other osteochondrodysplasias**
   EXCLUDES 2   *congenital myotonic chondrodystrophy (G71.13)*

Q78.0 Osteogenesis imperfecta `CC`
   Fragilitas ossium
   Osteopsathyrosis
   CC Excl: PDX collection 1104

Q78.1 Polyostotic fibrous dysplasia
   Albright(-McCune)(-Sternberg) syndrome

Q78.2 Osteopetrosis `CC`
   Albers-Schönberg syndrome
   Osteosclerosis NOS
   DEF: Rare congenital condition in which the bones are excessively dense, resulting from a discrepancy in the formation and breakdown of bone.
   CC Excl: PDX collection 1104

Q78.3 Progressive diaphyseal dysplasia
   Camurati-Engelmann syndrome

Q78.4 Enchondromatosis
   Maffucci's syndrome
   Ollier's disease

Q78.5 Metaphyseal dysplasia
   Pyle's syndrome

Q78.6 Multiple congenital exostoses
   Diaphyseal aclasis

Q78.8 Other specified osteochondrodysplasias
   Osteopoikilosis

Q78.9 Osteochondrodysplasia, unspecified
   Chondrodystrophy NOS
   Osteodystrophy NOS

✔4ᵗʰ **Q79 Congenital malformations of musculoskeletal system, not elsewhere classified**
   EXCLUDES 2   *congenital (sternomastoid) torticollis (Q68.0)*
   CC Excl: For MCC codes in category Q79, unless otherwise noted: PDX collection 1106

Q79.0 Congenital diaphragmatic hernia `MCC`
   EXCLUDES 1   *congenital hiatus hernia (Q40.1)*
   CC Excl: PDX collection 1105

Q79.1 Other congenital malformations of diaphragm `MCC`
   Absence of diaphragm
   Congenital malformation of diaphragm NOS
   Eventration of diaphragm
   CC Excl: PDX collection 1105

Q79.2 Exomphalos `MCC`
   Omphalocele
   EXCLUDES 1   *umbilical hernia (K42.-)*

Q79.3 Gastroschisis `MCC`

Gastroschisis

Herniated small bowel (gastroschisis)

Rectus abdominus m.

Umbilicus

skin

distal

proximal

Defect

Q79.4 Prune belly syndrome `CC`
   Congenital prolapse of bladder mucosa
   Eagle-Barrett syndrome

✔5ᵗʰ **Q79.5 Other congenital malformations of abdominal wall**
   EXCLUDES 1   *umbilical hernia (K42.-)*

Q79.51 Congenital hernia of bladder `CC`

Q79.59 Other congenital malformations of abdominal wall `CC`

▲ ✔5ᵗʰ **Q79.6 Ehlers-Danlos syndromes**
   DEF: Connective tissue disorder that causes hyperextended skin and joints and results in fragile blood vessels with bleeding, poor wound healing, and subcutaneous pseudotumors.

● **Q79.60 Ehlers-Danlos syndrome, unspecified**

● **Q79.61 Classical Ehlers-Danlos syndrome**
   Classical EDS (cEDS)

● **Q79.62 Hypermobile Ehlers-Danlos syndrome**
   Hypermobile EDS (hEDS)

● **Q79.63 Vascular Ehlers-Danlos syndrome**
   Vascular EDS (vEDS)

● **Q79.69 Other Ehlers-Danlos syndromes**

Q79.8 Other congenital malformations of musculoskeletal system
   Absence of muscle
   Absence of tendon
   Accessory muscle
   Amyotrophia congenita
   Congenital constricting bands
   Congenital shortening of tendon
   Poland syndrome

Q79.9 Congenital malformation of musculoskeletal system, unspecified
   Congenital anomaly of musculoskeletal system NOS
   Congenital deformity of musculoskeletal system NOS

Other congenital malformations (Q80-Q89)

✔4ᵗʰ **Q80 Congenital ichthyosis**
   EXCLUDES 1   *Refsum's disease (G60.1)*
   DEF: Excessive production of skin cells resulting in red, dry, scaly skin.

Q80.0 Ichthyosis vulgaris

Q80.1 X-linked ichthyosis

Q80.2 Lamellar ichthyosis
   Collodion baby

Q80.3 Congenital bullous ichthyosiform erythroderma

Q80.4 Harlequin fetus

Q80.8 Other congenital ichthyosis

Q80.9 Congenital ichthyosis, unspecified

✔4ᵗʰ **Q81 Epidermolysis bullosa**

Q81.0 Epidermolysis bullosa simplex
   EXCLUDES 1   *Cockayne's syndrome ▶(Q87.19)◀*

Q81.1 Epidermolysis bullosa letalis
   Herlitz' syndrome

Q81.2 Epidermolysis bullosa dystrophica

Q81.8 Other epidermolysis bullosa

Q81.9 Epidermolysis bullosa, unspecified

✓4ᵗʰ Q82　Other congenital malformations of skin

> **EXCLUDES 1**　acrodermatitis enteropathica (E83.2)
>
> congenital erythropoietic porphyria (E80.0)
>
> pilonidal cyst or sinus (L05.-)
>
> Sturge-Weber (-Dimitri) syndrome (Q85.8)

Q82.0　Hereditary lymphedema

Q82.1　Xeroderma pigmentosum

Q82.2　Congenital cutaneous mastocytosis

　　Congenital diffuse cutaneous mastocytosis

　　Congenital maculopapular cutaneous mastocytosis

　　Congenital urticaria pigmentosa

> **EXCLUDES 1**　cutaneous mastocytosis NOS (D47.01)
>
> diffuse cutaneous mastocytosis (with onset after newborn period) (D47.01)
>
> malignant mastocytosis (C96.2-)
>
> systemic mastocytosis (D47.02)
>
> urticaria pigmentosa (non-congenital) (with onset after newborn period) (D47.01)

　　AHA: 2017,4Q,5

Q82.3　Incontinentia pigmenti

Q82.4　Ectodermal dysplasia (anhidrotic)

> **EXCLUDES 1**　Ellis-van Creveld syndrome (Q77.6)

Q82.5　Congenital non-neoplastic nevus

　　Birthmark NOS

　　Flammeus Nevus

　　Portwine Nevus

　　Sanguineous Nevus

　　Strawberry Nevus

　　Vascular Nevus NOS

　　Verrucous Nevus

> **EXCLUDES 2**　araneus nevus (I78.1)
>
> Café au lait spots (L81.3)
>
> lentigo (L81.4)
>
> melanocytic nevus (D22.-)
>
> nevus NOS (D22.-)
>
> pigmented nevus (D22.-)
>
> spider nevus (I78.1)
>
> stellar nevus (I78.1)

Q82.6　Congenital sacral dimple

　　Parasacral dimple

> **EXCLUDES 2**　pilonidal cyst with abscess (L05.01)
>
> pilonidal cyst without abscess (L05.91)

　　AHA: 2016,4Q,60

Q82.8　Other specified congenital malformations of skin

　　Abnormal palmar creases

　　Accessory skin tags

　　Benign familial pemphigus [Hailey-Hailey]

　　Congenital poikiloderma

　　Cutis laxa (hyperelastica)

　　Dermatoglyphic anomalies

　　Inherited keratosis palmaris et plantaris

　　Keratosis follicularis [Darier-White]

> **EXCLUDES 1**　Ehlers-Danlos syndrome ▶(Q79.6-)◀

　　AHA: 2016,1Q,17

Q82.9　Congenital malformation of skin, unspecified

✓4ᵗʰ Q83　Congenital malformations of breast

> **EXCLUDES 2**　absence of pectoral muscle (Q79.8)
>
> hypoplasia of breast (N64.82)
>
> micromastia (N64.82)

Q83.0　Congenital absence of breast with absent nipple

Q83.1　Accessory breast

　　Supernumerary breast

Q83.2　Absent nipple

Q83.3　Accessory nipple

　　Supernumerary nipple

Q83.8　Other congenital malformations of breast

Q83.9　Congenital malformation of breast, unspecified

✓4ᵗʰ Q84　Other congenital malformations of integument

Q84.0　Congenital alopecia

　　Congenital atrichosis

Q84.1　Congenital morphological disturbances of hair, not elsewhere classified

　　Beaded hair

　　Monilethrix

　　Pili annulati

> **EXCLUDES 1**　Menkes' kinky hair syndrome (E83.0)

Q84.2　Other congenital malformations of hair

　　Congenital hypertrichosis

　　Congenital malformation of hair NOS

　　Persistent lanugo

Q84.3　Anonychia

> **EXCLUDES 1**　nail patella syndrome (Q87.2)

Q84.4　Congenital leukonychia

Q84.5　Enlarged and hypertrophic nails

　　Congenital onychauxis

　　Pachyonychia

Q84.6　Other congenital malformations of nails

　　Congenital clubnail

　　Congenital koilonychia

　　Congenital malformation of nail NOS

Q84.8　Other specified congenital malformations of integument

　　Aplasia cutis congenita

Q84.9　Congenital malformation of integument, unspecified

　　Congenital anomaly of integument NOS

　　Congenital deformity of integument NOS

✓4ᵗʰ Q85　Phakomatoses, not elsewhere classified

> **EXCLUDES 1**　ataxia telangiectasia [Louis-Bar] (G11.3)
>
> familial dysautonomia [Riley-Day] (G90.1)

✓5ᵗʰ Q85.0　Neurofibromatosis (nonmalignant)

　　Q85.00　Neurofibromatosis, unspecified　HCC

　　Q85.01　Neurofibromatosis, type 1　HCC

　　　　Von Recklinghausen disease

　　Q85.02　Neurofibromatosis, type 2　HCC

　　　　Acoustic neurofibromatosis

　　　　DEF: Inherited condition with cutaneous lesions, benign tumors of peripheral nerves, and bilateral 8th nerve masses.

　　Q85.03　Schwannomatosis　HCC

　　　　DEF: Genetic mutation (SMARCB1/INI1) causing multiple benign tumors along the nerve pathways, except on the 8th cranial (vestibular) nerve.

　　Q85.09　Other neurofibromatosis　HCC

Q85.1　Tuberous sclerosis　CC HCC

　　Bourneville's disease

　　Epiloia

　　CC Excl: PDX collection 1108

Q85.8　Other phakomatoses, not elsewhere classified　CC HCC

　　Peutz-Jeghers Syndrome

　　Sturge-Weber(-Dimitri) syndrome

　　von Hippel-Lindau syndrome

> **EXCLUDES 1**　Meckel-Gruber syndrome (Q61.9)

　　CC Excl: PDX collection 1109

Q85.9　Phakomatosis, unspecified　CC HCC

　　Hamartosis NOS

　　CC Excl: PDX collection 1109

✓4ᵗʰ Q86　Congenital malformation syndromes due to known exogenous causes, not elsewhere classified

> **EXCLUDES 2**　iodine-deficiency-related hypothyroidism (E00-E02)
>
> nonteratogenic effects of substances transmitted via placenta or breast milk (P04.-)

Q86.0　Fetal alcohol syndrome (dysmorphic)

Q86.1　Fetal hydantoin syndrome

　　Meadow's syndrome

Q86.2　Dysmorphism due to warfarin

Q86.8　Other congenital malformation syndromes due to known exogenous causes

✓ Additional Character Required　✓x7ᵗʰ Placeholder　Unacceptable PDx　Questionable PDx　Manifestation　Unspecified Dx　H1-H14 HAC　HCC CMS-HCC Dx　HIV HIV Dx

ICD-10-CM 2020

949

Chapter 17. Congenital Malformations, Deformations and Chromosomal Abnormalities

_Q82–Q86.8_

Chapter 17. Congenital Malformations, Deformations and Chromosomal Abnormalities

Q87–Q91.7

☑4ᵗʰ **Q87 Other specified congenital malformation syndromes affecting multiple systems**

Use additional code(s) to identify all associated manifestations

Q87.0 Congenital malformation syndromes predominantly affecting facial appearance

Acrocephalopolysyndactyly

Acrocephalosyndactyly [Apert]

Cryptophthalmos syndrome

Cyclopia

Goldenhar syndrome

Moebius syndrome

Oro-facial-digital syndrome

Robin syndrome

Whistling face

▲ ☑5ᵗʰ **Q87.1 Congenital malformation syndromes predominantly associated with short stature**

~~Aarskog syndrome~~

~~Cockayne syndrome~~

~~De Lange syndrome~~

~~Dubowitz syndrome~~

~~Noonan syndrome~~

~~Prader-Willi syndrome~~

~~Robinow-Silverman-Smith syndrome~~

~~Russell-Silver syndrome~~

~~Seckel syndrome~~

EXCLUDES 1   *Ellis-van Creveld syndrome (Q77.6)*

Smith-Lemli-Opitz syndrome (E78.72)

● **Q87.11 Prader-Willi syndrome**

● **Q87.19 Other congenital malformation syndromes predominantly associated with short stature**

Aarskog syndrome

Cockayne syndrome

De Lange syndrome

Dubowitz syndrome

Noonan syndrome

Robinow-Silverman-Smith syndrome

Russell-Silver syndrome

Seckel syndrome

Q87.2 Congenital malformation syndromes predominantly involving limbs

Holt-Oram syndrome

Klippel-Trenaunay-Weber syndrome

Nail patella syndrome

Rubinstein-Taybi syndrome

Sirenomelia syndrome

Thrombocytopenia with absent radius [TAR] syndrome

VATER syndrome

Q87.3 Congenital malformation syndromes involving early overgrowth

Beckwith-Wiedemann syndrome

Sotos syndrome

Weaver syndrome

☑5ᵗʰ **Q87.4 Marfan's syndrome**

DEF: Disorder that affects the connective tissue of multiple systems, including disproportionally long or abnormal bone structure and eye and cardiovascular complications.

CC Excl: For CC codes in subcategory Q87.4: PDX collection 1110

Q87.40 Marfan's syndrome, unspecified   CC

☑6ᵗʰ **Q87.41 Marfan's syndrome with cardiovascular manifestations**   CC

Q87.410 Marfan's syndrome with aortic dilation   CC

Q87.418 Marfan's syndrome with other cardiovascular manifestations   CC

Q87.42 Marfan's syndrome with ocular manifestations   CC

Q87.43 Marfan's syndrome with skeletal manifestation   CC

Q87.5 Other congenital malformation syndromes with other skeletal changes   CC

CC Excl: PDX collection 540

☑5ᵗʰ **Q87.8 Other specified congenital malformation syndromes, not elsewhere classified**

EXCLUDES 1   *Zellweger syndrome (E71.510)*

Q87.81 Alport syndrome

Use additional code to identify stage of chronic kidney disease (N18.1-N18.6)

Q87.82 Arterial tortuosity syndrome

AHA: 2016,4Q,60-61

Q87.89 Other specified congenital malformation syndromes, not elsewhere classified

Laurence-Moon (-Bardet)-Biedl syndrome

☑4ᵗʰ **Q89 Other congenital malformations, not elsewhere classified**

☑5ᵗʰ **Q89.0 Congenital absence and malformations of spleen**

EXCLUDES 1   *isomerism of atrial appendages (with asplenia or polysplenia) (Q20.6)*

Q89.01 Asplenia (congenital)

Q89.09 Congenital malformations of spleen

Congenital splenomegaly

Q89.1 Congenital malformations of adrenal gland

EXCLUDES 1   *adrenogenital disorders (E25.-)*

congenital adrenal hyperplasia (E25.0)

Q89.2 Congenital malformations of other endocrine glands

Congenital malformation of parathyroid or thyroid gland

Persistent thyroglossal duct

Thyroglossal cyst

EXCLUDES 1   *congenital goiter (E03.0)*

congenital hypothyroidism (E03.1)

Q89.3 Situs inversus

Dextrocardia with situs inversus

Mirror-image atrial arrangement with situs inversus

Situs inversus or transversus abdominalis

Situs inversus or transversus thoracis

Transposition of abdominal viscera

Transposition of thoracic viscera

EXCLUDES 1   *dextrocardia NOS (Q24.0)*

DEF: Congenital anomaly in which the internal thoracic and abdominal organs are transposed laterally and found on the opposite side from the normal position.

Q89.4 Conjoined twins   MCC

Craniopagus

Dicephaly

Pygopagus

Thoracopagus

CC Excl: PDX collection 1113

Q89.7 Multiple congenital malformations, not elsewhere classified

Multiple congenital anomalies NOS

Multiple congenital deformities NOS

EXCLUDES 1   *congenital malformation syndromes affecting multiple systems (Q87.-)*

Q89.8 Other specified congenital malformations

Use additional code(s) to identify all associated manifestations

Q89.9 Congenital malformation, unspecified

Congenital anomaly NOS

Congenital deformity NOS

Chromosomal abnormalities, not elsewhere classified (Q90-Q99)

EXCLUDES 2   *mitochondrial metabolic disorders (E88.4-)*

☑4ᵗʰ **Q90 Down syndrome**

Use additional code(s) to identify any associated physical conditions and degree of intellectual disabilities (F70-F79)

Q90.0 Trisomy 21, nonmosaicism (meiotic nondisjunction)

Q90.1 Trisomy 21, mosaicism (mitotic nondisjunction)

Q90.2 Trisomy 21, translocation

Q90.9 Down syndrome, unspecified

Trisomy 21 NOS

☑4ᵗʰ **Q91 Trisomy 18 and Trisomy 13**

Q91.0 Trisomy 18, nonmosaicism (meiotic nondisjunction)

Q91.1 Trisomy 18, mosaicism (mitotic nondisjunction)

Q91.2 Trisomy 18, translocation

Q91.3 Trisomy 18, unspecified

Q91.4 Trisomy 13, nonmosaicism (meiotic nondisjunction)

Q91.5 Trisomy 13, mosaicism (mitotic nondisjunction)

Q91.6 Trisomy 13, translocation

Q91.7 Trisomy 13, unspecified

N Newborn: 0   P Pediatric: 0-17   M Maternity: 9-64   A Adult: 15-124   MCC Major Complication/Comorbidity   CC Complication/Comorbidity   SW Severe Wound Dx

950   ICD-10-CM 2020

☑4ᵗʰ **Q92** **Other trisomies and partial trisomies of the autosomes, not elsewhere classified**

    INCLUDES unbalanced translocations and insertions

    EXCLUDES 1 *trisomies of chromosomes 13, 18, 21 (Q90-Q91)*

    Q92.0 **Whole chromosome trisomy, nonmosaicism (meiotic nondisjunction)**

    Q92.1 **Whole chromosome trisomy, mosaicism (mitotic nondisjunction)**

    Q92.2 **Partial trisomy**

        Less than whole arm duplicated

        Whole arm or more duplicated

        EXCLUDES 1 *partial trisomy due to unbalanced translocation (Q92.5)*

    Q92.5 **Duplications with other complex rearrangements**

        Partial trisomy due to unbalanced translocations

        Code also any associated deletions due to unbalanced translocations, inversions and insertions (Q93.7)

    ☑5ᵗʰ **Q92.6** **Marker chromosomes**

        Trisomies due to dicentrics

        Trisomies due to extra rings

        Trisomies due to isochromosomes

        Individual with marker heterochromatin

        Q92.61 **Marker chromosomes in normal individual**

        Q92.62 **Marker chromosomes in abnormal individual**

    Q92.7 **Triploidy and polyploidy**

    Q92.8 **Other specified trisomies and partial trisomies of autosomes**

        Duplications identified by fluorescence in situ hybridization (FISH)

        Duplications identified by in situ hybridization (ISH)

        Duplications seen only at prometaphase

    Q92.9 **Trisomy and partial trisomy of autosomes, unspecified**

☑4ᵗʰ **Q93** **Monosomies and deletions from the autosomes, not elsewhere classified**

    Q93.0 **Whole chromosome monosomy, nonmosaicism (meiotic nondisjunction)**

    Q93.1 **Whole chromosome monosomy, mosaicism (mitotic nondisjunction)**

    Q93.2 **Chromosome replaced with ring, dicentric or isochromosome**

    Q93.3 **Deletion of short arm of chromosome 4**

        Wolff-Hirschorn syndrome

    Q93.4 **Deletion of short arm of chromosome 5**

        Cri-du-chat syndrome

    ☑5ᵗʰ **Q93.5** **Other deletions of part of a chromosome**

        AHA: 2018,4Q,28

        Q93.51 **Angelman syndrome** `CC`

            CC Excl: PDX collection 1114

        Q93.59 **Other deletions of part of a chromosome** `CC`

            CC Excl: PDX collection 1114

    Q93.7 **Deletions with other complex rearrangements**

        Deletions due to unbalanced translocations, inversions and insertions

        Code also any associated duplications due to unbalanced translocations, inversions and insertions (Q92.5)

    ☑6ᵗʰ **Q93.8** **Other deletions from the autosomes**

        Q93.81 **Velo-cardio-facial syndrome** `CC`

            Deletion 22q11.2

            DEF: Microdeletion syndrome affecting multiple organs characterized by a cleft palate, heart defects, an elongated face with almond-shaped eyes, wide nose, small ears, weak immune system, weak musculature, hypothyroidism, short stature, and scoliosis. The deletion occurs at q11.2 on the long arm of the chromosome 22.

        Q93.82 **Williams syndrome** `CC`

            AHA: 2018,4Q,28-29

            CC Excl: PDX collection 1114

        Q93.88 **Other microdeletions** `CC`

            Miller-Dieker syndrome

            Smith-Magenis syndrome

            CC Excl: PDX collection 1118

        Q93.89 **Other deletions from the autosomes** `CC`

            Deletions identified by fluorescence in situ hybridization (FISH)

            Deletions identified by in situ hybridization (ISH)

            Deletions seen only at prometaphase

            CC Excl: PDX collection 1115

    Q93.9 **Deletion from autosomes, unspecified** `CC`

        CC Excl: PDX collection 1115

☑4ᵗʰ **Q95** **Balanced rearrangements and structural markers, not elsewhere classified**

    INCLUDES Robertsonian and balanced reciprocal translocations and insertions

    Q95.0 **Balanced translocation and insertion in normal individual**

    Q95.1 **Chromosome inversion in normal individual**

    Q95.2 **Balanced autosomal rearrangement in abnormal individual**

    Q95.3 **Balanced sex/autosomal rearrangement in abnormal individual**

    Q95.5 **Individual with autosomal fragile site**

    Q95.8 **Other balanced rearrangements and structural markers**

    Q95.9 **Balanced rearrangement and structural marker, unspecified**

☑4ᵗʰ **Q96** **Turner's syndrome**

    EXCLUDES 1 *Noonan syndrome ▶(Q87.19)◀*

    Q96.0 **Karyotype 45, X** ♀

    Q96.1 **Karyotype 46, X iso (Xq)** ♀

        Karyotype 46, isochromosome Xq

    Q96.2 **Karyotype 46, X with abnormal sex chromosome, except iso (Xq)** ♀

        Karyotype 46, X with abnormal sex chromosome, except isochromosome Xq

    Q96.3 **Mosaicism, 45, X/46, XX or XY** ♀

    Q96.4 **Mosaicism, 45, X/other cell line(s) with abnormal sex chromosome** ♀

    Q96.8 **Other variants of Turner's syndrome** ♀

    Q96.9 **Turner's syndrome, unspecified** ♀

☑4ᵗʰ **Q97** **Other sex chromosome abnormalities, female phenotype, not elsewhere classified**

    EXCLUDES 1 *Turner's syndrome (Q96.-)*

    Q97.0 **Karyotype 47, XXX** ♀

    Q97.1 **Female with more than three X chromosomes** ♀

    Q97.2 **Mosaicism, lines with various numbers of X chromosomes** ♀

    Q97.3 **Female with 46, XY karyotype** ♀

    Q97.8 **Other specified sex chromosome abnormalities, female phenotype** ♀

    Q97.9 **Sex chromosome abnormality, female phenotype, unspecified** ♀

☑4ᵗʰ **Q98** **Other sex chromosome abnormalities, male phenotype, not elsewhere classified**

    Q98.0 **Klinefelter syndrome karyotype 47, XXY** ♂

    Q98.1 **Klinefelter syndrome, male with more than two X chromosomes** ♂

    Q98.3 **Other male with 46, XX karyotype** ♂

    Q98.4 **Klinefelter syndrome, unspecified** ♂

    Q98.5 **Karyotype 47, XYY**

    Q98.6 **Male with structurally abnormal sex chromosome**

    Q98.7 **Male with sex chromosome mosaicism** ♂

    Q98.8 **Other specified sex chromosome abnormalities, male phenotype** ♂

    Q98.9 **Sex chromosome abnormality, male phenotype, unspecified** ♂

☑4ᵗʰ **Q99** **Other chromosome abnormalities, not elsewhere classified**

    Q99.0 **Chimera 46, XX/46, XY**

        Chimera 46, XX/46, XY true hermaphrodite

    Q99.1 **46, XX true hermaphrodite**

        46, XX with streak gonads

        46, XY with streak gonads

        Pure gonadal dysgenesis

    Q99.2 **Fragile X chromosome**

        Fragile X syndrome

    Q99.8 **Other specified chromosome abnormalities**

    Q99.9 **Chromosomal abnormality, unspecified**

☑ Additional Character Required   ☑7ᵗʰ Placeholder   Unacceptable PDx   Questionable PDx   Manifestation   Unspecified Dx   H1-H14 HAC   HCC CMS-HCC Dx   HIV HIV Dx

ICD-10-CM 2020

951

Chapter 18. Symptoms, Signs and Abnormal Clinical and Laboratory Findings, Not Elsewhere Classified (RØØ–R99)

Chapter-specific Guidelines with Coding Examples

The chapter-specific guidelines from the ICD-10-CM Official Guidelines for Coding and Reporting have been provided below. Along with these guidelines are coding examples, contained in the shaded boxes, that have been developed to help illustrate the coding and/or sequencing guidance found in these guidelines.

Chapter 18 includes symptoms, signs, abnormal results of clinical or other investigative procedures, and ill-defined conditions regarding which no diagnosis classifiable elsewhere is recorded. Signs and symptoms that point to a specific diagnosis have been assigned to a category in other chapters of the classification.

a. Use of symptom codes

Codes that describe symptoms and signs are acceptable for reporting purposes when a related definitive diagnosis has not been established (confirmed) by the provider.

Chest pain of unknown origin

RØ7.9   Chest pain, unspecified

Explanation: Codes that describe symptoms such as chest pain are acceptable for reporting purposes when the provider has not established (confirmed) a related definitive diagnosis.

---

b. Use of a symptom code with a definitive diagnosis code

Codes for signs and symptoms may be reported in addition to a related definitive diagnosis when the sign or symptom is not routinely associated with that diagnosis, such as the various signs and symptoms associated with complex syndromes. The definitive diagnosis code should be sequenced before the symptom code.

Signs or symptoms that are associated routinely with a disease process should not be assigned as additional codes, unless otherwise instructed by the classification.

Pneumonia with hemoptysis

J18.9   Pneumonia, unspecified organism

RØ4.2   Hemoptysis

Explanation: Codes for signs and symptoms may be reported in addition to a related definitive diagnosis when the sign or symptom is not routinely associated with that diagnosis.

Abdominal pain due to acute appendicitis

K35.8Ø   Unspecified acute appendicitis

Explanation: Codes for signs or symptoms routinely associated with a disease process should not be assigned unless the classification instructs otherwise.

---

c. Combination codes that include symptoms

ICD-10-CM contains a number of combination codes that identify both the definitive diagnosis and common symptoms of that diagnosis. When using one of these combination codes, an additional code should not be assigned for the symptom.

Acute gastritis with hemorrhage

K29.Ø1   Acute gastritis with bleeding

Explanation: When a combination code identifies both the definitive diagnosis and the symptom, an additional code should not be assigned for the symptom.

---

d. Repeated falls

Code R29.6, Repeated falls, is for use for encounters when a patient has recently fallen and the reason for the fall is being investigated.

Code Z91.81, History of falling, is for use when a patient has fallen in the past and is at risk for future falls. When appropriate, both codes R29.6 and Z91.81 may be assigned together.

e. Coma scale

The coma scale codes (R4Ø.2-) can be used in conjunction with traumatic brain injury codes, acute cerebrovascular disease or sequelae of cerebrovascular disease codes. These codes are primarily for use by trauma registries, but they may be used in any setting where this information is collected. The coma scale may also be used to assess the status of the central nervous system for other non-trauma conditions, such as monitoring patients in the intensive care unit regardless of medical condition. The coma scale codes should be sequenced after the diagnosis code(s).

These codes, one from each subcategory, are needed to complete the scale. The 7th character indicates when the scale was recorded. The 7th character should match for all three codes.

At a minimum, report the initial score documented on presentation at your facility. This may be a score from the emergency medicine technician (EMT) or in the emergency department. If desired, a facility may choose to capture multiple coma scale scores.

Assign code R4Ø.24, Glasgow coma scale, total score, when only the total score is documented in the medical record and not the individual score(s).

Do not report codes for individual or total Glasgow coma scale scores for a patient with a medically induced coma or a sedated patient.

See Section I.B.14 for coma scale documentation by clinicians other than patient's provider

---

23-year-old man found down after unknown injury with skull fracture and with concussion and loss of consciousness of unknown duration. EMS evaluated the patient in the field and reported the individual Glasgow coma scores:

Eye opening response—3: eyes open to speech

Verbal response—4: confused but coherent speech

Motor response—6: obeys commands fully

SØ2.ØXXA   Fracture of vault of skull, initial encounter for closed fracture

SØ6.ØX9A   Concussion with loss of consciousness of unspecified duration, initial encounter

R4Ø.2131   Coma scale, eyes open, to sound, in the field [EMT or ambulance]

R4Ø.2241   Coma scale, best verbal response, confused conversation, in the field [EMT or ambulance]

R4Ø.2361   Coma scale, best motor response, obeys commands, in the field [EMT or ambulance]

Explanation: When individual scores for the Glasgow coma scale are documented, one code from each category is needed to complete the scale. The seventh character indicates when the scale was recorded and should match for all three codes. Assign a code from subcategory R4Ø.24- Glasgow coma scale, total score, when only the total and not the individual score(s) is documented.

Patient with intractable epilepsy with status epilepticus arrives to ED with alteration of consciousness. Coma scale performed en route by EMT documented total coma score as 11. Another coma score was performed upon hospital admission that was documented as 14.

G4Ø.911   Epilepsy, unspecified, intractable, with status epilepticus

R4Ø.2421   Glasgow coma scale score 9-12, in the field [EMT or ambulance]

R4Ø.2413   Glasgow coma scale score 13-15, at hospital admission

Explanation: Coma scores may be used to assess mental status in non-trauma conditions. Use only code R4Ø.24- Glasgow coma scale, total scores when individual scores are unavailable. Multiple scores may be reported with the seventh character representing where or when the assessment was made.

---

f. Functional quadriplegia

GUIDELINE HAS BEEN DELETED EFFECTIVE OCTOBER 1, 2Ø17

g.   SIRS due to non-infectious process

The systemic inflammatory response syndrome (SIRS) can develop as a result of certain non-infectious disease processes, such as trauma, malignant neoplasm, or pancreatitis. When SIRS is documented with a noninfectious condition, and no subsequent infection is documented, the code for the underlying condition, such as an injury, should be assigned, followed by code R65.10, Systemic inflammatory response syndrome (SIRS) of non-infectious origin without acute organ dysfunction, or code R65.11, Systemic inflammatory response syndrome (SIRS) of non-infectious origin with acute organ dysfunction. If an associated acute organ dysfunction is documented, the appropriate code(s) for the specific type of organ dysfunction(s) should be assigned in addition to code R65.11. If acute organ dysfunction is documented, but it cannot be determined if the acute organ dysfunction is associated with SIRS or due to another condition (e.g., directly due to the trauma), the provider should be queried.

Systemic inflammatory response syndrome (SIRS) due to acute gallstone pancreatitis

K85.10   Biliary acute pancreatitis without necrosis or infection

R65.10   Systemic inflammatory response syndrome [SIRS] of non-infectious origin without acute organ dysfunction

Explanation: When SIRS is documented with a non-infectious condition without subsequent infection documented, the code for the underlying condition such as pancreatitis should be assigned followed by the appropriate code for SIRS of noninfectious origin, either with or without associated organ dysfunction.

h.   Death NOS

Code R99, Ill-defined and unknown cause of mortality, is only for use in the very limited circumstance when a patient who has already died is brought into an emergency department or other healthcare facility and is pronounced dead upon arrival. It does not represent the discharge disposition of death.

i.   NIHSS stroke scale

The NIH stroke scale (NIHSS) codes (R29.7- -) can be used in conjunction with acute stroke codes (I63) to identify the patient's neurological status and the severity of the stroke. The stroke scale codes should be sequenced after the acute stroke diagnosis code(s).

At a minimum, report the initial score documented. If desired, a facility may choose to capture multiple stroke scale scores.

See Section I.B.14 for NIHSS stroke scale documentation by clinicians other than patient's provider

Patient admitted with CVA seen by neurology consult who documents moderate to severe stroke, 17 on NIHSS stroke scale.

I63.9   Cerebral infarction, unspecified

R29.717   NIHSS score 17

Explanation: Unspecified cerebral vascular accident (CVA) is sequenced before the NIHSS stroke scale score code. The stroke scale is an assessment tool to help measure stroke-related neurological deficits. Fifteen items are evaluated by trained observers and include such conditions as levels of consciousness, language, dysarthria, ataxia, and sensory loss. A facility may report multiple stroke scale scores if it wants to.

Chapter 18. Symptoms, Signs and Abnormal Clinical and Laboratory Findings, Not Elsewhere Classified (R00-R99)

NOTE This chapter includes symptoms, signs, abnormal results of clinical or other investigative procedures, and ill-defined conditions regarding which no diagnosis classifiable elsewhere is recorded.

Signs and symptoms that point rather definitely to a given diagnosis have been assigned to a category in other chapters of the classification. In general, categories in this chapter include the less well-defined conditions and symptoms that, without the necessary study of the case to establish a final diagnosis, point perhaps equally to two or more diseases or to two or more systems of the body. Practically all categories in the chapter could be designated 'not otherwise specified', 'unknown etiology' or 'transient'. The Alphabetical Index should be consulted to determine which symptoms and signs are to be allocated here and which to other chapters. The residual subcategories, numbered .8, are generally provided for other relevant symptoms that cannot be allocated elsewhere in the classification.

The conditions and signs or symptoms included in categories R00-R94 consist of:

(a) cases for which no more specific diagnosis can be made even after all the facts bearing on the case have been investigated;

(b) signs or symptoms existing at the time of initial encounter that proved to be transient and whose causes could not be determined;

(c) provisional diagnosis in a patient who failed to return for further investigation or care;

(d) cases referred elsewhere for investigation or treatment before the diagnosis was made;

(e) cases in which a more precise diagnosis was not available for any other reason;

(f) certain symptoms, for which supplementary information is provided, that represent important problems in medical care in their own right.

EXCLUDES 2 *abnormal findings on antenatal screening of mother (O28.-)*
certain conditions originating in the perinatal period (P04-P96)
signs and symptoms classified in the body system chapters
signs and symptoms of breast (N63, N64.5)

AHA: 2017,1Q,6,7

This chapter contains the following blocks:

R00-R09   Symptoms and signs involving the circulatory and respiratory systems
R10-R19   Symptoms and signs involving the digestive system and abdomen
R20-R23   Symptoms and signs involving the skin and subcutaneous tissue
R25-R29   Symptoms and signs involving the nervous and musculoskeletal systems
R30-R39   Symptoms and signs involving the genitourinary system
R40-R46   Symptoms and signs involving cognition, perception, emotional state and behavior
R47-R49   Symptoms and signs involving speech and voice
R50-R69   General symptoms and signs
R70-R79   Abnormal findings on examination of blood, without diagnosis
R80-R82   Abnormal findings on examination of urine, without diagnosis
R83-R89   Abnormal findings on examination of other body fluids, substances and tissues, without diagnosis
R90-R94   Abnormal findings on diagnostic imaging and in function studies, without diagnosis
R97   Abnormal tumor markers
R99   Ill-defined and unknown cause of mortality

Symptoms and signs involving the circulatory and respiratory systems (R00-R09)

☑4ᵗʰ R00 Abnormalities of heart beat

EXCLUDES 1 *abnormalities originating in the perinatal period (P29.1-)*
EXCLUDES 2 *specified arrhythmias (I47-I49)*

R00.0 Tachycardia, unspecified
Rapid heart beat
Sinoauricular tachycardia NOS
Sinus [sinusal] tachycardia NOS

EXCLUDES 1 *neonatal tachycardia (P29.11)*
paroxysmal tachycardia (I47.-)

DEF: Excessively rapid heart rate of more than 100 beats per minute.

R00.1 Bradycardia, unspecified
Sinoatrial bradycardia
Sinus bradycardia
Slow heart beat
Vagal bradycardia
Use additional code for adverse effect, if applicable, to identify drug (T36-T50 with fifth or sixth character 5)

EXCLUDES 1 *neonatal bradycardia (P29.12)*

DEF: Slowed heartbeat, usually defined as a rate fewer than 60 beats per minute. Heart rhythm may be slow as a result of a congenital defect or an acquired problem.

R00.2 Palpitations
Awareness of heart beat

R00.8 Other abnormalities of heart beat

R00.9 Unspecified abnormalities of heart beat

☑4ᵗʰ R01 Cardiac murmurs and other cardiac sounds

EXCLUDES 1 *cardiac murmurs and sounds originating in the perinatal period (P29.8)*

R01.0 Benign and innocent cardiac murmurs
Functional cardiac murmur

R01.1 Cardiac murmur, unspecified
Cardiac bruit NOS
Heart murmur NOS
Systolic murmur NOS

R01.2 Other cardiac sounds
Cardiac dullness, increased or decreased
Precordial friction

☑4ᵗʰ R03 Abnormal blood-pressure reading, without diagnosis

R03.0 Elevated blood-pressure reading, without diagnosis of hypertension

NOTE This category is to be used to record an episode of elevated blood pressure in a patient in whom no formal diagnosis of hypertension has been made, or as an isolated incidental finding.

R03.1 Nonspecific low blood-pressure reading

EXCLUDES 1 *hypotension (I95.-)*
maternal hypotension syndrome (O26.5-)
neurogenic orthostatic hypotension (G90.3)

☑4ᵗʰ R04 Hemorrhage from respiratory passages

CC Excl: For CC codes in category R04: PDX collection 1119

R04.0 Epistaxis   **CC**
Hemorrhage from nose
Nosebleed

R04.1 Hemorrhage from throat   **CC**
EXCLUDES 2 *hemoptysis (R04.2)*

R04.2 Hemoptysis   **CC**
Blood-stained sputum
Cough with hemorrhage
AHA: 2013,4Q,118

☑5ᵗʰ R04.8 Hemorrhage from other sites in respiratory passages

R04.81 Acute idiopathic pulmonary hemorrhage in infants   **CC P**
AIPHI
Acute idiopathic hemorrhage in infants over 28 days old
EXCLUDES 1 *perinatal pulmonary hemorrhage (P26.-)*
von Willebrand's disease (D68.0)

R04.89 Hemorrhage from other sites in respiratory passages   **CC**
Pulmonary hemorrhage NOS

R04.9 Hemorrhage from respiratory passages, unspecified   **CC**

R05 Cough
EXCLUDES 1 *cough with hemorrhage (R04.2)*
smoker's cough (J41.0)
AHA: 2016,2Q,33

Chapter 18. Symptoms, Signs and Abnormal Clinical and Laboratory Findings

R06–R09.89

☑4ᵗʰ **R06 Abnormalities of breathing**

     EXCLUDES 1   *acute respiratory distress syndrome (J80)*
            respiratory arrest (R09.2)
            respiratory arrest of newborn (P28.81)
            respiratory distress syndrome of newborn (P22.-)
            respiratory failure (J96.-)
            respiratory failure of newborn (P28.5)

☑5ᵗʰ **R06.0 Dyspnea**

     EXCLUDES 1   *tachypnea NOS (R06.82)*
            transient tachypnea of newborn (P22.1)

     R06.00 Dyspnea, unspecified
         AHA: 2017,1Q,26

     R06.01 Orthopnea

     R06.02 Shortness of breath

     R06.03 Acute respiratory distress
         AHA: 2017,4Q,23

     R06.09 Other forms of dyspnea

R06.1 Stridor

     EXCLUDES 1   *congenital laryngeal stridor (P28.89)*
            laryngismus (stridulus) (J38.5)

     DEF: Certain type of wheezing described as a loud, constant, musical sound produced when breathing with an obstructed airway, like the inspiratory sound heard when laryngeal or esophageal obstruction is present.

R06.2 Wheezing

     EXCLUDES 1   *asthma (J45.-)*

     AHA: 2016,2Q,33
     DEF: High-pitched whistling sound during breathing due to stenosis of the respiratory passageway. Wheezing is associated with asthma, sleep apnea, bronchiectasis, bronchiolitis, COPD, and pleural effusion.

R06.3 Periodic breathing   CC

     Cheyne-Stokes breathing
     CC Excl: PDX collection 1120

R06.4 Hyperventilation

     EXCLUDES 1   *psychogenic hyperventilation (F45.8)*

R06.5 Mouth breathing

     EXCLUDES 2   *dry mouth NOS (R68.2)*

R06.6 Hiccough

     EXCLUDES 1   *psychogenic hiccough (F45.8)*

R06.7 Sneezing

☑5ᵗʰ **R06.8 Other abnormalities of breathing**

     R06.81 Apnea, not elsewhere classified
         Apnea NOS
         EXCLUDES 1   *apnea (of) newborn (P28.4)*
                sleep apnea (G47.3-)
                sleep apnea of newborn (primary) (P28.3)

     R06.82 Tachypnea, not elsewhere classified
         Tachypnea NOS
         EXCLUDES 1   *transitory tachypnea of newborn (P22.1)*

     R06.83 Snoring

     R06.89 Other abnormalities of breathing
         Breath-holding (spells)
         Sighing

     R06.9 Unspecified abnormalities of breathing

☑4ᵗʰ **R07 Pain in throat and chest**

     EXCLUDES 1   *epidemic myalgia (B33.0)*
     EXCLUDES 2   *jaw pain R68.84*
            pain in breast (N64.4)

R07.0 Pain in throat

     EXCLUDES 1   *chronic sore throat (J31.2)*
            sore throat (acute) NOS (J02.9)
     EXCLUDES 2   *dysphagia (R13.1-)*
            pain in neck (M54.2)

R07.1 Chest pain on breathing
     Painful respiration

R07.2 Precordial pain
     DEF: Pain felt in the anterior (front) chest wall over the region of the heart. This type of pain is generally felt slightly to the left of the sternum, but may also extend into the surrounding chest wall region.

☑5ᵗʰ **R07.8 Other chest pain**

     R07.81 Pleurodynia
         Pleurodynia NOS
         EXCLUDES 1   *epidemic pleurodynia (B33.0)*

     R07.82 Intercostal pain

     R07.89 Other chest pain
         Anterior chest-wall pain NOS

     R07.9 Chest pain, unspecified

☑4ᵗʰ **R09 Other symptoms and signs involving the circulatory and respiratory system**

     EXCLUDES 1   *acute respiratory distress syndrome (J80)*
            respiratory arrest of newborn (P28.81)
            respiratory distress syndrome of newborn (P22.0)
            respiratory failure (J96.-)
            respiratory failure of newborn (P28.5)

☑5ᵗʰ **R09.0 Asphyxia and hypoxemia**

     EXCLUDES 1   *asphyxia due to carbon monoxide (T58.-)*
            asphyxia due to foreign body in respiratory tract (T17.-)
            birth (intrauterine) asphyxia (P84)
            hyperventilation (R06.4)
            traumatic asphyxia (T71.-)
     EXCLUDES 2   *hypercapnia (R06.89)*

     R09.01 Asphyxia   CC
         DEF: Interference of oxygen intake due to obstruction or injury of airways resulting in a lack of oxygen perfusion to the tissues or excessive carbon dioxide in the blood. Can cause unconsciousness or death.
         CC Excl: PDX collection 1121

     R09.02 Hypoxemia
         DEF: Insufficient oxygen in the arterial blood resulting in inadequate delivery of oxygen to the body tissues.

R09.1 Pleurisy

     EXCLUDES 1   *pleurisy with effusion (J90)*

¹ **R09.2 Respiratory arrest**   MCC HCC

     Cardiorespiratory failure
     EXCLUDES 1   *cardiac arrest (I46.-)*
            respiratory arrest of newborn (P28.81)
            respiratory distress of newborn (P22.0)
            respiratory failure (J96.-)
            respiratory failure of newborn (P28.5)
            respiratory insufficiency (R06.89)
            respiratory insufficiency of newborn (P28.5)

     CC Excl: PDX collection 1121

R09.3 Abnormal sputum
     Abnormal amount of sputum
     Abnormal color of sputum
     Abnormal odor of sputum
     Excessive sputum
     EXCLUDES 1   *blood-stained sputum (R04.2)*

☑5ᵗʰ **R09.8 Other specified symptoms and signs involving the circulatory and respiratory systems**

     R09.81 Nasal congestion

     R09.82 Postnasal drip

     R09.89 Other specified symptoms and signs involving the circulatory and respiratory systems
         Abnormal chest percussion
         Bruit (arterial)
         Chest tympany
         Choking sensation
         Feeling of foreign body in throat
         Friction sounds in chest
         Rales
         Weak pulse
         EXCLUDES 2   *foreign body in throat (T17.2-)*
                wheezing (R06.2)

Ⓝ Newborn: 0   Ⓟ Pediatric: 0-17   Ⓜ Maternity: 9-64   Ⓐ Adult: 15-124   MCC Major Complication/Comorbidity   CC Complication/Comorbidity   SW Severe Wound Dx

956   ICD-10-CM 2020

Symptoms and signs involving the digestive system and abdomen (R10–R19)

> **EXCLUDES 2**　congenital or infantile pylorospasm (Q40.0)
> gastrointestinal hemorrhage (K92.0-K92.2)
> intestinal obstruction (K56.-)
> newborn gastrointestinal hemorrhage (P54.0-P54.3)
> newborn intestinal obstruction (P76.-)
> pylorospasm (K31.3)
> signs and symptoms involving the urinary system (R30-R39)
> symptoms referable to female genital organs (N94.-)
> symptoms referable to male genital organs (N48-N50)

✓4th **R10　Abdominal and pelvic pain**

> **EXCLUDES 1**　renal colic (N23)
> **EXCLUDES 2**　dorsalgia (M54.-)
> flatulence and related conditions (R14.-)

R10.0　Acute abdomen
Severe abdominal pain (generalized) (with abdominal rigidity)
> **EXCLUDES 1**　abdominal rigidity NOS (R19.3)
> generalized abdominal pain NOS (R10.84)
> localized abdominal pain (R10.1-R10.3-)

✓5th **R10.1　Pain localized to upper abdomen**

　　R10.10　Upper abdominal pain, unspecified
　　R10.11　Right upper quadrant pain
　　R10.12　Left upper quadrant pain
　　R10.13　Epigastric pain
　　　　Dyspepsia
> 　　　　**EXCLUDES 1**　functional dyspepsia (K30)

Abdominal Pain

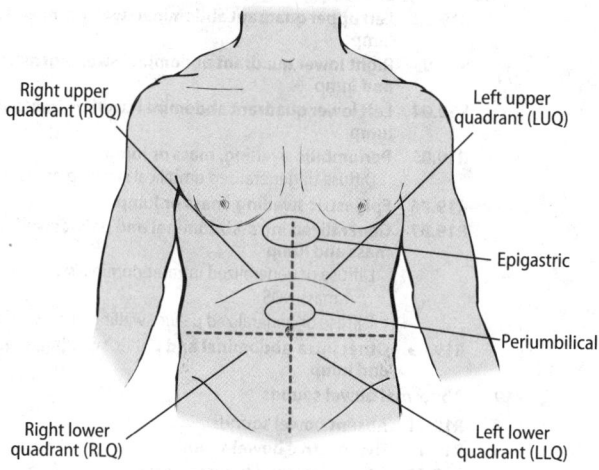

Right upper quadrant (RUQ)
Left upper quadrant (LUQ)
Epigastric
Periumbilical
Right lower quadrant (RLQ)
Left lower quadrant (LLQ)

R10.2　Pelvic and perineal pain
> **EXCLUDES 1**　vulvodynia (N94.81)

✓5th **R10.3　Pain localized to other parts of lower abdomen**

　　R10.30　Lower abdominal pain, unspecified
　　R10.31　Right lower quadrant pain
　　R10.32　Left lower quadrant pain
　　R10.33　Periumbilical pain

✓5th **R10.8　Other abdominal pain**

✓6th 　R10.81　Abdominal tenderness
　　　　Abdominal tenderness NOS
　　　　R10.811　Right upper quadrant abdominal tenderness
　　　　R10.812　Left upper quadrant abdominal tenderness
　　　　R10.813　Right lower quadrant abdominal tenderness
　　　　R10.814　Left lower quadrant abdominal tenderness
　　　　R10.815　Periumbilic abdominal tenderness
　　　　R10.816　Epigastric abdominal tenderness
　　　　R10.817　Generalized abdominal tenderness
　　　　R10.819　Abdominal tenderness, unspecified site

✓6th 　R10.82　Rebound abdominal tenderness
　　　　R10.821　Right upper quadrant rebound abdominal tenderness

　　　　R10.822　Left upper quadrant rebound abdominal tenderness
　　　　R10.823　Right lower quadrant rebound abdominal tenderness
　　　　R10.824　Left lower quadrant rebound abdominal tenderness
　　　　R10.825　Periumbilic rebound abdominal tenderness
　　　　R10.826　Epigastric rebound abdominal tenderness
　　　　R10.827　Generalized rebound abdominal tenderness
　　　　R10.829　Rebound abdominal tenderness, unspecified site

　R10.83　Colic　　　　　　　　　　　　　 P
　　　Colic NOS
　　　Infantile colic
> 　　　**EXCLUDES 1**　colic in adult and child over 12 months old (R10.84)

　　　DEF: Inconsolable crying in an otherwise well-fed and healthy infant for more than three hours a day, three days a week, for more than three weeks.

　R10.84　Generalized abdominal pain
> 　　　**EXCLUDES 1**　generalized abdominal pain associated with acute abdomen (R10.0)

R10.9　Unspecified abdominal pain

✓4th **R11　Nausea and vomiting**

> **EXCLUDES 1**　cyclical vomiting associated with migraine (G43.A-)
> excessive vomiting in pregnancy (O21.-)
> hematemesis (K92.0)
> neonatal hematemesis (P54.0)
> newborn vomiting (P92.0-)
> psychogenic vomiting (F50.89)
> vomiting associated with bulimia nervosa (F50.2)
> vomiting following gastrointestinal surgery (K91.0)

AHA: 2017,1Q,28
TIP: Assign a code from this category along with K31.89 Other diseases of stomach and duodenum, to describe cyclical vomiting not due to migraine.

R11.0　Nausea
　　Nausea NOS
　　Nausea without vomiting

✓5th **R11.1　Vomiting**

　　R11.10　Vomiting, unspecified
　　　　Vomiting NOS
　　R11.11　Vomiting without nausea
　　R11.12　Projectile vomiting
　　R11.13　Vomiting of fecal matter
　　R11.14　Bilious vomiting
　　　　Bilious emesis
　　R11.15　Cyclical vomiting syndrome unrelated to migraine
　　　　Cyclic vomiting syndrome NOS
　　　　Persistent vomiting
> 　　　　**EXCLUDES 1**　cyclical vomiting in migraine (G43.A-)
> 　　　　**EXCLUDES 2**　bulimia nervosa (F50.2)
> 　　　　diabetes mellitus due to underlying condition (E08.-)

R11.2　Nausea with vomiting, unspecified
　　Persistent nausea with vomiting NOS

R12　Heartburn
> **EXCLUDES 1**　dyspepsia NOS (R10.13)
> functional dyspepsia (K30)

✓4th **R13　Aphagia and dysphagia**

R13.0　Aphagia　　　　　　　　　　　　 CC
　　Inability to swallow
> 　　**EXCLUDES 1**　psychogenic aphagia (F50.9)

✓5th R13.1 Dysphagia

Code first, if applicable, dysphagia following cerebrovascular disease (I69. with final characters -91)

EXCLUDES 1   *psychogenic dysphagia (F45.8)*

Swallowing Function

Oral phase

Oropharyngeal phase

Pharyngeal phase

Pharyngoesophageal phase

R13.10   **Dysphagia, unspecified**
Difficulty in swallowing NOS

R13.11   **Dysphagia, oral phase**

R13.12   **Dysphagia, oropharyngeal phase**

R13.13   **Dysphagia, pharyngeal phase**

R13.14   **Dysphagia, pharyngoesophageal phase**

R13.19   **Other dysphagia**
Cervical dysphagia
Neurogenic dysphagia

✓4th R14 Flatulence and related conditions

EXCLUDES 1   *psychogenic aerophagy (F45.8)*

R14.0   **Abdominal distension (gaseous)**
Bloating
Tympanites (abdominal) (intestinal)

R14.1   **Gas pain**

R14.2   **Eructation**

R14.3   **Flatulence**

✓4th R15 Fecal incontinence

INCLUDES   encopresis NOS

EXCLUDES 1   *fecal incontinence of nonorganic origin (F98.1)*

R15.0   **Incomplete defecation**
EXCLUDES 1   *constipation (K59.0-)*
fecal impaction (K56.41)

R15.1   **Fecal smearing**
Fecal soiling

R15.2   **Fecal urgency**

R15.9   **Full incontinence of feces**
Fecal incontinence NOS

✓4th R16 Hepatomegaly and splenomegaly, not elsewhere classified

R16.0   **Hepatomegaly, not elsewhere classified**
Hepatomegaly NOS

R16.1   **Splenomegaly, not elsewhere classified**
Splenomegaly NOS

R16.2   **Hepatomegaly with splenomegaly, not elsewhere classified**
Hepatosplenomegaly NOS

R17 Unspecified jaundice   CC

EXCLUDES 1   *neonatal jaundice (P55, P57-P59)*

CC Excl: PDX collection 1122

✓4th R18 Ascites

INCLUDES   fluid in peritoneal cavity

EXCLUDES 1   *ascites in alcoholic cirrhosis (K70.31)*
ascites in alcoholic hepatitis (K70.11)
ascites in toxic liver disease with chronic active hepatitis (K71.51)

DEF: Abnormal accumulation of free fluid in the abdominal cavity, causing distention and tightness in addition to shortness of breath as the fluid accumulates. Ascites is usually an underlying disorder and can be a manifestation of any number of diseases.

R18.0   **Malignant ascites**   CC
Code first malignancy, such as:
malignant neoplasm of ovary (C56.-)
secondary malignant neoplasm of retroperitoneum and peritoneum (C78.6)
CC Excl: PDX collection 1123

R18.8   **Other ascites**   CC
Ascites NOS
Peritoneal effusion (chronic)
AHA: 2018,1Q,4
CC Excl: PDX collection 1123

✓4th R19 Other symptoms and signs involving the digestive system and abdomen

EXCLUDES 1   *acute abdomen (R10.0)*

✓5th R19.0   **Intra-abdominal and pelvic swelling, mass and lump**
EXCLUDES 1   *abdominal distension (gaseous) (R14.-)*
ascites (R18.-)

R19.00   **Intra-abdominal and pelvic swelling, mass and lump, unspecified site**

R19.01   **Right upper quadrant abdominal swelling, mass and lump**

R19.02   **Left upper quadrant abdominal swelling, mass and lump**

R19.03   **Right lower quadrant abdominal swelling, mass and lump**

R19.04   **Left lower quadrant abdominal swelling, mass and lump**

R19.05   **Periumbilic swelling, mass or lump**
Diffuse or generalized umbilical swelling or mass

R19.06   **Epigastric swelling, mass or lump**

R19.07   **Generalized intra-abdominal and pelvic swelling, mass and lump**
Diffuse or generalized intra-abdominal swelling or mass NOS
Diffuse or generalized pelvic swelling or mass NOS

R19.09   **Other intra-abdominal and pelvic swelling, mass and lump**

✓5th R19.1   **Abnormal bowel sounds**

R19.11   **Absent bowel sounds**

R19.12   **Hyperactive bowel sounds**

R19.15   **Other abnormal bowel sounds**
Abnormal bowel sounds NOS

R19.2   **Visible peristalsis**
Hyperperistalsis
DEF: Visible movements of muscular attempts to move food through the digestive tract due to pyloric obstruction, stomach obstruction, or intestinal obstruction.

✓5th R19.3   **Abdominal rigidity**
EXCLUDES 1   *abdominal rigidity with severe abdominal pain (R10.0)*

R19.30   **Abdominal rigidity, unspecified site**

R19.31   **Right upper quadrant abdominal rigidity**

R19.32   **Left upper quadrant abdominal rigidity**

R19.33   **Right lower quadrant abdominal rigidity**

R19.34   **Left lower quadrant abdominal rigidity**

R19.35   **Periumbilic abdominal rigidity**

R19.36   **Epigastric abdominal rigidity**

R19.37   **Generalized abdominal rigidity**

R19.4   **Change in bowel habit**
EXCLUDES 1   *constipation (K59.0-)*
functional diarrhea (K59.1)

N Newborn: 0   P Pediatric: 0-17   M Maternity: 9-64   A Adult: 15-124   MCC Major Complication/Comorbidity   CC Complication/Comorbidity   SW Severe Wound Dx

958   ICD-10-CM 2020

R19.5 **Other fecal abnormalities**
Abnormal stool color
Bulky stools
Mucus in stools
Occult blood in feces
Occult blood in stools
> EXCLUDES 1   *melena (K92.1)*
>   *neonatal melena (P54.1)*
AHA: 2019,1Q,32

R19.6 **Halitosis**

R19.7 **Diarrhea, unspecified**
Diarrhea NOS
> EXCLUDES 1   *functional diarrhea (K59.1)*
>   *neonatal diarrhea (P78.3)*
>   *psychogenic diarrhea (F45.8)*

R19.8 **Other specified symptoms and signs involving the digestive system and abdomen**

Symptoms and signs involving the skin and subcutaneous tissue (R20-R23)

> EXCLUDES 2   *symptoms relating to breast (N64.4-N64.5)*

☑4ᵗʰ **R20** **Disturbances of skin sensation**
> EXCLUDES 1   *dissociative anesthesia and sensory loss (F44.6)*
>   *psychogenic disturbances (F45.8)*

R20.0 **Anesthesia** of skin
R20.1 **Hypoesthesia** of skin
R20.2 **Paresthesia** of skin
Formication
Pins and needles
Tingling skin
> EXCLUDES 1   *acroparesthesia (I73.8)*

R20.3 **Hyperesthesia**
R20.8 **Other disturbances of skin sensation**
R20.9 **Unspecified disturbances of skin sensation**

R21 **Rash and other nonspecific skin eruption**
> INCLUDES   rash NOS
> EXCLUDES 1   *specified type of rash — code to condition*
>   *vesicular eruption (R23.8)*

☑4ᵗʰ **R22** **Localized swelling, mass and lump of skin and subcutaneous tissue**
> INCLUDES   subcutaneous nodules (localized)(superficial)
> EXCLUDES 1   *abnormal findings on diagnostic imaging (R90-R93)*
>   *edema (R60.-)*
>   *enlarged lymph nodes (R59.-)*
>   *localized adiposity (E65)*
>   *swelling of joint (M25.4-)*

R22.0 **Localized swelling, mass and lump, head**
R22.1 **Localized swelling, mass and lump, neck**
R22.2 **Localized swelling, mass and lump, trunk**
> EXCLUDES 1   *intra-abdominal or pelvic mass and lump (R19.0-)*
>   *intra-abdominal or pelvic swelling (R19.0-)*
> EXCLUDES 2   *breast mass and lump (N63)*

☑5ᵗʰ **R22.3** **Localized swelling, mass and lump, upper limb**
     R22.30 **Localized swelling, mass and lump, unspecified upper limb**
     R22.31 **Localized swelling, mass and lump, right upper limb**
     R22.32 **Localized swelling, mass and lump, left upper limb**
     R22.33 **Localized swelling, mass and lump, upper limb, bilateral**

☑5ᵗʰ **R22.4** **Localized swelling, mass and lump, lower limb**
     R22.40 **Localized swelling, mass and lump, unspecified lower limb**
     R22.41 **Localized swelling, mass and lump, right lower limb**
     R22.42 **Localized swelling, mass and lump, left lower limb**
     R22.43 **Localized swelling, mass and lump, lower limb, bilateral**

R22.9 **Localized swelling, mass and lump, unspecified**

☑4ᵗʰ **R23** **Other skin changes**
R23.0 **Cyanosis**
> EXCLUDES 1   *acrocyanosis (I73.8)*
>   *cyanotic attacks of newborn (P28.2)*
DEF: Bluish or purplish discoloration of the skin due to an inadequate oxygen blood level.

R23.1 **Pallor**
Clammy skin
R23.2 **Flushing**
Excessive blushing
Code first, if applicable, menopausal and female climacteric states (N95.1)
R23.3 **Spontaneous ecchymoses**
Petechiae
> EXCLUDES 1   *ecchymoses of newborn (P54.5)*
>   *purpura (D69.-)*
R23.4 **Changes in skin texture**
Desquamation of skin
Induration of skin
Scaling of skin
> EXCLUDES 1   *epidermal thickening NOS (L85.9)*
R23.8 **Other skin changes**
R23.9 **Unspecified skin changes**

Symptoms and signs involving the nervous and musculoskeletal systems (R25-R29)

☑4ᵗʰ **R25** **Abnormal involuntary movements**
> EXCLUDES 1   *specific movement disorders (G20-G26)*
>   *stereotyped movement disorders (F98.4)*
>   *tic disorders (F95.-)*

R25.0 **Abnormal head movements**
R25.1 **Tremor, unspecified**
> EXCLUDES 1   *chorea NOS (G25.5)*
>   *essential tremor (G25.0)*
>   *hysterical tremor (F44.4)*
>   *intention tremor (G25.2)*
R25.2 **Cramp and spasm**
> EXCLUDES 2   *carpopedal spasm (R29.0)*
>   *charley-horse (M62.831)*
>   *infantile spasms (G40.4-)*
>   *muscle spasm of back (M62.830)*
>   *muscle spasm of calf (M62.831)*
R25.3 **Fasciculation**
Twitching NOS
R25.8 **Other abnormal involuntary movements**
R25.9 **Unspecified abnormal involuntary movements**

☑4ᵗʰ **R26** **Abnormalities of gait and mobility**
> EXCLUDES 1   *ataxia NOS (R27.0)*
>   *hereditary ataxia (G11.-)*
>   *locomotor (syphilitic) ataxia (A52.11)*
>   *immobility syndrome (paraplegic) (M62.3)*

R26.0 **Ataxic gait**
Staggering gait
R26.1 **Paralytic gait**
Spastic gait
R26.2 **Difficulty in walking, not elsewhere classified**
> EXCLUDES 1   *falling (R29.6)*
>   *unsteadiness on feet (R26.81)*
AHA: 2016,2Q,7

☑5ᵗʰ **R26.8** **Other abnormalities of gait and mobility**
     R26.81 **Unsteadiness on feet**
     R26.89 **Other abnormalities of gait and mobility**
R26.9 **Unspecified abnormalities of gait and mobility**

☑4ᵗʰ **R27** **Other lack of coordination**
> EXCLUDES 1   *ataxic gait (R26.0)*
>   *hereditary ataxia (G11.-)*
>   *vertigo NOS (R42)*

R27.0 **Ataxia, unspecified**
> EXCLUDES 1   *ataxia following cerebrovascular disease (I69. with final characters -93)*
R27.8 **Other lack of coordination**
R27.9 **Unspecified lack of coordination**

✓4th **R29 Other symptoms and signs involving the nervous and musculoskeletal systems**

R29.0 Tetany   **CC**

   Carpopedal spasm

    EXCLUDES 1   *hysterical tetany (F44.5)*

         neonatal tetany (P71.3)

         parathyroid tetany (E20.9)

         post-thyroidectomy tetany (E89.2)

   DEF: Calcium or other mineral imbalance causing voluntary muscles such as hands, feet, or larynx to spasm rhythmically.

   CC Excl: PDX collection 1124

R29.1 Meningismus   **CC**

   CC Excl: PDX collection 1125

R29.2 Abnormal reflex

    EXCLUDES 2   *abnormal pupillary reflex (H57.0)*

         hyperactive gag reflex (J39.2)

         vasovagal reaction or syncope (R55)

R29.3 Abnormal posture

R29.4 Clicking hip

    EXCLUDES 1   *congenital deformities of hip (Q65.-)*

R29.5 Transient paralysis   **CC**

   Code first any associated spinal cord injury (S14.0, S14.1-, S24.0, S24.1-, S34.0-, S34.1-)

    EXCLUDES 1   *transient ischemic attack (G45.9)*

   CC Excl: PDX collection 1126

R29.6 Repeated falls

   Falling

   Tendency to fall

    EXCLUDES 2   *at risk for falling (Z91.81)*

         history of falling (Z91.81)

   AHA: 2016,2Q,6

   TIP: Code in addition to Parkinson's disease (G20), when documented.

✓5th **R29.7 National Institutes of Health Stroke Scale (NIHSS) score**

   Code first the type of cerebral infarction (I63.-)

   AHA: 2016,4Q,61-62

   TIP: Codes from this subcategory may be assigned based on medical record documentation from clinicians who are not the patient's provider.

   ✓6th **R29.70 NIHSS score 0-9**

     R29.700 NIHSS score 0

     R29.701 NIHSS score 1

     R29.702 NIHSS score 2

     R29.703 NIHSS score 3

     R29.704 NIHSS score 4

     R29.705 NIHSS score 5

     R29.706 NIHSS score 6

     R29.707 NIHSS score 7

     R29.708 NIHSS score 8

     R29.709 NIHSS score 9

   ✓6th **R29.71 NIHSS score 10-19**

     R29.710 NIHSS score 10

     R29.711 NIHSS score 11

     R29.712 NIHSS score 12

     R29.713 NIHSS score 13

     R29.714 NIHSS score 14

     R29.715 NIHSS score 15

     R29.716 NIHSS score 16

     R29.717 NIHSS score 17

     R29.718 NIHSS score 18

     R29.719 NIHSS score 19

   ✓6th **R29.72 NIHSS score 20-29**

     R29.720 NIHSS score 20

     R29.721 NIHSS score 21

     R29.722 NIHSS score 22

     R29.723 NIHSS score 23

     R29.724 NIHSS score 24

     R29.725 NIHSS score 25

     R29.726 NIHSS score 26

     R29.727 NIHSS score 27

     R29.728 NIHSS score 28

     R29.729 NIHSS score 29

   ✓6th **R29.73 NIHSS score 30-39**

     R29.730 NIHSS score 30

     R29.731 NIHSS score 31

     R29.732 NIHSS score 32

     R29.733 NIHSS score 33

     R29.734 NIHSS score 34

     R29.735 NIHSS score 35

     R29.736 NIHSS score 36

     R29.737 NIHSS score 37

     R29.738 NIHSS score 38

     R29.739 NIHSS score 39

   ✓6th **R29.74 NIHSS score 40-42**

     R29.740 NIHSS score 40

     R29.741 NIHSS score 41

     R29.742 NIHSS score 42

✓5th **R29.8 Other symptoms and signs involving the nervous and musculoskeletal systems**

   ✓6th **R29.81 Other symptoms and signs involving the nervous system**

     R29.810 Facial weakness

       Facial droop

        EXCLUDES 1   *Bell's palsy (G51.0)*

          facial weakness following cerebrovascular disease (I69. with final characters -92)

     R29.818 Other symptoms and signs involving the nervous system

   ✓6th **R29.89 Other symptoms and signs involving the musculoskeletal system**

     EXCLUDES 2   *pain in limb (M79.6-)*

     R29.890 Loss of height

        EXCLUDES 1   *osteoporosis (M80-M81)*

     R29.891 Ocular torticollis

        EXCLUDES 1   *congenital (sternomastoid) torticollis Q68.0*

         psychogenic torticollis (F45.8)

         spasmodic torticollis (G24.3)

         torticollis due to birth injury (P15.8)

         torticollis NOS M43.6

       DEF: Abnormal head posture as a result of a contracted state of cervical muscles to correct a visual disturbance, either double vision or a visual field defect.

     R29.898 Other symptoms and signs involving the musculoskeletal system

✓5th **R29.9 Unspecified symptoms and signs involving the nervous and musculoskeletal systems**

   R29.90 Unspecified symptoms and signs involving the nervous system

   R29.91 Unspecified symptoms and signs involving the musculoskeletal system

Symptoms and signs involving the genitourinary system (R30-R39)

✓4th **R30 Pain associated with micturition**

    EXCLUDES 1   *psychogenic pain associated with micturition (F45.8)*

R30.0 Dysuria

   Strangury

R30.1 Vesical tenesmus

   DEF: Feeling of a full bladder even when there is little or no urine in the bladder.

R30.9 Painful micturition, unspecified

   Painful urination NOS

✓4th **R31 Hematuria**

    EXCLUDES 1   *hematuria included with underlying conditions, such as:*

       acute cystitis with hematuria (N30.01)

       recurrent and persistent hematuria in glomerular diseases (N02.-)

   AHA: 2017,1Q,17

R31.0 Gross hematuria

R31.1 Benign essential microscopic hematuria

✓5th **R31.2 Other microscopic hematuria**

   AHA: 2016,4Q,62

   R31.21 Asymptomatic microscopic hematuria

     AMH

   R31.29 Other microscopic hematuria

R31.9 Hematuria, unspecified

N Newborn: 0   **P** Pediatric: 0-17   **M** Maternity: 9-64   **A** Adult: 15-124   **MCC** Major Complication/Comorbidity   **CC** Complication/Comorbidity   **SW** Severe Wound Dx

960   ICD-10-CM 2020

R32 **Unspecified urinary incontinence**
Enuresis NOS
EXCLUDES 1   *functional urinary incontinence (R39.81)*
nonorganic enuresis (F98.Ø)
stress incontinence and other specified urinary incontinence (N39.3-N39.4-)
urinary incontinence associated with cognitive impairment (R39.81)

√4ᵗʰ **R33** **Retention of urine**
EXCLUDES 1   *psychogenic retention of urine (F45.8)*
R33.Ø **Drug induced retention of urine**
Use additional code for adverse effect, if applicable, to identify drug (T36-T5Ø with fifth or sixth character 5)
R33.8 **Other retention of urine**
Code first, if applicable, any causal condition, such as:
enlarged prostate (N4Ø.1)
AHA: 2018,4Q,55
R33.9 **Retention of urine, unspecified**

R34 **Anuria and oliguria**
EXCLUDES 1   *anuria and oliguria complicating abortion or ectopic or molar pregnancy (O00-O07, O08.4)*
anuria and oliguria complicating pregnancy (O26.83-)
anuria and oliguria complicating the puerperium (O90.4)

√4ᵗʰ **R35** **Polyuria**
Code first, if applicable, any causal condition, such as:
enlarged prostate (N4Ø.1)
EXCLUDES 1   *psychogenic polyuria (F45.8)*
R35.Ø **Frequency of micturition**
R35.1 **Nocturia**
R35.8 **Other polyuria**
Polyuria NOS

√4ᵗʰ **R36** **Urethral discharge**
R36.Ø **Urethral discharge without blood**
R36.1 **Hematospermia** ♂
R36.9 **Urethral discharge, unspecified**
Penile discharge NOS
Urethrorrhea

R37 **Sexual dysfunction, unspecified**

√4ᵗʰ **R39** **Other and unspecified symptoms and signs involving the genitourinary system**
R39.Ø **Extravasation of urine** CC
CC Excl: PDX collection 1127
√5ᵗʰ **R39.1** **Other difficulties with micturition**
Code first, if applicable, any causal condition, such as:
enlarged prostate (N4Ø.1)
R39.11 **Hesitancy of micturition**
R39.12 **Poor urinary stream**
Weak urinary steam
R39.13 **Splitting of urinary stream**
R39.14 **Feeling of incomplete bladder emptying**
R39.15 **Urgency of urination**
EXCLUDES 1   *urge incontinence (N39.41, N39.46)*
R39.16 **Straining to void**
√6ᵗʰ **R39.19** **Other difficulties with micturition**
AHA: 2016,4Q,63
R39.191 **Need to immediately re-void**
R39.192 **Position dependent micturition**
R39.198 **Other difficulties with micturition**
R39.2 **Extrarenal uremia**
Prerenal uremia
EXCLUDES 1   *uremia NOS (N19)*
√5ᵗʰ **R39.8** **Other symptoms and signs involving the genitourinary system**
AHA: 2017,4Q,22-23
R39.81 **Functional urinary incontinence**
Urinary incontinence due to cognitive impairment, or severe physical disability or immobility
EXCLUDES 1   *stress incontinence and other specified urinary incontinence (N39.3-N39.4-)*
urinary incontinence NOS (R32)
R39.82 **Chronic bladder pain**
AHA: 2016,4Q,64
R39.83 **Unilateral non-palpable testicle** ♂
R39.84 **Bilateral non-palpable testicles** ♂

R39.89 **Other symptoms and signs involving the genitourinary system**
R39.9 **Unspecified symptoms and signs involving the genitourinary system**

Symptoms and signs involving cognition, perception, emotional state and behavior (R40-R46)

EXCLUDES 2   *symptoms and signs constituting part of a pattern of mental disorder (FØ1-F99)*

√4ᵗʰ **R40** **Somnolence, stupor and coma**
EXCLUDES 1   *neonatal coma (P91.5)*
somnolence, stupor and coma in diabetes (EØ8-E13)
somnolence, stupor and coma in hepatic failure (K72.-)
somnolence, stupor and coma in hypoglycemia (nondiabetic) (E15)
R40.Ø **Somnolence**
Drowsiness
EXCLUDES 1   *coma (R40.2-)*
R40.1 **Stupor**
Catatonic stupor
Semicoma
EXCLUDES 1   *catatonic schizophrenia (F2Ø.2)*
coma (R40.2-)
depressive stupor (F31-F33)
dissociative stupor (F44.2)
manic stupor (F3Ø.2)
√5ᵗʰ **R40.2** **Coma**
Code first any associated:
fracture of skull (SØ2.-)
intracranial injury (SØ6.-)
NOTE   One code from each subcategory, R40.21-R40.23, is required to complete the coma scale
AHA: 2019,2Q,12; 2018,4Q,70; 2017,4Q,23-25,95; 2015,2Q,17; 2014,1Q,19
TIP: Codes for individual (R40.21-, R40.22, R40.23-) or total (R40.24-) coma scale scores may be assigned based on medical record documentation from clinicians who are not the patient's provider.
TIP: It is not appropriate to assign individual (R40.21-, R40.22-, R40.23-) or total (R40.24-) coma scale score codes for patients who are sedated or in medically induced comas.
CC Excl: For MCC codes in subcategory R40.2: PDX collection 515
R40.20 **Unspecified coma** MCC HCC
Coma NOS
Unconsciousness NOS
√6ᵗʰ **R40.21** **Coma scale, eyes open**

The following appropriate 7th character is to be added to subcategory R40.21-, R40.22-, R40.23-, and R40.24-.
Ø   unspecified time
1   in the field [EMT or ambulance]
2   at arrival to emergency department
3   at hospital admission
4   24 hours or more after hospital admission

√7ᵗʰ **R40.211** **Coma scale, eyes open, never** MCC HCC
Coma scale eye opening score of 1
√7ᵗʰ **R40.212** **Coma scale, eyes open, to pain** MCC HCC
Coma scale eye opening score of 2
√7ᵗʰ **R40.213** **Coma scale, eyes open, to sound**
Coma scale eye opening score of 3
√7ᵗʰ **R40.214** **Coma scale, eyes open, spontaneous**
Coma scale eye opening score of 4
√6ᵗʰ **R40.22** **Coma scale, best verbal response**
√7ᵗʰ **R40.221** **Coma scale, best verbal response, none** MCC HCC
Coma scale verbal score of 1

Chapter 18. Symptoms, Signs and Abnormal Clinical and Laboratory Findings

R40.222–R43.1

✓7ᵗʰ **R40.222 Coma scale, best verbal response, incomprehensible words** `MCC` `HCC`
  Coma scale verbal score of 2
  Incomprehensible sounds (2-5 years of age)
  Moans/grunts to pain; restless (< 2 years old)

✓7ᵗʰ **R40.223 Coma scale, best verbal response, inappropriate words**
  Coma scale verbal score of 3
  Inappropriate crying or screaming (< 2 years of age)
  Screaming (2-5 years of age)

✓7ᵗʰ **R40.224 Coma scale, best verbal response, confused conversation**
  Coma scale verbal score of 4
  Inappropriate words (2-5 years of age)
  Irritable cries (< 2 years of age)

✓7ᵗʰ **R40.225 Coma scale, best verbal response, oriented**
  Coma scale verbal score of 5
  Cooing or babbling or crying appropriately (< 2 years of age)
  Uses appropriate words (2-5 years of age)

✓6ᵗʰ **R40.23 Coma scale, best motor response**

✓7ᵗʰ **R40.231 Coma scale, best motor response, none** `MCC` `HCC`
  Coma scale motor score of 1

✓7ᵗʰ **R40.232 Coma scale, best motor response, extension** `MCC` `HCC`
  Abnormal extensor posturing to pain or noxious stimuli (< 2 years of age)
  Coma scale motor score of 2
  Extensor posturing to pain or noxious stimuli (2-5 years of age)

✓7ᵗʰ **R40.233 Coma scale, best motor response, abnormal flexion**
  Abnormal flexure posturing to pain or noxious stimuli (2-5 years of age)
  Coma scale motor score of 3
  Flexion/decorticate posturing (< 2 years of age)

✓7ᵗʰ **R40.234 Coma scale, best motor response, flexion withdrawal** `MCC` `HCC`
  Coma scale motor score of 4
  Withdraws from pain or noxious stimuli (2-5 years of age)

✓7ᵗʰ **R40.235 Coma scale, best motor response, localizes pain**
  Coma scale motor score of 5
  Localizes pain (2-5 years of age)
  Withdraws to touch (< 2 years of age)

✓7ᵗʰ **R40.236 Coma scale, best motor response, obeys commands**
  Coma scale motor score of 6
  Normal or spontaneous movement (< 2 years of age)
  Obeys commands (2-5 years of age)

✓6ᵗʰ **R40.24 Glasgow coma scale, total score**

  `NOTE` Assign a code from subcategory R40.24, when only the total coma score is documented

  AHA: 2016,4Q,64-65

✓7ᵗʰ **R40.241 Glasgow coma scale score 13-15**

✓7ᵗʰ **R40.242 Glasgow coma scale score 9-12**

✓7ᵗʰ **R40.243 Glasgow coma scale score 3-8** `HCC`

✓7ᵗʰ **R40.244 Other coma, without documented Glasgow coma scale score, or with partial score reported** `HCC`

R40.3 Persistent vegetative state `CC` `HCC`
  DEF: Persistent wakefulness without consciousness due to a nonfunctioning cerebral cortex.
  CC Excl: PDX collection 515

R40.4 Transient alteration of awareness

✓4ᵗʰ **R41 Other symptoms and signs involving cognitive functions and awareness**
  `EXCLUDES 1` dissociative [conversion] disorders (F44.-)
    mild cognitive impairment, so stated (G31.84)

R41.0 Disorientation, unspecified
  Confusion NOS
  Delirium NOS
  AHA: 2019,2Q,34

R41.1 Anterograde amnesia

R41.2 Retrograde amnesia

R41.3 Other amnesia
  Amnesia NOS
  Memory loss NOS
  `EXCLUDES 1` amnestic disorder due to known physiologic condition (F04)
    amnestic syndrome due to psychoactive substance use (F10-F19 with 5th character .6)
    mild memory disturbance due to known physiological condition (F06.8)
    transient global amnesia (G45.4)

R41.4 Neurologic neglect syndrome `CC`
  Asomatognosia
  Hemi-akinesia
  Hemi-inattention
  Hemispatial neglect
  Left-sided neglect
  Sensory neglect
  Visuospatial neglect
  `EXCLUDES 1` visuospatial deficit (R41.842)
  CC Excl: PDX collection 1128

✓5ᵗʰ **R41.8 Other symptoms and signs involving cognitive functions and awareness**

R41.81 Age-related cognitive decline `A`
  Senility NOS

R41.82 Altered mental status, unspecified
  Change in mental status NOS
  `EXCLUDES 1` altered level of consciousness (R40.-)
    altered mental status due to known condition — code to condition
    delirium NOS (R41.0)
  AHA: 2012,4Q,97

R41.83 Borderline intellectual functioning
  IQ level 71 to 84
  `EXCLUDES 1` intellectual disabilities (F70-F79)

✓6ᵗʰ **R41.84 Other specified cognitive deficit**
  `EXCLUDES 1` cognitive deficits as sequelae of cerebrovascular disease (I69.01-, I69.11-, I69.21-, I69.31-, I69.81-, I69.91-)

  R41.840 Attention and concentration deficit
    `EXCLUDES 1` attention-deficit hyperactivity disorders (F90.-)

  R41.841 Cognitive communication deficit
  R41.842 Visuospatial deficit
  R41.843 Psychomotor deficit
  R41.844 Frontal lobe and executive function deficit

R41.89 Other symptoms and signs involving cognitive functions and awareness
  Anosognosia

R41.9 Unspecified symptoms and signs involving cognitive functions and awareness
  Unspecified neurocognitive disorder

R42 Dizziness and giddiness
  Light-headedness
  Vertigo NOS
  `EXCLUDES 1` vertiginous syndromes (H81.-)
    vertigo from infrasound (T75.23)

✓4ᵗʰ **R43 Disturbances of smell and taste**

R43.0 Anosmia
  DEF: Permanent or transient absence of smell that may be congenital or acquired.

R43.1 Parosmia
  DEF: Abnormal perception of smell usually triggered by environmental odors.

R43.2 Parageusia
DEF: Abnormal perception of taste.

R43.8 Other disturbances of smell and taste
Mixed disturbance of smell and taste

R43.9 Unspecified disturbances of smell and taste

✓4ᵗʰ **R44 Other symptoms and signs involving general sensations and perceptions**
EXCLUDES 1   alcoholic hallucinations (F1.5)
hallucinations in drug psychosis (F11-F19 with .5)
hallucinations in mood disorders with psychotic symptoms (F30.2, F31.5, F32.3, F33.3)
hallucinations in schizophrenia, schizotypal and delusional disorders (F20-F29)
EXCLUDES 2   disturbances of skin sensation (R20.-)
CC Excl: For CC codes in category R44: PDX collection 1129

R44.0 Auditory hallucinations   CC

R44.1 Visual hallucinations

R44.2 Other hallucinations   CC

R44.3 Hallucinations, unspecified   CC

R44.8 Other symptoms and signs involving general sensations and perceptions

R44.9 Unspecified symptoms and signs involving general sensations and perceptions

✓4ᵗʰ **R45 Symptoms and signs involving emotional state**

R45.0 Nervousness
Nervous tension

R45.1 Restlessness and agitation

R45.2 Unhappiness

R45.3 Demoralization and apathy
EXCLUDES 1   anhedonia (R45.84)

R45.4 Irritability and anger

R45.5 Hostility

R45.6 Violent behavior

R45.7 State of emotional shock and stress, unspecified

✓5ᵗʰ **R45.8 Other symptoms and signs involving emotional state**

   R45.81 Low self-esteem

   R45.82 Worries

   R45.83 Excessive crying of child, adolescent or adult
     EXCLUDES 1   excessive crying of infant (baby) R68.11

   R45.84 Anhedonia

✓6ᵗʰ   **R45.85 Homicidal and suicidal ideations**
     EXCLUDES 1   suicide attempt (T14.91)
       R45.850 Homicidal ideations
       R45.851 Suicidal ideations   CC
          DEF: Thoughts of committing suicide but no actual attempt of suicide has been made.
          CC Excl: PDX collection 1130

   R45.86 Emotional lability

   R45.87 Impulsiveness

   R45.89 Other symptoms and signs involving emotional state

✓4ᵗʰ **R46 Symptoms and signs involving appearance and behavior**
EXCLUDES 1   appearance and behavior in schizophrenia, schizotypal and delusional disorders (F20-F29)
mental and behavioral disorders (F01-F99)

R46.0 Very low level of personal hygiene

R46.1 Bizarre personal appearance

R46.2 Strange and inexplicable behavior

R46.3 Overactivity

R46.4 Slowness and poor responsiveness
EXCLUDES 1   stupor (R40.1)

R46.5 Suspiciousness and marked evasiveness

R46.6 Undue concern and preoccupation with stressful events

R46.7 Verbosity and circumstantial detail obscuring reason for contact

✓5ᵗʰ **R46.8 Other symptoms and signs involving appearance and behavior**

   R46.81 Obsessive-compulsive behavior
     EXCLUDES 1   obsessive-compulsive disorder (F42-)

   R46.89 Other symptoms and signs involving appearance and behavior

Symptoms and signs involving speech and voice (R47-R49)

✓4ᵗʰ **R47 Speech disturbances, not elsewhere classified**
EXCLUDES 1   autism (F84.0)
cluttering (F80.81)
specific developmental disorders of speech and language (F80.-)
stuttering (F80.81)

✓5ᵗʰ **R47.0 Dysphasia and aphasia**

   R47.01 Aphasia   CC
     EXCLUDES 1   aphasia following cerebrovascular disease (I69. with final characters -20)
progressive isolated aphasia (G31.01)
     CC Excl: PDX collection 1131

   R47.02 Dysphasia
     EXCLUDES 1   dysphasia following cerebrovascular disease (I69. with final characters -21)

R47.1 Dysarthria and anarthria
EXCLUDES 1   dysarthria following cerebrovascular disease (I69. with final characters -22)

✓5ᵗʰ **R47.8 Other speech disturbances**
EXCLUDES 1   dysarthria following cerebrovascular disease (I69. with final characters -28)

   R47.81 Slurred speech

   R47.82 Fluency disorder in conditions classified elsewhere
     Stuttering in conditions classified elsewhere
     Code first underlying disease or condition, such as:
     Parkinson's disease (G20)
     EXCLUDES 1   adult onset fluency disorder (F98.5)
childhood onset fluency disorder (F80.81)
fluency disorder (stuttering) following cerebrovascular disease (I69. with final characters -23)

   R47.89 Other speech disturbances

R47.9 Unspecified speech disturbances

✓4ᵗʰ **R48 Dyslexia and other symbolic dysfunctions, not elsewhere classified**
EXCLUDES 1   specific developmental disorders of scholastic skills (F81.-)

R48.0 Dyslexia and alexia

R48.1 Agnosia
Astereognosia (astereognosis)
Autotopagnosia
EXCLUDES 1   visual object agnosia (R48.3)
DEF: Inability to recognize common things such as faces, objects, smells, or voices.

R48.2 Apraxia
EXCLUDES 1   apraxia following cerebrovascular disease (I69. with final characters -90)

R48.3 Visual agnosia
Prosopagnosia
Simultanagnosia (asimultagnosia)

R48.8 Other symbolic dysfunctions
Acalculia
Agraphia
AHA: 2017, 1Q, 27

R48.9 Unspecified symbolic dysfunctions

✓4ᵗʰ **R49 Voice and resonance disorders**
EXCLUDES 1   psychogenic voice and resonance disorders (F44.4)

R49.0 Dysphonia
Hoarseness

R49.1 Aphonia
Loss of voice

✓5ᵗʰ **R49.2 Hypernasality and hyponasality**

   R49.21 Hypernasality

   R49.22 Hyponasality

R49.8 Other voice and resonance disorders

R49.9 Unspecified voice and resonance disorder
Change in voice NOS
Resonance disorder NOS

Chapter 18. Symptoms, Signs and Abnormal Clinical and Laboratory Findings

General symptoms and signs (R50-R69)

✓4ᵗʰ **R50** **Fever of other and unknown origin**
- EXCLUDES 1   *chills without fever (R68.83)*
  - *febrile convulsions (R56.0-)*
  - *fever of unknown origin during labor (O75.2)*
  - *fever of unknown origin in newborn (P81.9)*
  - *hypothermia due to illness (R68.0)*
  - *malignant hyperthermia due to anesthesia (T88.3)*
  - *puerperal pyrexia NOS (O86.4)*

R50.2 **Drug induced fever**   CC
- Use additional code for adverse effect, if applicable, to identify drug (T36-T50 with fifth or sixth character 5)
- EXCLUDES 1   *postvaccination (postimmunization) fever (R50.83)*

✓5ᵗʰ **R50.8** **Other specified fever**

    R50.81 ***Fever presenting with conditions classified elsewhere***
- Code first underlying condition when associated fever is present, such as with:
  - leukemia (C91-C95)
  - neutropenia (D70.-)
  - sickle-cell disease (D57.-)
- **AHA:** 2014,4Q,22

    R50.82 **Postprocedural fever**   CC
- EXCLUDES 1   *postprocedural infection (T81.4-)*
  - *posttransfusion fever (R50.84)*
  - *postvaccination (postimmunization) fever (R50.83)*

    R50.83 **Postvaccination fever**
- Postimmunization fever

    R50.84 **Febrile nonhemolytic transfusion reaction**
- FNHTR
- Posttransfusion fever

R50.9 **Fever, unspecified**
- Fever NOS
- Fever of unknown origin [FUO]
- Fever with chills
- Fever with rigors
- Hyperpyrexia NOS
- Persistent fever
- Pyrexia NOS

R51 **Headache**
- Facial pain NOS
- EXCLUDES 1   *atypical face pain (G50.1)*
  - *migraine and other headache syndromes (G43-G44)*
  - *trigeminal neuralgia (G50.0)*

R52 **Pain, unspecified**
- Acute pain NOS
- Generalized pain NOS
- Pain NOS
- EXCLUDES 1   *acute and chronic pain, not elsewhere classified (G89.-)*
  - *localized pain, unspecified type — code to pain by site, such as:*
    - *abdomen pain (R10.-)*
    - *back pain (M54.9)*
    - *breast pain (N64.4)*
    - *chest pain (R07.1-R07.9)*
    - *ear pain (H92.0-)*
    - *eye pain (H57.1)*
    - *headache (R51)*
    - *joint pain (M25.5-)*
    - *limb pain (M79.6-)*
    - *lumbar region pain (M54.5)*
    - *pelvic and perineal pain (R10.2)*
    - *renal colic (N23)*
    - *shoulder pain (M25.51-)*
    - *spine pain (M54.-)*
    - *throat pain (R07.0)*
    - *tongue pain (K14.6)*
    - *tooth pain (K08.8)*
  - *pain disorders exclusively related to psychological factors (F45.41)*

✓4ᵗʰ **R53** **Malaise and fatigue**

R53.0 **Neoplastic (malignant) related fatigue**
- Code first associated neoplasm

R53.1 **Weakness**
- Asthenia NOS
- EXCLUDES 1   *age-related weakness (R54)*
  - *muscle weakness (M62.8-)*
  - *sarcopenia (M62.84)*
  - *senile asthenia (R54)*
- **AHA:** 2017,1Q,7; 2015,1Q,25

R53.2 **Functional quadriplegia**   MCC   HCC
- Complete immobility due to severe physical disability or frailty
- EXCLUDES 1   *frailty NOS (R54)*
  - *hysterical paralysis (F44.4)*
  - *immobility syndrome (M62.3)*
  - *neurologic quadriplegia (G82.5-)*
  - *quadriplegia (G82.50)*
- **AHA:** 2016,2Q,6
- **DEF:** Inability to move due to a nonphysiological condition, such as dementia. The patient has no mental ability to move independently.
- **CC Excl:** PDX collection 595

✓5ᵗʰ **R53.8** **Other malaise and fatigue**
- EXCLUDES 1   *combat exhaustion and fatigue (F43.0)*
  - *congenital debility (P96.9)*
  - *exhaustion and fatigue due to excessive exertion (T73.3)*
  - *exhaustion and fatigue due to exposure (T73.2)*
  - *exhaustion and fatigue due to heat (T67.-)*
  - *exhaustion and fatigue due to pregnancy (O26.8-)*
  - *exhaustion and fatigue due to recurrent depressive episode (F33)*
  - *exhaustion and fatigue due to senile debility (R54)*

    R53.81 **Other malaise**
- Chronic debility
- Debility NOS
- General physical deterioration
- Malaise NOS
- Nervous debility
- EXCLUDES 1   *age-related physical debility (R54)*

    R53.82 **Chronic fatigue, unspecified**
- Chronic fatigue syndrome NOS
- EXCLUDES 1   *postviral fatigue syndrome (G93.3)*

    R53.83 **Other fatigue**
- Fatigue NOS
- Lack of energy
- Lethargy
- Tiredness
- EXCLUDES 2   *exhaustion and fatigue due to depressive episode (F32.-)*

R54 **Age-related physical debility**   A
- Frailty
- Old age
- Senescence
- Senile asthenia
- Senile debility
- EXCLUDES 1   *age-related cognitive decline (R41.81)*
  - *sarcopenia (M62.84)*
  - *senile psychosis (F03)*
  - *senility NOS (R41.81)*

R55 Syncope and collapse
    Blackout
    Fainting
    Vasovagal attack
    EXCLUDES 1   *cardiogenic shock (R57.0)*
       carotid sinus syncope (G90.01)
       heat syncope (T67.1)
       neurocirculatory asthenia (F45.8)
       neurogenic orthostatic hypotension (G90.3)
       orthostatic hypotension (I95.1)
       postprocedural shock (T81.1-)
       psychogenic syncope (F48.8)
       shock NOS (R57.9)
       shock complicating or following abortion or ectopic or molar pregnancy (O00-O07, O08.3)
       shock complicating or following labor and delivery (O75.1)
       Stokes-Adams attack (I45.9)
       unconsciousness NOS (R40.2-)

✓4ᵗʰ R56 Convulsions, not elsewhere classified
    EXCLUDES 1   *dissociative convulsions and seizures (F44.5)*
       epileptic convulsions and seizures (G40.-)
       newborn convulsions and seizures (P90)

   ✓5ᵗʰ R56.0 Febrile convulsions

     R56.00 Simple febrile convulsions   CC HCC
       Febrile convulsion NOS
       Febrile seizure NOS
       CC Excl: PDX collection 1132

     R56.01 Complex febrile convulsions   CC HCC
       Atypical febrile seizure
       Complex febrile seizure
       Complicated febrile seizure
       EXCLUDES 1   *status epilepticus (G40.901)*
       CC Excl: PDX collection 1132

   R56.1 Post traumatic seizures   CC HCC
       EXCLUDES 1   *post traumatic epilepsy (G40.-)*
       CC Excl: PDX collection 582

   R56.9 Unspecified convulsions   HCC
       Convulsion disorder
       Fit NOS
       Recurrent convulsions
       Seizure(s) (convulsive) NOS
       AHA: 2019,1Q,19

✓4ᵗʰ R57 Shock, not elsewhere classified
    EXCLUDES 1   *anaphylactic shock NOS (T78.2)*
       anaphylactic reaction or shock due to adverse food reaction (T78.0-)
       anaphylactic shock due to adverse effect of correct drug or medicament properly administered (T88.6)
       anaphylactic shock due to serum (T80.5-)
       anesthetic shock (T88.3)
       electric shock (T75.4)
       obstetric shock (O75.1)
       postprocedural shock (T81.1-)
       psychic shock (F43.0)
       shock complicating or following ectopic or molar pregnancy (O00-O07, O08.3)
       shock due to lightning (T75.01)
       traumatic shock (T79.4)
       toxic shock syndrome (A48.3)
    CC Excl: For CC/MCC codes in category R57: PDX collection 1133

   ¹ R57.0 Cardiogenic shock   MCC HCC
       EXCLUDES 2   *septic shock (R65.21)*
       DEF: Associated with myocardial infarction, cardiac tamponade, and massive pulmonary embolism. Symptoms include mental confusion, reduced blood pressure, tachycardia, pallor, and cold, clammy skin.

   ¹ R57.1 Hypovolemic shock   MCC HCC
       AHA: 2019,2Q,7

   ¹ R57.8 Other shock   MCC HCC

   R57.9 Shock, unspecified   CC HCC
       Failure of peripheral circulation NOS

R58 Hemorrhage, not elsewhere classified   CC
    Hemorrhage NOS
    EXCLUDES 1   *hemorrhage included with underlying conditions, such as:*
       acute duodenal ulcer with hemorrhage (K26.0)
       acute gastritis with bleeding (K29.01)
       ulcerative enterocolitis with rectal bleeding (K51.01)

✓4ᵗʰ R59 Enlarged lymph nodes
    INCLUDES   swollen glands
    EXCLUDES 1   *acute lymphadenitis (L04.-)*
       chronic lymphadenitis (I88.1)
       lymphadenitis NOS (I88.9)
       mesenteric (acute) (chronic) lymphadenitis (I88.0)

   R59.0 Localized enlarged lymph nodes
   R59.1 Generalized enlarged lymph nodes
       Lymphadenopathy NOS

   R59.9 Enlarged lymph nodes, unspecified

✓4ᵗʰ R60 Edema, not elsewhere classified
    EXCLUDES 1   *angioneurotic edema (T78.3)*
       ascites (R18.-)
       cerebral edema (G93.6)
       cerebral edema due to birth injury (P11.0)
       edema of larynx (J38.4)
       edema of nasopharynx (J39.2)
       edema of pharynx (J39.2)
       gestational edema (O12.0-)
       hereditary edema (Q82.0)
       hydrops fetalis NOS (P83.2)
       hydrothorax (J94.8)
       hydrops fetalis NOS (P83.2)
       newborn edema (P83.3)
       pulmonary edema (J81.-)

   R60.0 Localized edema
   R60.1 Generalized edema   CC
       EXCLUDES 2   *nutritional edema (E40-E46)*

   R60.9 Edema, unspecified
       Fluid retention NOS

R61 Generalized hyperhidrosis
    Excessive sweating
    Night sweats
    Secondary hyperhidrosis
    Code first, if applicable, menopausal and female climacteric states (N95.1)
    EXCLUDES 1   *focal (primary) (secondary) hyperhidrosis (L74.5-)*
       Frey's syndrome (L74.52)
       localized (primary) (secondary) hyperhidrosis (L74.5-)

✓4ᵗʰ R62 Lack of expected normal physiological development in childhood and adults
    EXCLUDES 1   *delayed puberty (E30.0)*
       gonadal dysgenesis (Q99.1)
       hypopituitarism (E23.0)

   R62.0 Delayed milestone in childhood   P
       Delayed attainment of expected physiological developmental stage
       Late talker
       Late walker

   ✓5ᵗʰ R62.5 Other and unspecified lack of expected normal physiological development in childhood
       EXCLUDES 1   *HIV disease resulting in failure to thrive (B20)*
         physical retardation due to malnutrition (E45)

     R62.50 Unspecified lack of expected normal physiological development in childhood
       Infantilism NOS

     R62.51 Failure to thrive (child)   P
       Failure to gain weight
       EXCLUDES 1   *failure to thrive in child under 28 days old (P92.6)*
       AHA: 2018,4Q,82
       DEF: Organic failure to thrive (FTT): Acute or chronic illness that interferes with nutritional intake, absorption, metabolism excretion, and energy requirements.
       DEF: Nonorganic failure to thrive (FTT): Symptom of neglect or abuse.

Chapter 18. Symptoms, Signs and Abnormal Clinical and Laboratory Findings

R62.52 **Short stature (child)**
Lack of growth
Physical retardation
Short stature NOS
EXCLUDES 1   *short stature due to endocrine disorder (E34.3)*

R62.59 **Other lack of expected normal physiological development in childhood**

R62.7 **Adult failure to thrive**   CC A

R63 **Symptoms and signs concerning food and fluid intake**
EXCLUDES 1   *bulimia NOS (F50.2)*
eating disorders of nonorganic origin (F50.-)
malnutrition (E40-E46)

R63.0 **Anorexia**
Loss of appetite
EXCLUDES 1   *anorexia nervosa (F50.0-)*
loss of appetite of nonorganic origin (F50.89)
AHA: 2018,4Q,82
TIP: Assign an additional code from category Z68 when BMI is documented. BMI can be based on documentation from clinicians who are not the patient's provider.

R63.1 **Polydipsia**
Excessive thirst

R63.2 **Polyphagia**
Excessive eating
Hyperalimentation NOS

R63.3 **Feeding difficulties**   CC
Feeding problem (elderly) (infant) NOS
Picky eater
EXCLUDES 1   *eating disorders (F50.-)*
feeding problems of newborn (P92.-)
infant feeding disorder of nonorganic origin (F98.2-)
AHA: 2017,1Q,28; 2016,3Q,19
TIP: Do not assign for feeding problems in a patient greater than 28 days old if the feeding problem was initially diagnosed between day 0 and day 28; use a code from category P92 instead.

R63.4 **Abnormal weight loss**
AHA: 2018,4Q,82
TIP: Assign an additional code from category Z68 when BMI is documented. BMI can be based on documentation from clinicians who are not the patient's provider.

R63.5 **Abnormal weight gain**
EXCLUDES 1   *excessive weight gain in pregnancy (O26.0-)*
obesity (E66.-)
AHA: 2018,4Q,82
TIP: Assign an additional code from category Z68 when BMI is documented. BMI can be based on documentation from clinicians who are not the patient's provider.

R63.6 **Underweight**
Use additional code to identify body mass index (BMI), if known (Z68.-)
EXCLUDES 1   *abnormal weight loss (R63.4)*
anorexia nervosa (F50.0-)
malnutrition (E40-E46)
AHA: 2018,4Q,82

R63.8 **Other symptoms and signs concerning food and fluid intake**

R64 **Cachexia**   CC HCC
Wasting syndrome
Code first underlying condition, if known
EXCLUDES 1   *abnormal weight loss (R63.4)*
nutritional marasmus (E41)
AHA: 2018,4Q,82; 2017,3Q,24
CC Excl: PDX collection 1134

R65 **Symptoms and signs specifically associated with systemic inflammation and infection**
AHA: 2019,2Q,38
TIP: When documentation states SIRS with an infection, assign only a code for the infection. ICD-10-CM does not offer a code for SIRS due to infectious process. If sepsis is suspected, query the provider.
CC Excl: For CC/MCC codes in category R65, unless otherwise noted: PDX collection 71

R65.1 **Systemic inflammatory response syndrome [SIRS] of non-infectious origin**
Code first underlying condition, such as:
heatstroke ▶(T67.0-)◀
injury and trauma (S00-T88)
EXCLUDES 1   *sepsis — code to infection*
severe sepsis (R65.2)

R65.10 **Systemic inflammatory response syndrome [SIRS] of non-infectious origin without acute organ dysfunction**   CC HCC
Systemic inflammatory response syndrome (SIRS) NOS
AHA: 2019,2Q,24

R65.11 **Systemic inflammatory response syndrome [SIRS] of non-infectious origin with acute organ dysfunction**   CC HCC
Use additional code to identify specific acute organ dysfunction, such as:
acute kidney failure (N17.-)
acute respiratory failure (J96.0-)
critical illness myopathy (G72.81)
critical illness polyneuropathy (G62.81)
disseminated intravascular coagulopathy [DIC] (D65)
encephalopathy (metabolic) (septic) (G93.41)
hepatic failure (K72.0-)

R65.2 **Severe sepsis**
Infection with associated acute organ dysfunction
Sepsis with acute organ dysfunction
Sepsis with multiple organ dysfunction
Systemic inflammatory response syndrome due to infectious process with acute organ dysfunction
Code first underlying infection, such as:
infection following a procedure (T81.4-)
infections following infusion, transfusion and therapeutic injection (T80.2-)
puerperal sepsis (O85)
sepsis following complete or unspecified spontaneous abortion (O03.87)
sepsis following ectopic and molar pregnancy (O08.82)
sepsis following incomplete spontaneous abortion (O03.37)
sepsis following (induced) termination of pregnancy (O04.87)
sepsis NOS (A41.9)
Use additional code to identify specific acute organ dysfunction, such as:
acute kidney failure (N17.-)
acute respiratory failure (J96.0-)
critical illness myopathy (G72.81)
critical illness polyneuropathy (G62.81)
disseminated intravascular coagulopathy [DIC] (D65)
encephalopathy (metabolic) (septic) (G93.41)
hepatic failure (K72.0-)
AHA: 2018,4Q,62-63; 2017,4Q,98-99; 2016,3Q,8

R65.20 **Severe sepsis without septic shock**   MCC HCC
Severe sepsis NOS
AHA: 2016,3Q,14; 2013,4Q,119

R65.21 **Severe sepsis with septic shock**   MCC HCC
AHA: 2018,4Q,63
CC Excl: PDX collection 1133

R68 **Other general symptoms and signs**

R68.0 **Hypothermia, not associated with low environmental temperature**
EXCLUDES 1   *hypothermia NOS (accidental) (T68)*
hypothermia due to anesthesia (T88.51)
hypothermia due to low environmental temperature (T68)
newborn hypothermia (P80.-)

✓5ᵗʰ **R68.1　Nonspecific symptoms peculiar to infancy**
　　　　　EXCLUDES 1　*colic, infantile (R10.83)*
　　　　　　　　　neonatal cerebral irritability (P91.3)
　　　　　　　　　teething syndrome (K00.7)
　　R68.11　Excessive crying of infant (baby)　　　P
　　　　　EXCLUDES 1　*excessive crying of child, adolescent, or adult (R45.83)*
　　R68.12　Fussy infant (baby)　　　P
　　　　　Irritable infant
　　R68.13　Apparent life threatening event in infant (ALTE)　　　P
　　　　　Apparent life threatening event in newborn
　　　　　Brief resolved unexplained event (BRUE)
　　　　　Code first confirmed diagnosis, if known
　　　　　Use additional code(s) for associated signs and symptoms if no confirmed diagnosis established, or if signs and symptoms are not associated routinely with confirmed diagnosis, or provide additional information for cause of ALTE
　　R68.19　Other nonspecific symptoms peculiar to infancy　　　P
R68.2　Dry mouth, unspecified
　　　　　EXCLUDES 1　*dry mouth due to dehydration (E86.0)*
　　　　　　　　　dry mouth due to sicca syndrome [Sjögren] (M35.0-)
　　　　　　　　　salivary gland hyposecretion (K11.7)
R68.3　Clubbing of fingers
　　　　　Clubbing of nails
　　　　　EXCLUDES 1　*congenital clubfinger (Q68.1)*
　　　　　DEF: Enlarged soft tissue of the distal fingers that usually occurs in heart and lung diseases.
✓5ᵗʰ **R68.8　Other general symptoms and signs**
　　R68.81　Early satiety
　　　　　DEF: Premature feeling of being full after eating only a small amount of food. The mechanism of satiety is multifactorial.
　　R68.82　Decreased libido　　　A
　　　　　Decreased sexual desire
　　R68.83　Chills (without fever)
　　　　　Chills NOS
　　　　　EXCLUDES 1　*chills with fever (R50.9)*
　　R68.84　Jaw pain
　　　　　Mandibular pain
　　　　　Maxilla pain
　　　　　EXCLUDES 1　*temporomandibular joint arthralgia (M26.62-)*
　　R68.89　Other general symptoms and signs
R69　Illness, unspecified
　　　　　Unknown and unspecified cases of morbidity

Abnormal findings on examination of blood, without diagnosis (R70-R79)

EXCLUDES 2　*abnormal findings on antenatal screening of mother (O28.-)*
　　　　abnormalities of lipids (E78.-)
　　　　abnormalities of platelets and thrombocytes (D69.-)
　　　　abnormalities of white blood cells classified elsewhere (D70-D72)
　　　　coagulation hemorrhagic disorders (D65-D68)
　　　　diagnostic abnormal findings classified elsewhere — see Alphabetical Index
　　　　hemorrhagic and hematological disorders of newborn (P50-P61)

✓4ᵗʰ **R70　Elevated erythrocyte sedimentation rate and abnormality of plasma viscosity**
　　R70.0　Elevated erythrocyte sedimentation rate
　　R70.1　Abnormal plasma viscosity

✓4ᵗʰ **R71　Abnormality of red blood cells**
　　　　　EXCLUDES 1　*anemias (D50-D64)*
　　　　　　　　　anemia of premature infant (P61.2)
　　　　　　　　　benign (familial) polycythemia (D75.0)
　　　　　　　　　congenital anemias (P61.2-P61.4)
　　　　　　　　　newborn anemia due to isoimmunization (P55.-)
　　　　　　　　　polycythemia neonatorum (P61.1)
　　　　　　　　　polycythemia NOS (D75.1)
　　　　　　　　　polycythemia vera (D45)
　　　　　　　　　secondary polycythemia (D75.1)
　　R71.0　Precipitous drop in hematocrit　　　CC
　　　　　Drop (precipitous) in hemoglobin
　　　　　Drop in hematocrit
　　　　　CC Excl: PDX collection 1135
　　R71.8　Other abnormality of red blood cells
　　　　　Abnormal red-cell morphology NOS
　　　　　Abnormal red-cell volume NOS
　　　　　Anisocytosis
　　　　　Poikilocytosis

✓4ᵗʰ **R73　Elevated blood glucose level**
　　　　　EXCLUDES 1　*diabetes mellitus (E08-E13)*
　　　　　　　　　diabetes mellitus in pregnancy, childbirth and the puerperium (O24.-)
　　　　　　　　　neonatal disorders (P70.0-P70.2)
　　　　　　　　　postsurgical hypoinsulinemia (E89.1)
　　✓5ᵗʰ **R73.0　Abnormal glucose**
　　　　　EXCLUDES 1　*abnormal glucose in pregnancy (O99.81-)*
　　　　　　　　　diabetes mellitus (E08-E13)
　　　　　　　　　dysmetabolic syndrome X (E88.81)
　　　　　　　　　gestational diabetes (O24.4-)
　　　　　　　　　glycosuria (R81)
　　　　　　　　　hypoglycemia (E16.2)
　　　　R73.01　Impaired fasting glucose
　　　　　　Elevated fasting glucose
　　　　R73.02　Impaired glucose tolerance (oral)
　　　　　　Elevated glucose tolerance
　　　　R73.03　Prediabetes
　　　　　　Latent diabetes
　　　　　　AHA: 2016,4Q,65
　　　　R73.09　Other abnormal glucose
　　　　　　Abnormal glucose NOS
　　　　　　Abnormal non-fasting glucose tolerance
　　R73.9　Hyperglycemia, unspecified

✓4ᵗʰ **R74　Abnormal serum enzyme levels**
　　R74.0　Nonspecific elevation of levels of transaminase and lactic acid dehydrogenase [LDH]
　　R74.8　Abnormal levels of other serum enzymes
　　　　　Abnormal level of acid phosphatase
　　　　　Abnormal level of alkaline phosphatase
　　　　　Abnormal level of amylase
　　　　　Abnormal level of lipase [triacylglycerol lipase]
　　　　　AHA: 2019,2Q,6
　　R74.9　Abnormal serum enzyme level, unspecified

R75　Inconclusive laboratory evidence of human immunodeficiency virus [HIV]
　　　　　Nonconclusive HIV-test finding in infants
　　　　　EXCLUDES 1　*asymptomatic human immunodeficiency virus [HIV] infection status (Z21)*
　　　　　　　　　human immunodeficiency virus [HIV] disease (B20)
　　　　　TIP: Do not assign for patients previously diagnosed with an HIV-related illness; assign code B20 instead.

✓4ᵗʰ **R76　Other abnormal immunological findings in serum**
　　R76.0　Raised antibody titer
　　　　　EXCLUDES 1　*isoimmunization in pregnancy (O36.0-O36.1)*
　　　　　　　　　isoimmunization affecting newborn (P55.-)

Chapter 18. Symptoms, Signs and Abnormal Clinical and Laboratory Findings

✓5ᵗʰ R76.1 Nonspecific reaction to test for tuberculosis

R76.11 Nonspecific reaction to tuberculin skin test without active tuberculosis
Abnormal result of Mantoux test
PPD positive
Tuberculin (skin test) positive
Tuberculin (skin test) reactor
> EXCLUDES 1   *nonspecific reaction to cell mediated immunity measurement of gamma interferon antigen response without active tuberculosis (R76.12)*

R76.12 Nonspecific reaction to cell mediated immunity measurement of gamma interferon antigen response without active tuberculosis
Nonspecific reaction to QuantiFERON-TB test (QFT) without active tuberculosis
> EXCLUDES 1   *nonspecific reaction to tuberculin skin test without active tuberculosis (R76.11)*
> *positive tuberculin skin test (R76.11)*

R76.8 Other specified abnormal immunological findings in serum
Raised level of immunoglobulins NOS

R76.9 Abnormal immunological finding in serum, unspecified

✓4ᵗʰ R77 Other abnormalities of plasma proteins
> EXCLUDES 1   *disorders of plasma-protein metabolism (E88.0-)*

R77.0 Abnormality of albumin
R77.1 Abnormality of globulin
Hyperglobulinemia NOS
R77.2 Abnormality of alphafetoprotein
R77.8 Other specified abnormalities of plasma proteins
R77.9 Abnormality of plasma protein, unspecified
AHA: 2019,2Q,6

✓4ᵗʰ R78 Findings of drugs and other substances, not normally found in blood
Use additional code to identify the any retained foreign body, if applicable (Z18.-)
> EXCLUDES 1   *mental or behavioral disorders due to psychoactive substance use (F10-F19)*

R78.0 Finding of alcohol in blood
Use additional external cause code (Y90.-), for detail regarding alcohol level
R78.1 Finding of opiate drug in blood
R78.2 Finding of cocaine in blood
R78.3 Finding of hallucinogen in blood
R78.4 Finding of other drugs of addictive potential in blood
R78.5 Finding of other psychotropic drug in blood
R78.6 Finding of steroid agent in blood
✓5ᵗʰ R78.7 Finding of abnormal level of heavy metals in blood
R78.71 Abnormal lead level in blood
> EXCLUDES 1   *lead poisoning (T56.0-)*
R78.79 Finding of abnormal level of heavy metals in blood
✓5ᵗʰ R78.8 Finding of other specified substances, not normally found in blood
R78.81 Bacteremia   **MCC**
> EXCLUDES 1   *sepsis — code to specified infection*
DEF: Laboratory finding of bacteria in the blood in the absence of two or more signs of sepsis. Transient in nature, it can progress to septicemia with a severe infectious process.
R78.89 Finding of other specified substances, not normally found in blood
Finding of abnormal level of lithium in blood
R78.9 Finding of unspecified substance, not normally found in blood

✓4ᵗʰ R79 Other abnormal findings of blood chemistry
Use additional code to identify any retained foreign body, if applicable (Z18.-)
> EXCLUDES 1   *asymptomatic hyperuricemia (E79.0)*
> *hyperglycemia NOS (R73.9)*
> *hypoglycemia NOS (E16.2)*
> *neonatal hypoglycemia (P70.3-P70.4)*
> *specific findings indicating disorder of amino-acid metabolism (E70-E72)*
> *specific findings indicating disorder of carbohydrate metabolism (E73-E74)*
> *specific findings indicating disorder of lipid metabolism (E75.-)*

R79.0 Abnormal level of blood mineral
Abnormal blood level of cobalt
Abnormal blood level of copper
Abnormal blood level of iron
Abnormal blood level of magnesium
Abnormal blood level of mineral NEC
Abnormal blood level of zinc
> EXCLUDES 1   *abnormal level of lithium (R78.89)*
> *disorders of mineral metabolism (E83.-)*
> *neonatal hypomagnesemia (P71.2)*
> *nutritional mineral deficiency (E58-E61)*

R79.1 Abnormal coagulation profile
Abnormal or prolonged bleeding time
Abnormal or prolonged coagulation time
Abnormal or prolonged partial thromboplastin time [PTT]
Abnormal or prolonged prothrombin time [PT]
> EXCLUDES 1   *coagulation defects (D68.-)*
> EXCLUDES 2   *abnormality of fluid, electrolyte or acid-base balance (E86-E87)*

✓5ᵗʰ R79.8 Other specified abnormal findings of blood chemistry
R79.81 Abnormal blood-gas level
R79.82 Elevated C-reactive protein [CRP]
R79.89 Other specified abnormal findings of blood chemistry
AHA: 2019,2Q,6
TIP: Assign for documented abnormal or elevated troponin level when a definitive diagnosis has not been established.
TIP: Assign for positive Coombs test when not further clarified in the documentation.

R79.9 Abnormal finding of blood chemistry, unspecified

Abnormal findings on examination of urine, without diagnosis (R80-R82)
> EXCLUDES 1   *abnormal findings on antenatal screening of mother (O28.-)*
> *diagnostic abnormal findings classified elsewhere — see Alphabetical Index*
> *specific findings indicating disorder of amino-acid metabolism (E70-E72)*
> *specific findings indicating disorder of carbohydrate metabolism (E73-E74)*

✓4ᵗʰ R80 Proteinuria
> EXCLUDES 1   *gestational proteinuria (O12.1-)*

R80.0 Isolated proteinuria
Idiopathic proteinuria
> EXCLUDES 1   *isolated proteinuria with specific morphological lesion (N06.-)*
R80.1 Persistent proteinuria, unspecified
R80.2 Orthostatic proteinuria, unspecified
Postural proteinuria
R80.3 Bence Jones proteinuria
R80.8 Other proteinuria
R80.9 Proteinuria, unspecified
Albuminuria NOS

R81 Glycosuria
> EXCLUDES 1   *renal glycosuria (E74.8)*

N Newborn: 0   P Pediatric: 0-17   M Maternity: 9-64   A Adult: 15-124   MCC Major Complication/Comorbidity   CC Complication/Comorbidity   SW Severe Wound Dx

968   ICD-10-CM 2020

✓4ᵗʰ **R82   Other and unspecified abnormal findings in urine**

INCLUDES   chromoabnormalities in urine

Use additional code to identify any retained foreign body, if applicable (Z18.-)

EXCLUDES 2   *hematuria (R31.-)*

R82.0   Chyluria   cc

EXCLUDES 1   *filarial chyluria (B74.-)*

CC Excl: PDX collection 1137

R82.1   Myoglobinuria   cc

CC Excl: PDX collection 1138

R82.2   Biliuria

R82.3   Hemoglobinuria

EXCLUDES 1   *hemoglobinuria due to hemolysis from external causes NEC (D59.6)*

hemoglobinuria due to paroxysmal nocturnal [Marchiafava-Micheli] (D59.5)

DEF: Free hemoglobin in blood due to rapid hemolysis of red blood cells. Causes include burns, crushed injury, sickle cell anemia, thalassemia, parasitic infections, or kidney infections.

R82.4   Acetonuria

Ketonuria

DEF: Excessive excretion of acetone in urine that commonly occurs in diabetic acidosis.

R82.5   Elevated urine levels of drugs, medicaments and biological substances

Elevated urine levels of catecholamines

Elevated urine levels of indoleacetic acid

Elevated urine levels of 17-ketosteroids

Elevated urine levels of steroids

R82.6   Abnormal urine levels of substances chiefly nonmedicinal as to source

Abnormal urine level of heavy metals

✓5ᵗʰ **R82.7   Abnormal findings on microbiological examination of urine**

EXCLUDES 1   *colonization status (Z22.-)*

AHA: 2016,4Q,65

R82.71   Bacteriuria

R82.79   Other abnormal findings on microbiological examination of urine

Positive culture findings of urine

▲ ✓5ᵗʰ **R82.8   Abnormal findings on cytological and histological examination of urine**

● **R82.81   Pyuria**

Sterile pyuria

● **R82.89   Other abnormal findings on cytological and histological examination of urine**

✓5ᵗʰ **R82.9   Other and unspecified abnormal findings in urine**

R82.90   Unspecified abnormal findings in urine

R82.91   Other chromoabnormalities of urine

Chromoconversion (dipstick)

Idiopathic dipstick converts positive for blood with no cellular forms in sediment

EXCLUDES 1   *hemoglobinuria (R82.3)*

myoglobinuria (R82.1)

✓6ᵗʰ **R82.99   Other abnormal findings in urine**

AHA: 2018,4Q,29-30

R82.991   Hypocitraturia

R82.992   Hyperoxaluria

EXCLUDES 1   *primary hyperoxaluria (E72.53)*

▲ **R82.993   Hyperuricosuria**

R82.994   Hypercalciuria

Idiopathic hypercalciuria

R82.998   Other abnormal findings in urine

Cells and casts in urine

Crystalluria

Melanuria

Abnormal findings on examination of other body fluids, substances and tissues, without diagnosis (R83-R89)

EXCLUDES 1   *abnormal findings on antenatal screening of mother (O28.-)*

diagnostic abnormal findings classified elsewhere — see Alphabetical Index

EXCLUDES 2   *abnormal findings on examination of blood, without diagnosis (R70-R79)*

abnormal findings on examination of urine, without diagnosis (R80-R82)

abnormal tumor markers (R97.-)

✓4ᵗʰ **R83   Abnormal findings in cerebrospinal fluid**

Cerebrospinal Fluid

Ventricles

Cerebrospinal fluid

Spinal cord

R83.0   Abnormal level of enzymes in cerebrospinal fluid

R83.1   Abnormal level of hormones in cerebrospinal fluid

R83.2   Abnormal level of other drugs, medicaments and biological substances in cerebrospinal fluid

R83.3   Abnormal level of substances chiefly nonmedicinal as to source in cerebrospinal fluid

R83.4   Abnormal immunological findings in cerebrospinal fluid

R83.5   Abnormal microbiological findings in cerebrospinal fluid

Positive culture findings in cerebrospinal fluid

EXCLUDES 1   *colonization status (Z22.-)*

R83.6   Abnormal cytological findings in cerebrospinal fluid

R83.8   Other abnormal findings in cerebrospinal fluid

Abnormal chromosomal findings in cerebrospinal fluid

R83.9   Unspecified abnormal finding in cerebrospinal fluid

✓4ᵗʰ **R84   Abnormal findings in specimens from respiratory organs and thorax**

INCLUDES   abnormal findings in bronchial washings

abnormal findings in nasal secretions

abnormal findings in pleural fluid

abnormal findings in sputum

abnormal findings in throat scrapings

EXCLUDES 1   *blood-stained sputum (R04.2)*

R84.0   Abnormal level of enzymes in specimens from respiratory organs and thorax

R84.1   Abnormal level of hormones in specimens from respiratory organs and thorax

R84.2   Abnormal level of other drugs, medicaments and biological substances in specimens from respiratory organs and thorax

R84.3   Abnormal level of substances chiefly nonmedicinal as to source in specimens from respiratory organs and thorax

R84.4   Abnormal immunological findings in specimens from respiratory organs and thorax

✔ Additional Character Required   ✓x7ᵗʰ Placeholder   Unacceptable PDx   Questionable PDx   Manifestation   Unspecified Dx   H1-H14 HAC   HCC CMS-HCC Dx   HIV HIV Dx

ICD-10-CM 2020   **969**

R84.5   **Abnormal microbiological findings in specimens from respiratory organs and thorax**
    Positive culture findings in specimens from respiratory organs and thorax
    EXCLUDES 1   *colonization status (Z22.-)*

R84.6   **Abnormal cytological findings in specimens from respiratory organs and thorax**

R84.7   **Abnormal histological findings in specimens from respiratory organs and thorax**

R84.8   **Other abnormal findings in specimens from respiratory organs and thorax**
    Abnormal chromosomal findings in specimens from respiratory organs and thorax

R84.9   **Unspecified abnormal finding in specimens from respiratory organs and thorax**

✓4ᵗʰ **R85**   **Abnormal findings in specimens from digestive organs and abdominal cavity**
    INCLUDES   abnormal findings in peritoneal fluid
        abnormal findings in saliva
    EXCLUDES 1   *cloudy peritoneal dialysis effluent (R88.0)*
        fecal abnormalities (R19.5)

R85.0   **Abnormal level of enzymes in specimens from digestive organs and abdominal cavity**

R85.1   **Abnormal level of hormones in specimens from digestive organs and abdominal cavity**

R85.2   **Abnormal level of other drugs, medicaments and biological substances in specimens from digestive organs and abdominal cavity**

R85.3   **Abnormal level of substances chiefly nonmedicinal as to source in specimens from digestive organs and abdominal cavity**

R85.4   **Abnormal immunological findings in specimens from digestive organs and abdominal cavity**

R85.5   **Abnormal microbiological findings in specimens from digestive organs and abdominal cavity**
    Positive culture findings in specimens from digestive organs and abdominal cavity
    EXCLUDES 1   *colonization status (Z22.-)*

✓5ᵗʰ **R85.6**   **Abnormal cytological findings in specimens from digestive organs and abdominal cavity**

✓6ᵗʰ   **R85.61**   **Abnormal cytologic smear of anus**
       EXCLUDES 1   *abnormal cytological findings in specimens from other digestive organs and abdominal cavity (R85.69)*
           anal intraepithelial neoplasia I [AIN I] (K62.82)
           anal intraepithelial neoplasia II [AIN II] (K62.82)
           anal intraepithelial neoplasia III [AIN III] (D01.3)
           carcinoma in situ of anus (histologically confirmed) (D01.3)
           dysplasia (mild) (moderate) of anus (histologically confirmed) (K62.82)
           severe dysplasia of anus (histologically confirmed) (D01.3)
       EXCLUDES 2   *anal high risk human papillomavirus (HPV) DNA test positive (R85.81)*
           anal low risk human papillomavirus (HPV) DNA test positive (R85.82)

      R85.610   **Atypical squamous cells of undetermined significance on cytologic smear of anus [ASC-US]**

      R85.611   **Atypical squamous cells cannot exclude high grade squamous intraepithelial lesion on cytologic smear of anus [ASC-H]**

      R85.612   **Low grade squamous intraepithelial lesion on cytologic smear of anus [LGSIL]**

      R85.613   **High grade squamous intraepithelial lesion on cytologic smear of anus [HGSIL]**

      R85.614   **Cytologic evidence of malignancy on smear of anus**

      R85.615   **Unsatisfactory cytologic smear of anus**
           Inadequate sample of cytologic smear of anus

      R85.616   **Satisfactory anal smear but lacking transformation zone**

      R85.618   **Other abnormal cytological findings on specimens from anus**

      R85.619   **Unspecified abnormal cytological findings in specimens from anus**
           Abnormal anal cytology NOS
           Atypical glandular cells of anus NOS

   R85.69   **Abnormal cytological findings in specimens from other digestive organs and abdominal cavity**

R85.7   **Abnormal histological findings in specimens from digestive organs and abdominal cavity**

✓5ᵗʰ **R85.8**   **Other abnormal findings in specimens from digestive organs and abdominal cavity**

   R85.81   **Anal high risk human papillomavirus [HPV] DNA test positive**
       EXCLUDES 1   *anogenital warts due to human papillomavirus (HPV) (A63.0)*
           condyloma acuminatum (A63.0)

   R85.82   **Anal low risk human papillomavirus [HPV] DNA test positive**
       Use additional code for associated human papillomavirus (B97.7)

   R85.89   **Other abnormal findings in specimens from digestive organs and abdominal cavity**
       Abnormal chromosomal findings in specimens from digestive organs and abdominal cavity

R85.9   **Unspecified abnormal finding in specimens from digestive organs and abdominal cavity**

✓4ᵗʰ **R86**   **Abnormal findings in specimens from male genital organs**
    INCLUDES   abnormal findings in prostatic secretions
        abnormal findings in semen, seminal fluid
        abnormal spermatozoa
    EXCLUDES 1   *azoospermia (N46.0-)*
        oligospermia (N46.1-)

R86.0   **Abnormal level of enzymes in specimens from male genital organs** ♂

R86.1   **Abnormal level of hormones in specimens from male genital organs** ♂

R86.2   **Abnormal level of other drugs, medicaments and biological substances in specimens from male genital organs** ♂

R86.3   **Abnormal level of substances chiefly nonmedicinal as to source in specimens from male genital organs** ♂

R86.4   **Abnormal immunological findings in specimens from male genital organs** ♂

R86.5   **Abnormal microbiological findings in specimens from male genital organs** ♂
    Positive culture findings in specimens from male genital organs
    EXCLUDES 1   *colonization status (Z22.-)*

R86.6   **Abnormal cytological findings in specimens from male genital organs** ♂

R86.7   **Abnormal histological findings in specimens from male genital organs** ♂

R86.8   **Other abnormal findings in specimens from male genital organs** ♂
    Abnormal chromosomal findings in specimens from male genital organs

R86.9   **Unspecified abnormal finding in specimens from male genital organs** ♂

✓4ᵗʰ **R87**   **Abnormal findings in specimens from female genital organs**
    INCLUDES   abnormal findings in secretion and smears from cervix uteri
        abnormal findings in secretion and smears from vagina
        abnormal findings in secretion and smears from vulva

R87.0   **Abnormal level of enzymes in specimens from female genital organs** ♀

R87.1   **Abnormal level of hormones in specimens from female genital organs** ♀

R87.2   **Abnormal level of other drugs, medicaments and biological substances in specimens from female genital organs** ♀

R87.3   **Abnormal level of substances chiefly nonmedicinal as to source in specimens from female genital organs** ♀

R87.4   **Abnormal immunological findings in specimens from female genital organs** ♀

R87.5   **Abnormal microbiological findings in specimens from female genital organs** ♀
    Positive culture findings in specimens from female genital organs
    EXCLUDES 1   *colonization status (Z22.-)*

✓5ᵗʰ **R87.6 Abnormal cytological findings in specimens from female genital organs**

✓6ᵗʰ **R87.61 Abnormal cytological findings in specimens from cervix uteri**

EXCLUDES 1   abnormal cytological findings in specimens from other female genital organs (R87.69)

abnormal cytological findings in specimens from vagina (R87.62-)

carcinoma in situ of cervix uteri (histologically confirmed) (D06.-)

cervical intraepithelial neoplasia I [CIN I] (N87.0)

cervical intraepithelial neoplasia II [CIN II] (N87.1)

cervical intraepithelial neoplasia III [CIN III] (D06.-)

dysplasia (mild) (moderate) of cervix uteri (histologically confirmed) (N87.-)

severe dysplasia of cervix uteri (histologically confirmed) (D06.-)

EXCLUDES 2   cervical high risk human papillomavirus (HPV) DNA test positive (R87.810)

cervical low risk human papillomavirus (HPV) DNA test positive (R87.820)

R87.610 Atypical squamous cells of undetermined significance on cytologic smear of cervix [ASC-US] ♀

R87.611 Atypical squamous cells cannot exclude high grade squamous intraepithelial lesion on cytologic smear of cervix [ASC-H] ♀

R87.612 Low grade squamous intraepithelial lesion on cytologic smear of cervix [LGSIL] ♀

R87.613 High grade squamous intraepithelial lesion on cytologic smear of cervix [HGSIL] ♀

R87.614 Cytologic evidence of malignancy on smear of cervix ♀

R87.615 Unsatisfactory cytologic smear of cervix ♀

Inadequate sample of cytologic smear of cervix

R87.616 Satisfactory cervical smear but lacking transformation zone ♀

R87.618 Other abnormal cytological findings on specimens from cervix uteri ♀

R87.619 Unspecified abnormal cytological findings in specimens from cervix uteri ♀

Abnormal cervical cytology NOS

Abnormal Papanicolaou smear of cervix NOS

Abnormal thin preparation smear of cervix NOS

Atypical endocervial cells of cervix NOS

Atypical endometrial cells of cervix NOS

Atypical glandular cells of cervix NOS

✓6ᵗʰ **R87.62 Abnormal cytological findings in specimens from vagina**

Use additional code to identify acquired absence of uterus and cervix, if applicable (Z90.71-)

EXCLUDES 1   abnormal cytological findings in specimens from cervix uteri (R87.61-)

abnormal cytological findings in specimens from other female genital organs (R87.69)

carcinoma in situ of vagina (histologically confirmed) (D07.2)

dysplasia (mild) (moderate) of vagina (histologically confirmed) (N89.-)

severe dysplasia of vagina (histologically confirmed) (D07.2)

vaginal intraepithelial neoplasia I [VAIN I] (N89.0)

vaginal intraepithelial neoplasia II [VAIN II] (N89.1)

vaginal intraepithelial neoplasia III [VAIN III] (D07.2)

EXCLUDES 2   vaginal high risk human papillomavirus (HPV) DNA test positive (R87.811)

vaginal low risk human papillomavirus (HPV) DNA test positive (R87.821)

R87.620 Atypical squamous cells of undetermined significance on cytologic smear of vagina [ASC-US] ♀

R87.621 Atypical squamous cells cannot exclude high grade squamous intraepithelial lesion on cytologic smear of vagina [ASC-H] ♀

R87.622 Low grade squamous intraepithelial lesion on cytologic smear of vagina [LGSIL] ♀

R87.623 High grade squamous intraepithelial lesion on cytologic smear of vagina [HGSIL] ♀

R87.624 Cytologic evidence of malignancy on smear of vagina ♀

R87.625 Unsatisfactory cytologic smear of vagina ♀

Inadequate sample of cytologic smear of vagina

R87.628 Other abnormal cytological findings on specimens from vagina ♀

R87.629 Unspecified abnormal cytological findings in specimens from vagina ♀

Abnormal Papanicolaou smear of vagina NOS

Abnormal thin preparation smear of vagina NOS

Abnormal vaginal cytology NOS

Atypical endocervical cells of vagina NOS

Atypical endometrial cells of vagina NOS

Atypical glandular cells of vagina NOS

R87.69 Abnormal cytological findings in specimens from other female genital organs ♀

Abnormal cytological findings in specimens from female genital organs NOS

EXCLUDES 1   dysplasia of vulva (histologically confirmed) (N90.0-N90.3)

✔ Additional Character Required   ✓x7ᵗʰ Placeholder   Unacceptable PDx   Questionable PDx   Manifestation   Unspecified Dx   H1 - H14 HAC   HCC CMS-HCC Dx   HIV HIV Dx

ICD-10-CM 2020   971

Chapter 18. Symptoms, Signs and Abnormal Clinical and Laboratory Findings

R87.7   **Abnormal histological findings in specimens from female genital organs**   ♀
> EXCLUDES 1   *carcinoma in situ (histologically confirmed) of female genital organs (D06-D07.3)*
> *cervical intraepithelial neoplasia I [CIN I] (N87.0)*
> *cervical intraepithelial neoplasia II [CIN II] (N87.1)*
> *cervical intraepithelial neoplasia III [CIN III] (D06.-)*
> *dysplasia (mild) (moderate) of cervix uteri (histologically confirmed) (N87.-)*
> *dysplasia (mild) (moderate) of vagina (histologically confirmed) (N89.-)*
> *severe dysplasia of cervix uteri (histologically confirmed) (D06.-)*
> *severe dysplasia of vagina (histologically confirmed) (D07.2)*
> *vaginal intraepithelial neoplasia I [VAIN I] (N89.0)*
> *vaginal intraepithelial neoplasia II [VAIN II] (N89.1)*
> *vaginal intraepithelial neoplasia III [VAIN III] (D07.2)*

✓6ᵗʰ R87.8   **Other abnormal findings in specimens from female genital organs**

✓6ᵗʰ R87.81   **High risk human papillomavirus [HPV] DNA test positive from female genital organs**
> EXCLUDES 1   *anogenital warts due to human papillomavirus (HPV) (A63.0)*
> *condyloma acuminatum (A63.0)*

R87.810   **Cervical high risk human papillomavirus [HPV] DNA test positive**   ♀

R87.811   **Vaginal high risk human papillomavirus [HPV] DNA test positive**   ♀

✓6ᵗʰ R87.82   **Low risk human papillomavirus [HPV] DNA test positive from female genital organs**
> Use additional code for associated human papillomavirus (B97.7)

R87.820   **Cervical low risk human papillomavirus [HPV] DNA test positive**   ♀

R87.821   **Vaginal low risk human papillomavirus [HPV] DNA test positive**   ♀

R87.89   **Other abnormal findings in specimens from female genital organs**   ♀
> Abnormal chromosomal findings in specimens from female genital organs

R87.9   **Unspecified abnormal finding in specimens from female genital organs**   ♀

✓4ᵗʰ R88   **Abnormal findings in other body fluids and substances**

R88.0   **Cloudy (hemodialysis) (peritoneal) dialysis effluent**

R88.8   **Abnormal findings in other body fluids and substances**

✓4ᵗʰ R89   **Abnormal findings in specimens from other organs, systems and tissues**
> INCLUDES   abnormal findings in nipple discharge
> abnormal findings in synovial fluid
> abnormal findings in wound secretions

R89.0   **Abnormal level of enzymes in specimens from other organs, systems and tissues**

R89.1   **Abnormal level of hormones in specimens from other organs, systems and tissues**

R89.2   **Abnormal level of other drugs, medicaments and biological substances in specimens from other organs, systems and tissues**

R89.3   **Abnormal level of substances chiefly nonmedicinal as to source in specimens from other organs, systems and tissues**

R89.4   **Abnormal immunological findings in specimens from other organs, systems and tissues**

R89.5   **Abnormal microbiological findings in specimens from other organs, systems and tissues**
> Positive culture findings in specimens from other organs, systems and tissues
> EXCLUDES 1   *colonization status (Z22.-)*

R89.6   **Abnormal cytological findings in specimens from other organs, systems and tissues**

R89.7   **Abnormal histological findings in specimens from other organs, systems and tissues**

R89.8   **Other abnormal findings in specimens from other organs, systems and tissues**
> Abnormal chromosomal findings in specimens from other organs, systems and tissues

R89.9   **Unspecified abnormal finding in specimens from other organs, systems and tissues**

Abnormal findings on diagnostic imaging and in function studies, without diagnosis (R90-R94)

> INCLUDES   nonspecific abnormal findings on diagnostic imaging by computerized axial tomography [CAT scan]
> nonspecific abnormal findings on diagnostic imaging by magnetic resonance imaging [MRI][NMR]
> nonspecific abnormal findings on diagnostic imaging by positron emission tomography [PET scan]
> nonspecific abnormal findings on diagnostic imaging by thermography
> nonspecific abnormal findings on diagnostic imaging by ultrasound [echogram]
> nonspecific abnormal findings on diagnostic imaging by X-ray examination
> EXCLUDES 1   *abnormal findings on antenatal screening of mother (O28.-)*
> *diagnostic abnormal findings classified elsewhere — see Alphabetical Index*

✓4ᵗʰ R90   **Abnormal findings on diagnostic imaging of central nervous system**

R90.0   **Intracranial space-occupying lesion found on diagnostic imaging of central nervous system**

✓5ᵗʰ R90.8   **Other abnormal findings on diagnostic imaging of central nervous system**

R90.81   **Abnormal echoencephalogram**

R90.82   **White matter disease, unspecified**

R90.89   **Other abnormal findings on diagnostic imaging of central nervous system**
> Other cerebrovascular abnormality found on diagnostic imaging of central nervous system

✓4ᵗʰ R91   **Abnormal findings on diagnostic imaging of lung**

R91.1   **Solitary pulmonary nodule**
> Coin lesion lung
> Solitary pulmonary nodule, subsegmental branch of the bronchial tree

R91.8   **Other nonspecific abnormal finding of lung field**
> Lung mass NOS found on diagnostic imaging of lung
> Pulmonary infiltrate NOS
> Shadow, lung

✓4ᵗʰ R92   **Abnormal and inconclusive findings on diagnostic imaging of breast**

R92.0   **Mammographic microcalcification found on diagnostic imaging of breast**
> EXCLUDES 2   *mammographic calcification (calculus) found on diagnostic imaging of breast (R92.1)*
> **DEF:** Calcium and cellular debris deposits in the breast that cannot be felt but can be detected on a mammogram. The deposits can be a sign of cancer, benign conditions, or changes in the breast tissue as a result of inflammation, injury, or an obstructed duct.

R92.1   **Mammographic calcification found on diagnostic imaging of breast**
> Mammographic calculus found on diagnostic imaging of breast

R92.2   **Inconclusive mammogram**
> Dense breasts NOS
> Inconclusive mammogram NEC
> Inconclusive mammography due to dense breasts
> Inconclusive mammography NEC
> AHA: 2015,1Q,24

R92.8   **Other abnormal and inconclusive findings on diagnostic imaging of breast**

✓4ᵗʰ R93   **Abnormal findings on diagnostic imaging of other body structures**

R93.0   **Abnormal findings on diagnostic imaging of skull and head, not elsewhere classified**
> EXCLUDES 1   *intracranial space-occupying lesion found on diagnostic imaging (R90.0)*

R93.1   **Abnormal findings on diagnostic imaging of heart and coronary circulation**
> Abnormal echocardiogram NOS
> Abnormal heart shadow

R93.2   **Abnormal findings on diagnostic imaging of liver and biliary tract**
> Nonvisualization of gallbladder

R93.3   **Abnormal findings on diagnostic imaging of other parts of digestive tract**

✓5ᵗʰ R93.4   **Abnormal findings on diagnostic imaging of** urinary organs
> EXCLUDES 2   *hypertrophy of kidney (N28.81)*
> AHA: 2016,4Q,66

      R93.41   **Abnormal radiologic findings on diagnostic imaging of** renal pelvis, ureter, or bladder
> Filling defect of bladder found on diagnostic imaging
> Filling defect of renal pelvis found on diagnostic imaging
> Filling defect of ureter found on diagnostic imaging

      ✓6ᵗʰ R93.42   **Abnormal radiologic findings on diagnostic imaging of kidney**

         R93.421   **Abnormal radiologic findings on diagnostic imaging of** right **kidney**

         R93.422   **Abnormal radiologic findings on diagnostic imaging of** left **kidney**

         R93.429   **Abnormal radiologic findings on diagnostic imaging of unspecified kidney**

      R93.49   **Abnormal radiologic findings on diagnostic imaging of other urinary organs**

R93.5   **Abnormal findings on diagnostic imaging of other abdominal regions, including retroperitoneum**

R93.6   **Abnormal findings on diagnostic imaging of** limbs
> EXCLUDES 2   *abnormal finding in skin and subcutaneous tissue (R93.8-)*

R93.7   **Abnormal findings on diagnostic imaging of other parts of musculoskeletal system**
> EXCLUDES 2   *abnormal findings on diagnostic imaging of skull (R93.0)*

✓5ᵗʰ R93.8   **Abnormal findings on diagnostic imaging of other specified body structures**
> AHA: 2018,4Q,30

      ✓6ᵗʰ R93.81   **Abnormal radiologic findings on diagnostic imaging of** testis

         R93.811   **Abnormal radiologic findings on diagnostic imaging of** right **testicle**   ♂

         R93.812   **Abnormal radiologic findings on diagnostic imaging of** left **testicle**   ♂

         R93.813   **Abnormal radiologic findings on diagnostic imaging of testicles, bilateral**   ♂

         R93.819   **Abnormal radiologic findings on diagnostic imaging of unspecified testicle**   ♂

      R93.89   **Abnormal findings on diagnostic imaging of other specified body structures**
> Abnormal finding by radioisotope localization of placenta
> Abnormal radiological finding in skin and subcutaneous tissue
> Mediastinal shift

R93.9   **Diagnostic imaging inconclusive due to** excess body fat **of patient**

✓4ᵗʰ **R94**   **Abnormal results of function studies**
> INCLUDES   abnormal results of radionuclide [radioisotope] uptake studies
> abnormal results of scintigraphy

✓5ᵗʰ R94.0   **Abnormal results of function studies of** central nervous system

      R94.01   **Abnormal** electroencephalogram [EEG]

      R94.02   **Abnormal** brain scan

      R94.09   **Abnormal results of other function studies of central nervous system**

✓5ᵗʰ R94.1   **Abnormal results of function studies of** peripheral nervous system and special senses

      ✓6ᵗʰ R94.11   **Abnormal results of function studies of** eye

         R94.110   **Abnormal** electro-oculogram [EOG]

         R94.111   **Abnormal** electroretinogram [ERG]
> Abnormal retinal function study

         R94.112   **Abnormal** visually evoked potential [VEP]

         R94.113   **Abnormal** oculomotor **study**

         R94.118   **Abnormal results of other function studies of eye**

      ✓6ᵗʰ R94.12   **Abnormal results of function studies of** ear and other special senses
> AHA: 2016,3Q,17

         R94.120   **Abnormal** auditory **function study**

         R94.121   **Abnormal** vestibular **function study**

         R94.128   **Abnormal results of other function studies of ear and other special senses**

      ✓6ᵗʰ R94.13   **Abnormal results of function studies of** peripheral nervous system

         R94.130   **Abnormal response to nerve stimulation, unspecified**

         R94.131   **Abnormal** electromyogram [EMG]
> EXCLUDES 1   *electromyogram of eye (R94.113)*

         R94.138   **Abnormal results of other function studies of peripheral nervous system**

R94.2   **Abnormal results of** pulmonary function **studies**
> Reduced ventilatory capacity
> Reduced vital capacity

✓5ᵗʰ R94.3   **Abnormal results of** cardiovascular function **studies**

      R94.30   **Abnormal result of cardiovascular function study, unspecified**

      R94.31   **Abnormal** electrocardiogram [ECG] [EKG]
> EXCLUDES 1   *long QT syndrome (I45.81)*

      R94.39   **Abnormal result of other cardiovascular function study**
> Abnormal electrophysiological intracardiac studies
> Abnormal phonocardiogram
> Abnormal vectorcardiogram

R94.4   **Abnormal results of** kidney function **studies**
> Abnormal renal function test

R94.5   **Abnormal results of** liver function **studies**

R94.6   **Abnormal results of** thyroid function **studies**

R94.7   **Abnormal results of other endocrine function studies**
> EXCLUDES 2   *abnormal glucose (R73.0-)*

R94.8   **Abnormal results of function studies of other organs and systems**
> Abnormal basal metabolic rate [BMR]
> Abnormal bladder function test
> Abnormal splenic function test

Abnormal tumor markers (R97)

✓4ᵗʰ **R97**   **Abnormal tumor markers**
> Elevated tumor associated antigens [TAA]
> Elevated tumor specific antigens [TSA]

R97.0   **Elevated carcinoembryonic antigen [CEA]**

R97.1   **Elevated cancer antigen 125 [CA 125]**

✓5ᵗʰ R97.2   **Elevated prostate specific antigen [PSA]**
> AHA: 2016,4Q,66

      R97.20   **Elevated prostate specific antigen [PSA]**   🅰♂

      R97.21   **Rising PSA following treatment for malignant neoplasm of prostate**   🅰♂

R97.8   **Other abnormal tumor markers**

Ill-defined and unknown cause of mortality (R99)

R99   **Ill-defined and unknown cause of mortality**
> Death (unexplained) NOS
> Unspecified cause of mortality

✔ Additional Character Required   ✔x7ᵗʰ Placeholder   Unacceptable PDx   Questionable PDx   Manifestation   Unspecified Dx   H1-H14 HAC   HCC CMS-HCC Dx   HIV HIV Dx

ICD-10-CM 2020   973

Chapter 19. Injury, Poisoning and Certain Other Consequences of External Causes (S00–T88)

Chapter-specific Guidelines with Coding Examples

The chapter-specific guidelines from the ICD-10-CM Official Guidelines for Coding and Reporting have been provided below. Along with these guidelines are coding examples, contained in the shaded boxes, that have been developed to help illustrate the coding and/or sequencing guidance found in these guidelines.

a. Application of 7th characters in Chapter 19

Most categories in chapter 19 have a 7th character requirement for each applicable code. Most categories in this chapter have three 7th character values (with the exception of fractures): A, initial encounter, D, subsequent encounter and S, sequela. Categories for traumatic fractures have additional 7th character values. While the patient may be seen by a new or different provider over the course of treatment for an injury, assignment of the 7th character is based on whether the patient is undergoing active treatment and not whether the provider is seeing the patient for the first time.

For complication codes, active treatment refers to treatment for the condition described by the code, even though it may be related to an earlier precipitating problem. For example, code T84.50XA, Infection and inflammatory reaction due to unspecified internal joint prosthesis, initial encounter, is used when active treatment is provided for the infection, even though the condition relates to the prosthetic device, implant or graft that was placed at a previous encounter.

7th character "A", initial encounter is used for each encounter where the patient is receiving active treatment for the condition.

> Patient admitted after fall from a skateboard onto the sidewalk, x-rays identify a nondisplaced fracture to the distal pole of the right scaphoid bone. The patient is placed in a cast.
>
> **S62.014A**   **Nondisplaced fracture of distal pole of navicular [scaphoid] bone of right wrist, initial encounter for closed fracture**
>
> **V00.131A**   **Fall from skateboard, initial encounter**
>
> **Y92.480**   **Sidewalk as the place of occurrence of the external cause**
>
> **Y93.51**   **Activity, roller skating (inline) and skateboarding**
>
> **Y99.8**   **Other external cause status**
>
> *Explanation:* This fracture would be coded with a seventh character A for initial encounter because the patient received x-rays to identify the site of the fracture and treatment was rendered; this would be considered active treatment.

7th character "D" subsequent encounter is used for encounters after the patient has completed active treatment of the condition and is receiving routine care for the condition during the healing or recovery phase.

> Patient admitted after fall from a skateboard onto the sidewalk resulted in casting of the right arm. X-rays are taken to evaluate how well the nondisplaced fracture to the distal pole of the right scaphoid bone is healing. The physician feels the fracture is healing appropriately; no adjustments to the cast are made.
>
> **S62.014D**   **Nondisplaced fracture of distal pole of navicular [scaphoid] bone of right wrist, subsequent encounter for fracture with routine healing**
>
> **V00.131D**   **Fall from skateboard, subsequent encounter**
>
> *Explanation:* This fracture would be coded with a seventh character D for subsequent encounter, whether the same physician who provided the initial cast application or a different physician is now seeing the patient. Although the patient received x-rays, the intent of the x-rays was to assess how the fracture was healing. There was no active treatment rendered and the visit is therefore considered a subsequent encounter.

The aftercare Z codes should not be used for aftercare for conditions such as injuries or poisonings, where 7th characters are provided to identify subsequent care. For example, for aftercare of an injury, assign the acute injury code with the 7th character "D" (subsequent encounter).

7th character "S", sequela, is for use for complications or conditions that arise as a direct result of a condition, such as scar formation after a burn. The scars are sequelae of the burn. When using 7th character "S", it is

necessary to use both the injury code that precipitated the sequela and the code for the sequela itself. The "S" is added only to the injury code, not the sequela code. The 7th character "S" identifies the injury responsible for the sequela. The specific type of sequela (e.g. scar) is sequenced first, followed by the injury code.

See Section I.B.10 Sequelae, (Late Effects)

> Patient with a history of a nondisplaced fracture to the distal pole of the right scaphoid bone due to a fall from a skateboard is admitted for evaluation of arthritis to the right wrist that has developed as a consequence of the traumatic fracture.
>
> **M12.531**   **Traumatic arthropathy, right wrist**
>
> **S62.014S**   **Nondisplaced fracture of distal pole of navicular [scaphoid] bone of right wrist, sequela**
>
> **V00.131S**   **Fall from skateboard, sequela**
>
> *Explanation:* The code identifying the specific sequela condition (traumatic arthritis) should be coded first followed by the injury that instigated the development of the sequela (fracture). The scaphoid fracture injury code is given a 7th character S for sequela to represent its role as the inciting injury. The fracture has healed and is not being managed or treated on this admit and therefore is not applicable as a first listed or principal diagnosis. However, it is directly related to the development of the arthritis and should be appended as a secondary code to signify this cause and effect relationship.

b. Coding of injuries

When coding injuries, assign separate codes for each injury unless a combination code is provided, in which case the combination code is assigned. Codes from category T07, Unspecified multiple injuries should not be assigned in the inpatient setting unless information for a more specific code is not available. Traumatic injury codes (S00–T14.9) are not to be used for normal, healing surgical wounds or to identify complications of surgical wounds.

The code for the most serious injury, as determined by the provider and the focus of treatment, is sequenced first.

1) Superficial injuries

Superficial injuries such as abrasions or contusions are not coded when associated with more severe injuries of the same site.

2) Primary injury with damage to nerves/blood vessels

When a primary injury results in minor damage to peripheral nerves or blood vessels, the primary injury is sequenced first with additional code(s) for injuries to nerves and spinal cord (such as category S04), and/or injury to blood vessels (such as category S15). When the primary injury is to the blood vessels or nerves, that injury should be sequenced first.

3) Iatrogenic injuries

Injury codes from Chapter 19 should not be assigned for injuries that occur during, or as a result of, a medical intervention. Assign the appropriate complication code(s).

c. Coding of traumatic fractures

The principles of multiple coding of injuries should be followed in coding fractures. Fractures of specified sites are coded individually by site in accordance with both the provisions within categories S02, S12, S22, S32, S42, S49, S52, S59, S62, S72, S79, S82, S89, S92 and the level of detail furnished by medical record content.

A fracture not indicated as open or closed should be coded to closed. A fracture not indicated whether displaced or not displaced should be coded to displaced.

More specific guidelines are as follows:

1) Initial vs. subsequent encounter for fractures

Traumatic fractures are coded using the appropriate 7th character for initial encounter (A, B, C) for each encounter where the patient is receiving active treatment for the fracture. The appropriate 7th character for initial encounter should also be assigned for a patient who delayed seeking treatment for the fracture or nonunion. Fractures are coded using the appropriate 7th character for subsequent care for encounters after the patient has completed active treatment of the fracture and is receiving routine care for the fracture during the healing or recovery phase.

Care for complications of surgical treatment for fracture repairs during the healing or recovery phase should be coded with the appropriate complication codes.

Care of complications of fractures, such as malunion and nonunion, should be reported with the appropriate 7th character for subsequent care with nonunion (K, M, N,) or subsequent care with malunion (P, Q, R).

Malunion/nonunion: The appropriate 7th character for initial encounter should also be assigned for a patient who delayed seeking treatment for the fracture or nonunion.

Female patient fell during a forest hiking excursion almost six months ago and until recently did not feel she needed to seek medical attention for her left ankle pain; x-rays show nonunion of lateral malleolus and surgery has been scheduled

S82.62XA	**Displaced fracture of lateral malleolus of left fibula, initial encounter for closed fracture**
W01.0XXA	**Fall on same level from slipping, tripping and stumbling without subsequent striking against object, initial encounter**
Y92.821	**Forest as place of occurrence of the external cause**
Y93.01	**Activity, walking, marching and hiking**
Y99.8	**Other external cause status**

Explanation: A seventh character of A is used for the lateral malleolus nonunion fracture to signify that the fracture is receiving active treatment. The delayed care for the fracture has resulted in a nonunion, but capturing the nonunion in the seventh character is trumped by the provision of active care.

The open fracture designations in the assignment of the 7th character for fractures of the forearm, femur and lower leg, including ankle are based on the Gustilo open fracture classification. When the Gustilo classification type is not specified for an open fracture, the 7th character for open fracture type I or II should be assigned (B, E, H, M, Q).

A 17-year-old arrives at the trauma center with open, displaced right forearm fracture with extensive soft tissue damage. He fell while being tackled playing football for his high school team. On-call orthopaedic specialist documents segmental type IIIA fracture of radial shaft with no need for plastic consult.

S52.361C	**Displaced segmental fracture of shaft of radius, right arm, initial encounter for open fracture type IIIA, IIIB, or IIIC**
W03.XXXA	**Other fall on same level due to collision with another person, initial encounter**
Y92.321	**Football field as the place of occurrence of the external cause**
Y93.61	**Activity, American tackle football**

Explanation: The seventh character for forearm fractures capture the type of encounter and whether the fracture is open or closed; open fractures are broken down further by the type of fracture based on the Gustilo classification. The Gustilo classification describes the severity of open fracture and soft tissue injury. Type IIIA describes an open fracture with extensive soft tissue injury but adequate soft tissue remaining for wound coverage. A segmental fracture means that the bone is broken in two places, leaving at least one segment unattached to the bone. There is no need to report an additional code for the soft tissue injury as it is captured in the fracture code.

A code from category M80, not a traumatic fracture code, should be used for any patient with known osteoporosis who suffers a fracture, even if the patient had a minor fall or trauma, if that fall or trauma would not usually break a normal, healthy bone.

See Section I.C.13. Osteoporosis.

The aftercare Z codes should not be used for aftercare for traumatic fractures. For aftercare of a traumatic fracture, assign the acute fracture code with the appropriate 7th character.

2) Multiple fractures sequencing

Multiple fractures are sequenced in accordance with the severity of the fracture.

3) Physeal fractures

For physeal fractures, assign only the code identifying the type of physeal fracture. Do not assign a separate code to identify the specific bone that is fractured.

d. Coding of burns and corrosions

The ICD-10-CM makes a distinction between burns and corrosions. The burn codes are for thermal burns, except sunburns, that come from a heat source, such as a fire or hot appliance. The burn codes are also for burns resulting from electricity and radiation. Corrosions are burns due to chemicals. The guidelines are the same for burns and corrosions.

Current burns (T20-T25) are classified by depth, extent and by agent (X code). Burns are classified by depth as first degree (erythema), second degree (blistering), and third degree (full-thickness involvement). Burns of the eye and internal organs (T26-T28) are classified by site, but not by degree.

1) Sequencing of burn and related condition codes

Sequence first the code that reflects the highest degree of burn when more than one burn is present.

    a. When the reason for the admission or encounter is for treatment of external multiple burns, sequence first the code that reflects the burn of the highest degree.

    b. When a patient has both internal and external burns, the circumstances of admission govern the selection of the principal diagnosis or first-listed diagnosis.

    c. When a patient is admitted for burn injuries and other related conditions such as smoke inhalation and/or respiratory failure, the circumstances of admission govern the selection of the principal or first-listed diagnosis.

Patient admitted with minor first-degree burns to multiple sites of her right and left hands as well as severe smoke inhalation. While she was sleeping at home, a candle on her dresser lit the bedroom curtains on fire.

T59.811A	**Toxic effect of smoke, accidental (unintentional), initial encounter**
J70.5	**Respiratory conditions due to smoke inhalation**
T23.191A	**Burn of first degree of multiple sites of right wrist and hand, initial encounter**
T23.192A	**Burn of first degree of multiple sites of left wrist and hand, initial encounter**
X08.8XXA	**Exposure to other specified smoke, fire and flames, initial encounter**
Y92.003	**Bedroom of unspecified non-institutional (private) residence as the place of occurrence of the external cause**
Y93.84	**Activity, sleeping**

Explanation: Based on the documentation, the inhalation injury is more severe than the first-degree burns and is sequenced first. The burns to the hands are appended as secondary diagnoses.

---

2) Burns of the same anatomic site

Classify burns of the same anatomic site and on the same side but of different degrees to the subcategory identifying the highest degree recorded in the diagnosis (e.g., for second and third degree burns of right thigh, assign only code T24.311-).

3) Non-healing burns

Non-healing burns are coded as acute burns.

Necrosis of burned skin should be coded as a non-healed burn.

4) Infected burn

For any documented infected burn site, use an additional code for the infection.

5) Assign separate codes for each burn site

When coding burns, assign separate codes for each burn site. Category T30, Burn and corrosion, body region unspecified is extremely vague and should rarely be used.

Codes for burns of "multiple sites" should only be assigned when the medical record documentation does not specify the individual sites.

> Patient is admitted with third-degree burns of the scalp as well as second-degree burns to the back of the right hand
>
> **T20.35XA** **Burn of third degree of scalp [any part], initial encounter**
>
> **T23.261A** **Burn of second degree of back of right hand, initial encounter**
>
> *Explanation:* Two codes may be reported as the hand and face represent distinct burn sites.

6) **Burns and corrosions classified according to extent of body surface involved**

Assign codes from category T31, Burns classified according to extent of body surface involved, or T32, Corrosions classified according to extent of body surface involved, when the site of the burn is not specified or when there is a need for additional data. It is advisable to use category T31 as additional coding when needed to provide data for evaluating burn mortality, such as that needed by burn units. It is also advisable to use category T31 as an additional code for reporting purposes when there is mention of a third-degree burn involving 20 percent or more of the body surface.

Categories T31 and T32 are based on the classic "rule of nines" in estimating body surface involved: head and neck are assigned nine percent, each arm nine percent, each leg 18 percent, the anterior trunk 18 percent, posterior trunk 18 percent, and genitalia one percent. Providers may change these percentage assignments where necessary to accommodate infants and children who have proportionately larger heads than adults, and patients who have large buttocks, thighs, or abdomen that involve burns.

> Patient seen in burn unit for dressing change after he accidentally spilled acetic acid on himself two days ago. The second-degree burns to his right thigh, covering about 3 percent of his body surface, are healing appropriately.
>
> **T54.2X1D** **Toxic effect of corrosive acids and acid-like substances, accidental (unintentional), subsequent encounter**
>
> **T24.611D** **Corrosion of second degree of right thigh, subsequent encounter**
>
> **T32.0** **Corrosions involving less than 10% of body surface**
>
> *Explanation:* Code T32.0 provides additional information as to how much of the patient's body was affected by the corrosive substance.

7) **Encounters for treatment of sequela of burns**

Encounters for the treatment of the late effects of burns or corrosions (i.e., scars or joint contractures) should be coded with a burn or corrosion code with the 7th character "S" for sequela.

8) **Sequelae with a late effect code and current burn**

When appropriate, both a code for a current burn or corrosion with 7th character "A" or "D" and a burn or corrosion code with 7th character "S" may be assigned on the same record (when both a current burn and sequelae of an old burn exist). Burns and corrosions do not heal at the same rate and a current healing wound may still exist with sequela of a healed burn or corrosion.

See Section I.B.10 Sequela (Late Effects)

> Female patient seen in ED for second-degree burn to the left ear; she also has significant scarring on her left elbow from a third-degree burn from childhood
>
> **T20.212A** **Burn of second degree of left ear [any part, except ear drum], initial encounter**
>
> **L90.5** **Scar conditions and fibrosis of skin**
>
> **T22.322S** **Burn of third degree of left elbow, sequela**
>
> *Explanation:* The patient is being seen for management of a current second-degree burn, which is reflected in the code by appending the seventh character of A, indicating active treatment or management of this burn. The elbow scarring is a sequela of a previous third-degree burn. The sequela condition precedes the original burn injury, which is appended with a seventh character of S.

9) **Use of an external cause code with burns and corrosions**

An external cause code should be used with burns and corrosions to identify the source and intent of the burn, as well as the place where it occurred.

e. **Adverse effects, poisoning, underdosing and toxic effects**

Codes in categories T36-T65 are combination codes that include the substance that was taken as well as the intent. No additional external cause code is required for poisonings, toxic effects, adverse effects and underdosing codes.

1) **Do not code directly from the Table of Drugs**

Do not code directly from the Table of Drugs and Chemicals. Always refer back to the Tabular List.

2) **Use as many codes as necessary to describe**

Use as many codes as necessary to describe completely all drugs, medicinal or biological substances.

3) **If the same code would describe the causative agent**

If the same code would describe the causative agent for more than one adverse reaction, poisoning, toxic effect or underdosing, assign the code only once.

4) **If two or more drugs, medicinal or biological substances**

If two or more drugs, medicinal or biological substances are **taken**, code each individually unless a combination code is listed in the Table of Drugs and Chemicals.

If multiple unspecified drugs, medicinal or biological substances were taken, assign the appropriate code from subcategory T50.91, Poisoning by, adverse effect of and underdosing of multiple unspecified drugs, medicaments and biological substances.

5) **The occurrence of drug toxicity is classified in ICD-10-CM as follows:**
(a) **Adverse effect**

When coding an adverse effect of a drug that has been correctly prescribed and properly administered, assign the appropriate code for the nature of the adverse effect followed by the appropriate code for the adverse effect of the drug (T36-T50). The code for the drug should have a 5th or 6th character "5" (for example T36.0X5-) Examples of the nature of an adverse effect are tachycardia, delirium, gastrointestinal hemorrhaging, vomiting, hypokalemia, hepatitis, renal failure, or respiratory failure.

> Patient admitted for stomach pain and jaundice, indicated by physician as possible side-effects of Inderal, recently started for hypertension. Inderal was discontinued and the patient switched to Atenolol instead.
>
> **R10.9** **Unspecified abdominal pain**
>
> **R17** **Unspecified jaundice**
>
> **T44.7X5A** **Adverse effect of beta-adrenoreceptor antagonists, initial encounter**
>
> **I10** **Essential (primary) hypertension**
>
> *Explanation:* The side-effects caused by the drug are listed first, followed by the code for the adverse effect of the drug to capture the specific drug that was used.

(b) **Poisoning**

When coding a poisoning or reaction to the improper use of a medication (e.g., overdose, wrong substance given or taken in error, wrong route of administration), first assign the appropriate code from categories T36-T50. The poisoning codes have an associated intent as their 5th or 6th character (accidental, intentional self-harm, assault and undetermined. If the intent of the poisoning is unknown or unspecified, code the intent as accidental intent. The undetermined intent is only for use if the documentation in the record specifies that the intent cannot be determined. Use additional code(s) for all manifestations of poisonings.

A 55-year-old female status post recent left knee replacement is admitted due to confusion, dizziness, and nausea. Her spouse brought in her prescribed Xanax, Ambien, and Percocet bottles but has no idea how many she took. It is suspected that her symptoms are due to an overdose of these medications.

T42.4X1A	**Poisoning by benzodiazepines, accidental (unintentional), initial encounter**
T42.6X1A	**Poisoning by other antiepileptic and sedative-hypnotic drugs, accidental (unintentional), initial encounter**
T40.2X1A	**Poisoning by other opioids, accidental (unintentional), initial encounter**
R41.0	**Disorientation, unspecified**
R42	**Dizziness and giddiness**
R11.0	**Nausea**

Explanation: It was not documented whether the overdose of the drugs was accidental or intentional; therefore the correct reporting of the poisoning codes is accidental intent. The poisoning codes are sequenced first, followed by manifestations of the poisoning.

If there is also a diagnosis of abuse or dependence of the substance, the abuse or dependence is assigned as an additional code.

Examples of poisoning include:

(i)   Error was made in drug prescription

Errors made in drug prescription or in the administration of the drug by provider, nurse, patient, or other person.

(ii)   Overdose of a drug intentionally taken

If an overdose of a drug was intentionally taken or administered and resulted in drug toxicity, it would be coded as a poisoning.

(iii)   Nonprescribed drug taken with correctly prescribed and properly administered drug

If a nonprescribed drug or medicinal agent was taken in combination with a correctly prescribed and properly administered drug, any drug toxicity or other reaction resulting from the interaction of the two drugs would be classified as a poisoning.

(iv)   Interaction of drug(s) and alcohol

When a reaction results from the interaction of a drug(s) and alcohol, this would be classified as poisoning.

See Section I.C.4. if poisoning is the result of insulin pump malfunctions.

(c) Underdosing

Underdosing refers to taking less of a medication than is prescribed by a provider or a manufacturer's instruction. Discontinuing the use of a prescribed medication on the patient's own initiative (not directed by the patient's provider) is also classified as an underdosing. For underdosing, assign the code from categories T36-T50 (fifth or sixth character "6").

Codes for underdosing should never be assigned as principal or first-listed codes. If a patient has a relapse or exacerbation of the medical condition for which the drug is prescribed because of the reduction in dose, then the medical condition itself should be coded.

Noncompliance (Z91.12-, Z91.13- and Z91.14-) or complication of care (Y63.6-Y63.9) codes are to be used with an underdosing code to indicate intent, if known.

Patient admitted for atrial fibrillation with history of chronic atrial fibrillation for which she is prescribed amiodarone. Financial concerns have left the patient unable to pay for her prescriptions and she has been skipping her amiodarone dose every other day to offset the cost.

I48.20	**Chronic atrial fibrillation, unspecified**
T46.2X6A	**Underdosing of other antidysrhythmic drugs, initial encounter**
Z91.120	**Patient's intentional underdosing of medication regimen due to financial hardship**

Explanation: By skipping her amiodarone pill every other day, the patient's atrial fibrillation returned. The condition for which the drug was being taken is reported first, followed by an underdosing code to show that the patient was not adhering to her prescription regimen. The Z code helps elaborate on the patient's social and/or economic circumstances that led to the patient taking less then what she was prescribed.

(d) Toxic effects

When a harmful substance is ingested or comes in contact with a person, this is classified as a toxic effect. The toxic effect codes are in categories T51-T65.

Toxic effect codes have an associated intent: accidental, intentional self-harm, assault and undetermined.

f.   Adult and child abuse, neglect and other maltreatment

Sequence first the appropriate code from categories T74.- (Adult and child abuse, neglect and other maltreatment, confirmed) or T76.- (Adult and child abuse, neglect and other maltreatment, suspected) for abuse, neglect and other maltreatment, followed by any accompanying mental health or injury code(s).

If the documentation in the medical record states abuse or neglect it is coded as confirmed (T74.-). It is coded as suspected if it is documented as suspected (T76.-).

For cases of confirmed abuse or neglect an external cause code from the assault section (X92-Y09) should be added to identify the cause of any physical injuries. A perpetrator code (Y07) should be added when the perpetrator of the abuse is known. For suspected cases of abuse or neglect, do not report external cause or perpetrator code.

If a suspected case of abuse, neglect or mistreatment is ruled out during an encounter code Z04.71, Encounter for examination and observation following alleged physical adult abuse, ruled out, or code Z04.72, Encounter for examination and observation following alleged child physical abuse, ruled out, should be used, not a code from T76.

If a suspected case of alleged rape or sexual abuse is ruled out during an encounter code Z04.41, Encounter for examination and observation following alleged adult rape or code Z04.42, Encounter for examination and observation following alleged child rape, should be used, not a code from T76.

If a suspected case of forced sexual exploitation or forced labor exploitation is ruled out during an encounter, code Z04.81, Encounter for examination and observation of victim following forced sexual exploitation, or code Z04.82, Encounter for examination and observation of victim following forced labor exploitation, should be used, not a code from T76.

See Section I.C.15. Abuse in a pregnant patient.

g. Complications of care

1) General guidelines for complications of care
(a) Documentation of complications of care

See Section I.B.16. for information on documentation of complications of care.

2) Pain due to medical devices

Pain associated with devices, implants or grafts left in a surgical site (for example painful hip prosthesis) is assigned to the appropriate code(s) found in Chapter 19, Injury, poisoning, and certain other consequences of external causes. Specific codes for pain due to medical devices are found in the T code section of the ICD-10-CM. Use additional code(s) from category G89 to identify acute or chronic pain due to presence of the device, implant or graft (G89.18 or G89.28).

Chronic left breast pain secondary to breast implant

T85.848A	**Pain due to other internal prosthetic devices, implants and grafts, initial encounter**
N64.4	**Mastodynia**
G89.28	**Other chronic postprocedural pain**

Explanation: As the pain is a complication related to the breast implant, the complication code is sequenced first. The T code does not describe the site or type of pain, so additional codes may be appended to indicate that the patient is experiencing chronic pain in the breast.

3) Transplant complications

(a) Transplant complications other than kidney

Codes under category T86, Complications of transplanted organs and tissues, are for use for both complications and rejection of transplanted organs. A transplant complication code is only assigned if the complication affects the function of the transplanted organ. Two codes are required to fully describe a transplant complication: the appropriate code from category T86 and a secondary code that identifies the complication.

Pre-existing conditions or conditions that develop after the transplant are not coded as complications unless they affect the function of the transplanted organs.

See I.C.21. for transplant organ removal status

See I.C.2. for malignant neoplasm associated with transplanted organ.

(b) Kidney transplant complications

Patients who have undergone kidney transplant may still have some form of chronic kidney disease (CKD) because the kidney transplant may not fully restore kidney function. Code T86.1- should be assigned for documented complications of a kidney transplant, such as transplant failure or rejection or other transplant complication. Code T86.1- should not be assigned for post kidney transplant patients who have chronic kidney (CKD) unless a transplant complication such as transplant failure or rejection is documented. If the documentation is unclear as to whether the patient has a complication of the transplant, query the provider.

Conditions that affect the function of the transplanted kidney, other than CKD, should be assigned a code from subcategory T86.1, Complications of transplanted organ, Kidney, and a secondary code that identifies the complication.

For patients with CKD following a kidney transplant, but who do not have a complication such as failure or rejection, *see section I.C.14. Chronic kidney disease and kidney transplant status.*

Patient with chronic kidney disease stage 2; history of successful kidney transplant with no complications identified

N18.2	**Chronic kidney disease, stage 2 (mild)**
Z94.0	**Kidney transplant status**

Explanation: This patient's stage 2 CKD is not indicated as being due to the transplanted kidney but instead is just the residual disease the patient had prior to the transplant.

4) Complication codes that include the external cause

As with certain other T codes, some of the complications of care codes have the external cause included in the code. The code includes the nature of the complication as well as the type of procedure that caused the complication. No external cause code indicating the type of procedure is necessary for these codes.

5) Complications of care codes within the body system chapters

Intraoperative and postprocedural complication codes are found within the body system chapters with codes specific to the organs and structures of that body system. These codes should be sequenced first, followed by a code(s) for the specific complication, if applicable.

Complication codes from the body system chapters should be assigned for intraoperative and postprocedural complications (e.g., the appropriate complication code from chapter 9 would be assigned for a vascular intraoperative or postprocedural complication) unless the complication is specifically indexed to a T code in chapter 19.

During a spinal fusion procedure, the surgeon inadvertently punctured the dura. The midline durotomy was repaired, and the fusion procedure was completed.

G97.41	**Accidental puncture or laceration of dura during a procedure**

Explanation: The accidental durotomy is not coded to an injury code in chapter 19 but instead is categorized to the nervous system chapter.

Muscle/Tendon Table

ICD-10-CM categorizes certain muscles and tendons in the upper and lower extremities by their action (e.g., extension, flexion), their anatomical location (e.g., posterior, anterior), and/or whether they are intrinsic or extrinsic to a certain anatomical area. The Muscle/Tendon Table is provided at the beginning of chapters 13 and 19 as a resource to help users when code selection depends on one or more of these characteristics. Please note that this table is not all-inclusive, and proper code assignment should be based on the provider's documentation.

Body Region	Muscle	Extensor Tendon	Flexor Tendon	Other Tendon
Shoulder				
	Deltoid	Posterior deltoid	Anterior deltoid	
	Rotator cuff			
	Infraspinatus			Infraspinatus
	Subscapularis			Subscapularis
	Supraspinatus			Supraspinatus
	Teres minor			Teres minor
	Teres major	Teres major		
Upper arm				
	Anterior muscles			
	Biceps brachii — long head		Biceps brachii — long head	
	Biceps brachii — short head		Biceps brachii — short head	
	Brachialis		Brachialis	
	Coracobrachialis		Coracobrachialis	
	Posterior muscles			
	Triceps brachii	Triceps brachii		
Forearm				
	Anterior muscles			
	Flexors			
	Deep			
	Flexor digitorum profundus		Flexor digitorum profundus	
	Flexor pollicis longus		Flexor pollicis longus	
	Intermediate			
	Flexor digitorum superficialis		Flexor digitorum superficialis	
	Superficial			
	Flexor carpi radialis		Flexor carpi radialis	
	Flexor carpi ulnaris		Flexor carpi ulnaris	
	Palmaris longus		Palmaris longus	
	Pronators			
	Pronator quadratus			Pronator quadratus
	Pronator teres			Pronator teres
	Posterior muscles			
	Extensors			
	Deep			
	Abductor pollicis longus			Abductor pollicis longus
	Extensor indicis	Extensor indicis		
	Extensor pollicis brevis	Extensor pollicis brevis		
	Extensor pollicis longus	Extensor pollicis longus		
	Superficial			
	Brachioradialis			Brachioradialis
	Extensor carpi radialis brevis	Extensor carpi radialis brevis		
	Extensor carpi radialis longus	Extensor carpi radialis longus		
	Extensor carpi ulnaris	Extensor carpi ulnaris		
	Extensor digiti minimi	Extensor digiti minimi		
	Extensor digitorum	Extensor digitorum		
	Anconeus	Anconeus		
	Supinator			Supinator

Body Region	Muscle	Extensor Tendon	Flexor Tendon	Other Tendon
Hand				
Extrinsic — attach to a site in the forearm as well as a site in the hand with action related to hand movement at the wrist				
	Extensor carpi radialis brevis	Extensor carpi radialis brevis		
	Extensor carpi radialis longus	Extensor carpie radialis longus		
	Extensor carpi ulnaris	Extensor carpi ulnaris		
	Flexor carpi radialis		Flexor carpi radialis	
	Flexor carpi ulnaris		Flexor carpi ulnaris	
	Flexor digitorum superficialis		Flexor digitorum superficialis	
	Palmaris longus		Palmaris longus	
Extrinsic — attach to a site in the forearm as well as a site in the hand with action in the hand related to finger movement				
	Adductor pollicis longus			Adductor pollicis longus
	Extensor digiti minimi	Extensor digiti minimi		
	Extensor digitorum	Extensor digitorum		
	Extensor indicis	Extensor indicis		
	Flexor digitorum profundus		Flexor digitorum profundus	
	Flexor digitorum superficialis		Flexor digitorum superficialis	
Extrinsic — attach to a site in the forearm as well as a site in the hand with action in the hand related to thumb movement				
	Extensor pollicis brevis	Extensor pollicis brevis		
	Extensor pollicis longus	Extensor pollicis longus		
	Flexor pollicis longus		Flexor pollicis longus	
Intrinsic — found within the hand only				
	Adductor pollicis			Adductor pollicis
	Dorsal interossei	Dorsal interossei	Dorsal interossei	
	Lumbricals	Lumbricals	Lumbricals	
	Palmaris brevis			Palmaris brevis
	Palmar interossei	Palmar interossei	Palmar interossei	
	Hypothenar muscles			
	Abductor digiti minimi			Abductor digiti minimi
	Flexor digiti minimi brevis		Flexor digiti minimi brevis	
	Oppenens digiti minimi		Oppenens digiti minimi	
	Thenar muscles			
	Abductor pollicis brevis			Abductor pollicis brevis
	Flexor pollicis brevis		Flexor pollicis brevis	
	Oppenens pollicis		Oppenens pollicis	
Thigh				
	Anterior muscles			
	Iliopsoas		Iliopsoas	
	Pectineus		Pectineus	
	Quadriceps	Quadriceps		
	Rectus femoris	Rectus femoris — Extends knee	Rectus femoris — Flexes hip	
	Vastus intermedius	Vastus intermedius		
	Vastus lateralis	Vastus lateralis		
	Vastus medialis	Vastus medialis		
	Sartorius		Sartorius	
	Medial muscles			
	Adductor brevis			Adductor brevis
	Adductor longus			Adductor longus
	Adductor magnus			Adductor magnus
	Gracilis			Gracilis
	Obturator externus			Obturator externus
	Posterior muscles			
	Hamstring	Hamstring — Extends hip	Hamstring — Flexes knee	
	Biceps femoris	Biceps femoris	Biceps femoris	
	Semimembranosus	Semimembranosus	Semimembranosus	
	Semitendinosus	Semitendinosus	Semitendinosus	

Chapter 19. Injury, Poisoning and Certain Other Consequences of External Causes

Body Region	Muscle	Extensor Tendon	Flexor Tendon	Other Tendon
Lower leg				
	Anterior muscles			
	Extensor digitorum longus	Extensor digitorum longus		
	Extensor hallucis longus	Extensor hallucis longus		
	Fibularis (peroneus) tertius	Fibularis (peroneus) tertius		
	Tibialis anterior	Tibialis anterior		Tibialis anterior
	Lateral muscles			
	Fibularis (peroneus) brevis		Fibularis (peroneus) brevis	
	Fibularis (peroneus) longus		Fibularis (peroneus) longus	
	Posterior muscles			
	Deep			
	Flexor digitorum longus		Flexor digitorum longus	
	Flexor hallucis longus		Flexor hallucis longus	
	Popliteus		Popliteus	
	Tibialis posterior		Tibialis posterior	
	Superficial			
	Gastrocnemius		Gastrocnemius	
	Plantaris		Plantaris	
	Soleus		Soleus	
				Calcaneal (Achilles)
Ankle/Foot				
Extrinsic — attach to a site in the lower leg as well as a site in the foot with action related to foot movement at the ankle				
	Plantaris		Plantaris	
	Soleus		Soleus	
	Tibialis anterior	Tibialis anterior		
	Tibialis posterior		Tibialis posterior	
Extrinsic — attach to a site in the lower leg as well as a site in the foot with action in the foot related to toe movement				
	Extensor digitorum longus	Extensor digitorum longus		
	Extensor hallicus longus	Extensor hallicus longus		
	Flexor digitorum longus		Flexor digitorum longus	
	Flexor hallucis longus		Flexor hallucis longus	
Intrinsic — found within the ankle/foot only				
	Dorsal muscles			
	Extensor digitorum brevis	Extensor digitorum brevis		
	Extensor hallucis brevis	Extensor hallucis brevis		
	Plantar muscles			
	Abductor digiti minimi		Abductor digiti minimi	
	Abductor hallucis		Abductor hallucis	
	Dorsal interossei	Dorsal interossei	Dorsal interossei	
	Flexor digiti minimi brevis		Flexor digiti minimi brevis	
	Flexor digitorum brevis		Flexor digitorum brevis	
	Flexor hallucis brevis		Flexor hallucis brevis	
	Lumbricals	Lumbricals	Lumbricals	
	Quadratus plantae		Quadratus plantae	
	Plantar interossei	Plantar interossei	Plantar interossei	

Chapter 19. Injury, Poisoning and Certain Other Consequences of External Causes (S00-T88)

NOTE   Use secondary code(s) from Chapter 20, External causes of morbidity, to indicate cause of injury. Codes within the T section that include the external cause do not require an additional external cause code.

Use additional code to identify any retained foreign body, if applicable (Z18.-)

EXCLUDES 1   birth trauma (P10-P15)
         obstetric trauma (O70-O71)

NOTE   The chapter uses the S-section for coding different types of injuries related to single body regions and the T-section to cover injuries to unspecified body regions as well as poisoning and certain other consequences of external causes.

AHA: 2016,2Q,3-7; 2015,4Q,35-38; 2015,3Q,37-39,40; 2015,2Q,6; 2015,1Q,3-21
TIP: The specific site of an injury can be determined from the radiology report when authenticated by a radiologist and available at the time of code assignment.

This chapter contains the following blocks:

S00-S09	Injuries to the head
S10-S19	Injuries to the neck
S20-S29	Injuries to the thorax
S30-S39	Injuries to the abdomen, lower back, lumbar spine, pelvis and external genitals
S40-S49	Injuries to the shoulder and upper arm
S50-S59	Injuries to the elbow and forearm
S60-S69	Injuries to the wrist, hand and fingers
S70-S79	Injuries to the hip and thigh
S80-S89	Injuries to the knee and lower leg
S90-S99	Injuries to the ankle and foot
T07	Injuries involving multiple body regions
T14	Injury of unspecified body region
T15-T19	Effects of foreign body entering through natural orifice
T20-T25	Burns and corrosions of external body surface, specified by site
T26-T28	Burns and corrosions confined to eye and internal organs
T30-T32	Burns and corrosions of multiple and unspecified body regions
T33-T34	Frostbite
T36-T50	Poisoning by, adverse effect of and underdosing of drugs, medicaments and biological substances
T51-T65	Toxic effects of substances chiefly nonmedicinal as to source
T66-T78	Other and unspecified effects of external causes
T79	Certain early complications of trauma
T80-T88	Complications of surgical and medical care, not elsewhere classified

Injuries to the head (S00-S09)

INCLUDES   injuries of ear
       injuries of eye
       injuries of face [any part]
       injuries of gum
       injuries of jaw
       injuries of oral cavity
       injuries of palate
       injuries of periocular area
       injuries of scalp
       injuries of temporomandibular joint area
       injuries of tongue
       injuries of tooth

Code also for any associated infection
EXCLUDES 2   burns and corrosions (T20-T32)
       effects of foreign body in ear (T16)
       effects of foreign body in larynx (T17.3)
       effects of foreign body in mouth NOS (T18.0)
       effects of foreign body in nose (T17.0-T17.1)
       effects of foreign body in pharynx (T17.2)
       effects of foreign body on external eye (T15.-)
       frostbite (T33-T34)
       insect bite or sting, venomous (T63.4)

√4ᵗʰ S00 Superficial injury of head

    EXCLUDES 1   diffuse cerebral contusion (S06.2-)
            focal cerebral contusion (S06.3-)
            injury of eye and orbit (S05.-)
            open wound of head (S01.-)

> The appropriate 7th character is to be added to each code from category S00.
> A   initial encounter
> D   subsequent encounter
> S   sequela

√5ᵗʰ S00.0 Superficial injury of scalp

    √x7ᵗʰ S00.00   Unspecified superficial injury of scalp

    √x7ᵗʰ S00.01   Abrasion of scalp

    √x7ᵗʰ S00.02   Blister (nonthermal) of scalp

    √x7ᵗʰ S00.03   Contusion of scalp
              Bruise of scalp
              Hematoma of scalp

    √x7ᵗʰ S00.04   External constriction of part of scalp

    √x7ᵗʰ S00.05   Superficial foreign body of scalp
              Splinter in the scalp

    √x7ᵗʰ S00.06   Insect bite (nonvenomous) of scalp

    √x7ᵗʰ S00.07   Other superficial bite of scalp
       EXCLUDES 1   open bite of scalp (S01.05)

√5ᵗʰ S00.1 Contusion of eyelid and periocular area
       Black eye
       EXCLUDES 2   contusion of eyeball and orbital tissues (S05.1)

    √x7ᵗʰ S00.10   Contusion of unspecified eyelid and periocular area

    √x7ᵗʰ S00.11   Contusion of right eyelid and periocular area

    √x7ᵗʰ S00.12   Contusion of left eyelid and periocular area

√5ᵗʰ S00.2 Other and unspecified superficial injuries of eyelid and periocular area
       EXCLUDES 2   superficial injury of conjunctiva and cornea (S05.0-)

    √6ᵗʰ S00.20   Unspecified superficial injury of eyelid and periocular area

       √7ᵗʰ S00.201   Unspecified superficial injury of right eyelid and periocular area

       √7ᵗʰ S00.202   Unspecified superficial injury of left eyelid and periocular area

       √7ᵗʰ S00.209   Unspecified superficial injury of unspecified eyelid and periocular area

    √6ᵗʰ S00.21   Abrasion of eyelid and periocular area

       √7ᵗʰ S00.211   Abrasion of right eyelid and periocular area

       √7ᵗʰ S00.212   Abrasion of left eyelid and periocular area

       √7ᵗʰ S00.219   Abrasion of unspecified eyelid and periocular area

    √6ᵗʰ S00.22   Blister (nonthermal) of eyelid and periocular area

       √7ᵗʰ S00.221   Blister (nonthermal) of right eyelid and periocular area

       √7ᵗʰ S00.222   Blister (nonthermal) of left eyelid and periocular area

       √7ᵗʰ S00.229   Blister (nonthermal) of unspecified eyelid and periocular area

    √6ᵗʰ S00.24   External constriction of eyelid and periocular area

       √7ᵗʰ S00.241   External constriction of right eyelid and periocular area

       √7ᵗʰ S00.242   External constriction of left eyelid and periocular area

       √7ᵗʰ S00.249   External constriction of unspecified eyelid and periocular area

    √6ᵗʰ S00.25   Superficial foreign body of eyelid and periocular area
         Splinter of eyelid and periocular area
         EXCLUDES 2   retained foreign body in eyelid (H02.81-)

       √7ᵗʰ S00.251   Superficial foreign body of right eyelid and periocular area

       √7ᵗʰ S00.252   Superficial foreign body of left eyelid and periocular area

       √7ᵗʰ S00.259   Superficial foreign body of unspecified eyelid and periocular area

    √6ᵗʰ S00.26   Insect bite (nonvenomous) of eyelid and periocular area

       √7ᵗʰ S00.261   Insect bite (nonvenomous) of right eyelid and periocular area

       √7ᵗʰ S00.262   Insect bite (nonvenomous) of left eyelid and periocular area

       √7ᵗʰ S00.269   Insect bite (nonvenomous) of unspecified eyelid and periocular area

    √6ᵗʰ S00.27   Other superficial bite of eyelid and periocular area
       EXCLUDES 1   open bite of eyelid and periocular area (S01.15)

       √7ᵗʰ S00.271   Other superficial bite of right eyelid and periocular area

       √7ᵗʰ S00.272   Other superficial bite of left eyelid and periocular area

       √7ᵗʰ S00.279   Other superficial bite of unspecified eyelid and periocular area

√5ᵗʰ S00.3 Superficial injury of nose

    √x7ᵗʰ S00.30   Unspecified superficial injury of nose

    √x7ᵗʰ S00.31   Abrasion of nose

    √x7ᵗʰ S00.32   Blister (nonthermal) of nose

√x7th **S00.33** Contusion **of nose**
Bruise of nose
Hematoma of nose

√x7th **S00.34** External constriction **of nose**

√x7th **S00.35** Superficial foreign body **of nose**
Splinter in the nose

√x7th **S00.36** Insect bite (nonvenomous) **of nose**

√x7th **S00.37** Other superficial bite **of nose**
EXCLUDES 1   *open bite of nose (S01.25)*

√5th **S00.4** Superficial injury of ear

  √6th **S00.40** Unspecified superficial injury of ear

    √7th **S00.401** Unspecified superficial injury of right ear

    √7th **S00.402** Unspecified superficial injury of left ear

    √7th **S00.409** Unspecified superficial injury of unspecified ear

  √6th **S00.41** Abrasion **of ear**

    √7th **S00.411** Abrasion of right ear

    √7th **S00.412** Abrasion of left ear

    √7th **S00.419** Abrasion of unspecified ear

  √6th **S00.42** Blister (nonthermal) **of ear**

    √7th **S00.421** Blister (nonthermal) of right ear

    √7th **S00.422** Blister (nonthermal) of left ear

    √7th **S00.429** Blister (nonthermal) of unspecified ear

  √6th **S00.43** Contusion **of ear**
Bruise of ear
Hematoma of ear

    √7th **S00.431** Contusion of right ear

    √7th **S00.432** Contusion of left ear

    √7th **S00.439** Contusion of unspecified ear

  √6th **S00.44** External constriction **of ear**

    √7th **S00.441** External constriction of right ear

    √7th **S00.442** External constriction of left ear

    √7th **S00.449** External constriction of unspecified ear

  √6th **S00.45** Superficial foreign body **of ear**
Splinter in the ear

    √7th **S00.451** Superficial foreign body of right ear

    √7th **S00.452** Superficial foreign body of left ear

    √7th **S00.459** Superficial foreign body of unspecified ear

  √6th **S00.46** Insect bite (nonvenomous) **of ear**

    √7th **S00.461** Insect bite (nonvenomous) of right ear

    √7th **S00.462** Insect bite (nonvenomous) of left ear

    √7th **S00.469** Insect bite (nonvenomous) of unspecified ear

  √6th **S00.47** Other superficial bite **of ear**
EXCLUDES 1   *open bite of ear (S01.35)*

    √7th **S00.471** Other superficial bite of right ear

    √7th **S00.472** Other superficial bite of left ear

    √7th **S00.479** Other superficial bite of unspecified ear

√5th **S00.5** Superficial injury of lip and oral cavity

  √6th **S00.50** Unspecified superficial injury of lip and oral cavity

    √7th **S00.501** Unspecified superficial injury of lip

    √7th **S00.502** Unspecified superficial injury of oral cavity

  √6th **S00.51** Abrasion **of lip and oral cavity**

    √7th **S00.511** Abrasion of lip

    √7th **S00.512** Abrasion of oral cavity

  √6th **S00.52** Blister (nonthermal) **of lip and oral cavity**

    √7th **S00.521** Blister (nonthermal) of lip

    √7th **S00.522** Blister (nonthermal) of oral cavity

  √6th **S00.53** Contusion **of lip and oral cavity**

    √7th **S00.531** Contusion of lip
Bruise of lip
Hematoma of lip

    √7th **S00.532** Contusion of oral cavity
Bruise of oral cavity
Hematoma of oral cavity

  √6th **S00.54** External constriction **of lip and oral cavity**

    √7th **S00.541** External constriction of lip

    √7th **S00.542** External constriction of oral cavity

  √6th **S00.55** Superficial foreign body **of lip and oral cavity**

    √7th **S00.551** Superficial foreign body of lip
Splinter of lip and oral cavity

    √7th **S00.552** Superficial foreign body of oral cavity
Splinter of lip and oral cavity

  √6th **S00.56** Insect bite (nonvenomous) **of lip and oral cavity**

    √7th **S00.561** Insect bite (nonvenomous) of lip

    √7th **S00.562** Insect bite (nonvenomous) of oral cavity

  √6th **S00.57** Other superficial bite **of lip and oral cavity**

    √7th **S00.571** Other superficial bite of lip
EXCLUDES 1   *open bite of lip (S01.551)*

    √7th **S00.572** Other superficial bite of oral cavity
EXCLUDES 1   *open bite of oral cavity (S01.552)*

√5th **S00.8** Superficial injury of other parts of head
Superficial injuries of face [any part]

√x7th **S00.80** Unspecified superficial injury of other part of head

√x7th **S00.81** Abrasion **of other part of head**

√x7th **S00.82** Blister (nonthermal) **of other part of head**

√x7th **S00.83** Contusion **of other part of head**
Bruise of other part of head
Hematoma of other part of head

√x7th **S00.84** External constriction **of other part of head**

√x7th **S00.85** Superficial foreign body **of other part of head**
Splinter in other part of head

√x7th **S00.86** Insect bite (nonvenomous) **of other part of head**

√x7th **S00.87** Other superficial bite **of other part of head**
EXCLUDES 1   *open bite of other part of head (S01.85)*

√5th **S00.9** Superficial injury of unspecified part of head

√x7th **S00.90** Unspecified superficial injury of unspecified part of head

√x7th **S00.91** Abrasion **of unspecified part of head**

√x7th **S00.92** Blister (nonthermal) **of unspecified part of head**

√x7th **S00.93** Contusion **of unspecified part of head**
Bruise of head
Hematoma of head

√x7th **S00.94** External constriction **of unspecified part of head**

√x7th **S00.95** Superficial foreign body **of unspecified part of head**
Splinter of head

√x7th **S00.96** Insect bite (nonvenomous) **of unspecified part of head**

√x7th **S00.97** Other superficial bite **of unspecified part of head**
EXCLUDES 1   *open bite of head (S01.95)*

√4th **S01** Open wound of head
Code also any associated:
  injury of cranial nerve (S04.-)
  injury of muscle and tendon of head (S09.1-)
  intracranial injury (S06.-)
  wound infection
EXCLUDES 1   *open skull fracture (S02.- with 7th character B)*
EXCLUDES 2   *injury of eye and orbit (S05.-)*
       traumatic amputation of part of head (S08.-)

The appropriate 7th character is to be added to each code from category S01.
A initial encounter
D subsequent encounter
S sequela

√5th **S01.0** Open wound of scalp
EXCLUDES 1   *avulsion of scalp (S08.0)*

√x7th **S01.00** Unspecified open wound of scalp

√x7th **S01.01** Laceration without foreign body **of scalp**

√x7th **S01.02** Laceration with foreign body **of scalp**

√x7th **S01.03** Puncture wound without foreign body **of scalp**

√x7th **S01.04** Puncture wound with foreign body **of scalp**

√x7th **S01.05** Open bite **of scalp**
Bite of scalp NOS
EXCLUDES 1   *superficial bite of scalp (S00.06, S00.07-)*

N Newborn: 0   P Pediatric: 0-17   M Maternity: 9-64   A Adult: 15-124   MCC Major Complication/Comorbidity   CC Complication/Comorbidity   SW Severe Wound Dx

984   ICD-10-CM 2020

√5ᵗʰ **S01.1 Open wound of eyelid and periocular area**

Open wound of eyelid and periocular area with or without involvement of lacrimal passages

√6ᵗʰ **S01.10 Unspecified open wound of eyelid and periocular area**

CC Excl: For CC codes in subcategory S01.10: PDX collection 1139

√7ᵗʰ **S01.101 Unspecified open wound of right eyelid and periocular area**   `CC`

√7ᵗʰ **S01.102 Unspecified open wound of left eyelid and periocular area**   `CC`

√7ᵗʰ **S01.109 Unspecified open wound of unspecified eyelid and periocular area**   `CC`

√6ᵗʰ **S01.11 Laceration without foreign body of eyelid and periocular area**

√7ᵗʰ **S01.111 Laceration without foreign body of right eyelid and periocular area**

√7ᵗʰ **S01.112 Laceration without foreign body of left eyelid and periocular area**

√7ᵗʰ **S01.119 Laceration without foreign body of unspecified eyelid and periocular area**

√6ᵗʰ **S01.12 Laceration with foreign body of eyelid and periocular area**

√7ᵗʰ **S01.121 Laceration with foreign body of right eyelid and periocular area**

√7ᵗʰ **S01.122 Laceration with foreign body of left eyelid and periocular area**

√7ᵗʰ **S01.129 Laceration with foreign body of unspecified eyelid and periocular area**

√6ᵗʰ **S01.13 Puncture wound without foreign body of eyelid and periocular area**

√7ᵗʰ **S01.131 Puncture wound without foreign body of right eyelid and periocular area**

√7ᵗʰ **S01.132 Puncture wound without foreign body of left eyelid and periocular area**

√7ᵗʰ **S01.139 Puncture wound without foreign body of unspecified eyelid and periocular area**

√6ᵗʰ **S01.14 Puncture wound with foreign body of eyelid and periocular area**

√7ᵗʰ **S01.141 Puncture wound with foreign body of right eyelid and periocular area**

√7ᵗʰ **S01.142 Puncture wound with foreign body of left eyelid and periocular area**

√7ᵗʰ **S01.149 Puncture wound with foreign body of unspecified eyelid and periocular area**

√6ᵗʰ **S01.15 Open bite of eyelid and periocular area**

Bite of eyelid and periocular area NOS

EXCLUDES 1 superficial bite of eyelid and periocular area (S00.26, S00.27)

√7ᵗʰ **S01.151 Open bite of right eyelid and periocular area**

√7ᵗʰ **S01.152 Open bite of left eyelid and periocular area**

√7ᵗʰ **S01.159 Open bite of unspecified eyelid and periocular area**

√5ᵗʰ **S01.2 Open wound of nose**

√x7ᵗʰ **S01.20 Unspecified open wound of nose**

√x7ᵗʰ **S01.21 Laceration without foreign body of nose**

√x7ᵗʰ **S01.22 Laceration with foreign body of nose**

√x7ᵗʰ **S01.23 Puncture wound without foreign body of nose**

√x7ᵗʰ **S01.24 Puncture wound with foreign body of nose**

√x7ᵗʰ **S01.25 Open bite of nose**

Bite of nose NOS

EXCLUDES 1 superficial bite of nose (S00.36, S00.37)

√5ᵗʰ **S01.3 Open wound of ear**

√6ᵗʰ **S01.30 Unspecified open wound of ear**

√7ᵗʰ **S01.301 Unspecified open wound of right ear**

√7ᵗʰ **S01.302 Unspecified open wound of left ear**

√7ᵗʰ **S01.309 Unspecified open wound of unspecified ear**

√6ᵗʰ **S01.31 Laceration without foreign body of ear**

√7ᵗʰ **S01.311 Laceration without foreign body of right ear**

√7ᵗʰ **S01.312 Laceration without foreign body of left ear**

√7ᵗʰ **S01.319 Laceration without foreign body of unspecified ear**

√6ᵗʰ **S01.32 Laceration with foreign body of ear**

√7ᵗʰ **S01.321 Laceration with foreign body of right ear**

√7ᵗʰ **S01.322 Laceration with foreign body of left ear**

√7ᵗʰ **S01.329 Laceration with foreign body of unspecified ear**

√6ᵗʰ **S01.33 Puncture wound without foreign body of ear**

√7ᵗʰ **S01.331 Puncture wound without foreign body of right ear**

√7ᵗʰ **S01.332 Puncture wound without foreign body of left ear**

√7ᵗʰ **S01.339 Puncture wound without foreign body of unspecified ear**

√6ᵗʰ **S01.34 Puncture wound with foreign body of ear**

√7ᵗʰ **S01.341 Puncture wound with foreign body of right ear**

√7ᵗʰ **S01.342 Puncture wound with foreign body of left ear**

√7ᵗʰ **S01.349 Puncture wound with foreign body of unspecified ear**

√6ᵗʰ **S01.35 Open bite of ear**

Bite of ear NOS

EXCLUDES 1 superficial bite of ear (S00.46, S00.47)

√7ᵗʰ **S01.351 Open bite of right ear**

√7ᵗʰ **S01.352 Open bite of left ear**

√7ᵗʰ **S01.359 Open bite of unspecified ear**

√5ᵗʰ **S01.4 Open wound of cheek and temporomandibular area**

√6ᵗʰ **S01.40 Unspecified open wound of cheek and temporomandibular area**

√7ᵗʰ **S01.401 Unspecified open wound of right cheek and temporomandibular area**

√7ᵗʰ **S01.402 Unspecified open wound of left cheek and temporomandibular area**

√7ᵗʰ **S01.409 Unspecified open wound of unspecified cheek and temporomandibular area**

√6ᵗʰ **S01.41 Laceration without foreign body of cheek and temporomandibular area**

√7ᵗʰ **S01.411 Laceration without foreign body of right cheek and temporomandibular area**

√7ᵗʰ **S01.412 Laceration without foreign body of left cheek and temporomandibular area**

√7ᵗʰ **S01.419 Laceration without foreign body of unspecified cheek and temporomandibular area**

√6ᵗʰ **S01.42 Laceration with foreign body of cheek and temporomandibular area**

√7ᵗʰ **S01.421 Laceration with foreign body of right cheek and temporomandibular area**

√7ᵗʰ **S01.422 Laceration with foreign body of left cheek and temporomandibular area**

√7ᵗʰ **S01.429 Laceration with foreign body of unspecified cheek and temporomandibular area**

√6ᵗʰ **S01.43 Puncture wound without foreign body of cheek and temporomandibular area**

√7ᵗʰ **S01.431 Puncture wound without foreign body of right cheek and temporomandibular area**

√7ᵗʰ **S01.432 Puncture wound without foreign body of left cheek and temporomandibular area**

√7ᵗʰ **S01.439 Puncture wound without foreign body of unspecified cheek and temporomandibular area**

√6ᵗʰ **S01.44 Puncture wound with foreign body of cheek and temporomandibular area**

√7ᵗʰ **S01.441 Puncture wound with foreign body of right cheek and temporomandibular area**

√7ᵗʰ **S01.442 Puncture wound with foreign body of left cheek and temporomandibular area**

√7ᵗʰ **S01.449 Puncture wound with foreign body of unspecified cheek and temporomandibular area**

√6ᵗʰ **S01.45 Open bite of cheek and temporomandibular area**

Bite of cheek and temporomandibular area NOS

EXCLUDES 2 superficial bite of cheek and temporomandibular area (S00.86, S00.87)

√7ᵗʰ **S01.451 Open bite of right cheek and temporomandibular area**

☑ Additional Character Required   √x7ᵗʰ Placeholder   Unacceptable PDx   Questionable PDx   Manifestation   Unspecified Dx   H1 - H14 HAC   HCC CMS-HCC Dx   HIV HIV Dx

ICD-10-CM 2020

985

Chapter 19. Injury, Poisoning and Certain Other Consequences of External Causes *(side tab)*

✓7ᵗʰ **S01.452** Open bite of **left** cheek and **temporomandibular** area

✓7ᵗʰ **S01.459** Open bite of **unspecified** cheek and **temporomandibular** area

✓5ᵗʰ **S01.5** **Open wound** of **lip and oral cavity**

> EXCLUDES 2   tooth dislocation (S03.2)
>   tooth fracture (S02.5)

  ✓6ᵗʰ **S01.50** **Unspecified open wound of lip and oral cavity**

    ✓7ᵗʰ **S01.501** **Unspecified open wound of lip**

    ✓7ᵗʰ **S01.502** **Unspecified open wound of oral cavity**

  ✓6ᵗʰ **S01.51** **Laceration of lip and oral cavity without foreign body**

    ✓7ᵗʰ **S01.511** **Laceration without foreign body of lip**

    ✓7ᵗʰ **S01.512** **Laceration without foreign body of oral cavity**

  ✓6ᵗʰ **S01.52** **Laceration of lip and oral cavity with foreign body**

    ✓7ᵗʰ **S01.521** **Laceration with foreign body of lip**

    ✓7ᵗʰ **S01.522** **Laceration with foreign body of oral cavity**

  ✓6ᵗʰ **S01.53** **Puncture wound of lip and oral cavity without foreign body**

    ✓7ᵗʰ **S01.531** **Puncture wound without foreign body of lip**

    ✓7ᵗʰ **S01.532** **Puncture wound without foreign body of oral cavity**

  ✓6ᵗʰ **S01.54** **Puncture wound of lip and oral cavity with foreign body**

    ✓7ᵗʰ **S01.541** **Puncture wound with foreign body of lip**

    ✓7ᵗʰ **S01.542** **Puncture wound with foreign body of oral cavity**

  ✓6ᵗʰ **S01.55** **Open bite of lip and oral cavity**

    ✓7ᵗʰ **S01.551** **Open bite of lip**

         Bite of lip NOS

> EXCLUDES 1   superficial bite of lip (S00.571)

    ✓7ᵗʰ **S01.552** **Open bite of oral cavity**

         Bite of oral cavity NOS

> EXCLUDES 1   superficial bite of oral cavity (S00.572)

✓5ᵗʰ **S01.8** **Open wound of other parts of head**

  ✓7ᵗʰ **S01.80** **Unspecified open wound of other part of head**

  ✓7ᵗʰ **S01.81** **Laceration without foreign body of other part of head**

  ✓7ᵗʰ **S01.82** **Laceration with foreign body of other part of head**

  ✓7ᵗʰ **S01.83** **Puncture wound without foreign body of other part of head**

  ✓7ᵗʰ **S01.84** **Puncture wound with foreign body of other part of head**

  ✓7ᵗʰ **S01.85** **Open bite of other part of head**

         Bite of other part of head NOS

> EXCLUDES 1   superficial bite of other part of head (S00.87)

✓5ᵗʰ **S01.9** **Open wound of unspecified part of head**

  ✓7ᵗʰ **S01.90** **Unspecified open wound of unspecified part of head**

  ✓7ᵗʰ **S01.91** **Laceration without foreign body of unspecified part of head**

  ✓7ᵗʰ **S01.92** **Laceration with foreign body of unspecified part of head**

  ✓7ᵗʰ **S01.93** **Puncture wound without foreign body of unspecified part of head**

  ✓7ᵗʰ **S01.94** **Puncture wound with foreign body of unspecified part of head**

  ✓7ᵗʰ **S01.95** **Open bite of unspecified part of head**

         Bite of head NOS

> EXCLUDES 1   superficial bite of head NOS (S00.97)

✓4ᵗʰ **S02** **Fracture of skull and facial bones**

> **NOTE**   A fracture not indicated as open or closed should be coded to closed.

Code also any associated intracranial injury (S06.-)

AHA: 2017,1Q,42; 2016,4Q,66-67

> The appropriate 7th character is to be added to each code from category S02.
> A   initial encounter for closed fracture
> B   initial encounter for open fracture
> D   subsequent encounter for fracture with routine healing
> G   subsequent encounter for fracture with delayed healing
> K   subsequent encounter for fracture with nonunion
> S   sequela

2,3,7 ✓x7ᵗʰ **S02.0** **Fracture of vault of skull**   MCC CC H5 HCC

     Fracture of frontal bone
     Fracture of parietal bone

> **CC Excl:** For codes in subcategory S02.0:
> **CC with 7th character A or MCC with 7th character B:** PDX collection 1140
> **CC with 7th character K:** PDX collection 897

✓5ᵗʰ **S02.1** **Fracture of base of skull**

> EXCLUDES 1   orbit NOS (S02.8)
> EXCLUDES 2   ▶lateral orbital wall (S02.84-)◀
>   ▶medial orbital wall (S02.83-)◀
>   orbital floor (S02.3-)

> **CC Excl:** For codes in subcategory S02.1:
> **CC with 7th character A or MCC with 7th character B:** PDX collection 1140
> **CC with 7th character K:** PDX collection 897

  ✓6ᵗʰ **S02.10** **Unspecified fracture of base of skull**

  2,3,7 ✓7ᵗʰ **S02.101** **Fracture of base of skull, right side**   MCC CC H5 HCC

  2,3,7 ✓7ᵗʰ **S02.102** **Fracture of base of skull, left side**   MCC CC H5 HCC

  2,3,7 ✓7ᵗʰ **S02.109** **Fracture of base of skull, unspecified side**   MCC CC H5 HCC

  ✓6ᵗʰ **S02.11** **Fracture of occiput**

  2,3,7 ✓7ᵗʰ **S02.110** **Type I occipital condyle fracture, unspecified side**   MCC CC H5 HCC

  2,3,7 ✓7ᵗʰ **S02.111** **Type II occipital condyle fracture, unspecified side**   MCC CC H5 HCC

  2,3,7 ✓7ᵗʰ **S02.112** **Type III occipital condyle fracture, unspecified side**   MCC CC H5 HCC

  2,3,7 ✓7ᵗʰ **S02.113** **Unspecified occipital condyle fracture**   MCC CC H5 HCC

  2,3,7 ✓7ᵗʰ **S02.118** **Other fracture of occiput, unspecified side**   MCC CC H5 HCC

  2,3,7 ✓7ᵗʰ **S02.119** **Unspecified fracture of occiput**   MCC CC H5 HCC

  2,3,7 ✓7ᵗʰ **S02.11A** **Type I occipital condyle fracture, right side**   MCC CC H5 HCC

  2,3,7 ✓7ᵗʰ **S02.11B** **Type I occipital condyle fracture, left side**   MCC CC H5 HCC

  2,3,7 ✓7ᵗʰ **S02.11C** **Type II occipital condyle fracture, right side**   MCC CC H5 HCC

  2,3,7 ✓7ᵗʰ **S02.11D** **Type II occipital condyle fracture, left side**   MCC CC H5 HCC

  2,3,7 ✓7ᵗʰ **S02.11E** **Type III occipital condyle fracture, right side**   MCC CC H5 HCC

  2,3,7 ✓7ᵗʰ **S02.11F** **Type III occipital condyle fracture, left side**   MCC CC H5 HCC

  2,3,7 ✓7ᵗʰ **S02.11G** **Other fracture of occiput, right side**   MCC CC H5 HCC

  2,3,7 ✓7ᵗʰ **S02.11H** **Other fracture of occiput, left side**   MCC CC H5 HCC

  ● ✓6ᵗʰ **S02.12** **Fracture of orbital roof**

  ● 2,3 ✓7ᵗʰ **S02.121** **Fracture of orbital roof, right side**   MCC CC

  ● 2,3 ✓7ᵗʰ **S02.122** **Fracture of orbital roof, left side**   MCC CC

  ● 2,3 ✓7ᵗʰ **S02.129** **Fracture of orbital roof, unspecified side**   MCC CC

N Newborn: 0   **P** Pediatric: 0-17   **M** Maternity: 9-64   **A** Adult: 15-124   **MCC** Major Complication/Comorbidity   **CC** Complication/Comorbidity   **SW** Severe Wound Dx

986   ICD-10-CM 2020

2,3,7 √x7ᵗʰ **S02.19** **Other fracture of base of skull** `MCC` `CC` `H5` `HCC`

Fracture of anterior fossa of base of skull
Fracture of ethmoid sinus
Fracture of frontal sinus
Fracture of middle fossa of base of skull
~~Fracture of orbital roof~~
Fracture of posterior fossa of base of skull
Fracture of sphenoid
Fracture of temporal bone

3 √x7ᵗʰ **S02.2** **Fracture of** nasal bones `CC` `H5`

CC Excl: CC with 7th character B: PDX collection 1141
CC Excl: CC with 7th character K: PDX collection 897

√5ᵗʰ **S02.3** **Fracture of** orbital floor

▶Fracture of inferior orbital wall◀
EXCLUDES 1   orbit NOS ▶(S02.85)◀
EXCLUDES 2 ▶lateral orbital wall (S02.84-)◀
▶medial orbital wall (S02.83-) ◀
orbital roof (S02.1-)

CC Excl: For codes in subcategory S02.3:
CC with 7th character A or B: PDX collection 1142
CC with 7th character K: PDX collection 897

3,7 √x7ᵗʰ **S02.30** **Fracture of orbital floor, unspecified side** `CC` `H5` `HCC`

3,7 √x7ᵗʰ **S02.31** **Fracture of orbital floor, right side** `CC` `H5` `HCC`

3,7 √x7ᵗʰ **S02.32** **Fracture of orbital floor, left side** `CC` `H5` `HCC`

√5ᵗʰ **S02.4** **Fracture of** malar, maxillary and zygoma bones

Fracture of superior maxilla
Fracture of upper jaw (bone)
Fracture of zygomatic process of temporal bone

CC Excl: For codes in subcategory S02.4, unless otherwise noted:
CC with 7th character A or B: PDX collection 1143
CC with 7th character K: PDX collection 897

√6ᵗʰ **S02.40** **Fracture of malar, maxillary and zygoma bones, unspecified**

3,7 √7ᵗʰ **S02.400** **Malar fracture, unspecified side** `CC` `H5` `HCC`

3,7 √7ᵗʰ **S02.401** **Maxillary fracture, unspecified side** `CC` `H5` `HCC`

3,7 √7ᵗʰ **S02.402** **Zygomatic fracture, unspecified side** `CC` `H5` `HCC`

3,7 √7ᵗʰ **S02.40A** **Malar fracture, right side** `CC` `H5` `HCC`

3,7 √7ᵗʰ **S02.40B** **Malar fracture, left side** `CC` `H5` `HCC`

3,7 √7ᵗʰ **S02.40C** **Maxillary fracture, right side** `CC` `H5` `HCC`

3,7 √7ᵗʰ **S02.40D** **Maxillary fracture, left side** `CC` `H5` `HCC`

3,7 √7ᵗʰ **S02.40E** **Zygomatic fracture, right side** `CC` `H5` `HCC`

3,7 √7ᵗʰ **S02.40F** **Zygomatic fracture, left side** `CC` `H5` `HCC`

√6ᵗʰ **S02.41** **LeFort fracture**

DEF: Named for Rene Le Fort, these fractures describe different combinations of multiple fractures that occur from significant force to the midface. A common denominator in all three types of LeFort fractures is fracture of the pterygoid processes, which are two bony plates resembling wings that extend downward from the sphenoid bone.

LeFort Fracture Types

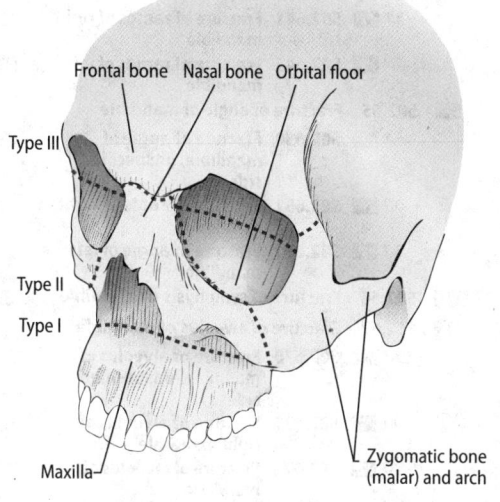

Frontal bone   Nasal bone   Orbital floor
Type III
Type II
Type I
Maxilla
Zygomatic bone (malar) and arch

3,7 √7ᵗʰ **S02.411** **LeFort I fracture** `CC` `H5` `HCC`

3,7 √7ᵗʰ **S02.412** **LeFort II fracture** `CC` `H5` `HCC`

3,7 √7ᵗʰ **S02.413** **LeFort III fracture** `CC` `H5` `HCC`

3,7 √x7ᵗʰ **S02.42** **Fracture of alveolus of maxilla** `CC` `H5` `HCC`

CC Excl: CC with 7th character B: PDX collection 1141
CC Excl: CC with 7th character K: PDX collection 897

4 √x7ᵗʰ **S02.5** **Fracture of tooth (traumatic)** `CC`

Broken tooth
EXCLUDES 1   cracked tooth (nontraumatic) (K03.81)
CC Excl: CC with 7th character K: PDX collection 897

√5ᵗʰ **S02.6** **Fracture of** mandible

Fracture of lower jaw (bone)
CC Excl: For codes in subcategory S02.6:
CC with 7th character A or B: PDX collection 1143
CC with 7th character K: PDX collection 897

√6ᵗʰ **S02.60** **Fracture of mandible, unspecified**

3,7 √7ᵗʰ **S02.600** **Fracture of unspecified part of body of mandible, unspecified side** `CC` `H5` `HCC`

3,7 √7ᵗʰ **S02.601** **Fracture of unspecified part of body of right mandible** `CC` `H5` `HCC`

3,7 √7ᵗʰ **S02.602** **Fracture of unspecified part of body of left mandible** `CC` `H5` `HCC`

3,7 √7ᵗʰ **S02.609** **Fracture of mandible, unspecified** `CC` `H5` `HCC`

√6ᵗʰ **S02.61** **Fracture of condylar process of mandible**

3,7 √7ᵗʰ **S02.610** **Fracture of condylar process of mandible, unspecified side** `CC` `H5` `HCC`

3,7 √7ᵗʰ **S02.611** **Fracture of condylar process of right mandible** `CC` `H5` `HCC`

3,7 √7ᵗʰ **S02.612** **Fracture of condylar process of left mandible** `CC` `H5` `HCC`

√6ᵗʰ **S02.62** **Fracture of subcondylar process of mandible**

3,7 √7ᵗʰ **S02.620** **Fracture of subcondylar process of mandible, unspecified side** `CC` `H5` `HCC`

3,7 √7ᵗʰ **S02.621** **Fracture of subcondylar process of right mandible** `CC` `H5` `HCC`

3,7 √7ᵗʰ **S02.622** **Fracture of subcondylar process of left mandible** `CC` `H5` `HCC`

☑ Additional Character Required   √7ᵗʰ Placeholder   Unacceptable PDx   Questionable PDx   Manifestation   Unspecified Dx   `H1`-`H14` HAC   `HCC` CMS-HCC Dx   `HIV` HIV Dx

ICD-10-CM 2020

987

√6ᵗʰ **S02.63 Fracture of coronoid process of mandible**

3,7 √7ᵗʰ **S02.630 Fracture of coronoid process of mandible, unspecified side** `CC` `H5` `HCC`

3,7 √7ᵗʰ **S02.631 Fracture of coronoid process of right mandible** `CC` `H5` `HCC`

3,7 √7ᵗʰ **S02.632 Fracture of coronoid process of left mandible** `CC` `H5` `HCC`

√6ᵗʰ **S02.64 Fracture of ramus of mandible**

3,7 √7ᵗʰ **S02.640 Fracture of ramus of mandible, unspecified side** `CC` `H5` `HCC`

3,7 √7ᵗʰ **S02.641 Fracture of ramus of right mandible** `CC` `H5` `HCC`

3,7 √7ᵗʰ **S02.642 Fracture of ramus of left mandible** `CC` `H5` `HCC`

√6ᵗʰ **S02.65 Fracture of angle of mandible**

3,7 √7ᵗʰ **S02.650 Fracture of angle of mandible, unspecified side** `CC` `H5` `HCC`

3,7 √7ᵗʰ **S02.651 Fracture of angle of right mandible** `CC` `H5` `HCC`

3,7 √7ᵗʰ **S02.652 Fracture of angle of left mandible** `CC` `H5` `HCC`

3,7 √x7ᵗʰ **S02.66 Fracture of symphysis of mandible** `CC` `H5` `HCC`

√6ᵗʰ **S02.67 Fracture of alveolus of mandible**

3,7 √7ᵗʰ **S02.670 Fracture of alveolus of mandible, unspecified side** `CC` `H5` `HCC`

3,7 √7ᵗʰ **S02.671 Fracture of alveolus of right mandible** `CC` `H5` `HCC`

3,7 √7ᵗʰ **S02.672 Fracture of alveolus of left mandible** `CC` `H5` `HCC`

3,7 √x7ᵗʰ **S02.69 Fracture of mandible of other specified site** `CC` `H5` `HCC`

√6ᵗʰ **S02.8 Fractures of other specified skull and facial bones**

Fracture of orbit NOS

Fracture of palate

EXCLUDES 1   *fracture of orbital floor (S02.3-)*
          fracture of orbital roof (S02.1-)

EXCLUDES 2   ▸*fracture of orbital floor (S02.3-)*◂
          ▸*fracture of orbital roof (S02.12-)*◂

CC Excl: For codes in subcategory S02.8:
CC with 7th character A or B: PDX collection 1142
CC with 7th character K: PDX collection 897

3,7 √x7ᵗʰ **S02.80 Fracture of other specified skull and facial bones, unspecified side** `CC` `H5` `HCC`

3,7 √x7ᵗʰ **S02.81 Fracture of other specified skull and facial bones, right side** `CC` `H5` `HCC`

3,7 √x7ᵗʰ **S02.82 Fracture of other specified skull and facial bones, left side** `CC` `H5` `HCC`

● √6ᵗʰ **S02.83 Fracture of medial orbital wall**

EXCLUDES 2   *orbital floor (S02.3-)*
          orbital roof (S02.12-)

● 3 √7ᵗʰ **S02.831 Fracture of medial orbital wall, right side** `CC`

● 3 √7ᵗʰ **S02.832 Fracture of medial orbital wall, left side** `CC`

● 3 √7ᵗʰ **S02.839 Fracture of medial orbital wall, unspecified side** `CC`

● √6ᵗʰ **S02.84 Fracture of lateral orbital wall**

EXCLUDES 2   *orbital floor (S02.3-)*
          orbital roof (S02.12-)

● 3 √7ᵗʰ **S02.841 Fracture of lateral orbital wall, right side** `CC`

● 3 √7ᵗʰ **S02.842 Fracture of lateral orbital wall, left side** `CC`

● 3 √7ᵗʰ **S02.849 Fracture of lateral orbital wall, unspecified side** `CC`

● 3 √x7ᵗʰ **S02.85 Fracture of orbit, unspecified** `CC`

Fracture of orbit NOS

Fracture of orbit wall NOS

EXCLUDES 1   *lateral orbital wall (S02.84-)*
          medial orbital wall (S02.83-)
          orbital floor (S02.3-)
          orbital roof (S02.12-)

√5ᵗʰ **S02.9 Fracture of unspecified skull and facial bones**

2,3,7 √x7ᵗʰ **S02.91 Unspecified fracture of skull** `MCC` `CC` `H5` `HCC`

CC Excl: CC with 7th character A or MCC with 7th character B: PDX collection 1140
CC Excl: CC with 7th character K: PDX collection 897

3,7 √x7ᵗʰ **S02.92 Unspecified fracture of facial bones** `CC` `H5` `HCC`

CC Excl: CC with 7th character A or B: PDX collection 1142
CC Excl: CC with 7th character K: PDX collection 897

√4ᵗʰ **S03 Dislocation and sprain of joints and ligaments of head**

INCLUDES   avulsion of joint (capsule) or ligament of head
          laceration of cartilage, joint (capsule) or ligament of head
          sprain of cartilage, joint (capsule) or ligament of head
          traumatic hemarthrosis of joint or ligament of head
          traumatic rupture of joint or ligament of head
          traumatic subluxation of joint or ligament of head
          traumatic tear of joint or ligament of head

Code also any associated open wound

EXCLUDES 2   *strain of muscle or tendon of head (S09.1)*

The appropriate 7th character is to be added to each code from category S03.
A   initial encounter
D   subsequent encounter
S   sequela

√5ᵗʰ **S03.0 Dislocation of jaw**

Dislocation of jaw (cartilage) (meniscus)
Dislocation of mandible
Dislocation of temporomandibular (joint)
AHA: 2016,4Q,67

√x7ᵗʰ **S03.00 Dislocation of jaw, unspecified side**

√x7ᵗʰ **S03.01 Dislocation of jaw, right side**

√x7ᵗʰ **S03.02 Dislocation of jaw, left side**

√x7ᵗʰ **S03.03 Dislocation of jaw, bilateral**

√x7ᵗʰ **S03.1 Dislocation of septal cartilage of nose**

√x7ᵗʰ **S03.2 Dislocation of tooth**

√5ᵗʰ **S03.4 Sprain of jaw**

Sprain of temporomandibular (joint) (ligament)
AHA: 2016,4Q,67

√x7ᵗʰ **S03.40 Sprain of jaw, unspecified side**

√x7ᵗʰ **S03.41 Sprain of jaw, right side**

√x7ᵗʰ **S03.42 Sprain of jaw, left side**

√x7ᵗʰ **S03.43 Sprain of jaw, bilateral**

√x7ᵗʰ **S03.8 Sprain of joints and ligaments of other parts of head**

√x7ᵗʰ **S03.9 Sprain of joints and ligaments of unspecified parts of head**

√4ᵗʰ **S04 Injury of cranial nerve**

The selection of side should be based on the side of the body being affected
Code first any associated intracranial injury (S06.-)
Code also any associated:
   open wound of head (S01.-)
   skull fracture (S02.-)

The appropriate 7th character is to be added to each code from category S04.
A   initial encounter
D   subsequent encounter
S   sequela

√5ᵗʰ **S04.0 Injury of optic nerve and pathways**

Use additional code to identify any visual field defect or blindness (H53.4-, H54.-)

CC Excl: For CC codes in subcategory S04.0: PDX collection 1144

√6ᵗʰ **S04.01 Injury of optic nerve**

Injury of 2nd cranial nerve

√7ᵗʰ **S04.011 Injury of optic nerve, right eye** `CC`

√7ᵗʰ **S04.012 Injury of optic nerve, left eye** `CC`

√7ᵗʰ **S04.019 Injury of optic nerve, unspecified eye** `CC`

Injury of optic nerve NOS

√x7ᵗʰ **S04.02 Injury of optic chiasm** `CC`

`N` Newborn: 0   `P` Pediatric: 0-17   `M` Maternity: 9-64   `A` Adult: 15-124   `MCC` Major Complication/Comorbidity   `CC` Complication/Comorbidity   `SW` Severe Wound Dx

988   ICD-10-CM 2020

√6ᵗʰ **S04.03** **Injury of optic** tract and pathways

Injury of optic radiation

√7ᵗʰ **S04.031** **Injury of optic tract and pathways, right** side   CC

√7ᵗʰ **S04.032** **Injury of optic tract and pathways, left** side   CC

√7ᵗʰ **S04.039** **Injury of optic tract and pathways, unspecified side**   CC

Injury of optic tract and pathways NOS

√6ᵗʰ **S04.04** **Injury of** visual cortex

√7ᵗʰ **S04.041** **Injury of visual cortex, right** side   CC

√7ᵗʰ **S04.042** **Injury of visual cortex, left** side   CC

√7ᵗʰ **S04.049** **Injury of visual cortex, unspecified side**   CC

Injury of visual cortex NOS

√5ᵗʰ **S04.1** **Injury of** oculomotor nerve

Injury of 3rd cranial nerve

CC Excl: For CC codes in subcategory S04.1: PDX collection 1145

√x7ᵗʰ **S04.10** **Injury of oculomotor nerve, unspecified side**   CC

√x7ᵗʰ **S04.11** **Injury of oculomotor nerve, right** side   CC

√x7ᵗʰ **S04.12** **Injury of oculomotor nerve, left** side   CC

√5ᵗʰ **S04.2** **Injury of** trochlear nerve

Injury of 4th cranial nerve

CC Excl: For CC codes in subcategory S04.2: PDX collection 1146

√x7ᵗʰ **S04.20** **Injury of trochlear nerve, unspecified side**   CC

√x7ᵗʰ **S04.21** **Injury of trochlear nerve, right** side   CC

√x7ᵗʰ **S04.22** **Injury of trochlear nerve, left** side   CC

√5ᵗʰ **S04.3** **Injury of** trigeminal nerve

Injury of 5th cranial nerve

CC Excl: For CC codes in subcategory S04.3: PDX collection 1147

√x7ᵗʰ **S04.30** **Injury of trigeminal nerve, unspecified side**   CC

√x7ᵗʰ **S04.31** **Injury of trigeminal nerve, right** side   CC

√x7ᵗʰ **S04.32** **Injury of trigeminal nerve, left** side   CC

√5ᵗʰ **S04.4** **Injury of** abducent nerve

Injury of 6th cranial nerve

CC Excl: For CC codes in subcategory S04.4: PDX collection 1148

√x7ᵗʰ **S04.40** **Injury of abducent nerve, unspecified side**   CC

√x7ᵗʰ **S04.41** **Injury of abducent nerve, right** side   CC

√x7ᵗʰ **S04.42** **Injury of abducent nerve, left** side   CC

√5ᵗʰ **S04.5** **Injury of** facial nerve

Injury of 7th cranial nerve

CC Excl: For CC codes in subcategory S04.5: PDX collection 1149

√x7ᵗʰ **S04.50** **Injury of facial nerve, unspecified side**   CC

√x7ᵗʰ **S04.51** **Injury of facial nerve, right** side   CC

√x7ᵗʰ **S04.52** **Injury of facial nerve, left** side   CC

√5ᵗʰ **S04.6** **Injury of** acoustic nerve

Injury of auditory nerve

Injury of 8th cranial nerve

CC Excl: For CC codes in subcategory S04.6: PDX collection 1150

√x7ᵗʰ **S04.60** **Injury of acoustic nerve, unspecified side**   CC

√x7ᵗʰ **S04.61** **Injury of acoustic nerve, right** side   CC

√x7ᵗʰ **S04.62** **Injury of acoustic nerve, left** side   CC

√5ᵗʰ **S04.7** **Injury of** accessory nerve

Injury of 11th cranial nerve

CC Excl: For CC codes in subcategory S04.7: PDX collection 1151

√x7ᵗʰ **S04.70** **Injury of accessory nerve, unspecified side**   CC

√x7ᵗʰ **S04.71** **Injury of accessory nerve, right** side   CC

√x7ᵗʰ **S04.72** **Injury of accessory nerve, left** side   CC

√5ᵗʰ **S04.8** **Injury of other cranial nerves**

CC Excl: For CC codes in subcategory S04.8: PDX collection 1152

√6ᵗʰ **S04.81** **Injury of** olfactory [1st] nerve

√7ᵗʰ **S04.811** **Injury of olfactory [1st] nerve, right** side   CC

√7ᵗʰ **S04.812** **Injury of olfactory [1st] nerve, left** side   CC

√7ᵗʰ **S04.819** **Injury of olfactory [1st] nerve, unspecified side**   CC

√6ᵗʰ **S04.89** **Injury of other cranial nerves**

Injury of vagus [10th] nerve

√7ᵗʰ **S04.891** **Injury of other cranial nerves, right** side   CC

√7ᵗʰ **S04.892** **Injury of other cranial nerves, left** side   CC

√7ᵗʰ **S04.899** **Injury of other cranial nerves, unspecified side**   CC

√x7ᵗʰ **S04.9** **Injury of unspecified cranial nerve**   CC

CC Excl: PDX collection 1152

√4ᵗʰ **S05** **Injury of eye and orbit**

INCLUDES   open wound of eye and orbit

EXCLUDES 2   2nd cranial [optic] nerve injury (S04.0-)

3rd cranial [oculomotor] nerve injury (S04.1-)

open wound of eyelid and periocular area (S01.1-)

orbital bone fracture (S02.1-, S02.3-, S02.8-)

superficial injury of eyelid (S00.1-S00.2)

The appropriate 7th character is to be added to each code from category S05.

A   initial encounter

D   subsequent encounter

S   sequela

CC Excl: For CC codes in category S05, unless otherwise noted: PDX collection 1139

√5ᵗʰ **S05.0** **Injury of conjunctiva and corneal abrasion** without foreign body

EXCLUDES 1   foreign body in conjunctival sac (T15.1)

foreign body in cornea (T15.0)

√x7ᵗʰ **S05.00** **Injury of conjunctiva and corneal abrasion without foreign body, unspecified eye**

√x7ᵗʰ **S05.01** **Injury of conjunctiva and corneal abrasion without foreign body, right eye**

√x7ᵗʰ **S05.02** **Injury of conjunctiva and corneal abrasion without foreign body, left eye**

√5ᵗʰ **S05.1** **Contusion of eyeball and orbital tissues**

Traumatic hyphema

EXCLUDES 2   black eye NOS (S00.1)

contusion of eyelid and periocular area (S00.1)

√x7ᵗʰ **S05.10** **Contusion of eyeball and orbital tissues, unspecified eye**

√x7ᵗʰ **S05.11** **Contusion of eyeball and orbital tissues, right** eye

√x7ᵗʰ **S05.12** **Contusion of eyeball and orbital tissues, left** eye

√5ᵗʰ **S05.2** **Ocular laceration and rupture** with prolapse or loss of intraocular tissue

√x7ᵗʰ **S05.20** **Ocular laceration and rupture with prolapse or loss of intraocular tissue, unspecified eye**   CC

√x7ᵗʰ **S05.21** **Ocular laceration and rupture with prolapse or loss of intraocular tissue, right eye**   CC

√x7ᵗʰ **S05.22** **Ocular laceration and rupture with prolapse or loss of intraocular tissue, left eye**   CC

√5ᵗʰ **S05.3** **Ocular laceration** without prolapse or loss of intraocular tissue

Laceration of eye NOS

DEF: Tear in ocular tissue without displacing structures that is due to blunt trauma. It is characterized by pain, redness, and decreased vision.

√x7ᵗʰ **S05.30** **Ocular laceration without prolapse or loss of intraocular tissue, unspecified eye**   CC

√x7ᵗʰ **S05.31** **Ocular laceration without prolapse or loss of intraocular tissue, right** eye   CC

√x7ᵗʰ **S05.32** **Ocular laceration without prolapse or loss of intraocular tissue, left** eye   CC

☑ Additional Character Required   √x7ᵗʰ Placeholder   Unacceptable PDx   Questionable PDx   Manifestation   Unspecified Dx   H1 - H14 HAC   HCC CMS-HCC Dx   HIV HIV Dx

ICD-10-CM 2020   989

√5ᵗʰ **S05.4** Penetrating wound of orbit with or without foreign body

> EXCLUDES 2   *retained (old) foreign body following penetrating wound in orbit (H05.5-)*

√x7ᵗʰ **S05.40** Penetrating wound of orbit with or without foreign body, **unspecified eye**   CC

√x7ᵗʰ **S05.41** Penetrating wound of orbit with or without foreign body, **right** eye   CC

√x7ᵗʰ **S05.42** Penetrating wound of orbit with or without foreign body, **left** eye   CC

√5ᵗʰ **S05.5** Penetrating wound with foreign body of eyeball

> EXCLUDES 2   *retained (old) intraocular foreign body (H44.6-, H44.7)*

> **CC Excl:** For CC Codes in subcategory S05.5: PDX collection 1153

√x7ᵗʰ **S05.50** Penetrating wound with foreign body of **unspecified eyeball**   CC

√x7ᵗʰ **S05.51** Penetrating wound with foreign body of **right** eyeball   CC

√x7ᵗʰ **S05.52** Penetrating wound with foreign body of **left** eyeball   CC

√5ᵗʰ **S05.6** Penetrating wound without foreign body of eyeball

> Ocular penetration NOS

√x7ᵗʰ **S05.60** Penetrating wound without foreign body of **unspecified eyeball**   CC

√x7ᵗʰ **S05.61** Penetrating wound without foreign body of **right** eyeball   CC

√x7ᵗʰ **S05.62** Penetrating wound without foreign body of **left** eyeball   CC

√5ᵗʰ **S05.7** Avulsion of eye

> Traumatic enucleation

√x7ᵗʰ **S05.70** Avulsion of **unspecified** eye   CC

√x7ᵗʰ **S05.71** Avulsion of **right** eye   CC

√x7ᵗʰ **S05.72** Avulsion of **left** eye   CC

√5ᵗʰ **S05.8** Other injuries of eye and orbit

> Lacrimal duct injury

√6ᵗʰ **S05.8X** Other injuries of eye and orbit

√7ᵗʰ **S05.8X1** Other injuries of **right** eye and orbit   CC

√7ᵗʰ **S05.8X2** Other injuries of **left** eye and orbit   CC

√7ᵗʰ **S05.8X9** Other injuries of **unspecified** eye and orbit   CC

√5ᵗʰ **S05.9** Unspecified injury of eye and orbit

> Injury of eye NOS

√x7ᵗʰ **S05.90** Unspecified injury of **unspecified** eye and orbit

√x7ᵗʰ **S05.91** Unspecified injury of **right** eye and orbit   CC

√x7ᵗʰ **S05.92** Unspecified injury of **left** eye and orbit   CC

√4ᵗʰ **S06** Intracranial injury

> **NOTE**   7th characters D and S do not apply to codes in category S06 with 6th character 7 – death due to brain injury prior to regaining consciousness, or 8 – death due to other cause prior to regaining consciousness.

> INCLUDES   traumatic brain injury

> Code also any associated:
> open wound of head (S01.-)
> skull fracture (S02.-)

> EXCLUDES 1   *head injury NOS (S09.90)*

> **AHA:** 2017,4Q,25; 2017,1Q,42; 2015,3Q,37

> **TIP:** Do not assign Z87.820 Personal history of traumatic brain injury, when residual conditions persist after an intracranial injury. The codes for the residual conditions should be first listed, followed by a code from category S06 using seventh character S to identify sequelae.

> The appropriate 7th character is to be added to each code from category S06.
> A   initial encounter
> D   subsequent encounter
> S   sequela

> **CC Excl:** For CC/MCC codes in category S06, unless otherwise noted: PDX collection 1154

√5ᵗʰ **S06.0** Concussion

> Commotio cerebri

> EXCLUDES 1   *concussion with other intracranial injuries classified in subcategories S06.1- to S06.6- , S06.81- and S06.82- — code to specified intracranial injury*

> **AHA:** 2016,4Q,67-68

√6ᵗʰ **S06.0X** Concussion

8 √7ᵗʰ **S06.0X0** **Concussion** without loss of consciousness   CC HCC

8 √7ᵗʰ **S06.0X1** **Concussion** with loss of consciousness of 30 minutes or less   CC H5 HCC

8 √7ᵗʰ **S06.0X9** **Concussion** with loss of consciousness of unspecified duration
> Concussion NOS   CC H5 HCC

√5ᵗʰ **S06.1** Traumatic cerebral edema

> Diffuse traumatic cerebral edema
> Focal traumatic cerebral edema

> **CC Excl:** For MCC codes in category S06.1, unless otherwise noted: PDX collection 1155

√6ᵗʰ **S06.1X** Traumatic cerebral edema

7 √7ᵗʰ **S06.1X0** Traumatic cerebral edema without loss of consciousness   MCC HCC
> **CC Excl:** PDX collection 612

7 √7ᵗʰ **S06.1X1** Traumatic cerebral edema with loss of consciousness of 30 minutes or less   MCC H5 HCC

7 √7ᵗʰ **S06.1X2** Traumatic cerebral edema with loss of consciousness of 31 minutes to 59 minutes   MCC H5 HCC

7 √7ᵗʰ **S06.1X3** Traumatic cerebral edema with loss of consciousness of 1 hour to 5 hours 59 minutes   MCC H5 HCC

7 √7ᵗʰ **S06.1X4** Traumatic cerebral edema with loss of consciousness of 6 hours to 24 hours   MCC H5 HCC

7 √7ᵗʰ **S06.1X5** Traumatic cerebral edema with loss of consciousness greater than 24 hours with return to pre-existing conscious level   MCC H5 HCC

7 √7ᵗʰ **S06.1X6** Traumatic cerebral edema with loss of consciousness greater than 24 hours without return to pre-existing conscious level with patient surviving   MCC H5 HCC
> **CC Excl:** PDX collection 1154

√7ᵗʰ **S06.1X7** **Traumatic cerebral edema with loss of consciousness of** any duration with death due to brain injury prior to regaining consciousness   `MCC` `H5`
CC Excl: PDX collection 1154

√7ᵗʰ **S06.1X8** **Traumatic cerebral edema with loss of consciousness of** any duration with death due to other cause prior to regaining consciousness   `MCC` `H5`
CC Excl: PDX collection 1154

7 √7ᵗʰ **S06.1X9** **Traumatic cerebral edema with loss of consciousness of unspecified duration**   `MCC` `H5` `HCC`
Traumatic cerebral edema NOS

√5ᵗʰ **S06.2** **Diffuse traumatic brain injury**
Diffuse axonal brain injury
EXCLUDES 1   *traumatic diffuse cerebral edema (S06.1X-)*

√6ᵗʰ **S06.2X** Diffuse traumatic brain injury

7 √7ᵗʰ **S06.2X0** **Diffuse traumatic brain injury** without loss of consciousness   `HCC`

7 √7ᵗʰ **S06.2X1** **Diffuse traumatic brain injury with loss of consciousness of** 30 minutes or less   `CC` `H5` `HCC`

7 √7ᵗʰ **S06.2X2** **Diffuse traumatic brain injury with loss of consciousness of** 31 minutes to 59 minutes   `CC` `H5` `HCC`

7 √7ᵗʰ **S06.2X3** **Diffuse traumatic brain injury with loss of consciousness of** 1 hour to 5 hours 59 minutes   `CC` `H5` `HCC`

7 √7ᵗʰ **S06.2X4** **Diffuse traumatic brain injury with loss of consciousness of** 6 hours to 24 hours   `CC` `H5` `HCC`

7 √7ᵗʰ **S06.2X5** **Diffuse traumatic brain injury with loss of consciousness** greater than 24 hours with return to pre-existing conscious levels   `CC` `H5` `HCC`

7 √7ᵗʰ **S06.2X6** **Diffuse traumatic brain injury with loss of consciousness** greater than 24 hours without return to pre-existing conscious level with patient surviving   `MCC` `H5` `HCC`

√7ᵗʰ **S06.2X7** **Diffuse traumatic brain injury with loss of consciousness of** any duration with death due to brain injury prior to regaining consciousness   `MCC` `H5`

√7ᵗʰ **S06.2X8** **Diffuse traumatic brain injury with loss of consciousness of** any duration with death due to other cause prior to regaining consciousness   `MCC` `H5`

7 √7ᵗʰ **S06.2X9** **Diffuse traumatic brain injury with loss of consciousness of unspecified duration**   `CC` `H5` `HCC`
Diffuse traumatic brain injury NOS

√5ᵗʰ **S06.3** Focal traumatic brain injury
EXCLUDES 1   any condition classifiable to S06.4-S06.6
focal cerebral edema (S06.1)

√6ᵗʰ **S06.30** Unspecified focal traumatic brain injury

7 √7ᵗʰ **S06.300** **Unspecified focal traumatic brain injury** without loss of consciousness   `HCC`

7 √7ᵗʰ **S06.301** **Unspecified focal traumatic brain injury with loss of consciousness of** 30 minutes or less   `CC` `H5` `HCC`

7 √7ᵗʰ **S06.302** **Unspecified focal traumatic brain injury with loss of consciousness of** 31 minutes to 59 minutes   `CC` `H5` `HCC`

7 √7ᵗʰ **S06.303** **Unspecified focal traumatic brain injury with loss of consciousness of** 1 hour to 5 hours 59 minutes   `CC` `H5` `HCC`

7 √7ᵗʰ **S06.304** **Unspecified focal traumatic brain injury with loss of consciousness of** 6 hours to 24 hours   `CC` `H5` `HCC`

7 √7ᵗʰ **S06.305** **Unspecified focal traumatic brain injury with loss of consciousness** greater than 24 hours with return to pre-existing conscious level   `CC` `H5` `HCC`

7 √7ᵗʰ **S06.306** **Unspecified focal traumatic brain injury with loss of consciousness** greater than 24 hours without return to pre-existing conscious level with patient surviving   `MCC` `H5` `HCC`

√7ᵗʰ **S06.307** **Unspecified focal traumatic brain injury with loss of consciousness of** any duration with death due to brain injury prior to regaining consciousness   `MCC` `H5`

√7ᵗʰ **S06.308** **Unspecified focal traumatic brain injury with loss of consciousness of** any duration with death due to other cause prior to regaining consciousness   `MCC` `H5`

7 √7ᵗʰ **S06.309** **Unspecified focal traumatic brain injury with loss of consciousness of unspecified duration**   `CC` `H5` `HCC`
Unspecified focal traumatic brain injury NOS

√6ᵗʰ **S06.31** Contusion and laceration of right cerebrum

7 √7ᵗʰ **S06.310** **Contusion and laceration of right cerebrum** without loss of consciousness   `MCC` `H5` `HCC`

7 √7ᵗʰ **S06.311** **Contusion and laceration of right cerebrum with loss of consciousness of** 30 minutes or less   `MCC` `H5` `HCC`

7 √7ᵗʰ **S06.312** **Contusion and laceration of right cerebrum with loss of consciousness of** 31 minutes to 59 minutes   `MCC` `H5` `HCC`

7 √7ᵗʰ **S06.313** **Contusion and laceration of right cerebrum with loss of consciousness of** 1 hour to 5 hours 59 minutes   `MCC` `H5` `HCC`

7 √7ᵗʰ **S06.314** **Contusion and laceration of right cerebrum with loss of consciousness of** 6 hours to 24 hours   `MCC` `H5` `HCC`

7 √7ᵗʰ **S06.315** **Contusion and laceration of right cerebrum with loss of consciousness** greater than 24 hours with return to pre-existing conscious level   `MCC` `H5` `HCC`

7 √7ᵗʰ **S06.316** **Contusion and laceration of right cerebrum with loss of consciousness** greater than 24 hours without return to pre-existing conscious level with patient surviving   `MCC` `H5` `HCC`

√7ᵗʰ **S06.317** Contusion and laceration of right cerebrum with loss of consciousness of any duration with death due to brain injury prior to regaining consciousness   `MCC` `H5`

√7ᵗʰ **S06.318** Contusion and laceration of right cerebrum with loss of consciousness of any duration with death due to **other** cause prior to regaining consciousness   `MCC` `H5`

7 √7ᵗʰ **S06.319** Contusion and laceration of right cerebrum with loss of consciousness of unspecified duration   `MCC` `H5` `HCC`

Contusion and laceration of right cerebrum NOS

√6ᵗʰ **S06.32** Contusion and laceration of left cerebrum

7 √7ᵗʰ **S06.320** Contusion and laceration of left cerebrum without loss of consciousness   `MCC` `H5` `HCC`

7 √7ᵗʰ **S06.321** Contusion and laceration of left cerebrum with loss of consciousness of 30 minutes or less   `MCC` `H5` `HCC`

7 √7ᵗʰ **S06.322** Contusion and laceration of left cerebrum with loss of consciousness of 31 minutes to 59 minutes   `MCC` `H5` `HCC`

7 √7ᵗʰ **S06.323** Contusion and laceration of left cerebrum with loss of consciousness of 1 hour to 5 hours 59 minutes   `MCC` `H5` `HCC`

7 √7ᵗʰ **S06.324** Contusion and laceration of left cerebrum with loss of consciousness of 6 hours to 24 hours   `MCC` `H5` `HCC`

7 √7ᵗʰ **S06.325** Contusion and laceration of left cerebrum with loss of consciousness greater than 24 hours with return to pre-existing conscious level   `MCC` `H5` `HCC`

7 √7ᵗʰ **S06.326** Contusion and laceration of left cerebrum with loss of consciousness greater than 24 hours without return to pre-existing conscious level with patient surviving   `MCC` `H5` `HCC`

√7ᵗʰ **S06.327** Contusion and laceration of left cerebrum with loss of consciousness of any duration with death due to brain injury prior to regaining consciousness   `MCC` `H5`

√7ᵗʰ **S06.328** Contusion and laceration of left cerebrum with loss of consciousness of any duration with death due to **other** cause prior to regaining consciousness   `MCC` `H5`

7 √7ᵗʰ **S06.329** Contusion and laceration of left cerebrum with loss of consciousness of unspecified duration   `MCC` `H5` `HCC`

Contusion and laceration of left cerebrum NOS

√6ᵗʰ **S06.33** Contusion and laceration of cerebrum, unspecified

7 √7ᵗʰ **S06.330** Contusion and laceration of cerebrum, unspecified, without loss of consciousness   `MCC` `H5` `HCC`

7 √7ᵗʰ **S06.331** Contusion and laceration of cerebrum, unspecified, with loss of consciousness of 30 minutes or less   `MCC` `H5` `HCC`

7 √7ᵗʰ **S06.332** Contusion and laceration of cerebrum, unspecified, with loss of consciousness of 31 minutes to 59 minutes   `MCC` `H5` `HCC`

7 √7ᵗʰ **S06.333** Contusion and laceration of cerebrum, unspecified, with loss of consciousness of 1 hour to 5 hours 59 minutes   `MCC` `H5` `HCC`

7 √7ᵗʰ **S06.334** Contusion and laceration of cerebrum, unspecified, with loss of consciousness of 6 hours to 24 hours   `MCC` `H5` `HCC`

7 √7ᵗʰ **S06.335** Contusion and laceration of cerebrum, unspecified, with loss of consciousness greater than 24 hours with return to pre-existing conscious level   `MCC` `H5` `HCC`

7 √7ᵗʰ **S06.336** Contusion and laceration of cerebrum, unspecified, with loss of consciousness greater than 24 hours without return to pre-existing conscious level with patient surviving   `MCC` `H5` `HCC`

√7ᵗʰ **S06.337** Contusion and laceration of cerebrum, unspecified, with loss of consciousness of any duration with death due to brain injury prior to regaining consciousness   `MCC` `H5`

√7ᵗʰ **S06.338** Contusion and laceration of cerebrum, unspecified, with loss of consciousness of any duration with death due to **other** cause prior to regaining consciousness   `MCC` `H5`

7 √7ᵗʰ **S06.339** Contusion and laceration of cerebrum, unspecified, with loss of consciousness of unspecified duration   `MCC` `H5` `HCC`

Contusion and laceration of cerebrum NOS

√6ᵗʰ **S06.34** Traumatic hemorrhage of right cerebrum

Traumatic intracerebral hemorrhage and hematoma of right cerebrum

7 √7ᵗʰ **S06.340** Traumatic hemorrhage of right cerebrum without loss of consciousness   `MCC` `H5` `HCC`

7 √7ᵗʰ **S06.341** Traumatic hemorrhage of right cerebrum with loss of consciousness of 30 minutes or less   `MCC` `H5` `HCC`

7 √7ᵗʰ **S06.342** Traumatic hemorrhage of right cerebrum with loss of consciousness of 31 minutes to 59 minutes   `MCC` `H5` `HCC`

7 √7ᵗʰ **S06.343** Traumatic hemorrhage of right cerebrum with loss of consciousness of 1 hours to 5 hours 59 minutes   `MCC` `H5` `HCC`

7 √7ᵗʰ **S06.344** Traumatic hemorrhage of right cerebrum with loss of consciousness of 6 hours to 24 hours   `MCC` `H5` `HCC`

7 √7ᵗʰ **S06.345** Traumatic hemorrhage of right cerebrum with loss of consciousness greater than 24 hours with return to pre-existing conscious level   `MCC` `H5` `HCC`

7 √7ᵗʰ **S06.346** Traumatic hemorrhage of right cerebrum with loss of consciousness greater than 24 hours without return to pre-existing conscious level with patient surviving   `MCC` `H5` `HCC`

√7ᵗʰ **S06.347** Traumatic hemorrhage of right cerebrum with loss of consciousness of any duration with death due to brain injury prior to regaining consciousness   `MCC` `H5`

N Newborn: 0   P Pediatric: 0-17   M Maternity: 9-64   A Adult: 15-124   `MCC` Major Complication/Comorbidity   `CC` Complication/Comorbidity   `SW` Severe Wound Dx

992   ICD-10-CM 2020

√7ᵗʰ **S06.348** **Traumatic hemorrhage of right cerebrum with loss of consciousness of** any **duration with death due to** other **cause prior to regaining consciousness** `MCC` `H5`

7 √7ᵗʰ **S06.349** **Traumatic hemorrhage of right cerebrum with loss of consciousness of unspecified duration** `MCC` `H5` `HCC`
> Traumatic hemorrhage of right cerebrum NOS

√6ᵗʰ **S06.35** **Traumatic hemorrhage of** left cerebrum
> Traumatic intracerebral hemorrhage and hematoma of left cerebrum

7 √7ᵗʰ **S06.350** **Traumatic hemorrhage of left cerebrum** without loss of consciousness `MCC` `H5` `HCC`

7 √7ᵗʰ **S06.351** **Traumatic hemorrhage of left cerebrum with loss of consciousness of** 30 minutes or less `MCC` `H5` `HCC`

7 √7ᵗʰ **S06.352** **Traumatic hemorrhage of left cerebrum with loss of consciousness of** 31 minutes to 59 minutes `MCC` `H5` `HCC`

7 √7ᵗʰ **S06.353** **Traumatic hemorrhage of left cerebrum with loss of consciousness of** 1 hours to 5 hours 59 minutes `MCC` `H5` `HCC`

7 √7ᵗʰ **S06.354** **Traumatic hemorrhage of left cerebrum with loss of consciousness of** 6 hours to 24 hours `MCC` `H5` `HCC`

7 √7ᵗʰ **S06.355** **Traumatic hemorrhage of left cerebrum with loss of consciousness** greater than 24 hours with return to pre-existing conscious level `MCC` `H5` `HCC`

7 √7ᵗʰ **S06.356** **Traumatic hemorrhage of left cerebrum with loss of consciousness** greater than 24 hours without return to pre-existing conscious level with patient surviving `MCC` `H5` `HCC`

√7ᵗʰ **S06.357** **Traumatic hemorrhage of left cerebrum with loss of consciousness of** any duration with death due to brain injury prior to regaining consciousness `MCC` `H5`

√7ᵗʰ **S06.358** **Traumatic hemorrhage of left cerebrum with loss of consciousness of** any duration with death due to other cause prior to regaining consciousness `MCC` `H5`

7 √7ᵗʰ **S06.359** **Traumatic hemorrhage of left cerebrum with loss of consciousness of unspecified duration** `MCC` `H5` `HCC`
> Traumatic hemorrhage of left cerebrum NOS

√6ᵗʰ **S06.36** **Traumatic hemorrhage of cerebrum, unspecified**
> Traumatic intracerebral hemorrhage and hematoma, unspecified

7 √7ᵗʰ **S06.360** **Traumatic hemorrhage of cerebrum, unspecified,** without loss of consciousness `MCC` `H5` `HCC`

7 √7ᵗʰ **S06.361** **Traumatic hemorrhage of cerebrum, unspecified, with loss of consciousness of** 30 minutes or less `MCC` `H5` `HCC`

7 √7ᵗʰ **S06.362** **Traumatic hemorrhage of cerebrum, unspecified, with loss of consciousness of** 31 minutes to 59 minutes `MCC` `H5` `HCC`

7 √7ᵗʰ **S06.363** **Traumatic hemorrhage of cerebrum, unspecified, with loss of consciousness of** 1 hours to 5 hours 59 minutes `MCC` `H5` `HCC`

7 √7ᵗʰ **S06.364** **Traumatic hemorrhage of cerebrum, unspecified, with loss of consciousness of** 6 hours to 24 hours `MCC` `H5` `HCC`

7 √7ᵗʰ **S06.365** **Traumatic hemorrhage of cerebrum, unspecified, with loss of consciousness** greater than 24 hours with return to pre-existing conscious level `MCC` `H5` `HCC`

7 √7ᵗʰ **S06.366** **Traumatic hemorrhage of cerebrum, unspecified, with loss of consciousness** greater than 24 hours without return to pre-existing conscious level with patient surviving `MCC` `H5` `HCC`

√7ᵗʰ **S06.367** **Traumatic hemorrhage of cerebrum, unspecified, with loss of consciousness of** any duration with death due to brain injury prior to regaining consciousness `MCC` `H5`

√7ᵗʰ **S06.368** **Traumatic hemorrhage of cerebrum, unspecified, with loss of consciousness of** any duration with death due to other cause prior to regaining consciousness `MCC` `H5`

7 √7ᵗʰ **S06.369** **Traumatic hemorrhage of cerebrum, unspecified, with loss of consciousness of unspecified duration** `MCC` `H5` `HCC`
> Traumatic hemorrhage of cerebrum NOS

√6ᵗʰ **S06.37** **Contusion, laceration, and hemorrhage of cerebellum**

7 √7ᵗʰ **S06.370** **Contusion, laceration, and hemorrhage of cerebellum** without loss of consciousness `MCC` `H5` `HCC`
> CC Excl: No Excl

7 √7ᵗʰ **S06.371** **Contusion, laceration, and hemorrhage of cerebellum with loss of consciousness of** 30 minutes or less `CC` `H5` `HCC`

7 √7ᵗʰ **S06.372** **Contusion, laceration, and hemorrhage of cerebellum with loss of consciousness of** 31 minutes to 59 minutes `CC` `H5` `HCC`

7 √7ᵗʰ **S06.373** **Contusion, laceration, and hemorrhage of cerebellum with loss of consciousness of** 1 hour to 5 hours 59 minutes `CC` `H5` `HCC`

7 √7ᵗʰ **S06.374** **Contusion, laceration, and hemorrhage of cerebellum with loss of consciousness of** 6 hours to 24 hours `CC` `H5` `HCC`

7 √7ᵗʰ **S06.375** **Contusion, laceration, and hemorrhage of cerebellum with loss of consciousness** greater than 24 hours with return to pre-existing conscious level `CC` `H5` `HCC`

7 √7ᵗʰ **S06.376** **Contusion, laceration, and hemorrhage of cerebellum with loss of consciousness** greater than 24 hours without return to pre-existing conscious level with patient surviving `MCC` `H5` `HCC`

√7ᵗʰ **S06.377** **Contusion, laceration, and hemorrhage of cerebellum with loss of consciousness of** any duration with death due to brain injury prior to regaining consciousness `MCC` `H5`

√7ᵗʰ **S06.378 Contusion, laceration, and hemorrhage of cerebellum with loss of consciousness of** any duration with death due to **other** cause prior to regaining consciousness   `MCC` `H5`

7 √7ᵗʰ **S06.379 Contusion, laceration, and hemorrhage of cerebellum with loss of consciousness of unspecified duration**   `CC` `H5` `HCC`
Contusion, laceration, and hemorrhage of cerebellum NOS

√6ᵗʰ **S06.38 Contusion, laceration, and hemorrhage of brainstem**

7 √7ᵗʰ **S06.380 Contusion, laceration, and hemorrhage of brainstem** without loss of consciousness   `MCC` `H5` `HCC`
CC Excl: No Excl

7 √7ᵗʰ **S06.381 Contusion, laceration, and hemorrhage of brainstem with loss of consciousness of** 30 minutes or less   `CC` `H5` `HCC`

7 √7ᵗʰ **S06.382 Contusion, laceration, and hemorrhage of brainstem with loss of consciousness of** 31 minutes to 59 minutes   `CC` `H5` `HCC`

7 √7ᵗʰ **S06.383 Contusion, laceration, and hemorrhage of brainstem with loss of consciousness of** 1 hour to 5 hours 59 minutes   `CC` `H5` `HCC`

7 √7ᵗʰ **S06.384 Contusion, laceration, and hemorrhage of brainstem with loss of consciousness of** 6 hours to 24 hours   `CC` `H5` `HCC`

7 √7ᵗʰ **S06.385 Contusion, laceration, and hemorrhage of brainstem with loss of consciousness** greater than 24 hours with return to pre-existing conscious level   `CC` `H5` `HCC`

7 √7ᵗʰ **S06.386 Contusion, laceration, and hemorrhage of brainstem with loss of consciousness** greater than 24 hours without return to pre-existing conscious level with patient surviving   `MCC` `H5` `HCC`

√7ᵗʰ **S06.387 Contusion, laceration, and hemorrhage of brainstem with loss of consciousness of** any duration with death due to brain injury prior to regaining consciousness   `MCC` `H5`

√7ᵗʰ **S06.388 Contusion, laceration, and hemorrhage of brainstem with loss of consciousness of** any duration with death due to **other** cause prior to regaining consciousness   `MCC` `H5`

7 √7ᵗʰ **S06.389 Contusion, laceration, and hemorrhage of brainstem with loss of consciousness of unspecified duration**   `CC` `H5` `HCC`
Contusion, laceration, and hemorrhage of brainstem NOS

√5ᵗʰ **S06.4 Epidural hemorrhage**
Extradural hemorrhage NOS
Extradural hemorrhage (traumatic)
DEF: Epidural space: Space between the endosteum of the cranium (skull) and the dura mater, the outermost layer of a three-layer membrane that covers the brain.

√6ᵗʰ **S06.4X Epidural hemorrhage**

7 √7ᵗʰ **S06.4X0 Epidural hemorrhage** without loss of consciousness   `MCC` `H5` `HCC`

7 √7ᵗʰ **S06.4X1 Epidural hemorrhage with loss of consciousness of** 30 minutes or less   `MCC` `H5` `HCC`

7 √7ᵗʰ **S06.4X2 Epidural hemorrhage with loss of consciousness of** 31 minutes to 59 minutes   `MCC` `H5` `HCC`

7 √7ᵗʰ **S06.4X3 Epidural hemorrhage with loss of consciousness of** 1 hour to 5 hours 59 minutes   `MCC` `H5` `HCC`

7 √7ᵗʰ **S06.4X4 Epidural hemorrhage with loss of consciousness of** 6 hours to 24 hours   `MCC` `H5` `HCC`

7 √7ᵗʰ **S06.4X5 Epidural hemorrhage with loss of consciousness** greater than 24 hours with return to pre-existing conscious level   `MCC` `H5` `HCC`

7 √7ᵗʰ **S06.4X6 Epidural hemorrhage with loss of consciousness** greater than 24 hours without return to pre-existing conscious level with patient surviving   `MCC` `H5` `HCC`

√7ᵗʰ **S06.4X7 Epidural hemorrhage with loss of consciousness of** any duration with death due to brain injury prior to regaining consciousness   `MCC` `H5`

√7ᵗʰ **S06.4X8 Epidural hemorrhage with loss of consciousness of** any duration with death due to **other** causes prior to regaining consciousness   `MCC` `H5`

7 √7ᵗʰ **S06.4X9 Epidural hemorrhage with loss of consciousness of unspecified duration**   `MCC` `H5` `HCC`
Epidural hemorrhage NOS

√5ᵗʰ **S06.5 Traumatic subdural hemorrhage**
DEF: Subdural: Potential space between the dura mater and arachnoid membrane around the brain.

√6ᵗʰ **S06.5X Traumatic subdural hemorrhage**

7 √7ᵗʰ **S06.5X0 Traumatic subdural hemorrhage** without loss of consciousness   `MCC` `H5` `HCC`

7 √7ᵗʰ **S06.5X1 Traumatic subdural hemorrhage with loss of consciousness of** 30 minutes or less   `MCC` `H5` `HCC`

7 √7ᵗʰ **S06.5X2 Traumatic subdural hemorrhage with loss of consciousness of** 31 minutes to 59 minutes   `MCC` `H5` `HCC`

7 √7ᵗʰ **S06.5X3 Traumatic subdural hemorrhage with loss of consciousness of** 1 hour to 5 hours 59 minutes   `MCC` `H5` `HCC`

7 √7ᵗʰ **S06.5X4 Traumatic subdural hemorrhage with loss of consciousness of** 6 hours to 24 hours   `MCC` `H5` `HCC`

7 √7ᵗʰ **S06.5X5 Traumatic subdural hemorrhage with loss of consciousness** greater than 24 hours with return to pre-existing conscious level   `MCC` `H5` `HCC`

7 √7ᵗʰ **S06.5X6 Traumatic subdural hemorrhage with loss of consciousness** greater than 24 hours without return to pre-existing conscious level with patient surviving   `MCC` `H5` `HCC`

√7ᵗʰ **S06.5X7 Traumatic subdural hemorrhage with loss of consciousness of** any duration with death due to brain injury before regaining consciousness   `MCC` `H5`

√7ᵗʰ **S06.5X8 Traumatic subdural hemorrhage with loss of consciousness of** any duration with death due to **other** cause before regaining consciousness   `MCC` `H5`

7 √7th **S06.5X9** Traumatic subdural
hemorrhage with loss of
consciousness of
unspecified duration   `MCC` `H5` `HCC`
Traumatic subdural hemorrhage NOS

√5th **S06.6** Traumatic subarachnoid hemorrhage
DEF: Subarachnoid: Space located between the arachnoid
membrane and the pia mater that contains cerebrospinal fluid.

√6th **S06.6X** Traumatic subarachnoid hemorrhage

7 √7th **S06.6X0** Traumatic subarachnoid
hemorrhage without loss
of consciousness   `MCC` `H5` `HCC`

7 √7th **S06.6X1** Traumatic subarachnoid
hemorrhage with loss of
consciousness of 30
minutes or less   `MCC` `H5` `HCC`

7 √7th **S06.6X2** Traumatic subarachnoid
hemorrhage with loss of
consciousness of 31
minutes to 59 minutes   `MCC` `H5` `HCC`

7 √7th **S06.6X3** Traumatic subarachnoid
hemorrhage with loss of
consciousness of 1 hour to
5 hours 59 minutes   `MCC` `H5` `HCC`

7 √7th **S06.6X4** Traumatic subarachnoid
hemorrhage with loss of
consciousness of 6 hours
to 24 hours   `MCC` `H5` `HCC`

7 √7th **S06.6X5** Traumatic subarachnoid
hemorrhage with loss of
consciousness greater
than 24 hours with return
to pre-existing conscious
level   `MCC` `H5` `HCC`

7 √7th **S06.6X6** Traumatic subarachnoid
hemorrhage with loss of
consciousness greater
than 24 hours without
return to pre-existing
conscious level with
patient surviving   `MCC` `H5` `HCC`

√7th **S06.6X7** Traumatic subarachnoid
hemorrhage with loss of
consciousness of any
duration with death due
to brain injury prior to
regaining consciousness   `MCC` `H5`

√7th **S06.6X8** Traumatic subarachnoid
hemorrhage with loss of
consciousness of any
duration with death due
to other cause prior to
regaining consciousness   `MCC` `H5`

7 √7th **S06.6X9** Traumatic subarachnoid
hemorrhage with loss of
consciousness of
unspecified duration   `MCC` `H5` `HCC`
Traumatic subarachnoid hemorrhage NOS

√5th **S06.8** Other specified intracranial injuries

√6th **S06.81** Injury of right internal carotid artery, intracranial
portion, not elsewhere classified

7 √7th **S06.810** Injury of right internal
carotid artery, intracranial
portion, not elsewhere
classified without loss of
consciousness   `HCC`

7 √7th **S06.811** Injury of right internal
carotid artery, intracranial
portion, not elsewhere
classified with loss of
consciousness of 30
minutes or less   `CC` `H5` `HCC`

7 √7th **S06.812** Injury of right internal
carotid artery, intracranial
portion, not elsewhere
classified with loss of
consciousness of 31
minutes to 59 minutes   `CC` `H5` `HCC`

7 √7th **S06.813** Injury of right internal
carotid artery, intracranial
portion, not elsewhere
classified with loss of
consciousness of 1 hour to
5 hours 59 minutes   `CC` `H5` `HCC`

7 √7th **S06.814** Injury of right internal
carotid artery, intracranial
portion, not elsewhere
classified with loss of
consciousness of 6 hours
to 24 hours   `CC` `H5` `HCC`

7 √7th **S06.815** Injury of right internal
carotid artery, intracranial
portion, not elsewhere
classified with loss of
consciousness greater
than 24 hours with return
to pre-existing conscious
level   `CC` `H5` `HCC`

7 √7th **S06.816** Injury of right internal
carotid artery, intracranial
portion, not elsewhere
classified with loss of
consciousness greater
than 24 hours without
return to pre-existing
conscious level with
patient surviving   `MCC` `H5` `HCC`

√7th **S06.817** Injury of right internal
carotid artery, intracranial
portion, not elsewhere
classified with loss of
consciousness of any
duration with death due
to brain injury prior to
regaining consciousness   `MCC` `H5`

√7th **S06.818** Injury of right internal
carotid artery, intracranial
portion, not elsewhere
classified with loss of
consciousness of any
duration with death due
to other cause prior to
regaining consciousness   `MCC` `H5`

7 √7th **S06.819** Injury of right internal
carotid artery, intracranial
portion, not elsewhere
classified with loss of
consciousness of
unspecified duration   `CC` `H5` `HCC`
Injury of right internal carotid artery,
intracranial portion, not elsewhere
classified NOS

√6th **S06.82** Injury of left internal carotid artery, intracranial
portion, not elsewhere classified

7 √7th **S06.820** Injury of left internal
carotid artery, intracranial
portion, not elsewhere
classified without loss of
consciousness   `HCC`

7 √7th **S06.821** Injury of left internal
carotid artery, intracranial
portion, not elsewhere
classified with loss of
consciousness of 30
minutes or less   `CC` `H5` `HCC`

7 √7th **S06.822** Injury of left internal
carotid artery, intracranial
portion, not elsewhere
classified with loss of
consciousness of 31
minutes to 59 minutes   `CC` `H5` `HCC`

7 √7th **S06.823** Injury of left internal
carotid artery, intracranial
portion, not elsewhere
classified with loss of
consciousness of 1 hour to
5 hours 59 minutes   `CC` `H5` `HCC`

7 √7th **S06.824** Injury of left internal
carotid artery, intracranial
portion, not elsewhere
classified with loss of
consciousness of 6 hours
to 24 hours   `CC` `H5` `HCC`

7 √7th **S06.825** Injury of left internal
carotid artery, intracranial
portion, not elsewhere
classified with loss of
consciousness greater
than 24 hours with return
to pre-existing conscious
level   `CC` `H5` `HCC`

7 √7ᵗʰ **S06.826 Injury of left internal carotid artery, intracranial portion, not elsewhere classified with loss of consciousness** greater than 24 hours without return to pre-existing conscious level with patient surviving   `MCC` `H5` `HCC`

√7ᵗʰ **S06.827 Injury of left internal carotid artery, intracranial portion, not elsewhere classified with loss of consciousness of** any duration with death due to brain injury prior to regaining consciousness   `MCC` `H5`

√7ᵗʰ **S06.828 Injury of left internal carotid artery, intracranial portion, not elsewhere classified with loss of consciousness of** any duration with death due to **other** cause prior to regaining consciousness   `MCC` `H5`

7 √7ᵗʰ **S06.829 Injury of left internal carotid artery, intracranial portion, not elsewhere classified with loss of consciousness of unspecified duration**   `CC` `H5` `HCC`

     Injury of left internal carotid artery, intracranial portion, not elsewhere classified NOS

√6ᵗʰ **S06.89 Other specified intracranial injury**

     EXCLUDES 1   concussion (S06.0X-)

7 √7ᵗʰ **S06.890 Other specified intracranial injury** without loss of consciousness   `HCC`

7 √7ᵗʰ **S06.891 Other specified intracranial injury with loss of consciousness of** 30 minutes or less   `CC` `H5` `HCC`

7 √7ᵗʰ **S06.892 Other specified intracranial injury with loss of consciousness of** 31 minutes to 59 minutes   `CC` `H5` `HCC`

7 √7ᵗʰ **S06.893 Other specified intracranial injury with loss of consciousness of** 1 hour to 5 hours 59 minutes   `CC` `H5` `HCC`

7 √7ᵗʰ **S06.894 Other specified intracranial injury with loss of consciousness of** 6 hours to 24 hours   `CC` `H5` `HCC`

7 √7ᵗʰ **S06.895 Other specified intracranial injury with loss of consciousness** greater than 24 hours with return to pre-existing conscious level   `CC` `H5` `HCC`

7 √7ᵗʰ **S06.896 Other specified intracranial injury with loss of consciousness** greater than 24 hours without return to pre-existing conscious level with patient surviving   `MCC` `H5` `HCC`

√7ᵗʰ **S06.897 Other specified intracranial injury with loss of consciousness of** any duration with death due to brain injury prior to regaining consciousness   `MCC` `H5`

√7ᵗʰ **S06.898 Other specified intracranial injury with loss of consciousness of** any duration with death due to **other** cause prior to regaining consciousness   `MCC` `H5`

7 √7ᵗʰ **S06.899 Other specified intracranial injury with loss of consciousness of unspecified duration**   `CC` `H5` `HCC`

√5ᵗʰ **S06.9 Unspecified intracranial injury**

     Brain injury NOS

     Head injury NOS with loss of consciousness

     Traumatic brain injury NOS

     EXCLUDES 1   conditions classifiable to S06.0- to S06.8- code to specified intracranial injury

               head injury NOS (S09.90)

√6ᵗʰ **S06.9X Unspecified intracranial injury**

7 √7ᵗʰ **S06.9X0 Unspecified intracranial injury** without loss of consciousness   `HCC`

7 √7ᵗʰ **S06.9X1 Unspecified intracranial injury with loss of consciousness of** 30 minutes or less   `CC` `H5` `HCC`

7 √7ᵗʰ **S06.9X2 Unspecified intracranial injury with loss of consciousness of** 31 minutes to 59 minutes   `CC` `H5` `HCC`

7 √7ᵗʰ **S06.9X3 Unspecified intracranial injury with loss of consciousness of** 1 hour to 5 hours 59 minutes   `CC` `H5` `HCC`

7 √7ᵗʰ **S06.9X4 Unspecified intracranial injury with loss of consciousness of** 6 hours to 24 hours   `CC` `H5` `HCC`

7 √7ᵗʰ **S06.9X5 Unspecified intracranial injury with loss of consciousness** greater than 24 hours with return to pre-existing conscious level   `CC` `H5` `HCC`

7 √7ᵗʰ **S06.9X6 Unspecified intracranial injury with loss of consciousness** greater than 24 hours without return to pre-existing conscious level with patient surviving   `MCC` `H5` `HCC`

√7ᵗʰ **S06.9X7 Unspecified intracranial injury with loss of consciousness of** any duration with death due to brain injury prior to regaining consciousness   `MCC` `H5`

√7ᵗʰ **S06.9X8 Unspecified intracranial injury with loss of consciousness of** any duration with death due to **other** cause prior to regaining consciousness   `MCC` `H5`

7 √7ᵗʰ **S06.9X9 Unspecified intracranial injury with loss of consciousness of unspecified duration**   `CC` `H5` `HCC`

√4ᵗʰ **S07 Crushing injury of head**

     Use additional code for all associated injuries, such as:

        intracranial injuries (S06.-)

        skull fractures (S02.-)

> The appropriate 7th character is to be added to each code from category S07.
> A   initial encounter
> D   subsequent encounter
> S   sequela

> **CC Excl: For CC codes in category S07:** PDX collection 1156

√ₓ7ᵗʰ **S07.0 Crushing injury of** face   `CC` `H5`

√ₓ7ᵗʰ **S07.1 Crushing injury of** skull   `CC` `H5`

√ₓ7ᵗʰ **S07.8 Crushing injury of other parts of head**   `CC` `H5`

√ₓ7ᵗʰ **S07.9 Crushing injury of head, part unspecified**   `CC` `H5`

√4ᵗʰ **S08 Avulsion and traumatic amputation of part of head**

     An amputation not identified as partial or complete should be coded to complete

> The appropriate 7th character is to be added to each code from category S08.
> A   initial encounter
> D   subsequent encounter
> S   sequela

√ₓ7ᵗʰ **S08.0 Avulsion of** scalp

N Newborn: 0   P Pediatric: 0-17   M Maternity: 9-64   A Adult: 15-124   `MCC` Major Complication/Comorbidity   `CC` Complication/Comorbidity   `SW` Severe Wound Dx

996   ICD-10-CM 2020

√5th **S08.1** **Traumatic amputation of** ear

    √6th **S08.11** **Complete** **traumatic amputation of ear**

       √7th **S08.111** **Complete traumatic amputation of** right **ear**

       √7th **S08.112** **Complete traumatic amputation of** left **ear**

       √7th **S08.119** **Complete traumatic amputation of unspecified ear**

    √6th **S08.12** **Partial** **traumatic amputation of ear**

       √7th **S08.121** **Partial traumatic amputation of** right **ear**

       √7th **S08.122** **Partial traumatic amputation of** left **ear**

       √7th **S08.129** **Partial traumatic amputation of unspecified ear**

√5th **S08.8** **Traumatic amputation of other parts of head**

    √6th **S08.81** **Traumatic amputation of** nose

       √7th **S08.811** **Complete** **traumatic amputation of nose**

       √7th **S08.812** **Partial** **traumatic amputation of nose**

    √x7th **S08.89** **Traumatic amputation of other parts of head**

√4th **S09** **Other and unspecified injuries of head**

> The appropriate 7th character is to be added to each code from category S09.
> A   initial encounter
> D   subsequent encounter
> S   sequela

CC Excl: For CC codes in category S09, unless otherwise noted: PDX collection 1158

    √x7th **S09.0** **Injury of** blood vessels **of head, not elsewhere classified**   CC

       EXCLUDES 1   injury of cerebral blood vessels (S06.-)

                   injury of precerebral blood vessels (S15.-)

       CC Excl: PDX collection 1157

    √5th **S09.1** **Injury of** muscle and tendon **of head**

       Code also any associated open wound (S01.-)

       EXCLUDES 2   sprain to joints and ligament of head (S03.9)

       √x7th **S09.10** **Unspecified injury of muscle and tendon of head**

          Injury of muscle and tendon of head NOS

       √x7th **S09.11** **Strain** **of muscle and tendon of head**

       √x7th **S09.12** **Laceration** **of muscle and tendon of head**

       √x7th **S09.19** **Other specified injury of muscle and tendon of head**

    √5th **S09.2** **Traumatic rupture of** ear drum

       EXCLUDES 1   traumatic rupture of ear drum due to blast injury (S09.31-)

       √x7th **S09.20** **Traumatic rupture of unspecified ear drum**   CC

       √x7th **S09.21** **Traumatic rupture of** right **ear drum**   CC

       √x7th **S09.22** **Traumatic rupture of** left **ear drum**   CC

    √5th **S09.3** **Other specified and unspecified injury of middle and inner ear**

       EXCLUDES 1   injury to ear NOS (S09.91-)

       EXCLUDES 2   injury to external ear (S00.4-, S01.3-, S08.1-)

       √6th **S09.30** **Unspecified injury of** middle and inner ear

          √7th **S09.301** **Unspecified injury of** right **middle and inner ear**   CC

          √7th **S09.302** **Unspecified injury of** left **middle and inner ear**   CC

          √7th **S09.309** **Unspecified injury of unspecified middle and inner ear**   CC

       √6th **S09.31** **Primary** blast injury **of ear**

          Blast injury of ear NOS

          √7th **S09.311** **Primary blast injury of** right **ear**   CC

          √7th **S09.312** **Primary blast injury of** left **ear**   CC

          √7th **S09.313** **Primary blast injury of ear, bilateral**   CC

          √7th **S09.319** **Primary blast injury of unspecified ear**   CC

       √6th **S09.39** **Other specified injury of middle and inner ear**

          Secondary blast injury to ear

          √7th **S09.391** **Other specified injury of** right **middle and inner ear**   CC

          √7th **S09.392** **Other specified injury of** left **middle and inner ear**   CC

          √7th **S09.399** **Other specified injury of unspecified middle and inner ear**   CC

    √x7th **S09.8** **Other specified injuries of head**

    √5th **S09.9** **Unspecified injury of face and head**

       √x7th **S09.90** **Unspecified injury of** head

          Head injury NOS

          EXCLUDES 1   brain injury NOS (S06.9-)

                   head injury NOS with loss of consciousness (S06.9-)

                   intracranial injury NOS (S06.9-)

       √x7th **S09.91** **Unspecified injury of** ear

          Injury of ear NOS

       √x7th **S09.92** **Unspecified injury of** nose

          Injury of nose NOS

       √x7th **S09.93** **Unspecified injury of** face

          Injury of face NOS

          AHA: 2019,2Q,23

Injuries to the neck (S10-S19)

INCLUDES   injuries of nape

             injuries of supraclavicular region

             injuries of throat

EXCLUDES 2   burns and corrosions (T20-T32)

             effects of foreign body in esophagus (T18.1)

             effects of foreign body in larynx (T17.3)

             effects of foreign body in pharynx (T17.2)

             effects of foreign body in trachea (T17.4)

             frostbite (T33-T34)

             insect bite or sting, venomous (T63.4)

√4th **S10** **Superficial injury of neck**

> The appropriate 7th character is to be added to each code from category S10.
> A   initial encounter
> D   subsequent encounter
> S   sequela

    √x7th **S10.0** **Contusion of throat**

       Contusion of cervical esophagus

       Contusion of larynx

       Contusion of pharynx

       Contusion of trachea

    √5th **S10.1** **Other and unspecified superficial injuries of throat**

       √x7th **S10.10** **Unspecified superficial injuries of throat**

       √x7th **S10.11** **Abrasion of throat**

       √x7th **S10.12** **Blister (nonthermal) of throat**

       √x7th **S10.14** **External constriction of part of throat**

       √x7th **S10.15** **Superficial** foreign body **of throat**

          Splinter in the throat

       √x7th **S10.16** **Insect bite (nonvenomous) of throat**

       √x7th **S10.17** **Other superficial** bite **of throat**

          EXCLUDES 1   open bite of throat (S11.85)

    √5th **S10.8** **Superficial injury of other specified parts of neck**

       √x7th **S10.80** **Unspecified superficial injury of other specified part of neck**

       √x7th **S10.81** **Abrasion of other specified part of neck**

       √x7th **S10.82** **Blister (nonthermal) of other specified part of neck**

       √x7th **S10.83** **Contusion of other specified part of neck**

       √x7th **S10.84** **External constriction of other specified part of neck**

       √x7th **S10.85** **Superficial** foreign body **of other specified part of neck**

          Splinter in other specified part of neck

       √x7th **S10.86** **Insect bite of other specified part of neck**

       √x7th **S10.87** **Other superficial** bite **of other specified part of neck**

          EXCLUDES 1   open bite of other specified parts of neck (S11.85)

    √5th **S10.9** **Superficial injury of unspecified part of neck**

       √x7th **S10.90** **Unspecified superficial injury of unspecified part of neck**

       √x7th **S10.91** **Abrasion of unspecified part of neck**

       √x7th **S10.92** **Blister (nonthermal) of unspecified part of neck**

       √x7th **S10.93** **Contusion of unspecified part of neck**

       √x7th **S10.94** **External constriction of unspecified part of neck**

✓x7ᵗʰ **S10.95** Superficial foreign body of unspecified part of neck

✓x7ᵗʰ **S10.96** Insect bite of unspecified part of neck

✓x7ᵗʰ **S10.97** Other superficial bite of unspecified part of neck

✓4ᵗʰ **S11 Open wound of neck**

Code also any associated:
spinal cord injury (S14.0, S14.1-)
wound infection

EXCLUDES 2   *open fracture of vertebra (S12.- with 7th character B)*

The appropriate 7th character is to be added to each code from category S11.
A   initial encounter
D   subsequent encounter
S   sequela

✓5ᵗʰ **S11.0 Open wound of larynx and trachea**

CC Excl: For MCC codes in subcategory S11.0: PDX collection 1159

✓6ᵗʰ **S11.01 Open wound of larynx**

EXCLUDES 2   *open wound of vocal cord (S11.03)*

✓7ᵗʰ **S11.011 Laceration without foreign body of larynx**   MCC

✓7ᵗʰ **S11.012 Laceration with foreign body of larynx**   MCC

✓7ᵗʰ **S11.013 Puncture wound without foreign body of larynx**   MCC

✓7ᵗʰ **S11.014 Puncture wound with foreign body of larynx**   MCC

✓7ᵗʰ **S11.015 Open bite of larynx**   MCC

Bite of larynx NOS

✓7ᵗʰ **S11.019 Unspecified open wound of larynx**   MCC

✓6ᵗʰ **S11.02 Open wound of trachea**

Open wound of cervical trachea
Open wound of trachea NOS

EXCLUDES 2   *open wound of thoracic trachea (S27.5-)*

✓7ᵗʰ **S11.021 Laceration without foreign body of trachea**   MCC

✓7ᵗʰ **S11.022 Laceration with foreign body of trachea**   MCC

✓7ᵗʰ **S11.023 Puncture wound without foreign body of trachea**   MCC

✓7ᵗʰ **S11.024 Puncture wound with foreign body of trachea**   MCC

✓7ᵗʰ **S11.025 Open bite of trachea**   MCC

Bite of trachea NOS

✓7ᵗʰ **S11.029 Unspecified open wound of trachea**   MCC

✓6ᵗʰ **S11.03 Open wound of vocal cord**

✓7ᵗʰ **S11.031 Laceration without foreign body of vocal cord**   MCC

✓7ᵗʰ **S11.032 Laceration with foreign body of vocal cord**   MCC

✓7ᵗʰ **S11.033 Puncture wound without foreign body of vocal cord**   MCC

✓7ᵗʰ **S11.034 Puncture wound with foreign body of vocal cord**   MCC

✓7ᵗʰ **S11.035 Open bite of vocal cord**   MCC

Bite of vocal cord NOS

✓7ᵗʰ **S11.039 Unspecified open wound of vocal cord**   MCC

✓5ᵗʰ **S11.1 Open wound of thyroid gland**

CC Excl: For CC codes in subcategory S11.1, unless otherwise noted: PDX collection 1160

✓x7ᵗʰ **S11.10 Unspecified open wound of thyroid gland**   CC

✓x7ᵗʰ **S11.11 Laceration without foreign body of thyroid gland**   CC

✓x7ᵗʰ **S11.12 Laceration with foreign body of thyroid gland**   CC

CC Excl: PDX collection 1161

✓x7ᵗʰ **S11.13 Puncture wound without foreign body of thyroid gland**   CC

✓x7ᵗʰ **S11.14 Puncture wound with foreign body of thyroid gland**   CC

CC Excl: PDX collection 1161

✓x7ᵗʰ **S11.15 Open bite of thyroid gland**   CC

Bite of thyroid gland NOS

✓5ᵗʰ **S11.2 Open wound of pharynx and cervical esophagus**

EXCLUDES 1   *open wound of esophagus NOS (S27.8-)*

CC Excl: For CC codes in subcategory S11.2, unless otherwise noted: PDX collection 1162

✓7ᵗʰ **S11.20 Unspecified open wound of pharynx and cervical esophagus**   CC

✓7ᵗʰ **S11.21 Laceration without foreign body of pharynx and cervical esophagus**   CC

✓7ᵗʰ **S11.22 Laceration with foreign body of pharynx and cervical esophagus**   CC

CC Excl: PDX collection 1163

✓7ᵗʰ **S11.23 Puncture wound without foreign body of pharynx and cervical esophagus**   CC

✓7ᵗʰ **S11.24 Puncture wound with foreign body of pharynx and cervical esophagus**   CC

CC Excl: PDX collection 1163

✓7ᵗʰ **S11.25 Open bite of pharynx and cervical esophagus**   CC

Bite of pharynx and cervical esophagus NOS

✓5ᵗʰ **S11.8 Open wound of other specified parts of neck**

✓x7ᵗʰ **S11.80 Unspecified open wound of other specified part of neck**

✓x7ᵗʰ **S11.81 Laceration without foreign body of other specified part of neck**

✓x7ᵗʰ **S11.82 Laceration with foreign body of other specified part of neck**

✓x7ᵗʰ **S11.83 Puncture wound without foreign body of other specified part of neck**

✓x7ᵗʰ **S11.84 Puncture wound with foreign body of other specified part of neck**

✓x7ᵗʰ **S11.85 Open bite of other specified part of neck**

Bite of other specified part of neck NOS

EXCLUDES 1   *superficial bite of other specified part of neck (S10.87)*

✓x7ᵗʰ **S11.89 Other open wound of other specified part of neck**

✓5ᵗʰ **S11.9 Open wound of unspecified part of neck**

✓x7ᵗʰ **S11.90 Unspecified open wound of unspecified part of neck**

✓x7ᵗʰ **S11.91 Laceration without foreign body of unspecified part of neck**

✓x7ᵗʰ **S11.92 Laceration with foreign body of unspecified part of neck**

✓x7ᵗʰ **S11.93 Puncture wound without foreign body of unspecified part of neck**

✓x7ᵗʰ **S11.94 Puncture wound with foreign body of unspecified part of neck**

✓x7ᵗʰ **S11.95 Open bite of unspecified part of neck**

Bite of neck NOS

EXCLUDES 1   *superficial bite of neck (S10.97)*

Ⓝ Newborn: 0   Ⓟ Pediatric: 0-17   Ⓜ Maternity: 9-64   Ⓐ Adult: 15-124   **MCC** Major Complication/Comorbidity   **CC** Complication/Comorbidity   **SW** Severe Wound Dx

998   ICD-10-CM 2020

✓4ᵗʰ **S12 Fracture of cervical vertebra and other parts of neck**

NOTE A fracture not indicated as displaced or nondisplaced should be coded to displaced.

A fracture not indicated as open or closed should be coded to closed.

INCLUDES fracture of cervical neural arch
fracture of cervical spine
fracture of cervical spinous process
fracture of cervical transverse process
fracture of cervical vertebral arch
fracture of neck

Code first any associated cervical spinal cord injury (S14.0, S14.1-)
AHA: 2018,2Q,12; 2015,3Q,37-39

The appropriate 7th character is to be added to all codes from subcategories S12.0-S12.6.
A   initial encounter for closed fracture
B   initial encounter for open fracture
D   subsequent encounter for fracture with routine healing
G   subsequent encounter for fracture with delayed healing
K   subsequent encounter for fracture with nonunion
S   sequela

CC Excl: For codes in category S12, unless otherwise noted:
CC with 7th character A or MCC with 7th character B: PDX collection 1164
CC with 7th character K: PDX collection 897

✓5ᵗʰ **S12.0 Fracture of first cervical vertebra**
Atlas

✓6ᵗʰ **S12.00 Unspecified fracture of first cervical vertebra**

2,3,6 ✓7ᵗʰ **S12.000 Unspecified displaced fracture of first cervical vertebra** MCC CC H5 HCC

2,3,6 ✓7ᵗʰ **S12.001 Unspecified nondisplaced fracture of first cervical vertebra** MCC CC H5 HCC

2,3,6 ✓x7ᵗʰ **S12.01 Stable burst fracture of first cervical vertebra** MCC CC H5 HCC

2,3,6 ✓x7ᵗʰ **S12.02 Unstable burst fracture of first cervical vertebra** MCC CC H5 HCC

✓6ᵗʰ **S12.03 Posterior arch fracture of first cervical vertebra**

2,3,6 ✓7ᵗʰ **S12.030 Displaced posterior arch fracture of first cervical vertebra** MCC CC H5 HCC

2,3,6 ✓7ᵗʰ **S12.031 Nondisplaced posterior arch fracture of first cervical vertebra** MCC CC H5 HCC

✓6ᵗʰ **S12.04 Lateral mass fracture of first cervical vertebra**

2,3,6 ✓7ᵗʰ **S12.040 Displaced lateral mass fracture of first cervical vertebra** MCC CC H5 HCC

2,3,6 ✓7ᵗʰ **S12.041 Nondisplaced lateral mass fracture of first cervical vertebra** MCC CC H5 HCC

✓6ᵗʰ **S12.09 Other fracture of first cervical vertebra**

2,3,6 ✓7ᵗʰ **S12.090 Other displaced fracture of first cervical vertebra** MCC CC H5 HCC

2,3,6 ✓7ᵗʰ **S12.091 Other nondisplaced fracture of first cervical vertebra** MCC CC H5 HCC

✓5ᵗʰ **S12.1 Fracture of second cervical vertebra**
Axis

✓6ᵗʰ **S12.10 Unspecified fracture of second cervical vertebra**

2,3,6 ✓7ᵗʰ **S12.100 Unspecified displaced fracture of second cervical vertebra** MCC CC H5 HCC

2,3,6 ✓7ᵗʰ **S12.101 Unspecified nondisplaced fracture of second cervical vertebra** MCC CC H5 HCC

✓6ᵗʰ **S12.11 Type II dens fracture**

2,3,6 ✓7ᵗʰ **S12.110 Anterior displaced Type II dens fracture** MCC CC H5 HCC

2,3,6 ✓7ᵗʰ **S12.111 Posterior displaced Type II dens fracture** MCC CC H5 HCC

2,3,6 ✓7ᵗʰ **S12.112 Nondisplaced Type II dens fracture** MCC CC H5 HCC

✓6ᵗʰ **S12.12 Other dens fracture**

2,3,6 ✓7ᵗʰ **S12.120 Other displaced dens fracture** MCC CC H5 HCC

2,3,6 ✓7ᵗʰ **S12.121 Other nondisplaced dens fracture** MCC CC H5 HCC

✓6ᵗʰ **S12.13 Unspecified traumatic spondylolisthesis of second cervical vertebra**

2,3,6 ✓7ᵗʰ **S12.130 Unspecified traumatic displaced spondylolisthesis of second cervical vertebra** MCC CC H5 HCC

2,3,6 ✓7ᵗʰ **S12.131 Unspecified traumatic nondisplaced spondylolisthesis of second cervical vertebra** MCC CC H5 HCC

2,3,6 ✓x7ᵗʰ **S12.14 Type III traumatic spondylolisthesis of second cervical vertebra** MCC CC H5 HCC

✓6ᵗʰ **S12.15 Other traumatic spondylolisthesis of second cervical vertebra**

2,3,6 ✓7ᵗʰ **S12.150 Other traumatic displaced spondylolisthesis of second cervical vertebra** MCC CC H5 HCC

2,3,6 ✓7ᵗʰ **S12.151 Other traumatic nondisplaced spondylolisthesis of second cervical vertebra** MCC CC H5 HCC

✓6ᵗʰ **S12.19 Other fracture of second cervical vertebra**

2,3,6 ✓7ᵗʰ **S12.190 Other displaced fracture of second cervical vertebra** MCC CC H5 HCC

2,3,6 ✓7ᵗʰ **S12.191 Other nondisplaced fracture of second cervical vertebra** MCC CC H5 HCC

✓5ᵗʰ **S12.2 Fracture of third cervical vertebra**

✓6ᵗʰ **S12.20 Unspecified fracture of third cervical vertebra**

2,3,6 ✓7ᵗʰ **S12.200 Unspecified displaced fracture of third cervical vertebra** MCC CC H5 HCC

2,3,6 ✓7ᵗʰ **S12.201 Unspecified nondisplaced fracture of third cervical vertebra** MCC CC H5 HCC

✓6ᵗʰ **S12.23 Unspecified traumatic spondylolisthesis of third cervical vertebra**

2,3,6 ✓7ᵗʰ **S12.230 Unspecified traumatic displaced spondylolisthesis of third cervical vertebra** MCC CC H5 HCC

2,3,6 ✓7ᵗʰ **S12.231 Unspecified traumatic nondisplaced spondylolisthesis of third cervical vertebra** MCC CC H5 HCC

2,3,6 ✓x7ᵗʰ **S12.24 Type III traumatic spondylolisthesis of third cervical vertebra** MCC CC H5 HCC

✓6ᵗʰ **S12.25 Other traumatic spondylolisthesis of third cervical vertebra**

2,3,6 ✓7ᵗʰ **S12.250 Other traumatic displaced spondylolisthesis of third cervical vertebra** MCC CC H5 HCC

2,3,6 ✓7ᵗʰ **S12.251 Other traumatic nondisplaced spondylolisthesis of third cervical vertebra** MCC CC H5 HCC

✓6ᵗʰ **S12.29 Other fracture of third cervical vertebra**

2,3,6 ✓7ᵗʰ **S12.290 Other displaced fracture of third cervical vertebra** MCC CC H5 HCC

2,3,6 ✓7ᵗʰ **S12.291 Other nondisplaced fracture of third cervical vertebra** MCC CC H5 HCC

✓5ᵗʰ **S12.3 Fracture of fourth cervical vertebra**

✓6ᵗʰ **S12.30 Unspecified fracture of fourth cervical vertebra**

2,3,6 ✓7ᵗʰ **S12.300 Unspecified displaced fracture of fourth cervical vertebra** MCC CC H5 HCC

2,3,6 ✓7ᵗʰ **S12.301 Unspecified nondisplaced fracture of fourth cervical vertebra** MCC CC H5 HCC

✓6ᵗʰ **S12.33 Unspecified traumatic spondylolisthesis of fourth cervical vertebra**

2,3,6 ✓7ᵗʰ **S12.330 Unspecified traumatic displaced spondylolisthesis of fourth cervical vertebra** MCC CC H5 HCC

2,3,6 ✓7ᵗʰ **S12.331 Unspecified traumatic nondisplaced spondylolisthesis of fourth cervical vertebra** MCC CC H5 HCC

✓ Additional Character Required   ✓x7ᵗʰ Placeholder   Unacceptable PDx   Questionable PDx   Manifestation   Unspecified Dx   H1-H14 HAC   HCC CMS-HCC Dx   HIV HIV Dx

Chapter 19. Injury, Poisoning and Certain Other Consequences of External Causes

2,3,6 √x7th **S12.34** Type III traumatic spondylolisthesis MCC CC H5 HCC of fourth cervical vertebra

√6th **S12.35** Other traumatic spondylolisthesis of fourth cervical vertebra

  2,3,6 √7th **S12.350** Other traumatic displaced MCC CC H5 HCC spondylolisthesis of fourth cervical vertebra

  2,3,6 √7th **S12.351** Other traumatic MCC CC H5 HCC nondisplaced spondylolisthesis of fourth cervical vertebra

√6th **S12.39** Other fracture of fourth cervical vertebra

  2,3,6 √7th **S12.390** Other displaced fracture MCC CC H5 HCC of fourth cervical vertebra

  2,3,6 √7th **S12.391** Other nondisplaced MCC CC H5 HCC fracture of fourth cervical vertebra

√5th **S12.4** Fracture of fifth cervical vertebra

√6th **S12.40** Unspecified fracture of fifth cervical vertebra

  2,3,6 √7th **S12.400** Unspecified displaced MCC CC H5 HCC fracture of fifth cervical vertebra

  2,3,6 √7th **S12.401** Unspecified nondisplaced MCC CC H5 HCC fracture of fifth cervical vertebra

√6th **S12.43** Unspecified traumatic spondylolisthesis of fifth cervical vertebra

  2,3,6 √7th **S12.430** Unspecified traumatic MCC CC H5 HCC displaced spondylolisthesis of fifth cervical vertebra

  2,3,6 √7th **S12.431** Unspecified traumatic MCC CC H5 HCC nondisplaced spondylolisthesis of fifth cervical vertebra

2,3,6 √x7th **S12.44** Type III traumatic spondylolisthesis MCC CC H5 HCC of fifth cervical vertebra

√6th **S12.45** Other traumatic spondylolisthesis of fifth cervical vertebra

  2,3,6 √7th **S12.450** Other traumatic displaced MCC CC H5 HCC spondylolisthesis of fifth cervical vertebra

  2,3,6 √7th **S12.451** Other traumatic MCC CC H5 HCC nondisplaced spondylolisthesis of fifth cervical vertebra

√6th **S12.49** Other fracture of fifth cervical vertebra

  2,3,6 √7th **S12.490** Other displaced fracture MCC CC H5 HCC of fifth cervical vertebra

  2,3,6 √7th **S12.491** Other nondisplaced MCC CC H5 HCC fracture of fifth cervical vertebra

√5th **S12.5** Fracture of sixth cervical vertebra

√6th **S12.50** Unspecified fracture of sixth cervical vertebra

  2,3,6 √7th **S12.500** Unspecified displaced MCC CC H5 HCC fracture of sixth cervical vertebra

  2,3,6 √7th **S12.501** Unspecified nondisplaced MCC CC H5 HCC fracture of sixth cervical vertebra

√6th **S12.53** Unspecified traumatic spondylolisthesis of sixth cervical vertebra

  2,3,6 √7th **S12.530** Unspecified traumatic MCC CC H5 HCC displaced spondylolisthesis of sixth cervical vertebra

  2,3,6 √7th **S12.531** Unspecified traumatic MCC CC H5 HCC nondisplaced spondylolisthesis of sixth cervical vertebra

2,3,6 √x7th **S12.54** Type III traumatic spondylolisthesis MCC CC H5 HCC of sixth cervical vertebra

√6th **S12.55** Other traumatic spondylolisthesis of sixth cervical vertebra

  2,3,6 √7th **S12.550** Other traumatic displaced MCC CC H5 HCC spondylolisthesis of sixth cervical vertebra

  2,3,6 √7th **S12.551** Other traumatic MCC CC H5 HCC nondisplaced spondylolisthesis of sixth cervical vertebra

√6th **S12.59** Other fracture of sixth cervical vertebra

  2,3,6 √7th **S12.590** Other displaced fracture MCC CC H5 HCC of sixth cervical vertebra

  2,3,6 √7th **S12.591** Other nondisplaced MCC CC H5 HCC fracture of sixth cervical vertebra

√5th **S12.6** Fracture of seventh cervical vertebra

√6th **S12.60** Unspecified fracture of seventh cervical vertebra

  2,3,6 √7th **S12.600** Unspecified displaced MCC CC H5 HCC fracture of seventh cervical vertebra

  2,3,6 √7th **S12.601** Unspecified nondisplaced MCC CC H5 HCC fracture of seventh cervical vertebra

√6th **S12.63** Unspecified traumatic spondylolisthesis of seventh cervical vertebra

  2,3,6 √7th **S12.630** Unspecified traumatic MCC CC H5 HCC displaced spondylolisthesis of seventh cervical vertebra

  2,3,6 √7th **S12.631** Unspecified traumatic MCC CC H5 HCC nondisplaced spondylolisthesis of seventh cervical vertebra

2,3,6 √x7th **S12.64** Type III traumatic spondylolisthesis MCC CC H5 HCC of seventh cervical vertebra

√6th **S12.65** Other traumatic spondylolisthesis of seventh cervical vertebra

  2,3,6 √7th **S12.650** Other traumatic displaced MCC CC H5 HCC spondylolisthesis of seventh cervical vertebra

  2,3,6 √7th **S12.651** Other traumatic MCC CC H5 HCC nondisplaced spondylolisthesis of seventh cervical vertebra

√6th **S12.69** Other fracture of seventh cervical vertebra

  2,3,6 √7th **S12.690** Other displaced fracture MCC CC H5 HCC of seventh cervical vertebra

  2,3,6 √7th **S12.691** Other nondisplaced MCC CC H5 HCC fracture of seventh cervical vertebra

6 √x7th **S12.8** Fracture of other parts of neck MCC H5 HCC

Hyoid bone
Larynx
Thyroid cartilage
Trachea

> The appropriate 7th character is to be added to code S12.8.
> A initial encounter
> D subsequent encounter
> S sequela

CC Excl: PDX collection 1165

6 √x7th **S12.9** Fracture of neck, unspecified CC H5 HCC

Fracture of neck NOS
Fracture of cervical spine NOS
Fracture of cervical vertebra NOS

> The appropriate 7th character is to be added to code S12.9.
> A initial encounter
> D subsequent encounter
> S sequela

CC Excl: PDX collection 1164

N Newborn: 0   P Pediatric: 0-17   M Maternity: 9-64   A Adult: 15-124   MCC Major Complication/Comorbidity   CC Complication/Comorbidity   SW Severe Wound Dx

1000   ICD-10-CM 2020

✓4ᵗʰ **S13 Dislocation and sprain of joints and ligaments at neck level**

INCLUDES avulsion of joint or ligament at neck level
laceration of cartilage, joint or ligament at neck level
sprain of cartilage, joint or ligament at neck level
traumatic hemarthrosis of joint or ligament at neck level
traumatic rupture of joint or ligament at neck level
traumatic subluxation of joint or ligament at neck level
traumatic tear of joint or ligament at neck level

Code also any associated open wound

EXCLUDES 2 *strain of muscle or tendon at neck level (S16.1)*

The appropriate 7th character is to be added to each code from category S13.
A   initial encounter
D   subsequent encounter
S   sequela

CC Excl: For CC codes in category S13: PDX collection 913

✓x7ᵗʰ **S13.0 Traumatic rupture of cervical intervertebral disc**   CC H5

EXCLUDES 1 *rupture or displacement (nontraumatic) of cervical intervertebral disc NOS (M50.-)*

✓5ᵗʰ **S13.1 Subluxation and dislocation of cervical vertebrae**

Code also any associated:
open wound of neck (S11.-)
spinal cord injury (S14.1-)

EXCLUDES 2 *fracture of cervical vertebrae (S12.0-S12.3-)*

✓6ᵗʰ **S13.10 Subluxation and dislocation of unspecified cervical vertebrae**

✓7ᵗʰ **S13.100 Subluxation of unspecified cervical vertebrae**   CC H5

✓7ᵗʰ **S13.101 Dislocation of unspecified cervical vertebrae**   CC H5

✓6ᵗʰ **S13.11 Subluxation and dislocation of C0/C1 cervical vertebrae**

Subluxation and dislocation of atlantooccipital joint
Subluxation and dislocation of atloidooccipital joint
Subluxation and dislocation of occipitoatloid joint

✓7ᵗʰ **S13.110 Subluxation of C0/C1 cervical vertebrae**   CC H5

✓7ᵗʰ **S13.111 Dislocation of C0/C1 cervical vertebrae**   CC H5

✓6ᵗʰ **S13.12 Subluxation and dislocation of C1/C2 cervical vertebrae**

Subluxation and dislocation of atlantoaxial joint

✓7ᵗʰ **S13.120 Subluxation of C1/C2 cervical vertebrae**   CC H5

✓7ᵗʰ **S13.121 Dislocation of C1/C2 cervical vertebrae**   CC H5

✓6ᵗʰ **S13.13 Subluxation and dislocation of C2/C3 cervical vertebrae**

✓7ᵗʰ **S13.130 Subluxation of C2/C3 cervical vertebrae**   CC H5

✓7ᵗʰ **S13.131 Dislocation of C2/C3 cervical vertebrae**   CC H5

✓6ᵗʰ **S13.14 Subluxation and dislocation of C3/C4 cervical vertebrae**

✓7ᵗʰ **S13.140 Subluxation of C3/C4 cervical vertebrae**   CC H5

✓7ᵗʰ **S13.141 Dislocation of C3/C4 cervical vertebrae**   CC H5

✓6ᵗʰ **S13.15 Subluxation and dislocation of C4/C5 cervical vertebrae**

✓7ᵗʰ **S13.150 Subluxation of C4/C5 cervical vertebrae**   CC H5

✓7ᵗʰ **S13.151 Dislocation of C4/C5 cervical vertebrae**   CC H5

✓6ᵗʰ **S13.16 Subluxation and dislocation of C5/C6 cervical vertebrae**

✓7ᵗʰ **S13.160 Subluxation of C5/C6 cervical vertebrae**   CC H5

✓7ᵗʰ **S13.161 Dislocation of C5/C6 cervical vertebrae**   CC H5

✓6ᵗʰ **S13.17 Subluxation and dislocation of C6/C7 cervical vertebrae**

✓7ᵗʰ **S13.170 Subluxation of C6/C7 cervical vertebrae**   CC H5

✓7ᵗʰ **S13.171 Dislocation of C6/C7 cervical vertebrae**   CC H5

✓6ᵗʰ **S13.18 Subluxation and dislocation of C7/T1 cervical vertebrae**

✓7ᵗʰ **S13.180 Subluxation of C7/T1 cervical vertebrae**   CC H5

✓7ᵗʰ **S13.181 Dislocation of C7/T1 cervical vertebrae**   CC H5

✓5ᵗʰ **S13.2 Dislocation of other and unspecified parts of neck**

✓x7ᵗʰ **S13.20 Dislocation of unspecified parts of neck**   CC H5

✓x7ᵗʰ **S13.29 Dislocation of other parts of neck**   CC H5

✓x7ᵗʰ **S13.4 Sprain of ligaments of cervical spine**

Sprain of anterior longitudinal (ligament), cervical
Sprain of atlanto-axial (joints)
Sprain of atlanto-occipital (joints)
Whiplash injury of cervical spine

✓x7ᵗʰ **S13.5 Sprain of thyroid region**

Sprain of cricoarytenoid (joint) (ligament)
Sprain of cricothyroid (joint) (ligament)
Sprain of thyroid cartilage

✓x7ᵗʰ **S13.8 Sprain of joints and ligaments of other parts of neck**

✓x7ᵗʰ **S13.9 Sprain of joints and ligaments of unspecified parts of neck**

✓4ᵗʰ **S14 Injury of nerves and spinal cord at neck level**

NOTE Code to highest level of cervical cord injury

Code also any associated:
fracture of cervical vertebra (S12.0- — S12.6.-)
open wound of neck (S11.-)
transient paralysis (R29.5)

The appropriate 7th character is to be added to each code from category S14.
A   initial encounter
D   subsequent encounter
S   sequela

CC Excl: For MCC codes in category S14: PDX collection 1166

✓x7ᵗʰ **S14.0 Concussion and edema of cervical spinal cord**   MCC HCC

✓5ᵗʰ **S14.1 Other and unspecified injuries of cervical spinal cord**

✓6ᵗʰ **S14.10 Unspecified injury of cervical spinal cord**

✓7ᵗʰ **S14.101 Unspecified injury at C1 level of cervical spinal cord**   MCC H5 HCC

✓7ᵗʰ **S14.102 Unspecified injury at C2 level of cervical spinal cord**   MCC H5 HCC

✓7ᵗʰ **S14.103 Unspecified injury at C3 level of cervical spinal cord**   MCC H5 HCC

✓7ᵗʰ **S14.104 Unspecified injury at C4 level of cervical spinal cord**   MCC H5 HCC

✓7ᵗʰ **S14.105 Unspecified injury at C5 level of cervical spinal cord**   MCC H5 HCC

✓7ᵗʰ **S14.106 Unspecified injury at C6 level of cervical spinal cord**   MCC H5 HCC

✓7ᵗʰ **S14.107 Unspecified injury at C7 level of cervical spinal cord**   MCC H5 HCC

✓7ᵗʰ **S14.108 Unspecified injury at C8 level of cervical spinal cord**   MCC HCC

✓7ᵗʰ **S14.109 Unspecified injury at unspecified level of cervical spinal cord**   HCC

Injury of cervical spinal cord NOS

✓6ᵗʰ **S14.11 Complete lesion of cervical spinal cord**

✓7ᵗʰ **S14.111 Complete lesion at C1 level of cervical spinal cord**   MCC H5 HCC

✓7ᵗʰ **S14.112 Complete lesion at C2 level of cervical spinal cord**   MCC H5 HCC

✓7ᵗʰ **S14.113 Complete lesion at C3 level of cervical spinal cord**   MCC H5 HCC

✓7ᵗʰ **S14.114 Complete lesion at C4 level of cervical spinal cord**   MCC H5 HCC

☑ Additional Character Required   ✓x7ᵗʰ Placeholder   Unacceptable PDx   Questionable PDx   Manifestation   Unspecified Dx   H1 -H14 HAC   HCC CMS-HCC Dx   HIV HIV Dx

ICD-10-CM 2020

1001

- ✓7ᵗʰ **S14.115** **Complete lesion at C5 level** of cervical spinal cord   `MCC` `H5` `HCC`
- ✓7ᵗʰ **S14.116** **Complete lesion at C6 level** of cervical spinal cord   `MCC` `H5` `HCC`
- ✓7ᵗʰ **S14.117** **Complete lesion at C7 level** of cervical spinal cord   `MCC` `H5` `HCC`
- ✓7ᵗʰ **S14.118** **Complete lesion at C8 level** of cervical spinal cord   `MCC` `HCC`
- ✓7ᵗʰ **S14.119** **Complete lesion at unspecified level of cervical spinal cord**   `HCC`
- ✓6ᵗʰ **S14.12** Central cord syndrome of cervical spinal cord
  - ✓7ᵗʰ **S14.121** **Central cord syndrome at C1 level** of cervical spinal cord   `MCC` `H5` `HCC`
  - ✓7ᵗʰ **S14.122** **Central cord syndrome at C2 level** of cervical spinal cord   `MCC` `H5` `HCC`
  - ✓7ᵗʰ **S14.123** **Central cord syndrome at C3 level** of cervical spinal cord   `MCC` `H5` `HCC`
  - ✓7ᵗʰ **S14.124** **Central cord syndrome at C4 level** of cervical spinal cord   `MCC` `H5` `HCC`
  - ✓7ᵗʰ **S14.125** **Central cord syndrome at C5 level** of cervical spinal cord   `MCC` `H5` `HCC`
  - ✓7ᵗʰ **S14.126** **Central cord syndrome at C6 level** of cervical spinal cord   `MCC` `H5` `HCC`
  - ✓7ᵗʰ **S14.127** **Central cord syndrome at C7 level** of cervical spinal cord   `MCC` `H5` `HCC`
  - ✓7ᵗʰ **S14.128** **Central cord syndrome at C8 level** of cervical spinal cord   `MCC` `HCC`
  - ✓7ᵗʰ **S14.129** **Central cord syndrome at unspecified level of cervical spinal cord**   `HCC`
- ✓6ᵗʰ **S14.13** Anterior cord syndrome of cervical spinal cord
  - ✓7ᵗʰ **S14.131** **Anterior cord syndrome at C1 level** of cervical spinal cord   `MCC` `H5` `HCC`
  - ✓7ᵗʰ **S14.132** **Anterior cord syndrome at C2 level** of cervical spinal cord   `MCC` `H5` `HCC`
  - ✓7ᵗʰ **S14.133** **Anterior cord syndrome at C3 level** of cervical spinal cord   `MCC` `H5` `HCC`
  - ✓7ᵗʰ **S14.134** **Anterior cord syndrome at C4 level** of cervical spinal cord   `MCC` `H5` `HCC`
  - ✓7ᵗʰ **S14.135** **Anterior cord syndrome at C5 level** of cervical spinal cord   `MCC` `H5` `HCC`
  - ✓7ᵗʰ **S14.136** **Anterior cord syndrome at C6 level** of cervical spinal cord   `MCC` `H5` `HCC`
  - ✓7ᵗʰ **S14.137** **Anterior cord syndrome at C7 level** of cervical spinal cord   `MCC` `H5` `HCC`
  - ✓7ᵗʰ **S14.138** **Anterior cord syndrome at C8 level** of cervical spinal cord   `MCC` `HCC`
  - ✓7ᵗʰ **S14.139** **Anterior cord syndrome at unspecified level of cervical spinal cord**   `HCC`
- ✓6ᵗʰ **S14.14** Brown-Séquard syndrome of cervical spinal cord
  - ✓7ᵗʰ **S14.141** **Brown-Séquard syndrome at C1 level** of cervical spinal cord   `MCC` `HCC`
  - ✓7ᵗʰ **S14.142** **Brown-Séquard syndrome at C2 level** of cervical spinal cord   `MCC` `HCC`
  - ✓7ᵗʰ **S14.143** **Brown-Séquard syndrome at C3 level** of cervical spinal cord   `MCC` `HCC`
  - ✓7ᵗʰ **S14.144** **Brown-Séquard syndrome at C4 level** of cervical spinal cord   `MCC` `HCC`

- ✓7ᵗʰ **S14.145** **Brown-Séquard syndrome at C5 level** of cervical spinal cord   `MCC` `HCC`
- ✓7ᵗʰ **S14.146** **Brown-Séquard syndrome at C6 level** of cervical spinal cord   `MCC` `HCC`
- ✓7ᵗʰ **S14.147** **Brown-Séquard syndrome at C7 level** of cervical spinal cord   `MCC` `HCC`
- ✓7ᵗʰ **S14.148** **Brown-Séquard syndrome at C8 level** of cervical spinal cord   `MCC` `HCC`
- ✓7ᵗʰ **S14.149** **Brown-Séquard syndrome at unspecified level of cervical spinal cord**   `HCC`
- ✓6ᵗʰ **S14.15** Other incomplete lesions of cervical spinal cord

  Incomplete lesion of cervical spinal cord NOS
  Posterior cord syndrome of cervical spinal cord
  - ✓7ᵗʰ **S14.151** **Other incomplete lesion at C1 level** of cervical spinal cord   `MCC` `H5` `HCC`
  - ✓7ᵗʰ **S14.152** **Other incomplete lesion at C2 level** of cervical spinal cord   `MCC` `H5` `HCC`
  - ✓7ᵗʰ **S14.153** **Other incomplete lesion at C3 level** of cervical spinal cord   `MCC` `H5` `HCC`
  - ✓7ᵗʰ **S14.154** **Other incomplete lesion at C4 level** of cervical spinal cord   `MCC` `H5` `HCC`
  - ✓7ᵗʰ **S14.155** **Other incomplete lesion at C5 level** of cervical spinal cord   `MCC` `H5` `HCC`
  - ✓7ᵗʰ **S14.156** **Other incomplete lesion at C6 level** of cervical spinal cord   `MCC` `H5` `HCC`
  - ✓7ᵗʰ **S14.157** **Other incomplete lesion at C7 level** of cervical spinal cord   `MCC` `H5` `HCC`
  - ✓7ᵗʰ **S14.158** **Other incomplete lesion at C8 level** of cervical spinal cord   `MCC` `HCC`
  - ✓7ᵗʰ **S14.159** **Other incomplete lesion at unspecified level of cervical spinal cord**   `HCC`
- ✓x7ᵗʰ **S14.2** Injury of nerve root of cervical spine
- ✓x7ᵗʰ **S14.3** Injury of brachial plexus
- ✓x7ᵗʰ **S14.4** Injury of peripheral nerves of neck
- ✓x7ᵗʰ **S14.5** Injury of cervical sympathetic nerves
- ✓x7ᵗʰ **S14.8** Injury of other specified nerves of neck
- ✓x7ᵗʰ **S14.9** Injury of unspecified nerves of neck

- ✓4ᵗʰ **S15** Injury of blood vessels at neck level

  Code also any associated open wound (S11.-)

  > The appropriate 7th character is to be added to each code from category S15.
  > A   initial encounter
  > D   subsequent encounter
  > S   sequela

  CC Excl: For CC codes in category S15, unless otherwise noted: PDX collection 1157

  - ✓5ᵗʰ **S15.0** Injury of carotid artery of neck

    Injury of carotid artery (common) (external) (internal, extracranial portion)
    Injury of carotid artery NOS
    > *EXCLUDES 1*   injury of internal carotid artery, intracranial portion (S06.8)

    CC Excl: For CC codes in subcategory S15.0: PDX collection 1167

    - ✓6ᵗʰ **S15.00** Unspecified injury of carotid artery
      - ✓7ᵗʰ **S15.001** **Unspecified injury of right carotid artery**   `CC`
      - ✓7ᵗʰ **S15.002** **Unspecified injury of left carotid artery**   `CC`
      - ✓7ᵗʰ **S15.009** **Unspecified injury of unspecified carotid artery**   `CC`

✓6ᵗʰ **S15.Ø1** Minor laceration of carotid artery

    Incomplete transection of carotid artery
    Laceration of carotid artery NOS
    Superficial laceration of carotid artery

    ✓7ᵗʰ **S15.Ø11** Minor laceration of right carotid artery   CC

    ✓7ᵗʰ **S15.Ø12** Minor laceration of left carotid artery   CC

    ✓7ᵗʰ **S15.Ø19** Minor laceration of unspecified carotid artery   CC

✓6ᵗʰ **S15.Ø2** Major laceration of carotid artery

    Complete transection of carotid artery
    Traumatic rupture of carotid artery

    ✓7ᵗʰ **S15.Ø21** Major laceration of right carotid artery   CC

    ✓7ᵗʰ **S15.Ø22** Major laceration of left carotid artery   CC

    ✓7ᵗʰ **S15.Ø29** Major laceration of unspecified carotid artery   CC

✓6ᵗʰ **S15.Ø9** Other specified injury of carotid artery

    ✓7ᵗʰ **S15.Ø91** Other specified injury of right carotid artery   CC

    ✓7ᵗʰ **S15.Ø92** Other specified injury of left carotid artery   CC

    ✓7ᵗʰ **S15.Ø99** Other specified injury of unspecified carotid artery   CC

✓5ᵗʰ **S15.1** Injury of vertebral artery

    ✓6ᵗʰ **S15.1Ø** Unspecified injury of vertebral artery

      ✓7ᵗʰ **S15.1Ø1** Unspecified injury of right vertebral artery   CC

      ✓7ᵗʰ **S15.1Ø2** Unspecified injury of left vertebral artery   CC

      ✓7ᵗʰ **S15.1Ø9** Unspecified injury of unspecified vertebral artery   CC

    ✓6ᵗʰ **S15.11** Minor laceration of vertebral artery

      Incomplete transection of vertebral artery
      Laceration of vertebral artery NOS
      Superficial laceration of vertebral artery

      ✓7ᵗʰ **S15.111** Minor laceration of right vertebral artery   CC

      ✓7ᵗʰ **S15.112** Minor laceration of left vertebral artery   CC

      ✓7ᵗʰ **S15.119** Minor laceration of unspecified vertebral artery   CC

    ✓6ᵗʰ **S15.12** Major laceration of vertebral artery

      Complete transection of vertebral artery
      Traumatic rupture of vertebral artery

      ✓7ᵗʰ **S15.121** Major laceration of right vertebral artery   CC

      ✓7ᵗʰ **S15.122** Major laceration of left vertebral artery   CC

      ✓7ᵗʰ **S15.129** Major laceration of unspecified vertebral artery   CC

    ✓6ᵗʰ **S15.19** Other specified injury of vertebral artery

      ✓7ᵗʰ **S15.191** Other specified injury of right vertebral artery   CC

      ✓7ᵗʰ **S15.192** Other specified injury of left vertebral artery   CC

      ✓7ᵗʰ **S15.199** Other specified injury of unspecified vertebral artery   CC

✓5ᵗʰ **S15.2** Injury of external jugular vein

    ✓6ᵗʰ **S15.2Ø** Unspecified injury of external jugular vein

      ✓7ᵗʰ **S15.2Ø1** Unspecified injury of right external jugular vein   CC

      ✓7ᵗʰ **S15.2Ø2** Unspecified injury of left external jugular vein   CC

      ✓7ᵗʰ **S15.2Ø9** Unspecified injury of unspecified external jugular vein   CC

    ✓6ᵗʰ **S15.21** Minor laceration of external jugular vein

      Incomplete transection of external jugular vein
      Laceration of external jugular vein NOS
      Superficial laceration of external jugular vein

      ✓7ᵗʰ **S15.211** Minor laceration of right external jugular vein   CC

      ✓7ᵗʰ **S15.212** Minor laceration of left external jugular vein   CC

      ✓7ᵗʰ **S15.219** Minor laceration of unspecified external jugular vein   CC

    ✓6ᵗʰ **S15.22** Major laceration of external jugular vein

      Complete transection of external jugular vein
      Traumatic rupture of external jugular vein

      ✓7ᵗʰ **S15.221** Major laceration of right external jugular vein   CC

      ✓7ᵗʰ **S15.222** Major laceration of left external jugular vein   CC

      ✓7ᵗʰ **S15.229** Major laceration of unspecified external jugular vein   CC

    ✓6ᵗʰ **S15.29** Other specified injury of external jugular vein

      ✓7ᵗʰ **S15.291** Other specified injury of right external jugular vein   CC

      ✓7ᵗʰ **S15.292** Other specified injury of left external jugular vein   CC

      ✓7ᵗʰ **S15.299** Other specified injury of unspecified external jugular vein   CC

✓5ᵗʰ **S15.3** Injury of internal jugular vein

    ✓6ᵗʰ **S15.3Ø** Unspecified injury of internal jugular vein

      ✓7ᵗʰ **S15.3Ø1** Unspecified injury of right internal jugular vein   CC

      ✓7ᵗʰ **S15.3Ø2** Unspecified injury of left internal jugular vein   CC

      ✓7ᵗʰ **S15.3Ø9** Unspecified injury of unspecified internal jugular vein   CC

    ✓6ᵗʰ **S15.31** Minor laceration of internal jugular vein

      Incomplete transection of internal jugular vein
      Laceration of internal jugular vein NOS
      Superficial laceration of internal jugular vein

      ✓7ᵗʰ **S15.311** Minor laceration of right internal jugular vein   CC

      ✓7ᵗʰ **S15.312** Minor laceration of left internal jugular vein   CC

      ✓7ᵗʰ **S15.319** Minor laceration of unspecified internal jugular vein   CC

    ✓6ᵗʰ **S15.32** Major laceration of internal jugular vein

      Complete transection of internal jugular vein
      Traumatic rupture of internal jugular vein

      ✓7ᵗʰ **S15.321** Major laceration of right internal jugular vein   CC

      ✓7ᵗʰ **S15.322** Major laceration of left internal jugular vein   CC

      ✓7ᵗʰ **S15.329** Major laceration of unspecified internal jugular vein   CC

    ✓6ᵗʰ **S15.39** Other specified injury of internal jugular vein

      ✓7ᵗʰ **S15.391** Other specified injury of right internal jugular vein   CC

      ✓7ᵗʰ **S15.392** Other specified injury of left internal jugular vein   CC

      ✓7ᵗʰ **S15.399** Other specified injury of unspecified internal jugular vein   CC

✓x7ᵗʰ **S15.8** Injury of other specified blood vessels at neck level   CC

✓x7ᵗʰ **S15.9** Injury of unspecified blood vessel at neck level   CC

✓4ᵗʰ **S16** Injury of muscle, fascia and tendon at neck level

    Code also any associated open wound (S11.-)

    EXCLUDES 2   sprain of joint or ligament at neck level (S13.9)

    The appropriate 7th character is to be added to each code from category S16.
    A   initial encounter
    D   subsequent encounter
    S   sequela

✓x7ᵗʰ **S16.1** Strain of muscle, fascia and tendon at neck level

✓x7ᵗʰ **S16.2** Laceration of muscle, fascia and tendon at neck level

✓x7ᵗʰ **S16.8** Other specified injury of muscle, fascia and tendon at neck level

✓x7ᵗʰ **S16.9** Unspecified injury of muscle, fascia and tendon at neck level

☑ Additional Character Required   ✓x7ᵗʰ Placeholder   Unacceptable PDx   Questionable PDx   Manifestation   Unspecified Dx   H1-H4 HAC   HCC CMS-HCC Dx   HIV HIV Dx

ICD-10-CM 2020

1003

S17 Crushing injury of neck

Use additional code for all associated injuries, such as:
injury of blood vessels (S15.-)
open wound of neck (S11.-)
spinal cord injury (S14.0, S14.1-)
vertebral fracture (S12.0- — S12.3-)

The appropriate 7th character is to be added to each code from category S17.
A   initial encounter
D   subsequent encounter
S   sequela

CC Excl: For CC codes in category S17: PDX collection 1156

√x7ᵗʰ	**S17.0** Crushing injury of larynx and trachea	CC H5
√x7ᵗʰ	**S17.8** Crushing injury of other specified parts of neck	CC H5
√x7ᵗʰ	**S17.9** Crushing injury of neck, part unspecified	CC H5

S19 Other specified and unspecified injuries of neck

The appropriate 7th character is to be added to each code from category S19.
A   initial encounter
D   subsequent encounter
S   sequela

S19.8 Other specified injuries of neck

√x7ᵗʰ   **S19.80** Other specified injuries of unspecified part of neck

√x7ᵗʰ   **S19.81** Other specified injuries of larynx

√x7ᵗʰ   **S19.82** Other specified injuries of cervical trachea

> *EXCLUDES 2*   other specified injury of thoracic trachea (S27.5-)

√x7ᵗʰ   **S19.83** Other specified injuries of vocal cord

√x7ᵗʰ   **S19.84** Other specified injuries of thyroid gland

√x7ᵗʰ   **S19.85** Other specified injuries of pharynx and cervical esophagus

√x7ᵗʰ   **S19.89** Other specified injuries of other specified part of neck

√x7ᵗʰ   **S19.9** Unspecified injury of neck

Injuries to the thorax (S20–S29)

INCLUDES	injuries of breast
	injuries of chest (wall)
	injuries of interscapular area
EXCLUDES 2	burns and corrosions (T20-T32)
	effects of foreign body in bronchus (T17.5)
	effects of foreign body in esophagus (T18.1)
	effects of foreign body in lung (T17.8)
	effects of foreign body in trachea (T17.4)
	frostbite (T33-T34)
	injuries of axilla
	injuries of clavicle
	injuries of scapular region
	injuries of shoulder
	insect bite or sting, venomous (T63.4)

S20 Superficial injury of thorax

The appropriate 7th character is to be added to each code from category S20.
A   initial encounter
D   subsequent encounter
S   sequela

S20.0 Contusion of breast

√x7ᵗʰ   **S20.00** Contusion of breast, unspecified breast

√x7ᵗʰ   **S20.01** Contusion of right breast

√x7ᵗʰ   **S20.02** Contusion of left breast

S20.1 Other and unspecified superficial injuries of breast

√6ᵗʰ   **S20.10** Unspecified superficial injuries of breast

√7ᵗʰ   **S20.101** Unspecified superficial injuries of breast, right breast

√7ᵗʰ   **S20.102** Unspecified superficial injuries of breast, left breast

√7ᵗʰ   **S20.109** Unspecified superficial injuries of breast, unspecified breast

√6ᵗʰ   **S20.11** Abrasion of breast

√7ᵗʰ   **S20.111** Abrasion of breast, right breast

√7ᵗʰ   **S20.112** Abrasion of breast, left breast

√7ᵗʰ   **S20.119** Abrasion of breast, unspecified breast

√6ᵗʰ   **S20.12** Blister (nonthermal) of breast

√7ᵗʰ   **S20.121** Blister (nonthermal) of breast, right breast

√7ᵗʰ   **S20.122** Blister (nonthermal) of breast, left breast

√7ᵗʰ   **S20.129** Blister (nonthermal) of breast, unspecified breast

√6ᵗʰ   **S20.14** External constriction of part of breast

√7ᵗʰ   **S20.141** External constriction of part of breast, right breast

√7ᵗʰ   **S20.142** External constriction of part of breast, left breast

√7ᵗʰ   **S20.149** External constriction of part of breast, unspecified breast

√6ᵗʰ   **S20.15** Superficial foreign body of breast

Splinter in the breast

√7ᵗʰ   **S20.151** Superficial foreign body of breast, right breast

√7ᵗʰ   **S20.152** Superficial foreign body of breast, left breast

√7ᵗʰ   **S20.159** Superficial foreign body of breast, unspecified breast

√6ᵗʰ   **S20.16** Insect bite (nonvenomous) of breast

√7ᵗʰ   **S20.161** Insect bite (nonvenomous) of breast, right breast

√7ᵗʰ   **S20.162** Insect bite (nonvenomous) of breast, left breast

√7ᵗʰ   **S20.169** Insect bite (nonvenomous) of breast, unspecified breast

√6ᵗʰ   **S20.17** Other superficial bite of breast

> *EXCLUDES 1*   open bite of breast (S21.05-)

√7ᵗʰ   **S20.171** Other superficial bite of breast, right breast

√7ᵗʰ   **S20.172** Other superficial bite of breast, left breast

√7ᵗʰ   **S20.179** Other superficial bite of breast, unspecified breast

S20.2 Contusion of thorax

√x7ᵗʰ   **S20.20** Contusion of thorax, unspecified

√6ᵗʰ   **S20.21** Contusion of front wall of thorax

√7ᵗʰ   **S20.211** Contusion of right front wall of thorax

√7ᵗʰ   **S20.212** Contusion of left front wall of thorax

√7ᵗʰ   **S20.219** Contusion of unspecified front wall of thorax

√6ᵗʰ   **S20.22** Contusion of back wall of thorax

√7ᵗʰ   **S20.221** Contusion of right back wall of thorax

√7ᵗʰ   **S20.222** Contusion of left back wall of thorax

√7ᵗʰ   **S20.229** Contusion of unspecified back wall of thorax

S20.3 Other and unspecified superficial injuries of front wall of thorax

√6ᵗʰ   **S20.30** Unspecified superficial injuries of front wall of thorax

√7ᵗʰ   **S20.301** Unspecified superficial injuries of right front wall of thorax

√7ᵗʰ   **S20.302** Unspecified superficial injuries of left front wall of thorax

√7ᵗʰ   **S20.309** Unspecified superficial injuries of unspecified front wall of thorax

√6ᵗʰ   **S20.31** Abrasion of front wall of thorax

√7ᵗʰ   **S20.311** Abrasion of right front wall of thorax

√7ᵗʰ   **S20.312** Abrasion of left front wall of thorax

√7ᵗʰ   **S20.319** Abrasion of unspecified front wall of thorax

√6ᵗʰ   **S20.32** Blister (nonthermal) of front wall of thorax

√7ᵗʰ   **S20.321** Blister (nonthermal) of right front wall of thorax

√7ᵗʰ   **S20.322** Blister (nonthermal) of left front wall of thorax

√7ᵗʰ   **S20.329** Blister (nonthermal) of unspecified front wall of thorax

√6ᵗʰ   **S20.34** External constriction of front wall of thorax

√7ᵗʰ   **S20.341** External constriction of right front wall of thorax

√7ᵗʰ   **S20.342** External constriction of left front wall of thorax

√7ᵗʰ   **S20.349** External constriction of unspecified front wall of thorax

Ⓝ Newborn: 0   Ⓟ Pediatric: 0-17   Ⓜ Maternity: 9-64   Ⓐ Adult: 15-124   MCC Major Complication/Comorbidity   CC Complication/Comorbidity   SW Severe Wound Dx

1004   ICD-10-CM 2020

√6ᵗʰ **S20.35** **Superficial foreign body of front wall of thorax**
Splinter in front wall of thorax

√7ᵗʰ **S20.351** **Superficial foreign body of right front wall of thorax**

√7ᵗʰ **S20.352** **Superficial foreign body of left front wall of thorax**

√7ᵗʰ **S20.359** **Superficial foreign body of unspecified front wall of thorax**

√6ᵗʰ **S20.36** **Insect bite (nonvenomous) of front wall of thorax**

√7ᵗʰ **S20.361** **Insect bite (nonvenomous) of right front wall of thorax**

√7ᵗʰ **S20.362** **Insect bite (nonvenomous) of left front wall of thorax**

√7ᵗʰ **S20.369** **Insect bite (nonvenomous) of unspecified front wall of thorax**

√6ᵗʰ **S20.37** **Other superficial bite of front wall of thorax**
EXCLUDES 1   *open bite of front wall of thorax (S21.15)*

√7ᵗʰ **S20.371** **Other superficial bite of right front wall of thorax**

√7ᵗʰ **S20.372** **Other superficial bite of left front wall of thorax**

√7ᵗʰ **S20.379** **Other superficial bite of unspecified front wall of thorax**

√5ᵗʰ **S20.4** **Other and unspecified superficial injuries of back wall of thorax**

√6ᵗʰ **S20.40** **Unspecified superficial injuries of back wall of thorax**

√7ᵗʰ **S20.401** **Unspecified superficial injuries of right back wall of thorax**

√7ᵗʰ **S20.402** **Unspecified superficial injuries of left back wall of thorax**

√7ᵗʰ **S20.409** **Unspecified superficial injuries of unspecified back wall of thorax**

√6ᵗʰ **S20.41** **Abrasion of back wall of thorax**

√7ᵗʰ **S20.411** **Abrasion of right back wall of thorax**

√7ᵗʰ **S20.412** **Abrasion of left back wall of thorax**

√7ᵗʰ **S20.419** **Abrasion of unspecified back wall of thorax**

√6ᵗʰ **S20.42** **Blister (nonthermal) of back wall of thorax**

√7ᵗʰ **S20.421** **Blister (nonthermal) of right back wall of thorax**

√7ᵗʰ **S20.422** **Blister (nonthermal) of left back wall of thorax**

√7ᵗʰ **S20.429** **Blister (nonthermal) of unspecified back wall of thorax**

√6ᵗʰ **S20.44** **External constriction of back wall of thorax**

√7ᵗʰ **S20.441** **External constriction of right back wall of thorax**

√7ᵗʰ **S20.442** **External constriction of left back wall of thorax**

√7ᵗʰ **S20.449** **External constriction of unspecified back wall of thorax**

√6ᵗʰ **S20.45** **Superficial foreign body of back wall of thorax**
Splinter of back wall of thorax

√7ᵗʰ **S20.451** **Superficial foreign body of right back wall of thorax**

√7ᵗʰ **S20.452** **Superficial foreign body of left back wall of thorax**

√7ᵗʰ **S20.459** **Superficial foreign body of unspecified back wall of thorax**

√6ᵗʰ **S20.46** **Insect bite (nonvenomous) of back wall of thorax**

√7ᵗʰ **S20.461** **Insect bite (nonvenomous) of right back wall of thorax**

√7ᵗʰ **S20.462** **Insect bite (nonvenomous) of left back wall of thorax**

√7ᵗʰ **S20.469** **Insect bite (nonvenomous) of unspecified back wall of thorax**

√6ᵗʰ **S20.47** **Other superficial bite of back wall of thorax**
EXCLUDES 1   *open bite of back wall of thorax (S21.25)*

√7ᵗʰ **S20.471** **Other superficial bite of right back wall of thorax**

√7ᵗʰ **S20.472** **Other superficial bite of left back wall of thorax**

√7ᵗʰ **S20.479** **Other superficial bite of unspecified back wall of thorax**

√5ᵗʰ **S20.9** **Superficial injury of unspecified parts of thorax**
EXCLUDES 1   *contusion of thorax NOS (S20.20)*

√x7ᵗʰ **S20.90** **Unspecified superficial injury of unspecified parts of thorax**
Superficial injury of thoracic wall NOS

√x7ᵗʰ **S20.91** **Abrasion of unspecified parts of thorax**

√x7ᵗʰ **S20.92** **Blister (nonthermal) of unspecified parts of thorax**

√x7ᵗʰ **S20.94** **External constriction of unspecified parts of thorax**

√x7ᵗʰ **S20.95** **Superficial foreign body of unspecified parts of thorax**
Splinter in thorax NOS

√x7ᵗʰ **S20.96** **Insect bite (nonvenomous) of unspecified parts of thorax**

√x7ᵗʰ **S20.97** **Other superficial bite of unspecified parts of thorax**
EXCLUDES 1   *open bite of thorax NOS (S21.95)*

√4ᵗʰ **S21** **Open wound of thorax**
Code also any associated injury, such as:
injury of heart (S26.-)
injury of intrathoracic organs (S27.-)
rib fracture (S22.3-, S22.4-)
spinal cord injury (S24.0-, S24.1-)
traumatic hemopneumothorax (S27.3)
traumatic hemothorax (S27.1)
traumatic pneumothorax (S27.0)
wound infection
EXCLUDES 1   *traumatic amputation (partial) of thorax (S28.1)*

The appropriate 7th character is to be added to each code from category S21.
A   initial encounter
D   subsequent encounter
S   sequela

CC Excl: For codes in category S21:
For MCC codes, unless otherwise noted: PDX collection 1169
For CC codes: PDX collection 1168

√5ᵗʰ **S21.0** **Open wound of breast**

√6ᵗʰ **S21.00** **Unspecified open wound of breast**

√7ᵗʰ **S21.001** **Unspecified open wound of right breast**

√7ᵗʰ **S21.002** **Unspecified open wound of left breast**

√7ᵗʰ **S21.009** **Unspecified open wound of unspecified breast**

√6ᵗʰ **S21.01** **Laceration without foreign body of breast**

√7ᵗʰ **S21.011** **Laceration without foreign body of right breast**

√7ᵗʰ **S21.012** **Laceration without foreign body of left breast**

√7ᵗʰ **S21.019** **Laceration without foreign body of unspecified breast**

√6ᵗʰ **S21.02** **Laceration with foreign body of breast**

√7ᵗʰ **S21.021** **Laceration with foreign body of right breast**

√7ᵗʰ **S21.022** **Laceration with foreign body of left breast**

√7ᵗʰ **S21.029** **Laceration with foreign body of unspecified breast**

√6ᵗʰ **S21.03** **Puncture wound without foreign body of breast**

√7ᵗʰ **S21.031** **Puncture wound without foreign body of right breast**

√7ᵗʰ **S21.032** **Puncture wound without foreign body of left breast**

√7ᵗʰ **S21.039** **Puncture wound without foreign body of unspecified breast**

√6ᵗʰ **S21.04** **Puncture wound with foreign body of breast**

√7ᵗʰ **S21.041** **Puncture wound with foreign body of right breast**

√7ᵗʰ **S21.042** **Puncture wound with foreign body of left breast**

√7ᵗʰ **S21.049** **Puncture wound with foreign body of unspecified breast**

√6ᵗʰ **S21.05** **Open bite of breast**
Bite of breast NOS
EXCLUDES 1   *superficial bite of breast (S20.17)*

√7ᵗʰ **S21.051** **Open bite of right breast**

√7ᵗʰ **S21.052** **Open bite of left breast**

√7ᵗʰ **S21.059** **Open bite of unspecified breast**

√5ᵗʰ **S21.1** **Open wound of** front wall of thorax without penetration **into thoracic cavity**

> Open wound of chest without penetration into thoracic cavity

√6ᵗʰ **S21.10** **Unspecified open wound of front wall of thorax without penetration into thoracic cavity**

√7ᵗʰ **S21.101** Unspecified open wound of right front wall of thorax without penetration into thoracic cavity   **cc**

√7ᵗʰ **S21.102** Unspecified open wound of left front wall of thorax without penetration into thoracic cavity   **cc**

√7ᵗʰ **S21.109** Unspecified open wound of unspecified front wall of thorax without penetration into thoracic cavity   **cc**

√6ᵗʰ **S21.11** Laceration without foreign body of front wall of thorax without penetration into thoracic cavity

√7ᵗʰ **S21.111** Laceration without foreign body of right front wall of thorax without penetration into thoracic cavity   **cc**

√7ᵗʰ **S21.112** Laceration without foreign body of left front wall of thorax without penetration into thoracic cavity   **cc**

√7ᵗʰ **S21.119** Laceration without foreign body of unspecified front wall of thorax without penetration into thoracic cavity   **cc**

√6ᵗʰ **S21.12** Laceration with foreign body of front wall of thorax without penetration into thoracic cavity

√7ᵗʰ **S21.121** Laceration with foreign body of right front wall of thorax without penetration into thoracic cavity   **cc**

√7ᵗʰ **S21.122** Laceration with foreign body of left front wall of thorax without penetration into thoracic cavity   **cc**

√7ᵗʰ **S21.129** Laceration with foreign body of unspecified front wall of thorax without penetration into thoracic cavity   **cc**

√6ᵗʰ **S21.13** Puncture wound without foreign body of front wall of thorax without penetration into thoracic cavity

√7ᵗʰ **S21.131** Puncture wound without foreign body of right front wall of thorax without penetration into thoracic cavity   **cc**

√7ᵗʰ **S21.132** Puncture wound without foreign body of left front wall of thorax without penetration into thoracic cavity   **cc**

√7ᵗʰ **S21.139** Puncture wound without foreign body of unspecified front wall of thorax without penetration into thoracic cavity   **cc**

√6ᵗʰ **S21.14** Puncture wound with foreign body of front wall of thorax without penetration into thoracic cavity

√7ᵗʰ **S21.141** Puncture wound with foreign body of right front wall of thorax without penetration into thoracic cavity   **cc**

√7ᵗʰ **S21.142** Puncture wound with foreign body of left front wall of thorax without penetration into thoracic cavity   **cc**

√7ᵗʰ **S21.149** Puncture wound with foreign body of unspecified front wall of thorax without penetration into thoracic cavity   **cc**

√6ᵗʰ **S21.15** Open bite **of front wall of thorax without penetration into thoracic cavity**

> Bite of front wall of thorax NOS

EXCLUDES 1   superficial bite of front wall of thorax (S20.37)

√7ᵗʰ **S21.151** Open bite of right front wall of thorax without penetration into thoracic cavity   **cc**

√7ᵗʰ **S21.152** Open bite of left front wall of thorax without penetration into thoracic cavity   **cc**

√7ᵗʰ **S21.159** Open bite of unspecified front wall of thorax without penetration into thoracic cavity   **cc**

√5ᵗʰ **S21.2** **Open wound of** back wall of thorax without penetration **into thoracic cavity**

√6ᵗʰ **S21.20** **Unspecified open wound of back wall of thorax without penetration into thoracic cavity**

√7ᵗʰ **S21.201** Unspecified open wound of right back wall of thorax without penetration into thoracic cavity

√7ᵗʰ **S21.202** Unspecified open wound of left back wall of thorax without penetration into thoracic cavity

√7ᵗʰ **S21.209** Unspecified open wound of unspecified back wall of thorax without penetration into thoracic cavity

√6ᵗʰ **S21.21** Laceration without foreign body of back wall of thorax without penetration into thoracic cavity

√7ᵗʰ **S21.211** Laceration without foreign body of right back wall of thorax without penetration into thoracic cavity

√7ᵗʰ **S21.212** Laceration without foreign body of left back wall of thorax without penetration into thoracic cavity

√7ᵗʰ **S21.219** Laceration without foreign body of unspecified back wall of thorax without penetration into thoracic cavity

√6ᵗʰ **S21.22** Laceration with foreign body of back wall of thorax without penetration into thoracic cavity

√7ᵗʰ **S21.221** Laceration with foreign body of right back wall of thorax without penetration into thoracic cavity

√7ᵗʰ **S21.222** Laceration with foreign body of left back wall of thorax without penetration into thoracic cavity

√7ᵗʰ **S21.229** Laceration with foreign body of unspecified back wall of thorax without penetration into thoracic cavity

√6ᵗʰ **S21.23** Puncture wound without foreign body of back wall of thorax without penetration into thoracic cavity

√7ᵗʰ **S21.231** Puncture wound without foreign body of right back wall of thorax without penetration into thoracic cavity

√7ᵗʰ **S21.232** Puncture wound without foreign body of left back wall of thorax without penetration into thoracic cavity

√7ᵗʰ **S21.239** Puncture wound without foreign body of unspecified back wall of thorax without penetration into thoracic cavity

√6ᵗʰ **S21.24** Puncture wound with foreign body of back wall of thorax without penetration into thoracic cavity

√7ᵗʰ **S21.241** Puncture wound with foreign body of right back wall of thorax without penetration into thoracic cavity

√7ᵗʰ **S21.242** Puncture wound with foreign body of left back wall of thorax without penetration into thoracic cavity

√7ᵗʰ **S21.249** Puncture wound with foreign body of unspecified back wall of thorax without penetration into thoracic cavity

N Newborn: 0   **P** Pediatric: 0-17   **M** Maternity: 9-64   **A** Adult: 15-124   **MCC** Major Complication/Comorbidity   **CC** Complication/Comorbidity   **SW** Severe Wound Dx

1006   ICD-10-CM 2020

✓6ᵗʰ **S21.25** Open bite of back wall of thorax without penetration into thoracic cavity
    Bite of back wall of thorax NOS
    EXCLUDES 1   *superficial bite of back wall of thorax (S20.47)*

    ✓7ᵗʰ **S21.251** Open bite of right back wall of thorax without penetration into thoracic cavity
    ✓7ᵗʰ **S21.252** Open bite of left back wall of thorax without penetration into thoracic cavity
    ✓7ᵗʰ **S21.259** Open bite of unspecified back wall of thorax without penetration into thoracic cavity

✓5ᵗʰ **S21.3** Open wound of front wall of thorax with penetration into thoracic cavity
    Open wound of chest with penetration into thoracic cavity

    ✓6ᵗʰ **S21.30** Unspecified open wound of front wall of thorax with penetration into thoracic cavity

        ✓7ᵗʰ **S21.301** Unspecified open wound of right front wall of thorax with penetration into thoracic cavity   `MCC`
        ✓7ᵗʰ **S21.302** Unspecified open wound of left front wall of thorax with penetration into thoracic cavity   `MCC`
        ✓7ᵗʰ **S21.309** Unspecified open wound of unspecified front wall of thorax with penetration into thoracic cavity   `MCC`
            CC Excl: PDX collection 1170

    ✓6ᵗʰ **S21.31** Laceration without foreign body of front wall of thorax with penetration into thoracic cavity

        ✓7ᵗʰ **S21.311** Laceration without foreign body of right front wall of thorax with penetration into thoracic cavity   `MCC`
        ✓7ᵗʰ **S21.312** Laceration without foreign body of left front wall of thorax with penetration into thoracic cavity   `MCC`
        ✓7ᵗʰ **S21.319** Laceration without foreign body of unspecified front wall of thorax with penetration into thoracic cavity   `MCC`

    ✓6ᵗʰ **S21.32** Laceration with foreign body of front wall of thorax with penetration into thoracic cavity

        ✓7ᵗʰ **S21.321** Laceration with foreign body of right front wall of thorax with penetration into thoracic cavity   `MCC`
        ✓7ᵗʰ **S21.322** Laceration with foreign body of left front wall of thorax with penetration into thoracic cavity   `MCC`
        ✓7ᵗʰ **S21.329** Laceration with foreign body of unspecified front wall of thorax with penetration into thoracic cavity   `MCC`

    ✓6ᵗʰ **S21.33** Puncture wound without foreign body of front wall of thorax with penetration into thoracic cavity

        ✓7ᵗʰ **S21.331** Puncture wound without foreign body of right front wall of thorax with penetration into thoracic cavity   `MCC`
        ✓7ᵗʰ **S21.332** Puncture wound without foreign body of left front wall of thorax with penetration into thoracic cavity   `MCC`
        ✓7ᵗʰ **S21.339** Puncture wound without foreign body of unspecified front wall of thorax with penetration into thoracic cavity   `MCC`

✓6ᵗʰ **S21.34** Puncture wound with foreign body of front wall of thorax with penetration into thoracic cavity

    ✓7ᵗʰ **S21.341** Puncture wound with foreign body of right front wall of thorax with penetration into thoracic cavity   `MCC`
    ✓7ᵗʰ **S21.342** Puncture wound with foreign body of left front wall of thorax with penetration into thoracic cavity   `MCC`
    ✓7ᵗʰ **S21.349** Puncture wound with foreign body of unspecified front wall of thorax with penetration into thoracic cavity   `MCC`

✓6ᵗʰ **S21.35** Open bite of front wall of thorax with penetration into thoracic cavity
    EXCLUDES 1   *superficial bite of front wall of thorax (S20.37)*

    ✓7ᵗʰ **S21.351** Open bite of right front wall of thorax with penetration into thoracic cavity   `MCC`
    ✓7ᵗʰ **S21.352** Open bite of left front wall of thorax with penetration into thoracic cavity   `MCC`
    ✓7ᵗʰ **S21.359** Open bite of unspecified front wall of thorax with penetration into thoracic cavity   `MCC`

✓5ᵗʰ **S21.4** Open wound of back wall of thorax with penetration into thoracic cavity

    ✓6ᵗʰ **S21.40** Unspecified open wound of back wall of thorax with penetration into thoracic cavity

        ✓7ᵗʰ **S21.401** Unspecified open wound of right back wall of thorax with penetration into thoracic cavity   `MCC`
        ✓7ᵗʰ **S21.402** Unspecified open wound of left back wall of thorax with penetration into thoracic cavity   `MCC`
        ✓7ᵗʰ **S21.409** Unspecified open wound of unspecified back wall of thorax with penetration into thoracic cavity   `MCC`

    ✓6ᵗʰ **S21.41** Laceration without foreign body of back wall of thorax with penetration into thoracic cavity

        ✓7ᵗʰ **S21.411** Laceration without foreign body of right back wall of thorax with penetration into thoracic cavity   `MCC`
        ✓7ᵗʰ **S21.412** Laceration without foreign body of left back wall of thorax with penetration into thoracic cavity   `MCC`
        ✓7ᵗʰ **S21.419** Laceration without foreign body of unspecified back wall of thorax with penetration into thoracic cavity   `MCC`

    ✓6ᵗʰ **S21.42** Laceration with foreign body of back wall of thorax with penetration into thoracic cavity

        ✓7ᵗʰ **S21.421** Laceration with foreign body of right back wall of thorax with penetration into thoracic cavity   `MCC`
        ✓7ᵗʰ **S21.422** Laceration with foreign body of left back wall of thorax with penetration into thoracic cavity   `MCC`
        ✓7ᵗʰ **S21.429** Laceration with foreign body of unspecified back wall of thorax with penetration into thoracic cavity   `MCC`

✅ Additional Character Required   ✓x7ᵗʰ Placeholder   Unacceptable PDx   Questionable PDx   Manifestation   Unspecified Dx   **H1**-**H14** HAC   **HCC** CMS-HCC Dx   **HIV** HIV Dx

✓6ᵗʰ **S21.43** Puncture wound without foreign body of back wall of thorax with penetration into thoracic cavity

    ✓7ᵗʰ **S21.431** Puncture wound without foreign body of right back wall of thorax with penetration into thoracic cavity   `MCC`

    ✓7ᵗʰ **S21.432** Puncture wound without foreign body of left back wall of thorax with penetration into thoracic cavity   `MCC`

    ✓7ᵗʰ **S21.439** Puncture wound without foreign body of unspecified back wall of thorax with penetration into thoracic cavity   `MCC`

✓6ᵗʰ **S21.44** Puncture wound with foreign body of back wall of thorax with penetration into thoracic cavity

    ✓7ᵗʰ **S21.441** Puncture wound with foreign body of right back wall of thorax with penetration into thoracic cavity   `MCC`

    ✓7ᵗʰ **S21.442** Puncture wound with foreign body of left back wall of thorax with penetration into thoracic cavity   `MCC`

    ✓7ᵗʰ **S21.449** Puncture wound with foreign body of unspecified back wall of thorax with penetration into thoracic cavity   `MCC`

✓6ᵗʰ **S21.45** Open bite of back wall of thorax with penetration into thoracic cavity

Bite of back wall of thorax NOS

    EXCLUDES 1   superficial bite of back wall of thorax (S20.47)

    ✓7ᵗʰ **S21.451** Open bite of right back wall of thorax with penetration into thoracic cavity   `MCC`

    ✓7ᵗʰ **S21.452** Open bite of left back wall of thorax with penetration into thoracic cavity   `MCC`

    ✓7ᵗʰ **S21.459** Open bite of unspecified back wall of thorax with penetration into thoracic cavity   `MCC`

✓5ᵗʰ **S21.9** Open wound of unspecified part of thorax

Open wound of thoracic wall NOS

    ✓7ᵗʰ **S21.90** Unspecified open wound of unspecified part of thorax   `CC`

    ✓x7ᵗʰ **S21.91** Laceration without foreign body of unspecified part of thorax   `CC`

    ✓x7ᵗʰ **S21.92** Laceration with foreign body of unspecified part of thorax   `CC`

    ✓x7ᵗʰ **S21.93** Puncture wound without foreign body of unspecified part of thorax   `CC`

    ✓x7ᵗʰ **S21.94** Puncture wound with foreign body of unspecified part of thorax   `CC`

    ✓x7ᵗʰ **S21.95** Open bite of unspecified part of thorax   `CC`

      EXCLUDES 1   superficial bite of thorax (S20.97)

✓4ᵗʰ **S22** Fracture of rib(s), sternum and thoracic spine

`NOTE`   A fracture not indicated as displaced or nondisplaced should be coded to displaced

    A fracture not indicated as open or closed should be coded to closed

`INCLUDES`   fracture of thoracic neural arch
    fracture of thoracic spinous process
    fracture of thoracic transverse process
    fracture of thoracic vertebra
    fracture of thoracic vertebral arch

Code first any associated:
    injury of intrathoracic organ (S27.-)
    spinal cord injury (S24.0-, S24.1-)

EXCLUDES 1   transection of thorax (S28.1)

EXCLUDES 2   fracture of clavicle (S42.0-)
      fracture of scapula (S42.1-)

AHA: 2018,2Q,12; 2015,3Q,37-39

The appropriate 7th character is to be added to each code from category S22.
A   initial encounter for closed fracture
B   initial encounter for open fracture
D   subsequent encounter for fracture with routine healing
G   subsequent encounter for fracture with delayed healing
K   subsequent encounter for fracture with nonunion
S   sequela

✓5ᵗʰ **S22.0** Fracture of thoracic vertebra

CC Excl: For codes in subcategory S22.0:
CC with 7th character A or MCC with 7th character B: PDX collection 1171
CC with 7th character K: PDX collection 897

✓6ᵗʰ **S22.00** Fracture of unspecified thoracic vertebra

    2,3,6 ✓7ᵗʰ **S22.000** Wedge compression fracture of unspecified thoracic vertebra   `MCC` `CC` `H5` `HCC`

    2,3,6 ✓7ᵗʰ **S22.001** Stable burst fracture of unspecified thoracic vertebra   `MCC` `CC` `H5` `HCC`

    2,3,6 ✓7ᵗʰ **S22.002** Unstable burst fracture of unspecified thoracic vertebra   `MCC` `CC` `H5` `HCC`

    2,3,6 ✓7ᵗʰ **S22.008** Other fracture of unspecified thoracic vertebra   `MCC` `CC` `H5` `HCC`

    2,3,6 ✓7ᵗʰ **S22.009** Unspecified fracture of unspecified thoracic vertebra   `MCC` `CC` `H5` `HCC`

✓6ᵗʰ **S22.01** Fracture of first thoracic vertebra

    2,3,6 ✓7ᵗʰ **S22.010** Wedge compression fracture of first thoracic vertebra   `MCC` `CC` `H5` `HCC`

    2,3,6 ✓7ᵗʰ **S22.011** Stable burst fracture of first thoracic vertebra   `MCC` `CC` `H5` `HCC`

    2,3,6 ✓7ᵗʰ **S22.012** Unstable burst fracture of first thoracic vertebra   `MCC` `CC` `H5` `HCC`

    2,3,6 ✓7ᵗʰ **S22.018** Other fracture of first thoracic vertebra   `MCC` `CC` `H5` `HCC`

    2,3,6 ✓7ᵗʰ **S22.019** Unspecified fracture of first thoracic vertebra   `MCC` `CC` `H5` `HCC`

✓6ᵗʰ **S22.02** Fracture of second thoracic vertebra

    2,3,6 ✓7ᵗʰ **S22.020** Wedge compression fracture of second thoracic vertebra   `MCC` `CC` `H5` `HCC`

    2,3,6 ✓7ᵗʰ **S22.021** Stable burst fracture of second thoracic vertebra   `MCC` `CC` `H5` `HCC`

    2,3,6 ✓7ᵗʰ **S22.022** Unstable burst fracture of second thoracic vertebra   `MCC` `CC` `H5` `HCC`

    2,3,6 ✓7ᵗʰ **S22.028** Other fracture of second thoracic vertebra   `MCC` `CC` `H5` `HCC`

    2,3,6 ✓7ᵗʰ **S22.029** Unspecified fracture of second thoracic vertebra   `MCC` `CC` `H5` `HCC`

✓6ᵗʰ **S22.03** Fracture of third thoracic vertebra

    2,3,6 ✓7ᵗʰ **S22.030** Wedge compression fracture of third thoracic vertebra   `MCC` `CC` `H5` `HCC`

    2,3,6 ✓7ᵗʰ **S22.031** Stable burst fracture of third thoracic vertebra   `MCC` `CC` `H5` `HCC`

    2,3,6 ✓7ᵗʰ **S22.032** Unstable burst fracture of third thoracic vertebra   `MCC` `CC` `H5` `HCC`

N Newborn: 0   P Pediatric: 0-17   M Maternity: 9-64   A Adult: 15-124   `MCC` Major Complication/Comorbidity   `CC` Complication/Comorbidity   `SW` Severe Wound Dx

1008   ICD-10-CM 2020

2,3,6 √7th **S22.038** **Other fracture of third thoracic vertebra** `MCC` `CC` `H5` `HCC`

2,3,6 √7th **S22.039** **Unspecified fracture of third thoracic vertebra** `MCC` `CC` `H5` `HCC`

√6th **S22.04** **Fracture of fourth thoracic vertebra**

2,3,6 √7th **S22.040** **Wedge compression fracture of fourth thoracic vertebra** `MCC` `CC` `H5` `HCC`

2,3,6 √7th **S22.041** **Stable burst fracture of fourth thoracic vertebra** `MCC` `CC` `H5` `HCC`

2,3,6 √7th **S22.042** **Unstable burst fracture of fourth thoracic vertebra** `MCC` `CC` `H5` `HCC`

2,3,6 √7th **S22.048** **Other fracture of fourth thoracic vertebra** `MCC` `CC` `H5` `HCC`

2,3,6 √7th **S22.049** **Unspecified fracture of fourth thoracic vertebra** `MCC` `CC` `H5` `HCC`

√6th **S22.05** **Fracture of T5-T6 vertebra**

2,3,6 √7th **S22.050** **Wedge compression fracture of T5-T6 vertebra** `MCC` `CC` `H5` `HCC`

2,3,6 √7th **S22.051** **Stable burst fracture of T5-T6 vertebra** `MCC` `CC` `H5` `HCC`

2,3,6 √7th **S22.052** **Unstable burst fracture of T5-T6 vertebra** `MCC` `CC` `H5` `HCC`

2,3,6 √7th **S22.058** **Other fracture of T5-T6 vertebra** `MCC` `CC` `H5` `HCC`

2,3,6 √7th **S22.059** **Unspecified fracture of T5-T6 vertebra** `MCC` `CC` `H5` `HCC`

√6th **S22.06** **Fracture of T7-T8 vertebra**

2,3,6 √7th **S22.060** **Wedge compression fracture of T7-T8 vertebra** `MCC` `CC` `H5` `HCC`

2,3,6 √7th **S22.061** **Stable burst fracture of T7-T8 vertebra** `MCC` `CC` `H5` `HCC`

2,3,6 √7th **S22.062** **Unstable burst fracture of T7-T8 vertebra** `MCC` `CC` `H5` `HCC`

2,3,6 √7th **S22.068** **Other fracture of T7-T8 thoracic vertebra** `MCC` `CC` `H5` `HCC`

2,3,6 √7th **S22.069** **Unspecified fracture of T7-T8 vertebra** `MCC` `CC` `H5` `HCC`

√6th **S22.07** **Fracture of T9-T10 vertebra**

2,3,6 √7th **S22.070** **Wedge compression fracture of T9-T10 vertebra** `MCC` `CC` `H5` `HCC`

2,3,6 √7th **S22.071** **Stable burst fracture of T9-T10 vertebra** `MCC` `CC` `H5` `HCC`

2,3,6 √7th **S22.072** **Unstable burst fracture of T9-T10 vertebra** `MCC` `CC` `H5` `HCC`

2,3,6 √7th **S22.078** **Other fracture of T9-T10 vertebra** `MCC` `CC` `H5` `HCC`

2,3,6 √7th **S22.079** **Unspecified fracture of T9-T10 vertebra** `MCC` `CC` `H5` `HCC`

√6th **S22.08** **Fracture of T11-T12 vertebra**

2,3,6 √7th **S22.080** **Wedge compression fracture of T11-T12 vertebra** `MCC` `CC` `H5` `HCC`

2,3,6 √7th **S22.081** **Stable burst fracture of T11-T12 vertebra** `MCC` `CC` `H5` `HCC`

2,3,6 √7th **S22.082** **Unstable burst fracture of T11-T12 vertebra** `MCC` `CC` `H5` `HCC`

2,3,6 √7th **S22.088** **Other fracture of T11-T12 vertebra** `MCC` `CC` `H5` `HCC`

2,3,6 √7th **S22.089** **Unspecified fracture of T11-T12 vertebra** `MCC` `CC` `H5` `HCC`

√5th **S22.2** **Fracture of sternum**

> **DEF:** Break in flat bone (breast bone) in the anterior thorax caused by blunt trauma to the anterior chest.
> **CC Excl: For codes in subcategory S22.2:**
> **CC with 7th character A or MCC with 7th character B:** PDX collection 1172
> **CC with 7th character K:** PDX collection 897

2,4 √x7th **S22.20** **Unspecified fracture of sternum** `MCC` `CC` `H5`

2,3 √x7th **S22.21** **Fracture of manubrium** `MCC` `CC` `H5`

2,3 √x7th **S22.22** **Fracture of body of sternum** `MCC` `CC` `H5`

2,3 √x7th **S22.23** **Sternal manubrial dissociation** `MCC` `CC` `H5`

2,3 √x7th **S22.24** **Fracture of xiphoid process** `MCC` `CC` `H5`

√5th **S22.3** **Fracture of one rib**

> **CC Excl: For codes in subcategory S22.3:**
> **CC with 7th character A:** PDX collection 1173
> **MCC with 7th character B:** PDX collection 1174
> **CC with 7th character K:** PDX collection 897

2,3 √x7th **S22.31** **Fracture of one rib, right side** `MCC` `CC` `H5`

2,3 √x7th **S22.32** **Fracture of one rib, left side** `MCC` `CC` `H5`

2,3 √x7th **S22.39** **Fracture of one rib, unspecified side** `MCC` `CC` `H5`

√5th **S22.4** **Multiple fractures of ribs**

> Fractures of two or more ribs
> `EXCLUDES 1`　flail chest (S22.5-)
> **CC Excl: For codes in subcategory S22.4, unless otherwise noted:**
> **CC with 7th character A or or MCC with 7th character B:** PDX collection 1174
> **CC with 7th character K:** PDX collection 897

2,3 √x7th **S22.41** **Multiple fractures of ribs, right side** `MCC` `CC` `H5`

2,3 √x7th **S22.42** **Multiple fractures of ribs, left side** `MCC` `CC` `H5`

2,3 √x7th **S22.43** **Multiple fractures of ribs, bilateral** `MCC` `CC` `H5`

2,3 √x7th **S22.49** **Multiple fractures of ribs, unspecified side** `MCC` `CC` `H5`

> **CC Excl: CC with 7th character A:** PDX collection 1174
> **CC Excl: MCC with 7th character B:** No Excl
> **CC Excl: CC with 7th character K:** PDX collection 897

4 √x7th **S22.5** **Flail chest** `MCC` `CC` `H5`

> **CC Excl: MCC with 7th character A or B:** PDX collection 1175
> **CC Excl: CC with 7th character K:** PDX collection 897

2,3 √x7th **S22.9** **Fracture of bony thorax, part unspecified** `MCC` `CC` `H5`

> **CC Excl: CC with 7th character A or MCC with 7th character B:** PDX collection 1176
> **CC Excl: CC with 7th character K:** PDX collection 897

√4th **S23** **Dislocation and sprain of joints and ligaments of thorax**

> `INCLUDES`　avulsion of joint or ligament of thorax
> laceration of cartilage, joint or ligament of thorax
> sprain of cartilage, joint or ligament of thorax
> traumatic hemarthrosis of joint or ligament of thorax
> traumatic rupture of joint or ligament of thorax
> traumatic subluxation of joint or ligament of thorax
> traumatic tear of joint or ligament of thorax
> Code also any associated open wound
> `EXCLUDES 2`　dislocation, sprain of sternoclavicular joint (S43.2, S43.6)
> strain of muscle or tendon of thorax (S29.01-)

> The appropriate 7th character is to be added to each code from category S23.
> A　initial encounter
> D　subsequent encounter
> S　sequela

√x7th **S23.0** **Traumatic rupture of thoracic intervertebral disc**

> `EXCLUDES 1`　rupture or displacement (nontraumatic) of thoracic intervertebral disc NOS (M51.- with fifth character 4)

√5th **S23.1** **Subluxation and dislocation of thoracic vertebra**

> Code also any associated:
> open wound of thorax (S21.-)
> spinal cord injury (S24.0-, S24.1-)
> `EXCLUDES 2`　fracture of thoracic vertebrae (S22.0-)

√6th **S23.10** **Subluxation and dislocation of unspecified thoracic vertebra**

√7th **S23.100** **Subluxation of unspecified thoracic vertebra**

√7th **S23.101** **Dislocation of unspecified thoracic vertebra**

√6th **S23.11** **Subluxation and dislocation of T1/T2 thoracic vertebra**

√7th **S23.110** **Subluxation of T1/T2 thoracic vertebra**

√7th **S23.111** **Dislocation of T1/T2 thoracic vertebra**

√6th **S23.12** **Subluxation and dislocation of T2/T3-T3/T4 thoracic vertebra**

√7th **S23.120** **Subluxation of T2/T3 thoracic vertebra**

√7th **S23.121** **Dislocation of T2/T3 thoracic vertebra**

√7th **S23.122** **Subluxation of T3/T4 thoracic vertebra**

√7th **S23.123** **Dislocation of T3/T4 thoracic vertebra**

√6ᵗʰ **S23.13** Subluxation and dislocation of T4/T5-T5/T6 thoracic vertebra
- √7ᵗʰ **S23.130** Subluxation of T4/T5 thoracic vertebra
- √7ᵗʰ **S23.131** Dislocation of T4/T5 thoracic vertebra
- √7ᵗʰ **S23.132** Subluxation of T5/T6 thoracic vertebra
- √7ᵗʰ **S23.133** Dislocation of T5/T6 thoracic vertebra

√6ᵗʰ **S23.14** Subluxation and dislocation of T6/T7-T7/T8 thoracic vertebra
- √7ᵗʰ **S23.140** Subluxation of T6/T7 thoracic vertebra
- √7ᵗʰ **S23.141** Dislocation of T6/T7 thoracic vertebra
- √7ᵗʰ **S23.142** Subluxation of T7/T8 thoracic vertebra
- √7ᵗʰ **S23.143** Dislocation of T7/T8 thoracic vertebra

√6ᵗʰ **S23.15** Subluxation and dislocation of T8/T9-T9/T10 thoracic vertebra
- √7ᵗʰ **S23.150** Subluxation of T8/T9 thoracic vertebra
- √7ᵗʰ **S23.151** Dislocation of T8/T9 thoracic vertebra
- √7ᵗʰ **S23.152** Subluxation of T9/T10 thoracic vertebra
- √7ᵗʰ **S23.153** Dislocation of T9/T10 thoracic vertebra

√6ᵗʰ **S23.16** Subluxation and dislocation of T10/T11-T11/T12 thoracic vertebra
- √7ᵗʰ **S23.160** Subluxation of T10/T11 thoracic vertebra
- √7ᵗʰ **S23.161** Dislocation of T10/T11 thoracic vertebra
- √7ᵗʰ **S23.162** Subluxation of T11/T12 thoracic vertebra
- √7ᵗʰ **S23.163** Dislocation of T11/T12 thoracic vertebra

√6ᵗʰ **S23.17** Subluxation and dislocation of T12/L1 thoracic vertebra
- √7ᵗʰ **S23.170** Subluxation of T12/L1 thoracic vertebra
- √7ᵗʰ **S23.171** Dislocation of T12/L1 thoracic vertebra

√5ᵗʰ **S23.2** Dislocation of other and unspecified parts of thorax
- √x7ᵗʰ **S23.20** Dislocation of unspecified part of thorax
- √x7ᵗʰ **S23.29** Dislocation of other parts of thorax

√x7ᵗʰ **S23.3** Sprain of ligaments of thoracic spine

√5ᵗʰ **S23.4** Sprain of ribs and sternum
- √x7ᵗʰ **S23.41** Sprain of ribs
- √6ᵗʰ **S23.42** Sprain of sternum
  - √7ᵗʰ **S23.420** Sprain of sternoclavicular (joint) (ligament)
  - √7ᵗʰ **S23.421** Sprain of chondrosternal joint
  - √7ᵗʰ **S23.428** Other sprain of sternum
  - √7ᵗʰ **S23.429** Unspecified sprain of sternum

√x7ᵗʰ **S23.8** Sprain of other specified parts of thorax

√x7ᵗʰ **S23.9** Sprain of unspecified parts of thorax

√4ᵗʰ **S24** Injury of nerves and spinal cord at thorax level

> **NOTE** Code to highest level of thoracic spinal cord injury.
> Injuries to the spinal cord (S24.0 and S24.1) refer to the cord level and not bone level injury, and can affect nerve roots at and below the level given.

Code also any associated:
  fracture of thoracic vertebra (S22.0-)
  open wound of thorax (S21.-)
  transient paralysis (R29.5)

EXCLUDES 2   injury of brachial plexus (S14.3)

The appropriate 7th character is to be added to each code from category S24.
- A initial encounter
- D subsequent encounter
- S sequela

CC Excl: For MCC codes in category S24: PDX collection 1177

√x7ᵗʰ **S24.0** Concussion and edema of thoracic spinal cord   MCC HCC

√5ᵗʰ **S24.1** Other and unspecified injuries of thoracic spinal cord
- √6ᵗʰ **S24.10** Unspecified injury of thoracic spinal cord
  - √7ᵗʰ **S24.101** Unspecified injury at T1 level of thoracic spinal cord   MCC H5 HCC
  - √7ᵗʰ **S24.102** Unspecified injury at T2-T6 level of thoracic spinal cord   MCC H5 HCC
  - √7ᵗʰ **S24.103** Unspecified injury at T7-T10 level of thoracic spinal cord   MCC H5 HCC
  - √7ᵗʰ **S24.104** Unspecified injury at T11-T12 level of thoracic spinal cord   MCC H5 HCC
  - √7ᵗʰ **S24.109** Unspecified injury at unspecified level of thoracic spinal cord   HCC
    Injury of thoracic spinal cord NOS

√6ᵗʰ **S24.11** Complete lesion of thoracic spinal cord
- √7ᵗʰ **S24.111** Complete lesion at T1 level of thoracic spinal cord   MCC H5 HCC
- √7ᵗʰ **S24.112** Complete lesion at T2-T6 level of thoracic spinal cord   MCC H5 HCC
- √7ᵗʰ **S24.113** Complete lesion at T7-T10 level of thoracic spinal cord   MCC H5 HCC
- √7ᵗʰ **S24.114** Complete lesion at T11-T12 level of thoracic spinal cord   MCC H5 HCC
- √7ᵗʰ **S24.119** Complete lesion at unspecified level of thoracic spinal cord   HCC

√6ᵗʰ **S24.13** Anterior cord syndrome of thoracic spinal cord
- √7ᵗʰ **S24.131** Anterior cord syndrome at T1 level of thoracic spinal cord   MCC H5 HCC
- √7ᵗʰ **S24.132** Anterior cord syndrome at T2-T6 level of thoracic spinal cord   MCC H5 HCC
- √7ᵗʰ **S24.133** Anterior cord syndrome at T7-T10 level of thoracic spinal cord   MCC H5 HCC
- √7ᵗʰ **S24.134** Anterior cord syndrome at T11-T12 level of thoracic spinal cord   MCC H5 HCC
- √7ᵗʰ **S24.139** Anterior cord syndrome at unspecified level of thoracic spinal cord   HCC

√6ᵗʰ **S24.14** Brown-Séquard syndrome of thoracic spinal cord
- √7ᵗʰ **S24.141** Brown-Séquard syndrome at T1 level of thoracic spinal cord   MCC HCC
- √7ᵗʰ **S24.142** Brown-Séquard syndrome at T2-T6 level of thoracic spinal cord   MCC HCC
- √7ᵗʰ **S24.143** Brown-Séquard syndrome at T7-T10 level of thoracic spinal cord   MCC HCC
- √7ᵗʰ **S24.144** Brown-Séquard syndrome at T11-T12 level of thoracic spinal cord   MCC HCC
- √7ᵗʰ **S24.149** Brown-Séquard syndrome at unspecified level of thoracic spinal cord   HCC

√6ᵗʰ **S24.15** Other incomplete lesions of thoracic spinal cord
  Incomplete lesion of thoracic spinal cord NOS
  Posterior cord syndrome of thoracic spinal cord
- √7ᵗʰ **S24.151** Other incomplete lesion at T1 level of thoracic spinal cord   MCC H5 HCC
- √7ᵗʰ **S24.152** Other incomplete lesion at T2-T6 level of thoracic spinal cord   MCC H5 HCC
- √7ᵗʰ **S24.153** Other incomplete lesion at T7-T10 level of thoracic spinal cord   MCC H5 HCC
- √7ᵗʰ **S24.154** Other incomplete lesion at T11-T12 level of thoracic spinal cord   MCC H5 HCC
- √7ᵗʰ **S24.159** Other incomplete lesion at unspecified level of thoracic spinal cord   HCC

√x7ᵗʰ **S24.2** Injury of nerve root of thoracic spine

√x7ᵗʰ **S24.3** Injury of peripheral nerves of thorax

√x7ᵗʰ **S24.4** Injury of thoracic sympathetic nervous system
  Injury of cardiac plexus
  Injury of esophageal plexus
  Injury of pulmonary plexus
  Injury of stellate ganglion
  Injury of thoracic sympathetic ganglion

√x7ᵗʰ **S24.8** Injury of other specified nerves of thorax

☑x 7ᵗʰ **S24.9** **Injury of unspecified nerve of thorax**

☑4ᵗʰ **S25** **Injury of blood vessels of thorax**

> Code also any associated open wound (S21.-)

> The appropriate 7th character is to be added to each code from category S25.
> A   initial encounter
> D   subsequent encounter
> S   sequela

☑5ᵗʰ **S25.0** **Injury of thoracic aorta**

> Injury of aorta NOS
> **CC Excl: For MCC codes in subcategory S25.0:** PDX collection 1178

☑x 7ᵗʰ **S25.00** **Unspecified injury of thoracic aorta**   `MCC`

☑x 7ᵗʰ **S25.01** **Minor laceration of thoracic aorta**   `MCC`

> Incomplete transection of thoracic aorta
> Laceration of thoracic aorta NOS
> Superficial laceration of thoracic aorta

☑x 7ᵗʰ **S25.02** **Major laceration of thoracic aorta**   `MCC`

> Complete transection of thoracic aorta
> Traumatic rupture of thoracic aorta

☑x 7ᵗʰ **S25.09** **Other specified injury of thoracic aorta**   `MCC`

☑5ᵗʰ **S25.1** **Injury of innominate or subclavian artery**

> **CC Excl: For MCC codes in subcategory S25.1:** PDX collection 1179

☑6ᵗʰ **S25.10** **Unspecified injury of innominate or subclavian artery**

☑7ᵗʰ **S25.101** **Unspecified injury of right innominate or subclavian artery**   `MCC`

☑7ᵗʰ **S25.102** **Unspecified injury of left innominate or subclavian artery**   `MCC`

☑7ᵗʰ **S25.109** **Unspecified injury of unspecified innominate or subclavian artery**   `MCC`

☑6ᵗʰ **S25.11** **Minor laceration of innominate or subclavian artery**

> Incomplete transection of innominate or subclavian artery
> Laceration of innominate or subclavian artery NOS
> Superficial laceration of innominate or subclavian artery

☑7ᵗʰ **S25.111** **Minor laceration of right innominate or subclavian artery**   `MCC`

☑7ᵗʰ **S25.112** **Minor laceration of left innominate or subclavian artery**   `MCC`

☑7ᵗʰ **S25.119** **Minor laceration of unspecified innominate or subclavian artery**   `MCC`

☑6ᵗʰ **S25.12** **Major laceration of innominate or subclavian artery**

> Complete transection of innominate or subclavian artery
> Traumatic rupture of innominate or subclavian artery

☑7ᵗʰ **S25.121** **Major laceration of right innominate or subclavian artery**   `MCC`

☑7ᵗʰ **S25.122** **Major laceration of left innominate or subclavian artery**   `MCC`

☑7ᵗʰ **S25.129** **Major laceration of unspecified innominate or subclavian artery**   `MCC`

☑6ᵗʰ **S25.19** **Other specified injury of innominate or subclavian artery**

☑7ᵗʰ **S25.191** **Other specified injury of right innominate or subclavian artery**   `MCC`

☑7ᵗʰ **S25.192** **Other specified injury of left innominate or subclavian artery**   `MCC`

☑7ᵗʰ **S25.199** **Other specified injury of unspecified innominate or subclavian artery**   `MCC`

☑5ᵗʰ **S25.2** **Injury of superior vena cava**

> Injury of vena cava NOS
> **CC Excl: For MCC codes in subcategory S25.2:** PDX collection 1180

☑x 7ᵗʰ **S25.20** **Unspecified injury of superior vena cava**   `MCC`

☑x 7ᵗʰ **S25.21** **Minor laceration of superior vena cava**   `MCC`

> Incomplete transection of superior vena cava
> Laceration of superior vena cava NOS
> Superficial laceration of superior vena cava

☑x 7ᵗʰ **S25.22** **Major laceration of superior vena cava**   `MCC`

> Complete transection of superior vena cava
> Traumatic rupture of superior vena cava

☑x 7ᵗʰ **S25.29** **Other specified injury of superior vena cava**   `MCC`

☑5ᵗʰ **S25.3** **Injury of innominate or subclavian vein**

> **CC Excl: For MCC codes in subcategory S25.3:** PDX collection 1181

☑6ᵗʰ **S25.30** **Unspecified injury of innominate or subclavian vein**

☑7ᵗʰ **S25.301** **Unspecified injury of right innominate or subclavian vein**   `MCC`

☑7ᵗʰ **S25.302** **Unspecified injury of left innominate or subclavian vein**   `MCC`

☑7ᵗʰ **S25.309** **Unspecified injury of unspecified innominate or subclavian vein**   `MCC`

☑6ᵗʰ **S25.31** **Minor laceration of innominate or subclavian vein**

> Incomplete transection of innominate or subclavian vein
> Laceration of innominate or subclavian vein NOS
> Superficial laceration of innominate or subclavian vein

☑7ᵗʰ **S25.311** **Minor laceration of right innominate or subclavian vein**   `MCC`

☑7ᵗʰ **S25.312** **Minor laceration of left innominate or subclavian vein**   `MCC`

☑7ᵗʰ **S25.319** **Minor laceration of unspecified innominate or subclavian vein**   `MCC`

☑6ᵗʰ **S25.32** **Major laceration of innominate or subclavian vein**

> Complete transection of innominate or subclavian vein
> Traumatic rupture of innominate or subclavian vein

☑7ᵗʰ **S25.321** **Major laceration of right innominate or subclavian vein**   `MCC`

☑7ᵗʰ **S25.322** **Major laceration of left innominate or subclavian vein**   `MCC`

☑7ᵗʰ **S25.329** **Major laceration of unspecified innominate or subclavian vein**   `MCC`

☑6ᵗʰ **S25.39** **Other specified injury of innominate or subclavian vein**

☑7ᵗʰ **S25.391** **Other specified injury of right innominate or subclavian vein**   `MCC`

☑7ᵗʰ **S25.392** **Other specified injury of left innominate or subclavian vein**   `MCC`

☑7ᵗʰ **S25.399** **Other specified injury of unspecified innominate or subclavian vein**   `MCC`

☑5ᵗʰ **S25.4** **Injury of pulmonary blood vessels**

> **CC Excl: For MCC codes in subcategory S25.4, unless otherwise noted:** PDX collection 1182

☑6ᵗʰ **S25.40** **Unspecified injury of pulmonary blood vessels**

☑7ᵗʰ **S25.401** **Unspecified injury of right pulmonary blood vessels**   `MCC`

☑7ᵗʰ **S25.402** **Unspecified injury of left pulmonary blood vessels**   `MCC`

☑7ᵗʰ **S25.409** **Unspecified injury of unspecified pulmonary blood vessels**   `MCC`

☑ Additional Character Required   ☑x 7ᵗʰ Placeholder   Unacceptable PDx   Questionable PDx   Manifestation   Unspecified Dx   H1 - H14 HAC   HCC CMS-HCC Dx   HIV HIV Dx
ICD-10-CM 2020

1011

√6ᵗʰ **S25.41** Minor laceration **of pulmonary blood vessels**

Incomplete transection of pulmonary blood vessels
Laceration of pulmonary blood vessels NOS
Superficial laceration of pulmonary blood vessels

√7ᵗʰ **S25.411 Minor laceration of** right **pulmonary blood vessels** `MCC`

√7ᵗʰ **S25.412 Minor laceration of** left **pulmonary blood vessels** `MCC`

√7ᵗʰ **S25.419 Minor laceration of unspecified pulmonary blood vessels** `MCC`

√6ᵗʰ **S25.42** Major laceration **of pulmonary blood vessels**

Complete transection of pulmonary blood vessels
Traumatic rupture of pulmonary blood vessels

√7ᵗʰ **S25.421 Major laceration of** right **pulmonary blood vessels** `MCC`
     CC Excl: PDX collection 1183

√7ᵗʰ **S25.422 Major laceration of** left **pulmonary blood vessels** `MCC`

√7ᵗʰ **S25.429 Major laceration of unspecified pulmonary blood vessels** `MCC`

√6ᵗʰ **S25.49 Other specified injury of pulmonary blood vessels**

√7ᵗʰ **S25.491 Other specified injury of** right **pulmonary blood vessels** `MCC`

√7ᵗʰ **S25.492 Other specified injury of** left **pulmonary blood vessels** `MCC`

√7ᵗʰ **S25.499 Other specified injury of unspecified pulmonary blood vessels** `MCC`

√5ᵗʰ **S25.5 Injury of** intercostal blood vessels
     CC Excl: For CC codes in subcategory S25.5: PDX collection 1184

√6ᵗʰ **S25.50 Unspecified injury of intercostal blood vessels**

√7ᵗʰ **S25.501 Unspecified injury of intercostal blood vessels,** right **side** `CC`

√7ᵗʰ **S25.502 Unspecified injury of intercostal blood vessels,** left **side** `CC`

√7ᵗʰ **S25.509 Unspecified injury of intercostal blood vessels, unspecified side** `CC`

√6ᵗʰ **S25.51** Laceration **of intercostal blood vessels**

√7ᵗʰ **S25.511 Laceration of intercostal blood vessels,** right **side** `CC`

√7ᵗʰ **S25.512 Laceration of intercostal blood vessels,** left **side** `CC`

√7ᵗʰ **S25.519 Laceration of intercostal blood vessels, unspecified side** `CC`

√6ᵗʰ **S25.59 Other specified injury of intercostal blood vessels**

√7ᵗʰ **S25.591 Other specified injury of intercostal blood vessels,** right **side** `CC`

√7ᵗʰ **S25.592 Other specified injury of intercostal blood vessels,** left **side** `CC`

√7ᵗʰ **S25.599 Other specified injury of intercostal blood vessels, unspecified side** `CC`

√5ᵗʰ **S25.8 Injury of other blood vessels of thorax**

Injury of azygos vein
Injury of mammary artery or vein
CC Excl: For CC codes in subcategory S25.8: PDX collection 1185

√6ᵗʰ **S25.80 Unspecified injury of other blood vessels of thorax**

√7ᵗʰ **S25.801 Unspecified injury of other blood vessels of thorax,** right **side** `CC`

√7ᵗʰ **S25.802 Unspecified injury of other blood vessels of thorax,** left **side** `CC`

√7ᵗʰ **S25.809 Unspecified injury of other blood vessels of thorax, unspecified side** `CC`

√6ᵗʰ **S25.81** Laceration **of other blood vessels of thorax**

√7ᵗʰ **S25.811 Laceration of other blood vessels of thorax,** right **side** `CC`

√7ᵗʰ **S25.812 Laceration of other blood vessels of thorax,** left **side** `CC`

√7ᵗʰ **S25.819 Laceration of other blood vessels of thorax, unspecified side** `CC`

√6ᵗʰ **S25.89 Other specified injury of other blood vessels of thorax**

√7ᵗʰ **S25.891 Other specified injury of other blood vessels of thorax,** right **side** `CC`

√7ᵗʰ **S25.892 Other specified injury of other blood vessels of thorax,** left **side** `CC`

√7ᵗʰ **S25.899 Other specified injury of other blood vessels of thorax, unspecified side** `CC`

√5ᵗʰ **S25.9 Injury of unspecified blood vessel of thorax**
     CC Excl: For CC codes in subcategory S25.9: PDX collection 1185

√x7ᵗʰ **S25.90 Unspecified injury of unspecified blood vessel of thorax** `CC`

√x7ᵗʰ **S25.91** Laceration **of unspecified blood vessel of thorax** `CC`

√x7ᵗʰ **S25.99 Other specified injury of unspecified blood vessel of thorax** `CC`

√4ᵗʰ **S26 Injury of heart**

Code also any associated:
   open wound of thorax (S21.-)
   traumatic hemopneumothorax (S27.2)
   traumatic hemothorax (S27.1)
   traumatic pneumothorax (S27.0)

The appropriate 7th character is to be added to each code from category S26.
A   initial encounter
D   subsequent encounter
S   sequela

CC Excl: For codes in category S26:
For MCC codes: PDX collection 1187
For CC codes, unless otherwise noted: PDX collection 1186

√5ᵗʰ **S26.0 Injury of heart with hemopericardium**

√x7ᵗʰ **S26.00 Unspecified injury of heart with hemopericardium** `CC`

√x7ᵗʰ **S26.01 Contusion of heart with hemopericardium** `CC`
     CC Excl: PDX collection 1187

√6ᵗʰ **S26.02** Laceration **of heart with hemopericardium**

√7ᵗʰ **S26.020 Mild laceration of heart with hemopericardium** `MCC`
     Laceration of heart without penetration of heart chamber

√7ᵗʰ **S26.021 Moderate laceration of heart with hemopericardium** `MCC`
     Laceration of heart with penetration of heart chamber

√7ᵗʰ **S26.022 Major laceration of heart with hemopericardium** `MCC`
     Laceration of heart with penetration of multiple heart chambers

√x7ᵗʰ **S26.09 Other injury of heart with hemopericardium** `CC`

√5ᵗʰ **S26.1 Injury of heart** without hemopericardium

√x7ᵗʰ **S26.10 Unspecified injury of heart without hemopericardium** `CC`

√x7ᵗʰ **S26.11 Contusion of heart without hemopericardium** `CC`

√x7ᵗʰ **S26.12 Laceration of heart without hemopericardium** `MCC`

√x7ᵗʰ **S26.19 Other injury of heart without hemopericardium** `CC`

√5ᵗʰ **S26.9 Injury of heart, unspecified with or without hemopericardium**

√x7ᵗʰ **S26.90 Unspecified injury of heart, unspecified with or without hemopericardium** `CC`

N Newborn: 0   P Pediatric: 0-17   M Maternity: 9-64   A Adult: 15-124   MCC Major Complication/Comorbidity   CC Complication/Comorbidity   SW Severe Wound Dx

1012   ICD-10-CM 2020

√x7ᵗʰ **S26.91 Contusion** of heart, unspecified with or without hemopericardium   CC
> **DEF:** Bruising within the heart muscle, with no mention of an open wound, usually caused by blunt chest trauma in motor vehicle accidents, falling from great heights, or receiving CPR.

√x7ᵗʰ **S26.92 Laceration** of heart, unspecified with or without hemopericardium   MCC
> Laceration of heart NOS
> **AHA:** 2019,2Q,24

√x7ᵗʰ **S26.99 Other injury** of heart, unspecified with or without hemopericardium   CC

√4ᵗʰ **S27 Injury of other and unspecified intrathoracic organs**
> Code also any associated open wound of thorax (S21.-)
> EXCLUDES 2   injury of cervical esophagus (S10-S19)
>   injury of trachea (cervical) (S10-S19)

> The appropriate 7th character is to be added to each code from category S27.
> A   initial encounter
> D   subsequent encounter
> S   sequela

√x7ᵗʰ **S27.0 Traumatic pneumothorax**   CC
> EXCLUDES 1   spontaneous pneumothorax (J93.-)
> **CC Excl:** PDX collection 1188

√x7ᵗʰ **S27.1 Traumatic hemothorax**   MCC
> **CC Excl:** PDX collection 1188

√x7ᵗʰ **S27.2 Traumatic hemopneumothorax**   MCC
> **CC Excl:** PDX collection 1188

√5ᵗʰ **S27.3 Other and unspecified injuries of lung**
> **CC Excl: For codes in subcategory S27.3:**
> **MCC codes:** PDX collection 1190
> **CC codes:** PDX collection 1189

√6ᵗʰ **S27.30 Unspecified injury of lung**
> √7ᵗʰ **S27.301 Unspecified injury of lung, unilateral**   CC
> √7ᵗʰ **S27.302 Unspecified injury of lung, bilateral**   CC
> √7ᵗʰ **S27.309 Unspecified injury of lung, unspecified**   CC

√6ᵗʰ **S27.31 Primary blast injury of lung**
> Blast injury of lung NOS
> √7ᵗʰ **S27.311 Primary blast injury of lung, unilateral**   CC
> √7ᵗʰ **S27.312 Primary blast injury of lung, bilateral**   CC
> √7ᵗʰ **S27.319 Primary blast injury of lung, unspecified**   CC

√6ᵗʰ **S27.32 Contusion of lung**
> **DEF:** Bruising of the lung without mention of an open wound.
> √7ᵗʰ **S27.321 Contusion of lung, unilateral**   CC
> √7ᵗʰ **S27.322 Contusion of lung, bilateral**   CC
> √7ᵗʰ **S27.329 Contusion of lung, unspecified**   CC

√6ᵗʰ **S27.33 Laceration of lung**
> √7ᵗʰ **S27.331 Laceration of lung, unilateral**   MCC
> √7ᵗʰ **S27.332 Laceration of lung, bilateral**   MCC
> √7ᵗʰ **S27.339 Laceration of lung, unspecified**   MCC

√6ᵗʰ **S27.39 Other injuries of lung**
> Secondary blast injury of lung
> √7ᵗʰ **S27.391 Other injuries of lung, unilateral**   CC
> √7ᵗʰ **S27.392 Other injuries of lung, bilateral**   CC
> √7ᵗʰ **S27.399 Other injuries of lung, unspecified**   CC

√5ᵗʰ **S27.4 Injury of bronchus**
> **CC Excl: For MCC codes in subcategory S27.4:** PDX collection 1191

√6ᵗʰ **S27.40 Unspecified injury of bronchus**
> √7ᵗʰ **S27.401 Unspecified injury of bronchus, unilateral**   MCC

> √7ᵗʰ **S27.402 Unspecified injury of bronchus, bilateral**   MCC
> √7ᵗʰ **S27.409 Unspecified injury of bronchus, unspecified**   MCC

√6ᵗʰ **S27.41 Primary blast injury of bronchus**
> Blast injury of bronchus NOS
> √7ᵗʰ **S27.411 Primary blast injury of bronchus, unilateral**   MCC
> √7ᵗʰ **S27.412 Primary blast injury of bronchus, bilateral**   MCC
> √7ᵗʰ **S27.419 Primary blast injury of bronchus, unspecified**   MCC

√6ᵗʰ **S27.42 Contusion of bronchus**
> √7ᵗʰ **S27.421 Contusion of bronchus, unilateral**   MCC
> √7ᵗʰ **S27.422 Contusion of bronchus, bilateral**   MCC
> √7ᵗʰ **S27.429 Contusion of bronchus, unspecified**   MCC

√6ᵗʰ **S27.43 Laceration of bronchus**
> √7ᵗʰ **S27.431 Laceration of bronchus, unilateral**   MCC
> √7ᵗʰ **S27.432 Laceration of bronchus, bilateral**   MCC
> √7ᵗʰ **S27.439 Laceration of bronchus, unspecified**   MCC

√6ᵗʰ **S27.49 Other injury of bronchus**
> Secondary blast injury of bronchus
> √7ᵗʰ **S27.491 Other injury of bronchus, unilateral**   MCC
> √7ᵗʰ **S27.492 Other injury of bronchus, bilateral**   MCC
> √7ᵗʰ **S27.499 Other injury of bronchus, unspecified**   MCC

√5ᵗʰ **S27.5 Injury of thoracic trachea**
> **CC Excl: For CC codes in subcategory S27.5:** PDX collection 1169

√x7ᵗʰ **S27.50 Unspecified injury of thoracic trachea**   CC
√x7ᵗʰ **S27.51 Primary blast injury of thoracic trachea**   CC
> Blast injury of thoracic trachea NOS
√x7ᵗʰ **S27.52 Contusion of thoracic trachea**   CC
√x7ᵗʰ **S27.53 Laceration of thoracic trachea**   CC
√x7ᵗʰ **S27.59 Other injury of thoracic trachea**   CC
> Secondary blast injury of thoracic trachea

√5ᵗʰ **S27.6 Injury of pleura**
> **CC Excl: For CC codes in subcategory S27.6:** PDX collection 1169

√x7ᵗʰ **S27.60 Unspecified injury of pleura**   CC
√x7ᵗʰ **S27.63 Laceration of pleura**   CC
√x7ᵗʰ **S27.69 Other injury of pleura**   CC

√5ᵗʰ **S27.8 Injury of other specified intrathoracic organs**
√6ᵗʰ **S27.80 Injury of diaphragm**
> **CC Excl: For CC codes in subcategory S27.80:** PDX collection 1192
> √7ᵗʰ **S27.802 Contusion of diaphragm**   CC
> √7ᵗʰ **S27.803 Laceration of diaphragm**   CC
> √7ᵗʰ **S27.808 Other injury of diaphragm**   CC
> √7ᵗʰ **S27.809 Unspecified injury of diaphragm**   CC

√6ᵗʰ **S27.81 Injury of esophagus (thoracic part)**
> **CC Excl: For MCC codes in subcategory S27.81:** PDX collection 1193
> √7ᵗʰ **S27.812 Contusion of esophagus (thoracic part)**   MCC
> √7ᵗʰ **S27.813 Laceration of esophagus (thoracic part)**   MCC
> √7ᵗʰ **S27.818 Other injury of esophagus (thoracic part)**   MCC
> √7ᵗʰ **S27.819 Unspecified injury of esophagus (thoracic part)**   MCC

√6ᵗʰ **S27.89** **Injury of other specified intrathoracic organs**

Injury of lymphatic thoracic duct

Injury of thymus gland

CC Excl: For CC codes in subcategory S27.89: PDX collection 1169

√7ᵗʰ **S27.892** **Contusion** of other specified intrathoracic organs   **CC**

√7ᵗʰ **S27.893** **Laceration** of other specified intrathoracic organs   **CC**

√7ᵗʰ **S27.898** **Other injury** of other specified intrathoracic organs   **CC**

√7ᵗʰ **S27.899** **Unspecified injury** of other specified intrathoracic organs   **CC**

√x7ᵗʰ **S27.9** **Injury of unspecified intrathoracic organ**   **CC**

CC Excl: PDX collection 1194

√4ᵗʰ **S28** **Crushing injury of thorax, and traumatic amputation of part of thorax**

The appropriate 7th character is to be added to each code from category S28.

A   initial encounter

D   subsequent encounter

S   sequela

√x7ᵗʰ **S28.0** **Crushed chest**

Use additional code for all associated injuries

EXCLUDES 1   flail chest (S22.5)

√x7ᵗʰ **S28.1** **Traumatic amputation (partial) of** part of thorax, except breast   **CC**

CC Excl: PDX collection 1168

√5ᵗʰ **S28.2** **Traumatic amputation of** breast

√6ᵗʰ **S28.21** **Complete** traumatic amputation of breast

Traumatic amputation of breast NOS

√7ᵗʰ **S28.211** **Complete traumatic amputation of** right breast

√7ᵗʰ **S28.212** **Complete traumatic amputation of** left breast

√7ᵗʰ **S28.219** **Complete traumatic amputation of** unspecified breast

√6ᵗʰ **S28.22** **Partial** traumatic amputation of breast

√7ᵗʰ **S28.221** **Partial traumatic amputation of** right breast

√7ᵗʰ **S28.222** **Partial traumatic amputation of** left breast

√7ᵗʰ **S28.229** **Partial traumatic amputation of** unspecified breast

√4ᵗʰ **S29** **Other and unspecified injuries of thorax**

Code also any associated open wound (S21.-)

The appropriate 7th character is to be added to each code from category S29.

A   initial encounter

D   subsequent encounter

S   sequela

√5ᵗʰ **S29.0** **Injury of muscle and tendon at thorax level**

√6ᵗʰ **S29.00** **Unspecified injury of muscle and tendon of thorax**

√7ᵗʰ **S29.001** **Unspecified injury of muscle and tendon of** front wall of thorax

√7ᵗʰ **S29.002** **Unspecified injury of muscle and tendon of** back wall of thorax

√7ᵗʰ **S29.009** **Unspecified injury of muscle and tendon of** unspecified wall of thorax

√6ᵗʰ **S29.01** **Strain of muscle and tendon of thorax**

√7ᵗʰ **S29.011** **Strain of muscle and tendon of** front wall of thorax

√7ᵗʰ **S29.012** **Strain of muscle and tendon of** back wall of thorax

√7ᵗʰ **S29.019** **Strain of muscle and tendon of** unspecified wall of thorax

√6ᵗʰ **S29.02** **Laceration of muscle and tendon of thorax**

√7ᵗʰ **S29.021** **Laceration of muscle and tendon of** front wall of thorax   **CC**

CC Excl: PDX collection 1168

√7ᵗʰ **S29.022** **Laceration of muscle and tendon of** back wall of thorax

√7ᵗʰ **S29.029** **Laceration of muscle and tendon of** unspecified wall of thorax   **CC**

CC Excl: PDX collection 1168

√6ᵗʰ **S29.09** **Other injury of muscle and tendon of thorax**

√7ᵗʰ **S29.091** **Other injury of muscle and tendon of** front wall of thorax

√7ᵗʰ **S29.092** **Other injury of muscle and tendon of** back wall of thorax

√7ᵗʰ **S29.099** **Other injury of muscle and tendon of** unspecified wall of thorax

√x7ᵗʰ **S29.8** **Other specified injuries of thorax**

√x7ᵗʰ **S29.9** **Unspecified injury of thorax**

Injuries to the abdomen, lower back, lumbar spine, pelvis and external genitals (S30-S39)

INCLUDES   injuries to the abdominal wall

injuries to the anus

injuries to the buttock

injuries to the external genitalia

injuries to the flank

injuries to the groin

EXCLUDES 2   burns and corrosions (T20-T32)

effects of foreign body in anus and rectum (T18.5)

effects of foreign body in genitourinary tract (T19.-)

effects of foreign body in stomach, small intestine and colon (T18.2-T18.4)

frostbite (T33-T34)

insect bite or sting, venomous (T63.4)

√4ᵗʰ **S30** **Superficial injury of abdomen, lower back, pelvis and external genitals**

EXCLUDES 2   superficial injury of hip (S70.-)

The appropriate 7th character is to be added to each code from category S30.

A   initial encounter

D   subsequent encounter

S   sequela

√x7ᵗʰ **S30.0** **Contusion of lower back and pelvis**

Contusion of buttock

√x7ᵗʰ **S30.1** **Contusion of abdominal wall**

Contusion of flank

Contusion of groin

√5ᵗʰ **S30.2** **Contusion of** external genital organs

√6ᵗʰ **S30.20** **Contusion of unspecified external genital organ**

√7ᵗʰ **S30.201** **Contusion of unspecified external genital organ, male**   ♂

√7ᵗʰ **S30.202** **Contusion of unspecified external genital organ, female**   ♀

√x7ᵗʰ **S30.21** **Contusion of** penis   ♂

√x7ᵗʰ **S30.22** **Contusion of** scrotum and testes   ♂

√x7ᵗʰ **S30.23** **Contusion of** vagina and vulva   ♀

√x7ᵗʰ **S30.3** **Contusion of** anus

√5ᵗʰ **S30.8** **Other superficial injuries of abdomen, lower back, pelvis and external genitals**

√6ᵗʰ **S30.81** **Abrasion** of abdomen, lower back, pelvis and external genitals

√7ᵗʰ **S30.810** **Abrasion of** lower back and pelvis

√7ᵗʰ **S30.811** **Abrasion of** abdominal wall

√7ᵗʰ **S30.812** **Abrasion of** penis   ♂

√7ᵗʰ **S30.813** **Abrasion of** scrotum and testes   ♂

√7ᵗʰ **S30.814** **Abrasion of** vagina and vulva   ♀

√7ᵗʰ **S30.815** **Abrasion of unspecified** external genital organs, male   ♂

√7ᵗʰ **S30.816** **Abrasion of unspecified** external genital organs, female   ♀

√7ᵗʰ **S30.817** **Abrasion of** anus

√6ᵗʰ **S30.82** **Blister** (nonthermal) of abdomen, lower back, pelvis and external genitals

√7ᵗʰ **S30.820** **Blister (nonthermal) of** lower back and pelvis

√7ᵗʰ **S30.821** **Blister (nonthermal) of** abdominal wall

Ⓝ Newborn: 0   Ⓟ Pediatric: 0-17   Ⓜ Maternity: 9-64   Ⓐ Adult: 15-124   **MCC** Major Complication/Comorbidity   **CC** Complication/Comorbidity   **SW** Severe Wound Dx

1014   ICD-10-CM 2020

√7ᵗʰ **S30.822** Blister (nonthermal) of
penis ♂

√7ᵗʰ **S30.823** Blister (nonthermal) of
scrotum and testes ♂

√7ᵗʰ **S30.824** Blister (nonthermal) of
vagina and vulva ♀

√7ᵗʰ **S30.825** Blister (nonthermal) of
unspecified external
genital organs, male ♂

√7ᵗʰ **S30.826** Blister (nonthermal) of
unspecified external
genital organs, female ♀

√7ᵗʰ **S30.827** Blister (nonthermal) of anus

√6ᵗʰ **S30.84** External constriction of abdomen, lower back,
pelvis and external genitals

√7ᵗʰ **S30.840** External constriction of lower back and
pelvis

√7ᵗʰ **S30.841** External constriction of abdominal wall

√7ᵗʰ **S30.842** External constriction of
penis ♂

Hair tourniquet syndrome of penis
Use additional cause code to identify the
constricting item (W49.0-)

√7ᵗʰ **S30.843** External constriction of
scrotum and testes ♂

√7ᵗʰ **S30.844** External constriction of
vagina and vulva ♀

√7ᵗʰ **S30.845** External constriction of
unspecified external
genital organs, male ♂

√7ᵗʰ **S30.846** External constriction of
unspecified external
genital organs, female ♀

√6ᵗʰ **S30.85** Superficial foreign body of abdomen, lower back,
pelvis and external genitals

Splinter in the abdomen, lower back, pelvis and
external genitals

√7ᵗʰ **S30.850** Superficial foreign body of lower back
and pelvis

√7ᵗʰ **S30.851** Superficial foreign body of abdominal
wall

√7ᵗʰ **S30.852** Superficial foreign body
of penis ♂

√7ᵗʰ **S30.853** Superficial foreign body
of scrotum and testes ♂

√7ᵗʰ **S30.854** Superficial foreign body
of vagina and vulva ♀

√7ᵗʰ **S30.855** Superficial foreign body
of unspecified external
genital organs, male ♂

√7ᵗʰ **S30.856** Superficial foreign body
of unspecified external
genital organs, female ♀

√7ᵗʰ **S30.857** Superficial foreign body of anus

√6ᵗʰ **S30.86** Insect bite (nonvenomous) of abdomen, lower back,
pelvis and external genitals

√7ᵗʰ **S30.860** Insect bite (nonvenomous) of lower back
and pelvis

√7ᵗʰ **S30.861** Insect bite (nonvenomous) of abdominal
wall

√7ᵗʰ **S30.862** Insect bite (nonvenomous)
of penis ♂

√7ᵗʰ **S30.863** Insect bite (nonvenomous)
of scrotum and testes ♂

√7ᵗʰ **S30.864** Insect bite (nonvenomous)
of vagina and vulva ♀

√7ᵗʰ **S30.865** Insect bite (nonvenomous)
of unspecified external
genital organs, male ♂

√7ᵗʰ **S30.866** Insect bite (nonvenomous)
of unspecified external
genital organs, female ♀

√7ᵗʰ **S30.867** Insect bite (nonvenomous) of anus

√6ᵗʰ **S30.87** Other superficial bite of abdomen, lower back,
pelvis and external genitals

EXCLUDES 1 open bite of abdomen, lower back, pelvis
and external genitals (S31.05, S31.15,
S31.25, S31.35, S31.45, S31.55)

√7ᵗʰ **S30.870** Other superficial bite of lower back and
pelvis

√7ᵗʰ **S30.871** Other superficial bite of abdominal wall

√7ᵗʰ **S30.872** Other superficial bite of
penis ♂

√7ᵗʰ **S30.873** Other superficial bite of
scrotum and testes ♂

√7ᵗʰ **S30.874** Other superficial bite of
vagina and vulva ♀

√7ᵗʰ **S30.875** Other superficial bite of
unspecified external
genital organs, male ♂

√7ᵗʰ **S30.876** Other superficial bite of
unspecified external
genital organs, female ♀

√7ᵗʰ **S30.877** Other superficial bite of anus

√5ᵗʰ **S30.9** Unspecified superficial injury of abdomen, lower back, pelvis
and external genitals

√x7ᵗʰ **S30.91** Unspecified superficial injury of lower back and
pelvis

√x7ᵗʰ **S30.92** Unspecified superficial injury of abdominal wall

√x7ᵗʰ **S30.93** Unspecified superficial injury of
penis ♂

√x7ᵗʰ **S30.94** Unspecified superficial injury of
scrotum and testes ♂

√x7ᵗʰ **S30.95** Unspecified superficial injury of
vagina and vulva ♀

√x7ᵗʰ **S30.96** Unspecified superficial injury of
unspecified external genital organs,
male ♂

√x7ᵗʰ **S30.97** Unspecified superficial injury of
unspecified external genital organs,
female ♀

√x7ᵗʰ **S30.98** Unspecified superficial injury of anus

√4ᵗʰ **S31** Open wound of abdomen, lower back, pelvis and external genitals

Code also any associated:
spinal cord injury (S24.0, S24.1-, S34.0-, S34.1-)
wound infection

EXCLUDES 1 traumatic amputation of part of abdomen, lower back and
pelvis (S38.2-, S38.3)

EXCLUDES 2 open wound of hip (S71.00-S71.02)
open fracture of pelvis (S32.1- – S32.9 with 7th character B)

The appropriate 7th character is to be added to each code from
category S31.
A   initial encounter
D   subsequent encounter
S   sequela

CC Excl: For MCC codes in category S31: PDX collection 1195

√5ᵗʰ **S31.0** Open wound of lower back and pelvis

√6ᵗʰ **S31.00** Unspecified open wound of lower back and pelvis

√7ᵗʰ **S31.000** Unspecified open wound of lower back
and pelvis without penetration into
retroperitoneum

Unspecified open wound of lower back
and pelvis NOS

√7ᵗʰ **S31.001** Unspecified open wound   **MCC**
of lower back and pelvis
with penetration into
retroperitoneum

√6ᵗʰ **S31.01** Laceration without foreign body of lower back and
pelvis

√7ᵗʰ **S31.010** Laceration without foreign body of lower
back and pelvis without penetration into
retroperitoneum

Laceration without foreign body of lower
back and pelvis NOS

√7ᵗʰ **S31.011** Laceration without   **MCC**
foreign body of lower back
and pelvis with
penetration into
retroperitoneum

√6ᵗʰ **S31.02** Laceration with foreign body of lower back and
pelvis

√7ᵗʰ **S31.020** Laceration with foreign body of lower
back and pelvis without penetration into
retroperitoneum

Laceration with foreign body of lower
back and pelvis NOS

√7ᵗʰ **S31.021** Laceration with foreign   **MCC**
body of lower back and
pelvis with penetration
into retroperitoneum

✓6ᵗʰ **S31.Ø3** Puncture wound without foreign body of lower back and pelvis

  ✓7ᵗʰ **S31.Ø3Ø** Puncture wound without foreign body of lower back and pelvis without penetration into retroperitoneum
    Puncture wound without foreign body of lower back and pelvis NOS

  ✓7ᵗʰ **S31.Ø31** Puncture wound without foreign body of lower back and pelvis with penetration into retroperitoneum   MCC

✓6ᵗʰ **S31.Ø4** Puncture wound with foreign body of lower back and pelvis

  ✓7ᵗʰ **S31.Ø4Ø** Puncture wound with foreign body of lower back and pelvis without penetration into retroperitoneum
    Puncture wound with foreign body of lower back and pelvis NOS

  ✓7ᵗʰ **S31.Ø41** Puncture wound with foreign body of lower back and pelvis with penetration into retroperitoneum   MCC

✓6ᵗʰ **S31.Ø5** Open bite of lower back and pelvis
    Bite of lower back and pelvis NOS
    EXCLUDES 1 *superficial bite of lower back and pelvis (S3Ø.86Ø, S3Ø.87Ø)*

  ✓7ᵗʰ **S31.Ø5Ø** Open bite of lower back and pelvis without penetration into retroperitoneum
    Open bite of lower back and pelvis NOS

  ✓7ᵗʰ **S31.Ø51** Open bite of lower back and pelvis with penetration into retroperitoneum   MCC

✓5ᵗʰ **S31.1** Open wound of abdominal wall without penetration into peritoneal cavity
    Open wound of abdominal wall NOS
    EXCLUDES 2 *open wound of abdominal wall with penetration into peritoneal cavity (S31.6-)*

  ✓6ᵗʰ **S31.1Ø** Unspecified open wound of abdominal wall without penetration into peritoneal cavity

    ✓7ᵗʰ **S31.1ØØ** Unspecified open wound of abdominal wall, right upper quadrant without penetration into peritoneal cavity

    ✓7ᵗʰ **S31.1Ø1** Unspecified open wound of abdominal wall, left upper quadrant without penetration into peritoneal cavity

    ✓7ᵗʰ **S31.1Ø2** Unspecified open wound of abdominal wall, epigastric region without penetration into peritoneal cavity

    ✓7ᵗʰ **S31.1Ø3** Unspecified open wound of abdominal wall, right lower quadrant without penetration into peritoneal cavity

    ✓7ᵗʰ **S31.1Ø4** Unspecified open wound of abdominal wall, left lower quadrant without penetration into peritoneal cavity

    ✓7ᵗʰ **S31.1Ø5** Unspecified open wound of abdominal wall, periumbilic region without penetration into peritoneal cavity

    ✓7ᵗʰ **S31.1Ø9** Unspecified open wound of abdominal wall, unspecified quadrant without penetration into peritoneal cavity
      Unspecified open wound of abdominal wall NOS

  ✓6ᵗʰ **S31.11** Laceration without foreign body of abdominal wall without penetration into peritoneal cavity

    ✓7ᵗʰ **S31.11Ø** Laceration without foreign body of abdominal wall, right upper quadrant without penetration into peritoneal cavity

    ✓7ᵗʰ **S31.111** Laceration without foreign body of abdominal wall, left upper quadrant without penetration into peritoneal cavity

    ✓7ᵗʰ **S31.112** Laceration without foreign body of abdominal wall, epigastric region without penetration into peritoneal cavity

    ✓7ᵗʰ **S31.113** Laceration without foreign body of abdominal wall, right lower quadrant without penetration into peritoneal cavity

    ✓7ᵗʰ **S31.114** Laceration without foreign body of abdominal wall, left lower quadrant without penetration into peritoneal cavity

    ✓7ᵗʰ **S31.115** Laceration without foreign body of abdominal wall, periumbilic region without penetration into peritoneal cavity

    ✓7ᵗʰ **S31.119** Laceration without foreign body of abdominal wall, unspecified quadrant without penetration into peritoneal cavity

  ✓6ᵗʰ **S31.12** Laceration with foreign body of abdominal wall without penetration into peritoneal cavity

    ✓7ᵗʰ **S31.12Ø** Laceration of abdominal wall with foreign body, right upper quadrant without penetration into peritoneal cavity

    ✓7ᵗʰ **S31.121** Laceration of abdominal wall with foreign body, left upper quadrant without penetration into peritoneal cavity

    ✓7ᵗʰ **S31.122** Laceration of abdominal wall with foreign body, epigastric region without penetration into peritoneal cavity

    ✓7ᵗʰ **S31.123** Laceration of abdominal wall with foreign body, right lower quadrant without penetration into peritoneal cavity

    ✓7ᵗʰ **S31.124** Laceration of abdominal wall with foreign body, left lower quadrant without penetration into peritoneal cavity

    ✓7ᵗʰ **S31.125** Laceration of abdominal wall with foreign body, periumbilic region without penetration into peritoneal cavity

    ✓7ᵗʰ **S31.129** Laceration of abdominal wall with foreign body, unspecified quadrant without penetration into peritoneal cavity

  ✓6ᵗʰ **S31.13** Puncture wound of abdominal wall without foreign body without penetration into peritoneal cavity

    ✓7ᵗʰ **S31.13Ø** Puncture wound of abdominal wall without foreign body, right upper quadrant without penetration into peritoneal cavity

    ✓7ᵗʰ **S31.131** Puncture wound of abdominal wall without foreign body, left upper quadrant without penetration into peritoneal cavity

    ✓7ᵗʰ **S31.132** Puncture wound of abdominal wall without foreign body, epigastric region without penetration into peritoneal cavity

    ✓7ᵗʰ **S31.133** Puncture wound of abdominal wall without foreign body, right lower quadrant without penetration into peritoneal cavity

    ✓7ᵗʰ **S31.134** Puncture wound of abdominal wall without foreign body, left lower quadrant without penetration into peritoneal cavity

    ✓7ᵗʰ **S31.135** Puncture wound of abdominal wall without foreign body, periumbilic region without penetration into peritoneal cavity

    ✓7ᵗʰ **S31.139** Puncture wound of abdominal wall without foreign body, unspecified quadrant without penetration into peritoneal cavity

  ✓6ᵗʰ **S31.14** Puncture wound of abdominal wall with foreign body without penetration into peritoneal cavity

    ✓7ᵗʰ **S31.14Ø** Puncture wound of abdominal wall with foreign body, right upper quadrant without penetration into peritoneal cavity

    ✓7ᵗʰ **S31.141** Puncture wound of abdominal wall with foreign body, left upper quadrant without penetration into peritoneal cavity

    ✓7ᵗʰ **S31.142** Puncture wound of abdominal wall with foreign body, epigastric region without penetration into peritoneal cavity

    ✓7ᵗʰ **S31.143** Puncture wound of abdominal wall with foreign body, right lower quadrant without penetration into peritoneal cavity

    ✓7ᵗʰ **S31.144** Puncture wound of abdominal wall with foreign body, left lower quadrant without penetration into peritoneal cavity

N Newborn: 0 P Pediatric: 0-17 M Maternity: 9-64 A Adult: 15-124 MCC Major Complication/Comorbidity CC Complication/Comorbidity SW Severe Wound Dx

1016 ICD-10-CM 2020

√7ᵗʰ **S31.145** Puncture wound of abdominal wall with foreign body, periumbilic region without penetration into peritoneal cavity

√7ᵗʰ **S31.149** Puncture wound of abdominal wall with foreign body, unspecified quadrant without penetration into peritoneal cavity

√6ᵗʰ **S31.15** Open bite of abdominal wall without penetration into peritoneal cavity

Bite of abdominal wall NOS

EXCLUDES 1 superficial bite of abdominal wall (S30.871)

√7ᵗʰ **S31.150** Open bite of abdominal wall, right upper quadrant without penetration into peritoneal cavity

√7ᵗʰ **S31.151** Open bite of abdominal wall, left upper quadrant without penetration into peritoneal cavity

√7ᵗʰ **S31.152** Open bite of abdominal wall, epigastric region without penetration into peritoneal cavity

√7ᵗʰ **S31.153** Open bite of abdominal wall, right lower quadrant without penetration into peritoneal cavity

√7ᵗʰ **S31.154** Open bite of abdominal wall, left lower quadrant without penetration into peritoneal cavity

√7ᵗʰ **S31.155** Open bite of abdominal wall, periumbilic region without penetration into peritoneal cavity

√7ᵗʰ **S31.159** Open bite of abdominal wall, unspecified quadrant without penetration into peritoneal cavity

√5ᵗʰ **S31.2** Open wound of penis

√x7ᵗʰ **S31.20** Unspecified open wound of penis ♂

√x7ᵗʰ **S31.21** Laceration without foreign body of penis ♂

√x7ᵗʰ **S31.22** Laceration with foreign body of penis ♂

√x7ᵗʰ **S31.23** Puncture wound without foreign body of penis ♂

√x7ᵗʰ **S31.24** Puncture wound with foreign body of penis ♂

√x7ᵗʰ **S31.25** Open bite of penis ♂

Bite of penis NOS

EXCLUDES 1 superficial bite of penis (S30.862, S30.872)

√5ᵗʰ **S31.3** Open wound of scrotum and testes

√x7ᵗʰ **S31.30** Unspecified open wound of scrotum and testes ♂

√x7ᵗʰ **S31.31** Laceration without foreign body of scrotum and testes ♂

√x7ᵗʰ **S31.32** Laceration with foreign body of scrotum and testes ♂

√x7ᵗʰ **S31.33** Puncture wound without foreign body of scrotum and testes ♂

√x7ᵗʰ **S31.34** Puncture wound with foreign body of scrotum and testes ♂

√x7ᵗʰ **S31.35** Open bite of scrotum and testes ♂

Bite of scrotum and testes NOS

EXCLUDES 1 superficial bite of scrotum and testes (S30.863, S30.873)

√5ᵗʰ **S31.4** Open wound of vagina and vulva

EXCLUDES 1 injury to vagina and vulva during delivery (O70.-, O71.4)

√x7ᵗʰ **S31.40** Unspecified open wound of vagina and vulva ♀

√x7ᵗʰ **S31.41** Laceration without foreign body of vagina and vulva ♀

√x7ᵗʰ **S31.42** Laceration with foreign body of vagina and vulva ♀

√x7ᵗʰ **S31.43** Puncture wound without foreign body of vagina and vulva ♀

√x7ᵗʰ **S31.44** Puncture wound with foreign body of vagina and vulva ♀

√x7ᵗʰ **S31.45** Open bite of vagina and vulva ♀

Bite of vagina and vulva NOS

EXCLUDES 1 superficial bite of vagina and vulva (S30.864, S30.874)

√5ᵗʰ **S31.5** Open wound of unspecified external genital organs

EXCLUDES 1 traumatic amputation of external genital organs (S38.21, S38.22)

√6ᵗʰ **S31.50** Unspecified open wound of unspecified external genital organs

√7ᵗʰ **S31.501** Unspecified open wound of unspecified external genital organs, male ♂

√7ᵗʰ **S31.502** Unspecified open wound of unspecified external genital organs, female ♀

√6ᵗʰ **S31.51** Laceration without foreign body of unspecified external genital organs

√7ᵗʰ **S31.511** Laceration without foreign body of unspecified external genital organs, male ♂

√7ᵗʰ **S31.512** Laceration without foreign body of unspecified external genital organs, female ♀

√6ᵗʰ **S31.52** Laceration with foreign body of unspecified external genital organs

√7ᵗʰ **S31.521** Laceration with foreign body of unspecified external genital organs, male ♂

√7ᵗʰ **S31.522** Laceration with foreign body of unspecified external genital organs, female ♀

√6ᵗʰ **S31.53** Puncture wound without foreign body of unspecified external genital organs

√7ᵗʰ **S31.531** Puncture wound without foreign body of unspecified external genital organs, male ♂

√7ᵗʰ **S31.532** Puncture wound without foreign body of unspecified external genital organs, female ♀

√6ᵗʰ **S31.54** Puncture wound with foreign body of unspecified external genital organs

√7ᵗʰ **S31.541** Puncture wound with foreign body of unspecified external genital organs, male ♂

√7ᵗʰ **S31.542** Puncture wound with foreign body of unspecified external genital organs, female ♀

√6ᵗʰ **S31.55** Open bite of unspecified external genital organs

Bite of unspecified external genital organs NOS

EXCLUDES 1 superficial bite of unspecified external genital organs (S30.865, S30.866, S30.875, S30.876)

√7ᵗʰ **S31.551** Open bite of unspecified external genital organs, male ♂

√7ᵗʰ **S31.552** Open bite of unspecified external genital organs, female ♀

√5ᵗʰ **S31.6** Open wound of abdominal wall with penetration into peritoneal cavity

√6ᵗʰ **S31.60** Unspecified open wound of abdominal wall with penetration into peritoneal cavity

√7ᵗʰ **S31.600** Unspecified open wound of abdominal wall, right upper quadrant with penetration into peritoneal cavity MCC

√7ᵗʰ **S31.601** Unspecified open wound of abdominal wall, left upper quadrant with penetration into peritoneal cavity MCC

√7ᵗʰ **S31.602** Unspecified open wound of abdominal wall, epigastric region with penetration into peritoneal cavity MCC

☑ Additional Character Required   √x7ᵗʰ Placeholder   Unacceptable PDx   Questionable PDx   Manifestation   Unspecified Dx   H1-H14 HAC   HCC CMS-HCC Dx   HIV HIV Dx

ICD-10-CM 2020

1017

√7ᵗʰ **S31.603** Unspecified open wound of abdominal wall, right lower quadrant with penetration into peritoneal cavity `MCC`

√7ᵗʰ **S31.604** Unspecified open wound of abdominal wall, left lower quadrant with penetration into peritoneal cavity `MCC`

√7ᵗʰ **S31.605** Unspecified open wound of abdominal wall, periumbilic region with penetration into peritoneal cavity `MCC`

√7ᵗʰ **S31.609** Unspecified open wound of abdominal wall, unspecified quadrant with penetration into peritoneal cavity `MCC`

√6ᵗʰ **S31.61** Laceration without foreign body of abdominal wall with penetration into peritoneal cavity

√7ᵗʰ **S31.610** Laceration without foreign body of abdominal wall, right upper quadrant with penetration into peritoneal cavity `MCC`

√7ᵗʰ **S31.611** Laceration without foreign body of abdominal wall, left upper quadrant with penetration into peritoneal cavity `MCC`

√7ᵗʰ **S31.612** Laceration without foreign body of abdominal wall, epigastric region with penetration into peritoneal cavity `MCC`

√7ᵗʰ **S31.613** Laceration without foreign body of abdominal wall, right lower quadrant with penetration into peritoneal cavity `MCC`

√7ᵗʰ **S31.614** Laceration without foreign body of abdominal wall, left lower quadrant with penetration into peritoneal cavity `MCC`

√7ᵗʰ **S31.615** Laceration without foreign body of abdominal wall, periumbilic region with penetration into peritoneal cavity `MCC`

√7ᵗʰ **S31.619** Laceration without foreign body of abdominal wall, unspecified quadrant with penetration into peritoneal cavity `MCC`

√6ᵗʰ **S31.62** Laceration with foreign body of abdominal wall with penetration into peritoneal cavity

√7ᵗʰ **S31.620** Laceration with foreign body of abdominal wall, right upper quadrant with penetration into peritoneal cavity `MCC`

√7ᵗʰ **S31.621** Laceration with foreign body of abdominal wall, left upper quadrant with penetration into peritoneal cavity `MCC`

√7ᵗʰ **S31.622** Laceration with foreign body of abdominal wall, epigastric region with penetration into peritoneal cavity `MCC`

√7ᵗʰ **S31.623** Laceration with foreign body of abdominal wall, right lower quadrant with penetration into peritoneal cavity `MCC`

√7ᵗʰ **S31.624** Laceration with foreign body of abdominal wall, left lower quadrant with penetration into peritoneal cavity `MCC`

√7ᵗʰ **S31.625** Laceration with foreign body of abdominal wall, periumbilic region with penetration into peritoneal cavity `MCC`

√7ᵗʰ **S31.629** Laceration with foreign body of abdominal wall, unspecified quadrant with penetration into peritoneal cavity `MCC`

√6ᵗʰ **S31.63** Puncture wound without foreign body of abdominal wall with penetration into peritoneal cavity

√7ᵗʰ **S31.630** Puncture wound without foreign body of abdominal wall, right upper quadrant with penetration into peritoneal cavity `MCC`

√7ᵗʰ **S31.631** Puncture wound without foreign body of abdominal wall, left upper quadrant with penetration into peritoneal cavity `MCC`

√7ᵗʰ **S31.632** Puncture wound without foreign body of abdominal wall, epigastric region with penetration into peritoneal cavity `MCC`

√7ᵗʰ **S31.633** Puncture wound without foreign body of abdominal wall, right lower quadrant with penetration into peritoneal cavity `MCC`

√7ᵗʰ **S31.634** Puncture wound without foreign body of abdominal wall, left lower quadrant with penetration into peritoneal cavity `MCC`

√7ᵗʰ **S31.635** Puncture wound without foreign body of abdominal wall, periumbilic region with penetration into peritoneal cavity `MCC`

√7ᵗʰ **S31.639** Puncture wound without foreign body of abdominal wall, unspecified quadrant with penetration into peritoneal cavity `MCC`

√6ᵗʰ **S31.64** Puncture wound with foreign body of abdominal wall with penetration into peritoneal cavity

√7ᵗʰ **S31.640** Puncture wound with foreign body of abdominal wall, right upper quadrant with penetration into peritoneal cavity `MCC`

√7ᵗʰ **S31.641** Puncture wound with foreign body of abdominal wall, left upper quadrant with penetration into peritoneal cavity `MCC`

√7ᵗʰ **S31.642** Puncture wound with foreign body of abdominal wall, epigastric region with penetration into peritoneal cavity `MCC`

√7ᵗʰ **S31.643** Puncture wound with foreign body of abdominal wall, right lower quadrant with penetration into peritoneal cavity `MCC`

√7ᵗʰ **S31.644** Puncture wound with foreign body of abdominal wall, left lower quadrant with penetration into peritoneal cavity `MCC`

√7ᵗʰ **S31.645** Puncture wound with foreign body of abdominal wall, periumbilic region with penetration into peritoneal cavity `MCC`

√7ᵗʰ **S31.649** Puncture wound with foreign body of abdominal wall, unspecified quadrant with penetration into peritoneal cavity `MCC`

N Newborn: 0   **P** Pediatric: 0-17   **M** Maternity: 9-64   **A** Adult: 15-124   `MCC` Major Complication/Comorbidity   `CC` Complication/Comorbidity   `SW` Severe Wound Dx

1018

S31.603–S31.649

ICD-10-CM 2020

√6ᵗʰ **S31.65** Open bite of abdominal wall with penetration into peritoneal cavity

> EXCLUDES 1 superficial bite of abdominal wall (S30.861, S30.871)

√7ᵗʰ **S31.650** Open bite of abdominal wall, right upper quadrant with penetration into peritoneal cavity MCC

√7ᵗʰ **S31.651** Open bite of abdominal wall, left upper quadrant with penetration into peritoneal cavity MCC

√7ᵗʰ **S31.652** Open bite of abdominal wall, epigastric region with penetration into peritoneal cavity MCC

√7ᵗʰ **S31.653** Open bite of abdominal wall, right lower quadrant with penetration into peritoneal cavity MCC

√7ᵗʰ **S31.654** Open bite of abdominal wall, left lower quadrant with penetration into peritoneal cavity MCC

√7ᵗʰ **S31.655** Open bite of abdominal wall, periumbilic region with penetration into peritoneal cavity MCC

√7ᵗʰ **S31.659** Open bite of abdominal wall, unspecified quadrant with penetration into peritoneal cavity MCC

√5ᵗʰ **S31.8** Open wound of other parts of abdomen, lower back and pelvis

√6ᵗʰ **S31.80** Open wound of unspecified buttock

√7ᵗʰ **S31.801** Laceration without foreign body of unspecified buttock

√7ᵗʰ **S31.802** Laceration with foreign body of unspecified buttock

√7ᵗʰ **S31.803** Puncture wound without foreign body of unspecified buttock

√7ᵗʰ **S31.804** Puncture wound with foreign body of unspecified buttock

√7ᵗʰ **S31.805** Open bite of unspecified buttock

> Bite of buttock NOS
>
> EXCLUDES 1 superficial bite of buttock (S30.870)

√7ᵗʰ **S31.809** Unspecified open wound of unspecified buttock

√6ᵗʰ **S31.81** Open wound of right buttock

√7ᵗʰ **S31.811** Laceration without foreign body of right buttock

√7ᵗʰ **S31.812** Laceration with foreign body of right buttock

√7ᵗʰ **S31.813** Puncture wound without foreign body of right buttock

√7ᵗʰ **S31.814** Puncture wound with foreign body of right buttock

√7ᵗʰ **S31.815** Open bite of right buttock

> Bite of right buttock NOS
>
> EXCLUDES 1 superficial bite of buttock (S30.870)

√7ᵗʰ **S31.819** Unspecified open wound of right buttock

√6ᵗʰ **S31.82** Open wound of left buttock

√7ᵗʰ **S31.821** Laceration without foreign body of left buttock

√7ᵗʰ **S31.822** Laceration with foreign body of left buttock

√7ᵗʰ **S31.823** Puncture wound without foreign body of left buttock

√7ᵗʰ **S31.824** Puncture wound with foreign body of left buttock

√7ᵗʰ **S31.825** Open bite of left buttock

> Bite of left buttock NOS
>
> EXCLUDES 1 superficial bite of buttock (S30.870)

√7ᵗʰ **S31.829** Unspecified open wound of left buttock

√6ᵗʰ **S31.83** Open wound of anus

√7ᵗʰ **S31.831** Laceration without foreign body of anus

√7ᵗʰ **S31.832** Laceration with foreign body of anus

√7ᵗʰ **S31.833** Puncture wound without foreign body of anus

√7ᵗʰ **S31.834** Puncture wound with foreign body of anus

√7ᵗʰ **S31.835** Open bite of anus

> Bite of anus NOS
>
> EXCLUDES 1 superficial bite of anus (S30.877)

√7ᵗʰ **S31.839** Unspecified open wound of anus

√4ᵗʰ **S32** Fracture of lumbar spine and pelvis

> **NOTE** A fracture not indicated as displaced or nondisplaced should be coded to displaced.
>
> A fracture not indicated as opened or closed should be coded to closed.

> **INCLUDES** fracture of lumbosacral neural arch
> fracture of lumbosacral spinous process
> fracture of lumbosacral transverse process
> fracture of lumbosacral vertebra
> fracture of lumbosacral vertebral arch

Code first any associated spinal cord and spinal nerve injury (S34.-)

> EXCLUDES 1 transection of abdomen (S38.3)
> EXCLUDES 2 fracture of hip NOS (S72.0-)

AHA: 2018,2Q,12; 2015,3Q,37-39; 2012,4Q,93

> The appropriate 7th character is to be added to each code from category S32.
> A initial encounter for closed fracture
> B initial encounter for open fracture
> D subsequent encounter for fracture with routine healing
> G subsequent encounter for fracture with delayed healing
> K subsequent encounter for fracture with nonunion
> S sequela

√5ᵗʰ **S32.0** Fracture of lumbar vertebra

> Fracture of lumbar spine NOS
>
> **CC Excl: For codes in subcategory S32.0:**
> **CC with 7th character A or MCC with 7th character B:** PDX collection 1196
> **CC with 7th character K:** PDX collection 897

√6ᵗʰ **S32.00** Fracture of unspecified lumbar vertebra

2,3,6 √7ᵗʰ **S32.000** Wedge compression fracture of unspecified lumbar vertebra MCC CC H5 HCC

2,3,6 √7ᵗʰ **S32.001** Stable burst fracture of unspecified lumbar vertebra MCC CC H5 HCC

2,3,6 √7ᵗʰ **S32.002** Unstable burst fracture of unspecified lumbar vertebra MCC CC H5 HCC

2,3,6 √7ᵗʰ **S32.008** Other fracture of unspecified lumbar vertebra MCC CC H5 HCC

2,3,6 √7ᵗʰ **S32.009** Unspecified fracture of unspecified lumbar vertebra MCC CC H5 HCC

√6ᵗʰ **S32.01** Fracture of first lumbar vertebra

2,3,6 √7ᵗʰ **S32.010** Wedge compression fracture of first lumbar vertebra MCC CC H5 HCC

2,3,6 √7ᵗʰ **S32.011** Stable burst fracture of first lumbar vertebra MCC CC H5 HCC

2,3,6 √7ᵗʰ **S32.012** Unstable burst fracture of first lumbar vertebra MCC CC H5 HCC

2,3,6 √7ᵗʰ **S32.018** Other fracture of first lumbar vertebra MCC CC H5 HCC

2,3,6 √7ᵗʰ **S32.019** Unspecified fracture of first lumbar vertebra MCC CC H5 HCC

√6ᵗʰ **S32.02** Fracture of second lumbar vertebra

2,3,6 √7ᵗʰ **S32.020** Wedge compression fracture of second lumbar vertebra MCC CC H5 HCC

2,3,6 √7ᵗʰ **S32.021** Stable burst fracture of second lumbar vertebra MCC CC H5 HCC

2,3,6 √7ᵗʰ **S32.022** Unstable burst fracture of second lumbar vertebra MCC CC H5 HCC

2,3,6 √7ᵗʰ **S32.028** Other fracture of second lumbar vertebra MCC CC H5 HCC

2,3,6 √7ᵗʰ **S32.029** Unspecified fracture of second lumbar vertebra MCC CC H5 HCC

√6ᵗʰ **S32.Ø3 Fracture of third lumbar vertebra**

2,3,6 √7ᵗʰ **S32.Ø3Ø Wedge compression fracture of third lumbar vertebra** MCC CC H5 HCC

2,3,6 √7ᵗʰ **S32.Ø31 Stable burst fracture of third lumbar vertebra** MCC CC H5 HCC

2,3,6 √7ᵗʰ **S32.Ø32 Unstable burst fracture of third lumbar vertebra** MCC CC H5 HCC

2,3,6 √7ᵗʰ **S32.Ø38 Other fracture of third lumbar vertebra** MCC CC H5 HCC

2,3,6 √7ᵗʰ **S32.Ø39 Unspecified fracture of third lumbar vertebra** MCC CC H5 HCC

√6ᵗʰ **S32.Ø4 Fracture of fourth lumbar vertebra**

2,3,6 √7ᵗʰ **S32.Ø4Ø Wedge compression fracture of fourth lumbar vertebra** MCC CC H5 HCC

2,3,6 √7ᵗʰ **S32.Ø41 Stable burst fracture of fourth lumbar vertebra** MCC CC H5 HCC

2,3,6 √7ᵗʰ **S32.Ø42 Unstable burst fracture of fourth lumbar vertebra** MCC CC H5 HCC

2,3,6 √7ᵗʰ **S32.Ø48 Other fracture of fourth lumbar vertebra** MCC CC H5 HCC

2,3,6 √7ᵗʰ **S32.Ø49 Unspecified fracture of fourth lumbar vertebra** MCC CC H5 HCC

√6ᵗʰ **S32.Ø5 Fracture of fifth lumbar vertebra**

2,3,6 √7ᵗʰ **S32.Ø5Ø Wedge compression fracture of fifth lumbar vertebra** MCC CC H5 HCC

2,3,6 √7ᵗʰ **S32.Ø51 Stable burst fracture of fifth lumbar vertebra** MCC CC H5 HCC

2,3,6 √7ᵗʰ **S32.Ø52 Unstable burst fracture of fifth lumbar vertebra** MCC CC H5 HCC

2,3,6 √7ᵗʰ **S32.Ø58 Other fracture of fifth lumbar vertebra** MCC CC H5 HCC

2,3,6 √7ᵗʰ **S32.Ø59 Unspecified fracture of fifth lumbar vertebra** MCC CC H5 HCC

√5ᵗʰ **S32.1 Fracture of sacrum**

NOTE   For vertical fractures, code to most medial fracture extension

Use two codes if both a vertical and transverse fracture are present

Code also any associated fracture of pelvic ring (S32.8-)

CC Excl: For codes in subcategory S32.1:
CC with 7th character A or MCC with 7th character B: PDX collection 1197
CC with 7th character K: PDX collection 897

2,3,6 √x7ᵗʰ **S32.1Ø Unspecified fracture of sacrum** MCC CC H5 HCC

√6ᵗʰ **S32.11 Zone I fracture of sacrum**

Vertical sacral ala fracture of sacrum

Vertical Sacral Fracture Zones

Zones: ① ② ③

2,3,6 √7ᵗʰ **S32.11Ø Nondisplaced Zone I fracture of sacrum** MCC CC H5 HCC

2,3,6 √7ᵗʰ **S32.111 Minimally displaced Zone I fracture of sacrum** MCC CC H5 HCC

2,3,6 √7ᵗʰ **S32.112 Severely displaced Zone I fracture of sacrum** MCC CC H5 HCC

2,3,6 √7ᵗʰ **S32.119 Unspecified Zone I fracture of sacrum** MCC CC H5 HCC

√6ᵗʰ **S32.12 Zone II fracture of sacrum**

Vertical foraminal region fracture of sacrum

2,3,6 √7ᵗʰ **S32.12Ø Nondisplaced Zone II fracture of sacrum** MCC CC H5 HCC

2,3,6 √7ᵗʰ **S32.121 Minimally displaced Zone II fracture of sacrum** MCC CC H5 HCC

2,3,6 √7ᵗʰ **S32.122 Severely displaced Zone II fracture of sacrum** MCC CC H5 HCC

2,3,6 √7ᵗʰ **S32.129 Unspecified Zone II fracture of sacrum** MCC CC H5 HCC

√6ᵗʰ **S32.13 Zone III fracture of sacrum**

Vertical fracture into spinal canal region of sacrum

2,3,6 √7ᵗʰ **S32.13Ø Nondisplaced Zone III fracture of sacrum** MCC CC H5 HCC

2,3,6 √7ᵗʰ **S32.131 Minimally displaced Zone III fracture of sacrum** MCC CC H5 HCC

2,3,6 √7ᵗʰ **S32.132 Severely displaced Zone III fracture of sacrum** MCC CC H5 HCC

2,3,6 √7ᵗʰ **S32.139 Unspecified Zone III fracture of sacrum** MCC CC H5 HCC

Transverse Sacral Fracture Types

Type 1   Type 2   Type 3   Type 4

2,3,6 √x7ᵗʰ **S32.14 Type 1 fracture of sacrum** MCC CC H5 HCC

Transverse flexion fracture of sacrum without displacement

2,3,6 √x7ᵗʰ **S32.15 Type 2 fracture of sacrum** MCC CC H5 HCC

Transverse flexion fracture of sacrum with posterior displacement

2,3,6 √x7ᵗʰ **S32.16 Type 3 fracture of sacrum** MCC CC H5 HCC

Transverse extension fracture of sacrum with anterior displacement

2,3,6 √x7ᵗʰ **S32.17 Type 4 fracture of sacrum** MCC CC H5 HCC

Transverse segmental comminution of upper sacrum

2,3,6 √x7ᵗʰ **S32.19 Other fracture of sacrum** MCC CC H5 HCC

2,3,6 √x7ᵗʰ **S32.2 Fracture of coccyx** MCC CC H5 HCC

CC Excl: See code S32.1

√5ᵗʰ **S32.3 Fracture of ilium**

EXCLUDES 1   fracture of ilium with associated disruption of pelvic ring (S32.8-)

CC Excl: For codes in subcategory S32.3:
CC with 7th character A: PDX collection 1176
MCC with 7th character B: PDX collection 1198
CC with 7th character K: PDX collection 897

√6ᵗʰ **S32.3Ø Unspecified fracture of ilium**

2,3,6 √7ᵗʰ **S32.3Ø1 Unspecified fracture of right ilium** MCC CC H5 HCC

2,3,6 √7ᵗʰ **S32.3Ø2 Unspecified fracture of left ilium** MCC CC H5 HCC

2,3,6 √7ᵗʰ **S32.3Ø9 Unspecified fracture of unspecified ilium** MCC CC H5 HCC

√6ᵗʰ **S32.31 Avulsion fracture of ilium**

2,3,6 √7ᵗʰ **S32.311 Displaced avulsion fracture of right ilium** MCC CC H5 HCC

2,3,6 √7ᵗʰ **S32.312 Displaced avulsion fracture of left ilium** MCC CC H5 HCC

2,3,6 √7ᵗʰ **S32.313 Displaced avulsion fracture of unspecified ilium** MCC CC H5 HCC

2,3,6 √7ᵗʰ **S32.314 Nondisplaced avulsion fracture of right ilium** MCC CC H5 HCC

2,3,6 √7ᵗʰ **S32.315 Nondisplaced avulsion fracture of left ilium** MCC CC H5 HCC

2,3,6 √7ᵗʰ **S32.316 Nondisplaced avulsion fracture of unspecified ilium** MCC CC H5 HCC

√6ᵗʰ **S32.39 Other fracture of ilium**

     2,3,6 √7ᵗʰ **S32.391 Other fracture of right ilium** `MCC` `CC` `H5` `HCC`

     2,3,6 √7ᵗʰ **S32.392 Other fracture of left ilium** `MCC` `CC` `H5` `HCC`

     2,3,6 √7ᵗʰ **S32.399 Other fracture of unspecified ilium** `MCC` `CC` `H5` `HCC`

√5ᵗʰ **S32.4 Fracture of acetabulum**

> Code also any associated fracture of pelvic ring (S32.8-)
> AHA: 2016,3Q,16
> CC Excl: For codes in subcategory S32.4:
> MCC with 7th character A: PDX collection 1199
> MCC with 7th character B: PDX collection 1200
> CC with 7th character K: PDX collection 897

√6ᵗʰ **S32.40 Unspecified fracture of acetabulum**

     2,3,6 √7ᵗʰ **S32.401 Unspecified fracture of right acetabulum** `MCC` `CC` `H5` `HCC`

     2,3,6 √7ᵗʰ **S32.402 Unspecified fracture of left acetabulum** `MCC` `CC` `H5` `HCC`

     2,3,6 √7ᵗʰ **S32.409 Unspecified fracture of unspecified acetabulum** `MCC` `CC` `H5` `HCC`

√6ᵗʰ **S32.41 Fracture of anterior wall of acetabulum**

     4,6 √7ᵗʰ **S32.411 Displaced fracture of anterior wall of right acetabulum** `MCC` `CC` `H5` `HCC`

     4,6 √7ᵗʰ **S32.412 Displaced fracture of anterior wall of left acetabulum** `MCC` `CC` `H5` `HCC`

     4,6 √7ᵗʰ **S32.413 Displaced fracture of anterior wall of unspecified acetabulum** `MCC` `CC` `H5` `HCC`

     4,6 √7ᵗʰ **S32.414 Nondisplaced fracture of anterior wall of right acetabulum** `MCC` `CC` `H5` `HCC`

     4,6 √7ᵗʰ **S32.415 Nondisplaced fracture of anterior wall of left acetabulum** `MCC` `CC` `H5` `HCC`

     4,6 √7ᵗʰ **S32.416 Nondisplaced fracture of anterior wall of unspecified acetabulum** `MCC` `CC` `H5` `HCC`

√6ᵗʰ **S32.42 Fracture of posterior wall of acetabulum**

     4,6 √7ᵗʰ **S32.421 Displaced fracture of posterior wall of right acetabulum** `MCC` `CC` `H5` `HCC`

     4,6 √7ᵗʰ **S32.422 Displaced fracture of posterior wall of left acetabulum** `MCC` `CC` `H5` `HCC`

     4,6 √7ᵗʰ **S32.423 Displaced fracture of posterior wall of unspecified acetabulum** `MCC` `CC` `H5` `HCC`

     4,6 √7ᵗʰ **S32.424 Nondisplaced fracture of posterior wall of right acetabulum** `MCC` `CC` `H5` `HCC`

     4,6 √7ᵗʰ **S32.425 Nondisplaced fracture of posterior wall of left acetabulum** `MCC` `CC` `H5` `HCC`

     4,6 √7ᵗʰ **S32.426 Nondisplaced fracture of posterior wall of unspecified acetabulum** `MCC` `CC` `H5` `HCC`

√6ᵗʰ **S32.43 Fracture of anterior column [iliopubic] of acetabulum**

     4,6 √7ᵗʰ **S32.431 Displaced fracture of anterior column [iliopubic] of right acetabulum** `MCC` `CC` `H5` `HCC`

     4,6 √7ᵗʰ **S32.432 Displaced fracture of anterior column [iliopubic] of left acetabulum** `MCC` `CC` `H5` `HCC`

     4,6 √7ᵗʰ **S32.433 Displaced fracture of anterior column [iliopubic] of unspecified acetabulum** `MCC` `CC` `H5` `HCC`

     4,6 √7ᵗʰ **S32.434 Nondisplaced fracture of anterior column [iliopubic] of right acetabulum** `MCC` `CC` `H5` `HCC`

     4,6 √7ᵗʰ **S32.435 Nondisplaced fracture of anterior column [iliopubic] of left acetabulum** `MCC` `CC` `H5` `HCC`

     4,6 √7ᵗʰ **S32.436 Nondisplaced fracture of anterior column [iliopubic] of unspecified acetabulum** `MCC` `CC` `H5` `HCC`

√6ᵗʰ **S32.44 Fracture of posterior column [ilioischial] of acetabulum**

     4,6 √7ᵗʰ **S32.441 Displaced fracture of posterior column [ilioischial] of right acetabulum** `MCC` `CC` `H5` `HCC`

     4,6 √7ᵗʰ **S32.442 Displaced fracture of posterior column [ilioischial] of left acetabulum** `MCC` `CC` `H5` `HCC`

     4,6 √7ᵗʰ **S32.443 Displaced fracture of posterior column [ilioischial] of unspecified acetabulum** `MCC` `CC` `H5` `HCC`

     4,6 √7ᵗʰ **S32.444 Nondisplaced fracture of posterior column [ilioischial] of right acetabulum** `MCC` `CC` `H5` `HCC`

     4,6 √7ᵗʰ **S32.445 Nondisplaced fracture of posterior column [ilioischial] of left acetabulum** `MCC` `CC` `H5` `HCC`

     4,6 √7ᵗʰ **S32.446 Nondisplaced fracture of posterior column [ilioischial] of unspecified acetabulum** `MCC` `CC` `H5` `HCC`

√6ᵗʰ **S32.45 Transverse fracture of acetabulum**

     4,6 √7ᵗʰ **S32.451 Displaced transverse fracture of right acetabulum** `MCC` `CC` `H5` `HCC`

     4,6 √7ᵗʰ **S32.452 Displaced transverse fracture of left acetabulum** `MCC` `CC` `H5` `HCC`

     4,6 √7ᵗʰ **S32.453 Displaced transverse fracture of unspecified acetabulum** `MCC` `CC` `H5` `HCC`

     4,6 √7ᵗʰ **S32.454 Nondisplaced transverse fracture of right acetabulum** `MCC` `CC` `H5` `HCC`

     4,6 √7ᵗʰ **S32.455 Nondisplaced transverse fracture of left acetabulum** `MCC` `CC` `H5` `HCC`

     4,6 √7ᵗʰ **S32.456 Nondisplaced transverse fracture of unspecified acetabulum** `MCC` `CC` `H5` `HCC`

√6ᵗʰ **S32.46 Associated transverse-posterior fracture of acetabulum**

     4,6 √7ᵗʰ **S32.461 Displaced associated transverse-posterior fracture of right acetabulum** `MCC` `CC` `H5` `HCC`

     4,6 √7ᵗʰ **S32.462 Displaced associated transverse-posterior fracture of left acetabulum** `MCC` `CC` `H5` `HCC`

     4,6 √7ᵗʰ **S32.463 Displaced associated transverse-posterior fracture of unspecified acetabulum** `MCC` `CC` `H5` `HCC`

     4,6 √7ᵗʰ **S32.464 Nondisplaced associated transverse-posterior fracture of right acetabulum** `MCC` `CC` `H5` `HCC`

     4,6 √7ᵗʰ **S32.465 Nondisplaced associated transverse-posterior fracture of left acetabulum** `MCC` `CC` `H5` `HCC`

     4,6 √7ᵗʰ **S32.466 Nondisplaced associated transverse-posterior fracture of unspecified acetabulum** `MCC` `CC` `H5` `HCC`

√6ᵗʰ **S32.47 Fracture of medial wall of acetabulum**

     4,6 √7ᵗʰ **S32.471 Displaced fracture of medial wall of right acetabulum** `MCC` `CC` `H5` `HCC`

     4,6 √7ᵗʰ **S32.472 Displaced fracture of medial wall of left acetabulum** `MCC` `CC` `H5` `HCC`

     4,6 √7ᵗʰ **S32.473 Displaced fracture of medial wall of unspecified acetabulum** `MCC` `CC` `H5` `HCC`

     4,6 √7ᵗʰ **S32.474 Nondisplaced fracture of medial wall of right acetabulum** `MCC` `CC` `H5` `HCC`

4,6 √7ᵗʰ **S32.475** **Nondisplaced** fracture of MCC CC H5 HCC
medial wall of left acetabulum

4,6 √7ᵗʰ **S32.476** **Nondisplaced** fracture of MCC CC H5 HCC
medial wall of unspecified acetabulum

√6ᵗʰ **S32.48** **Dome fracture** of acetabulum

4,6 √7ᵗʰ **S32.481** **Displaced dome** fracture MCC CC H5 HCC
of **right** acetabulum

4,6 √7ᵗʰ **S32.482** **Displaced dome** fracture MCC CC H5 HCC
of **left** acetabulum

4,6 √7ᵗʰ **S32.483** **Displaced dome** fracture MCC CC H5 HCC
of **unspecified** acetabulum

4,6 √7ᵗʰ **S32.484** **Nondisplaced dome** MCC CC H5 HCC
fracture of right acetabulum

4,6 √7ᵗʰ **S32.485** **Nondisplaced dome** MCC CC H5 HCC
fracture of left acetabulum

4,6 √7ᵗʰ **S32.486** **Nondisplaced dome** MCC CC H5 HCC
fracture of unspecified acetabulum

√6ᵗʰ **S32.49** **Other specified fracture** of acetabulum

4,6 √7ᵗʰ **S32.491** **Other specified fracture of** MCC CC H5 HCC
right acetabulum

4,6 √7ᵗʰ **S32.492** **Other specified fracture of** MCC CC H5 HCC
left acetabulum

4,6 √7ᵗʰ **S32.499** **Other specified fracture of** MCC CC H5 HCC
unspecified acetabulum

√5ᵗʰ **S32.5** **Fracture of pubis**

EXCLUDES 1   *fracture of pubis with associated disruption of pelvic ring (S32.8-)*

CC Excl: For codes in subcategory S32.5:
MCC with 7th character B: PDX collection 1201

√6ᵗʰ **S32.50** **Unspecified fracture of pubis**

2,6 √7ᵗʰ **S32.501** **Unspecified fracture of** MCC H5 HCC
right pubis

2,6 √7ᵗʰ **S32.502** **Unspecified fracture of left** MCC H5 HCC
pubis

2,6 √7ᵗʰ **S32.509** **Unspecified fracture of** MCC H5 HCC
unspecified pubis

√6ᵗʰ **S32.51** **Fracture of superior rim** of pubis

2,6 √7ᵗʰ **S32.511** **Fracture of superior rim of** MCC H5 HCC
right pubis

2,6 √7ᵗʰ **S32.512** **Fracture of superior rim of** MCC H5 HCC
left pubis

2,6 √7ᵗʰ **S32.519** **Fracture of superior rim of** MCC H5 HCC
unspecified pubis

√6ᵗʰ **S32.59** **Other specified fracture** of pubis

2,6 √7ᵗʰ **S32.591** **Other specified fracture of** MCC H5 HCC
right pubis

2,6 √7ᵗʰ **S32.592** **Other specified fracture of** MCC H5 HCC
left pubis

2,6 √7ᵗʰ **S32.599** **Other specified fracture of** MCC H5 HCC
unspecified pubis

√5ᵗʰ **S32.6** **Fracture of ischium**

EXCLUDES 1   *fracture of ischium with associated disruption of pelvic ring (S32.8-)*

CC Excl: For codes in subcategory S32.6:
CC with 7th character A: PDX collection 1202
MCC with 7th character B: PDX collection 1203
CC with 7th character K: PDX collection 897

√6ᵗʰ **S32.60** **Unspecified fracture of ischium**

2,3,6 √7ᵗʰ **S32.601** **Unspecified fracture of** MCC CC H5 HCC
right ischium

2,3,6 √7ᵗʰ **S32.602** **Unspecified fracture of left** MCC CC H5 HCC
ischium

2,3,6 √7ᵗʰ **S32.609** **Unspecified fracture of** MCC CC H5 HCC
unspecified ischium

√6ᵗʰ **S32.61** **Avulsion** fracture of ischium

2,3,6 √7ᵗʰ **S32.611** **Displaced avulsion** MCC CC H5 HCC
fracture of right ischium

2,3,6 √7ᵗʰ **S32.612** **Displaced avulsion** MCC CC H5 HCC
fracture of left ischium

2,3,6 √7ᵗʰ **S32.613** **Displaced avulsion** MCC CC H5 HCC
fracture of unspecified ischium

2,3,6 √7ᵗʰ **S32.614** **Nondisplaced avulsion** MCC CC H5 HCC
fracture of right ischium

2,3,6 √7ᵗʰ **S32.615** **Nondisplaced avulsion** MCC CC H5 HCC
fracture of left ischium

2,3,6 √7ᵗʰ **S32.616** **Nondisplaced avulsion** MCC CC H5 HCC
fracture of unspecified ischium

√6ᵗʰ **S32.69** **Other specified fracture** of ischium

2,3,6 √7ᵗʰ **S32.691** **Other specified fracture of** MCC CC H5 HCC
right ischium

2,3,6 √7ᵗʰ **S32.692** **Other specified fracture of** MCC CC H5 HCC
left ischium

2,3,6 √7ᵗʰ **S32.699** **Other specified fracture of** MCC CC H5 HCC
unspecified ischium

√5ᵗʰ **S32.8** **Fracture of other parts of pelvis**

Code also any associated:
fracture of acetabulum (S32.4-)
sacral fracture (S32.1-)

Fractures Disrupting Pelvic Circle

√6ᵗʰ **S32.81** **Multiple fractures of pelvis** with disruption of pelvic ring

Multiple pelvic fractures with disruption of pelvic circle

CC Excl: For codes in subcategory S32.81:
CC with 7th character A or MCC with 7th character
B: PDX collection 1204
CC with 7th character K: PDX collection 897

2,3,6 √7ᵗʰ **S32.810** **Multiple fractures of pelvis** MCC CC H5 HCC
with **stable** disruption of pelvic ring

2,3,6 √7ᵗʰ **S32.811** **Multiple fractures of pelvis** MCC CC H5 HCC
with **unstable** disruption of pelvic ring

2,3,6 √x7ᵗʰ **S32.82** **Multiple fractures of pelvis** without MCC CC H5 HCC
disruption of pelvic ring

Multiple pelvic fractures without disruption of pelvic circle

CC Excl: CC with 7th character A or MCC with 7th
character B: PDX collection 1205
CC Excl: CC with 7th character K: PDX collection 897

2,3,6 √x7ᵗʰ **S32.89** **Fracture of other parts of pelvis** MCC CC H5 HCC

CC Excl: CC with 7th character A or MCC with 7th
character B: PDX collection 1206
CC Excl: CC with 7th character K: PDX collection 897

2,3,6 √x7ᵗʰ **S32.9** **Fracture of unspecified parts of lumbosacral** MCC CC H5 HCC
spine and pelvis

Fracture of lumbosacral spine NOS
Fracture of pelvis NOS
AHA: 2012,4Q,93
CC Excl: CC with 7th character A or MCC with 7th character
B: PDX collection 1204
CC Excl: CC with 7th character K: PDX collection 897

N Newborn: 0   P Pediatric: 0-17   M Maternity: 9-64   A Adult: 15-124   MCC Major Complication/Comorbidity   CC Complication/Comorbidity   SW Severe Wound Dx

1022   ICD-10-CM 2020

√4ᵗʰ **S33 Dislocation and sprain of joints and ligaments of lumbar spine and pelvis**

     INCLUDES avulsion of joint or ligament of lumbar spine and pelvis

     laceration of cartilage, joint or ligament of lumbar spine and pelvis

     sprain of cartilage, joint or ligament of lumbar spine and pelvis

     traumatic hemarthrosis of joint or ligament of lumbar spine and pelvis

     traumatic rupture of joint or ligament of lumbar spine and pelvis

     traumatic subluxation of joint or ligament of lumbar spine and pelvis

     traumatic tear of joint or ligament of lumbar spine and pelvis

Code also any associated open wound

     EXCLUDES 1 *nontraumatic rupture or displacement of lumbar intervertebral disc NOS (M51.-)*

     obstetric damage to pelvic joints and ligaments (O71.6)

     EXCLUDES 2 *dislocation and sprain of joints and ligaments of hip (S73.-)*

     strain of muscle of lower back and pelvis (S39.01-)

> The appropriate 7th character is to be added to each code from category S33.
> A   initial encounter
> D   subsequent encounter
> S   sequela

√x7ᵗʰ **S33.0 Traumatic rupture of lumbar intervertebral disc**

     EXCLUDES 1 *rupture or displacement (nontraumatic) of lumbar intervertebral disc NOS (M51.- with fifth character 6)*

√5ᵗʰ **S33.1 Subluxation and dislocation of lumbar vertebra**

     Code also any associated:

     open wound of abdomen, lower back and pelvis (S31)

     spinal cord injury (S24.0, S24.1-, S34.0-, S34.1-)

     EXCLUDES 2 *fracture of lumbar vertebrae (S32.0-)*

     √6ᵗʰ **S33.10 Subluxation and dislocation of unspecified lumbar vertebra**

         √7ᵗʰ **S33.100 Subluxation of unspecified lumbar vertebra**

         √7ᵗʰ **S33.101 Dislocation of unspecified lumbar vertebra**

     √6ᵗʰ **S33.11 Subluxation and dislocation of L1/L2 lumbar vertebra**

         √7ᵗʰ **S33.110 Subluxation of L1/L2 lumbar vertebra**

         √7ᵗʰ **S33.111 Dislocation of L1/L2 lumbar vertebra**

     √6ᵗʰ **S33.12 Subluxation and dislocation of L2/L3 lumbar vertebra**

         √7ᵗʰ **S33.120 Subluxation of L2/L3 lumbar vertebra**

         √7ᵗʰ **S33.121 Dislocation of L2/L3 lumbar vertebra**

     √6ᵗʰ **S33.13 Subluxation and dislocation of L3/L4 lumbar vertebra**

         √7ᵗʰ **S33.130 Subluxation of L3/L4 lumbar vertebra**

         √7ᵗʰ **S33.131 Dislocation of L3/L4 lumbar vertebra**

     √6ᵗʰ **S33.14 Subluxation and dislocation of L4/L5 lumbar vertebra**

         √7ᵗʰ **S33.140 Subluxation of L4/L5 lumbar vertebra**

         √7ᵗʰ **S33.141 Dislocation of L4/L5 lumbar vertebra**

√x7ᵗʰ **S33.2 Dislocation of sacroiliac and sacrococcygeal joint**

√5ᵗʰ **S33.3 Dislocation of other and unspecified parts of lumbar spine and pelvis**

     √x7ᵗʰ **S33.30 Dislocation of unspecified parts of lumbar spine and pelvis**

     √x7ᵗʰ **S33.39 Dislocation of other parts of lumbar spine and pelvis**

√x7ᵗʰ **S33.4 Traumatic rupture of symphysis pubis**

√x7ᵗʰ **S33.5 Sprain of ligaments of lumbar spine**

√x7ᵗʰ **S33.6 Sprain of sacroiliac joint**

√x7ᵗʰ **S33.8 Sprain of other parts of lumbar spine and pelvis**

√x7ᵗʰ **S33.9 Sprain of unspecified parts of lumbar spine and pelvis**

√4ᵗʰ **S34 Injury of lumbar and sacral spinal cord and nerves at abdomen, lower back and pelvis level**

     NOTE Code to highest level of lumbar cord injury.

     Injuries to the spinal cord (S34.0 and S34.1) refer to the cord level and not bone level injury, and can affect nerve roots at and below the level given.

Code also any associated:

     fracture of vertebra (S22.0-, S32.0-)

     open wound of abdomen, lower back and pelvis (S31.-)

     transient paralysis (R29.5)

> The appropriate 7th character is to be added to each code from category S34.
> A   initial encounter
> D   subsequent encounter
> S   sequela

CC Excl: For MCC codes in category S34, unless otherwise noted: PDX collection 1207

√5ᵗʰ **S34.0 Concussion and edema of lumbar and sacral spinal cord**

     √x7ᵗʰ **S34.01 Concussion and edema of lumbar spinal cord** `MCC` `HCC`

     √x7ᵗʰ **S34.02 Concussion and edema of sacral spinal cord** `MCC` `HCC`

         Concussion and edema of conus medullaris

         CC Excl: PDX collection 1208

√5ᵗʰ **S34.1 Other and unspecified injury of lumbar and sacral spinal cord**

     √6ᵗʰ **S34.10 Unspecified injury to lumbar spinal cord**

         √7ᵗʰ **S34.101 Unspecified injury to L1 level of lumbar spinal cord** `MCC` `H5` `HCC`

         Unspecified injury to lumbar spinal cord level 1

         √7ᵗʰ **S34.102 Unspecified injury to L2 level of lumbar spinal cord** `MCC` `H5` `HCC`

         Unspecified injury to lumbar spinal cord level 2

         √7ᵗʰ **S34.103 Unspecified injury to L3 level of lumbar spinal cord** `MCC` `H5` `HCC`

         Unspecified injury to lumbar spinal cord level 3

         √7ᵗʰ **S34.104 Unspecified injury to L4 level of lumbar spinal cord** `MCC` `H5` `HCC`

         Unspecified injury to lumbar spinal cord level 4

         √7ᵗʰ **S34.105 Unspecified injury to L5 level of lumbar spinal cord** `MCC` `H5` `HCC`

         Unspecified injury to lumbar spinal cord level 5

         √7ᵗʰ **S34.109 Unspecified injury to unspecified level of lumbar spinal cord** `MCC` `H5` `HCC`

     √6ᵗʰ **S34.11 Complete lesion of lumbar spinal cord**

         √7ᵗʰ **S34.111 Complete lesion of L1 level of lumbar spinal cord** `MCC` `H5` `HCC`

         Complete lesion of lumbar spinal cord level 1

         √7ᵗʰ **S34.112 Complete lesion of L2 level of lumbar spinal cord** `MCC` `H5` `HCC`

         Complete lesion of lumbar spinal cord level 2

         √7ᵗʰ **S34.113 Complete lesion of L3 level of lumbar spinal cord** `MCC` `H5` `HCC`

         Complete lesion of lumbar spinal cord level 3

         √7ᵗʰ **S34.114 Complete lesion of L4 level of lumbar spinal cord** `MCC` `H5` `HCC`

         Complete lesion of lumbar spinal cord level 4

         √7ᵗʰ **S34.115 Complete lesion of L5 level of lumbar spinal cord** `MCC` `H5` `HCC`

         Complete lesion of lumbar spinal cord level 5

         √7ᵗʰ **S34.119 Complete lesion of unspecified level of lumbar spinal cord** `MCC` `H5` `HCC`

☑ Additional Character Required   √x7ᵗʰ Placeholder   Unacceptable PDx   Questionable PDx   Manifestation   Unspecified Dx   H1-H14 HAC   HCC CMS-HCC Dx   HIV HIV Dx

ICD-10-CM 2020   1023

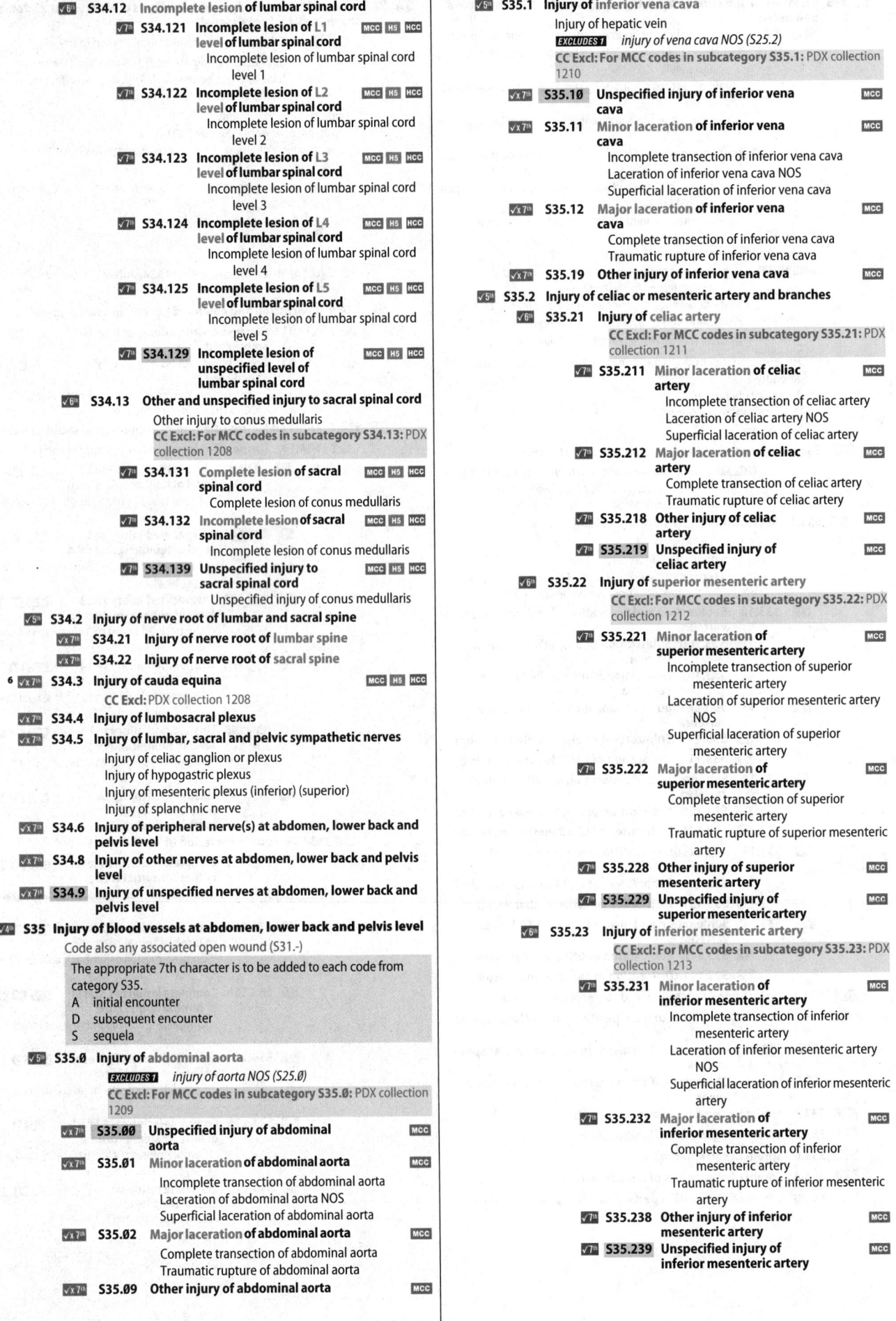

Chapter 19. Injury, Poisoning and Certain Other Consequences of External Causes

S34.12   Incomplete lesion of lumbar spinal cord

S34.121   Incomplete lesion of L1 level of lumbar spinal cord   MCC H5 HCC
    Incomplete lesion of lumbar spinal cord level 1

S34.122   Incomplete lesion of L2 level of lumbar spinal cord   MCC H5 HCC
    Incomplete lesion of lumbar spinal cord level 2

S34.123   Incomplete lesion of L3 level of lumbar spinal cord   MCC H5 HCC
    Incomplete lesion of lumbar spinal cord level 3

S34.124   Incomplete lesion of L4 level of lumbar spinal cord   MCC H5 HCC
    Incomplete lesion of lumbar spinal cord level 4

S34.125   Incomplete lesion of L5 level of lumbar spinal cord   MCC H5 HCC
    Incomplete lesion of lumbar spinal cord level 5

S34.129   Incomplete lesion of unspecified level of lumbar spinal cord   MCC H5 HCC

S34.13   Other and unspecified injury to sacral spinal cord
    Other injury to conus medullaris
    CC Excl: For MCC codes in subcategory S34.13: PDX collection 1208

S34.131   Complete lesion of sacral spinal cord   MCC H5 HCC
    Complete lesion of conus medullaris

S34.132   Incomplete lesion of sacral spinal cord   MCC H5 HCC
    Incomplete lesion of conus medullaris

S34.139   Unspecified injury to sacral spinal cord   MCC H5 HCC
    Unspecified injury of conus medullaris

S34.2   Injury of nerve root of lumbar and sacral spine

S34.21   Injury of nerve root of lumbar spine

S34.22   Injury of nerve root of sacral spine

S34.3   Injury of cauda equina   MCC H5 HCC
    CC Excl: PDX collection 1208

S34.4   Injury of lumbosacral plexus

S34.5   Injury of lumbar, sacral and pelvic sympathetic nerves
    Injury of celiac ganglion or plexus
    Injury of hypogastric plexus
    Injury of mesenteric plexus (inferior) (superior)
    Injury of splanchnic nerve

S34.6   Injury of peripheral nerve(s) at abdomen, lower back and pelvis level

S34.8   Injury of other nerves at abdomen, lower back and pelvis level

S34.9   Injury of unspecified nerves at abdomen, lower back and pelvis level

S35   Injury of blood vessels at abdomen, lower back and pelvis level
    Code also any associated open wound (S31.-)

The appropriate 7th character is to be added to each code from category S35.
    A   initial encounter
    D   subsequent encounter
    S   sequela

S35.0   Injury of abdominal aorta
    EXCLUDES 1   injury of aorta NOS (S25.0)
    CC Excl: For MCC codes in subcategory S35.0: PDX collection 1209

S35.00   Unspecified injury of abdominal aorta   MCC

S35.01   Minor laceration of abdominal aorta   MCC
    Incomplete transection of abdominal aorta
    Laceration of abdominal aorta NOS
    Superficial laceration of abdominal aorta

S35.02   Major laceration of abdominal aorta   MCC
    Complete transection of abdominal aorta
    Traumatic rupture of abdominal aorta

S35.09   Other injury of abdominal aorta   MCC

S35.1   Injury of inferior vena cava
    Injury of hepatic vein
    EXCLUDES 1   injury of vena cava NOS (S25.2)
    CC Excl: For MCC codes in subcategory S35.1: PDX collection 1210

S35.10   Unspecified injury of inferior vena cava   MCC

S35.11   Minor laceration of inferior vena cava   MCC
    Incomplete transection of inferior vena cava
    Laceration of inferior vena cava NOS
    Superficial laceration of inferior vena cava

S35.12   Major laceration of inferior vena cava   MCC
    Complete transection of inferior vena cava
    Traumatic rupture of inferior vena cava

S35.19   Other injury of inferior vena cava   MCC

S35.2   Injury of celiac or mesenteric artery and branches

S35.21   Injury of celiac artery
    CC Excl: For MCC codes in subcategory S35.21: PDX collection 1211

S35.211   Minor laceration of celiac artery   MCC
    Incomplete transection of celiac artery
    Laceration of celiac artery NOS
    Superficial laceration of celiac artery

S35.212   Major laceration of celiac artery   MCC
    Complete transection of celiac artery
    Traumatic rupture of celiac artery

S35.218   Other injury of celiac artery   MCC

S35.219   Unspecified injury of celiac artery   MCC

S35.22   Injury of superior mesenteric artery
    CC Excl: For MCC codes in subcategory S35.22: PDX collection 1212

S35.221   Minor laceration of superior mesenteric artery   MCC
    Incomplete transection of superior mesenteric artery
    Laceration of superior mesenteric artery NOS
    Superficial laceration of superior mesenteric artery

S35.222   Major laceration of superior mesenteric artery   MCC
    Complete transection of superior mesenteric artery
    Traumatic rupture of superior mesenteric artery

S35.228   Other injury of superior mesenteric artery   MCC

S35.229   Unspecified injury of superior mesenteric artery   MCC

S35.23   Injury of inferior mesenteric artery
    CC Excl: For MCC codes in subcategory S35.23: PDX collection 1213

S35.231   Minor laceration of inferior mesenteric artery   MCC
    Incomplete transection of inferior mesenteric artery
    Laceration of inferior mesenteric artery NOS
    Superficial laceration of inferior mesenteric artery

S35.232   Major laceration of inferior mesenteric artery   MCC
    Complete transection of inferior mesenteric artery
    Traumatic rupture of inferior mesenteric artery

S35.238   Other injury of inferior mesenteric artery   MCC

S35.239   Unspecified injury of inferior mesenteric artery   MCC

N Newborn: 0   P Pediatric: 0-17   M Maternity: 9-64   A Adult: 15-124   MCC Major Complication/Comorbidity   CC Complication/Comorbidity   SW Severe Wound Dx

1024   ICD-10-CM 2020

√6ᵗʰ S35.29 Injury of branches of celiac and mesenteric artery
Injury of gastric artery
Injury of gastroduodenal artery
Injury of hepatic artery
Injury of splenic artery

√7ᵗʰ S35.291 Minor laceration of branches of celiac and mesenteric artery `MCC`
Incomplete transection of branches of celiac and mesenteric artery
Laceration of branches of celiac and mesenteric artery NOS
Superficial laceration of branches of celiac and mesenteric artery
CC Excl: PDX collection 1214

√7ᵗʰ S35.292 Major laceration of branches of celiac and mesenteric artery `MCC`
Complete transection of branches of celiac and mesenteric artery
Traumatic rupture of branches of celiac and mesenteric artery
CC Excl: PDX collection 1215

√7ᵗʰ S35.298 Other injury of branches of celiac and mesenteric artery `MCC`
CC Excl: PDX collection 1215

√7ᵗʰ S35.299 Unspecified injury of branches of celiac and mesenteric artery `MCC`
CC Excl: PDX collection 1216

√5ᵗʰ S35.3 Injury of portal or splenic vein and branches

√6ᵗʰ S35.31 Injury of portal vein
CC Excl: For MCC codes in subcategory S35.31: PDX collection 1217

√7ᵗʰ S35.311 Laceration of portal vein `MCC`
√7ᵗʰ S35.318 Other specified injury of portal vein `MCC`
√7ᵗʰ S35.319 Unspecified injury of portal vein `MCC`

√6ᵗʰ S35.32 Injury of splenic vein
CC Excl: For MCC codes in subcategory S35.32: PDX collection 1218

√7ᵗʰ S35.321 Laceration of splenic vein `MCC`
√7ᵗʰ S35.328 Other specified injury of splenic vein `MCC`
√7ᵗʰ S35.329 Unspecified injury of splenic vein `MCC`

√6ᵗʰ S35.33 Injury of superior mesenteric vein
CC Excl: For MCC codes in subcategory S35.33: PDX collection 1219

√7ᵗʰ S35.331 Laceration of superior mesenteric vein `MCC`
√7ᵗʰ S35.338 Other specified injury of superior mesenteric vein `MCC`
√7ᵗʰ S35.339 Unspecified injury of superior mesenteric vein `MCC`

√6ᵗʰ S35.34 Injury of inferior mesenteric vein
CC Excl: For MCC codes in subcategory S35.34: PDX collection 1220

√7ᵗʰ S35.341 Laceration of inferior mesenteric vein `MCC`
√7ᵗʰ S35.348 Other specified injury of inferior mesenteric vein `MCC`
√7ᵗʰ S35.349 Unspecified injury of inferior mesenteric vein `MCC`

√5ᵗʰ S35.4 Injury of renal blood vessels
CC Excl: For MCC codes in subcategory S35.4, unless otherwise noted: PDX collection 1221

√6ᵗʰ S35.40 Unspecified injury of renal blood vessel
√7ᵗʰ S35.401 Unspecified injury of right renal artery `MCC`
√7ᵗʰ S35.402 Unspecified injury of left renal artery `MCC`
√7ᵗʰ S35.403 Unspecified injury of unspecified renal artery `MCC`
√7ᵗʰ S35.404 Unspecified injury of right renal vein `MCC`
CC Excl: PDX collection 1222
√7ᵗʰ S35.405 Unspecified injury of left renal vein `MCC`
CC Excl: PDX collection 1222
√7ᵗʰ S35.406 Unspecified injury of unspecified renal vein `MCC`
CC Excl: PDX collection 1222

√6ᵗʰ S35.41 Laceration of renal blood vessel
√7ᵗʰ S35.411 Laceration of right renal artery `MCC`
√7ᵗʰ S35.412 Laceration of left renal artery `MCC`
√7ᵗʰ S35.413 Laceration of unspecified renal artery `MCC`
√7ᵗʰ S35.414 Laceration of right renal vein `MCC`
CC Excl: PDX collection 1222
√7ᵗʰ S35.415 Laceration of left renal vein `MCC`
CC Excl: PDX collection 1222
√7ᵗʰ S35.416 Laceration of unspecified renal vein `MCC`
CC Excl: PDX collection 1222

√6ᵗʰ S35.49 Other specified injury of renal blood vessel
√7ᵗʰ S35.491 Other specified injury of right renal artery `MCC`
√7ᵗʰ S35.492 Other specified injury of left renal artery `MCC`
√7ᵗʰ S35.493 Other specified injury of unspecified renal artery `MCC`
√7ᵗʰ S35.494 Other specified injury of right renal vein `MCC`
CC Excl: PDX collection 1222
√7ᵗʰ S35.495 Other specified injury of left renal vein `MCC`
CC Excl: PDX collection 1222
√7ᵗʰ S35.496 Other specified injury of unspecified renal vein `MCC`
CC Excl: PDX collection 1222

√5ᵗʰ S35.5 Injury of iliac blood vessels
√x7ᵗʰ S35.50 Injury of unspecified iliac blood vessel(s) `MCC`
CC Excl: PDX collection 1223

√6ᵗʰ S35.51 Injury of iliac artery or vein
Injury of hypogastric artery or vein
√7ᵗʰ S35.511 Injury of right iliac artery `MCC`
CC Excl: PDX collection 1224
√7ᵗʰ S35.512 Injury of left iliac artery `MCC`
CC Excl: PDX collection 1224
√7ᵗʰ S35.513 Injury of unspecified iliac artery `MCC`
CC Excl: PDX collection 1224
√7ᵗʰ S35.514 Injury of right iliac vein `MCC`
CC Excl: PDX collection 1225
√7ᵗʰ S35.515 Injury of left iliac vein `MCC`
CC Excl: PDX collection 1225
√7ᵗʰ S35.516 Injury of unspecified iliac vein `MCC`
CC Excl: PDX collection 1225

√6ᵗʰ S35.53 Injury of uterine artery or vein
√7ᵗʰ S35.531 Injury of right uterine artery `CC` ♀
CC Excl: PDX collection 1226
√7ᵗʰ S35.532 Injury of left uterine artery `CC` ♀
CC Excl: PDX collection 1226
√7ᵗʰ S35.533 Injury of unspecified uterine artery `CC` ♀
CC Excl: PDX collection 1226
√7ᵗʰ S35.534 Injury of right uterine vein `CC` ♀
CC Excl: PDX collection 1227
√7ᵗʰ S35.535 Injury of left uterine vein `CC` ♀
CC Excl: PDX collection 1227
√7ᵗʰ S35.536 Injury of unspecified uterine vein `CC` ♀
CC Excl: PDX collection 1227

√x7ᵗʰ S35.59 Injury of other iliac blood vessels `MCC`
CC Excl: PDX collection 1223

Chapter 19. Injury, Poisoning and Certain Other Consequences of External Causes

S35.8–S36.241

√5ᵗʰ **S35.8** **Injury of other blood vessels at abdomen, lower back and pelvis level**
     Injury of ovarian artery or vein

√6ᵗʰ **S35.8X** **Injury of other blood vessels at abdomen, lower back and pelvis level**
     CC Excl: For CC codes in subcategory S35.8X: PDX collection 1228

√7ᵗʰ **S35.8X1** Laceration of other blood vessels at abdomen, lower back and pelvis level   `CC`

√7ᵗʰ **S35.8X8** Other specified injury of other blood vessels at abdomen, lower back and pelvis level   `CC`

√7ᵗʰ **S35.8X9** Unspecified injury of other blood vessels at abdomen, lower back and pelvis level   `CC`

√5ᵗʰ **S35.9** **Injury of unspecified blood vessel at abdomen, lower back and pelvis level**
     CC Excl: For CC codes in subcategory S35.9: PDX collection 1229

√x7ᵗʰ **S35.90** **Unspecified injury of unspecified blood vessel at abdomen, lower back and pelvis level**   `CC`

√x7ᵗʰ **S35.91** **Laceration of unspecified blood vessel at abdomen, lower back and pelvis level**   `CC`

√x7ᵗʰ **S35.99** **Other specified injury of unspecified blood vessel at abdomen, lower back and pelvis level**   `CC`

√4ᵗʰ **S36** **Injury of intra-abdominal organs**
     Code also any associated open wound (S31.-)

     The appropriate 7th character is to be added to each code from category S36.
     A   initial encounter
     D   subsequent encounter
     S   sequela

√5ᵗʰ **S36.0** **Injury of spleen**
     AHA: 2015,2Q,36; 2015,1Q,10
     CC Excl: For CC/MCC codes in subcategory S36.0: PDX collection 1230

√x7ᵗʰ **S36.00** **Unspecified injury of spleen**   `CC`

√6ᵗʰ **S36.02** **Contusion of spleen**
     TIP: When both traumatic splenic laceration and contusion are documented in the same encounter, code only the laceration, as contusions are not coded when they occur with a more severe injury in the same body site.

√7ᵗʰ **S36.020** Minor contusion of spleen   `CC`
     Contusion of spleen less than 2 cm

√7ᵗʰ **S36.021** Major contusion of spleen   `CC`
     Contusion of spleen greater than 2 cm

√7ᵗʰ **S36.029** Unspecified contusion of spleen   `CC`

√6ᵗʰ **S36.03** **Laceration of spleen**
     TIP: When both traumatic splenic laceration and contusion are documented in the same encounter, code only the laceration, as contusions are not coded when they occur with a more severe injury in the same body site.

√7ᵗʰ **S36.030** Superficial (capsular) laceration of spleen   `CC`
     Laceration of spleen less than 1 cm
     Minor laceration of spleen

√7ᵗʰ **S36.031** Moderate laceration of spleen   `MCC`
     Laceration of spleen 1 to 3 cm

√7ᵗʰ **S36.032** Major laceration of spleen   `MCC`
     Avulsion of spleen
     Laceration of spleen greater than 3 cm
     Massive laceration of spleen
     Multiple moderate lacerations of spleen
     Stellate laceration of spleen

√7ᵗʰ **S36.039** Unspecified laceration of spleen   `CC`

√x7ᵗʰ **S36.09** **Other injury of spleen**   `CC`

√5ᵗʰ **S36.1** **Injury of liver and gallbladder and bile duct**

√6ᵗʰ **S36.11** **Injury of liver**
     CC Excl: For CC/MCC codes in subcategory S36.11: PDX collection 1231

√7ᵗʰ **S36.112** Contusion of liver   `CC`

√7ᵗʰ **S36.113** Laceration of liver, unspecified degree   `CC`

√7ᵗʰ **S36.114** Minor laceration of liver   `CC`
     Laceration involving capsule only, or, without significant involvement of hepatic parenchyma [i.e., less than 1 cm deep]

√7ᵗʰ **S36.115** Moderate laceration of liver   `MCC`
     Laceration involving parenchyma but without major disruption of parenchyma [i.e., less than 10 cm long and less than 3 cm deep]

√7ᵗʰ **S36.116** Major laceration of liver   `MCC`
     Laceration with significant disruption of hepatic parenchyma [i.e., greater than 10 cm long and 3 cm deep]
     Multiple moderate lacerations, with or without hematoma
     Stellate laceration of liver

√7ᵗʰ **S36.118** Other injury of liver   `CC`

√7ᵗʰ **S36.119** Unspecified injury of liver   `CC`

√6ᵗʰ **S36.12** **Injury of gallbladder**
     CC Excl: For CC codes in subcategory S36.12: PDX collection 1232

√7ᵗʰ **S36.122** Contusion of gallbladder   `CC`

√7ᵗʰ **S36.123** Laceration of gallbladder   `CC`

√7ᵗʰ **S36.128** Other injury of gallbladder   `CC`

√7ᵗʰ **S36.129** Unspecified injury of gallbladder   `CC`

√x7ᵗʰ **S36.13** **Injury of bile duct**   `CC`
     CC Excl: PDX collection 1232

√5ᵗʰ **S36.2** **Injury of pancreas**
     CC Excl: For CC codes in subcategory S36.2: PDX collection 1233

√6ᵗʰ **S36.20** **Unspecified injury of pancreas**

√7ᵗʰ **S36.200** Unspecified injury of head of pancreas   `CC`

√7ᵗʰ **S36.201** Unspecified injury of body of pancreas   `CC`

√7ᵗʰ **S36.202** Unspecified injury of tail of pancreas   `CC`

√7ᵗʰ **S36.209** Unspecified injury of unspecified part of pancreas   `CC`

√6ᵗʰ **S36.22** **Contusion of pancreas**

√7ᵗʰ **S36.220** Contusion of head of pancreas   `CC`

√7ᵗʰ **S36.221** Contusion of body of pancreas   `CC`

√7ᵗʰ **S36.222** Contusion of tail of pancreas   `CC`

√7ᵗʰ **S36.229** Contusion of unspecified part of pancreas   `CC`

√6ᵗʰ **S36.23** **Laceration of pancreas, unspecified degree**

√7ᵗʰ **S36.230** Laceration of head of pancreas, unspecified degree   `CC`

√7ᵗʰ **S36.231** Laceration of body of pancreas, unspecified degree   `CC`

√7ᵗʰ **S36.232** Laceration of tail of pancreas, unspecified degree   `CC`

√7ᵗʰ **S36.239** Laceration of unspecified part of pancreas, unspecified degree   `CC`

√6ᵗʰ **S36.24** **Minor laceration of pancreas**

√7ᵗʰ **S36.240** Minor laceration of head of pancreas   `CC`

√7ᵗʰ **S36.241** Minor laceration of body of pancreas   `CC`

√7ᵗʰ **S36.242** Minor laceration of tail of pancreas CC

√7ᵗʰ **S36.249** Minor laceration of unspecified part of pancreas CC

√6ᵗʰ **S36.25** Moderate laceration of pancreas

√7ᵗʰ **S36.250** Moderate laceration of head of pancreas CC

√7ᵗʰ **S36.251** Moderate laceration of body of pancreas CC

√7ᵗʰ **S36.252** Moderate laceration of tail of pancreas CC

√7ᵗʰ **S36.259** Moderate laceration of unspecified part of pancreas CC

√6ᵗʰ **S36.26** Major laceration of pancreas

√7ᵗʰ **S36.260** Major laceration of head of pancreas CC

√7ᵗʰ **S36.261** Major laceration of body of pancreas CC

√7ᵗʰ **S36.262** Major laceration of tail of pancreas CC

√7ᵗʰ **S36.269** Major laceration of unspecified part of pancreas CC

√6ᵗʰ **S36.29** Other injury of pancreas

√7ᵗʰ **S36.290** Other injury of head of pancreas CC

√7ᵗʰ **S36.291** Other injury of body of pancreas CC

√7ᵗʰ **S36.292** Other injury of tail of pancreas CC

√7ᵗʰ **S36.299** Other injury of unspecified part of pancreas CC

√5ᵗʰ **S36.3** Injury of stomach

CC Excl: For CC codes in subcategory S36.3: PDX collection 1234

√x7ᵗʰ **S36.30** Unspecified injury of stomach CC

√x7ᵗʰ **S36.32** Contusion of stomach CC

√x7ᵗʰ **S36.33** Laceration of stomach CC

√x7ᵗʰ **S36.39** Other injury of stomach CC

√5ᵗʰ **S36.4** Injury of small intestine

CC Excl: For CC codes in subcategory S36.4: PDX collection 1235

√6ᵗʰ **S36.40** Unspecified injury of small intestine

√7ᵗʰ **S36.400** Unspecified injury of duodenum CC

√7ᵗʰ **S36.408** Unspecified injury of other part of small intestine CC

√7ᵗʰ **S36.409** Unspecified injury of unspecified part of small intestine CC

√6ᵗʰ **S36.41** Primary blast injury of small intestine

Blast injury of small intestine NOS

√7ᵗʰ **S36.410** Primary blast injury of duodenum CC

√7ᵗʰ **S36.418** Primary blast injury of other part of small intestine CC

√7ᵗʰ **S36.419** Primary blast injury of unspecified part of small intestine CC

√6ᵗʰ **S36.42** Contusion of small intestine

√7ᵗʰ **S36.420** Contusion of duodenum CC

√7ᵗʰ **S36.428** Contusion of other part of small intestine CC

√7ᵗʰ **S36.429** Contusion of unspecified part of small intestine CC

√6ᵗʰ **S36.43** Laceration of small intestine

√7ᵗʰ **S36.430** Laceration of duodenum CC

√7ᵗʰ **S36.438** Laceration of other part of small intestine CC

√7ᵗʰ **S36.439** Laceration of unspecified part of small intestine CC

√6ᵗʰ **S36.49** Other injury of small intestine

√7ᵗʰ **S36.490** Other injury of duodenum CC

√7ᵗʰ **S36.498** Other injury of other part of small intestine CC

√7ᵗʰ **S36.499** Other injury of unspecified part of small intestine CC

√5ᵗʰ **S36.5** Injury of colon

EXCLUDES 2 injury of rectum (S36.6-)

CC Excl: For CC codes in subcategory S36.5: PDX collection 1236

√6ᵗʰ **S36.50** Unspecified injury of colon

√7ᵗʰ **S36.500** Unspecified injury of ascending [right] colon CC

√7ᵗʰ **S36.501** Unspecified injury of transverse colon CC

√7ᵗʰ **S36.502** Unspecified injury of descending [left] colon CC

√7ᵗʰ **S36.503** Unspecified injury of sigmoid colon CC

√7ᵗʰ **S36.508** Unspecified injury of other part of colon CC

√7ᵗʰ **S36.509** Unspecified injury of unspecified part of colon CC

√6ᵗʰ **S36.51** Primary blast injury of colon

Blast injury of colon NOS

√7ᵗʰ **S36.510** Primary blast injury of ascending [right] colon CC

√7ᵗʰ **S36.511** Primary blast injury of transverse colon CC

√7ᵗʰ **S36.512** Primary blast injury of descending [left] colon CC

√7ᵗʰ **S36.513** Primary blast injury of sigmoid colon CC

√7ᵗʰ **S36.518** Primary blast injury of other part of colon CC

√7ᵗʰ **S36.519** Primary blast injury of unspecified part of colon CC

√6ᵗʰ **S36.52** Contusion of colon

√7ᵗʰ **S36.520** Contusion of ascending [right] colon CC

√7ᵗʰ **S36.521** Contusion of transverse colon CC

√7ᵗʰ **S36.522** Contusion of descending [left] colon CC

√7ᵗʰ **S36.523** Contusion of sigmoid colon CC

√7ᵗʰ **S36.528** Contusion of other part of colon CC

√7ᵗʰ **S36.529** Contusion of unspecified part of colon CC

√6ᵗʰ **S36.53** Laceration of colon

√7ᵗʰ **S36.530** Laceration of ascending [right] colon CC

√7ᵗʰ **S36.531** Laceration of transverse colon CC

√7ᵗʰ **S36.532** Laceration of descending [left] colon CC

√7ᵗʰ **S36.533** Laceration of sigmoid colon CC

√7ᵗʰ **S36.538** Laceration of other part of colon CC

√7ᵗʰ **S36.539** Laceration of unspecified part of colon CC

√6ᵗʰ **S36.59** Other injury of colon

Secondary blast injury of colon

√7ᵗʰ **S36.590** Other injury of ascending [right] colon CC

√7ᵗʰ **S36.591** Other injury of transverse colon CC

√7ᵗʰ **S36.592** Other injury of descending [left] colon CC

√7ᵗʰ **S36.593** Other injury of sigmoid colon CC

√7ᵗʰ **S36.598** Other injury of other part of colon CC

√7ᵗʰ **S36.599** Other injury of unspecified part of colon CC

√5ᵗʰ **S36.6** Injury of rectum

CC Excl: For CC codes in subcategory S36.6: PDX collection 1236

√x7ᵗʰ **S36.60** Unspecified injury of rectum CC

√x7ᵗʰ **S36.61** Primary blast injury of rectum CC

Blast injury of rectum NOS

√x7ᵗʰ **S36.62** Contusion of rectum CC

☑ Additional Character Required √x7ᵗʰ Placeholder Unacceptable PDx Questionable PDx Manifestation Unspecified Dx H1 -H14 HAC HCC CMS-HCC Dx HIV HIV Dx

√x7ᵗʰ **S36.63** Laceration of rectum   `CC`

√x7ᵗʰ **S36.69** Other injury of rectum   `CC`

    Secondary blast injury of rectum

√6ᵗʰ **S36.8** Injury of other intra-abdominal organs

> **CC Excl:** For CC codes in subcategory S36.8: PDX collection 1195

√x7ᵗʰ **S36.81** Injury of peritoneum   `CC`

√6ᵗʰ **S36.89** Injury of other intra-abdominal organs

    Injury of retroperitoneum

√7ᵗʰ **S36.892** Contusion of other intra-abdominal organs   `CC`

√7ᵗʰ **S36.893** Laceration of other intra-abdominal organs   `CC`

√7ᵗʰ **S36.898** Other injury of other intra-abdominal organs   `CC`

√7ᵗʰ **S36.899** Unspecified injury of other intra-abdominal organs   `CC`

√5ᵗʰ **S36.9** Injury of unspecified intra-abdominal organ

> **CC Excl:** For CC codes in subcategory S36.9: PDX collection 1195

√x7ᵗʰ **S36.90** Unspecified injury of unspecified intra-abdominal organ   `CC`

√x7ᵗʰ **S36.92** Contusion of unspecified intra-abdominal organ   `CC`

√x7ᵗʰ **S36.93** Laceration of unspecified intra-abdominal organ   `CC`

√x7ᵗʰ **S36.99** Other injury of unspecified intra-abdominal organ   `CC`

√4ᵗʰ **S37** **Injury of urinary and pelvic organs**

    Code also any associated open wound (S31.-)

> **EXCLUDES 1**   obstetric trauma to pelvic organs (O71.-)
> **EXCLUDES 2**   injury of peritoneum (S36.81)
>   injury of retroperitoneum (S36.89-)

> The appropriate 7th character is to be added to each code from category S37.
> A   initial encounter
> D   subsequent encounter
> S   sequela

√5ᵗʰ **S37.0** Injury of kidney

> **EXCLUDES 2**   acute kidney injury (nontraumatic) (N17.9)
> **CC Excl:** For CC/MCC codes in subcategory S37.0: PDX collection 1237

√6ᵗʰ **S37.00** Unspecified injury of kidney

√7ᵗʰ **S37.001** Unspecified injury of right kidney   `CC`

√7ᵗʰ **S37.002** Unspecified injury of left kidney   `CC`

√7ᵗʰ **S37.009** Unspecified injury of unspecified kidney   `CC`

√6ᵗʰ **S37.01** Minor contusion of kidney

    Contusion of kidney less than 2 cm
    Contusion of kidney NOS

√7ᵗʰ **S37.011** Minor contusion of right kidney   `CC`

√7ᵗʰ **S37.012** Minor contusion of left kidney   `CC`

√7ᵗʰ **S37.019** Minor contusion of unspecified kidney   `CC`

√6ᵗʰ **S37.02** Major contusion of kidney

    Contusion of kidney greater than 2 cm

√7ᵗʰ **S37.021** Major contusion of right kidney   `CC`

√7ᵗʰ **S37.022** Major contusion of left kidney   `CC`

√7ᵗʰ **S37.029** Major contusion of unspecified kidney   `CC`

√6ᵗʰ **S37.03** Laceration of kidney, unspecified degree

√7ᵗʰ **S37.031** Laceration of right kidney, unspecified degree   `CC`

√7ᵗʰ **S37.032** Laceration of left kidney, unspecified degree   `CC`

√7ᵗʰ **S37.039** Laceration of unspecified kidney, unspecified degree   `CC`

√6ᵗʰ **S37.04** Minor laceration of kidney

    Laceration of kidney less than 1 cm

√7ᵗʰ **S37.041** Minor laceration of right kidney   `CC`

√7ᵗʰ **S37.042** Minor laceration of left kidney   `CC`

√7ᵗʰ **S37.049** Minor laceration of unspecified kidney   `CC`

√6ᵗʰ **S37.05** Moderate laceration of kidney

    Laceration of kidney 1 to 3 cm

√7ᵗʰ **S37.051** Moderate laceration of right kidney   `CC`

√7ᵗʰ **S37.052** Moderate laceration of left kidney   `CC`

√7ᵗʰ **S37.059** Moderate laceration of unspecified kidney   `CC`

√6ᵗʰ **S37.06** Major laceration of kidney

    Avulsion of kidney
    Laceration of kidney greater than 3 cm
    Massive laceration of kidney
    Multiple moderate lacerations of kidney
    Stellate laceration of kidney

√7ᵗʰ **S37.061** Major laceration of right kidney   `MCC`

√7ᵗʰ **S37.062** Major laceration of left kidney   `MCC`

√7ᵗʰ **S37.069** Major laceration of unspecified kidney   `MCC`

√6ᵗʰ **S37.09** Other injury of kidney

√7ᵗʰ **S37.091** Other injury of right kidney   `MCC`

√7ᵗʰ **S37.092** Other injury of left kidney   `MCC`

√7ᵗʰ **S37.099** Other injury of unspecified kidney   `MCC`

√5ᵗʰ **S37.1** Injury of ureter

> **CC Excl:** For CC codes in subcategory S37.1: PDX collection 1238

√x7ᵗʰ **S37.10** Unspecified injury of ureter   `CC`

√x7ᵗʰ **S37.12** Contusion of ureter   `CC`

√x7ᵗʰ **S37.13** Laceration of ureter   `CC`

√x7ᵗʰ **S37.19** Other injury of ureter   `CC`

√5ᵗʰ **S37.2** Injury of bladder

> **CC Excl:** For CC codes in subcategory S37.2: PDX collection 1239

√x7ᵗʰ **S37.20** Unspecified injury of bladder   `CC`

√x7ᵗʰ **S37.22** Contusion of bladder   `CC`

√x7ᵗʰ **S37.23** Laceration of bladder   `CC`

√x7ᵗʰ **S37.29** Other injury of bladder   `CC`

√5ᵗʰ **S37.3** Injury of urethra

> **CC Excl:** For CC codes in subcategory S37.3: PDX collection 1239

√x7ᵗʰ **S37.30** Unspecified injury of urethra   `CC`

√x7ᵗʰ **S37.32** Contusion of urethra   `CC`

√x7ᵗʰ **S37.33** Laceration of urethra   `CC`

√x7ᵗʰ **S37.39** Other injury of urethra   `CC`

√5ᵗʰ **S37.4** Injury of ovary

√6ᵗʰ **S37.40** Unspecified injury of ovary

√7ᵗʰ **S37.401** Unspecified injury of ovary, unilateral   ♀

√7ᵗʰ **S37.402** Unspecified injury of ovary, bilateral   ♀

√7ᵗʰ **S37.409** Unspecified injury of ovary, unspecified   ♀

√6ᵗʰ **S37.42** Contusion of ovary

√7ᵗʰ **S37.421** Contusion of ovary, unilateral   ♀

√7ᵗʰ **S37.422** Contusion of ovary, bilateral   ♀

√7ᵗʰ **S37.429** Contusion of ovary, unspecified   ♀

√6ᵗʰ **S37.43** Laceration of ovary

√7ᵗʰ **S37.431** Laceration of ovary, unilateral   ♀

√7ᵗʰ **S37.432** Laceration of ovary, bilateral   ♀

N Newborn: 0   **P** Pediatric: 0-17   **M** Maternity: 9-64   **A** Adult: 15-124   **MCC** Major Complication/Comorbidity   **CC** Complication/Comorbidity   **SW** Severe Wound Dx

1028   ICD-10-CM 2020

     √7ᵗʰ **S37.439** Laceration of ovary, unspecified ♀

   √6ᵗʰ **S37.49** Other injury of ovary

     √7ᵗʰ **S37.491** Other injury of ovary, unilateral ♀

     √7ᵗʰ **S37.492** Other injury of ovary, bilateral ♀

     √7ᵗʰ **S37.499** Other injury of ovary, unspecified ♀

√5ᵗʰ **S37.5** Injury of fallopian tube

   √6ᵗʰ **S37.50** Unspecified injury of fallopian tube

     √7ᵗʰ **S37.501** Unspecified injury of fallopian tube, unilateral ♀

     √7ᵗʰ **S37.502** Unspecified injury of fallopian tube, bilateral ♀

     √7ᵗʰ **S37.509** Unspecified injury of fallopian tube, unspecified ♀

   √6ᵗʰ **S37.51** Primary blast injury of fallopian tube

     Blast injury of fallopian tube NOS

     √7ᵗʰ **S37.511** Primary blast injury of fallopian tube, unilateral ♀

     √7ᵗʰ **S37.512** Primary blast injury of fallopian tube, bilateral ♀

     √7ᵗʰ **S37.519** Primary blast injury of fallopian tube, unspecified ♀

   √6ᵗʰ **S37.52** Contusion of fallopian tube

     √7ᵗʰ **S37.521** Contusion of fallopian tube, unilateral ♀

     √7ᵗʰ **S37.522** Contusion of fallopian tube, bilateral ♀

     √7ᵗʰ **S37.529** Contusion of fallopian tube, unspecified ♀

   √6ᵗʰ **S37.53** Laceration of fallopian tube

     √7ᵗʰ **S37.531** Laceration of fallopian tube, unilateral ♀

     √7ᵗʰ **S37.532** Laceration of fallopian tube, bilateral ♀

     √7ᵗʰ **S37.539** Laceration of fallopian tube, unspecified ♀

   √6ᵗʰ **S37.59** Other injury of fallopian tube

     Secondary blast injury of fallopian tube

     √7ᵗʰ **S37.591** Other injury of fallopian tube, unilateral ♀

     √7ᵗʰ **S37.592** Other injury of fallopian tube, bilateral ♀

     √7ᵗʰ **S37.599** Other injury of fallopian tube, unspecified ♀

√5ᵗʰ **S37.6** Injury of uterus

   EXCLUDES 1 injury to gravid uterus (O9A.2-)

     injury to uterus during delivery (O71.-)

   CC Excl: For CC codes in subcategory S37.6: PDX collection 1240

   √x7ᵗʰ **S37.60** Unspecified injury of uterus CC ♀

   √x7ᵗʰ **S37.62** Contusion of uterus CC ♀

   √x7ᵗʰ **S37.63** Laceration of uterus CC ♀

   √x7ᵗʰ **S37.69** Other injury of uterus CC ♀

√5ᵗʰ **S37.8** Injury of other urinary and pelvic organs

   √6ᵗʰ **S37.81** Injury of adrenal gland

     CC Excl: For CC codes in subcategory S37.81: PDX collection 1241

     √7ᵗʰ **S37.812** Contusion of adrenal gland CC

     √7ᵗʰ **S37.813** Laceration of adrenal gland CC

     √7ᵗʰ **S37.818** Other injury of adrenal gland CC

     √7ᵗʰ **S37.819** Unspecified injury of adrenal gland CC

   √6ᵗʰ **S37.82** Injury of prostate

     √7ᵗʰ **S37.822** Contusion of prostate ♂

     √7ᵗʰ **S37.823** Laceration of prostate ♂

     √7ᵗʰ **S37.828** Other injury of prostate ♂

     √7ᵗʰ **S37.829** Unspecified injury of prostate ♂

   √6ᵗʰ **S37.89** Injury of other urinary and pelvic organ

     CC Excl: For CC codes in subcategory S37.89: PDX collection 1242

     √7ᵗʰ **S37.892** Contusion of other urinary and pelvic organ CC

     √7ᵗʰ **S37.893** Laceration of other urinary and pelvic organ CC

     √7ᵗʰ **S37.898** Other injury of other urinary and pelvic organ CC

     √7ᵗʰ **S37.899** Unspecified injury of other urinary and pelvic organ CC

√5ᵗʰ **S37.9** Injury of unspecified urinary and pelvic organ

   CC Excl: For CC codes in subcategory S37.9: PDX collection 1242

   √x7ᵗʰ **S37.90** Unspecified injury of unspecified urinary and pelvic organ CC

   √x7ᵗʰ **S37.92** Contusion of unspecified urinary and pelvic organ CC

   √x7ᵗʰ **S37.93** Laceration of unspecified urinary and pelvic organ CC

   √x7ᵗʰ **S37.99** Other injury of unspecified urinary and pelvic organ CC

√4ᵗʰ **S38** Crushing injury and traumatic amputation of abdomen, lower back, pelvis and external genitals

   NOTE An amputation not identified as partial or complete should be coded to complete

   The appropriate 7th character is to be added to each code from category S38.

   A   initial encounter

   D   subsequent encounter

   S   sequela

√5ᵗʰ **S38.0** Crushing injury of external genital organs

   Use additional code for any associated injuries

   √6ᵗʰ **S38.00** Crushing injury of unspecified external genital organs

     √7ᵗʰ **S38.001** Crushing injury of unspecified external genital organs, male ♂

     √7ᵗʰ **S38.002** Crushing injury of unspecified external genital organs, female ♀

   √x7ᵗʰ **S38.01** Crushing injury of penis ♂

   √x7ᵗʰ **S38.02** Crushing injury of scrotum and testis ♂

   √x7ᵗʰ **S38.03** Crushing injury of vulva ♀

√x7ᵗʰ **S38.1** Crushing injury of abdomen, lower back, and pelvis

   Use additional code for all associated injuries, such as:

     fracture of thoracic or lumbar spine and pelvis (S22.0-, S32.-)

     injury to intra-abdominal organs (S36.-)

     injury to urinary and pelvic organs (S37.-)

     open wound of abdominal wall (S31.-)

     spinal cord injury (S34.0, S34.1-)

   EXCLUDES 2 crushing injury of external genital organs (S38.0-)

√6ᵗʰ **S38.2** Traumatic amputation of external genital organs

   √6ᵗʰ **S38.21** Traumatic amputation of female external genital organs

     Traumatic amputation of clitoris

     Traumatic amputation of labium (majus) (minus)

     Traumatic amputation of vulva

     √7ᵗʰ **S38.211** Complete traumatic amputation of female external genital organs ♀

     √7ᵗʰ **S38.212** Partial traumatic amputation of female external genital organs ♀

   √6ᵗʰ **S38.22** Traumatic amputation of penis

     √7ᵗʰ **S38.221** Complete traumatic amputation of penis ♂

     √7ᵗʰ **S38.222** Partial traumatic amputation of penis ♂

   √6ᵗʰ **S38.23** Traumatic amputation of scrotum and testis

     √7ᵗʰ **S38.231** Complete traumatic amputation of scrotum and testis ♂

     √7ᵗʰ **S38.232** Partial traumatic amputation of scrotum and testis ♂

√x7ᵗʰ **S38.3** Transection (partial) of abdomen

✔ Additional Character Required   √x7ᵗʰ Placeholder   Unacceptable PDx   Questionable PDx   Manifestation   Unspecified Dx   H1-H4 HAC   HCC CMS-HCC Dx   HIV HIV Dx

√4ᵗʰ **S39 Other and unspecified injuries of abdomen, lower back, pelvis and external genitals**

Code also any associated open wound (S31.-)

EXCLUDES 2   *sprain of joints and ligaments of lumbar spine and pelvis (S33.-)*

The appropriate 7th character is to be added to each code from category S39.
A   initial encounter
D   subsequent encounter
S   sequela

√5ᵗʰ **S39.0 Injury of muscle, fascia and tendon of abdomen, lower back and pelvis**

√6ᵗʰ   **S39.00 Unspecified injury of muscle, fascia and tendon of abdomen, lower back and pelvis**

    √7ᵗʰ **S39.001** Unspecified injury of muscle, fascia and tendon of abdomen

    √7ᵗʰ **S39.002** Unspecified injury of muscle, fascia and tendon of lower back

    √7ᵗʰ **S39.003** Unspecified injury of muscle, fascia and tendon of pelvis

√6ᵗʰ   **S39.01 Strain of muscle, fascia and tendon of abdomen, lower back and pelvis**

    √7ᵗʰ **S39.011** Strain of muscle, fascia and tendon of abdomen

    √7ᵗʰ **S39.012** Strain of muscle, fascia and tendon of lower back

    √7ᵗʰ **S39.013** Strain of muscle, fascia and tendon of pelvis

√6ᵗʰ   **S39.02 Laceration of muscle, fascia and tendon of abdomen, lower back and pelvis**

    √7ᵗʰ **S39.021** Laceration of muscle, fascia and tendon of abdomen

    √7ᵗʰ **S39.022** Laceration of muscle, fascia and tendon of lower back

    √7ᵗʰ **S39.023** Laceration of muscle, fascia and tendon of pelvis

√6ᵗʰ   **S39.09 Other injury of muscle, fascia and tendon of abdomen, lower back and pelvis**

    √7ᵗʰ **S39.091** Other injury of muscle, fascia and tendon of abdomen

    √7ᵗʰ **S39.092** Other injury of muscle, fascia and tendon of lower back

    √7ᵗʰ **S39.093** Other injury of muscle, fascia and tendon of pelvis

√5ᵗʰ **S39.8 Other specified injuries of abdomen, lower back, pelvis and external genitals**

√×7ᵗʰ   **S39.81 Other specified injuries of abdomen**

√×7ᵗʰ   **S39.82 Other specified injuries of lower back**

√×7ᵗʰ   **S39.83 Other specified injuries of pelvis**

√6ᵗʰ   **S39.84 Other specified injuries of external genitals**

    √7ᵗʰ **S39.840 Fracture of corpus cavernosum penis** ♂

    √7ᵗʰ **S39.848 Other specified injuries of external genitals**

      TIP: Assign for traumatic rupture of testis.

√5ᵗʰ **S39.9 Unspecified injury of abdomen, lower back, pelvis and external genitals**

√×7ᵗʰ   **S39.91 Unspecified injury of abdomen**

√×7ᵗʰ   **S39.92 Unspecified injury of lower back**

√×7ᵗʰ   **S39.93 Unspecified injury of pelvis**

√×7ᵗʰ   **S39.94 Unspecified injury of external genitals**

Injuries to the shoulder and upper arm (S40-S49)

INCLUDES   injuries of axilla
    injuries of scapular region

EXCLUDES 2   *burns and corrosions (T20-T32)*
    frostbite (T33-T34)
    injuries of elbow (S50-S59)
    insect bite or sting, venomous (T63.4)

√4ᵗʰ **S40 Superficial injury of shoulder and upper arm**

The appropriate 7th character is to be added to each code from category S40.
A   initial encounter
D   subsequent encounter
S   sequela

√5ᵗʰ **S40.0 Contusion of shoulder and upper arm**

√6ᵗʰ   **S40.01 Contusion of shoulder**

    √7ᵗʰ **S40.011** Contusion of right shoulder

    √7ᵗʰ **S40.012** Contusion of left shoulder

    √7ᵗʰ **S40.019** Contusion of unspecified shoulder

√6ᵗʰ   **S40.02 Contusion of upper arm**

    √7ᵗʰ **S40.021** Contusion of right upper arm

    √7ᵗʰ **S40.022** Contusion of left upper arm

    √7ᵗʰ **S40.029** Contusion of unspecified upper arm

√5ᵗʰ **S40.2 Other superficial injuries of shoulder**

√6ᵗʰ   **S40.21 Abrasion of shoulder**

    √7ᵗʰ **S40.211** Abrasion of right shoulder

    √7ᵗʰ **S40.212** Abrasion of left shoulder

    √7ᵗʰ **S40.219** Abrasion of unspecified shoulder

√6ᵗʰ   **S40.22 Blister (nonthermal) of shoulder**

    √7ᵗʰ **S40.221** Blister (nonthermal) of right shoulder

    √7ᵗʰ **S40.222** Blister (nonthermal) of left shoulder

    √7ᵗʰ **S40.229** Blister (nonthermal) of unspecified shoulder

√6ᵗʰ   **S40.24 External constriction of shoulder**

    √7ᵗʰ **S40.241** External constriction of right shoulder

    √7ᵗʰ **S40.242** External constriction of left shoulder

    √7ᵗʰ **S40.249** External constriction of unspecified shoulder

√6ᵗʰ   **S40.25 Superficial foreign body of shoulder**

     Splinter in the shoulder

    √7ᵗʰ **S40.251** Superficial foreign body of right shoulder

    √7ᵗʰ **S40.252** Superficial foreign body of left shoulder

    √7ᵗʰ **S40.259** Superficial foreign body of unspecified shoulder

√6ᵗʰ   **S40.26 Insect bite (nonvenomous) of shoulder**

    √7ᵗʰ **S40.261** Insect bite (nonvenomous) of right shoulder

    √7ᵗʰ **S40.262** Insect bite (nonvenomous) of left shoulder

    √7ᵗʰ **S40.269** Insect bite (nonvenomous) of unspecified shoulder

√6ᵗʰ   **S40.27 Other superficial bite of shoulder**

     EXCLUDES 1   *open bite of shoulder (S41.05)*

    √7ᵗʰ **S40.271** Other superficial bite of right shoulder

    √7ᵗʰ **S40.272** Other superficial bite of left shoulder

    √7ᵗʰ **S40.279** Other superficial bite of unspecified shoulder

√5ᵗʰ **S40.8 Other superficial injuries of upper arm**

√6ᵗʰ   **S40.81 Abrasion of upper arm**

    √7ᵗʰ **S40.811** Abrasion of right upper arm

    √7ᵗʰ **S40.812** Abrasion of left upper arm

    √7ᵗʰ **S40.819** Abrasion of unspecified upper arm

√6ᵗʰ   **S40.82 Blister (nonthermal) of upper arm**

    √7ᵗʰ **S40.821** Blister (nonthermal) of right upper arm

    √7ᵗʰ **S40.822** Blister (nonthermal) of left upper arm

    √7ᵗʰ **S40.829** Blister (nonthermal) of unspecified upper arm

√6ᵗʰ   **S40.84 External constriction of upper arm**

    √7ᵗʰ **S40.841** External constriction of right upper arm

    √7ᵗʰ **S40.842** External constriction of left upper arm

N Newborn: 0   P Pediatric: 0-17   M Maternity: 9-64   A Adult: 15-124   MCC Major Complication/Comorbidity   CC Complication/Comorbidity   SW Severe Wound Dx

1030   ICD-10-CM 2020

√7ᵗʰ **S40.849** External constriction of unspecified upper arm

√6ᵗʰ **S40.85** Superficial foreign body of upper arm

Splinter in the upper arm

√7ᵗʰ **S40.851** Superficial foreign body of right upper arm

√7ᵗʰ **S40.852** Superficial foreign body of left upper arm

√7ᵗʰ **S40.859** Superficial foreign body of unspecified upper arm

√6ᵗʰ **S40.86** Insect bite (nonvenomous) of upper arm

√7ᵗʰ **S40.861** Insect bite (nonvenomous) of right upper arm

√7ᵗʰ **S40.862** Insect bite (nonvenomous) of left upper arm

√7ᵗʰ **S40.869** Insect bite (nonvenomous) of unspecified upper arm

√6ᵗʰ **S40.87** Other superficial bite of upper arm

EXCLUDES 1   *open bite of upper arm (S41.14)*

EXCLUDES 2   *other superficial bite of shoulder (S40.27-)*

√7ᵗʰ **S40.871** Other superficial bite of right upper arm

√7ᵗʰ **S40.872** Other superficial bite of left upper arm

√7ᵗʰ **S40.879** Other superficial bite of unspecified upper arm

√5ᵗʰ **S40.9** Unspecified superficial injury of shoulder and upper arm

√6ᵗʰ **S40.91** Unspecified superficial injury of shoulder

√7ᵗʰ **S40.911** Unspecified superficial injury of right shoulder

√7ᵗʰ **S40.912** Unspecified superficial injury of left shoulder

√7ᵗʰ **S40.919** Unspecified superficial injury of unspecified shoulder

√6ᵗʰ **S40.92** Unspecified superficial injury of upper arm

√7ᵗʰ **S40.921** Unspecified superficial injury of right upper arm

√7ᵗʰ **S40.922** Unspecified superficial injury of left upper arm

√7ᵗʰ **S40.929** Unspecified superficial injury of unspecified upper arm

√4ᵗʰ **S41 Open wound of shoulder and upper arm**

Code also any associated wound infection

EXCLUDES 1   *traumatic amputation of shoulder and upper arm (S48.-)*

EXCLUDES 2   *open fracture of shoulder and upper arm (S42.- with 7th character B or C)*

The appropriate 7th character is to be added to each code from category S41.
A   initial encounter
D   subsequent encounter
S   sequela

√5ᵗʰ **S41.0** Open wound of shoulder

√6ᵗʰ **S41.00** Unspecified open wound of shoulder

√7ᵗʰ **S41.001** Unspecified open wound of right shoulder

√7ᵗʰ **S41.002** Unspecified open wound of left shoulder

√7ᵗʰ **S41.009** Unspecified open wound of unspecified shoulder

√6ᵗʰ **S41.01** Laceration without foreign body of shoulder

√7ᵗʰ **S41.011** Laceration without foreign body of right shoulder

√7ᵗʰ **S41.012** Laceration without foreign body of left shoulder

√7ᵗʰ **S41.019** Laceration without foreign body of unspecified shoulder

√6ᵗʰ **S41.02** Laceration with foreign body of shoulder

√7ᵗʰ **S41.021** Laceration with foreign body of right shoulder

√7ᵗʰ **S41.022** Laceration with foreign body of left shoulder

√7ᵗʰ **S41.029** Laceration with foreign body of unspecified shoulder

√6ᵗʰ **S41.03** Puncture wound without foreign body of shoulder

√7ᵗʰ **S41.031** Puncture wound without foreign body of right shoulder

√7ᵗʰ **S41.032** Puncture wound without foreign body of left shoulder

√7ᵗʰ **S41.039** Puncture wound without foreign body of unspecified shoulder

√6ᵗʰ **S41.04** Puncture wound with foreign body of shoulder

√7ᵗʰ **S41.041** Puncture wound with foreign body of right shoulder

√7ᵗʰ **S41.042** Puncture wound with foreign body of left shoulder

√7ᵗʰ **S41.049** Puncture wound with foreign body of unspecified shoulder

√6ᵗʰ **S41.05** Open bite of shoulder

Bite of shoulder NOS

EXCLUDES 1   *superficial bite of shoulder (S40.27)*

√7ᵗʰ **S41.051** Open bite of right shoulder

√7ᵗʰ **S41.052** Open bite of left shoulder

√7ᵗʰ **S41.059** Open bite of unspecified shoulder

√5ᵗʰ **S41.1** Open wound of upper arm

√6ᵗʰ **S41.10** Unspecified open wound of upper arm

AHA: 2016,3Q,24

√7ᵗʰ **S41.101** Unspecified open wound of right upper arm

√7ᵗʰ **S41.102** Unspecified open wound of left upper arm

√7ᵗʰ **S41.109** Unspecified open wound of unspecified upper arm

√6ᵗʰ **S41.11** Laceration without foreign body of upper arm

√7ᵗʰ **S41.111** Laceration without foreign body of right upper arm

√7ᵗʰ **S41.112** Laceration without foreign body of left upper arm

√7ᵗʰ **S41.119** Laceration without foreign body of unspecified upper arm

√6ᵗʰ **S41.12** Laceration with foreign body of upper arm

√7ᵗʰ **S41.121** Laceration with foreign body of right upper arm

√7ᵗʰ **S41.122** Laceration with foreign body of left upper arm

√7ᵗʰ **S41.129** Laceration with foreign body of unspecified upper arm

√6ᵗʰ **S41.13** Puncture wound without foreign body of upper arm

AHA: 2016,3Q,24

√7ᵗʰ **S41.131** Puncture wound without foreign body of right upper arm

√7ᵗʰ **S41.132** Puncture wound without foreign body of left upper arm

√7ᵗʰ **S41.139** Puncture wound without foreign body of unspecified upper arm

√6ᵗʰ **S41.14** Puncture wound with foreign body of upper arm

AHA: 2016,3Q,24

√7ᵗʰ **S41.141** Puncture wound with foreign body of right upper arm

√7ᵗʰ **S41.142** Puncture wound with foreign body of left upper arm

√7ᵗʰ **S41.149** Puncture wound with foreign body of unspecified upper arm

√6ᵗʰ **S41.15** Open bite of upper arm

Bite of upper arm NOS

EXCLUDES 1   *superficial bite of upper arm (S40.87)*

√7ᵗʰ **S41.151** Open bite of right upper arm

√7ᵗʰ **S41.152** Open bite of left upper arm

√7ᵗʰ **S41.159** Open bite of unspecified upper arm

√4ᵗʰ S42   Fracture of shoulder and upper arm

> **NOTE**   A fracture not indicated as displaced or nondisplaced should be coded to displaced
>
> A fracture not indicated as open or closed should be coded to closed

EXCLUDES 1   traumatic amputation of shoulder and upper arm (S48.-)

AHA: 2018,2Q,12; 2015,3Q,37-39

DEF: Diaphysis: Central shaft of a long bone.

DEF: Epiphysis: Proximal and distal rounded ends of a long bone, communicates with the joint.

DEF: Metaphysis: Section of a long bone located between the epiphysis and diaphysis at the proximal and distal ends.

DEF: Physis (growth plate): Narrow zone of cartilaginous tissue between the epiphysis and metaphysis at each end of a long bone. In childhood, proliferation of cells in this zone lengthens the bone. As the bone matures, this area thins, ossification eventually fusing into solid bone and growth stops. *Synonyms: Epiphyseal plate.*

The appropriate 7th character is to be added to all codes from category S42 [unless otherwise indicated].

- A   initial encounter for closed fracture
- B   initial encounter for open fracture
- D   subsequent encounter for fracture with routine healing
- G   subsequent encounter for fracture with delayed healing
- K   subsequent encounter for fracture with nonunion
- P   subsequent encounter for fracture with malunion
- S   sequela

√5ᵗʰ S42.0   Fracture of clavicle

CC Excl: For codes in subcategory S42.0:
CC with 7th character B: PDX collection 1243
CC with 7th character K or P: PDX collection 897

√6ᵗʰ S42.00   Fracture of unspecified part of clavicle

- ³ √7ᵗʰ **S42.001**   Fracture of unspecified part of right clavicle   CC H5
- ³ √7ᵗʰ **S42.002**   Fracture of unspecified part of left clavicle   CC H5
- ³ √7ᵗʰ **S42.009**   Fracture of unspecified part of unspecified clavicle   CC H5
  - **AHA:** 2012,4Q,93

√6ᵗʰ S42.01   Fracture of sternal end of clavicle

- ³ √7ᵗʰ **S42.011**   Anterior displaced fracture of sternal end of right clavicle   CC H5
- ³ √7ᵗʰ **S42.012**   Anterior displaced fracture of sternal end of left clavicle   CC H5
- ³ √7ᵗʰ **S42.013**   Anterior displaced fracture of sternal end of unspecified clavicle   CC H5
  - Displaced fracture of sternal end of clavicle NOS
- ³ √7ᵗʰ **S42.014**   Posterior displaced fracture of sternal end of right clavicle   CC H5
- ³ √7ᵗʰ **S42.015**   Posterior displaced fracture of sternal end of left clavicle   CC H5
- ³ √7ᵗʰ **S42.016**   Posterior displaced fracture of sternal end of unspecified clavicle   CC H5
- ³ √7ᵗʰ **S42.017**   Nondisplaced fracture of sternal end of right clavicle   CC H5
- ³ √7ᵗʰ **S42.018**   Nondisplaced fracture of sternal end of left clavicle   CC H5
- ³ √7ᵗʰ **S42.019**   Nondisplaced fracture of sternal end of unspecified clavicle   CC H5

√6ᵗʰ S42.02   Fracture of shaft of clavicle

- ³ √7ᵗʰ **S42.021**   Displaced fracture of shaft of right clavicle   CC H5
- ³ √7ᵗʰ **S42.022**   Displaced fracture of shaft of left clavicle   CC H5
- ³ √7ᵗʰ **S42.023**   Displaced fracture of shaft of unspecified clavicle   CC H5
- ³ √7ᵗʰ **S42.024**   Nondisplaced fracture of shaft of right clavicle   CC H5
- ³ √7ᵗʰ **S42.025**   Nondisplaced fracture of shaft of left clavicle   CC H5
- ³ √7ᵗʰ **S42.026**   Nondisplaced fracture of shaft of unspecified clavicle   CC H5

√6ᵗʰ S42.03   Fracture of lateral end of clavicle

Fracture of acromial end of clavicle

- ³ √7ᵗʰ **S42.031**   Displaced fracture of lateral end of right clavicle   CC H5
- ³ √7ᵗʰ **S42.032**   Displaced fracture of lateral end of left clavicle   CC H5
- ³ √7ᵗʰ **S42.033**   Displaced fracture of lateral end of unspecified clavicle   CC H5
- ³ √7ᵗʰ **S42.034**   Nondisplaced fracture of lateral end of right clavicle   CC H5
- ³ √7ᵗʰ **S42.035**   Nondisplaced fracture of lateral end of left clavicle   CC H5
- ³ √7ᵗʰ **S42.036**   Nondisplaced fracture of lateral end of unspecified clavicle   CC H5

√5ᵗʰ S42.1   Fracture of scapula

CC Excl: For codes in subcategory S42.1:
CC with 7th character B: PDX collection 1244
CC with 7th character K or P: PDX collection 897

√6ᵗʰ S42.10   Fracture of unspecified part of scapula

- ³ √7ᵗʰ **S42.101**   Fracture of unspecified part of scapula, right shoulder   CC H5
- ³ √7ᵗʰ **S42.102**   Fracture of unspecified part of scapula, left shoulder   CC H5
- ³ √7ᵗʰ **S42.109**   Fracture of unspecified part of scapula, unspecified shoulder   CC H5

√6ᵗʰ S42.11   Fracture of body of scapula

- ³ √7ᵗʰ **S42.111**   Displaced fracture of body of scapula, right shoulder   CC H5
- ³ √7ᵗʰ **S42.112**   Displaced fracture of body of scapula, left shoulder   CC H5
- ³ √7ᵗʰ **S42.113**   Displaced fracture of body of scapula, unspecified shoulder   CC H5
- ³ √7ᵗʰ **S42.114**   Nondisplaced fracture of body of scapula, right shoulder   CC H5
- ³ √7ᵗʰ **S42.115**   Nondisplaced fracture of body of scapula, left shoulder   CC H5
- ³ √7ᵗʰ **S42.116**   Nondisplaced fracture of body of scapula, unspecified shoulder   CC H5

√6ᵗʰ S42.12   Fracture of acromial process

- ³ √7ᵗʰ **S42.121**   Displaced fracture of acromial process, right shoulder   CC H5
- ³ √7ᵗʰ **S42.122**   Displaced fracture of acromial process, left shoulder   CC H5
- ³ √7ᵗʰ **S42.123**   Displaced fracture of acromial process, unspecified shoulder   CC H5
- ³ √7ᵗʰ **S42.124**   Nondisplaced fracture of acromial process, right shoulder   CC H5
- ³ √7ᵗʰ **S42.125**   Nondisplaced fracture of acromial process, left shoulder   CC H5
- ³ √7ᵗʰ **S42.126**   Nondisplaced fracture of acromial process, unspecified shoulder   CC H5

√6ᵗʰ S42.13   Fracture of coracoid process

- ³ √7ᵗʰ **S42.131**   Displaced fracture of coracoid process, right shoulder   CC H5
- ³ √7ᵗʰ **S42.132**   Displaced fracture of coracoid process, left shoulder   CC H5
- ³ √7ᵗʰ **S42.133**   Displaced fracture of coracoid process, unspecified shoulder   CC H5
- ³ √7ᵗʰ **S42.134**   Nondisplaced fracture of coracoid process, right shoulder   CC H5

N Newborn: 0   **P** Pediatric: 0-17   **M** Maternity: 9-64   **A** Adult: 15-124   **MCC** Major Complication/Comorbidity   **CC** Complication/Comorbidity   **SW** Severe Wound Dx

1032   ICD-10-CM 2020

3 √7ᵗʰ **S42.135** Nondisplaced fracture of coracoid process, **left** shoulder   CC H5

3 √7ᵗʰ **S42.136** Nondisplaced fracture of coracoid process, unspecified shoulder   CC H5

√6ᵗʰ **S42.14** Fracture of glenoid cavity of scapula

3 √7ᵗʰ **S42.141** Displaced fracture of glenoid cavity of scapula, **right** shoulder   CC H5

3 √7ᵗʰ **S42.142** Displaced fracture of glenoid cavity of scapula, **left** shoulder   CC H5

3 √7ᵗʰ **S42.143** Displaced fracture of glenoid cavity of scapula, unspecified shoulder   CC H5

3 √7ᵗʰ **S42.144** Nondisplaced fracture of glenoid cavity of scapula, **right** shoulder   CC H5

3 √7ᵗʰ **S42.145** Nondisplaced fracture of glenoid cavity of scapula, **left** shoulder   CC H5

3 √7ᵗʰ **S42.146** Nondisplaced fracture of glenoid cavity of scapula, unspecified shoulder   CC H5

√6ᵗʰ **S42.15** Fracture of neck of scapula

3 √7ᵗʰ **S42.151** Displaced fracture of neck of scapula, **right** shoulder   CC H5

3 √7ᵗʰ **S42.152** Displaced fracture of neck of scapula, **left** shoulder   CC H5

3 √7ᵗʰ **S42.153** Displaced fracture of neck of scapula, unspecified shoulder   CC H5

3 √7ᵗʰ **S42.154** Nondisplaced fracture of neck of scapula, **right** shoulder   CC H5

3 √7ᵗʰ **S42.155** Nondisplaced fracture of neck of scapula, **left** shoulder   CC H5

3 √7ᵗʰ **S42.156** Nondisplaced fracture of neck of scapula, unspecified shoulder   CC H5

√6ᵗʰ **S42.19** Fracture of other part of scapula

3 √7ᵗʰ **S42.191** Fracture of other part of scapula, **right** shoulder   CC H5

3 √7ᵗʰ **S42.192** Fracture of other part of scapula, **left** shoulder   CC H5

3 √7ᵗʰ **S42.199** Fracture of other part of scapula, unspecified shoulder   CC H5

√5ᵗʰ **S42.2** Fracture of upper end of humerus

Fracture of proximal end of humerus

EXCLUDES 2   fracture of shaft of humerus (S42.3-)

physeal fracture of upper end of humerus (S49.0-)

CC Excl: For CC/MCC codes in subcategory S42.2, unless otherwise noted:
Right side: See code S42.201
Left side: See code S42.202
Unspecified side: See code S42.209

√6ᵗʰ **S42.20** Unspecified fracture of upper end of humerus

2,3 √7ᵗʰ **S42.201** Unspecified fracture of upper end of **right** humerus   MCC CC H5

CC Excl: CC with 7th character A: PDX collection 1245
CC Excl: MCC with 7th character B: PDX collection 1246
CC Excl: CC with 7th character K or P: PDX collection 897

2,3 √7ᵗʰ **S42.202** Unspecified fracture of upper end of **left** humerus   MCC CC H5

CC Excl: CC with 7th character A: PDX collection 1247
CC Excl: MCC with 7th character B: PDX collection 1246
CC Excl: CC with 7th character K or P: PDX collection 897

2,3 √7ᵗʰ **S42.209** Unspecified fracture of upper end of unspecified humerus   MCC CC H5

CC Excl: CC with 7th character A: PDX collection 1248
CC Excl: MCC with 7th character B: PDX collection 1246
CC Excl: CC with 7th character K or P: PDX collection 897

√6ᵗʰ **S42.21** Unspecified fracture of surgical neck of humerus

Fracture of neck of humerus NOS

2,3 √7ᵗʰ **S42.211** Unspecified displaced fracture of surgical neck of **right** humerus   MCC CC H5

2,3 √7ᵗʰ **S42.212** Unspecified displaced fracture of surgical neck of **left** humerus   MCC CC H5

2,3 √7ᵗʰ **S42.213** Unspecified displaced fracture of surgical neck of unspecified humerus   MCC CC H5

2,3 √7ᵗʰ **S42.214** Unspecified nondisplaced fracture of surgical neck of **right** humerus   MCC CC H5

2,3 √7ᵗʰ **S42.215** Unspecified nondisplaced fracture of surgical neck of **left** humerus   MCC CC H5

2,3 √7ᵗʰ **S42.216** Unspecified nondisplaced fracture of surgical neck of unspecified humerus   MCC CC H5

√6ᵗʰ **S42.22** 2-part fracture of surgical neck of humerus

2,3 √7ᵗʰ **S42.221** 2-part displaced fracture of surgical neck of **right** humerus   MCC CC H5

2,3 √7ᵗʰ **S42.222** 2-part displaced fracture of surgical neck of **left** humerus   MCC CC H5

2,3 √7ᵗʰ **S42.223** 2-part displaced fracture of surgical neck of unspecified humerus   MCC CC H5

2,3 √7ᵗʰ **S42.224** 2-part nondisplaced fracture of surgical neck of **right** humerus   MCC CC H5

2,3 √7ᵗʰ **S42.225** 2-part nondisplaced fracture of surgical neck of **left** humerus   MCC CC H5

2,3 √7ᵗʰ **S42.226** 2-part nondisplaced fracture of surgical neck of unspecified humerus   MCC CC H5

√6ᵗʰ **S42.23** 3-part fracture of surgical neck of humerus

2,3 √7ᵗʰ **S42.231** 3-part fracture of surgical neck of **right** humerus   MCC CC H5

2,3 √7ᵗʰ **S42.232** 3-part fracture of surgical neck of **left** humerus   MCC CC H5

2,3 √7ᵗʰ **S42.239** 3-part fracture of surgical neck of unspecified humerus   MCC CC H5

√6ᵗʰ **S42.24** 4-part fracture of surgical neck of humerus

2,3 √7ᵗʰ **S42.241** 4-part fracture of surgical neck of **right** humerus   MCC CC H5

2,3 √7ᵗʰ **S42.242** 4-part fracture of surgical neck of **left** humerus   MCC CC H5

2,3 √7ᵗʰ **S42.249** 4-part fracture of surgical neck of unspecified humerus   MCC CC H5

√6ᵗʰ **S42.25** Fracture of greater tuberosity of humerus

2,3 √7ᵗʰ **S42.251** Displaced fracture of greater tuberosity of **right** humerus   MCC CC H5

2,3 √7ᵗʰ **S42.252** Displaced fracture of greater tuberosity of **left** humerus   MCC CC H5

2,3 √7ᵗʰ **S42.253** Displaced fracture of greater tuberosity of unspecified humerus   MCC CC H5

2,3 √7ᵗʰ **S42.254** Nondisplaced fracture of greater tuberosity of **right** humerus   MCC CC H5

2,3 √7ᵗʰ **S42.255** Nondisplaced fracture of greater tuberosity of **left** humerus   MCC CC H5

2,3 √7ᵗʰ **S42.256** Nondisplaced fracture of greater tuberosity of unspecified humerus   MCC H5

✔ Additional Character Required   √x7ᵗʰ Placeholder   Unacceptable PDx   Questionable PDx   Manifestation   Unspecified Dx   H1 -H14 HAC   HCC CMS-HCC Dx   HIV HIV Dx

ICD-10-CM 2020   1033

√6ᵗʰ **S42.26 Fracture of lesser tuberosity of humerus**

2,3 √7ᵗʰ **S42.261 Displaced fracture of lesser tuberosity of right humerus** `MCC` `CC` `H5`

2,3 √7ᵗʰ **S42.262 Displaced fracture of lesser tuberosity of left humerus** `MCC` `CC` `H5`

2,3 √7ᵗʰ **S42.263 Displaced fracture of lesser tuberosity of unspecified humerus** `MCC` `CC` `H5`

2,3 √7ᵗʰ **S42.264 Nondisplaced fracture of lesser tuberosity of right humerus** `MCC` `CC` `H5`

2,3 √7ᵗʰ **S42.265 Nondisplaced fracture of lesser tuberosity of left humerus** `MCC` `CC` `H5`

2,3 √7ᵗʰ **S42.266 Nondisplaced fracture of lesser tuberosity of unspecified humerus** `MCC` `CC` `H5`

√6ᵗʰ **S42.27 Torus fracture of upper end of humerus**

> The appropriate 7th character is to be added to all codes in subcategory S42.27
> A   initial encounter for closed fracture
> D   subsequent encounter for fracture with routine healing
> G   subsequent encounter for fracture with delayed healing
> K   subsequent encounter for fracture with nonunion
> P   subsequent encounter for fracture with malunion
> S   sequela

3 √7ᵗʰ **S42.271 Torus fracture of upper end of right humerus** `CC` `H5`
    CC Excl: CC with 7th character A: PDX collection 1245
    CC Excl: CC with 7th character K or P: PDX collection 897

3 √7ᵗʰ **S42.272 Torus fracture of upper end of left humerus** `CC` `H5`
    CC Excl: CC with 7th character A: PDX collection 1247
    CC Excl: CC with 7th character K or P: PDX collection 897

3 √7ᵗʰ **S42.279 Torus fracture of upper end of unspecified humerus** `CC` `H5`
    CC Excl: CC with 7th character A: PDX collection 1248
    CC Excl: CC with 7th character K or P: PDX collection 897

√6ᵗʰ **S42.29 Other fracture of upper end of humerus**

Fracture of anatomical neck of humerus
Fracture of articular head of humerus
AHA: 2019,1Q,18

2,3 √7ᵗʰ **S42.291 Other displaced fracture of upper end of right humerus** `MCC` `CC` `H5`

2,3 √7ᵗʰ **S42.292 Other displaced fracture of upper end of left humerus** `MCC` `CC` `H5`

2,3 √7ᵗʰ **S42.293 Other displaced fracture of upper end of unspecified humerus** `MCC` `CC` `H5`

2,3 √7ᵗʰ **S42.294 Other nondisplaced fracture of upper end of right humerus** `MCC` `CC` `H5`

2,3 √7ᵗʰ **S42.295 Other nondisplaced fracture of upper end of left humerus** `MCC` `CC` `H5`

2,3 √7ᵗʰ **S42.296 Other nondisplaced fracture of upper end of unspecified humerus** `MCC` `CC` `H5`

√5ᵗʰ **S42.3 Fracture of shaft of humerus**

Fracture of humerus NOS
Fracture of upper arm NOS
EXCLUDES 2 physeal fractures of upper end of humerus (S49.0-)
physeal fractures of lower end of humerus (S49.1-)
CC Excl: For CC/MCC codes in subcategory S42.3, unless otherwise noted:
Right side: See code S42.321
Left side: See code S42.322
Unspecified side: See code S42.323

√6ᵗʰ **S42.30 Unspecified fracture of shaft of humerus**

2,3 √7ᵗʰ **S42.301 Unspecified fracture of shaft of humerus, right arm** `MCC` `CC` `H5`

2,3 √7ᵗʰ **S42.302 Unspecified fracture of shaft of humerus, left arm** `MCC` `CC` `H5`

2,3 √7ᵗʰ **S42.309 Unspecified fracture of shaft of humerus, unspecified arm** `MCC` `CC` `H5`

√6ᵗʰ **S42.31 Greenstick fracture of shaft of humerus**

> The appropriate 7th character is to be added to all codes in subcategory S42.31
> A   initial encounter for closed fracture
> D   subsequent encounter for fracture with routine healing
> G   subsequent encounter for fracture with delayed healing
> K   subsequent encounter for fracture with nonunion
> P   subsequent encounter for fracture with malunion
> S   sequela

3 √7ᵗʰ **S42.311 Greenstick fracture of shaft of humerus, right arm** `CC` `H5`
    CC Excl: CC with 7th character A: PDX collection 1249
    CC Excl: CC with 7th character K or P: PDX collection 897

3 √7ᵗʰ **S42.312 Greenstick fracture of shaft of humerus, left arm** `CC` `H5`
    CC Excl: CC with 7th character A: PDX collection 1250
    CC Excl: CC with 7th character K or P: PDX collection 897

3 √7ᵗʰ **S42.319 Greenstick fracture of shaft of humerus, unspecified arm** `CC` `H5`
    CC Excl: CC with 7th character A: PDX collection 1251
    CC Excl: CC with 7th character K or P: PDX collection 897

√6ᵗʰ **S42.32 Transverse fracture of shaft of humerus**

2,3 √7ᵗʰ **S42.321 Displaced transverse fracture of shaft of humerus, right arm** `MCC` `CC` `H5`
    CC Excl: CC with 7th character A: PDX collection 1249
    CC Excl: MCC with 7th character B: PDX collection 1246
    CC Excl: CC with 7th character K or P: PDX collection 897

2,3 √7ᵗʰ **S42.322 Displaced transverse fracture of shaft of humerus, left arm** `MCC` `CC` `H5`
    CC Excl: CC with 7th character A: PDX collection 1250
    CC Excl: MCC with 7th character B: PDX collection 1246
    CC Excl: CC with 7th character K or P: PDX collection 897

2,3 √7ᵗʰ **S42.323 Displaced transverse fracture of shaft of humerus, unspecified arm** `MCC` `CC` `H5`
    CC Excl: CC with 7th character A: PDX collection 1251
    CC Excl: MCC with 7th character B: PDX collection 1246
    CC Excl: CC with 7th character K or P: PDX collection 897

2,3 ✓7th **S42.324** Nondisplaced transverse fracture of shaft of humerus, right arm   MCC CC H5

2,3 ✓7th **S42.325** Nondisplaced transverse fracture of shaft of humerus, left arm   MCC CC H5

2,3 ✓7th **S42.326** Nondisplaced transverse fracture of shaft of humerus, unspecified arm   MCC CC H5

✓6th **S42.33** Oblique fracture of shaft of humerus

2,3 ✓7th **S42.331** Displaced oblique fracture of shaft of humerus, right arm   MCC CC H5

2,3 ✓7th **S42.332** Displaced oblique fracture of shaft of humerus, left arm   MCC CC H5

2,3 ✓7th **S42.333** Displaced oblique fracture of shaft of humerus, unspecified arm   MCC CC H5

2,3 ✓7th **S42.334** Nondisplaced oblique fracture of shaft of humerus, right arm   MCC CC H5

2,3 ✓7th **S42.335** Nondisplaced oblique fracture of shaft of humerus, left arm   MCC CC H5

2,3 ✓7th **S42.336** Nondisplaced oblique fracture of shaft of humerus, unspecified arm   MCC CC H5

✓6th **S42.34** Spiral fracture of shaft of humerus

2,3 ✓7th **S42.341** Displaced spiral fracture of shaft of humerus, right arm   MCC CC H5

2,3 ✓7th **S42.342** Displaced spiral fracture of shaft of humerus, left arm   MCC CC H5

2,3 ✓7th **S42.343** Displaced spiral fracture of shaft of humerus, unspecified arm   MCC CC H5

2,3 ✓7th **S42.344** Nondisplaced spiral fracture of shaft of humerus, right arm   MCC CC H5

2,3 ✓7th **S42.345** Nondisplaced spiral fracture of shaft of humerus, left arm   MCC CC H5

2,3 ✓7th **S42.346** Nondisplaced spiral fracture of shaft of humerus, unspecified arm   MCC CC H5

✓6th **S42.35** Comminuted fracture of shaft of humerus

2,3 ✓7th **S42.351** Displaced comminuted fracture of shaft of humerus, right arm   MCC CC H5

2,3 ✓7th **S42.352** Displaced comminuted fracture of shaft of humerus, left arm   MCC CC H5

2,3 ✓7th **S42.353** Displaced comminuted fracture of shaft of humerus, unspecified arm   MCC CC H5

2,3 ✓7th **S42.354** Nondisplaced comminuted fracture of shaft of humerus, right arm   MCC CC H5

2,3 ✓7th **S42.355** Nondisplaced comminuted fracture of shaft of humerus, left arm   MCC CC H5

2,3 ✓7th **S42.356** Nondisplaced comminuted fracture of shaft of humerus, unspecified arm   MCC CC H5

✓6th **S42.36** Segmental fracture of shaft of humerus

2,3 ✓7th **S42.361** Displaced segmental fracture of shaft of humerus, right arm   MCC CC H5

2,3 ✓7th **S42.362** Displaced segmental fracture of shaft of humerus, left arm   MCC CC H5

2,3 ✓7th **S42.363** Displaced segmental fracture of shaft of humerus, unspecified arm   MCC CC H5

2,3 ✓7th **S42.364** Nondisplaced segmental fracture of shaft of humerus, right arm   MCC CC H5

2,3 ✓7th **S42.365** Nondisplaced segmental fracture of shaft of humerus, left arm   MCC CC H5

2,3 ✓7th **S42.366** Nondisplaced segmental fracture of shaft of humerus, unspecified arm   MCC CC H5

✓6th **S42.39** Other fracture of shaft of humerus

2,3 ✓7th **S42.391** Other fracture of shaft of right humerus   MCC CC H5

2,3 ✓7th **S42.392** Other fracture of shaft of left humerus   MCC CC H5

2,3 ✓7th **S42.399** Other fracture of shaft of unspecified humerus   MCC CC H5

✓5th **S42.4** Fracture of lower end of humerus

Fracture of distal end of humerus

EXCLUDES 2   fracture of shaft of humerus (S42.3-)

physeal fracture of lower end of humerus (S49.1-)

CC Excl: For CC/MCC codes in subcategory S42.4, unless otherwise noted:
Right side: See code S42.201
Left side: See code S42.202
Unspecified side: See code S42.209

✓6th **S42.40** Unspecified fracture of lower end of humerus

Fracture of elbow NOS

2,3 ✓7th **S42.401** Unspecified fracture of lower end of right humerus   MCC CC H5

2,3 ✓7th **S42.402** Unspecified fracture of lower end of left humerus   MCC CC H5

2,3 ✓7th **S42.409** Unspecified fracture of lower end of unspecified humerus   MCC CC H5

✓6th **S42.41** Simple supracondylar fracture without intercondylar fracture of humerus

2,3 ✓7th **S42.411** Displaced simple supracondylar fracture without intercondylar fracture of right humerus   MCC CC H5

2,3 ✓7th **S42.412** Displaced simple supracondylar fracture without intercondylar fracture of left humerus   MCC CC H5

2,3 ✓7th **S42.413** Displaced simple supracondylar fracture without intercondylar fracture of unspecified humerus   MCC CC H5

2,3 ✓7th **S42.414** Nondisplaced simple supracondylar fracture without intercondylar fracture of right humerus   MCC CC H5

2,3 ✓7th **S42.415** Nondisplaced simple supracondylar fracture without intercondylar fracture of left humerus   MCC CC H5

2,3 ✓7th **S42.416** Nondisplaced simple supracondylar fracture without intercondylar fracture of unspecified humerus   MCC CC H5

✓6th **S42.42** Comminuted supracondylar fracture without intercondylar fracture of humerus

2,3 ✓7th **S42.421** Displaced comminuted supracondylar fracture without intercondylar fracture of right humerus   MCC CC H5

2,3 ✓7th **S42.422** Displaced comminuted supracondylar fracture without intercondylar fracture of left humerus   MCC CC H5

2,3 ✓7th **S42.423** Displaced comminuted supracondylar fracture without intercondylar fracture of unspecified humerus   MCC CC H5

2,3 ✓7th **S42.424** Nondisplaced comminuted supracondylar fracture without intercondylar fracture of right humerus   MCC CC H5

2,3 ✓7th **S42.425** Nondisplaced comminuted supracondylar fracture without intercondylar fracture of left humerus   MCC CC H5

2,3 √7ᵗʰ **S42.426** Nondisplaced comminuted supracondylar fracture without intercondylar fracture of unspecified humerus   MCC CC H5

√6ᵗʰ **S42.43** Fracture (avulsion) of lateral epicondyle of humerus

2,3 √7ᵗʰ **S42.431** Displaced fracture (avulsion) of lateral epicondyle of right humerus   MCC CC H5

2,3 √7ᵗʰ **S42.432** Displaced fracture (avulsion) of lateral epicondyle of left humerus   MCC CC H5

2,3 √7ᵗʰ **S42.433** Displaced fracture (avulsion) of lateral epicondyle of unspecified humerus   MCC CC H5

2,3 √7ᵗʰ **S42.434** Nondisplaced fracture (avulsion) of lateral epicondyle of right humerus   MCC CC H5

2,3 √7ᵗʰ **S42.435** Nondisplaced fracture (avulsion) of lateral epicondyle of left humerus   MCC CC H5

2,3 √7ᵗʰ **S42.436** Nondisplaced fracture (avulsion) of lateral epicondyle of unspecified humerus   MCC CC H5

√6ᵗʰ **S42.44** Fracture (avulsion) of medial epicondyle of humerus

2,3 √7ᵗʰ **S42.441** Displaced fracture (avulsion) of medial epicondyle of right humerus   MCC CC H5

2,3 √7ᵗʰ **S42.442** Displaced fracture (avulsion) of medial epicondyle of left humerus   MCC CC H5

2,3 √7ᵗʰ **S42.443** Displaced fracture (avulsion) of medial epicondyle of unspecified humerus   MCC CC H5

2,3 √7ᵗʰ **S42.444** Nondisplaced fracture (avulsion) of medial epicondyle of right humerus   MCC CC H5

2,3 √7ᵗʰ **S42.445** Nondisplaced fracture (avulsion) of medial epicondyle of left humerus   MCC CC H5

2,3 √7ᵗʰ **S42.446** Nondisplaced fracture (avulsion) of medial epicondyle of unspecified humerus   MCC CC H5

2,3 √7ᵗʰ **S42.447** Incarcerated fracture (avulsion) of medial epicondyle of right humerus   MCC CC H5

2,3 √7ᵗʰ **S42.448** Incarcerated fracture (avulsion) of medial epicondyle of left humerus   MCC CC H5

2,3 √7ᵗʰ **S42.449** Incarcerated fracture (avulsion) of medial epicondyle of unspecified humerus   MCC CC H5

√6ᵗʰ **S42.45** Fracture of lateral condyle of humerus
    Fracture of capitellum of humerus

2,3 √7ᵗʰ **S42.451** Displaced fracture of lateral condyle of right humerus   MCC CC H5

2,3 √7ᵗʰ **S42.452** Displaced fracture of lateral condyle of left humerus   MCC CC H5

2,3 √7ᵗʰ **S42.453** Displaced fracture of lateral condyle of unspecified humerus   MCC CC H5

2,3 √7ᵗʰ **S42.454** Nondisplaced fracture of lateral condyle of right humerus   MCC CC H5

2,3 √7ᵗʰ **S42.455** Nondisplaced fracture of lateral condyle of left humerus   MCC CC H5

2,3 √7ᵗʰ **S42.456** Nondisplaced fracture of lateral condyle of unspecified humerus   MCC CC H5

√6ᵗʰ **S42.46** Fracture of medial condyle of humerus
    Trochlea fracture of humerus

2,3 √7ᵗʰ **S42.461** Displaced fracture of medial condyle of right humerus   MCC CC H5

2,3 √7ᵗʰ **S42.462** Displaced fracture of medial condyle of left humerus   MCC CC H5

2,3 √7ᵗʰ **S42.463** Displaced fracture of medial condyle of unspecified humerus   MCC CC H5

2,3 √7ᵗʰ **S42.464** Nondisplaced fracture of medial condyle of right humerus   MCC CC H5

2,3 √7ᵗʰ **S42.465** Nondisplaced fracture of medial condyle of left humerus   MCC CC H5

2,3 √7ᵗʰ **S42.466** Nondisplaced fracture of medial condyle of unspecified humerus   MCC CC H5

√6ᵗʰ **S42.47** Transcondylar fracture of humerus

2,3 √7ᵗʰ **S42.471** Displaced transcondylar fracture of right humerus   MCC CC H5

2,3 √7ᵗʰ **S42.472** Displaced transcondylar fracture of left humerus   MCC CC H5

2,3 √7ᵗʰ **S42.473** Displaced transcondylar fracture of unspecified humerus   MCC CC H5

2,3 √7ᵗʰ **S42.474** Nondisplaced transcondylar fracture of right humerus   MCC CC H5

2,3 √7ᵗʰ **S42.475** Nondisplaced transcondylar fracture of left humerus   MCC CC H5

2,3 √7ᵗʰ **S42.476** Nondisplaced transcondylar fracture of unspecified humerus   MCC CC H5

√6ᵗʰ **S42.48** Torus fracture of lower end of humerus

> The appropriate 7th character is to be added to all codes in subcategory S42.48.
> A   initial encounter for closed fracture
> D   subsequent encounter for fracture with routine healing
> G   subsequent encounter for fracture with delayed healing
> K   subsequent encounter for fracture with nonunion
> P   subsequent encounter for fracture with malunion
> S   sequela

3 √7ᵗʰ **S42.481** Torus fracture of lower end of right humerus   CC H5
    CC Excl: CC with 7th character A: PDX collection 1245
    CC Excl: CC with 7th character K or P: PDX collection 897

3 √7ᵗʰ **S42.482** Torus fracture of lower end of left humerus   CC H5
    CC Excl: CC with 7th character A: PDX collection 1247
    CC Excl: CC with 7th character K or P: PDX collection 897

3 √7ᵗʰ **S42.489** Torus fracture of lower end of unspecified humerus   CC H5
    CC Excl: CC with 7th character A: PDX collection 1248
    CC Excl: CC with 7th character K or P: PDX collection 897

√6ᵗʰ **S42.49** Other fracture of lower end of humerus

2,3 √7ᵗʰ **S42.491** Other displaced fracture of lower end of right humerus   MCC CC H5

2,3 √7ᵗʰ **S42.492** Other displaced fracture of lower end of left humerus   MCC CC H5

2,3 √7ᵗʰ **S42.493** Other displaced fracture of lower end of unspecified humerus   MCC CC H5

N Newborn: 0   P Pediatric: 0-17   M Maternity: 9-64   A Adult: 15-124   MCC Major Complication/Comorbidity   CC Complication/Comorbidity   SW Severe Wound Dx

2,3 √7ᵗʰ **S42.494** Other nondisplaced fracture of lower end of right humerus   MCC CC H5

2,3 √7ᵗʰ **S42.495** Other nondisplaced fracture of lower end of left humerus   MCC CC H5

2,3 √7ᵗʰ **S42.496** Other nondisplaced fracture of lower end of unspecified humerus   MCC CC H5

√5ᵗʰ **S42.9** Fracture of shoulder girdle, part unspecified

Fracture of shoulder NOS

CC Excl: For CC/MCC codes in subcategory S42.9: See code S42.209

2,3 √x7ᵗʰ **S42.90** Fracture of unspecified shoulder girdle, part unspecified   MCC CC H5

2,3 √x7ᵗʰ **S42.91** Fracture of right shoulder girdle, part unspecified   MCC CC H5

2,3 √x7ᵗʰ **S42.92** Fracture of left shoulder girdle, part unspecified   MCC CC H5

√4ᵗʰ **S43** Dislocation and sprain of joints and ligaments of shoulder girdle

INCLUDES   avulsion of joint or ligament of shoulder girdle

laceration of cartilage, joint or ligament of shoulder girdle

sprain of cartilage, joint or ligament of shoulder girdle

traumatic hemarthrosis of joint or ligament of shoulder girdle

traumatic rupture of joint or ligament of shoulder girdle

traumatic subluxation of joint or ligament of shoulder girdle

traumatic tear of joint or ligament of shoulder girdle

Code also any associated open wound

EXCLUDES 2   strain of muscle, fascia and tendon of shoulder and upper arm (S46.-)

The appropriate 7th character is to be added to each code from category S43.
A   initial encounter
D   subsequent encounter
S   sequela

√5ᵗʰ **S43.0** Subluxation and dislocation of shoulder joint

Dislocation of glenohumeral joint

Subluxation of glenohumeral joint

√6ᵗʰ **S43.00** Unspecified subluxation and dislocation of shoulder joint

Dislocation of humerus NOS

Subluxation of humerus NOS

√7ᵗʰ **S43.001** Unspecified subluxation of right shoulder joint

√7ᵗʰ **S43.002** Unspecified subluxation of left shoulder joint

√7ᵗʰ **S43.003** Unspecified subluxation of unspecified shoulder joint

√7ᵗʰ **S43.004** Unspecified dislocation of right shoulder joint

√7ᵗʰ **S43.005** Unspecified dislocation of left shoulder joint

√7ᵗʰ **S43.006** Unspecified dislocation of unspecified shoulder joint

√6ᵗʰ **S43.01** Anterior subluxation and dislocation of humerus

√7ᵗʰ **S43.011** Anterior subluxation of right humerus

√7ᵗʰ **S43.012** Anterior subluxation of left humerus

√7ᵗʰ **S43.013** Anterior subluxation of unspecified humerus

√7ᵗʰ **S43.014** Anterior dislocation of right humerus

√7ᵗʰ **S43.015** Anterior dislocation of left humerus

√7ᵗʰ **S43.016** Anterior dislocation of unspecified humerus

√6ᵗʰ **S43.02** Posterior subluxation and dislocation of humerus

√7ᵗʰ **S43.021** Posterior subluxation of right humerus

√7ᵗʰ **S43.022** Posterior subluxation of left humerus

√7ᵗʰ **S43.023** Posterior subluxation of unspecified humerus

√7ᵗʰ **S43.024** Posterior dislocation of right humerus

√7ᵗʰ **S43.025** Posterior dislocation of left humerus

√7ᵗʰ **S43.026** Posterior dislocation of unspecified humerus

√6ᵗʰ **S43.03** Inferior subluxation and dislocation of humerus

√7ᵗʰ **S43.031** Inferior subluxation of right humerus

√7ᵗʰ **S43.032** Inferior subluxation of left humerus

√7ᵗʰ **S43.033** Inferior subluxation of unspecified humerus

√7ᵗʰ **S43.034** Inferior dislocation of right humerus

√7ᵗʰ **S43.035** Inferior dislocation of left humerus

√7ᵗʰ **S43.036** Inferior dislocation of unspecified humerus

√6ᵗʰ **S43.08** Other subluxation and dislocation of shoulder joint

√7ᵗʰ **S43.081** Other subluxation of right shoulder joint

√7ᵗʰ **S43.082** Other subluxation of left shoulder joint

√7ᵗʰ **S43.083** Other subluxation of unspecified shoulder joint

√7ᵗʰ **S43.084** Other dislocation of right shoulder joint

√7ᵗʰ **S43.085** Other dislocation of left shoulder joint

√7ᵗʰ **S43.086** Other dislocation of unspecified shoulder joint

√5ᵗʰ **S43.1** Subluxation and dislocation of acromioclavicular joint

√6ᵗʰ **S43.10** Unspecified dislocation of acromioclavicular joint

√7ᵗʰ **S43.101** Unspecified dislocation of right acromioclavicular joint

√7ᵗʰ **S43.102** Unspecified dislocation of left acromioclavicular joint

√7ᵗʰ **S43.109** Unspecified dislocation of unspecified acromioclavicular joint

√6ᵗʰ **S43.11** Subluxation of acromioclavicular joint

√7ᵗʰ **S43.111** Subluxation of right acromioclavicular joint

√7ᵗʰ **S43.112** Subluxation of left acromioclavicular joint

√7ᵗʰ **S43.119** Subluxation of unspecified acromioclavicular joint

√6ᵗʰ **S43.12** Dislocation of acromioclavicular joint, 100%-200% displacement

√7ᵗʰ **S43.121** Dislocation of right acromioclavicular joint, 100%-200% displacement

√7ᵗʰ **S43.122** Dislocation of left acromioclavicular joint, 100%-200% displacement

√7ᵗʰ **S43.129** Dislocation of unspecified acromioclavicular joint, 100%-200% displacement

√6ᵗʰ **S43.13** Dislocation of acromioclavicular joint, greater than 200% displacement

√7ᵗʰ **S43.131** Dislocation of right acromioclavicular joint, greater than 200% displacement

√7ᵗʰ **S43.132** Dislocation of left acromioclavicular joint, greater than 200% displacement

√7ᵗʰ **S43.139** Dislocation of unspecified acromioclavicular joint, greater than 200% displacement

√6ᵗʰ **S43.14** Inferior dislocation of acromioclavicular joint

√7ᵗʰ **S43.141** Inferior dislocation of right acromioclavicular joint

√7ᵗʰ **S43.142** Inferior dislocation of left acromioclavicular joint

√7ᵗʰ **S43.149** Inferior dislocation of unspecified acromioclavicular joint

√6ᵗʰ **S43.15** Posterior dislocation of acromioclavicular joint

√7ᵗʰ **S43.151** Posterior dislocation of right acromioclavicular joint

√7ᵗʰ **S43.152** Posterior dislocation of left acromioclavicular joint

√7ᵗʰ **S43.159** Posterior dislocation of unspecified acromioclavicular joint

√5ᵗʰ **S43.2** Subluxation and dislocation of sternoclavicular joint

CC Excl: For CC codes in subcategory S43.2:
Right side: PDX collection 1252
Left side: PDX collection 1253
Unspecified side: PDX collection 914

√6ᵗʰ **S43.20** Unspecified subluxation and dislocation of sternoclavicular joint

√7ᵗʰ **S43.201** Unspecified subluxation of right sternoclavicular joint   CC H5

√7ᵗʰ **S43.202** Unspecified subluxation of left sternoclavicular joint   CC H5

√7ᵗʰ **S43.203** Unspecified subluxation of unspecified sternoclavicular joint   CC H5

√7ᵗʰ **S43.204** Unspecified dislocation of right sternoclavicular joint   CC H5

✓ Additional Character Required   √x7ᵗʰ Placeholder   Unacceptable PDx   Questionable PDx   Manifestation   Unspecified Dx   H1 -H14 HAC   HCC CMS-HCC Dx   HIV HIV Dx

ICD-10-CM 2020   1037

√7th **S43.205** Unspecified dislocation of left sternoclavicular joint `CC` `H5`

√7th **S43.206** Unspecified dislocation of unspecified sternoclavicular joint `CC` `H5`

√6th **S43.21** Anterior subluxation and dislocation of sternoclavicular joint

√7th **S43.211** Anterior subluxation of right sternoclavicular joint `CC` `H5`

√7th **S43.212** Anterior subluxation of left sternoclavicular joint `CC` `H5`

√7th **S43.213** Anterior subluxation of unspecified sternoclavicular joint `CC` `H5`

√7th **S43.214** Anterior dislocation of right sternoclavicular joint `CC` `H5`

√7th **S43.215** Anterior dislocation of left sternoclavicular joint `CC` `H5`

√7th **S43.216** Anterior dislocation of unspecified sternoclavicular joint `CC` `H5`

√6th **S43.22** Posterior subluxation and dislocation of sternoclavicular joint

√7th **S43.221** Posterior subluxation of right sternoclavicular joint `CC` `H5`

√7th **S43.222** Posterior subluxation of left sternoclavicular joint `CC` `H5`

√7th **S43.223** Posterior subluxation of unspecified sternoclavicular joint `CC` `H5`

√7th **S43.224** Posterior dislocation of right sternoclavicular joint `CC` `H5`

√7th **S43.225** Posterior dislocation of left sternoclavicular joint `CC` `H5`

√7th **S43.226** Posterior dislocation of unspecified sternoclavicular joint `CC` `H5`

√5th **S43.3** Subluxation and dislocation of other and unspecified parts of shoulder girdle

√6th **S43.30** Subluxation and dislocation of unspecified parts of shoulder girdle

Dislocation of shoulder girdle NOS
Subluxation of shoulder girdle NOS

√7th **S43.301** Subluxation of unspecified parts of right shoulder girdle

√7th **S43.302** Subluxation of unspecified parts of left shoulder girdle

√7th **S43.303** Subluxation of unspecified parts of unspecified shoulder girdle

√7th **S43.304** Dislocation of unspecified parts of right shoulder girdle

√7th **S43.305** Dislocation of unspecified parts of left shoulder girdle

√7th **S43.306** Dislocation of unspecified parts of unspecified shoulder girdle

√6th **S43.31** Subluxation and dislocation of scapula

√7th **S43.311** Subluxation of right scapula

√7th **S43.312** Subluxation of left scapula

√7th **S43.313** Subluxation of unspecified scapula

√7th **S43.314** Dislocation of right scapula

√7th **S43.315** Dislocation of left scapula

√7th **S43.316** Dislocation of unspecified scapula

√6th **S43.39** Subluxation and dislocation of other parts of shoulder girdle

√7th **S43.391** Subluxation of other parts of right shoulder girdle

√7th **S43.392** Subluxation of other parts of left shoulder girdle

√7th **S43.393** Subluxation of other parts of unspecified shoulder girdle

√7th **S43.394** Dislocation of other parts of right shoulder girdle

√7th **S43.395** Dislocation of other parts of left shoulder girdle

√7th **S43.396** Dislocation of other parts of unspecified shoulder girdle

√5th **S43.4** Sprain of shoulder joint

√6th **S43.40** Unspecified sprain of shoulder joint

√7th **S43.401** Unspecified sprain of right shoulder joint

√7th **S43.402** Unspecified sprain of left shoulder joint

√7th **S43.409** Unspecified sprain of unspecified shoulder joint

√6th **S43.41** Sprain of coracohumeral (ligament)

√7th **S43.411** Sprain of right coracohumeral (ligament)

√7th **S43.412** Sprain of left coracohumeral (ligament)

√7th **S43.419** Sprain of unspecified coracohumeral (ligament)

√6th **S43.42** Sprain of rotator cuff capsule

`EXCLUDES 1` rotator cuff syndrome (complete) (incomplete), not specified as traumatic (M75.1-)

`EXCLUDES 2` injury of tendon of rotator cuff (S46.0-)

√7th **S43.421** Sprain of right rotator cuff capsule

√7th **S43.422** Sprain of left rotator cuff capsule

√7th **S43.429** Sprain of unspecified rotator cuff capsule

√6th **S43.43** Superior glenoid labrum lesion

SLAP lesion
AHA: 2019,2Q,26
DEF: Detachment injury of the superior aspect of the glenoid labrum, which is the ring of fibrocartilage attached to the rim of the glenoid cavity of the scapula.

√7th **S43.431** Superior glenoid labrum lesion of right shoulder

√7th **S43.432** Superior glenoid labrum lesion of left shoulder

√7th **S43.439** Superior glenoid labrum lesion of unspecified shoulder

√6th **S43.49** Other sprain of shoulder joint

√7th **S43.491** Other sprain of right shoulder joint

√7th **S43.492** Other sprain of left shoulder joint

√7th **S43.499** Other sprain of unspecified shoulder joint

√5th **S43.5** Sprain of acromioclavicular joint

Sprain of acromioclavicular ligament

√x7th **S43.50** Sprain of unspecified acromioclavicular joint

√x7th **S43.51** Sprain of right acromioclavicular joint

√x7th **S43.52** Sprain of left acromioclavicular joint

√5th **S43.6** Sprain of sternoclavicular joint

√x7th **S43.60** Sprain of unspecified sternoclavicular joint

√x7th **S43.61** Sprain of right sternoclavicular joint

√x7th **S43.62** Sprain of left sternoclavicular joint

√5th **S43.8** Sprain of other specified parts of shoulder girdle

√x7th **S43.80** Sprain of other specified parts of unspecified shoulder girdle

√x7th **S43.81** Sprain of other specified parts of right shoulder girdle

√x7th **S43.82** Sprain of other specified parts of left shoulder girdle

√5th **S43.9** Sprain of unspecified parts of shoulder girdle

√x7th **S43.90** Sprain of unspecified parts of unspecified shoulder girdle

Sprain of shoulder girdle NOS

√x7th **S43.91** Sprain of unspecified parts of right shoulder girdle

√x7th **S43.92** Sprain of unspecified parts of left shoulder girdle

√4th **S44** Injury of nerves at shoulder and upper arm level

Code also any associated open wound (S41.-)

`EXCLUDES 2` injury of brachial plexus (S14.3-)

The appropriate 7th character is to be added to each code from category S44.
A initial encounter
D subsequent encounter
S sequela

√5th **S44.0** Injury of ulnar nerve at upper arm level

`EXCLUDES 1` ulnar nerve NOS (S54.0)

√x7th **S44.00** Injury of ulnar nerve at upper arm level, unspecified arm

√x7th **S44.01** Injury of ulnar nerve at upper arm level, right arm

√x7th **S44.02** Injury of ulnar nerve at upper arm level, left arm

√5th **S44.1** Injury of median nerve at upper arm level

`EXCLUDES 1` median nerve NOS (S54.1)

√x7th **S44.10** Injury of median nerve at upper arm level, unspecified arm

√x7th **S44.11** Injury of median nerve at upper arm level, right arm

`N` Newborn: 0 　`P` Pediatric: 0-17 　`M` Maternity: 9-64 　`A` Adult: 15-124 　`MCC` Major Complication/Comorbidity 　`CC` Complication/Comorbidity 　`SW` Severe Wound Dx

1038 　ICD-10-CM 2020

✓x7ᵗʰ **S44.12** Injury of median nerve at upper arm level, left arm

✓5ᵗʰ **S44.2** Injury of radial nerve at upper arm level

     EXCLUDES 1   radial nerve NOS (S54.2)

   ✓x7ᵗʰ **S44.20** Injury of radial nerve at upper arm level, unspecified arm

   ✓x7ᵗʰ **S44.21** Injury of radial nerve at upper arm level, right arm

   ✓x7ᵗʰ **S44.22** Injury of radial nerve at upper arm level, left arm

✓5ᵗʰ **S44.3** Injury of axillary nerve

   ✓x7ᵗʰ **S44.30** Injury of axillary nerve, unspecified arm

   ✓x7ᵗʰ **S44.31** Injury of axillary nerve, right arm

   ✓x7ᵗʰ **S44.32** Injury of axillary nerve, left arm

✓5ᵗʰ **S44.4** Injury of musculocutaneous nerve

   ✓x7ᵗʰ **S44.40** Injury of musculocutaneous nerve, unspecified arm

   ✓x7ᵗʰ **S44.41** Injury of musculocutaneous nerve, right arm

   ✓x7ᵗʰ **S44.42** Injury of musculocutaneous nerve, left arm

✓5ᵗʰ **S44.5** Injury of cutaneous sensory nerve at shoulder and upper arm level

   ✓x7ᵗʰ **S44.50** Injury of cutaneous sensory nerve at shoulder and upper arm level, unspecified arm

   ✓x7ᵗʰ **S44.51** Injury of cutaneous sensory nerve at shoulder and upper arm level, right arm

   ✓x7ᵗʰ **S44.52** Injury of cutaneous sensory nerve at shoulder and upper arm level, left arm

✓5ᵗʰ **S44.8** Injury of other nerves at shoulder and upper arm level

   ✓6ᵗʰ **S44.8X** Injury of other nerves at shoulder and upper arm level

     ✓7ᵗʰ **S44.8X1** Injury of other nerves at shoulder and upper arm level, right arm

     ✓7ᵗʰ **S44.8X2** Injury of other nerves at shoulder and upper arm level, left arm

     ✓7ᵗʰ **S44.8X9** Injury of other nerves at shoulder and upper arm level, unspecified arm

✓5ᵗʰ **S44.9** Injury of unspecified nerve at shoulder and upper arm level

   ✓x7ᵗʰ **S44.90** Injury of unspecified nerve at shoulder and upper arm level, unspecified arm

   ✓x7ᵗʰ **S44.91** Injury of unspecified nerve at shoulder and upper arm level, right arm

   ✓x7ᵗʰ **S44.92** Injury of unspecified nerve at shoulder and upper arm level, left arm

✓4ᵗʰ **S45** Injury of blood vessels at shoulder and upper arm level

   Code also any associated open wound (S41.-)

   EXCLUDES 2   injury of subclavian artery (S25.1)
                  injury of subclavian vein (S25.3)

   The appropriate 7th character is to be added to each code from category S45.
   A   initial encounter
   D   subsequent encounter
   S   sequela

✓5ᵗʰ **S45.0** Injury of axillary artery

   CC Excl: For MCC codes in subcategory S45.0:
   Right side: PDX collection 1254
   Left side: PDX collection 1255
   Unspecified side: PDX collection 1256

   ✓6ᵗʰ **S45.00** Unspecified injury of axillary artery

     ✓7ᵗʰ **S45.001** Unspecified injury of axillary artery, right side   `MCC`

     ✓7ᵗʰ **S45.002** Unspecified injury of axillary artery, left side   `MCC`

     ✓7ᵗʰ **S45.009** Unspecified injury of axillary artery, unspecified side   `MCC`

   ✓6ᵗʰ **S45.01** Laceration of axillary artery

     ✓7ᵗʰ **S45.011** Laceration of axillary artery, right side   `MCC`

     ✓7ᵗʰ **S45.012** Laceration of axillary artery, left side   `MCC`

     ✓7ᵗʰ **S45.019** Laceration of axillary artery, unspecified side   `MCC`

   ✓6ᵗʰ **S45.09** Other specified injury of axillary artery

     ✓7ᵗʰ **S45.091** Other specified injury of axillary artery, right side   `MCC`

     ✓7ᵗʰ **S45.092** Other specified injury of axillary artery, left side   `MCC`

     ✓7ᵗʰ **S45.099** Other specified injury of axillary artery, unspecified side   `MCC`

✓5ᵗʰ **S45.1** Injury of brachial artery

   CC Excl: For CC codes in subcategory S45.1:
   Right side: PDX collection 1257
   Left side: PDX collection 1258
   Unspecified side: PDX collection 1259

   ✓6ᵗʰ **S45.10** Unspecified injury of brachial artery

     ✓7ᵗʰ **S45.101** Unspecified injury of brachial artery, right side   `CC`

     ✓7ᵗʰ **S45.102** Unspecified injury of brachial artery, left side   `CC`

     ✓7ᵗʰ **S45.109** Unspecified injury of brachial artery, unspecified side   `CC`

   ✓6ᵗʰ **S45.11** Laceration of brachial artery

     ✓7ᵗʰ **S45.111** Laceration of brachial artery, right side   `CC`

     ✓7ᵗʰ **S45.112** Laceration of brachial artery, left side   `CC`

     ✓7ᵗʰ **S45.119** Laceration of brachial artery, unspecified side   `CC`

   ✓6ᵗʰ **S45.19** Other specified injury of brachial artery

     ✓7ᵗʰ **S45.191** Other specified injury of brachial artery, right side   `CC`

     ✓7ᵗʰ **S45.192** Other specified injury of brachial artery, left side   `CC`

     ✓7ᵗʰ **S45.199** Other specified injury of brachial artery, unspecified side   `CC`

✓5ᵗʰ **S45.2** Injury of axillary or brachial vein

   CC Excl: For CC codes in subcategory S45.2:
   Right side: PDX collection 1257
   Left side: PDX collection 1258
   Unspecified side: PDX collection 1259

   ✓6ᵗʰ **S45.20** Unspecified injury of axillary or brachial vein

     ✓7ᵗʰ **S45.201** Unspecified injury of axillary or brachial vein, right side   `CC`

     ✓7ᵗʰ **S45.202** Unspecified injury of axillary or brachial vein, left side   `CC`

     ✓7ᵗʰ **S45.209** Unspecified injury of axillary or brachial vein, unspecified side   `CC`

   ✓6ᵗʰ **S45.21** Laceration of axillary or brachial vein

     ✓7ᵗʰ **S45.211** Laceration of axillary or brachial vein, right side   `CC`

     ✓7ᵗʰ **S45.212** Laceration of axillary or brachial vein, left side   `CC`

     ✓7ᵗʰ **S45.219** Laceration of axillary or brachial vein, unspecified side   `CC`

   ✓6ᵗʰ **S45.29** Other specified injury of axillary or brachial vein

     ✓7ᵗʰ **S45.291** Other specified injury of axillary or brachial vein, right side   `CC`

     ✓7ᵗʰ **S45.292** Other specified injury of axillary or brachial vein, left side   `CC`

     ✓7ᵗʰ **S45.299** Other specified injury of axillary or brachial vein, unspecified side   `CC`

✓5ᵗʰ **S45.3** Injury of superficial vein at shoulder and upper arm level

   CC Excl: For CC codes in subcategory S45.3:
   Right side: PDX collection 1260
   Left side: PDX collection 1261
   Unspecified side: PDX collection 1262

   ✓6ᵗʰ **S45.30** Unspecified injury of superficial vein at shoulder and upper arm level

     ✓7ᵗʰ **S45.301** Unspecified injury of superficial vein at shoulder and upper arm level, right arm   `CC`

     ✓7ᵗʰ **S45.302** Unspecified injury of superficial vein at shoulder and upper arm level, left arm   `CC`

     ✓7ᵗʰ **S45.309** Unspecified injury of superficial vein at shoulder and upper arm level, unspecified arm   `CC`

✅ Additional Character Required   ✓x7ᵗʰ Placeholder   Unacceptable PDx   Questionable PDx   Manifestation   Unspecified Dx   `H1`-`H14` HAC   `HCC` CMS-HCC Dx   `HIV` HIV Dx

ICD-10-CM 2020

1039

√6ᵗʰ **S45.31** Laceration of superficial vein at shoulder and upper arm level

√7ᵗʰ **S45.311** Laceration of superficial vein at shoulder and upper arm level, **right** arm   `CC`

√7ᵗʰ **S45.312** Laceration of superficial vein at shoulder and upper arm level, **left** arm   `CC`

√7ᵗʰ **S45.319** Laceration of superficial vein at shoulder and upper arm level, unspecified arm   `CC`

√6ᵗʰ **S45.39** Other specified injury of superficial vein at shoulder and upper arm level

√7ᵗʰ **S45.391** Other specified injury of superficial vein at shoulder and upper arm level, **right** arm   `CC`

√7ᵗʰ **S45.392** Other specified injury of superficial vein at shoulder and upper arm level, **left** arm   `CC`

√7ᵗʰ **S45.399** Other specified injury of superficial vein at shoulder and upper arm level, unspecified arm   `CC`

√5ᵗʰ **S45.8** Injury of other specified blood vessels at shoulder and upper arm level

CC Excl: For CC codes in subcategory S45.8:
Right side: PDX collection 1260
Left side: PDX collection 1261
Unspecified side: PDX collection 1262

√6ᵗʰ **S45.80** Unspecified injury of other specified blood vessels at shoulder and upper arm level

√7ᵗʰ **S45.801** Unspecified injury of other specified blood vessels at shoulder and upper arm level, **right** arm   `CC`

√7ᵗʰ **S45.802** Unspecified injury of other specified blood vessels at shoulder and upper arm level, **left** arm   `CC`

√7ᵗʰ **S45.809** Unspecified injury of other specified blood vessels at shoulder and upper arm level, unspecified arm   `CC`

√6ᵗʰ **S45.81** Laceration of other specified blood vessels at shoulder and upper arm level

√7ᵗʰ **S45.811** Laceration of other specified blood vessels at shoulder and upper arm level, **right** arm   `CC`

√7ᵗʰ **S45.812** Laceration of other specified blood vessels at shoulder and upper arm level, **left** arm   `CC`

√7ᵗʰ **S45.819** Laceration of other specified blood vessels at shoulder and upper arm level, unspecified arm   `CC`

√6ᵗʰ **S45.89** Other specified injury of other specified blood vessels at shoulder and upper arm level

√7ᵗʰ **S45.891** Other specified injury of other specified blood vessels at shoulder and upper arm level, **right** arm   `CC`

√7ᵗʰ **S45.892** Other specified injury of other specified blood vessels at shoulder and upper arm level, **left** arm   `CC`

√7ᵗʰ **S45.899** Other specified injury of other specified blood vessels at shoulder and upper arm level, unspecified arm   `CC`

√5ᵗʰ **S45.9** Injury of unspecified blood vessel at shoulder and upper arm level

CC Excl: For CC codes in subcategory S45.9:
Right side: PDX collection 1260
Left side: PDX collection 1261
Unspecified side: PDX collection 1262

√6ᵗʰ **S45.90** Unspecified injury of unspecified blood vessel at shoulder and upper arm level

√7ᵗʰ **S45.901** Unspecified injury of unspecified blood vessel at shoulder and upper arm level, **right** arm   `CC`

√7ᵗʰ **S45.902** Unspecified injury of unspecified blood vessel at shoulder and upper arm level, **left** arm   `CC`

√7ᵗʰ **S45.909** Unspecified injury of unspecified blood vessel at shoulder and upper arm level, unspecified arm   `CC`

√6ᵗʰ **S45.91** Laceration of unspecified blood vessel at shoulder and upper arm level

√7ᵗʰ **S45.911** Laceration of unspecified blood vessel at shoulder and upper arm level, **right** arm   `CC`

√7ᵗʰ **S45.912** Laceration of unspecified blood vessel at shoulder and upper arm level, **left** arm   `CC`

√7ᵗʰ **S45.919** Laceration of unspecified blood vessel at shoulder and upper arm level, unspecified arm   `CC`

√6ᵗʰ **S45.99** Other specified injury of unspecified blood vessel at shoulder and upper arm level

√7ᵗʰ **S45.991** Other specified injury of unspecified blood vessel at shoulder and upper arm level, **right** arm   `CC`

√7ᵗʰ **S45.992** Other specified injury of unspecified blood vessel at shoulder and upper arm level, **left** arm   `CC`

√7ᵗʰ **S45.999** Other specified injury of unspecified blood vessel at shoulder and upper arm level, unspecified arm   `CC`

√4ᵗʰ **S46** Injury of muscle, fascia and tendon at shoulder and upper arm level

Code also any associated open wound (S41.-)

EXCLUDES 2   *injury of muscle, fascia and tendon at elbow (S56.-)*
sprain of joints and ligaments of shoulder girdle (S43.9)

TIP: Refer to the Muscle/Tendon table at the beginning of this chapter.

The appropriate 7th character is to be added to each code from category S46.
A   initial encounter
D   subsequent encounter
S   sequela

CC Excl: For CC codes in category S46:
Right side: PDX collection 1263
Left side: PDX collection 1264
Unspecified side: PDX collection 1265

√5ᵗʰ **S46.0** Injury of muscle(s) and tendon(s) of the rotator cuff of shoulder

√6ᵗʰ **S46.00** Unspecified injury of muscle(s) and tendon(s) of the rotator cuff of shoulder

√7ᵗʰ **S46.001** Unspecified injury of muscle(s) and tendon(s) of the rotator cuff of **right** shoulder

√7ᵗʰ **S46.002** Unspecified injury of muscle(s) and tendon(s) of the rotator cuff of **left** shoulder

√7ᵗʰ **S46.009** Unspecified injury of muscle(s) and tendon(s) of the rotator cuff of unspecified shoulder

√6ᵗʰ **S46.01** Strain of muscle(s) and tendon(s) of the rotator cuff of shoulder

√7ᵗʰ **S46.011** Strain of muscle(s) and tendon(s) of the rotator cuff of **right** shoulder

√7ᵗʰ **S46.012** Strain of muscle(s) and tendon(s) of the rotator cuff of **left** shoulder

√7ᵗʰ **S46.019** Strain of muscle(s) and tendon(s) of the rotator cuff of unspecified shoulder

√6ᵗʰ **S46.02** Laceration of muscle(s) and tendon(s) of the rotator cuff of shoulder

     √7ᵗʰ **S46.021** Laceration of muscle(s) and tendon(s) of the rotator cuff of right shoulder   cc

     √7ᵗʰ **S46.022** Laceration of muscle(s) and tendon(s) of the rotator cuff of left shoulder   cc

     √7ᵗʰ **S46.029** Laceration of muscle(s) and tendon(s) of the rotator cuff of unspecified shoulder   cc

√6ᵗʰ **S46.09** Other injury of muscle(s) and tendon(s) of the rotator cuff of shoulder

     √7ᵗʰ **S46.091** Other injury of muscle(s) and tendon(s) of the rotator cuff of right shoulder

     √7ᵗʰ **S46.092** Other injury of muscle(s) and tendon(s) of the rotator cuff of left shoulder

     √7ᵗʰ **S46.099** Other injury of muscle(s) and tendon(s) of the rotator cuff of unspecified shoulder

√5ᵗʰ **S46.1** Injury of muscle, fascia and tendon of long head of biceps

√6ᵗʰ **S46.10** Unspecified injury of muscle, fascia and tendon of long head of biceps

     √7ᵗʰ **S46.101** Unspecified injury of muscle, fascia and tendon of long head of biceps, right arm

     √7ᵗʰ **S46.102** Unspecified injury of muscle, fascia and tendon of long head of biceps, left arm

     √7ᵗʰ **S46.109** Unspecified injury of muscle, fascia and tendon of long head of biceps, unspecified arm

√6ᵗʰ **S46.11** Strain of muscle, fascia and tendon of long head of biceps

     AHA: 2019,2Q,27

     √7ᵗʰ **S46.111** Strain of muscle, fascia and tendon of long head of biceps, right arm

     √7ᵗʰ **S46.112** Strain of muscle, fascia and tendon of long head of biceps, left arm

     √7ᵗʰ **S46.119** Strain of muscle, fascia and tendon of long head of biceps, unspecified arm

√6ᵗʰ **S46.12** Laceration of muscle, fascia and tendon of long head of biceps

     √7ᵗʰ **S46.121** Laceration of muscle, fascia and tendon of long head of biceps, right arm   cc

     √7ᵗʰ **S46.122** Laceration of muscle, fascia and tendon of long head of biceps, left arm   cc

     √7ᵗʰ **S46.129** Laceration of muscle, fascia and tendon of long head of biceps, unspecified arm   cc

√6ᵗʰ **S46.19** Other injury of muscle, fascia and tendon of long head of biceps

     √7ᵗʰ **S46.191** Other injury of muscle, fascia and tendon of long head of biceps, right arm

     √7ᵗʰ **S46.192** Other injury of muscle, fascia and tendon of long head of biceps, left arm

     √7ᵗʰ **S46.199** Other injury of muscle, fascia and tendon of long head of biceps, unspecified arm

√5ᵗʰ **S46.2** Injury of muscle, fascia and tendon of other parts of biceps

√6ᵗʰ **S46.20** Unspecified injury of muscle, fascia and tendon of other parts of biceps

     √7ᵗʰ **S46.201** Unspecified injury of muscle, fascia and tendon of other parts of biceps, right arm

     √7ᵗʰ **S46.202** Unspecified injury of muscle, fascia and tendon of other parts of biceps, left arm

     √7ᵗʰ **S46.209** Unspecified injury of muscle, fascia and tendon of other parts of biceps, unspecified arm

√6ᵗʰ **S46.21** Strain of muscle, fascia and tendon of other parts of biceps

     √7ᵗʰ **S46.211** Strain of muscle, fascia and tendon of other parts of biceps, right arm

     √7ᵗʰ **S46.212** Strain of muscle, fascia and tendon of other parts of biceps, left arm

     √7ᵗʰ **S46.219** Strain of muscle, fascia and tendon of other parts of biceps, unspecified arm

√6ᵗʰ **S46.22** Laceration of muscle, fascia and tendon of other parts of biceps

     √7ᵗʰ **S46.221** Laceration of muscle, fascia and tendon of other parts of biceps, right arm   cc

     √7ᵗʰ **S46.222** Laceration of muscle, fascia and tendon of other parts of biceps, left arm   cc

     √7ᵗʰ **S46.229** Laceration of muscle, fascia and tendon of other parts of biceps, unspecified arm   cc

√6ᵗʰ **S46.29** Other injury of muscle, fascia and tendon of other parts of biceps

     √7ᵗʰ **S46.291** Other injury of muscle, fascia and tendon of other parts of biceps, right arm

     √7ᵗʰ **S46.292** Other injury of muscle, fascia and tendon of other parts of biceps, left arm

     √7ᵗʰ **S46.299** Other injury of muscle, fascia and tendon of other parts of biceps, unspecified arm

√5ᵗʰ **S46.3** Injury of muscle, fascia and tendon of triceps

√6ᵗʰ **S46.30** Unspecified injury of muscle, fascia and tendon of triceps

     √7ᵗʰ **S46.301** Unspecified injury of muscle, fascia and tendon of triceps, right arm

     √7ᵗʰ **S46.302** Unspecified injury of muscle, fascia and tendon of triceps, left arm

     √7ᵗʰ **S46.309** Unspecified injury of muscle, fascia and tendon of triceps, unspecified arm

√6ᵗʰ **S46.31** Strain of muscle, fascia and tendon of triceps

     √7ᵗʰ **S46.311** Strain of muscle, fascia and tendon of triceps, right arm

     √7ᵗʰ **S46.312** Strain of muscle, fascia and tendon of triceps, left arm

     √7ᵗʰ **S46.319** Strain of muscle, fascia and tendon of triceps, unspecified arm

√6ᵗʰ **S46.32** Laceration of muscle, fascia and tendon of triceps

     √7ᵗʰ **S46.321** Laceration of muscle, fascia and tendon of triceps, right arm   cc

     √7ᵗʰ **S46.322** Laceration of muscle, fascia and tendon of triceps, left arm   cc

     √7ᵗʰ **S46.329** Laceration of muscle, fascia and tendon of triceps, unspecified arm   cc

√6ᵗʰ **S46.39** Other injury of muscle, fascia and tendon of triceps

     √7ᵗʰ **S46.391** Other injury of muscle, fascia and tendon of triceps, right arm

     √7ᵗʰ **S46.392** Other injury of muscle, fascia and tendon of triceps, left arm

     √7ᵗʰ **S46.399** Other injury of muscle, fascia and tendon of triceps, unspecified arm

√5ᵗʰ **S46.8** Injury of other muscles, fascia and tendons at shoulder and upper arm level

√6ᵗʰ **S46.80** Unspecified injury of other muscles, fascia and tendons at shoulder and upper arm level

     √7ᵗʰ **S46.801** Unspecified injury of other muscles, fascia and tendons at shoulder and upper arm level, right arm

     √7ᵗʰ **S46.802** Unspecified injury of other muscles, fascia and tendons at shoulder and upper arm level, left arm

     √7ᵗʰ **S46.809** Unspecified injury of other muscles, fascia and tendons at shoulder and upper arm level, unspecified arm

√6ᵗʰ **S46.81** Strain of other muscles, fascia and tendons at shoulder and upper arm level

     √7ᵗʰ **S46.811** Strain of other muscles, fascia and tendons at shoulder and upper arm level, right arm

     √7ᵗʰ **S46.812** Strain of other muscles, fascia and tendons at shoulder and upper arm level, left arm

     √7ᵗʰ **S46.819** Strain of other muscles, fascia and tendons at shoulder and upper arm level, unspecified arm

√6ᵗʰ **S46.82** Laceration of other muscles, fascia and tendons at shoulder and upper arm level

     √7ᵗʰ **S46.821** Laceration of other muscles, fascia and tendons at shoulder and upper arm level, right arm   cc

☑ Additional Character Required   √x7ᵗʰ Placeholder   Unacceptable PDx   Questionable PDx   Manifestation   Unspecified Dx   HI-HIV HAC   HCC CMS-HCC Dx   HIV HIV Dx

ICD-10-CM 2020   1041

√7ᵗʰ **S46.822** Laceration of other muscles, fascia and tendons at shoulder and upper arm level, left arm   `CC`

√7ᵗʰ **S46.829** Laceration of other muscles, fascia and tendons at shoulder and upper arm level, unspecified arm   `CC`

√6ᵗʰ **S46.89** Other injury of other muscles, fascia and tendons at shoulder and upper arm level

√7ᵗʰ **S46.891** Other injury of other muscles, fascia and tendons at shoulder and upper arm level, right arm

√7ᵗʰ **S46.892** Other injury of other muscles, fascia and tendons at shoulder and upper arm level, left arm

√7ᵗʰ **S46.899** Other injury of other muscles, fascia and tendons at shoulder and upper arm level, unspecified arm

√6ᵗʰ **S46.9** Injury of unspecified muscle, fascia and tendon at shoulder and upper arm level

√6ᵗʰ **S46.90** Unspecified injury of unspecified muscle, fascia and tendon at shoulder and upper arm level

√7ᵗʰ **S46.901** Unspecified injury of unspecified muscle, fascia and tendon at shoulder and upper arm level, right arm

√7ᵗʰ **S46.902** Unspecified injury of unspecified muscle, fascia and tendon at shoulder and upper arm level, left arm

√7ᵗʰ **S46.909** Unspecified injury of unspecified muscle, fascia and tendon at shoulder and upper arm level, unspecified arm

√6ᵗʰ **S46.91** Strain of unspecified muscle, fascia and tendon at shoulder and upper arm level

√7ᵗʰ **S46.911** Strain of unspecified muscle, fascia and tendon at shoulder and upper arm level, right arm

√7ᵗʰ **S46.912** Strain of unspecified muscle, fascia and tendon at shoulder and upper arm level, left arm

√7ᵗʰ **S46.919** Strain of unspecified muscle, fascia and tendon at shoulder and upper arm level, unspecified arm

√6ᵗʰ **S46.92** Laceration of unspecified muscle, fascia and tendon at shoulder and upper arm level

√7ᵗʰ **S46.921** Laceration of unspecified muscle, fascia and tendon at shoulder and upper arm level, right arm   `CC`

√7ᵗʰ **S46.922** Laceration of unspecified muscle, fascia and tendon at shoulder and upper arm level, left arm   `CC`

√7ᵗʰ **S46.929** Laceration of unspecified muscle, fascia and tendon at shoulder and upper arm level, unspecified arm   `CC`

√6ᵗʰ **S46.99** Other injury of unspecified muscle, fascia and tendon at shoulder and upper arm level

√7ᵗʰ **S46.991** Other injury of unspecified muscle, fascia and tendon at shoulder and upper arm level, right arm

√7ᵗʰ **S46.992** Other injury of unspecified muscle, fascia and tendon at shoulder and upper arm level, left arm

√7ᵗʰ **S46.999** Other injury of unspecified muscle, fascia and tendon at shoulder and upper arm level, unspecified arm

√4ᵗʰ **S47** Crushing injury of shoulder and upper arm

Use additional code for all associated injuries

`EXCLUDES 2`   crushing injury of elbow (S57.0-)

The appropriate 7th character is to be added to each code from category S47.
A   initial encounter
D   subsequent encounter
S   sequela

√ˣ7ᵗʰ **S47.1** Crushing injury of right shoulder and upper arm

√ˣ7ᵗʰ **S47.2** Crushing injury of left shoulder and upper arm

√ˣ7ᵗʰ **S47.9** Crushing injury of shoulder and upper arm, unspecified arm

√4ᵗʰ **S48** Traumatic amputation of shoulder and upper arm

An amputation not identified as partial or complete should be coded to complete

`EXCLUDES 1`   traumatic amputation at elbow level (S58.0)

The appropriate 7th character is to be added to each code from category S48.
A   initial encounter
D   subsequent encounter
S   sequela

CC Excl: For CC codes in category S48:
Right side: PDX collection 1266
Left side: PDX collection 1267
Unspecified side: PDX collection 1268

√5ᵗʰ **S48.0** Traumatic amputation at shoulder joint

√6ᵗʰ **S48.01** Complete traumatic amputation at shoulder joint

7 √7ᵗʰ **S48.011** Complete traumatic amputation at right shoulder joint   `CC` `HCC`

7 √7ᵗʰ **S48.012** Complete traumatic amputation at left shoulder joint   `CC` `HCC`

7 √7ᵗʰ **S48.019** Complete traumatic amputation at unspecified shoulder joint   `CC` `HCC`

√6ᵗʰ **S48.02** Partial traumatic amputation at shoulder joint

7 √7ᵗʰ **S48.021** Partial traumatic amputation at right shoulder joint   `CC` `HCC`

7 √7ᵗʰ **S48.022** Partial traumatic amputation at left shoulder joint   `CC` `HCC`

7 √7ᵗʰ **S48.029** Partial traumatic amputation at unspecified shoulder joint   `CC` `HCC`

√5ᵗʰ **S48.1** Traumatic amputation at level between shoulder and elbow

√6ᵗʰ **S48.11** Complete traumatic amputation at level between shoulder and elbow

7 √7ᵗʰ **S48.111** Complete traumatic amputation at level between right shoulder and elbow   `CC` `HCC`

7 √7ᵗʰ **S48.112** Complete traumatic amputation at level between left shoulder and elbow   `CC` `HCC`

7 √7ᵗʰ **S48.119** Complete traumatic amputation at level between unspecified shoulder and elbow   `CC` `HCC`

√6ᵗʰ **S48.12** Partial traumatic amputation at level between shoulder and elbow

7 √7ᵗʰ **S48.121** Partial traumatic amputation at level between right shoulder and elbow   `CC` `HCC`

7 √7ᵗʰ **S48.122** Partial traumatic amputation at level between left shoulder and elbow   `CC` `HCC`

7 √7ᵗʰ **S48.129** Partial traumatic amputation at level between unspecified shoulder and elbow   `CC` `HCC`

√5ᵗʰ **S48.9** Traumatic amputation of shoulder and upper arm, level unspecified

√6ᵗʰ **S48.91** Complete traumatic amputation of shoulder and upper arm, level unspecified

7 √7ᵗʰ **S48.911** Complete traumatic amputation of right shoulder and upper arm, level unspecified   `CC` `HCC`

7 √7ᵗʰ **S48.912** Complete traumatic amputation of left shoulder and upper arm, level unspecified   `CC` `HCC`

7 √7ᵗʰ **S48.919** Complete traumatic amputation of unspecified shoulder and upper arm, level unspecified   `CC` `HCC`

✓6th **S48.92** Partial traumatic amputation of shoulder and upper arm, level unspecified

    7 ✓7th **S48.921** Partial traumatic amputation of right shoulder and upper arm, level unspecified   `CC` `HCC`

    7 ✓7th **S48.922** Partial traumatic amputation of left shoulder and upper arm, level unspecified   `CC` `HCC`

    7 ✓7th **S48.929** Partial traumatic amputation of unspecified shoulder and upper arm, level unspecified   `CC` `HCC`

✓4th **S49** Other and unspecified injuries of shoulder and upper arm

    AHA: 2018,2Q,12; 2018,1Q,3

    The appropriate 7th character is to be added to each code from subcategories S49.0 and S49.1.
    A   initial encounter for closed fracture
    D   subsequent encounter for fracture with routine healing
    G   subsequent encounter for fracture with delayed healing
    K   subsequent encounter for fracture with nonunion
    P   subsequent encounter for fracture with malunion
    S   sequela

    CC Excl: For CC codes in category S49:
    Right side: See code S49.001
    Left side: See code S49.002
    Unspecified side: See code S49.009

✓5th **S49.0** Physeal fracture of upper end of humerus

    ✓6th **S49.00** Unspecified physeal fracture of upper end of humerus

      3 ✓7th **S49.001** Unspecified physeal fracture of upper end of humerus, right arm   `CC` `H5`
        CC Excl: CC with 7th character A: PDX collection 1245
        CC Excl: CC with 7th character K or P: PDX collection 897

      3 ✓7th **S49.002** Unspecified physeal fracture of upper end of humerus, left arm   `CC` `H5`
        CC Excl: CC with 7th character A: PDX collection 1247
        CC Excl: CC with 7th character K or P: PDX collection 897

      3 ✓7th **S49.009** Unspecified physeal fracture of upper end of humerus, unspecified arm   `CC` `H5`
        CC Excl: CC with 7th character A: PDX collection 1248
        CC Excl: CC with 7th character K or P: PDX collection 897

    ✓6th **S49.01** Salter-Harris Type I physeal fracture of upper end of humerus

      3 ✓7th **S49.011** Salter-Harris Type I physeal fracture of upper end of humerus, right arm   `CC` `H5`

      3 ✓7th **S49.012** Salter-Harris Type I physeal fracture of upper end of humerus, left arm   `CC` `H5`

      3 ✓7th **S49.019** Salter-Harris Type I physeal fracture of upper end of humerus, unspecified arm   `CC` `H5`

    ✓6th **S49.02** Salter-Harris Type II physeal fracture of upper end of humerus

      3 ✓7th **S49.021** Salter-Harris Type II physeal fracture of upper end of humerus, right arm   `CC` `H5`

      3 ✓7th **S49.022** Salter-Harris Type II physeal fracture of upper end of humerus, left arm   `CC` `H5`

      3 ✓7th **S49.029** Salter-Harris Type II physeal fracture of upper end of humerus, unspecified arm   `CC` `H5`

    ✓6th **S49.03** Salter-Harris Type III physeal fracture of upper end of humerus

      3 ✓7th **S49.031** Salter-Harris Type III physeal fracture of upper end of humerus, right arm   `CC` `H5`

      3 ✓7th **S49.032** Salter-Harris Type III physeal fracture of upper end of humerus, left arm   `CC` `H5`

      3 ✓7th **S49.039** Salter-Harris Type III physeal fracture of upper end of humerus, unspecified arm   `CC` `H5`

    ✓6th **S49.04** Salter-Harris Type IV physeal fracture of upper end of humerus

      3 ✓7th **S49.041** Salter-Harris Type IV physeal fracture of upper end of humerus, right arm   `CC` `H5`

      3 ✓7th **S49.042** Salter-Harris Type IV physeal fracture of upper end of humerus, left arm   `CC` `H5`

      3 ✓7th **S49.049** Salter-Harris Type IV physeal fracture of upper end of humerus, unspecified arm   `CC` `H5`

    ✓6th **S49.09** Other physeal fracture of upper end of humerus

      3 ✓7th **S49.091** Other physeal fracture of upper end of humerus, right arm   `CC` `H5`

      3 ✓7th **S49.092** Other physeal fracture of upper end of humerus, left arm   `CC` `H5`

      3 ✓7th **S49.099** Other physeal fracture of upper end of humerus, unspecified arm   `CC` `H5`

✓5th **S49.1** Physeal fracture of lower end of humerus

    ✓6th **S49.10** Unspecified physeal fracture of lower end of humerus

      3 ✓7th **S49.101** Unspecified physeal fracture of lower end of humerus, right arm   `CC` `H5`

      3 ✓7th **S49.102** Unspecified physeal fracture of lower end of humerus, left arm   `CC` `H5`

      3 ✓7th **S49.109** Unspecified physeal fracture of lower end of humerus, unspecified arm   `CC` `H5`

    ✓6th **S49.11** Salter-Harris Type I physeal fracture of lower end of humerus

      3 ✓7th **S49.111** Salter-Harris Type I physeal fracture of lower end of humerus, right arm   `CC` `H5`

      3 ✓7th **S49.112** Salter-Harris Type I physeal fracture of lower end of humerus, left arm   `CC` `H5`

      3 ✓7th **S49.119** Salter-Harris Type I physeal fracture of lower end of humerus, unspecified arm   `CC` `H5`

    ✓6th **S49.12** Salter-Harris Type II physeal fracture of lower end of humerus

      3 ✓7th **S49.121** Salter-Harris Type II physeal fracture of lower end of humerus, right arm   `CC` `H5`

      3 ✓7th **S49.122** Salter-Harris Type II physeal fracture of lower end of humerus, left arm   `CC` `H5`

      3 ✓7th **S49.129** Salter-Harris Type II physeal fracture of lower end of humerus, unspecified arm   `CC` `H5`

    ✓6th **S49.13** Salter-Harris Type III physeal fracture of lower end of humerus

      3 ✓7th **S49.131** Salter-Harris Type III physeal fracture of lower end of humerus, right arm   `CC` `H5`

      3 ✓7th **S49.132** Salter-Harris Type III physeal fracture of lower end of humerus, left arm   `CC` `H5`

      3 ✓7th **S49.139** Salter-Harris Type III physeal fracture of lower end of humerus, unspecified arm   `CC` `H5`

    ✓6th **S49.14** Salter-Harris Type IV physeal fracture of lower end of humerus

      3 ✓7th **S49.141** Salter-Harris Type IV physeal fracture of lower end of humerus, right arm   `CC` `H5`

3 √7ᵗʰ **S49.142 Salter-Harris Type IV physeal fracture of lower end of humerus, left arm** CC H5

3 √7ᵗʰ **S49.149 Salter-Harris Type IV physeal fracture of lower end of humerus, unspecified arm** CC H5

√6ᵗʰ **S49.19 Other physeal fracture of lower end of humerus**

3 √7ᵗʰ **S49.191 Other physeal fracture of lower end of humerus, right arm** CC H5

3 √7ᵗʰ **S49.192 Other physeal fracture of lower end of humerus, left arm** CC H5

3 √7ᵗʰ **S49.199 Other physeal fracture of lower end of humerus, unspecified arm** CC H5

√5ᵗʰ **S49.8 Other specified injuries of shoulder and upper arm**

The appropriate 7th character is to be added to each code in subcategory S49.8.
A initial encounter
D subsequent encounter
S sequela

√x7ᵗʰ **S49.80 Other specified injuries of shoulder and upper arm, unspecified arm**

√x7ᵗʰ **S49.81 Other specified injuries of right shoulder and upper arm**

√x7ᵗʰ **S49.82 Other specified injuries of left shoulder and upper arm**

√5ᵗʰ **S49.9 Unspecified injury of shoulder and upper arm**

The appropriate 7th character is to be added to each code in subcategory S49.9.
A initial encounter
D subsequent encounter
S sequela

√x7ᵗʰ **S49.90 Unspecified injury of shoulder and upper arm, unspecified arm**

√x7ᵗʰ **S49.91 Unspecified injury of right shoulder and upper arm**

√x7ᵗʰ **S49.92 Unspecified injury of left shoulder and upper arm**

Injuries to the elbow and forearm (S50-S59)

EXCLUDES 2 burns and corrosions (T20-T32)
frostbite (T33-T34)
injuries of wrist and hand (S60-S69)
insect bite or sting, venomous (T63.4)

√4ᵗʰ **S50 Superficial injury of elbow and forearm**

EXCLUDES 2 superficial injury of wrist and hand (S60.-)

The appropriate 7th character is to be added to each code from category S50.
A initial encounter
D subsequent encounter
S sequela

√5ᵗʰ **S50.0 Contusion of elbow**

√x7ᵗʰ **S50.00 Contusion of unspecified elbow**

√x7ᵗʰ **S50.01 Contusion of right elbow**

√x7ᵗʰ **S50.02 Contusion of left elbow**

√5ᵗʰ **S50.1 Contusion of forearm**

√x7ᵗʰ **S50.10 Contusion of unspecified forearm**

√x7ᵗʰ **S50.11 Contusion of right forearm**

√x7ᵗʰ **S50.12 Contusion of left forearm**

√5ᵗʰ **S50.3 Other superficial injuries of elbow**

√6ᵗʰ **S50.31 Abrasion of elbow**

√7ᵗʰ **S50.311 Abrasion of right elbow**

√7ᵗʰ **S50.312 Abrasion of left elbow**

√7ᵗʰ **S50.319 Abrasion of unspecified elbow**

√6ᵗʰ **S50.32 Blister (nonthermal) of elbow**

√7ᵗʰ **S50.321 Blister (nonthermal) of right elbow**

√7ᵗʰ **S50.322 Blister (nonthermal) of left elbow**

√7ᵗʰ **S50.329 Blister (nonthermal) of unspecified elbow**

√6ᵗʰ **S50.34 External constriction of elbow**

√7ᵗʰ **S50.341 External constriction of right elbow**

√7ᵗʰ **S50.342 External constriction of left elbow**

√7ᵗʰ **S50.349 External constriction of unspecified elbow**

√6ᵗʰ **S50.35 Superficial foreign body of elbow**

Splinter in the elbow

√7ᵗʰ **S50.351 Superficial foreign body of right elbow**

√7ᵗʰ **S50.352 Superficial foreign body of left elbow**

√7ᵗʰ **S50.359 Superficial foreign body of unspecified elbow**

√6ᵗʰ **S50.36 Insect bite (nonvenomous) of elbow**

√7ᵗʰ **S50.361 Insect bite (nonvenomous) of right elbow**

√7ᵗʰ **S50.362 Insect bite (nonvenomous) of left elbow**

√7ᵗʰ **S50.369 Insect bite (nonvenomous) of unspecified elbow**

√6ᵗʰ **S50.37 Other superficial bite of elbow**

EXCLUDES 1 open bite of elbow (S51.05)

√7ᵗʰ **S50.371 Other superficial bite of right elbow**

√7ᵗʰ **S50.372 Other superficial bite of left elbow**

√7ᵗʰ **S50.379 Other superficial bite of unspecified elbow**

√5ᵗʰ **S50.8 Other superficial injuries of forearm**

√6ᵗʰ **S50.81 Abrasion of forearm**

√7ᵗʰ **S50.811 Abrasion of right forearm**

√7ᵗʰ **S50.812 Abrasion of left forearm**

√7ᵗʰ **S50.819 Abrasion of unspecified forearm**

√6ᵗʰ **S50.82 Blister (nonthermal) of forearm**

√7ᵗʰ **S50.821 Blister (nonthermal) of right forearm**

√7ᵗʰ **S50.822 Blister (nonthermal) of left forearm**

√7ᵗʰ **S50.829 Blister (nonthermal) of unspecified forearm**

√6ᵗʰ **S50.84 External constriction of forearm**

√7ᵗʰ **S50.841 External constriction of right forearm**

√7ᵗʰ **S50.842 External constriction of left forearm**

√7ᵗʰ **S50.849 External constriction of unspecified forearm**

√6ᵗʰ **S50.85 Superficial foreign body of forearm**

Splinter in the forearm

√7ᵗʰ **S50.851 Superficial foreign body of right forearm**

√7ᵗʰ **S50.852 Superficial foreign body of left forearm**

√7ᵗʰ **S50.859 Superficial foreign body of unspecified forearm**

√6ᵗʰ **S50.86 Insect bite (nonvenomous) of forearm**

√7ᵗʰ **S50.861 Insect bite (nonvenomous) of right forearm**

√7ᵗʰ **S50.862 Insect bite (nonvenomous) of left forearm**

√7ᵗʰ **S50.869 Insect bite (nonvenomous) of unspecified forearm**

√6ᵗʰ **S50.87 Other superficial bite of forearm**

EXCLUDES 1 open bite of forearm (S51.85)

√7ᵗʰ **S50.871 Other superficial bite of right forearm**

√7ᵗʰ **S50.872 Other superficial bite of left forearm**

√7ᵗʰ **S50.879 Other superficial bite of unspecified forearm**

√5ᵗʰ **S50.9 Unspecified superficial injury of elbow and forearm**

√6ᵗʰ **S50.90 Unspecified superficial injury of elbow**

√7ᵗʰ **S50.901 Unspecified superficial injury of right elbow**

√7ᵗʰ **S50.902 Unspecified superficial injury of left elbow**

√7ᵗʰ **S50.909 Unspecified superficial injury of unspecified elbow**

√6ᵗʰ **S50.91 Unspecified superficial injury of forearm**

√7ᵗʰ **S50.911 Unspecified superficial injury of right forearm**

√7ᵗʰ **S50.912 Unspecified superficial injury of left forearm**

√7ᵗʰ **S50.919 Unspecified superficial injury of unspecified forearm**

N Newborn: 0   P Pediatric: 0-17   M Maternity: 9-64   A Adult: 15-124   MCC Major Complication/Comorbidity   CC Complication/Comorbidity   SW Severe Wound Dx

1044
ICD-10-CM 2020

☑4ᵗʰ **S51 Open wound of elbow and forearm**

Code also any associated wound infection

EXCLUDES 1   open fracture of elbow and forearm (S52.- with open fracture 7th character)

traumatic amputation of elbow and forearm (S58.-)

EXCLUDES 2   open wound of wrist and hand (S61.-)

The appropriate 7th character is to be added to each code from category S51.
A   initial encounter
D   subsequent encounter
S   sequela

☑5ᵗʰ **S51.0 Open wound of elbow**

  ☑6ᵗʰ **S51.00 Unspecified open wound of elbow**

    ☑7ᵗʰ **S51.001 Unspecified open wound of right elbow**

      AHA: 2012,4Q,108

    ☑7ᵗʰ **S51.002 Unspecified open wound of left elbow**

    ☑7ᵗʰ **S51.009 Unspecified open wound of unspecified elbow**

      Open wound of elbow NOS

  ☑6ᵗʰ **S51.01 Laceration without foreign body of elbow**

    ☑7ᵗʰ **S51.011 Laceration without foreign body of right elbow**

    ☑7ᵗʰ **S51.012 Laceration without foreign body of left elbow**

    ☑7ᵗʰ **S51.019 Laceration without foreign body of unspecified elbow**

  ☑6ᵗʰ **S51.02 Laceration with foreign body of elbow**

    ☑7ᵗʰ **S51.021 Laceration with foreign body of right elbow**

    ☑7ᵗʰ **S51.022 Laceration with foreign body of left elbow**

    ☑7ᵗʰ **S51.029 Laceration with foreign body of unspecified elbow**

  ☑6ᵗʰ **S51.03 Puncture wound without foreign body of elbow**

    ☑7ᵗʰ **S51.031 Puncture wound without foreign body of right elbow**

    ☑7ᵗʰ **S51.032 Puncture wound without foreign body of left elbow**

    ☑7ᵗʰ **S51.039 Puncture wound without foreign body of unspecified elbow**

  ☑6ᵗʰ **S51.04 Puncture wound with foreign body of elbow**

    ☑7ᵗʰ **S51.041 Puncture wound with foreign body of right elbow**

    ☑7ᵗʰ **S51.042 Puncture wound with foreign body of left elbow**

    ☑7ᵗʰ **S51.049 Puncture wound with foreign body of unspecified elbow**

  ☑6ᵗʰ **S51.05 Open bite of elbow**

    Bite of elbow NOS

    EXCLUDES 1   superficial bite of elbow (S50.36, S50.37)

    ☑7ᵗʰ **S51.051 Open bite, right elbow**

    ☑7ᵗʰ **S51.052 Open bite, left elbow**

    ☑7ᵗʰ **S51.059 Open bite, unspecified elbow**

☑5ᵗʰ **S51.8 Open wound of forearm**

  EXCLUDES 2   open wound of elbow (S51.0-)

  ☑6ᵗʰ **S51.80 Unspecified open wound of forearm**

    AHA: 2016,3Q,24

    ☑7ᵗʰ **S51.801 Unspecified open wound of right forearm**

    ☑7ᵗʰ **S51.802 Unspecified open wound of left forearm**

    ☑7ᵗʰ **S51.809 Unspecified open wound of unspecified forearm**

      Open wound of forearm NOS

  ☑6ᵗʰ **S51.81 Laceration without foreign body of forearm**

    ☑7ᵗʰ **S51.811 Laceration without foreign body of right forearm**

    ☑7ᵗʰ **S51.812 Laceration without foreign body of left forearm**

    ☑7ᵗʰ **S51.819 Laceration without foreign body of unspecified forearm**

  ☑6ᵗʰ **S51.82 Laceration with foreign body of forearm**

    ☑7ᵗʰ **S51.821 Laceration with foreign body of right forearm**

    ☑7ᵗʰ **S51.822 Laceration with foreign body of left forearm**

    ☑7ᵗʰ **S51.829 Laceration with foreign body of unspecified forearm**

  ☑6ᵗʰ **S51.83 Puncture wound without foreign body of forearm**

    AHA: 2016,3Q,24

    ☑7ᵗʰ **S51.831 Puncture wound without foreign body of right forearm**

    ☑7ᵗʰ **S51.832 Puncture wound without foreign body of left forearm**

    ☑7ᵗʰ **S51.839 Puncture wound without foreign body of unspecified forearm**

  ☑6ᵗʰ **S51.84 Puncture wound with foreign body of forearm**

    AHA: 2016,3Q,24

    ☑7ᵗʰ **S51.841 Puncture wound with foreign body of right forearm**

    ☑7ᵗʰ **S51.842 Puncture wound with foreign body of left forearm**

    ☑7ᵗʰ **S51.849 Puncture wound with foreign body of unspecified forearm**

  ☑6ᵗʰ **S51.85 Open bite of forearm**

    Bite of forearm NOS

    EXCLUDES 1   superficial bite of forearm (S50.86, S50.87)

    ☑7ᵗʰ **S51.851 Open bite of right forearm**

    ☑7ᵗʰ **S51.852 Open bite of left forearm**

    ☑7ᵗʰ **S51.859 Open bite of unspecified forearm**

☑ Additional Character Required   ☑x7ᵗʰ Placeholder   Unacceptable PDx   Questionable PDx   Manifestation   Unspecified Dx   H1-H14 HAC   HCC CMS-HCC Dx   HIV HIV Dx

√4ᵗʰ S52 Fracture of forearm

NOTE   A fracture not indicated as displaced or nondisplaced should be coded to displaced.

A fracture not indicated as open or closed should be coded to closed.

The open fracture designations are based on the Gustilo open fracture classification.

EXCLUDES 1   traumatic amputation of forearm (S58.-)
EXCLUDES 2   fracture at wrist and hand level (S62.-)

AHA: 2018,2Q,12; 2016,1Q,33; 2015,3Q,37-39
DEF: Diaphysis: Central shaft of a long bone.
DEF: Epiphysis: Proximal and distal rounded ends of a long bone, communicates with the joint.
DEF: Metaphysis: Section of a long bone located between the epiphysis and diaphysis at the proximal and distal ends.
DEF: Physis (growth plate): Narrow zone of cartilaginous tissue between the epiphysis and metaphysis at each end of a long bone. In childhood, proliferation of cells in this zone lengthens the bone. As the bone matures, this area thins, ossification eventually fusing into solid bone and growth stops. *Synonyms: Epiphyseal plate.*

The appropriate 7th character is to be added to all codes from category S52 [unless otherwise indicated].
A   initial encounter for closed fracture
B   initial encounter for open fracture type I or II
    initial encounter for open fracture NOS
C   initial encounter for open fracture type IIIA, IIIB, or IIIC
D   subsequent encounter for closed fracture with routine healing
E   subsequent encounter for open fracture type I or II with routine healing
F   subsequent encounter for open fracture type IIIA, IIIB, or IIIC with routine healing
G   subsequent encounter for closed fracture with delayed healing
H   subsequent encounter for open fracture type I or II with delayed healing
J   subsequent encounter for open fracture type IIIA, IIIB, or IIIC with delayed healing
K   subsequent encounter for closed fracture with nonunion
M   subsequent encounter for open fracture type I or II with nonunion
N   subsequent encounter for open fracture type IIIA, IIIB, or IIIC with nonunion
P   subsequent encounter for closed fracture with malunion
Q   subsequent encounter for open fracture type I or II with malunion
R   subsequent encounter for open fracture type IIIA, IIIB, or IIIC with malunion
S   sequela

√5ᵗʰ S52.0 Fracture of upper end of ulna

Fracture of proximal end of ulna
EXCLUDES 2   fracture of elbow NOS (S42.40-)
               fractures of shaft of ulna (S52.2-)

√6ᵗʰ S52.00 Unspecified fracture of upper end of ulna

CC Excl: For codes in subcategory S52.00:
MCC with 7th character B or C: PDX collection 1296
CC with 7th character K, M, N, P, Q, or R: PDX collection 897

2,4 √7ᵗʰ **S52.001** Unspecified fracture of upper end of **right** ulna   MCC CC H5

2,4 √7ᵗʰ **S52.002** Unspecified fracture of upper end of **left** ulna   MCC CC H5

2,4 √7ᵗʰ **S52.009** Unspecified fracture of upper end of unspecified ulna   MCC CC H5

√6ᵗʰ S52.01 **Torus** fracture of upper end of ulna

The appropriate 7th character is to be added to all codes in subcategory S52.01
A   initial encounter for closed fracture
D   subsequent encounter for fracture with routine healing
G   subsequent encounter for fracture with delayed healing
K   subsequent encounter for fracture with nonunion
P   subsequent encounter for fracture with malunion
S   sequela

3 √7ᵗʰ **S52.011** Torus fracture of upper end of **right** ulna   CC H5
CC Excl: CC with 7th character A: PDX collection 1270
CC Excl: CC with 7th character K or P: PDX collection 897

3 √7ᵗʰ **S52.012** Torus fracture of upper end of **left** ulna   CC H5
CC Excl: CC with 7th character A: PDX collection 1271
CC Excl: CC with 7th character K or P: PDX collection 897

3 √7ᵗʰ **S52.019** Torus fracture of upper end of unspecified ulna   CC H5
CC Excl: CC with 7th character A: PDX collection 1272
CC Excl: CC with 7th character K or P: PDX collection 897

√6ᵗʰ S52.02 Fracture of olecranon process without intraarticular extension of ulna

CC Excl: For codes in subcategory S52.02:
MCC with 7th character B or C: PDX collection 1273
CC with 7th character K, M, N, P, Q, or R: PDX collection 897

2,4 √7ᵗʰ **S52.021** Displaced fracture of olecranon process without intraarticular extension of **right** ulna   MCC CC H5

2,4 √7ᵗʰ **S52.022** Displaced fracture of olecranon process without intraarticular extension of **left** ulna   MCC CC H5

2,4 √7ᵗʰ **S52.023** Displaced fracture of olecranon process without intraarticular extension of unspecified ulna   MCC CC H5

2,4 √7ᵗʰ **S52.024** Nondisplaced fracture of olecranon process without intraarticular extension of **right** ulna   MCC CC H5

2,4 √7ᵗʰ **S52.025** Nondisplaced fracture of olecranon process without intraarticular extension of **left** ulna   MCC CC H5

2,4 √7ᵗʰ **S52.026** Nondisplaced fracture of olecranon process without intraarticular extension of unspecified ulna   MCC CC H5

√6ᵗʰ S52.03 Fracture of olecranon process with intraarticular extension of ulna

CC Excl: For codes in subcategory S52.03:
MCC with 7th character B or C: PDX collection 1273
CC with 7th character K, M, N, P, Q, or R: PDX collection 897

2,4 √7ᵗʰ **S52.031** Displaced fracture of olecranon process with intraarticular extension of **right** ulna   MCC CC H5

2,4 √7ᵗʰ **S52.032** Displaced fracture of olecranon process with intraarticular extension of **left** ulna   MCC CC H5

2,4 √7ᵗʰ **S52.033** Displaced fracture of olecranon process with intraarticular extension of unspecified ulna   MCC CC H5

2,4 √7ᵗʰ **S52.034** Nondisplaced fracture of olecranon process with intraarticular extension of **right** ulna   MCC CC H5

2,4 √7ᵗʰ **S52.035** Nondisplaced fracture of olecranon process with intraarticular extension of left ulna `MCC` `CC` `H5`

2,4 √7ᵗʰ **S52.036** Nondisplaced fracture of olecranon process with intraarticular extension of unspecified ulna `MCC` `CC` `H5`

√6ᵗʰ **S52.04** Fracture of coronoid process of ulna

CC Excl: For codes in subcategory S52.04:
MCC with 7th character B or C: PDX collection 1269
CC with 7th character K, M, N, P, Q, or R: PDX collection 897

2,4 √7ᵗʰ **S52.041** Displaced fracture of coronoid process of right ulna `MCC` `CC` `H5`

2,4 √7ᵗʰ **S52.042** Displaced fracture of coronoid process of left ulna `MCC` `CC` `H5`

2,4 √7ᵗʰ **S52.043** Displaced fracture of coronoid process of unspecified ulna `MCC` `CC` `H5`

2,4 √7ᵗʰ **S52.044** Nondisplaced fracture of coronoid process of right ulna `MCC` `CC` `H5`

2,4 √7ᵗʰ **S52.045** Nondisplaced fracture of coronoid process of left ulna `MCC` `CC` `H5`

2,4 √7ᵗʰ **S52.046** Nondisplaced fracture of coronoid process of unspecified ulna `MCC` `CC` `H5`

√6ᵗʰ **S52.09** Other fracture of upper end of ulna

CC Excl: For codes in subcategory S52.09:
MCC with 7th character B or C: PDX collection 1269
CC with 7th character K, M, N, P, Q, or R: PDX collection 897

2,4 √7ᵗʰ **S52.091** Other fracture of upper end of right ulna `MCC` `CC` `H5`

2,4 √7ᵗʰ **S52.092** Other fracture of upper end of left ulna `MCC` `CC` `H5`

2,4 √7ᵗʰ **S52.099** Other fracture of upper end of unspecified ulna `MCC` `CC` `H5`

√5ᵗʰ **S52.1** Fracture of upper end of radius

Fracture of proximal end of radius

EXCLUDES 2   physeal fractures of upper end of radius (S59.2-)
fracture of shaft of radius (S52.3-)

CC Excl: For codes in subcategory S52.1, unless otherwise noted:
MCC with 7th character B or C: PDX collection 1269
CC with 7th character K, M, N, P, Q, or R: PDX collection 897

√6ᵗʰ **S52.10** Unspecified fracture of upper end of radius

2,4 √7ᵗʰ **S52.101** Unspecified fracture of upper end of right radius `MCC` `CC` `H5`

2,4 √7ᵗʰ **S52.102** Unspecified fracture of upper end of left radius `MCC` `CC` `H5`

2,4 √7ᵗʰ **S52.109** Unspecified fracture of upper end of unspecified radius `MCC` `CC` `H5`

√6ᵗʰ **S52.11** Torus fracture of upper end of radius

The appropriate 7th character is to be added to all codes in subcategory S52.11
A   initial encounter for closed fracture
D   subsequent encounter for fracture with routine healing
G   subsequent encounter for fracture with delayed healing
K   subsequent encounter for fracture with nonunion
P   subsequent encounter for fracture with malunion
S   sequela

3 √7ᵗʰ **S52.111** Torus fracture of upper end of right radius `CC` `H5`
CC Excl: CC with 7th character A: PDX collection 1270
CC Excl: CC with 7th character K or P: PDX collection 897

3 √7ᵗʰ **S52.112** Torus fracture of upper end of left radius `CC` `H5`
CC Excl: CC with 7th character A: PDX collection 1271
CC Excl: CC with 7th character K or P: PDX collection 897

3 √7ᵗʰ **S52.119** Torus fracture of upper end of unspecified radius `CC` `H5`
CC Excl: CC with 7th character A: PDX collection 1272
CC Excl: CC with 7th character K or P: PDX collection 897

√6ᵗʰ **S52.12** Fracture of head of radius

2,4 √7ᵗʰ **S52.121** Displaced fracture of head of right radius `MCC` `CC` `H5`

2,4 √7ᵗʰ **S52.122** Displaced fracture of head of left radius `MCC` `CC` `H5`

2,4 √7ᵗʰ **S52.123** Displaced fracture of head of unspecified radius `MCC` `CC` `H5`

2,4 √7ᵗʰ **S52.124** Nondisplaced fracture of head of right radius `MCC` `CC` `H5`

2,4 √7ᵗʰ **S52.125** Nondisplaced fracture of head of left radius `MCC` `CC` `H5`

2,4 √7ᵗʰ **S52.126** Nondisplaced fracture of head of unspecified radius `MCC` `CC` `H5`

√6ᵗʰ **S52.13** Fracture of neck of radius

2,4 √7ᵗʰ **S52.131** Displaced fracture of neck of right radius `MCC` `CC` `H5`

2,4 √7ᵗʰ **S52.132** Displaced fracture of neck of left radius `MCC` `CC` `H5`

2,4 √7ᵗʰ **S52.133** Displaced fracture of neck of unspecified radius `MCC` `CC` `H5`

2,4 √7ᵗʰ **S52.134** Nondisplaced fracture of neck of right radius `MCC` `CC` `H5`

2,4 √7ᵗʰ **S52.135** Nondisplaced fracture of neck of left radius `MCC` `CC` `H5`

2,4 √7ᵗʰ **S52.136** Nondisplaced fracture of neck of unspecified radius `MCC` `CC` `H5`

√6ᵗʰ **S52.18** Other fracture of upper end of radius

2,4 √7ᵗʰ **S52.181** Other fracture of upper end of right radius `MCC` `CC` `H5`

2,4 √7ᵗʰ **S52.182** Other fracture of upper end of left radius `MCC` `CC` `H5`

2,4 √7ᵗʰ **S52.189** Other fracture of upper end of unspecified radius `MCC` `CC` `H5`

√5ᵗʰ **S52.2** Fracture of shaft of ulna

CC Excl: For CC/MCC codes in subcategory S52.2, unless otherwise noted:
Right side: See code S52.201
Left side: See code S52.202
Unspecified side: See code S52.209

√6ᵗʰ **S52.20** Unspecified fracture of shaft of ulna

Fracture of ulna NOS

2,3 √7ᵗʰ **S52.201** Unspecified fracture of shaft of right ulna `MCC` `CC` `H5`
CC Excl: CC with 7th character A: PDX collection 1270
CC Excl: MCC with 7th character B or C: PDX collection 1269
CC Excl: CC with 7th character K, M, N, P, Q, or R: PDX collection 897

2,3 √7ᵗʰ **S52.202** Unspecified fracture of shaft of left ulna `MCC` `CC` `H5`
CC Excl: CC with 7th character A: PDX collection 1271
CC Excl: MCC with 7th character B or C: PDX collection 1269
CC Excl: CC with 7th character K, M, N, P, Q, or R: PDX collection 897

2,3 √7ᵗʰ **S52.209** Unspecified fracture of shaft of unspecified ulna `MCC` `CC` `H5`
CC Excl: CC with 7th character A: PDX collection 1272
CC Excl: MCC with 7th character B or C: PDX collection 1269
CC Excl: CC with 7th character K, M, N, P, Q, or R: PDX collection 897

√6ᵗʰ S52.21 Greenstick fracture of shaft of ulna

> The appropriate 7th character is to be added to all codes in subcategory S52.21
> A   initial encounter for closed fracture
> D   subsequent encounter for fracture with routine healing
> G   subsequent encounter for fracture with delayed healing
> K   subsequent encounter for fracture with nonunion
> P   subsequent encounter for fracture with malunion
> S   sequela

3 √7ᵗʰ **S52.211 Greenstick fracture of shaft of right ulna**   CC H5
    CC Excl: CC with 7th character A: PDX collection 1270
    CC Excl: CC with 7th character K or P: PDX collection 897

3 √7ᵗʰ **S52.212 Greenstick fracture of shaft of left ulna**   CC H5
    CC Excl: CC with 7th character A: PDX collection 1271
    CC Excl: CC with 7th character K or P: PDX collection 897

3 √7ᵗʰ **S52.219 Greenstick fracture of shaft of unspecified ulna**   CC H5
    CC Excl: CC with 7th character A: PDX collection 1272
    CC Excl: CC with 7th character K or P: PDX collection 897

√6ᵗʰ S52.22 Transverse fracture of shaft of ulna

2,3 √7ᵗʰ **S52.221 Displaced transverse fracture of shaft of right ulna**   MCC CC H5

2,3 √7ᵗʰ **S52.222 Displaced transverse fracture of shaft of left ulna**   MCC CC H5

2,3 √7ᵗʰ **S52.223 Displaced transverse fracture of shaft of unspecified ulna**   MCC CC H5

2,3 √7ᵗʰ **S52.224 Nondisplaced transverse fracture of shaft of right ulna**   MCC CC H5

2,3 √7ᵗʰ **S52.225 Nondisplaced transverse fracture of shaft of left ulna**   MCC CC H5

2,3 √7ᵗʰ **S52.226 Nondisplaced transverse fracture of shaft of unspecified ulna**   MCC CC H5

√6ᵗʰ S52.23 Oblique fracture of shaft of ulna

2,3 √7ᵗʰ **S52.231 Displaced oblique fracture of shaft of right ulna**   MCC CC H5

2,3 √7ᵗʰ **S52.232 Displaced oblique fracture of shaft of left ulna**   MCC CC H5

2,3 √7ᵗʰ **S52.233 Displaced oblique fracture of shaft of unspecified ulna**   MCC CC H5

2,3 √7ᵗʰ **S52.234 Nondisplaced oblique fracture of shaft of right ulna**   MCC CC H5

2,3 √7ᵗʰ **S52.235 Nondisplaced oblique fracture of shaft of left ulna**   MCC CC H5

2,3 √7ᵗʰ **S52.236 Nondisplaced oblique fracture of shaft of unspecified ulna**   MCC CC H5

√6ᵗʰ S52.24 Spiral fracture of shaft of ulna

2,3 √7ᵗʰ **S52.241 Displaced spiral fracture of shaft of ulna, right arm**   MCC CC H5

2,3 √7ᵗʰ **S52.242 Displaced spiral fracture of shaft of ulna, left arm**   MCC CC H5

2,3 √7ᵗʰ **S52.243 Displaced spiral fracture of shaft of ulna, unspecified arm**   MCC CC H5

2,3 √7ᵗʰ **S52.244 Nondisplaced spiral fracture of shaft of ulna, right arm**   MCC CC H5

2,3 √7ᵗʰ **S52.245 Nondisplaced spiral fracture of shaft of ulna, left arm**   MCC CC H5

2,3 √7ᵗʰ **S52.246 Nondisplaced spiral fracture of shaft of ulna, unspecified arm**   MCC CC H5

√6ᵗʰ S52.25 Comminuted fracture of shaft of ulna

2,3 √7ᵗʰ **S52.251 Displaced comminuted fracture of shaft of ulna, right arm**   MCC CC H5

2,3 √7ᵗʰ **S52.252 Displaced comminuted fracture of shaft of ulna, left arm**   MCC CC H5

2,3 √7ᵗʰ **S52.253 Displaced comminuted fracture of shaft of ulna, unspecified arm**   MCC CC H5

2,3 √7ᵗʰ **S52.254 Nondisplaced comminuted fracture of shaft of ulna, right arm**   MCC CC H5

2,3 √7ᵗʰ **S52.255 Nondisplaced comminuted fracture of shaft of ulna, left arm**   MCC CC H5

2,3 √7ᵗʰ **S52.256 Nondisplaced comminuted fracture of shaft of ulna, unspecified arm**   MCC CC H5

√6ᵗʰ S52.26 Segmental fracture of shaft of ulna

2,3 √7ᵗʰ **S52.261 Displaced segmental fracture of shaft of ulna, right arm**   MCC CC H5

2,3 √7ᵗʰ **S52.262 Displaced segmental fracture of shaft of ulna, left arm**   MCC CC H5

2,3 √7ᵗʰ **S52.263 Displaced segmental fracture of shaft of ulna, unspecified arm**   MCC CC H5

2,3 √7ᵗʰ **S52.264 Nondisplaced segmental fracture of shaft of ulna, right arm**   MCC CC H5

2,3 √7ᵗʰ **S52.265 Nondisplaced segmental fracture of shaft of ulna, left arm**   MCC CC H5

2,3 √7ᵗʰ **S52.266 Nondisplaced segmental fracture of shaft of ulna, unspecified arm**   MCC CC H5

√6ᵗʰ S52.27 Monteggia's fracture of ulna

> Fracture of upper shaft of ulna with dislocation of radial head
> CC Excl: For codes in subcategory S52.27:
> MCC with 7th character B or C: PDX collection 1269
> CC with 7th character K, M, N, P, Q, or R: PDX collection 897

2,4 √7ᵗʰ **S52.271 Monteggia's fracture of right ulna**   MCC CC H5

2,4 √7ᵗʰ **S52.272 Monteggia's fracture of left ulna**   MCC CC H5

2,4 √7ᵗʰ **S52.279 Monteggia's fracture of unspecified ulna**   MCC CC H5

√6ᵗʰ S52.28 Bent bone of ulna

2,3 √7ᵗʰ **S52.281 Bent bone of right ulna**   MCC CC H5

2,3 √7ᵗʰ **S52.282 Bent bone of left ulna**   MCC CC H5

2,3 √7ᵗʰ **S52.283 Bent bone of unspecified ulna**   MCC CC H5

√6ᵗʰ S52.29 Other fracture of shaft of ulna

2,3 √7ᵗʰ **S52.291 Other fracture of shaft of right ulna**   MCC CC H5

2,3 √7ᵗʰ **S52.292 Other fracture of shaft of left ulna**   MCC CC H5

2,3 √7ᵗʰ **S52.299 Other fracture of shaft of unspecified ulna**   MCC CC H5

√5ᵗʰ S52.3 Fracture of shaft of radius

> CC Excl: For CC/MCC codes in subcategory S52.3, unless otherwise noted:
> Right side: See code S52.201
> Left side: See code S52.202
> Unspecified side: See code S52.209

√6ᵗʰ S52.30 Unspecified fracture of shaft of radius

2,3 √7ᵗʰ **S52.301 Unspecified fracture of shaft of right radius**   MCC CC H5

2,3 √7ᵗʰ **S52.302 Unspecified fracture of shaft of left radius**   MCC CC H5

2,3 √7ᵗʰ **S52.309 Unspecified fracture of shaft of unspecified radius**   MCC CC H5

√6ᵗʰ **S52.31** Greenstick **fracture of shaft of radius**

The appropriate 7th character is to be added to all codes in subcategory S52.31.
A   initial encounter for closed fracture
D   subsequent encounter for fracture with routine healing
G   subsequent encounter for fracture with delayed healing
K   subsequent encounter for fracture with nonunion
P   subsequent encounter for fracture with malunion
S   sequela

³ √7ᵗʰ **S52.311** Greenstick fracture of shaft of radius, right arm   CC H5
     CC Excl: See code S52.211

³ √7ᵗʰ **S52.312** Greenstick fracture of shaft of radius, left arm   CC H5
     CC Excl: See code S52.212

³ √7ᵗʰ **S52.319** Greenstick fracture of shaft of radius, unspecified arm   CC H5
     CC Excl: See code S52.219

√6ᵗʰ **S52.32** Transverse **fracture of shaft of radius**

2,3 √7ᵗʰ **S52.321** Displaced transverse fracture of shaft of right radius   MCC CC H5

2,3 √7ᵗʰ **S52.322** Displaced transverse fracture of shaft of left radius   MCC CC H5

2,3 √7ᵗʰ **S52.323** Displaced transverse fracture of shaft of unspecified radius   MCC CC H5

2,3 √7ᵗʰ **S52.324** Nondisplaced transverse fracture of shaft of right radius   MCC CC H5

2,3 √7ᵗʰ **S52.325** Nondisplaced transverse fracture of shaft of left radius   MCC CC H5

2,3 √7ᵗʰ **S52.326** Nondisplaced transverse fracture of shaft of unspecified radius   MCC CC H5

√6ᵗʰ **S52.33** Oblique **fracture of shaft of radius**

2,3 √7ᵗʰ **S52.331** Displaced oblique fracture of shaft of right radius   MCC CC H5

2,3 √7ᵗʰ **S52.332** Displaced oblique fracture of shaft of left radius   MCC CC H5

2,3 √7ᵗʰ **S52.333** Displaced oblique fracture of shaft of unspecified radius   MCC CC H5

2,3 √7ᵗʰ **S52.334** Nondisplaced oblique fracture of shaft of right radius   MCC CC H5

2,3 √7ᵗʰ **S52.335** Nondisplaced oblique fracture of shaft of left radius   MCC CC H5

2,3 √7ᵗʰ **S52.336** Nondisplaced oblique fracture of shaft of unspecified radius   MCC CC H5

√6ᵗʰ **S52.34** Spiral **fracture of shaft of radius**

2,3 √7ᵗʰ **S52.341** Displaced spiral fracture of shaft of radius, right arm   MCC CC H5

2,3 √7ᵗʰ **S52.342** Displaced spiral fracture of shaft of radius, left arm   MCC CC H5

2,3 √7ᵗʰ **S52.343** Displaced spiral fracture of shaft of radius, unspecified arm   MCC CC H5

2,3 √7ᵗʰ **S52.344** Nondisplaced spiral fracture of shaft of radius, right arm   MCC CC H5

2,3 √7ᵗʰ **S52.345** Nondisplaced spiral fracture of shaft of radius, left arm   MCC CC H5

2,3 √7ᵗʰ **S52.346** Nondisplaced spiral fracture of shaft of radius, unspecified arm   MCC CC H5

√6ᵗʰ **S52.35** Comminuted **fracture of shaft of radius**

2,3 √7ᵗʰ **S52.351** Displaced comminuted fracture of shaft of radius, right arm   MCC CC H5

2,3 √7ᵗʰ **S52.352** Displaced comminuted fracture of shaft of radius, left arm   MCC CC H5

2,3 √7ᵗʰ **S52.353** Displaced comminuted fracture of shaft of radius, unspecified arm   MCC CC H5

2,3 √7ᵗʰ **S52.354** Nondisplaced comminuted fracture of shaft of radius, right arm   MCC CC H5

2,3 √7ᵗʰ **S52.355** Nondisplaced comminuted fracture of shaft of radius, left arm   MCC CC H5

2,3 √7ᵗʰ **S52.356** Nondisplaced comminuted fracture of shaft of radius, unspecified arm   MCC CC H5

√6ᵗʰ **S52.36** Segmental **fracture of shaft of radius**

2,3 √7ᵗʰ **S52.361** Displaced segmental fracture of shaft of radius, right arm   MCC CC H5

2,3 √7ᵗʰ **S52.362** Displaced segmental fracture of shaft of radius, left arm   MCC CC H5

2,3 √7ᵗʰ **S52.363** Displaced segmental fracture of shaft of radius, unspecified arm   MCC CC H5

2,3 √7ᵗʰ **S52.364** Nondisplaced segmental fracture of shaft of radius, right arm   MCC CC H5

2,3 √7ᵗʰ **S52.365** Nondisplaced segmental fracture of shaft of radius, left arm   MCC CC H5

2,3 √7ᵗʰ **S52.366** Nondisplaced segmental fracture of shaft of radius, unspecified arm   MCC CC H5

√6ᵗʰ **S52.37** Galeazzi's **fracture**

Fracture of lower shaft of radius with radioulnar joint dislocation

2,3 √7ᵗʰ **S52.371** Galeazzi's fracture of right radius   MCC CC H5

2,3 √7ᵗʰ **S52.372** Galeazzi's fracture of left radius   MCC CC H5

2,3 √7ᵗʰ **S52.379** Galeazzi's fracture of unspecified radius   MCC CC H5

√6ᵗʰ **S52.38** Bent bone **of radius**

2,3 √7ᵗʰ **S52.381** Bent bone of right radius   MCC CC H5

2,3 √7ᵗʰ **S52.382** Bent bone of left radius   MCC CC H5

2,3 √7ᵗʰ **S52.389** Bent bone of unspecified radius   MCC CC H5

√6ᵗʰ **S52.39** Other **fracture of shaft of radius**

2,3 √7ᵗʰ **S52.391** Other fracture of shaft of radius, right arm   MCC CC H5

2,3 √7ᵗʰ **S52.392** Other fracture of shaft of radius, left arm   MCC CC H5

2,3 √7ᵗʰ **S52.399** Other fracture of shaft of radius, unspecified arm   MCC CC H5

√5ᵗʰ **S52.5** **Fracture of lower end of radius**

Fracture of distal end of radius

EXCLUDES 2   *physeal fractures of lower end of radius (S59.2-)*

DEF: Fracture of the distal end of the radius above the wrist, most commonly caused by a fall onto an outstretched hand.

CC Excl: For CC/MCC codes in subcategory S52.5, unless otherwise noted:
Right side: See code S52.201
Left side: See code S52.202
Unspecified side: See code S52.209

√6ᵗʰ **S52.50** Unspecified **fracture of the lower end of radius**

2,3 √7ᵗʰ **S52.501** Unspecified fracture of the lower end of right radius   MCC CC H5

2,3 √7ᵗʰ **S52.502** Unspecified fracture of the lower end of left radius   MCC CC H5

2,3 √7ᵗʰ **S52.509** Unspecified fracture of the lower end of unspecified radius   MCC CC H5

√6ᵗʰ **S52.51** Fracture **of radial styloid process**

2,3 √7ᵗʰ **S52.511** Displaced fracture of right radial styloid process   MCC CC H5

2,3 √7ᵗʰ **S52.512** Displaced fracture of left radial styloid process   MCC CC H5

2,3 ✓7ᵗʰ **S52.513 Displaced fracture of** `MCC` `CC` `H5`
unspecified radial styloid
process

2,3 ✓7ᵗʰ **S52.514 Nondisplaced fracture of** `MCC` `CC` `H5`
right radial styloid process

2,3 ✓7ᵗʰ **S52.515 Nondisplaced fracture of** `MCC` `CC` `H5`
left radial styloid process

2,3 ✓7ᵗʰ **S52.516 Nondisplaced fracture of** `MCC` `CC` `H5`
unspecified radial styloid
process

✓6ᵗʰ **S52.52 Torus fracture of lower end of radius**

> The appropriate 7th character is to be added to all
> codes in subcategory S52.52.
> A   initial encounter for closed fracture
> D   subsequent encounter for fracture with routine
>   healing
> G   subsequent encounter for fracture with delayed
>   healing
> K   subsequent encounter for fracture with
>   nonunion
> P   subsequent encounter for fracture with
>   malunion
> S   sequela

3 ✓7ᵗʰ **S52.521 Torus fracture of lower** `CC` `H5`
end of right radius
     CC Excl: See code S52.211

3 ✓7ᵗʰ **S52.522 Torus fracture of lower** `CC` `H5`
end of left radius
     CC Excl: See code S52.212

3 ✓7ᵗʰ **S52.529 Torus fracture of lower** `CC` `H5`
end of unspecified radius
     CC Excl: See code S52.219

✓6ᵗʰ **S52.53 Colles' fracture**

AHA: 2016,2Q,4
DEF: Fracture of the radius at the wrist in which the
distal fragment is pushed posteriorly. The dorsal
angulation of the fragment results in the wrist cocking
up.

2,3 ✓7ᵗʰ **S52.531 Colles' fracture of right** `MCC` `CC` `H5`
radius

2,3 ✓7ᵗʰ **S52.532 Colles' fracture of left** `MCC` `CC` `H5`
radius

2,3 ✓7ᵗʰ **S52.539 Colles' fracture of** `MCC` `CC` `H5`
unspecified radius

✓6ᵗʰ **S52.54 Smith's fracture**

2,3 ✓7ᵗʰ **S52.541 Smith's fracture of right** `MCC` `CC` `H5`
radius

2,3 ✓7ᵗʰ **S52.542 Smith's fracture of left** `MCC` `CC` `H5`
radius

2,3 ✓7ᵗʰ **S52.549 Smith's fracture of** `MCC` `CC` `H5`
unspecified radius

✓6ᵗʰ **S52.55 Other extraarticular fracture of lower end of radius**

2,3 ✓7ᵗʰ **S52.551 Other extraarticular** `MCC` `CC` `H5`
fracture of lower end of
right radius

2,3 ✓7ᵗʰ **S52.552 Other extraarticular** `MCC` `CC` `H5`
fracture of lower end of
left radius

2,3 ✓7ᵗʰ **S52.559 Other extraarticular** `MCC` `CC` `H5`
fracture of lower end of
unspecified radius

✓6ᵗʰ **S52.56 Barton's fracture**

2,3 ✓7ᵗʰ **S52.561 Barton's fracture of right** `MCC` `CC` `H5`
radius

2,3 ✓7ᵗʰ **S52.562 Barton's fracture of left** `MCC` `CC` `H5`
radius

2,3 ✓7ᵗʰ **S52.569 Barton's fracture of** `MCC` `CC` `H5`
unspecified radius

✓6ᵗʰ **S52.57 Other intraarticular fracture of lower end of radius**

2,3 ✓7ᵗʰ **S52.571 Other intraarticular** `MCC` `CC` `H5`
fracture of lower end of
right radius

2,3 ✓7ᵗʰ **S52.572 Other intraarticular** `MCC` `CC` `H5`
fracture of lower end of
left radius

2,3 ✓7ᵗʰ **S52.579 Other intraarticular** `MCC` `CC` `H5`
fracture of lower end of
unspecified radius

✓6ᵗʰ **S52.59 Other fractures of lower end of radius**

2,3 ✓7ᵗʰ **S52.591 Other fractures of lower** `MCC` `CC` `H5`
end of right radius

2,3 ✓7ᵗʰ **S52.592 Other fractures of lower** `MCC` `CC` `H5`
end of left radius

2,3 ✓7ᵗʰ **S52.599 Other fractures of lower** `MCC` `CC` `H5`
end of unspecified radius

✓5ᵗʰ **S52.6 Fracture of lower end of ulna**

> **CC Excl: For CC/MCC codes in subcategory S52.6, unless**
> **otherwise noted:**
> **Right side:** See code S52.201
> **Left side:** See code S52.202
> **Unspecified side:** See code S52.209

✓6ᵗʰ **S52.60 Unspecified fracture of lower end of ulna**

2,3 ✓7ᵗʰ **S52.601 Unspecified fracture of** `MCC` `CC` `H5`
lower end of right ulna

2,3 ✓7ᵗʰ **S52.602 Unspecified fracture of** `MCC` `CC` `H5`
lower end of left ulna

2,3 ✓7ᵗʰ **S52.609 Unspecified fracture of** `MCC` `CC` `H5`
lower end of unspecified
ulna

✓6ᵗʰ **S52.61 Fracture of ulna styloid process**

2,3 ✓7ᵗʰ **S52.611 Displaced fracture of right** `MCC` `CC` `H5`
ulna styloid process

2,3 ✓7ᵗʰ **S52.612 Displaced fracture of left** `MCC` `CC` `H5`
ulna styloid process

2,3 ✓7ᵗʰ **S52.613 Displaced fracture of** `MCC` `CC` `H5`
unspecified ulna styloid
process

2,3 ✓7ᵗʰ **S52.614 Nondisplaced fracture of** `MCC` `CC` `H5`
right ulna styloid process

2,3 ✓7ᵗʰ **S52.615 Nondisplaced fracture of** `MCC` `CC` `H5`
left ulna styloid process

2,3 ✓7ᵗʰ **S52.616 Nondisplaced fracture of** `MCC` `CC` `H5`
unspecified ulna styloid
process

✓6ᵗʰ **S52.62 Torus fracture of lower end of ulna**

> The appropriate 7th character is to be added to all
> codes in subcategory S52.62.
> A   initial encounter for closed fracture
> D   subsequent encounter for fracture with routine
>   healing
> G   subsequent encounter for fracture with delayed
>   healing
> K   subsequent encounter for fracture with
>   nonunion
> P   subsequent encounter for fracture with
>   malunion
> S   sequela

3 ✓7ᵗʰ **S52.621 Torus fracture of lower** `CC` `H5`
end of right ulna
     CC Excl: See code S52.211

3 ✓7ᵗʰ **S52.622 Torus fracture of lower** `CC` `H5`
end of left ulna
     CC Excl: See code S52.212

3 ✓7ᵗʰ **S52.629 Torus fracture of lower** `CC` `H5`
end of unspecified ulna
     CC Excl: See code S52.219

✓6ᵗʰ **S52.69 Other fracture of lower end of ulna**

2,3 ✓7ᵗʰ **S52.691 Other fracture of lower** `MCC` `CC` `H5`
end of right ulna

2,3 ✓7ᵗʰ **S52.692 Other fracture of lower** `MCC` `CC` `H5`
end of left ulna

2,3 ✓7ᵗʰ **S52.699 Other fracture of lower** `MCC` `CC` `H5`
end of unspecified ulna

✓5ᵗʰ **S52.9 Unspecified fracture of forearm**

> **CC Excl: For CC/MCC codes in subcategory S52.9:** See code
> S52.209

2,3 ✓×7ᵗʰ **S52.90 Unspecified fracture of unspecified** `MCC` `CC` `H5`
forearm

2,3 ✓×7ᵗʰ **S52.91 Unspecified fracture of right forearm** `MCC` `CC` `H5`

2,3 ✓×7ᵗʰ **S52.92 Unspecified fracture of left forearm** `MCC` `CC` `H5`

Ⓝ Newborn: 0   Ⓟ Pediatric: 0-17   Ⓜ Maternity: 9-64   Ⓐ Adult: 15-124   `MCC` Major Complication/Comorbidity   `CC` Complication/Comorbidity   `SW` Severe Wound Dx

1050   ICD-10-CM 2020

√4ᵗʰ S53 Dislocation and sprain of joints and ligaments of elbow

INCLUDES   avulsion of joint or ligament of elbow
laceration of cartilage, joint or ligament of elbow
sprain of cartilage, joint or ligament of elbow
traumatic hemarthrosis of joint or ligament of elbow
traumatic rupture of joint or ligament of elbow
traumatic subluxation of joint or ligament of elbow
traumatic tear of joint or ligament of elbow

Code also any associated open wound

EXCLUDES 2   strain of muscle, fascia and tendon at forearm level (S56.-)

The appropriate 7th character is to be added to each code from category S53.
A   initial encounter
D   subsequent encounter
S   sequela

√5ᵗʰ S53.0 Subluxation and dislocation of radial head

Dislocation of radiohumeral joint
Subluxation of radiohumeral joint

EXCLUDES 1   Monteggia's fracture-dislocation (S52.27-)

√6ᵗʰ S53.00 Unspecified subluxation and dislocation of radial head

√7ᵗʰ **S53.001** Unspecified subluxation of right radial head

√7ᵗʰ **S53.002** Unspecified subluxation of left radial head

√7ᵗʰ **S53.003** Unspecified subluxation of unspecified radial head

√7ᵗʰ **S53.004** Unspecified dislocation of right radial head

√7ᵗʰ **S53.005** Unspecified dislocation of left radial head

√7ᵗʰ **S53.006** Unspecified dislocation of unspecified radial head

√6ᵗʰ S53.01 Anterior subluxation and dislocation of radial head

Anteriomedial subluxation and dislocation of radial head

√7ᵗʰ **S53.011** Anterior subluxation of right radial head

√7ᵗʰ **S53.012** Anterior subluxation of left radial head

√7ᵗʰ **S53.013** Anterior subluxation of unspecified radial head

√7ᵗʰ **S53.014** Anterior dislocation of right radial head

√7ᵗʰ **S53.015** Anterior dislocation of left radial head

√7ᵗʰ **S53.016** Anterior dislocation of unspecified radial head

√6ᵗʰ S53.02 Posterior subluxation and dislocation of radial head

Posteriolateral subluxation and dislocation of radial head

√7ᵗʰ **S53.021** Posterior subluxation of right radial head

√7ᵗʰ **S53.022** Posterior subluxation of left radial head

√7ᵗʰ **S53.023** Posterior subluxation of unspecified radial head

√7ᵗʰ **S53.024** Posterior dislocation of right radial head

√7ᵗʰ **S53.025** Posterior dislocation of left radial head

√7ᵗʰ **S53.026** Posterior dislocation of unspecified radial head

√6ᵗʰ S53.03 Nursemaid's elbow

√7ᵗʰ **S53.031** Nursemaid's elbow, right elbow

√7ᵗʰ **S53.032** Nursemaid's elbow, left elbow

√7ᵗʰ **S53.033** Nursemaid's elbow, unspecified elbow

√6ᵗʰ S53.09 Other subluxation and dislocation of radial head

√7ᵗʰ **S53.091** Other subluxation of right radial head

√7ᵗʰ **S53.092** Other subluxation of left radial head

√7ᵗʰ **S53.093** Other subluxation of unspecified radial head

√7ᵗʰ **S53.094** Other dislocation of right radial head

√7ᵗʰ **S53.095** Other dislocation of left radial head

√7ᵗʰ **S53.096** Other dislocation of unspecified radial head

√5ᵗʰ S53.1 Subluxation and dislocation of ulnohumeral joint

Subluxation and dislocation of elbow NOS

EXCLUDES 1   dislocation of radial head alone (S53.0-)

√6ᵗʰ S53.10 Unspecified subluxation and dislocation of ulnohumeral joint

√7ᵗʰ **S53.101** Unspecified subluxation of right ulnohumeral joint

√7ᵗʰ **S53.102** Unspecified subluxation of left ulnohumeral joint

√7ᵗʰ **S53.103** Unspecified subluxation of unspecified ulnohumeral joint

√7ᵗʰ **S53.104** Unspecified dislocation of right ulnohumeral joint

√7ᵗʰ **S53.105** Unspecified dislocation of left ulnohumeral joint

√7ᵗʰ **S53.106** Unspecified dislocation of unspecified ulnohumeral joint

√6ᵗʰ S53.11 Anterior subluxation and dislocation of ulnohumeral joint

√7ᵗʰ **S53.111** Anterior subluxation of right ulnohumeral joint

√7ᵗʰ **S53.112** Anterior subluxation of left ulnohumeral joint

√7ᵗʰ **S53.113** Anterior subluxation of unspecified ulnohumeral joint

√7ᵗʰ **S53.114** Anterior dislocation of right ulnohumeral joint

AHA: 2012,4Q,108

√7ᵗʰ **S53.115** Anterior dislocation of left ulnohumeral joint

√7ᵗʰ **S53.116** Anterior dislocation of unspecified ulnohumeral joint

√6ᵗʰ S53.12 Posterior subluxation and dislocation of ulnohumeral joint

√7ᵗʰ **S53.121** Posterior subluxation of right ulnohumeral joint

√7ᵗʰ **S53.122** Posterior subluxation of left ulnohumeral joint

√7ᵗʰ **S53.123** Posterior subluxation of unspecified ulnohumeral joint

√7ᵗʰ **S53.124** Posterior dislocation of right ulnohumeral joint

√7ᵗʰ **S53.125** Posterior dislocation of left ulnohumeral joint

√7ᵗʰ **S53.126** Posterior dislocation of unspecified ulnohumeral joint

√6ᵗʰ S53.13 Medial subluxation and dislocation of ulnohumeral joint

√7ᵗʰ **S53.131** Medial subluxation of right ulnohumeral joint

√7ᵗʰ **S53.132** Medial subluxation of left ulnohumeral joint

√7ᵗʰ **S53.133** Medial subluxation of unspecified ulnohumeral joint

√7ᵗʰ **S53.134** Medial dislocation of right ulnohumeral joint

√7ᵗʰ **S53.135** Medial dislocation of left ulnohumeral joint

√7ᵗʰ **S53.136** Medial dislocation of unspecified ulnohumeral joint

√6ᵗʰ S53.14 Lateral subluxation and dislocation of ulnohumeral joint

√7ᵗʰ **S53.141** Lateral subluxation of right ulnohumeral joint

√7ᵗʰ **S53.142** Lateral subluxation of left ulnohumeral joint

√7ᵗʰ **S53.143** Lateral subluxation of unspecified ulnohumeral joint

√7ᵗʰ **S53.144** Lateral dislocation of right ulnohumeral joint

√7ᵗʰ **S53.145** Lateral dislocation of left ulnohumeral joint

√7ᵗʰ **S53.146** Lateral dislocation of unspecified ulnohumeral joint

√6ᵗʰ S53.19 Other subluxation and dislocation of ulnohumeral joint

√7ᵗʰ **S53.191** Other subluxation of right ulnohumeral joint

√7ᵗʰ **S53.192** Other subluxation of left ulnohumeral joint

√7ᵗʰ **S53.193** Other subluxation of unspecified ulnohumeral joint

√7ᵗʰ **S53.194** Other dislocation of right ulnohumeral joint

√7ᵗʰ **S53.195** Other dislocation of left ulnohumeral joint

√7ᵗʰ **S53.196** Other dislocation of unspecified ulnohumeral joint

√5ᵗʰ **S53.2 Traumatic rupture of radial collateral ligament**
> EXCLUDES 1   *sprain of radial collateral ligament NOS (S53.43-)*

√x7ᵗʰ **S53.20 Traumatic rupture of unspecified radial collateral ligament**

√x7ᵗʰ **S53.21 Traumatic rupture of right radial collateral ligament**

√x7ᵗʰ **S53.22 Traumatic rupture of left radial collateral ligament**

√6ᵗʰ **S53.3 Traumatic rupture of ulnar collateral ligament**
> EXCLUDES 1   *sprain of ulnar collateral ligament (S53.44-)*

√x7ᵗʰ **S53.30 Traumatic rupture of unspecified ulnar collateral ligament**

√x7ᵗʰ **S53.31 Traumatic rupture of right ulnar collateral ligament**

√x7ᵗʰ **S53.32 Traumatic rupture of left ulnar collateral ligament**

√5ᵗʰ **S53.4 Sprain of elbow**
> EXCLUDES 2   *traumatic rupture of radial collateral ligament (S53.2-)*
> *traumatic rupture of ulnar collateral ligament (S53.3-)*

√6ᵗʰ **S53.40 Unspecified sprain of elbow**

7ᵗʰ **S53.401 Unspecified sprain of right elbow**

7ᵗʰ **S53.402 Unspecified sprain of left elbow**

7ᵗʰ **S53.409 Unspecified sprain of unspecified elbow**
Sprain of elbow NOS

√6ᵗʰ **S53.41 Radiohumeral (joint) sprain**

7ᵗʰ **S53.411 Radiohumeral (joint) sprain of right elbow**

7ᵗʰ **S53.412 Radiohumeral (joint) sprain of left elbow**

7ᵗʰ **S53.419 Radiohumeral (joint) sprain of unspecified elbow**

√6ᵗʰ **S53.42 Ulnohumeral (joint) sprain**

7ᵗʰ **S53.421 Ulnohumeral (joint) sprain of right elbow**

7ᵗʰ **S53.422 Ulnohumeral (joint) sprain of left elbow**

7ᵗʰ **S53.429 Ulnohumeral (joint) sprain of unspecified elbow**

√6ᵗʰ **S53.43 Radial collateral ligament sprain**

7ᵗʰ **S53.431 Radial collateral ligament sprain of right elbow**

7ᵗʰ **S53.432 Radial collateral ligament sprain of left elbow**

7ᵗʰ **S53.439 Radial collateral ligament sprain of unspecified elbow**

√6ᵗʰ **S53.44 Ulnar collateral ligament sprain**

7ᵗʰ **S53.441 Ulnar collateral ligament sprain of right elbow**

7ᵗʰ **S53.442 Ulnar collateral ligament sprain of left elbow**

7ᵗʰ **S53.449 Ulnar collateral ligament sprain of unspecified elbow**

√6ᵗʰ **S53.49 Other sprain of elbow**

7ᵗʰ **S53.491 Other sprain of right elbow**

7ᵗʰ **S53.492 Other sprain of left elbow**

7ᵗʰ **S53.499 Other sprain of unspecified elbow**

√4ᵗʰ **S54 Injury of nerves at forearm level**
Code also any associated open wound (S51.-)
> EXCLUDES 2   *injury of nerves at wrist and hand level (S64.-)*

The appropriate 7th character is to be added to each code from category S54.
A   initial encounter
D   subsequent encounter
S   sequela

√5ᵗʰ **S54.0 Injury of ulnar nerve at forearm level**
Injury of ulnar nerve NOS

√x7ᵗʰ **S54.00 Injury of ulnar nerve at forearm level, unspecified arm**

√x7ᵗʰ **S54.01 Injury of ulnar nerve at forearm level, right arm**

√x7ᵗʰ **S54.02 Injury of ulnar nerve at forearm level, left arm**

√5ᵗʰ **S54.1 Injury of median nerve at forearm level**
Injury of median nerve NOS

√x7ᵗʰ **S54.10 Injury of median nerve at forearm level, unspecified arm**

√x7ᵗʰ **S54.11 Injury of median nerve at forearm level, right arm**

√x7ᵗʰ **S54.12 Injury of median nerve at forearm level, left arm**

√5ᵗʰ **S54.2 Injury of radial nerve at forearm level**
Injury of radial nerve NOS

√x7ᵗʰ **S54.20 Injury of radial nerve at forearm level, unspecified arm**

√x7ᵗʰ **S54.21 Injury of radial nerve at forearm level, right arm**

√x7ᵗʰ **S54.22 Injury of radial nerve at forearm level, left arm**

√5ᵗʰ **S54.3 Injury of cutaneous sensory nerve at forearm level**

√x7ᵗʰ **S54.30 Injury of cutaneous sensory nerve at forearm level, unspecified arm**

√x7ᵗʰ **S54.31 Injury of cutaneous sensory nerve at forearm level, right arm**

√x7ᵗʰ **S54.32 Injury of cutaneous sensory nerve at forearm level, left arm**

√5ᵗʰ **S54.8 Injury of other nerves at forearm level**

√6ᵗʰ **S54.8X Injury of other nerves at forearm level**

7ᵗʰ **S54.8X1 Injury of other nerves at forearm level, right arm**

7ᵗʰ **S54.8X2 Injury of other nerves at forearm level, left arm**

7ᵗʰ **S54.8X9 Injury of other nerves at forearm level, unspecified arm**

√5ᵗʰ **S54.9 Injury of unspecified nerve at forearm level**

√x7ᵗʰ **S54.90 Injury of unspecified nerve at forearm level, unspecified arm**

√x7ᵗʰ **S54.91 Injury of unspecified nerve at forearm level, right arm**

√x7ᵗʰ **S54.92 Injury of unspecified nerve at forearm level, left arm**

√4ᵗʰ **S55 Injury of blood vessels at forearm level**
Code also any associated open wound (S51.-)
> EXCLUDES 2   *injury of blood vessels at wrist and hand level (S65.-)*
> *injury of brachial vessels (S45.1-S45.2)*

The appropriate 7th character is to be added to each code from category S55.
A   initial encounter
D   subsequent encounter
S   sequela

√5ᵗʰ **S55.0 Injury of ulnar artery at forearm level**
> CC Excl: For CC codes in subcategory S55.0:
> Right side: PDX collection 1274
> Left side: PDX collection 1275
> Unspecified side: PDX collection 1276

√6ᵗʰ **S55.00 Unspecified injury of ulnar artery at forearm level**

7ᵗʰ **S55.001 Unspecified injury of ulnar artery at forearm level, right arm**   CC

7ᵗʰ **S55.002 Unspecified injury of ulnar artery at forearm level, left arm**   CC

7ᵗʰ **S55.009 Unspecified injury of ulnar artery at forearm level, unspecified arm**   CC

√6ᵗʰ **S55.01 Laceration of ulnar artery at forearm level**

7ᵗʰ **S55.011 Laceration of ulnar artery at forearm level, right arm**   CC

7ᵗʰ **S55.012 Laceration of ulnar artery at forearm level, left arm**   CC

7ᵗʰ **S55.019 Laceration of ulnar artery at forearm level, unspecified arm**   CC

√6ᵗʰ **S55.09 Other specified injury of ulnar artery at forearm level**

7ᵗʰ **S55.091 Other specified injury of ulnar artery at forearm level, right arm**   CC

7ᵗʰ **S55.092 Other specified injury of ulnar artery at forearm level, left arm**   CC

7ᵗʰ **S55.099 Other specified injury of ulnar artery at forearm level, unspecified arm**   CC

N Newborn: 0   P Pediatric: 0-17   M Maternity: 9-64   A Adult: 15-124   MCC Major Complication/Comorbidity   CC Complication/Comorbidity   SW Severe Wound Dx

1052   ICD-10-CM 2020

√5ᵗʰ S55.1 Injury of radial artery at forearm level

> **CC Excl:** For CC codes in subcategory S55.1:
> **Right side:** PDX collection 1277
> **Left side:** PDX collection 1278
> **Unspecified side:** PDX collection 1279

√6ᵗʰ S55.10 Unspecified injury of radial artery at forearm level

√7ᵗʰ **S55.101** Unspecified injury of radial artery at forearm level, **right** arm   CC

√7ᵗʰ **S55.102** Unspecified injury of radial artery at forearm level, **left** arm   CC

√7ᵗʰ **S55.109** Unspecified injury of radial artery at forearm level, unspecified arm   CC

√6ᵗʰ S55.11 Laceration of radial artery at forearm level

√7ᵗʰ **S55.111** Laceration of radial artery at forearm level, **right** arm   CC

√7ᵗʰ **S55.112** Laceration of radial artery at forearm level, **left** arm   CC

√7ᵗʰ **S55.119** Laceration of radial artery at forearm level, unspecified arm   CC

√6ᵗʰ S55.19 Other specified injury of radial artery at forearm level

√7ᵗʰ **S55.191** Other specified injury of radial artery at forearm level, **right** arm   CC

√7ᵗʰ **S55.192** Other specified injury of radial artery at forearm level, **left** arm   CC

√7ᵗʰ **S55.199** Other specified injury of radial artery at forearm level, unspecified arm   CC

√5ᵗʰ S55.2 Injury of vein at forearm level

> **CC Excl:** For CC codes in subcategory S55.2:
> **Right side:** PDX collection 1260
> **Left side:** PDX collection 1261
> **Unspecified side:** PDX collection 1262

√6ᵗʰ S55.20 Unspecified injury of vein at forearm level

√7ᵗʰ **S55.201** Unspecified injury of vein at forearm level, **right** arm   CC

√7ᵗʰ **S55.202** Unspecified injury of vein at forearm level, **left** arm   CC

√7ᵗʰ **S55.209** Unspecified injury of vein at forearm level, unspecified arm   CC

√6ᵗʰ S55.21 Laceration of vein at forearm level

√7ᵗʰ **S55.211** Laceration of vein at forearm level, **right** arm   CC

√7ᵗʰ **S55.212** Laceration of vein at forearm level, **left** arm   CC

√7ᵗʰ **S55.219** Laceration of vein at forearm level, unspecified arm   CC

√6ᵗʰ S55.29 Other specified injury of vein at forearm level

√7ᵗʰ **S55.291** Other specified injury of vein at forearm level, **right** arm   CC

√7ᵗʰ **S55.292** Other specified injury of vein at forearm level, **left** arm   CC

√7ᵗʰ **S55.299** Other specified injury of vein at forearm level, unspecified arm   CC

√5ᵗʰ S55.8 Injury of other blood vessels at forearm level

> **CC Excl:** For CC codes in subcategory S55.8:
> **Right side:** PDX collection 1260
> **Left side:** PDX collection 1261
> **Unspecified side:** PDX collection 1262

√6ᵗʰ S55.80 Unspecified injury of other blood vessels at forearm level

√7ᵗʰ **S55.801** Unspecified injury of other blood vessels at forearm level, **right** arm   CC

√7ᵗʰ **S55.802** Unspecified injury of other blood vessels at forearm level, **left** arm   CC

√7ᵗʰ **S55.809** Unspecified injury of other blood vessels at forearm level, unspecified arm   CC

√6ᵗʰ S55.81 Laceration of other blood vessels at forearm level

√7ᵗʰ **S55.811** Laceration of other blood vessels at forearm level, **right** arm   CC

√7ᵗʰ **S55.812** Laceration of other blood vessels at forearm level, **left** arm   CC

√7ᵗʰ **S55.819** Laceration of other blood vessels at forearm level, unspecified arm   CC

√6ᵗʰ S55.89 Other specified injury of other blood vessels at forearm level

√7ᵗʰ **S55.891** Other specified injury of other blood vessels at forearm level, **right** arm   CC

√7ᵗʰ **S55.892** Other specified injury of other blood vessels at forearm level, **left** arm   CC

√7ᵗʰ **S55.899** Other specified injury of other blood vessels at forearm level, unspecified arm   CC

√5ᵗʰ S55.9 Injury of unspecified blood vessel at forearm level

> **CC Excl:** For CC codes in subcategory S55.9:
> **Right side:** PDX collection 1260
> **Left side:** PDX collection 1261
> **Unspecified side:** PDX collection 1262

√6ᵗʰ S55.90 Unspecified injury of unspecified blood vessel at forearm level

√7ᵗʰ **S55.901** Unspecified injury of unspecified blood vessel at forearm level, **right** arm   CC

√7ᵗʰ **S55.902** Unspecified injury of unspecified blood vessel at forearm level, **left** arm   CC

√7ᵗʰ **S55.909** Unspecified injury of unspecified blood vessel at forearm level, unspecified arm   CC

√6ᵗʰ S55.91 Laceration of unspecified blood vessel at forearm level

√7ᵗʰ **S55.911** Laceration of unspecified blood vessel at forearm level, **right** arm   CC

√7ᵗʰ **S55.912** Laceration of unspecified blood vessel at forearm level, **left** arm   CC

√7ᵗʰ **S55.919** Laceration of unspecified blood vessel at forearm level, unspecified arm   CC

√6ᵗʰ S55.99 Other specified injury of unspecified blood vessel at forearm level

√7ᵗʰ **S55.991** Other specified injury of unspecified blood vessel at forearm level, **right** arm   CC

√7ᵗʰ **S55.992** Other specified injury of unspecified blood vessel at forearm level, **left** arm   CC

√7ᵗʰ **S55.999** Other specified injury of unspecified blood vessel at forearm level, unspecified arm   CC

✔ Additional Character Required   √x7ᵗʰ Placeholder   Unacceptable PDx   Questionable PDx   Manifestation   Unspecified Dx   H1-H14 HAC   HCC CMS-HCC Dx   HIV HIV Dx

✔4ᵗʰ **S56 Injury of muscle, fascia and tendon at forearm level**

Code also any associated open wound (S51.-)

EXCLUDES 2   *injury of muscle, fascia and tendon at or below wrist (S66.-)*
sprain of joints and ligaments of elbow (S53.4-)

TIP: Refer to the Muscle/Tendon table at the beginning of this chapter

The appropriate 7th character is to be added to each code from category S56.
A   initial encounter
D   subsequent encounter
S   sequela

CC Excl: For CC codes in category S56:
Right side: PDX collection 1280
Left side: PDX collection 1281
Unspecified side: PDX collection 1282

✔5ᵗʰ **S56.0 Injury of** flexor **muscle, fascia and tendon of** thumb **at forearm level**

✔6ᵗʰ **S56.00 Unspecified injury of flexor muscle, fascia and tendon of thumb at forearm level**

✔7ᵗʰ **S56.001 Unspecified injury of flexor muscle, fascia and tendon of** right thumb **at forearm level**

✔7ᵗʰ **S56.002 Unspecified injury of flexor muscle, fascia and tendon of** left thumb **at forearm level**

✔7ᵗʰ **S56.009 Unspecified injury of flexor muscle, fascia and tendon of unspecified thumb at forearm level**

✔6ᵗʰ **S56.01 Strain of flexor muscle, fascia and tendon of thumb at forearm level**

✔7ᵗʰ **S56.011 Strain of flexor muscle, fascia and tendon of** right thumb **at forearm level**

✔7ᵗʰ **S56.012 Strain of flexor muscle, fascia and tendon of** left thumb **at forearm level**

✔7ᵗʰ **S56.019 Strain of flexor muscle, fascia and tendon of unspecified thumb at forearm level**

✔6ᵗʰ **S56.02 Laceration of flexor muscle, fascia and tendon of thumb at forearm level**

✔7ᵗʰ **S56.021 Laceration of flexor muscle, fascia and tendon of** right thumb **at forearm level** `CC`

✔7ᵗʰ **S56.022 Laceration of flexor muscle, fascia and tendon of** left thumb **at forearm level** `CC`

✔7ᵗʰ **S56.029 Laceration of flexor muscle, fascia and tendon of unspecified thumb at forearm level** `CC`

✔6ᵗʰ **S56.09 Other injury of flexor muscle, fascia and tendon of thumb at forearm level**

✔7ᵗʰ **S56.091 Other injury of flexor muscle, fascia and tendon of** right thumb **at forearm level**

✔7ᵗʰ **S56.092 Other injury of flexor muscle, fascia and tendon of** left thumb **at forearm level**

✔7ᵗʰ **S56.099 Other injury of flexor muscle, fascia and tendon of unspecified thumb at forearm level**

✔5ᵗʰ **S56.1 Injury of** flexor **muscle, fascia and tendon of other and unspecified** finger **at forearm level**

✔6ᵗʰ **S56.10 Unspecified injury of flexor muscle, fascia and tendon of other and unspecified finger at forearm level**

✔7ᵗʰ **S56.101 Unspecified injury of flexor muscle, fascia and tendon of** right index finger **at forearm level**

✔7ᵗʰ **S56.102 Unspecified injury of flexor muscle, fascia and tendon of** left index finger **at forearm level**

✔7ᵗʰ **S56.103 Unspecified injury of flexor muscle, fascia and tendon of** right middle finger **at forearm level**

✔7ᵗʰ **S56.104 Unspecified injury of flexor muscle, fascia and tendon of** left middle finger **at forearm level**

✔7ᵗʰ **S56.105 Unspecified injury of flexor muscle, fascia and tendon of** right ring finger **at forearm level**

✔7ᵗʰ **S56.106 Unspecified injury of flexor muscle, fascia and tendon of** left ring finger **at forearm level**

✔7ᵗʰ **S56.107 Unspecified injury of flexor muscle, fascia and tendon of** right little finger **at forearm level**

✔7ᵗʰ **S56.108 Unspecified injury of flexor muscle, fascia and tendon of** left little finger **at forearm level**

✔7ᵗʰ **S56.109 Unspecified injury of flexor muscle, fascia and tendon of unspecified finger at forearm level**

✔6ᵗʰ **S56.11 Strain of flexor muscle, fascia and tendon of other and unspecified finger at forearm level**

✔7ᵗʰ **S56.111 Strain of flexor muscle, fascia and tendon of** right index finger **at forearm level**

✔7ᵗʰ **S56.112 Strain of flexor muscle, fascia and tendon of** left index finger **at forearm level**

✔7ᵗʰ **S56.113 Strain of flexor muscle, fascia and tendon of** right middle finger **at forearm level**

✔7ᵗʰ **S56.114 Strain of flexor muscle, fascia and tendon of** left middle finger **at forearm level**

✔7ᵗʰ **S56.115 Strain of flexor muscle, fascia and tendon of** right ring finger **at forearm level**

✔7ᵗʰ **S56.116 Strain of flexor muscle, fascia and tendon of** left ring finger **at forearm level**

✔7ᵗʰ **S56.117 Strain of flexor muscle, fascia and tendon of** right little finger **at forearm level**

✔7ᵗʰ **S56.118 Strain of flexor muscle, fascia and tendon of** left little finger **at forearm level**

✔7ᵗʰ **S56.119 Strain of flexor muscle, fascia and tendon of finger of unspecified finger at forearm level**

✔6ᵗʰ **S56.12 Laceration of flexor muscle, fascia and tendon of other and unspecified finger at forearm level**

✔7ᵗʰ **S56.121 Laceration of flexor muscle, fascia and tendon of** right index finger **at forearm level** `CC`

✔7ᵗʰ **S56.122 Laceration of flexor muscle, fascia and tendon of** left index finger **at forearm level** `CC`

✔7ᵗʰ **S56.123 Laceration of flexor muscle, fascia and tendon of** right middle finger **at forearm level** `CC`

✔7ᵗʰ **S56.124 Laceration of flexor muscle, fascia and tendon of** left middle finger **at forearm level** `CC`

✔7ᵗʰ **S56.125 Laceration of flexor muscle, fascia and tendon of** right ring finger **at forearm level** `CC`

✔7ᵗʰ **S56.126 Laceration of flexor muscle, fascia and tendon of** left ring finger **at forearm level** `CC`

✔7ᵗʰ **S56.127 Laceration of flexor muscle, fascia and tendon of** right little finger **at forearm level** `CC`

✔7ᵗʰ **S56.128 Laceration of flexor muscle, fascia and tendon of** left little finger **at forearm level** `CC`

✔7ᵗʰ **S56.129 Laceration of flexor muscle, fascia and tendon of unspecified finger at forearm level** `CC`

✔6ᵗʰ **S56.19 Other injury of flexor muscle, fascia and tendon of other and unspecified finger at forearm level**

✔7ᵗʰ **S56.191 Other injury of flexor muscle, fascia and tendon of** right index finger **at forearm level**

✔7ᵗʰ **S56.192 Other injury of flexor muscle, fascia and tendon of** left index finger **at forearm level**

✔7ᵗʰ **S56.193 Other injury of flexor muscle, fascia and tendon of** right middle finger **at forearm level**

✔7ᵗʰ **S56.194 Other injury of flexor muscle, fascia and tendon of** left middle finger **at forearm level**

✔7ᵗʰ **S56.195 Other injury of flexor muscle, fascia and tendon of** right ring finger **at forearm level**

✔7ᵗʰ **S56.196 Other injury of flexor muscle, fascia and tendon of** left ring finger **at forearm level**

N Newborn: 0   P Pediatric: 0-17   M Maternity: 9-64   A Adult: 15-124   MCC Major Complication/Comorbidity   CC Complication/Comorbidity   SW Severe Wound Dx

1054   ICD-10-CM 2020

✓7ᵗʰ S56.197 Other injury of flexor muscle, fascia and tendon of right little finger at forearm level

✓7ᵗʰ S56.198 Other injury of flexor muscle, fascia and tendon of left little finger at forearm level

✓7ᵗʰ S56.199 Other injury of flexor muscle, fascia and tendon of unspecified finger at forearm level

✓5ᵗʰ S56.2 Injury of other flexor muscle, fascia and tendon at forearm level

✓6ᵗʰ S56.20 Unspecified injury of other flexor muscle, fascia and tendon at forearm level

✓7ᵗʰ S56.201 Unspecified injury of other flexor muscle, fascia and tendon at forearm level, right arm

✓7ᵗʰ S56.202 Unspecified injury of other flexor muscle, fascia and tendon at forearm level, left arm

✓7ᵗʰ S56.209 Unspecified injury of other flexor muscle, fascia and tendon at forearm level, unspecified arm

✓6ᵗʰ S56.21 Strain of other flexor muscle, fascia and tendon at forearm level

✓7ᵗʰ S56.211 Strain of other flexor muscle, fascia and tendon at forearm level, right arm

✓7ᵗʰ S56.212 Strain of other flexor muscle, fascia and tendon at forearm level, left arm

✓7ᵗʰ S56.219 Strain of other flexor muscle, fascia and tendon at forearm level, unspecified arm

✓6ᵗʰ S56.22 Laceration of other flexor muscle, fascia and tendon at forearm level

✓7ᵗʰ S56.221 Laceration of other flexor muscle, fascia and tendon at forearm level, right arm   `CC`

✓7ᵗʰ S56.222 Laceration of other flexor muscle, fascia and tendon at forearm level, left arm   `CC`

✓7ᵗʰ S56.229 Laceration of other flexor muscle, fascia and tendon at forearm level, unspecified arm   `CC`

✓6ᵗʰ S56.29 Other injury of other flexor muscle, fascia and tendon at forearm level

✓7ᵗʰ S56.291 Other injury of other flexor muscle, fascia and tendon at forearm level, right arm

✓7ᵗʰ S56.292 Other injury of other flexor muscle, fascia and tendon at forearm level, left arm

✓7ᵗʰ S56.299 Other injury of other flexor muscle, fascia and tendon at forearm level, unspecified arm

✓5ᵗʰ S56.3 Injury of extensor or abductor muscles, fascia and tendons of thumb at forearm level

✓6ᵗʰ S56.30 Unspecified injury of extensor or abductor muscles, fascia and tendons of thumb at forearm level

✓7ᵗʰ S56.301 Unspecified injury of extensor or abductor muscles, fascia and tendons of right thumb at forearm level

✓7ᵗʰ S56.302 Unspecified injury of extensor or abductor muscles, fascia and tendons of left thumb at forearm level

✓7ᵗʰ S56.309 Unspecified injury of extensor or abductor muscles, fascia and tendons of unspecified thumb at forearm level

✓6ᵗʰ S56.31 Strain of extensor or abductor muscles, fascia and tendons of thumb at forearm level

✓7ᵗʰ S56.311 Strain of extensor or abductor muscles, fascia and tendons of right thumb at forearm level

✓7ᵗʰ S56.312 Strain of extensor or abductor muscles, fascia and tendons of left thumb at forearm level

✓7ᵗʰ S56.319 Strain of extensor or abductor muscles, fascia and tendons of unspecified thumb at forearm level

✓6ᵗʰ S56.32 Laceration of extensor or abductor muscles, fascia and tendons of thumb at forearm level

✓7ᵗʰ S56.321 Laceration of extensor or abductor muscles, fascia and tendons of right thumb at forearm level   `CC`

✓7ᵗʰ S56.322 Laceration of extensor or abductor muscles, fascia and tendons of left thumb at forearm level   `CC`

✓7ᵗʰ S56.329 Laceration of extensor or abductor muscles, fascia and tendons of unspecified thumb at forearm level   `CC`

✓6ᵗʰ S56.39 Other injury of extensor or abductor muscles, fascia and tendons of thumb at forearm level

✓7ᵗʰ S56.391 Other injury of extensor or abductor muscles, fascia and tendons of right thumb at forearm level

✓7ᵗʰ S56.392 Other injury of extensor or abductor muscles, fascia and tendons of left thumb at forearm level

✓7ᵗʰ S56.399 Other injury of extensor or abductor muscles, fascia and tendons of unspecified thumb at forearm level

✓5ᵗʰ S56.4 Injury of extensor muscle, fascia and tendon of other and unspecified finger at forearm level

✓6ᵗʰ S56.40 Unspecified injury of extensor muscle, fascia and tendon of other and unspecified finger at forearm level

✓7ᵗʰ S56.401 Unspecified injury of extensor muscle, fascia and tendon of right index finger at forearm level

✓7ᵗʰ S56.402 Unspecified injury of extensor muscle, fascia and tendon of left index finger at forearm level

✓7ᵗʰ S56.403 Unspecified injury of extensor muscle, fascia and tendon of right middle finger at forearm level

✓7ᵗʰ S56.404 Unspecified injury of extensor muscle, fascia and tendon of left middle finger at forearm level

✓7ᵗʰ S56.405 Unspecified injury of extensor muscle, fascia and tendon of right ring finger at forearm level

✓7ᵗʰ S56.406 Unspecified injury of extensor muscle, fascia and tendon of left ring finger at forearm level

✓7ᵗʰ S56.407 Unspecified injury of extensor muscle, fascia and tendon of right little finger at forearm level

✓7ᵗʰ S56.408 Unspecified injury of extensor muscle, fascia and tendon of left little finger at forearm level

✓7ᵗʰ S56.409 Unspecified injury of extensor muscle, fascia and tendon of unspecified finger at forearm level

✓6ᵗʰ S56.41 Strain of extensor muscle, fascia and tendon of other and unspecified finger at forearm level

✓7ᵗʰ S56.411 Strain of extensor muscle, fascia and tendon of right index finger at forearm level

✓7ᵗʰ S56.412 Strain of extensor muscle, fascia and tendon of left index finger at forearm level

✓7ᵗʰ S56.413 Strain of extensor muscle, fascia and tendon of right middle finger at forearm level

✓7ᵗʰ S56.414 Strain of extensor muscle, fascia and tendon of left middle finger at forearm level

✓7ᵗʰ S56.415 Strain of extensor muscle, fascia and tendon of right ring finger at forearm level

✓7ᵗʰ S56.416 Strain of extensor muscle, fascia and tendon of left ring finger at forearm level

✓7ᵗʰ S56.417 Strain of extensor muscle, fascia and tendon of right little finger at forearm level

✓7ᵗʰ S56.418 Strain of extensor muscle, fascia and tendon of left little finger at forearm level

✓7ᵗʰ S56.419 Strain of extensor muscle, fascia and tendon of finger, unspecified finger at forearm level

✓6ᵗʰ S56.42 Laceration of extensor muscle, fascia and tendon of other and unspecified finger at forearm level

✓7ᵗʰ S56.421 Laceration of extensor muscle, fascia and tendon of right index finger at forearm level   `CC`

✓7ᵗʰ S56.422 Laceration of extensor muscle, fascia and tendon of left index finger at forearm level   `CC`

✓ Additional Character Required   ✓ₓ7ᵗʰ Placeholder   Unacceptable PDx   Questionable PDx   Manifestation   Unspecified Dx   H1–H14 HAC   HCC CMS-HCC Dx   HIV HIV Dx

ICD-10-CM 2020   1055

√7th **S56.423** Laceration of extensor muscle, fascia and tendon of right middle finger at forearm level   **cc**

√7th **S56.424** Laceration of extensor muscle, fascia and tendon of left middle finger at forearm level   **cc**

√7th **S56.425** Laceration of extensor muscle, fascia and tendon of right ring finger at forearm level   **cc**

√7th **S56.426** Laceration of extensor muscle, fascia and tendon of left ring finger at forearm level   **cc**

√7th **S56.427** Laceration of extensor muscle, fascia and tendon of right little finger at forearm level   **cc**

√7th **S56.428** Laceration of extensor muscle, fascia and tendon of left little finger at forearm level   **cc**

√7th **S56.429** Laceration of extensor muscle, fascia and tendon of unspecified finger at forearm level   **cc**

√6th **S56.49** Other injury of extensor muscle, fascia and tendon of other and unspecified finger at forearm level

√7th **S56.491** Other injury of extensor muscle, fascia and tendon of right index finger at forearm level

√7th **S56.492** Other injury of extensor muscle, fascia and tendon of left index finger at forearm level

√7th **S56.493** Other injury of extensor muscle, fascia and tendon of right middle finger at forearm level

√7th **S56.494** Other injury of extensor muscle, fascia and tendon of left middle finger at forearm level

√7th **S56.495** Other injury of extensor muscle, fascia and tendon of right ring finger at forearm level

√7th **S56.496** Other injury of extensor muscle, fascia and tendon of left ring finger at forearm level

√7th **S56.497** Other injury of extensor muscle, fascia and tendon of right little finger at forearm level

√7th **S56.498** Other injury of extensor muscle, fascia and tendon of left little finger at forearm level

√7th **S56.499** Other injury of extensor muscle, fascia and tendon of unspecified finger at forearm level

√5th **S56.5** Injury of other extensor muscle, fascia and tendon at forearm level

√6th **S56.50** Unspecified injury of other extensor muscle, fascia and tendon at forearm level

√7th **S56.501** Unspecified injury of other extensor muscle, fascia and tendon at forearm level, right arm

√7th **S56.502** Unspecified injury of other extensor muscle, fascia and tendon at forearm level, left arm

√7th **S56.509** Unspecified injury of other extensor muscle, fascia and tendon at forearm level, unspecified arm

√6th **S56.51** Strain of other extensor muscle, fascia and tendon at forearm level

√7th **S56.511** Strain of other extensor muscle, fascia and tendon at forearm level, right arm

√7th **S56.512** Strain of other extensor muscle, fascia and tendon at forearm level, left arm

√7th **S56.519** Strain of other extensor muscle, fascia and tendon at forearm level, unspecified arm

√6th **S56.52** Laceration of other extensor muscle, fascia and tendon at forearm level

√7th **S56.521** Laceration of other extensor muscle, fascia and tendon at forearm level, right arm   **cc**

√7th **S56.522** Laceration of other extensor muscle, fascia and tendon at forearm level, left arm   **cc**

√7th **S56.529** Laceration of other extensor muscle, fascia and tendon at forearm level, unspecified arm   **cc**

√6th **S56.59** Other injury of other extensor muscle, fascia and tendon at forearm level

√7th **S56.591** Other injury of other extensor muscle, fascia and tendon at forearm level, right arm

√7th **S56.592** Other injury of other extensor muscle, fascia and tendon at forearm level, left arm

√7th **S56.599** Other injury of other extensor muscle, fascia and tendon at forearm level, unspecified arm

√5th **S56.8** Injury of other muscles, fascia and tendons at forearm level

√6th **S56.80** Unspecified injury of other muscles, fascia and tendons at forearm level

√7th **S56.801** Unspecified injury of other muscles, fascia and tendons at forearm level, right arm

√7th **S56.802** Unspecified injury of other muscles, fascia and tendons at forearm level, left arm

√7th **S56.809** Unspecified injury of other muscles, fascia and tendons at forearm level, unspecified arm

√6th **S56.81** Strain of other muscles, fascia and tendons at forearm level

√7th **S56.811** Strain of other muscles, fascia and tendons at forearm level, right arm

√7th **S56.812** Strain of other muscles, fascia and tendons at forearm level, left arm

√7th **S56.819** Strain of other muscles, fascia and tendons at forearm level, unspecified arm

√6th **S56.82** Laceration of other muscles, fascia and tendons at forearm level

√7th **S56.821** Laceration of other muscles, fascia and tendons at forearm level, right arm   **cc**

√7th **S56.822** Laceration of other muscles, fascia and tendons at forearm level, left arm   **cc**

√7th **S56.829** Laceration of other muscles, fascia and tendons at forearm level, unspecified arm   **cc**

√6th **S56.89** Other injury of other muscles, fascia and tendons at forearm level

√7th **S56.891** Other injury of other muscles, fascia and tendons at forearm level, right arm

√7th **S56.892** Other injury of other muscles, fascia and tendons at forearm level, left arm

√7th **S56.899** Other injury of other muscles, fascia and tendons at forearm level, unspecified arm

√5th **S56.9** Injury of unspecified muscles, fascia and tendons at forearm level

√6th **S56.90** Unspecified injury of unspecified muscles, fascia and tendons at forearm level

√7th **S56.901** Unspecified injury of unspecified muscles, fascia and tendons at forearm level, right arm

√7th **S56.902** Unspecified injury of unspecified muscles, fascia and tendons at forearm level, left arm

√7th **S56.909** Unspecified injury of unspecified muscles, fascia and tendons at forearm level, unspecified arm

√6th **S56.91** Strain of unspecified muscles, fascia and tendons at forearm level

√7th **S56.911** Strain of unspecified muscles, fascia and tendons at forearm level, right arm

√7th **S56.912** Strain of unspecified muscles, fascia and tendons at forearm level, left arm

√7th **S56.919** Strain of unspecified muscles, fascia and tendons at forearm level, unspecified arm

N Newborn: 0   **P** Pediatric: 0-17   **M** Maternity: 9-64   **A** Adult: 15-124   **MCC** Major Complication/Comorbidity   **CC** Complication/Comorbidity   **SW** Severe Wound Dx

1056   ICD-10-CM 2020

√6ᵗʰ **S56.92 Laceration** of unspecified muscles, fascia and tendons at forearm level

√7ᵗʰ **S56.921 Laceration** of unspecified muscles, fascia and tendons at forearm level, **right arm** `CC`

√7ᵗʰ **S56.922 Laceration** of unspecified muscles, fascia and tendons at forearm level, **left arm** `CC`

√7ᵗʰ **S56.929 Laceration** of unspecified muscles, fascia and tendons at forearm level, unspecified arm `CC`

√6ᵗʰ **S56.99 Other injury** of unspecified muscles, fascia and tendons at forearm level

√7ᵗʰ **S56.991 Other injury** of unspecified muscles, fascia and tendons at forearm level, **right arm**

√7ᵗʰ **S56.992 Other injury** of unspecified muscles, fascia and tendons at forearm level, **left arm**

√7ᵗʰ **S56.999 Other injury** of unspecified muscles, fascia and tendons at forearm level, unspecified arm

√4ᵗʰ **S57 Crushing injury** of elbow and forearm

Use additional code(s) for all associated injuries

EXCLUDES 2 crushing injury of wrist and hand (S67.-)

The appropriate 7th character is to be added to each code from category S57.
A initial encounter
D subsequent encounter
S sequela

√5ᵗʰ **S57.0 Crushing injury** of elbow

√x7ᵗʰ **S57.00 Crushing injury** of unspecified elbow

√x7ᵗʰ **S57.01 Crushing injury** of **right** elbow

√x7ᵗʰ **S57.02 Crushing injury** of **left** elbow

√5ᵗʰ **S57.8 Crushing injury** of forearm

√x7ᵗʰ **S57.80 Crushing injury** of unspecified forearm

√x7ᵗʰ **S57.81 Crushing injury** of **right** forearm

√x7ᵗʰ **S57.82 Crushing injury** of **left** forearm

√4ᵗʰ **S58 Traumatic amputation** of elbow and forearm

An amputation not identified as partial or complete should be coded to complete

EXCLUDES 1 traumatic amputation of wrist and hand (S68.-)

The appropriate 7th character is to be added to each code from category S58.
A initial encounter
D subsequent encounter
S sequela

CC Excl: For CC codes in category S58:
Right side: PDX collection 1266
Left side: PDX collection 1267
Unspecified side: PDX collection 1268

√5ᵗʰ **S58.0 Traumatic amputation** at elbow level

√6ᵗʰ **S58.01 Complete** traumatic amputation at elbow level

√7ᵗʰ **S58.011 Complete** traumatic amputation at elbow level, **right arm** `CC` `HCC`

√7ᵗʰ **S58.012 Complete** traumatic amputation at elbow level, **left arm** `CC` `HCC`

√7ᵗʰ **S58.019 Complete** traumatic amputation at elbow level, unspecified arm `CC` `HCC`

√6ᵗʰ **S58.02 Partial** traumatic amputation at elbow level

√7ᵗʰ **S58.021 Partial** traumatic amputation at elbow level, **right arm** `CC` `HCC`

√7ᵗʰ **S58.022 Partial** traumatic amputation at elbow level, **left arm** `CC` `HCC`

√7ᵗʰ **S58.029 Partial** traumatic amputation at elbow level, unspecified arm `CC` `HCC`

√5ᵗʰ **S58.1 Traumatic amputation** at level between elbow and wrist

√6ᵗʰ **S58.11 Complete** traumatic amputation at level between elbow and wrist

√7ᵗʰ **S58.111 Complete** traumatic amputation at level between elbow and wrist, **right arm** `CC` `HCC`

√7ᵗʰ **S58.112 Complete** traumatic amputation at level between elbow and wrist, **left arm** `CC` `HCC`

√7ᵗʰ **S58.119 Complete** traumatic amputation at level between elbow and wrist, unspecified arm `CC` `HCC`

√6ᵗʰ **S58.12 Partial** traumatic amputation at level between elbow and wrist

√7ᵗʰ **S58.121 Partial** traumatic amputation at level between elbow and wrist, **right arm** `CC` `HCC`

√7ᵗʰ **S58.122 Partial** traumatic amputation at level between elbow and wrist, **left arm** `CC` `HCC`

√7ᵗʰ **S58.129 Partial** traumatic amputation at level between elbow and wrist, unspecified arm `CC` `HCC`

√5ᵗʰ **S58.9 Traumatic amputation** of forearm, level unspecified

EXCLUDES 1 traumatic amputation of wrist (S68.-)

√6ᵗʰ **S58.91 Complete** traumatic amputation of forearm, level unspecified

√7ᵗʰ **S58.911 Complete** traumatic amputation of **right** forearm, level unspecified `CC` `HCC`

√7ᵗʰ **S58.912 Complete** traumatic amputation of **left** forearm, level unspecified `CC` `HCC`

√7ᵗʰ **S58.919 Complete** traumatic amputation of unspecified forearm, level unspecified `CC` `HCC`

√6ᵗʰ **S58.92 Partial** traumatic amputation of forearm, level unspecified

√7ᵗʰ **S58.921 Partial** traumatic amputation of **right** forearm, level unspecified `CC` `HCC`

√7ᵗʰ **S58.922 Partial** traumatic amputation of **left** forearm, level unspecified `CC` `HCC`

√7ᵗʰ **S58.929 Partial** traumatic amputation of unspecified forearm, level unspecified `CC` `HCC`

√4ᵗʰ **S59 Other and unspecified injuries** of elbow and forearm

EXCLUDES 2 other and unspecified injuries of wrist and hand (S69.-)

AHA: 2018,2Q,12; 2018,1Q,3; 2015,3Q,37-39

The appropriate 7th character is to be added to each code from subcategories S59.0, S59.1, and S59.2.
A initial encounter for closed fracture
D subsequent encounter for fracture with routine healing
G subsequent encounter for fracture with delayed healing
K subsequent encounter for fracture with nonunion
P subsequent encounter for fracture with malunion
S sequela

√5ᵗʰ **S59.0 Physeal fracture** of lower end of ulna

CC Excl: For CC/MCC codes in subcategory S59.0:
Right side: See code S59.001
Left side: See code S59.002
Unspecified side: See code S59.009

√6ᵗʰ **S59.00 Unspecified physeal fracture** of lower end of ulna

√7ᵗʰ **S59.001 Unspecified physeal fracture** of lower end of ulna, **right arm** `CC` `H5`
CC Excl: CC with 7th character A: PDX collection 1270
CC Excl: CC with 7th character K or P: PDX collection 897

3 √7ᵗʰ **S59.002** Unspecified physeal fracture of lower end of ulna, **left arm**   `CC` `H5`
    CC Excl: CC with 7th character A: PDX collection 1271
    CC Excl: CC with 7th character K or P: PDX collection 897

3 √7ᵗʰ **S59.009** Unspecified physeal fracture of lower end of ulna, **unspecified arm**   `CC` `H5`
    CC Excl: CC with 7th character A: PDX collection 1272
    CC Excl: CC with 7th character K or P: PDX collection 897

√6ᵗʰ **S59.01** Salter-Harris Type I physeal fracture of lower end of ulna

    3 √7ᵗʰ **S59.011** Salter-Harris Type I physeal fracture of lower end of ulna, **right arm**   `CC` `H5`

    3 √7ᵗʰ **S59.012** Salter-Harris Type I physeal fracture of lower end of ulna, **left arm**   `CC` `H5`

    3 √7ᵗʰ **S59.019** Salter-Harris Type I physeal fracture of lower end of ulna, **unspecified arm**   `CC` `H5`

√6ᵗʰ **S59.02** Salter-Harris Type II physeal fracture of lower end of ulna

    3 √7ᵗʰ **S59.021** Salter-Harris Type II physeal fracture of lower end of ulna, **right arm**   `CC` `H5`

    3 √7ᵗʰ **S59.022** Salter-Harris Type II physeal fracture of lower end of ulna, **left arm**   `CC` `H5`

    3 √7ᵗʰ **S59.029** Salter-Harris Type II physeal fracture of lower end of ulna, **unspecified arm**   `CC` `H5`

√6ᵗʰ **S59.03** Salter-Harris Type III physeal fracture of lower end of ulna

    3 √7ᵗʰ **S59.031** Salter-Harris Type III physeal fracture of lower end of ulna, **right arm**   `CC` `H5`

    3 √7ᵗʰ **S59.032** Salter-Harris Type III physeal fracture of lower end of ulna, **left arm**   `CC` `H5`

    3 √7ᵗʰ **S59.039** Salter-Harris Type III physeal fracture of lower end of ulna, **unspecified arm**   `CC` `H5`

√6ᵗʰ **S59.04** Salter-Harris Type IV physeal fracture of lower end of ulna

    3 √7ᵗʰ **S59.041** Salter-Harris Type IV physeal fracture of lower end of ulna, **right arm**   `CC` `H5`

    3 √7ᵗʰ **S59.042** Salter-Harris Type IV physeal fracture of lower end of ulna, **left arm**   `CC` `H5`

    3 √7ᵗʰ **S59.049** Salter-Harris Type IV physeal fracture of lower end of ulna, **unspecified arm**   `CC` `H5`

√6ᵗʰ **S59.09** Other physeal fracture of lower end of ulna

    3 √7ᵗʰ **S59.091** Other physeal fracture of lower end of ulna, **right arm**   `CC` `H5`

    3 √7ᵗʰ **S59.092** Other physeal fracture of lower end of ulna, **left arm**   `CC` `H5`

    3 √7ᵗʰ **S59.099** Other physeal fracture of lower end of ulna, **unspecified arm**   `CC` `H5`

√5ᵗʰ **S59.1** Physeal fracture of upper end of radius
    CC Excl: For CC codes in subcategory S59.1:
    CC with 7th character K or P: PDX collection 897

    √6ᵗʰ **S59.10** Unspecified physeal fracture of upper end of radius

      4 √7ᵗʰ **S59.101** Unspecified physeal fracture of upper end of radius, **right arm**   `CC`

      4 √7ᵗʰ **S59.102** Unspecified physeal fracture of upper end of radius, **left arm**   `CC`

      4 √7ᵗʰ **S59.109** Unspecified physeal fracture of upper end of radius, **unspecified arm**   `CC`

√6ᵗʰ **S59.11** Salter-Harris Type I physeal fracture of upper end of radius

    4 √7ᵗʰ **S59.111** Salter-Harris Type I physeal fracture of upper end of radius, **right arm**   `CC`

    4 √7ᵗʰ **S59.112** Salter-Harris Type I physeal fracture of upper end of radius, **left arm**   `CC`

    4 √7ᵗʰ **S59.119** Salter-Harris Type I physeal fracture of upper end of radius, **unspecified arm**   `CC`

√6ᵗʰ **S59.12** Salter-Harris Type II physeal fracture of upper end of radius

    4 √7ᵗʰ **S59.121** Salter-Harris Type II physeal fracture of upper end of radius, **right arm**   `CC`

    4 √7ᵗʰ **S59.122** Salter-Harris Type II physeal fracture of upper end of radius, **left arm**   `CC`

    4 √7ᵗʰ **S59.129** Salter-Harris Type II physeal fracture of upper end of radius, **unspecified arm**   `CC`

√6ᵗʰ **S59.13** Salter-Harris Type III physeal fracture of upper end of radius

    4 √7ᵗʰ **S59.131** Salter-Harris Type III physeal fracture of upper end of radius, **right arm**   `CC`

    4 √7ᵗʰ **S59.132** Salter-Harris Type III physeal fracture of upper end of radius, **left arm**   `CC`

    4 √7ᵗʰ **S59.139** Salter-Harris Type III physeal fracture of upper end of radius, **unspecified arm**   `CC`

√6ᵗʰ **S59.14** Salter-Harris Type IV physeal fracture of upper end of radius

    4 √7ᵗʰ **S59.141** Salter-Harris Type IV physeal fracture of upper end of radius, **right arm**   `CC`

    4 √7ᵗʰ **S59.142** Salter-Harris Type IV physeal fracture of upper end of radius, **left arm**   `CC`

    4 √7ᵗʰ **S59.149** Salter-Harris Type IV physeal fracture of upper end of radius, **unspecified arm**   `CC`

√6ᵗʰ **S59.19** Other physeal fracture of upper end of radius

    4 √7ᵗʰ **S59.191** Other physeal fracture of upper end of radius, **right**   `CC`

    4 √7ᵗʰ **S59.192** Other physeal fracture of upper end of radius, **left arm**   `CC`

    4 √7ᵗʰ **S59.199** Other physeal fracture of upper end of radius, **unspecified arm**   `CC`

√5ᵗʰ **S59.2** Physeal fracture of lower end of radius
    CC Excl: For CC codes in subcategory S59.2:
    Right side: See code S59.201
    Left side: See code S59.202
    Unspecified side: See code S59.209

    √6ᵗʰ **S59.20** Unspecified physeal fracture of lower end of radius

      3 √7ᵗʰ **S59.201** Unspecified physeal fracture of lower end of radius, **right arm**   `CC` `H5`
        CC Excl: CC with 7th character A: PDX collection 1270
        CC Excl: CC with 7th character K or P: PDX collection 897

      3 √7ᵗʰ **S59.202** Unspecified physeal fracture of lower end of radius, **left arm**   `CC` `H5`
        CC Excl: CC with 7th character A: PDX collection 1271
        CC Excl: CC with 7th character K or P: PDX collection 897

³ √7ᵗʰ **S59.209** Unspecified physeal fracture of lower end of radius, unspecified arm   CC H5
     CC Excl: CC with 7th character A: PDX collection 1272
     CC Excl: CC with 7th character K or P: PDX collection 897

√6ᵗʰ **S59.21** Salter-Harris Type I physeal fracture of lower end of radius

     ³ √7ᵗʰ **S59.211** Salter-Harris Type I physeal fracture of lower end of radius, right arm   CC H5

     ³ √7ᵗʰ **S59.212** Salter-Harris Type I physeal fracture of lower end of radius, left arm   CC H5

     ³ √7ᵗʰ **S59.219** Salter-Harris Type I physeal fracture of lower end of radius, unspecified arm   CC H5

√6ᵗʰ **S59.22** Salter-Harris Type II physeal fracture of lower end of radius

     ³ √7ᵗʰ **S59.221** Salter-Harris Type II physeal fracture of lower end of radius, right arm   CC H5

     ³ √7ᵗʰ **S59.222** Salter-Harris Type II physeal fracture of lower end of radius, left arm   CC H5

     ³ √7ᵗʰ **S59.229** Salter-Harris Type II physeal fracture of lower end of radius, unspecified arm   CC H5

√6ᵗʰ **S59.23** Salter-Harris Type III physeal fracture of lower end of radius

     ³ √7ᵗʰ **S59.231** Salter-Harris Type III physeal fracture of lower end of radius, right arm   CC H5

     ³ √7ᵗʰ **S59.232** Salter-Harris Type III physeal fracture of lower end of radius, left arm   CC H5

     ³ √7ᵗʰ **S59.239** Salter-Harris Type III physeal fracture of lower end of radius, unspecified arm   CC H5

√6ᵗʰ **S59.24** Salter-Harris Type IV physeal fracture of lower end of radius

     ³ √7ᵗʰ **S59.241** Salter-Harris Type IV physeal fracture of lower end of radius, right arm   CC H5

     ³ √7ᵗʰ **S59.242** Salter-Harris Type IV physeal fracture of lower end of radius, left arm   CC H5

     ³ √7ᵗʰ **S59.249** Salter-Harris Type IV physeal fracture of lower end of radius, unspecified arm   CC H5

√6ᵗʰ **S59.29** Other physeal fracture of lower end of radius

     ³ √7ᵗʰ **S59.291** Other physeal fracture of lower end of radius, right arm   CC H5

     ³ √7ᵗʰ **S59.292** Other physeal fracture of lower end of radius, left arm   CC H5

     ³ √7ᵗʰ **S59.299** Other physeal fracture of lower end of radius, unspecified arm   CC H5

√5ᵗʰ **S59.8** Other specified injuries of elbow and forearm

     The appropriate 7th character is to be added to each code in subcategory S59.8.
     A   initial encounter
     D   subsequent encounter
     S   sequela

√6ᵗʰ **S59.80** Other specified injuries of elbow

     √7ᵗʰ **S59.801** Other specified injuries of right elbow

     √7ᵗʰ **S59.802** Other specified injuries of left elbow

     √7ᵗʰ **S59.809** Other specified injuries of unspecified elbow

√6ᵗʰ **S59.81** Other specified injuries of forearm

     √7ᵗʰ **S59.811** Other specified injuries right forearm

     √7ᵗʰ **S59.812** Other specified injuries left forearm

     √7ᵗʰ **S59.819** Other specified injuries unspecified forearm

√5ᵗʰ **S59.9** Unspecified injury of elbow and forearm

     The appropriate 7th character is to be added to each code in subcategory S59.9.
     A   initial encounter
     D   subsequent encounter
     S   sequela

√6ᵗʰ **S59.90** Unspecified injury of elbow

     √7ᵗʰ **S59.901** Unspecified injury of right elbow

     √7ᵗʰ **S59.902** Unspecified injury of left elbow

     √7ᵗʰ **S59.909** Unspecified injury of unspecified elbow

√6ᵗʰ **S59.91** Unspecified injury of forearm

     √7ᵗʰ **S59.911** Unspecified injury of right forearm

     √7ᵗʰ **S59.912** Unspecified injury of left forearm

     √7ᵗʰ **S59.919** Unspecified injury of unspecified forearm

Injuries to the wrist, hand and fingers (S60-S69)

EXCLUDES 2   burns and corrosions (T20-T32)
       frostbite (T33-T34)
       insect bite or sting, venomous (T63.4)

√4ᵗʰ **S60** Superficial injury of wrist, hand and fingers

     The appropriate 7th character is to be added to each code from category S60.
     A   initial encounter
     D   subsequent encounter
     S   sequela

√5ᵗʰ **S60.0** Contusion of finger without damage to nail

     EXCLUDES 1   contusion involving nail (matrix) (S60.1)

√x7ᵗʰ **S60.00** Contusion of unspecified finger without damage to nail
     Contusion of finger(s) NOS

√6ᵗʰ **S60.01** Contusion of thumb without damage to nail

     √7ᵗʰ **S60.011** Contusion of right thumb without damage to nail

     √7ᵗʰ **S60.012** Contusion of left thumb without damage to nail

     √7ᵗʰ **S60.019** Contusion of unspecified thumb without damage to nail

√6ᵗʰ **S60.02** Contusion of index finger without damage to nail

     √7ᵗʰ **S60.021** Contusion of right index finger without damage to nail

     √7ᵗʰ **S60.022** Contusion of left index finger without damage to nail

     √7ᵗʰ **S60.029** Contusion of unspecified index finger without damage to nail

√6ᵗʰ **S60.03** Contusion of middle finger without damage to nail

     √7ᵗʰ **S60.031** Contusion of right middle finger without damage to nail

     √7ᵗʰ **S60.032** Contusion of left middle finger without damage to nail

     √7ᵗʰ **S60.039** Contusion of unspecified middle finger without damage to nail

√6ᵗʰ **S60.04** Contusion of ring finger without damage to nail

     √7ᵗʰ **S60.041** Contusion of right ring finger without damage to nail

     √7ᵗʰ **S60.042** Contusion of left ring finger without damage to nail

     √7ᵗʰ **S60.049** Contusion of unspecified ring finger without damage to nail

√6ᵗʰ **S60.05** Contusion of little finger without damage to nail

     √7ᵗʰ **S60.051** Contusion of right little finger without damage to nail

     √7ᵗʰ **S60.052** Contusion of left little finger without damage to nail

     √7ᵗʰ **S60.059** Contusion of unspecified little finger without damage to nail

√5ᵗʰ **S60.1** Contusion of finger with damage to nail

√x7ᵗʰ **S60.10** Contusion of unspecified finger with damage to nail

√6ᵗʰ **S60.11** Contusion of thumb with damage to nail

     √7ᵗʰ **S60.111** Contusion of right thumb with damage to nail

     √7ᵗʰ **S60.112** Contusion of left thumb with damage to nail

     √7ᵗʰ **S60.119** Contusion of unspecified thumb with damage to nail

- √6ᵗʰ **S60.12** Contusion of index finger with damage to nail
  - √7ᵗʰ **S60.121** Contusion of right index finger with damage to nail
  - √7ᵗʰ **S60.122** Contusion of left index finger with damage to nail
  - √7ᵗʰ **S60.129** Contusion of unspecified index finger with damage to nail
- √6ᵗʰ **S60.13** Contusion of middle finger with damage to nail
  - √7ᵗʰ **S60.131** Contusion of right middle finger with damage to nail
  - √7ᵗʰ **S60.132** Contusion of left middle finger with damage to nail
  - √7ᵗʰ **S60.139** Contusion of unspecified middle finger with damage to nail
- √6ᵗʰ **S60.14** Contusion of ring finger with damage to nail
  - √7ᵗʰ **S60.141** Contusion of right ring finger with damage to nail
  - √7ᵗʰ **S60.142** Contusion of left ring finger with damage to nail
  - √7ᵗʰ **S60.149** Contusion of unspecified ring finger with damage to nail
- √6ᵗʰ **S60.15** Contusion of little finger with damage to nail
  - √7ᵗʰ **S60.151** Contusion of right little finger with damage to nail
  - √7ᵗʰ **S60.152** Contusion of left little finger with damage to nail
  - √7ᵗʰ **S60.159** Contusion of unspecified little finger with damage to nail
- √5ᵗʰ **S60.2** Contusion of wrist and hand
  - EXCLUDES 2   contusion of fingers (S60.0-, S60.1-)
  - √6ᵗʰ **S60.21** Contusion of wrist
    - √7ᵗʰ **S60.211** Contusion of right wrist
    - √7ᵗʰ **S60.212** Contusion of left wrist
    - √7ᵗʰ **S60.219** Contusion of unspecified wrist
  - √6ᵗʰ **S60.22** Contusion of hand
    - √7ᵗʰ **S60.221** Contusion of right hand
    - √7ᵗʰ **S60.222** Contusion of left hand
    - √7ᵗʰ **S60.229** Contusion of unspecified hand
- √5ᵗʰ **S60.3** Other superficial injuries of thumb
  - √6ᵗʰ **S60.31** Abrasion of thumb
    - √7ᵗʰ **S60.311** Abrasion of right thumb
    - √7ᵗʰ **S60.312** Abrasion of left thumb
    - √7ᵗʰ **S60.319** Abrasion of unspecified thumb
  - √6ᵗʰ **S60.32** Blister (nonthermal) of thumb
    - √7ᵗʰ **S60.321** Blister (nonthermal) of right thumb
    - √7ᵗʰ **S60.322** Blister (nonthermal) of left thumb
    - √7ᵗʰ **S60.329** Blister (nonthermal) of unspecified thumb
  - √6ᵗʰ **S60.34** External constriction of thumb
    - Hair tourniquet syndrome of thumb
    - Use additional cause code to identify the constricting item (W49.0-)
    - √7ᵗʰ **S60.341** External constriction of right thumb
    - √7ᵗʰ **S60.342** External constriction of left thumb
    - √7ᵗʰ **S60.349** External constriction of unspecified thumb
  - √6ᵗʰ **S60.35** Superficial foreign body of thumb
    - Splinter in the thumb
    - √7ᵗʰ **S60.351** Superficial foreign body of right thumb
    - √7ᵗʰ **S60.352** Superficial foreign body of left thumb
    - √7ᵗʰ **S60.359** Superficial foreign body of unspecified thumb
  - √6ᵗʰ **S60.36** Insect bite (nonvenomous) of thumb
    - √7ᵗʰ **S60.361** Insect bite (nonvenomous) of right thumb
    - √7ᵗʰ **S60.362** Insect bite (nonvenomous) of left thumb
    - √7ᵗʰ **S60.369** Insect bite (nonvenomous) of unspecified thumb
  - √6ᵗʰ **S60.37** Other superficial bite of thumb
    - EXCLUDES 1   open bite of thumb (S61.05-, S61.15-)
    - √7ᵗʰ **S60.371** Other superficial bite of right thumb
    - √7ᵗʰ **S60.372** Other superficial bite of left thumb
    - √7ᵗʰ **S60.379** Other superficial bite of unspecified thumb

- √6ᵗʰ **S60.39** Other superficial injuries of thumb
  - √7ᵗʰ **S60.391** Other superficial injuries of right thumb
  - √7ᵗʰ **S60.392** Other superficial injuries of left thumb
  - √7ᵗʰ **S60.399** Other superficial injuries of unspecified thumb
- √5ᵗʰ **S60.4** Other superficial injuries of other fingers
  - √6ᵗʰ **S60.41** Abrasion of fingers
    - √7ᵗʰ **S60.410** Abrasion of right index finger
    - √7ᵗʰ **S60.411** Abrasion of left index finger
    - √7ᵗʰ **S60.412** Abrasion of right middle finger
    - √7ᵗʰ **S60.413** Abrasion of left middle finger
    - √7ᵗʰ **S60.414** Abrasion of right ring finger
    - √7ᵗʰ **S60.415** Abrasion of left ring finger
    - √7ᵗʰ **S60.416** Abrasion of right little finger
    - √7ᵗʰ **S60.417** Abrasion of left little finger
    - √7ᵗʰ **S60.418** Abrasion of other finger
      - Abrasion of specified finger with unspecified laterality
    - √7ᵗʰ **S60.419** Abrasion of unspecified finger
  - √6ᵗʰ **S60.42** Blister (nonthermal) of fingers
    - √7ᵗʰ **S60.420** Blister (nonthermal) of right index finger
    - √7ᵗʰ **S60.421** Blister (nonthermal) of left index finger
    - √7ᵗʰ **S60.422** Blister (nonthermal) of right middle finger
    - √7ᵗʰ **S60.423** Blister (nonthermal) of left middle finger
    - √7ᵗʰ **S60.424** Blister (nonthermal) of right ring finger
    - √7ᵗʰ **S60.425** Blister (nonthermal) of left ring finger
    - √7ᵗʰ **S60.426** Blister (nonthermal) of right little finger
    - √7ᵗʰ **S60.427** Blister (nonthermal) of left little finger
    - √7ᵗʰ **S60.428** Blister (nonthermal) of other finger
      - Blister (nonthermal) of specified finger with unspecified laterality
    - √7ᵗʰ **S60.429** Blister (nonthermal) of unspecified finger
  - √6ᵗʰ **S60.44** External constriction of fingers
    - Hair tourniquet syndrome of finger
    - Use additional cause code to identify the constricting item (W49.0-)
    - √7ᵗʰ **S60.440** External constriction of right index finger
    - √7ᵗʰ **S60.441** External constriction of left index finger
    - √7ᵗʰ **S60.442** External constriction of right middle finger
    - √7ᵗʰ **S60.443** External constriction of left middle finger
    - √7ᵗʰ **S60.444** External constriction of right ring finger
    - √7ᵗʰ **S60.445** External constriction of left ring finger
    - √7ᵗʰ **S60.446** External constriction of right little finger
    - √7ᵗʰ **S60.447** External constriction of left little finger
    - √7ᵗʰ **S60.448** External constriction of other finger
      - External constriction of specified finger with unspecified laterality
    - √7ᵗʰ **S60.449** External constriction of unspecified finger
  - √6ᵗʰ **S60.45** Superficial foreign body of fingers
    - Splinter in the finger(s)
    - √7ᵗʰ **S60.450** Superficial foreign body of right index finger
    - √7ᵗʰ **S60.451** Superficial foreign body of left index finger
    - √7ᵗʰ **S60.452** Superficial foreign body of right middle finger
    - √7ᵗʰ **S60.453** Superficial foreign body of left middle finger
    - √7ᵗʰ **S60.454** Superficial foreign body of right ring finger
    - √7ᵗʰ **S60.455** Superficial foreign body of left ring finger
    - √7ᵗʰ **S60.456** Superficial foreign body of right little finger
    - √7ᵗʰ **S60.457** Superficial foreign body of left little finger
    - √7ᵗʰ **S60.458** Superficial foreign body of other finger
      - Superficial foreign body of specified finger with unspecified laterality
    - √7ᵗʰ **S60.459** Superficial foreign body of unspecified finger

N Newborn: 0   P Pediatric: 0-17   M Maternity: 9-64   A Adult: 15-124   MCC Major Complication/Comorbidity   CC Complication/Comorbidity   SW Severe Wound Dx

1060   ICD-10-CM 2020

√6ᵗʰ **S60.46** Insect bite (nonvenomous) of fingers
    √7ᵗʰ **S60.460** Insect bite (nonvenomous) of right index finger
    √7ᵗʰ **S60.461** Insect bite (nonvenomous) of left index finger
    √7ᵗʰ **S60.462** Insect bite (nonvenomous) of right middle finger
    √7ᵗʰ **S60.463** Insect bite (nonvenomous) of left middle finger
    √7ᵗʰ **S60.464** Insect bite (nonvenomous) of right ring finger
    √7ᵗʰ **S60.465** Insect bite (nonvenomous) of left ring finger
    √7ᵗʰ **S60.466** Insect bite (nonvenomous) of right little finger
    √7ᵗʰ **S60.467** Insect bite (nonvenomous) of left little finger
    √7ᵗʰ **S60.468** Insect bite (nonvenomous) of other finger
       Insect bite (nonvenomous) of specified finger with unspecified laterality
    √7ᵗʰ **S60.469** Insect bite (nonvenomous) of unspecified finger

√6ᵗʰ **S60.47** Other superficial bite of fingers
    EXCLUDES 1   open bite of fingers (S61.25-, S61.35-)
    √7ᵗʰ **S60.470** Other superficial bite of right index finger
    √7ᵗʰ **S60.471** Other superficial bite of left index finger
    √7ᵗʰ **S60.472** Other superficial bite of right middle finger
    √7ᵗʰ **S60.473** Other superficial bite of left middle finger
    √7ᵗʰ **S60.474** Other superficial bite of right ring finger
    √7ᵗʰ **S60.475** Other superficial bite of left ring finger
    √7ᵗʰ **S60.476** Other superficial bite of right little finger
    √7ᵗʰ **S60.477** Other superficial bite of left little finger
    √7ᵗʰ **S60.478** Other superficial bite of other finger
       Other superficial bite of specified finger with unspecified laterality
    √7ᵗʰ **S60.479** Other superficial bite of unspecified finger

√5ᵗʰ **S60.5** Other superficial injuries of hand
    EXCLUDES 2   superficial injuries of fingers (S60.3-, S60.4-)

√6ᵗʰ **S60.51** Abrasion of hand
    √7ᵗʰ **S60.511** Abrasion of right hand
    √7ᵗʰ **S60.512** Abrasion of left hand
    √7ᵗʰ **S60.519** Abrasion of unspecified hand

√6ᵗʰ **S60.52** Blister (nonthermal) of hand
    √7ᵗʰ **S60.521** Blister (nonthermal) of right hand
    √7ᵗʰ **S60.522** Blister (nonthermal) of left hand
    √7ᵗʰ **S60.529** Blister (nonthermal) of unspecified hand

√6ᵗʰ **S60.54** External constriction of hand
    √7ᵗʰ **S60.541** External constriction of right hand
    √7ᵗʰ **S60.542** External constriction of left hand
    √7ᵗʰ **S60.549** External constriction of unspecified hand

√6ᵗʰ **S60.55** Superficial foreign body of hand
    Splinter in the hand
    √7ᵗʰ **S60.551** Superficial foreign body of right hand
    √7ᵗʰ **S60.552** Superficial foreign body of left hand
    √7ᵗʰ **S60.559** Superficial foreign body of unspecified hand

√6ᵗʰ **S60.56** Insect bite (nonvenomous) of hand
    √7ᵗʰ **S60.561** Insect bite (nonvenomous) of right hand
    √7ᵗʰ **S60.562** Insect bite (nonvenomous) of left hand
    √7ᵗʰ **S60.569** Insect bite (nonvenomous) of unspecified hand

√6ᵗʰ **S60.57** Other superficial bite of hand
    EXCLUDES 1   open bite of hand (S61.45-)
    √7ᵗʰ **S60.571** Other superficial bite of hand of right hand
    √7ᵗʰ **S60.572** Other superficial bite of hand of left hand
    √7ᵗʰ **S60.579** Other superficial bite of hand of unspecified hand

√5ᵗʰ **S60.8** Other superficial injuries of wrist

√6ᵗʰ **S60.81** Abrasion of wrist
    √7ᵗʰ **S60.811** Abrasion of right wrist
    √7ᵗʰ **S60.812** Abrasion of left wrist
    √7ᵗʰ **S60.819** Abrasion of unspecified wrist

√6ᵗʰ **S60.82** Blister (nonthermal) of wrist
    √7ᵗʰ **S60.821** Blister (nonthermal) of right wrist
    √7ᵗʰ **S60.822** Blister (nonthermal) of left wrist
    √7ᵗʰ **S60.829** Blister (nonthermal) of unspecified wrist

√6ᵗʰ **S60.84** External constriction of wrist
    √7ᵗʰ **S60.841** External constriction of right wrist
    √7ᵗʰ **S60.842** External constriction of left wrist
    √7ᵗʰ **S60.849** External constriction of unspecified wrist

√6ᵗʰ **S60.85** Superficial foreign body of wrist
    Splinter in the wrist
    √7ᵗʰ **S60.851** Superficial foreign body of right wrist
    √7ᵗʰ **S60.852** Superficial foreign body of left wrist
    √7ᵗʰ **S60.859** Superficial foreign body of unspecified wrist

√6ᵗʰ **S60.86** Insect bite (nonvenomous) of wrist
    √7ᵗʰ **S60.861** Insect bite (nonvenomous) of right wrist
    √7ᵗʰ **S60.862** Insect bite (nonvenomous) of left wrist
    √7ᵗʰ **S60.869** Insect bite (nonvenomous) of unspecified wrist

√6ᵗʰ **S60.87** Other superficial bite of wrist
    EXCLUDES 1   open bite of wrist (S61.55)
    √7ᵗʰ **S60.871** Other superficial bite of right wrist
    √7ᵗʰ **S60.872** Other superficial bite of left wrist
    √7ᵗʰ **S60.879** Other superficial bite of unspecified wrist

√5ᵗʰ **S60.9** Unspecified superficial injury of wrist, hand and fingers

√6ᵗʰ **S60.91** Unspecified superficial injury of wrist
    √7ᵗʰ **S60.911** Unspecified superficial injury of right wrist
    √7ᵗʰ **S60.912** Unspecified superficial injury of left wrist
    √7ᵗʰ **S60.919** Unspecified superficial injury of unspecified wrist

√6ᵗʰ **S60.92** Unspecified superficial injury of hand
    √7ᵗʰ **S60.921** Unspecified superficial injury of right hand
    √7ᵗʰ **S60.922** Unspecified superficial injury of left hand
    √7ᵗʰ **S60.929** Unspecified superficial injury of unspecified hand

√6ᵗʰ **S60.93** Unspecified superficial injury of thumb
    √7ᵗʰ **S60.931** Unspecified superficial injury of right thumb
    √7ᵗʰ **S60.932** Unspecified superficial injury of left thumb
    √7ᵗʰ **S60.939** Unspecified superficial injury of unspecified thumb

√6ᵗʰ **S60.94** Unspecified superficial injury of other fingers
    √7ᵗʰ **S60.940** Unspecified superficial injury of right index finger
    √7ᵗʰ **S60.941** Unspecified superficial injury of left index finger
    √7ᵗʰ **S60.942** Unspecified superficial injury of right middle finger
    √7ᵗʰ **S60.943** Unspecified superficial injury of left middle finger
    √7ᵗʰ **S60.944** Unspecified superficial injury of right ring finger
    √7ᵗʰ **S60.945** Unspecified superficial injury of left ring finger
    √7ᵗʰ **S60.946** Unspecified superficial injury of right little finger
    √7ᵗʰ **S60.947** Unspecified superficial injury of left little finger
    √7ᵗʰ **S60.948** Unspecified superficial injury of other finger
       Unspecified superficial injury of specified finger with unspecified laterality
    √7ᵗʰ **S60.949** Unspecified superficial injury of unspecified finger

☑4ᵗʰ S61   Open wound of wrist, hand and fingers

Code also any associated wound infection

EXCLUDES 1   open fracture of wrist, hand and finger (S62.- with 7th character B)

traumatic amputation of wrist and hand (S68.-)

The appropriate 7th character is to be added to each code from category S61.

A   initial encounter
D   subsequent encounter
S   sequela

☑5ᵗʰ S61.0   Open wound of thumb without damage to nail

EXCLUDES 1   open wound of thumb with damage to nail (S61.1-)

☑6ᵗʰ S61.00   Unspecified open wound of thumb without damage to nail

- ☑7ᵗʰ **S61.001** Unspecified open wound of right thumb without damage to nail
- ☑7ᵗʰ **S61.002** Unspecified open wound of left thumb without damage to nail
- ☑7ᵗʰ **S61.009** Unspecified open wound of unspecified thumb without damage to nail

☑6ᵗʰ S61.01   Laceration without foreign body of thumb without damage to nail

- ☑7ᵗʰ **S61.011** Laceration without foreign body of right thumb without damage to nail
- ☑7ᵗʰ **S61.012** Laceration without foreign body of left thumb without damage to nail
- ☑7ᵗʰ **S61.019** Laceration without foreign body of unspecified thumb without damage to nail

☑6ᵗʰ S61.02   Laceration with foreign body of thumb without damage to nail

- ☑7ᵗʰ **S61.021** Laceration with foreign body of right thumb without damage to nail
- ☑7ᵗʰ **S61.022** Laceration with foreign body of left thumb without damage to nail
- ☑7ᵗʰ **S61.029** Laceration with foreign body of unspecified thumb without damage to nail

☑6ᵗʰ S61.03   Puncture wound without foreign body of thumb without damage to nail

- ☑7ᵗʰ **S61.031** Puncture wound without foreign body of right thumb without damage to nail
- ☑7ᵗʰ **S61.032** Puncture wound without foreign body of left thumb without damage to nail
- ☑7ᵗʰ **S61.039** Puncture wound without foreign body of unspecified thumb without damage to nail

☑6ᵗʰ S61.04   Puncture wound with foreign body of thumb without damage to nail

- ☑7ᵗʰ **S61.041** Puncture wound with foreign body of right thumb without damage to nail
- ☑7ᵗʰ **S61.042** Puncture wound with foreign body of left thumb without damage to nail
- ☑7ᵗʰ **S61.049** Puncture wound with foreign body of unspecified thumb without damage to nail

☑6ᵗʰ S61.05   Open bite of thumb without damage to nail

Bite of thumb NOS

EXCLUDES 1   superficial bite of thumb (S60.36-, S60.37-)

- ☑7ᵗʰ **S61.051** Open bite of right thumb without damage to nail
- ☑7ᵗʰ **S61.052** Open bite of left thumb without damage to nail
- ☑7ᵗʰ **S61.059** Open bite of unspecified thumb without damage to nail

☑5ᵗʰ S61.1   Open wound of thumb with damage to nail

☑6ᵗʰ S61.10   Unspecified open wound of thumb with damage to nail

- ☑7ᵗʰ **S61.101** Unspecified open wound of right thumb with damage to nail
- ☑7ᵗʰ **S61.102** Unspecified open wound of left thumb with damage to nail
- ☑7ᵗʰ **S61.109** Unspecified open wound of unspecified thumb with damage to nail

☑6ᵗʰ S61.11   Laceration without foreign body of thumb with damage to nail

- ☑7ᵗʰ **S61.111** Laceration without foreign body of right thumb with damage to nail
- ☑7ᵗʰ **S61.112** Laceration without foreign body of left thumb with damage to nail

☑7ᵗʰ **S61.119** Laceration without foreign body of unspecified thumb with damage to nail

☑6ᵗʰ S61.12   Laceration with foreign body of thumb with damage to nail

- ☑7ᵗʰ **S61.121** Laceration with foreign body of right thumb with damage to nail
- ☑7ᵗʰ **S61.122** Laceration with foreign body of left thumb with damage to nail
- ☑7ᵗʰ **S61.129** Laceration with foreign body of unspecified thumb with damage to nail

☑6ᵗʰ S61.13   Puncture wound without foreign body of thumb with damage to nail

- ☑7ᵗʰ **S61.131** Puncture wound without foreign body of right thumb with damage to nail
- ☑7ᵗʰ **S61.132** Puncture wound without foreign body of left thumb with damage to nail
- ☑7ᵗʰ **S61.139** Puncture wound without foreign body of unspecified thumb with damage to nail

☑6ᵗʰ S61.14   Puncture wound with foreign body of thumb with damage to nail

- ☑7ᵗʰ **S61.141** Puncture wound with foreign body of right thumb with damage to nail
- ☑7ᵗʰ **S61.142** Puncture wound with foreign body of left thumb with damage to nail
- ☑7ᵗʰ **S61.149** Puncture wound with foreign body of unspecified thumb with damage to nail

☑6ᵗʰ S61.15   Open bite of thumb with damage to nail

Bite of thumb with damage to nail NOS

EXCLUDES 1   superficial bite of thumb (S60.36-, S60.37-)

- ☑7ᵗʰ **S61.151** Open bite of right thumb with damage to nail
- ☑7ᵗʰ **S61.152** Open bite of left thumb with damage to nail
- ☑7ᵗʰ **S61.159** Open bite of unspecified thumb with damage to nail

☑5ᵗʰ S61.2   Open wound of other finger without damage to nail

EXCLUDES 1   open wound of finger involving nail (matrix) (S61.3-)

EXCLUDES 2   open wound of thumb without damage to nail (S61.0-)

☑6ᵗʰ S61.20   Unspecified open wound of other finger without damage to nail

- ☑7ᵗʰ **S61.200** Unspecified open wound of right index finger without damage to nail
- ☑7ᵗʰ **S61.201** Unspecified open wound of left index finger without damage to nail
- ☑7ᵗʰ **S61.202** Unspecified open wound of right middle finger without damage to nail
- ☑7ᵗʰ **S61.203** Unspecified open wound of left middle finger without damage to nail
- ☑7ᵗʰ **S61.204** Unspecified open wound of right ring finger without damage to nail
- ☑7ᵗʰ **S61.205** Unspecified open wound of left ring finger without damage to nail
- ☑7ᵗʰ **S61.206** Unspecified open wound of right little finger without damage to nail
- ☑7ᵗʰ **S61.207** Unspecified open wound of left little finger without damage to nail
- ☑7ᵗʰ **S61.208** Unspecified open wound of other finger without damage to nail

Unspecified open wound of specified finger with unspecified laterality without damage to nail

- ☑7ᵗʰ **S61.209** Unspecified open wound of unspecified finger without damage to nail

☑6ᵗʰ S61.21   Laceration without foreign body of finger without damage to nail

- ☑7ᵗʰ **S61.210** Laceration without foreign body of right index finger without damage to nail
- ☑7ᵗʰ **S61.211** Laceration without foreign body of left index finger without damage to nail
- ☑7ᵗʰ **S61.212** Laceration without foreign body of right middle finger without damage to nail
- ☑7ᵗʰ **S61.213** Laceration without foreign body of left middle finger without damage to nail
- ☑7ᵗʰ **S61.214** Laceration without foreign body of right ring finger without damage to nail
- ☑7ᵗʰ **S61.215** Laceration without foreign body of left ring finger without damage to nail
- ☑7ᵗʰ **S61.216** Laceration without foreign body of right little finger without damage to nail
- ☑7ᵗʰ **S61.217** Laceration without foreign body of left little finger without damage to nail

N Newborn: 0   P Pediatric: 0-17   M Maternity: 9-64   A Adult: 15-124   MCC Major Complication/Comorbidity   CC Complication/Comorbidity   SW Severe Wound Dx

1062   ICD-10-CM 2020

√7ᵗʰ **S61.218** **Laceration without foreign body of other finger without damage to nail**
Laceration without foreign body of specified finger with unspecified laterality without damage to nail

√7ᵗʰ **S61.219** **Laceration without foreign body of unspecified finger without damage to nail**

√6ᵗʰ **S61.22** Laceration with foreign body of finger without damage to nail

√7ᵗʰ **S61.220** **Laceration with foreign body of right index finger without damage to nail**

√7ᵗʰ **S61.221** **Laceration with foreign body of left index finger without damage to nail**

√7ᵗʰ **S61.222** **Laceration with foreign body of right middle finger without damage to nail**

√7ᵗʰ **S61.223** **Laceration with foreign body of left middle finger without damage to nail**

√7ᵗʰ **S61.224** **Laceration with foreign body of right ring finger without damage to nail**

√7ᵗʰ **S61.225** **Laceration with foreign body of left ring finger without damage to nail**

√7ᵗʰ **S61.226** **Laceration with foreign body of right little finger without damage to nail**

√7ᵗʰ **S61.227** **Laceration with foreign body of left little finger without damage to nail**

√7ᵗʰ **S61.228** **Laceration with foreign body of other finger without damage to nail**
Laceration with foreign body of specified finger with unspecified laterality without damage to nail

√7ᵗʰ **S61.229** **Laceration with foreign body of unspecified finger without damage to nail**

√6ᵗʰ **S61.23** Puncture wound without foreign body of finger without damage to nail

√7ᵗʰ **S61.230** **Puncture wound without foreign body of right index finger without damage to nail**

√7ᵗʰ **S61.231** **Puncture wound without foreign body of left index finger without damage to nail**

√7ᵗʰ **S61.232** **Puncture wound without foreign body of right middle finger without damage to nail**

√7ᵗʰ **S61.233** **Puncture wound without foreign body of left middle finger without damage to nail**

√7ᵗʰ **S61.234** **Puncture wound without foreign body of right ring finger without damage to nail**

√7ᵗʰ **S61.235** **Puncture wound without foreign body of left ring finger without damage to nail**

√7ᵗʰ **S61.236** **Puncture wound without foreign body of right little finger without damage to nail**

√7ᵗʰ **S61.237** **Puncture wound without foreign body of left little finger without damage to nail**

√7ᵗʰ **S61.238** **Puncture wound without foreign body of other finger without damage to nail**
Puncture wound without foreign body of specified finger with unspecified laterality without damage to nail

√7ᵗʰ **S61.239** **Puncture wound without foreign body of unspecified finger without damage to nail**

√6ᵗʰ **S61.24** Puncture wound with foreign body of finger without damage to nail

√7ᵗʰ **S61.240** **Puncture wound with foreign body of right index finger without damage to nail**

√7ᵗʰ **S61.241** **Puncture wound with foreign body of left index finger without damage to nail**

√7ᵗʰ **S61.242** **Puncture wound with foreign body of right middle finger without damage to nail**

√7ᵗʰ **S61.243** **Puncture wound with foreign body of left middle finger without damage to nail**

√7ᵗʰ **S61.244** **Puncture wound with foreign body of right ring finger without damage to nail**

√7ᵗʰ **S61.245** **Puncture wound with foreign body of left ring finger without damage to nail**

√7ᵗʰ **S61.246** **Puncture wound with foreign body of right little finger without damage to nail**

√7ᵗʰ **S61.247** **Puncture wound with foreign body of left little finger without damage to nail**

√7ᵗʰ **S61.248** **Puncture wound with foreign body of other finger without damage to nail**
Puncture wound with foreign body of specified finger with unspecified laterality without damage to nail

√7ᵗʰ **S61.249** **Puncture wound with foreign body of unspecified finger without damage to nail**

√6ᵗʰ **S61.25** Open bite of finger without damage to nail
Bite of finger without damage to nail NOS
EXCLUDES 1   superficial bite of finger (S60.46-, S60.47-)

√7ᵗʰ **S61.250** **Open bite of right index finger without damage to nail**

√7ᵗʰ **S61.251** **Open bite of left index finger without damage to nail**

√7ᵗʰ **S61.252** **Open bite of right middle finger without damage to nail**

√7ᵗʰ **S61.253** **Open bite of left middle finger without damage to nail**

√7ᵗʰ **S61.254** **Open bite of right ring finger without damage to nail**

√7ᵗʰ **S61.255** **Open bite of left ring finger without damage to nail**

√7ᵗʰ **S61.256** **Open bite of right little finger without damage to nail**

√7ᵗʰ **S61.257** **Open bite of left little finger without damage to nail**

√7ᵗʰ **S61.258** **Open bite of other finger without damage to nail**
Open bite of specified finger with unspecified laterality without damage to nail

√7ᵗʰ **S61.259** **Open bite of unspecified finger without damage to nail**

√5ᵗʰ **S61.3** Open wound of other finger with damage to nail

√6ᵗʰ **S61.30** Unspecified open wound of finger with damage to nail

√7ᵗʰ **S61.300** **Unspecified open wound of right index finger with damage to nail**

√7ᵗʰ **S61.301** **Unspecified open wound of left index finger with damage to nail**

√7ᵗʰ **S61.302** **Unspecified open wound of right middle finger with damage to nail**

√7ᵗʰ **S61.303** **Unspecified open wound of left middle finger with damage to nail**

√7ᵗʰ **S61.304** **Unspecified open wound of right ring finger with damage to nail**

√7ᵗʰ **S61.305** **Unspecified open wound of left ring finger with damage to nail**

√7ᵗʰ **S61.306** **Unspecified open wound of right little finger with damage to nail**

√7ᵗʰ **S61.307** **Unspecified open wound of left little finger with damage to nail**

√7ᵗʰ **S61.308** **Unspecified open wound of other finger with damage to nail**
Unspecified open wound of specified finger with unspecified laterality with damage to nail

√7ᵗʰ **S61.309** **Unspecified open wound of unspecified finger with damage to nail**

√6ᵗʰ **S61.31** Laceration without foreign body of finger with damage to nail

√7ᵗʰ **S61.310** **Laceration without foreign body of right index finger with damage to nail**

√7ᵗʰ **S61.311** **Laceration without foreign body of left index finger with damage to nail**

√7ᵗʰ **S61.312** **Laceration without foreign body of right middle finger with damage to nail**

√7ᵗʰ **S61.313** **Laceration without foreign body of left middle finger with damage to nail**

√7ᵗʰ **S61.314** **Laceration without foreign body of right ring finger with damage to nail**

√7ᵗʰ **S61.315** **Laceration without foreign body of left ring finger with damage to nail**

√7ᵗʰ **S61.316** **Laceration without foreign body of right little finger with damage to nail**

√7ᵗʰ **S61.317** **Laceration without foreign body of left little finger with damage to nail**

☑ Additional Character Required   √x7ᵗʰ Placeholder   Unacceptable PDx   Questionable PDx   Manifestation   Unspecified Dx   H1-H14 HAC   HCC CMS-HCC Dx   HIV HIV Dx

ICD-10-CM 2020

1063

√7ᵗʰ **S61.318** **Laceration without foreign body of other finger with damage to nail**
Laceration without foreign body of specified finger with unspecified laterality with damage to nail

√7ᵗʰ **S61.319** **Laceration without foreign body of unspecified finger with damage to nail**

√6ᵗʰ **S61.32** **Laceration with foreign body of finger with damage to nail**

√7ᵗʰ **S61.320** **Laceration with foreign body of right index finger with damage to nail**

√7ᵗʰ **S61.321** **Laceration with foreign body of left index finger with damage to nail**

√7ᵗʰ **S61.322** **Laceration with foreign body of right middle finger with damage to nail**

√7ᵗʰ **S61.323** **Laceration with foreign body of left middle finger with damage to nail**

√7ᵗʰ **S61.324** **Laceration with foreign body of right ring finger with damage to nail**

√7ᵗʰ **S61.325** **Laceration with foreign body of left ring finger with damage to nail**

√7ᵗʰ **S61.326** **Laceration with foreign body of right little finger with damage to nail**

√7ᵗʰ **S61.327** **Laceration with foreign body of left little finger with damage to nail**

√7ᵗʰ **S61.328** **Laceration with foreign body of other finger with damage to nail**
Laceration with foreign body of specified finger with unspecified laterality with damage to nail

√7ᵗʰ **S61.329** **Laceration with foreign body of unspecified finger with damage to nail**

√6ᵗʰ **S61.33** **Puncture wound without foreign body of finger with damage to nail**

√7ᵗʰ **S61.330** **Puncture wound without foreign body of right index finger with damage to nail**

√7ᵗʰ **S61.331** **Puncture wound without foreign body of left index finger with damage to nail**

√7ᵗʰ **S61.332** **Puncture wound without foreign body of right middle finger with damage to nail**

√7ᵗʰ **S61.333** **Puncture wound without foreign body of left middle finger with damage to nail**

√7ᵗʰ **S61.334** **Puncture wound without foreign body of right ring finger with damage to nail**

√7ᵗʰ **S61.335** **Puncture wound without foreign body of left ring finger with damage to nail**

√7ᵗʰ **S61.336** **Puncture wound without foreign body of right little finger with damage to nail**

√7ᵗʰ **S61.337** **Puncture wound without foreign body of left little finger with damage to nail**

√7ᵗʰ **S61.338** **Puncture wound without foreign body of other finger with damage to nail**
Puncture wound without foreign body of specified finger with unspecified laterality with damage to nail

√7ᵗʰ **S61.339** **Puncture wound without foreign body of unspecified finger with damage to nail**

√6ᵗʰ **S61.34** **Puncture wound with foreign body of finger with damage to nail**

√7ᵗʰ **S61.340** **Puncture wound with foreign body of right index finger with damage to nail**

√7ᵗʰ **S61.341** **Puncture wound with foreign body of left index finger with damage to nail**

√7ᵗʰ **S61.342** **Puncture wound with foreign body of right middle finger with damage to nail**

√7ᵗʰ **S61.343** **Puncture wound with foreign body of left middle finger with damage to nail**

√7ᵗʰ **S61.344** **Puncture wound with foreign body of right ring finger with damage to nail**

√7ᵗʰ **S61.345** **Puncture wound with foreign body of left ring finger with damage to nail**

√7ᵗʰ **S61.346** **Puncture wound with foreign body of right little finger with damage to nail**

√7ᵗʰ **S61.347** **Puncture wound with foreign body of left little finger with damage to nail**

√7ᵗʰ **S61.348** **Puncture wound with foreign body of other finger with damage to nail**
Puncture wound with foreign body of specified finger with unspecified laterality with damage to nail

√7ᵗʰ **S61.349** **Puncture wound with foreign body of unspecified finger with damage to nail**

√6ᵗʰ **S61.35** **Open bite of finger with damage to nail**
Bite of finger with damage to nail NOS
EXCLUDES 1 *superficial bite of finger (S60.46-, S60.47-)*

√7ᵗʰ **S61.350** **Open bite of right index finger with damage to nail**

√7ᵗʰ **S61.351** **Open bite of left index finger with damage to nail**

√7ᵗʰ **S61.352** **Open bite of right middle finger with damage to nail**

√7ᵗʰ **S61.353** **Open bite of left middle finger with damage to nail**

√7ᵗʰ **S61.354** **Open bite of right ring finger with damage to nail**

√7ᵗʰ **S61.355** **Open bite of left ring finger with damage to nail**

√7ᵗʰ **S61.356** **Open bite of right little finger with damage to nail**

√7ᵗʰ **S61.357** **Open bite of left little finger with damage to nail**

√7ᵗʰ **S61.358** **Open bite of other finger with damage to nail**
Open bite of specified finger with unspecified laterality with damage to nail

√7ᵗʰ **S61.359** **Open bite of unspecified finger with damage to nail**

√5ᵗʰ **S61.4** **Open wound of hand**

√6ᵗʰ **S61.40** **Unspecified open wound of hand**

√7ᵗʰ **S61.401** **Unspecified open wound of right hand**

√7ᵗʰ **S61.402** **Unspecified open wound of left hand**

√7ᵗʰ **S61.409** **Unspecified open wound of unspecified hand**

√6ᵗʰ **S61.41** **Laceration without foreign body of hand**

√7ᵗʰ **S61.411** **Laceration without foreign body of right hand**

√7ᵗʰ **S61.412** **Laceration without foreign body of left hand**

√7ᵗʰ **S61.419** **Laceration without foreign body of unspecified hand**

√6ᵗʰ **S61.42** **Laceration with foreign body of hand**

√7ᵗʰ **S61.421** **Laceration with foreign body of right hand**

√7ᵗʰ **S61.422** **Laceration with foreign body of left hand**

√7ᵗʰ **S61.429** **Laceration with foreign body of unspecified hand**

√6ᵗʰ **S61.43** **Puncture wound without foreign body of hand**

√7ᵗʰ **S61.431** **Puncture wound without foreign body of right hand**

√7ᵗʰ **S61.432** **Puncture wound without foreign body of left hand**

√7ᵗʰ **S61.439** **Puncture wound without foreign body of unspecified hand**

√6ᵗʰ **S61.44** **Puncture wound with foreign body of hand**

√7ᵗʰ **S61.441** **Puncture wound with foreign body of right hand**

√7ᵗʰ **S61.442** **Puncture wound with foreign body of left hand**

√7ᵗʰ **S61.449** **Puncture wound with foreign body of unspecified hand**

√6ᵗʰ **S61.45** **Open bite of hand**
Bite of hand NOS
EXCLUDES 1 *superficial bite of hand (S60.56-, S60.57-)*

√7ᵗʰ **S61.451** **Open bite of right hand**

√7ᵗʰ **S61.452** **Open bite of left hand**

√7ᵗʰ **S61.459** **Open bite of unspecified hand**

√5ᵗʰ **S61.5** **Open wound of wrist**

√6ᵗʰ **S61.50** **Unspecified open wound of wrist**

√7ᵗʰ **S61.501** **Unspecified open wound of right wrist**

√7ᵗʰ **S61.502** **Unspecified open wound of left wrist**

√7ᵗʰ **S61.509** **Unspecified open wound of unspecified wrist**

√6ᵗʰ **S61.51** **Laceration without foreign body of wrist**

√7ᵗʰ **S61.511** **Laceration without foreign body of right wrist**

√7ᵗʰ **S61.512** **Laceration without foreign body of left wrist**

√7ᵗʰ **S61.519** **Laceration without foreign body of unspecified wrist**

√6ᵗʰ **S61.52** Laceration with foreign body of wrist

√7ᵗʰ **S61.521** Laceration with foreign body of right wrist

√7ᵗʰ **S61.522** Laceration with foreign body of left wrist

√7ᵗʰ **S61.529** Laceration with foreign body of unspecified wrist

√6ᵗʰ **S61.53** Puncture wound without foreign body of wrist

√7ᵗʰ **S61.531** Puncture wound without foreign body of right wrist

√7ᵗʰ **S61.532** Puncture wound without foreign body of left wrist

√7ᵗʰ **S61.539** Puncture wound without foreign body of unspecified wrist

√6ᵗʰ **S61.54** Puncture wound with foreign body of wrist

√7ᵗʰ **S61.541** Puncture wound with foreign body of right wrist

√7ᵗʰ **S61.542** Puncture wound with foreign body of left wrist

√7ᵗʰ **S61.549** Puncture wound with foreign body of unspecified wrist

√6ᵗʰ **S61.55** Open bite of wrist

Bite of wrist NOS

> EXCLUDES 1   superficial bite of wrist (S60.86-, S60.87-)

√7ᵗʰ **S61.551** Open bite of right wrist

√7ᵗʰ **S61.552** Open bite of left wrist

√7ᵗʰ **S61.559** Open bite of unspecified wrist

√4ᵗʰ **S62** **Fracture at wrist and hand level**

NOTE   A fracture not indicated as displaced or nondisplaced should be coded to displaced

A fracture not indicated as open or closed should be coded to closed

EXCLUDES 1   traumatic amputation of wrist and hand (S68.-)

EXCLUDES 2   fracture of distal parts of ulna and radius (S52.-)

AHA: 2018,2Q,12; 2015,3Q,37-39

> The appropriate 7th character is to be added to each code from category S62.
> A   initial encounter for closed fracture
> B   initial encounter for open fracture
> D   subsequent encounter for fracture with routine healing
> G   subsequent encounter for fracture with delayed healing
> K   subsequent encounter for fracture with nonunion
> P   subsequent encounter for fracture with malunion
> S   sequela

√5ᵗʰ **S62.0** Fracture of navicular [scaphoid] bone of wrist

> **CC Excl: For codes in subcategory S62.0:**
> **CC with 7th character B:** PDX collection 1283
> **CC with 7th character K or P:** PDX collection 897

√6ᵗʰ **S62.00** **Unspecified fracture of navicular [scaphoid] bone of wrist**

³ √7ᵗʰ **S62.001** Unspecified fracture of navicular [scaphoid] bone of right wrist   CC H5

³ √7ᵗʰ **S62.002** Unspecified fracture of navicular [scaphoid] bone of left wrist   CC H5

AHA: 2012,4Q,106

³ √7ᵗʰ **S62.009** Unspecified fracture of navicular [scaphoid] bone of unspecified wrist   CC H5

√6ᵗʰ **S62.01** **Fracture of distal pole of navicular [scaphoid] bone of wrist**

Fracture of volar tuberosity of navicular [scaphoid] bone of wrist

³ √7ᵗʰ **S62.011** Displaced fracture of distal pole of navicular [scaphoid] bone of right wrist   CC H5

³ √7ᵗʰ **S62.012** Displaced fracture of distal pole of navicular [scaphoid] bone of left wrist   CC H5

³ √7ᵗʰ **S62.013** Displaced fracture of distal pole of navicular [scaphoid] bone of unspecified wrist   CC H5

³ √7ᵗʰ **S62.014** Nondisplaced fracture of distal pole of navicular [scaphoid] bone of right wrist   CC H5

³ √7ᵗʰ **S62.015** Nondisplaced fracture of distal pole of navicular [scaphoid] bone of left wrist   CC H5

³ √7ᵗʰ **S62.016** Nondisplaced fracture of distal pole of navicular [scaphoid] bone of unspecified wrist   CC H5

√6ᵗʰ **S62.02** Fracture of middle third of navicular [scaphoid] bone of wrist

³ √7ᵗʰ **S62.021** Displaced fracture of middle third of navicular [scaphoid] bone of right wrist   CC H5

³ √7ᵗʰ **S62.022** Displaced fracture of middle third of navicular [scaphoid] bone of left wrist   CC H5

³ √7ᵗʰ **S62.023** Displaced fracture of middle third of navicular [scaphoid] bone of unspecified wrist   CC H5

³ √7ᵗʰ **S62.024** Nondisplaced fracture of middle third of navicular [scaphoid] bone of right wrist   CC H5

³ √7ᵗʰ **S62.025** Nondisplaced fracture of middle third of navicular [scaphoid] bone of left wrist   CC H5

³ √7ᵗʰ **S62.026** Nondisplaced fracture of middle third of navicular [scaphoid] bone of unspecified wrist   CC H5

√6ᵗʰ **S62.03** Fracture of proximal third of navicular [scaphoid] bone of wrist

³ √7ᵗʰ **S62.031** Displaced fracture of proximal third of navicular [scaphoid] bone of right wrist   CC H5

³ √7ᵗʰ **S62.032** Displaced fracture of proximal third of navicular [scaphoid] bone of left wrist   CC H5

³ √7ᵗʰ **S62.033** Displaced fracture of proximal third of navicular [scaphoid] bone of unspecified wrist   CC H5

³ √7ᵗʰ **S62.034** Nondisplaced fracture of proximal third of navicular [scaphoid] bone of right wrist   CC H5

³ √7ᵗʰ **S62.035** Nondisplaced fracture of proximal third of navicular [scaphoid] bone of left wrist   CC H5

³ √7ᵗʰ **S62.036** Nondisplaced fracture of proximal third of navicular [scaphoid] bone of unspecified wrist   CC H5

√5ᵗʰ **S62.1** Fracture of other and unspecified carpal bone(s)

EXCLUDES 2   fracture of scaphoid of wrist (S62.0-)

> **CC Excl: For codes in subcategory S62.1:**
> **CC with 7th character B:** PDX collection 1283
> **CC with 7th character K or P:** PDX collection 897

√6ᵗʰ **S62.10** **Fracture of unspecified carpal bone**

Fracture of wrist NOS

³ √7ᵗʰ **S62.101** Fracture of unspecified carpal bone, right wrist   CC H5

³ √7ᵗʰ **S62.102** Fracture of unspecified carpal bone, left wrist   CC H5

AHA: 2012,4Q,95

³ √7ᵗʰ **S62.109** Fracture of unspecified carpal bone, unspecified wrist   CC H5

√6ᵗʰ **S62.11** Fracture of triquetrum [cuneiform] bone of wrist

³ √7ᵗʰ **S62.111** Displaced fracture of triquetrum [cuneiform] bone, right wrist   CC H5

3 √7ᵗʰ **S62.112** Displaced fracture of triquetrum [cuneiform] bone, left wrist   `CC` `H5`

3 √7ᵗʰ **S62.113** Displaced fracture of triquetrum [cuneiform] bone, unspecified wrist   `CC` `H5`

3 √7ᵗʰ **S62.114** Nondisplaced fracture of triquetrum [cuneiform] bone, right wrist   `CC` `H5`

3 √7ᵗʰ **S62.115** Nondisplaced fracture of triquetrum [cuneiform] bone, left wrist   `CC` `H5`

3 √7ᵗʰ **S62.116** Nondisplaced fracture of triquetrum [cuneiform] bone, unspecified wrist   `CC` `H5`

√6ᵗʰ **S62.12** Fracture of lunate [semilunar]

3 √7ᵗʰ **S62.121** Displaced fracture of lunate [semilunar], right wrist   `CC` `H5`

3 √7ᵗʰ **S62.122** Displaced fracture of lunate [semilunar], left wrist   `CC` `H5`

3 √7ᵗʰ **S62.123** Displaced fracture of lunate [semilunar], unspecified wrist   `CC` `H5`

3 √7ᵗʰ **S62.124** Nondisplaced fracture of lunate [semilunar], right wrist   `CC` `H5`

3 √7ᵗʰ **S62.125** Nondisplaced fracture of lunate [semilunar], left wrist   `CC` `H5`

3 √7ᵗʰ **S62.126** Nondisplaced fracture of lunate [semilunar], unspecified wrist   `CC` `H5`

√6ᵗʰ **S62.13** Fracture of capitate [os magnum] bone

3 √7ᵗʰ **S62.131** Displaced fracture of capitate [os magnum] bone, right wrist   `CC` `H5`

3 √7ᵗʰ **S62.132** Displaced fracture of capitate [os magnum] bone, left wrist   `CC` `H5`

3 √7ᵗʰ **S62.133** Displaced fracture of capitate [os magnum] bone, unspecified wrist   `CC` `H5`

3 √7ᵗʰ **S62.134** Nondisplaced fracture of capitate [os magnum] bone, right wrist   `CC` `H5`

3 √7ᵗʰ **S62.135** Nondisplaced fracture of capitate [os magnum] bone, left wrist   `CC` `H5`

3 √7ᵗʰ **S62.136** Nondisplaced fracture of capitate [os magnum] bone, unspecified wrist   `CC` `H5`

√6ᵗʰ **S62.14** Fracture of body of hamate [unciform] bone

Fracture of hamate [unciform] bone NOS

3 √7ᵗʰ **S62.141** Displaced fracture of body of hamate [unciform] bone, right wrist   `CC` `H5`

3 √7ᵗʰ **S62.142** Displaced fracture of body of hamate [unciform] bone, left wrist   `CC` `H5`

3 √7ᵗʰ **S62.143** Displaced fracture of body of hamate [unciform] bone, unspecified wrist   `CC` `H5`

3 √7ᵗʰ **S62.144** Nondisplaced fracture of body of hamate [unciform] bone, right wrist   `CC` `H5`

3 √7ᵗʰ **S62.145** Nondisplaced fracture of body of hamate [unciform] bone, left wrist   `CC` `H5`

3 √7ᵗʰ **S62.146** Nondisplaced fracture of body of hamate [unciform] bone, unspecified wrist   `CC` `H5`

√6ᵗʰ **S62.15** Fracture of hook process of hamate [unciform] bone

Fracture of unciform process of hamate [unciform] bone

3 √7ᵗʰ **S62.151** Displaced fracture of hook process of hamate [unciform] bone, right wrist   `CC` `H5`

3 √7ᵗʰ **S62.152** Displaced fracture of hook process of hamate [unciform] bone, left wrist   `CC` `H5`

3 √7ᵗʰ **S62.153** Displaced fracture of hook process of hamate [unciform] bone, unspecified wrist   `CC` `H5`

3 √7ᵗʰ **S62.154** Nondisplaced fracture of hook process of hamate [unciform] bone, right wrist   `CC` `H5`

3 √7ᵗʰ **S62.155** Nondisplaced fracture of hook process of hamate [unciform] bone, left wrist   `CC` `H5`

3 √7ᵗʰ **S62.156** Nondisplaced fracture of hook process of hamate [unciform] bone, unspecified wrist   `CC` `H5`

√6ᵗʰ **S62.16** Fracture of pisiform

3 √7ᵗʰ **S62.161** Displaced fracture of pisiform, right wrist   `CC` `H5`

3 √7ᵗʰ **S62.162** Displaced fracture of pisiform, left wrist   `CC` `H5`

3 √7ᵗʰ **S62.163** Displaced fracture of pisiform, unspecified wrist   `CC` `H5`

3 √7ᵗʰ **S62.164** Nondisplaced fracture of pisiform, right wrist   `CC` `H5`

3 √7ᵗʰ **S62.165** Nondisplaced fracture of pisiform, left wrist   `CC` `H5`

3 √7ᵗʰ **S62.166** Nondisplaced fracture of pisiform, unspecified wrist   `CC` `H5`

√6ᵗʰ **S62.17** Fracture of trapezium [larger multangular]

3 √7ᵗʰ **S62.171** Displaced fracture of trapezium [larger multangular], right wrist   `CC` `H5`

3 √7ᵗʰ **S62.172** Displaced fracture of trapezium [larger multangular], left wrist   `CC` `H5`

3 √7ᵗʰ **S62.173** Displaced fracture of trapezium [larger multangular], unspecified wrist   `CC` `H5`

3 √7ᵗʰ **S62.174** Nondisplaced fracture of trapezium [larger multangular], right wrist   `CC` `H5`

3 √7ᵗʰ **S62.175** Nondisplaced fracture of trapezium [larger multangular], left wrist   `CC` `H5`

3 √7ᵗʰ **S62.176** Nondisplaced fracture of trapezium [larger multangular], unspecified wrist   `CC` `H5`

√6ᵗʰ **S62.18** Fracture of trapezoid [smaller multangular]

3 √7ᵗʰ **S62.181** Displaced fracture of trapezoid [smaller multangular], right wrist   `CC` `H5`

3 √7ᵗʰ **S62.182** Displaced fracture of trapezoid [smaller multangular], left wrist   `CC` `H5`

3 √7ᵗʰ **S62.183** Displaced fracture of trapezoid [smaller multangular], unspecified wrist   `CC` `H5`

3 √7ᵗʰ **S62.184** Nondisplaced fracture of trapezoid [smaller multangular], right wrist   `CC` `H5`

3 √7ᵗʰ **S62.185** Nondisplaced fracture of trapezoid [smaller multangular], left wrist   `CC` `H5`

3 √7ᵗʰ **S62.186** Nondisplaced fracture of trapezoid [smaller multangular], unspecified wrist   `CC` `H5`

√5ᵗʰ **S62.2** Fracture of first metacarpal bone

CC Excl: For codes in subcategory S62.2:
CC with 7th character B: PDX collection 1284
CC with 7th character K or P: PDX collection 897

√6ᵗʰ **S62.20** Unspecified fracture of first metacarpal bone

3 √7ᵗʰ **S62.201** Unspecified fracture of first metacarpal bone, right hand   `CC` `H5`

3 √7ᵗʰ **S62.202** Unspecified fracture of first metacarpal bone, left hand   `CC` `H5`

`N` Newborn: 0   `P` Pediatric: 0-17   `M` Maternity: 9-64   `A` Adult: 15-124   `MCC` Major Complication/Comorbidity   `CC` Complication/Comorbidity   `SW` Severe Wound Dx

1066   ICD-10-CM 2020

³ √7ᵗʰ **S62.209** Unspecified fracture of first metacarpal bone, unspecified hand   `CC` `H5`

√6ᵗʰ **S62.21** Bennett's fracture

    DEF: Intra-articular, two-part fracture at the base of the first metacarpal bone (thumb) on the ulnar side at the carpometacarpal (CMC) joint.

³ √7ᵗʰ **S62.211** Bennett's fracture, right hand   `CC` `H5`

³ √7ᵗʰ **S62.212** Bennett's fracture, left hand   `CC` `H5`

³ √7ᵗʰ **S62.213** Bennett's fracture, unspecified hand   `CC` `H5`

√6ᵗʰ **S62.22** Rolando's fracture

    DEF: Comminuted, three part intra-articular fracture at the base of the thumb metacarpal.

³ √7ᵗʰ **S62.221** Displaced Rolando's fracture, right hand   `CC` `H5`

³ √7ᵗʰ **S62.222** Displaced Rolando's fracture, left hand   `CC` `H5`

³ √7ᵗʰ **S62.223** Displaced Rolando's fracture, unspecified hand   `CC` `H5`

³ √7ᵗʰ **S62.224** Nondisplaced Rolando's fracture, right hand   `CC` `H5`

³ √7ᵗʰ **S62.225** Nondisplaced Rolando's fracture, left hand   `CC` `H5`

³ √7ᵗʰ **S62.226** Nondisplaced Rolando's fracture, unspecified hand   `CC` `H5`

√6ᵗʰ **S62.23** Other fracture of base of first metacarpal bone

³ √7ᵗʰ **S62.231** Other displaced fracture of base of first metacarpal bone, right hand   `CC` `H5`

³ √7ᵗʰ **S62.232** Other displaced fracture of base of first metacarpal bone, left hand   `CC` `H5`

³ √7ᵗʰ **S62.233** Other displaced fracture of base of first metacarpal bone, unspecified hand   `CC` `H5`

³ √7ᵗʰ **S62.234** Other nondisplaced fracture of base of first metacarpal bone, right hand   `CC` `H5`

³ √7ᵗʰ **S62.235** Other nondisplaced fracture of base of first metacarpal bone, left hand   `CC` `H5`

³ √7ᵗʰ **S62.236** Other nondisplaced fracture of base of first metacarpal bone, unspecified hand   `CC` `H5`

√6ᵗʰ **S62.24** Fracture of shaft of first metacarpal bone

³ √7ᵗʰ **S62.241** Displaced fracture of shaft of first metacarpal bone, right hand   `CC` `H5`

³ √7ᵗʰ **S62.242** Displaced fracture of shaft of first metacarpal bone, left hand   `CC` `H5`

³ √7ᵗʰ **S62.243** Displaced fracture of shaft of first metacarpal bone, unspecified hand   `CC` `H5`

³ √7ᵗʰ **S62.244** Nondisplaced fracture of shaft of first metacarpal bone, right hand   `CC` `H5`

³ √7ᵗʰ **S62.245** Nondisplaced fracture of shaft of first metacarpal bone, left hand   `CC` `H5`

³ √7ᵗʰ **S62.246** Nondisplaced fracture of shaft of first metacarpal bone, unspecified hand   `CC` `H5`

√6ᵗʰ **S62.25** Fracture of neck of first metacarpal bone

³ √7ᵗʰ **S62.251** Displaced fracture of neck of first metacarpal bone, right hand   `CC` `H5`

³ √7ᵗʰ **S62.252** Displaced fracture of neck of first metacarpal bone, left hand   `CC` `H5`

³ √7ᵗʰ **S62.253** Displaced fracture of neck of first metacarpal bone, unspecified hand   `CC` `H5`

³ √7ᵗʰ **S62.254** Nondisplaced fracture of neck of first metacarpal bone, right hand   `CC` `H5`

³ √7ᵗʰ **S62.255** Nondisplaced fracture of neck of first metacarpal bone, left hand   `CC` `H5`

³ √7ᵗʰ **S62.256** Nondisplaced fracture of neck of first metacarpal bone, unspecified hand   `CC` `H5`

√6ᵗʰ **S62.29** Other fracture of first metacarpal bone

³ √7ᵗʰ **S62.291** Other fracture of first metacarpal bone, right hand   `CC` `H5`

³ √7ᵗʰ **S62.292** Other fracture of first metacarpal bone, left hand   `CC` `H5`

³ √7ᵗʰ **S62.299** Other fracture of first metacarpal bone, unspecified hand   `CC` `H5`

√5ᵗʰ **S62.3** Fracture of other and unspecified metacarpal bone

    EXCLUDES 2   *fracture of first metacarpal bone (S62.2-)*

    CC Excl: For codes in subcategory S62.3:
    CC with 7th character B: PDX collection 1284
    CC with 7th character K or P: PDX collection 897

√6ᵗʰ **S62.30** Unspecified fracture of other metacarpal bone

³ √7ᵗʰ **S62.300** Unspecified fracture of second metacarpal bone, right hand   `CC` `H5`

³ √7ᵗʰ **S62.301** Unspecified fracture of second metacarpal bone, left hand   `CC` `H5`

³ √7ᵗʰ **S62.302** Unspecified fracture of third metacarpal bone, right hand   `CC` `H5`

³ √7ᵗʰ **S62.303** Unspecified fracture of third metacarpal bone, left hand   `CC` `H5`

³ √7ᵗʰ **S62.304** Unspecified fracture of fourth metacarpal bone, right hand   `CC` `H5`

³ √7ᵗʰ **S62.305** Unspecified fracture of fourth metacarpal bone, left hand   `CC` `H5`

³ √7ᵗʰ **S62.306** Unspecified fracture of fifth metacarpal bone, right hand   `CC` `H5`

³ √7ᵗʰ **S62.307** Unspecified fracture of fifth metacarpal bone, left hand   `CC` `H5`

³ √7ᵗʰ **S62.308** Unspecified fracture of other metacarpal bone   `CC` `H5`

    Unspecified fracture of specified metacarpal bone with unspecified laterality

³ √7ᵗʰ **S62.309** Unspecified fracture of unspecified metacarpal bone   `CC` `H5`

√6ᵗʰ **S62.31** Displaced fracture of base of other metacarpal bone

³ √7ᵗʰ **S62.310** Displaced fracture of base of second metacarpal bone, right hand   `CC` `H5`

³ √7ᵗʰ **S62.311** Displaced fracture of base of second metacarpal bone, left hand   `CC` `H5`

³ √7ᵗʰ **S62.312** Displaced fracture of base of third metacarpal bone, right hand   `CC` `H5`

³ √7ᵗʰ **S62.313** Displaced fracture of base of third metacarpal bone, left hand   `CC` `H5`

³ √7ᵗʰ **S62.314** Displaced fracture of base of fourth metacarpal bone, right hand   `CC` `H5`

³ √7ᵗʰ **S62.315** Displaced fracture of base of fourth metacarpal bone, left hand   `CC` `H5`

³ √7ᵗʰ **S62.316** Displaced fracture of base of fifth metacarpal bone, right hand   `CC` `H5`

³ √7ᵗʰ **S62.317** Displaced fracture of base of fifth metacarpal bone, left hand   `CC` `H5`

☑ Additional Character Required   √x7ᵗʰ Placeholder   Unacceptable PDx   Questionable PDx   Manifestation   Unspecified Dx   `H1`-`H14` HAC   `HCC` CMS-HCC Dx   `HIV` HIV Dx

ICD-10-CM 2020   1067

Chapter 19. Injury, Poisoning and Certain Other Consequences of External Causes

3 √7ᵗʰ **S62.318** Displaced fracture of base of other metacarpal bone   `CC` `H5`
  Displaced fracture of base of specified metacarpal bone with unspecified laterality

3 √7ᵗʰ **S62.319** Displaced fracture of base of unspecified metacarpal bone   `CC` `H5`

√6ᵗʰ **S62.32** Displaced fracture of shaft of other metacarpal bone

3 √7ᵗʰ **S62.320** Displaced fracture of shaft of second metacarpal bone, right hand   `CC` `H5`

3 √7ᵗʰ **S62.321** Displaced fracture of shaft of second metacarpal bone, left hand   `CC` `H5`

3 √7ᵗʰ **S62.322** Displaced fracture of shaft of third metacarpal bone, right hand   `CC` `H5`

3 √7ᵗʰ **S62.323** Displaced fracture of shaft of third metacarpal bone, left hand   `CC` `H5`

3 √7ᵗʰ **S62.324** Displaced fracture of shaft of fourth metacarpal bone, right hand   `CC` `H5`

3 √7ᵗʰ **S62.325** Displaced fracture of shaft of fourth metacarpal bone, left hand   `CC` `H5`

3 √7ᵗʰ **S62.326** Displaced fracture of shaft of fifth metacarpal bone, right hand   `CC` `H5`

3 √7ᵗʰ **S62.327** Displaced fracture of shaft of fifth metacarpal bone, left hand   `CC` `H5`

3 √7ᵗʰ **S62.328** Displaced fracture of shaft of other metacarpal bone   `CC` `H5`
  Displaced fracture of shaft of specified metacarpal bone with unspecified laterality

3 √7ᵗʰ **S62.329** Displaced fracture of shaft of unspecified metacarpal bone   `CC` `H5`

√6ᵗʰ **S62.33** Displaced fracture of neck of other metacarpal bone

3 √7ᵗʰ **S62.330** Displaced fracture of neck of second metacarpal bone, right hand   `CC` `H5`

3 √7ᵗʰ **S62.331** Displaced fracture of neck of second metacarpal bone, left hand   `CC` `H5`

3 √7ᵗʰ **S62.332** Displaced fracture of neck of third metacarpal bone, right hand   `CC` `H5`

3 √7ᵗʰ **S62.333** Displaced fracture of neck of third metacarpal bone, left hand   `CC` `H5`

3 √7ᵗʰ **S62.334** Displaced fracture of neck of fourth metacarpal bone, right hand   `CC` `H5`

3 √7ᵗʰ **S62.335** Displaced fracture of neck of fourth metacarpal bone, left hand   `CC` `H5`

3 √7ᵗʰ **S62.336** Displaced fracture of neck of fifth metacarpal bone, right hand   `CC` `H5`

3 √7ᵗʰ **S62.337** Displaced fracture of neck of fifth metacarpal bone, left hand   `CC` `H5`

3 √7ᵗʰ **S62.338** Displaced fracture of neck of other metacarpal bone   `CC` `H5`
  Displaced fracture of neck of specified metacarpal bone with unspecified laterality

3 √7ᵗʰ **S62.339** Displaced fracture of neck of unspecified metacarpal bone   `CC` `H5`

√6ᵗʰ **S62.34** Nondisplaced fracture of base of other metacarpal bone

3 √7ᵗʰ **S62.340** Nondisplaced fracture of base of second metacarpal bone, right hand   `CC` `H5`

3 √7ᵗʰ **S62.341** Nondisplaced fracture of base of second metacarpal bone, left hand   `CC` `H5`

3 √7ᵗʰ **S62.342** Nondisplaced fracture of base of third metacarpal bone, right hand   `CC` `H5`

3 √7ᵗʰ **S62.343** Nondisplaced fracture of base of third metacarpal bone, left hand   `CC` `H5`

3 √7ᵗʰ **S62.344** Nondisplaced fracture of base of fourth metacarpal bone, right hand   `CC` `H5`

3 √7ᵗʰ **S62.345** Nondisplaced fracture of base of fourth metacarpal bone, left hand   `CC` `H5`

3 √7ᵗʰ **S62.346** Nondisplaced fracture of base of fifth metacarpal bone, right hand   `CC` `H5`

3 √7ᵗʰ **S62.347** Nondisplaced fracture of base of fifth metacarpal bone, left hand   `CC` `H5`

3 √7ᵗʰ **S62.348** Nondisplaced fracture of base of other metacarpal bone   `CC` `H5`
  Nondisplaced fracture of base of specified metacarpal bone with unspecified laterality

3 √7ᵗʰ **S62.349** Nondisplaced fracture of base of unspecified metacarpal bone   `CC` `H5`

√6ᵗʰ **S62.35** Nondisplaced fracture of shaft of other metacarpal bone

3 √7ᵗʰ **S62.350** Nondisplaced fracture of shaft of second metacarpal bone, right hand   `CC` `H5`

3 √7ᵗʰ **S62.351** Nondisplaced fracture of shaft of second metacarpal bone, left hand   `CC` `H5`

3 √7ᵗʰ **S62.352** Nondisplaced fracture of shaft of third metacarpal bone, right hand   `CC` `H5`

3 √7ᵗʰ **S62.353** Nondisplaced fracture of shaft of third metacarpal bone, left hand   `CC` `H5`

3 √7ᵗʰ **S62.354** Nondisplaced fracture of shaft of fourth metacarpal bone, right hand   `CC` `H5`

3 √7ᵗʰ **S62.355** Nondisplaced fracture of shaft of fourth metacarpal bone, left hand   `CC` `H5`

3 √7ᵗʰ **S62.356** Nondisplaced fracture of shaft of fifth metacarpal bone, right hand   `CC` `H5`

3 √7ᵗʰ **S62.357** Nondisplaced fracture of shaft of fifth metacarpal bone, left hand   `CC` `H5`

3 √7ᵗʰ **S62.358** Nondisplaced fracture of shaft of other metacarpal bone   `CC` `H5`
  Nondisplaced fracture of shaft of specified metacarpal bone with unspecified laterality

3 √7ᵗʰ **S62.359** Nondisplaced fracture of shaft of unspecified metacarpal bone   `CC` `H5`

√6ᵗʰ **S62.36** Nondisplaced fracture of neck of other metacarpal bone

3 √7ᵗʰ **S62.360** Nondisplaced fracture of neck of second metacarpal bone, right hand   `CC` `H5`

3 √7ᵗʰ **S62.361** Nondisplaced fracture of neck of second metacarpal bone, left hand   `CC` `H5`

3 √7ᵗʰ **S62.362** Nondisplaced fracture of neck of third metacarpal bone, right hand   `CC` `H5`

3 √7ᵗʰ **S62.363** Nondisplaced fracture of neck of third metacarpal bone, left hand   `CC` `H5`

3 √7ᵗʰ **S62.364** Nondisplaced fracture of neck of fourth metacarpal bone, right hand   `CC` `H5`

3 √7ᵗʰ **S62.365** Nondisplaced fracture of neck of fourth metacarpal bone, left hand   `CC` `H5`

`N` Newborn: 0   `P` Pediatric: 0-17   `M` Maternity: 9-64   `A` Adult: 15-124   `MCC` Major Complication/Comorbidity   `CC` Complication/Comorbidity   `SW` Severe Wound Dx

1068   ICD-10-CM 2020

³ √7ᵗʰ **S62.366** **Nondisplaced fracture of neck of fifth metacarpal bone, right hand** `CC` `H5`

³ √7ᵗʰ **S62.367** **Nondisplaced fracture of neck of fifth metacarpal bone, left hand** `CC` `H5`

³ √7ᵗʰ **S62.368** **Nondisplaced fracture of neck of other metacarpal bone** `CC` `H5`

Nondisplaced fracture of neck of specified metacarpal bone with unspecified laterality

³ √7ᵗʰ **S62.369** **Nondisplaced fracture of neck of unspecified metacarpal bone** `CC` `H5`

√6ᵗʰ **S62.39** **Other fracture of other metacarpal bone**

³ √7ᵗʰ **S62.390** **Other fracture of second metacarpal bone, right hand** `CC` `H5`

³ √7ᵗʰ **S62.391** **Other fracture of second metacarpal bone, left hand** `CC` `H5`

³ √7ᵗʰ **S62.392** **Other fracture of third metacarpal bone, right hand** `CC` `H5`

³ √7ᵗʰ **S62.393** **Other fracture of third metacarpal bone, left hand** `CC` `H5`

³ √7ᵗʰ **S62.394** **Other fracture of fourth metacarpal bone, right hand** `CC` `H5`

³ √7ᵗʰ **S62.395** **Other fracture of fourth metacarpal bone, left hand** `CC` `H5`

³ √7ᵗʰ **S62.396** **Other fracture of fifth metacarpal bone, right hand** `CC` `H5`

³ √7ᵗʰ **S62.397** **Other fracture of fifth metacarpal bone, left hand** `CC` `H5`

³ √7ᵗʰ **S62.398** **Other fracture of other metacarpal bone** `CC` `H5`

Other fracture of specified metacarpal bone with unspecified laterality

³ √7ᵗʰ **S62.399** **Other fracture of unspecified metacarpal bone** `CC` `H5`

√5ᵗʰ **S62.5** **Fracture of thumb**

CC Excl: For codes in subcategory S62.5:
CC with 7th character B: PDX collection 1285
CC with 7th character K or P: PDX collection 897

√6ᵗʰ **S62.50** **Fracture of unspecified phalanx of thumb**

³ √7ᵗʰ **S62.501** **Fracture of unspecified phalanx of right thumb** `CC` `H5`

³ √7ᵗʰ **S62.502** **Fracture of unspecified phalanx of left thumb** `CC` `H5`

³ √7ᵗʰ **S62.509** **Fracture of unspecified phalanx of unspecified thumb** `CC` `H5`

√6ᵗʰ **S62.51** **Fracture of proximal phalanx of thumb**

³ √7ᵗʰ **S62.511** **Displaced fracture of proximal phalanx of right thumb** `CC` `H5`

³ √7ᵗʰ **S62.512** **Displaced fracture of proximal phalanx of left thumb** `CC` `H5`

³ √7ᵗʰ **S62.513** **Displaced fracture of proximal phalanx of unspecified thumb** `CC` `H5`

³ √7ᵗʰ **S62.514** **Nondisplaced fracture of proximal phalanx of right thumb** `CC` `H5`

³ √7ᵗʰ **S62.515** **Nondisplaced fracture of proximal phalanx of left thumb** `CC` `H5`

³ √7ᵗʰ **S62.516** **Nondisplaced fracture of proximal phalanx of unspecified thumb** `CC` `H5`

√6ᵗʰ **S62.52** **Fracture of distal phalanx of thumb**

³ √7ᵗʰ **S62.521** **Displaced fracture of distal phalanx of right thumb** `CC` `H5`

³ √7ᵗʰ **S62.522** **Displaced fracture of distal phalanx of left thumb** `CC` `H5`

³ √7ᵗʰ **S62.523** **Displaced fracture of distal phalanx of unspecified thumb** `CC` `H5`

³ √7ᵗʰ **S62.524** **Nondisplaced fracture of distal phalanx of right thumb** `CC` `H5`

³ √7ᵗʰ **S62.525** **Nondisplaced fracture of distal phalanx of left thumb** `CC` `H5`

³ √7ᵗʰ **S62.526** **Nondisplaced fracture of distal phalanx of unspecified thumb** `CC` `H5`

√5ᵗʰ **S62.6** **Fracture of other and unspecified finger(s)**

EXCLUDES 2   fracture of thumb (S62.5-)

CC Excl: For codes in subcategory S62.6:
CC with 7th character B: PDX collection 1285
CC with 7th character K or P: PDX collection 897

√6ᵗʰ **S62.60** **Fracture of unspecified phalanx of finger**

³ √7ᵗʰ **S62.600** **Fracture of unspecified phalanx of right index finger** `CC` `H5`

³ √7ᵗʰ **S62.601** **Fracture of unspecified phalanx of left index finger** `CC` `H5`

³ √7ᵗʰ **S62.602** **Fracture of unspecified phalanx of right middle finger** `CC` `H5`

³ √7ᵗʰ **S62.603** **Fracture of unspecified phalanx of left middle finger** `CC` `H5`

³ √7ᵗʰ **S62.604** **Fracture of unspecified phalanx of right ring finger** `CC` `H5`

³ √7ᵗʰ **S62.605** **Fracture of unspecified phalanx of left ring finger** `CC` `H5`

³ √7ᵗʰ **S62.606** **Fracture of unspecified phalanx of right little finger** `CC` `H5`

³ √7ᵗʰ **S62.607** **Fracture of unspecified phalanx of left little finger** `CC` `H5`

³ √7ᵗʰ **S62.608** **Fracture of unspecified phalanx of other finger** `CC` `H5`

Fracture of unspecified phalanx of specified finger with unspecified laterality

³ √7ᵗʰ **S62.609** **Fracture of unspecified phalanx of unspecified finger** `CC` `H5`

√6ᵗʰ **S62.61** **Displaced fracture of proximal phalanx of finger**

³ √7ᵗʰ **S62.610** **Displaced fracture of proximal phalanx of right index finger** `CC` `H5`

³ √7ᵗʰ **S62.611** **Displaced fracture of proximal phalanx of left index finger** `CC` `H5`

³ √7ᵗʰ **S62.612** **Displaced fracture of proximal phalanx of right middle finger** `CC` `H5`

³ √7ᵗʰ **S62.613** **Displaced fracture of proximal phalanx of left middle finger** `CC` `H5`

³ √7ᵗʰ **S62.614** **Displaced fracture of proximal phalanx of right ring finger** `CC` `H5`

³ √7ᵗʰ **S62.615** **Displaced fracture of proximal phalanx of left ring finger** `CC` `H5`

³ √7ᵗʰ **S62.616** **Displaced fracture of proximal phalanx of right little finger** `CC` `H5`

³ √7ᵗʰ **S62.617** **Displaced fracture of proximal phalanx of left little finger** `CC` `H5`

³ √7ᵗʰ **S62.618** **Displaced fracture of proximal phalanx of other finger** `CC` `H5`

Displaced fracture of proximal phalanx of specified finger with unspecified laterality

✔ Additional Character Required   √x7ᵗʰ Placeholder   Unacceptable PDx   Questionable PDx   Manifestation   Unspecified Dx   H1 - H14 HAC   HCC CMS-HCC Dx   HIV HIV Dx

ICD-10-CM 2020   1069

3 √7th **S62.619 Displaced fracture of proximal phalanx of unspecified finger** `CC` `H5`

√6th **S62.62** Displaced fracture of middle phalanx of finger

3 √7th **S62.620 Displaced fracture of middle phalanx of right index finger** `CC` `H5`

3 √7th **S62.621 Displaced fracture of middle phalanx of left index finger** `CC` `H5`

3 √7th **S62.622 Displaced fracture of middle phalanx of right middle finger** `CC` `H5`

3 √7th **S62.623 Displaced fracture of middle phalanx of left middle finger** `CC` `H5`

3 √7th **S62.624 Displaced fracture of middle phalanx of right ring finger** `CC` `H5`

3 √7th **S62.625 Displaced fracture of middle phalanx of left ring finger** `CC` `H5`

3 √7th **S62.626 Displaced fracture of middle phalanx of right little finger** `CC` `H5`

3 √7th **S62.627 Displaced fracture of middle phalanx of left little finger** `CC` `H5`

3 √7th **S62.628 Displaced fracture of middle phalanx of other finger** `CC` `H5`

Displaced fracture of middle phalanx of specified finger with unspecified laterality

3 √7th **S62.629 Displaced fracture of middle phalanx of unspecified finger** `CC` `H5`

√6th **S62.63** Displaced fracture of distal phalanx of finger

3 √7th **S62.630 Displaced fracture of distal phalanx of right index finger** `CC` `H5`

3 √7th **S62.631 Displaced fracture of distal phalanx of left index finger** `CC` `H5`

3 √7th **S62.632 Displaced fracture of distal phalanx of right middle finger** `CC` `H5`

3 √7th **S62.633 Displaced fracture of distal phalanx of left middle finger** `CC` `H5`

3 √7th **S62.634 Displaced fracture of distal phalanx of right ring finger** `CC` `H5`

3 √7th **S62.635 Displaced fracture of distal phalanx of left ring finger** `CC` `H5`

3 √7th **S62.636 Displaced fracture of distal phalanx of right little finger** `CC` `H5`

3 √7th **S62.637 Displaced fracture of distal phalanx of left little finger** `CC` `H5`

3 √7th **S62.638 Displaced fracture of distal phalanx of other finger** `CC` `H5`

Displaced fracture of distal phalanx of specified finger with unspecified laterality

3 √7th **S62.639 Displaced fracture of distal phalanx of unspecified finger** `CC` `H5`

√6th **S62.64** Nondisplaced fracture of proximal phalanx of finger

3 √7th **S62.640 Nondisplaced fracture of proximal phalanx of right index finger** `CC` `H5`

3 √7th **S62.641 Nondisplaced fracture of proximal phalanx of left index finger** `CC` `H5`

3 √7th **S62.642 Nondisplaced fracture of proximal phalanx of right middle finger** `CC` `H5`

3 √7th **S62.643 Nondisplaced fracture of proximal phalanx of left middle finger** `CC` `H5`

3 √7th **S62.644 Nondisplaced fracture of proximal phalanx of right ring finger** `CC` `H5`

3 √7th **S62.645 Nondisplaced fracture of proximal phalanx of left ring finger** `CC` `H5`

3 √7th **S62.646 Nondisplaced fracture of proximal phalanx of right little finger** `CC` `H5`

3 √7th **S62.647 Nondisplaced fracture of proximal phalanx of left little finger** `CC` `H5`

3 √7th **S62.648 Nondisplaced fracture of proximal phalanx of other finger** `CC` `H5`

Nondisplaced fracture of proximal phalanx of specified finger with unspecified laterality

3 √7th **S62.649 Nondisplaced fracture of proximal phalanx of unspecified finger** `CC` `H5`

√6th **S62.65** Nondisplaced fracture of middle phalanx of finger

3 √7th **S62.650 Nondisplaced fracture of middle phalanx of right index finger** `CC` `H5`

3 √7th **S62.651 Nondisplaced fracture of middle phalanx of left index finger** `CC` `H5`

3 √7th **S62.652 Nondisplaced fracture of middle phalanx of right middle finger** `CC` `H5`

3 √7th **S62.653 Nondisplaced fracture of middle phalanx of left middle finger** `CC` `H5`

3 √7th **S62.654 Nondisplaced fracture of middle phalanx of right ring finger** `CC` `H5`

3 √7th **S62.655 Nondisplaced fracture of middle phalanx of left ring finger** `CC` `H5`

3 √7th **S62.656 Nondisplaced fracture of middle phalanx of right little finger** `CC` `H5`

3 √7th **S62.657 Nondisplaced fracture of middle phalanx of left little finger** `CC` `H5`

3 √7th **S62.658 Nondisplaced fracture of middle phalanx of other finger** `CC` `H5`

Nondisplaced fracture of middle phalanx of specified finger with unspecified laterality

3 √7th **S62.659 Nondisplaced fracture of middle phalanx of unspecified finger** `CC` `H5`

√6th **S62.66** Nondisplaced fracture of distal phalanx of finger

3 √7th **S62.660 Nondisplaced fracture of distal phalanx of right index finger** `CC` `H5`

3 √7th **S62.661 Nondisplaced fracture of distal phalanx of left index finger** `CC` `H5`

3 √7th **S62.662 Nondisplaced fracture of distal phalanx of right middle finger** `CC` `H5`

3 √7th **S62.663 Nondisplaced fracture of distal phalanx of left middle finger** `CC` `H5`

3 √7th **S62.664 Nondisplaced fracture of distal phalanx of right ring finger** `CC` `H5`

3 √7th **S62.665 Nondisplaced fracture of distal phalanx of left ring finger** `CC` `H5`

3 √7th **S62.666 Nondisplaced fracture of distal phalanx of right little finger** `CC` `H5`

3 √7th **S62.667 Nondisplaced fracture of distal phalanx of left little finger** `CC` `H5`

³ ✓7ᵗʰ **S62.668** **Nondisplaced fracture of distal phalanx of other finger** `CC` `H5`

Nondisplaced fracture of distal phalanx of specified finger with unspecified laterality

³ ✓7ᵗʰ **S62.669** **Nondisplaced fracture of distal phalanx of unspecified finger** `CC` `H5`

✓5ᵗʰ **S62.9** **Unspecified fracture of wrist and hand**

³ ✓x7ᵗʰ **S62.90** **Unspecified fracture of unspecified wrist and hand** `CC` `H5`

CC Excl: CC with 7th character B: PDX collection 1286
CC Excl: CC with 7th character K or P: PDX collection 897

³ ✓x7ᵗʰ **S62.91** **Unspecified fracture of right wrist and hand** `CC` `H5`

CC Excl: CC with 7th character B: PDX collection 1287
CC Excl: CC with 7th character K or P: PDX collection 897

³ ✓x7ᵗʰ **S62.92** **Unspecified fracture of left wrist and hand** `CC` `H5`

CC Excl: CC with 7th character B: PDX collection 1287
CC Excl: CC with 7th character K or P: PDX collection 897

✓4ᵗʰ **S63** **Dislocation and sprain of joints and ligaments at wrist and hand level**

     `INCLUDES`   avulsion of joint or ligament at wrist and hand level
laceration of cartilage, joint or ligament at wrist and hand level
sprain of cartilage, joint or ligament at wrist and hand level
traumatic hemarthrosis of joint or ligament at wrist and hand level
traumatic rupture of joint or ligament at wrist and hand level
traumatic subluxation of joint or ligament at wrist and hand level
traumatic tear of joint or ligament at wrist and hand level

Code also any associated open wound

     `EXCLUDES 2`   *strain of muscle, fascia and tendon of wrist and hand (S66.-)*

The appropriate 7th character is to be added to each code from category S63.
A   initial encounter
D   subsequent encounter
S   sequela

✓5ᵗʰ **S63.0** **Subluxation and dislocation of wrist and hand joints**

✓6ᵗʰ **S63.00** **Unspecified subluxation and dislocation of wrist and hand**

Dislocation of carpal bone NOS
Dislocation of distal end of radius NOS
Subluxation of carpal bone NOS
Subluxation of distal end of radius NOS

✓7ᵗʰ **S63.001** **Unspecified subluxation of right wrist and hand**

✓7ᵗʰ **S63.002** **Unspecified subluxation of left wrist and hand**

✓7ᵗʰ **S63.003** **Unspecified subluxation of unspecified wrist and hand**

✓7ᵗʰ **S63.004** **Unspecified dislocation of right wrist and hand**

✓7ᵗʰ **S63.005** **Unspecified dislocation of left wrist and hand**

✓7ᵗʰ **S63.006** **Unspecified dislocation of unspecified wrist and hand**

✓6ᵗʰ **S63.01** **Subluxation and dislocation of distal radioulnar joint**

✓7ᵗʰ **S63.011** **Subluxation of distal radioulnar joint of right wrist**

✓7ᵗʰ **S63.012** **Subluxation of distal radioulnar joint of left wrist**

✓7ᵗʰ **S63.013** **Subluxation of distal radioulnar joint of unspecified wrist**

✓7ᵗʰ **S63.014** **Dislocation of distal radioulnar joint of right wrist**

✓7ᵗʰ **S63.015** **Dislocation of distal radioulnar joint of left wrist**

✓7ᵗʰ **S63.016** **Dislocation of distal radioulnar joint of unspecified wrist**

✓6ᵗʰ **S63.02** **Subluxation and dislocation of radiocarpal joint**

✓7ᵗʰ **S63.021** **Subluxation of radiocarpal joint of right wrist**

✓7ᵗʰ **S63.022** **Subluxation of radiocarpal joint of left wrist**

✓7ᵗʰ **S63.023** **Subluxation of radiocarpal joint of unspecified wrist**

✓7ᵗʰ **S63.024** **Dislocation of radiocarpal joint of right wrist**

✓7ᵗʰ **S63.025** **Dislocation of radiocarpal joint of left wrist**

✓7ᵗʰ **S63.026** **Dislocation of radiocarpal joint of unspecified wrist**

✓6ᵗʰ **S63.03** **Subluxation and dislocation of midcarpal joint**

✓7ᵗʰ **S63.031** **Subluxation of midcarpal joint of right wrist**

✓7ᵗʰ **S63.032** **Subluxation of midcarpal joint of left wrist**

✓7ᵗʰ **S63.033** **Subluxation of midcarpal joint of unspecified wrist**

✓7ᵗʰ **S63.034** **Dislocation of midcarpal joint of right wrist**

✓7ᵗʰ **S63.035** **Dislocation of midcarpal joint of left wrist**

✓7ᵗʰ **S63.036** **Dislocation of midcarpal joint of unspecified wrist**

✓6ᵗʰ **S63.04** **Subluxation and dislocation of carpometacarpal joint of thumb**

     `EXCLUDES 2`   *interphalangeal subluxation and dislocation of thumb (S63.1-)*

✓7ᵗʰ **S63.041** **Subluxation of carpometacarpal joint of right thumb**

✓7ᵗʰ **S63.042** **Subluxation of carpometacarpal joint of left thumb**

✓7ᵗʰ **S63.043** **Subluxation of carpometacarpal joint of unspecified thumb**

✓7ᵗʰ **S63.044** **Dislocation of carpometacarpal joint of right thumb**

✓7ᵗʰ **S63.045** **Dislocation of carpometacarpal joint of left thumb**

✓7ᵗʰ **S63.046** **Dislocation of carpometacarpal joint of unspecified thumb**

✓6ᵗʰ **S63.05** **Subluxation and dislocation of other carpometacarpal joint**

     `EXCLUDES 2`   *subluxation and dislocation of carpometacarpal joint of thumb (S63.04-)*

✓7ᵗʰ **S63.051** **Subluxation of other carpometacarpal joint of right hand**

✓7ᵗʰ **S63.052** **Subluxation of other carpometacarpal joint of left hand**

✓7ᵗʰ **S63.053** **Subluxation of other carpometacarpal joint of unspecified hand**

✓7ᵗʰ **S63.054** **Dislocation of other carpometacarpal joint of right hand**

✓7ᵗʰ **S63.055** **Dislocation of other carpometacarpal joint of left hand**

✓7ᵗʰ **S63.056** **Dislocation of other carpometacarpal joint of unspecified hand**

✓6ᵗʰ **S63.06** **Subluxation and dislocation of metacarpal (bone), proximal end**

✓7ᵗʰ **S63.061** **Subluxation of metacarpal (bone), proximal end of right hand**

✓7ᵗʰ **S63.062** **Subluxation of metacarpal (bone), proximal end of left hand**

✓7ᵗʰ **S63.063** **Subluxation of metacarpal (bone), proximal end of unspecified hand**

✓7ᵗʰ **S63.064** **Dislocation of metacarpal (bone), proximal end of right hand**

✓7ᵗʰ **S63.065** **Dislocation of metacarpal (bone), proximal end of left hand**

✓7ᵗʰ **S63.066** **Dislocation of metacarpal (bone), proximal end of unspecified hand**

✓6ᵗʰ **S63.07** **Subluxation and dislocation of distal end of ulna**

✓7ᵗʰ **S63.071** **Subluxation of distal end of right ulna**

✓7ᵗʰ **S63.072** **Subluxation of distal end of left ulna**

✓7ᵗʰ **S63.073** **Subluxation of distal end of unspecified ulna**

✓7ᵗʰ **S63.074** **Dislocation of distal end of right ulna**

✓7ᵗʰ **S63.075** **Dislocation of distal end of left ulna**

✓7ᵗʰ **S63.076** **Dislocation of distal end of unspecified ulna**

✓ Additional Character Required   ✓x7ᵗʰ Placeholder   Unacceptable PDx   Questionable PDx   Manifestation   Unspecified Dx   `H1`-`H14` HAC   `HCC` CMS-HCC Dx   `HIV` HIV Dx

ICD-10-CM 2020

1071

√6ᵗʰ **S63.09** Other subluxation and dislocation of wrist and hand
- √7ᵗʰ **S63.091** Other subluxation of right wrist and hand
- √7ᵗʰ **S63.092** Other subluxation of left wrist and hand
- √7ᵗʰ **S63.093** Other subluxation of unspecified wrist and hand
- √7ᵗʰ **S63.094** Other dislocation of right wrist and hand
- √7ᵗʰ **S63.095** Other dislocation of left wrist and hand
- √7ᵗʰ **S63.096** Other dislocation of unspecified wrist and hand

√5ᵗʰ **S63.1** Subluxation and dislocation of thumb
- √6ᵗʰ **S63.10** Unspecified subluxation and dislocation of thumb
  - √7ᵗʰ **S63.101** Unspecified subluxation of right thumb
  - √7ᵗʰ **S63.102** Unspecified subluxation of left thumb
  - √7ᵗʰ **S63.103** Unspecified subluxation of unspecified thumb
  - √7ᵗʰ **S63.104** Unspecified dislocation of right thumb
  - √7ᵗʰ **S63.105** Unspecified dislocation of left thumb
  - √7ᵗʰ **S63.106** Unspecified dislocation of unspecified thumb
- √6ᵗʰ **S63.11** Subluxation and dislocation of metacarpophalangeal joint of thumb
  - √7ᵗʰ **S63.111** Subluxation of metacarpophalangeal joint of right thumb
  - √7ᵗʰ **S63.112** Subluxation of metacarpophalangeal joint of left thumb
  - √7ᵗʰ **S63.113** Subluxation of metacarpophalangeal joint of unspecified thumb
  - √7ᵗʰ **S63.114** Dislocation of metacarpophalangeal joint of right thumb
  - √7ᵗʰ **S63.115** Dislocation of metacarpophalangeal joint of left thumb
  - √7ᵗʰ **S63.116** Dislocation of metacarpophalangeal joint of unspecified thumb
- √6ᵗʰ **S63.12** Subluxation and dislocation of interphalangeal joint of thumb
  - √7ᵗʰ **S63.121** Subluxation of interphalangeal joint of right thumb
  - √7ᵗʰ **S63.122** Subluxation of interphalangeal joint of left thumb
  - √7ᵗʰ **S63.123** Subluxation of interphalangeal joint of unspecified thumb
  - √7ᵗʰ **S63.124** Dislocation of interphalangeal joint of right thumb
  - √7ᵗʰ **S63.125** Dislocation of interphalangeal joint of left thumb
  - √7ᵗʰ **S63.126** Dislocation of interphalangeal joint of unspecified thumb

√5ᵗʰ **S63.2** Subluxation and dislocation of other finger(s)
> **EXCLUDES 2**   *subluxation and dislocation of thumb (S63.1-)*
- √6ᵗʰ **S63.20** Unspecified subluxation of other finger
  - √7ᵗʰ **S63.200** Unspecified subluxation of right index finger
  - √7ᵗʰ **S63.201** Unspecified subluxation of left index finger
  - √7ᵗʰ **S63.202** Unspecified subluxation of right middle finger
  - √7ᵗʰ **S63.203** Unspecified subluxation of left middle finger
  - √7ᵗʰ **S63.204** Unspecified subluxation of right ring finger
  - √7ᵗʰ **S63.205** Unspecified subluxation of left ring finger
  - √7ᵗʰ **S63.206** Unspecified subluxation of right little finger
  - √7ᵗʰ **S63.207** Unspecified subluxation of left little finger
  - √7ᵗʰ **S63.208** Unspecified subluxation of other finger
    Unspecified subluxation of specified finger with unspecified laterality
  - √7ᵗʰ **S63.209** Unspecified subluxation of unspecified finger
- √6ᵗʰ **S63.21** Subluxation of metacarpophalangeal joint of finger
  - √7ᵗʰ **S63.210** Subluxation of metacarpophalangeal joint of right index finger
  - √7ᵗʰ **S63.211** Subluxation of metacarpophalangeal joint of left index finger
  - √7ᵗʰ **S63.212** Subluxation of metacarpophalangeal joint of right middle finger
  - √7ᵗʰ **S63.213** Subluxation of metacarpophalangeal joint of left middle finger
  - √7ᵗʰ **S63.214** Subluxation of metacarpophalangeal joint of right ring finger
  - √7ᵗʰ **S63.215** Subluxation of metacarpophalangeal joint of left ring finger
  - √7ᵗʰ **S63.216** Subluxation of metacarpophalangeal joint of right little finger
  - √7ᵗʰ **S63.217** Subluxation of metacarpophalangeal joint of left little finger
  - √7ᵗʰ **S63.218** Subluxation of metacarpophalangeal joint of other finger
    Subluxation of metacarpophalangeal joint of specified finger with unspecified laterality
  - √7ᵗʰ **S63.219** Subluxation of metacarpophalangeal joint of unspecified finger
- √6ᵗʰ **S63.22** Subluxation of unspecified interphalangeal joint of finger
  - √7ᵗʰ **S63.220** Subluxation of unspecified interphalangeal joint of right index finger
  - √7ᵗʰ **S63.221** Subluxation of unspecified interphalangeal joint of left index finger
  - √7ᵗʰ **S63.222** Subluxation of unspecified interphalangeal joint of right middle finger
  - √7ᵗʰ **S63.223** Subluxation of unspecified interphalangeal joint of left middle finger
  - √7ᵗʰ **S63.224** Subluxation of unspecified interphalangeal joint of right ring finger
  - √7ᵗʰ **S63.225** Subluxation of unspecified interphalangeal joint of left ring finger
  - √7ᵗʰ **S63.226** Subluxation of unspecified interphalangeal joint of right little finger
  - √7ᵗʰ **S63.227** Subluxation of unspecified interphalangeal joint of left little finger
  - √7ᵗʰ **S63.228** Subluxation of unspecified interphalangeal joint of other finger
    Subluxation of unspecified interphalangeal joint of specified finger with unspecified laterality
  - √7ᵗʰ **S63.229** Subluxation of unspecified interphalangeal joint of unspecified finger
- √6ᵗʰ **S63.23** Subluxation of proximal interphalangeal joint of finger
  - √7ᵗʰ **S63.230** Subluxation of proximal interphalangeal joint of right index finger
  - √7ᵗʰ **S63.231** Subluxation of proximal interphalangeal joint of left index finger
  - √7ᵗʰ **S63.232** Subluxation of proximal interphalangeal joint of right middle finger
  - √7ᵗʰ **S63.233** Subluxation of proximal interphalangeal joint of left middle finger
  - √7ᵗʰ **S63.234** Subluxation of proximal interphalangeal joint of right ring finger
  - √7ᵗʰ **S63.235** Subluxation of proximal interphalangeal joint of left ring finger
  - √7ᵗʰ **S63.236** Subluxation of proximal interphalangeal joint of right little finger
  - √7ᵗʰ **S63.237** Subluxation of proximal interphalangeal joint of left little finger
  - √7ᵗʰ **S63.238** Subluxation of proximal interphalangeal joint of other finger
    Subluxation of proximal interphalangeal joint of specified finger with unspecified laterality
  - √7ᵗʰ **S63.239** Subluxation of proximal interphalangeal joint of unspecified finger
- √6ᵗʰ **S63.24** Subluxation of distal interphalangeal joint of finger
  - √7ᵗʰ **S63.240** Subluxation of distal interphalangeal joint of right index finger
  - √7ᵗʰ **S63.241** Subluxation of distal interphalangeal joint of left index finger
  - √7ᵗʰ **S63.242** Subluxation of distal interphalangeal joint of right middle finger
  - √7ᵗʰ **S63.243** Subluxation of distal interphalangeal joint of left middle finger
  - √7ᵗʰ **S63.244** Subluxation of distal interphalangeal joint of right ring finger
  - √7ᵗʰ **S63.245** Subluxation of distal interphalangeal joint of left ring finger
  - √7ᵗʰ **S63.246** Subluxation of distal interphalangeal joint of right little finger

√7ᵗʰ **S63.247** Subluxation of distal interphalangeal joint of left little finger

√7ᵗʰ **S63.248** Subluxation of distal interphalangeal joint of other finger

Subluxation of distal interphalangeal joint of specified finger with unspecified laterality

√7ᵗʰ **S63.249** Subluxation of distal interphalangeal joint of unspecified finger

√6ᵗʰ **S63.25** Unspecified dislocation of other finger

√7ᵗʰ **S63.250** Unspecified dislocation of right index finger

√7ᵗʰ **S63.251** Unspecified dislocation of left index finger

√7ᵗʰ **S63.252** Unspecified dislocation of right middle finger

√7ᵗʰ **S63.253** Unspecified dislocation of left middle finger

√7ᵗʰ **S63.254** Unspecified dislocation of right ring finger

√7ᵗʰ **S63.255** Unspecified dislocation of left ring finger

√7ᵗʰ **S63.256** Unspecified dislocation of right little finger

√7ᵗʰ **S63.257** Unspecified dislocation of left little finger

√7ᵗʰ **S63.258** Unspecified dislocation of other finger

Unspecified dislocation of specified finger with unspecified laterality

√7ᵗʰ **S63.259** Unspecified dislocation of unspecified finger

Unspecified dislocation of unspecified finger with unspecified laterality

√6ᵗʰ **S63.26** Dislocation of metacarpophalangeal joint of finger

√7ᵗʰ **S63.260** Dislocation of metacarpophalangeal joint of right index finger

√7ᵗʰ **S63.261** Dislocation of metacarpophalangeal joint of left index finger

√7ᵗʰ **S63.262** Dislocation of metacarpophalangeal joint of right middle finger

√7ᵗʰ **S63.263** Dislocation of metacarpophalangeal joint of left middle finger

√7ᵗʰ **S63.264** Dislocation of metacarpophalangeal joint of right ring finger

√7ᵗʰ **S63.265** Dislocation of metacarpophalangeal joint of left ring finger

√7ᵗʰ **S63.266** Dislocation of metacarpophalangeal joint of right little finger

√7ᵗʰ **S63.267** Dislocation of metacarpophalangeal joint of left little finger

√7ᵗʰ **S63.268** Dislocation of metacarpophalangeal joint of other finger

Dislocation of metacarpophalangeal joint of specified finger with unspecified laterality

√7ᵗʰ **S63.269** Dislocation of metacarpophalangeal joint of unspecified finger

√6ᵗʰ **S63.27** Dislocation of unspecified interphalangeal joint of finger

√7ᵗʰ **S63.270** Dislocation of unspecified interphalangeal joint of right index finger

√7ᵗʰ **S63.271** Dislocation of unspecified interphalangeal joint of left index finger

√7ᵗʰ **S63.272** Dislocation of unspecified interphalangeal joint of right middle finger

√7ᵗʰ **S63.273** Dislocation of unspecified interphalangeal joint of left middle finger

√7ᵗʰ **S63.274** Dislocation of unspecified interphalangeal joint of right ring finger

√7ᵗʰ **S63.275** Dislocation of unspecified interphalangeal joint of left ring finger

√7ᵗʰ **S63.276** Dislocation of unspecified interphalangeal joint of right little finger

√7ᵗʰ **S63.277** Dislocation of unspecified interphalangeal joint of left little finger

√7ᵗʰ **S63.278** Dislocation of unspecified interphalangeal joint of other finger

Dislocation of unspecified interphalangeal joint of specified finger with unspecified laterality

√7ᵗʰ **S63.279** Dislocation of unspecified interphalangeal joint of unspecified finger

Dislocation of unspecified interphalangeal joint of unspecified finger without specified laterality

√6ᵗʰ **S63.28** Dislocation of proximal interphalangeal joint of finger

√7ᵗʰ **S63.280** Dislocation of proximal interphalangeal joint of right index finger

√7ᵗʰ **S63.281** Dislocation of proximal interphalangeal joint of left index finger

√7ᵗʰ **S63.282** Dislocation of proximal interphalangeal joint of right middle finger

√7ᵗʰ **S63.283** Dislocation of proximal interphalangeal joint of left middle finger

√7ᵗʰ **S63.284** Dislocation of proximal interphalangeal joint of right ring finger

√7ᵗʰ **S63.285** Dislocation of proximal interphalangeal joint of left ring finger

√7ᵗʰ **S63.286** Dislocation of proximal interphalangeal joint of right little finger

√7ᵗʰ **S63.287** Dislocation of proximal interphalangeal joint of left little finger

√7ᵗʰ **S63.288** Dislocation of proximal interphalangeal joint of other finger

Dislocation of proximal interphalangeal joint of specified finger with unspecified laterality

√7ᵗʰ **S63.289** Dislocation of proximal interphalangeal joint of unspecified finger

√6ᵗʰ **S63.29** Dislocation of distal interphalangeal joint of finger

√7ᵗʰ **S63.290** Dislocation of distal interphalangeal joint of right index finger

√7ᵗʰ **S63.291** Dislocation of distal interphalangeal joint of left index finger

√7ᵗʰ **S63.292** Dislocation of distal interphalangeal joint of right middle finger

√7ᵗʰ **S63.293** Dislocation of distal interphalangeal joint of left middle finger

√7ᵗʰ **S63.294** Dislocation of distal interphalangeal joint of right ring finger

√7ᵗʰ **S63.295** Dislocation of distal interphalangeal joint of left ring finger

√7ᵗʰ **S63.296** Dislocation of distal interphalangeal joint of right little finger

√7ᵗʰ **S63.297** Dislocation of distal interphalangeal joint of left little finger

√7ᵗʰ **S63.298** Dislocation of distal interphalangeal joint of other finger

Dislocation of distal interphalangeal joint of specified finger with unspecified laterality

√7ᵗʰ **S63.299** Dislocation of distal interphalangeal joint of unspecified finger

√5ᵗʰ **S63.3** Traumatic rupture of ligament of wrist

√6ᵗʰ **S63.30** Traumatic rupture of unspecified ligament of wrist

√7ᵗʰ **S63.301** Traumatic rupture of unspecified ligament of right wrist

√7ᵗʰ **S63.302** Traumatic rupture of unspecified ligament of left wrist

√7ᵗʰ **S63.309** Traumatic rupture of unspecified ligament of unspecified wrist

√6ᵗʰ **S63.31** Traumatic rupture of collateral ligament of wrist

√7ᵗʰ **S63.311** Traumatic rupture of collateral ligament of right wrist

√7ᵗʰ **S63.312** Traumatic rupture of collateral ligament of left wrist

√7ᵗʰ **S63.319** Traumatic rupture of collateral ligament of unspecified wrist

√6ᵗʰ **S63.32** Traumatic rupture of radiocarpal ligament

√7ᵗʰ **S63.321** Traumatic rupture of right radiocarpal ligament

√7ᵗʰ **S63.322** Traumatic rupture of left radiocarpal ligament

√7ᵗʰ **S63.329** Traumatic rupture of unspecified radiocarpal ligament

√6ᵗʰ **S63.33** Traumatic rupture of ulnocarpal (palmar) ligament

√7ᵗʰ **S63.331** Traumatic rupture of right ulnocarpal (palmar) ligament

√7ᵗʰ **S63.332** Traumatic rupture of left ulnocarpal (palmar) ligament

√7ᵗʰ **S63.339** Traumatic rupture of unspecified ulnocarpal (palmar) ligament

√6ᵗʰ **S63.39** Traumatic rupture of other ligament of wrist

√7ᵗʰ **S63.391** Traumatic rupture of other ligament of right wrist

√7ᵗʰ **S63.392** Traumatic rupture of other ligament of left wrist

√7ᵗʰ **S63.399** Traumatic rupture of other ligament of unspecified wrist

√5ᵗʰ **S63.4** Traumatic rupture of ligament of finger at metacarpophalangeal and interphalangeal joint(s)

√6ᵗʰ **S63.40** Traumatic rupture of unspecified ligament of finger at metacarpophalangeal and interphalangeal joint

√7ᵗʰ **S63.400** Traumatic rupture of unspecified ligament of right index finger at metacarpophalangeal and interphalangeal joint

√7ᵗʰ **S63.401** Traumatic rupture of unspecified ligament of left index finger at metacarpophalangeal and interphalangeal joint

√7ᵗʰ **S63.402** Traumatic rupture of unspecified ligament of right middle finger at metacarpophalangeal and interphalangeal joint

√7ᵗʰ **S63.403** Traumatic rupture of unspecified ligament of left middle finger at metacarpophalangeal and interphalangeal joint

√7ᵗʰ **S63.404** Traumatic rupture of unspecified ligament of right ring finger at metacarpophalangeal and interphalangeal joint

√7ᵗʰ **S63.405** Traumatic rupture of unspecified ligament of left ring finger at metacarpophalangeal and interphalangeal joint

√7ᵗʰ **S63.406** Traumatic rupture of unspecified ligament of right little finger at metacarpophalangeal and interphalangeal joint

√7ᵗʰ **S63.407** Traumatic rupture of unspecified ligament of left little finger at metacarpophalangeal and interphalangeal joint

√7ᵗʰ **S63.408** Traumatic rupture of unspecified ligament of other finger at metacarpophalangeal and interphalangeal joint

     Traumatic rupture of unspecified ligament of specified finger with unspecified laterality at metacarpophalangeal and interphalangeal joint

√7ᵗʰ **S63.409** Traumatic rupture of unspecified ligament of unspecified finger at metacarpophalangeal and interphalangeal joint

√6ᵗʰ **S63.41** Traumatic rupture of collateral ligament of finger at metacarpophalangeal and interphalangeal joint

√7ᵗʰ **S63.410** Traumatic rupture of collateral ligament of right index finger at metacarpophalangeal and interphalangeal joint

√7ᵗʰ **S63.411** Traumatic rupture of collateral ligament of left index finger at metacarpophalangeal and interphalangeal joint

√7ᵗʰ **S63.412** Traumatic rupture of collateral ligament of right middle finger at metacarpophalangeal and interphalangeal joint

√7ᵗʰ **S63.413** Traumatic rupture of collateral ligament of left middle finger at metacarpophalangeal and interphalangeal joint

√7ᵗʰ **S63.414** Traumatic rupture of collateral ligament of right ring finger at metacarpophalangeal and interphalangeal joint

√7ᵗʰ **S63.415** Traumatic rupture of collateral ligament of left ring finger at metacarpophalangeal and interphalangeal joint

√7ᵗʰ **S63.416** Traumatic rupture of collateral ligament of right little finger at metacarpophalangeal and interphalangeal joint

√7ᵗʰ **S63.417** Traumatic rupture of collateral ligament of left little finger at metacarpophalangeal and interphalangeal joint

√7ᵗʰ **S63.418** Traumatic rupture of collateral ligament of other finger at metacarpophalangeal and interphalangeal joint

     Traumatic rupture of collateral ligament of specified finger with unspecified laterality at metacarpophalangeal and interphalangeal joint

√7ᵗʰ **S63.419** Traumatic rupture of collateral ligament of unspecified finger at metacarpophalangeal and interphalangeal joint

√6ᵗʰ **S63.42** Traumatic rupture of palmar ligament of finger at metacarpophalangeal and interphalangeal joint

√7ᵗʰ **S63.420** Traumatic rupture of palmar ligament of right index finger at metacarpophalangeal and interphalangeal joint

√7ᵗʰ **S63.421** Traumatic rupture of palmar ligament of left index finger at metacarpophalangeal and interphalangeal joint

√7ᵗʰ **S63.422** Traumatic rupture of palmar ligament of right middle finger at metacarpophalangeal and interphalangeal joint

√7ᵗʰ **S63.423** Traumatic rupture of palmar ligament of left middle finger at metacarpophalangeal and interphalangeal joint

√7ᵗʰ **S63.424** Traumatic rupture of palmar ligament of right ring finger at metacarpophalangeal and interphalangeal joint

√7ᵗʰ **S63.425** Traumatic rupture of palmar ligament of left ring finger at metacarpophalangeal and interphalangeal joint

√7ᵗʰ **S63.426** Traumatic rupture of palmar ligament of right little finger at metacarpophalangeal and interphalangeal joint

√7ᵗʰ **S63.427** Traumatic rupture of palmar ligament of left little finger at metacarpophalangeal and interphalangeal joint

√7ᵗʰ **S63.428** Traumatic rupture of palmar ligament of other finger at metacarpophalangeal and interphalangeal joint

     Traumatic rupture of palmar ligament of specified finger with unspecified laterality at metacarpophalangeal and interphalangeal joint

√7ᵗʰ **S63.429** Traumatic rupture of palmar ligament of unspecified finger at metacarpophalangeal and interphalangeal joint

√6ᵗʰ **S63.43** Traumatic rupture of volar plate of finger at metacarpophalangeal and interphalangeal joint

√7ᵗʰ **S63.430** Traumatic rupture of volar plate of right index finger at metacarpophalangeal and interphalangeal joint

√7ᵗʰ **S63.431** Traumatic rupture of volar plate of left index finger at metacarpophalangeal and interphalangeal joint

√7ᵗʰ **S63.432** Traumatic rupture of volar plate of right middle finger at metacarpophalangeal and interphalangeal joint

√7ᵗʰ **S63.433** Traumatic rupture of volar plate of left middle finger at metacarpophalangeal and interphalangeal joint

√7ᵗʰ **S63.434** Traumatic rupture of volar plate of right ring finger at metacarpophalangeal and interphalangeal joint

√7ᵗʰ **S63.435** Traumatic rupture of volar plate of left ring finger at metacarpophalangeal and interphalangeal joint

√7ᵗʰ **S63.436** Traumatic rupture of volar plate of right little finger at metacarpophalangeal and interphalangeal joint

√7ᵗʰ **S63.437** Traumatic rupture of volar plate of left little finger at metacarpophalangeal and interphalangeal joint

N Newborn: 0   P Pediatric: 0-17   M Maternity: 9-64   A Adult: 15-124   MCC Major Complication/Comorbidity   CC Complication/Comorbidity   SW Severe Wound Dx

1074   ICD-10-CM 2020

√7ᵗʰ **S63.438** Traumatic rupture of volar plate of other finger at metacarpophalangeal and interphalangeal joint

    Traumatic rupture of volar plate of specified finger with unspecified laterality at metacarpophalangeal and interphalangeal joint

√7ᵗʰ **S63.439** Traumatic rupture of volar plate of unspecified finger at metacarpophalangeal and interphalangeal joint

√6ᵗʰ **S63.49** Traumatic rupture of other ligament of finger at metacarpophalangeal and interphalangeal joint

√7ᵗʰ **S63.490** Traumatic rupture of other ligament of right index finger at metacarpophalangeal and interphalangeal joint

√7ᵗʰ **S63.491** Traumatic rupture of other ligament of left index finger at metacarpophalangeal and interphalangeal joint

√7ᵗʰ **S63.492** Traumatic rupture of other ligament of right middle finger at metacarpophalangeal and interphalangeal joint

√7ᵗʰ **S63.493** Traumatic rupture of other ligament of left middle finger at metacarpophalangeal and interphalangeal joint

√7ᵗʰ **S63.494** Traumatic rupture of other ligament of right ring finger at metacarpophalangeal and interphalangeal joint

√7ᵗʰ **S63.495** Traumatic rupture of other ligament of left ring finger at metacarpophalangeal and interphalangeal joint

√7ᵗʰ **S63.496** Traumatic rupture of other ligament of right little finger at metacarpophalangeal and interphalangeal joint

√7ᵗʰ **S63.497** Traumatic rupture of other ligament of left little finger at metacarpophalangeal and interphalangeal joint

√7ᵗʰ **S63.498** Traumatic rupture of other ligament of other finger at metacarpophalangeal and interphalangeal joint

    Traumatic rupture of ligament of specified finger with unspecified laterality at metacarpophalangeal and interphalangeal joint

√7ᵗʰ **S63.499** Traumatic rupture of other ligament of unspecified finger at metacarpophalangeal and interphalangeal joint

√5ᵗʰ **S63.5** Other and unspecified sprain of wrist

√6ᵗʰ **S63.50** Unspecified sprain of wrist

√7ᵗʰ **S63.501** Unspecified sprain of right wrist

√7ᵗʰ **S63.502** Unspecified sprain of left wrist

√7ᵗʰ **S63.509** Unspecified sprain of unspecified wrist

√6ᵗʰ **S63.51** Sprain of carpal (joint)

√7ᵗʰ **S63.511** Sprain of carpal joint of right wrist

√7ᵗʰ **S63.512** Sprain of carpal joint of left wrist

√7ᵗʰ **S63.519** Sprain of carpal joint of unspecified wrist

√6ᵗʰ **S63.52** Sprain of radiocarpal joint

EXCLUDES 1   traumatic rupture of radiocarpal ligament (S63.32-)

√7ᵗʰ **S63.521** Sprain of radiocarpal joint of right wrist

√7ᵗʰ **S63.522** Sprain of radiocarpal joint of left wrist

√7ᵗʰ **S63.529** Sprain of radiocarpal joint of unspecified wrist

√6ᵗʰ **S63.59** Other specified sprain of wrist

√7ᵗʰ **S63.591** Other specified sprain of right wrist

√7ᵗʰ **S63.592** Other specified sprain of left wrist

√7ᵗʰ **S63.599** Other specified sprain of unspecified wrist

√5ᵗʰ **S63.6** Other and unspecified sprain of finger(s)

EXCLUDES 1   traumatic rupture of ligament of finger at metacarpophalangeal and interphalangeal joint(s) (S63.4-)

√6ᵗʰ **S63.60** Unspecified sprain of thumb

√7ᵗʰ **S63.601** Unspecified sprain of right thumb

√7ᵗʰ **S63.602** Unspecified sprain of left thumb

√7ᵗʰ **S63.609** Unspecified sprain of unspecified thumb

√6ᵗʰ **S63.61** Unspecified sprain of other and unspecified finger(s)

√7ᵗʰ **S63.610** Unspecified sprain of right index finger

√7ᵗʰ **S63.611** Unspecified sprain of left index finger

√7ᵗʰ **S63.612** Unspecified sprain of right middle finger

√7ᵗʰ **S63.613** Unspecified sprain of left middle finger

√7ᵗʰ **S63.614** Unspecified sprain of right ring finger

√7ᵗʰ **S63.615** Unspecified sprain of left ring finger

√7ᵗʰ **S63.616** Unspecified sprain of right little finger

√7ᵗʰ **S63.617** Unspecified sprain of left little finger

√7ᵗʰ **S63.618** Unspecified sprain of other finger

    Unspecified sprain of specified finger with unspecified laterality

√7ᵗʰ **S63.619** Unspecified sprain of unspecified finger

√6ᵗʰ **S63.62** Sprain of interphalangeal joint of thumb

√7ᵗʰ **S63.621** Sprain of interphalangeal joint of right thumb

√7ᵗʰ **S63.622** Sprain of interphalangeal joint of left thumb

√7ᵗʰ **S63.629** Sprain of interphalangeal joint of unspecified thumb

√6ᵗʰ **S63.63** Sprain of interphalangeal joint of other and unspecified finger(s)

√7ᵗʰ **S63.630** Sprain of interphalangeal joint of right index finger

√7ᵗʰ **S63.631** Sprain of interphalangeal joint of left index finger

√7ᵗʰ **S63.632** Sprain of interphalangeal joint of right middle finger

√7ᵗʰ **S63.633** Sprain of interphalangeal joint of left middle finger

√7ᵗʰ **S63.634** Sprain of interphalangeal joint of right ring finger

√7ᵗʰ **S63.635** Sprain of interphalangeal joint of left ring finger

√7ᵗʰ **S63.636** Sprain of interphalangeal joint of right little finger

√7ᵗʰ **S63.637** Sprain of interphalangeal joint of left little finger

√7ᵗʰ **S63.638** Sprain of interphalangeal joint of other finger

√7ᵗʰ **S63.639** Sprain of interphalangeal joint of unspecified finger

√6ᵗʰ **S63.64** Sprain of metacarpophalangeal joint of thumb

√7ᵗʰ **S63.641** Sprain of metacarpophalangeal joint of right thumb

√7ᵗʰ **S63.642** Sprain of metacarpophalangeal joint of left thumb

√7ᵗʰ **S63.649** Sprain of metacarpophalangeal joint of unspecified thumb

√6ᵗʰ **S63.65** Sprain of metacarpophalangeal joint of other and unspecified finger(s)

√7ᵗʰ **S63.650** Sprain of metacarpophalangeal joint of right index finger

√7ᵗʰ **S63.651** Sprain of metacarpophalangeal joint of left index finger

√7ᵗʰ **S63.652** Sprain of metacarpophalangeal joint of right middle finger

√7ᵗʰ **S63.653** Sprain of metacarpophalangeal joint of left middle finger

√7ᵗʰ **S63.654** Sprain of metacarpophalangeal joint of right ring finger

√7ᵗʰ **S63.655** Sprain of metacarpophalangeal joint of left ring finger

√7ᵗʰ **S63.656** Sprain of metacarpophalangeal joint of right little finger

√7ᵗʰ **S63.657** Sprain of metacarpophalangeal joint of left little finger

√7ᵗʰ **S63.658** Sprain of metacarpophalangeal joint of other finger

    Sprain of metacarpophalangeal joint of specified finger with unspecified laterality

√7ᵗʰ **S63.659** Sprain of metacarpophalangeal joint of unspecified finger

√6ᵗʰ **S63.68** Other sprain of thumb

√7ᵗʰ **S63.681** Other sprain of right thumb

✔ Additional Character Required   √x7ᵗʰ Placeholder   Unacceptable PDx   Questionable PDx   Manifestation   Unspecified Dx   H1-H14 HAC   HCC CMS-HCC Dx   HIV HIV Dx

ICD-10-CM 2020   1075

√7ᵗʰ **S63.682** Other sprain of left thumb

√7ᵗʰ **S63.689** Other sprain of unspecified thumb

√6ᵗʰ **S63.69** Other sprain of other and unspecified finger(s)

√7ᵗʰ **S63.690** Other sprain of right index finger

√7ᵗʰ **S63.691** Other sprain of left index finger

√7ᵗʰ **S63.692** Other sprain of right middle finger

√7ᵗʰ **S63.693** Other sprain of left middle finger

√7ᵗʰ **S63.694** Other sprain of right ring finger

√7ᵗʰ **S63.695** Other sprain of left ring finger

√7ᵗʰ **S63.696** Other sprain of right little finger

√7ᵗʰ **S63.697** Other sprain of left little finger

√7ᵗʰ **S63.698** Other sprain of other finger
Other sprain of specified finger with unspecified laterality

√7ᵗʰ **S63.699** Other sprain of unspecified finger

√5ᵗʰ **S63.8** Sprain of other part of wrist and hand

√6ᵗʰ **S63.8X** Sprain of other part of wrist and hand

√7ᵗʰ **S63.8X1** Sprain of other part of right wrist and hand

√7ᵗʰ **S63.8X2** Sprain of other part of left wrist and hand

√7ᵗʰ **S63.8X9** Sprain of other part of unspecified wrist and hand

√5ᵗʰ **S63.9** Sprain of unspecified part of wrist and hand

√x7ᵗʰ **S63.90** Sprain of unspecified part of unspecified wrist and hand

√x7ᵗʰ **S63.91** Sprain of unspecified part of right wrist and hand

√x7ᵗʰ **S63.92** Sprain of unspecified part of left wrist and hand

√4ᵗʰ **S64 Injury of nerves at wrist and hand level**

Code also any associated open wound (S61.-)

The appropriate 7th character is to be added to each code from category S64.
A   initial encounter
D   subsequent encounter
S   sequela

√5ᵗʰ **S64.0** Injury of ulnar nerve at wrist and hand level

√x7ᵗʰ **S64.00** Injury of ulnar nerve at wrist and hand level of unspecified arm

√x7ᵗʰ **S64.01** Injury of ulnar nerve at wrist and hand level of right arm

√x7ᵗʰ **S64.02** Injury of ulnar nerve at wrist and hand level of left arm

√5ᵗʰ **S64.1** Injury of median nerve at wrist and hand level

√x7ᵗʰ **S64.10** Injury of median nerve at wrist and hand level of unspecified arm

√x7ᵗʰ **S64.11** Injury of median nerve at wrist and hand level of right arm

√x7ᵗʰ **S64.12** Injury of median nerve at wrist and hand level of left arm

√5ᵗʰ **S64.2** Injury of radial nerve at wrist and hand level

√x7ᵗʰ **S64.20** Injury of radial nerve at wrist and hand level of unspecified arm

√x7ᵗʰ **S64.21** Injury of radial nerve at wrist and hand level of right arm

√x7ᵗʰ **S64.22** Injury of radial nerve at wrist and hand level of left arm

√5ᵗʰ **S64.3** Injury of digital nerve of thumb

√x7ᵗʰ **S64.30** Injury of digital nerve of unspecified thumb

√x7ᵗʰ **S64.31** Injury of digital nerve of right thumb

√x7ᵗʰ **S64.32** Injury of digital nerve of left thumb

√5ᵗʰ **S64.4** Injury of digital nerve of other and unspecified finger

√x7ᵗʰ **S64.40** Injury of digital nerve of unspecified finger

√6ᵗʰ **S64.49** Injury of digital nerve of other finger

√7ᵗʰ **S64.490** Injury of digital nerve of right index finger

√7ᵗʰ **S64.491** Injury of digital nerve of left index finger

√7ᵗʰ **S64.492** Injury of digital nerve of right middle finger

√7ᵗʰ **S64.493** Injury of digital nerve of left middle finger

√7ᵗʰ **S64.494** Injury of digital nerve of right ring finger

√7ᵗʰ **S64.495** Injury of digital nerve of left ring finger

√7ᵗʰ **S64.496** Injury of digital nerve of right little finger

√7ᵗʰ **S64.497** Injury of digital nerve of left little finger

√7ᵗʰ **S64.498** Injury of digital nerve of other finger
Injury of digital nerve of specified finger with unspecified laterality

√5ᵗʰ **S64.8** Injury of other nerves at wrist and hand level

√6ᵗʰ **S64.8X** Injury of other nerves at wrist and hand level

√7ᵗʰ **S64.8X1** Injury of other nerves at wrist and hand level of right arm

√7ᵗʰ **S64.8X2** Injury of other nerves at wrist and hand level of left arm

√7ᵗʰ **S64.8X9** Injury of other nerves at wrist and hand level of unspecified arm

√5ᵗʰ **S64.9** Injury of unspecified nerve at wrist and hand level

√x7ᵗʰ **S64.90** Injury of unspecified nerve at wrist and hand level of unspecified arm

√x7ᵗʰ **S64.91** Injury of unspecified nerve at wrist and hand level of right arm

√x7ᵗʰ **S64.92** Injury of unspecified nerve at wrist and hand level of left arm

√4ᵗʰ **S65 Injury of blood vessels at wrist and hand level**

Code also any associated open wound (S61.-)

The appropriate 7th character is to be added to each code from category S65.
A   initial encounter
D   subsequent encounter
S   sequela

√5ᵗʰ **S65.0** Injury of ulnar artery at wrist and hand level

CC Excl: For CC codes in subcategory S65.0:
Right side: PDX collection 1274
Left side: PDX collection 1275
Unspecified side: PDX collection 1276

√6ᵗʰ **S65.00** Unspecified injury of ulnar artery at wrist and hand level

√7ᵗʰ **S65.001** Unspecified injury of ulnar artery at wrist and hand level of right arm   CC

√7ᵗʰ **S65.002** Unspecified injury of ulnar artery at wrist and hand level of left arm   CC

√7ᵗʰ **S65.009** Unspecified injury of ulnar artery at wrist and hand level of unspecified arm   CC

√6ᵗʰ **S65.01** Laceration of ulnar artery at wrist and hand level

√7ᵗʰ **S65.011** Laceration of ulnar artery at wrist and hand level of right arm   CC

√7ᵗʰ **S65.012** Laceration of ulnar artery at wrist and hand level of left arm   CC

√7ᵗʰ **S65.019** Laceration of ulnar artery at wrist and hand level of unspecified arm   CC

√6ᵗʰ **S65.09** Other specified injury of ulnar artery at wrist and hand level

√7ᵗʰ **S65.091** Other specified injury of ulnar artery at wrist and hand level of right arm   CC

√7ᵗʰ **S65.092** Other specified injury of ulnar artery at wrist and hand level of left arm   CC

√7ᵗʰ **S65.099** Other specified injury of ulnar artery at wrist and hand level of unspecified arm   CC

√5ᵗʰ **S65.1** Injury of radial artery at wrist and hand level

CC Excl: For CC codes in subcategory S65.1:
Right side: PDX collection 1277
Left side: PDX collection 1278
Unspecified side: PDX collection 1279

√6ᵗʰ **S65.10** Unspecified injury of radial artery at wrist and hand level

√7ᵗʰ **S65.101** Unspecified injury of radial artery at wrist and hand level of right arm   CC

√7ᵗʰ **S65.102** Unspecified injury of radial artery at wrist and hand level of left arm   CC

N Newborn: 0   P Pediatric: 0-17   M Maternity: 9-64   A Adult: 15-124   MCC Major Complication/Comorbidity   CC Complication/Comorbidity   SW Severe Wound Dx

1076   ICD-10-CM 2020

√7ᵗʰ **S65.109** Unspecified injury of radial artery at wrist and hand level of unspecified arm   CC

√6ᵗʰ **S65.11** Laceration of radial artery at wrist and hand level

  √7ᵗʰ **S65.111** Laceration of radial artery at wrist and hand level of right arm   CC

  √7ᵗʰ **S65.112** Laceration of radial artery at wrist and hand level of left arm   CC

  √7ᵗʰ **S65.119** Laceration of radial artery at wrist and hand level of unspecified arm   CC

√6ᵗʰ **S65.19** Other specified injury of radial artery at wrist and hand level

  √7ᵗʰ **S65.191** Other specified injury of radial artery at wrist and hand level of right arm   CC

  √7ᵗʰ **S65.192** Other specified injury of radial artery at wrist and hand level of left arm   CC

  √7ᵗʰ **S65.199** Other specified injury of radial artery at wrist and hand level of unspecified arm   CC

√5ᵗʰ **S65.2** Injury of superficial palmar arch

> **CC Excl: For CC codes in subcategory S65.2:**
> **Right side:** PDX collection 1288
> **Left side:** PDX collection 1289
> **Unspecified side:** PDX collection 1290

√6ᵗʰ **S65.20** Unspecified injury of superficial palmar arch

  √7ᵗʰ **S65.201** Unspecified injury of superficial palmar arch of right hand   CC

  √7ᵗʰ **S65.202** Unspecified injury of superficial palmar arch of left hand   CC

  √7ᵗʰ **S65.209** Unspecified injury of superficial palmar arch of unspecified hand   CC

√6ᵗʰ **S65.21** Laceration of superficial palmar arch

  √7ᵗʰ **S65.211** Laceration of superficial palmar arch of right hand   CC

  √7ᵗʰ **S65.212** Laceration of superficial palmar arch of left hand   CC

  √7ᵗʰ **S65.219** Laceration of superficial palmar arch of unspecified hand   CC

√6ᵗʰ **S65.29** Other specified injury of superficial palmar arch

  √7ᵗʰ **S65.291** Other specified injury of superficial palmar arch of right hand   CC

  √7ᵗʰ **S65.292** Other specified injury of superficial palmar arch of left hand   CC

  √7ᵗʰ **S65.299** Other specified injury of superficial palmar arch of unspecified hand   CC

√5ᵗʰ **S65.3** Injury of deep palmar arch

> **CC Excl: For CC codes in subcategory S65.3:**
> **Right side:** PDX collection 1288
> **Left side:** PDX collection 1289
> **Unspecified side:** PDX collection 1290

√6ᵗʰ **S65.30** Unspecified injury of deep palmar arch

  √7ᵗʰ **S65.301** Unspecified injury of deep palmar arch of right hand   CC

  √7ᵗʰ **S65.302** Unspecified injury of deep palmar arch of left hand   CC

  √7ᵗʰ **S65.309** Unspecified injury of deep palmar arch of unspecified hand   CC

√6ᵗʰ **S65.31** Laceration of deep palmar arch

  √7ᵗʰ **S65.311** Laceration of deep palmar arch of right hand   CC

  √7ᵗʰ **S65.312** Laceration of deep palmar arch of left hand   CC

  √7ᵗʰ **S65.319** Laceration of deep palmar arch of unspecified hand   CC

√6ᵗʰ **S65.39** Other specified injury of deep palmar arch

  √7ᵗʰ **S65.391** Other specified injury of deep palmar arch of right hand   CC

  √7ᵗʰ **S65.392** Other specified injury of deep palmar arch of left hand   CC

  √7ᵗʰ **S65.399** Other specified injury of deep palmar arch of unspecified hand   CC

√5ᵗʰ **S65.4** Injury of blood vessel of thumb

> **CC Excl: For CC codes in subcategory S65.4:**
> **Right side:** PDX collection 1291
> **Left side:** PDX collection 1292
> **Unspecified side:** PDX collection 1293

√6ᵗʰ **S65.40** Unspecified injury of blood vessel of thumb

  √7ᵗʰ **S65.401** Unspecified injury of blood vessel of right thumb   CC

  √7ᵗʰ **S65.402** Unspecified injury of blood vessel of left thumb   CC

  √7ᵗʰ **S65.409** Unspecified injury of blood vessel of unspecified thumb   CC

√6ᵗʰ **S65.41** Laceration of blood vessel of thumb

  √7ᵗʰ **S65.411** Laceration of blood vessel of right thumb   CC

  √7ᵗʰ **S65.412** Laceration of blood vessel of left thumb   CC

  √7ᵗʰ **S65.419** Laceration of blood vessel of unspecified thumb   CC

√6ᵗʰ **S65.49** Other specified injury of blood vessel of thumb

  √7ᵗʰ **S65.491** Other specified injury of blood vessel of right thumb   CC

  √7ᵗʰ **S65.492** Other specified injury of blood vessel of left thumb   CC

  √7ᵗʰ **S65.499** Other specified injury of blood vessel of unspecified thumb   CC

√5ᵗʰ **S65.5** Injury of blood vessel of other and unspecified finger

> **CC Excl: For CC codes in subcategory S65.5:**
> **Right side:** PDX collection 1291
> **Left side:** PDX collection 1292
> **Unspecified side:** PDX collection 1293

√6ᵗʰ **S65.50** Unspecified injury of blood vessel of other and unspecified finger

  √7ᵗʰ **S65.500** Unspecified injury of blood vessel of right index finger   CC

  √7ᵗʰ **S65.501** Unspecified injury of blood vessel of left index finger   CC

  √7ᵗʰ **S65.502** Unspecified injury of blood vessel of right middle finger   CC

  √7ᵗʰ **S65.503** Unspecified injury of blood vessel of left middle finger   CC

  √7ᵗʰ **S65.504** Unspecified injury of blood vessel of right ring finger   CC

  √7ᵗʰ **S65.505** Unspecified injury of blood vessel of left ring finger   CC

  √7ᵗʰ **S65.506** Unspecified injury of blood vessel of right little finger   CC

  √7ᵗʰ **S65.507** Unspecified injury of blood vessel of left little finger   CC

  √7ᵗʰ **S65.508** Unspecified injury of blood vessel of other finger   CC

      Unspecified injury of blood vessel of specified finger with unspecified laterality

  √7ᵗʰ **S65.509** Unspecified injury of blood vessel of unspecified finger   CC

☑ Additional Character Required   √x7ᵗʰ Placeholder   Unacceptable PDx   Questionable PDx   Manifestation   Unspecified Dx   H1-H14 HAC   HCC CMS-HCC Dx   HIV HIV Dx

ICD-10-CM 2020   1077

√6ᵗʰ   **S65.51**   Laceration of blood vessel of other and unspecified finger

    √7ᵗʰ   **S65.510**   Laceration of blood vessel of right index finger   `CC`

    √7ᵗʰ   **S65.511**   Laceration of blood vessel of left index finger   `CC`

    √7ᵗʰ   **S65.512**   Laceration of blood vessel of right middle finger   `CC`

    √7ᵗʰ   **S65.513**   Laceration of blood vessel of left middle finger   `CC`

    √7ᵗʰ   **S65.514**   Laceration of blood vessel of right ring finger   `CC`

    √7ᵗʰ   **S65.515**   Laceration of blood vessel of left ring finger   `CC`

    √7ᵗʰ   **S65.516**   Laceration of blood vessel of right little finger   `CC`

    √7ᵗʰ   **S65.517**   Laceration of blood vessel of left little finger   `CC`

    √7ᵗʰ   **S65.518**   Laceration of blood vessel of other finger   `CC`
       Laceration of blood vessel of specified finger with unspecified laterality

    √7ᵗʰ   **S65.519**   Laceration of blood vessel of unspecified finger   `CC`

√6ᵗʰ   **S65.59**   Other specified injury of blood vessel of other and unspecified finger

    √7ᵗʰ   **S65.590**   Other specified injury of blood vessel of right index finger   `CC`

    √7ᵗʰ   **S65.591**   Other specified injury of blood vessel of left index finger   `CC`

    √7ᵗʰ   **S65.592**   Other specified injury of blood vessel of right middle finger   `CC`

    √7ᵗʰ   **S65.593**   Other specified injury of blood vessel of left middle finger   `CC`

    √7ᵗʰ   **S65.594**   Other specified injury of blood vessel of right ring finger   `CC`

    √7ᵗʰ   **S65.595**   Other specified injury of blood vessel of left ring finger   `CC`

    √7ᵗʰ   **S65.596**   Other specified injury of blood vessel of right little finger   `CC`

    √7ᵗʰ   **S65.597**   Other specified injury of blood vessel of left little finger   `CC`

    √7ᵗʰ   **S65.598**   Other specified injury of blood vessel of other finger   `CC`
       Other specified injury of blood vessel of specified finger with unspecified laterality

    √7ᵗʰ   **S65.599**   Other specified injury of blood vessel of unspecified finger   `CC`

√5ᵗʰ   **S65.8**   Injury of other blood vessels at wrist and hand level

> **CC Excl: For CC codes in subcategory S65.8:**
> **Right side:** PDX collection 1260
> **Left side:** PDX collection 1261
> **Unspecified side:** PDX collection 1262

√6ᵗʰ   **S65.80**   Unspecified injury of other blood vessels at wrist and hand level

    √7ᵗʰ   **S65.801**   Unspecified injury of other blood vessels at wrist and hand level of right arm   `CC`

    √7ᵗʰ   **S65.802**   Unspecified injury of other blood vessels at wrist and hand level of left arm   `CC`

    √7ᵗʰ   **S65.809**   Unspecified injury of other blood vessels at wrist and hand level of unspecified arm   `CC`

√6ᵗʰ   **S65.81**   Laceration of other blood vessels at wrist and hand level

    √7ᵗʰ   **S65.811**   Laceration of other blood vessels at wrist and hand level of right arm   `CC`

    √7ᵗʰ   **S65.812**   Laceration of other blood vessels at wrist and hand level of left arm   `CC`

    √7ᵗʰ   **S65.819**   Laceration of other blood vessels at wrist and hand level of unspecified arm   `CC`

√6ᵗʰ   **S65.89**   Other specified injury of other blood vessels at wrist and hand level

    √7ᵗʰ   **S65.891**   Other specified injury of other blood vessels at wrist and hand level of right arm   `CC`

    √7ᵗʰ   **S65.892**   Other specified injury of other blood vessels at wrist and hand level of left arm   `CC`

    √7ᵗʰ   **S65.899**   Other specified injury of other blood vessels at wrist and hand level of unspecified arm   `CC`

√5ᵗʰ   **S65.9**   Injury of unspecified blood vessel at wrist and hand level

> **CC Excl: For CC codes in subcategory S65.9:**
> **Right side:** PDX collection 1260
> **Left side:** PDX collection 1261
> **Unspecified side:** PDX collection 1262

√6ᵗʰ   **S65.90**   Unspecified injury of unspecified blood vessel at wrist and hand level

    √7ᵗʰ   **S65.901**   Unspecified injury of unspecified blood vessel at wrist and hand level of right arm   `CC`

    √7ᵗʰ   **S65.902**   Unspecified injury of unspecified blood vessel at wrist and hand level of left arm   `CC`

    √7ᵗʰ   **S65.909**   Unspecified injury of unspecified blood vessel at wrist and hand level of unspecified arm   `CC`

√6ᵗʰ   **S65.91**   Laceration of unspecified blood vessel at wrist and hand level

    √7ᵗʰ   **S65.911**   Laceration of unspecified blood vessel at wrist and hand level of right arm   `CC`

    √7ᵗʰ   **S65.912**   Laceration of unspecified blood vessel at wrist and hand level of left arm   `CC`

    √7ᵗʰ   **S65.919**   Laceration of unspecified blood vessel at wrist and hand level of unspecified arm   `CC`

√6ᵗʰ   **S65.99**   Other specified injury of unspecified blood vessel at wrist and hand level

    √7ᵗʰ   **S65.991**   Other specified injury of unspecified blood vessel at wrist and hand of right arm   `CC`

    √7ᵗʰ   **S65.992**   Other specified injury of unspecified blood vessel at wrist and hand of left arm   `CC`

    √7ᵗʰ   **S65.999**   Other specified injury of unspecified blood vessel at wrist and hand of unspecified arm   `CC`

√4ᵗʰ   **S66**   **Injury of muscle, fascia and tendon at wrist and hand level**

    Code also any associated open wound (S61.-)

    EXCLUDES 2   *sprain of joints and ligaments of wrist and hand (S63.-)*

    TIP: Refer to the Muscle/Tendon table at the beginning of this chapter.

> The appropriate 7th character is to be added to each code from category S66.
> A   initial encounter
> D   subsequent encounter
> S   sequela

> **CC Excl: For CC codes in category S66:**
> **Right side:** PDX collection 1294
> **Left side:** PDX collection 1295
> **Unspecified side:** PDX collection 1296

√5ᵗʰ   **S66.0**   Injury of long flexor muscle, fascia and tendon of thumb at wrist and hand level

√6ᵗʰ   **S66.00**   Unspecified injury of long flexor muscle, fascia and tendon of thumb at wrist and hand level

    √7ᵗʰ   **S66.001**   Unspecified injury of long flexor muscle, fascia and tendon of right thumb at wrist and hand level

N Newborn: 0   P Pediatric: 0-17   M Maternity: 9-64   A Adult: 15-124   `MCC` Major Complication/Comorbidity   `CC` Complication/Comorbidity   `SW` Severe Wound Dx

1078   ICD-10-CM 2020

√7ᵗʰ **S66.002** Unspecified injury of long flexor muscle, fascia and tendon of left thumb at wrist and hand level

√7ᵗʰ **S66.009** Unspecified injury of long flexor muscle, fascia and tendon of unspecified thumb at wrist and hand level

√6ᵗʰ **S66.01** Strain of long flexor muscle, fascia and tendon of thumb at wrist and hand level

√7ᵗʰ **S66.011** Strain of long flexor muscle, fascia and tendon of right thumb at wrist and hand level

√7ᵗʰ **S66.012** Strain of long flexor muscle, fascia and tendon of left thumb at wrist and hand level

√7ᵗʰ **S66.019** Strain of long flexor muscle, fascia and tendon of unspecified thumb at wrist and hand level

√6ᵗʰ **S66.02** Laceration of long flexor muscle, fascia and tendon of thumb at wrist and hand level

√7ᵗʰ **S66.021** Laceration of long flexor muscle, fascia and tendon of right thumb at wrist and hand level   CC

√7ᵗʰ **S66.022** Laceration of long flexor muscle, fascia and tendon of left thumb at wrist and hand level   CC

√7ᵗʰ **S66.029** Laceration of long flexor muscle, fascia and tendon of unspecified thumb at wrist and hand level   CC

√6ᵗʰ **S66.09** Other specified injury of long flexor muscle, fascia and tendon of thumb at wrist and hand level

√7ᵗʰ **S66.091** Other specified injury of long flexor muscle, fascia and tendon of right thumb at wrist and hand level

√7ᵗʰ **S66.092** Other specified injury of long flexor muscle, fascia and tendon of left thumb at wrist and hand level

√7ᵗʰ **S66.099** Other specified injury of long flexor muscle, fascia and tendon of unspecified thumb at wrist and hand level

√5ᵗʰ **S66.1** Injury of flexor muscle, fascia and tendon of other and unspecified finger at wrist and hand level

> EXCLUDES 2   injury of long flexor muscle, fascia and tendon of thumb at wrist and hand level (S66.0-)

√6ᵗʰ **S66.10** Unspecified injury of flexor muscle, fascia and tendon of other and unspecified finger at wrist and hand level

√7ᵗʰ **S66.100** Unspecified injury of flexor muscle, fascia and tendon of right index finger at wrist and hand level

√7ᵗʰ **S66.101** Unspecified injury of flexor muscle, fascia and tendon of left index finger at wrist and hand level

√7ᵗʰ **S66.102** Unspecified injury of flexor muscle, fascia and tendon of right middle finger at wrist and hand level

√7ᵗʰ **S66.103** Unspecified injury of flexor muscle, fascia and tendon of left middle finger at wrist and hand level

√7ᵗʰ **S66.104** Unspecified injury of flexor muscle, fascia and tendon of right ring finger at wrist and hand level

√7ᵗʰ **S66.105** Unspecified injury of flexor muscle, fascia and tendon of left ring finger at wrist and hand level

√7ᵗʰ **S66.106** Unspecified injury of flexor muscle, fascia and tendon of right little finger at wrist and hand level

√7ᵗʰ **S66.107** Unspecified injury of flexor muscle, fascia and tendon of left little finger at wrist and hand level

√7ᵗʰ **S66.108** Unspecified injury of flexor muscle, fascia and tendon of other finger at wrist and hand level

> Unspecified injury of flexor muscle, fascia and tendon of specified finger with unspecified laterality at wrist and hand level

√7ᵗʰ **S66.109** Unspecified injury of flexor muscle, fascia and tendon of unspecified finger at wrist and hand level

√6ᵗʰ **S66.11** Strain of flexor muscle, fascia and tendon of other and unspecified finger at wrist and hand level

√7ᵗʰ **S66.110** Strain of flexor muscle, fascia and tendon of right index finger at wrist and hand level

√7ᵗʰ **S66.111** Strain of flexor muscle, fascia and tendon of left index finger at wrist and hand level

√7ᵗʰ **S66.112** Strain of flexor muscle, fascia and tendon of right middle finger at wrist and hand level

√7ᵗʰ **S66.113** Strain of flexor muscle, fascia and tendon of left middle finger at wrist and hand level

√7ᵗʰ **S66.114** Strain of flexor muscle, fascia and tendon of right ring finger at wrist and hand level

√7ᵗʰ **S66.115** Strain of flexor muscle, fascia and tendon of left ring finger at wrist and hand level

√7ᵗʰ **S66.116** Strain of flexor muscle, fascia and tendon of right little finger at wrist and hand level

√7ᵗʰ **S66.117** Strain of flexor muscle, fascia and tendon of left little finger at wrist and hand level

√7ᵗʰ **S66.118** Strain of flexor muscle, fascia and tendon of other finger at wrist and hand level

> Strain of flexor muscle, fascia and tendon of specified finger with unspecified laterality at wrist and hand level

√7ᵗʰ **S66.119** Strain of flexor muscle, fascia and tendon of unspecified finger at wrist and hand level

√6ᵗʰ **S66.12** Laceration of flexor muscle, fascia and tendon of other and unspecified finger at wrist and hand level

√7ᵗʰ **S66.120** Laceration of flexor muscle, fascia and tendon of right index finger at wrist and hand level   CC

√7ᵗʰ **S66.121** Laceration of flexor muscle, fascia and tendon of left index finger at wrist and hand level   CC

√7ᵗʰ **S66.122** Laceration of flexor muscle, fascia and tendon of right middle finger at wrist and hand level   CC

√7ᵗʰ **S66.123** Laceration of flexor muscle, fascia and tendon of left middle finger at wrist and hand level   CC

√7ᵗʰ **S66.124** Laceration of flexor muscle, fascia and tendon of right ring finger at wrist and hand level   CC

√7ᵗʰ **S66.125** Laceration of flexor muscle, fascia and tendon of left ring finger at wrist and hand level   CC

√7ᵗʰ **S66.126** Laceration of flexor muscle, fascia and tendon of right little finger at wrist and hand level   CC

√7ᵗʰ **S66.127** Laceration of flexor muscle, fascia and tendon of left little finger at wrist and hand level   CC

√7ᵗʰ **S66.128** Laceration of flexor muscle, fascia and tendon of other finger at wrist and hand level   CC

> Laceration of flexor muscle, fascia and tendon of specified finger with unspecified laterality at wrist and hand level

√7ᵗʰ **S66.129** Laceration of flexor muscle, fascia and tendon of unspecified finger at wrist and hand level   CC

√6ᵗʰ **S66.19** Other injury of flexor muscle, fascia and tendon of other and unspecified finger at wrist and hand level

√7ᵗʰ **S66.190** Other injury of flexor muscle, fascia and tendon of right index finger at wrist and hand level

√7ᵗʰ **S66.191** Other injury of flexor muscle, fascia and tendon of left index finger at wrist and hand level

☑ Additional Character Required   √x7ᵗʰ Placeholder   Unacceptable PDx   Questionable PDx   Manifestation   Unspecified Dx   H1-H14 HAC   HCC CMS-HCC Dx   HIV HIV Dx

ICD-10-CM 2020

1079

Chapter 19. Injury, Poisoning and Certain Other Consequences of External Causes

S66.002–S66.191

Chapter 19. Injury, Poisoning and Certain Other Consequences of External Causes

√7ᵗʰ **S66.192** Other injury of flexor muscle, fascia and tendon of **right middle** finger at wrist and hand level

√7ᵗʰ **S66.193** Other injury of flexor muscle, fascia and tendon of **left middle** finger at wrist and hand level

√7ᵗʰ **S66.194** Other injury of flexor muscle, fascia and tendon of **right ring** finger at wrist and hand level

√7ᵗʰ **S66.195** Other injury of flexor muscle, fascia and tendon of **left ring** finger at wrist and hand level

√7ᵗʰ **S66.196** Other injury of flexor muscle, fascia and tendon of **right little** finger at wrist and hand level

√7ᵗʰ **S66.197** Other injury of flexor muscle, fascia and tendon of **left little** finger at wrist and hand level

√7ᵗʰ **S66.198** Other injury of flexor muscle, fascia and tendon of other finger at wrist and hand level

Other injury of flexor muscle, tendon of specified finger with unspecified laterality at wrist and hand level

√7ᵗʰ **S66.199** Other injury of flexor muscle, fascia and tendon of unspecified finger at wrist and hand level

√5ᵗʰ **S66.2** Injury of **extensor** muscle, fascia and tendon of **thumb** at wrist and hand level

√6ᵗʰ **S66.20** Unspecified injury of extensor muscle, fascia and tendon of thumb at wrist and hand level

√7ᵗʰ **S66.201** Unspecified injury of extensor muscle, fascia and tendon of **right** thumb at wrist and hand level

√7ᵗʰ **S66.202** Unspecified injury of extensor muscle, fascia and tendon of **left** thumb at wrist and hand level

√7ᵗʰ **S66.209** Unspecified injury of extensor muscle, fascia and tendon of unspecified thumb at wrist and hand level

√6ᵗʰ **S66.21** Strain of extensor muscle, fascia and tendon of thumb at wrist and hand level

√7ᵗʰ **S66.211** Strain of extensor muscle, fascia and tendon of **right** thumb at wrist and hand level

√7ᵗʰ **S66.212** Strain of extensor muscle, fascia and tendon of **left** thumb at wrist and hand level

√7ᵗʰ **S66.219** Strain of extensor muscle, fascia and tendon of unspecified thumb at wrist and hand level

√6ᵗʰ **S66.22** Laceration of extensor muscle, fascia and tendon of thumb at wrist and hand level

√7ᵗʰ **S66.221** Laceration of extensor muscle, fascia and tendon of **right** thumb at wrist and hand level   `CC`

√7ᵗʰ **S66.222** Laceration of extensor muscle, fascia and tendon of **left** thumb at wrist and hand level   `CC`

√7ᵗʰ **S66.229** Laceration of extensor muscle, fascia and tendon of unspecified thumb at wrist and hand level   `CC`

√6ᵗʰ **S66.29** Other specified injury of extensor muscle, fascia and tendon of thumb at wrist and hand level

√7ᵗʰ **S66.291** Other specified injury of extensor muscle, fascia and tendon of **right** thumb at wrist and hand level

√7ᵗʰ **S66.292** Other specified injury of extensor muscle, fascia and tendon of **left** thumb at wrist and hand level

√7ᵗʰ **S66.299** Other specified injury of extensor muscle, fascia and tendon of unspecified thumb at wrist and hand level

√5ᵗʰ **S66.3** Injury of **extensor** muscle, fascia and tendon of other and unspecified **finger** at wrist and hand level

EXCLUDES 2   injury of extensor muscle, fascia and tendon of thumb at wrist and hand level (S66.2-)

√6ᵗʰ **S66.30** Unspecified injury of extensor muscle, fascia and tendon of other and unspecified finger at wrist and hand level

√7ᵗʰ **S66.300** Unspecified injury of extensor muscle, fascia and tendon of **right index** finger at wrist and hand level

√7ᵗʰ **S66.301** Unspecified injury of extensor muscle, fascia and tendon of **left index** finger at wrist and hand level

√7ᵗʰ **S66.302** Unspecified injury of extensor muscle, fascia and tendon of **right middle** finger at wrist and hand level

√7ᵗʰ **S66.303** Unspecified injury of extensor muscle, fascia and tendon of **left middle** finger at wrist and hand level

√7ᵗʰ **S66.304** Unspecified injury of extensor muscle, fascia and tendon of **right ring** finger at wrist and hand level

√7ᵗʰ **S66.305** Unspecified injury of extensor muscle, fascia and tendon of **left ring** finger at wrist and hand level

√7ᵗʰ **S66.306** Unspecified injury of extensor muscle, fascia and tendon of **right little** finger at wrist and hand level

√7ᵗʰ **S66.307** Unspecified injury of extensor muscle, fascia and tendon of **left little** finger at wrist and hand level

√7ᵗʰ **S66.308** Unspecified injury of extensor muscle, fascia and tendon of other finger at wrist and hand level

Unspecified injury of extensor muscle, fascia and tendon of specified finger with unspecified laterality at wrist and hand level

√7ᵗʰ **S66.309** Unspecified injury of extensor muscle, fascia and tendon of unspecified finger at wrist and hand level

√6ᵗʰ **S66.31** Strain of extensor muscle, fascia and tendon of other and unspecified finger at wrist and hand level

√7ᵗʰ **S66.310** Strain of extensor muscle, fascia and tendon of **right index** finger at wrist and hand level

√7ᵗʰ **S66.311** Strain of extensor muscle, fascia and tendon of **left index** finger at wrist and hand level

√7ᵗʰ **S66.312** Strain of extensor muscle, fascia and tendon of **right middle** finger at wrist and hand level

√7ᵗʰ **S66.313** Strain of extensor muscle, fascia and tendon of **left middle** finger at wrist and hand level

√7ᵗʰ **S66.314** Strain of extensor muscle, fascia and tendon of **right ring** finger at wrist and hand level

√7ᵗʰ **S66.315** Strain of extensor muscle, fascia and tendon of **left ring** finger at wrist and hand level

√7ᵗʰ **S66.316** Strain of extensor muscle, fascia and tendon of **right little** finger at wrist and hand level

√7ᵗʰ **S66.317** Strain of extensor muscle, fascia and tendon of **left little** finger at wrist and hand level

√7ᵗʰ **S66.318** Strain of extensor muscle, fascia and tendon of other finger at wrist and hand level

Strain of extensor muscle, fascia and tendon of specified finger with unspecified laterality at wrist and hand level

√7ᵗʰ **S66.319** Strain of extensor muscle, fascia and tendon of unspecified finger at wrist and hand level

√6ᵗʰ **S66.32** Laceration of extensor muscle, fascia and tendon of other and unspecified finger at wrist and hand level

√7ᵗʰ **S66.320** Laceration of extensor muscle, fascia and tendon of **right index** finger at wrist and hand level   `CC`

N Newborn: 0   P Pediatric: 0-17   M Maternity: 9-64   A Adult: 15-124   **MCC** Major Complication/Comorbidity   **CC** Complication/Comorbidity   **SW** Severe Wound Dx

1080   ICD-10-CM 2020

√7ᵗʰ **S66.321** Laceration of extensor muscle, fascia and tendon of **left index** finger at wrist and hand level   CC

√7ᵗʰ **S66.322** Laceration of extensor muscle, fascia and tendon of **right middle** finger at wrist and hand level   CC

√7ᵗʰ **S66.323** Laceration of extensor muscle, fascia and tendon of **left middle** finger at wrist and hand level   CC

√7ᵗʰ **S66.324** Laceration of extensor muscle, fascia and tendon of **right ring** finger at wrist and hand level   CC

√7ᵗʰ **S66.325** Laceration of extensor muscle, fascia and tendon of **left ring** finger at wrist and hand level   CC

√7ᵗʰ **S66.326** Laceration of extensor muscle, fascia and tendon of **right little** finger at wrist and hand level   CC

√7ᵗʰ **S66.327** Laceration of extensor muscle, fascia and tendon of **left little** finger at wrist and hand level   CC

√7ᵗʰ **S66.328** Laceration of extensor muscle, fascia and tendon of **other finger** at wrist and hand level   CC

     Laceration of extensor muscle, fascia and tendon of specified finger with unspecified laterality at wrist and hand level

√7ᵗʰ **S66.329** Laceration of extensor muscle, fascia and tendon of **unspecified finger** at wrist and hand level   CC

√6ᵗʰ **S66.39** Other injury of extensor muscle, fascia and tendon of other and unspecified finger at wrist and hand level

√7ᵗʰ **S66.390** Other injury of extensor muscle, fascia and tendon of **right index** finger at wrist and hand level

√7ᵗʰ **S66.391** Other injury of extensor muscle, fascia and tendon of **left index** finger at wrist and hand level

√7ᵗʰ **S66.392** Other injury of extensor muscle, fascia and tendon of **right middle** finger at wrist and hand level

√7ᵗʰ **S66.393** Other injury of extensor muscle, fascia and tendon of **left middle** finger at wrist and hand level

√7ᵗʰ **S66.394** Other injury of extensor muscle, fascia and tendon of **right ring** finger at wrist and hand level

√7ᵗʰ **S66.395** Other injury of extensor muscle, fascia and tendon of **left ring** finger at wrist and hand level

√7ᵗʰ **S66.396** Other injury of extensor muscle, fascia and tendon of **right little** finger at wrist and hand level

√7ᵗʰ **S66.397** Other injury of extensor muscle, fascia and tendon of **left little** finger at wrist and hand level

√7ᵗʰ **S66.398** Other injury of extensor muscle, fascia and tendon of **other finger** at wrist and hand level

     Other injury of extensor muscle, fascia and tendon of specified finger with unspecified laterality at wrist and hand level

√7ᵗʰ **S66.399** Other injury of extensor muscle, fascia and tendon of **unspecified finger** at wrist and hand level

√5ᵗʰ **S66.4** Injury of **intrinsic** muscle, fascia and tendon of **thumb** at wrist and hand level

√6ᵗʰ **S66.40** Unspecified injury of intrinsic muscle, fascia and tendon of thumb at wrist and hand level

√7ᵗʰ **S66.401** Unspecified injury of intrinsic muscle, fascia and tendon of **right** thumb at wrist and hand level

√7ᵗʰ **S66.402** Unspecified injury of intrinsic muscle, fascia and tendon of **left** thumb at wrist and hand level

√7ᵗʰ **S66.409** Unspecified injury of intrinsic muscle, fascia and tendon of **unspecified** thumb at wrist and hand level

√6ᵗʰ **S66.41** Strain of intrinsic muscle, fascia and tendon of thumb at wrist and hand level

√7ᵗʰ **S66.411** Strain of intrinsic muscle, fascia and tendon of **right** thumb at wrist and hand level

√7ᵗʰ **S66.412** Strain of intrinsic muscle, fascia and tendon of **left** thumb at wrist and hand level

√7ᵗʰ **S66.419** Strain of intrinsic muscle, fascia and tendon of **unspecified** thumb at wrist and hand level

√6ᵗʰ **S66.42** Laceration of intrinsic muscle, fascia and tendon of thumb at wrist and hand level

√7ᵗʰ **S66.421** Laceration of intrinsic muscle, fascia and tendon of **right** thumb at wrist and hand level   CC

√7ᵗʰ **S66.422** Laceration of intrinsic muscle, fascia and tendon of **left** thumb at wrist and hand level   CC

√7ᵗʰ **S66.429** Laceration of intrinsic muscle, fascia and tendon of **unspecified** thumb at wrist and hand level   CC

√6ᵗʰ **S66.49** Other specified injury of intrinsic muscle, fascia and tendon of thumb at wrist and hand level

√7ᵗʰ **S66.491** Other specified injury of intrinsic muscle, fascia and tendon of **right** thumb at wrist and hand level

√7ᵗʰ **S66.492** Other specified injury of intrinsic muscle, fascia and tendon of **left** thumb at wrist and hand level

√7ᵗʰ **S66.499** Other specified injury of intrinsic muscle, fascia and tendon of **unspecified** thumb at wrist and hand level

√5ᵗʰ **S66.5** Injury of **intrinsic** muscle, fascia and tendon of other and unspecified **finger** at wrist and hand level

     EXCLUDES 2   *injury of intrinsic muscle, fascia and tendon of thumb at wrist and hand level (S66.4-)*

√6ᵗʰ **S66.50** Unspecified injury of intrinsic muscle, fascia and tendon of other and unspecified finger at wrist and hand level

√7ᵗʰ **S66.500** Unspecified injury of intrinsic muscle, fascia and tendon of **right index** finger at wrist and hand level

√7ᵗʰ **S66.501** Unspecified injury of intrinsic muscle, fascia and tendon of **left index** finger at wrist and hand level

√7ᵗʰ **S66.502** Unspecified injury of intrinsic muscle, fascia and tendon of **right middle** finger at wrist and hand level

√7ᵗʰ **S66.503** Unspecified injury of intrinsic muscle, fascia and tendon of **left middle** finger at wrist and hand level

√7ᵗʰ **S66.504** Unspecified injury of intrinsic muscle, fascia and tendon of **right ring** finger at wrist and hand level

√7ᵗʰ **S66.505** Unspecified injury of intrinsic muscle, fascia and tendon of **left ring** finger at wrist and hand level

√7ᵗʰ **S66.506** Unspecified injury of intrinsic muscle, fascia and tendon of **right little** finger at wrist and hand level

√7ᵗʰ **S66.507** Unspecified injury of intrinsic muscle, fascia and tendon of **left little** finger at wrist and hand level

√7ᵗʰ **S66.508** Unspecified injury of intrinsic muscle, fascia and tendon of **other finger** at wrist and hand level

     Unspecified injury of intrinsic muscle, fascia and tendon of specified finger with unspecified laterality at wrist and hand level

√7ᵗʰ **S66.509** Unspecified injury of intrinsic muscle, fascia and tendon of **unspecified finger** at wrist and hand level

✔ Additional Character Required   √×7ᵗʰ Placeholder   Unacceptable PDx   Questionable PDx   Manifestation   Unspecified Dx   H1-H14 HAC   HCC CMS-HCC Dx   HIV HIV Dx

ICD-10-CM 2020   1081

✓6ᵗʰ **S66.51** Strain of intrinsic muscle, fascia and tendon of other and unspecified finger at wrist and hand level

     ✓7ᵗʰ **S66.510** Strain of intrinsic muscle, fascia and tendon of right index finger at wrist and hand level

     ✓7ᵗʰ **S66.511** Strain of intrinsic muscle, fascia and tendon of left index finger at wrist and hand level

     ✓7ᵗʰ **S66.512** Strain of intrinsic muscle, fascia and tendon of right middle finger at wrist and hand level

     ✓7ᵗʰ **S66.513** Strain of intrinsic muscle, fascia and tendon of left middle finger at wrist and hand level

     ✓7ᵗʰ **S66.514** Strain of intrinsic muscle, fascia and tendon of right ring finger at wrist and hand level

     ✓7ᵗʰ **S66.515** Strain of intrinsic muscle, fascia and tendon of left ring finger at wrist and hand level

     ✓7ᵗʰ **S66.516** Strain of intrinsic muscle, fascia and tendon of right little finger at wrist and hand level

     ✓7ᵗʰ **S66.517** Strain of intrinsic muscle, fascia and tendon of left little finger at wrist and hand level

     ✓7ᵗʰ **S66.518** Strain of intrinsic muscle, fascia and tendon of other finger at wrist and hand level

        Strain of intrinsic muscle, fascia and tendon of specified finger with unspecified laterality at wrist and hand level

     ✓7ᵗʰ **S66.519** Strain of intrinsic muscle, fascia and tendon of unspecified finger at wrist and hand level

✓6ᵗʰ **S66.52** Laceration of intrinsic muscle, fascia and tendon of other and unspecified finger at wrist and hand level

     ✓7ᵗʰ **S66.520** Laceration of intrinsic muscle, fascia and tendon of right index finger at wrist and hand level   CC

     ✓7ᵗʰ **S66.521** Laceration of intrinsic muscle, fascia and tendon of left index finger at wrist and hand level   CC

     ✓7ᵗʰ **S66.522** Laceration of intrinsic muscle, fascia and tendon of right middle finger at wrist and hand level   CC

     ✓7ᵗʰ **S66.523** Laceration of intrinsic muscle, fascia and tendon of left middle finger at wrist and hand level   CC

     ✓7ᵗʰ **S66.524** Laceration of intrinsic muscle, fascia and tendon of right ring finger at wrist and hand level   CC

     ✓7ᵗʰ **S66.525** Laceration of intrinsic muscle, fascia and tendon of left ring finger at wrist and hand level   CC

     ✓7ᵗʰ **S66.526** Laceration of intrinsic muscle, fascia and tendon of right little finger at wrist and hand level   CC

     ✓7ᵗʰ **S66.527** Laceration of intrinsic muscle, fascia and tendon of left little finger at wrist and hand level   CC

     ✓7ᵗʰ **S66.528** Laceration of intrinsic muscle, fascia and tendon of other finger at wrist and hand level   CC

        Laceration of intrinsic muscle, fascia and tendon of specified finger with unspecified laterality at wrist and hand level

     ✓7ᵗʰ **S66.529** Laceration of intrinsic muscle, fascia and tendon of unspecified finger at wrist and hand level   CC

✓6ᵗʰ **S66.59** Other injury of intrinsic muscle, fascia and tendon of other and unspecified finger at wrist and hand level

     ✓7ᵗʰ **S66.590** Other injury of intrinsic muscle, fascia and tendon of right index finger at wrist and hand level

     ✓7ᵗʰ **S66.591** Other injury of intrinsic muscle, fascia and tendon of left index finger at wrist and hand level

     ✓7ᵗʰ **S66.592** Other injury of intrinsic muscle, fascia and tendon of right middle finger at wrist and hand level

     ✓7ᵗʰ **S66.593** Other injury of intrinsic muscle, fascia and tendon of left middle finger at wrist and hand level

     ✓7ᵗʰ **S66.594** Other injury of intrinsic muscle, fascia and tendon of right ring finger at wrist and hand level

     ✓7ᵗʰ **S66.595** Other injury of intrinsic muscle, fascia and tendon of left ring finger at wrist and hand level

     ✓7ᵗʰ **S66.596** Other injury of intrinsic muscle, fascia and tendon of right little finger at wrist and hand level

     ✓7ᵗʰ **S66.597** Other injury of intrinsic muscle, fascia and tendon of left little finger at wrist and hand level

     ✓7ᵗʰ **S66.598** Other injury of intrinsic muscle, fascia and tendon of other finger at wrist and hand level

        Other injury of intrinsic muscle, fascia and tendon of specified finger with unspecified laterality at wrist and hand level

     ✓7ᵗʰ **S66.599** Other injury of intrinsic muscle, fascia and tendon of unspecified finger at wrist and hand level

✓5ᵗʰ **S66.8** Injury of other specified muscles, fascia and tendons at wrist and hand level

     ✓6ᵗʰ **S66.80** Unspecified injury of other specified muscles, fascia and tendons at wrist and hand level

        ✓7ᵗʰ **S66.801** Unspecified injury of other specified muscles, fascia and tendons at wrist and hand level, right hand

        ✓7ᵗʰ **S66.802** Unspecified injury of other specified muscles, fascia and tendons at wrist and hand level, left hand

        ✓7ᵗʰ **S66.809** Unspecified injury of other specified muscles, fascia and tendons at wrist and hand level, unspecified hand

     ✓6ᵗʰ **S66.81** Strain of other specified muscles, fascia and tendons at wrist and hand level

        ✓7ᵗʰ **S66.811** Strain of other specified muscles, fascia and tendons at wrist and hand level, right hand

        ✓7ᵗʰ **S66.812** Strain of other specified muscles, fascia and tendons at wrist and hand level, left hand

        ✓7ᵗʰ **S66.819** Strain of other specified muscles, fascia and tendons at wrist and hand level, unspecified hand

     ✓6ᵗʰ **S66.82** Laceration of other specified muscles, fascia and tendons at wrist and hand level

        ✓7ᵗʰ **S66.821** Laceration of other specified muscles, fascia and tendons at wrist and hand level, right hand   CC

        ✓7ᵗʰ **S66.822** Laceration of other specified muscles, fascia and tendons at wrist and hand level, left hand   CC

        ✓7ᵗʰ **S66.829** Laceration of other specified muscles, fascia and tendons at wrist and hand level, unspecified hand   CC

     ✓6ᵗʰ **S66.89** Other injury of other specified muscles, fascia and tendons at wrist and hand level

        ✓7ᵗʰ **S66.891** Other injury of other specified muscles, fascia and tendons at wrist and hand level, right hand

        ✓7ᵗʰ **S66.892** Other injury of other specified muscles, fascia and tendons at wrist and hand level, left hand

N Newborn: 0   P Pediatric: 0-17   M Maternity: 9-64   A Adult: 15-124   MCC Major Complication/Comorbidity   CC Complication/Comorbidity   SW Severe Wound Dx

1082   ICD-10-CM 2020

✓7ᵗʰ **S66.899** Other injury of other specified muscles, fascia and tendons at wrist and hand level, unspecified hand

✓5ᵗʰ **S66.9** Injury of unspecified muscle, fascia and tendon at wrist and hand level

✓6ᵗʰ **S66.90** Unspecified injury of unspecified muscle, fascia and tendon at wrist and hand level

✓7ᵗʰ **S66.901** Unspecified injury of unspecified muscle, fascia and tendon at wrist and hand level, right hand

✓7ᵗʰ **S66.902** Unspecified injury of unspecified muscle, fascia and tendon at wrist and hand level, left hand

✓7ᵗʰ **S66.909** Unspecified injury of unspecified muscle, fascia and tendon at wrist and hand level, unspecified hand

✓6ᵗʰ **S66.91** Strain of unspecified muscle, fascia and tendon at wrist and hand level

✓7ᵗʰ **S66.911** Strain of unspecified muscle, fascia and tendon at wrist and hand level, right hand

✓7ᵗʰ **S66.912** Strain of unspecified muscle, fascia and tendon at wrist and hand level, left hand

✓7ᵗʰ **S66.919** Strain of unspecified muscle, fascia and tendon at wrist and hand level, unspecified hand

✓6ᵗʰ **S66.92** Laceration of unspecified muscle, fascia and tendon at wrist and hand level

✓7ᵗʰ **S66.921** Laceration of unspecified muscle, fascia and tendon at wrist and hand level, right hand　CC

✓7ᵗʰ **S66.922** Laceration of unspecified muscle, fascia and tendon at wrist and hand level, left hand　CC

✓7ᵗʰ **S66.929** Laceration of unspecified muscle, fascia and tendon at wrist and hand level, unspecified hand　CC

✓6ᵗʰ **S66.99** Other injury of unspecified muscle, fascia and tendon at wrist and hand level

✓7ᵗʰ **S66.991** Other injury of unspecified muscle, fascia and tendon at wrist and hand level, right hand

✓7ᵗʰ **S66.992** Other injury of unspecified muscle, fascia and tendon at wrist and hand level, left hand

✓7ᵗʰ **S66.999** Other injury of unspecified muscle, fascia and tendon at wrist and hand level, unspecified hand

✓4ᵗʰ **S67** Crushing injury of wrist, hand and fingers

Use additional code for all associated injuries, such as:
　fracture of wrist and hand (S62.-)
　open wound of wrist and hand (S61.-)

The appropriate 7th character is to be added to each code from category S67.
A　initial encounter
D　subsequent encounter
S　sequela

✓5ᵗʰ **S67.0** Crushing injury of thumb

✓x7ᵗʰ **S67.00** Crushing injury of unspecified thumb

✓x7ᵗʰ **S67.01** Crushing injury of right thumb

✓x7ᵗʰ **S67.02** Crushing injury of left thumb

✓5ᵗʰ **S67.1** Crushing injury of other and unspecified finger(s)

　　EXCLUDES 2　crushing injury of thumb (S67.0-)

✓x7ᵗʰ **S67.10** Crushing injury of unspecified finger(s)

✓6ᵗʰ **S67.19** Crushing injury of other finger(s)

✓7ᵗʰ **S67.190** Crushing injury of right index finger

✓7ᵗʰ **S67.191** Crushing injury of left index finger

✓7ᵗʰ **S67.192** Crushing injury of right middle finger

✓7ᵗʰ **S67.193** Crushing injury of left middle finger

✓7ᵗʰ **S67.194** Crushing injury of right ring finger

✓7ᵗʰ **S67.195** Crushing injury of left ring finger

✓7ᵗʰ **S67.196** Crushing injury of right little finger

✓7ᵗʰ **S67.197** Crushing injury of left little finger

✓7ᵗʰ **S67.198** Crushing injury of other finger
　　　Crushing injury of specified finger with unspecified laterality

✓5ᵗʰ **S67.2** Crushing injury of hand

　　EXCLUDES 2　crushing injury of fingers (S67.1-)
　　　　　crushing injury of thumb (S67.0-)

✓x7ᵗʰ **S67.20** Crushing injury of unspecified hand

✓x7ᵗʰ **S67.21** Crushing injury of right hand

✓x7ᵗʰ **S67.22** Crushing injury of left hand

✓5ᵗʰ **S67.3** Crushing injury of wrist

✓x7ᵗʰ **S67.30** Crushing injury of unspecified wrist

✓x7ᵗʰ **S67.31** Crushing injury of right wrist

✓x7ᵗʰ **S67.32** Crushing injury of left wrist

✓5ᵗʰ **S67.4** Crushing injury of wrist and hand

　　EXCLUDES 1　crushing injury of hand alone (S67.2-)
　　　　　crushing injury of wrist alone (S67.3-)
　　EXCLUDES 2　crushing injury of fingers (S67.1-)
　　　　　crushing injury of thumb (S67.0-)

✓x7ᵗʰ **S67.40** Crushing injury of unspecified wrist and hand

✓x7ᵗʰ **S67.41** Crushing injury of right wrist and hand

✓x7ᵗʰ **S67.42** Crushing injury of left wrist and hand

✓5ᵗʰ **S67.9** Crushing injury of unspecified part(s) of wrist, hand and fingers

✓x7ᵗʰ **S67.90** Crushing injury of unspecified part(s) of unspecified wrist, hand and fingers

✓x7ᵗʰ **S67.91** Crushing injury of unspecified part(s) of right wrist, hand and fingers

✓x7ᵗʰ **S67.92** Crushing injury of unspecified part(s) of left wrist, hand and fingers

✓4ᵗʰ **S68** Traumatic amputation of wrist, hand and fingers

An amputation not identified as partial or complete should be coded to complete.

The appropriate 7th character is to be added to each code from category S68.
A　initial encounter
D　subsequent encounter
S　sequela

CC Excl: For CC codes in category S68:
Right side: PDX collection 1266
Left side: PDX collection 1267
Unspecified side: PDX collection 1268

✓5ᵗʰ **S68.0** Traumatic metacarpophalangeal amputation of thumb
　　　Traumatic amputation of thumb NOS

✓6ᵗʰ **S68.01** Complete traumatic metacarpophalangeal amputation of thumb

8 ✓7ᵗʰ **S68.011** Complete traumatic metacarpophalangeal amputation of right thumb　HCC

8 ✓7ᵗʰ **S68.012** Complete traumatic metacarpophalangeal amputation of left thumb　HCC

8 ✓7ᵗʰ **S68.019** Complete traumatic metacarpophalangeal amputation of unspecified thumb　HCC

✓6ᵗʰ **S68.02** Partial traumatic metacarpophalangeal amputation of thumb

8 ✓7ᵗʰ **S68.021** Partial traumatic metacarpophalangeal amputation of right thumb　HCC

8 ✓7ᵗʰ **S68.022** Partial traumatic metacarpophalangeal amputation of left thumb　HCC

8 ✓7ᵗʰ **S68.029** Partial traumatic metacarpophalangeal amputation of unspecified thumb　HCC

Chapter 19. Injury, Poisoning and Certain Other Consequences of External Causes

S68.1–S68.613

√5ᵗʰ **S68.1** **Traumatic metacarpophalangeal amputation of other and unspecified finger**

Traumatic amputation of finger NOS

EXCLUDES 2   *traumatic metacarpophalangeal amputation of thumb (S68.0-)*

√6ᵗʰ **S68.11** **Complete traumatic metacarpophalangeal amputation of other and unspecified finger**

8 √7ᵗʰ **S68.110** Complete traumatic metacarpophalangeal amputation of right index finger   HCC

8 √7ᵗʰ **S68.111** Complete traumatic metacarpophalangeal amputation of left index finger   HCC

8 √7ᵗʰ **S68.112** Complete traumatic metacarpophalangeal amputation of right middle finger   HCC

8 √7ᵗʰ **S68.113** Complete traumatic metacarpophalangeal amputation of left middle finger   HCC

8 √7ᵗʰ **S68.114** Complete traumatic metacarpophalangeal amputation of right ring finger   HCC

8 √7ᵗʰ **S68.115** Complete traumatic metacarpophalangeal amputation of left ring finger   HCC

8 √7ᵗʰ **S68.116** Complete traumatic metacarpophalangeal amputation of right little finger   HCC

8 √7ᵗʰ **S68.117** Complete traumatic metacarpophalangeal amputation of left little finger   HCC

8 √7ᵗʰ **S68.118** Complete traumatic metacarpophalangeal amputation of other finger   HCC

Complete traumatic metacarpophalangeal amputation of specified finger with unspecified laterality

8 √7ᵗʰ **S68.119** Complete traumatic metacarpophalangeal amputation of unspecified finger   HCC

√6ᵗʰ **S68.12** **Partial traumatic metacarpophalangeal amputation of other and unspecified finger**

8 √7ᵗʰ **S68.120** Partial traumatic metacarpophalangeal amputation of right index finger   HCC

8 √7ᵗʰ **S68.121** Partial traumatic metacarpophalangeal amputation of left index finger   HCC

8 √7ᵗʰ **S68.122** Partial traumatic metacarpophalangeal amputation of right middle finger   HCC

8 √7ᵗʰ **S68.123** Partial traumatic metacarpophalangeal amputation of left middle finger   HCC

8 √7ᵗʰ **S68.124** Partial traumatic metacarpophalangeal amputation of right ring finger   HCC

8 √7ᵗʰ **S68.125** Partial traumatic metacarpophalangeal amputation of left ring finger   HCC

8 √7ᵗʰ **S68.126** Partial traumatic metacarpophalangeal amputation of right little finger   HCC

8 √7ᵗʰ **S68.127** Partial traumatic metacarpophalangeal amputation of left little finger   HCC

8 √7ᵗʰ **S68.128** Partial traumatic metacarpophalangeal amputation of other finger   HCC

Partial traumatic metacarpophalangeal amputation of specified finger with unspecified laterality

8 √7ᵗʰ **S68.129** Partial traumatic metacarpophalangeal amputation of unspecified finger   HCC

√5ᵗʰ **S68.4** **Traumatic amputation of hand at wrist level**

Traumatic amputation of hand NOS
Traumatic amputation of wrist

√6ᵗʰ **S68.41** **Complete traumatic amputation of hand at wrist level**

7 √7ᵗʰ **S68.411** Complete traumatic amputation of right hand at wrist level   CC HCC

7 √7ᵗʰ **S68.412** Complete traumatic amputation of left hand at wrist level   CC HCC

7 √7ᵗʰ **S68.419** Complete traumatic amputation of unspecified hand at wrist level   CC HCC

√6ᵗʰ **S68.42** **Partial traumatic amputation of hand at wrist level**

7 √7ᵗʰ **S68.421** Partial traumatic amputation of right hand at wrist level   CC HCC

7 √7ᵗʰ **S68.422** Partial traumatic amputation of left hand at wrist level   CC HCC

7 √7ᵗʰ **S68.429** Partial traumatic amputation of unspecified hand at wrist level   CC HCC

√5ᵗʰ **S68.5** **Traumatic transphalangeal amputation of thumb**

Traumatic interphalangeal joint amputation of thumb

√6ᵗʰ **S68.51** **Complete traumatic transphalangeal amputation of thumb**

8 √7ᵗʰ **S68.511** Complete traumatic transphalangeal amputation of right thumb   HCC

8 √7ᵗʰ **S68.512** Complete traumatic transphalangeal amputation of left thumb   HCC

8 √7ᵗʰ **S68.519** Complete traumatic transphalangeal amputation of unspecified thumb   HCC

√6ᵗʰ **S68.52** **Partial traumatic transphalangeal amputation of thumb**

8 √7ᵗʰ **S68.521** Partial traumatic transphalangeal amputation of right thumb   HCC

8 √7ᵗʰ **S68.522** Partial traumatic transphalangeal amputation of left thumb   HCC

8 √7ᵗʰ **S68.529** Partial traumatic transphalangeal amputation of unspecified thumb   HCC

√5ᵗʰ **S68.6** **Traumatic transphalangeal amputation of other and unspecified finger**

√6ᵗʰ **S68.61** **Complete traumatic transphalangeal amputation of other and unspecified finger(s)**

8 √7ᵗʰ **S68.610** Complete traumatic transphalangeal amputation of right index finger   HCC

8 √7ᵗʰ **S68.611** Complete traumatic transphalangeal amputation of left index finger   HCC

8 √7ᵗʰ **S68.612** Complete traumatic transphalangeal amputation of right middle finger   HCC

8 √7ᵗʰ **S68.613** Complete traumatic transphalangeal amputation of left middle finger   HCC

N Newborn: 0   P Pediatric: 0-17   M Maternity: 9-64   A Adult: 15-124   MCC Major Complication/Comorbidity   CC Complication/Comorbidity   SW Severe Wound Dx

1084   ICD-10-CM 2020

8 √7ᵗʰ **S68.614 Complete traumatic transphalangeal amputation of** right ring finger   `HCC`

8 √7ᵗʰ **S68.615 Complete traumatic transphalangeal amputation of** left ring finger   `HCC`

8 √7ᵗʰ **S68.616 Complete traumatic transphalangeal amputation of** right little finger   `HCC`

8 √7ᵗʰ **S68.617 Complete traumatic transphalangeal amputation of** left little finger   `HCC`

8 √7ᵗʰ **S68.618 Complete traumatic transphalangeal amputation of other** finger   `HCC`

Complete traumatic transphalangeal amputation of specified finger with unspecified laterality

8 √7ᵗʰ **S68.619 Complete traumatic transphalangeal amputation of unspecified** finger   `HCC`

√6ᵗʰ **S68.62 Partial traumatic transphalangeal amputation of other and unspecified finger**

8 √7ᵗʰ **S68.620 Partial traumatic transphalangeal amputation of** right index finger   `HCC`

8 √7ᵗʰ **S68.621 Partial traumatic transphalangeal amputation of** left index finger   `HCC`

8 √7ᵗʰ **S68.622 Partial traumatic transphalangeal amputation of** right middle finger   `HCC`

8 √7ᵗʰ **S68.623 Partial traumatic transphalangeal amputation of** left middle finger   `HCC`

8 √7ᵗʰ **S68.624 Partial traumatic transphalangeal amputation of** right ring finger   `HCC`

8 √7ᵗʰ **S68.625 Partial traumatic transphalangeal amputation of** left ring finger   `HCC`

8 √7ᵗʰ **S68.626 Partial traumatic transphalangeal amputation of** right little finger   `HCC`

8 √7ᵗʰ **S68.627 Partial traumatic transphalangeal amputation of** left little finger   `HCC`

8 √7ᵗʰ **S68.628 Partial traumatic transphalangeal amputation of other** finger   `HCC`

Partial traumatic transphalangeal amputation of specified finger with unspecified laterality

8 √7ᵗʰ **S68.629 Partial traumatic transphalangeal amputation of unspecified** finger   `HCC`

√5ᵗʰ **S68.7 Traumatic transmetacarpal amputation of hand**

√6ᵗʰ **S68.71 Complete traumatic transmetacarpal amputation of hand**

7 √7ᵗʰ **S68.711 Complete traumatic transmetacarpal amputation of** right hand   `CC` `HCC`

7 √7ᵗʰ **S68.712 Complete traumatic transmetacarpal amputation of** left hand   `CC` `HCC`

7 √7ᵗʰ **S68.719 Complete traumatic transmetacarpal amputation of unspecified hand**   `CC` `HCC`

√6ᵗʰ **S68.72 Partial traumatic transmetacarpal amputation of hand**

7 √7ᵗʰ **S68.721 Partial traumatic transmetacarpal amputation of** right hand   `CC` `HCC`

7 √7ᵗʰ **S68.722 Partial traumatic transmetacarpal amputation of** left hand   `CC` `HCC`

7 √7ᵗʰ **S68.729 Partial traumatic transmetacarpal amputation of unspecified hand**   `CC` `HCC`

√4ᵗʰ **S69 Other and unspecified injuries of wrist, hand and finger(s)**

The appropriate 7th character is to be added to each code from category S69.
A   initial encounter
D   subsequent encounter
S   sequela

√5ᵗʰ **S69.8 Other specified injuries of wrist, hand and finger(s)**

√x7ᵗʰ **S69.80 Other specified injuries of unspecified wrist, hand and finger(s)**

√x7ᵗʰ **S69.81 Other specified injuries of** right **wrist, hand and finger(s)**

√x7ᵗʰ **S69.82 Other specified injuries of** left **wrist, hand and finger(s)**

√5ᵗʰ **S69.9 Unspecified injury of wrist, hand and finger(s)**

√x7ᵗʰ **S69.90 Unspecified injury of unspecified wrist, hand and finger(s)**

√x7ᵗʰ **S69.91 Unspecified injury of** right **wrist, hand and finger(s)**

√x7ᵗʰ **S69.92 Unspecified injury of** left **wrist, hand and finger(s)**

Injuries to the hip and thigh (S70-S79)

`EXCLUDES 2`   *burns and corrosions (T20-T32)*
frostbite (T33-T34)
snake bite (T63.0-)
venomous insect bite or sting (T63.4-)

√4ᵗʰ **S70 Superficial injury of hip and thigh**

The appropriate 7th character is to be added to each code from category S70.
A   initial encounter
D   subsequent encounter
S   sequela

√5ᵗʰ **S70.0 Contusion of hip**

√x7ᵗʰ **S70.00 Contusion of unspecified hip**

√x7ᵗʰ **S70.01 Contusion of** right **hip**

√x7ᵗʰ **S70.02 Contusion of** left **hip**

√5ᵗʰ **S70.1 Contusion of thigh**

√x7ᵗʰ **S70.10 Contusion of unspecified thigh**

√x7ᵗʰ **S70.11 Contusion of** right **thigh**

√x7ᵗʰ **S70.12 Contusion of** left **thigh**

√5ᵗʰ **S70.2 Other superficial injuries of hip**

√6ᵗʰ **S70.21 Abrasion of hip**

√7ᵗʰ **S70.211 Abrasion,** right **hip**

√7ᵗʰ **S70.212 Abrasion,** left **hip**

√7ᵗʰ **S70.219 Abrasion, unspecified hip**

√6ᵗʰ **S70.22 Blister (nonthermal) of hip**

√7ᵗʰ **S70.221 Blister (nonthermal),** right **hip**

√7ᵗʰ **S70.222 Blister (nonthermal),** left **hip**

√7ᵗʰ **S70.229 Blister (nonthermal), unspecified hip**

√6ᵗʰ **S70.24 External constriction of hip**

√7ᵗʰ **S70.241 External constriction,** right **hip**

√7ᵗʰ **S70.242 External constriction,** left **hip**

√7ᵗʰ **S70.249 External constriction, unspecified hip**

√6ᵗʰ **S70.25 Superficial foreign body of hip**

Splinter in the hip

√7ᵗʰ **S70.251 Superficial foreign body,** right **hip**

√7ᵗʰ **S70.252 Superficial foreign body,** left **hip**

√7ᵗʰ **S70.259 Superficial foreign body, unspecified hip**

√6ᵗʰ **S70.26 Insect bite (nonvenomous) of hip**

√7ᵗʰ **S70.261 Insect bite (nonvenomous),** right **hip**

√7ᵗʰ **S70.262 Insect bite (nonvenomous),** left **hip**

√7ᵗʰ **S70.269** Insect bite (nonvenomous), unspecified hip

√6ᵗʰ **S70.27** Other superficial **bite** of hip

    EXCLUDES 1   *open bite of hip (S71.05-)*

√7ᵗʰ **S70.271** Other superficial bite of hip, right hip

√7ᵗʰ **S70.272** Other superficial bite of hip, left hip

√7ᵗʰ **S70.279** Other superficial bite of hip, unspecified hip

√5ᵗʰ **S70.3** Other superficial injuries of thigh

√6ᵗʰ **S70.31** Abrasion of thigh

√7ᵗʰ **S70.311** Abrasion, right thigh

√7ᵗʰ **S70.312** Abrasion, left thigh

√7ᵗʰ **S70.319** Abrasion, unspecified thigh

√6ᵗʰ **S70.32** Blister (nonthermal) of thigh

√7ᵗʰ **S70.321** Blister (nonthermal), right thigh

√7ᵗʰ **S70.322** Blister (nonthermal), left thigh

√7ᵗʰ **S70.329** Blister (nonthermal), unspecified thigh

√6ᵗʰ **S70.34** External constriction of thigh

√7ᵗʰ **S70.341** External constriction, right thigh

√7ᵗʰ **S70.342** External constriction, left thigh

√7ᵗʰ **S70.349** External constriction, unspecified thigh

√6ᵗʰ **S70.35** Superficial foreign body of thigh

    Splinter in the thigh

√7ᵗʰ **S70.351** Superficial foreign body, right thigh

√7ᵗʰ **S70.352** Superficial foreign body, left thigh

√7ᵗʰ **S70.359** Superficial foreign body, unspecified thigh

√6ᵗʰ **S70.36** Insect bite (nonvenomous) of thigh

√7ᵗʰ **S70.361** Insect bite (nonvenomous), right thigh

√7ᵗʰ **S70.362** Insect bite (nonvenomous), left thigh

√7ᵗʰ **S70.369** Insect bite (nonvenomous), unspecified thigh

√6ᵗʰ **S70.37** Other superficial **bite** of thigh

    EXCLUDES 1   *open bite of thigh (S71.15)*

√7ᵗʰ **S70.371** Other superficial bite of right thigh

√7ᵗʰ **S70.372** Other superficial bite of left thigh

√7ᵗʰ **S70.379** Other superficial bite of unspecified thigh

√5ᵗʰ **S70.9** Unspecified superficial injury of hip and thigh

√6ᵗʰ **S70.91** Unspecified superficial injury of hip

√7ᵗʰ **S70.911** Unspecified superficial injury of right hip

√7ᵗʰ **S70.912** Unspecified superficial injury of left hip

√7ᵗʰ **S70.919** Unspecified superficial injury of unspecified hip

√6ᵗʰ **S70.92** Unspecified superficial injury of thigh

√7ᵗʰ **S70.921** Unspecified superficial injury of right thigh

√7ᵗʰ **S70.922** Unspecified superficial injury of left thigh

√7ᵗʰ **S70.929** Unspecified superficial injury of unspecified thigh

√4ᵗʰ **S71** Open wound of hip and thigh

    Code also any associated wound infection

    EXCLUDES 1   *open fracture of hip and thigh (S72.-)*

               traumatic amputation of hip and thigh (S78.-)

    EXCLUDES 2   *bite of venomous animal (T63.-)*

               open wound of ankle, foot and toes (S91.-)

               open wound of knee and lower leg (S81.-)

> The appropriate 7th character is to be added to each code from category S71.
> A   initial encounter
> D   subsequent encounter
> S   sequela

√5ᵗʰ **S71.0** Open wound of hip

√6ᵗʰ **S71.00** Unspecified open wound of hip

√7ᵗʰ **S71.001** Unspecified open wound, right hip

√7ᵗʰ **S71.002** Unspecified open wound, left hip

√7ᵗʰ **S71.009** Unspecified open wound, unspecified hip

√6ᵗʰ **S71.01** Laceration without foreign body of hip

√7ᵗʰ **S71.011** Laceration without foreign body, right hip

√7ᵗʰ **S71.012** Laceration without foreign body, left hip

√7ᵗʰ **S71.019** Laceration without foreign body, unspecified hip

√6ᵗʰ **S71.02** Laceration with foreign body of hip

√7ᵗʰ **S71.021** Laceration with foreign body, right hip

√7ᵗʰ **S71.022** Laceration with foreign body, left hip

√7ᵗʰ **S71.029** Laceration with foreign body, unspecified hip

√6ᵗʰ **S71.03** Puncture wound without foreign body of hip

√7ᵗʰ **S71.031** Puncture wound without foreign body, right hip

√7ᵗʰ **S71.032** Puncture wound without foreign body, left hip

√7ᵗʰ **S71.039** Puncture wound without foreign body, unspecified hip

√6ᵗʰ **S71.04** Puncture wound with foreign body of hip

√7ᵗʰ **S71.041** Puncture wound with foreign body, right hip

√7ᵗʰ **S71.042** Puncture wound with foreign body, left hip

√7ᵗʰ **S71.049** Puncture wound with foreign body, unspecified hip

√6ᵗʰ **S71.05** Open bite of hip

    Bite of hip NOS

    EXCLUDES 1   *superficial bite of hip (S70.26, S70.27)*

√7ᵗʰ **S71.051** Open bite, right hip

√7ᵗʰ **S71.052** Open bite, left hip

√7ᵗʰ **S71.059** Open bite, unspecified hip

√5ᵗʰ **S71.1** Open wound of thigh

√6ᵗʰ **S71.10** Unspecified open wound of thigh

    AHA: 2016,3Q,24

√7ᵗʰ **S71.101** Unspecified open wound, right thigh

√7ᵗʰ **S71.102** Unspecified open wound, left thigh

√7ᵗʰ **S71.109** Unspecified open wound, unspecified thigh

√6ᵗʰ **S71.11** Laceration without foreign body of thigh

√7ᵗʰ **S71.111** Laceration without foreign body, right thigh

√7ᵗʰ **S71.112** Laceration without foreign body, left thigh

√7ᵗʰ **S71.119** Laceration without foreign body, unspecified thigh

√6ᵗʰ **S71.12** Laceration with foreign body of thigh

√7ᵗʰ **S71.121** Laceration with foreign body, right thigh

√7ᵗʰ **S71.122** Laceration with foreign body, left thigh

√7ᵗʰ **S71.129** Laceration with foreign body, unspecified thigh

√6ᵗʰ **S71.13** Puncture wound without foreign body of thigh

    AHA: 2016,3Q,24

√7ᵗʰ **S71.131** Puncture wound without foreign body, right thigh

√7ᵗʰ **S71.132** Puncture wound without foreign body, left thigh

√7ᵗʰ **S71.139** Puncture wound without foreign body, unspecified thigh

√6ᵗʰ **S71.14** Puncture wound with foreign body of thigh

    AHA: 2016,3Q,24

√7ᵗʰ **S71.141** Puncture wound with foreign body, right thigh

√7ᵗʰ **S71.142** Puncture wound with foreign body, left thigh

√7ᵗʰ **S71.149** Puncture wound with foreign body, unspecified thigh

√6ᵗʰ **S71.15** Open bite of thigh

    Bite of thigh NOS

    EXCLUDES 1   *superficial bite of thigh (S70.37-)*

√7ᵗʰ **S71.151** Open bite, right thigh

√7ᵗʰ **S71.152** Open bite, left thigh

√7ᵗʰ **S71.159** Open bite, unspecified thigh

N Newborn: 0   P Pediatric: 0-17   M Maternity: 9-64   A Adult: 15-124   MCC Major Complication/Comorbidity   CC Complication/Comorbidity   SW Severe Wound Dx

1086   ICD-10-CM 2020

✓4th S72 Fracture of femur

NOTE   A fracture not indicated as displaced or nondisplaced should be coded to displaced.

A fracture not indicated as open or closed should be coded to closed.

The open fracture designations are based on the Gustilo open fracture classification.

EXCLUDES 1   traumatic amputation of hip and thigh (S78.-)
EXCLUDES 2   fracture of lower leg and ankle (S82.-)
    fracture of foot (S92.-)
    periprosthetic fracture of prosthetic implant of hip (M97.0-)

AHA: 2018,2Q,12; 2016,1Q,33; 2015,3Q,37-39; 2015,1Q,17; 2013,4Q,128
DEF: Diaphysis: Central shaft of a long bone.
DEF: Epiphysis: Proximal and distal rounded ends of a long bone communicates with the joint.
DEF: Metaphysis: Section of a long bone located between the epiphysis and diaphysis at the proximal and distal ends.
DEF: Physis (growth plate): Narrow zone of cartilaginous tissue between the epiphysis and metaphysis at each end of a long bone. In childhood, proliferation of cells in this zone lengthens the bone. As the bone matures, this area thins, ossification eventually fusing into solid bone and growth stops. *Synonyms: Epiphyseal plate.*

The appropriate 7th character is to be added to all codes from category S72 [unless otherwise indicated].
A   initial encounter for closed fracture
B   initial encounter for open fracture type I or II
    initial encounter for open fracture NOS
C   initial encounter for open fracture type IIIA, IIIB, or IIIC
D   subsequent encounter for closed fracture with routine healing
E   subsequent encounter for open fracture type I or II with routine healing
F   subsequent encounter for open fracture type IIIA, IIIB, or IIIC with routine healing
G   subsequent encounter for closed fracture with delayed healing
H   subsequent encounter for open fracture type I or II with delayed healing
J   subsequent encounter for open fracture type IIIA, IIIB, or IIIC with delayed healing
K   subsequent encounter for closed fracture with nonunion
M   subsequent encounter for open fracture type I or II with nonunion
N   subsequent encounter for open fracture type IIIA, IIIB, or IIIC with nonunion
P   subsequent encounter for closed fracture with malunion
Q   subsequent encounter for open fracture type I or II with malunion
R   subsequent encounter for open fracture type IIIA, IIIB, or IIIC with malunion
S   sequela

✓5th S72.0 Fracture of head and neck of femur

EXCLUDES 2   physeal fracture of upper end of femur (S79.0-)
AHA: 2016,3Q,16
CC Excl: For CC/MCC codes in subcategory S72.0:
Right side: See code S72.001
Left side: See code S72.002
Unspecified side: See code S72.009

✓6th S72.00 Fracture of unspecified part of neck of femur

Fracture of hip NOS
Fracture of neck of femur NOS

4,6 ✓7th **S72.001** Fracture of unspecified   MCC CC H5 HCC
part of neck of right femur
CC Excl: MCC with 7th character A: PDX collection 1297
CC Excl: MCC with 7th character B or C: PDX collection 1298
CC Excl: CC with 7th character K, M, N, P, Q, or R: PDX collection 897

4,6 ✓7th **S72.002** Fracture of unspecified   MCC CC H5 HCC
part of neck of left femur
CC Excl: MCC with 7th character A: PDX collection 1299
CC Excl: MCC with 7th character B or C: PDX collection 1298
CC Excl: CC with 7th character K, M, N, P, Q, or R: PDX collection 897

4,6 ✓7th **S72.009** Fracture of unspecified   MCC CC H5 HCC
part of neck of unspecified femur
CC Excl: MCC with 7th character A, B or C: PDX collection 1298
CC Excl: CC with 7th character K, M, N, P, Q, or R: PDX collection 897

✓6th S72.01 Unspecified intracapsular fracture of femur

Subcapital fracture of femur

2,3,6 ✓7th **S72.011** Unspecified intracapsular MCC CC H5 HCC
fracture of right femur

2,3,6 ✓7th **S72.012** Unspecified intracapsular MCC CC H5 HCC
fracture of left femur

2,3,6 ✓7th **S72.019** Unspecified intracapsular MCC CC H5 HCC
fracture of unspecified femur

✓6th S72.02 Fracture of epiphysis (separation) (upper) of femur

Transepiphyseal fracture of femur
EXCLUDES 1   capital femoral epiphyseal fracture (pediatric) of femur (S79.01-)
    Salter-Harris Type I physeal fracture of upper end of femur (S79.01-)

4,6 ✓7th **S72.021** Displaced fracture of   MCC CC H5 HCC
epiphysis (separation) (upper) of right femur

4,6 ✓7th **S72.022** Displaced fracture of   MCC CC H5 HCC
epiphysis (separation) (upper) of left femur

4,6 ✓7th **S72.023** Displaced fracture of   MCC CC H5 HCC
epiphysis (separation) (upper) of unspecified femur

4,6 ✓7th **S72.024** Nondisplaced fracture of MCC CC H5 HCC
epiphysis (separation) (upper) of right femur

4,6 ✓7th **S72.025** Nondisplaced fracture of MCC CC H5 HCC
epiphysis (separation) (upper) of left femur

4,6 ✓7th **S72.026** Nondisplaced fracture of MCC CC H5 HCC
epiphysis (separation) (upper) of unspecified femur

✓6th S72.03 Midcervical fracture of femur

Transcervical fracture of femur NOS

4,6 ✓7th **S72.031** Displaced midcervical   MCC CC H5 HCC
fracture of right femur

4,6 ✓7th **S72.032** Displaced midcervical   MCC CC H5 HCC
fracture of left femur

4,6 ✓7th **S72.033** Displaced midcervical   MCC CC H5 HCC
fracture of unspecified femur

4,6 ✓7th **S72.034** Nondisplaced midcervical MCC CC H5 HCC
fracture of right femur

4,6 ✓7th **S72.035** Nondisplaced midcervical MCC CC H5 HCC
fracture of left femur

4,6 ✓7th **S72.036** Nondisplaced midcervical MCC CC H5 HCC
fracture of unspecified femur

✓6th S72.04 Fracture of base of neck of femur

Cervicotrochanteric fracture of femur

4,6 ✓7th **S72.041** Displaced fracture of base MCC CC H5 HCC
of neck of right femur

4,6 ✓7th **S72.042** Displaced fracture of base MCC CC H5 HCC
of neck of left femur

4,6 ✓7th **S72.043** Displaced fracture of base MCC CC H5 HCC
of neck of unspecified femur

4,6 ✓7th **S72.044** Nondisplaced fracture of MCC CC H5 HCC
base of neck of right femur

4,6 ✓7th **S72.045** Nondisplaced fracture of MCC CC H5 HCC
base of neck of left femur

4,6 ✓7th **S72.046** Nondisplaced fracture of MCC CC H5 HCC
base of neck of unspecified femur

✓6th S72.05 Unspecified fracture of head of femur

Fracture of head of femur NOS

4,6 ✓7th **S72.051** Unspecified fracture of   MCC CC H5 HCC
head of right femur

4,6 ✓7th **S72.052** Unspecified fracture of   MCC CC H5 HCC
head of left femur

Chapter 19. Injury, Poisoning and Certain Other Consequences of External Causes

4,6 √7ᵗʰ **S72.059** Unspecified fracture of head of unspecified femur `MCC` `CC` `H5` `HCC`

√6ᵗʰ **S72.06** Articular fracture of head of femur

4,6 √7ᵗʰ **S72.061** Displaced articular fracture of head of right femur `MCC` `CC` `H5` `HCC`

4,6 √7ᵗʰ **S72.062** Displaced articular fracture of head of left femur `MCC` `CC` `H5` `HCC`

4,6 √7ᵗʰ **S72.063** Displaced articular fracture of head of unspecified femur `MCC` `CC` `H5` `HCC`

4,6 √7ᵗʰ **S72.064** Nondisplaced articular fracture of head of right femur `MCC` `CC` `H5` `HCC`

4,6 √7ᵗʰ **S72.065** Nondisplaced articular fracture of head of left femur `MCC` `CC` `H5` `HCC`

4,6 √7ᵗʰ **S72.066** Nondisplaced articular fracture of head of unspecified femur `MCC` `CC` `H5` `HCC`

√6ᵗʰ **S72.09** Other fracture of head and neck of femur

4,6 √7ᵗʰ **S72.091** Other fracture of head and neck of right femur `MCC` `CC` `H5` `HCC`

4,6 √7ᵗʰ **S72.092** Other fracture of head and neck of left femur `MCC` `CC` `H5` `HCC`

4,6 √7ᵗʰ **S72.099** Other fracture of head and neck of unspecified femur `MCC` `CC` `H5` `HCC`

√5ᵗʰ **S72.1** Pertrochanteric fracture

> **AHA:** 2016,3Q,16
>
> **CC Excl: For CC/MCC codes in subcategory S72.1:**
> **Right side:** See code S72.001
> **Left side:** See code S72.002
> **Unspecified side:** See code S72.009

√6ᵗʰ **S72.10** Unspecified trochanteric fracture of femur

Fracture of trochanter NOS

4,6 √7ᵗʰ **S72.101** Unspecified trochanteric fracture of right femur `MCC` `CC` `H5` `HCC`

4,6 √7ᵗʰ **S72.102** Unspecified trochanteric fracture of left femur `MCC` `CC` `H5` `HCC`

4,6 √7ᵗʰ **S72.109** Unspecified trochanteric fracture of unspecified femur `MCC` `CC` `H5` `HCC`

√6ᵗʰ **S72.11** Fracture of greater trochanter of femur

2,3,6 √7ᵗʰ **S72.111** Displaced fracture of greater trochanter of right femur `MCC` `CC` `H5` `HCC`

2,3,6 √7ᵗʰ **S72.112** Displaced fracture of greater trochanter of left femur `MCC` `CC` `H5` `HCC`

2,3,6 √7ᵗʰ **S72.113** Displaced fracture of greater trochanter of unspecified femur `MCC` `CC` `H5` `HCC`

2,3,6 √7ᵗʰ **S72.114** Nondisplaced fracture of greater trochanter of right femur `MCC` `CC` `H5` `HCC`

2,3,6 √7ᵗʰ **S72.115** Nondisplaced fracture of greater trochanter of left femur `MCC` `CC` `H5` `HCC`

2,3,6 √7ᵗʰ **S72.116** Nondisplaced fracture of greater trochanter of unspecified femur `MCC` `CC` `H5` `HCC`

√6ᵗʰ **S72.12** Fracture of lesser trochanter of femur

2,3,6 √7ᵗʰ **S72.121** Displaced fracture of lesser trochanter of right femur `MCC` `CC` `H5` `HCC`

2,3,6 √7ᵗʰ **S72.122** Displaced fracture of lesser trochanter of left femur `MCC` `CC` `H5` `HCC`

2,3,6 √7ᵗʰ **S72.123** Displaced fracture of lesser trochanter of unspecified femur `MCC` `CC` `H5` `HCC`

2,3,6 √7ᵗʰ **S72.124** Nondisplaced fracture of lesser trochanter of right femur `MCC` `CC` `H5` `HCC`

2,3,6 √7ᵗʰ **S72.125** Nondisplaced fracture of lesser trochanter of left femur `MCC` `CC` `H5` `HCC`

2,3,6 √7ᵗʰ **S72.126** Nondisplaced fracture of lesser trochanter of unspecified femur `MCC` `CC` `H5` `HCC`

√6ᵗʰ **S72.13** Apophyseal fracture of femur

> **EXCLUDES 1**   chronic (nontraumatic) slipped upper femoral epiphysis (M93.0-)

2,3,6 √7ᵗʰ **S72.131** Displaced apophyseal fracture of right femur `MCC` `CC` `H5` `HCC`

2,3,6 √7ᵗʰ **S72.132** Displaced apophyseal fracture of left femur `MCC` `CC` `H5` `HCC`

2,3,6 √7ᵗʰ **S72.133** Displaced apophyseal fracture of unspecified femur `MCC` `CC` `H5` `HCC`

2,3,6 √7ᵗʰ **S72.134** Nondisplaced apophyseal fracture of right femur `MCC` `CC` `H5` `HCC`

2,3,6 √7ᵗʰ **S72.135** Nondisplaced apophyseal fracture of left femur `MCC` `CC` `H5` `HCC`

2,3,6 √7ᵗʰ **S72.136** Nondisplaced apophyseal fracture of unspecified femur `MCC` `CC` `H5` `HCC`

√6ᵗʰ **S72.14** Intertrochanteric fracture of femur

2,3,6 √7ᵗʰ **S72.141** Displaced intertrochanteric fracture of right femur `MCC` `CC` `H5` `HCC`

2,3,6 √7ᵗʰ **S72.142** Displaced intertrochanteric fracture of left femur `MCC` `CC` `H5` `HCC`

2,3,6 √7ᵗʰ **S72.143** Displaced intertrochanteric fracture of unspecified femur `MCC` `CC` `H5` `HCC`

2,3,6 √7ᵗʰ **S72.144** Nondisplaced intertrochanteric fracture of right femur `MCC` `CC` `H5` `HCC`

2,3,6 √7ᵗʰ **S72.145** Nondisplaced intertrochanteric fracture of left femur `MCC` `CC` `H5` `HCC`

2,3,6 √7ᵗʰ **S72.146** Nondisplaced intertrochanteric fracture of unspecified femur `MCC` `CC` `H5` `HCC`

√5ᵗʰ **S72.2** Subtrochanteric fracture of femur

> **CC Excl: For CC/MCC codes in subcategory S72.0:** See code S72.009

2,3,6 √x7ᵗʰ **S72.21** Displaced subtrochanteric fracture of right femur `MCC` `CC` `H5` `HCC`

2,3,6 √x7ᵗʰ **S72.22** Displaced subtrochanteric fracture of left femur `MCC` `CC` `H5` `HCC`

2,3,6 √x7ᵗʰ **S72.23** Displaced subtrochanteric fracture of unspecified femur `MCC` `CC` `H5` `HCC`

2,3,6 √x7ᵗʰ **S72.24** Nondisplaced subtrochanteric fracture of right femur `MCC` `CC` `H5` `HCC`

2,3,6 √x7ᵗʰ **S72.25** Nondisplaced subtrochanteric fracture of left femur `MCC` `CC` `H5` `HCC`

2,3,6 √x7ᵗʰ **S72.26** Nondisplaced subtrochanteric fracture of unspecified femur `MCC` `CC` `H5` `HCC`

√5ᵗʰ **S72.3** Fracture of shaft of femur

> **CC Excl: For CC/MCC codes in subcategory S72.3:**
> **Right side:** See code S72.001
> **Left side:** See code S72.002
> **Unspecified side:** See code S72.009

√6ᵗʰ **S72.30** Unspecified fracture of shaft of femur

2,3,6 √7ᵗʰ **S72.301** Unspecified fracture of shaft of right femur `MCC` `CC` `H5` `HCC`

2,3,6 √7ᵗʰ **S72.302** Unspecified fracture of shaft of left femur `MCC` `CC` `H5` `HCC`

2,3,6 √7ᵗʰ **S72.309** Unspecified fracture of shaft of unspecified femur `MCC` `CC` `H5` `HCC`

√6ᵗʰ **S72.32** Transverse fracture of shaft of femur

4,6 √7ᵗʰ **S72.321** Displaced transverse fracture of shaft of right femur `MCC` `CC` `H5` `HCC`

4,6 √7ᵗʰ **S72.322** Displaced transverse fracture of shaft of left femur `MCC` `CC` `H5` `HCC`

4,6 √7ᵗʰ **S72.323** Displaced transverse fracture of shaft of unspecified femur `MCC` `CC` `H5` `HCC`

4,6 √7ᵗʰ **S72.324** Nondisplaced transverse fracture of shaft of right femur `MCC` `CC` `H5` `HCC`

4,6 √7ᵗʰ **S72.325** Nondisplaced transverse fracture of shaft of left femur `MCC` `CC` `H5` `HCC`

4,6 √7ᵗʰ **S72.326** Nondisplaced transverse fracture of shaft of unspecified femur `MCC` `CC` `H5` `HCC`

`N` Newborn: 0   `P` Pediatric: 0-17   `M` Maternity: 9-64   `A` Adult: 15-124   `MCC` Major Complication/Comorbidity   `CC` Complication/Comorbidity   `SW` Severe Wound Dx

1088   ICD-10-CM 2020

√6ᵗʰ **S72.33**   Oblique **fracture of shaft of femur**

    4,6 √7ᵗʰ **S72.331** Displaced **oblique fracture** MCC CC H5 HCC **of shaft of right femur**

    4,6 √7ᵗʰ **S72.332** Displaced **oblique fracture** MCC CC H5 HCC **of shaft of left femur**

    4,6 √7ᵗʰ **S72.333** Displaced **oblique fracture** MCC CC H5 HCC **of shaft of unspecified femur**

    4,6 √7ᵗʰ **S72.334** Nondisplaced **oblique** MCC CC H5 HCC **fracture of shaft of right femur**

    4,6 √7ᵗʰ **S72.335** Nondisplaced **oblique** MCC CC H5 HCC **fracture of shaft of left femur**

    4,6 √7ᵗʰ **S72.336** Nondisplaced **oblique** MCC CC H5 HCC **fracture of shaft of unspecified femur**

√6ᵗʰ **S72.34**   Spiral **fracture of shaft of femur**

    4,6 √7ᵗʰ **S72.341** Displaced **spiral fracture** MCC CC H5 HCC **of shaft of right femur**

    4,6 √7ᵗʰ **S72.342** Displaced **spiral fracture** MCC CC H5 HCC **of shaft of left femur**

    4,6 √7ᵗʰ **S72.343** Displaced **spiral fracture** MCC CC H5 HCC **of shaft of unspecified femur**

    4,6 √7ᵗʰ **S72.344** Nondisplaced **spiral** MCC CC H5 HCC **fracture of shaft of right femur**

    4,6 √7ᵗʰ **S72.345** Nondisplaced **spiral** MCC CC H5 HCC **fracture of shaft of left femur**

    4,6 √7ᵗʰ **S72.346** Nondisplaced **spiral** MCC CC H5 HCC **fracture of shaft of unspecified femur**

√6ᵗʰ **S72.35**   Comminuted **fracture of shaft of femur**

    4,6 √7ᵗʰ **S72.351** Displaced **comminuted fracture of shaft of right femur** MCC CC H5 HCC

    4,6 √7ᵗʰ **S72.352** Displaced **comminuted fracture of shaft of left femur** MCC CC H5 HCC

    4,6 √7ᵗʰ **S72.353** Displaced **comminuted fracture of shaft of unspecified femur** MCC CC H5 HCC

    4,6 √7ᵗʰ **S72.354** Nondisplaced **comminuted fracture of shaft of right femur** MCC CC H5 HCC

    4,6 √7ᵗʰ **S72.355** Nondisplaced **comminuted fracture of shaft of left femur** MCC CC H5 HCC

    4,6 √7ᵗʰ **S72.356** Nondisplaced **comminuted fracture of shaft of unspecified femur** MCC CC H5 HCC

√6ᵗʰ **S72.36**   Segmental **fracture of shaft of femur**

    4,6 √7ᵗʰ **S72.361** Displaced **segmental fracture of shaft of right femur** MCC CC H5 HCC

    4,6 √7ᵗʰ **S72.362** Displaced **segmental fracture of shaft of left femur** MCC CC H5 HCC

    4,6 √7ᵗʰ **S72.363** Displaced **segmental fracture of shaft of unspecified femur** MCC CC H5 HCC

    4,6 √7ᵗʰ **S72.364** Nondisplaced **segmental fracture of shaft of right femur** MCC CC H5 HCC

    4,6 √7ᵗʰ **S72.365** Nondisplaced **segmental fracture of shaft of left femur** MCC CC H5 HCC

    4,6 √7ᵗʰ **S72.366** Nondisplaced **segmental fracture of shaft of unspecified femur** MCC CC H5 HCC

√6ᵗʰ **S72.39**   Other **fracture of shaft of femur**

    4,6 √7ᵗʰ **S72.391** Other **fracture of shaft of right femur** MCC CC H5 HCC

    4,6 √7ᵗʰ **S72.392** Other **fracture of shaft of left femur** MCC CC H5 HCC

    4,6 √7ᵗʰ **S72.399** Other **fracture of shaft of unspecified femur** MCC CC H5 HCC

√5ᵗʰ **S72.4**   Fracture of lower end of femur

    Fracture of distal end of femur

    EXCLUDES 2   *fracture of shaft of femur (S72.3-)*
             physeal fracture of lower end of femur (S79.1-)

    AHA: 2016,4Q,42

    CC Excl: For CC/MCC codes in subcategory S72.4, unless otherwise noted:
    Right side: See code S72.401
    Left side: See code S72.402
    Unspecified side: See code S72.409

√6ᵗʰ **S72.40**   Unspecified **fracture of lower end of femur**

    AHA: 2018,1Q,21; 2016,4Q,42

    2,3,6 √7ᵗʰ **S72.401** Unspecified **fracture of lower end of right femur** MCC CC H5 HCC
             CC Excl: CC with 7th character A: PDX collection 1300
             CC Excl: MCC with 7th character B or C: PDX collection 1301
             CC Excl: CC with 7th character K, M, N, P, Q, or R: PDX collection 897

    2,3,6 √7ᵗʰ **S72.402** Unspecified **fracture of lower end of left femur** MCC CC H5 HCC
             CC Excl: CC with 7th character A: PDX collection 1302
             CC Excl: MCC with 7th character B or C: PDX collection 1301
             CC Excl: CC with 7th character K, M, N, P, Q, or R: PDX collection 897

    2,3,6 √7ᵗʰ **S72.409** Unspecified **fracture of lower end of unspecified femur** MCC CC H5 HCC
             CC Excl: CC with 7th character A or MCC with 7th character B or C: PDX collection 1301
             CC Excl: CC with 7th character K, M, N, P, Q, or R: PDX collection 897

√6ᵗʰ **S72.41**   Unspecified condyle **fracture of lower end of femur**

    Condyle fracture of femur NOS

    2,3,6 √7ᵗʰ **S72.411** Displaced **unspecified condyle fracture of lower end of right femur** MCC CC H5 HCC

    2,3,6 √7ᵗʰ **S72.412** Displaced **unspecified condyle fracture of lower end of left femur** MCC CC H5 HCC

    2,3,6 √7ᵗʰ **S72.413** Displaced **unspecified condyle fracture of lower end of unspecified femur** MCC CC H5 HCC

    2,3,6 √7ᵗʰ **S72.414** Nondisplaced **unspecified** MCC CC H5 HCC **condyle fracture of lower end of right femur**

    2,3,6 √7ᵗʰ **S72.415** Nondisplaced **unspecified** MCC CC H5 HCC **condyle fracture of lower end of left femur**

    2,3,6 √7ᵗʰ **S72.416** Nondisplaced **unspecified** MCC CC H5 HCC **condyle fracture of lower end of unspecified femur**

√6ᵗʰ **S72.42**   Fracture of lateral condyle **of femur**

    2,3,6 √7ᵗʰ **S72.421** Displaced **fracture of lateral condyle of right femur** MCC CC H5 HCC

    2,3,6 √7ᵗʰ **S72.422** Displaced **fracture of lateral condyle of left femur** MCC CC H5 HCC

    2,3,6 √7ᵗʰ **S72.423** Displaced **fracture of lateral condyle of unspecified femur** MCC CC H5 HCC

    2,3,6 √7ᵗʰ **S72.424** Nondisplaced **fracture of** MCC CC H5 HCC **lateral condyle of right femur**

    2,3,6 √7ᵗʰ **S72.425** Nondisplaced **fracture of** MCC CC H5 HCC **lateral condyle of left femur**

    2,3,6 √7ᵗʰ **S72.426** Nondisplaced **fracture of** MCC CC H5 HCC **lateral condyle of unspecified femur**

√6ᵗʰ **S72.43**   Fracture of medial condyle **of femur**

    2,3,6 √7ᵗʰ **S72.431** Displaced **fracture of medial condyle of right femur** MCC CC H5 HCC

    2,3,6 √7ᵗʰ **S72.432** Displaced **fracture of medial condyle of left femur** MCC CC H5 HCC

Chapter 19. Injury, Poisoning and Certain Other Consequences of External Causes

2,3,6 √7ᵗʰ S72.433 Displaced **fracture of** medial condyle of unspecified **femur** `MCC` `CC` `H5` `HCC`

2,3,6 √7ᵗʰ S72.434 Nondisplaced **fracture of** medial condyle of right **femur** `MCC` `CC` `H5` `HCC`

2,3,6 √7ᵗʰ S72.435 Nondisplaced **fracture of** medial condyle of left **femur** `MCC` `CC` `H5` `HCC`

2,3,6 √7ᵗʰ S72.436 Nondisplaced **fracture of** medial condyle of unspecified **femur** `MCC` `CC` `H5` `HCC`

√6ᵗʰ S72.44 Fracture of lower epiphysis (separation) of femur

> **EXCLUDES 1**   *Salter-Harris Type I physeal fracture of lower end of femur (S79.11-)*

2,3,6 √7ᵗʰ S72.441 Displaced **fracture of** lower epiphysis (separation) of right **femur** `MCC` `CC` `H5` `HCC`

2,3,6 √7ᵗʰ S72.442 Displaced **fracture of** lower epiphysis (separation) of left **femur** `MCC` `CC` `H5` `HCC`

2,3,6 √7ᵗʰ S72.443 Displaced **fracture of** lower epiphysis (separation) of unspecified **femur** `MCC` `CC` `H5` `HCC`

2,3,6 √7ᵗʰ S72.444 Nondisplaced **fracture of** lower epiphysis (separation) of right **femur** `MCC` `CC` `H5` `HCC`

2,3,6 √7ᵗʰ S72.445 Nondisplaced **fracture of** lower epiphysis (separation) of left **femur** `MCC` `CC` `H5` `HCC`

2,3,6 √7ᵗʰ S72.446 Nondisplaced **fracture of** lower epiphysis (separation) of unspecified **femur** `MCC` `CC` `H5` `HCC`

√6ᵗʰ S72.45 Supracondylar fracture without intracondylar extension of lower end of femur

Supracondylar fracture of lower end of femur NOS

> **EXCLUDES 1**   *supracondylar fracture with intracondylar extension of lower end of femur (S72.46-)*

2,3,6 √7ᵗʰ S72.451 Displaced **supracondylar fracture without intracondylar extension of** lower end of right **femur** `MCC` `CC` `H5` `HCC`

2,3,6 √7ᵗʰ S72.452 Displaced **supracondylar fracture without intracondylar extension of** lower end of left **femur** `MCC` `CC` `H5` `HCC`

2,3,6 √7ᵗʰ S72.453 Displaced **supracondylar fracture without intracondylar extension of** lower end of unspecified **femur** `MCC` `CC` `H5` `HCC`

2,3,6 √7ᵗʰ S72.454 Nondisplaced supracondylar fracture without intracondylar extension of lower end of right **femur** `MCC` `CC` `H5` `HCC`

2,3,6 √7ᵗʰ S72.455 Nondisplaced supracondylar fracture without intracondylar extension of lower end of left **femur** `MCC` `CC` `H5` `HCC`

2,3,6 √7ᵗʰ S72.456 Nondisplaced supracondylar fracture without intracondylar extension of lower end of unspecified **femur** `MCC` `CC` `H5` `HCC`

√6ᵗʰ S72.46 Supracondylar fracture with intracondylar extension of lower end of femur

> **EXCLUDES 1**   *supracondylar fracture without intracondylar extension of lower end of femur (S72.45-)*

2,3,6 √7ᵗʰ S72.461 Displaced **supracondylar fracture with intracondylar extension of** lower end of right **femur** `MCC` `CC` `H5` `HCC`

2,3,6 √7ᵗʰ S72.462 Displaced **supracondylar fracture with intracondylar extension of** lower end of left **femur** `MCC` `CC` `H5` `HCC`

2,3,6 √7ᵗʰ S72.463 Displaced **supracondylar fracture with intracondylar extension of** lower end of unspecified **femur** `MCC` `CC` `H5` `HCC`

2,3,6 √7ᵗʰ S72.464 Nondisplaced supracondylar fracture with intracondylar extension of lower end of right **femur** `MCC` `CC` `H5` `HCC`

2,3,6 √7ᵗʰ S72.465 Nondisplaced supracondylar fracture with intracondylar extension of lower end of left **femur** `MCC` `CC` `H5` `HCC`

2,3,6 √7ᵗʰ S72.466 Nondisplaced supracondylar fracture with intracondylar extension of lower end of unspecified **femur** `MCC` `CC` `H5` `HCC`

√6ᵗʰ S72.47 Torus fracture of lower end of femur

> The appropriate 7th character is to be added to all codes in subcategory S72.47.
> A   initial encounter for closed fracture
> D   subsequent encounter for fracture with routine healing
> G   subsequent encounter for fracture with delayed healing
> K   subsequent encounter for fracture with nonunion
> P   subsequent encounter for fracture with malunion
> S   sequela

3,6 √7ᵗʰ S72.471 Torus fracture of lower end of right **femur** `CC` `H5` `HCC`

   CC Excl: CC with 7th character A: PDX collection 1300

   CC Excl: CC with 7th character K or P: PDX collection 897

3,6 √7ᵗʰ S72.472 Torus fracture of lower end of left **femur** `CC` `H5` `HCC`

   CC Excl: CC with 7th character A: PDX collection 1302

   CC Excl: CC with 7th character K or P: PDX collection 897

3,6 √7ᵗʰ S72.479 Torus fracture of lower end of unspecified **femur** `CC` `H5` `HCC`

   CC Excl: CC with 7th character A: PDX collection 1301

   CC Excl: CC with 7th character K or P: PDX collection 897

√6ᵗʰ S72.49 Other fracture of lower end of femur

2,3,6 √7ᵗʰ S72.491 Other fracture of lower end of right **femur** `MCC` `CC` `H5` `HCC`

   CC Excl: CC with 7th character A: PDX collection 1300

   CC Excl: MCC with 7th character B or C: PDX collection 1303

   CC Excl: CC with 7th character K, M, N, P, Q, or R: PDX collection 897

2,3,6 √7ᵗʰ S72.492 Other fracture of lower end of left **femur** `MCC` `CC` `H5` `HCC`

   CC Excl: CC with 7th character A: PDX collection 1302

   CC Excl: MCC with 7th character B or C: PDX collection 1303

   CC Excl: CC with 7th character K, M, N, P, Q, or R: PDX collection 897

2,3,6 √7ᵗʰ S72.499 Other fracture of lower end of unspecified **femur** `MCC` `CC` `H5` `HCC`

   CC Excl: CC with 7th character A: PDX collection 1301

   CC Excl: MCC with 7th character B or C: PDX collection 1303

   CC Excl: CC with 7th character K, M, N, P, Q, or R: PDX collection 897

Ⓝ Newborn: 0   Ⓟ Pediatric: 0-17   Ⓜ Maternity: 9-64   Ⓐ Adult: 15-124   `MCC` Major Complication/Comorbidity   `CC` Complication/Comorbidity   `SW` Severe Wound Dx

1090   ICD-10-CM 2020

√5ᵗʰ S72.8 Other fracture of femur

    √6ᵗʰ S72.8X Other fracture of femur

> **CC Excl: For codes in subcategory S72.8X:**
> MCC with 7th character A, B or C: PDX collection 1298
> CC with 7th character K, M, N, P, Q, or R: PDX collection 897

    4,6 √7ᵗʰ **S72.8X1 Other fracture of** right femur   MCC CC H5 HCC

    4,6 √7ᵗʰ **S72.8X2 Other fracture of** left femur   MCC CC H5 HCC

    4,6 √7ᵗʰ **S72.8X9 Other fracture of** unspecified femur   MCC CC H5 HCC

√5ᵗʰ S72.9 Unspecified fracture of femur

Fracture of thigh NOS
Fracture of upper leg NOS
EXCLUDES 1   *fracture of hip NOS (S72.00-, S72.01-)*

> **CC Excl: For codes in subcategory S72.9:**
> MCC with 7th character A, B or C: PDX collection 1298
> CC with 7th character K, M, N, P, Q, or R: PDX collection 897

    4,6 √x 7ᵗʰ **S72.90 Unspecified fracture of unspecified femur**   MCC CC H5 HCC

        AHA: 2012,4Q,93

    4,6 √x 7ᵗʰ **S72.91 Unspecified fracture of** right femur   MCC CC H5 HCC

    4,6 √x 7ᵗʰ **S72.92 Unspecified fracture of** left femur   MCC CC H5 HCC

√4ᵗʰ S73 Dislocation and sprain of joint and ligaments of hip

INCLUDES   avulsion of joint or ligament of hip
laceration of cartilage, joint or ligament of hip
sprain of cartilage, joint or ligament of hip
traumatic hemarthrosis of joint or ligament of hip
traumatic rupture of joint or ligament of hip
traumatic subluxation of joint or ligament of hip
traumatic tear of joint or ligament of hip

Code also any associated open wound
EXCLUDES 2   *strain of muscle, fascia and tendon of hip and thigh (S76.-)*

> The appropriate 7th character is to be added to each code from category S73.
> A   initial encounter
> D   subsequent encounter
> S   sequela

√5ᵗʰ S73.0 Subluxation and dislocation of hip

    EXCLUDES 2   *dislocation and subluxation of hip prosthesis (T84.020, T84.021)*

    √6ᵗʰ S73.00 Unspecified subluxation and dislocation of hip

Dislocation of hip NOS
Subluxation of hip NOS

> **CC Excl: For CC codes in subcategory S73.00:**
> **Right side:** PDX collection 1304
> **Left side:** PDX collection 1305
> **Unspecified side:** PDX collection 1306

    6 √7ᵗʰ **S73.001 Unspecified subluxation of right hip**   CC H5 HCC

    6 √7ᵗʰ **S73.002 Unspecified subluxation of left hip**   CC H5 HCC

    6 √7ᵗʰ **S73.003 Unspecified subluxation of unspecified hip**   CC H5 HCC

    6 √7ᵗʰ **S73.004 Unspecified dislocation of right hip**   CC H5 HCC

    6 √7ᵗʰ **S73.005 Unspecified dislocation of left hip**   CC H5 HCC

    6 √7ᵗʰ **S73.006 Unspecified dislocation of unspecified hip**   CC H5 HCC

    √6ᵗʰ S73.01 Posterior subluxation and dislocation of hip

> **CC Excl: For CC codes in subcategory S73.01:**
> **Right side:** PDX collection 1307
> **Left side:** PDX collection 1308
> **Unspecified side:** PDX collection 1309

    6 √7ᵗʰ **S73.011 Posterior subluxation of right hip**   CC H5 HCC

    6 √7ᵗʰ **S73.012 Posterior subluxation of left hip**   CC H5 HCC

    6 √7ᵗʰ **S73.013 Posterior subluxation of unspecified hip**   CC H5 HCC

    6 √7ᵗʰ **S73.014 Posterior dislocation of right hip**   CC H5 HCC

    6 √7ᵗʰ **S73.015 Posterior dislocation of left hip**   CC H5 HCC

    6 √7ᵗʰ **S73.016 Posterior dislocation of unspecified hip**   CC H5 HCC

√6ᵗʰ S73.02 Obturator subluxation and dislocation of hip

> **CC Excl: For CC codes in subcategory S73.02:**
> **Right side:** PDX collection 1310
> **Left side:** PDX collection 1311
> **Unspecified side:** PDX collection 1312

    6 √7ᵗʰ **S73.021 Obturator subluxation of right hip**   CC H5 HCC

    6 √7ᵗʰ **S73.022 Obturator subluxation of left hip**   CC H5 HCC

    6 √7ᵗʰ **S73.023 Obturator subluxation of unspecified hip**   CC H5 HCC

    6 √7ᵗʰ **S73.024 Obturator dislocation of right hip**   CC H5 HCC

    6 √7ᵗʰ **S73.025 Obturator dislocation of left hip**   CC H5 HCC

    6 √7ᵗʰ **S73.026 Obturator dislocation of unspecified hip**   CC H5 HCC

√6ᵗʰ S73.03 Other anterior subluxation and dislocation of hip

> **CC Excl: For CC codes in subcategory S73.03:**
> **Right side:** PDX collection 1313
> **Left side:** PDX collection 1314
> **Unspecified side:** PDX collection 1315

    6 √7ᵗʰ **S73.031 Other anterior subluxation of right hip**   CC H5 HCC

    6 √7ᵗʰ **S73.032 Other anterior subluxation of left hip**   CC H5 HCC

    6 √7ᵗʰ **S73.033 Other anterior subluxation of unspecified hip**   CC H5 HCC

    6 √7ᵗʰ **S73.034 Other anterior dislocation of right hip**   CC H5 HCC

    6 √7ᵗʰ **S73.035 Other anterior dislocation of left hip**   CC H5 HCC

    6 √7ᵗʰ **S73.036 Other anterior dislocation of unspecified hip**   CC H5 HCC

√6ᵗʰ S73.04 Central subluxation and dislocation of hip

> **CC Excl: For CC codes in subcategory S73.04:**
> **Right side:** PDX collection 1304
> **Left side:** PDX collection 1305
> **Unspecified side:** PDX collection 1306

    6 √7ᵗʰ **S73.041 Central subluxation of right hip**   CC H5 HCC

    6 √7ᵗʰ **S73.042 Central subluxation of left hip**   CC H5 HCC

    6 √7ᵗʰ **S73.043 Central subluxation of unspecified hip**   CC H5 HCC

    6 √7ᵗʰ **S73.044 Central dislocation of right hip**   CC H5 HCC

    6 √7ᵗʰ **S73.045 Central dislocation of left hip**   CC H5 HCC

    6 √7ᵗʰ **S73.046 Central dislocation of unspecified hip**   CC H5 HCC

√5ᵗʰ S73.1 Sprain of hip

    AHA: 2014,4Q,25

    √6ᵗʰ S73.10 Unspecified sprain of hip

    √7ᵗʰ **S73.101 Unspecified sprain of** right hip

    √7ᵗʰ **S73.102 Unspecified sprain of** left hip

    √7ᵗʰ **S73.109 Unspecified sprain of unspecified hip**

    √6ᵗʰ S73.11 Iliofemoral ligament sprain of hip

    √7ᵗʰ **S73.111 Iliofemoral ligament sprain of** right hip

    √7ᵗʰ **S73.112 Iliofemoral ligament sprain of** left hip

    √7ᵗʰ **S73.119 Iliofemoral ligament sprain of unspecified hip**

    √6ᵗʰ S73.12 Ischiocapsular (ligament) sprain of hip

    √7ᵗʰ **S73.121 Ischiocapsular ligament sprain of** right hip

    √7ᵗʰ **S73.122 Ischiocapsular ligament sprain of** left hip

    √7ᵗʰ **S73.129 Ischiocapsular ligament sprain of unspecified hip**

    √6ᵗʰ S73.19 Other sprain of hip

    √7ᵗʰ **S73.191 Other sprain of** right hip

    √7ᵗʰ **S73.192 Other sprain of** left hip

    √7ᵗʰ **S73.199 Other sprain of unspecified hip**

√4ᵗʰ **S74 Injury of nerves at hip and thigh level**

Code also any associated open wound (S71.-)

EXCLUDES 2   injury of nerves at ankle and foot level (S94.-)
          injury of nerves at lower leg level (S84.-)

The appropriate 7th character is to be added to each code from category S74.
A   initial encounter
D   subsequent encounter
S   sequela

√5ᵗʰ **S74.0 Injury of sciatic nerve at hip and thigh level**

√x7ᵗʰ **S74.00** Injury of sciatic nerve at hip and thigh level, unspecified leg

√x7ᵗʰ **S74.01** Injury of sciatic nerve at hip and thigh level, **right** leg

√x7ᵗʰ **S74.02** Injury of sciatic nerve at hip and thigh level, **left** leg

√5ᵗʰ **S74.1 Injury of femoral nerve at hip and thigh level**

√x7ᵗʰ **S74.10** Injury of femoral nerve at hip and thigh level, unspecified leg

√x7ᵗʰ **S74.11** Injury of femoral nerve at hip and thigh level, **right** leg

√x7ᵗʰ **S74.12** Injury of femoral nerve at hip and thigh level, **left** leg

√5ᵗʰ **S74.2 Injury of cutaneous sensory nerve at hip and thigh level**

√x7ᵗʰ **S74.20** Injury of cutaneous sensory nerve at hip and thigh level, unspecified leg

√x7ᵗʰ **S74.21** Injury of cutaneous sensory nerve at hip and high level, **right** leg

√x7ᵗʰ **S74.22** Injury of cutaneous sensory nerve at hip and thigh level, **left** leg

√5ᵗʰ **S74.8 Injury of other nerves at hip and thigh level**

√6ᵗʰ **S74.8X** Injury of other nerves at hip and thigh level

√7ᵗʰ **S74.8X1** Injury of other nerves at hip and thigh level, **right** leg

√7ᵗʰ **S74.8X2** Injury of other nerves at hip and thigh level, **left** leg

√7ᵗʰ **S74.8X9** Injury of other nerves at hip and thigh level, unspecified leg

√5ᵗʰ **S74.9 Injury of unspecified nerve at hip and thigh level**

√x7ᵗʰ **S74.90** Injury of unspecified nerve at hip and thigh level, unspecified leg

√x7ᵗʰ **S74.91** Injury of unspecified nerve at hip and thigh level, **right** leg

√x7ᵗʰ **S74.92** Injury of unspecified nerve at hip and thigh level, **left** leg

√4ᵗʰ **S75 Injury of blood vessels at hip and thigh level**

Code also any associated open wound (S71.-)

EXCLUDES 2   injury of blood vessels at lower leg level (S85.-)
          injury of popliteal artery (S85.0)

The appropriate 7th character is to be added to each code from category S75.
A   initial encounter
D   subsequent encounter
S   sequela

√5ᵗʰ **S75.0 Injury of femoral artery**

CC Excl: For MCC codes in subcategory S75.0:
Right side: PDX collection 1316
Left side: PDX collection 1317
Unspecified side: PDX collection 1318

√6ᵗʰ **S75.00** Unspecified injury of femoral artery

√7ᵗʰ **S75.001** Unspecified injury of femoral artery, **right** leg   MCC

√7ᵗʰ **S75.002** Unspecified injury of femoral artery, **left** leg   MCC

√7ᵗʰ **S75.009** Unspecified injury of femoral artery, unspecified leg   MCC

√6ᵗʰ **S75.01** Minor laceration of femoral artery

Incomplete transection of femoral artery
Laceration of femoral artery NOS
Superficial laceration of femoral artery

√7ᵗʰ **S75.011** Minor laceration of femoral artery, **right** leg   MCC

√7ᵗʰ **S75.012** Minor laceration of femoral artery, **left** leg   MCC

√7ᵗʰ **S75.019** Minor laceration of femoral artery, unspecified leg   MCC

√6ᵗʰ **S75.02** Major laceration of femoral artery

Complete transection of femoral artery
Traumatic rupture of femoral artery

√7ᵗʰ **S75.021** Major laceration of femoral artery, **right** leg   MCC

√7ᵗʰ **S75.022** Major laceration of femoral artery, **left** leg   MCC

√7ᵗʰ **S75.029** Major laceration of femoral artery, unspecified leg   MCC

√6ᵗʰ **S75.09** Other specified injury of femoral artery

√7ᵗʰ **S75.091** Other specified injury of femoral artery, **right** leg   MCC

√7ᵗʰ **S75.092** Other specified injury of femoral artery, **left** leg   MCC

√7ᵗʰ **S75.099** Other specified injury of femoral artery, unspecified leg   MCC

√5ᵗʰ **S75.1 Injury of femoral vein at hip and thigh level**

CC Excl: For MCC codes in subcategory S75.1:
Right side: PDX collection 1319
Left side: PDX collection 1320
Unspecified side: PDX collection 1321

√6ᵗʰ **S75.10** Unspecified injury of femoral vein at hip and thigh level

√7ᵗʰ **S75.101** Unspecified injury of femoral vein at hip and thigh level, **right** leg   MCC

√7ᵗʰ **S75.102** Unspecified injury of femoral vein at hip and thigh level, **left** leg   MCC

√7ᵗʰ **S75.109** Unspecified injury of femoral vein at hip and thigh level, unspecified leg   MCC

√6ᵗʰ **S75.11** Minor laceration of femoral vein at hip and thigh level

Incomplete transection of femoral vein at hip and thigh level
Laceration of femoral vein at hip and thigh level NOS
Superficial laceration of femoral vein at hip and thigh level

√7ᵗʰ **S75.111** Minor laceration of femoral vein at hip and thigh level, **right** leg   MCC

√7ᵗʰ **S75.112** Minor laceration of femoral vein at hip and thigh level, **left** leg   MCC

√7ᵗʰ **S75.119** Minor laceration of femoral vein at hip and thigh level, unspecified leg   MCC

√6ᵗʰ **S75.12** Major laceration of femoral vein at hip and thigh level

Complete transection of femoral vein at hip and thigh level
Traumatic rupture of femoral vein at hip and thigh level

√7ᵗʰ **S75.121** Major laceration of femoral vein at hip and thigh level, **right** leg   MCC

√7ᵗʰ **S75.122** Major laceration of femoral vein at hip and thigh level, **left** leg   MCC

√7ᵗʰ **S75.129** Major laceration of femoral vein at hip and thigh level, unspecified leg   MCC

√6ᵗʰ **S75.19** Other specified injury of femoral vein at hip and thigh level

√7ᵗʰ **S75.191** Other specified injury of femoral vein at hip and thigh level, **right** leg   MCC

√7ᵗʰ **S75.192** Other specified injury of femoral vein at hip and thigh level, **left** leg   MCC

√7ᵗʰ **S75.199** Other specified injury of femoral vein at hip and thigh level, unspecified leg   MCC

N Newborn: 0   P Pediatric: 0-17   M Maternity: 9-64   A Adult: 15-124   MCC Major Complication/Comorbidity   CC Complication/Comorbidity   SW Severe Wound Dx

1092   ICD-10-CM 2020

√5ᵗʰ **S75.2** **Injury of** greater saphenous vein **at hip and thigh level**

> EXCLUDES 1   greater saphenous vein NOS (S85.3)

> **CC Excl: For CC codes in subcategory S75.2:**
> **Right side:** PDX collection 1322
> **Left side:** PDX collection 1323
> **Unspecified side:** PDX collection 1324

√6ᵗʰ   **S75.20**   **Unspecified injury of greater saphenous vein at hip and thigh level**

√7ᵗʰ   **S75.201**   **Unspecified injury of greater saphenous vein at hip and thigh level,** right **leg**   CC

√7ᵗʰ   **S75.202**   **Unspecified injury of greater saphenous vein at hip and thigh level,** left **leg**   CC

√7ᵗʰ   **S75.209**   **Unspecified injury of greater saphenous vein at hip and thigh level, unspecified leg**   CC

√6ᵗʰ   **S75.21**   Minor laceration **of greater saphenous vein at hip and thigh level**

> Incomplete transection of greater saphenous vein at hip and thigh level
> Laceration of greater saphenous vein at hip and thigh level NOS
> Superficial laceration of greater saphenous vein at hip and thigh level

√7ᵗʰ   **S75.211**   **Minor laceration of greater saphenous vein at hip and thigh level,** right **leg**   CC

√7ᵗʰ   **S75.212**   **Minor laceration of greater saphenous vein at hip and thigh level,** left **leg**   CC

√7ᵗʰ   **S75.219**   **Minor laceration of greater saphenous vein at hip and thigh level, unspecified leg**   CC

√6ᵗʰ   **S75.22**   Major laceration **of greater saphenous vein at hip and thigh level**

> Complete transection of greater saphenous vein at hip and thigh level
> Traumatic rupture of greater saphenous vein at hip and thigh level

√7ᵗʰ   **S75.221**   **Major laceration of greater saphenous vein at hip and thigh level,** right **leg**   CC

√7ᵗʰ   **S75.222**   **Major laceration of greater saphenous vein at hip and thigh level,** left **leg**   CC

√7ᵗʰ   **S75.229**   **Major laceration of greater saphenous vein at hip and thigh level, unspecified leg**   CC

√6ᵗʰ   **S75.29**   **Other specified injury of greater saphenous vein at hip and thigh level**

√7ᵗʰ   **S75.291**   **Other specified injury of greater saphenous vein at hip and thigh level,** right **leg**   CC

√7ᵗʰ   **S75.292**   **Other specified injury of greater saphenous vein at hip and thigh level,** left **leg**   CC

√7ᵗʰ   **S75.299**   **Other specified injury of greater saphenous vein at hip and thigh level, unspecified leg**   CC

√5ᵗʰ **S75.8** **Injury of other blood vessels at hip and thigh level**

> **CC Excl: For CC codes in subcategory S75.8:**
> **Right side:** PDX collection 1325
> **Left side:** PDX collection 1326
> **Unspecified side:** PDX collection 1327

√6ᵗʰ   **S75.80**   **Unspecified injury of other blood vessels at hip and thigh level**

√7ᵗʰ   **S75.801**   **Unspecified injury of other blood vessels at hip and thigh level,** right **leg**   CC

√7ᵗʰ   **S75.802**   **Unspecified injury of other blood vessels at hip and thigh level,** left **leg**   CC

√7ᵗʰ   **S75.809**   **Unspecified injury of other blood vessels at hip and thigh level, unspecified leg**   CC

√6ᵗʰ   **S75.81**   Laceration **of other blood vessels at hip and thigh level**

√7ᵗʰ   **S75.811**   **Laceration of other blood vessels at hip and thigh level,** right **leg**   CC

√7ᵗʰ   **S75.812**   **Laceration of other blood vessels at hip and thigh level,** left **leg**   CC

√7ᵗʰ   **S75.819**   **Laceration of other blood vessels at hip and thigh level, unspecified leg**   CC

√6ᵗʰ   **S75.89**   **Other specified injury of other blood vessels at hip and thigh level**

√7ᵗʰ   **S75.891**   **Other specified injury of other blood vessels at hip and thigh level,** right **leg**   CC

√7ᵗʰ   **S75.892**   **Other specified injury of other blood vessels at hip and thigh level,** left **leg**   CC

√7ᵗʰ   **S75.899**   **Other specified injury of other blood vessels at hip and thigh level, unspecified leg**   CC

√5ᵗʰ **S75.9** **Injury of unspecified blood vessel at hip and thigh level**

> **CC Excl: For CC codes in subcategory S75.9:**
> **Right side:** PDX collection 1325
> **Left side:** PDX collection 1326
> **Unspecified side:** PDX collection 1327

√6ᵗʰ   **S75.90**   **Unspecified injury of unspecified blood vessel at hip and thigh level**

√7ᵗʰ   **S75.901**   **Unspecified injury of unspecified blood vessel at hip and thigh level,** right **leg**   CC

√7ᵗʰ   **S75.902**   **Unspecified injury of unspecified blood vessel at hip and thigh level,** left **leg**   CC

√7ᵗʰ   **S75.909**   **Unspecified injury of unspecified blood vessel at hip and thigh level, unspecified leg**   CC

√6ᵗʰ   **S75.91**   Laceration **of unspecified blood vessel at hip and thigh level**

√7ᵗʰ   **S75.911**   **Laceration of unspecified blood vessel at hip and thigh level,** right **leg**   CC

√7ᵗʰ   **S75.912**   **Laceration of unspecified blood vessel at hip and thigh level,** left **leg**   CC

√7ᵗʰ   **S75.919**   **Laceration of unspecified blood vessel at hip and thigh level, unspecified leg**   CC

√6ᵗʰ   **S75.99**   **Other specified injury of unspecified blood vessel at hip and thigh level**

√7ᵗʰ   **S75.991**   **Other specified injury of unspecified blood vessel at hip and thigh level,** right **leg**   CC

√7ᵗʰ   **S75.992**   **Other specified injury of unspecified blood vessel at hip and thigh level,** left **leg**   CC

√7ᵗʰ   **S75.999**   **Other specified injury of unspecified blood vessel at hip and thigh level, unspecified leg**   CC

✔ Additional Character Required   √x7ᵗʰ Placeholder   Unacceptable PDx   Questionable PDx   Manifestation   Unspecified Dx   H1-H14 HAC   HCC CMS-HCC Dx   HIV HIV Dx

ICD-10-CM 2020   1093

S75.2–S75.999

√4ᵗʰ **S76 Injury of muscle, fascia and tendon at hip and thigh level**

Code also any associated open wound (S71.-)

EXCLUDES 2   *injury of muscle, fascia and tendon at lower leg level (S86)*

            sprain of joint and ligament of hip (S73.1)

TIP: Refer to the Muscle/Tendon table at the beginning of this chapter.

> The appropriate 7th character is to be added to each code from category S76.
> A   initial encounter
> D   subsequent encounter
> S   sequela

CC Excl: For CC codes in category S76:
Right side: PDX collection 1328
Left side: PDX collection 1329
Unspecified side: PDX collection 1330

√5ᵗʰ **S76.0 Injury of muscle, fascia and tendon of hip**

  √6ᵗʰ **S76.00 Unspecified injury of muscle, fascia and tendon of hip**

    √7ᵗʰ **S76.001** Unspecified injury of muscle, fascia and tendon of right hip

    √7ᵗʰ **S76.002** Unspecified injury of muscle, fascia and tendon of left hip

    √7ᵗʰ **S76.009** Unspecified injury of muscle, fascia and tendon of unspecified hip

  √6ᵗʰ **S76.01 Strain of muscle, fascia and tendon of hip**

    √7ᵗʰ **S76.011** Strain of muscle, fascia and tendon of right hip

    √7ᵗʰ **S76.012** Strain of muscle, fascia and tendon of left hip

    √7ᵗʰ **S76.019** Strain of muscle, fascia and tendon of unspecified hip

  √6ᵗʰ **S76.02 Laceration of muscle, fascia and tendon of hip**

    √7ᵗʰ **S76.021** Laceration of muscle, fascia and tendon of right hip   CC

    √7ᵗʰ **S76.022** Laceration of muscle, fascia and tendon of left hip   CC

    √7ᵗʰ **S76.029** Laceration of muscle, fascia and tendon of unspecified hip   CC

  √6ᵗʰ **S76.09 Other specified injury of muscle, fascia and tendon of hip**

    √7ᵗʰ **S76.091** Other specified injury of muscle, fascia and tendon of right hip

    √7ᵗʰ **S76.092** Other specified injury of muscle, fascia and tendon of left hip

    √7ᵗʰ **S76.099** Other specified injury of muscle, fascia and tendon of unspecified hip

√5ᵗʰ **S76.1 Injury of quadriceps muscle, fascia and tendon**

  Injury of patellar ligament (tendon)

  √6ᵗʰ **S76.10 Unspecified injury of quadriceps muscle, fascia and tendon**

    √7ᵗʰ **S76.101** Unspecified injury of right quadriceps muscle, fascia and tendon

    √7ᵗʰ **S76.102** Unspecified injury of left quadriceps muscle, fascia and tendon

    √7ᵗʰ **S76.109** Unspecified injury of unspecified quadriceps muscle, fascia and tendon

  √6ᵗʰ **S76.11 Strain of quadriceps muscle, fascia and tendon**

    √7ᵗʰ **S76.111** Strain of right quadriceps muscle, fascia and tendon

    √7ᵗʰ **S76.112** Strain of left quadriceps muscle, fascia and tendon

    √7ᵗʰ **S76.119** Strain of unspecified quadriceps muscle, fascia and tendon

  √6ᵗʰ **S76.12 Laceration of quadriceps muscle, fascia and tendon**

    √7ᵗʰ **S76.121** Laceration of right quadriceps muscle, fascia and tendon   CC

    √7ᵗʰ **S76.122** Laceration of left quadriceps muscle, fascia and tendon   CC

    √7ᵗʰ **S76.129** Laceration of unspecified quadriceps muscle, fascia and tendon   CC

  √6ᵗʰ **S76.19 Other specified injury of quadriceps muscle, fascia and tendon**

    √7ᵗʰ **S76.191** Other specified injury of right quadriceps muscle, fascia and tendon

    √7ᵗʰ **S76.192** Other specified injury of left quadriceps muscle, fascia and tendon

    √7ᵗʰ **S76.199** Other specified injury of unspecified quadriceps muscle, fascia and tendon

√5ᵗʰ **S76.2 Injury of adductor muscle, fascia and tendon of thigh**

  √6ᵗʰ **S76.20 Unspecified injury of adductor muscle, fascia and tendon of thigh**

    √7ᵗʰ **S76.201** Unspecified injury of adductor muscle, fascia and tendon of right thigh

    √7ᵗʰ **S76.202** Unspecified injury of adductor muscle, fascia and tendon of left thigh

    √7ᵗʰ **S76.209** Unspecified injury of adductor muscle, fascia and tendon of unspecified thigh

  √6ᵗʰ **S76.21 Strain of adductor muscle, fascia and tendon of thigh**

    √7ᵗʰ **S76.211** Strain of adductor muscle, fascia and tendon of right thigh

    √7ᵗʰ **S76.212** Strain of adductor muscle, fascia and tendon of left thigh

    √7ᵗʰ **S76.219** Strain of adductor muscle, fascia and tendon of unspecified thigh

  √6ᵗʰ **S76.22 Laceration of adductor muscle, fascia and tendon of thigh**

    √7ᵗʰ **S76.221** Laceration of adductor muscle, fascia and tendon of right thigh   CC

    √7ᵗʰ **S76.222** Laceration of adductor muscle, fascia and tendon of left thigh   CC

    √7ᵗʰ **S76.229** Laceration of adductor muscle, fascia and tendon of unspecified thigh   CC

  √6ᵗʰ **S76.29 Other injury of adductor muscle, fascia and tendon of thigh**

    √7ᵗʰ **S76.291** Other injury of adductor muscle, fascia and tendon of right thigh

    √7ᵗʰ **S76.292** Other injury of adductor muscle, fascia and tendon of left thigh

    √7ᵗʰ **S76.299** Other injury of adductor muscle, fascia and tendon of unspecified thigh

√5ᵗʰ **S76.3 Injury of muscle, fascia and tendon of the posterior muscle group at thigh level**

  √6ᵗʰ **S76.30 Unspecified injury of muscle, fascia and tendon of the posterior muscle group at thigh level**

    √7ᵗʰ **S76.301** Unspecified injury of muscle, fascia and tendon of the posterior muscle group at thigh level, right thigh

    √7ᵗʰ **S76.302** Unspecified injury of muscle, fascia and tendon of the posterior muscle group at thigh level, left thigh

    √7ᵗʰ **S76.309** Unspecified injury of muscle, fascia and tendon of the posterior muscle group at thigh level, unspecified thigh

  √6ᵗʰ **S76.31 Strain of muscle, fascia and tendon of the posterior muscle group at thigh level**

    √7ᵗʰ **S76.311** Strain of muscle, fascia and tendon of the posterior muscle group at thigh level, right thigh

    √7ᵗʰ **S76.312** Strain of muscle, fascia and tendon of the posterior muscle group at thigh level, left thigh

    √7ᵗʰ **S76.319** Strain of muscle, fascia and tendon of the posterior muscle group at thigh level, unspecified thigh

  √6ᵗʰ **S76.32 Laceration of muscle, fascia and tendon of the posterior muscle group at thigh level**

    √7ᵗʰ **S76.321** Laceration of muscle, fascia and tendon of the posterior muscle group at thigh level, right thigh   CC

    √7ᵗʰ **S76.322** Laceration of muscle, fascia and tendon of the posterior muscle group at thigh level, left thigh   CC

    √7ᵗʰ **S76.329** Laceration of muscle, fascia and tendon of the posterior muscle group at thigh level, unspecified thigh   CC

  √6ᵗʰ **S76.39 Other specified injury of muscle, fascia and tendon of the posterior muscle group at thigh level**

    √7ᵗʰ **S76.391** Other specified injury of muscle, fascia and tendon of the posterior muscle group at thigh level, right thigh

Ⓝ Newborn: 0   Ⓟ Pediatric: 0-17   Ⓜ Maternity: 9-64   Ⓐ Adult: 15-124   **MCC** Major Complication/Comorbidity   **CC** Complication/Comorbidity   **SW** Severe Wound Dx

1094   ICD-10-CM 2020

√7ᵗʰ **S76.392** Other specified injury of muscle, fascia and tendon of the posterior muscle group at thigh level, left thigh

√7ᵗʰ **S76.399** Other specified injury of muscle, fascia and tendon of the posterior muscle group at thigh level, unspecified thigh

√5ᵗʰ **S76.8** Injury of other specified muscles, fascia and tendons at thigh level

√6ᵗʰ **S76.80** Unspecified injury of other specified muscles, fascia and tendons at thigh level

√7ᵗʰ **S76.801** Unspecified injury of other specified muscles, fascia and tendons at thigh level, right thigh

√7ᵗʰ **S76.802** Unspecified injury of other specified muscles, fascia and tendons at thigh level, left thigh

√7ᵗʰ **S76.809** Unspecified injury of other specified muscles, fascia and tendons at thigh level, unspecified thigh

√6ᵗʰ **S76.81** Strain of other specified muscles, fascia and tendons at thigh level

√7ᵗʰ **S76.811** Strain of other specified muscles, fascia and tendons at thigh level, right thigh

√7ᵗʰ **S76.812** Strain of other specified muscles, fascia and tendons at thigh level, left thigh

√7ᵗʰ **S76.819** Strain of other specified muscles, fascia and tendons at thigh level, unspecified thigh

√6ᵗʰ **S76.82** Laceration of other specified muscles, fascia and tendons at thigh level

√7ᵗʰ **S76.821** Laceration of other specified muscles, fascia and tendons at thigh level, right thigh   `CC`

√7ᵗʰ **S76.822** Laceration of other specified muscles, fascia and tendons at thigh level, left thigh   `CC`

√7ᵗʰ **S76.829** Laceration of other specified muscles, fascia and tendons at thigh level, unspecified thigh   `CC`

√6ᵗʰ **S76.89** Other injury of other specified muscles, fascia and tendons at thigh level

√7ᵗʰ **S76.891** Other injury of other specified muscles, fascia and tendons at thigh level, right thigh

√7ᵗʰ **S76.892** Other injury of other specified muscles, fascia and tendons at thigh level, left thigh

√7ᵗʰ **S76.899** Other injury of other specified muscles, fascia and tendons at thigh level, unspecified thigh

√5ᵗʰ **S76.9** Injury of unspecified muscles, fascia and tendons at thigh level

√6ᵗʰ **S76.90** Unspecified injury of unspecified muscles, fascia and tendons at thigh level

√7ᵗʰ **S76.901** Unspecified injury of unspecified muscles, fascia and tendons at thigh level, right thigh

√7ᵗʰ **S76.902** Unspecified injury of unspecified muscles, fascia and tendons at thigh level, left thigh

√7ᵗʰ **S76.909** Unspecified injury of unspecified muscles, fascia and tendons at thigh level, unspecified thigh

√6ᵗʰ **S76.91** Strain of unspecified muscles, fascia and tendons at thigh level

√7ᵗʰ **S76.911** Strain of unspecified muscles, fascia and tendons at thigh level, right thigh

√7ᵗʰ **S76.912** Strain of unspecified muscles, fascia and tendons at thigh level, left thigh

√7ᵗʰ **S76.919** Strain of unspecified muscles, fascia and tendons at thigh level, unspecified thigh

√6ᵗʰ **S76.92** Laceration of unspecified muscles, fascia and tendons at thigh level

√7ᵗʰ **S76.921** Laceration of unspecified muscles, fascia and tendons at thigh level, right thigh   `CC`

√7ᵗʰ **S76.922** Laceration of unspecified muscles, fascia and tendons at thigh level, left thigh   `CC`

√7ᵗʰ **S76.929** Laceration of unspecified muscles, fascia and tendons at thigh level, unspecified thigh   `CC`

√6ᵗʰ **S76.99** Other specified injury of unspecified muscles, fascia and tendons at thigh level

√7ᵗʰ **S76.991** Other specified injury of unspecified muscles, fascia and tendons at thigh level, right thigh

√7ᵗʰ **S76.992** Other specified injury of unspecified muscles, fascia and tendons at thigh level, left thigh

√7ᵗʰ **S76.999** Other specified injury of unspecified muscles, fascia and tendons at thigh level, unspecified thigh

√4ᵗʰ **S77** Crushing injury of hip and thigh

Use additional code(s) for all associated injuries

EXCLUDES 2   crushing injury of ankle and foot (S97.-)
              crushing injury of lower leg (S87.-)

The appropriate 7th character is to be added to each code from category S77.
A   initial encounter
D   subsequent encounter
S   sequela

√5ᵗʰ **S77.0** Crushing injury of hip

CC Excl: For CC codes in subcategory S77.0: PDX collection 1331

√x7ᵗʰ **S77.00** Crushing injury of unspecified hip   `CC` `H5`

√x7ᵗʰ **S77.01** Crushing injury of right hip   `CC` `H5`

√x7ᵗʰ **S77.02** Crushing injury of left hip   `CC` `H5`

√5ᵗʰ **S77.1** Crushing injury of thigh

CC Excl: For CC codes in subcategory S77.1: PDX collection 1332

√x7ᵗʰ **S77.10** Crushing injury of unspecified thigh   `CC` `H5`

√x7ᵗʰ **S77.11** Crushing injury of right thigh   `CC` `H5`

√x7ᵗʰ **S77.12** Crushing injury of left thigh   `CC` `H5`

√5ᵗʰ **S77.2** Crushing injury of hip with thigh

√x7ᵗʰ **S77.20** Crushing injury of unspecified hip with thigh

√x7ᵗʰ **S77.21** Crushing injury of right hip with thigh

√x7ᵗʰ **S77.22** Crushing injury of left hip with thigh

√4ᵗʰ **S78** Traumatic amputation of hip and thigh

An amputation not identified as partial or complete should be coded to complete

EXCLUDES 1   traumatic amputation of knee (S88.0-)

The appropriate 7th character is to be added to each code from category S78.
A   initial encounter
D   subsequent encounter
S   sequela

CC Excl: For CC codes in category S78:
Right side: PDX collection 1333
Left side: PDX collection 1334
Unspecified side: PDX collection 1335

√5ᵗʰ **S78.0** Traumatic amputation at hip joint

√6ᵗʰ **S78.01** Complete traumatic amputation at hip joint

√7ᵗʰ **S78.011** Complete traumatic amputation at right hip joint   `CC` `HCC`

√7ᵗʰ **S78.012** Complete traumatic amputation at left hip joint   `CC` `HCC`

√7ᵗʰ **S78.019** Complete traumatic amputation at unspecified hip joint   `CC` `HCC`

√6ᵗʰ **S78.02** Partial traumatic amputation at hip joint

√7ᵗʰ **S78.021** Partial traumatic amputation at right hip joint   `CC` `HCC`

√7ᵗʰ **S78.022** Partial traumatic amputation at left hip joint   `CC` `HCC`

√7ᵗʰ **S78.029** Partial traumatic amputation at unspecified hip joint   `CC` `HCC`

✔ Additional Character Required   √x7ᵗʰ Placeholder   Unacceptable PDx   Questionable PDx   Manifestation   Unspecified Dx   `H1`-`H14` HAC   `HCC` CMS-HCC Dx   `HIV` HIV Dx

ICD-10-CM 2020

1095

S76.392–S78.029

Chapter 19. Injury, Poisoning and Certain Other Consequences of External Causes

Chapter 19. Injury, Poisoning and Certain Other Consequences of External Causes

√5ᵗʰ **S78.1** Traumatic amputation at level between hip and knee
> EXCLUDES 1   traumatic amputation of knee (S88.Ø-)

√6ᵗʰ **S78.11** Complete traumatic amputation at level between hip and knee

     √7ᵗʰ **S78.111** Complete traumatic amputation at level between right hip and knee   `CC` `HCC`

     √7ᵗʰ **S78.112** Complete traumatic amputation at level between left hip and knee   `CC` `HCC`

     √7ᵗʰ **S78.119** Complete traumatic amputation at level between unspecified hip and knee   `CC` `HCC`

√6ᵗʰ **S78.12** Partial traumatic amputation at level between hip and knee

     √7ᵗʰ **S78.121** Partial traumatic amputation at level between right hip and knee   `CC` `HCC`

     √7ᵗʰ **S78.122** Partial traumatic amputation at level between left hip and knee   `CC` `HCC`

     √7ᵗʰ **S78.129** Partial traumatic amputation at level between unspecified hip and knee   `CC` `HCC`

√5ᵗʰ **S78.9** Traumatic amputation of hip and thigh, level unspecified

√6ᵗʰ **S78.91** Complete traumatic amputation of hip and thigh, level unspecified

     √7ᵗʰ **S78.911** Complete traumatic amputation of right hip and thigh, level unspecified   `CC` `HCC`

     √7ᵗʰ **S78.912** Complete traumatic amputation of left hip and thigh, level unspecified   `CC` `HCC`

     √7ᵗʰ **S78.919** Complete traumatic amputation of unspecified hip and thigh, level unspecified   `CC` `HCC`

√6ᵗʰ **S78.92** Partial traumatic amputation of hip and thigh, level unspecified

     √7ᵗʰ **S78.921** Partial traumatic amputation of right hip and thigh, level unspecified   `CC` `HCC`

     √7ᵗʰ **S78.922** Partial traumatic amputation of left hip and thigh, level unspecified   `CC` `HCC`

     √7ᵗʰ **S78.929** Partial traumatic amputation of unspecified hip and thigh, level unspecified   `CC` `HCC`

√4ᵗʰ **S79** Other and unspecified injuries of hip and thigh

> `NOTE`   A fracture not indicated as open or closed should be coded to closed

AHA: 2018,2Q,12; 2018,1Q,3; 2015,3Q,37-39

The appropriate 7th character is to be added to each code from subcategories S79.Ø and S79.1.
A   initial encounter for closed fracture
D   subsequent encounter for fracture with routine healing
G   subsequent encounter for fracture with delayed healing
K   subsequent encounter for fracture with nonunion
P   subsequent encounter for fracture with malunion
S   sequela

√5ᵗʰ **S79.Ø** Physeal fracture of upper end of femur
> EXCLUDES 1   apophyseal fracture of upper end of femur (S72.13-)
>   nontraumatic slipped upper femoral epiphysis (M93.Ø-)

CC Excl: For CC/MCC codes in subcategory S79.Ø:
Right side: See code S79.001
Left side: See code S79.002
Unspecified side: See code S79.009

√6ᵗʰ **S79.ØØ** Unspecified physeal fracture of upper end of femur

     4,6 √7ᵗʰ **S79.001** Unspecified physeal fracture of upper end of right femur   `MCC` `CC` `H5` `HCC`
     CC Excl: MCC with 7th character A: PDX collection 1297
     CC Excl: CC with 7th character K or P: PDX collection 897

     4,6 √7ᵗʰ **S79.002** Unspecified physeal fracture of upper end of left femur   `MCC` `CC` `H5` `HCC`
     CC Excl: MCC with 7th character A: PDX collection 1299
     CC Excl: CC with 7th character K or P: PDX collection 897

     4,6 √7ᵗʰ **S79.009** Unspecified physeal fracture of upper end of unspecified femur   `MCC` `CC` `H5` `HCC`
     CC Excl: MCC with 7th character A: PDX collection 1298
     CC Excl: CC with 7th character K or P: PDX collection 897

√6ᵗʰ **S79.01** Salter-Harris Type I physeal fracture of upper end of femur
   Acute on chronic slipped capital femoral epiphysis (traumatic)
   Acute slipped capital femoral epiphysis (traumatic)
   Capital femoral epiphyseal fracture
> EXCLUDES 1   chronic slipped upper femoral epiphysis (nontraumatic) (M93.Ø2-)

     4,6 √7ᵗʰ **S79.011** Salter-Harris Type I physeal fracture of upper end of right femur   `MCC` `CC` `H5` `HCC`

     4,6 √7ᵗʰ **S79.012** Salter-Harris Type I physeal fracture of upper end of left femur   `MCC` `CC` `H5` `HCC`

     4,6 √7ᵗʰ **S79.019** Salter-Harris Type I physeal fracture of upper end of unspecified femur   `MCC` `CC` `H5` `HCC`

√6ᵗʰ **S79.09** Other physeal fracture of upper end of femur

     4,6 √7ᵗʰ **S79.091** Other physeal fracture of upper end of right femur   `MCC` `CC` `H5` `HCC`

     4,6 √7ᵗʰ **S79.092** Other physeal fracture of upper end of left femur   `MCC` `CC` `H5` `HCC`

     4,6 √7ᵗʰ **S79.099** Other physeal fracture of upper end of unspecified femur   `MCC` `CC` `H5` `HCC`

N Newborn: 0   P Pediatric: 0-17   M Maternity: 9-64   A Adult: 15-124   `MCC` Major Complication/Comorbidity   `CC` Complication/Comorbidity   `SW` Severe Wound Dx

1096   ICD-10-CM 2020

✓5ᵗʰ **S79.1** **Physeal fracture of** lower end of femur

CC Excl: For CC/MCC codes in subcategory S79.1:
Right side: See code S79.101
Left side: See code S79.102
Unspecified side: See code S79.109

✓6ᵗʰ **S79.10** **Unspecified physeal fracture of lower end of femur**

3,6 ✓7ᵗʰ **S79.101** **Unspecified physeal fracture of lower end of right femur**   CC H5 HCC
CC Excl: CC with 7th character A: PDX collection 1300
CC Excl: CC with 7th character K or P: PDX collection 897

3,6 ✓7ᵗʰ **S79.102** **Unspecified physeal fracture of lower end of left femur**   CC H5 HCC
CC Excl: CC with 7th character A: PDX collection 1302
CC Excl: CC with 7th character K or P: PDX collection 897

3,6 ✓7ᵗʰ **S79.109** **Unspecified physeal fracture of lower end of unspecified femur**   CC H5 HCC
CC Excl: CC with 7th character A: PDX collection 1301
CC Excl: CC with 7th character K or P: PDX collection 897

✓6ᵗʰ **S79.11** **Salter-Harris Type I physeal fracture of lower end of femur**

3,6 ✓7ᵗʰ **S79.111** **Salter-Harris Type I physeal fracture of lower end of right femur**   CC H5 HCC

3,6 ✓7ᵗʰ **S79.112** **Salter-Harris Type I physeal fracture of lower end of left femur**   CC H5 HCC

3,6 ✓7ᵗʰ **S79.119** **Salter-Harris Type I physeal fracture of lower end of unspecified femur**   CC H5 HCC

✓6ᵗʰ **S79.12** **Salter-Harris Type II physeal fracture of lower end of femur**

3,6 ✓7ᵗʰ **S79.121** **Salter-Harris Type II physeal fracture of lower end of right femur**   CC H5 HCC

3,6 ✓7ᵗʰ **S79.122** **Salter-Harris Type II physeal fracture of lower end of left femur**   CC H5 HCC

3,6 ✓7ᵗʰ **S79.129** **Salter-Harris Type II physeal fracture of lower end of unspecified femur**   CC H5 HCC

✓6ᵗʰ **S79.13** **Salter-Harris Type III physeal fracture of lower end of femur**

3,6 ✓7ᵗʰ **S79.131** **Salter-Harris Type III physeal fracture of lower end of right femur**   CC H5 HCC

3,6 ✓7ᵗʰ **S79.132** **Salter-Harris Type III physeal fracture of lower end of left femur**   CC H5 HCC

3,6 ✓7ᵗʰ **S79.139** **Salter-Harris Type III physeal fracture of lower end of unspecified femur**   CC H5 HCC

✓6ᵗʰ **S79.14** **Salter-Harris Type IV physeal fracture of lower end of femur**

3,6 ✓7ᵗʰ **S79.141** **Salter-Harris Type IV physeal fracture of lower end of right femur**   CC H5 HCC

3,6 ✓7ᵗʰ **S79.142** **Salter-Harris Type IV physeal fracture of lower end of left femur**   CC H5 HCC

3,6 ✓7ᵗʰ **S79.149** **Salter-Harris Type IV physeal fracture of lower end of unspecified femur**   CC H5 HCC

✓6ᵗʰ **S79.19** **Other physeal fracture of lower end of femur**

3,6 ✓7ᵗʰ **S79.191** **Other physeal fracture of lower end of right femur**   CC H5 HCC

3,6 ✓7ᵗʰ **S79.192** **Other physeal fracture of lower end of left femur**   CC H5 HCC

3,6 ✓7ᵗʰ **S79.199** **Other physeal fracture of lower end of unspecified femur**   CC H5 HCC

✓5ᵗʰ **S79.8** **Other specified injuries of hip and thigh**

The appropriate 7th character is to be added to each code in subcategory S79.8.
A   initial encounter
D   subsequent encounter
S   sequela

✓6ᵗʰ **S79.81** **Other specified injuries of** hip

✓7ᵗʰ **S79.811** **Other specified injuries of** right hip

✓7ᵗʰ **S79.812** **Other specified injuries of** left hip

✓7ᵗʰ **S79.819** **Other specified injuries of unspecified hip**

✓6ᵗʰ **S79.82** **Other specified injuries of** thigh

✓7ᵗʰ **S79.821** **Other specified injuries of** right thigh

✓7ᵗʰ **S79.822** **Other specified injuries of** left thigh

✓7ᵗʰ **S79.829** **Other specified injuries of unspecified thigh**

✓5ᵗʰ **S79.9** **Unspecified injury of hip and thigh**

The appropriate 7th character is to be added to each code in subcategory S79.9.
A   initial encounter
D   subsequent encounter
S   sequela

✓6ᵗʰ **S79.91** **Unspecified injury of** hip

✓7ᵗʰ **S79.911** **Unspecified injury of** right hip

✓7ᵗʰ **S79.912** **Unspecified injury of** left hip

✓7ᵗʰ **S79.919** **Unspecified injury of unspecified hip**

✓6ᵗʰ **S79.92** **Unspecified injury of** thigh

✓7ᵗʰ **S79.921** **Unspecified injury of** right thigh

✓7ᵗʰ **S79.922** **Unspecified injury of** left thigh

✓7ᵗʰ **S79.929** **Unspecified injury of unspecified thigh**

Injuries to the knee and lower leg (S80-S89)

EXCLUDES 2   burns and corrosions (T20-T32)
frostbite (T33-T34)
injuries of ankle and foot, except fracture of ankle and malleolus (S90-S99)
insect bite or sting, venomous (T63.4)

✓4ᵗʰ **S80** **Superficial injury of knee and lower leg**

EXCLUDES 2   superficial injury of ankle and foot (S90.-)

The appropriate 7th character is to be added to each code from category S80.
A   initial encounter
D   subsequent encounter
S   sequela

✓5ᵗʰ **S80.0** **Contusion of** knee

✓x7ᵗʰ **S80.00** **Contusion of unspecified knee**

✓x7ᵗʰ **S80.01** **Contusion of** right knee

✓x7ᵗʰ **S80.02** **Contusion of** left knee

✓5ᵗʰ **S80.1** **Contusion of** lower leg

✓x7ᵗʰ **S80.10** **Contusion of unspecified lower leg**

✓x7ᵗʰ **S80.11** **Contusion of** right lower leg

✓x7ᵗʰ **S80.12** **Contusion of** left lower leg

✓5ᵗʰ **S80.2** **Other superficial injuries of** knee

✓6ᵗʰ **S80.21** **Abrasion of knee**

✓7ᵗʰ **S80.211** **Abrasion,** right knee

✓7ᵗʰ **S80.212** **Abrasion,** left knee

✓7ᵗʰ **S80.219** **Abrasion, unspecified knee**

✓6ᵗʰ **S80.22** **Blister (nonthermal) of knee**

✓7ᵗʰ **S80.221** **Blister (nonthermal),** right knee

✓7ᵗʰ **S80.222** **Blister (nonthermal),** left knee

✓7ᵗʰ **S80.229** **Blister (nonthermal), unspecified knee**

✓6ᵗʰ **S80.24** **External constriction of knee**

✓7ᵗʰ **S80.241** **External constriction,** right knee

✓7ᵗʰ **S80.242** **External constriction,** left knee

✓7ᵗʰ **S80.249** **External constriction, unspecified knee**

✓6ᵗʰ **S80.25** **Superficial foreign body of knee**

Splinter in the knee

✓7ᵗʰ **S80.251** **Superficial foreign body,** right knee

✓7ᵗʰ **S80.252** **Superficial foreign body,** left knee

        ✓7ᵗʰ **S80.259**   Superficial foreign body, unspecified knee

      ✓6ᵗʰ **S80.26**   Insect bite (nonvenomous) of knee

        ✓7ᵗʰ **S80.261**   Insect bite (nonvenomous), right knee

        ✓7ᵗʰ **S80.262**   Insect bite (nonvenomous), left knee

        ✓7ᵗʰ **S80.269**   Insect bite (nonvenomous), unspecified knee

      ✓6ᵗʰ **S80.27**   Other superficial bite of knee

         EXCLUDES 1   *open bite of knee (S81.05-)*

        ✓7ᵗʰ **S80.271**   Other superficial bite of right knee

        ✓7ᵗʰ **S80.272**   Other superficial bite of left knee

        ✓7ᵗʰ **S80.279**   Other superficial bite of unspecified knee

    ✓5ᵗʰ **S80.8**   Other superficial injuries of lower leg

      ✓6ᵗʰ **S80.81**   Abrasion of lower leg

        ✓7ᵗʰ **S80.811**   Abrasion, right lower leg

        ✓7ᵗʰ **S80.812**   Abrasion, left lower leg

        ✓7ᵗʰ **S80.819**   Abrasion, unspecified lower leg

      ✓6ᵗʰ **S80.82**   Blister (nonthermal) of lower leg

        ✓7ᵗʰ **S80.821**   Blister (nonthermal), right lower leg

        ✓7ᵗʰ **S80.822**   Blister (nonthermal), left lower leg

        ✓7ᵗʰ **S80.829**   Blister (nonthermal), unspecified lower leg

      ✓6ᵗʰ **S80.84**   External constriction of lower leg

        ✓7ᵗʰ **S80.841**   External constriction, right lower leg

        ✓7ᵗʰ **S80.842**   External constriction, left lower leg

        ✓7ᵗʰ **S80.849**   External constriction, unspecified lower leg

      ✓6ᵗʰ **S80.85**   Superficial foreign body of lower leg

         Splinter in the lower leg

        ✓7ᵗʰ **S80.851**   Superficial foreign body, right lower leg

        ✓7ᵗʰ **S80.852**   Superficial foreign body, left lower leg

        ✓7ᵗʰ **S80.859**   Superficial foreign body, unspecified lower leg

      ✓6ᵗʰ **S80.86**   Insect bite (nonvenomous) of lower leg

        ✓7ᵗʰ **S80.861**   Insect bite (nonvenomous), right lower leg

        ✓7ᵗʰ **S80.862**   Insect bite (nonvenomous), left lower leg

        ✓7ᵗʰ **S80.869**   Insect bite (nonvenomous), unspecified lower leg

      ✓6ᵗʰ **S80.87**   Other superficial bite of lower leg

         EXCLUDES 1   *open bite of lower leg (S81.85-)*

        ✓7ᵗʰ **S80.871**   Other superficial bite, right lower leg

        ✓7ᵗʰ **S80.872**   Other superficial bite, left lower leg

        ✓7ᵗʰ **S80.879**   Other superficial bite, unspecified lower leg

    ✓5ᵗʰ **S80.9**   Unspecified superficial injury of knee and lower leg

      ✓6ᵗʰ **S80.91**   Unspecified superficial injury of knee

        ✓7ᵗʰ **S80.911**   Unspecified superficial injury of right knee

        ✓7ᵗʰ **S80.912**   Unspecified superficial injury of left knee

        ✓7ᵗʰ **S80.919**   Unspecified superficial injury of unspecified knee

      ✓6ᵗʰ **S80.92**   Unspecified superficial injury of lower leg

        ✓7ᵗʰ **S80.921**   Unspecified superficial injury of right lower leg

        ✓7ᵗʰ **S80.922**   Unspecified superficial injury of left lower leg

        ✓7ᵗʰ **S80.929**   Unspecified superficial injury of unspecified lower leg

✓4ᵗʰ **S81**   Open wound of knee and lower leg

    Code also any associated wound infection

    EXCLUDES 1   *open fracture of knee and lower leg (S82.-)*

             traumatic amputation of lower leg (S88.-)

    EXCLUDES 2   *open wound of ankle and foot (S91.-)*

The appropriate 7th character is to be added to each code from category S81.

   A   initial encounter

   D   subsequent encounter

   S   sequela

    ✓5ᵗʰ **S81.0**   Open wound of knee

      ✓6ᵗʰ **S81.00**   Unspecified open wound of knee

        ✓7ᵗʰ **S81.001**   Unspecified open wound, right knee

        ✓7ᵗʰ **S81.002**   Unspecified open wound, left knee

        ✓7ᵗʰ **S81.009**   Unspecified open wound, unspecified knee

      ✓6ᵗʰ **S81.01**   Laceration without foreign body of knee

        ✓7ᵗʰ **S81.011**   Laceration without foreign body, right knee

        ✓7ᵗʰ **S81.012**   Laceration without foreign body, left knee

        ✓7ᵗʰ **S81.019**   Laceration without foreign body, unspecified knee

      ✓6ᵗʰ **S81.02**   Laceration with foreign body of knee

        ✓7ᵗʰ **S81.021**   Laceration with foreign body, right knee

        ✓7ᵗʰ **S81.022**   Laceration with foreign body, left knee

        ✓7ᵗʰ **S81.029**   Laceration with foreign body, unspecified knee

      ✓6ᵗʰ **S81.03**   Puncture wound without foreign body of knee

        ✓7ᵗʰ **S81.031**   Puncture wound without foreign body, right knee

        ✓7ᵗʰ **S81.032**   Puncture wound without foreign body, left knee

        ✓7ᵗʰ **S81.039**   Puncture wound without foreign body, unspecified knee

      ✓6ᵗʰ **S81.04**   Puncture wound with foreign body of knee

        ✓7ᵗʰ **S81.041**   Puncture wound with foreign body, right knee

        ✓7ᵗʰ **S81.042**   Puncture wound with foreign body, left knee

        ✓7ᵗʰ **S81.049**   Puncture wound with foreign body, unspecified knee

      ✓6ᵗʰ **S81.05**   Open bite of knee

         Bite of knee NOS

         EXCLUDES 1   *superficial bite of knee (S80.27-)*

        ✓7ᵗʰ **S81.051**   Open bite, right knee

        ✓7ᵗʰ **S81.052**   Open bite, left knee

        ✓7ᵗʰ **S81.059**   Open bite, unspecified knee

    ✓5ᵗʰ **S81.8**   Open wound of lower leg

      ✓6ᵗʰ **S81.80**   Unspecified open wound of lower leg

         AHA: 2016,3Q,24

        ✓7ᵗʰ **S81.801**   Unspecified open wound, right lower leg

        ✓7ᵗʰ **S81.802**   Unspecified open wound, left lower leg

        ✓7ᵗʰ **S81.809**   Unspecified open wound, unspecified lower leg

      ✓6ᵗʰ **S81.81**   Laceration without foreign body of lower leg

        ✓7ᵗʰ **S81.811**   Laceration without foreign body, right lower leg

        ✓7ᵗʰ **S81.812**   Laceration without foreign body, left lower leg

        ✓7ᵗʰ **S81.819**   Laceration without foreign body, unspecified lower leg

      ✓6ᵗʰ **S81.82**   Laceration with foreign body of lower leg

        ✓7ᵗʰ **S81.821**   Laceration with foreign body, right lower leg

        ✓7ᵗʰ **S81.822**   Laceration with foreign body, left lower leg

        ✓7ᵗʰ **S81.829**   Laceration with foreign body, unspecified lower leg

      ✓6ᵗʰ **S81.83**   Puncture wound without foreign body of lower leg

         AHA: 2016,3Q,24

        ✓7ᵗʰ **S81.831**   Puncture wound without foreign body, right lower leg

        ✓7ᵗʰ **S81.832**   Puncture wound without foreign body, left lower leg

        ✓7ᵗʰ **S81.839**   Puncture wound without foreign body, unspecified lower leg

      ✓6ᵗʰ **S81.84**   Puncture wound with foreign body of lower leg

         AHA: 2016,3Q,24

        ✓7ᵗʰ **S81.841**   Puncture wound with foreign body, right lower leg

        ✓7ᵗʰ **S81.842**   Puncture wound with foreign body, left lower leg

        ✓7ᵗʰ **S81.849**   Puncture wound with foreign body, unspecified lower leg

      ✓6ᵗʰ **S81.85**   Open bite of lower leg

         Bite of lower leg NOS

         EXCLUDES 1   *superficial bite of lower leg (S80.86-, S80.87-)*

        ✓7ᵗʰ **S81.851**   Open bite, right lower leg

N Newborn: 0   P Pediatric: 0-17   M Maternity: 9-64   A Adult: 15-124   MCC Major Complication/Comorbidity   CC Complication/Comorbidity   SW Severe Wound Dx

1098   ICD-10-CM 2020

√7ᵗʰ **S81.852** Open bite, left lower leg

√7ᵗʰ **S81.859** Open bite, unspecified lower leg

√4ᵗʰ **S82** **Fracture of lower leg, including ankle**

> **NOTE** A fracture not indicated as displaced or nondisplaced should be coded to displaced
>
> A fracture not indicated as open or closed should be coded to closed
>
> The open fracture designations are based on the Gustilo open fracture classification.

INCLUDES fracture of malleolus

EXCLUDES 1 *traumatic amputation of lower leg (S88.-)*

EXCLUDES 2 *fracture of foot, except ankle (S92.-)*

periprosthetic fracture of prosthetic implant of knee (M97.0-)

AHA: 2018,2Q,12; 2016,1Q,33; 2015,3Q,37-39

DEF: Diaphysis: Central shaft of a long bone.

DEF: Epiphysis: Proximal and distal rounded ends of a long bone, communicates with the joint.

DEF: Metaphysis: Section of a long bone located between the epiphysis and diaphysis at the proximal and distal ends.

DEF: Physis (growth plate): Narrow zone of cartilaginous tissue between the epiphysis and metaphysis at each end of a long bone. In childhood, proliferation of cells in this zone lengthens the bone. As the bone matures, this area thins, ossification eventually fusing into solid bone and growth stops. *Synonyms:* Epiphyseal plate.

> The appropriate 7th character is to be added to all codes from category S82 [unless otherwise indicated].
>
> A   initial encounter for closed fracture
> B   initial encounter for open fracture type I or II
>   initial encounter for open fracture NOS
> C   initial encounter for open fracture type IIIA, IIIB, or IIIC
> D   subsequent encounter for closed fracture with routine healing
> E   subsequent encounter for open fracture type I or II with routine healing
> F   subsequent encounter for open fracture type IIIA, IIIB, or IIIC with routine healing
> G   subsequent encounter for closed fracture with delayed healing
> H   subsequent encounter for open fracture type I or II with delayed healing
> J   subsequent encounter for open fracture type IIIA, IIIB, or IIIC with delayed healing
> K   subsequent encounter for closed fracture with nonunion
> M   subsequent encounter for open fracture type I or II with nonunion
> N   subsequent encounter for open fracture type IIIA, IIIB, or IIIC with nonunion
> P   subsequent encounter for closed fracture with malunion
> Q   subsequent encounter for open fracture type I or II with malunion
> R   subsequent encounter for open fracture type IIIA, IIIB, or IIIC with malunion
> S   sequela

√5ᵗʰ **S82.0** **Fracture of** patella

Knee cap

> **CC Excl: For CC codes in subcategory S82.0:**
> **Right side:** See code S82.001
> **Left side:** See code S82.002
> **Unspecified side:** See code S82.009

√6ᵗʰ **S82.00** **Unspecified fracture of patella**

³ √7ᵗʰ **S82.001** Unspecified fracture of right patella   CC H5

> CC Excl: CC with 7th character A: PDX collection 1336
> CC Excl: CC with 7th character B or C: PDX collection 1337
> CC Excl: CC with 7th character K, M, N, P, Q, or R: PDX collection 897

³ √7ᵗʰ **S82.002** Unspecified fracture of left patella   CC H5

> CC Excl: CC with 7th character A: PDX collection 1338
> CC Excl: CC with 7th character B or C: PDX collection 1337
> CC Excl: CC with 7th character K, M, N, P, Q, or R: PDX collection 897

³ √7ᵗʰ **S82.009** Unspecified fracture of unspecified patella   CC H5

> CC Excl: CC with 7th character A: PDX collection 1339
> CC Excl: CC with 7th character B or C: PDX collection 1337
> CC Excl: CC with 7th character K, M, N, P, Q, or R: PDX collection 897

√6ᵗʰ **S82.01** **Osteochondral fracture of patella**

³ √7ᵗʰ **S82.011** Displaced osteochondral fracture of right patella   CC H5

³ √7ᵗʰ **S82.012** Displaced osteochondral fracture of left patella   CC H5

³ √7ᵗʰ **S82.013** Displaced osteochondral fracture of unspecified patella   CC H5

³ √7ᵗʰ **S82.014** Nondisplaced osteochondral fracture of right patella   CC H5

³ √7ᵗʰ **S82.015** Nondisplaced osteochondral fracture of left patella   CC H5

³ √7ᵗʰ **S82.016** Nondisplaced osteochondral fracture of unspecified patella   CC H5

√6ᵗʰ **S82.02** **Longitudinal fracture of patella**

³ √7ᵗʰ **S82.021** Displaced longitudinal fracture of right patella   CC H5

³ √7ᵗʰ **S82.022** Displaced longitudinal fracture of left patella   CC H5

³ √7ᵗʰ **S82.023** Displaced longitudinal fracture of unspecified patella   CC H5

³ √7ᵗʰ **S82.024** Nondisplaced longitudinal fracture of right patella   CC H5

³ √7ᵗʰ **S82.025** Nondisplaced longitudinal fracture of left patella   CC H5

³ √7ᵗʰ **S82.026** Nondisplaced longitudinal fracture of unspecified patella   CC H5

√6ᵗʰ **S82.03** **Transverse fracture of patella**

³ √7ᵗʰ **S82.031** Displaced transverse fracture of right patella   CC H5

³ √7ᵗʰ **S82.032** Displaced transverse fracture of left patella   CC H5

³ √7ᵗʰ **S82.033** Displaced transverse fracture of unspecified patella   CC H5

³ √7ᵗʰ **S82.034** Nondisplaced transverse fracture of right patella   CC H5

³ √7ᵗʰ **S82.035** Nondisplaced transverse fracture of left patella   CC H5

³ √7ᵗʰ **S82.036** Nondisplaced transverse fracture of unspecified patella   CC H5

√6ᵗʰ **S82.04** **Comminuted fracture of patella**

³ √7ᵗʰ **S82.041** Displaced comminuted fracture of right patella   CC H5

³ √7ᵗʰ **S82.042** Displaced comminuted fracture of left patella   CC H5

³ √7ᵗʰ **S82.043** Displaced comminuted fracture of unspecified patella   CC H5

³ √7ᵗʰ **S82.044** Nondisplaced comminuted fracture of right patella   CC H5

³ √7ᵗʰ **S82.045** Nondisplaced comminuted fracture of left patella   CC H5

³ √7ᵗʰ **S82.046** Nondisplaced comminuted fracture of unspecified patella   CC H5

√6ᵗʰ **S82.09** **Other fracture of patella**

³ √7ᵗʰ **S82.091** Other fracture of right patella   CC H5

³ √7ᵗʰ **S82.092** Other fracture of left patella   CC H5

³ √7ᵗʰ **S82.099** Other fracture of unspecified patella   CC H5

Chapter 19. Injury, Poisoning and Certain Other Consequences of External Causes

√5ᵗʰ **S82.1** **Fracture of** upper end of tibia

Fracture of proximal end of tibia

EXCLUDES 2   *fracture of shaft of tibia (S82.2-)*

physeal fracture of upper end of tibia (S89.0-)

CC Excl: For CC/MCC codes in subcategory S82.1:
Right side: See code S82.101
Left side: See code S82.102
Unspecified side: See code S82.109

√6ᵗʰ **S82.10** **Unspecified fracture of upper end of tibia**

2,3 √7ᵗʰ **S82.101** **Unspecified fracture of upper end of** right **tibia**   MCC CC H5

CC Excl: CC with 7th character A: PDX collection 1340
CC Excl: MCC with 7th character B or C: PDX collection 1341
CC Excl: CC with 7th character K, M, N, P, Q, or R: PDX collection 897

2,3 √7ᵗʰ **S82.102** **Unspecified fracture of upper end of left tibia**   MCC CC H5

CC Excl: CC with 7th character A: PDX collection 1342
CC Excl: MCC with 7th character B or C: PDX collection 1341
CC Excl: CC with 7th character K, M, N, P, Q, or R: PDX collection 897

2,3 √7ᵗʰ **S82.109** **Unspecified fracture of upper end of unspecified tibia**   MCC CC H5

CC Excl: CC or MCC with 7th character A, B, or C: PDX collection 1341
CC Excl: CC with 7th character K, M, N, P, Q, or R: PDX collection 897

√6ᵗʰ **S82.11** **Fracture of** tibial spine

2,3 √7ᵗʰ **S82.111** **Displaced fracture of** right **tibial spine**   MCC CC H5

2,3 √7ᵗʰ **S82.112** **Displaced fracture of** left **tibial spine**   MCC CC H5

2,3 √7ᵗʰ **S82.113** **Displaced fracture of unspecified tibial spine**   MCC CC H5

2,3 √7ᵗʰ **S82.114** **Nondisplaced fracture of** right **tibial spine**   MCC CC H5

2,3 √7ᵗʰ **S82.115** **Nondisplaced fracture of** left **tibial spine**   MCC CC H5

2,3 √7ᵗʰ **S82.116** **Nondisplaced fracture of unspecified tibial spine**   MCC CC H5

√6ᵗʰ **S82.12** **Fracture of** lateral condyle of tibia

2,3 √7ᵗʰ **S82.121** **Displaced fracture of lateral condyle of** right **tibia**   MCC CC H5

2,3 √7ᵗʰ **S82.122** **Displaced fracture of lateral condyle of** left **tibia**   MCC CC H5

2,3 √7ᵗʰ **S82.123** **Displaced fracture of lateral condyle of unspecified tibia**   MCC CC H5

2,3 √7ᵗʰ **S82.124** **Nondisplaced fracture of lateral condyle of** right **tibia**   MCC CC H5

2,3 √7ᵗʰ **S82.125** **Nondisplaced fracture of lateral condyle of** left **tibia**   MCC CC H5

2,3 √7ᵗʰ **S82.126** **Nondisplaced fracture of lateral condyle of unspecified tibia**   MCC CC H5

√6ᵗʰ **S82.13** **Fracture of** medial condyle of tibia

2,3 √7ᵗʰ **S82.131** **Displaced fracture of medial condyle of** right **tibia**   MCC CC H5

2,3 √7ᵗʰ **S82.132** **Displaced fracture of medial condyle of** left **tibia**   MCC CC H5

2,3 √7ᵗʰ **S82.133** **Displaced fracture of medial condyle of unspecified tibia**   MCC CC H5

2,3 √7ᵗʰ **S82.134** **Nondisplaced fracture of medial condyle of** right **tibia**   MCC CC H5

2,3 √7ᵗʰ **S82.135** **Nondisplaced fracture of medial condyle of** left **tibia**   MCC CC H5

2,3 √7ᵗʰ **S82.136** **Nondisplaced fracture of medial condyle of unspecified tibia**   MCC CC H5

√6ᵗʰ **S82.14** **Bicondylar fracture of tibia**

Fracture of tibial plateau NOS

2,3 √7ᵗʰ **S82.141** **Displaced bicondylar fracture of** right **tibia**   MCC CC H5

2,3 √7ᵗʰ **S82.142** **Displaced bicondylar fracture of** left **tibia**   MCC CC H5

2,3 √7ᵗʰ **S82.143** **Displaced bicondylar fracture of unspecified tibia**   MCC CC H5

2,3 √7ᵗʰ **S82.144** **Nondisplaced bicondylar fracture of** right **tibia**   MCC CC H5

2,3 √7ᵗʰ **S82.145** **Nondisplaced bicondylar fracture of** left **tibia**   MCC CC H5

2,3 √7ᵗʰ **S82.146** **Nondisplaced bicondylar fracture of unspecified tibia**   MCC CC H5

√6ᵗʰ **S82.15** **Fracture of** tibial tuberosity

2,3 √7ᵗʰ **S82.151** **Displaced fracture of** right **tibial tuberosity**   MCC CC H5

2,3 √7ᵗʰ **S82.152** **Displaced fracture of** left **tibial tuberosity**   MCC CC H5

2,3 √7ᵗʰ **S82.153** **Displaced fracture of unspecified tibial tuberosity**   MCC CC H5

2,3 √7ᵗʰ **S82.154** **Nondisplaced fracture of** right **tibial tuberosity**   MCC CC H5

2,3 √7ᵗʰ **S82.155** **Nondisplaced fracture of** left **tibial tuberosity**   MCC CC H5

2,3 √7ᵗʰ **S82.156** **Nondisplaced fracture of unspecified tibial tuberosity**   MCC CC H5

√6ᵗʰ **S82.16** **Torus fracture of upper end of tibia**

The appropriate 7th character is to be added to all codes in subcategory S82.16.
A   initial encounter for closed fracture
D   subsequent encounter for fracture with routine healing
G   subsequent encounter for fracture with delayed healing
K   subsequent encounter for fracture with nonunion
P   subsequent encounter for fracture with malunion
S   sequela

3 √7ᵗʰ **S82.161** **Torus fracture of upper end of** right **tibia**   CC H5

CC Excl: CC with 7th character A: PDX collection 1343
CC Excl: CC with 7th character K or P: PDX collection 897

3 √7ᵗʰ **S82.162** **Torus fracture of upper end of** left **tibia**   CC H5

CC Excl: CC with 7th character A: PDX collection 1344
CC Excl: CC with 7th character K or P: PDX collection 897

3 √7ᵗʰ **S82.169** **Torus fracture of upper end of unspecified tibia**   CC H5

CC Excl: CC with 7th character A: PDX collection 1345
CC Excl: CC with 7th character K or P: PDX collection 897

√6ᵗʰ **S82.19** **Other fracture of upper end of tibia**

2,3 √7ᵗʰ **S82.191** **Other fracture of upper end of** right **tibia**   MCC CC H5

2,3 √7ᵗʰ **S82.192** **Other fracture of upper end of** left **tibia**   MCC CC H5

2,3 √7ᵗʰ **S82.199** **Other fracture of upper end of unspecified tibia**   MCC CC H5

N Newborn: 0   P Pediatric: 0-17   M Maternity: 9-64   A Adult: 15-124   MCC Major Complication/Comorbidity   CC Complication/Comorbidity   SW Severe Wound Dx

1100   ICD-10-CM 2020

✓5th **S82.2** **Fracture of** shaft of tibia

CC Excl: For CC/MCC codes in subcategory S82.2:
Right side: See code S82.101
Left side: See code S82.102
Unspecified side: See code S82.109

✓6th **S82.20** **Unspecified fracture of shaft of tibia**
Fracture of tibia NOS

2,3 ✓7th **S82.201** **Unspecified fracture of shaft of right tibia** `MCC` `CC` `H5`
CC Excl: CC with 7th character A: PDX collection 1346
CC Excl: MCC with 7th character B or C: PDX collection 1341
CC Excl: CC with 7th character K, M, N, P, Q, or R: PDX collection 897

2,3 ✓7th **S82.202** **Unspecified fracture of shaft of left tibia** `MCC` `CC` `H5`
CC Excl: CC with 7th character A: PDX collection 1342
CC Excl: MCC with 7th character B or C: PDX collection 1341
CC Excl: CC with 7th character K, M, N, P, Q, or R: PDX collection 897

2,3 ✓7th **S82.209** **Unspecified fracture of shaft of unspecified tibia** `MCC` `CC` `H5`
CC Excl: CC or MCC with 7th character A, B, or C: PDX collection 1341
CC Excl: CC with 7th character K, M, N, P, Q, or R: PDX collection 897

✓6th **S82.22** **Transverse fracture of shaft of tibia**

2,3 ✓7th **S82.221** **Displaced transverse fracture of shaft of right tibia** `MCC` `CC` `H5`

2,3 ✓7th **S82.222** **Displaced transverse fracture of shaft of left tibia** `MCC` `CC` `H5`

2,3 ✓7th **S82.223** **Displaced transverse fracture of shaft of unspecified tibia** `MCC` `CC` `H5`

2,3 ✓7th **S82.224** **Nondisplaced transverse fracture of shaft of right tibia** `MCC` `CC` `H5`

2,3 ✓7th **S82.225** **Nondisplaced transverse fracture of shaft of left tibia** `MCC` `CC` `H5`

2,3 ✓7th **S82.226** **Nondisplaced transverse fracture of shaft of unspecified tibia** `MCC` `CC` `H5`

✓6th **S82.23** **Oblique fracture of shaft of tibia**

2,3 ✓7th **S82.231** **Displaced oblique fracture of shaft of right tibia** `MCC` `CC` `H5`

2,3 ✓7th **S82.232** **Displaced oblique fracture of shaft of left tibia** `MCC` `CC` `H5`

2,3 ✓7th **S82.233** **Displaced oblique fracture of shaft of unspecified tibia** `MCC` `CC` `H5`

2,3 ✓7th **S82.234** **Nondisplaced oblique fracture of shaft of right tibia** `MCC` `CC` `H5`

2,3 ✓7th **S82.235** **Nondisplaced oblique fracture of shaft of left tibia** `MCC` `CC` `H5`

2,3 ✓7th **S82.236** **Nondisplaced oblique fracture of shaft of unspecified tibia** `MCC` `CC` `H5`

✓6th **S82.24** **Spiral fracture of shaft of tibia**
Toddler fracture

2,3 ✓7th **S82.241** **Displaced spiral fracture of shaft of right tibia** `MCC` `CC` `H5`

2,3 ✓7th **S82.242** **Displaced spiral fracture of shaft of left tibia** `MCC` `CC` `H5`

2,3 ✓7th **S82.243** **Displaced spiral fracture of shaft of unspecified tibia** `MCC` `CC` `H5`

2,3 ✓7th **S82.244** **Nondisplaced spiral fracture of shaft of right tibia** `MCC` `CC` `H5`

2,3 ✓7th **S82.245** **Nondisplaced spiral fracture of shaft of left tibia** `MCC` `CC` `H5`

2,3 ✓7th **S82.246** **Nondisplaced spiral fracture of shaft of unspecified tibia** `MCC` `CC` `H5`

✓6th **S82.25** **Comminuted fracture of shaft of tibia**

2,3 ✓7th **S82.251** **Displaced comminuted fracture of shaft of right tibia** `MCC` `CC` `H5`

2,3 ✓7th **S82.252** **Displaced comminuted fracture of shaft of left tibia** `MCC` `CC` `H5`

2,3 ✓7th **S82.253** **Displaced comminuted fracture of shaft of unspecified tibia** `MCC` `CC` `H5`

2,3 ✓7th **S82.254** **Nondisplaced comminuted fracture of shaft of right tibia** `MCC` `CC` `H5`

2,3 ✓7th **S82.255** **Nondisplaced comminuted fracture of shaft of left tibia** `MCC` `CC` `H5`

2,3 ✓7th **S82.256** **Nondisplaced comminuted fracture of shaft of unspecified tibia** `MCC` `CC` `H5`

✓6th **S82.26** **Segmental fracture of shaft of tibia**

2,3 ✓7th **S82.261** **Displaced segmental fracture of shaft of right tibia** `MCC` `CC` `H5`

2,3 ✓7th **S82.262** **Displaced segmental fracture of shaft of left tibia** `MCC` `CC` `H5`

2,3 ✓7th **S82.263** **Displaced segmental fracture of shaft of unspecified tibia** `MCC` `CC` `H5`

2,3 ✓7th **S82.264** **Nondisplaced segmental fracture of shaft of right tibia** `MCC` `CC` `H5`

2,3 ✓7th **S82.265** **Nondisplaced segmental fracture of shaft of left tibia** `MCC` `CC` `H5`

2,3 ✓7th **S82.266** **Nondisplaced segmental fracture of shaft of unspecified tibia** `MCC` `CC` `H5`

✓6th **S82.29** **Other fracture of shaft of tibia**

2,3 ✓7th **S82.291** **Other fracture of shaft of right tibia** `MCC` `CC` `H5`

2,3 ✓7th **S82.292** **Other fracture of shaft of left tibia** `MCC` `CC` `H5`

2,3 ✓7th **S82.299** **Other fracture of shaft of unspecified tibia** `MCC` `CC` `H5`

✓5th **S82.3** **Fracture of** lower end of tibia

EXCLUDES 1 bimalleolar fracture of lower leg (S82.84-)
fracture of medial malleolus alone (S82.5-)
Maisonneuve's fracture (S82.86-)
pilon fracture of distal tibia (S82.87-)
trimalleolar fractures of lower leg (S82.85-)

✓6th **S82.30** **Unspecified fracture of lower end of tibia**

CC Excl: For codes in subcategory S82.30:
CC with 7th character B or C: PDX collection 1347
CC with 7th character K, M, N, P, Q, or R: PDX collection 897

3 ✓7th **S82.301** **Unspecified fracture of lower end of right tibia** `CC` `H5`

3 ✓7th **S82.302** **Unspecified fracture of lower end of left tibia** `CC` `H5`

3 ✓7th **S82.309** **Unspecified fracture of lower end of unspecified tibia** `CC` `H5`

✓ Additional Character Required   ✓x7th Placeholder   Unacceptable PDx   Questionable PDx   Manifestation   Unspecified Dx   `H1`-`H14` HAC   `HCC` CMS-HCC Dx   `HIV` HIV Dx

√6ᵗʰ **S82.31**   Torus **fracture of lower end of tibia**

> The appropriate 7th character is to be added to all codes in subcategory S82.31.
> A   initial encounter for closed fracture
> D   subsequent encounter for fracture with routine healing
> G   subsequent encounter for fracture with delayed healing
> K   subsequent encounter for fracture with nonunion
> P   subsequent encounter for fracture with malunion
> S   sequela

3 √7ᵗʰ **S82.311**   Torus **fracture of lower end of** right **tibia**   `CC` `H5`
> CC Excl: CC with 7th character A: PDX collection 1343
> CC Excl: CC with 7th character K or P: PDX collection 897

3 √7ᵗʰ **S82.312**   Torus **fracture of lower end of** left **tibia**   `CC` `H5`
> CC Excl: CC with 7th character A: PDX collection 1344
> CC Excl: CC with 7th character K or P: PDX collection 897

3 √7ᵗʰ **S82.319**   Torus **fracture of lower end of unspecified tibia**   `CC` `H5`
> CC Excl: CC with 7th character A: PDX collection 1345
> CC Excl: CC with 7th character K or P: PDX collection 897

√6ᵗʰ **S82.39**   Other **fracture of lower end of tibia**
> AHA: 2015,1Q,25
> CC Excl: For codes in subcategory S82.39:
> CC with 7th character B or C: PDX collection 1347
> CC with 7th character K, M, N, P, Q, or R: PDX collection 897

3 √7ᵗʰ **S82.391**   Other **fracture of lower end of** right **tibia**   `CC` `H5`

3 √7ᵗʰ **S82.392**   Other **fracture of lower end of** left **tibia**   `CC` `H5`

3 √7ᵗʰ **S82.399**   Other **fracture of lower end of unspecified tibia**   `CC` `H5`

√5ᵗʰ **S82.4**   **Fracture of** shaft **of fibula**
> EXCLUDES 2   *fracture of lateral malleolus alone (S82.6-)*
> CC Excl: For codes in subcategory S82.4:
> MCC with 7th character B or C: PDX collection 1341
> CC with 7th character K, M, N, P, Q, or R: PDX collection 897

√6ᵗʰ **S82.40**   **Unspecified fracture of shaft of fibula**

2,4 √7ᵗʰ **S82.401**   **Unspecified fracture of shaft of** right **fibula**   `MCC` `CC` `H5`

2,4 √7ᵗʰ **S82.402**   **Unspecified fracture of shaft of** left **fibula**   `MCC` `CC` `H5`

2,4 √7ᵗʰ **S82.409**   **Unspecified fracture of shaft of unspecified fibula**   `MCC` `CC` `H5`

√6ᵗʰ **S82.42**   Transverse **fracture of shaft of fibula**

2,4 √7ᵗʰ **S82.421**   Displaced transverse **fracture of shaft of** right **fibula**   `MCC` `CC` `H5`

2,4 √7ᵗʰ **S82.422**   Displaced transverse **fracture of shaft of** left **fibula**   `MCC` `CC` `H5`

2,4 √7ᵗʰ **S82.423**   Displaced transverse **fracture of shaft of unspecified fibula**   `MCC` `CC` `H5`

2,4 √7ᵗʰ **S82.424**   Nondisplaced transverse **fracture of shaft of** right **fibula**   `MCC` `CC` `H5`

2,4 √7ᵗʰ **S82.425**   Nondisplaced transverse **fracture of shaft of** left **fibula**   `MCC` `CC` `H5`

2,4 √7ᵗʰ **S82.426**   Nondisplaced transverse **fracture of shaft of unspecified fibula**   `MCC` `CC` `H5`

√6ᵗʰ **S82.43**   Oblique **fracture of shaft of fibula**

2,4 √7ᵗʰ **S82.431**   Displaced oblique **fracture of shaft of** right **fibula**   `MCC` `CC` `H5`

2,4 √7ᵗʰ **S82.432**   Displaced oblique **fracture of shaft of** left **fibula**   `MCC` `CC` `H5`

2,4 √7ᵗʰ **S82.433**   Displaced oblique **fracture of shaft of unspecified fibula**   `MCC` `CC` `H5`

2,4 √7ᵗʰ **S82.434**   Nondisplaced oblique **fracture of shaft of** right **fibula**   `MCC` `CC` `H5`

2,4 √7ᵗʰ **S82.435**   Nondisplaced oblique **fracture of shaft of** left **fibula**   `MCC` `CC` `H5`

2,4 √7ᵗʰ **S82.436**   Nondisplaced oblique **fracture of shaft of unspecified fibula**   `MCC` `CC` `H5`

√6ᵗʰ **S82.44**   Spiral **fracture of shaft of fibula**

2,4 √7ᵗʰ **S82.441**   Displaced spiral fracture **of shaft of** right **fibula**   `MCC` `CC` `H5`

2,4 √7ᵗʰ **S82.442**   Displaced spiral fracture **of shaft of** left **fibula**   `MCC` `CC` `H5`

2,4 √7ᵗʰ **S82.443**   Displaced spiral fracture **of shaft of unspecified fibula**   `MCC` `CC` `H5`

2,4 √7ᵗʰ **S82.444**   Nondisplaced spiral **fracture of shaft of** right **fibula**   `MCC` `CC` `H5`

2,4 √7ᵗʰ **S82.445**   Nondisplaced spiral **fracture of shaft of** left **fibula**   `MCC` `CC` `H5`

2,4 √7ᵗʰ **S82.446**   Nondisplaced spiral **fracture of shaft of unspecified fibula**   `MCC` `CC` `H5`

√6ᵗʰ **S82.45**   Comminuted **fracture of shaft of fibula**

2,4 √7ᵗʰ **S82.451**   Displaced comminuted **fracture of shaft of** right **fibula**   `MCC` `CC` `H5`

2,4 √7ᵗʰ **S82.452**   Displaced comminuted **fracture of shaft of** left **fibula**   `MCC` `CC` `H5`

2,4 √7ᵗʰ **S82.453**   Displaced comminuted **fracture of shaft of unspecified fibula**   `MCC` `CC` `H5`

2,4 √7ᵗʰ **S82.454**   Nondisplaced comminuted fracture of **shaft of** right **fibula**   `MCC` `CC` `H5`

2,4 √7ᵗʰ **S82.455**   Nondisplaced comminuted fracture of **shaft of** left **fibula**   `MCC` `CC` `H5`

2,4 √7ᵗʰ **S82.456**   Nondisplaced comminuted fracture of **shaft of unspecified fibula**   `MCC` `CC` `H5`

√6ᵗʰ **S82.46**   Segmental **fracture of shaft of fibula**

2,4 √7ᵗʰ **S82.461**   Displaced segmental **fracture of shaft of** right **fibula**   `MCC` `CC` `H5`

2,4 √7ᵗʰ **S82.462**   Displaced segmental **fracture of shaft of** left **fibula**   `MCC` `CC` `H5`

2,4 √7ᵗʰ **S82.463**   Displaced segmental **fracture of shaft of unspecified fibula**   `MCC` `CC` `H5`

2,4 √7ᵗʰ **S82.464**   Nondisplaced segmental **fracture of shaft of** right **fibula**   `MCC` `CC` `H5`

2,4 √7ᵗʰ **S82.465**   Nondisplaced segmental **fracture of shaft of** left **fibula**   `MCC` `CC` `H5`

2,4 √7ᵗʰ **S82.466**   Nondisplaced segmental **fracture of shaft of unspecified fibula**   `MCC` `CC` `H5`

√6ᵗʰ **S82.49**   Other **fracture of shaft of fibula**

2,4 √7ᵗʰ **S82.491**   Other **fracture of shaft of** right **fibula**   `MCC` `CC` `H5`

2,4 √7ᵗʰ **S82.492**   Other **fracture of shaft of** left **fibula**   `MCC` `CC` `H5`

2,4 √7ᵗʰ **S82.499**   Other **fracture of shaft of unspecified fibula**   `MCC` `CC` `H5`

√5ᵗʰ **S82.5**   **Fracture of** medial **malleolus**
> EXCLUDES 1   *pilon fracture of distal tibia (S82.87-)*
> *Salter-Harris type III of lower end of tibia (S89.13-)*
> *Salter-Harris type IV of lower end of tibia (S89.14-)*
> CC Excl: For codes in subcategory S82.5:
> CC with 7th character B or C: PDX collection 1347
> CC with 7th character K, M, N, P, Q, or R: PDX collection 897

3 √x7ᵗʰ **S82.51**   Displaced **fracture of medial malleolus of** right **tibia**   `CC` `H5`

`N` Newborn: 0   `P` Pediatric: 0-17   `M` Maternity: 9-64   `A` Adult: 15-124   `MCC` Major Complication/Comorbidity   `CC` Complication/Comorbidity   `SW` Severe Wound Dx

1102   ICD-10-CM 2020

3 ✓x7ᵗʰ **S82.52** Displaced fracture of medial malleolus of left tibia   `CC` `H5`

3 ✓x7ᵗʰ **S82.53** Displaced fracture of medial malleolus of unspecified tibia   `CC` `H5`

3 ✓x7ᵗʰ **S82.54** Nondisplaced fracture of medial malleolus of right tibia   `CC` `H5`

3 ✓x7ᵗʰ **S82.55** Nondisplaced fracture of medial malleolus of left tibia   `CC` `H5`

3 ✓x7ᵗʰ **S82.56** Nondisplaced fracture of medial malleolus of unspecified tibia   `CC` `H5`

✓5ᵗʰ **S82.6 Fracture of lateral malleolus**

> EXCLUDES 1   pilon fracture of distal tibia (S82.87-)
>
> CC Excl: For codes in subcategory S82.6:
> CC with 7th character B or C: PDX collection 1347
> CC with 7th character K, M, N, P, Q, or R: PDX collection 897

3 ✓x7ᵗʰ **S82.61** Displaced fracture of lateral malleolus of right fibula   `CC` `H5`

3 ✓x7ᵗʰ **S82.62** Displaced fracture of lateral malleolus of left fibula   `CC` `H5`

3 ✓x7ᵗʰ **S82.63** Displaced fracture of lateral malleolus of unspecified fibula   `CC` `H5`

3 ✓x7ᵗʰ **S82.64** Nondisplaced fracture of lateral malleolus of right fibula   `CC` `H5`

3 ✓x7ᵗʰ **S82.65** Nondisplaced fracture of lateral malleolus of left fibula   `CC` `H5`

3 ✓x7ᵗʰ **S82.66** Nondisplaced fracture of lateral malleolus of unspecified fibula   `CC` `H5`

✓5ᵗʰ **S82.8 Other fractures of lower leg**

   ✓6ᵗʰ **S82.81** Torus fracture of upper end of fibula

> The appropriate 7th character is to be added to all codes in subcategory S82.81
> A   initial encounter for closed fracture
> D   subsequent encounter for fracture with routine healing
> G   subsequent encounter for fracture with delayed healing
> K   subsequent encounter for fracture with nonunion
> P   subsequent encounter for fracture with malunion
> S   sequela
>
> CC Excl: For codes in subcategory S82.81:
> CC with 7th character K or P: PDX collection 897

     4 ✓7ᵗʰ **S82.811** Torus fracture of upper end of right fibula   `CC`

     4 ✓7ᵗʰ **S82.812** Torus fracture of upper end of left fibula   `CC`

     4 ✓7ᵗʰ **S82.819** Torus fracture of upper end of unspecified fibula   `CC`

   ✓6ᵗʰ **S82.82** Torus fracture of lower end of fibula

> The appropriate 7th character is to be added to all codes in subcategory S82.82.
> A   initial encounter for closed fracture
> D   subsequent encounter for fracture with routine healing
> G   subsequent encounter for fracture with delayed healing
> K   subsequent encounter for fracture with nonunion
> P   subsequent encounter for fracture with malunion
> S   sequela
>
> CC Excl: For codes in subcategory S82.82:
> CC with 7th character K or P: PDX collection 897

     4 ✓7ᵗʰ **S82.821** Torus fracture of lower end of right fibula   `CC`

     4 ✓7ᵗʰ **S82.822** Torus fracture of lower end of left fibula   `CC`

     4 ✓7ᵗʰ **S82.829** Torus fracture of lower end of unspecified fibula   `CC`

   ✓6ᵗʰ **S82.83** Other fracture of upper and lower end of fibula

> AHA: 2015,1Q,25
> CC Excl: For codes in subcategory S82.83:
> MCC with 7th character B or C: PDX collection 1341
> CC with 7th character K, M, N, P, Q, or R: PDX collection 897

     2,4 ✓7ᵗʰ **S82.831** Other fracture of upper and lower end of right fibula   `MCC` `CC` `H5`

     2,4 ✓7ᵗʰ **S82.832** Other fracture of upper and lower end of left fibula   `MCC` `CC` `H5`

     2,4 ✓7ᵗʰ **S82.839** Other fracture of upper and lower end of unspecified fibula   `MCC` `CC` `H5`

   ✓6ᵗʰ **S82.84** Bimalleolar fracture of lower leg

> CC Excl: For codes in subcategory S82.84:
> CC with 7th character B or C: PDX collection 1347
> CC with 7th character K, M, N, P, Q, or R: PDX collection 897

Right Bimalleolar Fracture

Labels: Patella, Tibial plateau, Tibial tubercle, Fibula, Tibia, Fracture medial malleolus, Fracture lateral malleolus, Talus, Medial (tibial) malleolus, Lateral (fibular) malleolus

     3 ✓7ᵗʰ **S82.841** Displaced bimalleolar fracture of right lower leg   `CC` `H5`

     3 ✓7ᵗʰ **S82.842** Displaced bimalleolar fracture of left lower leg   `CC` `H5`

     3 ✓7ᵗʰ **S82.843** Displaced bimalleolar fracture of unspecified lower leg   `CC` `H5`

     3 ✓7ᵗʰ **S82.844** Nondisplaced bimalleolar fracture of right lower leg   `CC` `H5`

     3 ✓7ᵗʰ **S82.845** Nondisplaced bimalleolar fracture of left lower leg   `CC` `H5`

     3 ✓7ᵗʰ **S82.846** Nondisplaced bimalleolar fracture of unspecified lower leg   `CC` `H5`

   ✓6ᵗʰ **S82.85** Trimalleolar fracture of lower leg

> CC Excl: For codes in subcategory S82.85:
> CC with 7th character B or C: PDX collection 1347
> CC with 7th character K, M, N, P, Q, or R: PDX collection 897

     3 ✓7ᵗʰ **S82.851** Displaced trimalleolar fracture of right lower leg   `CC` `H5`

     3 ✓7ᵗʰ **S82.852** Displaced trimalleolar fracture of left lower leg   `CC` `H5`

     3 ✓7ᵗʰ **S82.853** Displaced trimalleolar fracture of unspecified lower leg   `CC` `H5`

     3 ✓7ᵗʰ **S82.854** Nondisplaced trimalleolar fracture of right lower leg   `CC` `H5`

     3 ✓7ᵗʰ **S82.855** Nondisplaced trimalleolar fracture of left lower leg   `CC` `H5`

✓ Additional Character Required   ✓x7ᵗʰ Placeholder   Unacceptable PDx   Questionable PDx   Manifestation   Unspecified Dx   H1-H14 HAC   HCC CMS-HCC Dx   HIV HIV Dx

ICD-10-CM 2020   1103

3 √7th **S82.856** Nondisplaced **trimalleolar fracture of unspecified lower leg** [CC] [H5]

√6th **S82.86** **Maisonneuve's fracture**

> CC Excl: For codes in subcategory S82.86:
> MCC with 7th character B or C: PDX collection 1341
> CC with 7th character K, M, N, P, Q, or R: PDX collection 897

2,4 √7th **S82.861** Displaced **Maisonneuve's fracture of right leg** [MCC] [CC] [H5]

2,4 √7th **S82.862** Displaced **Maisonneuve's fracture of left leg** [MCC] [CC] [H5]

2,4 √7th **S82.863** Displaced **Maisonneuve's fracture of unspecified leg** [MCC] [CC] [H5]

2,4 √7th **S82.864** Nondisplaced **Maisonneuve's fracture of right leg** [MCC] [CC] [H5]

2,4 √7th **S82.865** Nondisplaced **Maisonneuve's fracture of left leg** [MCC] [CC] [H5]

2,4 √7th **S82.866** Nondisplaced **Maisonneuve's fracture of unspecified leg** [MCC] [CC] [H5]

√6th **S82.87** **Pilon fracture of tibia**

> CC Excl: For codes in subcategory S82.87:
> CC with 7th character B or C: PDX collection 1347
> CC with 7th character K, M, N, P, Q, or R: PDX collection 897

3 √7th **S82.871** Displaced **pilon fracture of right tibia** [CC] [H5]

3 √7th **S82.872** Displaced **pilon fracture of left tibia** [CC] [H5]

3 √7th **S82.873** Displaced **pilon fracture of unspecified tibia** [CC] [H5]

3 √7th **S82.874** Nondisplaced **pilon fracture of right tibia** [CC] [H5]

3 √7th **S82.875** Nondisplaced **pilon fracture of left tibia** [CC] [H5]

3 √7th **S82.876** Nondisplaced **pilon fracture of unspecified tibia** [CC] [H5]

√6th **S82.89** **Other fractures of lower leg**

> Fracture of ankle NOS

> CC Excl: For codes in subcategory S82.89:
> CC with 7th character B or C: PDX collection 1347
> CC with 7th character K, M, N, P, Q, or R: PDX collection 897

3 √7th **S82.891** Other fracture of **right lower leg** [CC] [H5]

3 √7th **S82.892** Other fracture of **left lower leg** [CC] [H5]

3 √7th **S82.899** Other fracture of **unspecified lower leg** [CC] [H5]

√5th **S82.9** **Unspecified fracture of lower leg**

> CC Excl: For codes in subcategory S82.9:
> CC with 7th character B or C: PDX collection 1348
> CC with 7th character K, M, N, P, Q, or R: PDX collection 897

3 √x7th **S82.90** Unspecified fracture of unspecified **lower leg** [CC] [H5]

3 √x7th **S82.91** Unspecified fracture of **right lower leg** [CC] [H5]

3 √x7th **S82.92** Unspecified fracture of **left lower leg** [CC] [H5]

√4th **S83** **Dislocation and sprain of joints and ligaments of knee**

> [INCLUDES] avulsion of joint or ligament of knee
> laceration of cartilage, joint or ligament of knee
> sprain of cartilage, joint or ligament of knee
> traumatic hemarthrosis of joint or ligament of knee
> traumatic rupture of joint or ligament of knee
> traumatic subluxation of joint or ligament of knee
> traumatic tear of joint or ligament of knee

Code also any associated open wound

> [EXCLUDES 1] derangement of patella (M22.0-M22.3)
> injury of patellar ligament (tendon) (S76.1-)
> internal derangement of knee (M23.-)
> old dislocation of knee (M23.8X)
> pathological dislocation of knee (M24.36)
> recurrent dislocation of knee (M22.0)

> [EXCLUDES 2] strain of muscle, fascia and tendon of lower leg (S86.-)

> The appropriate 7th character is to be added to each code from category S83.
> A initial encounter
> D subsequent encounter
> S sequela

√5th **S83.0** **Subluxation and dislocation of patella**

√6th **S83.00** **Unspecified subluxation and dislocation of patella**

√7th **S83.001** Unspecified **subluxation** of **right patella**

√7th **S83.002** Unspecified **subluxation** of **left patella**

√7th **S83.003** Unspecified **subluxation** of **unspecified patella**

√7th **S83.004** Unspecified **dislocation** of **right patella**

√7th **S83.005** Unspecified **dislocation** of **left patella**

√7th **S83.006** Unspecified **dislocation** of **unspecified patella**

√6th **S83.01** **Lateral subluxation and dislocation of patella**

√7th **S83.011** Lateral **subluxation** of **right patella**

√7th **S83.012** Lateral **subluxation** of **left patella**

√7th **S83.013** Lateral **subluxation** of unspecified patella

√7th **S83.014** Lateral **dislocation** of **right patella**

√7th **S83.015** Lateral **dislocation** of **left patella**

√7th **S83.016** Lateral **dislocation** of unspecified patella

√6th **S83.09** **Other subluxation and dislocation of patella**

√7th **S83.091** Other **subluxation** of **right patella**

√7th **S83.092** Other **subluxation** of **left patella**

√7th **S83.093** Other **subluxation** of **unspecified patella**

√7th **S83.094** Other **dislocation** of **right patella**

√7th **S83.095** Other **dislocation** of **left patella**

√7th **S83.096** Other **dislocation** of **unspecified patella**

√5th **S83.1** **Subluxation and dislocation of knee**

> [EXCLUDES 2] instability of knee prosthesis (T84.022, T84.023)

√6th **S83.10** **Unspecified subluxation and dislocation of knee**

√7th **S83.101** Unspecified **subluxation** of **right knee**

√7th **S83.102** Unspecified **subluxation** of **left knee**

√7th **S83.103** Unspecified **subluxation** of **unspecified knee**

√7th **S83.104** Unspecified **dislocation** of **right knee**

√7th **S83.105** Unspecified **dislocation** of **left knee**

√7th **S83.106** Unspecified **dislocation** of **unspecified knee**

√6th **S83.11** **Anterior subluxation and dislocation of proximal end of tibia**

> Posterior subluxation and dislocation of distal end of femur

√7th **S83.111** Anterior **subluxation** of proximal end of tibia, **right knee**

√7th **S83.112** Anterior **subluxation** of proximal end of tibia, **left knee**

√7th **S83.113** Anterior **subluxation** of proximal end of tibia, **unspecified knee**

√7th **S83.114** Anterior **dislocation** of proximal end of tibia, **right knee**

√7th **S83.115** Anterior **dislocation** of proximal end of tibia, **left knee**

√7th **S83.116** Anterior **dislocation** of proximal end of tibia, **unspecified knee**

[N] Newborn: 0   [P] Pediatric: 0-17   [M] Maternity: 9-64   [A] Adult: 15-124   [MCC] Major Complication/Comorbidity   [CC] Complication/Comorbidity   [SW] Severe Wound Dx

1104   ICD-10-CM 2020

✓6th **S83.12** **Posterior** subluxation and dislocation of proximal end of tibia
Anterior dislocation of distal end of femur

  ✓7th **S83.121** **Posterior** subluxation of proximal end of tibia, **right** knee

  ✓7th **S83.122** **Posterior** subluxation of proximal end of tibia, **left** knee

  ✓7th **S83.123** **Posterior** subluxation of proximal end of tibia, unspecified knee

  ✓7th **S83.124** **Posterior** dislocation of proximal end of tibia, **right** knee

  ✓7th **S83.125** **Posterior** dislocation of proximal end of tibia, **left** knee

  ✓7th **S83.126** **Posterior** dislocation of proximal end of tibia, unspecified knee

✓6th **S83.13** **Medial** subluxation and dislocation of proximal end of tibia

  ✓7th **S83.131** **Medial** subluxation of proximal end of tibia, **right** knee

  ✓7th **S83.132** **Medial** subluxation of proximal end of tibia, **left** knee

  ✓7th **S83.133** **Medial** subluxation of proximal end of tibia, unspecified knee

  ✓7th **S83.134** **Medial** dislocation of proximal end of tibia, **right** knee

  ✓7th **S83.135** **Medial** dislocation of proximal end of tibia, **left** knee

  ✓7th **S83.136** **Medial** dislocation of proximal end of tibia, unspecified knee

✓6th **S83.14** **Lateral** subluxation and dislocation of proximal end of tibia

  ✓7th **S83.141** **Lateral** subluxation of proximal end of tibia, **right** knee

  ✓7th **S83.142** **Lateral** subluxation of proximal end of tibia, **left** knee

  ✓7th **S83.143** **Lateral** subluxation of proximal end of tibia, unspecified knee

  ✓7th **S83.144** **Lateral** dislocation of proximal end of tibia, **right** knee

  ✓7th **S83.145** **Lateral** dislocation of proximal end of tibia, **left** knee

  ✓7th **S83.146** **Lateral** dislocation of proximal end of tibia, unspecified knee

✓6th **S83.19** **Other** subluxation and dislocation of knee

  ✓7th **S83.191** Other subluxation of **right** knee

  ✓7th **S83.192** Other subluxation of **left** knee

  ✓7th **S83.193** Other subluxation of unspecified knee

  ✓7th **S83.194** Other dislocation of **right** knee

  ✓7th **S83.195** Other dislocation of **left** knee

  ✓7th **S83.196** Other dislocation of unspecified knee

✓5th **S83.2** **Tear of meniscus, current injury**

  EXCLUDES 1 old bucket-handle tear (M23.2)

  AHA: 2019,2Q,26

✓6th **S83.20** **Tear of unspecified meniscus, current injury**
Tear of meniscus of knee NOS

  ✓7th **S83.200** **Bucket-handle** tear of unspecified meniscus, current injury, **right** knee

  ✓7th **S83.201** **Bucket-handle** tear of unspecified meniscus, current injury, **left** knee

  ✓7th **S83.202** **Bucket-handle** tear of unspecified meniscus, current injury, unspecified knee

  ✓7th **S83.203** Other tear of unspecified meniscus, current injury, **right** knee

  ✓7th **S83.204** Other tear of unspecified meniscus, current injury, **left** knee

  ✓7th **S83.205** Other tear of unspecified meniscus, current injury, unspecified knee

  ✓7th **S83.206** Unspecified tear of unspecified meniscus, current injury, **right** knee

  ✓7th **S83.207** Unspecified tear of unspecified meniscus, current injury, **left** knee

  ✓7th **S83.209** Unspecified tear of unspecified meniscus, current injury, unspecified knee

✓6th **S83.21** **Bucket-handle** tear of **medial** meniscus, current injury

  ✓7th **S83.211** Bucket-handle tear of medial meniscus, current injury, **right** knee

  ✓7th **S83.212** Bucket-handle tear of medial meniscus, current injury, **left** knee

  ✓7th **S83.219** Bucket-handle tear of medial meniscus, current injury, unspecified knee

✓6th **S83.22** **Peripheral** tear of **medial** meniscus, current injury

  ✓7th **S83.221** **Peripheral** tear of medial meniscus, current injury, **right** knee

  ✓7th **S83.222** **Peripheral** tear of medial meniscus, current injury, **left** knee

  ✓7th **S83.229** **Peripheral** tear of medial meniscus, current injury, unspecified knee

✓6th **S83.23** **Complex** tear of **medial** meniscus, current injury

  ✓7th **S83.231** Complex tear of medial meniscus, current injury, **right** knee

  ✓7th **S83.232** Complex tear of medial meniscus, current injury, **left** knee

  ✓7th **S83.239** Complex tear of medial meniscus, current injury, unspecified knee

✓6th **S83.24** **Other** tear of **medial** meniscus, current injury

  ✓7th **S83.241** Other tear of medial meniscus, current injury, **right** knee

  ✓7th **S83.242** Other tear of medial meniscus, current injury, **left** knee

  ✓7th **S83.249** Other tear of medial meniscus, current injury, unspecified knee

✓6th **S83.25** **Bucket-handle** tear of **lateral** meniscus, current injury

  ✓7th **S83.251** Bucket-handle tear of lateral meniscus, current injury, **right** knee

  ✓7th **S83.252** Bucket-handle tear of lateral meniscus, current injury, **left** knee

  ✓7th **S83.259** Bucket-handle tear of lateral meniscus, current injury, unspecified knee

✓6th **S83.26** **Peripheral** tear of **lateral** meniscus, current injury

  ✓7th **S83.261** Peripheral tear of lateral meniscus, current injury, **right** knee

  ✓7th **S83.262** Peripheral tear of lateral meniscus, current injury, **left** knee

  ✓7th **S83.269** Peripheral tear of lateral meniscus, current injury, unspecified knee

✓6th **S83.27** **Complex** tear of **lateral** meniscus, current injury

  ✓7th **S83.271** Complex tear of lateral meniscus, current injury, **right** knee

  ✓7th **S83.272** Complex tear of lateral meniscus, current injury, **left** knee

  ✓7th **S83.279** Complex tear of lateral meniscus, current injury, unspecified knee

✓6th **S83.28** **Other** tear of **lateral** meniscus, current injury

  ✓7th **S83.281** Other tear of lateral meniscus, current injury, **right** knee

  ✓7th **S83.282** Other tear of lateral meniscus, current injury, **left** knee

  ✓7th **S83.289** Other tear of lateral meniscus, current injury, unspecified knee

✓5th **S83.3** **Tear of articular cartilage** of knee, current

  ✓x 7th **S83.30** Tear of articular cartilage of unspecified knee, current

  ✓x 7th **S83.31** Tear of articular cartilage of **right** knee, current

  ✓x 7th **S83.32** Tear of articular cartilage of **left** knee, current

✓5th **S83.4** **Sprain of collateral ligament of knee**

  ✓6th **S83.40** Sprain of unspecified collateral ligament of knee

    ✓7th **S83.401** Sprain of unspecified collateral ligament of **right** knee

    ✓7th **S83.402** Sprain of unspecified collateral ligament of **left** knee

    ✓7th **S83.409** Sprain of unspecified collateral ligament of unspecified knee

  ✓6th **S83.41** Sprain of **medial** collateral ligament of knee
Sprain of tibial collateral ligament

    ✓7th **S83.411** Sprain of medial collateral ligament of **right** knee

    ✓7th **S83.412** Sprain of medial collateral ligament of **left** knee

    ✓7th **S83.419** Sprain of medial collateral ligament of unspecified knee

  ✓6th **S83.42** Sprain of **lateral** collateral ligament of knee
Sprain of fibular collateral ligament

    ✓7th **S83.421** Sprain of lateral collateral ligament of **right** knee

    ✓7th **S83.422** Sprain of lateral collateral ligament of **left** knee

☑ Additional Character Required ✓x7th Placeholder **Unacceptable PDx** Questionable PDx Manifestation **Unspecified Dx** H1-H15 HAC HCC CMS-HCC Dx HIV HIV Dx

ICD-10-CM 2020

1105

☑7ᵗʰ S83.429 Sprain of lateral collateral ligament of unspecified knee

☑5ᵗʰ S83.5 Sprain of cruciate ligament of knee

    AHA: 2016,2Q,3

  ☑6ᵗʰ S83.50 Sprain of unspecified cruciate ligament of knee

    ☑7ᵗʰ S83.501 Sprain of unspecified cruciate ligament of right knee

    ☑7ᵗʰ S83.502 Sprain of unspecified cruciate ligament of left knee

    ☑7ᵗʰ S83.509 Sprain of unspecified cruciate ligament of unspecified knee

  ☑6ᵗʰ S83.51 Sprain of anterior cruciate ligament of knee

    ☑7ᵗʰ S83.511 Sprain of anterior cruciate ligament of right knee

    ☑7ᵗʰ S83.512 Sprain of anterior cruciate ligament of left knee

    ☑7ᵗʰ S83.519 Sprain of anterior cruciate ligament of unspecified knee

  ☑6ᵗʰ S83.52 Sprain of posterior cruciate ligament of knee

    ☑7ᵗʰ S83.521 Sprain of posterior cruciate ligament of right knee

    ☑7ᵗʰ S83.522 Sprain of posterior cruciate ligament of left knee

    ☑7ᵗʰ S83.529 Sprain of posterior cruciate ligament of unspecified knee

☑5ᵗʰ S83.6 Sprain of the superior tibiofibular joint and ligament

  ☑x7ᵗʰ S83.60 Sprain of the superior tibiofibular joint and ligament, unspecified knee

  ☑x7ᵗʰ S83.61 Sprain of the superior tibiofibular joint and ligament, right knee

  ☑x7ᵗʰ S83.62 Sprain of the superior tibiofibular joint and ligament, left knee

☑5ᵗʰ S83.8 Sprain of other specified parts of knee

  ☑6ᵗʰ S83.8X Sprain of other specified parts of knee

    ☑7ᵗʰ S83.8X1 Sprain of other specified parts of right knee

    ☑7ᵗʰ S83.8X2 Sprain of other specified parts of left knee

    ☑7ᵗʰ S83.8X9 Sprain of other specified parts of unspecified knee

☑5ᵗʰ S83.9 Sprain of unspecified site of knee

  ☑x7ᵗʰ S83.90 Sprain of unspecified site of unspecified knee

  ☑x7ᵗʰ S83.91 Sprain of unspecified site of right knee

  ☑x7ᵗʰ S83.92 Sprain of unspecified site of left knee

☑4ᵗʰ S84 Injury of nerves at lower leg level

    Code also any associated open wound (S81.-)

    EXCLUDES 2   injury of nerves at ankle and foot level (S94.-)

    The appropriate 7th character is to be added to each code from category S84.
    A   initial encounter
    D   subsequent encounter
    S   sequela

☑5ᵗʰ S84.0 Injury of tibial nerve at lower leg level

  ☑x7ᵗʰ S84.00 Injury of tibial nerve at lower leg level, unspecified leg

  ☑x7ᵗʰ S84.01 Injury of tibial nerve at lower leg level, right leg

  ☑x7ᵗʰ S84.02 Injury of tibial nerve at lower leg level, left leg

☑5ᵗʰ S84.1 Injury of peroneal nerve at lower leg level

  ☑x7ᵗʰ S84.10 Injury of peroneal nerve at lower leg level, unspecified leg

  ☑x7ᵗʰ S84.11 Injury of peroneal nerve at lower leg level, right leg

  ☑x7ᵗʰ S84.12 Injury of peroneal nerve at lower leg level, left leg

☑5ᵗʰ S84.2 Injury of cutaneous sensory nerve at lower leg level

  ☑x7ᵗʰ S84.20 Injury of cutaneous sensory nerve at lower leg level, unspecified leg

  ☑x7ᵗʰ S84.21 Injury of cutaneous sensory nerve at lower leg level, right leg

  ☑x7ᵗʰ S84.22 Injury of cutaneous sensory nerve at lower leg level, left leg

☑5ᵗʰ S84.8 Injury of other nerves at lower leg level

  ☑6ᵗʰ S84.80 Injury of other nerves at lower leg level

    ☑7ᵗʰ S84.801 Injury of other nerves at lower leg level, right leg

    ☑7ᵗʰ S84.802 Injury of other nerves at lower leg level, left leg

    ☑7ᵗʰ S84.809 Injury of other nerves at lower leg level, unspecified leg

☑5ᵗʰ S84.9 Injury of unspecified nerve at lower leg level

  ☑x7ᵗʰ S84.90 Injury of unspecified nerve at lower leg level, unspecified leg

  ☑x7ᵗʰ S84.91 Injury of unspecified nerve at lower leg level, right leg

  ☑x7ᵗʰ S84.92 Injury of unspecified nerve at lower leg level, left leg

☑4ᵗʰ S85 Injury of blood vessels at lower leg level

    Code also any associated open wound (S81.-)

    EXCLUDES 2   injury of blood vessels at ankle and foot level (S95.-)

    The appropriate 7th character is to be added to each code from category S85.
    A   initial encounter
    D   subsequent encounter
    S   sequela

☑5ᵗʰ S85.0 Injury of popliteal artery

    CC Excl: For MCC codes in subcategory S85.0:
    Right side: PDX collection 1349
    Left side: PDX collection 1350
    Unspecified side: PDX collection 1351

  ☑6ᵗʰ S85.00 Unspecified injury of popliteal artery

    ☑7ᵗʰ S85.001 Unspecified injury of popliteal artery, right leg   MCC

    ☑7ᵗʰ S85.002 Unspecified injury of popliteal artery, left leg   MCC

    ☑7ᵗʰ S85.009 Unspecified injury of popliteal artery, unspecified leg   MCC

  ☑6ᵗʰ S85.01 Laceration of popliteal artery

    ☑7ᵗʰ S85.011 Laceration of popliteal artery, right leg   MCC

    ☑7ᵗʰ S85.012 Laceration of popliteal artery, left leg   MCC

    ☑7ᵗʰ S85.019 Laceration of popliteal artery, unspecified leg   MCC

  ☑6ᵗʰ S85.09 Other specified injury of popliteal artery

    ☑7ᵗʰ S85.091 Other specified injury of popliteal artery, right leg   MCC

    ☑7ᵗʰ S85.092 Other specified injury of popliteal artery, left leg   MCC

    ☑7ᵗʰ S85.099 Other specified injury of popliteal artery, unspecified leg   MCC

☑5ᵗʰ S85.1 Injury of tibial artery

  ☑6ᵗʰ S85.10 Unspecified injury of unspecified tibial artery

    Injury of tibial artery NOS

    ☑7ᵗʰ S85.101 Unspecified injury of unspecified tibial artery, right leg   CC
        CC Excl: PDX collection 1352

    ☑7ᵗʰ S85.102 Unspecified injury of unspecified tibial artery, left leg   CC
        CC Excl: PDX collection 1353

    ☑7ᵗʰ S85.109 Unspecified injury of unspecified tibial artery, unspecified leg   CC
        CC Excl: PDX collection 1354

  ☑6ᵗʰ S85.11 Laceration of unspecified tibial artery

    ☑7ᵗʰ S85.111 Laceration of unspecified tibial artery, right leg   CC
        CC Excl: PDX collection 1352

    ☑7ᵗʰ S85.112 Laceration of unspecified tibial artery, left leg   CC
        CC Excl: PDX collection 1353

    ☑7ᵗʰ S85.119 Laceration of unspecified tibial artery, unspecified leg   CC
        CC Excl: PDX collection 1354

  ☑6ᵗʰ S85.12 Other specified injury of unspecified tibial artery

    ☑7ᵗʰ S85.121 Other specified injury of unspecified tibial artery, right leg   CC
        CC Excl: PDX collection 1352

N Newborn: 0   P Pediatric: 0-17   M Maternity: 9-64   A Adult: 15-124   MCC Major Complication/Comorbidity   CC Complication/Comorbidity   SW Severe Wound Dx

1106   ICD-10-CM 2020

✓7ᵗʰ **S85.122** Other specified injury of unspecified tibial artery, **left** leg   CC
     CC Excl: PDX collection 1353

✓7ᵗʰ **S85.129** Other specified injury of unspecified tibial artery, **unspecified** leg   CC
     CC Excl: PDX collection 1354

✓6ᵗʰ **S85.13** Unspecified injury of **anterior** tibial artery

✓7ᵗʰ **S85.131** Unspecified injury of anterior tibial artery, **right** leg   CC
     CC Excl: PDX collection 1355

✓7ᵗʰ **S85.132** Unspecified injury of anterior tibial artery, **left** leg   CC
     CC Excl: PDX collection 1356

✓7ᵗʰ **S85.139** Unspecified injury of anterior tibial artery, **unspecified** leg   CC
     CC Excl: PDX collection 1357

✓6ᵗʰ **S85.14** Laceration of **anterior** tibial artery

✓7ᵗʰ **S85.141** Laceration of anterior tibial artery, **right** leg   CC
     CC Excl: PDX collection 1355

✓7ᵗʰ **S85.142** Laceration of anterior tibial artery, **left** leg   CC
     CC Excl: PDX collection 1356

✓7ᵗʰ **S85.149** Laceration of anterior tibial artery, **unspecified** leg   CC
     CC Excl: PDX collection 1357

✓6ᵗʰ **S85.15** Other specified injury of **anterior** tibial artery

✓7ᵗʰ **S85.151** Other specified injury of anterior tibial artery, **right** leg   CC
     CC Excl: PDX collection 1355

✓7ᵗʰ **S85.152** Other specified injury of anterior tibial artery, **left** leg   CC
     CC Excl: PDX collection 1356

✓7ᵗʰ **S85.159** Other specified injury of anterior tibial artery, **unspecified** leg   CC
     CC Excl: PDX collection 1357

✓6ᵗʰ **S85.16** Unspecified injury of **posterior** tibial artery

✓7ᵗʰ **S85.161** Unspecified injury of posterior tibial artery, **right** leg   CC
     CC Excl: PDX collection 1358

✓7ᵗʰ **S85.162** Unspecified injury of posterior tibial artery, **left** leg   CC
     CC Excl: PDX collection 1359

✓7ᵗʰ **S85.169** Unspecified injury of posterior tibial artery, **unspecified** leg   CC
     CC Excl: PDX collection 1360

✓6ᵗʰ **S85.17** Laceration of **posterior** tibial artery

✓7ᵗʰ **S85.171** Laceration of posterior tibial artery, **right** leg   CC
     CC Excl: PDX collection 1358

✓7ᵗʰ **S85.172** Laceration of posterior tibial artery, **left** leg   CC
     CC Excl: PDX collection 1359

✓7ᵗʰ **S85.179** Laceration of posterior tibial artery, **unspecified** leg   CC
     CC Excl: PDX collection 1360

✓6ᵗʰ **S85.18** Other specified injury of **posterior** tibial artery

✓7ᵗʰ **S85.181** Other specified injury of posterior tibial artery, **right** leg   CC
     CC Excl: PDX collection 1358

✓7ᵗʰ **S85.182** Other specified injury of posterior tibial artery, **left** leg   CC
     CC Excl: PDX collection 1359

✓7ᵗʰ **S85.189** Other specified injury of posterior tibial artery, **unspecified** leg   CC
     CC Excl: PDX collection 1360

✓5ᵗʰ **S85.2** Injury of **peroneal** artery
     CC Excl: For CC codes in subcategory S85.2:
     Right side: PDX collection 1325
     Left side: PDX collection 1326
     Unspecified side: PDX collection 1327

✓6ᵗʰ **S85.20** Unspecified injury of peroneal artery

✓7ᵗʰ **S85.201** Unspecified injury of peroneal artery, **right** leg   CC

✓7ᵗʰ **S85.202** Unspecified injury of peroneal artery, **left** leg   CC

✓7ᵗʰ **S85.209** Unspecified injury of peroneal artery, **unspecified** leg   CC

✓6ᵗʰ **S85.21** Laceration of peroneal artery

✓7ᵗʰ **S85.211** Laceration of peroneal artery, **right** leg   CC

✓7ᵗʰ **S85.212** Laceration of peroneal artery, **left** leg   CC

✓7ᵗʰ **S85.219** Laceration of peroneal artery, unspecified leg   CC

✓6ᵗʰ **S85.29** Other specified injury of peroneal artery

✓7ᵗʰ **S85.291** Other specified injury of peroneal artery, **right** leg   CC

✓7ᵗʰ **S85.292** Other specified injury of peroneal artery, **left** leg   CC

✓7ᵗʰ **S85.299** Other specified injury of peroneal artery, **unspecified** leg   CC

✓5ᵗʰ **S85.3** Injury of **greater saphenous vein** at lower leg level
     Injury of greater saphenous vein NOS
     Injury of saphenous vein NOS
     CC Excl: For CC codes in subcategory S85.3:
     Right side: PDX collection 1322
     Left side: PDX collection 1323
     Unspecified side: PDX collection 1324

✓6ᵗʰ **S85.30** Unspecified injury of greater saphenous vein at lower leg level

✓7ᵗʰ **S85.301** Unspecified injury of greater saphenous vein at lower leg level, **right** leg   CC

✓7ᵗʰ **S85.302** Unspecified injury of greater saphenous vein at lower leg level, **left** leg   CC

✓7ᵗʰ **S85.309** Unspecified injury of greater saphenous vein at lower leg level, unspecified leg   CC

✓6ᵗʰ **S85.31** Laceration of greater saphenous vein at lower leg level

✓7ᵗʰ **S85.311** Laceration of greater saphenous vein at lower leg level, **right** leg   CC

✓7ᵗʰ **S85.312** Laceration of greater saphenous vein at lower leg level, **left** leg   CC

✓7ᵗʰ **S85.319** Laceration of greater saphenous vein at lower leg level, unspecified leg   CC

✓6ᵗʰ **S85.39** Other specified injury of greater saphenous vein at lower leg level

✓7ᵗʰ **S85.391** Other specified injury of greater saphenous vein at lower leg level, **right** leg   CC

✓7ᵗʰ **S85.392** Other specified injury of greater saphenous vein at lower leg level, **left** leg   CC

✓7ᵗʰ **S85.399** Other specified injury of greater saphenous vein at lower leg level, unspecified leg   CC

✓5ᵗʰ **S85.4** Injury of **lesser saphenous vein** at lower leg level
     CC Excl: For CC codes in subcategory S85.4:
     Right side: PDX collection 1322
     Left side: PDX collection 1323
     Unspecified side: PDX collection 1324

✓6ᵗʰ **S85.40** Unspecified injury of lesser saphenous vein at lower leg level

✓7ᵗʰ **S85.401** Unspecified injury of lesser saphenous vein at lower leg level, **right** leg   CC

Chapter 19. Injury, Poisoning and Certain Other Consequences of External Causes

S85.402–S86.012

√7ᵗʰ **S85.402** Unspecified injury of lesser saphenous vein at lower leg level, **left** leg   CC

√7ᵗʰ **S85.409** Unspecified injury of lesser saphenous vein at lower leg level, unspecified leg   CC

√6ᵗʰ **S85.41** Laceration of lesser saphenous vein at lower leg level

√7ᵗʰ **S85.411** Laceration of lesser saphenous vein at lower leg level, **right** leg   CC

√7ᵗʰ **S85.412** Laceration of lesser saphenous vein at lower leg level, **left** leg   CC

√7ᵗʰ **S85.419** Laceration of lesser saphenous vein at lower leg level, unspecified leg   CC

√6ᵗʰ **S85.49** Other specified injury of lesser saphenous vein at lower leg level

√7ᵗʰ **S85.491** Other specified injury of lesser saphenous vein at lower leg level, **right** leg   CC

√7ᵗʰ **S85.492** Other specified injury of lesser saphenous vein at lower leg level, **left** leg   CC

√7ᵗʰ **S85.499** Other specified injury of lesser saphenous vein at lower leg level, unspecified leg   CC

√5ᵗʰ **S85.5** Injury of popliteal vein

CC Excl: For MCC codes in subcategory S85.5:
Right side: PDX collection 1361
Left side: PDX collection 1362
Unspecified side: PDX collection 1363

√6ᵗʰ **S85.50** Unspecified injury of popliteal vein

√7ᵗʰ **S85.501** Unspecified injury of popliteal vein, **right** leg   MCC

√7ᵗʰ **S85.502** Unspecified injury of popliteal vein, **left** leg   MCC

√7ᵗʰ **S85.509** Unspecified injury of popliteal vein, unspecified leg   MCC

√6ᵗʰ **S85.51** Laceration of popliteal vein

√7ᵗʰ **S85.511** Laceration of popliteal vein, **right** leg   MCC

√7ᵗʰ **S85.512** Laceration of popliteal vein, **left** leg   MCC

√7ᵗʰ **S85.519** Laceration of popliteal vein, unspecified leg   MCC

√6ᵗʰ **S85.59** Other specified injury of popliteal vein

√7ᵗʰ **S85.591** Other specified injury of popliteal vein, **right** leg   MCC

√7ᵗʰ **S85.592** Other specified injury of popliteal vein, **left** leg   MCC

√7ᵗʰ **S85.599** Other specified injury of popliteal vein, unspecified leg   MCC

√5ᵗʰ **S85.8** Injury of other blood vessels at lower leg level

CC Excl: For CC codes in subcategory S85.8:
Right side: PDX collection 1325
Left side: PDX collection 1326
Unspecified side: PDX collection 1327

√6ᵗʰ **S85.80** Unspecified injury of other blood vessels at lower leg level

√7ᵗʰ **S85.801** Unspecified injury of other blood vessels at lower leg level, **right** leg   CC

√7ᵗʰ **S85.802** Unspecified injury of other blood vessels at lower leg level, **left** leg   CC

√7ᵗʰ **S85.809** Unspecified injury of other blood vessels at lower leg level, unspecified leg   CC

√6ᵗʰ **S85.81** Laceration of other blood vessels at lower leg level

√7ᵗʰ **S85.811** Laceration of other blood vessels at lower leg level, **right** leg   CC

√7ᵗʰ **S85.812** Laceration of other blood vessels at lower leg level, **left** leg   CC

√7ᵗʰ **S85.819** Laceration of other blood vessels at lower leg level, unspecified leg   CC

√6ᵗʰ **S85.89** Other specified injury of other blood vessels at lower leg level

√7ᵗʰ **S85.891** Other specified injury of other blood vessels at lower leg level, **right** leg   CC

√7ᵗʰ **S85.892** Other specified injury of other blood vessels at lower leg level, **left** leg   CC

√7ᵗʰ **S85.899** Other specified injury of other blood vessels at lower leg level, unspecified leg   CC

√5ᵗʰ **S85.9** Injury of unspecified blood vessel at lower leg level

CC Excl: For CC codes in subcategory S85.9:
Right side: PDX collection 1325
Left side: PDX collection 1326
Unspecified side: PDX collection 1327

√6ᵗʰ **S85.90** Unspecified injury of unspecified blood vessel at lower leg level

√7ᵗʰ **S85.901** Unspecified injury of unspecified blood vessel at lower leg level, **right** leg   CC

√7ᵗʰ **S85.902** Unspecified injury of unspecified blood vessel at lower leg level, **left** leg   CC

√7ᵗʰ **S85.909** Unspecified injury of unspecified blood vessel at lower leg level, unspecified leg   CC

√6ᵗʰ **S85.91** Laceration of unspecified blood vessel at lower leg level

√7ᵗʰ **S85.911** Laceration of unspecified blood vessel at lower leg level, **right** leg   CC

√7ᵗʰ **S85.912** Laceration of unspecified blood vessel at lower leg level, **left** leg   CC

√7ᵗʰ **S85.919** Laceration of unspecified blood vessel at lower leg level, unspecified leg   CC

√6ᵗʰ **S85.99** Other specified injury of unspecified blood vessel at lower leg level

√7ᵗʰ **S85.991** Other specified injury of unspecified blood vessel at lower leg level, **right** leg   CC

√7ᵗʰ **S85.992** Other specified injury of unspecified blood vessel at lower leg level, **left** leg   CC

√7ᵗʰ **S85.999** Other specified injury of unspecified blood vessel at lower leg level, unspecified leg   CC

√4ᵗʰ **S86** Injury of muscle, fascia and tendon at lower leg level

Code also any associated open wound (S81.-)

EXCLUDES 2   *injury of muscle, fascia and tendon at ankle (S96.-)*
injury of patellar ligament (tendon) (S76.1-)
sprain of joints and ligaments of knee (S83.-)

TIP: Refer to the Muscle/Tendon table at the beginning of this chapter.

The appropriate 7th character is to be added to each code from category S86.
A   initial encounter
D   subsequent encounter
S   sequela

CC Excl: For CC codes in category S86:
Right side: PDX collection 1364
Left side: PDX collection 1365
Unspecified side: PDX collection 1366

√5ᵗʰ **S86.0** Injury of Achilles tendon

√6ᵗʰ **S86.00** Unspecified injury of Achilles tendon

√7ᵗʰ **S86.001** Unspecified injury of **right** Achilles tendon

√7ᵗʰ **S86.002** Unspecified injury of **left** Achilles tendon

√7ᵗʰ **S86.009** Unspecified injury of unspecified Achilles tendon

√6ᵗʰ **S86.01** Strain of Achilles tendon

√7ᵗʰ **S86.011** Strain of **right** Achilles tendon

√7ᵗʰ **S86.012** Strain of **left** Achilles tendon

N Newborn: 0   P Pediatric: 0-17   M Maternity: 9-64   A Adult: 15-124   MCC Major Complication/Comorbidity   CC Complication/Comorbidity   SW Severe Wound Dx

1108   ICD-10-CM 2020

     √7ᵗʰ S86.019 Strain of unspecified Achilles tendon

√6ᵗʰ S86.02 **Laceration** of Achilles tendon

     √7ᵗʰ S86.021 Laceration of right Achilles tendon   `cc`

     √7ᵗʰ S86.022 Laceration of left Achilles tendon   `cc`

     √7ᵗʰ S86.029 Laceration of unspecified Achilles tendon   `cc`

√6ᵗʰ S86.09 Other specified injury of Achilles tendon

     √7ᵗʰ S86.091 Other specified injury of right Achilles tendon

     √7ᵗʰ S86.092 Other specified injury of left Achilles tendon

     √7ᵗʰ S86.099 Other specified injury of unspecified Achilles tendon

√5ᵗʰ S86.1 Injury of other muscle(s) and tendon(s) of posterior muscle group at lower leg level

√6ᵗʰ S86.10 Unspecified injury of other muscle(s) and tendon(s) of posterior muscle group at lower leg level

     √7ᵗʰ S86.101 Unspecified injury of other muscle(s) and tendon(s) of posterior muscle group at lower leg level, right leg

     √7ᵗʰ S86.102 Unspecified injury of other muscle(s) and tendon(s) of posterior muscle group at lower leg level, left leg

     √7ᵗʰ S86.109 Unspecified injury of other muscle(s) and tendon(s) of posterior muscle group at lower leg level, unspecified leg

√6ᵗʰ S86.11 **Strain** of other muscle(s) and tendon(s) of posterior muscle group at lower leg level

     √7ᵗʰ S86.111 Strain of other muscle(s) and tendon(s) of posterior muscle group at lower leg level, right leg

     √7ᵗʰ S86.112 Strain of other muscle(s) and tendon(s) of posterior muscle group at lower leg level, left leg

     √7ᵗʰ S86.119 Strain of other muscle(s) and tendon(s) of posterior muscle group at lower leg level, unspecified leg

√6ᵗʰ S86.12 **Laceration** of other muscle(s) and tendon(s) of posterior muscle group at lower leg level

     √7ᵗʰ S86.121 Laceration of other muscle(s) and tendon(s) of posterior muscle group at lower leg level, right leg   `cc`

     √7ᵗʰ S86.122 Laceration of other muscle(s) and tendon(s) of posterior muscle group at lower leg level, left leg   `cc`

     √7ᵗʰ S86.129 Laceration of other muscle(s) and tendon(s) of posterior muscle group at lower leg level, unspecified leg   `cc`

√6ᵗʰ S86.19 Other injury of other muscle(s) and tendon(s) of posterior muscle group at lower leg level

     √7ᵗʰ S86.191 Other injury of other muscle(s) and tendon(s) of posterior muscle group at lower leg level, right leg

     √7ᵗʰ S86.192 Other injury of other muscle(s) and tendon(s) of posterior muscle group at lower leg level, left leg

     √7ᵗʰ S86.199 Other injury of other muscle(s) and tendon(s) of posterior muscle group at lower leg level, unspecified leg

√5ᵗʰ S86.2 Injury of muscle(s) and tendon(s) of anterior muscle group at lower leg level

√6ᵗʰ S86.20 Unspecified injury of muscle(s) and tendon(s) of anterior muscle group at lower leg level

     √7ᵗʰ S86.201 Unspecified injury of muscle(s) and tendon(s) of anterior muscle group at lower leg level, right leg

     √7ᵗʰ S86.202 Unspecified injury of muscle(s) and tendon(s) of anterior muscle group at lower leg level, left leg

     √7ᵗʰ S86.209 Unspecified injury of muscle(s) and tendon(s) of anterior muscle group at lower leg level, unspecified leg

√6ᵗʰ S86.21 **Strain** of muscle(s) and tendon(s) of anterior muscle group at lower leg level

     √7ᵗʰ S86.211 Strain of muscle(s) and tendon(s) of anterior muscle group at lower leg level, right leg

     √7ᵗʰ S86.212 Strain of muscle(s) and tendon(s) of anterior muscle group at lower leg level, left leg

     √7ᵗʰ S86.219 Strain of muscle(s) and tendon(s) of anterior muscle group at lower leg level, unspecified leg

√6ᵗʰ S86.22 **Laceration** of muscle(s) and tendon(s) of anterior muscle group at lower leg level

     √7ᵗʰ S86.221 Laceration of muscle(s) and tendon(s) of anterior muscle group at lower leg level, right leg   `cc`

     √7ᵗʰ S86.222 Laceration of muscle(s) and tendon(s) of anterior muscle group at lower leg level, left leg   `cc`

     √7ᵗʰ S86.229 Laceration of muscle(s) and tendon(s) of anterior muscle group at lower leg level, unspecified leg   `cc`

√6ᵗʰ S86.29 Other injury of muscle(s) and tendon(s) of anterior muscle group at lower leg level

     √7ᵗʰ S86.291 Other injury of muscle(s) and tendon(s) of anterior muscle group at lower leg level, right leg

     √7ᵗʰ S86.292 Other injury of muscle(s) and tendon(s) of anterior muscle group at lower leg level, left leg

     √7ᵗʰ S86.299 Other injury of muscle(s) and tendon(s) of anterior muscle group at lower leg level, unspecified leg

√5ᵗʰ S86.3 Injury of muscle(s) and tendon(s) of peroneal muscle group at lower leg level

√6ᵗʰ S86.30 Unspecified injury of muscle(s) and tendon(s) of peroneal muscle group at lower leg level

     √7ᵗʰ S86.301 Unspecified injury of muscle(s) and tendon(s) of peroneal muscle group at lower leg level, right leg

     √7ᵗʰ S86.302 Unspecified injury of muscle(s) and tendon(s) of peroneal muscle group at lower leg level, left leg

     √7ᵗʰ S86.309 Unspecified injury of muscle(s) and tendon(s) of peroneal muscle group at lower leg level, unspecified leg

√6ᵗʰ S86.31 **Strain** of muscle(s) and tendon(s) of peroneal muscle group at lower leg level

     √7ᵗʰ S86.311 Strain of muscle(s) and tendon(s) of peroneal muscle group at lower leg level, right leg

     √7ᵗʰ S86.312 Strain of muscle(s) and tendon(s) of peroneal muscle group at lower leg level, left leg

     √7ᵗʰ S86.319 Strain of muscle(s) and tendon(s) of peroneal muscle group at lower leg level, unspecified leg

√6ᵗʰ S86.32 **Laceration** of muscle(s) and tendon(s) of peroneal muscle group at lower leg level

     √7ᵗʰ S86.321 Laceration of muscle(s) and tendon(s) of peroneal muscle group at lower leg level, right leg   `cc`

     √7ᵗʰ S86.322 Laceration of muscle(s) and tendon(s) of peroneal muscle group at lower leg level, left leg   `cc`

     √7ᵗʰ S86.329 Laceration of muscle(s) and tendon(s) of peroneal muscle group at lower leg level, unspecified leg   `cc`

√6ᵗʰ S86.39 Other injury of muscle(s) and tendon(s) of peroneal muscle group at lower leg level

     √7ᵗʰ S86.391 Other injury of muscle(s) and tendon(s) of peroneal muscle group at lower leg level, right leg

     √7ᵗʰ S86.392 Other injury of muscle(s) and tendon(s) of peroneal muscle group at lower leg level, left leg

     √7ᵗʰ S86.399 Other injury of muscle(s) and tendon(s) of peroneal muscle group at lower leg level, unspecified leg

√5ᵗʰ S86.8 Injury of other muscles and tendons at lower leg level

√6ᵗʰ S86.80 Unspecified injury of other muscles and tendons at lower leg level

     √7ᵗʰ S86.801 Unspecified injury of other muscle(s) and tendon(s) at lower leg level, right leg

☑ Additional Character Required   √x7ᵗʰ Placeholder   Unacceptable PDx   Questionable PDx   Manifestation   Unspecified Dx   H1 - H14 HAC   HCC CMS-HCC Dx   HIV HIV Dx

ICD-10-CM 2020   1109

√7th **S86.802** Unspecified injury of other muscle(s) and tendon(s) at lower leg level, **left** leg

√7th **S86.809** Unspecified injury of other muscle(s) and tendon(s) at lower leg level, unspecified leg

√6th **S86.81** Strain of other muscles and tendons at lower leg level

√7th **S86.811** Strain of other muscle(s) and tendon(s) at lower leg level, **right** leg

√7th **S86.812** Strain of other muscle(s) and tendon(s) at lower leg level, **left** leg

√7th **S86.819** Strain of other muscle(s) and tendon(s) at lower leg level, unspecified leg

√6th **S86.82** Laceration of other muscles and tendons at lower leg level

√7th **S86.821** Laceration of other muscle(s) and tendon(s) at lower leg level, **right** leg `CC`

√7th **S86.822** Laceration of other muscle(s) and tendon(s) at lower leg level, **left** leg `CC`

√7th **S86.829** Laceration of other muscle(s) and tendon(s) at lower leg level, unspecified leg `CC`

√6th **S86.89** Other injury of other muscles and tendons at lower leg level

√7th **S86.891** Other injury of other muscle(s) and tendon(s) at lower leg level, **right** leg

√7th **S86.892** Other injury of other muscle(s) and tendon(s) at lower leg level, **left** leg

√7th **S86.899** Other injury of other muscle(s) and tendon(s) at lower leg level, unspecified leg

√5th **S86.9** Injury of unspecified muscle and tendon at lower leg level

√6th **S86.90** Unspecified injury of unspecified muscle and tendon at lower leg level

√7th **S86.901** Unspecified injury of unspecified muscle(s) and tendon(s) at lower leg level, **right** leg

√7th **S86.902** Unspecified injury of unspecified muscle(s) and tendon(s) at lower leg level, **left** leg

√7th **S86.909** Unspecified injury of unspecified muscle(s) and tendon(s) at lower leg level, unspecified leg

√6th **S86.91** Strain of unspecified muscle and tendon at lower leg level

√7th **S86.911** Strain of unspecified muscle(s) and tendon(s) at lower leg level, **right** leg

√7th **S86.912** Strain of unspecified muscle(s) and tendon(s) at lower leg level, **left** leg

√7th **S86.919** Strain of unspecified muscle(s) and tendon(s) at lower leg level, unspecified leg

√6th **S86.92** Laceration of unspecified muscle and tendon at lower leg level

√7th **S86.921** Laceration of unspecified muscle(s) and tendon(s) at lower leg level, **right** leg `CC`

√7th **S86.922** Laceration of unspecified muscle(s) and tendon(s) at lower leg level, **left** leg `CC`

√7th **S86.929** Laceration of unspecified muscle(s) and tendon(s) at lower leg level, unspecified leg `CC`

√6th **S86.99** Other injury of unspecified muscle and tendon at lower leg level

√7th **S86.991** Other injury of unspecified muscle(s) and tendon(s) at lower leg level, **right** leg

√7th **S86.992** Other injury of unspecified muscle(s) and tendon(s) at lower leg level, **left** leg

√7th **S86.999** Other injury of unspecified muscle(s) and tendon(s) at lower leg level, unspecified leg

√4th **S87 Crushing injury of lower leg**

Use additional code(s) for all associated injuries

EXCLUDES 2 crushing injury of ankle and foot (S97.-)

The appropriate 7th character is to be added to each code from category S87.
A initial encounter
D subsequent encounter
S sequela

√5th **S87.0** Crushing injury of knee

√x7th **S87.00** Crushing injury of unspecified knee

√x7th **S87.01** Crushing injury of **right** knee

√x7th **S87.02** Crushing injury of **left** knee

√5th **S87.8** Crushing injury of lower leg

√x7th **S87.80** Crushing injury of unspecified lower leg

√x7th **S87.81** Crushing injury of **right** lower leg

√x7th **S87.82** Crushing injury of **left** lower leg

√4th **S88 Traumatic amputation of lower leg**

An amputation not identified as partial or complete should be coded to complete

EXCLUDES 1 traumatic amputation of ankle and foot (S98.-)

The appropriate 7th character is to be added to each code from category S88.
A initial encounter
D subsequent encounter
S sequela

CC Excl: For CC codes in category S88:
Right side: PDX collection 1333
Left side: PDX collection 1334
Unspecified side: PDX collection 1335

√5th **S88.0** Traumatic amputation at knee level

√6th **S88.01** Complete traumatic amputation at knee level

√7th **S88.011** Complete traumatic amputation at knee level, **right** lower leg `CC` `HCC`

√7th **S88.012** Complete traumatic amputation at knee level, **left** lower leg `CC` `HCC`

√7th **S88.019** Complete traumatic amputation at knee level, unspecified lower leg `CC` `HCC`

√6th **S88.02** Partial traumatic amputation at knee level

√7th **S88.021** Partial traumatic amputation at knee level, **right** lower leg `CC` `HCC`

√7th **S88.022** Partial traumatic amputation at knee level, **left** lower leg `CC` `HCC`

√7th **S88.029** Partial traumatic amputation at knee level, unspecified lower leg `CC` `HCC`

√5th **S88.1** Traumatic amputation at level between knee and ankle

√6th **S88.11** Complete traumatic amputation at level between knee and ankle

√7th **S88.111** Complete traumatic amputation at level between knee and ankle, **right** lower leg `CC` `HCC`

√7th **S88.112** Complete traumatic amputation at level between knee and ankle, **left** lower leg `CC` `HCC`

√7th **S88.119** Complete traumatic amputation at level between knee and ankle, unspecified lower leg `CC` `HCC`

√6th **S88.12** Partial traumatic amputation at level between knee and ankle

√7th **S88.121** Partial traumatic amputation at level between knee and ankle, **right** lower leg `CC` `HCC`

√7th **S88.122** Partial traumatic amputation at level between knee and ankle, **left** lower leg `CC` `HCC`

N Newborn: 0   P Pediatric: 0-17   M Maternity: 9-64   A Adult: 15-124   MCC Major Complication/Comorbidity   CC Complication/Comorbidity   SW Severe Wound Dx

1110   ICD-10-CM 2020

√7ᵗʰ **S88.129** Partial traumatic amputation at level between knee and ankle, unspecified lower leg   `CC` `HCC`

√5ᵗʰ **S88.9** Traumatic amputation of lower leg, level unspecified

√6ᵗʰ **S88.91** Complete traumatic amputation of lower leg, level unspecified

√7ᵗʰ **S88.911** Complete traumatic amputation of right lower leg, level unspecified   `CC` `HCC`

√7ᵗʰ **S88.912** Complete traumatic amputation of left lower leg, level unspecified   `CC` `HCC`

√7ᵗʰ **S88.919** Complete traumatic amputation of unspecified lower leg, level unspecified   `CC` `HCC`

√6ᵗʰ **S88.92** Partial traumatic amputation of lower leg, level unspecified

√7ᵗʰ **S88.921** Partial traumatic amputation of right lower leg, level unspecified   `CC` `HCC`

√7ᵗʰ **S88.922** Partial traumatic amputation of left lower leg, level unspecified   `CC` `HCC`

√7ᵗʰ **S88.929** Partial traumatic amputation of unspecified lower leg, level unspecified   `CC` `HCC`

√4ᵗʰ **S89** Other and unspecified injuries of lower leg

NOTE   A fracture not indicated as open or closed should be coded to closed.

EXCLUDES 2   other and unspecified injuries of ankle and foot (S99.-)

AHA: 2018,2Q,12; 2018,1Q,3; 2015,3Q,37-39

The appropriate 7th character is to be added to each code from subcategories S89.0, S89.1, S89.2, and S89.3.
A initial encounter for closed fracture
D subsequent encounter for fracture with routine healing
G subsequent encounter for fracture with delayed healing
K subsequent encounter for fracture with nonunion
P subsequent encounter for fracture with malunion
S sequela

√5ᵗʰ **S89.0** Physeal fracture of upper end of tibia

CC Excl: For CC codes in subcategory S89.0:
Right side: See code S89.001
Left side: See code S89.002
Unspecified side: See code S89.009

√6ᵗʰ **S89.00** Unspecified physeal fracture of upper end of tibia

3 √7ᵗʰ **S89.001** Unspecified physeal fracture of upper end of right tibia   `CC` `H5`

CC Excl: CC with 7th character A: PDX collection 1340
CC Excl: CC with 7th character K or P: PDX collection 897

3 √7ᵗʰ **S89.002** Unspecified physeal fracture of upper end of left tibia   `CC` `H5`

CC Excl: CC with 7th character A: PDX collection 1342
CC Excl: CC with 7th character K or P: PDX collection 897

3 √7ᵗʰ **S89.009** Unspecified physeal fracture of upper end of unspecified tibia   `CC` `H5`

CC Excl: CC with 7th character A: PDX collection 1341
CC Excl: CC with 7th character K or P: PDX collection 897

√6ᵗʰ **S89.01** Salter-Harris Type I physeal fracture of upper end of tibia

3 √7ᵗʰ **S89.011** Salter-Harris Type I physeal fracture of upper end of right tibia   `CC` `H5`

3 √7ᵗʰ **S89.012** Salter-Harris Type I physeal fracture of upper end of left tibia   `CC` `H5`

3 √7ᵗʰ **S89.019** Salter-Harris Type I physeal fracture of upper end of unspecified tibia   `CC` `H5`

√6ᵗʰ **S89.02** Salter-Harris Type II physeal fracture of upper end of tibia

3 √7ᵗʰ **S89.021** Salter-Harris Type II physeal fracture of upper end of right tibia   `CC` `H5`

3 √7ᵗʰ **S89.022** Salter-Harris Type II physeal fracture of upper end of left tibia   `CC` `H5`

3 √7ᵗʰ **S89.029** Salter-Harris Type II physeal fracture of upper end of unspecified tibia   `CC` `H5`

√6ᵗʰ **S89.03** Salter-Harris Type III physeal fracture of upper end of tibia

3 √7ᵗʰ **S89.031** Salter-Harris Type III physeal fracture of upper end of right tibia   `CC` `H5`

3 √7ᵗʰ **S89.032** Salter-Harris Type III physeal fracture of upper end of left tibia   `CC` `H5`

3 √7ᵗʰ **S89.039** Salter-Harris Type III physeal fracture of upper end of unspecified tibia   `CC` `H5`

√6ᵗʰ **S89.04** Salter-Harris Type IV physeal fracture of upper end of tibia

3 √7ᵗʰ **S89.041** Salter-Harris Type IV physeal fracture of upper end of right tibia   `CC` `H5`

3 √7ᵗʰ **S89.042** Salter-Harris Type IV physeal fracture of upper end of left tibia   `CC` `H5`

3 √7ᵗʰ **S89.049** Salter-Harris Type IV physeal fracture of upper end of unspecified tibia   `CC` `H5`

√6ᵗʰ **S89.09** Other physeal fracture of upper end of tibia

3 √7ᵗʰ **S89.091** Other physeal fracture of upper end of right tibia   `CC` `H5`

3 √7ᵗʰ **S89.092** Other physeal fracture of upper end of left tibia   `CC` `H5`

3 √7ᵗʰ **S89.099** Other physeal fracture of upper end of unspecified tibia   `CC` `H5`

√5ᵗʰ **S89.1** Physeal fracture of lower end of tibia

CC Excl: For codes in subcategory S89.1:
CC with 7th character K or P: PDX collection 897

√6ᵗʰ **S89.10** Unspecified physeal fracture of lower end of tibia

4 √7ᵗʰ **S89.101** Unspecified physeal fracture of lower end of right tibia   `CC`

4 √7ᵗʰ **S89.102** Unspecified physeal fracture of lower end of left tibia   `CC`

4 √7ᵗʰ **S89.109** Unspecified physeal fracture of lower end of unspecified tibia   `CC`

√6ᵗʰ **S89.11** Salter-Harris Type I physeal fracture of lower end of tibia

4 √7ᵗʰ **S89.111** Salter-Harris Type I physeal fracture of lower end of right tibia   `CC`

4 √7ᵗʰ **S89.112** Salter-Harris Type I physeal fracture of lower end of left tibia   `CC`

4 √7ᵗʰ **S89.119** Salter-Harris Type I physeal fracture of lower end of unspecified tibia   `CC`

√6ᵗʰ **S89.12** Salter-Harris Type II physeal fracture of lower end of tibia

4 √7ᵗʰ **S89.121** Salter-Harris Type II physeal fracture of lower end of right tibia   `CC`

4 √7ᵗʰ **S89.122** Salter-Harris Type II physeal fracture of lower end of left tibia   `CC`

4 √7ᵗʰ **S89.129** Salter-Harris Type II physeal fracture of lower end of unspecified tibia   `CC`

√6ᵗʰ **S89.13** Salter-Harris Type III physeal fracture of lower end of tibia

EXCLUDES 1   fracture of medial malleolus (adult) (S82.5-)

4 √7ᵗʰ **S89.131** Salter-Harris Type III physeal fracture of lower end of right tibia   `CC`

4 ✓7ᵗʰ **S89.132** Salter-Harris Type III physeal fracture of lower end of left tibia   `CC`

4 ✓7ᵗʰ **S89.139** Salter-Harris Type III physeal fracture of lower end of unspecified tibia   `CC`

✓6ᵗʰ **S89.14** Salter-Harris Type IV physeal fracture of lower end of tibia

    `EXCLUDES 1`   *fracture of medial malleolus (adult) (S82.5-)*

4 ✓7ᵗʰ **S89.141** Salter-Harris Type IV physeal fracture of lower end of right tibia   `CC`

4 ✓7ᵗʰ **S89.142** Salter-Harris Type IV physeal fracture of lower end of left tibia   `CC`

4 ✓7ᵗʰ **S89.149** Salter-Harris Type IV physeal fracture of lower end of unspecified tibia   `CC`

✓6ᵗʰ **S89.19** Other physeal fracture of lower end of tibia

4 ✓7ᵗʰ **S89.191** Other physeal fracture of lower end of right tibia   `CC`

4 ✓7ᵗʰ **S89.192** Other physeal fracture of lower end of left tibia   `CC`

4 ✓7ᵗʰ **S89.199** Other physeal fracture of lower end of unspecified tibia   `CC`

✓5ᵗʰ **S89.2** Physeal fracture of upper end of fibula

    CC Excl: For codes in subcategory S89.2:
    CC with 7th character K or P: PDX collection 897

✓6ᵗʰ **S89.20** Unspecified physeal fracture of upper end of fibula

4 ✓7ᵗʰ **S89.201** Unspecified physeal fracture of upper end of right fibula   `CC`

4 ✓7ᵗʰ **S89.202** Unspecified physeal fracture of upper end of left fibula   `CC`

4 ✓7ᵗʰ **S89.209** Unspecified physeal fracture of upper end of unspecified fibula   `CC`

✓6ᵗʰ **S89.21** Salter-Harris Type I physeal fracture of upper end of fibula

4 ✓7ᵗʰ **S89.211** Salter-Harris Type I physeal fracture of upper end of right fibula   `CC`

4 ✓7ᵗʰ **S89.212** Salter-Harris Type I physeal fracture of upper end of left fibula   `CC`

4 ✓7ᵗʰ **S89.219** Salter-Harris Type I physeal fracture of upper end of unspecified fibula   `CC`

✓6ᵗʰ **S89.22** Salter-Harris Type II physeal fracture of upper end of fibula

4 ✓7ᵗʰ **S89.221** Salter-Harris Type II physeal fracture of upper end of right fibula   `CC`

4 ✓7ᵗʰ **S89.222** Salter-Harris Type II physeal fracture of upper end of left fibula   `CC`

4 ✓7ᵗʰ **S89.229** Salter-Harris Type II physeal fracture of upper end of unspecified fibula   `CC`

✓6ᵗʰ **S89.29** Other physeal fracture of upper end of fibula

4 ✓7ᵗʰ **S89.291** Other physeal fracture of upper end of right fibula   `CC`

4 ✓7ᵗʰ **S89.292** Other physeal fracture of upper end of left fibula   `CC`

4 ✓7ᵗʰ **S89.299** Other physeal fracture of upper end of unspecified fibula   `CC`

✓5ᵗʰ **S89.3** Physeal fracture of lower end of fibula

    CC Excl: For codes in subcategory S89.3:
    CC with 7th character K or P: PDX collection 897

✓6ᵗʰ **S89.30** Unspecified physeal fracture of lower end of fibula

4 ✓7ᵗʰ **S89.301** Unspecified physeal fracture of lower end of right fibula   `CC`

4 ✓7ᵗʰ **S89.302** Unspecified physeal fracture of lower end of left fibula   `CC`

4 ✓7ᵗʰ **S89.309** Unspecified physeal fracture of lower end of unspecified fibula   `CC`

✓6ᵗʰ **S89.31** Salter-Harris Type I physeal fracture of lower end of fibula

4 ✓7ᵗʰ **S89.311** Salter-Harris Type I physeal fracture of lower end of right fibula   `CC`

4 ✓7ᵗʰ **S89.312** Salter-Harris Type I physeal fracture of lower end of left fibula   `CC`

4 ✓7ᵗʰ **S89.319** Salter-Harris Type I physeal fracture of lower end of unspecified fibula   `CC`

✓6ᵗʰ **S89.32** Salter-Harris Type II physeal fracture of lower end of fibula

4 ✓7ᵗʰ **S89.321** Salter-Harris Type II physeal fracture of lower end of right fibula   `CC`

4 ✓7ᵗʰ **S89.322** Salter-Harris Type II physeal fracture of lower end of left fibula   `CC`

4 ✓7ᵗʰ **S89.329** Salter-Harris Type II physeal fracture of lower end of unspecified fibula   `CC`

✓6ᵗʰ **S89.39** Other physeal fracture of lower end of fibula

4 ✓7ᵗʰ **S89.391** Other physeal fracture of lower end of right fibula   `CC`

4 ✓7ᵗʰ **S89.392** Other physeal fracture of lower end of left fibula   `CC`

4 ✓7ᵗʰ **S89.399** Other physeal fracture of lower end of unspecified fibula   `CC`

✓5ᵗʰ **S89.8** Other specified injuries of lower leg

    The appropriate 7th character is to be added to each code in subcategory S89.8.
    A   initial encounter
    D   subsequent encounter
    S   sequela

✓x7ᵗʰ **S89.80** Other specified injuries of unspecified lower leg

✓x7ᵗʰ **S89.81** Other specified injuries of right lower leg

✓x7ᵗʰ **S89.82** Other specified injuries of left lower leg

✓5ᵗʰ **S89.9** Unspecified injury of lower leg

    The appropriate 7th character is to be added to each code in subcategory S89.9.
    A   initial encounter
    D   subsequent encounter
    S   sequela

✓x7ᵗʰ **S89.90** Unspecified injury of unspecified lower leg

✓x7ᵗʰ **S89.91** Unspecified injury of right lower leg

✓x7ᵗʰ **S89.92** Unspecified injury of left lower leg

Injuries to the ankle and foot (S90-S99)

`EXCLUDES 2`   *burns and corrosions (T20-T32)*
          fracture of ankle and malleolus (S82.-)
          frostbite (T33-T34)
          insect bite or sting, venomous (T63.4)

✓4ᵗʰ **S90** Superficial injury of ankle, foot and toes

    The appropriate 7th character is to be added to each code from category S90.
    A   initial encounter
    D   subsequent encounter
    S   sequela

✓5ᵗʰ **S90.0** Contusion of ankle

✓x7ᵗʰ **S90.00** Contusion of unspecified ankle

✓x7ᵗʰ **S90.01** Contusion of right ankle

✓x7ᵗʰ **S90.02** Contusion of left ankle

✓5ᵗʰ **S90.1** Contusion of toe without damage to nail

✓6ᵗʰ **S90.11** Contusion of great toe without damage to nail

✓7ᵗʰ **S90.111** Contusion of right great toe without damage to nail

✓7ᵗʰ **S90.112** Contusion of left great toe without damage to nail

✓7ᵗʰ **S90.119** Contusion of unspecified great toe without damage to nail

√6ᵗʰ **S90.12** **Contusion of** lesser **toe without damage to nail**

    √7ᵗʰ **S90.121** Contusion of right lesser toe(s) without damage to nail

    √7ᵗʰ **S90.122** Contusion of left lesser toe(s) without damage to nail

    √7ᵗʰ **S90.129** Contusion of unspecified lesser toe(s) without damage to nail
         Contusion of toe NOS

√5ᵗʰ **S90.2** **Contusion of** toe with damage to nail

  √6ᵗʰ **S90.21** **Contusion of** great **toe with damage to nail**

    √7ᵗʰ **S90.211** Contusion of right great toe with damage to nail

    √7ᵗʰ **S90.212** Contusion of left great toe with damage to nail

    √7ᵗʰ **S90.219** Contusion of unspecified great toe with damage to nail

  √6ᵗʰ **S90.22** **Contusion of** lesser **toe with damage to nail**

    √7ᵗʰ **S90.221** Contusion of right lesser toe(s) with damage to nail

    √7ᵗʰ **S90.222** Contusion of left lesser toe(s) with damage to nail

    √7ᵗʰ **S90.229** Contusion of unspecified lesser toe(s) with damage to nail

√5ᵗʰ **S90.3** **Contusion of** foot

    EXCLUDES 2   *contusion of toes (S90.1-, S90.2-)*

  √x7ᵗʰ **S90.30** **Contusion of unspecified foot**
         Contusion of foot NOS

  √x7ᵗʰ **S90.31** **Contusion of** right **foot**

  √x7ᵗʰ **S90.32** **Contusion of** left **foot**

√5ᵗʰ **S90.4** **Other superficial injuries of** toe

  √6ᵗʰ **S90.41** Abrasion **of toe**

    √7ᵗʰ **S90.411** Abrasion, right great toe

    √7ᵗʰ **S90.412** Abrasion, left great toe

    √7ᵗʰ **S90.413** Abrasion, unspecified great toe

    √7ᵗʰ **S90.414** Abrasion, right lesser toe(s)

    √7ᵗʰ **S90.415** Abrasion, left lesser toe(s)

    √7ᵗʰ **S90.416** Abrasion, unspecified lesser toe(s)

  √6ᵗʰ **S90.42** Blister (nonthermal) **of toe**

    √7ᵗʰ **S90.421** Blister (nonthermal), right great toe

    √7ᵗʰ **S90.422** Blister (nonthermal), left great toe

    √7ᵗʰ **S90.423** Blister (nonthermal), unspecified great toe

    √7ᵗʰ **S90.424** Blister (nonthermal), right lesser toe(s)

    √7ᵗʰ **S90.425** Blister (nonthermal), left lesser toe(s)

    √7ᵗʰ **S90.426** Blister (nonthermal), unspecified lesser toe(s)

  √6ᵗʰ **S90.44** External constriction **of toe**
         Hair tourniquet syndrome of toe

    √7ᵗʰ **S90.441** External constriction, right great toe

    √7ᵗʰ **S90.442** External constriction, left great toe

    √7ᵗʰ **S90.443** External constriction, unspecified great toe

    √7ᵗʰ **S90.444** External constriction, right lesser toe(s)

    √7ᵗʰ **S90.445** External constriction, left lesser toe(s)

    √7ᵗʰ **S90.446** External constriction, unspecified lesser toe(s)

  √6ᵗʰ **S90.45** **Superficial** foreign body **of toe**
         Splinter in the toe

    √7ᵗʰ **S90.451** Superficial foreign body, right great toe

    √7ᵗʰ **S90.452** Superficial foreign body, left great toe

    √7ᵗʰ **S90.453** Superficial foreign body, unspecified great toe

    √7ᵗʰ **S90.454** Superficial foreign body, right lesser toe(s)

    √7ᵗʰ **S90.455** Superficial foreign body, left lesser toe(s)

    √7ᵗʰ **S90.456** Superficial foreign body, unspecified lesser toe(s)

  √6ᵗʰ **S90.46** Insect bite (nonvenomous) **of toe**

    √7ᵗʰ **S90.461** Insect bite (nonvenomous), right great toe

    √7ᵗʰ **S90.462** Insect bite (nonvenomous), left great toe

    √7ᵗʰ **S90.463** Insect bite (nonvenomous), unspecified great toe

    √7ᵗʰ **S90.464** Insect bite (nonvenomous), right lesser toe(s)

    √7ᵗʰ **S90.465** Insect bite (nonvenomous), left lesser toe(s)

    √7ᵗʰ **S90.466** Insect bite (nonvenomous), unspecified lesser toe(s)

  √6ᵗʰ **S90.47** **Other superficial** bite **of toe**
    EXCLUDES 1   *open bite of toe (S91.15-, S91.25-)*

    √7ᵗʰ **S90.471** Other superficial bite of right great toe

    √7ᵗʰ **S90.472** Other superficial bite of left great toe

    √7ᵗʰ **S90.473** Other superficial bite of unspecified great toe

    √7ᵗʰ **S90.474** Other superficial bite of right lesser toe(s)

    √7ᵗʰ **S90.475** Other superficial bite of left lesser toe(s)

    √7ᵗʰ **S90.476** Other superficial bite of unspecified lesser toe(s)

√5ᵗʰ **S90.5** **Other superficial injuries of** ankle

  √6ᵗʰ **S90.51** Abrasion **of ankle**

    √7ᵗʰ **S90.511** Abrasion, right ankle

    √7ᵗʰ **S90.512** Abrasion, left ankle

    √7ᵗʰ **S90.519** Abrasion, unspecified ankle

  √6ᵗʰ **S90.52** Blister (nonthermal) **of ankle**

    √7ᵗʰ **S90.521** Blister (nonthermal), right ankle

    √7ᵗʰ **S90.522** Blister (nonthermal), left ankle

    √7ᵗʰ **S90.529** Blister (nonthermal), unspecified ankle

  √6ᵗʰ **S90.54** External constriction **of ankle**

    √7ᵗʰ **S90.541** External constriction, right ankle

    √7ᵗʰ **S90.542** External constriction, left ankle

    √7ᵗʰ **S90.549** External constriction, unspecified ankle

  √6ᵗʰ **S90.55** **Superficial** foreign body **of ankle**
         Splinter in the ankle

    √7ᵗʰ **S90.551** Superficial foreign body, right ankle

    √7ᵗʰ **S90.552** Superficial foreign body, left ankle

    √7ᵗʰ **S90.559** Superficial foreign body, unspecified ankle

  √6ᵗʰ **S90.56** Insect bite (nonvenomous) **of ankle**

    √7ᵗʰ **S90.561** Insect bite (nonvenomous), right ankle

    √7ᵗʰ **S90.562** Insect bite (nonvenomous), left ankle

    √7ᵗʰ **S90.569** Insect bite (nonvenomous), unspecified ankle

  √6ᵗʰ **S90.57** **Other superficial** bite **of ankle**
    EXCLUDES 1   *open bite of ankle (S91.05-)*

    √7ᵗʰ **S90.571** Other superficial bite of ankle, right ankle

    √7ᵗʰ **S90.572** Other superficial bite of ankle, left ankle

    √7ᵗʰ **S90.579** Other superficial bite of ankle, unspecified ankle

√5ᵗʰ **S90.8** **Other superficial injuries of** foot

  √6ᵗʰ **S90.81** Abrasion **of foot**

    √7ᵗʰ **S90.811** Abrasion, right foot

    √7ᵗʰ **S90.812** Abrasion, left foot

    √7ᵗʰ **S90.819** Abrasion, unspecified foot

  √6ᵗʰ **S90.82** Blister (nonthermal) **of foot**

    √7ᵗʰ **S90.821** Blister (nonthermal), right foot

    √7ᵗʰ **S90.822** Blister (nonthermal), left foot

    √7ᵗʰ **S90.829** Blister (nonthermal), unspecified foot

  √6ᵗʰ **S90.84** External constriction **of foot**

    √7ᵗʰ **S90.841** External constriction, right foot

    √7ᵗʰ **S90.842** External constriction, left foot

    √7ᵗʰ **S90.849** External constriction, unspecified foot

  √6ᵗʰ **S90.85** **Superficial** foreign body **of foot**
         Splinter in the foot

    √7ᵗʰ **S90.851** Superficial foreign body, right foot

    √7ᵗʰ **S90.852** Superficial foreign body, left foot

    √7ᵗʰ **S90.859** Superficial foreign body, unspecified foot

  √6ᵗʰ **S90.86** Insect bite (nonvenomous) **of foot**

    √7ᵗʰ **S90.861** Insect bite (nonvenomous), right foot

    √7ᵗʰ **S90.862** Insect bite (nonvenomous), left foot

    √7ᵗʰ **S90.869** Insect bite (nonvenomous), unspecified foot

---

√6ᵗʰ **S90.87**   **Other superficial** bite **of foot**
> EXCLUDES 1   *open bite of foot (S91.35-)*

     √7ᵗʰ **S90.871**   Other superficial bite of right foot
     √7ᵗʰ **S90.872**   Other superficial bite of left foot
     √7ᵗʰ **S90.879**   Other superficial bite of unspecified foot

√5ᵗʰ **S90.9**   **Unspecified superficial injury of ankle, foot and toe**

   √6ᵗʰ **S90.91**   **Unspecified superficial injury of** ankle
     √7ᵗʰ **S90.911**   Unspecified superficial injury of right ankle
     √7ᵗʰ **S90.912**   Unspecified superficial injury of left ankle
     √7ᵗʰ **S90.919**   Unspecified superficial injury of unspecified ankle

   √6ᵗʰ **S90.92**   **Unspecified superficial injury of** foot
     √7ᵗʰ **S90.921**   Unspecified superficial injury of right foot
     √7ᵗʰ **S90.922**   Unspecified superficial injury of left foot
     √7ᵗʰ **S90.929**   Unspecified superficial injury of unspecified foot

   √6ᵗʰ **S90.93**   **Unspecified superficial injury of** toes
     √7ᵗʰ **S90.931**   Unspecified superficial injury of right great toe
     √7ᵗʰ **S90.932**   Unspecified superficial injury of left great toe
     √7ᵗʰ **S90.933**   Unspecified superficial injury of unspecified great toe
     √7ᵗʰ **S90.934**   Unspecified superficial injury of right lesser toe(s)
     √7ᵗʰ **S90.935**   Unspecified superficial injury of left lesser toe(s)
     √7ᵗʰ **S90.936**   Unspecified superficial injury of unspecified lesser toe(s)

√4ᵗʰ **S91**   **Open wound of ankle, foot and toes**
Code also any associated wound infection
> EXCLUDES 1   *open fracture of ankle, foot and toes (S92.- with 7th character B)*
> *traumatic amputation of ankle and foot (S98.-)*

The appropriate 7th character is to be added to each code from category S91.
A   initial encounter
D   subsequent encounter
S   sequela

√5ᵗʰ **S91.0**   **Open wound of ankle**

   √6ᵗʰ **S91.00**   **Unspecified open wound of ankle**
     √7ᵗʰ **S91.001**   Unspecified open wound, right ankle
     √7ᵗʰ **S91.002**   Unspecified open wound, left ankle
     √7ᵗʰ **S91.009**   Unspecified open wound, unspecified ankle

   √6ᵗʰ **S91.01**   **Laceration without foreign body of ankle**
     √7ᵗʰ **S91.011**   Laceration without foreign body, right ankle
     √7ᵗʰ **S91.012**   Laceration without foreign body, left ankle
     √7ᵗʰ **S91.019**   Laceration without foreign body, unspecified ankle

   √6ᵗʰ **S91.02**   **Laceration with foreign body of ankle**
     √7ᵗʰ **S91.021**   Laceration with foreign body, right ankle
     √7ᵗʰ **S91.022**   Laceration with foreign body, left ankle
     √7ᵗʰ **S91.029**   Laceration with foreign body, unspecified ankle

   √6ᵗʰ **S91.03**   **Puncture wound without foreign body of ankle**
     √7ᵗʰ **S91.031**   Puncture wound without foreign body, right ankle
     √7ᵗʰ **S91.032**   Puncture wound without foreign body, left ankle
     √7ᵗʰ **S91.039**   Puncture wound without foreign body, unspecified ankle

   √6ᵗʰ **S91.04**   **Puncture wound with foreign body of ankle**
     √7ᵗʰ **S91.041**   Puncture wound with foreign body, right ankle
     √7ᵗʰ **S91.042**   Puncture wound with foreign body, left ankle
     √7ᵗʰ **S91.049**   Puncture wound with foreign body, unspecified ankle

   √6ᵗʰ **S91.05**   **Open bite of ankle**
> EXCLUDES 1   *superficial bite of ankle (S90.56-, S90.57-)*

     √7ᵗʰ **S91.051**   Open bite, right ankle

     √7ᵗʰ **S91.052**   Open bite, left ankle
     √7ᵗʰ **S91.059**   Open bite, unspecified ankle

√5ᵗʰ **S91.1**   **Open wound of** toe without damage to nail

   √6ᵗʰ **S91.10**   **Unspecified open wound of toe without damage to nail**
     √7ᵗʰ **S91.101**   Unspecified open wound of right great toe without damage to nail
     √7ᵗʰ **S91.102**   Unspecified open wound of left great toe without damage to nail
     √7ᵗʰ **S91.103**   Unspecified open wound of unspecified great toe without damage to nail
     √7ᵗʰ **S91.104**   Unspecified open wound of right lesser toe(s) without damage to nail
     √7ᵗʰ **S91.105**   Unspecified open wound of left lesser toe(s) without damage to nail
     √7ᵗʰ **S91.106**   Unspecified open wound of unspecified lesser toe(s) without damage to nail
     √7ᵗʰ **S91.109**   Unspecified open wound of unspecified toe(s) without damage to nail

   √6ᵗʰ **S91.11**   **Laceration without foreign body of toe without damage to nail**
     √7ᵗʰ **S91.111**   Laceration without foreign body of right great toe without damage to nail
     √7ᵗʰ **S91.112**   Laceration without foreign body of left great toe without damage to nail
     √7ᵗʰ **S91.113**   Laceration without foreign body of unspecified great toe without damage to nail
     √7ᵗʰ **S91.114**   Laceration without foreign body of right lesser toe(s) without damage to nail
     √7ᵗʰ **S91.115**   Laceration without foreign body of left lesser toe(s) without damage to nail
     √7ᵗʰ **S91.116**   Laceration without foreign body of unspecified lesser toe(s) without damage to nail
     √7ᵗʰ **S91.119**   Laceration without foreign body of unspecified toe without damage to nail

   √6ᵗʰ **S91.12**   **Laceration with foreign body of toe without damage to nail**
     √7ᵗʰ **S91.121**   Laceration with foreign body of right great toe without damage to nail
     √7ᵗʰ **S91.122**   Laceration with foreign body of left great toe without damage to nail
     √7ᵗʰ **S91.123**   Laceration with foreign body of unspecified great toe without damage to nail
     √7ᵗʰ **S91.124**   Laceration with foreign body of right lesser toe(s) without damage to nail
     √7ᵗʰ **S91.125**   Laceration with foreign body of left lesser toe(s) without damage to nail
     √7ᵗʰ **S91.126**   Laceration with foreign body of unspecified lesser toe(s) without damage to nail
     √7ᵗʰ **S91.129**   Laceration with foreign body of unspecified toe(s) without damage to nail

   √6ᵗʰ **S91.13**   **Puncture wound without foreign body of toe without damage to nail**
     √7ᵗʰ **S91.131**   Puncture wound without foreign body of right great toe without damage to nail
     √7ᵗʰ **S91.132**   Puncture wound without foreign body of left great toe without damage to nail
     √7ᵗʰ **S91.133**   Puncture wound without foreign body of unspecified great toe without damage to nail
     √7ᵗʰ **S91.134**   Puncture wound without foreign body of right lesser toe(s) without damage to nail
     √7ᵗʰ **S91.135**   Puncture wound without foreign body of left lesser toe(s) without damage to nail
     √7ᵗʰ **S91.136**   Puncture wound without foreign body of unspecified lesser toe(s) without damage to nail
     √7ᵗʰ **S91.139**   Puncture wound without foreign body of unspecified toe(s) without damage to nail

   √6ᵗʰ **S91.14**   **Puncture wound with foreign body of toe without damage to nail**
     √7ᵗʰ **S91.141**   Puncture wound with foreign body of right great toe without damage to nail
     √7ᵗʰ **S91.142**   Puncture wound with foreign body of left great toe without damage to nail
     √7ᵗʰ **S91.143**   Puncture wound with foreign body of unspecified great toe without damage to nail

N Newborn: 0   P Pediatric: 0-17   M Maternity: 9-64   A Adult: 15-124   MCC Major Complication/Comorbidity   CC Complication/Comorbidity   SW Severe Wound Dx

1114   ICD-10-CM 2020

√7ᵗʰ **S91.144** Puncture wound with foreign body of right lesser toe(s) without damage to nail

√7ᵗʰ **S91.145** Puncture wound with foreign body of left lesser toe(s) without damage to nail

√7ᵗʰ **S91.146** Puncture wound with foreign body of unspecified lesser toe(s) without damage to nail

√7ᵗʰ **S91.149** Puncture wound with foreign body of unspecified toe(s) without damage to nail

√6ᵗʰ **S91.15** Open bite of toe without damage to nail

Bite of toe NOS

EXCLUDES 1   superficial bite of toe (S90.46-, S90.47-)

√7ᵗʰ **S91.151** Open bite of right great toe without damage to nail

√7ᵗʰ **S91.152** Open bite of left great toe without damage to nail

√7ᵗʰ **S91.153** Open bite of unspecified great toe without damage to nail

√7ᵗʰ **S91.154** Open bite of right lesser toe(s) without damage to nail

√7ᵗʰ **S91.155** Open bite of left lesser toe(s) without damage to nail

√7ᵗʰ **S91.156** Open bite of unspecified lesser toe(s) without damage to nail

√7ᵗʰ **S91.159** Open bite of unspecified toe(s) without damage to nail

√5ᵗʰ **S91.2** Open wound of toe with damage to nail

√6ᵗʰ **S91.20** Unspecified open wound of toe with damage to nail

√7ᵗʰ **S91.201** Unspecified open wound of right great toe with damage to nail

√7ᵗʰ **S91.202** Unspecified open wound of left great toe with damage to nail

√7ᵗʰ **S91.203** Unspecified open wound of unspecified great toe with damage to nail

√7ᵗʰ **S91.204** Unspecified open wound of right lesser toe(s) with damage to nail

√7ᵗʰ **S91.205** Unspecified open wound of left lesser toe(s) with damage to nail

√7ᵗʰ **S91.206** Unspecified open wound of unspecified lesser toe(s) with damage to nail

√7ᵗʰ **S91.209** Unspecified open wound of unspecified toe(s) with damage to nail

√6ᵗʰ **S91.21** Laceration without foreign body of toe with damage to nail

√7ᵗʰ **S91.211** Laceration without foreign body of right great toe with damage to nail

√7ᵗʰ **S91.212** Laceration without foreign body of left great toe with damage to nail

√7ᵗʰ **S91.213** Laceration without foreign body of unspecified great toe with damage to nail

√7ᵗʰ **S91.214** Laceration without foreign body of right lesser toe(s) with damage to nail

√7ᵗʰ **S91.215** Laceration without foreign body of left lesser toe(s) with damage to nail

√7ᵗʰ **S91.216** Laceration without foreign body of unspecified lesser toe(s) with damage to nail

√7ᵗʰ **S91.219** Laceration without foreign body of unspecified toe(s) with damage to nail

√6ᵗʰ **S91.22** Laceration with foreign body of toe with damage to nail

√7ᵗʰ **S91.221** Laceration with foreign body of right great toe with damage to nail

√7ᵗʰ **S91.222** Laceration with foreign body of left great toe with damage to nail

√7ᵗʰ **S91.223** Laceration with foreign body of unspecified great toe with damage to nail

√7ᵗʰ **S91.224** Laceration with foreign body of right lesser toe(s) with damage to nail

√7ᵗʰ **S91.225** Laceration with foreign body of left lesser toe(s) with damage to nail

√7ᵗʰ **S91.226** Laceration with foreign body of unspecified lesser toe(s) with damage to nail

√7ᵗʰ **S91.229** Laceration with foreign body of unspecified toe(s) with damage to nail

√6ᵗʰ **S91.23** Puncture wound without foreign body of toe with damage to nail

√7ᵗʰ **S91.231** Puncture wound without foreign body of right great toe with damage to nail

√7ᵗʰ **S91.232** Puncture wound without foreign body of left great toe with damage to nail

√7ᵗʰ **S91.233** Puncture wound without foreign body of unspecified great toe with damage to nail

√7ᵗʰ **S91.234** Puncture wound without foreign body of right lesser toe(s) with damage to nail

√7ᵗʰ **S91.235** Puncture wound without foreign body of left lesser toe(s) with damage to nail

√7ᵗʰ **S91.236** Puncture wound without foreign body of unspecified lesser toe(s) with damage to nail

√7ᵗʰ **S91.239** Puncture wound without foreign body of unspecified toe(s) with damage to nail

√6ᵗʰ **S91.24** Puncture wound with foreign body of toe with damage to nail

√7ᵗʰ **S91.241** Puncture wound with foreign body of right great toe with damage to nail

√7ᵗʰ **S91.242** Puncture wound with foreign body of left great toe with damage to nail

√7ᵗʰ **S91.243** Puncture wound with foreign body of unspecified great toe with damage to nail

√7ᵗʰ **S91.244** Puncture wound with foreign body of right lesser toe(s) with damage to nail

√7ᵗʰ **S91.245** Puncture wound with foreign body of left lesser toe(s) with damage to nail

√7ᵗʰ **S91.246** Puncture wound with foreign body of unspecified lesser toe(s) with damage to nail

√7ᵗʰ **S91.249** Puncture wound with foreign body of unspecified toe(s) with damage to nail

√6ᵗʰ **S91.25** Open bite of toe with damage to nail

Bite of toe with damage to nail NOS

EXCLUDES 1   superficial bite of toe (S90.46-, S90.47-)

√7ᵗʰ **S91.251** Open bite of right great toe with damage to nail

√7ᵗʰ **S91.252** Open bite of left great toe with damage to nail

√7ᵗʰ **S91.253** Open bite of unspecified great toe with damage to nail

√7ᵗʰ **S91.254** Open bite of right lesser toe(s) with damage to nail

√7ᵗʰ **S91.255** Open bite of left lesser toe(s) with damage to nail

√7ᵗʰ **S91.256** Open bite of unspecified lesser toe(s) with damage to nail

√7ᵗʰ **S91.259** Open bite of unspecified toe(s) with damage to nail

√5ᵗʰ **S91.3** Open wound of foot

√6ᵗʰ **S91.30** Unspecified open wound of foot

√7ᵗʰ **S91.301** Unspecified open wound, right foot

√7ᵗʰ **S91.302** Unspecified open wound, left foot

√7ᵗʰ **S91.309** Unspecified open wound, unspecified foot

√6ᵗʰ **S91.31** Laceration without foreign body of foot

√7ᵗʰ **S91.311** Laceration without foreign body, right foot

√7ᵗʰ **S91.312** Laceration without foreign body, left foot

√7ᵗʰ **S91.319** Laceration without foreign body, unspecified foot

√6ᵗʰ **S91.32** Laceration with foreign body of foot

√7ᵗʰ **S91.321** Laceration with foreign body, right foot

√7ᵗʰ **S91.322** Laceration with foreign body, left foot

√7ᵗʰ **S91.329** Laceration with foreign body, unspecified foot

√6ᵗʰ **S91.33** Puncture wound without foreign body of foot

√7ᵗʰ **S91.331** Puncture wound without foreign body, right foot

√7ᵗʰ **S91.332** Puncture wound without foreign body, left foot

√7ᵗʰ **S91.339** Puncture wound without foreign body, unspecified foot

√6ᵗʰ **S91.34** Puncture wound with foreign body of foot

√7ᵗʰ **S91.341** Puncture wound with foreign body, right foot

√7ᵗʰ **S91.342** Puncture wound with foreign body, left foot

√7ᵗʰ **S91.349** Puncture wound with foreign body, unspecified foot

√6ᵗʰ **S91.35** Open bite of foot

EXCLUDES 1   superficial bite of foot (S90.86-, S90.87-)

√7ᵗʰ **S91.351** Open bite, right foot

✔ Additional Character Required   √ˣ7ᵗʰ Placeholder   Unacceptable PDx   Questionable PDx   Manifestation   Unspecified Dx   H1-H1d HAC   HCC CMS-HCC Dx   HIV HIV Dx

ICD-10-CM 2020

1115

√7ᵗʰ **S91.352** Open bite, left foot

√7ᵗʰ **S91.359** Open bite, unspecified foot

√4ᵗʰ **S92 Fracture of foot and toe, except ankle**

NOTE   A fracture not indicated as displaced or nondisplaced should be coded to displaced

A fracture not indicated as open or closed should be coded to closed.

EXCLUDES 1   traumatic amputation of ankle and foot (S98.-)

EXCLUDES 2   fracture of ankle (S82.-)

fracture of malleolus (S82.-)

AHA: 2018,2Q,12; 2015,3Q,37-39

The appropriate 7th character is to be added to each code from category S92.

A   initial encounter for closed fracture

B   initial encounter for open fracture

D   subsequent encounter for fracture with routine healing

G   subsequent encounter for fracture with delayed healing

K   subsequent encounter for fracture with nonunion

P   subsequent encounter for fracture with malunion

S   sequela

√5ᵗʰ **S92.0 Fracture of calcaneus**

Heel bone

Os calcis

EXCLUDES 2   physeal fracture of calcaneus (S99.0-)

CC Excl: For codes in subcategory S92.0:
CC with 7th character B: PDX collection 1367
CC with 7th character K or P: PDX collection 897

√6ᵗʰ **S92.00**   **Unspecified fracture of calcaneus**

3 √7ᵗʰ **S92.001** Unspecified fracture of right calcaneus   CC H5

3 √7ᵗʰ **S92.002** Unspecified fracture of left calcaneus   CC H5

3 √7ᵗʰ **S92.009** Unspecified fracture of unspecified calcaneus   CC H5

√6ᵗʰ **S92.01**   **Fracture of body of calcaneus**

3 √7ᵗʰ **S92.011** Displaced fracture of body of right calcaneus   CC H5

3 √7ᵗʰ **S92.012** Displaced fracture of body of left calcaneus   CC H5

3 √7ᵗʰ **S92.013** Displaced fracture of body of unspecified calcaneus   CC H5

3 √7ᵗʰ **S92.014** Nondisplaced fracture of body of right calcaneus   CC H5

3 √7ᵗʰ **S92.015** Nondisplaced fracture of body of left calcaneus   CC H5

3 √7ᵗʰ **S92.016** Nondisplaced fracture of body of unspecified calcaneus   CC H5

√6ᵗʰ **S92.02**   **Fracture of anterior process of calcaneus**

3 √7ᵗʰ **S92.021** Displaced fracture of anterior process of right calcaneus   CC H5

3 √7ᵗʰ **S92.022** Displaced fracture of anterior process of left calcaneus   OO H5

3 √7ᵗʰ **S92.023** Displaced fracture of anterior process of unspecified calcaneus   CC H5

3 √7ᵗʰ **S92.024** Nondisplaced fracture of anterior process of right calcaneus   CC H5

3 √7ᵗʰ **S92.025** Nondisplaced fracture of anterior process of left calcaneus   CC H5

3 √7ᵗʰ **S92.026** Nondisplaced fracture of anterior process of unspecified calcaneus   CC H5

√6ᵗʰ **S92.03**   **Avulsion fracture of tuberosity of calcaneus**

3 √7ᵗʰ **S92.031** Displaced avulsion fracture of tuberosity of right calcaneus   CC H5

3 √7ᵗʰ **S92.032** Displaced avulsion fracture of tuberosity of left calcaneus   CC H5

3 √7ᵗʰ **S92.033** Displaced avulsion fracture of tuberosity of unspecified calcaneus   CC H5

3 √7ᵗʰ **S92.034** Nondisplaced avulsion fracture of tuberosity of right calcaneus   CC H5

3 √7ᵗʰ **S92.035** Nondisplaced avulsion fracture of tuberosity of left calcaneus   CC H5

3 √7ᵗʰ **S92.036** Nondisplaced avulsion fracture of tuberosity of unspecified calcaneus   CC H5

√6ᵗʰ **S92.04**   **Other fracture of tuberosity of calcaneus**

3 √7ᵗʰ **S92.041** Displaced other fracture of tuberosity of right calcaneus   CC H5

3 √7ᵗʰ **S92.042** Displaced other fracture of tuberosity of left calcaneus   CC H5

3 √7ᵗʰ **S92.043** Displaced other fracture of tuberosity of unspecified calcaneus   CC H5

3 √7ᵗʰ **S92.044** Nondisplaced other fracture of tuberosity of right calcaneus   CC H5

3 √7ᵗʰ **S92.045** Nondisplaced other fracture of tuberosity of left calcaneus   CC H5

3 √7ᵗʰ **S92.046** Nondisplaced other fracture of tuberosity of unspecified calcaneus   CC H5

√6ᵗʰ **S92.05**   **Other extraarticular fracture of calcaneus**

3 √7ᵗʰ **S92.051** Displaced other extraarticular fracture of right calcaneus   CC H5

3 √7ᵗʰ **S92.052** Displaced other extraarticular fracture of left calcaneus   CC H5

3 √7ᵗʰ **S92.053** Displaced other extraarticular fracture of unspecified calcaneus   CC H5

3 √7ᵗʰ **S92.054** Nondisplaced other extraarticular fracture of right calcaneus   CC H5

3 √7ᵗʰ **S92.055** Nondisplaced other extraarticular fracture of left calcaneus   CC H5

3 √7ᵗʰ **S92.056** Nondisplaced other extraarticular fracture of unspecified calcaneus   CC H5

√6ᵗʰ **S92.06**   **Intraarticular fracture of calcaneus**

3 √7ᵗʰ **S92.061** Displaced intraarticular fracture of right calcaneus   CC H5

3 √7ᵗʰ **S92.062** Displaced intraarticular fracture of left calcaneus   CC H5

3 √7ᵗʰ **S92.063** Displaced intraarticular fracture of unspecified calcaneus   CC H5

3 √7ᵗʰ **S92.064** Nondisplaced intraarticular fracture of right calcaneus   CC H5

3 √7ᵗʰ **S92.065** Nondisplaced intraarticular fracture of left calcaneus   CC H5

3 √7ᵗʰ **S92.066** Nondisplaced intraarticular fracture of unspecified calcaneus   CC H5

√5ᵗʰ **S92.1 Fracture of talus**

Astragalus

CC Excl: For codes in subcategory S92.1:
CC with 7th character B: PDX collection 1368
CC with 7th character K or P: PDX collection 897

√6ᵗʰ **S92.10**   **Unspecified fracture of talus**

3 √7ᵗʰ **S92.101** Unspecified fracture of right talus   CC H5

3 √7ᵗʰ **S92.102** Unspecified fracture of left talus   CC H5

3 √7ᵗʰ **S92.109** Unspecified fracture of unspecified talus   CC H5

√6ᵗʰ **S92.11**   **Fracture of neck of talus**

3 √7ᵗʰ **S92.111** Displaced fracture of neck of right talus   CC H5

3 √7ᵗʰ **S92.112** Displaced fracture of neck of left talus   CC H5

3 √7ᵗʰ **S92.113** Displaced fracture of neck of unspecified talus   CC H5

N Newborn: 0   P Pediatric: 0-17   M Maternity: 9-64   A Adult: 15-124   MCC Major Complication/Comorbidity   CC Complication/Comorbidity   SW Severe Wound Dx

1116   ICD-10-CM 2020

3 √7ᵗʰ **S92.114** Nondisplaced fracture of neck of right talus   `CC` `H5`

3 √7ᵗʰ **S92.115** Nondisplaced fracture of neck of left talus   `CC` `H5`

3 √7ᵗʰ **S92.116** Nondisplaced fracture of neck of unspecified talus   `CC` `H5`

√6ᵗʰ **S92.12** Fracture of body of talus

3 √7ᵗʰ **S92.121** Displaced fracture of body of right talus   `CC` `H5`

3 √7ᵗʰ **S92.122** Displaced fracture of body of left talus   `CC` `H5`

3 √7ᵗʰ **S92.123** Displaced fracture of body of unspecified talus   `CC` `H5`

3 √7ᵗʰ **S92.124** Nondisplaced fracture of body of right talus   `CC` `H5`

3 √7ᵗʰ **S92.125** Nondisplaced fracture of body of left talus   `CC` `H5`

3 √7ᵗʰ **S92.126** Nondisplaced fracture of body of unspecified talus   `CC` `H5`

√6ᵗʰ **S92.13** Fracture of posterior process of talus

3 √7ᵗʰ **S92.131** Displaced fracture of posterior process of right talus   `CC` `H5`

3 √7ᵗʰ **S92.132** Displaced fracture of posterior process of left talus   `CC` `H5`

3 √7ᵗʰ **S92.133** Displaced fracture of posterior process of unspecified talus   `CC` `H5`

3 √7ᵗʰ **S92.134** Nondisplaced fracture of posterior process of right talus   `CC` `H5`

3 √7ᵗʰ **S92.135** Nondisplaced fracture of posterior process of left talus   `CC` `H5`

3 √7ᵗʰ **S92.136** Nondisplaced fracture of posterior process of unspecified talus   `CC` `H5`

√6ᵗʰ **S92.14** Dome fracture of talus

EXCLUDES 1   osteochondritis dissecans (M93.2)

3 √7ᵗʰ **S92.141** Displaced dome fracture of right talus   `CC` `H5`

3 √7ᵗʰ **S92.142** Displaced dome fracture of left talus   `CC` `H5`

3 √7ᵗʰ **S92.143** Displaced dome fracture of unspecified talus   `CC` `H5`

3 √7ᵗʰ **S92.144** Nondisplaced dome fracture of right talus   `CC` `H5`

3 √7ᵗʰ **S92.145** Nondisplaced dome fracture of left talus   `CC` `H5`

3 √7ᵗʰ **S92.146** Nondisplaced dome fracture of unspecified talus   `CC` `H5`

√6ᵗʰ **S92.15** Avulsion fracture (chip fracture) of talus

3 √7ᵗʰ **S92.151** Displaced avulsion fracture (chip fracture) of right talus   `CC` `H5`

3 √7ᵗʰ **S92.152** Displaced avulsion fracture (chip fracture) of left talus   `CC` `H5`

3 √7ᵗʰ **S92.153** Displaced avulsion fracture (chip fracture) of unspecified talus   `CC` `H5`

3 √7ᵗʰ **S92.154** Nondisplaced avulsion fracture (chip fracture) of right talus   `CC` `H5`

3 √7ᵗʰ **S92.155** Nondisplaced avulsion fracture (chip fracture) of left talus   `CC` `H5`

3 √7ᵗʰ **S92.156** Nondisplaced avulsion fracture (chip fracture) of unspecified talus   `CC` `H5`

√6ᵗʰ **S92.19** Other fracture of talus

3 √7ᵗʰ **S92.191** Other fracture of right talus   `CC` `H5`

3 √7ᵗʰ **S92.192** Other fracture of left talus   `CC` `H5`

3 √7ᵗʰ **S92.199** Other fracture of unspecified talus   `CC` `H5`

√5ᵗʰ **S92.2** Fracture of other and unspecified tarsal bone(s)

CC Excl: For codes in subcategory S92.2, unless otherwise noted:
CC with 7th character B: PDX collection 1368
CC with 7th character K or P: PDX collection 897

√6ᵗʰ **S92.20** Fracture of unspecified tarsal bone(s)

CC Excl: For codes in subcategory S92.20:
CC with 7th character B: PDX collection 1369

3 √7ᵗʰ **S92.201** Fracture of unspecified tarsal bone(s) of right foot   `CC` `H5`

3 √7ᵗʰ **S92.202** Fracture of unspecified tarsal bone(s) of left foot   `CC` `H5`

3 √7ᵗʰ **S92.209** Fracture of unspecified tarsal bone(s) of unspecified foot   `CC` `H5`

√6ᵗʰ **S92.21** Fracture of cuboid bone

3 √7ᵗʰ **S92.211** Displaced fracture of cuboid bone of right foot   `CC` `H5`

3 √7ᵗʰ **S92.212** Displaced fracture of cuboid bone of left foot   `CC` `H5`

3 √7ᵗʰ **S92.213** Displaced fracture of cuboid bone of unspecified foot   `CC` `H5`

3 √7ᵗʰ **S92.214** Nondisplaced fracture of cuboid bone of right foot   `CC` `H5`

3 √7ᵗʰ **S92.215** Nondisplaced fracture of cuboid bone of left foot   `CC` `H5`

3 √7ᵗʰ **S92.216** Nondisplaced fracture of cuboid bone of unspecified foot   `CC` `H5`

√6ᵗʰ **S92.22** Fracture of lateral cuneiform

3 √7ᵗʰ **S92.221** Displaced fracture of lateral cuneiform of right foot   `CC` `H5`

3 √7ᵗʰ **S92.222** Displaced fracture of lateral cuneiform of left foot   `CC` `H5`

3 √7ᵗʰ **S92.223** Displaced fracture of lateral cuneiform of unspecified foot   `CC` `H5`

3 √7ᵗʰ **S92.224** Nondisplaced fracture of lateral cuneiform of right foot   `CC` `H5`

3 √7ᵗʰ **S92.225** Nondisplaced fracture of lateral cuneiform of left foot   `CC` `H5`

3 √7ᵗʰ **S92.226** Nondisplaced fracture of lateral cuneiform of unspecified foot   `CC` `H5`

√6ᵗʰ **S92.23** Fracture of intermediate cuneiform

3 √7ᵗʰ **S92.231** Displaced fracture of intermediate cuneiform of right foot   `CC` `H5`

3 √7ᵗʰ **S92.232** Displaced fracture of intermediate cuneiform of left foot   `CC` `H5`

3 √7ᵗʰ **S92.233** Displaced fracture of intermediate cuneiform of unspecified foot   `CC` `H5`

3 √7ᵗʰ **S92.234** Nondisplaced fracture of intermediate cuneiform of right foot   `CC` `H5`

3 √7ᵗʰ **S92.235** Nondisplaced fracture of intermediate cuneiform of left foot   `CC` `H5`

3 √7ᵗʰ **S92.236** Nondisplaced fracture of intermediate cuneiform of unspecified foot   `CC` `H5`

√6ᵗʰ **S92.24** Fracture of medial cuneiform

3 √7ᵗʰ **S92.241** Displaced fracture of medial cuneiform of right foot   `CC` `H5`

3 √7ᵗʰ **S92.242** Displaced fracture of medial cuneiform of left foot   `CC` `H5`

3 √7ᵗʰ **S92.243** Displaced fracture of medial cuneiform of unspecified foot   `CC` `H5`

3 √7ᵗʰ **S92.244** Nondisplaced fracture of medial cuneiform of right foot   `CC` `H5`

S92.245 Nondisplaced fracture of medial cuneiform of left foot `CC` `H5`

S92.246 Nondisplaced fracture of medial cuneiform of unspecified foot `CC` `H5`

√6ᵗʰ **S92.25 Fracture of navicular [scaphoid] of foot**

S92.251 Displaced fracture of navicular [scaphoid] of right foot `CC` `H5`

S92.252 Displaced fracture of navicular [scaphoid] of left foot `CC` `H5`

S92.253 Displaced fracture of navicular [scaphoid] of unspecified foot `CC` `H5`

S92.254 Nondisplaced fracture of navicular [scaphoid] of right foot `CC` `H5`

S92.255 Nondisplaced fracture of navicular [scaphoid] of left foot `CC` `H5`

S92.256 Nondisplaced fracture of navicular [scaphoid] of unspecified foot `CC` `H5`

√5ᵗʰ **S92.3 Fracture of metatarsal bone(s)**

EXCLUDES 2   physeal fracture of metatarsal (S99.1-)

AHA: 2018,1Q,3

CC Excl: For codes in subcategory S92.3:
CC with 7th character B: PDX collection 1368
CC with 7th character K or P: PDX collection 897

√6ᵗʰ **S92.30 Fracture of unspecified metatarsal bone(s)**

S92.301 Fracture of unspecified metatarsal bone(s), right foot `CC` `H5`

S92.302 Fracture of unspecified metatarsal bone(s), left foot `CC` `H5`

S92.309 Fracture of unspecified metatarsal bone(s), unspecified foot `CC` `H5`

√6ᵗʰ **S92.31 Fracture of first metatarsal bone**

S92.311 Displaced fracture of first metatarsal bone, right foot `CC` `H5`

S92.312 Displaced fracture of first metatarsal bone, left foot `CC` `H5`

S92.313 Displaced fracture of first metatarsal bone, unspecified foot `CC` `H5`

S92.314 Nondisplaced fracture of first metatarsal bone, right foot `CC` `H5`

S92.315 Nondisplaced fracture of first metatarsal bone, left foot `CC` `H5`

S92.316 Nondisplaced fracture of first metatarsal bone, unspecified foot `CC` `H5`

√6ᵗʰ **S92.32 Fracture of second metatarsal bone**

S92.321 Displaced fracture of second metatarsal bone, right foot `CC` `H5`

S92.322 Displaced fracture of second metatarsal bone, left foot `CC` `H5`

S92.323 Displaced fracture of second metatarsal bone, unspecified foot `CC` `H5`

S92.324 Nondisplaced fracture of second metatarsal bone, right foot `CC` `H5`

S92.325 Nondisplaced fracture of second metatarsal bone, left foot `CC` `H5`

S92.326 Nondisplaced fracture of second metatarsal bone, unspecified foot `CC` `H5`

√6ᵗʰ **S92.33 Fracture of third metatarsal bone**

S92.331 Displaced fracture of third metatarsal bone, right foot `CC` `H5`

S92.332 Displaced fracture of third metatarsal bone, left foot `CC` `H5`

S92.333 Displaced fracture of third metatarsal bone, unspecified foot `CC` `H5`

S92.334 Nondisplaced fracture of third metatarsal bone, right foot `CC` `H5`

S92.335 Nondisplaced fracture of third metatarsal bone, left foot `CC` `H5`

S92.336 Nondisplaced fracture of third metatarsal bone, unspecified foot `CC` `H5`

√6ᵗʰ **S92.34 Fracture of fourth metatarsal bone**

S92.341 Displaced fracture of fourth metatarsal bone, right foot `CC` `H5`

S92.342 Displaced fracture of fourth metatarsal bone, left foot `CC` `H5`

S92.343 Displaced fracture of fourth metatarsal bone, unspecified foot `CC` `H5`

S92.344 Nondisplaced fracture of fourth metatarsal bone, right foot `CC` `H5`

S92.345 Nondisplaced fracture of fourth metatarsal bone, left foot `CC` `H5`

S92.346 Nondisplaced fracture of fourth metatarsal bone, unspecified foot `CC` `H5`

√6ᵗʰ **S92.35 Fracture of fifth metatarsal bone**

S92.351 Displaced fracture of fifth metatarsal bone, right foot `CC` `H5`

S92.352 Displaced fracture of fifth metatarsal bone, left foot `CC` `H5`

S92.353 Displaced fracture of fifth metatarsal bone, unspecified foot `CC` `H5`

S92.354 Nondisplaced fracture of fifth metatarsal bone, right foot `CC` `H5`

S92.355 Nondisplaced fracture of fifth metatarsal bone, left foot `CC` `H5`

S92.356 Nondisplaced fracture of fifth metatarsal bone, unspecified foot `CC` `H5`

√5ᵗʰ **S92.4 Fracture of great toe**

EXCLUDES 2   physeal fracture of phalanx of toe (S99.2-)

CC Excl: For codes in subcategory S92.4:
CC with 7th character K or P: PDX collection 897

√6ᵗʰ **S92.40 Unspecified fracture of great toe**

S92.401 Displaced unspecified fracture of right great toe `CC`

S92.402 Displaced unspecified fracture of left great toe `CC`

S92.403 Displaced unspecified fracture of unspecified great toe `CC`

S92.404 Nondisplaced unspecified fracture of right great toe `CC`

S92.405 Nondisplaced unspecified fracture of left great toe `CC`

S92.406 Nondisplaced unspecified fracture of unspecified great toe `CC`

√6ᵗʰ **S92.41 Fracture of proximal phalanx of great toe**

S92.411 Displaced fracture of proximal phalanx of right great toe `CC`

S92.412 Displaced fracture of proximal phalanx of left great toe `CC`

S92.413 Displaced fracture of proximal phalanx of unspecified great toe `CC`

S92.414 Nondisplaced fracture of proximal phalanx of right great toe `CC`

`N` Newborn: 0   `P` Pediatric: 0-17   `M` Maternity: 9-64   `A` Adult: 15-124   `MCC` Major Complication/Comorbidity   `CC` Complication/Comorbidity   `SW` Severe Wound Dx

1118   ICD-10-CM 2020

4 √7ᵗʰ **S92.415** Nondisplaced fracture of proximal phalanx of left great toe   CC

4 √7ᵗʰ **S92.416** Nondisplaced fracture of proximal phalanx of unspecified great toe   CC

√6ᵗʰ **S92.42** Fracture of distal phalanx of great toe

4 √7ᵗʰ **S92.421** Displaced fracture of distal phalanx of right great toe   CC

4 √7ᵗʰ **S92.422** Displaced fracture of distal phalanx of left great toe   CC

4 √7ᵗʰ **S92.423** Displaced fracture of distal phalanx of unspecified great toe   CC

4 √7ᵗʰ **S92.424** Nondisplaced fracture of distal phalanx of right great toe   CC

4 √7ᵗʰ **S92.425** Nondisplaced fracture of distal phalanx of left great toe   CC

4 √7ᵗʰ **S92.426** Nondisplaced fracture of distal phalanx of unspecified great toe   CC

√6ᵗʰ **S92.49** Other fracture of great toe

4 √7ᵗʰ **S92.491** Other fracture of right great toe   CC

4 √7ᵗʰ **S92.492** Other fracture of left great toe   CC

4 √7ᵗʰ **S92.499** Other fracture of unspecified great toe   CC

√5ᵗʰ **S92.5** Fracture of lesser toe(s)

EXCLUDES 2   physeal fracture of phalanx of toe (S99.2-)

CC Excl: For codes in subcategory S92.5:
CC with 7th character K or P: PDX collection 897

√6ᵗʰ **S92.50** Unspecified fracture of lesser toe(s)

4 √7ᵗʰ **S92.501** Displaced unspecified fracture of right lesser toe(s)   CC

4 √7ᵗʰ **S92.502** Displaced unspecified fracture of left lesser toe(s)   CC

4 √7ᵗʰ **S92.503** Displaced unspecified fracture of unspecified lesser toe(s)   CC

4 √7ᵗʰ **S92.504** Nondisplaced unspecified fracture of right lesser toe(s)   CC

4 √7ᵗʰ **S92.505** Nondisplaced unspecified fracture of left lesser toe(s)   CC

4 √7ᵗʰ **S92.506** Nondisplaced unspecified fracture of unspecified lesser toe(s)   CC

√6ᵗʰ **S92.51** Fracture of proximal phalanx of lesser toe(s)

4 √7ᵗʰ **S92.511** Displaced fracture of proximal phalanx of right lesser toe(s)   CC

4 √7ᵗʰ **S92.512** Displaced fracture of proximal phalanx of left lesser toe(s)   CC

4 √7ᵗʰ **S92.513** Displaced fracture of proximal phalanx of unspecified lesser toe(s)   CC

4 √7ᵗʰ **S92.514** Nondisplaced fracture of proximal phalanx of right lesser toe(s)   CC

4 √7ᵗʰ **S92.515** Nondisplaced fracture of proximal phalanx of left lesser toe(s))   CC

4 √7ᵗʰ **S92.516** Nondisplaced fracture of proximal phalanx of unspecified lesser toe(s)   CC

√6ᵗʰ **S92.52** Fracture of middle phalanx of lesser toe(s)

4 √7ᵗʰ **S92.521** Displaced fracture of middle phalanx of right lesser toe(s)   CC

4 √7ᵗʰ **S92.522** Displaced fracture of middle phalanx of left lesser toe(s)   CC

4 √7ᵗʰ **S92.523** Displaced fracture of middle phalanx of unspecified lesser toe(s)   CC

4 √7ᵗʰ **S92.524** Nondisplaced fracture of middle phalanx of right lesser toe(s)   CC

4 √7ᵗʰ **S92.525** Nondisplaced fracture of middle phalanx of left lesser toe(s)   CC

4 √7ᵗʰ **S92.526** Nondisplaced fracture of middle phalanx of unspecified lesser toe(s)   CC

√6ᵗʰ **S92.53** Fracture of distal phalanx of lesser toe(s)

4 √7ᵗʰ **S92.531** Displaced fracture of distal phalanx of right lesser toe(s)   CC

4 √7ᵗʰ **S92.532** Displaced fracture of distal phalanx of left lesser toe(s)   CC

4 √7ᵗʰ **S92.533** Displaced fracture of distal phalanx of unspecified lesser toe(s)   CC

4 √7ᵗʰ **S92.534** Nondisplaced fracture of distal phalanx of right lesser toe(s)   CC

4 √7ᵗʰ **S92.535** Nondisplaced fracture of distal phalanx of left lesser toe(s)   CC

4 √7ᵗʰ **S92.536** Nondisplaced fracture of distal phalanx of unspecified lesser toe(s)   CC

√6ᵗʰ **S92.59** Other fracture of lesser toe(s)

4 √7ᵗʰ **S92.591** Other fracture of right lesser toe(s)   CC

4 √7ᵗʰ **S92.592** Other fracture of left lesser toe(s)   CC

4 √7ᵗʰ **S92.599** Other fracture of unspecified lesser toe(s)   CC

√5ᵗʰ **S92.8** Other fracture of foot, except ankle

√6ᵗʰ **S92.81** Other fracture of foot

Sesamoid fracture of foot
AHA: 2016,4Q,68

CC Excl: For codes in subcategory S92.81:
CC with 7th character B: PDX collection 1369
CC with 7th character K or P: PDX collection 897

3 √7ᵗʰ **S92.811** Other fracture of right foot   CC H5

3 √7ᵗʰ **S92.812** Other fracture of left foot   CC H5

3 √7ᵗʰ **S92.819** Other fracture of unspecified foot   CC H5

√5ᵗʰ **S92.9** Unspecified fracture of foot and toe

CC Excl: For codes in subcategory S92.9, unless otherwise noted:
CC with 7th character K or P: PDX collection 897

√6ᵗʰ **S92.90** Unspecified fracture of foot

CC Excl: For codes in subcategory S92.90:
CC with 7th character B: PDX collection 1369

3 √7ᵗʰ **S92.901** Unspecified fracture of right foot   CC H5

3 √7ᵗʰ **S92.902** Unspecified fracture of left foot   CC H5

3 √7ᵗʰ **S92.909** Unspecified fracture of unspecified foot   CC H5

√6ᵗʰ **S92.91** Unspecified fracture of toe

4 √7ᵗʰ **S92.911** Unspecified fracture of right toe(s)   CC

4 √7ᵗʰ **S92.912** Unspecified fracture of left toe(s)   CC

4 √7ᵗʰ **S92.919** Unspecified fracture of unspecified toe(s)   CC

Chapter 19. Injury, Poisoning and Certain Other Consequences of External Causes

S92.415–S92.919

√4ᵗʰ S93 Dislocation and sprain of joints and ligaments at ankle, foot and toe level

INCLUDES   avulsion of joint or ligament of ankle, foot and toe

laceration of cartilage, joint or ligament of ankle, foot and toe

sprain of cartilage, joint or ligament of ankle, foot and toe

traumatic hemarthrosis of joint or ligament of ankle, foot and toe

traumatic rupture of joint or ligament of ankle, foot and toe

traumatic subluxation of joint or ligament of ankle, foot and toe

traumatic tear of joint or ligament of ankle, foot and toe

Code also any associated open wound

EXCLUDES 2   *strain of muscle and tendon of ankle and foot (S96.-)*

The appropriate 7th character is to be added to each code from category S93.
A   initial encounter
D   subsequent encounter
S   sequela

√5ᵗʰ S93.0 Subluxation and dislocation of ankle joint

Subluxation and dislocation of astragalus
Subluxation and dislocation of fibula, lower end
Subluxation and dislocation of talus
Subluxation and dislocation of tibia, lower end

√x7ᵗʰ   **S93.01 Subluxation of right ankle joint**
√x7ᵗʰ   **S93.02 Subluxation of left ankle joint**
√x7ᵗʰ   **S93.03 Subluxation of unspecified ankle joint**
√x7ᵗʰ   **S93.04 Dislocation of right ankle joint**
√x7ᵗʰ   **S93.05 Dislocation of left ankle joint**
√x7ᵗʰ   **S93.06 Dislocation of unspecified ankle joint**

√5ᵗʰ S93.1 Subluxation and dislocation of toe

√6ᵗʰ S93.10 Unspecified subluxation and dislocation of toe

Dislocation of toe NOS
Subluxation of toe NOS

√7ᵗʰ   **S93.101 Unspecified subluxation of right toe(s)**
√7ᵗʰ   **S93.102 Unspecified subluxation of left toe(s)**
√7ᵗʰ   **S93.103 Unspecified subluxation of unspecified toe(s)**
√7ᵗʰ   **S93.104 Unspecified dislocation of right toe(s)**
√7ᵗʰ   **S93.105 Unspecified dislocation of left toe(s)**
√7ᵗʰ   **S93.106 Unspecified dislocation of unspecified toe(s)**

√6ᵗʰ S93.11 Dislocation of interphalangeal joint

√7ᵗʰ   **S93.111 Dislocation of interphalangeal joint of right great toe**
√7ᵗʰ   **S93.112 Dislocation of interphalangeal joint of left great toe**
√7ᵗʰ   **S93.113 Dislocation of interphalangeal joint of unspecified great toe**
√7ᵗʰ   **S93.114 Dislocation of interphalangeal joint of right lesser toe(s)**
√7ᵗʰ   **S93.115 Dislocation of interphalangeal joint of left lesser toe(s)**
√7ᵗʰ   **S93.116 Dislocation of interphalangeal joint of unspecified lesser toe(s)**
√7ᵗʰ   **S93.119 Dislocation of interphalangeal joint of unspecified toe(s)**

√6ᵗʰ S93.12 Dislocation of metatarsophalangeal joint

√7ᵗʰ   **S93.121 Dislocation of metatarsophalangeal joint of right great toe**
√7ᵗʰ   **S93.122 Dislocation of metatarsophalangeal joint of left great toe**
√7ᵗʰ   **S93.123 Dislocation of metatarsophalangeal joint of unspecified great toe**
√7ᵗʰ   **S93.124 Dislocation of metatarsophalangeal joint of right lesser toe(s)**
√7ᵗʰ   **S93.125 Dislocation of metatarsophalangeal joint of left lesser toe(s)**
√7ᵗʰ   **S93.126 Dislocation of metatarsophalangeal joint of unspecified lesser toe(s)**
√7ᵗʰ   **S93.129 Dislocation of metatarsophalangeal joint of unspecified toe(s)**

√6ᵗʰ S93.13 Subluxation of interphalangeal joint

√7ᵗʰ   **S93.131 Subluxation of interphalangeal joint of right great toe**

√7ᵗʰ   **S93.132 Subluxation of interphalangeal joint of left great toe**
√7ᵗʰ   **S93.133 Subluxation of interphalangeal joint of unspecified great toe**
√7ᵗʰ   **S93.134 Subluxation of interphalangeal joint of right lesser toe(s)**
√7ᵗʰ   **S93.135 Subluxation of interphalangeal joint of left lesser toe(s)**
√7ᵗʰ   **S93.136 Subluxation of interphalangeal joint of unspecified lesser toe(s)**
√7ᵗʰ   **S93.139 Subluxation of interphalangeal joint of unspecified toe(s)**

√6ᵗʰ S93.14 Subluxation of metatarsophalangeal joint

√7ᵗʰ   **S93.141 Subluxation of metatarsophalangeal joint of right great toe**
√7ᵗʰ   **S93.142 Subluxation of metatarsophalangeal joint of left great toe**
√7ᵗʰ   **S93.143 Subluxation of metatarsophalangeal joint of unspecified great toe**
√7ᵗʰ   **S93.144 Subluxation of metatarsophalangeal joint of right lesser toe(s)**
√7ᵗʰ   **S93.145 Subluxation of metatarsophalangeal joint of left lesser toe(s)**
√7ᵗʰ   **S93.146 Subluxation of metatarsophalangeal joint of unspecified lesser toe(s)**
√7ᵗʰ   **S93.149 Subluxation of metatarsophalangeal joint of unspecified toe(s)**

√5ᵗʰ S93.3 Subluxation and dislocation of foot

EXCLUDES 2   *dislocation of toe (S93.1-)*

√6ᵗʰ S93.30 Unspecified subluxation and dislocation of foot

Dislocation of foot NOS
Subluxation of foot NOS

√7ᵗʰ   **S93.301 Unspecified subluxation of right foot**
√7ᵗʰ   **S93.302 Unspecified subluxation of left foot**
√7ᵗʰ   **S93.303 Unspecified subluxation of unspecified foot**
√7ᵗʰ   **S93.304 Unspecified dislocation of right foot**
√7ᵗʰ   **S93.305 Unspecified dislocation of left foot**
√7ᵗʰ   **S93.306 Unspecified dislocation of unspecified foot**

√6ᵗʰ S93.31 Subluxation and dislocation of tarsal joint

√7ᵗʰ   **S93.311 Subluxation of tarsal joint of right foot**
√7ᵗʰ   **S93.312 Subluxation of tarsal joint of left foot**
√7ᵗʰ   **S93.313 Subluxation of tarsal joint of unspecified foot**
√7ᵗʰ   **S93.314 Dislocation of tarsal joint of right foot**
√7ᵗʰ   **S93.315 Dislocation of tarsal joint of left foot**
√7ᵗʰ   **S93.316 Dislocation of tarsal joint of unspecified foot**

√6ᵗʰ S93.32 Subluxation and dislocation of tarsometatarsal joint

√7ᵗʰ   **S93.321 Subluxation of tarsometatarsal joint of right foot**
√7ᵗʰ   **S93.322 Subluxation of tarsometatarsal joint of left foot**
√7ᵗʰ   **S93.323 Subluxation of tarsometatarsal joint of unspecified foot**
√7ᵗʰ   **S93.324 Dislocation of tarsometatarsal joint of right foot**
√7ᵗʰ   **S93.325 Dislocation of tarsometatarsal joint of left foot**
√7ᵗʰ   **S93.326 Dislocation of tarsometatarsal joint of unspecified foot**

√6ᵗʰ S93.33 Other subluxation and dislocation of foot

√7ᵗʰ   **S93.331 Other subluxation of right foot**
√7ᵗʰ   **S93.332 Other subluxation of left foot**
√7ᵗʰ   **S93.333 Other subluxation of unspecified foot**
√7ᵗʰ   **S93.334 Other dislocation of right foot**
√7ᵗʰ   **S93.335 Other dislocation of left foot**
√7ᵗʰ   **S93.336 Other dislocation of unspecified foot**

√5ᵗʰ S93.4 Sprain of ankle

EXCLUDES 2   *injury of Achilles tendon (S86.0-)*

√6ᵗʰ S93.40 Sprain of unspecified ligament of ankle

Sprain of ankle NOS
Sprained ankle NOS

√7ᵗʰ   **S93.401 Sprain of unspecified ligament of right ankle**

N Newborn: 0   P Pediatric: 0-17   M Maternity: 9-64   A Adult: 15-124   MCC Major Complication/Comorbidity   CC Complication/Comorbidity   SW Severe Wound Dx

1120   ICD-10-CM 2020

☑7ᵗʰ **S93.402** Sprain of unspecified ligament of left ankle

☑7ᵗʰ **S93.409** Sprain of unspecified ligament of unspecified ankle

☑6ᵗʰ **S93.41** Sprain of calcaneofibular ligament

☑7ᵗʰ **S93.411** Sprain of calcaneofibular ligament of right ankle

☑7ᵗʰ **S93.412** Sprain of calcaneofibular ligament of left ankle

☑7ᵗʰ **S93.419** Sprain of calcaneofibular ligament of unspecified ankle

☑6ᵗʰ **S93.42** Sprain of deltoid ligament

☑7ᵗʰ **S93.421** Sprain of deltoid ligament of right ankle

☑7ᵗʰ **S93.422** Sprain of deltoid ligament of left ankle

☑7ᵗʰ **S93.429** Sprain of deltoid ligament of unspecified ankle

☑6ᵗʰ **S93.43** Sprain of tibiofibular ligament

☑7ᵗʰ **S93.431** Sprain of tibiofibular ligament of right ankle

☑7ᵗʰ **S93.432** Sprain of tibiofibular ligament of left ankle

☑7ᵗʰ **S93.439** Sprain of tibiofibular ligament of unspecified ankle

☑6ᵗʰ **S93.49** Sprain of other ligament of ankle
Sprain of internal collateral ligament
Sprain of talofibular ligament

☑7ᵗʰ **S93.491** Sprain of other ligament of right ankle

☑7ᵗʰ **S93.492** Sprain of other ligament of left ankle

☑7ᵗʰ **S93.499** Sprain of other ligament of unspecified ankle

☑5ᵗʰ **S93.5** Sprain of toe

☑6ᵗʰ **S93.50** Unspecified sprain of toe

☑7ᵗʰ **S93.501** Unspecified sprain of right great toe

☑7ᵗʰ **S93.502** Unspecified sprain of left great toe

☑7ᵗʰ **S93.503** Unspecified sprain of unspecified great toe

☑7ᵗʰ **S93.504** Unspecified sprain of right lesser toe(s)

☑7ᵗʰ **S93.505** Unspecified sprain of left lesser toe(s)

☑7ᵗʰ **S93.506** Unspecified sprain of unspecified lesser toe(s)

☑7ᵗʰ **S93.509** Unspecified sprain of unspecified toe(s)

☑6ᵗʰ **S93.51** Sprain of interphalangeal joint of toe

☑7ᵗʰ **S93.511** Sprain of interphalangeal joint of right great toe

☑7ᵗʰ **S93.512** Sprain of interphalangeal joint of left great toe

☑7ᵗʰ **S93.513** Sprain of interphalangeal joint of unspecified great toe

☑7ᵗʰ **S93.514** Sprain of interphalangeal joint of right lesser toe(s)

☑7ᵗʰ **S93.515** Sprain of interphalangeal joint of left lesser toe(s)

☑7ᵗʰ **S93.516** Sprain of interphalangeal joint of unspecified lesser toe(s)

☑7ᵗʰ **S93.519** Sprain of interphalangeal joint of unspecified toe(s)

☑6ᵗʰ **S93.52** Sprain of metatarsophalangeal joint of toe

☑7ᵗʰ **S93.521** Sprain of metatarsophalangeal joint of right great toe

☑7ᵗʰ **S93.522** Sprain of metatarsophalangeal joint of left great toe

☑7ᵗʰ **S93.523** Sprain of metatarsophalangeal joint of unspecified great toe

☑7ᵗʰ **S93.524** Sprain of metatarsophalangeal joint of right lesser toe(s)

☑7ᵗʰ **S93.525** Sprain of metatarsophalangeal joint of left lesser toe(s)

☑7ᵗʰ **S93.526** Sprain of metatarsophalangeal joint of unspecified lesser toe(s)

☑7ᵗʰ **S93.529** Sprain of metatarsophalangeal joint of unspecified toe(s)

☑5ᵗʰ **S93.6** Sprain of foot

EXCLUDES 2 sprain of metatarsophalangeal joint of toe (S93.52-)
sprain of toe (S93.5-)

☑6ᵗʰ **S93.60** Unspecified sprain of foot

☑7ᵗʰ **S93.601** Unspecified sprain of right foot

☑7ᵗʰ **S93.602** Unspecified sprain of left foot

☑7ᵗʰ **S93.609** Unspecified sprain of unspecified foot

☑6ᵗʰ **S93.61** Sprain of tarsal ligament of foot

☑7ᵗʰ **S93.611** Sprain of tarsal ligament of right foot

☑7ᵗʰ **S93.612** Sprain of tarsal ligament of left foot

☑7ᵗʰ **S93.619** Sprain of tarsal ligament of unspecified foot

☑6ᵗʰ **S93.62** Sprain of tarsometatarsal ligament of foot

☑7ᵗʰ **S93.621** Sprain of tarsometatarsal ligament of right foot

☑7ᵗʰ **S93.622** Sprain of tarsometatarsal ligament of left foot

☑7ᵗʰ **S93.629** Sprain of tarsometatarsal ligament of unspecified foot

☑6ᵗʰ **S93.69** Other sprain of foot

☑7ᵗʰ **S93.691** Other sprain of right foot

☑7ᵗʰ **S93.692** Other sprain of left foot

☑7ᵗʰ **S93.699** Other sprain of unspecified foot

☑4ᵗʰ **S94** Injury of nerves at ankle and foot level
Code also any associated open wound (S91.-)

The appropriate 7th character is to be added to each code from category S94.
A initial encounter
D subsequent encounter
S sequela

☑5ᵗʰ **S94.0** Injury of lateral plantar nerve

☑×7ᵗʰ **S94.00** Injury of lateral plantar nerve, unspecified leg

☑×7ᵗʰ **S94.01** Injury of lateral plantar nerve, right leg

☑×7ᵗʰ **S94.02** Injury of lateral plantar nerve, left leg

☑5ᵗʰ **S94.1** Injury of medial plantar nerve

☑×7ᵗʰ **S94.10** Injury of medial plantar nerve, unspecified leg

☑×7ᵗʰ **S94.11** Injury of medial plantar nerve, right leg

☑×7ᵗʰ **S94.12** Injury of medial plantar nerve, left leg

☑5ᵗʰ **S94.2** Injury of deep peroneal nerve at ankle and foot level
Injury of terminal, lateral branch of deep peroneal nerve

☑×7ᵗʰ **S94.20** Injury of deep peroneal nerve at ankle and foot level, unspecified leg

☑×7ᵗʰ **S94.21** Injury of deep peroneal nerve at ankle and foot level, right leg

☑×7ᵗʰ **S94.22** Injury of deep peroneal nerve at ankle and foot level, left leg

☑5ᵗʰ **S94.3** Injury of cutaneous sensory nerve at ankle and foot level

☑×7ᵗʰ **S94.30** Injury of cutaneous sensory nerve at ankle and foot level, unspecified leg

☑×7ᵗʰ **S94.31** Injury of cutaneous sensory nerve at ankle and foot level, right leg

☑×7ᵗʰ **S94.32** Injury of cutaneous sensory nerve at ankle and foot level, left leg

☑5ᵗʰ **S94.8** Injury of other nerves at ankle and foot level

☑6ᵗʰ **S94.8X** Injury of other nerves at ankle and foot level

☑7ᵗʰ **S94.8X1** Injury of other nerves at ankle and foot level, right leg

☑7ᵗʰ **S94.8X2** Injury of other nerves at ankle and foot level, left leg

☑7ᵗʰ **S94.8X9** Injury of other nerves at ankle and foot level, unspecified leg

☑5ᵗʰ **S94.9** Injury of unspecified nerve at ankle and foot level

☑×7ᵗʰ **S94.90** Injury of unspecified nerve at ankle and foot level, unspecified leg

☑×7ᵗʰ **S94.91** Injury of unspecified nerve at ankle and foot level, right leg

☑×7ᵗʰ **S94.92** Injury of unspecified nerve at ankle and foot level, left leg

Chapter 19. Injury, Poisoning and Certain Other Consequences of External Causes

S95-S95.992

√4ᵗʰ **S95 Injury of blood vessels at ankle and foot level**

Code also any associated open wound (S91.-)

EXCLUDES 2   injury of posterior tibial artery and vein (S85.1-, S85.8-)

The appropriate 7th character is to be added to each code from category S95.

A   initial encounter
D   subsequent encounter
S   sequela

CC Excl: For CC codes in category S95, unless otherwise noted:
Right side: PDX collection 1325
Left side: PDX collection 1326
Unspecified side: PDX collection 1327

√5ᵗʰ **S95.0 Injury of dorsal artery of foot**

√6ᵗʰ   **S95.00 Unspecified injury of dorsal artery of foot**

     √7ᵗʰ **S95.001 Unspecified injury of dorsal artery of right foot**   CC

     √7ᵗʰ **S95.002 Unspecified injury of dorsal artery of left foot**   CC

     √7ᵗʰ **S95.009 Unspecified injury of dorsal artery of unspecified foot**

√6ᵗʰ   **S95.01 Laceration of dorsal artery of foot**

     √7ᵗʰ **S95.011 Laceration of dorsal artery of right foot**   CC

     √7ᵗʰ **S95.012 Laceration of dorsal artery of left foot**   CC

     √7ᵗʰ **S95.019 Laceration of dorsal artery of unspecified foot**   CC

√6ᵗʰ   **S95.09 Other specified injury of dorsal artery of foot**

     √7ᵗʰ **S95.091 Other specified injury of dorsal artery of right foot**   CC

     √7ᵗʰ **S95.092 Other specified injury of dorsal artery of left foot**   CC

     √7ᵗʰ **S95.099 Other specified injury of dorsal artery of unspecified foot**   CC

√5ᵗʰ **S95.1 Injury of plantar artery of foot**

CC Excl: For CC codes in subcategory S95.1:
Right side: PDX collection 1370
Left side: PDX collection 1371
Unspecified side: PDX collection 1372

√6ᵗʰ   **S95.10 Unspecified injury of plantar artery of foot**

     √7ᵗʰ **S95.101 Unspecified injury of plantar artery of right foot**   CC

     √7ᵗʰ **S95.102 Unspecified injury of plantar artery of left foot**   CC

     √7ᵗʰ **S95.109 Unspecified injury of plantar artery of unspecified foot**   CC

√6ᵗʰ   **S95.11 Laceration of plantar artery of foot**

     √7ᵗʰ **S95.111 Laceration of plantar artery of right foot**   CC

     √7ᵗʰ **S95.112 Laceration of plantar artery of left foot**   CC

     √7ᵗʰ **S95.119 Laceration of plantar artery of unspecified foot**   CC

√6ᵗʰ   **S95.19 Other specified injury of plantar artery of foot**

     √7ᵗʰ **S95.191 Other specified injury of plantar artery of right foot**   CC

     √7ᵗʰ **S95.192 Other specified injury of plantar artery of left foot**   CC

     √7ᵗʰ **S95.199 Other specified injury of plantar artery of unspecified foot**   CC

√5ᵗʰ **S95.2 Injury of dorsal vein of foot**

√6ᵗʰ   **S95.20 Unspecified injury of dorsal vein of foot**

     √7ᵗʰ **S95.201 Unspecified injury of dorsal vein of right foot**   CC

     √7ᵗʰ **S95.202 Unspecified injury of dorsal vein of left foot**   CC

     √7ᵗʰ **S95.209 Unspecified injury of dorsal vein of unspecified foot**   CC

√6ᵗʰ   **S95.21 Laceration of dorsal vein of foot**

     √7ᵗʰ **S95.211 Laceration of dorsal vein of right foot**   CC

     √7ᵗʰ **S95.212 Laceration of dorsal vein of left foot**   CC

     √7ᵗʰ **S95.219 Laceration of dorsal vein of unspecified foot**   CC

√6ᵗʰ   **S95.29 Other specified injury of dorsal vein of foot**

     √7ᵗʰ **S95.291 Other specified injury of dorsal vein of right foot**   CC

     √7ᵗʰ **S95.292 Other specified injury of dorsal vein of left foot**   CC

     √7ᵗʰ **S95.299 Other specified injury of dorsal vein of unspecified foot**   CC

√5ᵗʰ **S95.8 Injury of other blood vessels at ankle and foot level**

√6ᵗʰ   **S95.80 Unspecified injury of other blood vessels at ankle and foot level**

     √7ᵗʰ **S95.801 Unspecified injury of other blood vessels at ankle and foot level, right leg**   CC

     √7ᵗʰ **S95.802 Unspecified injury of other blood vessels at ankle and foot level, left leg**   CC

     √7ᵗʰ **S95.809 Unspecified injury of other blood vessels at ankle and foot level, unspecified leg**   CC

√6ᵗʰ   **S95.81 Laceration of other blood vessels at ankle and foot level**

     √7ᵗʰ **S95.811 Laceration of other blood vessels at ankle and foot level, right leg**   CC

     √7ᵗʰ **S95.812 Laceration of other blood vessels at ankle and foot level, left leg**   CC

     √7ᵗʰ **S95.819 Laceration of other blood vessels at ankle and foot level, unspecified leg**   CC

√6ᵗʰ   **S95.89 Other specified injury of other blood vessels at ankle and foot level**

     √7ᵗʰ **S95.891 Other specified injury of other blood vessels at ankle and foot level, right leg**   CC

     √7ᵗʰ **S95.892 Other specified injury of other blood vessels at ankle and foot level, left leg**   CC

     √7ᵗʰ **S95.899 Other specified injury of other blood vessels at ankle and foot level, unspecified leg**   CC

√5ᵗʰ **S95.9 Injury of unspecified blood vessel at ankle and foot level**

√6ᵗʰ   **S95.90 Unspecified injury of unspecified blood vessel at ankle and foot level**

     √7ᵗʰ **S95.901 Unspecified injury of unspecified blood vessel at ankle and foot level, right leg**   CC

     √7ᵗʰ **S95.902 Unspecified injury of unspecified blood vessel at ankle and foot level, left leg**   CC

     √7ᵗʰ **S95.909 Unspecified injury of unspecified blood vessel at ankle and foot level, unspecified leg**   CC

√6ᵗʰ   **S95.91 Laceration of unspecified blood vessel at ankle and foot level**

     √7ᵗʰ **S95.911 Laceration of unspecified blood vessel at ankle and foot level, right leg**   CC

     √7ᵗʰ **S95.912 Laceration of unspecified blood vessel at ankle and foot level, left leg**   CC

     √7ᵗʰ **S95.919 Laceration of unspecified blood vessel at ankle and foot level, unspecified leg**   CC

√6ᵗʰ   **S95.99 Other specified injury of unspecified blood vessel at ankle and foot level**

     √7ᵗʰ **S95.991 Other specified injury of unspecified blood vessel at ankle and foot level, right leg**   CC

     √7ᵗʰ **S95.992 Other specified injury of unspecified blood vessel at ankle and foot level, left leg**   CC

N Newborn: 0   P Pediatric: 0-17   M Maternity: 9-64   A Adult: 15-124   MCC Major Complication/Comorbidity   CC Complication/Comorbidity   SW Severe Wound Dx

1122   ICD-10-CM 2020

√7ᵗʰ **S95.999** Other specified injury of unspecified blood vessel at ankle and foot level, unspecified leg   cc

√4ᵗʰ **S96 Injury of muscle and tendon at ankle and foot level**

Code also any associated open wound (S91.-)

EXCLUDES 2   injury of Achilles tendon (S86.0-)

sprain of joints and ligaments of ankle and foot (S93.-)

TIP: Refer to the Muscle/Tendon table at the beginning of this chapter,

The appropriate 7th character is to be added to each code from category S96.

A   initial encounter

D   subsequent encounter

S   sequela

CC Excl: For CC codes in category S96:
Right side: PDX collection 1364
Left side: PDX collection 1365
Unspecified side: PDX collection 1366

√5ᵗʰ **S96.0 Injury of muscle and tendon of long flexor muscle of toe at ankle and foot level**

√6ᵗʰ **S96.00** Unspecified injury of muscle and tendon of long flexor muscle of toe at ankle and foot level

√7ᵗʰ **S96.001** Unspecified injury of muscle and tendon of long flexor muscle of toe at ankle and foot level, right foot

√7ᵗʰ **S96.002** Unspecified injury of muscle and tendon of long flexor muscle of toe at ankle and foot level, left foot

√7ᵗʰ **S96.009** Unspecified injury of muscle and tendon of long flexor muscle of toe at ankle and foot level, unspecified foot

√6ᵗʰ **S96.01** Strain of muscle and tendon of long flexor muscle of toe at ankle and foot level

√7ᵗʰ **S96.011** Strain of muscle and tendon of long flexor muscle of toe at ankle and foot level, right foot

√7ᵗʰ **S96.012** Strain of muscle and tendon of long flexor muscle of toe at ankle and foot level, left foot

√7ᵗʰ **S96.019** Strain of muscle and tendon of long flexor muscle of toe at ankle and foot level, unspecified foot

√6ᵗʰ **S96.02** Laceration of muscle and tendon of long flexor muscle of toe at ankle and foot level

√7ᵗʰ **S96.021** Laceration of muscle and tendon of long flexor muscle of toe at ankle and foot level, right foot   cc

√7ᵗʰ **S96.022** Laceration of muscle and tendon of long flexor muscle of toe at ankle and foot level, left foot   cc

√7ᵗʰ **S96.029** Laceration of muscle and tendon of long flexor muscle of toe at ankle and foot level, unspecified foot   cc

√6ᵗʰ **S96.09** Other injury of muscle and tendon of long flexor muscle of toe at ankle and foot level

√7ᵗʰ **S96.091** Other injury of muscle and tendon of long flexor muscle of toe at ankle and foot level, right foot

√7ᵗʰ **S96.092** Other injury of muscle and tendon of long flexor muscle of toe at ankle and foot level, left foot

√7ᵗʰ **S96.099** Other injury of muscle and tendon of long flexor muscle of toe at ankle and foot level, unspecified foot

√5ᵗʰ **S96.1 Injury of muscle and tendon of long extensor muscle of toe at ankle and foot level**

√6ᵗʰ **S96.10** Unspecified injury of muscle and tendon of long extensor muscle of toe at ankle and foot level

√7ᵗʰ **S96.101** Unspecified injury of muscle and tendon of long extensor muscle of toe at ankle and foot level, right foot

√7ᵗʰ **S96.102** Unspecified injury of muscle and tendon of long extensor muscle of toe at ankle and foot level, left foot

√7ᵗʰ **S96.109** Unspecified injury of muscle and tendon of long extensor muscle of toe at ankle and foot level, unspecified foot

√6ᵗʰ **S96.11** Strain of muscle and tendon of long extensor muscle of toe at ankle and foot level

√7ᵗʰ **S96.111** Strain of muscle and tendon of long extensor muscle of toe at ankle and foot level, right foot

√7ᵗʰ **S96.112** Strain of muscle and tendon of long extensor muscle of toe at ankle and foot level, left foot

√7ᵗʰ **S96.119** Strain of muscle and tendon of long extensor muscle of toe at ankle and foot level, unspecified foot

√6ᵗʰ **S96.12** Laceration of muscle and tendon of long extensor muscle of toe at ankle and foot level

√7ᵗʰ **S96.121** Laceration of muscle and tendon of long extensor muscle of toe at ankle and foot level, right foot   cc

√7ᵗʰ **S96.122** Laceration of muscle and tendon of long extensor muscle of toe at ankle and foot level, left foot   cc

√7ᵗʰ **S96.129** Laceration of muscle and tendon of long extensor muscle of toe at ankle and foot level, unspecified foot   cc

√6ᵗʰ **S96.19** Other specified injury of muscle and tendon of long extensor muscle of toe at ankle and foot level

√7ᵗʰ **S96.191** Other specified injury of muscle and tendon of long extensor muscle of toe at ankle and foot level, right foot

√7ᵗʰ **S96.192** Other specified injury of muscle and tendon of long extensor muscle of toe at ankle and foot level, left foot

√7ᵗʰ **S96.199** Other specified injury of muscle and tendon of long extensor muscle of toe at ankle and foot level, unspecified foot

√5ᵗʰ **S96.2 Injury of intrinsic muscle and tendon at ankle and foot level**

√6ᵗʰ **S96.20** Unspecified injury of intrinsic muscle and tendon at ankle and foot level

√7ᵗʰ **S96.201** Unspecified injury of intrinsic muscle and tendon at ankle and foot level, right foot

√7ᵗʰ **S96.202** Unspecified injury of intrinsic muscle and tendon at ankle and foot level, left foot

√7ᵗʰ **S96.209** Unspecified injury of intrinsic muscle and tendon at ankle and foot level, unspecified foot

√6ᵗʰ **S96.21** Strain of intrinsic muscle and tendon at ankle and foot level

√7ᵗʰ **S96.211** Strain of intrinsic muscle and tendon at ankle and foot level, right foot

√7ᵗʰ **S96.212** Strain of intrinsic muscle and tendon at ankle and foot level, left foot

√7ᵗʰ **S96.219** Strain of intrinsic muscle and tendon at ankle and foot level, unspecified foot

√6ᵗʰ **S96.22** Laceration of intrinsic muscle and tendon at ankle and foot level

√7ᵗʰ **S96.221** Laceration of intrinsic muscle and tendon at ankle and foot level, right foot   cc

√7ᵗʰ **S96.222** Laceration of intrinsic muscle and tendon at ankle and foot level, left foot   cc

√7ᵗʰ **S96.229** Laceration of intrinsic muscle and tendon at ankle and foot level, unspecified foot   cc

√6ᵗʰ **S96.29** Other specified injury of intrinsic muscle and tendon at ankle and foot level

√7ᵗʰ **S96.291** Other specified injury of intrinsic muscle and tendon at ankle and foot level, right foot

√7ᵗʰ **S96.292** Other specified injury of intrinsic muscle and tendon at ankle and foot level, left foot

√7ᵗʰ **S96.299** Other specified injury of intrinsic muscle and tendon at ankle and foot level, unspecified foot

√5ᵗʰ S96.8 Injury of other specified muscles and tendons at ankle and foot level

   √6ᵗʰ S96.80 Unspecified injury of other specified muscles and tendons at ankle and foot level

     √7ᵗʰ S96.801 Unspecified injury of other specified muscles and tendons at ankle and foot level, right foot

     √7ᵗʰ S96.802 Unspecified injury of other specified muscles and tendons at ankle and foot level, left foot

     √7ᵗʰ S96.809 Unspecified injury of other specified muscles and tendons at ankle and foot level, unspecified foot

   √6ᵗʰ S96.81 Strain of other specified muscles and tendons at ankle and foot level

     √7ᵗʰ S96.811 Strain of other specified muscles and tendons at ankle and foot level, right foot

     √7ᵗʰ S96.812 Strain of other specified muscles and tendons at ankle and foot level, left foot

     √7ᵗʰ S96.819 Strain of other specified muscles and tendons at ankle and foot level, unspecified foot

   √6ᵗʰ S96.82 Laceration of other specified muscles and tendons at ankle and foot level

     √7ᵗʰ S96.821 Laceration of other specified muscles and tendons at ankle and foot level, right foot   CC

     √7ᵗʰ S96.822 Laceration of other specified muscles and tendons at ankle and foot level, left foot   CC

     √7ᵗʰ S96.829 Laceration of other specified muscles and tendons at ankle and foot level, unspecified foot   CC

   √6ᵗʰ S96.89 Other specified injury of other specified muscles and tendons at ankle and foot level

     √7ᵗʰ S96.891 Other specified injury of other specified muscles and tendons at ankle and foot level, right foot

     √7ᵗʰ S96.892 Other specified injury of other specified muscles and tendons at ankle and foot level, left foot

     √7ᵗʰ S96.899 Other specified injury of other specified muscles and tendons at ankle and foot level, unspecified foot

√5ᵗʰ S96.9 Injury of unspecified muscle and tendon at ankle and foot level

   √6ᵗʰ S96.90 Unspecified injury of unspecified muscle and tendon at ankle and foot level

     √7ᵗʰ S96.901 Unspecified injury of unspecified muscle and tendon at ankle and foot level, right foot

     √7ᵗʰ S96.902 Unspecified injury of unspecified muscle and tendon at ankle and foot level, left foot

     √7ᵗʰ S96.909 Unspecified injury of unspecified muscle and tendon at ankle and foot level, unspecified foot

   √6ᵗʰ S96.91 Strain of unspecified muscle and tendon at ankle and foot level

     √7ᵗʰ S96.911 Strain of unspecified muscle and tendon at ankle and foot level, right foot

     √7ᵗʰ S96.912 Strain of unspecified muscle and tendon at ankle and foot level, left foot

     √7ᵗʰ S96.919 Strain of unspecified muscle and tendon at ankle and foot level, unspecified foot

   √6ᵗʰ S96.92 Laceration of unspecified muscle and tendon at ankle and foot level

     √7ᵗʰ S96.921 Laceration of unspecified muscle and tendon at ankle and foot level, right foot   CC

     √7ᵗʰ S96.922 Laceration of unspecified muscle and tendon at ankle and foot level, left foot   CC

     √7ᵗʰ S96.929 Laceration of unspecified muscle and tendon at ankle and foot level, unspecified foot   CC

   √6ᵗʰ S96.99 Other specified injury of unspecified muscle and tendon at ankle and foot level

     √7ᵗʰ S96.991 Other specified injury of unspecified muscle and tendon at ankle and foot level, right foot

     √7ᵗʰ S96.992 Other specified injury of unspecified muscle and tendon at ankle and foot level, left foot

     √7ᵗʰ S96.999 Other specified injury of unspecified muscle and tendon at ankle and foot level, unspecified foot

√4ᵗʰ S97 Crushing injury of ankle and foot

Use additional code(s) for all associated injuries

The appropriate 7th character is to be added to each code from category S97.
A   initial encounter
D   subsequent encounter
S   sequela

√5ᵗʰ S97.0 Crushing injury of ankle

   √x7ᵗʰ S97.00 Crushing injury of unspecified ankle

   √x7ᵗʰ S97.01 Crushing injury of right ankle

   √x7ᵗʰ S97.02 Crushing injury of left ankle

√5ᵗʰ S97.1 Crushing injury of toe

   √6ᵗʰ S97.10 Crushing injury of unspecified toe(s)

     √7ᵗʰ S97.101 Crushing injury of unspecified right toe(s)

     √7ᵗʰ S97.102 Crushing injury of unspecified left toe(s)

     √7ᵗʰ S97.109 Crushing injury of unspecified toe(s)
       Crushing injury of toe NOS

   √6ᵗʰ S97.11 Crushing injury of great toe

     √7ᵗʰ S97.111 Crushing injury of right great toe

     √7ᵗʰ S97.112 Crushing injury of left great toe

     √7ᵗʰ S97.119 Crushing injury of unspecified great toe

   √6ᵗʰ S97.12 Crushing injury of lesser toe(s)

     √7ᵗʰ S97.121 Crushing injury of right lesser toe(s)

     √7ᵗʰ S97.122 Crushing injury of left lesser toe(s)

     √7ᵗʰ S97.129 Crushing injury of unspecified lesser toe(s)

√5ᵗʰ S97.8 Crushing injury of foot

   √x7ᵗʰ S97.80 Crushing injury of unspecified foot
     Crushing injury of foot NOS

   √x7ᵗʰ S97.81 Crushing injury of right foot

   √x7ᵗʰ S97.82 Crushing injury of left foot

√4ᵗʰ S98 Traumatic amputation of ankle and foot

An amputation not identified as partial or complete should be coded to complete

The appropriate 7th character is to be added to each code from category S98.
A   initial encounter
D   subsequent encounter
S   sequela

CC Excl: For CC codes in category S98:
Right side: PDX collection 1333
Left side: PDX collection 1334
Unspecified side: PDX collection 1335

√5ᵗʰ S98.0 Traumatic amputation of foot at ankle level

   √6ᵗʰ S98.01 Complete traumatic amputation of foot at ankle level

     √7ᵗʰ S98.011 Complete traumatic amputation of right foot at ankle level   CC HCC

     √7ᵗʰ S98.012 Complete traumatic amputation of left foot at ankle level   CC HCC

     √7ᵗʰ S98.019 Complete traumatic amputation of unspecified foot at ankle level   CC HCC

   √6ᵗʰ S98.02 Partial traumatic amputation of foot at ankle level

     √7ᵗʰ S98.021 Partial traumatic amputation of right foot at ankle level   CC HCC

     √7ᵗʰ S98.022 Partial traumatic amputation of left foot at ankle level   CC HCC

√7ᵗʰ **S98.029** Partial traumatic amputation of unspecified foot at ankle level `CC` `HCC`

√5ᵗʰ **S98.1** Traumatic amputation of one toe

  √6ᵗʰ **S98.11** Complete traumatic amputation of great toe

    √7ᵗʰ **S98.111** Complete traumatic amputation of right great toe `HCC`

    √7ᵗʰ **S98.112** Complete traumatic amputation of left great toe `HCC`

    √7ᵗʰ **S98.119** Complete traumatic amputation of unspecified great toe `HCC`

  √6ᵗʰ **S98.12** Partial traumatic amputation of great toe

    √7ᵗʰ **S98.121** Partial traumatic amputation of right great toe `HCC`

    √7ᵗʰ **S98.122** Partial traumatic amputation of left great toe `HCC`

    √7ᵗʰ **S98.129** Partial traumatic amputation of unspecified great toe `HCC`

  √6ᵗʰ **S98.13** Complete traumatic amputation of one lesser toe
Traumatic amputation of toe NOS

    √7ᵗʰ **S98.131** Complete traumatic amputation of one right lesser toe `HCC`

    √7ᵗʰ **S98.132** Complete traumatic amputation of one left lesser toe `HCC`

    √7ᵗʰ **S98.139** Complete traumatic amputation of one unspecified lesser toe `HCC`

  √6ᵗʰ **S98.14** Partial traumatic amputation of one lesser toe

    √7ᵗʰ **S98.141** Partial traumatic amputation of one right lesser toe `HCC`

    √7ᵗʰ **S98.142** Partial traumatic amputation of one left lesser toe `HCC`

    √7ᵗʰ **S98.149** Partial traumatic amputation of one unspecified lesser toe `HCC`

√5ᵗʰ **S98.2** Traumatic amputation of two or more lesser toes

  √6ᵗʰ **S98.21** Complete traumatic amputation of two or more lesser toes

    √7ᵗʰ **S98.211** Complete traumatic amputation of two or more right lesser toes `HCC`

    √7ᵗʰ **S98.212** Complete traumatic amputation of two or more left lesser toes `HCC`

    √7ᵗʰ **S98.219** Complete traumatic amputation of two or more unspecified lesser toes `HCC`

  √6ᵗʰ **S98.22** Partial traumatic amputation of two or more lesser toes

    √7ᵗʰ **S98.221** Partial traumatic amputation of two or more right lesser toes `HCC`

    √7ᵗʰ **S98.222** Partial traumatic amputation of two or more left lesser toes `HCC`

    √7ᵗʰ **S98.229** Partial traumatic amputation of two or more unspecified lesser toes `HCC`

√5ᵗʰ **S98.3** Traumatic amputation of midfoot

  √6ᵗʰ **S98.31** Complete traumatic amputation of midfoot

    √7ᵗʰ **S98.311** Complete traumatic amputation of right midfoot `CC` `HCC`

    √7ᵗʰ **S98.312** Complete traumatic amputation of left midfoot `CC` `HCC`

    √7ᵗʰ **S98.319** Complete traumatic amputation of unspecified midfoot `CC` `HCC`

  √6ᵗʰ **S98.32** Partial traumatic amputation of midfoot

    √7ᵗʰ **S98.321** Partial traumatic amputation of right midfoot `CC` `HCC`

    √7ᵗʰ **S98.322** Partial traumatic amputation of left midfoot `CC` `HCC`

    √7ᵗʰ **S98.329** Partial traumatic amputation of unspecified midfoot `CC` `HCC`

√5ᵗʰ **S98.9** Traumatic amputation of foot, level unspecified

  √6ᵗʰ **S98.91** Complete traumatic amputation of foot, level unspecified

    √7ᵗʰ **S98.911** Complete traumatic amputation of right foot, level unspecified `CC` `HCC`

    √7ᵗʰ **S98.912** Complete traumatic amputation of left foot, level unspecified `CC` `HCC`

    √7ᵗʰ **S98.919** Complete traumatic amputation of unspecified foot, level unspecified `CC` `HCC`

  √6ᵗʰ **S98.92** Partial traumatic amputation of foot, level unspecified

    √7ᵗʰ **S98.921** Partial traumatic amputation of right foot, level unspecified `CC` `HCC`

    √7ᵗʰ **S98.922** Partial traumatic amputation of left foot, level unspecified `CC` `HCC`

    √7ᵗʰ **S98.929** Partial traumatic amputation of unspecified foot, level unspecified `CC` `HCC`

√4ᵗʰ **S99** Other and unspecified injuries of ankle and foot
AHA: 2018,2Q,12; 2018,1Q,3; 2016,4Q,68-69

√5ᵗʰ **S99.0** Physeal fracture of calcaneus

> The appropriate 7th character is to be added to each code from subcategory S99.0.
> A initial encounter for closed fracture
> B initial encounter for open fracture
> D subsequent encounter for fracture with routine healing
> G subsequent encounter for fracture with delayed healing
> K subsequent encounter for fracture with nonunion
> P subsequent encounter for fracture with malunion
> S sequela

  √6ᵗʰ **S99.00** Unspecified physeal fracture of calcaneus

    √7ᵗʰ **S99.001** Unspecified physeal fracture of right calcaneus

    √7ᵗʰ **S99.002** Unspecified physeal fracture of left calcaneus

    √7ᵗʰ **S99.009** Unspecified physeal fracture of unspecified calcaneus

  √6ᵗʰ **S99.01** Salter-Harris Type I physeal fracture of calcaneus

    √7ᵗʰ **S99.011** Salter-Harris Type I physeal fracture of right calcaneus

    √7ᵗʰ **S99.012** Salter-Harris Type I physeal fracture of left calcaneus

    √7ᵗʰ **S99.019** Salter-Harris Type I physeal fracture of unspecified calcaneus

  √6ᵗʰ **S99.02** Salter-Harris Type II physeal fracture of calcaneus

    √7ᵗʰ **S99.021** Salter-Harris Type II physeal fracture of right calcaneus

    √7ᵗʰ **S99.022** Salter-Harris Type II physeal fracture of left calcaneus

    √7ᵗʰ **S99.029** Salter-Harris Type II physeal fracture of unspecified calcaneus

  √6ᵗʰ **S99.03** Salter-Harris Type III physeal fracture of calcaneus

    √7ᵗʰ **S99.031** Salter-Harris Type III physeal fracture of right calcaneus

    √7ᵗʰ **S99.032** Salter-Harris Type III physeal fracture of left calcaneus

    √7ᵗʰ **S99.039** Salter-Harris Type III physeal fracture of unspecified calcaneus

  √6ᵗʰ **S99.04** Salter-Harris Type IV physeal fracture of calcaneus

    √7ᵗʰ **S99.041** Salter-Harris Type IV physeal fracture of right calcaneus

    √7ᵗʰ **S99.042** Salter-Harris Type IV physeal fracture of left calcaneus

    √7ᵗʰ **S99.049** Salter-Harris Type IV physeal fracture of unspecified calcaneus

√6ᵗʰ S99.09 Other physeal fracture of calcaneus
- **√7ᵗʰ S99.091** Other physeal fracture of right calcaneus
- **√7ᵗʰ S99.092** Other physeal fracture of left calcaneus
- **√7ᵗʰ S99.099** Other physeal fracture of unspecified calcaneus

√5ᵗʰ S99.1 Physeal fracture of metatarsal

> The appropriate 7th character is to be added to each code from subcategory S99.1
> A   initial encounter for closed fracture
> B   initial encounter for open fracture
> D   subsequent encounter for fracture with routine healing
> G   subsequent encounter for fracture with delayed healing
> K   subsequent encounter for fracture with nonunion
> P   subsequent encounter for fracture with malunion
> S   sequela

√6ᵗʰ S99.10 Unspecified physeal fracture of metatarsal
- **√7ᵗʰ S99.101** Unspecified physeal fracture of right metatarsal
- **√7ᵗʰ S99.102** Unspecified physeal fracture of left metatarsal
- **√7ᵗʰ S99.109** Unspecified physeal fracture of unspecified metatarsal

√6ᵗʰ S99.11 Salter-Harris Type I physeal fracture of metatarsal
- **√7ᵗʰ S99.111** Salter-Harris Type I physeal fracture of right metatarsal
- **√7ᵗʰ S99.112** Salter-Harris Type I physeal fracture of left metatarsal
- **√7ᵗʰ S99.119** Salter-Harris Type I physeal fracture of unspecified metatarsal

√6ᵗʰ S99.12 Salter-Harris Type II physeal fracture of metatarsal
- **√7ᵗʰ S99.121** Salter-Harris Type II physeal fracture of right metatarsal
- **√7ᵗʰ S99.122** Salter-Harris Type II physeal fracture of left metatarsal
- **√7ᵗʰ S99.129** Salter-Harris Type II physeal fracture of unspecified metatarsal

√6ᵗʰ S99.13 Salter-Harris Type III physeal fracture of metatarsal
- **√7ᵗʰ S99.131** Salter-Harris Type III physeal fracture of right metatarsal
- **√7ᵗʰ S99.132** Salter-Harris Type III physeal fracture of left metatarsal
- **√7ᵗʰ S99.139** Salter-Harris Type III physeal fracture of unspecified metatarsal

√6ᵗʰ S99.14 Salter-Harris Type IV physeal fracture of metatarsal
- **√7ᵗʰ S99.141** Salter-Harris Type IV physeal fracture of right metatarsal
- **√7ᵗʰ S99.142** Salter-Harris Type IV physeal fracture of left metatarsal
- **√7ᵗʰ S99.149** Salter-Harris Type IV physeal fracture of unspecified metatarsal

√6ᵗʰ S99.19 Other physeal fracture of metatarsal
- **√7ᵗʰ S99.191** Other physeal fracture of right metatarsal
- **√7ᵗʰ S99.192** Other physeal fracture of left metatarsal
- **√7ᵗʰ S99.199** Other physeal fracture of unspecified metatarsal

√5ᵗʰ S99.2 Physeal fracture of phalanx of toe

> The appropriate 7th character is to be added to each code from subcategories S99.2.
> A   initial encounter for closed fracture
> B   initial encounter for open fracture
> D   subsequent encounter for fracture with routine healing
> G   subsequent encounter for fracture with delayed healing
> K   subsequent encounter for fracture with nonunion
> P   subsequent encounter for fracture with malunion
> S   sequela

√6ᵗʰ S99.20 Unspecified physeal fracture of phalanx of toe
- **√7ᵗʰ S99.201** Unspecified physeal fracture of phalanx of right toe
- **√7ᵗʰ S99.202** Unspecified physeal fracture of phalanx of left toe
- **√7ᵗʰ S99.209** Unspecified physeal fracture of phalanx of unspecified toe

√6ᵗʰ S99.21 Salter-Harris Type I physeal fracture of phalanx of toe
- **√7ᵗʰ S99.211** Salter-Harris Type I physeal fracture of phalanx of right toe

- **√7ᵗʰ S99.212** Salter-Harris Type I physeal fracture of phalanx of left toe
- **√7ᵗʰ S99.219** Salter-Harris Type I physeal fracture of phalanx of unspecified toe

√6ᵗʰ S99.22 Salter-Harris Type II physeal fracture of phalanx of toe
- **√7ᵗʰ S99.221** Salter-Harris Type II physeal fracture of phalanx of right toe
- **√7ᵗʰ S99.222** Salter-Harris Type II physeal fracture of phalanx of left toe
- **√7ᵗʰ S99.229** Salter-Harris Type II physeal fracture of phalanx of unspecified toe

√6ᵗʰ S99.23 Salter-Harris Type III physeal fracture of phalanx of toe
- **√7ᵗʰ S99.231** Salter-Harris Type III physeal fracture of phalanx of right toe
- **√7ᵗʰ S99.232** Salter-Harris Type III physeal fracture of phalanx of left toe
- **√7ᵗʰ S99.239** Salter-Harris Type III physeal fracture of phalanx of unspecified toe

√6ᵗʰ S99.24 Salter-Harris Type IV physeal fracture of phalanx of toe
- **√7ᵗʰ S99.241** Salter-Harris Type IV physeal fracture of phalanx of right toe
- **√7ᵗʰ S99.242** Salter-Harris Type IV physeal fracture of phalanx of left toe
- **√7ᵗʰ S99.249** Salter-Harris Type IV physeal fracture of phalanx of unspecified toe

√6ᵗʰ S99.29 Other physeal fracture of phalanx of toe
- **√7ᵗʰ S99.291** Other physeal fracture of phalanx of right toe
- **√7ᵗʰ S99.292** Other physeal fracture of phalanx of left toe
- **√7ᵗʰ S99.299** Other physeal fracture of phalanx of unspecified toe

√5ᵗʰ S99.8 Other specified injuries of ankle and foot

> The appropriate 7th character is to be added to each code from subcategory S99.8.
> A   initial encounter
> D   subsequent encounter
> S   sequela

√6ᵗʰ S99.81 Other specified injuries of ankle
- **√7ᵗʰ S99.811** Other specified injuries of right ankle
- **√7ᵗʰ S99.812** Other specified injuries of left ankle
- **√7ᵗʰ S99.819** Other specified injuries of unspecified ankle

√6ᵗʰ S99.82 Other specified injuries of foot
- **√7ᵗʰ S99.821** Other specified injuries of right foot
- **√7ᵗʰ S99.822** Other specified injuries of left foot
- **√7ᵗʰ S99.829** Other specified injuries of unspecified foot

√5ᵗʰ S99.9 Unspecified injury of ankle and foot

> The appropriate 7th character is to be added to each code from subcategory S99.9.
> A   initial encounter
> D   subsequent encounter
> S   sequela

√6ᵗʰ S99.91 Unspecified injury of ankle
- **√7ᵗʰ S99.911** Unspecified injury of right ankle
- **√7ᵗʰ S99.912** Unspecified injury of left ankle
- **√7ᵗʰ S99.919** Unspecified injury of unspecified ankle

√6ᵗʰ S99.92 Unspecified injury of foot
- **√7ᵗʰ S99.921** Unspecified injury of right foot
- **√7ᵗʰ S99.922** Unspecified injury of left foot
- **√7ᵗʰ S99.929** Unspecified injury of unspecified foot

N Newborn: 0   **P** Pediatric: 0-17   **M** Maternity: 9-64   **A** Adult: 15-124   **MCC** Major Complication/Comorbidity   **CC** Complication/Comorbidity   **SW** Severe Wound Dx

1126   ICD-10-CM 2020

INJURY, POISONING AND CERTAIN OTHER CONSEQUENCES OF EXTERNAL CAUSES (T07-T88)

Injuries involving multiple body regions (T07)

EXCLUDES 1   burns and corrosions (T20-T32)
frostbite (T33-T34)
insect bite or sting, venomous (T63.4)
sunburn (L55.-)

√x7ᵗʰ **T07   Unspecified multiple injuries**

EXCLUDES 1   injury NOS (T14.90)

AHA: 2017,4Q,26

The appropriate 7th character is to be added to code T07.
A   initial encounter
D   subsequent encounter
S   sequela

Injury of unspecified body region (T14)

√4ᵗʰ **T14   Injury of unspecified body region**

EXCLUDES 1   multiple unspecified injuries (T07)

AHA: 2017,4Q,26

The appropriate 7th character is to be added to each code from category T14.
A   initial encounter
D   subsequent encounter
S   sequela

√x7ᵗʰ **T14.8   Other injury of unspecified body region**
Abrasion NOS
Contusion NOS
Crush injury NOS
Fracture NOS
Skin injury NOS
Vascular injury NOS
Wound NOS

√5ᵗʰ **T14.9   Unspecified injury**

√x7ᵗʰ **T14.90   Injury, unspecified**
Injury NOS

√x7ᵗʰ **T14.91   Suicide attempt**   **HCC**
Attempted suicide NOS

Effects of foreign body entering through natural orifice (T15-T19)

EXCLUDES 2   foreign body accidentally left in operation wound (T81.5-)
foreign body in penetrating wound — see open wound by body region
residual foreign body in soft tissue (M79.5)
splinter, without open wound — see superficial injury by body region

√4ᵗʰ **T15   Foreign body on external eye**

EXCLUDES 2   foreign body in penetrating wound of orbit and eye ball (S05.4-, S05.5-)
open wound of eyelid and periocular area (S01.1-)
retained foreign body in eyelid (H02.8-)
retained (old) foreign body in penetrating wound of orbit and eye ball (H05.5-, H44.6-, H44.7-)
superficial foreign body of eyelid and periocular area (S00.25-)

The appropriate 7th character is to be added to each code from category T15.
A   initial encounter
D   subsequent encounter
S   sequela

√5ᵗʰ **T15.0   Foreign body in cornea**

√x7ᵗʰ **T15.00   Foreign body in cornea, unspecified eye**

√x7ᵗʰ **T15.01   Foreign body in cornea, right eye**

√x7ᵗʰ **T15.02   Foreign body in cornea, left eye**

√5ᵗʰ **T15.1   Foreign body in conjunctival sac**

√x7ᵗʰ **T15.10   Foreign body in conjunctival sac, unspecified eye**

√x7ᵗʰ **T15.11   Foreign body in conjunctival sac, right eye**

√x7ᵗʰ **T15.12   Foreign body in conjunctival sac, left eye**

√5ᵗʰ **T15.8   Foreign body in other and multiple parts of external eye**
Foreign body in lacrimal punctum

√x7ᵗʰ **T15.80   Foreign body in other and multiple parts of external eye, unspecified eye**

√x7ᵗʰ **T15.81   Foreign body in other and multiple parts of external eye, right eye**

√x7ᵗʰ **T15.82   Foreign body in other and multiple parts of external eye, left eye**

√5ᵗʰ **T15.9   Foreign body on external eye, part unspecified**

√x7ᵗʰ **T15.90   Foreign body on external eye, part unspecified, unspecified eye**

√x7ᵗʰ **T15.91   Foreign body on external eye, part unspecified, right eye**

√x7ᵗʰ **T15.92   Foreign body on external eye, part unspecified, left eye**

√4ᵗʰ **T16   Foreign body in ear**

INCLUDES   foreign body in auditory canal

The appropriate 7th character is to be added to each code from category T16.
A   initial encounter
D   subsequent encounter
S   sequela

√x7ᵗʰ **T16.1   Foreign body in right ear**

√x7ᵗʰ **T16.2   Foreign body in left ear**

√x7ᵗʰ **T16.9   Foreign body in ear, unspecified ear**

√4ᵗʰ **T17   Foreign body in respiratory tract**

The appropriate 7th character is to be added to each code from category T17.
A   initial encounter
D   subsequent encounter
S   sequela

CC Excl: For CC codes in category T17, unless otherwise noted: PDX collection 1374

√x7ᵗʰ **T17.0   Foreign body in nasal sinus**

√x7ᵗʰ **T17.1   Foreign body in nostril**
Foreign body in nose NOS

√5ᵗʰ **T17.2   Foreign body in pharynx**
Foreign body in nasopharynx
Foreign body in throat NOS

√6ᵗʰ **T17.20   Unspecified foreign body in pharynx**

√7ᵗʰ **T17.200   Unspecified foreign body in pharynx causing asphyxiation**

√7ᵗʰ **T17.208   Unspecified foreign body in pharynx causing other injury**

√6ᵗʰ **T17.21   Gastric contents in pharynx**
Aspiration of gastric contents into pharynx
Vomitus in pharynx

√7ᵗʰ **T17.210   Gastric contents in pharynx causing asphyxiation**

√7ᵗʰ **T17.218   Gastric contents in pharynx causing other injury**

√6ᵗʰ **T17.22   Food in pharynx**
Bones in pharynx
Seeds in pharynx

√7ᵗʰ **T17.220   Food in pharynx causing asphyxiation**

√7ᵗʰ **T17.228   Food in pharynx causing other injury**

√6ᵗʰ **T17.29   Other foreign object in pharynx**

√7ᵗʰ **T17.290   Other foreign object in pharynx causing asphyxiation**

√7ᵗʰ **T17.298   Other foreign object in pharynx causing other injury**

√5ᵗʰ **T17.3   Foreign body in larynx**

√6ᵗʰ **T17.30   Unspecified foreign body in larynx**

√7ᵗʰ **T17.300   Unspecified foreign body in larynx causing asphyxiation**

√7ᵗʰ **T17.308   Unspecified foreign body in larynx causing other injury**

√6ᵗʰ **T17.31   Gastric contents in larynx**
Aspiration of gastric contents into larynx
Vomitus in larynx

√7ᵗʰ **T17.310   Gastric contents in larynx causing asphyxiation**

√7ᵗʰ **T17.318   Gastric contents in larynx causing other injury**

√6ᵗʰ **T17.32   Food in larynx**
Bones in larynx
Seeds in larynx

√7ᵗʰ **T17.320   Food in larynx causing asphyxiation**

√7ᵗʰ **T17.328** Food in larynx causing other injury

√6ᵗʰ **T17.39** Other foreign object in larynx
- √7ᵗʰ **T17.390** Other foreign object in larynx causing asphyxiation
- √7ᵗʰ **T17.398** Other foreign object in larynx causing other injury

√5ᵗʰ **T17.4** Foreign body in trachea

CC Excl: For CC codes in subcategory T17.4: PDX collection 1373

√6ᵗʰ **T17.40** Unspecified foreign body in trachea
- √7ᵗʰ **T17.400** Unspecified foreign body in trachea causing asphyxiation   CC
- √7ᵗʰ **T17.408** Unspecified foreign body in trachea causing other injury   CC

√6ᵗʰ **T17.41** Gastric contents in trachea
Aspiration of gastric contents into trachea
Vomitus in trachea
- √7ᵗʰ **T17.410** Gastric contents in trachea causing asphyxiation   CC
- √7ᵗʰ **T17.418** Gastric contents in trachea causing other injury   CC

√6ᵗʰ **T17.42** Food in trachea
Bones in trachea
Seeds in trachea
- √7ᵗʰ **T17.420** Food in trachea causing asphyxiation   CC
- √7ᵗʰ **T17.428** Food in trachea causing other injury   CC

√6ᵗʰ **T17.49** Other foreign object in trachea
- √7ᵗʰ **T17.490** Other foreign object in trachea causing asphyxiation   CC
- √7ᵗʰ **T17.498** Other foreign object in trachea causing other injury   CC

√5ᵗʰ **T17.5** Foreign body in bronchus

√6ᵗʰ **T17.50** Unspecified foreign body in bronchus
- √7ᵗʰ **T17.500** Unspecified foreign body in bronchus causing asphyxiation   CC
- √7ᵗʰ **T17.508** Unspecified foreign body in bronchus causing other injury   CC

√6ᵗʰ **T17.51** Gastric contents in bronchus
Aspiration of gastric contents into bronchus
Vomitus in bronchus
- √7ᵗʰ **T17.510** Gastric contents in bronchus causing asphyxiation   CC
- √7ᵗʰ **T17.518** Gastric contents in bronchus causing other injury   CC

√0ᵗʰ **T17.52** Food in bronchus
Bones in bronchus
Seeds in bronchus
- √7ᵗʰ **T17.520** Food in bronchus causing asphyxiation   CC
- √7ᵗʰ **T17.528** Food in bronchus causing other injury   CC

√6ᵗʰ **T17.59** Other foreign object in bronchus
- √7ᵗʰ **T17.590** Other foreign object in bronchus causing asphyxiation   CC
- √7ᵗʰ **T17.598** Other foreign object in bronchus causing other injury   CC

√5ᵗʰ **T17.8** Foreign body in other parts of respiratory tract
Foreign body in bronchioles
Foreign body in lung

√6ᵗʰ **T17.80** Unspecified foreign body in other parts of respiratory tract
- √7ᵗʰ **T17.800** Unspecified foreign body in other parts of respiratory tract causing asphyxiation   CC

√7ᵗʰ **T17.808** Unspecified foreign body in other parts of respiratory tract causing other injury   CC

√6ᵗʰ **T17.81** Gastric contents in other parts of respiratory tract
Aspiration of gastric contents into other parts of respiratory tract
Vomitus in other parts of respiratory tract
- √7ᵗʰ **T17.810** Gastric contents in other parts of respiratory tract causing asphyxiation   CC
- √7ᵗʰ **T17.818** Gastric contents in other parts of respiratory tract causing other injury   CC

√6ᵗʰ **T17.82** Food in other parts of respiratory tract
Bones in other parts of respiratory tract
Seeds in other parts of respiratory tract
- √7ᵗʰ **T17.820** Food in other parts of respiratory tract causing asphyxiation   CC
- √7ᵗʰ **T17.828** Food in other parts of respiratory tract causing other injury   CC

√6ᵗʰ **T17.89** Other foreign object in other parts of respiratory tract
- √7ᵗʰ **T17.890** Other foreign object in other parts of respiratory tract causing asphyxiation   CC
- √7ᵗʰ **T17.898** Other foreign object in other parts of respiratory tract causing other injury   CC

√5ᵗʰ **T17.9** Foreign body in respiratory tract, part unspecified

√6ᵗʰ **T17.90** Unspecified foreign body in respiratory tract, part unspecified
- √7ᵗʰ **T17.900** Unspecified foreign body in respiratory tract, part unspecified causing asphyxiation   CC
- √7ᵗʰ **T17.908** Unspecified foreign body in respiratory tract, part unspecified causing other injury

√6ᵗʰ **T17.91** Gastric contents in respiratory tract, part unspecified
Aspiration of gastric contents into respiratory tract, part unspecified
Vomitus in trachea respiratory tract, part unspecified
- √7ᵗʰ **T17.910** Gastric contents in respiratory tract, part unspecified causing asphyxiation   CC
- √7ᵗʰ **T17.918** Gastric contents in respiratory tract, part unspecified causing other injury

√6ᵗʰ **T17.92** Food in respiratory tract, part unspecified
Bones in respiratory tract, part unspecified
Seeds in respiratory tract, part unspecified
- √7ᵗʰ **T17.920** Food in respiratory tract, part unspecified causing asphyxiation   CC
- √7ᵗʰ **T17.928** Food in respiratory tract, part unspecified causing other injury

√6ᵗʰ **T17.99** Other foreign object in respiratory tract, part unspecified
- √7ᵗʰ **T17.990** Other foreign object in respiratory tract, part unspecified in causing asphyxiation   CC
- √7ᵗʰ **T17.998** Other foreign object in respiratory tract, part unspecified causing other injury

√4ᵗʰ **T18** Foreign body in alimentary tract

EXCLUDES 2   foreign body in pharynx (T17.2-)

The appropriate 7th character is to be added to each code from category T18.
A   initial encounter
D   subsequent encounter
S   sequela

√x7ᵗʰ **T18.0** Foreign body in mouth

√5ᵗʰ **T18.1** **Foreign body in** esophagus

    EXCLUDES 2   *foreign body in respiratory tract (T17.-)*

√6ᵗʰ **T18.10** **Unspecified foreign body in esophagus**

    √7ᵗʰ **T18.100** **Unspecified foreign body in esophagus causing compression of trachea**

         Unspecified foreign body in esophagus causing obstruction of respiration

    √7ᵗʰ **T18.108** **Unspecified foreign body in esophagus causing other injury**

√6ᵗʰ **T18.11** **Gastric contents in esophagus**

     Vomitus in esophagus

    √7ᵗʰ **T18.110** **Gastric contents in esophagus** causing compression of trachea

         Gastric contents in esophagus causing obstruction of respiration

    √7ᵗʰ **T18.118** **Gastric contents in esophagus** causing other injury

√6ᵗʰ **T18.12** Food in esophagus

     Bones in esophagus
     Seeds in esophagus

    √7ᵗʰ **T18.120** **Food in esophagus** causing compression of trachea

         Food in esophagus causing obstruction of respiration

    √7ᵗʰ **T18.128** **Food in esophagus** causing other injury

√6ᵗʰ **T18.19** **Other foreign object in esophagus**

     AHA: 2015,1Q,23

    √7ᵗʰ **T18.190** **Other foreign object in esophagus** causing compression of trachea   CC

         Other foreign body in esophagus causing obstruction of respiration

         TIP: Any foreign object lodged in the esophagus requires immediate treatment and is considered an injury. Assign this code when there is respiratory compromise or compression.

    √7ᵗʰ **T18.198** **Other foreign object in esophagus causing other injury**

         TIP: Any foreign object lodged in the esophagus requires immediate treatment and is considered an injury. Assign this code when there is no respiratory compromise or compression.

√ₓ7ᵗʰ **T18.2** **Foreign body in** stomach   CC

√ₓ7ᵗʰ **T18.3** **Foreign body in** small intestine

√ₓ7ᵗʰ **T18.4** **Foreign body in** colon

√ₓ7ᵗʰ **T18.5** **Foreign body in** anus and rectum

     Foreign body in rectosigmoid (junction)

√ₓ7ᵗʰ **T18.8** **Foreign body in other parts of alimentary tract**

√ₓ7ᵗʰ **T18.9** **Foreign body of alimentary tract, part unspecified**

     Foreign body in digestive system NOS
     Swallowed foreign body NOS

√4ᵗʰ **T19** **Foreign body in genitourinary tract**

    EXCLUDES 2   *complications due to implanted mesh (T83.7-)*

         mechanical complications of contraceptive device (intrauterine) (vaginal) (T83.3-)

         presence of contraceptive device (intrauterine) (vaginal) (Z97.5)

The appropriate 7th character is to be added to each code from category T19.
A   initial encounter
D   subsequent encounter
S   sequela

√ₓ7ᵗʰ **T19.0** **Foreign body in** urethra

√ₓ7ᵗʰ **T19.1** **Foreign body in** bladder

√ₓ7ᵗʰ **T19.2** **Foreign body in** vulva and vagina   ♀

√ₓ7ᵗʰ **T19.3** **Foreign body in** uterus   ♀

√ₓ7ᵗʰ **T19.4** **Foreign body in** penis   ♂

√ₓ7ᵗʰ **T19.8** **Foreign body in other parts of genitourinary tract**

√ₓ7ᵗʰ **T19.9** **Foreign body in genitourinary tract, part unspecified**

BURNS AND CORROSIONS (T20-T32)

INCLUDES   burns (thermal) from electrical heating appliances
     burns (thermal) from electricity
     burns (thermal) from flame
     burns (thermal) from friction
     burns (thermal) from hot air and hot gases
     burns (thermal) from hot objects
     burns (thermal) from lightning
     burns (thermal) from radiation
     chemical burn [corrosion] (external) (internal)
     scalds

EXCLUDES 2   *erythema [dermatitis] ab igne (L59.0)*
     radiation-related disorders of the skin and subcutaneous tissue (L55-L59)
     sunburn (L55.-)

AHA: 2016,2Q,4

Burns and corrosions of external body surface, specified by site (T20-T25)

INCLUDES   burns and corrosions of first degree [erythema]
     burns and corrosions of second degree [blisters] [epidermal loss]
     burns and corrosions of third degree [deep necrosis of underlying tissue] [full-thickness skin loss]

Use additional code from category T31 or T32 to identify extent of body surface involved

√4ᵗʰ **T20** **Burn and corrosion of head, face, and neck**

    EXCLUDES 2   *burn and corrosion of ear drum (T28.41, T28.91)*

         burn and corrosion of eye and adnexa (T26.-)

         burn and corrosion of mouth and pharynx (T28.0)

     AHA: 2015,1Q,18-19

The appropriate 7th character is to be added to each code from category T20.
A   initial encounter
D   subsequent encounter
S   sequela

√5ᵗʰ **T20.0** **Burn of unspecified degree of head, face, and neck**

     Use additional external cause code to identify the source, place and intent of the burn (X00-X19, X75-X77, X96-X98, Y92)

    √ₓ7ᵗʰ **T20.00** **Burn of unspecified degree of head, face, and neck, unspecified site**

    √6ᵗʰ **T20.01** **Burn of unspecified degree of ear [any part, except ear drum]**

        EXCLUDES 2   *burn of ear drum (T28.41-)*

        √7ᵗʰ **T20.011** **Burn of unspecified degree of** right ear [any part, except ear drum]

        √7ᵗʰ **T20.012** **Burn of unspecified degree of** left ear [any part, except ear drum]

        √7ᵗʰ **T20.019** **Burn of unspecified degree of** unspecified ear [any part, except ear drum]

    √ₓ7ᵗʰ **T20.02** **Burn of unspecified degree of** lip(s)

    √ₓ7ᵗʰ **T20.03** **Burn of unspecified degree of** chin

    √ₓ7ᵗʰ **T20.04** **Burn of unspecified degree of** nose (septum)

    √ₓ7ᵗʰ **T20.05** **Burn of unspecified degree of** scalp [any part]

    √ₓ7ᵗʰ **T20.06** **Burn of unspecified degree of** forehead and cheek

    √ₓ7ᵗʰ **T20.07** **Burn of unspecified degree of** neck

    √ₓ7ᵗʰ **T20.09** **Burn of unspecified degree of** multiple sites of head, face, and neck

√5ᵗʰ **T20.1** **Burn of** first degree **of head, face, and neck**

     Use additional external cause code to identify the source, place and intent of the burn (X00-X19, X75-X77, X96-X98, Y92)

    √ₓ7ᵗʰ **T20.10** **Burn of first degree of head, face, and neck, unspecified site**

    √6ᵗʰ **T20.11** **Burn of first degree of** ear [any part, except ear drum]

        EXCLUDES 2   *burn of ear drum (T28.41-)*

        √7ᵗʰ **T20.111** **Burn of first degree of** right ear [any part, except ear drum]

        √7ᵗʰ **T20.112** **Burn of first degree of** left ear [any part, except ear drum]

        √7ᵗʰ **T20.119** **Burn of first degree of** unspecified ear [any part, except ear drum]

    √ₓ7ᵗʰ **T20.12** **Burn of first degree of** lip(s)

    √ₓ7ᵗʰ **T20.13** **Burn of first degree of** chin

    √ₓ7ᵗʰ **T20.14** **Burn of first degree of** nose (septum)

    √ₓ7ᵗʰ **T20.15** **Burn of first degree of** scalp [any part]

    √ₓ7ᵗʰ **T20.16** **Burn of first degree of** forehead and cheek

√x7ᵗʰ **T20.17** Burn of first degree of neck

√x7ᵗʰ **T20.19** Burn of first degree of multiple sites of head, face, and neck

Degree of Burns

Epidermis
Dermis
Subcutaneous

Normal   First Degree Burn

Epidermis
Dermis
Subcutaneous

Second Degree Burn   Third Degree Burn

√5ᵗʰ **T20.2** Burn of second degree of head, face, and neck

Use additional external cause code to identify the source, place and intent of the burn (X00-X19, X75-X77, X96-X98, Y92)

√x7ᵗʰ **T20.20** Burn of second degree of head, face, and neck, unspecified site

√6ᵗʰ **T20.21** Burn of second degree of ear [any part, except ear drum]

EXCLUDES 2   burn of ear drum (T28.41-)

√7ᵗʰ **T20.211** Burn of second degree of right ear [any part, except ear drum]

√7ᵗʰ **T20.212** Burn of second degree of left ear [any part, except ear drum]

√7ᵗʰ **T20.219** Burn of second degree of unspecified ear [any part, except ear drum]

√x7ᵗʰ **T20.22** Burn of second degree of lip(s)

√x7ᵗʰ **T20.23** Burn of second degree of chin

√x7ᵗʰ **T20.24** Burn of second degree of nose (septum)

√x7ᵗʰ **T20.25** Burn of second degree of scalp [any part]

√x7ᵗʰ **T20.26** Burn of second degree of forehead and cheek

√x7ᵗʰ **T20.27** Burn of second degree of neck

√x7ᵗʰ **T20.29** Burn of second degree of multiple sites of head, face, and neck

√5ᵗʰ **T20.3** Burn of third degree of head, face, and neck

Use additional external cause code to identify the source, place and intent of the burn (X00-X19, X75-X77, X96-X98, Y92)

√x7ᵗʰ **T20.30** Burn of third degree of head, face, and neck, unspecified site   CC H5 SW

CC Excl: PDX collection 1375

√6ᵗʰ **T20.31** Burn of third degree of ear [any part, except ear drum]

EXCLUDES 2   burn of ear drum (T28.41-)

AHA: 2015,1Q,18

CC Excl: For CC codes in subcategory T20.31: PDX collection 1376

√7ᵗʰ **T20.311** Burn of third degree of right ear [any part, except ear drum]   CC H5 SW

√7ᵗʰ **T20.312** Burn of third degree of left ear [any part, except ear drum]   CC H5 SW

√7ᵗʰ **T20.319** Burn of third degree of unspecified ear [any part, except ear drum]   CC H5 SW

√x7ᵗʰ **T20.32** Burn of third degree of lip(s)   CC H5 SW

CC Excl: PDX collection 1377

√x7ᵗʰ **T20.33** Burn of third degree of chin   CC H5 SW

CC Excl: PDX collection 1378

√x7ᵗʰ **T20.34** Burn of third degree of nose (septum)   CC H5 SW

CC Excl: PDX collection 1379

√x7ᵗʰ **T20.35** Burn of third degree of scalp [any part]   CC H5 SW

CC Excl: PDX collection 1380

√x7ᵗʰ **T20.36** Burn of third degree of forehead and cheek   CC H5 SW

CC Excl: PDX collection 1381

√x7ᵗʰ **T20.37** Burn of third degree of neck   CC H5 SW

CC Excl: PDX collection 1382

√x7ᵗʰ **T20.39** Burn of third degree of multiple sites of head, face, and neck   CC H5 SW

CC Excl: PDX collection 1383

√5ᵗʰ **T20.4** Corrosion of unspecified degree of head, face, and neck

Code first (T51-T65) to identify chemical and intent
Use additional external cause code to identify place (Y92)

√x7ᵗʰ **T20.40** Corrosion of unspecified degree of head, face, and neck, unspecified site

√6ᵗʰ **T20.41** Corrosion of unspecified degree of ear [any part, except ear drum]

EXCLUDES 2   corrosion of ear drum (T28.91-)

√7ᵗʰ **T20.411** Corrosion of unspecified degree of right ear [any part, except ear drum]

√7ᵗʰ **T20.412** Corrosion of unspecified degree of left ear [any part, except ear drum]

√7ᵗʰ **T20.419** Corrosion of unspecified degree of unspecified ear [any part, except ear drum]

√x7ᵗʰ **T20.42** Corrosion of unspecified degree of lip(s)

√x7ᵗʰ **T20.43** Corrosion of unspecified degree of chin

√x7ᵗʰ **T20.44** Corrosion of unspecified degree of nose (septum)

√x7ᵗʰ **T20.45** Corrosion of unspecified degree of scalp [any part]

√x7ᵗʰ **T20.46** Corrosion of unspecified degree of forehead and cheek

√x7ᵗʰ **T20.47** Corrosion of unspecified degree of neck

√x7ᵗʰ **T20.49** Corrosion of unspecified degree of multiple sites of head, face, and neck

√5ᵗʰ **T20.5** Corrosion of first degree of head, face, and neck

Code first (T51-T65) to identify chemical and intent
Use additional external cause code to identify place (Y92)

√x7ᵗʰ **T20.50** Corrosion of first degree of head, face, and neck, unspecified site

√6ᵗʰ **T20.51** Corrosion of first degree of ear [any part, except ear drum]

EXCLUDES 2   corrosion of ear drum (T28.91-)

√7ᵗʰ **T20.511** Corrosion of first degree of right ear [any part, except ear drum]

√7ᵗʰ **T20.512** Corrosion of first degree of left ear [any part, except ear drum]

√7ᵗʰ **T20.519** Corrosion of first degree of unspecified ear [any part, except ear drum]

√x7ᵗʰ **T20.52** Corrosion of first degree of lip(s)

√x7ᵗʰ **T20.53** Corrosion of first degree of chin

√x7ᵗʰ **T20.54** Corrosion of first degree of nose (septum)

√x7ᵗʰ **T20.55** Corrosion of first degree of scalp [any part]

√x7ᵗʰ **T20.56** Corrosion of first degree of forehead and cheek

√x7ᵗʰ **T20.57** Corrosion of first degree of neck

√x7ᵗʰ **T20.59** Corrosion of first degree of multiple sites of head, face, and neck

√5ᵗʰ **T20.6** Corrosion of second degree of head, face, and neck

Code first (T51-T65) to identify chemical and intent
Use additional external cause code to identify place (Y92)

√x7ᵗʰ **T20.60** Corrosion of second degree of head, face, and neck, unspecified site

√6ᵗʰ **T20.61** Corrosion of second degree of ear [any part, except ear drum]

EXCLUDES 2   corrosion of ear drum (T28.91-)

√7ᵗʰ **T20.611** Corrosion of second degree of right ear [any part, except ear drum]

√7ᵗʰ **T20.612** Corrosion of second degree of left ear [any part, except ear drum]

√7ᵗʰ **T20.619** Corrosion of second degree of unspecified ear [any part, except ear drum]

√x7ᵗʰ **T20.62** Corrosion of second degree of lip(s)

√x7ᵗʰ **T20.63** Corrosion of second degree of chin

√x7ᵗʰ **T20.64** Corrosion of second degree of nose (septum)

N Newborn: 0   P Pediatric: 0-17   M Maternity: 9-64   A Adult: 15-124   MCC Major Complication/Comorbidity   CC Complication/Comorbidity   SW Severe Wound Dx

1130   ICD-10-CM 2020

√x 7ᵗʰ **T20.65** Corrosion of second degree of scalp [any part]

√x 7ᵗʰ **T20.66** Corrosion of second degree of forehead and cheek

√x 7ᵗʰ **T20.67** Corrosion of second degree of neck

√x 7ᵗʰ **T20.69** Corrosion of second degree of multiple sites of head, face, and neck

√ 5ᵗʰ **T20.7** Corrosion of third degree of head, face, and neck

Code first (T51-T65) to identify chemical and intent

Use additional external cause code to identify place (Y92)

√x 7ᵗʰ **T20.70** Corrosion of third degree of head, face, and neck, unspecified site `CC` `H5` `SW`

CC Excl: PDX collection 1375

√ 6ᵗʰ **T20.71** Corrosion of third degree of ear [any part, except ear drum]

EXCLUDES 2 *corrosion of ear drum (T28.91-)*

CC Excl: For CC codes in subcategory T20.71: PDX collection 1376

√ 7ᵗʰ **T20.711** Corrosion of third degree of right ear [any part, except ear drum] `CC` `H5` `SW`

√ 7ᵗʰ **T20.712** Corrosion of third degree of left ear [any part, except ear drum] `CC` `H5` `SW`

√ 7ᵗʰ **T20.719** Corrosion of third degree of unspecified ear [any part, except ear drum] `CC` `H5` `SW`

√x 7ᵗʰ **T20.72** Corrosion of third degree of lip(s) `CC` `H5` `SW`

CC Excl: PDX collection 1377

√x 7ᵗʰ **T20.73** Corrosion of third degree of chin `CC` `H5` `SW`

CC Excl: PDX collection 1378

√x 7ᵗʰ **T20.74** Corrosion of third degree of nose (septum) `CC` `H5` `SW`

CC Excl: PDX collection 1379

√x 7ᵗʰ **T20.75** Corrosion of third degree of scalp [any part] `CC` `H5` `SW`

CC Excl: PDX collection 1380

√x 7ᵗʰ **T20.76** Corrosion of third degree of forehead and cheek `CC` `H5` `SW`

CC Excl: PDX collection 1381

√x 7ᵗʰ **T20.77** Corrosion of third degree of neck `CC` `H5` `SW`

CC Excl: PDX collection 1382

√x 7ᵗʰ **T20.79** Corrosion of third degree of multiple sites of head, face, and neck `CC` `H5` `SW`

CC Excl: PDX collection 1383

√ 4ᵗʰ **T21** Burn and corrosion of trunk

INCLUDES burns and corrosion of hip region

EXCLUDES 2 *burns and corrosion of axilla (T22.- with fifth character 4)*

burns and corrosion of scapular region (T22.- with fifth character 6)

burns and corrosion of shoulder (T22.- with fifth character 5)

The appropriate 7th character is to be added to each code from category T21.

A initial encounter
D subsequent encounter
S sequela

√ 5ᵗʰ **T21.0** Burn of unspecified degree of trunk

Use additional external cause code to identify the source, place and intent of the burn (X00-X19, X75-X77, X96-X98, Y92)

√x 7ᵗʰ **T21.00** Burn of unspecified degree of trunk, unspecified site

√x 7ᵗʰ **T21.01** Burn of unspecified degree of chest wall

Burn of unspecified degree of breast

√x 7ᵗʰ **T21.02** Burn of unspecified degree of abdominal wall

Burn of unspecified degree of flank
Burn of unspecified degree of groin

√x 7ᵗʰ **T21.03** Burn of unspecified degree of upper back

Burn of unspecified degree of interscapular region

√x 7ᵗʰ **T21.04** Burn of unspecified degree of lower back

√x 7ᵗʰ **T21.05** Burn of unspecified degree of buttock

Burn of unspecified degree of anus

√x 7ᵗʰ **T21.06** Burn of unspecified degree of male genital region ♂

Burn of unspecified degree of penis
Burn of unspecified degree of scrotum
Burn of unspecified degree of testis

√x 7ᵗʰ **T21.07** Burn of unspecified degree of female genital region ♀

Burn of unspecified degree of labium (majus) (minus)
Burn of unspecified degree of perineum
Burn of unspecified degree of vulva

EXCLUDES 2 *burn of vagina (T28.3)*

√x 7ᵗʰ **T21.09** Burn of unspecified degree of other site of trunk

√ 5ᵗʰ **T21.1** Burn of first degree of trunk

Use additional external cause code to identify the source, place and intent of the burn (X00-X19, X75-X77, X96-X98, Y92)

√x 7ᵗʰ **T21.10** Burn of first degree of trunk, unspecified site

√x 7ᵗʰ **T21.11** Burn of first degree of chest wall

Burn of first degree of breast

√x 7ᵗʰ **T21.12** Burn of first degree of abdominal wall

Burn of first degree of flank
Burn of first degree of groin

√x 7ᵗʰ **T21.13** Burn of first degree of upper back

Burn of first degree of interscapular region

√x 7ᵗʰ **T21.14** Burn of first degree of lower back

√x 7ᵗʰ **T21.15** Burn of first degree of buttock

Burn of first degree of anus

√x 7ᵗʰ **T21.16** Burn of first degree of male genital region ♂

Burn of first degree of penis
Burn of first degree of scrotum
Burn of first degree of testis

√x 7ᵗʰ **T21.17** Burn of first degree of female genital region ♀

Burn of first degree of labium (majus) (minus)
Burn of first degree of perineum
Burn of first degree of vulva

EXCLUDES 2 *burn of vagina (T28.3)*

√x 7ᵗʰ **T21.19** Burn of first degree of other site of trunk

√ 5ᵗʰ **T21.2** Burn of second degree of trunk

Use additional external cause code to identify the source, place and intent of the burn (X00-X19, X75-X77, X96-X98, Y92)

√x 7ᵗʰ **T21.20** Burn of second degree of trunk, unspecified site

√x 7ᵗʰ **T21.21** Burn of second degree of chest wall

Burn of second degree of breast

√x 7ᵗʰ **T21.22** Burn of second degree of abdominal wall

Burn of second degree of flank
Burn of second degree of groin

√x 7ᵗʰ **T21.23** Burn of second degree of upper back

Burn of second degree of interscapular region

√x 7ᵗʰ **T21.24** Burn of second degree of lower back

√x 7ᵗʰ **T21.25** Burn of second degree of buttock

Burn of second degree of anus

√x 7ᵗʰ **T21.26** Burn of second degree of male genital region ♂

Burn of second degree of penis
Burn of second degree of scrotum
Burn of second degree of testis

√x 7ᵗʰ **T21.27** Burn of second degree of female genital region ♀

Burn of second degree of labium (majus) (minus)
Burn of second degree of perineum
Burn of second degree of vulva

EXCLUDES 2 *burn of vagina (T28.3)*

√x 7ᵗʰ **T21.29** Burn of second degree of other site of trunk

√ 5ᵗʰ **T21.3** Burn of third degree of trunk

Use additional external cause code to identify the source, place and intent of the burn (X00-X19, X75-X77, X96-X98, Y92)

√x 7ᵗʰ **T21.30** Burn of third degree of trunk, unspecified site `CC` `H5` `SW`

CC Excl: PDX collection 1384

√x 7ᵗʰ **T21.31** Burn of third degree of chest wall `CC` `H5` `SW`

Burn of third degree of breast

AHA: 2016,2Q,5

CC Excl: PDX collection 1385

√x 7ᵗʰ **T21.32** Burn of third degree of abdominal wall `CC` `H5` `SW`

Burn of third degree of flank
Burn of third degree of groin

CC Excl: PDX collection 1386

✔ Additional Character Required √x 7ᵗʰ Placeholder Unacceptable PDx Questionable PDx Manifestation Unspecified Dx H1-H14 HAC HCC CMS-HCC Dx HIV HIV Dx

ICD-10-CM 2020   1131

√x7th **T21.33** **Burn of third degree of upper back** CC H5 SW

Burn of third degree of interscapular region
CC Excl: PDX collection 1387

√x7th **T21.34** **Burn of third degree of lower back** CC H5 SW

CC Excl: PDX collection 1387

√x7th **T21.35** **Burn of third degree of buttock** CC H5 SW

Burn of third degree of anus
CC Excl: PDX collection 1387

√x7th **T21.36** **Burn of third degree of male genital region** CC H5 SW ♂

Burn of third degree of penis
Burn of third degree of scrotum
Burn of third degree of testis
CC Excl: PDX collection 1388

√x7th **T21.37** **Burn of third degree of female genital region** CC H5 SW ♀

Burn of third degree of labium (majus) (minus)
Burn of third degree of perineum
Burn of third degree of vulva
EXCLUDES 2 *burn of vagina (T28.3)*
CC Excl: PDX collection 1388

√x7th **T21.39** **Burn of third degree of other site of trunk** CC H5 SW

CC Excl: PDX collection 1384

√5th **T21.4** **Corrosion of unspecified degree of trunk**

Code first (T51-T65) to identify chemical and intent
Use additional external cause code to identify place (Y92)

√x7th **T21.40** **Corrosion of unspecified degree of trunk, unspecified site**

√x7th **T21.41** **Corrosion of unspecified degree of chest wall**

Corrosion of unspecified degree of breast

√x7th **T21.42** **Corrosion of unspecified degree of abdominal wall**

Corrosion of unspecified degree of flank
Corrosion of unspecified degree of groin

√x7th **T21.43** **Corrosion of unspecified degree of upper back**

Corrosion of unspecified degree of interscapular region

√x7th **T21.44** **Corrosion of unspecified degree of lower back**

√x7th **T21.45** **Corrosion of unspecified degree of buttock**

Corrosion of unspecified degree of anus

√x7th **T21.46** **Corrosion of unspecified degree of male genital region** ♂

Corrosion of unspecified degree of penis
Corrosion of unspecified degree of scrotum
Corrosion of unspecified degree of testis

√x7th **T21.47** **Corrosion of unspecified degree of female genital region** ♀

Corrosion of unspecified degree of labium (majus) (minus)
Corrosion of unspecified degree of perineum
Corrosion of unspecified degree of vulva
EXCLUDES 2 *corrosion of vagina (T28.8)*

√x7th **T21.49** **Corrosion of unspecified degree of other site of trunk**

√5th **T21.5** **Corrosion of first degree of trunk**

Code first (T51-T65) to identify chemical and intent
Use additional external cause code to identify place (Y92)

√x7th **T21.50** **Corrosion of first degree of trunk, unspecified site**

√x7th **T21.51** **Corrosion of first degree of chest wall**

Corrosion of first degree of breast

√x7th **T21.52** **Corrosion of first degree of abdominal wall**

Corrosion of first degree of flank
Corrosion of first degree of groin

√x7th **T21.53** **Corrosion of first degree of upper back**

Corrosion of first degree of interscapular region

√x7th **T21.54** **Corrosion of first degree of lower back**

√x7th **T21.55** **Corrosion of first degree of buttock**

Corrosion of first degree of anus

√x7th **T21.56** **Corrosion of first degree of male genital region** ♂

Corrosion of first degree of penis
Corrosion of first degree of scrotum
Corrosion of first degree of testis

√x7th **T21.57** **Corrosion of first degree of female genital region** ♀

Corrosion of first degree of labium (majus) (minus)
Corrosion of first degree of perineum
Corrosion of first degree of vulva
EXCLUDES 2 *corrosion of vagina (T28.8)*

√x7th **T21.59** **Corrosion of first degree of other site of trunk**

√5th **T21.6** **Corrosion of second degree of trunk**

Code first (T51-T65) to identify chemical and intent
Use additional external cause code to identify place (Y92)

√x7th **T21.60** **Corrosion of second degree of trunk, unspecified site**

√x7th **T21.61** **Corrosion of second degree of chest wall**

Corrosion of second degree of breast

√x7th **T21.62** **Corrosion of second degree of abdominal wall**

Corrosion of second degree of flank
Corrosion of second degree of groin

√x7th **T21.63** **Corrosion of second degree of upper back**

Corrosion of second degree of interscapular region

√x7th **T21.64** **Corrosion of second degree of lower back**

√x7th **T21.65** **Corrosion of second degree of buttock**

Corrosion of second degree of anus

√x7th **T21.66** **Corrosion of second degree of male genital region** ♂

Corrosion of second degree of penis
Corrosion of second degree of scrotum
Corrosion of second degree of testis

√x7th **T21.67** **Corrosion of second degree of female genital region** ♀

Corrosion of second degree of labium (majus) (minus)
Corrosion of second degree of perineum
Corrosion of second degree of vulva
EXCLUDES 2 *corrosion of vagina (T28.8)*

√x7th **T21.69** **Corrosion of second degree of other site of trunk**

√5th **T21.7** **Corrosion of third degree of trunk**

Code first (T51-T65) to identify chemical and intent
Use additional external cause code to identify place (Y92)

√x7th **T21.70** **Corrosion of third degree of trunk, unspecified site** CC H5 SW

CC Excl: PDX collection 1384

√x7th **T21.71** **Corrosion of third degree of chest wall** CC H5 SW

Corrosion of third degree of breast
CC Excl: PDX collection 1385

√x7th **T21.72** **Corrosion of third degree of abdominal wall** CC H5 SW

Corrosion of third degree of flank
Corrosion of third degree of groin
CC Excl: PDX collection 1386

√x7th **T21.73** **Corrosion of third degree of upper back** CC H5 SW

Corrosion of third degree of interscapular region
CC Excl: PDX collection 1387

√x7th **T21.74** **Corrosion of third degree of lower back** CC H5 SW

CC Excl: PDX collection 1387

√x7th **T21.75** **Corrosion of third degree of buttock** CC H5 SW

Corrosion of third degree of anus
CC Excl: PDX collection 1387

√x7th **T21.76** **Corrosion of third degree of male genital region** CC H5 SW ♂

Corrosion of third degree of penis
Corrosion of third degree of scrotum
Corrosion of third degree of testis
CC Excl: PDX collection 1388

√x7th **T21.77** **Corrosion of third degree of female genital region** CC H5 SW ♀

Corrosion of third degree of labium (majus) (minus)
Corrosion of third degree of perineum
Corrosion of third degree of vulva
EXCLUDES 2 *corrosion of vagina (T28.8)*
CC Excl: PDX collection 1388

√x7th **T21.79** **Corrosion of third degree of other site of trunk** CC H5 SW

CC Excl: PDX collection 1384

☑4ᵗʰ **T22 Burn and corrosion of shoulder and upper limb, except wrist and hand**

> EXCLUDES 2   *burn and corrosion of interscapular region (T21.-)*
> *burn and corrosion of wrist and hand (T23.-)*

> The appropriate 7th character is to be added to each code from category T22.
> A   initial encounter
> D   subsequent encounter
> S   sequela

☑5ᵗʰ **T22.0 Burn of unspecified degree of shoulder and upper limb, except wrist and hand**

> Use additional external cause code to identify the source, place and intent of the burn (X00-X19, X75-X77, X96-X98, Y92)

   ☑x7ᵗʰ **T22.00** Burn of unspecified degree of shoulder and upper limb, except wrist and hand, unspecified site

   ☑6ᵗʰ **T22.01** Burn of unspecified degree of forearm
      ☑7ᵗʰ **T22.011** Burn of unspecified degree of right forearm
      ☑7ᵗʰ **T22.012** Burn of unspecified degree of left forearm
      ☑7ᵗʰ **T22.019** Burn of unspecified degree of unspecified forearm

   ☑6ᵗʰ **T22.02** Burn of unspecified degree of elbow
      ☑7ᵗʰ **T22.021** Burn of unspecified degree of right elbow
      ☑7ᵗʰ **T22.022** Burn of unspecified degree of left elbow
      ☑7ᵗʰ **T22.029** Burn of unspecified degree of unspecified elbow

   ☑6ᵗʰ **T22.03** Burn of unspecified degree of upper arm
      ☑7ᵗʰ **T22.031** Burn of unspecified degree of right upper arm
      ☑7ᵗʰ **T22.032** Burn of unspecified degree of left upper arm
      ☑7ᵗʰ **T22.039** Burn of unspecified degree of unspecified upper arm

   ☑6ᵗʰ **T22.04** Burn of unspecified degree of axilla
      ☑7ᵗʰ **T22.041** Burn of unspecified degree of right axilla
      ☑7ᵗʰ **T22.042** Burn of unspecified degree of left axilla
      ☑7ᵗʰ **T22.049** Burn of unspecified degree of unspecified axilla

   ☑6ᵗʰ **T22.05** Burn of unspecified degree of shoulder
      ☑7ᵗʰ **T22.051** Burn of unspecified degree of right shoulder
      ☑7ᵗʰ **T22.052** Burn of unspecified degree of left shoulder
      ☑7ᵗʰ **T22.059** Burn of unspecified degree of unspecified shoulder

   ☑6ᵗʰ **T22.06** Burn of unspecified degree of scapular region
      ☑7ᵗʰ **T22.061** Burn of unspecified degree of right scapular region
      ☑7ᵗʰ **T22.062** Burn of unspecified degree of left scapular region
      ☑7ᵗʰ **T22.069** Burn of unspecified degree of unspecified scapular region

   ☑6ᵗʰ **T22.09** Burn of unspecified degree of multiple sites of shoulder and upper limb, except wrist and hand
      ☑7ᵗʰ **T22.091** Burn of unspecified degree of multiple sites of right shoulder and upper limb, except wrist and hand
      ☑7ᵗʰ **T22.092** Burn of unspecified degree of multiple sites of left shoulder and upper limb, except wrist and hand
      ☑7ᵗʰ **T22.099** Burn of unspecified degree of multiple sites of unspecified shoulder and upper limb, except wrist and hand

☑5ᵗʰ **T22.1 Burn of first degree of shoulder and upper limb, except wrist and hand**

> Use additional external cause code to identify the source, place and intent of the burn (X00-X19, X75-X77, X96-X98, Y92)

   ☑x7ᵗʰ **T22.10** Burn of first degree of shoulder and upper limb, except wrist and hand, unspecified site

   ☑6ᵗʰ **T22.11** Burn of first degree of forearm
      ☑7ᵗʰ **T22.111** Burn of first degree of right forearm
      ☑7ᵗʰ **T22.112** Burn of first degree of left forearm
      ☑7ᵗʰ **T22.119** Burn of first degree of unspecified forearm

   ☑6ᵗʰ **T22.12** Burn of first degree of elbow
      ☑7ᵗʰ **T22.121** Burn of first degree of right elbow
      ☑7ᵗʰ **T22.122** Burn of first degree of left elbow
      ☑7ᵗʰ **T22.129** Burn of first degree of unspecified elbow

   ☑6ᵗʰ **T22.13** Burn of first degree of upper arm
      ☑7ᵗʰ **T22.131** Burn of first degree of right upper arm
      ☑7ᵗʰ **T22.132** Burn of first degree of left upper arm
      ☑7ᵗʰ **T22.139** Burn of first degree of unspecified upper arm

   ☑6ᵗʰ **T22.14** Burn of first degree of axilla
      ☑7ᵗʰ **T22.141** Burn of first degree of right axilla
      ☑7ᵗʰ **T22.142** Burn of first degree of left axilla
      ☑7ᵗʰ **T22.149** Burn of first degree of unspecified axilla

   ☑6ᵗʰ **T22.15** Burn of first degree of shoulder
      ☑7ᵗʰ **T22.151** Burn of first degree of right shoulder
      ☑7ᵗʰ **T22.152** Burn of first degree of left shoulder
      ☑7ᵗʰ **T22.159** Burn of first degree of unspecified shoulder

   ☑6ᵗʰ **T22.16** Burn of first degree of scapular region
      ☑7ᵗʰ **T22.161** Burn of first degree of right scapular region
      ☑7ᵗʰ **T22.162** Burn of first degree of left scapular region
      ☑7ᵗʰ **T22.169** Burn of first degree of unspecified scapular region

   ☑6ᵗʰ **T22.19** Burn of first degree of multiple sites of shoulder and upper limb, except wrist and hand
      ☑7ᵗʰ **T22.191** Burn of first degree of multiple sites of right shoulder and upper limb, except wrist and hand
      ☑7ᵗʰ **T22.192** Burn of first degree of multiple sites of left shoulder and upper limb, except wrist and hand
      ☑7ᵗʰ **T22.199** Burn of first degree of multiple sites of unspecified shoulder and upper limb, except wrist and hand

☑5ᵗʰ **T22.2 Burn of second degree of shoulder and upper limb, except wrist and hand**

> Use additional external cause code to identify the source, place and intent of the burn (X00-X19, X75-X77, X96-X98, Y92)

   ☑x7ᵗʰ **T22.20** Burn of second degree of shoulder and upper limb, except wrist and hand, unspecified site

   ☑6ᵗʰ **T22.21** Burn of second degree of forearm
      ☑7ᵗʰ **T22.211** Burn of second degree of right forearm
      ☑7ᵗʰ **T22.212** Burn of second degree of left forearm
      ☑7ᵗʰ **T22.219** Burn of second degree of unspecified forearm

   ☑6ᵗʰ **T22.22** Burn of second degree of elbow
      ☑7ᵗʰ **T22.221** Burn of second degree of right elbow
      ☑7ᵗʰ **T22.222** Burn of second degree of left elbow
      ☑7ᵗʰ **T22.229** Burn of second degree of unspecified elbow

   ☑6ᵗʰ **T22.23** Burn of second degree of upper arm
      ☑7ᵗʰ **T22.231** Burn of second degree of right upper arm
      ☑7ᵗʰ **T22.232** Burn of second degree of left upper arm
      ☑7ᵗʰ **T22.239** Burn of second degree of unspecified upper arm

   ☑6ᵗʰ **T22.24** Burn of second degree of axilla
      ☑7ᵗʰ **T22.241** Burn of second degree of right axilla
      ☑7ᵗʰ **T22.242** Burn of second degree of left axilla
      ☑7ᵗʰ **T22.249** Burn of second degree of unspecified axilla

   ☑6ᵗʰ **T22.25** Burn of second degree of shoulder
      ☑7ᵗʰ **T22.251** Burn of second degree of right shoulder
      ☑7ᵗʰ **T22.252** Burn of second degree of left shoulder
      ☑7ᵗʰ **T22.259** Burn of second degree of unspecified shoulder

   ☑6ᵗʰ **T22.26** Burn of second degree of scapular region
      ☑7ᵗʰ **T22.261** Burn of second degree of right scapular region
      ☑7ᵗʰ **T22.262** Burn of second degree of left scapular region
      ☑7ᵗʰ **T22.269** Burn of second degree of unspecified scapular region

   ☑6ᵗʰ **T22.29** Burn of second degree of multiple sites of shoulder and upper limb, except wrist and hand
      ☑7ᵗʰ **T22.291** Burn of second degree of multiple sites of right shoulder and upper limb, except wrist and hand

☑ Additional Character Required   ☑x7ᵗʰ Placeholder   Unacceptable PDx   Questionable PDx   Manifestation   Unspecified Dx   H1-H14 HAC   HCC CMS-HCC Dx   HIV HIV Dx

ICD-10-CM 2020   1133

√7ᵗʰ **T22.292** Burn of second degree of multiple sites of left shoulder and upper limb, except wrist and hand

√7ᵗʰ **T22.299** Burn of second degree of multiple sites of unspecified shoulder and upper limb, except wrist and hand

√5ᵗʰ **T22.3** Burn of third degree of shoulder and upper limb, except wrist and hand

Use additional external cause code to identify the source, place and intent of the burn (X00-X19, X75-X77, X96-X98, Y92)

√x7ᵗʰ **T22.30** Burn of third degree of shoulder and upper limb, except wrist and hand, unspecified site   CC H5 SW

CC Excl: PDX collection 1389

√6ᵗʰ **T22.31** Burn of third degree of forearm

CC Excl: For CC codes in subcategory T22.31: PDX collection 1390

√7ᵗʰ **T22.311** Burn of third degree of right forearm   CC H5 SW

√7ᵗʰ **T22.312** Burn of third degree of left forearm   CC H5 SW

√7ᵗʰ **T22.319** Burn of third degree of unspecified forearm   CC H5 SW

√6ᵗʰ **T22.32** Burn of third degree of elbow

CC Excl: For CC codes in subcategory T22.32: PDX collection 1391

√7ᵗʰ **T22.321** Burn of third degree of right elbow   CC H5 SW

√7ᵗʰ **T22.322** Burn of third degree of left elbow   CC H5 SW

√7ᵗʰ **T22.329** Burn of third degree of unspecified elbow   CC H5 SW

√6ᵗʰ **T22.33** Burn of third degree of upper arm

CC Excl: For CC codes in subcategory T22.32: PDX collection 1392

√7ᵗʰ **T22.331** Burn of third degree of right upper arm   CC H5 SW

√7ᵗʰ **T22.332** Burn of third degree of left upper arm   CC H5 SW

√7ᵗʰ **T22.339** Burn of third degree of unspecified upper arm   CC H5 SW

√6ᵗʰ **T22.34** Burn of third degree of axilla

CC Excl: For CC codes in subcategory T22.34: PDX collection 1393

√7ᵗʰ **T22.341** Burn of third degree of right axilla   CC H5 SW

√7ᵗʰ **T22.342** Burn of third degree of left axilla   CC H5 SW

√7ᵗʰ **T22.349** Burn of third degree of unspecified axilla   CC H5 SW

√6ᵗʰ **T22.35** Burn of third degree of shoulder

CC Excl: For CC codes in subcategory T22.35: PDX collection 1394

√7ᵗʰ **T22.351** Burn of third degree of right shoulder   CC H5 SW

√7ᵗʰ **T22.352** Burn of third degree of left shoulder   CC H5 SW

√7ᵗʰ **T22.359** Burn of third degree of unspecified shoulder   CC H5 SW

√6ᵗʰ **T22.36** Burn of third degree of scapular region

CC Excl: For CC codes in subcategory T22.36: PDX collection 1395

√7ᵗʰ **T22.361** Burn of third degree of right scapular region   CC H5 SW

√7ᵗʰ **T22.362** Burn of third degree of left scapular region   CC H5 SW

√7ᵗʰ **T22.369** Burn of third degree of unspecified scapular region   CC H5 SW

√6ᵗʰ **T22.39** Burn of third degree of multiple sites of shoulder and upper limb, except wrist and hand

CC Excl: For CC codes in subcategory T22.39: PDX collection 1389

√7ᵗʰ **T22.391** Burn of third degree of multiple sites of right shoulder and upper limb, except wrist and hand   CC H5 SW

√7ᵗʰ **T22.392** Burn of third degree of multiple sites of left shoulder and upper limb, except wrist and hand   CC H5 SW

√7ᵗʰ **T22.399** Burn of third degree of multiple sites of unspecified shoulder and upper limb, except wrist and hand   CC H5 SW

√5ᵗʰ **T22.4** Corrosion of unspecified degree of shoulder and upper limb, except wrist and hand

Code first (T51-T65) to identify chemical and intent

Use additional external cause code to identify place (Y92)

√x7ᵗʰ **T22.40** Corrosion of unspecified degree of shoulder and upper limb, except wrist and hand, unspecified site

√6ᵗʰ **T22.41** Corrosion of unspecified degree of forearm

√7ᵗʰ **T22.411** Corrosion of unspecified degree of right forearm

√7ᵗʰ **T22.412** Corrosion of unspecified degree of left forearm

√7ᵗʰ **T22.419** Corrosion of unspecified degree of unspecified forearm

√6ᵗʰ **T22.42** Corrosion of unspecified degree of elbow

√7ᵗʰ **T22.421** Corrosion of unspecified degree of right elbow

√7ᵗʰ **T22.422** Corrosion of unspecified degree of left elbow

√7ᵗʰ **T22.429** Corrosion of unspecified degree of unspecified elbow

√6ᵗʰ **T22.43** Corrosion of unspecified degree of upper arm

√7ᵗʰ **T22.431** Corrosion of unspecified degree of right upper arm

√7ᵗʰ **T22.432** Corrosion of unspecified degree of left upper arm

√7ᵗʰ **T22.439** Corrosion of unspecified degree of unspecified upper arm

√6ᵗʰ **T22.44** Corrosion of unspecified degree of axilla

√7ᵗʰ **T22.441** Corrosion of unspecified degree of right axilla

√7ᵗʰ **T22.442** Corrosion of unspecified degree of left axilla

√7ᵗʰ **T22.449** Corrosion of unspecified degree of unspecified axilla

√6ᵗʰ **T22.45** Corrosion of unspecified degree of shoulder

√7ᵗʰ **T22.451** Corrosion of unspecified degree of right shoulder

√7ᵗʰ **T22.452** Corrosion of unspecified degree of left shoulder

√7ᵗʰ **T22.459** Corrosion of unspecified degree of unspecified shoulder

√6ᵗʰ **T22.46** Corrosion of unspecified degree of scapular region

√7ᵗʰ **T22.461** Corrosion of unspecified degree of right scapular region

√7ᵗʰ **T22.462** Corrosion of unspecified degree of left scapular region

√7ᵗʰ **T22.469** Corrosion of unspecified degree of unspecified scapular region

√6ᵗʰ **T22.49** Corrosion of unspecified degree of multiple sites of shoulder and upper limb, except wrist and hand

√7ᵗʰ **T22.491** Corrosion of unspecified degree of multiple sites of right shoulder and upper limb, except wrist and hand

√7ᵗʰ **T22.492** Corrosion of unspecified degree of multiple sites of left shoulder and upper limb, except wrist and hand

√7ᵗʰ **T22.499** Corrosion of unspecified degree of multiple sites of unspecified shoulder and upper limb, except wrist and hand

√5ᵗʰ **T22.5** Corrosion of first degree of shoulder and upper limb, except wrist and hand

Code first (T51-T65) to identify chemical and intent

Use additional external cause code to identify place (Y92)

√x7ᵗʰ **T22.50** Corrosion of first degree of shoulder and upper limb, except wrist and hand unspecified site

√6ᵗʰ **T22.51** Corrosion of first degree of forearm

√7ᵗʰ **T22.511** Corrosion of first degree of right forearm

√7ᵗʰ **T22.512** Corrosion of first degree of left forearm

√7ᵗʰ **T22.519** Corrosion of first degree of unspecified forearm

√6ᵗʰ **T22.52** Corrosion of first degree of elbow

√7ᵗʰ **T22.521** Corrosion of first degree of right elbow

√7ᵗʰ **T22.522** Corrosion of first degree of left elbow

√7ᵗʰ **T22.529** Corrosion of first degree of unspecified elbow

N Newborn: 0   P Pediatric: 0-17   M Maternity: 9-64   A Adult: 15-124   MCC Major Complication/Comorbidity   CC Complication/Comorbidity   SW Severe Wound Dx

1134   ICD-10-CM 2020

☑6ᵗʰ **T22.53** **Corrosion of first degree of** upper arm
- ☑7ᵗʰ **T22.531** **Corrosion of first degree of** right upper arm
- ☑7ᵗʰ **T22.532** **Corrosion of first degree of** left upper arm
- ☑7ᵗʰ **T22.539** **Corrosion of first degree of unspecified upper arm**

☑6ᵗʰ **T22.54** **Corrosion of first degree of** axilla
- ☑7ᵗʰ **T22.541** **Corrosion of first degree of** right axilla
- ☑7ᵗʰ **T22.542** **Corrosion of first degree of** left axilla
- ☑7ᵗʰ **T22.549** **Corrosion of first degree of unspecified axilla**

☑6ᵗʰ **T22.55** **Corrosion of first degree of** shoulder
- ☑7ᵗʰ **T22.551** **Corrosion of first degree of** right shoulder
- ☑7ᵗʰ **T22.552** **Corrosion of first degree of** left shoulder
- ☑7ᵗʰ **T22.559** **Corrosion of first degree of unspecified shoulder**

☑6ᵗʰ **T22.56** **Corrosion of first degree of** scapular region
- ☑7ᵗʰ **T22.561** **Corrosion of first degree of** right scapular region
- ☑7ᵗʰ **T22.562** **Corrosion of first degree of** left scapular region
- ☑7ᵗʰ **T22.569** **Corrosion of first degree of unspecified scapular region**

☑6ᵗʰ **T22.59** **Corrosion of first degree of** multiple sites of shoulder and upper limb, except wrist and hand
- ☑7ᵗʰ **T22.591** **Corrosion of first degree of multiple sites of** right shoulder and upper limb, except wrist and hand
- ☑7ᵗʰ **T22.592** **Corrosion of first degree of multiple sites of** left shoulder and upper limb, except wrist and hand
- ☑7ᵗʰ **T22.599** **Corrosion of first degree of multiple sites of unspecified shoulder and upper limb, except wrist and hand**

☑5ᵗʰ **T22.6** **Corrosion of** second degree **of shoulder and upper limb, except wrist and hand**
> Code first (T51-T65) to identify chemical and intent
> Use additional external cause code to identify place (Y92)

☑x7ᵗʰ **T22.60** **Corrosion of second degree of shoulder and upper limb, except wrist and hand, unspecified site**

☑6ᵗʰ **T22.61** **Corrosion of second degree of** forearm
- ☑7ᵗʰ **T22.611** **Corrosion of second degree of** right forearm
- ☑7ᵗʰ **T22.612** **Corrosion of second degree of** left forearm
- ☑7ᵗʰ **T22.619** **Corrosion of second degree of unspecified forearm**

☑6ᵗʰ **T22.62** **Corrosion of second degree of** elbow
- ☑7ᵗʰ **T22.621** **Corrosion of second degree of** right elbow
- ☑7ᵗʰ **T22.622** **Corrosion of second degree of** left elbow
- ☑7ᵗʰ **T22.629** **Corrosion of second degree of unspecified elbow**

☑6ᵗʰ **T22.63** **Corrosion of second degree of** upper arm
- ☑7ᵗʰ **T22.631** **Corrosion of second degree of** right upper arm
- ☑7ᵗʰ **T22.632** **Corrosion of second degree of** left upper arm
- ☑7ᵗʰ **T22.639** **Corrosion of second degree of unspecified upper arm**

☑6ᵗʰ **T22.64** **Corrosion of second degree of** axilla
- ☑7ᵗʰ **T22.641** **Corrosion of second degree of** right axilla
- ☑7ᵗʰ **T22.642** **Corrosion of second degree of** left axilla
- ☑7ᵗʰ **T22.649** **Corrosion of second degree of unspecified axilla**

☑6ᵗʰ **T22.65** **Corrosion of second degree of** shoulder
- ☑7ᵗʰ **T22.651** **Corrosion of second degree of** right shoulder
- ☑7ᵗʰ **T22.652** **Corrosion of second degree of** left shoulder
- ☑7ᵗʰ **T22.659** **Corrosion of second degree of unspecified shoulder**

☑6ᵗʰ **T22.66** **Corrosion of second degree of** scapular region
- ☑7ᵗʰ **T22.661** **Corrosion of second degree of** right scapular region
- ☑7ᵗʰ **T22.662** **Corrosion of second degree of** left scapular region
- ☑7ᵗʰ **T22.669** **Corrosion of second degree of unspecified scapular region**

☑6ᵗʰ **T22.69** **Corrosion of second degree of** multiple sites of shoulder and upper limb, except wrist and hand
- ☑7ᵗʰ **T22.691** **Corrosion of second degree of multiple sites of** right shoulder and upper limb, except wrist and hand
- ☑7ᵗʰ **T22.692** **Corrosion of second degree of multiple sites of** left shoulder and upper limb, except wrist and hand
- ☑7ᵗʰ **T22.699** **Corrosion of second degree of multiple sites of unspecified shoulder and upper limb, except wrist and hand**

☑5ᵗʰ **T22.7** **Corrosion of** third degree **of shoulder and upper limb, except wrist and hand**
> Code first (T51-T65) to identify chemical and intent
> Use additional external cause code to identify place (Y92)

☑x7ᵗʰ **T22.70** **Corrosion of third degree of shoulder and upper limb, except wrist and hand, unspecified site**   CC H5 SW
> CC Excl: PDX collection 1389

☑6ᵗʰ **T22.71** **Corrosion of third degree of** forearm
> CC Excl: For CC codes in subcategory T22.71: PDX collection 1390
- ☑7ᵗʰ **T22.711** **Corrosion of third degree of** right forearm   CC H5 SW
- ☑7ᵗʰ **T22.712** **Corrosion of third degree of** left forearm   CC H5 SW
- ☑7ᵗʰ **T22.719** **Corrosion of third degree of unspecified forearm**   CC H5 SW

☑6ᵗʰ **T22.72** **Corrosion of third degree of** elbow
> CC Excl: For CC codes in subcategory T22.72: PDX collection 1391
- ☑7ᵗʰ **T22.721** **Corrosion of third degree of** right elbow   CC H5 SW
- ☑7ᵗʰ **T22.722** **Corrosion of third degree of** left elbow   CC H5 SW
- ☑7ᵗʰ **T22.729** **Corrosion of third degree of unspecified elbow**   CC H5 SW

☑6ᵗʰ **T22.73** **Corrosion of third degree of** upper arm
> CC Excl: For CC codes in subcategory T22.73: PDX collection 1392
- ☑7ᵗʰ **T22.731** **Corrosion of third degree of** right upper arm   CC H5 SW
- ☑7ᵗʰ **T22.732** **Corrosion of third degree of** left upper arm   CC H5 SW
- ☑7ᵗʰ **T22.739** **Corrosion of third degree of unspecified upper arm**   CC H5 SW

☑6ᵗʰ **T22.74** **Corrosion of third degree of** axilla
> CC Excl: For CC codes in subcategory T22.74: PDX collection 1393
- ☑7ᵗʰ **T22.741** **Corrosion of third degree of** right axilla   CC H5 SW
- ☑7ᵗʰ **T22.742** **Corrosion of third degree of** left axilla   CC H5 SW
- ☑7ᵗʰ **T22.749** **Corrosion of third degree of unspecified axilla**   CC H5 SW

☑6ᵗʰ **T22.75** **Corrosion of third degree of** shoulder
> CC Excl: For CC codes in subcategory T22.75: PDX collection 1394
- ☑7ᵗʰ **T22.751** **Corrosion of third degree of** right shoulder   CC H5 SW
- ☑7ᵗʰ **T22.752** **Corrosion of third degree of** left shoulder   CC H5 SW
- ☑7ᵗʰ **T22.759** **Corrosion of third degree of unspecified shoulder**   CC H5 SW

☑6ᵗʰ **T22.76** **Corrosion of third degree of** scapular region
> CC Excl: For CC codes in subcategory T22.76: PDX collection 1395
- ☑7ᵗʰ **T22.761** **Corrosion of third degree of** right scapular region   CC H5 SW
- ☑7ᵗʰ **T22.762** **Corrosion of third degree of** left scapular region   CC H5 SW
- ☑7ᵗʰ **T22.769** **Corrosion of third degree of unspecified scapular region**   CC H5 SW

☑ Additional Character Required   ☑x7ᵗʰ Placeholder   Unacceptable PDx   Questionable PDx   Manifestation   Unspecified Dx   H1-H14 HAC   HCC CMS-HCC Dx   HIV HIV Dx

Chapter 19. Injury, Poisoning and Certain Other Consequences of External Causes

T22.79–T23.199

√6ᵗʰ **T22.79** **Corrosion of third degree of** multiple sites **of shoulder and upper limb, except wrist and hand**
> **CC Excl: For CC codes in subcategory T22.79:** PDX collection 1389

√7ᵗʰ **T22.791** Corrosion of third degree of multiple sites of right shoulder and upper limb, except wrist and hand   `CC` `H5` `SW`

√7ᵗʰ **T22.792** Corrosion of third degree of multiple sites of left shoulder and upper limb, except wrist and hand   `CC` `H5` `SW`

√7ᵗʰ **T22.799** Corrosion of third degree of multiple sites of unspecified shoulder and upper limb, except wrist and hand   `CC` `H5` `SW`

√4ᵗʰ **T23** **Burn and corrosion of wrist and hand**
> **AHA:** 2015,1Q,19

> The appropriate 7th character is to be added to each code from category T23.
> A   initial encounter
> D   subsequent encounter
> S   sequela

√5ᵗʰ **T23.0** **Burn of unspecified degree of wrist and hand**
> Use additional external cause code to identify the source, place and intent of the burn (X00-X19, X75-X77, X96-X98, Y92)

√6ᵗʰ **T23.00** **Burn of unspecified degree of hand, unspecified site**

√7ᵗʰ **T23.001** Burn of unspecified degree of right hand, unspecified site

√7ᵗʰ **T23.002** Burn of unspecified degree of left hand, unspecified site

√7ᵗʰ **T23.009** Burn of unspecified degree of unspecified hand, unspecified site

√6ᵗʰ **T23.01** **Burn of unspecified degree of** thumb (nail)

√7ᵗʰ **T23.011** Burn of unspecified degree of right thumb (nail)

√7ᵗʰ **T23.012** Burn of unspecified degree of left thumb (nail)

√7ᵗʰ **T23.019** Burn of unspecified degree of unspecified thumb (nail)

√6ᵗʰ **T23.02** **Burn of unspecified degree of** single finger (nail) **except thumb**

√7ᵗʰ **T23.021** Burn of unspecified degree of single right finger (nail) except thumb

√7ᵗʰ **T23.022** Burn of unspecified degree of single left finger (nail) except thumb

√7ᵗʰ **T23.029** Burn of unspecified degree of unspecified single finger (nail) except thumb

√6ᵗʰ **T23.03** **Burn of unspecified degree of** multiple fingers (nail), not including thumb

√7ᵗʰ **T23.031** Burn of unspecified degree of multiple right fingers (nail), not including thumb

√7ᵗʰ **T23.032** Burn of unspecified degree of multiple left fingers (nail), not including thumb

√7ᵗʰ **T23.039** Burn of unspecified degree of unspecified multiple fingers (nail), not including thumb

√6ᵗʰ **T23.04** **Burn of unspecified degree of** multiple fingers (nail), including thumb

√7ᵗʰ **T23.041** Burn of unspecified degree of multiple right fingers (nail), including thumb

√7ᵗʰ **T23.042** Burn of unspecified degree of multiple left fingers (nail), including thumb

√7ᵗʰ **T23.049** Burn of unspecified degree of unspecified multiple fingers (nail), including thumb

√6ᵗʰ **T23.05** **Burn of unspecified degree of** palm

√7ᵗʰ **T23.051** Burn of unspecified degree of right palm

√7ᵗʰ **T23.052** Burn of unspecified degree of left palm

√7ᵗʰ **T23.059** Burn of unspecified degree of unspecified palm

√6ᵗʰ **T23.06** **Burn of unspecified degree of** back of hand

√7ᵗʰ **T23.061** Burn of unspecified degree of back of right hand

√7ᵗʰ **T23.062** Burn of unspecified degree of back of left hand

√7ᵗʰ **T23.069** Burn of unspecified degree of back of unspecified hand

√6ᵗʰ **T23.07** **Burn of unspecified degree of** wrist

√7ᵗʰ **T23.071** Burn of unspecified degree of right wrist

√7ᵗʰ **T23.072** Burn of unspecified degree of left wrist

√7ᵗʰ **T23.079** Burn of unspecified degree of unspecified wrist

√6ᵗʰ **T23.09** **Burn of unspecified degree of** multiple sites **of wrist and hand**

√7ᵗʰ **T23.091** Burn of unspecified degree of multiple sites of right wrist and hand

√7ᵗʰ **T23.092** Burn of unspecified degree of multiple sites of left wrist and hand

√7ᵗʰ **T23.099** Burn of unspecified degree of multiple sites of unspecified wrist and hand

√5ᵗʰ **T23.1** **Burn of** first degree **of wrist and hand**
> Use additional external cause code to identify the source, place and intent of the burn (X00-X19, X75-X77, X96-X98, Y92)

√6ᵗʰ **T23.10** **Burn of first degree of hand, unspecified site**

√7ᵗʰ **T23.101** Burn of first degree of right hand, unspecified site

√7ᵗʰ **T23.102** Burn of first degree of left hand, unspecified site

√7ᵗʰ **T23.109** Burn of first degree of unspecified hand, unspecified site

√6ᵗʰ **T23.11** **Burn of first degree of** thumb (nail)

√7ᵗʰ **T23.111** Burn of first degree of right thumb (nail)

√7ᵗʰ **T23.112** Burn of first degree of left thumb (nail)

√7ᵗʰ **T23.119** Burn of first degree of unspecified thumb (nail)

√6ᵗʰ **T23.12** **Burn of first degree of** single finger (nail) except **thumb**

√7ᵗʰ **T23.121** Burn of first degree of single right finger (nail) except thumb

√7ᵗʰ **T23.122** Burn of first degree of single left finger (nail) except thumb

√7ᵗʰ **T23.129** Burn of first degree of unspecified single finger (nail) except thumb

√6ᵗʰ **T23.13** **Burn of first degree of** multiple fingers (nail), not including thumb

√7ᵗʰ **T23.131** Burn of first degree of multiple right fingers (nail), not including thumb

√7ᵗʰ **T23.132** Burn of first degree of multiple left fingers (nail), not including thumb

√7ᵗʰ **T23.139** Burn of first degree of unspecified multiple fingers (nail), not including thumb

√6ᵗʰ **T23.14** **Burn of first degree of** multiple fingers (nail), including thumb

√7ᵗʰ **T23.141** Burn of first degree of multiple right fingers (nail), including thumb

√7ᵗʰ **T23.142** Burn of first degree of multiple left fingers (nail), including thumb

√7ᵗʰ **T23.149** Burn of first degree of unspecified multiple fingers (nail), including thumb

√6ᵗʰ **T23.15** **Burn of first degree of** palm

√7ᵗʰ **T23.151** Burn of first degree of right palm

√7ᵗʰ **T23.152** Burn of first degree of left palm

√7ᵗʰ **T23.159** Burn of first degree of unspecified palm

√6ᵗʰ **T23.16** **Burn of first degree of** back of hand

√7ᵗʰ **T23.161** Burn of first degree of back of right hand

√7ᵗʰ **T23.162** Burn of first degree of back of left hand

√7ᵗʰ **T23.169** Burn of first degree of back of unspecified hand

√6ᵗʰ **T23.17** **Burn of first degree of** wrist

√7ᵗʰ **T23.171** Burn of first degree of right wrist

√7ᵗʰ **T23.172** Burn of first degree of left wrist

√7ᵗʰ **T23.179** Burn of first degree of unspecified wrist

√6ᵗʰ **T23.19** **Burn of first degree of** multiple sites **of wrist and hand**

√7ᵗʰ **T23.191** Burn of first degree of multiple sites of right wrist and hand

√7ᵗʰ **T23.192** Burn of first degree of multiple sites of left wrist and hand

√7ᵗʰ **T23.199** Burn of first degree of multiple sites of unspecified wrist and hand

`N` Newborn: 0   `P` Pediatric: 0-17   `M` Maternity: 9-64   `A` Adult: 15-124   `MCC` Major Complication/Comorbidity   `CC` Complication/Comorbidity   `SW` Severe Wound Dx

1136   ICD-10-CM 2020

✓5ᵗʰ T23.2 Burn of second degree **of wrist and hand**

Use additional external cause code to identify the source, place and intent of the burn (X00-X19, X75-X77, X96-X98, Y92)

✓6ᵗʰ T23.20 Burn of second degree of hand, unspecified site

✓7ᵗʰ T23.201 Burn of second degree of right **hand, unspecified site**

✓7ᵗʰ T23.202 Burn of second degree of left **hand, unspecified site**

✓7ᵗʰ T23.209 Burn of second degree of unspecified hand, unspecified site

✓6ᵗʰ T23.21 Burn of second degree of thumb **(nail)**

✓7ᵗʰ T23.211 Burn of second degree of right **thumb (nail)**

✓7ᵗʰ T23.212 Burn of second degree of left **thumb (nail)**

✓7ᵗʰ T23.219 Burn of second degree of unspecified thumb (nail)

✓6ᵗʰ T23.22 Burn of second degree of single finger **(nail) except thumb**

✓7ᵗʰ T23.221 Burn of second degree of single right **finger (nail) except thumb**

✓7ᵗʰ T23.222 Burn of second degree of single left **finger (nail) except thumb**

✓7ᵗʰ T23.229 Burn of second degree of unspecified single finger (nail) except thumb

✓6ᵗʰ T23.23 Burn of second degree of multiple fingers **(nail),** not including thumb

✓7ᵗʰ T23.231 Burn of second degree of multiple right **fingers (nail), not including thumb**

✓7ᵗʰ T23.232 Burn of second degree of multiple left **fingers (nail), not including thumb**

✓7ᵗʰ T23.239 Burn of second degree of unspecified multiple fingers (nail), not including thumb

✓6ᵗʰ T23.24 Burn of second degree of multiple fingers **(nail),** including thumb

✓7ᵗʰ T23.241 Burn of second degree of multiple right **fingers (nail), including thumb**

✓7ᵗʰ T23.242 Burn of second degree of multiple left **fingers (nail), including thumb**

✓7ᵗʰ T23.249 Burn of second degree of unspecified multiple fingers (nail), including thumb

✓6ᵗʰ T23.25 Burn of second degree of palm

✓7ᵗʰ T23.251 Burn of second degree of right **palm**

✓7ᵗʰ T23.252 Burn of second degree of left **palm**

✓7ᵗʰ T23.259 Burn of second degree of unspecified palm

✓6ᵗʰ T23.26 Burn of second degree of back of hand

✓7ᵗʰ T23.261 Burn of second degree of back of right **hand**

✓7ᵗʰ T23.262 Burn of second degree of back of left **hand**

✓7ᵗʰ T23.269 Burn of second degree of back of unspecified hand

✓6ᵗʰ T23.27 Burn of second degree of wrist

✓7ᵗʰ T23.271 Burn of second degree of right **wrist**

✓7ᵗʰ T23.272 Burn of second degree of left **wrist**

✓7ᵗʰ T23.279 Burn of second degree of unspecified wrist

✓6ᵗʰ T23.29 Burn of second degree of multiple sites **of wrist and hand**

✓7ᵗʰ T23.291 Burn of second degree of multiple sites of right **wrist and hand**

✓7ᵗʰ T23.292 Burn of second degree of multiple sites of left **wrist and hand**

✓7ᵗʰ T23.299 Burn of second degree of multiple sites of unspecified wrist and hand

✓5ᵗʰ T23.3 Burn of third degree **of wrist and hand**

Use additional external cause code to identify the source, place and intent of the burn (X00-X19, X75-X77, X96-X98, Y92)

✓6ᵗʰ T23.30 Burn of third degree of hand, unspecified site

AHA: 2016,2Q,5
CC Excl: For CC codes in subcategory T23.30: PDX collection 1396

✓7ᵗʰ T23.301 Burn of third degree of right **hand, unspecified site** `CC` `H5` `SW`

✓7ᵗʰ T23.302 Burn of third degree of left **hand, unspecified site** `CC` `H5` `SW`

✓7ᵗʰ T23.309 Burn of third degree of unspecified hand, unspecified site `CC` `H5` `SW`

✓6ᵗʰ T23.31 Burn of third degree of thumb **(nail)**

CC Excl: For CC codes in subcategory T23.31: PDX collection 1397

✓7ᵗʰ T23.311 Burn of third degree of right **thumb (nail)** `CC` `H5` `SW`

✓7ᵗʰ T23.312 Burn of third degree of left **thumb (nail)** `CC` `H5` `SW`

✓7ᵗʰ T23.319 Burn of third degree of unspecified thumb (nail) `CC` `H5` `SW`

✓6ᵗʰ T23.32 Burn of third degree of single finger **(nail) except thumb**

CC Excl: For CC codes in subcategory T23.32: PDX collection 1398

✓7ᵗʰ T23.321 Burn of third degree of single right **finger (nail) except thumb** `CC` `H5` `SW`

✓7ᵗʰ T23.322 Burn of third degree of single left **finger (nail) except thumb** `CC` `H5` `SW`

✓7ᵗʰ T23.329 Burn of third degree of unspecified single finger (nail) except thumb `CC` `H5` `SW`

✓6ᵗʰ T23.33 Burn of third degree of multiple fingers **(nail),** not including thumb

CC Excl: For CC codes in subcategory T23.33: PDX collection 1399

✓7ᵗʰ T23.331 Burn of third degree of multiple right **fingers (nail), not including thumb** `CC` `H5` `SW`

✓7ᵗʰ T23.332 Burn of third degree of multiple left **fingers (nail), not including thumb** `CC` `H5` `SW`

✓7ᵗʰ T23.339 Burn of third degree of unspecified multiple fingers (nail), not including thumb `CC` `H5` `SW`

✓6ᵗʰ T23.34 Burn of third degree of multiple fingers **(nail),** including thumb

CC Excl: For CC codes in subcategory T23.34: PDX collection 1400

✓7ᵗʰ T23.341 Burn of third degree of multiple right **fingers (nail), including thumb** `CC` `H5` `SW`

✓7ᵗʰ T23.342 Burn of third degree of multiple left **fingers (nail), including thumb** `CC` `H5` `SW`

✓7ᵗʰ T23.349 Burn of third degree of unspecified multiple fingers (nail), including thumb `CC` `H5` `SW`

✓6ᵗʰ T23.35 Burn of third degree of palm

CC Excl: For CC codes in subcategory T23.35: PDX collection 1401

✓7ᵗʰ T23.351 Burn of third degree of right **palm** `CC` `H5` `SW`

✓7ᵗʰ T23.352 Burn of third degree of left **palm** `CC` `H5` `SW`

✓7ᵗʰ T23.359 Burn of third degree of unspecified palm `CC` `H5` `SW`

✓6ᵗʰ T23.36 Burn of third degree of back of hand

CC Excl: For CC codes in subcategory T23.36: PDX collection 1402

✓7ᵗʰ T23.361 Burn of third degree of back of right **hand** `CC` `H5` `SW`

✓7ᵗʰ T23.362 Burn of third degree of back of left **hand** `CC` `H5` `SW`

✓7ᵗʰ T23.369 Burn of third degree of back of unspecified hand `CC` `H5` `SW`

✓6ᵗʰ T23.37 Burn of third degree of wrist

CC Excl: For CC codes in subcategory T23.37: PDX collection 1403

✓7ᵗʰ T23.371 Burn of third degree of right **wrist** `CC` `H5` `SW`

✓7ᵗʰ T23.372 Burn of third degree of left **wrist** `CC` `H5` `SW`

✓7ᵗʰ T23.379 Burn of third degree of unspecified wrist `CC` `H5` `SW`

√6ᵗʰ T23.39 Burn of third degree of multiple sites of wrist and hand

> CC Excl: For CC codes in subcategory T23.39: PDX collection 1396

     √7ᵗʰ T23.391 Burn of third degree of multiple sites of right wrist and hand   CC H5 SW

     √7ᵗʰ T23.392 Burn of third degree of multiple sites of left wrist and hand   CC H5 SW

     √7ᵗʰ T23.399 Burn of third degree of multiple sites of unspecified wrist and hand   CC H5 SW

√5ᵗʰ T23.4 Corrosion of unspecified degree of wrist and hand

> Code first (T51-T65) to identify chemical and intent
> Use additional external cause code to identify place (Y92)

√6ᵗʰ T23.40 Corrosion of unspecified degree of hand, unspecified site

     √7ᵗʰ T23.401 Corrosion of unspecified degree of right hand, unspecified site

     √7ᵗʰ T23.402 Corrosion of unspecified degree of left hand, unspecified site

     √7ᵗʰ T23.409 Corrosion of unspecified degree of unspecified hand, unspecified site

√6ᵗʰ T23.41 Corrosion of unspecified degree of thumb (nail)

     √7ᵗʰ T23.411 Corrosion of unspecified degree of right thumb (nail)

     √7ᵗʰ T23.412 Corrosion of unspecified degree of left thumb (nail)

     √7ᵗʰ T23.419 Corrosion of unspecified degree of unspecified thumb (nail)

√6ᵗʰ T23.42 Corrosion of unspecified degree of single finger (nail) except thumb

     √7ᵗʰ T23.421 Corrosion of unspecified degree of single right finger (nail) except thumb

     √7ᵗʰ T23.422 Corrosion of unspecified degree of single left finger (nail) except thumb

     √7ᵗʰ T23.429 Corrosion of unspecified degree of unspecified single finger (nail) except thumb

√6ᵗʰ T23.43 Corrosion of unspecified degree of multiple fingers (nail), not including thumb

     √7ᵗʰ T23.431 Corrosion of unspecified degree of multiple right fingers (nail), not including thumb

     √7ᵗʰ T23.432 Corrosion of unspecified degree of multiple left fingers (nail), not including thumb

     √7ᵗʰ T23.439 Corrosion of unspecified degree of unspecified multiple fingers (nail), not including thumb

√6ᵗʰ T23.44 Corrosion of unspecified degree of multiple fingers (nail), including thumb

     √7ᵗʰ T23.441 Corrosion of unspecified degree of multiple right fingers (nail), including thumb

     √7ᵗʰ T23.442 Corrosion of unspecified degree of multiple left fingers (nail), including thumb

     √7ᵗʰ T23.449 Corrosion of unspecified degree of unspecified multiple fingers (nail), including thumb

√6ᵗʰ T23.45 Corrosion of unspecified degree of palm

     √7ᵗʰ T23.451 Corrosion of unspecified degree of right palm

     √7ᵗʰ T23.452 Corrosion of unspecified degree of left palm

     √7ᵗʰ T23.459 Corrosion of unspecified degree of unspecified palm

√6ᵗʰ T23.46 Corrosion of unspecified degree of back of hand

     √7ᵗʰ T23.461 Corrosion of unspecified degree of back of right hand

     √7ᵗʰ T23.462 Corrosion of unspecified degree of back of left hand

     √7ᵗʰ T23.469 Corrosion of unspecified degree of back of unspecified hand

√6ᵗʰ T23.47 Corrosion of unspecified degree of wrist

     √7ᵗʰ T23.471 Corrosion of unspecified degree of right wrist

     √7ᵗʰ T23.472 Corrosion of unspecified degree of left wrist

     √7ᵗʰ T23.479 Corrosion of unspecified degree of unspecified wrist

√6ᵗʰ T23.49 Corrosion of unspecified degree of multiple sites of wrist and hand

     √7ᵗʰ T23.491 Corrosion of unspecified degree of multiple sites of right wrist and hand

     √7ᵗʰ T23.492 Corrosion of unspecified degree of multiple sites of left wrist and hand

     √7ᵗʰ T23.499 Corrosion of unspecified degree of multiple sites of unspecified wrist and hand

√5ᵗʰ T23.5 Corrosion of first degree of wrist and hand

> Code first (T51-T65) to identify chemical and intent
> Use additional external cause code to identify place (Y92)

√6ᵗʰ T23.50 Corrosion of first degree of hand, unspecified site

     √7ᵗʰ T23.501 Corrosion of first degree of right hand, unspecified site

     √7ᵗʰ T23.502 Corrosion of first degree of left hand, unspecified site

     √7ᵗʰ T23.509 Corrosion of first degree of unspecified hand, unspecified site

√6ᵗʰ T23.51 Corrosion of first degree of thumb (nail)

     √7ᵗʰ T23.511 Corrosion of first degree of right thumb (nail)

     √7ᵗʰ T23.512 Corrosion of first degree of left thumb (nail)

     √7ᵗʰ T23.519 Corrosion of first degree of unspecified thumb (nail)

√6ᵗʰ T23.52 Corrosion of first degree of single finger (nail) except thumb

     √7ᵗʰ T23.521 Corrosion of first degree of single right finger (nail) except thumb

     √7ᵗʰ T23.522 Corrosion of first degree of single left finger (nail) except thumb

     √7ᵗʰ T23.529 Corrosion of first degree of unspecified single finger (nail) except thumb

√6ᵗʰ T23.53 Corrosion of first degree of multiple fingers (nail), not including thumb

     √7ᵗʰ T23.531 Corrosion of first degree of multiple right fingers (nail), not including thumb

     √7ᵗʰ T23.532 Corrosion of first degree of multiple left fingers (nail), not including thumb

     √7ᵗʰ T23.539 Corrosion of first degree of unspecified multiple fingers (nail), not including thumb

√6ᵗʰ T23.54 Corrosion of first degree of multiple fingers (nail), including thumb

     √7ᵗʰ T23.541 Corrosion of first degree of multiple right fingers (nail), including thumb

     √7ᵗʰ T23.542 Corrosion of first degree of multiple left fingers (nail), including thumb

     √7ᵗʰ T23.549 Corrosion of first degree of unspecified multiple fingers (nail), including thumb

√6ᵗʰ T23.55 Corrosion of first degree of palm

     √7ᵗʰ T23.551 Corrosion of first degree of right palm

     √7ᵗʰ T23.552 Corrosion of first degree of left palm

     √7ᵗʰ T23.559 Corrosion of first degree of unspecified palm

√6ᵗʰ T23.56 Corrosion of first degree of back of hand

     √7ᵗʰ T23.561 Corrosion of first degree of back of right hand

     √7ᵗʰ T23.562 Corrosion of first degree of back of left hand

     √7ᵗʰ T23.569 Corrosion of first degree of back of unspecified hand

√6ᵗʰ T23.57 Corrosion of first degree of wrist

     √7ᵗʰ T23.571 Corrosion of first degree of right wrist

     √7ᵗʰ T23.572 Corrosion of first degree of left wrist

     √7ᵗʰ T23.579 Corrosion of first degree of unspecified wrist

√6ᵗʰ T23.59 Corrosion of first degree of multiple sites of wrist and hand

     √7ᵗʰ T23.591 Corrosion of first degree of multiple sites of right wrist and hand

     √7ᵗʰ T23.592 Corrosion of first degree of multiple sites of left wrist and hand

     √7ᵗʰ T23.599 Corrosion of first degree of multiple sites of unspecified wrist and hand

N Newborn: 0   P Pediatric: 0-17   M Maternity: 9-64   A Adult: 15-124   MCC Major Complication/Comorbidity   CC Complication/Comorbidity   SW Severe Wound Dx

1138   ICD-10-CM 2020

✓5ᵗʰ **T23.6** **Corrosion** of second degree **of wrist and hand**

Code first (T51-T65) to identify chemical and intent
Use additional external cause code to identify place (Y92)

✓6ᵗʰ **T23.60** **Corrosion of second degree of hand, unspecified site**

✓7ᵗʰ **T23.601** **Corrosion of second degree of right hand, unspecified site**

✓7ᵗʰ **T23.602** **Corrosion of second degree of left hand, unspecified site**

✓7ᵗʰ **T23.609** **Corrosion of second degree of unspecified hand, unspecified site**

✓6ᵗʰ **T23.61** **Corrosion of second degree of thumb (nail)**

✓7ᵗʰ **T23.611** **Corrosion of second degree of right thumb (nail)**

✓7ᵗʰ **T23.612** **Corrosion of second degree of left thumb (nail)**

✓7ᵗʰ **T23.619** **Corrosion of second degree of unspecified thumb (nail)**

✓6ᵗʰ **T23.62** **Corrosion of second degree of single finger (nail) except thumb**

✓7ᵗʰ **T23.621** **Corrosion of second degree of single right finger (nail) except thumb**

✓7ᵗʰ **T23.622** **Corrosion of second degree of single left finger (nail) except thumb**

✓7ᵗʰ **T23.629** **Corrosion of second degree of unspecified single finger (nail) except thumb**

✓6ᵗʰ **T23.63** **Corrosion of second degree of multiple fingers (nail), not including thumb**

✓7ᵗʰ **T23.631** **Corrosion of second degree of multiple right fingers (nail), not including thumb**

✓7ᵗʰ **T23.632** **Corrosion of second degree of multiple left fingers (nail), not including thumb**

✓7ᵗʰ **T23.639** **Corrosion of second degree of unspecified multiple fingers (nail), not including thumb**

✓6ᵗʰ **T23.64** **Corrosion of second degree of multiple fingers (nail), including thumb**

✓7ᵗʰ **T23.641** **Corrosion of second degree of multiple right fingers (nail), including thumb**

✓7ᵗʰ **T23.642** **Corrosion of second degree of multiple left fingers (nail), including thumb**

✓7ᵗʰ **T23.649** **Corrosion of second degree of unspecified multiple fingers (nail), including thumb**

✓6ᵗʰ **T23.65** **Corrosion of second degree of palm**

✓7ᵗʰ **T23.651** **Corrosion of second degree of right palm**

✓7ᵗʰ **T23.652** **Corrosion of second degree of left palm**

✓7ᵗʰ **T23.659** **Corrosion of second degree of unspecified palm**

✓6ᵗʰ **T23.66** **Corrosion of second degree of back of hand**

✓7ᵗʰ **T23.661** **Corrosion of second degree back of right hand**

✓7ᵗʰ **T23.662** **Corrosion of second degree back of left hand**

✓7ᵗʰ **T23.669** **Corrosion of second degree back of unspecified hand**

✓6ᵗʰ **T23.67** **Corrosion of second degree of wrist**

✓7ᵗʰ **T23.671** **Corrosion of second degree of right wrist**

✓7ᵗʰ **T23.672** **Corrosion of second degree of left wrist**

✓7ᵗʰ **T23.679** **Corrosion of second degree of unspecified wrist**

✓6ᵗʰ **T23.69** **Corrosion of second degree of multiple sites of wrist and hand**

✓7ᵗʰ **T23.691** **Corrosion of second degree of multiple sites of right wrist and hand**

✓7ᵗʰ **T23.692** **Corrosion of second degree of multiple sites of left wrist and hand**

✓7ᵗʰ **T23.699** **Corrosion of second degree of multiple sites of unspecified wrist and hand**

✓5ᵗʰ **T23.7** **Corrosion** of third degree **of wrist and hand**

Code first (T51-T65) to identify chemical and intent
Use additional external cause code to identify place (Y92)

✓6ᵗʰ **T23.70** **Corrosion of third degree of hand, unspecified site**

CC Excl: For CC codes in subcategory T23.70: PDX collection 1396

✓7ᵗʰ **T23.701** **Corrosion of third degree of right hand, unspecified site** CC H5 SW

✓7ᵗʰ **T23.702** **Corrosion of third degree of left hand, unspecified site** CC H5 SW

✓7ᵗʰ **T23.709** **Corrosion of third degree of unspecified hand, unspecified site** CC H5 SW

✓6ᵗʰ **T23.71** **Corrosion of third degree of thumb (nail)**

CC Excl: For CC codes in subcategory T23.71: PDX collection 1397

✓7ᵗʰ **T23.711** **Corrosion of third degree of right thumb (nail)** CC H5 SW

✓7ᵗʰ **T23.712** **Corrosion of third degree of left thumb (nail)** CC H5 SW

✓7ᵗʰ **T23.719** **Corrosion of third degree of unspecified thumb (nail)** CC H5 SW

✓6ᵗʰ **T23.72** **Corrosion of third degree of single finger (nail) except thumb**

CC Excl: For CC codes in subcategory T23.72: PDX collection 1398

✓7ᵗʰ **T23.721** **Corrosion of third degree of single right finger (nail) except thumb** CC H5 SW

✓7ᵗʰ **T23.722** **Corrosion of third degree of single left finger (nail) except thumb** CC H5 SW

✓7ᵗʰ **T23.729** **Corrosion of third degree of unspecified single finger (nail) except thumb** CC H5 SW

✓6ᵗʰ **T23.73** **Corrosion of third degree of multiple fingers (nail), not including thumb**

CC Excl: For CC codes in subcategory T23.73: PDX collection 1399

✓7ᵗʰ **T23.731** **Corrosion of third degree of multiple right fingers (nail), not including thumb** CC H5 SW

✓7ᵗʰ **T23.732** **Corrosion of third degree of multiple left fingers (nail), not including thumb** CC H5 SW

✓7ᵗʰ **T23.739** **Corrosion of third degree of unspecified multiple fingers (nail), not including thumb** CC H5 SW

✓6ᵗʰ **T23.74** **Corrosion of third degree of multiple fingers (nail), including thumb**

CC Excl: For CC codes in subcategory T23.74: PDX collection 1400

✓7ᵗʰ **T23.741** **Corrosion of third degree of multiple right fingers (nail), including thumb** CC H5 SW

✓7ᵗʰ **T23.742** **Corrosion of third degree of multiple left fingers (nail), including thumb** CC H5 SW

✓7ᵗʰ **T23.749** **Corrosion of third degree of unspecified multiple fingers (nail), including thumb** CC H5 SW

✓6ᵗʰ **T23.75** **Corrosion of third degree of palm**

CC Excl: For CC codes in subcategory T23.75: PDX collection 1401

✓7ᵗʰ **T23.751** **Corrosion of third degree of right palm** CC H5 SW

✓7ᵗʰ **T23.752** **Corrosion of third degree of left palm** CC H5 SW

✓7ᵗʰ **T23.759** **Corrosion of third degree of unspecified palm** CC H5 SW

✓6ᵗʰ **T23.76** **Corrosion of third degree of back of hand**

CC Excl: For CC codes in subcategory T23.76: PDX collection 1402

✓7ᵗʰ **T23.761** **Corrosion of third degree of back of right hand** CC H5 SW

✓7ᵗʰ **T23.762** **Corrosion of third degree of back of left hand** CC H5 SW

✓7ᵗʰ **T23.769** **Corrosion of third degree back of unspecified hand** CC H5 SW

✓6ᵗʰ **T23.77** **Corrosion of third degree of wrist**

CC Excl: For CC codes in subcategory T23.77: PDX collection 1403

✓7ᵗʰ **T23.771** **Corrosion of third degree of right wrist** CC H5 SW

✓7ᵗʰ **T23.772** **Corrosion of third degree of left wrist** CC H5 SW

✓7ᵗʰ **T23.779** **Corrosion of third degree of unspecified wrist** CC H5 SW

Chapter 19. Injury, Poisoning and Certain Other Consequences of External Causes

T23.79–T24.309

√6ᵗʰ **T23.79** Corrosion of third degree of multiple sites of wrist and hand
> **CC Excl: For CC codes in subcategory T23.79:** PDX collection 1396

√7ᵗʰ **T23.791** Corrosion of third degree of multiple sites of right wrist and hand   `CC` `H5` `SW`

√7ᵗʰ **T23.792** Corrosion of third degree of multiple sites of left wrist and hand   `CC` `H5` `SW`

√7ᵗʰ **T23.799** Corrosion of third degree of multiple sites of unspecified wrist and hand   `CC` `H5` `SW`

√4ᵗʰ **T24** **Burn and corrosion of lower limb, except ankle and foot**

> EXCLUDES 2   burn and corrosion of ankle and foot (T25.-)
> burn and corrosion of hip region (T21.-)

> The appropriate 7th character is to be added to each code from category T24.
> A   initial encounter
> D   subsequent encounter
> S   sequela

√5ᵗʰ **T24.0** Burn of unspecified degree of lower limb, except ankle and foot
> Use additional external cause code to identify the source, place and intent of the burn (X00-X19, X75-X77, X96-X98, Y92)

√6ᵗʰ **T24.00** Burn of unspecified degree of unspecified site of lower limb, except ankle and foot

√7ᵗʰ **T24.001** Burn of unspecified degree of unspecified site of right lower limb, except ankle and foot

√7ᵗʰ **T24.002** Burn of unspecified degree of unspecified site of left lower limb, except ankle and foot

√7ᵗʰ **T24.009** Burn of unspecified degree of unspecified site of unspecified lower limb, except ankle and foot

√6ᵗʰ **T24.01** Burn of unspecified degree of thigh

√7ᵗʰ **T24.011** Burn of unspecified degree of right thigh

√7ᵗʰ **T24.012** Burn of unspecified degree of left thigh

√7ᵗʰ **T24.019** Burn of unspecified degree of unspecified thigh

√6ᵗʰ **T24.02** Burn of unspecified degree of knee

√7ᵗʰ **T24.021** Burn of unspecified degree of right knee

√7ᵗʰ **T24.022** Burn of unspecified degree of left knee

√7ᵗʰ **T24.029** Burn of unspecified degree of unspecified knee

√6ᵗʰ **T24.03** Burn of unspecified degree of lower leg

√7ᵗʰ **T24.031** Burn of unspecified degree of right lower leg

√7ᵗʰ **T24.032** Burn of unspecified degree of left lower leg

√7ᵗʰ **T24.039** Burn of unspecified degree of unspecified lower leg

√6ᵗʰ **T24.09** Burn of unspecified degree of multiple sites of lower limb, except ankle and foot

√7ᵗʰ **T24.091** Burn of unspecified degree of multiple sites of right lower limb, except ankle and foot

√7ᵗʰ **T24.092** Burn of unspecified degree of multiple sites of left lower limb, except ankle and foot

√7ᵗʰ **T24.099** Burn of unspecified degree of multiple sites of unspecified lower limb, except ankle and foot

√5ᵗʰ **T24.1** Burn of first degree of lower limb, except ankle and foot
> Use additional external cause code to identify the source, place and intent of the burn (X00-X19, X75-X77, X96-X98, Y92)

√6ᵗʰ **T24.10** Burn of first degree of unspecified site of lower limb, except ankle and foot

√7ᵗʰ **T24.101** Burn of first degree of unspecified site of right lower limb, except ankle and foot

√7ᵗʰ **T24.102** Burn of first degree of unspecified site of left lower limb, except ankle and foot

√7ᵗʰ **T24.109** Burn of first degree of unspecified site of unspecified lower limb, except ankle and foot

√6ᵗʰ **T24.11** Burn of first degree of thigh

√7ᵗʰ **T24.111** Burn of first degree of right thigh

√7ᵗʰ **T24.112** Burn of first degree of left thigh

√7ᵗʰ **T24.119** Burn of first degree of unspecified thigh

√6ᵗʰ **T24.12** Burn of first degree of knee

√7ᵗʰ **T24.121** Burn of first degree of right knee

√7ᵗʰ **T24.122** Burn of first degree of left knee

√7ᵗʰ **T24.129** Burn of first degree of unspecified knee

√6ᵗʰ **T24.13** Burn of first degree of lower leg

√7ᵗʰ **T24.131** Burn of first degree of right lower leg

√7ᵗʰ **T24.132** Burn of first degree of left lower leg

√7ᵗʰ **T24.139** Burn of first degree of unspecified lower leg

√6ᵗʰ **T24.19** Burn of first degree of multiple sites of lower limb, except ankle and foot

√7ᵗʰ **T24.191** Burn of first degree of multiple sites of right lower limb, except ankle and foot

√7ᵗʰ **T24.192** Burn of first degree of multiple sites of left lower limb, except ankle and foot

√7ᵗʰ **T24.199** Burn of first degree of multiple sites of unspecified lower limb, except ankle and foot

√5ᵗʰ **T24.2** Burn of second degree of lower limb, except ankle and foot
> Use additional external cause code to identify the source, place and intent of the burn (X00-X19, X75-X77, X96-X98, Y92)

√6ᵗʰ **T24.20** Burn of second degree of unspecified site of lower limb, except ankle and foot

√7ᵗʰ **T24.201** Burn of second degree of unspecified site of right lower limb, except ankle and foot

√7ᵗʰ **T24.202** Burn of second degree of unspecified site of left lower limb, except ankle and foot

√7ᵗʰ **T24.209** Burn of second degree of unspecified site of unspecified lower limb, except ankle and foot

√6ᵗʰ **T24.21** Burn of second degree of thigh

√7ᵗʰ **T24.211** Burn of second degree of right thigh

√7ᵗʰ **T24.212** Burn of second degree of left thigh

√7ᵗʰ **T24.219** Burn of second degree of unspecified thigh

√6ᵗʰ **T24.22** Burn of second degree of knee

√7ᵗʰ **T24.221** Burn of second degree of right knee

√7ᵗʰ **T24.222** Burn of second degree of left knee

√7ᵗʰ **T24.229** Burn of second degree of unspecified knee

√6ᵗʰ **T24.23** Burn of second degree of lower leg

√7ᵗʰ **T24.231** Burn of second degree of right lower leg

√7ᵗʰ **T24.232** Burn of second degree of left lower leg

√7ᵗʰ **T24.239** Burn of second degree of unspecified lower leg

√6ᵗʰ **T24.29** Burn of second degree of multiple sites of lower limb, except ankle and foot

√7ᵗʰ **T24.291** Burn of second degree of multiple sites of right lower limb, except ankle and foot

√7ᵗʰ **T24.292** Burn of second degree of multiple sites of left lower limb, except ankle and foot

√7ᵗʰ **T24.299** Burn of second degree of multiple sites of unspecified lower limb, except ankle and foot

√5ᵗʰ **T24.3** Burn of third degree of lower limb, except ankle and foot
> Use additional external cause code to identify the source, place and intent of the burn (X00-X19, X75-X77, X96-X98, Y92)

√6ᵗʰ **T24.30** Burn of third degree of unspecified site of lower limb, except ankle and foot
> **CC Excl: For CC codes in subcategory T24.30:** PDX collection 1404

√7ᵗʰ **T24.301** Burn of third degree of unspecified site of right lower limb, except ankle and foot   `CC` `H5` `SW`

√7ᵗʰ **T24.302** Burn of third degree of unspecified site of left lower limb, except ankle and foot   `CC` `H5` `SW`

√7ᵗʰ **T24.309** Burn of third degree of unspecified site of unspecified lower limb, except ankle and foot   `CC` `H5` `SW`

√6ᵗʰ **T24.31** Burn of third degree of thigh

     CC Excl: For CC codes in subcategory T24.31: PDX collection 1405

     √7ᵗʰ **T24.311** Burn of third degree of right thigh   `CC` `H5` `SW`

     √7ᵗʰ **T24.312** Burn of third degree of left thigh   `CC` `H5` `SW`

     √7ᵗʰ **T24.319** Burn of third degree of unspecified thigh   `CC` `H5` `SW`

√6ᵗʰ **T24.32** Burn of third degree of knee

     CC Excl: For CC codes in subcategory T24.32: PDX collection 1406

     √7ᵗʰ **T24.321** Burn of third degree of right knee   `CC` `H5` `SW`

     √7ᵗʰ **T24.322** Burn of third degree of left knee   `CC` `H5` `SW`

     √7ᵗʰ **T24.329** Burn of third degree of unspecified knee   `CC` `H5` `SW`

√6ᵗʰ **T24.33** Burn of third degree of lower leg

     CC Excl: For CC codes in subcategory T24.33: PDX collection 1407

     √7ᵗʰ **T24.331** Burn of third degree of right lower leg   `CC` `H5` `SW`

     √7ᵗʰ **T24.332** Burn of third degree of left lower leg   `CC` `H5` `SW`

     √7ᵗʰ **T24.339** Burn of third degree of unspecified lower leg   `CC` `H5` `SW`

√6ᵗʰ **T24.39** Burn of third degree of multiple sites of lower limb, except ankle and foot

     AHA: 2016,2Q,4

     CC Excl: For CC codes in subcategory T24.39: PDX collection 1404

     √7ᵗʰ **T24.391** Burn of third degree of multiple sites of right lower limb, except ankle and foot   `CC` `H5` `SW`

     √7ᵗʰ **T24.392** Burn of third degree of multiple sites of left lower limb, except ankle and foot   `CC` `H5` `SW`

     √7ᵗʰ **T24.399** Burn of third degree of multiple sites of unspecified lower limb, except ankle and foot   `CC` `H5` `SW`

√5ᵗʰ **T24.4** Corrosion of unspecified degree of lower limb, except ankle and foot

     Code first (T51-T65) to identify chemical and intent

     Use additional external cause code to identify place (Y92)

     √6ᵗʰ **T24.40** Corrosion of unspecified degree of unspecified site of lower limb, except ankle and foot

         √7ᵗʰ **T24.401** Corrosion of unspecified degree of unspecified site of right lower limb, except ankle and foot

         √7ᵗʰ **T24.402** Corrosion of unspecified degree of unspecified site of left lower limb, except ankle and foot

         √7ᵗʰ **T24.409** Corrosion of unspecified degree of unspecified site of unspecified lower limb, except ankle and foot

     √6ᵗʰ **T24.41** Corrosion of unspecified degree of thigh

         √7ᵗʰ **T24.411** Corrosion of unspecified degree of right thigh

         √7ᵗʰ **T24.412** Corrosion of unspecified degree of left thigh

         √7ᵗʰ **T24.419** Corrosion of unspecified degree of unspecified thigh

     √6ᵗʰ **T24.42** Corrosion of unspecified degree of knee

         √7ᵗʰ **T24.421** Corrosion of unspecified degree of right knee

         √7ᵗʰ **T24.422** Corrosion of unspecified degree of left knee

         √7ᵗʰ **T24.429** Corrosion of unspecified degree of unspecified knee

     √6ᵗʰ **T24.43** Corrosion of unspecified degree of lower leg

         √7ᵗʰ **T24.431** Corrosion of unspecified degree of right lower leg

         √7ᵗʰ **T24.432** Corrosion of unspecified degree of left lower leg

         √7ᵗʰ **T24.439** Corrosion of unspecified degree of unspecified lower leg

√6ᵗʰ **T24.49** Corrosion of unspecified degree of multiple sites of lower limb, except ankle and foot

     √7ᵗʰ **T24.491** Corrosion of unspecified degree of multiple sites of right lower limb, except ankle and foot

     √7ᵗʰ **T24.492** Corrosion of unspecified degree of multiple sites of left lower limb, except ankle and foot

     √7ᵗʰ **T24.499** Corrosion of unspecified degree of multiple sites of unspecified lower limb, except ankle and foot

√5ᵗʰ **T24.5** Corrosion of first degree of lower limb, except ankle and foot

     Code first (T51-T65) to identify chemical and intent

     Use additional external cause code to identify place (Y92)

     √6ᵗʰ **T24.50** Corrosion of first degree of unspecified site of lower limb, except ankle and foot

         √7ᵗʰ **T24.501** Corrosion of first degree of unspecified site of right lower limb, except ankle and foot

         √7ᵗʰ **T24.502** Corrosion of first degree of unspecified site of left lower limb, except ankle and foot

         √7ᵗʰ **T24.509** Corrosion of first degree of unspecified site of unspecified lower limb, except ankle and foot

     √6ᵗʰ **T24.51** Corrosion of first degree of thigh

         √7ᵗʰ **T24.511** Corrosion of first degree of right thigh

         √7ᵗʰ **T24.512** Corrosion of first degree of left thigh

         √7ᵗʰ **T24.519** Corrosion of first degree of unspecified thigh

     √6ᵗʰ **T24.52** Corrosion of first degree of knee

         √7ᵗʰ **T24.521** Corrosion of first degree of right knee

         √7ᵗʰ **T24.522** Corrosion of first degree of left knee

         √7ᵗʰ **T24.529** Corrosion of first degree of unspecified knee

     √6ᵗʰ **T24.53** Corrosion of first degree of lower leg

         √7ᵗʰ **T24.531** Corrosion of first degree of right lower leg

         √7ᵗʰ **T24.532** Corrosion of first degree of left lower leg

         √7ᵗʰ **T24.539** Corrosion of first degree of unspecified lower leg

     √6ᵗʰ **T24.59** Corrosion of first degree of multiple sites of lower limb, except ankle and foot

         √7ᵗʰ **T24.591** Corrosion of first degree of multiple sites of right lower limb, except ankle and foot

         √7ᵗʰ **T24.592** Corrosion of first degree of multiple sites of left lower limb, except ankle and foot

         √7ᵗʰ **T24.599** Corrosion of first degree of multiple sites of unspecified lower limb, except ankle and foot

√5ᵗʰ **T24.6** Corrosion of second degree of lower limb, except ankle and foot

     Code first (T51-T65) to identify chemical and intent

     Use additional external cause code to identify place (Y92)

     √6ᵗʰ **T24.60** Corrosion of second degree of unspecified site of lower limb, except ankle and foot

         √7ᵗʰ **T24.601** Corrosion of second degree of unspecified site of right lower limb, except ankle and foot

         √7ᵗʰ **T24.602** Corrosion of second degree of unspecified site of left lower limb, except ankle and foot

         √7ᵗʰ **T24.609** Corrosion of second degree of unspecified site of unspecified lower limb, except ankle and foot

     √6ᵗʰ **T24.61** Corrosion of second degree of thigh

         √7ᵗʰ **T24.611** Corrosion of second degree of right thigh

         √7ᵗʰ **T24.612** Corrosion of second degree of left thigh

         √7ᵗʰ **T24.619** Corrosion of second degree of unspecified thigh

     √6ᵗʰ **T24.62** Corrosion of second degree of knee

         √7ᵗʰ **T24.621** Corrosion of second degree of right knee

         √7ᵗʰ **T24.622** Corrosion of second degree of left knee

         √7ᵗʰ **T24.629** Corrosion of second degree of unspecified knee

     √6ᵗʰ **T24.63** Corrosion of second degree of lower leg

         √7ᵗʰ **T24.631** Corrosion of second degree of right lower leg

---

☑ Additional Character Required   √ˣ7ᵗʰ Placeholder   Unacceptable PDx   Questionable PDx   Manifestation   Unspecified Dx   `H1`-`H14` HAC   `HCC` CMS-HCC Dx   `HIV` HIV Dx

Chapter 19. Injury, Poisoning and Certain Other Consequences of External Causes

T24.632–T25.222

☑7ᵗʰ **T24.632** Corrosion of second degree of left lower leg

☑7ᵗʰ **T24.639** Corrosion of second degree of unspecified lower leg

☑6ᵗʰ **T24.69** Corrosion of second degree of multiple sites of lower limb, except ankle and foot

☑7ᵗʰ **T24.691** Corrosion of second degree of multiple sites of right lower limb, except ankle and foot

☑7ᵗʰ **T24.692** Corrosion of second degree of multiple sites of left lower limb, except ankle and foot

☑7ᵗʰ **T24.699** Corrosion of second degree of multiple sites of unspecified lower limb, except ankle and foot

☑5ᵗʰ **T24.7** Corrosion of third degree of lower limb, except ankle and foot

Code first (T51-T65) to identify chemical and intent
Use additional external cause code to identify place (Y92)

☑6ᵗʰ **T24.70** Corrosion of third degree of unspecified site of lower limb, except ankle and foot

CC Excl: For CC codes in subcategory T24.70: PDX collection 1404

☑7ᵗʰ **T24.701** Corrosion of third degree of unspecified site of right lower limb, except ankle and foot   CC H5 SW

☑7ᵗʰ **T24.702** Corrosion of third degree of unspecified site of left lower limb, except ankle and foot   CC H5 SW

☑7ᵗʰ **T24.709** Corrosion of third degree of unspecified site of unspecified lower limb, except ankle and foot   CC H5 SW

☑6ᵗʰ **T24.71** Corrosion of third degree of thigh

CC Excl: For CC codes in subcategory T24.71: PDX collection 1405

☑7ᵗʰ **T24.711** Corrosion of third degree of right thigh   CC H5 SW

☑7ᵗʰ **T24.712** Corrosion of third degree of left thigh   CC H5 SW

☑7ᵗʰ **T24.719** Corrosion of third degree of unspecified thigh   CC H5 SW

☑6ᵗʰ **T24.72** Corrosion of third degree of knee

CC Excl: For CC codes in subcategory T24.72: PDX collection 1406

☑7ᵗʰ **T24.721** Corrosion of third degree of right knee   CC H5 SW

☑7ᵗʰ **T24.722** Corrosion of third degree of left knee   CC H5 SW

☑7ᵗʰ **T24.729** Corrosion of third degree of unspecified knee   CC H5 SW

☑6ᵗʰ **T24.73** Corrosion of third degree of lower leg

CC Excl: For CC codes in subcategory T24.73: PDX collection 1407

☑7ᵗʰ **T24.731** Corrosion of third degree of right lower leg   CC H5 SW

☑7ᵗʰ **T24.732** Corrosion of third degree of left lower leg   CC H5 SW

☑7ᵗʰ **T24.739** Corrosion of third degree of unspecified lower leg   CC H5 SW

☑6ᵗʰ **T24.79** Corrosion of third degree of multiple sites of lower limb, except ankle and foot

CC Excl: For CC codes in subcategory T24.79: PDX collection 1404

☑7ᵗʰ **T24.791** Corrosion of third degree of multiple sites of right lower limb, except ankle and foot   CC H5 SW

☑7ᵗʰ **T24.792** Corrosion of third degree of multiple sites of left lower limb, except ankle and foot   CC H5 SW

☑7ᵗʰ **T24.799** Corrosion of third degree of multiple sites of unspecified lower limb, except ankle and foot   CC H5 SW

☑4ᵗʰ **T25** Burn and corrosion of ankle and foot

The appropriate 7th character is to be added to each code from category T25.
A   initial encounter
D   subsequent encounter
S   sequela

☑5ᵗʰ **T25.0** Burn of unspecified degree of ankle and foot

Use additional external cause code to identify the source, place and intent of the burn (X00-X19, X75-X77, X96-X98, Y92)

☑6ᵗʰ **T25.01** Burn of unspecified degree of ankle

☑7ᵗʰ **T25.011** Burn of unspecified degree of right ankle

☑7ᵗʰ **T25.012** Burn of unspecified degree of left ankle

☑7ᵗʰ **T25.019** Burn of unspecified degree of unspecified ankle

☑6ᵗʰ **T25.02** Burn of unspecified degree of foot

EXCLUDES 2   burn of unspecified degree of toe(s) (nail) (T25.03-)

☑7ᵗʰ **T25.021** Burn of unspecified degree of right foot

☑7ᵗʰ **T25.022** Burn of unspecified degree of left foot

☑7ᵗʰ **T25.029** Burn of unspecified degree of unspecified foot

☑6ᵗʰ **T25.03** Burn of unspecified degree of toe(s) (nail)

☑7ᵗʰ **T25.031** Burn of unspecified degree of right toe(s) (nail)

☑7ᵗʰ **T25.032** Burn of unspecified degree of left toe(s) (nail)

☑7ᵗʰ **T25.039** Burn of unspecified degree of unspecified toe(s) (nail)

☑6ᵗʰ **T25.09** Burn of unspecified degree of multiple sites of ankle and foot

☑7ᵗʰ **T25.091** Burn of unspecified degree of multiple sites of right ankle and foot

☑7ᵗʰ **T25.092** Burn of unspecified degree of multiple sites of left ankle and foot

☑7ᵗʰ **T25.099** Burn of unspecified degree of multiple sites of unspecified ankle and foot

☑5ᵗʰ **T25.1** Burn of first degree of ankle and foot

Use additional external cause code to identify the source, place and intent of the burn (X00-X19, X75-X77, X96-X98, Y92)

☑6ᵗʰ **T25.11** Burn of first degree of ankle

☑7ᵗʰ **T25.111** Burn of first degree of right ankle

☑7ᵗʰ **T25.112** Burn of first degree of left ankle

☑7ᵗʰ **T25.119** Burn of first degree of unspecified ankle

☑6ᵗʰ **T25.12** Burn of first degree of foot

EXCLUDES 2   burn of first degree of toe(s) (nail) (T25.13-)

☑7ᵗʰ **T25.121** Burn of first degree of right foot

☑7ᵗʰ **T25.122** Burn of first degree of left foot

☑7ᵗʰ **T25.129** Burn of first degree of unspecified foot

☑6ᵗʰ **T25.13** Burn of first degree of toe(s) (nail)

☑7ᵗʰ **T25.131** Burn of first degree of right toe(s) (nail)

☑7ᵗʰ **T25.132** Burn of first degree of left toe(s) (nail)

☑7ᵗʰ **T25.139** Burn of first degree of unspecified toe(s) (nail)

☑6ᵗʰ **T25.19** Burn of first degree of multiple sites of ankle and foot

☑7ᵗʰ **T25.191** Burn of first degree of multiple sites of right ankle and foot

☑7ᵗʰ **T25.192** Burn of first degree of multiple sites of left ankle and foot

☑7ᵗʰ **T25.199** Burn of first degree of multiple sites of unspecified ankle and foot

☑5ᵗʰ **T25.2** Burn of second degree of ankle and foot

Use additional external cause code to identify the source, place and intent of the burn (X00-X19, X75-X77, X96-X98, Y92)

☑6ᵗʰ **T25.21** Burn of second degree of ankle

☑7ᵗʰ **T25.211** Burn of second degree of right ankle

☑7ᵗʰ **T25.212** Burn of second degree of left ankle

☑7ᵗʰ **T25.219** Burn of second degree of unspecified ankle

☑6ᵗʰ **T25.22** Burn of second degree of foot

EXCLUDES 2   burn of second degree of toe(s) (nail) (T25.23-)

☑7ᵗʰ **T25.221** Burn of second degree of right foot

☑7ᵗʰ **T25.222** Burn of second degree of left foot

√7ᵗʰ **T25.229** Burn of second degree of unspecified foot

√6ᵗʰ **T25.23** Burn of second degree of toe(s) (nail)

√7ᵗʰ **T25.231** Burn of second degree of right toe(s) (nail)

√7ᵗʰ **T25.232** Burn of second degree of left toe(s) (nail)

√7ᵗʰ **T25.239** Burn of second degree of unspecified toe(s) (nail)

√6ᵗʰ **T25.29** Burn of second degree of multiple sites of ankle and foot

√7ᵗʰ **T25.291** Burn of second degree of multiple sites of right ankle and foot

√7ᵗʰ **T25.292** Burn of second degree of multiple sites of left ankle and foot

√7ᵗʰ **T25.299** Burn of second degree of multiple sites of unspecified ankle and foot

√5ᵗʰ **T25.3** Burn of third degree of ankle and foot

Use additional external cause code to identify the source, place and intent of the burn (X00-X19, X75-X77, X96-X98, Y92)

√6ᵗʰ **T25.31** Burn of third degree of ankle

CC Excl: For CC codes in subcategory T25.31: PDX collection 1408

√7ᵗʰ **T25.311** Burn of third degree of right ankle   CC H5 SW

√7ᵗʰ **T25.312** Burn of third degree of left ankle   CC H5 SW

√7ᵗʰ **T25.319** Burn of third degree of unspecified ankle   CC H5 SW

√6ᵗʰ **T25.32** Burn of third degree of foot

EXCLUDES 2   burn of third degree of toe(s) (nail) (T25.33-)

CC Excl: For CC codes in subcategory T25.32: PDX collection 1409

√7ᵗʰ **T25.321** Burn of third degree of right foot   CC H5 SW

√7ᵗʰ **T25.322** Burn of third degree of left foot   CC H5 SW

√7ᵗʰ **T25.329** Burn of third degree of unspecified foot   CC H5 SW

√6ᵗʰ **T25.33** Burn of third degree of toe(s) (nail)

CC Excl: For CC codes in subcategory T25.33: PDX collection 1410

√7ᵗʰ **T25.331** Burn of third degree of right toe(s) (nail)   CC H5 SW

√7ᵗʰ **T25.332** Burn of third degree of left toe(s) (nail)   CC H5 SW

√7ᵗʰ **T25.339** Burn of third degree of unspecified toe(s) (nail)   CC H5 SW

√6ᵗʰ **T25.39** Burn of third degree of multiple sites of ankle and foot

CC Excl: For CC codes in subcategory T25.39: PDX collection 1404

√7ᵗʰ **T25.391** Burn of third degree of multiple sites of right ankle and foot   CC H5 SW

√7ᵗʰ **T25.392** Burn of third degree of multiple sites of left ankle and foot   CC H5 SW

√7ᵗʰ **T25.399** Burn of third degree of multiple sites of unspecified ankle and foot   CC H5 SW

√5ᵗʰ **T25.4** Corrosion of unspecified degree of ankle and foot

Code first (T51-T65) to identify chemical and intent

Use additional external cause code to identify place (Y92)

√6ᵗʰ **T25.41** Corrosion of unspecified degree of ankle

√7ᵗʰ **T25.411** Corrosion of unspecified degree of right ankle

√7ᵗʰ **T25.412** Corrosion of unspecified degree of left ankle

√7ᵗʰ **T25.419** Corrosion of unspecified degree of unspecified ankle

√6ᵗʰ **T25.42** Corrosion of unspecified degree of foot

EXCLUDES 2   corrosion of unspecified degree of toe(s) (nail) (T25.43-)

√7ᵗʰ **T25.421** Corrosion of unspecified degree of right foot

√7ᵗʰ **T25.422** Corrosion of unspecified degree of left foot

√7ᵗʰ **T25.429** Corrosion of unspecified degree of unspecified foot

√6ᵗʰ **T25.43** Corrosion of unspecified degree of toe(s) (nail)

√7ᵗʰ **T25.431** Corrosion of unspecified degree of right toe(s) (nail)

√7ᵗʰ **T25.432** Corrosion of unspecified degree of left toe(s) (nail)

√7ᵗʰ **T25.439** Corrosion of unspecified degree of unspecified toe(s) (nail)

√6ᵗʰ **T25.49** Corrosion of unspecified degree of multiple sites of ankle and foot

√7ᵗʰ **T25.491** Corrosion of unspecified degree of multiple sites of right ankle and foot

√7ᵗʰ **T25.492** Corrosion of unspecified degree of multiple sites of left ankle and foot

√7ᵗʰ **T25.499** Corrosion of unspecified degree of multiple sites of unspecified ankle and foot

√5ᵗʰ **T25.5** Corrosion of first degree of ankle and foot

Code first (T51-T65) to identify chemical and intent

Use additional external cause code to identify place (Y92)

√6ᵗʰ **T25.51** Corrosion of first degree of ankle

√7ᵗʰ **T25.511** Corrosion of first degree of right ankle

√7ᵗʰ **T25.512** Corrosion of first degree of left ankle

√7ᵗʰ **T25.519** Corrosion of first degree of unspecified ankle

√6ᵗʰ **T25.52** Corrosion of first degree of foot

EXCLUDES 2   corrosion of first degree of toe(s) (nail) (T25.53-)

√7ᵗʰ **T25.521** Corrosion of first degree of right foot

√7ᵗʰ **T25.522** Corrosion of first degree of left foot

√7ᵗʰ **T25.529** Corrosion of first degree of unspecified foot

√6ᵗʰ **T25.53** Corrosion of first degree of toe(s) (nail)

√7ᵗʰ **T25.531** Corrosion of first degree of right toe(s) (nail)

√7ᵗʰ **T25.532** Corrosion of first degree of left toe(s) (nail)

√7ᵗʰ **T25.539** Corrosion of first degree of unspecified toe(s) (nail)

√6ᵗʰ **T25.59** Corrosion of first degree of multiple sites of ankle and foot

√7ᵗʰ **T25.591** Corrosion of first degree of multiple sites of right ankle and foot

√7ᵗʰ **T25.592** Corrosion of first degree of multiple sites of left ankle and foot

√7ᵗʰ **T25.599** Corrosion of first degree of multiple sites of unspecified ankle and foot

√5ᵗʰ **T25.6** Corrosion of second degree of ankle and foot

Code first (T51-T65) to identify chemical and intent

Use additional external cause code to identify place (Y92)

√6ᵗʰ **T25.61** Corrosion of second degree of ankle

√7ᵗʰ **T25.611** Corrosion of second degree of right ankle

√7ᵗʰ **T25.612** Corrosion of second degree of left ankle

√7ᵗʰ **T25.619** Corrosion of second degree of unspecified ankle

√6ᵗʰ **T25.62** Corrosion of second degree of foot

EXCLUDES 2   corrosion of second degree of toe(s) (nail) (T25.63-)

√7ᵗʰ **T25.621** Corrosion of second degree of right foot

√7ᵗʰ **T25.622** Corrosion of second degree of left foot

√7ᵗʰ **T25.629** Corrosion of second degree of unspecified foot

√6ᵗʰ **T25.63** Corrosion of second degree of toe(s) (nail)

√7ᵗʰ **T25.631** Corrosion of second degree of right toe(s) (nail)

√7ᵗʰ **T25.632** Corrosion of second degree of left toe(s) (nail)

√7ᵗʰ **T25.639** Corrosion of second degree of unspecified toe(s) (nail)

√6ᵗʰ **T25.69** Corrosion of second degree of multiple sites of ankle and foot

√7ᵗʰ **T25.691** Corrosion of second degree of right ankle and foot

√7ᵗʰ **T25.692** Corrosion of second degree of left ankle and foot

√7ᵗʰ **T25.699** Corrosion of second degree of unspecified ankle and foot

✔ Additional Character Required   √x7ᵗʰ Placeholder   Unacceptable PDx   Questionable PDx   Manifestation   Unspecified Dx   H1-H14 HAC   HCC CMS-HCC Dx   HIV HIV Dx

ICD-10-CM 2020   1143

√5ᵗʰ T25.7 Corrosion of third degree of ankle and foot

Code first (T51-T65) to identify chemical and intent
Use additional external cause code to identify place (Y92)

√6ᵗʰ T25.71 Corrosion of third degree of ankle

CC Excl: For CC codes in subcategory T25.71: PDX collection 1408

√7ᵗʰ **T25.711 Corrosion of third degree of right ankle** `CC` `H5` `SW`

√7ᵗʰ **T25.712 Corrosion of third degree of left ankle** `CC` `H5` `SW`

√7ᵗʰ **T25.719 Corrosion of third degree of unspecified ankle** `CC` `H5` `SW`

√6ᵗʰ T25.72 Corrosion of third degree of foot

EXCLUDES 2   corrosion of third degree of toe(s) (nail) (T25.73-)

CC Excl: For CC codes in subcategory T25.72: PDX collection 1409

√7ᵗʰ **T25.721 Corrosion of third degree of right foot** `CC` `H5` `SW`

√7ᵗʰ **T25.722 Corrosion of third degree of left foot** `CC` `H5` `SW`

√7ᵗʰ **T25.729 Corrosion of third degree of unspecified foot** `CC` `H5` `SW`

√6ᵗʰ T25.73 Corrosion of third degree of toe(s) (nail)

CC Excl: For CC codes in subcategory T25.73: PDX collection 1410

√7ᵗʰ **T25.731 Corrosion of third degree of right toe(s) (nail)** `CC` `H5` `SW`

√7ᵗʰ **T25.732 Corrosion of third degree of left toe(s) (nail)** `CC` `H5` `SW`

√7ᵗʰ **T25.739 Corrosion of third degree of unspecified toe(s) (nail)** `CC` `H5` `SW`

√6ᵗʰ T25.79 Corrosion of third degree of multiple sites of ankle and foot

CC Excl: For CC codes in subcategory T25.79: PDX collection 1404

√7ᵗʰ **T25.791 Corrosion of third degree of multiple sites of right ankle and foot** `CC` `H5` `SW`

√7ᵗʰ **T25.792 Corrosion of third degree of multiple sites of left ankle and foot** `CC` `H5` `SW`

√7ᵗʰ **T25.799 Corrosion of third degree of multiple sites of unspecified ankle and foot** `CC` `H5` `SW`

Burns and corrosions confined to eye and internal organs (T26-T28)

√4ᵗʰ T26 Burn and corrosion confined to eye and adnexa

The appropriate 7th character is to be added to each code from category T26.
A   initial encounter
D   subsequent encounter
S   sequela

√5ᵗʰ T26.0 Burn of eyelid and periocular area

Use additional external cause code to identify the source, place and intent of the burn (X00-X19, X75-X77, X96-X98, Y92)

√x7ᵗʰ **T26.00 Burn of unspecified eyelid and periocular area**

√x7ᵗʰ **T26.01 Burn of right eyelid and periocular area**

√x7ᵗʰ **T26.02 Burn of left eyelid and periocular area**

√5ᵗʰ T26.1 Burn of cornea and conjunctival sac

Use additional external cause code to identify the source, place and intent of the burn (X00-X19, X75-X77, X96-X98, Y92)

√x7ᵗʰ **T26.10 Burn of cornea and conjunctival sac, unspecified eye**

√x7ᵗʰ **T26.11 Burn of cornea and conjunctival sac, right eye**

√x7ᵗʰ **T26.12 Burn of cornea and conjunctival sac, left eye**

√5ᵗʰ T26.2 Burn with resulting rupture and destruction of eyeball

Use additional external cause code to identify the source, place and intent of the burn (X00-X19, X75-X77, X96-X98, Y92)

√x7ᵗʰ **T26.20 Burn with resulting rupture and destruction of unspecified eyeball** `CC` `H5`
CC Excl: No Excl

√x7ᵗʰ **T26.21 Burn with resulting rupture and destruction of right eyeball** `CC` `H5`
CC Excl: No Excl

√x7ᵗʰ **T26.22 Burn with resulting rupture and destruction of left eyeball** `CC` `H5`
CC Excl: No Excl

√5ᵗʰ T26.3 Burns of other specified parts of eye and adnexa

Use additional external cause code to identify the source, place and intent of the burn (X00-X19, X75-X77, X96-X98, Y92)

√x7ᵗʰ **T26.30 Burns of other specified parts of unspecified eye and adnexa**

√x7ᵗʰ **T26.31 Burns of other specified parts of right eye and adnexa**

√x7ᵗʰ **T26.32 Burns of other specified parts of left eye and adnexa**

√5ᵗʰ T26.4 Burn of eye and adnexa, part unspecified

Use additional external cause code to identify the source, place and intent of the burn (X00-X19, X75-X77, X96-X98, Y92)

√x7ᵗʰ **T26.40 Burn of unspecified eye and adnexa, part unspecified**

√x7ᵗʰ **T26.41 Burn of right eye and adnexa, part unspecified**

√x7ᵗʰ **T26.42 Burn of left eye and adnexa, part unspecified**

√5ᵗʰ T26.5 Corrosion of eyelid and periocular area

Code first (T51-T65) to identify chemical and intent
Use additional external cause code to identify place (Y92)

√x7ᵗʰ **T26.50 Corrosion of unspecified eyelid and periocular area**

√x7ᵗʰ **T26.51 Corrosion of right eyelid and periocular area**

√x7ᵗʰ **T26.52 Corrosion of left eyelid and periocular area**

√5ᵗʰ T26.6 Corrosion of cornea and conjunctival sac

Code first (T51-T65) to identify chemical and intent
Use additional external cause code to identify place (Y92)

√x7ᵗʰ **T26.60 Corrosion of cornea and conjunctival sac, unspecified eye**

√x7ᵗʰ **T26.61 Corrosion of cornea and conjunctival sac, right eye**

√x7ᵗʰ **T26.62 Corrosion of cornea and conjunctival sac, left eye**

√5ᵗʰ T26.7 Corrosion with resulting rupture and destruction of eyeball

Code first (T51-T65) to identify chemical and intent
Use additional external cause code to identify place (Y92)

√x7ᵗʰ **T26.70 Corrosion with resulting rupture and destruction of unspecified eyeball** `CC` `H5`
CC Excl: No Excl

√x7ᵗʰ **T26.71 Corrosion with resulting rupture and destruction of right eyeball** `CC` `H5`
CC Excl: No Excl

√x7ᵗʰ **T26.72 Corrosion with resulting rupture and destruction of left eyeball** `CC` `H5`
CC Excl: No Excl

√5ᵗʰ T26.8 Corrosions of other specified parts of eye and adnexa

Code first (T51-T65) to identify chemical and intent
Use additional external cause code to identify place (Y92)

√x7ᵗʰ **T26.80 Corrosions of other specified parts of unspecified eye and adnexa**

√x7ᵗʰ **T26.81 Corrosions of other specified parts of right eye and adnexa**

√x7ᵗʰ **T26.82 Corrosions of other specified parts of left eye and adnexa**

√5ᵗʰ T26.9 Corrosion of eye and adnexa, part unspecified

Code first (T51-T65) to identify chemical and intent
Use additional external cause code to identify place (Y92)

√x7ᵗʰ **T26.90 Corrosion of unspecified eye and adnexa, part unspecified**

√x7ᵗʰ **T26.91 Corrosion of right eye and adnexa, part unspecified**

√x7ᵗʰ **T26.92 Corrosion of left eye and adnexa, part unspecified**

√4ᵗʰ T27 Burn and corrosion of respiratory tract

Use additional external cause code to identify the source and intent of the burn (X00-X19, X75-X77, X96-X98)
Use additional external cause code to identify place (Y92)

The appropriate 7th character is to be added to each code from category T27.
A   initial encounter
D   subsequent encounter
S   sequela

CC Excl: For CC codes in category T27: PDX collection 1411

√x7ᵗʰ **T27.0 Burn of larynx and trachea** `CC` `H5`

√x7ᵗʰ **T27.1 Burn involving larynx and trachea with lung** `CC` `H5`

√x7ᵗʰ **T27.2 Burn of other parts of respiratory tract** `CC` `H5`

Burn of thoracic cavity

√x7ᵗʰ **T27.3 Burn of respiratory tract, part unspecified** `CC` `H5`

`N` Newborn: 0   `P` Pediatric: 0-17   `M` Maternity: 9-64   `A` Adult: 15-124   `MCC` Major Complication/Comorbidity   `CC` Complication/Comorbidity   `SW` Severe Wound Dx

1144   ICD-10-CM 2020

√x7ᵗʰ **T27.4** **Corrosion** of **larynx and trachea**   CC H5
     Code first (T51-T65) to identify chemical and intent

√x7ᵗʰ **T27.5** **Corrosion involving** **larynx and trachea with**   CC H5
     lung
     ▶Code first (T51-T65) to identify chemical and intent◀

√x7ᵗʰ **T27.6** **Corrosion** of **other parts of respiratory tract**   CC H5
     Code first (T51-T65) to identify chemical and intent

√x7ᵗʰ **T27.7** **Corrosion** of **respiratory tract, part**   CC H5
     unspecified
     Code first (T51-T65) to identify chemical and intent

√4ᵗʰ **T28** **Burn and corrosion of other internal organs**
     Use additional external cause code to identify the source and intent of
         the burn (X00-X19, X75-X77, X96-X98)
     Use additional external cause code to identify place (Y92)

     The appropriate 7th character is to be added to each code from
     category T28.
     A   initial encounter
     D   subsequent encounter
     S   sequela

√x7ᵗʰ **T28.0** **Burn** of **mouth and pharynx**

√x7ᵗʰ **T28.1** **Burn** of **esophagus**   CC H5
     CC Excl: PDX collection 1412

√x7ᵗʰ **T28.2** **Burn** of **other parts of alimentary tract**   CC H5
     CC Excl: PDX collection 1413

√x7ᵗʰ **T28.3** **Burn** of **internal genitourinary organs**

√5ᵗʰ **T28.4** **Burns** of **other and unspecified internal organs**
     Code first (T51-T65) to identify chemical and intent

     √x7ᵗʰ **T28.40** **Burn of unspecified internal organ**

     √6ᵗʰ **T28.41** **Burn** of **ear drum**

         √7ᵗʰ **T28.411** **Burn of right ear drum**

         √7ᵗʰ **T28.412** **Burn of left ear drum**

         √7ᵗʰ **T28.419** **Burn of unspecified ear drum**

     √x7ᵗʰ **T28.49** **Burn of other internal organ**

√x7ᵗʰ **T28.5** **Corrosion** of **mouth and pharynx**
     Code first (T51-T65) to identify chemical and intent

√x7ᵗʰ **T28.6** **Corrosion** of **esophagus**   CC H5
     Code first (T51-T65) to identify chemical and intent
     CC Excl: PDX collection 1412

√x7ᵗʰ **T28.7** **Corrosion** of **other parts of alimentary tract**   CC H5
     Code first (T51-T65) to identify chemical and intent
     CC Excl: PDX collection 1413

√x7ᵗʰ **T28.8** **Corrosion** of **internal genitourinary organs**
     Code first (T51-T65) to identify chemical and intent

√5ᵗʰ **T28.9** **Corrosions** of **other and unspecified internal organs**
     Code first (T51-T65) to identify chemical and intent

     √x7ᵗʰ **T28.90** **Corrosions of unspecified internal organs**

     √6ᵗʰ **T28.91** **Corrosions** of **ear drum**

         √7ᵗʰ **T28.911** **Corrosions of right ear drum**

         √7ᵗʰ **T28.912** **Corrosions of left ear drum**

         √7ᵗʰ **T28.919** **Corrosions of unspecified ear drum**

     √x7ᵗʰ **T28.99** **Corrosions of other internal organs**

Burns and corrosions of multiple and unspecified body regions (T30-T32)

CC Excl: For CC/MCC codes in categories T30-T32: PDX collection 1414

√4ᵗʰ **T30** **Burn and corrosion, body region unspecified**

     T30.0 **Burn** of **unspecified body region, unspecified degree**
         This code is not for inpatient use. Code to specified site and
             degree of burns
         Burn NOS
         Multiple burns NOS

     T30.4 **Corrosion** of **unspecified body region, unspecified degree**
         This code is not for inpatient use. Code to specified site and
             degree of corrosion
         Corrosion NOS
         Multiple corrosion NOS

√4ᵗʰ **T31** **Burns classified according to extent of body surface involved**

     NOTE   This category is to be used as the primary code only when
         the site of the burn is unspecified. It should be used as a
         supplementary code with categories T20-T25 when the site
         is specified.

     T31.0 **Burns involving less than 10% of body surface**

     √5ᵗʰ **T31.1** **Burns involving 10-19% of body surface**

         T31.10 **Burns involving 10-19% of body**   CC H5
             surface with 0% to 9% third degree
             burns
                 Burns involving 10-19% of body surface NOS

         T31.11 **Burns involving 10-19% of body**   CC H5 HCC
             surface with 10-19% third degree
             burns

     √5ᵗʰ **T31.2** **Burns involving 20-29% of body surface**

         T31.20 **Burns involving 20-29% of body**   CC H5
             surface with 0% to 9% third degree
             burns
                 Burns involving 20-29% of body surface NOS

         T31.21 **Burns involving 20-29% of body**   MCC H5 HCC
             surface with 10-19% third degree
             burns

         T31.22 **Burns involving 20-29% of body**   MCC H5 HCC
             surface with 20-29% third degree
             burns

     √5ᵗʰ **T31.3** **Burns involving 30-39% of body surface**

         T31.30 **Burns involving 30-39% of body**   CC H5
             surface with 0% to 9% third degree
             burns
                 Burns involving 30-39% of body surface NOS

         T31.31 **Burns involving 30-39% of body**   MCC H5 HCC
             surface with 10-19% third degree
             burns

         T31.32 **Burns involving 30-39% of body**   MCC H5 HCC
             surface with 20-29% third degree
             burns

         T31.33 **Burns involving 30-39% of body**   MCC H5 HCC
             surface with 30-39% third degree
             burns

     √5ᵗʰ **T31.4** **Burns involving 40-49% of body surface**

         T31.40 **Burns involving 40-49% of body**   CC H5
             surface with 0% to 9% third degree
             burns
                 Burns involving 40-49% of body surface NOS

         T31.41 **Burns involving 40-49% of body**   MCC H5 HCC
             surface with 10-19% third degree
             burns

         T31.42 **Burns involving 40-49% of body**   MCC H5 HCC
             surface with 20-29% third degree
             burns

         T31.43 **Burns involving 40-49% of body**   MCC H5 HCC
             surface with 30-39% third degree
             burns

         T31.44 **Burns involving 40-49% of body**   MCC H5 HCC
             surface with 40-49% third degree
             burns

     √5ᵗʰ **T31.5** **Burns involving 50-59% of body surface**

         T31.50 **Burns involving 50-59% of body**   CC H5
             surface with 0% to 9% third degree
             burns
                 Burns involving 50-59% of body surface NOS

         T31.51 **Burns involving 50-59% of body**   MCC H5 HCC
             surface with 10-19% third degree
             burns

         T31.52 **Burns involving 50-59% of body**   MCC H5 HCC
             surface with 20-29% third degree
             burns

         T31.53 **Burns involving 50-59% of body**   MCC H5 HCC
             surface with 30-39% third degree
             burns

         T31.54 **Burns involving 50-59% of body**   MCC H5 HCC
             surface with 40-49% third degree
             burns

         T31.55 **Burns involving 50-59% of body**   MCC H5 HCC
             surface with 50-59% third degree
             burns

✓5th **T31.6** Burns involving 60-69% of body surface

T31.60 Burns involving 60-69% of body surface with 0% to 9% third degree burns   CC H5
  Burns involving 60-69% of body surface NOS

T31.61 Burns involving 60-69% of body surface with 10-19% third degree burns   MCC H5 HCC

T31.62 Burns involving 60-69% of body surface with 20-29% third degree burns   MCC H5 HCC

T31.63 Burns involving 60-69% of body surface with 30-39% third degree burns   MCC H5 HCC

T31.64 Burns involving 60-69% of body surface with 40-49% third degree burns   MCC H5 HCC

T31.65 Burns involving 60-69% of body surface with 50-59% third degree burns   MCC H5 HCC

T31.66 Burns involving 60-69% of body surface with 60-69% third degree burns   MCC H5 HCC

✓5th **T31.7** Burns involving 70-79% of body surface

T31.70 Burns involving 70-79% of body surface with 0% to 9% third degree burns   CC H5
  Burns involving 70-79% of body surface NOS

T31.71 Burns involving 70-79% of body surface with 10-19% third degree burns   MCC H5 HCC

T31.72 Burns involving 70-79% of body surface with 20-29% third degree burns   MCC H5 HCC

T31.73 Burns involving 70-79% of body surface with 30-39% third degree burns   MCC H5 HCC

T31.74 Burns involving 70-79% of body surface with 40-49% third degree burns   MCC H5 HCC

T31.75 Burns involving 70-79% of body surface with 50-59% third degree burns   MCC H5 HCC

T31.76 Burns involving 70-79% of body surface with 60-69% third degree burns   MCC H5 HCC

T31.77 Burns involving 70-79% of body surface with 70-79% third degree burns   MCC H5 HCC

✓5th **T31.8** Burns involving 80-89% of body surface

T31.80 Burns involving 80-89% of body surface with 0% to 9% third degree burns   CC H5
  Burns involving 80-89% of body surface NOS

T31.81 Burns involving 80-89% of body surface with 10-19% third degree burns   MCC H5 HCC

T31.82 Burns involving 80-89% of body surface with 20-29% third degree burns   MCC H5 HCC

T31.83 Burns involving 80-89% of body surface with 30-39% third degree burns   MCC H5 HCC

T31.84 Burns involving 80-89% of body surface with 40-49% third degree burns   MCC H5 HCC

T31.85 Burns involving 80-89% of body surface with 50-59% third degree burns   MCC H5 HCC

T31.86 Burns involving 80-89% of body surface with 60-69% third degree burns   MCC H5 HCC

T31.87 Burns involving 80-89% of body surface with 70-79% third degree burns   MCC H5 HCC

T31.88 Burns involving 80-89% of body surface with 80-89% third degree burns   MCC H5 HCC

✓5th **T31.9** Burns involving 90% or more of body surface

T31.90 Burns involving 90% or more of body surface with 0% to 9% third degree burns   CC H5
  Burns involving 90% or more of body surface NOS

T31.91 Burns involving 90% or more of body surface with 10-19% third degree burns   MCC H5 HCC

T31.92 Burns involving 90% or more of body surface with 20-29% third degree burns   MCC H5 HCC

T31.93 Burns involving 90% or more of body surface with 30-39% third degree burns   MCC H5 HCC

T31.94 Burns involving 90% or more of body surface with 40-49% third degree burns   MCC H5 HCC

T31.95 Burns involving 90% or more of body surface with 50-59% third degree burns   MCC H5 HCC

T31.96 Burns involving 90% or more of body surface with 60-69% third degree burns   MCC H5 HCC

T31.97 Burns involving 90% or more of body surface with 70-79% third degree burns   MCC H5 HCC

T31.98 Burns involving 90% or more of body surface with 80-89% third degree burns   MCC H5 HCC

T31.99 Burns involving 90% or more of body surface with 90% or more third degree burns   MCC H5 HCC

Rule of Nines Estimation of Total Body Surface Burned

Head and neck 9%
Each arm 9%
Anterior trunk 18%
Genitalia 1%
Anterior leg 9%
Posterior trunk 18%
Posterior leg 9%

✓4th **T32** **Corrosions classified** according to extent of body surface involved

NOTE This category is to be used as the primary code only when the site of the corrosion is unspecified. It may be used as a supplementary code with categories T20-T25 when the site is specified.

T32.0 Corrosions involving less than 10% of body surface

✓5th **T32.1** Corrosions involving 10-19% of body surface

T32.10 Corrosions involving 10-19% of body surface with 0% to 9% third degree corrosion   CC H5
  Corrosions involving 10-19% of body surface NOS

T32.11 Corrosions involving 10-19% of body surface with 10-19% third degree corrosion   CC H5 HCC

✓5th **T32.2** Corrosions involving 20-29% of body surface

T32.20 Corrosions involving 20-29% of body surface with 0% to 9% third degree corrosion   CC H5

T32.21 Corrosions involving 20-29% of body surface with 10-19% third degree corrosion   MCC H5 HCC

T32.22 Corrosions involving 20-29% of body surface with 20-29% third degree corrosion   MCC H5 HCC

✓5ᵗʰ **T32.3 Corrosions involving 30-39% of body surface**

T32.30 Corrosions involving 30-39% of body surface with 0% to 9% third degree corrosion `CC` `H5`

T32.31 Corrosions involving 30-39% of body surface with 10-19% third degree corrosion `MCC` `H5` `HCC`

T32.32 Corrosions involving 30-39% of body surface with 20-29% third degree corrosion `MCC` `H5` `HCC`

T32.33 Corrosions involving 30-39% of body surface with 30-39% third degree corrosion `MCC` `H5` `HCC`

✓5ᵗʰ **T32.4 Corrosions involving 40-49% of body surface**

T32.40 Corrosions involving 40-49% of body surface with 0% to 9% third degree corrosion `CC` `H5`

T32.41 Corrosions involving 40-49% of body surface with 10-19% third degree corrosion `MCC` `H5` `HCC`

T32.42 Corrosions involving 40-49% of body surface with 20-29% third degree corrosion `MCC` `H5` `HCC`

T32.43 Corrosions involving 40-49% of body surface with 30-39% third degree corrosion `MCC` `H5` `HCC`

T32.44 Corrosions involving 40-49% of body surface with 40-49% third degree corrosion `MCC` `H5` `HCC`

✓5ᵗʰ **T32.5 Corrosions involving 50-59% of body surface**

T32.50 Corrosions involving 50-59% of body surface with 0% to 9% third degree corrosion `CC` `H5`

T32.51 Corrosions involving 50-59% of body surface with 10-19% third degree corrosion `MCC` `H5` `HCC`

T32.52 Corrosions involving 50-59% of body surface with 20-29% third degree corrosion `MCC` `H5` `HCC`

T32.53 Corrosions involving 50-59% of body surface with 30-39% third degree corrosion `MCC` `H5` `HCC`

T32.54 Corrosions involving 50-59% of body surface with 40-49% third degree corrosion `MCC` `H5` `HCC`

T32.55 Corrosions involving 50-59% of body surface with 50-59% third degree corrosion `MCC` `H5` `HCC`

✓5ᵗʰ **T32.6 Corrosions involving 60-69% of body surface**

T32.60 Corrosions involving 60-69% of body surface with 0% to 9% third degree corrosion `CC` `H5`

T32.61 Corrosions involving 60-69% of body surface with 10-19% third degree corrosion `MCC` `H5` `HCC`

T32.62 Corrosions involving 60-69% of body surface with 20-29% third degree corrosion `MCC` `H5` `HCC`

T32.63 Corrosions involving 60-69% of body surface with 30-39% third degree corrosion `MCC` `H5` `HCC`

T32.64 Corrosions involving 60-69% of body surface with 40-49% third degree corrosion `MCC` `H5` `HCC`

T32.65 Corrosions involving 60-69% of body surface with 50-59% third degree corrosion `MCC` `H5` `HCC`

T32.66 Corrosions involving 60-69% of body surface with 60-69% third degree corrosion `MCC` `H5` `HCC`

✓5ᵗʰ **T32.7 Corrosions involving 70-79% of body surface**

T32.70 Corrosions involving 70-79% of body surface with 0% to 9% third degree corrosion `CC` `H5`

T32.71 Corrosions involving 70-79% of body surface with 10-19% third degree corrosion `MCC` `H5` `HCC`

T32.72 Corrosions involving 70-79% of body surface with 20-29% third degree corrosion `MCC` `H5` `HCC`

T32.73 Corrosions involving 70-79% of body surface with 30-39% third degree corrosion `MCC` `H5` `HCC`

T32.74 Corrosions involving 70-79% of body surface with 40-49% third degree corrosion `MCC` `H5` `HCC`

T32.75 Corrosions involving 70-79% of body surface with 50-59% third degree corrosion `MCC` `H5` `HCC`

T32.76 Corrosions involving 70-79% of body surface with 60-69% third degree corrosion `MCC` `H5` `HCC`

T32.77 Corrosions involving 70-79% of body surface with 70-79% third degree corrosion `MCC` `H5` `HCC`

✓5ᵗʰ **T32.8 Corrosions involving 80-89% of body surface**

T32.80 Corrosions involving 80-89% of body surface with 0% to 9% third degree corrosion `CC` `H5`

T32.81 Corrosions involving 80-89% of body surface with 10-19% third degree corrosion `MCC` `H5` `HCC`

T32.82 Corrosions involving 80-89% of body surface with 20-29% third degree corrosion `MCC` `H5` `HCC`

T32.83 Corrosions involving 80-89% of body surface with 30-39% third degree corrosion `MCC` `H5` `HCC`

T32.84 Corrosions involving 80-89% of body surface with 40-49% third degree corrosion `MCC` `H5` `HCC`

T32.85 Corrosions involving 80-89% of body surface with 50-59% third degree corrosion `MCC` `H5` `HCC`

T32.86 Corrosions involving 80-89% of body surface with 60-69% third degree corrosion `MCC` `H5` `HCC`

T32.87 Corrosions involving 80-89% of body surface with 70-79% third degree corrosion `MCC` `H5` `HCC`

T32.88 Corrosions involving 80-89% of body surface with 80-89% third degree corrosion `MCC` `H5` `HCC`

✓5ᵗʰ **T32.9 Corrosions involving 90% or more of body surface**

T32.90 Corrosions involving 90% or more of body surface with 0% to 9% third degree corrosion `CC` `H5`

T32.91 Corrosions involving 90% or more of body surface with 10-19% third degree corrosion `MCC` `H5` `HCC`

T32.92 Corrosions involving 90% or more of body surface with 20-29% third degree corrosion `MCC` `H5` `HCC`

T32.93 Corrosions involving 90% or more of body surface with 30-39% third degree corrosion `MCC` `H5` `HCC`

T32.94 Corrosions involving 90% or more of body surface with 40-49% third degree corrosion `MCC` `H5` `HCC`

T32.95 Corrosions involving 90% or more of body surface with 50-59% third degree corrosion `MCC` `H5` `HCC`

T32.96 Corrosions involving 90% or more of body surface with 60-69% third degree corrosion `MCC` `H5` `HCC`

T32.97 Corrosions involving 90% or more of body surface with 70-79% third degree corrosion `MCC` `H5` `HCC`

T32.98 Corrosions involving 90% or more of body surface with 80-89% third degree corrosion `MCC` `H5` `HCC`

T32.99 Corrosions involving 90% or more of body surface with 90% or more third degree corrosion `MCC` `H5` `HCC`

☑ Additional Character Required   ✓x7ᵗʰ Placeholder   Unacceptable PDx   Questionable PDx   Manifestation   Unspecified Dx   `H1`-`H14` HAC   `HCC` CMS-HCC Dx   `HIV` HIV Dx

Frostbite (T33–T34)

EXCLUDES 2   hypothermia and other effects of reduced temperature (T68, T69.-)

✓4ᵗʰ **T33** **Superficial frostbite**

INCLUDES   frostbite with partial thickness skin loss

The appropriate 7th character is to be added to each code from category T33.
A   initial encounter
D   subsequent encounter
S   sequela

CC Excl: For CC codes in category T33, unless otherwise noted: PDX collection 1416

✓5ᵗʰ **T33.0** **Superficial frostbite of head**

CC Excl: For CC codes in subcategory T33.0: PDX collection 1415

    ✓6ᵗʰ **T33.01** **Superficial frostbite of ear**

      ✓7ᵗʰ **T33.011** **Superficial frostbite of right ear** CC H5

      ✓7ᵗʰ **T33.012** **Superficial frostbite of left ear** CC H5

      ✓7ᵗʰ **T33.019** **Superficial frostbite of unspecified ear** CC H5

    ✓x7ᵗʰ **T33.02** **Superficial frostbite of nose** CC H5

    ✓x7ᵗʰ **T33.09** **Superficial frostbite of other part of head** CC H5

   ✓x7ᵗʰ **T33.1** **Superficial frostbite of neck** CC H5

    CC Excl: PDX collection 1415

   ✓x7ᵗʰ **T33.2** **Superficial frostbite of thorax** CC H5

   ✓x7ᵗʰ **T33.3** **Superficial frostbite of abdominal wall, lower back and pelvis** CC H5

   ✓5ᵗʰ **T33.4** **Superficial frostbite of arm**

     EXCLUDES 2   superficial frostbite of wrist and hand (T33.5-)

    ✓x7ᵗʰ **T33.40** **Superficial frostbite of unspecified arm** CC H5

    ✓x7ᵗʰ **T33.41** **Superficial frostbite of right arm** CC H5

    ✓x7ᵗʰ **T33.42** **Superficial frostbite of left arm** CC H5

   ✓5ᵗʰ **T33.5** **Superficial frostbite of wrist, hand, and fingers**

    CC Excl: For CC codes in subcategory T33.5: PDX collection 1417

    ✓6ᵗʰ **T33.51** **Superficial frostbite of wrist**

      ✓7ᵗʰ **T33.511** **Superficial frostbite of right wrist** CC H5

      ✓7ᵗʰ **T33.512** **Superficial frostbite of left wrist** CC H5

      ✓7ᵗʰ **T33.519** **Superficial frostbite of unspecified wrist** CC H5

    ✓6ᵗʰ **T33.52** **Superficial frostbite of hand**

     EXCLUDES 2   superficial frostbite of fingers (T33.53-)

      ✓7ᵗʰ **T33.521** **Superficial frostbite of right hand** CC H5

      ✓7ᵗʰ **T33.522** **Superficial frostbite of left hand** CC H5

      ✓7ᵗʰ **T33.529** **Superficial frostbite of unspecified hand** CC H5

    ✓6ᵗʰ **T33.53** **Superficial frostbite of finger(s)**

      ✓7ᵗʰ **T33.531** **Superficial frostbite of right finger(s)** CC H5

      ✓7ᵗʰ **T33.532** **Superficial frostbite of left finger(s)** CC H5

      ✓7ᵗʰ **T33.539** **Superficial frostbite of unspecified finger(s)** CC H5

   ✓5ᵗʰ **T33.6** **Superficial frostbite of hip and thigh**

    ✓x7ᵗʰ **T33.60** **Superficial frostbite of unspecified hip and thigh** CC H5

    ✓x7ᵗʰ **T33.61** **Superficial frostbite of right hip and thigh** CC H5

    ✓x7ᵗʰ **T33.62** **Superficial frostbite of left hip and thigh** CC H5

   ✓5ᵗʰ **T33.7** **Superficial frostbite of knee and lower leg**

     EXCLUDES 2   superficial frostbite of ankle and foot (T33.8-)

    ✓x7ᵗʰ **T33.70** **Superficial frostbite of unspecified knee and lower leg** CC H5

    ✓x7ᵗʰ **T33.71** **Superficial frostbite of right knee and lower leg** CC H5

    ✓x7ᵗʰ **T33.72** **Superficial frostbite of left knee and lower leg** CC H5

   ✓5ᵗʰ **T33.8** **Superficial frostbite of ankle, foot, and toe(s)**

    CC Excl: For CC codes in subcategory T33.8: PDX collection 1418

    ✓6ᵗʰ **T33.81** **Superficial frostbite of ankle**

      ✓7ᵗʰ **T33.811** **Superficial frostbite of right ankle** CC H5

      ✓7ᵗʰ **T33.812** **Superficial frostbite of left ankle** CC H5

      ✓7ᵗʰ **T33.819** **Superficial frostbite of unspecified ankle** CC H5

    ✓6ᵗʰ **T33.82** **Superficial frostbite of foot**

      ✓7ᵗʰ **T33.821** **Superficial frostbite of right foot** CC H5

      ✓7ᵗʰ **T33.822** **Superficial frostbite of left foot** CC H5

      ✓7ᵗʰ **T33.829** **Superficial frostbite of unspecified foot** CC H5

    ✓6ᵗʰ **T33.83** **Superficial frostbite of toe(s)**

      ✓7ᵗʰ **T33.831** **Superficial frostbite of right toe(s)** CC H5

      ✓7ᵗʰ **T33.832** **Superficial frostbite of left toe(s)** CC H5

      ✓7ᵗʰ **T33.839** **Superficial frostbite of unspecified toe(s)** CC H5

   ✓5ᵗʰ **T33.9** **Superficial frostbite of other and unspecified sites**

    ✓x7ᵗʰ **T33.90** **Superficial frostbite of unspecified sites** CC H5

     Superficial frostbite NOS

    ✓x7ᵗʰ **T33.99** **Superficial frostbite of other sites** CC H5

     Superficial frostbite of leg NOS
     Superficial frostbite of trunk NOS

✓4ᵗʰ **T34** **Frostbite with tissue necrosis**

The appropriate 7th character is to be added to each code from category T34.
A   initial encounter
D   subsequent encounter
S   sequela

CC Excl: For CC codes in category T34, unless otherwise noted: PDX collection 1416

✓5ᵗʰ **T34.0** **Frostbite with tissue necrosis of head**

    CC Excl: For CC codes in subcategory T34.0: PDX collection 1415

    ✓6ᵗʰ **T34.01** **Frostbite with tissue necrosis of ear**

      ✓7ᵗʰ **T34.011** **Frostbite with tissue necrosis of right ear** CC H5

      ✓7ᵗʰ **T34.012** **Frostbite with tissue necrosis of left ear** CC H5

      ✓7ᵗʰ **T34.019** **Frostbite with tissue necrosis of unspecified ear** CC H5

    ✓x7ᵗʰ **T34.02** **Frostbite with tissue necrosis of nose** CC H5

    ✓x7ᵗʰ **T34.09** **Frostbite with tissue necrosis of other part of head** CC H5

   ✓x7ᵗʰ **T34.1** **Frostbite with tissue necrosis of neck** CC H5

    CC Excl: PDX collection 1415

   ✓x7ᵗʰ **T34.2** **Frostbite with tissue necrosis of thorax** CC H5

   ✓x7ᵗʰ **T34.3** **Frostbite with tissue necrosis of abdominal wall, lower back and pelvis** CC H5

   ✓5ᵗʰ **T34.4** **Frostbite with tissue necrosis of arm**

     EXCLUDES 2   frostbite with tissue necrosis of wrist and hand (T34.5-)

    ✓x7ᵗʰ **T34.40** **Frostbite with tissue necrosis of unspecified arm** CC H5

    ✓x7ᵗʰ **T34.41** **Frostbite with tissue necrosis of right arm** CC H5

    ✓x7ᵗʰ **T34.42** **Frostbite with tissue necrosis of left arm** CC H5

   ✓5ᵗʰ **T34.5** **Frostbite with tissue necrosis of wrist, hand, and finger(s)**

    CC Excl: For CC codes in subcategory T34.5: PDX collection 1417

    ✓6ᵗʰ **T34.51** **Frostbite with tissue necrosis of wrist**

      ✓7ᵗʰ **T34.511** **Frostbite with tissue necrosis of right wrist** CC H5

      ✓7ᵗʰ **T34.512** **Frostbite with tissue necrosis of left wrist** CC H5

      ✓7ᵗʰ **T34.519** **Frostbite with tissue necrosis of unspecified wrist** CC H5

N Newborn: 0   P Pediatric: 0-17   M Maternity: 9-64   A Adult: 15-124   MCC Major Complication/Comorbidity   CC Complication/Comorbidity   SW Severe Wound Dx

1148   ICD-10-CM 2020

√6ᵗʰ **T34.52** Frostbite with tissue necrosis of **hand**

EXCLUDES 2 *frostbite with tissue necrosis of finger(s) (T34.53-)*

√7ᵗʰ **T34.521 Frostbite with tissue necrosis of right hand**   CC H5

√7ᵗʰ **T34.522 Frostbite with tissue necrosis of left hand**   CC H5

√7ᵗʰ **T34.529 Frostbite with tissue necrosis of unspecified hand**   CC H5

√6ᵗʰ **T34.53** Frostbite with tissue necrosis of **finger(s)**

√7ᵗʰ **T34.531 Frostbite with tissue necrosis of right finger(s)**   CC H5

√7ᵗʰ **T34.532 Frostbite with tissue necrosis of left finger(s)**   CC H5

√7ᵗʰ **T34.539 Frostbite with tissue necrosis of unspecified finger(s)**   CC H5

√5ᵗʰ **T34.6** Frostbite with tissue necrosis of **hip and thigh**

√x7ᵗʰ **T34.60 Frostbite with tissue necrosis of unspecified hip and thigh**   CC H5

√x7ᵗʰ **T34.61 Frostbite with tissue necrosis of right hip and thigh**   CC H5

√x7ᵗʰ **T34.62 Frostbite with tissue necrosis of left hip and thigh**   CC H5

√5ᵗʰ **T34.7** Frostbite with tissue necrosis of **knee and lower leg**

EXCLUDES 2 *frostbite with tissue necrosis of ankle and foot (T34.8-)*

√x7ᵗʰ **T34.70 Frostbite with tissue necrosis of unspecified knee and lower leg**   CC H5

√x7ᵗʰ **T34.71 Frostbite with tissue necrosis of right knee and lower leg**   CC H5

√x7ᵗʰ **T34.72 Frostbite with tissue necrosis of left knee and lower leg**   CC H5

√5ᵗʰ **T34.8** Frostbite with tissue necrosis of **ankle, foot, and toe(s)**

CC Excl: For CC codes in subcategory T34.8: PDX collection 1418

√6ᵗʰ **T34.81** Frostbite with tissue necrosis of **ankle**

√7ᵗʰ **T34.811 Frostbite with tissue necrosis of right ankle**   CC H5

√7ᵗʰ **T34.812 Frostbite with tissue necrosis of left ankle**   CC H5

√7ᵗʰ **T34.819 Frostbite with tissue necrosis of unspecified ankle**   CC H5

√6ᵗʰ **T34.82** Frostbite with tissue necrosis of **foot**

√7ᵗʰ **T34.821 Frostbite with tissue necrosis of right foot**   CC H5

√7ᵗʰ **T34.822 Frostbite with tissue necrosis of left foot**   CC H5

√7ᵗʰ **T34.829 Frostbite with tissue necrosis of unspecified foot**   CC H5

√6ᵗʰ **T34.83** Frostbite with tissue necrosis of **toe(s)**

√7ᵗʰ **T34.831 Frostbite with tissue necrosis of right toe(s)**   CC H5

√7ᵗʰ **T34.832 Frostbite with tissue necrosis of left toe(s)**   CC H5

√7ᵗʰ **T34.839 Frostbite with tissue necrosis of unspecified toe(s)**   CC H5

√5ᵗʰ **T34.9** Frostbite with tissue necrosis of **other and unspecified sites**

√x7ᵗʰ **T34.90 Frostbite with tissue necrosis of unspecified sites**   CC H5
Frostbite with tissue necrosis NOS

√x7ᵗʰ **T34.99 Frostbite with tissue necrosis of other sites**   CC H5
Frostbite with tissue necrosis of leg NOS
Frostbite with tissue necrosis of trunk NOS

Poisoning by, adverse effects of and underdosing of drugs, medicaments and biological substances (T36-T50)

INCLUDES adverse effect of correct substance properly administered
poisoning by overdose of substance
poisoning by wrong substance given or taken in error
underdosing by (inadvertently) (deliberately) taking less substance than prescribed or instructed

Code first, for adverse effects, the nature of the adverse effect, such as:
adverse effect NOS (T88.7)
aspirin gastritis (K29.-)
blood disorders (D56-D76)
contact dermatitis (L23-L25)
dermatitis due to substances taken internally (L27.-)
nephropathy (N14.0-N14.2)

NOTE The drug giving rise to the adverse effect should be identified by use of codes from categories T36-T50 with fifth or sixth character 5.

Use additional code(s) to specify:
manifestations of poisoning
underdosing or failure in dosage during medical and surgical care (Y63.6, Y63.8-Y63.9)
underdosing of medication regimen (Z91.12-, Z91.13-)

EXCLUDES 1 *toxic reaction to local anesthesia in pregnancy (O29.3-)*
EXCLUDES 2 *abuse and dependence of psychoactive substances (F10-F19)*
abuse of non-dependence-producing substances (F55.-)
drug reaction and poisoning affecting newborn (P00-P96)
pathological drug intoxication (inebriation) (F10-F19)

AHA: 2018,4Q,71; 2016,2Q,8; 2015,3Q,22

√4ᵗʰ **T36** Poisoning by, adverse effect of and underdosing of systemic antibiotics

EXCLUDES 1 *antineoplastic antibiotics (T45.1-)*
locally applied antibiotic NEC (T49.0)
topically used antibiotic for ear, nose and throat (T49.6)
topically used antibiotic for eye (T49.5)

The appropriate 7th character is to be added to each code from category T36.
A initial encounter
D subsequent encounter
S sequela

√5ᵗʰ **T36.0** Poisoning by, adverse effect of and underdosing of penicillins

√6ᵗʰ **T36.0X** Poisoning by, adverse effect of and underdosing of **penicillins**

√7ᵗʰ **T36.0X1 Poisoning by penicillins, accidental (unintentional)**
Poisoning by penicillins NOS

7 √7ᵗʰ **T36.0X2 Poisoning by penicillins, intentional self-harm**   HCC

√7ᵗʰ **T36.0X3 Poisoning by penicillins, assault**

√7ᵗʰ **T36.0X4 Poisoning by penicillins, undetermined**

√7ᵗʰ **T36.0X5 Adverse effect of penicillins**

√7ᵗʰ **T36.0X6 Underdosing of penicillins**

√5ᵗʰ **T36.1** Poisoning by, adverse effect of and underdosing of cephalosporins and other beta-lactam antibiotics

√6ᵗʰ **T36.1X** Poisoning by, adverse effect of and underdosing of **cephalosporins and other beta-lactam antibiotics**

√7ᵗʰ **T36.1X1 Poisoning by cephalosporins and other beta-lactam antibiotics, accidental (unintentional)**
Poisoning by cephalosporins and other beta-lactam antibiotics NOS

7 √7ᵗʰ **T36.1X2 Poisoning by cephalosporins and other beta-lactam antibiotics, intentional self-harm**   HCC

√7ᵗʰ **T36.1X3 Poisoning by cephalosporins and other beta-lactam antibiotics, assault**

√7ᵗʰ **T36.1X4 Poisoning by cephalosporins and other beta-lactam antibiotics, undetermined**

√7ᵗʰ **T36.1X5 Adverse effect of cephalosporins and other beta-lactam antibiotics**

√7ᵗʰ **T36.1X6 Underdosing of cephalosporins and other beta-lactam antibiotics**

√5ᵗʰ **T36.2** Poisoning by, adverse effect of and underdosing of chloramphenicol group

√6ᵗʰ **T36.2X** Poisoning by, adverse effect of and underdosing of **chloramphenicol group**

√7ᵗʰ **T36.2X1 Poisoning by chloramphenicol group, accidental (unintentional)**
Poisoning by chloramphenicol group NOS

7 √7ᵗʰ **T36.2X2** Poisoning by chloramphenicol group, intentional self-harm **HCC**

√7ᵗʰ **T36.2X3** Poisoning by chloramphenicol group, assault

√7ᵗʰ **T36.2X4** Poisoning by chloramphenicol group, undetermined

√7ᵗʰ **T36.2X5** Adverse effect of chloramphenicol group

√7ᵗʰ **T36.2X6** Underdosing of chloramphenicol group

√5ᵗʰ **T36.3** Poisoning by, adverse effect of and underdosing of macrolides

√6ᵗʰ **T36.3X** Poisoning by, adverse effect of and underdosing of macrolides

√7ᵗʰ **T36.3X1** Poisoning by macrolides, accidental (unintentional)
Poisoning by macrolides NOS

7 √7ᵗʰ **T36.3X2** Poisoning by macrolides, intentional self-harm **HCC**

√7ᵗʰ **T36.3X3** Poisoning by macrolides, assault

√7ᵗʰ **T36.3X4** Poisoning by macrolides, undetermined

√7ᵗʰ **T36.3X5** Adverse effect of macrolides

√7ᵗʰ **T36.3X6** Underdosing of macrolides

√5ᵗʰ **T36.4** Poisoning by, adverse effect of and underdosing of tetracyclines

√6ᵗʰ **T36.4X** Poisoning by, adverse effect of and underdosing of tetracyclines

√7ᵗʰ **T36.4X1** Poisoning by tetracyclines, accidental (unintentional)
Poisoning by tetracyclines NOS

7 √7ᵗʰ **T36.4X2** Poisoning by tetracyclines, intentional self-harm **HCC**

√7ᵗʰ **T36.4X3** Poisoning by tetracyclines, assault

√7ᵗʰ **T36.4X4** Poisoning by tetracyclines, undetermined

√7ᵗʰ **T36.4X5** Adverse effect of tetracyclines

√7ᵗʰ **T36.4X6** Underdosing of tetracyclines

√5ᵗʰ **T36.5** Poisoning by, adverse effect of and underdosing of aminoglycosides
Poisoning by, adverse effect of and underdosing of streptomycin

√6ᵗʰ **T36.5X** Poisoning by, adverse effect of and underdosing of aminoglycosides

√7ᵗʰ **T36.5X1** Poisoning by aminoglycosides, accidental (unintentional)
Poisoning by aminoglycosides NOS

7 √7ᵗʰ **T36.5X2** Poisoning by aminoglycosides, intentional self-harm **HCC**

√7ᵗʰ **T36.5X3** Poisoning by aminoglycosides, assault

√7ᵗʰ **T36.5X4** Poisoning by aminoglycosides, undetermined

√7ᵗʰ **T36.5X5** Adverse effect of aminoglycosides

√7ᵗʰ **T36.5X6** Underdosing of aminoglycosides

√5ᵗʰ **T36.6** Poisoning by, adverse effect of and underdosing of rifampicins

√6ᵗʰ **T36.6X** Poisoning by, adverse effect of and underdosing of rifampicins

√7ᵗʰ **T36.6X1** Poisoning by rifampicins, accidental (unintentional)
Poisoning by rifampicins NOS

7 √7ᵗʰ **T36.6X2** Poisoning by rifampicins, intentional self-harm **HCC**

√7ᵗʰ **T36.6X3** Poisoning by rifampicins, assault

√7ᵗʰ **T36.6X4** Poisoning by rifampicins, undetermined

√7ᵗʰ **T36.6X5** Adverse effect of rifampicins

√7ᵗʰ **T36.6X6** Underdosing of rifampicins

√5ᵗʰ **T36.7** Poisoning by, adverse effect of and underdosing of antifungal antibiotics, systemically used

√6ᵗʰ **T36.7X** Poisoning by, adverse effect of and underdosing of antifungal antibiotics, systemically used

√7ᵗʰ **T36.7X1** Poisoning by antifungal antibiotics, systemically used, accidental (unintentional)
Poisoning by antifungal antibiotics, systemically used NOS

7 √7ᵗʰ **T36.7X2** Poisoning by antifungal antibiotics, systemically used, intentional self-harm **HCC**

√7ᵗʰ **T36.7X3** Poisoning by antifungal antibiotics, systemically used, assault

√7ᵗʰ **T36.7X4** Poisoning by antifungal antibiotics, systemically used, undetermined

√7ᵗʰ **T36.7X5** Adverse effect of antifungal antibiotics, systemically used

√7ᵗʰ **T36.7X6** Underdosing of antifungal antibiotics, systemically used

√5ᵗʰ **T36.8** Poisoning by, adverse effect of and underdosing of other systemic antibiotics

√6ᵗʰ **T36.8X** Poisoning by, adverse effect of and underdosing of other systemic antibiotics
AHA: 2017,1Q,39

√7ᵗʰ **T36.8X1** Poisoning by other systemic antibiotics, accidental (unintentional)
Poisoning by other systemic antibiotics NOS

7 √7ᵗʰ **T36.8X2** Poisoning by other systemic antibiotics, intentional self-harm **HCC**

√7ᵗʰ **T36.8X3** Poisoning by other systemic antibiotics, assault

√7ᵗʰ **T36.8X4** Poisoning by other systemic antibiotics, undetermined

√7ᵗʰ **T36.8X5** Adverse effect of other systemic antibiotics

√7ᵗʰ **T36.8X6** Underdosing of other systemic antibiotics

√5ᵗʰ **T36.9** Poisoning by, adverse effect of and underdosing of unspecified systemic antibiotic

√x7ᵗʰ **T36.91** Poisoning by unspecified systemic antibiotic, accidental (unintentional)
Poisoning by systemic antibiotic NOS

7 √x7ᵗʰ **T36.92** Poisoning by unspecified systemic antibiotic, intentional self-harm **HCC**

√x7ᵗʰ **T36.93** Poisoning by unspecified systemic antibiotic, assault

√x7ᵗʰ **T36.94** Poisoning by unspecified systemic antibiotic, undetermined

√x7ᵗʰ **T36.95** Adverse effect of unspecified systemic antibiotic

√x7ᵗʰ **T36.96** Underdosing of unspecified systemic antibiotic

√4ᵗʰ **T37** Poisoning by, adverse effect of and underdosing of other systemic anti-infectives and antiparasitics

EXCLUDES 1 anti-infectives topically used for ear, nose and throat (T49.6-)
anti-infectives topically used for eye (T49.5-)
locally applied anti-infectives NEC (T49.0-)

The appropriate 7th character is to be added to each code from category T37.
A   initial encounter
D   subsequent encounter
S   sequela

√5ᵗʰ **T37.0** Poisoning by, adverse effect of and underdosing of sulfonamides

√6ᵗʰ **T37.0X** Poisoning by, adverse effect of and underdosing of sulfonamides

√7ᵗʰ **T37.0X1** Poisoning by sulfonamides, accidental (unintentional)
Poisoning by sulfonamides NOS

7 √7ᵗʰ **T37.0X2** Poisoning by sulfonamides, intentional self-harm **HCC**

√7ᵗʰ **T37.0X3** Poisoning by sulfonamides, assault

√7ᵗʰ **T37.0X4** Poisoning by sulfonamides, undetermined

√7ᵗʰ **T37.0X5** Adverse effect of sulfonamides

√7ᵗʰ **T37.0X6** Underdosing of sulfonamides

√5ᵗʰ **T37.1** Poisoning by, adverse effect of and underdosing of antimycobacterial drugs

EXCLUDES 1 rifampicins (T36.6-)
streptomycin (T36.5-)

√6ᵗʰ **T37.1X** Poisoning by, adverse effect of and underdosing of antimycobacterial drugs

√7ᵗʰ **T37.1X1** Poisoning by antimycobacterial drugs, accidental (unintentional)
Poisoning by antimycobacterial drugs NOS

7 √7ᵗʰ **T37.1X2** Poisoning by antimycobacterial drugs, intentional self-harm **HCC**

√7ᵗʰ **T37.1X3** Poisoning by antimycobacterial drugs, assault

✓7ᵗʰ **T37.1X4** **Poisoning by antimycobacterial drugs, undetermined**

✓7ᵗʰ **T37.1X5** Adverse effect of antimycobacterial drugs

✓7ᵗʰ **T37.1X6** Underdosing of antimycobacterial drugs

✓5ᵗʰ **T37.2** **Poisoning by, adverse effect of and underdosing of antimalarials and drugs acting on other blood protozoa**

> EXCLUDES 1   hydroxyquinoline derivatives (T37.8-)

✓6ᵗʰ **T37.2X** **Poisoning by, adverse effect of and underdosing of antimalarials and drugs acting on other blood protozoa**

✓7ᵗʰ **T37.2X1** **Poisoning by antimalarials and drugs acting on other blood protozoa, accidental (unintentional)**

> Poisoning by antimalarials and drugs acting on other blood protozoa NOS

7 ✓7ᵗʰ **T37.2X2** **Poisoning by antimalarials and drugs acting on other blood protozoa, intentional self-harm**   HCC

✓7ᵗʰ **T37.2X3** **Poisoning by antimalarials and drugs acting on other blood protozoa, assault**

✓7ᵗʰ **T37.2X4** **Poisoning by antimalarials and drugs acting on other blood protozoa, undetermined**

✓7ᵗʰ **T37.2X5** Adverse effect of antimalarials and drugs acting on other blood protozoa

✓7ᵗʰ **T37.2X6** Underdosing of antimalarials and drugs acting on other blood protozoa

✓5ᵗʰ **T37.3** **Poisoning by, adverse effect of and underdosing of other antiprotozoal drugs**

✓6ᵗʰ **T37.3X** **Poisoning by, adverse effect of and underdosing of other antiprotozoal drugs**

✓7ᵗʰ **T37.3X1** **Poisoning by other antiprotozoal drugs, accidental (unintentional)**

> Poisoning by other antiprotozoal drugs NOS

7 ✓7ᵗʰ **T37.3X2** **Poisoning by other antiprotozoal drugs, intentional self-harm**   HCC

✓7ᵗʰ **T37.3X3** **Poisoning by other antiprotozoal drugs, assault**

✓7ᵗʰ **T37.3X4** **Poisoning by other antiprotozoal drugs, undetermined**

✓7ᵗʰ **T37.3X5** Adverse effect of other antiprotozoal drugs

✓7ᵗʰ **T37.3X6** Underdosing of other antiprotozoal drugs

✓5ᵗʰ **T37.4** **Poisoning by, adverse effect of and underdosing of anthelminthics**

✓6ᵗʰ **T37.4X** **Poisoning by, adverse effect of and underdosing of anthelminthics**

✓7ᵗʰ **T37.4X1** **Poisoning by anthelminthics, accidental (unintentional)**

> Poisoning by anthelminthics NOS

7 ✓7ᵗʰ **T37.4X2** **Poisoning by anthelminthics, intentional self-harm**   HCC

✓7ᵗʰ **T37.4X3** **Poisoning by anthelminthics, assault**

✓7ᵗʰ **T37.4X4** **Poisoning by anthelminthics, undetermined**

✓7ᵗʰ **T37.4X5** Adverse effect of anthelminthics

✓7ᵗʰ **T37.4X6** Underdosing of anthelminthics

✓5ᵗʰ **T37.5** **Poisoning by, adverse effect of and underdosing of antiviral drugs**

> EXCLUDES 1   amantadine (T42.8-)
> cytarabine (T45.1-)

✓6ᵗʰ **T37.5X** **Poisoning by, adverse effect of and underdosing of antiviral drugs**

✓7ᵗʰ **T37.5X1** **Poisoning by antiviral drugs, accidental (unintentional)**

> Poisoning by antiviral drugs NOS

7 ✓7ᵗʰ **T37.5X2** **Poisoning by antiviral drugs, intentional self-harm**   HCC

✓7ᵗʰ **T37.5X3** **Poisoning by antiviral drugs, assault**

✓7ᵗʰ **T37.5X4** **Poisoning by antiviral drugs, undetermined**

✓7ᵗʰ **T37.5X5** Adverse effect of antiviral drugs

✓7ᵗʰ **T37.5X6** Underdosing of antiviral drugs

✓5ᵗʰ **T37.8** **Poisoning by, adverse effect of and underdosing of other specified systemic anti-infectives and antiparasitics**

> Poisoning by, adverse effect of and underdosing of hydroxyquinoline derivatives
>
> EXCLUDES 1   antimalarial drugs (T37.2-)

✓6ᵗʰ **T37.8X** **Poisoning by, adverse effect of and underdosing of other specified systemic anti-infectives and antiparasitics**

✓7ᵗʰ **T37.8X1** **Poisoning by other specified systemic anti-infectives and antiparasitics, accidental (unintentional)**

> Poisoning by other specified systemic anti-infectives and antiparasitics NOS

7 ✓7ᵗʰ **T37.8X2** **Poisoning by other specified systemic anti-infectives and antiparasitics, intentional self-harm**   HCC

✓7ᵗʰ **T37.8X3** **Poisoning by other specified systemic anti-infectives and antiparasitics, assault**

✓7ᵗʰ **T37.8X4** **Poisoning by other specified systemic anti-infectives and antiparasitics, undetermined**

✓7ᵗʰ **T37.8X5** Adverse effect of other specified systemic anti-infectives and antiparasitics

✓7ᵗʰ **T37.8X6** Underdosing of other specified systemic anti-infectives and antiparasitics

✓5ᵗʰ **T37.9** **Poisoning by, adverse effect of and underdosing of unspecified systemic anti-infective and antiparasitics**

✓x7ᵗʰ **T37.91** **Poisoning by unspecified systemic anti-infective and antiparasitics, accidental (unintentional)**

> Poisoning by, adverse effect of and underdosing of systemic anti-infective and antiparasitics NOS

7 ✓x7ᵗʰ **T37.92** **Poisoning by unspecified systemic anti-infective and antiparasitics, intentional self-harm**   HCC

✓x7ᵗʰ **T37.93** **Poisoning by unspecified systemic anti-infective and antiparasitics, assault**

✓x7ᵗʰ **T37.94** **Poisoning by unspecified systemic anti-infective and antiparasitics, undetermined**

✓x7ᵗʰ **T37.95** Adverse effect of unspecified systemic anti-infective and antiparasitic

✓x7ᵗʰ **T37.96** Underdosing of unspecified systemic anti-infectives and antiparasitics

✓4ᵗʰ **T38** **Poisoning by, adverse effect of and underdosing of hormones and their synthetic substitutes and antagonists, not elsewhere classified**

> EXCLUDES 1   mineralocorticoids and their antagonists (T50.0-)
> oxytocic hormones (T48.0-)
> parathyroid hormones and derivatives (T50.9-)

> The appropriate 7th character is to be added to each code from category T38.
> A   initial encounter
> D   subsequent encounter
> S   sequela

✓5ᵗʰ **T38.0** **Poisoning by, adverse effect of and underdosing of glucocorticoids and synthetic analogues**

> EXCLUDES 1   glucocorticoids, topically used (T49.-)

✓6ᵗʰ **T38.0X** **Poisoning by, adverse effect of and underdosing of glucocorticoids and synthetic analogues**

✓7ᵗʰ **T38.0X1** **Poisoning by glucocorticoids and synthetic analogues, accidental (unintentional)**

> Poisoning by glucocorticoids and synthetic analogues NOS

7 ✓7ᵗʰ **T38.0X2** **Poisoning by glucocorticoids and synthetic analogues, intentional self-harm**   HCC

✓7ᵗʰ **T38.0X3** **Poisoning by glucocorticoids and synthetic analogues, assault**

✓7ᵗʰ **T38.0X4** **Poisoning by glucocorticoids and synthetic analogues, undetermined**

✓7ᵗʰ **T38.0X5** Adverse effect of glucocorticoids and synthetic analogues

✓7ᵗʰ **T38.0X6** Underdosing of glucocorticoids and synthetic analogues

☑ Additional Character Required   ✓x7ᵗʰ Placeholder   Unacceptable PDx   Questionable PDx   Manifestation   Unspecified Dx   H1-H4 HAC   HCC CMS-HCC Dx   HIV HIV Dx

ICD-10-CM 2020

1151

√6ᵗʰ **T38.1** **Poisoning by, adverse effect of and underdosing of thyroid hormones and substitutes**

√6ᵗʰ **T38.1X** Poisoning by, adverse effect of and underdosing of thyroid hormones and substitutes

√7ᵗʰ **T38.1X1** Poisoning by thyroid hormones and substitutes, accidental (unintentional)
Poisoning by thyroid hormones and substitutes NOS

7 √7ᵗʰ **T38.1X2** Poisoning by thyroid hormones and substitutes, intentional self-harm `HCC`

√7ᵗʰ **T38.1X3** Poisoning by thyroid hormones and substitutes, assault

√7ᵗʰ **T38.1X4** Poisoning by thyroid hormones and substitutes, undetermined

√7ᵗʰ **T38.1X5** Adverse effect of thyroid hormones and substitutes

√7ᵗʰ **T38.1X6** Underdosing of thyroid hormones and substitutes

√5ᵗʰ **T38.2** **Poisoning by, adverse effect of and underdosing of antithyroid drugs**

√6ᵗʰ **T38.2X** Poisoning by, adverse effect of and underdosing of antithyroid drugs

√7ᵗʰ **T38.2X1** Poisoning by antithyroid drugs, accidental (unintentional)
Poisoning by antithyroid drugs NOS

7 √7ᵗʰ **T38.2X2** Poisoning by antithyroid drugs, intentional self-harm `HCC`

√7ᵗʰ **T38.2X3** Poisoning by antithyroid drugs, assault

√7ᵗʰ **T38.2X4** Poisoning by antithyroid drugs, undetermined

√7ᵗʰ **T38.2X5** Adverse effect of antithyroid drugs

√7ᵗʰ **T38.2X6** Underdosing of antithyroid drugs

√5ᵗʰ **T38.3** **Poisoning by, adverse effect of and underdosing of insulin and oral hypoglycemic [antidiabetic] drugs**

√6ᵗʰ **T38.3X** Poisoning by, adverse effect of and underdosing of insulin and oral hypoglycemic [antidiabetic] drugs

√7ᵗʰ **T38.3X1** Poisoning by insulin and oral hypoglycemic [antidiabetic] drugs, accidental (unintentional)
Poisoning by insulin and oral hypoglycemic [antidiabetic] drugs NOS

7 √7ᵗʰ **T38.3X2** Poisoning by insulin and oral hypoglycemic [antidiabetic] drugs, intentional self-harm `HCC`

√7ᵗʰ **T38.3X3** Poisoning by insulin and oral hypoglycemic [antidiabetic] drugs, assault

√7ᵗʰ **T38.3X4** Poisoning by insulin and oral hypoglycemic [antidiabetic] drugs, undetermined

√7ᵗʰ **T38.3X5** Adverse effect of insulin and oral hypoglycemic [antidiabetic] drugs

√7ᵗʰ **T38.3X6** Underdosing of insulin and oral hypoglycemic [antidiabetic] drugs

√5ᵗʰ **T38.4** **Poisoning by, adverse effect of and underdosing of oral contraceptives**
Poisoning by, adverse effect of and underdosing of multiple- and single-ingredient oral contraceptive preparations

√6ᵗʰ **T38.4X** Poisoning by, adverse effect of and underdosing of oral contraceptives

√7ᵗʰ **T38.4X1** Poisoning by oral contraceptives, accidental (unintentional)
Poisoning by oral contraceptives NOS

7 √7ᵗʰ **T38.4X2** Poisoning by oral contraceptives, intentional self-harm `HCC`

√7ᵗʰ **T38.4X3** Poisoning by oral contraceptives, assault

√7ᵗʰ **T38.4X4** Poisoning by oral contraceptives, undetermined

√7ᵗʰ **T38.4X5** Adverse effect of oral contraceptives

√7ᵗʰ **T38.4X6** Underdosing of oral contraceptives

√5ᵗʰ **T38.5** **Poisoning by, adverse effect of and underdosing of other estrogens and progestogens**
Poisoning by, adverse effect of and underdosing of estrogens and progestogens mixtures and substitutes

√6ᵗʰ **T38.5X** Poisoning by, adverse effect of and underdosing of other estrogens and progestogens

√7ᵗʰ **T38.5X1** Poisoning by other estrogens and progestogens, accidental (unintentional)
Poisoning by other estrogens and progestogens NOS

7 √7ᵗʰ **T38.5X2** Poisoning by other estrogens and progestogens, intentional self-harm `HCC`

√7ᵗʰ **T38.5X3** Poisoning by other estrogens and progestogens, assault

√7ᵗʰ **T38.5X4** Poisoning by other estrogens and progestogens, undetermined

√7ᵗʰ **T38.5X5** Adverse effect of other estrogens and progestogens

√7ᵗʰ **T38.5X6** Underdosing of other estrogens and progestogens

√5ᵗʰ **T38.6** **Poisoning by, adverse effect of and underdosing of antigonadotrophins, antiestrogens, antiandrogens, not elsewhere classified**
Poisoning by, adverse effect of and underdosing of tamoxifen

√6ᵗʰ **T38.6X** Poisoning by, adverse effect of and underdosing of antigonadotrophins, antiestrogens, antiandrogens, not elsewhere classified

√7ᵗʰ **T38.6X1** Poisoning by antigonadotrophins, antiestrogens, antiandrogens, not elsewhere classified, accidental (unintentional)
Poisoning by antigonadotrophins, antiestrogens, antiandrogens, not elsewhere classified NOS

7 √7ᵗʰ **T38.6X2** Poisoning by antigonadotrophins, antiestrogens, antiandrogens, not elsewhere classified, intentional self-harm `HCC`

√7ᵗʰ **T38.6X3** Poisoning by antigonadotrophins, antiestrogens, antiandrogens, not elsewhere classified, assault

√7ᵗʰ **T38.6X4** Poisoning by antigonadotrophins, antiestrogens, antiandrogens, not elsewhere classified, undetermined

√7ᵗʰ **T38.6X5** Adverse effect of antigonadotrophins, antiestrogens, antiandrogens, not elsewhere classified

√7ᵗʰ **T38.6X6** Underdosing of antigonadotrophins, antiestrogens, antiandrogens, not elsewhere classified

√5ᵗʰ **T38.7** **Poisoning by, adverse effect of and underdosing of androgens and anabolic congeners**

√6ᵗʰ **T38.7X** Poisoning by, adverse effect of and underdosing of androgens and anabolic congeners

√7ᵗʰ **T38.7X1** Poisoning by androgens and anabolic congeners, accidental (unintentional)
Poisoning by androgens and anabolic congeners NOS

7 √7ᵗʰ **T38.7X2** Poisoning by androgens and anabolic congeners, intentional self-harm `HCC`

√7ᵗʰ **T38.7X3** Poisoning by androgens and anabolic congeners, assault

√7ᵗʰ **T38.7X4** Poisoning by androgens and anabolic congeners, undetermined

√7ᵗʰ **T38.7X5** Adverse effect of androgens and anabolic congeners

√7ᵗʰ **T38.7X6** Underdosing of androgens and anabolic congeners

√5ᵗʰ **T38.8** **Poisoning by, adverse effect of and underdosing of other and unspecified hormones and synthetic substitutes**

√6ᵗʰ **T38.80** Poisoning by, adverse effect of and underdosing of unspecified hormones and synthetic substitutes

√7ᵗʰ **T38.801** Poisoning by unspecified hormones and synthetic substitutes, accidental (unintentional)
Poisoning by unspecified hormones and synthetic substitutes NOS

⁷ ✓7ᵗʰ **T38.802** Poisoning by unspecified hormones and synthetic substitutes, intentional self-harm   HCC

✓7ᵗʰ **T38.803** Poisoning by unspecified hormones and synthetic substitutes, assault

✓7ᵗʰ **T38.804** Poisoning by unspecified hormones and synthetic substitutes, undetermined

✓7ᵗʰ **T38.805** Adverse effect of unspecified hormones and synthetic substitutes

✓7ᵗʰ **T38.806** Underdosing of unspecified hormones and synthetic substitutes

✓6ᵗʰ **T38.81** Poisoning by, adverse effect of and underdosing of anterior pituitary [adenohypophyseal] hormones

✓7ᵗʰ **T38.811** Poisoning by anterior pituitary [adenohypophyseal] hormones, accidental (unintentional)
Poisoning by anterior pituitary [adenohypophyseal] hormones NOS

⁷ ✓7ᵗʰ **T38.812** Poisoning by anterior pituitary [adenohypophyseal] hormones, intentional self-harm   HCC

✓7ᵗʰ **T38.813** Poisoning by anterior pituitary [adenohypophyseal] hormones, assault

✓7ᵗʰ **T38.814** Poisoning by anterior pituitary [adenohypophyseal] hormones, undetermined

✓7ᵗʰ **T38.815** Adverse effect of anterior pituitary [adenohypophyseal] hormones

✓7ᵗʰ **T38.816** Underdosing of anterior pituitary [adenohypophyseal] hormones

✓6ᵗʰ **T38.89** Poisoning by, adverse effect of and underdosing of other hormones and synthetic substitutes

✓7ᵗʰ **T38.891** Poisoning by other hormones and synthetic substitutes, accidental (unintentional)
Poisoning by other hormones and synthetic substitutes NOS

⁷ ✓7ᵗʰ **T38.892** Poisoning by other hormones and synthetic substitutes, intentional self-harm   HCC

✓7ᵗʰ **T38.893** Poisoning by other hormones and synthetic substitutes, assault

✓7ᵗʰ **T38.894** Poisoning by other hormones and synthetic substitutes, undetermined

✓7ᵗʰ **T38.895** Adverse effect of other hormones and synthetic substitutes

✓7ᵗʰ **T38.896** Underdosing of other hormones and synthetic substitutes

✓5ᵗʰ **T38.9** Poisoning by, adverse effect of and underdosing of other and unspecified hormone antagonists

✓6ᵗʰ **T38.90** Poisoning by, adverse effect of and underdosing of unspecified hormone antagonists

✓7ᵗʰ **T38.901** Poisoning by unspecified hormone antagonists, accidental (unintentional)
Poisoning by unspecified hormone antagonists NOS

⁷ ✓7ᵗʰ **T38.902** Poisoning by unspecified hormone antagonists, intentional self-harm   HCC

✓7ᵗʰ **T38.903** Poisoning by unspecified hormone antagonists, assault

✓7ᵗʰ **T38.904** Poisoning by unspecified hormone antagonists, undetermined

✓7ᵗʰ **T38.905** Adverse effect of unspecified hormone antagonists

✓7ᵗʰ **T38.906** Underdosing of unspecified hormone antagonists

✓6ᵗʰ **T38.99** Poisoning by, adverse effect of and underdosing of other hormone antagonists

✓7ᵗʰ **T38.991** Poisoning by other hormone antagonists, accidental (unintentional)
Poisoning by other hormone antagonists NOS

⁷ ✓7ᵗʰ **T38.992** Poisoning by other hormone antagonists, intentional self-harm   HCC

✓7ᵗʰ **T38.993** Poisoning by other hormone antagonists, assault

✓7ᵗʰ **T38.994** Poisoning by other hormone antagonists, undetermined

✓7ᵗʰ **T38.995** Adverse effect of other hormone antagonists

✓7ᵗʰ **T38.996** Underdosing of other hormone antagonists

✓4ᵗʰ **T39** Poisoning by, adverse effect of and underdosing of nonopioid analgesics, antipyretics and antirheumatics

The appropriate 7th character is to be added to each code from category T39.
A   initial encounter
D   subsequent encounter
S   sequela

✓5ᵗʰ **T39.0** Poisoning by, adverse effect of and underdosing of salicylates

✓6ᵗʰ **T39.01** Poisoning by, adverse effect of and underdosing of aspirin
Poisoning by, adverse effect of and underdosing of acetylsalicylic acid

✓7ᵗʰ **T39.011** Poisoning by aspirin, accidental (unintentional)

⁷ ✓7ᵗʰ **T39.012** Poisoning by aspirin, intentional self-harm   HCC

✓7ᵗʰ **T39.013** Poisoning by aspirin, assault

✓7ᵗʰ **T39.014** Poisoning by aspirin, undetermined

✓7ᵗʰ **T39.015** Adverse effect of aspirin
AHA: 2016,1Q,15

✓7ᵗʰ **T39.016** Underdosing of aspirin

✓6ᵗʰ **T39.09** Poisoning by, adverse effect of and underdosing of other salicylates

✓7ᵗʰ **T39.091** Poisoning by salicylates, accidental (unintentional)
Poisoning by salicylates NOS

⁷ ✓7ᵗʰ **T39.092** Poisoning by salicylates, intentional self-harm   HCC

✓7ᵗʰ **T39.093** Poisoning by salicylates, assault

✓7ᵗʰ **T39.094** Poisoning by salicylates, undetermined

✓7ᵗʰ **T39.095** Adverse effect of salicylates

✓7ᵗʰ **T39.096** Underdosing of salicylates

✓5ᵗʰ **T39.1** Poisoning by, adverse effect of and underdosing of 4-Aminophenol derivatives

✓6ᵗʰ **T39.1X** Poisoning by, adverse effect of and underdosing of 4-Aminophenol derivatives

✓7ᵗʰ **T39.1X1** Poisoning by 4-Aminophenol derivatives, accidental (unintentional)
Poisoning by 4-Aminophenol derivatives NOS

⁷ ✓7ᵗʰ **T39.1X2** Poisoning by 4-Aminophenol derivatives, intentional self-harm   HCC

✓7ᵗʰ **T39.1X3** Poisoning by 4-Aminophenol derivatives, assault

✓7ᵗʰ **T39.1X4** Poisoning by 4-Aminophenol derivatives, undetermined

✓7ᵗʰ **T39.1X5** Adverse effect of 4-Aminophenol derivatives

✓7ᵗʰ **T39.1X6** Underdosing of 4-Aminophenol derivatives

✓5ᵗʰ **T39.2** Poisoning by, adverse effect of and underdosing of pyrazolone derivatives

✓6ᵗʰ **T39.2X** Poisoning by, adverse effect of and underdosing of pyrazolone derivatives

✓7ᵗʰ **T39.2X1** Poisoning by pyrazolone derivatives, accidental (unintentional)
Poisoning by pyrazolone derivatives NOS

⁷ ✓7ᵗʰ **T39.2X2** Poisoning by pyrazolone derivatives, intentional self-harm   HCC

✓7ᵗʰ **T39.2X3** Poisoning by pyrazolone derivatives, assault

✓7ᵗʰ **T39.2X4** Poisoning by pyrazolone derivatives, undetermined

✓7ᵗʰ **T39.2X5** Adverse effect of pyrazolone derivatives

✓7ᵗʰ **T39.2X6** Underdosing of pyrazolone derivatives

✓5ᵗʰ **T39.3** **Poisoning by, adverse effect of and underdosing of other nonsteroidal anti-inflammatory drugs [NSAID]**

✓6ᵗʰ **T39.31** **Poisoning by, adverse effect of and underdosing of** propionic acid derivatives

Poisoning by, adverse effect of and underdosing of fenoprofen

Poisoning by, adverse effect of and underdosing of flurbiprofen

Poisoning by, adverse effect of and underdosing of ibuprofen

Poisoning by, adverse effect of and underdosing of ketoprofen

Poisoning by, adverse effect of and underdosing of naproxen

Poisoning by, adverse effect of and underdosing of oxaprozin

✓7ᵗʰ **T39.311** **Poisoning by propionic acid derivatives, accidental (unintentional)**

7 ✓7ᵗʰ **T39.312** **Poisoning by propionic acid derivatives, intentional self-harm** HCC

✓7ᵗʰ **T39.313** **Poisoning by propionic acid derivatives, assault**

✓7ᵗʰ **T39.314** **Poisoning by propionic acid derivatives, undetermined**

✓7ᵗʰ **T39.315** **Adverse effect of propionic acid derivatives**

✓7ᵗʰ **T39.316** **Underdosing of propionic acid derivatives**

✓6ᵗʰ **T39.39** **Poisoning by, adverse effect of and underdosing of other nonsteroidal anti-inflammatory drugs [NSAID]**

✓7ᵗʰ **T39.391** **Poisoning by other nonsteroidal anti-inflammatory drugs [NSAID], accidental (unintentional)**

Poisoning by other nonsteroidal anti-inflammatory drugs NOS

7 ✓7ᵗʰ **T39.392** **Poisoning by other nonsteroidal anti-inflammatory drugs [NSAID], intentional self-harm** HCC

✓7ᵗʰ **T39.393** **Poisoning by other nonsteroidal anti-inflammatory drugs [NSAID], assault**

✓7ᵗʰ **T39.394** **Poisoning by other nonsteroidal anti-inflammatory drugs [NSAID], undetermined**

✓7ᵗʰ **T39.395** **Adverse effect of other nonsteroidal anti-inflammatory drugs [NSAID]**

✓7ᵗʰ **T39.396** **Underdosing of other nonsteroidal anti-inflammatory drugs [NSAID]**

✓5ᵗʰ **T39.4** **Poisoning by, adverse effect of and underdosing of antirheumatics, not elsewhere classified**

EXCLUDES 1   *poisoning by, adverse effect of and underdosing of glucocorticoids (T38.0-)*

poisoning by, adverse effect of and underdosing of salicylates (T39.0-)

✓6ᵗʰ **T39.4X** **Poisoning by, adverse effect of and underdosing of antirheumatics, not elsewhere classified**

✓7ᵗʰ **T39.4X1** **Poisoning by antirheumatics, not elsewhere classified, accidental (unintentional)**

Poisoning by antirheumatics, not elsewhere classified NOS

7 ✓7ᵗʰ **T39.4X2** **Poisoning by antirheumatics, not elsewhere classified, intentional self-harm** HCC

✓7ᵗʰ **T39.4X3** **Poisoning by antirheumatics, not elsewhere classified, assault**

✓7ᵗʰ **T39.4X4** **Poisoning by antirheumatics, not elsewhere classified, undetermined**

✓7ᵗʰ **T39.4X5** **Adverse effect of antirheumatics, not elsewhere classified**

✓7ᵗʰ **T39.4X6** **Underdosing of antirheumatics, not elsewhere classified**

✓5ᵗʰ **T39.8** **Poisoning by, adverse effect of and underdosing of other nonopioid analgesics and antipyretics, not elsewhere classified**

✓6ᵗʰ **T39.8X** **Poisoning by, adverse effect of and underdosing of other nonopioid analgesics and antipyretics, not elsewhere classified**

✓7ᵗʰ **T39.8X1** **Poisoning by other nonopioid analgesics and antipyretics, not elsewhere classified, accidental (unintentional)**

Poisoning by other nonopioid analgesics and antipyretics, not elsewhere classified NOS

7 ✓7ᵗʰ **T39.8X2** **Poisoning by other nonopioid analgesics and antipyretics, not elsewhere classified, intentional self-harm** HCC

✓7ᵗʰ **T39.8X3** **Poisoning by other nonopioid analgesics and antipyretics, not elsewhere classified, assault**

✓7ᵗʰ **T39.8X4** **Poisoning by other nonopioid analgesics and antipyretics, not elsewhere classified, undetermined**

✓7ᵗʰ **T39.8X5** **Adverse effect of other nonopioid analgesics and antipyretics, not elsewhere classified**

✓7ᵗʰ **T39.8X6** **Underdosing of other nonopioid analgesics and antipyretics, not elsewhere classified**

✓5ᵗʰ **T39.9** **Poisoning by, adverse effect of and underdosing of unspecified nonopioid analgesic, antipyretic and antirheumatic**

✓×7ᵗʰ **T39.91** **Poisoning by unspecified nonopioid analgesic, antipyretic and antirheumatic, accidental (unintentional)**

Poisoning by nonopioid analgesic, antipyretic and antirheumatic NOS

7 ✓×7ᵗʰ **T39.92** **Poisoning by unspecified nonopioid analgesic, antipyretic and antirheumatic, intentional self-harm** HCC

✓×7ᵗʰ **T39.93** **Poisoning by unspecified nonopioid analgesic, antipyretic and antirheumatic, assault**

✓×7ᵗʰ **T39.94** **Poisoning by unspecified nonopioid analgesic, antipyretic and antirheumatic, undetermined**

✓×7ᵗʰ **T39.95** **Adverse effect of unspecified nonopioid analgesic, antipyretic and antirheumatic**

✓×7ᵗʰ **T39.96** **Underdosing of unspecified nonopioid analgesic, antipyretic and antirheumatic**

✓4ᵗʰ **T40** **Poisoning by, adverse effect of and underdosing of narcotics and psychodysleptics [hallucinogens]**

EXCLUDES 2   *drug dependence and related mental and behavioral disorders due to psychoactive substance use (F10.-F19.-)*

The appropriate 7th character is to be added to each code from category T40.
A   initial encounter
D   subsequent encounter
S   sequela

✓5ᵗʰ **T40.0** **Poisoning by, adverse effect of and underdosing of opium**

✓6ᵗʰ **T40.0X** **Poisoning by, adverse effect of and underdosing of** opium

6 ✓7ᵗʰ **T40.0X1** **Poisoning by opium, accidental (unintentional)** HCC

Poisoning by opium NOS

7 ✓7ᵗʰ **T40.0X2** **Poisoning by opium, intentional self-harm** HCC

✓7ᵗʰ **T40.0X3** **Poisoning by opium, assault**

6 ✓7ᵗʰ **T40.0X4** **Poisoning by opium, undetermined** HCC

✓7ᵗʰ **T40.0X5** **Adverse effect of opium**

✓7ᵗʰ **T40.0X6** **Underdosing of opium**

✓5ᵗʰ **T40.1** **Poisoning by and adverse effect of heroin**

✓6ᵗʰ **T40.1X** **Poisoning by and adverse effect of** heroin

6 ✓7ᵗʰ **T40.1X1** **Poisoning by heroin, accidental (unintentional)** HCC

Poisoning by heroin NOS

7 ✓7ᵗʰ **T40.1X2** **Poisoning by heroin, intentional self-harm** HCC

✓7ᵗʰ **T40.1X3** **Poisoning by heroin, assault**

6 ✓7ᵗʰ **T40.1X4** **Poisoning by heroin, undetermined** HCC

N Newborn: 0   P Pediatric: 0-17   M Maternity: 9-64   A Adult: 15-124   MCC Major Complication/Comorbidity   CC Complication/Comorbidity   SW Severe Wound Dx

1154   ICD-10-CM 2020

√5ᵗʰ **T40.2** Poisoning by, adverse effect of and underdosing of other opioids

  √6ᵗʰ **T40.2X** Poisoning by, adverse effect of and underdosing of other opioids

    6 √7ᵗʰ **T40.2X1** Poisoning by other opioids, accidental (unintentional) — HCC
      Poisoning by other opioids NOS

    7 √7ᵗʰ **T40.2X2** Poisoning by other opioids, intentional self-harm — HCC

    √7ᵗʰ **T40.2X3** Poisoning by other opioids, assault

    6 √7ᵗʰ **T40.2X4** Poisoning by other opioids, undetermined — HCC

    √7ᵗʰ **T40.2X5** Adverse effect of other opioids

    √7ᵗʰ **T40.2X6** Underdosing of other opioids

√5ᵗʰ **T40.3** Poisoning by, adverse effect of and underdosing of methadone

  √6ᵗʰ **T40.3X** Poisoning by, adverse effect of and underdosing of methadone

    6 √7ᵗʰ **T40.3X1** Poisoning by methadone, accidental (unintentional) — HCC
      Poisoning by methadone NOS

    7 √7ᵗʰ **T40.3X2** Poisoning by methadone, intentional self-harm — HCC

    √7ᵗʰ **T40.3X3** Poisoning by methadone, assault

    6 √7ᵗʰ **T40.3X4** Poisoning by methadone, undetermined — HCC

    √7ᵗʰ **T40.3X5** Adverse effect of methadone

    √7ᵗʰ **T40.3X6** Underdosing of methadone

√5ᵗʰ **T40.4** Poisoning by, adverse effect of and underdosing of other synthetic narcotics

  √6ᵗʰ **T40.4X** Poisoning by, adverse effect of and underdosing of other synthetic narcotics

    6 √7ᵗʰ **T40.4X1** Poisoning by other synthetic narcotics, accidental (unintentional) — HCC
      Poisoning by other synthetic narcotics NOS

    7 √7ᵗʰ **T40.4X2** Poisoning by other synthetic narcotics, intentional self-harm — HCC

    √7ᵗʰ **T40.4X3** Poisoning by other synthetic narcotics, assault

    6 √7ᵗʰ **T40.4X4** Poisoning by other synthetic narcotics, undetermined — HCC

    √7ᵗʰ **T40.4X5** Adverse effect of other synthetic narcotics

    √7ᵗʰ **T40.4X6** Underdosing of other synthetic narcotics

√5ᵗʰ **T40.5** Poisoning by, adverse effect of and underdosing of cocaine

  √6ᵗʰ **T40.5X** Poisoning by, adverse effect of and underdosing of cocaine

    6 √7ᵗʰ **T40.5X1** Poisoning by cocaine, accidental (unintentional) — HCC
      Poisoning by cocaine NOS
      AHA: 2016,2Q,8

    7 √7ᵗʰ **T40.5X2** Poisoning by cocaine, intentional self-harm — HCC

    √7ᵗʰ **T40.5X3** Poisoning by cocaine, assault

    6 √7ᵗʰ **T40.5X4** Poisoning by cocaine, undetermined — HCC

    √7ᵗʰ **T40.5X5** Adverse effect of cocaine

    √7ᵗʰ **T40.5X6** Underdosing of cocaine

√5ᵗʰ **T40.6** Poisoning by, adverse effect of and underdosing of other and unspecified narcotics

  √6ᵗʰ **T40.60** Poisoning by, adverse effect of and underdosing of unspecified narcotics

    6 √7ᵗʰ **T40.601** Poisoning by unspecified narcotics, accidental (unintentional) — HCC
      Poisoning by narcotics NOS

    7 √7ᵗʰ **T40.602** Poisoning by unspecified narcotics, intentional self-harm — HCC

    √7ᵗʰ **T40.603** Poisoning by unspecified narcotics, assault

    6 √7ᵗʰ **T40.604** Poisoning by unspecified narcotics, undetermined — HCC

    √7ᵗʰ **T40.605** Adverse effect of unspecified narcotics

    √7ᵗʰ **T40.606** Underdosing of unspecified narcotics

  √6ᵗʰ **T40.69** Poisoning by, adverse effect of and underdosing of other narcotics

    6 √7ᵗʰ **T40.691** Poisoning by other narcotics, accidental (unintentional) — HCC
      Poisoning by other narcotics NOS

    7 √7ᵗʰ **T40.692** Poisoning by other narcotics, intentional self-harm — HCC

    √7ᵗʰ **T40.693** Poisoning by other narcotics, assault

    6 √7ᵗʰ **T40.694** Poisoning by other narcotics, undetermined — HCC

    √7ᵗʰ **T40.695** Adverse effect of other narcotics

    √7ᵗʰ **T40.696** Underdosing of other narcotics

√5ᵗʰ **T40.7** Poisoning by, adverse effect of and underdosing of cannabis (derivatives)

  √6ᵗʰ **T40.7X** Poisoning by, adverse effect of and underdosing of cannabis (derivatives)

    √7ᵗʰ **T40.7X1** Poisoning by cannabis (derivatives), accidental (unintentional)
      Poisoning by cannabis NOS

    7 √7ᵗʰ **T40.7X2** Poisoning by cannabis (derivatives), intentional self-harm — HCC

    √7ᵗʰ **T40.7X3** Poisoning by cannabis (derivatives), assault

    √7ᵗʰ **T40.7X4** Poisoning by cannabis (derivatives), undetermined

    √7ᵗʰ **T40.7X5** Adverse effect of cannabis (derivatives)

    √7ᵗʰ **T40.7X6** Underdosing of cannabis (derivatives)

√5ᵗʰ **T40.8** Poisoning by and adverse effect of lysergide [LSD]

  √6ᵗʰ **T40.8X** Poisoning by and adverse effect of lysergide [LSD]

    6 √7ᵗʰ **T40.8X1** Poisoning by lysergide [LSD], accidental (unintentional) — HCC
      Poisoning by lysergide [LSD] NOS

    7 √7ᵗʰ **T40.8X2** Poisoning by lysergide [LSD], intentional self-harm — HCC

    √7ᵗʰ **T40.8X3** Poisoning by lysergide [LSD], assault

    6 √7ᵗʰ **T40.8X4** Poisoning by lysergide [LSD], undetermined — HCC

√5ᵗʰ **T40.9** Poisoning by, adverse effect of and underdosing of other and unspecified psychodysleptics [hallucinogens]

  √6ᵗʰ **T40.90** Poisoning by, adverse effect of and underdosing of unspecified psychodysleptics [hallucinogens]

    6 √7ᵗʰ **T40.901** Poisoning by unspecified psychodysleptics [hallucinogens], accidental (unintentional) — HCC

    7 √7ᵗʰ **T40.902** Poisoning by unspecified psychodysleptics [hallucinogens], intentional self-harm — HCC

    √7ᵗʰ **T40.903** Poisoning by unspecified psychodysleptics [hallucinogens], assault

    6 √7ᵗʰ **T40.904** Poisoning by unspecified psychodysleptics [hallucinogens], undetermined — HCC

    √7ᵗʰ **T40.905** Adverse effect of unspecified psychodysleptics [hallucinogens]

    √7ᵗʰ **T40.906** Underdosing of unspecified psychodysleptics [hallucinogens]

  √6ᵗʰ **T40.99** Poisoning by, adverse effect of and underdosing of other psychodysleptics [hallucinogens]

    6 √7ᵗʰ **T40.991** Poisoning by other psychodysleptics [hallucinogens], accidental (unintentional) — HCC
      Poisoning by other psychodysleptics [hallucinogens] NOS

    7 √7ᵗʰ **T40.992** Poisoning by other psychodysleptics [hallucinogens], intentional self-harm — HCC

    √7ᵗʰ **T40.993** Poisoning by other psychodysleptics [hallucinogens], assault

    6 √7ᵗʰ **T40.994** Poisoning by other psychodysleptics [hallucinogens], undetermined — HCC

☑7ᵗʰ **T40.995** Adverse effect of other psychodysleptics [hallucinogens]

☑7ᵗʰ **T40.996** Underdosing of other psychodysleptics [hallucinogens]

☑4ᵗʰ **T41 Poisoning by, adverse effect of and underdosing of anesthetics and therapeutic gases**

> EXCLUDES 1   benzodiazepines (T42.4-)
> cocaine (T40.5-)
> complications of anesthesia during labor and delivery (O74.-)
> complications of anesthesia during pregnancy (O29.-)
> complications of anesthesia during the puerperium (O89.-)
> opioids (T40.0-T40.2-)

> The appropriate 7th character is to be added to each code from category T41.
> A   initial encounter
> D   subsequent encounter
> S   sequela

☑5ᵗʰ **T41.0 Poisoning by, adverse effect of and underdosing of inhaled anesthetics**

> EXCLUDES 1   oxygen (T41.5-)

☑6ᵗʰ **T41.0X Poisoning by, adverse effect of and underdosing of inhaled anesthetics**

☑7ᵗʰ **T41.0X1 Poisoning by inhaled anesthetics, accidental (unintentional)**
> Poisoning by inhaled anesthetics NOS

7 ☑7ᵗʰ **T41.0X2 Poisoning by inhaled anesthetics, intentional self-harm**   HCC

☑7ᵗʰ **T41.0X3 Poisoning by inhaled anesthetics, assault**

☑7ᵗʰ **T41.0X4 Poisoning by inhaled anesthetics, undetermined**

☑7ᵗʰ **T41.0X5 Adverse effect of inhaled anesthetics**

☑7ᵗʰ **T41.0X6 Underdosing of inhaled anesthetics**

☑5ᵗʰ **T41.1 Poisoning by, adverse effect of and underdosing of intravenous anesthetics**
> Poisoning by, adverse effect of and underdosing of thiobarbiturates

☑6ᵗʰ **T41.1X Poisoning by, adverse effect of and underdosing of intravenous anesthetics**

☑7ᵗʰ **T41.1X1 Poisoning by intravenous anesthetics, accidental (unintentional)**
> Poisoning by intravenous anesthetics NOS

7 ☑7ᵗʰ **T41.1X2 Poisoning by intravenous anesthetics, intentional self-harm**   HCC

☑7ᵗʰ **T41.1X3 Poisoning by intravenous anesthetics, assault**

☑7ᵗʰ **T41.1X4 Poisoning by intravenous anesthetics, undetermined**

☑7ᵗʰ **T41.1X5 Adverse effect of intravenous anesthetics**

☑7ᵗʰ **T41.1X6 Underdosing of intravenous anesthetics**

☑5ᵗʰ **T41.2 Poisoning by, adverse effect of and underdosing of other and unspecified general anesthetics**

☑6ᵗʰ **T41.20 Poisoning by, adverse effect of and underdosing of unspecified general anesthetics**

☑7ᵗʰ **T41.201 Poisoning by unspecified general anesthetics, accidental (unintentional)**
> Poisoning by general anesthetics NOS

7 ☑7ᵗʰ **T41.202 Poisoning by unspecified general anesthetics, intentional self-harm**   HCC

☑7ᵗʰ **T41.203 Poisoning by unspecified general anesthetics, assault**

☑7ᵗʰ **T41.204 Poisoning by unspecified general anesthetics, undetermined**

☑7ᵗʰ **T41.205 Adverse effect of unspecified general anesthetics**
> AHA: 2016,4Q,73

☑7ᵗʰ **T41.206 Underdosing of unspecified general anesthetics**

☑6ᵗʰ **T41.29 Poisoning by, adverse effect of and underdosing of other general anesthetics**

☑7ᵗʰ **T41.291 Poisoning by other general anesthetics, accidental (unintentional)**
> Poisoning by other general anesthetics NOS

7 ☑7ᵗʰ **T41.292 Poisoning by other general anesthetics, intentional self-harm**   HCC

☑7ᵗʰ **T41.293 Poisoning by other general anesthetics, assault**

☑7ᵗʰ **T41.294 Poisoning by other general anesthetics, undetermined**

☑7ᵗʰ **T41.295 Adverse effect of other general anesthetics**

☑7ᵗʰ **T41.296 Underdosing of other general anesthetics**

☑5ᵗʰ **T41.3 Poisoning by, adverse effect of and underdosing of local anesthetics**
> Cocaine (topical)
> EXCLUDES 2   poisoning by cocaine used as a central nervous system stimulant (T40.5X1-T40.5X4)

☑6ᵗʰ **T41.3X Poisoning by, adverse effect of and underdosing of local anesthetics**

☑7ᵗʰ **T41.3X1 Poisoning by local anesthetics, accidental (unintentional)**
> Poisoning by local anesthetics NOS

7 ☑7ᵗʰ **T41.3X2 Poisoning by local anesthetics, intentional self-harm**   HCC

☑7ᵗʰ **T41.3X3 Poisoning by local anesthetics, assault**

☑7ᵗʰ **T41.3X4 Poisoning by local anesthetics, undetermined**

☑7ᵗʰ **T41.3X5 Adverse effect of local anesthetics**

☑7ᵗʰ **T41.3X6 Underdosing of local anesthetics**

☑5ᵗʰ **T41.4 Poisoning by, adverse effect of and underdosing of unspecified anesthetic**

☑x7ᵗʰ **T41.41 Poisoning by unspecified anesthetic, accidental (unintentional)**
> Poisoning by anesthetic NOS

7 ☑x7ᵗʰ **T41.42 Poisoning by unspecified anesthetic, intentional self-harm**   HCC

☑x7ᵗʰ **T41.43 Poisoning by unspecified anesthetic, assault**

☑x7ᵗʰ **T41.44 Poisoning by unspecified anesthetic, undetermined**

☑x7ᵗʰ **T41.45 Adverse effect of unspecified anesthetic**

☑x7ᵗʰ **T41.46 Underdosing of unspecified anesthetics**

☑5ᵗʰ **T41.5 Poisoning by, adverse effect of and underdosing of therapeutic gases**

☑6ᵗʰ **T41.5X Poisoning by, adverse effect of and underdosing of therapeutic gases**

☑7ᵗʰ **T41.5X1 Poisoning by therapeutic gases, accidental (unintentional)**
> Poisoning by therapeutic gases NOS

7 ☑7ᵗʰ **T41.5X2 Poisoning by therapeutic gases, intentional self-harm**   HCC

☑7ᵗʰ **T41.5X3 Poisoning by therapeutic gases, assault**

☑7ᵗʰ **T41.5X4 Poisoning by therapeutic gases, undetermined**

☑7ᵗʰ **T41.5X5 Adverse effect of therapeutic gases**

☑7ᵗʰ **T41.5X6 Underdosing of therapeutic gases**

☑4ᵗʰ **T42 Poisoning by, adverse effect of and underdosing of antiepileptic, sedative-hypnotic and antiparkinsonism drugs**

> EXCLUDES 2   drug dependence and related mental and behavioral disorders due to psychoactive substance use (F10.- – F19.-)

> The appropriate 7th character is to be added to each code from category T42.
> A   initial encounter
> D   subsequent encounter
> S   sequela

☑5ᵗʰ **T42.0 Poisoning by, adverse effect of and underdosing of hydantoin derivatives**

☑6ᵗʰ **T42.0X Poisoning by, adverse effect of and underdosing of hydantoin derivatives**

☑7ᵗʰ **T42.0X1 Poisoning by hydantoin derivatives, accidental (unintentional)**
> Poisoning by hydantoin derivatives NOS

7 ☑7ᵗʰ **T42.0X2 Poisoning by hydantoin derivatives, intentional self-harm**   HCC

☑7ᵗʰ **T42.0X3 Poisoning by hydantoin derivatives, assault**

☑7ᵗʰ **T42.0X4 Poisoning by hydantoin derivatives, undetermined**

☑7ᵗʰ **T42.0X5 Adverse effect of hydantoin derivatives**

☑7ᵗʰ **T42.0X6 Underdosing of hydantoin derivatives**

N Newborn: 0   **P** Pediatric: 0-17   **M** Maternity: 9-64   **A** Adult: 15-124   **MCC** Major Complication/Comorbidity   **CC** Complication/Comorbidity   **SW** Severe Wound Dx

1156   ICD-10-CM 2020

☑5ᵗʰ **T42.1** **Poisoning by, adverse effect of and underdosing of iminostilbenes**

Poisoning by, adverse effect of and underdosing of carbamazepine

    ☑6ᵗʰ **T42.1X** **Poisoning by, adverse effect of and underdosing of** iminostilbenes

        ☑7ᵗʰ **T42.1X1** **Poisoning by iminostilbenes,** accidental (unintentional)

Poisoning by iminostilbenes NOS

        7 ☑7ᵗʰ **T42.1X2** **Poisoning by iminostilbenes, intentional self-harm**   `HCC`

        ☑7ᵗʰ **T42.1X3** **Poisoning by iminostilbenes,** assault

        ☑7ᵗʰ **T42.1X4** **Poisoning by iminostilbenes, undetermined**

        ☑7ᵗʰ **T42.1X5** Adverse effect **of iminostilbenes**

        ☑7ᵗʰ **T42.1X6** Underdosing **of iminostilbenes**

☑5ᵗʰ **T42.2** **Poisoning by, adverse effect of and underdosing of succinimides and oxazolidinediones**

    ☑6ᵗʰ **T42.2X** **Poisoning by, adverse effect of and underdosing of** succinimides and oxazolidinediones

        ☑7ᵗʰ **T42.2X1** **Poisoning by succinimides and oxazolidinediones,** accidental (unintentional)

Poisoning by succinimides and oxazolidinediones NOS

        7 ☑7ᵗʰ **T42.2X2** **Poisoning by succinimides and oxazolidinediones, intentional self-harm**   `HCC`

        ☑7ᵗʰ **T42.2X3** **Poisoning by succinimides and oxazolidinediones,** assault

        ☑7ᵗʰ **T42.2X4** **Poisoning by succinimides and oxazolidinediones,** undetermined

        ☑7ᵗʰ **T42.2X5** Adverse effect **of succinimides and oxazolidinediones**

        ☑7ᵗʰ **T42.2X6** Underdosing **of succinimides and oxazolidinediones**

☑5ᵗʰ **T42.3** **Poisoning by, adverse effect of and underdosing of barbiturates**

EXCLUDES 1   poisoning by, adverse effect of and underdosing of thiobarbiturates (T41.1-)

    ☑6ᵗʰ **T42.3X** **Poisoning by, adverse effect of and underdosing of** barbiturates

        ☑7ᵗʰ **T42.3X1** **Poisoning by barbiturates,** accidental (unintentional)

Poisoning by barbiturates NOS

        7 ☑7ᵗʰ **T42.3X2** **Poisoning by barbiturates, intentional self-harm**   `HCC`

        ☑7ᵗʰ **T42.3X3** **Poisoning by barbiturates,** assault

        ☑7ᵗʰ **T42.3X4** **Poisoning by barbiturates,** undetermined

        ☑7ᵗʰ **T42.3X5** Adverse effect **of barbiturates**

        ☑7ᵗʰ **T42.3X6** Underdosing **of barbiturates**

☑5ᵗʰ **T42.4** **Poisoning by, adverse effect of and underdosing of benzodiazepines**

    ☑6ᵗʰ **T42.4X** **Poisoning by, adverse effect of and underdosing of** benzodiazepines

        ☑7ᵗʰ **T42.4X1** **Poisoning by benzodiazepines,** accidental (unintentional)

Poisoning by benzodiazepines NOS

        7 ☑7ᵗʰ **T42.4X2** **Poisoning by benzodiazepines, intentional self-harm**   `HCC`

        ☑7ᵗʰ **T42.4X3** **Poisoning by benzodiazepines,** assault

        ☑7ᵗʰ **T42.4X4** **Poisoning by benzodiazepines,** undetermined

        ☑7ᵗʰ **T42.4X5** Adverse effect **of benzodiazepines**

        ☑7ᵗʰ **T42.4X6** Underdosing **of benzodiazepines**

☑5ᵗʰ **T42.5** **Poisoning by, adverse effect of and underdosing of mixed antiepileptics**

    ☑6ᵗʰ **T42.5X** **Poisoning by, adverse effect of and underdosing of** antiepileptics

        ☑7ᵗʰ **T42.5X1** **Poisoning by mixed antiepileptics,** accidental (unintentional)

Poisoning by mixed antiepileptics NOS

        7 ☑7ᵗʰ **T42.5X2** **Poisoning by mixed antiepileptics,** intentional self-harm   `HCC`

        ☑7ᵗʰ **T42.5X3** **Poisoning by mixed antiepileptics,** assault

        ☑7ᵗʰ **T42.5X4** **Poisoning by mixed antiepileptics, undetermined**

        ☑7ᵗʰ **T42.5X5** Adverse effect **of mixed antiepileptics**

        ☑7ᵗʰ **T42.5X6** Underdosing **of mixed antiepileptics**

☑5ᵗʰ **T42.6** **Poisoning by, adverse effect of and underdosing of other antiepileptic and sedative-hypnotic drugs**

Poisoning by, adverse effect of and underdosing of methaqualone

Poisoning by, adverse effect of and underdosing of valproic acid

EXCLUDES 1   poisoning by, adverse effect of and underdosing of carbamazepine (T42.1-)

    ☑6ᵗʰ **T42.6X** **Poisoning by, adverse effect of and underdosing of other antiepileptic and sedative-hypnotic drugs**

        ☑7ᵗʰ **T42.6X1** **Poisoning by other antiepileptic and sedative-hypnotic drugs,** accidental (unintentional)

Poisoning by other antiepileptic and sedative-hypnotic drugs NOS

        7 ☑7ᵗʰ **T42.6X2** **Poisoning by other antiepileptic and sedative-hypnotic drugs, intentional self-harm**   `HCC`

        ☑7ᵗʰ **T42.6X3** **Poisoning by other antiepileptic and sedative-hypnotic drugs,** assault

        ☑7ᵗʰ **T42.6X4** **Poisoning by other antiepileptic and sedative-hypnotic drugs,** undetermined

        ☑7ᵗʰ **T42.6X5** Adverse effect **of other antiepileptic and sedative-hypnotic drugs**

        ☑7ᵗʰ **T42.6X6** Underdosing **of other antiepileptic and sedative-hypnotic drugs**

☑5ᵗʰ **T42.7** **Poisoning by, adverse effect of and underdosing of unspecified antiepileptic and sedative-hypnotic drugs**

    √x7ᵗʰ **T42.71** **Poisoning by unspecified antiepileptic and sedative-hypnotic drugs,** accidental (unintentional)

Poisoning by antiepileptic and sedative-hypnotic drugs NOS

    7 √x7ᵗʰ **T42.72** **Poisoning by unspecified antiepileptic and sedative-hypnotic drugs, intentional self-harm**   `HCC`

    √x7ᵗʰ **T42.73** **Poisoning by unspecified antiepileptic and sedative-hypnotic drugs,** assault

    √x7ᵗʰ **T42.74** **Poisoning by unspecified antiepileptic and sedative-hypnotic drugs,** undetermined

    √x7ᵗʰ **T42.75** Adverse effect **of unspecified antiepileptic and sedative-hypnotic drugs**

    √x7ᵗʰ **T42.76** Underdosing **of unspecified antiepileptic and sedative-hypnotic drugs**

☑5ᵗʰ **T42.8** **Poisoning by, adverse effect of and underdosing of antiparkinsonism drugs and other central muscle-tone depressants**

Poisoning by, adverse effect of and underdosing of amantadine

    ☑6ᵗʰ **T42.8X** **Poisoning by, adverse effect of and underdosing of** antiparkinsonism drugs and other central muscle-tone depressants

        ☑7ᵗʰ **T42.8X1** **Poisoning by antiparkinsonism drugs and other central muscle-tone depressants,** accidental (unintentional)

Poisoning by antiparkinsonism drugs and other central muscle-tone depressants NOS

        7 ☑7ᵗʰ **T42.8X2** **Poisoning by antiparkinsonism drugs and other central muscle-tone depressants, intentional self-harm**   `HCC`

        ☑7ᵗʰ **T42.8X3** **Poisoning by antiparkinsonism drugs and other central muscle-tone depressants,** assault

        ☑7ᵗʰ **T42.8X4** **Poisoning by antiparkinsonism drugs and other central muscle-tone depressants,** undetermined

        ☑7ᵗʰ **T42.8X5** Adverse effect **of antiparkinsonism drugs and other central muscle-tone depressants**

        ☑7ᵗʰ **T42.8X6** Underdosing **of antiparkinsonism drugs and other central muscle-tone depressants**

☑ Additional Character Required   √x7ᵗʰ Placeholder   Unacceptable PDx   Questionable PDx   Manifestation   Unspecified Dx   H1 - H14 HAC   HCC CMS-HCC Dx   HIV HIV Dx

ICD-10-CM 2020   1157

✓4th **T43 Poisoning by, adverse effect of and underdosing of psychotropic drugs, not elsewhere classified**

> EXCLUDES 1   appetite depressants (T50.5-)
> barbiturates (T42.3-)
> benzodiazepines (T42.4-)
> methaqualone (T42.6-)
> psychodysleptics [hallucinogens] (T40.7-T40.9-)
>
> EXCLUDES 2   drug dependence and related mental and behavioral disorders due to psychoactive substance use (F10.- – F19.-)

> The appropriate 7th character is to be added to each code from category T43.
> A   initial encounter
> D   subsequent encounter
> S   sequela

✓5th **T43.0 Poisoning by, adverse effect of and underdosing of tricyclic and tetracyclic antidepressants**

     ✓6th **T43.01 Poisoning by, adverse effect of and underdosing of tricyclic antidepressants**

         ✓7th **T43.011 Poisoning by tricyclic antidepressants, accidental (unintentional)**
             Poisoning by tricyclic antidepressants NOS

         7 ✓7th **T43.012 Poisoning by tricyclic antidepressants, intentional self-harm**   HCC

         ✓7th **T43.013 Poisoning by tricyclic antidepressants, assault**

         ✓7th **T43.014 Poisoning by tricyclic antidepressants, undetermined**

         ✓7th **T43.015 Adverse effect of tricyclic antidepressants**

         ✓7th **T43.016 Underdosing of tricyclic antidepressants**

     ✓6th **T43.02 Poisoning by, adverse effect of and underdosing of tetracyclic antidepressants**

         ✓7th **T43.021 Poisoning by tetracyclic antidepressants, accidental (unintentional)**
             Poisoning by tetracyclic antidepressants NOS

         7 ✓7th **T43.022 Poisoning by tetracyclic antidepressants, intentional self-harm**   HCC

         ✓7th **T43.023 Poisoning by tetracyclic antidepressants, assault**

         ✓7th **T43.024 Poisoning by tetracyclic antidepressants, undetermined**

         ✓7th **T43.025 Adverse effect of tetracyclic antidepressants**

         ✓7th **T43.026 Underdosing of tetracyclic antidepressants**

✓5th **T43.1 Poisoning by, adverse effect of and underdosing of monoamine-oxidase-inhibitor antidepressants**

     ✓6th **T43.1X Poisoning by, adverse effect of and underdosing of monoamine-oxidase-inhibitor antidepressants**

         ✓7th **T43.1X1 Poisoning by monoamine-oxidase-inhibitor antidepressants, accidental (unintentional)**
             Poisoning by monoamine oxidase inhibitor antidepressants NOS

         7 ✓7th **T43.1X2 Poisoning by monoamine-oxidase-inhibitor antidepressants, intentional self-harm**   HCC

         ✓7th **T43.1X3 Poisoning by monoamine-oxidase-inhibitor antidepressants, assault**

         ✓7th **T43.1X4 Poisoning by monoamine-oxidase-inhibitor antidepressants, undetermined**

         ✓7th **T43.1X5 Adverse effect of monoamine-oxidase-inhibitor antidepressants**

         ✓7th **T43.1X6 Underdosing of monoamine-oxidase-inhibitor antidepressants**

✓5th **T43.2 Poisoning by, adverse effect of and underdosing of other and unspecified antidepressants**

     ✓6th **T43.20 Poisoning by, adverse effect of and underdosing of unspecified antidepressants**

         ✓7th **T43.201 Poisoning by unspecified antidepressants, accidental (unintentional)**
             Poisoning by antidepressants NOS

         7 ✓7th **T43.202 Poisoning by unspecified antidepressants, intentional self-harm**   HCC

         ✓7th **T43.203 Poisoning by unspecified antidepressants, assault**

         ✓7th **T43.204 Poisoning by unspecified antidepressants, undetermined**

         ✓7th **T43.205 Adverse effect of unspecified antidepressants**
             Antidepressant discontinuation syndrome

         ✓7th **T43.206 Underdosing of unspecified antidepressants**

     ✓6th **T43.21 Poisoning by, adverse effect of and underdosing of selective serotonin and norepinephrine reuptake inhibitors**
         Poisoning by, adverse effect of and underdosing of SSNRI antidepressants

         ✓7th **T43.211 Poisoning by selective serotonin and norepinephrine reuptake inhibitors, accidental (unintentional)**

         7 ✓7th **T43.212 Poisoning by selective serotonin and norepinephrine reuptake inhibitors, intentional self-harm**   HCC

         ✓7th **T43.213 Poisoning by selective serotonin and norepinephrine reuptake inhibitors, assault**

         ✓7th **T43.214 Poisoning by selective serotonin and norepinephrine reuptake inhibitors, undetermined**

         ✓7th **T43.215 Adverse effect of selective serotonin and norepinephrine reuptake inhibitors**

         ✓7th **T43.216 Underdosing of selective serotonin and norepinephrine reuptake inhibitors**

     ✓6th **T43.22 Poisoning by, adverse effect of and underdosing of selective serotonin reuptake inhibitors**
         Poisoning by, adverse effect of and underdosing of SSRI antidepressants

         ✓7th **T43.221 Poisoning by selective serotonin reuptake inhibitors, accidental (unintentional)**

         7 ✓7th **T43.222 Poisoning by selective serotonin reuptake inhibitors, intentional self-harm**   HCC

         ✓7th **T43.223 Poisoning by selective serotonin reuptake inhibitors, assault**

         ✓7th **T43.224 Poisoning by selective serotonin reuptake inhibitors, undetermined**

         ✓7th **T43.225 Adverse effect of selective serotonin reuptake inhibitors**

         ✓7th **T43.226 Underdosing of selective serotonin reuptake inhibitors**

     ✓6th **T43.29 Poisoning by, adverse effect of and underdosing of other antidepressants**

         ✓7th **T43.291 Poisoning by other antidepressants, accidental (unintentional)**
             Poisoning by other antidepressants NOS

         7 ✓7th **T43.292 Poisoning by other antidepressants, intentional self-harm**   HCC

         ✓7th **T43.293 Poisoning by other antidepressants, assault**

         ✓7th **T43.294 Poisoning by other antidepressants, undetermined**

         ✓7th **T43.295 Adverse effect of other antidepressants**

         ✓7th **T43.296 Underdosing of other antidepressants**

√5ᵗʰ **T43.3** **Poisoning by, adverse effect of and underdosing of phenothiazine antipsychotics and neuroleptics**

√6ᵗʰ **T43.3X** **Poisoning by, adverse effect of and underdosing of phenothiazine antipsychotics and neuroleptics**

√7ᵗʰ **T43.3X1** **Poisoning by phenothiazine antipsychotics and neuroleptics, accidental (unintentional)**
Poisoning by phenothiazine antipsychotics and neuroleptics NOS

7 √7ᵗʰ **T43.3X2** **Poisoning by phenothiazine antipsychotics and neuroleptics, intentional self-harm** `HCC`

√7ᵗʰ **T43.3X3** **Poisoning by phenothiazine antipsychotics and neuroleptics, assault**

√7ᵗʰ **T43.3X4** **Poisoning by phenothiazine antipsychotics and neuroleptics, undetermined**

√7ᵗʰ **T43.3X5** **Adverse effect of phenothiazine antipsychotics and neuroleptics**

√7ᵗʰ **T43.3X6** **Underdosing of phenothiazine antipsychotics and neuroleptics**

√5ᵗʰ **T43.4** **Poisoning by, adverse effect of and underdosing of butyrophenone and thiothixene neuroleptics**

√6ᵗʰ **T43.4X** **Poisoning by, adverse effect of and underdosing of butyrophenone and thiothixene neuroleptics**

√7ᵗʰ **T43.4X1** **Poisoning by butyrophenone and thiothixene neuroleptics, accidental (unintentional)**
Poisoning by butyrophenone and thiothixene neuroleptics NOS

7 √7ᵗʰ **T43.4X2** **Poisoning by butyrophenone and thiothixene neuroleptics, intentional self-harm** `HCC`

√7ᵗʰ **T43.4X3** **Poisoning by butyrophenone and thiothixene neuroleptics, assault**

√7ᵗʰ **T43.4X4** **Poisoning by butyrophenone and thiothixene neuroleptics, undetermined**

√7ᵗʰ **T43.4X5** **Adverse effect of butyrophenone and thiothixene neuroleptics**

√7ᵗʰ **T43.4X6** **Underdosing of butyrophenone and thiothixene neuroleptics**

√5ᵗʰ **T43.5** **Poisoning by, adverse effect of and underdosing of other and unspecified antipsychotics and neuroleptics**

EXCLUDES 1   *poisoning by, adverse effect of and underdosing of rauwolfia (T46.5-)*

√6ᵗʰ **T43.50** **Poisoning by, adverse effect of and underdosing of unspecified antipsychotics and neuroleptics**

√7ᵗʰ **T43.501** **Poisoning by unspecified antipsychotics and neuroleptics, accidental (unintentional)**
Poisoning by antipsychotics and neuroleptics NOS

7 √7ᵗʰ **T43.502** **Poisoning by unspecified antipsychotics and neuroleptics, intentional self-harm** `HCC`

√7ᵗʰ **T43.503** **Poisoning by unspecified antipsychotics and neuroleptics, assault**

√7ᵗʰ **T43.504** **Poisoning by unspecified antipsychotics and neuroleptics, undetermined**

√7ᵗʰ **T43.505** **Adverse effect of unspecified antipsychotics and neuroleptics**

√7ᵗʰ **T43.506** **Underdosing of unspecified antipsychotics and neuroleptics**

√6ᵗʰ **T43.59** **Poisoning by, adverse effect of and underdosing of other antipsychotics and neuroleptics**
AHA: 2017,1Q,40

√7ᵗʰ **T43.591** **Poisoning by other antipsychotics and neuroleptics, accidental (unintentional)**
Poisoning by other antipsychotics and neuroleptics NOS

7 √7ᵗʰ **T43.592** **Poisoning by other antipsychotics and neuroleptics, intentional self-harm** `HCC`

√7ᵗʰ **T43.593** **Poisoning by other antipsychotics and neuroleptics, assault**

√7ᵗʰ **T43.594** **Poisoning by other antipsychotics and neuroleptics, undetermined**

√7ᵗʰ **T43.595** **Adverse effect of other antipsychotics and neuroleptics**

√7ᵗʰ **T43.596** **Underdosing of other antipsychotics and neuroleptics**

√5ᵗʰ **T43.6** **Poisoning by, adverse effect of and underdosing of psychostimulants**

EXCLUDES 1   *poisoning by, adverse effect of and underdosing of cocaine (T40.5-)*

√6ᵗʰ **T43.60** **Poisoning by, adverse effect of and underdosing of unspecified psychostimulant**

6 √7ᵗʰ **T43.601** **Poisoning by unspecified psychostimulants, accidental (unintentional)** `HCC`
Poisoning by psychostimulants NOS

7 √7ᵗʰ **T43.602** **Poisoning by unspecified psychostimulants, intentional self-harm** `HCC`

√7ᵗʰ **T43.603** **Poisoning by unspecified psychostimulants, assault**

6 √7ᵗʰ **T43.604** **Poisoning by unspecified psychostimulants, undetermined** `HCC`

√7ᵗʰ **T43.605** **Adverse effect of unspecified psychostimulants**

√7ᵗʰ **T43.606** **Underdosing of unspecified psychostimulants**

√6ᵗʰ **T43.61** **Poisoning by, adverse effect of and underdosing of caffeine**

6 √7ᵗʰ **T43.611** **Poisoning by caffeine, accidental (unintentional)** `HCC`
Poisoning by caffeine NOS

7 √7ᵗʰ **T43.612** **Poisoning by caffeine, intentional self-harm** `HCC`

√7ᵗʰ **T43.613** **Poisoning by caffeine, assault**

6 √7ᵗʰ **T43.614** **Poisoning by caffeine, undetermined** `HCC`

√7ᵗʰ **T43.615** **Adverse effect of caffeine**

√7ᵗʰ **T43.616** **Underdosing of caffeine**

√6ᵗʰ **T43.62** **Poisoning by, adverse effect of and underdosing of amphetamines**
Poisoning by, adverse effect of and underdosing of methamphetamines

6 √7ᵗʰ **T43.621** **Poisoning by amphetamines, accidental (unintentional)** `HCC`
Poisoning by amphetamines NOS

7 √7ᵗʰ **T43.622** **Poisoning by amphetamines, intentional self-harm** `HCC`

√7ᵗʰ **T43.623** **Poisoning by amphetamines, assault**

6 √7ᵗʰ **T43.624** **Poisoning by amphetamines, undetermined** `HCC`

√7ᵗʰ **T43.625** **Adverse effect of amphetamines**

√7ᵗʰ **T43.626** **Underdosing of amphetamines**

√6ᵗʰ **T43.63** **Poisoning by, adverse effect of and underdosing of methylphenidate**

6 √7ᵗʰ **T43.631** **Poisoning by methylphenidate, accidental (unintentional)** `HCC`
Poisoning by methylphenidate NOS

7 √7ᵗʰ **T43.632** **Poisoning by methylphenidate, intentional self-harm** `HCC`

√7ᵗʰ **T43.633** **Poisoning by methylphenidate, assault**

6 √7ᵗʰ **T43.634** **Poisoning by methylphenidate, undetermined** `HCC`

√7ᵗʰ **T43.635** **Adverse effect of methylphenidate**

√7ᵗʰ **T43.636** **Underdosing of methylphenidate**

√6ᵗʰ **T43.64** **Poisoning by ecstasy**
Poisoning by MDMA
Poisoning by 3,4-methylenedioxymethamphetamine
AHA: 2018,4Q,30-31

6 √7ᵗʰ **T43.641** **Poisoning by ecstasy, accidental (unintentional)** `HCC`
Poisoning by ecstasy NOS

7 √7ᵗʰ **T43.642** **Poisoning by ecstasy, intentional self-harm** `HCC`

√7ᵗʰ **T43.643** **Poisoning by ecstasy, assault**

☑ Additional Character Required   √x7ᵗʰ Placeholder   Unacceptable PDx   Questionable PDx   Manifestation   Unspecified Dx   H1-H14 HAC   HCC CMS-HCC Dx   HIV HIV Dx

ICD-10-CM 2020   **1159**

Chapter 19. Injury, Poisoning and Certain Other Consequences of External Causes

6 √7ᵗʰ **T43.644** **Poisoning by ecstasy,** undetermined   HCC

√6ᵗʰ **T43.69** **Poisoning by, adverse effect of and underdosing of other psychostimulants**

    6 √7ᵗʰ **T43.691** **Poisoning by other psychostimulants,** accidental (unintentional)   HCC
       Poisoning by other psychostimulants NOS

    7 √7ᵗʰ **T43.692** **Poisoning by other psychostimulants,** intentional self-harm   HCC

    √7ᵗʰ **T43.693** **Poisoning by other psychostimulants,** assault

    6 √7ᵗʰ **T43.694** **Poisoning by other psychostimulants,** undetermined   HCC

    √7ᵗʰ **T43.695** Adverse effect of other psychostimulants

    √7ᵗʰ **T43.696** Underdosing of other psychostimulants

√5ᵗʰ **T43.8** **Poisoning by, adverse effect of and underdosing of other psychotropic drugs**

√6ᵗʰ **T43.8X** **Poisoning by, adverse effect of and underdosing of other psychotropic drugs**

    √7ᵗʰ **T43.8X1** **Poisoning by other psychotropic drugs,** accidental (unintentional)
       Poisoning by other psychotropic drugs NOS

    7 √7ᵗʰ **T43.8X2** **Poisoning by other psychotropic drugs,** intentional self-harm   HCC

    √7ᵗʰ **T43.8X3** **Poisoning by other psychotropic drugs,** assault

    √7ᵗʰ **T43.8X4** **Poisoning by other psychotropic drugs,** undetermined

    √7ᵗʰ **T43.8X5** Adverse effect of other psychotropic drugs

    √7ᵗʰ **T43.8X6** Underdosing of other psychotropic drugs

√5ᵗʰ **T43.9** **Poisoning by, adverse effect of and underdosing of unspecified psychotropic drug**

    √x7ᵗʰ **T43.91** **Poisoning by unspecified psychotropic drug,** accidental (unintentional)
       Poisoning by psychotropic drug NOS

    7 √x7ᵗʰ **T43.92** **Poisoning by unspecified psychotropic drug,** intentional self-harm   HCC

    √x7ᵗʰ **T43.93** **Poisoning by unspecified psychotropic drug,** assault

    √x7ᵗʰ **T43.94** **Poisoning by unspecified psychotropic drug,** undetermined

    √x7ᵗʰ **T43.95** Adverse effect of unspecified psychotropic drug

    √x7ᵗʰ **T43.96** Underdosing of unspecified psychotropic drug

√4ᵗʰ **T44** **Poisoning by, adverse effect of and underdosing of drugs primarily affecting the autonomic nervous system**

The appropriate 7th character is to be added to each code from category T44.
A   initial encounter
D   subsequent encounter
S   sequela

√5ᵗʰ **T44.0** **Poisoning by, adverse effect of and underdosing of anticholinesterase agents**

√6ᵗʰ **T44.0X** **Poisoning by, adverse effect of and underdosing of anticholinesterase agents**

    √7ᵗʰ **T44.0X1** **Poisoning by anticholinesterase agents,** accidental (unintentional)
       Poisoning by anticholinesterase agents NOS

    7 √7ᵗʰ **T44.0X2** **Poisoning by anticholinesterase agents,** intentional self-harm   HCC

    √7ᵗʰ **T44.0X3** **Poisoning by anticholinesterase agents,** assault

    √7ᵗʰ **T44.0X4** **Poisoning by anticholinesterase agents,** undetermined

    √7ᵗʰ **T44.0X5** Adverse effect of anticholinesterase agents

    √7ᵗʰ **T44.0X6** Underdosing of anticholinesterase agents

√5ᵗʰ **T44.1** **Poisoning by, adverse effect of and underdosing of other parasympathomimetics [cholinergics]**

√6ᵗʰ **T44.1X** **Poisoning by, adverse effect of and underdosing of other parasympathomimetics [cholinergics]**

    √7ᵗʰ **T44.1X1** **Poisoning by other parasympathomimetics [cholinergics],** accidental (unintentional)
       Poisoning by other parasympathomimetics [cholinergics] NOS

    7 √7ᵗʰ **T44.1X2** **Poisoning by other parasympathomimetics [cholinergics], intentional self-harm**   HCC

    √7ᵗʰ **T44.1X3** **Poisoning by other parasympathomimetics [cholinergics], assault**

    √7ᵗʰ **T44.1X4** **Poisoning by other parasympathomimetics [cholinergics],** undetermined

    √7ᵗʰ **T44.1X5** Adverse effect of other parasympathomimetics [cholinergics]

    √7ᵗʰ **T44.1X6** Underdosing of other parasympathomimetics [cholinergics]

√5ᵗʰ **T44.2** **Poisoning by, adverse effect of and underdosing of ganglionic blocking drugs**

√6ᵗʰ **T44.2X** **Poisoning by, adverse effect of and underdosing of ganglionic blocking drugs**

    √7ᵗʰ **T44.2X1** **Poisoning by ganglionic blocking drugs,** accidental (unintentional)
       Poisoning by ganglionic blocking drugs NOS

    7 √7ᵗʰ **T44.2X2** **Poisoning by ganglionic blocking drugs, intentional self-harm**   HCC

    √7ᵗʰ **T44.2X3** **Poisoning by ganglionic blocking drugs,** assault

    √7ᵗʰ **T44.2X4** **Poisoning by ganglionic blocking drugs,** undetermined

    √7ᵗʰ **T44.2X5** Adverse effect of ganglionic blocking drugs

    √7ᵗʰ **T44.2X6** Underdosing of ganglionic blocking drugs

√5ᵗʰ **T44.3** **Poisoning by, adverse effect of and underdosing of other parasympatholytics [anticholinergics and antimuscarinics] and spasmolytics**
    Poisoning by, adverse effect of and underdosing of papaverine

√6ᵗʰ **T44.3X** **Poisoning by, adverse effect of and underdosing of other parasympatholytics [anticholinergics and antimuscarinics] and spasmolytics**

    √7ᵗʰ **T44.3X1** **Poisoning by other parasympatholytics [anticholinergics and antimuscarinics] and spasmolytics,** accidental (unintentional)
       Poisoning by other parasympatholytics [anticholinergics and antimuscarinics] and spasmolytics NOS

    7 √7ᵗʰ **T44.3X2** **Poisoning by other parasympatholytics [anticholinergics and antimuscarinics] and spasmolytics, intentional self-harm**   HCC

    √7ᵗʰ **T44.3X3** **Poisoning by other parasympatholytics [anticholinergics and antimuscarinics] and spasmolytics, assault**

    √7ᵗʰ **T44.3X4** **Poisoning by other parasympatholytics [anticholinergics and antimuscarinics] and spasmolytics,** undetermined

    √7ᵗʰ **T44.3X5** Adverse effect of other parasympatholytics [anticholinergics and antimuscarinics] and spasmolytics

    √7ᵗʰ **T44.3X6** Underdosing of other parasympatholytics [anticholinergics and antimuscarinics] and spasmolytics

N Newborn: 0   P Pediatric: 0-17   M Maternity: 9-64   A Adult: 15-124   MCC Major Complication/Comorbidity   CC Complication/Comorbidity   SW Severe Wound Dx

1160   ICD-10-CM 2020

√5ᵗʰ T44.4 Poisoning by, adverse effect of and underdosing of predominantly alpha-adrenoreceptor agonists
Poisoning by, adverse effect of and underdosing of metaraminol

√6ᵗʰ T44.4X Poisoning by, adverse effect of and underdosing of predominantly alpha-adrenoreceptor agonists

√7ᵗʰ **T44.4X1 Poisoning by predominantly alpha-adrenoreceptor agonists, accidental (unintentional)**
Poisoning by predominantly alpha-adrenoreceptor agonists NOS

7 √7ᵗʰ **T44.4X2 Poisoning by predominantly alpha-adrenoreceptor agonists, intentional self-harm**   HCC

√7ᵗʰ **T44.4X3 Poisoning by predominantly alpha-adrenoreceptor agonists, assault**

√7ᵗʰ **T44.4X4 Poisoning by predominantly alpha-adrenoreceptor agonists, undetermined**

√7ᵗʰ **T44.4X5 Adverse effect of predominantly alpha-adrenoreceptor agonists**

√7ᵗʰ **T44.4X6 Underdosing of predominantly alpha-adrenoreceptor agonists**

√5ᵗʰ T44.5 Poisoning by, adverse effect of and underdosing of predominantly beta-adrenoreceptor agonists
EXCLUDES 1   poisoning by, adverse effect of and underdosing of beta-adrenoreceptor agonists used in asthma therapy (T48.6-)

√6ᵗʰ T44.5X Poisoning by, adverse effect of and underdosing of predominantly beta-adrenoreceptor agonists

√7ᵗʰ **T44.5X1 Poisoning by predominantly beta-adrenoreceptor agonists, accidental (unintentional)**
Poisoning by predominantly beta-adrenoreceptor agonists NOS

7 √7ᵗʰ **T44.5X2 Poisoning by predominantly beta-adrenoreceptor agonists, intentional self-harm**   HCC

√7ᵗʰ **T44.5X3 Poisoning by predominantly beta-adrenoreceptor agonists, assault**

√7ᵗʰ **T44.5X4 Poisoning by predominantly beta-adrenoreceptor agonists, undetermined**

√7ᵗʰ **T44.5X5 Adverse effect of predominantly beta-adrenoreceptor agonists**

√7ᵗʰ **T44.5X6 Underdosing of predominantly beta-adrenoreceptor agonists**

√5ᵗʰ T44.6 Poisoning by, adverse effect of and underdosing of alpha-adrenoreceptor antagonists
EXCLUDES 1   poisoning by, adverse effect of and underdosing of ergot alkaloids (T48.0)

√6ᵗʰ T44.6X Poisoning by, adverse effect of and underdosing of alpha-adrenoreceptor antagonists

√7ᵗʰ **T44.6X1 Poisoning by alpha-adrenoreceptor antagonists, accidental (unintentional)**
Poisoning by alpha-adrenoreceptor antagonists NOS

7 √7ᵗʰ **T44.6X2 Poisoning by alpha-adrenoreceptor antagonists, intentional self-harm**   HCC

√7ᵗʰ **T44.6X3 Poisoning by alpha-adrenoreceptor antagonists, assault**

√7ᵗʰ **T44.6X4 Poisoning by alpha-adrenoreceptor antagonists, undetermined**

√7ᵗʰ **T44.6X5 Adverse effect of alpha-adrenoreceptor antagonists**

√7ᵗʰ **T44.6X6 Underdosing of alpha-adrenoreceptor antagonists**

√5ᵗʰ T44.7 Poisoning by, adverse effect of and underdosing of beta-adrenoreceptor antagonists

√6ᵗʰ T44.7X Poisoning by, adverse effect of and underdosing of beta-adrenoreceptor antagonists

√7ᵗʰ **T44.7X1 Poisoning by beta-adrenoreceptor antagonists, accidental (unintentional)**
Poisoning by beta-adrenoreceptor antagonists NOS

7 √7ᵗʰ **T44.7X2 Poisoning by beta-adrenoreceptor antagonists, intentional self-harm**   HCC

√7ᵗʰ **T44.7X3 Poisoning by beta-adrenoreceptor antagonists, assault**

√7ᵗʰ **T44.7X4 Poisoning by beta-adrenoreceptor antagonists, undetermined**

√7ᵗʰ **T44.7X5 Adverse effect of beta-adrenoreceptor antagonists**

√7ᵗʰ **T44.7X6 Underdosing of beta-adrenoreceptor antagonists**

√5ᵗʰ T44.8 Poisoning by, adverse effect of and underdosing of centrally-acting and adrenergic-neuron- blocking agents
EXCLUDES 1   poisoning by, adverse effect of and underdosing of clonidine (T46.5)
poisoning by, adverse effect of and underdosing of guanethidine (T46.5)

√6ᵗʰ T44.8X Poisoning by, adverse effect of and underdosing of centrally-acting and adrenergic- neuron-blocking agents

√7ᵗʰ **T44.8X1 Poisoning by centrally-acting and adrenergic-neuron-blocking agents, accidental (unintentional)**
Poisoning by centrally-acting and adrenergic-neuron-blocking agents NOS

7 √7ᵗʰ **T44.8X2 Poisoning by centrally-acting and adrenergic-neuron-blocking agents, intentional self-harm**   HCC

√7ᵗʰ **T44.8X3 Poisoning by centrally-acting and adrenergic-neuron-blocking agents, assault**

√7ᵗʰ **T44.8X4 Poisoning by centrally-acting and adrenergic-neuron-blocking agents, undetermined**

√7ᵗʰ **T44.8X5 Adverse effect of centrally-acting and adrenergic-neuron-blocking agents**

√7ᵗʰ **T44.8X6 Underdosing of centrally-acting and adrenergic-neuron-blocking agents**

√5ᵗʰ T44.9 Poisoning by, adverse effect of and underdosing of other and unspecified drugs primarily affecting the autonomic nervous system
Poisoning by, adverse effect of and underdosing of drug stimulating both alpha and beta-adrenoreceptors

√6ᵗʰ T44.90 Poisoning by, adverse effect of and underdosing of unspecified drugs primarily affecting the autonomic nervous system

√7ᵗʰ **T44.901 Poisoning by unspecified drugs primarily affecting the autonomic nervous system, accidental (unintentional)**
Poisoning by unspecified drugs primarily affecting the autonomic nervous system NOS

7 √7ᵗʰ **T44.902 Poisoning by unspecified drugs primarily affecting the autonomic nervous system, intentional self-harm**   HCC

√7ᵗʰ **T44.903 Poisoning by unspecified drugs primarily affecting the autonomic nervous system, assault**

√7ᵗʰ **T44.904 Poisoning by unspecified drugs primarily affecting the autonomic nervous system, undetermined**

√7ᵗʰ **T44.905 Adverse effect of unspecified drugs primarily affecting the autonomic nervous system**

√7ᵗʰ **T44.906 Underdosing of unspecified drugs primarily affecting the autonomic nervous system**

√6ᵗʰ T44.99 Poisoning by, adverse effect of and underdosing of other drugs primarily affecting the autonomic nervous system

√7ᵗʰ **T44.991 Poisoning by other drug primarily affecting the autonomic nervous system, accidental (unintentional)**
Poisoning by other drugs primarily affecting the autonomic nervous system NOS

Chapter 19. Injury, Poisoning and Certain Other Consequences of External Causes

T44.4–T44.991

7 ✓7ᵗʰ T44.992 Poisoning by other drug primarily affecting the autonomic nervous system, intentional self-harm   HCC

✓7ᵗʰ T44.993 Poisoning by other drug primarily affecting the autonomic nervous system, assault

✓7ᵗʰ T44.994 Poisoning by other drug primarily affecting the autonomic nervous system, undetermined

✓7ᵗʰ T44.995 Adverse effect of other drug primarily affecting the autonomic nervous system

✓7ᵗʰ T44.996 Underdosing of other drug primarily affecting the autonomic nervous system

✓4ᵗʰ T45 Poisoning by, adverse effect of and underdosing of primarily systemic and hematological agents, not elsewhere classified

The appropriate 7th character is to be added to each code from category T45.
- A   initial encounter
- D   subsequent encounter
- S   sequela

✓5ᵗʰ T45.0 Poisoning by, adverse effect of and underdosing of antiallergic and antiemetic drugs

> EXCLUDES 1   *poisoning by, adverse effect of and underdosing of phenothiazine-based neuroleptics (T43.3)*

✓6ᵗʰ T45.0X Poisoning by, adverse effect of and underdosing of antiallergic and antiemetic drugs

✓7ᵗʰ T45.0X1 Poisoning by antiallergic and antiemetic drugs, accidental (unintentional)
Poisoning by antiallergic and antiemetic drugs NOS

7 ✓7ᵗʰ T45.0X2 Poisoning by antiallergic and antiemetic drugs, intentional self-harm   HCC

✓7ᵗʰ T45.0X3 Poisoning by antiallergic and antiemetic drugs, assault

✓7ᵗʰ T45.0X4 Poisoning by antiallergic and antiemetic drugs, undetermined

✓7ᵗʰ T45.0X5 Adverse effect of antiallergic and antiemetic drugs

✓7ᵗʰ T45.0X6 Underdosing of antiallergic and antiemetic drugs

✓5ᵗʰ T45.1 Poisoning by, adverse effect of and underdosing of antineoplastic and immunosuppressive drugs

> EXCLUDES 1   *poisoning by, adverse effect of and underdosing of tamoxifen (T38.6)*

AHA: 2019,1Q,17,20; 2014,4Q,22

✓6ᵗʰ T45.1X Poisoning by, adverse effect of and underdosing of antineoplastic and immunosuppressive drugs

✓7ᵗʰ T45.1X1 Poisoning by antineoplastic and immunosuppressive drugs, accidental (unintentional)
Poisoning by antineoplastic and immunosuppressive drugs NOS

7 ✓7ᵗʰ T45.1X2 Poisoning by antineoplastic and immunosuppressive drugs, intentional self-harm   HCC

✓7ᵗʰ T45.1X3 Poisoning by antineoplastic and immunosuppressive drugs, assault

✓7ᵗʰ T45.1X4 Poisoning by antineoplastic and immunosuppressive drugs, undetermined

✓7ᵗʰ T45.1X5 Adverse effect of antineoplastic and immunosuppressive drugs

AHA: 2019,2Q,24,28

✓7ᵗʰ T45.1X6 Underdosing of antineoplastic and immunosuppressive drugs

✓5ᵗʰ T45.2 Poisoning by, adverse effect of and underdosing of vitamins

> EXCLUDES 2   *poisoning by, adverse effect of and underdosing of iron (T45.4)*
> *poisoning by, adverse effect of and underdosing of nicotinic acid (derivatives) (T46.7)*
> *poisoning by, adverse effect of and underdosing of vitamin K (T45.7)*

✓6ᵗʰ T45.2X Poisoning by, adverse effect of and underdosing of vitamins

✓7ᵗʰ T45.2X1 Poisoning by vitamins, accidental (unintentional)
Poisoning by vitamins NOS

7 ✓7ᵗʰ T45.2X2 Poisoning by vitamins, intentional self-harm   HCC

✓7ᵗʰ T45.2X3 Poisoning by vitamins, assault

✓7ᵗʰ T45.2X4 Poisoning by vitamins, undetermined

✓7ᵗʰ T45.2X5 Adverse effect of vitamins

✓7ᵗʰ T45.2X6 Underdosing of vitamins

> EXCLUDES 1   *vitamin deficiencies (E50-E56)*

✓5ᵗʰ T45.3 Poisoning by, adverse effect of and underdosing of enzymes

✓6ᵗʰ T45.3X Poisoning by, adverse effect of and underdosing of enzymes

✓7ᵗʰ T45.3X1 Poisoning by enzymes, accidental (unintentional)
Poisoning by enzymes NOS

7 ✓7ᵗʰ T45.3X2 Poisoning by enzymes, intentional self-harm   HCC

✓7ᵗʰ T45.3X3 Poisoning by enzymes, assault

✓7ᵗʰ T45.3X4 Poisoning by enzymes, undetermined

✓7ᵗʰ T45.3X5 Adverse effect of enzymes

✓7ᵗʰ T45.3X6 Underdosing of enzymes

✓5ᵗʰ T45.4 Poisoning by, adverse effect of and underdosing of iron and its compounds

✓6ᵗʰ T45.4X Poisoning by, adverse effect of and underdosing of iron and its compounds

✓7ᵗʰ T45.4X1 Poisoning by iron and its compounds, accidental (unintentional)
Poisoning by iron and its compounds NOS

7 ✓7ᵗʰ T45.4X2 Poisoning by iron and its compounds, intentional self-harm   HCC

✓7ᵗʰ T45.4X3 Poisoning by iron and its compounds, assault

✓7ᵗʰ T45.4X4 Poisoning by iron and its compounds, undetermined

✓7ᵗʰ T45.4X5 Adverse effect of iron and its compounds

✓7ᵗʰ T45.4X6 Underdosing of iron and its compounds

> EXCLUDES 1   *iron deficiency (E61.1)*

✓5ᵗʰ T45.5 Poisoning by, adverse effect of and underdosing of anticoagulants and antithrombotic drugs

✓6ᵗʰ T45.51 Poisoning by, adverse effect of and underdosing of anticoagulants

✓7ᵗʰ T45.511 Poisoning by anticoagulants, accidental (unintentional)
Poisoning by anticoagulants NOS

7 ✓7ᵗʰ T45.512 Poisoning by anticoagulants, intentional self-harm   HCC

✓7ᵗʰ T45.513 Poisoning by anticoagulants, assault

✓7ᵗʰ T45.514 Poisoning by anticoagulants, undetermined

✓7ᵗʰ T45.515 Adverse effect of anticoagulants

AHA: 2016,1Q,14; 2013,2Q,34

✓7ᵗʰ T45.516 Underdosing of anticoagulants

✓6ᵗʰ T45.52 Poisoning by, adverse effect of and underdosing of antithrombotic drugs
Poisoning by, adverse effect of and underdosing of antiplatelet drugs

> EXCLUDES 2   *poisoning by, adverse effect of and underdosing of aspirin (T39.0̸1-)*
> *poisoning by, adverse effect of and underdosing of acetylsalicylic acid (T39.0̸1-)*

✓7ᵗʰ T45.521 Poisoning by antithrombotic drugs, accidental (unintentional)
Poisoning by antithrombotic drug NOS

Ⓝ Newborn: 0   Ⓟ Pediatric: 0-17   Ⓜ Maternity: 9-64   Ⓐ Adult: 15-124   MCC Major Complication/Comorbidity   CC Complication/Comorbidity   SW Severe Wound Dx

1162   ICD-10-CM 2020

7 ✓7ᵗʰ **T45.522 Poisoning by antithrombotic drugs, intentional self-harm** HCC

✓7ᵗʰ **T45.523 Poisoning by antithrombotic drugs, assault**

✓7ᵗʰ **T45.524 Poisoning by antithrombotic drugs, undetermined**

✓7ᵗʰ **T45.525 Adverse effect of antithrombotic drugs**
     AHA: 2016,1Q,15

✓7ᵗʰ **T45.526 Underdosing of antithrombotic drugs**

✓5ᵗʰ **T45.6 Poisoning by, adverse effect of and underdosing of fibrinolysis-affecting drugs**

✓6ᵗʰ **T45.60 Poisoning by, adverse effect of and underdosing of unspecified fibrinolysis-affecting drugs**

✓7ᵗʰ **T45.601 Poisoning by unspecified fibrinolysis-affecting drugs, accidental (unintentional)**
     Poisoning by fibrinolysis-affecting drug NOS

7 ✓7ᵗʰ **T45.602 Poisoning by unspecified fibrinolysis-affecting drugs, intentional self-harm** HCC

✓7ᵗʰ **T45.603 Poisoning by unspecified fibrinolysis-affecting drugs, assault**

✓7ᵗʰ **T45.604 Poisoning by unspecified fibrinolysis-affecting drugs, undetermined**

✓7ᵗʰ **T45.605 Adverse effect of unspecified fibrinolysis-affecting drugs**

✓7ᵗʰ **T45.606 Underdosing of unspecified fibrinolysis-affecting drugs**

✓6ᵗʰ **T45.61 Poisoning by, adverse effect of and underdosing of thrombolytic drugs**

✓7ᵗʰ **T45.611 Poisoning by thrombolytic drug, accidental (unintentional)**
     Poisoning by thrombolytic drug NOS

7 ✓7ᵗʰ **T45.612 Poisoning by thrombolytic drug, intentional self-harm** HCC

✓7ᵗʰ **T45.613 Poisoning by thrombolytic drug, assault**

✓7ᵗʰ **T45.614 Poisoning by thrombolytic drug, undetermined**

✓7ᵗʰ **T45.615 Adverse effect of thrombolytic drugs**
     AHA: 2017,2Q,9

✓7ᵗʰ **T45.616 Underdosing of thrombolytic drugs**

✓6ᵗʰ **T45.62 Poisoning by, adverse effect of and underdosing of hemostatic drugs**

✓7ᵗʰ **T45.621 Poisoning by hemostatic drug, accidental (unintentional)**
     Poisoning by hemostatic drug NOS

7 ✓7ᵗʰ **T45.622 Poisoning by hemostatic drug, intentional self-harm** HCC

✓7ᵗʰ **T45.623 Poisoning by hemostatic drug, assault**

✓7ᵗʰ **T45.624 Poisoning by hemostatic drug, undetermined**

✓7ᵗʰ **T45.625 Adverse effect of hemostatic drug**

✓7ᵗʰ **T45.626 Underdosing of hemostatic drugs**

✓6ᵗʰ **T45.69 Poisoning by, adverse effect of and underdosing of other fibrinolysis-affecting drugs**

✓7ᵗʰ **T45.691 Poisoning by other fibrinolysis-affecting drugs, accidental (unintentional)**
     Poisoning by other fibrinolysis-affecting drug NOS

7 ✓7ᵗʰ **T45.692 Poisoning by other fibrinolysis-affecting drugs, intentional self-harm** HCC

✓7ᵗʰ **T45.693 Poisoning by other fibrinolysis-affecting drugs, assault**

✓7ᵗʰ **T45.694 Poisoning by other fibrinolysis-affecting drugs, undetermined**

✓7ᵗʰ **T45.695 Adverse effect of other fibrinolysis-affecting drugs**

✓7ᵗʰ **T45.696 Underdosing of other fibrinolysis-affecting drugs**

✓5ᵗʰ **T45.7 Poisoning by, adverse effect of and underdosing of anticoagulant antagonists, vitamin K and other coagulants**

✓6ᵗʰ **T45.7X Poisoning by, adverse effect of and underdosing of anticoagulant antagonists, vitamin K and other coagulants**

✓7ᵗʰ **T45.7X1 Poisoning by anticoagulant antagonists, vitamin K and other coagulants, accidental (unintentional)**
     Poisoning by anticoagulant antagonists, vitamin K and other coagulants NOS

7 ✓7ᵗʰ **T45.7X2 Poisoning by anticoagulant antagonists, vitamin K and other coagulants, intentional self-harm** HCC

✓7ᵗʰ **T45.7X3 Poisoning by anticoagulant antagonists, vitamin K and other coagulants, assault**

✓7ᵗʰ **T45.7X4 Poisoning by anticoagulant antagonists, vitamin K and other coagulants, undetermined**

✓7ᵗʰ **T45.7X5 Adverse effect of anticoagulant antagonists, vitamin K and other coagulants**

✓7ᵗʰ **T45.7X6 Underdosing of anticoagulant antagonist, vitamin K and other coagulants**
     EXCLUDES 1   vitamin K deficiency (E56.1)

✓5ᵗʰ **T45.8 Poisoning by, adverse effect of and underdosing of other primarily systemic and hematological agents**
     Poisoning by, adverse effect of and underdosing of liver preparations and other antianemic agents
     Poisoning by, adverse effect of and underdosing of natural blood and blood products
     Poisoning by, adverse effect of and underdosing of plasma substitute
     EXCLUDES 2   poisoning by, adverse effect of and underdosing of immunoglobulin (T50.Z1)
         poisoning by, adverse effect of and underdosing of iron (T45.4)
         transfusion reactions (T80.-)

✓6ᵗʰ **T45.8X Poisoning by, adverse effect of and underdosing of other primarily systemic and hematological agents**

✓7ᵗʰ **T45.8X1 Poisoning by other primarily systemic and hematological agents, accidental (unintentional)**
     Poisoning by other primarily systemic and hematological agents NOS

7 ✓7ᵗʰ **T45.8X2 Poisoning by other primarily systemic and hematological agents, intentional self-harm** HCC

✓7ᵗʰ **T45.8X3 Poisoning by other primarily systemic and hematological agents, assault**

✓7ᵗʰ **T45.8X4 Poisoning by other primarily systemic and hematological agents, undetermined**

✓7ᵗʰ **T45.8X5 Adverse effect of other primarily systemic and hematological agents**
     AHA: 2016,4Q,42

✓7ᵗʰ **T45.8X6 Underdosing of other primarily systemic and hematological agents**

✓5ᵗʰ **T45.9 Poisoning by, adverse effect of and underdosing of unspecified primarily systemic and hematological agent**

✓x7ᵗʰ **T45.91 Poisoning by unspecified primarily systemic and hematological agent, accidental (unintentional)**
     Poisoning by primarily systemic and hematological agent NOS

7 ✓x7ᵗʰ **T45.92 Poisoning by unspecified primarily systemic and hematological agent, intentional self-harm** HCC

✓x7ᵗʰ **T45.93 Poisoning by unspecified primarily systemic and hematological agent, assault**

✓x7ᵗʰ **T45.94 Poisoning by unspecified primarily systemic and hematological agent, undetermined**

✓x7ᵗʰ **T45.95 Adverse effect of unspecified primarily systemic and hematological agent**

✓x7ᵗʰ **T45.96 Underdosing of unspecified primarily systemic and hematological agent**

√4ᵗʰ **T46** **Poisoning by, adverse effect of and underdosing of agents primarily affecting the cardiovascular system**

> EXCLUDES 1   *poisoning by, adverse effect of and underdosing of metaraminol (T44.4)*

> The appropriate 7th character is to be added to each code from category T46.
> A   initial encounter
> D   subsequent encounter
> S   sequela

√5ᵗʰ **T46.0** **Poisoning by, adverse effect of and underdosing of cardiac-stimulant glycosides and drugs of similar action**

   √6ᵗʰ **T46.0X** **Poisoning by, adverse effect of and underdosing of cardiac-stimulant glycosides and drugs of similar action**

     √7ᵗʰ **T46.0X1** **Poisoning by cardiac-stimulant glycosides and drugs of similar action, accidental (unintentional)**

       Poisoning by cardiac-stimulant glycosides and drugs of similar action NOS

     7 √7ᵗʰ **T46.0X2** **Poisoning by cardiac-stimulant glycosides and drugs of similar action, intentional self-harm**   HCC

     √7ᵗʰ **T46.0X3** **Poisoning by cardiac-stimulant glycosides and drugs of similar action, assault**

     √7ᵗʰ **T46.0X4** **Poisoning by cardiac-stimulant glycosides and drugs of similar action, undetermined**

     √7ᵗʰ **T46.0X5** **Adverse effect of cardiac-stimulant glycosides and drugs of similar action**

     √7ᵗʰ **T46.0X6** **Underdosing of cardiac-stimulant glycosides and drugs of similar action**

√5ᵗʰ **T46.1** **Poisoning by, adverse effect of and underdosing of calcium-channel blockers**

   √6ᵗʰ **T46.1X** **Poisoning by, adverse effect of and underdosing of calcium-channel blockers**

     √7ᵗʰ **T46.1X1** **Poisoning by calcium-channel blockers, accidental (unintentional)**

       Poisoning by calcium-channel blockers NOS

     7 √7ᵗʰ **T46.1X2** **Poisoning by calcium-channel blockers, intentional self-harm**   HCC

     √7ᵗʰ **T46.1X3** **Poisoning by calcium-channel blockers, assault**

     √7ᵗʰ **T46.1X4** **Poisoning by calcium-channel blockers, undetermined**

     √7ᵗʰ **T46.1X5** **Adverse effect of calcium-channel blockers**

     √7ᵗʰ **T46.1X6** **Underdosing of calcium-channel blockers**

√5ᵗʰ **T46.2** **Poisoning by, adverse effect of and underdosing of other antidysrhythmic drugs, not elsewhere classified**

> EXCLUDES 1   *poisoning by, adverse effect of and underdosing of beta-adrenoreceptor antagonists (T44.7-)*

   √6ᵗʰ **T46.2X** **Poisoning by, adverse effect of and underdosing of other antidysrhythmic drugs**

     √7ᵗʰ **T46.2X1** **Poisoning by other antidysrhythmic drugs, accidental (unintentional)**

       Poisoning by other antidysrhythmic drugs NOS

     7 √7ᵗʰ **T46.2X2** **Poisoning by other antidysrhythmic drugs, intentional self-harm**   HCC

     √7ᵗʰ **T46.2X3** **Poisoning by other antidysrhythmic drugs, assault**

     √7ᵗʰ **T46.2X4** **Poisoning by other antidysrhythmic drugs, undetermined**

     √7ᵗʰ **T46.2X5** **Adverse effect of other antidysrhythmic drugs**

     √7ᵗʰ **T46.2X6** **Underdosing of other antidysrhythmic drugs**

√5ᵗʰ **T46.3** **Poisoning by, adverse effect of and underdosing of coronary vasodilators**

   Poisoning by, adverse effect of and underdosing of dipyridamole

> EXCLUDES 1   *poisoning by, adverse effect of and underdosing of calcium-channel blockers (T46.1)*

   √6ᵗʰ **T46.3X** **Poisoning by, adverse effect of and underdosing of coronary vasodilators**

     √7ᵗʰ **T46.3X1** **Poisoning by coronary vasodilators, accidental (unintentional)**

       Poisoning by coronary vasodilators NOS

     7 √7ᵗʰ **T46.3X2** **Poisoning by coronary vasodilators, intentional self-harm**   HCC

     √7ᵗʰ **T46.3X3** **Poisoning by coronary vasodilators, assault**

     √7ᵗʰ **T46.3X4** **Poisoning by coronary vasodilators, undetermined**

     √7ᵗʰ **T46.3X5** **Adverse effect of coronary vasodilators**

     √7ᵗʰ **T46.3X6** **Underdosing of coronary vasodilators**

√5ᵗʰ **T46.4** **Poisoning by, adverse effect of and underdosing of angiotensin-converting-enzyme inhibitors**

   √6ᵗʰ **T46.4X** **Poisoning by, adverse effect of and underdosing of angiotensin-converting-enzyme inhibitors**

     √7ᵗʰ **T46.4X1** **Poisoning by angiotensin-converting-enzyme inhibitors, accidental (unintentional)**

       Poisoning by angiotensin-converting-enzyme inhibitors NOS

     7 √7ᵗʰ **T46.4X2** **Poisoning by angiotensin-converting-enzyme inhibitors, intentional self-harm**   HCC

     √7ᵗʰ **T46.4X3** **Poisoning by angiotensin-converting-enzyme inhibitors, assault**

     √7ᵗʰ **T46.4X4** **Poisoning by angiotensin-converting-enzyme inhibitors, undetermined**

     √7ᵗʰ **T46.4X5** **Adverse effect of angiotensin-converting-enzyme inhibitors**

     √7ᵗʰ **T46.4X6** **Underdosing of angiotensin-converting-enzyme inhibitors**

√5ᵗʰ **T46.5** **Poisoning by, adverse effect of and underdosing of other antihypertensive drugs**

> EXCLUDES 2   *poisoning by, adverse effect of and underdosing of beta-adrenoreceptor antagonists (T44.7)*
> *poisoning by, adverse effect of and underdosing of calcium-channel blockers (T46.1)*
> *poisoning by, adverse effect of and underdosing of diuretics (T50.0-T50.2)*

   √6ᵗʰ **T46.5X** **Poisoning by, adverse effect of and underdosing of other antihypertensive drugs**

     √7ᵗʰ **T46.5X1** **Poisoning by other antihypertensive drugs, accidental (unintentional)**

       Poisoning by other antihypertensive drugs NOS

     7 √7ᵗʰ **T46.5X2** **Poisoning by other antihypertensive drugs, intentional self-harm**   HCC

     √7ᵗʰ **T46.5X3** **Poisoning by other antihypertensive drugs, assault**

     √7ᵗʰ **T46.5X4** **Poisoning by other antihypertensive drugs, undetermined**

     √7ᵗʰ **T46.5X5** **Adverse effect of other antihypertensive drugs**

     √7ᵗʰ **T46.5X6** **Underdosing of other antihypertensive drugs**

√5ᵗʰ **T46.6** **Poisoning by, adverse effect of and underdosing of antihyperlipidemic and antiarteriosclerotic drugs**

   √6ᵗʰ **T46.6X** **Poisoning by, adverse effect of and underdosing of antihyperlipidemic and antiarteriosclerotic drugs**

     √7ᵗʰ **T46.6X1** **Poisoning by antihyperlipidemic and antiarteriosclerotic drugs, accidental (unintentional)**

       Poisoning by antihyperlipidemic and antiarteriosclerotic drugs NOS

N Newborn: 0   P Pediatric: 0-17   M Maternity: 9-64   A Adult: 15-124   MCC Major Complication/Comorbidity   CC Complication/Comorbidity   SW Severe Wound Dx

1164   ICD-10-CM 2020

7 √7th **T46.6X2 Poisoning by antihyperlipidemic and antiarteriosclerotic drugs, intentional self-harm** `HCC`

√7th **T46.6X3 Poisoning by antihyperlipidemic and antiarteriosclerotic drugs, assault**

√7th **T46.6X4 Poisoning by antihyperlipidemic and antiarteriosclerotic drugs, undetermined**

√7th **T46.6X5 Adverse effect of antihyperlipidemic and antiarteriosclerotic drugs**

√7th **T46.6X6 Underdosing of antihyperlipidemic and antiarteriosclerotic drugs**

√5th **T46.7 Poisoning by, adverse effect of and underdosing of peripheral vasodilators**

Poisoning by, adverse effect of and underdosing of nicotinic acid (derivatives)

> **EXCLUDES 1**   poisoning by, adverse effect of and underdosing of papaverine (T44.3)

√6th **T46.7X Poisoning by, adverse effect of and underdosing of peripheral vasodilators**

√7th **T46.7X1 Poisoning by peripheral vasodilators, accidental (unintentional)**

Poisoning by peripheral vasodilators NOS

7 √7th **T46.7X2 Poisoning by peripheral vasodilators, intentional self-harm** `HCC`

√7th **T46.7X3 Poisoning by peripheral vasodilators, assault**

√7th **T46.7X4 Poisoning by peripheral vasodilators, undetermined**

√7th **T46.7X5 Adverse effect of peripheral vasodilators**

√7th **T46.7X6 Underdosing of peripheral vasodilators**

√5th **T46.8 Poisoning by, adverse effect of and underdosing of antivaricose drugs, including sclerosing agents**

√6th **T46.8X Poisoning by, adverse effect of and underdosing of antivaricose drugs, including sclerosing agents**

√7th **T46.8X1 Poisoning by antivaricose drugs, including sclerosing agents, accidental (unintentional)**

Poisoning by antivaricose drugs, including sclerosing agents NOS

7 √7th **T46.8X2 Poisoning by antivaricose drugs, including sclerosing agents, intentional self-harm** `HCC`

√7th **T46.8X3 Poisoning by antivaricose drugs, including sclerosing agents, assault**

√7th **T46.8X4 Poisoning by antivaricose drugs, including sclerosing agents, undetermined**

√7th **T46.8X5 Adverse effect of antivaricose drugs, including sclerosing agents**

√7th **T46.8X6 Underdosing of antivaricose drugs, including sclerosing agents**

√5th **T46.9 Poisoning by, adverse effect of and underdosing of other and unspecified agents primarily affecting the cardiovascular system**

√6th **T46.90 Poisoning by, adverse effect of and underdosing of unspecified agents primarily affecting the cardiovascular system**

√7th **T46.901 Poisoning by unspecified agents primarily affecting the cardiovascular system, accidental (unintentional)**

7 √7th **T46.902 Poisoning by unspecified agents primarily affecting the cardiovascular system, intentional self-harm** `HCC`

√7th **T46.903 Poisoning by unspecified agents primarily affecting the cardiovascular system, assault**

√7th **T46.904 Poisoning by unspecified agents primarily affecting the cardiovascular system, undetermined**

√7th **T46.905 Adverse effect of unspecified agents primarily affecting the cardiovascular system**

√7th **T46.906 Underdosing of unspecified agents primarily affecting the cardiovascular system**

√6th **T46.99 Poisoning by, adverse effect of and underdosing of other agents primarily affecting the cardiovascular system**

√7th **T46.991 Poisoning by other agents primarily affecting the cardiovascular system, accidental (unintentional)**

7 √7th **T46.992 Poisoning by other agents primarily affecting the cardiovascular system, intentional self-harm** `HCC`

√7th **T46.993 Poisoning by other agents primarily affecting the cardiovascular system, assault**

√7th **T46.994 Poisoning by other agents primarily affecting the cardiovascular system, undetermined**

√7th **T46.995 Adverse effect of other agents primarily affecting the cardiovascular system**

√7th **T46.996 Underdosing of other agents primarily affecting the cardiovascular system**

√4th **T47 Poisoning by, adverse effect of and underdosing of agents primarily affecting the gastrointestinal system**

> The appropriate 7th character is to be added to each code from category T47.
> A   initial encounter
> D   subsequent encounter
> S   sequela

√5th **T47.0 Poisoning by, adverse effect of and underdosing of histamine H2-receptor blockers**

√6th **T47.0X Poisoning by, adverse effect of and underdosing of histamine H2-receptor blockers**

√7th **T47.0X1 Poisoning by histamine H2-receptor blockers, accidental (unintentional)**

Poisoning by histamine H2-receptor blockers NOS

7 √7th **T47.0X2 Poisoning by histamine H2-receptor blockers, intentional self-harm** `HCC`

√7th **T47.0X3 Poisoning by histamine H2-receptor blockers, assault**

√7th **T47.0X4 Poisoning by histamine H2-receptor blockers, undetermined**

√7th **T47.0X5 Adverse effect of histamine H2-receptor blockers**

√7th **T47.0X6 Underdosing of histamine H2-receptor blockers**

√5th **T47.1 Poisoning by, adverse effect of and underdosing of other antacids and anti-gastric-secretion drugs**

√6th **T47.1X Poisoning by, adverse effect of and underdosing of other antacids and anti-gastric-secretion drugs**

√7th **T47.1X1 Poisoning by other antacids and anti-gastric-secretion drugs, accidental (unintentional)**

Poisoning by other antacids and anti-gastric-secretion drugs NOS

7 √7th **T47.1X2 Poisoning by other antacids and anti-gastric-secretion drugs, intentional self-harm** `HCC`

√7th **T47.1X3 Poisoning by other antacids and anti-gastric-secretion drugs, assault**

√7th **T47.1X4 Poisoning by other antacids and anti-gastric-secretion drugs, undetermined**

√7th **T47.1X5 Adverse effect of other antacids and anti-gastric-secretion drugs**

√7th **T47.1X6 Underdosing of other antacids and anti-gastric-secretion drugs**

√5th **T47.2 Poisoning by, adverse effect of and underdosing of stimulant laxatives**

√6th **T47.2X Poisoning by, adverse effect of and underdosing of stimulant laxatives**

√7th **T47.2X1 Poisoning by stimulant laxatives, accidental (unintentional)**

Poisoning by stimulant laxatives NOS

7 √7th **T47.2X2 Poisoning by stimulant laxatives, intentional self-harm** `HCC`

√7th **T47.2X3 Poisoning by stimulant laxatives, assault**

√7th **T47.2X4 Poisoning by stimulant laxatives, undetermined**

☑ Additional Character Required   √x7th Placeholder   Unacceptable PDx   Questionable PDx   Manifestation   Unspecified Dx   H1-H14 HAC   HCC CMS-HCC Dx   HIV HIV Dx

ICD-10-CM 2020   T46.6X2–T47.2X4   1165

✓7ᵗʰ **T47.2X5** Adverse effect of stimulant laxatives

✓7ᵗʰ **T47.2X6** Underdosing of stimulant laxatives

✓5ᵗʰ **T47.3** Poisoning by, adverse effect of and underdosing of saline and osmotic laxatives

✓6ᵗʰ **T47.3X** Poisoning by and adverse effect of saline and osmotic laxatives

✓7ᵗʰ **T47.3X1** Poisoning by saline and osmotic laxatives, accidental (unintentional)
Poisoning by saline and osmotic laxatives NOS

7 ✓7ᵗʰ **T47.3X2** Poisoning by saline and osmotic laxatives, intentional self-harm [HCC]

✓7ᵗʰ **T47.3X3** Poisoning by saline and osmotic laxatives, assault

✓7ᵗʰ **T47.3X4** Poisoning by saline and osmotic laxatives, undetermined

✓7ᵗʰ **T47.3X5** Adverse effect of saline and osmotic laxatives

✓7ᵗʰ **T47.3X6** Underdosing of saline and osmotic laxatives

✓5ᵗʰ **T47.4** Poisoning by, adverse effect of and underdosing of other laxatives

✓6ᵗʰ **T47.4X** Poisoning by, adverse effect of and underdosing of other laxatives

✓7ᵗʰ **T47.4X1** Poisoning by other laxatives, accidental (unintentional)
Poisoning by other laxatives NOS

7 ✓7ᵗʰ **T47.4X2** Poisoning by other laxatives, intentional self-harm [HCC]

✓7ᵗʰ **T47.4X3** Poisoning by other laxatives, assault

✓7ᵗʰ **T47.4X4** Poisoning by other laxatives, undetermined

✓7ᵗʰ **T47.4X5** Adverse effect of other laxatives

✓7ᵗʰ **T47.4X6** Underdosing of other laxatives

✓5ᵗʰ **T47.5** Poisoning by, adverse effect of and underdosing of digestants

✓6ᵗʰ **T47.5X** Poisoning by, adverse effect of and underdosing of digestants

✓7ᵗʰ **T47.5X1** Poisoning by digestants, accidental (unintentional)
Poisoning by digestants NOS

7 ✓7ᵗʰ **T47.5X2** Poisoning by digestants, intentional self-harm [HCC]

✓7ᵗʰ **T47.5X3** Poisoning by digestants, assault

✓7ᵗʰ **T47.5X4** Poisoning by digestants, undetermined

✓7ᵗʰ **T47.5X5** Adverse effect of digestants

✓7ᵗʰ **T47.5X6** Underdosing of digestants

✓5ᵗʰ **T47.6** Poisoning by, adverse effect of and underdosing of antidiarrheal drugs

EXCLUDES 2 poisoning by, adverse effect of and underdosing of systemic antibiotics and other anti-infectives (T36-T37)

✓6ᵗʰ **T47.6X** Poisoning by, adverse effect of and underdosing of antidiarrheal drugs

✓7ᵗʰ **T47.6X1** Poisoning by antidiarrheal drugs, accidental (unintentional)
Poisoning by antidiarrheal drugs NOS

7 ✓7ᵗʰ **T47.6X2** Poisoning by antidiarrheal drugs, intentional self-harm [HCC]

✓7ᵗʰ **T47.6X3** Poisoning by antidiarrheal drugs, assault

✓7ᵗʰ **T47.6X4** Poisoning by antidiarrheal drugs, undetermined

✓7ᵗʰ **T47.6X5** Adverse effect of antidiarrheal drugs

✓7ᵗʰ **T47.6X6** Underdosing of antidiarrheal drugs

✓5ᵗʰ **T47.7** Poisoning by, adverse effect of and underdosing of emetics

✓6ᵗʰ **T47.7X** Poisoning by, adverse effect of and underdosing of emetics

✓7ᵗʰ **T47.7X1** Poisoning by emetics, accidental (unintentional)
Poisoning by emetics NOS

7 ✓7ᵗʰ **T47.7X2** Poisoning by emetics, intentional self-harm [HCC]

✓7ᵗʰ **T47.7X3** Poisoning by emetics, assault

✓7ᵗʰ **T47.7X4** Poisoning by emetics, undetermined

✓7ᵗʰ **T47.7X5** Adverse effect of emetics

✓7ᵗʰ **T47.7X6** Underdosing of emetics

✓5ᵗʰ **T47.8** Poisoning by, adverse effect of and underdosing of other agents primarily affecting gastrointestinal system

✓6ᵗʰ **T47.8X** Poisoning by, adverse effect of and underdosing of other agents primarily affecting gastrointestinal system

✓7ᵗʰ **T47.8X1** Poisoning by other agents primarily affecting gastrointestinal system, accidental (unintentional)
Poisoning by other agents primarily affecting gastrointestinal system NOS

7 ✓7ᵗʰ **T47.8X2** Poisoning by other agents primarily affecting gastrointestinal system, intentional self-harm [HCC]

✓7ᵗʰ **T47.8X3** Poisoning by other agents primarily affecting gastrointestinal system, assault

✓7ᵗʰ **T47.8X4** Poisoning by other agents primarily affecting gastrointestinal system, undetermined

✓7ᵗʰ **T47.8X5** Adverse effect of other agents primarily affecting gastrointestinal system

✓7ᵗʰ **T47.8X6** Underdosing of other agents primarily affecting gastrointestinal system

✓5ᵗʰ **T47.9** Poisoning by, adverse effect of and underdosing of unspecified agents primarily affecting the gastrointestinal system

✓x7ᵗʰ **T47.91** Poisoning by unspecified agents primarily affecting the gastrointestinal system, accidental (unintentional)
Poisoning by agents primarily affecting the gastrointestinal system NOS

7 ✓x7ᵗʰ **T47.92** Poisoning by unspecified agents primarily affecting the gastrointestinal system, intentional self-harm [HCC]

✓x7ᵗʰ **T47.93** Poisoning by unspecified agents primarily affecting the gastrointestinal system, assault

✓x7ᵗʰ **T47.94** Poisoning by unspecified agents primarily affecting the gastrointestinal system, undetermined

✓x7ᵗʰ **T47.95** Adverse effect of unspecified agents primarily affecting the gastrointestinal system

✓x7ᵗʰ **T47.96** Underdosing of unspecified agents primarily affecting the gastrointestinal system

✓4ᵗʰ **T48** Poisoning by, adverse effect of and underdosing of agents primarily acting on smooth and skeletal muscles and the respiratory system

The appropriate 7th character is to be added to each code from category T48.
A initial encounter
D subsequent encounter
S sequela

✓5ᵗʰ **T48.0** Poisoning by, adverse effect of and underdosing of oxytocic drugs

EXCLUDES 1 poisoning by, adverse effect of and underdosing of estrogens, progestogens and antagonists (T38.4-T38.6)

✓6ᵗʰ **T48.0X** Poisoning by, adverse effect of and underdosing of oxytocic drugs

✓7ᵗʰ **T48.0X1** Poisoning by oxytocic drugs, accidental (unintentional)
Poisoning by oxytocic drugs NOS

7 ✓7ᵗʰ **T48.0X2** Poisoning by oxytocic drugs, intentional self-harm [HCC]

✓7ᵗʰ **T48.0X3** Poisoning by oxytocic drugs, assault

✓7ᵗʰ **T48.0X4** Poisoning by oxytocic drugs, undetermined

✓7ᵗʰ **T48.0X5** Adverse effect of oxytocic drugs

✓7ᵗʰ **T48.0X6** Underdosing of oxytocic drugs

✓5ᵗʰ **T48.1** Poisoning by, adverse effect of and underdosing of skeletal muscle relaxants [neuromuscular blocking agents]

✓6ᵗʰ **T48.1X** Poisoning by, adverse effect of and underdosing of skeletal muscle relaxants [neuromuscular blocking agents]

✓7ᵗʰ **T48.1X1** Poisoning by skeletal muscle relaxants [neuromuscular blocking agents], accidental (unintentional)
Poisoning by skeletal muscle relaxants [neuromuscular blocking agents] NOS

7 ✓7ᵗʰ **T48.1X2** **Poisoning by skeletal muscle relaxants [neuromuscular blocking agents], intentional self-harm**   HCC

✓7ᵗʰ **T48.1X3** **Poisoning by skeletal muscle relaxants [neuromuscular blocking agents], assault**

✓7ᵗʰ **T48.1X4** **Poisoning by skeletal muscle relaxants [neuromuscular blocking agents], undetermined**

✓7ᵗʰ **T48.1X5** **Adverse effect of skeletal muscle relaxants [neuromuscular blocking agents]**

✓7ᵗʰ **T48.1X6** **Underdosing of skeletal muscle relaxants [neuromuscular blocking agents]**

✓5ᵗʰ **T48.2** **Poisoning by, adverse effect of and underdosing of other and unspecified drugs acting on muscles**

✓6ᵗʰ **T48.20** **Poisoning by, adverse effect of and underdosing of unspecified drugs acting on muscles**

✓7ᵗʰ **T48.201** **Poisoning by unspecified drugs acting on muscles, accidental (unintentional)**
Poisoning by unspecified drugs acting on muscles NOS

7 ✓7ᵗʰ **T48.202** **Poisoning by unspecified drugs acting on muscles, intentional self-harm**   HCC

✓7ᵗʰ **T48.203** **Poisoning by unspecified drugs acting on muscles, assault**

✓7ᵗʰ **T48.204** **Poisoning by unspecified drugs acting on muscles, undetermined**

✓7ᵗʰ **T48.205** **Adverse effect of unspecified drugs acting on muscles**

✓7ᵗʰ **T48.206** **Underdosing of unspecified drugs acting on muscles**

✓6ᵗʰ **T48.29** **Poisoning by, adverse effect of and underdosing of other drugs acting on muscles**

✓7ᵗʰ **T48.291** **Poisoning by other drugs acting on muscles, accidental (unintentional)**
Poisoning by other drugs acting on muscles NOS

7 ✓7ᵗʰ **T48.292** **Poisoning by other drugs acting on muscles, intentional self-harm**   HCC

✓7ᵗʰ **T48.293** **Poisoning by other drugs acting on muscles, assault**

✓7ᵗʰ **T48.294** **Poisoning by other drugs acting on muscles, undetermined**

✓7ᵗʰ **T48.295** **Adverse effect of other drugs acting on muscles**

✓7ᵗʰ **T48.296** **Underdosing of other drugs acting on muscles**

✓5ᵗʰ **T48.3** **Poisoning by, adverse effect of and underdosing of antitussives**

✓6ᵗʰ **T48.3X** **Poisoning by, adverse effect of and underdosing of antitussives**

✓7ᵗʰ **T48.3X1** **Poisoning by antitussives, accidental (unintentional)**
Poisoning by antitussives NOS

7 ✓7ᵗʰ **T48.3X2** **Poisoning by antitussives, intentional self-harm**   HCC

✓7ᵗʰ **T48.3X3** **Poisoning by antitussives, assault**

✓7ᵗʰ **T48.3X4** **Poisoning by antitussives, undetermined**

✓7ᵗʰ **T48.3X5** **Adverse effect of antitussives**

✓7ᵗʰ **T48.3X6** **Underdosing of antitussives**

✓5ᵗʰ **T48.4** **Poisoning by, adverse effect of and underdosing of expectorants**

✓6ᵗʰ **T48.4X** **Poisoning by, adverse effect of and underdosing of expectorants**

✓7ᵗʰ **T48.4X1** **Poisoning by expectorants, accidental (unintentional)**
Poisoning by expectorants NOS

7 ✓7ᵗʰ **T48.4X2** **Poisoning by expectorants, intentional self-harm**   HCC

✓7ᵗʰ **T48.4X3** **Poisoning by expectorants, assault**

✓7ᵗʰ **T48.4X4** **Poisoning by expectorants, undetermined**

✓7ᵗʰ **T48.4X5** **Adverse effect of expectorants**

✓7ᵗʰ **T48.4X6** **Underdosing of expectorants**

✓5ᵗʰ **T48.5** **Poisoning by, adverse effect of and underdosing of other anti-common-cold drugs**
Poisoning by, adverse effect of and underdosing of decongestants
EXCLUDES 2   *poisoning by, adverse effect of and underdosing of antipyretics, NEC (T39.9-)*
poisoning by, adverse effect of and underdosing of non-steroidal antiinflammatory drugs (T39.3-)
poisoning by, adverse effect of and underdosing of salicylates (T39.0-)

✓6ᵗʰ **T48.5X** **Poisoning by, adverse effect of and underdosing of other anti-common-cold drugs**

✓7ᵗʰ **T48.5X1** **Poisoning by other anti-common-cold drugs, accidental (unintentional)**
Poisoning by other anti-common-cold drugs NOS

7 ✓7ᵗʰ **T48.5X2** **Poisoning by other anti-common-cold drugs, intentional self-harm**   HCC

✓7ᵗʰ **T48.5X3** **Poisoning by other anti-common-cold drugs, assault**

✓7ᵗʰ **T48.5X4** **Poisoning by other anti-common-cold drugs, undetermined**

✓7ᵗʰ **T48.5X5** **Adverse effect of other anti-common-cold drugs**

✓7ᵗʰ **T48.5X6** **Underdosing of other anti-common-cold drugs**

✓5ᵗʰ **T48.6** **Poisoning by, adverse effect of and underdosing of antiasthmatics, not elsewhere classified**
Poisoning by, adverse effect of and underdosing of beta-adrenoreceptor agonists used in asthma therapy
EXCLUDES 1   *poisoning by, adverse effect of and underdosing of anterior pituitary [adenohypophyseal] hormones (T38.8)*
poisoning by, adverse effect of and underdosing of beta-adrenoreceptor agonists not used in asthma therapy (T44.5)

✓6ᵗʰ **T48.6X** **Poisoning by, adverse effect of and underdosing of antiasthmatics**

✓7ᵗʰ **T48.6X1** **Poisoning by antiasthmatics, accidental (unintentional)**
Poisoning by antiasthmatics NOS

7 ✓7ᵗʰ **T48.6X2** **Poisoning by antiasthmatics, intentional self-harm**   HCC

✓7ᵗʰ **T48.6X3** **Poisoning by antiasthmatics, assault**

✓7ᵗʰ **T48.6X4** **Poisoning by antiasthmatics, undetermined**

✓7ᵗʰ **T48.6X5** **Adverse effect of antiasthmatics**

✓7ᵗʰ **T48.6X6** **Underdosing of antiasthmatics**

✓5ᵗʰ **T48.9** **Poisoning by, adverse effect of and underdosing of other and unspecified agents primarily acting on the respiratory system**

✓6ᵗʰ **T48.90** **Poisoning by, adverse effect of and underdosing of unspecified agents primarily acting on the respiratory system**

✓7ᵗʰ **T48.901** **Poisoning by unspecified agents primarily acting on the respiratory system, accidental (unintentional)**

7 ✓7ᵗʰ **T48.902** **Poisoning by unspecified agents primarily acting on the respiratory system, intentional self-harm**   HCC

✓7ᵗʰ **T48.903** **Poisoning by unspecified agents primarily acting on the respiratory system, assault**

✓7ᵗʰ **T48.904** **Poisoning by unspecified agents primarily acting on the respiratory system, undetermined**

✓7ᵗʰ **T48.905** **Adverse effect of unspecified agents primarily acting on the respiratory system**

✓7ᵗʰ **T48.906** **Underdosing of unspecified agents primarily acting on the respiratory system**

✓6ᵗʰ **T48.99** **Poisoning by, adverse effect of and underdosing of other agents primarily acting on the respiratory system**

✓7ᵗʰ **T48.991** **Poisoning by other agents primarily acting on the respiratory system, accidental (unintentional)**

7 ✓7ᵗʰ **T48.992 Poisoning by other agents primarily acting on the respiratory system, intentional self-harm** HCC

✓7ᵗʰ **T48.993 Poisoning by other agents primarily acting on the respiratory system, assault**

✓7ᵗʰ **T48.994 Poisoning by other agents primarily acting on the respiratory system, undetermined**

✓7ᵗʰ **T48.995 Adverse effect of other agents primarily acting on the respiratory system**

✓7ᵗʰ **T48.996 Underdosing of other agents primarily acting on the respiratory system**

✓4ᵗʰ **T49 Poisoning by, adverse effect of and underdosing of topical agents primarily affecting skin and mucous membrane and by ophthalmological, otorhinolaryngological and dental drugs**

INCLUDES   poisoning by, adverse effect of and underdosing of glucocorticoids, topically used

The appropriate 7th character is to be added to each code from category T49.
A   initial encounter
D   subsequent encounter
S   sequela

✓5ᵗʰ **T49.0 Poisoning by, adverse effect of and underdosing of local antifungal, anti-infective and anti-inflammatory drugs**

✓6ᵗʰ **T49.0X Poisoning by, adverse effect of and underdosing of local antifungal, anti-infective and anti-inflammatory drugs**

✓7ᵗʰ **T49.0X1 Poisoning by local antifungal, anti-infective and anti-inflammatory drugs, accidental (unintentional)**
Poisoning by local antifungal, anti-infective and anti-inflammatory drugs NOS

7 ✓7ᵗʰ **T49.0X2 Poisoning by local antifungal, anti-infective and anti-inflammatory drugs, intentional self-harm** HCC

✓7ᵗʰ **T49.0X3 Poisoning by local antifungal, anti-infective and anti-inflammatory drugs, assault**

✓7ᵗʰ **T49.0X4 Poisoning by local antifungal, anti-infective and anti-inflammatory drugs, undetermined**

✓7ᵗʰ **T49.0X5 Adverse effect of local antifungal, anti-infective and anti-inflammatory drugs**

✓7ᵗʰ **T49.0X6 Underdosing of local antifungal, anti-infective and anti-inflammatory drugs**

✓5ᵗʰ **T49.1 Poisoning by, adverse effect of and underdosing of antipruritics**

✓6ᵗʰ **T49.1X Poisoning by, adverse effect of and underdosing of antipruritics**

✓7ᵗʰ **T49.1X1 Poisoning by antipruritics, accidental (unintentional)**
Poisoning by antipruritics NOS

7 ✓7ᵗʰ **T49.1X2 Poisoning by antipruritics, intentional self-harm** HCC

✓7ᵗʰ **T49.1X3 Poisoning by antipruritics, assault**

✓7ᵗʰ **T49.1X4 Poisoning by antipruritics, undetermined**

✓7ᵗʰ **T49.1X5 Adverse effect of antipruritics**

✓7ᵗʰ **T49.1X6 Underdosing of antipruritics**

✓5ᵗʰ **T49.2 Poisoning by, adverse effect of and underdosing of local astringents and local detergents**

✓6ᵗʰ **T49.2X Poisoning by, adverse effect of and underdosing of local astringents and local detergents**

✓7ᵗʰ **T49.2X1 Poisoning by local astringents and local detergents, accidental (unintentional)**
Poisoning by local astringents and local detergents NOS

7 ✓7ᵗʰ **T49.2X2 Poisoning by local astringents and local detergents, intentional self-harm** HCC

✓7ᵗʰ **T49.2X3 Poisoning by local astringents and local detergents, assault**

✓7ᵗʰ **T49.2X4 Poisoning by local astringents and local detergents, undetermined**

✓7ᵗʰ **T49.2X5 Adverse effect of local astringents and local detergents**

✓7ᵗʰ **T49.2X6 Underdosing of local astringents and local detergents**

✓5ᵗʰ **T49.3 Poisoning by, adverse effect of and underdosing of emollients, demulcents and protectants**

✓6ᵗʰ **T49.3X Poisoning by, adverse effect of and underdosing of emollients, demulcents and protectants**

✓7ᵗʰ **T49.3X1 Poisoning by emollients, demulcents and protectants, accidental (unintentional)**
Poisoning by emollients, demulcents and protectants NOS

7 ✓7ᵗʰ **T49.3X2 Poisoning by emollients, demulcents and protectants, intentional self-harm** HCC

✓7ᵗʰ **T49.3X3 Poisoning by emollients, demulcents and protectants, assault**

✓7ᵗʰ **T49.3X4 Poisoning by emollients, demulcents and protectants, undetermined**

✓7ᵗʰ **T49.3X5 Adverse effect of emollients, demulcents and protectants**

✓7ᵗʰ **T49.3X6 Underdosing of emollients, demulcents and protectants**

✓5ᵗʰ **T49.4 Poisoning by, adverse effect of and underdosing of keratolytics, keratoplastics, and other hair treatment drugs and preparations**

✓6ᵗʰ **T49.4X Poisoning by, adverse effect of and underdosing of keratolytics, keratoplastics, and other hair treatment drugs and preparations**

✓7ᵗʰ **T49.4X1 Poisoning by keratolytics, keratoplastics, and other hair treatment drugs and preparations, accidental (unintentional)**
Poisoning by keratolytics, keratoplastics, and other hair treatment drugs and preparations NOS

7 ✓7ᵗʰ **T49.4X2 Poisoning by keratolytics, keratoplastics, and other hair treatment drugs and preparations, intentional self-harm** HCC

✓7ᵗʰ **T49.4X3 Poisoning by keratolytics, keratoplastics, and other hair treatment drugs and preparations, assault**

✓7ᵗʰ **T49.4X4 Poisoning by keratolytics, keratoplastics, and other hair treatment drugs and preparations, undetermined**

✓7ᵗʰ **T49.4X5 Adverse effect of keratolytics, keratoplastics, and other hair treatment drugs and preparations**

✓7ᵗʰ **T49.4X6 Underdosing of keratolytics, keratoplastics, and other hair treatment drugs and preparations**

✓5ᵗʰ **T49.5 Poisoning by, adverse effect of and underdosing of ophthalmological drugs and preparations**

✓6ᵗʰ **T49.5X Poisoning by, adverse effect of and underdosing of ophthalmological drugs and preparations**

✓7ᵗʰ **T49.5X1 Poisoning by ophthalmological drugs and preparations, accidental (unintentional)**
Poisoning by ophthalmological drugs and preparations NOS

7 ✓7ᵗʰ **T49.5X2 Poisoning by ophthalmological drugs and preparations, intentional self-harm** HCC

✓7ᵗʰ **T49.5X3 Poisoning by ophthalmological drugs and preparations, assault**

✓7ᵗʰ **T49.5X4 Poisoning by ophthalmological drugs and preparations, undetermined**

✓7ᵗʰ **T49.5X5 Adverse effect of ophthalmological drugs and preparations**

✓7ᵗʰ **T49.5X6 Underdosing of ophthalmological drugs and preparations**

✓5ᵗʰ **T49.6 Poisoning by, adverse effect of and underdosing of otorhinolaryngological drugs and preparations**

✓6ᵗʰ **T49.6X Poisoning by, adverse effect of and underdosing of otorhinolaryngological drugs and preparations**

✓7ᵗʰ **T49.6X1 Poisoning by otorhinolaryngological drugs and preparations, accidental (unintentional)**
Poisoning by otorhinolaryngological drugs and preparations NOS

7 ✓7ᵗʰ **T49.6X2 Poisoning by otorhinolaryngological drugs and preparations, intentional self-harm** HCC

N Newborn: 0   P Pediatric: 0-17   M Maternity: 9-64   A Adult: 15-124   MCC Major Complication/Comorbidity   CC Complication/Comorbidity   SW Severe Wound Dx

1168   ICD-10-CM 2020

√7th **T49.6X3** **Poisoning by otorhinolaryngological drugs and preparations,** assault

√7th **T49.6X4** **Poisoning by otorhinolaryngological drugs and preparations,** undetermined

√7th **T49.6X5** Adverse effect of otorhinolaryngological drugs and preparations

√7th **T49.6X6** Underdosing of otorhinolaryngological drugs and preparations

√5th **T49.7** **Poisoning by, adverse effect of and underdosing of dental drugs, topically applied**

√6th **T49.7X** **Poisoning by, adverse effect of and underdosing of dental drugs, topically applied**

√7th **T49.7X1** **Poisoning by dental drugs, topically applied,** accidental (unintentional)
Poisoning by dental drugs, topically applied NOS

7 √7th **T49.7X2** **Poisoning by dental drugs, topically applied,** intentional self-harm　HCC

√7th **T49.7X3** **Poisoning by dental drugs, topically applied,** assault

√7th **T49.7X4** **Poisoning by dental drugs, topically applied,** undetermined

√7th **T49.7X5** Adverse effect of dental drugs, topically applied

√7th **T49.7X6** Underdosing of dental drugs, topically applied

√5th **T49.8** **Poisoning by, adverse effect of and underdosing of other topical agents**
Poisoning by, adverse effect of and underdosing of spermicides

√6th **T49.8X** **Poisoning by, adverse effect of and underdosing of other topical agents**

√7th **T49.8X1** **Poisoning by other topical agents,** accidental (unintentional)
Poisoning by other topical agents NOS

7 √7th **T49.8X2** **Poisoning by other topical agents,** intentional self-harm　HCC

√7th **T49.8X3** **Poisoning by other topical agents,** assault

√7th **T49.8X4** **Poisoning by other topical agents,** undetermined

√7th **T49.8X5** Adverse effect of other topical agents

√7th **T49.8X6** Underdosing of other topical agents

√5th **T49.9** **Poisoning by, adverse effect of and underdosing of unspecified topical agent**

√x7th **T49.91** **Poisoning by unspecified topical agent,** accidental (unintentional)

7 √x7th **T49.92** **Poisoning by unspecified topical agent,** intentional self-harm　HCC

√x7th **T49.93** **Poisoning by unspecified topical agent,** assault

√x7th **T49.94** **Poisoning by unspecified topical agent,** undetermined

√x7th **T49.95** Adverse effect of unspecified topical agent

√x7th **T49.96** Underdosing of unspecified topical agent

√4th **T50** **Poisoning by, adverse effect of and underdosing of diuretics and other and unspecified drugs, medicaments and biological substances**

The appropriate 7th character is to be added to each code from category T50.
A　initial encounter
D　subsequent encounter
S　sequela

√5th **T50.0** **Poisoning by, adverse effect of and underdosing of mineralocorticoids and their antagonists**

√6th **T50.0X** **Poisoning by, adverse effect of and underdosing of mineralocorticoids and their antagonists**

√7th **T50.0X1** **Poisoning by mineralocorticoids and their antagonists,** accidental (unintentional)
Poisoning by mineralocorticoids and their antagonists NOS

7 √7th **T50.0X2** **Poisoning by mineralocorticoids and their antagonists,** intentional self-harm　HCC

√7th **T50.0X3** **Poisoning by mineralocorticoids and their antagonists,** assault

√7th **T50.0X4** **Poisoning by mineralocorticoids and their antagonists,** undetermined

√7th **T50.0X5** Adverse effect of mineralocorticoids and their antagonists

√7th **T50.0X6** Underdosing of mineralocorticoids and their antagonists

√5th **T50.1** **Poisoning by, adverse effect of and underdosing of loop [high-ceiling] diuretics**

√6th **T50.1X** **Poisoning by, adverse effect of and underdosing of loop [high-ceiling] diuretics**

√7th **T50.1X1** **Poisoning by loop [high-ceiling] diuretics,** accidental (unintentional)
Poisoning by loop [high-ceiling] diuretics NOS

7 √7th **T50.1X2** **Poisoning by loop [high-ceiling] diuretics,** intentional self-harm　HCC

√7th **T50.1X3** **Poisoning by loop [high-ceiling] diuretics,** assault

√7th **T50.1X4** **Poisoning by loop [high-ceiling] diuretics,** undetermined

√7th **T50.1X5** Adverse effect of loop [high-ceiling] diuretics

√7th **T50.1X6** Underdosing of loop [high-ceiling] diuretics

√5th **T50.2** **Poisoning by, adverse effect of and underdosing of carbonic-anhydrase inhibitors, benzothiadiazides and other diuretics**
Poisoning by, adverse effect of and underdosing of acetazolamide

√6th **T50.2X** **Poisoning by, adverse effect of and underdosing of carbonic-anhydrase inhibitors, benzothiadiazides and other diuretics**

√7th **T50.2X1** **Poisoning by carbonic-anhydrase inhibitors, benzothiadiazides and other diuretics,** accidental (unintentional)
Poisoning by carbonic-anhydrase inhibitors, benzothiadiazides and other diuretics NOS

7 √7th **T50.2X2** **Poisoning by carbonic-anhydrase inhibitors, benzothiadiazides and other diuretics,** intentional self-harm　HCC

√7th **T50.2X3** **Poisoning by carbonic-anhydrase inhibitors, benzothiadiazides and other diuretics,** assault

√7th **T50.2X4** **Poisoning by carbonic-anhydrase inhibitors, benzothiadiazides and other diuretics,** undetermined

√7th **T50.2X5** Adverse effect of carbonic-anhydrase inhibitors, benzothiadiazides and other diuretics

√7th **T50.2X6** Underdosing of carbonic-anhydrase inhibitors, benzothiadiazides and other diuretics

√5th **T50.3** **Poisoning by, adverse effect of and underdosing of electrolytic, caloric and water-balance agents**
Poisoning by, adverse effect of and underdosing of oral rehydration salts

√6th **T50.3X** **Poisoning by, adverse effect of and underdosing of electrolytic, caloric and water-balance agents**

√7th **T50.3X1** **Poisoning by electrolytic, caloric and water-balance agents,** accidental (unintentional)
Poisoning by electrolytic, caloric and water-balance agents NOS

7 √7th **T50.3X2** **Poisoning by electrolytic, caloric and water-balance agents,** intentional self-harm　HCC

√7th **T50.3X3** **Poisoning by electrolytic, caloric and water-balance agents,** assault

√7th **T50.3X4** **Poisoning by electrolytic, caloric and water-balance agents,** undetermined

√7th **T50.3X5** Adverse effect of electrolytic, caloric and water-balance agents

√7th **T50.3X6** Underdosing of electrolytic, caloric and water-balance agents

√5ᵗʰ **T50.4** **Poisoning by, adverse effect of and underdosing of drugs affecting uric acid metabolism**

    √6ᵗʰ **T50.4X** **Poisoning by, adverse effect of and underdosing of** drugs affecting uric acid metabolism

        √7ᵗʰ **T50.4X1** **Poisoning by drugs affecting uric acid metabolism,** accidental (unintentional)

             Poisoning by drugs affecting uric acid metabolism NOS

        7 √7ᵗʰ **T50.4X2** **Poisoning by drugs affecting uric acid metabolism,** intentional **self-harm**   HCC

        √7ᵗʰ **T50.4X3** **Poisoning by drugs affecting uric acid metabolism,** assault

        √7ᵗʰ **T50.4X4** **Poisoning by drugs affecting uric acid metabolism,** undetermined

        √7ᵗʰ **T50.4X5** Adverse effect **of drugs affecting uric acid metabolism**

        √7ᵗʰ **T50.4X6** Underdosing **of drugs affecting uric acid metabolism**

√5ᵗʰ **T50.5** **Poisoning by, adverse effect of and underdosing of appetite depressants**

    √6ᵗʰ **T50.5X** **Poisoning by, adverse effect of and underdosing of** appetite depressants

        √7ᵗʰ **T50.5X1** **Poisoning by appetite depressants,** accidental (unintentional)

             Poisoning by appetite depressants NOS

        7 √7ᵗʰ **T50.5X2** **Poisoning by appetite depressants,** intentional **self-harm**   HCC

        √7ᵗʰ **T50.5X3** **Poisoning by appetite depressants,** assault

        √7ᵗʰ **T50.5X4** **Poisoning by appetite depressants,** undetermined

        √7ᵗʰ **T50.5X5** Adverse effect **of appetite depressants**

        √7ᵗʰ **T50.5X6** Underdosing **of appetite depressants**

√5ᵗʰ **T50.6** **Poisoning by, adverse effect of and underdosing of antidotes and chelating agents**

     Poisoning by, adverse effect of and underdosing of alcohol deterrents

    √6ᵗʰ **T50.6X** **Poisoning by, adverse effect of and underdosing of** antidotes and chelating agents

        √7ᵗʰ **T50.6X1** **Poisoning by antidotes and chelating agents,** accidental (unintentional)

             Poisoning by antidotes and chelating agents NOS

        7 √7ᵗʰ **T50.6X2** **Poisoning by antidotes and chelating agents,** intentional self-harm   HCC

        √7ᵗʰ **T50.6X3** **Poisoning by antidotes and chelating agents,** assault

        √7ᵗʰ **T50.6X4** **Poisoning by antidotes and chelating agents,** undetermined

        √7ᵗʰ **T50.6X5** Adverse effect **of antidotes and chelating agents**

        √7ᵗʰ **T50.6X6** Underdosing **of antidotes and chelating agents**

√5ᵗʰ **T50.7** **Poisoning by, adverse effect of and underdosing of analeptics and opioid receptor antagonists**

    √6ᵗʰ **T50.7X** **Poisoning by, adverse effect of and underdosing of** analeptics and opioid receptor antagonists

        √7ᵗʰ **T50.7X1** **Poisoning by analeptics and opioid receptor antagonists,** accidental (unintentional)

             Poisoning by analeptics and opioid receptor antagonists NOS

        7 √7ᵗʰ **T50.7X2** **Poisoning by analeptics and opioid receptor antagonists,** intentional self-harm   HCC

        √7ᵗʰ **T50.7X3** **Poisoning by analeptics and opioid receptor antagonists,** assault

        √7ᵗʰ **T50.7X4** **Poisoning by analeptics and opioid receptor antagonists,** undetermined

        √7ᵗʰ **T50.7X5** Adverse effect **of analeptics and opioid receptor antagonists**

        √7ᵗʰ **T50.7X6** Underdosing **of analeptics and opioid receptor antagonists**

√5ᵗʰ **T50.8** **Poisoning by, adverse effect of and underdosing of diagnostic agents**

    √6ᵗʰ **T50.8X** **Poisoning by, adverse effect of and underdosing of** diagnostic agents

        √7ᵗʰ **T50.8X1** **Poisoning by diagnostic agents,** accidental (unintentional)

             Poisoning by diagnostic agents NOS

        7 √7ᵗʰ **T50.8X2** **Poisoning by diagnostic agents,** intentional **self-harm**   HCC

        √7ᵗʰ **T50.8X3** **Poisoning by diagnostic agents,** assault

        √7ᵗʰ **T50.8X4** **Poisoning by diagnostic agents,** undetermined

        √7ᵗʰ **T50.8X5** Adverse effect **of diagnostic agents**

        √7ᵗʰ **T50.8X6** Underdosing **of diagnostic agents**

√5ᵗʰ **T50.A** **Poisoning by, adverse effect of and underdosing of bacterial vaccines**

    √6ᵗʰ **T50.A1** **Poisoning by, adverse effect of and underdosing of** pertussis vaccine, including combinations with a pertussis component

        √7ᵗʰ **T50.A11** **Poisoning by pertussis vaccine, including combinations with a pertussis component,** accidental (unintentional)

        7 √7ᵗʰ **T50.A12** **Poisoning by pertussis vaccine, including combinations with a pertussis component,** intentional self-harm   HCC

        √7ᵗʰ **T50.A13** **Poisoning by pertussis vaccine, including combinations with a pertussis component,** assault

        √7ᵗʰ **T50.A14** **Poisoning by pertussis vaccine, including combinations with a pertussis component,** undetermined

        √7ᵗʰ **T50.A15** Adverse effect **of pertussis vaccine, including combinations with a pertussis component**

        √7ᵗʰ **T50.A16** Underdosing **of pertussis vaccine, including combinations with a pertussis component**

    √6ᵗʰ **T50.A2** **Poisoning by, adverse effect of and underdosing of** mixed bacterial vaccines without a pertussis component

        √7ᵗʰ **T50.A21** **Poisoning by mixed bacterial vaccines without a pertussis component,** accidental (unintentional)

        7 √7ᵗʰ **T50.A22** **Poisoning by mixed bacterial vaccines without a pertussis component,** intentional self-harm   HCC

        √7ᵗʰ **T50.A23** **Poisoning by mixed bacterial vaccines without a pertussis component,** assault

        √7ᵗʰ **T50.A24** **Poisoning by mixed bacterial vaccines without a pertussis component,** undetermined

        √7ᵗʰ **T50.A25** Adverse effect **of mixed bacterial vaccines without a pertussis component**

        √7ᵗʰ **T50.A26** Underdosing **of mixed bacterial vaccines without a pertussis component**

    √6ᵗʰ **T50.A9** **Poisoning by, adverse effect of and underdosing of other bacterial vaccines**

        √7ᵗʰ **T50.A91** **Poisoning by other bacterial vaccines,** accidental (unintentional)

        7 √7ᵗʰ **T50.A92** **Poisoning by other bacterial vaccines,** intentional self-harm   HCC

        √7ᵗʰ **T50.A93** **Poisoning by other bacterial vaccines,** assault

        √7ᵗʰ **T50.A94** **Poisoning by other bacterial vaccines,** undetermined

        √7ᵗʰ **T50.A95** Adverse effect **of other bacterial vaccines**

        √7ᵗʰ **T50.A96** Underdosing **of other bacterial vaccines**

√5ᵗʰ **T50.B** **Poisoning by, adverse effect of and underdosing of viral vaccines**

    √6ᵗʰ **T50.B1** **Poisoning by, adverse effect of and underdosing of** smallpox vaccines

        √7ᵗʰ **T50.B11** **Poisoning by smallpox vaccines,** accidental (unintentional)

        7 √7ᵗʰ **T50.B12** **Poisoning by smallpox vaccines,** intentional self-harm   HCC

        √7ᵗʰ **T50.B13** **Poisoning by smallpox vaccines,** assault

N Newborn: 0   P Pediatric: 0-17   M Maternity: 9-64   A Adult: 15-124   MCC Major Complication/Comorbidity   CC Complication/Comorbidity   SW Severe Wound Dx

1170   ICD-10-CM 2020

√7ᵗʰ **T50.B14** Poisoning by smallpox vaccines, undetermined

√7ᵗʰ **T50.B15** Adverse effect of smallpox vaccines

√7ᵗʰ **T50.B16** Underdosing of smallpox vaccines

√6ᵗʰ **T50.B9** Poisoning by, adverse effect of and underdosing of other viral vaccines

√7ᵗʰ **T50.B91** Poisoning by other viral vaccines, accidental (unintentional)

⁷ √7ᵗʰ **T50.B92** Poisoning by other viral vaccines, intentional self-harm   HCC

√7ᵗʰ **T50.B93** Poisoning by other viral vaccines, assault

√7ᵗʰ **T50.B94** Poisoning by other viral vaccines, undetermined

√7ᵗʰ **T50.B95** Adverse effect of other viral vaccines

√7ᵗʰ **T50.B96** Underdosing of other viral vaccines

√5ᵗʰ **T50.Z** Poisoning by, adverse effect of and underdosing of other vaccines and biological substances

√6ᵗʰ **T50.Z1** Poisoning by, adverse effect of and underdosing of immunoglobulin

√7ᵗʰ **T50.Z11** Poisoning by immunoglobulin, accidental (unintentional)

⁷ √7ᵗʰ **T50.Z12** Poisoning by immunoglobulin, intentional self-harm   HCC

√7ᵗʰ **T50.Z13** Poisoning by immunoglobulin, assault

√7ᵗʰ **T50.Z14** Poisoning by immunoglobulin, undetermined

√7ᵗʰ **T50.Z15** Adverse effect of immunoglobulin

√7ᵗʰ **T50.Z16** Underdosing of immunoglobulin

√6ᵗʰ **T50.Z9** Poisoning by, adverse effect of and underdosing of other vaccines and biological substances

√7ᵗʰ **T50.Z91** Poisoning by other vaccines and biological substances, accidental (unintentional)

⁷ √7ᵗʰ **T50.Z92** Poisoning by other vaccines and biological substances, intentional self-harm   HCC

√7ᵗʰ **T50.Z93** Poisoning by other vaccines and biological substances, assault

√7ᵗʰ **T50.Z94** Poisoning by other vaccines and biological substances, undetermined

√7ᵗʰ **T50.Z95** Adverse effect of other vaccines and biological substances

√7ᵗʰ **T50.Z96** Underdosing of other vaccines and biological substances

√5ᵗʰ **T50.9** Poisoning by, adverse effect of and underdosing of other and unspecified drugs, medicaments and biological substances

AHA: 2016,1Q,38; 2015,1Q,21

√6ᵗʰ **T50.90** Poisoning by, adverse effect of and underdosing of unspecified drugs, medicaments and biological substances

√7ᵗʰ **T50.901** Poisoning by unspecified drugs, medicaments and biological substances, accidental (unintentional)

⁷ √7ᵗʰ **T50.902** Poisoning by unspecified drugs, medicaments and biological substances, intentional self-harm   HCC

√7ᵗʰ **T50.903** Poisoning by unspecified drugs, medicaments and biological substances, assault

√7ᵗʰ **T50.904** Poisoning by unspecified drugs, medicaments and biological substances, undetermined

√7ᵗʰ **T50.905** Adverse effect of unspecified drugs, medicaments and biological substances

√7ᵗʰ **T50.906** Underdosing of unspecified drugs, medicaments and biological substances

√6ᵗʰ **T50.91** Poisoning by, adverse effect of and underdosing of multiple unspecified drugs, medicaments and biological substances

Multiple drug ingestion NOS

Code also any specific drugs, medicaments and biological substances

√7ᵗʰ **T50.911** Poisoning by multiple unspecified drugs, medicaments and biological substances, accidental (unintentional)

√7ᵗʰ **T50.912** Poisoning by multiple unspecified drugs, medicaments and biological substances, intentional self-harm

√7ᵗʰ **T50.913** Poisoning by multiple unspecified drugs, medicaments and biological substances, assault

√7ᵗʰ **T50.914** Poisoning by multiple unspecified drugs, medicaments and biological substances, undetermined

√7ᵗʰ **T50.915** Adverse effect of multiple unspecified drugs, medicaments and biological substances

√7ᵗʰ **T50.916** Underdosing of multiple unspecified drugs, medicaments and biological substances

√6ᵗʰ **T50.99** Poisoning by, adverse effect of and underdosing of other drugs, medicaments and biological substances

√7ᵗʰ **T50.991** Poisoning by other drugs, medicaments and biological substances, accidental (unintentional)

⁷ √7ᵗʰ **T50.992** Poisoning by other drugs, medicaments and biological substances, intentional self-harm   HCC

√7ᵗʰ **T50.993** Poisoning by other drugs, medicaments and biological substances, assault

√7ᵗʰ **T50.994** Poisoning by other drugs, medicaments and biological substances, undetermined

√7ᵗʰ **T50.995** Adverse effect of other drugs, medicaments and biological substances

√7ᵗʰ **T50.996** Underdosing of other drugs, medicaments and biological substances

Toxic effects of substances chiefly nonmedicinal as to source (T51-T65)

NOTE   When no intent is indicated code to accidental. Undetermined intent is only for use when there is specific documentation in the record that the intent of the toxic effect cannot be determined.

Use additional code(s) for all associated manifestations of toxic effect, such as:
personal history of foreign body fully removed (Z87.821)
respiratory conditions due to external agents (J60-J70)
to identify any retained foreign body, if applicable (Z18.-)

EXCLUDES 1   contact with and (suspected) exposure to toxic substances (Z77.-)

AHA: 2017,1Q,39-40

√4ᵗʰ **T51** **Toxic effect of alcohol**

> The appropriate 7th character is to be added to each code from category T51.
> A   initial encounter
> D   subsequent encounter
> S   sequela

√5ᵗʰ **T51.0** **Toxic effect of ethanol**

Toxic effect of ethyl alcohol

EXCLUDES 2   acute alcohol intoxication or "hangover" effects (F10.129, F10.229, F10.929)
drunkenness (F10.129, F10.229, F10.929)
pathological alcohol intoxication (F10.129, F10.229, F10.929)

√6ᵗʰ **T51.0X** **Toxic effect of ethanol**

⁶ √7ᵗʰ **T51.0X1** Toxic effect of ethanol, accidental (unintentional)   HCC
Toxic effect of ethanol NOS

⁷ √7ᵗʰ **T51.0X2** Toxic effect of ethanol, intentional self-harm   HCC

√7ᵗʰ **T51.0X3** Toxic effect of ethanol, assault

⁶ √7ᵗʰ **T51.0X4** Toxic effect of ethanol, undetermined   HCC

√5ᵗʰ **T51.1** **Toxic effect of methanol**

Toxic effect of methyl alcohol

√6ᵗʰ **T51.1X** **Toxic effect of methanol**

√7ᵗʰ **T51.1X1** Toxic effect of methanol, accidental (unintentional)
Toxic effect of methanol NOS

⁷ √7ᵗʰ **T51.1X2** Toxic effect of methanol, intentional self-harm   HCC

√7ᵗʰ **T51.1X3** Toxic effect of methanol, assault

√7ᵗʰ **T51.1X4** Toxic effect of methanol, undetermined

☑ Additional Character Required   √x7ᵗʰ Placeholder   Unacceptable PDx   Questionable PDx   Manifestation   Unspecified Dx   H1-H14 HAC   HCC CMS-HCC Dx   HIV HIV Dx

ICD-10-CM 2020   1171

✓5ᵗʰ T51.2 Toxic effect of 2-Propanol
Toxic effect of isopropyl alcohol

   ✓6ᵗʰ **T51.2X Toxic effect of 2-Propanol**

     ✓7ᵗʰ **T51.2X1 Toxic effect of 2-Propanol, accidental (unintentional)**
         Toxic effect of 2-Propanol NOS

     ⁷ ✓7ᵗʰ **T51.2X2 Toxic effect of 2-Propanol, intentional self-harm**   HCC

     ✓7ᵗʰ **T51.2X3 Toxic effect of 2-Propanol, assault**

     ✓7ᵗʰ **T51.2X4 Toxic effect of 2-Propanol, undetermined**

✓5ᵗʰ T51.3 Toxic effect of fusel oil
Toxic effect of amyl alcohol
Toxic effect of butyl [1-butanol] alcohol
Toxic effect of propyl [1-propanol] alcohol

   ✓6ᵗʰ **T51.3X Toxic effect of fusel oil**

     ✓7ᵗʰ **T51.3X1 Toxic effect of fusel oil, accidental (unintentional)**
         Toxic effect of fusel oil NOS

     ⁷ ✓7ᵗʰ **T51.3X2 Toxic effect of fusel oil, intentional self-harm**   HCC

     ✓7ᵗʰ **T51.3X3 Toxic effect of fusel oil, assault**

     ✓7ᵗʰ **T51.3X4 Toxic effect of fusel oil, undetermined**

✓5ᵗʰ T51.8 Toxic effect of other alcohols

   ✓6ᵗʰ **T51.8X Toxic effect of other alcohols**

     ✓7ᵗʰ **T51.8X1 Toxic effect of other alcohols, accidental (unintentional)**
         Toxic effect of other alcohols NOS

     ⁷ ✓7ᵗʰ **T51.8X2 Toxic effect of other alcohols, intentional self-harm**   HCC

     ✓7ᵗʰ **T51.8X3 Toxic effect of other alcohols, assault**

     ✓7ᵗʰ **T51.8X4 Toxic effect of other alcohols, undetermined**

✓5ᵗʰ T51.9 Toxic effect of unspecified alcohol

   ✓x7ᵗʰ **T51.91 Toxic effect of unspecified alcohol, accidental (unintentional)**

   ⁷ ✓x7ᵗʰ **T51.92 Toxic effect of unspecified alcohol, intentional self-harm**   HCC

   ✓x7ᵗʰ **T51.93 Toxic effect of unspecified alcohol, assault**

   ✓x7ᵗʰ **T51.94 Toxic effect of unspecified alcohol, undetermined**

✓4ᵗʰ T52 Toxic effect of organic solvents

    EXCLUDES 1   *halogen derivatives of aliphatic and aromatic hydrocarbons (T53.-)*

> The appropriate 7th character is to be added to each code from category T52.
> A   initial encounter
> D   subsequent encounter
> S   sequela

  ✓5ᵗʰ **T52.0 Toxic effects of petroleum products**
Toxic effects of ether petroleum
Toxic effects of gasoline [petrol]
Toxic effects of kerosene [paraffin oil]
Toxic effects of naphtha petroleum
Toxic effects of paraffin wax
Toxic effects of spirit petroleum

   ✓6ᵗʰ **T52.0X Toxic effects of petroleum products**

     ✓7ᵗʰ **T52.0X1 Toxic effect of petroleum products, accidental (unintentional)**
         Toxic effects of petroleum products NOS

     ⁷ ✓7ᵗʰ **T52.0X2 Toxic effect of petroleum products, intentional self-harm**   HCC

     ✓7ᵗʰ **T52.0X3 Toxic effect of petroleum products, assault**

     ✓7ᵗʰ **T52.0X4 Toxic effect of petroleum products, undetermined**

  ✓5ᵗʰ **T52.1 Toxic effects of benzene**

    EXCLUDES 1   *homologues of benzene (T52.2)*
          nitroderivatives and aminoderivatives of benzene and its homologues (T65.3)

   ✓6ᵗʰ **T52.1X Toxic effects of benzene**

     ✓7ᵗʰ **T52.1X1 Toxic effect of benzene, accidental (unintentional)**
         Toxic effects of benzene NOS

     ⁷ ✓7ᵗʰ **T52.1X2 Toxic effect of benzene, intentional self-harm**   HCC

     ✓7ᵗʰ **T52.1X3 Toxic effect of benzene, assault**

     ✓7ᵗʰ **T52.1X4 Toxic effect of benzene, undetermined**

  ✓5ᵗʰ **T52.2 Toxic effects of homologues of benzene**
Toxic effects of toluene [methylbenzene]
Toxic effects of xylene [dimethylbenzene]

   ✓6ᵗʰ **T52.2X Toxic effects of homologues of benzene**

     ✓7ᵗʰ **T52.2X1 Toxic effect of homologues of benzene, accidental (unintentional)**
         Toxic effects of homologues of benzene NOS

     ⁷ ✓7ᵗʰ **T52.2X2 Toxic effect of homologues of benzene, intentional self-harm**   HCC

     ✓7ᵗʰ **T52.2X3 Toxic effect of homologues of benzene, assault**

     ✓7ᵗʰ **T52.2X4 Toxic effect of homologues of benzene, undetermined**

  ✓5ᵗʰ **T52.3 Toxic effects of glycols**

   ✓6ᵗʰ **T52.3X Toxic effects of glycols**

     ✓7ᵗʰ **T52.3X1 Toxic effect of glycols, accidental (unintentional)**
         Toxic effects of glycols NOS

     ⁷ ✓7ᵗʰ **T52.3X2 Toxic effect of glycols, intentional self-harm**   HCC

     ✓7ᵗʰ **T52.3X3 Toxic effect of glycols, assault**

     ✓7ᵗʰ **T52.3X4 Toxic effect of glycols, undetermined**

  ✓5ᵗʰ **T52.4 Toxic effects of ketones**

   ✓6ᵗʰ **T52.4X Toxic effects of ketones**

     ✓7ᵗʰ **T52.4X1 Toxic effect of ketones, accidental (unintentional)**
         Toxic effects of ketones NOS

     ⁷ ✓7ᵗʰ **T52.4X2 Toxic effect of ketones, intentional self-harm**   HCC

     ✓7ᵗʰ **T52.4X3 Toxic effect of ketones, assault**

     ✓7ᵗʰ **T52.4X4 Toxic effect of ketones, undetermined**

  ✓5ᵗʰ **T52.8 Toxic effects of other organic solvents**

   ✓6ᵗʰ **T52.8X Toxic effects of other organic solvents**

     ✓7ᵗʰ **T52.8X1 Toxic effect of other organic solvents, accidental (unintentional)**
         Toxic effects of other organic solvents NOS

     ⁷ ✓7ᵗʰ **T52.8X2 Toxic effect of other organic solvents, intentional self-harm**   HCC

     ✓7ᵗʰ **T52.8X3 Toxic effect of other organic solvents, assault**

     ✓7ᵗʰ **T52.8X4 Toxic effect of other organic solvents, undetermined**

  ✓5ᵗʰ **T52.9 Toxic effects of unspecified organic solvent**

   ✓x7ᵗʰ **T52.91 Toxic effect of unspecified organic solvent, accidental (unintentional)**

   ⁷ ✓x7ᵗʰ **T52.92 Toxic effect of unspecified organic solvent, intentional self-harm**   HCC

   ✓x7ᵗʰ **T52.93 Toxic effect of unspecified organic solvent, assault**

   ✓x7ᵗʰ **T52.94 Toxic effect of unspecified organic solvent, undetermined**

✓4ᵗʰ T53 Toxic effect of halogen derivatives of aliphatic and aromatic hydrocarbons

> The appropriate 7th character is to be added to each code from category T53.
> A   initial encounter
> D   subsequent encounter
> S   sequela

  ✓5ᵗʰ **T53.0 Toxic effects of carbon tetrachloride**
Toxic effects of tetrachloromethane

   ✓6ᵗʰ **T53.0X Toxic effects of carbon tetrachloride**

     ✓7ᵗʰ **T53.0X1 Toxic effect of carbon tetrachloride, accidental (unintentional)**
         Toxic effects of carbon tetrachloride NOS

     ⁷ ✓7ᵗʰ **T53.0X2 Toxic effect of carbon tetrachloride, intentional self-harm**   HCC

     ✓7ᵗʰ **T53.0X3 Toxic effect of carbon tetrachloride, assault**

     ✓7ᵗʰ **T53.0X4 Toxic effect of carbon tetrachloride, undetermined**

ℕ Newborn: 0   ℙ Pediatric: 0-17   𝕄 Maternity: 9-64   𝔸 Adult: 15-124   MCC Major Complication/Comorbidity   CC Complication/Comorbidity   SW Severe Wound Dx

1172   ICD-10-CM 2020

✓5th **T53.1 Toxic effects of chloroform**
  Toxic effects of trichloromethane
  ✓6th **T53.1X Toxic effects of** chloroform
    ✓7th **T53.1X1 Toxic effect of chloroform, accidental (unintentional)**
      Toxic effects of chloroform NOS
    7 ✓7th **T53.1X2 Toxic effect of chloroform, intentional self-harm** HCC
    ✓7th **T53.1X3 Toxic effect of chloroform, assault**
    ✓7th **T53.1X4 Toxic effect of chloroform, undetermined**

✓5th **T53.2 Toxic effects of trichloroethylene**
  Toxic effects of trichloroethene
  ✓6th **T53.2X Toxic effects of** trichloroethylene
    ✓7th **T53.2X1 Toxic effect of trichloroethylene, accidental (unintentional)**
      Toxic effects of trichloroethylene NOS
    7 ✓7th **T53.2X2 Toxic effect of trichloroethylene, intentional self-harm** HCC
    ✓7th **T53.2X3 Toxic effect of trichloroethylene, assault**
    ✓7th **T53.2X4 Toxic effect of trichloroethylene, undetermined**

✓5th **T53.3 Toxic effects of tetrachloroethylene**
  Toxic effects of perchloroethylene
  Toxic effect of tetrachloroethene
  ✓6th **T53.3X Toxic effects of** tetrachloroethylene
    ✓7th **T53.3X1 Toxic effect of tetrachloroethylene, accidental (unintentional)**
      Toxic effects of tetrachloroethylene NOS
    7 ✓7th **T53.3X2 Toxic effect of tetrachloroethylene, intentional self-harm** HCC
    ✓7th **T53.3X3 Toxic effect of tetrachloroethylene, assault**
    ✓7th **T53.3X4 Toxic effect of tetrachloroethylene, undetermined**

✓5th **T53.4 Toxic effects of dichloromethane**
  Toxic effects of methylene chloride
  ✓6th **T53.4X Toxic effects of** dichloromethane
    ✓7th **T53.4X1 Toxic effect of dichloromethane, accidental (unintentional)**
      Toxic effects of dichloromethane NOS
    7 ✓7th **T53.4X2 Toxic effect of dichloromethane, intentional self-harm** HCC
    ✓7th **T53.4X3 Toxic effect of dichloromethane, assault**
    ✓7th **T53.4X4 Toxic effect of dichloromethane, undetermined**

✓5th **T53.5 Toxic effects of chlorofluorocarbons**
  ✓6th **T53.5X Toxic effects of** chlorofluorocarbons
    ✓7th **T53.5X1 Toxic effect of chlorofluorocarbons, accidental (unintentional)**
      Toxic effects of chlorofluorocarbons NOS
    7 ✓7th **T53.5X2 Toxic effect of chlorofluorocarbons, intentional self-harm** HCC
    ✓7th **T53.5X3 Toxic effect of chlorofluorocarbons, assault**
    ✓7th **T53.5X4 Toxic effect of chlorofluorocarbons, undetermined**

✓5th **T53.6 Toxic effects of other halogen derivatives of aliphatic hydrocarbons**
  ✓6th **T53.6X Toxic effects of** other halogen derivatives of aliphatic hydrocarbons
    ✓7th **T53.6X1 Toxic effect of other halogen derivatives of aliphatic hydrocarbons, accidental (unintentional)**
      Toxic effects of other halogen derivatives of aliphatic hydrocarbons NOS
    7 ✓7th **T53.6X2 Toxic effect of other halogen derivatives of aliphatic hydrocarbons, intentional self-harm** HCC
    ✓7th **T53.6X3 Toxic effect of other halogen derivatives of aliphatic hydrocarbons, assault**
    ✓7th **T53.6X4 Toxic effect of other halogen derivatives of aliphatic hydrocarbons, undetermined**

✓5th **T53.7 Toxic effects of other halogen derivatives of aromatic hydrocarbons**
  ✓6th **T53.7X Toxic effects of** other halogen derivatives of aromatic hydrocarbons
    ✓7th **T53.7X1 Toxic effect of other halogen derivatives of aromatic hydrocarbons, accidental (unintentional)**
      Toxic effects of other halogen derivatives of aromatic hydrocarbons NOS
    7 ✓7th **T53.7X2 Toxic effect of other halogen derivatives of aromatic hydrocarbons, intentional self-harm** HCC
    ✓7th **T53.7X3 Toxic effect of other halogen derivatives of aromatic hydrocarbons, assault**
    ✓7th **T53.7X4 Toxic effect of other halogen derivatives of aromatic hydrocarbons, undetermined**

✓5th **T53.9 Toxic effects of unspecified halogen derivatives of aliphatic and aromatic hydrocarbons**
  ✓x7th **T53.91 Toxic effect of unspecified halogen derivatives of aliphatic and aromatic hydrocarbons, accidental (unintentional)**
  7 ✓x7th **T53.92 Toxic effect of unspecified halogen derivatives of aliphatic and aromatic hydrocarbons, intentional self-harm** HCC
  ✓x7th **T53.93 Toxic effect of unspecified halogen derivatives of aliphatic and aromatic hydrocarbons, assault**
  ✓x7th **T53.94 Toxic effect of unspecified halogen derivatives of aliphatic and aromatic hydrocarbons, undetermined**

✓4th **T54 Toxic effect of corrosive substances**
  The appropriate 7th character is to be added to each code from category T54.
  A   initial encounter
  D   subsequent encounter
  S   sequela

✓5th **T54.0 Toxic effects of phenol and phenol homologues**
  ✓6th **T54.0X Toxic effects of** phenol and phenol homologues
    ✓7th **T54.0X1 Toxic effect of phenol and phenol homologues, accidental (unintentional)**
      Toxic effects of phenol and phenol homologues NOS
    7 ✓7th **T54.0X2 Toxic effect of phenol and phenol homologues, intentional self-harm** HCC
    ✓7th **T54.0X3 Toxic effect of phenol and phenol homologues, assault**
    ✓7th **T54.0X4 Toxic effect of phenol and phenol homologues, undetermined**

✓5th **T54.1 Toxic effects of other corrosive organic compounds**
  ✓6th **T54.1X Toxic effects of** other corrosive organic compounds
    ✓7th **T54.1X1 Toxic effect of other corrosive organic compounds, accidental (unintentional)**
      Toxic effects of other corrosive organic compounds NOS
    7 ✓7th **T54.1X2 Toxic effect of other corrosive organic compounds, intentional self-harm** HCC
    ✓7th **T54.1X3 Toxic effect of other corrosive organic compounds, assault**
    ✓7th **T54.1X4 Toxic effect of other corrosive organic compounds, undetermined**

✓5th **T54.2 Toxic effects of corrosive acids and acid-like substances**
  Toxic effects of hydrochloric acid
  Toxic effects of sulfuric acid
  ✓6th **T54.2X Toxic effects of** corrosive acids and acid-like substances
    ✓7th **T54.2X1 Toxic effect of corrosive acids and acid-like substances, accidental (unintentional)**
      Toxic effects of corrosive acids and acid-like substances NOS
    7 ✓7th **T54.2X2 Toxic effect of corrosive acids and acid-like substances, intentional self-harm** HCC
    ✓7th **T54.2X3 Toxic effect of corrosive acids and acid-like substances, assault**

☑7ᵗʰ **T54.2X4 Toxic effect of corrosive acids and acid-like substances,** undetermined

☑5ᵗʰ **T54.3 Toxic effects of corrosive alkalis and alkali-like substances**
  Toxic effects of potassium hydroxide
  Toxic effects of sodium hydroxide

  ☑6ᵗʰ **T54.3X Toxic effects of** corrosive alkalis and alkali-like substances

    ☑7ᵗʰ **T54.3X1 Toxic effect of corrosive alkalis and alkali-like substances,** accidental **(unintentional)**
      Toxic effects of corrosive alkalis and alkali-like substances NOS

    7 ☑7ᵗʰ **T54.3X2 Toxic effect of corrosive alkalis and alkali-like substances,** intentional self-harm   HCC

    ☑7ᵗʰ **T54.3X3 Toxic effect of corrosive alkalis and alkali-like substances,** assault

    ☑7ᵗʰ **T54.3X4 Toxic effect of corrosive alkalis and alkali-like substances,** undetermined

☑5ᵗʰ **T54.9 Toxic effects of unspecified corrosive substance**

  ☑x7ᵗʰ **T54.91 Toxic effect of unspecified corrosive substance,** accidental (unintentional)

  7 ☑x7ᵗʰ **T54.92 Toxic effect of unspecified corrosive substance,** intentional self-harm   HCC

  ☑x7ᵗʰ **T54.93 Toxic effect of unspecified corrosive substance,** assault

  ☑x7ᵗʰ **T54.94 Toxic effect of unspecified corrosive substance,** undetermined

☑4ᵗʰ **T55 Toxic effect of soaps and detergents**

> The appropriate 7th character is to be added to each code from category T55.
> A   initial encounter
> D   subsequent encounter
> S   sequela

☑5ᵗʰ **T55.0 Toxic effect of soaps**

  ☑6ᵗʰ **T55.0X Toxic effect of** soaps

    ☑7ᵗʰ **T55.0X1 Toxic effect of soaps,** accidental **(unintentional)**
      Toxic effect of soaps NOS

    7 ☑7ᵗʰ **T55.0X2 Toxic effect of soaps,** intentional self-harm   HCC

    ☑7ᵗʰ **T55.0X3 Toxic effect of soaps,** assault

    ☑7ᵗʰ **T55.0X4 Toxic effect of soaps,** undetermined

☑5ᵗʰ **T55.1 Toxic effect of detergents**

  ☑6ᵗʰ **T55.1X Toxic effect of** detergents

    ☑7ᵗʰ **T55.1X1 Toxic effect of detergents,** accidental **(unintentional)**
      Toxic effect of detergents NOS

    7 ☑7ᵗʰ **T55.1X2 Toxic effect of detergents,** intentional self-harm   HCC

    ☑7ᵗʰ **T55.1X3 Toxic effect of detergents,** assault

    ☑7ᵗʰ **T55.1X4 Toxic effect of detergents,** undetermined

☑4ᵗʰ **T56 Toxic effect of metals**

  INCLUDES   toxic effects of fumes and vapors of metals
  toxic effects of metals from all sources, except medicinal substances

  Use additional code to identify any retained metal foreign body, if applicable (Z18.0-, T18.1-)

  EXCLUDES 1   *arsenic and its compounds (T57.0)*
  manganese and its compounds (T57.2)

> The appropriate 7th character is to be added to each code from category T56.
> A   initial encounter
> D   subsequent encounter
> S   sequela

☑5ᵗʰ **T56.0 Toxic effects of lead and its compounds**

  ☑6ᵗʰ **T56.0X Toxic effects of** lead and its compounds

    ☑7ᵗʰ **T56.0X1 Toxic effect of lead and its compounds,** accidental **(unintentional)**
      Toxic effects of lead and its compounds NOS

    7 ☑7ᵗʰ **T56.0X2 Toxic effect of lead and its compounds,** intentional self-harm   HCC

☑7ᵗʰ **T56.0X3 Toxic effect of lead and its compounds,** assault

☑7ᵗʰ **T56.0X4 Toxic effect of lead and its compounds,** undetermined

☑5ᵗʰ **T56.1 Toxic effects of mercury and its compounds**

  ☑6ᵗʰ **T56.1X Toxic effects of** mercury and its compounds

    ☑7ᵗʰ **T56.1X1 Toxic effect of mercury and its compounds,** accidental **(unintentional)**
      Toxic effects of mercury and its compounds NOS

    7 ☑7ᵗʰ **T56.1X2 Toxic effect of mercury and its compounds,** intentional self-harm   HCC

    ☑7ᵗʰ **T56.1X3 Toxic effect of mercury and its compounds,** assault

    ☑7ᵗʰ **T56.1X4 Toxic effect of mercury and its compounds,** undetermined

☑5ᵗʰ **T56.2 Toxic effects of chromium and its compounds**

  ☑6ᵗʰ **T56.2X Toxic effects of** chromium and its compounds

    ☑7ᵗʰ **T56.2X1 Toxic effect of chromium and its compounds,** accidental **(unintentional)**
      Toxic effects of chromium and its compounds NOS

    7 ☑7ᵗʰ **T56.2X2 Toxic effect of chromium and its compounds,** intentional self-harm   HCC

    ☑7ᵗʰ **T56.2X3 Toxic effect of chromium and its compounds,** assault

    ☑7ᵗʰ **T56.2X4 Toxic effect of chromium and its compounds,** undetermined

☑5ᵗʰ **T56.3 Toxic effects of cadmium and its compounds**

  ☑6ᵗʰ **T56.3X Toxic effects of** cadmium and its compounds

    ☑7ᵗʰ **T56.3X1 Toxic effect of cadmium and its compounds,** accidental **(unintentional)**
      Toxic effects of cadmium and its compounds NOS

    7 ☑7ᵗʰ **T56.3X2 Toxic effect of cadmium and its compounds,** intentional self-harm   HCC

    ☑7ᵗʰ **T56.3X3 Toxic effect of cadmium and its compounds,** assault

    ☑7ᵗʰ **T56.3X4 Toxic effect of cadmium and its compounds,** undetermined

☑5ᵗʰ **T56.4 Toxic effects of copper and its compounds**

  ☑6ᵗʰ **T56.4X Toxic effects of** copper and its compounds

    ☑7ᵗʰ **T56.4X1 Toxic effect of copper and its compounds,** accidental **(unintentional)**
      Toxic effects of copper and its compounds NOS

    7 ☑7ᵗʰ **T56.4X2 Toxic effect of copper and its compounds,** intentional self-harm   HCC

    ☑7ᵗʰ **T56.4X3 Toxic effect of copper and its compounds,** assault

    ☑7ᵗʰ **T56.4X4 Toxic effect of copper and its compounds,** undetermined

☑5ᵗʰ **T56.5 Toxic effects of zinc and its compounds**

  ☑6ᵗʰ **T56.5X Toxic effects of** zinc and its compounds

    ☑7ᵗʰ **T56.5X1 Toxic effect of zinc and its compounds,** accidental **(unintentional)**
      Toxic effects of zinc and its compounds NOS

    7 ☑7ᵗʰ **T56.5X2 Toxic effect of zinc and its compounds,** intentional self-harm   HCC

    ☑7ᵗʰ **T56.5X3 Toxic effect of zinc and its compounds,** assault

    ☑7ᵗʰ **T56.5X4 Toxic effect of zinc and its compounds,** undetermined

☑5ᵗʰ **T56.6 Toxic effects of tin and its compounds**

  ☑6ᵗʰ **T56.6X Toxic effects of** tin and its compounds

    ☑7ᵗʰ **T56.6X1 Toxic effect of tin and its compounds,** accidental **(unintentional)**
      Toxic effects of tin and its compounds NOS

    7 ☑7ᵗʰ **T56.6X2 Toxic effect of tin and its compounds,** intentional self-harm   HCC

    ☑7ᵗʰ **T56.6X3 Toxic effect of tin and its compounds,** assault

N Newborn: 0   P Pediatric: 0-17   M Maternity: 9-64   A Adult: 15-124   MCC Major Complication/Comorbidity   CC Complication/Comorbidity   SW Severe Wound Dx

1174   ICD-10-CM 2020

√7ᵗʰ **T56.6X4** Toxic effect of tin and its compounds, undetermined

√5ᵗʰ **T56.7 Toxic effects of beryllium and its compounds**

  √6ᵗʰ **T56.7X** Toxic effects of beryllium and its compounds

    √7ᵗʰ **T56.7X1** Toxic effect of beryllium and its compounds, accidental (unintentional)
Toxic effects of beryllium and its compounds NOS

    7 √7ᵗʰ **T56.7X2** Toxic effect of beryllium and its compounds, intentional self-harm   HCC

    √7ᵗʰ **T56.7X3** Toxic effect of beryllium and its compounds, assault

    √7ᵗʰ **T56.7X4** Toxic effect of beryllium and its compounds, undetermined

√5ᵗʰ **T56.8 Toxic effects of other metals**

  √6ᵗʰ **T56.81** Toxic effect of thallium

    √7ᵗʰ **T56.811** Toxic effect of thallium, accidental (unintentional)
Toxic effect of thallium NOS

    7 √7ᵗʰ **T56.812** Toxic effect of thallium, intentional self-harm   HCC

    √7ᵗʰ **T56.813** Toxic effect of thallium, assault

    √7ᵗʰ **T56.814** Toxic effect of thallium, undetermined

  √6ᵗʰ **T56.89** Toxic effects of other metals

    √7ᵗʰ **T56.891** Toxic effect of other metals, accidental (unintentional)
Toxic effects of other metals NOS

    7 √7ᵗʰ **T56.892** Toxic effect of other metals, intentional self-harm   HCC

    √7ᵗʰ **T56.893** Toxic effect of other metals, assault

    √7ᵗʰ **T56.894** Toxic effect of other metals, undetermined

√5ᵗʰ **T56.9 Toxic effects of unspecified metal**

  √x7ᵗʰ **T56.91** Toxic effect of unspecified metal, accidental (unintentional)

  7 √x7ᵗʰ **T56.92** Toxic effect of unspecified metal, intentional self-harm   HCC

  √x7ᵗʰ **T56.93** Toxic effect of unspecified metal, assault

  √x7ᵗʰ **T56.94** Toxic effect of unspecified metal, undetermined

√4ᵗʰ **T57 Toxic effect of other inorganic substances**

The appropriate 7th character is to be added to each code from category T57.
A   initial encounter
D   subsequent encounter
S   sequela

√5ᵗʰ **T57.0 Toxic effect of arsenic and its compounds**

  √6ᵗʰ **T57.0X** Toxic effect of arsenic and its compounds

    √7ᵗʰ **T57.0X1** Toxic effect of arsenic and its compounds, accidental (unintentional)
Toxic effect of arsenic and its compounds NOS

    7 √7ᵗʰ **T57.0X2** Toxic effect of arsenic and its compounds, intentional self-harm   HCC

    √7ᵗʰ **T57.0X3** Toxic effect of arsenic and its compounds, assault

    √7ᵗʰ **T57.0X4** Toxic effect of arsenic and its compounds, undetermined

√5ᵗʰ **T57.1 Toxic effect of phosphorus and its compounds**

  EXCLUDES 1   organophosphate insecticides (T60.0)

  √6ᵗʰ **T57.1X** Toxic effect of phosphorus and its compounds

    √7ᵗʰ **T57.1X1** Toxic effect of phosphorus and its compounds, accidental (unintentional)
Toxic effect of phosphorus and its compounds NOS

    7 √7ᵗʰ **T57.1X2** Toxic effect of phosphorus and its compounds, intentional self-harm   HCC

    √7ᵗʰ **T57.1X3** Toxic effect of phosphorus and its compounds, assault

    √7ᵗʰ **T57.1X4** Toxic effect of phosphorus and its compounds, undetermined

√5ᵗʰ **T57.2 Toxic effect of manganese and its compounds**

  √6ᵗʰ **T57.2X** Toxic effect of manganese and its compounds

    √7ᵗʰ **T57.2X1** Toxic effect of manganese and its compounds, accidental (unintentional)
Toxic effect of manganese and its compounds NOS

    7 √7ᵗʰ **T57.2X2** Toxic effect of manganese and its compounds, intentional self-harm   HCC

    √7ᵗʰ **T57.2X3** Toxic effect of manganese and its compounds, assault

    √7ᵗʰ **T57.2X4** Toxic effect of manganese and its compounds, undetermined

√5ᵗʰ **T57.3 Toxic effect of hydrogen cyanide**

  √6ᵗʰ **T57.3X** Toxic effect of hydrogen cyanide

    √7ᵗʰ **T57.3X1** Toxic effect of hydrogen cyanide, accidental (unintentional)
Toxic effect of hydrogen cyanide NOS

    7 √7ᵗʰ **T57.3X2** Toxic effect of hydrogen cyanide, intentional self-harm   HCC

    √7ᵗʰ **T57.3X3** Toxic effect of hydrogen cyanide, assault

    √7ᵗʰ **T57.3X4** Toxic effect of hydrogen cyanide, undetermined

√5ᵗʰ **T57.8 Toxic effect of other specified inorganic substances**

  √6ᵗʰ **T57.8X** Toxic effect of other specified inorganic substances

    √7ᵗʰ **T57.8X1** Toxic effect of other specified inorganic substances, accidental (unintentional)
Toxic effect of other specified inorganic substances NOS

    7 √7ᵗʰ **T57.8X2** Toxic effect of other specified inorganic substances, intentional self-harm   HCC

    √7ᵗʰ **T57.8X3** Toxic effect of other specified inorganic substances, assault

    √7ᵗʰ **T57.8X4** Toxic effect of other specified inorganic substances, undetermined

√5ᵗʰ **T57.9 Toxic effect of unspecified inorganic substance**

  √x7ᵗʰ **T57.91** Toxic effect of unspecified inorganic substance, accidental (unintentional)

  7 √x7ᵗʰ **T57.92** Toxic effect of unspecified inorganic substance, intentional self-harm   HCC

  √x7ᵗʰ **T57.93** Toxic effect of unspecified inorganic substance, assault

  √x7ᵗʰ **T57.94** Toxic effect of unspecified inorganic substance, undetermined

√4ᵗʰ **T58 Toxic effect of carbon monoxide**

INCLUDES   asphyxiation from carbon monoxide
toxic effect of carbon monoxide from all sources

The appropriate 7th character is to be added to each code from category T58.
A   initial encounter
D   subsequent encounter
S   sequela

√5ᵗʰ **T58.0 Toxic effect of carbon monoxide from motor vehicle exhaust**

Toxic effect of exhaust gas from gas engine
Toxic effect of exhaust gas from motor pump

  √x7ᵗʰ **T58.01** Toxic effect of carbon monoxide from motor vehicle exhaust, accidental (unintentional)

  7 √x7ᵗʰ **T58.02** Toxic effect of carbon monoxide from motor vehicle exhaust, intentional self-harm   HCC

  √x7ᵗʰ **T58.03** Toxic effect of carbon monoxide from motor vehicle exhaust, assault

  √x7ᵗʰ **T58.04** Toxic effect of carbon monoxide from motor vehicle exhaust, undetermined

√5ᵗʰ **T58.1 Toxic effect of carbon monoxide from utility gas**

Toxic effect of acetylene
Toxic effect of gas NOS used for lighting, heating, cooking
Toxic effect of water gas

  √x7ᵗʰ **T58.11** Toxic effect of carbon monoxide from utility gas, accidental (unintentional)

  7 √x7ᵗʰ **T58.12** Toxic effect of carbon monoxide from utility gas, intentional self-harm   HCC

  √x7ᵗʰ **T58.13** Toxic effect of carbon monoxide from utility gas, assault

√x7ᵗʰ   **T58.14**   Toxic effect of carbon monoxide from utility gas, undetermined

√5ᵗʰ   **T58.2**   Toxic effect of carbon monoxide from incomplete combustion of other domestic fuels
     Toxic effect of carbon monoxide from incomplete combustion of coal, coke, kerosene, wood

√6ᵗʰ   **T58.2X**   Toxic effect of carbon monoxide from incomplete combustion of other domestic fuels

√7ᵗʰ   **T58.2X1**   Toxic effect of carbon monoxide from incomplete combustion of other domestic fuels, accidental (unintentional)

7 √7ᵗʰ   **T58.2X2**   Toxic effect of carbon monoxide from incomplete combustion of other domestic fuels, intentional self-harm   HCC

√7ᵗʰ   **T58.2X3**   Toxic effect of carbon monoxide from incomplete combustion of other domestic fuels, assault

√7ᵗʰ   **T58.2X4**   Toxic effect of carbon monoxide from incomplete combustion of other domestic fuels, undetermined

√5ᵗʰ   **T58.8**   Toxic effect of carbon monoxide from other source
     Toxic effect of carbon monoxide from blast furnace gas
     Toxic effect of carbon monoxide from fuels in industrial use
     Toxic effect of carbon monoxide from kiln vapor

√6ᵗʰ   **T58.8X**   Toxic effect of carbon monoxide from other source

√7ᵗʰ   **T58.8X1**   Toxic effect of carbon monoxide from other source, accidental (unintentional)

7 √7ᵗʰ   **T58.8X2**   Toxic effect of carbon monoxide from other source, intentional self-harm   HCC

√7ᵗʰ   **T58.8X3**   Toxic effect of carbon monoxide from other source, assault

√7ᵗʰ   **T58.8X4**   Toxic effect of carbon monoxide from other source, undetermined

√5ᵗʰ   **T58.9**   Toxic effect of carbon monoxide from unspecified source

√x7ᵗʰ   **T58.91**   Toxic effect of carbon monoxide from unspecified source, accidental (unintentional)

7 √x7ᵗʰ   **T58.92**   Toxic effect of carbon monoxide from unspecified source, intentional self-harm   HCC

√x7ᵗʰ   **T58.93**   Toxic effect of carbon monoxide from unspecified source, assault

√x7ᵗʰ   **T58.94**   Toxic effect of carbon monoxide from unspecified source, undetermined

√4ᵗʰ   **T59**   Toxic effect of other gases, fumes and vapors

INCLUDES   aerosol propellants
EXCLUDES 1   *chlorofluorocarbons (T53.5)*

The appropriate 7th character is to be added to each code from category T59.
A   initial encounter
D   subsequent encounter
S   sequela

√6ᵗʰ   **T59.0**   Toxic effect of nitrogen oxides

√6ᵗʰ   **T59.0X**   Toxic effect of nitrogen oxides

√7ᵗʰ   **T59.0X1**   Toxic effect of nitrogen oxides, accidental (unintentional)
     Toxic effect of nitrogen oxides NOS

7 √7ᵗʰ   **T59.0X2**   Toxic effect of nitrogen oxides, intentional self-harm   HCC

√7ᵗʰ   **T59.0X3**   Toxic effect of nitrogen oxides, assault

√7ᵗʰ   **T59.0X4**   Toxic effect of nitrogen oxides, undetermined

√5ᵗʰ   **T59.1**   Toxic effect of sulfur dioxide

√6ᵗʰ   **T59.1X**   Toxic effect of sulfur dioxide

√7ᵗʰ   **T59.1X1**   Toxic effect of sulfur dioxide, accidental (unintentional)
     Toxic effect of sulfur dioxide NOS

7 √7ᵗʰ   **T59.1X2**   Toxic effect of sulfur dioxide, intentional self-harm   HCC

√7ᵗʰ   **T59.1X3**   Toxic effect of sulfur dioxide, assault

√7ᵗʰ   **T59.1X4**   Toxic effect of sulfur dioxide, undetermined

√5ᵗʰ   **T59.2**   Toxic effect of formaldehyde

√6ᵗʰ   **T59.2X**   Toxic effect of formaldehyde

√7ᵗʰ   **T59.2X1**   Toxic effect of formaldehyde, accidental (unintentional)
     Toxic effect of formaldehyde NOS

7 √7ᵗʰ   **T59.2X2**   Toxic effect of formaldehyde, intentional self-harm   HCC

√7ᵗʰ   **T59.2X3**   Toxic effect of formaldehyde, assault

√7ᵗʰ   **T59.2X4**   Toxic effect of formaldehyde, undetermined

√5ᵗʰ   **T59.3**   Toxic effect of lacrimogenic gas
     Toxic effect of tear gas

√6ᵗʰ   **T59.3X**   Toxic effect of lacrimogenic gas

√7ᵗʰ   **T59.3X1**   Toxic effect of lacrimogenic gas, accidental (unintentional)
     Toxic effect of lacrimogenic gas NOS

7 √7ᵗʰ   **T59.3X2**   Toxic effect of lacrimogenic gas, intentional self-harm   HCC

√7ᵗʰ   **T59.3X3**   Toxic effect of lacrimogenic gas, assault

√7ᵗʰ   **T59.3X4**   Toxic effect of lacrimogenic gas, undetermined

√5ᵗʰ   **T59.4**   Toxic effect of chlorine gas

√6ᵗʰ   **T59.4X**   Toxic effect of chlorine gas

√7ᵗʰ   **T59.4X1**   Toxic effect of chlorine gas, accidental (unintentional)
     Toxic effect of chlorine gas NOS

7 √7ᵗʰ   **T59.4X2**   Toxic effect of chlorine gas, intentional self-harm   HCC

√7ᵗʰ   **T59.4X3**   Toxic effect of chlorine gas, assault

√7ᵗʰ   **T59.4X4**   Toxic effect of chlorine gas, undetermined

√5ᵗʰ   **T59.5**   Toxic effect of fluorine gas and hydrogen fluoride

√6ᵗʰ   **T59.5X**   Toxic effect of fluorine gas and hydrogen fluoride

√7ᵗʰ   **T59.5X1**   Toxic effect of fluorine gas and hydrogen fluoride, accidental (unintentional)
     Toxic effect of fluorine gas and hydrogen fluoride NOS

7 √7ᵗʰ   **T59.5X2**   Toxic effect of fluorine gas and hydrogen fluoride, intentional self-harm   HCC

√7ᵗʰ   **T59.5X3**   Toxic effect of fluorine gas and hydrogen fluoride, assault

√7ᵗʰ   **T59.5X4**   Toxic effect of fluorine gas and hydrogen fluoride, undetermined

√5ᵗʰ   **T59.6**   Toxic effect of hydrogen sulfide

√6ᵗʰ   **T59.6X**   Toxic effect of hydrogen sulfide

√7ᵗʰ   **T59.6X1**   Toxic effect of hydrogen sulfide, accidental (unintentional)
     Toxic effect of hydrogen sulfide NOS

7 √7ᵗʰ   **T59.6X2**   Toxic effect of hydrogen sulfide, intentional self-harm   HCC

√7ᵗʰ   **T59.6X3**   Toxic effect of hydrogen sulfide, assault

√7ᵗʰ   **T59.6X4**   Toxic effect of hydrogen sulfide, undetermined

√5ᵗʰ   **T59.7**   Toxic effect of carbon dioxide

√6ᵗʰ   **T59.7X**   Toxic effect of carbon dioxide

√7ᵗʰ   **T59.7X1**   Toxic effect of carbon dioxide, accidental (unintentional)
     Toxic effect of carbon dioxide NOS

7 √7ᵗʰ   **T59.7X2**   Toxic effect of carbon dioxide, intentional self-harm   HCC

√7ᵗʰ   **T59.7X3**   Toxic effect of carbon dioxide, assault

√7ᵗʰ   **T59.7X4**   Toxic effect of carbon dioxide, undetermined

N Newborn: 0   P Pediatric: 0-17   M Maternity: 9-64   A Adult: 15-124   MCC Major Complication/Comorbidity   CC Complication/Comorbidity   SW Severe Wound Dx

1176   ICD-10-CM 2020

√5ᵗʰ **T59.8 Toxic effect of other specified gases, fumes and vapors**

    √6ᵗʰ **T59.81 Toxic effect of** smoke
       Smoke inhalation
       EXCLUDES 2   *toxic effect of cigarette (tobacco) smoke (T65.22-)*

       √7ᵗʰ **T59.811 Toxic effect of smoke,** accidental (unintentional)
          Toxic effect of smoke NOS
          AHA: 2013,4Q,121

       7 √7ᵗʰ **T59.812 Toxic effect of smoke,** intentional self-harm   HCC

       √7ᵗʰ **T59.813 Toxic effect of smoke,** assault

       √7ᵗʰ **T59.814 Toxic effect of smoke,** undetermined

    √6ᵗʰ **T59.89 Toxic effect of other specified gases, fumes and vapors**

       √7ᵗʰ **T59.891 Toxic effect of other specified gases, fumes and vapors,** accidental (unintentional)

       7 √7ᵗʰ **T59.892 Toxic effect of other specified gases, fumes and vapors,** intentional self-harm   HCC

       √7ᵗʰ **T59.893 Toxic effect of other specified gases, fumes and vapors,** assault

       √7ᵗʰ **T59.894 Toxic effect of other specified gases, fumes and vapors,** undetermined

√5ᵗʰ **T59.9 Toxic effect of unspecified gases, fumes and vapors**

    √x7ᵗʰ **T59.91 Toxic effect of unspecified gases, fumes and vapors,** accidental (unintentional)

    7 √x7ᵗʰ **T59.92 Toxic effect of unspecified gases, fumes and vapors,** intentional self-harm   HCC

    √x7ᵗʰ **T59.93 Toxic effect of unspecified gases, fumes and vapors,** assault

    √x7ᵗʰ **T59.94 Toxic effect of unspecified gases, fumes and vapors,** undetermined

√4ᵗʰ **T60 Toxic effect of pesticides**

    INCLUDES   toxic effect of wood preservatives

    The appropriate 7th character is to be added to each code from category T60.
    A   initial encounter
    D   subsequent encounter
    S   sequela

√5ᵗʰ **T60.0 Toxic effect of organophosphate and carbamate insecticides**

    √6ᵗʰ **T60.0X Toxic effect of** organophosphate and carbamate insecticides

       √7ᵗʰ **T60.0X1 Toxic effect of organophosphate and carbamate insecticides,** accidental (unintentional)
          Toxic effect of organophosphate and carbamate insecticides NOS

       7 √7ᵗʰ **T60.0X2 Toxic effect of organophosphate and carbamate insecticides,** intentional self-harm   HCC

       √7ᵗʰ **T60.0X3 Toxic effect of organophosphate and carbamate insecticides,** assault

       √7ᵗʰ **T60.0X4 Toxic effect of organophosphate and carbamate insecticides,** undetermined

√5ᵗʰ **T60.1 Toxic effect of halogenated insecticides**

    EXCLUDES 1   *chlorinated hydrocarbon (T53.-)*

    √6ᵗʰ **T60.1X Toxic effect of** halogenated insecticides

       √7ᵗʰ **T60.1X1 Toxic effect of halogenated insecticides,** accidental (unintentional)
          Toxic effect of halogenated insecticides NOS

       7 √7ᵗʰ **T60.1X2 Toxic effect of halogenated insecticides,** intentional self-harm   HCC

       √7ᵗʰ **T60.1X3 Toxic effect of halogenated insecticides,** assault

       √7ᵗʰ **T60.1X4 Toxic effect of halogenated insecticides,** undetermined

√5ᵗʰ **T60.2 Toxic effect of other insecticides**

    √6ᵗʰ **T60.2X Toxic effect of** other insecticides

       √7ᵗʰ **T60.2X1 Toxic effect of other insecticides,** accidental (unintentional)
          Toxic effect of other insecticides NOS

       7 √7ᵗʰ **T60.2X2 Toxic effect of other insecticides,** intentional self-harm   HCC

       √7ᵗʰ **T60.2X3 Toxic effect of other insecticides,** assault

       √7ᵗʰ **T60.2X4 Toxic effect of other insecticides,** undetermined

√5ᵗʰ **T60.3 Toxic effect of herbicides and fungicides**

    √6ᵗʰ **T60.3X Toxic effect of** herbicides and fungicides

       √7ᵗʰ **T60.3X1 Toxic effect of herbicides and fungicides,** accidental (unintentional)
          Toxic effect of herbicides and fungicides NOS

       7 √7ᵗʰ **T60.3X2 Toxic effect of herbicides and fungicides,** intentional self-harm   HCC

       √7ᵗʰ **T60.3X3 Toxic effect of herbicides and fungicides,** assault

       √7ᵗʰ **T60.3X4 Toxic effect of herbicides and fungicides,** undetermined

√5ᵗʰ **T60.4 Toxic effect of rodenticides**

    EXCLUDES 1   *strychnine and its salts (T65.1)*
          thallium (T56.81-)

    √6ᵗʰ **T60.4X Toxic effect of** rodenticides

       √7ᵗʰ **T60.4X1 Toxic effect of rodenticides,** accidental (unintentional)
          Toxic effect of rodenticides NOS

       7 √7ᵗʰ **T60.4X2 Toxic effect of rodenticides,** intentional self-harm   HCC

       √7ᵗʰ **T60.4X3 Toxic effect of rodenticides,** assault

       √7ᵗʰ **T60.4X4 Toxic effect of rodenticides,** undetermined

√5ᵗʰ **T60.8 Toxic effect of other pesticides**

    √6ᵗʰ **T60.8X Toxic effect of other pesticides**

       √7ᵗʰ **T60.8X1 Toxic effect of other pesticides,** accidental (unintentional)
          Toxic effect of other pesticides NOS

       7 √7ᵗʰ **T60.8X2 Toxic effect of other pesticides,** intentional self-harm   HCC

       √7ᵗʰ **T60.8X3 Toxic effect of other pesticides,** assault

       √7ᵗʰ **T60.8X4 Toxic effect of other pesticides,** undetermined

√5ᵗʰ **T60.9 Toxic effect of unspecified pesticide**

    √x7ᵗʰ **T60.91 Toxic effect of unspecified pesticide,** accidental (unintentional)

    7 √x7ᵗʰ **T60.92 Toxic effect of unspecified pesticide,** intentional self-harm   HCC

    √x7ᵗʰ **T60.93 Toxic effect of unspecified pesticide,** assault

    √x7ᵗʰ **T60.94 Toxic effect of unspecified pesticide,** undetermined

✓4ᵗʰ **T61 Toxic effect of noxious substances eaten as seafood**

     EXCLUDES 1   *allergic reaction to food, such as:*
         anaphylactic reaction or shock due to adverse food reaction (T78.0-)
         bacterial foodborne intoxications (A05.-)
         dermatitis (L23.6, L25.4, L27.2)
         food protein-induced enterocolitis syndrome (K52.21)
         food protein-induced enteropathy (K52.22)
         gastroenteritis (noninfective) (K52.29)
     toxic effect of aflatoxin and other mycotoxins (T64)
     toxic effect of cyanides (T65.0-)
     toxic effect of harmful algae bloom (T65.82-)
     toxic effect of hydrogen cyanide (T57.3-)
     toxic effect of mercury (T56.1-)
     toxic effect of red tide (T65.82-)

> The appropriate 7th character is to be added to each code from category T61.
> A   initial encounter
> D   subsequent encounter
> S   sequela

✓5ᵗʰ **T61.0 Ciguatera fish poisoning**

   ✓x7ᵗʰ **T61.01 Ciguatera fish poisoning, accidental (unintentional)**

   7 ✓x7ᵗʰ **T61.02 Ciguatera fish poisoning, intentional self-harm** HCC

   ✓x7ᵗʰ **T61.03 Ciguatera fish poisoning, assault**

   ✓x7ᵗʰ **T61.04 Ciguatera fish poisoning, undetermined**

✓5ᵗʰ **T61.1 Scombroid fish poisoning**
     Histamine-like syndrome

   ✓x7ᵗʰ **T61.11 Scombroid fish poisoning, accidental (unintentional)**

   7 ✓x7ᵗʰ **T61.12 Scombroid fish poisoning, intentional self-harm** HCC

   ✓x7ᵗʰ **T61.13 Scombroid fish poisoning, assault**

   ✓x7ᵗʰ **T61.14 Scombroid fish poisoning, undetermined**

✓5ᵗʰ **T61.7 Other fish and shellfish poisoning**

   ✓6ᵗʰ **T61.77 Other fish poisoning**

     ✓7ᵗʰ **T61.771 Other fish poisoning, accidental (unintentional)**

     7 ✓7ᵗʰ **T61.772 Other fish poisoning, intentional self-harm** HCC

     ✓7ᵗʰ **T61.773 Other fish poisoning, assault**

     ✓7ᵗʰ **T61.774 Other fish poisoning, undetermined**

   ✓6ᵗʰ **T61.78 Other shellfish poisoning**

     ✓7ᵗʰ **T61.781 Other shellfish poisoning, accidental (unintentional)**

     7 ✓7ᵗʰ **T61.782 Other shellfish poisoning, intentional self-harm** HCC

     ✓7ᵗʰ **T61.783 Other shellfish poisoning, assault**

     ✓7ᵗʰ **T61.784 Other shellfish poisoning, undetermined**

✓5ᵗʰ **T61.8 Toxic effect of other seafood**

   ✓6ᵗʰ **T61.8X Toxic effect of other seafood**

     ✓7ᵗʰ **T61.8X1 Toxic effect of other seafood, accidental (unintentional)**

     7 ✓7ᵗʰ **T61.8X2 Toxic effect of other seafood, intentional self-harm** HCC

     ✓7ᵗʰ **T61.8X3 Toxic effect of other seafood, assault**

     ✓7ᵗʰ **T61.8X4 Toxic effect of other seafood, undetermined**

✓5ᵗʰ **T61.9 Toxic effect of unspecified seafood**

   ✓x7ᵗʰ **T61.91 Toxic effect of unspecified seafood, accidental (unintentional)**

   7 ✓x7ᵗʰ **T61.92 Toxic effect of unspecified seafood, intentional self-harm** HCC

   ✓x7ᵗʰ **T61.93 Toxic effect of unspecified seafood, assault**

   ✓x7ᵗʰ **T61.94 Toxic effect of unspecified seafood, undetermined**

✓4ᵗʰ **T62 Toxic effect of other noxious substances eaten as food**

     EXCLUDES 1   *allergic reaction to food, such as:*
         anaphylactic shock (reaction) due to adverse food reaction (T78.0-)
         bacterial food borne intoxications (A05.-)
         dermatitis (L23.6, L25.4, L27.2)
         food protein-induced enterocolitis syndrome (K52.21)
         food protein-induced enteropathy (K52.22)
         gastroenteritis (noninfective) (K52.29)
     toxic effect of aflatoxin and other mycotoxins (T64)
     toxic effect of cyanides (T65.0-)
     toxic effect of hydrogen cyanide (T57.3-)
     toxic effect of mercury (T56.1-)

> The appropriate 7th character is to be added to each code from category T62.
> A   initial encounter
> D   subsequent encounter
> S   sequela

✓5ᵗʰ **T62.0 Toxic effect of ingested mushrooms**

   ✓6ᵗʰ **T62.0X Toxic effect of ingested mushrooms**

     ✓7ᵗʰ **T62.0X1 Toxic effect of ingested mushrooms, accidental (unintentional)**
         Toxic effect of ingested mushrooms NOS

     7 ✓7ᵗʰ **T62.0X2 Toxic effect of ingested mushrooms, intentional self-harm** HCC

     ✓7ᵗʰ **T62.0X3 Toxic effect of ingested mushrooms, assault**

     ✓7ᵗʰ **T62.0X4 Toxic effect of ingested mushrooms, undetermined**

✓5ᵗʰ **T62.1 Toxic effect of ingested berries**

   ✓6ᵗʰ **T62.1X Toxic effect of ingested berries**

     ✓7ᵗʰ **T62.1X1 Toxic effect of ingested berries, accidental (unintentional)**
         Toxic effect of ingested berries NOS

     7 ✓7ᵗʰ **T62.1X2 Toxic effect of ingested berries, intentional self-harm** HCC

     ✓7ᵗʰ **T62.1X3 Toxic effect of ingested berries, assault**

     ✓7ᵗʰ **T62.1X4 Toxic effect of ingested berries, undetermined**

✓5ᵗʰ **T62.2 Toxic effect of other ingested (parts of) plant(s)**

   ✓6ᵗʰ **T62.2X Toxic effect of other ingested (parts of) plant(s)**

     ✓7ᵗʰ **T62.2X1 Toxic effect of other ingested (parts of) plant(s), accidental (unintentional)**
         Toxic effect of other ingested (parts of) plant(s) NOS

     7 ✓7ᵗʰ **T62.2X2 Toxic effect of other ingested (parts of) plant(s), intentional self-harm** HCC

     ✓7ᵗʰ **T62.2X3 Toxic effect of other ingested (parts of) plant(s), assault**

     ✓7ᵗʰ **T62.2X4 Toxic effect of other ingested (parts of) plant(s), undetermined**

✓5ᵗʰ **T62.8 Toxic effect of other specified noxious substances eaten as food**

   ✓6ᵗʰ **T62.8X Toxic effect of other specified noxious substances eaten as food**

     ✓7ᵗʰ **T62.8X1 Toxic effect of other specified noxious substances eaten as food, accidental (unintentional)**
         Toxic effect of other specified noxious substances eaten as food NOS

     7 ✓7ᵗʰ **T62.8X2 Toxic effect of other specified noxious substances eaten as food, intentional self-harm** HCC

     ✓7ᵗʰ **T62.8X3 Toxic effect of other specified noxious substances eaten as food, assault**

     ✓7ᵗʰ **T62.8X4 Toxic effect of other specified noxious substances eaten as food, undetermined**

✓5ᵗʰ **T62.9 Toxic effect of unspecified noxious substance eaten as food**

   ✓x7ᵗʰ **T62.91 Toxic effect of unspecified noxious substance eaten as food, accidental (unintentional)**
     Toxic effect of unspecified noxious substance eaten as food NOS

N Newborn: 0   P Pediatric: 0-17   M Maternity: 9-64   A Adult: 15-124   HCC Major Complication/Comorbidity   CC Complication/Comorbidity   SW Severe Wound Dx

1178   ICD-10-CM 2020

7 ✓x7ᵗʰ **T62.92** **Toxic effect of unspecified noxious substance eaten as food,** intentional self-harm   HCC

✓x7ᵗʰ **T62.93** **Toxic effect of unspecified noxious substance eaten as food,** assault

✓x7ᵗʰ **T62.94** **Toxic effect of unspecified noxious substance eaten as food,** undetermined

✓4ᵗʰ **T63** **Toxic effect of contact with venomous animals and plants**

INCLUDES   bite or touch of venomous animal
pricked or stuck by thorn or leaf

EXCLUDES 2   *ingestion of toxic animal or plant (T61.-, T62.-)*

The appropriate 7th character is to be added to each code from category T63.
A   initial encounter
D   subsequent encounter
S   sequela

✓5ᵗʰ **T63.0** **Toxic effect of** snake venom

✓6ᵗʰ **T63.00** **Toxic effect of unspecified snake venom**

✓7ᵗʰ **T63.001** **Toxic effect of unspecified snake venom,** accidental (unintentional)
Toxic effect of unspecified snake venom NOS

7 ✓7ᵗʰ **T63.002** **Toxic effect of unspecified snake venom,** intentional self-harm   HCC

✓7ᵗʰ **T63.003** **Toxic effect of unspecified snake venom,** assault

✓7ᵗʰ **T63.004** **Toxic effect of unspecified snake venom,** undetermined

✓6ᵗʰ **T63.01** **Toxic effect of** rattlesnake **venom**

✓7ᵗʰ **T63.011** **Toxic effect of rattlesnake venom,** accidental (unintentional)
Toxic effect of rattlesnake venom NOS

7 ✓7ᵗʰ **T63.012** **Toxic effect of rattlesnake venom,** intentional self-harm   HCC

✓7ᵗʰ **T63.013** **Toxic effect of rattlesnake venom,** assault

✓7ᵗʰ **T63.014** **Toxic effect of rattlesnake venom,** undetermined

✓6ᵗʰ **T63.02** **Toxic effect of** coral snake **venom**

✓7ᵗʰ **T63.021** **Toxic effect of coral snake venom,** accidental (unintentional)
Toxic effect of coral snake venom NOS

7 ✓7ᵗʰ **T63.022** **Toxic effect of coral snake venom,** intentional self-harm   HCC

✓7ᵗʰ **T63.023** **Toxic effect of coral snake venom,** assault

✓7ᵗʰ **T63.024** **Toxic effect of coral snake venom,** undetermined

✓6ᵗʰ **T63.03** **Toxic effect of** taipan **venom**

✓7ᵗʰ **T63.031** **Toxic effect of taipan venom,** accidental (unintentional)
Toxic effect of taipan venom NOS

7 ✓7ᵗʰ **T63.032** **Toxic effect of taipan venom,** intentional self-harm   HCC

✓7ᵗʰ **T63.033** **Toxic effect of taipan venom,** assault

✓7ᵗʰ **T63.034** **Toxic effect of taipan venom,** undetermined

✓6ᵗʰ **T63.04** **Toxic effect of** cobra **venom**

✓7ᵗʰ **T63.041** **Toxic effect of cobra venom,** accidental (unintentional)
Toxic effect of cobra venom NOS

7 ✓7ᵗʰ **T63.042** **Toxic effect of cobra venom,** intentional self-harm   HCC

✓7ᵗʰ **T63.043** **Toxic effect of cobra venom,** assault

✓7ᵗʰ **T63.044** **Toxic effect of cobra venom,** undetermined

✓6ᵗʰ **T63.06** **Toxic effect of venom of** other North and South American snake

T63.061 **Toxic effect of venom of other North and South American snake,** accidental (unintentional)
Toxic effect of venom of other North and South American snake NOS

✓7ᵗʰ **T63.062** **Toxic effect of venom of other North and South American snake,** intentional self-harm   HCC

✓7ᵗʰ **T63.063** **Toxic effect of venom of other North and South American snake,** assault

✓7ᵗʰ **T63.064** **Toxic effect of venom of other North and South American snake,** undetermined

✓6ᵗʰ **T63.07** **Toxic effect of venom of** other Australian snake

✓7ᵗʰ **T63.071** **Toxic effect of venom of other Australian snake,** accidental (unintentional)
Toxic effect of venom of other Australian snake NOS

7 ✓7ᵗʰ **T63.072** **Toxic effect of venom of other Australian snake,** intentional self-harm   HCC

✓7ᵗʰ **T63.073** **Toxic effect of venom of other Australian snake,** assault

✓7ᵗʰ **T63.074** **Toxic effect of venom of other Australian snake,** undetermined

✓6ᵗʰ **T63.08** **Toxic effect of venom of** other African and Asian snake

✓7ᵗʰ **T63.081** **Toxic effect of venom of other African and Asian snake,** accidental (unintentional)
Toxic effect of venom of other African and Asian snake NOS

7 ✓7ᵗʰ **T63.082** **Toxic effect of venom of other African and Asian snake,** intentional self-harm   HCC

✓7ᵗʰ **T63.083** **Toxic effect of venom of other African and Asian snake,** assault

✓7ᵗʰ **T63.084** **Toxic effect of venom of other African and Asian snake,** undetermined

✓6ᵗʰ **T63.09** **Toxic effect of venom of** other snake

✓7ᵗʰ **T63.091** **Toxic effect of venom of other snake,** accidental (unintentional)
Toxic effect of venom of other snake NOS

7 ✓7ᵗʰ **T63.092** **Toxic effect of venom of other snake,** intentional self-harm   HCC

✓7ᵗʰ **T63.093** **Toxic effect of venom of other snake,** assault

✓7ᵗʰ **T63.094** **Toxic effect of venom of other snake,** undetermined

✓5ᵗʰ **T63.1** **Toxic effect of venom of other reptiles**

✓6ᵗʰ **T63.11** **Toxic effect of venom of** gila monster

✓7ᵗʰ **T63.111** **Toxic effect of venom of gila monster,** accidental (unintentional)
Toxic effect of venom of gila monster NOS

7 ✓7ᵗʰ **T63.112** **Toxic effect of venom of gila monster,** intentional self-harm   HCC

✓7ᵗʰ **T63.113** **Toxic effect of venom of gila monster,** assault

✓7ᵗʰ **T63.114** **Toxic effect of venom of gila monster,** undetermined

✓6ᵗʰ **T63.12** **Toxic effect of venom of other venomous lizard**

✓7ᵗʰ **T63.121** **Toxic effect of venom of other venomous lizard,** accidental (unintentional)
Toxic effect of venom of other venomous lizard NOS

7 ✓7ᵗʰ **T63.122** **Toxic effect of venom of other venomous lizard,** intentional self-harm   HCC

✓7ᵗʰ **T63.123** **Toxic effect of venom of other venomous lizard,** assault

✓7ᵗʰ **T63.124** **Toxic effect of venom of other venomous lizard,** undetermined

✓6ᵗʰ **T63.19** **Toxic effect of venom of other reptiles**

✓7ᵗʰ **T63.191** **Toxic effect of venom of other reptiles,** accidental (unintentional)
Toxic effect of venom of other reptiles NOS

7 ✓7ᵗʰ **T63.192** **Toxic effect of venom of other reptiles,** intentional self-harm   HCC

✓7ᵗʰ **T63.193** **Toxic effect of venom of other reptiles,** assault

✓7ᵗʰ **T63.194** **Toxic effect of venom of other reptiles,** undetermined

✓ Additional Character Required   ✓x7ᵗʰ Placeholder   Unacceptable PDx   Questionable PDx   Manifestation   Unspecified Dx   H1–H14 HAC   HCC CMS-HCC Dx   HIV HIV Dx

ICD-10-CM 2020   1179

Chapter 19. Injury, Poisoning and Certain Other Consequences of External Causes

T63.2–T63.594

√5ᵗʰ **T63.2** Toxic effect of venom of scorpion

  √6ᵗʰ **T63.2X** Toxic effect of venom of scorpion

    √7ᵗʰ **T63.2X1** Toxic effect of venom of scorpion, accidental (unintentional)
        Toxic effect of venom of scorpion NOS

    ⁷ √7ᵗʰ **T63.2X2** Toxic effect of venom of scorpion, intentional self-harm   HCC

    √7ᵗʰ **T63.2X3** Toxic effect of venom of scorpion, assault

    √7ᵗʰ **T63.2X4** Toxic effect of venom of scorpion, undetermined

√5ᵗʰ **T63.3** Toxic effect of venom of spider

  √6ᵗʰ **T63.30** Toxic effect of unspecified spider venom

    √7ᵗʰ **T63.301** Toxic effect of unspecified spider venom, accidental (unintentional)

    ⁷ √7ᵗʰ **T63.302** Toxic effect of unspecified spider venom, intentional self-harm   HCC

    √7ᵗʰ **T63.303** Toxic effect of unspecified spider venom, assault

    √7ᵗʰ **T63.304** Toxic effect of unspecified spider venom, undetermined

  √6ᵗʰ **T63.31** Toxic effect of venom of black widow spider

    √7ᵗʰ **T63.311** Toxic effect of venom of black widow spider, accidental (unintentional)

    ⁷ √7ᵗʰ **T63.312** Toxic effect of venom of black widow spider, intentional self-harm   HCC

    √7ᵗʰ **T63.313** Toxic effect of venom of black widow spider, assault

    √7ᵗʰ **T63.314** Toxic effect of venom of black widow spider, undetermined

  √6ᵗʰ **T63.32** Toxic effect of venom of tarantula

    √7ᵗʰ **T63.321** Toxic effect of venom of tarantula, accidental (unintentional)

    ⁷ √7ᵗʰ **T63.322** Toxic effect of venom of tarantula, intentional self-harm   HCC

    √7ᵗʰ **T63.323** Toxic effect of venom of tarantula, assault

    √7ᵗʰ **T63.324** Toxic effect of venom of tarantula, undetermined

  √6ᵗʰ **T63.33** Toxic effect of venom of brown recluse spider

    √7ᵗʰ **T63.331** Toxic effect of venom of brown recluse spider, accidental (unintentional)

    ⁷ √7ᵗʰ **T63.332** Toxic effect of venom of brown recluse spider, intentional self-harm   HCC

    √7ᵗʰ **T63.333** Toxic effect of venom of brown recluse spider, assault

    √7ᵗʰ **T63.334** Toxic effect of venom of brown recluse spider, undetermined

  √6ᵗʰ **T63.39** Toxic effect of venom of other spider

    √7ᵗʰ **T63.391** Toxic effect of venom of other spider, accidental (unintentional)

    ⁷ √7ᵗʰ **T63.392** Toxic effect of venom of other spider, intentional self-harm   HCC

    √7ᵗʰ **T63.393** Toxic effect of venom of other spider, assault

    √7ᵗʰ **T63.394** Toxic effect of venom of other spider, undetermined

√5ᵗʰ **T63.4** Toxic effect of venom of other arthropods

  √6ᵗʰ **T63.41** Toxic effect of venom of centipedes and venomous millipedes

    √7ᵗʰ **T63.411** Toxic effect of venom of centipedes and venomous millipedes, accidental (unintentional)

    ⁷ √7ᵗʰ **T63.412** Toxic effect of venom of centipedes and venomous millipedes, intentional self-harm   HCC

    √7ᵗʰ **T63.413** Toxic effect of venom of centipedes and venomous millipedes, assault

    √7ᵗʰ **T63.414** Toxic effect of venom of centipedes and venomous millipedes, undetermined

  √6ᵗʰ **T63.42** Toxic effect of venom of ants

    √7ᵗʰ **T63.421** Toxic effect of venom of ants, accidental (unintentional)

    ⁷ √7ᵗʰ **T63.422** Toxic effect of venom of ants, intentional self-harm   HCC

    √7ᵗʰ **T63.423** Toxic effect of venom of ants, assault

    √7ᵗʰ **T63.424** Toxic effect of venom of ants, undetermined

  √6ᵗʰ **T63.43** Toxic effect of venom of caterpillars

    √7ᵗʰ **T63.431** Toxic effect of venom of caterpillars, accidental (unintentional)

    ⁷ √7ᵗʰ **T63.432** Toxic effect of venom of caterpillars, intentional self-harm   HCC

    √7ᵗʰ **T63.433** Toxic effect of venom of caterpillars, assault

    √7ᵗʰ **T63.434** Toxic effect of venom of caterpillars, undetermined

  √6ᵗʰ **T63.44** Toxic effect of venom of bees

    √7ᵗʰ **T63.441** Toxic effect of venom of bees, accidental (unintentional)

    ⁷ √7ᵗʰ **T63.442** Toxic effect of venom of bees, intentional self-harm   HCC

    √7ᵗʰ **T63.443** Toxic effect of venom of bees, assault

    √7ᵗʰ **T63.444** Toxic effect of venom of bees, undetermined

  √6ᵗʰ **T63.45** Toxic effect of venom of hornets

    √7ᵗʰ **T63.451** Toxic effect of venom of hornets, accidental (unintentional)

    ⁷ √7ᵗʰ **T63.452** Toxic effect of venom of hornets, intentional self-harm   HCC

    √7ᵗʰ **T63.453** Toxic effect of venom of hornets, assault

    √7ᵗʰ **T63.454** Toxic effect of venom of hornets, undetermined

  √6ᵗʰ **T63.46** Toxic effect of venom of wasps
    Toxic effect of yellow jacket

    √7ᵗʰ **T63.461** Toxic effect of venom of wasps, accidental (unintentional)

    ⁷ √7ᵗʰ **T63.462** Toxic effect of venom of wasps, intentional self-harm   HCC

    √7ᵗʰ **T63.463** Toxic effect of venom of wasps, assault

    √7ᵗʰ **T63.464** Toxic effect of venom of wasps, undetermined

  √6ᵗʰ **T63.48** Toxic effect of venom of other arthropod

    √7ᵗʰ **T63.481** Toxic effect of venom of other arthropod, accidental (unintentional)

    ⁷ √7ᵗʰ **T63.482** Toxic effect of venom of other arthropod, intentional self-harm   HCC

    √7ᵗʰ **T63.483** Toxic effect of venom of other arthropod, assault

    √7ᵗʰ **T63.484** Toxic effect of venom of other arthropod, undetermined

√5ᵗʰ **T63.5** Toxic effect of contact with venomous fish
    EXCLUDES 2   poisoning by ingestion of fish (T61.-)

  √6ᵗʰ **T63.51** Toxic effect of contact with stingray

    √7ᵗʰ **T63.511** Toxic effect of contact with stingray, accidental (unintentional)

    ⁷ √7ᵗʰ **T63.512** Toxic effect of contact with stingray, intentional self-harm   HCC

    √7ᵗʰ **T63.513** Toxic effect of contact with stingray, assault

    √7ᵗʰ **T63.514** Toxic effect of contact with stingray, undetermined

  √6ᵗʰ **T63.59** Toxic effect of contact with other venomous fish

    √7ᵗʰ **T63.591** Toxic effect of contact with other venomous fish, accidental (unintentional)

    ⁷ √7ᵗʰ **T63.592** Toxic effect of contact with other venomous fish, intentional self-harm   HCC

    √7ᵗʰ **T63.593** Toxic effect of contact with other venomous fish, assault

    √7ᵗʰ **T63.594** Toxic effect of contact with other venomous fish, undetermined

✓5ᵗʰ **T63.6** **Toxic effect of contact with other** venomous marine animals
> *EXCLUDES 1*   sea-snake venom (T63.Ø9)
> *EXCLUDES 2*   poisoning by ingestion of shellfish (T61.78-)

  ✓6ᵗʰ **T63.61** **Toxic effect of contact with** Portugese Man-o-war
     Toxic effect of contact with bluebottle

    ✓7ᵗʰ **T63.611** **Toxic effect of contact with Portugese Man-o-war,** accidental (unintentional)

    ⁷ ✓7ᵗʰ **T63.612** **Toxic effect of contact with Portugese Man-o-war,** intentional self-harm   HCC

    ✓7ᵗʰ **T63.613** **Toxic effect of contact with Portugese Man-o-war,** assault

    ✓7ᵗʰ **T63.614** **Toxic effect of contact with Portugese Man-o-war,** undetermined

  ✓6ᵗʰ **T63.62** **Toxic effect of contact with other jellyfish**

    ✓7ᵗʰ **T63.621** **Toxic effect of contact with other jellyfish,** accidental (unintentional)

    ⁷ ✓7ᵗʰ **T63.622** **Toxic effect of contact with other jellyfish,** intentional self-harm   HCC

    ✓7ᵗʰ **T63.623** **Toxic effect of contact with other jellyfish,** assault

    ✓7ᵗʰ **T63.624** **Toxic effect of contact with other jellyfish,** undetermined

  ✓6ᵗʰ **T63.63** **Toxic effect of contact with** sea anemone

    ✓7ᵗʰ **T63.631** **Toxic effect of contact with sea anemone,** accidental (unintentional)

    ⁷ ✓7ᵗʰ **T63.632** **Toxic effect of contact with sea anemone,** intentional self-harm   HCC

    ✓7ᵗʰ **T63.633** **Toxic effect of contact with sea anemone,** assault

    ✓7ᵗʰ **T63.634** **Toxic effect of contact with sea anemone,** undetermined

  ✓6ᵗʰ **T63.69** **Toxic effect of contact with other venomous marine animals**

    ✓7ᵗʰ **T63.691** **Toxic effect of contact with other venomous marine animals,** accidental (unintentional)

    ⁷ ✓7ᵗʰ **T63.692** **Toxic effect of contact with other venomous marine animals,** intentional self-harm   HCC

    ✓7ᵗʰ **T63.693** **Toxic effect of contact with other venomous marine animals,** assault

    ✓7ᵗʰ **T63.694** **Toxic effect of contact with other venomous marine animals,** undetermined

✓5ᵗʰ **T63.7** **Toxic effect of contact with** venomous plant

  ✓6ᵗʰ **T63.71** **Toxic effect of contact with venomous** marine **plant**

    ✓7ᵗʰ **T63.711** **Toxic effect of contact with venomous marine plant,** accidental (unintentional)

    ⁷ ✓7ᵗʰ **T63.712** **Toxic effect of contact with venomous marine plant,** intentional self-harm   HCC

    ✓7ᵗʰ **T63.713** **Toxic effect of contact with venomous marine plant,** assault

    ✓7ᵗʰ **T63.714** **Toxic effect of contact with venomous marine plant,** undetermined

  ✓6ᵗʰ **T63.79** **Toxic effect of contact with other venomous plant**

    ✓7ᵗʰ **T63.791** **Toxic effect of contact with other venomous plant,** accidental (unintentional)

    ⁷ ✓7ᵗʰ **T63.792** **Toxic effect of contact with other venomous plant,** intentional self-harm   HCC

    ✓7ᵗʰ **T63.793** **Toxic effect of contact with other venomous plant,** assault

    ✓7ᵗʰ **T63.794** **Toxic effect of contact with other venomous plant,** undetermined

✓5ᵗʰ **T63.8** **Toxic effect of contact with other venomous animals**

  ✓6ᵗʰ **T63.81** **Toxic effect of contact with venomous** frog
> *EXCLUDES 1*   contact with nonvenomous frog (W62.Ø)

    ✓7ᵗʰ **T63.811** **Toxic effect of contact with venomous frog,** accidental (unintentional)

    ⁷ ✓7ᵗʰ **T63.812** **Toxic effect of contact with venomous frog,** intentional self-harm   HCC

    ✓7ᵗʰ **T63.813** **Toxic effect of contact with venomous frog,** assault

    ✓7ᵗʰ **T63.814** **Toxic effect of contact with venomous frog,** undetermined

  ✓6ᵗʰ **T63.82** **Toxic effect of contact with venomous** toad
> *EXCLUDES 1*   contact with nonvenomous toad (W62.1)

    ✓7ᵗʰ **T63.821** **Toxic effect of contact with venomous toad,** accidental (unintentional)

    ⁷ ✓7ᵗʰ **T63.822** **Toxic effect of contact with venomous toad,** intentional self-harm   HCC

    ✓7ᵗʰ **T63.823** **Toxic effect of contact with venomous toad,** assault

    ✓7ᵗʰ **T63.824** **Toxic effect of contact with venomous toad,** undetermined

  ✓6ᵗʰ **T63.83** **Toxic effect of contact with other venomous amphibian**
> *EXCLUDES 1*   contact with nonvenomous amphibian (W62.9)

    ✓7ᵗʰ **T63.831** **Toxic effect of contact with other venomous amphibian,** accidental (unintentional)

    ⁷ ✓7ᵗʰ **T63.832** **Toxic effect of contact with other venomous amphibian,** intentional self-harm   HCC

    ✓7ᵗʰ **T63.833** **Toxic effect of contact with other venomous amphibian,** assault

    ✓7ᵗʰ **T63.834** **Toxic effect of contact with other venomous amphibian,** undetermined

  ✓6ᵗʰ **T63.89** **Toxic effect of contact with other venomous animals**

    ✓7ᵗʰ **T63.891** **Toxic effect of contact with other venomous animals,** accidental (unintentional)

    ⁷ ✓7ᵗʰ **T63.892** **Toxic effect of contact with other venomous animals,** intentional self-harm   HCC

    ✓7ᵗʰ **T63.893** **Toxic effect of contact with other venomous animals,** assault

    ✓7ᵗʰ **T63.894** **Toxic effect of contact with other venomous animals,** undetermined

✓5ᵗʰ **T63.9** **Toxic effect of contact with unspecified venomous animal**

  ✓x7ᵗʰ **T63.91** **Toxic effect of contact with unspecified venomous animal,** accidental (unintentional)

  ⁷ ✓x7ᵗʰ **T63.92** **Toxic effect of contact with unspecified venomous animal,** intentional self-harm   HCC

  ✓x7ᵗʰ **T63.93** **Toxic effect of contact with unspecified venomous animal,** assault

  ✓x7ᵗʰ **T63.94** **Toxic effect of contact with unspecified venomous animal,** undetermined

✓4ᵗʰ **T64** **Toxic effect of aflatoxin and other mycotoxin food contaminants**

> The appropriate 7th character is to be added to each code from category T64.
> A   initial encounter
> D   subsequent encounter
> S   sequela

✓5ᵗʰ **T64.Ø** **Toxic effect of** aflatoxin

  ✓x7ᵗʰ **T64.Ø1** **Toxic effect of aflatoxin,** accidental (unintentional)

  ⁷ ✓x7ᵗʰ **T64.Ø2** **Toxic effect of aflatoxin,** intentional self-harm   HCC

  ✓x7ᵗʰ **T64.Ø3** **Toxic effect of aflatoxin,** assault

  ✓x7ᵗʰ **T64.Ø4** **Toxic effect of aflatoxin,** undetermined

✓5ᵗʰ **T64.8** **Toxic effect of other mycotoxin food contaminants**

  ✓x7ᵗʰ **T64.81** **Toxic effect of other mycotoxin food contaminants,** accidental (unintentional)

  ⁷ ✓x7ᵗʰ **T64.82** **Toxic effect of other mycotoxin food contaminants,** intentional self-harm   HCC

  ✓x7ᵗʰ **T64.83** **Toxic effect of other mycotoxin food contaminants,** assault

  ✓x7ᵗʰ **T64.84** **Toxic effect of other mycotoxin food contaminants,** undetermined

☑ Additional Character Required   ✓x7ᵗʰ Placeholder   Unacceptable PDx   Questionable PDx   Manifestation   Unspecified Dx   H1-H4 HAC   HCC CMS-HCC Dx   HIV HIV Dx

ICD-10-CM 2020   1181

Chapter 19. Injury, Poisoning and Certain Other Consequences of External Causes

☑4ᵗʰ **T65** **Toxic effect of other and unspecified substances**

> The appropriate 7th character is to be added to each code from category T65.
> A initial encounter
> D subsequent encounter
> S sequela

☑5ᵗʰ **T65.0** **Toxic effect of cyanides**
> EXCLUDES 1   hydrogen cyanide (T57.3-)

  ☑6ᵗʰ **T65.0X** **Toxic effect of cyanides**

    ☑7ᵗʰ **T65.0X1** **Toxic effect of cyanides, accidental (unintentional)**
        Toxic effect of cyanides NOS

    7 ☑7ᵗʰ **T65.0X2** **Toxic effect of cyanides, intentional self-harm**   HCC

    ☑7ᵗʰ **T65.0X3** **Toxic effect of cyanides, assault**

    ☑7ᵗʰ **T65.0X4** **Toxic effect of cyanides, undetermined**

☑5ᵗʰ **T65.1** **Toxic effect of strychnine and its salts**

  ☑6ᵗʰ **T65.1X** **Toxic effect of strychnine and its salts**

    ☑7ᵗʰ **T65.1X1** **Toxic effect of strychnine and its salts, accidental (unintentional)**
        Toxic effect of strychnine and its salts NOS

    7 ☑7ᵗʰ **T65.1X2** **Toxic effect of strychnine and its salts, intentional self-harm**   HCC

    ☑7ᵗʰ **T65.1X3** **Toxic effect of strychnine and its salts, assault**

    ☑7ᵗʰ **T65.1X4** **Toxic effect of strychnine and its salts, undetermined**

☑5ᵗʰ **T65.2** **Toxic effect of tobacco and nicotine**
> EXCLUDES 2   nicotine dependence (F17.-)

  ☑6ᵗʰ **T65.21** **Toxic effect of chewing tobacco**

    ☑7ᵗʰ **T65.211** **Toxic effect of chewing tobacco, accidental (unintentional)**
        Toxic effect of chewing tobacco NOS

    7 ☑7ᵗʰ **T65.212** **Toxic effect of chewing tobacco, intentional self-harm**   HCC

    ☑7ᵗʰ **T65.213** **Toxic effect of chewing tobacco, assault**

    ☑7ᵗʰ **T65.214** **Toxic effect of chewing tobacco, undetermined**

  ☑6ᵗʰ **T65.22** **Toxic effect of tobacco cigarettes**
    Toxic effect of tobacco smoke
    Use additional code for exposure to second hand tobacco smoke (Z57.31, Z77.22)

    ☑7ᵗʰ **T65.221** **Toxic effect of tobacco cigarettes, accidental (unintentional)**
        Toxic effect of tobacco cigarettes NOS

    7 ☑7ᵗʰ **T65.222** **Toxic effect of tobacco cigarettes, intentional self-harm**   HCC

    ☑7ᵗʰ **T65.223** **Toxic effect of tobacco cigarettes, assault**

    ☑7ᵗʰ **T65.224** **Toxic effect of tobacco cigarettes, undetermined**

  ☑6ᵗʰ **T65.29** **Toxic effect of other tobacco and nicotine**

    ☑7ᵗʰ **T65.291** **Toxic effect of other tobacco and nicotine, accidental (unintentional)**
        Toxic effect of other tobacco and nicotine NOS

    7 ☑7ᵗʰ **T65.292** **Toxic effect of other tobacco and nicotine, intentional self-harm**   HCC

    ☑7ᵗʰ **T65.293** **Toxic effect of other tobacco and nicotine, assault**

    ☑7ᵗʰ **T65.294** **Toxic effect of other tobacco and nicotine, undetermined**

☑5ᵗʰ **T65.3** **Toxic effect of nitroderivatives and aminoderivatives of benzene and its homologues**
    Toxic effect of anilin [benzenamine]
    Toxic effect of nitrobenzene
    Toxic effect of trinitrotoluene

  ☑6ᵗʰ **T65.3X** **Toxic effect of nitroderivatives and aminoderivatives of benzene and its homologues**

    ☑7ᵗʰ **T65.3X1** **Toxic effect of nitroderivatives and aminoderivatives of benzene and its homologues, accidental (unintentional)**
        Toxic effect of nitroderivatives and aminoderivatives of benzene and its homologues NOS

    7 ☑7ᵗʰ **T65.3X2** **Toxic effect of nitroderivatives and aminoderivatives of benzene and its homologues, intentional self-harm**   HCC

    ☑7ᵗʰ **T65.3X3** **Toxic effect of nitroderivatives and aminoderivatives of benzene and its homologues, assault**

    ☑7ᵗʰ **T65.3X4** **Toxic effect of nitroderivatives and aminoderivatives of benzene and its homologues, undetermined**

☑5ᵗʰ **T65.4** **Toxic effect of carbon disulfide**

  ☑6ᵗʰ **T65.4X** **Toxic effect of carbon disulfide**

    ☑7ᵗʰ **T65.4X1** **Toxic effect of carbon disulfide, accidental (unintentional)**
        Toxic effect of carbon disulfide NOS

    7 ☑7ᵗʰ **T65.4X2** **Toxic effect of carbon disulfide, intentional self-harm**   HCC

    ☑7ᵗʰ **T65.4X3** **Toxic effect of carbon disulfide, assault**

    ☑7ᵗʰ **T65.4X4** **Toxic effect of carbon disulfide, undetermined**

☑5ᵗʰ **T65.5** **Toxic effect of nitroglycerin and other nitric acids and esters**
    Toxic effect of 1,2,3-Propanetriol trinitrate

  ☑6ᵗʰ **T65.5X** **Toxic effect of nitroglycerin and other nitric acids and esters**

    ☑7ᵗʰ **T65.5X1** **Toxic effect of nitroglycerin and other nitric acids and esters, accidental (unintentional)**
        Toxic effect of nitroglycerin and other nitric acids and esters NOS

    7 ☑7ᵗʰ **T65.5X2** **Toxic effect of nitroglycerin and other nitric acids and esters, intentional self-harm**   HCC

    ☑7ᵗʰ **T65.5X3** **Toxic effect of nitroglycerin and other nitric acids and esters, assault**

    ☑7ᵗʰ **T65.5X4** **Toxic effect of nitroglycerin and other nitric acids and esters, undetermined**

☑5ᵗʰ **T65.6** **Toxic effect of paints and dyes, not elsewhere classified**

  ☑6ᵗʰ **T65.6X** **Toxic effect of paints and dyes, not elsewhere classified**

    ☑7ᵗʰ **T65.6X1** **Toxic effect of paints and dyes, not elsewhere classified, accidental (unintentional)**
        Toxic effect of paints and dyes NOS

    7 ☑7ᵗʰ **T65.6X2** **Toxic effect of paints and dyes, not elsewhere classified, intentional self-harm**   HCC

    ☑7ᵗʰ **T65.6X3** **Toxic effect of paints and dyes, not elsewhere classified, assault**

    ☑7ᵗʰ **T65.6X4** **Toxic effect of paints and dyes, not elsewhere classified, undetermined**

☑5ᵗʰ **T65.8** **Toxic effect of other specified substances**

  ☑6ᵗʰ **T65.81** **Toxic effect of latex**

    ☑7ᵗʰ **T65.811** **Toxic effect of latex, accidental (unintentional)**
        Toxic effect of latex NOS

    7 ☑7ᵗʰ **T65.812** **Toxic effect of latex, intentional self-harm**   HCC

    ☑7ᵗʰ **T65.813** **Toxic effect of latex, assault**

    ☑7ᵗʰ **T65.814** **Toxic effect of latex, undetermined**

ℕ Newborn: 0   ℙ Pediatric: 0-17   𝕄 Maternity: 9-64   𝔸 Adult: 15-124   MCC Major Complication/Comorbidity   CC Complication/Comorbidity   SW Severe Wound Dx

1182   ICD-10-CM 2020

√6ᵗʰ **T65.82 Toxic effect of harmful algae and algae toxins**

    Toxic effect of (harmful) algae bloom NOS
    Toxic effect of blue-green algae bloom
    Toxic effect of brown tide
    Toxic effect of cyanobacteria bloom
    Toxic effect of Florida red tide
    Toxic effect of pfiesteria piscicida
    Toxic effect of red tide

    √7ᵗʰ **T65.821 Toxic effect of harmful algae and algae toxins, accidental (unintentional)**
        Toxic effect of harmful algae and algae toxins NOS

    ⁷ √7ᵗʰ **T65.822 Toxic effect of harmful algae and algae toxins, intentional self-harm**   HCC

    √7ᵗʰ **T65.823 Toxic effect of harmful algae and algae toxins, assault**

    √7ᵗʰ **T65.824 Toxic effect of harmful algae and algae toxins, undetermined**

√6ᵗʰ **T65.83 Toxic effect of fiberglass**

    √7ᵗʰ **T65.831 Toxic effect of fiberglass, accidental (unintentional)**
        Toxic effect of fiberglass NOS

    ⁷ √7ᵗʰ **T65.832 Toxic effect of fiberglass, intentional self-harm**   HCC

    √7ᵗʰ **T65.833 Toxic effect of fiberglass, assault**

    √7ᵗʰ **T65.834 Toxic effect of fiberglass, undetermined**

√6ᵗʰ **T65.89 Toxic effect of other specified substances**

    √7ᵗʰ **T65.891 Toxic effect of other specified substances, accidental (unintentional)**
        Toxic effect of other specified substances NOS
        AHA: 2018,1Q,5

    ⁷ √7ᵗʰ **T65.892 Toxic effect of other specified substances, intentional self-harm**   HCC

    √7ᵗʰ **T65.893 Toxic effect of other specified substances, assault**

    √7ᵗʰ **T65.894 Toxic effect of other specified substances, undetermined**

√5ᵗʰ **T65.9 Toxic effect of unspecified substance**

    √x7ᵗʰ **T65.91 Toxic effect of unspecified substance, accidental (unintentional)**
        Poisoning NOS

    ⁷ √x7ᵗʰ **T65.92 Toxic effect of unspecified substance, intentional self-harm**   HCC

    √x7ᵗʰ **T65.93 Toxic effect of unspecified substance, assault**

    √x7ᵗʰ **T65.94 Toxic effect of unspecified substance, undetermined**

Other and unspecified effects of external causes (T66-T78)

√x7ᵗʰ **T66 Radiation sickness, unspecified**

    EXCLUDES 1   specified adverse effects of radiation, such as:
            burns (T20-T31)
            leukemia (C91-C95)
            radiation gastroenteritis and colitis (K52.0)
            radiation pneumonitis (J70.0)
            radiation related disorders of the skin and subcutaneous tissue (L55-L59)
            radiation sunburn (L55.-)

    The appropriate 7th character is to be added to code T66.
    A   initial encounter
    D   subsequent encounter
    S   sequela

√4ᵗʰ **T67 Effects of heat and light**

    EXCLUDES 1   erythema [dermatitis] ab igne (L59.0)
            malignant hyperpyrexia due to anesthesia (T88.3)
            radiation-related disorders of the skin and subcutaneous tissue (L55-L59)
    EXCLUDES 2   burns (T20-T31)
            sunburn (L55.-)
            sweat disorder due to heat (L74-L75)

    The appropriate 7th character is to be added to each code from category T67.
    A   initial encounter
    D   subsequent encounter
    S   sequela

    √5ᵗʰ **T67.0 Heatstroke and sunstroke**

        ~~Heat apoplexy~~
        ~~Heat pyrexia~~
        ~~Siriasis~~
        ~~Thermoplegia~~
        Use additional code(s) to identify any associated complications of heatstroke, such as:
            coma and stupor (R40.-)
            ►rhabdomyolysis (M62.82)◄
            systemic inflammatory response syndrome (R65.1-)
        DEF: Headache, vertigo, cramps, and elevated body temperature due to prolonged exposure to high environmental temperatures that requires emergency intervention.

        √x7ᵗʰ **T67.01 Heatstroke and sunstroke**   CC
            Heat apoplexy
            Heat pyrexia
            Siriasis
            Thermoplegia

        √x7ᵗʰ **T67.02 Exertional heatstroke**   CC

        √x7ᵗʰ **T67.09 Other heatstroke and sunstroke**   CC

    √x7ᵗʰ **T67.1 Heat syncope**
        Heat collapse

    √x7ᵗʰ **T67.2 Heat cramp**

    √x7ᵗʰ **T67.3 Heat exhaustion, anhydrotic**
        Heat prostration due to water depletion
        EXCLUDES 1   heat exhaustion due to salt depletion (T67.4)

    √x7ᵗʰ **T67.4 Heat exhaustion due to salt depletion**
        Heat prostration due to salt (and water) depletion

    √x7ᵗʰ **T67.5 Heat exhaustion, unspecified**
        Heat prostration NOS

    √x7ᵗʰ **T67.6 Heat fatigue, transient**

    √x7ᵗʰ **T67.7 Heat edema**

    √x7ᵗʰ **T67.8 Other effects of heat and light**

    √x7ᵗʰ **T67.9 Effect of heat and light, unspecified**

√x7ᵗʰ **T68 Hypothermia**

    Accidental hypothermia
    Hypothermia NOS
    Use additional code to identify source of exposure:
        exposure to excessive cold of man-made origin (W93)
        exposure to excessive cold of natural origin (X31)
    EXCLUDES 1   hypothermia following anesthesia (T88.51)
            hypothermia not associated with low environmental temperature (R68.0)
            hypothermia of newborn (P80.-)
    EXCLUDES 2   frostbite (T33-T34)

    The appropriate 7th character is to be added to code T68.
    A   initial encounter
    D   subsequent encounter
    S   sequela

Chapter 19. Injury, Poisoning and Certain Other Consequences of External Causes

✓4th T69 Other effects of reduced temperature

Use additional code to identify source of exposure:
exposure to excessive cold of man-made origin (W93)
exposure to excessive cold of natural origin (X31)

EXCLUDES 2   frostbite (T33-T34)

The appropriate 7th character is to be added to each code from category T69.
- A   initial encounter
- D   subsequent encounter
- S   sequela

✓5th T69.0 Immersion hand and foot

✓6th T69.01 Immersion hand
- ✓7th T69.011 Immersion hand, right hand
- ✓7th T69.012 Immersion hand, left hand
- ✓7th T69.019 Immersion hand, unspecified hand

✓6th T69.02 Immersion foot
Trench foot
CC Excl: For CC codes in subcategory T69.02: PDX collection 1420
- ✓7th T69.021 Immersion foot, right foot   CC H5
- ✓7th T69.022 Immersion foot, left foot   CC H5
- ✓7th T69.029 Immersion foot, unspecified foot   CC H5

✓x7th T69.1 Chilblains
DEF: Red, swollen, itchy skin primarily affecting the fingers and toes, nose and ears, and legs. Chilblains follows damp-cold exposure, and can also be associated with pruritus and a burning feeling.

✓x7th T69.8 Other specified effects of reduced temperature

✓x7th T69.9 Effect of reduced temperature, unspecified

✓4th T70 Effects of air pressure and water pressure

The appropriate 7th character is to be added to each code from category T70.
- A   initial encounter
- D   subsequent encounter
- S   sequela

✓x7th T70.0 Otitic barotrauma
Aero-otitis media
Effects of change in ambient atmospheric pressure or water pressure on ears

✓x7th T70.1 Sinus barotrauma
Aerosinusitis
Effects of change in ambient atmospheric pressure on sinuses

✓5th T70.2 Other and unspecified effects of high altitude
EXCLUDES 2   polycythemia due to high altitude (D75.1)
- ✓x7th T70.20 Unspecified effects of high altitude
- ✓x7th T70.29 Other effects of high altitude
  Alpine sickness
  Anoxia due to high altitude
  Barotrauma NOS
  Hypobaropathy
  Mountain sickness

✓x7th T70.3 Caisson disease [decompression sickness]   CC H5
Compressed-air disease
Diver's palsy or paralysis
DEF: Rapid reduction in air pressure while breathing compressed air. Symptoms include skin lesions, joint pains, and respiratory and neurological problems.
CC Excl: PDX collection 1421

✓x7th T70.4 Effects of high-pressure fluids
Hydraulic jet injection (industrial)
Pneumatic jet injection (industrial)
Traumatic jet injection (industrial)

✓x7th T70.8 Other effects of air pressure and water pressure

✓x7th T70.9 Effect of air pressure and water pressure, unspecified

✓4th T71 Asphyxiation
Mechanical suffocation
Traumatic suffocation

EXCLUDES 1   acute respiratory distress (syndrome) (J80)
anoxia due to high altitude (T70.2)
asphyxia NOS (R09.01)
asphyxia from carbon monoxide (T58.-)
asphyxia from inhalation of food or foreign body (T17.-)
asphyxia from other gases, fumes and vapors (T59.-)
respiratory distress (syndrome) in newborn (P22.-)

The appropriate 7th character is to be added to each code from category T71.
- A   initial encounter
- D   subsequent encounter
- S   sequela

CC Excl: For CC codes in category T71: PDX collection 1422

✓5th T71.1 Asphyxiation due to mechanical threat to breathing
Suffocation due to mechanical threat to breathing

✓6th T71.11 Asphyxiation due to smothering under pillow
- ✓7th T71.111 Asphyxiation due to smothering under pillow, accidental   CC H5
  Asphyxiation due to smothering under pillow NOS
- 7 ✓7th T71.112 Asphyxiation due to smothering under pillow, intentional self-harm   CC H5 HCC
- ✓7th T71.113 Asphyxiation due to smothering under pillow, assault   CC H5
- ✓7th T71.114 Asphyxiation due to smothering under pillow, undetermined   CC H5

✓6th T71.12 Asphyxiation due to plastic bag
- ✓7th T71.121 Asphyxiation due to plastic bag, accidental   CC H5
  Asphyxiation due to plastic bag NOS
- 7 ✓7th T71.122 Asphyxiation due to plastic bag, intentional self-harm   CC H5 HCC
- ✓7th T71.123 Asphyxiation due to plastic bag, assault   CC H5
- ✓7th T71.124 Asphyxiation due to plastic bag, undetermined   CC H5

✓6th T71.13 Asphyxiation due to being trapped in bed linens
- ✓7th T71.131 Asphyxiation due to being trapped in bed linens, accidental   CC H5
  Asphyxiation due to being trapped in bed linens NOS
- 7 ✓7th T71.132 Asphyxiation due to being trapped in bed linens, intentional self-harm   CC H5 HCC
- ✓7th T71.133 Asphyxiation due to being trapped in bed linens, assault   CC H5
- ✓7th T71.134 Asphyxiation due to being trapped in bed linens, undetermined   CC H5

✓6th T71.14 Asphyxiation due to smothering under another person's body (in bed)
- ✓7th T71.141 Asphyxiation due to smothering under another person's body (in bed), accidental   CC H5
  Asphyxiation due to smothering under another person's body (in bed) NOS
- ✓7th T71.143 Asphyxiation due to smothering under another person's body (in bed), assault   CC H5
- ✓7th T71.144 Asphyxiation due to smothering under another person's body (in bed), undetermined   CC H5

√6ᵗʰ **T71.15** **Asphyxiation due to** smothering in furniture

     √7ᵗʰ **T71.151** **Asphyxiation due to smothering in furniture, accidental** `CC` `H5`

         Asphyxiation due to smothering in furniture NOS

     7 √7ᵗʰ **T71.152** **Asphyxiation due to smothering in furniture, intentional self-harm** `CC` `H5` `HCC`

     √7ᵗʰ **T71.153** **Asphyxiation due to smothering in furniture, assault** `CC` `H5`

     √7ᵗʰ **T71.154** **Asphyxiation due to smothering in furniture, undetermined** `CC` `H5`

√6ᵗʰ **T71.16** **Asphyxiation due to** hanging

     Hanging by window shade cord
     Use additional code for any associated injuries, such as:
         crushing injury of neck (S17.-)
         fracture of cervical vertebrae (S12.0-S12.2-)
         open wound of neck (S11.-)

     √7ᵗʰ **T71.161** **Asphyxiation due to hanging, accidental** `CC` `H5`

         Asphyxiation due to hanging NOS
         Hanging NOS

     7 √7ᵗʰ **T71.162** **Asphyxiation due to hanging, intentional self-harm** `CC` `H5` `HCC`

     √7ᵗʰ **T71.163** **Asphyxiation due to hanging, assault** `CC` `H5`

     √7ᵗʰ **T71.164** **Asphyxiation due to hanging, undetermined** `CC` `H5`

√6ᵗʰ **T71.19** **Asphyxiation due to mechanical threat to breathing due to other causes**

     √7ᵗʰ **T71.191** **Asphyxiation due to mechanical threat to breathing due to other causes, accidental** `CC` `H5`

         Asphyxiation due to other causes NOS

     7 √7ᵗʰ **T71.192** **Asphyxiation due to mechanical threat to breathing due to other causes, intentional self-harm** `CC` `H5` `HCC`

     √7ᵗʰ **T71.193** **Asphyxiation due to mechanical threat to breathing due to other causes, assault** `CC` `H5`

     √7ᵗʰ **T71.194** **Asphyxiation due to mechanical threat to breathing due to other causes, undetermined** `CC` `H5`

√5ᵗʰ **T71.2** **Asphyxiation due to** systemic oxygen deficiency due to low oxygen content in ambient air

     Suffocation due to systemic oxygen deficiency due to low oxygen content in ambient air

     √x7ᵗʰ **T71.20** **Asphyxiation due to systemic oxygen deficiency due to low oxygen content in ambient air due to unspecified cause** `CC` `H5`

     √x7ᵗʰ **T71.21** **Asphyxiation due to** cave-in or falling earth `CC` `H5`

         Use additional code for any associated cataclysm (X34-X38)

√6ᵗʰ **T71.22** **Asphyxiation due to** being trapped in a car trunk

     √7ᵗʰ **T71.221** **Asphyxiation due to being trapped in a car trunk, accidental** `CC`

     7 √7ᵗʰ **T71.222** **Asphyxiation due to being trapped in a car trunk, intentional self-harm** `CC` `HCC`

     √7ᵗʰ **T71.223** **Asphyxiation due to being trapped in a car trunk, assault** `CC`

     √7ᵗʰ **T71.224** **Asphyxiation due to being trapped in a car trunk, undetermined** `CC`

√6ᵗʰ **T71.23** **Asphyxiation due to being** trapped in a (discarded) refrigerator

     √7ᵗʰ **T71.231** **Asphyxiation due to being trapped in a (discarded) refrigerator, accidental** `CC`

     7 √7ᵗʰ **T71.232** **Asphyxiation due to being trapped in a (discarded) refrigerator, intentional self-harm** `CC` `HCC`

     √7ᵗʰ **T71.233** **Asphyxiation due to being trapped in a (discarded) refrigerator, assault** `CC`

     √7ᵗʰ **T71.234** **Asphyxiation due to being trapped in a (discarded) refrigerator, undetermined** `CC`

     √x7ᵗʰ **T71.29** **Asphyxiation due to being trapped in other low oxygen environment** `CC` `H5`

√x7ᵗʰ **T71.9** **Asphyxiation due to unspecified cause** `CC` `H5`

     Suffocation (by strangulation) due to unspecified cause
     Suffocation NOS
     Systemic oxygen deficiency due to low oxygen content in ambient air due to unspecified cause
     Systemic oxygen deficiency due to mechanical threat to breathing due to unspecified cause
     Traumatic asphyxia NOS

√4ᵗʰ **T73** **Effects of other deprivation**

> The appropriate 7th character is to be added to each code from category T73.
> A   initial encounter
> D   subsequent encounter
> S   sequela

√x7ᵗʰ **T73.0** **Starvation**

     Deprivation of food

√x7ᵗʰ **T73.1** **Deprivation of water**

√x7ᵗʰ **T73.2** **Exhaustion due to exposure**

√x7ᵗʰ **T73.3** **Exhaustion due to excessive exertion**

     Exhaustion due to overexertion

√x7ᵗʰ **T73.8** **Other effects of deprivation**

√x7ᵗʰ **T73.9** **Effect of deprivation, unspecified**

√4ᵗʰ **T74** **Adult and child abuse, neglect and other maltreatment,** confirmed

     Use additional code, if applicable, to identify any associated current injury
     Use additional external cause code to identify perpetrator, if known (Y07.-)

     EXCLUDES 1   abuse and maltreatment in pregnancy (O9A.3-, O9A.4-, O9A.5-)
         adult and child maltreatment, suspected (T76.-)

> The appropriate 7th character is to be added to each code from category T74.
> A   initial encounter
> D   subsequent encounter
> S   sequela

CC Excl: For CC codes in category T74, unless otherwise noted: PDX collection 2033

√5ᵗʰ **T74.0** **Neglect or abandonment, confirmed**

     √x7ᵗʰ **T74.01** Adult **neglect or abandonment, confirmed** `CC` `A`

     √x7ᵗʰ **T74.02** Child **neglect or abandonment, confirmed** `CC` `P`

√5ᵗʰ **T74.1** **Physical abuse, confirmed**

     EXCLUDES 2   sexual abuse (T74.2-)

     √x7ᵗʰ **T74.11** Adult **physical abuse, confirmed** `CC` `A`

     √x7ᵗʰ **T74.12** Child **physical abuse, confirmed** `CC` `P`

         EXCLUDES 2   shaken infant syndrome (T74.4)

√5ᵗʰ **T74.2** **Sexual abuse, confirmed**

     Rape, confirmed
     Sexual assault, confirmed

     √x7ᵗʰ **T74.21** Adult **sexual abuse, confirmed** `CC` `A`

     √x7ᵗʰ **T74.22** Child **sexual abuse, confirmed** `CC` `P`

√5ᵗʰ **T74.3** **Psychological abuse, confirmed**

     Bullying and intimidation, confirmed
     Intimidation through social media, confirmed

     √x7ᵗʰ **T74.31** Adult **psychological abuse, confirmed** `A`

     √x7ᵗʰ **T74.32** Child **psychological abuse, confirmed** `CC` `P`

√x7ᵗʰ **T74.4** **Shaken infant syndrome** `CC` `P`

☑ Additional Character Required   √x7ᵗʰ Placeholder   Unacceptable PDx   Questionable PDx   Manifestation   Unspecified Dx   `H1`-`H14` HAC   `HCC` CMS-HCC Dx   `HIV` HIV Dx

ICD-10-CM 2020   1185

√6ᵗʰ **T74.5 Forced sexual exploitation, confirmed**
  AHA: 2018,4Q,32-33,65
  √x7ᵗʰ **T74.51 Adult forced sexual exploitation, confirmed**   CC A
    CC Excl: PDX collection 1423
  √x7ᵗʰ **T74.52 Child sexual exploitation, confirmed**   CC P
    CC Excl: PDX collection 1423

√5ᵗʰ **T74.6 Forced labor exploitation, confirmed**
  AHA: 2018,4Q,32-33,65
  √x7ᵗʰ **T74.61 Adult forced labor exploitation, confirmed**   CC A
    CC Excl: PDX collection 2029
  √x7ᵗʰ **T74.62 Child forced labor exploitation, confirmed**   CC P
    CC Excl: PDX collection 2030

√5ᵗʰ **T74.9 Unspecified maltreatment, confirmed**
  √x7ᵗʰ **T74.91 Unspecified adult maltreatment, confirmed**   CC A
    CC Excl: PDX collection 1424
  √x7ᵗʰ **T74.92 Unspecified child maltreatment, confirmed**   CC P

√4ᵗʰ **T75 Other and unspecified effects of other external causes**
  EXCLUDES 1   adverse effects NEC (T78.-)
  EXCLUDES 2   burns (electric) (T20-T31)

  The appropriate 7th character is to be added to each code from category T75.
  A   initial encounter
  D   subsequent encounter
  S   sequela

  √5ᵗʰ **T75.0 Effects of lightning**
    Struck by lightning
    √x7ᵗʰ **T75.00 Unspecified effects of lightning**
      Struck by lightning NOS
    √x7ᵗʰ **T75.01 Shock due to being struck by lightning**
    √x7ᵗʰ **T75.09 Other effects of lightning**
      Use additional code for other effects of lightning

  √x7ᵗʰ **T75.1 Unspecified effects of drowning and nonfatal submersion**   CC H5
    Immersion
    EXCLUDES 1   specified effects of drowning — code to effects
    CC Excl: PDX collection 1425

  √5ᵗʰ **T75.2 Effects of vibration**
    √x7ᵗʰ **T75.20 Unspecified effects of vibration**
    √x7ᵗʰ **T75.21 Pneumatic hammer syndrome**
    √x7ᵗʰ **T75.22 Traumatic vasospastic syndrome**
    √x7ᵗʰ **T75.23 Vertigo from infrasound**
      EXCLUDES 1   vertigo NOS (R42)
    √x7ᵗʰ **T75.29 Other effects of vibration**

  √x7ᵗʰ **T75.3 Motion sickness**
    Airsickness
    Seasickness
    Travel sickness
    Use additional external cause code to identify vehicle or type of motion (Y92.81-, Y93.5-)

  √x7ᵗʰ **T75.4 Electrocution**
    Shock from electric current
    Shock from electroshock gun (taser)

  √5ᵗʰ **T75.8 Other specified effects of external causes**
    √x7ᵗʰ **T75.81 Effects of abnormal gravitation [G] forces**
    √x7ᵗʰ **T75.82 Effects of weightlessness**
    √x7ᵗʰ **T75.89 Other specified effects of external causes**

√4ᵗʰ **T76 Adult and child abuse, neglect and other maltreatment, suspected**
  Use additional code, if applicable, to identify any associated current injury
  EXCLUDES 1   adult and child maltreatment, confirmed (T74.-)
    suspected abuse and maltreatment in pregnancy (O9A.3-, O9A.4-, O9A.5-)
    suspected adult physical abuse, ruled out (Z04.71)
    suspected adult sexual abuse, ruled out (Z04.41)
    suspected child physical abuse, ruled out (Z04.72)
    suspected child sexual abuse, ruled out (Z04.42)
  AHA: 2018,4Q,72

  The appropriate 7th character is to be added to each code from category T76.
  A   initial encounter
  D   subsequent encounter
  S   sequela
  CC Excl: For CC codes in category T76, unless otherwise noted: PDX collection 2033

  √5ᵗʰ **T76.0 Neglect or abandonment, suspected**
    √x7ᵗʰ **T76.01 Adult neglect or abandonment, suspected**   CC A
    √x7ᵗʰ **T76.02 Child neglect or abandonment, suspected**   CC P

  √5ᵗʰ **T76.1 Physical abuse, suspected**
    √x7ᵗʰ **T76.11 Adult physical abuse, suspected**   CC A
    √x7ᵗʰ **T76.12 Child physical abuse, suspected**   CC P
      AHA: 2019,2Q,12

  √5ᵗʰ **T76.2 Sexual abuse, suspected**
    Rape, suspected
    EXCLUDES 1   alleged abuse, ruled out (Z04.7)
    √x7ᵗʰ **T76.21 Adult sexual abuse, suspected**   CC A
    √x7ᵗʰ **T76.22 Child sexual abuse, suspected**   CC P

  √5ᵗʰ **T76.3 Psychological abuse, suspected**
    Bullying and intimidation, suspected
    Intimidation through social media, suspected
    √x7ᵗʰ **T76.31 Adult psychological abuse, suspected**   A
    √x7ᵗʰ **T76.32 Child psychological abuse, suspected**   CC P

  √5ᵗʰ **T76.5 Forced sexual exploitation, suspected**
    AHA: 2018,4Q,32-33,65
    √x7ᵗʰ **T76.51 Adult forced sexual exploitation, suspected**   CC A
      CC Excl: PDX collection 1423
    √x7ᵗʰ **T76.52 Child sexual exploitation, suspected**   CC P
      CC Excl: PDX collection 1423

  √5ᵗʰ **T76.6 Forced labor exploitation, suspected**
    AHA: 2018,4Q,32-33,65
    √x7ᵗʰ **T76.61 Adult forced labor exploitation, suspected**   CC A
      CC Excl: PDX collection 2031
    √x7ᵗʰ **T76.62 Child forced labor exploitation, suspected**   CC P
      CC Excl: PDX collection 2032

  √5ᵗʰ **T76.9 Unspecified maltreatment, suspected**
    √x7ᵗʰ **T76.91 Unspecified adult maltreatment, suspected**   CC A
      CC Excl: PDX collection 1424
    √x7ᵗʰ **T76.92 Unspecified child maltreatment, suspected**   CC P

√4ᵗʰ **T78 Adverse effects, not elsewhere classified**
  EXCLUDES 2   complications of surgical and medical care NEC (T80-T88)

  The appropriate 7th character is to be added to each code from category T78.
  A   initial encounter
  D   subsequent encounter
  S   sequela
  CC Excl: For CC codes in category T78: PDX collection 1426

  √5ᵗʰ **T78.0 Anaphylactic reaction due to food**
    Anaphylactic reaction due to adverse food reaction
    Anaphylactic shock or reaction due to nonpoisonous foods
    Anaphylactoid reaction due to food
    √x7ᵗʰ **T78.00 Anaphylactic reaction due to unspecified food**   CC

√x7ᵗʰ **T78.01** **Anaphylactic reaction due to peanuts** `CC`

√x7ᵗʰ **T78.02** **Anaphylactic reaction due to shellfish (crustaceans)** `CC`

√x7ᵗʰ **T78.03** **Anaphylactic reaction due to other fish** `CC`

√x7ᵗʰ **T78.04** **Anaphylactic reaction due to fruits and vegetables** `CC`

√x7ᵗʰ **T78.05** **Anaphylactic reaction due to tree nuts and seeds** `CC`

EXCLUDES 2   anaphylactic reaction due to peanuts (T78.01)

√x7ᵗʰ **T78.06** **Anaphylactic reaction due to food additives** `CC`

√x7ᵗʰ **T78.07** **Anaphylactic reaction due to milk and dairy products** `CC`

√x7ᵗʰ **T78.08** **Anaphylactic reaction due to eggs** `CC`

√x7ᵗʰ **T78.09** **Anaphylactic reaction due to other food products** `CC`

√x7ᵗʰ **T78.1** **Other adverse food reactions, not elsewhere classified**

Use additional code to identify the type of reaction, if applicable

EXCLUDES 1   anaphylactic reaction or shock due to adverse food reaction (T78.0-)

anaphylactic reaction due to food (T78.0-)

bacterial food borne intoxications (A05.-)

EXCLUDES 2   allergic and dietetic gastroenteritis and colitis (K52.29)

allergic rhinitis due to food (J30.5)

dermatitis due to food in contact with skin (L23.6, L24.6, L25.4)

dermatitis due to ingested food (L27.2)

food protein-induced enterocolitis syndrome (K52.21)

food protein-induced enteropathy (K52.22)

√x7ᵗʰ **T78.2** **Anaphylactic shock, unspecified** `CC`

Allergic shock

Anaphylactic reaction

Anaphylaxis

EXCLUDES 1   anaphylactic reaction or shock due to adverse effect of correct medicinal substance properly administered (T88.6)

anaphylactic reaction or shock due to adverse food reaction (T78.0-)

anaphylactic reaction or shock due to serum (T80.5-)

√x7ᵗʰ **T78.3** **Angioneurotic edema**

Allergic angioedema

Giant urticaria

Quincke's edema

EXCLUDES 1   serum urticaria (T80.6-)

urticaria (L50.-)

√5ᵗʰ **T78.4** **Other and unspecified allergy**

EXCLUDES 1   specified types of allergic reaction such as:

allergic diarrhea (K52.29)

allergic gastroenteritis and colitis (K52.29)

dermatitis (L23-L25, L27.-)

food protein-induced enterocolitis syndrome (K52.21)

food protein-induced enteropathy (K52.22)

hay fever (J30.1)

√x7ᵗʰ **T78.40** **Allergy, unspecified**

Allergic reaction NOS

Hypersensitivity NOS

√x7ᵗʰ **T78.41** **Arthus phenomenon**

Arthus reaction

√x7ᵗʰ **T78.49** **Other allergy**

√x7ᵗʰ **T78.8** **Other adverse effects, not elsewhere classified**

Certain early complications of trauma (T79)

√4ᵗʰ **T79** **Certain early complications of trauma, not elsewhere classified**

EXCLUDES 2   acute respiratory distress syndrome (J80)

complications occurring during or following medical procedures (T80-T88)

complications of surgical and medical care NEC (T80-T88)

newborn respiratory distress syndrome (P22.0)

The appropriate 7th character is to be added to each code from category T79.

A   initial encounter

D   subsequent encounter

S   sequela

6 √x7ᵗʰ **T79.0** **Air embolism (traumatic)** `MCC` `HCC`

EXCLUDES 1   air embolism complicating abortion or ectopic or molar pregnancy (O00-O07, O08.2)

air embolism complicating pregnancy, childbirth and the puerperium (O88.0)

air embolism following infusion, transfusion, and therapeutic injection (T80.0)

air embolism following procedure NEC (T81.7-)

DEF: Arterial or venous obstruction due to the introduction of air bubbles into the blood vessels following surgery or trauma.

CC Excl: PDX collection 1427

6 √x7ᵗʰ **T79.1** **Fat embolism (traumatic)** `MCC` `HCC`

EXCLUDES 1   fat embolism complicating:

abortion or ectopic or molar pregnancy (O00-O07, O08.2)

pregnancy, childbirth and the puerperium (O88.8)

DEF: Arterial blockage due to the entrance of fat into the circulatory system after a fracture of the large bones or administration of corticosteroids.

CC Excl: PDX collection 1428

6 √x7ᵗʰ **T79.2** **Traumatic secondary and recurrent hemorrhage and seroma** `CC` `HCC`

CC Excl: PDX collection 1429

6 √x7ᵗʰ **T79.4** **Traumatic shock** `MCC` `HCC`

Shock (immediate) (delayed) following injury

EXCLUDES 1   anaphylactic shock due to adverse food reaction (T78.0-)

anaphylactic shock due to correct medicinal substance properly administered (T88.6)

anaphylactic shock due to serum (T80.5-)

anaphylactic shock NOS (T78.2)

anesthetic shock (T88.2)

electric shock (T75.4)

nontraumatic shock NEC (R57.-)

obstetric shock (O75.1)

postprocedural shock (T81.1-)

septic shock (R65.21)

shock complicating abortion or ectopic or molar pregnancy (O00-O07, O08.3)

shock due to lightning (T75.01)

shock NOS (R57.9)

CC Excl: PDX collection 1430

6 √x7ᵗʰ **T79.5** **Traumatic anuria** `MCC` `HCC`

Crush syndrome

Renal failure following crushing

CC Excl: PDX collection 1431

6 √x7ᵗʰ **T79.6** **Traumatic ischemia of muscle** `HCC`

Traumatic rhabdomyolysis

Volkmann's ischemic contracture

EXCLUDES 2   anterior tibial syndrome (M76.8)

compartment syndrome (traumatic) (T79.A-)

nontraumatic ischemia of muscle (M62.2-)

AHA: 2019,2Q,12

6 √x7ᵗʰ **T79.7** **Traumatic subcutaneous emphysema** `CC` `HCC`

EXCLUDES 1   emphysema NOS (J43)

emphysema (subcutaneous) resulting from a procedure (T81.82)

CC Excl: PDX collection 1432

☑ Additional Character Required   √x7ᵗʰ Placeholder   <u>Unacceptable PDx</u>   Questionable PDx   Manifestation   <u>Unspecified Dx</u>   `H1`-`H14` HAC   `HCC` CMS-HCC Dx   `HIV` HIV Dx

ICD-10-CM 2020   **1187**

Chapter 19. Injury, Poisoning and Certain Other Consequences of External Causes

√6ᵗʰ **T79.A Traumatic compartment syndrome**

     EXCLUDES 1   fibromyalgia (M79.7)
                   nontraumatic compartment syndrome (M79.A-)
                   ~~traumatic ischemic infarction of muscle (T79.6)~~

     EXCLUDES 2   ▶traumatic ischemic infarction of muscle (T79.6)◀

     DEF: Compression of nerves and blood vessels within an enclosed muscle space due to previous trauma, which leads to impaired blood flow and muscle and nerve damage.

6 √x7ᵗʰ **T79.A0 Compartment syndrome, unspecified**   CC HCC

     Compartment syndrome NOS
     CC Excl: PDX collection 896

√6ᵗʰ **T79.A1 Traumatic compartment syndrome of upper extremity**

     Traumatic compartment syndrome of shoulder, arm, forearm, wrist, hand, and fingers
     CC Excl: For CC codes in subcategory T79.A1: PDX collection 1433

6 √7ᵗʰ **T79.A11 Traumatic compartment syndrome of right upper extremity**   CC HCC

6 √7ᵗʰ **T79.A12 Traumatic compartment syndrome of left upper extremity**   CC HCC

6 √7ᵗʰ **T79.A19 Traumatic compartment syndrome of unspecified upper extremity**   CC HCC

√6ᵗʰ **T79.A2 Traumatic compartment syndrome of lower extremity**

     Traumatic compartment syndrome of hip, buttock, thigh, leg, foot, and toes
     CC Excl: For CC codes in subcategory T79.A2: PDX collection 1433

6 √7ᵗʰ **T79.A21 Traumatic compartment syndrome of right lower extremity**   CC HCC

6 √7ᵗʰ **T79.A22 Traumatic compartment syndrome of left lower extremity**   CC HCC

6 √7ᵗʰ **T79.A29 Traumatic compartment syndrome of unspecified lower extremity**   CC HCC

6 √x7ᵗʰ **T79.A3 Traumatic compartment syndrome of abdomen**   CC HCC

     CC Excl: PDX collection 1434

6 √x7ᵗʰ **T79.A9 Traumatic compartment syndrome of other sites**   CC HCC

     CC Excl: PDX collection 896

6 √x7ᵗʰ **T79.8 Other early complications of trauma**   HCC

6 √x7ᵗʰ **T79.9 Unspecified early complication of trauma**   HCC

Complications of surgical and medical care, not elsewhere classified (T80-T88)

Use additional code for adverse effect, if applicable, to identify drug (T36-T50 with fifth or sixth character 5)

Use additional code(s) to identify the specified condition resulting from the complication

Use additional code to identify devices involved and details of circumstances (Y62-Y82)

     EXCLUDES 2   any encounters with medical care for postprocedural conditions in which no complications are present, such as:
                   artificial opening status (Z93.-)
                   closure of external stoma (Z43.-)
                   fitting and adjustment of external prosthetic device (Z44.-)
           burns and corrosions from local applications and irradiation (T20-T32)
           complications of surgical procedures during pregnancy, childbirth and the puerperium (O00-O9A)
           mechanical complication of respirator [ventilator] (J95.850)
           poisoning and toxic effects of drugs and chemicals (T36-T65 with fifth or sixth character 1-4 or 6)
           postprocedural fever (R50.82)
           specified complications classified elsewhere, such as:
                   cerebrospinal fluid leak from spinal puncture (G97.0)
                   colostomy malfunction (K94.0-)
                   disorders of fluid and electrolyte imbalance (E86-E87)
                   functional disturbances following cardiac surgery (I97.0-I97.1)
                   intraoperative and postprocedural complications of specified body systems (D78.-, E36.-, E89.-, G97.3-, G97.4, H59.3-, H59.-, H95.2-, H95.3, I97.4-, I97.5, J95.6-, J95.7, K91.6-, L76.-, M96.-, N99.-)
                   ostomy complications (J95.0-, K94.-, N99.5-)
                   postgastric surgery syndromes (K91.1)
                   postlaminectomy syndrome NEC (M96.1)
                   postmastectomy lymphedema syndrome (I97.2)
                   postsurgical blind-loop syndrome (K91.2)
                   ventilator associated pneumonia (J95.851)

     AHA: 2015,1Q,15

√4ᵗʰ **T80 Complications following infusion, transfusion and therapeutic injection**

     INCLUDES   complications following perfusion

     EXCLUDES 2   bone marrow transplant rejection (T86.01)
                   febrile nonhemolytic transfusion reaction (R50.84)
                   fluid overload due to transfusion (E87.71)
                   posttransfusion purpura (D69.51)
                   transfusion associated circulatory overload (TACO) (E87.71)
                   transfusion (red blood cell) associated hemochromatosis (E83.111)
                   transfusion related acute lung injury (TRALI) (J95.84)

> The appropriate 7th character is to be added to each code from category T80.
> A   initial encounter
> D   subsequent encounter
> S   sequela

√x7ᵗʰ **T80.0 Air embolism following infusion, transfusion and therapeutic injection**   MCC H2

     CC Excl: PDX collection 1435

√x7ᵗʰ **T80.1 Vascular complications following infusion, transfusion and therapeutic injection**   CC

     Use additional code to identify the vascular complication

     EXCLUDES 2   extravasation of vesicant agent (T80.81-)
                   infiltration of vesicant agent (T80.81-)
                   postprocedural vascular complications (T81.7-)
                   vascular complications specified as due to prosthetic devices, implants and grafts (T82.8-, T83.8-, T84.8-, T85.8-)

     CC Excl: PDX collection 1436

N Newborn: 0   P Pediatric: 0-17   M Maternity: 9-64   A Adult: 15-124   MCC Major Complication/Comorbidity   CC Complication/Comorbidity   SW Severe Wound Dx

1188   ICD-10-CM 2020

T79.A–T80.1

√5ᵗʰ T80.2 Infections following infusion, transfusion and therapeutic injection

Use additional code to identify the specific infection, such as: sepsis (A41.9)

Use additional code (R65.2-) to identify severe sepsis, if applicable

EXCLUDES 2   *infections specified as due to prosthetic devices, implants and grafts (T82.6-T82.7, T83.5-T83.6, T84.5-T84.7, T85.7)*

postprocedural infections (T81.4-)

AHA: 2018,4Q,62

CC Excl: For CC codes in subcategory T80.2: PDX collection 948

√6ᵗʰ T80.21   Infection due to central venous catheter

Infection due to pulmonary artery catheter (Swan-Ganz catheter)

AHA: 2019,1Q,13-14

TIP: Only centrally placed catheters are captured with this subcategory. Infections resulting from catheters that are not central lines, including those used for hemodialysis, should be coded to T82.7-.

√7ᵗʰ T80.211   Bloodstream infection due to central venous catheter   CC H7

Catheter-related bloodstream infection (CRBSI) NOS

Central line-associated bloodstream infection (CLABSI)

Bloodstream infection due to Hickman catheter

Bloodstream infection due to peripherally inserted central catheter (PICC)

Bloodstream infection due to portacath (port-a-cath)

Bloodstream infection due to pulmonary artery catheter

Bloodstream infection due to triple lumen catheter

Bloodstream infection due to umbilical venous catheter

AHA: 2019,1Q,13,14; 2018,4Q,89

√7ᵗʰ T80.212   Local infection due to central venous catheter   CC H7

Exit or insertion site infection

Local infection due to Hickman catheter

Local infection due to peripherally inserted central catheter (PICC)

Local infection due to portacath (port-a-cath)

Local infection due to pulmonary artery catheter

Local infection due to triple lumen catheter

Local infection due to umbilical venous catheter

Port or reservoir infection

Tunnel infection

√7ᵗʰ T80.218   Other infection due to central venous catheter   CC H7

Other central line-associated infection

Other infection due to Hickman catheter

Other infection due to peripherally inserted central catheter (PICC)

Other infection due to portacath (port-a-cath)

Other infection due to pulmonary artery catheter

Other infection due to triple lumen catheter

Other infection due to umbilical venous catheter

√7ᵗʰ T80.219   Unspecified infection due to central venous catheter   CC H7

Central line-associated infection NOS

Unspecified infection due to Hickman catheter

Unspecified infection due to peripherally inserted central catheter (PICC)

Unspecified infection due to portacath (port-a-cath)

Unspecified infection due to pulmonary artery catheter

Unspecified infection due to triple lumen catheter

Unspecified infection due to umbilical venous catheter

√x7ᵗʰ T80.22   Acute infection following transfusion, infusion, or injection of blood and blood products   CC

√x7ᵗʰ T80.29   Infection following other infusion, transfusion and therapeutic injection   CC

√5ᵗʰ T80.3   ABO incompatibility reaction due to transfusion of blood or blood products

EXCLUDES 1   *minor blood group antigens reactions (Duffy) (E) (K) (Kell) (Kidd) (Lewis) (M) (N) (P) (S) (T80.A-)*

CC Excl: For CC codes in subcategory T80.3: PDX collection 1437

√x7ᵗʰ T80.30   ABO incompatibility reaction due to transfusion of blood or blood products, unspecified   CC H3

ABO incompatibility blood transfusion NOS

Reaction to ABO incompatibility from transfusion NOS

√6ᵗʰ T80.31   ABO incompatibility with hemolytic transfusion reaction

√7ᵗʰ T80.310   ABO incompatibility with acute hemolytic transfusion reaction   CC H3

ABO incompatibility with hemolytic transfusion reaction less than 24 hours after transfusion

Acute hemolytic transfusion reaction (AHTR) due to ABO incompatibility

√7ᵗʰ T80.311   ABO incompatibility with delayed hemolytic transfusion reaction   CC H3

ABO incompatibility with hemolytic transfusion reaction 24 hours or more after transfusion

Delayed hemolytic transfusion reaction (DHTR) due to ABO incompatibility

√7ᵗʰ T80.319   ABO incompatibility with hemolytic transfusion reaction, unspecified   CC H3

ABO incompatibility with hemolytic transfusion reaction at unspecified time after transfusion

Hemolytic transfusion reaction (HTR) due to ABO incompatibility NOS

√x7ᵗʰ T80.39   Other ABO incompatibility reaction due to transfusion of blood or blood products   CC H3

Delayed serologic transfusion reaction (DSTR) from ABO incompatibility

Other ABO incompatible blood transfusion

Other reaction to ABO incompatible blood transfusion

√5ᵗʰ T80.4   Rh incompatibility reaction due to transfusion of blood or blood products

Reaction due to incompatibility of Rh antigens (C) (c) (D) (E) (e)

CC Excl: For CC codes in subcategory T80.4, unless otherwise noted: PDX collection 1437

√x7ᵗʰ T80.40   Rh incompatibility reaction due to transfusion of blood or blood products, unspecified   CC

Reaction due to Rh factor in transfusion NOS

Rh incompatible blood transfusion NOS

✓ Additional Character Required   √x7ᵗʰ Placeholder   Unacceptable PDx   Questionable PDx   Manifestation   Unspecified Dx   H1 - H14 HAC   HCC CMS-HCC Dx   HIV HIV Dx

ICD-10-CM 2020   1189

√6ᵗʰ T80.41 Rh incompatibility with hemolytic transfusion reaction

√7ᵗʰ T80.410 Rh incompatibility with acute hemolytic transfusion reaction `CC`

Acute hemolytic transfusion reaction (AHTR) due to Rh incompatibility

Rh incompatibility with hemolytic transfusion reaction less than 24 hours after transfusion

√7ᵗʰ T80.411 Rh incompatibility with delayed hemolytic transfusion reaction `CC`

Delayed hemolytic transfusion reaction (DHTR) due to Rh incompatibility

Rh incompatibility with hemolytic transfusion reaction 24 hours or more after transfusion

√7ᵗʰ T80.419 Rh incompatibility with hemolytic transfusion reaction, unspecified `CC`

Rh incompatibility with hemolytic transfusion reaction at unspecified time after transfusion

Hemolytic transfusion reaction (HTR) due to Rh incompatibility NOS

√x7ᵗʰ T80.49 Other Rh incompatibility reaction due to transfusion of blood or blood products `CC`

Delayed serologic transfusion reaction (DSTR) from Rh incompatibility

Other reaction to Rh incompatible blood transfusion

CC Excl: PDX collection 1438

√5ᵗʰ T80.A Non-ABO incompatibility reaction due to transfusion of blood or blood products

Reaction due to incompatibility of minor antigens (Duffy) (Kell) (Kidd) (Lewis) (M) (N) (P) (S)

CC Excl: For CC codes in subcategory T80.A, unless otherwise noted: PDX collection 1438

√x7ᵗʰ T80.A0 Non-ABO incompatibility reaction due to transfusion of blood or blood products, unspecified `CC`

Non-ABO antigen incompatibility reaction from transfusion NOS

√6ᵗʰ T80.A1 Non-ABO incompatibility with hemolytic transfusion reaction

√7ᵗʰ T80.A10 Non-ABO incompatibility with acute hemolytic transfusion reaction `CC`

Acute hemolytic transfusion reaction (AHTR) due to non-ABO incompatibility

Non-ABO incompatibility with hemolytic transfusion reaction less than 24 hours after transfusion

√7ᵗʰ T80.A11 Non-ABO incompatibility with delayed hemolytic transfusion reaction `CC`

Delayed hemolytic transfusion reaction (DHTR) due to non-ABO incompatibility

Non-ABO incompatibility with hemolytic transfusion reaction 24 or more hours after transfusion

√7ᵗʰ T80.A19 Non-ABO incompatibility with hemolytic transfusion reaction, unspecified `CC`

Hemolytic transfusion reaction (HTR) due to non-ABO incompatibility NOS

Non-ABO incompatibility with hemolytic transfusion reaction at unspecified time after transfusion

√x7ᵗʰ T80.A9 Other non-ABO incompatibility reaction due to transfusion of blood or blood products `CC`

Delayed serologic transfusion reaction (DSTR) from non-ABO incompatibility

Other reaction to non-ABO incompatible blood transfusion

CC Excl: PDX collection 1437

√5ᵗʰ T80.5 Anaphylactic reaction due to serum

Allergic shock due to serum

Anaphylactic shock due to serum

Anaphylactoid reaction due to serum

Anaphylaxis due to serum

EXCLUDES 1   ABO incompatibility reaction due to transfusion of blood or blood products (T80.3-)

allergic reaction or shock NOS (T78.2)

anaphylactic reaction or shock NOS (T78.2)

anaphylactic reaction or shock due to adverse effect of correct medicinal substance properly administered (T88.6)

other serum reaction (T80.6-)

DEF: Life-threatening hypersensitivity to a foreign serum causing respiratory distress, vascular collapse, and shock.

CC Excl: For CC codes in subcategory T80.5: PDX collection 1439

√x7ᵗʰ T80.51 Anaphylactic reaction due to administration of blood and blood products `CC`

√x7ᵗʰ T80.52 Anaphylactic reaction due to vaccination `CC`

√x7ᵗʰ T80.59 Anaphylactic reaction due to other serum `CC`

√5ᵗʰ T80.6 Other serum reactions

Intoxication by serum

Protein sickness

Serum rash

Serum sickness

Serum urticaria

EXCLUDES 2   serum hepatitis (B16-B19)

DEF: Serum sickness: Hypersensitivity to a foreign serum that causes fever, hives, swelling, and lymphadenopathy.

CC Excl: For CC codes in subcategory T80.6: PDX collection 1439

√x7ᵗʰ T80.61 Other serum reaction due to administration of blood and blood products `CC`

√x7ᵗʰ T80.62 Other serum reaction due to vaccination `CC`

√x7ᵗʰ T80.69 Other serum reaction due to other serum `CC`

Code also, if applicable, arthropathy in hypersensitivity reactions classified elsewhere (M36.4)

CC Excl: PDX collection 1440

√5ᵗʰ T80.8 Other complications following infusion, transfusion and therapeutic injection

√6ᵗʰ T80.81 Extravasation of vesicant agent

Infiltration of vesicant agent

√7ᵗʰ T80.810 Extravasation of vesicant antineoplastic chemotherapy `CC`

Infiltration of vesicant antineoplastic chemotherapy

CC Excl: PDX collection 1436

√7ᵗʰ T80.818 Extravasation of other vesicant agent `CC`

Infiltration of other vesicant agent

CC Excl: PDX collection 1436

√x7ᵗʰ T80.89 Other complications following infusion, transfusion and therapeutic injection `CC`

Delayed serologic transfusion reaction (DSTR), unspecified incompatibility

Use additional code to identify graft-versus-host reaction, if applicable, (D89.81-)

√5ᵗʰ T80.9 Unspecified complication following infusion, transfusion and therapeutic injection

√x7ᵗʰ T80.90 Unspecified complication following infusion and therapeutic injection

N Newborn: 0   **P** Pediatric: 0-17   **M** Maternity: 9-64   **A** Adult: 15-124   **MCC** Major Complication/Comorbidity   **CC** Complication/Comorbidity   **SW** Severe Wound Dx

1190   ICD-10-CM 2020

☑6ᵗʰ **T80.91 Hemolytic transfusion reaction, unspecified incompatibility**

EXCLUDES 1 *ABO incompatibility with hemolytic transfusion reaction (T80.31-)*
non-ABO incompatibility with hemolytic transfusion reaction (T80.A1-)
Rh incompatibility with hemolytic transfusion reaction (T80.41-)

CC Excl: For CC codes in subcategory T80.91: PDX collection 1437

☑7ᵗʰ **T80.910 Acute hemolytic transfusion reaction, unspecified incompatibility** CC

☑7ᵗʰ **T80.911 Delayed hemolytic transfusion reaction, unspecified incompatibility** CC

☑7ᵗʰ **T80.919 Hemolytic transfusion reaction, unspecified incompatibility, unspecified as acute or delayed** CC
Hemolytic transfusion reaction NOS

☑x7ᵗʰ **T80.92 Unspecified transfusion reaction**
Transfusion reaction NOS

☑4ᵗʰ **T81 Complications of procedures, not elsewhere classified**

Use additional code for adverse effect, if applicable, to identify drug (T36-T50 with fifth or sixth character 5)

EXCLUDES 2 *complications following immunization (T88.0-T88.1)*
complications following infusion, transfusion and therapeutic injection (T80.-)
complications of transplanted organs and tissue (T86.-)
specified complications classified elsewhere, such as:
complication of prosthetic devices, implants and grafts (T82-T85)
dermatitis due to drugs and medicaments (L23.3, L24.4, L25.1, L27.0-L27.1)
endosseous dental implant failure (M27.6-)
floppy iris syndrome (IFIS) (intraoperative) (H21.81)
intraoperative and postprocedural complications of specific body system (D78.-, E36.-, E89.-, G97.3-, G97.4, H59.3-, H59.-, H95.2-, H95.3, I97.4-, I97.5, J95, K91.-, L76.-, M96.-, N99.-)
ostomy complications (J95.0-, K94.-, N99.5-)
plateau iris syndrome (post-iridectomy) (postprocedural) H21.82
poisoning and toxic effects of drugs and chemicals (T36-T65 with fifth or sixth character 1-4 or 6)

AHA: 2019,2Q,21

The appropriate 7th character is to be added to each code from category T81.
A initial encounter
D subsequent encounter
S sequela

☑5ᵗʰ **T81.1 Postprocedural shock**

Shock during or resulting from a procedure, not elsewhere classified

EXCLUDES 1 *anaphylactic shock due to correct substance properly administered (T88.6)*
anaphylactic shock due to serum (T80.5-)
anaphylactic shock NOS (T78.2)
anesthetic shock (T88.2)
electric shock (T75.4)
obstetric shock (O75.1)
septic shock (R65.21)
shock following abortion or ectopic or molar pregnancy (O00-O07, O08.3)
traumatic shock (T79.4)

CC Excl: For CC/MCC codes in subcategory T81.1: PDX collection 1441

☑x7ᵗʰ **T81.10 Postprocedural shock unspecified** CC
Collapse NOS during or resulting from a procedure, not elsewhere classified
Postprocedural failure of peripheral circulation
Postprocedural shock NOS

6 ☑x7ᵗʰ **T81.11 Postprocedural cardiogenic shock** MCC HCC

6 ☑x7ᵗʰ **T81.12 Postprocedural septic shock** MCC HCC
Postprocedural endotoxic shock resulting from a procedure, not elsewhere classified
Postprocedural gram-negative shock resulting from a procedure, not elsewhere classified
Code first underlying infection
Use additional code, to identify any associated acute organ dysfunction, if applicable
AHA: 2018,4Q,63

☑x7ᵗʰ **T81.19 Other postprocedural shock** MCC
Postprocedural hypovolemic shock

☑5ᵗʰ **T81.3 Disruption of wound, not elsewhere classified**

Disruption of any suture materials or other closure methods

EXCLUDES 1 *breakdown (mechanical) of permanent sutures (T85.612)*
displacement of permanent sutures (T85.622)
disruption of cesarean delivery wound (O90.0)
disruption of perineal obstetric wound (O90.1)
mechanical complication of permanent sutures NEC (T85.692)

AHA: 2014,1Q,23

CC Excl: For CC codes in subcategory T81.3: PDX collection 1442

☑x7ᵗʰ **T81.30 Disruption of wound, unspecified** CC SW
Disruption of wound NOS

☑x7ᵗʰ **T81.31 Disruption of external operation (surgical) wound, not elsewhere classified** CC SW
Dehiscence of operation wound NOS
Disruption of operation wound NOS
Disruption or dehiscence of closure of cornea
Disruption or dehiscence of closure of mucosa
Disruption or dehiscence of closure of skin and subcutaneous tissue
Full-thickness skin disruption or dehiscence
Superficial disruption or dehiscence of operation wound

EXCLUDES 1 *dehiscence of amputation stump (T87.81)*

☑x7ᵗʰ **T81.32 Disruption of internal operation (surgical) wound, not elsewhere classified** CC SW
Deep disruption or dehiscence of operation wound NOS
Disruption or dehiscence of closure of internal organ or other internal tissue
Disruption or dehiscence of closure of muscle or muscle flap
Disruption or dehiscence of closure of ribs or rib cage
Disruption or dehiscence of closure of skull or craniotomy
Disruption or dehiscence of closure of sternum or sternotomy
Disruption or dehiscence of closure of tendon or ligament
Disruption or dehiscence of closure of superficial or muscular fascia
AHA: 2017,3Q,4

☑x7ᵗʰ **T81.33 Disruption of traumatic injury wound repair** CC
Disruption or dehiscence of closure of traumatic laceration (external) (internal)

Chapter 19. Injury, Poisoning and Certain Other Consequences of External Causes

T81.4–T81.526

√5ᵗʰ **T81.4 Infection following a procedure**
> Wound abscess following a procedure
> Use additional code to identify infection
> Use additional code (R65.2-) to identify severe sepsis, if applicable
> EXCLUDES 2   bleb associated endophthalmitis (H59.4-)
> infection due to infusion, transfusion and therapeutic injection (T80.2-)
> infection due to prosthetic devices, implants and grafts (T82.6-T82.7, T83.5-T83.6, T84.5-T84.7, T85.7)
> obstetric surgical wound infection (O86.0-)
> postprocedural fever NOS (R50.82)
> postprocedural retroperitoneal abscess (K68.11)
> **AHA:** 2018,4Q,33-34,62; 2014,1Q,23
> **CC Excl: For CC codes in subcategory T81.4:** PDX collection 805

√x 7ᵗʰ **T81.40 Infection following a procedure, unspecified**   CC H11 H12 H13

√x 7ᵗʰ **T81.41 Infection following a procedure, superficial incisional surgical site**   CC H11 H12 H13
> Subcutaneous abscess following a procedure
> Stitch abscess following a procedure

√x 7ᵗʰ **T81.42 Infection following a procedure, deep incisional surgical site**   CC H11 H12 H13
> Intra-muscular abscess following a procedure

√x 7ᵗʰ **T81.43 Infection following a procedure, organ and space surgical site**   CC H11 H12 H13
> Intra-abdominal abscess following a procedure
> Subphrenic abscess following a procedure

6 √x 7ᵗʰ **T81.44 Sepsis following a procedure**   CC H11 H12 H13 HCC
> Use additional code to identify the sepsis

√x 7ᵗʰ **T81.49 Infection following a procedure, other surgical site**   CC H11 H12 H13

√5ᵗʰ **T81.5 Complications of foreign body accidentally left in body following procedure**
> **AHA:** 2014,4Q,24
> **CC Excl: For CC codes in subcategory T81.5:** PDX collection 1443

√6ᵗʰ **T81.50 Unspecified complication of foreign body accidentally left in body following procedure**

√7ᵗʰ **T81.500 Unspecified complication of foreign body accidentally left in body following surgical operation**   CC H1

√7ᵗʰ **T81.501 Unspecified complication of foreign body accidentally left in body following infusion or transfusion**   CC H1

√7ᵗʰ **T81.502 Unspecified complication of foreign body accidentally left in body following kidney dialysis**   CC H1 HCC

√7ᵗʰ **T81.503 Unspecified complication of foreign body accidentally left in body following injection or immunization**   CC H1

√7ᵗʰ **T81.504 Unspecified complication of foreign body accidentally left in body following endoscopic examination**   CC H1

√7ᵗʰ **T81.505 Unspecified complication of foreign body accidentally left in body following heart catheterization**   CC H1

√7ᵗʰ **T81.506 Unspecified complication of foreign body accidentally left in body following aspiration, puncture or other catheterization**   CC H1

√7ᵗʰ **T81.507 Unspecified complication of foreign body accidentally left in body following removal of catheter or packing**   CC H1

√7ᵗʰ **T81.508 Unspecified complication of foreign body accidentally left in body following other procedure**   CC H1

√7ᵗʰ **T81.509 Unspecified complication of foreign body accidentally left in body following unspecified procedure**   CC H1

√6ᵗʰ **T81.51 Adhesions due to foreign body accidentally left in body following procedure**

√7ᵗʰ **T81.510 Adhesions due to foreign body accidentally left in body following surgical operation**   CC H1

√7ᵗʰ **T81.511 Adhesions due to foreign body accidentally left in body following infusion or transfusion**   CC H1

√7ᵗʰ **T81.512 Adhesions due to foreign body accidentally left in body following kidney dialysis**   CC H1 HCC

√7ᵗʰ **T81.513 Adhesions due to foreign body accidentally left in body following injection or immunization**   CC H1

√7ᵗʰ **T81.514 Adhesions due to foreign body accidentally left in body following endoscopic examination**   CC H1

√7ᵗʰ **T81.515 Adhesions due to foreign body accidentally left in body following heart catheterization**   CC H1

√7ᵗʰ **T81.516 Adhesions due to foreign body accidentally left in body following aspiration, puncture or other catheterization**   CC H1

√7ᵗʰ **T81.517 Adhesions due to foreign body accidentally left in body following removal of catheter or packing**   CC H1

√7ᵗʰ **T81.518 Adhesions due to foreign body accidentally left in body following other procedure**   CC H1

√7ᵗʰ **T81.519 Adhesions due to foreign body accidentally left in body following unspecified procedure**   CC H1

√6ᵗʰ **T81.52 Obstruction due to foreign body accidentally left in body following procedure**

√7ᵗʰ **T81.520 Obstruction due to foreign body accidentally left in body following surgical operation**   CC H1

√7ᵗʰ **T81.521 Obstruction due to foreign body accidentally left in body following infusion or transfusion**   CC H1

√7ᵗʰ **T81.522 Obstruction due to foreign body accidentally left in body following kidney dialysis**   CC H1 HCC

√7ᵗʰ **T81.523 Obstruction due to foreign body accidentally left in body following injection or immunization**   CC H1

√7ᵗʰ **T81.524 Obstruction due to foreign body accidentally left in body following endoscopic examination**   CC H1

√7ᵗʰ **T81.525 Obstruction due to foreign body accidentally left in body following heart catheterization**   CC H1

√7ᵗʰ **T81.526 Obstruction due to foreign body accidentally left in body following aspiration, puncture or other catheterization**   CC H1

√7ᵗʰ **T81.527** Obstruction due to foreign body accidentally left in body following removal of catheter or packing   `CC` `H1`

√7ᵗʰ **T81.528** Obstruction due to foreign body accidentally left in body following other procedure   `CC` `H1`

√7ᵗʰ **T81.529** Obstruction due to foreign body accidentally left in body following unspecified procedure   `CC` `H1`

√6ᵗʰ **T81.53** Perforation due to foreign body accidentally left in body following procedure

√7ᵗʰ **T81.530** Perforation due to foreign body accidentally left in body following surgical operation   `CC` `H1`

√7ᵗʰ **T81.531** Perforation due to foreign body accidentally left in body following infusion or transfusion   `CC` `H1`

√7ᵗʰ **T81.532** Perforation due to foreign body accidentally left in body following kidney dialysis   `CC` `H1` `HCC`

√7ᵗʰ **T81.533** Perforation due to foreign body accidentally left in body following injection or immunization   `CC` `H1`

√7ᵗʰ **T81.534** Perforation due to foreign body accidentally left in body following endoscopic examination   `CC` `H1`

√7ᵗʰ **T81.535** Perforation due to foreign body accidentally left in body following heart catheterization   `CC` `H1`

√7ᵗʰ **T81.536** Perforation due to foreign body accidentally left in body following aspiration, puncture or other catheterization   `CC` `H1`

√7ᵗʰ **T81.537** Perforation due to foreign body accidentally left in body following removal of catheter or packing   `CC` `H1`

√7ᵗʰ **T81.538** Perforation due to foreign body accidentally left in body following other procedure   `CC` `H1`

√7ᵗʰ **T81.539** Perforation due to foreign body accidentally left in body following unspecified procedure   `CC` `H1`

√6ᵗʰ **T81.59** Other complications of foreign body accidentally left in body following procedure

> EXCLUDES 2   obstruction or perforation due to prosthetic devices and implants intentionally left in body (T82.0-T82.5, T83.0-T83.4, T83.7, T84.0-T84.4, T85.0-T85.6)

√7ᵗʰ **T81.590** Other complications of foreign body accidentally left in body following surgical operation   `CC` `H1`

√7ᵗʰ **T81.591** Other complications of foreign body accidentally left in body following infusion or transfusion   `CC` `H1`

√7ᵗʰ **T81.592** Other complications of foreign body accidentally left in body following kidney dialysis   `CC` `H1` `HCC`

√7ᵗʰ **T81.593** Other complications of foreign body accidentally left in body following injection or immunization   `CC` `H1`

√7ᵗʰ **T81.594** Other complications of foreign body accidentally left in body following endoscopic examination   `CC` `H1`

√7ᵗʰ **T81.595** Other complications of foreign body accidentally left in body following heart catheterization   `CC` `H1`

√7ᵗʰ **T81.596** Other complications of foreign body accidentally left in body following aspiration, puncture or other catheterization   `CC` `H1`

√7ᵗʰ **T81.597** Other complications of foreign body accidentally left in body following removal of catheter or packing   `CC` `H1`

√7ᵗʰ **T81.598** Other complications of foreign body accidentally left in body following other procedure   `CC` `H1`

√7ᵗʰ **T81.599** Other complications of foreign body accidentally left in body following unspecified procedure   `CC` `H1`

√5ᵗʰ **T81.6** Acute reaction to foreign substance accidentally left during a procedure

> EXCLUDES 2   complications of foreign body accidentally left in body cavity or operation wound following procedure (T81.5-)

CC Excl: For CC codes in subcategory T81.6: PDX collection 1444

√x7ᵗʰ **T81.60** Unspecified acute reaction to foreign substance accidentally left during a procedure   `CC` `H1`

√x7ᵗʰ **T81.61** Aseptic peritonitis due to foreign substance accidentally left during a procedure   `CC` `H1`
    Chemical peritonitis

√x7ᵗʰ **T81.69** Other acute reaction to foreign substance accidentally left during a procedure   `CC` `H1`

√5ᵗʰ **T81.7** Vascular complications following a procedure, not elsewhere classified
    Air embolism following procedure NEC
    Phlebitis or thrombophlebitis resulting from a procedure

> EXCLUDES 1   embolism complicating abortion or ectopic or molar pregnancy (O00-O07, O08.2)
>   embolism complicating pregnancy, childbirth and the puerperium (O88.-)
>   traumatic embolism (T79.0)

> EXCLUDES 2   embolism due to prosthetic devices, implants and grafts (T82.8-, T83.81, T84.8-, T85.81-)
>   embolism following infusion, transfusion and therapeutic injection (T80.0)

AHA: 2019,2Q,22

CC Excl: For CC codes in subcategory T81.7, unless otherwise stated: PDX collection 1446

√6ᵗʰ **T81.71** Complication of artery following a procedure, not elsewhere classified

√7ᵗʰ **T81.710** Complication of mesenteric artery following a procedure, not elsewhere classified   `CC`
    CC Excl: PDX collection 1445

√7ᵗʰ **T81.711** Complication of renal artery following a procedure, not elsewhere classified   `CC`
    CC Excl: PDX collection 1445

√7ᵗʰ **T81.718** Complication of other artery following a procedure, not elsewhere classified   `CC`
    AHA: 2019,2Q,21-22

√7ᵗʰ **T81.719** Complication of unspecified artery following a procedure, not elsewhere classified   `CC`

√x7ᵗʰ **T81.72** Complication of vein following a procedure, not elsewhere classified   `CC`

√5ᵗʰ **T81.8** Other complications of procedures, not elsewhere classified

> EXCLUDES 2   hypothermia following anesthesia (T88.51)
>   malignant hyperpyrexia due to anesthesia (T88.3)

√x7ᵗʰ **T81.81** Complication of inhalation therapy

√x7ᵗʰ **T81.82** Emphysema (subcutaneous) resulting from a procedure

√x7th **T81.83** **Persistent postprocedural fistula** CC SW

AHA: 2017,3Q,3-4
CC Excl: PDX collection 1447

√x7th **T81.89** **Other complications of procedures,** SW
not elsewhere classified

Use additional code to specify complication, such as:
postprocedural delirium (F05)
AHA: 2014,1Q,23

√x7th **T81.9** **Unspecified complication of procedure**

√4th **T82** **Complications of cardiac and vascular prosthetic devices, implants**
and grafts

EXCLUDES 2   *failure and rejection of transplanted organs and tissue (T86.-)*

The appropriate 7th character is to be added to each code from
category T82.
A   initial encounter
D   subsequent encounter
S   sequela

√5th **T82.0** **Mechanical complication of heart valve prosthesis**

Mechanical complication of artificial heart valve
EXCLUDES 1   *mechanical complication of biological heart valve*
graft (T82.22-)
CC Excl: For CC codes in subcategory T82.0: PDX collection
1448

√x7th **T82.01** **Breakdown (mechanical) of heart** CC
valve prosthesis

√x7th **T82.02** **Displacement of heart valve** CC
prosthesis
Malposition of heart valve prosthesis

√x7th **T82.03** **Leakage of heart valve prosthesis** CC

√x7th **T82.09** **Other mechanical complication of** CC
heart valve prosthesis
Obstruction (mechanical) of heart valve prosthesis
Perforation of heart valve prosthesis
Protrusion of heart valve prosthesis

√5th **T82.1** **Mechanical complication of cardiac electronic device**
CC Excl: For CC codes in subcategory T82.1, unless otherwise
noted: PDX collection 1449

√6th **T82.11** **Breakdown (mechanical) of cardiac electronic**
device

√7th **T82.110** **Breakdown (mechanical)** CC
of cardiac electrode

√7th **T82.111** **Breakdown (mechanical)** CC
of cardiac pulse generator
(battery)

√7th **T82.118** **Breakdown (mechanical)** CC
of other cardiac electronic
device
CC Excl: PDX collection 1450

√7th **T82.119** **Breakdown (mechanical)** CC
of unspecified cardiac
electronic device
CC Excl: No Excl

√6th **T82.12** **Displacement of cardiac electronic device**
Malposition of cardiac electronic device

√7th **T82.120** **Displacement of cardiac** CC
electrode

√7th **T82.121** **Displacement of cardiac** CC
pulse generator (battery)

√7th **T82.128** **Displacement of other** CC
cardiac electronic device
CC Excl: PDX collection 1450

√7th **T82.129** **Displacement of** CC
unspecified cardiac
electronic device
CC Excl: No Excl

√6th **T82.19** **Other mechanical complication of cardiac electronic**
device
Leakage of cardiac electronic device
Obstruction of cardiac electronic device
Perforation of cardiac electronic device
Protrusion of cardiac electronic device

√7th **T82.190** **Other mechanical** CC
complication of cardiac
electrode

√7th **T82.191** **Other mechanical** CC
complication of cardiac
pulse generator (battery)

√7th **T82.198** **Other mechanical** CC
complication of other
cardiac electronic device
CC Excl: PDX collection 1450

√7th **T82.199** **Other mechanical** CC
complication of
unspecified cardiac device
CC Excl: No Excl

√5th **T82.2** **Mechanical complication of coronary artery bypass graft and**
biological heart valve graft
EXCLUDES 1   *mechanical complication of artificial heart valve*
prosthesis (T82.0-)

√6th **T82.21** **Mechanical complication of coronary artery bypass**
graft
CC Excl: For CC codes in subcategory T82.21: PDX
collection 1451

√7th **T82.211** **Breakdown (mechanical)** CC
of coronary artery bypass
graft

√7th **T82.212** **Displacement of coronary** CC
artery bypass graft
Malposition of coronary artery bypass graft

√7th **T82.213** **Leakage of coronary** CC
artery bypass graft

√7th **T82.218** **Other mechanical** CC
complication of coronary
artery bypass graft
Obstruction, mechanical of coronary artery
bypass graft
Perforation of coronary artery bypass graft
Protrusion of coronary artery bypass graft

√6th **T82.22** **Mechanical complication of biological heart valve**
graft
CC Excl: For CC codes in subcategory T82.22: PDX
collection 1450

√7th **T82.221** **Breakdown (mechanical)** CC
of biological heart valve
graft

√7th **T82.222** **Displacement of biological** CC
heart valve graft
Malposition of biological heart valve graft

√7th **T82.223** **Leakage of biological** CC
heart valve graft

√7th **T82.228** **Other mechanical** CC
complication of biological
heart valve graft
Obstruction of biological heart valve graft
Perforation of biological heart valve graft
Protrusion of biological heart valve graft

√5th **T82.3** **Mechanical complication of other vascular grafts**
CC Excl: For CC codes in subcategory T82.3: PDX collection
1452

√6th **T82.31** **Breakdown (mechanical) of other vascular grafts**

6 √7th **T82.310** **Breakdown (mechanical)** CC HCC
of aortic (bifurcation) graft
(replacement)

6 √7th **T82.311** **Breakdown (mechanical)** CC HCC
of carotid arterial graft
(bypass)

6 √7th **T82.312** **Breakdown (mechanical)** CC HCC
of femoral arterial graft
(bypass)

6 √7th **T82.318** **Breakdown (mechanical)** CC HCC
of other vascular grafts

6 √7th **T82.319** **Breakdown (mechanical)** CC HCC
of unspecified vascular
grafts

√6th **T82.32** **Displacement of other vascular grafts**
Malposition of other vascular grafts

6 √7th **T82.320** **Displacement of aortic** CC HCC
(bifurcation) graft
(replacement)

6 √7th **T82.321** **Displacement of carotid** CC HCC
arterial graft (bypass)

6 √7th **T82.322** **Displacement of femoral** CC HCC
arterial graft (bypass)

6 √7th **T82.328** **Displacement of other** CC HCC
vascular grafts

6 √7th **T82.329** **Displacement of** CC HCC
unspecified vascular
grafts

N Newborn: 0   P Pediatric: 0-17   M Maternity: 9-64   A Adult: 15-124   MCC Major Complication/Comorbidity   CC Complication/Comorbidity   SW Severe Wound Dx

✓6ᵗʰ **T82.33** Leakage of other vascular grafts

  6 ✓7ᵗʰ **T82.330** Leakage of aortic (bifurcation) graft (replacement)   CC HCC

  6 ✓7ᵗʰ **T82.331** Leakage of carotid arterial graft (bypass)   CC HCC

  6 ✓7ᵗʰ **T82.332** Leakage of femoral arterial graft (bypass)   CC HCC

  6 ✓7ᵗʰ **T82.338** Leakage of other vascular grafts   CC HCC

  6 ✓7ᵗʰ **T82.339** Leakage of unspecified vascular graft   CC HCC

✓6ᵗʰ **T82.39** Other mechanical complication of other vascular grafts

  Obstruction (mechanical) of other vascular grafts

  Perforation of other vascular grafts

  Protrusion of other vascular grafts

  6 ✓7ᵗʰ **T82.390** Other mechanical complication of aortic (bifurcation) graft (replacement)   CC HCC

  6 ✓7ᵗʰ **T82.391** Other mechanical complication of carotid arterial graft (bypass)   CC HCC

  6 ✓7ᵗʰ **T82.392** Other mechanical complication of femoral arterial graft (bypass)   CC HCC

  6 ✓7ᵗʰ **T82.398** Other mechanical complication of other vascular grafts   CC HCC

  6 ✓7ᵗʰ **T82.399** Other mechanical complication of unspecified vascular grafts   CC HCC

✓5ᵗʰ **T82.4** Mechanical complication of vascular dialysis catheter

  Mechanical complication of hemodialysis catheter

    EXCLUDES 1   *mechanical complication of intraperitoneal dialysis catheter (T85.62)*

  CC Excl: For CC codes in subcategory T82.4: PDX collection 1452

  ✓x7ᵗʰ **T82.41** Breakdown (mechanical) of vascular dialysis catheter   CC HCC

  ✓x7ᵗʰ **T82.42** Displacement of vascular dialysis catheter   CC HCC

    Malposition of vascular dialysis catheter

  ✓x7ᵗʰ **T82.43** Leakage of vascular dialysis catheter   CC HCC

  ✓x7ᵗʰ **T82.49** Other complication of vascular dialysis catheter   CC HCC

    Obstruction (mechanical) of vascular dialysis catheter

    Perforation of vascular dialysis catheter

    Protrusion of vascular dialysis catheter

✓5ᵗʰ **T82.5** Mechanical complication of other cardiac and vascular devices and implants

    EXCLUDES 2   *mechanical complication of epidural and subdural infusion catheter (T85.61)*

  CC Excl: For CC codes in subcategory T82.5, unless otherwise noted: PDX collection 1452

  ✓6ᵗʰ **T82.51** Breakdown (mechanical) of other cardiac and vascular devices and implants

    6 ✓7ᵗʰ **T82.510** Breakdown (mechanical) of surgically created arteriovenous fistula   CC HCC

    6 ✓7ᵗʰ **T82.511** Breakdown (mechanical) of surgically created arteriovenous shunt   CC HCC

    ✓7ᵗʰ **T82.512** Breakdown (mechanical) of artificial heart   CC

      CC Excl: PDX collection 1450

    6 ✓7ᵗʰ **T82.513** Breakdown (mechanical) of balloon (counterpulsation) device   CC HCC

    6 ✓7ᵗʰ **T82.514** Breakdown (mechanical) of infusion catheter   CC HCC

    6 ✓7ᵗʰ **T82.515** Breakdown (mechanical) of umbrella device   CC HCC

    6 ✓7ᵗʰ **T82.518** Breakdown (mechanical) of other cardiac and vascular devices and implants   CC HCC

    ✓7ᵗʰ **T82.519** Breakdown (mechanical) of unspecified cardiac and vascular devices and implants   CC

      CC Excl: PDX collection 1453

✓6ᵗʰ **T82.52** Displacement of other cardiac and vascular devices and implants

  Malposition of other cardiac and vascular devices and implants

  6 ✓7ᵗʰ **T82.520** Displacement of surgically created arteriovenous fistula   CC HCC

  6 ✓7ᵗʰ **T82.521** Displacement of surgically created arteriovenous shunt   CC HCC

  ✓7ᵗʰ **T82.522** Displacement of artificial heart   CC

    CC Excl: PDX collection 1450

  6 ✓7ᵗʰ **T82.523** Displacement of balloon (counterpulsation) device   CC HCC

  6 ✓7ᵗʰ **T82.524** Displacement of infusion catheter   CC HCC

  6 ✓7ᵗʰ **T82.525** Displacement of umbrella device   CC HCC

  6 ✓7ᵗʰ **T82.528** Displacement of other cardiac and vascular devices and implants   CC HCC

  ✓7ᵗʰ **T82.529** Displacement of unspecified cardiac and vascular devices and implants   CC

✓6ᵗʰ **T82.53** Leakage of other cardiac and vascular devices and implants

  6 ✓7ᵗʰ **T82.530** Leakage of surgically created arteriovenous fistula   CC HCC

  6 ✓7ᵗʰ **T82.531** Leakage of surgically created arteriovenous shunt   CC HCC

  ✓7ᵗʰ **T82.532** Leakage of artificial heart   CC

    CC Excl: PDX collection 1450

  6 ✓7ᵗʰ **T82.533** Leakage of balloon (counterpulsation) device   CC HCC

  6 ✓7ᵗʰ **T82.534** Leakage of infusion catheter   CC HCC

  6 ✓7ᵗʰ **T82.535** Leakage of umbrella device   CC HCC

  6 ✓7ᵗʰ **T82.538** Leakage of other cardiac and vascular devices and implants   CC HCC

  ✓7ᵗʰ **T82.539** Leakage of unspecified cardiac and vascular devices and implants   CC

    CC Excl: PDX collection 1453

✓6ᵗʰ **T82.59** Other mechanical complication of other cardiac and vascular devices and implants

  Obstruction (mechanical) of other cardiac and vascular devices and implants

  Perforation of other cardiac and vascular devices and implants

  Protrusion of other cardiac and vascular devices and implants

  6 ✓7ᵗʰ **T82.590** Other mechanical complication of surgically created arteriovenous fistula   CC HCC

  6 ✓7ᵗʰ **T82.591** Other mechanical complication of surgically created arteriovenous shunt   CC HCC

  ✓7ᵗʰ **T82.592** Other mechanical complication of artificial heart   CC

    CC Excl: PDX collection 1450

  6 ✓7ᵗʰ **T82.593** Other mechanical complication of balloon (counterpulsation) device   CC HCC

  6 ✓7ᵗʰ **T82.594** Other mechanical complication of infusion catheter   CC HCC

    CC Excl: PDX collection 1450

  6 ✓7ᵗʰ **T82.595** Other mechanical complication of umbrella device   CC HCC

☑ Additional Character Required   ✓x7ᵗʰ Placeholder   Unacceptable PDx   Questionable PDx   Manifestation   Unspecified Dx   H1-H14 HAC   HCC CMS-HCC Dx   HIV HIV Dx

ICD-10-CM 2020

1195

Chapter 19. Injury, Poisoning and Certain Other Consequences of External Causes

T82.598–T83.030

6 √7ᵗʰ **T82.598 Other mechanical** `CC` `HCC`
complication of other
cardiac and vascular
devices and implants
CC Excl: PDX collection 1450

√7ᵗʰ **T82.599 Other mechanical** `CC`
complication of
unspecified cardiac and
vascular devices and
implants
CC Excl: PDX collection 1453

6 √x7ᵗʰ **T82.6 Infection and inflammatory reaction due to** `CC` `H13` `HCC`
cardiac valve prosthesis
Use additional code to identify infection
CC Excl: PDX collection 1454

6 √x7ᵗʰ **T82.7 Infection and inflammatory reaction due to** `CC` `H13` `HCC`
other cardiac and vascular devices, implants
and grafts
Use additional code to identify infection
AHA: 2019,1Q,13-14
TIP: Assign this code for infections and/or cellulitis resulting from
catheters that are not centrally placed (e.g., midline catheters).
CC Excl: PDX collection 1454

√5ᵗʰ **T82.8 Other specified complications of cardiac and vascular**
prosthetic devices, implants and grafts
AHA: 2016,4Q,70

√6ᵗʰ **T82.81 Embolism due to cardiac and vascular prosthetic**
devices, implants and grafts

√7ᵗʰ **T82.817 Embolism due to cardiac** `CC`
prosthetic devices,
implants and grafts
CC Excl: PDX collection 1455

6 √7ᵗʰ **T82.818 Embolism due to vascular** `CC` `HCC`
prosthetic devices,
implants and grafts
CC Excl: PDX collection 1454

√6ᵗʰ **T82.82 Fibrosis due to cardiac and vascular prosthetic**
devices, implants and grafts

√7ᵗʰ **T82.827 Fibrosis due to cardiac** `CC`
prosthetic devices,
implants and grafts
CC Excl: PDX collection 1455

6 √7ᵗʰ **T82.828 Fibrosis due vascular** `CC` `HCC`
prosthetic devices,
implants and grafts
CC Excl: PDX collection 1454

√6ᵗʰ **T82.83 Hemorrhage due to cardiac and vascular prosthetic**
devices, implants and grafts

√7ᵗʰ **T82.837 Hemorrhage due to** `CC`
cardiac prosthetic devices,
implants and grafts
CC Excl: PDX collection 1455

6 √7ᵗʰ **T82.838 Hemorrhage due to** `CC` `HCC`
vascular prosthetic
devices, implants and
grafts
CC Excl: PDX collection 1454

√6ᵗʰ **T82.84 Pain due to cardiac and vascular prosthetic devices,**
implants and grafts

√7ᵗʰ **T82.847 Pain due to cardiac** `CC`
prosthetic devices,
implants and grafts
CC Excl: PDX collection 1455

6 √7ᵗʰ **T82.848 Pain due to vascular** `CC` `HCC`
prosthetic devices,
implants and grafts
CC Excl: PDX collection 1454

√6ᵗʰ **T82.85 Stenosis due to cardiac and vascular prosthetic**
devices, implants and grafts

√7ᵗʰ **T82.855 Stenosis of coronary** `CC`
artery stent
In-stent stenosis (restenosis) of coronary
artery stent
Restenosis of coronary artery stent
CC Excl: PDX collection 1455

6 √7ᵗʰ **T82.856 Stenosis of peripheral** `CC` `HCC`
vascular stent
In-stent stenosis (restenosis) of peripheral
vascular stent
Restenosis of peripheral vascular stent
CC Excl: PDX collection 1454

√7ᵗʰ **T82.857 Stenosis of other cardiac** `CC`
prosthetic devices,
implants and grafts
CC Excl: PDX collection 1455

6 √7ᵗʰ **T82.858 Stenosis of other vascular** `CC` `HCC`
prosthetic devices,
implants and grafts
CC Excl: PDX collection 1454

√6ᵗʰ **T82.86 Thrombosis of cardiac and vascular prosthetic**
devices, implants and grafts

√7ᵗʰ **T82.867 Thrombosis due to cardiac** `CC`
prosthetic devices,
implants and grafts
CC Excl: PDX collection 1455

6 √7ᵗʰ **T82.868 Thrombosis due to** `CC` `HCC`
vascular prosthetic
devices, implants and
grafts
CC Excl: PDX collection 1454

√6ᵗʰ **T82.89 Other specified complication of cardiac and vascular**
prosthetic devices, implants and grafts

√7ᵗʰ **T82.897 Other specified** `CC`
complication of cardiac
prosthetic devices,
implants and grafts
AHA: 2019,2Q,33
CC Excl: PDX collection 1455

6 √7ᵗʰ **T82.898 Other specified** `CC` `HCC`
complication of vascular
prosthetic devices,
implants and grafts
CC Excl: PDX collection 1454

√x7ᵗʰ **T82.9 Unspecified complication of cardiac and** `CC`
vascular prosthetic device, implant and graft
CC Excl: PDX collection 1455

√4ᵗʰ **T83 Complications of genitourinary prosthetic devices, implants and**
grafts
EXCLUDES 2   *failure and rejection of transplanted organs and tissue (T86.-)*
AHA: 2016,4Q,70-71

The appropriate 7th character is to be added to each code from
category T83.
A   initial encounter
D   subsequent encounter
S   sequela

CC Excl: For CC codes in category T83, unless otherwise noted: PDX
collection 1456

√5ᵗʰ **T83.0 Mechanical complication of urinary catheter**
EXCLUDES 2   *complications of stoma of urinary tract (N99.5-)*

√6ᵗʰ **T83.01 Breakdown (mechanical) of urinary catheter**

6 √7ᵗʰ **T83.010 Breakdown (mechanical)** `CC` `HCC`
of cystostomy catheter

6 √7ᵗʰ **T83.011 Breakdown (mechanical)** `HCC`
of indwelling urethral
catheter

6 √7ᵗʰ **T83.012 Breakdown (mechanical)** `HCC`
of nephrostomy catheter

6 √7ᵗʰ **T83.018 Breakdown (mechanical)** `HCC`
of other urinary catheter
Breakdown (mechanical) of Hopkins
catheter
Breakdown (mechanical) of ileostomy
catheter
Breakdown (mechanical) urostomy
catheter

√6ᵗʰ **T83.02 Displacement of urinary catheter**
Malposition of urinary catheter

6 √7ᵗʰ **T83.020 Displacement of** `CC` `HCC`
cystostomy catheter

6 √7ᵗʰ **T83.021 Displacement of** `HCC`
indwelling urethral
catheter

6 √7ᵗʰ **T83.022 Displacement of** `HCC`
nephrostomy catheter

6 √7ᵗʰ **T83.028 Displacement of other** `HCC`
urinary catheter
Displacement of Hopkins catheter
Displacement of ileostomy catheter
Displacement of urostomy catheter

√6ᵗʰ **T83.03 Leakage of urinary catheter**

6 √7ᵗʰ **T83.030 Leakage of cystostomy** `CC` `HCC`
catheter

`N` Newborn: 0   `P` Pediatric: 0-17   `M` Maternity: 9-64   `A` Adult: 15-124   `MCC` Major Complication/Comorbidity   `CC` Complication/Comorbidity   `SW` Severe Wound Dx

1196   **ICD-10-CM 2020**

6 √7ᵗʰ **T83.031 Leakage of indwelling urethral catheter** HCC

6 √7ᵗʰ **T83.032 Leakage of nephrostomy catheter** HCC

6 √7ᵗʰ **T83.038 Leakage of other urinary catheter** HCC
Leakage of Hopkins catheter
Leakage of ileostomy catheter
Leakage of urostomy catheter

√6ᵗʰ **T83.09 Other mechanical complication of urinary catheter**
Obstruction (mechanical) of urinary catheter
Perforation of urinary catheter
Protrusion of urinary catheter

6 √7ᵗʰ **T83.090 Other mechanical complication of cystostomy catheter** CC HCC

6 √7ᵗʰ **T83.091 Other mechanical complication of indwelling urethral catheter** HCC

6 √7ᵗʰ **T83.092 Other mechanical complication of nephrostomy catheter** HCC

6 √7ᵗʰ **T83.098 Other mechanical complication of other urinary catheter** HCC
Other mechanical complication of Hopkins catheter
Other mechanical complication of ileostomy catheter
Other mechanical complication of urostomy catheter

√5ᵗʰ **T83.1 Mechanical complication of other urinary devices and implants**

√6ᵗʰ **T83.11 Breakdown (mechanical) of other urinary devices and implants**

6 √7ᵗʰ **T83.110 Breakdown (mechanical) of urinary electronic stimulator device** CC HCC
EXCLUDES 2   *breakdown (mechanical) of electrode (lead) for sacral nerve neurostimulator (T85.111)*
breakdown (mechanical) of implanted electronic sacral neurostimulator, pulse generator or receiver (T85.113)

6 √7ᵗʰ **T83.111 Breakdown (mechanical) of implanted urinary sphincter** CC HCC

6 √7ᵗʰ **T83.112 Breakdown (mechanical) of indwelling ureteral stent** CC HCC

6 √7ᵗʰ **T83.113 Breakdown (mechanical) of other urinary stents** CC HCC
Breakdown (mechanical) of ileal conduit stent
Breakdown (mechanical) of nephroureteral stent

6 √7ᵗʰ **T83.118 Breakdown (mechanical) of other urinary devices and implants** CC HCC

√6ᵗʰ **T83.12 Displacement of other urinary devices and implants**
Malposition of other urinary devices and implants

6 √7ᵗʰ **T83.120 Displacement of urinary electronic stimulator device** CC HCC
EXCLUDES 2   *displacement of electrode (lead) for sacral nerve neurostimulator (T85.121)*
displacement of implanted electronic sacral neurostimulator, pulse generator or receiver (T85.123)

6 √7ᵗʰ **T83.121 Displacement of implanted urinary sphincter** CC HCC

6 √7ᵗʰ **T83.122 Displacement of indwelling ureteral stent** CC HCC

6 √7ᵗʰ **T83.123 Displacement of other urinary stents** CC HCC
Displacement of ileal conduit stent
Displacement of nephroureteral stent

6 √7ᵗʰ **T83.128 Displacement of other urinary devices and implants** CC HCC

√6ᵗʰ **T83.19 Other mechanical complication of other urinary devices and implants**
Leakage of other urinary devices and implants
Obstruction (mechanical) of other urinary devices and implants
Perforation of other urinary devices and implants
Protrusion of other urinary devices and implants

6 √7ᵗʰ **T83.190 Other mechanical complication of urinary electronic stimulator device** CC HCC
EXCLUDES 2   *other mechanical complication of electrode (lead) for sacral nerve neurostimulator (T85.191)*
other mechanical complication of implanted electronic sacral neurostimulator, pulse generator or receiver (T85.193)

6 √7ᵗʰ **T83.191 Other mechanical complication of implanted urinary sphincter** CC HCC

6 √7ᵗʰ **T83.192 Other mechanical complication of indwelling ureteral stent** CC HCC

6 √7ᵗʰ **T83.193 Other mechanical complication of other urinary stent** CC HCC
Other mechanical complication of ileal conduit stent
Other mechanical complication of nephroureteral stent

6 √7ᵗʰ **T83.198 Other mechanical complication of other urinary devices and implants** CC HCC

√5ᵗʰ **T83.2 Mechanical complication of graft of urinary organ**

6 √x7ᵗʰ **T83.21 Breakdown (mechanical) of graft of urinary organ** CC HCC

6 √x7ᵗʰ **T83.22 Displacement of graft of urinary organ** CC HCC
Malposition of graft of urinary organ

6 √x7ᵗʰ **T83.23 Leakage of graft of urinary organ** CC HCC

6 √x7ᵗʰ **T83.24 Erosion of graft of urinary organ** CC HCC

6 √x7ᵗʰ **T83.25 Exposure of graft of urinary organ** CC HCC

6 √x7ᵗʰ **T83.29 Other mechanical complication of graft of urinary organ** CC HCC
Obstruction (mechanical) of graft of urinary organ
Perforation of graft of urinary organ
Protrusion of graft of urinary organ

√5ᵗʰ **T83.3 Mechanical complication of intrauterine contraceptive device**

√x7ᵗʰ **T83.31 Breakdown (mechanical) of intrauterine contraceptive device** ♀

√x7ᵗʰ **T83.32 Displacement of intrauterine contraceptive device** ♀
Malposition of intrauterine contraceptive device
Missing string of intrauterine contraceptive device
AHA: 2018,1Q,5

√x7ᵗʰ **T83.39 Other mechanical complication of intrauterine contraceptive device** ♀
Leakage of intrauterine contraceptive device
Obstruction (mechanical) of intrauterine contraceptive device
Perforation of intrauterine contraceptive device
Protrusion of intrauterine contraceptive device

Chapter 19. Injury, Poisoning and Certain Other Consequences of External Causes

√5ᵗʰ **T83.4** **Mechanical complication of other prosthetic devices, implants and grafts of genital tract**

  √6ᵗʰ **T83.41** Breakdown (mechanical) of other prosthetic devices, implants and grafts of genital tract

    6 √7ᵗʰ **T83.410** **Breakdown (mechanical) of implanted penile prosthesis**   CC HCC ♂

        Breakdown (mechanical) of penile prosthesis cylinder

        Breakdown (mechanical) of penile prosthesis pump

        Breakdown (mechanical) of penile prosthesis reservoir

    6 √7ᵗʰ **T83.411** **Breakdown (mechanical) of implanted testicular prosthesis**   CC HCC

    6 √7ᵗʰ **T83.418** **Breakdown (mechanical) of other prosthetic devices, implants and grafts of genital tract**   CC HCC

  √6ᵗʰ **T83.42** Displacement of other prosthetic devices, implants and grafts of genital tract

      Malposition of other prosthetic devices, implants and grafts of genital tract

    6 √7ᵗʰ **T83.420** **Displacement of implanted penile prosthesis**   CC HCC ♂

        Displacement of penile prosthesis cylinder

        Displacement of penile prosthesis pump

        Displacement of penile prosthesis reservoir

    6 √7ᵗʰ **T83.421** **Displacement of implanted testicular prosthesis**   CC HCC

    6 √7ᵗʰ **T83.428** **Displacement of other prosthetic devices, implants and grafts of genital tract**   CC HCC

        AHA: 2018,1Q,5

  √6ᵗʰ **T83.49** Other mechanical complication of other prosthetic devices, implants and grafts of genital tract

      Leakage of other prosthetic devices, implants and grafts of genital tract

      Obstruction, mechanical of other prosthetic devices, implants and grafts of genital tract

      Perforation of other prosthetic devices, implants and grafts of genital tract

      Protrusion of other prosthetic devices, implants and grafts of genital tract

    6 √7ᵗʰ **T83.490** **Other mechanical complication of implanted penile prosthesis**   CC HCC ♂

        Other mechanical complication of penile prosthesis cylinder

        Other mechanical complication of penile prosthesis pump

        Other mechanical complication of penile prosthesis reservoir

    6 √7ᵗʰ **T83.491** **Other mechanical complication of implanted testicular prosthesis**   CC HCC

    6 √7ᵗʰ **T83.498** **Other mechanical complication of other prosthetic devices, implants and grafts of genital tract**   CC HCC

√5ᵗʰ **T83.5** **Infection and inflammatory reaction due to prosthetic device, implant and graft in urinary system**

    Use additional code to identify infection

    CC Excl: For CC codes in subcategory T83.5, unless otherwise noted: PDX collection 1458

  √6ᵗʰ **T83.51** Infection and inflammatory reaction due to urinary catheter

      EXCLUDES 2   *complications of stoma of urinary tract (N99.5-)*

    6 √7ᵗʰ **T83.510** **Infection and inflammatory reaction due to cystostomy catheter**   CC HCC

    6 √7ᵗʰ **T83.511** **Infection and inflammatory reaction due to indwelling urethral catheter**   CC H6 HCC

        CC Excl: PDX collection 1457

    6 √7ᵗʰ **T83.512** **Infection and inflammatory reaction due to nephrostomy catheter**   CC HCC

    6 √7ᵗʰ **T83.518** **Infection and inflammatory reaction due to other urinary catheter**   CC H6 HCC

        Infection and inflammatory reaction due to Hopkins catheter

        Infection and inflammatory reaction due to ileostomy catheter

        Infection and inflammatory reaction due to urostomy catheter

  √6ᵗʰ **T83.59** Infection and inflammatory reaction due to prosthetic device, implant and graft in urinary system

    6 √7ᵗʰ **T83.590** **Infection and inflammatory reaction due to implanted urinary neurostimulation device**   CC HCC

        EXCLUDES 2   *infection and inflammatory reaction due to electrode lead of sacral nerve neurostimulator (T85.732)*

             infection and inflammatory reaction due to pulse generator or receiver of sacral nerve neurostimulator (T85.734)

    6 √7ᵗʰ **T83.591** **Infection and inflammatory reaction due to implanted urinary sphincter**   CC HCC

    6 √7ᵗʰ **T83.592** **Infection and inflammatory reaction due to indwelling ureteral stent**   CC HCC

    6 √7ᵗʰ **T83.593** **Infection and inflammatory reaction due to other urinary stents**   CC HCC

        Infection and inflammatory reaction due to ileal conduit stents

        Infection and inflammatory reaction due to nephroureteral stent

    6 √7ᵗʰ **T83.598** **Infection and inflammatory reaction due to other prosthetic device, implant and graft in urinary system**   CC HCC

√5ᵗʰ **T83.6** **Infection and inflammatory reaction due to prosthetic device, implant and graft in genital tract**

    Use additional code to identify infection

    CC Excl: For CC codes in subcategory T83.6: PDX collection 1458

  6 √x7ᵗʰ **T83.61** **Infection and inflammatory reaction due to implanted penile prosthesis**   CC HCC

      Infection and inflammatory reaction due to penile prosthesis cylinder

      Infection and inflammatory reaction due to penile prosthesis pump

      Infection and inflammatory reaction due to penile prosthesis reservoir

  6 √x7ᵗʰ **T83.62** **Infection and inflammatory reaction due to implanted testicular prosthesis**   CC HCC

  6 √x7ᵗʰ **T83.69** **Infection and inflammatory reaction due to other prosthetic device, implant and graft in genital tract**   CC HCC

N Newborn: 0   P Pediatric: 0-17   M Maternity: 9-64   A Adult: 15-124   MCC Major Complication/Comorbidity   CC Complication/Comorbidity   SW Severe Wound Dx

1198   ICD-10-CM 2020

✓5ᵗʰ T83.7 Complications due to implanted mesh and other prosthetic materials

✓6ᵗʰ T83.71 Erosion of implanted mesh and other prosthetic materials

6 ✓7ᵗʰ **T83.711 Erosion of implanted vaginal mesh to surrounding organ or tissue** `HCC` ♀

Erosion of implanted vaginal mesh into pelvic floor muscles

6 ✓7ᵗʰ **T83.712 Erosion of implanted urethral mesh to surrounding organ or tissue** `CC` `HCC`

Erosion of implanted female urethral sling

Erosion of implanted male urethral sling

Erosion of implanted urethral mesh into pelvic floor muscles

6 ✓7ᵗʰ **T83.713 Erosion of implanted urethral bulking agent to surrounding organ or tissue** `CC` `HCC`

6 ✓7ᵗʰ **T83.714 Erosion of implanted ureteral bulking agent to surrounding organ or tissue** `CC` `HCC`

6 ✓7ᵗʰ **T83.718 Erosion of other implanted mesh to organ or tissue** `CC` `HCC`

6 ✓7ᵗʰ **T83.719 Erosion of other prosthetic materials to surrounding organ or tissue** `CC` `HCC`

✓6ᵗʰ T83.72 Exposure of implanted mesh and other prosthetic materials into surrounding organ or tissue

Extrusion of implanted mesh

6 ✓7ᵗʰ **T83.721 Exposure of implanted vaginal mesh into vagina** `HCC` ♀

Exposure of implanted vaginal mesh through vaginal wall

6 ✓7ᵗʰ **T83.722 Exposure of implanted urethral mesh into urethra** `CC` `HCC`

Exposure of implanted female urethral sling

Exposure of implanted male urethral sling

Exposure of implanted urethral mesh through urethral wall

6 ✓7ᵗʰ **T83.723 Exposure of implanted urethral bulking agent into urethra** `CC` `HCC`

6 ✓7ᵗʰ **T83.724 Exposure of implanted ureteral bulking agent into ureter** `CC` `HCC`

6 ✓7ᵗʰ **T83.728 Exposure of other implanted mesh into organ or tissue** `CC` `HCC`

6 ✓7ᵗʰ **T83.729 Exposure of other prosthetic materials into organ or tissue** `CC` `HCC`

6 ✓x7ᵗʰ **T83.79 Other specified complications due to other genitourinary prosthetic materials** `CC` `HCC`

CC Excl: PDX collection 1458

✓5ᵗʰ T83.8 Other specified complications of genitourinary prosthetic devices, implants and grafts

CC Excl: For CC codes in subcategory T83.8: PDX collection 1458

6 ✓x7ᵗʰ **T83.81 Embolism due to genitourinary prosthetic devices, implants and grafts** `CC` `HCC`

6 ✓x7ᵗʰ **T83.82 Fibrosis due to genitourinary prosthetic devices, implants and grafts** `CC` `HCC`

6 ✓x7ᵗʰ **T83.83 Hemorrhage due to genitourinary prosthetic devices, implants and grafts** `CC` `HCC`

6 ✓x7ᵗʰ **T83.84 Pain due to genitourinary prosthetic devices, implants and grafts** `CC` `HCC`

6 ✓x7ᵗʰ **T83.85 Stenosis due to genitourinary prosthetic devices, implants and grafts** `CC` `HCC`

6 ✓x7ᵗʰ **T83.86 Thrombosis due to genitourinary prosthetic devices, implants and grafts** `CC` `HCC`

6 ✓x7ᵗʰ **T83.89 Other specified complication of genitourinary prosthetic devices, implants and grafts** `CC` `HCC`

6 ✓x7ᵗʰ **T83.9 Unspecified complication of genitourinary prosthetic device, implant and graft** `CC` `HCC`

CC Excl: PDX collection 1458

✓4ᵗʰ T84 Complications of internal orthopedic prosthetic devices, implants and grafts

EXCLUDES 2 failure and rejection of transplanted organs and tissues (T86.-)

fracture of bone following insertion of orthopedic implant, joint prosthesis or bone plate (M96.6)

The appropriate 7th character is to be added to each code from category T84.

A   initial encounter

D   subsequent encounter

S   sequela

CC Excl: For CC codes in category T84, unless otherwise noted: PDX collection 911

✓5ᵗʰ T84.0 Mechanical complication of internal joint prosthesis

✓6ᵗʰ T84.01 Broken internal joint prosthesis

Breakage (fracture) of prosthetic joint

Broken prosthetic joint implant

EXCLUDES 1 periprosthetic joint implant fracture (M97-)

AHA: 2016,4Q,42

6 ✓7ᵗʰ **T84.010 Broken internal right hip prosthesis** `CC` `HCC`

6 ✓7ᵗʰ **T84.011 Broken internal left hip prosthesis** `CC` `HCC`

6 ✓7ᵗʰ **T84.012 Broken internal right knee prosthesis** `CC` `HCC`

6 ✓7ᵗʰ **T84.013 Broken internal left knee prosthesis** `CC` `HCC`

6 ✓7ᵗʰ **T84.018 Broken internal joint prosthesis, other site** `CC` `HCC`

Use additional code to identify the joint (Z96.6-)

6 ✓7ᵗʰ **T84.019 Broken internal joint prosthesis, unspecified site** `CC` `HCC`

✓6ᵗʰ T84.02 Dislocation of internal joint prosthesis

Instability of internal joint prosthesis

Subluxation of internal joint prosthesis

AHA: 2019,2Q,27

6 ✓7ᵗʰ **T84.020 Dislocation of internal right hip prosthesis** `CC` `HCC`

6 ✓7ᵗʰ **T84.021 Dislocation of internal left hip prosthesis** `CC` `HCC`

6 ✓7ᵗʰ **T84.022 Instability of internal right knee prosthesis** `CC` `HCC`

6 ✓7ᵗʰ **T84.023 Instability of internal left knee prosthesis** `CC` `HCC`

6 ✓7ᵗʰ **T84.028 Dislocation of other internal joint prosthesis** `CC` `HCC`

Use additional code to identify the joint (Z96.6-)

6 ✓7ᵗʰ **T84.029 Dislocation of unspecified internal joint prosthesis** `CC` `HCC`

✓6ᵗʰ T84.03 Mechanical loosening of internal prosthetic joint

Aseptic loosening of prosthetic joint

6 ✓7ᵗʰ **T84.030 Mechanical loosening of internal right hip prosthetic joint** `CC` `HCC`

6 ✓7ᵗʰ **T84.031 Mechanical loosening of internal left hip prosthetic joint** `CC` `HCC`

6 ✓7ᵗʰ **T84.032 Mechanical loosening of internal right knee prosthetic joint** `CC` `HCC`

6 ✓7ᵗʰ **T84.033 Mechanical loosening of internal left knee prosthetic joint** `CC` `HCC`

6 ✓7ᵗʰ **T84.038 Mechanical loosening of other internal prosthetic joint** `CC` `HCC`

Use additional code to identify the joint (Z96.6-)

6 ✓7ᵗʰ **T84.039 Mechanical loosening of unspecified internal prosthetic joint** `CC` `HCC`

✅ Additional Character Required   ✓x7ᵗʰ Placeholder   Unacceptable PDx   Questionable PDx   Manifestation   Unspecified Dx   H1 - H14 HAC   HCC CMS-HCC Dx   HIV HIV Dx

ICD-10-CM 2020   1199

√6ᵗʰ T84.05 Periprosthetic osteolysis of internal prosthetic joint
Use additional code to identify major osseous defect, if applicable (M89.7-)

- 6 √7ᵗʰ **T84.050** Periprosthetic osteolysis of internal prosthetic **right hip joint** `CC` `HCC`
- 6 √7ᵗʰ **T84.051** Periprosthetic osteolysis of internal prosthetic **left hip joint** `CC` `HCC`
- 6 √7ᵗʰ **T84.052** Periprosthetic osteolysis of internal prosthetic **right knee joint** `CC` `HCC`
- 6 √7ᵗʰ **T84.053** Periprosthetic osteolysis of internal prosthetic **left knee joint** `CC` `HCC`
- 6 √7ᵗʰ **T84.058** Periprosthetic osteolysis of other internal prosthetic joint `CC` `HCC`
  Use additional code to identify the joint (Z96.6-)
- 6 √7ᵗʰ **T84.059** Periprosthetic osteolysis of unspecified internal prosthetic joint `CC` `HCC`

√6ᵗʰ T84.06 Wear of articular bearing surface of internal prosthetic joint

- 6 √7ᵗʰ **T84.060** Wear of articular bearing surface of internal prosthetic **right hip joint** `CC` `HCC`
- 6 √7ᵗʰ **T84.061** Wear of articular bearing surface of internal prosthetic **left hip joint** `CC` `HCC`
- 6 √7ᵗʰ **T84.062** Wear of articular bearing surface of internal prosthetic **right knee joint** `CC` `HCC`
- 6 √7ᵗʰ **T84.063** Wear of articular bearing surface of internal prosthetic **left knee joint** `CC` `HCC`
- 6 √7ᵗʰ **T84.068** Wear of articular bearing surface of other internal prosthetic joint `CC` `HCC`
  Use additional code to identify the joint (Z96.6-)
- 6 √7ᵗʰ **T84.069** Wear of articular bearing surface of unspecified internal prosthetic joint `CC` `HCC`

√6ᵗʰ T84.09 Other mechanical complication of internal joint prosthesis
Prosthetic joint implant failure NOS
AHA: 2019,1Q,20

- 6 √7ᵗʰ **T84.090** Other mechanical complication of internal **right hip prosthesis** `CC` `HCC`
- 6 √7ᵗʰ **T84.091** Other mechanical complication of internal **left hip prosthesis** `CC` `HCC`
- 6 √7ᵗʰ **T84.092** Other mechanical complication of internal **right knee prosthesis** `CC` `HCC`
- 6 √7ᵗʰ **T84.093** Other mechanical complication of internal **left knee prosthesis** `CC` `HCC`
- 6 √7ᵗʰ **T84.098** Other mechanical complication of other internal joint prosthesis `CC` `HCC`
  Use additional code to identify the joint (Z96.6-)
- 6 √7ᵗʰ **T84.099** Other mechanical complication of unspecified internal joint prosthesis `CC` `HCC`

√5ᵗʰ T84.1 Mechanical complication of internal fixation device of bones of limb

> *EXCLUDES 2*   mechanical complication of internal fixation device of bones of feet (T84.2-)
> mechanical complication of internal fixation device of bones of fingers (T84.2-)
> mechanical complication of internal fixation device of bones of hands (T84.2-)
> mechanical complication of internal fixation device of bones of toes (T84.2-)

√6ᵗʰ T84.11 Breakdown (mechanical) of internal fixation device of bones of limb

- 6 √7ᵗʰ **T84.110** Breakdown (mechanical) of internal fixation device of **right humerus** `CC` `HCC`
- 6 √7ᵗʰ **T84.111** Breakdown (mechanical) of internal fixation device of **left humerus** `CC` `HCC`
- 6 √7ᵗʰ **T84.112** Breakdown (mechanical) of internal fixation device of bone of **right forearm** `CC` `HCC`
- 6 √7ᵗʰ **T84.113** Breakdown (mechanical) of internal fixation device of bone of **left forearm** `CC` `HCC`
- 6 √7ᵗʰ **T84.114** Breakdown (mechanical) of internal fixation device of **right femur** `CC` `HCC`
- 6 √7ᵗʰ **T84.115** Breakdown (mechanical) of internal fixation device of **left femur** `CC` `HCC`
- 6 √7ᵗʰ **T84.116** Breakdown (mechanical) of internal fixation device of bone of **right lower leg** `CC` `HCC`
- 6 √7ᵗʰ **T84.117** Breakdown (mechanical) of internal fixation device of bone of **left lower leg** `CC` `HCC`
- 6 √7ᵗʰ **T84.119** Breakdown (mechanical) of internal fixation device of **unspecified bone of limb** `CC` `HCC`

√6ᵗʰ T84.12 Displacement of internal fixation device of bones of limb
Malposition of internal fixation device of bones of limb

- 6 √7ᵗʰ **T84.120** Displacement of internal fixation device of **right humerus** `CC` `HCC`
- 6 √7ᵗʰ **T84.121** Displacement of internal fixation device of **left humerus** `CC` `HCC`
- 6 √7ᵗʰ **T84.122** Displacement of internal fixation device of bone of **right forearm** `CC` `HCC`
- 6 √7ᵗʰ **T84.123** Displacement of internal fixation device of bone of **left forearm** `CC` `HCC`
- 6 √7ᵗʰ **T84.124** Displacement of internal fixation device of **right femur** `CC` `HCC`
- 6 √7ᵗʰ **T84.125** Displacement of internal fixation device of **left femur** `CC` `HCC`
- 6 √7ᵗʰ **T84.126** Displacement of internal fixation device of bone of **right lower leg** `CC` `HCC`
- 6 √7ᵗʰ **T84.127** Displacement of internal fixation device of bone of **left lower leg** `CC` `HCC`
- 6 √7ᵗʰ **T84.129** Displacement of internal fixation device of **unspecified bone of limb** `CC` `HCC`

√6ᵗʰ T84.19 Other mechanical complication of internal fixation device of bones of limb
Obstruction (mechanical) of internal fixation device of bones of limb
Perforation of internal fixation device of bones of limb
Protrusion of internal fixation device of bones of limb

- 6 √7ᵗʰ **T84.190** Other mechanical complication of internal fixation device of **right humerus** `CC` `HCC`

N Newborn: 0   P Pediatric: 0-17   M Maternity: 9-64   A Adult: 15-124   **MCC** Major Complication/Comorbidity   **CC** Complication/Comorbidity   **SW** Severe Wound Dx

1200   ICD-10-CM 2020

6 √7ᵗʰ **T84.191 Other mechanical complication of internal fixation device of** left humerus   `CC` `HCC`

6 √7ᵗʰ **T84.192 Other mechanical complication of internal fixation device of bone of** right forearm   `CC` `HCC`

6 √7ᵗʰ **T84.193 Other mechanical complication of internal fixation device of bone of** left forearm   `CC` `HCC`

6 √7ᵗʰ **T84.194 Other mechanical complication of internal fixation device of** right femur   `CC` `HCC`

6 √7ᵗʰ **T84.195 Other mechanical complication of internal fixation device of** left femur   `CC` `HCC`

6 √7ᵗʰ **T84.196 Other mechanical complication of internal fixation device of bone of** right lower leg   `CC` `HCC`

6 √7ᵗʰ **T84.197 Other mechanical complication of internal fixation device of bone of** left lower leg   `CC` `HCC`

6 √7ᵗʰ **T84.199 Other mechanical complication of internal fixation device of** unspecified bone of limb   `CC` `HCC`

√5ᵗʰ **T84.2 Mechanical complication of** internal fixation device **of** other bones

  √6ᵗʰ **T84.21 Breakdown (mechanical) of internal fixation device of other bones**

    6 √7ᵗʰ **T84.210 Breakdown (mechanical) of internal fixation device of bones of** hand and fingers   `CC` `HCC`

    6 √7ᵗʰ **T84.213 Breakdown (mechanical) of internal fixation device of bones of** foot and toes   `CC` `HCC`

    6 √7ᵗʰ **T84.216 Breakdown (mechanical) of internal fixation device of** vertebrae   `CC` `HCC`

    6 √7ᵗʰ **T84.218 Breakdown (mechanical) of internal fixation device of other bones**   `CC` `HCC`

  √6ᵗʰ **T84.22 Displacement of internal fixation device of other bones**

Malposition of internal fixation device of other bones

    6 √7ᵗʰ **T84.220 Displacement of internal fixation device of bones of** hand and fingers   `CC` `HCC`

    6 √7ᵗʰ **T84.223 Displacement of internal fixation device of bones of** foot and toes   `CC` `HCC`

    6 √7ᵗʰ **T84.226 Displacement of internal fixation device of** vertebrae   `CC` `HCC`

    6 √7ᵗʰ **T84.228 Displacement of internal fixation device of other bones**   `CC` `HCC`

  √6ᵗʰ **T84.29 Other mechanical complication of internal fixation device of other bones**

Obstruction (mechanical) of internal fixation device of other bones

Perforation of internal fixation device of other bones

Protrusion of internal fixation device of other bones

    6 √7ᵗʰ **T84.290 Other mechanical complication of internal fixation device of bones of** hand and fingers   `CC` `HCC`

    6 √7ᵗʰ **T84.293 Other mechanical complication of internal fixation device of bones of** foot and toes   `CC` `HCC`

    6 √7ᵗʰ **T84.296 Other mechanical complication of internal fixation device of** vertebrae   `CC` `HCC`

6 √7ᵗʰ **T84.298 Other mechanical complication of internal fixation device of other bones**   `CC` `HCC`

√5ᵗʰ **T84.3 Mechanical complication of other bone devices, implants and grafts**

  EXCLUDES 2 *other complications of bone graft (T86.83-)*

  √6ᵗʰ **T84.31 Breakdown (mechanical) of other bone devices, implants and grafts**

    6 √7ᵗʰ **T84.310 Breakdown (mechanical) of** electronic bone stimulator   `CC` `HCC`

    6 √7ᵗʰ **T84.318 Breakdown (mechanical) of other bone devices, implants and grafts**   `CC` `HCC`

  √6ᵗʰ **T84.32 Displacement of other bone devices, implants and grafts**

Malposition of other bone devices, implants and grafts

    6 √7ᵗʰ **T84.320 Displacement of** electronic bone stimulator   `CC` `HCC`

    6 √7ᵗʰ **T84.328 Displacement of other bone devices, implants and grafts**   `CC` `HCC`

      AHA: 2014,4Q,28

  √6ᵗʰ **T84.39 Other mechanical complication of other bone devices, implants and grafts**

Obstruction (mechanical) of other bone devices, implants and grafts

Perforation of other bone devices, implants and grafts

Protrusion of other bone devices, implants and grafts

    6 √7ᵗʰ **T84.390 Other mechanical complication of** electronic bone stimulator   `CC` `HCC`

    6 √7ᵗʰ **T84.398 Other mechanical complication of other bone devices, implants and grafts**   `CC` `HCC`

√5ᵗʰ **T84.4 Mechanical complication of other internal orthopedic devices, implants and grafts**

  √6ᵗʰ **T84.41 Breakdown (mechanical) of other internal orthopedic devices, implants and grafts**

    6 √7ᵗʰ **T84.410 Breakdown (mechanical) of** muscle and tendon graft   `CC` `HCC`

    6 √7ᵗʰ **T84.418 Breakdown (mechanical) of other internal orthopedic devices, implants and grafts**   `CC` `HCC`

  √6ᵗʰ **T84.42 Displacement of other internal orthopedic devices, implants and grafts**

Malposition of other internal orthopedic devices, implants and grafts

    6 √7ᵗʰ **T84.420 Displacement of** muscle and tendon graft   `CC` `HCC`

    6 √7ᵗʰ **T84.428 Displacement of other internal orthopedic devices, implants and grafts**   `CC` `HCC`

  √6ᵗʰ **T84.49 Other mechanical complication of other internal orthopedic devices, implants and grafts**

Mechanical complication of other internal orthopedic devices, implants and grafts NOS

Obstruction (mechanical) of other internal orthopedic devices, implants and grafts

Perforation of other internal orthopedic devices, implants and grafts

Protrusion of other internal orthopedic devices, implants and grafts

    6 √7ᵗʰ **T84.490 Other mechanical complication of** muscle and tendon graft   `CC` `HCC`

    6 √7ᵗʰ **T84.498 Other mechanical complication of other internal orthopedic devices, implants and grafts**   `CC` `HCC`

☑ Additional Character Required   √x7ᵗʰ Placeholder   Unacceptable PDx   Questionable PDx   Manifestation   Unspecified Dx   `H1`-`H14` HAC   `HCC` CMS-HCC Dx   `HIV` HIV Dx

ICD-10-CM 2020   1201

T84.5 Infection and inflammatory reaction due to internal joint prosthesis

Use additional code to identify infection

AHA: 2015,1Q,16

CC Excl: For CC codes in subcategory T84.5: PDX collection 1459

T84.50 Infection and inflammatory reaction due to unspecified internal joint prosthesis `CC` `HCC`

T84.51 Infection and inflammatory reaction due to internal right hip prosthesis `CC` `HCC`

T84.52 Infection and inflammatory reaction due to internal left hip prosthesis `CC` `HCC`

T84.53 Infection and inflammatory reaction due to internal right knee prosthesis `CC` `HCC`

T84.54 Infection and inflammatory reaction due to internal left knee prosthesis `CC` `HCC`

T84.59 Infection and inflammatory reaction due to other internal joint prosthesis `CC` `HCC`

T84.6 Infection and inflammatory reaction due to internal fixation device

Use additional code to identify infection

CC Excl: For CC codes in subcategory T84.6: PDX collection 1459

T84.60 Infection and inflammatory reaction due to internal fixation device of unspecified site `CC` `H12` `HCC`

T84.61 Infection and inflammatory reaction due to internal fixation device of arm

    T84.610 Infection and inflammatory reaction due to internal fixation device of right humerus `CC` `H12` `HCC`

    T84.611 Infection and inflammatory reaction due to internal fixation device of left humerus `CC` `H12` `HCC`

    T84.612 Infection and inflammatory reaction due to internal fixation device of right radius `CC` `H12` `HCC`

    T84.613 Infection and inflammatory reaction due to internal fixation device of left radius `CC` `H12` `HCC`

    T84.614 Infection and inflammatory reaction due to internal fixation device of right ulna `CC` `H12` `HCC`

    T84.615 Infection and inflammatory reaction due to internal fixation device of left ulna `CC` `H12` `HCC`

    T84.619 Infection and inflammatory reaction due to internal fixation device of unspecified bone of arm `CC` `H12` `HCC`

T84.62 Infection and inflammatory reaction due to internal fixation device of leg

    T84.620 Infection and inflammatory reaction due to internal fixation device of right femur `CC` `HCC`

    T84.621 Infection and inflammatory reaction due to internal fixation device of left femur `CC` `HCC`

    T84.622 Infection and inflammatory reaction due to internal fixation device of right tibia `CC` `HCC`

    T84.623 Infection and inflammatory reaction due to internal fixation device of left tibia `CC` `HCC`

    T84.624 Infection and inflammatory reaction due to internal fixation device of right fibula `CC` `HCC`

    T84.625 Infection and inflammatory reaction due to internal fixation device of left fibula `CC` `HCC`

    T84.629 Infection and inflammatory reaction due to internal fixation device of unspecified bone of leg `CC` `HCC`

T84.63 Infection and inflammatory reaction due to internal fixation device of spine `CC` `H12` `HCC`

T84.69 Infection and inflammatory reaction due to internal fixation device of other site `CC` `H12` `HCC`

T84.7 Infection and inflammatory reaction due to other internal orthopedic prosthetic devices, implants and grafts `CC` `H12` `HCC`

Use additional code to identify infection

CC Excl: PDX collection 1459

T84.8 Other specified complications of internal orthopedic prosthetic devices, implants and grafts

CC Excl: For CC codes in subcategory T84.8: PDX collection 1459

T84.81 Embolism due to internal orthopedic prosthetic devices, implants and grafts `CC` `HCC`

T84.82 Fibrosis due to internal orthopedic prosthetic devices, implants and grafts `CC` `HCC`

T84.83 Hemorrhage due to internal orthopedic prosthetic devices, implants and grafts `CC` `HCC`

T84.84 Pain due to internal orthopedic prosthetic devices, implants and grafts `CC` `HCC`

T84.85 Stenosis due to internal orthopedic prosthetic devices, implants and grafts `CC` `HCC`

T84.86 Thrombosis due to internal orthopedic prosthetic devices, implants and grafts `CC` `HCC`

T84.89 Other specified complication of internal orthopedic prosthetic devices, implants and grafts `CC` `HCC`

T84.9 Unspecified complication of internal orthopedic prosthetic device, implant and graft `CC` `HCC`

CC Excl: PDX collection 1459

T85 Complications of other internal prosthetic devices, implants and grafts

EXCLUDES 2   *failure and rejection of transplanted organs and tissue (T86.-)*

AHA: 2016,4Q,71-72

The appropriate 7th character is to be added to each code from category T85.
A   initial encounter
D   subsequent encounter
S   sequela

T85.0 Mechanical complication of ventricular intracranial (communicating) shunt

CC Excl: For CC codes in subcategory T85.0: PDX collection 1460

T85.01 Breakdown (mechanical) of ventricular intracranial (communicating) shunt `CC` `HCC`

T85.02 Displacement of ventricular intracranial (communicating) shunt `CC` `HCC`

Malposition of ventricular intracranial (communicating) shunt

T85.03 Leakage of ventricular intracranial (communicating) shunt `CC` `HCC`

T85.09 Other mechanical complication of ventricular intracranial (communicating) shunt `CC` `HCC`

Obstruction (mechanical) of ventricular intracranial (communicating) shunt

Perforation of ventricular intracranial (communicating) shunt

Protrusion of ventricular intracranial (communicating) shunt

N Newborn: 0   P Pediatric: 0-17   M Maternity: 9-64   A Adult: 15-124   MCC Major Complication/Comorbidity   CC Complication/Comorbidity   SW Severe Wound Dx

1202   ICD-10-CM 2020

✓5ᵗʰ **T85.1 Mechanical complication of** implanted electronic stimulator of nervous system

> **CC Excl: For CC codes in subcategory T85.1:** PDX collection 1460

✓6ᵗʰ **T85.11 Breakdown (mechanical) of implanted electronic stimulator of nervous system**

6 ✓7ᵗʰ **T85.110 Breakdown (mechanical) of implanted electronic neurostimulator** of brain electrode (lead)   `CC` `HCC`

6 ✓7ᵗʰ **T85.111 Breakdown (mechanical) of implanted electronic neurostimulator of** peripheral nerve electrode (lead)   `CC` `HCC`

> Breakdown of electrode (lead) for cranial nerve neurostimulators
> Breakdown of electrode (lead) for gastric neurostimulator
> Breakdown of electrode (lead) for sacral nerve neurostimulator
> Breakdown of electrode (lead) for vagal nerve neurostimulators

6 ✓7ᵗʰ **T85.112 Breakdown (mechanical) of implanted electronic neurostimulator of** spinal cord electrode (lead)   `CC` `HCC`

6 ✓7ᵗʰ **T85.113 Breakdown (mechanical) of implanted electronic neurostimulator,** generator   `CC` `HCC`

> Breakdown (mechanical) of implanted electronic neurostimulator generator, brain, peripheral, gastric, spinal
> Breakdown (mechanical) of implanted electronic sacral neurostimulator, pulse generator or receiver

6 ✓7ᵗʰ **T85.118 Breakdown (mechanical) of other implanted electronic stimulator of** nervous system   `CC` `HCC`

✓6ᵗʰ **T85.12 Displacement of implanted electronic stimulator of nervous system**

> Malposition of implanted electronic stimulator of nervous system

6 ✓7ᵗʰ **T85.120 Displacement of implanted electronic neurostimulator of** brain electrode (lead)   `CC` `HCC`

6 ✓7ᵗʰ **T85.121 Displacement of implanted electronic neurostimulator of** peripheral nerve electrode (lead)   `CC` `HCC`

> Displacement of electrode (lead) for cranial nerve neurostimulators
> Displacement of electrode (lead) for gastric neurostimulator
> Displacement of electrode (lead) for sacral nerve neurostimulator
> Displacement of electrode (lead) for vagal nerve neurostimulators

6 ✓7ᵗʰ **T85.122 Displacement of implanted electronic neurostimulator of** spinal cord electrode (lead)   `CC` `HCC`

6 ✓7ᵗʰ **T85.123 Displacement of implanted electronic neurostimulator,** generator   `CC` `HCC`

> Displacement of implanted electronic neurostimulator generator, brain, peripheral, gastric, spinal
> Displacement of implanted electronic sacral neurostimulator, pulse generator or receiver

6 ✓7ᵗʰ **T85.128 Displacement of other implanted electronic stimulator of nervous system**   `CC` `HCC`

✓6ᵗʰ **T85.19 Other mechanical complication of implanted electronic stimulator of nervous system**

> Leakage of implanted electronic stimulator of nervous system
> Obstruction (mechanical) of implanted electronic stimulator of nervous system
> Perforation of implanted electronic stimulator of nervous system
> Protrusion of implanted electronic stimulator of nervous system

6 ✓7ᵗʰ **T85.190 Other mechanical complication of implanted electronic neurostimulator** of brain electrode (lead)   `CC` `HCC`

6 ✓7ᵗʰ **T85.191 Other mechanical complication of implanted electronic neurostimulator** of peripheral nerve electrode (lead)   `CC` `HCC`

> Other mechanical complication of electrode (lead) for cranial nerve neurostimulators
> Other mechanical complication of electrode (lead) for gastric neurostimulator
> Other mechanical complication of electrode (lead) for sacral nerve neurostimulator
> Other mechanical complication of electrode (lead) for vagal nerve neurostimulators

6 ✓7ᵗʰ **T85.192 Other mechanical complication of implanted electronic neurostimulator** of spinal cord electrode (lead)   `CC` `HCC`

6 ✓7ᵗʰ **T85.193 Other mechanical complication of implanted electronic neurostimulator,** generator   `CC` `HCC`

> Other mechanical complication of implanted electronic neurostimulator generator, brain, peripheral, gastric, spinal
> Other mechanical complication of implanted electronic sacral neurostimulator, pulse generator or receiver

6 ✓7ᵗʰ **T85.199 Other mechanical complication of other implanted electronic stimulator of nervous system**   `CC` `HCC`

✓5ᵗʰ **T85.2 Mechanical complication of** intraocular lens

> **CC Excl: For CC codes in subcategory T85.2:** PDX collection 1461

✓x7ᵗʰ **T85.21 Breakdown (mechanical) of intraocular lens**   `CC`

✓x7ᵗʰ **T85.22 Displacement of intraocular lens**   `CC`

> Malposition of intraocular lens

✓x7ᵗʰ **T85.29 Other mechanical complication of intraocular lens**   `CC`

> Obstruction (mechanical) of intraocular lens
> Perforation of intraocular lens
> Protrusion of intraocular lens

✓5ᵗʰ **T85.3 Mechanical complication of other ocular prosthetic devices, implants and grafts**

> **EXCLUDES 2**   *other complications of corneal graft (T86.84-)*

> **CC Excl: For CC codes in subcategory T85.3:** PDX collection 1462

✓6ᵗʰ **T85.31 Breakdown (mechanical) of other ocular prosthetic devices, implants and grafts**

✓7ᵗʰ **T85.310 Breakdown (mechanical) of prosthetic orbit of** right eye   `CC`

✓7ᵗʰ **T85.311 Breakdown (mechanical) of prosthetic orbit of** left eye   `CC`

✓7ᵗʰ **T85.318 Breakdown (mechanical) of other ocular prosthetic devices, implants and grafts**

✔ Additional Character Required   ✓x7ᵗʰ Placeholder   Unacceptable PDx   Questionable PDx   Manifestation   Unspecified Dx   H1-H4 HAC   HCC CMS-HCC Dx   HIV HIV Dx

ICD-10-CM 2020

1203

Chapter 19. Injury, Poisoning and Certain Other Consequences of External Causes

T85.1–T85.318

Chapter 19. Injury, Poisoning and Certain Other Consequences of External Causes

T85.32–T85.618

√6ᵗʰ **T85.32** Displacement of other ocular prosthetic devices, implants and grafts
     Malposition of other ocular prosthetic devices, implants and grafts

     √7ᵗʰ **T85.320** Displacement of prosthetic orbit of right eye   `CC`

     √7ᵗʰ **T85.321** Displacement of prosthetic orbit of left eye

     √7ᵗʰ **T85.328** Displacement of other ocular prosthetic devices, implants and grafts

√6ᵗʰ **T85.39** Other mechanical complication of other ocular prosthetic devices, implants and grafts
     Obstruction (mechanical) of other ocular prosthetic devices, implants and grafts
     Perforation of other ocular prosthetic devices, implants and grafts
     Protrusion of other ocular prosthetic devices, implants and grafts

     √7ᵗʰ **T85.390** Other mechanical complication of prosthetic orbit of right eye   `CC`

     √7ᵗʰ **T85.391** Other mechanical complication of prosthetic orbit of left eye   `CC`

     √7ᵗʰ **T85.398** Other mechanical complication of other ocular prosthetic devices, implants and grafts

√5ᵗʰ **T85.4** Mechanical complication of breast prosthesis and implant

     CC Excl: For CC codes in subcategory T85.4: PDX collection 1463

√x7ᵗʰ **T85.41** Breakdown (mechanical) of breast prosthesis and implant   `CC`

√x7ᵗʰ **T85.42** Displacement of breast prosthesis and implant   `CC`
     Malposition of breast prosthesis and implant

√x7ᵗʰ **T85.43** Leakage of breast prosthesis and implant   `CC`

√x7ᵗʰ **T85.44** Capsular contracture of breast implant   `CC`

√x7ᵗʰ **T85.49** Other mechanical complication of breast prosthesis and implant   `CC`
     Obstruction (mechanical) of breast prosthesis and implant
     Perforation of breast prosthesis and implant
     Protrusion of breast prosthesis and implant

√5ᵗʰ **T85.5** Mechanical complication of gastrointestinal prosthetic devices, implants and grafts

     CC Excl: For CC codes in subcategory T85.5: PDX collection 1464

√6ᵗʰ **T85.51** Breakdown (mechanical) of gastrointestinal prosthetic devices, implants and grafts

     √7ᵗʰ **T85.510** Breakdown (mechanical) of bile duct prosthesis   `CC`

     √7ᵗʰ **T85.511** Breakdown (mechanical) of esophageal anti-reflux device   `CC`

     √7ᵗʰ **T85.518** Breakdown (mechanical) of other gastrointestinal prosthetic devices, implants and grafts   `CC`

√6ᵗʰ **T85.52** Displacement of gastrointestinal prosthetic devices, implants and grafts
     Malposition of gastrointestinal prosthetic devices, implants and grafts

     √7ᵗʰ **T85.520** Displacement of bile duct prosthesis   `CC`

     √7ᵗʰ **T85.521** Displacement of esophageal anti-reflux device   `CC`

     √7ᵗʰ **T85.528** Displacement of other gastrointestinal prosthetic devices, implants and grafts   `CC`

√6ᵗʰ **T85.59** Other mechanical complication of gastrointestinal prosthetic devices, implants and grafts
     Obstruction, mechanical of gastrointestinal prosthetic devices, implants and grafts
     Perforation of gastrointestinal prosthetic devices, implants and grafts
     Protrusion of gastrointestinal prosthetic devices, implants and grafts

     √7ᵗʰ **T85.590** Other mechanical complication of bile duct prosthesis   `CC`

     √7ᵗʰ **T85.591** Other mechanical complication of esophageal anti-reflux device   `CC`

     √7ᵗʰ **T85.598** Other mechanical complication of other gastrointestinal prosthetic devices, implants and grafts   `CC`

√5ᵗʰ **T85.6** Mechanical complication of other specified internal and external prosthetic devices, implants and grafts

√6ᵗʰ **T85.61** Breakdown (mechanical) of other specified internal prosthetic devices, implants and grafts

     √7ᵗʰ **T85.610** Breakdown (mechanical) of cranial or spinal infusion catheter   `CC`
         Breakdown (mechanical) of epidural infusion catheter
         Breakdown (mechanical) of intrathecal infusion catheter
         Breakdown (mechanical) of subarachnoid infusion catheter
         Breakdown (mechanical) of subdural infusion catheter
         CC Excl: PDX collection 1465

     √7ᵗʰ **T85.611** Breakdown (mechanical) of intraperitoneal dialysis catheter   `CC` `HCC`
         EXCLUDES 1 mechanical complication of vascular dialysis catheter (T82.4-)
         CC Excl: PDX collection 1466

     √7ᵗʰ **T85.612** Breakdown (mechanical) of permanent sutures   `CC`
         EXCLUDES 1 mechanical complication of permanent (wire) suture used in bone repair (T84.1-T84.2)
         CC Excl: PDX collection 1467

     √7ᵗʰ **T85.613** Breakdown (mechanical) of artificial skin graft and decellularized allodermis   `CC`
         Failure of artificial skin graft and decellularized allodermis
         Non-adherence of artificial skin graft and decellularized allodermis
         Poor incorporation of artificial skin graft and decellularized allodermis
         Shearing of artificial skin graft and decellularized allodermis
         CC Excl: PDX collection 1468

     √7ᵗʰ **T85.614** Breakdown (mechanical) of insulin pump   `CC`
         CC Excl: PDX collection 1469

     6 √7ᵗʰ **T85.615** Breakdown (mechanical) of other nervous system device, implant or graft   `CC` `HCC`
         Breakdown (mechanical) of intrathecal infusion pump
         CC Excl: PDX collection 1467

     √7ᵗʰ **T85.618** Breakdown (mechanical) of other specified internal prosthetic devices, implants and grafts   `CC`
         CC Excl: PDX collection 1467

N Newborn: 0   **P** Pediatric: 0-17   **M** Maternity: 9-64   **A** Adult: 15-124   **MCC** Major Complication/Comorbidity   **CC** Complication/Comorbidity   **SW** Severe Wound Dx

1204   ICD-10-CM 2020

√6ᵗʰ **T85.62** Displacement of other specified internal prosthetic devices, implants and grafts

Malposition of other specified internal prosthetic devices, implants and grafts

√7ᵗʰ **T85.620** Displacement of cranial or spinal infusion catheter   CC

Displacement of epidural infusion catheter

Displacement of intrathecal infusion catheter

Displacement of subarachnoid infusion catheter

Displacement of subdural infusion catheter

CC Excl: PDX collection 1465

√7ᵗʰ **T85.621** Displacement of intraperitoneal dialysis catheter   CC HCC

> EXCLUDES 1   mechanical complication of vascular dialysis catheter (T82.4-)

CC Excl: PDX collection 1466

√7ᵗʰ **T85.622** Displacement of permanent sutures   CC

> EXCLUDES 1   mechanical complication of permanent (wire) suture used in bone repair (T84.1-T84.2)

CC Excl: PDX collection 1467

√7ᵗʰ **T85.623** Displacement of artificial skin graft and decellularized allodermis   CC

Dislodgement of artificial skin graft and decellularized allodermis

CC Excl: PDX collection 1468

√7ᵗʰ **T85.624** Displacement of insulin pump   CC

CC Excl: PDX collection 1469

6 √7ᵗʰ **T85.625** Displacement of other nervous system device, implant or graft   CC HCC

Displacement of intrathecal infusion pump

CC Excl: PDX collection 1467

√7ᵗʰ **T85.628** Displacement of other specified internal prosthetic devices, implants and grafts   CC

CC Excl: PDX collection 1467

√6ᵗʰ **T85.63** Leakage of other specified internal prosthetic devices, implants and grafts

√7ᵗʰ **T85.630** Leakage of cranial or spinal infusion catheter   CC

Leakage of epidural infusion catheter

Leakage of intrathecal infusion catheter infusion catheter

Leakage of subdural infusion catheter

Leakage of subarachnoid infusion catheter

CC Excl: PDX collection 1465

√7ᵗʰ **T85.631** Leakage of intraperitoneal dialysis catheter   CC HCC

> EXCLUDES 1   mechanical complication of vascular dialysis catheter (T82.4)

CC Excl: PDX collection 1466

√7ᵗʰ **T85.633** Leakage of insulin pump   CC

CC Excl: PDX collection 1469

6 √7ᵗʰ **T85.635** Leakage of other nervous system device, implant or graft   CC HCC

Leakage of intrathecal infusion pump

CC Excl: PDX collection 1467

√7ᵗʰ **T85.638** Leakage of other specified internal prosthetic devices, implants and grafts   CC

CC Excl: PDX collection 1467

√6ᵗʰ **T85.69** Other mechanical complication of other specified internal prosthetic devices, implants and grafts

Obstruction, mechanical of other specified internal prosthetic devices, implants and grafts

Perforation of other specified internal prosthetic devices, implants and grafts

Protrusion of other specified internal prosthetic devices, implants and grafts

√7ᵗʰ **T85.690** Other mechanical complication of cranial or spinal infusion catheter   CC

Other mechanical complication of epidural infusion catheter

Other mechanical complication of intrathecal infusion catheter

Other mechanical complication of subarachnoid infusion catheter

Other mechanical complication of subdural infusion catheter

CC Excl: PDX collection 1465

√7ᵗʰ **T85.691** Other mechanical complication of intraperitoneal dialysis catheter   CC HCC

> EXCLUDES 1   mechanical complication of vascular dialysis catheter (T82.4)

CC Excl: PDX collection 1466

√7ᵗʰ **T85.692** Other mechanical complication of permanent sutures   CC

> EXCLUDES 1   mechanical complication of permanent (wire) suture used in bone repair (T84.1-T84.2)

CC Excl: PDX collection 1467

√7ᵗʰ **T85.693** Other mechanical complication of artificial skin graft and decellularized allodermis   CC

CC Excl: PDX collection 1468

√7ᵗʰ **T85.694** Other mechanical complication of insulin pump   CC

CC Excl: PDX collection 1469

6 √7ᵗʰ **T85.695** Other mechanical complication of other nervous system device, implant or graft   CC HCC

Other mechanical complication of intrathecal infusion pump

CC Excl: PDX collection 1467

√7ᵗʰ **T85.698** Other mechanical complication of other specified internal prosthetic devices, implants and grafts   CC

Mechanical complication of nonabsorbable surgical material NOS

CC Excl: PDX collection 1467

√5ᵗʰ **T85.7** Infection and inflammatory reaction due to other internal prosthetic devices, implants and grafts

Use additional code to identify infection

CC Excl: For CC codes in subcategory T85.7, unless otherwise noted: PDX collection 1470

√x7ᵗʰ **T85.71** Infection and inflammatory reaction due to peritoneal dialysis catheter   CC HCC

CC Excl: PDX collection 1467

6 √x7ᵗʰ **T85.72** Infection and inflammatory reaction due to insulin pump   CC HCC

√6ᵗʰ **T85.73** Infection and inflammatory reaction due to nervous system devices, implants and graft

6 √7ᵗʰ **T85.730** Infection and inflammatory reaction due to ventricular intracranial (communicating) shunt   CC HCC

6 √7ᵗʰ **T85.731** Infection and inflammatory reaction due to implanted electronic neurostimulator of brain, electrode (lead)   CC HCC

☑ Additional Character Required   √x7ᵗʰ Placeholder   Unacceptable PDx   Questionable PDx   Manifestation   Unspecified Dx   H1-H14 HAC   HCC CMS-HCC Dx   HIV HIV Dx

ICD-10-CM 2020   1205

6 ✓7ᵗʰ **T85.732 Infection and inflammatory reaction due to implanted electronic neurostimulator of peripheral nerve, electrode (lead)** CC HCC

> Infection and inflammatory reaction due to electrode (lead) for cranial nerve neurostimulators
>
> Infection and inflammatory reaction due to electrode (lead) for gastric neurostimulator
>
> Infection and inflammatory reaction due to electrode (lead) for sacral nerve neurostimulator
>
> Infection and inflammatory reaction due to electrode (lead) for vagal nerve neurostimulators

6 ✓7ᵗʰ **T85.733 Infection and inflammatory reaction due to implanted electronic neurostimulator of spinal cord, electrode (lead)** CC HCC

6 ✓7ᵗʰ **T85.734 Infection and inflammatory reaction due to implanted electronic neurostimulator, generator** CC HCC

> Generator pocket infection

6 ✓7ᵗʰ **T85.735 Infection and inflammatory reaction due to cranial or spinal infusion catheter** CC HCC

> Infection and inflammatory reaction due to epidural catheter
>
> Infection and inflammatory reaction due to intrathecal infusion catheter
>
> Infection and inflammatory reaction due to subarachnoid catheter
>
> Infection and inflammatory reaction due to subdural catheter

6 ✓7ᵗʰ **T85.738 Infection and inflammatory reaction due to other nervous system device, implant or graft** CC HCC

> Infection and inflammatory reaction due to intrathecal infusion pump

6 ✓×7ᵗʰ **T85.79 Infection and inflammatory reaction due to other internal prosthetic devices, implants and grafts** CC HCC

✓5ᵗʰ **T85.8 Other specified complications of internal prosthetic devices, implants and grafts, not elsewhere classified**

CC Excl: For codes in subcategory T85.8: CC with 7th character A or D: PDX collection 1470

✓6ᵗʰ **T85.81 Embolism due to internal prosthetic devices, implants and grafts, not elsewhere classified**

5,6 ✓7ᵗʰ **T85.810 Embolism due to nervous system prosthetic devices, implants and grafts** CC HCC

✓7ᵗʰ **T85.818 Embolism due to other internal prosthetic devices, implants and grafts**

✓6ᵗʰ **T85.82 Fibrosis due to internal prosthetic devices, implants and grafts, not elsewhere classified**

5,6 ✓7ᵗʰ **T85.820 Fibrosis due to nervous system prosthetic devices, implants and grafts** CC HCC

✓7ᵗʰ **T85.828 Fibrosis due to other internal prosthetic devices, implants and grafts**

✓6ᵗʰ **T85.83 Hemorrhage due to internal prosthetic devices, implants and grafts, not elsewhere classified**

5,6 ✓7ᵗʰ **T85.830 Hemorrhage due to nervous system prosthetic devices, implants and grafts** CC HCC

✓7ᵗʰ **T85.838 Hemorrhage due to other internal prosthetic devices, implants and grafts**

✓6ᵗʰ **T85.84 Pain due to internal prosthetic devices, implants and grafts, not elsewhere classified**

5,6 ✓7ᵗʰ **T85.840 Pain due to nervous system prosthetic devices, implants and grafts** CC HCC

✓7ᵗʰ **T85.848 Pain due to other internal prosthetic devices, implants and grafts**

✓6ᵗʰ **T85.85 Stenosis due to internal prosthetic devices, implants and grafts, not elsewhere classified**

5,6 ✓7ᵗʰ **T85.850 Stenosis due to nervous system prosthetic devices, implants and grafts** CC HCC

✓7ᵗʰ **T85.858 Stenosis due to other internal prosthetic devices, implants and grafts**

✓6ᵗʰ **T85.86 Thrombosis due to internal prosthetic devices, implants and grafts, not elsewhere classified**

5,6 ✓7ᵗʰ **T85.860 Thrombosis due to nervous system prosthetic devices, implants and grafts** CC HCC

✓7ᵗʰ **T85.868 Thrombosis due to other internal prosthetic devices, implants and grafts**

✓6ᵗʰ **T85.89 Other specified complication of internal prosthetic devices, implants and grafts, not elsewhere classified**

> Erosion or breakdown of subcutaneous device pocket

5,6 ✓7ᵗʰ **T85.890 Other specified complication of nervous system prosthetic devices, implants and grafts** CC HCC

✓7ᵗʰ **T85.898 Other specified complication of other internal prosthetic devices, implants and grafts**

✓×7ᵗʰ **T85.9 Unspecified complication of internal prosthetic device, implant and graft**

> Complication of internal prosthetic device, implant and graft NOS

✓4ᵗʰ **T86 Complications of transplanted organs and tissue**

> Use additional code to identify other transplant complications, such as:
> graft-versus-host disease (D89.81-)
> malignancy associated with organ transplant (C80.2)
> post-transplant lymphoproliferative disorders (PTLD) (D47.Z1)

✓5ᵗʰ **T86.0 Complications of bone marrow transplant**

CC Excl: For CC codes in subcategory T86.0: PDX collection 514

T86.00 Unspecified complication of bone marrow transplant CC HCC

T86.01 Bone marrow transplant rejection CC HCC

T86.02 Bone marrow transplant failure CC HCC

T86.03 Bone marrow transplant infection CC HCC

T86.09 Other complications of bone marrow transplant CC HCC

✓5ᵗʰ **T86.1 Complications of kidney transplant**

CC Excl: For CC codes in subcategory T86.1: PDX collection 1471

T86.10 Unspecified complication of kidney transplant CC

T86.11 Kidney transplant rejection CC

T86.12 Kidney transplant failure CC

AHA: 2013,1Q,24

T86.13 Kidney transplant infection CC

> Use additional code to specify infection

T86.19 Other complication of kidney transplant CC

AHA: 2019,2Q,7

✓5ᵗʰ **T86.2 Complications of heart transplant**

EXCLUDES 1 complication of:
artificial heart device (T82.5)
heart-lung transplant (T86.3)

CC Excl: For CC codes in subcategory T86.2: PDX collection 1472

T86.20 Unspecified complication of heart transplant CC HCC

T86.21 Heart transplant rejection CC HCC

T86.22 Heart transplant failure CC HCC

T86.23 Heart transplant infection CC HCC

> Use additional code to specify infection

✓6ᵗʰ **T86.29 Other complications of heart transplant**

T86.290 Cardiac allograft vasculopathy CC HCC

EXCLUDES 1 atherosclerosis of coronary arteries (I25.75-, I25.76-, I25.81-)

T86.298 Other complications of heart transplant CC HCC

N Newborn: 0 P Pediatric: 0-17 M Maternity: 9-64 A Adult: 15-124 MCC Major Complication/Comorbidity CC Complication/Comorbidity SW Severe Wound Dx

1206 ICD-10-CM 2020

√5ᵗʰ T86.3 Complications of heart-lung transplant

CC Excl: For CC codes in subcategory T86.3: PDX collection 1472

T86.30 Unspecified complication of heart-lung transplant `CC` `HCC`

T86.31 Heart-lung transplant rejection `CC` `HCC`

T86.32 Heart-lung transplant failure `CC` `HCC`

T86.33 Heart-lung transplant infection `CC` `HCC`
Use additional code to specify infection

T86.39 Other complications of heart-lung transplant `CC` `HCC`

√5ᵗʰ T86.4 Complications of liver transplant

CC Excl: For CC codes in subcategory T86.4: PDX collection 1473

T86.40 Unspecified complication of liver transplant `CC` `HCC`

T86.41 Liver transplant rejection `CC` `HCC`

T86.42 Liver transplant failure `CC` `HCC`

T86.43 Liver transplant infection `CC` `HCC`
Use additional code to identify infection, such as: cytomegalovirus (CMV) infection (B25.-)

T86.49 Other complications of liver transplant `CC` `HCC`

T86.5 Complications of stem cell transplant `CC` `HCC`
Complications from stem cells from peripheral blood
Complications from stem cells from umbilical cord
CC Excl: PDX collection 1474

√5ᵗʰ T86.8 Complications of other transplanted organs and tissues

√6ᵗʰ T86.81 Complications of lung transplant

EXCLUDES 1   complication of heart-lung transplant (T86.3-)

CC Excl: For CC codes in subcategory T86.81: PDX collection 1475

T86.810 Lung transplant rejection `CC` `HCC`

T86.811 Lung transplant failure `CC` `HCC`

T86.812 Lung transplant infection `CC` `HCC`
Use additional code to specify infection

T86.818 Other complications of lung transplant `CC` `HCC`
AHA: 2019,2Q,6

T86.819 Unspecified complication of lung transplant `CC` `HCC`

√6ᵗʰ T86.82 Complications of skin graft (allograft) (autograft)

EXCLUDES 2   complication of artificial skin graft (T85.693)

CC Excl: For CC codes in subcategory T86.82: PDX collection 1476

T86.820 Skin graft (allograft) rejection `CC`

T86.821 Skin graft (allograft) (autograft) failure `CC`

T86.822 Skin graft (allograft) (autograft) infection `CC`
Use additional code to specify infection

T86.828 Other complications of skin graft (allograft) (autograft) `CC`

T86.829 Unspecified complication of skin graft (allograft) (autograft) `CC`

√6ᵗʰ T86.83 Complications of bone graft

EXCLUDES 2   mechanical complications of bone graft (T84.3-)

CC Excl: For CC codes in subcategory T86.83: PDX collection 1477

T86.830 Bone graft rejection `CC`

T86.831 Bone graft failure `CC`

T86.832 Bone graft infection `CC`
Use additional code to specify infection

T86.838 Other complications of bone graft `CC`

T86.839 Unspecified complication of bone graft `CC`

√6ᵗʰ T86.84 Complications of corneal transplant

EXCLUDES 2   mechanical complications of corneal graft (T85.3-)

CC Excl: For CC codes in subcategory T86.84, unless otherwise noted: PDX collection 1479

T86.840 Corneal transplant rejection `CC`
CC Excl: PDX collection 1478

T86.841 Corneal transplant failure `CC`
CC Excl: PDX collection 1478

T86.842 Corneal transplant infection `CC` `HCC`
Use additional code to specify infection

T86.848 Other complications of corneal transplant `CC`

T86.849 Unspecified complication of corneal transplant `CC`

√6ᵗʰ T86.85 Complication of intestine transplant

CC Excl: For CC codes in subcategory T86.85: PDX collection 495

T86.850 Intestine transplant rejection `CC` `HCC`

T86.851 Intestine transplant failure `CC` `HCC`

T86.852 Intestine transplant infection `CC` `HCC`
Use additional code to specify infection

T86.858 Other complications of intestine transplant `CC` `HCC`

T86.859 Unspecified complication of intestine transplant `CC` `HCC`

√6ᵗʰ T86.89 Complications of other transplanted tissue
Transplant failure or rejection of pancreas

CC Excl: For CC codes in subcategory T86.89: PDX collection 1480

T86.890 Other transplanted tissue rejection `CC`

T86.891 Other transplanted tissue failure `CC`

T86.892 Other transplanted tissue infection `CC`
Use additional code to specify infection

T86.898 Other complications of other transplanted tissue `CC`

T86.899 Unspecified complication of other transplanted tissue `CC`

√5ᵗʰ T86.9 Complication of unspecified transplanted organ and tissue

CC Excl: For CC codes in subcategory T86.9: PDX collection 495

T86.90 Unspecified complication of unspecified transplanted organ and tissue `CC`

T86.91 Unspecified transplanted organ and tissue rejection `CC`

T86.92 Unspecified transplanted organ and tissue failure `CC`

T86.93 Unspecified transplanted organ and tissue infection `CC`
Use additional code to specify infection

T86.99 Other complications of unspecified transplanted organ and tissue `CC`

√4ᵗʰ T87 Complications peculiar to reattachment and amputation

√5ᵗʰ T87.0 Complications of reattached (part of) upper extremity

√6ᵗʰ T87.0X Complications of reattached (part of) upper extremity

CC Excl: For CC codes in subcategory T87.0X: PDX collection 1481

T87.0X1 Complications of reattached (part of) right upper extremity `CC` `HCC`

T87.0X2 Complications of reattached (part of) left upper extremity `CC` `HCC`

T87.0X9 Complications of reattached (part of) unspecified upper extremity `CC` `HCC`

✔ Additional Character Required   √xⁿᵗʰ Placeholder   **Unacceptable PDx**   Questionable PDx   Manifestation   Unspecified Dx   H1-H14 HAC   HCC CMS-HCC Dx   HIV HIV Dx

ICD-10-CM 2020   1207

Chapter 19. Injury, Poisoning and Certain Other Consequences of External Causes

T87.1–T88.6

√5ᵗʰ **T87.1** **Complications of reattached (part of) lower extremity**

     √6ᵗʰ **T87.1X** **Complications of reattached (part of) lower extremity**

         CC Excl: For CC codes in subcategory T87.1X: PDX collection 1482

         T87.1X1 **Complications of reattached (part of) right lower extremity**   CC HCC

         T87.1X2 **Complications of reattached (part of) left lower extremity**   CC HCC

         T87.1X9 **Complications of reattached (part of) unspecified lower extremity**   CC HCC

     T87.2 **Complications of other reattached body part**   CC HCC

         CC Excl: PDX collection 1483

√5ᵗʰ **T87.3** **Neuroma of amputation stump**

     DEF: Non-neoplastic tumor generated at the proximal end of severed, partially transected, or injured nerve following amputation.

     T87.30 **Neuroma of amputation stump, unspecified extremity**   HCC

     T87.31 **Neuroma of amputation stump, right upper extremity**   HCC

     T87.32 **Neuroma of amputation stump, left upper extremity**   HCC

     T87.33 **Neuroma of amputation stump, right lower extremity**   HCC

     T87.34 **Neuroma of amputation stump, left lower extremity**   HCC

√5ᵗʰ **T87.4** **Infection of amputation stump**

     CC Excl: For CC codes in subcategory T87.4: PDX collection 1484

     T87.40 **Infection of amputation stump, unspecified extremity**   CC HCC

     T87.41 **Infection of amputation stump, right upper extremity**   CC HCC

     T87.42 **Infection of amputation stump, left upper extremity**   CC HCC

     T87.43 **Infection of amputation stump, right lower extremity**   CC HCC

     T87.44 **Infection of amputation stump, left lower extremity**   CC HCC

√5ᵗʰ **T87.5** **Necrosis of amputation stump**

     T87.50 **Necrosis of amputation stump, unspecified extremity**   HCC

     T87.51 **Necrosis of amputation stump, right upper extremity**   HCC

     T87.52 **Necrosis of amputation stump, left upper extremity**   HCC

     T87.53 **Necrosis of amputation stump, right lower extremity**   HCC

     T87.54 **Necrosis of amputation stump, left lower extremity**   HCC

√5ᵗʰ **T87.8** **Other complications of amputation stump**

     T87.81 **Dehiscence of amputation stump**   HCC

     T87.89 **Other complications of amputation stump**   HCC

         Amputation stump contracture

         Amputation stump contracture of next proximal joint

         Amputation stump flexion

         Amputation stump edema

         Amputation stump hematoma

         EXCLUDES 2   *phantom limb syndrome (G54.6-G54.7)*

     T87.9 **Unspecified complications of amputation stump**   HCC

√4ᵗʰ **T88** **Other complications of surgical and medical care, not elsewhere classified**

     EXCLUDES 2   *complication following infusion, transfusion and therapeutic injection (T80.-)*

         complication following procedure NEC (T81.-)

         complications of anesthesia in labor and delivery (O74.-)

         complications of anesthesia in pregnancy (O29.-)

         complications of anesthesia in puerperium (O89.-)

         complications of devices, implants and grafts (T82-T85)

         complications of obstetric surgery and procedure (O75.4)

         dermatitis due to drugs and medicaments (L23.3, L24.4, L25.1, L27.0-L27.1)

         poisoning and toxic effects of drugs and chemicals (T36-T65 with fifth or sixth character 1-4 or 6)

         specified complications classified elsewhere

The appropriate 7th character is to be added to each code from category T88.

A   initial encounter

D   subsequent encounter

S   sequela

√x7ᵗʰ **T88.0** **Infection following immunization**   CC

     Sepsis following immunization

     AHA: 2018,4Q,62-63

     CC Excl: PDX collection 948

√x7ᵗʰ **T88.1** **Other complications following immunization, not elsewhere classified**   CC

     Generalized vaccinia

     Rash following immunization

     EXCLUDES 1   *vaccinia not from vaccine (B08.011)*

     EXCLUDES 2   *anaphylactic shock due to serum (T80.5-)*

         other serum reactions (T80.6-)

         postimmunization arthropathy (M02.2)

         postimmunization encephalitis (G04.02)

         postimmunization fever (R50.83)

     CC Excl: PDX collection 1485

√x7ᵗʰ **T88.2** **Shock due to anesthesia**   CC

     Use additional code for adverse effect, if applicable, to identify drug (T41.- with fifth or sixth character 5)

     EXCLUDES 1   *complications of anesthesia (in):*

         labor and delivery (O74.-)

         postprocedural shock NOS (T81.1-)

         pregnancy (O29.-)

         puerperium (O89.-)

     CC Excl: PDX collection 1441

√x7ᵗʰ **T88.3** **Malignant hyperthermia due to anesthesia**   CC

     Use additional code for adverse effect, if applicable, to identify drug (T41.- with fifth or sixth character 5)

     CC Excl: PDX collection 1486

√x7ᵗʰ **T88.4** **Failed or difficult intubation**

√5ᵗʰ **T88.5** **Other complications of anesthesia**

     Use additional code for adverse effect, if applicable, to identify drug (T41.- with fifth or sixth character 5)

     √x7ᵗʰ **T88.51** **Hypothermia following anesthesia**

     √x7ᵗʰ **T88.52** **Failed moderate sedation during procedure**

         Failed conscious sedation during procedure

         EXCLUDES 2   *personal history of failed moderate sedation (Z92.83)*

     √x7ᵗʰ **T88.53** **Unintended awareness under general anesthesia during procedure**

         EXCLUDES 2   *personal history of unintended awareness under general anesthesia (Z92.84)*

         AHA: 2016,4Q,72-73

     √x7ᵗʰ **T88.59** **Other complications of anesthesia**

√x7ᵗʰ **T88.6** **Anaphylactic reaction due to adverse effect of correct drug or medicament properly administered**   CC

     Anaphylactic shock due to adverse effect of correct drug or medicament properly administered

     Anaphylactoid reaction NOS

     Use additional code for adverse effect, if applicable, to identify drug (T36-T50 with fifth or sixth character 5)

     EXCLUDES 1   *anaphylactic reaction due to serum (T80.5-)*

         anaphylactic shock or reaction due to adverse food reaction (T78.0-)

     CC Excl: PDX collection 1426

N Newborn: 0   P Pediatric: 0-17   M Maternity: 9-64   A Adult: 15-124   MCC Major Complication/Comorbidity   CC Complication/Comorbidity   SW Severe Wound Dx

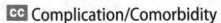

1208   **ICD-10-CM 2020**

✓x7ᵗʰ **T88.7** **Unspecified adverse effect of drug or medicament**

         Drug hypersensitivity NOS

         Drug reaction NOS

         Use additional code for adverse effect, if applicable, to identify drug (T36-T5Ø with fifth or sixth character 5)

         EXCLUDES 1   *specified adverse effects of drugs and medicaments (AØØ-R94 and T8Ø-T88.6, T88.8)*

✓x7ᵗʰ **T88.8** **Other specified complications of surgical and medical care, not elsewhere classified**

         Use additional code to identify the complication

✓x7ᵗʰ **T88.9** **Complication of surgical and medical care, unspecified**

✔ Additional Character Required   ✓x7ᵗʰ Placeholder   <u>Unacceptable PDx</u>   Questionable PDx   Manifestation   <u>Unspecified Dx</u>   H1-H14 HAC   HCC CMS-HCC Dx   HIV HIV Dx

ICD-10-CM 2020   **1209**

Chapter 20. External Causes of Morbidity (V00–Y99)

Chapter-specific Guidelines with Coding Examples

The chapter-specific guidelines from the ICD-10-CM Official Guidelines for Coding and Reporting have been provided below. Along with these guidelines are coding examples, contained in the shaded boxes, that have been developed to help illustrate the coding and/or sequencing guidance found in these guidelines.

The external causes of morbidity codes should never be sequenced as the first-listed or principal diagnosis.

External cause codes are intended to provide data for injury research and evaluation of injury prevention strategies. These codes capture how the injury or health condition happened (cause), the intent (unintentional or accidental; or intentional, such as suicide or assault), the place where the event occurred the activity of the patient at the time of the event, and the person's status (e.g., civilian, military).

There is no national requirement for mandatory ICD-10-CM external cause code reporting. Unless a provider is subject to a state-based external cause code reporting mandate or these codes are required by a particular payer, reporting of ICD-10-CM codes in Chapter 20, External Causes of Morbidity, is not required. In the absence of a mandatory reporting requirement, providers are encouraged to voluntarily report external cause codes, as they provide valuable data for injury research and evaluation of injury prevention strategies.

a. General external cause coding guidelines

1) Used with any code in the range of A00.0–T88.9, Z00–Z99

An external cause code may be used with any code in the range of A00.0–T88.9, Z00-Z99, classification that represents a health condition due to an external cause. Though they are most applicable to injuries, they are also valid for use with such things as infections or diseases due to an external source, and other health conditions, such as a heart attack that occurs during strenuous physical activity.

Actinic reticuloid due to tanning bed use	
L57.1	Actinic reticuloid
W89.1XXA	Exposure to tanning bed, initial encounter

Explanation: An external cause code may be used with any code in the range of A00.0–T88.9, Z00–Z99, classifications that describe health conditions due to an external cause. Code W89.1 Exposure to tanning bed requires a seventh character of A to report this initial encounter, with a placeholder X for the fifth and sixth characters.

2) External cause code used for length of treatment

Assign the external cause code, with the appropriate 7th character (initial encounter, subsequent encounter or sequela) for each encounter for which the injury or condition is being treated.

Most categories in chapter 20 have a 7th character requirement for each applicable code. Most categories in this chapter have three 7th character values: A, initial encounter, D, subsequent encounter and S, sequela. While the patient may be seen by a new or different provider over the course of treatment for an injury or condition, assignment of the 7th character for external cause should match the 7th character of the code assigned for the associated injury or condition for the encounter.

3) Use the full range of external cause codes

Use the full range of external cause codes to completely describe the cause, the intent, the place of occurrence, and if applicable, the activity of the patient at the time of the event, and the patient's status, for all injuries, and other health conditions due to an external cause.

4) Assign as many external cause codes as necessary

Assign as many external cause codes as necessary to fully explain each cause. If only one external code can be recorded, assign the code most related to the principal diagnosis.

5) The selection of the appropriate external cause code

The selection of the appropriate external cause code is guided by the Alphabetic Index of External Causes and by Inclusion and Exclusion notes in the Tabular List.

6) External cause code can never be a principal diagnosis

An external cause code can never be a principal (first-listed) diagnosis.

7) Combination external cause codes

Certain of the external cause codes are combination codes that identify sequential events that result in an injury, such as a fall which results in striking against an object. The injury may be due to either event or both.

The combination external cause code used should correspond to the sequence of events regardless of which caused the most serious injury.

Toddler tripped and fell while walking and struck his head on an end table, sustaining a scalp contusion	
S00.03XA	Contusion of scalp, initial encounter
W01.190A	Fall on same level from slipping, tripping and stumbling with subsequent striking against furniture, initial encounter

Explanation: Combination external cause codes identify sequential events that result in an injury, such as a fall resulting in striking against an object. The injury may be due to either or both events.

8) No external cause code needed in certain circumstances

No external cause code from Chapter 20 is needed if the external cause and intent are included in a code from another chapter (e.g. T36.0X1-Poisoning by penicillins, accidental (unintentional)).

b. Place of occurrence guideline

Codes from category Y92, Place of occurrence of the external cause, are secondary codes for use after other external cause codes to identify the location of the patient at the time of injury or other condition.

Generally, a place of occurrence code is assigned only once, at the initial encounter for treatment. However, in the rare instance that a new injury occurs during hospitalization, an additional place of occurrence code may be assigned. No 7th characters are used for Y92.

Do not use place of occurrence code Y92.9 if the place is not stated or is not applicable.

A farmer was working in his barn and sustained a foot contusion when the horse stepped on his left foot	
S90.32XA	Contusion of left foot, initial encounter
W55.19XA	Other contact with horse, initial encounter
Y92.71	Barn as the place of occurrence of the external cause

Explanation: A place-of-occurrence code from category Y92 is assigned at the initial encounter to identify the location of the patient at the time the injury occurred.

c. Activity code

Assign a code from category Y93, Activity code, to describe the activity of the patient at the time the injury or other health condition occurred.

An activity code is used only once, at the initial encounter for treatment. Only one code from Y93 should be recorded on a medical record.

The activity codes are not applicable to poisonings, adverse effects, misadventures or sequela.

Do not assign Y93.9, Unspecified activity, if the activity is not stated.

A code from category Y93 is appropriate for use with external cause and intent codes if identifying the activity provides additional information about the event.

Ranch hand who was grooming a horse sustained a foot contusion when the horse stepped on his left foot	
S90.32XA	Contusion of left foot, initial encounter
W55.19XA	Other contact with horse, initial encounter
Y93.K3	Activity, grooming and shearing an animal

Explanation: One activity code from category Y93 is assigned at the initial encounter only to describe the activity of the patient at the time the injury occurred.

d. Place of occurrence, activity, and status codes used with other external cause code

When applicable, place of occurrence, activity, and external cause status codes are sequenced after the main external cause code(s). Regardless of the number of external cause codes assigned, generally there should be only one place of occurrence code, one activity code, and one external cause status code assigned to an encounter. However, in the rare instance that a new injury occurs during hospitalization, an additional place of occurrence code may be assigned.

e. If the reporting format limits the number of external cause codes

If the reporting format limits the number of external cause codes that can be used in reporting clinical data, report the code for the cause/intent most related to the principal diagnosis. If the format permits capture of additional external cause codes, the cause/intent, including medical misadventures, of the additional events should be reported rather than the codes for place, activity, or external status.

f. Multiple external cause coding guidelines

More than one external cause code is required to fully describe the external cause of an illness or injury. The assignment of external cause codes should be sequenced in the following priority:

If two or more events cause separate injuries, an external cause code should be assigned for each cause. The first-listed external cause code will be selected in the following order:

External codes for child and adult abuse take priority over all other external cause codes.

See Section I.C.19., Child and Adult abuse guidelines.

External cause codes for terrorism events take priority over all other external cause codes except child and adult abuse.

External cause codes for cataclysmic events take priority over all other external cause codes except child and adult abuse and terrorism.

External cause codes for transport accidents take priority over all other external cause codes except cataclysmic events, child and adult abuse and terrorism.

Activity and external cause status codes are assigned following all causal (intent) external cause codes.

The first-listed external cause code should correspond to the cause of the most serious diagnosis due to an assault, accident, or self-harm, following the order of hierarchy listed above..

30-year-old man accidentally discharged his hunting rifle, sustaining an open gunshot wound to the right thigh, which caused him to fall down the stairs, resulting in closed displaced comminuted fracture of his left radial shaft	
S71.131A	**Puncture wound without foreign body, right thigh, initial encounter**
W33.02XA	**Accidental discharge of hunting rifle, initial encounter**
S52.352A	**Displaced comminuted fracture of shaft of radius, left arm, initial encounter for closed fracture**
W10.9XXA	**Fall (on) (from) unspecified stairs and steps, initial encounter**

Explanation: If two or more events cause separate injuries, an external cause code should be assigned for each cause.

g. Child and adult abuse guideline

Adult and child abuse, neglect and maltreatment are classified as assault. Any of the assault codes may be used to indicate the external cause of any injury resulting from the confirmed abuse.

For confirmed cases of abuse, neglect and maltreatment, when the perpetrator is known, a code from Y07, Perpetrator of maltreatment and neglect, should accompany any other assault codes.

See Section I.C.19. Adult and child abuse, neglect and other maltreatment

h. Unknown or undetermined intent guideline

If the intent (accident, self-harm, assault) of the cause of an injury or other condition is unknown or unspecified, code the intent as accidental intent. All transport accident categories assume accidental intent.

1) Use of undetermined intent

External cause codes for events of undetermined intent are only for use if the documentation in the record specifies that the intent cannot be determined.

i. Sequelae (late effects) of external cause guidelines

1) Sequelae external cause codes

Sequela are reported using the external cause code with the 7th character "S" for sequela. These codes should be used with any report of a late effect or sequela resulting from a previous injury.

See Section I.B.10 Sequela (Late Effects)

2) Sequela external cause code with a related current injury

A sequela external cause code should never be used with a related current nature of injury code.

3) Use of sequela external cause codes for subsequent visits

Use a late effect external cause code for subsequent visits when a late effect of the initial injury is being treated. Do not use a late effect external cause code for subsequent visits for follow-up care (e.g., to assess healing, to receive rehabilitative therapy) of the injury when no late effect of the injury has been documented.

j. Terrorism guidelines

1) Cause of injury identified by the Federal Government (FBI) as terrorism

When the cause of an injury is identified by the Federal Government (FBI) as terrorism, the first-listed external cause code should be a code from category Y38, Terrorism. The definition of terrorism employed by the FBI is found at the inclusion note at the beginning of category Y38. Use additional code for place of occurrence (Y92.-). More than one Y38 code may be assigned if the injury is the result of more than one mechanism of terrorism.

2) Cause of an injury is suspected to be the result of terrorism

When the cause of an injury is suspected to be the result of terrorism a code from category Y38 should not be assigned. Suspected cases should be classified as assault.

3) Code Y38.9, Terrorism, secondary effects

Assign code Y38.9, Terrorism, secondary effects, for conditions occurring subsequent to the terrorist event. This code should not be assigned for conditions that are due to the initial terrorist act.

It is acceptable to assign code Y38.9 with another code from Y38 if there is an injury due to the initial terrorist event and an injury that is a subsequent result of the terrorist event.

k. External cause status

A code from category Y99, External cause status, should be assigned whenever any other external cause code is assigned for an encounter, including an Activity code, except for the events noted below. Assign a code from category Y99, External cause status, to indicate the work status of the person at the time the event occurred. The status code indicates whether the event occurred during military activity, whether a non-military person was at work, whether an individual including a student or volunteer was involved in a non-work activity at the time of the causal event.

A code from Y99, External cause status, should be assigned, when applicable, with other external cause codes, such as transport accidents and falls. The external cause status codes are not applicable to poisonings, adverse effects, misadventures or late effects.

Do not assign a code from category Y99 if no other external cause codes (cause, activity) are applicable for the encounter.

An external cause status code is used only once, at the initial encounter for treatment. Only one code from Y99 should be recorded on a medical record.

Do not assign code Y99.9, Unspecified external cause status, if the status is not stated.

Chapter 20. External Causes of Morbidity (V00-Y99)

NOTE   This chapter permits the classification of environmental events and circumstances as the cause of injury, and other adverse effects. Where a code from this section is applicable, it is intended that it shall be used secondary to a code from another chapter of the Classification indicating the nature of the condition. Most often, the condition will be classifiable to Chapter 19, Injury, poisoning and certain other consequences of external causes (S00-T88). Other conditions that may be stated to be due to external causes are classified in Chapters I to XVIII. For these conditions, codes from Chapter 20 should be used to provide additional information as to the cause of the condition.

AHA: 2018,4Q,58-60

This chapter contains the following blocks:

V00-X58	Accidents
V00-V99	Transport accidents
V00-V09	Pedestrian injured in transport accident
V10-V19	Pedal cycle rider injured in transport accident
V20-V29	Motorcycle rider injured in transport accident
V30-V39	Occupant of three-wheeled motor vehicle injured in transport accident
V40-V49	Car occupant injured in transport accident
V50-V59	Occupant of pick-up truck or van injured in transport accident
V60-V69	Occupant of heavy transport vehicle injured in transport accident
V70-V79	Bus occupant injured in transport accident
V80-V89	Other land transport accidents
V90-V94	Water transport accidents
V95-V97	Air and space transport accidents
V98-V99	Other and unspecified transport accidents
W00-X58	Other external causes of accidental injury
W00-W19	Slipping, tripping, stumbling and falls
W20-W49	Exposure to inanimate mechanical forces
W50-W64	Exposure to animate mechanical forces
W65-W74	Accidental non-transport drowning and submersion
W85-W99	Exposure to electric current, radiation and extreme ambient air temperature and pressure
X00-X08	Exposure to smoke, fire and flames
X10-X19	Contact with heat and hot substances
X30-X39	Exposure to forces of nature
X50	Overexertion and strenuous or repetitive movements
X52-X58	Accidental exposure to other specified factors
X71-X83	Intentional self-harm
X92-Y09	Assault
Y21-Y33	Event of undetermined intent
Y35-Y38	Legal intervention, operations of war, military operations, and terrorism
Y62-Y84	Complications of medical and surgical care
Y62-Y69	Misadventures to patients during surgical and medical care
Y70-Y82	Medical devices associated with adverse incidents in diagnostic and therapeutic use
Y83-Y84	Surgical and other medical procedures as the cause of abnormal reaction of the patient, or of later complication, without mention of misadventure at the time of the procedure
Y90-Y99	Supplementary factors related to causes of morbidity classified elsewhere

ACCIDENTS (V00-X58)

AHA: 2018,2Q,7-8

Transport accidents (V00-V99)

NOTE   This section is structured in 12 groups. Those relating to land transport accidents (V00-V89) reflect the victim's mode of transport and are subdivided to identify the victim's 'counterpart' or the type of event. The vehicle of which the injured person is an occupant is identified in the first two characters since it is seen as the most important factor to identify for prevention purposes. A transport accident is one in which the vehicle involved must be moving or running or in use for transport purposes at the time of the accident.

Use additional code to identify:
airbag injury (W22.1)
type of street or road (Y92.4-)
use of cellular telephone and other electronic equipment at the time of the transport accident (Y93.C-)

EXCLUDES 1   *agricultural vehicles in stationary use or maintenance (W31.-)*
assault by crashing of motor vehicle (Y03.-)
automobile or motor cycle in stationary use or maintenance — code to type of accident
crashing of motor vehicle, undetermined intent (Y32)
intentional self-harm by crashing of motor vehicle (X82)
EXCLUDES 2   *transport accidents due to cataclysm (X34-X38)*
NOTE   Definitions related to transport accidents:

(a)   A transport accident (V00-V99) is any accident involving a device designed primarily for, or used at the time primarily for, conveying persons or good from one place to another.

(b)   A public highway [trafficway] or street is the entire width between property lines (or other boundary lines) of land open to the public as a matter of right or custom for purposes of moving persons or property from one place to another. A roadway is that part of the public highway designed, improved and customarily used for vehicular traffic.

(c)   A traffic accident is any vehicle accident occurring on the public highway [i.e. originating on, terminating on, or involving a vehicle partially on the highway]. A vehicle accident is assumed to have occurred on the public highway unless another place is specified, except in the case of accidents involving only off-road motor vehicles, which are classified as nontraffic accidents unless the contrary is stated.

(d)   A nontraffic accident is any vehicle accident that occurs entirely in any place other than a public highway.

(e)   A pedestrian is any person involved in an accident who was not at the time of the accident riding in or on a motor vehicle, railway train, streetcar or animal-drawn or other vehicle, or on a pedal cycle or animal. This includes, a person changing a tire, working on a parked car, or a person on foot. It also includes the user of a pedestrian conveyance such as a baby stroller, ice-skates, skis, sled, roller skates, a skateboard, nonmotorized or motorized wheelchair, motorized mobility scooter, or nonmotorized scooter.

(f)   A driver is an occupant of a transport vehicle who is operating or intending to operate it.

(g)   A passenger is any occupant of a transport vehicle other than the driver, except a person traveling on the outside of the vehicle.

(h)   A person on the outside of a vehicle is any person being transported by a vehicle but not occupying the space normally reserved for the driver or passengers, or the space intended for the transport of property. This includes a person travelling on the bodywork, bumper, fender, roof, running board or step of a vehicle, as well as, hanging on the outside of the vehicle.

(i)   A pedal cycle is any land transport vehicle operated solely by nonmotorized pedals including a bicycle or tricycle.

(j)   A pedal cyclist is any person riding a pedal cycle or in a sidecar or trailer attached to a pedal cycle.

(k)   A motorcycle is a two-wheeled motor vehicle with one or two riding saddles and sometimes with a third wheel for the support of a sidecar. The sidecar is considered part of the motorcycle. This includes a moped, motor scooter, or motorized bicycle.

(l)   A motorcycle rider is any person riding a motorcycle or in a sidecar or trailer attached to the motorcycle.

(m)   A three-wheeled motor vehicle is a motorized tricycle designed primarily for on-road use. This includes a motor-driven tricycle, a motorized rickshaw, or a three-wheeled motor car.

(n)   A car [automobile] is a four-wheeled motor vehicle designed primarily for carrying up to 7 persons. A trailer being towed by the car is considered part of the car. It does not include a van or minivan — see definition (o).

(o)   A pick-up truck or van is a four or six-wheeled motor vehicle designed for carrying passengers as well as property or cargo weighing less than the local limit for classification as a heavy goods vehicle, and not requiring a special driver's license. This includes a minivan and a sport-utility vehicle (SUV).

(p)   A heavy transport vehicle is a motor vehicle designed primarily for carrying property, meeting local criteria for classification as a heavy goods vehicle in terms of weight and requiring a special driver's license.

(q)   A bus (coach) is a motor vehicle designed or adapted primarily for carrying more than 10 passengers, and requiring a special driver's license.

(r)   A railway train or railway vehicle is any device, with or without freight or passenger cars couple to it, designed for traffic on a railway track. This includes subterranean (subways) or elevated trains.

(s)   A streetcar, is a device designed and used primarily for transporting passengers within a municipality, running on rails, usually subject to normal traffic control signals, and operated principally on a right-of-way that forms part of the roadway. This includes a tram or trolley that runs on rails. A trailer being towed by a streetcar is considered part of the streetcar.

(t)   A special vehicle mainly used on industrial premises is a motor vehicle designed primarily for use within the buildings and premises of industrial or commercial establishments. This includes battery-powered airport passenger vehicles or baggage/mail trucks, forklifts, coal-cars in a coal mine, logging cars and trucks used in mines or quarries.

(u)   A special vehicle mainly used in agriculture is a motor vehicle designed specifically for use in farming and agriculture

Chapter 20. External Causes of Morbidity

V00–V00.312

(horticulture), to work the land, tend and harvest crops and transport materials on the farm. This includes harvesters, farm machinery and tractor and trailers.

(v) A special construction vehicle is a motor vehicle designed specifically for use on construction and demolition sites. This includes bulldozers, diggers, earth levellers, dump trucks, backhoes, front-end loaders, pavers, and mechanical shovels.

(w) A special all-terrain vehicle is a motor vehicle of special design to enable it to negotiate over rough or soft terrain, snow or sand. Examples of special design are high construction, special wheels and tires, tracks, and support on a cushion of air. This includes snow mobiles, All-terrain vehicles (ATV), and dune buggies. It does not include passenger vehicle designated as Sport Utility Vehicles. (SUV)

(x) A watercraft is any device designed for transporting passengers or goods on water. This includes motor or sailboats, ships, and hovercraft.

(y) An aircraft is any device for transporting passengers or goods in the air. This includes hot-air balloons, gliders, helicopters and airplanes.

(z) A military vehicle is any motorized vehicle operating on a public roadway owned by the military and being operated by a member of the military.

Pedestrian injured in transport accident (V00-V09)

INCLUDES   person changing tire on transport vehicle
person examining engine of vehicle broken down in (on side of) road
EXCLUDES 1   fall due to non-transport collision with other person (W03)
pedestrian on foot falling (slipping) on ice and snow (W00.-)
struck or bumped by another person (W51)

The appropriate 7th character is to be added to each code from categories V00-V09.
A   initial encounter
D   subsequent encounter
S   sequela

✓4ᵗʰ **V00**   **Pedestrian conveyance accident**
Use additional place of occurrence and activity external cause codes, if known (Y92.-, Y93.-)
    EXCLUDES 1   collision with another person without fall (W51)
fall due to person on foot colliding with another person on foot (W03)
fall from non-moving wheelchair, nonmotorized scooter and motorized mobility scooter without collision (W05.-)
pedestrian (conveyance) collision with other land transport vehicle (V01-V09)
pedestrian on foot falling (slipping) on ice and snow (W00.-)

   ✓5ᵗʰ **V00.0**   **Pedestrian on foot injured in collision with pedestrian conveyance**
     ✓x 7ᵗʰ **V00.01**   **Pedestrian on foot injured in collision with roller-skater**
     ✓x 7ᵗʰ **V00.02**   **Pedestrian on foot injured in collision with skateboarder**
     ✓x 7ᵗʰ **V00.09**   **Pedestrian on foot injured in collision with other pedestrian conveyance**

   ✓5ᵗʰ **V00.1**   **Rolling-type pedestrian conveyance accident**
     EXCLUDES 1   accident with baby stroller (V00.82-)
accident with motorized mobility scooter (V00.83-)
accident with wheelchair (powered) (V00.81-)
     ✓6ᵗʰ **V00.11**   **In-line roller-skate accident**
       ✓7ᵗʰ **V00.111**   **Fall from in-line roller-skates**
       ✓7ᵗʰ **V00.112**   **In-line roller-skater colliding with stationary object**
       ✓7ᵗʰ **V00.118**   **Other in-line roller-skate accident**
         EXCLUDES 1   roller-skater collision with other land transport vehicle (V01-V09 with 5th character 1)
     ✓6ᵗʰ **V00.12**   **Non-in-line roller-skate accident**
       ✓7ᵗʰ **V00.121**   **Fall from non-in-line roller-skates**
       ✓7ᵗʰ **V00.122**   **Non-in-line roller-skater colliding with stationary object**
       ✓7ᵗʰ **V00.128**   **Other non-in-line roller-skating accident**
         EXCLUDES 1   roller-skater collision with other land transport vehicle (V01-V09 with 5th character 1)

     ✓6ᵗʰ **V00.13**   **Skateboard accident**
       ✓7ᵗʰ **V00.131**   **Fall from skateboard**
       ✓7ᵗʰ **V00.132**   **Skateboarder colliding with stationary object**
       ✓7ᵗʰ **V00.138**   **Other skateboard accident**
         EXCLUDES 1   skateboarder collision with other land transport vehicle (V01-V09 with 5th character 2)

     ✓6ᵗʰ **V00.14**   **Scooter (nonmotorized) accident**
       EXCLUDES 1   motor scooter accident (V20-V29)
       ✓7ᵗʰ **V00.141**   **Fall from scooter (nonmotorized)**
       ✓7ᵗʰ **V00.142**   **Scooter (nonmotorized) colliding with stationary object**
       ✓7ᵗʰ **V00.148**   **Other scooter (nonmotorized) accident**
         EXCLUDES 1   scooter (nonmotorized) collision with other land transport vehicle (V01-V09 with fifth character 9)

     ✓6ᵗʰ **V00.15**   **Heelies accident**
       Rolling shoe
       Wheeled shoe
       Wheelies accident
       ✓7ᵗʰ **V00.151**   **Fall from heelies**
       ✓7ᵗʰ **V00.152**   **Heelies colliding with stationary object**
       ✓7ᵗʰ **V00.158**   **Other heelies accident**
     ✓6ᵗʰ **V00.18**   **Accident on other rolling-type pedestrian conveyance**
       ✓7ᵗʰ **V00.181**   **Fall from other rolling-type pedestrian conveyance**
       ✓7ᵗʰ **V00.182**   **Pedestrian on other rolling-type pedestrian conveyance colliding with stationary object**
       ✓7ᵗʰ **V00.188**   **Other accident on other rolling-type pedestrian conveyance**

   ✓5ᵗʰ **V00.2**   **Gliding-type pedestrian conveyance accident**
     ✓6ᵗʰ **V00.21**   **Ice-skates accident**
       ✓7ᵗʰ **V00.211**   **Fall from ice-skates**
       ✓7ᵗʰ **V00.212**   **Ice-skater colliding with stationary object**
       ✓7ᵗʰ **V00.218**   **Other ice-skates accident**
         EXCLUDES 1   ice-skater collision with other land transport vehicle (V01-V09 with 5th character 9)

     ✓6ᵗʰ **V00.22**   **Sled accident**
       ✓7ᵗʰ **V00.221**   **Fall from sled**
       ✓7ᵗʰ **V00.222**   **Sledder colliding with stationary object**
       ✓7ᵗʰ **V00.228**   **Other sled accident**
         EXCLUDES 1   sled collision with other land transport vehicle (V01-V09 with 5th character 9)

     ✓6ᵗʰ **V00.28**   **Other gliding-type pedestrian conveyance accident**
       ✓7ᵗʰ **V00.281**   **Fall from other gliding-type pedestrian conveyance**
       ✓7ᵗʰ **V00.282**   **Pedestrian on other gliding-type pedestrian conveyance colliding with stationary object**
       ✓7ᵗʰ **V00.288**   **Other accident on other gliding-type pedestrian conveyance**
         EXCLUDES 1   gliding-type pedestrian conveyance collision with other land transport vehicle (V01-V09 with 5th character 9)

   ✓5ᵗʰ **V00.3**   **Flat-bottomed pedestrian conveyance accident**
     ✓6ᵗʰ **V00.31**   **Snowboard accident**
       ✓7ᵗʰ **V00.311**   **Fall from snowboard**
       ✓7ᵗʰ **V00.312**   **Snowboarder colliding with stationary object**

N Newborn: 0   **P** Pediatric: 0-17   **M** Maternity: 9-64   **A** Adult: 15-124   **MCC** Major Complication/Comorbidity   **CC** Complication/Comorbidity   **SW** Severe Wound Dx

1214   ICD-10-CM 2020

√7ᵗʰ **V00.318 Other snowboard accident**
> EXCLUDES 1　*snowboarder collision with other land transport vehicle (V01-V09 with 5th character 9)*

√6ᵗʰ **V00.32 Snow-ski accident**
> √7ᵗʰ **V00.321 Fall from snow-skis**
> √7ᵗʰ **V00.322 Snow-skier colliding with stationary object**
> √7ᵗʰ **V00.328 Other snow-ski accident**
> > EXCLUDES 1　*snow-skier collision with other land transport vehicle (V01-V09 with 5th character 9)*

√6ᵗʰ **V00.38 Other flat-bottomed pedestrian conveyance accident**
> √7ᵗʰ **V00.381 Fall from other flat-bottomed conveyance**
> √7ᵗʰ **V00.382 Pedestrian on other flat-bottomed pedestrian conveyance colliding with stationary object**
> √7ᵗʰ **V00.388 Other accident on other flat-bottomed pedestrian conveyance**

√5ᵗʰ **V00.8 Accident on other pedestrian conveyance**
> √6ᵗʰ **V00.81 Accident with wheelchair (powered)**
> > √7ᵗʰ **V00.811 Fall from moving wheelchair (powered)**
> > > EXCLUDES 1　*fall from non-moving wheelchair (W05.0)*
> > √7ᵗʰ **V00.812 Wheelchair (powered) colliding with stationary object**
> > √7ᵗʰ **V00.818 Other accident with wheelchair (powered)**
> √6ᵗʰ **V00.82 Accident with baby stroller**
> > √7ᵗʰ **V00.821 Fall from baby stroller**
> > √7ᵗʰ **V00.822 Baby stroller colliding with stationary object**
> > √7ᵗʰ **V00.828 Other accident with baby stroller**
> √6ᵗʰ **V00.83 Accident with motorized mobility scooter**
> > √7ᵗʰ **V00.831 Fall from motorized mobility scooter**
> > > EXCLUDES 1　*fall from non-moving motorized mobility scooter (W05.2)*
> > √7ᵗʰ **V00.832 Motorized mobility scooter colliding with stationary object**
> > √7ᵗʰ **V00.838 Other accident with motorized mobility scooter**
> √6ᵗʰ **V00.89 Accident on other pedestrian conveyance**
> > √7ᵗʰ **V00.891 Fall from other pedestrian conveyance**
> > √7ᵗʰ **V00.892 Pedestrian on other pedestrian conveyance colliding with stationary object**
> > √7ᵗʰ **V00.898 Other accident on other pedestrian conveyance**
> > > EXCLUDES 1　*other pedestrian (conveyance) collision with other land transport vehicle (V01-V09 with 5th character 9)*

√4ᵗʰ **V01 Pedestrian injured in collision with pedal cycle**

√5ᵗʰ **V01.0 Pedestrian injured in collision with pedal cycle in nontraffic accident**
> √x7ᵗʰ **V01.00 Pedestrian on foot injured in collision with pedal cycle in nontraffic accident**
> > Pedestrian NOS injured in collision with pedal cycle in nontraffic accident
> √x7ᵗʰ **V01.01 Pedestrian on roller-skates injured in collision with pedal cycle in nontraffic accident**
> √x7ᵗʰ **V01.02 Pedestrian on skateboard injured in collision with pedal cycle in nontraffic accident**

√x7ᵗʰ **V01.09 Pedestrian with other conveyance injured in collision with pedal cycle in nontraffic accident**
> Pedestrian with baby stroller injured in collision with pedal cycle in nontraffic accident
> Pedestrian on ice-skates injured in collision with pedal cycle in nontraffic accident
> Pedestrian on nonmotorized scooter injured in collision with pedal cycle in nontraffic accident
> Pedestrian on sled injured in collision with pedal cycle in nontraffic accident
> Pedestrian on snowboard injured in collision with pedal cycle in nontraffic accident
> Pedestrian on snow-skis injured in collision with pedal cycle in nontraffic accident
> Pedestrian in wheelchair (powered) injured in collision with pedal cycle in nontraffic accident
> Pedestrian in motorized mobility scooter injured in collision with pedal cycle in nontraffic accident

√5ᵗʰ **V01.1 Pedestrian injured in collision with pedal cycle in traffic accident**
> √x7ᵗʰ **V01.10 Pedestrian on foot injured in collision with pedal cycle in traffic accident**
> > Pedestrian NOS injured in collision with pedal cycle in traffic accident
> √x7ᵗʰ **V01.11 Pedestrian on roller-skates injured in collision with pedal cycle in traffic accident**
> √x7ᵗʰ **V01.12 Pedestrian on skateboard injured in collision with pedal cycle in traffic accident**
> √x7ᵗʰ **V01.19 Pedestrian with other conveyance injured in collision with pedal cycle in traffic accident**
> > Pedestrian with baby stroller injured in collision with pedal cycle in traffic accident
> > Pedestrian on ice-skates injured in collision with pedal cycle in traffic accident
> > Pedestrian on nonmotorized scooter injured in collision with pedal cycle in traffic accident
> > Pedestrian on sled injured in collision with pedal cycle in traffic accident
> > Pedestrian on snowboard injured in collision with pedal cycle in traffic accident
> > Pedestrian on snow-skis injured in collision with pedal cycle in traffic accident
> > Pedestrian in wheelchair (powered) injured in collision with pedal cycle in traffic accident
> > Pedestrian in motorized mobility scooter injured in collision with pedal cycle in traffic accident

√5ᵗʰ **V01.9 Pedestrian injured in collision with pedal cycle, unspecified whether traffic or nontraffic accident**
> √x7ᵗʰ **V01.90 Pedestrian on foot injured in collision with pedal cycle, unspecified whether traffic or nontraffic accident**
> > Pedestrian NOS injured in collision with pedal cycle, unspecified whether traffic or nontraffic accident
> √x7ᵗʰ **V01.91 Pedestrian on roller-skates injured in collision with pedal cycle, unspecified whether traffic or nontraffic accident**
> √x7ᵗʰ **V01.92 Pedestrian on skateboard injured in collision with pedal cycle, unspecified whether traffic or nontraffic accident**

✓x7ᵗʰ **V01.99** **Pedestrian with other conveyance injured in collision with pedal cycle, unspecified whether traffic or nontraffic accident**

Pedestrian with baby stroller injured in collision with pedal cycle, unspecified whether traffic or nontraffic accident

Pedestrian on ice-skates injured in collision with pedal cycle unspecified, whether traffic or nontraffic accident

Pedestrian on nonmotorized scooter injured in collision with pedal cycle, unspecified whether traffic or nontraffic accident

Pedestrian on sled injured in collision with pedal cycle unspecified, whether traffic or nontraffic accident

Pedestrian on snowboard injured in collision with pedal cycle, unspecified whether traffic or nontraffic accident

Pedestrian on snow-skis injured in collision with pedal cycle, unspecified whether traffic or nontraffic accident

Pedestrian in wheelchair (powered) injured in collision with pedal cycle, unspecified whether traffic or nontraffic accident

Pedestrian in motorized mobility scooter injured in collision with pedal cycle, unspecified whether traffic or nontraffic accident

✓4ᵗʰ **V02** **Pedestrian injured in collision with two- or three-wheeled motor vehicle**

✓5ᵗʰ **V02.0** **Pedestrian injured in collision with two- or three-wheeled motor vehicle in nontraffic accident**

✓x7ᵗʰ **V02.00** **Pedestrian on foot injured in collision with two- or three-wheeled motor vehicle in nontraffic accident**

Pedestrian NOS injured in collision with two- or three-wheeled motor vehicle in nontraffic accident

✓x7ᵗʰ **V02.01** **Pedestrian on roller-skates injured in collision with two- or three-wheeled motor vehicle in nontraffic accident**

✓x7ᵗʰ **V02.02** **Pedestrian on skateboard injured in collision with two- or three-wheeled motor vehicle in nontraffic accident**

✓x7ᵗʰ **V02.09** **Pedestrian with other conveyance injured in collision with two- or three-wheeled motor vehicle in nontraffic accident**

Pedestrian with baby stroller injured in collision with two- or three-wheeled motor vehicle in nontraffic accident

Pedestrian on ice-skates injured in collision with two- or three-wheeled motor vehicle in nontraffic accident

Pedestrian on nonmotorized scooter injured in collision with two- or three-wheeled motor vehicle in nontraffic accident

Pedestrian on sled injured in collision with two- or three-wheeled motor vehicle in nontraffic accident

Pedestrian on snowboard injured in collision with two- or three-wheeled motor vehicle in nontraffic accident

Pedestrian on snow-skis injured in collision with two- or three-wheeled motor vehicle in nontraffic accident

Pedestrian in wheelchair (powered) injured in collision with two- or three-wheeled motor vehicle in nontraffic accident

Pedestrian in motorized mobility scooter injured in collision with two- or three-wheeled motor vehicle in nontraffic accident

✓5ᵗʰ **V02.1** **Pedestrian injured in collision with two- or three-wheeled motor vehicle in traffic accident**

✓x7ᵗʰ **V02.10** **Pedestrian on foot injured in collision with two- or three-wheeled motor vehicle in traffic accident**

Pedestrian NOS injured in collision with two- or three-wheeled motor vehicle in traffic accident

✓x7ᵗʰ **V02.11** **Pedestrian on roller-skates injured in collision with two- or three-wheeled motor vehicle in traffic accident**

✓x7ᵗʰ **V02.12** **Pedestrian on skateboard injured in collision with two- or three-wheeled motor vehicle in traffic accident**

✓x7ᵗʰ **V02.19** **Pedestrian with other conveyance injured in collision with two- or three-wheeled motor vehicle in traffic accident**

Pedestrian with baby stroller injured in collision with two- or three-wheeled motor vehicle in traffic accident

Pedestrian on ice-skates injured in collision with two- or three-wheeled motor vehicle in traffic accident

Pedestrian on nonmotorized scooter injured in collision with two- or three-wheeled motor vehicle in traffic accident

Pedestrian on sled injured in collision with two- or three-wheeled motor vehicle in traffic accident

Pedestrian on snowboard injured in collision with two- or three-wheeled motor vehicle in traffic accident

Pedestrian on snow-skis injured in collision with two- or three-wheeled motor vehicle in traffic accident

Pedestrian in wheelchair (powered) injured in collision with two- or three-wheeled motor vehicle in traffic accident

Pedestrian in motorized mobility scooter injued in collision with two- or three-wheeled motor vehicle in traffic accident

✓5ᵗʰ **V02.9** **Pedestrian injured in collision with two- or three-wheeled motor vehicle, unspecified whether traffic or nontraffic accident**

✓x7ᵗʰ **V02.90** **Pedestrian on foot injured in collision with two- or three-wheeled motor vehicle, unspecified whether traffic or nontraffic accident**

Pedestrian NOS injured in collision with two- or three-wheeled motor vehicle, unspecified whether traffic or nontraffic accident

✓x7ᵗʰ **V02.91** **Pedestrian on roller-skates injured in collision with two- or three-wheeled motor vehicle, unspecified whether traffic or nontraffic accident**

✓x7ᵗʰ **V02.92** **Pedestrian on skateboard injured in collision with two- or three-wheeled motor vehicle, unspecified whether traffic or nontraffic accident**

✓x7ᵗʰ **V02.99** **Pedestrian with other conveyance injured in collision with two- or three-wheeled motor vehicle, unspecified whether traffic or nontraffic accident**

Pedestrian with baby stroller injured in collision with two- or three-wheeled motor vehicle, unspecified whether traffic or nontraffic accident

Pedestrian on ice-skates injured in collision with two- or three-wheeled motor vehicle, unspecified whether traffic or nontraffic accident

Pedestrian on nonmotorized scooter injured in collision with two- or three-wheeled motor vehicle, unspecified whether traffic or nontraffic accident

Pedestrian on sled injured in collision with two- or three-wheeled motor vehicle, unspecified whether traffic or nontraffic accident

Pedestrian on snowboard injured in collision with two- or three-wheeled motor vehicle, unspecified whether traffic or nontraffic accident

Pedestrian on snow-skis injured in collision with two- or three-wheeled motor vehicle, unspecified whether traffic or nontraffic accident

Pedestrian in wheelchair (powered) injured in collision with two- or three-wheeled motor vehicle, unspecified whether traffic or nontraffic accident

Pedestrian in motorized mobility scooter injured in collision with two- or three wheeled motor vehicle, unspecified whether traffic or nontraffic accident

✓4ᵗʰ **V03** **Pedestrian injured in collision with car, pick-up truck or van**

✓5ᵗʰ **V03.0** **Pedestrian injured in collision with car, pick-up truck or van in nontraffic accident**

✓x7ᵗʰ **V03.00** **Pedestrian on foot injured in collision with car, pick-up truck or van in nontraffic accident**

Pedestrian NOS injured in collision with car, pick-up truck or van in nontraffic accident

✓x7ᵗʰ **V03.01** **Pedestrian on roller-skates injured in collision with car, pick-up truck or van in nontraffic accident**

√x7th **V03.02** **Pedestrian** on skateboard **injured in collision with car, pick-up truck or van in nontraffic accident**

√x7th **V03.09** **Pedestrian with other conveyance injured in collision with car, pick-up truck or van in nontraffic accident**

Pedestrian with baby stroller injured in collision with car, pick-up truck or van in nontraffic accident

Pedestrian on ice-skates injured in collision with car, pick-up truck or van in nontraffic accident

Pedestrian on nonmotorized scooter injured in collision with car, pick-up truck or van in nontraffic accident

Pedestrian on sled injured in collision with car, pick-up truck or van in nontraffic accident

Pedestrian on snowboard injured in collision with car, pick-up truck or van in nontraffic accident

Pedestrian on snow-skis injured in collision with car, pick-up truck or van in nontraffic accident

Pedestrian in wheelchair (powered) injured in collision with car, pick-up truck or van in nontraffic accident

Pedestrian in motorized mobility scooter injured in collision with car, pick-up truck or van in nontraffic accident

√5th **V03.1** **Pedestrian injured in collision with car, pick-up truck or van in traffic accident**

√x7th **V03.10** **Pedestrian** on foot **injured in collision with car, pick-up truck or van in traffic accident**

Pedestrian NOS injured in collision with car, pick-up truck or van in traffic accident

√x7th **V03.11** **Pedestrian** on roller-skates **injured in collision with car, pick-up truck or van in traffic accident**

√x7th **V03.12** **Pedestrian** on skateboard **injured in collision with car, pick-up truck or van in traffic accident**

√x7th **V03.19** **Pedestrian with other conveyance injured in collision with car, pick-up truck or van in traffic accident**

Pedestrian with baby stroller injured in collision with car, pick-up truck or van in traffic accident

Pedestrian on ice-skates injured in collision with car, pick-up truck or van in traffic accident

Pedestrian on nonmotorized scooter injured in collision with car, pick-up truck or van in traffic accident

Pedestrian on sled injured in collision with car, pick-up truck or van in traffic accident

Pedestrian on snowboard injured in collision with car, pick-up truck or van in traffic accident

Pedestrian on snow-skis injured in collision with car, pick-up truck or van in traffic accident

Pedestrian in wheelchair (powered) injured in collision with car, pick-up truck or van in traffic accident

Pedestrian in motorized mobility scooter injured in collision with car, pick-up truck or van in nontraffic accident

√5th **V03.9** **Pedestrian injured in collision with car, pick-up truck or van, unspecified whether traffic or nontraffic accident**

√x7th **V03.90** **Pedestrian** on foot **injured in collision with car, pick-up truck or van, unspecified whether traffic or nontraffic accident**

Pedestrian NOS injured in collision with car, pick-up truck or van, unspecified whether traffic or nontraffic accident

√x7th **V03.91** **Pedestrian** on roller-skates **injured in collision with car, pick-up truck or van, unspecified whether traffic or nontraffic accident**

√x7th **V03.92** **Pedestrian** on skateboard **injured in collision with car, pick-up truck or van, unspecified whether traffic or nontraffic accident**

√x7th **V03.99** **Pedestrian with other conveyance injured in collision with car, pick-up truck or van, unspecified whether traffic or nontraffic accident**

Pedestrian with baby stroller injured in collision with car, pick-up truck or van, unspecified whether traffic or nontraffic accident

Pedestrian on ice-skates injured in collision with car, pick-up truck or van, unspecified whether traffic or nontraffic accident

Pedestrian on nonmotorized scooter injured in collision with car, pick-up truck or van, unspecified whether traffic or nontraffic accident

Pedestrian on sled injured in collision with car, pick-up truck or van in nontraffic accident

Pedestrian on snowboard injured in collision with car, pick-up truck or van, unspecified whether traffic or nontraffic accident

Pedestrian on snow-skis injured in collision with car, pick-up truck or van, unspecified whether traffic or nontraffic accident

Pedestrian in wheelchair (powered) injured in collision with car, pick-up truck or van, unspecified whether traffic or nontraffic accident

Pedestrian in motorized mobility scooter injured in collision with car, pick-up truck or van, unspecified whether traffic or nontraffic accident

√4th **V04** **Pedestrian injured in collision with heavy transport vehicle or bus**

EXCLUDES 1   *pedestrian injured in collision with military vehicle (V09.01, V09.21)*

√5th **V04.0** **Pedestrian injured in collision with heavy transport vehicle or bus in nontraffic accident**

√x7th **V04.00** **Pedestrian** on foot **injured in collision with heavy transport vehicle or bus in nontraffic accident**

Pedestrian NOS injured in collision with heavy transport vehicle or bus in nontraffic accident

√x7th **V04.01** **Pedestrian** on roller-skates **injured in collision with heavy transport vehicle or bus in nontraffic accident**

√x7th **V04.02** **Pedestrian** on skateboard **injured in collision with heavy transport vehicle or bus in nontraffic accident**

√x7th **V04.09** **Pedestrian with other conveyance injured in collision with heavy transport vehicle or bus in nontraffic accident**

Pedestrian with baby stroller injured in collision with heavy transport vehicle or bus in nontraffic accident

Pedestrian on ice-skates injured in collision with heavy transport vehicle or bus in nontraffic accident

Pedestrian on nonmotorized scooter injured in collision with heavy transport vehicle or bus in nontraffic accident

Pedestrian on sled injured in collision with heavy transport vehicle or bus in nontraffic accident

Pedestrian on snowboard injured in collision with heavy transport vehicle or bus in nontraffic accident

Pedestrian on snow-skis injured in collision with heavy transport vehicle or bus in nontraffic accident

Pedestrian in wheelchair (powered) injured in collision with heavy transport vehicle or bus in nontraffic accident

Pedestrian in motorized mobility scooter injured in collision with heavy transport vehicle or bus in nontraffic accident

√5th **V04.1** **Pedestrian injured in collision with heavy transport vehicle or bus in traffic accident**

√x7th **V04.10** **Pedestrian** on foot **injured in collision with heavy transport vehicle or bus in traffic accident**

Pedestrian NOS injured in collision with heavy transport vehicle or bus in traffic accident

√x7th **V04.11** **Pedestrian** on roller-skates **injured in collision with heavy transport vehicle or bus in traffic accident**

√x7th **V04.12** **Pedestrian** on skateboard **injured in collision with heavy transport vehicle or bus in traffic accident**

✔ Additional Char Req   √x7th Placeholder   Unacceptable PDx   Questionable PDx   Wrong Procedure   Manifestation   Unspecified Dx   H1–H14 HAC   HCC CMS-HCC Dx   HIV HIV Dx

ICD-10-CM 2020   1217

V03.02–V04.12

√x7ᵗʰ **V04.19 Pedestrian with other conveyance injured in collision with heavy transport vehicle or bus in traffic accident**

Pedestrian with baby stroller injured in collision with heavy transport vehicle or bus in traffic accident

Pedestrian on ice-skates injured in collision with heavy transport vehicle or bus in traffic accident

Pedestrian on nonmotorized scooter injured in collision with heavy transport vehicle or bus in traffic accident

Pedestrian on sled injured in collision with heavy transport vehicle or bus in traffic accident

Pedestrian on snowboard injured in collision with heavy transport vehicle or bus in traffic accident

Pedestrian on snow-skis injured in collision with heavy transport vehicle or bus in traffic accident

Pedestrian in wheelchair (powered) injured in collision with heavy transport vehicle or bus in traffic accident

Pedestrian in motorized mobility scooter injured in collision with heavy transport vehicle or bus in traffic accident

√5ᵗʰ **V04.9 Pedestrian injured in collision with heavy transport vehicle or bus, unspecified whether traffic or nontraffic accident**

√x7ᵗʰ **V04.90 Pedestrian on foot injured in collision with heavy transport vehicle or bus, unspecified whether traffic or nontraffic accident**

Pedestrian NOS injured in collision with heavy transport vehicle or bus, unspecified whether traffic or nontraffic accident

√x7ᵗʰ **V04.91 Pedestrian on roller-skates injured in collision with heavy transport vehicle or bus, unspecified whether traffic or nontraffic accident**

√x7ᵗʰ **V04.92 Pedestrian on skateboard injured in collision with heavy transport vehicle or bus, unspecified whether traffic or nontraffic accident**

√x7ᵗʰ **V04.99 Pedestrian with other conveyance injured in collision with heavy transport vehicle or bus, unspecified whether traffic or nontraffic accident**

Pedestrian with baby stroller injured in collision with heavy transport vehicle or bus, unspecified whether traffic or nontraffic accident

Pedestrian on ice-skates injured in collision with heavy transport vehicle or bus, unspecified whether traffic or nontraffic accident

Pedestrian on nonmotorized scooter injured in collision with heavy transport vehicle or bus, unspecified whether traffic or nontraffic accident

Pedestrian on sled injured in collision with heavy transport vehicle or bus, unspecified whether traffic or nontraffic accident

Pedestrian on snowboard injured in collision with heavy transport vehicle or bus, unspecified whether traffic or nontraffic accident

Pedestrian on snow-skis injured in collision with heavy transport vehicle or bus, unspecified whether traffic or nontraffic accident

Pedestrian in wheelchair (powered) injured in collision with heavy transport vehicle or bus, unspecified whether traffic or nontraffic accident

Pedestrian in motorized mobility scooter injured in collision with heavy transport vehicle or bus, unspecified whether traffic or nontraffic accident

√4ᵗʰ **V05 Pedestrian injured in collision with railway train or railway vehicle**

√5ᵗʰ **V05.0 Pedestrian injured in collision with railway train or railway vehicle in nontraffic accident**

√x7ᵗʰ **V05.00 Pedestrian on foot injured in collision with railway train or railway vehicle in nontraffic accident**

Pedestrian NOS injured in collision with railway train or railway vehicle in nontraffic accident

√x7ᵗʰ **V05.01 Pedestrian on roller-skates injured in collision with railway train or railway vehicle in nontraffic accident**

√x7ᵗʰ **V05.02 Pedestrian on skateboard injured in collision with railway train or railway vehicle in nontraffic accident**

√x7ᵗʰ **V05.09 Pedestrian with other conveyance injured in collision with railway train or railway vehicle in nontraffic accident**

Pedestrian with baby stroller injured in collision with railway train or railway vehicle in nontraffic accident

Pedestrian on ice-skates injured in collision with railway train or railway vehicle in nontraffic accident

Pedestrian on nonmotorized scooter injured in collision with railway train or railway vehicle in nontraffic accident

Pedestrian on sled injured in collision with railway train or railway vehicle in nontraffic accident

Pedestrian on snowboard injured in collision with railway train or railway vehicle in nontraffic accident

Pedestrian on snow-skis injured in collision with railway train or railway vehicle in nontraffic accident

Pedestrian in wheelchair (powered) injured in collision with railway train or railway vehicle in nontraffic accident

Pedestrian in motorized mobility scooter injured in collision with railway train or railway vehicle in nontraffic accident

√5ᵗʰ **V05.1 Pedestrian injured in collision with railway train or railway vehicle in traffic accident**

√x7ᵗʰ **V05.10 Pedestrian on foot injured in collision with railway train or railway vehicle in traffic accident**

Pedestrian NOS injured in collision with railway train or railway vehicle in traffic accident

√x7ᵗʰ **V05.11 Pedestrian on roller-skates injured in collision with railway train or railway vehicle in traffic accident**

√x7ᵗʰ **V05.12 Pedestrian on skateboard injured in collision with railway train or railway vehicle in traffic accident**

√x7ᵗʰ **V05.19 Pedestrian with other conveyance injured in collision with railway train or railway vehicle in traffic accident**

Pedestrian with baby stroller injured in collision with railway train or railway vehicle in traffic accident

Pedestrian on ice-skates injured in collision with railway train or railway vehicle in traffic accident

Pedestrian on nonmotorized scooter injured in collision with railway train or railway vehicle in traffic accident

Pedestrian on sled injured in collision with railway train or railway vehicle in traffic accident

Pedestrian on snowboard injured in collision with railway train or railway vehicle in traffic accident

Pedestrian on snow-skis injured in collision with railway train or railway vehicle in traffic accident

Pedestrian in wheelchair (powered) injured in collision with railway train or railway vehicle in traffic accident

Pedestrian in motorized mobility scooter injured in collision with railway train or railway vehicle in traffic accident

√5ᵗʰ **V05.9 Pedestrian injured in collision with railway train or railway vehicle, unspecified whether traffic or nontraffic accident**

√x7ᵗʰ **V05.90 Pedestrian on foot injured in collision with railway train or railway vehicle, unspecified whether traffic or nontraffic accident**

Pedestrian NOS injured in collision with railway train or railway vehicle, unspecified whether traffic or nontraffic accident

√x7ᵗʰ **V05.91 Pedestrian on roller-skates injured in collision with railway train or railway vehicle, unspecified whether traffic or nontraffic accident**

√x7ᵗʰ **V05.92 Pedestrian on skateboard injured in collision with railway train or railway vehicle, unspecified whether traffic or nontraffic accident**

Ⓝ Newborn: 0   Ⓟ Pediatric: 0-17   Ⓜ Maternity: 9-64   Ⓐ Adult: 15-124   MCC Major Complication/Comorbidity   CC Complication/Comorbidity   SW Severe Wound Dx

1218   ICD-10-CM 2020

V04.19–V05.92

✓x7ᵗʰ **V05.99** **Pedestrian with other conveyance injured in collision with railway train or railway vehicle, unspecified whether traffic or nontraffic accident**

Pedestrian with baby stroller injured in collision with railway train or railway vehicle, unspecified whether traffic or nontraffic

Pedestrian on ice-skates injured in collision with railway train or railway vehicle, unspecified whether traffic or nontraffic

Pedestrian on nonmotorized scooter injured in collision with railway train or railway vehicle, unspecified whether traffic or nontraffic

Pedestrian on sled injured in collision with railway train or railway vehicle, unspecified whether traffic or nontraffic

Pedestrian on snowboard injured in collision with railway train or railway vehicle, unspecified whether traffic or nontraffic

Pedestrian on snow-skis injured in collision with railway train or railway vehicle, unspecified whether traffic or nontraffic

Pedestrian in wheelchair (powered) injured in collision with railway train or railway vehicle, unspecified whether traffic or nontraffic

Pedestrian in motorized mobility scooter injured in collision with railway train or railway vehicle, unspecified whether traffic or nontraffic

✓4ᵗʰ **V06** **Pedestrian injured in collision with other nonmotor vehicle**

> **INCLUDES**   collision with animal-drawn vehicle, animal being ridden, nonpowered streetcar
> **EXCLUDES 1**   *pedestrian injured in collision with pedestrian conveyance (V00.0-)*

✓5ᵗʰ **V06.0** **Pedestrian injured in collision with other nonmotor vehicle in nontraffic accident**

✓x7ᵗʰ **V06.00** **Pedestrian on foot injured in collision with other nonmotor vehicle in nontraffic accident**

Pedestrian NOS injured in collision with other nonmotor vehicle in nontraffic accident

✓x7ᵗʰ **V06.01** **Pedestrian on roller-skates injured in collision with other nonmotor vehicle in nontraffic accident**

✓x7ᵗʰ **V06.02** **Pedestrian on skateboard injured in collision with other nonmotor vehicle in nontraffic accident**

✓x7ᵗʰ **V06.09** **Pedestrian with other conveyance injured in collision with other nonmotor vehicle in nontraffic accident**

Pedestrian with baby stroller injured in collision with other nonmotor vehicle in nontraffic accident

Pedestrian on ice-skates injured in collision with other nonmotor vehicle in nontraffic accident

Pedestrian on nonmotorized scooter injured in collision with other nonmotor vehicle in nontraffic accident

Pedestrian on sled injured in collision with other nonmotor vehicle in nontraffic accident

Pedestrian on snowboard injured in collision with other nonmotor vehicle in nontraffic accident

Pedestrian on snow-skis injured in collision with other nonmotor vehicle in nontraffic accident

Pedestrian in wheelchair (powered) injured in collision with other nonmotor vehicle in nontraffic accident

Pedestrian in motorized mobility scooter injured in collision with other nonmotor vehicle in nontraffic accident

✓5ᵗʰ **V06.1** **Pedestrian injured in collision with other nonmotor vehicle in traffic accident**

✓x7ᵗʰ **V06.10** **Pedestrian on foot injured in collision with other nonmotor vehicle in traffic accident**

Pedestrian NOS injured in collision with other nonmotor vehicle in traffic accident

✓x7ᵗʰ **V06.11** **Pedestrian on roller-skates injured in collision with other nonmotor vehicle in traffic accident**

✓x7ᵗʰ **V06.12** **Pedestrian on skateboard injured in collision with other nonmotor vehicle in traffic accident**

✓x7ᵗʰ **V06.19** **Pedestrian with other conveyance injured in collision with other nonmotor vehicle in traffic accident**

Pedestrian with baby stroller injured in collision with other nonmotor vehicle in nontraffic accident

Pedestrian on ice-skates injured in collision with other nonmotor vehicle in traffic accident

Pedestrian on nonmotorized scooter injured in collision with other nonmotor vehicle in traffic accident

Pedestrian on sled injured in collision with other nonmotor vehicle in traffic accident

Pedestrian on snowboard injured in collision with other nonmotor vehicle in traffic accident

Pedestrian on snow-skis injured in collision with other nonmotor vehicle in traffic accident

Pedestrian in wheelchair (powered) injured in collision with other nonmotor vehicle in traffic accident

Pedestrian in motorized mobility scooter injured in collision with other nonmotor vehicle in traffic accident

✓5ᵗʰ **V06.9** **Pedestrian injured in collision with other nonmotor vehicle, unspecified whether traffic or nontraffic accident**

✓x7ᵗʰ **V06.90** **Pedestrian on foot injured in collision with other nonmotor vehicle, unspecified whether traffic or nontraffic accident**

Pedestrian NOS injured in collision with other nonmotor vehicle, unspecified whether traffic or nontraffic accident

✓x7ᵗʰ **V06.91** **Pedestrian on roller-skates injured in collision with other nonmotor vehicle, unspecified whether traffic or nontraffic accident**

✓x7ᵗʰ **V06.92** **Pedestrian on skateboard injured in collision with other nonmotor vehicle, unspecified whether traffic or nontraffic accident**

✓x7ᵗʰ **V06.99** **Pedestrian with other conveyance injured in collision with other nonmotor vehicle, unspecified whether traffic or nontraffic accident**

Pedestrian with baby stroller injured in collision with other nonmotor vehicle, unspecified whether traffic or nontraffic accident

Pedestrian on ice-skates injured in collision with other nonmotor vehicle, unspecified whether traffic or nontraffic accident

Pedestrian on nonmotorized scooter injured in collision with other nonmotor vehicle, unspecified whether traffic or nontraffic accident

Pedestrian on sled injured in collision with other nonmotor vehicle, unspecified whether traffic or nontraffic accident

Pedestrian on snowboard injured in collision with other nonmotor vehicle, unspecified whether traffic or nontraffic accident

Pedestrian on snow-skis injured in collision with other nonmotor vehicle, unspecified whether traffic or nontraffic accident

Pedestrian in wheelchair (powered) injured in collision with other nonmotor vehicle, unspecified whether traffic or nontraffic accident

Pedestrian in motorized mobility scooter injured in collision with other nonmotorized vehicle, unspecified whether traffic or nontraffic accident

✓4ᵗʰ **V09** **Pedestrian injured in other and unspecified transport accidents**

✓5ᵗʰ **V09.0** **Pedestrian injured in nontraffic accident involving other and unspecified motor vehicles**

✓x7ᵗʰ **V09.00** **Pedestrian injured in nontraffic accident involving unspecified motor vehicles**

✓x7ᵗʰ **V09.01** **Pedestrian injured in nontraffic accident involving military vehicle**

✓x7ᵗʰ **V09.09** **Pedestrian injured in nontraffic accident involving other motor vehicles**

Pedestrian injured in nontraffic accident by special vehicle

✓x7ᵗʰ **V09.1** **Pedestrian injured in unspecified nontraffic accident**

✓5ᵗʰ **V09.2** **Pedestrian injured in traffic accident involving other and unspecified motor vehicles**

✓x7ᵗʰ **V09.20** **Pedestrian injured in traffic accident involving unspecified motor vehicles**

✓x7ᵗʰ **V09.21** **Pedestrian injured in traffic accident involving military vehicle**

Chapter 20. External Causes of Morbidity

√x7ᵗʰ **V09.29** Pedestrian injured in traffic accident involving other motor vehicles

√x7ᵗʰ **V09.3** Pedestrian injured in unspecified traffic accident

√x7ᵗʰ **V09.9** Pedestrian injured in unspecified transport accident

Pedal cycle rider injured in transport accident (V10-V19)

INCLUDES   any non-motorized vehicle, excluding an animal-drawn vehicle, or a sidecar or trailer attached to the pedal cycle

EXCLUDES 2   rupture of pedal cycle tire (W37.0)

The appropriate 7th character is to be added to each code from categories V10-V19.
A   initial encounter
D   subsequent encounter
S   sequela

√4ᵗʰ **V10** Pedal cycle rider injured in collision with pedestrian or animal

> **EXCLUDES 1**   pedal cycle rider collision with animal-drawn vehicle or animal being ridden (V16.-)

√x7ᵗʰ **V10.0** Pedal cycle driver injured in collision with pedestrian or animal in nontraffic accident

√x7ᵗʰ **V10.1** Pedal cycle passenger injured in collision with pedestrian or animal in nontraffic accident

√x7ᵗʰ **V10.2** Unspecified pedal cyclist injured in collision with pedestrian or animal in nontraffic accident

√x7ᵗʰ **V10.3** Person boarding or alighting a pedal cycle injured in collision with pedestrian or animal

√x7ᵗʰ **V10.4** Pedal cycle driver injured in collision with pedestrian or animal in traffic accident

√x7ᵗʰ **V10.5** Pedal cycle passenger injured in collision with pedestrian or animal in traffic accident

√x7ᵗʰ **V10.9** Unspecified pedal cyclist injured in collision with pedestrian or animal in traffic accident

√4ᵗʰ **V11** Pedal cycle rider injured in collision with other pedal cycle

√x7ᵗʰ **V11.0** Pedal cycle driver injured in collision with other pedal cycle in nontraffic accident

√x7ᵗʰ **V11.1** Pedal cycle passenger injured in collision with other pedal cycle in nontraffic accident

√x7ᵗʰ **V11.2** Unspecified pedal cyclist injured in collision with other pedal cycle in nontraffic accident

√x7ᵗʰ **V11.3** Person boarding or alighting a pedal cycle injured in collision with other pedal cycle

√x7ᵗʰ **V11.4** Pedal cycle driver injured in collision with other pedal cycle in traffic accident

√x7ᵗʰ **V11.5** Pedal cycle passenger injured in collision with other pedal cycle in traffic accident

√x7ᵗʰ **V11.9** Unspecified pedal cyclist injured in collision with other pedal cycle in traffic accident

√4ᵗʰ **V12** Pedal cycle rider injured in collision with two- or three-wheeled motor vehicle

√x7ᵗʰ **V12.0** Pedal cycle driver injured in collision with two- or three-wheeled motor vehicle in nontraffic accident

√x7ᵗʰ **V12.1** Pedal cycle passenger injured in collision with two- or three-wheeled motor vehicle in nontraffic accident

√x7ᵗʰ **V12.2** Unspecified pedal cyclist injured in collision with two- or three-wheeled motor vehicle in nontraffic accident

√x7ᵗʰ **V12.3** Person boarding or alighting a pedal cycle injured in collision with two- or three-wheeled motor vehicle

√x7ᵗʰ **V12.4** Pedal cycle driver injured in collision with two- or three-wheeled motor vehicle in traffic accident

√x7ᵗʰ **V12.5** Pedal cycle passenger injured in collision with two- or three-wheeled motor vehicle in traffic accident

√x7ᵗʰ **V12.9** Unspecified pedal cyclist injured in collision with two- or three-wheeled motor vehicle in traffic accident

√4ᵗʰ **V13** Pedal cycle rider injured in collision with car, pick-up truck or van

√x7ᵗʰ **V13.0** Pedal cycle driver injured in collision with car, pick-up truck or van in nontraffic accident

√x7ᵗʰ **V13.1** Pedal cycle passenger injured in collision with car, pick-up truck or van in nontraffic accident

√x7ᵗʰ **V13.2** Unspecified pedal cyclist injured in collision with car, pick-up truck or van in nontraffic accident

√x7ᵗʰ **V13.3** Person boarding or alighting a pedal cycle injured in collision with car, pick-up truck or van

√x7ᵗʰ **V13.4** Pedal cycle driver injured in collision with car, pick-up truck or van in traffic accident

√x7ᵗʰ **V13.5** Pedal cycle passenger injured in collision with car, pick-up truck or van in traffic accident

√x7ᵗʰ **V13.9** Unspecified pedal cyclist injured in collision with car, pick-up truck or van in traffic accident

√4ᵗʰ **V14** Pedal cycle rider injured in collision with heavy transport vehicle or bus

> **EXCLUDES 1**   pedal cycle rider injured in collision with military vehicle (V19.81)

√x7ᵗʰ **V14.0** Pedal cycle driver injured in collision with heavy transport vehicle or bus in nontraffic accident

√x7ᵗʰ **V14.1** Pedal cycle passenger injured in collision with heavy transport vehicle or bus in nontraffic accident

√x7ᵗʰ **V14.2** Unspecified pedal cyclist injured in collision with heavy transport vehicle or bus in nontraffic accident

√x7ᵗʰ **V14.3** Person boarding or alighting a pedal cycle injured in collision with heavy transport vehicle or bus

√x7ᵗʰ **V14.4** Pedal cycle driver injured in collision with heavy transport vehicle or bus in traffic accident

√x7ᵗʰ **V14.5** Pedal cycle passenger injured in collision with heavy transport vehicle or bus in traffic accident

√x7ᵗʰ **V14.9** Unspecified pedal cyclist injured in collision with heavy transport vehicle or bus in traffic accident

√4ᵗʰ **V15** Pedal cycle rider injured in collision with railway train or railway vehicle

√x7ᵗʰ **V15.0** Pedal cycle driver injured in collision with railway train or railway vehicle in nontraffic accident

√x7ᵗʰ **V15.1** Pedal cycle passenger injured in collision with railway train or railway vehicle in nontraffic accident

√x7ᵗʰ **V15.2** Unspecified pedal cyclist injured in collision with railway train or railway vehicle in nontraffic accident

√x7ᵗʰ **V15.3** Person boarding or alighting a pedal cycle injured in collision with railway train or railway vehicle

√x7ᵗʰ **V15.4** Pedal cycle driver injured in collision with railway train or railway vehicle in traffic accident

√x7ᵗʰ **V15.5** Pedal cycle passenger injured in collision with railway train or railway vehicle in traffic accident

√x7ᵗʰ **V15.9** Unspecified pedal cyclist injured in collision with railway train or railway vehicle in traffic accident

√4ᵗʰ **V16** Pedal cycle rider injured in collision with other nonmotor vehicle

> **INCLUDES**   collision with animal-drawn vehicle, animal being ridden, streetcar

√x7ᵗʰ **V16.0** Pedal cycle driver injured in collision with other nonmotor vehicle in nontraffic accident

√x7ᵗʰ **V16.1** Pedal cycle passenger injured in collision with other nonmotor vehicle in nontraffic accident

√x7ᵗʰ **V16.2** Unspecified pedal cyclist injured in collision with other nonmotor vehicle in nontraffic accident

√x7ᵗʰ **V16.3** Person boarding or alighting a pedal cycle injured in collision with other nonmotor vehicle in nontraffic accident

√x7ᵗʰ **V16.4** Pedal cycle driver injured in collision with other nonmotor vehicle in traffic accident

√x7ᵗʰ **V16.5** Pedal cycle passenger injured in collision with other nonmotor vehicle in traffic accident

√x7ᵗʰ **V16.9** Unspecified pedal cyclist injured in collision with other nonmotor vehicle in traffic accident

√4ᵗʰ **V17** Pedal cycle rider injured in collision with fixed or stationary object

√x7ᵗʰ **V17.0** Pedal cycle driver injured in collision with fixed or stationary object in nontraffic accident

√x7ᵗʰ **V17.1** Pedal cycle passenger injured in collision with fixed or stationary object in nontraffic accident

√x7ᵗʰ **V17.2** Unspecified pedal cyclist injured in collision with fixed or stationary object in nontraffic accident

√x7ᵗʰ **V17.3** Person boarding or alighting a pedal cycle injured in collision with fixed or stationary object

√x7ᵗʰ **V17.4** Pedal cycle driver injured in collision with fixed or stationary object in traffic accident

√x7ᵗʰ **V17.5** Pedal cycle passenger injured in collision with fixed or stationary object in traffic accident

√x7ᵗʰ **V17.9** Unspecified pedal cyclist injured in collision with fixed or stationary object in traffic accident

√4ᵗʰ **V18** Pedal cycle rider injured in noncollision transport accident

> **INCLUDES**   fall or thrown from pedal cycle (without antecedent collision)
> overturning pedal cycle NOS
> overturning pedal cycle without collision

√x7ᵗʰ **V18.0** Pedal cycle driver injured in noncollision transport accident in nontraffic accident

√x7ᵗʰ **V18.1** Pedal cycle passenger injured in noncollision transport accident in nontraffic accident

√x7ᵗʰ **V18.2** Unspecified pedal cyclist injured in noncollision transport accident in nontraffic accident

√x7ᵗʰ **V18.3** Person boarding or alighting a pedal cycle injured in noncollision transport accident

Ⓝ Newborn: 0   Ⓟ Pediatric: 0-17   Ⓜ Maternity: 9-64   Ⓐ Adult: 15-124   **MCC** Major Complication/Comorbidity   **CC** Complication/Comorbidity   **SW** Severe Wound Dx

1220   ICD-10-CM 2020

✓x7ᵗʰ **V18.4** **Pedal cycle** driver **injured in noncollision transport accident** in traffic accident

✓x7ᵗʰ **V18.5** **Pedal cycle** passenger **injured in noncollision transport accident** in traffic accident

✓x7ᵗʰ **V18.9** **Unspecified pedal cyclist injured in noncollision transport accident** in traffic accident

✓4ᵗʰ **V19** **Pedal cycle rider injured in other and unspecified transport accidents**

  ✓5ᵗʰ **V19.0** **Pedal cycle** driver **injured in collision with other and unspecified motor vehicles** in nontraffic accident

    ✓x7ᵗʰ **V19.00** **Pedal cycle driver injured in collision with unspecified motor vehicles in nontraffic accident**

    ✓x7ᵗʰ **V19.09** **Pedal cycle driver injured in collision with other motor vehicles in nontraffic accident**

  ✓5ᵗʰ **V19.1** **Pedal cycle** passenger **injured in collision with other and unspecified motor vehicles** in nontraffic accident

    ✓x7ᵗʰ **V19.10** **Pedal cycle passenger injured in collision with unspecified motor vehicles in nontraffic accident**

    ✓x7ᵗʰ **V19.19** **Pedal cycle passenger injured in collision with other motor vehicles in nontraffic accident**

  ✓5ᵗʰ **V19.2** **Unspecified pedal cyclist injured in collision with other and unspecified motor vehicles** in nontraffic accident

    ✓x7ᵗʰ **V19.20** **Unspecified pedal cyclist injured in collision with unspecified motor vehicles in nontraffic accident**
        Pedal cycle collision NOS, nontraffic

    ✓x7ᵗʰ **V19.29** **Unspecified pedal cyclist injured in collision with other motor vehicles in nontraffic accident**

  ✓x7ᵗʰ **V19.3** **Pedal cyclist (driver) (passenger) injured in unspecified nontraffic accident**
        Pedal cycle accident NOS, nontraffic
        Pedal cyclist injured in nontraffic accident NOS

  ✓5ᵗʰ **V19.4** **Pedal cycle** driver **injured in collision with other and unspecified motor vehicles** in traffic accident

    ✓x7ᵗʰ **V19.40** **Pedal cycle driver injured in collision with unspecified motor vehicles in traffic accident**

    ✓x7ᵗʰ **V19.49** **Pedal cycle driver injured in collision with other motor vehicles in traffic accident**

  ✓5ᵗʰ **V19.5** **Pedal cycle** passenger **injured in collision with other and unspecified motor vehicles** in traffic accident

    ✓x7ᵗʰ **V19.50** **Pedal cycle passenger injured in collision with unspecified motor vehicles in traffic accident**

    ✓x7ᵗʰ **V19.59** **Pedal cycle passenger injured in collision with other motor vehicles in traffic accident**

  ✓5ᵗʰ **V19.6** **Unspecified pedal cyclist injured in collision with other and unspecified motor vehicles** in traffic accident

    ✓x7ᵗʰ **V19.60** **Unspecified pedal cyclist injured in collision with unspecified motor vehicles in traffic accident**
        Pedal cycle collision NOS (traffic)

    ✓x7ᵗʰ **V19.69** **Unspecified pedal cyclist injured in collision with other motor vehicles in traffic accident**

  ✓5ᵗʰ **V19.8** **Pedal cyclist (driver) (passenger) injured in other specified transport accidents**

    ✓x7ᵗʰ **V19.81** **Pedal cyclist (driver) (passenger) injured in transport accident with** military vehicle

    ✓x7ᵗʰ **V19.88** **Pedal cyclist (driver) (passenger) injured in other specified transport accidents**

  ✓x7ᵗʰ **V19.9** **Pedal cyclist (driver) (passenger) injured in unspecified traffic accident**
        Pedal cycle accident NOS

Motorcycle rider injured in transport accident (V20-V29)

INCLUDES   moped
        motorcycle with sidecar
        motorized bicycle
        motor scooter

EXCLUDES 1   three-wheeled motor vehicle (V30-V39)

The appropriate 7th character is to be added to each code from categories V20-V29.
A   initial encounter
D   subsequent encounter
S   sequela

✓4ᵗʰ **V20** **Motorcycle rider injured in collision with pedestrian or animal**

  EXCLUDES 1   motorcycle rider collision with animal-drawn vehicle or animal being ridden (V26.-)

  ✓x7ᵗʰ **V20.0** **Motorcycle** driver **injured in collision with pedestrian or animal** in nontraffic accident

  ✓x7ᵗʰ **V20.1** **Motorcycle** passenger **injured in collision with pedestrian or animal** in nontraffic accident

  ✓x7ᵗʰ **V20.2** **Unspecified motorcycle rider injured in collision with pedestrian or animal** in nontraffic accident

  ✓x7ᵗʰ **V20.3** Person boarding or alighting **a motorcycle injured in collision with pedestrian or animal**

  ✓x7ᵗʰ **V20.4** **Motorcycle** driver **injured in collision with pedestrian or animal** in traffic accident

  ✓x7ᵗʰ **V20.5** **Motorcycle** passenger **injured in collision with pedestrian or animal** in traffic accident

  ✓x7ᵗʰ **V20.9** **Unspecified motorcycle rider injured in collision with pedestrian or animal** in traffic accident

✓4ᵗʰ **V21** **Motorcycle rider injured in collision with pedal cycle**

  ✓x7ᵗʰ **V21.0** **Motorcycle** driver **injured in collision with pedal cycle** in nontraffic accident

  ✓x7ᵗʰ **V21.1** **Motorcycle** passenger **injured in collision with pedal cycle** in nontraffic accident

  ✓x7ᵗʰ **V21.2** **Unspecified motorcycle rider injured in collision with pedal cycle** in nontraffic accident

  ✓x7ᵗʰ **V21.3** Person boarding or alighting **a motorcycle injured in collision with pedal cycle**

  ✓x7ᵗʰ **V21.4** **Motorcycle** driver **injured in collision with pedal cycle** in traffic accident

  ✓x7ᵗʰ **V21.5** **Motorcycle** passenger **injured in collision with pedal cycle** in traffic accident

  ✓x7ᵗʰ **V21.9** **Unspecified motorcycle rider injured in collision with pedal cycle** in traffic accident

✓4ᵗʰ **V22** **Motorcycle rider injured in collision with two- or three-wheeled motor vehicle**

  ✓x7ᵗʰ **V22.0** **Motorcycle** driver **injured in collision with two- or three-wheeled motor vehicle** in nontraffic accident

  ✓x7ᵗʰ **V22.1** **Motorcycle** passenger **injured in collision with two- or three-wheeled motor vehicle** in nontraffic accident

  ✓x7ᵗʰ **V22.2** **Unspecified motorcycle rider injured in collision with two- or three-wheeled motor vehicle** in nontraffic accident

  ✓x7ᵗʰ **V22.3** Person boarding or alighting **a motorcycle injured in collision with two- or three-wheeled motor vehicle**

  ✓x7ᵗʰ **V22.4** **Motorcycle** driver **injured in collision with two- or three-wheeled motor vehicle** in traffic accident

  ✓x7ᵗʰ **V22.5** **Motorcycle** passenger **injured in collision with two- or three-wheeled motor vehicle** in traffic accident

  ✓x7ᵗʰ **V22.9** **Unspecified motorcycle rider injured in collision with two- or three-wheeled motor vehicle** in traffic accident

✓4ᵗʰ **V23** **Motorcycle rider injured in collision with car, pick-up truck or van**

  ✓x7ᵗʰ **V23.0** **Motorcycle** driver **injured in collision with car, pick-up truck or van** in nontraffic accident

  ✓x7ᵗʰ **V23.1** **Motorcycle** passenger **injured in collision with car, pick-up truck or van** in nontraffic accident

  ✓x7ᵗʰ **V23.2** **Unspecified motorcycle rider injured in collision with car, pick-up truck or van** in nontraffic accident

  ✓x7ᵗʰ **V23.3** Person boarding or alighting **a motorcycle injured in collision with car, pick-up truck or van**

  ✓x7ᵗʰ **V23.4** **Motorcycle** driver **injured in collision with car, pick-up truck or van** in traffic accident

  ✓x7ᵗʰ **V23.5** **Motorcycle** passenger **injured in collision with car, pick-up truck or van** in traffic accident

  ✓x7ᵗʰ **V23.9** **Unspecified motorcycle rider injured in collision with car, pick-up truck or van** in traffic accident

✓4ᵗʰ **V24** **Motorcycle rider injured in collision with heavy transport vehicle or bus**

  EXCLUDES 1   motorcycle rider injured in collision with military vehicle (V29.81)

  ✓x7ᵗʰ **V24.0** **Motorcycle** driver **injured in collision with heavy transport vehicle or bus** in nontraffic accident

  ✓x7ᵗʰ **V24.1** **Motorcycle** passenger **injured in collision with heavy transport vehicle or bus** in nontraffic accident

  ✓x7ᵗʰ **V24.2** **Unspecified motorcycle rider injured in collision with heavy transport vehicle or bus** in nontraffic accident

  ✓x7ᵗʰ **V24.3** Person boarding or alighting **a motorcycle injured in collision with heavy transport vehicle or bus**

  ✓x7ᵗʰ **V24.4** **Motorcycle** driver **injured in collision with heavy transport vehicle or bus** in traffic accident

  ✓x7ᵗʰ **V24.5** **Motorcycle** passenger **injured in collision with heavy transport vehicle or bus** in traffic accident

  ✓x7ᵗʰ **V24.9** **Unspecified motorcycle rider injured in collision with heavy transport vehicle or bus** in traffic accident

✓4ᵗʰ **V25** **Motorcycle rider injured in collision with railway train or railway vehicle**

  ✓x7ᵗʰ **V25.0** **Motorcycle** driver **injured in collision with railway train or railway vehicle** in nontraffic accident

  ✓x7ᵗʰ **V25.1** **Motorcycle** passenger **injured in collision with railway train or railway vehicle** in nontraffic accident

✔ Additional Char Req   ✓x7ᵗʰ Placeholder   Unacceptable PDx   Questionable PDx   Wrong Procedure   Manifestation   Unspecified Dx   H1-H14 HAC   HCC CMS-HCC Dx   HIV HIV Dx

ICD-10-CM 2020   1221

√x7th **V25.2** Unspecified motorcycle rider injured in collision with railway train or railway vehicle in nontraffic accident

√x7th **V25.3** Person boarding or alighting a motorcycle injured in collision with railway train or railway vehicle

√x7th **V25.4** Motorcycle driver injured in collision with railway train or railway vehicle in traffic accident

√x7th **V25.5** Motorcycle passenger injured in collision with railway train or railway vehicle in traffic accident

√x7th **V25.9** Unspecified motorcycle rider injured in collision with railway train or railway vehicle in traffic accident

√4th **V26** Motorcycle rider injured in collision with other nonmotor vehicle

> INCLUDES collision with animal-drawn vehicle, animal being ridden, streetcar

√x7th **V26.0** Motorcycle driver injured in collision with other nonmotor vehicle in nontraffic accident

√x7th **V26.1** Motorcycle passenger injured in collision with other nonmotor vehicle in nontraffic accident

√x7th **V26.2** Unspecified motorcycle rider injured in collision with other nonmotor vehicle in nontraffic accident

√x7th **V26.3** Person boarding or alighting a motorcycle injured in collision with other nonmotor vehicle

√x7th **V26.4** Motorcycle driver injured in collision with other nonmotor vehicle in traffic accident

√x7th **V26.5** Motorcycle passenger injured in collision with other nonmotor vehicle in traffic accident

√x7th **V26.9** Unspecified motorcycle rider injured in collision with other nonmotor vehicle in traffic accident

√4th **V27** Motorcycle rider injured in collision with fixed or stationary object

√x7th **V27.0** Motorcycle driver injured in collision with fixed or stationary object in nontraffic accident

√x7th **V27.1** Motorcycle passenger injured in collision with fixed or stationary object in nontraffic accident

√x7th **V27.2** Unspecified motorcycle rider injured in collision with fixed or stationary object in nontraffic accident

√x7th **V27.3** Person boarding or alighting a motorcycle injured in collision with fixed or stationary object

√x7th **V27.4** Motorcycle driver injured in collision with fixed or stationary object in traffic accident

√x7th **V27.5** Motorcycle passenger injured in collision with fixed or stationary object in traffic accident

√x7th **V27.9** Unspecified motorcycle rider injured in collision with fixed or stationary object in traffic accident

√4th **V28** Motorcycle rider injured in noncollision transport accident

> INCLUDES fall or thrown from motorcycle (without antecedent collision)
> overturning motorcycle NOS
> overturning motorcycle without collision

√x7th **V28.0** Motorcycle driver injured in noncollision transport accident in nontraffic accident

√x7th **V28.1** Motorcycle passenger injured in noncollision transport accident in nontraffic accident

√x7th **V28.2** Unspecified motorcycle rider injured in noncollision transport accident in nontraffic accident

√x7th **V28.3** Person boarding or alighting a motorcycle injured in noncollision transport accident

√x7th **V28.4** Motorcycle driver injured in noncollision transport accident in traffic accident

√x7th **V28.5** Motorcycle passenger injured in noncollision transport accident in traffic accident

√x7th **V28.9** Unspecified motorcycle rider injured in noncollision transport accident in traffic accident

√4th **V29** Motorcycle rider injured in other and unspecified transport accidents

√5th **V29.0** Motorcycle driver injured in collision with other and unspecified motor vehicles in nontraffic accident

√x7th **V29.00** Motorcycle driver injured in collision with unspecified motor vehicles in nontraffic accident

√x7th **V29.09** Motorcycle driver injured in collision with other motor vehicles in nontraffic accident

√5th **V29.1** Motorcycle passenger injured in collision with other and unspecified motor vehicles in nontraffic accident

√x7th **V29.10** Motorcycle passenger injured in collision with unspecified motor vehicles in nontraffic accident

√x7th **V29.19** Motorcycle passenger injured in collision with other motor vehicles in nontraffic accident

√5th **V29.2** Unspecified motorcycle rider injured in collision with other and unspecified motor vehicles in nontraffic accident

√x7th **V29.20** Unspecified motorcycle rider injured in collision with unspecified motor vehicles in nontraffic accident
> Motorcycle collision NOS, nontraffic

√x7th **V29.29** Unspecified motorcycle rider injured in collision with other motor vehicles in nontraffic accident

√x7th **V29.3** Motorcycle rider (driver) (passenger) injured in unspecified nontraffic accident
> Motorcycle accident NOS, nontraffic
> Motorcycle rider injured in nontraffic accident NOS

√5th **V29.4** Motorcycle driver injured in collision with other and unspecified motor vehicles in traffic accident

√x7th **V29.40** Motorcycle driver injured in collision with unspecified motor vehicles in traffic accident

√x7th **V29.49** Motorcycle driver injured in collision with other motor vehicles in traffic accident

√5th **V29.5** Motorcycle passenger injured in collision with other and unspecified motor vehicles in traffic accident

√x7th **V29.50** Motorcycle passenger injured in collision with unspecified motor vehicles in traffic accident

√x7th **V29.59** Motorcycle passenger injured in collision with other motor vehicles in traffic accident

√5th **V29.6** Unspecified motorcycle rider injured in collision with other and unspecified motor vehicles in traffic accident

√x7th **V29.60** Unspecified motorcycle rider injured in collision with unspecified motor vehicles in traffic accident
> Motorcycle collision NOS (traffic)

√x7th **V29.69** Unspecified motorcycle rider injured in collision with other motor vehicles in traffic accident

√5th **V29.8** Motorcycle rider (driver) (passenger) injured in other specified transport accidents

√x7th **V29.81** Motorcycle rider (driver) (passenger) injured in transport accident with military vehicle

√x7th **V29.88** Motorcycle rider (driver) (passenger) injured in other specified transport accidents

√x7th **V29.9** Motorcycle rider (driver) (passenger) injured in unspecified traffic accident
> Motorcycle accident NOS

Occupant of three-wheeled motor vehicle injured in transport accident (V30-V39)

> INCLUDES motorized tricycle
> motorized rickshaw
> three-wheeled motor car
>
> EXCLUDES 1 *all-terrain vehicles (V86.-)*
> *motorcycle with sidecar (V20-V29)*
> *vehicle designed primarily for off-road use (V86.-)*

The appropriate 7th character is to be added to each code from categories V30-V39.
A   initial encounter
D   subsequent encounter
S   sequela

√4th **V30** Occupant of three-wheeled motor vehicle injured in collision with pedestrian or animal

> EXCLUDES 1 *three-wheeled motor vehicle collision with animal-drawn vehicle or animal being ridden (V36.-)*

√x7th **V30.0** Driver of three-wheeled motor vehicle injured in collision with pedestrian or animal in nontraffic accident

√x7th **V30.1** Passenger in three-wheeled motor vehicle injured in collision with pedestrian or animal in nontraffic accident

√x7th **V30.2** Person on outside of three-wheeled motor vehicle injured in collision with pedestrian or animal in nontraffic accident

√x7th **V30.3** Unspecified occupant of three-wheeled motor vehicle injured in collision with pedestrian or animal in nontraffic accident

√x7th **V30.4** Person boarding or alighting a three-wheeled motor vehicle injured in collision with pedestrian or animal

√x7th **V30.5** Driver of three-wheeled motor vehicle injured in collision with pedestrian or animal in traffic accident

√x7th **V30.6** Passenger in three-wheeled motor vehicle injured in collision with pedestrian or animal in traffic accident

√x7th **V30.7** Person on outside of three-wheeled motor vehicle injured in collision with pedestrian or animal in traffic accident

√x7th **V30.9** Unspecified occupant of three-wheeled motor vehicle injured in collision with pedestrian or animal in traffic accident

√4th **V31** Occupant of three-wheeled motor vehicle injured in collision with pedal cycle

√x7th **V31.0** Driver of three-wheeled motor vehicle injured in collision with pedal cycle in nontraffic accident

√x7ᵗʰ **V31.1** Passenger in three-wheeled motor vehicle injured in collision with pedal cycle in nontraffic accident

√x7ᵗʰ **V31.2** Person on outside of three-wheeled motor vehicle injured in collision with pedal cycle in nontraffic accident

√x7ᵗʰ **V31.3** Unspecified occupant of three-wheeled motor vehicle injured in collision with pedal cycle in nontraffic accident

√x7ᵗʰ **V31.4** Person boarding or alighting a three-wheeled motor vehicle injured in collision with pedal cycle

√x7ᵗʰ **V31.5** Driver of three-wheeled motor vehicle injured in collision with pedal cycle in traffic accident

√x7ᵗʰ **V31.6** Passenger in three-wheeled motor vehicle injured in collision with pedal cycle in traffic accident

√x7ᵗʰ **V31.7** Person on outside of three-wheeled motor vehicle injured in collision with pedal cycle in traffic accident

√x7ᵗʰ **V31.9** Unspecified occupant of three-wheeled motor vehicle injured in collision with pedal cycle in traffic accident

✓4ᵗʰ **V32** Occupant of three-wheeled motor vehicle injured in collision with two- or three-wheeled motor vehicle

√x7ᵗʰ **V32.0** Driver of three-wheeled motor vehicle injured in collision with two- or three-wheeled motor vehicle in nontraffic accident

√x7ᵗʰ **V32.1** Passenger in three-wheeled motor vehicle injured in collision with two- or three-wheeled motor vehicle in nontraffic accident

√x7ᵗʰ **V32.2** Person on outside of three-wheeled motor vehicle injured in collision with two- or three-wheeled motor vehicle in nontraffic accident

√x7ᵗʰ **V32.3** Unspecified occupant of three-wheeled motor vehicle injured in collision with two- or three-wheeled motor vehicle in nontraffic accident

√x7ᵗʰ **V32.4** Person boarding or alighting a three-wheeled motor vehicle injured in collision with two- or three-wheeled motor vehicle

√x7ᵗʰ **V32.5** Driver of three-wheeled motor vehicle injured in collision with two- or three-wheeled motor vehicle in traffic accident

√x7ᵗʰ **V32.6** Passenger in three-wheeled motor vehicle injured in collision with two- or three-wheeled motor vehicle in traffic accident

√x7ᵗʰ **V32.7** Person on outside of three-wheeled motor vehicle injured in collision with two- or three-wheeled motor vehicle in traffic accident

√x7ᵗʰ **V32.9** Unspecified occupant of three-wheeled motor vehicle injured in collision with two- or three-wheeled motor vehicle in traffic accident

✓4ᵗʰ **V33** Occupant of three-wheeled motor vehicle injured in collision with car, pick-up truck or van

√x7ᵗʰ **V33.0** Driver of three-wheeled motor vehicle injured in collision with car, pick-up truck or van in nontraffic accident

√x7ᵗʰ **V33.1** Passenger in three-wheeled motor vehicle injured in collision with car, pick-up truck or van in nontraffic accident

√x7ᵗʰ **V33.2** Person on outside of three-wheeled motor vehicle injured in collision with car, pick-up truck or van in nontraffic accident

√x7ᵗʰ **V33.3** Unspecified occupant of three-wheeled motor vehicle injured in collision with car, pick-up truck or van in nontraffic accident

√x7ᵗʰ **V33.4** Person boarding or alighting a three-wheeled motor vehicle injured in collision with car, pick-up truck or van

√x7ᵗʰ **V33.5** Driver of three-wheeled motor vehicle injured in collision with car, pick-up truck or van in traffic accident

√x7ᵗʰ **V33.6** Passenger in three-wheeled motor vehicle injured in collision with car, pick-up truck or van in traffic accident

√x7ᵗʰ **V33.7** Person on outside of three-wheeled motor vehicle injured in collision with car, pick-up truck or van in traffic accident

√x7ᵗʰ **V33.9** Unspecified occupant of three-wheeled motor vehicle injured in collision with car, pick-up truck or van in traffic accident

✓4ᵗʰ **V34** Occupant of three-wheeled motor vehicle injured in collision with heavy transport vehicle or bus

EXCLUDES 1   occupant of three-wheeled motor vehicle injured in collision with military vehicle (V39.81)

√x7ᵗʰ **V34.0** Driver of three-wheeled motor vehicle injured in collision with heavy transport vehicle or bus in nontraffic accident

√x7ᵗʰ **V34.1** Passenger in three-wheeled motor vehicle injured in collision with heavy transport vehicle or bus in nontraffic accident

√x7ᵗʰ **V34.2** Person on outside of three-wheeled motor vehicle injured in collision with heavy transport vehicle or bus in nontraffic accident

√x7ᵗʰ **V34.3** Unspecified occupant of three-wheeled motor vehicle injured in collision with heavy transport vehicle or bus in nontraffic accident

√x7ᵗʰ **V34.4** Person boarding or alighting a three-wheeled motor vehicle injured in collision with heavy transport vehicle or bus

√x7ᵗʰ **V34.5** Driver of three-wheeled motor vehicle injured in collision with heavy transport vehicle or bus in traffic accident

√x7ᵗʰ **V34.6** Passenger in three-wheeled motor vehicle injured in collision with heavy transport vehicle or bus in traffic accident

√x7ᵗʰ **V34.7** Person on outside of three-wheeled motor vehicle injured in collision with heavy transport vehicle or bus in traffic accident

√x7ᵗʰ **V34.9** Unspecified occupant of three-wheeled motor vehicle injured in collision with heavy transport vehicle or bus in traffic accident

✓4ᵗʰ **V35** Occupant of three-wheeled motor vehicle injured in collision with railway train or railway vehicle

√x7ᵗʰ **V35.0** Driver of three-wheeled motor vehicle injured in collision with railway train or railway vehicle in nontraffic accident

√x7ᵗʰ **V35.1** Passenger in three-wheeled motor vehicle injured in collision with railway train or railway vehicle in nontraffic accident

√x7ᵗʰ **V35.2** Person on outside of three-wheeled motor vehicle injured in collision with railway train or railway vehicle in nontraffic accident

√x7ᵗʰ **V35.3** Unspecified occupant of three-wheeled motor vehicle injured in collision with railway train or railway vehicle in nontraffic accident

√x7ᵗʰ **V35.4** Person boarding or alighting a three-wheeled motor vehicle injured in collision with railway train or railway vehicle

√x7ᵗʰ **V35.5** Driver of three-wheeled motor vehicle injured in collision with railway train or railway vehicle in traffic accident

√x7ᵗʰ **V35.6** Passenger in three-wheeled motor vehicle injured in collision with railway train or railway vehicle in traffic accident

√x7ᵗʰ **V35.7** Person on outside of three-wheeled motor vehicle injured in collision with railway train or railway vehicle in traffic accident

√x7ᵗʰ **V35.9** Unspecified occupant of three-wheeled motor vehicle injured in collision with railway train or railway vehicle in traffic accident

✓4ᵗʰ **V36** Occupant of three-wheeled motor vehicle injured in collision with other nonmotor vehicle

INCLUDES   collision with animal-drawn vehicle, animal being ridden, streetcar

√x7ᵗʰ **V36.0** Driver of three-wheeled motor vehicle injured in collision with other nonmotor vehicle in nontraffic accident

√x7ᵗʰ **V36.1** Passenger in three-wheeled motor vehicle injured in collision with other nonmotor vehicle in nontraffic accident

√x7ᵗʰ **V36.2** Person on outside of three-wheeled motor vehicle injured in collision with other nonmotor vehicle in nontraffic accident

√x7ᵗʰ **V36.3** Unspecified occupant of three-wheeled motor vehicle injured in collision with other nonmotor vehicle in nontraffic accident

√x7ᵗʰ **V36.4** Person boarding or alighting a three-wheeled motor vehicle injured in collision with other nonmotor vehicle

√x7ᵗʰ **V36.5** Driver of three-wheeled motor vehicle injured in collision with other nonmotor vehicle in traffic accident

√x7ᵗʰ **V36.6** Passenger in three-wheeled motor vehicle injured in collision with other nonmotor vehicle in traffic accident

√x7ᵗʰ **V36.7** Person on outside of three-wheeled motor vehicle injured in collision with other nonmotor vehicle in traffic accident

√x7ᵗʰ **V36.9** Unspecified occupant of three-wheeled motor vehicle injured in collision with other nonmotor vehicle in traffic accident

✓4ᵗʰ **V37** Occupant of three-wheeled motor vehicle injured in collision with fixed or stationary object

√x7ᵗʰ **V37.0** Driver of three-wheeled motor vehicle injured in collision with fixed or stationary object in nontraffic accident

√x7ᵗʰ **V37.1** Passenger in three-wheeled motor vehicle injured in collision with fixed or stationary object in nontraffic accident

√x7ᵗʰ **V37.2** Person on outside of three-wheeled motor vehicle injured in collision with fixed or stationary object in nontraffic accident

√x7ᵗʰ **V37.3** Unspecified occupant of three-wheeled motor vehicle injured in collision with fixed or stationary object in nontraffic accident

√x7ᵗʰ **V37.4** Person boarding or alighting a three-wheeled motor vehicle injured in collision with fixed or stationary object

√x7ᵗʰ **V37.5** Driver of three-wheeled motor vehicle injured in collision with fixed or stationary object in traffic accident

√x7ᵗʰ **V37.6** Passenger in three-wheeled motor vehicle injured in collision with fixed or stationary object in traffic accident

√x7ᵗʰ **V37.7** Person on outside of three-wheeled motor vehicle injured in collision with fixed or stationary object in traffic accident

√x7ᵗʰ **V37.9** Unspecified occupant of three-wheeled motor vehicle injured in collision with fixed or stationary object in traffic accident

✓ Additional Char Req   √x7ᵗʰ Placeholder   Unacceptable PDx   Questionable PDx   Wrong Procedure   Manifestation   Unspecified Dx   H1-H14 HAC   HCC CMS-HCC Dx   HIV HIV Dx

ICD-10-CM 2020   1223

Chapter 20. External Causes of Morbidity *(left margin)*

V38–V41.9 *(left margin)*

√4ᵗʰ **V38 Occupant of three-wheeled motor vehicle injured in noncollision transport accident**

INCLUDES   fall or thrown from three-wheeled motor vehicle
overturning of three-wheeled motor vehicle NOS
overturning of three-wheeled motor vehicle without collision

√x7ᵗʰ **V38.0** Driver of three-wheeled motor vehicle injured in noncollision transport accident in nontraffic accident

√x7ᵗʰ **V38.1** Passenger in three-wheeled motor vehicle injured in noncollision transport accident in nontraffic accident

√x7ᵗʰ **V38.2** Person on outside of three-wheeled motor vehicle injured in noncollision transport accident in nontraffic accident

√x7ᵗʰ **V38.3** Unspecified occupant of three-wheeled motor vehicle injured in noncollision transport accident in nontraffic accident

√x7ᵗʰ **V38.4** Person boarding or alighting a three-wheeled motor vehicle injured in noncollision transport accident

√x7ᵗʰ **V38.5** Driver of three-wheeled motor vehicle injured in noncollision transport accident in traffic accident

√x7ᵗʰ **V38.6** Passenger in three-wheeled motor vehicle injured in noncollision transport accident in traffic accident

√x7ᵗʰ **V38.7** Person on outside of three-wheeled motor vehicle injured in noncollision transport accident in traffic accident

√x7ᵗʰ **V38.9** Unspecified occupant of three-wheeled motor vehicle injured in noncollision transport accident in traffic accident

√4ᵗʰ **V39 Occupant of three-wheeled motor vehicle injured in other and unspecified transport accidents**

√5ᵗʰ **V39.0** Driver of three-wheeled motor vehicle injured in collision with other and unspecified motor vehicles in nontraffic accident

√x7ᵗʰ **V39.00** Driver of three-wheeled motor vehicle injured in collision with unspecified motor vehicles in nontraffic accident

√x7ᵗʰ **V39.09** Driver of three-wheeled motor vehicle injured in collision with other motor vehicles in nontraffic accident

√5ᵗʰ **V39.1** Passenger in three-wheeled motor vehicle injured in collision with other and unspecified motor vehicles in nontraffic accident

√x7ᵗʰ **V39.10** Passenger in three-wheeled motor vehicle injured in collision with unspecified motor vehicles in nontraffic accident

√x7ᵗʰ **V39.19** Passenger in three-wheeled motor vehicle injured in collision with other motor vehicles in nontraffic accident

√5ᵗʰ **V39.2** Unspecified occupant of three-wheeled motor vehicle injured in collision with other and unspecified motor vehicles in nontraffic accident

√x7ᵗʰ **V39.20** Unspecified occupant of three-wheeled motor vehicle injured in collision with unspecified motor vehicles in nontraffic accident
Collision NOS involving three-wheeled motor vehicle, nontraffic

√x7ᵗʰ **V39.29** Unspecified occupant of three-wheeled motor vehicle injured in collision with other motor vehicles in nontraffic accident

√x7ᵗʰ **V39.3** Occupant (driver) (passenger) of three-wheeled motor vehicle injured in unspecified nontraffic accident
Accident NOS involving three-wheeled motor vehicle, nontraffic
Occupant of three-wheeled motor vehicle injured in nontraffic accident NOS

√5ᵗʰ **V39.4** Driver of three-wheeled motor vehicle injured in collision with other and unspecified motor vehicles in traffic accident

√x7ᵗʰ **V39.40** Driver of three-wheeled motor vehicle injured in collision with unspecified motor vehicles in traffic accident

√x7ᵗʰ **V39.49** Driver of three-wheeled motor vehicle injured in collision with other motor vehicles in traffic accident

√5ᵗʰ **V39.5** Passenger in three-wheeled motor vehicle injured in collision with other and unspecified motor vehicles in traffic accident

√x7ᵗʰ **V39.50** Passenger in three-wheeled motor vehicle injured in collision with unspecified motor vehicles in traffic accident

√x7ᵗʰ **V39.59** Passenger in three-wheeled motor vehicle injured in collision with other motor vehicles in traffic accident

√5ᵗʰ **V39.6** Unspecified occupant of three-wheeled motor vehicle injured in collision with other and unspecified motor vehicles in traffic accident

√x7ᵗʰ **V39.60** Unspecified occupant of three-wheeled motor vehicle injured in collision with unspecified motor vehicles in traffic accident
Collision NOS involving three-wheeled motor vehicle (traffic)

√x7ᵗʰ **V39.69** Unspecified occupant of three-wheeled motor vehicle injured in collision with other motor vehicles in traffic accident

√5ᵗʰ **V39.8** Occupant (driver) (passenger) of three-wheeled motor vehicle injured in other specified transport accidents

√x7ᵗʰ **V39.81** Occupant (driver) (passenger) of three-wheeled motor vehicle injured in transport accident with military vehicle

√x7ᵗʰ **V39.89** Occupant (driver) (passenger) of three-wheeled motor vehicle injured in other specified transport accidents

√x7ᵗʰ **V39.9** Occupant (driver) (passenger) of three-wheeled motor vehicle injured in unspecified traffic accident
Accident NOS involving three-wheeled motor vehicle

Car occupant injured in transport accident (V40-V49)

INCLUDES   a four-wheeled motor vehicle designed primarily for carrying passengers
automobile (pulling a trailer or camper)

EXCLUDES 1   bus (V50-V59)
minibus (V50-V59)
minivan (V50-V59)
motorcoach (V70-V79)
pick-up truck (V50-V59)
sport utility vehicle (SUV) (V50-V59)

The appropriate 7th character is to be added to each code from categories V40-V49.
A   initial encounter
D   subsequent encounter
S   sequela

√4ᵗʰ **V40 Car occupant injured in collision with pedestrian or animal**

EXCLUDES 1   car collision with animal-drawn vehicle or animal being ridden (V46.-)

√x7ᵗʰ **V40.0** Car driver injured in collision with pedestrian or animal in nontraffic accident

√x7ᵗʰ **V40.1** Car passenger injured in collision with pedestrian or animal in nontraffic accident

√x7ᵗʰ **V40.2** Person on outside of car injured in collision with pedestrian or animal in nontraffic accident

√x7ᵗʰ **V40.3** Unspecified car occupant injured in collision with pedestrian or animal in nontraffic accident

√x7ᵗʰ **V40.4** Person boarding or alighting a car injured in collision with pedestrian or animal

√x7ᵗʰ **V40.5** Car driver injured in collision with pedestrian or animal in traffic accident

√x7ᵗʰ **V40.6** Car passenger injured in collision with pedestrian or animal in traffic accident

√x7ᵗʰ **V40.7** Person on outside of car injured in collision with pedestrian or animal in traffic accident

√x7ᵗʰ **V40.9** Unspecified car occupant injured in collision with pedestrian or animal in traffic accident

√4ᵗʰ **V41 Car occupant injured in collision with pedal cycle**

√x7ᵗʰ **V41.0** Car driver injured in collision with pedal cycle in nontraffic accident

√x7ᵗʰ **V41.1** Car passenger injured in collision with pedal cycle in nontraffic accident

√x7ᵗʰ **V41.2** Person on outside of car injured in collision with pedal cycle in nontraffic accident

√x7ᵗʰ **V41.3** Unspecified car occupant injured in collision with pedal cycle in nontraffic accident

√x7ᵗʰ **V41.4** Person boarding or alighting a car injured in collision with pedal cycle

√x7ᵗʰ **V41.5** Car driver injured in collision with pedal cycle in traffic accident

√x7ᵗʰ **V41.6** Car passenger injured in collision with pedal cycle in traffic accident

√x7ᵗʰ **V41.7** Person on outside of car injured in collision with pedal cycle in traffic accident

√x7ᵗʰ **V41.9** Unspecified car occupant injured in collision with pedal cycle in traffic accident

N Newborn: 0   P Pediatric: 0-17   M Maternity: 9-64   A Adult: 15-124   MCC Major Complication/Comorbidity   CC Complication/Comorbidity   SW Severe Wound Dx

1224   ICD-10-CM 2020

√4ᵗʰ **V42** Car occupant injured in collision with two- or three-wheeled motor vehicle

√x7ᵗʰ **V42.0** Car driver injured in collision with two- or three-wheeled motor vehicle in nontraffic accident

√x7ᵗʰ **V42.1** Car passenger injured in collision with two- or three-wheeled motor vehicle in nontraffic accident

√x7ᵗʰ **V42.2** Person on outside of car injured in collision with two- or three-wheeled motor vehicle in nontraffic accident

√x7ᵗʰ **V42.3** Unspecified car occupant injured in collision with two- or three-wheeled motor vehicle in nontraffic accident

√x7ᵗʰ **V42.4** Person boarding or alighting a car injured in collision with two- or three-wheeled motor vehicle

√x7ᵗʰ **V42.5** Car driver injured in collision with two- or three-wheeled motor vehicle in traffic accident

√x7ᵗʰ **V42.6** Car passenger injured in collision with two- or three-wheeled motor vehicle in traffic accident

√x7ᵗʰ **V42.7** Person on outside of car injured in collision with two- or three-wheeled motor vehicle in traffic accident

√x7ᵗʰ **V42.9** Unspecified car occupant injured in collision with two- or three-wheeled motor vehicle in traffic accident

√4ᵗʰ **V43** Car occupant injured in collision with car, pick-up truck or van

√5ᵗʰ **V43.0** Car driver injured in collision with car, pick-up truck or van in nontraffic accident

√x7ᵗʰ **V43.01** Car driver injured in collision with sport utility vehicle in nontraffic accident

√x7ᵗʰ **V43.02** Car driver injured in collision with other type car in nontraffic accident

√x7ᵗʰ **V43.03** Car driver injured in collision with pick-up truck in nontraffic accident

√x7ᵗʰ **V43.04** Car driver injured in collision with van in nontraffic accident

√5ᵗʰ **V43.1** Car passenger injured in collision with car, pick-up truck or van in nontraffic accident

√x7ᵗʰ **V43.11** Car passenger injured in collision with sport utility vehicle in nontraffic accident

√x7ᵗʰ **V43.12** Car passenger injured in collision with other type car in nontraffic accident

√x7ᵗʰ **V43.13** Car passenger injured in collision with pick-up truck in nontraffic accident

√x7ᵗʰ **V43.14** Car passenger injured in collision with van in nontraffic accident

√5ᵗʰ **V43.2** Person on outside of car injured in collision with car, pick-up truck or van in nontraffic accident

√x7ᵗʰ **V43.21** Person on outside of car injured in collision with sport utility vehicle in nontraffic accident

√x7ᵗʰ **V43.22** Person on outside of car injured in collision with other type car in nontraffic accident

√x7ᵗʰ **V43.23** Person on outside of car injured in collision with pick-up truck in nontraffic accident

√x7ᵗʰ **V43.24** Person on outside of car injured in collision with van in nontraffic accident

√5ᵗʰ **V43.3** Unspecified car occupant injured in collision with car, pick-up truck or van in nontraffic accident

√x7ᵗʰ **V43.31** Unspecified car occupant injured in collision with sport utility vehicle in nontraffic accident

√x7ᵗʰ **V43.32** Unspecified car occupant injured in collision with other type car in nontraffic accident

√x7ᵗʰ **V43.33** Unspecified car occupant injured in collision with pick-up truck in nontraffic accident

√x7ᵗʰ **V43.34** Unspecified car occupant injured in collision with van in nontraffic accident

√5ᵗʰ **V43.4** Person boarding or alighting a car injured in collision with car, pick-up truck or van

√x7ᵗʰ **V43.41** Person boarding or alighting a car injured in collision with sport utility vehicle

√x7ᵗʰ **V43.42** Person boarding or alighting a car injured in collision with other type car

√x7ᵗʰ **V43.43** Person boarding or alighting a car injured in collision with pick-up truck

√x7ᵗʰ **V43.44** Person boarding or alighting a car injured in collision with van

√5ᵗʰ **V43.5** Car driver injured in collision with car, pick-up truck or van in traffic accident

√x7ᵗʰ **V43.51** Car driver injured in collision with sport utility vehicle in traffic accident

√x7ᵗʰ **V43.52** Car driver injured in collision with other type car in traffic accident

√x7ᵗʰ **V43.53** Car driver injured in collision with pick-up truck in traffic accident

√x7ᵗʰ **V43.54** Car driver injured in collision with van in traffic accident

√5ᵗʰ **V43.6** Car passenger injured in collision with car, pick-up truck or van in traffic accident

√x7ᵗʰ **V43.61** Car passenger injured in collision with sport utility vehicle in traffic accident

√x7ᵗʰ **V43.62** Car passenger injured in collision with other type car in traffic accident

√x7ᵗʰ **V43.63** Car passenger injured in collision with pick-up truck in traffic accident

√x7ᵗʰ **V43.64** Car passenger injured in collision with van in traffic accident

√5ᵗʰ **V43.7** Person on outside of car injured in collision with car, pick-up truck or van in traffic accident

√x7ᵗʰ **V43.71** Person on outside of car injured in collision with sport utility vehicle in traffic accident

√x7ᵗʰ **V43.72** Person on outside of car injured in collision with other type car in traffic accident

√x7ᵗʰ **V43.73** Person on outside of car injured in collision with pick-up truck in traffic accident

√x7ᵗʰ **V43.74** Person on outside of car injured in collision with van in traffic accident

√5ᵗʰ **V43.9** Unspecified car occupant injured in collision with car, pick-up truck or van in traffic accident

√x7ᵗʰ **V43.91** Unspecified car occupant injured in collision with sport utility vehicle in traffic accident

√x7ᵗʰ **V43.92** Unspecified car occupant injured in collision with other type car in traffic accident

√x7ᵗʰ **V43.93** Unspecified car occupant injured in collision with pick-up truck in traffic accident

√x7ᵗʰ **V43.94** Unspecified car occupant injured in collision with van in traffic accident

√4ᵗʰ **V44** Car occupant injured in collision with heavy transport vehicle or bus

EXCLUDES 1   car occupant injured in collision with military vehicle (V49.81)

√x7ᵗʰ **V44.0** Car driver injured in collision with heavy transport vehicle or bus in nontraffic accident

√x7ᵗʰ **V44.1** Car passenger injured in collision with heavy transport vehicle or bus in nontraffic accident

√x7ᵗʰ **V44.2** Person on outside of car injured in collision with heavy transport vehicle or bus in nontraffic accident

√x7ᵗʰ **V44.3** Unspecified car occupant injured in collision with heavy transport vehicle or bus in nontraffic accident

√x7ᵗʰ **V44.4** Person boarding or alighting a car injured in collision with heavy transport vehicle or bus

√x7ᵗʰ **V44.5** Car driver injured in collision with heavy transport vehicle or bus in traffic accident

√x7ᵗʰ **V44.6** Car passenger injured in collision with heavy transport vehicle or bus in traffic accident

√x7ᵗʰ **V44.7** Person on outside of car injured in collision with heavy transport vehicle or bus in traffic accident

√x7ᵗʰ **V44.9** Unspecified car occupant injured in collision with heavy transport vehicle or bus in traffic accident

√4ᵗʰ **V45** Car occupant injured in collision with railway train or railway vehicle

√x7ᵗʰ **V45.0** Car driver injured in collision with railway train or railway vehicle in nontraffic accident

√x7ᵗʰ **V45.1** Car passenger injured in collision with railway train or railway vehicle in nontraffic accident

√x7ᵗʰ **V45.2** Person on outside of car injured in collision with railway train or railway vehicle in nontraffic accident

√x7ᵗʰ **V45.3** Unspecified car occupant injured in collision with railway train or railway vehicle in nontraffic accident

√x7ᵗʰ **V45.4** Person boarding or alighting a car injured in collision with railway train or railway vehicle

√x7ᵗʰ **V45.5** Car driver injured in collision with railway train or railway vehicle in traffic accident

√x7ᵗʰ **V45.6** Car passenger injured in collision with railway train or railway vehicle in traffic accident

√x7ᵗʰ **V45.7** Person on outside of car injured in collision with railway train or railway vehicle in traffic accident

√x7ᵗʰ **V45.9** Unspecified car occupant injured in collision with railway train or railway vehicle in traffic accident

√4ᵗʰ **V46** Car occupant injured in collision with other nonmotor vehicle

INCLUDES   collision with animal-drawn vehicle, animal being ridden, streetcar

√x7ᵗʰ **V46.0** Car driver injured in collision with other nonmotor vehicle in nontraffic accident

√x7ᵗʰ **V46.1** Car passenger injured in collision with other nonmotor vehicle in nontraffic accident

√x7ᵗʰ **V46.2** Person on outside of car injured in collision with other nonmotor vehicle in nontraffic accident

✓x7ᵗʰ **V46.3** Unspecified car occupant injured in collision with other nonmotor vehicle in nontraffic accident

✓x7ᵗʰ **V46.4** Person boarding or alighting a car injured in collision with other nonmotor vehicle

✓x7ᵗʰ **V46.5** Car driver injured in collision with other nonmotor vehicle in traffic accident

✓x7ᵗʰ **V46.6** Car passenger injured in collision with other nonmotor vehicle in traffic accident

✓x7ᵗʰ **V46.7** Person on outside of car injured in collision with other nonmotor vehicle in traffic accident

✓x7ᵗʰ **V46.9** Unspecified car occupant injured in collision with other nonmotor vehicle in traffic accident

✓4ᵗʰ **V47** Car occupant injured in collision with fixed or stationary object

     AHA: 2016,4Q,73

✓x7ᵗʰ **V47.0** Car driver injured in collision with fixed or stationary object in nontraffic accident

✓x7ᵗʰ **V47.1** Car passenger injured in collision with fixed or stationary object in nontraffic accident

✓x7ᵗʰ **V47.2** Person on outside of car injured in collision with fixed or stationary object in nontraffic accident

✓x7ᵗʰ **V47.3** Unspecified car occupant injured in collision with fixed or stationary object in nontraffic accident

✓x7ᵗʰ **V47.4** Person boarding or alighting a car injured in collision with fixed or stationary object

✓x7ᵗʰ **V47.5** Car driver injured in collision with fixed or stationary object in traffic accident

✓x7ᵗʰ **V47.6** Car passenger injured in collision with fixed or stationary object in traffic accident

✓x7ᵗʰ **V47.7** Person on outside of car injured in collision with fixed or stationary object in traffic accident

✓x7ᵗʰ **V47.9** Unspecified car occupant injured in collision with fixed or stationary object in traffic accident

✓4ᵗʰ **V48** Car occupant injured in noncollision transport accident

     INCLUDES   overturning car NOS

                 overturning car without collision

✓x7ᵗʰ **V48.0** Car driver injured in noncollision transport accident in nontraffic accident

✓x7ᵗʰ **V48.1** Car passenger injured in noncollision transport accident in nontraffic accident

✓x7ᵗʰ **V48.2** Person on outside of car injured in noncollision transport accident in nontraffic accident

✓x7ᵗʰ **V48.3** Unspecified car occupant injured in noncollision transport accident in nontraffic accident

✓x7ᵗʰ **V48.4** Person boarding or alighting a car injured in noncollision transport accident

✓x7ᵗʰ **V48.5** Car driver injured in noncollision transport accident in traffic accident

✓x7ᵗʰ **V48.6** Car passenger injured in noncollision transport accident in traffic accident

✓x7ᵗʰ **V48.7** Person on outside of car injured in noncollision transport accident in traffic accident

✓x7ᵗʰ **V48.9** Unspecified car occupant injured in noncollision transport accident in traffic accident

✓4ᵗʰ **V49** Car occupant injured in other and unspecified transport accidents

✓5ᵗʰ **V49.0** Driver injured in collision with other and unspecified motor vehicles in nontraffic accident

     ✓x7ᵗʰ **V49.00** Driver injured in collision with unspecified motor vehicles in nontraffic accident

     ✓x7ᵗʰ **V49.09** Driver injured in collision with other motor vehicles in nontraffic accident

✓5ᵗʰ **V49.1** Passenger injured in collision with other and unspecified motor vehicles in nontraffic accident

     ✓x7ᵗʰ **V49.10** Passenger injured in collision with unspecified motor vehicles in nontraffic accident

     ✓x7ᵗʰ **V49.19** Passenger injured in collision with other motor vehicles in nontraffic accident

✓5ᵗʰ **V49.2** Unspecified car occupant injured in collision with other and unspecified motor vehicles in nontraffic accident

     ✓x7ᵗʰ **V49.20** Unspecified car occupant injured in collision with unspecified motor vehicles in nontraffic accident

                Car collision NOS, nontraffic

     ✓x7ᵗʰ **V49.29** Unspecified car occupant injured in collision with other motor vehicles in nontraffic accident

✓x7ᵗʰ **V49.3** Car occupant (driver) (passenger) injured in unspecified nontraffic accident

         Car accident NOS, nontraffic

         Car occupant injured in nontraffic accident NOS

✓5ᵗʰ **V49.4** Driver injured in collision with other and unspecified motor vehicles in traffic accident

     ✓x7ᵗʰ **V49.40** Driver injured in collision with unspecified motor vehicles in traffic accident

     ✓x7ᵗʰ **V49.49** Driver injured in collision with other motor vehicles in traffic accident

✓5ᵗʰ **V49.5** Passenger injured in collision with other and unspecified motor vehicles in traffic accident

     ✓x7ᵗʰ **V49.50** Passenger injured in collision with unspecified motor vehicles in traffic accident

     ✓x7ᵗʰ **V49.59** Passenger injured in collision with other motor vehicles in traffic accident

✓5ᵗʰ **V49.6** Unspecified car occupant injured in collision with other and unspecified motor vehicles in traffic accident

     ✓x7ᵗʰ **V49.60** Unspecified car occupant injured in collision with unspecified motor vehicles in traffic accident

                Car collision NOS (traffic)

     ✓x7ᵗʰ **V49.69** Unspecified car occupant injured in collision with other motor vehicles in traffic accident

✓5ᵗʰ **V49.8** Car occupant (driver) (passenger) injured in other specified transport accidents

     ✓x7ᵗʰ **V49.81** Car occupant (driver) (passenger) injured in transport accident with military vehicle

     ✓x7ᵗʰ **V49.88** Car occupant (driver) (passenger) injured in other specified transport accidents

✓x7ᵗʰ **V49.9** Car occupant (driver) (passenger) injured in unspecified traffic accident

         Car accident NOS

Occupant of pick-up truck or van injured in transport accident (V50-V59)

     INCLUDES   a four or six wheel motor vehicle designed primarily for carrying passengers and property but weighing less than the local limit for classification as a heavy goods vehicle

            minibus

            minivan

            sport utility vehicle (SUV)

            truck

            van

     EXCLUDES 1   heavy transport vehicle (V60-V69)

The appropriate 7th character is to be added to each code from categories V50-V59.
A   initial encounter
D   subsequent encounter
S   sequela

✓4ᵗʰ **V50** Occupant of pick-up truck or van injured in collision with pedestrian or animal

     EXCLUDES 1   pick-up truck or van collision with animal-drawn vehicle or animal being ridden (V56.-)

✓x7ᵗʰ **V50.0** Driver of pick-up truck or van injured in collision with pedestrian or animal in nontraffic accident

✓x7ᵗʰ **V50.1** Passenger in pick-up truck or van injured in collision with pedestrian or animal in nontraffic accident

✓x7ᵗʰ **V50.2** Person on outside of pick-up truck or van injured in collision with pedestrian or animal in nontraffic accident

✓x7ᵗʰ **V50.3** Unspecified occupant of pick-up truck or van injured in collision with pedestrian or animal in nontraffic accident

✓x7ᵗʰ **V50.4** Person boarding or alighting a pick-up truck or van injured in collision with pedestrian or animal

✓x7ᵗʰ **V50.5** Driver of pick-up truck or van injured in collision with pedestrian or animal in traffic accident

✓x7ᵗʰ **V50.6** Passenger in pick-up truck or van injured in collision with pedestrian or animal in traffic accident

✓x7ᵗʰ **V50.7** Person on outside of pick-up truck or van injured in collision with pedestrian or animal in traffic accident

✓x7ᵗʰ **V50.9** Unspecified occupant of pick-up truck or van injured in collision with pedestrian or animal in traffic accident

✓4ᵗʰ **V51** Occupant of pick-up truck or van injured in collision with pedal cycle

✓x7ᵗʰ **V51.0** Driver of pick-up truck or van injured in collision with pedal cycle in nontraffic accident

✓x7ᵗʰ **V51.1** Passenger in pick-up truck or van injured in collision with pedal cycle in nontraffic accident

✓x7ᵗʰ **V51.2** Person on outside of pick-up truck or van injured in collision with pedal cycle in nontraffic accident

✓x7ᵗʰ **V51.3** Unspecified occupant of pick-up truck or van injured in collision with pedal cycle in nontraffic accident

✓x7ᵗʰ **V51.4** Person boarding or alighting a pick-up truck or van injured in collision with pedal cycle

✓x7ᵗʰ **V51.5** Driver of pick-up truck or van injured in collision with pedal cycle in traffic accident

N Newborn: 0   **P** Pediatric: 0-17   **M** Maternity: 9-64   **A** Adult: 15-124   **MCC** Major Complication/Comorbidity   **CC** Complication/Comorbidity   **SW** Severe Wound Dx

1226   ICD-10-CM 2020

Chapter 20. External Causes of Morbidity

√x7ᵗʰ **V51.6** Passenger in pick-up truck or van injured in collision with pedal cycle in traffic accident

√x7ᵗʰ **V51.7** Person on outside of pick-up truck or van injured in collision with pedal cycle in traffic accident

√x7ᵗʰ **V51.9** Unspecified occupant of pick-up truck or van injured in collision with pedal cycle in traffic accident

✓4ᵗʰ **V52** Occupant of pick-up truck or van injured in collision with two- or three-wheeled motor vehicle

√x7ᵗʰ **V52.0** Driver of pick-up truck or van injured in collision with two- or three-wheeled motor vehicle in nontraffic accident

√x7ᵗʰ **V52.1** Passenger in pick-up truck or van injured in collision with two- or three-wheeled motor vehicle in nontraffic accident

√x7ᵗʰ **V52.2** Person on outside of pick-up truck or van injured in collision with two- or three-wheeled motor vehicle in nontraffic accident

√x7ᵗʰ **V52.3** Unspecified occupant of pick-up truck or van injured in collision with two- or three-wheeled motor vehicle in nontraffic accident

√x7ᵗʰ **V52.4** Person boarding or alighting a pick-up truck or van injured in collision with two- or three-wheeled motor vehicle

√x7ᵗʰ **V52.5** Driver of pick-up truck or van injured in collision with two- or three-wheeled motor vehicle in traffic accident

√x7ᵗʰ **V52.6** Passenger in pick-up truck or van injured in collision with two- or three-wheeled motor vehicle in traffic accident

√x7ᵗʰ **V52.7** Person on outside of pick-up truck or van injured in collision with two- or three-wheeled motor vehicle in traffic accident

√x7ᵗʰ **V52.9** Unspecified occupant of pick-up truck or van injured in collision with two- or three-wheeled motor vehicle in traffic accident

✓4ᵗʰ **V53** Occupant of pick-up truck or van injured in collision with car, pick-up truck or van

√x7ᵗʰ **V53.0** Driver of pick-up truck or van injured in collision with car, pick-up truck or van in nontraffic accident

√x7ᵗʰ **V53.1** Passenger in pick-up truck or van injured in collision with car, pick-up truck or van in nontraffic accident

√x7ᵗʰ **V53.2** Person on outside of pick-up truck or van injured in collision with car, pick-up truck or van in nontraffic accident

√x7ᵗʰ **V53.3** Unspecified occupant of pick-up truck or van injured in collision with car, pick-up truck or van in nontraffic accident

√x7ᵗʰ **V53.4** Person boarding or alighting a pick-up truck or van injured in collision with car, pick-up truck or van

√x7ᵗʰ **V53.5** Driver of pick-up truck or van injured in collision with car, pick-up truck or van in traffic accident

√x7ᵗʰ **V53.6** Passenger in pick-up truck or van injured in collision with car, pick-up truck or van in traffic accident

√x7ᵗʰ **V53.7** Person on outside of pick-up truck or van injured in collision with car, pick-up truck or van in traffic accident

√x7ᵗʰ **V53.9** Unspecified occupant of pick-up truck or van injured in collision with car, pick-up truck or van in traffic accident

✓4ᵗʰ **V54** Occupant of pick-up truck or van injured in collision with heavy transport vehicle or bus

EXCLUDES 1   *occupant of pick-up truck or van injured in collision with military vehicle (V59.81)*

√x7ᵗʰ **V54.0** Driver of pick-up truck or van injured in collision with heavy transport vehicle or bus in nontraffic accident

√x7ᵗʰ **V54.1** Passenger in pick-up truck or van injured in collision with heavy transport vehicle or bus in nontraffic accident

√x7ᵗʰ **V54.2** Person on outside of pick-up truck or van injured in collision with heavy transport vehicle or bus in nontraffic accident

√x7ᵗʰ **V54.3** Unspecified occupant of pick-up truck or van injured in collision with heavy transport vehicle or bus in nontraffic accident

√x7ᵗʰ **V54.4** Person boarding or alighting a pick-up truck or van injured in collision with heavy transport vehicle or bus

√x7ᵗʰ **V54.5** Driver of pick-up truck or van injured in collision with heavy transport vehicle or bus in traffic accident

√x7ᵗʰ **V54.6** Passenger in pick-up truck or van injured in collision with heavy transport vehicle or bus in traffic accident

√x7ᵗʰ **V54.7** Person on outside of pick-up truck or van injured in collision with heavy transport vehicle or bus in traffic accident

√x7ᵗʰ **V54.9** Unspecified occupant of pick-up truck or van injured in collision with heavy transport vehicle or bus in traffic accident

✓4ᵗʰ **V55** Occupant of pick-up truck or van injured in collision with railway train or railway vehicle

√x7ᵗʰ **V55.0** Driver of pick-up truck or van injured in collision with railway train or railway vehicle in nontraffic accident

√x7ᵗʰ **V55.1** Passenger in pick-up truck or van injured in collision with railway train or railway vehicle in nontraffic accident

√x7ᵗʰ **V55.2** Person on outside of pick-up truck or van injured in collision with railway train or railway vehicle in nontraffic accident

√x7ᵗʰ **V55.3** Unspecified occupant of pick-up truck or van injured in collision with railway train or railway vehicle in nontraffic accident

√x7ᵗʰ **V55.4** Person boarding or alighting a pick-up truck or van injured in collision with railway train or railway vehicle

√x7ᵗʰ **V55.5** Driver of pick-up truck or van injured in collision with railway train or railway vehicle in traffic accident

√x7ᵗʰ **V55.6** Passenger in pick-up truck or van injured in collision with railway train or railway vehicle in traffic accident

√x7ᵗʰ **V55.7** Person on outside of pick-up truck or van injured in collision with railway train or railway vehicle in traffic accident

√x7ᵗʰ **V55.9** Unspecified occupant of pick-up truck or van injured in collision with railway train or railway vehicle in traffic accident

✓4ᵗʰ **V56** Occupant of pick-up truck or van injured in collision with other nonmotor vehicle

INCLUDES   collision with animal-drawn vehicle, animal being ridden, streetcar

√x7ᵗʰ **V56.0** Driver of pick-up truck or van injured in collision with other nonmotor vehicle in nontraffic accident

√x7ᵗʰ **V56.1** Passenger in pick-up truck or van injured in collision with other nonmotor vehicle in nontraffic accident

√x7ᵗʰ **V56.2** Person on outside of pick-up truck or van injured in collision with other nonmotor vehicle in nontraffic accident

√x7ᵗʰ **V56.3** Unspecified occupant of pick-up truck or van injured in collision with other nonmotor vehicle in nontraffic accident

√x7ᵗʰ **V56.4** Person boarding or alighting a pick-up truck or van injured in collision with other nonmotor vehicle

√x7ᵗʰ **V56.5** Driver of pick-up truck or van injured in collision with other nonmotor vehicle in traffic accident

√x7ᵗʰ **V56.6** Passenger in pick-up truck or van injured in collision with other nonmotor vehicle in traffic accident

√x7ᵗʰ **V56.7** Person on outside of pick-up truck or van injured in collision with other nonmotor vehicle in traffic accident

√x7ᵗʰ **V56.9** Unspecified occupant of pick-up truck or van injured in collision with other nonmotor vehicle in traffic accident

✓4ᵗʰ **V57** Occupant of pick-up truck or van injured in collision with fixed or stationary object

√x7ᵗʰ **V57.0** Driver of pick-up truck or van injured in collision with fixed or stationary object in nontraffic accident

√x7ᵗʰ **V57.1** Passenger in pick-up truck or van injured in collision with fixed or stationary object in nontraffic accident

√x7ᵗʰ **V57.2** Person on outside of pick-up truck or van injured in collision with fixed or stationary object in nontraffic accident

√x7ᵗʰ **V57.3** Unspecified occupant of pick-up truck or van injured in collision with fixed or stationary object in nontraffic accident

√x7ᵗʰ **V57.4** Person boarding or alighting a pick-up truck or van injured in collision with fixed or stationary object

√x7ᵗʰ **V57.5** Driver of pick-up truck or van injured in collision with fixed or stationary object in traffic accident

√x7ᵗʰ **V57.6** Passenger in pick-up truck or van injured in collision with fixed or stationary object in traffic accident

√x7ᵗʰ **V57.7** Person on outside of pick-up truck or van injured in collision with fixed or stationary object in traffic accident

√x7ᵗʰ **V57.9** Unspecified occupant of pick-up truck or van injured in collision with fixed or stationary object in traffic accident

✓4ᵗʰ **V58** Occupant of pick-up truck or van injured in noncollision transport accident

INCLUDES   overturning pick-up truck or van NOS
             overturning pick-up truck or van without collision

√x7ᵗʰ **V58.0** Driver of pick-up truck or van injured in noncollision transport accident in nontraffic accident

√x7ᵗʰ **V58.1** Passenger in pick-up truck or van injured in noncollision transport accident in nontraffic accident

√x7ᵗʰ **V58.2** Person on outside of pick-up truck or van injured in noncollision transport accident in nontraffic accident

√x7ᵗʰ **V58.3** Unspecified occupant of pick-up truck or van injured in noncollision transport accident in nontraffic accident

√x7ᵗʰ **V58.4** Person boarding or alighting a pick-up truck or van injured in noncollision transport accident

√x7ᵗʰ **V58.5** Driver of pick-up truck or van injured in noncollision transport accident in traffic accident

√x7ᵗʰ **V58.6** Passenger in pick-up truck or van injured in noncollision transport accident in traffic accident

√x7ᵗʰ **V58.7** Person on outside of pick-up truck or van injured in noncollision transport accident in traffic accident

√x7ᵗʰ **V58.9** Unspecified occupant of pick-up truck or van injured in noncollision transport accident in traffic accident

☑ Additional Char Req   √x7ᵗʰ Placeholder   Unacceptable PDx   Questionable PDx   Wrong Procedure   Manifestation   Unspecified Dx   H1-H14 HAC   HCC CMS-HCC Dx   HIV HIV Dx

ICD-10-CM 2020   1227

✓4ᵗʰ **V59 Occupant of pick-up truck or van injured in other and unspecified transport accidents**

  ✓5ᵗʰ **V59.0** Driver of pick-up truck or van injured in collision with other and unspecified motor vehicles in nontraffic accident

    ✓x7ᵗʰ **V59.00** Driver of pick-up truck or van injured in collision with unspecified motor vehicles in nontraffic accident

    ✓x7ᵗʰ **V59.09** Driver of pick-up truck or van injured in collision with other motor vehicles in nontraffic accident

  ✓5ᵗʰ **V59.1** Passenger in pick-up truck or van injured in collision with other and unspecified motor vehicles in nontraffic accident

    ✓x7ᵗʰ **V59.10** Passenger in pick-up truck or van injured in collision with unspecified motor vehicles in nontraffic accident

    ✓x7ᵗʰ **V59.19** Passenger in pick-up truck or van injured in collision with other motor vehicles in nontraffic accident

  ✓5ᵗʰ **V59.2** Unspecified occupant of pick-up truck or van injured in collision with other and unspecified motor vehicles in nontraffic accident

    ✓x7ᵗʰ **V59.20** Unspecified occupant of pick-up truck or van injured in collision with unspecified motor vehicles in nontraffic accident

      Collision NOS involving pick-up truck or van, nontraffic

    ✓x7ᵗʰ **V59.29** Unspecified occupant of pick-up truck or van injured in collision with other motor vehicles in nontraffic accident

  ✓x7ᵗʰ **V59.3** Occupant (driver) (passenger) of pick-up truck or van injured in unspecified nontraffic accident

    Accident NOS involving pick-up truck or van, nontraffic

    Occupant of pick-up truck or van injured in nontraffic accident NOS

  ✓5ᵗʰ **V59.4** Driver of pick-up truck or van injured in collision with other and unspecified motor vehicles in traffic accident

    ✓x7ᵗʰ **V59.40** Driver of pick-up truck or van injured in collision with unspecified motor vehicles in traffic accident

    ✓x7ᵗʰ **V59.49** Driver of pick-up truck or van injured in collision with other motor vehicles in traffic accident

  ✓5ᵗʰ **V59.5** Passenger in pick-up truck or van injured in collision with other and unspecified motor vehicles in traffic accident

    ✓x7ᵗʰ **V59.50** Passenger in pick-up truck or van injured in collision with unspecified motor vehicles in traffic accident

    ✓x7ᵗʰ **V59.59** Passenger in pick-up truck or van injured in collision with other motor vehicles in traffic accident

  ✓5ᵗʰ **V59.6** Unspecified occupant of pick-up truck or van injured in collision with other and unspecified motor vehicles in traffic accident

    ✓x7ᵗʰ **V59.60** Unspecified occupant of pick-up truck or van injured in collision with unspecified motor vehicles in traffic accident

      Collision NOS involving pick-up truck or van (traffic)

    ✓x7ᵗʰ **V59.69** Unspecified occupant of pick-up truck or van injured in collision with other motor vehicles in traffic accident

  ✓5ᵗʰ **V59.8** Occupant (driver) (passenger) of pick-up truck or van injured in other specified transport accidents

    ✓x7ᵗʰ **V59.81** Occupant (driver) (passenger) of pick-up truck or van injured in transport accident with military vehicle

    ✓x7ᵗʰ **V59.88** Occupant (driver) (passenger) of pick-up truck or van injured in other specified transport accidents

  ✓x7ᵗʰ **V59.9** Occupant (driver) (passenger) of pick-up truck or van injured in unspecified traffic accident

    Accident NOS involving pick-up truck or van

Occupant of heavy transport vehicle injured in transport accident (V60-V69)

> **INCLUDES** 18 wheeler
> armored car
> panel truck
>
> **EXCLUDES 1** bus
> motorcoach

The appropriate 7th character is to be added to each code from categories V60-V69.
A initial encounter
D subsequent encounter
S sequela

✓4ᵗʰ **V60 Occupant of heavy transport vehicle injured in collision with pedestrian or animal**

> **EXCLUDES 1** heavy transport vehicle collision with animal-drawn vehicle or animal being ridden (V66.-)

  ✓x7ᵗʰ **V60.0** Driver of heavy transport vehicle injured in collision with pedestrian or animal in nontraffic accident

  ✓x7ᵗʰ **V60.1** Passenger in heavy transport vehicle injured in collision with pedestrian or animal in nontraffic accident

  ✓x7ᵗʰ **V60.2** Person on outside of heavy transport vehicle injured in collision with pedestrian or animal in nontraffic accident

  ✓x7ᵗʰ **V60.3** Unspecified occupant of heavy transport vehicle injured in collision with pedestrian or animal in nontraffic accident

  ✓x7ᵗʰ **V60.4** Person boarding or alighting a heavy transport vehicle injured in collision with pedestrian or animal

  ✓x7ᵗʰ **V60.5** Driver of heavy transport vehicle injured in collision with pedestrian or animal in traffic accident

  ✓x7ᵗʰ **V60.6** Passenger in heavy transport vehicle injured in collision with pedestrian or animal in traffic accident

  ✓x7ᵗʰ **V60.7** Person on outside of heavy transport vehicle injured in collision with pedestrian or animal in traffic accident

  ✓x7ᵗʰ **V60.9** Unspecified occupant of heavy transport vehicle injured in collision with pedestrian or animal in traffic accident

✓4ᵗʰ **V61 Occupant of heavy transport vehicle injured in collision with pedal cycle**

  ✓x7ᵗʰ **V61.0** Driver of heavy transport vehicle injured in collision with pedal cycle in nontraffic accident

  ✓x7ᵗʰ **V61.1** Passenger in heavy transport vehicle injured in collision with pedal cycle in nontraffic accident

  ✓x7ᵗʰ **V61.2** Person on outside of heavy transport vehicle injured in collision with pedal cycle in nontraffic accident

  ✓x7ᵗʰ **V61.3** Unspecified occupant of heavy transport vehicle injured in collision with pedal cycle in nontraffic accident

  ✓x7ᵗʰ **V61.4** Person boarding or alighting a heavy transport vehicle injured in collision with pedal cycle while boarding or alighting

  ✓x7ᵗʰ **V61.5** Driver of heavy transport vehicle injured in collision with pedal cycle in traffic accident

  ✓x7ᵗʰ **V61.6** Passenger in heavy transport vehicle injured in collision with pedal cycle in traffic accident

  ✓x7ᵗʰ **V61.7** Person on outside of heavy transport vehicle injured in collision with pedal cycle in traffic accident

  ✓x7ᵗʰ **V61.9** Unspecified occupant of heavy transport vehicle injured in collision with pedal cycle in traffic accident

✓4ᵗʰ **V62 Occupant of heavy transport vehicle injured in collision with two- or three-wheeled motor vehicle**

  ✓x7ᵗʰ **V62.0** Driver of heavy transport vehicle injured in collision with two- or three-wheeled motor vehicle in nontraffic accident

  ✓x7ᵗʰ **V62.1** Passenger in heavy transport vehicle injured in collision with two- or three-wheeled motor vehicle in nontraffic accident

  ✓x7ᵗʰ **V62.2** Person on outside of heavy transport vehicle injured in collision with two- or three-wheeled motor vehicle in nontraffic accident

  ✓x7ᵗʰ **V62.3** Unspecified occupant of heavy transport vehicle injured in collision with two- or three-wheeled motor vehicle in nontraffic accident

  ✓x7ᵗʰ **V62.4** Person boarding or alighting a heavy transport vehicle injured in collision with two- or three-wheeled motor vehicle

  ✓x7ᵗʰ **V62.5** Driver of heavy transport vehicle injured in collision with two- or three-wheeled motor vehicle in traffic accident

  ✓x7ᵗʰ **V62.6** Passenger in heavy transport vehicle injured in collision with two- or three-wheeled motor vehicle in traffic accident

  ✓x7ᵗʰ **V62.7** Person on outside of heavy transport vehicle injured in collision with two- or three-wheeled motor vehicle in traffic accident

  ✓x7ᵗʰ **V62.9** Unspecified occupant of heavy transport vehicle injured in collision with two- or three-wheeled motor vehicle in traffic accident

N Newborn: 0   **P** Pediatric: 0-17   **M** Maternity: 9-64   **A** Adult: 15-124   **MCC** Major Complication/Comorbidity   **CC** Complication/Comorbidity   **SW** Severe Wound Dx

1228   ICD-10-CM 2020

✓4th **V63** **Occupant of heavy transport vehicle injured in collision with car, pick-up truck or van**

✓x7th **V63.0** Driver of heavy transport vehicle injured in collision with car, pick-up truck or van in nontraffic accident

✓x7th **V63.1** Passenger in heavy transport vehicle injured in collision with car, pick-up truck or van in nontraffic accident

✓x7th **V63.2** Person on outside of heavy transport vehicle injured in collision with car, pick-up truck or van in nontraffic accident

✓x7th **V63.3** Unspecified occupant of heavy transport vehicle injured in collision with car, pick-up truck or van in nontraffic accident

✓x7th **V63.4** Person boarding or alighting a heavy transport vehicle injured in collision with car, pick-up truck or van

✓x7th **V63.5** Driver of heavy transport vehicle injured in collision with car, pick-up truck or van in traffic accident

✓x7th **V63.6** Passenger in heavy transport vehicle injured in collision with car, pick-up truck or van in traffic accident

✓x7th **V63.7** Person on outside of heavy transport vehicle injured in collision with car, pick-up truck or van in traffic accident

✓x7th **V63.9** Unspecified occupant of heavy transport vehicle injured in collision with car, pick-up truck or van in traffic accident

✓4th **V64** **Occupant of heavy transport vehicle injured in collision with heavy transport vehicle or bus**

> EXCLUDES 1   occupant of heavy transport vehicle injured in collision with military vehicle (V69.81)

✓x7th **V64.0** Driver of heavy transport vehicle injured in collision with heavy transport vehicle or bus in nontraffic accident

✓x7th **V64.1** Passenger in heavy transport vehicle injured in collision with heavy transport vehicle or bus in nontraffic accident

✓x7th **V64.2** Person on outside of heavy transport vehicle injured in collision with heavy transport vehicle or bus in nontraffic accident

✓x7th **V64.3** Unspecified occupant of heavy transport vehicle injured in collision with heavy transport vehicle or bus in nontraffic accident

✓x7th **V64.4** Person boarding or alighting a heavy transport vehicle injured in collision with heavy transport vehicle or bus while boarding or alighting

✓x7th **V64.5** Driver of heavy transport vehicle injured in collision with heavy transport vehicle or bus in traffic accident

✓x7th **V64.6** Passenger in heavy transport vehicle injured in collision with heavy transport vehicle or bus in traffic accident

✓x7th **V64.7** Person on outside of heavy transport vehicle injured in collision with heavy transport vehicle or bus in traffic accident

✓x7th **V64.9** Unspecified occupant of heavy transport vehicle injured in collision with heavy transport vehicle or bus in traffic accident

✓4th **V65** **Occupant of heavy transport vehicle injured in collision with railway train or railway vehicle**

✓x7th **V65.0** Driver of heavy transport vehicle injured in collision with railway train or railway vehicle in nontraffic accident

✓x7th **V65.1** Passenger in heavy transport vehicle injured in collision with railway train or railway vehicle in nontraffic accident

✓x7th **V65.2** Person on outside of heavy transport vehicle injured in collision with railway train or railway vehicle in nontraffic accident

✓x7th **V65.3** Unspecified occupant of heavy transport vehicle injured in collision with railway train or railway vehicle in nontraffic accident

✓x7th **V65.4** Person boarding or alighting a heavy transport vehicle injured in collision with railway train or railway vehicle

✓x7th **V65.5** Driver of heavy transport vehicle injured in collision with railway train or railway vehicle in traffic accident

✓x7th **V65.6** Passenger in heavy transport vehicle injured in collision with railway train or railway vehicle in traffic accident

✓x7th **V65.7** Person on outside of heavy transport vehicle injured in collision with railway train or railway vehicle in traffic accident

✓x7th **V65.9** Unspecified occupant of heavy transport vehicle injured in collision with railway train or railway vehicle in traffic accident

✓4th **V66** **Occupant of heavy transport vehicle injured in collision with other nonmotor vehicle**

> INCLUDES   collision with animal-drawn vehicle, animal being ridden, streetcar

✓x7th **V66.0** Driver of heavy transport vehicle injured in collision with other nonmotor vehicle in nontraffic accident

✓x7th **V66.1** Passenger in heavy transport vehicle injured in collision with other nonmotor vehicle in nontraffic accident

✓x7th **V66.2** Person on outside of heavy transport vehicle injured in collision with other nonmotor vehicle in nontraffic accident

✓x7th **V66.3** Unspecified occupant of heavy transport vehicle injured in collision with other nonmotor vehicle in nontraffic accident

✓x7th **V66.4** Person boarding or alighting a heavy transport vehicle injured in collision with other nonmotor vehicle

✓x7th **V66.5** Driver of heavy transport vehicle injured in collision with other nonmotor vehicle in traffic accident

✓x7th **V66.6** Passenger in heavy transport vehicle injured in collision with other nonmotor vehicle in traffic accident

✓x7th **V66.7** Person on outside of heavy transport vehicle injured in collision with other nonmotor vehicle in traffic accident

✓x7th **V66.9** Unspecified occupant of heavy transport vehicle injured in collision with other nonmotor vehicle in traffic accident

✓4th **V67** **Occupant of heavy transport vehicle injured in collision with fixed or stationary object**

✓x7th **V67.0** Driver of heavy transport vehicle injured in collision with fixed or stationary object in nontraffic accident

✓x7th **V67.1** Passenger in heavy transport vehicle injured in collision with fixed or stationary object in nontraffic accident

✓x7th **V67.2** Person on outside of heavy transport vehicle injured in collision with fixed or stationary object in nontraffic accident

✓x7th **V67.3** Unspecified occupant of heavy transport vehicle injured in collision with fixed or stationary object in nontraffic accident

✓x7th **V67.4** Person boarding or alighting a heavy transport vehicle injured in collision with fixed or stationary object

✓x7th **V67.5** Driver of heavy transport vehicle injured in collision with fixed or stationary object in traffic accident

✓x7th **V67.6** Passenger in heavy transport vehicle injured in collision with fixed or stationary object in traffic accident

✓x7th **V67.7** Person on outside of heavy transport vehicle injured in collision with fixed or stationary object in traffic accident

✓x7th **V67.9** Unspecified occupant of heavy transport vehicle injured in collision with fixed or stationary object in traffic accident

✓4th **V68** **Occupant of heavy transport vehicle injured in noncollision transport accident**

> INCLUDES   overturning heavy transport vehicle NOS
> overturning heavy transport vehicle without collision

✓x7th **V68.0** Driver of heavy transport vehicle injured in noncollision transport accident in nontraffic accident

✓x7th **V68.1** Passenger in heavy transport vehicle injured in noncollision transport accident in nontraffic accident

✓x7th **V68.2** Person on outside of heavy transport vehicle injured in noncollision transport accident in nontraffic accident

✓x7th **V68.3** Unspecified occupant of heavy transport vehicle injured in noncollision transport accident in nontraffic accident

✓x7th **V68.4** Person boarding or alighting a heavy transport vehicle injured in noncollision transport accident

✓x7th **V68.5** Driver of heavy transport vehicle injured in noncollision transport accident in traffic accident

✓x7th **V68.6** Passenger in heavy transport vehicle injured in noncollision transport accident in traffic accident

✓x7th **V68.7** Person on outside of heavy transport vehicle injured in noncollision transport accident in traffic accident

✓x7th **V68.9** Unspecified occupant of heavy transport vehicle injured in noncollision transport accident in traffic accident

✓4th **V69** **Occupant of heavy transport vehicle injured in other and unspecified transport accidents**

✓5th **V69.0** Driver of heavy transport vehicle injured in collision with other and unspecified motor vehicles in nontraffic accident

✓x7th **V69.00** Driver of heavy transport vehicle injured in collision with unspecified motor vehicles in nontraffic accident

✓x7th **V69.09** Driver of heavy transport vehicle injured in collision with other motor vehicles in nontraffic accident

✓5th **V69.1** Passenger in heavy transport vehicle injured in collision with other and unspecified motor vehicles in nontraffic accident

✓x7th **V69.10** Passenger in heavy transport vehicle injured in collision with unspecified motor vehicles in nontraffic accident

✓x7th **V69.19** Passenger in heavy transport vehicle injured in collision with other motor vehicles in nontraffic accident

✓5th **V69.2** Unspecified occupant of heavy transport vehicle injured in collision with other and unspecified motor vehicles in nontraffic accident

✓x7th **V69.20** Unspecified occupant of heavy transport vehicle injured in collision with unspecified motor vehicles in nontraffic accident

> Collision NOS involving heavy transport vehicle, nontraffic

✓ Additional Char Req   ✓x7th Placeholder   Unacceptable PDx   Questionable PDx   Wrong Procedure   Manifestation   Unspecified Dx   H1-H14 HAC   HCC CMS-HCC Dx   HIV HIV Dx

ICD-10-CM 2020   1229

✓x7th **V69.29** Unspecified occupant of heavy transport vehicle injured in collision with other motor vehicles in nontraffic accident

✓x7th **V69.3** Occupant (driver) (passenger) of heavy transport vehicle injured in unspecified nontraffic accident

Accident NOS involving heavy transport vehicle, nontraffic

Occupant of heavy transport vehicle injured in nontraffic accident NOS

✓5th **V69.4** Driver of heavy transport vehicle injured in collision with other and unspecified motor vehicles in traffic accident

✓x7th **V69.40** Driver of heavy transport vehicle injured in collision with unspecified motor vehicles in traffic accident

✓x7th **V69.49** Driver of heavy transport vehicle injured in collision with other motor vehicles in traffic accident

✓5th **V69.5** Passenger in heavy transport vehicle injured in collision with other and unspecified motor vehicles in traffic accident

✓x7th **V69.50** Passenger in heavy transport vehicle injured in collision with unspecified motor vehicles in traffic accident

✓x7th **V69.59** Passenger in heavy transport vehicle injured in collision with other motor vehicles in traffic accident

✓5th **V69.6** Unspecified occupant of heavy transport vehicle injured in collision with other and unspecified motor vehicles in traffic accident

✓x7th **V69.60** Unspecified occupant of heavy transport vehicle injured in collision with unspecified motor vehicles in traffic accident

Collision NOS involving heavy transport vehicle (traffic)

✓x7th **V69.69** Unspecified occupant of heavy transport vehicle injured in collision with other motor vehicles in traffic accident

✓5th **V69.8** Occupant (driver) (passenger) of heavy transport vehicle injured in other specified transport accidents

✓x7th **V69.81** Occupant (driver) (passenger) of heavy transport vehicle injured in transport accidents with military vehicle

✓x7th **V69.88** Occupant (driver) (passenger) of heavy transport vehicle injured in other specified transport accidents

✓x7th **V69.9** Occupant (driver) (passenger) of heavy transport vehicle injured in unspecified traffic accident

Accident NOS involving heavy transport vehicle

Bus occupant injured in transport accident (V70-V79)

INCLUDES   motorcoach
EXCLUDES 1   minibus (V50-V59)

The appropriate 7th character is to be added to each code from categories V70-V79.
A   initial encounter
D   subsequent encounter
S   sequela

✓4th **V70** Bus occupant injured in collision with pedestrian or animal

EXCLUDES 1   bus collision with animal-drawn vehicle or animal being ridden (V76.-)

✓x7th **V70.0** Driver of bus injured in collision with pedestrian or animal in nontraffic accident

✓x7th **V70.1** Passenger on bus injured in collision with pedestrian or animal in nontraffic accident

✓x7th **V70.2** Person on outside of bus injured in collision with pedestrian or animal in nontraffic accident

✓x7th **V70.3** Unspecified occupant of bus injured in collision with pedestrian or animal in nontraffic accident

✓x7th **V70.4** Person boarding or alighting from bus injured in collision with pedestrian or animal

✓x7th **V70.5** Driver of bus injured in collision with pedestrian or animal in traffic accident

✓x7th **V70.6** Passenger on bus injured in collision with pedestrian or animal in traffic accident

✓x7th **V70.7** Person on outside of bus injured in collision with pedestrian or animal in traffic accident

✓x7th **V70.9** Unspecified occupant of bus injured in collision with pedestrian or animal in traffic accident

✓4th **V71** Bus occupant injured in collision with pedal cycle

✓x7th **V71.0** Driver of bus injured in collision with pedal cycle in nontraffic accident

✓x7th **V71.1** Passenger on bus injured in collision with pedal cycle in nontraffic accident

✓x7th **V71.2** Person on outside of bus injured in collision with pedal cycle in nontraffic accident

✓x7th **V71.3** Unspecified occupant of bus injured in collision with pedal cycle in nontraffic accident

✓x7th **V71.4** Person boarding or alighting from bus injured in collision with pedal cycle

✓x7th **V71.5** Driver of bus injured in collision with pedal cycle in traffic accident

✓x7th **V71.6** Passenger on bus injured in collision with pedal cycle in traffic accident

✓x7th **V71.7** Person on outside of bus injured in collision with pedal cycle in traffic accident

✓x7th **V71.9** Unspecified occupant of bus injured in collision with pedal cycle in traffic accident

✓4th **V72** Bus occupant injured in collision with two- or three-wheeled motor vehicle

✓x7th **V72.0** Driver of bus injured in collision with two- or three-wheeled motor vehicle in nontraffic accident

✓x7th **V72.1** Passenger on bus injured in collision with two- or three-wheeled motor vehicle in nontraffic accident

✓x7th **V72.2** Person on outside of bus injured in collision with two- or three-wheeled motor vehicle in nontraffic accident

✓x7th **V72.3** Unspecified occupant of bus injured in collision with two- or three-wheeled motor vehicle in nontraffic accident

✓x7th **V72.4** Person boarding or alighting from bus injured in collision with two- or three-wheeled motor vehicle

✓x7th **V72.5** Driver of bus injured in collision with two- or three-wheeled motor vehicle in traffic accident

✓x7th **V72.6** Passenger on bus injured in collision with two- or three-wheeled motor vehicle in traffic accident

✓x7th **V72.7** Person on outside of bus injured in collision with two- or three-wheeled motor vehicle in traffic accident

✓x7th **V72.9** Unspecified occupant of bus injured in collision with two- or three-wheeled motor vehicle in traffic accident

✓4th **V73** Bus occupant injured in collision with car, pick-up truck or van

✓x7th **V73.0** Driver of bus injured in collision with car, pick-up truck or van in nontraffic accident

✓x7th **V73.1** Passenger on bus injured in collision with car, pick-up truck or van in nontraffic accident

✓x7th **V73.2** Person on outside of bus injured in collision with car, pick-up truck or van in nontraffic accident

✓x7th **V73.3** Unspecified occupant of bus injured in collision with car, pick-up truck or van in nontraffic accident

✓x7th **V73.4** Person boarding or alighting from bus injured in collision with car, pick-up truck or van

✓x7th **V73.5** Driver of bus injured in collision with car, pick-up truck or van in traffic accident

✓x7th **V73.6** Passenger on bus injured in collision with car, pick-up truck or van in traffic accident

✓x7th **V73.7** Person on outside of bus injured in collision with car, pick-up truck or van in traffic accident

✓x7th **V73.9** Unspecified occupant of bus injured in collision with car, pick-up truck or van in traffic accident

✓4th **V74** Bus occupant injured in collision with heavy transport vehicle or bus

EXCLUDES 1   bus occupant injured in collision with military vehicle (V79.81)

✓x7th **V74.0** Driver of bus injured in collision with heavy transport vehicle or bus in nontraffic accident

✓x7th **V74.1** Passenger on bus injured in collision with heavy transport vehicle or bus in nontraffic accident

✓x7th **V74.2** Person on outside of bus injured in collision with heavy transport vehicle or bus in nontraffic accident

✓x7th **V74.3** Unspecified occupant of bus injured in collision with heavy transport vehicle or bus in nontraffic accident

✓x7th **V74.4** Person boarding or alighting from bus injured in collision with heavy transport vehicle or bus

✓x7th **V74.5** Driver of bus injured in collision with heavy transport vehicle or bus in traffic accident

✓x7th **V74.6** Passenger on bus injured in collision with heavy transport vehicle or bus in traffic accident

✓x7th **V74.7** Person on outside of bus injured in collision with heavy transport vehicle or bus in traffic accident

✓x7th **V74.9** Unspecified occupant of bus injured in collision with heavy transport vehicle or bus in traffic accident

✓4th **V75** Bus occupant injured in collision with railway train or railway vehicle

✓x7th **V75.0** Driver of bus injured in collision with railway train or railway vehicle in nontraffic accident

✓x7th **V75.1** Passenger on bus injured in collision with railway train or railway vehicle in nontraffic accident

✓x7th **V75.2** Person on outside of bus injured in collision with railway train or railway vehicle in nontraffic accident

Chapter 20. External Causes of Morbidity

✓x7ᵗʰ **V75.3** Unspecified occupant of bus injured in collision with railway train or railway vehicle **in nontraffic accident**

✓x7ᵗʰ **V75.4** Person boarding or alighting **from bus injured in collision with railway train or railway vehicle**

✓x7ᵗʰ **V75.5** Driver of bus injured in collision with railway train or railway vehicle **in traffic accident**

✓x7ᵗʰ **V75.6** Passenger on bus injured in collision with railway train or railway vehicle **in traffic accident**

✓x7ᵗʰ **V75.7** Person on outside of bus injured in collision with railway train or railway vehicle **in traffic accident**

✓x7ᵗʰ **V75.9** Unspecified occupant of bus injured in collision with railway train or railway vehicle **in traffic accident**

✓4ᵗʰ **V76 Bus occupant injured in collision with other nonmotor vehicle**

    INCLUDES   collision with animal-drawn vehicle, animal being ridden, streetcar

✓x7ᵗʰ **V76.0** Driver of bus injured in collision with other nonmotor vehicle **in nontraffic accident**

✓x7ᵗʰ **V76.1** Passenger on bus injured in collision with other nonmotor vehicle **in nontraffic accident**

✓x7ᵗʰ **V76.2** Person on outside of bus injured in collision with other nonmotor vehicle **in nontraffic accident**

✓x7ᵗʰ **V76.3** Unspecified occupant of bus injured in collision with other nonmotor vehicle **in nontraffic accident**

✓x7ᵗʰ **V76.4** Person boarding or alighting **from bus injured in collision with other nonmotor vehicle**

✓x7ᵗʰ **V76.5** Driver of bus injured in collision with other nonmotor vehicle **in traffic accident**

✓x7ᵗʰ **V76.6** Passenger on bus injured in collision with other nonmotor vehicle **in traffic accident**

✓x7ᵗʰ **V76.7** Person on outside of bus injured in collision with other nonmotor vehicle **in traffic accident**

✓x7ᵗʰ **V76.9** Unspecified occupant of bus injured in collision with other nonmotor vehicle **in traffic accident**

✓4ᵗʰ **V77 Bus occupant injured in collision with fixed or stationary object**

✓x7ᵗʰ **V77.0** Driver of bus injured in collision with fixed or stationary object **in nontraffic accident**

✓x7ᵗʰ **V77.1** Passenger on bus injured in collision with fixed or stationary object **in nontraffic accident**

✓x7ᵗʰ **V77.2** Person on outside of bus injured in collision with fixed or stationary object **in nontraffic accident**

✓x7ᵗʰ **V77.3** Unspecified occupant of bus injured in collision with fixed or stationary object **in nontraffic accident**

✓x7ᵗʰ **V77.4** Person boarding or alighting **from bus injured in collision with fixed or stationary object**

✓x7ᵗʰ **V77.5** Driver of bus injured in collision with fixed or stationary object **in traffic accident**

✓x7ᵗʰ **V77.6** Passenger on bus injured in collision with fixed or stationary object **in traffic accident**

✓x7ᵗʰ **V77.7** Person on outside of bus injured in collision with fixed or stationary object **in traffic accident**

✓x7ᵗʰ **V77.9** Unspecified occupant of bus injured in collision with fixed or stationary object **in traffic accident**

✓4ᵗʰ **V78 Bus occupant injured in noncollision transport accident**

    INCLUDES   overturning bus NOS
                 overturning bus without collision

✓x7ᵗʰ **V78.0** Driver of bus injured in noncollision transport accident **in nontraffic accident**

✓x7ᵗʰ **V78.1** Passenger on bus injured in noncollision transport accident **in nontraffic accident**

✓x7ᵗʰ **V78.2** Person on outside of bus injured in noncollision transport accident **in nontraffic accident**

✓x7ᵗʰ **V78.3** Unspecified occupant of bus injured in noncollision transport accident **in nontraffic accident**

✓x7ᵗʰ **V78.4** Person boarding or alighting **from bus injured in noncollision transport accident**

✓x7ᵗʰ **V78.5** Driver of bus injured in noncollision transport accident **in traffic accident**

✓x7ᵗʰ **V78.6** Passenger on bus injured in noncollision transport accident **in traffic accident**

✓x7ᵗʰ **V78.7** Person on outside of bus injured in noncollision transport accident **in traffic accident**

✓x7ᵗʰ **V78.9** Unspecified occupant of bus injured in noncollision transport accident **in traffic accident**

✓4ᵗʰ **V79 Bus occupant injured in other and unspecified transport accidents**

✓5ᵗʰ **V79.0** Driver of bus injured in collision with other and unspecified motor vehicle **in nontraffic accident**

✓x7ᵗʰ **V79.00** Driver of bus injured in collision with unspecified motor vehicles in nontraffic accident

✓x7ᵗʰ **V79.09** Driver of bus injured in collision with other motor vehicles in nontraffic accident

✓5ᵗʰ **V79.1** Passenger on bus injured in collision with other and unspecified motor vehicles **in nontraffic accident**

✓x7ᵗʰ **V79.10** Passenger on bus injured in collision with unspecified motor vehicles in nontraffic accident

✓x7ᵗʰ **V79.19** Passenger on bus injured in collision with other motor vehicles in nontraffic accident

✓5ᵗʰ **V79.2** Unspecified bus occupant injured in collision with other and unspecified motor vehicles **in nontraffic accident**

✓x7ᵗʰ **V79.20** Unspecified bus occupant injured in collision with unspecified motor vehicles in nontraffic accident
        Bus collision NOS, nontraffic

✓x7ᵗʰ **V79.29** Unspecified bus occupant injured in collision with other motor vehicles in nontraffic accident

✓x7ᵗʰ **V79.3** Bus occupant (driver) (passenger) injured in unspecified nontraffic accident
        Bus accident NOS, nontraffic
        Bus occupant injured in nontraffic accident NOS

✓5ᵗʰ **V79.4** Driver of bus injured in collision with other and unspecified motor vehicles **in traffic accident**

✓x7ᵗʰ **V79.40** Driver of bus injured in collision with unspecified motor vehicles in traffic accident

✓x7ᵗʰ **V79.49** Driver of bus injured in collision with other motor vehicles in traffic accident

✓5ᵗʰ **V79.5** Passenger on bus injured in collision with other and unspecified motor vehicles **in traffic accident**

✓x7ᵗʰ **V79.50** Passenger on bus injured in collision with unspecified motor vehicles in traffic accident

✓x7ᵗʰ **V79.59** Passenger on bus injured in collision with other motor vehicles in traffic accident

✓5ᵗʰ **V79.6** Unspecified bus occupant injured in collision with other and unspecified motor vehicles **in traffic accident**

✓x7ᵗʰ **V79.60** Unspecified bus occupant injured in collision with unspecified motor vehicles in traffic accident
        Bus collision NOS (traffic)

✓x7ᵗʰ **V79.69** Unspecified bus occupant injured in collision with other motor vehicles in traffic accident

✓5ᵗʰ **V79.8** Bus occupant (driver) (passenger) injured in other specified transport accidents

✓x7ᵗʰ **V79.81** Bus occupant (driver) (passenger) injured in transport accidents with **military vehicle**

✓x7ᵗʰ **V79.88** Bus occupant (driver) (passenger) injured in other specified transport accidents

✓x7ᵗʰ **V79.9** Bus occupant (driver) (passenger) injured in unspecified traffic accident
        Bus accident NOS

Other land transport accidents (V80-V89)

The appropriate 7th character is to be added to each code from categories V80-V89.
A   initial encounter
D   subsequent encounter
S   sequela

✓4ᵗʰ **V80 Animal-rider or occupant of animal-drawn vehicle injured in transport accident**

✓5ᵗʰ **V80.0** Animal-rider or occupant of animal drawn vehicle injured by fall from or being thrown from animal or animal-drawn vehicle in **noncollision accident**

✓6ᵗʰ **V80.01** Animal-rider injured by fall from or being thrown from animal in noncollision accident

✓7ᵗʰ **V80.010** Animal-rider injured by fall from or being thrown from **horse** in noncollision accident

✓7ᵗʰ **V80.018** Animal-rider injured by fall from or being thrown from other animal in noncollision accident

✓x7ᵗʰ **V80.02** Occupant of animal-drawn vehicle injured by fall from or being thrown from animal-drawn vehicle in noncollision accident
        Overturning animal-drawn vehicle NOS
        Overturning animal-drawn vehicle without collision

✓5ᵗʰ **V80.1** Animal-rider or occupant of animal-drawn vehicle injured in collision with **pedestrian or animal**

    EXCLUDES 1   *animal-rider or animal-drawn vehicle collision with animal-drawn vehicle or animal being ridden (V80.7)*

✓x7ᵗʰ **V80.11** Animal-rider injured in collision with pedestrian or animal

✓x7ᵗʰ **V80.12** Occupant of animal-drawn vehicle injured in collision with pedestrian or animal

---

√5ᵗʰ **V80.2** **Animal-rider or occupant of animal-drawn vehicle injured in collision with** pedal cycle

    √x7ᵗʰ **V80.21** Animal-rider **injured in collision with pedal cycle**

    √x7ᵗʰ **V80.22** Occupant **of animal-drawn vehicle injured in collision with pedal cycle**

√5ᵗʰ **V80.3** **Animal-rider or occupant of animal-drawn vehicle injured in collision with** two- or three-wheeled motor vehicle

    √x7ᵗʰ **V80.31** Animal-rider **injured in collision with two- or three-wheeled motor vehicle**

    √x7ᵗʰ **V80.32** Occupant **of animal-drawn vehicle injured in collision with two- or three-wheeled motor vehicle**

√5ᵗʰ **V80.4** **Animal-rider or occupant of animal-drawn vehicle injured in collision with** car, pick-up truck, van, heavy transport vehicle or bus

    EXCLUDES 1 *animal-rider injured in collision with military vehicle (V80.910)*

        occupant of animal-drawn vehicle injured in collision with military vehicle (V80.920)

    √x7ᵗʰ **V80.41** Animal-rider **injured in collision with car, pick-up truck, van, heavy transport vehicle or bus**

    √x7ᵗʰ **V80.42** Occupant **of animal-drawn vehicle injured in collision with car, pick-up truck, van, heavy transport vehicle or bus**

√5ᵗʰ **V80.5** **Animal-rider or occupant of animal-drawn vehicle injured in collision with** other specified motor vehicle

    √x7ᵗʰ **V80.51** Animal-rider **injured in collision with other specified motor vehicle**

    √x7ᵗʰ **V80.52** Occupant **of animal-drawn vehicle injured in collision with other specified motor vehicle**

√5ᵗʰ **V80.6** **Animal-rider or occupant of animal-drawn vehicle injured in collision with** railway train or railway vehicle

    √x7ᵗʰ **V80.61** Animal-rider **injured in collision with railway train or railway vehicle**

    √x7ᵗʰ **V80.62** Occupant **of animal-drawn vehicle injured in collision with railway train or railway vehicle**

√5ᵗʰ **V80.7** **Animal-rider or occupant of animal-drawn vehicle injured in collision with** other nonmotor vehicles

    √6ᵗʰ **V80.71** **Animal-rider or occupant of animal-drawn vehicle injured in collision with** animal being ridden

        √7ᵗʰ **V80.710** Animal-rider **injured in collision with other animal being ridden**

        √7ᵗʰ **V80.711** Occupant **of animal-drawn vehicle injured in collision with animal being ridden**

    √6ᵗʰ **V80.72** **Animal-rider or occupant of animal-drawn vehicle injured in collision with** other animal-drawn vehicle

        √7ᵗʰ **V80.720** Animal-rider **injured in collision with animal-drawn vehicle**

        √7ᵗʰ **V80.721** Occupant **of animal-drawn vehicle injured in collision with other animal-drawn vehicle**

    √6ᵗʰ **V80.73** **Animal-rider or occupant of animal-drawn vehicle injured in collision with** streetcar

        √7ᵗʰ **V80.730** Animal-rider **injured in collision with streetcar**

        √7ᵗʰ **V80.731** Occupant **of animal-drawn vehicle injured in collision with streetcar**

    √6ᵗʰ **V80.79** **Animal-rider or occupant of animal-drawn vehicle injured in collision with** other nonmotor vehicles

        √7ᵗʰ **V80.790** Animal-rider **injured in collision with other nonmotor vehicles**

        √7ᵗʰ **V80.791** Occupant **of animal-drawn vehicle injured in collision with other nonmotor vehicles**

√5ᵗʰ **V80.8** **Animal-rider or occupant of animal-drawn vehicle injured in collision with** fixed or stationary object

    √x7ᵗʰ **V80.81** Animal-rider **injured in collision with fixed or stationary object**

    √x7ᵗʰ **V80.82** Occupant **of animal-drawn vehicle injured in collision with fixed or stationary object**

√5ᵗʰ **V80.9** **Animal-rider or occupant of animal-drawn vehicle injured in other and unspecified transport accidents**

    √6ᵗʰ **V80.91** Animal-rider **injured in other and unspecified transport accidents**

        √7ᵗʰ **V80.910** **Animal-rider injured in transport accident with** military vehicle

        √7ᵗʰ **V80.918** **Animal-rider injured in other transport accident**

        √7ᵗʰ **V80.919** **Animal-rider injured in unspecified transport accident**

           Animal rider accident NOS

    √6ᵗʰ **V80.92** Occupant **of animal-drawn vehicle injured in other and unspecified transport accidents**

        √7ᵗʰ **V80.920** **Occupant of animal-drawn vehicle injured in transport accident with** military vehicle

        √7ᵗʰ **V80.928** **Occupant of animal-drawn vehicle injured in other transport accident**

        √7ᵗʰ **V80.929** **Occupant of animal-drawn vehicle injured in unspecified transport accident**

           Animal-drawn vehicle accident NOS

√4ᵗʰ **V81** **Occupant of railway train or railway vehicle injured in transport accident**

    INCLUDES derailment of railway train or railway vehicle

             person on outside of train

    EXCLUDES 1 *streetcar (V82.-)*

√x7ᵗʰ **V81.0** **Occupant of railway train or railway vehicle injured in collision with motor vehicle** in nontraffic accident

    EXCLUDES 1 *occupant of railway train or railway vehicle injured due to collision with military vehicle (V81.83)*

√x7ᵗʰ **V81.1** **Occupant of railway train or railway vehicle injured in collision with motor vehicle** in traffic accident

    EXCLUDES 1 *occupant of railway train or railway vehicle injured due to collision with military vehicle (V81.83)*

√x7ᵗʰ **V81.2** **Occupant of railway train or railway vehicle injured in collision with or** hit by rolling stock

√x7ᵗʰ **V81.3** **Occupant of railway train or railway vehicle injured in collision with other object**

    Railway collision NOS

√x7ᵗʰ **V81.4** **Person injured** while boarding or alighting **from railway train or railway vehicle**

√x7ᵗʰ **V81.5** **Occupant of railway train or railway vehicle injured by** fall in railway train **or railway vehicle**

√x7ᵗʰ **V81.6** **Occupant of railway train or railway vehicle injured by** fall from railway train **or railway vehicle**

√x7ᵗʰ **V81.7** **Occupant of railway train or railway vehicle injured in** derailment without antecedent collision

√5ᵗʰ **V81.8** **Occupant of railway train or railway vehicle injured in other specified railway accidents**

    √x7ᵗʰ **V81.81** **Occupant of railway train or railway vehicle injured due to** explosion or fire **on train**

    √x7ᵗʰ **V81.82** **Occupant of railway train or railway vehicle injured due to** object falling onto **train**

        Occupant of railway train or railway vehicle injured due to falling earth onto train

        Occupant of railway train or railway vehicle injured due to falling rocks onto train

        Occupant of railway train or railway vehicle injured due to falling snow onto train

        Occupant of railway train or railway vehicle injured due to falling trees onto train

    √x7ᵗʰ **V81.83** **Occupant of railway train or railway vehicle injured due to** collision with military vehicle

    √x7ᵗʰ **V81.89** **Occupant of railway train or railway vehicle injured due to other specified railway accident**

√x7ᵗʰ **V81.9** **Occupant of railway train or railway vehicle injured in unspecified railway accident**

    Railway accident NOS

√4ᵗʰ **V82** **Occupant of powered streetcar injured in transport accident**

    INCLUDES interurban electric car

             person on outside of streetcar

             tram (car)

             trolley (car)

    EXCLUDES 1 *bus (V70-V79)*

             motorcoach (V70-V79)

             nonpowered streetcar (V76.-)

             train (V81.-)

√x7ᵗʰ **V82.0** **Occupant of streetcar injured in collision with motor vehicle** in nontraffic accident

√x7ᵗʰ **V82.1** **Occupant of streetcar injured in collision with motor vehicle** in traffic accident

√x7ᵗʰ **V82.2** **Occupant of streetcar injured in collision with or** hit by rolling stock

√x7ᵗʰ **V82.3** **Occupant of streetcar injured in collision with other object**

    EXCLUDES 1 *collision with animal-drawn vehicle or animal being ridden (V82.8)*

√x7ᵗʰ **V82.4** **Person injured** while boarding or alighting **from streetcar**

N Newborn: 0   P Pediatric: 0-17   M Maternity: 9-64   A Adult: 15-124   MCC Major Complication/Comorbidity   CC Complication/Comorbidity   SW Severe Wound Dx

1232   ICD-10-CM 2020

√x7ᵗʰ **V82.5 Occupant of streetcar injured by** fall in streetcar

> EXCLUDES 1   *fall in streetcar:*
> *while boarding or alighting (V82.4)*
> *with antecedent collision (V82.0-V82.3)*

√x7ᵗʰ **V82.6 Occupant of streetcar injured by** fall from streetcar

> EXCLUDES 1   *fall from streetcar:*
> *while boarding or alighting (V82.4)*
> *with antecedent collision (V82.0-V82.3)*

√x7ᵗʰ **V82.7 Occupant of streetcar injured in** derailment without antecedent collision

> EXCLUDES 1   *occupant of streetcar injured in derailment with antecedent collision (V82.0-V82.3)*

√x7ᵗʰ **V82.8 Occupant of streetcar injured in other specified transport accidents**

> Streetcar collision with military vehicle
> Streetcar collision with train or nonmotor vehicles

√x7ᵗʰ **V82.9 Occupant of streetcar injured in unspecified traffic accident**

> Streetcar accident NOS

√4ᵗʰ **V83 Occupant of special vehicle mainly used on industrial premises injured in transport accident**

> INCLUDES   battery-powered airport passenger vehicle
> battery-powered truck (baggage) (mail)
> coal-car in mine
> forklift (truck)
> logging car
> self-propelled industrial truck
> station baggage truck (powered)
> tram, truck, or tub (powered) in mine or quarry

> EXCLUDES 1   *special construction vehicles (V85.-)*
> *special industrial vehicle in stationary use or maintenance (W31.-)*

√x7ᵗʰ **V83.0 Driver** of special industrial vehicle injured in traffic accident

√x7ᵗʰ **V83.1 Passenger** of special industrial vehicle injured in traffic accident

√x7ᵗʰ **V83.2 Person on outside** of special industrial vehicle injured in traffic accident

√x7ᵗʰ **V83.3 Unspecified occupant** of special industrial vehicle injured in traffic accident

√x7ᵗʰ **V83.4 Person injured while** boarding or alighting from special industrial vehicle

√x7ᵗʰ **V83.5 Driver** of special industrial vehicle injured in nontraffic accident

√x7ᵗʰ **V83.6 Passenger** of special industrial vehicle injured in nontraffic accident

√x7ᵗʰ **V83.7 Person on outside** of special industrial vehicle injured in nontraffic accident

√x7ᵗʰ **V83.9 Unspecified occupant** of special industrial vehicle injured in nontraffic accident

> Special-industrial-vehicle accident NOS

√4ᵗʰ **V84 Occupant of special vehicle mainly used in agriculture injured in transport accident**

> INCLUDES   self-propelled farm machinery
> tractor (and trailer)

> EXCLUDES 1   *animal-powered farm machinery accident (W30.8-)*
> *contact with combine harvester (W30.0)*
> *special agricultural vehicle in stationary use or maintenance (W30.-)*

√x7ᵗʰ **V84.0 Driver** of special agricultural vehicle injured in traffic accident

√x7ᵗʰ **V84.1 Passenger** of special agricultural vehicle injured in traffic accident

√x7ᵗʰ **V84.2 Person on outside** of special agricultural vehicle injured in traffic accident

√x7ᵗʰ **V84.3 Unspecified occupant** of special agricultural vehicle injured in traffic accident

√x7ᵗʰ **V84.4 Person injured while** boarding or alighting from special agricultural vehicle

√x7ᵗʰ **V84.5 Driver** of special agricultural vehicle injured in nontraffic accident

√x7ᵗʰ **V84.6 Passenger** of special agricultural vehicle injured in nontraffic accident

√x7ᵗʰ **V84.7 Person on outside** of special agricultural vehicle injured in nontraffic accident

√x7ᵗʰ **V84.9 Unspecified occupant** of special agricultural vehicle injured in nontraffic accident

> Special-agricultural vehicle accident NOS

√4ᵗʰ **V85 Occupant of special construction vehicle injured in transport accident**

> INCLUDES   bulldozer
> digger
> dump truck
> earth-leveller
> mechanical shovel
> road-roller

> EXCLUDES 1   *special industrial vehicle (V83.-)*
> *special construction vehicle in stationary use or maintenance (W31.-)*

√x7ᵗʰ **V85.0 Driver** of special construction vehicle injured in traffic accident

√x7ᵗʰ **V85.1 Passenger** of special construction vehicle injured in traffic accident

√x7ᵗʰ **V85.2 Person on outside** of special construction vehicle injured in traffic accident

√x7ᵗʰ **V85.3 Unspecified occupant** of special construction vehicle injured in traffic accident

√x7ᵗʰ **V85.4 Person injured while** boarding or alighting from special construction vehicle

√x7ᵗʰ **V85.5 Driver** of special construction vehicle injured in nontraffic accident

√x7ᵗʰ **V85.6 Passenger** of special construction vehicle injured in nontraffic accident

√x7ᵗʰ **V85.7 Person on outside** of special construction vehicle injured in nontraffic accident

√x7ᵗʰ **V85.9 Unspecified occupant** of special construction vehicle injured in nontraffic accident

> Special-construction-vehicle accident NOS

√4ᵗʰ **V86 Occupant of special all-terrain or other off-road motor vehicle, injured in transport accident**

> EXCLUDES 1   *special all-terrain vehicle in stationary use or maintenance (W31.-)*
> *sport-utility vehicle (V50-V59)*
> *three-wheeled motor vehicle designed for on-road use (V30-V39)*

> AHA: 2017,4Q,26

√5ᵗʰ **V86.0 Driver** of special all-terrain or other off-road motor vehicle injured in traffic accident

√x7ᵗʰ **V86.01 Driver of** ambulance or fire engine injured in traffic accident

√x7ᵗʰ **V86.02 Driver of** snowmobile injured in traffic accident

√x7ᵗʰ **V86.03 Driver of** dune buggy injured in traffic accident

√x7ᵗʰ **V86.04 Driver of** military vehicle injured in traffic accident

√x7ᵗʰ **V86.05 Driver of** 3- or 4- wheeled all-terrain vehicle (ATV) injured in traffic accident

√x7ᵗʰ **V86.06 Driver of** dirt bike or motor/cross bike injured in traffic accident

√x7ᵗʰ **V86.09 Driver of other special all-terrain or other off-road motor vehicle injured in traffic accident**

> ~~Driver of dirt bike injured in traffic accident~~
> Driver of go cart injured in traffic accident
> Driver of golf cart injured in traffic accident

√5ᵗʰ **V86.1 Passenger** of special all-terrain or other off-road motor vehicle injured in traffic accident

√x7ᵗʰ **V86.11 Passenger of** ambulance or fire engine injured in traffic accident

√x7ᵗʰ **V86.12 Passenger of** snowmobile injured in traffic accident

√x7ᵗʰ **V86.13 Passenger of** dune buggy injured in traffic accident

√x7ᵗʰ **V86.14 Passenger of** military vehicle injured in traffic accident

√x7ᵗʰ **V86.15 Passenger of** 3- or 4- wheeled all-terrain vehicle (ATV) injured in traffic accident

√x7ᵗʰ **V86.16 Passenger of** dirt bike or motor/cross bike injured in traffic accident

√x7ᵗʰ **V86.19 Passenger of other special all-terrain or other off-road motor vehicle injured in traffic accident**

> ~~Passenger of dirt bike injured in traffic accident~~
> Passenger of go cart injured in traffic accident
> Passenger of golf cart injured in traffic accident

√5ᵗʰ **V86.2 Person on outside** of special all-terrain or other off-road motor vehicle injured in traffic accident

√x7ᵗʰ **V86.21 Person on outside of** ambulance or fire engine injured in traffic accident

√x7ᵗʰ **V86.22 Person on outside of** snowmobile injured in traffic accident

√x7ᵗʰ **V86.23 Person on outside of** dune buggy injured in traffic accident

✓ Additional Char Req   √x7ᵗʰ Placeholder   Unacceptable PDx   Questionable PDx   Wrong Procedure   Manifestation   Unspecified Dx   H1-H14 HAC   HCC CMS-HCC Dx   HIV HIV Dx

ICD-10-CM 2020   1233

✓x7th **V86.24** Person on outside of military vehicle injured in traffic accident

✓x7th **V86.25** Person on outside of 3- or 4- wheeled all-terrain vehicle (ATV) injured in traffic accident

✓x7th **V86.26** Person on outside of dirt bike or motor/cross bike injured in traffic accident

✓x7th **V86.29** Person on outside of other special all-terrain or other off-road motor vehicle injured in traffic accident

~~Person on outside of dirt bike injured in traffic accident~~

Person on outside of go cart in traffic accident

Person on outside of golf cart injured in traffic accident

✓5th **V86.3** Unspecified occupant of special all-terrain or other off-road motor vehicle injured in traffic accident

✓x7th **V86.31** Unspecified occupant of ambulance or fire engine injured in traffic accident

✓x7th **V86.32** Unspecified occupant of snowmobile injured in traffic accident

✓x7th **V86.33** Unspecified occupant of dune buggy injured in traffic accident

✓x7th **V86.34** Unspecified occupant of military vehicle injured in traffic accident

✓x7th **V86.35** Unspecified occupant of 3- or 4- wheeled all-terrain vehicle (ATV) injured in traffic accident

✓x7th **V86.36** Unspecified occupant of dirt bike or motor/cross bike injured in traffic accident

✓x7th **V86.39** Unspecified occupant of other special all-terrain or other off-road motor vehicle injured in traffic accident

~~Unspecified occupant of dirt bike injured in traffic accident~~

Unspecified occupant of go cart injured in traffic accident

Unspecified occupant of golf cart injured in traffic accident

✓5th **V86.4** Person injured while boarding or alighting from special all-terrain or other off-road motor vehicle

✓x7th **V86.41** Person injured while boarding or alighting from ambulance or fire engine

✓x7th **V86.42** Person injured while boarding or alighting from snowmobile

✓x7th **V86.43** Person injured while boarding or alighting from dune buggy

✓x7th **V86.44** Person injured while boarding or alighting from military vehicle

✓x7th **V86.45** Person injured while boarding or alighting from a 3- or 4- wheeled all-terrain vehicle (ATV)

✓x7th **V86.46** Person injured while boarding or alighting from a dirt bike or motor/cross bike

✓x7th **V86.49** Person injured while boarding or alighting from other special all-terrain or other off-road motor vehicle

~~Person injured while boarding or alighting from dirt bike~~

Person injured while boarding or alighting from go cart

Person injured while boarding or alighting from golf cart

✓5th **V86.5** Driver of special all-terrain or other off-road motor vehicle injured in nontraffic accident

✓x7th **V86.51** Driver of ambulance or fire engine injured in nontraffic accident

✓x7th **V86.52** Driver of snowmobile injured in nontraffic accident

✓x7th **V86.53** Driver of dune buggy injured in nontraffic accident

✓x7th **V86.54** Driver of military vehicle injured in nontraffic accident

✓x7th **V86.55** Driver of 3- or 4- wheeled all-terrain vehicle (ATV) injured in nontraffic accident

✓x7th **V86.56** Driver of dirt bike or motor/cross bike injured in nontraffic accident

✓x7th **V86.59** Driver of other special all-terrain or other off-road motor vehicle injured in nontraffic accident

~~Driver of dirt bike injured in nontraffic accident~~

Driver of go cart injured in nontraffic accident

Driver of golf cart injured in nontraffic accident

✓5th **V86.6** Passenger of special all-terrain or other off-road motor vehicle injured in nontraffic accident

✓x7th **V86.61** Passenger of ambulance or fire engine injured in nontraffic accident

✓x7th **V86.62** Passenger of snowmobile injured in nontraffic accident

✓x7th **V86.63** Passenger of dune buggy injured in nontraffic accident

✓x7th **V86.64** Passenger of military vehicle injured in nontraffic accident

✓x7th **V86.65** Passenger of 3- or 4- wheeled all-terrain vehicle (ATV) injured in nontraffic accident

✓x7th **V86.66** Passenger of dirt bike or motor/cross bike injured in nontraffic accident

✓x7th **V86.69** Passenger of other special all-terrain or other off-road motor vehicle injured in nontraffic accident

~~Passenger of dirt bike injured in nontraffic accident~~

Passenger of go cart injured in nontraffic accident

Passenger of golf cart injured in nontraffic accident

✓5th **V86.7** Person on outside of special all-terrain or other off-road motor vehicle injured in nontraffic accident

✓x7th **V86.71** Person on outside of ambulance or fire engine injured in nontraffic accident

✓x7th **V86.72** Person on outside of snowmobile injured in nontraffic accident

✓x7th **V86.73** Person on outside of dune buggy injured in nontraffic accident

✓x7th **V86.74** Person on outside of military vehicle injured in nontraffic accident

✓x7th **V86.75** Person on outside of 3- or 4- wheeled all-terrain vehicle (ATV) injured in nontraffic accident

✓x7th **V86.76** Person on outside of dirt bike or motor/cross bike injured in nontraffic accident

✓x7th **V86.79** Person on outside of other special all-terrain or other off-road motor vehicles injured in nontraffic accident

~~Person on outside of dirt bike injured in nontraffic accident~~

Person on outside of go cart injured in nontraffic accident

Person on outside of golf cart injured in nontraffic accident

✓5th **V86.9** Unspecified occupant of special all-terrain or other off-road motor vehicle injured in nontraffic accident

✓x7th **V86.91** Unspecified occupant of ambulance or fire engine injured in nontraffic accident

✓x7th **V86.92** Unspecified occupant of snowmobile injured in nontraffic accident

✓x7th **V86.93** Unspecified occupant of dune buggy injured in nontraffic accident

✓x7th **V86.94** Unspecified occupant of military vehicle injured in nontraffic accident

✓x7th **V86.95** Unspecified occupant of 3- or 4- wheeled all-terrain vehicle (ATV) injured in nontraffic accident

✓x7th **V86.96** Unspecified occupant of dirt bike or motor/cross bike injured in nontraffic accident

✓x7th **V86.99** Unspecified occupant of other special all-terrain or other off-road motor vehicle injured in nontraffic accident

Off-road motor-vehicle accident NOS

Other motor-vehicle accident NOS

Unspecified occupant of go cart injured in nontraffic accident

Unspecified occupant of golf cart injured in nontraffic accident

✓4th **V87** Traffic accident of specified type but victim's mode of transport unknown

EXCLUDES 1 collision involving:

pedal cycle (V10-V19)

pedestrian (V01-V09)

✓x7th **V87.0** Person injured in collision between car and two- or three-wheeled powered vehicle (traffic)

✓x7th **V87.1** Person injured in collision between other motor vehicle and two- or three-wheeled motor vehicle (traffic)

✓x7th **V87.2** Person injured in collision between car and pick-up truck or van (traffic)

✓x7th **V87.3** Person injured in collision between car and bus (traffic)

✓x7th **V87.4** Person injured in collision between car and heavy transport vehicle (traffic)

✓x7th **V87.5** Person injured in collision between heavy transport vehicle and bus (traffic)

✓x7th **V87.6** Person injured in collision between railway train or railway vehicle and car (traffic)

✓x7th **V87.7** Person injured in collision between other specified motor vehicles (traffic)

N Newborn: 0   P Pediatric: 0-17   M Maternity: 9-64   A Adult: 15-124   MCC Major Complication/Comorbidity   CC Complication/Comorbidity   SW Severe Wound Dx

1234   ICD-10-CM 2020

☑x7ᵗʰ **V87.8**   **Person injured in other specified noncollision transport accidents involving motor vehicle (traffic)**

☑x7ᵗʰ **V87.9**   **Person injured in other specified (collision)(noncollision) transport accidents involving nonmotor vehicle (traffic)**

☑4ᵗʰ **V88**   **Nontraffic accident of specified type but victim's mode of transport unknown**

     EXCLUDES 1   collision involving:
            pedal cycle (V10-V19)
            pedestrian (V01-V09)

☑x7ᵗʰ **V88.0**   **Person injured in collision between car and two- or three-wheeled motor vehicle, nontraffic**

☑x7ᵗʰ **V88.1**   **Person injured in collision between other motor vehicle and two- or three-wheeled motor vehicle, nontraffic**

☑x7ᵗʰ **V88.2**   **Person injured in collision between car and pick-up truck or van, nontraffic**

☑x7ᵗʰ **V88.3**   **Person injured in collision between car and bus, nontraffic**

☑x7ᵗʰ **V88.4**   **Person injured in collision between car and heavy transport vehicle, nontraffic**

☑x7ᵗʰ **V88.5**   **Person injured in collision between heavy transport vehicle and bus, nontraffic**

☑x7ᵗʰ **V88.6**   **Person injured in collision between railway train or railway vehicle and car, nontraffic**

☑x7ᵗʰ **V88.7**   **Person injured in collision between other specified motor vehicle, nontraffic**

☑x7ᵗʰ **V88.8**   **Person injured in other specified noncollision transport accidents involving motor vehicle, nontraffic**

☑x7ᵗʰ **V88.9**   **Person injured in other specified (collision)(noncollision) transport accidents involving nonmotor vehicle, nontraffic**

☑4ᵗʰ **V89**   **Motor- or nonmotor-vehicle accident, type of vehicle unspecified**

☑x7ᵗʰ **V89.0**   **Person injured in unspecified motor-vehicle accident, nontraffic**
        Motor-vehicle accident NOS, nontraffic

☑x7ᵗʰ **V89.1**   **Person injured in unspecified nonmotor-vehicle accident, nontraffic**
        Nonmotor-vehicle accident NOS (nontraffic)

☑x7ᵗʰ **V89.2**   **Person injured in unspecified motor-vehicle accident, traffic**
        Motor-vehicle accident [MVA] NOS
        Road (traffic) accident [RTA] NOS

☑x7ᵗʰ **V89.3**   **Person injured in unspecified nonmotor-vehicle accident, traffic**
        Nonmotor-vehicle traffic accident NOS

☑x7ᵗʰ **V89.9**   **Person injured in unspecified vehicle accident**
        Collision NOS

Water transport accidents (V90-V94)

The appropriate 7th character is to be added to each code from categories V90-V94.
A   initial encounter
D   subsequent encounter
S   sequela

☑4ᵗʰ **V90**   **Drowning and submersion due to accident to watercraft**

     EXCLUDES 1   civilian water transport accident involving military watercraft (V94.81-)
            fall into water not from watercraft (W16.-)
            military watercraft accident in military or war operations (Y36.0-, Y37.0-)
            water-transport-related drowning or submersion without accident to watercraft (V92.-)

☑5ᵗʰ **V90.0**   **Drowning and submersion due to watercraft overturning**

☑x7ᵗʰ **V90.00**   **Drowning and submersion due to merchant ship overturning**

☑x7ᵗʰ **V90.01**   **Drowning and submersion due to passenger ship overturning**
        Drowning and submersion due to Ferry-boat overturning
        Drowning and submersion due to Liner overturning

☑x7ᵗʰ **V90.02**   **Drowning and submersion due to fishing boat overturning**

☑x7ᵗʰ **V90.03**   **Drowning and submersion due to other powered watercraft overturning**
        Drowning and submersion due to Hovercraft (on open water) overturning
        Drowning and submersion due to Jet ski overturning

☑x7ᵗʰ **V90.04**   **Drowning and submersion due to sailboat overturning**

☑x7ᵗʰ **V90.05**   **Drowning and submersion due to canoe or kayak overturning**

☑x7ᵗʰ **V90.06**   **Drowning and submersion due to (nonpowered) inflatable craft overturning**

☑x7ᵗʰ **V90.08**   **Drowning and submersion due to other unpowered watercraft overturning**
        Drowning and submersion due to windsurfer overturning

☑x7ᵗʰ **V90.09**   **Drowning and submersion due to unspecified watercraft overturning**
        Drowning and submersion due to boat NOS overturning
        Drowning and submersion due to ship NOS overturning
        Drowning and submersion due to watercraft NOS overturning

☑5ᵗʰ **V90.1**   **Drowning and submersion due to watercraft sinking**

☑x7ᵗʰ **V90.10**   **Drowning and submersion due to merchant ship sinking**

☑x7ᵗʰ **V90.11**   **Drowning and submersion due to passenger ship sinking**
        Drowning and submersion due to Ferry-boat sinking
        Drowning and submersion due to Liner sinking

☑x7ᵗʰ **V90.12**   **Drowning and submersion due to fishing boat sinking**

☑x7ᵗʰ **V90.13**   **Drowning and submersion due to other powered watercraft sinking**
        Drowning and submersion due to Hovercraft (on open water) sinking
        Drowning and submersion due to Jet ski sinking

☑x7ᵗʰ **V90.14**   **Drowning and submersion due to sailboat sinking**

☑x7ᵗʰ **V90.15**   **Drowning and submersion due to canoe or kayak sinking**

☑x7ᵗʰ **V90.16**   **Drowning and submersion due to (nonpowered) inflatable craft sinking**

☑x7ᵗʰ **V90.18**   **Drowning and submersion due to other unpowered watercraft sinking**

☑x7ᵗʰ **V90.19**   **Drowning and submersion due to unspecified watercraft sinking**
        Drowning and submersion due to boat NOS sinking
        Drowning and submersion due to ship NOS sinking
        Drowning and submersion due to watercraft NOS sinking

☑5ᵗʰ **V90.2**   **Drowning and submersion due to falling or jumping from burning watercraft**

☑x7ᵗʰ **V90.20**   **Drowning and submersion due to falling or jumping from burning merchant ship**

☑x7ᵗʰ **V90.21**   **Drowning and submersion due to falling or jumping from burning passenger ship**
        Drowning and submersion due to falling or jumping from burning Ferry-boat
        Drowning and submersion due to falling or jumping from burning Liner

☑x7ᵗʰ **V90.22**   **Drowning and submersion due to falling or jumping from burning fishing boat**

☑x7ᵗʰ **V90.23**   **Drowning and submersion due to falling or jumping from other burning powered watercraft**
        Drowning and submersion due to falling and jumping from burning Hovercraft (on open water)
        Drowning and submersion due to falling and jumping from burning Jet ski

☑x7ᵗʰ **V90.24**   **Drowning and submersion due to falling or jumping from burning sailboat**

☑x7ᵗʰ **V90.25**   **Drowning and submersion due to falling or jumping from burning canoe or kayak**

☑x7ᵗʰ **V90.26**   **Drowning and submersion due to falling or jumping from burning (nonpowered) inflatable craft**

☑x7ᵗʰ **V90.27**   **Drowning and submersion due to falling or jumping from burning water-skis**

☑x7ᵗʰ **V90.28**   **Drowning and submersion due to falling or jumping from other burning unpowered watercraft**
        Drowning and submersion due to falling and jumping from burning surf-board
        Drowning and submersion due to falling and jumping from burning windsurfer

☑ Additional Char Req   x7ᵗʰ Placeholder   Unacceptable PDx   Questionable PDx   Wrong Procedure   Manifestation   Unspecified Dx   H1-H14 HAC   HCC CMS-HCC Dx   HIV HIV Dx

ICD-10-CM 2020   1235

√x7ᵗʰ **V90.29 Drowning and submersion due to falling or jumping from unspecified burning watercraft**

Drowning and submersion due to falling or jumping from burning boat NOS

Drowning and submersion due to falling or jumping from burning ship NOS

Drowning and submersion due to falling or jumping from burning watercraft NOS

√5ᵗʰ **V90.3 Drowning and submersion due to falling or jumping from crushed watercraft**

√x7ᵗʰ **V90.30 Drowning and submersion due to falling or jumping from crushed merchant ship**

√x7ᵗʰ **V90.31 Drowning and submersion due to falling or jumping from crushed passenger ship**

Drowning and submersion due to falling and jumping from crushed Ferry boat

Drowning and submersion due to falling and jumping from crushed Liner

√x7ᵗʰ **V90.32 Drowning and submersion due to falling or jumping from crushed fishing boat**

√x7ᵗʰ **V90.33 Drowning and submersion due to falling or jumping from other crushed powered watercraft**

Drowning and submersion due to falling and jumping from crushed Hovercraft

Drowning and submersion due to falling and jumping from crushed Jet ski

√x7ᵗʰ **V90.34 Drowning and submersion due to falling or jumping from crushed sailboat**

√x7ᵗʰ **V90.35 Drowning and submersion due to falling or jumping from crushed canoe or kayak**

√x7ᵗʰ **V90.36 Drowning and submersion due to falling or jumping from crushed (nonpowered) inflatable craft**

√x7ᵗʰ **V90.37 Drowning and submersion due to falling or jumping from crushed water-skis**

√x7ᵗʰ **V90.38 Drowning and submersion due to falling or jumping from other crushed unpowered watercraft**

Drowning and submersion due to falling and jumping from crushed surf-board

Drowning and submersion due to falling and jumping from crushed windsurfer

√x7ᵗʰ **V90.39 Drowning and submersion due to falling or jumping from crushed unspecified watercraft**

Drowning and submersion due to falling and jumping from crushed boat NOS

Drowning and submersion due to falling and jumping from crushed ship NOS

Drowning and submersion due to falling and jumping from crushed watercraft NOS

√5ᵗʰ **V90.8 Drowning and submersion due to other accident to watercraft**

√x7ᵗʰ **V90.80 Drowning and submersion due to other accident to merchant ship**

√x7ᵗʰ **V90.81 Drowning and submersion due to other accident to passenger ship**

Drowning and submersion due to other accident to Ferry-boat

Drowning and submersion due to other accident to Liner

√x7ᵗʰ **V90.82 Drowning and submersion due to other accident to fishing boat**

√x7ᵗʰ **V90.83 Drowning and submersion due to other accident to other powered watercraft**

Drowning and submersion due to other accident to Hovercraft (on open water)

Drowning and submersion due to other accident to Jet ski

√x7ᵗʰ **V90.84 Drowning and submersion due to other accident to sailboat**

√x7ᵗʰ **V90.85 Drowning and submersion due to other accident to canoe or kayak**

√x7ᵗʰ **V90.86 Drowning and submersion due to other accident to (nonpowered) inflatable craft**

√x7ᵗʰ **V90.87 Drowning and submersion due to other accident to water-skis**

√x7ᵗʰ **V90.88 Drowning and submersion due to other accident to other unpowered watercraft**

Drowning and submersion due to other accident to surf-board

Drowning and submersion due to other accident to windsurfer

√x7ᵗʰ **V90.89 Drowning and submersion due to other accident to unspecified watercraft**

Drowning and submersion due to other accident to boat NOS

Drowning and submersion due to other accident to ship NOS

Drowning and submersion due to other accident to watercraft NOS

√4ᵗʰ **V91 Other injury due to accident to watercraft**

INCLUDES   any injury except drowning and submersion as a result of an accident to watercraft

EXCLUDES 1   civilian water transport accident involving military watercraft (V94.81-)

military watercraft accident in military or war operations (Y36, Y37.-)

EXCLUDES 2   drowning and submersion due to accident to watercraft (V90.-)

√5ᵗʰ **V91.0 Burn due to watercraft on fire**

EXCLUDES 1   burn from localized fire or explosion on board ship without accident to watercraft (V93.-)

√x7ᵗʰ **V91.00 Burn due to merchant ship on fire**

√x7ᵗʰ **V91.01 Burn due to passenger ship on fire**

Burn due to Ferry-boat on fire

Burn due to Liner on fire

√x7ᵗʰ **V91.02 Burn due to fishing boat on fire**

√x7ᵗʰ **V91.03 Burn due to other powered watercraft on fire**

Burn due to Hovercraft (on open water) on fire

Burn due to Jet ski on fire

√x7ᵗʰ **V91.04 Burn due to sailboat on fire**

√x7ᵗʰ **V91.05 Burn due to canoe or kayak on fire**

√x7ᵗʰ **V91.06 Burn due to (nonpowered) inflatable craft on fire**

√x7ᵗʰ **V91.07 Burn due to water-skis on fire**

√x7ᵗʰ **V91.08 Burn due to other unpowered watercraft on fire**

√x7ᵗʰ **V91.09 Burn due to unspecified watercraft on fire**

Burn due to boat NOS on fire

Burn due to ship NOS on fire

Burn due to watercraft NOS on fire

√5ᵗʰ **V91.1 Crushed between watercraft and other watercraft or other object due to collision**

Crushed by lifeboat after abandoning ship in a collision

NOTE   Select the specified type of watercraft that the victim was on at the time of the collision

√x7ᵗʰ **V91.10 Crushed between merchant ship and other watercraft or other object due to collision**

√x7ᵗʰ **V91.11 Crushed between passenger ship and other watercraft or other object due to collision**

Crushed between Ferry-boat and other watercraft or other object due to collision

Crushed between Liner and other watercraft or other object due to collision

√x7ᵗʰ **V91.12 Crushed between fishing boat and other watercraft or other object due to collision**

√x7ᵗʰ **V91.13 Crushed between other powered watercraft and other watercraft or other object due to collision**

Crushed between Hovercraft (on open water) and other watercraft or other object due to collision

Crushed between Jet ski and other watercraft or other object due to collision

√x7ᵗʰ **V91.14 Crushed between sailboat and other watercraft or other object due to collision**

√x7ᵗʰ **V91.15 Crushed between canoe or kayak and other watercraft or other object due to collision**

√x7ᵗʰ **V91.16 Crushed between (nonpowered) inflatable craft and other watercraft or other object due to collision**

N Newborn: 0   P Pediatric: 0-17   M Maternity: 9-64   A Adult: 15-124   MCC Major Complication/Comorbidity   CC Complication/Comorbidity   SW Severe Wound Dx

1236   ICD-10-CM 2020

√x7ᵗʰ **V91.18 Crushed between other** unpowered **watercraft and other watercraft or other object due to collision**
Crushed between surfboard and other watercraft or other object due to collision
Crushed between windsurfer and other watercraft or other object due to collision

√5ᵗʰ **V91.19 Crushed between unspecified watercraft and other watercraft or other object due to collision**
Crushed between boat NOS and other watercraft or other object due to collision
Crushed between ship NOS and other watercraft or other object due to collision
Crushed between watercraft NOS and other watercraft or other object due to collision

√5ᵗʰ **V91.2 Fall due to collision between watercraft and other watercraft or other object**
Fall while remaining on watercraft after collision

> **NOTE** Select the specified type of watercraft that the victim was on at the time of the collision

> **EXCLUDES 1** *crushed between watercraft and other watercraft and other object due to collision (V91.1-)*
> *drowning and submersion due to falling from crushed watercraft (V90.3-)*

√x7ᵗʰ **V91.20 Fall due to collision between** merchant ship **and other watercraft or other object**

√x7ᵗʰ **V91.21 Fall due to collision between** passenger ship **and other watercraft or other object**
Fall due to collision between Ferry-boat and other watercraft or other object
Fall due to collision between Liner and other watercraft or other object

√x7ᵗʰ **V91.22 Fall due to collision between** fishing boat **and other watercraft or other object**

√x7ᵗʰ **V91.23 Fall due to collision between other** powered **watercraft and other watercraft or other object**
Fall due to collision between Hovercraft (on open water) and other watercraft or other object
Fall due to collision between Jet ski and other watercraft or other object

√x7ᵗʰ **V91.24 Fall due to collision between** sailboat **and other watercraft or other object**

√x7ᵗʰ **V91.25 Fall due to collision between** canoe or kayak **and other watercraft or other object**

√x7ᵗʰ **V91.26 Fall due to collision between (nonpowered)** inflatable craft **and other watercraft or other object**

√x7ᵗʰ **V91.29 Fall due to collision between unspecified watercraft and other watercraft or other object**
Fall due to collision between boat NOS and other watercraft or other object
Fall due to collision between ship NOS and other watercraft or other object
Fall due to collision between watercraft NOS and other watercraft or other object

√5ᵗʰ **V91.3 Hit or struck by falling object due to accident to watercraft**
Hit or struck by falling object (part of damaged watercraft or other object) after falling or jumping from damaged watercraft

> **EXCLUDES 2** *drowning or submersion due to fall or jumping from damaged watercraft (V90.2-, V90.3-)*

√x7ᵗʰ **V91.30 Hit or struck by falling object due to accident to** merchant ship

√x7ᵗʰ **V91.31 Hit or struck by falling object due to accident to** passenger ship
Hit or struck by falling object due to accident to Ferry-boat
Hit or struck by falling object due to accident to Liner

√x7ᵗʰ **V91.32 Hit or struck by falling object due to accident to** fishing boat

√x7ᵗʰ **V91.33 Hit or struck by falling object due to accident to other** powered **watercraft**
Hit or struck by falling object due to accident to Hovercraft (on open water)
Hit or struck by falling object due to accident to Jet ski

√x7ᵗʰ **V91.34 Hit or struck by falling object due to accident to** sailboat

√x7ᵗʰ **V91.35 Hit or struck by falling object due to accident to** canoe or kayak

√x7ᵗʰ **V91.36 Hit or struck by falling object due to accident to (nonpowered)** inflatable craft

√x7ᵗʰ **V91.37 Hit or struck by falling object due to accident to** water-skis
Hit by water-skis after jumping off of waterskis

√x7ᵗʰ **V91.38 Hit or struck by falling object due to accident to other** unpowered **watercraft**
Hit or struck by surf-board after falling off damaged surf-board
Hit or struck by object after falling off damaged windsurfer

√x7ᵗʰ **V91.39 Hit or struck by falling object due to accident to unspecified watercraft**
Hit or struck by falling object due to accident to boat NOS
Hit or struck by falling object due to accident to ship NOS
Hit or struck by falling object due to accident to watercraft NOS

√5ᵗʰ **V91.8 Other injury due to other accident to watercraft**

√x7ᵗʰ **V91.80 Other injury due to other accident to** merchant ship

√x7ᵗʰ **V91.81 Other injury due to other accident to** passenger ship
Other injury due to other accident to Ferry-boat
Other injury due to other accident to Liner

√x7ᵗʰ **V91.82 Other injury due to other accident to** fishing boat

√x7ᵗʰ **V91.83 Other injury due to other accident to other** powered **watercraft**
Other injury due to other accident to Hovercraft (on open water)
Other injury due to other accident to Jet ski

√x7ᵗʰ **V91.84 Other injury due to other accident to** sailboat

√x7ᵗʰ **V91.85 Other injury due to other accident to** canoe or kayak

√x7ᵗʰ **V91.86 Other injury due to other accident to (nonpowered)** inflatable craft

√x7ᵗʰ **V91.87 Other injury due to other accident to** water-skis

√x7ᵗʰ **V91.88 Other injury due to other accident to other** unpowered **watercraft**
Other injury due to other accident to surf-board
Other injury due to other accident to windsurfer

√x7ᵗʰ **V91.89 Other injury due to other accident to unspecified watercraft**
Other injury due to other accident to boat NOS
Other injury due to other accident to ship NOS
Other injury due to other accident to watercraft NOS

√4ᵗʰ **V92 Drowning and submersion due to accident on board watercraft, without accident to watercraft**

> **EXCLUDES 1** *civilian water transport accident involving military watercraft (V94.81-)*
> *drowning or submersion due to accident to watercraft (V90-V91)*
> *drowning or submersion of diver who voluntarily jumps from boat not involved in an accident (W16.711, W16.721)*
> *fall into water without watercraft (W16.-)*
> *military watercraft accident in military or war operations (Y36, Y37)*

√5ᵗʰ **V92.0 Drowning and submersion due to** fall off **watercraft**
Drowning and submersion due to fall from gangplank of watercraft
Drowning and submersion due to fall overboard watercraft

> **EXCLUDES 2** *hitting head on object or bottom of body of water due to fall from watercraft (V94.0-)*

√x7ᵗʰ **V92.00 Drowning and submersion due to fall off** merchant ship

√x7ᵗʰ **V92.01 Drowning and submersion due to fall off** passenger ship
Drowning and submersion due to fall off Ferry-boat
Drowning and submersion due to fall off Liner

√x7ᵗʰ **V92.02 Drowning and submersion due to fall off** fishing boat

√x7ᵗʰ **V92.03 Drowning and submersion due to fall off other** powered **watercraft**
Drowning and submersion due to fall off Hovercraft (on open water)
Drowning and submersion due to fall off Jet ski

√x7ᵗʰ **V92.04 Drowning and submersion due to fall off** sailboat

√x7ᵗʰ **V92.05 Drowning and submersion due to fall off** canoe or kayak

√x7th V92.06 **Drowning and submersion due to fall off (nonpowered)** inflatable craft

√x7th V92.07 **Drowning and submersion due to fall off** water-skis

> *EXCLUDES 1*   *drowning and submersion due to falling off burning water-skis (V90.27)*
> *drowning and submersion due to falling off crushed water-skis (V90.37)*
> *hit by boat while water-skiing NOS (V94.X)*

√x7th V92.08 **Drowning and submersion due to fall off other unpowered watercraft**

Drowning and submersion due to fall off surf-board
Drowning and submersion due to fall off windsurfer

> *EXCLUDES 1*   *drowning and submersion due to fall off burning unpowered watercraft (V90.28)*
> *drowning and submersion due to fall off crushed unpowered watercraft (V90.38)*
> *drowning and submersion due to fall off damaged unpowered watercraft (V90.88)*
> *drowning and submersion due to rider of nonpowered watercraft being hit by other watercraft (V94.-)*
> *other injury due to rider of nonpowered watercraft being hit by other watercraft (V94.-)*

√x7th V92.09 **Drowning and submersion due to fall off unspecified watercraft**

Drowning and submersion due to fall off boat NOS
Drowning and submersion due to fall off ship
Drowning and submersion due to fall off watercraft NOS

√5th V92.1 **Drowning and submersion due to being** thrown overboard **by motion of watercraft**

> *EXCLUDES 1*   *drowning and submersion due to fall off surf-board (V92.08)*
> *drowning and submersion due to fall off water-skis (V92.07)*
> *drowning and submersion due to fall off windsurfer (V92.08)*

√x7th V92.10 **Drowning and submersion due to being thrown overboard by motion of** merchant ship

√x7th V92.11 **Drowning and submersion due to being thrown overboard by motion of** passenger ship

Drowning and submersion due to being thrown overboard by motion of Ferry-boat
Drowning and submersion due to being thrown overboard by motion of Liner

√x7th V92.12 **Drowning and submersion due to being thrown overboard by motion of** fishing boat

√x7th V92.13 **Drowning and submersion due to being thrown overboard by motion of other** powered **watercraft**

Drowning and submersion due to being thrown overboard by motion of Hovercraft

√x7th V92.14 **Drowning and submersion due to being thrown overboard by motion of** sailboat

√x7th V92.15 **Drowning and submersion due to being thrown overboard by motion of** canoe or kayak

√x7th V92.16 **Drowning and submersion due to being thrown overboard by motion of (nonpowered)** inflatable craft

√x7th V92.19 **Drowning and submersion due to being thrown overboard by motion of unspecified watercraft**

Drowning and submersion due to being thrown overboard by motion of boat NOS
Drowning and submersion due to being thrown overboard by motion of ship NOS
Drowning and submersion due to being thrown overboard by motion of watercraft NOS

√5th V92.2 **Drowning and submersion due to being** washed overboard **from watercraft**

Code first any associated cataclysm (X37.0-)

√x7th V92.20 **Drowning and submersion due to being washed overboard from** merchant ship

√x7th V92.21 **Drowning and submersion due to being washed overboard from** passenger ship

Drowning and submersion due to being washed overboard from Ferry-boat
Drowning and submersion due to being washed overboard from Liner

√x7th V92.22 **Drowning and submersion due to being washed overboard from** fishing boat

√x7th V92.23 **Drowning and submersion due to being washed overboard from other** powered **watercraft**

Drowning and submersion due to being washed overboard from Hovercraft (on open water)
Drowning and submersion due to being washed overboard from Jet ski

√x7th V92.24 **Drowning and submersion due to being washed overboard from** sailboat

√x7th V92.25 **Drowning and submersion due to being washed overboard from** canoe or kayak

√x7th V92.26 **Drowning and submersion due to being washed overboard from (nonpowered)** inflatable craft

√x7th V92.27 **Drowning and submersion due to being washed overboard from** water-skis

> *EXCLUDES 1*   *drowning and submersion due to fall off water-skis (V92.07)*

√x7th V92.28 **Drowning and submersion due to being washed overboard from other** unpowered **watercraft**

Drowning and submersion due to being washed overboard from surf-board
Drowning and submersion due to being washed overboard from windsurfer

√x7th V92.29 **Drowning and submersion due to being washed overboard from unspecified watercraft**

Drowning and submersion due to being washed overboard from boat NOS
Drowning and submersion due to being washed overboard from ship NOS
Drowning and submersion due to being washed overboard from watercraft NOS

√4th V93 **Other injury due to accident on board watercraft, without accident to watercraft**

> *EXCLUDES 1*   *civilian water transport accident involving military watercraft (V94.81-)*
> *other injury due to accident to watercraft (V91.-)*
> *military watercraft accident in military or war operations (Y36, Y37.-)*

> *EXCLUDES 2*   *drowning and submersion due to accident on board watercraft, without accident to watercraft (V92.-)*

√5th V93.0 **Burn due to localized fire on board watercraft**

> *EXCLUDES 1*   *burn due to watercraft on fire (V91.0-)*

√x7th V93.00 **Burn due to localized fire on board** merchant vessel

√x7th V93.01 **Burn due to localized fire on board** passenger vessel

Burn due to localized fire on board Ferry-boat
Burn due to localized fire on board Liner

√x7th V93.02 **Burn due to localized fire on board** fishing boat

√x7th V93.03 **Burn due to localized fire on board other** powered **watercraft**

Burn due to localized fire on board Hovercraft
Burn due to localized fire on board Jet ski

√x7th V93.04 **Burn due to localized fire on board** sailboat

√x7th V93.09 **Burn due to localized fire on board unspecified watercraft**

Burn due to localized fire on board boat NOS
Burn due to localized fire on board ship NOS
Burn due to localized fire on board watercraft NOS

√5th V93.1 **Other burn on board watercraft**

Burn due to source other than fire on board watercraft

> *EXCLUDES 1*   *burn due to watercraft on fire (V91.0-)*

√x7th V93.10 **Other burn on board** merchant vessel

√x7th V93.11 **Other burn on board** passenger vessel

Other burn on board Ferry-boat
Other burn on board Liner

√x7th V93.12 **Other burn on board** fishing boat

√x7th V93.13 **Other burn on board other** powered **watercraft**

Other burn on board Hovercraft
Other burn on board Jet ski

√x7th V93.14 **Other burn on board** sailboat

✓x7ᵗʰ **V93.19** **Other burn on board unspecified watercraft**

Other burn on board boat NOS

Other burn on board ship NOS

Other burn on board watercraft NOS

✓5ᵗʰ **V93.2** **Heat exposure on board watercraft**

EXCLUDES 1   *exposure to man-made heat not aboard watercraft (W92)*

exposure to natural heat while on board watercraft (X30)

exposure to sunlight while on board watercraft (X32)

EXCLUDES 2   *burn due to fire on board watercraft (V93.0-)*

✓x7ᵗʰ **V93.20** **Heat exposure on board merchant ship**

✓x7ᵗʰ **V93.21** **Heat exposure on board passenger ship**

Heat exposure on board Ferry-boat

Heat exposure on board Liner

✓x7ᵗʰ **V93.22** **Heat exposure on board fishing boat**

✓x7ᵗʰ **V93.23** **Heat exposure on board other powered watercraft**

Heat exposure on board hovercraft

✓x7ᵗʰ **V93.24** **Heat exposure on board sailboat**

✓x7ᵗʰ **V93.29** **Heat exposure on board unspecified watercraft**

Heat exposure on board boat NOS

Heat exposure on board ship NOS

Heat exposure on board watercraft NOS

✓5ᵗʰ **V93.3** **Fall on board watercraft**

EXCLUDES 1   *fall due to collision of watercraft (V91.2-)*

✓x7ᵗʰ **V93.30** **Fall on board merchant ship**

✓x7ᵗʰ **V93.31** **Fall on board passenger ship**

Fall on board Ferry-boat

Fall on board Liner

✓x7ᵗʰ **V93.32** **Fall on board fishing boat**

✓x7ᵗʰ **V93.33** **Fall on board other powered watercraft**

Fall on board Hovercraft (on open water)

Fall on board Jet ski

✓x7ᵗʰ **V93.34** **Fall on board sailboat**

✓x7ᵗʰ **V93.35** **Fall on board canoe or kayak**

✓x7ᵗʰ **V93.36** **Fall on board (nonpowered) inflatable craft**

✓x7ᵗʰ **V93.38** **Fall on board other unpowered watercraft**

✓x7ᵗʰ **V93.39** **Fall on board unspecified watercraft**

Fall on board boat NOS

Fall on board ship NOS

Fall on board watercraft NOS

✓5ᵗʰ **V93.4** **Struck by falling object on board watercraft**

Hit by falling object on board watercraft

EXCLUDES 1   *struck by falling object due to accident to watercraft (V91.3)*

✓x7ᵗʰ **V93.40** **Struck by falling object on merchant ship**

✓x7ᵗʰ **V93.41** **Struck by falling object on passenger ship**

Struck by falling object on Ferry-boat

Struck by falling object on Liner

✓x7ᵗʰ **V93.42** **Struck by falling object on fishing boat**

✓x7ᵗʰ **V93.43** **Struck by falling object on other powered watercraft**

Struck by falling object on Hovercraft

✓x7ᵗʰ **V93.44** **Struck by falling object on sailboat**

✓x7ᵗʰ **V93.48** **Struck by falling object on other unpowered watercraft**

✓x7ᵗʰ **V93.49** **Struck by falling object on unspecified watercraft**

✓5ᵗʰ **V93.5** **Explosion on board watercraft**

Boiler explosion on steamship

EXCLUDES 2   *fire on board watercraft (V93.0-)*

✓x7ᵗʰ **V93.50** **Explosion on board merchant ship**

✓x7ᵗʰ **V93.51** **Explosion on board passenger ship**

Explosion on board Ferry-boat

Explosion on board Liner

✓x7ᵗʰ **V93.52** **Explosion on board fishing boat**

✓x7ᵗʰ **V93.53** **Explosion on board other powered watercraft**

Explosion on board Hovercraft

Explosion on board Jet ski

✓x7ᵗʰ **V93.54** **Explosion on board sailboat**

✓x7ᵗʰ **V93.59** **Explosion on board unspecified watercraft**

Explosion on board boat NOS

Explosion on board ship NOS

Explosion on board watercraft NOS

✓5ᵗʰ **V93.6** **Machinery accident on board watercraft**

EXCLUDES 1   *machinery explosion on board watercraft (V93.4-)*

machinery fire on board watercraft (V93.0-)

✓x7ᵗʰ **V93.60** **Machinery accident on board merchant ship**

✓x7ᵗʰ **V93.61** **Machinery accident on board passenger ship**

Machinery accident on board Ferry-boat

Machinery accident on board Liner

✓x7ᵗʰ **V93.62** **Machinery accident on board fishing boat**

✓x7ᵗʰ **V93.63** **Machinery accident on board other powered watercraft**

Machinery accident on board Hovercraft

✓x7ᵗʰ **V93.64** **Machinery accident on board sailboat**

✓x7ᵗʰ **V93.69** **Machinery accident on board unspecified watercraft**

Machinery accident on board boat NOS

Machinery accident on board ship NOS

Machinery accident on board watercraft NOS

✓5ᵗʰ **V93.8** **Other injury due to other accident on board watercraft**

Accidental poisoning by gases or fumes on watercraft

✓x7ᵗʰ **V93.80** **Other injury due to other accident on board merchant ship**

✓x7ᵗʰ **V93.81** **Other injury due to other accident on board passenger ship**

Other injury due to other accident on board Ferry-boat

Other injury due to other accident on board Liner

✓x7ᵗʰ **V93.82** **Other injury due to other accident on board fishing boat**

✓x7ᵗʰ **V93.83** **Other injury due to other accident on board other powered watercraft**

Other injury due to other accident on board Hovercraft

Other injury due to other accident on board Jet ski

✓x7ᵗʰ **V93.84** **Other injury due to other accident on board sailboat**

✓x7ᵗʰ **V93.85** **Other injury due to other accident on board canoe or kayak**

✓x7ᵗʰ **V93.86** **Other injury due to other accident on board (nonpowered) inflatable craft**

✓x7ᵗʰ **V93.87** **Other injury due to other accident on board water-skis**

Hit or struck by object while waterskiing

✓x7ᵗʰ **V93.88** **Other injury due to other accident on board other unpowered watercraft**

Hit or struck by object while surfing

Hit or struck by object while on board windsurfer

✓x7ᵗʰ **V93.89** **Other injury due to other accident on board unspecified watercraft**

Other injury due to other accident on board boat NOS

Other injury due to other accident on board ship NOS

Other injury due to other accident on board watercraft NOS

✓4ᵗʰ **V94** **Other and unspecified water transport accidents**

EXCLUDES 1   *military watercraft accidents in military or war operations (Y36, Y37)*

✓x7ᵗʰ **V94.0** **Hitting object or bottom of body of water due to fall from watercraft**

EXCLUDES 2   *drowning and submersion due to fall from watercraft (V92.0-)*

✓5ᵗʰ **V94.1** **Bather struck by watercraft**

Swimmer hit by watercraft

✓x7ᵗʰ **V94.11** **Bather struck by powered watercraft**

✓x7ᵗʰ **V94.12** **Bather struck by nonpowered watercraft**

✓5ᵗʰ **V94.2** **Rider of nonpowered watercraft struck by other watercraft**

✓x7ᵗʰ **V94.21** **Rider of nonpowered watercraft struck by other nonpowered watercraft**

Canoer hit by other nonpowered watercraft

Surfer hit by other nonpowered watercraft

Windsurfer hit by other nonpowered watercraft

✓ Additional Char Req   ✓x7ᵗʰ Placeholder   Unacceptable PDx   Questionable PDx   Wrong Procedure   Manifestation   Unspecified Dx   H1-H14 HAC   HCC CMS-HCC Dx   HIV HIV Dx

ICD-10-CM 2020   1239

Chapter 20. External Causes of Morbidity

V93.19–V94.21

√x7ᵗʰ **V94.22 Rider of nonpowered watercraft struck by** powered **watercraft**
Canoer hit by motorboat
Surfer hit by motorboat
Windsurfer hit by motorboat

√5ᵗʰ **V94.3 Injury to rider of (inflatable) watercraft being pulled behind other watercraft**

√x7ᵗʰ **V94.31 Injury to rider of (inflatable)** recreational **watercraft being pulled behind other watercraft**
Injury to rider of inner-tube pulled behind motor boat

√x7ᵗʰ **V94.32 Injury to rider of** non-recreational **watercraft being pulled behind other watercraft**
Injury to occupant of dingy being pulled behind boat or ship
Injury to occupant of life-raft being pulled behind boat or ship

√x7ᵗʰ **V94.4 Injury to barefoot water-skier**
Injury to person being pulled behind boat or ship

√5ᵗʰ **V94.8 Other water transport accident**

√6ᵗʰ **V94.81 Water transport accident involving military watercraft**

√7ᵗʰ **V94.810 Civilian watercraft involved in water transport accident with military watercraft**
Passenger on civilian watercraft injured due to accident with military watercraft

√7ᵗʰ **V94.811 Civilian in water injured by military watercraft**

√7ᵗʰ **V94.818 Other water transport accident involving military watercraft**

√x7ᵗʰ **V94.89 Other water transport accident**

√x7ᵗʰ **V94.9 Unspecified water transport accident**
Water transport accident NOS

Air and space transport accidents (V95-V97)

EXCLUDES 1 *military aircraft accidents in military or war operations (Y36, Y37)*

The appropriate 7th character is to be added to each code from categories V95-V97.
A   initial encounter
D   subsequent encounter
S   sequela

√4ᵗʰ **V95 Accident to powered aircraft causing injury to occupant**

√5ᵗʰ **V95.0** Helicopter **accident injuring occupant**

√x7ᵗʰ **V95.00 Unspecified helicopter accident injuring occupant**

√x7ᵗʰ **V95.01 Helicopter** crash **injuring occupant**

√x7ᵗʰ **V95.02** Forced landing **of helicopter injuring occupant**

√x7ᵗʰ **V95.03 Helicopter** collision **injuring occupant**
Helicopter collision with any object, fixed, movable or moving

√x7ᵗʰ **V95.04 Helicopter** fire **injuring occupant**

√x7ᵗʰ **V95.05 Helicopter** explosion **injuring occupant**

√x7ᵗʰ **V95.09 Other helicopter accident injuring occupant**

√5ᵗʰ **V95.1** Ultralight, microlight or powered-glider **accident injuring occupant**

√x7ᵗʰ **V95.10 Unspecified ultralight, microlight or powered-glider accident injuring occupant**

√x7ᵗʰ **V95.11 Ultralight, microlight or powered-glider** crash **injuring occupant**

√x7ᵗʰ **V95.12** Forced landing **of ultralight, microlight or powered-glider injuring occupant**

√x7ᵗʰ **V95.13 Ultralight, microlight or powered-glider** collision **injuring occupant**
Ultralight, microlight or powered-glider collision with any object, fixed, movable or moving

√x7ᵗʰ **V95.14 Ultralight, microlight or powered-glider** fire **injuring occupant**

√x7ᵗʰ **V95.15 Ultralight, microlight or powered-glider** explosion **injuring occupant**

√x7ᵗʰ **V95.19 Other ultralight, microlight or powered-glider accident injuring occupant**

√5ᵗʰ **V95.2 Other private fixed-wing aircraft accident injuring occupant**

√x7ᵗʰ **V95.20 Unspecified accident to other private fixed-wing aircraft, injuring occupant**

√x7ᵗʰ **V95.21 Other private fixed-wing aircraft crash injuring occupant**

√x7ᵗʰ **V95.22** Forced landing **of other private fixed-wing aircraft injuring occupant**

√x7ᵗʰ **V95.23 Other private fixed-wing aircraft** collision **injuring occupant**
Other private fixed-wing aircraft collision with any object, fixed, movable or moving

√x7ᵗʰ **V95.24 Other private fixed-wing aircraft** fire **injuring occupant**

√x7ᵗʰ **V95.25 Other private fixed-wing aircraft** explosion **injuring occupant**

√x7ᵗʰ **V95.29 Other accident to other private fixed-wing aircraft injuring occupant**

√5ᵗʰ **V95.3** Commercial fixed-wing **aircraft accident injuring occupant**

√x7ᵗʰ **V95.30 Unspecified accident to commercial fixed-wing aircraft injuring occupant**

√x7ᵗʰ **V95.31 Commercial fixed-wing aircraft** crash **injuring occupant**

√x7ᵗʰ **V95.32** Forced landing **of commercial fixed-wing aircraft injuring occupant**

√x7ᵗʰ **V95.33 Commercial fixed-wing aircraft** collision **injuring occupant**
Commercial fixed-wing aircraft collision with any object, fixed, movable or moving

√x7ᵗʰ **V95.34 Commercial fixed-wing aircraft** fire **injuring occupant**

√x7ᵗʰ **V95.35 Commercial fixed-wing aircraft** explosion **injuring occupant**

√x7ᵗʰ **V95.39 Other accident to commercial fixed-wing aircraft injuring occupant**

√5ᵗʰ **V95.4** Spacecraft **accident injuring occupant**

√x7ᵗʰ **V95.40 Unspecified spacecraft accident injuring occupant**

√x7ᵗʰ **V95.41 Spacecraft** crash **injuring occupant**

√x7ᵗʰ **V95.42** Forced landing **of spacecraft injuring occupant**

√x7ᵗʰ **V95.43 Spacecraft** collision **injuring occupant**
Spacecraft collision with any object, fixed, moveable or moving

√x7ᵗʰ **V95.44 Spacecraft** fire **injuring occupant**

√x7ᵗʰ **V95.45 Spacecraft** explosion **injuring occupant**

√x7ᵗʰ **V95.49 Other spacecraft accident injuring occupant**

√x7ᵗʰ **V95.8 Other powered aircraft accidents injuring occupant**

√x7ᵗʰ **V95.9 Unspecified aircraft accident injuring occupant**
Aircraft accident NOS
Air transport accident NOS

√4ᵗʰ **V96 Accident to nonpowered aircraft causing injury to occupant**

√5ᵗʰ **V96.0** Balloon **accident injuring occupant**

√x7ᵗʰ **V96.00 Unspecified balloon accident injuring occupant**

√x7ᵗʰ **V96.01 Balloon** crash **injuring occupant**

√x7ᵗʰ **V96.02** Forced landing **of balloon injuring occupant**

√x7ᵗʰ **V96.03 Balloon** collision **injuring occupant**
Balloon collision with any object, fixed, moveable or moving

√x7ᵗʰ **V96.04 Balloon** fire **injuring occupant**

√x7ᵗʰ **V96.05 Balloon** explosion **injuring occupant**

√x7ᵗʰ **V96.09 Other balloon accident injuring occupant**

√5ᵗʰ **V96.1** Hang-glider **accident injuring occupant**

√x7ᵗʰ **V96.10 Unspecified hang-glider accident injuring occupant**

√x7ᵗʰ **V96.11 Hang-glider** crash **injuring occupant**

√x7ᵗʰ **V96.12** Forced landing **of hang-glider injuring occupant**

√x7ᵗʰ **V96.13 Hang-glider** collision **injuring occupant**
Hang-glider collision with any object, fixed, moveable or moving

√x7ᵗʰ **V96.14 Hang-glider** fire **injuring occupant**

√x7ᵗʰ **V96.15 Hang-glider** explosion **injuring occupant**

√x7ᵗʰ **V96.19 Other hang-glider accident injuring occupant**

√5ᵗʰ **V96.2** Glider (nonpowered) **accident injuring occupant**

√x7ᵗʰ **V96.20 Unspecified glider (nonpowered) accident injuring occupant**

√x7ᵗʰ **V96.21 Glider (nonpowered)** crash **injuring occupant**

√x7ᵗʰ **V96.22** Forced landing **of glider (nonpowered) injuring occupant**

✓x7ᵗʰ V96.23 Glider (nonpowered) collision injuring occupant
Glider (nonpowered) collision with any object, fixed, moveable or moving

✓x7ᵗʰ V96.24 Glider (nonpowered) fire injuring occupant

✓x7ᵗʰ V96.25 Glider (nonpowered) explosion injuring occupant

✓x7ᵗʰ V96.29 Other glider (nonpowered) accident injuring occupant

✓x7ᵗʰ V96.8 Other nonpowered-aircraft accidents injuring occupant
Kite carrying a person accident injuring occupant

✓x7ᵗʰ V96.9 Unspecified nonpowered-aircraft accident injuring occupant
Nonpowered-aircraft accident NOS

✓4ᵗʰ V97 Other specified air transport accidents

✓x7ᵗʰ V97.0 Occupant of aircraft injured in other specified air transport accidents
Fall in, on or from aircraft in air transport accident
    EXCLUDES 1   *accident while boarding or alighting aircraft (V97.1)*

✓x7ᵗʰ V97.1 Person injured while boarding or alighting from aircraft

✓5ᵗʰ V97.2 Parachutist accident

    ✓x7ᵗʰ V97.21 Parachutist entangled in object
       Parachutist landing in tree

    ✓x7ᵗʰ V97.22 Parachutist injured on landing

    ✓x7ᵗʰ V97.29 Other parachutist accident

✓5ᵗʰ V97.3 Person on ground injured in air transport accident

    ✓x7ᵗʰ V97.31 Hit by object falling from aircraft
       Hit by crashing aircraft
       Injured by aircraft hitting house
       Injured by aircraft hitting car

    ✓x7ᵗʰ V97.32 Injured by rotating propeller

    ✓x7ᵗʰ V97.33 Sucked into jet engine

    ✓x7ᵗʰ V97.39 Other injury to person on ground due to air transport accident

✓5ᵗʰ V97.8 Other air transport accidents, not elsewhere classified
    EXCLUDES 1   *aircraft accident NOS (V95.9)*
          exposure to changes in air pressure during ascent or descent (W94.-)

    ✓6ᵗʰ V97.81 Air transport accident involving military aircraft

       ✓7ᵗʰ V97.810 Civilian aircraft involved in air transport accident with military aircraft
          Passenger in civilian aircraft injured due to accident with military aircraft

       ✓7ᵗʰ V97.811 Civilian injured by military aircraft

       ✓7ᵗʰ V97.818 Other air transport accident involving military aircraft

    ✓x7ᵗʰ V97.89 Other air transport accidents, not elsewhere classified
       Injury from machinery on aircraft

Other and unspecified transport accidents (V98-V99)

   EXCLUDES 1   *vehicle accident, type of vehicle unspecified (V89.-)*

The appropriate 7th character is to be added to each code from categories V98-V99.
A   initial encounter
D   subsequent encounter
S   sequela

✓4ᵗʰ V98 Other specified transport accidents

    ✓x7ᵗʰ V98.0 Accident to, on or involving cable-car, not on rails
       Caught or dragged by cable-car, not on rails
       Fall or jump from cable-car, not on rails
       Object thrown from or in cable-car, not on rails

    ✓x7ᵗʰ V98.1 Accident to, on or involving land-yacht

    ✓x7ᵗʰ V98.2 Accident to, on or involving ice yacht

    ✓x7ᵗʰ V98.3 Accident to, on or involving ski lift
       Accident to, on or involving ski chair-lift
       Accident to, on or involving ski-lift with gondola

    ✓x7ᵗʰ V98.8 Other specified transport accidents

✓x7ᵗʰ V99 Unspecified transport accident

OTHER EXTERNAL CAUSES OF ACCIDENTAL INJURY (W00-X58)

Slipping, tripping, stumbling and falls (W00-W19)

   EXCLUDES 1   *assault involving a fall (Y01-Y02)*
          fall from animal (V80.-)
          fall (in) (from) machinery (in operation) (W28-W31)
          fall (in) (from) transport vehicle (V01-V99)
          intentional self-harm involving a fall (X80-X81)
   EXCLUDES 2   *at risk for fall (history of fall) Z91.81*
          fall (in) (from) burning building (X00.-)
          fall into fire (X00-X04, X08)

The appropriate 7th character is to be added to each code from categories W00-W19.
A   initial encounter
D   subsequent encounter
S   sequela

✓4ᵗʰ W00 Fall due to ice and snow

    INCLUDES   pedestrian on foot falling (slipping) on ice and snow
    EXCLUDES 1   *fall on (from) ice and snow involving pedestrian conveyance (V00.-)*
          fall from stairs and steps not due to ice and snow (W10.-)
    AHA: 2016,2Q,4

    ✓x7ᵗʰ W00.0 Fall on same level due to ice and snow

    ✓x7ᵗʰ W00.1 Fall from stairs and steps due to ice and snow

    ✓x7ᵗʰ W00.2 Other fall from one level to another due to ice and snow

    ✓x7ᵗʰ W00.9 Unspecified fall due to ice and snow

✓4ᵗʰ W01 Fall on same level from slipping, tripping and stumbling

    INCLUDES   fall on moving sidewalk
    EXCLUDES 1   *fall due to bumping (striking) against object (W18.0-)*
          fall in shower or bathtub (W18.2-)
          fall on same level NOS (W18.30)
          fall on same level from slipping, tripping and stumbling due to ice or snow (W00.0)
          fall off or from toilet (W18.1-)
          slipping, tripping and stumbling NOS (W18.40)
          slipping, tripping and stumbling without falling (W18.4-)

    ✓x7ᵗʰ W01.0 Fall on same level from slipping, tripping and stumbling without subsequent striking against object
       Falling over animal

    ✓5ᵗʰ W01.1 Fall on same level from slipping, tripping and stumbling with subsequent striking against object

       ✓x7ᵗʰ W01.10 Fall on same level from slipping, tripping and stumbling with subsequent striking against unspecified object

       ✓6ᵗʰ W01.11 Fall on same level from slipping, tripping and stumbling with subsequent striking against sharp object

          ✓7ᵗʰ W01.110 Fall on same level from slipping, tripping and stumbling with subsequent striking against sharp glass

          ✓7ᵗʰ W01.111 Fall on same level from slipping, tripping and stumbling with subsequent striking against power tool or machine

          ✓7ᵗʰ W01.118 Fall on same level from slipping, tripping and stumbling with subsequent striking against other sharp object

          ✓7ᵗʰ W01.119 Fall on same level from slipping, tripping and stumbling with subsequent striking against unspecified sharp object

       ✓6ᵗʰ W01.19 Fall on same level from slipping, tripping and stumbling with subsequent striking against other object

          ✓7ᵗʰ W01.190 Fall on same level from slipping, tripping and stumbling with subsequent striking against furniture

          ✓7ᵗʰ W01.198 Fall on same level from slipping, tripping and stumbling with subsequent striking against other object

Chapter 20. External Causes of Morbidity

W03–W16.212

√x7ᵗʰ **W03 Other fall on same level due to collision with another person**

Fall due to non-transport collision with other person

EXCLUDES 1   *collision with another person without fall (W51)*

crushed or pushed by a crowd or human stampede (W52)

fall involving pedestrian conveyance (V00-V09)

fall due to ice or snow (W00)

fall on same level NOS (W18.30)

AHA: 2012,4Q,108

√x7ᵗʰ **W04 Fall while being carried or supported by other persons**

Accidentally dropped while being carried

√4ᵗʰ **W05 Fall from non-moving wheelchair, nonmotorized scooter and motorized mobility scooter**

EXCLUDES 1   *fall from moving wheelchair (powered) (V00.811)*

fall from moving motorized mobility scooter (V00.831)

fall from nonmotorized scooter (V00.141)

√x7ᵗʰ **W05.0 Fall from non-moving wheelchair**

AHA: 2019,2Q,27

√x7ᵗʰ **W05.1 Fall from non-moving nonmotorized scooter**

√x7ᵗʰ **W05.2 Fall from non-moving motorized mobility scooter**

√x7ᵗʰ **W06 Fall from bed**

√x7ᵗʰ **W07 Fall from chair**

√x7ᵗʰ **W08 Fall from other furniture**

√4ᵗʰ **W09 Fall on and from playground equipment**

EXCLUDES 1   *fall involving recreational machinery (W31)*

√x7ᵗʰ **W09.0 Fall on or from playground slide**

√x7ᵗʰ **W09.1 Fall from playground swing**

√x7ᵗʰ **W09.2 Fall on or from jungle gym**

√x7ᵗʰ **W09.8 Fall on or from other playground equipment**

√4ᵗʰ **W10 Fall on and from stairs and steps**

EXCLUDES 1   *Fall from stairs and steps due to ice and snow (W00.1)*

√x7ᵗʰ **W10.0 Fall (on)(from) escalator**

√x7ᵗʰ **W10.1 Fall (on)(from) sidewalk curb**

√x7ᵗʰ **W10.2 Fall (on)(from) incline**

Fall (on) (from) ramp

√x7ᵗʰ **W10.8 Fall (on) (from) other stairs and steps**

√x7ᵗʰ **W10.9 Fall (on) (from) unspecified stairs and steps**

√x7ᵗʰ **W11 Fall on and from ladder**

√x7ᵗʰ **W12 Fall on and from scaffolding**

√4ᵗʰ **W13 Fall from, out of or through building or structure**

√x7ᵗʰ **W13.0 Fall from, out of or through balcony**

Fall from, out of or through railing

√x7ᵗʰ **W13.1 Fall from, out of or through bridge**

√x7ᵗʰ **W13.2 Fall from, out of or through roof**

√x7ᵗʰ **W13.3 Fall through floor**

√x7ᵗʰ **W13.4 Fall from, out of or through window**

EXCLUDES 2   *fall with subsequent striking against sharp glass (W01.110)*

√x7ᵗʰ **W13.8 Fall from, out of or through other building or structure**

Fall from, out of or through viaduct

Fall from, out of or through wall

Fall from, out of or through flag-pole

√x7ᵗʰ **W13.9 Fall from, out of or through building, not otherwise specified**

EXCLUDES 1   *collapse of a building or structure (W20.-)*

fall or jump from burning building or structure (X00.-)

√x7ᵗʰ **W14 Fall from tree**

√x7ᵗʰ **W15 Fall from cliff**

√4ᵗʰ **W16 Fall, jump or diving into water**

EXCLUDES 1   *accidental non-watercraft drowning and submersion not involving fall (W65-W74)*

effects of air pressure from diving (W94.-)

fall into water from watercraft (V90-V94)

hitting an object or against bottom when falling from watercraft (V94.0)

EXCLUDES 2   *striking or hitting diving board (W21.4)*

√5ᵗʰ **W16.0 Fall into swimming pool**

Fall into swimming pool NOS

EXCLUDES 1   *fall into empty swimming pool (W17.3)*

√6ᵗʰ **W16.01 Fall into swimming pool striking water surface**

√7ᵗʰ **W16.011 Fall into swimming pool striking water surface causing drowning and submersion**

EXCLUDES 1   *drowning and submersion while in swimming pool without fall (W67)*

√7ᵗʰ **W16.012 Fall into swimming pool striking water surface causing other injury**

√6ᵗʰ **W16.02 Fall into swimming pool striking bottom**

√7ᵗʰ **W16.021 Fall into swimming pool striking bottom causing drowning and submersion**

EXCLUDES 1   *drowning and submersion while in swimming pool without fall (W67)*

√7ᵗʰ **W16.022 Fall into swimming pool striking bottom causing other injury**

√6ᵗʰ **W16.03 Fall into swimming pool striking wall**

√7ᵗʰ **W16.031 Fall into swimming pool striking wall causing drowning and submersion**

EXCLUDES 1   *drowning and submersion while in swimming pool without fall (W67)*

√7ᵗʰ **W16.032 Fall into swimming pool striking wall causing other injury**

√5ᵗʰ **W16.1 Fall into natural body of water**

Fall into lake

Fall into open sea

Fall into river

Fall into stream

√6ᵗʰ **W16.11 Fall into natural body of water striking water surface**

√7ᵗʰ **W16.111 Fall into natural body of water striking water surface causing drowning and submersion**

EXCLUDES 1   *drowning and submersion while in natural body of water without fall (W69)*

√7ᵗʰ **W16.112 Fall into natural body of water striking water surface causing other injury**

√6ᵗʰ **W16.12 Fall into natural body of water striking bottom**

√7ᵗʰ **W16.121 Fall into natural body of water striking bottom causing drowning and submersion**

EXCLUDES 1   *drowning and submersion while in natural body of water without fall (W69)*

√7ᵗʰ **W16.122 Fall into natural body of water striking bottom causing other injury**

√6ᵗʰ **W16.13 Fall into natural body of water striking side**

√7ᵗʰ **W16.131 Fall into natural body of water striking side causing drowning and submersion**

EXCLUDES 1   *drowning and submersion while in natural body of water without fall (W69)*

√7ᵗʰ **W16.132 Fall into natural body of water striking side causing other injury**

√5ᵗʰ **W16.2 Fall in (into) filled bathtub or bucket of water**

√6ᵗʰ **W16.21 Fall in (into) filled bathtub**

EXCLUDES 1   *fall into empty bathtub (W18.2)*

√7ᵗʰ **W16.211 Fall in (into) filled bathtub causing drowning and submersion**

EXCLUDES 1   *drowning and submersion while in filled bathtub without fall (W65)*

√7ᵗʰ **W16.212 Fall in (into) filled bathtub causing other injury**

N Newborn: 0   P Pediatric: 0-17   M Maternity: 9-64   A Adult: 15-124   MCC Major Complication/Comorbidity   CC Complication/Comorbidity   SW Severe Wound Dx

1242   ICD-10-CM 2020

√6ᵗʰ **W16.22**   **Fall in (into)** bucket of water

     √7ᵗʰ **W16.221**   **Fall in (into) bucket of water causing** drowning and submersion

     √7ᵗʰ **W16.222**   **Fall in (into) bucket of water causing other injury**

√5ᵗʰ **W16.3**   **Fall into other water**

     Fall into fountain
     Fall into reservoir

     √6ᵗʰ **W16.31**   **Fall into other water** striking water surface

         √7ᵗʰ **W16.311**   **Fall into other water striking water surface causing** drowning and submersion

           EXCLUDES 1   *drowning and submersion while in other water without fall (W73)*

         √7ᵗʰ **W16.312**   **Fall into other water striking water surface causing other injury**

     √6ᵗʰ **W16.32**   **Fall into other water** striking bottom

         √7ᵗʰ **W16.321**   **Fall into other water striking bottom causing** drowning and submersion

           EXCLUDES 1   *drowning and submersion while in other water without fall (W73)*

         √7ᵗʰ **W16.322**   **Fall into other water striking bottom causing other injury**

     √6ᵗʰ **W16.33**   **Fall into other water** striking wall

         √7ᵗʰ **W16.331**   **Fall into other water striking wall causing** drowning and submersion

           EXCLUDES 1   *drowning and submersion while in other water without fall (W73)*

         √7ᵗʰ **W16.332**   **Fall into other water striking wall causing other injury**

√5ᵗʰ **W16.4**   **Fall into unspecified water**

     √×7ᵗʰ **W16.41**   **Fall into unspecified water causing** drowning and submersion

     √×7ᵗʰ **W16.42**   **Fall into unspecified water causing other injury**

√5ᵗʰ **W16.5**   **Jumping or diving into** swimming pool

     √6ᵗʰ **W16.51**   **Jumping or diving into swimming pool** striking water surface

         √7ᵗʰ **W16.511**   **Jumping or diving into swimming pool striking water surface causing** drowning and submersion

           EXCLUDES 1   *drowning and submersion while in swimming pool without jumping or diving (W67)*

         √7ᵗʰ **W16.512**   **Jumping or diving into swimming pool striking water surface causing other injury**

     √6ᵗʰ **W16.52**   **Jumping or diving into swimming pool** striking bottom

         √7ᵗʰ **W16.521**   **Jumping or diving into swimming pool striking bottom causing** drowning and submersion

           EXCLUDES 1   *drowning and submersion while in swimming pool without jumping or diving (W67)*

         √7ᵗʰ **W16.522**   **Jumping or diving into swimming pool striking bottom causing other injury**

     √6ᵗʰ **W16.53**   **Jumping or diving into swimming pool** striking wall

         √7ᵗʰ **W16.531**   **Jumping or diving into swimming pool striking wall causing** drowning and submersion

           EXCLUDES 1   *drowning and submersion while in swimming pool without jumping or diving (W67)*

         √7ᵗʰ **W16.532**   **Jumping or diving into swimming pool striking wall causing other injury**

√5ᵗʰ **W16.6**   **Jumping or diving into** natural body of water

     Jumping or diving into lake
     Jumping or diving into open sea
     Jumping or diving into river
     Jumping or diving into stream

     √6ᵗʰ **W16.61**   **Jumping or diving into natural body of water** striking water surface

         √7ᵗʰ **W16.611**   **Jumping or diving into natural body of water striking water surface causing** drowning and submersion

           EXCLUDES 1   *drowning and submersion while in natural body of water without jumping or diving (W69)*

         √7ᵗʰ **W16.612**   **Jumping or diving into natural body of water striking water surface causing other injury**

     √6ᵗʰ **W16.62**   **Jumping or diving into natural body of water** striking bottom

         √7ᵗʰ **W16.621**   **Jumping or diving into natural body of water striking bottom causing** drowning and submersion

           EXCLUDES 1   *drowning and submersion while in natural body of water without jumping or diving (W69)*

         √7ᵗʰ **W16.622**   **Jumping or diving into natural body of water striking bottom causing other injury**

√5ᵗʰ **W16.7**   **Jumping or diving** from boat

     EXCLUDES 1   *fall from boat into water — see watercraft accident (V90-V94)*

     √6ᵗʰ **W16.71**   **Jumping or diving from boat** striking water surface

         √7ᵗʰ **W16.711**   **Jumping or diving from boat striking water surface causing** drowning and submersion

         √7ᵗʰ **W16.712**   **Jumping or diving from boat striking water surface causing other injury**

     √6ᵗʰ **W16.72**   **Jumping or diving from boat** striking bottom

         √7ᵗʰ **W16.721**   **Jumping or diving from boat striking bottom causing** drowning and submersion

         √7ᵗʰ **W16.722**   **Jumping or diving from boat striking bottom causing other injury**

√5ᵗʰ **W16.8**   **Jumping or diving into** other water

     Jumping or diving into fountain
     Jumping or diving into reservoir

     √6ᵗʰ **W16.81**   **Jumping or diving into other water** striking water surface

         √7ᵗʰ **W16.811**   **Jumping or diving into other water striking water surface causing** drowning and submersion

           EXCLUDES 1   *drowning and submersion while in other water without jumping or diving (W73)*

         √7ᵗʰ **W16.812**   **Jumping or diving into other water striking water surface causing other injury**

     √6ᵗʰ **W16.82**   **Jumping or diving into other water** striking bottom

         √7ᵗʰ **W16.821**   **Jumping or diving into other water striking bottom causing** drowning and submersion

           EXCLUDES 1   *drowning and submersion while in other water without jumping or diving (W73)*

         √7ᵗʰ **W16.822**   **Jumping or diving into other water striking bottom causing other injury**

     √6ᵗʰ **W16.83**   **Jumping or diving into other water** striking wall

         √7ᵗʰ **W16.831**   **Jumping or diving into other water striking wall causing** drowning and submersion

           EXCLUDES 1   *drowning and submersion while in other water without jumping or diving (W73)*

         √7ᵗʰ **W16.832**   **Jumping or diving into other water striking wall causing other injury**

☑ Additional Char Req   √×7ᵗʰ Placeholder   Unacceptable PDx   Questionable PDx   Wrong Procedure   Manifestation   Unspecified Dx   H1-H14 HAC   HCC CMS-HCC Dx   HIV HIV Dx

ICD-10-CM 2020   1243

√5ᵗʰ **W16.9 Jumping or diving into unspecified water**

   √x7ᵗʰ **W16.91 Jumping or diving into unspecified water causing drowning and submersion**

   √x7ᵗʰ **W16.92 Jumping or diving into unspecified water causing other injury**

√4ᵗʰ **W17 Other fall from one level to another**

  √x7ᵗʰ **W17.0 Fall into well**

  √x7ᵗʰ **W17.1 Fall into storm drain or manhole**

  √x7ᵗʰ **W17.2 Fall into hole**
      Fall into pit

  √x7ᵗʰ **W17.3 Fall into empty swimming pool**
      EXCLUDES 1   fall into filled swimming pool (W16.0-)

  √x7ᵗʰ **W17.4 Fall from dock**

  √5ᵗʰ **W17.8 Other fall from one level to another**

   √x7ᵗʰ **W17.81 Fall down embankment (hill)**

   √x7ᵗʰ **W17.82 Fall from (out of) grocery cart**
      Fall due to grocery cart tipping over

   √x7ᵗʰ **W17.89 Other fall from one level to another**
      Fall from cherry picker
      Fall from lifting device
      Fall from mobile elevated work platform [MEWP]
      Fall from sky lift
      AHA: 2015,2Q,6

√4ᵗʰ **W18 Other slipping, tripping and stumbling and falls**

  √5ᵗʰ **W18.0 Fall due to bumping against object**
      Striking against object with subsequent fall
      EXCLUDES 1   fall on same level due to slipping, tripping, or stumbling with subsequent striking against object (W01.1-)

   √x7ᵗʰ **W18.00 Striking against unspecified object with subsequent fall**

   √x7ᵗʰ **W18.01 Striking against sports equipment with subsequent fall**

   √x7ᵗʰ **W18.02 Striking against glass with subsequent fall**

   √x7ᵗʰ **W18.09 Striking against other object with subsequent fall**

  √5ᵗʰ **W18.1 Fall from or off toilet**

   √x7ᵗʰ **W18.11 Fall from or off toilet without subsequent striking against object**
      Fall from (off) toilet NOS

   √x7ᵗʰ **W18.12 Fall from or off toilet with subsequent striking against object**

  √x7ᵗʰ **W18.2 Fall in (into) shower or empty bathtub**
      EXCLUDES 1   fall in full bathtub causing drowning or submersion (W16.21-)

  √5ᵗʰ **W18.3 Other and unspecified fall on same level**

   √x7ᵗʰ **W18.30 Fall on same level, unspecified**

   √x7ᵗʰ **W18.31 Fall on same level due to stepping on an object**
      Fall on same level due to stepping on an animal
      EXCLUDES 1   slipping, tripping and stumbling without fall due to stepping on animal (W18.41)

   √x7ᵗʰ **W18.39 Other fall on same level**

  √5ᵗʰ **W18.4 Slipping, tripping and stumbling without falling**
      EXCLUDES 1   collision with another person without fall (W51)

   √x7ᵗʰ **W18.40 Slipping, tripping and stumbling without falling, unspecified**

   √x7ᵗʰ **W18.41 Slipping, tripping and stumbling without falling due to stepping on object**
      Slipping, tripping and stumbling without falling due to stepping on animal
      EXCLUDES 1   slipping, tripping and stumbling with fall due to stepping on animal (W18.31)

   √x7ᵗʰ **W18.42 Slipping, tripping and stumbling without falling due to stepping into hole or opening**

   √x7ᵗʰ **W18.43 Slipping, tripping and stumbling without falling due to stepping from one level to another**

   √x7ᵗʰ **W18.49 Other slipping, tripping and stumbling without falling**

√x7ᵗʰ **W19 Unspecified fall**
    Accidental fall NOS
    AHA: 2012,4Q,95

Exposure to inanimate mechanical forces (W20-W49)

EXCLUDES 1   assault (X92-Y09)
    contact or collision with animals or persons (W50-W64)
    exposure to inanimate mechanical forces involving military or war operations (Y36.-, Y37.-)
    intentional self-harm (X71-X83)

The appropriate 7th character is to be added to each code from categories W20-W49.
A   initial encounter
D   subsequent encounter
S   sequela

√4ᵗʰ **W20 Struck by thrown, projected or falling object**
    Code first any associated:
    cataclysm (X34-X39)
    lightning strike (T75.00)
    EXCLUDES 1   falling object in machinery accident (W24, W28-W31)
      falling object in transport accident (V01-V99)
      object set in motion by explosion (W35-W40)
      object set in motion by firearm (W32-W34)
      struck by thrown sports equipment (W21.-)

  √x7ᵗʰ **W20.0 Struck by falling object in cave-in**
      EXCLUDES 2   asphyxiation due to cave-in (T71.21)

  √x7ᵗʰ **W20.1 Struck by object due to collapse of building**
      EXCLUDES 1   struck by object due to collapse of burning building (X00.2, X02.2)

  √x7ᵗʰ **W20.8 Other cause of strike by thrown, projected or falling object**
      EXCLUDES 1   struck by thrown sports equipment (W21.-)

√4ᵗʰ **W21 Striking against or struck by sports equipment**
    EXCLUDES 1   assault with sports equipment (Y08.0-)
      striking against or struck by sports equipment with subsequent fall (W18.01)

  √5ᵗʰ **W21.0 Struck by hit or thrown ball**

   √x7ᵗʰ **W21.00 Struck by hit or thrown ball, unspecified type**

   √x7ᵗʰ **W21.01 Struck by football**

   √x7ᵗʰ **W21.02 Struck by soccer ball**

   √x7ᵗʰ **W21.03 Struck by baseball**

   √x7ᵗʰ **W21.04 Struck by golf ball**

   √x7ᵗʰ **W21.05 Struck by basketball**

   √x7ᵗʰ **W21.06 Struck by volleyball**

   √x7ᵗʰ **W21.07 Struck by softball**

   √x7ᵗʰ **W21.09 Struck by other hit or thrown ball**

  √5ᵗʰ **W21.1 Struck by bat, racquet or club**

   √x7ᵗʰ **W21.11 Struck by baseball bat**

   √x7ᵗʰ **W21.12 Struck by tennis racquet**

   √x7ᵗʰ **W21.13 Struck by golf club**

   √x7ᵗʰ **W21.19 Struck by other bat, racquet or club**

  √5ᵗʰ **W21.2 Struck by hockey stick or puck**

   √6ᵗʰ **W21.21 Struck by hockey stick**

    √7ᵗʰ **W21.210 Struck by ice hockey stick**

    √7ᵗʰ **W21.211 Struck by field hockey stick**

   √6ᵗʰ **W21.22 Struck by hockey puck**

    √7ᵗʰ **W21.220 Struck by ice hockey puck**

    √7ᵗʰ **W21.221 Struck by field hockey puck**

  √5ᵗʰ **W21.3 Struck by sports foot wear**

   √x7ᵗʰ **W21.31 Struck by shoe cleats**
      Stepped on by shoe cleats

   √x7ᵗʰ **W21.32 Struck by skate blades**
      Skated over by skate blades

   √x7ᵗʰ **W21.39 Struck by other sports foot wear**

  √x7ᵗʰ **W21.4 Striking against diving board**
      Use additional code for subsequent falling into water, if applicable (W16.-)

  √5ᵗʰ **W21.8 Striking against or struck by other sports equipment**

   √x7ᵗʰ **W21.81 Striking against or struck by football helmet**

   √x7ᵗʰ **W21.89 Striking against or struck by other sports equipment**

  √x7ᵗʰ **W21.9 Striking against or struck by unspecified sports equipment**

☐ Newborn: 0   ☐ Pediatric: 0-17   ☐ Maternity: 9-64   ☐ Adult: 15-124   **MCC** Major Complication/Comorbidity   **CC** Complication/Comorbidity   **SW** Severe Wound Dx

1244   ICD-10-CM 2020

✓4ᵗʰ **W22 Striking against or struck by other objects**

    EXCLUDES 1   striking against or struck by object with subsequent fall (W18.09)

✓5ᵗʰ **W22.0 Striking against stationary object**

    EXCLUDES 1   striking against stationary sports equipment (W21.8)

✓x7ᵗʰ **W22.01 Walked into wall**

✓x7ᵗʰ **W22.02 Walked into lamppost**

✓x7ᵗʰ **W22.03 Walked into furniture**

✓6ᵗʰ **W22.04 Striking against wall of swimming pool**

✓7ᵗʰ **W22.041 Striking against wall of swimming pool causing drowning and submersion**

    EXCLUDES 1   drowning and submersion while swimming without striking against wall (W67)

✓7ᵗʰ **W22.042 Striking against wall of swimming pool causing other injury**

✓x7ᵗʰ **W22.09 Striking against other stationary object**

✓5ᵗʰ **W22.1 Striking against or struck by automobile airbag**

✓x7ᵗʰ **W22.10 Striking against or struck by unspecified automobile airbag**

✓x7ᵗʰ **W22.11 Striking against or struck by driver side automobile airbag**

✓x7ᵗʰ **W22.12 Striking against or struck by front passenger side automobile airbag**

✓x7ᵗʰ **W22.19 Striking against or struck by other automobile airbag**

✓x7ᵗʰ **W22.8 Striking against or struck by other objects**

    Striking against or struck by object NOS

    EXCLUDES 1   struck by thrown, projected or falling object (W20.-)

✓4ᵗʰ **W23 Caught, crushed, jammed or pinched in or between objects**

    EXCLUDES 1   injury caused by cutting or piercing instruments (W25-W27)

         injury caused by firearms malfunction (W32.1, W33.1-, W34.1-)

         injury caused by lifting and transmission devices (W24.-)

         injury caused by machinery (W28-W31)

         injury caused by nonpowered hand tools (W27.-)

         injury caused by transport vehicle being used as a means of transportation (V01-V99)

         injury caused by struck by thrown, projected or falling object (W20.-)

✓x7ᵗʰ **W23.0 Caught, crushed, jammed, or pinched between moving objects**

✓x7ᵗʰ **W23.1 Caught, crushed, jammed, or pinched between stationary objects**

✓4ᵗʰ **W24 Contact with lifting and transmission devices, not elsewhere classified**

    EXCLUDES 1   transport accidents (V01-V99)

✓x7ᵗʰ **W24.0 Contact with lifting devices, not elsewhere classified**

    Contact with chain hoist

    Contact with drive belt

    Contact with pulley (block)

✓x7ᵗʰ **W24.1 Contact with transmission devices, not elsewhere classified**

    Contact with transmission belt or cable

✓x7ᵗʰ **W25 Contact with sharp glass**

    Code first any associated:

    injury due to flying glass from explosion or firearm discharge (W32-W40)

    transport accident (V00-V99)

    EXCLUDES 1   fall on same level due to slipping, tripping and stumbling with subsequent striking against sharp glass ▶(W01.110)◀

         striking against sharp glass with subsequent fall (W18.02)

    EXCLUDES 2   glass embedded in skin (W45)

✓4ᵗʰ **W26 Contact with other sharp objects**

    EXCLUDES 2   sharp object(s) embedded in skin (W45)

    AHA: 2016,4Q,73

✓x7ᵗʰ **W26.0 Contact with knife**

    EXCLUDES 1   contact with electric knife (W29.1)

✓x7ᵗʰ **W26.1 Contact with sword or dagger**

✓x7ᵗʰ **W26.2 Contact with edge of stiff paper**

    Paper cut

✓x7ᵗʰ **W26.8 Contact with other sharp object(s), not elsewhere classified**

    Contact with tin can lid

✓x7ᵗʰ **W26.9 Contact with unspecified sharp object(s)**

✓4ᵗʰ **W27 Contact with nonpowered hand tool**

✓x7ᵗʰ **W27.0 Contact with workbench tool**

    Contact with auger

    Contact with axe

    Contact with chisel

    Contact with handsaw

    Contact with screwdriver

✓x7ᵗʰ **W27.1 Contact with garden tool**

    Contact with hoe

    Contact with nonpowered lawn mower

    Contact with pitchfork

    Contact with rake

✓x7ᵗʰ **W27.2 Contact with scissors**

✓x7ᵗʰ **W27.3 Contact with needle (sewing)**

    EXCLUDES 1   contact with hypodermic needle (W46.-)

✓x7ᵗʰ **W27.4 Contact with kitchen utensil**

    Contact with fork

    Contact with ice-pick

    Contact with can-opener NOS

✓x7ᵗʰ **W27.5 Contact with paper-cutter**

✓x7ᵗʰ **W27.8 Contact with other nonpowered hand tool**

    Contact with nonpowered sewing machine

    Contact with shovel

✓x7ᵗʰ **W28 Contact with powered lawn mower**

    Powered lawn mower (commercial) (residential)

    EXCLUDES 1   contact with nonpowered lawn mower (W27.1)

    EXCLUDES 2   exposure to electric current (W86.-)

✓4ᵗʰ **W29 Contact with other powered hand tools and household machinery**

    EXCLUDES 1   contact with commercial machinery (W31.82)

         contact with hot household appliance (X15)

         contact with nonpowered hand tool (W27.-)

         exposure to electric current (W86)

✓x7ᵗʰ **W29.0 Contact with powered kitchen appliance**

    Contact with blender

    Contact with can-opener

    Contact with garbage disposal

    Contact with mixer

✓x7ᵗʰ **W29.1 Contact with electric knife**

✓x7ᵗʰ **W29.2 Contact with other powered household machinery**

    Contact with electric fan

    Contact with powered dryer (clothes) (powered) (spin)

    Contact with washing-machine

    Contact with sewing machine

✓x7ᵗʰ **W29.3 Contact with powered garden and outdoor hand tools and machinery**

    Contact with chainsaw

    Contact with edger

    Contact with garden cultivator (tiller)

    Contact with hedge trimmer

    Contact with other powered garden tool

    EXCLUDES 1   contact with powered lawn mower (W28)

✓x7ᵗʰ **W29.4 Contact with nail gun**

✓x7ᵗʰ **W29.8 Contact with other powered hand tools and household machinery**

    Contact with do-it-yourself tool NOS

✓4ᵗʰ **W30 Contact with agricultural machinery**

    INCLUDES   animal-powered farm machine

    EXCLUDES 1   agricultural transport vehicle accident (V01-V99)

         explosion of grain store (W40.8)

         exposure to electric current (W86.-)

✓x7ᵗʰ **W30.0 Contact with combine harvester**

    Contact with reaper

    Contact with thresher

✓x7ᵗʰ **W30.1 Contact with power take-off devices (PTO)**

✓x7ᵗʰ **W30.2 Contact with hay derrick**

✓x7ᵗʰ **W30.3 Contact with grain storage elevator**

    EXCLUDES 1   explosion of grain store (W40.8)

Chapter 20. External Causes of Morbidity *(side tab)*

W30.8–W33.13 *(side tab)*

✓5ᵗʰ **W30.8 Contact with other specified agricultural machinery**

    ✓x7ᵗʰ **W30.81 Contact with agricultural transport vehicle in stationary use**

         Contact with agricultural transport vehicle under repair, not on public roadway

         EXCLUDES 1   *agricultural transport vehicle accident (V01-V99)*

    ✓x7ᵗʰ **W30.89 Contact with other specified agricultural machinery**

✓x7ᵗʰ **W30.9 Contact with unspecified agricultural machinery**

     Contact with farm machinery NOS

✓4ᵗʰ **W31 Contact with other and unspecified machinery**

     EXCLUDES 1   *contact with agricultural machinery (W30.-)*

         contact with machinery in transport under own power or being towed by a vehicle (V01-V99)

         exposure to electric current (W86)

✓x7ᵗʰ **W31.0 Contact with mining and earth-drilling machinery**

     Contact with bore or drill (land) (seabed)

     Contact with shaft hoist

     Contact with shaft lift

     Contact with undercutter

✓x7ᵗʰ **W31.1 Contact with metalworking machines**

     Contact with abrasive wheel

     Contact with forging machine

     Contact with lathe

     Contact with mechanical shears

     Contact with metal drilling machine

     Contact with milling machine

     Contact with power press

     Contact with rolling-mill

     Contact with metal sawing machine

✓x7ᵗʰ **W31.2 Contact with powered woodworking and forming machines**

     Contact with band saw

     Contact with bench saw

     Contact with circular saw

     Contact with molding machine

     Contact with overhead plane

     Contact with powered saw

     Contact with radial saw

     Contact with sander

     EXCLUDES 1   *nonpowered woodworking tools (W27.0)*

✓x7ᵗʰ **W31.3 Contact with prime movers**

     Contact with gas turbine

     Contact with internal combustion engine

     Contact with steam engine

     Contact with water driven turbine

✓5ᵗʰ **W31.8 Contact with other specified machinery**

    ✓x7ᵗʰ **W31.81 Contact with recreational machinery**

         Contact with roller coaster

    ✓x7ᵗʰ **W31.82 Contact with other commercial machinery**

         Contact with commercial electric fan

         Contact with commercial kitchen appliances

         Contact with commercial powered dryer (clothes) (powered) (spin)

         Contact with commercial washing-machine

         Contact with commercial sewing machine

         EXCLUDES 1   *contact with household machinery (W29.-)*

                 contact with powered lawn mower (W28)

    ✓x7ᵗʰ **W31.83 Contact with special construction vehicle in stationary use**

         Contact with special construction vehicle under repair, not on public roadway

         EXCLUDES 1   *special construction vehicle accident (V01-V99)*

    ✓x7ᵗʰ **W31.89 Contact with other specified machinery**

✓x7ᵗʰ **W31.9 Contact with unspecified machinery**

     Contact with machinery NOS

✓4ᵗʰ **W32 Accidental handgun discharge and malfunction**

     INCLUDES   accidental discharge and malfunction of gun for single hand use

         accidental discharge and malfunction of pistol

         accidental discharge and malfunction of revolver

         handgun discharge and malfunction NOS

     EXCLUDES 1   *accidental airgun discharge and malfunction (W34.010, W34.110)*

         accidental BB gun discharge and malfunction (W34.010, W34.110)

         accidental pellet gun discharge and malfunction (W34.010, W34.110)

         accidental shotgun discharge and malfunction (W33.01, W33.11)

         assault by handgun discharge (X93)

         handgun discharge involving legal intervention (Y35.0-)

         handgun discharge involving military or war operations (Y36.4-)

         intentional self-harm by handgun discharge (X72)

         Very pistol discharge and malfunction (W34.09, W34.19)

✓x7ᵗʰ **W32.0 Accidental handgun discharge**

✓x7ᵗʰ **W32.1 Accidental handgun malfunction**

     Injury due to explosion of handgun (parts)

     Injury due to malfunction of mechanism or component of handgun

     Injury due to recoil of handgun

     Powder burn from handgun

✓4ᵗʰ **W33 Accidental rifle, shotgun and larger firearm discharge and malfunction**

     INCLUDES   rifle, shotgun and larger firearm discharge and malfunction NOS

     EXCLUDES 1   *accidental airgun discharge and malfunction (W34.010, W34.110)*

         accidental BB gun discharge and malfunction (W34.010, W34.110)

         accidental handgun discharge and malfunction (W32.-)

         accidental pellet gun discharge and malfunction (W34.010, W34.110)

         assault by rifle, shotgun and larger firearm discharge (X94)

         firearm discharge involving legal intervention (Y35.0-)

         firearm discharge involving military or war operations (Y36.4-)

         intentional self-harm by rifle, shotgun and larger firearm discharge (X73)

✓5ᵗʰ **W33.0 Accidental rifle, shotgun and larger firearm discharge**

    ✓x7ᵗʰ **W33.00 Accidental discharge of unspecified larger firearm**

         Discharge of unspecified larger firearm NOS

    ✓x7ᵗʰ **W33.01 Accidental discharge of shotgun**

         Discharge of shotgun NOS

    ✓x7ᵗʰ **W33.02 Accidental discharge of hunting rifle**

         Discharge of hunting rifle NOS

    ✓x7ᵗʰ **W33.03 Accidental discharge of machine gun**

         Discharge of machine gun NOS

    ✓x7ᵗʰ **W33.09 Accidental discharge of other larger firearm**

         Discharge of other larger firearm NOS

✓5ᵗʰ **W33.1 Accidental rifle, shotgun and larger firearm malfunction**

     Injury due to explosion of rifle, shotgun and larger firearm (parts)

     Injury due to malfunction of mechanism or component of rifle, shotgun and larger firearm

     Injury due to piercing, cutting, crushing or pinching due to (by) slide trigger mechanism, scope or other gun part

     Injury due to recoil of rifle, shotgun and larger firearm

     Powder burn from rifle, shotgun and larger firearm

    ✓x7ᵗʰ **W33.10 Accidental malfunction of unspecified larger firearm**

         Malfunction of unspecified larger firearm NOS

    ✓x7ᵗʰ **W33.11 Accidental malfunction of shotgun**

         Malfunction of shotgun NOS

    ✓x7ᵗʰ **W33.12 Accidental malfunction of hunting rifle**

         Malfunction of hunting rifle NOS

    ✓x7ᵗʰ **W33.13 Accidental malfunction of machine gun**

         Malfunction of machine gun NOS

N Newborn: 0   P Pediatric: 0-17   M Maternity: 9-64   A Adult: 15-124   MCC Major Complication/Comorbidity   CC Complication/Comorbidity   SW Severe Wound Dx

1246   ICD-10-CM 2020

✓x 7th **W33.19** **Accidental malfunction of other larger firearm**
Malfunction of other larger firearm NOS

✓4th **W34** **Accidental discharge and malfunction from other and unspecified firearms and guns**

✓5th **W34.0** **Accidental discharge from other and unspecified firearms and guns**

✓x 7th **W34.00** **Accidental discharge from unspecified firearms or gun**
Discharge from firearm NOS
Gunshot wound NOS
Shot NOS

✓6th **W34.01** **Accidental discharge of gas, air or spring-operated guns**

✓7th **W34.010** **Accidental discharge of airgun**
Accidental discharge of BB gun
Accidental discharge of pellet gun

✓7th **W34.011** **Accidental discharge of paintball gun**
Accidental injury due to paintball discharge

✓7th **W34.018** **Accidental discharge of other gas, air or spring-operated gun**

✓x 7th **W34.09** **Accidental discharge from other specified firearms**
Accidental discharge from Very pistol [flare]

✓5th **W34.1** **Accidental malfunction from other and unspecified firearms and guns**

✓x 7th **W34.10** **Accidental malfunction from unspecified firearms or gun**
Firearm malfunction NOS

✓6th **W34.11** **Accidental malfunction of gas, air or spring-operated guns**

✓7th **W34.110** **Accidental malfunction of airgun**
Accidental malfunction of BB gun
Accidental malfunction of pellet gun

✓7th **W34.111** **Accidental malfunction of paintball gun**
Accidental injury due to paintball gun malfunction

✓7th **W34.118** **Accidental malfunction of other gas, air or spring-operated gun**

✓x 7th **W34.19** **Accidental malfunction from other specified firearms**
Accidental malfunction from Very pistol [flare]

✓x 7th **W35** **Explosion and rupture of boiler**
EXCLUDES 1   *explosion and rupture of boiler on watercraft (V93.4)*

✓4th **W36** **Explosion and rupture of gas cylinder**

✓x 7th **W36.1** **Explosion and rupture of aerosol can**

✓x 7th **W36.2** **Explosion and rupture of air tank**

✓x 7th **W36.3** **Explosion and rupture of pressurized-gas tank**

✓x 7th **W36.8** **Explosion and rupture of other gas cylinder**

✓x 7th **W36.9** **Explosion and rupture of unspecified gas cylinder**

✓4th **W37** **Explosion and rupture of pressurized tire, pipe or hose**

✓x 7th **W37.0** **Explosion of bicycle tire**

✓x 7th **W37.8** **Explosion and rupture of other pressurized tire, pipe or hose**

✓x 7th **W38** **Explosion and rupture of other specified pressurized devices**

✓x 7th **W39** **Discharge of firework**

✓4th **W40** **Explosion of other materials**
EXCLUDES 1   *assault by explosive material (X96)*
explosion involving legal intervention (Y35.1-)
explosion involving military or war operations (Y36.0-, Y36.2-)
intentional self-harm by explosive material (X75)

✓x 7th **W40.0** **Explosion of blasting material**
Explosion of blasting cap
Explosion of detonator
Explosion of dynamite
Explosion of explosive (any) used in blasting operations

✓x 7th **W40.1** **Explosion of explosive gases**
Explosion of acetylene
Explosion of butane
Explosion of coal gas
Explosion in mine NOS
Explosion of explosive gas
Explosion of fire damp
Explosion of gasoline fumes
Explosion of methane
Explosion of propane

✓x 7th **W40.8** **Explosion of other specified explosive materials**
Explosion in dump NOS
Explosion in factory NOS
Explosion in grain store
Explosion in munitions
EXCLUDES 1   *explosion involving legal intervention (Y35.1-)*
explosion involving military or war operations (Y36.0-, Y36.2-)

✓x 7th **W40.9** **Explosion of unspecified explosive materials**
Explosion NOS

✓4th **W42** **Exposure to noise**

✓x 7th **W42.0** **Exposure to supersonic waves**

✓x 7th **W42.9** **Exposure to other noise**
Exposure to sound waves NOS

✓4th **W45** **Foreign body or object entering through skin**
INCLUDES   foreign body or object embedded in skin
nail embedded in skin
EXCLUDES 2   *contact with hand tools (nonpowered) (powered) (W27-W29)*
contact with other sharp objects (W26.-)
contact with sharp glass (W25.-)
struck by objects (W20-W22)

✓x 7th **W45.0** **Nail entering through skin**

✓x 7th **W45.8** **Other foreign body or object entering through skin**
Splinter in skin NOS

✓4th **W46** **Contact with hypodermic needle**

✓x 7th **W46.0** **Contact with hypodermic needle**
Hypodermic needle stick NOS

✓x 7th **W46.1** **Contact with contaminated hypodermic needle**

✓4th **W49** **Exposure to other inanimate mechanical forces**
INCLUDES   exposure to abnormal gravitational [G] forces
exposure to inanimate mechanical forces NEC
EXCLUDES 1   *exposure to inanimate mechanical forces involving military or war operations (Y36.-, Y37.-)*

✓5th **W49.0** **Item causing external constriction**

✓x 7th **W49.01** **Hair causing external constriction**

✓x 7th **W49.02** **String or thread causing external constriction**

✓x 7th **W49.03** **Rubber band causing external constriction**

✓x 7th **W49.04** **Ring or other jewelry causing external constriction**

✓x 7th **W49.09** **Other specified item causing external constriction**

✓x 7th **W49.9** **Exposure to other inanimate mechanical forces**

Exposure to animate mechanical forces (W50-W64)

EXCLUDES 1   *toxic effect of contact with venomous animals and plants (T63.-)*

The appropriate 7th character is to be added to each code from categories W50-W64.
A   initial encounter
D   subsequent encounter
S   sequela

✓4th **W50** **Accidental hit, strike, kick, twist, bite or scratch by another person**
INCLUDES   hit, strike, kick, twist, bite, or scratch by another person NOS
EXCLUDES 1   *assault by bodily force (Y04)*
struck by objects (W20-W22)

✓x 7th **W50.0** **Accidental hit or strike by another person**
Hit or strike by another person NOS

✓x 7th **W50.1** **Accidental kick by another person**
Kick by another person NOS

✓x 7th **W50.2** **Accidental twist by another person**
Twist by another person NOS

√x7ᵗʰ **W50.3 Accidental bite by another person**
    Human bite
    Bite by another person NOS

√x7ᵗʰ **W50.4 Accidental scratch by another person**
    Scratch by another person NOS

√x7ᵗʰ **W51 Accidental striking against or bumped into by another person**
    EXCLUDES 1   *assault by striking against or bumping into by another person (Y04.2)*
            fall due to collision with another person (W03)

√x7ᵗʰ **W52 Crushed, pushed or stepped on by crowd or human stampede**
    Crushed, pushed or stepped on by crowd or human stampede with or without fall

√4ᵗʰ **W53 Contact with rodent**
    INCLUDES   contact with saliva, feces or urine of rodent

  √5ᵗʰ **W53.0 Contact with mouse**
    √x7ᵗʰ **W53.01 Bitten by mouse**
    √x7ᵗʰ **W53.09 Other contact with mouse**

  √5ᵗʰ **W53.1 Contact with rat**
    √x7ᵗʰ **W53.11 Bitten by rat**
    √x7ᵗʰ **W53.19 Other contact with rat**

  √5ᵗʰ **W53.2 Contact with squirrel**
    √x7ᵗʰ **W53.21 Bitten by squirrel**
    √x7ᵗʰ **W53.29 Other contact with squirrel**

  √5ᵗʰ **W53.8 Contact with other rodent**
    √x7ᵗʰ **W53.81 Bitten by other rodent**
    √x7ᵗʰ **W53.89 Other contact with other rodent**

√4ᵗʰ **W54 Contact with dog**
    INCLUDES   contact with saliva, feces or urine of dog

  √x7ᵗʰ **W54.0 Bitten by dog**
  √x7ᵗʰ **W54.1 Struck by dog**
    Knocked over by dog
  √x7ᵗʰ **W54.8 Other contact with dog**

√4ᵗʰ **W55 Contact with other mammals**
    INCLUDES   contact with saliva, feces or urine of mammal
    EXCLUDES 1   *animal being ridden — see transport accidents*
            bitten or struck by dog (W54)
            bitten or struck by rodent (W53.-)
            contact with marine mammals (W56.-)

  √5ᵗʰ **W55.0 Contact with cat**
    √x7ᵗʰ **W55.01 Bitten by cat**
    √x7ᵗʰ **W55.03 Scratched by cat**
    √x7ᵗʰ **W55.09 Other contact with cat**

  √5ᵗʰ **W55.1 Contact with horse**
    √x7ᵗʰ **W55.11 Bitten by horse**
    √x7ᵗʰ **W55.12 Struck by horse**
    √x7ᵗʰ **W55.19 Other contact with horse**

  √5ᵗʰ **W55.2 Contact with cow**
    Contact with bull
    √x7ᵗʰ **W55.21 Bitten by cow**
    √x7ᵗʰ **W55.22 Struck by cow**
        Gored by bull
    √x7ᵗʰ **W55.29 Other contact with cow**

  √5ᵗʰ **W55.3 Contact with other hoof stock**
    Contact with goats
    Contact with sheep
    √x7ᵗʰ **W55.31 Bitten by other hoof stock**
    √x7ᵗʰ **W55.32 Struck by other hoof stock**
        Gored by goat
        Gored by ram
    √x7ᵗʰ **W55.39 Other contact with other hoof stock**

  √5ᵗʰ **W55.4 Contact with pig**
    √x7ᵗʰ **W55.41 Bitten by pig**
    √x7ᵗʰ **W55.42 Struck by pig**
    √x7ᵗʰ **W55.49 Other contact with pig**

  √5ᵗʰ **W55.5 Contact with raccoon**
    √x7ᵗʰ **W55.51 Bitten by raccoon**

    √x7ᵗʰ **W55.52 Struck by raccoon**
    √x7ᵗʰ **W55.59 Other contact with raccoon**

  √5ᵗʰ **W55.8 Contact with other mammals**
    √x7ᵗʰ **W55.81 Bitten by other mammals**
    √x7ᵗʰ **W55.82 Struck by other mammals**
    √x7ᵗʰ **W55.89 Other contact with other mammals**

√4ᵗʰ **W56 Contact with nonvenomous marine animal**
    EXCLUDES 1   *contact with venomous marine animal (T63.-)*

  √5ᵗʰ **W56.0 Contact with dolphin**
    √x7ᵗʰ **W56.01 Bitten by dolphin**
    √x7ᵗʰ **W56.02 Struck by dolphin**
    √x7ᵗʰ **W56.09 Other contact with dolphin**

  √5ᵗʰ **W56.1 Contact with sea lion**
    √x7ᵗʰ **W56.11 Bitten by sea lion**
    √x7ᵗʰ **W56.12 Struck by sea lion**
    √x7ᵗʰ **W56.19 Other contact with sea lion**

  √5ᵗʰ **W56.2 Contact with orca**
    Contact with killer whale
    √x7ᵗʰ **W56.21 Bitten by orca**
    √x7ᵗʰ **W56.22 Struck by orca**
    √x7ᵗʰ **W56.29 Other contact with orca**

  √5ᵗʰ **W56.3 Contact with other marine mammals**
    √x7ᵗʰ **W56.31 Bitten by other marine mammals**
    √x7ᵗʰ **W56.32 Struck by other marine mammals**
    √x7ᵗʰ **W56.39 Other contact with other marine mammals**

  √5ᵗʰ **W56.4 Contact with shark**
    √x7ᵗʰ **W56.41 Bitten by shark**
    √x7ᵗʰ **W56.42 Struck by shark**
    √x7ᵗʰ **W56.49 Other contact with shark**

  √5ᵗʰ **W56.5 Contact with other fish**
    √x7ᵗʰ **W56.51 Bitten by other fish**
    √x7ᵗʰ **W56.52 Struck by other fish**
    √x7ᵗʰ **W56.59 Other contact with other fish**

  √5ᵗʰ **W56.8 Contact with other nonvenomous marine animals**
    √x7ᵗʰ **W56.81 Bitten by other nonvenomous marine animals**
    √x7ᵗʰ **W56.82 Struck by other nonvenomous marine animals**
    √x7ᵗʰ **W56.89 Other contact with other nonvenomous marine animals**

√x7ᵗʰ **W57 Bitten or stung by nonvenomous insect and other nonvenomous arthropods**
    EXCLUDES 1   *contact with venomous insects and arthropods (T63.2-, T63.3-, T63.4-)*

√4ᵗʰ **W58 Contact with crocodile or alligator**

  √5ᵗʰ **W58.0 Contact with alligator**
    √x7ᵗʰ **W58.01 Bitten by alligator**
    √x7ᵗʰ **W58.02 Struck by alligator**
    √x7ᵗʰ **W58.03 Crushed by alligator**
    √x7ᵗʰ **W58.09 Other contact with alligator**

  √5ᵗʰ **W58.1 Contact with crocodile**
    √x7ᵗʰ **W58.11 Bitten by crocodile**
    √x7ᵗʰ **W58.12 Struck by crocodile**
    √x7ᵗʰ **W58.13 Crushed by crocodile**
    √x7ᵗʰ **W58.19 Other contact with crocodile**

√4ᵗʰ **W59 Contact with other nonvenomous reptiles**
    EXCLUDES 1   *contact with venomous reptile (T63.0-, T63.1-)*

  √5ᵗʰ **W59.0 Contact with nonvenomous lizards**
    √x7ᵗʰ **W59.01 Bitten by nonvenomous lizards**
    √x7ᵗʰ **W59.02 Struck by nonvenomous lizards**
    √x7ᵗʰ **W59.09 Other contact with nonvenomous lizards**
        Exposure to nonvenomous lizards

  √5ᵗʰ **W59.1 Contact with nonvenomous snakes**
    √x7ᵗʰ **W59.11 Bitten by nonvenomous snake**
    √x7ᵗʰ **W59.12 Struck by nonvenomous snake**
    √x7ᵗʰ **W59.13 Crushed by nonvenomous snake**
    √x7ᵗʰ **W59.19 Other contact with nonvenomous snake**

Ⓝ Newborn: 0   Ⓟ Pediatric: 0-17   Ⓜ Maternity: 9-64   Ⓐ Adult: 15-124   MCC Major Complication/Comorbidity   CC Complication/Comorbidity   SW Severe Wound Dx

1248   ICD-10-CM 2020

√5ᵗʰ **W59.2 Contact with** turtles

     EXCLUDES 1   contact with tortoises (W59.8-)

√x7ᵗʰ **W59.21 Bitten by turtle**

√x7ᵗʰ **W59.22 Struck by turtle**

√x7ᵗʰ **W59.29 Other contact with turtle**

     Exposure to turtles

√5ᵗʰ **W59.8 Contact with other nonvenomous reptiles**

√x7ᵗʰ **W59.81 Bitten by other nonvenomous reptiles**

√x7ᵗʰ **W59.82 Struck by other nonvenomous reptiles**

√x7ᵗʰ **W59.83 Crushed by other nonvenomous reptiles**

√x7ᵗʰ **W59.89 Other contact with other nonvenomous reptiles**

√x7ᵗʰ **W60 Contact with nonvenomous plant thorns and spines and sharp leaves**

     EXCLUDES 1   contact with venomous plants (T63.7-)

√4ᵗʰ **W61 Contact with birds (domestic) (wild)**

     INCLUDES   contact with excreta of birds

√5ᵗʰ **W61.0 Contact with** parrot

√x7ᵗʰ **W61.01 Bitten by parrot**

√x7ᵗʰ **W61.02 Struck by parrot**

√x7ᵗʰ **W61.09 Other contact with parrot**

     Exposure to parrots

√5ᵗʰ **W61.1 Contact with** macaw

√x7ᵗʰ **W61.11 Bitten by macaw**

√x7ᵗʰ **W61.12 Struck by macaw**

√x7ᵗʰ **W61.19 Other contact with macaw**

     Exposure to macaws

√5ᵗʰ **W61.2 Contact with other** psittacines

√x7ᵗʰ **W61.21 Bitten by other psittacines**

√x7ᵗʰ **W61.22 Struck by other psittacines**

√x7ᵗʰ **W61.29 Other contact with other psittacines**

     Exposure to other psittacines

√5ᵗʰ **W61.3 Contact with** chicken

√x7ᵗʰ **W61.32 Struck by chicken**

√x7ᵗʰ **W61.33 Pecked by chicken**

√x7ᵗʰ **W61.39 Other contact with chicken**

     Exposure to chickens

√5ᵗʰ **W61.4 Contact with** turkey

√x7ᵗʰ **W61.42 Struck by turkey**

√x7ᵗʰ **W61.43 Pecked by turkey**

√x7ᵗʰ **W61.49 Other contact with turkey**

√5ᵗʰ **W61.5 Contact with** goose

√x7ᵗʰ **W61.51 Bitten by goose**

√x7ᵗʰ **W61.52 Struck by goose**

√x7ᵗʰ **W61.59 Other contact with goose**

√5ᵗʰ **W61.6 Contact with** duck

√x7ᵗʰ **W61.61 Bitten by duck**

√x7ᵗʰ **W61.62 Struck by duck**

√x7ᵗʰ **W61.69 Other contact with duck**

√5ᵗʰ **W61.9 Contact with other birds**

√x7ᵗʰ **W61.91 Bitten by other birds**

√x7ᵗʰ **W61.92 Struck by other birds**

√x7ᵗʰ **W61.99 Other contact with other birds**

     Contact with bird NOS

√4ᵗʰ **W62 Contact with nonvenomous amphibians**

     EXCLUDES 1   contact with venomous amphibians (T63.81-R63.83)

√x7ᵗʰ **W62.0 Contact with nonvenomous** frogs

√x7ᵗʰ **W62.1 Contact with nonvenomous** toads

√x7ᵗʰ **W62.9 Contact with other nonvenomous amphibians**

√x7ᵗʰ **W64 Exposure to other animate mechanical forces**

     INCLUDES   exposure to nonvenomous animal NOS

     EXCLUDES 1   contact with venomous animal (T63.-)

Accidental non-transport drowning and submersion (W65-W74)

     EXCLUDES 1   accidental drowning and submersion due to fall into water (W16.-)

            accidental drowning and submersion due to water transport accident (V90.-, V92.-)

     EXCLUDES 2   accidental drowning and submersion due to cataclysm (X34-X39)

The appropriate 7th character is to be added to each code from categories W65-W74.

A   initial encounter

D   subsequent encounter

S   sequela

√x7ᵗʰ **W65 Accidental drowning and submersion while in** bath-tub

     EXCLUDES 1   accidental drowning and submersion due to fall in (into) bathtub (W16.211)

√x7ᵗʰ **W67 Accidental drowning and submersion while in** swimming-pool

     EXCLUDES 1   accidental drowning and submersion due to fall into swimming pool (W16.011, W16.021, W16.031)

            accidental drowning and submersion due to striking into wall of swimming pool (W22.041)

√x7ᵗʰ **W69 Accidental drowning and submersion while in** natural water

     Accidental drowning and submersion while in lake

     Accidental drowning and submersion while in open sea

     Accidental drowning and submersion while in river

     Accidental drowning and submersion while in stream

     EXCLUDES 1   accidental drowning and submersion due to fall into natural body of water (W16.111, W16.121, W16.131)

√x7ᵗʰ **W73 Other specified cause of accidental non-transport drowning and submersion**

     Accidental drowning and submersion while in quenching tank

     Accidental drowning and submersion while in reservoir

     EXCLUDES 1   accidental drowning and submersion due to fall into other water (W16.311, W16.321, W16.331)

√x7ᵗʰ **W74 Unspecified cause of accidental drowning and submersion**

     Drowning NOS

Exposure to electric current, radiation and extreme ambient air temperature and pressure (W85-W99)

     EXCLUDES 1   exposure to:

            failure in dosage of radiation or temperature during surgical and medical care (Y63.2-Y63.5)

            lightning (T75.0-)

            natural cold (X31)

            natural heat (X30)

            natural radiation NOS (X39)

            radiological procedure and radiotherapy (Y84.2)

            sunlight (X32)

AHA: 2018,2Q,7-8

The appropriate 7th character is to be added to each code from categories W85-W99.

A   initial encounter

D   subsequent encounter

S   sequela

√x7ᵗʰ **W85 Exposure to electric transmission lines**

     Broken power line

√4ᵗʰ **W86 Exposure to other specified electric current**

√x7ᵗʰ **W86.0 Exposure to domestic wiring and appliances**

√x7ᵗʰ **W86.1 Exposure to industrial wiring, appliances and electrical machinery**

     Exposure to conductors

     Exposure to control apparatus

     Exposure to electrical equipment and machinery

     Exposure to transformers

√x7ᵗʰ **W86.8 Exposure to other electric current**

     Exposure to wiring and appliances in or on farm (not farmhouse)

     Exposure to wiring and appliances outdoors

     Exposure to wiring and appliances in or on public building

     Exposure to wiring and appliances in or on residential institutions

     Exposure to wiring and appliances in or on schools

√4ᵗʰ **W88 Exposure to ionizing radiation**

     EXCLUDES 1   exposure to sunlight (X32)

√x7ᵗʰ **W88.0 Exposure to** X-rays

√x7ᵗʰ **W88.1 Exposure to** radioactive isotopes

✔ Additional Char Req   √x7ᵗʰ Placeholder   Unacceptable PDx   Questionable PDx   Wrong Procedure   Manifestation   Unspecified Dx   H1-H14 HAC   HCC CMS-HCC Dx   HIV HIV Dx

ICD-10-CM 2020   1249

√x7ᵗʰ **W88.8 Exposure to other ionizing radiation**

✓4ᵗʰ **W89 Exposure to man-made visible and ultraviolet light**

INCLUDES   exposure to welding light (arc)
EXCLUDES 1   *exposure to sunlight (X32)*

√x7ᵗʰ **W89.0 Exposure to welding light (arc)**

√x7ᵗʰ **W89.1 Exposure to tanning bed**

√x7ᵗʰ **W89.8 Exposure to other man-made visible and ultraviolet light**

√x7ᵗʰ **W89.9 Exposure to unspecified man-made visible and ultraviolet light**

✓4ᵗʰ **W90 Exposure to other nonionizing radiation**

EXCLUDES 1   *exposure to sunlight (X32)*
AHA: 2019,1Q,21

√x7ᵗʰ **W90.0 Exposure to radiofrequency**

√x7ᵗʰ **W90.1 Exposure to infrared radiation**

√x7ᵗʰ **W90.2 Exposure to laser radiation**

√x7ᵗʰ **W90.8 Exposure to other nonionizing radiation**

√x7ᵗʰ **W92 Exposure to excessive heat of man-made origin**

✓4ᵗʰ **W93 Exposure to excessive cold of man-made origin**

√5ᵗʰ **W93.0 Contact with or inhalation of dry ice**

√x7ᵗʰ **W93.01 Contact with dry ice**

√x7ᵗʰ **W93.02 Inhalation of dry ice**

√5ᵗʰ **W93.1 Contact with or inhalation of liquid air**

√x7ᵗʰ **W93.11 Contact with liquid air**

Contact with liquid hydrogen
Contact with liquid nitrogen

√x7ᵗʰ **W93.12 Inhalation of liquid air**

Inhalation of liquid hydrogen
Inhalation of liquid nitrogen

√x7ᵗʰ **W93.2 Prolonged exposure in deep freeze unit or refrigerator**

√x7ᵗʰ **W93.8 Exposure to other excessive cold of man-made origin**

✓4ᵗʰ **W94 Exposure to high and low air pressure and changes in air pressure**

√x7ᵗʰ **W94.0 Exposure to prolonged high air pressure**

√5ᵗʰ **W94.1 Exposure to prolonged low air pressure**

√x7ᵗʰ **W94.11 Exposure to residence or prolonged visit at high altitude**

√x7ᵗʰ **W94.12 Exposure to other prolonged low air pressure**

√5ᵗʰ **W94.2 Exposure to rapid changes in air pressure during ascent**

√x7ᵗʰ **W94.21 Exposure to reduction in atmospheric pressure while surfacing from deep-water diving**

√x7ᵗʰ **W94.22 Exposure to reduction in atmospheric pressure while surfacing from underground**

√x7ᵗʰ **W94.23 Exposure to sudden change in air pressure in aircraft during ascent**

√x7ᵗʰ **W94.29 Exposure to other rapid changes in air pressure during ascent**

√5ᵗʰ **W94.3 Exposure to rapid changes in air pressure during descent**

√x7ᵗʰ **W94.31 Exposure to sudden change in air pressure in aircraft during descent**

√x7ᵗʰ **W94.32 Exposure to high air pressure from rapid descent in water**

√x7ᵗʰ **W94.39 Exposure to other rapid changes in air pressure during descent**

√x7ᵗʰ **W99 Exposure to other man-made environmental factors**

Exposure to smoke, fire and flames (X00-X08)

EXCLUDES 1   *arson (X97)*
EXCLUDES 2   *explosions (W35-W40)*
              lightning (T75.0-)
              transport accident (V01-V99)
AHA: 2018,2Q,7-8

The appropriate 7th character is to be added to each code from categories X00-X08.
A   initial encounter
D   subsequent encounter
S   sequela

✓4ᵗʰ **X00 Exposure to uncontrolled fire in building or structure**

INCLUDES   conflagration in building or structure
Code first any associated cataclysm
EXCLUDES 2   *exposure to ignition or melting of nightwear (X05)*
              exposure to ignition or melting of other clothing and apparel (X06.-)
              exposure to other specified smoke, fire and flames (X08.-)
AHA: 2016,2Q,5

√x7ᵗʰ **X00.0 Exposure to flames in uncontrolled fire in building or structure**

√x7ᵗʰ **X00.1 Exposure to smoke in uncontrolled fire in building or structure**

√x7ᵗʰ **X00.2 Injury due to collapse of burning building or structure in uncontrolled fire**

EXCLUDES 1   *injury due to collapse of building not on fire (W20.1)*

√x7ᵗʰ **X00.3 Fall from burning building or structure in uncontrolled fire**

√x7ᵗʰ **X00.4 Hit by object from burning building or structure in uncontrolled fire**

AHA: 2016,2Q,4

√x7ᵗʰ **X00.5 Jump from burning building or structure in uncontrolled fire**

√x7ᵗʰ **X00.8 Other exposure to uncontrolled fire in building or structure**

✓4ᵗʰ **X01 Exposure to uncontrolled fire, not in building or structure**

INCLUDES   exposure to forest fire

√x7ᵗʰ **X01.0 Exposure to flames in uncontrolled fire, not in building or structure**

√x7ᵗʰ **X01.1 Exposure to smoke in uncontrolled fire, not in building or structure**

√x7ᵗʰ **X01.3 Fall due to uncontrolled fire, not in building or structure**

√x7ᵗʰ **X01.4 Hit by object due to uncontrolled fire, not in building or structure**

√x7ᵗʰ **X01.8 Other exposure to uncontrolled fire, not in building or structure**

✓4ᵗʰ **X02 Exposure to controlled fire in building or structure**

INCLUDES   exposure to fire in fireplace
            exposure to fire in stove

√x7ᵗʰ **X02.0 Exposure to flames in controlled fire in building or structure**

√x7ᵗʰ **X02.1 Exposure to smoke in controlled fire in building or structure**

√x7ᵗʰ **X02.2 Injury due to collapse of burning building or structure in controlled fire**

EXCLUDES 1   *injury due to collapse of building not on fire (W20.1)*

√x7ᵗʰ **X02.3 Fall from burning building or structure in controlled fire**

√x7ᵗʰ **X02.4 Hit by object from burning building or structure in controlled fire**

√x7ᵗʰ **X02.5 Jump from burning building or structure in controlled fire**

√x7ᵗʰ **X02.8 Other exposure to controlled fire in building or structure**

✓4ᵗʰ **X03 Exposure to controlled fire, not in building or structure**

INCLUDES   exposure to bon fire
            exposure to camp-fire
            exposure to trash fire

√x7ᵗʰ **X03.0 Exposure to flames in controlled fire, not in building or structure**

√x7ᵗʰ **X03.1 Exposure to smoke in controlled fire, not in building or structure**

√x7ᵗʰ **X03.3 Fall due to controlled fire, not in building or structure**

√x7ᵗʰ **X03.4 Hit by object due to controlled fire, not in building or structure**

√x7ᵗʰ **X03.8 Other exposure to controlled fire, not in building or structure**

✓x7ᵗʰ **X04 Exposure to ignition of highly flammable material**

Exposure to ignition of gasoline
Exposure to ignition of kerosene
Exposure to ignition of petrol

EXCLUDES 2   *exposure to ignition or melting of nightwear (X05)*
exposure to ignition or melting of other clothing and apparel (X06)

AHA: 2016,2Q,4

✓x7ᵗʰ **X05 Exposure to ignition or melting of nightwear**

EXCLUDES 2   *exposure to uncontrolled fire in building or structure (X00.-)*
exposure to uncontrolled fire, not in building or structure (X01.-)
exposure to controlled fire in building or structure (X02.-)
exposure to controlled fire, not in building or structure (X03.-)
exposure to ignition of highly flammable materials (X04.-)

✓4ᵗʰ **X06 Exposure to ignition or melting of other clothing and apparel**

EXCLUDES 2   *exposure to uncontrolled fire in building or structure (X00.-)*
exposure to uncontrolled fire, not in building or structure (X01.-)
exposure to controlled fire in building or structure (X02.-)
exposure to controlled fire, not in building or structure (X03.-)
exposure to ignition of highly flammable materials (X04.-)

✓x7ᵗʰ **X06.0 Exposure to ignition of plastic jewelry**

✓x7ᵗʰ **X06.1 Exposure to melting of plastic jewelry**

✓x7ᵗʰ **X06.2 Exposure to ignition of other clothing and apparel**

✓x7ᵗʰ **X06.3 Exposure to melting of other clothing and apparel**

✓4ᵗʰ **X08 Exposure to other specified smoke, fire and flames**

✓5ᵗʰ **X08.0 Exposure to bed fire**

Exposure to mattress fire

✓x7ᵗʰ **X08.00 Exposure to bed fire due to unspecified burning material**

✓x7ᵗʰ **X08.01 Exposure to bed fire due to burning cigarette**

✓x7ᵗʰ **X08.09 Exposure to bed fire due to other burning material**

✓5ᵗʰ **X08.1 Exposure to sofa fire**

✓x7ᵗʰ **X08.10 Exposure to sofa fire due to unspecified burning material**

✓x7ᵗʰ **X08.11 Exposure to sofa fire due to burning cigarette**

✓x7ᵗʰ **X08.19 Exposure to sofa fire due to other burning material**

✓5ᵗʰ **X08.2 Exposure to other furniture fire**

✓x7ᵗʰ **X08.20 Exposure to other furniture fire due to unspecified burning material**

✓x7ᵗʰ **X08.21 Exposure to other furniture fire due to burning cigarette**

✓x7ᵗʰ **X08.29 Exposure to other furniture fire due to other burning material**

✓x7ᵗʰ **X08.8 Exposure to other specified smoke, fire and flames**

Contact with heat and hot substances (X10-X19)

EXCLUDES 1   *exposure to excessive natural heat (X30)*
exposure to fire and flames (X00-X08)

AHA: 2018,2Q,7-8

The appropriate 7th character is to be added to each code from categories X10-X19.
A   initial encounter
D   subsequent encounter
S   sequela

✓4ᵗʰ **X10 Contact with hot drinks, food, fats and cooking oils**

✓x7ᵗʰ **X10.0 Contact with hot drinks**

✓x7ᵗʰ **X10.1 Contact with hot food**

✓x7ᵗʰ **X10.2 Contact with fats and cooking oils**

✓4ᵗʰ **X11 Contact with hot tap-water**

INCLUDES   contact with boiling tap-water
contact with boiling water NOS

EXCLUDES 1   *contact with water heated on stove (X12)*

✓x7ᵗʰ **X11.0 Contact with hot water in bath or tub**

EXCLUDES 1   *contact with running hot water in bath or tub (X11.1)*

✓x7ᵗʰ **X11.1 Contact with running hot water**

Contact with hot water running out of hose
Contact with hot water running out of tap

✓x7ᵗʰ **X11.8 Contact with other hot tap-water**

Contact with hot water in bucket
Contact with hot tap-water NOS

✓x7ᵗʰ **X12 Contact with other hot fluids**

Contact with water heated on stove

EXCLUDES 1   *hot (liquid) metals (X18)*

✓4ᵗʰ **X13 Contact with steam and other hot vapors**

✓x7ᵗʰ **X13.0 Inhalation of steam and other hot vapors**

✓x7ᵗʰ **X13.1 Other contact with steam and other hot vapors**

✓4ᵗʰ **X14 Contact with hot air and other hot gases**

✓x7ᵗʰ **X14.0 Inhalation of hot air and gases**

✓x7ᵗʰ **X14.1 Other contact with hot air and other hot gases**

✓4ᵗʰ **X15 Contact with hot household appliances**

EXCLUDES 1   *contact with heating appliances (X16)*
contact with powered household appliances (W29.-)
exposure to controlled fire in building or structure due to household appliance (X02.8)
exposure to household appliances electrical current (W86.0)

✓x7ᵗʰ **X15.0 Contact with hot stove (kitchen)**

✓x7ᵗʰ **X15.1 Contact with hot toaster**

✓x7ᵗʰ **X15.2 Contact with hotplate**

✓x7ᵗʰ **X15.3 Contact with hot saucepan or skillet**

✓x7ᵗʰ **X15.8 Contact with other hot household appliances**

Contact with cooker
Contact with kettle
Contact with light bulbs

✓x7ᵗʰ **X16 Contact with hot heating appliances, radiators and pipes**

EXCLUDES 1   *contact with powered appliances (W29.-)*
exposure to controlled fire in building or structure due to appliance (X02.8)
exposure to industrial appliances electrical current (W86.1)

✓x7ᵗʰ **X17 Contact with hot engines, machinery and tools**

EXCLUDES 1   *contact with hot heating appliances, radiators and pipes (X16)*
contact with hot household appliances (X15)

✓x7ᵗʰ **X18 Contact with other hot metals**

Contact with liquid metal

✓x7ᵗʰ **X19 Contact with other heat and hot substances**

EXCLUDES 1   *objects that are not normally hot, e.g., an object made hot by a house fire (X00-X08)*

Exposure to forces of nature (X30-X39)

AHA: 2018,2Q,7-8

The appropriate 7th character is to be added to each code from categories X30-X39.
A   initial encounter
D   subsequent encounter
S   sequela

✓x7ᵗʰ **X30 Exposure to excessive natural heat**

Exposure to excessive heat as the cause of sunstroke
Exposure to heat NOS

EXCLUDES 1   *excessive heat of man-made origin (W92)*
exposure to man-made radiation (W89)
exposure to sunlight (X32)
exposure to tanning bed (W89)

✓x7ᵗʰ **X31 Exposure to excessive natural cold**

Excessive cold as the cause of chilblains NOS
Excessive cold as the cause of immersion foot or hand
Exposure to cold NOS
Exposure to weather conditions

EXCLUDES 1   *cold of man-made origin (W93.-)*
contact with or inhalation of dry ice (W93.-)
contact with or inhalation of liquefied gas (W93.-)

✓x7ᵗʰ **X32 Exposure to sunlight**

EXCLUDES 1   *man-made radiation (tanning bed) (W89)*

EXCLUDES 2   *radiation-related disorders of the skin and subcutaneous tissue (L55-L59)*

✓7ᵗʰ **X34 Earthquake**

> EXCLUDES 2   *tidal wave (tsunami) due to earthquake (X37.41)*

✓7ᵗʰ **X35 Volcanic eruption**

> EXCLUDES 2   *tidal wave (tsunami) due to volcanic eruption (X37.41)*

✓4ᵗʰ **X36 Avalanche, landslide and other earth movements**

> INCLUDES   victim of mudslide of cataclysmic nature
> EXCLUDES 1   *earthquake (X34)*
> EXCLUDES 2   *transport accident involving collision with avalanche or landslide not in motion (V01-V99)*

  ✓7ᵗʰ **X36.0 Collapse of dam or man-made structure causing earth movement**

  ✓7ᵗʰ **X36.1 Avalanche, landslide, or mudslide**

✓4ᵗʰ **X37 Cataclysmic storm**

  ✓7ᵗʰ **X37.0 Hurricane**

> Storm surge
> Typhoon

  ✓7ᵗʰ **X37.1 Tornado**

> Cyclone
> Twister

  ✓7ᵗʰ **X37.2 Blizzard (snow)(ice)**

  ✓7ᵗʰ **X37.3 Dust storm**

  ✓5ᵗʰ **X37.4 Tidalwave**

    ✓7ᵗʰ **X37.41 Tidal wave due to earthquake or volcanic eruption**

> Tidal wave NOS
> Tsunami

    ✓7ᵗʰ **X37.42 Tidal wave due to storm**

    ✓7ᵗʰ **X37.43 Tidal wave due to landslide**

  ✓7ᵗʰ **X37.8 Other cataclysmic storms**

> Cloudburst
> Torrential rain
> EXCLUDES 2   *flood (X38)*

  ✓7ᵗʰ **X37.9 Unspecified cataclysmic storm**

> Storm NOS
> EXCLUDES 1   *collapse of dam or man-made structure causing earth movement (X36.0)*

✓7ᵗʰ **X38 Flood**

> Flood arising from remote storm
> Flood of cataclysmic nature arising from melting snow
> Flood resulting directly from storm
> EXCLUDES 1   *collapse of dam or man-made structure causing earth movement (X36.0)*
> *tidal wave NOS (X37.41)*
> *tidal wave caused by storm (X37.42)*

✓4ᵗʰ **X39 Exposure to other forces of nature**

  ✓5ᵗʰ **X39.0 Exposure to natural radiation**

> EXCLUDES 1   *contact with and (suspected) exposure to radon and other naturally occurring radiation (Z77.123)*
> *exposure to man-made radiation (W88-W90)*
> *exposure to sunlight (X32)*

    ✓7ᵗʰ **X39.01 Exposure to radon**

    ✓7ᵗʰ **X39.08 Exposure to other natural radiation**

  ✓7ᵗʰ **X39.8 Other exposure to forces of nature**

Overexertion and strenuous or repetitive movements (X50)

✓4ᵗʰ **X50 Overexertion and strenuous or repetitive movements**

> **AHA:** 2018,2Q,7-8; 2016,4Q,73-74
>
> The appropriate 7th character is to be added to each code from category X50.
> A   initial encounter
> D   subsequent encounter
> S   sequela

  ✓7ᵗʰ **X50.0 Overexertion from strenuous movement or load**

> Lifting heavy objects
> Lifting weights

  ✓7ᵗʰ **X50.1 Overexertion from prolonged static or awkward postures**

> Prolonged bending
> Prolonged kneeling
> Prolonged reaching
> Prolonged sitting
> Prolonged standing
> Prolonged twisting
> Static bending
> Static kneeling
> Static reaching
> Static sitting
> Static standing
> Static twisting

  ✓7ᵗʰ **X50.3 Overexertion from repetitive movements**

> Use of hand as hammer
> EXCLUDES 2   *overuse from prolonged static or awkward postures (X50.1)*

  ✓7ᵗʰ **X50.9 Other and unspecified overexertion or strenuous movements or postures**

> Contact pressure
> Contact stress

Accidental exposure to other specified factors (X52-X58)

AHA: 2018,2Q,7-8

> The appropriate 7th character is to be added to each code from categories X52-X58.
> A   initial encounter
> D   subsequent encounter
> S   sequela

✓7ᵗʰ **X52 Prolonged stay in weightless environment**

> Weightlessness in spacecraft (simulator)

✓7ᵗʰ **X58 Exposure to other specified factors**

> Accident NOS
> Exposure NOS

Intentional self-harm (X71-X83)

Purposely self-inflicted injury
Suicide (attempted)

> The appropriate 7th character is to be added to each code from categories X71-X83.
> A   initial encounter
> D   subsequent encounter
> S   sequela

✓4ᵗʰ **X71 Intentional self-harm by drowning and submersion**

  ✓7ᵗʰ **X71.0 Intentional self-harm by drowning and submersion while in bathtub**   HCC

  ✓7ᵗʰ **X71.1 Intentional self-harm by drowning and submersion while in swimming pool**   HCC

  ✓7ᵗʰ **X71.2 Intentional self-harm by drowning and submersion after jump into swimming pool**   HCC

  ✓7ᵗʰ **X71.3 Intentional self-harm by drowning and submersion in natural water**   HCC

  ✓7ᵗʰ **X71.8 Other intentional self-harm by drowning and submersion**   HCC

  ✓7ᵗʰ **X71.9 Intentional self-harm by drowning and submersion, unspecified**   HCC

✓7ᵗʰ **X72 Intentional self-harm by handgun discharge**   HCC

> Intentional self-harm by gun for single hand use
> Intentional self-harm by pistol
> Intentional self-harm by revolver
> EXCLUDES 1   *Very pistol (X74.8)*

✓4ᵗʰ **X73 Intentional self-harm by rifle, shotgun and larger firearm discharge**

> EXCLUDES 1   *airgun (X74.01)*

  ✓7ᵗʰ **X73.0 Intentional self-harm by shotgun discharge**   HCC

  ✓7ᵗʰ **X73.1 Intentional self-harm by hunting rifle discharge**   HCC

  ✓7ᵗʰ **X73.2 Intentional self-harm by machine gun discharge**   HCC

  ✓7ᵗʰ **X73.8 Intentional self-harm by other larger firearm discharge**   HCC

  ✓7ᵗʰ **X73.9 Intentional self-harm by unspecified larger firearm discharge**   HCC

Ⓝ Newborn: 0   Ⓟ Pediatric: 0-17   Ⓜ Maternity: 9-64   Ⓐ Adult: 15-124   **MCC** Major Complication/Comorbidity   **CC** Complication/Comorbidity   **SW** Severe Wound Dx

1252   ICD-10-CM 2020

✓4th **X74** **Intentional self-harm by other and unspecified firearm and gun discharge**

✓5th **X74.0** **Intentional self-harm by gas, air or spring-operated guns**

✓x7th **X74.01** **Intentional self-harm by airgun**   HCC
Intentional self-harm by BB gun discharge
Intentional self-harm by pellet gun discharge

✓x7th **X74.02** **Intentional self-harm by paintball gun**   HCC

✓x7th **X74.09** **Intentional self-harm by other gas, air or spring-operated gun**   HCC

✓x7th **X74.8** **Intentional self-harm by other firearm discharge**   HCC
Intentional self-harm by Very pistol [flare] discharge

✓x7th **X74.9** **Intentional self-harm by unspecified firearm discharge**   HCC

✓x7th **X75** **Intentional self-harm by explosive material**   HCC

✓x7th **X76** **Intentional self-harm by smoke, fire and flames**   HCC

✓4th **X77** **Intentional self-harm by steam, hot vapors and hot objects**

✓x7th **X77.0** **Intentional self-harm by steam or hot vapors**   HCC

✓x7th **X77.1** **Intentional self-harm by hot tap water**   HCC

✓x7th **X77.2** **Intentional self-harm by other hot fluids**   HCC

✓x7th **X77.3** **Intentional self-harm by hot household appliances**   HCC

✓x7th **X77.8** **Intentional self-harm by other hot objects**   HCC

✓x7th **X77.9** **Intentional self-harm by unspecified hot objects**   HCC

✓4th **X78** **Intentional self-harm by sharp object**

✓x7th **X78.0** **Intentional self-harm by sharp glass**   HCC

✓x7th **X78.1** **Intentional self-harm by knife**   HCC

✓x7th **X78.2** **Intentional self-harm by sword or dagger**   HCC

✓x7th **X78.8** **Intentional self-harm by other sharp object**   HCC

✓x7th **X78.9** **Intentional self-harm by unspecified sharp object**   HCC

✓x7th **X79** **Intentional self-harm by blunt object**   HCC

✓x7th **X80** **Intentional self-harm by jumping from a high place**   HCC
Intentional fall from one level to another

✓4th **X81** **Intentional self-harm by jumping or lying in front of moving object**

✓x7th **X81.0** **Intentional self-harm by jumping or lying in front of motor vehicle**   HCC

✓x7th **X81.1** **Intentional self-harm by jumping or lying in front of (subway) train**   HCC

✓x7th **X81.8** **Intentional self-harm by jumping or lying in front of other moving object**   HCC

✓4th **X82** **Intentional self-harm by crashing of motor vehicle**

✓x7th **X82.0** **Intentional collision of motor vehicle with other motor vehicle**   HCC

✓x7th **X82.1** **Intentional collision of motor vehicle with train**   HCC

✓x7th **X82.2** **Intentional collision of motor vehicle with tree**   HCC

✓x7th **X82.8** **Other intentional self-harm by crashing of motor vehicle**   HCC

✓4th **X83** **Intentional self-harm by other specified means**

EXCLUDES 1   *intentional self-harm by poisoning or contact with toxic substance — see Table of Drugs and Chemicals*

✓x7th **X83.0** **Intentional self-harm by crashing of aircraft**   HCC

✓x7th **X83.1** **Intentional self-harm by electrocution**   HCC

✓x7th **X83.2** **Intentional self-harm by exposure to extremes of cold**   HCC

✓x7th **X83.8** **Intentional self-harm by other specified means**   HCC

Assault (X92-Y09)

INCLUDES   homicide
injuries inflicted by another person with intent to injure or kill, by any means

EXCLUDES 1   *injuries due to legal intervention (Y35.-)*
injuries due to operations of war (Y36.-)
injuries due to terrorism (Y38.-)

The appropriate 7th character is to be added to each code from categories X92-Y04 and Y08.
A   initial encounter
D   subsequent encounter
S   sequela

✓4th **X92** **Assault by drowning and submersion**

✓x7th **X92.0** **Assault by drowning and submersion while in bathtub**

✓x7th **X92.1** **Assault by drowning and submersion while in swimming pool**

✓x7th **X92.2** **Assault by drowning and submersion after push into swimming pool**

✓x7th **X92.3** **Assault by drowning and submersion in natural water**

✓x7th **X92.8** **Other assault by drowning and submersion**

✓x7th **X92.9** **Assault by drowning and submersion, unspecified**

✓x7th **X93** **Assault by handgun discharge**
Assault by discharge of gun for single hand use
Assault by discharge of pistol
Assault by discharge of revolver
EXCLUDES 1   *Very pistol (X95.8)*

✓4th **X94** **Assault by rifle, shotgun and larger firearm discharge**
EXCLUDES 1   *airgun (X95.01)*

✓x7th **X94.0** **Assault by shotgun**

✓x7th **X94.1** **Assault by hunting rifle**

✓x7th **X94.2** **Assault by machine gun**

✓x7th **X94.8** **Assault by other larger firearm discharge**

✓x7th **X94.9** **Assault by unspecified larger firearm discharge**

✓4th **X95** **Assault by other and unspecified firearm and gun discharge**

✓5th **X95.0** **Assault by gas, air or spring-operated guns**

✓x7th **X95.01** **Assault by airgun discharge**
Assault by BB gun discharge
Assault by pellet gun discharge

✓x7th **X95.02** **Assault by paintball gun discharge**

✓x7th **X95.09** **Assault by other gas, air or spring-operated gun**

✓x7th **X95.8** **Assault by other firearm discharge**
Assault by Very pistol [flare] discharge

✓x7th **X95.9** **Assault by unspecified firearm discharge**

✓4th **X96** **Assault by explosive material**
EXCLUDES 1   *incendiary device (X97)*
terrorism involving explosive material (Y38.2-)

✓x7th **X96.0** **Assault by antipersonnel bomb**
EXCLUDES 1   *antipersonnel bomb use in military or war (Y36.2-)*

✓x7th **X96.1** **Assault by gasoline bomb**

✓x7th **X96.2** **Assault by letter bomb**

✓x7th **X96.3** **Assault by fertilizer bomb**

✓x7th **X96.4** **Assault by pipe bomb**

✓x7th **X96.8** **Assault by other specified explosive**

✓x7th **X96.9** **Assault by unspecified explosive**

✓x7th **X97** **Assault by smoke, fire and flames**
Assault by arson
Assault by cigarettes
Assault by incendiary device

✓4th **X98** **Assault by steam, hot vapors and hot objects**

✓x7th **X98.0** **Assault by steam or hot vapors**

✓x7th **X98.1** **Assault by hot tap water**

✓x7th **X98.2** **Assault by hot fluids**

✓x7th **X98.3** **Assault by hot household appliances**

✓x7th **X98.8** **Assault by other hot objects**

✓x7th **X98.9** **Assault by unspecified hot objects**

✔ Additional Char Req   ✓x7th Placeholder   Unacceptable PDx   Questionable PDx   Wrong Procedure   Manifestation   Unspecified Dx   H1-H14 HAC   HCC CMS-HCC Dx   HIV HIV Dx

ICD-10-CM 2020   1253

☑4ᵗʰ **X99 Assault by sharp object**
> EXCLUDES 1   *assault by strike by sports equipment (Y08.0-)*

☑x7ᵗʰ **X99.0 Assault by sharp** glass

☑x7ᵗʰ **X99.1 Assault by** knife

☑x7ᵗʰ **X99.2 Assault by** sword or dagger

☑x7ᵗʰ **X99.8 Assault by other sharp object**

☑x7ᵗʰ **X99.9 Assault by unspecified sharp object**
> Assault by stabbing NOS

☑x7ᵗʰ **Y00 Assault by blunt object**
> EXCLUDES 1   *assault by strike by sports equipment (Y08.0-)*

☑x7ᵗʰ **Y01 Assault by pushing from high place**

☑4ᵗʰ **Y02 Assault by pushing or placing victim in front of moving object**

☑x7ᵗʰ **Y02.0 Assault by pushing or placing victim in front of** motor vehicle

☑x7ᵗʰ **Y02.1 Assault by pushing or placing victim in front of (subway) train**

☑x7ᵗʰ **Y02.8 Assault by pushing or placing victim in front of other moving object**

☑4ᵗʰ **Y03 Assault by crashing of motor vehicle**

☑x7ᵗʰ **Y03.0 Assault by being hit or run over by motor vehicle**

☑x7ᵗʰ **Y03.8 Other assault by crashing of motor vehicle**

☑4ᵗʰ **Y04 Assault by bodily force**
> EXCLUDES 1   *assault by:*
> *submersion (X92.-)*
> *use of weapon (X93-X95, X99, Y00)*

☑x7ᵗʰ **Y04.0 Assault by** unarmed brawl or fight

☑x7ᵗʰ **Y04.1 Assault by** human bite

☑x7ᵗʰ **Y04.2 Assault by** strike **against or bumped into by another person**

☑x7ᵗʰ **Y04.8 Assault by other bodily force**
> Assault by bodily force NOS

☑4ᵗʰ **Y07 Perpetrator of assault, maltreatment and neglect**
> **NOTE**   Codes from this category are for use only in cases of confirmed abuse (T74.-)
> Selection of the correct perpetrator code is based on the relationship between the perpetrator and the victim
> **INCLUDES**   perpetrator of abandonment
> perpetrator of emotional neglect
> perpetrator of mental cruelty
> perpetrator of physical abuse
> perpetrator of physical neglect
> perpetrator of sexual abuse
> perpetrator of torture

☑5ᵗʰ **Y07.0** Spouse or partner, **perpetrator of maltreatment and neglect**
> Spouse or partner, perpetrator of maltreatment and neglect against spouse or partner

    Y07.01 Husband, **perpetrator of maltreatment and neglect**

    Y07.02 Wife, **perpetrator of maltreatment and neglect**

    Y07.03 Male partner, **perpetrator of maltreatment and neglect**

    Y07.04 Female partner, **perpetrator of maltreatment and neglect**

☑5ᵗʰ **Y07.1** Parent (adoptive) (biological), **perpetrator of maltreatment and neglect**

    Y07.11 Biological father, **perpetrator of maltreatment and neglect**

    Y07.12 Biological mother, **perpetrator of maltreatment and neglect**

    Y07.13 Adoptive father, **perpetrator of maltreatment and neglect**

    Y07.14 Adoptive mother, **perpetrator of maltreatment and neglect**

☑5ᵗʰ **Y07.4 Other family member, perpetrator of maltreatment and neglect**

☑6ᵗʰ **Y07.41** Sibling, **perpetrator of maltreatment and neglect**
> EXCLUDES 1   *stepsibling, perpetrator of maltreatment and neglect (Y07.435, Y07.436)*

    Y07.410 Brother, **perpetrator of maltreatment and neglect**

    Y07.411 Sister, **perpetrator of maltreatment and neglect**

☑6ᵗʰ **Y07.42** Foster parent, **perpetrator of maltreatment and neglect**

    Y07.420 Foster father, **perpetrator of maltreatment and neglect**

    Y07.421 Foster mother, **perpetrator of maltreatment and neglect**

☑6ᵗʰ **Y07.43** Stepparent or stepsibling, **perpetrator of maltreatment and neglect**

    Y07.430 Stepfather, **perpetrator of maltreatment and neglect**

    Y07.432 Male friend of parent (co-residing in household), **perpetrator of maltreatment and neglect**

    Y07.433 Stepmother, **perpetrator of maltreatment and neglect**

    Y07.434 Female friend of parent (co-residing in household), **perpetrator of maltreatment and neglect**

    Y07.435 Stepbrother, **perpetrator or maltreatment and neglect**

    Y07.436 Stepsister, **perpetrator of maltreatment and neglect**

☑6ᵗʰ **Y07.49 Other family member, perpetrator of maltreatment and neglect**

    Y07.490 Male cousin, **perpetrator of maltreatment and neglect**

    Y07.491 Female cousin, **perpetrator of maltreatment and neglect**

    Y07.499 Other family member, **perpetrator of maltreatment and neglect**

☑5ᵗʰ **Y07.5** Non-family member, **perpetrator of maltreatment and neglect**

    Y07.50 Unspecified non-family member, perpetrator of maltreatment and neglect

☑6ᵗʰ **Y07.51** Daycare provider, **perpetrator of maltreatment and neglect**

    Y07.510 At-home childcare provider, **perpetrator of maltreatment and neglect**

    Y07.511 Daycare center childcare provider, **perpetrator of maltreatment and neglect**

    Y07.512 At-home adultcare provider, **perpetrator of maltreatment and neglect**

    Y07.513 Adultcare center provider, **perpetrator of maltreatment and neglect**

    Y07.519 Unspecified daycare provider, perpetrator of maltreatment and neglect

☑6ᵗʰ **Y07.52** Healthcare provider, **perpetrator of maltreatment and neglect**

    Y07.521 Mental health provider, **perpetrator of maltreatment and neglect**

    Y07.528 Other therapist or healthcare provider, **perpetrator of maltreatment and neglect**
> Nurse perpetrator of maltreatment and neglect
> Occupational therapist perpetrator of maltreatment and neglect
> Physical therapist perpetrator of maltreatment and neglect
> Speech therapist perpetrator of maltreatment and neglect

    Y07.529 Unspecified healthcare provider, perpetrator of maltreatment and neglect

    Y07.53 Teacher or instructor, **perpetrator of maltreatment and neglect**
> Coach, perpetrator of maltreatment and neglect

    Y07.59 Other non-family member, perpetrator of maltreatment and neglect

Y07.6 Multiple perpetrators of maltreatment and neglect
> AHA: 2018,4Q,32

Y07.9 Unspecified perpetrator of maltreatment and neglect

☑4ᵗʰ **Y08 Assault by other specified means**

☑5ᵗʰ **Y08.0 Assault by strike by** sport equipment

☑x7ᵗʰ **Y08.01 Assault by strike by** hockey stick

☑x7ᵗʰ **Y08.02 Assault by strike by** baseball bat

☑x7ᵗʰ **Y08.09 Assault by strike by other specified type of sport equipment**

☑5ᵗʰ **Y08.8 Assault by other specified means**

☑x7ᵗʰ **Y08.81 Assault by crashing of** aircraft

☑x7ᵗʰ **Y08.89 Assault by other specified means**

Y09   **Assault by unspecified means**
    Assassination (attempted) NOS
    Homicide (attempted) NOS
    Manslaughter (attempted) NOS
    Murder (attempted) NOS

Event of undetermined intent (Y21-Y33)

Undetermined intent is only for use when there is specific documentation in the record that the intent of the injury cannot be determined. If no such documentation is present, code to accidental (unintentional).

The appropriate 7th character is to be added to each code from categories Y21-Y33.
A   initial encounter
D   subsequent encounter
S   sequela

✓4ᵗʰ Y21   **Drowning and submersion, undetermined intent**

   ✓x7ᵗʰ Y21.Ø   **Drowning and submersion** while in bathtub, **undetermined intent**

   ✓x7ᵗʰ Y21.1   **Drowning and submersion** after fall into bathtub, **undetermined intent**

   ✓x7ᵗʰ Y21.2   **Drowning and submersion** while in swimming pool, **undetermined intent**

   ✓x7ᵗʰ Y21.3   **Drowning and submersion** after fall into swimming pool, **undetermined intent**

   ✓x7ᵗʰ Y21.4   **Drowning and submersion** in natural water, **undetermined intent**

   ✓x7ᵗʰ Y21.8   **Other drowning and submersion, undetermined intent**

   ✓x7ᵗʰ Y21.9   **Unspecified drowning and submersion, undetermined intent**

✓x7ᵗʰ Y22   **Handgun discharge, undetermined intent**
    Discharge of gun for single hand use, undetermined intent
    Discharge of pistol, undetermined intent
    Discharge of revolver, undetermined intent
    EXCLUDES 2   Very pistol (Y24.8)

✓4ᵗʰ Y23   **Rifle, shotgun and larger firearm discharge, undetermined intent**
    EXCLUDES 2   airgun (Y24.Ø)

   ✓x7ᵗʰ Y23.Ø   **Shotgun discharge, undetermined intent**

   ✓x7ᵗʰ Y23.1   **Hunting rifle discharge, undetermined intent**

   ✓x7ᵗʰ Y23.2   **Military firearm discharge, undetermined intent**

   ✓x7ᵗʰ Y23.3   **Machine gun discharge, undetermined intent**

   ✓x7ᵗʰ Y23.8   **Other larger firearm discharge, undetermined intent**

   ✓x7ᵗʰ Y23.9   **Unspecified larger firearm discharge, undetermined intent**

✓4ᵗʰ Y24   **Other and unspecified firearm discharge, undetermined intent**

   ✓x7ᵗʰ Y24.Ø   **Airgun discharge, undetermined intent**
       BB gun discharge, undetermined intent
       Pellet gun discharge, undetermined intent

   ✓x7ᵗʰ Y24.8   **Other firearm discharge, undetermined intent**
       Paintball gun discharge, undetermined intent
       Very pistol [flare] discharge, undetermined intent

   ✓x7ᵗʰ Y24.9   **Unspecified firearm discharge, undetermined intent**

✓x7ᵗʰ Y25   **Contact with explosive material, undetermined intent**

✓x7ᵗʰ Y26   **Exposure to smoke, fire and flames, undetermined intent**

✓4ᵗʰ Y27   **Contact with steam, hot vapors and hot objects, undetermined intent**

   ✓x7ᵗʰ Y27.Ø   **Contact with** steam and hot vapors, **undetermined intent**

   ✓x7ᵗʰ Y27.1   **Contact with hot** tap water, **undetermined intent**

   ✓x7ᵗʰ Y27.2   **Contact with hot** fluids, **undetermined intent**

   ✓x7ᵗʰ Y27.3   **Contact with hot** household appliance, **undetermined intent**

   ✓x7ᵗʰ Y27.8   **Contact with other hot** objects, **undetermined intent**

   ✓x7ᵗʰ Y27.9   **Contact with unspecified hot objects, undetermined intent**

✓4ᵗʰ Y28   **Contact with sharp object, undetermined intent**

   ✓x7ᵗʰ Y28.Ø   **Contact with sharp** glass, **undetermined intent**

   ✓x7ᵗʰ Y28.1   **Contact with** knife, **undetermined intent**

   ✓x7ᵗʰ Y28.2   **Contact with** sword or dagger, **undetermined intent**

   ✓x7ᵗʰ Y28.8   **Contact with other sharp object, undetermined intent**

   ✓x7ᵗʰ Y28.9   **Contact with unspecified sharp object, undetermined intent**

✓x7ᵗʰ Y29   **Contact with blunt object, undetermined intent**

✓x7ᵗʰ Y30   **Falling, jumping or pushed from a high place, undetermined intent**
    Victim falling from one level to another, undetermined intent

✓x7ᵗʰ Y31   **Falling, lying or running before or into moving object, undetermined intent**

✓x7ᵗʰ Y32   **Crashing of motor vehicle, undetermined intent**

✓x7ᵗʰ Y33   **Other specified events, undetermined intent**

Legal intervention, operations of war, military operations, and terrorism (Y35-Y38)

The appropriate 7th character is to be added to each code from categories Y35-Y38.
A   initial encounter
D   subsequent encounter
S   sequela

✓4ᵗʰ Y35   **Legal intervention**
   INCLUDES   any injury sustained as a result of an encounter with any law enforcement official, serving in any capacity at the time of the encounter, whether on-duty or off-duty. Includes injury to law enforcement official, suspect and bystander

   ✓5ᵗʰ Y35.Ø   **Legal intervention involving** firearm discharge

      ✓6ᵗʰ Y35.ØØ   **Legal intervention involving unspecified firearm discharge**
         Legal intervention involving gunshot wound
         Legal intervention involving shot NOS

         ✓7ᵗʰ Y35.ØØ1   **Legal intervention involving unspecified firearm discharge,** law enforcement official **injured**

         ✓7ᵗʰ Y35.ØØ2   **Legal intervention involving unspecified firearm discharge,** bystander **injured**

         ✓7ᵗʰ Y35.ØØ3   **Legal intervention involving unspecified firearm discharge,** suspect **injured**

         ✓7ᵗʰ Y35.ØØ9   **Legal intervention involving unspecified firearm discharge, unspecified person injured**

      ✓6ᵗʰ Y35.Ø1   **Legal intervention involving injury by** machine gun

         ✓7ᵗʰ Y35.Ø11   **Legal intervention involving injury by machine gun,** law enforcement official **injured**

         ✓7ᵗʰ Y35.Ø12   **Legal intervention involving injury by machine gun,** bystander **injured**

         ✓7ᵗʰ Y35.Ø13   **Legal intervention involving injury by machine gun,** suspect **injured**

         ✓7ᵗʰ Y35.Ø19   **Legal intervention involving injury by machine gun, unspecified person injured**

      ✓6ᵗʰ Y35.Ø2   **Legal intervention involving injury by** handgun

         ✓7ᵗʰ Y35.Ø21   **Legal intervention involving injury by handgun,** law enforcement official **injured**

         ✓7ᵗʰ Y35.Ø22   **Legal intervention involving injury by handgun,** bystander **injured**

         ✓7ᵗʰ Y35.Ø23   **Legal intervention involving injury by handgun,** suspect **injured**

         ✓7ᵗʰ Y35.Ø29   **Legal intervention involving injury by handgun, unspecified person injured**

      ✓6ᵗʰ Y35.Ø3   **Legal intervention involving injury by** rifle pellet

         ✓7ᵗʰ Y35.Ø31   **Legal intervention involving injury by rifle pellet,** law enforcement official **injured**

         ✓7ᵗʰ Y35.Ø32   **Legal intervention involving injury by rifle pellet,** bystander **injured**

         ✓7ᵗʰ Y35.Ø33   **Legal intervention involving injury by rifle pellet,** suspect **injured**

         ✓7ᵗʰ Y35.Ø39   **Legal intervention involving injury by rifle pellet, unspecified person injured**

      ✓6ᵗʰ Y35.Ø4   **Legal intervention involving injury by** rubber bullet

         ✓7ᵗʰ Y35.Ø41   **Legal intervention involving injury by rubber bullet,** law enforcement official **injured**

         ✓7ᵗʰ Y35.Ø42   **Legal intervention involving injury by rubber bullet,** bystander **injured**

         ✓7ᵗʰ Y35.Ø43   **Legal intervention involving injury by rubber bullet,** suspect **injured**

         ✓7ᵗʰ Y35.Ø49   **Legal intervention involving injury by rubber bullet, unspecified person injured**

      ✓6ᵗʰ Y35.Ø9   **Legal intervention involving other firearm discharge**

         ✓7ᵗʰ Y35.Ø91   **Legal intervention involving other firearm discharge,** law enforcement official **injured**

         ✓7ᵗʰ Y35.Ø92   **Legal intervention involving other firearm discharge,** bystander **injured**

✅ Additional Char Req   ✓x7ᵗʰ Placeholder   Unacceptable PDx   Questionable PDx   Wrong Procedure   Manifestation   Unspecified Dx   H1-H14 HAC   HCC CMS-HCC Dx   HIV HIV Dx

Chapter 20. External Causes of Morbidity

Y35.093–Y35.831

√7ᵗʰ **Y35.093** Legal intervention involving other firearm discharge, **suspect** injured

√7ᵗʰ **Y35.099** Legal intervention involving other firearm discharge, unspecified person injured

√5ᵗʰ **Y35.1** Legal intervention involving **explosives**

√6ᵗʰ **Y35.10** Legal intervention involving unspecified explosives

√7ᵗʰ **Y35.101** Legal intervention involving unspecified explosives, **law enforcement official** injured

√7ᵗʰ **Y35.102** Legal intervention involving unspecified explosives, **bystander** injured

√7ᵗʰ **Y35.103** Legal intervention involving unspecified explosives, **suspect** injured

√7ᵗʰ **Y35.109** Legal intervention involving unspecified explosives, unspecified person injured

√6ᵗʰ **Y35.11** Legal intervention involving injury by **dynamite**

√7ᵗʰ **Y35.111** Legal intervention involving injury by dynamite, **law enforcement official** injured

√7ᵗʰ **Y35.112** Legal intervention involving injury by dynamite, **bystander** injured

√7ᵗʰ **Y35.113** Legal intervention involving injury by dynamite, **suspect** injured

√7ᵗʰ **Y35.119** Legal intervention involving injury by dynamite, unspecified person injured

√6ᵗʰ **Y35.12** Legal intervention involving injury by **explosive shell**

√7ᵗʰ **Y35.121** Legal intervention involving injury by explosive shell, **law enforcement official** injured

√7ᵗʰ **Y35.122** Legal intervention involving injury by explosive shell, **bystander** injured

√7ᵗʰ **Y35.123** Legal intervention involving injury by explosive shell, **suspect** injured

√7ᵗʰ **Y35.129** Legal intervention involving injury by explosive shell, unspecified person injured

√6ᵗʰ **Y35.19** Legal intervention involving other explosives

Legal intervention involving injury by grenade
Legal intervention involving injury by mortar bomb

√7ᵗʰ **Y35.191** Legal intervention involving other explosives, **law enforcement official** injured

√7ᵗʰ **Y35.192** Legal intervention involving other explosives, **bystander** injured

√7ᵗʰ **Y35.193** Legal intervention involving other explosives, **suspect** injured

√7ᵗʰ **Y35.199** Legal intervention involving other explosives, unspecified person injured

√5ᵗʰ **Y35.2** Legal intervention involving **gas**

Legal intervention involving asphyxiation by gas
Legal intervention involving poisoning by gas

√6ᵗʰ **Y35.20** Legal intervention involving unspecified gas

√7ᵗʰ **Y35.201** Legal intervention involving unspecified gas, **law enforcement official** injured

√7ᵗʰ **Y35.202** Legal intervention involving unspecified gas, **bystander** injured

√7ᵗʰ **Y35.203** Legal intervention involving unspecified gas, **suspect** injured

√7ᵗʰ **Y35.209** Legal intervention involving unspecified gas, unspecified person injured

√6ᵗʰ **Y35.21** Legal intervention involving injury by **tear gas**

√7ᵗʰ **Y35.211** Legal intervention involving injury by tear gas, **law enforcement official** injured

√7ᵗʰ **Y35.212** Legal intervention involving injury by tear gas, **bystander** injured

√7ᵗʰ **Y35.213** Legal intervention involving injury by tear gas, **suspect** injured

√7ᵗʰ **Y35.219** Legal intervention involving injury by tear gas, unspecified person injured

√6ᵗʰ **Y35.29** Legal intervention involving other gas

√7ᵗʰ **Y35.291** Legal intervention involving other gas, **law enforcement official** injured

√7ᵗʰ **Y35.292** Legal intervention involving other gas, **bystander** injured

√7ᵗʰ **Y35.293** Legal intervention involving other gas, **suspect** injured

√7ᵗʰ **Y35.299** Legal intervention involving other gas, unspecified person injured

√5ᵗʰ **Y35.3** Legal intervention involving **blunt objects**

Legal intervention involving being hit or struck by blunt object

√6ᵗʰ **Y35.30** Legal intervention involving unspecified blunt objects

√7ᵗʰ **Y35.301** Legal intervention involving unspecified blunt objects, **law enforcement official** injured

√7ᵗʰ **Y35.302** Legal intervention involving unspecified blunt objects, **bystander** injured

√7ᵗʰ **Y35.303** Legal intervention involving unspecified blunt objects, **suspect** injured

√7ᵗʰ **Y35.309** Legal intervention involving unspecified blunt objects, unspecified person injured

√6ᵗʰ **Y35.31** Legal intervention involving **baton**

√7ᵗʰ **Y35.311** Legal intervention involving baton, **law enforcement official** injured

√7ᵗʰ **Y35.312** Legal intervention involving baton, **bystander** injured

√7ᵗʰ **Y35.313** Legal intervention involving baton, **suspect** injured

√7ᵗʰ **Y35.319** Legal intervention involving baton, unspecified person injured

√6ᵗʰ **Y35.39** Legal intervention involving other blunt objects

√7ᵗʰ **Y35.391** Legal intervention involving other blunt objects, **law enforcement official** injured

√7ᵗʰ **Y35.392** Legal intervention involving other blunt objects, **bystander** injured

√7ᵗʰ **Y35.393** Legal intervention involving other blunt objects, **suspect** injured

√7ᵗʰ **Y35.399** Legal intervention involving other blunt objects, unspecified person injured

√5ᵗʰ **Y35.4** Legal intervention involving **sharp objects**

Legal intervention involving being cut by sharp objects
Legal intervention involving being stabbed by sharp objects

√6ᵗʰ **Y35.40** Legal intervention involving unspecified sharp objects

√7ᵗʰ **Y35.401** Legal intervention involving unspecified sharp objects, **law enforcement official** injured

√7ᵗʰ **Y35.402** Legal intervention involving unspecified sharp objects, **bystander** injured

√7ᵗʰ **Y35.403** Legal intervention involving unspecified sharp objects, **suspect** injured

√7ᵗʰ **Y35.409** Legal intervention involving unspecified sharp objects, unspecified person injured

√6ᵗʰ **Y35.41** Legal intervention involving **bayonet**

√7ᵗʰ **Y35.411** Legal intervention involving bayonet, **law enforcement official** injured

√7ᵗʰ **Y35.412** Legal intervention involving bayonet, **bystander** injured

√7ᵗʰ **Y35.413** Legal intervention involving bayonet, **suspect** injured

√7ᵗʰ **Y35.419** Legal intervention involving bayonet, unspecified person injured

√6ᵗʰ **Y35.49** Legal intervention involving other sharp objects

√7ᵗʰ **Y35.491** Legal intervention involving other sharp objects, **law enforcement official** injured

√7ᵗʰ **Y35.492** Legal intervention involving other sharp objects, **bystander** injured

√7ᵗʰ **Y35.493** Legal intervention involving other sharp objects, **suspect** injured

√7ᵗʰ **Y35.499** Legal intervention involving other sharp objects, unspecified person injured

√5ᵗʰ **Y35.8** Legal intervention involving other specified means

√6ᵗʰ **Y35.81** Legal intervention involving **manhandling**

√7ᵗʰ **Y35.811** Legal intervention involving manhandling, **law enforcement official** injured

√7ᵗʰ **Y35.812** Legal intervention involving manhandling, **bystander** injured

√7ᵗʰ **Y35.813** Legal intervention involving manhandling, **suspect** injured

√7ᵗʰ **Y35.819** Legal intervention involving manhandling, unspecified person injured

√6ᵗʰ **Y35.83** Legal intervention involving a **conducted energy device**

Electroshock device (taser)
Stun gun

√7ᵗʰ **Y35.831** Legal intervention involving a conducted energy device, **law enforcement official** injured

- ☑7ᵗʰ **Y35.832** Legal intervention involving a conducted energy device, bystander injured
- ☑7ᵗʰ **Y35.833** Legal intervention involving a conducted energy device, suspect injured
- ☑7ᵗʰ **Y35.839** Legal intervention involving a conducted energy device, unspecified person injured

✓6ᵗʰ **Y35.89** Legal intervention involving other specified means

    ☑7ᵗʰ **Y35.891** Legal intervention involving other specified means, law enforcement official injured

    ☑7ᵗʰ **Y35.892** Legal intervention involving other specified means, bystander injured

    ☑7ᵗʰ **Y35.893** Legal intervention involving other specified means, suspect injured

       AHA: 2018,1Q,5

✓5ᵗʰ **Y35.9** Legal intervention, means unspecified

    ✓x7ᵗʰ **Y35.91** Legal intervention, means unspecified, law enforcement official injured

    ✓x7ᵗʰ **Y35.92** Legal intervention, means unspecified, bystander injured

    ✓x7ᵗʰ **Y35.93** Legal intervention, means unspecified, suspect injured

- ✓x7ᵗʰ **Y35.99** Legal intervention, means unspecified, unspecified person injured

✓4ᵗʰ **Y36 Operations of war**

    INCLUDES injuries to military personnel and civilians caused by war, civil insurrection, and peacekeeping missions

    EXCLUDES 1 injury to military personnel occurring during peacetime military operations (Y37.-)

        military vehicles involved in transport accidents with non-military vehicle during peacetime (V09.01, V09.21, V19.81, V29.81, V39.81, V49.81, V59.81, V69.81, V79.81)

    AHA: 2014,3Q,4

✓5ᵗʰ **Y36.0** War operations involving explosion of marine weapons

    ✓6ᵗʰ **Y36.00** War operations involving explosion of unspecified marine weapon

        War operations involving underwater blast NOS

      ☑7ᵗʰ **Y36.000** War operations involving explosion of unspecified marine weapon, military personnel

      ☑7ᵗʰ **Y36.001** War operations involving explosion of unspecified marine weapon, civilian

    ✓6ᵗʰ **Y36.01** War operations involving explosion of depth-charge

      ☑7ᵗʰ **Y36.010** War operations involving explosion of depth-charge, military personnel

      ☑7ᵗʰ **Y36.011** War operations involving explosion of depth-charge, civilian

    ✓6ᵗʰ **Y36.02** War operations involving explosion of marine mine

        War operations involving explosion of marine mine, at sea or in harbor

      ☑7ᵗʰ **Y36.020** War operations involving explosion of marine mine, military personnel

      ☑7ᵗʰ **Y36.021** War operations involving explosion of marine mine, civilian

    ✓6ᵗʰ **Y36.03** War operations involving explosion of sea-based artillery shell

      ☑7ᵗʰ **Y36.030** War operations involving explosion of sea-based artillery shell, military personnel

      ☑7ᵗʰ **Y36.031** War operations involving explosion of sea-based artillery shell, civilian

    ✓6ᵗʰ **Y36.04** War operations involving explosion of torpedo

      ☑7ᵗʰ **Y36.040** War operations involving explosion of torpedo, military personnel

      ☑7ᵗʰ **Y36.041** War operations involving explosion of torpedo, civilian

    ✓6ᵗʰ **Y36.05** War operations involving accidental detonation of onboard marine weapons

      ☑7ᵗʰ **Y36.050** War operations involving accidental detonation of onboard marine weapons, military personnel

      ☑7ᵗʰ **Y36.051** War operations involving accidental detonation of onboard marine weapons, civilian

    ✓6ᵗʰ **Y36.09** War operations involving explosion of other marine weapons

      ☑7ᵗʰ **Y36.090** War operations involving explosion of other marine weapons, military personnel

      ☑7ᵗʰ **Y36.091** War operations involving explosion of other marine weapons, civilian

✓5ᵗʰ **Y36.1** War operations involving destruction of aircraft

    ✓6ᵗʰ **Y36.10** War operations involving unspecified destruction of aircraft

      ☑7ᵗʰ **Y36.100** War operations involving unspecified destruction of aircraft, military personnel

      ☑7ᵗʰ **Y36.101** War operations involving unspecified destruction of aircraft, civilian

    ✓6ᵗʰ **Y36.11** War operations involving destruction of aircraft due to enemy fire or explosives

        War operations involving destruction of aircraft due to air to air missile

        War operations involving destruction of aircraft due to explosive placed on aircraft

        War operations involving destruction of aircraft due to rocket propelled grenade [RPG]

        War operations involving destruction of aircraft due to small arms fire

        War operations involving destruction of aircraft due to surface to air missile

      ☑7ᵗʰ **Y36.110** War operations involving destruction of aircraft due to enemy fire or explosives, military personnel

      ☑7ᵗʰ **Y36.111** War operations involving destruction of aircraft due to enemy fire or explosives, civilian

    ✓6ᵗʰ **Y36.12** War operations involving destruction of aircraft due to collision with other aircraft

      ☑7ᵗʰ **Y36.120** War operations involving destruction of aircraft due to collision with other aircraft, military personnel

      ☑7ᵗʰ **Y36.121** War operations involving destruction of aircraft due to collision with other aircraft, civilian

    ✓6ᵗʰ **Y36.13** War operations involving destruction of aircraft due to onboard fire

      ☑7ᵗʰ **Y36.130** War operations involving destruction of aircraft due to onboard fire, military personnel

      ☑7ᵗʰ **Y36.131** War operations involving destruction of aircraft due to onboard fire, civilian

    ✓6ᵗʰ **Y36.14** War operations involving destruction of aircraft due to accidental detonation of onboard munitions and explosives

      ☑7ᵗʰ **Y36.140** War operations involving destruction of aircraft due to accidental detonation of onboard munitions and explosives, military personnel

      ☑7ᵗʰ **Y36.141** War operations involving destruction of aircraft due to accidental detonation of onboard munitions and explosives, civilian

    ✓6ᵗʰ **Y36.19** War operations involving other destruction of aircraft

      ☑7ᵗʰ **Y36.190** War operations involving other destruction of aircraft, military personnel

      ☑7ᵗʰ **Y36.191** War operations involving other destruction of aircraft, civilian

✓5ᵗʰ **Y36.2** War operations involving other explosions and fragments

    EXCLUDES 1 war operations involving explosion of aircraft (Y36.1-)

        war operations involving explosion of marine weapons (Y36.0-)

        war operations involving explosion of nuclear weapons (Y36.5-)

        war operations involving explosion occurring after cessation of hostilities (Y36.8-)

    ✓6ᵗʰ **Y36.20** War operations involving unspecified explosion and fragments

        War operations involving air blast NOS

        War operations involving blast NOS

        War operations involving blast fragments NOS

        War operations involving blast wave NOS

        War operations involving blast wind NOS

        War operations involving explosion NOS

        War operations involving explosion of bomb NOS

      ☑7ᵗʰ **Y36.200** War operations involving unspecified explosion and fragments, military personnel

      ☑7ᵗʰ **Y36.201** War operations involving unspecified explosion and fragments, civilian

✅Additional Char Req   ✓x7ᵗʰ Placeholder   Unacceptable PDx   Questionable PDx   Wrong Procedure   Manifestation   Unspecified Dx   H1-H14 HAC   HCC CMS-HCC Dx   HIV HIV Dx

ICD-10-CM 2020   1257

√6ᵗʰ **Y36.21** War operations involving explosion of aerial bomb

√7ᵗʰ **Y36.210** **War operations involving explosion of aerial bomb, military personnel**

√7ᵗʰ **Y36.211** **War operations involving explosion of aerial bomb, civilian**

√6ᵗʰ **Y36.22** War operations involving explosion of guided missile

√7ᵗʰ **Y36.220** **War operations involving explosion of guided missile, military personnel**

√7ᵗʰ **Y36.221** **War operations involving explosion of guided missile, civilian**

√6ᵗʰ **Y36.23** War operations involving explosion of improvised explosive device [IED]

War operations involving explosion of person-borne improvised explosive device [IED]

War operations involving explosion of vehicle-borne improvised explosive device [IED]

War operations involving explosion of roadside improvised explosive device [IED]

√7ᵗʰ **Y36.230** **War operations involving explosion of improvised explosive device [IED], military personnel**

√7ᵗʰ **Y36.231** **War operations involving explosion of improvised explosive device [IED], civilian**

√6ᵗʰ **Y36.24** War operations involving explosion due to accidental detonation and discharge of own munitions or munitions launch device

√7ᵗʰ **Y36.240** **War operations involving explosion due to accidental detonation and discharge of own munitions or munitions launch device, military personnel**

√7ᵗʰ **Y36.241** **War operations involving explosion due to accidental detonation and discharge of own munitions or munitions launch device, civilian**

√6ᵗʰ **Y36.25** War operations involving fragments from munitions

√7ᵗʰ **Y36.250** **War operations involving fragments from munitions, military personnel**

√7ᵗʰ **Y36.251** **War operations involving fragments from munitions, civilian**

√6ᵗʰ **Y36.26** War operations involving fragments of improvised explosive device [IED]

War operations involving fragments of person-borne improvised explosive device [IED]

War operations involving fragments of vehicle-borne improvised explosive device [IED]

War operations involving fragments of roadside improvised explosive device [IED]

√7ᵗʰ **Y36.260** **War operations involving fragments of improvised explosive device [IED], military personnel**

√7ᵗʰ **Y36.261** **War operations involving fragments of improvised explosive device [IED], civilian**

√6ᵗʰ **Y36.27** War operations involving fragments from weapons

√7ᵗʰ **Y36.270** **War operations involving fragments from weapons, military personnel**

√7ᵗʰ **Y36.271** **War operations involving fragments from weapons, civilian**

√6ᵗʰ **Y36.29** War operations involving other explosions and fragments

War operations involving explosion of grenade

War operations involving explosions of land mine

War operations involving shrapnel NOS

√7ᵗʰ **Y36.290** **War operations involving other explosions and fragments, military personnel**

√7ᵗʰ **Y36.291** **War operations involving other explosions and fragments, civilian**

√5ᵗʰ **Y36.3** War operations involving fires, conflagrations and hot substances

War operations involving smoke, fumes, and heat from fires, conflagrations and hot substances

EXCLUDES 1 *war operations involving fires and conflagrations aboard military aircraft (Y36.1-)*

war operations involving fires and conflagrations aboard military watercraft (Y36.0-)

war operations involving fires and conflagrations caused indirectly by conventional weapons (Y36.2-)

war operations involving fires and thermal effects of nuclear weapons (Y36.53-)

√6ᵗʰ **Y36.30** War operations involving unspecified fire, conflagration and hot substance

√7ᵗʰ **Y36.300** **War operations involving unspecified fire, conflagration and hot substance, military personnel**

√7ᵗʰ **Y36.301** **War operations involving unspecified fire, conflagration and hot substance, civilian**

√6ᵗʰ **Y36.31** War operations involving gasoline bomb

War operations involving incendiary bomb

War operations involving petrol bomb

√7ᵗʰ **Y36.310** **War operations involving gasoline bomb, military personnel**

√7ᵗʰ **Y36.311** **War operations involving gasoline bomb, civilian**

√6ᵗʰ **Y36.32** War operations involving incendiary bullet

√7ᵗʰ **Y36.320** **War operations involving incendiary bullet, military personnel**

√7ᵗʰ **Y36.321** **War operations involving incendiary bullet, civilian**

√6ᵗʰ **Y36.33** War operations involving flamethrower

√7ᵗʰ **Y36.330** **War operations involving flamethrower, military personnel**

√7ᵗʰ **Y36.331** **War operations involving flamethrower, civilian**

√6ᵗʰ **Y36.39** War operations involving other fires, conflagrations and hot substances

√7ᵗʰ **Y36.390** **War operations involving other fires, conflagrations and hot substances, military personnel**

√7ᵗʰ **Y36.391** **War operations involving other fires, conflagrations and hot substances, civilian**

√5ᵗʰ **Y36.4** War operations involving firearm discharge and other forms of conventional warfare

√6ᵗʰ **Y36.41** War operations involving rubber bullets

√7ᵗʰ **Y36.410** **War operations involving rubber bullets, military personnel**

√7ᵗʰ **Y36.411** **War operations involving rubber bullets, civilian**

√6ᵗʰ **Y36.42** War operations involving firearms pellets

√7ᵗʰ **Y36.420** **War operations involving firearms pellets, military personnel**

√7ᵗʰ **Y36.421** **War operations involving firearms pellets, civilian**

√6ᵗʰ **Y36.43** War operations involving other firearms discharge

War operations involving bullets NOS

EXCLUDES 1 *war operations involving munitions fragments (Y36.25-)*

war operations involving incendiary bullets (Y36.32-)

√7ᵗʰ **Y36.430** **War operations involving other firearms discharge, military personnel**

√7ᵗʰ **Y36.431** **War operations involving other firearms discharge, civilian**

√6ᵗʰ **Y36.44** War operations involving unarmed hand to hand combat

EXCLUDES 1 *war operations involving combat using blunt or piercing object (Y36.45-)*

war operations involving intentional restriction of air and airway (Y36.46-)

war operations involving unintentional restriction of air and airway (Y36.47-)

√7ᵗʰ **Y36.440** **War operations involving unarmed hand to hand combat, military personnel**

√7ᵗʰ **Y36.441** **War operations involving unarmed hand to hand combat, civilian**

🅝 Newborn: 0   🅟 Pediatric: 0-17   🅜 Maternity: 9-64   🅐 Adult: 15-124   ᴹᶜᶜ Major Complication/Comorbidity   ᶜᶜ Complication/Comorbidity   ˢᵂ Severe Wound Dx

1258   ICD-10-CM 2020

☑6ᵗʰ **Y36.45** **War operations involving combat using** blunt or piercing object
- ☑7ᵗʰ **Y36.450** **War operations involving combat using blunt or piercing object,** military personnel
- ☑7ᵗʰ **Y36.451** **War operations involving combat using blunt or piercing object,** civilian

☑6ᵗʰ **Y36.46** **War operations involving** intentional restriction of air and airway
- ☑7ᵗʰ **Y36.460** **War operations involving intentional restriction of air and airway,** military personnel
- ☑7ᵗʰ **Y36.461** **War operations involving intentional restriction of air and airway,** civilian

☑6ᵗʰ **Y36.47** **War operations involving** unintentional restriction of air and airway
- ☑7ᵗʰ **Y36.470** **War operations involving unintentional restriction of air and airway,** military personnel
- ☑7ᵗʰ **Y36.471** **War operations involving unintentional restriction of air and airway,** civilian

☑6ᵗʰ **Y36.49** **War operations involving other forms of conventional warfare**
- ☑7ᵗʰ **Y36.490** **War operations involving other forms of conventional warfare,** military personnel
- ☑7ᵗʰ **Y36.491** **War operations involving other forms of conventional warfare,** civilian

☑5ᵗʰ **Y36.5** **War operations involving** nuclear weapons

War operations involving dirty bomb NOS

☑6ᵗʰ **Y36.50** **War operations involving unspecified effect of nuclear weapon**
- ☑7ᵗʰ **Y36.500** **War operations involving unspecified effect of nuclear weapon,** military personnel
- ☑7ᵗʰ **Y36.501** **War operations involving unspecified effect of nuclear weapon,** civilian

☑6ᵗʰ **Y36.51** **War operations involving** direct blast **effect of nuclear weapon**

War operations involving blast pressure of nuclear weapon
- ☑7ᵗʰ **Y36.510** **War operations involving direct blast effect of nuclear weapon,** military personnel
- ☑7ᵗʰ **Y36.511** **War operations involving direct blast effect of nuclear weapon,** civilian

☑6ᵗʰ **Y36.52** **War operations involving** indirect blast **effect of nuclear weapon**

War operations involving being thrown by blast of nuclear weapon

War operations involving being struck or crushed by blast debris of nuclear weapon
- ☑7ᵗʰ **Y36.520** **War operations involving indirect blast effect of nuclear weapon,** military personnel
- ☑7ᵗʰ **Y36.521** **War operations involving indirect blast effect of nuclear weapon,** civilian

☑6ᵗʰ **Y36.53** **War operations involving** thermal radiation **effect of nuclear weapon**

War operations involving direct heat from nuclear weapon

War operation involving fireball effects from nuclear weapon
- ☑7ᵗʰ **Y36.530** **War operations involving thermal radiation effect of nuclear weapon,** military personnel
- ☑7ᵗʰ **Y36.531** **War operations involving thermal radiation effect of nuclear weapon,** civilian

☑6ᵗʰ **Y36.54** **War operation involving** nuclear radiation **effects of nuclear weapon**

War operation involving acute radiation exposure from nuclear weapon

War operation involving exposure to immediate ionizing radiation from nuclear weapon

War operation involving fallout exposure from nuclear weapon

War operation involving secondary effects of nuclear weapons
- ☑7ᵗʰ **Y36.540** **War operation involving nuclear radiation effects of nuclear weapon,** military personnel

- ☑7ᵗʰ **Y36.541** **War operation involving nuclear radiation effects of nuclear weapon,** civilian

☑6ᵗʰ **Y36.59** **War operation involving other effects of nuclear weapons**
- ☑7ᵗʰ **Y36.590** **War operation involving other effects of nuclear weapons,** military personnel
- ☑7ᵗʰ **Y36.591** **War operation involving other effects of nuclear weapons,** civilian

☑5ᵗʰ **Y36.6** **War operations involving biological weapons**

☑6ᵗʰ **Y36.6X** **War operations involving** biological weapons
- ☑7ᵗʰ **Y36.6X0** **War operations involving biological weapons,** military personnel
- ☑7ᵗʰ **Y36.6X1** **War operations involving biological weapons,** civilian

☑5ᵗʰ **Y36.7** **War operations involving chemical weapons and other forms of unconventional warfare**

> EXCLUDES 1   war operations involving incendiary devices (Y36.3-, Y36.5-)

☑6ᵗʰ **Y36.7X** **War operations involving** chemical weapons and other forms of unconventional warfare
- ☑7ᵗʰ **Y36.7X0** **War operations involving chemical weapons and other forms of unconventional warfare,** military personnel
- ☑7ᵗʰ **Y36.7X1** **War operations involving chemical weapons and other forms of unconventional warfare,** civilian

☑5ᵗʰ **Y36.8** **War operations occurring** after cessation of hostilities

War operations classifiable to categories Y36.0-Y36.8 but occurring after cessation of hostilities

☑6ᵗʰ **Y36.81** **Explosion of** mine **placed during war operations but exploding after cessation of hostilities**
- ☑7ᵗʰ **Y36.810** **Explosion of mine placed during war operations but exploding after cessation of hostilities,** military personnel
- ☑7ᵗʰ **Y36.811** **Explosion of mine placed during war operations but exploding after cessation of hostilities,** civilian

☑6ᵗʰ **Y36.82** **Explosion of** bomb **placed during war operations but exploding after cessation of hostilities**
- ☑7ᵗʰ **Y36.820** **Explosion of bomb placed during war operations but exploding after cessation of hostilities,** military personnel
- ☑7ᵗʰ **Y36.821** **Explosion of bomb placed during war operations but exploding after cessation of hostilities,** civilian

☑6ᵗʰ **Y36.88** **Other war operations occurring after cessation of hostilities**
- ☑7ᵗʰ **Y36.880** **Other war operations occurring after cessation of hostilities,** military personnel
- ☑7ᵗʰ **Y36.881** **Other war operations occurring after cessation of hostilities,** civilian

☑6ᵗʰ **Y36.89** **Unspecified war operations occurring after cessation of hostilities**
- ☑7ᵗʰ **Y36.890** **Unspecified war operations occurring after cessation of hostilities,** military personnel
- ☑7ᵗʰ **Y36.891** **Unspecified war operations occurring after cessation of hostilities,** civilian

☑5ᵗʰ **Y36.9** **Other and unspecified war operations**

☑x7ᵗʰ **Y36.90** **War operations, unspecified**

☑x7ᵗʰ **Y36.91** **War operations involving unspecified** weapon of mass destruction [WMD]

☑x7ᵗʰ **Y36.92** **War operations involving** friendly fire

☑ Additional Char Req   ☑x7ᵗʰ Placeholder   Unacceptable PDx   Questionable PDx   Wrong Procedure   Manifestation   Unspecified Dx   H1-H14 HAC   HCC CMS-HCC Dx   HIV HIV Dx

ICD-10-CM 2020   1259

Chapter 20. External Causes of Morbidity

Y37-Y37.220

✓4ᵗʰ **Y37** **Military operations**

INCLUDES   injuries to military personnel and civilians occurring during peacetime on military property and during routine military exercises and operations

EXCLUDES 1   *military aircraft involved in aircraft accident with civilian aircraft (V97.81-)*

military vehicles involved in transport accident with civilian vehicle (V09.01, V09.21, V19.81, V29.81, V39.81, V49.81, V59.81, V69.81, V79.81)

military watercraft involved in water transport accident with civilian watercraft (V94.81-)

war operations (Y36.-)

✓5ᵗʰ **Y37.0** **Military operations involving** explosion of marine weapons

✓6ᵗʰ **Y37.00** **Military operations involving explosion of unspecified marine weapon**

Military operations involving underwater blast NOS

✓7ᵗʰ **Y37.000** **Military operations involving explosion of unspecified marine weapon, military personnel**

✓7ᵗʰ **Y37.001** **Military operations involving explosion of unspecified marine weapon, civilian**

✓6ᵗʰ **Y37.01** **Military operations involving explosion of depth-charge**

✓7ᵗʰ **Y37.010** **Military operations involving explosion of depth-charge, military personnel**

✓7ᵗʰ **Y37.011** **Military operations involving explosion of depth-charge, civilian**

✓6ᵗʰ **Y37.02** **Military operations involving explosion of marine mine**

Military operations involving explosion of marine mine, at sea or in harbor

✓7ᵗʰ **Y37.020** **Military operations involving explosion of marine mine, military personnel**

✓7ᵗʰ **Y37.021** **Military operations involving explosion of marine mine, civilian**

✓6ᵗʰ **Y37.03** **Military operations involving explosion of sea-based artillery shell**

✓7ᵗʰ **Y37.030** **Military operations involving explosion of sea-based artillery shell, military personnel**

✓7ᵗʰ **Y37.031** **Military operations involving explosion of sea-based artillery shell, civilian**

✓6ᵗʰ **Y37.04** **Military operations involving explosion of torpedo**

✓7ᵗʰ **Y37.040** **Military operations involving explosion of torpedo, military personnel**

✓7ᵗʰ **Y37.041** **Military operations involving explosion of torpedo, civilian**

✓6ᵗʰ **Y37.05** **Military operations involving accidental detonation of onboard marine weapons**

✓7ᵗʰ **Y37.050** **Military operations involving accidental detonation of onboard marine weapons, military personnel**

✓7ᵗʰ **Y37.051** **Military operations involving accidental detonation of onboard marine weapons, civilian**

✓6ᵗʰ **Y37.09** **Military operations involving explosion of other marine weapons**

✓7ᵗʰ **Y37.090** **Military operations involving explosion of other marine weapons, military personnel**

✓7ᵗʰ **Y37.091** **Military operations involving explosion of other marine weapons, civilian**

✓5ᵗʰ **Y37.1** **Military operations involving** destruction of aircraft

✓6ᵗʰ **Y37.10** **Military operations involving unspecified destruction of aircraft**

✓7ᵗʰ **Y37.100** **Military operations involving unspecified destruction of aircraft, military personnel**

✓7ᵗʰ **Y37.101** **Military operations involving unspecified destruction of aircraft, civilian**

✓6ᵗʰ **Y37.11** **Military operations involving destruction of aircraft due to enemy fire or explosives**

Military operations involving destruction of aircraft due to air to air missile

Military operations involving destruction of aircraft due to explosive placed on aircraft

Military operations involving destruction of aircraft due to rocket propelled grenade [RPG]

Military operations involving destruction of aircraft due to small arms fire

Military operations involving destruction of aircraft due to surface to air missile

✓7ᵗʰ **Y37.110** **Military operations involving destruction of aircraft due to enemy fire or explosives, military personnel**

✓7ᵗʰ **Y37.111** **Military operations involving destruction of aircraft due to enemy fire or explosives, civilian**

✓6ᵗʰ **Y37.12** **Military operations involving destruction of aircraft due to collision with other aircraft**

✓7ᵗʰ **Y37.120** **Military operations involving destruction of aircraft due to collision with other aircraft, military personnel**

✓7ᵗʰ **Y37.121** **Military operations involving destruction of aircraft due to collision with other aircraft, civilian**

✓6ᵗʰ **Y37.13** **Military operations involving destruction of aircraft due to onboard fire**

✓7ᵗʰ **Y37.130** **Military operations involving destruction of aircraft due to onboard fire, military personnel**

✓7ᵗʰ **Y37.131** **Military operations involving destruction of aircraft due to onboard fire, civilian**

✓6ᵗʰ **Y37.14** **Military operations involving destruction of aircraft due to** accidental detonation of onboard munitions and explosives

✓7ᵗʰ **Y37.140** **Military operations involving destruction of aircraft due to accidental detonation of onboard munitions and explosives, military personnel**

✓7ᵗʰ **Y37.141** **Military operations involving destruction of aircraft due to accidental detonation of onboard munitions and explosives, civilian**

✓6ᵗʰ **Y37.19** **Military operations involving other destruction of aircraft**

✓7ᵗʰ **Y37.190** **Military operations involving other destruction of aircraft, military personnel**

✓7ᵗʰ **Y37.191** **Military operations involving other destruction of aircraft, civilian**

✓5ᵗʰ **Y37.2** **Military operations involving** other explosions and fragments

EXCLUDES 1   *military operations involving explosion of aircraft (Y37.1-)*

military operations involving explosion of marine weapons (Y37.0-)

military operations involving explosion of nuclear weapons (Y37.5-)

✓6ᵗʰ **Y37.20** **Military operations involving unspecified explosion and fragments**

Military operations involving air blast NOS

Military operations involving blast NOS

Military operations involving blast fragments NOS

Military operations involving blast wave NOS

Military operations involving blast wind NOS

Military operations involving explosion NOS

Military operations involving explosion of bomb NOS

✓7ᵗʰ **Y37.200** **Military operations involving unspecified explosion and fragments, military personnel**

✓7ᵗʰ **Y37.201** **Military operations involving unspecified explosion and fragments, civilian**

✓6ᵗʰ **Y37.21** **Military operations involving explosion of aerial bomb**

✓7ᵗʰ **Y37.210** **Military operations involving explosion of aerial bomb, military personnel**

✓7ᵗʰ **Y37.211** **Military operations involving explosion of aerial bomb, civilian**

✓6ᵗʰ **Y37.22** **Military operations involving explosion of guided missile**

✓7ᵗʰ **Y37.220** **Military operations involving explosion of guided missile, military personnel**

Ⓝ Newborn: 0   Ⓟ Pediatric: 0-17   Ⓜ Maternity: 9-64   Ⓐ Adult: 15-124   MCC Major Complication/Comorbidity   CC Complication/Comorbidity   SW Severe Wound Dx

1260   ICD-10-CM 2020

☑7ᵗʰ **Y37.221 Military operations involving explosion of guided missile, civilian**

☑6ᵗʰ **Y37.23 Military operations involving explosion of improvised explosive device [IED]**

Military operations involving explosion of person-borne improvised explosive device [IED]

Military operations involving explosion of vehicle-borne improvised explosive device [IED]

Military operations involving explosion of roadside improvised explosive device [IED]

☑7ᵗʰ **Y37.230 Military operations involving explosion of improvised explosive device [IED], military personnel**

☑7ᵗʰ **Y37.231 Military operations involving explosion of improvised explosive device [IED], civilian**

☑6ᵗʰ **Y37.24 Military operations involving explosion due to accidental detonation and discharge of own munitions or munitions launch device**

☑7ᵗʰ **Y37.240 Military operations involving explosion due to accidental detonation and discharge of own munitions or munitions launch device, military personnel**

☑7ᵗʰ **Y37.241 Military operations involving explosion due to accidental detonation and discharge of own munitions or munitions launch device, civilian**

☑6ᵗʰ **Y37.25 Military operations involving fragments from munitions**

☑7ᵗʰ **Y37.250 Military operations involving fragments from munitions, military personnel**

☑7ᵗʰ **Y37.251 Military operations involving fragments from munitions, civilian**

☑6ᵗʰ **Y37.26 Military operations involving fragments of improvised explosive device [IED]**

Military operations involving fragments of person-borne improvised explosive device [IED]

Military operations involving fragments of vehicle-borne improvised explosive device [IED]

Military operations involving fragments of roadside improvised explosive device [IED]

☑7ᵗʰ **Y37.260 Military operations involving fragments of improvised explosive device [IED], military personnel**

☑7ᵗʰ **Y37.261 Military operations involving fragments of improvised explosive device [IED], civilian**

☑6ᵗʰ **Y37.27 Military operations involving fragments from weapons**

☑7ᵗʰ **Y37.270 Military operations involving fragments from weapons, military personnel**

☑7ᵗʰ **Y37.271 Military operations involving fragments from weapons, civilian**

☑6ᵗʰ **Y37.29 Military operations involving other explosions and fragments**

Military operations involving explosion of grenade

Military operations involving explosions of land mine

Military operations involving shrapnel NOS

☑7ᵗʰ **Y37.290 Military operations involving other explosions and fragments, military personnel**

☑7ᵗʰ **Y37.291 Military operations involving other explosions and fragments, civilian**

☑5ᵗʰ **Y37.3 Military operations involving fires, conflagrations and hot substances**

Military operations involving smoke, fumes, and heat from fires, conflagrations and hot substances

EXCLUDES 1 *military operations involving fires and conflagrations aboard military aircraft (Y37.1-)*

military operations involving fires and conflagrations aboard military watercraft (Y37.0-)

military operations involving fires and conflagrations caused indirectly by conventional weapons (Y37.2-)

military operations involving fires and thermal effects of nuclear weapons (Y36.53-)

☑6ᵗʰ **Y37.30 Military operations involving unspecified fire, conflagration and hot substance**

☑7ᵗʰ **Y37.300 Military operations involving unspecified fire, conflagration and hot substance, military personnel**

☑7ᵗʰ **Y37.301 Military operations involving unspecified fire, conflagration and hot substance, civilian**

☑6ᵗʰ **Y37.31 Military operations involving gasoline bomb**

Military operations involving incendiary bomb

Military operations involving petrol bomb

☑7ᵗʰ **Y37.310 Military operations involving gasoline bomb, military personnel**

☑7ᵗʰ **Y37.311 Military operations involving gasoline bomb, civilian**

☑6ᵗʰ **Y37.32 Military operations involving incendiary bullet**

☑7ᵗʰ **Y37.320 Military operations involving incendiary bullet, military personnel**

☑7ᵗʰ **Y37.321 Military operations involving incendiary bullet, civilian**

☑6ᵗʰ **Y37.33 Military operations involving flamethrower**

☑7ᵗʰ **Y37.330 Military operations involving flamethrower, military personnel**

☑7ᵗʰ **Y37.331 Military operations involving flamethrower, civilian**

☑6ᵗʰ **Y37.39 Military operations involving other fires, conflagrations and hot substances**

☑7ᵗʰ **Y37.390 Military operations involving other fires, conflagrations and hot substances, military personnel**

☑7ᵗʰ **Y37.391 Military operations involving other fires, conflagrations and hot substances, civilian**

☑5ᵗʰ **Y37.4 Military operations involving firearm discharge and other forms of conventional warfare**

☑6ᵗʰ **Y37.41 Military operations involving rubber bullets**

☑7ᵗʰ **Y37.410 Military operations involving rubber bullets, military personnel**

☑7ᵗʰ **Y37.411 Military operations involving rubber bullets, civilian**

☑6ᵗʰ **Y37.42 Military operations involving firearms pellets**

☑7ᵗʰ **Y37.420 Military operations involving firearms pellets, military personnel**

☑7ᵗʰ **Y37.421 Military operations involving firearms pellets, civilian**

☑6ᵗʰ **Y37.43 Military operations involving other firearms discharge**

Military operations involving bullets NOS

EXCLUDES 1 *military operations involving munitions fragments (Y37.25-)*

military operations involving incendiary bullets (Y37.32-)

☑7ᵗʰ **Y37.430 Military operations involving other firearms discharge, military personnel**

☑7ᵗʰ **Y37.431 Military operations involving other firearms discharge, civilian**

☑6ᵗʰ **Y37.44 Military operations involving unarmed hand to hand combat**

EXCLUDES 1 *military operations involving combat using blunt or piercing object (Y37.45-)*

military operations involving intentional restriction of air and airway (Y37.46-)

military operations involving unintentional restriction of air and airway (Y37.47-)

☑7ᵗʰ **Y37.440 Military operations involving unarmed hand to hand combat, military personnel**

☑7ᵗʰ **Y37.441 Military operations involving unarmed hand to hand combat, civilian**

☑6ᵗʰ **Y37.45 Military operations involving combat using blunt or piercing object**

☑7ᵗʰ **Y37.450 Military operations involving combat using blunt or piercing object, military personnel**

☑7ᵗʰ **Y37.451 Military operations involving combat using blunt or piercing object, civilian**

☑6ᵗʰ **Y37.46 Military operations involving intentional restriction of air and airway**

☑7ᵗʰ **Y37.460 Military operations involving intentional restriction of air and airway, military personnel**

☑7ᵗʰ **Y37.461 Military operations involving intentional restriction of air and airway, civilian**

☑ Additional Char Req   ☑x7ᵗʰ Placeholder   Unacceptable PDx   Questionable PDx   Wrong Procedure   Manifestation   Unspecified Dx   H1-HIC HAC   HCC CMS-HCC Dx   HIV HIV Dx

ICD-10-CM 2020   1261

☑6ᵗʰ **Y37.47** **Military operations involving** unintentional restriction of air and airway

☑7ᵗʰ **Y37.470** **Military operations involving unintentional restriction of air and airway,** military personnel

☑7ᵗʰ **Y37.471** **Military operations involving unintentional restriction of air and airway,** civilian

☑6ᵗʰ **Y37.49** **Military operations involving other forms of conventional warfare**

☑7ᵗʰ **Y37.490** **Military operations involving other forms of conventional warfare,** military personnel

☑7ᵗʰ **Y37.491** **Military operations involving other forms of conventional warfare,** civilian

☑5ᵗʰ **Y37.5** **Military operations involving** nuclear weapons

Military operation involving dirty bomb NOS

☑6ᵗʰ **Y37.50** **Military operations involving unspecified effect of nuclear weapon**

☑7ᵗʰ **Y37.500** **Military operations involving unspecified effect of nuclear weapon,** military personnel

☑7ᵗʰ **Y37.501** **Military operations involving unspecified effect of nuclear weapon,** civilian

☑6ᵗʰ **Y37.51** **Military operations involving** direct blast effect **of nuclear weapon**

Military operations involving blast pressure of nuclear weapon

☑7ᵗʰ **Y37.510** **Military operations involving direct blast effect of nuclear weapon,** military personnel

☑7ᵗʰ **Y37.511** **Military operations involving direct blast effect of nuclear weapon,** civilian

☑6ᵗʰ **Y37.52** **Military operations involving** indirect blast effect **of nuclear weapon**

Military operations involving being thrown by blast of nuclear weapon

Military operations involving being struck or crushed by blast debris of nuclear weapon

☑7ᵗʰ **Y37.520** **Military operations involving indirect blast effect of nuclear weapon,** military personnel

☑7ᵗʰ **Y37.521** **Military operations involving indirect blast effect of nuclear weapon,** civilian

☑6ᵗʰ **Y37.53** **Military operations involving** thermal radiation effect **of nuclear weapon**

Military operations involving direct heat from nuclear weapon

Military operation involving fireball effects from nuclear weapon

☑7ᵗʰ **Y37.530** **Military operations involving thermal radiation effect of nuclear weapon,** military personnel

☑7ᵗʰ **Y37.531** **Military operations involving thermal radiation effect of nuclear weapon,** civilian

☑6ᵗʰ **Y37.54** **Military operation involving** nuclear radiation effects of nuclear weapon

Military operation involving acute radiation exposure from nuclear weapon

Military operation involving exposure to immediate ionizing radiation from nuclear weapon

Military operation involving fallout exposure from nuclear weapon

Military operation involving secondary effects of nuclear weapons

☑7ᵗʰ **Y37.540** **Military operation involving nuclear radiation effects of nuclear weapon,** military personnel

☑7ᵗʰ **Y37.541** **Military operation involving nuclear radiation effects of nuclear weapon,** civilian

☑6ᵗʰ **Y37.59** **Military operation involving other effects of nuclear weapons**

☑7ᵗʰ **Y37.590** **Military operation involving other effects of nuclear weapons,** military personnel

☑7ᵗʰ **Y37.591** **Military operation involving other effects of nuclear weapons,** civilian

☑5ᵗʰ **Y37.6** **Military operations involving** biological weapons

☑6ᵗʰ **Y37.6X** **Military operations involving biological weapons**

☑7ᵗʰ **Y37.6X0** **Military operations involving biological weapons,** military personnel

☑7ᵗʰ **Y37.6X1** **Military operations involving biological weapons,** civilian

☑5ᵗʰ **Y37.7** **Military operations involving chemical weapons and other forms of unconventional warfare**

EXCLUDES 1   military operations involving incendiary devices (Y36.3-, Y36.5-)

☑6ᵗʰ **Y37.7X** **Military operations involving** chemical weapons and other forms of unconventional warfare

☑7ᵗʰ **Y37.7X0** **Military operations involving chemical weapons and other forms of unconventional warfare,** military personnel

☑7ᵗʰ **Y37.7X1** **Military operations involving chemical weapons and other forms of unconventional warfare,** civilian

☑5ᵗʰ **Y37.9** **Other and unspecified military operations**

☑x7ᵗʰ **Y37.90** **Military operations, unspecified**

☑x7ᵗʰ **Y37.91** **Military operations involving unspecified** weapon of mass destruction [WMD]

☑x7ᵗʰ **Y37.92** **Military operations involving** friendly fire

☑4ᵗʰ **Y38** **Terrorism**

NOTE   These codes are for use to identify injuries resulting from the unlawful use of force or violence against persons or property to intimidate or coerce a Government, the civilian population, or any segment thereof, in furtherance of political or social objective

Use additional code for place of occurrence (Y92.-)

☑5ᵗʰ **Y38.0** **Terrorism involving explosion of marine weapons**

Terrorism involving depth-charge

Terrorism involving marine mine

Terrorism involving mine NOS, at sea or in harbor

Terrorism involving sea-based artillery shell

Terrorism involving torpedo

Terrorism involving underwater blast

☑6ᵗʰ **Y38.0X** **Terrorism involving explosion of** marine weapons

☑7ᵗʰ **Y38.0X1** **Terrorism involving explosion of marine weapons,** public safety official injured

☑7ᵗʰ **Y38.0X2** **Terrorism involving explosion of marine weapons,** civilian injured

☑7ᵗʰ **Y38.0X3** **Terrorism involving explosion of marine weapons,** terrorist injured

☑5ᵗʰ **Y38.1** **Terrorism involving destruction of aircraft**

Terrorism involving aircraft burned

Terrorism involving aircraft exploded

Terrorism involving aircraft being shot down

Terrorism involving aircraft used as a weapon

☑6ᵗʰ **Y38.1X** **Terrorism involving** destruction of aircraft

☑7ᵗʰ **Y38.1X1** **Terrorism involving destruction of aircraft,** public safety official injured

☑7ᵗʰ **Y38.1X2** **Terrorism involving destruction of aircraft,** civilian injured

☑7ᵗʰ **Y38.1X3** **Terrorism involving destruction of aircraft,** terrorist injured

☑5ᵗʰ **Y38.2** **Terrorism involving other explosions and fragments**

Terrorism involving antipersonnel (fragments) bomb

Terrorism involving blast NOS

Terrorism involving explosion NOS

Terrorism involving explosion of breech block

Terrorism involving explosion of cannon block

Terrorism involving explosion (fragments) of artillery shell

Terrorism involving explosion (fragments) of bomb

Terrorism involving explosion (fragments) of grenade

Terrorism involving explosion (fragments) of guided missile

Terrorism involving explosion (fragments) of land mine

Terrorism involving explosion of mortar bomb

Terrorism involving explosion of munitions

Terrorism involving explosion (fragments) of rocket

Terrorism involving explosion (fragments) of shell

Terrorism involving shrapnel

Terrorism involving mine NOS, on land

EXCLUDES 1   terrorism involving explosion of nuclear weapon (Y38.5)

terrorism involving suicide bomber (Y38.81)

☑6ᵗʰ **Y38.2X** **Terrorism involving other explosions and fragments**

☑7ᵗʰ **Y38.2X1** **Terrorism involving other explosions and fragments,** public safety official injured

☑7ᵀᴴ **Y38.2X2 Terrorism involving other explosions and fragments,** civilian **injured**

☑7ᵀᴴ **Y38.2X3 Terrorism involving other explosions and fragments,** terrorist **injured**

☑5ᵗʰ **Y38.3 Terrorism involving fires, conflagration and hot substances**

Terrorism involving conflagration NOS
Terrorism involving fire NOS
Terrorism involving petrol bomb

EXCLUDES 1 *terrorism involving fire or heat of nuclear weapon (Y38.5)*

☑6ᵗʰ **Y38.3X Terrorism involving** fires, conflagration and hot substances

☑7ᵀᴴ **Y38.3X1 Terrorism involving fires, conflagration and hot substances,** public safety official injured

☑7ᵀᴴ **Y38.3X2 Terrorism involving fires, conflagration and hot substances,** civilian **injured**

☑7ᵀᴴ **Y38.3X3 Terrorism involving fires, conflagration and hot substances,** terrorist **injured**

☑5ᵗʰ **Y38.4 Terrorism involving firearms**

Terrorism involving carbine bullet
Terrorism involving machine gun bullet
Terrorism involving pellets (shotgun)
Terrorism involving pistol bullet
Terrorism involving rifle bullet
Terrorism involving rubber (rifle) bullet

☑6ᵗʰ **Y38.4X Terrorism involving** firearms

☑7ᵀᴴ **Y38.4X1 Terrorism involving firearms,** public safety official **injured**

☑7ᵀᴴ **Y38.4X2 Terrorism involving firearms,** civilian **injured**

☑7ᵀᴴ **Y38.4X3 Terrorism involving firearms,** terrorist **injured**

☑5ᵗʰ **Y38.5 Terrorism involving nuclear weapons**

Terrorism involving blast effects of nuclear weapon
Terrorism involving exposure to ionizing radiation from nuclear weapon
Terrorism involving fireball effect of nuclear weapon
Terrorism involving heat from nuclear weapon

☑6ᵗʰ **Y38.5X Terrorism involving** nuclear weapons

☑7ᵀᴴ **Y38.5X1 Terrorism involving nuclear weapons,** public safety official **injured**

☑7ᵀᴴ **Y38.5X2 Terrorism involving nuclear weapons,** civilian **injured**

☑7ᵀᴴ **Y38.5X3 Terrorism involving nuclear weapons,** terrorist **injured**

☑5ᵗʰ **Y38.6 Terrorism involving biological weapons**

Terrorism involving anthrax
Terrorism involving cholera
Terrorism involving smallpox

☑6ᵗʰ **Y38.6X Terrorism involving** biological weapons

☑7ᵀᴴ **Y38.6X1 Terrorism involving biological weapons,** public safety official **injured**

☑7ᵀᴴ **Y38.6X2 Terrorism involving biological weapons,** civilian **injured**

☑7ᵀᴴ **Y38.6X3 Terrorism involving biological weapons,** terrorist **injured**

☑5ᵗʰ **Y38.7 Terrorism involving chemical weapons**

Terrorism involving gases, fumes, chemicals
Terrorism involving hydrogen cyanide
Terrorism involving phosgene
Terrorism involving sarin

☑6ᵗʰ **Y38.7X Terrorism involving** chemical weapons

☑7ᵀᴴ **Y38.7X1 Terrorism involving chemical weapons,** public safety official **injured**

☑7ᵀᴴ **Y38.7X2 Terrorism involving chemical weapons,** civilian **injured**

☑7ᵀᴴ **Y38.7X3 Terrorism involving chemical weapons,** terrorist **injured**

☑5ᵗʰ **Y38.8 Terrorism involving other and unspecified means**

☑x7ᵀᴴ **Y38.80 Terrorism involving unspecified means**

Terrorism NOS

☑6ᵗʰ **Y38.81 Terrorism involving** suicide bomber

☑7ᵀᴴ **Y38.811 Terrorism involving suicide bomber,** public safety official **injured**

☑7ᵀᴴ **Y38.812 Terrorism involving suicide bomber,** civilian **injured**

☑6ᵗʰ **Y38.89 Terrorism involving other means**

Terrorism involving drowning and submersion
Terrorism involving lasers
Terrorism involving piercing or stabbing instruments

☑7ᵀᴴ **Y38.891 Terrorism involving other means,** public safety official **injured**

☑7ᵀᴴ **Y38.892 Terrorism involving other means,** civilian **injured**

☑7ᵀᴴ **Y38.893 Terrorism involving other means,** terrorist **injured**

☑5ᵗʰ **Y38.9 Terrorism, secondary effects**

NOTE This code is for use to identify conditions occurring subsequent to a terrorist attack not those that are due to the initial terrorist attack

☑6ᵗʰ **Y38.9X Terrorism,** secondary effects

☑7ᵀᴴ **Y38.9X1 Terrorism, secondary effects,** public safety official **injured**

☑7ᵀᴴ **Y38.9X2 Terrorism, secondary effects,** civilian **injured**

COMPLICATIONS OF MEDICAL AND SURGICAL CARE (Y62-Y84)

INCLUDES complications of medical devices
surgical and medical procedures as the cause of abnormal reaction of the patient, or of later complication, without mention of misadventure at the time of the procedure

Misadventures to patients during surgical and medical care (Y62-Y69)

EXCLUDES 1 *surgical and medical procedures as the cause of abnormal reaction of the patient, without mention of misadventure at the time of the procedure (Y83-Y84)*

EXCLUDES 2 *breakdown or malfunctioning of medical device (during procedure) (after implantation) (ongoing use) (Y70-Y82)*

☑4ᵗʰ **Y62 Failure of** sterile precautions **during surgical and medical care**

Y62.0 Failure of sterile precautions during surgical operation

Y62.1 Failure of sterile precautions during infusion or transfusion

Y62.2 Failure of sterile precautions during kidney **HCC** dialysis and other perfusion

Y62.3 Failure of sterile precautions during injection or immunization

Y62.4 Failure of sterile precautions during endoscopic examination

Y62.5 Failure of sterile precautions during heart catheterization

Y62.6 Failure of sterile precautions during aspiration, puncture and other catheterization

Y62.8 Failure of sterile precautions during other surgical and medical care

Y62.9 Failure of sterile precautions during unspecified surgical and medical care

☑4ᵗʰ **Y63 Failure in** dosage **during surgical and medical care**

EXCLUDES 2 *accidental overdose of drug or wrong drug given in error (T36-T50)*

Y63.0 Excessive amount of blood or other fluid given during transfusion or infusion

Y63.1 Incorrect dilution of fluid used during infusion

Y63.2 Overdose of radiation given during therapy

Y63.3 Inadvertent exposure of patient to radiation during medical care

Y63.4 Failure in dosage in electroshock or insulin-shock therapy

Y63.5 Inappropriate temperature in local application and packing

Y63.6 Underdosing and nonadministration of necessary drug, medicament or biological substance
AHA: 2018,4Q,72

Y63.8 Failure in dosage during other surgical and medical care
AHA: 2018,4Q,72

Y63.9 Failure in dosage during unspecified surgical and medical care
AHA: 2018,4Q,72

☑4ᵗʰ **Y64 Contaminated medical or biological** substances

Y64.0 Contaminated medical or biological substance, transfused or infused

Y64.1 Contaminated medical or biological substance, injected or used for immunization

Y64.8 Contaminated medical or biological substance administered by other means

☑ Additional Char Req   ☑x7ᵀᴴ Placeholder   Unacceptable PDx   Questionable PDx   Wrong Procedure   Manifestation   Unspecified Dx   H1-H14 HAC   HCC CMS-HCC Dx   HIV HIV Dx

ICD-10-CM 2020   1263

Y64.9 Contaminated medical or biological substance administered by unspecified means

Administered contaminated medical or biological substance NOS

✓4ᵗʰ Y65 Other misadventures during surgical and medical care

Y65.0 Mismatched blood in transfusion

Y65.1 Wrong fluid used in infusion

Y65.2 Failure in suture or ligature during surgical operation

Y65.3 Endotracheal tube wrongly placed during anesthetic procedure

Y65.4 Failure to introduce or to remove other tube or instrument

✓5ᵗʰ **Y65.5** Performance of wrong procedure (operation)

     Y65.51 Performance of wrong procedure (operation) on correct patient

         Wrong device implanted into correct surgical site

         EXCLUDES 1   *performance of correct procedure (operation) on wrong side or body part (Y65.53)*

     Y65.52 Performance of procedure (operation) on patient not scheduled for surgery

         Performance of procedure (operation) intended for another patient

         Performance of procedure (operation) on wrong patient

     Y65.53 Performance of correct procedure (operation) on wrong side or body part

         Performance of correct procedure (operation) on wrong side

         Performance of correct procedure (operation) on wrong site

Y65.8 Other specified misadventures during surgical and medical care

     AHA: 2019,2Q,23-24

Y66 Nonadministration of surgical and medical care

Premature cessation of surgical and medical care

EXCLUDES 1   *DNR status (Z66)*
            palliative care (Z51.5)

Y69 Unspecified misadventure during surgical and medical care

Medical devices associated with adverse incidents in diagnostic and therapeutic use (Y70-Y82)

INCLUDES   breakdown or malfunction of medical devices (during use) (after implantation) (ongoing use)

EXCLUDES 2   *later complications following use of medical devices without breakdown or malfunctioning of device (Y83-Y84)*

            misadventure to patients during surgical and medical care, classifiable to (Y62-Y69)

            surgical and other medical procedures as the cause of abnormal reaction of the patient, or of later complication, without mention of misadventure at the time of the procedure (Y83-Y84)

✓4ᵗʰ Y70 Anesthesiology devices associated with adverse incidents

Y70.0 Diagnostic and monitoring anesthesiology devices associated with adverse incidents

Y70.1 Therapeutic (nonsurgical) and rehabilitative anesthesiology devices associated with adverse incidents

Y70.2 Prosthetic and other implants, materials and accessory anesthesiology devices associated with adverse incidents

Y70.3 Surgical instruments, materials and anesthesiology devices (including sutures) associated with adverse incidents

Y70.8 Miscellaneous anesthesiology devices associated with adverse incidents, not elsewhere classified

✓4ᵗʰ Y71 Cardiovascular devices associated with adverse incidents

Y71.0 Diagnostic and monitoring cardiovascular devices associated with adverse incidents

Y71.1 Therapeutic (nonsurgical) and rehabilitative cardiovascular devices associated with adverse incidents

Y71.2 Prosthetic and other implants, materials and accessory cardiovascular devices associated with adverse incidents

Y71.3 Surgical instruments, materials and cardiovascular devices (including sutures) associated with adverse incidents

Y71.8 Miscellaneous cardiovascular devices associated with adverse incidents, not elsewhere classified

✓4ᵗʰ Y72 Otorhinolaryngological devices associated with adverse incidents

Y72.0 Diagnostic and monitoring otorhinolaryngological devices associated with adverse incidents

Y72.1 Therapeutic (nonsurgical) and rehabilitative otorhinolaryngological devices associated with adverse incidents

Y72.2 Prosthetic and other implants, materials and accessory otorhinolaryngological devices associated with adverse incidents

Y72.3 Surgical instruments, materials and otorhinolaryngological devices (including sutures) associated with adverse incidents

Y72.8 Miscellaneous otorhinolaryngological devices associated with adverse incidents, not elsewhere classified

✓4ᵗʰ Y73 Gastroenterology and urology devices associated with adverse incidents

Y73.0 Diagnostic and monitoring gastroenterology and urology devices associated with adverse incidents

Y73.1 Therapeutic (nonsurgical) and rehabilitative gastroenterology and urology devices associated with adverse incidents

Y73.2 Prosthetic and other implants, materials and accessory gastroenterology and urology devices associated with adverse incidents

Y73.3 Surgical instruments, materials and gastroenterology and urology devices (including sutures) associated with adverse incidents

Y73.8 Miscellaneous gastroenterology and urology devices associated with adverse incidents, not elsewhere classified

✓4ᵗʰ Y74 General hospital and personal-use devices associated with adverse incidents

Y74.0 Diagnostic and monitoring general hospital and personal-use devices associated with adverse incidents

Y74.1 Therapeutic (nonsurgical) and rehabilitative general hospital and personal-use devices associated with adverse incidents

Y74.2 Prosthetic and other implants, materials and accessory general hospital and personal-use devices associated with adverse incidents

Y74.3 Surgical instruments, materials and general hospital and personal-use devices (including sutures) associated with adverse incidents

Y74.8 Miscellaneous general hospital and personal-use devices associated with adverse incidents, not elsewhere classified

✓4ᵗʰ Y75 Neurological devices associated with adverse incidents

Y75.0 Diagnostic and monitoring neurological devices associated with adverse incidents

Y75.1 Therapeutic (nonsurgical) and rehabilitative neurological devices associated with adverse incidents

Y75.2 Prosthetic and other implants, materials and neurological devices associated with adverse incidents

Y75.3 Surgical instruments, materials and neurological devices (including sutures) associated with adverse incidents

Y75.8 Miscellaneous neurological devices associated with adverse incidents, not elsewhere classified

✓4ᵗʰ Y76 Obstetric and gynecological devices associated with adverse incidents

Y76.0 Diagnostic and monitoring obstetric and gynecological devices associated with adverse incidents ♀

Y76.1 Therapeutic (nonsurgical) and rehabilitative obstetric and gynecological devices associated with adverse incidents ♀

Y76.2 Prosthetic and other implants, materials and accessory obstetric and gynecological devices associated with adverse incidents ♀

Y76.3 Surgical instruments, materials and obstetric and gynecological devices (including sutures) associated with adverse incidents ♀

Y76.8 Miscellaneous obstetric and gynecological devices associated with adverse incidents, not elsewhere classified ♀

✓4ᵗʰ Y77 Ophthalmic devices associated with adverse incidents

Y77.0 Diagnostic and monitoring ophthalmic devices associated with adverse incidents

Y77.1 Therapeutic (nonsurgical) and rehabilitative ophthalmic devices associated with adverse incidents

Y77.2 Prosthetic and other implants, materials and accessory ophthalmic devices associated with adverse incidents

Y77.3 Surgical instruments, materials and ophthalmic devices (including sutures) associated with adverse incidents

Y77.8 Miscellaneous ophthalmic devices associated with adverse incidents, not elsewhere classified

✓4ᵗʰ Y78 Radiological devices associated with adverse incidents

Y78.0 Diagnostic and monitoring radiological devices associated with adverse incidents

Y78.1 Therapeutic (nonsurgical) and rehabilitative radiological devices associated with adverse incidents

N Newborn: 0   P Pediatric: 0-17   M Maternity: 9-64   A Adult: 15-124   MCC Major Complication/Comorbidity   CC Complication/Comorbidity   SW Severe Wound Dx

1264   ICD-10-CM 2020

Y78.2 Prosthetic and other implants, materials and accessory radiological devices associated with adverse incidents

Y78.3 Surgical instruments, materials and radiological devices (including sutures) associated with adverse incidents

Y78.8 Miscellaneous radiological devices associated with adverse incidents, not elsewhere classified

✓4ᵗʰ **Y79 Orthopedic devices associated with adverse incidents**

Y79.0 Diagnostic and monitoring orthopedic devices associated with adverse incidents

Y79.1 Therapeutic (nonsurgical) and rehabilitative orthopedic devices associated with adverse incidents

Y79.2 Prosthetic and other implants, materials and accessory orthopedic devices associated with adverse incidents

Y79.3 Surgical instruments, materials and orthopedic devices (including sutures) associated with adverse incidents

Y79.8 Miscellaneous orthopedic devices associated with adverse incidents, not elsewhere classified

✓4ᵗʰ **Y80 Physical medicine devices associated with adverse incidents**

Y80.0 Diagnostic and monitoring physical medicine devices associated with adverse incidents

Y80.1 Therapeutic (nonsurgical) and rehabilitative physical medicine devices associated with adverse incidents

Y80.2 Prosthetic and other implants, materials and accessory physical medicine devices associated with adverse incidents

Y80.3 Surgical instruments, materials and physical medicine devices (including sutures) associated with adverse incidents

Y80.8 Miscellaneous physical medicine devices associated with adverse incidents, not elsewhere classified

✓4ᵗʰ **Y81 General- and plastic-surgery devices associated with adverse incidents**

Y81.0 Diagnostic and monitoring general- and plastic-surgery devices associated with adverse incidents

Y81.1 Therapeutic (nonsurgical) and rehabilitative general- and plastic-surgery devices associated with adverse incidents

Y81.2 Prosthetic and other implants, materials and accessory general- and plastic-surgery devices associated with adverse incidents

Y81.3 Surgical instruments, materials and general- and plastic-surgery devices (including sutures) associated with adverse incidents

Y81.8 Miscellaneous general- and plastic-surgery devices associated with adverse incidents, not elsewhere classified

✓4ᵗʰ **Y82 Other and unspecified medical devices associated with adverse incidents**

Y82.8 Other medical devices associated with adverse incidents

Y82.9 Unspecified medical devices associated with adverse incidents

Surgical and other medical procedures as the cause of abnormal reaction of the patient, or of later complication, without mention of misadventure at the time of the procedure (Y83-Y84)

EXCLUDES 1   misadventures to patients during surgical and medical care, classifiable to (Y62-Y69)

EXCLUDES 2   breakdown or malfunctioning of medical device (during procedure) (after implantation) (ongoing use) (Y70-Y82)

✓4ᵗʰ **Y83 Surgical operation and other surgical procedures as the cause of abnormal reaction of the patient, or of later complication, without mention of misadventure at the time of the procedure**

Y83.0 Surgical operation with transplant of whole organ as the cause of abnormal reaction of the patient, or of later complication, without mention of misadventure at the time of the procedure

Y83.1 Surgical operation with implant of artificial internal device as the cause of abnormal reaction of the patient, or of later complication, without mention of misadventure at the time of the procedure

Y83.2 Surgical operation with anastomosis, bypass or graft as the cause of abnormal reaction of the patient, or of later complication, without mention of misadventure at the time of the procedure

Y83.3 Surgical operation with formation of external stoma as the cause of abnormal reaction of the patient, or of later complication, without mention of misadventure at the time of the procedure

Y83.4 Other reconstructive surgery as the cause of abnormal reaction of the patient, or of later complication, without mention of misadventure at the time of the procedure

Y83.5 Amputation of limb(s) as the cause of abnormal reaction of the patient, or of later complication, without mention of misadventure at the time of the procedure

Y83.6 Removal of other organ (partial) (total) as the cause of abnormal reaction of the patient, or of later complication, without mention of misadventure at the time of the procedure

Y83.8 Other surgical procedures as the cause of abnormal reaction of the patient, or of later complication, without mention of misadventure at the time of the procedure

Y83.9 Surgical procedure, unspecified as the cause of abnormal reaction of the patient, or of later complication, without mention of misadventure at the time of the procedure

✓4ᵗʰ **Y84 Other medical procedures as the cause of abnormal reaction of the patient, or of later complication, without mention of misadventure at the time of the procedure**

Y84.0 Cardiac catheterization as the cause of abnormal reaction of the patient, or of later complication, without mention of misadventure at the time of the procedure

Y84.1 Kidney dialysis as the cause of abnormal reaction of the patient, or of later complication, without mention of misadventure at the time of the procedure

Y84.2 Radiological procedure and radiotherapy as the cause of abnormal reaction of the patient, or of later complication, without mention of misadventure at the time of the procedure
AHA: 2019,1Q,21; 2017,1Q,33

Y84.3 Shock therapy as the cause of abnormal reaction of the patient, or of later complication, without mention of misadventure at the time of the procedure

Y84.4 Aspiration of fluid as the cause of abnormal reaction of the patient, or of later complication, without mention of misadventure at the time of the procedure

Y84.5 Insertion of gastric or duodenal sound as the cause of abnormal reaction of the patient, or of later complication, without mention of misadventure at the time of the procedure

Y84.6 Urinary catheterization as the cause of abnormal reaction of the patient, or of later complication, without mention of misadventure at the time of the procedure

Y84.7 Blood-sampling as the cause of abnormal reaction of the patient, or of later complication, without mention of misadventure at the time of the procedure

Y84.8 Other medical procedures as the cause of abnormal reaction of the patient, or of later complication, without mention of misadventure at the time of the procedure
AHA: 2014,4Q,24

Y84.9 Medical procedure, unspecified as the cause of abnormal reaction of the patient, or of later complication, without mention of misadventure at the time of the procedure

Supplementary factors related to causes of morbidity classified elsewhere (Y90-Y99)

NOTE These categories may be used to provide supplementary information concerning causes of morbidity. They are not to be used for single-condition coding.

✓4ᵗʰ **Y90 Evidence of alcohol involvement determined by blood alcohol level**

Code first any associated alcohol related disorders (F10)

Y90.0 Blood alcohol level of less than 20 mg/100 ml

Y90.1 Blood alcohol level of 20-39 mg/100 ml

Y90.2 Blood alcohol level of 40-59 mg/100 ml

Y90.3 Blood alcohol level of 60-79 mg/100 ml

Y90.4 Blood alcohol level of 80-99 mg/100 ml

Y90.5 Blood alcohol level of 100-119 mg/100 ml

Y90.6 Blood alcohol level of 120-199 mg/100 ml

Y90.7 Blood alcohol level of 200-239 mg/100 ml

Y90.8 Blood alcohol level of 240 mg/100 ml or more

Y90.9 Presence of alcohol in blood, level not specified

Chapter 20. External Causes of Morbidity

✓4ᵗʰ Y92 Place of occurrence of the external cause

The following category is for use, when relevant, to identify the place of occurrence of the external cause. Use in conjunction with an activity code.

Place of occurrence should be recorded only at the initial encounter for treatment

✓5ᵗʰ Y92.0 Non-institutional (private) residence as the place of occurrence of the external cause

EXCLUDES 1   *abandoned or derelict house (Y92.89)*

home under construction but not yet occupied (Y92.6-)

institutional place of residence (Y92.1-)

✓6ᵗʰ Y92.00 Unspecified non-institutional (private) residence as the place of occurrence of the external cause

Y92.000 **Kitchen** of unspecified non-institutional (private) residence as the place of occurrence of the external cause

Y92.001 **Dining room** of unspecified non-institutional (private) residence as the place of occurrence of the external cause

Y92.002 **Bathroom** of unspecified non-institutional (private) residence single-family (private) house as the place of occurrence of the external cause

Y92.003 **Bedroom** of unspecified non-institutional (private) residence as the place of occurrence of the external cause

Y92.007 **Garden or yard** of unspecified non-institutional (private) residence as the place of occurrence of the external cause

Y92.008 **Other place** in unspecified non-institutional (private) residence as the place of occurrence of the external cause

Y92.009 **Unspecified place** in unspecified non-institutional (private) residence as the place of occurrence of the external cause

Home (NOS) as the place of occurrence of the external cause

✓6ᵗʰ Y92.01 Single-family non-institutional (private) house as the place of occurrence of the external cause

Farmhouse as the place of occurrence of the external cause

EXCLUDES 1   *barn (Y92.71)*

chicken coop or hen house (Y92.72)

farm field (Y92.73)

orchard (Y92.74)

single family mobile home or trailer (Y92.02-)

slaughter house (Y92.86)

Y92.010 **Kitchen** of single-family (private) house as the place of occurrence of the external cause

Y92.011 **Dining room** of single-family (private) house as the place of occurrence of the external cause

Y92.012 **Bathroom** of single-family (private) house as the place of occurrence of the external cause

Y92.013 **Bedroom** of single-family (private) house as the place of occurrence of the external cause

Y92.014 **Private driveway** to single-family (private) house as the place of occurrence of the external cause

Y92.015 **Private garage** of single-family (private) house as the place of occurrence of the external cause

Y92.016 **Swimming-pool** in single-family (private) house or garden as the place of occurrence of the external cause

Y92.017 **Garden or yard** in single-family (private) house as the place of occurrence of the external cause

Y92.018 **Other place** in single-family (private) house as the place of occurrence of the external cause

Y92.019 **Unspecified place** in single-family (private) house as the place of occurrence of the external cause

✓6ᵗʰ Y92.02 Mobile home as the place of occurrence of the external cause

Y92.020 **Kitchen** in mobile home as the place of occurrence of the external cause

Y92.021 **Dining room** in mobile home as the place of occurrence of the external cause

Y92.022 **Bathroom** in mobile home as the place of occurrence of the external cause

Y92.023 **Bedroom** in mobile home as the place of occurrence of the external cause

Y92.024 **Driveway** of mobile home as the place of occurrence of the external cause

Y92.025 **Garage** of mobile home as the place of occurrence of the external cause

Y92.026 **Swimming-pool** of mobile home as the place of occurrence of the external cause

Y92.027 **Garden or yard** of mobile home as the place of occurrence of the external cause

Y92.028 **Other place** in mobile home as the place of occurrence of the external cause

Y92.029 **Unspecified place** in mobile home as the place of occurrence of the external cause

✓6ᵗʰ Y92.03 Apartment as the place of occurrence of the external cause

Condominium as the place of occurrence of the external cause

Co-op apartment as the place of occurrence of the external cause

Y92.030 **Kitchen** in apartment as the place of occurrence of the external cause

Y92.031 **Bathroom** in apartment as the place of occurrence of the external cause

Y92.032 **Bedroom** in apartment as the place of occurrence of the external cause

Y92.038 **Other place** in apartment as the place of occurrence of the external cause

Y92.039 **Unspecified place** in apartment as the place of occurrence of the external cause

✓6ᵗʰ Y92.04 Boarding-house as the place of occurrence of the external cause

Y92.040 **Kitchen** in boarding-house as the place of occurrence of the external cause

Y92.041 **Bathroom** in boarding-house as the place of occurrence of the external cause

Y92.042 **Bedroom** in boarding-house as the place of occurrence of the external cause

Y92.043 **Driveway** of boarding-house as the place of occurrence of the external cause

Y92.044 **Garage** of boarding-house as the place of occurrence of the external cause

Y92.045 **Swimming-pool** of boarding-house as the place of occurrence of the external cause

Y92.046 **Garden or yard** of boarding-house as the place of occurrence of the external cause

Y92.048 **Other place** in boarding-house as the place of occurrence of the external cause

Y92.049 **Unspecified place** in boarding-house as the place of occurrence of the external cause

✓6ᵗʰ Y92.09 Other non-institutional residence as the place of occurrence of the external cause

AHA: 2017,2Q,10

Y92.090 **Kitchen** in other non-institutional residence as the place of occurrence of the external cause

Y92.091 **Bathroom** in other non-institutional residence as the place of occurrence of the external cause

Y92.092 **Bedroom** in other non-institutional residence as the place of occurrence of the external cause

Y92.093 **Driveway** of other non-institutional residence as the place of occurrence of the external cause

Y92.094 **Garage** of other non-institutional residence as the place of occurrence of the external cause

Y92.095 **Swimming-pool** of other non-institutional residence as the place of occurrence of the external cause

Y92.096 **Garden or yard** of other non-institutional residence as the place of occurrence of the external cause

N Newborn: 0   P Pediatric: 0-17   M Maternity: 9-64   A Adult: 15-124   MCC Major Complication/Comorbidity   CC Complication/Comorbidity   SW Severe Wound Dx

1266   ICD-10-CM 2020

Y92.Ø98 Other place in other non-institutional residence as the place of occurrence of the external cause

Y92.Ø99 Unspecified place in other non-institutional residence as the place of occurrence of the external cause

✓5ᵗʰ **Y92.1** Institutional (nonprivate) residence as the place of occurrence of the external cause

Y92.1Ø Unspecified residential institution as the place of occurrence of the external cause

✓6ᵗʰ **Y92.11** Children's home and orphanage as the place of occurrence of the external cause

Y92.11Ø Kitchen in children's home and orphanage as the place of occurrence of the external cause

Y92.111 Bathroom in children's home and orphanage as the place of occurrence of the external cause

Y92.112 Bedroom in children's home and orphanage as the place of occurrence of the external cause

Y92.113 Driveway of children's home and orphanage as the place of occurrence of the external cause

Y92.114 Garage of children's home and orphanage as the place of occurrence of the external cause

Y92.115 Swimming-pool of children's home and orphanage as the place of occurrence of the external cause

Y92.116 Garden or yard of children's home and orphanage as the place of occurrence of the external cause

Y92.118 Other place in children's home and orphanage as the place of occurrence of the external cause

Y92.119 Unspecified place in children's home and orphanage as the place of occurrence of the external cause

✓6ᵗʰ **Y92.12** Nursing home as the place of occurrence of the external cause

Home for the sick as the place of occurrence of the external cause

Hospice as the place of occurrence of the external cause

AHA: 2017,2Q,10

Y92.12Ø Kitchen in nursing home as the place of occurrence of the external cause

Y92.121 Bathroom in nursing home as the place of occurrence of the external cause

Y92.122 Bedroom in nursing home as the place of occurrence of the external cause

Y92.123 Driveway of nursing home as the place of occurrence of the external cause

Y92.124 Garage of nursing home as the place of occurrence of the external cause

Y92.125 Swimming-pool of nursing home as the place of occurrence of the external cause

Y92.126 Garden or yard of nursing home as the place of occurrence of the external cause

Y92.128 Other place in nursing home as the place of occurrence of the external cause

Y92.129 Unspecified place in nursing home as the place of occurrence of the external cause

✓6ᵗʰ **Y92.13** Military base as the place of occurrence of the external cause

EXCLUDES 1　　military training grounds (Y92.84)

Y92.13Ø Kitchen on military base as the place of occurrence of the external cause

Y92.131 Mess hall on military base as the place of occurrence of the external cause

Y92.133 Barracks on military base as the place of occurrence of the external cause

Y92.135 Garage on military base as the place of occurrence of the external cause

Y92.136 Swimming-pool on military base as the place of occurrence of the external cause

Y92.137 Garden or yard on military base as the place of occurrence of the external cause

Y92.138 Other place on military base as the place of occurrence of the external cause

Y92.139 Unspecified place military base as the place of occurrence of the external cause

✓6ᵗʰ **Y92.14** Prison as the place of occurrence of the external cause

Y92.14Ø Kitchen in prison as the place of occurrence of the external cause

Y92.141 Dining room in prison as the place of occurrence of the external cause

Y92.142 Bathroom in prison as the place of occurrence of the external cause

Y92.143 Cell of prison as the place of occurrence of the external cause

Y92.146 Swimming-pool of prison as the place of occurrence of the external cause

Y92.147 Courtyard of prison as the place of occurrence of the external cause

Y92.148 Other place in prison as the place of occurrence of the external cause

Y92.149 Unspecified place in prison as the place of occurrence of the external cause

✓6ᵗʰ **Y92.15** Reform school as the place of occurrence of the external cause

Y92.15Ø Kitchen in reform school as the place of occurrence of the external cause

Y92.151 Dining room in reform school as the place of occurrence of the external cause

Y92.152 Bathroom in reform school as the place of occurrence of the external cause

Y92.153 Bedroom in reform school as the place of occurrence of the external cause

Y92.154 Driveway of reform school as the place of occurrence of the external cause

Y92.155 Garage of reform school as the place of occurrence of the external cause

Y92.156 Swimming-pool of reform school as the place of occurrence of the external cause

Y92.157 Garden or yard of reform school as the place of occurrence of the external cause

Y92.158 Other place in reform school as the place of occurrence of the external cause

Y92.159 Unspecified place in reform school as the place of occurrence of the external cause

✓6ᵗʰ **Y92.16** School dormitory as the place of occurrence of the external cause

EXCLUDES 1　　reform school as the place of occurrence of the external cause (Y92.15-)

school buildings and grounds as the place of occurrence of the external cause (Y92.2-)

school sports and athletic areas as the place of occurrence of the external cause (Y92.3-)

Y92.16Ø Kitchen in school dormitory as the place of occurrence of the external cause

Y92.161 Dining room in school dormitory as the place of occurrence of the external cause

Y92.162 Bathroom in school dormitory as the place of occurrence of the external cause

Y92.163 Bedroom in school dormitory as the place of occurrence of the external cause

Y92.168 Other place in school dormitory as the place of occurrence of the external cause

Y92.169 Unspecified place in school dormitory as the place of occurrence of the external cause

✓6ᵗʰ **Y92.19** Other specified residential institution as the place of occurrence of the external cause

AHA: 2017,2Q,10

Y92.19Ø Kitchen in other specified residential institution as the place of occurrence of the external cause

Y92.191 Dining room in other specified residential institution as the place of occurrence of the external cause

Y92.192 Bathroom in other specified residential institution as the place of occurrence of the external cause

Y92.193 Bedroom in other specified residential institution as the place of occurrence of the external cause

Y92.194 Driveway of other specified residential institution as the place of occurrence of the external cause

Y92.195   **Garage** of other specified residential institution as the place of occurrence of the external cause

Y92.196   **Pool** of other specified residential institution as the place of occurrence of the external cause

Y92.197   **Garden or yard** of other specified residential institution as the place of occurrence of the external cause

Y92.198   **Other place** in other specified residential institution as the place of occurrence of the external cause

Y92.199   Unspecified place in other specified residential institution as the place of occurrence of the external cause

√5ᵗʰ   **Y92.2**   **School, other institution and public administrative area as the place of occurrence of the external cause**
Building and adjacent grounds used by the general public or by a particular group of the public

> EXCLUDES 1   *building under construction as the place of occurrence of the external cause (Y92.6)*
> *residential institution as the place of occurrence of the external cause (Y92.1)*
> *school dormitory as the place of occurrence of the external cause (Y92.16-)*
> *sports and athletics area of schools as the place of occurrence of the external cause (Y92.3-)*

√6ᵗʰ   **Y92.21**   **School (private) (public) (state) as the place of occurrence of the external cause**

Y92.210   **Daycare** center as the place of occurrence of the external cause

Y92.211   **Elementary school** as the place of occurrence of the external cause
Kindergarten as the place of occurrence of the external cause

Y92.212   **Middle school** as the place of occurrence of the external cause

Y92.213   **High school** as the place of occurrence of the external cause
AHA: 2012,4Q,108

Y92.214   **College** as the place of occurrence of the external cause
University as the place of occurrence of the external cause

Y92.215   **Trade school** as the place of occurrence of the external cause

Y92.218   **Other school** as the place of occurrence of the external cause

Y92.219   Unspecified school as the place of occurrence of the external cause

Y92.22   **Religious institution** as the place of occurrence of the external cause
Church as the place of occurrence of the external cause
Mosque as the place of occurrence of the external cause
Synagogue as the place of occurrence of the external cause

√6ᵗʰ   **Y92.23**   **Hospital** as the place of occurrence of the external cause

> EXCLUDES 1   *ambulatory (outpatient) health services establishments (Y92.53-)*
> *home for the sick as the place of occurrence of the external cause (Y92.12-)*
> *hospice as the place of occurrence of the external cause (Y92.12-)*
> *nursing home as the place of occurrence of the external cause (Y92.12-)*

Y92.230   **Patient room** in hospital as the place of occurrence of the external cause

Y92.231   **Patient bathroom** in hospital as the place of occurrence of the external cause

Y92.232   **Corridor** of hospital as the place of occurrence of the external cause

Y92.233   **Cafeteria** of hospital as the place of occurrence of the external cause

Y92.234   **Operating room** of hospital as the place of occurrence of the external cause

Y92.238   **Other place** in hospital as the place of occurrence of the external cause

Y92.239   Unspecified place in hospital as the place of occurrence of the external cause

√6ᵗʰ   **Y92.24**   **Public administrative building as the place of occurrence of the external cause**

Y92.240   **Courthouse** as the place of occurrence of the external cause

Y92.241   **Library** as the place of occurrence of the external cause

Y92.242   **Post office** as the place of occurrence of the external cause

Y92.243   **City hall** as the place of occurrence of the external cause

Y92.248   **Other** public administrative building as the place of occurrence of the external cause

√6ᵗʰ   **Y92.25**   **Cultural building** as the place of occurrence of the external cause

Y92.250   **Art Gallery** as the place of occurrence of the external cause

Y92.251   **Museum** as the place of occurrence of the external cause

Y92.252   **Music hall** as the place of occurrence of the external cause

Y92.253   **Opera house** as the place of occurrence of the external cause

Y92.254   **Theater (live)** as the place of occurrence of the external cause

Y92.258   **Other cultural** public building as the place of occurrence of the external cause

Y92.26   **Movie house or cinema** as the place of occurrence of the external cause

Y92.29   **Other specified public building** as the place of occurrence of the external cause
Assembly hall as the place of occurrence of the external cause
Clubhouse as the place of occurrence of the external cause

√5ᵗʰ   **Y92.3**   **Sports and athletics area as the place of occurrence of the external cause**

√6ᵗʰ   **Y92.31**   **Athletic court** as the place of occurrence of the external cause

> EXCLUDES 1   *tennis court in private home or garden (Y92.09)*

Y92.310   **Basketball** court as the place of occurrence of the external cause

Y92.311   **Squash** court as the place of occurrence of the external cause

Y92.312   **Tennis** court as the place of occurrence of the external cause

Y92.318   **Other athletic court** as the place of occurrence of the external cause

√6ᵗʰ   **Y92.32**   **Athletic field** as the place of occurrence of the external cause

Y92.320   **Baseball** field as the place of occurrence of the external cause

Y92.321   **Football** field as the place of occurrence of the external cause

Y92.322   **Soccer** field as the place of occurrence of the external cause

Y92.328   **Other athletic field** as the place of occurrence of the external cause
Cricket field as the place of occurrence of the external cause
Hockey field as the place of occurrence of the external cause

√6ᵗʰ   **Y92.33**   **Skating rink** as the place of occurrence of the external cause

Y92.330   **Ice skating** rink (indoor) (outdoor) as the place of occurrence of the external cause

Y92.331   **Roller skating** rink as the place of occurrence of the external cause

Y92.34   **Swimming pool (public)** as the place of occurrence of the external cause

> EXCLUDES 1   *swimming pool in private home or garden (Y92.016)*

N Newborn: 0   P Pediatric: 0-17   M Maternity: 9-64   A Adult: 15-124   MCC Major Complication/Comorbidity   CC Complication/Comorbidity   SW Severe Wound Dx

1268   ICD-10-CM 2020

Y92.39   **Other specified sports and athletic area as the place of occurrence of the external cause**
> Golf-course as the place of occurrence of the external cause
> Gymnasium as the place of occurrence of the external cause
> Riding-school as the place of occurrence of the external cause
> Stadium as the place of occurrence of the external cause

√5ᵗʰ Y92.4   **Street, highway and other paved roadways as the place of occurrence of the external cause**
> **EXCLUDES 1**   *private driveway of residence (Y92.014, Y92.024, Y92.043, Y92.093, Y92.113, Y92.123, Y92.154, Y92.194)*

√6ᵗʰ Y92.41   **Street and highway as the place of occurrence of the external cause**

Y92.410   **Unspecified street and highway as the place of occurrence of the external cause**
> Road NOS as the place of occurrence of the external cause

Y92.411   **Interstate highway as the place of occurrence of the external cause**
> Freeway as the place of occurrence of the external cause
> Motorway as the place of occurrence of the external cause

Y92.412   **Parkway as the place of occurrence of the external cause**

Y92.413   **State road as the place of occurrence of the external cause**

Y92.414   **Local residential or business street as the place of occurrence of the external cause**

Y92.415   **Exit ramp or entrance ramp of street or highway as the place of occurrence of the external cause**

√6ᵗʰ Y92.48   **Other paved roadways as the place of occurrence of the external cause**

Y92.480   **Sidewalk as the place of occurrence of the external cause**

Y92.481   **Parking lot as the place of occurrence of the external cause**

Y92.482   **Bike path as the place of occurrence of the external cause**

Y92.488   **Other paved roadways as the place of occurrence of the external cause**

√5ᵗʰ Y92.5   **Trade and service area as the place of occurrence of the external cause**
> **EXCLUDES 1**   *garage in private home (Y92.015)*
> *schools and other public administration buildings (Y92.2-)*

√6ᵗʰ Y92.51   **Private commercial establishments as the place of occurrence of the external cause**

Y92.510   **Bank as the place of occurrence of the external cause**

Y92.511   **Restaurant or café as the place of occurrence of the external cause**

Y92.512   **Supermarket, store or market as the place of occurrence of the external cause**

Y92.513   **Shop (commercial) as the place of occurrence of the external cause**

√6ᵗʰ Y92.52   **Service areas as the place of occurrence of the external cause**

Y92.520   **Airport as the place of occurrence of the external cause**

Y92.521   **Bus station as the place of occurrence of the external cause**

Y92.522   **Railway station as the place of occurrence of the external cause**

Y92.523   **Highway rest stop as the place of occurrence of the external cause**

Y92.524   **Gas station as the place of occurrence of the external cause**
> Petroleum station as the place of occurrence of the external cause
> Service station as the place of occurrence of the external cause

√6ᵗʰ Y92.53   **Ambulatory health services establishments as the place of occurrence of the external cause**

Y92.530   **Ambulatory surgery center as the place of occurrence of the external cause**
> Outpatient surgery center, including that connected with a hospital as the place of occurrence of the external cause
> Same day surgery center, including that connected with a hospital as the place of occurrence of the external cause

Y92.531   **Health care provider office as the place of occurrence of the external cause**
> Physician office as the place of occurrence of the external cause

Y92.532   **Urgent care center as the place of occurrence of the external cause**

Y92.538   **Other ambulatory health services establishments as the place of occurrence of the external cause**
> **AHA:** 2019,1Q,21

Y92.59   **Other trade areas as the place of occurrence of the external cause**
> Office building as the place of occurrence of the external cause
> Casino as the place of occurrence of the external cause
> Garage (commercial) as the place of occurrence of the external cause
> Hotel as the place of occurrence of the external cause
> Radio or television station as the place of occurrence of the external cause
> Shopping mall as the place of occurrence of the external cause
> Warehouse as the place of occurrence of the external cause

√5ᵗʰ Y92.6   **Industrial and construction area as the place of occurrence of the external cause**

Y92.61   **Building [any] under construction as the place of occurrence of the external cause**

Y92.62   **Dock or shipyard as the place of occurrence of the external cause**
> Dockyard as the place of occurrence of the external cause
> Dry dock as the place of occurrence of the external cause
> Shipyard as the place of occurrence of the external cause

Y92.63   **Factory as the place of occurrence of the external cause**
> Factory building as the place of occurrence of the external cause
> Factory premises as the place of occurrence of the external cause
> Industrial yard as the place of occurrence of the external cause

Y92.64   **Mine or pit as the place of occurrence of the external cause**
> Mine as the place of occurrence of the external cause

Y92.65   **Oil rig as the place of occurrence of the external cause**
> Pit (coal) (gravel) (sand) as the place of occurrence of the external cause

Y92.69   **Other specified industrial and construction area as the place of occurrence of the external cause**
> Gasworks as the place of occurrence of the external cause
> Power-station (coal) (nuclear) (oil) as the place of occurrence of the external cause
> Tunnel under construction as the place of occurrence of the external cause
> Workshop as the place of occurrence of the external cause

√5ᵗʰ Y92.7   **Farm as the place of occurrence of the external cause**
> Ranch as the place of occurrence of the external cause
> **EXCLUDES 1**   *farmhouse and home premises of farm (Y92.01-)*

Y92.71   **Barn as the place of occurrence of the external cause**

✔ Additional Char Req   √x7ᵗʰ Placeholder   Unacceptable PDx   Questionable PDx   Wrong Procedure   Manifestation   Unspecified Dx   H1-Htd HAC   HCC CMS-HCC Dx   HIV HIV Dx

ICD-10-CM 2020   1269

Chapter 20. External Causes of Morbidity

Y92.39–Y92.71

Y92.72   Chicken coop as the place of occurrence of the external cause
    Hen house as the place of occurrence of the external cause

Y92.73   Farm field as the place of occurrence of the external cause

Y92.74   Orchard as the place of occurrence of the external cause

Y92.79   Other farm location as the place of occurrence of the external cause

✓5ᵗʰ **Y92.8**   Other places as the place of occurrence of the external cause

   ✓6ᵗʰ **Y92.81**   Transport vehicle as the place of occurrence of the external cause
     EXCLUDES 1   transport accidents (V00-V99)

Y92.810   Car as the place of occurrence of the external cause

Y92.811   Bus as the place of occurrence of the external cause

Y92.812   Truck as the place of occurrence of the external cause

Y92.813   Airplane as the place of occurrence of the external cause

Y92.814   Boat as the place of occurrence of the external cause

Y92.815   Train as the place of occurrence of the external cause

Y92.816   Subway car as the place of occurrence of the external cause

Y92.818   Other transport vehicle as the place of occurrence of the external cause

   ✓6ᵗʰ **Y92.82**   Wilderness area

Y92.820   Desert as the place of occurrence of the external cause

Y92.821   Forest as the place of occurrence of the external cause

Y92.828   Other wilderness area as the place of occurrence of the external cause
    Swamp as the place of occurrence of the external cause
    Mountain as the place of occurrence of the external cause
    Marsh as the place of occurrence of the external cause
    Prairie as the place of occurrence of the external cause

   ✓6ᵗʰ **Y92.83**   Recreation area as the place of occurrence of the external cause

Y92.830   Public park as the place of occurrence of the external cause

Y92.831   Amusement park as the place of occurrence of the external cause

Y92.832   Beach as the place of occurrence of the external cause
    Seashore as the place of occurrence of the external cause

Y92.833   Campsite as the place of occurrence of the external cause

Y92.834   Zoological garden (Zoo) as the place of occurrence of the external cause

Y92.838   Other recreation area as the place of occurrence of the external cause

Y92.84   Military training ground as the place of occurrence of the external cause

Y92.85   Railroad track as the place of occurrence of the external cause

Y92.86   Slaughter house as the place of occurrence of the external cause

Y92.89   Other specified places as the place of occurrence of the external cause
    Derelict house as the place of occurrence of the external cause

Y92.9   Unspecified place or not applicable

✓4ᵗʰ **Y93**   **Activity codes**

NOTE   Category Y93 is provided for use to indicate the activity of the person seeking healthcare for an injury or health condition, such as a heart attack while shoveling snow, which resulted from, or was contributed to, by the activity. These codes are appropriate for use for both acute injuries, such as those from chapter 19, and conditions that are due to the long-term, cumulative effects of an activity, such as those from chapter 13. They are also appropriate for use with external cause codes for cause and intent if identifying the activity provides additional information on the event. These codes should be used in conjunction with codes for external cause status (Y99) and place of occurrence (Y92).

This section contains the following broad activity categories:

Y93.0	Activities involving walking and running
Y93.1	Activities involving water and water craft
Y93.2	Activities involving ice and snow
Y93.3	Activities involving climbing, rappelling, and jumping off
Y93.4	Activities involving dancing and other rhythmic movement
Y93.5	Activities involving other sports and athletics played individually
Y93.6	Activities involving other sports and athletics played as a team or group
Y93.7	Activities involving other specified sports and athletics
Y93.A	Activities involving other cardiorespiratory exercise
Y93.B	Activities involving other muscle strengthening exercises
Y93.C	Activities involving computer technology and electronic devices
Y93.D	Activities involving arts and handcrafts
Y93.E	Activities involving personal hygiene and interior property and clothing maintenance
Y93.F	Activities involving caregiving
Y93.G	Activities involving food preparation, cooking and grilling
Y93.H	Activities involving exterior property and land maintenance, building and construction
Y93.I	Activities involving roller coasters and other types of external motion
Y93.J	Activities involving playing musical instrument
Y93.K	Activities involving animal care
Y93.8	Activities, other specified
Y93.9	Activity, unspecified

✓5ᵗʰ **Y93.0**   **Activities involving walking and running**
   EXCLUDES 1   activity, walking an animal (Y93.K1)
             activity, walking or running on a treadmill (Y93.A1)

Y93.01   Activity, walking, marching and hiking
    Activity, walking, marching and hiking on level or elevated terrain
    EXCLUDES 1   activity, mountain climbing (Y93.31)

Y93.02   Activity, running

✓5ᵗʰ **Y93.1**   **Activities involving water and water craft**
   EXCLUDES 1   activities involving ice (Y93.2-)

Y93.11   Activity, swimming

Y93.12   Activity, springboard and platform diving

Y93.13   Activity, water polo

Y93.14   Activity, water aerobics and water exercise

Y93.15   Activity, underwater diving and snorkeling
    Activity, SCUBA diving

Y93.16   Activity, rowing, canoeing, kayaking, rafting and tubing
    Activity, canoeing, kayaking, rafting and tubing in calm and turbulent water

Y93.17   Activity, water skiing and wake boarding

Y93.18   Activity, surfing, windsurfing and boogie boarding
    Activity, water sliding

Y93.19   Activity, other involving water and watercraft
    Activity involving water NOS
    Activity, parasailing
    Activity, water survival training and testing

Ⓝ Newborn: 0   Ⓟ Pediatric: 0-17   Ⓜ Maternity: 9-64   Ⓐ Adult: 15-124   **MCC** Major Complication/Comorbidity   **CC** Complication/Comorbidity   **SW** Severe Wound Dx

1270   ICD-10-CM 2020

✓5ᵗʰ **Y93.2 Activities involving ice and snow**
> **EXCLUDES 1** *activity, shoveling ice and snow (Y93.H1)*

Y93.21 Activity, ice skating
Activity, figure skating (singles) (pairs)
Activity, ice dancing
> **EXCLUDES 1** *activity, ice hockey (Y93.22)*

Y93.22 Activity, ice hockey

Y93.23 Activity, snow (alpine) (downhill) skiing, snowboarding, sledding, tobogganing and snow tubing
> **EXCLUDES 1** *activity, cross country skiing (Y93.24)*

Y93.24 Activity, cross country skiing
Activity, nordic skiing

Y93.29 Activity, other involving ice and snow
Activity involving ice and snow NOS

✓5ᵗʰ **Y93.3 Activities involving climbing, rappelling and jumping off**
> **EXCLUDES 1** *activity, hiking on level or elevated terrain (Y93.Ø1)*
> *activity, jumping rope (Y93.56)*
> *activity, trampoline jumping (Y93.44)*

Y93.31 Activity, mountain climbing, rock climbing and wall climbing

Y93.32 Activity, rappelling

Y93.33 Activity, BASE jumping
Activity, Building, Antenna, Span, Earth jumping

Y93.34 Activity, bungee jumping

Y93.35 Activity, hang gliding

Y93.39 Activity, other involving climbing, rappelling and jumping off

✓5ᵗʰ **Y93.4 Activities involving dancing and other rhythmic movement**
> **EXCLUDES 1** *activity, martial arts (Y93.75)*

Y93.41 Activity, dancing
AHA: 2012,4Q,108

Y93.42 Activity, yoga

Y93.43 Activity, gymnastics
Activity, rhythmic gymnastics
> **EXCLUDES 1** *activity, trampolining (Y93.44)*

Y93.44 Activity, trampolining

Y93.45 Activity, cheerleading

Y93.49 Activity, other involving dancing and other rhythmic movements

✓5ᵗʰ **Y93.5 Activities involving other sports and athletics played individually**
> **EXCLUDES 1** *activity, dancing (Y93.41)*
> *activity, gymnastic (Y93.43)*
> *activity, trampolining (Y93.44)*
> *activity, yoga (Y93.42)*

Y93.51 Activity, roller skating (inline) and skateboarding

Y93.52 Activity, horseback riding

Y93.53 Activity, golf

Y93.54 Activity, bowling

Y93.55 Activity, bike riding

Y93.56 Activity, jumping rope

Y93.57 Activity, non-running track and field events
> **EXCLUDES 1** *activity, running (any form) (Y93.Ø2)*

Y93.59 Activity, other involving other sports and athletics played individually
> **EXCLUDES 1** *activities involving climbing, rappelling, and jumping (Y93.3-)*
> *activities involving ice and snow (Y93.2-)*
> *activities involving walking and running (Y93.Ø-)*
> *activities involving water and watercraft (Y93.1-)*

✓5ᵗʰ **Y93.6 Activities involving other sports and athletics played as a team or group**
> **EXCLUDES 1** *activity, ice hockey (Y93.22)*
> *activity, water polo (Y93.13)*

Y93.61 Activity, American tackle football
Activity, football NOS

Y93.62 Activity, American flag or touch football

Y93.63 Activity, rugby

Y93.64 Activity, baseball
Activity, softball

Y93.65 Activity, lacrosse and field hockey

Y93.66 Activity, soccer

Y93.67 Activity, basketball

Y93.68 Activity, volleyball (beach) (court)

Y93.6A Activity, physical games generally associated with school recess, summer camp and children
Activity, capture the flag
Activity, dodge ball
Activity, four square
Activity, kickball

Y93.69 Activity, other involving other sports and athletics played as a team or group
Activity, cricket

✓5ᵗʰ **Y93.7 Activities involving other specified sports and athletics**

Y93.71 Activity, boxing

Y93.72 Activity, wrestling

Y93.73 Activity, racquet and hand sports
Activity, handball
Activity, racquetball
Activity, squash
Activity, tennis

Y93.74 Activity, frisbee
Activity, ultimate frisbee

Y93.75 Activity, martial arts
Activity, combatives

Y93.79 Activity, other specified sports and athletics
> **EXCLUDES 1** *sports and athletics activities specified in categories Y93.Ø-Y93.6*

✓5ᵗʰ **Y93.A Activities involving other cardiorespiratory exercise**
Activities involving physical training

Y93.A1 Activity, exercise machines primarily for cardiorespiratory conditioning
Activity, elliptical and stepper machines
Activity, stationary bike
Activity, treadmill

Y93.A2 Activity, calisthenics
Activity, jumping jacks
Activity, warm up and cool down

Y93.A3 Activity, aerobic and step exercise

Y93.A4 Activity, circuit training

Y93.A5 Activity, obstacle course
Activity, challenge course
Activity, confidence course

Y93.A6 Activity, grass drills
Activity, guerilla drills

Y93.A9 Activity, other involving cardiorespiratory exercise
> **EXCLUDES 1** *activities involving cardiorespiratory exercise specified in categories Y93.Ø-Y93.7*

✓5ᵗʰ **Y93.B Activities involving other muscle strengthening exercises**

Y93.B1 Activity, exercise machines primarily for muscle strengthening

Y93.B2 Activity, push-ups, pull-ups, sit-ups

Y93.B3 Activity, free weights
Activity, barbells
Activity, dumbbells

Y93.B4 Activity, pilates

Y93.B9 Activity, other involving muscle strengthening exercises
> **EXCLUDES 1** *activities involving muscle strengthening specified in categories Y93.Ø-Y93.A*

✓5ᵗʰ **Y93.C Activities involving computer technology and electronic devices**
> **EXCLUDES 1** *activity, electronic musical keyboard or instruments (Y93.J-)*

Y93.C1 Activity, computer keyboarding
Activity, electronic game playing using keyboard or other stationary device

Y93.C2 Activity, hand held interactive electronic device
Activity, cellular telephone and communication device
Activity, electronic game playing using interactive device
> **EXCLUDES 1** *activity, electronic game playing using keyboard or other stationary device (Y93.C1)*

Y93.C9 Activity, other involving computer technology and electronic devices

✓5ᵗʰ **Y93.D Activities involving arts and handcrafts**
> **EXCLUDES 1** *activities involving playing musical instrument (Y93.J-)*

Y93.D1 Activity, knitting and crocheting

Y93.D2   Activity, sewing

Y93.D3   Activity, furniture building and finishing

Activity, furniture repair

Y93.D9   Activity, other involving arts and handcrafts

√5ᵗʰ **Y93.E**   Activities involving personal hygiene and interior property and clothing maintenance

> EXCLUDES 1   activities involving cooking and grilling (Y93.G-)
> activities involving exterior property and land maintenance, building and construction (Y93.H-)
> activities involving caregiving (Y93.F-)
> activity, dishwashing (Y93.G1)
> activity, food preparation (Y93.G1)
> activity, gardening (Y93.H2)

Y93.E1   Activity, personal bathing and showering

Y93.E2   Activity, laundry

Y93.E3   Activity, vacuuming

Y93.E4   Activity, ironing

Y93.E5   Activity, floor mopping and cleaning

Y93.E6   Activity, residential relocation

Activity, packing up and unpacking involved in moving to a new residence

Y93.E8   Activity, other personal hygiene

Y93.E9   Activity, other interior property and clothing maintenance

√5ᵗʰ **Y93.F**   Activities involving caregiving

Activity involving the provider of caregiving

Y93.F1   Activity, caregiving, bathing

Y93.F2   Activity, caregiving, lifting

Y93.F9   Activity, other caregiving

√5ᵗʰ **Y93.G**   Activities involving food preparation, cooking and grilling

Y93.G1   Activity, food preparation and clean up

Activity, dishwashing

Y93.G2   Activity, grilling and smoking food

Y93.G3   Activity, cooking and baking

Activity, use of stove, oven and microwave oven

Y93.G9   Activity, other involving cooking and grilling

√5ᵗʰ **Y93.H**   Activities involving exterior property and land maintenance, building and construction

Y93.H1   Activity, digging, shoveling and raking

Activity, dirt digging

Activity, raking leaves

Activity, snow shoveling

Y93.H2   Activity, gardening and landscaping

Activity, pruning, trimming shrubs, weeding

Y93.H3   Activity, building and construction

Y93.H9   Activity, other involving exterior property and land maintenance, building and construction

√5ᵗʰ **Y93.I**   Activities involving roller coasters and other types of external motion

Y93.I1   Activity, rollercoaster riding

Y93.I9   Activity, other involving external motion

√5ᵗʰ **Y93.J**   Activities involving playing musical instrument

Activity involving playing electric musical instrument

Y93.J1   Activity, piano playing

Activity, musical keyboard (electronic) playing

Y93.J2   Activity, drum and other percussion instrument playing

Y93.J3   Activity, string instrument playing

Y93.J4   Activity, winds and brass instrument playing

√5ᵗʰ **Y93.K**   Activities involving animal care

> EXCLUDES 1   activity, horseback riding (Y93.52)

Y93.K1   Activity, walking an animal

Y93.K2   Activity, milking an animal

Y93.K3   Activity, grooming and shearing an animal

Y93.K9   Activity, other involving animal care

√5ᵗʰ **Y93.8**   Activities, other specified

Y93.81   Activity, refereeing a sports activity

Y93.82   Activity, spectator at an event

Y93.83   Activity, rough housing and horseplay

Y93.84   Activity, sleeping

Y93.85   Activity, choking game

Activity, blackout game

Activity, fainting game

Activity, pass out game

AHA: 2016,4Q,74-76

Y93.89   Activity, other specified

Y93.9   Activity, unspecified

Y95   Nosocomial condition

AHA: 2013,4Q,119

√4ᵗʰ **Y99**   External cause status

> NOTE   A single code from category Y99 should be used in conjunction with the external cause code(s) assigned to a record to indicate the status of the person at the time the event occurred.

Y99.0   Civilian activity done for income or pay

Civilian activity done for financial or other compensation

> EXCLUDES 1   military activity (Y99.1)
> volunteer activity (Y99.2)

Y99.1   Military activity

> EXCLUDES 1   activity of off duty military personnel (Y99.8)

Y99.2   Volunteer activity

> EXCLUDES 1   activity of child or other family member assisting in compensated work of other family member (Y99.8)

Y99.8   Other external cause status

Activity NEC

Activity of child or other family member assisting in compensated work of other family member

Hobby not done for income

Leisure activity

Off-duty activity of military personnel

Recreation or sport not for income or while a student

Student activity

> EXCLUDES 1   civilian activity done for income or compensation (Y99.0)
> military activity (Y99.1)

AHA: 2012,4Q,108

Y99.9   Unspecified external cause status

N Newborn: 0   P Pediatric: 0-17   M Maternity: 9-64   A Adult: 15-124   MCC Major Complication/Comorbidity   CC Complication/Comorbidity   SW Severe Wound Dx

1272   ICD-10-CM 2020

Chapter 21. Factors Influencing Health Status and Contact with Health Services (Z00–Z99)

Chapter-specific Guidelines with Coding Examples

The chapter-specific guidelines from the ICD-10-CM Official Guidelines for Coding and Reporting have been provided below. Along with these guidelines are coding examples, contained in the shaded boxes, that have been developed to help illustrate the coding and/or sequencing guidance found in these guidelines.

Note: The chapter-specific guidelines provide additional information about the use of Z codes for specified encounters.

a. Use of Z Codes in any healthcare setting

Z codes are for use in any healthcare setting. Z codes may be used as either a first-listed (principal diagnosis code in the inpatient setting) or secondary code, depending on the circumstances of the encounter. Certain Z codes may only be used as first-listed or principal diagnosis.

Patient with middle lobe lung cancer admitted for initiation of chemotherapy

Z51.11   **Encounter for antineoplastic chemotherapy**

C34.2   **Malignant neoplasm of middle lobe, bronchus or lung**

Explanation: A Z code can be used as first-listed in this situation based on guidelines in this chapter as well as chapter 2, "Neoplasms."

b. Z Codes indicate a reason for an encounter

Z codes are not procedure codes. A corresponding procedure code must accompany a Z code to describe any procedure performed.

c. Categories of Z Codes

1) Contact/exposure

Category Z20 indicates contact with, and suspected exposure to, communicable diseases. These codes are for patients who do not show any sign or symptom of a disease but are suspected to have been exposed to it by close personal contact with an infected individual or are in an area where a disease is epidemic.

Category Z77, Other contact with and (suspected) exposures hazardous to health, indicates contact with and suspected exposures hazardous to health.

Contact/exposure codes may be used as a first-listed code to explain an encounter for testing, or, more commonly, as a secondary code to identify a potential risk.

2) Inoculations and vaccinations

Code Z23 is for encounters for inoculations and vaccinations. It indicates that a patient is being seen to receive a prophylactic inoculation against a disease. Procedure codes are required to identify the actual administration of the injection and the type(s) of immunizations given. Code Z23 may be used as a secondary code if the inoculation is given as a routine part of preventive health care, such as a well-baby visit.

3) Status

Status codes indicate that a patient is either a carrier of a disease or has the sequelae or residual of a past disease or condition. This includes such things as the presence of prosthetic or mechanical devices resulting from past treatment. A status code is informative, because the status may affect the course of treatment and its outcome. A status code is distinct from a history code. The history code indicates that the patient no longer has the condition.

A status code should not be used with a diagnosis code from one of the body system chapters, if the diagnosis code includes the information provided by the status code. For example, code Z94.1, Heart transplant status, should not be used with a code from subcategory T86.2, Complications of heart transplant. The status code does not provide additional information. The complication code indicates that the patient is a heart transplant patient.

For encounters for weaning from a mechanical ventilator, assign a code from subcategory J96.1, Chronic respiratory failure, followed by code Z99.11, Dependence on respirator [ventilator] status.

The status Z codes/categories are:

     Z14   Genetic carrier

         Genetic carrier status indicates that a person carries a gene, associated with a particular disease, which may be passed to offspring who may develop that disease. The person does not have the disease and is not at risk of developing the disease.

     Z15   Genetic susceptibility to disease

         Genetic susceptibility indicates that a person has a gene that increases the risk of that person developing the disease.

         Codes from category Z15 should not be used as principal or first-listed codes. If the patient has the condition to which he/she is susceptible, and that condition is the reason for the encounter, the code for the current condition should be sequenced first. If the patient is being seen for follow-up after completed treatment for this condition, and the condition no longer exists, a follow-up code should be sequenced first, followed by the appropriate personal history and genetic susceptibility codes. If the purpose of the encounter is genetic counseling associated with procreative management, code Z31.5, Encounter for genetic counseling, should be assigned as the first-listed code, followed by a code from category Z15. Additional codes should be assigned for any applicable family or personal history.

     Z16   Resistance to antimicrobial drugs

         This code indicates that a patient has a condition that is resistant to antimicrobial drug treatment. Sequence the infection code first.

Penicillin resistant streptococcus pneumoniae meningitis

G00.1   **Pneumococcal meningitis**

Z16.11   **Resistance to penicillins**

Explanation: The status Z code is used to describe the presence of a drug-resistant organism that most likely altered how the meningitis was treated.

     Z17   Estrogen receptor status

     Z18   Retained foreign body fragments

     Z19   Hormone sensitivity malignancy status

     Z21   Asymptomatic HIV infection status

         This code indicates that a patient has tested positive for HIV but has manifested no signs or symptoms of the disease.

     Z22   Carrier of infectious disease

         Carrier status indicates that a person harbors the specific organisms of a disease without manifest symptoms and is capable of transmitting the infection.

     Z28.3   Underimmunization status

     Z33.1   Pregnant state, incidental

         This code is a secondary code only for use when the pregnancy is in no way complicating the reason for visit. Otherwise, a code from the obstetric chapter is required.

     Z66   Do not resuscitate

         This code may be used when it is documented by the provider that a patient is on do not resuscitate status at any time during the stay.

     Z67   Blood type

     Z68   Body mass index (BMI)

         BMI codes should only be assigned when **there is an associated, reportable diagnosis (such as obesity).** Do not assign BMI codes during pregnancy.

         See Section I.B.14 for BMI documentation by clinicians other than the patient's provider.

     Z74.01   Bed confinement status

     Z76.82   Awaiting organ transplant status

     Z78   Other specified health status

         Code Z78.1, Physical restraint status, may be used when it is documented by the provider that a patient has been put in restraints during the current encounter. Please note that this code should not be reported when it is documented by the provider that a patient is temporarily restrained during a procedure.

Chapter 21. Factors Influencing Health Status and Contact with Health Services *(left margin)*

Z79   Long-term (current) drug therapy

Codes from this category indicate a patient's continuous use of a prescribed drug (including such things as aspirin therapy) for the long-term treatment of a condition or for prophylactic use. It is not for use for patients who have addictions to drugs. This subcategory is not for use of medications for detoxification or maintenance programs to prevent withdrawal symptoms in patients with drug dependence (e.g., methadone maintenance for opiate dependence). Assign the appropriate code for the drug dependence instead.

Assign a code from Z79 if the patient is receiving a medication for an extended period as a prophylactic measure (such as for the prevention of deep vein thrombosis) or as treatment of a chronic condition (such as arthritis) or a disease requiring a lengthy course of treatment (such as cancer). Do not assign a code from category Z79 for medication being administered for a brief period of time to treat an acute illness or injury (such as a course of antibiotics to treat acute bronchitis).

Z88   Allergy status to drugs, medicaments and biological substances

Except: Z88.9, Allergy status to unspecified drugs, medicaments and biological substances status

Z89   Acquired absence of limb

Z90   Acquired absence of organs, not elsewhere classified

Z91.0-   Allergy status, other than to drugs and biological substances

Z92.82   Status post administration of tPA (rtPA) in a different facility within the last 24 hours prior to admission to a current facility

Assign code Z92.82, Status post administration of tPA (rtPA) in a different facility within the last 24 hours prior to admission to current facility, as a secondary diagnosis when a patient is received by transfer into a facility and documentation indicates they were administered tissue plasminogen activator (tPA) within the last 24 hours prior to admission to the current facility.

This guideline applies even if the patient is still receiving the tPA at the time they are received into the current facility.

The appropriate code for the condition for which the tPA was administered (such as cerebrovascular disease or myocardial infarction) should be assigned first.

Code Z92.82 is only applicable to the receiving facility record and not to the transferring facility record.

Z93   Artificial opening status

Z94   Transplanted organ and tissue status

Z95   Presence of cardiac and vascular implants and grafts

Z96   Presence of other functional implants

Z97   Presence of other devices

Z98   Other postprocedural states

Assign code Z98.85, Transplanted organ removal status, to indicate that a transplanted organ has been previously removed. This code should not be assigned for the encounter in which the transplanted organ is removed. The complication necessitating removal of the transplant organ should be assigned for that encounter.

See section I.C.19. for information on the coding of organ transplant complications.

Z99   Dependence on enabling machines and devices, not elsewhere classified

Note: Categories Z89-Z90 and Z93-Z99 are for use only if there are no complications or malfunctions of the organ or tissue replaced, the amputation site or the equipment on which the patient is dependent.

4) History (of)

There are two types of history Z codes, personal and family. Personal history codes explain a patient's past medical condition that no longer exists and is not receiving any treatment, but that has the potential for recurrence, and therefore may require continued monitoring.

Family history codes are for use when a patient has a family member(s) who has had a particular disease that causes the patient to be at higher risk of also contracting the disease.

Personal history codes may be used in conjunction with follow-up codes and family history codes may be used in conjunction with screening codes to explain the need for a test or procedure. History codes are also acceptable on any medical record regardless of the reason for visit. A history of an illness, even if no longer present, is important information that may alter the type of treatment ordered.

The history Z code categories are:

Z80   Family history of primary malignant neoplasm

Z81   Family history of mental and behavioral disorders

Z82   Family history of certain disabilities and chronic diseases (leading to disablement)

Z83   Family history of other specific disorders

Z84   Family history of other conditions

Z85   Personal history of malignant neoplasm

Z86   Personal history of certain other diseases

Z87   Personal history of other diseases and conditions

Z91.4-   Personal history of psychological trauma, not elsewhere classified

Z91.5   Personal history of self-harm

Z91.81   History of falling

Z91.82   Personal history of military deployment

Z92   Personal history of medical treatment

Except: Z92.0, Personal history of contraception

Except: Z92.82, Status post administration of tPA (rtPA) in a different facility within the last 24 hours prior to admission to a current facility

Patient has chronic lymphocytic leukemia for which the patient had previous chemotherapy and is now in remission

C91.11   **Chronic lymphocytic leukemia of B-cell type in remission**

Z92.21   **Personal history of antineoplastic chemotherapy**

Explanation: The personal history Z code is used to describe a secondary (supplementary) diagnosis to identify that this patient has had chemotherapy in the past.

5) Screening

Screening is the testing for disease or disease precursors in seemingly well individuals so that early detection and treatment can be provided for those who test positive for the disease (e.g., screening mammogram).

The testing of a person to rule out or confirm a suspected diagnosis because the patient has some sign or symptom is a diagnostic examination, not a screening. In these cases, the sign or symptom is used to explain the reason for the test.

A screening code may be a first-listed code if the reason for the visit is specifically the screening exam. It may also be used as an additional code if the screening is done during an office visit for other health problems. A screening code is not necessary if the screening is inherent to a routine examination, such as a pap smear done during a routine pelvic examination.

Should a condition be discovered during the screening then the code for the condition may be assigned as an additional diagnosis.

The Z code indicates that a screening exam is planned. A procedure code is required to confirm that the screening was performed.

The screening Z codes/categories:

Z11   Encounter for screening for infectious and parasitic diseases

Z12   Encounter for screening for malignant neoplasms

Z13   Encounter for screening for other diseases and disorders

Except: Z13.9, Encounter for screening, unspecified

Z36   Encounter for antenatal screening for mother

6) Observation

There are three observation Z code categories. They are for use in very limited circumstances when a person is being observed for a suspected condition that is ruled out. The observation codes are not for use if an injury or illness or any signs or symptoms related to the suspected condition are present. In such cases the diagnosis/symptom code is used with the corresponding external cause code.

The observation codes are to be used as principal diagnosis only. The only exception to this is when the principal diagnosis is required to be a code from category Z38, Liveborn infants according to place of birth and type of delivery. Then a code from category Z05, Encounter for observation and evaluation of newborn for suspected diseases and conditions ruled out, is sequenced after the Z38 code. Additional codes may be used in addition to the observation code but only if they are unrelated to the suspected condition being observed.

Codes from subcategory Z03.7, Encounter for suspected maternal and fetal conditions ruled out, may either be used as a first-listed or as an additional code assignment depending on the case. They are for use in very limited circumstances on a maternal record when an encounter is for a suspected maternal or fetal condition that is ruled out during that encounter (for example, a maternal or fetal condition may be suspected due to an abnormal test result). These codes should not be used when the condition is confirmed. In those cases, the confirmed condition should be coded. In addition, these codes are not for use if an illness or any signs or symptoms related to the suspected condition or problem are present. In such cases the diagnosis/symptom code is used.

Additional codes may be used in addition to the code from subcategory Z03.7, but only if they are unrelated to the suspected condition being evaluated.

Codes from subcategory Z03.7 may not be used for encounters for antenatal screening of mother. *See Section I.C.21. Screening*.

For encounters for suspected fetal condition that are inconclusive following testing and evaluation, assign the appropriate code from category O35, O36, O40 or O41.

The observation Z code categories:

Z03	Encounter for medical observation for suspected diseases and conditions ruled out
Z04	Encounter for examination and observation for other reasons
	Except: Z04.9, Encounter for examination and observation for unspecified reason
Z05	Encounter for observation and evaluation of newborn for suspected diseases and conditions ruled out

Upon initial examination, a heart murmur was heard in a newborn infant delivered vaginally in the hospital; however, after further observation, any serious cardiac conditions were ruled out.

Z38.00	**Single liveborn infant, delivered vaginally**
Z05.0	**Observation and evaluation of newborn for suspected cardiac condition ruled out**

Explanation: Normally an observation code is used as the principal diagnosis except when the patient is a newborn. A code from category Z38 Liveborn infants according to place of birth and type of delivery code would be sequenced first, followed by the encounter for observation and evaluation of newborn for suspected diseases and conditions ruled out.

7) Aftercare

Aftercare visit codes cover situations when the initial treatment of a disease has been performed and the patient requires continued care during the healing or recovery phase, or for the long-term consequences of the disease. The aftercare Z code should not be used if treatment is directed at a current, acute disease. The diagnosis code is to be used in these cases. Exceptions to this rule are codes Z51.0, Encounter for antineoplastic radiation therapy, and codes from subcategory Z51.1, Encounter for antineoplastic chemotherapy and immunotherapy. These codes are to be first-listed, followed by the diagnosis code when a patient's encounter is solely to receive radiation therapy, chemotherapy, or immunotherapy for the treatment of a neoplasm. If the reason for the encounter is more than one type of antineoplastic therapy, code Z51.0 and a code from subcategory Z51.1 may be assigned together, in which case one of these codes would be reported as a secondary diagnosis.

The aftercare Z codes should also not be used for aftercare for injuries. For aftercare of an injury, assign the acute injury code with the appropriate 7th character (for subsequent encounter).

The aftercare codes are generally first-listed to explain the specific reason for the encounter. An aftercare code may be used as an additional code when some type of aftercare is provided in addition to the reason for admission and no diagnosis code is applicable. An example of this would be the closure of a colostomy during an encounter for treatment of another condition.

Aftercare codes should be used in conjunction with other aftercare codes or diagnosis codes to provide better detail on the specifics of an aftercare encounter visit, unless otherwise directed by the classification. The sequencing of multiple aftercare codes depends on the circumstances of the encounter.

Certain aftercare Z code categories need a secondary diagnosis code to describe the resolving condition or sequelae. For others, the condition is included in the code title.

Additional Z code aftercare category terms include fitting and adjustment, and attention to artificial openings.

Status Z codes may be used with aftercare Z codes to indicate the nature of the aftercare. For example code Z95.1, Presence of aortocoronary bypass graft, may be used with code Z48.812, Encounter for surgical aftercare following surgery on the circulatory system, to indicate the surgery for which the aftercare is being performed. A status code should not be used when the aftercare code indicates the type of status, such as using Z43.0, Encounter for attention to tracheostomy, with Z93.0, Tracheostomy status.

The aftercare Z category/codes:

Z42	Encounter for plastic and reconstructive surgery following medical procedure or healed injury
Z43	Encounter for attention to artificial openings
Z44	Encounter for fitting and adjustment of external prosthetic device
Z45	Encounter for adjustment and management of implanted device
Z46	Encounter for fitting and adjustment of other devices
Z47	Orthopedic aftercare
Z48	Encounter for other postprocedural aftercare
Z49	Encounter for care involving renal dialysis
Z51	Encounter for other aftercare and medical care

8) Follow-up

The follow-up codes are used to explain continuing surveillance following completed treatment of a disease, condition, or injury. They imply that the condition has been fully treated and no longer exists. They should not be confused with aftercare codes, or injury codes with a 7th character for subsequent encounter, that explain ongoing care of a healing condition or its sequelae. Follow-up codes may be used in conjunction with history codes to provide the full picture of the healed condition and its treatment. The follow-up code is sequenced first, followed by the history code.

A follow-up code may be used to explain multiple visits. Should a condition be found to have recurred on the follow-up visit, then the diagnosis code for the condition should be assigned in place of the follow-up code.

The follow-up Z code categories:

Z08	Encounter for follow-up examination after completed treatment for malignant neoplasm
Z09	Encounter for follow-up examination after completed treatment for conditions other than malignant neoplasm
Z39	Encounter for maternal postpartum care and examination

9) Donor

Codes in category Z52, Donors of organs and tissues, are used for living individuals who are donating blood or other body tissue. These codes are only for individuals donating for others, not for self-donations. They are not used to identify cadaveric donations.

10) Counseling

Counseling Z codes are used when a patient or family member receives assistance in the aftermath of an illness or injury, or when support is required in coping with family or social problems.

The counseling Z codes/categories:

Z30.0-	Encounter for general counseling and advice on contraception
Z31.5	Encounter for procreative genetic counseling
Z31.6-	Encounter for general counseling and advice on procreation
Z32.2	Encounter for childbirth instruction
Z32.3	Encounter for childcare instruction
Z69	Encounter for mental health services for victim and perpetrator of abuse
Z70	Counseling related to sexual attitude, behavior and orientation
Z71	Persons encountering health services for other counseling and medical advice, not elsewhere classified
	Note: Code Z71.84, Encounter for health counseling related to travel, is to be used for health risk and safety counseling for future travel purposes.
Z76.81	Expectant mother prebirth pediatrician visit

11) Encounters for obstetrical and reproductive services

See Section I.C.15. Pregnancy, Childbirth, and the Puerperium, for further instruction on the use of these codes.

Z codes for pregnancy are for use in those circumstances when none of the problems or complications included in the codes from the Obstetrics chapter exist (a routine prenatal visit or postpartum care). Codes in category Z34, Encounter for supervision of normal pregnancy, are always first-listed and are not to be used with any other code from the OB chapter.

Codes in category Z3A, Weeks of gestation, may be assigned to provide additional information about the pregnancy. Category Z3A codes should not be assigned for pregnancies with abortive outcomes (categories O00-O08), elective termination of pregnancy (code Z33.2), nor for postpartum conditions, as category Z3A is not applicable to these conditions. The date of the admission should be used to determine weeks of gestation for inpatient admissions that encompass more than one gestational week.

The outcome of delivery, category Z37, should be included on all maternal delivery records. It is always a secondary code. Codes in category Z37 should not be used on the newborn record.

Z codes for family planning (contraceptive) or procreative management and counseling should be included on an obstetric record either during the pregnancy or the postpartum stage, if applicable.

Z codes/categories for obstetrical and reproductive services:

Z30	Encounter for contraceptive management
Z31	Encounter for procreative management
Z32.2	Encounter for childbirth instruction
Z32.3	Encounter for childcare instruction
Z33	Pregnant state
Z34	Encounter for supervision of normal pregnancy
Z36	Encounter for antenatal screening of mother
Z3A	Weeks of gestation
Z37	Outcome of delivery
Z39	Encounter for maternal postpartum care and examination
Z76.81	Expectant mother prebirth pediatrician visit

12) Newborns and infants

See Section I.C.16. Newborn (Perinatal) Guidelines, for further instruction on the use of these codes.

Newborn Z codes/categories:

Z76.1	Encounter for health supervision and care of foundling
Z00.1-	Encounter for routine child health examination
Z38	Liveborn infants according to place of birth and type of delivery

13) Routine and administrative examinations

The Z codes allow for the description of encounters for routine examinations, such as, a general check-up, or, examinations for administrative purposes, such as, a pre-employment physical. The codes are not to be used if the examination is for diagnosis of a suspected condition or for treatment purposes. In such cases the diagnosis code is used. During a routine exam, should a diagnosis or condition be discovered, it should be coded as an additional code. Pre-existing and chronic conditions and history codes may also be included as additional codes as long as the examination is for administrative purposes and not focused on any particular condition.

Some of the codes for routine health examinations distinguish between "with" and "without" abnormal findings. Code assignment depends on the information that is known at the time the encounter is being coded. For example, if no abnormal findings were found during the examination, but the encounter is being coded before test results are back, it is acceptable to assign the code for "without abnormal findings." When assigning a code for "with abnormal findings," additional code(s) should be assigned to identify the specific abnormal finding(s).

Pre-operative examination and pre-procedural laboratory examination Z codes are for use only in those situations when a patient is being cleared for a procedure or surgery and no treatment is given.

The Z codes/categories for routine and administrative examinations:

Z00	Encounter for general examination without complaint, suspected or reported diagnosis
Z01	Encounter for other special examination without complaint, suspected or reported diagnosis
Z02	Encounter for administrative examination
	Except: Z02.9, Encounter for administrative examinations, unspecified
Z32.0-	Encounter for pregnancy test

14) Miscellaneous Z codes

The miscellaneous Z codes capture a number of other health care encounters that do not fall into one of the other categories. Certain of these codes identify the reason for the encounter; others are for use as additional codes that provide useful information on circumstances that may affect a patient's care and treatment.

Prophylactic organ removal

For encounters specifically for prophylactic removal of an organ (such as prophylactic removal of breasts due to a genetic susceptibility to cancer or a family history of cancer), the principal or first-listed code should be a code from category Z40, Encounter for prophylactic surgery, followed by the appropriate codes to identify the associated risk factor (such as genetic susceptibility or family history).

If the patient has a malignancy of one site and is having prophylactic removal at another site to prevent either a new primary malignancy or metastatic disease, a code for the malignancy should also be assigned in addition to a code from subcategory Z40.0, Encounter for prophylactic surgery for risk factors related to malignant neoplasms. A Z40.0 code should not be assigned if the patient is having organ removal for treatment of a malignancy, such as the removal of the testes for the treatment of prostate cancer.

Female patient with cancer in lower inner quadrant of right breast and positive BRCA 1 noted on testing is admitted for mastectomy of right breast and prophylactic removal of left breast

C50.311	Malignant neoplasm of lower-inner quadrant of right female breast
Z40.01	Encounter for prophylactic removal of breast
Z15.01	Genetic susceptibility to malignant neoplasm of breast

Explanation: Removal of the current neoplastic disease in the right breast was the focus of treatment for this admission and is sequenced first. The removal of the left breast was not required to treat a current disease process but as a means of prevention. The two Z codes are informational; they capture the reason behind the removal of what is currently a healthy left breast.

Miscellaneous Z codes/categories:

Z28	Immunization not carried out
	Except: Z28.3, Underimmunization status
Z29	Encounter for other prophylactic measures
Z40	Encounter for prophylactic surgery
Z41	Encounter for procedures for purposes other than remedying health state
	Except: Z41.9, Encounter for procedure for purposes other than remedying health state, unspecified
Z53	Persons encountering health services for specific procedures and treatment, not carried out
Z55	Problems related to education and literacy
Z56	Problems related to employment and unemployment
Z57	Occupational exposure to risk factors
Z58	Problems related to physical environment
Z59	Problems related to housing and economic circumstances
Z60	Problems related to social environment
Z62	Problems related to upbringing
Z63	Other problems related to primary support group, including family circumstances
Z64	Problems related to certain psychosocial circumstances
Z65	Problems related to other psychosocial circumstances
Z72	Problems related to lifestyle
	Note: These codes should be assigned only when the documentation specifies that the patient has an associated problem
Z73	Problems related to life management difficulty
Z74	Problems related to care provider dependency
	Except: Z74.01, Bed confinement status
Z75	Problems related to medical facilities and other health care
Z76.0	Encounter for issue of repeat prescription
Z76.3	Healthy person accompanying sick person
Z76.4	Other boarder to healthcare facility
Z76.5	Malingerer [conscious simulation]
Z91.1-	Patient's noncompliance with medical treatment and regimen
Z91.83	Wandering in diseases classified elsewhere
Z91.84-	Oral health risk factors
Z91.89	Other specified personal risk factors, not elsewhere classified

See Section I.B.14 for Z55-Z65 Persons with potential health hazards related to socioeconomic and psychosocial circumstances, documentation by clinicians other than the patient's provider

15) Nonspecific Z codes

Certain Z codes are so non-specific, or potentially redundant with other codes in the classification, that there can be little justification for their use in the inpatient setting. Their use in the outpatient setting should be limited to those instances when there is no further documentation to permit more precise coding. Otherwise, any sign or symptom or any other reason for visit that is captured in another code should be used.

Nonspecific Z codes/categories:

Z02.9   Encounter for administrative examinations, unspecified

Z04.9   Encounter for examination and observation for unspecified reason

Z13.9   Encounter for screening, unspecified

Z41.9   Encounter for procedure for purposes other than remedying health state, unspecified

Z52.9   Donor of unspecified organ or tissue

Z86.59   Personal history of other mental and behavioral disorders

Z88.9   Allergy status to unspecified drugs, medicaments and biological substances status

Z92.0   Personal history of contraception

16) Z codes that may only be principal/first-listed diagnosis

The following Z codes/categories may only be reported as the principal/first-listed diagnosis, except when there are multiple encounters on the same day and the medical records for the encounters are combined:

Z00   Encounter for general examination without complaint, suspected or reported diagnosis

     Except: Z00.6

Z01   Encounter for other special examination without complaint, suspected or reported diagnosis

Z02   Encounter for administrative examination

Z03   Encounter for medical observation for suspected diseases and conditions ruled out

Z04   Encounter for examination and observation for other reasons

Z33.2   Encounter for elective termination of pregnancy

Z31.81   Encounter for male factor infertility in female patient

Z31.83   Encounter for assisted reproductive fertility procedure cycle

Z31.84   Encounter for fertility preservation procedure

Z34   Encounter for supervision of normal pregnancy

Z39   Encounter for maternal postpartum care and examination

Z38   Liveborn infants according to place of birth and type of delivery

Z40   Encounter for prophylactic surgery

Z42   Encounter for plastic and reconstructive surgery following medical procedure or healed injury

Z51.0   Encounter for antineoplastic radiation therapy

Z51.1-   Encounter for antineoplastic chemotherapy and immunotherapy

Z52   Donors of organs and tissues

     Except: Z52.9, Donor of unspecified organ or tissue

Z76.1   Encounter for health supervision and care of foundling

Z76.2   Encounter for health supervision and care of other healthy infant and child

Z99.12   Encounter for respirator [ventilator] dependence during power failure

Chapter 21. Factors Influencing Health Status and Contact With Health Services (Z00-Z99)

NOTE Z codes represent reasons for encounters. A corresponding procedure code must accompany a Z code if a procedure is performed. Categories Z00-Z99 are provided for occasions when circumstances other than a disease, injury or external cause classifiable to categories A00-Y89 are recorded as "diagnoses" or "problems." This can arise in two main ways:

(a) When a person who may or may not be sick encounters the health services for some specific purpose, such as to receive limited care or service for a current condition, to donate an organ or tissue, to receive prophylactic vaccination (immunization), or to discuss a problem which is in itself not a disease or injury.

(b) When some circumstance or problem is present which influences the person's health status but is not in itself a current illness or injury.

AHA: 2018,4Q,60-61

This chapter contains the following blocks:

Z00-Z13   Persons encountering health services for examinations
Z14-Z15   Genetic carrier and genetic susceptibility to disease
Z16   Resistance to antimicrobial drugs
Z17   Estrogen receptor status
Z18   Retained foreign body fragments
Z19   Hormone sensitivity malignancy status
Z20-Z29   Persons with potential health hazards related to communicable diseases
Z30-Z39   Persons encountering health services in circumstances related to reproduction
Z40-Z53   Encounters for other specific health care
Z55-Z65   Persons with potential health hazards related to socioeconomic and psychosocial circumstances
Z66   Do not resuscitate status
Z67   Blood type
Z68   Body mass index (BMI)
Z69-Z76   Persons encountering health services in other circumstances
Z77-Z99   Persons with potential health hazards related to family and personal history and certain conditions influencing health status

Persons encountering health services for examinations (Z00-Z13)

NOTE Nonspecific abnormal findings disclosed at the time of these examinations are classified to categories R70-R94.

EXCLUDES 1 examinations related to pregnancy and reproduction (Z30-Z36, Z39.-)

√4ᵗʰ Z00 Encounter for general examination without complaint, suspected or reported diagnosis

    EXCLUDES 1 encounter for examination for administrative purposes (Z02.-)
    EXCLUDES 2 encounter for pre-procedural examinations (Z01.81-)
        special screening examinations (Z11-Z13)

    AHA: 2017,4Q,95

   √5ᵗʰ Z00.0 Encounter for general adult medical examination

Encounter for adult periodic examination (annual) (physical) and any associated laboratory and radiologic examinations

    EXCLUDES 1 encounter for examination of sign or symptom — code to sign or symptom
        general health check-up of infant or child (Z00.12.-)

    Z00.00 Encounter for general adult medical examination without abnormal findings   A

Encounter for adult health check-up NOS
AHA: 2016,1Q,36

    Z00.01 Encounter for general adult medical examination with abnormal findings   A

Use additional code to identify abnormal findings
AHA: 2016,1Q,35-36

   √5ᵗʰ Z00.1 Encounter for newborn, infant and child health examinations

    √6ᵗʰ Z00.11 Newborn health examination

Health check for child under 29 days old
Use additional code to identify any abnormal findings
    EXCLUDES 1 health check for child over 28 days old (Z00.12-)

     Z00.110 Health examination for newborn under 8 days old   N

Health check for newborn under 8 days old

     Z00.111 Health examination for newborn 8 to 28 days old   N

Health check for newborn 8 to 28 days old
Newborn weight check

    √6ᵗʰ Z00.12 Encounter for routine child health examination

Health check (routine) for child over 28 days old
Immunizations appropriate for age
Routine developmental screening of infant or child
Routine vison and hearing testing
    EXCLUDES 1 health check for child under 29 days old (Z00.11-)
        health supervision of foundling or other healthy infant or child (Z76.1-Z76.2)
        newborn health examination (Z00.11-)

    AHA: 2018,4Q,36

    Z00.121 Encounter for routine child health examination with abnormal findings   P

Use additional code to identify abnormal findings
AHA: 2016,1Q,34-35

    Z00.129 Encounter for routine child health examination without abnormal findings   P

Encounter for routine child health examination NOS
AHA: 2016,1Q,34

  Z00.2 Encounter for examination for period of rapid growth in childhood   P

  Z00.3 Encounter for examination for adolescent development state   P

Encounter for puberty development state

  Z00.5 Encounter for examination of potential donor of organ and tissue

  Z00.6 Encounter for examination for normal comparison and control in clinical research program

Examination of participant or control in clinical research program

  √5ᵗʰ Z00.7 Encounter for examination for period of delayed growth in childhood

    Z00.70 Encounter for examination for period of delayed growth in childhood without abnormal findings   P

    Z00.71 Encounter for examination for period of delayed growth in childhood with abnormal findings   P

Use additional code to identify abnormal findings

  Z00.8 Encounter for other general examination

Encounter for health examination in population surveys

√4ᵗʰ Z01 Encounter for other special examination without complaint, suspected or reported diagnosis

    INCLUDES routine examination of specific system

    NOTE Codes from category Z01 represent the reason for the encounter. A separate procedure code is required to identify any examinations or procedures performed

    EXCLUDES 1 encounter for examination for administrative purposes (Z02.-)
        encounter for examination for suspected conditions, proven not to exist (Z03.-)
        encounter for laboratory and radiologic examinations as a component of general medical examinations (Z00.0-)
        encounter for laboratory, radiologic and imaging examinations for sign(s) and symptom(s) — code to the sign(s) or symptom(s)

    EXCLUDES 2 screening examinations (Z11-Z13)

   √5ᵗʰ Z01.0 Encounter for examination of eyes and vision

    EXCLUDES 1 examination for driving license (Z02.4)

    Z01.00 Encounter for examination of eyes and vision without abnormal findings

Encounter for examination of eyes and vision NOS

    Z01.01 Encounter for examination of eyes and vision with abnormal findings

Use additional code to identify abnormal findings
AHA: 2016,4Q,21

N Newborn: 0   P Pediatric: 0-17   M Maternity: 9-64   A Adult: 15-124   MCC Major Complication/Comorbidity   CC Complication/Comorbidity   SW Severe Wound Dx

1278   ICD-10-CM 2020

● ✓6ᵗʰ **Z01.02** **Encounter for examination of eyes and vision following failed vision screening**
> EXCLUDES 1   *examination for examination of eyes and vision with abnormal findings (Z01.01)*
> *examination for examination of eyes and vision without abnormal findings (Z01.00)*

● **Z01.020** **Encounter for examination of eyes and vision following failed vision screening without abnormal findings**

● **Z01.021** **Encounter for examination of eyes and vision following failed vision screening with abnormal findings**
> Use additional code to identify abnormal findings

✓5ᵗʰ **Z01.1** **Encounter for examination of ears and hearing**

Z01.10 **Encounter for examination of ears and hearing without abnormal findings**
> Encounter for examination of ears and hearing NOS
> **AHA:** 2016,4Q,24

✓6ᵗʰ **Z01.11** **Encounter for examination of ears and hearing with abnormal findings**
> **AHA:** 2016,3Q,17-18

Z01.110 **Encounter for hearing examination following failed hearing screening**

Z01.118 **Encounter for examination of ears and hearing with other abnormal findings**
> Use additional code to identify abnormal findings

Z01.12 **Encounter for hearing conservation and treatment**

✓5ᵗʰ **Z01.2** **Encounter for dental examination and cleaning**

Z01.20 **Encounter for dental examination and cleaning without abnormal findings**
> Encounter for dental examination and cleaning NOS

Z01.21 **Encounter for dental examination and cleaning with abnormal findings**
> Use additional code to identify abnormal findings

✓5ᵗʰ **Z01.3** **Encounter for examination of blood pressure**

Z01.30 **Encounter for examination of blood pressure without abnormal findings**
> Encounter for examination of blood pressure NOS

Z01.31 **Encounter for examination of blood pressure with abnormal findings**
> Use additional code to identify abnormal findings

✓5ᵗʰ **Z01.4** **Encounter for gynecological examination**
> EXCLUDES 2   *pregnancy examination or test (Z32.0-)*
> *routine examination for contraceptive maintenance (Z30.4-)*

✓6ᵗʰ **Z01.41** **Encounter for routine gynecological examination**
> Encounter for general gynecological examination with or without cervical smear
> Encounter for gynecological examination (general) (routine) NOS
> Encounter for pelvic examination (annual) (periodic)
> Use additional code:
> for screening for human papillomavirus, if applicable, (Z11.51)
> for screening vaginal pap smear, if applicable (Z12.72)
> to identify acquired absence of uterus, if applicable (Z90.71-)
> EXCLUDES 1   *gynecologic examination status-post hysterectomy for malignant condition (Z08)*
> *screening cervical pap smear not a part of a routine gynecological examination (Z12.4)*

Z01.411 **Encounter for gynecological examination (general) (routine) with abnormal findings**   ♀
> Use additional code to identify abnormal findings

Z01.419 **Encounter for gynecological examination (general) (routine) without abnormal findings**   ♀

Z01.42 **Encounter for cervical smear to confirm findings of recent normal smear following initial abnormal smear**   ♀

✓5ᵗʰ **Z01.8** **Encounter for other specified special examinations**

✓6ᵗʰ **Z01.81** **Encounter for preprocedural examinations**
> Encounter for preoperative examinations
> Encounter for radiological and imaging examinations as part of preprocedural examination

Z01.810 **Encounter for preprocedural cardiovascular examination**

Z01.811 **Encounter for preprocedural respiratory examination**

Z01.812 **Encounter for preprocedural laboratory examination**
> Blood and urine tests prior to treatment or procedure

Z01.818 **Encounter for other preprocedural examination**
> Encounter for preprocedural examination NOS
> Encounter for examinations prior to antineoplastic chemotherapy

Z01.82 **Encounter for allergy testing**
> EXCLUDES 1   *encounter for antibody response examination (Z01.84)*

Z01.83 **Encounter for blood typing**
> Encounter for Rh typing

Z01.84 **Encounter for antibody response examination**
> Encounter for immunity status testing
> EXCLUDES 1   *encounter for allergy testing (Z01.82)*

Z01.89 **Encounter for other specified special examinations**

✓4ᵗʰ **Z02** **Encounter for administrative examination**

Z02.0 **Encounter for examination for admission to educational institution**
> Encounter for examination for admission to preschool (education)
> Encounter for examination for re-admission to school following illness or medical treatment

Z02.1 **Encounter for pre-employment examination**

Z02.2 **Encounter for examination for admission to residential institution**
> EXCLUDES 1   *examination for admission to prison (Z02.89)*

Z02.3 **Encounter for examination for recruitment to armed forces**

Z02.4 **Encounter for examination for driving license**

Z02.5 **Encounter for examination for participation in sport**
> EXCLUDES 1   *blood-alcohol and blood-drug test (Z02.83)*

Z02.6 **Encounter for examination for insurance purposes**

✓5ᵗʰ **Z02.7** **Encounter for issue of medical certificate**
> EXCLUDES 1   *encounter for general medical examination (Z00-Z01, Z02.0-Z02.6, Z02.8-Z02.9)*

Z02.71 **Encounter for disability determination**
> Encounter for issue of medical certificate of incapacity
> Encounter for issue of medical certificate of invalidity

Z02.79 **Encounter for issue of other medical certificate**

✓5ᵗʰ **Z02.8** **Encounter for other administrative examinations**

Z02.81 **Encounter for paternity testing**

Z02.82 **Encounter for adoption services**

Z02.83 **Encounter for blood-alcohol and blood-drug test**
> Use additional code for findings of alcohol or drugs in blood (R78.-)

Z02.89 **Encounter for other administrative examinations**
> Encounter for examination for admission to prison
> Encounter for examination for admission to summer camp
> Encounter for immigration examination
> Encounter for naturalization examination
> Encounter for premarital examination
> EXCLUDES 1   *health supervision of foundling or other healthy infant or child (Z76.1-Z76.2)*

Z02.9 **Encounter for administrative examinations, unspecified**

☑ Additional Character Required   ✓x7ᵗʰ Placeholder   Unacceptable PDx   Questionable PDx   Manifestation   Unspecified Dx   H1 - H14 HAC   HCC CMS-HCC Dx   HIV HIV Dx

ICD-10-CM 2020   **1279**

☑4ᵗʰ **Z03 Encounter for** medical observation **for suspected diseases and conditions ruled out**

This category is to be used when a person without a diagnosis is suspected of having an abnormal condition, without signs or symptoms, which requires study, but after examination and observation, is ruled out. This category is also for use for administrative and legal observation status.

> EXCLUDES 1   *contact with and (suspected) exposures hazardous to health (Z77.-)*
> *encounter for observation and evaluation of newborn for suspected diseases and conditions ruled out (Z05.-)*
> *person with feared complaint in whom no diagnosis is made (Z71.1)*
> *signs or symptoms under study — code to signs or symptoms*

AHA: 2018,2Q,7-8; 2017,4Q,27

Z03.6 Encounter for observation for suspected toxic effect from ingested substance **ruled out**

Encounter for observation for suspected adverse effect from drug

Encounter for observation for suspected poisoning

☑5ᵗʰ **Z03.7 Encounter for suspected** maternal and fetal conditions **ruled out**

Encounter for suspected maternal and fetal conditions not found

> EXCLUDES 1   *known or suspected fetal anomalies affecting management of mother, not ruled out (O26.-, O35.-, O36.-, O40.-, O41.-)*

   Z03.71 Encounter for suspected problem with amniotic cavity and membrane ruled out   Ⓜ ♀

Encounter for suspected oligohydramnios ruled out

Encounter for suspected polyhydramnios ruled out

   Z03.72 Encounter for suspected placental **problem ruled out**   Ⓜ ♀

   Z03.73 Encounter for suspected fetal anomaly **ruled out**   Ⓜ ♀

   Z03.74 Encounter for suspected problem with fetal growth **ruled out**   Ⓜ ♀

   Z03.75 Encounter for suspected cervical shortening **ruled out**   Ⓜ ♀

   Z03.79 Encounter for other suspected maternal and fetal conditions ruled out   Ⓜ ♀

☑5ᵗʰ **Z03.8 Encounter for** observation **for other suspected diseases and conditions ruled out**

   ☑6ᵗʰ **Z03.81 Encounter for observation for suspected** exposure to biological agents **ruled out**

     Z03.810 Encounter for observation for suspected exposure to anthrax **ruled out**

     Z03.818 Encounter for observation for suspected exposure to other biological agents ruled out

   Z03.89 Encounter for observation for other suspected diseases and conditions ruled out

☑4ᵗʰ **Z04 Encounter for examination and observation for other reasons**

> INCLUDES   encounter for examination for medicolegal reasons

This category is to be used when a person without a diagnosis is suspected of having an abnormal condition, without signs or symptoms, which requires study, but after examination and observation, is ruled-out. This category is also for use for administrative and legal observation status.

AHA: 2018,2Q,7-8

Z04.1 Encounter for examination and observation following transport accident

> EXCLUDES 1   *encounter for examination and observation following work accident (Z04.2)*

AHA: 2019,2Q,11; 2018,2Q,8

Z04.2 Encounter for examination and observation following work accident

Z04.3 Encounter for examination and observation following other accident

☑5ᵗʰ **Z04.4 Encounter for examination and observation following** alleged rape

Encounter for examination and observation of victim following alleged rape

Encounter for examination and observation of victim following alleged sexual abuse

   Z04.41 Encounter for examination and observation following alleged adult **rape**   Ⓐ

Suspected adult rape, ruled out

Suspected adult sexual abuse, ruled out

   Z04.42 Encounter for examination and observation following alleged child **rape**   Ⓟ

Suspected child rape, ruled out

Suspected child sexual abuse, ruled out

Z04.6 Encounter for general psychiatric examination, requested by authority

☑5ᵗʰ **Z04.7 Encounter for examination and observation following** alleged physical abuse

   Z04.71 Encounter for examination and observation following alleged adult physical abuse   Ⓐ

Suspected adult physical abuse, ruled out

> EXCLUDES 1   *confirmed case of adult physical abuse (T74.-)*
> *encounter for examination and observation following alleged adult sexual abuse (Z04.41)*
> *suspected case of adult physical abuse, not ruled out (T76.-)*

   Z04.72 Encounter for examination and observation following alleged child physical abuse   Ⓟ

Suspected child physical abuse, ruled out

> EXCLUDES 1   *confirmed case of child physical abuse (T74.-)*
> *encounter for examination and observation following alleged child sexual abuse (Z04.42)*
> *suspected case of child physical abuse, not ruled out (T76.-)*

☑5ᵗʰ **Z04.8 Encounter for examination and observation for** other specified reasons

Encounter for examination and observation for request for expert evidence

AHA: 2018,4Q,32,35,72

   Z04.81 Encounter for examination and observation of victim following forced sexual exploitation

   Z04.82 Encounter for examination and observation of victim following forced labor exploitation

   Z04.89 Encounter for examination and observation for other specified reasons

Z04.9 Encounter for examination and observation for unspecified reason

Encounter for observation NOS

☑4ᵗʰ **Z05 Encounter for observation and evaluation of newborn for** suspected diseases and conditions ruled out

This category is to be used for newborns, within the neonatal period (the first 28 days of life), who are suspected of having an abnormal condition, but without signs or symptoms, and which, after examination and observation, is ruled out.

AHA: 2017,4Q,27; 2016,4Q,77

Z05.0 Observation and evaluation of newborn for suspected cardiac **condition ruled out**   Ⓝ

Z05.1 Observation and evaluation of newborn for suspected infectious **condition ruled out**   Ⓝ

AHA: 2019,2Q,10

Z05.2 Observation and evaluation of newborn for suspected neurological **condition ruled out**   Ⓝ

Z05.3 Observation and evaluation of newborn for suspected respiratory **condition ruled out**   Ⓝ

☑5ᵗʰ **Z05.4 Observation and evaluation of newborn for suspected** genetic, metabolic or immunologic **condition ruled out**

   Z05.41 Observation and evaluation of newborn for suspected genetic **condition ruled out**   Ⓝ

AHA: 2016,4Q,55

   Z05.42 Observation and evaluation of newborn for suspected metabolic **condition ruled out**   Ⓝ

Ⓝ Newborn: 0   Ⓟ Pediatric: 0-17   Ⓜ Maternity: 9-64   Ⓐ Adult: 15-124   MCC Major Complication/Comorbidity   CC Complication/Comorbidity   SW Severe Wound Dx

1280   ICD-10-CM 2020

Z05.43 Observation and evaluation of newborn for suspected immunologic condition ruled out   N

Z05.5 Observation and evaluation of newborn for suspected gastrointestinal condition ruled out   N

Z05.6 Observation and evaluation of newborn for suspected genitourinary condition ruled out   N

✓5ᵗʰ **Z05.7** Observation and evaluation of newborn for suspected skin, subcutaneous, musculoskeletal and connective tissue condition ruled out

     Z05.71 Observation and evaluation of newborn for suspected skin and subcutaneous tissue condition ruled out   N

     Z05.72 Observation and evaluation of newborn for suspected musculoskeletal condition ruled out   N

     Z05.73 Observation and evaluation of newborn for suspected connective tissue condition ruled out   N

Z05.8 Observation and evaluation of newborn for other specified suspected condition ruled out   N

Z05.9 Observation and evaluation of newborn for unspecified suspected condition ruled out   N

Z08 Encounter for follow-up examination after completed treatment for malignant neoplasm
     Medical surveillance following completed treatment
     Use additional code to identify any acquired absence of organs (Z90.-)
     Use additional code to identify the personal history of malignant neoplasm (Z85.-)
     EXCLUDES 1   aftercare following medical care (Z43-Z49, Z51)

Z09 Encounter for follow-up examination after completed treatment for conditions other than malignant neoplasm
     Medical surveillance following completed treatment
     Use additional code to identify any applicable history of disease code (Z86.-. Z87.-)
     EXCLUDES 1   aftercare following medical care (Z43-Z49, Z51)
                surveillance of contraception (Z30.4-)
                surveillance of prosthetic and other medical devices (Z44-Z46)
     AHA: 2017,1Q,9; 2015,1Q,8

✓4ᵗʰ **Z11** Encounter for screening for infectious and parasitic diseases
     Screening is the testing for disease or disease precursors in asymptomatic individuals so that early detection and treatment can be provided for those who test positive for the disease.
     EXCLUDES 1   encounter for diagnostic examination — code to sign or symptom

Z11.0 Encounter for screening for intestinal infectious diseases

Z11.1 Encounter for screening for respiratory tuberculosis
     ▶Encounter for screening for active tuberculosis disease◀

Z11.2 Encounter for screening for other bacterial diseases

Z11.3 Encounter for screening for infections with a predominantly sexual mode of transmission
     EXCLUDES 2   encounter for screening for human immunodeficiency virus [HIV] (Z11.4)
                encounter for screening for human papillomavirus (Z11.51)

Z11.4 Encounter for screening for human immunodeficiency virus [HIV]

✓5ᵗʰ **Z11.5** Encounter for screening for other viral diseases
     EXCLUDES 2   encounter for screening for viral intestinal disease (Z11.0)

     Z11.51 Encounter for screening for human papillomavirus (HPV)

     Z11.59 Encounter for screening for other viral diseases

Z11.6 Encounter for screening for other protozoal diseases and helminthiases
     EXCLUDES 2   encounter for screening for protozoal intestinal disease (Z11.0)

● **Z11.7** Encounter for testing for latent tuberculosis infection

Z11.8 Encounter for screening for other infectious and parasitic diseases
     Encounter for screening for chlamydia
     Encounter for screening for rickettsial
     Encounter for screening for spirochetal
     Encounter for screening for mycoses

Z11.9 Encounter for screening for infectious and parasitic diseases, unspecified

✓4ᵗʰ **Z12** Encounter for screening for malignant neoplasms
     Screening is the testing for disease or disease precursors in asymptomatic individuals so that early detection and treatment can be provided for those who test positive for the disease.
     Use additional code to identify any family history of malignant neoplasm (Z80.-)
     EXCLUDES 1   encounter for diagnostic examination — code to sign or symptom

Z12.0 Encounter for screening for malignant neoplasm of stomach

✓5ᵗʰ **Z12.1** Encounter for screening for malignant neoplasm of intestinal tract
     AHA: 2017,1Q,8,9

     Z12.10 Encounter for screening for malignant neoplasm of intestinal tract, unspecified

     Z12.11 Encounter for screening for malignant neoplasm of colon
            Encounter for screening colonoscopy NOS
            AHA: 2019,1Q,32-33; 2018,1Q,6

     Z12.12 Encounter for screening for malignant neoplasm of rectum
            AHA: 2018,1Q,6

     Z12.13 Encounter for screening for malignant neoplasm of small intestine

Z12.2 Encounter for screening for malignant neoplasm of respiratory organs

✓5ᵗʰ **Z12.3** Encounter for screening for malignant neoplasm of breast

     Z12.31 Encounter for screening mammogram for malignant neoplasm of breast
            EXCLUDES 1   inconclusive mammogram (R92.2)
            AHA: 2015,1Q,24

     Z12.39 Encounter for other screening for malignant neoplasm of breast

Z12.4 Encounter for screening for malignant neoplasm of cervix   ♀
     Encounter for screening pap smear for malignant neoplasm of cervix
     EXCLUDES 1   when screening is part of general gynecological examination (Z01.4-)
     EXCLUDES 2   encounter for screening for human papillomavirus (Z11.51)

Z12.5 Encounter for screening for malignant neoplasm of prostate   ♂

Z12.6 Encounter for screening for malignant neoplasm of bladder

✓5ᵗʰ **Z12.7** Encounter for screening for malignant neoplasm of other genitourinary organs

     Z12.71 Encounter for screening for malignant neoplasm of testis   ♂

     Z12.72 Encounter for screening for malignant neoplasm of vagina   ♀
            Vaginal pap smear status-post hysterectomy for non-malignant condition
            Use additional code to identify acquired absence of uterus (Z90.71-)
            EXCLUDES 1   vaginal pap smear status-post hysterectomy for malignant conditions (Z08)

     Z12.73 Encounter for screening for malignant neoplasm of ovary   ♀

     Z12.79 Encounter for screening for malignant neoplasm of other genitourinary organs

✓5ᵗʰ **Z12.8** Encounter for screening for malignant neoplasm of other sites

     Z12.81 Encounter for screening for malignant neoplasm of oral cavity

     Z12.82 Encounter for screening for malignant neoplasm of nervous system

     Z12.83 Encounter for screening for malignant neoplasm of skin

     Z12.89 Encounter for screening for malignant neoplasm of other sites

Z12.9 Encounter for screening for malignant neoplasm, site unspecified

√4ᵗʰ **Z13 Encounter for screening for other diseases and disorders**

Screening is the testing for disease or disease precursors in asymptomatic individuals so that early detection and treatment can be provided for those who test positive for the disease.

> EXCLUDES 1   *encounter for diagnostic examination — code to sign or symptom*

Z13.0 Encounter for screening for diseases of the blood and blood-forming organs and certain disorders involving the immune mechanism

Z13.1 Encounter for screening for diabetes mellitus

√5ᵗʰ **Z13.2 Encounter for screening for nutritional, metabolic and other endocrine disorders**

    Z13.21 Encounter for screening for nutritional disorder

√6ᵗʰ   **Z13.22 Encounter for screening for metabolic disorder**

        Z13.220 Encounter for screening for lipoid disorders

        Encounter for screening for cholesterol level

        Encounter for screening for hypercholesterolemia

        Encounter for screening for hyperlipidemia

        Z13.228 Encounter for screening for other metabolic disorders

    Z13.29 Encounter for screening for other suspected endocrine disorder

> EXCLUDES 1   *encounter for screening for diabetes mellitus (Z13.1)*

√5ᵗʰ **Z13.3 Encounter for screening examination for mental health and behavioral disorders**

    AHA: 2018,4Q,35-36

    Z13.30 Encounter for screening examination for mental health and behavioral disorders, unspecified

    Z13.31 Encounter for screening for depression

    Encounter for screening for depression, adult

    Encounter for screening for depression for child or adolescent

    Z13.32 Encounter for screening for maternal depression ♀

    Encounter for screening for perinatal depression

    Z13.39 Encounter for screening examination for other mental health and behavioral disorders

    Encounter for screening for alcoholism

    Encounter for screening for intellectual disabilities

√5ᵗʰ **Z13.4 Encounter for screening for certain developmental disorders in childhood**

    Encounter for development testing of infant or child

    Encounter for screening for developmental handicaps in early childhood

> EXCLUDES 2   *encounter for routine child health examination (Z00.12-)*

    AHA: 2018,4Q,36

    Z13.40 Encounter for screening for unspecified developmental delays

    Z13.41 Encounter for autism screening

    Z13.42 Encounter for screening for global developmental delays (milestones)

    Encounter for screening for developmental handicaps in early childhood

    Z13.49 Encounter for screening for other developmental delays

Z13.5 Encounter for screening for eye and ear disorders

> EXCLUDES 2   *encounter for general hearing examination (Z01.1-)*
> *encounter for general vision examination (Z01.0-)*

    AHA: 2016,3Q,17

Z13.6 Encounter for screening for cardiovascular disorders

√5ᵗʰ **Z13.7 Encounter for screening for genetic and chromosomal anomalies**

> EXCLUDES 1   *genetic testing for procreative management (Z31.4-)*

    Z13.71 Encounter for nonprocreative screening for genetic disease carrier status

    Z13.79 Encounter for other screening for genetic and chromosomal anomalies

√5ᵗʰ **Z13.8 Encounter for screening for other specified diseases and disorders**

> EXCLUDES 2   *screening for malignant neoplasms (Z12.-)*

√6ᵗʰ   **Z13.81 Encounter for screening for digestive system disorders**

        Z13.810 Encounter for screening for upper gastrointestinal disorder

        Z13.811 Encounter for screening for lower gastrointestinal disorder

> EXCLUDES 1   *encounter for screening for intestinal infectious disease (Z11.0)*

        Z13.818 Encounter for screening for other digestive system disorders

√6ᵗʰ   **Z13.82 Encounter for screening for musculoskeletal disorder**

        Z13.820 Encounter for screening for osteoporosis

        Z13.828 Encounter for screening for other musculoskeletal disorder

    Z13.83 Encounter for screening for respiratory disorder NEC

> EXCLUDES 1   *encounter for screening for respiratory tuberculosis (Z11.1)*

    Z13.84 Encounter for screening for dental disorders

√6ᵗʰ   **Z13.85 Encounter for screening for nervous system disorders**

        Z13.850 Encounter for screening for traumatic brain injury

        Z13.858 Encounter for screening for other nervous system disorders

    Z13.88 Encounter for screening for disorder due to exposure to contaminants

> EXCLUDES 1   *those exposed to contaminants without suspected disorders (Z57.-, Z77.-)*

    Z13.89 Encounter for screening for other disorder

    Encounter for screening for genitourinary disorders

Z13.9 Encounter for screening, unspecified

Genetic carrier and genetic susceptibility to disease (Z14-Z15)

√4ᵗʰ **Z14 Genetic carrier**

> **DEF:** Individuals carrying a gene mutation associated with a certain disease that typically do not develop the disease but are able to pass the mutated genes to offspring.

√5ᵗʰ **Z14.0 Hemophilia A carrier**

    Z14.01 Asymptomatic hemophilia A carrier

    Z14.02 Symptomatic hemophilia A carrier

Z14.1 Cystic fibrosis carrier

Z14.8 Genetic carrier of other disease

√4ᵗʰ **Z15 Genetic susceptibility to disease**

> INCLUDES   confirmed abnormal gene

Use additional code, if applicable, for any associated family history of the disease (Z80-Z84)

> EXCLUDES 1   *chromosomal anomalies (Q90-Q99)*

√5ᵗʰ **Z15.0 Genetic susceptibility to malignant neoplasm**

Code first, if applicable, any current malignant neoplasm (C00-C75, C81-C96)

Use additional code, if applicable, for any personal history of malignant neoplasm (Z85.-)

    Z15.01 Genetic susceptibility to malignant neoplasm of breast

    Z15.02 Genetic susceptibility to malignant neoplasm of ovary ♀

    Z15.03 Genetic susceptibility to malignant neoplasm of prostate ♂

    Z15.04 Genetic susceptibility to malignant neoplasm of endometrium ♀

    Z15.09 Genetic susceptibility to other malignant neoplasm

√5ᵗʰ **Z15.8 Genetic susceptibility to other disease**

    Z15.81 Genetic susceptibility to multiple endocrine neoplasia [MEN]

> EXCLUDES 1   *multiple endocrine neoplasia [MEN] syndromes (E31.2-)*

> **DEF:** Group of conditions in which several endocrine glands grow excessively (such as in adenomatous hyperplasia) and/or develop benign or malignant tumors. Tumors and hyperplasia associated with MEN often produce excess hormones, which impede normal physiology. There is no comprehensive cure known for MEN syndrome. Treatment is directed at the hyperplasia or tumors in each individual gland. Tumors are usually surgically removed and oral medications or hormonal injections are used to correct hormone imbalances.

    Z15.89 Genetic susceptibility to other disease

Resistance to antimicrobial drugs (Z16)

Z16 Resistance to antimicrobial drugs

> **NOTE** The codes in this category are provided for use as additional codes to identify the resistance and non-responsiveness of a condition to antimicrobial drugs.
>
> Code first the infection
> **EXCLUDES 1** Methicillin resistant Staphylococcus aureus infection (A49.02)
> Methicillin resistant Staphylococcus aureus pneumonia (J15.212)
> sepsis due to Methicillin resistant Staphylococcus aureus (A41.02)

Z16.1 Resistance to beta lactam antibiotics

- **Z16.10 Resistance to unspecified beta lactam antibiotics**
- **Z16.11 Resistance to penicillins**
  Resistance to amoxicillin
  Resistance to ampicillin
- **Z16.12 Extended spectrum beta lactamase (ESBL) resistance** cc
  - **EXCLUDES 2** Methicillin resistant Staphylococcus aureus infection in diseases classified elsewhere (B95.62)
- **Z16.19 Resistance to other specified beta lactam antibiotics**
  Resistance to cephalosporins

Z16.2 Resistance to other antibiotics

- **Z16.20 Resistance to unspecified antibiotic**
  Resistance to antibiotics NOS
- **Z16.21 Resistance to vancomycin** cc
- **Z16.22 Resistance to vancomycin related antibiotics**
- **Z16.23 Resistance to quinolones and fluoroquinolones**
- **Z16.24 Resistance to multiple antibiotics** cc
- **Z16.29 Resistance to other single specified antibiotic**
  Resistance to aminoglycosides
  Resistance to macrolides
  Resistance to sulfonamides
  Resistance to tetracyclines

Z16.3 Resistance to other antimicrobial drugs

- **EXCLUDES 1** resistance to antibiotics (Z16.1-, Z16.2-)
- **Z16.30 Resistance to unspecified antimicrobial drugs**
  Drug resistance NOS
- **Z16.31 Resistance to antiparasitic drug(s)**
  Resistance to quinine and related compounds
- **Z16.32 Resistance to antifungal drug(s)**
- **Z16.33 Resistance to antiviral drug(s)**
- **Z16.34 Resistance to antimycobacterial drug(s)**
  Resistance to tuberculostatics
  - **Z16.341 Resistance to single antimycobacterial drug**
    Resistance to antimycobacterial drug NOS
  - **Z16.342 Resistance to multiple antimycobacterial drugs**
- **Z16.35 Resistance to multiple antimicrobial drugs**
  - **EXCLUDES 1** resistance to multiple antibiotics only (Z16.24)
- **Z16.39 Resistance to other specified antimicrobial drug** cc

Estrogen receptor status (Z17)

Z17 Estrogen receptor status

> Code first malignant neoplasm of breast (C50.-)
> **DEF:** Receptor status of breast cancer cells for the hormone estrogen that is used to help determine treatment and evaluate prognosis. ER+ breast cancer responds to hormone therapies while ER- breast cancer does not.

Z17.0 Estrogen receptor positive status [ER+]
Z17.1 Estrogen receptor negative status [ER-]

Retained foreign body fragments (Z18)

Z18 Retained foreign body fragments

> **INCLUDES** embedded fragment (status)
> embedded splinter (status)
> retained foreign body status
> **EXCLUDES 1** artificial joint prosthesis status (Z96.6-)
> foreign body accidentally left during a procedure (T81.5-)
> foreign body entering through orifice (T15-T19)
> in situ cardiac device (Z95.-)
> organ or tissue replaced by means other than transplant (Z96.-, Z97.-)
> organ or tissue replaced by transplant (Z94.-)
> personal history of retained foreign body fully removed Z87.821
> superficial foreign body (non-embedded splinter) — code to superficial foreign body, by site
> **DEF:** Embedded or retained fragment, splinter, or foreign body, natural or synthetic that can cause infection.

Z18.0 Retained radioactive fragments
- **Z18.01 Retained depleted uranium fragments**
- **Z18.09 Other retained radioactive fragments**
  Other retained depleted isotope fragments
  Retained nontherapeutic radioactive fragments

Z18.1 Retained metal fragments
- **EXCLUDES 1** retained radioactive metal fragments (Z18.01-Z18.09)
- **Z18.10 Retained metal fragments, unspecified**
  Retained metal fragment NOS
- **Z18.11 Retained magnetic metal fragments**
- **Z18.12 Retained nonmagnetic metal fragments**

Z18.2 Retained plastic fragments
  Acrylics fragments
  Diethylhexyl phthalates fragments
  Isocyanate fragments

Z18.3 Retained organic fragments
- **Z18.31 Retained animal quills or spines**
- **Z18.32 Retained tooth**
- **Z18.33 Retained wood fragments**
- **Z18.39 Other retained organic fragments**

Z18.8 Other specified retained foreign body
- **Z18.81 Retained glass fragments**
- **Z18.83 Retained stone or crystalline fragments**
  Retained concrete or cement fragments
- **Z18.89 Other specified retained foreign body fragments**

Z18.9 Retained foreign body fragments, unspecified material

Hormone sensitivity malignancy status (Z19)

Z19 Hormone sensitivity malignancy status

> Code first malignant neoplasm — see Table of Neoplasms, by site, malignant
> **AHA:** 2016,4Q,76

Z19.1 Hormone sensitive malignancy status
Z19.2 Hormone resistant malignancy status
  Castrate resistant prostate malignancy status

Persons with potential health hazards related to communicable diseases (Z20-Z29)

Z20 Contact with and (suspected) exposure to communicable diseases

> **EXCLUDES 1** carrier of infectious disease (Z22.-)
> diagnosed current infectious or parasitic disease — see Alphabetic Index
> **EXCLUDES 2** personal history of infectious and parasitic diseases (Z86.1-)

Z20.0 Contact with and (suspected) exposure to intestinal infectious diseases
- **Z20.01 Contact with and (suspected) exposure to intestinal infectious diseases due to Escherichia coli (E. coli)**
- **Z20.09 Contact with and (suspected) exposure to other intestinal infectious diseases**

Z20.1 Contact with and (suspected) exposure to tuberculosis
Z20.2 Contact with and (suspected) exposure to infections with a predominantly sexual mode of transmission
Z20.3 Contact with and (suspected) exposure to rabies
Z20.4 Contact with and (suspected) exposure to rubella

Chapter 21. Factors Influencing Health Status and Contact With Health Services

Z20.5 Contact with and (suspected) exposure to viral hepatitis

Z20.6 Contact with and (suspected) exposure to human immunodeficiency virus [HIV]
> EXCLUDES 1   asymptomatic human immunodeficiency virus [HIV] HIV infection status (Z21)

Z20.7 Contact with and (suspected) exposure to pediculosis, acariasis and other infestations

✓5ᵗʰ **Z20.8** Contact with and (suspected) exposure to other communicable diseases

    ✓6ᵗʰ **Z20.81** Contact with and (suspected) exposure to other bacterial communicable diseases

       Z20.810 Contact with and (suspected) exposure to anthrax

       Z20.811 Contact with and (suspected) exposure to meningococcus

       Z20.818 Contact with and (suspected) exposure to other bacterial communicable diseases
         AHA: 2019,2Q,10

    ✓6ᵗʰ **Z20.82** Contact with and (suspected) exposure to other viral communicable diseases

       Z20.820 Contact with and (suspected) exposure to varicella

       Z20.821 Contact with and (suspected) exposure to Zika virus
         AHA: 2018,4Q,35,64

       Z20.828 Contact with and (suspected) exposure to other viral communicable diseases

    Z20.89 Contact with and (suspected) exposure to other communicable diseases

   Z20.9 Contact with and (suspected) exposure to unspecified communicable disease

Z21 Asymptomatic human immunodeficiency virus [HIV] infection status   HCC
   HIV positive NOS
   Code first human immunodeficiency virus [HIV] disease complicating pregnancy, childbirth and the puerperium, if applicable (O98.7-)
> EXCLUDES 1   acquired immunodeficiency syndrome (B20)
> contact with human immunodeficiency virus [HIV] (Z20.6)
> exposure to human immunodeficiency virus [HIV] (Z20.6)
> human immunodeficiency virus [HIV] disease (B20)
> inconclusive laboratory evidence of human immunodeficiency virus [HIV] (R75)

   AHA: 2019,1Q,8-11
   DEF: Phase of human immunodeficiency virus (HIV) infection with no clinical symptoms. This phase may last for 10 years or more.

✓4ᵗʰ **Z22** Carrier of infectious disease
> INCLUDES   colonization status
> suspected carrier
> EXCLUDES 2   carrier of viral hepatitis (B18.-)

   Z22.0 Carrier of typhoid

   Z22.1 Carrier of other intestinal infectious diseases

   Z22.2 Carrier of diphtheria

   ✓5ᵗʰ **Z22.3** Carrier of other specified bacterial diseases

    Z22.31 Carrier of bacterial disease due to meningococci

    ✓6ᵗʰ **Z22.32** Carrier of bacterial disease due to staphylococci

       Z22.321 Carrier or suspected carrier of Methicillin susceptible Staphylococcus aureus
         MSSA colonization

       Z22.322 Carrier or suspected carrier of Methicillin resistant Staphylococcus aureus
         MRSA colonization
         DEF: Carriers (colonization) of methicillin resistant Staphylococcus aureus (MRSA) have MRSA on their skin or in their body but do not exhibit signs of infection. These individuals are able to pass MRSA on to others who may develop an infection.

    ✓6ᵗʰ **Z22.33** Carrier of bacterial disease due to streptococci

       Z22.330 Carrier of Group B streptococcus
> EXCLUDES 1   carrier of streptococcus group B (GBS) complicating pregnancy, childbirth and the puerperium (O99.82-)

       Z22.338 Carrier of other streptococcus

    Z22.39 Carrier of other specified bacterial diseases

   Z22.4 Carrier of infections with a predominantly sexual mode of transmission

   Z22.6 Carrier of human T-lymphotropic virus type-1 [HTLV-1] infection

● **Z22.7** Latent tuberculosis
   Latent tuberculosis infection (LTBI)
> EXCLUDES 1   nonspecific reaction to cell mediated immunity measurement of gamma interferon antigen response without active tuberculosis (R76.12)
> nonspecific reaction to tuberculin skin test without active tuberculosis (R76.11)

   Z22.8 Carrier of other infectious diseases

   Z22.9 Carrier of infectious disease, unspecified

Z23 Encounter for immunization
   Code first any routine childhood examination
> NOTE   Procedure codes are required to identify the types of immunizations given

✓4ᵗʰ **Z28** Immunization not carried out and underimmunization status
> INCLUDES   vaccination not carried out

   ✓5ᵗʰ **Z28.0** Immunization not carried out because of contraindication
     DEF: Contraindication: Situation where a drug, surgery, or other procedure may negatively affect or cause harm to a patient.

    Z28.01 Immunization not carried out because of acute illness of patient

    Z28.02 Immunization not carried out because of chronic illness or condition of patient

    Z28.03 Immunization not carried out because of immune compromised state of patient

    Z28.04 Immunization not carried out because of patient allergy to vaccine or component

    Z28.09 Immunization not carried out because of other contraindication

   Z28.1 Immunization not carried out because of patient decision for reasons of belief or group pressure
     Immunization not carried out because of religious belief

   ✓5ᵗʰ **Z28.2** Immunization not carried out because of patient decision for other and unspecified reason

    Z28.20 Immunization not carried out because of patient decision for unspecified reason

    Z28.21 Immunization not carried out because of patient refusal

    Z28.29 Immunization not carried out because of patient decision for other reason

   Z28.3 Underimmunization status
     Delinquent immunization status
     Lapsed immunization schedule status

   ✓5ᵗʰ **Z28.8** Immunization not carried out for other reason

    Z28.81 Immunization not carried out due to patient having had the disease

    Z28.82 Immunization not carried out because of caregiver refusal
     Immunization not carried out because of guardian refusal
     Immunization not carried out because of parent refusal
> EXCLUDES 1   immunization not carried out because of caregiver refusal because of religious belief (Z28.1)

    Z28.83 Immunization not carried out due to unavailability of vaccine
     Delay in delivery of vaccine
     Lack of availability of vaccine
     Manufacturer delay of vaccine
     AHA: 2018,4Q,36

    Z28.89 Immunization not carried out for other reason

   Z28.9 Immunization not carried out for unspecified reason

✓4ᵗʰ **Z29** Encounter for other prophylactic measures
> EXCLUDES 1   desensitization to allergens (Z51.6)
> prophylactic surgery (Z40.-)

   AHA: 2016,4Q,78-79

   ✓5ᵗʰ **Z29.1** Encounter for prophylactic immunotherapy
     Encounter for administration of immunoglobulin

    Z29.11 Encounter for prophylactic immunotherapy for respiratory syncytial virus (RSV)

    Z29.12 Encounter for prophylactic antivenin

    Z29.13 Encounter for prophylactic Rho(D) immune globulin

    Z29.14 Encounter for prophylactic rabies immune globin

   Z29.3 Encounter for prophylactic fluoride administration

   Z29.8 Encounter for other specified prophylactic measures

   Z29.9 Encounter for prophylactic measures, unspecified

Persons encountering health services in circumstances related to reproduction (Z30–Z39)

☑4ᵗʰ **Z30 Encounter for contraceptive management**
     AHA: 2016,4Q,78
     DEF: Contraceptive management to prevent pregnancy. Methods include oral medications, intrauterine devices, and surgical procedures for males and females (sterilization).

☑5ᵗʰ **Z30.0 Encounter for general counseling and advice on contraception**

☑6ᵗʰ   **Z30.01 Encounter for initial prescription of contraceptives**
     EXCLUDES 1   *encounter for surveillance of contraceptives (Z30.4-)*

     Z30.011 Encounter for initial prescription of contraceptive pills ♀

     Z30.012 Encounter for prescription of emergency contraception ♀
       Encounter for postcoital contraception

     Z30.013 Encounter for initial prescription of injectable contraceptive ♀

     Z30.014 Encounter for initial prescription of intrauterine contraceptive device ♀
       EXCLUDES 1   *encounter for insertion of intrauterine contraceptive device (Z30.430, Z30.432)*

     Z30.015 Encounter for initial prescription of vaginal ring hormonal contraceptive ♀

     Z30.016 Encounter for initial prescription of transdermal patch hormonal contraceptive device ♀

     Z30.017 Encounter for initial prescription of implantable subdermal contraceptive ♀

     Z30.018 Encounter for initial prescription of other contraceptives ♀
       Encounter for initial prescription of barrier contraception
       Encounter for initial prescription of diaphragm

     Z30.019 Encounter for initial prescription of contraceptives, unspecified ♀

   Z30.02 Counseling and instruction in natural family planning to avoid pregnancy

   Z30.09 Encounter for other general counseling and advice on contraception
     Encounter for family planning advice NOS

Z30.2 Encounter for sterilization

☑5ᵗʰ **Z30.4 Encounter for surveillance of contraceptives**

   Z30.40 Encounter for surveillance of contraceptives, unspecified

   Z30.41 Encounter for surveillance of contraceptive pills ♀
     Encounter for repeat prescription for contraceptive pill

   Z30.42 Encounter for surveillance of injectable contraceptive ♀

☑6ᵗʰ   **Z30.43 Encounter for surveillance of intrauterine contraceptive device**

     Z30.430 Encounter for insertion of intrauterine contraceptive device ♀

     Z30.431 Encounter for routine checking of intrauterine contraceptive device ♀

     Z30.432 Encounter for removal of intrauterine contraceptive device ♀

     Z30.433 Encounter for removal and reinsertion of intrauterine contraceptive device ♀
       Encounter for replacement of intrauterine contraceptive device

   Z30.44 Encounter for surveillance of vaginal ring hormonal contraceptive device ♀

   Z30.45 Encounter for surveillance of transdermal patch hormonal contraceptive device ♀

   Z30.46 Encounter for surveillance of implantable subdermal contraceptive ♀
     Encounter for checking, reinsertion or removal of implantable subdermal contraceptive

   Z30.49 Encounter for surveillance of other contraceptives ♀
     Encounter for surveillance of barrier contraception
     Encounter for surveillance of diaphragm

Z30.8 Encounter for other contraceptive management
     Encounter for postvasectomy sperm count
     Encounter for routine examination for contraceptive maintenance
     EXCLUDES 1   *sperm count following sterilization reversal (Z31.42)*
             sperm count for fertility testing (Z31.41)

Z30.9 Encounter for contraceptive management, unspecified

☑4ᵗʰ **Z31 Encounter for procreative management**
     EXCLUDES 1   *complications associated with artificial fertilization (N98.-)*
             female infertility (N97.-)
             male infertility (N46.-)

Z31.0 Encounter for reversal of previous sterilization

☑5ᵗʰ **Z31.4 Encounter for procreative investigation and testing**
     EXCLUDES 1   *postvasectomy sperm count (Z30.8)*

   Z31.41 Encounter for fertility testing
     Encounter for fallopian tube patency testing
     Encounter for sperm count for fertility testing

   Z31.42 Aftercare following sterilization reversal
     Sperm count following sterilization reversal

☑6ᵗʰ   **Z31.43 Encounter for genetic testing of female for procreative management**
     Use additional code for recurrent pregnancy loss, if applicable (N96, O26.2-)
     EXCLUDES 1   *nonprocreative genetic testing (Z13.7-)*

     Z31.430 Encounter of female for testing for genetic disease carrier status for procreative management ♀

     Z31.438 Encounter for other genetic testing of female for procreative management ♀

☑6ᵗʰ   **Z31.44 Encounter for genetic testing of male for procreative management**
     EXCLUDES 1   *nonprocreative genetic testing (Z13.7-)*

     Z31.440 Encounter of male for testing for genetic disease carrier status for procreative management ♂

     Z31.441 Encounter for testing of male partner of patient with recurrent pregnancy loss Ⓐ ♂

     Z31.448 Encounter for other genetic testing of male for procreative management Ⓐ ♂

   Z31.49 Encounter for other procreative investigation and testing

Z31.5 Encounter for procreative genetic counseling
     AHA: 2017,4Q,27

☑5ᵗʰ **Z31.6 Encounter for general counseling and advice on procreation**

   Z31.61 Procreative counseling and advice using natural family planning

   Z31.62 Encounter for fertility preservation counseling
     Encounter for fertility preservation counseling prior to cancer therapy
     Encounter for fertility preservation counseling prior to surgical removal of gonads

   Z31.69 Encounter for other general counseling and advice on procreation

Z31.7 Encounter for procreative management and counseling for gestational carrier ♀
     EXCLUDES 1   *pregnant state, gestational carrier (Z33.3)*
     AHA: 2016,4Q,78

☑5ᵗʰ **Z31.8 Encounter for other procreative management**

   Z31.81 Encounter for male factor infertility in female patient ♀

   Z31.82 Encounter for Rh incompatibility status ♀
     AHA: 2015,3Q,40; 2014,4Q,17

Z31.83 Encounter for assisted reproductive fertility procedure cycle ♀

Patient undergoing in vitro fertilization cycle

Use additional code to identify the type of infertility

EXCLUDES 1   *pre-cycle diagnosis and testing — code to reason for encounter*

Z31.84 Encounter for fertility preservation **procedure**

Encounter for fertility preservation procedure prior to cancer therapy

Encounter for fertility preservation procedure prior to surgical removal of gonads

Z31.89 Encounter for other procreative management

Z31.9 Encounter for procreative management, unspecified

✓4ᵗʰ **Z32 Encounter for pregnancy test and childbirth and childcare instruction**

✓5ᵗʰ **Z32.Ø Encounter for** pregnancy test

Z32.ØØ Encounter for pregnancy test, result unknown ♀

Encounter for pregnancy test NOS

Z32.Ø1 Encounter for pregnancy test, result positive Ⓜ ♀

Z32.Ø2 Encounter for pregnancy test, result negative ♀

Z32.2 Encounter for childbirth instruction

Z32.3 Encounter for childcare instruction

Encounter for prenatal or postpartum childcare instruction

✓4ᵗʰ **Z33 Pregnant state**

Z33.1 Pregnant state, incidental Ⓜ ♀

Pregnant state NOS

EXCLUDES 1   *complications of pregnancy (OØØ-O9A)*

pregnant state, gestational carrier (Z33.3)

Z33.2 Encounter for elective termination of pregnancy Ⓜ ♀

EXCLUDES 1   *early fetal death with retention of dead fetus (OØ2.1)*

late fetal death (O36.4)

spontaneous abortion (OØ3)

TIP: Do not assign a code from category Z3A with this code.

Z33.3 Pregnant state, gestational carrier Ⓜ ♀

EXCLUDES 1   *encounter for procreative management and counseling for gestational carrier (Z31.7)*

AHA: 2016,4Q,78

✓4ᵗʰ **Z34 Encounter for supervision of normal pregnancy**

EXCLUDES 1   *any complication of pregnancy (OØØ-O9A)*

encounter for pregnancy test (Z32.Ø-)

encounter for supervision of high risk pregnancy (OØ9.-)

AHA: 2014,4Q,17

✓5ᵗʰ **Z34.Ø Encounter for supervision of normal** first **pregnancy**

Z34.ØØ Encounter for supervision of normal first pregnancy, unspecified trimester Ⓜ ♀

Z34.Ø1 Encounter for supervision of normal first pregnancy, first trimester Ⓜ ♀

Z34.Ø2 Encounter for supervision of normal first pregnancy, second trimester Ⓜ ♀

Z34.Ø3 Encounter for supervision of normal first pregnancy, third trimester Ⓜ ♀

✓5ᵗʰ **Z34.8 Encounter for supervision of other normal pregnancy**

Z34.8Ø Encounter for supervision of other normal pregnancy, unspecified trimester Ⓜ ♀

Z34.81 Encounter for supervision of other normal pregnancy, first trimester Ⓜ ♀

Z34.82 Encounter for supervision of other normal pregnancy, second trimester Ⓜ ♀

Z34.83 Encounter for supervision of other normal pregnancy, third trimester Ⓜ ♀

✓5ᵗʰ **Z34.9 Encounter for supervision of normal pregnancy, unspecified**

Z34.9Ø Encounter for supervision of normal pregnancy, unspecified, unspecified trimester Ⓜ ♀

Z34.91 Encounter for supervision of normal pregnancy, unspecified, first trimester Ⓜ ♀

Z34.92 Encounter for supervision of normal pregnancy, unspecified, second trimester Ⓜ ♀

Z34.93 Encounter for supervision of normal pregnancy, unspecified, third trimester Ⓜ ♀

✓4ᵗʰ **Z36 Encounter for** antenatal screening **of mother**

INCLUDES   encounter for placental sample (taken vaginally)

screening is the testing for disease or disease precursors in asymptomatic individuals so that early detection and treatment can be provided for those who test positive for the disease.

EXCLUDES 1   *diagnostic examination — code to sign or symptom*

encounter for suspected maternal and fetal conditions ruled out (ZØ3.7-)

suspected fetal condition affecting management of pregnancy — code to condition in Chapter 15

EXCLUDES 2   *abnormal findings on antenatal screening of mother (O28.-)*

genetic counseling and testing (Z31.43-, Z31.5)

routine prenatal care (Z34)

AHA: 2017,4Q,28

Z36.Ø Encounter for antenatal screening for chromosomal anomalies Ⓜ ♀

Z36.1 Encounter for antenatal screening for raised alphafetoprotein level Ⓜ ♀

Encounter for antenatal screening for elevated maternal serum alphafetoprotein level

DEF: High levels of alpha-fetoprotein (AFP) that may indicate a possibility of spina bifida and other neural tube defects, anencephaly, or omphalocele in the fetus.

Z36.2 Encounter for other antenatal screening follow-up Ⓜ ♀

Non-visualized anatomy on a previous scan

Z36.3 Encounter for antenatal screening for malformations Ⓜ ♀

Screening for a suspected anomaly

Z36.4 Encounter for antenatal screening for fetal growth retardation Ⓜ ♀

Intrauterine growth restriction (IUGR)/small-for-dates

Z36.5 Encounter for antenatal screening for isoimmunization Ⓜ ♀

✓5ᵗʰ **Z36.8 Encounter for other antenatal screening**

Z36.81 Encounter for antenatal screening for hydrops fetalis Ⓜ ♀

DEF: Hydrops fetalis: Abnormal accumulation of fluid in two or more parts of the fetus, such as ascites, effusion of the pleural or pericardial tissues, or edema.

Z36.82 Encounter for antenatal screening for nuchal translucency Ⓜ ♀

Z36.83 Encounter for fetal screening for congenital cardiac abnormalities Ⓜ ♀

Z36.84 Encounter for antenatal screening for fetal lung maturity Ⓜ ♀

Z36.85 Encounter for antenatal screening for Streptococcus B Ⓜ ♀

Z36.86 Encounter for antenatal screening for cervical length Ⓜ ♀

Screening for risk of pre-term labor

Z36.87 Encounter for antenatal screening for uncertain dates Ⓜ ♀

Z36.88 Encounter for antenatal screening for fetal macrosomia Ⓜ ♀

Screening for large-for-dates

Z36.89 Encounter for other specified antenatal screening Ⓜ ♀

Z36.8A Encounter for antenatal screening for other genetic defects Ⓜ ♀

Z36.9 Encounter for antenatal screening, unspecified Ⓜ ♀

✓4ᵗʰ **Z3A Weeks of gestation**

NOTE   Codes from category Z3A are for use, only on the maternal record, to indicate the weeks of gestation of the pregnancy, if known.

Code first complications of pregnancy, childbirth and the puerperium (OØ9-O9A)

AHA: 2019,2Q,11; 2016,2Q,34; 2014,3Q,17; 2014,2Q,9; 2013,2Q,33

TIP: Do not assign a code from this category with codes from categories OØØ-OØ8 or code Z33.2.

✓5ᵗʰ **Z3A.Ø Weeks of gestation of pregnancy,** unspecified or less than 10 weeks

Z3A.ØØ Weeks of gestation of pregnancy not specified Ⓜ ♀

Z3A.Ø1 Less than 8 weeks **gestation of pregnancy** Ⓜ ♀

Z3A.Ø8 8 weeks **gestation of pregnancy** Ⓜ ♀

Z3A.Ø9 9 weeks **gestation of pregnancy** Ⓜ ♀

Ⓝ Newborn: 0   Ⓟ Pediatric: 0-17   Ⓜ Maternity: 9-64   Ⓐ Adult: 15-124   MCC Major Complication/Comorbidity   CC Complication/Comorbidity   SW Severe Wound Dx

1286   ICD-10-CM 2020

✓5ᵗʰ **Z3A.1 Weeks of gestation of pregnancy, weeks 10-19**

Z3A.10 10 weeks gestation of pregnancy M ♀

Z3A.11 11 weeks gestation of pregnancy M ♀

Z3A.12 12 weeks gestation of pregnancy M ♀

Z3A.13 13 weeks gestation of pregnancy M ♀

Z3A.14 14 weeks gestation of pregnancy M ♀

Z3A.15 15 weeks gestation of pregnancy M ♀

Z3A.16 16 weeks gestation of pregnancy M ♀

Z3A.17 17 weeks gestation of pregnancy M ♀

Z3A.18 18 weeks gestation of pregnancy M ♀

Z3A.19 19 weeks gestation of pregnancy M ♀

✓5ᵗʰ **Z3A.2 Weeks of gestation of pregnancy, weeks 20-29**

Z3A.20 20 weeks gestation of pregnancy M ♀

Z3A.21 21 weeks gestation of pregnancy M ♀

Z3A.22 22 weeks gestation of pregnancy M ♀

Z3A.23 23 weeks gestation of pregnancy M ♀

Z3A.24 24 weeks gestation of pregnancy M ♀

Z3A.25 25 weeks gestation of pregnancy M ♀

Z3A.26 26 weeks gestation of pregnancy M ♀

Z3A.27 27 weeks gestation of pregnancy M ♀

Z3A.28 28 weeks gestation of pregnancy M ♀

Z3A.29 29 weeks gestation of pregnancy M ♀

✓5ᵗʰ **Z3A.3 Weeks of gestation of pregnancy, weeks 30-39**

Z3A.30 30 weeks gestation of pregnancy M ♀

Z3A.31 31 weeks gestation of pregnancy M ♀

Z3A.32 32 weeks gestation of pregnancy M ♀

Z3A.33 33 weeks gestation of pregnancy M ♀

Z3A.34 34 weeks gestation of pregnancy M ♀

Z3A.35 35 weeks gestation of pregnancy M ♀

Z3A.36 36 weeks gestation of pregnancy M ♀

Z3A.37 37 weeks gestation of pregnancy M ♀

Z3A.38 38 weeks gestation of pregnancy M ♀

Z3A.39 39 weeks gestation of pregnancy M ♀

✓5ᵗʰ **Z3A.4 Weeks of gestation of pregnancy, weeks 40 or greater**

AHA: 2014,4Q,23

Z3A.40 40 weeks gestation of pregnancy M ♀

Z3A.41 41 weeks gestation of pregnancy M ♀

Z3A.42 42 weeks gestation of pregnancy M ♀

Z3A.49 Greater than 42 weeks gestation of pregnancy M ♀

✓4ᵗʰ **Z37 Outcome of delivery**

This category is intended for use as an additional code to identify the outcome of delivery on the mother's record. It is not for use on the newborn record.

EXCLUDES 1 stillbirth (P95)

Z37.0 Single live birth M ♀

AHA: 2016,2Q,34; 2014,2Q,9

Z37.1 Single stillbirth M ♀

Z37.2 Twins, both liveborn M ♀

Z37.3 Twins, one liveborn and one stillborn M ♀

Z37.4 Twins, both stillborn M ♀

✓5ᵗʰ **Z37.5 Other multiple births, all liveborn**

Z37.50 Multiple births, unspecified, all liveborn M ♀

Z37.51 Triplets, all liveborn M ♀

Z37.52 Quadruplets, all liveborn M ♀

Z37.53 Quintuplets, all liveborn M ♀

Z37.54 Sextuplets, all liveborn M ♀

Z37.59 Other multiple births, all liveborn M ♀

✓5ᵗʰ **Z37.6 Other multiple births, some liveborn**

Z37.60 Multiple births, unspecified, some liveborn M ♀

Z37.61 Triplets, some liveborn M ♀

Z37.62 Quadruplets, some liveborn M ♀

Z37.63 Quintuplets, some liveborn M ♀

Z37.64 Sextuplets, some liveborn M ♀

Z37.69 Other multiple births, some liveborn M ♀

Z37.7 Other multiple births, all stillborn M ♀

Z37.9 Outcome of delivery, unspecified M ♀

Multiple birth NOS

Single birth NOS

✓4ᵗʰ **Z38 Liveborn infants according to place of birth and type of delivery**

This category is for use as the principal code on the initial record of a newborn baby. It is to be used for the initial birth record only. It is not to be used on the mother's record.

AHA: 2017,2Q,5-7; 2016,3Q,18; 2015,2Q,15

✓5ᵗʰ **Z38.0 Single liveborn infant, born in hospital**

Single liveborn infant, born in birthing center or other health care facility

Z38.00 Single liveborn infant, delivered vaginally N

Z38.01 Single liveborn infant, delivered by cesarean N

Z38.1 Single liveborn infant, born outside hospital N

Z38.2 Single liveborn infant, unspecified as to place of birth N

Single liveborn infant NOS

✓5ᵗʰ **Z38.3 Twin liveborn infant, born in hospital**

Z38.30 Twin liveborn infant, delivered vaginally N

Z38.31 Twin liveborn infant, delivered by cesarean N

Z38.4 Twin liveborn infant, born outside hospital N

Z38.5 Twin liveborn infant, unspecified as to place of birth N

✓5ᵗʰ **Z38.6 Other multiple liveborn infant, born in hospital**

Z38.61 Triplet liveborn infant, delivered vaginally N

Z38.62 Triplet liveborn infant, delivered by cesarean N

Z38.63 Quadruplet liveborn infant, delivered vaginally N

Z38.64 Quadruplet liveborn infant, delivered by cesarean N

Z38.65 Quintuplet liveborn infant, delivered vaginally N

Z38.66 Quintuplet liveborn infant, delivered by cesarean N

Z38.68 Other multiple liveborn infant, delivered vaginally N

Z38.69 Other multiple liveborn infant, delivered by cesarean N

Z38.7 Other multiple liveborn infant, born outside hospital N

Z38.8 Other multiple liveborn infant, unspecified as to place of birth N

✓4ᵗʰ **Z39 Encounter for maternal postpartum care and examination**

Z39.0 Encounter for care and examination of mother immediately after delivery M ♀

Care and observation in uncomplicated cases when the delivery occurs outside a healthcare facility

EXCLUDES 1 care for postpartum complication — see Alphabetic Index

Z39.1 Encounter for care and examination of lactating mother M ♀

Encounter for supervision of lactation

EXCLUDES 1 disorders of lactation (O92.-)

Z39.2 Encounter for routine postpartum follow-up M ♀

✔ Additional Character Required   ✓x7ᵗʰ Placeholder   Unacceptable PDx   Questionable PDx   Manifestation   Unspecified Dx   H1-H14 HAC   HCC CMS-HCC Dx   HIV HIV Dx

ICD-10-CM 2020

1287

Chapter 21. Factors Influencing Health Status and Contact With Health Services

Z40–Z44.129

Encounters for other specific health care (Z40–Z53)

Categories Z40-Z53 are intended for use to indicate a reason for care. They may be used for patients who have already been treated for a disease or injury, but who are receiving aftercare or prophylactic care, or care to consolidate the treatment, or to deal with a residual state

EXCLUDES 2   *follow-up examination for medical surveillance after treatment (Z08-Z09)*

✓4ᵗʰ **Z40**   **Encounter for prophylactic surgery**

   EXCLUDES 1   *organ donations (Z52.-)*

          therapeutic organ removal — code to condition

   DEF: Agent or treatment measure intended to prevent or ward off a disease condition.

✓5ᵗʰ **Z40.0**   **Encounter for prophylactic surgery for risk factors related to malignant neoplasms**

     Admission for prophylactic organ removal

     Use additional code to identify risk factor

     AHA: 2017,4Q,28-29

     Z40.00   **Encounter for prophylactic removal of unspecified organ**

     Z40.01   **Encounter for prophylactic removal of breast**

     Z40.02   **Encounter for prophylactic removal of ovary(s)** ♀

         Encounter for prophylactic removal of ovary(s) and fallopian tube(s)

     Z40.03   **Encounter for prophylactic removal of fallopian tube(s)** ♀

     Z40.09   **Encounter for prophylactic removal of other organ**

   Z40.8   **Encounter for other prophylactic surgery**

   Z40.9   **Encounter for prophylactic surgery, unspecified**

✓4ᵗʰ **Z41**   **Encounter for procedures for purposes other than remedying health state**

   Z41.1   **Encounter for cosmetic surgery**

     Encounter for cosmetic breast implant

     Encounter for cosmetic procedure

     EXCLUDES 1   *encounter for plastic and reconstructive surgery following medical procedure or healed injury (Z42.-)*

          encounter for post-mastectomy breast implantation (Z42.1)

   Z41.2   **Encounter for routine and ritual male circumcision** ♂

     AHA: 2018,3Q,15

     TIP: Do not report this code when circumcision is performed during the birth admission.

   Z41.3   **Encounter for ear piercing**

   Z41.8   **Encounter for other procedures for purposes other than remedying health state**

   Z41.9   **Encounter for procedure for purposes other than remedying health state, unspecified**

✓4ᵗʰ **Z42**   **Encounter for plastic and reconstructive surgery following medical procedure or healed injury**

   EXCLUDES 1   *encounter for cosmetic plastic surgery (Z41.1)*

     encounter for plastic surgery for treatment of current injury — code to relevent injury

   Z42.1   **Encounter for breast reconstruction following mastectomy** 🅰

     EXCLUDES 1   *deformity and disproportion of reconstructed breast (N65.1-)*

   Z42.8   **Encounter for other plastic and reconstructive surgery following medical procedure or healed injury**

     AHA: 2017,1Q,42

✓4ᵗʰ **Z43**   **Encounter for attention to artificial openings**

   INCLUDES   closure of artificial openings

     passage of sounds or bougies through artificial openings

     reforming artificial openings

     removal of catheter from artificial openings

     toilet or cleansing of artificial openings

   EXCLUDES 1   *complications of external stoma (J95.0-, K94.-, N99.5-)*

   EXCLUDES 2   *fitting and adjustment of prosthetic and other devices (Z44-Z46)*

   AHA: 2019,2Q,33

   Z43.0   **Encounter for attention to tracheostomy** HCC

   Z43.1   **Encounter for attention to gastrostomy** HCC

     EXCLUDES 2   *artificial opening status only, without need for care (Z93.-)*

   Z43.2   **Encounter for attention to ileostomy** HCC

   Z43.3   **Encounter for attention to colostomy** HCC

   Z43.4   **Encounter for attention to other artificial openings of digestive tract** HCC

   Z43.5   **Encounter for attention to cystostomy** HCC

   Z43.6   **Encounter for attention to other artificial openings of urinary tract** HCC

     Encounter for attention to nephrostomy

     Encounter for attention to ureterostomy

     Encounter for attention to urethrostomy

   Z43.7   **Encounter for attention to artificial vagina**

   Z43.8   **Encounter for attention to other artificial openings** HCC

   Z43.9   **Encounter for attention to unspecified artificial opening** HCC

✓4ᵗʰ **Z44**   **Encounter for fitting and adjustment of external prosthetic device**

   INCLUDES   removal or replacement of external prosthetic device

   EXCLUDES 1   *malfunction or other complications of device — see Alphabetical Index*

     presence of prosthetic device (Z97.-)

✓5ᵗʰ **Z44.0**   **Encounter for fitting and adjustment of artificial arm**

   ✓6ᵗʰ **Z44.00**   **Encounter for fitting and adjustment of unspecified artificial arm**

     Z44.001   **Encounter for fitting and adjustment of unspecified right artificial arm**

     Z44.002   **Encounter for fitting and adjustment of unspecified left artificial arm**

     Z44.009   **Encounter for fitting and adjustment of unspecified artificial arm, unspecified arm**

   ✓6ᵗʰ **Z44.01**   **Encounter for fitting and adjustment of complete artificial arm**

     Z44.011   **Encounter for fitting and adjustment of complete right artificial arm**

     Z44.012   **Encounter for fitting and adjustment of complete left artificial arm**

     Z44.019   **Encounter for fitting and adjustment of complete artificial arm, unspecified arm**

   ✓6ᵗʰ **Z44.02**   **Encounter for fitting and adjustment of partial artificial arm**

     Z44.021   **Encounter for fitting and adjustment of partial artificial right arm**

     Z44.022   **Encounter for fitting and adjustment of partial artificial left arm**

     Z44.029   **Encounter for fitting and adjustment of partial artificial arm, unspecified arm**

✓5ᵗʰ **Z44.1**   **Encounter for fitting and adjustment of artificial leg**

   ✓6ᵗʰ **Z44.10**   **Encounter for fitting and adjustment of unspecified artificial leg**

     Z44.101   **Encounter for fitting and adjustment of unspecified right artificial leg** HCC

     Z44.102   **Encounter for fitting and adjustment of unspecified left artificial leg** HCC

     Z44.109   **Encounter for fitting and adjustment of unspecified artificial leg, unspecified leg** HCC

   ✓6ᵗʰ **Z44.11**   **Encounter for fitting and adjustment of complete artificial leg**

     Z44.111   **Encounter for fitting and adjustment of complete right artificial leg** HCC

     Z44.112   **Encounter for fitting and adjustment of complete left artificial leg** HCC

     Z44.119   **Encounter for fitting and adjustment of complete artificial leg, unspecified leg** HCC

   ✓6ᵗʰ **Z44.12**   **Encounter for fitting and adjustment of partial artificial leg**

     Z44.121   **Encounter for fitting and adjustment of partial artificial right leg** HCC

     Z44.122   **Encounter for fitting and adjustment of partial artificial left leg** HCC

     Z44.129   **Encounter for fitting and adjustment of partial artificial leg, unspecified leg** HCC

🅝 Newborn: 0   🅟 Pediatric: 0-17   🅜 Maternity: 9-64   🅐 Adult: 15-124   MCC Major Complication/Comorbidity   CC Complication/Comorbidity   SW Severe Wound Dx

1288   ICD-10-CM 2020

√5th **Z44.2** **Encounter for fitting and adjustment of** artificial eye

    EXCLUDES 1   *mechanical complication of ocular prosthesis (T85.3)*

    Z44.20 **Encounter for fitting and adjustment of artificial eye, unspecified**

    Z44.21 **Encounter for fitting and adjustment of artificial** right **eye**

    Z44.22 **Encounter for fitting and adjustment of artificial** left **eye**

√5th **Z44.3** **Encounter for fitting and adjustment of** external breast prosthesis

    EXCLUDES 1   *complications of breast implant (T85.4-)*

         encounter for adjustment or removal of breast implant (Z45.81-)

         encounter for initial breast implant insertion for cosmetic breast augmentation (Z41.1)

         encounter for breast reconstruction following mastectomy (Z42.1)

    Z44.30 **Encounter for fitting and adjustment of external breast prosthesis, unspecified breast**

    Z44.31 **Encounter for fitting and adjustment of external** right **breast prosthesis**

    Z44.32 **Encounter for fitting and adjustment of external** left **breast prosthesis**

Z44.8 **Encounter for fitting and adjustment of other external prosthetic devices**

Z44.9 **Encounter for fitting and adjustment of unspecified external prosthetic device**

√4th **Z45** **Encounter for adjustment and management of implanted device**

    INCLUDES   removal or replacement of implanted device

    EXCLUDES 1   *malfunction or other complications of device — see Alphabetical Index*

    EXCLUDES 2   *encounter for fitting and adjustment of non-implanted device (Z46.-)*

√5th **Z45.0** **Encounter for adjustment and management of** cardiac device

    √6th **Z45.01** **Encounter for adjustment and management of cardiac** pacemaker

         Encounter for adjustment and management of cardiac resynchronization therapy pacemaker (CRT-P)

         EXCLUDES 1   *encounter for adjustment and management of automatic implantable cardiac defibrillator with synchronous cardiac pacemaker (Z45.02)*

         Z45.010 **Encounter for checking and testing of cardiac pacemaker** pulse generator **[battery]**

            Encounter for replacing cardiac pacemaker pulse generator [battery]

         Z45.018 **Encounter for adjustment and management of other part of cardiac pacemaker**

            EXCLUDES 1   ▶*presence of other part of cardiac pacemaker (Z95.0)*◀

            EXCLUDES 2   *presence of prosthetic and other devices* ▶*(Z95.1-Z95.5, Z95.811-Z97)*◀

    Z45.02 **Encounter for adjustment and management of** automatic implantable cardiac defibrillator

         Encounter for adjustment and management of automatic implantable cardiac defibrillator with synchronous cardiac pacemaker

         Encounter for adjustment and management of cardiac resynchronization therapy defibrillator (CRT-D)

    Z45.09 **Encounter for adjustment and management of other cardiac device**

Z45.1 **Encounter for adjustment and management of** infusion pump

Z45.2 **Encounter for adjustment and management of** vascular access device

    Encounter for adjustment and management of vascular catheters

    EXCLUDES 1   *encounter for adjustment and management of renal dialysis catheter (Z49.01)*

    AHA: 2018,3Q,20

√5th **Z45.3** **Encounter for adjustment and management of implanted** devices of the special senses

    Z45.31 **Encounter for adjustment and management of implanted** visual **substitution device**

√6th **Z45.32** **Encounter for adjustment and management of implanted** hearing **device**

    EXCLUDES 1   *encounter for fitting and adjustment of hearing aide (Z46.1)*

    Z45.320 **Encounter for adjustment and management of** bone conduction **device**

    Z45.321 **Encounter for adjustment and management of** cochlear **device**

    Z45.328 **Encounter for adjustment and management of other implanted hearing device**

√5th **Z45.4** **Encounter for adjustment and management of implanted** nervous system device

    Z45.41 **Encounter for adjustment and management of** cerebrospinal fluid drainage **device**

         Encounter for adjustment and management of cerebral ventricular (communicating) shunt

    Z45.42 **Encounter for adjustment and management of** neurostimulator

         ▶Encounter for adjustment and management of brain neurostimulator◀

         ▶Encounter for adjustment and management of gastric neurostimulator◀

         ▶Encounter for adjustment and management of peripheral nerve neurostimulator◀

         ▶Encounter for adjustment and management of sacral nerve neurostimulator◀

         ▶Encounter for adjustment and management of spinal cord neurostimulator◀

         ▶Encounter for adjustment and management of vagus nerve neurostimulator◀

    Z45.49 **Encounter for adjustment and management of other implanted nervous system device**

         AHA: 2014,3Q,19

√5th **Z45.8** **Encounter for adjustment and management of other implanted devices**

    √6th **Z45.81** **Encounter for adjustment or** removal of breast implant

         Encounter for elective implant exchange (different material) (different size)

         ▶Encounter removal of tissue expander with or without synchronous insertion of permanent implant◀

         EXCLUDES 1   *complications of breast implant (T85.4-)*

            encounter for initial breast implant insertion for cosmetic breast augmentation (Z41.1)

            encounter for breast reconstruction following mastectomy (Z42.1)

    Z45.811 **Encounter for adjustment or removal of** right **breast implant**

    Z45.812 **Encounter for adjustment or removal of** left **breast implant**

    Z45.819 **Encounter for adjustment or removal of unspecified breast implant**

    Z45.82 **Encounter for** adjustment or removal of myringotomy device **(stent) (tube)**

    Z45.89 **Encounter for adjustment and management of other implanted devices**

         AHA: 2014,4Q,26-28

Z45.9 **Encounter for adjustment and management of unspecified implanted device**

√4th **Z46** **Encounter for fitting and adjustment of other devices**

    INCLUDES   removal or replacement of other device

    EXCLUDES 1   *malfunction or other complications of device — see Alphabetical Index*

    EXCLUDES 2   *encounter for fitting and management of implanted devices (Z45.-)*

         issue of repeat prescription only (Z76.0)

         presence of prosthetic and other devices (Z95-Z97)

Z46.0 **Encounter for fitting and adjustment of** spectacles and contact lenses

Z46.1 **Encounter for fitting and adjustment of** hearing aid

    EXCLUDES 1   *encounter for adjustment and management of implanted hearing device (Z45.32-)*

☑ Additional Character Required   √x7th Placeholder   Unacceptable PDx   Questionable PDx   Manifestation   Unspecified Dx   H1-H14 HAC   HCC CMS-HCC Dx   HIV HIV Dx

ICD-10-CM 2020   1289

Chapter 21. Factors Influencing Health Status and Contact With Health Services

Z44.2–Z46.1

Z46.2   **Encounter for fitting and adjustment of other devices related to nervous system and special senses**
> *EXCLUDES 2*   *encounter for adjustment and management of implanted nervous system device (Z45.4-)*
> *encounter for adjustment and management of implanted visual substitution device (Z45.31)*

Z46.3   **Encounter for fitting and adjustment of dental prosthetic device**
> Encounter for fitting and adjustment of dentures

Z46.4   **Encounter for fitting and adjustment of orthodontic device**

✓5ᵗʰ **Z46.5**   **Encounter for fitting and adjustment of other gastrointestinal appliance and device**
> *EXCLUDES 1*   *encounter for attention to artificial openings of digestive tract (Z43.1-Z43.4)*

    Z46.51   **Encounter for fitting and adjustment of gastric lap band**

    Z46.59   **Encounter for fitting and adjustment of other gastrointestinal appliance and device**

Z46.6   **Encounter for fitting and adjustment of urinary device**
> *EXCLUDES 2*   *attention to artificial openings of urinary tract (Z43.5, Z43.6)*

✓5ᵗʰ **Z46.8**   **Encounter for fitting and adjustment of other specified devices**

    Z46.81   **Encounter for fitting and adjustment of insulin pump**
> Encounter for insulin pump instruction and training
> Encounter for insulin pump titration

    Z46.82   **Encounter for fitting and adjustment of non-vascular catheter**

    Z46.89   **Encounter for fitting and adjustment of other specified devices**
> Encounter for fitting and adjustment of wheelchair

Z46.9   **Encounter for fitting and adjustment of unspecified device**

✓4ᵗʰ **Z47**   **Orthopedic aftercare**
> *EXCLUDES 1*   *aftercare for healing fracture — code to fracture with 7th character D*

Z47.1   **Aftercare following joint replacement surgery**
> Use additional code to identify the joint (Z96.6-)

Z47.2   **Encounter for removal of internal fixation device**
> *EXCLUDES 1*   *encounter for adjustment of internal fixation device for fracture treatment — code to fracture with appropriate 7th character*
> *encounter for removal of external fixation device — code to fracture with 7th character D*
> *infection or inflammatory reaction to internal fixation device (T84.6-)*
> *mechanical complication of internal fixation device (T84.1-)*

✓5ᵗʰ **Z47.3**   **Aftercare following explantation of joint prosthesis**
> Aftercare following explantation of joint prosthesis, staged procedure
> Encounter for joint prosthesis insertion following prior explantation of joint prosthesis
> **AHA:** 2015,1Q,16

    Z47.31   **Aftercare following explantation of shoulder joint prosthesis**
> *EXCLUDES 1*   *acquired absence of shoulder joint following prior explantation of shoulder joint prosthesis (Z89.23-)*
> *shoulder joint prosthesis explantation status (Z89.23-)*

    Z47.32   **Aftercare following explantation of hip joint prosthesis**
> *EXCLUDES 1*   *acquired absence of hip joint following prior explantation of hip joint prosthesis (Z89.62-)*
> *hip joint prosthesis explantation status (Z89.62-)*

    Z47.33   **Aftercare following explantation of knee joint prosthesis**
> *EXCLUDES 1*   *acquired absence of knee joint following prior explantation of knee prosthesis (Z89.52-)*
> *knee joint prosthesis explantation status (Z89.52-)*

✓5ᵗʰ **Z47.8**   **Encounter for other orthopedic aftercare**

    Z47.81   **Encounter for orthopedic aftercare following surgical amputation**
> Use additional code to identify the limb amputated (Z89.-)

    Z47.82   **Encounter for orthopedic aftercare following scoliosis surgery**

    Z47.89   **Encounter for other orthopedic aftercare**
> **AHA:** 2015,1Q,8

✓4ᵗʰ **Z48**   **Encounter for other postprocedural aftercare**
> *EXCLUDES 1*   *encounter for aftercare following injury — code to Injury, by site, with appropriate 7th character for subsequent encounter*
> *encounter for follow-up examination after completed treatment (Z08-Z09)*
> *EXCLUDES 2*   *encounter for attention to artificial openings (Z43.-)*
> *encounter for fitting and adjustment of prosthetic and other devices (Z44-Z46)*
> **AHA:** 2015,4Q,38; 2015,1Q,6-7

✓5ᵗʰ **Z48.0**   **Encounter for attention to dressings, sutures and drains**
> *EXCLUDES 1*   *encounter for planned postprocedural wound closure (Z48.1)*

    Z48.00   **Encounter for change or removal of nonsurgical wound dressing**
> Encounter for change or removal of wound dressing NOS

    Z48.01   **Encounter for change or removal of surgical wound dressing**
> **AHA:** 2019,2Q,33

    Z48.02   **Encounter for removal of sutures**
> Encounter for removal of staples

    Z48.03   **Encounter for change or removal of drains**
> **AHA:** 2019,2Q,33

Z48.1   **Encounter for planned postprocedural wound closure**
> *EXCLUDES 1*   *encounter for attention to dressings and sutures (Z48.0-)*

✓5ᵗʰ **Z48.2**   **Encounter for aftercare following organ transplant**

    Z48.21   **Encounter for aftercare following heart transplant**   `CC` `HCC`
> **CC Excl:** PDX collection 1488

    Z48.22   **Encounter for aftercare following kidney transplant**   `CC`
> **CC Excl:** PDX collection 1489

    Z48.23   **Encounter for aftercare following liver transplant**   `CC` `HCC`
> **CC Excl:** PDX collection 1490

    Z48.24   **Encounter for aftercare following lung transplant**   `CC` `HCC`
> **CC Excl:** PDX collection 1491

✓6ᵗʰ **Z48.28**   **Encounter for aftercare following multiple organ transplant**

      Z48.280   **Encounter for aftercare following heart-lung transplant**   `CC` `HCC`
> **CC Excl:** PDX collection 1488

      Z48.288   **Encounter for aftercare following multiple organ transplant**

✓6ᵗʰ **Z48.29**   **Encounter for aftercare following other organ transplant**

      Z48.290   **Encounter for aftercare following bone marrow transplant**   `CC` `HCC`
> **CC Excl:** PDX collection 1492

      Z48.298   **Encounter for aftercare following other organ transplant**

Z48.3   **Aftercare following surgery for neoplasm**
> Use additional code to identify the neoplasm

N Newborn: 0   P Pediatric: 0-17   M Maternity: 9-64   A Adult: 15-124   MCC Major Complication/Comorbidity   CC Complication/Comorbidity   SW Severe Wound Dx

1290   ICD-10-CM 2020

√5ᵗʰ **Z48.8** **Encounter for other specified postprocedural aftercare**

√6ᵗʰ **Z48.81** **Encounter for surgical aftercare following** surgery on specified body systems

These codes identify the body system requiring aftercare. They are for use in conjunction with other aftercare codes to fully explain the aftercare encounter. The condition treated should also be coded if still present.

> *EXCLUDES 1*   aftercare for injury — code the injury with 7th character D
> aftercare following surgery for neoplasm (Z48.3)
>
> *EXCLUDES 2*   aftercare following organ transplant (Z48.2-)
> orthopedic aftercare (Z47.-)

AHA: 2015,4Q,38

Z48.810 **Encounter for surgical aftercare following surgery on the** sense organs

Z48.811 **Encounter for surgical aftercare following surgery on the** nervous system

> *EXCLUDES 2*   encounter for surgical aftercare following surgery on the sense organs (Z48.810)

Z48.812 **Encounter for surgical aftercare following surgery on the** circulatory system
AHA: 2012,4Q,96

Z48.813 **Encounter for surgical aftercare following surgery on the** respiratory system
AHA: 2019,2Q,33

Z48.814 **Encounter for surgical aftercare following surgery on the** teeth or oral cavity

Z48.815 **Encounter for surgical aftercare following surgery on the** digestive system

Z48.816 **Encounter for surgical aftercare following surgery on the** genitourinary system

> *EXCLUDES 1*   encounter for aftercare following sterilization reversal (Z31.42)

Z48.817 **Encounter for surgical aftercare following surgery on the** skin and subcutaneous tissue

Z48.89 **Encounter for other specified surgical aftercare**

√4ᵗʰ **Z49** **Encounter for care involving renal dialysis**

Code also associated end stage renal disease (N18.6)

√5ᵗʰ **Z49.0** **Preparatory care for renal dialysis**

Encounter for dialysis instruction and training

Z49.01 **Encounter for fitting and adjustment of extracorporeal dialysis catheter** `HCC`

Removal or replacement of renal dialysis catheter
Toilet or cleansing of renal dialysis catheter

Z49.02 **Encounter for fitting and adjustment of peritoneal dialysis catheter** `HCC`

√5ᵗʰ **Z49.3** **Encounter for adequacy testing for dialysis**

Z49.31 **Encounter for adequacy testing for hemodialysis** `HCC`

Z49.32 **Encounter for adequacy testing for peritoneal dialysis** `HCC`

Encounter for peritoneal equilibration test

√4ᵗʰ **Z51** **Encounter for other aftercare and medical care**

Code also condition requiring care

> *EXCLUDES 1*   follow-up examination after treatment (Z08-Z09)

Z51.0 **Encounter for antineoplastic** radiation therapy
AHA: 2017,4Q,103
TIP: Do not assign when admission is for insertion/implantation of radioactive elements. Assign a code for the malignancy instead. Any complications related to the radioactive elements should be assigned as secondary diagnoses.

√5ᵗʰ **Z51.1** **Encounter for antineoplastic chemotherapy and immunotherapy**

> *EXCLUDES 2*   encounter for chemotherapy and immunotherapy for nonneoplastic condition — code to condition

Z51.11 **Encounter for antineoplastic** chemotherapy
AHA: 2015,3Q,19

Z51.12 **Encounter for antineoplastic** immunotherapy

Z51.5 **Encounter for** palliative care
AHA: 2017,1Q,48

Z51.6 **Encounter for** desensitization to allergens
AHA: 2016,4Q,77

√5ᵗʰ **Z51.8** **Encounter for other specified aftercare**

> *EXCLUDES 1*   holiday relief care (Z75.5)

Z51.81 **Encounter for** therapeutic drug level **monitoring**
Code also any long-term (current) drug therapy (Z79.-)

> *EXCLUDES 1*   encounter for blood-drug test for administrative or medicolegal reasons (Z02.83)

DEF: Drug monitoring: Measurement of the level of a specific drug in the body or measurement of a specific function to assess effectiveness of a drug.

Z51.89 **Encounter for other specified aftercare**
AHA: 2012,4Q,95-97

√4ᵗʰ **Z52** **Donors of organs and tissues**

> *INCLUDES*   autologous and other living donors
> *EXCLUDES 1*   cadaveric donor - omit code
> examination of potential donor (Z00.5)

AHA: 2012,4Q,99

√5ᵗʰ **Z52.0** **Blood** donor

√6ᵗʰ **Z52.00** **Unspecified blood donor**

Z52.000 **Unspecified donor,** whole **blood**
Z52.001 **Unspecified donor,** stem cells
Z52.008 **Unspecified donor, other blood**

√6ᵗʰ **Z52.01** **Autologous** blood donor

Z52.010 **Autologous donor,** whole blood
Z52.011 **Autologous donor,** stem cells
Z52.018 **Autologous donor, other blood**

√6ᵗʰ **Z52.09** **Other blood donor**

Volunteer donor

Z52.090 **Other blood donor,** whole blood
Z52.091 **Other blood donor,** stem cells
Z52.098 **Other blood donor, other blood**

√5ᵗʰ **Z52.1** **Skin** donor

Z52.10 **Skin donor, unspecified**
Z52.11 **Skin donor,** autologous
Z52.19 **Skin donor, other**

√5ᵗʰ **Z52.2** **Bone** donor

Z52.20 **Bone donor, unspecified**
Z52.21 **Bone donor,** autologous
Z52.29 **Bone donor, other**

Z52.3 **Bone marrow** donor

Z52.4 **Kidney** donor

Z52.5 **Cornea** donor

Z52.6 **Liver** donor

√5ᵗʰ **Z52.8** **Donor of other specified organs or tissues**

√6ᵗʰ **Z52.81** **Egg (Oocyte)** donor

Z52.810 **Egg (Oocyte) donor** under age 35, anonymous **recipient** ♀
Egg donor under age 35 NOS

Z52.811 **Egg (Oocyte) donor** under age 35, designated **recipient** ♀

Z52.812 **Egg (Oocyte) donor** age 35 and over, anonymous **recipient** ♀
Egg donor age 35 and over NOS

Z52.813 **Egg (Oocyte) donor** age 35 and over, designated **recipient** ♀

Z52.819 **Egg (Oocyte) donor, unspecified** ♀

Z52.89 **Donor of other specified organs or tissues**

Z52.9 **Donor of unspecified organ or tissue**
Donor NOS

√4ᵗʰ **Z53** **Persons encountering health services for specific procedures and treatment, not carried out**

√5ᵗʰ **Z53.0** **Procedure and treatment not carried out because of contraindication**

Z53.01 **Procedure and treatment not carried out due to patient smoking**

Z53.09 **Procedure and treatment not carried out because of other contraindication**

Z53.1 **Procedure and treatment not carried out because of patient's decision for** reasons of belief and group pressure

√5ᵗʰ **Z53.2** **Procedure and treatment not carried out because of patient's decision for other and unspecified reasons**

Z53.20 **Procedure and treatment not carried out because of patient's decision for unspecified reasons**

☑ Additional Character Required   √x7ᵗʰ Placeholder   Unacceptable PDx   Questionable PDx   Manifestation   Unspecified Dx   H1-H14 HAC   HCC CMS-HCC Dx   HIV HIV Dx

ICD-10-CM 2020   **1291**

Z53.21   Procedure and treatment not carried out due to patient leaving prior to being seen by health care provider

Z53.29   Procedure and treatment not carried out because of patient's decision for other reasons

✓5ᵗʰ **Z53.3**   Procedure converted to open procedure
AHA: 2016,4Q,79

Z53.31   Laparoscopic surgical procedure converted to open procedure

Z53.32   Thoracoscopic surgical procedure converted to open procedure

Z53.33   Arthroscopic surgical procedure converted to open procedure

Z53.39   Other specified procedure converted to open procedure

Z53.8   Procedure and treatment not carried out for other reasons

Z53.9   Procedure and treatment not carried out, unspecified reason

Persons with potential health hazards related to socioeconomic and psychosocial circumstances (Z55-Z65)

AHA: 2018,4Q,58,73; 2018,1Q,18
TIP: Codes from this code block can be assigned based on documentation from clinicians other than the diagnosing provider.

✓4ᵗʰ **Z55**   Problems related to education and literacy
EXCLUDES 1   disorders of psychological development (F80-F89)

Z55.0   Illiteracy and low-level literacy

Z55.1   Schooling unavailable and unattainable

Z55.2   Failed school examinations

Z55.3   Underachievement in school

Z55.4   Educational maladjustment and discord with teachers and classmates

Z55.8   Other problems related to education and literacy
Problems related to inadequate teaching

Z55.9   Problems related to education and literacy, unspecified
Academic problems NOS

✓4ᵗʰ **Z56**   Problems related to employment and unemployment
EXCLUDES 2   occupational exposure to risk factors (Z57.-)
problems related to housing and economic circumstances (Z59.-)

Z56.0   Unemployment, unspecified

Z56.1   Change of job   A

Z56.2   Threat of job loss

Z56.3   Stressful work schedule

Z56.4   Discord with boss and workmates

Z56.5   Uncongenial work environment
Difficult conditions at work

Z56.6   Other physical and mental strain related to work

✓5ᵗʰ **Z56.8**   Other problems related to employment

Z56.81   Sexual harassment on the job

Z56.82   Military deployment status
Individual (civilian or military) currently deployed in theater or in support of military war, peacekeeping and humanitarian operations

Z56.89   Other problems related to employment

Z56.9   Unspecified problems related to employment
Occupational problems NOS

✓4ᵗʰ **Z57**   Occupational exposure to risk factors

Z57.0   Occupational exposure to noise

Z57.1   Occupational exposure to radiation

Z57.2   Occupational exposure to dust

✓5ᵗʰ **Z57.3**   Occupational exposure to other air contaminants

Z57.31   Occupational exposure to environmental tobacco smoke
EXCLUDES 2   exposure to environmental tobacco smoke (Z77.22)

Z57.39   Occupational exposure to other air contaminants

Z57.4   Occupational exposure to toxic agents in agriculture
Occupational exposure to solids, liquids, gases or vapors in agriculture

Z57.5   Occupational exposure to toxic agents in other industries
Occupational exposure to solids, liquids, gases or vapors in other industries

Z57.6   Occupational exposure to extreme temperature

Z57.7   Occupational exposure to vibration

Z57.8   Occupational exposure to other risk factors

Z57.9   Occupational exposure to unspecified risk factor

✓4ᵗʰ **Z59**   Problems related to housing and economic circumstances
EXCLUDES 2   problems related to upbringing (Z62.-)

Z59.0   Homelessness   CC

Z59.1   Inadequate housing
Lack of heating
Restriction of space
Technical defects in home preventing adequate care
Unsatisfactory surroundings
EXCLUDES 1   problems related to the natural and physical environment (Z77.1-)

Z59.2   Discord with neighbors, lodgers and landlord

Z59.3   Problems related to living in residential institution
Boarding-school resident
EXCLUDES 1   institutional upbringing (Z62.2)

Z59.4   Lack of adequate food and safe drinking water
Inadequate drinking water supply
EXCLUDES 1   effects of hunger (T73.0)
inappropriate diet or eating habits (Z72.4)
malnutrition (E40-E46)

Z59.5   Extreme poverty

Z59.6   Low income

Z59.7   Insufficient social insurance and welfare support

Z59.8   Other problems related to housing and economic circumstances
Foreclosure on loan
Isolated dwelling
Problems with creditors

Z59.9   Problem related to housing and economic circumstances, unspecified

✓4ᵗʰ **Z60**   Problems related to social environment

Z60.0   Problems of adjustment to life-cycle transitions
Empty nest syndrome
Phase of life problem
Problem with adjustment to retirement [pension]

Z60.2   Problems related to living alone

Z60.3   Acculturation difficulty
Problem with migration
Problem with social transplantation
DEF: Problem adapting to a different culture or environment not based on any coexisting mental disorder.

Z60.4   Social exclusion and rejection
Exclusion and rejection on the basis of personal characteristics, such as unusual physical appearance, illness or behavior.
EXCLUDES 1   target of adverse discrimination such as for racial or religious reasons (Z60.5)

Z60.5   Target of (perceived) adverse discrimination and persecution
EXCLUDES 1   social exclusion and rejection (Z60.4)

Z60.8   Other problems related to social environment

Z60.9   Problem related to social environment, unspecified

✓4ᵗʰ **Z62**   Problems related to upbringing
INCLUDES   current and past negative life events in childhood
current and past problems of a child related to upbringing
EXCLUDES 2   maltreatment syndrome (T74.-)
problems related to housing and economic circumstances (Z59.-)

Z62.0   Inadequate parental supervision and control

Z62.1   Parental overprotection

✓5ᵗʰ **Z62.2**   Upbringing away from parents
EXCLUDES 1   problems with boarding school (Z59.3)

Z62.21   Child in welfare custody   P
Child in care of non-parental family member
Child in foster care
EXCLUDES 2   problem for parent due to child in welfare custody (Z63.5)

Z62.22   Institutional upbringing
Child living in orphanage or group home

Z62.29   Other upbringing away from parents

Z62.3   Hostility towards and scapegoating of child   P

Z62.6   Inappropriate (excessive) parental pressure

☑5ᵗʰ **Z62.8 Other specified problems related to upbringing**

☑6ᵗʰ **Z62.81 Personal history of abuse in childhood**

Z62.810 Personal history of physical and sexual abuse in childhood
EXCLUDES 1 current child physical abuse (T74.12, T76.12)
current child sexual abuse (T74.22, T76.22)

Z62.811 Personal history of psychological abuse in childhood
EXCLUDES 1 current child psychological abuse (T74.32, T76.32)

Z62.812 Personal history of neglect in childhood
EXCLUDES 1 current child neglect (T74.02, T76.02)

Z62.813 Personal history of forced labor or sexual exploitation in childhood
AHA: 2018,4Q,32,35

Z62.819 Personal history of unspecified abuse in childhood
EXCLUDES 1 current child abuse NOS (T74.92, T76.92)

☑6ᵗʰ **Z62.82 Parent-child conflict**

Z62.820 Parent-biological child conflict
Parent-child problem NOS

Z62.821 Parent-adopted child conflict

Z62.822 Parent-foster child conflict

☑6ᵗʰ **Z62.89 Other specified problems related to upbringing**

Z62.890 Parent-child estrangement NEC

Z62.891 Sibling rivalry

Z62.898 Other specified problems related to upbringing

Z62.9 Problem related to upbringing, unspecified

☑4ᵗʰ **Z63 Other problems related to primary support group, including family circumstances**
EXCLUDES 2 maltreatment syndrome (T74.-, T76)
parent-child problems (Z62.-)
problems related to negative life events in childhood (Z62.-)
problems related to upbringing (Z62.-)

Z63.0 Problems in relationship with spouse or partner
Relationship distress with spouse or intimate partner
EXCLUDES 1 counseling for spousal or partner abuse problems (Z69.1)
counseling related to sexual attitude, behavior, and orientation (Z70.-)

Z63.1 Problems in relationship with in-laws

☑5ᵗʰ **Z63.3 Absence of family member**
EXCLUDES 1 absence of family member due to disappearance and death (Z63.4)
absence of family member due to separation and divorce (Z63.5)

Z63.31 Absence of family member due to military deployment
Individual or family affected by other family member being on military deployment
EXCLUDES 1 family disruption due to return of family member from military deployment (Z63.71)

Z63.32 Other absence of family member

Z63.4 Disappearance and death of family member
Assumed death of family member
Bereavement
AHA: 2014,1Q,25

Z63.5 Disruption of family by separation and divorce
Marital estrangement

Z63.6 Dependent relative needing care at home

☑5ᵗʰ **Z63.7 Other stressful life events affecting family and household**

Z63.71 Stress on family due to return of family member from military deployment
Individual or family affected by family member having returned from military deployment (current or past conflict)

Z63.72 Alcoholism and drug addiction in family

Z63.79 Other stressful life events affecting family and household
Anxiety (normal) about sick person in family
Health problems within family
Ill or disturbed family member
Isolated family

Z63.8 Other specified problems related to primary support group
Family discord NOS
Family estrangement NOS
High expressed emotional level within family
Inadequate family support NOS
Inadequate or distorted communication within family

Z63.9 Problem related to primary support group, unspecified
Relationship disorder NOS

☑4ᵗʰ **Z64 Problems related to certain psychosocial circumstances**

Z64.0 Problems related to unwanted pregnancy   ♀

Z64.1 Problems related to multiparity   ♀

Z64.4 Discord with counselors
Discord with probation officer
Discord with social worker

☑4ᵗʰ **Z65 Problems related to other psychosocial circumstances**

Z65.0 Conviction in civil and criminal proceedings without imprisonment

Z65.1 Imprisonment and other incarceration

Z65.2 Problems related to release from prison

Z65.3 Problems related to other legal circumstances
Arrest
Child custody or support proceedings
Litigation
Prosecution

Z65.4 Victim of crime and terrorism
Victim of torture

Z65.5 Exposure to disaster, war and other hostilities
EXCLUDES 1 target of perceived discrimination or persecution (Z60.5)

Z65.8 Other specified problems related to psychosocial circumstances
Religious or spiritual problem

Z65.9 Problem related to unspecified psychosocial circumstances

Do not resuscitate status (Z66)

Z66 Do not resuscitate
DNR status
DEF: Medical order written by a physician that instructs others not to perform cardiopulmonary resuscitation (CPR), intubation, or advanced life support (ACLS). It prevents unnecessary invasive treatment to prolong life should breathing stop or cardiac arrest occur.

Blood type (Z67)

✓4ᵗʰ Z67 Blood type
AHA: 2015,3Q,40

Blood Types

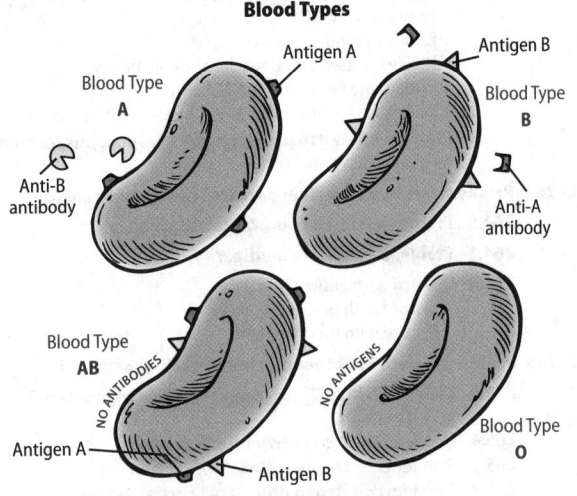

Antigen A — Blood Type A — Antigen B — Blood Type B
Anti-B antibody — Anti-A antibody
Blood Type AB — NO ANTIBODIES — NO ANTIGENS — Blood Type O
Antigen A — Antigen B

✓5ᵗʰ Z67.1 Type A blood

| Z67.1Ø | Type A blood, Rh positive |
| Z67.11 | Type A blood, Rh negative |

✓5ᵗʰ Z67.2 Type B blood

| Z67.2Ø | Type B blood, Rh positive |
| Z67.21 | Type B blood, Rh negative |

✓5ᵗʰ Z67.3 Type AB blood

| Z67.3Ø | Type AB blood, Rh positive |
| Z67.31 | Type AB blood, Rh negative |

✓5ᵗʰ Z67.4 Type O blood

| Z67.4Ø | Type O blood, Rh positive |
| Z67.41 | Type O blood, Rh negative |

✓5ᵗʰ Z67.9 Unspecified blood type

| Z67.9Ø | Unspecified blood type, Rh positive |
| Z67.91 | Unspecified blood type, Rh negative |

Body mass index [BMI] (Z68)

✓4ᵗʰ Z68 Body mass index [BMI]
Kilograms per meters squared

> **NOTE** ▶BMI adult codes are for use for persons 2Ø years of age or older◀
> ▶BMI pediatric codes are for use for persons 2-19 years of age.◀
> ▶These percentiles are based on the growth charts published by the Centers for Disease Control and Prevention (CDC)◀

AHA: 2018,4Q,73,77-83; 2017,1Q,39
DEF: Index used to help determine whether an individual is underweight, a healthy weight, overweight, or obese.
TIP: A BMI code may be assigned to support an associated condition based on medical record documentation from clinicians who are not the patient's provider.
TIP: Do not assign when used in association with fluctuations in body fluid during an encounter, such as fluid overload or fluid retention.
TIP: In order to assign a BMI code, the associated condition must meet the definition of a reportable diagnosis for nonoutpatient encounters, per section III of the *ICD-10-CM Official Guidelines for Coding and Reporting*.

| Z68.1 | Body mass index [BMI] 19.9 or less, adult | A |

✓5ᵗʰ Z68.2 Body mass index [BMI] 2Ø-29, adult

Z68.2Ø	Body mass index [BMI] 2Ø.Ø-2Ø.9, adult	A
Z68.21	Body mass index [BMI] 21.Ø-21.9, adult	A
Z68.22	Body mass index [BMI] 22.Ø-22.9, adult	A
Z68.23	Body mass index [BMI] 23.Ø-23.9, adult	A
Z68.24	Body mass index [BMI] 24.Ø-24.9, adult	A
Z68.25	Body mass index [BMI] 25.Ø-25.9, adult	A
Z68.26	Body mass index [BMI] 26.Ø-26.9, adult	A
Z68.27	Body mass index [BMI] 27.Ø-27.9, adult	A

| Z68.28 | Body mass index [BMI] 28.Ø-28.9, adult | A |
| Z68.29 | Body mass index [BMI] 29.Ø-29.9, adult | A |

✓5ᵗʰ Z68.3 Body mass index [BMI] 3Ø-39, adult

Z68.3Ø	Body mass index [BMI] 3Ø.Ø-3Ø.9, adult	A
Z68.31	Body mass index [BMI] 31.Ø-31.9, adult	A
Z68.32	Body mass index [BMI] 32.Ø-32.9, adult	A
Z68.33	Body mass index [BMI] 33.Ø-33.9, adult	A
Z68.34	Body mass index [BMI] 34.Ø-34.9, adult	A
Z68.35	Body mass index [BMI] 35.Ø-35.9, adult	A
Z68.36	Body mass index [BMI] 36.Ø-36.9, adult	A
Z68.37	Body mass index [BMI] 37.Ø-37.9, adult	A
Z68.38	Body mass index [BMI] 38.Ø-38.9, adult	A
Z68.39	Body mass index [BMI] 39.Ø-39.9, adult	A

✓5ᵗʰ Z68.4 Body mass index [BMI] 4Ø or greater, adult
CC Excl: For CC codes in subcategory Z68.4: PDX collection 1494

Z68.41	Body mass index [BMI] 4Ø.Ø-44.9, adult	HCC A
Z68.42	Body mass index [BMI] 45.Ø-49.9, adult	HCC A
Z68.43	Body mass index [BMI] 5Ø.Ø-59.9, adult	CC HCC A
Z68.44	Body mass index [BMI] 6Ø.Ø-69.9, adult	CC HCC A
Z68.45	Body mass index [BMI] 7Ø or greater, adult	CC HCC A

✓5ᵗʰ Z68.5 Body mass index [BMI] pediatric
AHA: 2018,4Q,81-82

Z68.51	Body mass index [BMI] pediatric, less than 5th percentile for age
Z68.52	Body mass index [BMI] pediatric, 5th percentile to less than 85th percentile for age
Z68.53	Body mass index [BMI] pediatric, 85th percentile to less than 95th percentile for age
Z68.54	Body mass index [BMI] pediatric, greater than or equal to 95th percentile for age

Persons encountering health services in other circumstances (Z69-Z76)

✓4ᵗʰ Z69 Encounter for mental health services for victim and perpetrator of abuse
> **INCLUDES** counseling for victims and perpetrators of abuse

✓5ᵗʰ Z69.Ø Encounter for mental health services for child abuse problems

✓6ᵗʰ Z69.Ø1 Encounter for mental health services for parental child abuse

Z69.Ø1Ø Encounter for mental health services for victim of parental child abuse   P
> Encounter for mental health services for victim of child abuse by parent
> Encounter for mental health services for victim of child neglect by parent
> Encounter for mental health services for victim of child psychological abuse by parent
> Encounter for mental health services for victim of child sexual abuse by parent

Z69.Ø11 Encounter for mental health services for perpetrator of parental child abuse
> Encounter for mental health services for perpetrator of parental child neglect
> Encounter for mental health services for perpetrator of parental child psychological abuse
> Encounter for mental health services for perpetrator of parental child sexual abuse

> **EXCLUDES 1** encounter for mental health services for non-parental child abuse (Z69.Ø2-)

☑6ᵗʰ Z69.02 Encounter for mental health services for non-parental child abuse

Z69.020 Encounter for mental health services for victim of non-parental child abuse   Ⓟ

Encounter for mental health services for victim of non-parental child neglect

Encounter for mental health services for victim of non-parental child psychological abuse

Encounter for mental health services for victim of non-parental child sexual abuse

Z69.021 Encounter for mental health services for perpetrator of non-parental child abuse

Encounter for mental health services for perpetrator of non-parental child neglect

Encounter for mental health services for perpetrator of non-parental child psychological abuse

Encounter for mental health services for perpetrator of non-parental child sexual abuse

☑5ᵗʰ Z69.1 Encounter for mental health services for spousal or partner abuse problems

Z69.11 Encounter for mental health services for victim of spousal or partner abuse

Encounter for mental health services for victim of spouse or partner neglect

Encounter for mental health services for victim of spouse or partner psychological abuse

Encounter for mental health services for victim of spouse or partner violence, physical

Z69.12 Encounter for mental health services for perpetrator of spousal or partner abuse

Encounter for mental health services for perpetrator of spouse or partner neglect

Encounter for mental health services for perpetrator of spouse or partner psychological abuse

Encounter for mental health services for perpetrator of spouse or partner violence, physical

Encounter for mental health services for perpetrator of spouse or partner violence, sexual

☑5ᵗʰ Z69.8 Encounter for mental health services for victim or perpetrator of other abuse

Z69.81 Encounter for mental health services for victim of other abuse

~~Encounter for mental health services for perpetrator of non-spousal adult abuse~~

Encounter for mental health services for victim of non-spousal adult abuse

Encounter for mental health services for victim of spouse or partner violence, sexual

Encounter for rape victim counseling

Z69.82 Encounter for mental health services for perpetrator of other abuse

▶Encounter for mental health services for perpetrator of non-spousal adult abuse◀

☑4ᵗʰ Z70 Counseling related to sexual attitude, behavior and orientation

INCLUDES encounter for mental health services for sexual attitude, behavior and orientation

EXCLUDES 2 contraceptive or procreative counseling (Z30-Z31)

Z70.0 Counseling related to sexual attitude

Z70.1 Counseling related to patient's sexual behavior and orientation

Patient concerned regarding impotence

Patient concerned regarding non-responsiveness

Patient concerned regarding promiscuity

Patient concerned regarding sexual orientation

Z70.2 Counseling related to sexual behavior and orientation of third party

Advice sought regarding sexual behavior and orientation of child

Advice sought regarding sexual behavior and orientation of partner

Advice sought regarding sexual behavior and orientation of spouse

Z70.3 Counseling related to combined concerns regarding sexual attitude, behavior and orientation

Z70.8 Other sex counseling

Encounter for sex education

Z70.9 Sex counseling, unspecified

☑4ᵗʰ Z71 Persons encountering health services for other counseling and medical advice, not elsewhere classified

EXCLUDES 2 contraceptive or procreation counseling (Z30-Z31)

sex counseling (Z70.-)

Z71.0 Person encountering health services to consult on behalf of another person

Person encountering health services to seek advice or treatment for non-attending third party

EXCLUDES 2 anxiety (normal) about sick person in family (Z63.7)

expectant (adoptive) parent(s) pre-birth pediatrician visit (Z76.81)

Z71.1 Person with feared health complaint in whom no diagnosis is made

Person encountering health services with feared condition which was not demonstrated

Person encountering health services in which problem was normal state

"Worried well"

EXCLUDES 1 medical observation for suspected diseases and conditions proven not to exist (Z03.-)

Z71.2 Person consulting for explanation of examination or test findings

Z71.3 Dietary counseling and surveillance

Use additional code for any associated underlying medical condition

Use additional code to identify body mass index (BMI), if known (Z68.-)

☑5ᵗʰ Z71.4 Alcohol abuse counseling and surveillance

Use additional code for alcohol abuse or dependence (F10.-)

Z71.41 Alcohol abuse counseling and surveillance of alcoholic

Z71.42 Counseling for family member of alcoholic

Counseling for significant other, partner, or friend of alcoholic

☑5ᵗʰ Z71.5 Drug abuse counseling and surveillance

Use additional code for drug abuse or dependence (F11-F16, F18-F19)

Z71.51 Drug abuse counseling and surveillance of drug abuser

Z71.52 Counseling for family member of drug abuser

Counseling for significant other, partner, or friend of drug abuser

Z71.6 Tobacco abuse counseling

Use additional code for nicotine dependence (F17.-)

Z71.7 Human immunodeficiency virus [HIV] counseling

☑5ᵗʰ Z71.8 Other specified counseling

EXCLUDES 2 counseling for contraception (Z30.0-)

AHA: 2017,4Q,27

Z71.81 Spiritual or religious counseling

Z71.82 Exercise counseling

Z71.83 Encounter for nonprocreative genetic counseling

EXCLUDES 1 counseling for procreative genetics (Z31.5)

counseling for procreative management (Z31.6)

Z71.84 Encounter for health counseling related to travel

Encounter for health risk and safety counseling for (international) travel

Code also, if applicable, encounter for immunization (Z23)

EXCLUDES 2 encounter for administrative examination (Z02.-)

encounter for other special examination without complaint, suspected or reported diagnosis (Z01.-)

Z71.89 Other specified counseling

Z71.9 Counseling, unspecified

Encounter for medical advice NOS

☑ Additional Character Required   ✓x7ᵗʰ Placeholder   Unacceptable PDx   Questionable PDx   Manifestation   Unspecified Dx   H1-H14 HAC   HCC CMS-HCC Dx   HIV HIV Dx

ICD-10-CM 2020   1295

Z72 Problems related to lifestyle
- EXCLUDES 2: problems related to life-management difficulty (Z73.-)
- problems related to socioeconomic and psychosocial circumstances (Z55-Z65)

Z72.0 Tobacco use
Tobacco use NOS
- EXCLUDES 1: history of tobacco dependence (Z87.891)
- nicotine dependence (F17.2-)
- tobacco dependence (F17.2-)
- tobacco use during pregnancy (O99.33-)

Z72.3 Lack of physical exercise

Z72.4 Inappropriate diet and eating habits
- EXCLUDES 1: behavioral eating disorders of infancy or childhood (F98.2-F98.3)
- eating disorders (F50.-)
- lack of adequate food (Z59.4)
- malnutrition and other nutritional deficiencies (E40-E64)

Z72.5 High risk sexual behavior
Promiscuity
- EXCLUDES 1: paraphilias (F65)
- **Z72.51 High risk heterosexual behavior**
- **Z72.52 High risk homosexual behavior**
- **Z72.53 High risk bisexual behavior**

Z72.6 Gambling and betting
- EXCLUDES 1: compulsive or pathological gambling (F63.0)

Z72.8 Other problems related to lifestyle
- **Z72.81 Antisocial behavior**
  - EXCLUDES 1: conduct disorders (F91.-)
  - **Z72.810 Child and adolescent antisocial behavior** P
    - Antisocial behavior (child) (adolescent) without manifest psychiatric disorder
    - Delinquency NOS
    - Group delinquency
    - Offenses in the context of gang membership
    - Stealing in company with others
    - Truancy from school
  - **Z72.811 Adult antisocial behavior** A
    - Adult antisocial behavior without manifest psychiatric disorder
- **Z72.82 Problems related to sleep**
  - **Z72.820 Sleep deprivation**
    - Lack of adequate sleep
    - EXCLUDES 1: insomnia (G47.0-)
  - **Z72.821 Inadequate sleep hygiene**
    - Bad sleep habits
    - Irregular sleep habits
    - Unhealthy sleep wake schedule
    - EXCLUDES 1: insomnia (F51.0-, G47.0-)
- **Z72.89 Other problems related to lifestyle**
  - Self-damaging behavior

Z72.9 Problem related to lifestyle, unspecified

Z73 Problems related to life management difficulty
- EXCLUDES 2: problems related to socioeconomic and psychosocial circumstances (Z55-Z65)
- DEF: State of emotional, mental, and physical exhaustion causing difficulties in managing personal, school, or work circumstances. It is usually due to prolonged stress or poor interpersonal relationship skills or parenting skills.

Z73.0 Burn-out

Z73.1 Type A behavior pattern

Z73.2 Lack of relaxation and leisure

Z73.3 Stress, not elsewhere classified
- Physical and mental strain NOS
- EXCLUDES 1: stress related to employment or unemployment (Z56.-)

Z73.4 Inadequate social skills, not elsewhere classified

Z73.5 Social role conflict, not elsewhere classified

Z73.6 Limitation of activities due to disability
- EXCLUDES 1: care-provider dependency (Z74.-)

Z73.8 Other problems related to life management difficulty
- **Z73.81 Behavioral insomnia of childhood**
  - DEF: Behaviors on the part of the child or caregivers that cause negative compliance with a child's sleep schedule resulting in lack of adequate sleep.
  - **Z73.810 Behavioral insomnia of childhood, sleep-onset association type** P
  - **Z73.811 Behavioral insomnia of childhood, limit setting type** P
  - **Z73.812 Behavioral insomnia of childhood, combined type** P
  - **Z73.819 Behavioral insomnia of childhood, unspecified type** P
- **Z73.82 Dual sensory impairment**
- **Z73.89 Other problems related to life management difficulty**

Z73.9 Problem related to life management difficulty, unspecified

Z74 Problems related to care provider dependency
- EXCLUDES 2: dependence on enabling machines or devices NEC (Z99.-)

Z74.0 Reduced mobility
- **Z74.01 Bed confinement status**
  - Bedridden
- **Z74.09 Other reduced mobility**
  - Chair ridden
  - Reduced mobility NOS
  - EXCLUDES 2: wheelchair dependence (Z99.3)

Z74.1 Need for assistance with personal care

Z74.2 Need for assistance at home and no other household member able to render care

Z74.3 Need for continuous supervision

Z74.8 Other problems related to care provider dependency

Z74.9 Problem related to care provider dependency, unspecified

Z75 Problems related to medical facilities and other health care

Z75.0 Medical services not available in home
- EXCLUDES 1: no other household member able to render care (Z74.2)

Z75.1 Person awaiting admission to adequate facility elsewhere

Z75.2 Other waiting period for investigation and treatment

Z75.3 Unavailability and inaccessibility of health-care facilities
- EXCLUDES 1: bed unavailable (Z75.1)

Z75.4 Unavailability and inaccessibility of other helping agencies

Z75.5 Holiday relief care

Z75.8 Other problems related to medical facilities and other health care

Z75.9 Unspecified problem related to medical facilities and other health care

Z76 Persons encountering health services in other circumstances

Z76.0 Encounter for issue of repeat prescription
- Encounter for issue of repeat prescription for appliance
- Encounter for issue of repeat prescription for medicaments
- Encounter for issue of repeat prescription for spectacles
- EXCLUDES 2: issue of medical certificate (Z02.7)
- repeat prescription for contraceptive (Z30.4-)

Z76.1 Encounter for health supervision and care of foundling

Z76.2 Encounter for health supervision and care of other healthy infant and child P
- Encounter for medical or nursing care or supervision of healthy infant under circumstances such as adverse socioeconomic conditions at home
- Encounter for medical or nursing care or supervision of healthy infant under circumstances such as awaiting foster or adoptive placement
- Encounter for medical or nursing care or supervision of healthy infant under circumstances such as maternal illness
- Encounter for medical or nursing care or supervision of healthy infant under circumstances such as number of children at home preventing or interfering with normal care

Z76.3 Healthy person accompanying sick person

Z76.4 Other boarder to healthcare facility
- EXCLUDES 1: homelessness (Z59.0)

Z76.5 Malingerer [conscious simulation]
Person feigning illness (with obvious motivation)
> EXCLUDES 1   *factitious disorder (F68.1-, F68.A)*
> *peregrinating patient (F68.1-)*

DEF: Act of intentionally exaggerating an illness or disability in order to receive personal gain or to avoid punishment or responsibility.

√5ᵗʰ **Z76.8 Persons encountering health services in other specified circumstances**

Z76.81 Expectant parent(s) prebirth pediatrician visit
Pre-adoption pediatrician visit for adoptive parent(s)

Z76.82 Awaiting organ transplant status
Patient waiting for organ availability

Z76.89 Persons encountering health services in other specified circumstances
Persons encountering health services NOS
AHA: 2014,2Q,10

Persons with potential health hazards related to family and personal history and certain conditions influencing health status (Z77-Z99)

Code also any follow-up examination (Z08-Z09)

√4ᵗʰ **Z77 Other contact with and (suspected) exposures hazardous to health**
> INCLUDES   contact with and (suspected) exposures to potential hazards to health
> EXCLUDES 2   *contact with and (suspected) exposure to communicable diseases (Z20.-)*
> *exposure to (parental) (environmental) tobacco smoke in the perinatal period (P96.81)*
> *newborn affected by noxious substances transmitted via placenta or breast milk (P04.-)*
> *occupational exposure to risk factors (Z57.-)*
> *retained foreign body (Z18.-)*
> *retained foreign body fully removed (Z87.821)*
> *toxic effects of substances chiefly nonmedicinal as to source (T51-T65)*

√5ᵗʰ **Z77.0 Contact with and (suspected) exposure to hazardous, chiefly nonmedicinal, chemicals**

√6ᵗʰ **Z77.01 Contact with and (suspected) exposure to hazardous metals**

Z77.010 Contact with and (suspected) exposure to arsenic

Z77.011 Contact with and (suspected) exposure to lead

Z77.012 Contact with and (suspected) exposure to uranium
> EXCLUDES 1   *retained depleted uranium fragments (Z18.01)*

Z77.018 Contact with and (suspected) exposure to other hazardous metals
Contact with and (suspected) exposure to chromium compounds
Contact with and (suspected) exposure to nickel dust

√6ᵗʰ **Z77.02 Contact with and (suspected) exposure to hazardous aromatic compounds**

Z77.020 Contact with and (suspected) exposure to aromatic amines

Z77.021 Contact with and (suspected) exposure to benzene

Z77.028 Contact with and (suspected) exposure to other hazardous aromatic compounds
Aromatic dyes NOS
Polycyclic aromatic hydrocarbons

√6ᵗʰ **Z77.09 Contact with and (suspected) exposure to other hazardous, chiefly nonmedicinal, chemicals**

Z77.090 Contact with and (suspected) exposure to asbestos

Z77.098 Contact with and (suspected) exposure to other hazardous, chiefly nonmedicinal, chemicals
Dyes NOS

√5ᵗʰ **Z77.1 Contact with and (suspected) exposure to environmental pollution and hazards in the physical environment**

√6ᵗʰ **Z77.11 Contact with and (suspected) exposure to environmental pollution**

Z77.110 Contact with and (suspected) exposure to air pollution

Z77.111 Contact with and (suspected) exposure to water pollution

Z77.112 Contact with and (suspected) exposure to soil pollution

Z77.118 Contact with and (suspected) exposure to other environmental pollution

√6ᵗʰ **Z77.12 Contact with and (suspected) exposure to hazards in the physical environment**

Z77.120 Contact with and (suspected) exposure to mold (toxic)

Z77.121 Contact with and (suspected) exposure to harmful algae and algae toxins
Contact with and (suspected) exposure to (harmful) algae bloom NOS
Contact with and (suspected) exposure to blue-green algae bloom
Contact with and (suspected) exposure to brown tide
Contact with and (suspected) exposure to cyanobacteria bloom
Contact with and (suspected) exposure to Florida red tide
Contact with and (suspected) exposure to pfiesteria piscicida
Contact with and (suspected) exposure to red tide

Z77.122 Contact with and (suspected) exposure to noise

Z77.123 Contact with and (suspected) exposure to radon and other naturally occurring radiation
> EXCLUDES 2   *radiation exposure as the cause of a confirmed condition (W88-W90, X39.0-)*
> *radiation sickness NOS (T66)*

Z77.128 Contact with and (suspected) exposure to other hazards in the physical environment

√5ᵗʰ **Z77.2 Contact with and (suspected) exposure to other hazardous substances**

Z77.21 Contact with and (suspected) exposure to potentially hazardous body fluids

Z77.22 Contact with and (suspected) exposure to environmental tobacco smoke (acute) (chronic)
Exposure to second hand tobacco smoke (acute) (chronic)
Passive smoking (acute) (chronic)
> EXCLUDES 1   *nicotine dependence (F17.-)*
> *tobacco use (Z72.0)*
> EXCLUDES 2   *occupational exposure to environmental tobacco smoke (Z57.31)*

Z77.29 Contact with and (suspected) exposure to other hazardous substances
AHA: 2016,2Q,33

Z77.9 Other contact with and (suspected) exposures hazardous to health

√4ᵗʰ **Z78 Other specified health status**
> EXCLUDES 2   *asymptomatic human immunodeficiency virus [HIV] infection status (Z21)*
> *postprocedural status (Z93-Z99)*
> *sex reassignment status (Z87.890)*

Z78.0 Asymptomatic menopausal state   A ♀
Menopausal state NOS
Postmenopausal status NOS
> EXCLUDES 2   *symptomatic menopausal state (N95.1)*

Z78.1 Physical restraint status
> EXCLUDES 1   *physical restraint due to a procedure — omit code*

DEF: Application of mechanical restraining devices or manual restraints to limit physical mobility of a patient.

Z78.9 Other specified health status

Chapter 21. Factors Influencing Health Status and Contact With Health Services

Z76.5–Z78.9

Chapter 21. Factors Influencing Health Status and Contact With Health Services

Z79 Long term (current) drug therapy

> INCLUDES   long term (current) drug use for prophylactic purposes
>
> Code also any therapeutic drug level monitoring (Z51.81)
>
> EXCLUDES 2   *drug abuse and dependence (F11-F19)*
>
> *drug use complicating pregnancy, childbirth, and the puerperium (O99.32-)*
>
> *long term (current) use of oral antidiabetic drugs (Z79.84)*
>
> *long term (current) use of oral hypoglycemic drugs (Z79.84)*

Z79.0 Long term (current) use of anticoagulants and antithrombotics/antiplatelets

> EXCLUDES 2   *long term (current) use of aspirin (Z79.82)*

Z79.01 Long term (current) use of anticoagulants

Z79.02 Long term (current) use of antithrombotics/antiplatelets

Z79.1 Long term (current) use of non-steroidal anti-inflammatories (NSAID)

> EXCLUDES 2   *long term (current) use of aspirin (Z79.82)*

Z79.2 Long term (current) use of antibiotics

Z79.3 Long term (current) use of hormonal contraceptives

> Long term (current) use of birth control pill or patch

Z79.4 Long term (current) use of insulin   HCC

> **TIP:** When both long-term (current) insulin and long-term (current) oral hypoglycemic use is documented, assign only a code for the long-term insulin use.

Z79.5 Long term (current) use of steroids

Z79.51 Long term (current) use of inhaled steroids

Z79.52 Long term (current) use of systemic steroids

Z79.8 Other long term (current) drug therapy

Z79.81 Long term (current) use of agents affecting estrogen receptors and estrogen levels

> Code first, if applicable:
>
> malignant neoplasm of breast (C50.-)
>
> malignant neoplasm of prostate (C61)
>
> Use additional code, if applicable, to identify:
>
> estrogen receptor positive status (Z17.0)
>
> family history of breast cancer (Z80.3)
>
> genetic susceptibility to malignant neoplasm (cancer) (Z15.0-)
>
> personal history of breast cancer (Z85.3)
>
> personal history of prostate cancer (Z85.46)
>
> postmenopausal status (Z78.0)
>
> EXCLUDES 1   *hormone replacement therapy (Z79.890)*

Z79.810 Long term (current) use of selective estrogen receptor modulators (SERMs)

> Long term (current) use of raloxifene (Evista)
>
> Long term (current) use of tamoxifen (Nolvadex)
>
> Long term (current) use of toremifene (Fareston)

Z79.811 Long term (current) use of aromatase inhibitors

> Long term (current) use of anastrozole (Arimidex)
>
> Long term (current) use of exemestane (Aromasin)
>
> Long term (current) use of letrozole (Femara)

Z79.818 Long term (current) use of other agents affecting estrogen receptors and estrogen levels

> Long term (current) use of estrogen receptor downregulators
>
> Long term (current) use of fulvestrant (Faslodex)
>
> Long term (current) use of gonadotropin-releasing hormone (GnRH) agonist
>
> Long term (current) use of goserelin acetate (Zoladex)
>
> Long term (current) use of leuprolide acetate (leuprorelin) (Lupron)
>
> Long term (current) use of megestrol acetate (Megace)

Z79.82 Long term (current) use of aspirin

Z79.83 Long term (current) use of bisphosphonates

> AHA: 2016,4Q,42

Z79.84 Long term (current) use of oral hypoglycemic drugs

> Long term (current) use of oral antidiabetic drugs
>
> EXCLUDES 2   *long term (current) use of insulin (Z79.4)*
>
> AHA: 2016,4Q,76
>
> **TIP:** When both long-term (current) insulin and long-term (current) oral hypoglycemic use is documented, assign only code Z79.4 for the long-term insulin use.

Z79.89 Other long term (current) drug therapy

Z79.890 Hormone replacement therapy

Z79.891 Long term (current) use of opiate analgesic

> Long term (current) use of methadone for pain management
>
> EXCLUDES 1   *methadone use NOS (F11.9-)*
>
> *use of methadone for treatment of heroin addiction (F11.2-)*

Z79.899 Other long term (current) drug therapy

> AHA: 2015,4Q,34; 2015,3Q,21

Z80 Family history of primary malignant neoplasm

Z80.0 Family history of malignant neoplasm of digestive organs

> Conditions classifiable to C15-C26
>
> AHA: 2018,1Q,6

Z80.1 Family history of malignant neoplasm of trachea, bronchus and lung

> Conditions classifiable to C33-C34

Z80.2 Family history of malignant neoplasm of other respiratory and intrathoracic organs

> Conditions classifiable to C30-C32, C37-C39

Z80.3 Family history of malignant neoplasm of breast

> Conditions classifiable to C50.-

Z80.4 Family history of malignant neoplasm of genital organs

> Conditions classifiable to C51-C63

Z80.41 Family history of malignant neoplasm of ovary

Z80.42 Family history of malignant neoplasm of prostate

Z80.43 Family history of malignant neoplasm of testis

Z80.49 Family history of malignant neoplasm of other genital organs

Z80.5 Family history of malignant neoplasm of urinary tract

> Conditions classifiable to C64-C68

Z80.51 Family history of malignant neoplasm of kidney

Z80.52 Family history of malignant neoplasm of bladder

Z80.59 Family history of malignant neoplasm of other urinary tract organ

Z80.6 Family history of leukemia

> Conditions classifiable to C91-C95

Z80.7 Family history of other malignant neoplasms of lymphoid, hematopoietic and related tissues

> Conditions classifiable to C81-C90, C96.-

Z80.8 Family history of malignant neoplasm of other organs or systems

> Conditions classifiable to C00-C14, C40-C49, C69-C79

Z80.9 Family history of malignant neoplasm, unspecified

> Conditions classifiable to C80.1

Z81 Family history of mental and behavioral disorders

Z81.0 Family history of intellectual disabilities

> Conditions classifiable to F70-F79

Z81.1 Family history of alcohol abuse and dependence

> Conditions classifiable to F10.-

Z81.2 Family history of tobacco abuse and dependence

> Conditions classifiable to F17.-

Z81.3 Family history of other psychoactive substance abuse and dependence

> Conditions classifiable to F11-F16, F18-F19

Z81.4 Family history of other substance abuse and dependence

> Conditions classifiable to F55

Z81.8 Family history of other mental and behavioral disorders

> Conditions classifiable elsewhere in F01-F99

Z82 Family history of certain disabilities and chronic diseases (leading to disablement)

Z82.0 Family history of epilepsy and other diseases of the nervous system

> Conditions classifiable to G00-G99

Z82.1 Family history of blindness and visual loss

> Conditions classifiable to H54.-

N Newborn: 0   P Pediatric: 0-17   M Maternity: 9-64   A Adult: 15-124   MCC Major Complication/Comorbidity   CC Complication/Comorbidity   SW Severe Wound Dx

1298   ICD-10-CM 2020

Z82.2   **Family history of** deafness and hearing loss
Conditions classifiable to H90-H91

Z82.3   **Family history of** stroke
Conditions classifiable to I60-I64

✓5ᵗʰ **Z82.4**   **Family history of ischemic heart disease and other diseases of the circulatory system**
Conditions classifiable to I00-I52, I65-I99

    Z82.41   **Family history of** sudden cardiac death

    Z82.49   **Family history of** ischemic heart disease **and other diseases of the circulatory system**

Z82.5   **Family history of** asthma **and other chronic lower respiratory diseases**
Conditions classifiable to J40-J47
    EXCLUDES 2   *family history of other diseases of the respiratory system (Z83.6)*

✓5ᵗʰ **Z82.6**   **Family history of arthritis and other diseases of the musculoskeletal system and connective tissue**
Conditions classifiable to M00-M99

    Z82.61   **Family history of** arthritis

    Z82.62   **Family history of** osteoporosis

    Z82.69   **Family history of other diseases of the musculoskeletal system and connective tissue**

✓5ᵗʰ **Z82.7**   **Family history of congenital malformations, deformations and chromosomal abnormalities**
Conditions classifiable to Q00-Q99

    Z82.71   **Family history of** polycystic kidney

    Z82.79   **Family history of other congenital malformations, deformations and chromosomal abnormalities**

Z82.8   **Family history of other disabilities and chronic diseases leading to disablement, not elsewhere classified**

✓4ᵗʰ **Z83**   **Family history of other specific disorders**
    EXCLUDES 2   *contact with and (suspected) exposure to communicable disease in the family (Z20.-)*

Z83.0   **Family history of** human immunodeficiency virus [HIV] **disease**
Conditions classifiable to B20

Z83.1   **Family history of other infectious and parasitic diseases**
Conditions classifiable to A00-B19, B25-B94, B99

Z83.2   **Family history of diseases of the** blood and blood-forming organs **and certain disorders involving the immune mechanism**
Conditions classifiable to D50-D89

Z83.3   **Family history of** diabetes mellitus
Conditions classifiable to E08-E13

✓5ᵗʰ **Z83.4**   **Family history of other endocrine, nutritional and metabolic diseases**
Conditions classifiable to E00-E07, E15-E88

    Z83.41   **Family history of** multiple endocrine neoplasia [MEN] syndrome

    Z83.42   **Family history of** familial hypercholesterolemia
      AHA: 2016,4Q,77

    ✓6ᵗʰ **Z83.43**   **Family history of other disorder of lipoprotein metabolism and other lipidemias**
      AHA: 2018,4Q,6,35

      Z83.430   **Family history of** elevated lipoprotein(a)
        Family history of elevated Lp(a)

      Z83.438   **Family history of other disorder of lipoprotein metabolism and other lipidemia**
        Family history of familial combined hyperlipidemia

    Z83.49   **Family history of other endocrine, nutritional and metabolic diseases**

✓5ᵗʰ **Z83.5**   **Family history of eye and ear disorders**

    ✓6ᵗʰ **Z83.51**   **Family history of** eye **disorders**
      Conditions classifiable to H00-H53, H55-H59
      EXCLUDES 2   *family history of blindness and visual loss (Z82.1)*

      Z83.511   **Family history of** glaucoma

      Z83.518   **Family history of other specified eye disorder**

    Z83.52   **Family history of** ear **disorders**
      Conditions classifiable to H60-H83, H92-H95
      EXCLUDES 2   *family history of deafness and hearing loss (Z82.2)*

Z83.6   **Family history of other diseases of the** respiratory system
Conditions classifiable to J00-J39, J60-J99
    EXCLUDES 2   *family history of asthma and other chronic lower respiratory diseases (Z82.5)*

✓5ᵗʰ **Z83.7**   **Family history of diseases of the digestive system**
Conditions classifiable to K00-K93

    Z83.71   **Family history of** colonic polyps
      EXCLUDES 2   *family history of malignant neoplasm of digestive organs (Z80.0)*

    Z83.79   **Family history of other diseases of the digestive system**

✓4ᵗʰ **Z84**   **Family history of other conditions**

Z84.0   **Family history of diseases of the** skin and subcutaneous tissue
Conditions classifiable to L00-L99

Z84.1   **Family history of disorders of** kidney and ureter
Conditions classifiable to N00-N29

Z84.2   **Family history of other diseases of the** genitourinary system
Conditions classifiable to N30-N99

Z84.3   **Family history of** consanguinity

✓5ᵗʰ **Z84.8**   **Family history of other specified conditions**

    Z84.81   **Family history of carrier of** genetic disease

    Z84.82   **Family history of** sudden infant death syndrome
      Family history of SIDS
      AHA: 2016,4Q,77

    Z84.89   **Family history of other specified conditions**

✓4ᵗʰ **Z85**   **Personal history of malignant neoplasm**
Code first any follow-up examination after treatment of malignant neoplasm (Z08)
Use additional code to identify:
   alcohol use and dependence (F10.-)
   exposure to environmental tobacco smoke (Z77.22)
   history of tobacco dependence (Z87.891)
   occupational exposure to environmental tobacco smoke (Z57.31)
   tobacco dependence (F17.-)
   tobacco use (Z72.0)
    EXCLUDES 2   *personal history of benign neoplasm (Z86.01-)*
            personal history of carcinoma-in-situ (Z86.00-)
AHA: 2018,4Q,64

✓5ᵗʰ **Z85.0**   **Personal history of malignant neoplasm of** digestive organs
    AHA: 2017,1Q,9

    Z85.00   **Personal history of malignant neoplasm of unspecified digestive organ**

    Z85.01   **Personal history of malignant neoplasm of** esophagus
      Conditions classifiable to C15

    ✓6ᵗʰ **Z85.02**   **Personal history of malignant neoplasm of** stomach

      Z85.020   **Personal history of malignant** carcinoid tumor **of stomach**
        Conditions classifiable to C7A.092

      Z85.028   **Personal history of other malignant neoplasm of stomach**
        Conditions classifiable to C16

    ✓6ᵗʰ **Z85.03**   **Personal history of malignant neoplasm of** large intestine

      Z85.030   **Personal history of malignant** carcinoid tumor **of large intestine**
        Conditions classifiable to C7A.022-C7A.025, C7A.029

      Z85.038   **Personal history of other malignant neoplasm of large intestine**
        Conditions classifiable to C18

    ✓6ᵗʰ **Z85.04**   **Personal history of malignant neoplasm of** rectum, rectosigmoid junction, and anus

      Z85.040   **Personal history of malignant** carcinoid tumor **of rectum**
        Conditions classifiable to C7A.026

      Z85.048   **Personal history of other malignant neoplasm of rectum, rectosigmoid junction, and anus**
        Conditions classifiable to C19-C21

    Z85.05   **Personal history of malignant neoplasm of** liver
      Conditions classifiable to C22

✓6ᵗʰ **Z85.06** **Personal history of malignant neoplasm of** small intestine

     Z85.060 **Personal history of malignant** carcinoid tumor **of small intestine**
       Conditions classifiable to C7A.01-

     Z85.068 **Personal history of other malignant neoplasm of small intestine**
       Conditions classifiable to C17

Z85.07 **Personal history of malignant neoplasm of** pancreas
     Conditions classifiable to C25

Z85.09 **Personal history of malignant neoplasm of other digestive organs**

✓5ᵗʰ **Z85.1** **Personal history of malignant neoplasm of** trachea, bronchus and lung

     ✓6ᵗʰ **Z85.11** **Personal history of malignant neoplasm of** bronchus and lung

       Z85.110 **Personal history of malignant** carcinoid tumor **of bronchus and lung**
         Conditions classifiable to C7A.090

       Z85.118 **Personal history of other malignant neoplasm of bronchus and lung**
         Conditions classifiable to C34

     Z85.12 **Personal history of malignant neoplasm of** trachea
       Conditions classifiable to C33

✓5ᵗʰ **Z85.2** **Personal history of malignant neoplasm of other** respiratory and intrathoracic organs

     Z85.20 **Personal history of malignant neoplasm of unspecified respiratory organ**

     Z85.21 **Personal history of malignant neoplasm of** larynx
       Conditions classifiable to C32

     Z85.22 **Personal history of malignant neoplasm of** nasal cavities, middle ear, and accessory sinuses
       Conditions classifiable to C30-C31

     ✓6ᵗʰ **Z85.23** **Personal history of malignant neoplasm of** thymus

       Z85.230 **Personal history of malignant** carcinoid tumor **of thymus**
         Conditions classifiable to C7A.091

       Z85.238 **Personal history of other malignant neoplasm of thymus**
         Conditions classifiable to C37

     Z85.29 **Personal history of malignant neoplasm of other respiratory and intrathoracic organs**

Z85.3 **Personal history of malignant neoplasm of** breast
     Conditions classifiable to C50.-

✓5ᵗʰ **Z85.4** **Personal history of malignant neoplasm of** genital organs
     Conditions classifiable to C51-C63

     Z85.40 **Personal history of malignant neoplasm of unspecified** female **genital organ** ♀

     Z85.41 **Personal history of malignant neoplasm of** cervix uteri ♀

     Z85.42 **Personal history of malignant neoplasm of other parts of uterus** ♀

     Z85.43 **Personal history of malignant neoplasm of** ovary ♀

     Z85.44 **Personal history of malignant neoplasm of other** female **genital organs** ♀

     Z85.45 **Personal history of malignant neoplasm of unspecified** male **genital organ** ♂

     Z85.46 **Personal history of malignant neoplasm of** prostate ♂

     Z85.47 **Personal history of malignant neoplasm of** testis ♂

     Z85.48 **Personal history of malignant neoplasm of** epididymis ♂

     Z85.49 **Personal history of malignant neoplasm of other** male **genital organs** ♂

✓5ᵗʰ **Z85.5** **Personal history of malignant neoplasm of** urinary tract
     Conditions classifiable to C64-C68

     Z85.50 **Personal history of malignant neoplasm of unspecified urinary tract organ**

     Z85.51 **Personal history of malignant neoplasm of** bladder

     ✓6ᵗʰ **Z85.52** **Personal history of malignant neoplasm of** kidney

       EXCLUDES 1   *personal history of malignant neoplasm of renal pelvis (Z85.53)*

       Z85.520 **Personal history of malignant** carcinoid tumor **of kidney**
         Conditions classifiable to C7A.093

       Z85.528 **Personal history of other malignant neoplasm of kidney**
         Conditions classifiable to C64

     Z85.53 **Personal history of malignant neoplasm of** renal pelvis

     Z85.54 **Personal history of malignant neoplasm of** ureter

     Z85.59 **Personal history of malignant neoplasm of other urinary tract organ**

Z85.6 **Personal history of** leukemia
     Conditions classifiable to C91-C95

     EXCLUDES 1   *leukemia in remission C91.0-C95.9 with 5th character 1*

✓5ᵗʰ **Z85.7** **Personal history of other malignant neoplasms of lymphoid, hematopoietic and related tissues**

     Z85.71 **Personal history of** Hodgkin lymphoma
       Conditions classifiable to C81

     Z85.72 **Personal history of** non-Hodgkin lymphomas
       Conditions classifiable to C82-C85

     Z85.79 **Personal history of other malignant neoplasms of lymphoid, hematopoietic and related tissues**
       Conditions classifiable to C88-C90, C96

       EXCLUDES 1   *multiple myeloma in remission (C90.01)*
            plasma cell leukemia in remission (C90.11)
            plasmacytoma in remission (C90.21)

✓5ᵗʰ **Z85.8** **Personal history of malignant neoplasms of other organs and systems**
     Conditions classifiable to C00-C14, C40-C49, C69-C75, C7A.098, C76-C79

     ✓6ᵗʰ **Z85.81** **Personal history of malignant neoplasm of** lip, oral cavity, and pharynx

       Z85.810 **Personal history of malignant neoplasm of** tongue

       Z85.818 **Personal history of malignant neoplasm of other sites of lip, oral cavity, and pharynx**

       Z85.819 **Personal history of malignant neoplasm of unspecified site of lip, oral cavity, and pharynx**

     ✓6ᵗʰ **Z85.82** **Personal history of malignant neoplasm of** skin

       Z85.820 **Personal history of malignant** melanoma **of skin**
         Conditions classifiable to C43

       Z85.821 **Personal history of** Merkel cell carcinoma
         Conditions classifiable to C4A

       Z85.828 **Personal history of other malignant neoplasm of skin**
         Conditions classifiable to C44

     ✓6ᵗʰ **Z85.83** **Personal history of malignant neoplasm of** bone and soft tissue

       Z85.830 **Personal history of malignant neoplasm of** bone

       Z85.831 **Personal history of malignant neoplasm of** soft tissue

         EXCLUDES 2   *personal history of malignant neoplasm of skin (Z85.82-)*

     ✓6ᵗʰ **Z85.84** **Personal history of malignant neoplasm of** eye and nervous tissue

       Z85.840 **Personal history of malignant neoplasm of** eye

       Z85.841 **Personal history of malignant neoplasm of** brain

       Z85.848 **Personal history of malignant neoplasm of other parts of nervous tissue**

     ✓6ᵗʰ **Z85.85** **Personal history of malignant neoplasm of** endocrine glands

       Z85.850 **Personal history of malignant neoplasm of** thyroid

       Z85.858 **Personal history of malignant neoplasm of other endocrine glands**

     Z85.89 **Personal history of malignant neoplasm of other organs and systems**

Z85.9 **Personal history of malignant neoplasm, unspecified**
     Conditions classifiable to C7A.00, C80.1

N Newborn: 0   P Pediatric: 0-17   M Maternity: 9-64   A Adult: 15-124   MCC Major Complication/Comorbidity   CC Complication/Comorbidity   SW Severe Wound Dx

1300   ICD-10-CM 2020

✓4ᵗʰ Z86 Personal history of certain other diseases

Code first any follow-up examination after treatment (Z09)

✓5ᵗʰ Z86.0 Personal history of in-situ and benign neoplasms and neoplasms of uncertain behavior

    EXCLUDES 2   personal history of malignant neoplasms (Z85.-)

    AHA: 2017,1Q,9

✓6ᵗʰ Z86.00 Personal history of in-situ neoplasm

    Conditions classifiable to D00-D09

Z86.000 Personal history of in-situ neoplasm of breast

    ►Conditions classifiable to D05◄

Z86.001 Personal history of in-situ neoplasm of cervix uteri   ♀

    ►Conditions classifiable to D06◄

    Personal history of cervical intraepithelial neoplasia III [CIN III]

Z86.002 Personal history of in-situ neoplasm of other and unspecified genital organs

    Conditions classifiable to D07

    Personal history of high-grade prostatic intraepithelial neoplasia III [HGPIN III]

    Personal history of vaginal intraepithelial neoplasia III [VAIN III]

    Personal history of vulvar intraepithelial neoplasia III [VIN III]

Z86.003 Personal history of in-situ neoplasm of oral cavity, esophagus and stomach

    Conditions classifiable to D00

Z86.004 Personal history of in-situ neoplasm of other and unspecified digestive organs

    Conditions classifiable to D01

    Personal history of anal intraepithelial neoplasia (AIN III)

Z86.005 Personal history of in-situ neoplasm of middle ear and respiratory system

    Conditions classifiable to D02

Z86.006 Personal history of melanoma in-situ

    Conditions classifiable to D03

    EXCLUDES 2   sites other than skin — code to personal history of in-situ neoplasm of the site

Z86.007 Personal history of in-situ neoplasm of skin

    Conditions classifiable to D04

    Personal history of carcinoma in situ of skin

Z86.008 Personal history of in-situ neoplasm of other site

    ►Conditions classifiable to D09◄

    ~~Personal history of vaginal intraepithelial neoplasia III [VAIN III]~~

    ~~Personal history of vulvar intraepithelial neoplasia III [VIN III]~~

✓6ᵗʰ Z86.01 Personal history of benign neoplasm

Z86.010 Personal history of colonic polyps

    AHA: 2017,1Q,14

Z86.011 Personal history of benign neoplasm of the brain

Z86.012 Personal history of benign carcinoid tumor

Z86.018 Personal history of other benign neoplasm

    AHA: 2017,1Q,14

Z86.03 Personal history of neoplasm of uncertain behavior

✓5ᵗʰ Z86.1 Personal history of infectious and parasitic diseases

    Conditions classifiable to A00-B89, B99

    EXCLUDES 1   personal history of infectious diseases specific to a body system

    sequelae of infectious and parasitic diseases (B90-B94)

Z86.11 Personal history of tuberculosis

Z86.12 Personal history of poliomyelitis

Z86.13 Personal history of malaria

Z86.14 Personal history of Methicillin resistant Staphylococcus aureus infection

    Personal history of MRSA infection

Z86.15 Personal history of latent tuberculosis infection

Z86.19 Personal history of other infectious and parasitic diseases

Z86.2 Personal history of diseases of the blood and blood-forming organs and certain disorders involving the immune mechanism

    Conditions classifiable to D50-D89

✓6ᵗʰ Z86.3 Personal history of endocrine, nutritional and metabolic diseases

    Conditions classifiable to E00-E88

Z86.31 Personal history of diabetic foot ulcer

    EXCLUDES 2   current diabetic foot ulcer (E08.621, E09.621, E10.621, E11.621, E13.621)

Z86.32 Personal history of gestational diabetes   ♀

    Personal history of conditions classifiable to O24.4-

    EXCLUDES 1   gestational diabetes mellitus in current pregnancy (O24.4-)

Z86.39 Personal history of other endocrine, nutritional and metabolic disease

✓5ᵗʰ Z86.5 Personal history of mental and behavioral disorders

    Conditions classifiable to F40-F59

Z86.51 Personal history of combat and operational stress reaction   A

Z86.59 Personal history of other mental and behavioral disorders

✓5ᵗʰ Z86.6 Personal history of diseases of the nervous system and sense organs

    Conditions classifiable to G00-G99, H00-H95

Z86.61 Personal history of infections of the central nervous system

    Personal history of encephalitis

    Personal history of meningitis

Z86.69 Personal history of other diseases of the nervous system and sense organs

    AHA: 2016,4Q,24

✓5ᵗʰ Z86.7 Personal history of diseases of the circulatory system

    Conditions classifiable to I00-I99

    EXCLUDES 2   old myocardial infarction (I25.2)

    personal history of anaphylactic shock (Z87.892)

    postmyocardial infarction syndrome (I24.1)

✓6ᵗʰ Z86.71 Personal history of venous thrombosis and embolism

Z86.711 Personal history of pulmonary embolism

Z86.718 Personal history of other venous thrombosis and embolism

Z86.72 Personal history of thrombophlebitis

Z86.73 Personal history of transient ischemic attack (TIA), and cerebral infarction without residual deficits

    Personal history of prolonged reversible ischemic neurological deficit (PRIND)

    Personal history of stroke NOS without residual deficits

    EXCLUDES 1   personal history of traumatic brain injury (Z87.820)

    sequelae of cerebrovascular disease (I69.-)

    AHA: 2012,4Q,92

Z86.74 Personal history of sudden cardiac arrest

    Personal history of sudden cardiac death successfully resuscitated

Z86.79 Personal history of other diseases of the circulatory system

✓4ᵗʰ Z87 Personal history of other diseases and conditions

Code first any follow-up examination after treatment (Z09)

✓5ᵗʰ Z87.0 Personal history of diseases of the respiratory system

    Conditions classifiable to J00-J99

Z87.01 Personal history of pneumonia (recurrent)

Z87.09 Personal history of other diseases of the respiratory system

✓5ᵗʰ Z87.1 Personal history of diseases of the digestive system

    Conditions classifiable to K00-K93

Z87.11 Personal history of peptic ulcer disease

Z87.19 Personal history of other diseases of the digestive system

    AHA: 2017,1Q,14

Z87.2 Personal history of diseases of the skin and subcutaneous tissue

    Conditions classifiable to L00-L99

    EXCLUDES 2   personal history of diabetic foot ulcer (Z86.31)

✔ Additional Character Required   ✓x7ᵗʰ Placeholder   Unacceptable PDx   Questionable PDx   Manifestation   Unspecified Dx   H1-H14 HAC   HCC CMS-HCC Dx   HIV HIV Dx

ICD-10-CM 2020   1301

√5ᵗʰ **Z87.3** **Personal history of diseases of the musculoskeletal system and connective tissue**
Conditions classifiable to M00-M99
EXCLUDES 2   *personal history of (healed) traumatic fracture (Z87.81)*

√6ᵗʰ **Z87.31** **Personal history of (healed) nontraumatic fracture**

Z87.310 **Personal history of (healed) osteoporosis fracture**
Personal history of (healed) fragility fracture
Personal history of (healed) collapsed vertebra due to osteoporosis
TIP: Assign for history of osteoporosis fractures that have resolved, even when a code from category M80 indicating current osteoporosis fracture is also reported.

Z87.311 **Personal history of (healed) other pathological fracture**
Personal history of (healed) collapsed vertebra NOS
EXCLUDES 2   *personal history of osteoporosis fracture (Z87.310)*

Z87.312 **Personal history of (healed) stress fracture**
Personal history of (healed) fatigue fracture

Z87.39 **Personal history of other diseases of the musculoskeletal system and connective tissue**

√5ᵗʰ **Z87.4** **Personal history of diseases of the genitourinary system**
Conditions classifiable to N00-N99

√6ᵗʰ **Z87.41** **Personal history of dysplasia of the female genital tract**
EXCLUDES 1   *personal history of intraepithelial neoplasia III of female genital tract (Z86.001, Z86.008)*
personal history of malignant neoplasm of female genital tract (Z85.40-Z85.44)

Z87.410 **Personal history of cervical dysplasia** ♀

Z87.411 **Personal history of vaginal dysplasia** ♀

Z87.412 **Personal history of vulvar dysplasia** ♀

Z87.42 **Personal history of other diseases of the female genital tract** ♀

√6ᵗʰ **Z87.43** **Personal history of diseases of the male genital organs**

Z87.430 **Personal history of prostatic dysplasia** ♂
EXCLUDES 1   *personal history of malignant neoplasm of prostate (Z85.46)*

Z87.438 **Personal history of other diseases of male genital organs** ♂

√6ᵗʰ **Z87.44** **Personal history of diseases of the urinary system**
EXCLUDES 1   *personal history of malignant neoplasm of cervix uteri (Z85.41)*

Z87.440 **Personal history of urinary (tract) infections**

Z87.441 **Personal history of nephrotic syndrome**

Z87.442 **Personal history of urinary calculi**
Personal history of kidney stones

Z87.448 **Personal history of other diseases of urinary system**

√5ᵗʰ **Z87.5** **Personal history of complications of pregnancy, childbirth and the puerperium**
Conditions classifiable to O00-O9A
EXCLUDES 2   *recurrent pregnancy loss (N96)*

Z87.51 **Personal history of pre-term labor** ♀
EXCLUDES 1   *current pregnancy with history of pre-term labor (O09.21-)*

Z87.59 **Personal history of other complications of pregnancy, childbirth and the puerperium** ♀
Personal history of trophoblastic disease

√5ᵗʰ **Z87.7** **Personal history of (corrected) congenital malformations**
Conditions classifiable to Q00-Q89 that have been repaired or corrected
EXCLUDES 1   *congenital malformations that have been partially corrected or repair but which still require medical treatment — code to condition*
EXCLUDES 2   *other postprocedural states (Z98.-)*
personal history of medical treatment (Z92.-)
presence of cardiac and vascular implants and grafts (Z95.-)
presence of other devices (Z97.-)
presence of other functional implants (Z96.-)
transplanted organ and tissue status (Z94.-)

√6ᵗʰ **Z87.71** **Personal history of (corrected) congenital malformations of genitourinary system**

Z87.710 **Personal history of (corrected) hypospadias** ♂

Z87.718 **Personal history of other specified (corrected) congenital malformations of genitourinary system**

√6ᵗʰ **Z87.72** **Personal history of (corrected) congenital malformations of nervous system and sense organs**

Z87.720 **Personal history of (corrected) congenital malformations of eye**

Z87.721 **Personal history of (corrected) congenital malformations of ear**

Z87.728 **Personal history of other specified (corrected) congenital malformations of nervous system and sense organs**

√6ᵗʰ **Z87.73** **Personal history of (corrected) congenital malformations of digestive system**

Z87.730 **Personal history of (corrected) cleft lip and palate**

Z87.738 **Personal history of other specified (corrected) congenital malformations of digestive system**

Z87.74 **Personal history of (corrected) congenital malformations of heart and circulatory system**

Z87.75 **Personal history of (corrected) congenital malformations of respiratory system**

Z87.76 **Personal history of (corrected) congenital malformations of integument, limbs and musculoskeletal system**

√6ᵗʰ **Z87.79** **Personal history of other (corrected) congenital malformations**

Z87.790 **Personal history of (corrected) congenital malformations of face and neck**

Z87.798 **Personal history of other (corrected) congenital malformations**

√5ᵗʰ **Z87.8** **Personal history of other specified conditions**
EXCLUDES 2   *personal history of self harm (Z91.5)*

Z87.81 **Personal history of (healed) traumatic fracture**
EXCLUDES 2   *personal history of (healed) nontraumatic fracture (Z87.31-)*

√6ᵗʰ **Z87.82** **Personal history of other (healed) physical injury and trauma**
Conditions classifiable to S00-T88, except traumatic fractures

Z87.820 **Personal history of traumatic brain injury**
EXCLUDES 1   *personal history of transient ischemic attack (TIA), and cerebral infarction without residual deficits (Z86.73)*

Z87.821 **Personal history of retained foreign body fully removed**

Z87.828 **Personal history of other (healed) physical injury and trauma**

√6ᵗʰ **Z87.89** **Personal history of other specified conditions**

Z87.890 **Personal history of sex reassignment**

Z87.891 **Personal history of nicotine dependence**
EXCLUDES 1   *current nicotine dependence (F17.2-)*

AHA: 2017,2Q,27

Z87.892 Personal history of anaphylaxis
Code also allergy status such as:
allergy status to drugs, medicaments and biological substances (Z88.-)
allergy status, other than to drugs and biological substances (Z91.0-)

Z87.898 Personal history of other specified conditions
AHA: 2013,1Q,21

√4th **Z88** Allergy status to drugs, medicaments and biological substances
EXCLUDES 2   allergy status, other than to drugs and biological substances (Z91.0-)
AHA: 2015,3Q,23

Z88.0 Allergy status to penicillin
Z88.1 Allergy status to other antibiotic agents status
Z88.2 Allergy status to sulfonamides status
Z88.3 Allergy status to other anti-infective agents status
Z88.4 Allergy status to anesthetic agent status
Z88.5 Allergy status to narcotic agent status
Z88.6 Allergy status to analgesic agent status
Z88.7 Allergy status to serum and vaccine status
Z88.8 Allergy status to other drugs, medicaments and biological substances status
Z88.9 Allergy status to unspecified drugs, medicaments and biological substances status

√4th **Z89** Acquired absence of limb
INCLUDES   amputation status
postprocedural loss of limb
post-traumatic loss of limb
EXCLUDES 1   acquired deformities of limbs (M20-M21)
congenital absence of limbs (Q71-Q73)

√5th **Z89.0** Acquired absence of thumb and other finger(s)

√6th **Z89.01** Acquired absence of thumb
Z89.011 Acquired absence of right thumb
Z89.012 Acquired absence of left thumb
Z89.019 Acquired absence of unspecified thumb

√6th **Z89.02** Acquired absence of other finger(s)
EXCLUDES 2   acquired absence of thumb (Z89.01-)
Z89.021 Acquired absence of right finger(s)
Z89.022 Acquired absence of left finger(s)
Z89.029 Acquired absence of unspecified finger(s)

√5th **Z89.1** Acquired absence of hand and wrist

√6th **Z89.11** Acquired absence of hand
Z89.111 Acquired absence of right hand
Z89.112 Acquired absence of left hand
Z89.119 Acquired absence of unspecified hand

√6th **Z89.12** Acquired absence of wrist
Disarticulation at wrist
Z89.121 Acquired absence of right wrist
Z89.122 Acquired absence of left wrist
Z89.129 Acquired absence of unspecified wrist

√5th **Z89.2** Acquired absence of upper limb above wrist

√6th **Z89.20** Acquired absence of upper limb, unspecified level
Z89.201 Acquired absence of right upper limb, unspecified level
Z89.202 Acquired absence of left upper limb, unspecified level
Z89.209 Acquired absence of unspecified upper limb, unspecified level
Acquired absence of arm NOS

√6th **Z89.21** Acquired absence of upper limb below elbow
Z89.211 Acquired absence of right upper limb below elbow
Z89.212 Acquired absence of left upper limb below elbow
Z89.219 Acquired absence of unspecified upper limb below elbow

√6th **Z89.22** Acquired absence of upper limb above elbow
Disarticulation at elbow
Z89.221 Acquired absence of right upper limb above elbow
Z89.222 Acquired absence of left upper limb above elbow
Z89.229 Acquired absence of unspecified upper limb above elbow

√6th **Z89.23** Acquired absence of shoulder
Acquired absence of shoulder joint following explantation of shoulder joint prosthesis, with or without presence of antibiotic-impregnated cement spacer
Z89.231 Acquired absence of right shoulder
Z89.232 Acquired absence of left shoulder
Z89.239 Acquired absence of unspecified shoulder

√5th **Z89.4** Acquired absence of toe(s), foot, and ankle

√6th **Z89.41** Acquired absence of great toe
Z89.411 Acquired absence of right great toe   HCC
Z89.412 Acquired absence of left great toe   HCC
Z89.419 Acquired absence of unspecified great toe   HCC

√6th **Z89.42** Acquired absence of other toe(s)
EXCLUDES 2   acquired absence of great toe (Z89.41-)
Z89.421 Acquired absence of other right toe(s)   HCC
Z89.422 Acquired absence of other left toe(s)   HCC
Z89.429 Acquired absence of other toe(s), unspecified side   HCC

√6th **Z89.43** Acquired absence of foot
Z89.431 Acquired absence of right foot   HCC
Z89.432 Acquired absence of left foot   HCC
Z89.439 Acquired absence of unspecified foot   HCC

√6th **Z89.44** Acquired absence of ankle
Disarticulation of ankle
Z89.441 Acquired absence of right ankle   HCC
Z89.442 Acquired absence of left ankle   HCC
Z89.449 Acquired absence of unspecified ankle   HCC

√5th **Z89.5** Acquired absence of leg below knee

√6th **Z89.51** Acquired absence of leg below knee
Z89.511 Acquired absence of right leg below knee   HCC
Z89.512 Acquired absence of left leg below knee   HCC
Z89.519 Acquired absence of unspecified leg below knee   HCC

√6th **Z89.52** Acquired absence of knee
Acquired absence of knee joint following explantation of knee joint prosthesis, with or without presence of antibiotic-impregnated cement spacer
Z89.521 Acquired absence of right knee
Z89.522 Acquired absence of left knee
Z89.529 Acquired absence of unspecified knee

√5th **Z89.6** Acquired absence of leg above knee

√6th **Z89.61** Acquired absence of leg above knee
Acquired absence of leg NOS
Disarticulation at knee
Z89.611 Acquired absence of right leg above knee   HCC
Z89.612 Acquired absence of left leg above knee   HCC
Z89.619 Acquired absence of unspecified leg above knee   HCC

√6th **Z89.62** Acquired absence of hip
Acquired absence of hip joint following explantation of hip joint prosthesis, with or without presence of antibiotic-impregnated cement spacer
Disarticulation at hip
Z89.621 Acquired absence of right hip joint
Z89.622 Acquired absence of left hip joint
Z89.629 Acquired absence of unspecified hip joint

Z89.9 Acquired absence of limb, unspecified

√4th **Z90** Acquired absence of organs, not elsewhere classified
INCLUDES   postprocedural or post-traumatic loss of body part NEC
EXCLUDES 1   congenital absence — see Alphabetical Index
EXCLUDES 2   postprocedural absence of endocrine glands (E89.-)

√5th **Z90.0** Acquired absence of part of head and neck
Z90.01 Acquired absence of eye

Z90.02 Acquired absence of larynx
Z90.09 Acquired absence of other part of head and neck
   Acquired absence of nose
   EXCLUDES 2 teeth (K08.1)
√5ᵗʰ **Z90.1** Acquired absence of breast and nipple
   Z90.10 Acquired absence of unspecified breast and nipple
   Z90.11 Acquired absence of right breast and nipple
   Z90.12 Acquired absence of left breast and nipple
   Z90.13 Acquired absence of bilateral breasts and nipples
Z90.2 Acquired absence of lung [part of]
Z90.3 Acquired absence of stomach [part of]
√5ᵗʰ **Z90.4** Acquired absence of other specified parts of digestive tract
   √6ᵗʰ **Z90.41** Acquired absence of pancreas
      Code also exocrine pancreatic insufficiency (K86.81)
      Use additional code to identify any associated:
         diabetes mellitus, postpancreatectomy (E13.-)
         insulin use (Z79.4)
      Z90.410 Acquired total absence of pancreas
         Acquired absence of pancreas NOS
      Z90.411 Acquired partial absence of pancreas
   Z90.49 Acquired absence of other specified parts of digestive tract
Z90.5 Acquired absence of kidney
Z90.6 Acquired absence of other parts of urinary tract
   Acquired absence of bladder
√5ᵗʰ **Z90.7** Acquired absence of genital organ(s)
   EXCLUDES 1 personal history of sex reassignment (Z87.890)
   EXCLUDES 2 female genital mutilation status (N90.81-)
   √6ᵗʰ **Z90.71** Acquired absence of cervix and uterus
      Z90.710 Acquired absence of both cervix and uterus   ♀
         Acquired absence of uterus NOS
         Status post total hysterectomy
      Z90.711 Acquired absence of uterus with remaining cervical stump   ♀
         Status post partial hysterectomy with remaining cervical stump
      Z90.712 Acquired absence of cervix with remaining uterus   ♀
   √6ᵗʰ **Z90.72** Acquired absence of ovaries
      Z90.721 Acquired absence of ovaries, unilateral   ♀
      Z90.722 Acquired absence of ovaries, bilateral   ♀
   Z90.79 Acquired absence of other genital organ(s)
√5ᵗʰ **Z90.8** Acquired absence of other organs
   Z90.81 Acquired absence of spleen
   Z90.89 Acquired absence of other organs

√4ᵗʰ **Z91** Personal risk factors, not elsewhere classified
   EXCLUDES 2 contact with and (suspected) exposures hazardous to health (Z77.-)
      exposure to pollution and other problems related to physical environment (Z77.1-)
      female genital mutilation status (N90.81-)
      personal history of physical injury and trauma (Z87.81, Z87.82-)
      occupational exposure to risk factors (Z57.-)
√5ᵗʰ **Z91.0** Allergy status, other than to drugs and biological substances
   EXCLUDES 2 allergy status to drugs, medicaments, and biological substances (Z88.-)
   √6ᵗʰ **Z91.01** Food allergy status
      EXCLUDES 2 food additives allergy status (Z91.02)
      Z91.010 Allergy to peanuts
      Z91.011 Allergy to milk products
         EXCLUDES 1 lactose intolerance (E73.-)
      Z91.012 Allergy to eggs
      Z91.013 Allergy to seafood
         Allergy to shellfish
         Allergy to octopus or squid ink
      Z91.018 Allergy to other foods
         Allergy to nuts other than peanuts
   Z91.02 Food additives allergy status
   √6ᵗʰ **Z91.03** Insect allergy status
      Z91.030 Bee allergy status
      Z91.038 Other insect allergy status

√6ᵗʰ **Z91.04** Nonmedicinal substance allergy status
   Z91.040 Latex allergy status
      Latex sensitivity status
   Z91.041 Radiographic dye allergy status
      Allergy status to contrast media used for diagnostic X-ray procedure
   Z91.048 Other nonmedicinal substance allergy status
Z91.09 Other allergy status, other than to drugs and biological substances
√5ᵗʰ **Z91.1** Patient's noncompliance with medical treatment and regimen
   Z91.11 Patient's noncompliance with dietary regimen
   √6ᵗʰ **Z91.12** Patient's intentional underdosing of medication regimen
      Code first underdosing of medication (T36-T50) with fifth or sixth character 6
      EXCLUDES 1 adverse effect of prescribed drug taken as directed — code to adverse effect
         poisoning (overdose) — code to poisoning
      AHA: 2018,4Q,72
      Z91.120 Patient's intentional underdosing of medication regimen due to financial hardship
      Z91.128 Patient's intentional underdosing of medication regimen for other reason
   √6ᵗʰ **Z91.13** Patient's unintentional underdosing of medication regimen
      Code first underdosing of medication (T36-T50) with fifth or sixth character 6
      EXCLUDES 1 adverse effect of prescribed drug taken as directed — code to adverse effect
         poisoning (overdose) — code to poisoning
      AHA: 2018,4Q,72
      Z91.130 Patient's unintentional underdosing of medication regimen due to age-related debility
      Z91.138 Patient's unintentional underdosing of medication regimen for other reason
   Z91.14 Patient's other noncompliance with medication regimen
      Patient's underdosing of medication NOS
      AHA: 2018,4Q,72
   Z91.15 Patient's noncompliance with renal dialysis   HCC
   Z91.19 Patient's noncompliance with other medical treatment and regimen
      Nonadherence to medical treatment
√5ᵗʰ **Z91.4** Personal history of psychological trauma, not elsewhere classified
   √6ᵗʰ **Z91.41** Personal history of adult abuse
      EXCLUDES 2 personal history of abuse in childhood (Z62.81-)
      Z91.410 Personal history of adult physical and sexual abuse   A
         EXCLUDES 1 current adult physical abuse (T74.11, T76.11)
            current adult sexual abuse (T74.21, T76.11)
      Z91.411 Personal history of adult psychological abuse   A
      Z91.412 Personal history of adult neglect   A
         EXCLUDES 1 current adult neglect (T74.01, T76.01)
      Z91.419 Personal history of unspecified adult abuse   A
   Z91.42 Personal history of forced labor or sexual exploitation
      AHA: 2018,4Q,32,35
   Z91.49 Other personal history of psychological trauma, not elsewhere classified
Z91.5 Personal history of self-harm
   Personal history of parasuicide
   Personal history of self-poisoning
   Personal history of suicide attempt
√5ᵗʰ **Z91.8** Other specified personal risk factors, not elsewhere classified
   Z91.81 History of falling
      At risk for falling

N Newborn: 0   P Pediatric: 0-17   M Maternity: 9-64   A Adult: 15-124   MCC Major Complication/Comorbidity   CC Complication/Comorbidity   SW Severe Wound Dx

1304

ICD-10-CM 2020

Z91.82 Personal history of military deployment [A]
> Individual (civilian or military) with past history of military war, peacekeeping and humanitarian deployment (current or past conflict)
> Returned from military deployment

Z91.83 *Wandering in diseases classified elsewhere*
> Code first underlying disorder such as:
> Alzheimer's disease (G30.-)
> autism or pervasive developmental disorder (F84.-)
> intellectual disabilities (F70-F79)
> unspecified dementia with behavioral disturbance (F03.9-)

√6ᵗʰ **Z91.84** Oral health risk factors
> **AHA:** 2017,4Q,29
>
> **Z91.841** Risk for dental caries, low
> **Z91.842** Risk for dental caries, moderate
> **Z91.843** Risk for dental caries, high
> **Z91.849** Unspecified risk for dental caries

Z91.89 Other specified personal risk factors, not elsewhere classified
> **AHA:** 2017,1Q,45

√4ᵗʰ **Z92** Personal history of medical treatment
> EXCLUDES 2   *postprocedural states (Z98.-)*

Z92.0 Personal history of contraception
> EXCLUDES 1   *counseling or management of current contraceptive practices (Z30.-)*
> *long term (current) use of contraception (Z79.3)*
> *presence of (intrauterine) contraceptive device (Z97.5)*

√5ᵗʰ **Z92.2** Personal history of drug therapy
> EXCLUDES 2   *long term (current) drug therapy (Z79.-)*
>
> **Z92.21** Personal history of antineoplastic chemotherapy
> **Z92.22** Personal history of monoclonal drug therapy
> **Z92.23** Personal history of estrogen therapy
> √6ᵗʰ **Z92.24** Personal history of steroid therapy
>> **Z92.240** Personal history of inhaled steroid therapy
>> **Z92.241** Personal history of systemic steroid therapy
>>> Personal history of steroid therapy NOS
>
> **Z92.25** Personal history of immunosupression therapy
>> EXCLUDES 2   *personal history of steroid therapy (Z92.24)*
>
> **Z92.29** Personal history of other drug therapy

Z92.3 Personal history of irradiation
> Personal history of exposure to therapeutic radiation
> EXCLUDES 1   *exposure to radiation in the physical environment (Z77.12)*
> *occupational exposure to radiation (Z57.1)*

√5ᵗʰ **Z92.8** Personal history of other medical treatment
> **Z92.81** Personal history of extracorporeal membrane oxygenation (ECMO)
> **Z92.82** Status post administration of tPA (rtPA) in a different facility within the last 24 hours prior to admission to current facility
>> Code first condition requiring tPA administration, such as:
>> acute cerebral infarction (I63.-)
>> acute myocardial infarction (I21.-, I22.-)
>> **AHA:** 2013,4Q,124
>
> **Z92.83** Personal history of failed moderate sedation
>> Personal history of failed conscious sedation
>> EXCLUDES 2   *failed moderate sedation during procedure (T88.52)*
>
> **Z92.84** Personal history of unintended awareness under general anesthesia
>> EXCLUDES 2   *unintended awareness under general anesthesia during procedure (T88.53)*
>> **AHA:** 2016,4Q,72-73,77
>
> **Z92.89** Personal history of other medical treatment

√4ᵗʰ **Z93** Artificial opening status
> EXCLUDES 1   *artificial openings requiring attention or management (Z43.-)*
> *complications of external stoma (J95.0-, K94.-, N99.5-)*

Z93.0 Tracheostomy status [HCC]
> **AHA:** 2013,4Q,129

Z93.1 Gastrostomy status [HCC]

Z93.2 Ileostomy status [HCC]
Z93.3 Colostomy status [HCC]
Z93.4 Other artificial openings of gastrointestinal tract status [HCC]

√6ᵗʰ **Z93.5** Cystostomy status
> **Z93.50** Unspecified cystostomy status [HCC]
> **Z93.51** Cutaneous-vesicostomy status [HCC]
> **Z93.52** Appendico-vesicostomy status [HCC]
> **Z93.59** Other cystostomy status [HCC]

Z93.6 Other artificial openings of urinary tract status [HCC]
> Nephrostomy status
> Ureterostomy status
> Urethrostomy status

Z93.8 Other artificial opening status [HCC]
Z93.9 Artificial opening status, unspecified [HCC]

√4ᵗʰ **Z94** Transplanted organ and tissue status
> INCLUDES   organ or tissue replaced by heterogenous or homogenous transplant
> EXCLUDES 1   *complications of transplanted organ or tissue — see Alphabetical Index*
> EXCLUDES 2   *presence of vascular grafts (Z95.-)*

Z94.0 Kidney transplant status
Z94.1 Heart transplant status [HCC]
> EXCLUDES 1   *artificial heart status (Z95.812)*
> *heart-valve replacement status (Z95.2-Z95.4)*

Z94.2 Lung transplant status [HCC]
Z94.3 Heart and lungs transplant status [HCC]
Z94.4 Liver transplant status [HCC]
Z94.5 Skin transplant status
> Autogenous skin transplant status

Z94.6 Bone transplant status
Z94.7 Corneal transplant status

√5ᵗʰ **Z94.8** Other transplanted organ and tissue status
> **Z94.81** Bone marrow transplant status [HCC]
> **Z94.82** Intestine transplant status [HCC]
> **Z94.83** Pancreas transplant status [HCC]
> **Z94.84** Stem cells transplant status [HCC]
> **Z94.89** Other transplanted organ and tissue status

Z94.9 Transplanted organ and tissue status, unspecified

√4ᵗʰ **Z95** Presence of cardiac and vascular implants and grafts
> EXCLUDES 2   *complications of cardiac and vascular devices, implants and grafts (T82.-)*

Z95.0 Presence of cardiac pacemaker
> Presence of cardiac resynchronization therapy (CRT-P) pacemaker
> EXCLUDES 1   *adjustment or management of cardiac device (Z45.0-)*
> *adjustment or management of cardiac pacemaker (Z45.0)*
> *presence of automatic (implantable) cardiac defibrillator with synchronous cardiac pacemaker (Z95.810)*
> **AHA:** 2019,1Q,33

Z95.1 Presence of aortocoronary bypass graft
> Presence of coronary artery bypass graft

Z95.2 Presence of prosthetic heart valve
> Presence of heart valve NOS

Z95.3 Presence of xenogenic heart valve
Z95.4 Presence of other heart-valve replacement
Z95.5 Presence of coronary angioplasty implant and graft
> EXCLUDES 1   *coronary angioplasty status without implant and graft (Z98.61)*

✓5ᵗʰ **Z95.8 Presence of other cardiac and vascular implants and grafts**

  ✓6ᵗʰ **Z95.81 Presence of other cardiac implants and grafts**

    Z95.810 Presence of automatic (implantable) cardiac defibrillator

      Presence of automatic (implantable) cardiac defibrillator with synchronous cardiac pacemaker

      Presence of cardiac resynchronization therapy defibrillator (CRT-D)

      Presence of cardioverter-defibrillator (ICD)

    Z95.811 Presence of heart assist device `HCC`

    Z95.812 Presence of fully implantable artificial heart `HCC`

    Z95.818 Presence of other cardiac implants and grafts

  ✓6ᵗʰ **Z95.82 Presence of other vascular implants and grafts**

    Z95.820 Peripheral vascular angioplasty status with implants and grafts

      EXCLUDES 1 *peripheral vascular angioplasty without implant and graft (Z98.62)*

    Z95.828 Presence of other vascular implants and grafts

      Presence of intravascular prosthesis NEC

Z95.9 Presence of cardiac and vascular implant and graft, unspecified

✓4ᵗʰ **Z96 Presence of other functional implants**

  EXCLUDES 2 *complications of internal prosthetic devices, implants and grafts (T82-T85)*

    fitting and adjustment of prosthetic and other devices (Z44-Z46)

Z96.0 Presence of urogenital implants

Z96.1 Presence of intraocular lens

  Presence of pseudophakia

✓5ᵗʰ **Z96.2 Presence of otological and audiological implants**

  Z96.20 Presence of otological and audiological implant, unspecified

  Z96.21 Cochlear implant status

  Z96.22 Myringotomy tube(s) status

  Z96.29 Presence of other otological and audiological implants

    Presence of bone-conduction hearing device

    Presence of eustachian tube stent

    Stapes replacement

Z96.3 Presence of artificial larynx

✓5ᵗʰ **Z96.4 Presence of endocrine implants**

  Z96.41 Presence of insulin pump (external) (internal)

  Z96.49 Presence of other endocrine implants

Z96.5 Presence of tooth-root and mandibular implants

✓5ᵗʰ **Z96.6 Presence of orthopedic joint implants**

  Z96.60 Presence of unspecified orthopedic joint implant

  ✓6ᵗʰ **Z96.61 Presence of artificial shoulder joint**

    Z96.611 Presence of right artificial shoulder joint

    Z96.612 Presence of left artificial shoulder joint

    Z96.619 Presence of unspecified artificial shoulder joint

  ✓6ᵗʰ **Z96.62 Presence of artificial elbow joint**

    Z96.621 Presence of right artificial elbow joint

    Z96.622 Presence of left artificial elbow joint

    Z96.629 Presence of unspecified artificial elbow joint

  ✓6ᵗʰ **Z96.63 Presence of artificial wrist joint**

    Z96.631 Presence of right artificial wrist joint

    Z96.632 Presence of left artificial wrist joint

    Z96.639 Presence of unspecified artificial wrist joint

  ✓6ᵗʰ **Z96.64 Presence of artificial hip joint**

    Hip-joint replacement (partial) (total)

    Z96.641 Presence of right artificial hip joint

    Z96.642 Presence of left artificial hip joint

    Z96.643 Presence of artificial hip joint, bilateral

    Z96.649 Presence of unspecified artificial hip joint

  ✓6ᵗʰ **Z96.65 Presence of artificial knee joint**

    Z96.651 Presence of right artificial knee joint

    Z96.652 Presence of left artificial knee joint

    Z96.653 Presence of artificial knee joint, bilateral

    Z96.659 Presence of unspecified artificial knee joint

  ✓6ᵗʰ **Z96.66 Presence of artificial ankle joint**

    Z96.661 Presence of right artificial ankle joint

    Z96.662 Presence of left artificial ankle joint

    Z96.669 Presence of unspecified artificial ankle joint

  ✓6ᵗʰ **Z96.69 Presence of other orthopedic joint implants**

    Z96.691 Finger-joint replacement of right hand

    Z96.692 Finger-joint replacement of left hand

    Z96.693 Finger-joint replacement, bilateral

    Z96.698 Presence of other orthopedic joint implants

Z96.7 Presence of other bone and tendon implants

  Presence of skull plate

✓5ᵗʰ **Z96.8 Presence of other specified functional implants**

  Z96.81 Presence of artificial skin

  Z96.82 Presence of neurostimulator

    Presence of brain neurostimulator

    Presence of gastric neurostimulator

    Presence of peripheral nerve neurostimulator

    Presence of sacral nerve neurostimulator

    Presence of spinal cord neurostimulator

    Presence of vagus nerve neurostimulator

  Z96.89 Presence of other specified functional implants

Z96.9 Presence of functional implant, unspecified

✓4ᵗʰ **Z97 Presence of other devices**

  EXCLUDES 1 *complications of internal prosthetic devices, implants and grafts (T82-T85)*

    ~~*fitting and adjustment of prosthetic and other devices (Z44-Z46)*~~

  EXCLUDES 2 ▶*fitting and adjustment of prosthetic and other devices (Z44-Z46)*◀

    presence of cerebrospinal fluid drainage device (Z98.2)

Z97.0 Presence of artificial eye

✓5ᵗʰ **Z97.1 Presence of artificial limb (complete) (partial)**

  Z97.10 Presence of artificial limb (complete) (partial), unspecified

  Z97.11 Presence of artificial right arm (complete) (partial)

  Z97.12 Presence of artificial left arm (complete) (partial)

  Z97.13 Presence of artificial right leg (complete) (partial)

  Z97.14 Presence of artificial left leg (complete) (partial)

  Z97.15 Presence of artificial arms, bilateral (complete) (partial)

  Z97.16 Presence of artificial legs, bilateral (complete) (partial)

Z97.2 Presence of dental prosthetic device (complete) (partial)

  Presence of dentures (complete) (partial)

Z97.3 Presence of spectacles and contact lenses

Z97.4 Presence of external hearing-aid

Z97.5 Presence of (intrauterine) contraceptive device ♀

  EXCLUDES 1 *checking, reinsertion or removal of implantable subdermal contraceptive (Z30.46)*

    checking, reinsertion or removal of intrauterine contraceptive device (Z30.43-)

Z97.8 Presence of other specified devices

✓4ᵗʰ **Z98 Other postprocedural states**

  EXCLUDES 2 *aftercare (Z43-Z49, Z51)*

    follow-up medical care (Z08-Z09)

    postprocedural complication — see Alphabetical Index

Z98.0 Intestinal bypass and anastomosis status

  EXCLUDES 2 *bariatric surgery status (Z98.84)*

    gastric bypass status (Z98.84)

    obesity surgery status (Z98.84)

Z98.1 Arthrodesis status

Z98.2 Presence of cerebrospinal fluid drainage device

  Presence of CSF shunt

Z98.3 Post therapeutic collapse of lung status

  Code first underlying disease

✓5ᵗʰ **Z98.4 Cataract extraction status**

  Use additional code to identify intraocular lens implant status (Z96.1)

  EXCLUDES 1 *aphakia (H27.0)*

  Z98.41 Cataract extraction status, right eye

N Newborn: 0   P Pediatric: 0-17   M Maternity: 9-64   A Adult: 15-124   MCC Major Complication/Comorbidity   CC Complication/Comorbidity   SW Severe Wound Dx

1306   ICD-10-CM 2020

Z98.42 **Cataract extraction status,** left eye
Z98.49 **Cataract extraction status, unspecified eye**
✓5ᵗʰ **Z98.5** **Sterilization status**
　　EXCLUDES 1　female infertility (N97.-)
　　　　male infertility (N46.-)
Z98.51 **Tubal ligation status**　　　　　♀
Z98.52 **Vasectomy status**　　　　　Ⓐ♂
✓5ᵗʰ **Z98.6** **Angioplasty status**
Z98.61 **Coronary angioplasty status**
　　EXCLUDES 1　coronary angioplasty status with implant
　　　　and graft (Z95.5)
Z98.62 **Peripheral vascular angioplasty status**
　　EXCLUDES 1　peripheral vascular angioplasty status
　　　　with implant and graft (Z95.820)
✓5ᵗʰ **Z98.8** **Other specified postprocedural states**
✓6ᵗʰ **Z98.81** **Dental procedure status**
Z98.810 **Dental sealant status**
Z98.811 **Dental restoration status**
　　　　Dental crown status
　　　　Dental fillings status
Z98.818 **Other dental procedure status**
Z98.82 **Breast implant status**
　　EXCLUDES 1　breast implant removal status (Z98.86)
Z98.83 **Filtering (vitreous) bleb after glaucoma surgery
status**
　　EXCLUDES 1　inflammation (infection) of postprocedural
　　　　bleb (H59.4-)
Z98.84 **Bariatric surgery status**
　　Gastric banding status
　　Gastric bypass status for obesity
　　Obesity surgery status
　　EXCLUDES 1　bariatric surgery status complicating
　　　　pregnancy, childbirth, or the
　　　　puerperium (O99.84)
　　EXCLUDES 2　intestinal bypass and anastomosis status
　　　　(Z98.0)
Z98.85 **Transplanted organ removal status**
　　Transplanted organ previously removed due to
　　　complication, failure, rejection or infection
　　EXCLUDES 1　encounter for removal of transplanted
　　　　organ — code to complication of
　　　　transplanted organ (T86.-)
Z98.86 **Personal history of breast implant removal**
✓6ᵗʰ **Z98.87** **Personal history of** in utero procedure
Z98.870 **Personal history of in utero**　　　♀
procedure during pregnancy
　　　　EXCLUDES 2　complications from in utero
　　　　　procedure for current
　　　　　pregnancy (O35.7)
　　　　supervision of current
　　　　　pregnancy with history of
　　　　　in utero procedure during
　　　　　previous pregnancy
　　　　　(O09.82-)
Z98.871 **Personal history of in utero procedure**
while a fetus
✓6ᵗʰ **Z98.89** **Other specified postprocedural states**
Z98.890 **Other specified postprocedural states**
　　　　Personal history of surgery, not elsewhere
　　　　classified
Z98.891 **History of uterine scar from**　　　♀
previous surgery
　　　　EXCLUDES 1　maternal care due to uterine
　　　　　scar from previous surgery
　　　　　(O34.2-)
　　AHA: 2016,4Q,51-52,76
✓4ᵗʰ **Z99** **Dependence on enabling machines and devices, not elsewhere
classified**
　　EXCLUDES 1　cardiac pacemaker status (Z95.0)
Z99.0 **Dependence on** aspirator
✓5ᵗʰ **Z99.1** **Dependence on** respirator
　　Dependence on ventilator
Z99.11 **Dependence on respirator [ventilator]**　　ʜᴄᴄ
status
　　AHA: 2015,1Q,21

Z99.12 **Encounter for respirator [ventilator]**　　ʜᴄᴄ
dependence during power failure
　　EXCLUDES 1　mechanical complication of respirator
　　　　[ventilator] (J95.850)
Z99.2 **Dependence on** renal dialysis　　　　ʜᴄᴄ
　　Hemodialysis status
　　Peritoneal dialysis status
　　Presence of arteriovenous shunt for dialysis
　　Renal dialysis status NOS
　　EXCLUDES 1　encounter for fitting and adjustment of dialysis
　　　　catheter (Z49.0-)
　　EXCLUDES 2　noncompliance with renal dialysis (Z91.15)
　　AHA: 2016,1Q,12; 2013,4Q,125
Z99.3 **Dependence on** wheelchair
　　Wheelchair confinement status
　　Code first cause of dependence, such as:
　　　muscular dystrophy (G71.0-)
　　　obesity (E66.-)
✓5ᵗʰ **Z99.8** **Dependence on other enabling machines and devices**
Z99.81 **Dependence on** supplemental oxygen
　　　　Dependence on long-term oxygen
　　　　AHA: 2013,4Q,129
Z99.89 **Dependence on other enabling machines and
devices**
　　　　Dependence on machine or device NOS

Illustrations

Chapter 3. Diseases of the Blood and Blood-forming Organs and Certain Disorders Involving the Immune Mechanism (D50–D89)

Red Blood Cells

White Blood Cell

Platelet

Coagulation

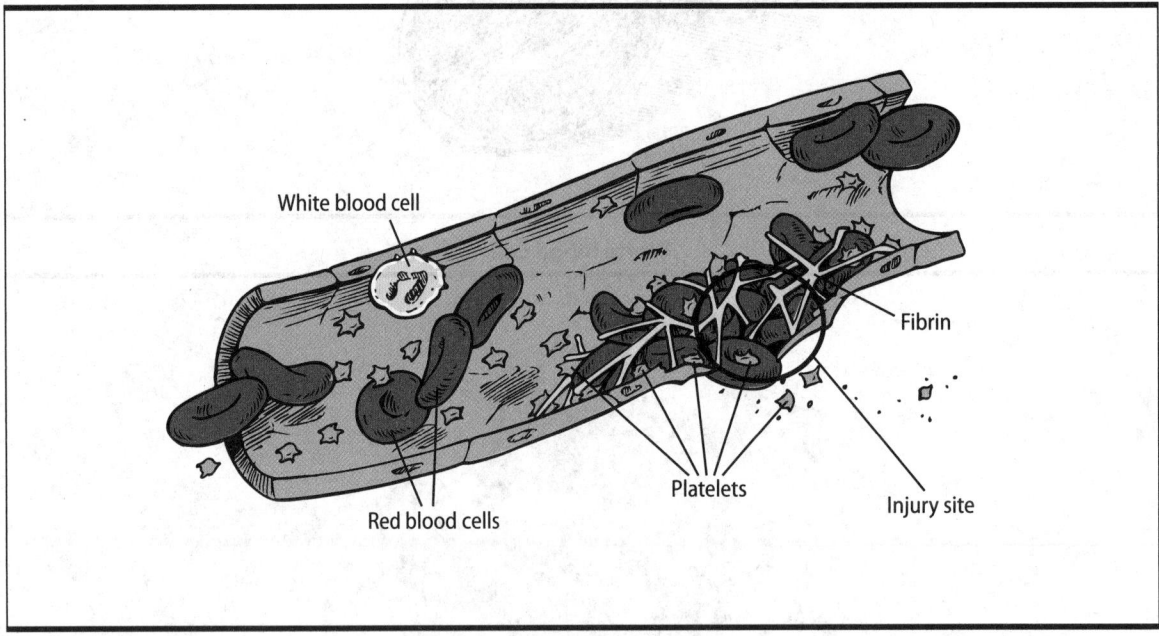

White blood cell

Fibrin

Platelets

Red blood cells

Injury site

Spleen Anatomical Location and External Structures

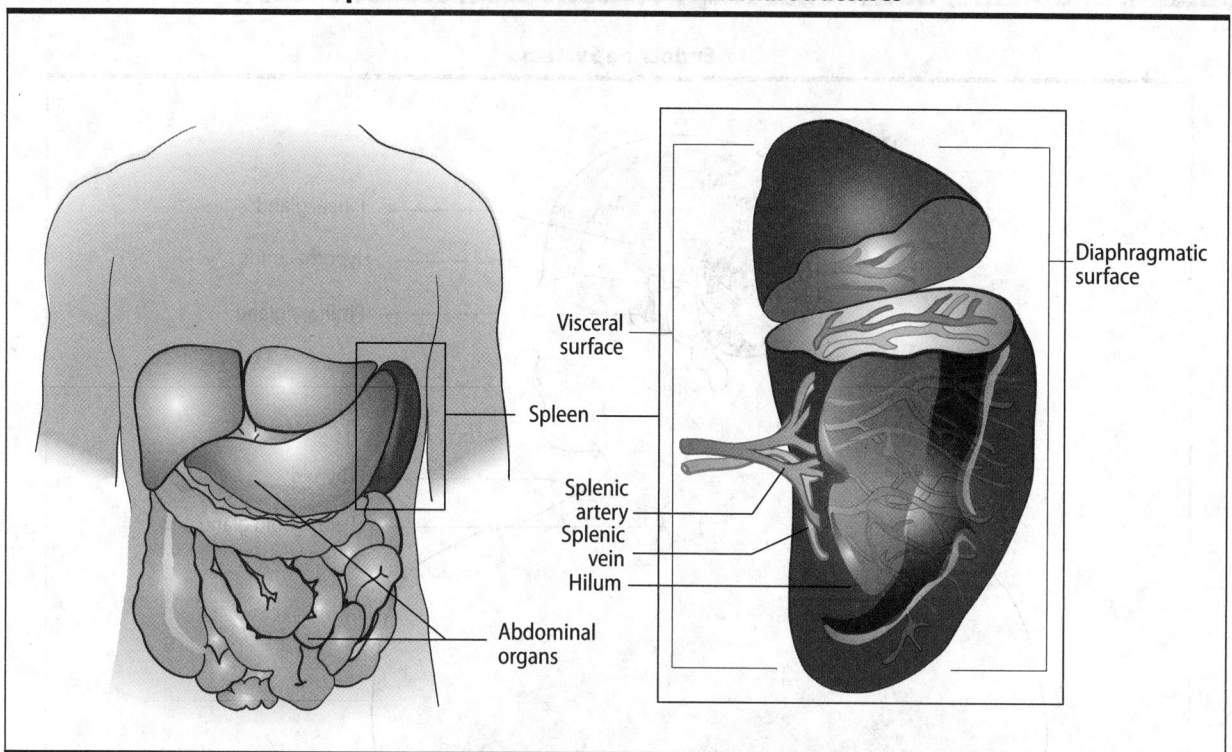

Spleen Interior Structures

Chapter 4. Endocrine, Nutritional and Metabolic Diseases (E00–E89)

Endocrine System

Thyroid

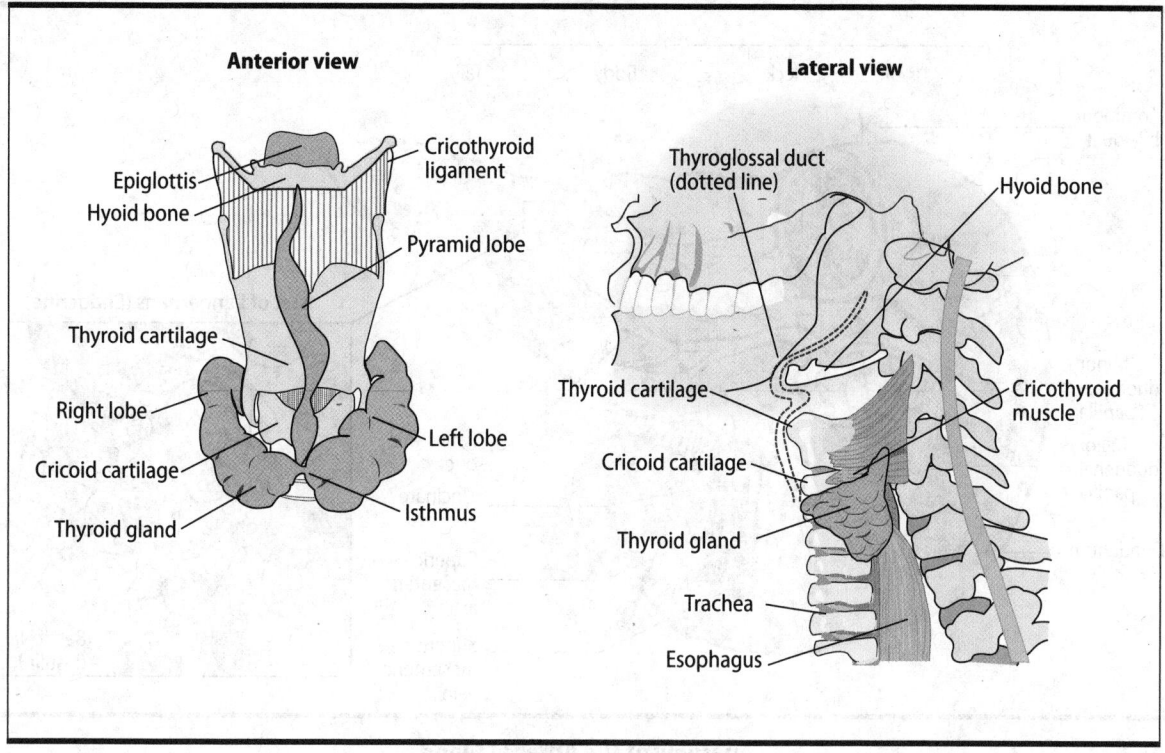

Anterior view

Lateral view

Thyroid and Parathyroid Glands

Posterior view

Pancreas

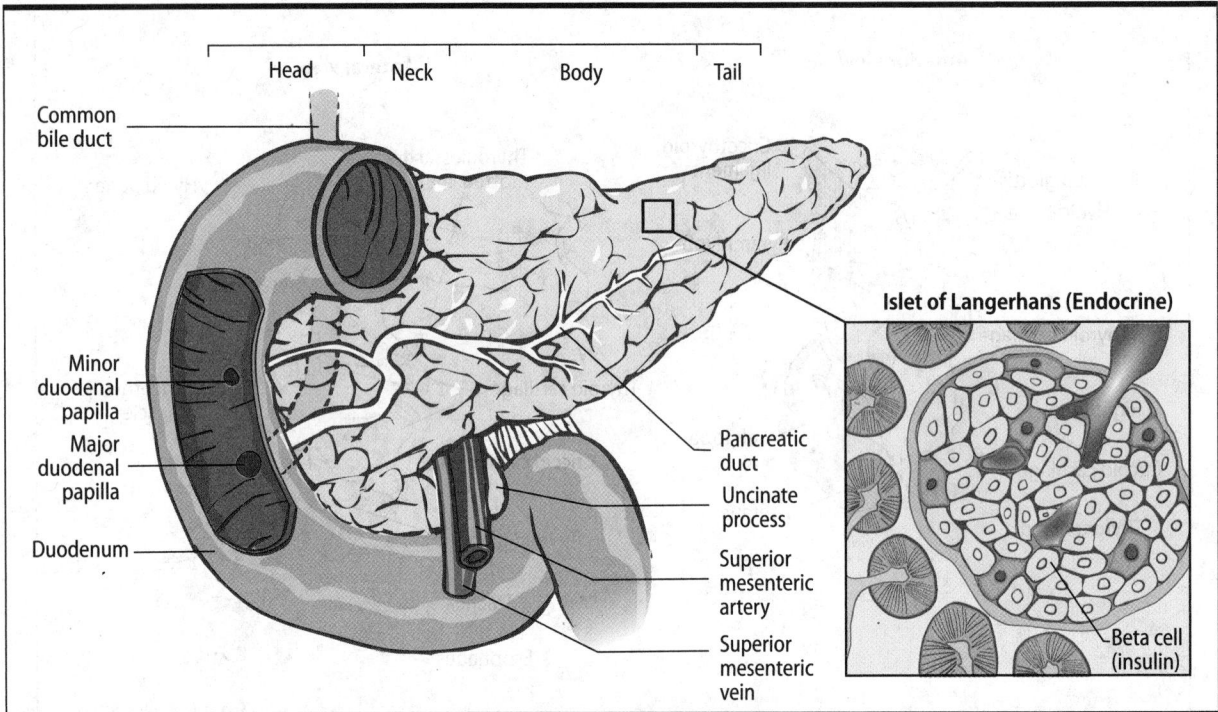

Islet of Langerhans (Endocrine)

Anatomy of the Adrenal Gland

Structure of an Ovary

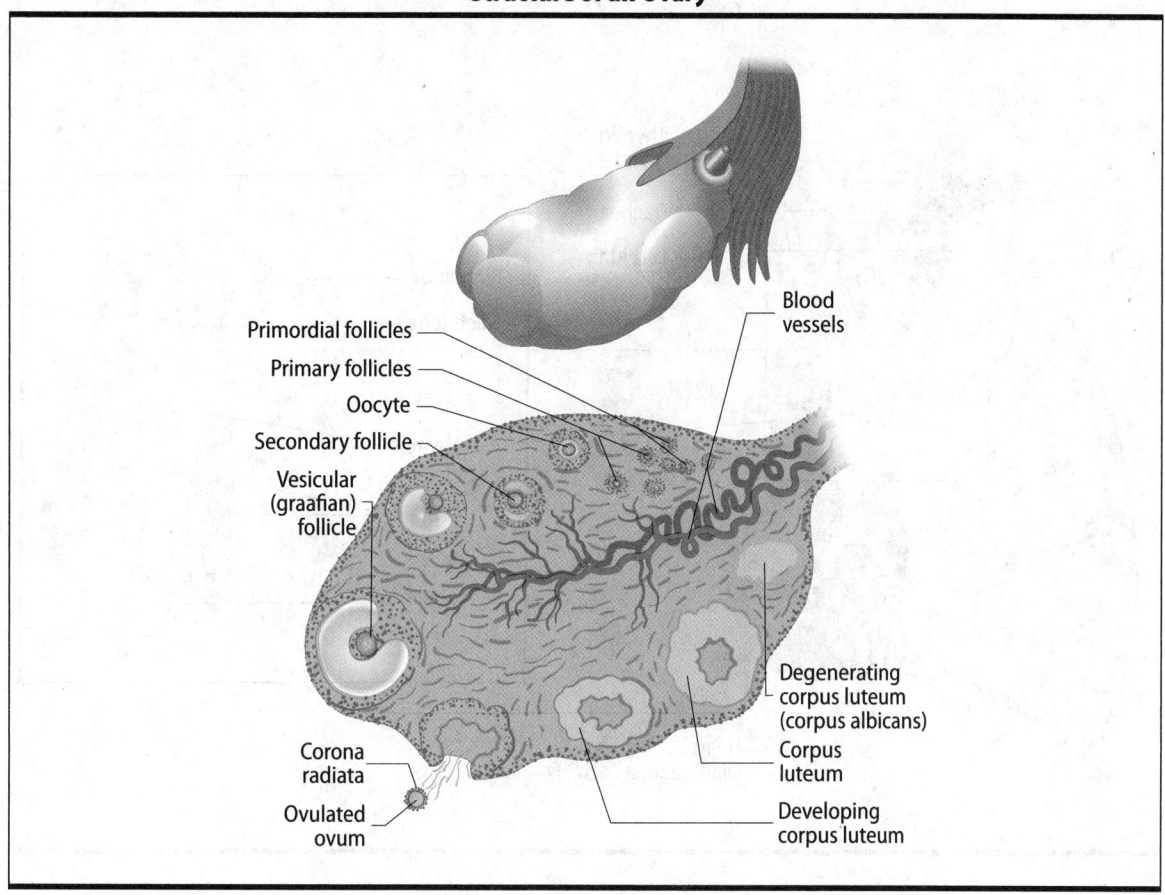

Testis and Associated Structures

Thymus

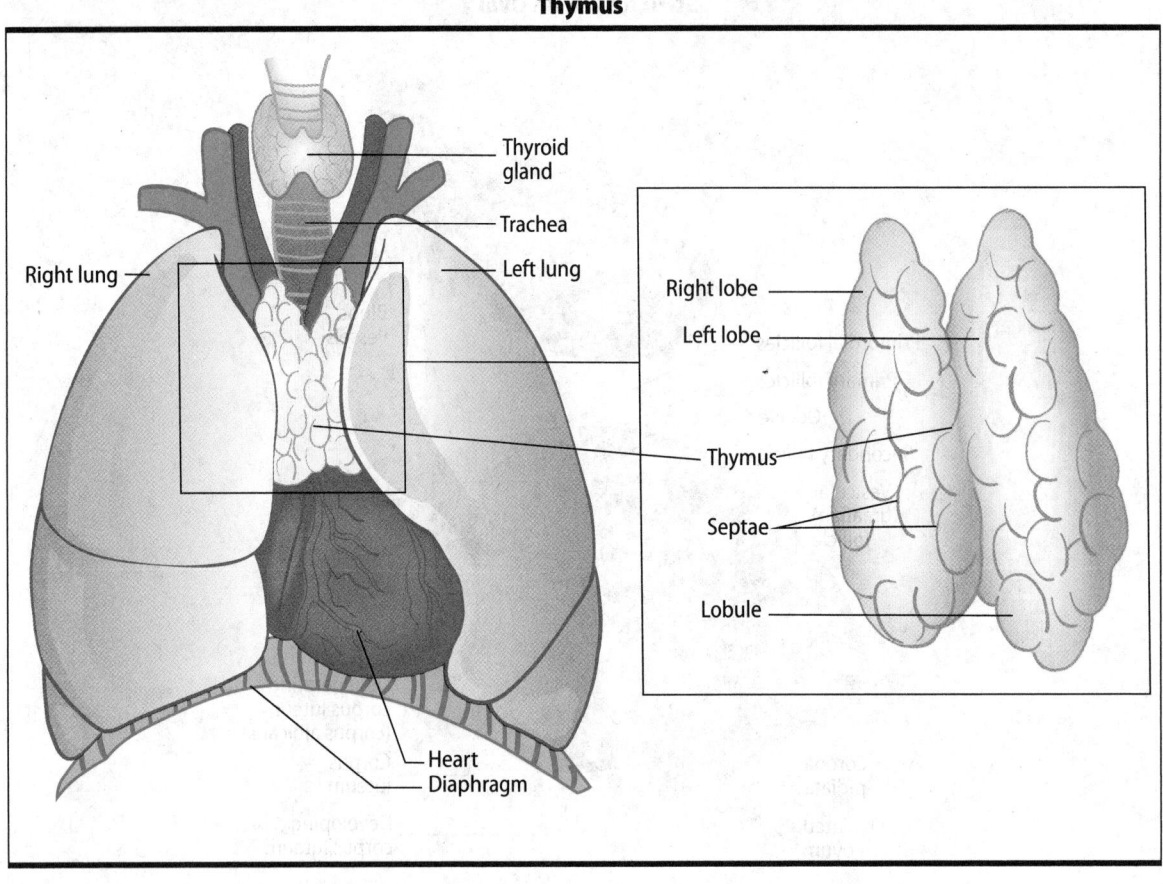

Chapter 6. Diseases of the Nervous System (G00–G99)

Brain

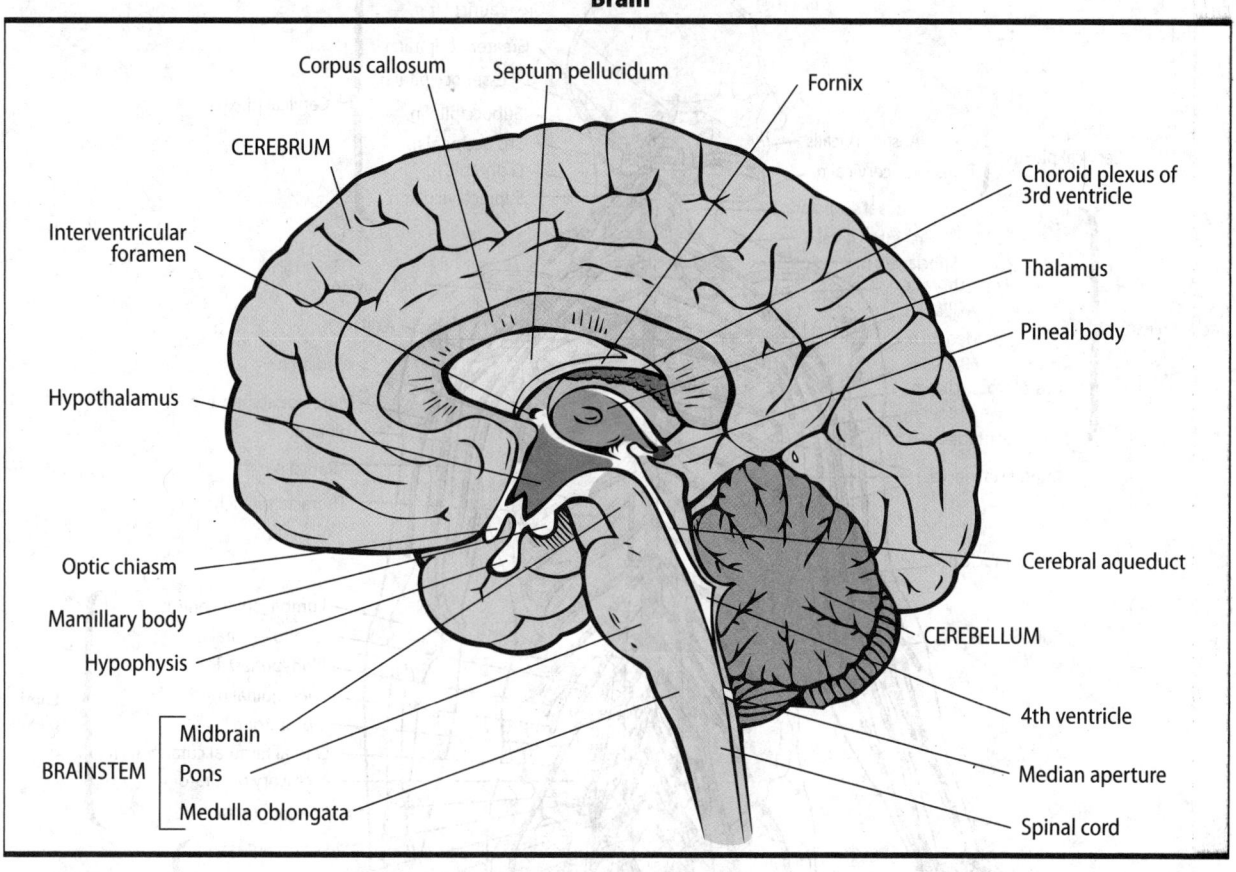

- Corpus callosum
- Septum pellucidum
- Fornix
- CEREBRUM
- Choroid plexus of 3rd ventricle
- Thalamus
- Pineal body
- Interventricular foramen
- Hypothalamus
- Optic chiasm
- Mamillary body
- Hypophysis
- BRAINSTEM
  - Midbrain
  - Pons
  - Medulla oblongata
- Cerebral aqueduct
- CEREBELLUM
- 4th ventricle
- Median aperture
- Spinal cord

Cranial Nerves

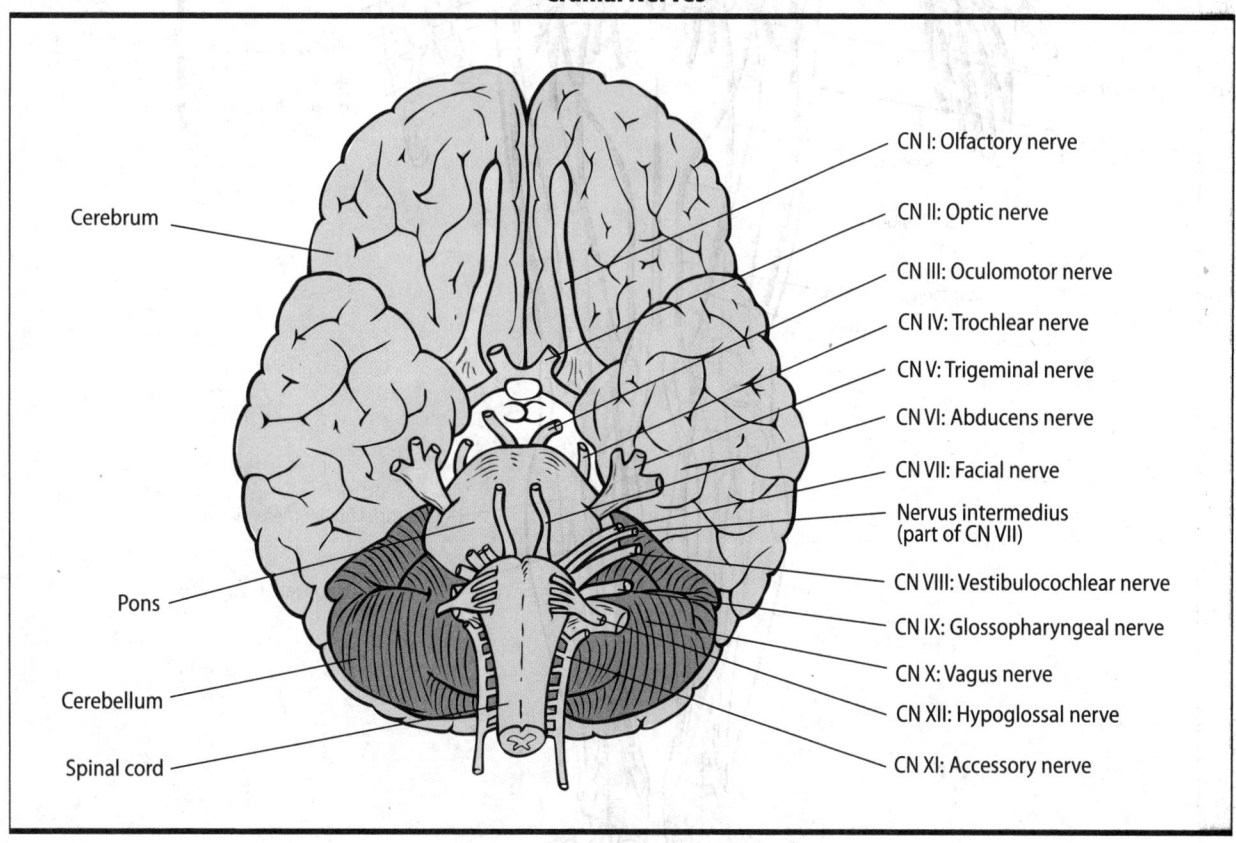

- Cerebrum
- Pons
- Cerebellum
- Spinal cord
- CN I: Olfactory nerve
- CN II: Optic nerve
- CN III: Oculomotor nerve
- CN IV: Trochlear nerve
- CN V: Trigeminal nerve
- CN VI: Abducens nerve
- CN VII: Facial nerve
- Nervus intermedius (part of CN VII)
- CN VIII: Vestibulocochlear nerve
- CN IX: Glossopharyngeal nerve
- CN X: Vagus nerve
- CN XII: Hypoglossal nerve
- CN XI: Accessory nerve

Peripheral Nervous System

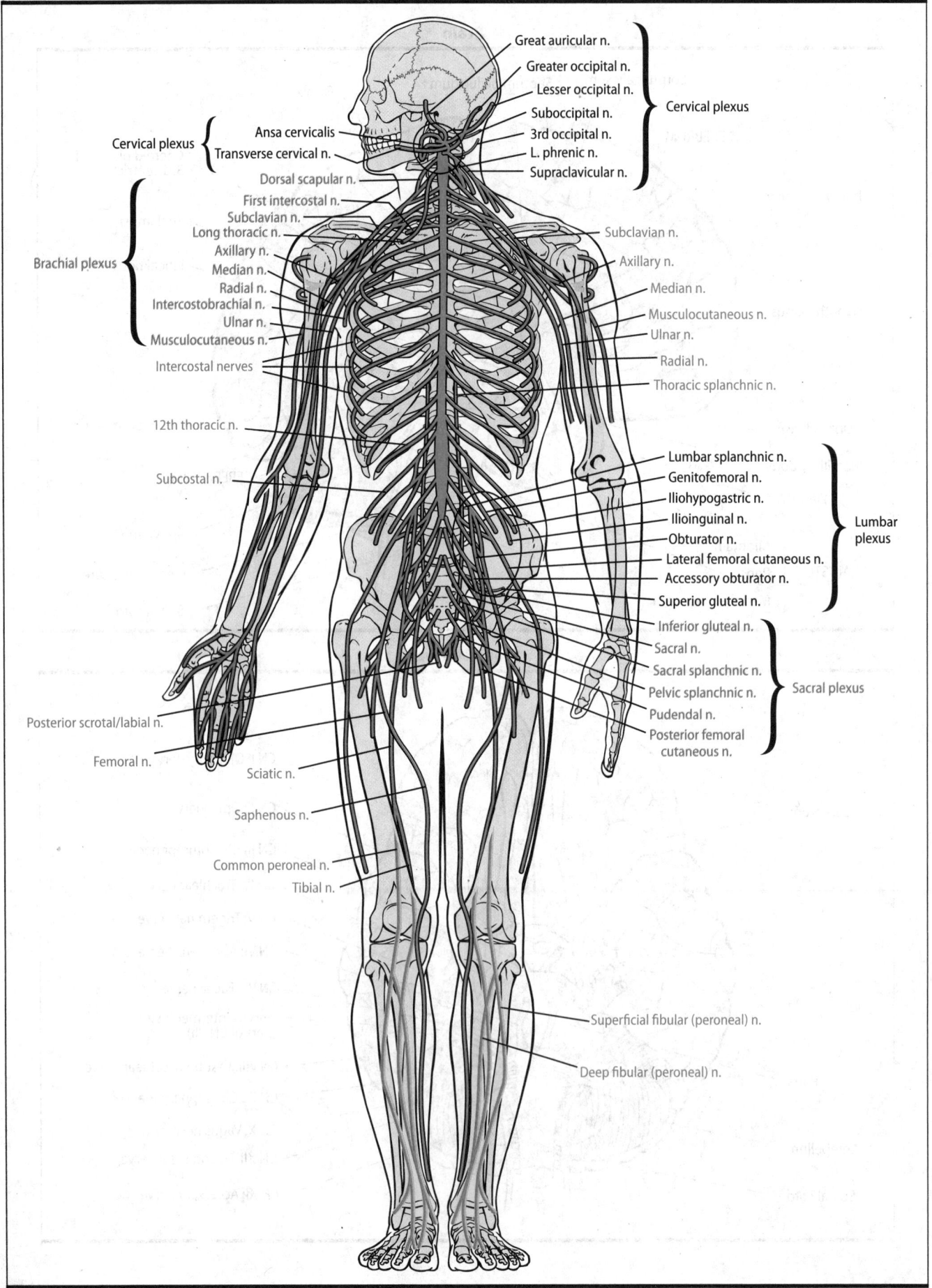

Great auricular n.
Greater occipital n.
Lesser occipital n.
Suboccipital n.
3rd occipital n.
L. phrenic n.
Supraclavicular n.

Cervical plexus

Cervical plexus
Ansa cervicalis
Transverse cervical n.
Dorsal scapular n.
First intercostal n.
Subclavian n.
Long thoracic n.
Axillary n.
Median n.
Radial n.
Intercostobrachial n.
Ulnar n.
Musculocutaneous n.
Intercostal nerves
12th thoracic n.
Subcostal n.

Brachial plexus

Subclavian n.
Axillary n.
Median n.
Musculocutaneous n.
Ulnar n.
Radial n.
Thoracic splanchnic n.

Lumbar splanchnic n.
Genitofemoral n.
Iliohypogastric n.
Ilioinguinal n.
Obturator n.
Lateral femoral cutaneous n.
Accessory obturator n.
Superior gluteal n.

Lumbar plexus

Inferior gluteal n.
Sacral n.
Sacral splanchnic n.
Pelvic splanchnic n.
Pudendal n.
Posterior femoral cutaneous n.

Sacral plexus

Posterior scrotal/labial n.
Femoral n.
Sciatic n.
Saphenous n.
Common peroneal n.
Tibial n.

Superficial fibular (peroneal) n.

Deep fibular (peroneal) n.

Peripheral Nervous System

Spinal Cord and Spinal Nerves

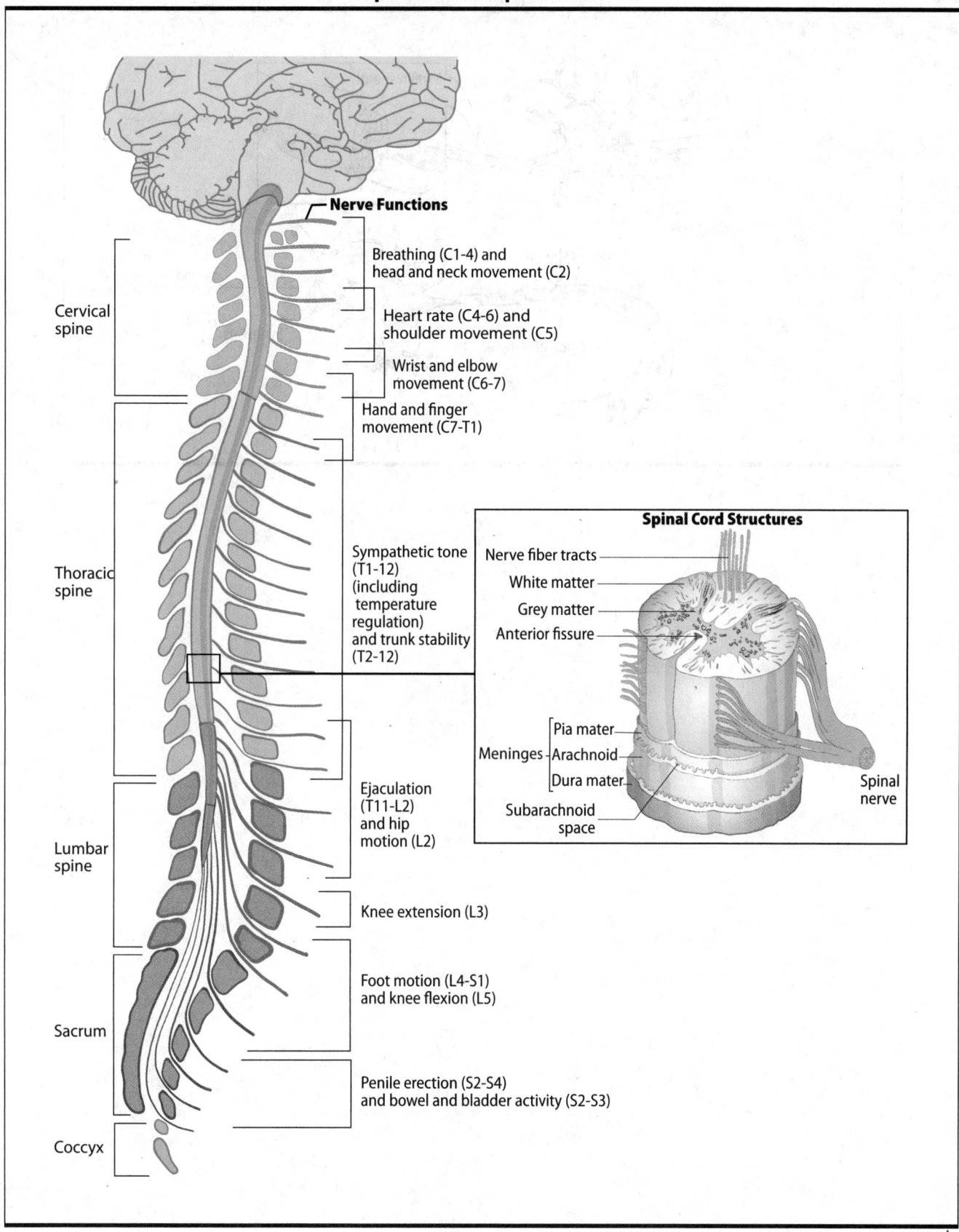

Nerve Functions

Breathing (C1-4) and
head and neck movement (C2)

Heart rate (C4-6) and
shoulder movement (C5)

Wrist and elbow
movement (C6-7)

Hand and finger
movement (C7-T1)

Sympathetic tone
(T1-12)
(including
temperature
regulation)
and trunk stability
(T2-12)

Ejaculation
(T11-L2)
and hip
motion (L2)

Knee extension (L3)

Foot motion (L4-S1)
and knee flexion (L5)

Penile erection (S2-S4)
and bowel and bladder activity (S2-S3)

Cervical spine

Thoracic spine

Lumbar spine

Sacrum

Coccyx

Spinal Cord Structures

Nerve fiber tracts

White matter

Grey matter

Anterior fissure

Meninges — Pia mater
Arachnoid
Dura mater

Subarachnoid space

Spinal nerve

Nerve Cell

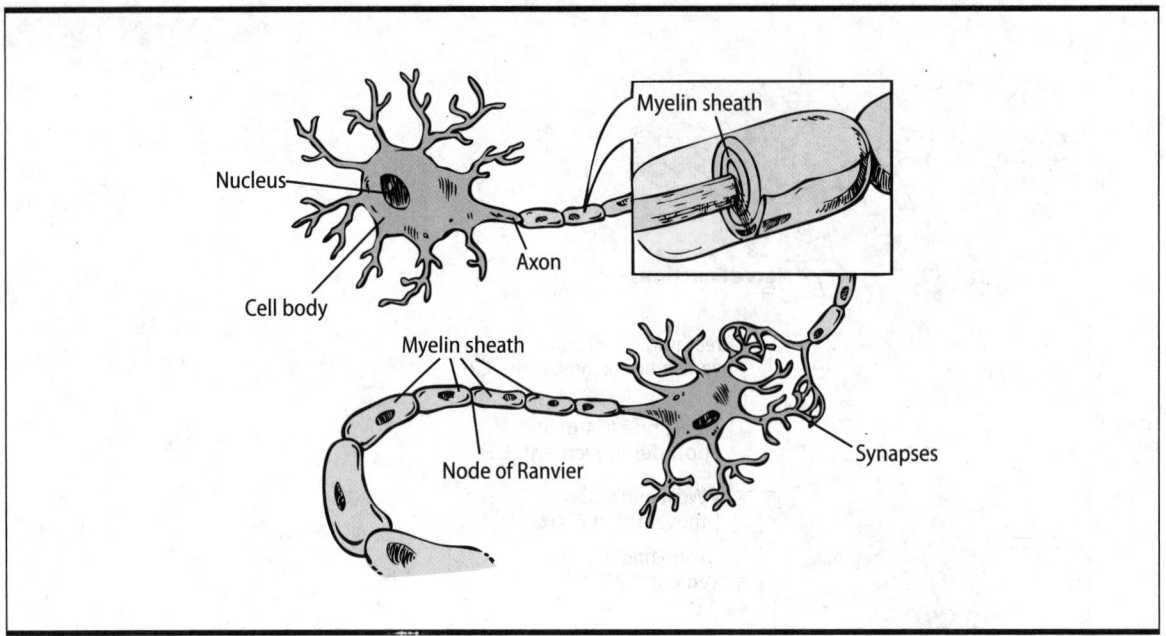

Chapter 7. Diseases of the Eye and Adnexa (H00–H59)

Eye

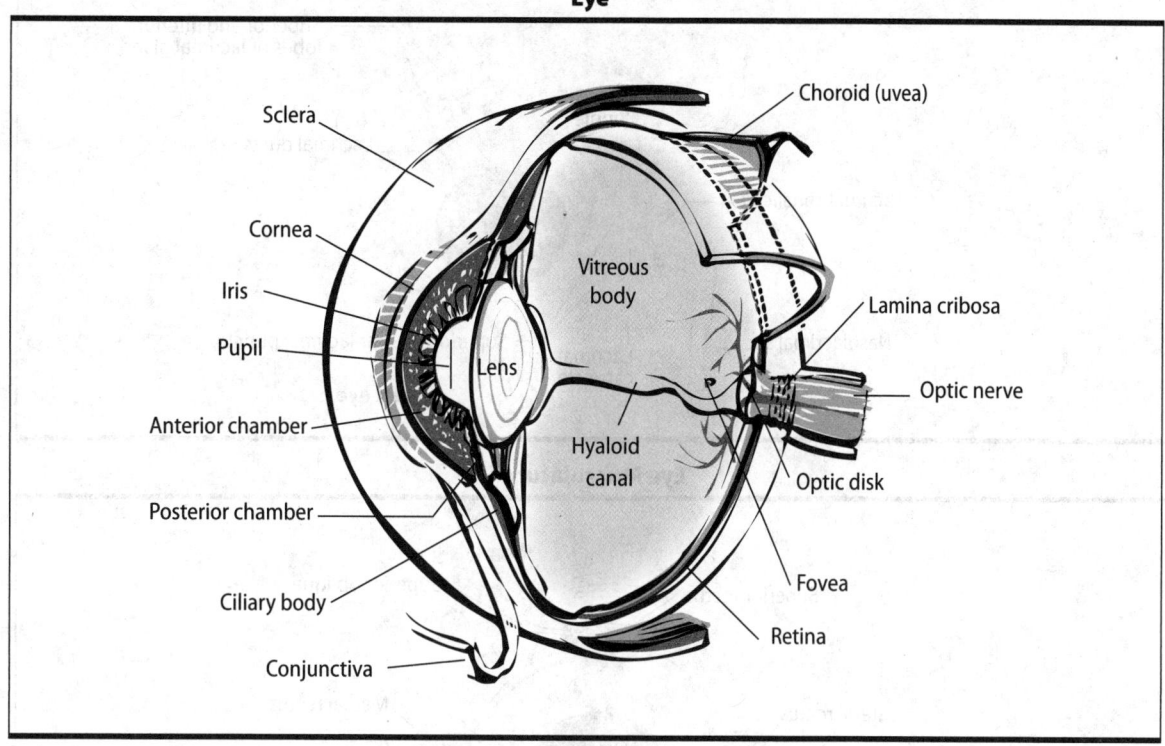

Posterior Pole of Globe/Flow of Aqueous Humor

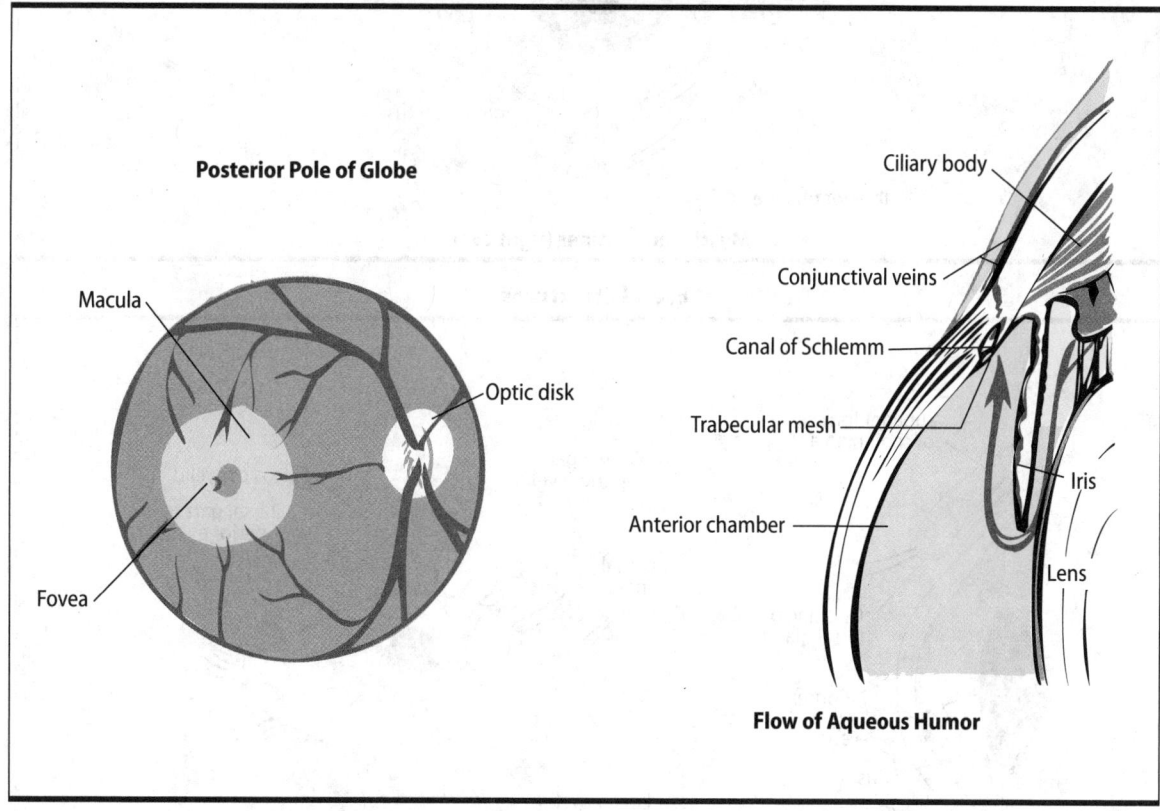

Posterior Pole of Globe

Flow of Aqueous Humor

Lacrimal System

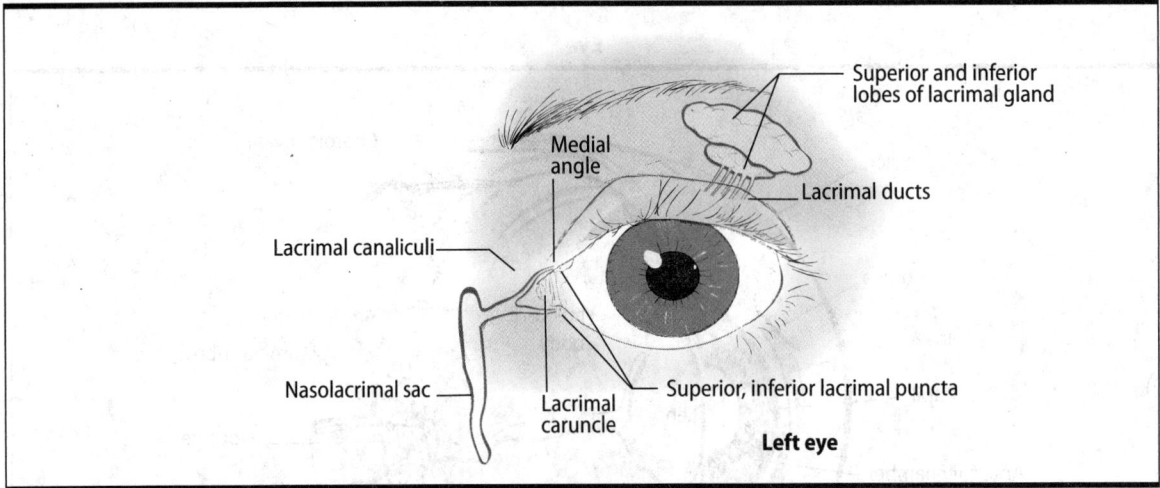

Superior and inferior lobes of lacrimal gland

Medial angle

Lacrimal ducts

Lacrimal canaliculi

Nasolacrimal sac

Lacrimal caruncle

Superior, inferior lacrimal puncta

Left eye

Eye Musculature

Superior rectus

Superior oblique

Lateral rectus

Medial rectus

Inferior rectus

Inferior oblique

Muscles and actions (right eye)

Eyelid Structures

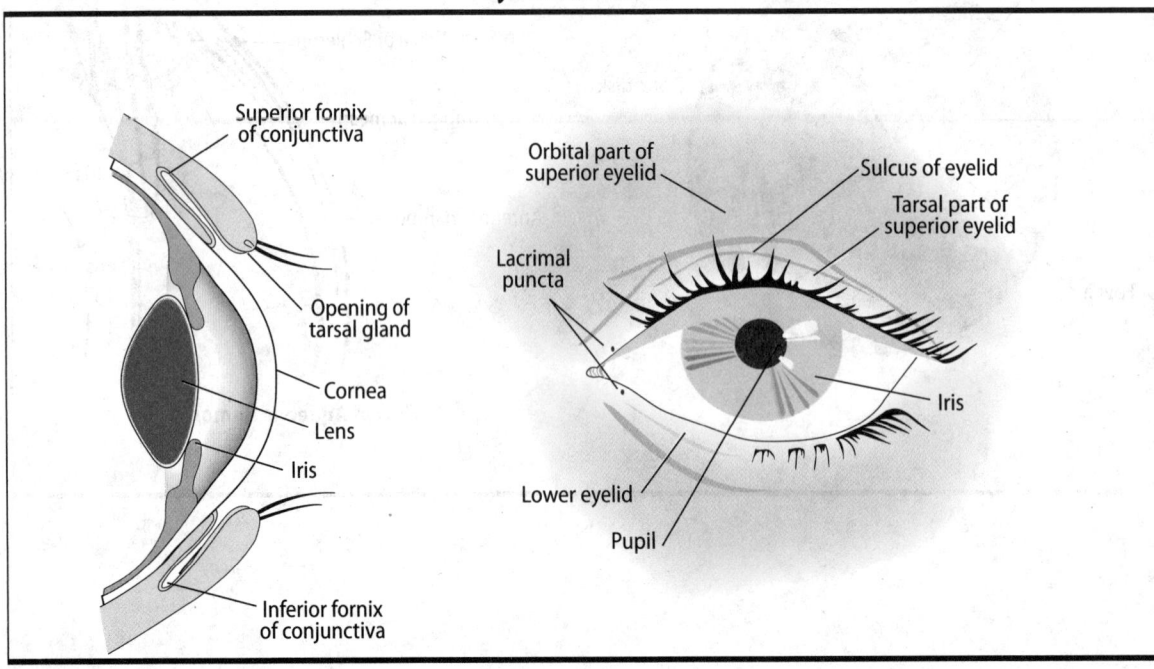

Superior fornix of conjunctiva

Opening of tarsal gland

Cornea

Lens

Iris

Inferior fornix of conjunctiva

Orbital part of superior eyelid

Sulcus of eyelid

Tarsal part of superior eyelid

Lacrimal puncta

Lower eyelid

Pupil

Iris

Chapter 8. Diseases of the Ear and Mastoid Process (H60–H95)

Ear Anatomy

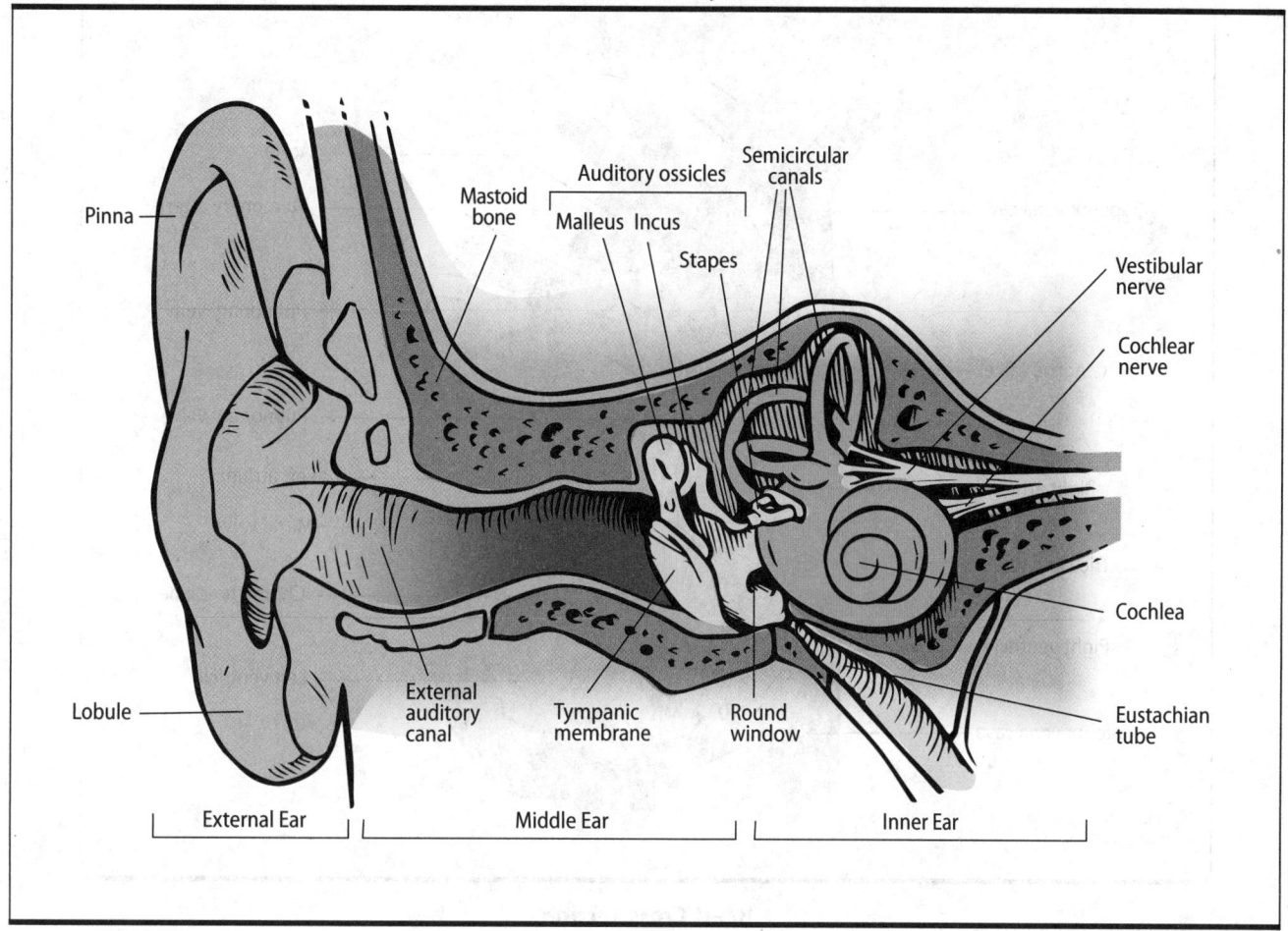

Chapter 9. Diseases of the Circulatory System (I00–I99)

Anatomy of the Heart

Heart Cross Section

Heart Valves

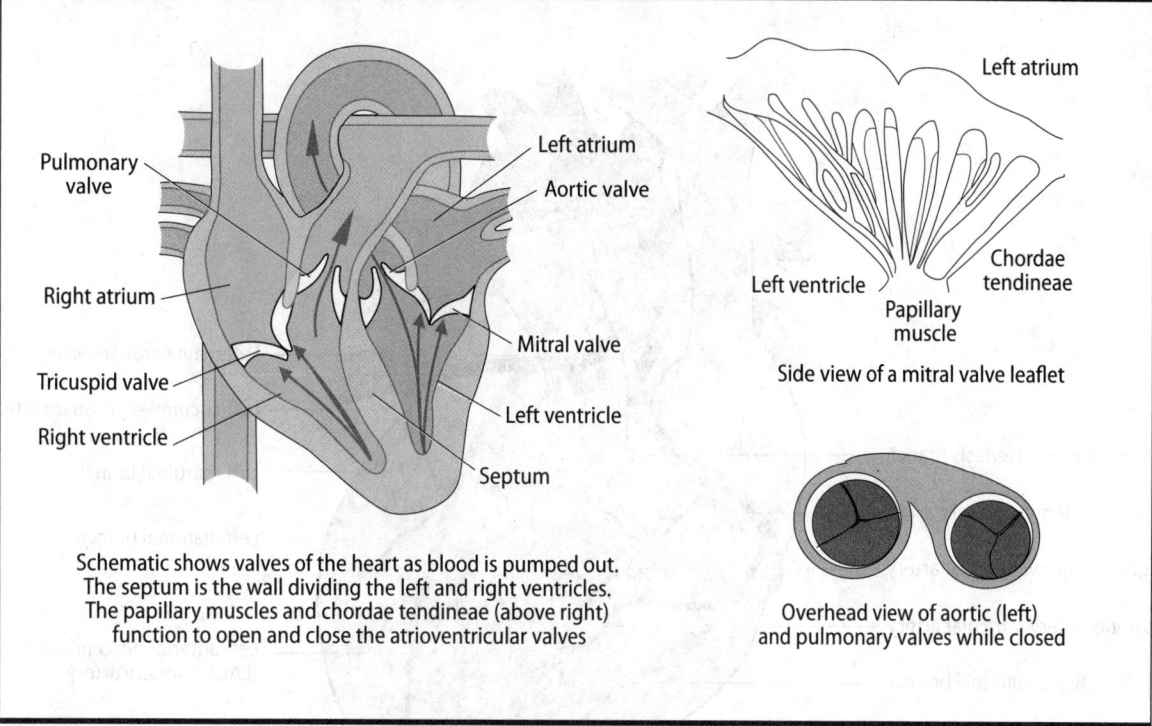

Pulmonary valve
Left atrium
Aortic valve
Right atrium
Tricuspid valve
Right ventricle
Mitral valve
Left ventricle
Septum

Left atrium
Chordae tendineae
Left ventricle
Papillary muscle

Side view of a mitral valve leaflet

Schematic shows valves of the heart as blood is pumped out.
The septum is the wall dividing the left and right ventricles.
The papillary muscles and chordae tendineae (above right)
function to open and close the atrioventricular valves

Overhead view of aortic (left)
and pulmonary valves while closed

Heart Conduction System

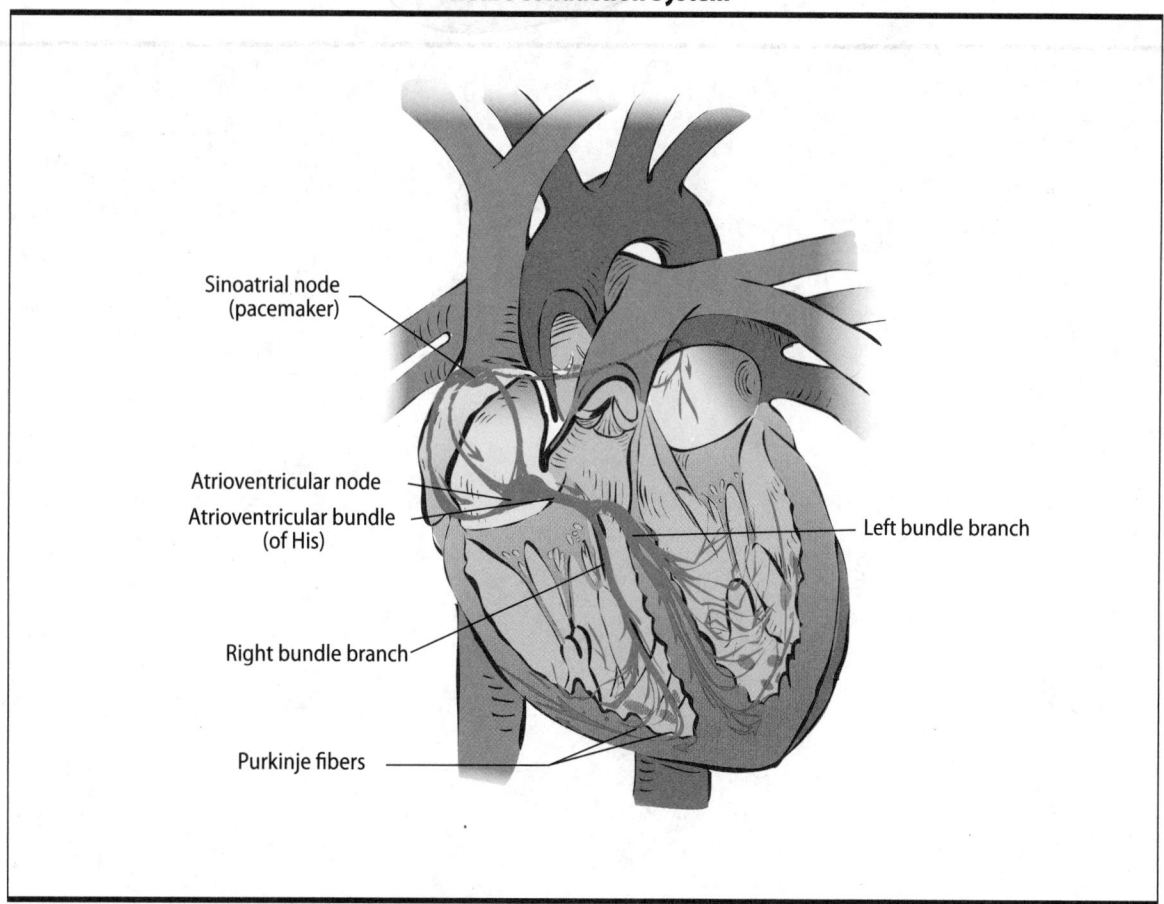

Sinoatrial node
(pacemaker)

Atrioventricular node
Atrioventricular bundle
(of His)

Right bundle branch

Purkinje fibers

Left bundle branch

Coronary Arteries

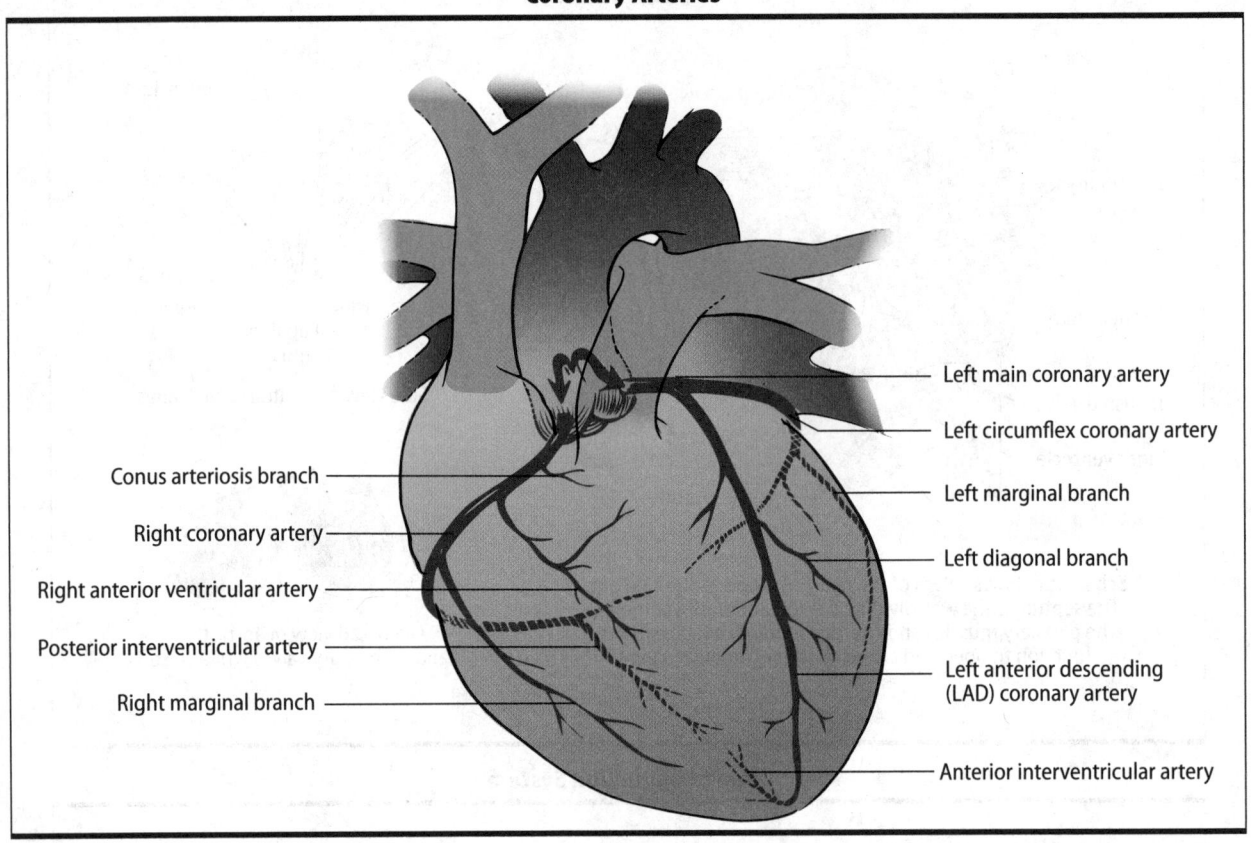

Left main coronary artery

Left circumflex coronary artery

Left marginal branch

Left diagonal branch

Left anterior descending (LAD) coronary artery

Anterior interventricular artery

Conus arteriosis branch

Right coronary artery

Right anterior ventricular artery

Posterior interventricular artery

Right marginal branch

Arteries

Veins

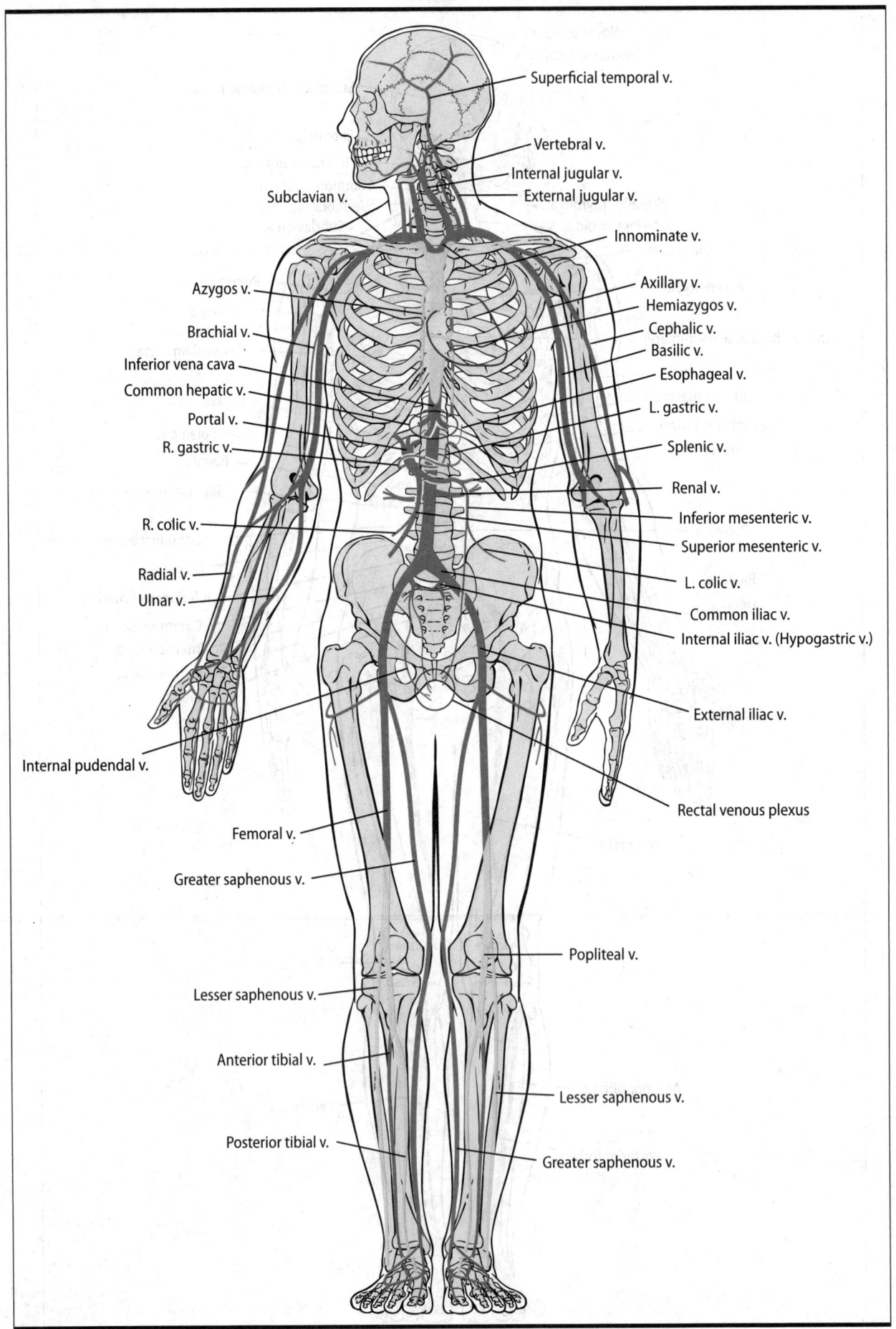

Superficial temporal v.

Vertebral v.

Internal jugular v.

External jugular v.

Innominate v.

Subclavian v.

Azygos v.

Brachial v.

Inferior vena cava

Common hepatic v.

Portal v.

R. gastric v.

R. colic v.

Radial v.

Ulnar v.

Internal pudendal v.

Axillary v.

Hemiazygos v.

Cephalic v.

Basilic v.

Esophageal v.

L. gastric v.

Splenic v.

Renal v.

Inferior mesenteric v.

Superior mesenteric v.

L. colic v.

Common iliac v.

Internal iliac v. (Hypogastric v.)

External iliac v.

Rectal venous plexus

Femoral v.

Greater saphenous v.

Popliteal v.

Lesser saphenous v.

Anterior tibial v.

Lesser saphenous v.

Posterior tibial v.

Greater saphenous v.

Internal Carotid and Vertebral Arteries and Branches

Side View

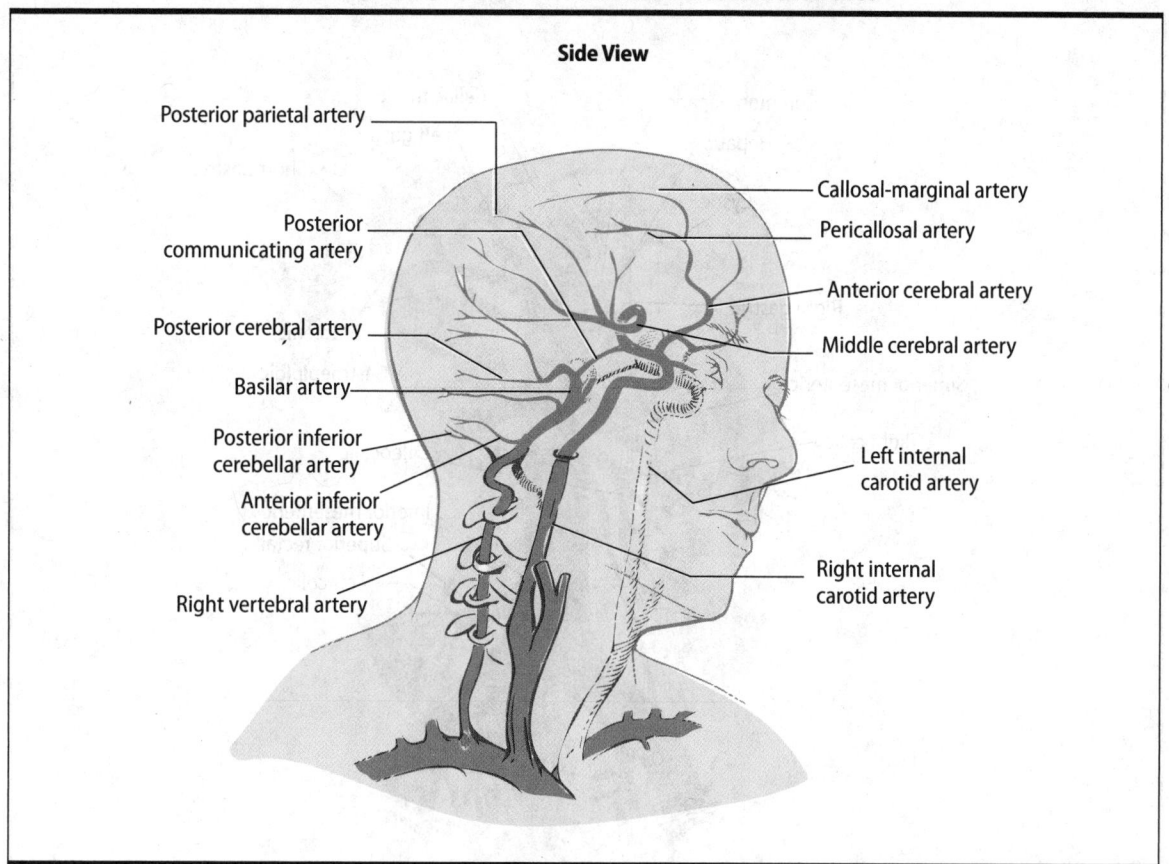

Posterior parietal artery

Posterior communicating artery

Posterior cerebral artery

Basilar artery

Posterior inferior cerebellar artery

Anterior inferior cerebellar artery

Right vertebral artery

Callosal-marginal artery

Pericallosal artery

Anterior cerebral artery

Middle cerebral artery

Left internal carotid artery

Right internal carotid artery

External Carotid Artery and Branches

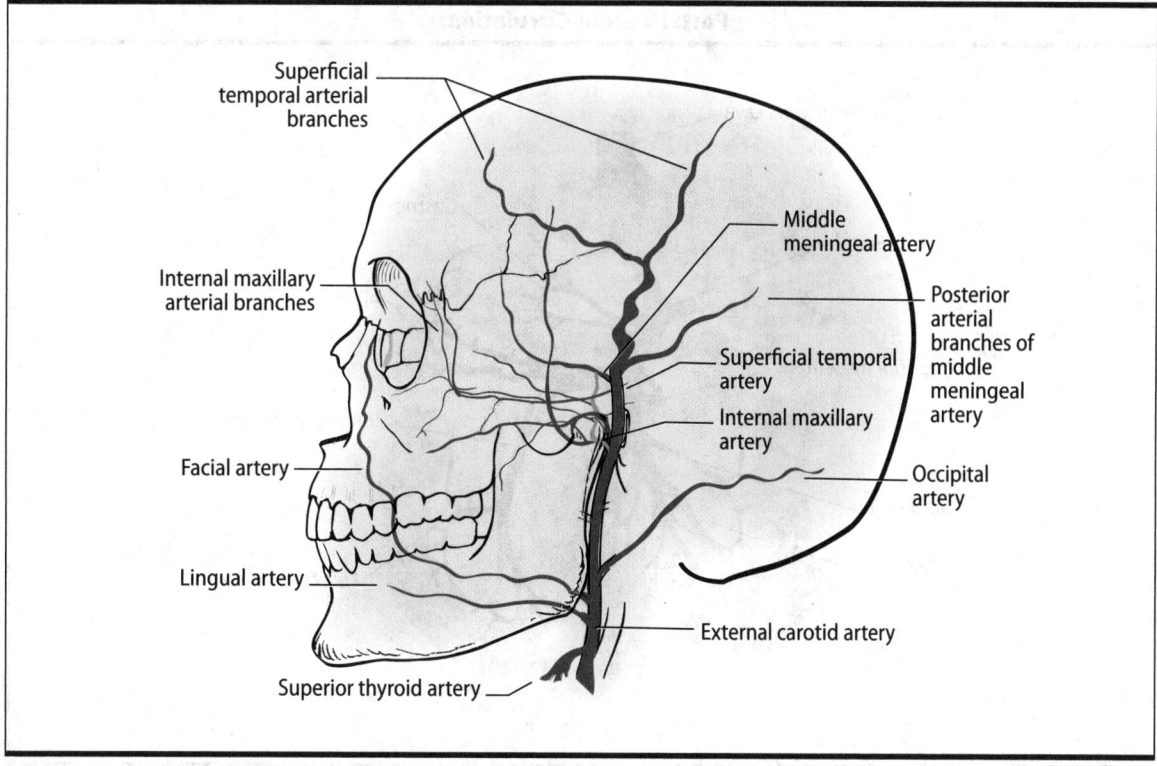

Superficial temporal arterial branches

Internal maxillary arterial branches

Facial artery

Lingual artery

Superior thyroid artery

Middle meningeal artery

Superficial temporal artery

Internal maxillary artery

Posterior arterial branches of middle meningeal artery

Occipital artery

External carotid artery

Branches of Abdominal Aorta

Portal Venous Circulation

Lymphatic System

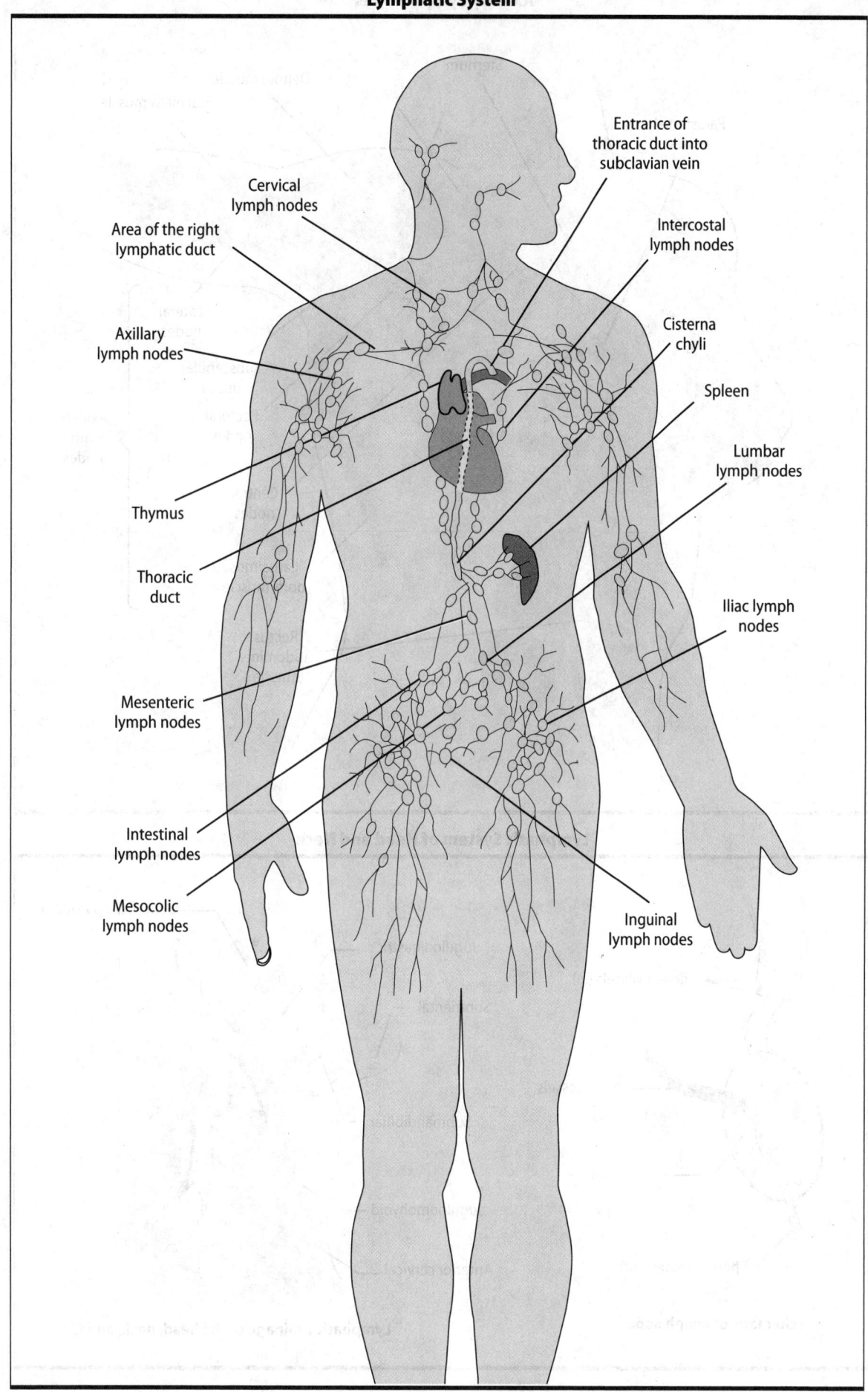

Axillary Lymph Nodes

Sternum

Clavicle

Deltoid muscle

Brachialis muscle

Parasternal nodes

Lateral nodes

Subscapular nodes

Pectoral nodes

Axillary lymph nodes

Central nodes

Latissimus dorsi muscle

Rectus abdominis muscle

Lymphatic System of Head and Neck

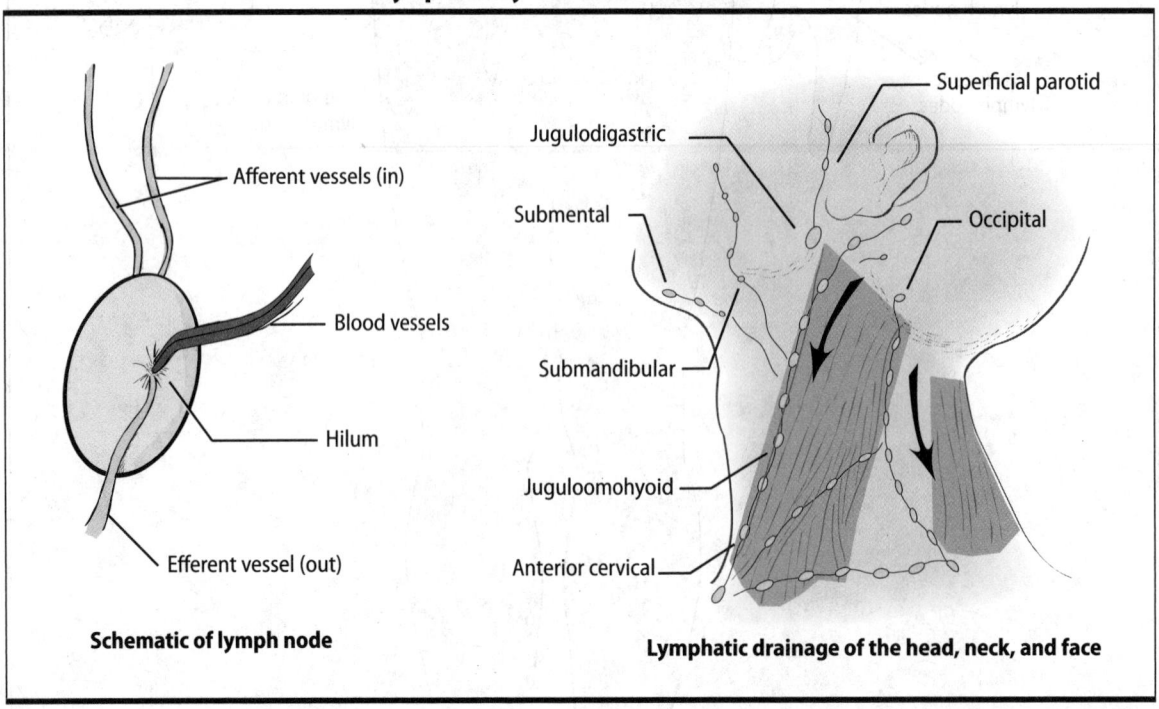

Afferent vessels (in)

Blood vessels

Hilum

Efferent vessel (out)

Schematic of lymph node

Superficial parotid

Jugulodigastric

Submental

Occipital

Submandibular

Juguloomohyoid

Anterior cervical

Lymphatic drainage of the head, neck, and face

Lymphatic Capillaries

Schematic of lymphatic capillaries

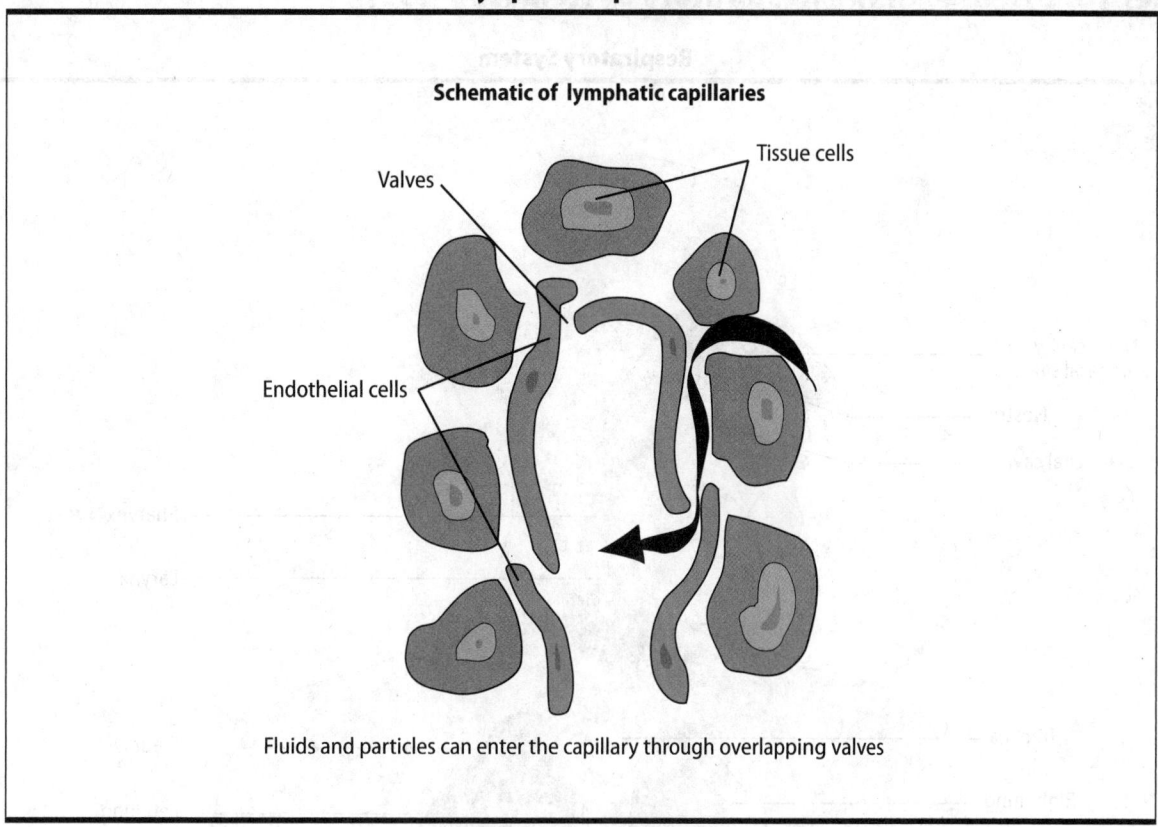

Valves

Tissue cells

Endothelial cells

Fluids and particles can enter the capillary through overlapping valves

Lymphatic Drainage

Lymphatic drainage of the colon follows blood supply

Middle colic nodes

Paracolic nodes

Left colic nodes

Ascending colon

Cecum

Rectum

Chapter 10. Diseases of the Respiratory System (J00–J99)

Respiratory System

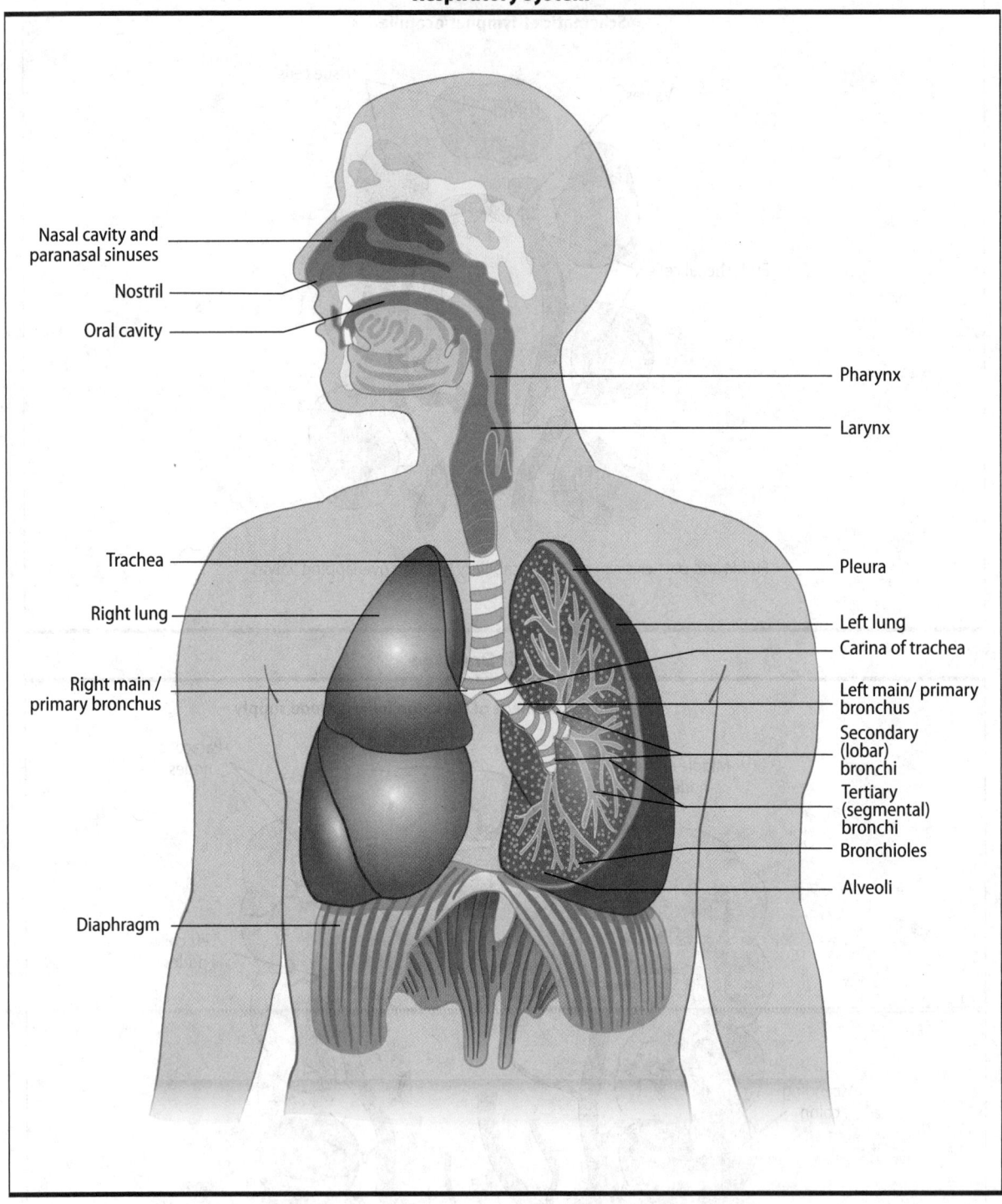

Nasal cavity and paranasal sinuses

Nostril

Oral cavity

Pharynx

Larynx

Trachea

Pleura

Right lung

Left lung

Carina of trachea

Right main / primary bronchus

Left main/ primary bronchus

Secondary (lobar) bronchi

Tertiary (segmental) bronchi

Bronchioles

Alveoli

Diaphragm

Upper Respiratory System

Lower Respiratory System

Paranasal Sinuses

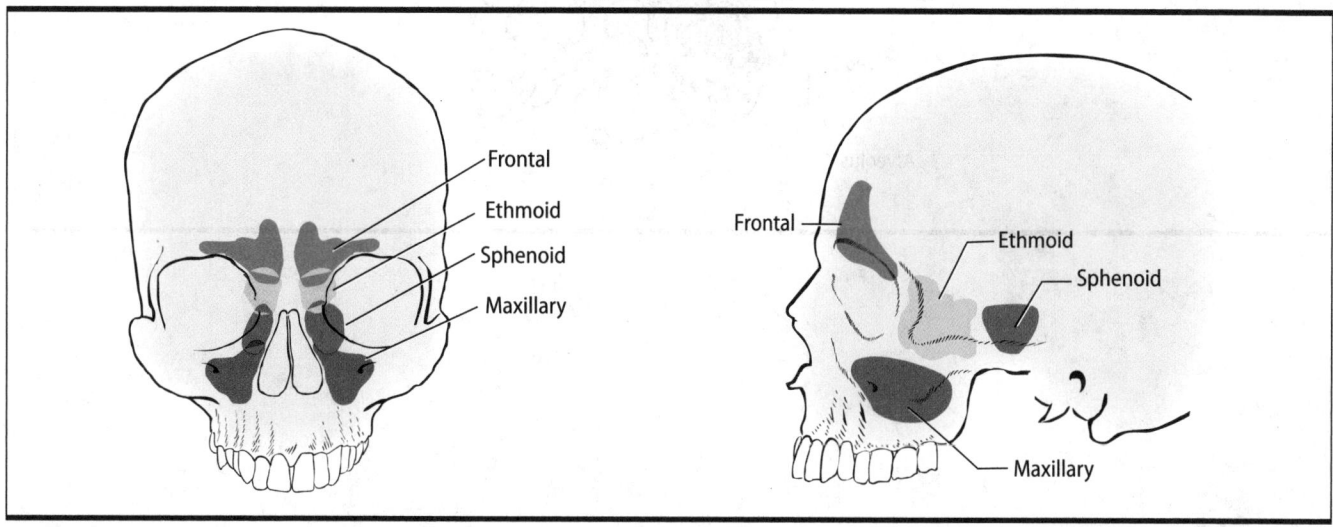

Lung Segments

Right lung   Left lung

Apical segment

Apical-posterior segment

Anterior segment

Superior lobe

Posterior segment

Superior lingular segment

Anterior segment

Inferior lingular segment

Superior lobe

Medial basal segment

Superior basal segment

Lateral segment

Superior segment

Lateral basal segment

Middle lobe

Posterior basal segment

Inferior lobe

Anterior medial segment

Inferior lobe

Anterior basal segment

Horizontal fissure

Oblique fissures

Alveoli

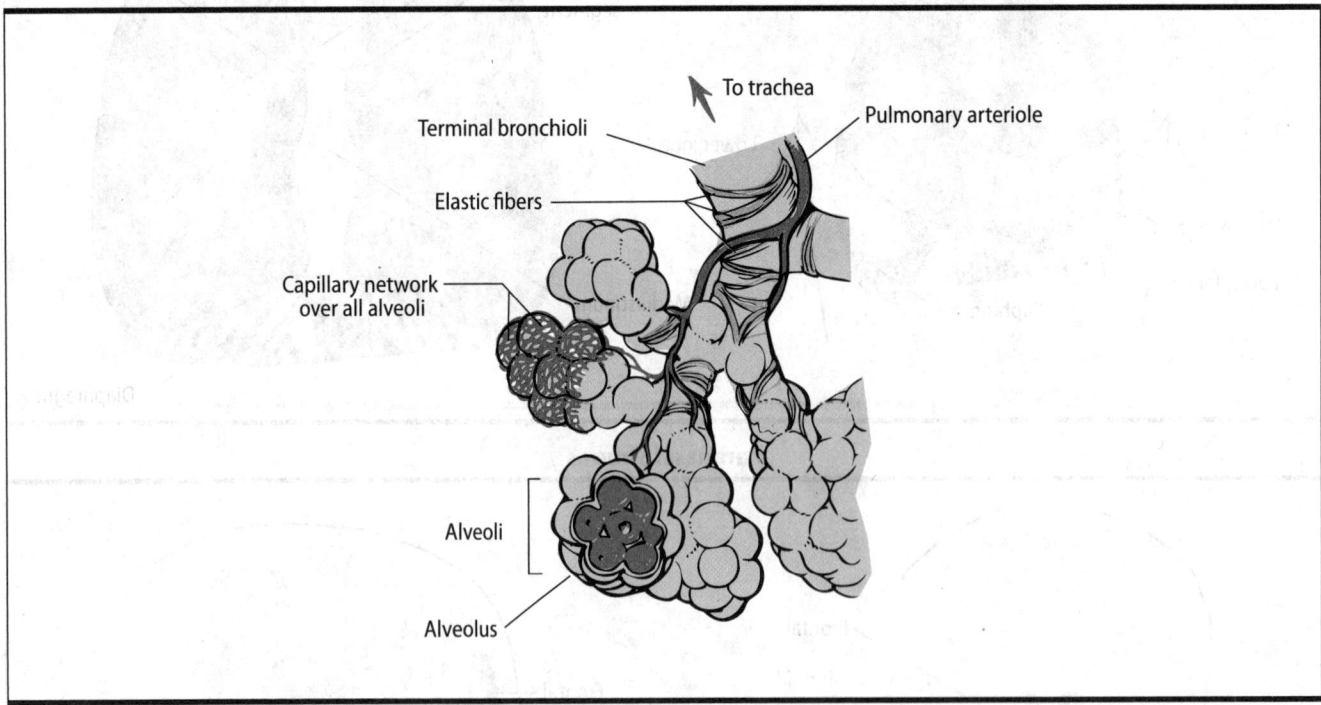

To trachea

Terminal bronchioli

Pulmonary arteriole

Elastic fibers

Capillary network over all alveoli

Alveoli

Alveolus

Chapter 11. Diseases of the Digestive System (K00–K95)

Digestive System

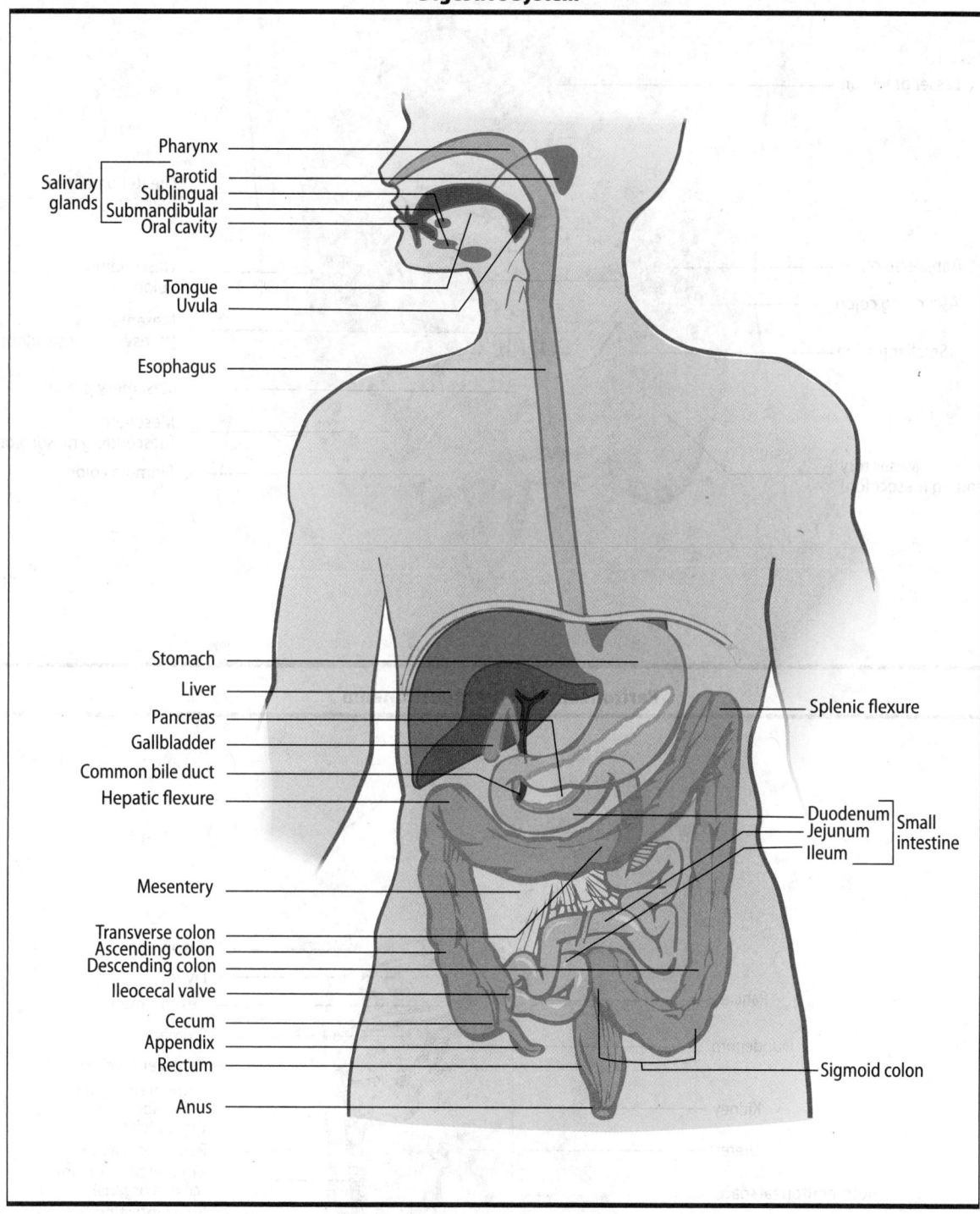

Omentum and Mesentery

Lesser omentum

Greater omentum
(cut edge)

Transverse colon

Descending
colon

Ascending colon

Mesentery
(transverse mesocolon)

Small intestine

Mesentery proper

Mesentery
(descending mesocolon)

Mesentery
(ascending mesocolon)

Sigmoid colon

Peritoneum and Retroperitoneum

Diaphragm

Liver

Pancreas

Lesser omentum

Duodenum

Stomach

Transverse colon

Kidney

Parietal peritoneum
(lines abdomen
and pelvis)

Ureter

Peritoneal cavity

Retroperitoneal space

Visceral peritoneum
(covers organs)

Small intestine

Mesentery

Greater omentum

Sigmoid colon

Bladder

Rectum

Chapter 12. Diseases of the Skin and Subcutaneous Tissue (L00–L99)

Nail Anatomy

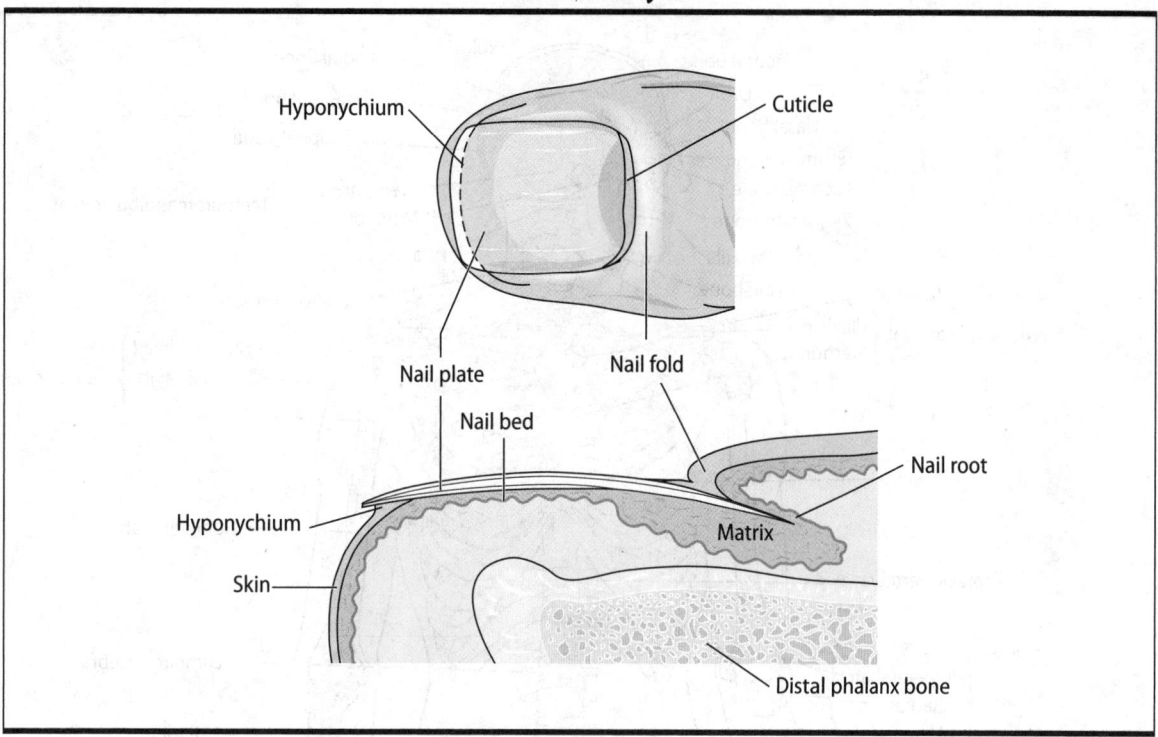

Skin and Subcutaneous Tissue

Chapter 13. Diseases of the Musculoskeletal System and Connective Tissue (M00–M99)

Bones and Joints

Shoulder Anterior View

Shoulder Posterior View

Elbow Anterior View

Elbow Posterior View

Hand

Hip Anterior View

Hip Posterior View

Knee Anterior View

Knee Posterior View

Foot

Muscles

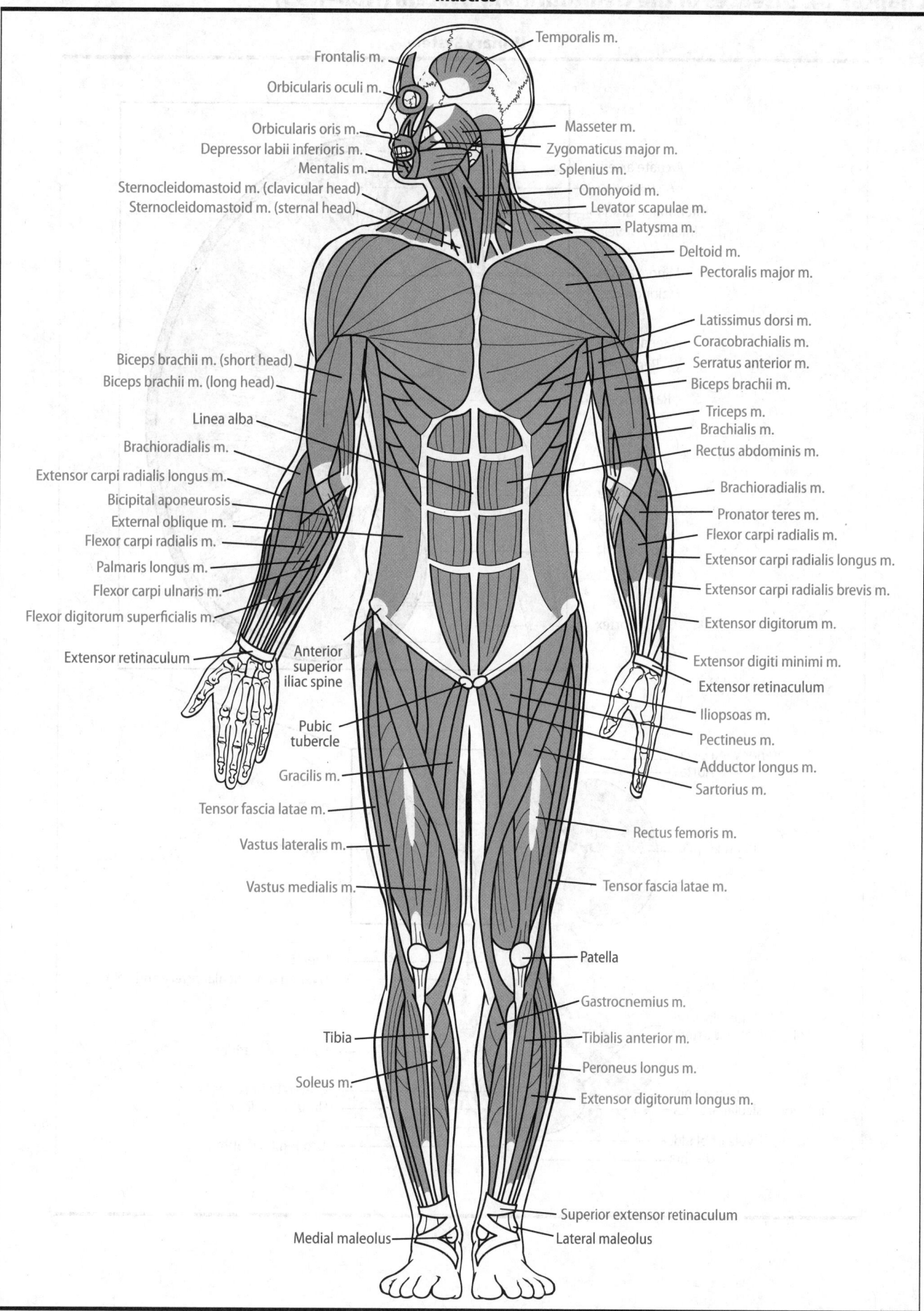

Frontalis m.

Temporalis m.

Orbicularis oculi m.

Orbicularis oris m.

Masseter m.

Depressor labii inferioris m.

Zygomaticus major m.

Mentalis m.

Splenius m.

Sternocleidomastoid m. (clavicular head)

Omohyoid m.

Sternocleidomastoid m. (sternal head)

Levator scapulae m.

Platysma m.

Deltoid m.

Pectoralis major m.

Latissimus dorsi m.

Coracobrachialis m.

Biceps brachii m. (short head)

Serratus anterior m.

Biceps brachii m. (long head)

Biceps brachii m.

Triceps m.

Linea alba

Brachialis m.

Brachioradialis m.

Rectus abdominis m.

Extensor carpi radialis longus m.

Brachioradialis m.

Bicipital aponeurosis

Pronator teres m.

External oblique m.

Flexor carpi radialis m.

Flexor carpi radialis m.

Extensor carpi radialis longus m.

Palmaris longus m.

Extensor carpi radialis brevis m.

Flexor carpi ulnaris m.

Extensor digitorum m.

Flexor digitorum superficialis m.

Extensor digiti minimi m.

Extensor retinaculum

Extensor retinaculum

Anterior superior iliac spine

Iliopsoas m.

Pectineus m.

Pubic tubercle

Adductor longus m.

Gracilis m.

Sartorius m.

Tensor fascia latae m.

Rectus femoris m.

Vastus lateralis m.

Vastus medialis m.

Tensor fascia latae m.

Patella

Gastrocnemius m.

Tibia

Tibialis anterior m.

Peroneus longus m.

Soleus m.

Extensor digitorum longus m.

Superior extensor retinaculum

Medial maleolus

Lateral maleolus

Chapter 14. Diseases of the Genitourinary System (N00–N99)

Urinary System

Male Genitourinary System

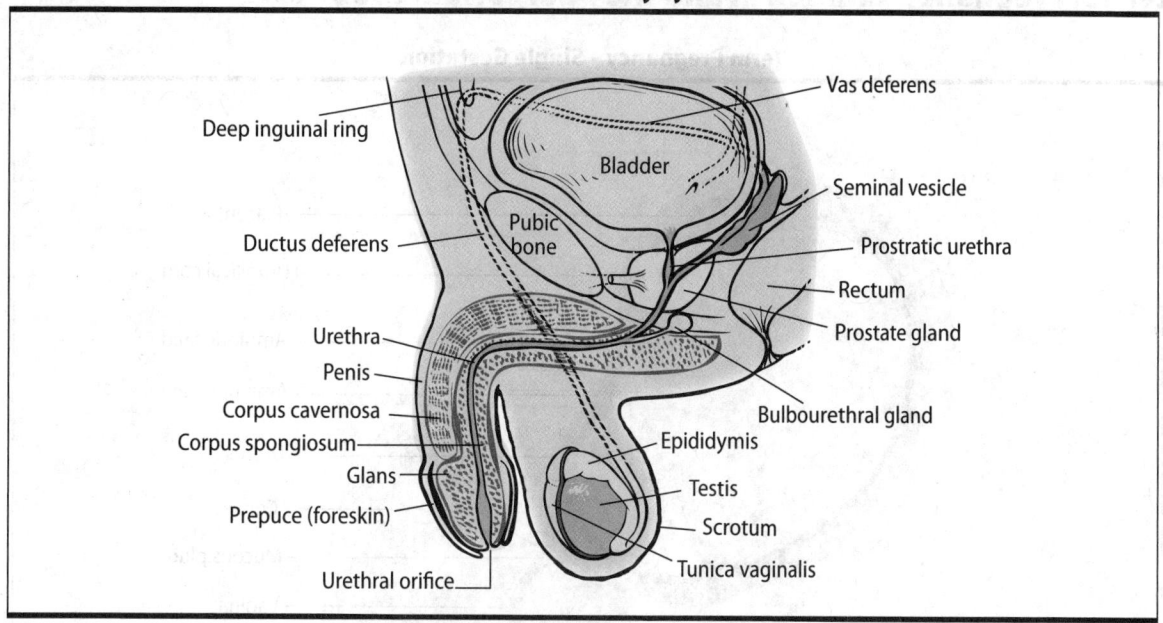

- Deep inguinal ring
- Vas deferens
- Bladder
- Seminal vesicle
- Pubic bone
- Ductus deferens
- Prostratic urethra
- Rectum
- Prostate gland
- Urethra
- Bulbourethral gland
- Penis
- Corpus cavernosa
- Epididymis
- Corpus spongiosum
- Glans
- Testis
- Prepuce (foreskin)
- Scrotum
- Urethral orifice
- Tunica vaginalis

Female Internal Genitalia

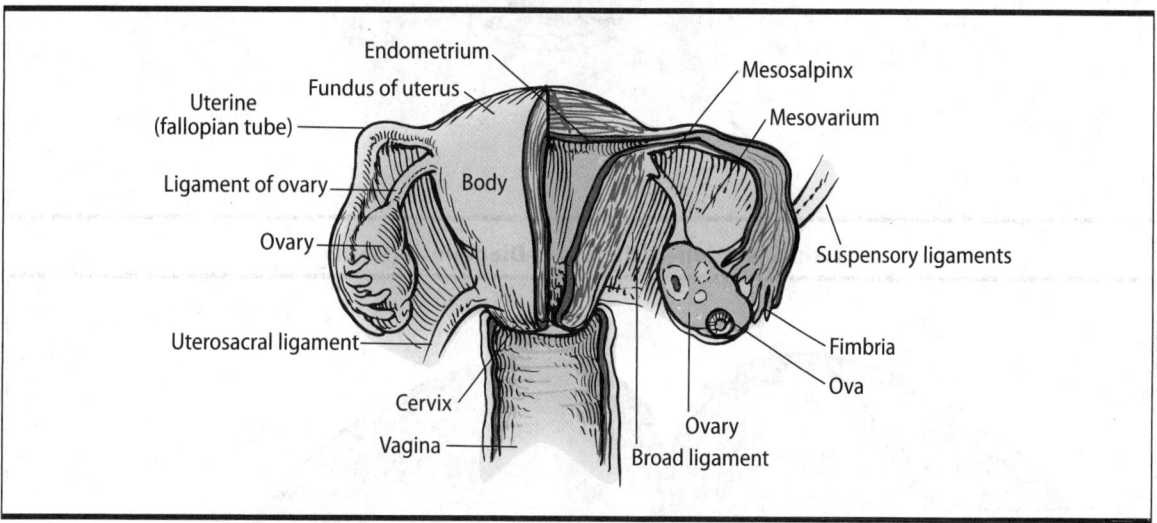

- Endometrium
- Mesosalpinx
- Fundus of uterus
- Mesovarium
- Uterine (fallopian tube)
- Ligament of ovary
- Body
- Ovary
- Suspensory ligaments
- Uterosacral ligament
- Fimbria
- Ova
- Cervix
- Ovary
- Vagina
- Broad ligament

Female Genitourinary Tract Lateral View

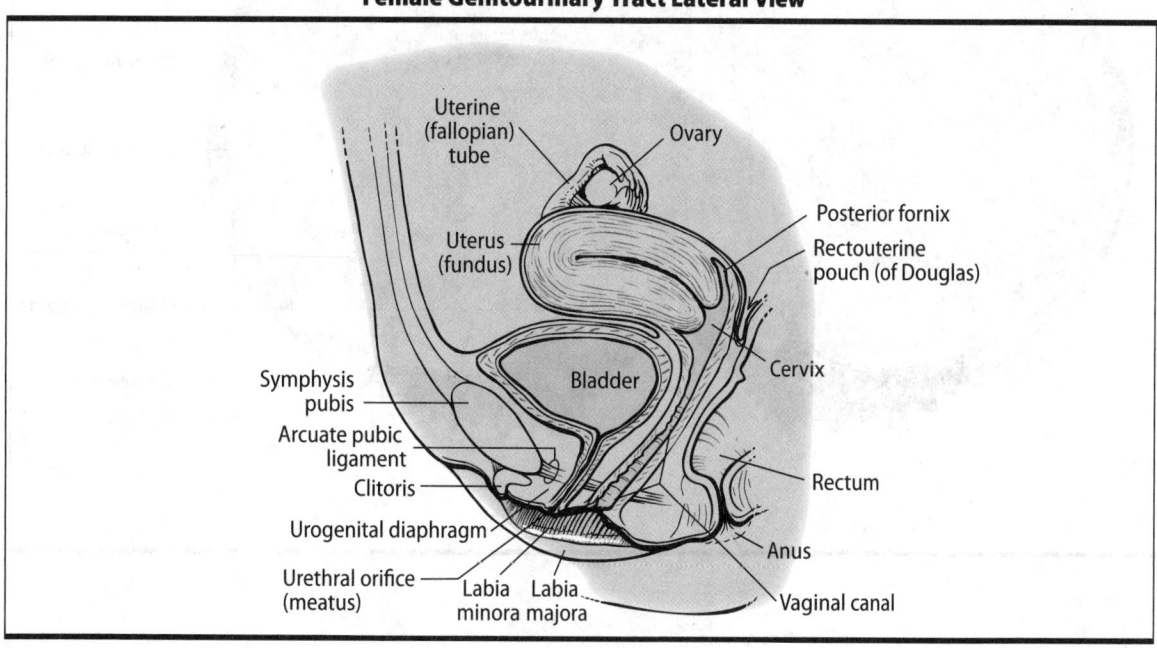

- Uterine (fallopian) tube
- Ovary
- Uterus (fundus)
- Posterior fornix
- Rectouterine pouch (of Douglas)
- Symphysis pubis
- Bladder
- Cervix
- Arcuate pubic ligament
- Clitoris
- Rectum
- Urogenital diaphragm
- Anus
- Urethral orifice (meatus)
- Labia minora
- Labia majora
- Vaginal canal

5. Pregnancy, Childbirth and the Puerperium (O00–O9A)

Term Pregnancy – Single Gestation

- Placenta
- Umbilical cord
- Amniotic fluid
- Amniotic sac
- Uterus
- Cervix
- Mucous plug
- Vagina
- Pubic bone

Twin Gestation–Dichorionic–Diamniotic (DI-DI)

- 2 Chorionic sacs
- 2 Amniotic sacs
- 2 Fetuses
- 2 Umbilical cords
- 2 Placentas

Twin Gestation–Monochorionic–Diamniotic (MO-DI)

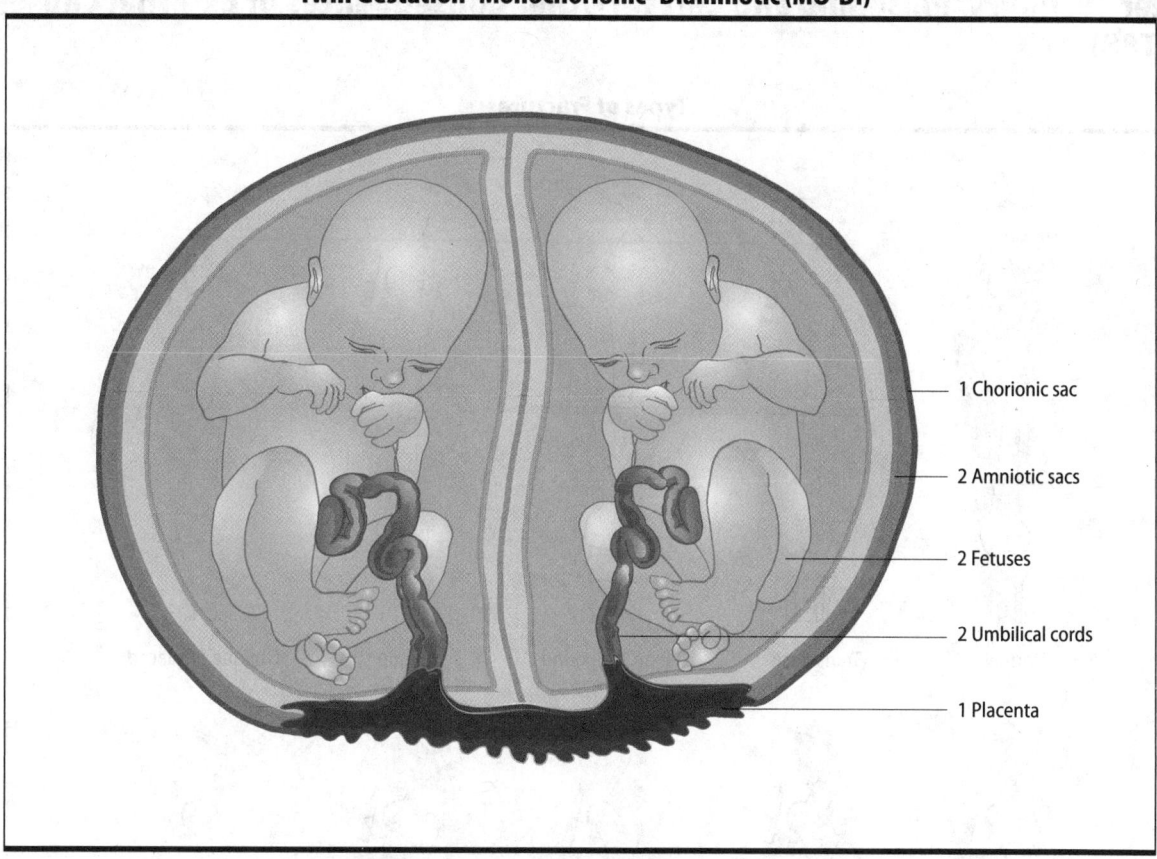

- 1 Chorionic sac
- 2 Amniotic sacs
- 2 Fetuses
- 2 Umbilical cords
- 1 Placenta

Twin Gestation–Monochorionic–Monoamniotic (MO-MO)

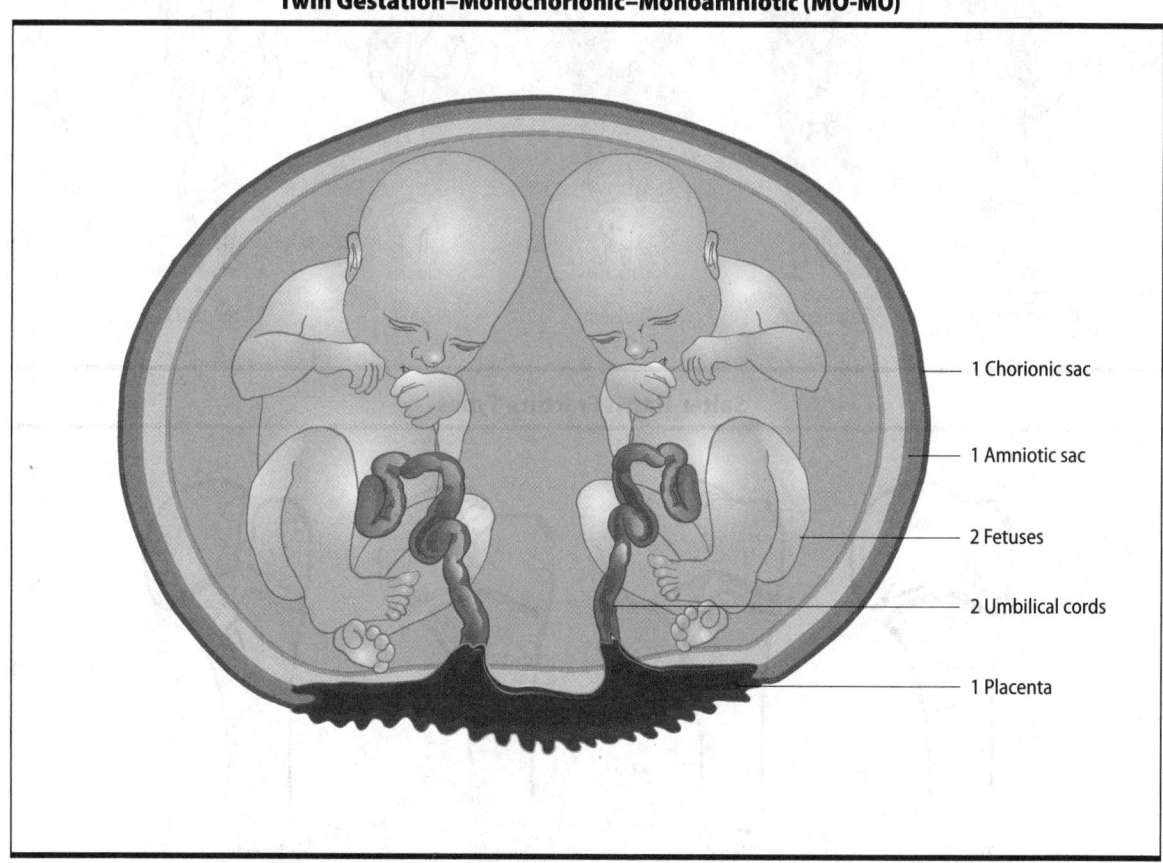

- 1 Chorionic sac
- 1 Amniotic sac
- 2 Fetuses
- 2 Umbilical cords
- 1 Placenta

Types of Fractures

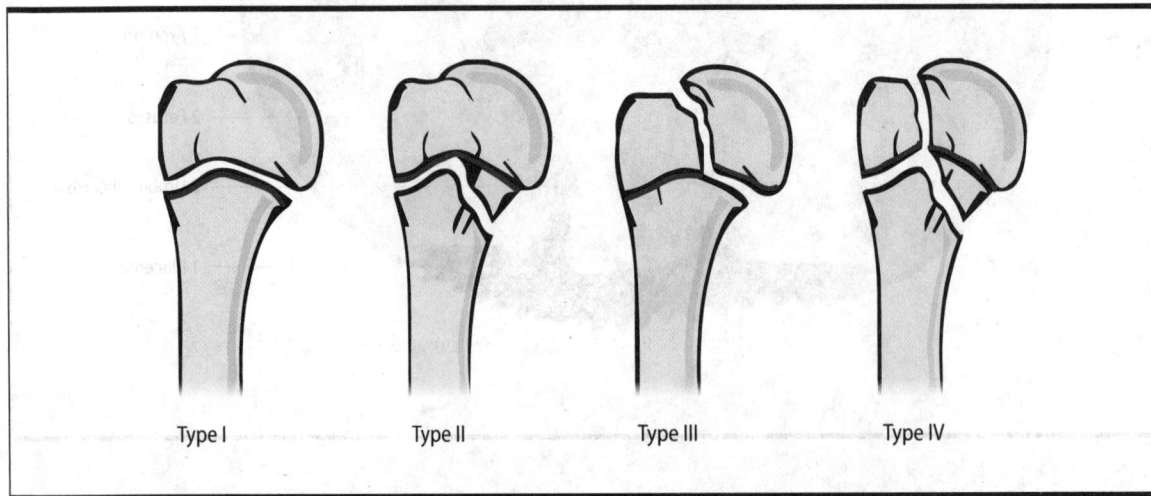

| Normal | Transverse | Open/Compound | Oblique | Oblique displaced |

| Comminuted | Segmental | Avulsed | Spiral | Greenstick |

Salter-Harris Fracture Types

| Type I | Type II | Type III | Type IV |